OXFORD MEDICAL PUBLICATIONS

OXFORD
TEXTBOOK OF
MEDICINE

OXFORD TEXTBOOK OF MEDICINE

SECOND EDITION

Edited by

D. J. WEATHERALL
Nuffield Professor of Clinical Medicine, University of Oxford

J. G. G. LEDINGHAM
May Reader in Medicine, Nuffield Department of Clinical Medicine, University of Oxford

D. A. WARRELL
*Professor of Tropical Medicine and Infectious Diseases,
University of Oxford*

VOLUME 2

Sections 13–28, Appendix, and Index

Oxford   Melbourne   New York
OXFORD UNIVERSITY PRESS

Oxford University Press, Walton Street, Oxford OX2 6DP
Oxford New York Toronto
Delhi Bombay Calcutta Madras Karachi
Petaling Jaya Singapore Hong Kong Tokyo
Nairobi Dar es Salaam Cape Town
Melbourne Auckland
and associated companies in
Beirut Berlin Ibadan Nicosia

Oxford is a trade mark of Oxford University Press

Published in the United States
by Oxford University Press, New York

First published 1983
Reprinted 1983 (with corrections), 1984, 1985
Second edition 1987
Reprinted (with corrections) 1988

First published in
paperback 1988

British Library Cataloguing in Publication Data
Oxford textbook of medicine.—2nd ed.—
(Oxford medical publications)
1. Pathology 2. Medicine
I. Weatherall, D. J. II. Ledingham, J. G. G.
III. Warrell, D. A.
616 RB111
ISBN 0–19–261551–3
ISBN 0–19–261720–6 (Pbk)

Library of Congress Cataloging in Publication Data
Oxford textbook of medicine.
(Oxford medical publications)
Includes bibliographies and indexes.
1. Internal medicine. I. Weatherall, D. J.
II. Ledingham, J. G. G. III. Warrell, D. A. IV. Series.
[DNLM: 1. Medicine. WB 100 0988]
RC46.0995 1987 616 86–31161
ISBN 0–19–261551–3 (set)
ISBN 0–19–261720–6 (set) (Pbk)

Printed in Great Britain by
Butler and Tanner Ltd, Frome, Somerset

Preface to the second edition

The four years that have passed since the first edition of the *Oxford Textbook of Medicine* was published has been a time of mixed fortunes for clinical medicine. A series of climatic catastrophies leading to years of drought and famine, together with our continued inability to control some of the major bacterial and parasitic illnesses which afflict many of the world's populations, have highlighted the intractable problems of medical care in the Third World. A time of economic recession together with the increasing costs and complexity of medical care, and the social problems that have resulted from an unpredicted increase in the size of the elderly population, have put an immense strain on the medical services of wealthier countries. Furthermore, most of the major causes of morbidity and mortality in western societies – rheumatism, the common cancers, and degenerative vascular disorders – continue to cause problems in management. Perhaps because of this, or for other reasons, there is a prevailing mood of disillusionment with conventional medical practice and a move towards 'alternative medicine'. Yet at the same time remarkable developments have occurred in the fields of cell and molecular biology that promise to make the next decade the most exciting period so far in the development of the medical sciences. The discovery of the causative agent of AIDS, a condition which was only just recognized as the first edition was going to press and which has since reached epidemic proportions, is just one example of the remarkable power of the application of the new techniques of the basic sciences to clinical practice.

Since a major objective of this *Textbook* is to provide a more global picture of disease than is usually given in books of this type many of the changes that appear in the second edition reflect these new problems in clinical practice, both in developed and underdeveloped countries. While we are convinced that the basic principles of a sound grasp of pathophysiology, communication, history taking, and clinical examination are applicable to all branches of clinical care, regardless of where and by whom it is carried out, we have added several new sections which examine the ethical and pastoral aspects of modern medicine and the problems of primary care, both in the developed and developing countries. Some of these topics are highly controversial. For example, we do not always agree with some of the conclusions about the relationships between the basic and clinical sciences or with some of the political aspects of Third World medicine which are presented in these sections. On the other hand we believe that these subjects are of such importance that debates of this kind constitute a vital part of the thinking and training of modern-day students and physicians. In an attempt to further broaden our rather narrow north European view of clinical practice we have added to many of the major sections of the book a series of essays by practitioners in different parts of the world describing the importance and peculiarities of the relevant diseases in their populations. We are particularly grateful to our many colleagues around the world for helping us in this way and for being so patient in the face of editorial foibles.

Though the reviewers of the first edition were remarkably kind, we are well aware of its deficiencies. Many sections have been completely rewritten and expanded and careful note has been taken of the numerous omissions ranging from AIDS to the management of hiccup. We are grateful to many of our readers who took the time and trouble to write to us to point out the errors of our ways. No textbook of this type can ever be all-embracing but we hope that this new edition will provide both students and practitioners with a reasonable account of most of the disorders that they will meet in day-to-day practice and an entrée to the rarer conditions together with a guide as to where more information can be found.

We are particularly sad to record the deaths of four of our authors, W. C. Marshall, Sister Mary Aquinas, M. Rachmilewitz, and E. G. Lee. Manny Lee was a particularly close colleague and friend, and his death at the peak of his surgical career has been a personal loss to each of us and a major tragedy for the Oxford Clinical School.

The Editors are grateful to the following persons who acted as sectional editors or advisers: Dr Roger Smith (Sections 8, 9, and 17), Dr Chris Redman (Section 11), Dr Derek Jewell (Section 12), Dr Derek Gibson (Section 13), Dr Ron Bradley (Section 14), Dr Don Lane (Section 15), Dr Terence Ryan (Section 20), Professor David Marsden (Section 21), Sir John Walton (Section 22), Mr David Spalton (Section 23), and Professor Michael Gelder (Section 25). Oxford University Press has shown its faith in this project by providing us with a full-time editor for this edition; we should like to record our thanks to the Press, and to Mairwen Lloyd-Williams for taking on this immense task and for her patience and forebearance with three increasingly irascible editors. As before, we are also particularly grateful to our secretaries Janet Watt, Judith Last, Eunice Berry, and Patchari Prakongpan for their excellent work in compiling this edition and in chasing many errant authors. The first Nuffield Professor of Clinical Medicine at Oxford, Leslie Witts, wrote that textbooks are usually written by those who have unsatisfactory marriages. We are happy to record that the marriages of the three editors have survived another edition; we are particularly grateful to our wives for their extreme forebearance and for proving that even Oxford professors are sometimes wrong.

Oxford, August 1986

D. J. WEATHERALL
J. G. G. LEDINGHAM
D. A. WARRELL

Preface to the first edition

The *Oxford Textbook of Medicine* is the reincarnation of 'Price' which, after 60 years as the major British postgraduate textbook of medicine, has been laid to rest by the Oxford University Press. The first edition of a *Textbook of the Practice of Medicine (including Sections on Diseases of the Skin and Psychological Medicine)* edited by Frederick Price was published in 1922. There were 26 contributors, all from London teaching hospitals. The book was updated roughly every four years up to the ninth edition (1957); for the tenth edition (1966) Sir Ronald Bodley Scott took over as editor. The last (twelfth) edition was published in 1978. Sir Ronald did much to modernize and expand the book during his time as editor and it is sad to record that his tragic death in an accident in 1982 prevented his seeing its successor.

When Sir Ronald Bodley Scott retired as editor of 'Price' in 1978, Oxford University Press approached us with the idea of producing a completely new textbook to replace it. This was a daunting proposal. There were several excellent American postgraduate textbooks of medicine already available and the undergraduate was well served on both sides of the Atlantic. Furthermore, although many of the reviewers of the twelfth edition of 'Price' were quite complimentary, others raised doubts about whether there was a place in the 1980s for a general textbook of medicine of its size and scope. Among the most critical reviews was a characteristically acerbic piece by J. R. A. Mitchell. After weighing the book he reminded us that dinosaurs became extinct because of their sheer bulk. 'Price' would suffer the same fate; it could not be lifted and therefore it could not be read! In addition, Professor Mitchell and other reviewers voiced the often-heard criticism that big textbooks are out of date before they are published, and suggested that smaller paperback textbooks, together with occasional forays into specialist monographs, provide the most economical and accessible guidance for students and general practitioners, while postgraduates are best served by specialist monographs and up-to-date review journals.

After considering these arguments very carefully we came to the conclusion that there is still an important role for a larger textbook of medicine. Certainly, the basic and clinical sciences are moving so fast that no textbook of medicine can hope to be absolutely up to date. However, relatively few of the advances in these fields lead to major changes in patient-care, and those that do require several years of critical evaluation before they become an integral part of routine clinical practice. Although we agree that the specialist monograph is often the best source of information in any particular area of medicine, the very breadth of the subject and the tendency to overspecialization means that few students and practitioners have immediate access to monographs on every branch of the subject, and even when they are available they are not always written by clinicians who are used to evaluating their patients in a general medical setting. Another reason for retaining at least a few broadly based textbooks of medicine is that medical practice varies very much in different parts of the world. Although it is important for students and practitioners to appreciate these differences as part of their general education, there is a more pragmatic reason for stressing this aspect of modern medicine. With increasing international travel and massive movement of refugee populations no practitioner can be sure that he will not be expected to deal with diseases with which he is unfamiliar and which may present in a variety of unexpected ways. The steadily rising number of deaths from malaria in the United Kingdom in the last few years is just one example of this new phenomenon.

Thus we believe that the rapid expansion of knowledge, increasing specialization, and the blossoming of narrow specialist monographs have, if anything, strengthened the case for the general reference book. Therefore we have attempted to produce a reference book of internal medicine which we hope will reflect current British practice, but which also includes the views of an international group of authors. We have also tried to present some of the problems of clinical practice in the developing countries and to describe how the pattern of disease varies in different parts of the world. We have included some background chapters describing how some of the important basic clinical sciences such as microbiology, genetics, immunology, epidemiology, and oncology are contributing to an understanding of the pathogenesis of the diseases which are described in the book. With Professor Mitchell's criticisms of 'Price' in mind, we have remembered the frail and divided the book into two volumes.

For whom is this book intended? The short answer is anyone who is studying or practising clinical medicine. Our overall aim has been to provide a bird's eye view of the subject; the book is designed primarily for general practitioners and specialists as a first reference source. In addition, we hope that it will provide medical students and postgraduates with an adequate guide to the more important clinical disorders and point them in the right direction when looking up the rarities. It is an impossible task to produce a balanced reference book of general medicine first time round and we are only too aware of the shortcomings of our first effort. However, we hope that we have laid a basis on which future editions can develop a more mature and balanced view of this increasingly complicated field.

We cannot acknowledge everyone who has helped us in this enterprise. Several of the major sections were planned with a sub-editor. These are: Nutrition: Dr Roger Smith; Reproductive medicine: Dr C. W. G. Redman; Gastroenterology: Dr D. P. Jewell; Cardiology: Dr D. G. Gibson; Respiratory disease: Dr D. J. Lane; Neurology: Professor W. B. Matthews; Psychiatry: Professor M. G. Gelder. We were cajoled into this impossible task by Richard Charkin of Oxford University Press. His colleagues at the Press, particularly Alison Langton, Nicholas Dunton, and Christopher Riches have managed to see it to a conclusion despite innumerable difficulties caused by errant authors and a typesetting process which, in the best traditions of an ancient University, persisted in producing sections of the book in ancient Greek. On a more personal note we take particular pleasure in acknowledging the help of our secretaries, Janet Watt, Jenny Stephens, Jeanne Packer, Sheila Hatton, Judith Last, Jacqueline Teodorczyx, Eunice Berry, and Patchari Prakongpan. Finally, we are happy to record that the marriages of the three editors have survived the production of this book; the forbearance of our wives during its difficult gestation is the major reason for its ever seeing the light of day.

Oxford, August 1982

D. J. WEATHERALL
J. G. G. LEDINGHAM
D. A. WARRELL

Contents

SECTION 6. Chemical and physical injuries, climatic and occupational diseases

Contents

SECTION 13. Cardiovascular disease

Contents

List of contributors

E. B. ADAMS, Emeritus Professor of Medicine, University of Natal, South Africa

K. G. M. M. ALBERTI, Professor of Clinical Biochemistry, University of Newcastle upon Tyne, Royal Victoria Infirmary, Newcastle upon Tyne, UK

M. P. ALPERS, Papua New Guinea Institute of Medical Research, Goroka, Papua New Guinea

D. S. AMORIM, Faculdade de Medicina de Ribeirao Preta, Universidade de Sao Paulo, Brasil

R. H. ANDERSON, Joseph Levy Professor of Paediatric Cardiac Morphology, Department of Paediatrics, Cardiothoracic Institute, University of London, Brompton Hospital, London, UK

M. J. ANDERSON, Senior Lecturer in Medical Microbiology, University College London and the Middlesex Hospital Medical School, London, UK

M. AQUINAS OBE (deceased), Honorary Clinical Lecturer in Medicine (Tuberculosis), University of Hong Kong

J. K. ARONSON, Clinical Reader (Wellcome Lecturer) and Honorary Consultant in Clinical Pharmacology, MRC Unit and University Department of Clinical Pharmacology, Radcliffe Infirmary, Oxford, UK

A. W. ASSCHER, Professor of Renal Medicine, University of Wales College of Medicine, Royal Infirmary, Cardiff, UK

R. M. ATKINS, Clinical Lecturer in Orthopaedic Surgery, University of Oxford, Nuffield Orthopaedic Centre, Oxford, UK

O. BADEMOSI, Professor, College of Medicine, University of Ibadan, Nigeria

L. R. I. BAKER, Consultant Physician, Nephrologist, and Director, Smithfield Renal Unit, St Bartholomew's Hospital, London, UK

R. BALCON, Consultant Cardiologist, The London Chest Hospital, London, UK

P. A. J. BALL, The Wellcome Trust, London, UK

SIR ROGER BANNISTER, Master, Pembroke College, Oxford; Honorary Consultant Neurologist, Oxford Regional Hospital Authority, Oxford, UK

SIR RICHARD BAYLISS, KCVO, Honorary Consultant Physician and Endocrinologist, Westminster Hospital, London; Consulting Physician, King Edward VII's Hospital for Officers, London, UK

P. B. BEESON, Emeritus Professor of Medicine, University of Washington, Seattle, USA

D. R. BELL, Reader in Tropical Medicine, Liverpool School of Tropical Medicine, Liverpool, UK

D. H. BENNETT, Regional Cardiac Centre, Wythenshawe Hospital, Manchester, UK

M. K. BENSON, Consultant Physician, Chest Clinic, Churchill Hospital, Oxford, UK

R. J. BERRY, Professor of Oncology, Middlesex Hospital Medical School, London, UK

F. W. BESWICK, Deputy Director, Chemical Defence Establishment, Salisbury, UK

SIR DOUGLAS BLACK, Emeritus Professor of Medicine, University of Manchester; Past President, Royal College of Physicians; Past President, British Medical Association

E. L. BLAIR, Professor of Physiology and Head of Department of Physiological Sciences, The University, Newcastle upon Tyne, UK

S. R. BLOOM, Professor of Endocrinology and Honorary Consultant Physician, Royal Postgraduate Medical School, Hammersmith Hospital, London, UK

B. S. BLUMBERG, Associate Director for Clinical Research, Fox Chase Cancer Center, Philadelphia; Professor of Medicine and Anthropology, University of Pennsylvania, Philadelphia, USA

R. T. BOOTH, Professor of Occupational Health and Safety, University of Aston in Birmingham, UK

SOMCHAI BOVORNKITTI, Professor of Medicine, Chief, Division of Respiratory Disease and Tubercules, Siriraj Hospital, Mahidol University, Bangkok, Thailand

E. T. W. BOWEN, Acting Director, PHLS Centre for Applied Microbiology and Research, Special Pathogens Reference Laboratory, Porton Down, Salisbury, UK

D. J. BRADLEY, Professor of Tropical Medicine, Director of the Ross Institute, and Chairman, Division of Communicable and Tropical Diseases, London School of Hygiene and Tropical Medicine, London, UK

R. D. BRADLEY, Consultant Physician, Intensive Therapy Unit, St Thomas' Hospital, London, UK

C. M. P. BRADSTREET, Formerly Director, Standards Laboratory for Serological Reagents, Central Public Health Laboratory, London, UK

J. M. BRAGANZA, Senior Lecturer in Gastroenterology, Manchester Royal Infirmary, Manchester, UK

A. M. BRECKENRIDGE, Professor of Clinical Pharmacology, University of Liverpool, UK

V A. BROADBENT, Senior Registrar in Paediatrics, Addenbrooke's Hospital, Cambridge, UK

M. J. BRODIE, Consultant Clinical Pharmacologist and Honorary Clinical Lecturer, Clinical Pharmacology Unit, University Department of Medicine, Western Infirmary, Glasgow, UK

A. D. M. BRYCESON, Consultant Physician, Hospital for Tropical Diseases, London, UK

C. BUNCH, Clinical Reader and Honorary Consultant Physician, Nuffield Department of Clinical Medicine, University of Oxford, John Radcliffe Hospital, Oxford, UK

DANAI BUNNAG, Director, Bangkok Hospital for Tropical Diseases; Head, Department of Clinical Tropical Medicine, Mahidol University, Bangkok, Thailand

W. BURGDORFER, Research Entomologist (Medical), Laboratory of Pathology, Rocky Mountain Laboratories, USA

C. W. BURKE, Consultant Physician, Department of Endocrinology, Radcliffe Infirmary, Oxford, UK

M. A. BYRON, Senior Registrar, Department of Rheumatology, Nuffield Orthopaedic Centre; and Fibrinolysis Research Group, John Radcliffe Hospital, Oxford, UK

F. I. CAIRD, David Cargill Professor of Geriatric Medicine, University of Glasgow, Southern General Hospital, Glasgow, UK

S. T. E. CALLENDER, Formerly Clinical Reader and Honorary Consultant Physician, Nuffield Department of Clinical Medicine, University of Oxford, John Radcliffe Hospital, Oxford, UK

J. S. CAMERON, Professor of Renal Medicine, Guy's Hospital Medical School, London, UK

D. M. CAMPBELL, Senior Lecturer in Obstetrics and Gynaecology and Reproductive Physiology, University of Aberdeen, UK

C. C. J. CARPENTER, Chairman, Department of Medicine, Case Western Reserve University, Cleveland, Ohio, USA

R. W. CARRELL, Professor of Haematology, University of Cambridge, Addenbrooke's Hospital, Cambridge, UK

D. CATOVSKY, Senior Lecturer in Haematology/Medicine, Royal Postgraduate Medical School, and Medical Research Council Leukaemia Unit, Hammersmith Hospital, London, UK

C. CHANTLER, Professor of Paediatric Nephrology, Evelina Children's Hospital, United Medical and Dental Schools of Guy's and St Thomas's Hospitals, London, UK

H. M. CHAPEL, Consultant Immunologist, John Radcliffe Hospital, Oxford, UK

K. CHATTERJEE, Professor of Medicine; Luciestern Professor of Cardiology; Associate Chief, Cardiovascular Division; Director of Coronary Care Unit, University of California, School of Medicine, San Francisco, USA

C. N. CHESTERMAN, Professor of Medicine, University of New South Wales, St George Hospital, Sydney, Australia

S.-Y. CHO, Associate Professor of Parasitology, College of Medicine, Chung-Aug University, Korea

A. B. CHRISTIE, Honorary Consultant, Fazakerley Hospital, Liverpool, UK

K. M. CITRON, Consultant Physician, Brompton Hospital, London, UK

M. L. CLARK, Consultant Physician, Hackney and St Bartholomew's Hospitals, London, UK

M. J. CLARKSON, Professor of Farm Animal Medicine, University of Liverpool, UK

R. D. COHEN, Professor of Medicine, London Hospital Medical College, London, UK

G. C. COOK, Honorary Consultant Physician, University College Hospital and the Hospital for Tropical Diseases, London, UK

A. M. COOKE, Honorary Consulting Physician to the United Oxford Hospitals; Emeritus Fellow of Merton College, Oxford, UK

P. J. COWEN, Medical Research Council Clinical Scientist, Research Unit, Littlemore Hospital, Oxford, UK

W. I. CRANSTON, Professor, Division of Medicine, United Medical and Dental Schools, Guy's and St Thomas's Hospitals, London, UK

SIR JOHN CROFTON, Emeritus Professor of Respiratory Diseases, University of Edinburgh, UK

G. W. CSONKA, Honorary Consultant Venereologist, Praed Street Clinic, and John Hunter Clinic, St Stephen's Hospital, London, UK

SIR JOHN DACIE, Emeritus Professor of Haematology, University of London, UK

A. G. DALGLEISH, Consultant Medical Oncologist, Northwick Park Hospital; Honorary Senior Lecturer in Oncology, Hammersmith Hospital, London, UK

S. DAROUGAR, Professor of Public Health Ophthamology, Head of the Subdepartment of Virology, Institute of Ophthalmology, London; Honorary Consultant, Moorfields Eye Hospital, London, UK

J. A. DAVIES, Senior Lecturer, University Department of Medicine and Consultant Physician, The General Infirmary, Leeds, UK

M. J. DAVIES, BHF Professor of Cardiovascular Pathology, St George's Hospital Medical School, London, UK

M. DAVIS, Consultant Physician, Royal United Hospital, Bath, UK

J. M. DAVISON, Member of the Scientific Staff, MRC Human Reproduction Group, Princess Mary Hospital, Newcastle upon Tyne, UK

D. M. DENISON, Professor of Clinical Physiology, Cardiothoracic Institute, University of London, UK

R. DICK, Consultant in Diagnostic Radiology, Royal Free Hospital, London, UK

P. DIEPPE, Senior Lecturer in Rheumatology, University of Bristol, Bristol Infirmary, Bristol, UK

SIR RICHARD DOLL, Emeritus Regius Professor of Medicine, University of Oxford; Honorary Consultant, Imperial Cancer Research Fund Cancer Epidemiology Unit, Radcliffe Infirmary, Oxford, UK

B. O. L. DUKE, Chief, Filarial Infections, Parasitic Diseases Programme, World Health Organization, Geneva, Switzerland

K. R. DUMBELL, Emeritus Professor of Virology, University of London, UK; Consultant Virologist, Department of Medical Microbiology, University of Cape Town, South Africa

M. S. DUNNILL, Consultant Pathologist, Histopathology Department, John Radcliffe Hospital, Oxford, UK

R. B. DUTHIE, Nuffield Professor of Orthopaedic Surgery, University of Oxford, Nuffield Orthopaedic Centre, Oxford, UK

M. DE SWIET, Consultant Physician, Queen Charlotte's Hospital for Women; Honorary Consultant Physician, University College Hospital and Brompton Hospital; Senior Lecturer, Cardiothoracic Institute and University College London, UK

M. A. EASTWOOD, Consultant Physician, Gastrointestinal Unit, Western General Hospital, Edinburgh, UK

A. L. W. F. EDDLESTON, Professor of Liver Immunology and Honorary Consultant Physician, Liver Unit, King's College Hospital, London, UK

C. W. R. EDWARDS, Professor of Clinical Medicine, University of Edinburgh; Chairman, Department of Medicine, Western General Hospital, Edinburgh, UK

M. ELIAKIM, Professor of Medicine, Hebrew University, Hadassah Medical School; Chairman, Department of Medicine A, Hadassah University Hospital, Jerusalem, Israel

E. ELIAS, Consultant Physician and Honorary Senior Clinical Lecturer, Queen Elizabeth Hospital, Birmingham, UK

T. A. H. ENGLISH, Consultant Cardiothoracic Surgeon, Papworth and Addenbrooke's Hospitals, Cambridge, UK

D. B. EVANS, Consultant Physician and Nephrologist, Addenbrooke's Hospital, Cambridge, UK

S. J. EYKYN, Reader in Clinical Microbiology, United Medical and Dental Schools of Guy's and St Thomas's Hospitals, London, UK

C. H. FANTA, Associate Physician, Brigham and Women's Hospital; Assistant Professor of Medicine, Harvard Medical School, Boston, USA

A. FISHER, Consultant Anaesthetist and Clinical Lecturer, Intensive Care Unit, John Radcliffe Hospital, Oxford, UK

R. A. FISHMAN, Professor and Chairman, Department of Neurology, School of Medicine, University of California, San Francisco, USA

A. F. FLEMING, Deputy Director, Tropical Diseases Research Centre, PMB 71769, Ndola, Zambia; Formerly Professor of Haematology, Ahmadu Bello University, Zaria, Nigeria

E. W. L. FLETCHER, Consultant Radiologist, John Radcliffe Hospital, Oxford, UK

P. FOEX, Clinical Reader and Honorary Consultant, Nuffield Department of Anaesthetics, University of Oxford, Radcliffe Infirmary, Oxford, UK

J. B. FOSTER, Honorary Reader in Neurology, University of Newcastle upon Tyne; Senior Neurologist, Newcastle General Hospital, UK

G. H. FOWLER, General Practitioner, Oxford; Clinical Reader in General Practice, University Department of Community Medicine and General Practice, Radcliffe Infirmary, Oxford, UK

D. A. G. GALTON, Professor of Haematology, University of London; Honorary Director, MRC Leukaemia Unit, Royal Postgraduate Medical School, Hammersmith Hospital, London, UK

S. D. GARDNER, Consultant Virologist, Virus Reference Laboratory, Central Public Health Laboratory, London, UK

D. GARDNER-MEDWIN, Paediatric Neurologist, Newcastle General Hospital, Newcastle upon Tyne, UK

D. H. Gath, Clinical Reader in Psychiatry, University Department of Psychiatry, Warneford Hospital, Oxford, UK

K. C. Gatter, Wellcome Senior Research Fellow in Clinical Science, John Radcliffe Hospital, Oxford, UK

D. M. Geddes, Consultant Physician, Brompton and London Chest Hospitals, London, UK

M. G. Gelder, Professor of Psychiatry, University of Oxford, Warneford Hospital, Oxford, UK

G. J. Gibson, Consultant Physician, Freeman Hospital, Newcastle upon Tyne, UK

D. G. Gibson, Consultant Cardiologist, National Heart and Chest Hospitals and The Brompton Hospital, London, UK

A. Giles, Chief Medical Laboratory Scientific Officer, Department of Clinical Biochemistry, John Radcliffe Hospital, Oxford, UK

R. W. Gilliatt, Professor of Clinical Neurology, Institute of Neurology; Honorary Consultant Neurologist, National Hospital for Nervous Diseases, London, UK

D. J. Girling, Member of Scientific Staff, MRC Tuberculosis and Chest Diseases Unit, Brompton Hospital, London, UK

D. H. Glaister, Consultant in Aviation Medicine, RAF Institute of Aviation Medicine, Farnborough

M. J. Goldacre, Lecturer, Department of Community Medicine and General Practice, University of Oxford, Radcliffe Infirmary, Oxford, UK

Sir Abraham Goldberg, Regius Professor of the Practice of Medicine, The University Department of Medicine, Gardiner Institute, Western Infirmary, Glasgow, UK

M. H. N. Golden, Wellcome Senior Lecturer, AG Director, Tropical Metabolism Research Unit, University of the West Indies, Mona, Kingston, Jamaica

L. G. Goodwin, Formerly Director of Science, The Zoological Society of London, UK

E. C. Gordon-Smith, Senior Lecturer and Honorary Consultant, Royal Postgraduate Medical School, Hammersmith Hospital, London, UK

R. Goulding, Formerly Director Poisons Unit, Guy's Hospital, London, UK

I. W. B. Grant, Formerly Consultant Physician, Respiratory Unit, Northern General Hospital, Edinburgh, UK

B. M. Greenwood, Director, MRC Laboratories, Fajara, Banjul, The Gambia, West Africa

D. M. Grennan, Consultant Physician, Hope Hospital, Salford; Senior Lecturer, Department of Rheumatology, University of Manchester, UK

B. Gribbin, Consultant Cardiologist, John Radcliffe Hospital, Oxford, UK

N. R. Grist, Emeritus Professor of Infectious Diseases, University of Glasgow; Formerly Head, Regional Virus Laboratory, Ruchill Hospital, Glasgow, UK

H. H. Gunson, Director, North Western Regional Transfusion Service; Reader in Human Serology, University of Manchester, UK

A. Guz, Professor of Medicine, Head, Department of Medicine, Charing Cross and Westminster Medical Schools, University of London, UK

R. Hall, Professor of Medicine, Welsh National School of Medicine, Cardiff, UK

A. M. Halliday, Consultant in Clinical Neurophysiology, National Hospital for Nervous Diseases, London; Member of the External Staff of the Medical Research Council, UK

Khunying Tranakchit Harinasuta, Emeritus Professor, Faculty of Tropical Medicine, Mahidol University, Bangkok, Thailand

H. Harris, Regius Professor of Medicine and Head of the Sir William Dunn School of Pathology, University of Oxford, UK

M. J. G. Harrison, Francis and Renee Hock Director of Research, Reta Lila Weston Institute of Neurological Studies, The Middlesex Hospital Medical School, London, UK

A. Harvey, Senior Registrar in Rheumatology, Yorkshire Regional Health Authority, UK

I. Haslock, Consultant Rheumatologist, Middlesbrough General Hospital, Middlesbrough, UK

Sant Hathirat, Associate Professor of Medicine, Ramathibodi Hospital, Mahidol University, Bangkok, Thailand

K. Hawton, Consultant Psychiatrist, Warneford Hospital; Clinical Lecturer, University of Oxford, UK

R. J. Hay, Consultant Dermatologist, St John's Hospital for Diseases of the Skin, London, UK

B. L. Hazleman, Associate Lecturer, Department of Medicine, University of Cambridge; Fellow of Corpus Christie College, Cambridge; Consultant Rheumatologist, Addenbrooke's Hospital, Cambridge and Newmarket Hospital; Honorary Consultant, Strangeways Research Laboratory, Cambridge, UK

D. J. Hendrick, Consultant Physician, Newcastle General Hospital; Honorary Lecturer in Medicine, University of Newcastle upon Tyne, UK

T. D. R. Hockaday, Consultant Physician, Radcliffe Infirmary, Oxford, UK

H. J. F. Hodgson, Senior Lecturer and Consultant Physician, Department of Medicine, Royal Postgraduate Medical School, Hammersmith Hospital, London, UK

A. V. Hoffbrand, Professor of Haematology, Royal Free Hospital School of Medicine, London, UK

Sir Raymond Hoffenberg, Formerly Professor of Medicine, University of Birmingham; President of the Royal College of Physicians, UK

J. M. Hopkin, Consultant Physician, Churchill and John Radcliffe Hospitals, Oxford; Clinical Lecturer, University of Oxford, UK

A. Hopkins, Physician in Charge, Department of Neurological Sciences, St Bartholomew's Hospital, London, UK

N. W. Horne, Formerly Consultant Physician, City Hospital, Edinburgh; Senior Lecturer, Department of Respiratory Medicine, University of Edinburgh, UK

D. F. Horrobin, Director, Efamol Research Institute, Kentville, Nova Scotia, Canada

M. D. Hourihan, Consultant Neuroradiologist, University Hospital of Wales, Cardiff, UK

J. B. L. Howell, Dean and Professor of Medicine, University of Southampton, Southampton General Hospital, Southampton, UK

T. A. Howlett, Lecturer in Endocrinology, St Bartholomew's Hospital, London, UK

W. T. Hughes, Chairman, Department of Child Science, St Jude Children's Research Hospital; Professor of Pediatrics, University of Tennessee Centre for Health Science, Memphis, USA

G. R. V. Hughes, Senior Lecturer in Medicine, Royal Postgraduate Medical School, Hammersmith Hospital, London, UK

R. Hurley, Professor of Microbiology, Institute of Obstetrics and Gynaecology, University of London, Queen Charlotte's Maternity Hospital, London, UK

M. S. R. Hutt, Emeritus Professor of Geographical Pathology, St Thomas's Hospital Medical School, London, UK

F. E. Hytten, Editor, British Journal of Obstetrics and Gynaecology, Formerly Professor, Division of Perinatal Medicine, Clinical Research Centre, Harrow, UK

I. Isherwood, Professor of Diagnostic Radiology, University of Manchester, UK

K. Ishikawa, Lecturer, Faculty of Medicine, Kyoto University, Kyoto, Japan

Surapol Issaragrisil, Associate Professor, Siriraj Hospital, Mahidol University, Bangkok, Thailand

A. A. Jackson, Professor of Human Nutrition, School of Biochemical and Physiological Sciences, University of Southampton, UK

A. Jacobs, Professor of Haematology, University of Wales College of Medicine, Cardiff, UK

W. P. T. James, Professor, Director, Rowett Research Institute, Aberdeen, UK

M. I. V. JAYSON, Professor of Rheumatology, University of Manchester, Rheumatic Diseases Centre, Hope Hospital, Salford, UK

B. JENNETT, Professor of Neurosurgery, Institute of Neurological Sciences, Glasgow, UK

D. P. JEWELL, Consultant Physician, John Radcliffe Hospital, Oxford, UK

B. E. JUEL-JENSEN, Consultant Physician (Communicable Diseases), Nuffield Department of Medicine, John Radcliffe Hospital, Oxford, UK

J. A. KANIS, Reader in Human Metabolism, Department of Human Metabolism and Clinical Biochemistry, University of Sheffield Medical School, Sheffield, UK

T. KAWASAKI, Director, Department of Pediatrics, Japanese Red Cross Medical Center, Tokyo, Japan

G. KAZANTZIS, Reader in Occupational Medicine, London School of Hygiene and Tropical Medicine; Honorary Consultant Physician, The Middlesex Hospital, London, UK

W. R. KEATINGE, Professor of Physiology, London Hospital Medical College, London, UK

D. N. S. KERR, Dean, Royal Postgraduate Medical School, Hammersmith Hospital, London, UK

R. H. KESTELOOT, Professor, Department of Cardiology, St Rafael, University Hospital, Leuven, Belgium

M. H. KING, Senior Lecturer, Department of Community Medicine, The University of Leeds, Leeds, UK

R. KNIGHT, Senior Lecturer, Department of Community Health, Faculty of Medicine, University of Nairobi; Parasitologist, Medical Research Centre, Kenya Medical Research Institute, Nairobi, Kenya

W. KWANTES, Formerly Director, Public Health Laboratory, Swansea, UK

K. S. L. LAM, Lecturer in Medicine, Department of Medicine, University of Hong Kong

D. J. LANE, Consultant Chest Physician, Churchill Hospital, Oxford, UK

H. E. LARSON, Member of the MRC Scientific Staff, Division of Communicable Diseases, Clinical Research Centre, Harrow, UK

P. J. LAWTHER, Emeritus Professor of Environmental and Preventive Medicine, St Bartholomew's and London Hospital Medical College, London, UK

N. F. LAWTON, Honorary Senior Lecturer in Neurology, University of Southampton; Consultant Neurologist, Wessex Neurological Centre, Southampton, UK

J. G. G. LEDINGHAM, Formerly Director of Clinical Studies, May Reader in Medicine, Nuffield Department of Clinical Medicine, University of Oxford; Honorary Consultant Physician, John Radcliffe Hospital, Oxford, UK

E. C. G. LEE (deceased), Consultant Surgeon, Department of Surgery, Radcliffe Infirmary, Oxford, UK

G. de J LEE, Honorary Consulting Physician, Oxford District Health Authority; Honorary Lecturer in Clinical Medicine, University of Oxford, UK

J. P. LEFF, Assistant Director, MRC Social Psychiatry Unit, Friern Hospital, London; Reader in Social and Cultural Psychiatry, University of London, UK

T. LEHNER, Head, Department of Immunology, United Medical and Dental Schools of Guy's and St Thomas's Hospitals, London, UK

E. A. LETSKY, Consultant Haematologist, Queen Charlotte's Hospital, London, UK

B. LEWIS, Professor of Chemical Pathology and Metabolic Disorders, United Medical and Dental Schools of Guy's and St Thomas's Hospitals, London, UK

S. M. LEWIS, Reader in Haematology, Royal Postgraduate Medical School; Consultant Haematologist, Hammersmith Hospital, London, UK

C. C. LINNEMANN Jr, Professor of Medicine, Division of Infectious Diseases, University of Cincinnati, Ohio, USA

M. J. LIPTON, Professor of Radiology and Medicine; Chief, Cardiovascular Imaging Section, University of California, San Francisco, USA

W. A. LISHMAN, Professor of Neuropsychiatry, Institute of Psychiatry, University of London, UK

A. LLANOS-CUENTAS, Instituto de Medicina Tropical Alexander von Humboldt, Universidad Peruana Cayetano Heredia; and Centro de Investigacion en Salud, Instituto Nacional de Salud, Peru

J. W. LLOYD, Director, Oxford Regional Pain Relief Unit, Oxford, UK

D. R. LONDON, Consultant Physician, Queen Elizabeth Hospital, Birmingham; Honorary Professor of Medicine, University of Birmingham, UK

R. G. LONG, Consultant Physician, Department of Gastroenterology, City Hospital, Nottingham, UK

M. S. LOSOWSKY, Professor of Medicine, University of Leeds, St James Hospital, Leeds, UK

W. S. LUND, Consultant ENT Surgeon, Radcliffe Infirmary, Oxford, UK

J. T. MACFARLANE, Consultant in General and Respiratory Medicine, Department of Thoracic Medicine, City Hospital, Nottingham, UK

B. MACGILLIVRAY, Physician in Clinical Neurophysiology, Royal Free Hospital and National Hospital for Nervous Diseases, London, UK

P. C. B. MACKINNON, Lecturer, Department of Human Anatomy, University of Oxford, UK

D. W. R. MACKENZIE, Director, Mycological Reference Library, Central Public Health Laboratory, London, UK

C. R. MADELEY, Professor of Clinical Virology, University of Newcastle upon Tyne, Royal Victoria Infirmary, Newcastle upon Tyne, UK

N. S. MAIR, Formerly Honorary Reader in Microbiology, School of Medicine and School of Biological Sciences, University of Leicester, UK

J. I. MANN, University Lecturer in Social Medicine and Honorary Consultant Physician, Department of Community Medicine and General Practice, University of Oxford, Radcliffe Infirmary and John Radcliffe Hospital, Oxford, UK

M. G. MARMOT, Professor of Community Medicine, University College London and The Middlesex Hospital Medical School, London, UK

C. D. MARSDEN, Professor of Clinical Neurology, King's College Hospital Medical School, London, UK

P. D. MARSDEN, Professor of Tropical Medicine, University of Brasilia, Brazil

F. P. MARSH, Consultant Nephrologist, The London Hospital, and Senior Lecturer in Medicine, The London Hospital Medical College, UK

V. J. MARTLEW, Consultant Haematologist, Regional Transfusion Service, Manchester, UK

W. C. MARSHALL (deceased), Senior Lecturer, Department of Microbiology, Institute of Child Health, University of London, UK

D. Y. MASON, University Lecturer and Honorary Consultant, Department of Haemotology, John Radcliffe Hospital, Oxford, UK

A. D. MASON Jr, Chief Laboratory Division, US Army Institute of Surgical Research, Brooke Army Medical Center, Fort Sam Houston, USA

V. I. MATHAN, Professor, Department of Gastroenterology, Wellcome Research Unit, Christian Medical College Hospital, Vellore, India

W. B. MATTHEWS, Professor of Clinical Neurology, University of Oxford, Radcliffe Infirmary, Oxford, UK

R. S. MAURICE-WILLIAMS, Consultant Neurosurgeon, Royal Free Hospital, London, UK

R. L. MAYNARD, Superintendent Medical Division, Chemical Defence Establishment, Salisbury, UK

R. A. MAYOU, Clinical Reader and Honorary Consultant Psychiatrist, University Department of Psychiatry, Warneford Hospital, Oxford, UK

K. E. L. MCCOLL, Senior Lecturer in Medicine and Honorary Consultant, The University Department of Medicine, Gardiner Institute, Western Infirmary, Glasgow, UK

N. MCINTYRE, Professor of Medicine, Royal Free Hospital and School of Medicine, London, UK

A. J. MCMICHAEL, MRC Clinical Research Professor of Immunology, John Radcliffe Hospital, Oxford, UK

B. C. MEHTA, Professor and Head, Dr J. C. Patel Department of Hematology, Seth G. S. Medical College and K. E. M. Hospital; Honorary Hematologist, Nanavati Hospital and Research Centre; Honorary Director, Blood Research Centre, Bombay, India

T. J. MEREDITH, Senior Registrar in Medicine, Guy's and Lewisham Hospitals, London, UK

G. A. H. MILLER, Consultant Cardiologist and Director, Cardiac Laboratories, Brompton Hospital, London, UK

P. R. MILLS, Associate Professor, Division of Gastroenterology, Medical College of Virginia, Richmond, USA

F. J. MILNE, Professor of Medicine, Coronation Hospital, University of the Witwatersrand Medical School, Johannesburg, South Africa

J. J. MISIEWICZ, Consultant Physician, Department of Gastroenterology and Nutrition, Central Middlesex Hospital, London, UK

R. G. MITCHELL, Consultant Microbiologist, Department of Medical Microbiology. John Radcliffe Hospital, Oxford, UK

M. MITCHESON, Consultant Psychiatrist, Formerly of the Drug Dependence Clinic, University College London, UK

S. MIWA, Professor, Department of Internal Medicine, Institute of Medical Science, University of Tokyo, Japan

HLA MON, Consulant Nephrologist, Rangoon General Hospital, Rangoon, Burma

M. A. MONNICKENDAM, Lecturer, Subdepartment of Virology, Institute of Ophthalmology, London, UK

M. R. MOORE, Senior Lecturer in Medicine, University Department of Medicine, Gardiner Institute, Western Infirmary, Glasgow, UK

H. G. MORGAN, Professor of Mental Health, University of Bristol, UK

P. J. MORRIS, Nuffield Professor of Surgery, University of Oxford, John Radcliffe Hospital, Oxford, UK

R. B. I. MORRISON, Consultant Physician, Renal Unit, Wellington Hospital, New Zealand

A. G. MOWAT, Clinical Lecturer in Rheumatology, University of Oxford; Consultant Rheumatologist, Nuffield Orthopaedic Centre, Oxford, UK

A. P. MOWAT, Consultant Paediatrician, Department of Child Health, King's College Hospital Medical School, London

M. F. MUERS, Consultant Physician and Honorary Clinical Lecturer, St James's University Hospital and Killingbeck Hospital, Leeds, UK

P. A. MURPHY, Professor of Medicine, Department of Microbiology, The Johns Hopkins University School of Medicine, Baltimore, USA

I. M. MURRAY-LYON, Consultant Physician and Gastroenterologist, Charing Cross Hospital, London, UK

J. NAGINGTON, Formerly Consultant Virologist, Addenbrooke's Hospital, Cambridge, UK

K. NAKAE, Associate Professor, Department of Public Health, Dokkyo University School of Medicine, Japan; Member of the SMON Research Committee of Japan

D. G. NATHAN, Physician-in-Chief, The Children's Hospital, Boston, and Robert A. Stranahan Professor of Paediatrics, Harvard Medical School, USA

P. NATHAN, Honorary Consultant in Clinical Neurophysiology, National Hospital for Nervous Diseases; Honorary Consultant Neurologist, Royal National Orthopaedic Hospital; and Honorary Consultant Neurologist, City Migraine Clinic, London, UK

G. NEALE, Consultant Physician, Addenbrooke's Hospital, Cambridge, UK

G. H. NEILD, Senior Lecturer, Institute of Urology and Honorary Consultant Physician, St Peter's Group of Hospitals, St Philip's Hospital, London, UK

J. M. NEUTZE, Cardiologist-in-Charge, Green Lane Hospital; Clinical Reader, School of Medicine, Auckland University, New Zealand

C. I. NEWBOLD, University Lecturer, Nuffield Department of Clinical Medicine, John Radcliffe Hospital, Oxford, UK

E. A. NEWSHOLME, Fellow and Tutor in Biochemistry, Merton College, Oxford; Lecturer in Biochemistry, University of Oxford, UK

J. NEWSOM-DAVIS, Professor of Neurology, Royal Free Hospital School of Medicine and the Institute of Neurology, London, UK

SUCHITRA NIMMANNITYA, Chief, Infectious Disease Unit, Children's Hospital, Bangkok, Thailand

D. J. NOLAN, Consultant Radiologist, John Radcliffe Hospital, Oxford, UK

G. NUKI, Professor of Rheumatology, University of Edinburgh; Consultant Rheumatologist, Rheumatic Diseases Unit, Northern General Hospital, Edinburgh, UK

C. M. OAKLEY, Consultant Cardiologist, Royal Postgraduate Medical School, Hammersmith Hospital, London, UK

C. OGILVIE, Consultant Physician, Royal Liverpool Hospital, Liverpool Cardiothoracic Centre and The King Edward VIIth Hospital, Midhurst, UK

D. O. OLIVER, Consultant Nephrologist, The Renal Unit, Churchill Hospital, Oxford, UK

M. L'E. ORME, Professor of Pharmacology and Therapeutics, University of Liverpool, UK

J. M. OXBURY, Consultant Neurologist, Department of Neurology, Radcliffe Infirmary, UK

G. S. PANAYI, Professor of Rheumatology, United Medical and Dental Schools of Guy's and St Thomas's Hospitals, London, UK

M. T. PARKER, Formerly Director, Cross Infection Reference Laboratory, Central Public Health Laboratory, London, UK

E. H. O. PARRY, Director, Wellcome Tropical Institute, London, UK

D. S. PARSONS, Emeritus University Reader in Physiological Biochemistry, University of Oxford; Emeritus Professorial Fellow, Merton College, Oxford, UK

J. R. PATTISON, Professor of Medical Microbiology, University College London and the Middlesex Hospital Medical School, London, UK

J. PAYAN, Consultant in clinical electromyography to Guy's and King's College Hospitals and the Hospital for Sick Children, London, UK

J. M. S. PEARCE, Consultant Neurologist, Hull Royal Infirmary, UK

M. E. PEMBREY, Senior Lecturer, Mothercare Unit of Paediatrics, Institute of Child Health; Honorary Consultant in Clinical Genetics, The Hospital for Sick Children, Great Ormond Street, London, UK

J. E. PENNINGTON, Associate Professor of Medicine, Harvard Medical School and Brigham and Women's Hospital, Boston, USA

B. L. PENTECOST, Consultant Physician, United Birmingham Hospitals; Senior Clinical Lecturer, University of Birmingham, UK

M. B. PEPYS, Professor of Immunological Medicine, MRC Acute Phase Protein Research Group, Immunological Medicine Unit, Department of Medicine, Royal Postgraduate Medical School, London, UK

P. L. PERINE, Professor and Director, Division of Tropical Public Health, Department of Preventative Medicine/Biometrics, Uniformed Services University of the Health Sciences, Bethesda, Maryland, USA

D. K. PETERS, Professor of Medicine, Royal Postgraduate Medical School, Hammersmith Hospital, London, UK

R. PETO, Imperial Cancer Research Fund Reader in Cancer Studies, Nuffield Department of Clinical Medicine, University of Oxford, Radcliffe Infirmary, Oxford, UK

I. PHILLIPS, Professor of Microbiology, United Medical and Dental Schools of Guy's and St Thomas's Hospitals, London, UK

PRIDA PHUAPRADIT, Assistant Professor, Department of Medicine, Ramathibodi Hospital, Mahidol University, Bangkok, Thailand

ANONG PIANKIJAGUM, Professor, Siriraj Hospital, Mahidol University, Bangkok, Thailand

M. J. PIPPARD, Consultant Haematologist, Northwick Park Hospital and Clinical Research Centre, Harrow, UK

J. M. POLAK, Professor of Endocrine Pathology, Department of Histochemistry, Royal Postgraduate Medical School, Hammersmith Hospital, London, UK

P. A. POOLE-WILSON, Professor of Cardiology, Department of Cardiac Medicine, The Cardiothoracic Institute; Honorary Consultant Physician, National Heart Hospital, London, UK

J. S. PORTERFIELD, Reader in Bacteriology, Sir William Dunn School of Pathology, University of Oxford, UK

R. E. POUNDER, Reader in Medicine, Royal Free Hospital Medical School, London, UK

F. S. PRESTON, Director, Medical Services, British Airways, London, UK

A. B. PRICE, Consultant Histopathologist, Northwick Park Hospital, Harrow, UK

E. W. PRICE, Formerly Research Fellow, Department of Clinical and Tropical Medicine, London School of Hygiene and Tropical Medicine, London, UK

J. S. PRICHARD, Associate Professor of Medicine, Trinity College, Dublin; Consultant Physician, St James's Hospital, Dublin, Eire

N. B. PRIDE, Senior Lecturer in Medicine, St Mary's Hospital and Royal Postgraduate Medical Schools, London, UK

J. PRITCHARD, Consultant and Senior Lecturer in Paediatric Oncology, Hospital for Sick Children, Great Ormond Street, London, UK

A. T. PROUDFOOT, Consultant Physician, Regional Poisoning Treatment Centre, Royal Infirmary, Edinburgh, UK

B. A. PRUITT Jr, Commander and Director, US Army Institute of Surgical Research, Brooke Army Medical Center, Fort Sam Houston, USA

SOMPONNE PUNYAGUPTA, Medical Director, Vichaiyut Hospital, and Consultant Physician, Phra Mongkutklao Medical School, Vajira Municipality Hospital and Bamras Naradura Hospital for Infectious Diseases, Bangkok, Thailand

M. RACHMILEWITZ (deceased), Professor Emeritus, Hebrew University, Hadassah Medical School, Jerusalem, Israel

A. J. RADFORD, Professor of Primary Care and Community Medicine, Flinders Medical Centre, The Flinders University of South Australia, Australia

B. RAJAGOPALAN, Nuffield Department of Medicine and Medical Research Council Clinical Magnetic Resonance Facility, John Radcliffe Hospital, Oxford, UK

C. W. G. REDMAN, Lecturer in Obstetric Medicine, Nuffield Department of Obstetrics and Gynaecology, University of Oxford, John Radcliffe Hospital, Oxford, UK

L. H. REES, Professor of Chemical Endocrinology, St Bartholomew's Hospital, London, UK

R. S. O. REES, Consultant Radiologist, St Bartholomew's Hospital and National Heart Hospital, London, UK

D. RENNIE, Professor of Medicine, Rush Medical College, Chicago; Chairman, Department of Medicine, West Suburban Hospital Medical Center, Oak Park, USA

M. RIGATTO, Docent and Associate Professor of Internal Medicine, Universidade Federal do Rio Grande do Sul; Senior Researcher, National Research Council, Brazil

A. ROMPALO, Senior Fellow, University of Washington School of Medicine, Division of Infectious Diseases, Harborview Medical Center, Seattle, USA

B. D. ROSS, Honorary Consultant Physician, Nuffield Department of Clinical Medicine, John Radcliffe Hospital, Oxford, UK

R. W. ROSS RUSSELL, Physician to St Thomas's Hospital, National Hospital and Moorfield's Eye Hospital, London, UK

D. J. ROWLANDS, Consultant Cardiologist, Manchester Area Health Authority; Lecturer in Cardiology, University of Manchester, UK

D. RUBENSTEIN, Physician, Addenbrooke's Hospital, Cambridge; Associate Lecturer, University of Cambridge, UK

P. RUDGE, Consultant Neurologist, The National Hospital and Northwick Park Hospital; Consultant Neurologist, Medical Research Council, Neuro-otology Unit, The National Hospital, London, UK

T. K. RUEBUSH II, Medical Officer, Malaria Branch, Division of Parasitic Diseases, Center for Infectious Diseases, Center for Disease Control, Public Health Service, US Department of Health and Human Services, Atlanta, USA

G. RUIZ REYES, Laboratoris Clinior de Puebla, Puebla, Peru

G. F. M. RUSSELL, Professor of Psychiatry, Institute of Psychiatry, University of London, Bethlem Royal and Maudsley Hospitals, London, UK

R. I. RUSSELL, Gastroenterology Unit, Royal Infirmary, Glasgow, UK

T. J. RYAN, Consultant Dermatologist, The Slade Hospital, Oxford, UK

L. SANCHEZ MEDAL, Fundacion de Investigaciones Sociales, Mexico City

DAME CICELY SAUNDERS CBE, Medical Director, St Christopher's Hospice, London, UK

J. G. SCADDING, Emeritus Professor of Medicine, University of London; Honorary Consulting Physician, Brompton Hospital and Hammersmith Hospital, London, UK

A. SEATON, Director, Institute of Occupational Medicine, Edinburgh, UK

J. L. SEGGIE, Senior Physician/Senior Lecturer, University of the Witwatersrand Medical School, Johannesburg, South Africa

E. A. SHINEBOURNE, Consultant Paediatric Cardiologist, Brompton Hospital, London, UK

J. R. SILVER, Consultant in Spinal Injuries, National Spinal Injuries Centre, Stoke Mandeville Hospital; Formerly Consultant in Charge, Liverpool Regional Paraplegic Centre and Lecturer in Surgery, Liverpool University, UK

D. I. H. SIMPSON, Professor of Microbiology, The Queen's University of Belfast, Northern Ireland

VISITH SITPRIJA, Professor of Medicine and Associate Dean, Division of Nephrology, Department of Medicine, Chulalongkorn Hospital, Bangkok, Thailand

M. B. SKIRROW, Consultant Microbiologist, Department of Pathology (Microbiology), Worcester Royal Infirmary, Worcester, UK

M. P. E. SLACK, Lecturer in Bacteriology, University of Oxford; Honorary Consultant Microbiologist, John Radcliffe Hospital, Oxford, UK

P. SLEIGHT, Field Marshall Alexander Professor of Cardiovascular Medicine, University of Oxford, Department of Cardiology, John Radcliffe Hospital, Oxford, UK

J. C. SMITH, Consultant Urological Surgeon, Churchill Hospital, Oxford, UK

R. SMITH, Consultant Physician and Consultant in Metabolic Medicine, John Radcliffe Hospital and Nuffield Orthopaedic Centre, Oxford, UK

M. L. SNAITH, Consultant Rheumatologist and Honorary Senior

Lecturer in Medicine, Faculty of Clinical Sciences, University College London, UK

J. SOMERVILLE, Consultant Physician in Congenital Heart Disease, National Heart Hospital; Honorary Consultant Physician, Hospital for Sick Children, Great Ormond Street, London, UK

W. SOMERVILLE CBE, Consultant Physician, Department of Cardiology, The Middlesex Hospital, London, UK

D. J. SPALTON, Consultant Ophthalmic Surgeon and Consultant Ophthalmologist to the Medical Eye Unit, St Thomas's Hospital; Senior Lecturer in Clinical Pharmacology, United Medical and Dental Schools of Guy's and St Thomas's Hospitals, London, UK

S. G. SPIRO, Consultant Physician, University College Hospital, The Middlesex Hospital and Brompton Hospital, London, UK

W. E. STAMM, Professor of Medicine, University of Washington, School of Medicine; Head, Division of Infectious Diseases, Harborview Medical Center, Seattle, USA

G. STORES, Consultant Neuropsychiatrist, The Park Hospital for Children, Oxford, UK

J. R. STRADLING, Wellcome Senior Research Fellow and Honorary Consultant, Osler Chest Unit, Churchill Hospital, Oxford, UK

J. A. SUMMERFIELD, Senior Lecturer in Medicine, Department of Medicine, Royal Free Hospital School of Medicine, London, UK

PRAVAN SUNTHARASAMAI, Associate Professor, Department of Clinical Tropical Medicine and the Hospital for Tropical Diseases, Faculty of Tropical Medicine, Mahidol University, Bangkok, Thailand

R. SUTTON, Consultant Cardiologist, Westminster Hospital, London, UK

K. B. TAYLOR, George DeForest Barnett Professor of Medicine, Stanford University School of Medicine, California, USA

D. TAYLOR-ROBINSON, Head, Division of Sexually Transmitted Diseases, Clinical Research Centre, Harrow, UK

G. TEASDALE, Professor of Neurosurgery, Institute of Neurological Sciences, Southern General Hospital, Glasgow, UK

P. J. TEDDY, Consultant Neurosurgeon, Radcliffe Infirmary, Oxford, UK

B. TEKLU, Associate Professor of Medicine, Addis Ababa University Medical Faculty; Attending Physician, Tikur Anbessa Hospital, Addis Ababa, Ethiopia

P. K. THOMAS, Professor of Neurology, Royal Free Hospital School of Medicine and Institute of Neurology, London, UK

H. C. THOMAS, Professor of Medicine and Honorary Consultant Physician, Royal Free Hospital and Medical School, London, UK

J. O'H TOBIN, Formerly Demonstrator in Pathology, Sir William Dunn School of Pathology, University of Oxford; Honorary Consultant Virologist, John Radcliffe Hospital, Oxford, UK

D. TODD OBE, Professor of Medicine, University of Hong Kong, Queen Mary Hospital, Hong Kong

A. M. TOMKINS, Department of Clinical Tropical Medicine and Department of Human Nutrition, London School of Hygiene and Tropical Medicine, London, UK

T. A. TRAILL, Assistant Professor of Medicine, The Johns Hopkins Hospital, Baltimore, USA

J. D. TREHARNE, Senior Lecturer in Virology, Subdepartment of Virology, Institute of Ophthalmology, London, UK

J. O. TRELLES, Emeritus Professor of Neurology, Lima, Peru

L. TRELLES, Professor of Neurology, Lima; Head of the Neurological and Research Department, Santo Toribio Neurological Hospital, Lima, Peru

S. C. TRUELOVE, Formerly Reader in Clinical Medicine, University of Oxford; Consultant Physician, Nuffield Department of Clinical Medicine, John Radcliffe Hospital, Oxford, UK

E. TUDDENHAM, Senior Lecturer in Haematology, Co-Director, Haemophilia Centre, Royal Free Hospital Medical School, London, UK

D. C. TURK, Formerly Consultant Microbiologist, Public Health Laboratory, Northern General Hospital, Sheffield, UK

L. A. TURNBERG, Professor of Medicine, University of Manchester; Honorary Consultant Physician, Hope Hospital, Salford, UK

R. C. TURNER, Clinical Reader and Honorary Consultant Physician, Nuffield Department of Clinical Medicine, Radcliffe Infirmary, Oxford, UK

M. E. H. TURNER-WARWICK, Dean and Professor of Medicine, The Cardiothoracic Institute, London, UK

D. A. J. TYRRELL, Director, MRC Common Cold Unit, Salisbury, UK

J. A. VALE, Director, West Midlands Poisons Unit, Birmingham; Senior Clinical Lecturer, University of Birmingham, UK

R. I. VANHEGAN, Consultant Histopathologist, Princess Margaret Hospital, Swindon, UK

ATHASIT VEJJAJIVA, Senior Neurologist, Professor and Chairman, Department of Medicine, Faculty of Medicine, Ramathibodi Hospital, Mahidol University, Bangkok, Thailand

M. P. VESSEY, Professor of Social and Community Medicine, Department of Community Medicine and General Practice, University of Oxford, UK

VIKIT VIRANUVATTI, Professor and Consultant, Siriraj Hospital, Mahidol University, Bangkok, Thailand

G. N. VOLANS, Director, National Poisons Unit, New Cross Hospital, London, UK

N. H. WADIA, Director of Neurology, Jaslok Hospital and Research Centre; Consultant Neurologist and Retired Professor of Neurology, J. J. Group of Hospitals and Grant Medical College; Visiting Neurologist, B. D. Petit Parsee General Hospital, Bombay, India

J. A. WALKER-SMITH, Professor of Paediatric Gastroenterology, St Bartholomew's Hospital, London, UK

J. M. WALSHE, Reader in Metabolic Diseases, University of Cambridge Clinical School; Honorary Consultant Physician, Addenbrooke's Hospital, Cambridge, UK

SIR JOHN WALTON, Warden, Green College, Oxford; Formerly Professor of Neurology, University of Newcastle upon Tyne, UK

C. P. WARLOW, Clinical Reader in Neurology, University of Oxford, UK

D. A. WARRELL, Professor of Tropical Medicine and Infectious Diseases, Nuffield Department of Clinical Medicine, University of Oxford, and Honorary Consultant Physician, John Radcliffe Hospital, Oxford, UK. Formerly Director, Wellcome-Mahidol University Oxford, Tropical Medicine Research Programme, Bangkok, Thailand

K. S. WARREN, Director, Health Sciences Division, The Rockefeller Foundation, New York, USA

PRAWASE WASI, Professor of Medicine, Head, Department of Medicine, Siriraj Hospital, Mahidol University, Bangkok, Thailand

M. F. R. WATERS OBE, Consultant Leprologist, Hospital for Tropical Diseases, London; Member of the Medical Research Council External Scientific Staff, Middlesex Hospital, London, UK

R. W. E. WATTS, Head, Division of Inherited Metabolic Diseases, Medical Research Council Clinical Research Centre; Consultant Physician, Northwick Park Hospital; Assistant Director (Clinical), Medical Research Council Clinical Research Centre, Harrow, UK

SIR DAVID WEATHERALL, Nuffield Professor of Clinical Medicine, University of Oxford, Nuffield Department of Clinical Medicine, John Radcliffe Hospital, Oxford, UK

A. D. B. WEBSTER, Consultant Physician, Northwick Park Hospital, Harrow, Middlesex, UK

R. A. WEISS, Director, Institute of Cancer Research, London, UK

N. J. WHITE, Director, Wellcome-Mahidol University, Oxford

Tropical Medicine Research Programme, Faculty of Tropical Medicine, Bangkok, Mahidol University, Thailand

H. C. WHITTLE, Senior Scientist, Medical Research Council Laboratories, Fajara, The Gambia

B. WIDDOP, Consultant Biochemist, Poisons Unit, Guy's Hospital, London, UK

D. E. L. WILCKEN, Associate Professor of Medicine, University of New South Wales, The Prince Henry Hospital, Sydney, Australia

C. M. WILES, Consultant Neurologist, The National Hospital for Nervous Diseases and St Thomas's Hospital, London, UK

C. B. WILLIAMS, Consultant Physician, St Mark's and St Bartholomew's Hospitals, London, UK

D. G. WILLIAMS, Consultant Nephrologist and Senior Lecturer in Medicine, Guy's Hospital and United Medical and Dental Schools of Guy's and St Thomas's Hospitals, London, UK

E. WILLIAMS, Consultant Physician, Withybush General Hospital, Haverfordwest, UK

R. WILLIAMS, Consultant Physician and Director, Liver Unit, King's College Hospital, London, UK

S. J. WILLIAMS, Consultant Physician, Chest Department, Stoke Mandeville Hospital, Aylesbury, UK

D. H. WILLIAMSON, Member of the Medical Research Council External Scientific Staff, Metabolic Research Laboratories, Radcliffe Infirmary, Oxford, UK

KYAW WIN, Lt Col., Burma Army Medical Corps; Consultant Physician, No. 2, Military Hospital, Rangoon, Burma

A. J. WING, Consultant Physician, St Thomas's Hospital, London, UK

D. L. WINGATE, Reader in Gastroenterology, University of London; Director, Gastrointestinal Science Research Unit, London Hospital Medical College; Honorary Consultant Gastroenterologist, The London Hospital, Whitechapel, London, UK

H. F. WOODS, Professor of Therapeutics, University of Sheffield, The Royal Hallamshire Hospital, Sheffield, UK

T. E. WOODWARD, Emeritus Professor of Medicine, University of Maryland School of Medicine and Hospital Veterans Administration Medical Center, Baltimore, USA

A. J. WOOLCOCK, Professor of Respiratory Medicine, University of Sydney, New South Wales, Australia

K. G. WORMSLEY, Consultant Physician, Ninewells Hospital, Dundee, UK

F. W. WRIGHT, Consultant Radiologist, Clinical Lecturer in Radiology, Department of Radiology, Churchill Hospital, Oxford, UK

R. WRIGHT, Professor of Medicine, University of Southampton Medical School and Medical Unit; Honorary Consultant Physician, Southampton General Hospital, Southampton, UK

S. G. WRIGHT, Associate Professor, Department of Medicine, College of Medicine, King Saud University, Riyadh, Saudi Arabia

V. WRIGHT, Professor of Rheumatology, University of Leeds; Consultant Physician in Rheumatology, Leeds Western District Health Authority and Yorkshire Regional Health Authority, UK

V. M. WRIGHT, Consultant Paediatric Surgeon, Queen Elizabeth Hospital for Children, London, UK

MARIA A. WYKE, Senior Lecturer in Neuropsychology, Institute of Psychiatry, London, UK

R. T. T. YEUNG, Professor of Medicine, Department of Medicine, University of Hong Kong

A. YOUNG, Consultant Physician in Geriatric Medicine, Royal Free Hospital, London, UK

V. ZAMAN, Professor of Parasitology, Faculty of Medicine, University of Singapore

A. J. ZUCKERMAN, Professor of Microbiology, University of London; Director of the Department of Medical Microbiology and of the World Health Organization Collaborating Centre for Reference and Research on Viral Hepatitis, London School of Hygiene and Tropical Medicine; Honorary Consultant in Medical Microbiology

SECTION 13
CARDIOVASCULAR DISEASE

Biochemistry and cellular physiology of heart muscle and membranes

P. A. POOLE-WILSON

Structure of the myocardial cell

The heart of normal man weighs 250–300 g, contracts at a rate of 70–75 beats/min at rest and pumps 5 l/min. On exercise the heart rate may increase to 200 beats/min and the cardiac output to 20 l/min. The organ is made up of many different cell types. Some cells such as those in the sinoatrial node, the atrioventricular node, the bundle of His, and Purkinje fibres are specialized for the purpose of initiating a heart beat and transmitting this signal in a regular and co-ordinated manner to the heart muscle in atria and ventricles. By volume the most common cells are myocardial cells (myocytes). These provide the contractile force needed for the ejection of blood from the right and the left ventricles. The myocardial cell is approximately 100 μm long and 15 μm wide (Fig. 1). The cell branches and interdigitates with adjacent cells and is surrounded by a rich capillary network. At its ends each cell is in contact with another cell through a characteristic area of cell membrane called the intercalated disc. The intercalated disc contains several specialized structures, the fascia adherens, macula adherens (desmosome), and gap junctions (nexus). The fascia adherens are mechanical links so that force can be transmitted between cells when the heart contracts. The macula adherens (desmosome) are the sites where cytoplasmic filaments, which provide a lattice structure for the cell, attach to the cell membrane. The gap junctions are the areas of the intercalated disc where the membranes of adjacent cells are particularly close and the permeability of the cell membrane to ions is low so that an electrical signal can pass easily between cells.

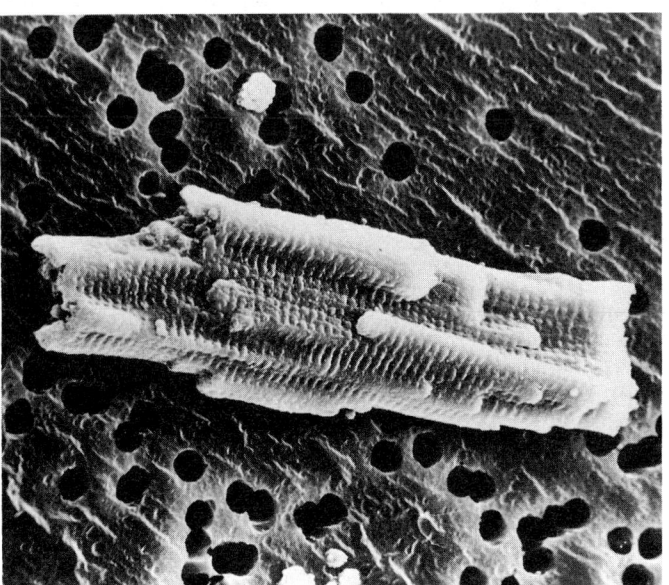

Fig. 1 A single myocardial cell (myocyte). The picture was obtained by scanning electron microscopy. The black holes in the background are part of the supporting material on which the cell has been placed. The cell is approximately 100 μm in length. (Provided by courtesy of Professor N. Woolf and Dr E. M. Steen, Middlesex Hospital.)

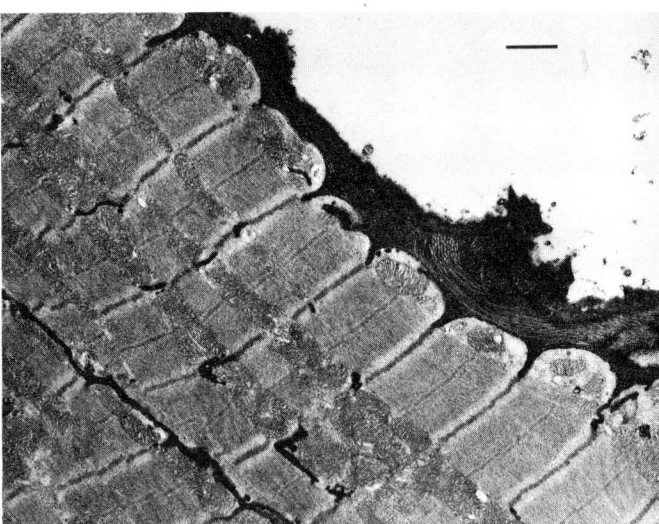

Fig. 2 Electron micrograph of part of a single myocardial cell. The glycocalyx (surface coat) and the T-tubules have been stained with potassium ferrocyanide and appear black. Note that the T-tubules penetrate deep into the cells, are connected to the extracellular space, and are aligned with the Z-lines of the sarcomeres. Scale bar: 1 μm.

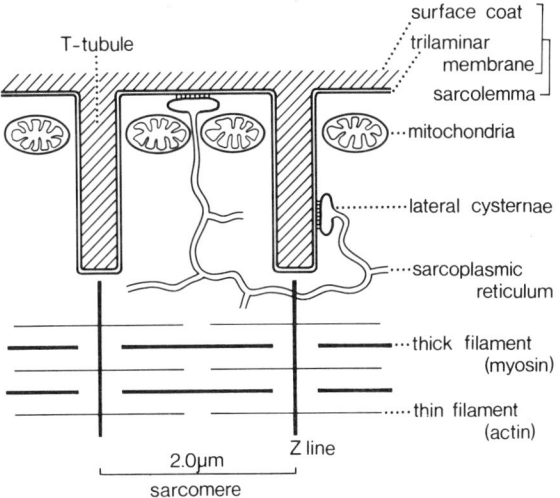

Fig. 3 Diagrammatic representation of organelles in a myocardial cell.

Each cell contains bundles of myofibrils (approximately 1 μm in diameter and 150 per cell). The myofibrils run the length of the cell and are made up of a repeating basic unit of contraction, the sarcomere (2 μm in length). The sarcomeres in adjacent myofibrils are aligned at the Z line. This gives heart muscle its striated appearance under both the light and electron microscopes (Fig. 2).

The myocardial cell is surrounded by a cell membrane (the sarcolemma). The sarcolemma is made up of a trilaminar membrane (10 nm thick) and an outer layer (70 nm thick) called the surface coat or glycocalyx (Fig. 3). The trilaminar membrane consists of two layers of lipid molecules which align themselves so that the polar heads of the molecules are facing outwards and the lipid tails

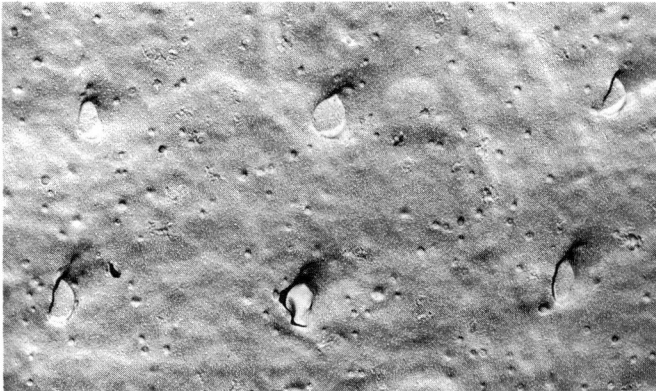

Fig. 4 Picture of the surface of a single myocardial cell viewed from the extracellular space. The openings of six T-tubules can be seen arranged in a regular pattern. The T-tubules are approximately 2 μm apart. The smaller dimples are caveolae. In the background very small particles can be seen. These are individual proteins in the trilaminar cell membrane.

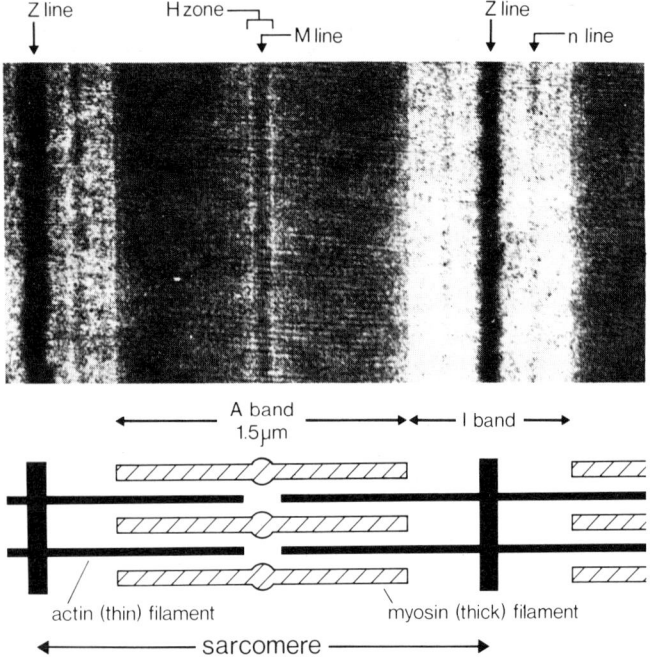

Fig. 5 An electron micrograph of a single sarcomere, the basic contractile unit of heart muscle. Below is a diagrammatic interpretation of how the thick and thin filaments interdigitate. The heads protruding from the thick filament are not shown.

are within (the meat in the sandwich). The characteristic pattern seen under the electron microscope (dark–pale–dark) is made up of polar heads–lipid–polar heads (hence 'trilaminar' membrane). The trilaminar membrane is not a static structure but has liquid properties. Numerous different proteins are located in the cell membrane and move freely in it (Fig. 4). These are the channels for the passage of ions through the membrane and receptor sites for hormones and pharmacologically active substances. Outside the trilaminar membrane but attached to it is the glycocalyx (surface coat, external lamina). The glycocalyx is made up of glycoproteins, glycolipids, and polysacharrides.

Most of the volume of a myocardial cell is taken up by cell water and myofibrils but 30 per cent of the volume is mitochondria. The numerous mitochondria provide the energy necessary for cardiac contraction in the form of adenosine triphosphate (ATP) and are the reason why the heart is so dependent on maintained coronary blood flow and the availability of oxygen.

The myocardial cell has wide T-tubules and an extensive sarcoplasmic reticulum (Figs 2–4). The T-tubules are invaginations from the cell surface with openings up to 200 nm in diameter (Fig. 4). The tubules are regularly spaced (approximately 2 μm apart) so that one T-tubule goes down to each Z line in each myofibril. The T-tubules allow the electrical signal for contraction and the passage of calcium across the cell membrane to be in close proximity to the Z line. The sarcoplasmic reticulum is a lace-like tubular structure (30 nm in diameter) spreading over the myofibrils and throughout the whole cell. Where the sarcoplasmic reticulum comes close to the surface membrane or T-tubules swellings develop called lateral cysternae. Feet, seen as dark opacities under the electron microscope, connect the lateral cysternae to the trilaminar membrane. The sarcoplasmic reticulum is a sink for the uptake of calcium within the cell, thus maintaining the low intracellular calcium concentration in diastole. The release of calcium from the sarcoplasmic reticulum contributes to the initiation of contraction.

The myocardial cell has a nucleus, Golgi apparatus, and ribosomes. These structures are concerned with cell repair and protein synthesis. The ability of myocardial cells to divide is lost early in life. Cardiac hypertrophy in adults is the result of protein synthesis and increase in the size of each cell not cell division.

Contraction of the heart is brought about by shortening of the sarcomeres within each cell. The contraction requires energy generated by the mitochondria in the form of ATP (adenosine triphosphate) and is triggered by a sudden increase of the calcium concentration in the region of the myofibrils.

The sarcomere and contractile proteins
The sarcomere at rest is between 1.8 and 2.0 μm in length from Z line to Z line (Figs 2 and 5). Under the electron microscope bands of differing density can be seen. These bands have names as in Fig. 5.

The sarcomere is made up of two interdigitating filaments, a thick filament made of the protein myosin and a thin filament made of actin (Figs 5 and 6). The thick filament (A band) is 15 nm across and 1.5 μm in length and is comprised of 400 myosin molecules (MW = 460 000). Each myosin molecule is 160 nm in length. The molecule has a long body consisting of two intertwining α-helical peptide molecules (heavy chains). At the end of each peptide is a head made up of two further peptide chains. The myosin molecules are aligned with their bodies longitudinally so that at any point the thick filament contains 18 myosin molecules in cross-section. The heads of the myosin molecule protrude from the thick filament in opposed pairs every 14.3 nm and are staggered around the filament to repeat every 43 nm. Thus, six heads are available in every 43 nm to connect with the actin molecules in the thin filaments (Fig. 7). The myosin head contains the enzyme myofibrillar ATPase which breaks down ATP to provide the energy for contraction.

The thin filament (6 nm thick, 1 μm long) is a more complex structure (Fig. 6). The actin molecule (MW = 42 000) is a small globular protein which polymerizes to form chains of molecules. Two chains of actin molecules form a helical structure such that one revolution occurs every 39 nm and contains seven actin mole-

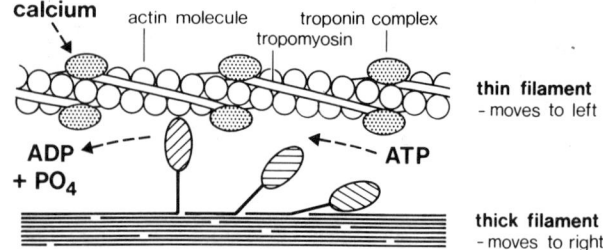

Fig. 6 Diagrammatic representation of the contractile proteins. The thick filament is made from myosin, the thin filament from actin.

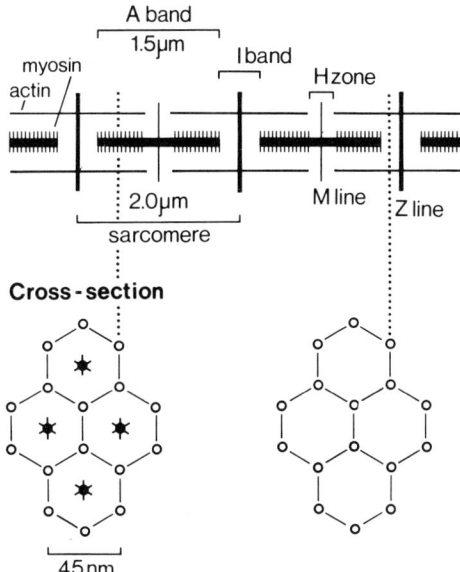

Fig. 7 Diagrammatic representation of the structure of the contractile proteins in longitudinal and transverse sections.

cules in each of the two strands. In the grooves of the helix runs a second molecule tropomyosin (MW = 68 000). Tropomyosin probably maintains the structure of the actin chain and by moving in the groove transmits information to all seven actin molecules in each revolution of the molecule. Attached to every seventh actin molecule is a further protein troponin. This protein has three parts. Troponin C (MW = 18 000) binds calcium with a high affinity and initiates contraction. Troponin I (MW = 28 0000) prevents an interaction between actin and myosin and is under the control of troponin C. Troponin T (MW = 41 000) binds the troponin complex to tropomyosin.

The exact mechanism by which movement occurs between actin and myosin molecules in cardiac muscle is not fully understood. Certainly the process is initiated by the binding of calcium to troponin C which then no longer causes troponin I to prevent an interaction between actin and myosin. The muscle shortens and ATP is broken down to ADP and phosphate. One possible sequence of events is the following. ATP combines with the myosin head. Under these conditions the muscle is relaxed and pliable. Calcium combines with troponin C which releases the inhibitor protein troponin I permitting the tropomyosin molecule to move, and thus allowing actin molecules to form a link with a myosin head. The muscle is now relaxed but stiff. A mechanical change in the angle at which the myosin head is attached to the body of the myosin molecule occurs spontaneously causing the two filaments to move (Fig. 6). The muscle is now contracted and stiff. ADP and phosphate are released. When ATP combines with myosin the actin–myosin bond is broken and the muscle returns to its relaxed and pliable state. The process repeats itself until the calcium is released from troponin C. Thus, muscle shortening is brought about by a ratchet mechanism. Alternative theories have been put forward. One point to note is that according to this hypothesis ATP is required both to bring about contraction and to permit relaxation.

Energy for contraction

In normal humans at rest the coronary blood flow is 0.8 ml/min/g, the arterial oxygen content is 180 ml/l and the coronary sinus oxygen content is 68 ml/l (equivalent to an oxygen saturation of 37 per cent and P_{O_2} of approximately 25 mmHg). The heart weighs 300 g. The oxygen consumption is, therefore, 27 ml/min for the whole heart or 0.09 ml/min/g. Oxygen is utilized in the mitochond-

ria by the process of oxidative phosphorylation to generate ATP. This is transported across the mitochondrial membrane to cytosolic sites.

The major substrates for the heart are fatty acids, glucose, and lactate. At rest and in the fasting state 60 per cent of the total oxygen consumption of the heart is utilized by the metabolism of fatty acids, 28 per cent by glucose, 11 per cent by lactate, and 1 per cent by pyruvate. On exercise the metabolism of fatty acids is increased whilst in the hypoxic or ischaemic myocardium the main substrate is either glucose of extracellular origin or intracellular glycogen.

Fatty acids are transported in the blood either bound to albumin or as triglycerides. Triglycerides are broken down by lipoprotein lipase in the capillary cell wall to form free fatty acids. The fatty acids cross the cell membrane and in the cytosol react with coenzyme-A (CoA) to form acyl CoA. This reaction consumes one molecule of ATP and is one reason why in conditions such as ischaemia, where there is a lack of ATP, fatty acid utilization is reduced. Acyl CoA may either form lipid droplets or cross the mitochondrial cell membrane by combining with carnitine. In the mitochondria degradation occurs by β-oxidation. The initial uptake of fatty acids by the heart is largely determined by the arterial concentration and does not have a threshold.

Glucose crosses the myocardial cell membrane by a carrier mechanism which depends largely on the intra- and extracellular concentrations. The threshold arterial concentration for glucose is 4 mmol/l. The threshold is lowered by insulin and the uptake is increased. Each molecule of glucose is degraded to pyruvate and then to acetyl CoA by the enzyme pyruvate dehydrogenase. Acetyl CoA enters the Krebs cycle in the mitochondria and generates by oxidative phosphorylation 36 ATP for each glucose molecule (aerobic metabolism). The breakdown to pyruvate (glycolysis) can also occur in the absence of oxygen (anaerobic metabolism) and generates two ATP molecules for each molecule of glucose. Thus only two of the possible 38 ATP molecules from each glucose molecule can be generated without oxidative phosphorylation. In hypoxic conditions the rate of glycolysis is increased (Pasteur effect) but cannot increase 18-fold, the rate which would be necessary for ATP production to be equal to that provided by oxidative phosphorylation.

The mechanisms by which lactate crosses the cell membrane are not understood. Lactate is converted to pyruvate by lactate dehydrogenase. Pyruvate is converted to acetyl CoA which enters the citric acid cycle. The normal heart consumes lactate. The production of lactate by the heart is an indication of a pathological condition since it implies an abnormal increase of anaerobic metabolism. Glucose or glycogen are metabolized to pyruvate by the glycolytic enzymes and instead of pyruvate forming acetyl CoA and entering the citric acid cycle, lactate is generated as an end product.

The control of substrate utilization in the myocardium is complex. Free fatty acids are the major substrate because the production of acetyl CoA from fats inhibits pyruvate dehydrogenase, the last enzyme in the glycolytic pathway for the metabolism of glucose or lactate. The production of citrate in the Krebs cycle inhibits phosphofructokinase, one of the rate-limiting enzymes in the glycolytic pathway. Given the concentrations in blood of free fatty acids, glucose and lactate, free fatty acids are the major fuel for the heart. In the presence of hypoxia little ATP is available to form acetyl CoA from fats but the glycolytic pathway is stimulated (Pasteur effect). Nevertheless, the increased glycolytic flux is insufficient to maintain sufficient ATP for myocardial cell function. Early in ischaemia a similar increase of glycolytic flux is observed. However, after only a few minutes of ischaemia glycolytic flux is reduced because two enzymes, phosphofructokinase and glyceraldehyde 3-phosphate dehydrogenase, are inhibited by the development of acidosis.

The metabolic pathways for fatty acids and carbohydrate are efficient, releasing between 40 and 60 per cent of the potential free energy in the form of ATP. Fatty acids generate eight ATP molecules per carbon atom and glucose six ATP molecules. On a weight basis the breakdown of fatty acids generates 2.5 times as many ATP molecules as glucose metabolism.

Energy in the form of ATP is used to maintain the integrity of cell structures, to fuel the pumps for maintenance of ionic gradients, and to provide energy for muscle shortening. The overall efficiency of the heart is the energy required to eject a volume of blood against the arterial pressure expressed as a percentage of energy which could be released from the uptake of oxygen in a given time. Efficiency at rest is about 12 per cent and on exercise can increase to between 18 and 25 per cent.

Calcium – initiator of contraction

Provided sufficient ATP is present, contraction of cardiac muscle is brought about by changes in the concentration of calcium within the cell. As the calcium concentration in the region of the myofibrils rises calcium binds to troponin C causing contraction. Later calcium is released and tension declines. The calcium concentration in the cytosol in resting cardiac muscle is approximately 10^{-7}M. For the development of half maximal tension the concentration must rise to 10^{-6}M. Such a concentration change would require only 1 μmol of calcium per litre of cell water. However, the total amount of calcium needed to bring about contraction is substantially greater because an appreciable quantity of calcium is bound to troponin C. The overall requirement for half maximal tension is 40 μmol/kg wet tissue.

The problem arises as to the origin of this calcium. During the action potential calcium enters the cell as the calcium current (see below) which accounts for 10 μmol/kg wet tissue. In order to maintain a steady state an equal quantity of calcium must be ejected from the cell during diastole. The extracellular space contains 400–1200 μmol/kg and the sarcoplasmic reticulum 150–350 μmol/kg. A large quantity of calcium (80–200 μmol/kg wet tissue) is bound to the cell membrane, some of it to the carbohydrate in the glycocalyx and some to the lipids in the trilaminar membrane.

Two theories have been put forward to account for calcium activation of the contractile proteins. The first is sometimes referred to as the 'trigger hypothesis'. Calcium entering the myocardial cell as the slow calcium current of the action potential is presumed to trigger a further release of calcium from the sarcoplasmic reticulum within the cell. A process of amplification occurs. During relaxation calcium is taken up again by the sarcoplasmic reticulum. The second theory (nicknamed the 'one way street hypothesis') proposes that calcium bound to the cell membrane is released into the cell with the slow calcium current during each heart beat. After release from troponin the calcium is taken up by the sarcoplasmic reticulum and returned to the outside of the cell or rebound to the cell membrane. The two theories are not mutually exclusive and may exist to different degrees in different species. For example, frog and rabbit heart muscle depend more on the transmembrane movement of calcium than the rat where most calcium for contraction seems to arise from the sarcoplasmic reticulum. It is also possible that calcium can be released for contraction from the specialized areas of the sarcoplasmic reticulum, lateral cysternae, near the cell surface and that the remainder of the sarcoplasmic reticulum is concerned only with calcium removal from the cytosol.

Recent studies with the calcium-sensitive light-emitting substance aequorin have shown that the calcium concentration in the cell rises rapidly after the start of the action potential and has returned to the resting value before the end of the action potential and before tension has started to fall. Relaxation of cardiac muscle is not determined by the rate of fall of the cytosolic calcium concentration but by other factors such as the rate of release of calcium from troponin C. Furthermore, the terminal part of the plateau of the action potential cannot be related simply to an inward calcium current.

A sodium–calcium (3 Na⁺ for 1 Ca²⁺) exchange mechanism in the cell membrane is an important mechanism for the extrusion of

Calcium exchange in heart muscle

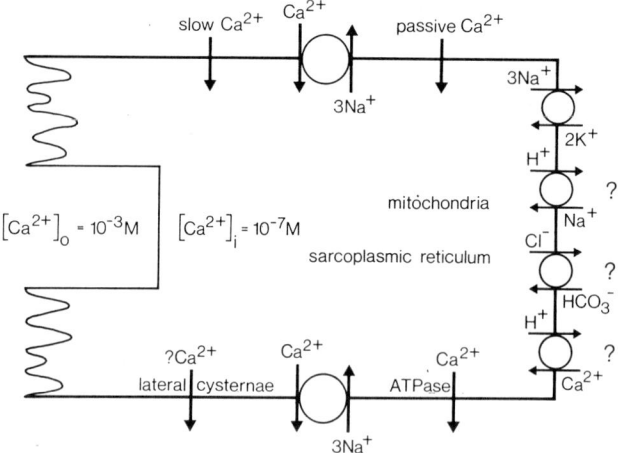

Fig. 8 Calcium exchange in heart muscle. Note the two intracellular stores in the mitochondria and sarcoplasmic reticulum. Three methods for influx and efflux of calcium are shown.

calcium from the cell and functioning in the reverse direction may under some circumstances contribute to the inward movement of calcium (Fig. 8). Calcium can also be pumped out of the cell by calcium ATPase. Such systems are necessary to maintain the large gradient between the extracellular calcium concentration (10^{-3}M) and the intracellular concentration (10^{-7}M) (Fig. 8) and to remove the small amount of calcium entering the cell with each heart beat.

Cardiac glycosides (e.g. digoxin) inhibit the sodium pump (the sodium–potassium ATPase). An increase of heart rate increases the frequency of cardiac depolarization and the sodium influx per unit time. Under both conditions the intracellular sodium rises. The rise of sodium decreases calcium efflux and probably increases calcium influx. More calcium enters the cell and is taken up by the sarcoplasmic reticulum and other stores. More calcium is available during each heart beat and an increased force of contraction results.

Electrophysiology

Each heart beat is initiated by a spontaneous electrical discharge in the sinoatrial node. The electrical signal passes across the atria to the atrioventricular node, through the bundle of His, and down the Purkinje fibres to the ventricular myocardium. These electrical events in the atria and the ventricle can be recorded on the surface of the chest as the electrocardiogram. The electrocardiogram is the sum of the electrical events in all the individual cells of the heart.

Within a ventricular cell the concentration of potassium and sodium ions are 140 and 10 mmol/l of cell water respectively. Negative changes are found on proteins which cannot permeate the cell membrane. In the extracellular fluid the concentrations of potassium and sodium are 4.0 and 140 mmol/l respectively, and the major negatively charged ions are chloride (110 mmol/l) and bicarbonate (24 mmol/l). In the resting state the cell membrane is more permeable to potassium than any other ion. Potassium, therefore, passes down the concentration gradient to the outside of the cell. Since potassium is positively charged and proteins remain in the cell, the inside of the cell becomes negatively charged. An equilibrium is reached where the electrical forces retaining potassium in the cell are balanced by the tendency to diffuse out of the cell down the concentration gradient. The electrical potential is then the equilibrium potential for that ion. It can be calculated from the Nernst equation.

$$E = \frac{RT}{zF} \ln \left(\frac{\text{Concentration outside}}{\text{Concentration inside}} \right)$$

where E is the equilibrium potential in mV, T is ⟨...⟩ perature, R is the gas constant, F is the Faraday constant, and Z is valency.

For potassium

$$E_{k^+} = 61.5 \log_{10}\left(\frac{4}{140}\right) = -95 \text{ mV}$$

The calculated equilibrium potential for sodium is $+70$ mV and for calcium is $+120$ mV.

In resting cardiac muscle (diastole) the membrane is permeable to potassium and the intracellular potential is -80 mV (Figs 9 and 10). The difference between this value and the equilibration potential for potassium (-95 mV) is accounted for by a small leakage of other ions and differences between activity and concentration of intracellular ions. The sodium pump (3 Na^+ for 2 K^+) is electrogenic and also contributes to the resting membrane potential. The pump maintains the intracellular ion concentrations despite small leakage currents. When a cell is electrically excited, the cell membrane allows sodium ions to enter the cell. The potential increases to approximately $+20$ mV (phase 0 in Fig. 9). The rate of change of the potential is related to the propagation velocity of the action potential across the heart. The increase in sodium conductance lasts only a few milliseconds ('fast' channel current) and is followed by a transient outward current probably carried by potassium (phase 1). Phase 2 is caused largely by the 'slow' inward current sometimes called the 'second' inward cur-

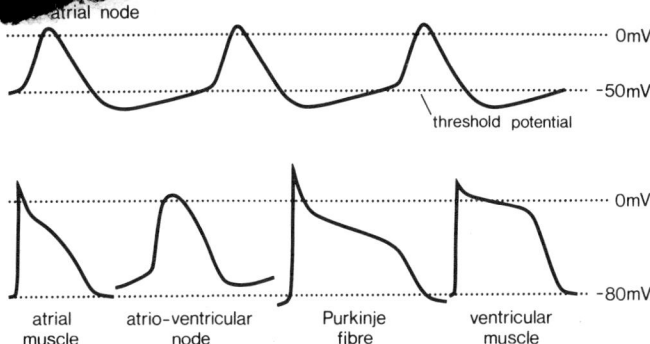

Fig. 11 The action potential has a different configuration in different parts of the heart. In the sinoatrial and atrioventricular nodes the cell spontaneously depolarizes during diastole (phase 4 depolarization). When the voltage reaches the threshold potential a complete action potential is initiated. Thus, the sinoatrial node with the fastest phase 4 depolarization acts as the primary pacemaker for the heart.

rent. This current is made up predominantly of calcium ions but there are some sodium ions (Fig. 9). At the same time the conductance to potassium is reduced so that despite depolarization a large outward potassium current does not occur (anomalous rectification). Phase 2 of the cardiac action potential is referred to as the plateau and is not present in skeletal muscle which has a much shorter action potential. Finally the cell repolarizes (phase 3). Repolarization occurs because of an increase in potassium conductance and termination of the calcium current.

In specialized cardiac tissue (sinoatrial node, atrioventricular node) and in damaged myocardial cells the resting membrane spontaneously depolarizes (phase 4). This is mainly due to a decrease of potassium conductance although sodium and calcium conductance may increase. When the membrane potential reaches a value of approximately -50 mV (threshold voltage) the cell spontaneously depolarizes and an action potential is initiated (Fig. 11).

The configuration of the action potential differs in different cardiac tissues (Fig. 11). The longest action potential is in Purkinje fibres. They act as a gate preventing retrograde activation by depolarization of adjacent ventricular muscle cells. The action potential is longer in the epicardium than endocardium and apex than base of the heart. The reason is not clear but the discrepancy is the probable explanation for the upright rather than inverted T wave on the electrocardiogram.

Electrical disequilibrium in the heart leads to arrhythmias. There are at least three cellular mechanisms. The first is called 'automaticity'. Injured myocardial cells or Purkinje fibres develop spontaneous phase 4 depolarization. Conditions which make the resting membrane potential less negative, the threshold voltage more negative or increase the rate of phase 4 depolarization favour automaticity.

The second mechanism is 're-entry'. The requirements for re-entry are undirectional block of an electrical impulse and slow propagation of the action potential. Under these circumstances the electrical wavefront may pass round diseased tissue through the block retrogradely and stimulate again cells which have had sufficient time to repolarize and not be refractory. A circus movement is established.

The third mechanism relates to after potentials and the slow calcium current. Injured cells are often partly depolarized and particularly in ischaemic tissue where the extracellular potassium can be high (up to 18 mmol/l) due to leakage of the ion out of the cell. Under these conditions spontaneous depolarization can occur and is often caused by calcium currents. It can be initiated by mechanical stretching of injured myocardium. If the phenomenon occurs in sufficient cells then the current density can be large enough to bring about depolarization of adjacent healthy cells and initiate an ectopic heart beat.

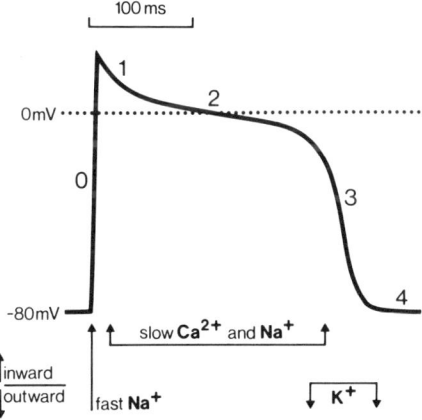

Fig. 9 Action potential of ventricular myocardium. The action potential is the voltage measured between a microelectrode inserted into the intracellular fluid (cytosol) of a myocardial cell and a reference electrode in the extracellular fluid. The action potential is recorded after the muscle has been stimulated by an electrical impulse.

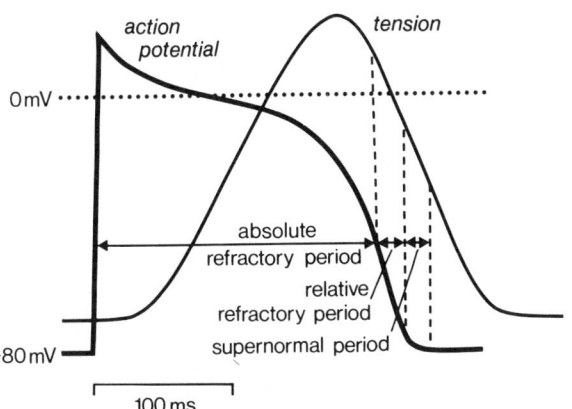

Fig. 10 The relation of the action potential to the generation of tension. The absolute refractory period is the period when a second electrical stimulus will elicit no response.

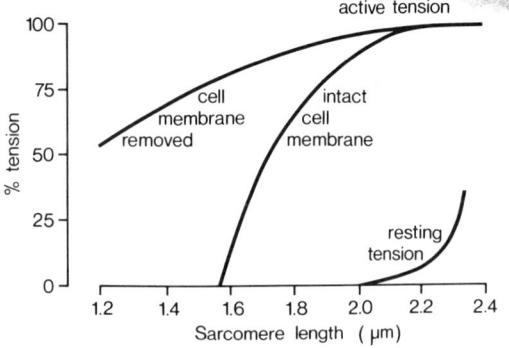

Fig. 12 Resting and active tension in isolated cardiac muscle at different initial sarcomere lengths. In intact tissue the sarcomere length at the end of systole (maximal contraction) is determined by the end systolic tension against which the muscle contracts and shortens. This relation at end systole is shown by the middle curve.

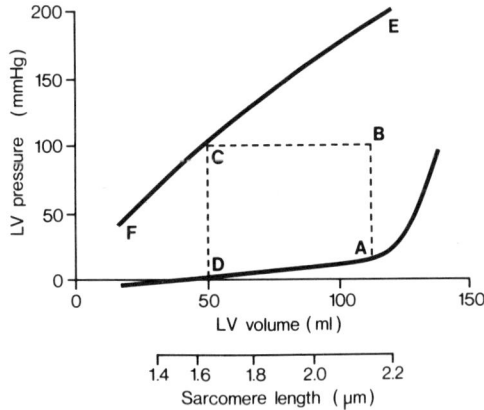

Fig. 13 The pressure–volume relation in the intact heart. A single heart beat is represented by the dotted line ABCD. EF is the line showing the end systolic relation between pressure and volume. The relation is almost constant provided myocardial contractility is unaltered.

The exact cause of an arrhythmia in an individual patient is rarely known and the classification of anti-arrhythmic drugs (page 13.132) is based on electrophysiological and pharmacological observations. At present a complete understanding of the interrelation between the aetiology of arrhythmias, the electrophysiological properties of drugs in single cells, and the effectiveness of any drug as an anti-arrhythmic agent, is only possible under some special circumstances.

Mechanics

The basic unit of contraction in cardiac muscle is the sarcomere. In resting muscle the sarcomere length is between 1.8 and 2.0 μm. If the pressure at the end of diastole (the left ventricular filling pressure) is increased as in acute heart failure, the volume of the ventricle is increased and the sarcomere lengthens to a maximum of 2.3 μm. Only when acute dilatation of the ventricle occurs, for example, by accident during cardiac surgery, is the sarcomere length increased beyond 2.3 μm. This is associated with tearing of the muscle and irreversible damage. The enlargement of the heart which occurs in severe chronic heart failure is due to slippage of the myofibrils and adjacent myocardial cells and is not due to excessive elongation of the sarcomere.

Recent techniques using diffraction patterns from laser beams have allowed the measurement of sarcomere length, and resting and developed tension during a single heart beat in which either sarcomere length is maintained constant or shortening is allowed to occur. Some of the results are shown in Fig. 12. Regardless of

the muscle or whether the muscle shortens against an afterload there is a constant relationship between maximum developed tension and the minimum sarcomere length. This generalization is not precisely true since shortening and stretch of myocardial cells can both bring about a small reduction in the duration of the action potential and the degree of activation of myofibrils. The relation between tension and minimum sarcomere length is analogous to the relation in the whole heart between pressure and volume (Fig. 13). There is an almost fixed relationship between end systolic volume and end systolic pressure. The relation is altered by inotropic agents and by the extracellular calcium concentration.

The extent to which the sarcomere can shorten determines the stroke volume. During severe exercise or in the presence of powerful inotropic drugs the sarcomere length at end systole may be only 1.4 μm. At this length cardiac muscle recoils. A negative pressure is present during early diastole and filling of the ventricle is partly due to suction. With zero filling pressure the sarcomere length is about 1.6 μm. Under normal resting conditions in humans the ventricle is filled by a positive pressure and the sarcomere length is between 1.8 and 2.0 μm.

From Figs 12 and 13 it is apparent that as the initial sarcomere length is increased the greater is the degree of shortening which occurs for a given afterload (tension or blood pressure). Since the greater degree of shortening occurs in a similar time, the velocity of contraction is also increased. If no shortening is permitted (isometric contraction) then the maximum developed tension increases with increasing resting sarcomere length. These observations form a basis for understanding the well-known Frank–Starling mechanism. Frank showed that the systolic pressure in systole increased in isovolumic hearts as end diastolic volume increased. Starling showed that an increase in atrial pressure resulted in an increase in end diastolic volume and cardiac output. This latter effect is often referred to as 'heterometric' regulation of the cardiac output, since resting sarcomere length is altered. In cardiac muscle the slope of the Starling curve (see Fig. 12) is much greater than in skeletal muscle. In skeletal muscle the mechanism for the increased developed force on increasing resting length is believed to be related to the greater overlap of the contractile proteins. In cardiac muscle the curve is too steep for this explanation to be possible. The increased developed tension is probably related to an increased calcium sensitivity of the contractile apparatus as the muscle is stretched.

A second intrinsic mechanism by which heart muscle increases the force of contraction is referred to as 'homeometric' regulation or the Anrep effect. After a sudden increase in afterload, end diastolic pressure and ventricular volume rise but decrease again over several minutes so that the heart finally ejects against an increased afterload from almost the initial end diastolic volume. The mechanism of this effect is probably related to intracellular control mechanisms for calcium. The effect is only of slight importance in humans.

The third intrinsic mechanism by which the heart can increase the force of contraction is by an increase of heart rate (Bowditch effect, rate-staircase, interval–strength relationship). If stroke volume remains constant an increase of heart rate will cause an increase of cardiac output. But experiments in isolated muscle show that in addition the strength of contraction is increased. The phenomenon is present in humans but is weak. A possible mechanism is that the increased number of depolarizations per minute increase the entry of sodium into the cell. The sodium pump reaches a new equilibrium when the intracellular sodium is slightly increased. The raised intracellular sodium concentration increases the net calcium movement into the myocardial cell and more calcium is available during each contraction.

Positive inotropic substances

No drug currently used in clinical practice increases the force of contraction by a direct effect on the myofibrils or troponin complex. Caffeine and other phosphodiesterase inhibitors affect the ability of the sarcoplasmic reticulum to sequester calcium and this may account for part of their clinical effect. All other drugs act primarily on the cell membrane. Cardiac glycosides (e.g. digoxin) inhibit the $Na^+–K^+$ ATPase. The resulting rise in intracellular sodium probably increases net calcium influx into the cell and thus contractility. Catecholamines (adrenaline and isoprenaline) react with β_1 receptors which interact with a modulator protein causing stimulation of the enzyme adenyl cyclase. Adenyl cyclase brings about the conversion of ATP to cyclic AMP. Cyclic AMP has many effects in the cell, but two are to increase calcium influx during the action potential and to augment calcium uptake by the sarcoplasmic reticulum. Both contraction and the rate of relaxation of cardiac muscle are increased. The 'calcium antagonists' (verapamil, nifedipine, diltiazem) have the property of inhibiting the slow calcium channel of the action potential and thus causing a fall in contractility, relaxation of smooth muscle, and reduced conduction in the atrioventricular node.

Ischaemia

Whatever the initiating mechanism for acute myocardial ischaemia, the three important consequences are a failure of contraction, arrhythmias, and cell death.

Myocardial ischaemia is traditionally regarded as that state which exists when myocardial oxygen supply is less than demand. Oxygen demand is more accurately the rate of consumption of ATP and oxygen supply is related to blood flow. Furthermore, blood flow not only provides a source of oxygen and substrate for heart muscle but also removes the products of metabolism. Two key products are heat and carbon dioxide. Ischaemia is better defined as an imbalance between ATP consumption and blood flow or as the state which exists when anaerobic metabolism occurs because of a low blood flow.

Total ischaemia results in cessation of contraction within 60 s. An important but not the sole mechanism is the rapid development of an intracellular acidosis. An intracellular rise in the concentration of the phosphate ion from the breakdown of ATP is another contributory factor. Total tissue ATP does not decline within 60 s but the rapid fall of tissue creatine phosphate is suggestive that ATP in some compartment within the cell does fall rapidly. A low ATP might affect contraction if insufficient ATP were available to maintain the normal functioning of ionic channels in the cell membrane or to allow shortening of the contractile proteins.

The exact mechanism of cell death is at present unknown. Under normal resting conditions the myocardium will recover almost completely after 10–15 min of ischaemia. More prolonged periods of ischaemia cause the cell membrane to become permeable to cations and recovery is reduced. If limited blood flow is present from collateral coronary arteries or from 'stuttering' ischaemia in the native coronary artery the cell gains sodium and loses potassium. After 60–90 min of ischaemia the cell membrane is destroyed. This can be attributed to a low tissue ATP, acidosis, activation of phospholipases, and lysosomal activity.

Reperfusion of ischaemic heart muscle results in further damage. There is an immediate swelling of the cell, release of intracellular enzymes and a large influx of calcium. Calcium is taken up by the mitochondria and can be seen as dark granules under the electron microscope. A large gain of calcium is an indicator of cell death since it prevents the normal functioning of mitochondria and the regeneration of ATP. Many theories exist to explain the sudden influx of calcium. A popular hypothesis is that the reintroduction of oxygen causes an increased generation of oxygen radicals which damage the cell membrane and in particular render the membrane permeable to calcium. The normal mechanisms within the cell for the removal of radicals are partly destroyed during the period of ischaemia. Recovery from a period of ischaemia is slow. This is partly because the myocardium loses nucleotides. ATP is broken down to ADP and AMP which in turn are broken down to inosine and adenosine. These latter are lost from the cell. Regeneration of nucleotides takes several days and is the probable reason why even if a cell does not die total recovery may take days even weeks.

At the present time drugs which are used in an attempt to reduce the size of a myocardial infarction act either by reducing ATP consumption (cardioplegic solutions, hypothermia, afterload reduction, negative inotropic agents) or by increasing coronary flow (afterload reduction, coronary vasodilators) through collaterals or the native coronary. The recent introduction of thrombolytic therapy for selected patients with myocardial infarction should reduce infarct size if the occlusion is due to thrombus, if the thrombus can be dissolved, and if the occlusion has not been present for much more than one hour. No drug has been shown to benefit the ischaemic myocardial cell by a mechanism which acts directly on the cell structure or cell metabolism with the possible exceptions of insulin, glucose and potassium therapy, corticosteroids, and hyaluronidase. Hypothermia is effective partly because metabolic pathways are inactivated.

Mechanism of heart failure

Acute heart failure is most commonly caused by reduced myocardial contractility secondary to ischaemia (e.g. acute myocardial infarction). More rarely the cause is associated with a high ATP consumption and an increased requirement for force development (e.g. aortic stenosis, malignant hypertension). Reduction of cardiac function due to structural derangement of the heart as a pump (e.g. acute mitral regurgitation) is another cause.

The cause of chronic heart failure is more puzzling since coronary blood flow, oxygen supply, and removal of metabolites are often normal and no initiating haemodynamic factor is present. Under these circumstances (e.g. cardiomyopathies, heart failure with chronic coronary artery disease) abnormalities have been reported in the cell membrane, sarcolemma, and myofibrils. Whether these abnormalities are primary or merely secondary to reduced contractility is unclear. The primary cellular event is different in the cardiomyopathies of varying aetiologies (e.g. cobalt, iron overload, myocarditis, and Adriamycin therapy). Nevertheless in many forms of chronic heart failure the activity of myofibrillar ATPase measured *in vitro* is reduced. In the animal kingdom the activity of this enzyme is related to resting heart rate and the speed of muscle shortening. Structural changes in the enzyme and a changed amino acid sequence may be an adaptive and potentially reversible cause of reduced contractility in chronic heart failure.

References

Folkow, B. and Neil, E. (1971). *Circulation*. Oxford University Press, Oxford.

Hearse, D. J. and Yellon, S. M. (1984). *Therapeutic approaches to myocardial infarct size limitation*. Raven Press, New York.

Katz, A. M. (1977). *Physiology of the heart*. Raven Press, New York.

Noble, D. (1979). *The initiation of the heart beat*. Clarendon Press, Oxford.

Opie, L. (1985). *The heart*. Grune and Stratten, New York.

Parratt, J. R. (1985). *Control and manipulation of calcium movement*. Raven Press, New York.

Clinical physiology of the normal heart

D. E. L. WILCKEN

Introduction

The function of the heart is to pump sufficient oxygenated blood containing nutrients, metabolites, and hormones to meet moment-to-moment metabolic needs and preserve a constant internal milieu. The heart has two essential characteristics, contractility and rhythmicity. The nervous system and neurohumoral agents modulate relationships between the venous return to the heart,

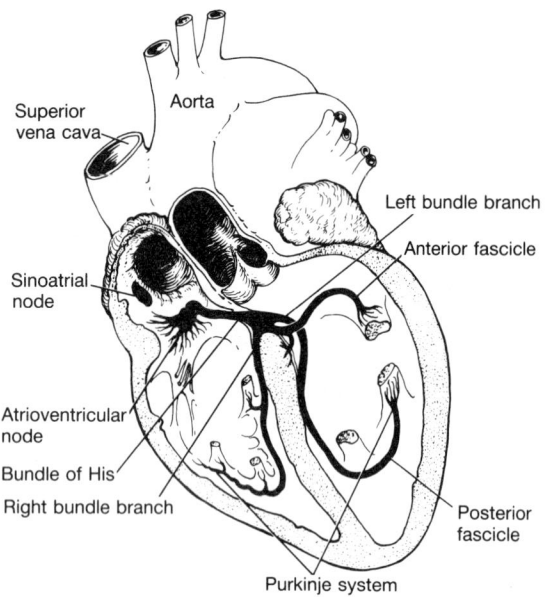

Fig. 1 Diagram of the heart showing the impulse-generating and impulse conducting system. (Reproduced from Junqueira, Carneiro and Contopoulos, 1977, *Basic histology* 2nd edn, Lange, with permission.)

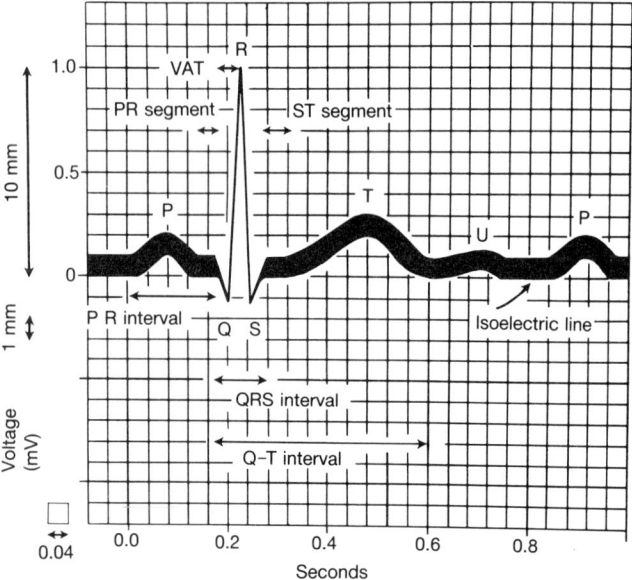

Fig. 2 Diagram of electrocardiographic complexes, intervals, and segments. VAT = ventricular activation time. (Reproduced from Goldman, 1976, *Principles of electrical cardiography* 9th edn, Lange, with permission.)

the outflow resistance against which it contracts, the frequency of contraction, and its inotropic state, and there are in addition instrinsic cardiac autoregulatory mechanisms. This section describes normal cardiac function and discusses the principal mechanisms contributing to its regulation.

The cardiac cycle

Electrical events initiate the cardiac cycle with depolarization of the sinoatrial node in the upper right atrium near the orifice of the superior vena cava (Fig. 1). Cardiac muscle acts as a functional syncytium. Cell-to-cell conduction is possible because the intercalated discs offer a low electrical resistance. The action potential in an active cell causes current flow which depolarizes the adjacent cells. The generated action potential spreads from the sinoatrial

node across the functional syncytium at a speed of 1.0 to 1.2 m/s. The first mechanical response is atrial systole.

The valvular attachments and connective tissue in the atrioventricular groove normally prevent cell-to-cell conduction of the electrical impulse from atrium to ventricle. This conduction occurs only through the specialized cells of the atrioventricular node (Fig. 1). The atrioventricular node is a region of slow conductance, from 0.02 to 0.1 m/s. This delays activation of the cells of the bundle of His and allows time for completion of ventricular filling. The conduction velocity in the bundle of His is from 1.2 to 2.0 m/s. The impulse passes via the right bundle branch and the two branches of the left bundle, and spreads rapidly (2.0 to 4.0 m/s) through the Purkinje fibres and each muscle cell to produce an orderly sequence of ventricular contraction (Fig. 1). Atrial and ventricular depolarization (P wave and a QRS complex) and repolarization (T wave) can be recorded on the electrocardiogram as the summation of the spread of the electrical potentials over all the cells of the heart (Fig. 2). Electrocardiography is considered on page 13.21.

The specialized cells of pacemaker tissue have an inherent rhythmicity which is shared by the sinoatrial node, the atrioventricular node, and Purkinje tissue. Unlike other myocardial cells these cells do not maintain a diastolic intracellular potential of about −90 mV but tend to depolarize spontaneously. Because the sinoatrial node has the fastest inherent discharge (depolarization) rate, and because there is a brief period after depolarization of the whole heart during which a further stimulus is ineffective – the absolute refractory period – the sinoatrial node is normally the pacesetter for the heart. However, if for some reason this does not function, pacemaker tissue in the atrioventricular node, bundle of His, or Purkinje system, will assume this role. The heart rate is then considerably slower.

Mechanical events

See page 13.53. The mechanical events following depolarization of atrial and ventricular muscle and their timing in relation to the electrocardiogram, to pressure and flow changes, and to heart sounds are shown in five phases in Fig. 3. After the P wave, and coinciding with atrial systole, 'a' waves appears in left atrial and right atrial pressure tracings due to atrial contraction, and an 'a' wave can be seen in the jugular venous pulse. Atrial contraction increases ventricular filling by about 10 per cent cent (phase 1).

The onset of ventricular contraction coincides with the peak of the R wave of the electrocardiogram and there is a rapid rise in intraventricular pressure which closes the mitral and tricuspid valves. The first heart sound is heard at the time of maximum displacement of these valves as they reach their closing positions. During this short isovolumetric period (phase 2 of Fig. 3) the pressure rises rapidly in the ventricle, which changes in shape but not in volume. When ventricular pressures exceed those in the pulmonary artery and aorta, the outflow valves open and ventricular ejection follows, with the highest flow rate occurring in early systole, and pressures in the aorta and pulmonary artery rise. Normally between 50 and 70 per cent of the ventricular volume is ejected during systole, and this can be seen in the volume curve included in Fig. 3 (phase 3).

The jugular venous pulse during ventricular contraction has a positive deflection in early systole, the 'c' wave, due to right ventricular contraction and bulging of the tricuspid valve into the right atrium. Descent of the tricuspid ring caused by ventricular contraction then produces a negative 'x' descent, but as atrial inflow continues the pressure rises in the atria and great veins, producing the 'v' wave. This reaches its peak just before the opening of the tricuspid valve, declining during early ventricular filling as the negative 'y' descent. The changes in the pulmonary veins and left atrium are similar.

As the strength of ventricular contraction declines, and coinciding with the end of the T wave of the electrocardiogram, the aortic and pulmonary valves close, producing the dicrotic notch seen on

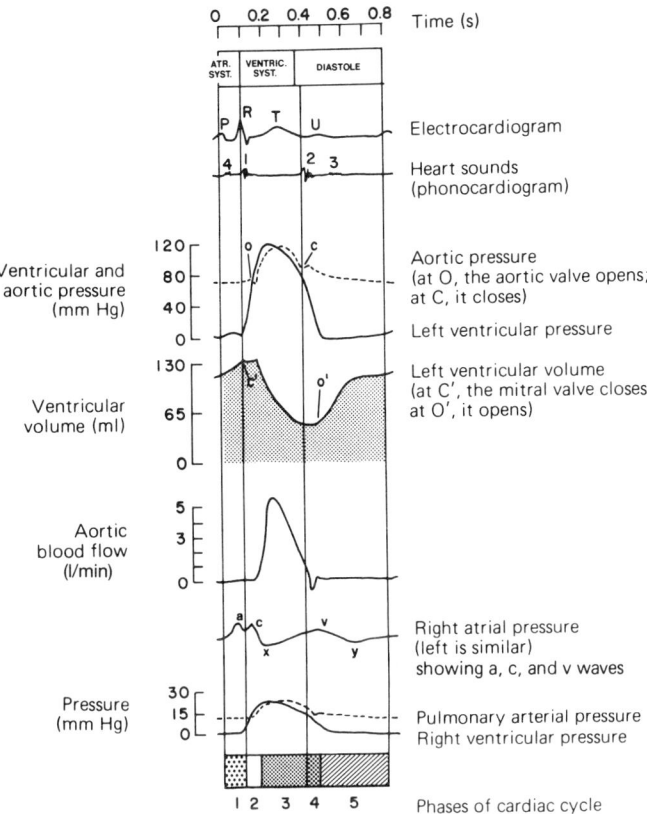

Fig. 3 Events of the cardiac cycle at a heart rate of 75 beats/min. The phases of the cardiac cycle identified by the numbers at the bottom are: (1) atrial systole, (2) isovolumetric ventricular contraction, (3) ventricular ejection, (4) isovolumetric ventricular relaxation, (5) ventricular filling. Note that late in systole, aortic pressure actually exceeds left ventricular pressure. However, the momentum of the blood keeps it flowing out of the ventricle for a short time. The pressure relationships in the right ventricle and pulmonary artery are similar. The jugular venous pulse is similar in form to that seen in the right atrial pressure tracing. The 'c' wave interrupts the 'x' descent of the 'a' wave. The decline in pressure from the peak of the 'v' is the 'y' descent; the rate of decline reflects speed of ventricular filling. Atr. Syst = atrial systole. Ventric. Syst. = ventricular systole. (Modified from Ganong, 1979, *Review of medical physiology* 9th edn, Lange, with permission.)

both aortic and pulmonary artery pressure tracings in Fig. 3. Aortic closure slightly precedes pulmonary closure, and together these are responsible for the two components of the second heart sound. A short period of further rapid decline in ventricular pressure ensues without changing ventricular volume (the period of isovolumetric ventricular relaxation, phase 4) and at the end of this the mitral and tricuspid valves open. There is a pressure gradient from atrium to ventricle so that a period of rapid ventricular filling follows, which coincides with the timing of the third heart sound. The rapid ventricular filling is reflected in the shape of the ventricular volume curve, and is followed by a period of slower filling (phase 5) with a final sudden small increment from the next atrial contraction as diastole ends (phase 1).

Third heart sounds are audible with the stethoscope in normal children and young adults. The hearing of these sounds in patients over the age of about 40 years, however, usually indicates elevation of ventricular end-diastolic pressure (most frequently in the left ventricle). This is probably because the myocardium and valvular structures become stiffer with aging, and large increases in ventricular end-diastolic pressure are then required to tense valvular structures and generate audible vibrations. The hearing of a fourth heart sound almost always indicates abnormal ventricular function. The end-diastolic pressure in the affected ventricle

Table 1 Normal resting values for pressures in the heart and great vessels

Site	Systolic pressure (mmHg)	Diastolic pressure (mmHg)	Mean pressure (mmHg)
Right atrium	'a' up to 7 'v' up to 5	'x' up to 3 'y' up to 3	Less than 5
Right ventricle	Up to 25	End pressure before 'a' up to 3; End pressure on 'a' up to 7	Not applicable
Pulmonary artery	Up to 25	Up to 15	Up to 18
Left atrium (direct or indirect pulmonary capillary wedge)	'a' up to 12 'v' up to 10	'x' up to 7 'y' up to 7	Up to 10
Left ventricle	120	End pressure up to 7; End pressure on 'a' up to 12	Not applicable

(usually the left) is increased, and the already stretched inflow valve responds to atrial systole and further filling with oscillations, producing a low pitched sound often palpable, as well as audible, at the cardiac apex. A fourth heart sound precedes the Q wave of the electrocardiogram and must be distinguished from a normal splitting of the two components of the first heart sound. The latter occurs after the Q wave (Figs 2 and 3).

Normal volumes, pressures, and flows
The blood volume in normal adults is about 5 litres (haematocrit 45 per cent) and of this about 1.5 litres are in the heart and lungs: the central blood volume. The pulmonary arteries, capillaries, and veins contain about 0.9 litres and at any one instant only about 75 ml are in the pulmonary capillaries. The volume of blood in the heart is about 0.6 litres. Left ventricular end-diastolic volume (EDV) is about 140 ml, the stroke volume (SV) about 90 ml so that the end-systolic volume is around 50 ml, and the ejection fraction (SV/EDV) from 50 to 70 per cent. Right ventricular ejection fraction is of the same order of magnitude.

Of the 3.5 litres in the systemic circulation most, at least 60 per cent of the total blood volume, is in the veins. The term 'mean circulatory pressure' introduced by Guyton is useful and refers to the equilibrium pressure measured in the entire circulation within a few seconds of stopping the heart. In dogs this is about 7 mmHg. The systemic veins containing most of the blood volume are easily distensible, and input of blood into the contracting heart is associated with only small changes in venous pressure. Ejection of blood into the much less distensible arterial tree, on the other hand, produces large pressure changes.

The normal values for pressures generated in the heart and great vessels during the cardiac cycle are shown in Table 1. Pressures are measured with reference to a zero pressure arbitrarily set at 5 cm below the sternal angle with the patient recumbent. 'Normal' arterial blood pressure is considered later (see page 13.360).

Cardiac output is the product of stroke volume and heart rate. It is related to body size and is best expressed as l/min/m² of body surface area: the 'cardiac index'. Mean cardiac index under resting and relaxed conditions is 3.5 l/min/m², and values below 2 and above 5 are abnormal. The cardiac index declines with age. In persons of average size, resting oxygen consumption is about 240 ml/min, and the difference in oxygen content between arterial and mixed venous blood about 40 ml/l (arteriovenous oxygen difference), giving a basal cardiac output of 6 l/min from the direct Fick equation. In normal subjects, arteriovenous difference at rest is

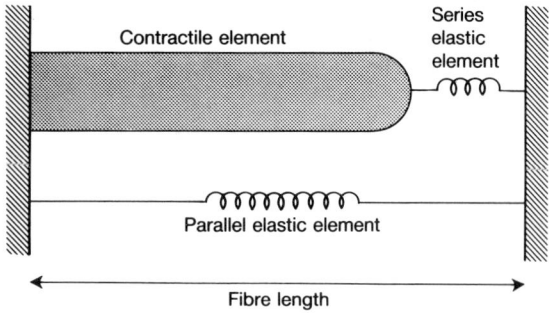

Fig. 4 A representation of the model A. V. Hill used to illustrate the three mechanical components of functioning muscle.

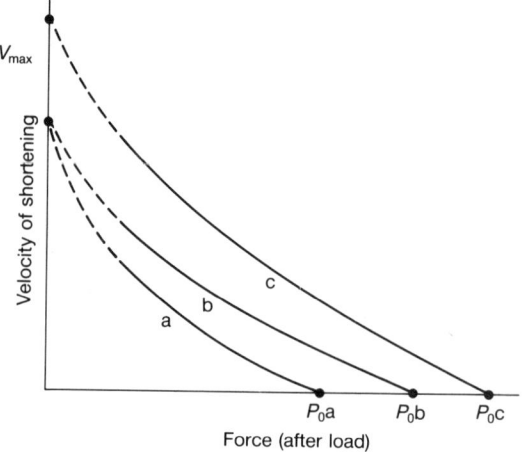

Fig. 5 Idealized relationships between velocity of fibre shortening and afterload or force developed during contraction of a strip of cardiac muscle under three different conditions. Curves 'a' and 'b' were obtained with the muscle in the same inotropic state but with a longer initial fibre length (greater preload) for curve 'b'. Curves 'b' and 'c' were obtained with initial fibre length the same but with contractility increased in 'c' by the addition of a drug producing a positive inotropic effect. The terms V_{max} and P_O were used by Hill to describe, respectively, a hypothetical maximum shortening velocity in the absence of any load (hence the broken lines), and the force developed in an isometric contraction. An increase in initial fibre length increases P_O but not V_{max}; a positive inotropic change increases both P_O and V_{max}.

maintained within narrow limits, from 35 to 45 ml/l; values of 55 ml/l and above are always abnormal.

Pulmonary or systemic vascular resistance is estimated by dividing the difference between mean inflow pressure (pulmonary artery or aortic) and mean outflow pressure (left atrial or right atrial) in mmHg by the flow in l/min through the respective circulations. In normal subjects and patients without intracardiac shunts this flow is the cardiac output. Normal pulmonary vascular resistance is less than 2 mmHg/l/min (160 dyne/s/cm^5) and normal systemic resistance less than 20 mmHg/l/min (1600 dyne/s/cm^5). Arterial blood pressure is the product of cardiac output and total peripheral resistance.

Stroke work is the integral of instantaneous ventricular pressure with respect to stroke volume but is usually estimated as the product of stroke volume and mean ejection pressure. The orderly sequence of contraction in the normal heart beat co-ordinates changes in instantaneous pressure and flow, so maximizing the transfer of energy to the circulation. Normal left ventricular work output at rest is about 6 kg m/min.

Myocardial mechanics

A more rational approach to the understanding of cardiac muscle contraction and altered performance in disease states has come from renewed interest in the results of classical experiments in skeletal muscle physiology. The three-component model for muscular contraction proposed by Hill in 1938 (Fig. 4) comprises firstly, a contractile element which, when activated, develops force and shortens; secondly, a series elastic element which is passively stretched during shortening and produces a dampening effect; and, thirdly, a parallel elastic element which supports resting tension. The latter together with the series elastic element, is responsible for the extensibility or compliance of relaxed muscle. It is not known which structures are responsible for the series elastic and parellel elastic components, but of their functional significance there is no doubt.

When a muscle is activated to contract, it develops a potential for doing work. In isolated skeletal and heart muscle preparations (for example, frog sartorius or cat papillary muscle) the stretching force applied to the muscle, and therefore the length of the muscle, can be varied before contraction. This is the preload. The activated muscle will begin to shorten when it has generated a force sufficient to overcome that exerted by the attached weight or load against which it is caused to contract. When the force exerted by the load is so arranged that it is not applied to the relaxed muscle and is applied only after the muscle has begun to develop tension, this force is termed the afterload. If the load is so large that the activated muscle is unable to overcome it and shorten, the contraction produces tension only, and the contraction is then isometric. When shortening does occur, external work is done. If the load is constant during the shortening, the contraction is said to be isotonic; if it changes it is auxotonic.

It is known that the tension produced by both skeletal and cardiac muscle during contraction depends on initial fibre length;

also, that during afterloaded isotonic contractions from a particular length, the amount and the speed of fibre shortening and the tension developed all depend upon the afterload. Over a range of loads the initial velocity of muscle shortening is most rapid when the load is smallest and least rapid with the largest load. The most extensive shortening occurs with the smallest load and the least with the load just less than that which would cause the contraction to be isometric.

The inverse relationship between initial velocity of fibre shortening and load in an isotonic contraction is a fundamental one for both skeletal and cardiac muscle (Fig. 5). There is, however, a major difference between the two types of muscle in that the relationship at any one length is constant in a skeletal muscle, whereas in cardiac muscle there are variations in inotropic state which are accompanied by considerable changes in the force–velocity relationship. A positive inotropic effect produces a more extensive contraction from the same initial length and afterload, and a faster maximum velocity of shortening (V_{max}). An increase in initial fibre length with no increase in inotropic state increases the force of contraction but does not, however, change V_{max}. This is illustrated in Fig. 5.

The contraction of the intact heart can be visualized as being similar mechanically to the afterloaded contraction of an isolated muscle strip. For the left ventricle, the preload is the distending force which stretches the muscle fibres in end-diastole, and the initial afterload is the force the ventricle must generate in order to open the aortic valve and eject blood. At the end of ejection, the ventricular muscle is isolated from the peripheral circulation, as the afterload is then supported by the competent aortic valve, and the muscle relaxes against a comparatively small force. Relaxation of the heart is an active process due to withdrawal of calcium ions from the cytoplasm surrounding the myofibrils. The relaxation rate is faster with smaller than with larger loads. 'Active' relaxation is still proceeding in the ventricular wall when the atrioventricular valves open, and, if it is delayed, as in the hypoxic heart, it increases the stiffness of the ventricular wall and reduces filling. Wall thickness is also a determinant of relaxation rate and compliance. For this reason filling pressures are higher for the thicker

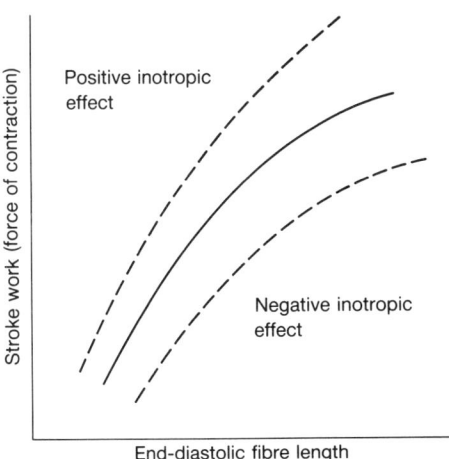

Fig. 6 The relation between left ventricular end diastolic fibre length and left ventricular stroke work showing displacement to the left with an increase in contractility and to the right with a reduction in contractility. Similar but not identical curves are obtained by plotting left ventricular stroke work as one measure of the force of contraction against ventricular end-diastolic pressure or volume. Similar function curves may be obtained from both ventricles and both atria.

and stiffer left ventricle than for the thinner and more distensible right ventricle (Table 1).

Regulation of cardiac function

There are four essential factors determining the performance of the heart. These are venous return, outflow resistance, inotropic state or contractility, and heart rate. Changes in cardiac performance are accomplished by mechanisms which alter these four determinants.

Venous return, preload, and the Frank–Starling relationship

The relationship described independently by Frank and Starling between end-diastolic fibre length and force of contraction is shown in Fig. 6. When the right or left ventricle ejects against a constant pressure, variations in venous return alter the degree of stretch of the muscle fibres in diastole, and this determines contraction strength. The number of active force-generating sites in each fibre increases as it lengthens so that, within limits, force of contraction and end-diastolic fibre length are positively related.

The relationship is curvilinear and for any particular heart at any particular time depends upon certain factors:

1. The intrinsic state of the muscle itself, i.e. the nature of its own biochemistry and contractile machinery.

2. The prevailing neurohumoral state. For instance, increased sympathetic outflow produces a more forceful contraction at any end-diastolic fibre length and shifts the curve to the left.

3. Extrinsic inotropic influences. Digitalis preparations, for example, have a positive inotropic effect and shift the curve to the left (at least in the short term), whereas myocardial depressants such as barbiturates in high blood concentration have a negative inotropic effect and shift the curve to the right.

End-diastolic fibre length is determined by the force distending the ventricle in end-diastole, and end-diastolic pressure provides a reasonable indication of this force when the ventricle has normal distensibility or compliance; this is the preload. The systemic venous return and the elastic properties of the myocardium produce the end-diastolic distending pressure for the right ventricle, and the pulmonary venous return and myocardial elasticity that for the left ventricle. For clinical purposes it is convenient to equate venous return with preload because, as it changes from beat to beat, it adjusts the strength of the subsequent ventricular (and atrial) contraction by varying the force stretching the relaxed cardiac muscle and changing end-diastolic fibre length.

Outflow resistance or afterload

The pressure which the ventricle must develop to exceed that in the pulmonary artery and the aorta and open the pulmonary and aortic valves is determined largely by the pulmonary and systemic vascular resistances. These resistances, together with an inertial component dependent upon the physical characteristics of each vascular tree and the fact that the flow is pulsatile, constitute the impedance to ventricular outflow. It is the load against which the ventricle must contract and shorten. As this load is not applied in diastole to the relaxed muscle, it then being supported by competent aortic and pulmonary valves, it is usefully described clinically as the afterload; it becomes applied to the muscle only after the ventricle has begun to develop tension.

Ventricular volume has a major effect on afterload. This can be illustrated quite simply by considering that pressure is force per unit area. The force acting radially on the inner surface of the whole ventricle at any time during systole is the product of the intraventricular pressure and surface area at that time. If the left ventricle is assumed to be a sphere (surface area $= \pi d^2$), the force opposing ejection at any time during contraction is the product of the intracavity pressure and πd^2 at that time. Thus, a change in left ventricular diameter from a normal value of 5 cm to one of 10 cm would result in a four-fold increase in the force opposing ejection for the same intracavity systolic pressure; the ventricle would need to develop greatly increased wall tension to overcome that force. Even taking into account the oversimplification of the spherical model, the contraction clearly will be much less efficient in the larger heart for the same stroke volume and ejection pressure (stroke work), since wall tension developed during systole is the major determinant of myocardial oxygen consumption.

During a normal heart beat the afterload is greatest at the beginning of ejection (rapid rise in pressure and maximum volume, Fig. 3), but thereafter decreases as the pressure plateaus and then declines as the ventricle becomes smaller. There is therefore a matching of the afterload to the declining intensity of the contraction as it proceeds to completion, and fibres shorten at a relatively constant rate. This is less obvious in a large heart where the volume change during ejection is a smaller proportion of the total ventricular volume.

The end-diastolic volume is influenced by preload, afterload, circulating blood volume, the inotropic state of the ventricle, heart rate, and neurohumoral influences. For example, it is smaller in the erect than in the horizontal position because of reduced venous return, and it decreases with a moderate increase in heart rate because of an associated positive inotropic effect. The proportion of end-diastolic volume ejected during systole, the ratio of stroke volume to end-diastole volume (SV/EDV), is the ejection fraction (normal 50–70 per cent). It is a useful index of overall left ventricular function, which is easily measured non-invasively by gated blood pool scanning and, more recently, by two-dimensional echocardiographic techniques. The ejection fraction increases with exercise and with positive inotropic interventions. Values for right ventricular ejection fraction are of the same order as those for the left side of the heart.

Myocardial contractility and inotropic state

Myocardial function is greatly altered by changes in inotropic state or contractility. Positive inotropic effects are thought to be mediated by activation of excitation–contraction coupling mechanisms and are associated with an increased influx of calcium ions into myocardial cells and a more powerful contraction. Changes in the intensity of excitation–contraction coupling are independent of the Frank–Starling mechanism, with increases shifting the curve to the left and decreases to the right (Fig. 6). With a positive inotropic effect the force of contraction, however measured, is increased for a given end-diastolic fibre length, and, if the afterload is the same, the initial velocity of fibre shortening is also increased (Fig. 5). In the intact heart there is more complete emptying during systole. Increased sympathetic stimulation, digitalis, and other drugs, and an increase in heart rate itself (the staircase or Bowditch phenomenon; postectopic potentiation, see below) have positive inotropic effects. Myocardial depressants, such as hypoxia and most anaesthetic drugs, have negative inotropic effects. Increased parasympathetic stimulation produces acetylcholine-mediated negative inotropic effects which are confined almost entirely to the atria, because of the anatomical distribution of vagal endings in the myocardium.

It is difficult to measure inotropic changes accurately in the human heart because changes in the intensity of excitation–contraction coupling and changes in the Frank–Starling relationship, though separate, are nevertheless closely linked. Whilst Hill's classic model (Fig. 4) has been important conceptually, attempts to define contractility as predicted by the model – by deriving an extrapolated maximum velocity of fibre shortening which would obtain with the muscle contracting against zero load – have not been rewarding. Peak rate of change of intraventricular pressure (peak dp/dt) is a useful index of change in contractility provided that preload, afterload, and heart rate remain constant. This index is less sensitive to changes in preload and afterload than those which relate it to intraventricular pressure, either at or before peak dp/dt, or to the area under the intraventricular pressure curve from the onset of contraction to peak dp/dt (Fig. 3). But an important new approach apparently insensitive to preload and afterload changes is that of Suga and Sagawa using the ventricular pressure–volume loop diagram.

There is a linear relationship between end-systolic pressure (or wall stress) and end-systolic volume in the physiological range of the human left ventricle. Increased contractility shifts the relationship to the left, as illustrated in Fig. 7, allowing the separation of enhanced from reduced contractility in the same heart, and poorly contracting from normally contracting ventricles. Stroke volume is shown on the abscissa as the difference between end-diastolic and end-systolic volumes. The efficacy of afterload reduction in assisting reduced ventricular function is also easily explained from the diagram. With a reduced afterload the aortic valve opens at a lower pressure and a greater stroke volume is ejected; a new end-systolic volume pressure point is reached which is shifted downwards on the same linear relationship. There has been no change in contractile state.

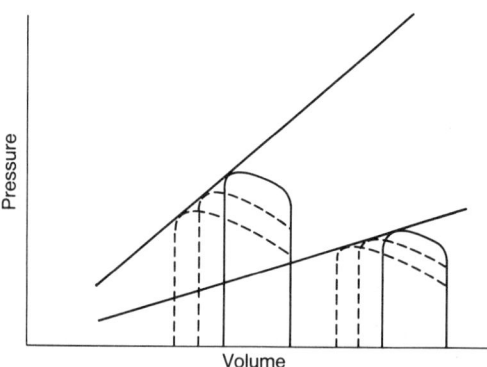

Fig. 7 Diagrammatic representation of intraventricular pressure and volume relationships during the cardiac cycle at two levels of myocardial contractility; three separate beats with the same end-diastolic volume are shown for each. The loops on the left of the diagram were obtained when contractility is increased and those on the right when it is reduced. There is a linear end-systolic pressure–volume relationship with different afterloads (pressures) for each level of contractility. The slope of the end-systolic pressure–volume relationship for any inotropic state is insensitive to a wide range of changes in afterload and preload, although changes in preload are not shown in this diagram. The volume change seen on the horizontal axis for each beat is the stroke volume. This increases with reduction in pressure (afterload).

Heart rate

Frequency of contraction is the fourth essential determinant of cardiac performance. Heart rate during rest and exertion may vary from 45 to 200 beats/min in the healthy young adult and as changes can occur within seconds, an increase in heart rate is the usual and most effective way of producing a rapid increase in cardiac output. It plays the major role in these responses. Stroke volume does increase on exercise, more so in athletes and when in the erect rather than the supine postion, but the changes are less marked. In addition, an increase in contraction frequency itself produces a positive inotropic effect, as already mentioned. The force of contraction increases and reaches a new steady state within a few beats. This is termed the 'positive staircase', Treppe, or Bowditch effect. It may be a consequence of an augmented movement of calcium ions into myocardial cells with increased frequency of action potentials, combined with diminished time for outward movement of calcium between beats. More forceful contractions also follow premature beats – the phenomenon of postextrasystolic potentiation – and the mechanism is probably the same. The extrasystole occurring prematurely is a weak contraction because of decreased filling time and an unco-ordinated activation of the ventricle when the ectopic focus is within the ventricle. The next beat is delayed because of the refractory period of the extrasystolic beat but is a more powerful contraction because of increased filling time and ventricular volume, and increased contractility. Calcium-dependent changes similar to those of the Bowditch effect are probably responsible for the latter.

Coronary blood flow

Coronary blood flow accounts for about 4 per cent of the cardiac output. The heart extracts most (70 per cent) of the oxygen carried in the coronary circulation; the arteriovenous difference for oxygen across the heart is about 110 ml/l whilst that for the whole body is only about 40 ml/l under resting conditions. Therefore, large increases in myocardial oxygen requirements must be met largely by increases in coronary blood flow and this may increase five- or six-fold during strenuous exercise. The greater part of this flow is to the left ventricle, of which at least two-thirds occurs during diastole, because of the throttling effect systole has on myocardial perfusion. The main coronary arteries are on the superficial surface of the heart, and because of this, and the hindrance to coronary flow during systole, the subendocardial region of the left ventricle is more vulnerable to perfusion deficits in relation to oxygen need than the outer two-thirds of the muscle wall. Despite these mechanical problems flow is normally evenly distributed throughout the myocardium so that, when regional coronary blood flow is measured using injected radioactive microspheres (in dogs), the ratio of endocardial to epicardial flow is approximately unity. In fact the inner layers of the heart probably receive slightly more blood (up to 10 per cent) than the outer layers, which is consistent with the subendocardium developing more tension than the subepicardium, and is evidence for a greater rate of myocardial oxygen consumption in the inner layers.

Regulation of coronary blood flow

Myocardial oxygen requirements and coronary blood flow are finely adjusted. The mechanisms are incompletely understood, but it is clear that the control resides largely in the heart itself. The major determinants are aortic pressure, myocardial extravascular compression, myocardial metabolism, and neurohumoral control.

Pressure gradients and extravascular compression As with any vascular bed, the available pressure gradient is a determinant of blood flow. The aortic pressure is the input pressure and the heart requires an adequate coronary blood flow to generate an adequate systemic arterial pressure. As already mentioned, myocardial extravascular compression with each left ventricular contraction nearly stops coronary blood flow during systole. Coronary inflow occurs mostly during diastole, probably entirely so in the subendocardial layers. Thus high diastolic intramyocardial pressure, secondary to elevated intraventricular (cavity) pressure, may restrict flow, particularly to the inner layers. The effective coronary perfusing pressure is the coronary pressure (aortic pressure) minus the outflow pressure. This may be the intramyocardial pressure or the coronary venous pressure or the diastolic zero flow pressure (see below) whichever is the largest. There is doubt about the reason(s) for the diastolic zero flow pressure. In dogs, end-diastolic flow at slow heart rates may be zero in the circumflex coronary artery when coronary pressure at the moment of zero flow may be between 20 and 50 mmHg, the lower pressures occurring with maximal coronary vasodilation. In conscious humans, distal coronary artery diastolic pressures at zero flow, determined during complete occlusion of the left anterior descending coronary artery at percutaneous transluminal angioplasty, are usually between 10 and 20 mmHg. The significance of these zero flow pressures is uncertain but they may reflect collateral flow. Extravascular factors are responsible for up to 50 per cent of hindrance to flow and, however, are largely systolic.

Autoregulation A relative constancy of coronary blood flow in relation to changes in driving pressure is readily demonstrated in isolated animal heart preparations; changes in coronary perfusion pressure ranging from 40 to 200 mmHg result in a return of coronary blood flow to approximately control levels in 30 to 60 s indicating that alterations in arteriolar calibre may occur through intrinsic mechanisms. This may be brought about by adjustments to local release of vasodilator metabolites which are increased when myocardial P_{O_2} falls. The ensuing vasodilation restores myocardial oxygenation and reduces local vasodilator metabolite release. Intrinsic coronary vascular smooth muscle stretch mechanisms may also contribute by adjusting vessel calibre in response to changes in coronary transmural pressure, although this is difficult to establish. However, similar myogenic mechanisms do operate in the peripheral circulation. The myogenic hypothesis suggests that elevation of vascular transmural pressure stretches arteriolar smooth muscle cells, inducing lengthened myofibrils to contract more forcefully, and that the ensuing vasoconstriction keeps contained a potential increase in blood flow, a mechanism which stems from the work of Bayliss in 1902.

Metabolic regulation Myocardial metabolism is, however, the main factor in the local control of the coronary circulation. An increase in cardiac metabolism is accompanied by functional coronary vasodilation. With an increase in heart rate and ventricular pressure, there is an increase in cardiac metabolism and local release of vasodilator metabolites. Almost any cardiovascular response will alter coronary blood flow secondary to a change in myocardial metabolism. There is a linear relationship between coronary blood flow and myocardial oxygen consumption, and a hyperbolic relationship with coronary venous oxygen content (which reflects myocardial oxygen partial pressure). Sharp increases in flow occur when coronary venous oxygen content falls below 5 ml per 100 ml. The mechanism of this vasodilation is unknown. Although oxygen itself might have a direct effect, it is unlikely that a change in coronary perivascular oxygen tension alone is the principal mechanism for metabolically induced vasodilation.

A number of vasoactive substances link coronary blood flow to the metabolic requirements of the heart, and Feigl has recently reviewed the evidence for and against the various putative coupling agents. A role for dissolved carbon dioxide is likely, since arterial hypercapnia results in coronary vasodilation independent of changes in myocardial oxygen consumption: a 1 mmHg increase in coronary venous carbon dioxide tension reduces coronary vascular resistance by about half that occurring with a 1 mmHg decrease in coronary venous oxygen tension. Potassium ions produce coronary vasodilation in a concentration of 1 to 10 mM. Potassium release may be involved in the initial vasodilation seen with an increase in heart rate. Carbon dioxide and locally released

potassium may act as vasodilator mediators under certain circumstances, without fully accounting for responses. There is also evidence favouring a vasodilator role for prostaglandins in human coronary flow regulation. Adenosine, however, has been most extensively investigated as a possible regulatory metabolite.

Berne and his associates have provided impressive evidence that adenosine is an important metabolic coupling agent linking coronary blood flow to myocardial oxygen demand. Adenosine monophosphate production reflects the degree of adenosine triphosphate utilization and hence the energy state of the cell. The enzyme which dephosphorylates adenosine monophosphate to adenosine, 5′-nucleotidase, appears to be conveniently situated at the cell membrane, in the T tubules, and in the cells surrounding capillaries, the pericytes. Adenosine moves quickly through cell membranes into the interstitial space. There it may dilate arterioles and enhance oxygen delivery, which then reduces the production of adenosine monophosphate and adenosine. Additional adenosine may re-enter the cell or be deaminated in red cells by adenosine deaminase. The evidence for the adenosine hypothesis is best for hypoxic conditions and remains to be established for normal conditions. Indeed recent direct measurement of left ventricular interstitial adenosine in relation to metabolic changes have failed to reproduce the expected correlations, suggesting that adenosine may be less of a coupling agent and more 'a fellow traveller'.

Considering the importance of metabolic vasodilation for normal cardiac function, a unitary theory of regulation of coronary blood flow with a single vasodilator would seem to lack built-in safety factors and flexibility. It is unlikely that there is any one sole mediator of every kind of physiological coronary vasodilation. Evidence is accumulating for interrelations between naturally occurring coronary vasodilators, with important links provided by prostaglandins.

Neurohumoral control Whilst metabolic factors, however mediated, are undoubtedly the principal mechanisms operating to adjust coronary flow to oxygen needs, it has become clear in recent years that stimulation of alpha-adrenoreceptors and beta-2 receptors in coronary vascular smooth muscle cells does play a subsidiary role in the regulation of the coronary circulation. These receptors mediate, respectively, vasoconstriction and vasodilation. Large epicardial and small coronary arteries have a similar density of innervated vasoconstrictor alpha-receptors. Stimulation of these receptors limits local metabolic vasodilatation by about 30 per cent in animal experiments. Adrenergic alpha-receptor coronary vasoconstriction may be unmasked by beta-receptor blockade. There is parasympathetic coronary innervation restricted apparently to small vessels distal to the epicardial arteries, which produces vasodilation, but at present the functional significance is uncertain. In animals such nerves mediate reflex coronary vasodilation resulting from stimulation of chemoreceptors in the carotid body.

Alterations of adrenergic vasoconstrictor tone also occur via the carotid sinus reflex. With carotid sinus hypotension there is a coronary vasoconstrictor effect. However, this is usually masked by the metabolic effects of the accompanying hypertension and tachycardia. There is evidence, too, for the presence of an alpha-sympathetic coronary vasoconstrictor influence restricting coronary vasodilation, even during strenuous exercise (in animals). Both of these conclusions are difficult to understand teleologically. Deep inspiration on the other hand reduces alpha-adrenergic stimulation and produces coronary vasodilation. There is also a coronary baroreceptor reflex which presumably functions in concert with baroreceptor reflexes from the carotid sinus.

Whilst the functional significance of reflex activity in the coronary circulation remains uncertain, changes in reflexly mediated alpha-adrenergic receptor activity may be responsible for periodic spontaneous increases seen in coronary blood flow (up to twofold). This has been documented in sleeping baboons without changes in heart rate or aortic blood pressure. Alterations in sympathetic discharge may also be relevant to the pathogenesis of coronary artery spasm, which is now known to occur in a subset of patients whose coronary arteries may or may not have detectable fixed atherosclerotic luminal obstructions. The functional integrity of endothelium may also be important in this regard since the endothelium itself produces vasodilators.

Endothelium-induced vasodilation The endothelial cells release at least two powerful vasodilator substances. Vane showed that prostacyclin is synthesized in endothelial cells by the cyclo-oxygenase pathway, and that it is both a vasodilator and also an inhibitor of platelet aggregation. It opposes the vasoconstrictor effects of thromboxane, released locally from platelets aggregating at sites of endothelial damage, and is discussed elsewhere (see page 13.139). Recently, Furchgott has identified another locally acting vasodilator, endothelial-derived relaxing factor, or EDRF. It is released from endothelium by the vasodilators acetylcholine, substance P, bradykinin, and adenosine triphosphate. It has a half-life of about 1 min, and its chemical structure and role in local blood flow regulation both await further study.

Myocardial oxygen supply and demand
At present it is difficult to measure myocardial oxygen supply and demand directly in humans. However, the product of systolic pressure and heart rate is a useful index of myocardial oxygen requirement at rest and on exercise. Also, Hoffman and his colleagues have derived an index of left ventricular oxygen supply in relation to demand, by dividing the area under the diastolic aortic pressure trace by the area enclosed by the left ventricular pressure trace (Fig. 3). This ratio is normally about 0.9, and a value below 0.5 is associated with subendocardial ischaemia in dogs. This is almost certainly true in humans also, in the absence of coronary atherosclerosis. The rationale for using coronary perfusion pressure to estimate myocardial oxygen supply depends upon the assumption that flow is primarily pressure dependent when the coronary vasculature becomes maximally dilated, as a level of 0.5 is approached. Obviously, coronary obstructions producing local pressure gradients could result in subendocardial ischaemia with values above 0.5.

The nervous system and the heart
The heart is richly supplied with adrenergic nerves. Terminals reach atrial and ventricular muscle fibres and impinge upon all pacemaker tissue: both sinoatrial and atrioventicular nodes and Purkinje fibres as well. Sympathetic stimulation leads to an increase in myocardial contractility and heart rate, and in the rate of spread of the activation wave through the atrioventricular node and the Purkinje system. This is mediated by local noradrenaline release which interacts with beta-adrenergic receptors. The key elements in these regulatory mechanisms are calcium ions and cyclic AMP. The activated beta-receptor increases adenylcyclase activity and conversion of ATP to cyclic AMP. Peptide co-transmitters released with noradrenaline and acetylcholine have been recently isolated, and probably also influence autonomic function: neuropeptide Y, released with sympathetic stimulation, appears to augment noradrenaline effects.

The distribution of parasympathetic fibres is much more limited, being confined to the sinoatrial and atrioventricular nodes and the atria, with few if any fibres reaching the ventricles in humans, except perhaps in relation to coronary arteries. The effects of parasympathetic nerve stimulation are mediated by local acetylcholine release which slows the heart rate and speed of conduction through the atrioventricular node and Purkinje tissue, and depresses atrial contractility. The negative inotropic effects are associated with a lowering of intracellular cyclic AMP concentration.

The effect of the nervous system on the heart at any one time is the sum of the activities of these two opposing control systems. They usually vary reciprocally. Under resting conditions, vagal inhibitory effects predominate, maintaining a slow heart rate, there being virtually no sympathetic outflow. With exercise, there is withdrawal of vagal activity and an increase in sympathetic outflow. Afferents from stretch receptors in the carotid sinus and aortic arch – the baroreceptors – also have a considerable effect on cardiac performance, this effect being mediated via the adrenergic nervous system. A fall in blood pressure reduces carotid sinus stretch and inhibitory afferent traffic so that sympathetic outflow increases. As a consequence there is a quickening of the heart rate within one or two beats, a positive inotropic effect on the heart and also a constriction of veins and arterioles which increases preload and afterload. Elevation of carotid sinus pressure has the reverse effects.

There are also mechanoreceptors in all four chambers of the heart and in the coronary vessels which give rise to depressor reflexes. Their clinical relevance is uncertain, but they may contribute, for example, to the bradycardia and hypotension occurring in some patients with acute myocardial infarction. Vagal afferents from reflexogenic areas in the infarcting left ventricle may also be responsible for the gastric distension, nausea, and vomiting which frequently occur with the onset of infarction. The cardiac receptors connected to afferent fibres running in cardiac sympathetic nerves, however, are very important because they are responsible for the impulses which are perceived as cardiac pain. Receptors have also been identified (in animals) at the junction of pulmonary veins with the atrial wall. These respond to mechanical distension with increased sympathetic outflow to the sinus node and inhibition of antidiuretic hormone secretion from the posterior lobe of the pituitary gland. The result is quickening of the heart rate and a diuresis, effects which could contribute to the regulation of cardiac volume.

Atrial natriuretic factor The discovery of natriuretic granules which resemble secretory tissue in the atria of the heart also has important implications for the regulation of blood volume. These granules produce atrial natriuretic factor which inhibits the reabsorption of sodium in the distal tubule of the kidney. It has a vasodilator action and opposes the constricting effects of noradrenaline and angiotensin II and depresses plasma aldosterone concentration, either directly or through effects on angiotensin II. The peptide nature and amino acid content have been determined. Atrial natriuretic factor is present in the circulation, concentrations increasing during volume expansion. Release is thought to result from atrial distension and may depend upon an intact vagus although this is not certain. The right atrium contains about 2–4 times as much activity as the left. Atrial natriuretic factor has stimulated much recent research, and whilst its overall effect is to produce a diuresis, and reduce cardiac and circulating blood volume, its precise regulator role in cardiovascular homeostasis awaits further study (page 13.82).

Autonomic efferent activity The autonomic outflow to the heart is controlled by multiple integrative sites within the central nervous system, with complex interactions between afferent and central inputs. Autonomic responses are mediated through suprapontine and bulbo-spinal pathways, both those arising 'reflexly' and those arising from various types of central 'command'. Nevertheless, intrinsic mechanisms are sufficient for adequate cardiac function in the absence of autonomic control, as prolonged survival after cardiac transplantation has shown. But in the denervated heart there is blunting of the normally rapid physiological adjustments mediated by the autonomic nervous system.

Exercise and the heart: cardiac reserve
The heart responds to exercise with an increase in cardiac output, and values of 30 l/min may be achieved in a trained athlete. Exercising muscles extract more oxygen from the blood perfusing them but the cardiac output response is the ultimate determinant of oxygen delivery to tissues and is the limiting factor for aerobic exercise.

The cardiac response to exercise involves all the mechanisms already discussed. Interaction within the central nervous system between higher and autonomic centres augments sympathetic discharge and there is a withdrawal of parasympathetic outflow. The heart rate increases immediately, and redistribution of peripheral flow increases venous return and preload. There is venoconstriction, particularly in the large-volume splanchnic circulation, and vasoconstriction and increased oxygen extraction in non-active parts. In active parts there is vasodilation. This is most evident in the vascular beds of the exercising skeletal muscles and of the heart. The overall effect is a marked lowering of total peripheral vascular resistance, which reduces afterload and encourages greater systolic emptying of the left ventricle. Stroke volume increases during exercise in the upright position. During light to moderate exercise, up to about 80 per cent of maximum exercise capacity, there is an almost linear relationship between work intensity and heart rate response, cardiac output, and oxygen uptake. With further exercise the heart rate and cardiac output responses level off whilst additional increases in oxygen consumption (about 500 ml) occur by increased oxygen extraction and a greater widening of the arteriovenous difference for oxygen.

The venous return increases in relation to the elevated cardiac output. Vasodilation in the working muscles which receive the bulk of the redirected blood permits high flow rates into the capacitance vessels. Because of adrenergically mediated venoconstriction the capacity of this system is reduced, so that blood moves rapidly into the right atrium. Venous return is also enhanced by an increase in intra-abdominal pressure, a decrease in intrathoracic pressure with forced inspiration, and by the pumping action of the rhythmically contracting working muscles. The augmented pulmonary blood flow results in only slight increases in pulmonary artery pressure (page 13.326) due to the distensibility of the large pulmonary arteries, an increase in the area of the pulmonary capillary bed due to the recruitment of more capillaries, and the low resistance offered by the normal pulmonary circulation (Table 1).

Because of the elevated cardiac output and larger stroke volume, systolic blood pressure and pulse pressure increase even though the afterload itself is reduced. Enhanced neurohumoral activity from adrenergic stimulation of the heart and the suprarenal glands (increased circulating adrenaline and noradrenaline) effect positive inotropic changes, to which tachycardia also contributes because of the Bowditch effect. There is a shift in the Frank–Starling relationship to the left accompanied by greater speed and force of cardiac contraction which tends to elevate further the ejection fraction and stroke volume. Peak dp/dt is increased and there is a rapid rise in coronary blood flow to meet myocardial oxygen requirements which increase linearly with the product of systolic blood pressure and heart rate. During moderate exercise these changes together result in a decreased or unaltered end-diastolic volume and, as mentioned, a decreased end-systolic volume. With severe exercise, end-diastolic dimensions and end-diastolic fibre length are slightly increased and the Frank–Starling mechanism then operates and augments further the force of contraction.

The haemodynamic and ventilatory responses evoked by an increase to a new steady work load take about 2–3 min to equilibrate and adjust oxygen supply to the greater demand. Protocols for exercise testing are therefore usually based on work increments at 3 min intervals to allow time for a new 'steady state' to occur as, for example, in the standard Bruce Protocol. A steady state becomes progressively more difficult to maintain as maximal exercise capacity is approached. Glycogen is used by the working muscles as a source of stored energy and the anaerobic metabolism which ensues produces lactic acidosis which further increases ventilation. As all cardiopulmonary transport mechanisms reach maximum levels, shortness of breath, fatigue, and muscle pain become limiting symptoms; motivation is then the final determinant of duration of exercise. Aging reduces the efficacy of cardiopulmonary transport mechanisms and, of course, exercise capacity. The heart rate response at peak exercise reflects this. In healthy individuals aged 20 years it is about 200 beats/min and at 65 years about 170 beats/min.

When exercise stops, the cardiopulmonary and metabolic changes return rapidly to resting levels, the rate following an exponential pattern in the first few minutes; the excretion of lactate and other metabolites and the dissipation of heat generated take longer (time constant of about 15 min or more). Reduced circulatory function slows the recovery rate. The mechanisms responsible for dyspnoea and ventilatory responses to exercise are considered in a later section.

Training effects

Regular exercise to about 60 per cent of maximal heart rate for 20 to 30 min three times a week is the minimum requirement for a training effect. The resting heart rate becomes slower whilst the cardiac output is maintained by an increased end-diastolic volume and ejection fraction, and therefore stroke volume. In a 'trained' exercizing individual there is a reduced heart rate response to a standard submaximal work load, and systemic blood flow is more effectively distributed away from visceral and skin circulations to working muscles. Adaptive changes in muscle mitochondria occur, permitting improved oxygen extraction from perfusing blood so that maximum oxygen consumption increases. There is suggestive evidence for prolonged endurance training increasing the calibre of coronary arteries and enlarging capillary surface area relative to cardiac muscle mass (in animals). Myocardial protein synthesis increases. Adrenergic mechanisms appear to be involved in mediating this response. It should be noted that rhythmic exercise (e.g. running) and isometric exercise (e.g. weight lifting) have different physiological effects. The blood pressure rises disproportionately during the latter. The mechanisms are partly reflex, and partly mechanical from the contracting muscles. Isometric exercise training is not recommended for cardiac patients because of the increased afterload it imposes on the heart.

Hormonal responses to exercise (see page 9.175)

In addition to substantial elevations of circulating noradrenaline and adrenaline in acute exercise, other diverse hormonal responses occur. Plasma insulin declines but there are marked transient increases in growth hormone, glucagon, plasma renin activity, and aldosterone, and small increases in cortisol, prolactin, luteinizing hormone, follicle-stimulating hormone, and, in males, testosterone. Values usually return to control levels within an hour of stopping. Reports of exercise-induced mood changes are difficult to validate scientifically, although feelings of wellbeing seem to occur. There is evidence, however, for increased concentrations of circulating β-endorphin during exercise, and recent studies with naloxone to block the effects of opioid peptides suggest that β-endorphin release may reduce exercise-induced adrenaline and noradrenaline responses (page 10.111 *et seq.*). Regular exercise lowers blood pressure in normotensive and mildly hypertensive subjects, and modulation of catecholamine release by changes in endogenous opioid peptide secretion may be a possible contributing mechanism.

To summarize, changes in the four essential determinants of cardiac function – preload, afterload, heart rate, and contractility – combine to augment cardiac output and oxygen delivery during exercise. Measurement of the cardiovascular response to exercise is essential for the objective assessment of cardiac function and is the subject of a later section (see page 13.159).

References

Braunwald, E. and Ross, J. (1979). Control of cardiac performance. *Handbook of physiology of the American Physiological Society* Section 2, Vol. 1, pp. 533–580. American Physiological Society, Bethesda, Maryland.

—— and —— (1984). Contraction of the normal heart. In *Heart disease* 2nd edn (ed. E. Braunwald), pp. 409–446. W. B. Saunders, Philadelphia.

Ellestad, M. R. (1980). *Stress testing*, 2nd edn. F. A. Davis, Philadelphia.

Feigl, E. O. (1983). Coronary physiology. *Physiol. Rev.* **63**, 1–205.

Hill, A. V. (1970). *First and last experiments in muscle mechanics.* Cambridge University Press, Cambridge.

Kalsner, S. (ed.) (1982). *The coronary artery.* Croom Helm Ltd, London.

O'Rouke, M. F. (1982). *Arterial function in health and disease.* Churchill Livingstone, Edinburgh.

Schlant, R. C. and Sonnenblick, E. H. (1986). Normal physiology of the cardiovascular system. In *The heart* 6th edn (ed. J. W. Hurst), pp. 37–73. McGraw-Hill, New York.

Shepherd, J. T. and Vanhoutte, P. M. (1979). *The human cardiovascular system, facts and concepts.* Raven Press, New York.

CLINICAL ASSESSMENT OF CARDIOVASCULAR FUNCTION

The chest X-ray in heart disease

R. S. O. REES

In a patient with suspected heart disease, the views employed as a routine are standard and penetrated postero-anterior with right lateral at the first attendance, and standard postero-anterior only at subsequent visits. An alternative, which has economic advantages, is a standard postero-anterior only, with the addition of penetrated and lateral if the radiographer observes a large heart or suspects any other abnormality.

Radiographic anatomy

About two-thirds of the cardiac shadow is to the left and one-third to the right of the midline. The right border is composed of three contours, which from above downwards are (a) the innominate vein and its continuation into the superior vena cava; (b) the superior vena cava or, in older individuals, the ascending aorta; and (c) the right atrium. The left border also has three main contours which are formed from above downward by (a) the aortic arch (aortic knuckle or knob) continuing into the descending aorta; (b) the pulmonary trunk; and (c) the left ventricle.

The main branches of the right and left pulmonary arteries form the hilar arteries, the right vessels being situated at a slightly lower level than the left. The normal pulmonary arterial branches arborize into approximately equal but smaller branches of gradually diminishing calibre in proportion to the branches from which they arise, and on a correctly exposed film, are visible well into the periphery. Some of the pulmonary veins may be distinguished from arteries at segmental level in the right lung. In the upper zone, the most lateral ascending vessel is generally a vein, and in the lower zone, veins pursue a more horizontal course compared to arteries. On the left side, differentiation of veins from arteries is more difficult.

The appearance of the chest radiograph has a considerable range of normal variation, depending on the age, sex, height and weight of the patient, shape of the bony thorax, phase of respiration, position of the diaphragm, and phase of the cardiac cycle. In obese persons with a short, broad, rounded chest and elevated diaphragm, the cardiac shadow tends to be short, wide, and situated transversely, and the apex appears to be displaced to the left. The pulmonary trunk segment is relatively short forming a distinct waist, with long prominent left ventricular contour below, the lower portion of which is often obscured by the diaphragm or by a fat pad. A similar transverse position of the heart simulating cardiac enlargement may be due to a high diaphragm, such as in expiration, hepatic enlargement, ascites, or pregnancy. In thin persons with a long flat narrow chest, the cardiac shadow is long and narrow, and its major contours only slightly convex. The pulmonary trunk segment is relatively long and prominent. A vertical cardiac shadow tends to be seen in deep inspiration, in the erect as compared to the recumbent position, and in patients with pulmonary emphysema. Apparent cardiac enlargement with such a chest shape is usually due to sternal depression (pectus excavatum, funnel chest) or a straight thoracic spine with a narrow anteroposterior diameter (straight back syndrome). In infants and young children the chest is rounder, the diaphragm higher and more horizontal, and the cardiac shadow more centrally located than in the adult. Widening of the superior mediastinum due to physiological thymic enlargement is a common normal finding in infants, and must not be confused with abnormal superior mediastinal or vascular widening. In the elderly, the size of the heart relative to the thorax as a whole tends to increase, but this is due more to shrinkage of the thorax than to an absolute increase in heart size. The cardiac cycle might be thought to have a profound effect on the size of the heart as seen on the chest radiograph. The variation from systole to diastole in the normal subject, is however, quite small, certainly less than 1 cm in the transverse diameter; the probable explanation is that the total volume of blood in all four chambers varies much less than that in any individual chamber, particularly of course, the ventricles. Similar but small variations between systole and diastole may also be observed in the pulmonary trunk, aorta, and proximal pulmonary vessels.

On the lateral view the anterior heart border, which is in contact with the sternum for a variable distance above the diaphragm, is formed by the right ventricle below and is continuous above with the pulmonary trunk, which arches backwards and disappears into the mediastinum. Posteriorly, the entry of the pulmonary veins into the left atrium renders this border indistinct, but below, the posterior edge of the left ventricle forms a clear-cut border curving anteriorly as it descends to cross the diaphragm. The inferior vena cava is seen crossing the left ventricular border obliquely. Other structures which may be visible are the ascending and descending aorta, but the extent to which these are seen depends upon how much they are indenting adjacent lung; they are therefore more apparent in the older person with an elongated or unfolded aorta. The right and left pulmonary arteries are also often visible. The right artery appears as a dense round shadow just below and in front of the carina, whereas the upper border of the left may be discerned as it arches backwards over the left bronchus.

Cardiac enlargement

Cardiac enlargement may involve the entire heart, as in various toxic, infective, and metabolic diseases, severe anaemias, and certain forms of combined left-and right-sided heart failure, but in some of the most common and important lesions, especially in their less advanced stages, enlargement is confined to a single chamber or to two chambers. Cardiac enlargement may also be due to pericardial effusion but this can only be differentiated from chamber dilatation with certainty by echocardiography.

For the assessment of overall heart size, three methods are in general use, the first being simply subjective and based on the visual impression of an experienced observer. This is the one most commonly used, the measurements described below only being employed in cases of doubt.

The second is assessment based on measurement of the transverse cardiac diameter, either as a simple figure or expressed as the cardiothoracic ratio. Although it is true that in 95 per cent of adults the transverse diameter is 15.5 cm or less, this is of limited help in the diagnosis or exclusion of cardiac enlargement in smaller persons whose normal diameter may be as little as 7 cm, or indeed in the very large male. Measurement of the transverse diameter is of more practical use when expressed in relation to the

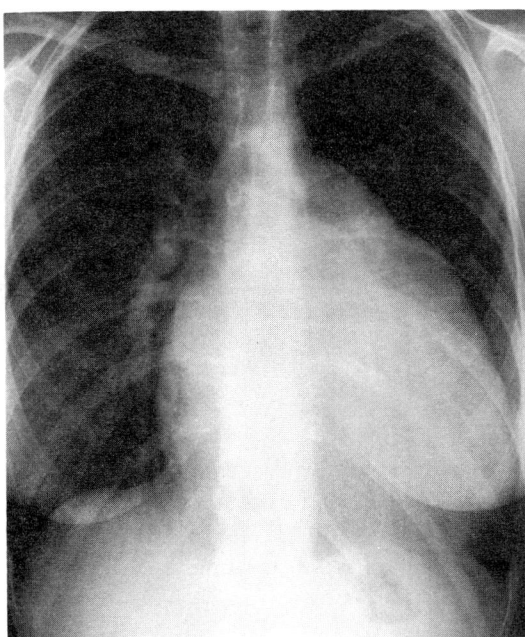

Fig. 1 Left atrial enlargement. Centre of heart dense. Double edge within right heart border. Elevated left bronchus.

internal diameter of the chest at its widest point just above the level of the diaphragm. If the ratio exceeds 50 per cent, it is assumed that there is cardiac enlargement, but even this is only a rough guide, as the relationship between the diameter of the heart and that of the chest varies considerably.

The third method of assessing heart size is a volume measurement based on the assumption that the form of the heart is an ellipsoid. The volume equals length × width × depth × 0.63. Corrected for magnification, the average volume for all adults is about 450 ml per square metre of body surface area with a standard deviation of about 80 ml. Since males have slightly larger hearts than females, the upper limits of normal for practical purposes may be taken as 500 ml per square metre of body surface for females and 550 for males.

It is important to note that when taking measurements of the heart, pads of fat around the apex should be recognized and ignored. If in doubt on the standard view, the differing radiographic density of fat compared to other soft tissue is usually obvious on the penetrated view.

Enlargement of the heart to the right is a difficult sign to analyse, as it may occur from dilatation of either atrium or the right ventricle. Isolated enlargement of the right atrium is rare, and is only seen in tricuspid stenosis without significant regurgitation, so that, with a normal-sized left atrium, enlargement to the right can be assumed to be due to dilatation of the right heart. If the prominence of the right border extends to involve the superior vena cava, enlargement of the right atrium is likely. Right atrial enlargement is a feature of any lesion affecting the right ventricle such as tricuspid regurgitation and right-sided heart failure. Dilatation is not very great in the common shunts, such as atrial septal defect, but may be marked in conditions where the flow is very high, such as total anomalous pulmonary venous drainage.

When the left atrium enlarges, it does so initially posteriorly and to the right, with enlargement of the appendix being visible to the left (Fig. 1). Slight left atrial enlargement is best seen on the penetrated postero-anterior and lateral views. On the penetrated view, posterior enlargement with increase in depth can be detected by an increase in radiographic density of the middle of the heart, slight indentation of the left bronchus which assumes a bowed shape convex to the left, and the appearance of a curved edge,

convex to the right within the right heart border, representing the right posterior edge of the left atrium indenting the lung. The enlarged appendix is visible as a small localized bulge between the pulmonary trunk and left ventricular segments on the left heart border. On the lateral view, posterior enlargement is reflected in increased depth of the upper half of the heart, although the posterior border remains indistinct. Slight indentation of the left bronchus may also be seen on the lateral view. Moderate left atrial enlargement is present when the signs described become obvious, with the right edge approaching or coinciding with the right heart border, the left bronchus obviously elevated, and the centre of the heart very dense. Gross enlargement may be to the left or the right, more commonly the right, and in some cases of giant left atrium the chamber may reach either lateral chest wall. Left atrial enlargement is a feature of mitral valve disease and of any lesion involving the left ventricle, whether causing hypertrophy or dilatation; gross enlargement is only seen in chronic rheumatic mitral valve disease or severe congenital mitral regurgitation. Slight enlargement is also a feature of left-to-right shunts at ventricular or aortopulmonary levels and atrial arrhythmias.

Enlargement of the heart to the left indicates enlargement of one or both ventricles. In considering ventricular enlargement distinction must be made between hypertrophy and dilatation, although the two may coexist. Hypertrophy is an increase in wall thickness in which the volume of the cavity does not increase and may actually decrease, so that hypertrophy alone may not be seen as enlargement radiologically unless very extreme, or until the terminal stages when the heart begins to fail and the chamber dilates. With dilatation the overall volume of the cavity is increased, so that chamber enlargement is readily appreciated radiologically.

Enlargement of the right ventricle is difficult to diagnose in its early stages, as it is usually anterior and does not cause the chamber to reach the cardiac border. On the postero-anterior view the subtle change in shape produced by early right as opposed to left ventricular enlargement is that the left border of the heart becomes straight and the apex slightly high. With generalized cardiac enlargement, this different shape may enable right ventricular enlargement to be distinguished from left, but owing to the great individual variation, such a distinction is not often of great practical value. On the lateral view, a large right ventricle renders the anterior border of the heart in contact with the sternum above the normal level; in the absence of thoracic deformity, right ventricular enlargement is probably present if the upper point of contact is above the mid-point between the diaphragm and the sternal angle.

Right ventricular hypertrophy is a feature of all types of right ventricular outflow tract obstruction and pulmonary arterial hypertension, whereas dilatation is seen in shunts at atrial or ventricular level, regurgitation of the right-sided valves and right-sided heart failure.

The earliest sign of left ventricular enlargement on the postero-anterior view is increased convexity of the left ventricular border which may be maximal anywhere from the mid-border to the apex. Such a change, which is difficult to establish with certainty, is not accompanied initially by any measurable increase in heart size. With obvious enlargement, the curve of the left heart border tends to be long and smooth with no abrupt changes in the arc of curvature. The most lateral point is above the diaphragm with a vertical heart, and lower with a horizontal heart. Left ventricular enlargement is seen on the lateral view as a prominent convexity of the lower posterior cardiac border behind the inferior vena cava.

Left ventricular hypertrophy is a feature of systemic hypertension, hypertrophic cardiomyopathy, and all types of left ventricular outflow tract obstruction, whereas dilatation is seen in regurgitation of the left-sided valves, ischaemic heart disease, congestive cardiomyopathy, shunts at ventricular or aortopulmonary level, and left heart failure from any other cause.

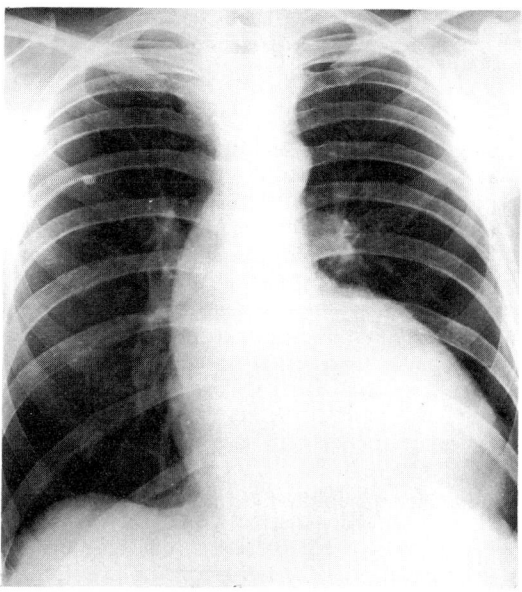

Fig. 2 Marfan's syndrome with aortic regurgitation. Gross dilatation of ascending aorta and left ventricle.

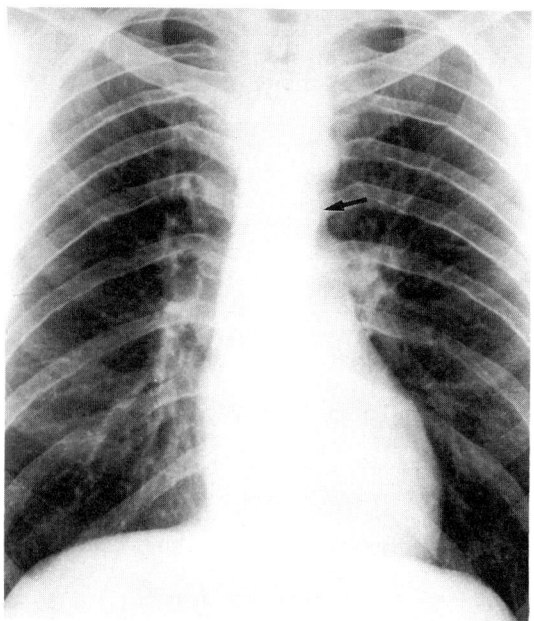

Fig. 3 Co-arctation of the aorta. Rib notching, itself a non-specific sign of co-arctation. Arrow points to bulge below aortic knuckle formed by post-stenotic dilatation.

The great vessels

The thoracic aorta undergoes a gradual increase in length and diameter as age advances, but with considerable individual variation. In early adult life, the right upper cardiac border is formed by the superior vena cava, but in the average person, by the age of 40, this edge assumes a slightly convex shape and is formed by the ascending aorta. The diameter of the aortic knuckle also increases gradually, and by middle age, it is common to see a rim of calcification around its lower margin, which does not necessarily indicate the presence of generalized atherosclerosis. Elongation of the descending aorta usually appears as increased convexity to the left on the penetrated view, although in some cases, greater tortuosity with an addional curve to the right may be present. In systemic hypertension, these changes are more obvious and may be seen at

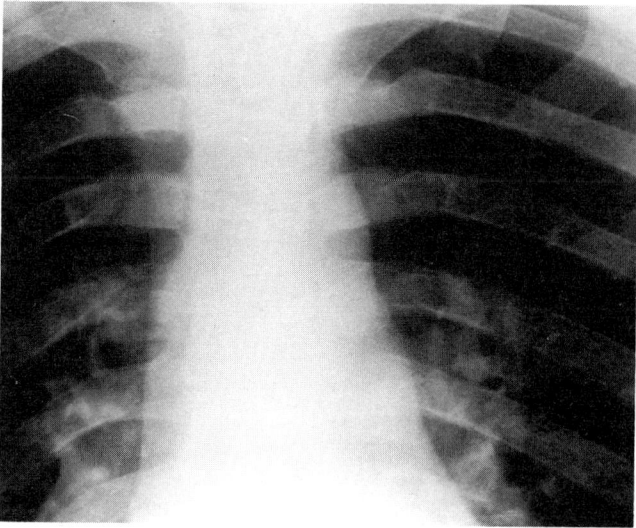

Fig. 4 Ductus arteriosus. The long flat aortic knuckle typical of this condition.

a younger age, and generalized calcific atherosclerosis is common.

Localized or generalized dilatation of the aorta is a feature of many conditions. Differentiation of dilatation from elongation on postero-anterior or lateral views is often difficult, because it is not always possible to obtain a clear view of both sides of the aortic wall in one projection, one side usually being continuous with the mediastinum. The observer should bear this in mind before giving a firm opinion. Localized dilatation of the ascending aorta is a feature of bicuspid aortic valve and aortic stenosis. This post-stenotic dilatation is variable in degree and bears no relationship to the severity of obstruction. On the postero-anterior view it appears as a convex bulge on the right upper cardiovascular border, which may be distinguished from elongation if the rest of the aorta appears normal for the patient's age. More pronounced localized dilatation is a feature of Marfan's syndrome (Fig. 2). In long-standing aortic regurgitation primarily due to cusp disease, the whole thoracic aorta is dilated, similar to that seen in systemic hypertension. It is also very pulsatile, and appears significantly larger in systole than in diastole. Aortic aneurysms are most commonly due to dissection, trauma, syphilis, or atherosclerosis, and are usually seen on both postero-anterior and lateral views as a well-defined mass continuous with a part of the thoracic aorta. Oblique views may help to localize and distinguish the lesion from other conditions, such as bronchial carcinoma, but other investigations may be necessary to establish the diagnosis with certainty.

In co-arctation of the aorta the ascending portion is prominent, very often due to a bicuspid valve. The patterns seen in the aortic arch are variable. The commonest is a flat knuckle continuous above with a straight superior mediastinal edge, which is formed by a large left subclavian artery. Below, a slight bulge convex to the left may be visible, particularly on the penetrated view, representing the poststenotic dilatation of the descending aorta distal to the obstruction (Fig. 3). Other varieties include a prominent bulge of the arch above the obstruction, resembling a high aortic knuckle, a prominent poststenotic dilatation below a flat segment, resembling a low aortic knuckle, or a double knuckle. Notching on the inferior borders of the ribs is a common feature of co-arctation, being due to tortuosity of the intercostal arteries. In persistent ductus arteriosus, the aortic knuckle usually has an abnormal shape. The arc is elongated and represents the localized dilatation characteristically present at the aortic end of the ductus (Fig. 4). This sign is not constant and is not visible in small children. Its value is to alert the clinician to the possibility of a lesion other than a ductus when the aortic knuckle appears normal in a patient with a continuous murmur.

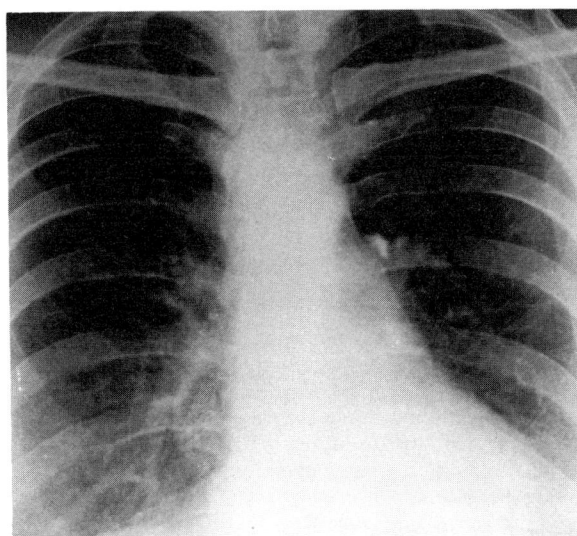

Fig. 5 Right-sided aortic arch.

In cyanosed patients, enlargement of the aorta, particularly the ascending portion and arch, is a feature of Fallot's tetralogy, pulmonary atresia, and truncus arteriosus, in all of which the incidence of right aortic arch is high (25–50 per cent). Right aortic arch may also occur as an isolated anomaly. Its recognition on the chest radiograph is important and is not always easy, unless both standard and penetrated postero-anterior views are available (Fig. 5). If the actual convexity of the knuckle is not visible, then the side of the arch can be established by observation of the relative width of the mediastinum on either side of the trachea, of the tracheal impression just above the carina, or of the lateral border of the descending aorta.

A small aortic knuckle with an inconspicuous ascending aorta are features of atrial septal defect, long-standing rheumatic mitral valve disease, particularly mitral stenosis, and supravalvar aortic stenosis.

The pulmonary trunk may enlarge from increased pressure, increased flow, or poststenotic dilatation. An enlarged pulmonary trunk is visible on the postero-anterior view as a convex segment on the left border joining the bottom of the aortic knuckle to the upper end of the left ventricular border. Its maximal convexity is in the middle except in poststenotic dilatation, where it tends to be higher, beneath the aortic knuckle. Increased flow in the pulmonary trunk is present in all types of left-to-right shunt, but with comparable levels of flow, the pulmonary trunk appears consistently larger in atrial compared to ventricular shunts. In pulmonary hypertension, dilatation is also a typical feature. Particularly gross dilatation is seen in the Eisenmenger syndrome with the shunt at atrial or aortopulmonary levels, but paradoxically may be slight or absent when the defect is interventricular. In left-sided lesions, and particularly mitral valve disease, a dilated pulmonary trunk is a reliable indicator of an elevated pulmonary vascular resistance. Other rare causes of a dilated pulmonary trunk include pulmonary regurgitation and aneurysm. Dilatation without obvious cause is usually described as idiopathic. Provided the patient is not a female under 25, such an appearance is most likely due to a minor pulmonary valve abnormality, which produces dilatation in the same way as a bicuspid aortic valve does in the ascending aorta.

The lungs

Alterations in pulmonary haemodynamics are a feature of many types of heart disease. They fall into four groups, each of which gives a particular pattern of radiological change. These are pulmonary venous hypertension, increased pulmonary flow, pulmonary arterial hypertension, and decreased pulmonary flow.

Elevation of the pulmonary venous pressure may result from any lesion of the left heart. Whatever the cause, the radiological changes are similar, and modified more by the rate of change and duration of the pressure rise than by the underlying aetiology. Whether acute or chronic, elevation of the pulmonary venous pressure causes a relative diversion of blood flow from the lower to the upper zones of the lungs in the erect position, and is reflected in an increase in the calibre of the upper vessels. Normally they are smaller than the lower vessels. With pulmonary venous hypertension, they enlarge to equal or exceed the calibre of vessels in the lower zones at a comparable distance from the hilum. In very long-standing pulmonary venous hypertension, after surgical correction of the left heart lesion, or in a rapidly varying acute situation, the presence of upper vessel dilatation may not necessarily indicate pulmonary venous hypertension at the time of the radiograph, although it is clear evidence that this abnormality was present at some time. Absence of upper vessel dilatation, however, is a reliable indication of a normal pressure, provided the pulmonary vessels are not obliterated by pulmonary disease, such as old tuberculosis or emphysema.

Haemodynamically mild lesions may result in pulmonary venous hypertension which shows only as upper vessel dilatation. However, more severe elevation of the pressure, either acute or chronic, results in pulmonary oedema in the interstitial or alveolar spaces or both. Acute pulmonary oedema may show on the chest radiograph in a variety of ways. In its severest form, large volumes of fluid accumulate in the alveolar spaces, causing extensive, but often rapidly variable ill-defined shadows. The hila are enlarged, often greatly so, and surrounded by a hazy indistinct edge ('bat's wing oedema'). Less dramatic changes include blurring of the clear-cut edges of the vessels, vague generalized loss of translucency, and widespread small ill-defined shadows ('mottling'): these may be difficult to appreciate, but become obvious in retrospect when the film is compared to a later one taken after treatment. Pleural effusions are common and for reasons unknown, are seen more often on the right side than the left. They may loculate against the chest wall or in the fissures.

These radiological changes are often non-specific and differentiation from pneumonia or pulmonary embolism may not be poss-

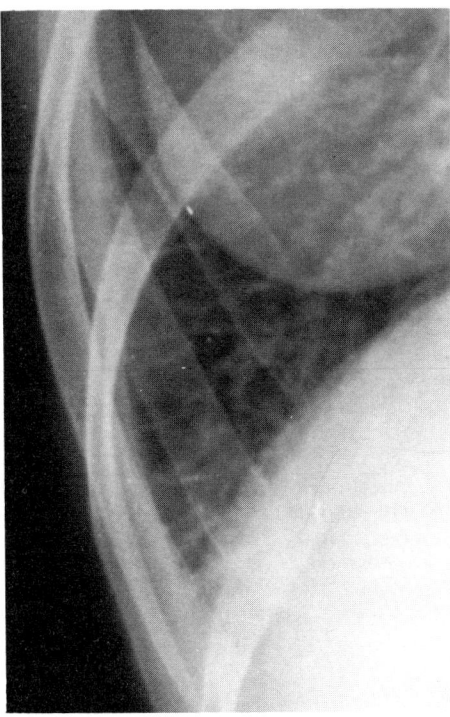

Fig. 6 Septal lines and parietal effusion.

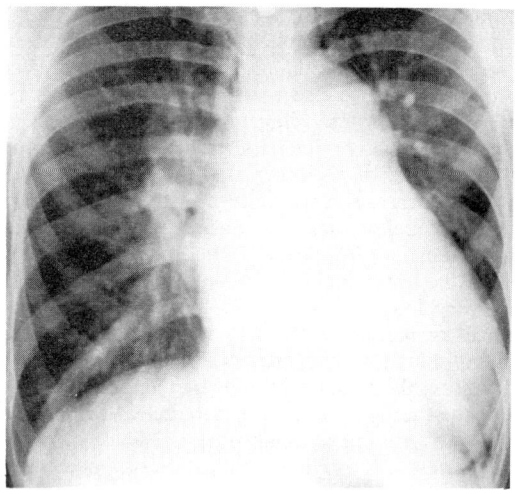

Fig. 7 Hyperkinetic pulmonary hypertension.

ible. There are, however, more specific signs of pulmonary oedema which should always be sought in order to establish the diagnosis. These are septal lines and parietal effusions (Fig. 6). Septal lines are fine dense lines in the lung, generally most easily visible in the costophrenic angles where they are horizontal (Kerley B lines), but also in other parts of the lower and less often upper zones where they run in haphazard directions and are of variable length. Their radiographic characteristics strongly suggest that they represent fluid lying within potential spaces, probably interlobular tissue planes, within the lung. Parietal effusions, so named to distinguish them from pleural effusions, are thin collections of fluid lying at the bases against the lateral chest wall and are also manifest by thickening of the fissures. They represent fluid in the subpleural space in potential communication with the interstitial space, and this accounts for their distribution and radiological appearances being different to fluid lying free in the pleural space.

Septal lines and parietal effusions are not only seen with pulmonary venous hypertension but may occur in lymphoma, acute leukaemia, and lymphangitis carcinomatosa. Septal lines have also been reported in sarcoidosis and occupational lung disease.

In acute pulmonary venous hypertension, any or all of the above features may be seen, but septal lines at the bases may be inconspicuous or absent; a careful search, however, will usually reveal them in other parts of the lungs. In long-standing pulmonary venous hypertension, most typically seen in untreated mitral stenosis, pulmonary oedema shows mainly as septal lines and parietal effusions, and the other more non-specific signs are less of a feature. In this group too, haemosiderosis (widespread low-density mottling) and bone deposits (dense lesions of varying size in the lower zones) are occasionally encountered.

Any communication between the systemic and pulmonary circulations, unless accompanied by obstruction in the right heart downstream from the defect, results in an increase in pulmonary flow, and is reflected radiologically by a generalized increase in pulmonary vessel size (pulmonary plethora). Cyanosis is absent if the vascular connections of the heart are normal, but is a feature of conditions with abnormal connections, such as total anomalous pulmonary venous drainage, transposition, and truncus arteriosus. Unlike pulmonary venous hypertension, there is no relative variation in vessel calibre. The degree of plethora, whether obvious or slight and questionably present, roughly parallels the magnitude of the flow providing the pulmonary arterial pressure remains normal.

Elevation of the pulmonary arterial pressure may result from various causes, and these causes are largely responsible for the differing pulmonary vascular patterns seen radiologically. When coexistent with a high pulmonary flow, such as is typically seen with a large ventricular shunt, pulmonary plethora is obvious and the generalized vessel dilatation extends at least to involve the distal segmental branches (hyperkinetic pulmonary hypertension) (Fig. 7). These patients may present with heart failure, in which case gross plethora is associated with pulmonary oedema.

Extreme irreversible pulmonary hypertension (Eisenmenger syndrome) may complicate any shunt whether at atrial, ventricular, or aortopulmonary levels. The pulmonary flow is normal or low and there is a right-to-left shunt. The pulmonary vascular pattern is variable. With atrial defects, pulmonary hypertension is of late onset, usually in patients in their 20s or after, the central vessels are huge, and there is an abrupt reduction in vessel calibre at midsegmental level with normal or small peripheral vessels. With ventricular shunts, the pulmonary hypertension is usually established in early childhood, and the vessel dilatation may be unimpressive; in Down's syndrome with Eisenmenger atrioventricular canal, the appearances may even be normal. With an Eisenmenger ductus, the appearance of the hilar and peripheral vessels are similar to ventricular shunts.

Pulmonary arterial hypertension with an elevated pulmonary vascular resistance may also be secondary to pulmonary venous hypertension. In a chronic situation, the relative difference between the calibre of the upper and lower vessels is exaggerated by reduction in size of the lower segmental branches, and the hilar arteries are prominent. Accurate prediction of an elevated pulmonary vascular resistance secondary to pulmonary venous hypertension from the radiograph is not always possible, although the presence of a large pulmonary trunk together with the features mentioned above make it highly likely. Elevation of the pulmonary artery pressure is often quite marked with acute left ventricular failure, but the established signs described above do not have time to develop so that prediction from the chest radiograph is difficult.

Pulmonary hypertension of unknown cause (primary) or due to multiple small thrombo-emboli may be impossible to distinguish radiologically. In both conditions, there is dilatation of the central pulmonary arteries with reduction in peripheral vessel calibre. Similar changes are encountered in other rare causes, such as arteritis. In the occasional case, thromboembolism is suggested by uneven vascular obliteration and infarct scars in the lungs.

Another important cause of pulmonary hypertension is respiratory disease (cor pulmonale). In some patients the pulmonary hypertension is permanent and irreversible, in others intermittent and present only during the acute phase of right-sided heart failure. Irreversible pulmonary hypertension secondary to chronic airways obstruction is uncommon and typically occurs in the patient with emphysema rather than bronchitis. It is difficult to predict from the radiograph as the characteristic thin vertical heart, prominent pulmonary trunk segment, and hilar vessels with small peripheral vessels are features of the long, thin chest with hyperinflated lungs seen in emphysema. Only if there is unequivocal cardiac enlargement should pulmonary hypertension be suggested. The patient with bronchitis may have a barrel-shaped chest, but often the radiograph is otherwise relatively normal apart from some irregular peripheral vascular obliteration. Acute exacerbations of the bronchitis are accompanied by a sudden obvious increase in heart size and a generalized increase in pulmonary vessel calibre, resembling plethora. Measurement of the pulmonary artery pressure during this acute phase of right-sided heart failure shows at least moderate and often severe elevation of the pulmonary artery pressure.

Obstruction at, above or below the pulmonary valve may cause reduction in total pulmonary flow, particularly when associated with a right-to-left shunt. As with increased flow, the reduction in vessel size roughly parallels the flow, and is best assessed by observation of the hilar arteries rather than those in the periphery whose size is more difficult to determine. Small pulmonary vessels due to decreased flow (pulmonary oligaemia) is almost invariably accompanied by cyanosis, the commonest cause being Fallot's tetralogy.

References

Jefferson, K. and Rees, S. (1980). *Clinical cardiac radiology*, 2nd edn. Butterworths, London.

The electrocardiogram

D. J. ROWLANDS

Electrocardiography developed empirically and its basic diagnostic criteria remain empirical. The criteria given here represent a reasonable compromise between sensitivity and specificity.

Normal electrocardiographic appearances

The basic ECG waveform

The basic ECG waveform consists of three recognizable deflections. These were termed 'P wave', 'QRS complex', and 'T wave' by Einthoven (Fig. 1). He allocated sequential alphabetical lettering to the waves because he did not know their origins and did not wish to suggest any interpretation by the labelling. The P wave and T wave are relatively simple shapes and they exhibit few variations in shape. The QRS complexes exhibit more readily recognizable differences in pattern in different leads within the same ECG.

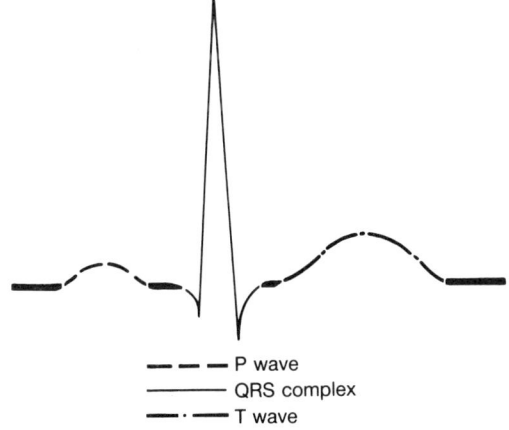

Fig. 1 The basic ECG waveform.

QRS waveform nomenclature

All sharp, pointed deflections resulting from electrical activation of the ventricles are called 'QRS complexes' whatever their configuration. The presence and relative size of the several possible components of the QRS complex may be indicated by a convention using combinations of the letters q, r, s, Q, R, S (Fig. 2). If a given component is considered to be large an upper case letter is used, if it is considered to be small a lower case letter is used.

Six limb leads (frontal plane leads) The orientation around the heart of the six limb leads is illustrated in Fig. 3.

Augmented limb leads All current ECG machines use augmented limb leads, i.e. they record aVL, aVF and aVR and not L, F, and R.

Leads I, II, and III are bipolar and leads aVL, aVF, and aVR are unipolar leads.

Precordial leads (chest leads) For each precordial lead, the positive (recording) terminal of the galvanometer is connected to an electrode at an agreed site on the chest wall. Since the connection

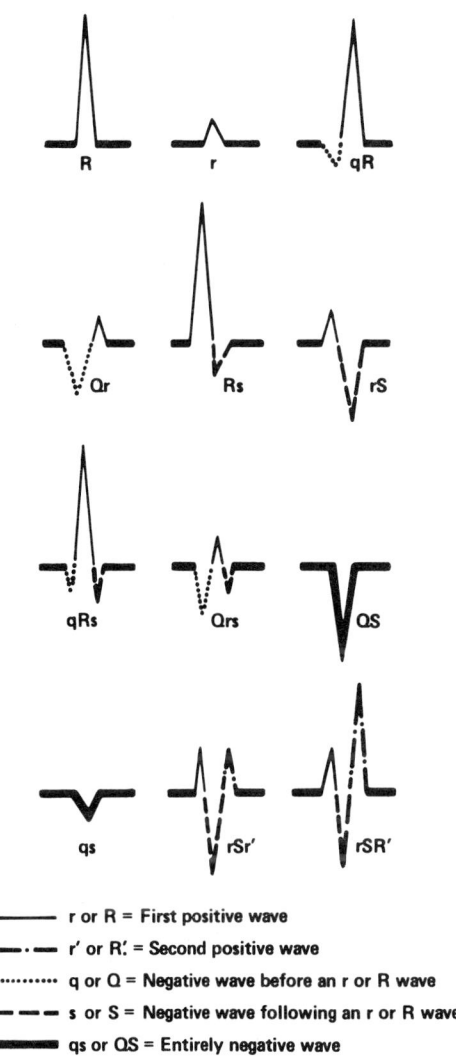

r or R = First positive wave

r' or R' = Second positive wave

q or Q = Negative wave before an r or R wave

s or S = Negative wave following an r or R wave

qs or QS = Entirely negative wave

Fig. 2 QRS waveform nomenclature.

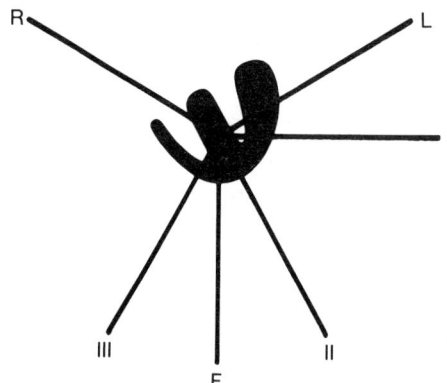

Fig. 3 The frontal plane leads. Note that leads II, III, and F are inferior to the heart, I and L are anterolateral to the heart, and R looks into the cavity of the heart.

to the negative terminal of the recorder is the 'indifferent' one formed by joining together leads R, L, and F, the chest leads are 'V' leads and are designated V_1, V_2, V_3, V_4, V_5, and V_6. A standard anatomical siting of the precordial electrodes has been agreed between the British Cardiac Society and the American Heart Association and is shown in Fig. 4. Figure 5 shows the

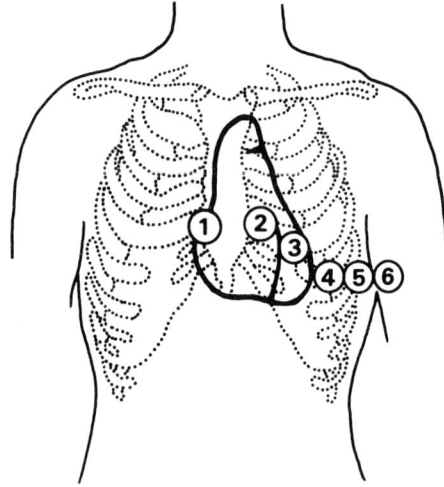

Fig. 4 The precordial lead V_1 is located at the right sternal margin in the fourth intercostal space, V_2 at the left sternal margin at the fourth intercostal space, V_4 at the intersection of the left mid-clavicular line and left fifth intercostal space, V_3 mid-way between V_2 and V_4, V_5 at the intersection of the left anterior axillary line with a horizontal line through V_4, and V_6 at the intersection of the left mid-axillary line with a horizontal line through V_4 and V_5.

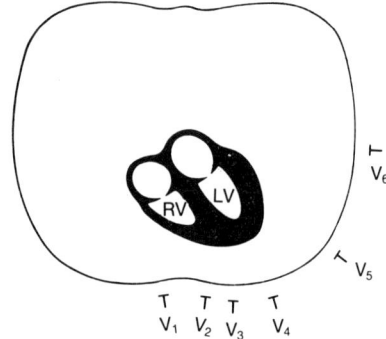

Fig. 5 The precordial leads. Their anatomical relationship to the main cardiac chambers.

important relationship of the precordial leads to the cardiac chambers.

Twelve conventional ECG leads Figure 6 shows the relationship of the 12 conventional electrocardiographic leads to one another and to the heart.

Recognizing the normal electrocardiogram

This is the most difficult and the most important aspect of understanding the electrocardiogram. The electrocardiogram is recognized as being within or beyond normal limits by the normality or otherwise of the shape and dimensions of its various substituent deflections, and the frequency of the deflections and their relationship in time to the deflections preceding and succeeding them.

This introduction to the subject considers only morphological normality or abnormality. The presence of sinus rhythm will be assumed. The criteria for normality of the P waves obtain in any rhythm where atrial depolarization is of sinus origin (sinus tachycardia, sinus bradycardia, sinus arrhythmia, first, second, or third degree heart block). Those for the QRS complexes, ST segments, and T waves obtain in any rhythm of supraventricular origin, provided the rate is not so rapid as to induce functional bundle branch block.

Normal QRS appearances in the precordial leads

The QRS complex in V_1 typically shows a small initial positive wave followed by a larger negative wave, and in V_6 a small initial

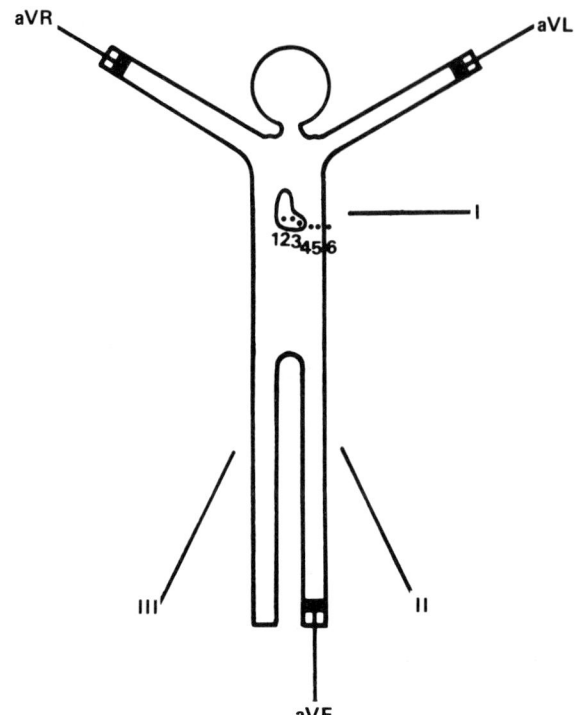

Fig. 6 The conventional 12 ECG leads and their relationships to the heart.

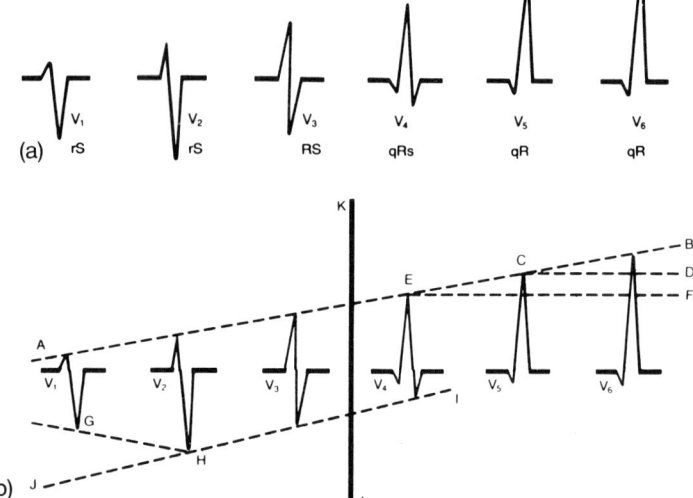

Fig. 7 (a) Typical normal QRS morphology of the precordial leads. (b) Normal variations of R wave amplitude and S wave depth in the precordial leads. The R wave in each precordial lead is usually larger than in the lead preceding in the series from V_1–V_6 (line AB). However, it is quite normal for the R wave in V_6 to be smaller than that in V_5 (line CD) or for the R wave in V_5 to be smaller than that in V_4 provided that the R wave in V_6 is also smaller than that in V_5 (line EF). The size of the S wave diminishes progressively across the precordial leads (line JI) although the S wave in V_2 is often greater than that in V_1 (line GHI). Leads before line KL have an initial deflection which is positive and those after line KL have an initial deflection which is negative.

negative wave followed by a large positive wave (Fig. 7a). In general the size of the initial positive wave (r or R wave) increases progressively from V_1–V_6. However, certain normal variations are possible (Fig. 7b). The direction of the initial part of the QRS is upward (i.e. positive) in V_1–V_3, but downward (i.e. negative) in

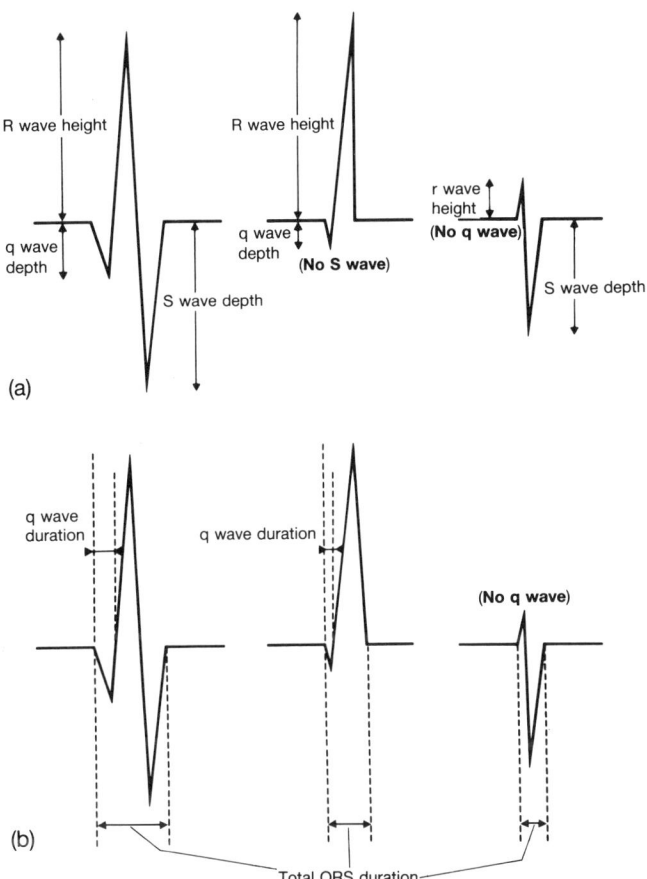

Fig. 8 The dimensions of constituent waves within QRS complexes. (a) Voltage requirements. (b) Wave duration measurements.

V_4–V_6. That is, V_1–V_3 show initial r waves and V_4–V_6 initial q waves. Leads showing an rS complex are being primarily influenced by right ventricular myocardium and leads showing a qR complex by left ventricular myocardium. The transition zone between right and left ventricular epicardial leads is seen (Fig. 7) to be between V_2 and V_4. When the transition zone falls outside this region the heart is said to be *rotated*. If the transition zone occurs further to the left of the precordial series (for example between V_5 and V_6) then the heart is said to be clockwise rotated. Conversely if the transition zone is moved to the right in the precordial series, the heart is said to be counter-clockwise rotated. Clockwise and counter-clockwise rotation refer to a normal state of variability between one subject and another and are not in themselves indicative of abnormality. For a detailed understanding of clockwise and counter-clockwise rotation, more extensive works should be consulted.

The dimensions of the individual waves making up each part of the precordial QRS complexes are of crucial importance in determining normality or otherwise. Figure 8 shows how measurements within the QRS complexes are obtained. The criteria for normality of these individual waves are: (*a*) minimum voltage: at least one R wave in the precordial leads must exceed 8 mm in height; (*b*) maximum voltage: (i) the tallest R wave in the left precordial leads must not exceed 27 mm, (ii) the deepest S wave in the right precordial leads must not exceed 30 mm, (iii) the sum of the tallest R wave in the left precordial leads and the deepest S wave in the right precordial leads must not exceed 40 mm; (*c*) maximum duration: the total QRS duration in any one precordial lead must not exceed 0.10 s ($2\frac{1}{2}$ small squares); (*d*) q wave criteria: (i) precordial q waves must not equal or exceed 0.04 (one small square), (ii) precordial q waves must not have a depth greater than a

quarter of the height of the R wave in the same lead; and (*e*) ventricular activation time, also known as 'intrinsic deflection time': in leads facing the left ventricle (i.e. showing qR complexes) must not exceed 0.04 (one small square).

Normal precordial T waves
The criteria given below for normality of the T waves are applicable to adults only.

V_1. Eighty per cent of normal adults have upright T waves, 20 per cent have flat or inverted T waves. Therefore, the finding of an inverted T wave in V_1 cannot be considered an abnormality (unless it was upright in a previous ECG).

V_2. About 95 per cent of normal adults show upright T waves and 5 per cent have flat or inverted T waves in V_2. Therefore there is a 1 in 20 possibility of inverted T waves in V_2 occurring by chance and not indicating an abnormality. However, if the T wave in V_2 is inverted when it was formerly upright, it is abnormal. Further, if there is T wave inversion in V_2 with an upright T wave in V_1 it is abnormal.

V_3–V_6. The T wave is normally upright in these leads. T wave inversion in V_4, V_5, or V_6 is always abnormal. T wave inversion in V_3, as well as in V_1 and V_2 may rarely be found in healthy young adults.

There are no strict criteria for T-wave size. In general the tallest precordial T wave is found in V_3 or V_4, and the smallest in V_1 and V_2 and, as a general rule, the T wave should not be less than 1/8 and not more than 2/3 of the height of the preceding R wave in each of the leads V_3–V_6.

Normal precordial ST segments
There is one rule for normality of the ST segment. It must not deviate by more than 1 mm above or below the iso-electric line in any precordial lead. The iso-electric line is that vertical position of the ECG recording when no part of the heart is being depolarized or repolarized (i.e. the interval between the end of one T wave and the beginning of the next P wave).

Normal precordial P waves
The P waves are usually upright from V_4–V_6. Upright or biphasic P waves may occur in V_1 and V_2. If the P waves are biphasic, the negative (terminal) component of the P wave must have a smaller area than the positive (initial) component.

Normal limb lead QRS complexes
Only three criteria need to be applied to the limb leads to determine normality of the QRS complexes: the size of any q waves in aVL, I, II, or aVF, the size of the R waves in aVL and aVF, and the electrical axis of the heart.

Any q wave present in lead I, II or aVF must not exceed one quarter the height of the ensuing R wave and must not equal or exceed 0.04s. Any q wave present in aVR or lead III should be ignored irrespective of its size. Q waves present in aVL should fulfil the same criteria as those in leads I, II, or aVF unless the frontal plane QRS axis is more positive than +60°, in which case large q waves in aVL are acceptable, since aVL is then a cavity lead.

The R wave in aVL must not exceed 13 mm and that in aVF must not exceed 20 mm.

The electrical axis of the heart must not lie outside the limits of −30° to +90°. The significance and technique of determination of the electrical axis are described in larger texts (see Rowlands, 1978, 1981).

Normal limb lead ST segments
Normal ST segments do not deviate above or below the iso-electric line by more than 1 mm.

Normal limb lead T waves
In general, the T waves and QRS complexes in the limb leads are concordant, i.e. when the QRS complexes are upright, the T waves are upright, and when the QRS complexes are negative the

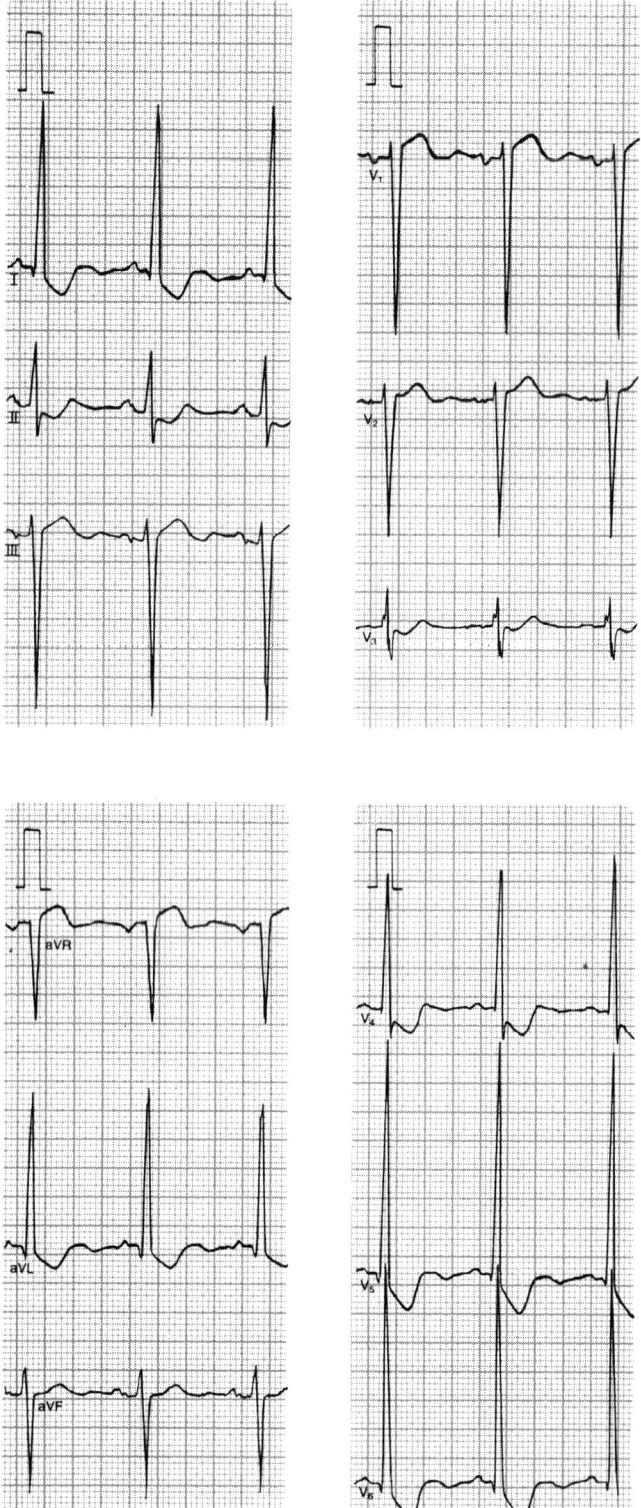

Fig. 9 Left ventricular hypertrophy. There is also left atrial hypertrophy.

deflections is close to zero, the T wave may be positive or negative (though small in either case) or iso-electric (flat); and (*d*) the normal T wave is always upright in leads I and II.

Normal limb lead P waves
The limb lead which normally best shows the P wave is lead II. In this lead the normal P wave does not exceed 0.12 s and its height does not exceed 2.5 mm.

All the above criteria are dependent upon a normal (standard) calibration and a normal paper recording speed.

Ventricular hypertrophy
Appreciable hypertrophy of the right or left ventricle produces characteristic changes in the electrocardiogram. Lesser degrees of hypertrophy may be present without ECG changes or with only non-specific changes. This is more often true of right than of left ventricular hypertrophy.

Left ventricular hypertrophy
The increased bulk of the left ventricle increases the voltage induced during left ventricular depolarization. This gives rise to taller R waves in the left precordial leads and deeper S waves in the right precordial leads. The increased ventricular bulk also prolongs the time taken to travel from endocardium to epicardium, i.e. in the ventricular activation time. In addition, secondary changes in depolarization occur changing the ST segments and T waves.

The electrocardiographic criteria for left ventricular hypertrophy are: (*a*) at least one R wave in the left precordial leads exceeds 27 mm; (*b*) at least one S wave in the right precordial leads exceeds 30 mm; (*c*) the sum of the tallest R wave voltage and the deepest S wave voltage in the precordial leads exceeds 40 mm; (*d*) the largest positive or negative deflection in the limb exceeds 20 mm; (*e*) the intrinsic deflection time (ventricular activation time) exceeds 0.04 s; and (*f*) ST segment depression and T wave inversion may occur in the left precordial leads and in those limb leads which face the left ventricle.

In addition to one or more of the above criteria, it is also necessary that the total QRS duration must not exceed 0.10 s.

Left ventricular hypertrophy is a graded, rather than an all-or-none diagnosis. The greater the number of criteria fulfilled, the more confident one can be of the diagnosis. The voltage criteria are the most sensitive and the intrinsic deflection time the most specific. An example is shown in Fig. 9.

Right ventricular hypertrophy
Increased bulk of the right ventricle gives rise to higher voltages during right ventricular depolarization, increasing the size of the positive deflection in the right precordial leads. In addition, it shifts the electrical axis towards the right and changes the ST segments and T waves, in leads facing the right ventricle, because of secondary changes in the repolarization process.

The electrocardiographic criteria for right ventricular hypertrophy are: (*a*) a dominant positive deflection in V$_1$ (Rs, qR, rR′) in the presence of a normal total QRS duration; (*b*) a mean frontal plane QRS axis more positive than +90°; and (*c*) ST segment depression and T wave inversion in right precordial leads.

The more features present, the more convincing is the electrocardiographic evidence for right ventricular hypertrophy but, in general, the combination of a dominant positive deflection of the QRS in V$_1$ and an abnormal degree of right axis deviation (axis more positive than +90°) establishes the diagnosis. Examples are shown in Fig. 10a and b. In both examples there is abnormal right axis deviation and a dominant R wave in V$_1$. Figure 10a shows an Rs complex in V$_1$ and Fig. 10b shows a qR complex. Figure 10b

T waves are negative. A normal T wave will always be negative in aVR and positive in I and II. T waves can be positive or negative in aVL, aVF, and II without necessarily indicating abnormality.

A rough guide to assess normality of the T waves in the limb leads is: (*a*) in any lead in which the QRS is predominantly upright, the T wave must be clearly upright; (*b*) in any lead in which the QRS is predominantly negative, the T wave should be clearly negative; (*c*) in any lead in which the algebraic sum of QRS

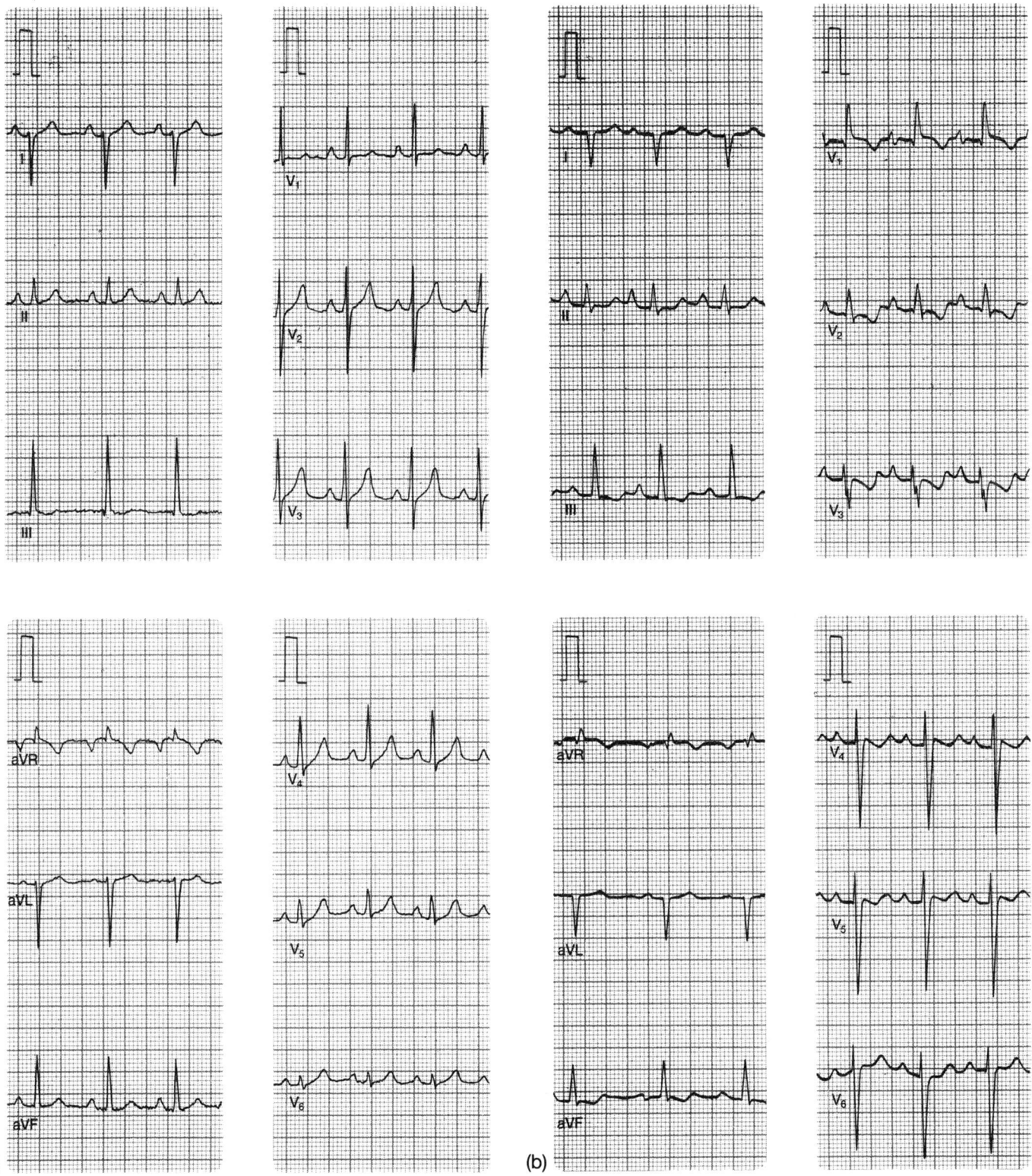

Fig. 10 Two examples of ECG evidence of right ventricular hypertrophy. There is also right atrial hypertrophy.

also shows pronounced clockwise cardiac rotation, which often accompanies right ventricular hypertrophy.

Atrial hypertrophy

The electrocardiographic changes produced by left atrial hypertrophy are those produced by an increase in the voltage and duration of the left atrial depolarization wave. Since the terminal part of the normal P wave is produced by left atrial depolarization, it follows that the total P wave duration is prolonged in left atrial hypertrophy. In addition, the P wave tends to be bifid in lead II and biphasic in V_1. In V_1 the area of the (terminal) negative component exceeds the area of the (initial) positive component (Fig. 11).

Bundle branch block

Total failure of conduction in the right or left branches of the bundle of His (bundle branch block) can only be diagnosed with confidence from the appearances in the precordial leads although there are necessarily changes in the appearances in the limb leads too.

Right bundle branch block

In right bundle branch block, the primary change induced is a delay in depolarization in the right ventricular free wall. This results in the development of a second positive wave in right ventricular leads (and a second negative wave in left ventricular leads), and prolongs the total QRS duration.

The essential electrocardiographic features of right bundle branch block are: (*a*) a total QRS duration of 0.12 s or more; and (*b*) the presence of a secondary positive wave in V_1 (rsR′, rR′).

In addition, secondary changes occur, but these are not in themselves essential for the definitive diagnosis. These include: (*c*) deep and slurred S waves in lead I, aVL, and V_4–V_6; and (*d*) secondary ST, T wave changes in leads V_1–V_3.

An example of the appearances in right bundle branch block is shown in Fig. 12.

Left bundle branch block

Left bundle branch block induces more extensive changes in the electrocardiographic appearance than does right bundle branch block. Not only is depolarization of the free wall of the left ventricle delayed (a precise corollary of the changes in right bundle branch block), but also the direction of depolarization of the interventricular septum is from right to left instead of from left to right as is the case in the normal electrocardiogram. This reversal of the direction of septal depolarization gives rise to widespread and major alterations in the QRS complexes in every lead of the electrocardiogram.

The diagnostic criteria for left bundle branch block are: (*a*) a total QRS duration equal to or in excess of 0.12 s; (*b*) absence of the normal (septal) q waves in lead I, aVL, and V_4–V_6; and (*c*) in order not to confuse the finding of right bundle branch block (which gives a QRS deviation of 0.12 s or more) in the presence of pronounced clockwise cardiac rotation (which gives loss of q waves in left ventricular leads) into left bundle branch block, the latter diagnosis also requires that one does not have a secondary r wave in V_1. The observation of a secondary r wave in V_1 excludes right bundle branch block.

Secondary changes also inevitably occur but these are not part of the diagnostic process. These include: (*c*) secondary ST depression and T wave inversion in leads I, aVL, and V_4–V_6; (*d*) broad QS waves in V_1–V_3; (*e*) notching of the R waves giving rise to rsR′, 'M-shape'; and (*f*) broad, R waves in leads I, aVL, and V_4–V_6.

An example of the ECG appearances in left bundle branch block is shown in Fig. 13.

The changes in left bundle branch block so disturb the normal pattern of the ECG that none of the usual criteria can be applied for determining any other abnormality of the QRS complexes, ST segments, or P waves. When left bundle branch block is present, a diagnosis of right or left ventricular hypertrophy, myocardial ischaemia or infarction, or non-specific changes in the ST segments and T waves cannot easily or reliably be made.

The electrocardiogram in ischaemic heart disease

ECG changes in ischaemic heart disease are very variable depending on the site and severity of the ischaemic damage. Certain patterns are, however, commonly produced.

Myocardial infarction

QRS changes

Two QRS changes are indicative of myocardial infarction. These are: (*a*) inappropriately low R wave voltage in a local area; and (*b*) abnormal q waves.

These two changes represent parts of the same process. The development of increased negativity in the precordial leads

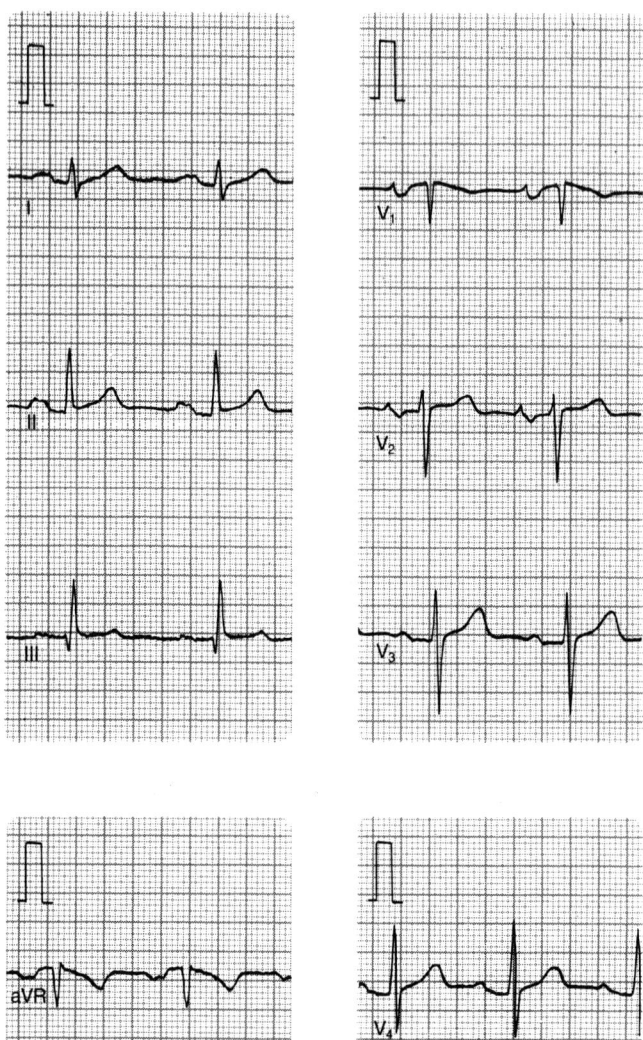

Fig. 11 Left atrial hypertrophy. Broad, bifid P waves in lead II. Biphasic P waves in V_1, with dominant negative component.

(abnormal q waves) and the reduction in the normal positivity of the precordial leads each results from a loss of underlying muscle with reduction in the normally generated positive voltage. When there is full thickness (transmural) myocardial infarction in an area of myocardium underlying the precordial leads there is total loss of the positive deflection. In this situation a totally negative wave (QS complex) occurs. This totally negative wave occurs as a result of depolarization of the posterior wall of the ventricle travelling from endocardium to epicardium in the normal way and no longer swamped by the usual simultaneous and dominant depolarization towards the exploring electrode of the anterior wall of the ventricle.

The *normal precordial QRS complexes* show a progressive increase in the R wave height from V_1–V_6 (Fig. 14). The positive

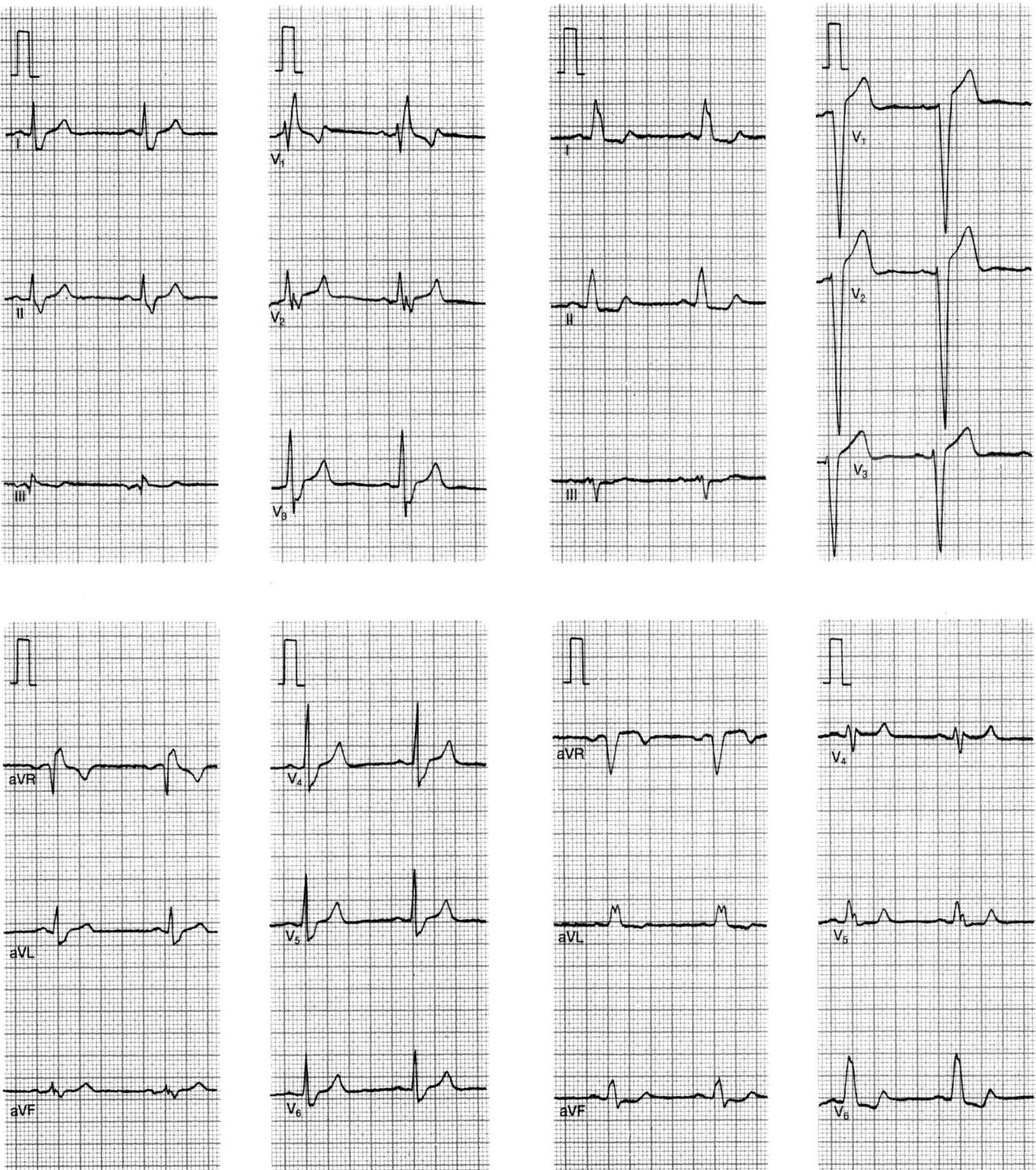

Fig. 12 Right bundle branch block.   **Fig. 13** Left bundle branch block.

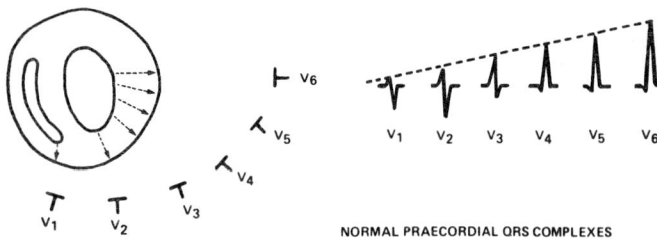

NORMAL PRAECORDIAL QRS COMPLEXES

Fig. 14 Normal R wave progression in the precordial series.

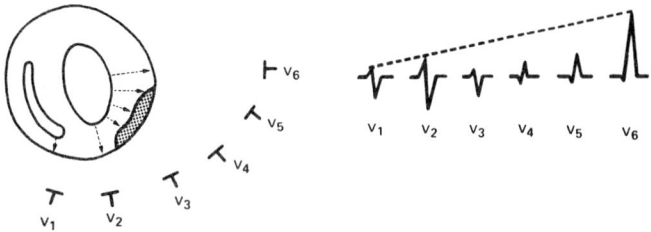

MYOCARDIAL INFARCTION : LOSS OF R WAVES

Fig. 15 Loss of R waves in myocardial infarction. The R wave height is reduced from V_3 to V_5.

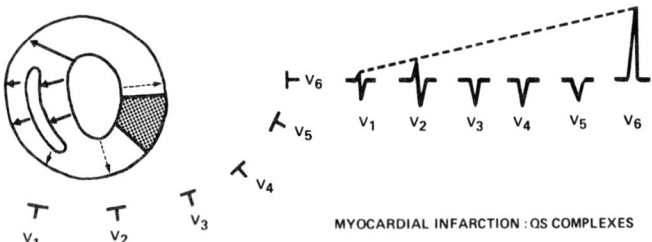

MYOCARDIAL INFARCTION : QS COMPLEXES

Fig. 16 Transmural myocardial infarction. QS complexes are seen from V_3 to V_5.

part of a deflection in each precordial lead is predominantly the result of depolarization from underlying endocardium to epicardium.

In the presence of *infarction of part of the left ventricle*, the positive waves overlying the necrotic area will be reduced in size (Fig. 15). Loss in R wave height can only be used as a criterion for myocardial infarction either if larger, normal R waves are visible on both sides of the infarcted zone or if previous ECGs are available demonstrating the normal R wave height for that particular lead in that particular subject.

If a *major part of the thickness of the myocardial wall is infarcted*, the positive wave generated by any remaining viable left ventricular myocardium underlying the electrode is insufficient to overcome the negative deflection induced by the normal depolarization of the interventricular septum from left to right and of the free wall of the right ventricle from endocardium to epicardium. In this situation an abnormal q wave will develop. In the precordial leads, a q wave is abnormal if its duration is equal to or in excess of 0.04 s or if its depth is equal to or greater than a quarter the height of the ensuing R wave in that lead. In Fig. 15, the q wave in V_4 satisfies this criterion. If the infarction involves the full thickness of the ventricular wall (transmural infarction), no R wave is generated at all and an entirely negative (QS) wave develops (Fig. 16).

Figure 17 shows (in diagrammatic form) the appearances produced in the precordial leads when infarcts of varying thickness occur under each of three precordial electrodes. The QRS complex in V_3 is of QS type and indicates transmural infarction at this site. The appearances in V_4 indicate a substantial loss of myocardium underlying that electrode. The q wave is abnormal in

duration and depth. The appearances in V_5 indicate a thinner zone of infarction. The q wave is not, in itself, abnormal but the R wave height is less than would be predicted from the height of the R waves present in V_2 and V_6.

The criteria for the diagnosis of myocardial infarction in the limb leads depend entirely on the presence of abnormal q waves. Q waves of any size may be seen in the normal ECG in aVR and in lead III. In leads I, II, and aVF q waves which are equal to or greater than 0.04 s in duration or which have a depth in excess of a quarter the height of the ensuing R wave are abnormal and, unless a defect of intraventricular conduction is known to be present, indicate myocardial infarction. The same is also true of abnormal q waves in aVL except when the mean frontal plane QRS axis is more positive than +60°, for in this situation aVL becomes a cavity lead like aVR.

ST segment changes of infarction

Only changes in the QRS complexes provide definitive evidence of infarction, but in the acute stages of myocardial infarction ST segment shift occurs. Strictly speaking this shift is evidence of injury to, rather than infarction of, the myocardium. Thus, although in the vast majority of cases the development of typical ST segment changes is followed by the development of definitive QRS changes, occasionally the ECG with ST segment changes of myocardial injury will revert to normal within days. This does not happen if definitive QRS changes of infarction are also present.

The essential change of myocardial injury is deviation of the ST segment above the iso-electric line. The ST segment shift must be in excess of 1 mm to be significant. Minor degrees of ST segment elevation in the right precordial leads are very common and ST segment elevation of up to 2 mm may be accepted as within normal limits in V_1 and V_2.

Significant ST segment elevation occurs in transmural and sub-epicardial infarction in leads facing the infarct. ST segment depression occurs in leads facing the infarct when it is subendocardial. ST segment depression also occurs as a reciprocal change (see below) in leads opposite to those showing the primary changes of acute infarction.

T wave changes of infarction

A variety of T wave changes occurs in association with myocardial infarction. These include flattened, diphasic, and inverted (nega-

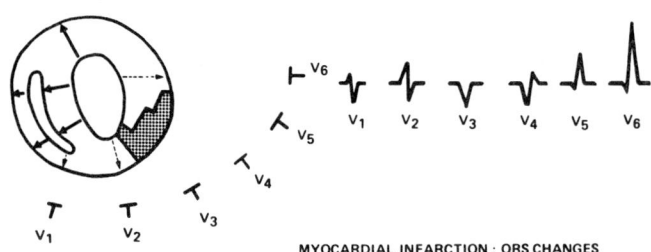

MYOCARDIAL INFARCTION : QRS CHANGES

Fig. 17 Variable thickness infarction.

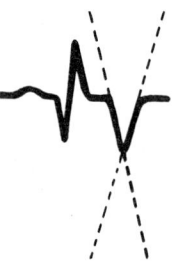

Fig. 18 Deep symmetrical T wave inversion typically found in association with myocardial infarction.

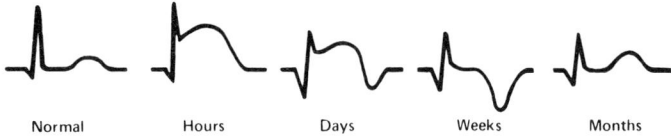

Fig. 19 Sequential changes in acute myocardial infarction.

Table 1

Location of infarction	Leads showing primary changes
	Typical changes
Anteroseptal	V_1, V_2, V_3.
Anterior	V_2, V_3, V_4.
Anterolateral	V_4, V_5, V_6, I, aVL.
Extensive anterior	V_1, V_2, V_3, V_4, V_5, V_6, I, aVL.
High lateral	aVL (plus high precordial leads)
Inferior	II, III, aVF.
Inferolateral (apical)	II, III, aVF, V_5, V_6, I, aVL.
Inferoseptal	II, III, aVF, V_1, V_2, V_3.
	Other changes
Posterior	V_1, V_2
Subendocardial	any lead (usually multiple leads)

tive) T waves. None of these changes is specific. Whilst they are always abnormal in leads V_4–V_6 and in those limb leads showing clearly upright QRS complexes, they may be caused by factors other than infarction or ischaemia, including electrolyte changes, digitalis effects, pericarditis, myocarditis, changes in body position, and changes in oesophageal temperature. T wave changes are never in themselves reliable indicators of infarction although characteristic T wave changes do occur in relation to the latter. The most typical T wave change associated with infarction is the deep, symmetrically inverted T wave (Fig. 18).

The sequence of ECG changes in infarction
Any combination of the QRS, ST segment, and T wave changes described above may occur in relation to acute infarction of the myocardium but commonly a typical sequence of changes can be recognized (Fig. 19). Typically, ST segment elevation (which is convex upwards) appears within hours of the onset of symptoms. At this stage no change in the QRS complex can be recognized. Within one to three days reduction in the R wave height occurs, abnormally deep and broad q waves develop, some reduction in the extent of ST segment elevation occurs, and there is development of T wave inversion. After the first few days the ST segment elevation disappears completely. The deep, symmetrical T wave inversion typically persists for weeks before reverting to normal. The changes in the QRS complex are usually permanent. The QRS changes may occasionally disappear altogether if the infarct is small and the myocardial scar subsequently shrinks.

Location of ECG changes in myocardial infarction
Primary ECG changes of the type described above occur in leads facing the infarct. It follows that the leads in which such primary changes occur indicate the location of the infarct (Table 1).

Reciprocal changes
In addition to the primary changes, 'reciprocal' changes occur in leads opposite those facing the infarction. Reciprocal changes are the inverse of primary changes (e.g. ST segment depression instead of ST segment elevation and tall, pointed T waves instead of symmetrical T wave inversion).

The inferior limb leads (II, III, and aVF) are reciprocal to the anterior leads (the precordial leads, lead I and aVL) and vice versa. Examples of recent and of old anterior and inferior infarctions are shown in Figs 20–24.

Subendocardial infarction does not always produce recognizable changes on the ECG, and such changes as are present are usually apparent only in the ST segments or T waves. Persistent deep symmetrical T wave inversion or persistent flat ST segment depression may be found.

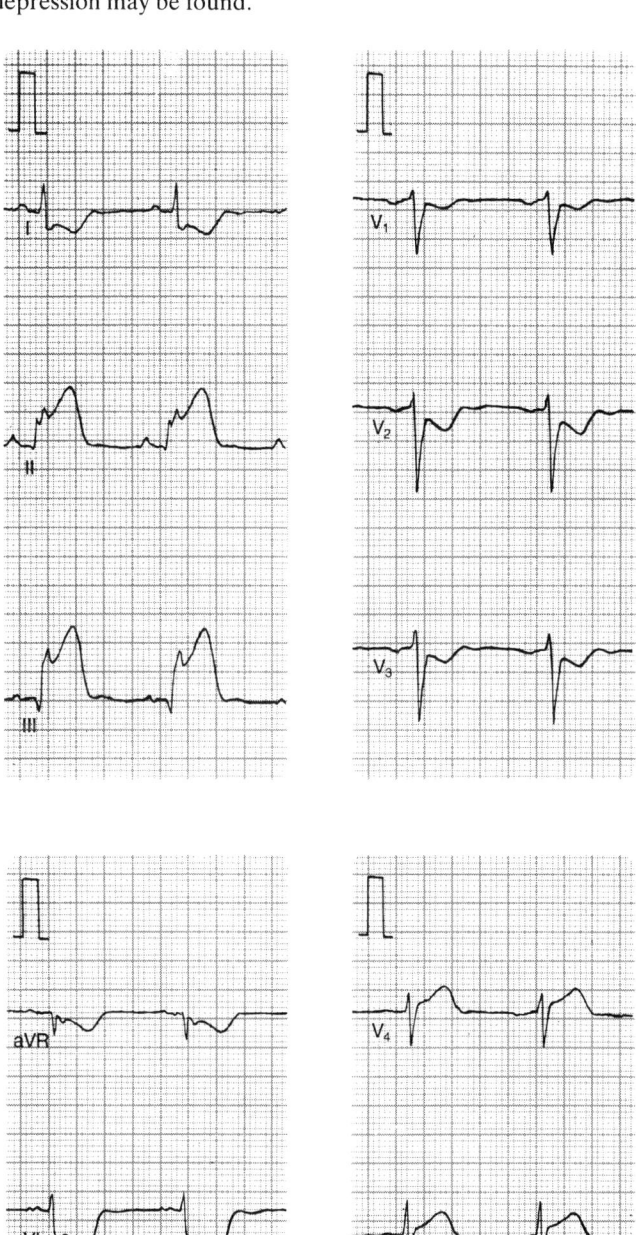

Fig. 20 Acute inferior myocardial ischaemic damage. Primary ST elevation is visible in leads II, III, and aVF. ST elevation is also visible in V_4–V_6, indicating that the damage extends over the lateral wall of the ventricle. There is reciprocal ST segment depression in I, aVL, aVR, and from V_1–V_3.

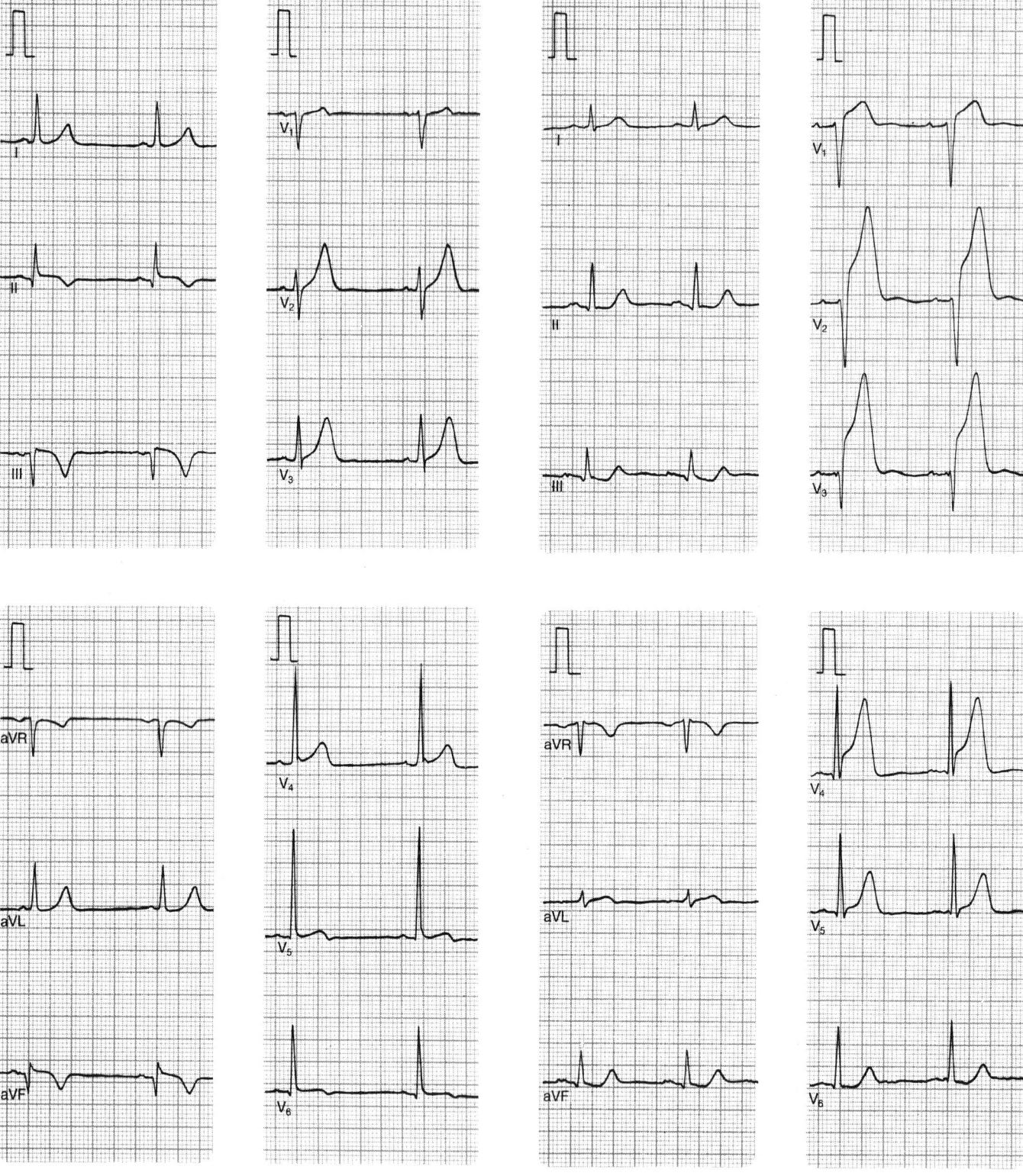

Fig. 21 Inferior myocardial infarction of intermediate age. The Q waves are abnormal in aVF (and also in III) and the q waves in II are borderline abnormal. There is T inversion in II, III, and aVF. The ST segments are still minimally elevated in these leads. There is inversion of the terminal part of the T wave and V_5 and V_6 suggesting that the ischaemic area extends to the lateral wall of the ventricle. The T waves are strikingly tall in V_2 and V_3. This is not necessarily abnormal but could indicate true posterior ischaemia.

Fig. 22 Acute anteroseptal infarction. There is obvious ST elevation in V_1–V_4 with minimal reciprocal ST depression in III and aVF. There is obvious loss of initial R wave height in V_2 and V_3.

Pitfalls in the diagnosis of myocardial infarction

Left bundle branch block so distorts the normal ECG that the usual criteria for the diagnosis of myocardial infarction are no longer applicable. Although it is *possible* to diagnose myocardial infarction in the presence of left bundle branch block, such diagnoses should be left for experts to make. In the presence of ventricular pre-excitation neither left branch bundle block nor myocardial infarction should be diagnosed by the non-expert.

Miscellaneous abnormalities of the electrocardiogram

Abnormalities associated with digitalis, hypokalaemia, hyperkalaemia, pericarditis, hypothyroidism, and ventricular pre-excitation are discussed in other parts of this text.

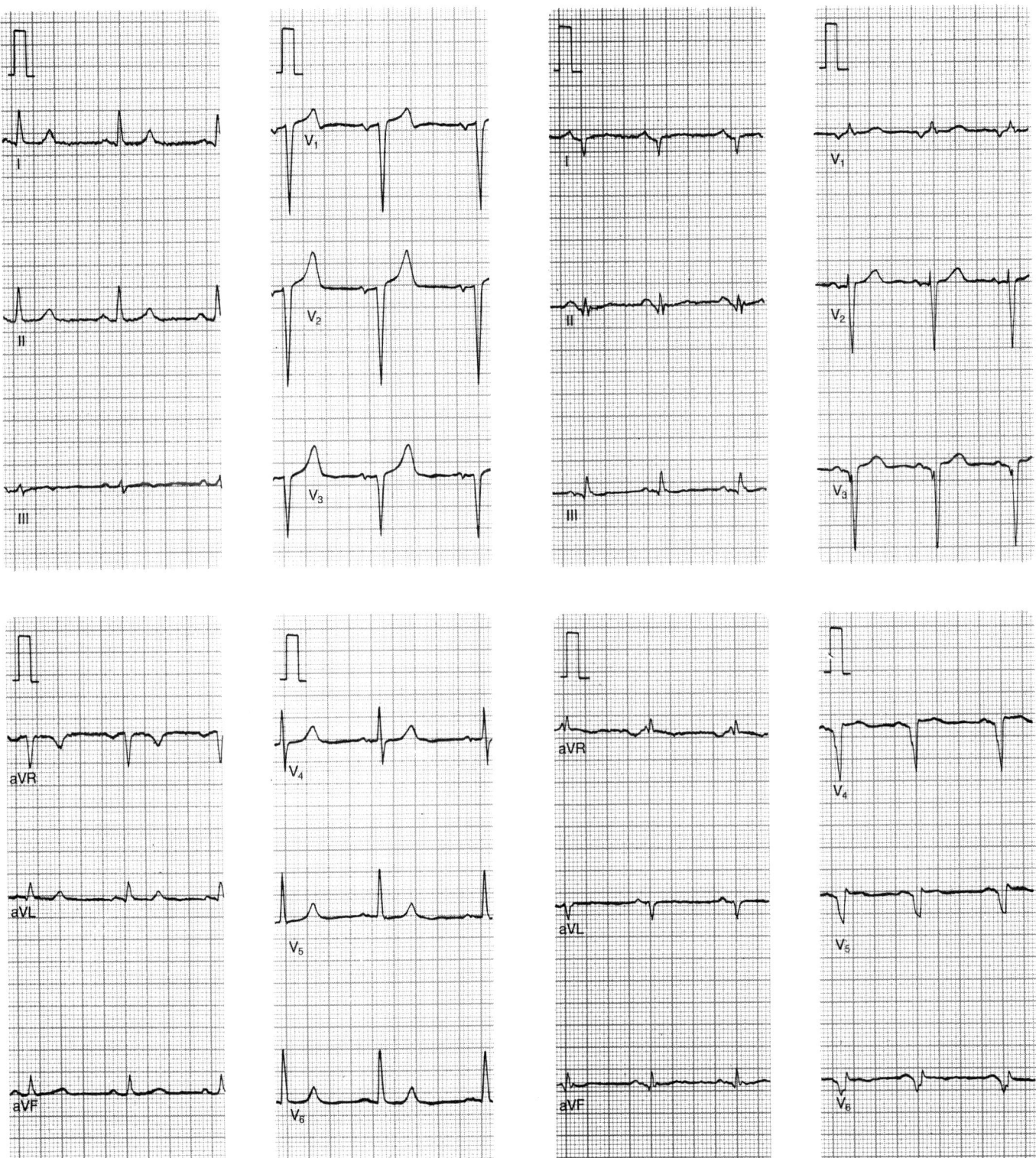

Fig. 23 Old anterior myocardial infarction. There are QS complexes in V_2 and V_3.

Fig. 24 Extensive anterior infarction. There are abnormally wide, abnormally deep Q waves from V_3–V_6 and in I. The T waves are of low voltage in most leads. This latter abnormality is non-specific.

References

Schamroth, L. (1976). *An introduction to electrocardiography*. Blackwell Scientific Publications, Oxford.

Goldman, M. J. (1979). *Principles of clinical electrocardiography*. Longe Medical Publications, Los Altos, California.

Rowlands, D. J. (1978). The electrified axis. *Br. J. Hosp. Med.* **19**, 472–481.

—— (1981). *Understanding the electrocardiogram*. Vols I and II. Gower Medical Publishing, London.

Ambulatory electrocardiography

The technique of ambulatory electrocardiographic monitoring was first introduced by Holter in 1961 and is still sometimes referred to as Holter monitoring. It is a technique designed to permit long-term electrocardiographic recording in patients during their normal, everyday activity. It is useful in the diagnosis and quantification of arrhythmias, the evaluation of anti-arrhythmic therapy, and in detecting pacemaker malfunction. It may also be useful in the recognition of the intermittent myocardial ischaemia from changes in the configuration of the ST segments and T waves.

Equipment used, recording technique, play-back technique

Several manufacturers now produce a range of equipment for ambulatory monitoring, most of which will be adequate for the recording of the cardiac rhythm. However, high specifications are needed for the recording system if reliable assessments of ST segment and T wave changes are to be made and more complex play-back equipment is needed if the assessment of the resulting record is to be automated or semi-automated.

The most commonly used type of equipment is the battery operated continuous ECG recorder (using the AM or the FM recording mode). The recording box is about the same size as a 'Walkman' type of recorder and is worn strapped under the patient's clothing. The ECG electrodes are connected to the patient via gel-type patch electrodes. The siting of the leads determines the size of normal and abnormal P waves and QRS complexes on the resulting recording. Sometimes it is worthwhile selecting a lead to give a maximum monophasic QRS amplitude (by inspecting the subject's resting 12-lead ECG). Typically, electrodes are placed in the V_1 and V_6 position with an indifferent electrode in the suprasternal area (electrode positions should avoid large muscle masses since the ECG signals have to compete with intermittent EMG signals from skeletal muscle). The ECG scanner or play-back unit either provides a full printout in miniaturized form of 24 hours of recording (one sheet per hour) or it permits a technician to view the ECG signal on an oscilloscope screen at 60 to 120 times natural speed. In the former system the clinician sees (albeit with difficulty) the entire recording. In the latter system the technician may, noticing a deviation from normal, obtain a 'natural' speed printout of the relevant parts of the record. Computer-assisted techniques are now becoming available to provide further help in the tedious, time-consuming, and error-fraught techniques of analysis.

In addition to the commonly used continuous recording systems there are systems available for the brief recording of the ECG following the recognition by the patient of some significant event. In one variety the patient carries a pocket-sized device which contains a solid state memory capable of recording the ECG for a limited period (typically 30 s). The device has metal 'feet' which are applied directly to the bare chest and also has a button to activate the recording. All the patient has to do is to open his shirt, place the device on his chest with the 'feet' electrodes touching the skin, and then press the button. The recording takes place automatically. The memory is non-volatile (though it can be overwritten, if required, by a further push on the button) and the equipment is taken to the recording centre for subsequent analysis (or if the appropriate model is available the contents of the memory can be transmitted via a telephone to the recording centre). Such intermittent devices are useful when arrhythmias are associated with symptoms (especially palpitation or tachycardia, but occasionally dizziness), but this technique is not useful when the patient presents with syncope.

Patient diary

A very important part of ambulatory monitoring is the daily log kept by patients of all relevant activities and symptoms and the times when various medications (especially anti-arrhythmic drugs) are taken. Most recorders are equipped with an event marker which the patient should be instructed to press when any relevant symptoms occur. Events coincidental with these symptoms and the timing of these symptoms should simultaneously be logged in the patient diary.

Normal database

The ECG in the normal subject varies much more than once realized. Normal, healthy subjects at rest (and especially during sleep) not uncommonly demonstrate profound sinus bradycardia (35 to 40 per min), sinus arrhythmia with R–R intervals of up to 2 s, the Wenckebach phenomenon (Möbitz type I second degree atrioventricular block), junctional escape beats, and occasional atrial and ventricular premature beats. However some arrhythmias are not known to occur in normal subjects. Their recognition is always significant. These include Möbitz type II second degree atrioventricular block. ST segment shifts may be artefactual unless the low frequency response of the recording equipment is of the highest calibre, but with top class equipment primary, ischaemic ST segment shift can be recognized.

Artefacts

Artefactual 'arrhythmias' may occur from inadequate skin preparation, poor electrode localization or securement or from inadequate recorder or play-back quality. Most systems record two ECG channels simultaneously and this minimizes the problem. However, the clinician using this technique should be alert to the possibility that a transient loss of signal (as a result of electrode movement) can mimic asystole and that sinus pauses and intermittent heartblock can be mimicked by transient slowing or sticking of the tape during play-back. In addition, pseudotachycardia can occur because of slowing of the tape speed during recording in cases of battery depletion. These pseudotachycardias can usually be recognized as such because the heart rate progressively increases towards the end of the recording and because the P waves, QRS complexes and T waves all become progressively narrower at the same rate as the R–R interval appears to shorten.

Ambulatory monitoring for palpitation

Palpitation, or unusual awareness of the cardiac action, frequently disturbs patients and often constitutes an indication for ambulatory monitoring in the hope that an electrocardiographic explanation of the symptoms will become apparent and that suitable treatment will then be possible. Examples of rhythm strips obtained from 24-hour ambulatory records used in this way are shown in Figs 25–30

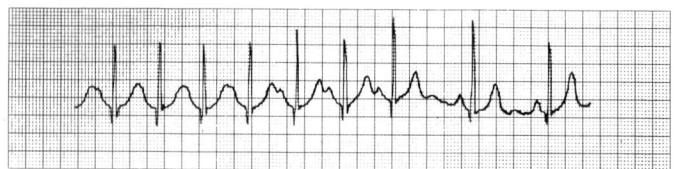

Fig. 25 Sinus rhythm. Varying sinus rate. The first four complexes show a very rapid sinus rate (approximately 115 per minute) with each P wave superimposed on the preceding T wave. The sinus rate then slows spontaneously and rapidly. This patient complained of pounding of the heart. Treatment with a beta-blocker suppressed the symptoms.

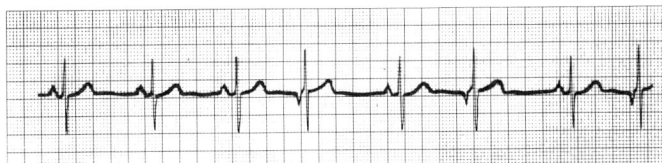

Fig. 26 Sinus rhythm with three junctional ('nodal') premature beats. The fourth, sixth, and eighth beats are junctional ('nodal') premature beats. The patient complained of occasional irregularity of the heart. No treatment was necessary.

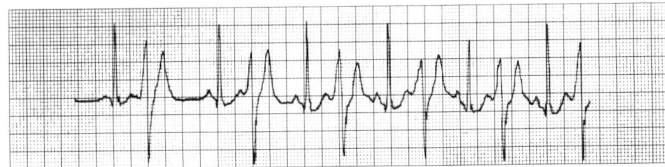

Fig. 27 Sinus rhythm with unifocal, coupled 'interpolated' ventricular premature beats. Such an arrhythmia is likely to result in symptoms. Hypokalaemia and digitalis toxicity should be considered.

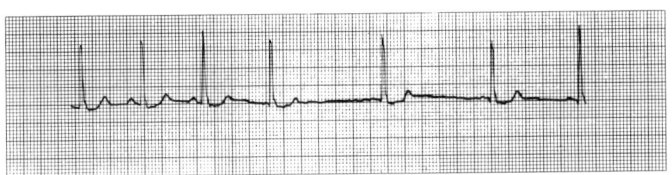

Fig. 28 Onset of atrial fibrillation. The first three beats are sinus beats. The remainder of the strip shows atrial fibrillation. The patient complained of repeated attacks of irregularity of the heart which he found disturbing. Treatment with digitalis or quinidine might be helpful in suppressing the arrhythmia and would be indicated if the symptoms were sufficiently disturbing. However, the ventricular rate during atrial fibrillation is surprisingly slow and one needs to take care that any anti-dysrrhythmic drugs prescribed do not induce dizziness.

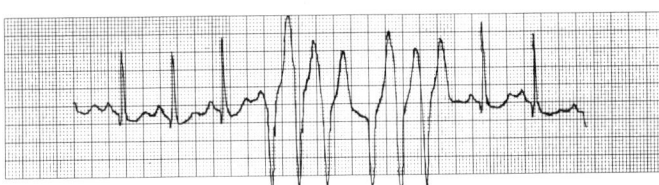

Fig. 29 Sinus rhythm with a run of wide QRS complex tachycardia, suggesting ventricular tachycardia. The P wave rhythm appears undisturbed (supporting this diagnosis) but it is difficult to follow the P waves through the QRS complexes and the ventricular rate is very irregular. An alternative explanation of the wide QRS tachycardia would be a burst of rapid atrial fibrillation with aberrant intraventricular conduction, but the long R–R interval during the wide QRS tachycardia is not followed by a more normal QRS which is a little against aberration as an explanation of the wide QRS complexes. This illustrates the difficulty of interpretation often found with ambulatory records. The correct diagnosis is probably ventricular tachycardia.

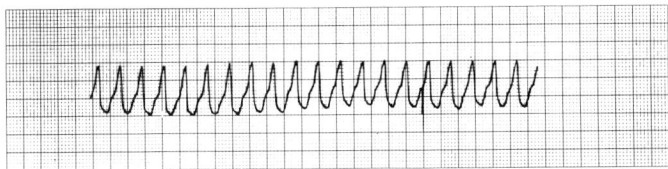

Fig. 30 Sustained wide QRS complex tachycardia. Probable ventricular tachycardia, though one would need to see the P waves (to demonstrate atrioventricular dissociation) to be sure of this.

Ambulatory monitoring for dizziness or syncope

Palpitation, occurring in association with frequent premature beats or with episodic tachydysrhythmias, is often symptomatically disturbing to patients but symptoms of dizziness or syncope are potentially of much greater importance since they can be indicative of serious or even life-threatening arrhythmias. Complaints of transient lightheadedness or of feelings of impending loss of consciousness or episodes of actual blackout may all be cardiac in origin. Equally, of course, they may not. A full clinical history and examination and appropriate investigations other than electrocardiography are required in addition to one or more periods of 24-hour ambulatory ECG recording.

The use of *ad hoc* transient recording techniques with short-term memory devices (applied by patients to their own chests) is inappropriate in the context of this symptom. Only when the patient experiences typical symptoms at the precise time when there are definitive electrocardiographic appearances in the ambulatory recording does the 24-hour ECG recording contribute to management. Definitive ECG appearances can be defined as (*a*) a cardiac rhythm likely to be, or inevitably, associated with loss of consciousness or (*b*) a cardiac rhythm which could not possibly *cause* loss of consciousness (although it might occur in association with or in response to a loss of consciousness). Examples of the former group include ventricular fibrillation, rapid ventricular tachycardia, profound bradycardia or asystole and of the latter group examples include sinus rhythm with rates of 60 or more, sinus rhythm with occasional atrial or ventricular ectopic beats, and first degree heartblock. Unfortunately there will be many occasions when the electrocardiogram is not definitive (e.g. when it shows atrial fibrillation with a rapid ventricular rate, short bursts of supraventricular or ventricular tachycardia, pauses of 1 to 3 s etc.). In such situations it may not be possible to reach a definitive conclusion about the possible role of the rhythm in producing the symptoms. If the symptoms of dizziness or syncope do not occur during the monitoring period and if no significant arrhythmia occurs, the investigation makes no significant contribution to diagnosis.

Although a 24-hour ambulatory record represents a considerable advance in the magnitude of data collection compared with a 12 lead ECG it still represents a very small time window and has, for example, only a 1 in 30 chance of catching an event which occurs monthly. Even so it has proved to be a very useful advance and examples of its value in the investigation of patients with dizzy spells are shown in Figs 31–34.

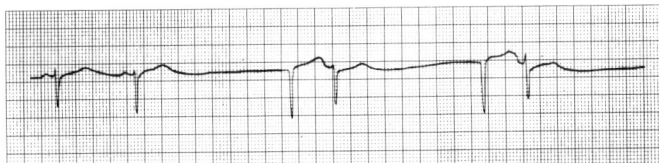

Fig. 31 The first two beats are sinus beats, followed by sinus arrest. The pause is ended by a junctional escape beat. The fourth beat is an echo beat followed by sinus arrest, a junctional escape beat and a further echo beat. The record leaves little doubt that the sino-atrial and atrioventricular nodes are diseased.

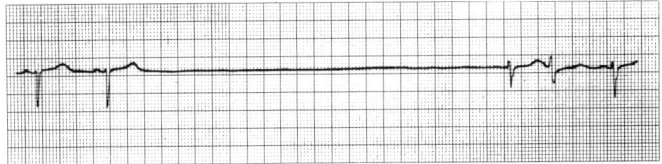

Fig. 32 The first two beats are sinus beats. There is then a period of atrial and junctional arrest for more than 4.5 s before a junctional escape beat occurred. The tracing coincided with syncope; permanent pacing was necessary.

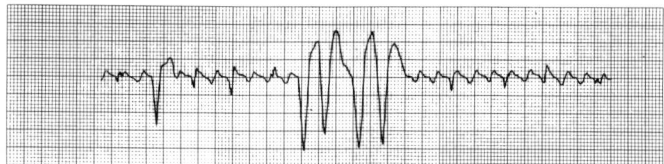

Fig. 33 Atrial flutter with 3 to 1 A/V block and a short run of ventricular tachycardia. A single ventricular premature beat is seen near the beginning of the trace and there is a run of four beats of ventricular tachycardia.

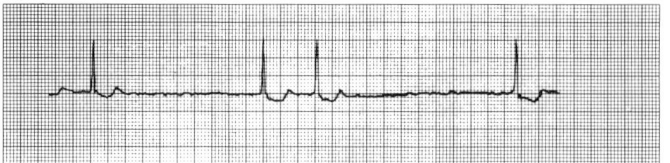

Fig. 34 Atrial fibrillation with a slow mean ventricular rate. Two pauses of 2 s each are seen in a short segment of trace.

Innocent arrhythmias recorded by ambulatory monitoring

Ambulatory electrocardiographic recordings from subjects with no overt evidence of ischaemic heart disease have demonstrated that a wide range of arrhythmias may occur. Occasional atrial or ventricular premature beats are found in 25–50 per cent of normal young subjects and in 60–70 per cent of subjects in the older age groups. Profound bradycardia (Fig. 35) is usual during sleep. Transient Wenckebach (Möbitz type I) second degree atrioventricular block is occasionally seen in normal subjects, especially those with an active vagus. When it occurs, it commonly presents against the background of a slow sinus rate as during sleep (Fig. 36).

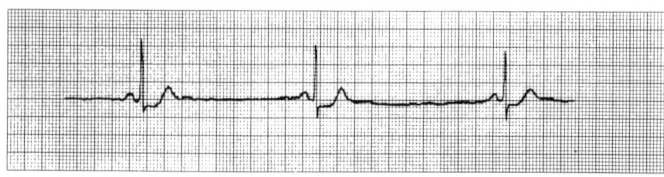

Fig. 35 Sinus bradycardia; rate 30 per minute; not abnormal during sleep.

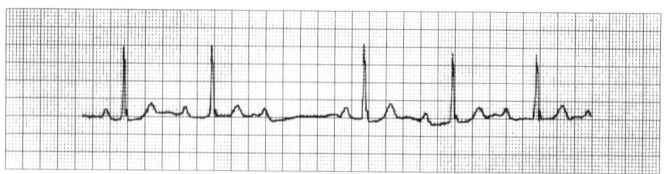

Fig. 36 Wenckebach type second degree atrioventricular block. The first two beats show atrioventricular conduction with increasing P–R interval. The third P wave is not followed by a QRS. The fourth P wave is followed by a QRS at a normal P–R interval. Subsequent cycles once more show progressive prolongation of the P–R interval.

Ambulatory monitoring in ischaemic heart disease

Subjects with ischaemic heart disease and symptoms suggestive of cardiac arrhythmias are also candidates for ambulatory monitoring which is sometimes of value in demonstrating electrocardio-

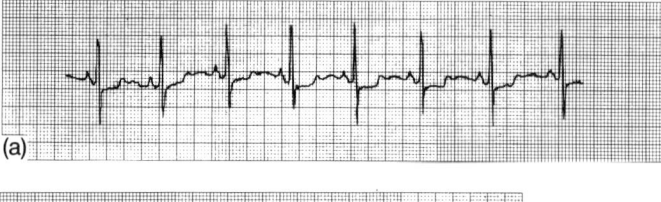

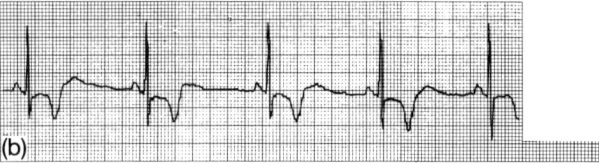

Fig. 37 Electrocardiographic appearances in a patient experiencing spontaneous (non-exercise induced) angina. (a) Control record in the absence of pain. (b) Record taken during an anginal episode. There is marked T wave inversion in the absence of a tachycardia.

graphic evidence of ischaemia. In the absence of increases in heart rate or blood pressure such changes are often thought to be indicative of coronary artery spasm (Fig. 37a and b).

Ambulatory monitoring in pacemaker patients

Pacemaker malfunction may be intermittent and in suspected cases ambulatory monitoring can demonstrate intermittent failure of capture of the pacing stimulus or intermittent failure of sensing (in the case of pacemakers with demand function). The ambulatory electrocardiographic recording can also be useful in showing *absence* of pacing malfunction at the time the patient experiences symptoms.

Acknowledgements

Figures 1–13 and 20–36 are reproduced with permission from Rowlands (1981). *Understanding the electrocardiogram.* Gower Medical Publishing, London. Copyright ICI PLC. The author is grateful to the Department of Medical Illustration of the Manchester Royal Infirmary for the reproduction of Figs 14–19.

Echocardiography

D. G. GIBSON

Physical principles

The clinical value of ultrasound in cardiology was first demonstrated by Edler in 1954, and the method has since developed into a major instrument of diagnosis. Ultrasound waves have frequencies greater than the highest appreciable by the human ear (18–20 kHz). They are propagated as longitudinal vibrations at a velocity determined by the physical properties of the material through which they pass. They are generated by materials with the property of piezo-electricity, that is, of undergoing deformation when an electric potential is applied across them; in cardiological work, frequencies of 2.5–5 MHz are used. As ultrasound passes through a homogeneous medium, it is absorbed and scattered to an extent dependent on the exact nature of the material in question. At a boundary between two materials with different physical properties, such as blood and endocardium or blood and valve, a proportion of the incident energy is reflected, depending on the difference in density and in the velocity of sound across the interface. Such reflection, for which the angle of incidence is equal to the angle of reflection, resembles that of light at a mirror, and so is termed 'specular'. This is the mechanism of image generation by structures that are large compared with the wavelength of the ultrasound used, such as the anterior cusp of the mitral valve. If the target is small, incident ultrasound is scattered rather than reflected, and the amplitude of the returning signal is much less sensitive to the orientation of the ultrasound beam. This process is described as back-scattering, and is the dominant mechanism by which targets within the myocardium are demonstrated.

Echocardiography

Echocardiography is a pulse–echo technique, in which the transducer is activated, not continuously, but in short pulses each lasting approximately 1 μs. These pulses are directed into the tissue to be studied, where they interact with it, returning to the transducer after a time interval which depends on the distance they have travelled, the path length, and the velocity of sound within the medium. Piezo-electric materials not only emit ultrasound when an electric potential is applied across them, but generate a potential when ultrasound impinges on them, so that the same transducer acts as a receiver as well as an emitter of ultrasound. The amplitude of the returning echo depends not only on the characteristics of the interface giving rise to it, but also, in view of the progressive absorption of ultrasound, on its depth. This effect of pathlength, which makes deeper structures give rise to weaker echoes, can be allowed for by using a method termed time compensated gain. Since echoes from deeper structures return later than those from more superficial ones, they can be selectively amplified by progressively increasing the gain after the emission of each pulse from the transducer. Interfaces with similar properties thus give rise to comparable deflections on the final trace, regardless of their depth.

The maximum repetition rate of an echocardiograph is limited by the time taken for impulses to pass from the transducer to the deepest structures to be examined and back again, i.e. on pathlength (approximately 30 cm) and the velocity of sound, 1500 m/s. This results in a maximum repetition rate of the order of 3000/s. These 3000 pulses can be used either to examine a single region of the heart with high frequency, and thus to detect motion with great sensitivity (M-mode), or to build up a two-dimensional image (cross-sectional echocardiography). With the latter approach, each image requires approximately 100 lines, giving a frame rate of 30/s in adults, or more in infants or children where the path length is shorter. Both methods have been found to have considerable clinical potential.

Of the two methods described above, anatomy is best studied using the cross-sectional technique. The ultrasound beam may be steered mechanically or electrically. The former is simpler, and is achieved by using a rotating head with three or four crystals mounted on it, giving a sector angle of more than 80°, and at the same time avoiding mechanical vibration. Alternatively, the beam may be steered electronically, using the phased array principle. This technique also gives a sector angle of up to 90°, but with a smaller transducer. It is also possible to vary focus with depth, a manoeuvre termed dynamic focusing, which improves image quality. This is offset to some extent by the presence of side lobes to the ultrasound beam, a limitation implicit in the phased array principle, which interferes with definition. Overall, phased array is more expensive than mechanical, but both techniques are in common use, and in clinical practice both have proved satisfactory. Both give resolution of the order of 1 mm along the axis of the ultrasound beam (range resolution), and of 2–3 mm perpendicular to it (lateral resolution).

The heart can be studied from only a limited number of directions, since the lung forms a virtually impenetrable barrier to ultrasound. In the normal adult, it is possible to obtain satisfactory images from the parasternal position, the apex, from beneath the ribs in the region of the xiphisternum (subcostal view), and from the suprasternal notch. A series of views from each of these four positions have been standardized which form the basis of any description of two-dimensional echocardiography.

Parasternal views

The parasternal long axis view of the normal left ventricle is shown in Fig. 1b with a corresponding anatomical specimen in Fig. 1a. In this view, the interventricular septum is shown anteriorly, continuous with the anterior wall of the aorta. The posterior wall of the aorta is continuous with the anterior cusp of the mitral valve, and the subvalvular apparatus, the chordae tendineae, and papillary muscles can readily be identified. Behind the aorta is the cavity of the left atrium. If the transducer is rotated through 90°, a series of minor axis views of the left ventricle can be obtained. Figure 2a shows a minor axis view at the level of the insertion of the papillary muscles, and Fig. 2b one at the level of the mitral valve. The latter view was timed early in diastole, when the mitral valve cusps were in their fully open position. In Fig. 2c, the transducer was moved higher, to the level of the aorta, which is seen here in cross-section. This view is particularly valuable for studying the outflow tract of the right ventricle, which can be seen to wrap round the aorta, with the tricuspid valve on the left side of the display and the pulmonary valve on the right. Beyond the pulmonary valve, the pulmonary artery can be seen to bifurcate into its right and left branches.

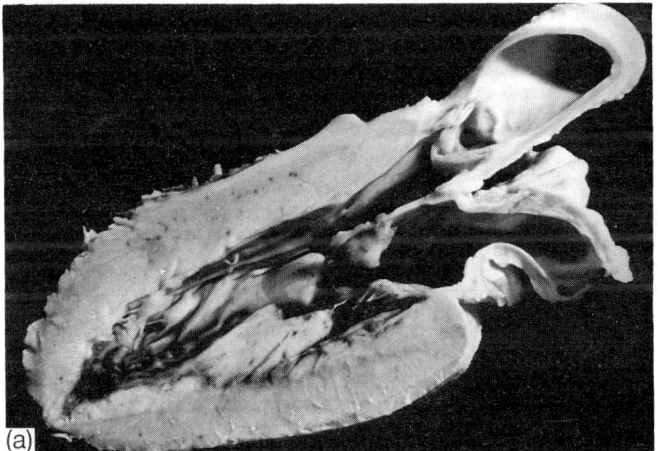

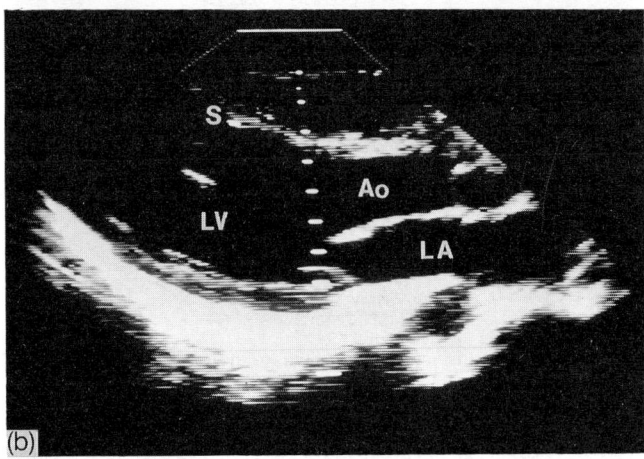

Fig. 1 (a) Longitudinal section of normal heart. (b) Two-dimensional echocardiogram showing normal long axis view. LA, left atrium; LV, left ventricle; S, interventricular septum; Ao, aortic root.

Apical views

The most useful view obtainable from this position is the apical four-chamber view (Fig. 3). Here both ventricles and both atria are demonstrated, with mitral and tricuspid valves. Normally, right and left ventricles are approximately equal in size in this view, although the right ventricle can readily be identified by the

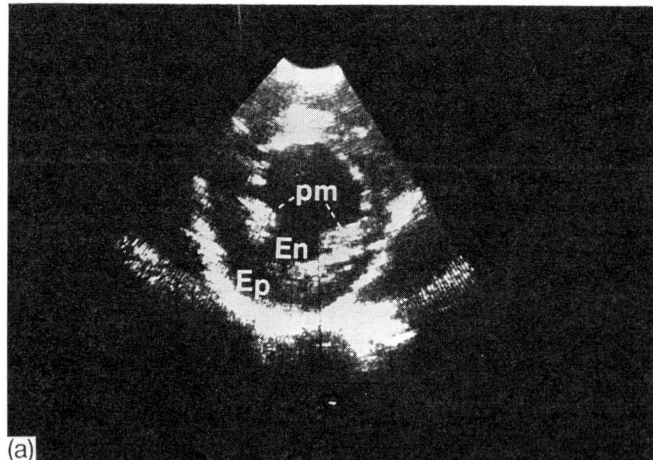

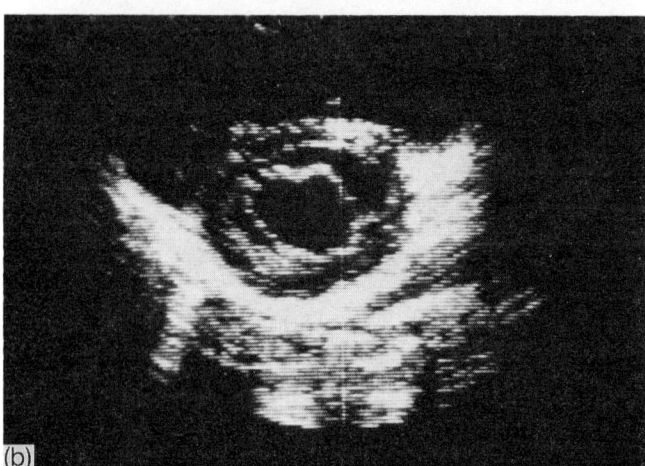

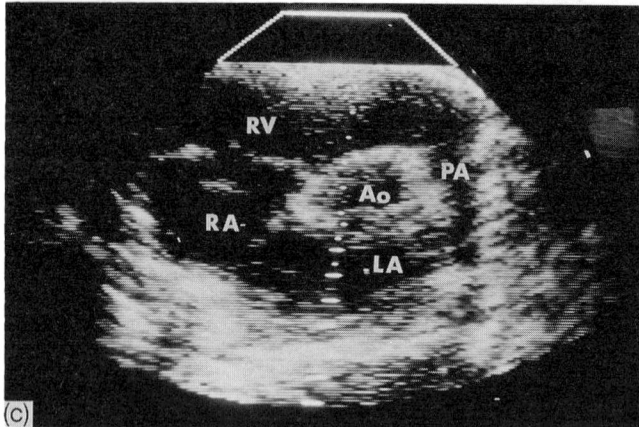

Fig. 2 (a) Two-dimensional echocardiogram, minor axis view of left ventricle at the level of the papillary muscles: PM, insertion of papillary muscles; En, endocardium; Ep, epicardium. (b) Minor axis view of left ventricle at the level of the mitral valve cusps. The mitral valve is in its fully open position early in diastole. (c) Minor axis view at the level of the aorta: Ao, aorta; LA, left atrium; RA, right atrium; RV, right ventricle; PA, pulmonary artery.

presence of the moderator band towards its apex. It can also be seen that the tricuspid valve is inserted a little further towards the apex than the mitral valve, so that there is a small region in which the left ventricle and right atrium are in direct contact with one another, the atrioventricular septum. This view also demonstrates the atrial septum well, except that even in normal subjects, an apparent discontinuity may be present in the region of the fossa

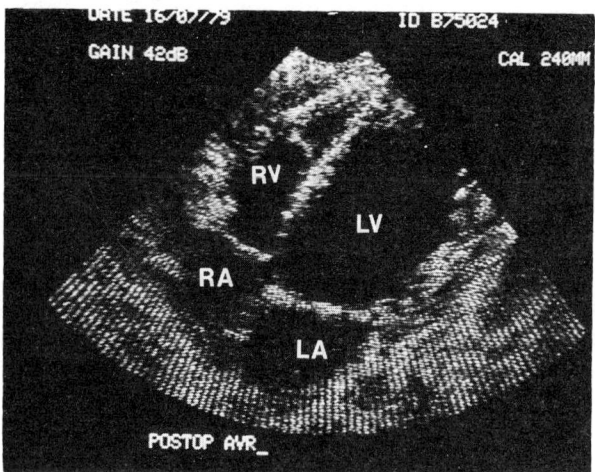

Fig. 3 Apical four-chamber view: LA, left atrium; LV, left ventricle; RA, right atrium; RV, right ventricle.

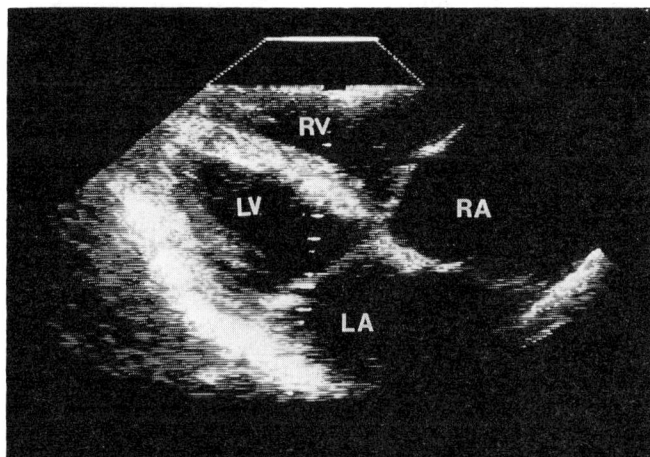

Fig. 4 Subcostal four-chamber view. Abbreviations as in Fig. 3.

ovalis. This is an example of the phenomenon of 'drop-out' in which structures parallel to the ultrasound beam are not well demonstrated. It frequently occurs in the region of the fossa ovalis, and is not to be taken as evidence of an atrial septal defect. The apical four-chamber view effectively demonstrates abnormal anatomy in patients with complex congenital heart disease, since it delineates the relation of the atrioventricular valves to the interventricular septum, as well as being the view of choice for showing defects in the inlet ventricular septum, or the lower part of the atrial septum (atrioventricular defects). If the transducer is rotated through 90° in this position, the mitral valve and aorta can be demonstrated in a view similar to the RAO view of the left ventricle, familiar from angiography.

Subcostal views

Here the transducer is applied to the epigastrium, and the heart is viewed from beneath, through the liver. In some adults this may not be possible, particularly in those in whom the heart is horizontal in position. However, in those with emphysema, excellent views may be obtained, even when parasternal approach proves unsatisfactory. In congenital heart disease it is probably the position of choice to start the examination. A subcostal four-chamber view is shown in Fig. 4, showing both atria and both ventricles from a direction approximately perpendicular to that obtained from the apex. This position can also be used to study the right ventricular outflow tract, the pulmonary artery to its bifurcation, as well as the left ventricular outflow tract, and aortic root and arch. The subcostal position is frequently the most satisfactory one for studying the apex of the left ventricle in order to confirm or exclude an apical aneurysm. As with the parasternal position, a series of subcostal minor axis views can be obtained.

Suprasternal views

From this position, it is possible to obtain excellent views of the great vessels. The aortic arch and its branches can be defined, as well as its characteristic relations with the pulmonary artery and left atrium. In infants and children, the presence of abnormalities such as coarctation of the aorta or persistent ductus can be confirmed or excluded.

M-mode echocardiography

An M-mode echocardiogram is obtained when the beam direction is fixed. It is used to study the motion of cardiac structures, and its great advantage is the greatly increased repetition rate compared with that obtained with the cross-sectional technique – 1000/s compared with 30/s. Simultaneous pulse and phonocardiographic traces can also be recorded, so the technique is a powerful one for investigating left ventricular physiology. Originally, M-mode echocardiograms were recorded using a single, hand-held crystal directed from anatomical landmarks. It has proved more satisfactory to determine the direction of the beam from the two-dimensional display, so that its exact position with respect to intracardiac anatomy can be recorded. M-mode echocardiography is traditionally performed from the left parasternal region, but excellent records can also be obtained from the subcostal approach. In the parasternal view, three standard levels are used. A record made at the level of the aorta and left atrium, is shown in Fig. 5. Here the aortic root is shown as two parallel lines, with the left atrial cavity behind it. It can be seen that the aortic root moves forward during systole, as the left atrium fills, and backwards during diastole following opening of the mitral valve. Within the aortic root the aortic valve cusps are visible. They show a characteristic box-like configuration, opening during systole, and closing at the onset of diastole, coincident with the aortic component of the second sound. In front of the aorta is a small portion of the outflow tract of the right ventricle. This view is used to measure left atrial size, the diameter of the aortic root, and to study movement of the aortic valve cusps.

Figure 6 shows an M-mode echocardiogram at the level of the anterior cusp of the mitral valve, shown at the centre of the display. Anterior to the valve is the interventricular septum, and

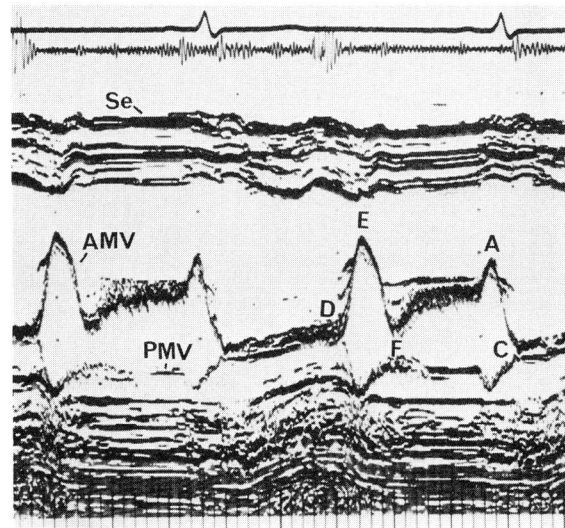

Fig. 6 M-mode echocardiogram at the level of the mitral valve showing anterior (AMV) and posterior (PMV) cusps. Se, septum. For description of mitral valve cusp motion, see text.

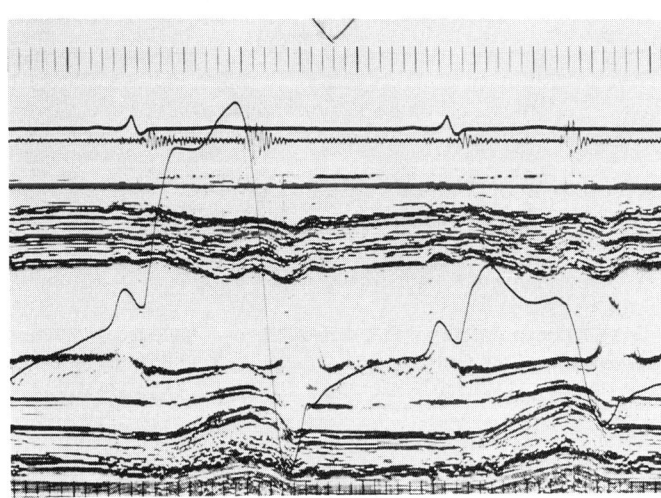

Fig. 7 M-mode echocardiogram of normal left ventricular cavity at the level of the tips of the mitral leaflets. Simultaneous phono- and apexcardiograms have been recorded.

posterior is the atrioventricular junction. The motion of the normal anterior cusp is characteristic. With atrial systole, there is a forward or opening movement (A), but by the onset of ventricular systole it has returned to its closed position (B). As ventricular pressure rises, there may be further posterior movement (C), but during ejection, the whole mitral valve is carried forwards as ventricular volume drops (D). As ventricular filling starts, the valve opens abruptly (E), and then during mid-diastole moves back towards its closed position, as flow rate into the left ventricle drops (F). This mid-diastolic closure is very characteristic of the normal anterior cusp, and depends both on normal physical characteristics of the cusp and also a normal flow pattern into the ventricle. The posterior mitral valve cusp can also be visualized. Its direction of motion is the reverse of that of the normal anterior cusp, and its amplitude is significantly less. The motion pattern of the normal tricuspid valve is identical to that of the mitral valve.

This view has proved extremely valuable in detecting abnormalities of mitral cusp motion which are described in detail elsewhere (page 13.284).

The third level corresponds to a transverse view across the left ventricular cavity (Fig. 7). It has been standardized to include part

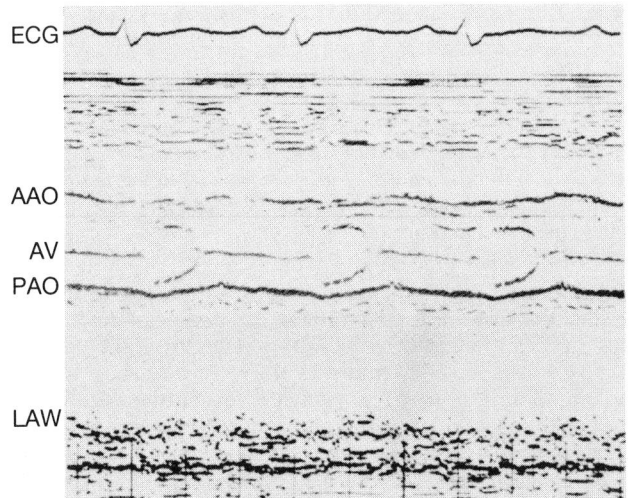

Fig. 5 Normal aortic valve echocardiogram, showing systolic separation of the cusps to form a box-like appearance. Diastolic closure leads to the appearance of a single line mid-way between the anterior (AAO) and posterior (PAO) walls.

Table 1 Normal M-mode measurements

Left ventricular dimension	
End-diastole	4.6 ± 0.9 cm
End-systole	3.1 ± 0.7 cm
Left ventricular posterior wall thickness†	1.0 ± 0.2 cm
Septal thickness†	0.9 ± 0.3 cm
Left atrial dimension	3.0 ± 1.1 cm
Aortic root dimension	2.9 ± 0.9 cm
Shortening fraction	32 ± 7%

† End diastole.
Mean values ± 95 per cent confidence limits.

of the subvalvular apparatus of the mitral valve. Movement of the interventricular septum is characteristic in the normal, showing posterior motion during systole as cavity size falls, and anterior motion during filling. Anterior to the septum is part of the right ventricular outflow tract. This view allows the transverse left ventricular dimension to be estimated, which gives useful information about cavity size. In addition, it is possible to estimate the thickness of the septum and posterior wall, and to observe the manner in which thickness changes with time. This view is useful in studying the anatomy and function of the left ventricle particularly when M-modes directed from the cross-sectional display are used to localize the exact position of the ultrasound beam.

In addition to recording views at these three levels, it is customary to perform an M-mode sweep, in which the transducer is moved from the direction of the aortic root to that of the left ventricle as the recording is being made at a slow paper speed.

Measurement of M-mode echocardiograms
Criteria have been established to standardize measurements made from M-mode echocardiograms.

1. Only high quality records, at paper speeds of 50–100 mm/s should be used.
2. All measurements are made from the leading edge of echoes.
3. End-diastolic measurements are synchronous with the onset of the q wave of the ECG in lead II. The timing of end-systole has not been defined, and, in disease, is frequently asynchronous in different parts of the left ventricle. Instead, end-ejection or the timing of A2 or aortic valve closure is measured from the phonocardiogram. All measurements of the left ventricle are taken at the level of the tips of the mitral leaflets or that of the chordae.
4. Left atrial and aortic root dimensions are measured at the level of the aortic valve cusps.
5. Measurements of right ventricular cavity size are affected by posture and refer to part of the outflow tract only. They have not been validated, and should probably be disregarded unless they are widely different from normal.

Normal measurements are given in Table 1.

Doppler cardiography
The Doppler technique makes use of the alteration in frequency of a reflected wave when the target is moving with respect to the observer, being increased if the two are approaching, and reduced if they are receding from one another. The change in frequency (Δf) depends on the velocity of sound (c), the relative velocity of the target and source (V), and the angle between the direction of motion and the ultrasound beam (θ), given by the relation:

$$\Delta f = \frac{2fv \cos \theta}{c}$$

The technique may be used in several ways in cardiology. A continuous source allows peak velocities within the heart to be measured, however high they are, a technique referred to as continuous wave (CW) Doppler. When combined with M-mode or

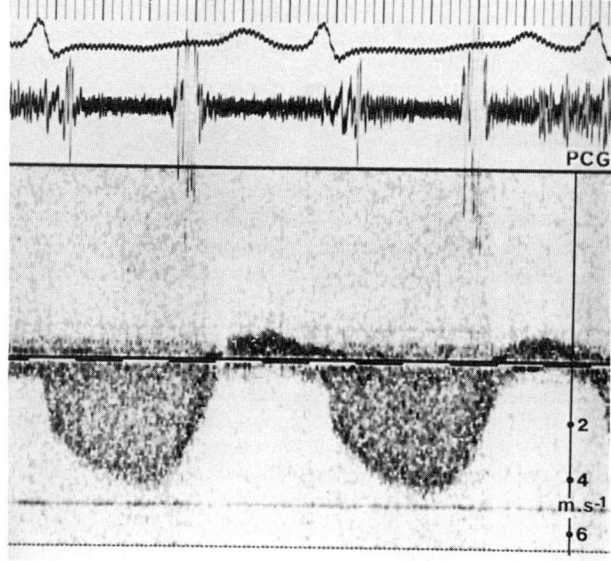

Fig. 8 Continuous wave Doppler cardiogram of retrograde blood flow velocity across the tricuspid valve in a patient with severe pulmonary hypertension. Peak velocity is approximately 4 m/s, which corresponds to a pressure drop of 64 mm Hg between right ventricle and right atrium during systole. Pulmonary valve closure is accentuated on the phonocardiogram (PCG).

two-dimensional echocardiography, pulsed Doppler, it may be used to make measurements of blood velocity in clearly defined regions of the heart. Finally, blood flow patterns, either towards or away from the transducer can be colour coded and superimposed on a cross-sectional display, a technique referred to as colour flow mapping.

Continuous wave Doppler
In continuous wave Doppler, a double transducer is used, so that ultrasound is emitted and received continuously. It is not a pulse–echo method, and it is not possible to locate the depth, but only the direction from which velocities are recorded. However, it has the advantage over pulsed Doppler that higher frequency shifts, and therefore higher velocities can be recorded. This allows the severity of stenoses to be estimated, since there is a relation, given by the Bernouilli equation between peak blood velocity and peak pressure gradient across a stenosis, which, for clinical purposes simplifies to:

$$\Delta P = 4V^2$$

where the pressure gradient (ΔP) is measured in mm Hg and peak velocity (V) in m/s. Thus a peak velocity of 1 m/s corresponds to a gradient of 4 mm Hg, and 4 m/s of 64 mm Hg. This information can be used in a number of ways:

1. Peak valve gradients can be estimated. Continuous wave Doppler has proved very successful in estimating peak systolic gradients across aortic and pulmonary, and peak diastolic gradients across mitral and tricuspid valves (Fig. 9b). It should be noted that peak instantaneous gradients are measured. These are not the same as those routinely reported at cardiac catheterization which are 'peak-to-peak' gradients, i.e. the difference between the values of peak pressure on either side of the obstruction regardless of the time during systole or diastole at which they occur. These estimates are also sensitive to the angle between the direction of blood flow and the ultrasound beam. Nevertheless, the method is potentially reliable since an increase in velocity is as fundamental a reflection of the disturbance to flow caused by a stenosis as a pressure difference.

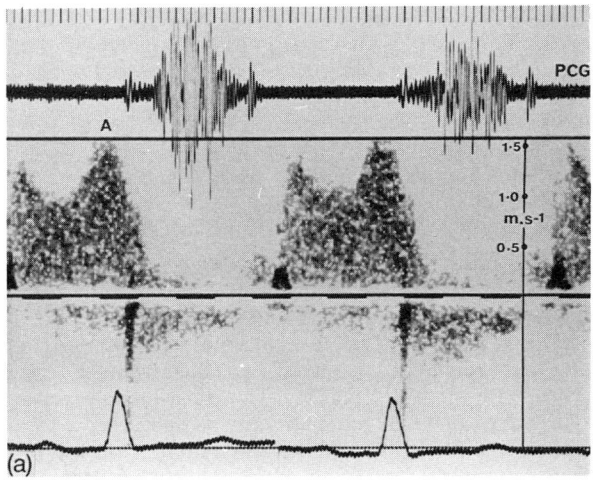

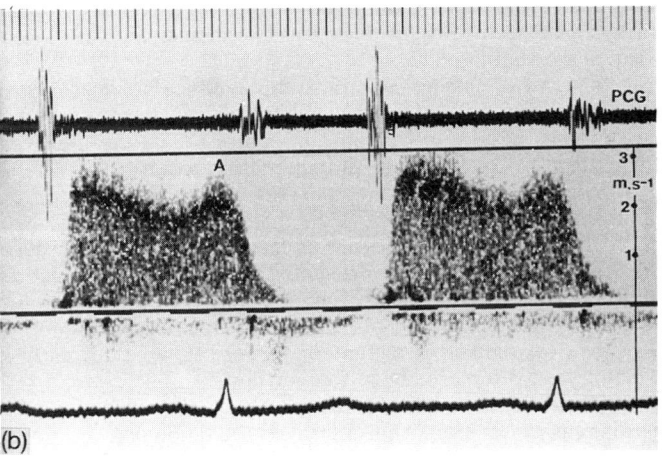

Fig. 9 (a) Continuous wave Doppler cardiogram of blood flow velocity across the normal mitral valve of a patient with aortic stenosis. Peak flow velocity (1.5 m/s) occurs during atrial systole (A). An ejection systolic murmur is demonstrated on the phonocardiogram (PCG). (b) Continuous wave Doppler cardiogram of blood flow velocity across the mitral valve in a patient with severe rheumatic mitral stenosis. Peak velocity is considerably increased to approximately 3 m/s, corresponding to an instantaneous pressure gradient of 36 mm Hg. Flow velocity declines during mid-diastole, but increases again with left atrial systole (A). PCG, phonocardiogram.

2. Valve area. If flow across a valve is passive, as in the case of the mitral valve during diastole, then pressure difference will fall exponentially, with a time constant dependent on valve area, and independent of blood flow. Since pressure gradient is proportional to the square of peak velocity, $t_{1/2}$, the pressure half-time, can be calculated as the time taken for velocity to fall to 70 per cent of its peak value. Effective valve area is calculated from the formula:

$$\text{Valve area} = (220)/t_{1/2}$$

where valve area is expressed in cm^2, and $t_{1/2}$ in ms. This approach gives useful estimates of effective valve area of mitral and tricuspid valves, or of prostheses in these positions.

3. Reverse pressure gradients. The peak velocity of retrograde flow across a regurgitant valve is related to pressure gradient in exactly the same way as for forward flow. Thus in patients with tricuspid regurgitation, right ventricular pressure can be calculated as the sum of right atrial pressure and the systolic pressure difference across the tricuspid valve (Fig. 8). Similarly, in mitral regurgitation, left atrial pressure can be derived from peak retrograde velocity and peak left ventricular pressure, measured as systolic arterial pressure. The same principles apply for aortic and pulmonary regurgitation.

Pulsed Doppler

Pulsed Doppler allows flow to be measured at levels within the heart defined from an M-mode or cross-sectional display. Its main advantage is the accurate localization of abnormal flow within the heart. Peak flow velocities can also be determined, provided they are not greatly increased. At high flow rates, such as occur across stenotic valves, however, pulsed Doppler records become ambiguous, a phenomenon referred to as 'aliasing', which reduces their value. Subject to this limitation, pulsed Doppler can be used to establish:

1. The direction of flow. Retrograde flow is characteristic of valvular regurgitation. Aortic regurgitation, for example, can be detected by reversed flow in the left ventricular outflow tract, and mitral regurgitation from systolic flow into the left atrium. The distribution of this abnormal flow can be mapped, but this is a time-consuming procedure.

2. The presence of abnormal flow, for example, through a persistent ductus arteriosus or ventricular septal defect.

3. The peak velocity of blood flow in the absence of significant valvular gradients. Characteristic patterns can be recorded from the ascending and descending aortas. Peak velocity, at rest, in the normal adult is in the range 40–80 cm/s, and significantly higher in infants and children. Values are also increased by drugs or sympathetic stimulation, and reduced in disease. Such measurements have been used to follow the progress of patients in the intensive care unit and to monitor the effects of treatment.

4. Measurement of blood flow. It must be stressed that Doppler methods measure blood velocity rather than blood flow, although the two may be closely related. In order to calculate flow from velocity it is necessary to know the cross-sectional area of the vessel through which flow occurs, and the flow profile, i.e. the change in velocity across its diameter. Cross-sectional area can be estimated from M-mode or cross-sectional echocardiography at a number of sites within the circulation, including the roots of both great arteries, and mitral and tricuspid valve rings. At all sites, the

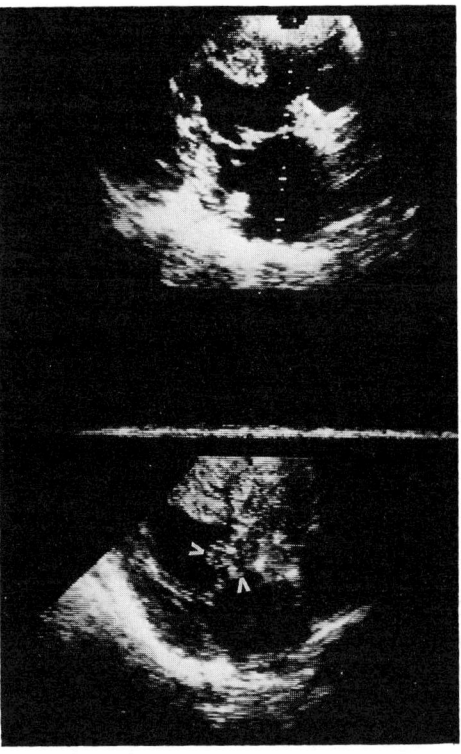

Fig. 10 Demonstration of right-to-left shunt by contrast echocardiography in a patient with an Eisenmenger VSD. Top panel, control. Lower panel shows opacification of right ventricle by dense contrast, with additional contrast, marked by arrow, passing into the left ventricle.

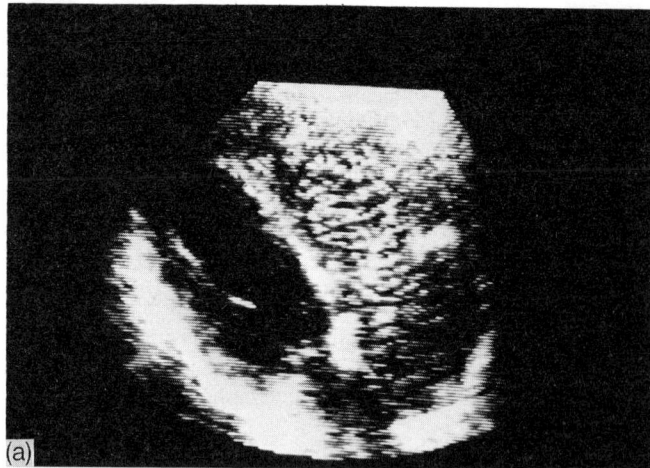

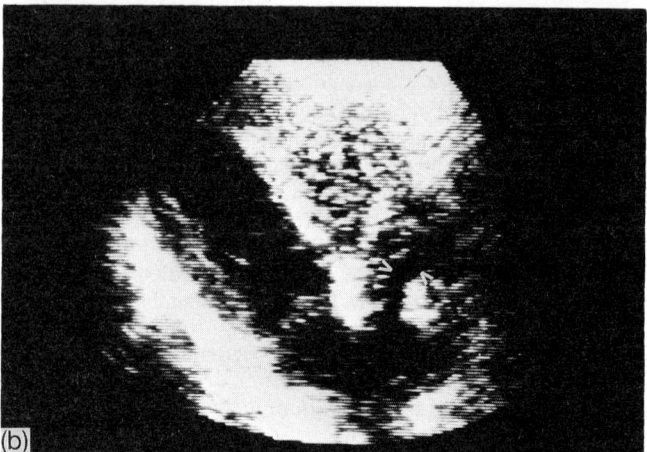

Fig. 11 (a) Opacification of right atrium and right ventricle by contrast in a patient with ostium secundum ASD. (b) Demonstration of left-to-right shunt at atrial level by the appearance of a 'negative jet', marked by arrows.

flow profile appears to be uniform, so that stroke volume can be estimated at any of these sites from cross-sectional area and the time integral of blood velocity. Shunts can be detected when estimates made on the right side of the heart differ significantly from those on the left.

Colour flow mapping

This technique has recently been introduced in order to display the direction of blood flow, either towards or away from the transducer in colour on a two-dimensional display. Although flow velocities are not available quantitatively, patterns of flow are readily apparent. It thus becomes possible to detect small VSDs, and to appreciate abnormal regurgitant jets which might not be apparent with conventional pulsed Doppler mapping techniques. It is also possible to assess the angle between the ultrasound beam and the jet across a stenotic or regurgitant valve, so that the two can be optimally aligned. It has become apparent that such jets are not always orientated directly perpendicular to the valve in question. The method has also demonstrated abnormal flow patterns within the dilated left ventricle during filling and ejection. The technique is a complex one, so that equipment is expensive and not generally available, while the clinical significance of much of the information it provides has yet to be determined.

Contrast echocardiography

Contrast echocardiography makes use of the appearance of a cloud of echoes within the circulation following rapid injection of

fluid, probably due to small air bubbles becoming entrained with the fluid. These bubbles are carried with the circulation, until they are cleared from it by either the systemic or the pulmonary capillary bed. The simplest method is to inject approximately 5 ml of fluid, e.g. saline or 5 per cent dextrose into a peripheral vein. This can be observed to pass through the chambers of the right heart, using either M-mode or two-dimensional methods, in 5 to 10 beats. The method is thus cheap and widely available. It can give useful information in a variety of circumstances:

1. In the presence of a right-to-left shunt, contrast can be seen to pass into the left heart. Both the presence and the site of the shunt can be localized from appropriate views (Fig. 10).

2. In the presence of a left-to-right shunt, contrast in right heart chambers is washed out by contrast-free blood from the left side of the heart, a 'negative jet' (Fig. 11). This is particularly well seen in patients with ostium secundum atrial septal defect.

3. With significant tricuspid regurgitation, contrast injected from an arm vein can be seen to enter hepatic veins. If an M-mode record is recorded from the inferior vena cava, contrast appearance can be seen to occur during systole, coinciding with the 'v' wave of the venous pulse.

4. The rate of passage of contrast through the right heart gives a semiquantitative idea of the circulation time, and hence of the cardiac output. Failure of clearance of contrast from the right ventricle suggests significant impairment of its function.

5. Very characteristic flow patterns can be recorded on M-mode contrast echograms from the main pulmonary artery. Normally the bubble trajectories are directed away from a transducer on the anterior chest wall throughout right ventricular ejection, their slopes on the M-mode record being vectors representing velocity. When pulmonary resistance is greatly raised, this normal forward flow pattern is disrupted; forward flow ceases early in ejection, and is replaced by retrograde flow.

6. Contrast can be introduced elsewhere in the circulation using cardiac catheterization. Thus, mitral regurgitation or a ventricular septal defect can be diagnosed following an injection into the left ventricle, a technique that may be useful in patients intolerant of angiographic contrast medium. Contrast can also be introduced into the left heart following injection through a catheter wedged in the pulmonary circulation. In these circumstances, the normal clearance of contrast by the lung does not occur. Contrast agents that pass through the pulmonary bed from a peripheral venous injection are available experimentally.

7. In experimental animals, contrast injected into the aortic root passes down the coronary arteries and opacifies the myocardium, thus outlining tissue perfusion. Coronary occlusion is associated with loss of myocardial opacification in the affected area. Agents are becoming available which will allow this method to be used in humans.

Tissue characterization

Tissue characterization represents the attempt to make deductions about the physical characteristics of structures within the heart by quantifying various aspects of the returning echoes, either individually, or from their variation in space or time. It is a complex and rapidly growing field, but even at this early stage, a number of trends have become apparent. The method appears applicable mainly to echoes arising by back scattering rather than by specular reflection, and so applies to those from myocardium rather than structures such as valve cusps or endocardium. Unfortunately, back scattering is a very complex process whose physical basis remains poorly understood. Nevertheless, semiquantitative estimates of echo amplitude have proved informative. Even with relatively simple methods of standardization, major differences in myocardial echo intensity can be demonstrated between patients. Important causes of increased amplitude are calcification, fibrosis, oedema, and inflammation. The distribution of values of echo intensity also contains informaton of clinical value. An increase in the spread of amplitude values about the mean (increased kurtosis) may be early evidence of myocardial ischaemia. The scatter of values in space, referred to as texture, may be abnormal in conditions such as myocardial amyloid or hypertrophic cardiomyopathy.

Major problems remain, however, including rather poor reproducibility from beat to beat. Development of these methods is limited by lack of understanding of the nature of the interaction between ultrasound and tissue, and hence of image generation in humans. These processes appear to be more complex than those with electromagnetic radiation, so that methods such as those underlying computerized tomographic scanning are not yet available, and techniques of image analysis remain largely empirical.

References

Edler, I. and Gustafson, A. (1957). Ultrasonic cardiogram in mitral stenosis. *Acta med. Scand.* **159**, 85–90.

Feigenbaum, H. (1986). *Echocardiography* 4th edn. Lea and Febiger. Philadelphia.

Hatle, L. and Angelsen, B. (1982). *Doppler ultrasound in cardiology*. Lea and Febiger, Philadelphia.

Henry W. L., DeMaria, A., Gramiak, R., King D. L., Kisslo, J. A., Popp, R. L., Sahn, D. J., Schiller, N., Tajik, A. and Teicholz, L. E. (1980). Report of the American Society of Echocardiography committee on nomenclature and standards in two dimensional echocardiography. *Circulation* **62**, 212–218.

——, Ware, J., Gardin, J. M., Hepner, S. I., McKay, J. and Weiner, M. (1978). Echocardiographic measurements in normal subjects. Growth related changes between infancy and early adulthood. *Circulation* **57**, 278–285.

Popp, R. L. (1976). Echocardiographic assessment of cardiac disease. *Circulation* **54**, 538.

Roelandt, J., van Dorp, W. G., Bom, N., Laird, J. D. and Hugenholtz, P. G. (1976). Resolution problems in echocardiology: a source of interpretation problems. *Am. J. Cardiol.* **37**, 256–262.

Roelandt, J. and Gibson, D. G. (1980). Recommendations for standardization of measurements from M-mode echocardiograms. *Eur. Heart. J.* **1**, 375–378.

Tajik, A. J., Seward, J. B., Hagler, D. J., Mair, D. D. and Lie, J. T. (1978). Two-dimensional real-time ultrasonic imaging of the heart and great vessels; technique, image orientation, structure identification and validation. *Mayo Clin. Proc.* **53**, 271–303.

Nuclear techniques

D. J. ROWLANDS

Nuclear imaging of the heart offers a relatively new approach to cardiac investigation. Techniques are currently available to demonstrate the extent and distribution of viable myocardium, localized areas of ischaemia induced by exercise or by drugs, recent myocardial cell damage, and global and regional left ventricular function. These investigations involve very low invasiveness and little discomfort or inconvenience to the patient. However, there are limitations inherent in the resolving power of nuclear techniques in general. Tissues less than one cubic centimetre in volume are not demonstrable with reliability, infarcts involving less than 3–7 g of myocardium are unlikely to be shown, and edge detection is less reliably accomplished with nuclear angiography than with contrast radiography. Nuclear techniques currently provide a very useful complement to rather than a substitute for electrocardiography, plane chest radiography, and cardiac catheterization.

Imaging in the diagnosis of myocardial infarction

Two general approaches have been used for the detection of myocardial infarction or ischaemia.

1. Recent myocardial damage may be demonstrated using radio-pharmaceuticals which concentrate selectively in acutely injured cells. This is called positive imaging, infarct-avid imaging, or 'hot-spot' scanning.

2. Ionic tracers which behave in a fashion similar to the potassium ion, accumulate in viable, perfused myocardium but are not taken up by infarcted myocardium and are taken up to a less than normal extent by ischaemic myocardium. This is called negative imaging, ionic tracer scanning, or 'cold-spot' scanning.

Hot-spot scanning

A large number of agents have been used for hot-spot scanning of myocardial infarction but the one most extensively used to date has been $^{99}Tc^m$-stannous pyrophosphate. The observation that calcium is deposited in irreversibly damaged myocardial cells led to the idea of using $^{99}Tc^m$-stannous pyrophosphate, a bone scanning agent, as a means of demonstrating myocardial necrosis.

The cellular death of myocardial infarction is accompanied by an influx of calcium ions which are deposited in crystalline and sub-crystalline form within mitochondria. It has been suggested that calcium accumulation in this way might be used as an index of irreversible myocardial cell damage after ischaemia, However, it may be that the tracer is associated with cytoplasmic denatured macromolecules rather than with mitrochondrial hydroxyapatite.

The three most important determinants of the uptake of $^{99}Tc^m$-stannous pyrophosphate by the myocardium are:

The presence of myocardial necrosis (at least 3 g of necrotic tissue seem to be necessary for a positive scan).

Persistent residual collateral coronary blood flow into the area of irreversible myocardial damage (something of the order of 20–40 per cent of the normal flow being required).

The time interval between the clinical onset of infarction and the scanning Scans are unlikely to be positive in the first 12 hours and the optimum scanning time is 24–96 hours. Ideally two or more scans should be undertaken within this time. Scans may occasionally be positive two weeks after an isolated episode of infarction.

Between 200 and 600 MB_q (approximately 5–15 mCi) of $^{99}Tc^m$-stannous pyrophosphate are given intravenously. Scanning is undertaken 60–90 minutes following the injection of radionuclide. Scans taken earlier than this are obscured by appreciable residual radioactivity in the cardiac blood pool. Scans taken much later demonstrate marked skeletal uptake. An example of a negative (normal) and of a positive (abnormal) $^{99}Tc^m$-stannous pyrophosphate scan is shown in Fig. 1. The ribs and sternum normally take up the isotope and are always apparent in both normal and abnormal $^{99}Tc^m$-stannous pyrophosphate scans.

Diagnosis of infarction

False negative and false positive results occur. In 14 different series involving 562 patients with acute myocardial infarction by all the usual criteria the false negative rate was 6 per cent. A further group of 15 different series involving 1083 patients with no evidence of acute infarction showed a false positive rate of 17 per cent. The 'efficiency' of the procedure (i.e. its overall ability correctly to classify patients as to whether or not they had acute infarctions) is 86 per cent. The recorded causes of false positive $^{99}Tc^m$-stannous pyrophosphate scans include unstable angina, left ventricular aneurysms, cardiomyopathy, valvular calcification, myocardial contusion, persistent blood pool activity, rib fractures, breast tumours, calcified costal cartilages, skeletal muscle damage, and cardioversion (giving skeletal muscle or myocardial damage).

Localization of infarction

In general, infarct localization by hot-spot scanning agrees with electrocardiographic localization when the infarct is transmural.

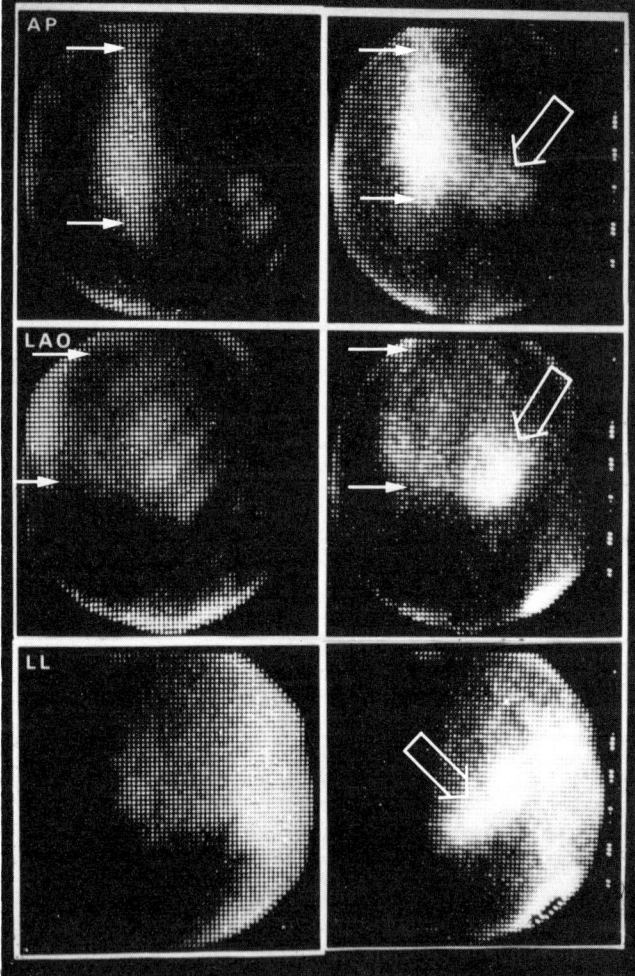

Fig. 1 $^{99}Tc^{m}$-stannous pyrophosphate scans. The left-hand column shows a normal scan in the anterior (AP), left anterior oblique (LAO), and lateral (LL) views. The upper and lower limits of the sternum are indicated in the AP and LAO views (small arrows). Normal activity in the obliquely running ribs can be seen to the left of the sternum (in the AP view) and posterior to it (LAO and LL views).

The right-hand column shows an abnormal scan. The sternum is recognizable (small arrows). There is a dense zone of abnormal activity in the region of the fresh infarct (chunky arrows).

Subendocardial infarction cannot be accurately localized. Posterior extension of infarction is more commonly found by hot-spot scanning than would be suggested by standard electrocardiographic criteria.

Sizing of infarction

Although experimental work shows a good correlation between the scintigraphic estimate of infarct size and histological post-mortem examination, *in vivo* scintigraphic studies in man do not permit accurate sizing because of the limited resolution of scintigraphic images and the complex geometry of infarction.

Cold-spot scanning (see also page 13.161)

For many years it has been known that radio-isotopes of potassium and of some of its homologues from Group I of the periodic table are actively taken up by myocardial cells. Extensive work has been done on isotopes of potassium, caesium, and rubidium. At present perfusion studies of the myocardium are usually performed with ^{201}Tl. Although thallium is not in the same group of the periodic table as potassium, its biological behaviour is analogous to that of potassium because of the similarity in size of the

hydrated ions. ^{201}Thallium appears the most suitable isotope for myocardial scanning at present because of its physical characterisics. It has a long physical half-life (72 hours) providing a longer shelf-life than ^{43}K but the total body radiation dose involved is less.

Thallium is cleared rapidly from the blood. Five minutes after intravenous injection the plasma activity has decreased to 50 per cent of its initial maximum. The myocardial extraction efficiency is high (80 per cent) but since the coronary artery blood flow is only 5 per cent of the total cardiac output, only some 5–10 per cent (after several circulations) of the administered dose is concentrated in the myocardium, most of the rest being taken up by kidneys, liver, stomach, and skeletal muscle.

Thallium uptake is dependent both upon *perfusion* and upon *viability* of myocardial cells and its concentration in the myocardium depends not only upon normal blood flow distribution but also upon the integrity of the myocardial cell membrane. Defects in the normal distribution of thallium may thus indicate infarction or ischaemia. Experience has shown that defects in scans obtained with the patient at rest indicate infarction, and that defects found on scanning during exercise and which are not present on scanning at rest indicate local myocardial ischaemia. In fact, both studies can be undertaken with a single injection, if the injection is given during exercise and the scan taken both immediately and also several hours later when redistribution of the thallium has occurred. The immediate (exercise-related) scan reflects myocardial blood flow (for this is what determines the initial thallium distribution), the subsequent scan reflects the potassium mass of the myocardium. Exercise is usually carried out on a bicycle or treadmill to the point of onset of angina pectoris or fatigue. At this stage 50–75 MB_q (approximately 1.5–2 mCi) of ^{201}Tl are given intravenously through an indwelling cannula and the exercise is continued for one or two minutes. After 5–10 minutes images are obtained, usually in the anterior, left anterior oblique, and lateral views.

An example of a normal myocardial perfusion scan is shown in Fig. 2. The scan shows a doughnut-shaped outline of the left ventricular mass with an area of lesser activity indicating the left ventricular cavity. The cavity is best delineated in the anterior and left anterior oblique view. The myocardium of the atria and right ventricle is not normally visualized because the mass of myocardium involved per unit area of scan is much less than is the case with the left ventricle. The use of three or more views permits separate visualization of most of the regions of the left ventricular myocardium. (Fig. 2)

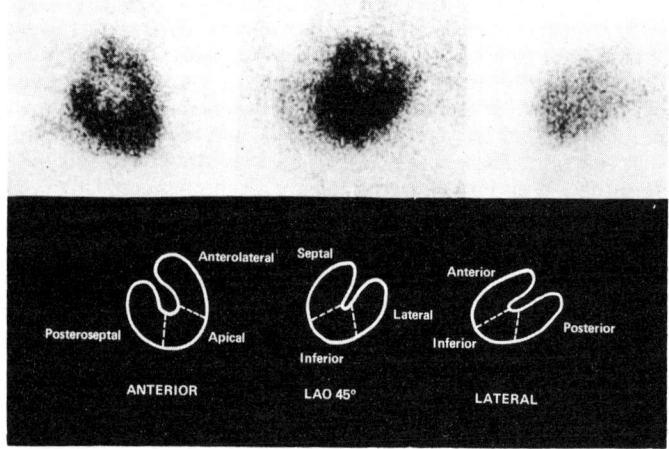

Fig. 2 Normal ^{201}Thallium scan. The upper row shows the thallium scans in the anterior, left anterior oblique, and left lateral views. The horse-shoe shaped zone of uptake in the left ventricular myocardium is seen (less well in the lateral view, as is typical). The lower row shows diagrammatically how the use of three views permits the visualization of different regions of the left ventricle.

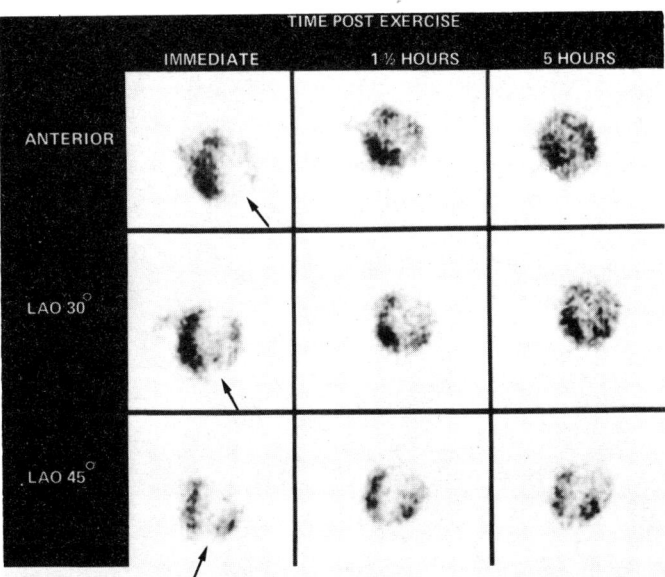

Fig. 3 [201]Thallium scans showing regional ischaemia on exercise. The left column shows the [201]Thallium scan in three views immediately after completion of exercise (with thallium injection during exercise). A defect (arrowed) is seen involving the apical region on the anterior view. The left anterior oblique views show that the defect involves the inferior wall also. After 1½ hours, considerable redistribution of thallium has occurred with significant uptake in those areas where initial uptake was defective. After 5 hours the thallium distribution is normal, indicating viability of the myocardium involved and confirms that the earlier defect was the result of ischaemia. Had the defect persisted unchanged it would have indicated infarction.

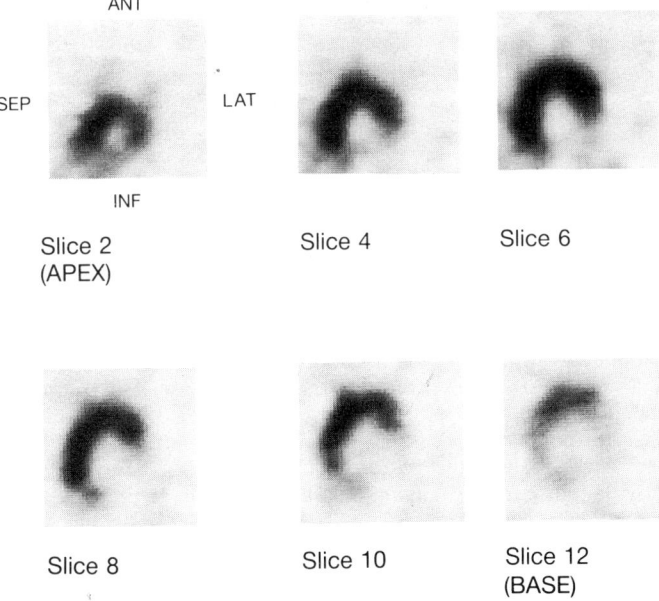

Slice 2 (APEX) Slice 4 Slice 6

Slice 8 Slice 10 Slice 12 (BASE)

Fig. 4 Emission computed thallium tomography, illustrating infero-lateral myocardial infarction. Anterior (ant), septal (sep), inferior (inf), and lateral (lat) left ventricular walls are indicated. Thallium uptake is defective in the infero-lateral walls.

Scans from a patient with exercise-induced myocardial ischaemia are shown in Fig. 3. A defect in tracer uptake is seen (arrow) on the immediate post-exercise scan. In the course of the next few hours, redistribution of thallium occurs within myocardium (as the ischaemic but viable area continues to take up thallium from residual blood pool activity). The ultimate normality of uptake indicates the uniform viability of the myocardium and the immediate post-exercise deficit is thus seen to be indicative of ischaemia.

Diagnosis of infarction

The sensitivity of thallium scintiscanning in the diagnosis of myocardial infarction is related to the size and age of the infarct. Infarcts involving less than 7 g of myocardium may be missed. It is claimed that no false negatives occur if the scans are undertaken within six hours of the onset of symptoms. With increasing intervals between the time of onset of symptoms of infarction and the time of scanning there is a moderate reduction in the sensitivity for detection of transmural infarcts and appreciable reduction in the sensitivity for detecting subendocardial infarcts.

Localization of infarction

The use of multiple views with thallium scans permits the localization of defects (whether the defect be an infarct or ischaemia). The scans have a tendency to underestimate the incidence of inferior infarction (compared with the electrocardiogram) but are more likely to diagnose true posterior infarcts than the standard ECG.

Sizing of infarction

No reliable clinical method currently exists for the assessment of infarct size. Early hopes that cold-spot scanning would provide such an estimate have not been sustained. There is certainly a correlation between the size of infarction as assessed isotopically and that assessed by electrocardiography or by serial enzyme estimation, but precise sizing of infarcts by this technique is not possible.

Emission computed tomography

Recently the technique of emission computed tomography has been applied to thallium studies which allow images of slices of the heart to be obtained. The tomographic 'cuts' are obtained perpendicular to the long axis of the heart. The gamma camera rotates around the patient producing 32 images over 180°. The data are fed into a dedicated computer and the slice images are constructed. An example of the images obtained in this way is shown in Fig. 4. This study was obtained from a patient with inferolateral myocardial infarction.

Scintigraphic determination of left ventricular function

The assessment of left ventricular function is one of the most important aspects of the evaluation of the cardiac status. Traditionally, left ventricular performance is evaluated by the determination of cardiac output and left ventricular end-diastolic pressure, and by cine-angiography following the injection of contrast material into the left ventricular cavity. These are all highly invasive investigations. Scintigraphic approaches now provide the possibility of obtaining some information on left ventricular performance by non-invasive means. This information consists of:

1. Estimates of left ventricular ejection fraction (the fraction of the ventricular end-diastolic volume ejected per beat), which is an *overall* measure of left ventricular performance.

2. Estimates of *regional* ventricular performance by observation of the movements of the margins of the ventricle.

Contrast radiology provides the same two classes of information. Each of these two separate items of information may be obtained by two totally different scintigraphic approaches – the *'first pass technique'* and the *'equilibrium'* method.

Both methods involve the intravenous injection of a radioactive tracer bound to an intravascular agent. ^{99}Tc^{m} is almost universally used as the tracer and this may be bound to human serum albumin or, nowadays more commonly, to the patient's own red blood cells.

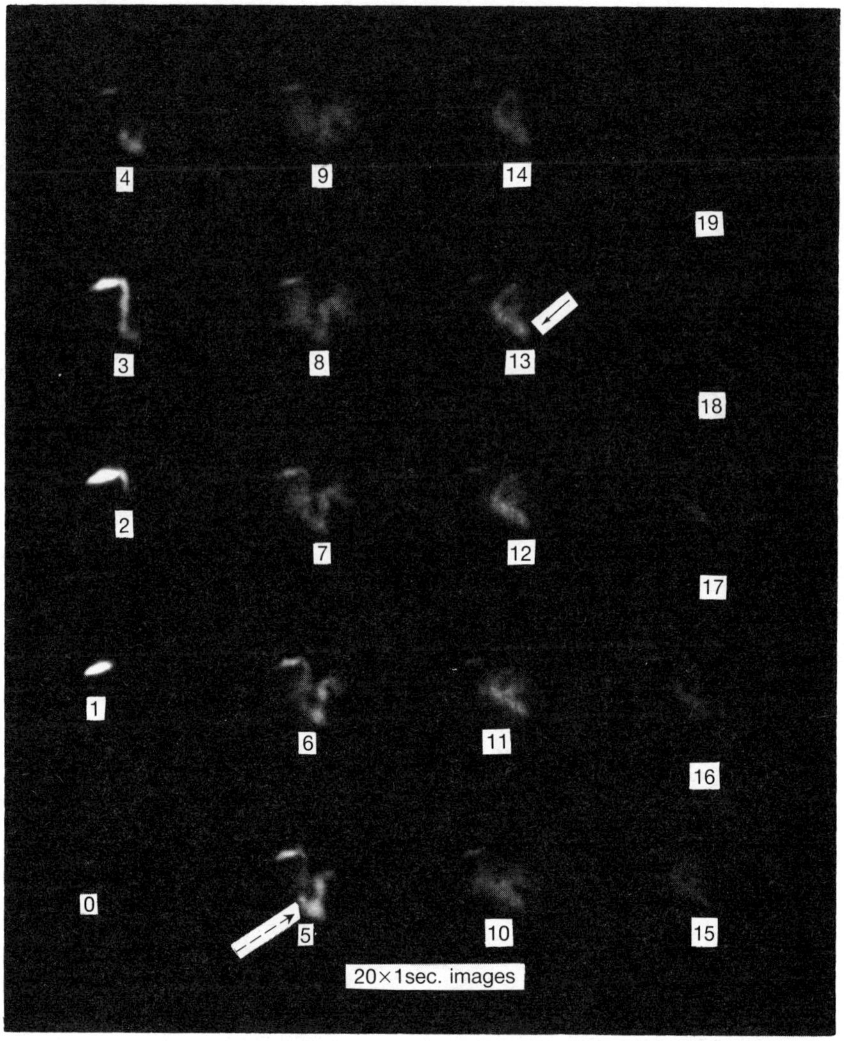

Fig. 5 Sequential blood pool images in the RAO view during the first passage through the central circulation of intravenously administered $^{99}Tc^m$-labelled red blood cells. Consecutive images are shown at one second intervals. The arrow points to the left ventricular image and the interrupted arrow to the right ventricular image. In frames 14–18 the descending aorta is visible. (Reproduced from *Advanced medicine* (1981). Pitman, London, by permission.)

The first-pass technique

In this technique the first passage of the radioactive bolus though the central circulation is studied. Since sequential images follow the passage of the tracer through the central circulation, the right and left ventricular images are separated in time, and because of this any desired view of the ventricles can be obtained without the problem of overlap of the two ventricular images. The single most useful view is probably the right anterior oblique which is the projection of choice in single plane contrast radiography of the left ventricle. With a gamma camera positioned over the patient in the right anterior oblique projection, sequential images are obtained after the administration of the tracer and are stored in the computer. Figure 5 shows a sequence of twenty such images obtained at one second intervals. In the first frame activity is seen in the subclavian vein. In subsequent frames it is seen descending in the superior vena cava, passing through the right heart, the pulmonary circulation, the left heart, and the aorta. The right ventricular image is well seen at 4–7 seconds (interrupted arrow) and the left ventricular image at 11–14 seconds (arrow). The pulmonary circulation is well shown at 9 seconds and the aorta at 14–18 seconds.

Determination of ejection fraction by the first-pass technique

Using the computer display of stored data a region of interest (ROI) over the left ventricle is outlined (for example with a light pen) and a high frequency activity-time curve for that ROI plotted. Each point on the curve represents accumulated counts for a period of 0.04 s. The amount of radioactivity in the heart is pro-

portional to the volume of blood in the cavities. Thus, the change in precordial count rate reflects the cyclical volume changes in the heart. A second ROI is taken (usually as a horse-shoe shaped region surrounding the left ventricular ROI) to sample the background activity variation with time. Digital smoothing processes are applied to the background curve to minimize statistical noise components. The background curve is then 'normalized' to the left ventricular curve (to correct for the different areas of the two). This normalized, smoothed background curve is then subtracted point-for-point from the high frequency left ventricular activity–time curve to give the corrected high frequency left venticular activity–time curve. An example is shown in Fig. 6. Ejection fraction is then obtained as:

$$\frac{ED_c - ES_c}{ED_c} \tag{1}$$

where ED_c is the background-corrected count of end-diastole and ES_c the background-corrected count of end-systole.

Although up to 10 or 12 cycles may be available for analysis, it is usual to take 4–6 cycles around the peak of the left ventricular curve and average the calculated ejection fractions from these cycles.

Regional wall motion studies by the first-pass technique

If the first pass data are acquired together with timing pulses from the electrocardiogram, the data may subsequently be reassembled to produce a 'representative cine-cycle' comprising a sequence of images within the representative cycle, each one of which consists

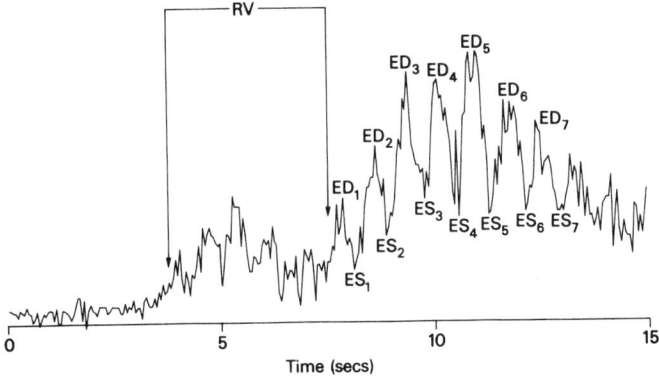

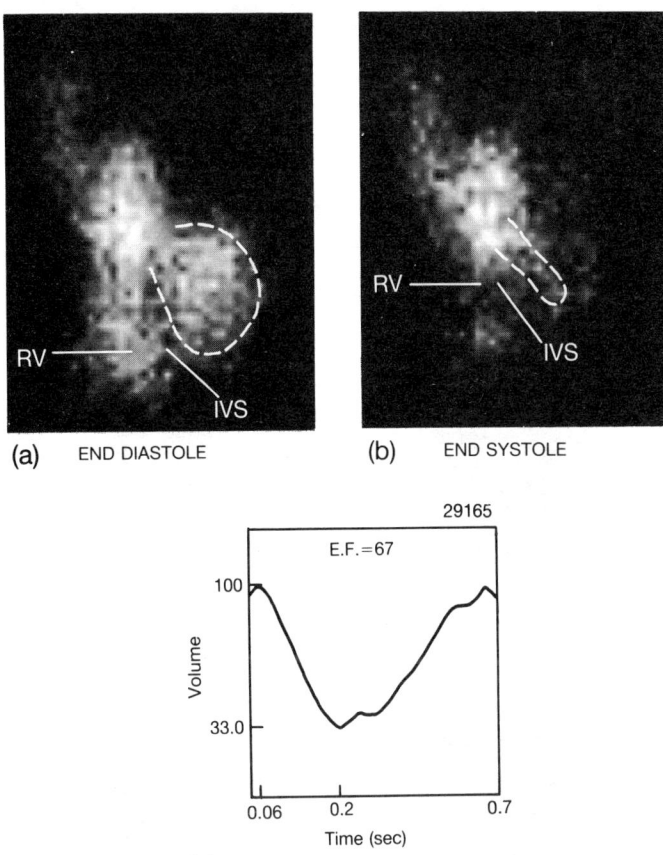

Fig. 6 High frequency activity–time curve recorded from the region of the left ventricle during the first passage of radioactive tracer through the central circulation. The time, in seconds, after the injection is shown on the abscissa. The ordinate displays scintillation counting rate on a linear scale, after background correction.

The early hump shows scattered radiation during the passage of the tracer through the right ventricle (RV). The later, larger hump shows the count rate during the passage through the left ventricle. Peaks and troughs are visible in relation to each cardiac cycle. Estimates of ejection fraction can be made for each cardiac cycle: $(ED_1–ES_1)/ED_1$, $(ED_2–ES_2)/ED_2$, etc.

Fig. 8 Normal resting MUGA scan in LAO 45° view. (a) End-diastolic and (b) end-systolic images are shown. The interrupted line indicates the outline of the left ventricular cavity. Arrows point to the right ventricular cavity (RV) and to the interventricular septum (IVS). All regions of the left ventricular wall contract well. In (c) the background-corrected activity–time curve obtained from the area of the left ventricle is shown with the end-diastolic volume normalized to 100 per cent. The ejection fraction is normal at 67 per cent.

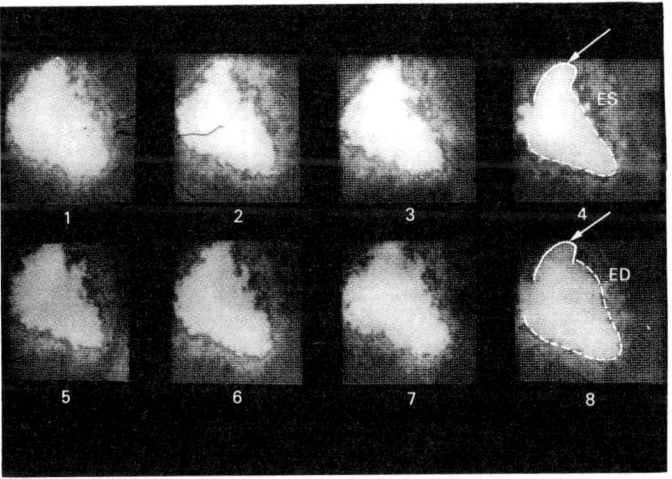

Fig. 7 Regional wall motion studies by the first-pass technique. Eight consecutive frames which between them represent a cardiac cycle, each frame containing summed data from several cardiac cycles. The fourth frame represents an end-systolic (ES) frame and the eighth an end-diastolic (ED) frame. The left ventricular outline is shown as the interrupted line. The aortic outline is shown as the continuous line (arrowed). The gap in the perimeter between the lower end of the aortic edge and the left end of the left ventricular edge is the region of the mitral valve. The images are all seen in the right anterior oblique view.

of summed data from the corresponding part of several successive cycles. (Summation of several cycles in this way is necessary, for the total count accumulation within the subdivision of a single cycle would not be sufficient to give an adequate image.) An example of such a representative cine-cycle is shown in Fig. 7. Once the sequence of left ventricular outlines representing the cine-cycle is obtained, it is a simple matter to display them consecutively in rapid succession as an endless loop to produce a cine effect.

The equilibrium technique

This techique is also referred to as gated cardiac blood pool imaging, or more recently as multigated acquisition (MUGA) imaging. It depends upon complete mixing of the marker throughout the

circulating volume and it therefore requires a marker which remains intravascular. Formerly $^{99}Tc^m$-HSA was used but difficulties with the labelling and instability of this marker have led to increasing use of $^{99}Tc^m$-labelled red blood cells. Currently the cells do not have to be removed from the patient for labelling, for the 'in vivo labelling' technique may be used. This involves predisposing the patient's red cells to accept the technetium label by the administration, 30 minutes prior to the technetium, of non-active stannous pyrophosphate. Subsequently, 600–750 MB$_q$ (approximately 15–20 mCi) of $^{99}Tc^m$ pertechnetate are injected intravenously and imaging is begun after a further 10 minutes or so. Since there is complete mixing of the marker throughout the blood volume, all four cardiac chambers are seen simultaneously and various degrees of superimposition of the chambers inevitably occurs. Proper alignment of the gamma camera is therefore crucial for the optimal separation of the cardiac chambers. In general, maximal separation of the right and left ventricles is achieved in the left anterior oblique view, to which a caudal tilt of 15° may be added.

Determination of ejection fraction by the equilibrium technique

A region of interest over the left ventricle and a second 'horseshoe' shaped region around the left ventricle for background correction are assigned in the same manner as for the first-pass technique. A background-corrected activity–time curve of the left ventricular area is obtained (Fig. 8c, normal, and Fig. 9c, abnormal). With the equilibrium technique this is usually displayed as a single cycle representative activity–time curve being produced as a composite of many (typically hundreds) consecutive cycles, synchronization of the cycles being achieved by means of the R wave

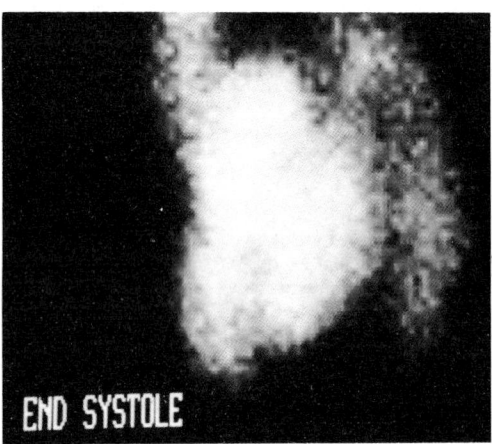

(a)

(b)

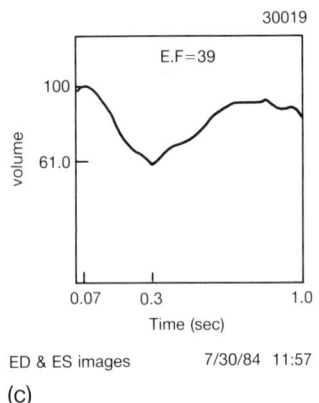

30019

E.F=39

(c)

Fig. 9 Abnormal resting MUGA scan from a patient with congestive cardiomyopathy. (a) The end-diastolic volume of the left ventricle (and to lesser extent the right ventricle) is increased (compare with Fig. 8a). (b) The left ventricular end-systolic volume is substantially increased (compare with Fig. 8b). All parts of the left ventricular wall show reduced contraction. (c) The overall left ventricular ejection fraction is diminished. Similar appearances may be found after multiple infarctions in three-vessel coronary disease.

of the ECG. Since the count rate is proportional to the ventricular volume, the ejection fraction can be determined in the same way as with the first-pass procedures:

$$EF = \frac{ED_c - ES_c}{ED_c} \tag{2}$$

Regional wall motion studies by the equilibrium technique

Left ventricular images are collected for each of many short time intervals and the images from corresponding parts of numerous cardiac cycles are summed to produce a composite. Typically, the 'exposure' time for each individual image collection might be 0.05 seconds so that if the heart rate were 80 per minute (i.e. R–R interval = 0.75 seconds), there would be 15 images per cardiac cycle. The summed image would typically be collected from several hundred cardiac cycles. In this way 15 'frames' of a 'representative cine-cycle' (i.e. representative of the several hundred actual cycles which occupied the data collection period) are produced. Figure 8 shows an example of end-diastolic and end-systolic 'frames' of such a representative cine-cycle, obtained from the normal heart in the LAO view. The zone of decreased activity between the two ventricles is arrowed. The interrupted line indicates the outline of the left ventricular cavity. Comparison of the end-diastolic and end-systolic ventricular boundaries permits the assessment of regional ventricular contractile performance. (In this example there is uniform contraction of those parts of the ventricular wall which are displayed in this view.) Figure 9 shows (a) end-systolic and (b) end-diastolic frames from a patient with congestive cardiomyopathy. There is uniformly reduced myocardial contraction.

Relative advantages and drawbacks of 'first-pass' and 'equilibrium' scintigraphic ventriculography

The first-pass procedure is superior to the equilibrium technique in the following ways:

1. Because of the temporal separation of right and left ventricular studies, it is possible to use the RAO view for the analysis of regional left ventricular function. This is the projection of choice for single plane contrast cine-angiography (where, of course, any view could be chosen).

2. The first-pass technique can also provide information on mean transit times between various sections of the circulation and it permits the production of indicator-dilution curves and of shunt ratios. Since absolute cardiac output (from which stroke volume is easily calculated) can be measured from the indicator dilution curves and since the ejection fraction is determined, the ventricular end-diastolic volume can easily be calculated from the equation which defines ejection fraction:

$$EF = \frac{SV}{EDV} \tag{3}$$

The end-diastolic volume (EDV) is easily calculated when the ejection fraction (EF) and the stroke volume (SV) are known.

3. The procedure is brief, the complete data being collected from the patient within a minute of the injection. This means that the procedure is less exacting for the patient and it is, of course, more likely that the heart rate will remain regular for a brief period than for a long period.

The equilibrium procedure is superior to the first-pass technique in two ways:

1. The injection technique is not critical since studies are undertaken only after a state of equilibrium is achieved in relation to intravascular radioactivity.

2. The technique allows sequential measurements of global and ventricular function to be obtained after a single tracer injection. For example, repeated measurements before, during, and after exercise, or before and after drug administration can be made

following the equilibration within the blood stream of a single administered isotope dose.

A combination of both procedures gives most information and this can easily be achieved using a non-diffusable marker (e.g. $^{99}Tc^m$-labelled red blood cells) for the first-pass technique so that the same tracer can be used for subsequent equilibrium studies.

Acknowledgement
The author wishes to acknowledge the help and expert advice of Dr H. J. Testa.

References
Willerson, J. T., Parkey, R. W., Buja, L. M., and Bonte, F. J. (1979). In *Nuclear cardiology*, (*Cardiovascular clinics*) (ed. J. T. Willerson). F. A. Davis, Philadelphia.
Wynne, J., Holman, B. L., and Lesch, M. (1978). Myocardial scintigraphy by infarct-avid radiotracers. *Prog. card. Dis.* **20**, 243–266.

Magnetic resonance imaging and spectroscopy

B. RAJAGOPALAN

Introduction
The physical principles of nuclear magnetic resonance were first demonstrated by Bloch and Purcell in 1946 and the technique has been extensively used in physics and chemistry since. In the last decade it has emerged as a novel non-invasive method for studying metabolism and anatomical structure in biological systems. Currently these methods can provide images of the human body similar to those produced by X-ray computed tomography (magnetic resonance imaging or MRI) as well as estimate levels of phosphorus metabolites in human tissues (magnetic resonance spectroscopy or MRS). MRI has been extensively used in the investigation of the nervous system and has proved to be clinically useful. Currently its usefulness in the study of the structure and function of the human heart is under clinical evaluation in several centres. Although spectroscopy has been successfully used in the study of the biochemistry of animal myocardium, its application to the human heart requires development of new techniques.

Physical principles
Certain atomic nuclei, such as hydrogen, phosphorus, and sodium, behave as tiny bar magnets spinning along their axes. If samples of such nuclei (such as water in the case of H) are placed in a powerful magnetic field within a magnet (conventionally known as the B_0 field), the 'magnets' align themselves along the axis of this B_0 field. Unlike conventional bar magnets, due to quantum mechanical principles, some of the nuclear magnets line up spinning parallel and the rest antiparallel to the imposed field. The difference between these two populations is typically 1 in 10^4. This net difference can be visualized as a tiny bar magnet spinning around the axis of the B_0 field. This magnetic property of the sample can be detected by applying a brief radiofrequency pulse (of the order of ms or less) at right angles to the B_0 field. This pulse acts as a magnetic field (known as the B_1 field) and tips the nuclear magnets to a plane at right angles to the original field. (The B_0 field is conventionally labelled the z-axis so that the nuclei now spin in the xy plane.) These spinning magnets can be detected by measuring the sinusoidal voltage they induce in a coil of wire placed near a sample (just as in a dynamo). This voltage is transformed by the mathematical technique of Fourier transform to a peak which has a magnitude (the height) and frequency (x-axis).

The magnitude of the voltage is proportional to the concentration of the nuclei. The rate at which the nuclear magnets spin is uniquely determined by the chemical species and the strength of the magnetic field. Thus, in a magnet 1.9 T in strength, (the earth's magnetic field is 5×10^{-5} T), protons spin at 80.5 MHz and phosphorus at 32.5 MHz. At 0.1 T protons spin at 4.3 MHz and phosphorus at 1.7 MHz. The rate of spin is a very sensitive index of the exact magnetic field experienced by the nucleus and is influenced by the chemical environments of individual nuclei in a molecule. Thus, the frequencies of spin of γ, α, and β phosphates of ATP are of the order of 160 Hz and 300 Hz apart at 1.9 T. At 0.1 T, the differences in frequencies are only of the order of 10–15 Hz. Thus, to resolve the phosphates of ATP, higher magnetic fields (1.5 T or greater) are necessary to obtain a signal from one species only. For just hydrogen in tissues much lower fields are adequate.

The signal generated in the xy plane by the nuclear magnets will die away as the B_1 field is turned off due to mechanisms known as relaxation. The magnet we imagine to be generating the signal in the xy plane is clearly made up of many individual nuclear magnets. Due to inhomogeneities in the magnetic field in the sample, and differences in its chemical environment, as well as flow and diffusion of nuclei, individual nuclear magnets will spin at slightly different frequencies. The single magnet envisaged earlier slowly changes into many small nuclear magnets spread around the xy plane like the spokes of a wheel. The net signal decreases to zero. This is known as spin–spin relaxation and is measured by the relaxation time T2.

At the same time, as the B_1 field was applied only briefly, the nuclear magnets will slowly return to the axis of the B_0 field and no longer produce a voltage in the coil. This is known as spin lattice relaxation and is measured by T1. Thus, the magnetic resonance experiment can give information about the concentration, chemical environments, and relaxation properties of nuclei such as hydrogen or phosphorus. Specific nuclei can be chosen for study as nuclei only respond when the B_1 field is of about the same frequency as the resonant frequency of a nuclei at the given B_0 field.

The strength of the nuclear magnets which can be studied is only 1 part in 10^4 of the total concentration, so that magnetic resonance is an inherently insensitive technique. This is less of a problem when hydrogen in tissues is the issue as the effective concentration of protons is 110 M. Phosphorus metabolities are only present in mM concentrations so that signal averaging over minutes is required to obtain adequate signal in relation to 'noise'.

Magnetic resonance imaging
The dependence of the frequency of spins on magnetic fields is of practical value as it can be used to determine the spatial distribution of nuclear magnets. For example, if during the collection of signal from the sample, a linearly increasing magnetic field is applied along the x-axis, the frequency of spins will increase with distance. The amplitude of signal will be proportional to the concentration so that the map of concentration of the nuclei in slices along the x-axis can be obtained. By repeating the measurements with gradients along different axes, a two-dimensional map of concentrations can be calculated by methods such as those used in computerized tomography scanners. Currently most imaging systems use a technique known as two-dimensional Fourier transformation to generate the images. In general, to obtain a two-dimensional image containing n times n picture elements (pixels), n^2 pieces of information or data blocks are required. By repeating the process along different axes a three-dimensional image can be constructed. The acquisition of data can be triggered by the electrocardiogram so that end-diastolic, end-systolic, and images in between of the heart can be obtained.

Most current imaging systems produce images 128×128 pixels in size, so that resolution of less than 2 mm can be obtained in less than 20 min. These images clearly represent the density of protons in different points in space in the volume under investigation. As discussed earlier, the relaxation times also affect the signal. There is a correlation between water content and T1 so that oedematous tissues have prolonged T1 times. In acute haemorrhage T1 is

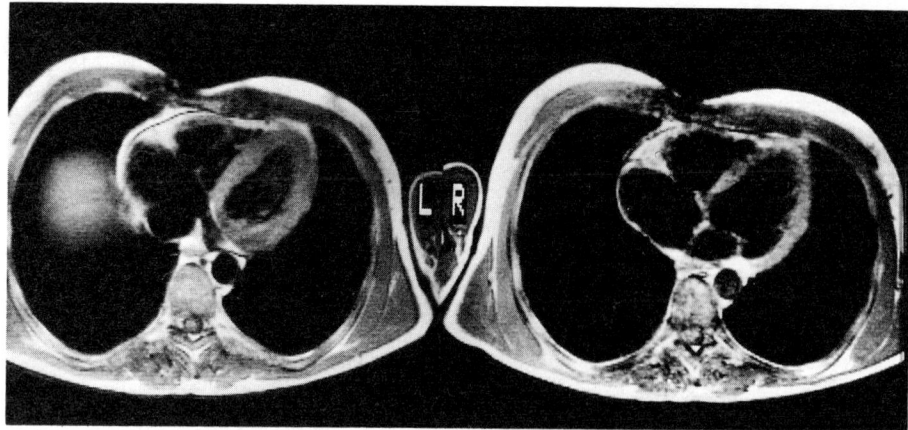

Fig. 1 Images of transverse sections of an adult human heart obtained in systole (left) and diastole (right) by magnetic resonance imaging techniques. (Figure reproduced by kind permission of Dr P. van Dijk and Philips Medical Systems.)

reduced while T2 may be normal or long. With time, both T1 and T2 increase in an infarcted zone. Thus the potential of MRI compared to other forms of imaging is that it is possible to obtain images which contain information about the distribution of T1 and T2, which are related to physiological and pathological changes. By altering the way in which the B_1 radiofrequency is applied, the images can be weighted so that they are more affected either by T1 or T2 so that specific information about the proton density or T1 or T2 can be obtained. Thus images obtained using a sequence of pulses called 'saturation recovery' reflect proton density. Inversion recovery sequences highlight T1 changes whilst an echo image shows changes in T2. As T2 is also affected by flow, it may be possible to measure blood flow by using appropriate pulse sequences. Preliminary data indicate that this may be practical in humans. Currently, the interpretation of images obtained using different frequencies is still empirical though with experience it should be possible to interpret these changes in terms of chemical environments and perhaps function. Certain paramagnetic ions cause changes in relaxation times and have been used as contrast agents. Gadolinium, for example, reduces relaxation times and after an intravenous injection can demonstrate regions of reduced myocardial perfusion in animals.

Clinical results

Images of the human heart showing remarkable detail have been obtained using MRI. A sequence of end-diastolic and end-systolic images from one such imaging system are shown in Fig. l. The images were reconstructed from MR image slices of the chest. By obtaining images throughout the cardiac cycle, a cineangiogram showing regional wall motion can be constructed.

Calibration of distances is relatively easy in magnetic resonance. Several groups have now demonstrated that stroke volumes, end-diastolic and end-systolic volumes, and regional wall motion can be accurately measured. Studies in phantoms suggest that these measurements are likely to be very good estimates of the true dimensions of the heart *in vivo*.

Preliminary studies after acute myocardial infarction in humans show that thinning of the abnormal myocardium is an early sign of damage as demonstrated in animal experiments. As predicted earlier, relaxation times have been shown to change as early as two hours after the onset of chest pain in myocardial infarction. What the optimum methods are for the differentiation of infarcted from normal and ischaemic myocardium, however, requires further research.

As the anatomy of the heart can be reconstructed in any plane from MRI data, myocardial hypertrophy and some congenital heart lesions have been successfully identified. The technique, however, has some limitations in that in small babies current resolution is inadequate to delineate complicated anatomy that may occur.

One of the early techniques of imaging which is also capable of

allowing real-time images of the heart to be obtained, known as echoplanar imaging, can produce an image of the heart in less than 35 ms. This technique is obviously suited for the study of small children with congenital heart disease as a complete image set can be generated in less than 5 min from which cross-sections, sagittal or coronal views can be reconstructed.

Experience of magnetic resonance imaging of the heart in clinical work is still anecdotal. More studies are required in the general population before the real potential and limitations of such imaging of the heart can be determined.

Magnetic resonance spectroscopy

Magnetic resonance can also provide information about the biochemistry of tissues including heart muscle. Current methods can be used to calculate relative concentrations of phosphocreatine, ATP, and inorganic phosphate as well as pH in a volume of cardiac muscle. Due to the low concentrations of phosphorus metabolites in tissues, information is currently only obtainable from a cylinder of muscle 5–6 cm in diameter, usually taking between 5 and 10 min. Animal studies in both open chest and intact animals suggest that it is possible to follow the biochemical changes of high energy phosphates following acute coronary occlusion. Though spectra of the human heart have been obtained non-invasively, there is no information as yet in pathological conditions. It is hoped that the technique can be extended in humans to allow the clinical investigation of the biochemical changes in both cardiomyopathies and ischaemic heart disease.

Safety of magnetic resonance measurements

A magnetic resonance examination requires the subject to lie in a static magnetic field and be subjected to both rapidly changing fields (the gradients used during imaging) and radiofrequency pulses.

The effect of static magnetic fields have been studied on enzyme systems, cell-suspensions, and animals. No mutagenic effects have been demonstrated in any experimental system, and no clearcut pathological abnormalities have been demonstrated in tissues of animals exposed to fields of up to 1.2 T. Physicists and technicians working in fields of up to 2 T in nuclear physics laboratories have not shown any demonstrable adverse effects. Clearly, however, follow-up studies are essential to exclude any small effects in the future.

The rapidly changing magnetic fields during imaging can induce currents in tissues which in theory could generate depolarization of cell membranes. The National Radiological Protection Board has advised that gradients should be less than 20 T/s. Calculations suggest that below this level, currents induced in muscle will be well below the threshold required to produce ventricular fibrillation in the heart.

The absorption of energy from radiofrequency pulses needed to generate the B_1 field can cause local heating. In most tissues, during imaging or phosphorus spectroscopy this is not a problem as the heat generated can be easily removed by blood flow and conduction. Current levels of radiofrequency power do not seem to have any pathological effects in humans. However, caution must be exercized in study of tissues with low or no blood flow such as the lens of the eye.

Magnetic fields affect pacemaker function at quite low levels. The behaviour of individual pacemakers in the magnetic field vary and current advice is that patients with pacemakers should not be studied in magnets.

The magnetic properties of metal prostheses are less clear. There is no standardization of the magnetic properties of prostheses. Many, such as artificial hips and orthopaedic pins, have been shown not be particularly magnetic *in vitro*. Patients with such implants have been imaged, but until further data is available it is prudent to be cautious in these cases. Surgeons use various forms of metal clips, for instance, in intracranial aneurysm surgery and it is possible that some of these are magnetic. A clip on an intracranial aneurysm could be subject to quite a significant force in a high magnetic field with the risk of twisting or even avulsion.

Thus, the main concern about safety in the NMR examinations at present is about magnetic objects in or around the patient but provided simple precautions are taken, there is considerable potential for the clinician to obtain new and unique information in disease.

Reference

Steiner, R. E. and Radda, G. K. (eds) (1984). Nuclear magnetic resonance and its clinical applications. *Br. Med. Bull.* **40**, no. 2.

Cardiac catheterization

G. A. H. MILLER

Introduction

From its early development in the 1940s cardiac catheterization has placed a powerful diagnostic tool in the hands of the cardiologist. Developments in cardiac surgery would not have been possible without the precision of diagnosis provided by this technique. At the same time catheterization has provided a yardstick against which the significance and accuracy of clinical and other diagnostic techniques could be checked, so that in many instances it has then been possible to dispense with catheterization. The indications for the investigation are constantly changing and differ from centre to centre and from country to country. At present by far the commonest reason for performing cardiac catheterization is the investigation of coronary artery disease (see section on coronary arteriography, page 13.162). Other indications of the investigation include valvular heart disease, congenital heart disease, and a miscellaneous group of acquired cardiac disease (aortic dissection, cardiomyopathy, etc).

The procedure involves the insertion of a long, hollow, radio-opaque tube (catheter) into an artery or vein and its manipulation within the heart and great vessels under fluoroscopic (X-ray) control. Vessels commonly used for the insertion of catheters include the antecubital vein and the brachial vein and artery in the arm and the saphenous and femoral vein and femoral artery in the leg. The vessels may be exposed by a 'cut-down' or may be entered percutaneously by passing the catheter over a guide-wire inserted through a needle. The use of an 'introducer' consisting of a guide wire, vessel dilator and thin-walled sheath permits percutaneous entry to the femoral artery and vein without the need for a cut-down and allows repeated use of the vessels. The sheath allows a variety of catheters to be inserted – including ones without an end-hole (angiographic catheters). Introducers may incorporate a one-way valve allowing arterial use or the introduction of catheters of varying sizes without blood loss. The availability of such intro-ducers has virtually eliminated the need for surgical exposure of the saphenous vein or femoral vessels in all but the smallest infants. In neonates and infants the axillary artery and vein may sometimes be used and the exposure of these vessels is surprisingly easy; naturally, meticulous repair is mandatory whenever an artery is opened by a cut-down. In adults local anaesthesia, with or without a light premedication, is all that is required. In infants and children the procedure may also be performed under sedation alone. Alternatively general anaesthesia with endotracheal intubation provides a more stable situation with better control of ventilation.

Manipulation of the catheter is achieved by causing its tip to impinge on the myocardium when further advancement will cause a loop to form. Rotation and either further advancement or withdrawal then allow the operator to manipulate the catheter tip to the desired site within the heart or great vessels. All catheter manipulation is performed under fluoroscopic control and with continuous monitoring of the electrocardiogram and of the pressure being recorded through the catheter tip. A change of pressure or wave form indicates to the operator that a new site has been entered within the heart.

There are many different types of catheter; each suitable for a particular purpose. For preliminary haemodynamic exploration of the heart a 'Goodale–Lubin' catheter with an end-hole and two side-holes is probably the most useful. Most catheters designed for angiography have a closed end and multiple, opposed side-holes to minimize recoil and movement during the high-pressure injection of contrast medium. Many catheters are pre-shaped for a particular purpose. Thus pre-shaped catheters make selective coronary arteriography a very simple procedure since they are designed to 'seek out' the coronary ostia. Balloon-tipped catheters (such as the 'Swan-Ganz') which are carried forward by the blood stream may permit entry to otherwise inaccessible sites as well as providing the facility for bed-side catheterization and wedge pressure monitoring without fluoroscopic control. Other catheters have been designed for therapeutic purposes. Thus, in complete transposition of the great arteries mixing is improved and survival ensured by the use of a balloon-tipped catheter which is pulled back across the foramen ovale to create an atrial septal defect ('balloon atrial septostomy'). Recently it has been shown that pulmonary and aortic valvotomy and dilation of coarctations and other stenotic lesions can be achieved by the forcible inflation of suitable balloon catheters during catheterization. Such varied balloon procedures have become increasingly common following their successful use in dilating stenotic coronary artery lesions (percutaneous transluminal coronary angioplasty, PTCA). Further developments can be expected in this field which allows surgery to be avoided or postponed in many cases of congenital as well as acquired heart disease.

The right atrium is entered from the superior or inferior vena cava, and the right ventricle and pulmonary artery entered by advancing the catheter anterogradely through the tricuspid and pulmonary valves. The left heart may be entered if the catheter crosses a patent foramen ovale or atrial septal defect and this is more easily achieved from the inferior vena cava. Alternatively the left heart may be entered by advancing the catheter from an artery so that it crosses the aortic valve in retrograde fashion. Other techniques for entering the left side of the heart include direct puncture of the left ventricle from its apex, and 'transseptal puncture' in which a long needle advanced from the femoral vein is used to puncture the atrial septum and the catheter is advanced over this needle so as to enter the left atrium and ventricle. In most cases an adequate record of left atrial pressure can be obtained by advancing a catheter through the pulmonary artery until it 'wedges' in a branch of the pulmonary artery, thus stopping all flow through a segment of the pulmonary circulation. At this moment the pressure being transmitted changes from a pulmonary arterial pressure to a pressure and wave form which closely reflects left atrial pressure: the so-called 'wedge-pressure'.

Techniques

Three techniques are employed to obtain diagnostic information.

1. Measurement of the pressure at the catheter tip transmitted to an external manometer (strain-gauge transducer). Where high fidelity pressure records are required, a special catheter may be used which has a miniature pressure manometer mounted at its tip. Pressure records obtained with such catheter-tip manometers avoid the artefact caused by motion of the long column of fluid contained within the catheter in conventional recording using an external manometer.

2. The measurement of oxygen saturation of samples drawn through the catheter from selected sites within the heart and great vessels. Oxygen saturation of such samples is usually measured colorimetrically using a photo-cell and filters sensitive to red/blue (oximetry).

3. The injection of a radio-opaque contrast medium through the catheter into selected sites within the heart or great vessels (selective angiocardiography).

Many other techniques have been developed (e.g. indicator dilution techniques) but these three procedures are all that are required to obtain a diagnosis in the majority of cases.

Pressure measurement

Diagnostic information is obtained from intracardiac pressure recording in three ways (Fig. 1).

1. Wave form. This allows the operator to identify the chamber that the catheter is in (atrium, ventricle, or artery). Abnormalities

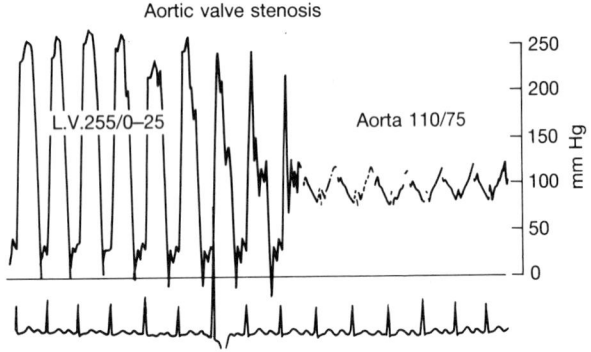

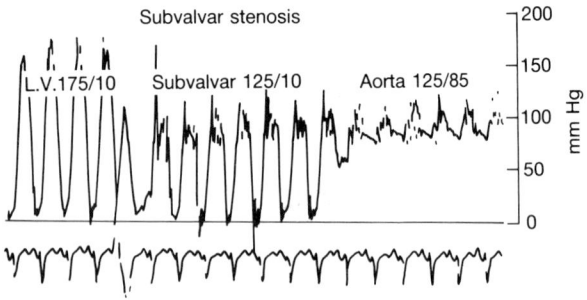

Fig. 1 Diagnostic use of pressure measurement. In the upper panel the record was made while the catheter was being withdrawn from the cavity of the left ventricle to the aorta. There is a fall in pressure (gradient) at the moment when the wave form changes from a ventricular pressure (low diastolic) to an arterial pressure. Thus the site of obstruction is located at the level of the aortic valve and the severity is indicated by the abnormally high left ventricular pressure and the pressure gradient. In the lower panel the same procedure was followed (in a different patient). The fall in pressure (gradient) occurs at a time when the wave form is still ventricular in character, indicating that the site of obstruction is within the ventricular cavity (suvalvar stenosis).

of wave form may give diagnostic information: for example the large 'v' wave of atrioventricular valve regurgitation.

2. Absolute magnitude of the recorded pressure; for example the elevated right ventricular and pulmonary artery pressure in pulmonary hypertension.

3. Comparison between the pressures at two sites – pressure 'gradients': for example the high right ventricular and low pulmonary artery pressure in pulmonary valve stenosis.

Measurement of oxygen saturation

This provides information in two ways.

1. The site at which an increase in oxygen saturation is detected in the right side of the heart (or a decrease in the left side) provides evidence about the presence and site of an intracardiac communication (e.g. atrial or ventricular septal defect, patent ductus arteriosus, etc.).

2. By measuring the oxygen content of blood entering and leaving the pulmonary or systemic circulation and knowing the simultaneous oxygen consumption, the flow in the two circulations can be measured. This, the direct 'Fick' principle is expressed as:

$$\text{Cardiac output} = \frac{\text{Oxygen consumption}}{\text{Arteriovenous oxygen difference}}$$

Where the pulmonary and systemic flows are different (due to a left-to-right or right-to-left shunt) the difference between the two flows is a measure of shunt size.

By combining the measurement of pressure and flow it is possible to calculate the 'resistance' to flow through the (pulmonary) circulation using the relationship:

$$R \text{ (resistance)} = P \text{ (pressure)}/Q \text{ (flow)}$$

The expression $R = P/Q$ may be modified to give a measure of the resistance to flow due to the pulmonary vascular tree: the so-called 'pulmonary arteriolar resistance' (Rp_a). The expression is modified:

$$Rp_a = Pp_a - Pl_a/Qp$$

where Pp_a is the mean pulmonary artery pressure, Pl_a is the mean left atrial (or 'wedge') pressure, and Qp is the pulmonary flow.

Selective angiocardiography

A mechanically driven injection syringe is used to force a relatively large volume of radio-opaque contrast medium through the catheter and into the appropriate site within the heart or great vessels. 35 mm cine-film recording is usually employed at a frame speed of up to 50 c.p.s. and analysis of the films provides iinformation of two kinds (Fig. 2).

Anatomical The contrast medium outlines the structure of the heart and, with appropriate projections, outlines structural abnormalities.

Physiological An angiocardiogram is, in effect, an indicator dilution (time/concentration) curve and provides similar information. Thus when contrast injected distal to a valve appears in the chamber proximal to that valve, there is evidence of valvar regurgitation. The severity of regurgitation can be estimated from the density and speed of opacification of the proximal chamber.

Since the size of a vessel or cardiac chamber is proportional to the flow through it, the outlining of vessel or chamber size by radio-opaque contrast also provides 'haemodynamic' information: an estimate of the volume load (e.g. shunt size) affecting that chamber or vessel.

Angiocardiography requires sophisticated and expensive radiological equipment. A high quality image-intensification system is required which must be capable of both being rotated around the patient and being angulated in a second plane at the same time so as to provide multiple projections of cardiac structures. For the examination of complex congenital anomalies a second image-

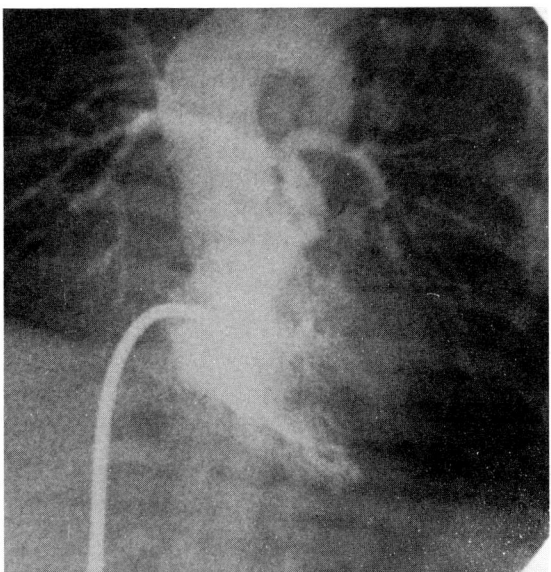

Fig. 2 Angiocardiography. Single frame from 35 mm cine film. Antero-posterior projection. Radio-opaque contrast medium has been injected into the right ventricle in a patient with tetralogy of Fallot. The narrowed right ventricular outflow tract (infundibular stenosis) and small pulmonary arteries are seen. The aorta has also filled with contrast indicating the presence of a ventricular septal defect and right-to-left shunting.

intensification system is required to provide simultaneous filming in two projections.

Recently computer techniques for image enhancement have been applied to angiography – digital subtraction angiography (DSA). Where there is no movement of the structure being imaged (as in carotid arteriography) these techniques allow excellent visualization following injection of contrast medium into a peripheral vein. It remains to be seen how useful such techniques will be when applied to the moving heart.

Analysis of results

Pulmonary hypertension, in the sense that pulmonary artery pressure is abnormally high, provides a good example of the way in which data obtained at cardiac catheterization is analysed to provide an anatomical and physiological diagnosis. Pulmonary hypertension can result from three distinct mechanisms. (a) Downstream pressure (left atrial or pulmonary vein pressure) is elevated with a secondary elevation of pulmonary artery pressure to maintain a gradient across the pulmonary circulation. An example of this mechanism is provided by mitral valve stenosis. (b) There is obstruction to flow within the pulmonary circulation so that while downstream pressure is normal, the pulmonary artery pressure is raised to 'overcome' this obstruction. An example of this mechanism is provided by pulmonary vascular disease as in the 'Eisenmenger reaction'. (c) There is increased flow through the pulmonary circulation. An example of this mechanism is provided by a left-to-right shunting ventricular septal defect.

In each case the relationship between pressure, resistance, and flow can be used to describe the findings

$$Rp_a = Pp_a - Pl_a / Qp$$

(see above).

In the first instance the primary abnormality is an elevation of Pl_a, in the second is an elevation of Rp_a, and in the third it is an increase in Qp.

In our first example the finding of a high downstream pressure (usually measured as high 'wedge' pressure – see above) without an increased flow or resistance requires that we establish the cause of the high downstream pressure. If this is due to mitral valve stenosis there will be a pressure *gradient* between the left atrium and

ventricle during diastole. Alternatively the high left atrial pressure may be due to a high left ventricular filling pressure (end-diastolic pressure) due to a 'stiff' or non-compliant left ventricle. Again a cause has to be found for this. Possible causes would include left ventricular hypertrophy due to hypertension or aortic stenosis, or poor left ventricular function due to primary disease of the left ventricular myocardium. Poor left ventricular function can be demonstrated in a number of ways. Perhaps the simplest depends on the relationship between the end-diastolic volume of the ventricle and its stroke volume. In a normally functioning ventricle this is such that the ventricule ejects about 70 per cent of its end-diastolic volume at each beat: the so-called 'ejection fraction'. When left ventricular function is impaired, the end-diastolic volume rises and the ejection fraction falls. This can be measured by determining the volume of the ventricle from left ventricular angiograms, and is easily detected by eye. Other methods for determining left ventricular volumes and ejection fraction include echocardiography and indicator dilution techniques. Where the disease of the left ventricule is non-uniform, as in coronary artery disease, this too can be detected by analysis of the shape change of left ventricular angiograms during the cardiac cycle, and the cause of the abnormality confirmed by demonstrating the presence of coronary artery disease by coronary arteriography.

Other techniques for analysing left ventricular function include measurement of indices of function such as the rate of pressure rise of the ventricle or the acceleration of blood in the aorta. Both techniques require left heart catheterization. Left ventricular muscle can be biopsied at catheterization using a long, flexible biotome passed through a catheter sheath lying within the ventricle.

In the second example of pulmonary hypertension the finding of a high pulmonary artery pressure without an increased flow and with a normal downstream ('wedge') pressure indicates that there is obstruction to flow somewhere in the pulmonary circulation. This might have a simple mechanical cause such as pulmonary emboli which can be demonstrated angiographically. More commonly it is due to changes in the pulmonary arterioles: 'pulmonary vascular disease' (e.g. the Eisenmenger reaction, primary pulmonary hypertension, cor pulmonale). Where pulmonary vascular disease has resulted from a long-standing left-to-right shunt (the Eisenmenger reaction) the anatomical defect responsible may be identified, such as a ventricular septal defect. In this situation the degree and potential reversibility of the pulmonary vascular disease may have to be determined accurately to decide on the operability of the primary abnormality. Accurate measurement of pulmonary arteriolar resistance demands measurement of oxygen consumption (otherwise frequently assumed from tables of normal values). Techniques such as spirometry and mass-spectrometry exist in catheterization laboratories for this purpose.

Finally, in the third example of pulmonary hypertension due to a high flow, the site of the left-to-right shunt needs to be demonstrated.

Catheterization in congenital heart disease

Recent developments in two-dimensional echocardiography have revolutionized the diagnosis of congenital heart disease. In many cases it is now possible to dispense with catheterization altogether; in others the operator starts with a much clearer knowledge of the abnormal anatomy present than was previously the case. Nonetheless, catheterization is still frequently necessary. It may be required to confirm the anatomy suggested by echocardiography or to demonstrate or exclude additional lesions not clearly seen on the echocardiogram. It may be required for therapy, for example, balloon atrial septostomy, or it may be required to quantify shunt size or pulmonary arteriolar resistance. It is increasingly common for palliative surgery (e.g. aortopulmonary shunt in tetralogy of Fallot) to be performed in a sick neonate on the basis of the echocardiogram alone while reserving catheterization until complete correction is contemplated when the surgeon may need to know

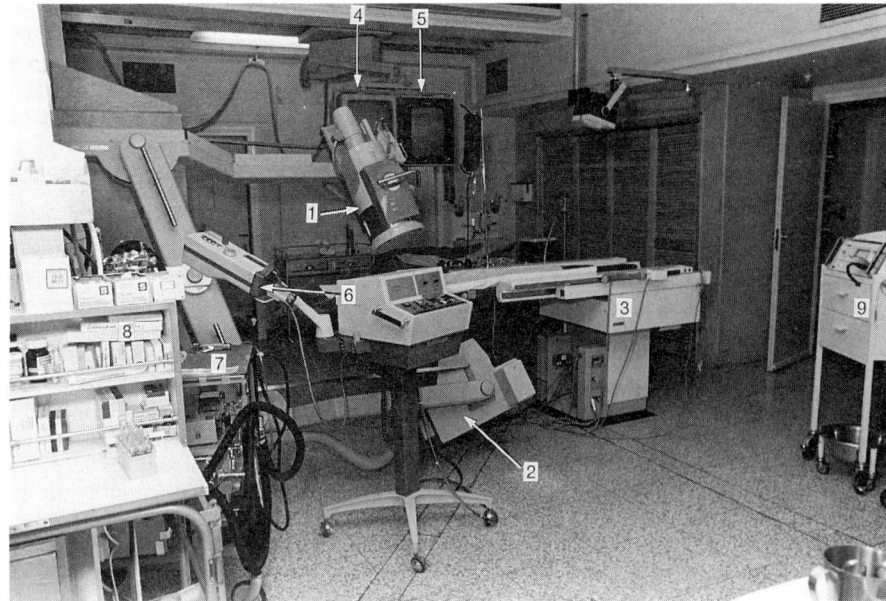

Fig. 3 A catheterization laboratory: (1) Image intensifer and cine camera mounted with the X-ray tube (2) so that it can be rotated and angulated; (3) moveable table for patient; (4) television monitor for display of fluoroscopic image, and (5) oscilloscope for display of ECG and intracardiac pressures; (6) injection syringe and controls for angiography; (7) anaesthetic trolley; (8) drugs for anaesthesia/resuscitation; (9) defibrillator.

the detailed anatomy (e.g. number and site of VSD(s), pulmonary artery size etc.).

Catheterization in cases of congenital heart disease requires that the operators possess particular skills; they must have considerable manipulative dexterity and complete familiarity with the discipline of paediatric cardiology and cardiac surgery so that they will recognize the abnormalities likely to be present and the answers that will be required for proper management. Catheterization in acquired heart disease in the adult is largely, and coronary arteriography almost entirely, a technical challenge. This is not so in congenital heart disease where there is a considerable additional intellectual challenge. In particular the operator must be able to 'think on his feet'. As catherization proceeds items of information are acquired (pressure, saturation, catheter position, and so on), each of which makes one set of diagnostic possibilities more likely and another less likely or impossible. These items of information will indicate which further pieces of information are required and which need be sought no longer. In this way the operator builds up an increasingly complete picture of the abnormalities present. The final stage is likely to be the performance of one, or several, angiocardiograms. Successful angiocardiography requires that the appropriate projections are used and appropriate volume of contrast medium injected. To profile the ventricular septum and visualize a ventricular septal defect requires that an angiographic projection combining a left oblique with craniocaudal tilt is used while the right ventricular outflow tract is best seen in the right oblique projection. Similarly, adequate opacification of a large, volume loaded ventricle (e.g. univentricular A/V connection with high pulmonary flow) requires 1.5 to 2.0 ml/kg of contrast medium to be injected – a volume that might well be fatal if injected into the minute right ventricle of a neonate with pulmonary atresia and intact ventricular septum. It follows that angiocardiography, though frequently providing most, or all, of the information required, tends to be performed at the end of the procedure when the haemodynamic findings have already provided a clear idea of the abnormalities present.

Cardiac catheterization in the neonate or infant carries a higher risk than catheterization in the adult. Much of this increased risk relates to the already poor condition of many patients with severe forms of congenital heart disease. It follows that the risk must be minimized by good precatheter preperation (or resuscitation). Of major importance is the use of E2 prostaglandins to dilate the ductus arteriosus in neonates with duct-dependent pulmonary or systemic circulations. Other measures include correction of acidosis,

hypoglycaemia, and hypothermia. Blood loss of small amounts can be significant in the small neonate and must be minimized by careful operative technique and the use of sampling techniques which require minimal amounts of blood (0.4 ml). Radio-opaque contrast media have adverse haemodynamic effects and the total volume given should probably not exceed 4.0 ml/kg. In the very sick neonate is is probably advisable to use one of the so-called non-ionic media. Although many centres perform catheterization under sedation alone it is the author's opinion that general anaesthesia with intubation and controlled ventilation is preferable, provided the services of a skilled anaesthetist are available. Such a policy avoids the dangers of hypoventilation liable to occur in a sedated infant and provides a stable haemodynamic situation easier to interpret than when the infant is alternating between crying and hypoventilation with consequent rise in pulmonary vascular resistance. Of greatest importance is the duration of the study; a prolonged study undoubtedly results in a worsened clinical state with hypothermia and hypoglycaemia contributing importantly. The duration of a study and the amount of catheter manipulation is reduced by clear and quick thinking as the procedure progresses as well as by manipulative skill. No study should take longer than an hour and the vast majority of cases of even the most complex congenital heart disease can be studied in far less time than this. No one should undertake cardiac catheterization unless fully trained or supervised, no laboratory should perform studies without full resuscitation and monitoring facilities and, most importantly, unless it can perform an adequate number of studies each year to maintain expertise and provide adequate experience for its staff – probably at least 50 to 1000 cases per year.

A catheterization laboratory (Fig. 3) is fully equipped with monitoring and resuscitation equipment with facilities for anaesthesia and endotracheal intubation, D/C countershock, and so on. The risks of catheterization in a properly equipped laboratory and in experienced hands should be very small. For adult patients the mortality should be less than 0.05 per cent, and even for sick neonates with complex congenital heart disease mortality should be well under 5.0 per cent.

Reference

Verel, D. and Grainger, R. D. (1978). *Cardiac catheterization and angiography* 3rd edn. Churchill Livingstone, Edinburgh.

Phonocardiography and mechanocardiography

H. KESTELOOT

Phonocardiography

Introduction

Phonocardiography (PCG) encompasses the graphic registration of heart sounds and murmurs in the frequency spectrum between 15 and 800 Hz. As the frequency content of the heart sounds and murmurs in this range has diagnostic significance, filter systems are used to divide the whole spectrum into a number of limited frequency bands. These filters are characterized by their high and low cut-off points delimiting the frequency range recorded, and by their attenuation properties outside the desired range. The attenuation varies in most cases between -12 and -24 decibel per octave. The normal frequencies of the recorded bands are generally 35, 70, 140, and 400 Hz.

The advantages of a phonocardiographic registration over auscultation are numerous:

1. PCG makes auscultation objective and permits sequential observations,

2. PCG allows the measurement of time intervals, for instance, A_2–P_2, Q–A_2, A_2–OS etc. Respiratory variation of the A_2–P_2 interval can also be measured accurately (A_2, P_2 represent the beginning of the high frequency components of the aortic and pulmonary components of the second heart sound; OS, opening snap; Q1, Q wave on ECG.)

3. The PCG can be recorded simultaneously with mechanocardiographic tracings, allowing the measurement of additional time intervals. A reversed splitting of the second heart sound can also be demonstrated by the relationship existing between the second sounds and the incisura of the carotid artery tracing.

4. It allows the study of the frequency content of heart sounds and murmurs together with an accurate assessment of their localization and morphology. In aortic and pulmonary stenosis, for instance, the later the maximum of the murmur in systole the more severe the disease. It demonstrates whether a murmur is pansystolic or not. The morphology of a murmur of infundibular pulmonary stenosis is different from that of valvular pulmonary stenosis.

5. It allows the recording of added sounds. For instance when the P–R interval is short or the first heart sound is barely audible, the differentiation between a split first heart sound and a presystolic gallop sound is often impossible by auscultation alone.

Heart sounds

The origin of heart sounds is still controversial. They are determined by several factors:

1. The abrupt halting of the movement of the valves
2. The arrested momentum of blood flow during valve closure or opening when the valve is stenotic
3. The speed of movement of the valves.

When the high frequency compounds (> 140 Hz) of the first and second heart sounds are recorded, there can be no doubt that the valve movement plays an important role in their genesis, as now documented by echocardiography. Abrupt distention of the aorta or pulmonary artery probably can also generate high frequency sounds, especially when they are dilated.

The first heart sound is often split, the first part coinciding with mitral closure, the second part with tricuspid closure. A third component can often be observed coinciding with the abrupt distention of the root of the aorta or pulmonary artery. An alternative theory explains this sound by an abrupt halting of the opening of the aortic or pulmonary valve.

The second heart sound has an aortic (A_2) and pulmonary (P_2) component coinciding with the closure of the respective valves in early diastole. The A_2–P_2 interval increases in pulmonary artery stenosis and the interval is proportional to the degree of stenosis. The A_2–P_2 interval is independent of respiration in patients with a large atrial septal defect.

Ejection clicks can be recorded in cases of valvular aortic and pulmonary stenosis due to sudden arrest of the opening movement of the valve due to the stenosis. They do not occur when valvular movement is very restricted, as in calcific aortic stenosis.

Mid-systolic clicks are often recorded in the syndrome due to valvular prolapse called the 'mid-systolic click-telesystolic murmur syndrome'. The click is probably caused by an abrupt arrest of the movement of the prolapsed valve.

Opening snaps (OS) occur in early diastole in mitral and tricuspid stenosis. The shorter the distance A_2–OS, the more severe the stenosis. They are absent when valvular movement is severely impaired as in calcific stenosis. Normal valves can cause opening snaps whenever the surface of the valve is enlarged and the opening is very abrupt due to a large flow over the valve. This is often the case for the tricuspid valve in the presence of large atrial septal defects.

The fourth heart sound is a low frequency sound (<35 Hz) with a presystolic localization. It occurs whenever the compliance of the ventricle is reduced and the speed of atrial contraction is high. More details on the origin and importance of this are given in the section on mechanocardiography. In younger people normal hearts can also generate fourth heart sounds.

The third heart sound occurs in early diastole and is due to a rapid filling of the left ventricle as occurs in severe mitral insufficiency. Speed of relaxation of the ventricle and myocardial compliance also play a role. A third heart sound occurs whenever an important viscoelastic element is present in early relaxation causing a rapid increase in early diastolic pressure which is coincident with a rapid decrease in ventricular inflow. It also occurs simultaneously with a reversal of the atrioventricular pressure gradient in early diastole. In younger subjects a physiological third heart sound is often present.

Heart murmurs

Pansystolic murmurs occur whenever a gradient is present throughout systole as in ventricular septal defects with low right ventricular pressure or in mitral and tricuspid regurgitation. They are normally of high frequency. When the left atrium is small and the mitral regurgitation large as in rupture of chordae tendineae, the murmur may not be pansystolic (Fig. 1).

Ejection murmurs are of low to medium frequency and often diamond shaped. They occur in aortic and pulmonary artery stenosis. A purely mid-systolic murmur is typical of infundibular hypertrophic aortic stenosis.

Telesystolic murmurs are a sign of a mitral valve prolapse accompanied by a slight mitral insufficiency.

Physiological murmurs often occur in younger subjects, especially when their cardiac output is high. They are of the ejection type, occur early in systole, practically always lasting less than 100 ms, and less than half of systole.

Diastolic murmurs can be of high frequency, as in aortic insufficiency where they start close to A_2, or low frequency diastolic rumbles, as in mitral and tricuspid valve stenosis. Short diastolic rumbles can be recorded when the flow over normal A–V valves is high as in atrial or ventricular septal defects, or in severe mitral regurgitation.

Continuous murmurs can be recorded whenever a systolic–diastolic pressure gradient exists as in cases with an open ductus with low pressure in the pulmonary artery or in arterio-venous shunts.

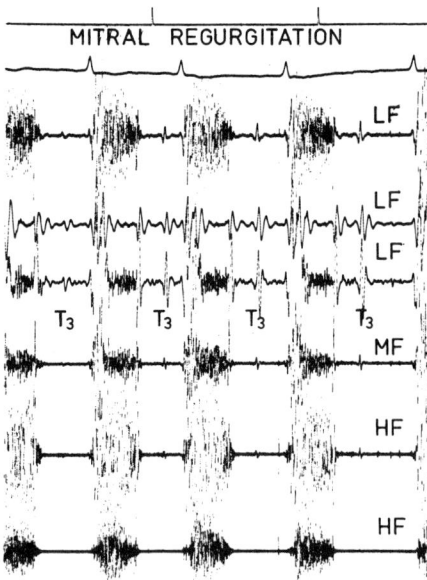

Fig. 1 Pansystolic murmur due to mitral regurgitation in the presence of atrial fibrillation. Low (LF), middle (MF), and high frequency (HF) filters are used. A third heart sound is present in the LF and MF tracings but invisible in the HF tracing. The high-frequency murmur is invisible in LF tracing with the lowest pass filter (second tracing).

Vascular murmurs (bruits)

Bruits can also be recorded over *peripheral arteries* whenever they are stenotic. When the stenosis is severe a systolic–diastolic pressure gradient will exist over the stenosis and the murmur will continue into diastole. The recording of these murmurs may thus allow an evaluation of the severity of the stenosis. When the murmur is short and only heard in early systole, the stenosis is not haemodynamically important. In the limbs, stenotic murmurs are greatly accentuated by exercise. Physiological vascular murmurs can be recorded particularly over the carotid arteries in young subjects; they can be loud but are always of short duration (100 ms and less than half of the systole).

Mechanocardiography

Introduction

The term mechanocardiography describes external, atraumatic recordings of all low-frequency pulsations due to the mechanical action of the heart. Recordings are made both for diagnostic purposes and for the determination of the severity of the underlying heart disease. The importance of mechanocardiography has increased since the demonstration that intracardiac or intravascular pressures are the major determinants of the time course and morphology of apexcardiograms, and of carotid artery and jugular venous pulse tracings. A major advantage of the method is that the examination can be repeated at will, with a minimum of inconvenience for the patient. The cost of the examination is low and the recordings can be made by trained technicians.

Historically the names of Chauveau (1855), Marey (1860), Garrod (1871), Mackenzie (1901), and Blumberger (1940) are connected with the development of the method.

Methodology

Until recently only uncalibrated methods have been used. In most cases the capsule of Marey was connected by air transmission via rubber tubing to a piezo-electric transducer. Good tracings can be obtained by this method as long as the time constant is more than 1.5 s and preferably more than 3 s (thus limiting the phase shifts

due to the time constant) and as long as the tubing length is not more than 30 cm in order to limit the delay time due to air transmission. Transducers with an infinite time constant are now also available at low cost. These tracings can be used for diagnostic purposes, for the measurement of time intervals (e.g. with the phonocardiogram and electrocardiogram) and for morphologic interpretation.

Calibrated methods have now been introduced allowing a quantitative interpretation. Essentially two methods have been used. In the first, a rubber membrane covers a water-filled chamber connected via a water-filled catheter to a pressure transducer. The chamber is pressed on the thoracic surface at the site of the apex beat until maximum amplitude of the tracing is obtained. The recorded pressure is measured directly in mm Hg. The quality of the tracings obtained by this method is often not optimal and resonance can to a certain extent deform the tracings. Another method consists of measuring the displacement of the chest wall due to the action of the heart, by measuring pressure changes in an applied air chamber. The resulting signal is then calibrated by electronic means. Thus an index is obtained, similar to $dp/dt/p$, which will be discussed later.

The electronic signal can also be calibrated in mm^3 displaced by means of a volume calibrating device. Fundamentally the first method records the pressure changes obtained on the thoracic wall due to the action of the heart, while the second measures the apical displacement. In most cases the tracings obtained are very similar. The major advantage of the displacement method is that it allows the recording of all mechanocardiographic tracings while the pressure method is essentially only suitable for the recording of the apexcardiogram. New pressure transducers are being developed; the most promising is a pixie-beam transducer. By appropriate filtering, the phonocardiogram can also be obtained from these transducers and from the rim of the device a precordial electrocardiogram can be recorded.

The different mechanocardiographic tracings which are of value for the clinician will now be reviewed.

The jugular venous pulse tracing

The jugular venous pulse tracing (JVPT) is one of the forgotten tools of cardiology and does not receive the attention it merits. The JVPT is optimally recorded in the subclavicular region, just lateral to the point of attachment of the sternocleidomastoid muscle. The great importance of the JVPT lies in the fact that it is very similar in morphology to the pressure tracing obtained from the right atrium and identical to the pressure obtained in the jugular vein existing at the site of the recording. It has, however, an important delay due to the transmission time of the pressure wave in the superior caval vein. The most important determinants of the transmission time and of the morphological differences are:

1. The distance between the right atrium and the site of registration
2. The elasticity of the veins
3. The inertia (and mass) of the blood column between right atrium and recording site
4. The direction of the flow in the superior vena caval vein at each moment
5. The fundamental frequency of each component of the pulse tracing (the lower the frequency, the greater the transmission time).

The a, v, and h waves have a mean transmission time of 40–60 ms and the x and y depression of 50–80 ms. As a result of this variable delay the JVPT cannot be used as a reference tracing for the phonocardiogram. The morphology of the JVPT is determined by the difference between the amount of blood arriving and leaving the site of the recording; a horizontal line thus can mean that an equal amount is arriving and leaving the place of recording or that no change is taking place.

The JVPT consists of a, v, c, and h waves and an x and y

depression. Calibration of the JVPT is still not used although much information is present in the speed of rise and decline of its different waves.

The *a wave* is due to right atrial contraction. Its height is essentially determined by the amount of resistance to filling of the right ventricle. This resistance is increased by disorders of the right ventricle. Left ventricular hypertrophy can, by encroachment, reduce the volume of the right ventricle resulting in an increased resistance to filling of this ventricle (the Bernheim effect). The resistance is also increased in tricuspid stenosis and during extrasystoles with atrioventricular conduction defects where the atrium contracts against closed atrioventricular valves. The height of the a wave is thus not an indicator of the contractility of the right atrium. Even with an increased contractility, the a wave may be small if ventricular compliance is high as in atrial septal defect or tricuspid insufficiency without pulmonary hypertension. A high and rapidly increasing a wave is always present whenever a right-sided fourth heart sound is recorded.

The *v wave* is recorded during the filling of the right atrium at the time the a–v valves are closed by ventricular contraction. The localization of the summit of the v wave is influenced by the isovolumetric relaxation of the right ventricle, probably by causing a slight depression of the level of the A–V valve during this period. After the summit, a rapid descent is often visible and this is due to the opening of the A–V valves. Due to dampening and time-lag, however, this phenomenon cannot be used to determine the exact moment of the opening of the right A–V valve in early diastole. This time-lag, however, still permits a differentiation between high right ventricular pressure due to pulmonary hypertension or to pulmonary stenosis. In pulmonary hypertension the time interval between the summit of the v wave and P_2 is 80–120 ms, while in pulmonary stenosis it is 10–30 ms, and in normal subjects about 60 ms. This disparity is due to the differences existing between the height of the right atrial pressure and the pulmonary artery pressure at the time of P_2 in these different conditions.

The *c wave* is nearly always due to a transmission of the pulsation of the carotid artery. It can also partially be due to a bulging of the A–V valves into the right atrium during isovolumetric right ventricular contraction.

The *h wave* records the end of the ascending limb of the y depression. It signals the end of the rapid passive filling of the right ventricle. It can only be seen in normal subjects when the heart rate is below 60 beats/min.

The *x depression* is largely due to atrial relaxation. At the end of atrial contraction, atrial pressure is at its lowest level. As a result of the elasticity of the ventricular wall, blood will be moved towards the atrium and thus contribute to the closure of the A–V valves. The higher the a wave, the deeper the x depression, because the more blood is moved by the atrial contraction, the lower the pressure will be within a given length–tension relation. The lowering of the level of the A–V valves during ventricular contraction is of minor importance in the genesis of the x depression, which is absent or barely present in cases of atrial fibrillation.

The *y depression* is due to the emptying of the atrium during ventricular diastole. Its depth is determined by the resistance to filling of the ventricle. All diseases influencing the diastolic compliance of the right ventricle will thus influence the depth of the y depression. The higher the resistance to filling, the smaller the y depression which is nearly always absent in cases of tricuspid stenosis. Left ventricular hypertrophy, by means of the Bernheim effect, can also reduce the depth of the y trough.

The normal jugular venous pulse tracing

In the normal JVPT the a wave is always the highest wave, while the x descent is always deeper than the y descent. The normal P_2-summit v wave time interval is 56 ± 12 ms and the normal mean Q–h interval is 740 ms (Figs. 2 and 3). The ratio of the summit of the a wave to the summit of the v wave, measured from the nadir

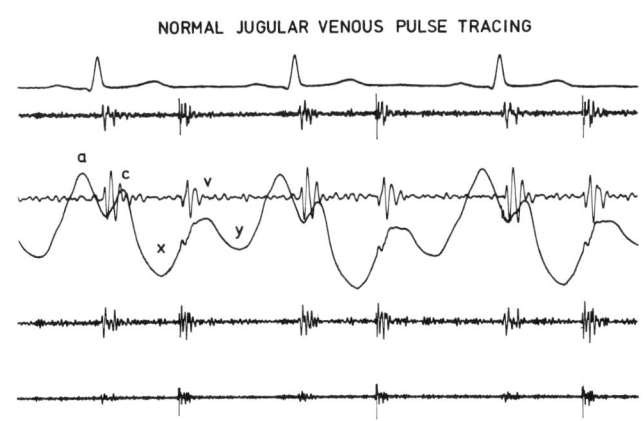

Fig. 2 Normal jugular venous pulse tracing. The a wave is the highest wave and the x depression is deeper than the y depression.

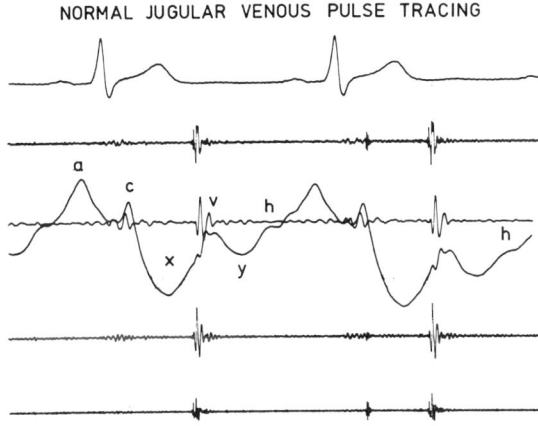

Fig. 3 Normal jugular venous pulse tracing. Due to the slow heart rate the h wave is visible.

of the x depression, is 1.8 ± 0.32. A pronounced c wave and a nadir of the x depression close to the aortic component of the second sound are signs of carotid contamination of the JVPT. Only in subjects with pectus excavatum and normal hearts can the y depression be deeper than the x depression.

The JVPT in specific cardiac diseases will now be discussed.

Right ventricular hypertrophy

In right ventricular hypertrophy due to systolic overload, right ventricular compliance is low, resulting in a dominant a wave followed by a marked x depression and a shallow y depression. The typical morphological change in the JVPT occurs whatever the origin of the hypertrophy might be (Fig. 4). The distance of the summit of the v wave to P_2, however, is significantly shorter in cases with pulmonary hypertension and this time interval depends on the height of the early diastolic pulmonary artery pressure. When the right ventricular hypertrophy is due to volume overload, compliance is high. In atrial septal defect the JVPT is either within normal limits or the v wave is higher than normal due to an increased right atrial filling during ventricular systole.

Bernheim effect

The morphologic changes of the Bernheim effect in the JVPT are due to a reduction of right ventricular dimensions as a consequence of left ventricular hypertrophy which causes the septum to bulge into the right ventricle. This reduces the compliance of the right ventricle and results in a JVPT which is very similar to that of right ventricular hypertrophy due to systolic overload with a high a wave, a deep x depression and a shallow y depression.

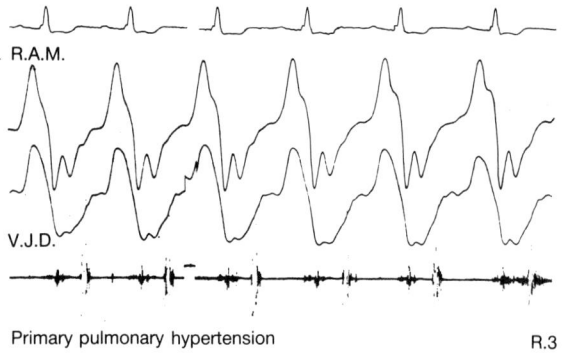

Fig. 4 Simultaneous recording of the jugular venous pulse tracing (JVPT) and right atrial pressure in right ventricular hypertrophy. Note the similarity between the two tracings (see text).

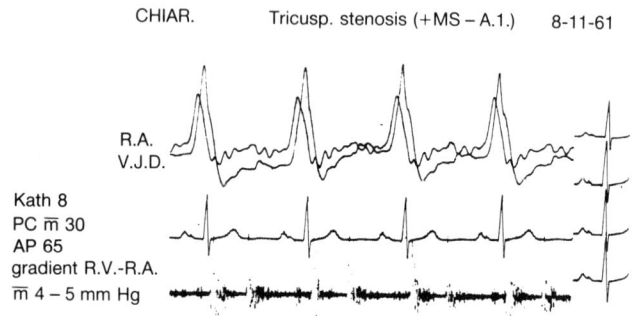

Fig. 5 Simultaneous recording of the jugular venous pulse tracing and right atrial pressure in tricuspid stenosis. Note the similarity between the two tracings (see text).

Tricuspid stenosis

In sinus rhythm the morphology of the JVPT is very similar to that of right ventricular hypertrophy of the systolic type. The a wave is then by far the dominant wave (Fig. 5). Diagnosis, is more difficult in cases with atrial fibrillation. Due to a slow emptying of the atrium in diastole, the q–h time interval is markedly increased and in most cases exceeds 1000 ms. This can only be established if the R–R interval is sufficiently long. This increase also exists in cases of combined tricuspid stenosis and regurgitation (Fig. 5).

Tricuspid regurgitation

In sinus rhythm the y depression is always the deepest depression and the v wave is in most cases the highest wave except in cases where a high a wave co-exists due to right ventricular concentric hypertrophy. In severe cases the x depression is completely absent and is replaced by a systolic square wave (Fig. 6). The higher the systolic pressure in the right atrium, the shorter the distance P_2-summit v wave (Fig. 6).

In atrial fibrillation the diagnosis of tricuspid insufficiency is made whenever the systolic wave exceeds the telediastolic level, and the 'c' wave can be replaced by a j wave which occurs somewhat earlier and is higher than the normal c wave. This wave also occurs during ventricular extrasystoles and is due to the failure of the A–V valves to close at the start of ventricular contraction in these two conditions. The presence of a j wave is thus not a reliable sign of tricuspid regurgitation.

During rapid heart rates it is often not possible to discern clinically between the rising limb of the y depression and a systolic wave due to tricuspid regurgitation. Only a recording after a longer diastolic interval will allow the differentiation. In atrial flutter and even atrial fibrillation, effective atrial contractions can still occur and during systole they may mimic tricuspid regurgitation. Careful inspection will reveal the relationship between the systolic waves and the flutter waves.

Constrictive pericarditis

The dominant feature of the JVPT in this disease is the steep and narrow y depression which is often nearly symmetrical. The q–h distance is less than 600 ms. The shorter the q–h interval, the higher the mean right atrial pressure. Constrictive *epicarditis*, however, results in a completely different morphology of the JVPT which then resembles the tracings obtained in right ventricular concentric hypertrophy. This difference is because early filling is unimpeded in constrictive pericarditis while early diastolic compliance is low in epicarditis. The JVPT in cases of constrictive pericarditis, complicated by pericardial effusion, may simulate constrictive epicarditis.

Apexcardiogram

Interest in the left apexcardiogram (LAC) is increasing as evidence accumulates that intraventricular pressure is one of its major determinants (Fig. 7). This concept originated when the morphology of the right apexcardiogram (RAC) and of the simultaneously recorded right ventricular pressure (RVP) were compared and found to be closely related. Moreover, it has been shown that during arrhythmias the percentual surface of RAC and RVP during systole, which for both corresponds to a pressure–time index, correlate highly significantly. Calibrated apexcardiography (QLAC) has shown that the LAC is well suited for the timing of intracardiac events especially for the determination of the point of the start of the pressure rise in the left ventricle.

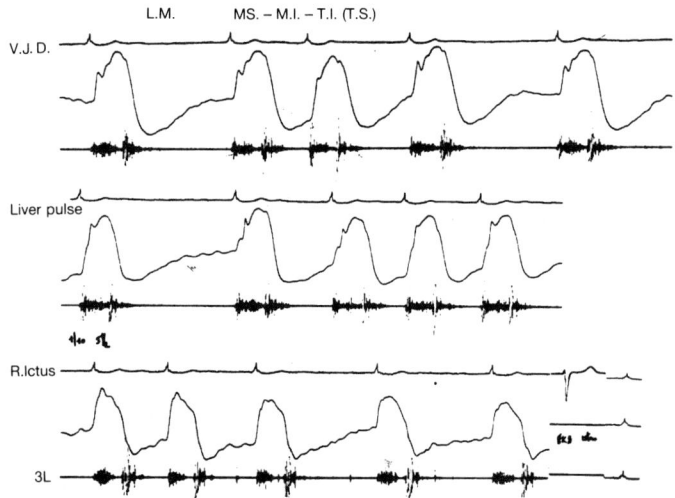

Fig. 6 Severe tricuspid regurgitation. Recording of the jugular venous pulse and the right apexcardiogram. All tracings are very similar and the right apexcardiogram could be due to systolic right auricular dilation. The q–H interval is prolonged due to relative tricuspid stenosis (see text).

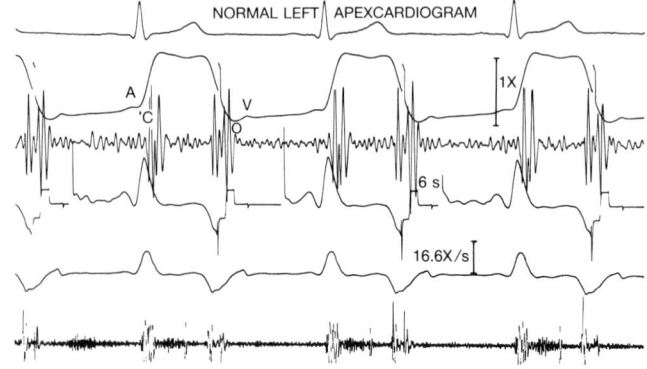

Fig. 7 The normal left apexcardiogram together with its normalized first derivative using total displacement (s^{-1}) and its first derivative (X/s). A high- and low-frequency phonocardiogram are also recorded.

Table 1 Relationship between total amplitude (S) and peak first derivative (dS) during isovolumic contraction in normal subjects and in patients with ischaemic heart disease: local hypokinesia is defined as 25–75 per cent of the ventricular wall showing dyskinesia or akinesia.

		N	r	p
Normals	peak dS = 14.5 S − 0.95	39	0.97	<0.001
Local hypokinesia	= 11.4 S − 0.32	14	0.95	<0.001
Diffuse hypokinesia	= 8.0 S + 2.94	12	0.96	<0.001

Table 2 Multiple regression analysis of the relationship between apexcardiographic parameters and systolic time intervals and invasive parameters of ventricular function

		Peak $(dD/dt/Dt)$	PEP/LVET	r,R
EF	= 0.50	+0.0012 (3.92)	−0.699 (−3.12)	0.77
Peak dP/dt	= 1,444	+32.5 (3.97)	−1.958 (−3.22)	0.78
Mean VCF	= −0.26	+0.043 (3.55)	—	0.61
Peak $(dP/dt/Pt)$	= 3.67	+0.94 (4.63)	—	0.71

EF = ejection fraction (per cent); VCF = peak velocity of circumferential fibre shortening obtained from LV angiogram expressed in circumferences/s. All pressure values obtained from catheter-tipped micromanometers. t-values are indicated in parentheses (N = 23). Dt and Pt: using total amplitude and total pressure.

Experimental work has shown that a highly significant correlation exists between the peak dp/dt obtained from LVP and peak dD/dt (speed of displacement of pressure rise) obtained from QLAC. Normalized indices of contractility can be calculated from QLAC and LVP (dD/dt/D versus dP/dt/P) using either total or developed pressure. The derived indices peak VCE (velocity of contractile clearcut shortening) and V_{max} (maximum velocity of shortening of the contractile elements) can be calculated both from LVP and QLAC and a highly significant correlation is found.

The a wave of the left apexcardiogram is an expression of the compliance of the left ventricle and to a minor extent of the contractility of the atrium. Experimental studies and clinical observations have shown that the speed of rise of the a wave and not its total height is the major determinant of the presence of a fourth heart sound. Small a waves but with a maximum speed of rise are always accompanied by a fourth heart sound. Paradoxically, the functionally most impaired ventricles, which do not allow a rapid rise of LVP during atrial contraction, are not accompanied by a presystolic gallop sound, even if the total height of the a wave is markedly increased.

The slope of the log–log relation between pressure development, obtained from LAC, and dimensional changes obtained from the echocardiogram, during atrial contraction, are significantly correlated with left ventricular compliance.

During the ejection phase, major differences exist between the plateau of QLAC and LVP. The systolic plateau phase is markedly influenced by dimensional changes of the left ventricle during systole. The time course of QLAC is closely correlated with the time course of left ventricular wall tension, as calculated from Laplace's law, during systole. A rapidly decreasing plateau phase is also correlated with a high ejection fraction and the reverse holds true for a rising plateau phase. Rounded left apexcardiograms with a late systolic maximum are a reliable sign of markedly impaired left ventricular function.

In normal individuals, a nearly constant relationship exists between the total height of QLAC and the maximum speed of rise during isovolumic contraction.

At a constant height of the QLAC, dD/dt max is lower when ventricular function is impaired and the degree of the decrease is proportional to the severity of the disease (Table 1).

From Table 2 it appears that contractility indices derived both from apexcardiographic tracings and from systolic time intervals are independent significant predictors of left ventricular function.

Diagnostic value of the apexcardiogram

The presence in sinus rhythm of a definite a wave in the LAC excludes the diagnosis of haemodynamically significant mitral stenosis. The same is true when a normal rapid filling wave is present. A peaked rapid filling wave is significantly correlated with the presence of a third heart sound. A short peak of rapid filling is often recorded in ventricular dysfunction and a longer one (40 ms between the O and V points) in mitral regurgitation (Figs. 8–10). These signs are important whenever diagnosis is difficult because of multivalvular disease. The duration of ventricular systole can also be calculated from LAC although the O-point of LAC precedes the nadir of LVP by 10–20 ms.

Systolic pulsations recorded at a site of QS or Qr morphology in the electrocardiogram indicate an akinetic zone or myocardial

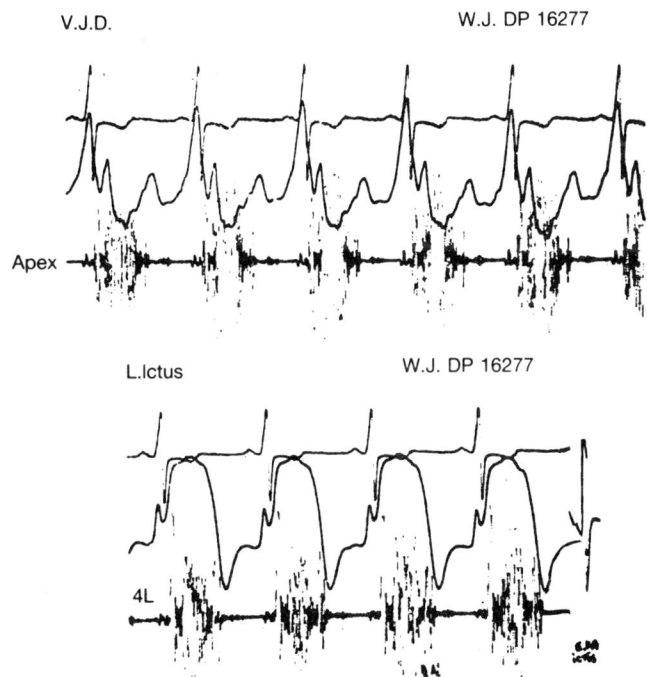

Fig. 8 Jugular venous pulse tracing (VJD) and left apexcardiogram in left ventricular hypertrophy. Note the sharp a wave in the left apexcardiogram and the high a wave in the VJD.

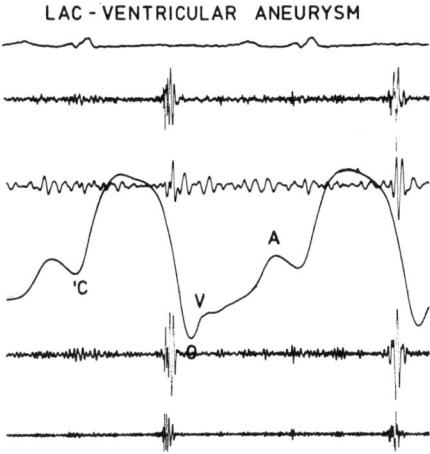

Fig. 9 Left apexcardiogram in a case of left ventricular aneurysm. Note the rounded a wave and systolic wave (see text).

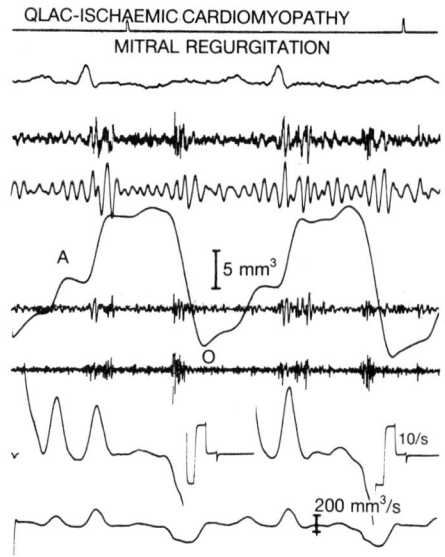

Fig. 10 Left apexcardiogram in a case of ischaemic cardiomyopathy. The a wave is high and rounded and the plateau phase shows a late systolic upstroke. The normalized peak upstroke of the a wave is as high as the iso-volumic systolic wave.

aneurysm. In right ventricular hypertrophy a right apexcardio-gram can often be recorded left of the sternal border. A heightened a wave in RAC is a sign of reduced ventricular compliance. In cases of constrictive pericarditis the apexcardiogram is usually negative. The end of the rising limb of this apexcardiogram in early diastole coincides with the end of the rapid filling of the ventricle. In severe aortic insufficiency LAC has a typical morphology with a rapidly increasing diastolic phase and a small contribution of ventricular systole to the total height of LAC.

Systolic time intervals

Systolic time intervals (STI) can be obtained from the simultaneous recording of the carotid artery tracing, the phonocardiogram and the electrocardiogram. The intervals most commonly used are the left ventricular ejection time (LVET), the interval q-aortic component of the second sound ($q-A_2$) and the pre-ejection period (PEP), where PEP is measured as $(q-A_2) - (LVET)$.

Several methodological problems arise. The exact moment of the upstroke of the carotid artery tracing (CAT) is often difficult to determine. The best method is to draw a straight line through the diastolic part of the trace of the preceding beat and through the systolic upstroke and to take the intersection of both lines as the beginning of the carotid artery upstroke. The LVET measurement from the CAT is nearly identical to the LVET obtained from the aortic pressure tracing obtained just distally from the aortic valve. Some minor differences exist, however, since the transmission time for the upstroke and incisura from the aortic valve to the carotid artery is not equal and this difference is heart-rate dependent. The determination of the beginning of the aortic component can also be difficult as it can depend on the frequency band and the filter system used. It is best measured in a high frequency band (>140 Hz).

The most useful of the STI is the PEP which can be considered equivalent to the mean dp/dt of the isovolumic contraction period. It is the least heart-rate dependent of the three intervals. Positive inotropic interventions shorten the PEP and negative ones prolong it. In general, the better the heart function, the shorter the PEP. The PEP interval also contains the electromechanical interval and thus can be influenced by conduction changes in the heart. More important is the fact that it is very sensitive to changes in preload and afterload. The PEP interval will be short when end-diastolic aortic pressure is low or end-diastolic left ventricular pressure is high and can thus lead to false conclusions regarding

Table 3 Regression equations between STI (ms) and heart rate (bpm) in normal subjects

				r	R
LVET	(a)	=	$377.4 - 1.161\,HR$	-0.83	
	(b)	=	$688.7 - 92.6\,\ln HR$	-0.84	
	(c)	=	$440.4 - 2.483\,HR + 0.0063\,HR^2$		0.94
MS		=	$1{,}192 - 174\,\ln HR$	-0.93	
$q-A_2$	(a)	=	$493.3 - 1.150\,HR$	-0.84	
	(b)	=	$892.85 - 119.25\,\ln HR$	-0.84	
q-U		=	$152.5 - 0.457\,HR$	-0.54	

(a) Linear equation, (b) exponential equation, (c) polynomial equation.
MS: mechanical systole from beginning upstroke to 0-point LAC.
q-U: q-upstroke CAT.
HR: heart rate.
Equations valid for both sexes.

the haemodynamic state of the heart. Another problem is that the PEP depends on a correct measurement of both LVET and $q-A_2$.

The LVET depends on numerous factors and is highly dependent on the preceding R-R interval. The maximum correlation coefficient for the relation between LVET and heart rate is about 0.85 (Table 3). As a result a rather high degree of imprecision remains when the equation between LVET and heart rate is applied to individual subjects. The LVET shortens during positive inotropic interventions; it is less dependent on preload and afterload but is sensitive to changes in stroke volume.

The exact nature of the relationship between LVET and heart rate is still unknown: a linear relationship is adequate at rest but non-linear relationships might be superior. This is an important consideration whenever LVET must be adjusted for heart rate, e.g. for the evaluation of interventions that can influence both.

The use of one universal regression coefficient for the adjustment of LVET for heart-rate changes is at the moment impossible and unwarranted. The best approach is to use the regression coefficients of the equation correlating LVET and heart rate obtained in each centre and adjusted for each study and to extrapolate not to heart rate zero but to the mean heart rate obtained during the experiment. There is no doubt, however, that LVET, expressed as a percentage of a normal value, derived from one of the many published regression equations gives clinically useful information, as values between 60 and 130 per cent can be obtained. The shortening of LVET in patients with cardiac failure is a function of the diminished stroke volume and its prolongation in cases of aortic stenosis is an indication of the severity of the disease.

The $q-A_2$ interval, containing both PEP and LVET, is very sensitive to interventions which can change PEP and LVET in the same direction but insensitive to those which do the opposite. For example, when a decrease in contractility leads to a decreased cardiac output, the PEP will increase, the LVET decrease, and the net result, $q-A_2$, will change very little.

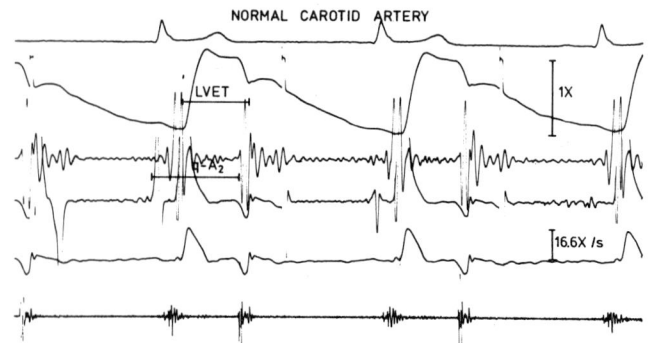

Fig. 11 Normal carotid artery tracing together with an LF and HF phonocardiogram. The first derivative and normalized derivative are also recorded.

Other time intervals, such as the q-upstroke interval (q–U) or the duration of mechanical systole (MS) derived from the C–O points on LAC are less commonly used. Several ratios have also been developed, such as q–U/LVET, PEP/LVET, and MS/LVET. All these have the advantage of being relatively insensitive to changes in heart rate so that correction is not necessary when the fluctuation is less than 20 beats/min. The ratio MS/LVET is the only one to make use of the isovolumic relaxation period of the heart and is useful for detecting ventricular failure. The ratio PEP/LVET may also reflect changes in the functional state of the heart, but may lead to false conclusions when both variables change in the same direction.

Carotid artery tracing

The morphology of the indirect carotid artery tracing can also be used for diagnostic purposes, apart from its measurement of LVET. It is useful for the diagnosis of valvular aortic stenosis and one glance is often sufficient to determine whether the stenosis is severe or not depending on the velocity of the upstroke and the extent of the carotid shudder. A typical carotid shudder, however, is only found when stroke volume is low due to ventricular dysfunction (Figs. 11–13). In aortic regurgitation the dicrotic wave will progressively disappear depending on the severity of the disease. In very severe cases, such as abrupt rupture of the aortic valve in bacterial endocarditis, this can lead to a 'ventricularized' morphology of the carotid artery tracing. In cases of muscular subaortic stenosis (IHSS), the typical pattern is of a rapid upstroke followed by a rapid downstroke and a small tidal wave. In cases with cardiac failure and a low stroke volume, both upstroke and downstroke of the systolic part are slow, and the dicrotic wave is large; LVET will be shortened proportionally to the severity of the disease.

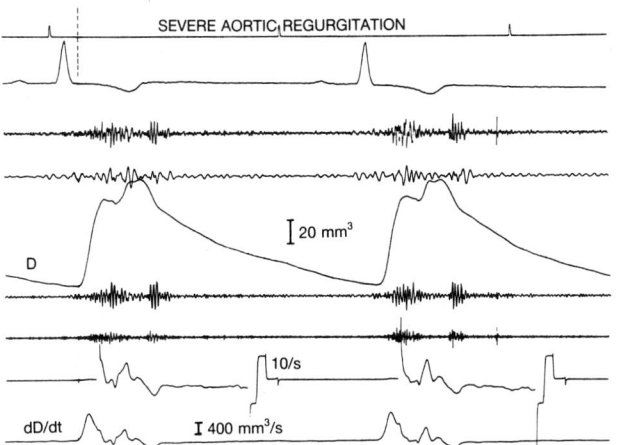

Fig. 12 The carotid artery tracing in severe aortic regurgitation. The dicrotic wave is nearly absent.

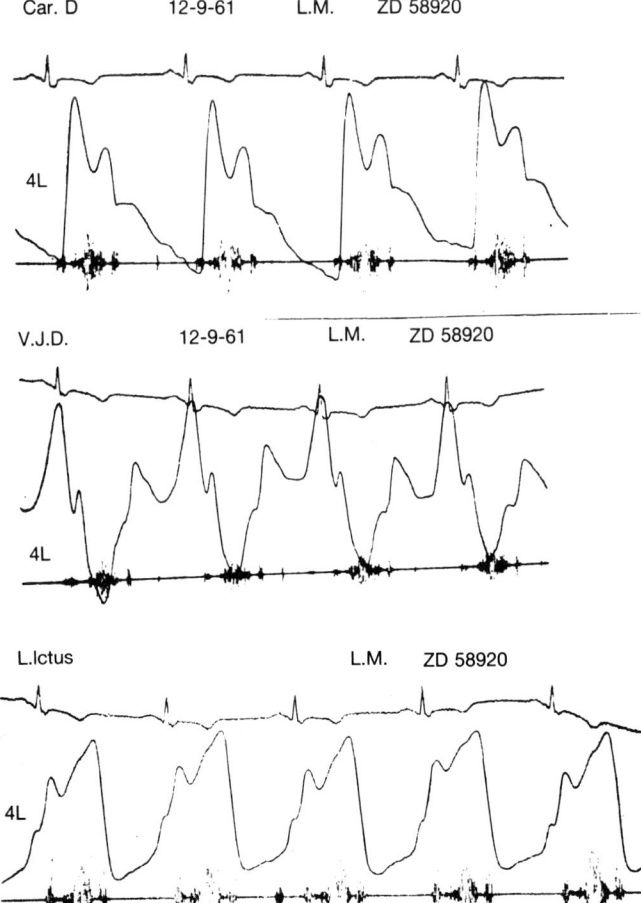

Fig. 13 The carotid artery tracing, together with the jugular venous pulse tracing, and the left apexcardiogram and phonocardiogram in a case of idiopathic hypertrophic subaortic stenosis (IHSS). The carotid artery tracing shows a typical morphology, the JVPT is typical for the Bernheim effect, and the LAC for left ventricular hypertrophy. The midsystolic murmur is typical for IHSS.

References

Phonocardiography

Baragan, J., Fernandez, F. and Thiron J. M. (1976). Phonocardiologie dynamique. Contribution des drogues vaso-actives au diagnostic des cardiopathies. *J. Baillière.*

Günther, K. H. (1969). *Vergleichende extrakardiale und intrakardiale Phonokardiographie auf haemodynamischer Grundlage.* Akademie-Verlag, Berlin.

Holldack, K. and Wolf, D. (1962). *Atlas und kurzgefasstes Lehrbuch der Phonokardiographie und verwandter Untersuchungsmethoden.* Thieme-Verlag, Stuttgart.

Tavel, M. E. (1978). *Clinical phonocardiography and external pulse recording.* Year Book Medical Publishers, Chicago.

Wood, P. (1958). Aortic stenosis. *Am. J. Cardiol*, **1**, 553–560.

Jugular venous pulse

Hartman, H. (1960). The jugular venous tracing. *Am. Heart J.* **59**, 698–703.

Kesteloot, H. (1963). *Functie-onderzoek van rechterhart door pols- en ictuskurven.* Arscia, Brussels.

Apexcardiography

Denef, B., Popeye, R., De Geest, H. and Kesteloot, H. (1975). On the clinical value of calibrated displacement apexcardiography. *Circulation* **51**, 541–551.

Denef, B., Van de Werf, F., De Geest, H. and Kesteloot, H. (1976). Calibrated apexcardiography and assessment of left ventricular dynamics in man. *Eur. J. Cardiol.* **4**, 143–152.

Kesteloot, H. (1977). Assessment of left ventricular function by means of calibrated apexcardiography. *Arch. Inst. Cardiol. Mèx.* **47**, 499–508.

Sutton, G. C. and Craige, E. (1967). Quantitation of precordial movements. *Circulation* **35**, 476–480.

Sutton, G. C., Prewitt, T. A. and Craige, E. (1970). Relationship between quantitated precordial movement and left ventricular function. *Circulation* **41**, 179–185.

Van de Werf, F., Piessens, J., De Geest, H. and Kesteloot, H. (1976). Normalized first derivative of the left apexcardiogram in the assessment of left ventricular function. *Am. J. Cardiol.* **37**, 1059–1064.

Willems, J. (1973). *The normal apexcardiogram*, P. 212. Arscia, Brussels.

Systolic time intervals

Lombard, W. P. and Cope, O. M. (1926). The duration of the systole of the left ventricle in man. *Am. J. Physiol.* **77**, 263–270.

Spodick, D. H. and Kumar, S. (1968). Left ventricular ejection period. *Am. Heart J.* **76**, 498–555.

—— and —— (1968). Left ventricular ejection period. Measurement by atraumatic techniques: results in normal young men and comparison of methods of calculation. *Am. Heart J.* **76**, 70–76.

Weissler, A. M., Harris, W. S. and Schoenfeld, C. D. (1968). Systolic time intervals in heart failure. *Circulation* **37**, 149–155.

Weissler, A. M., Harris, L. C. and White, G. D. (1963). Left ventricular ejection time index in man. *J. Appl. Physiol.* **18**, 919–925.

Weissler, A. M., Peeler, G. and Roehl JR, H. (1961). Relationship between left ventricular ejection time, stroke volume and heart rate in normal individuals and patients with cardiovascular disease. *Am. Heart J.* **62**, 367–371.

Willems, J., Roelandt, J., De Geest, H., Kesteloot, H. and Joossens, J. V. (1970). The left ventricular ejection time in elderly subjects. *Circulation* **42**, 37–42.

Computerized tomographic scanning of the heart

M. J. LIPTON

Introduction

Remarkable advances in the electronic industry during the past decade have resulted among other things in revolutionary imaging techniques. The first of these occurred in 1973 with the introduction of computed transmission tomography (CT). This technique involved a new concept, namely, imaging by the direct interaction of an X-ray machine with a computer. The computer in CT scanners not only guides the data acquisition, which involves the precise transmission of a thin beam of X-rays through the patient in a specific plane from many angles, but also it reconstructs the CT data obtained and displays it in the form of a cross-sectional image on a television monitor. The transmitted fan beam of radiation exiting through the patient is received by an array of X-ray detectors; this is in the form of an analogue signal which is then converted into digital form so that it can be manipulated by the computer. The CT image is displayed on a digital matrix, the grid size of which determines the spatial resolution. The contrast of the various tissues is expressed in the form of a gray scale of density. The units of density are known as Hounsfeld units named after one of the physicists who pioneered the mathematics of CT back projection imaging. Computed transmission axial tomography (CT) was the first of a series of advanced imaging modalities which share in common digital processing and imaging. The others are positron emission tomography (PET), digital subtraction angiography (DSA), and magnetic resonance imaging (MRI). All these digital imaging techniques possess a remarkable potential for direct quantification and, therefore, are of special interest for cardiovascular diagnosis.

This chapter describes the current clinical applications of cardiac CT scanning, using presently available equipment. The future prospects for greatly improved imaging with recently developed high-speed CT systems will also be addressed.

Technical requirements for cardiac imaging

Technical requirements are greater for imaging the heart than other organ systems because of the importance of the assessment of cardiac motion and function as well as of structure. Cineangiography has shown that cardiac diagnosis requires high sampling speeds of at least 16 frames per second in order to stop cardiac motion in systole and diastole. Furthermore, the whole heart must be imaged during the same phases of the cardiac cycle. Very few techniques completely satisfy such stringent demands and none is ideal. Cineangiography has emerged as the most successful method to date, but even this technique has the disadvantage of projection imaging as well as other limitations of invasive risk and expense. Conventional X-ray cinematography film, however, does provide one very important requirement for cardiac diagnosis,

namely, high spatial resolution (5 line pairs per mm) which is vastly superior to all competing modalities.

Strengths and limitations of CT in the heart

Computed transmission tomography by virtue of cross-sectional imaging offers a significantly different three-dimensional approach

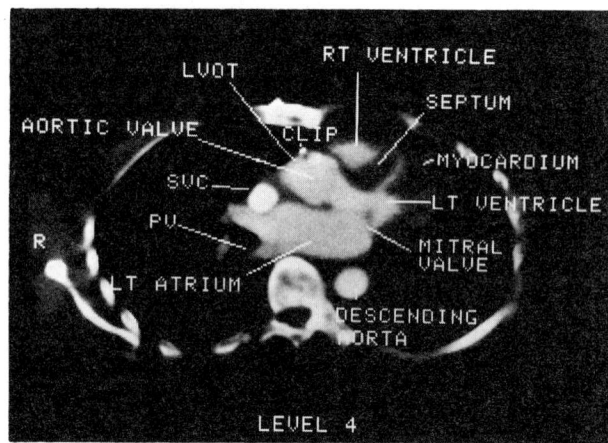

Fig. 1 An example of a 1 cm thick CT scan obtained during held inspiration and intravenous contrast enhancement of both the left (LT) and right (RT) sided cardiac structures. Note a radio-opaque clip from prior surgery, and the well-defined mitral valve plane at this level. This scan was obtained with the most recently developed high-speed (50 ms exposure) electron beam CT scanner. The orientation of CT scans is with the patient lying supine with the feet towards the observer, hence the right side of the patient is to the left side on this illustration.

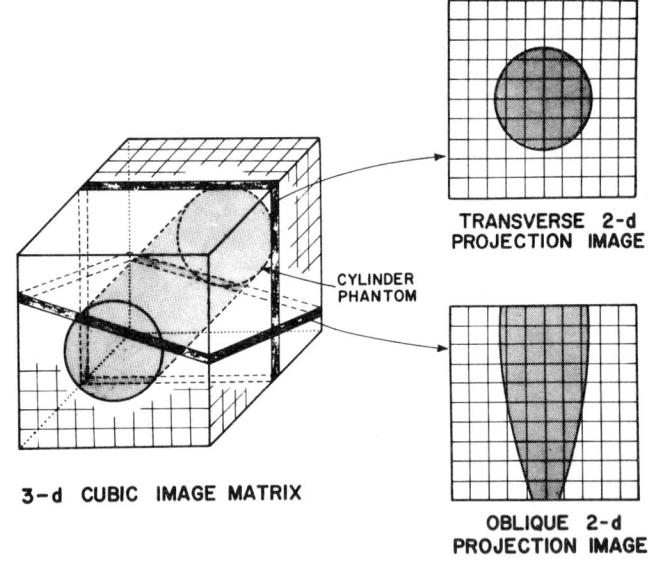

Fig. 2 (Left) Three-dimensional matrix image of a cylinder. (Right) Typical two-dimensional projector images of a transverse section and an oblique section are illustrated. Once a cubic matrix of CT scan data has been acquired by multilevel scanning any plane may be reconstructed. (Reproduced from Boyd, 1981, with permission.)

Table 1 Cine-CT capability

1 Rapid scan time, 50 ms
2 Multislice capability, eight or more simultaneously
3 Repeat multislice study at 1 s (or faster) during passage of contrast bolus
4 3D transformations into sagittal, coronal, and oblique images
5 Quantitative analysis software
6 Subtraction
7 Functional imaging analysis and display

which is not possible with either angiography or digital subtraction angiography. It is this aspect of CT which makes it attractive for cardiac diagnosis. Present whole body CT scanners were primarily designed to image organs other than the heart where motion is minimal or absent. Initial CT scan exposure times were accordingly long, and, in 1973, were the order of 5 min. Advances in CT technology have been rapid and by 1976 this was reduced to between 2 and 5 s. Further major limitations of CT for cardiac imaging to date have been the single slice capability together with a relatively long interscan delay time of aproximately 1 s. Equally restrictive is that the number of rapid sequential scans is limited, usually to 10, because the conventional X-ray tube source must then be rested for safety reasons owing to excessive heat production. Contrast medium is another essential requirement for cardiac CT in order to enhance the density of the blood pool compared with cardiac tissue. Fortunately, small, peripheral intravenous injections are adequate for this purpose unlike angiocardiography, mainly because CT has vastly superior density resolution and is tomographic thereby avoiding superimposition of structures. Figure 1 illustrates a contrast enhanced CT scan. This three-dimensional capability of CT has the potential to provide any projection image once the CT data has been acquired by dynamic multilevel scanning. The imaging planes are flexible and unlimited once a volume image has been acquired (Fig. 2). This is a unique advantage of CT compared with echocardiography or regular X-ray film-based techniques. Initial cardiac CT feasibility studies defined the requirements for future cardiac CT imaging. These requirements are summarized in Table 1 and have been subsequently incorporated in high-speed cine-CT scanners, specifically designed for cardiac diagnosis.

Clinical utility

CT scanning of the heart should be considered as a greatly modified angiographic procedure. It requires attention to simple but important details which greatly influence the quality and diagnostic utility of the study. Technical considerations involved in CT scanning will now be discussed.

Scan registration to define anatomical levels

The need to keep procedure time short and yet obtain an adequate diagnostic study requires accurate and rapid localization of the appropriate anatomical scan levels. This is particularly important with a technique which has only a single slice capability for each exposure and, in addition, requires temporally co-ordinated contrast medium enhancement. Anatomical localization is performed prior to any injections by obtaining a computed radiograph of the chest. This image is a digital radiograph produced by the CT scanner and provides essentially a chest X-ray together with a precise longitudinal 1 cm scale which is used for scan level registration. An example of a digital computed CT radiograph is illustrated in Fig. 3. This technique has greatly improved the precision of scan

selection which was initially based on surface anatomy. The CT computer registers each slice level in memory and, provided the patient does not move during the procedure, it enables the same level to be re-located accurately when necessary at some later time during the study. This is otherwise impossible. Furthermore, it ensures that all adjacent CT scanning levels are correctly registered. The thickness of the scans is determined by the operator and can be varied from 2 mm to 2 cm depending on the CT system. Usually 1 cm or 0.5 cm slices are most useful in the heart.

Contrast medium and dynamic scanning

The density of the blood and myocardium is so similar that some form of contrast enhancement is necessary for CT to distinguish between these structures. An important consideration for optimal CT imaging is the use of agents containing high concentrations of iodine (40 per cent) such as Renographin 76 or Conray 400. Studies should not be performed with more dilute agents – a common error – because this frequently results in suboptimal imaging. Suitable blood levels are achieved using a drip infusion of 1–1.5 ml/kg body weight, which allows the necessary time (5–10 min) for volume imaging. Several different levels are sequentially scanned in this technique which results in the enhancement level being similar for all the scans. This will provide smoother images when transformed by the CT computer into other planes.

Bolus injection is the other intravenous method of contrast administration. This is usually performed using approximately 20–25 ml in adults and is injected at a flow rate of 4 or 5 ml/s either by hand or power injector. This requires a suitably sized intracath (18 or 16 gauge) in a peripheral vein, either a large basilic tributary in the antecubital fossa or an external jugular vein. A common mistake is the placement of a small diameter needle useful only for drip infusion. The advantage of the approach recommended in conjunction with rapid sequential scanning at one level is that regional vascular anatomy can be defined. This technique is also termed dynamic CT, and provides useful information concerning blood flow in terms of transit times, and is the basis for quantitative CT flow analysis.

A variety of cardiac disorders has been identified in which CT scanning has a useful clinical diagnostic role. In general, CT is greatly underutilized for cardiac diagnosis even when a whole body CT scanner is available. The reasons for this are varied, but reflect, at least to some extent, the interest, experience, and enthusiasm of physicians for this technique.

Evaluation of aortic lesions by CT

True aneurysms

True aneurysms of the aorta have a similar appearance whether they occur in the mediastinum or in the abdomen. Curvilinear areas of calcification, when present, define the outer boundaries of these lesions and may or may not be seen on plain chest radio-

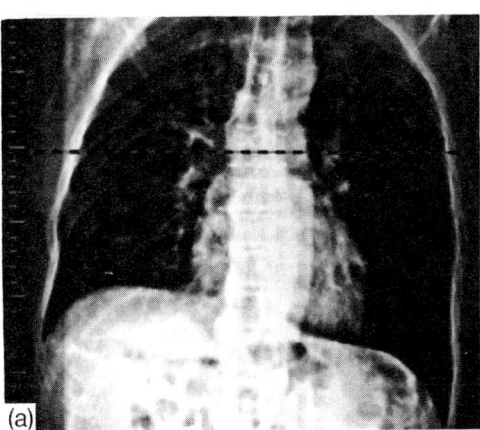
(a)

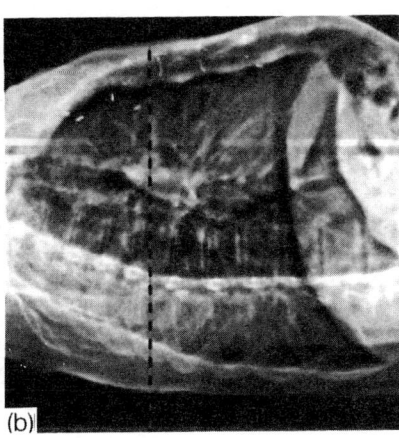
(b)

Fig. 3 Computed radiographs obtained by transporting the patient through the pulsed X-ray fan beam while the tube is kept stationary. The scanner is being used as a slit-digital radiographic system, and the resulting image has a wide dynamic range and it allows precise slice registration. Three radiopaque surgical clips placed on the ascending aorta can be seen. The dotted line illustrates a suitable scan-level for scanning coronary artery bypass grafts. This technique is rapid (15–30 s) and frontal and oblique projections are readily acquired.

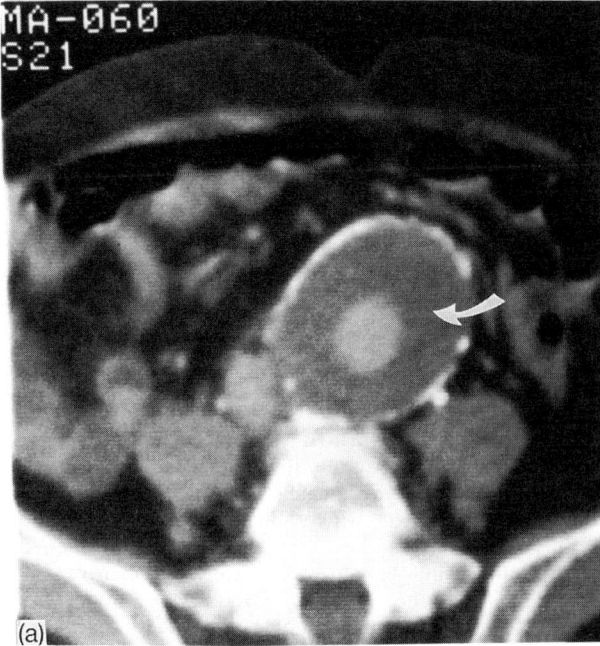

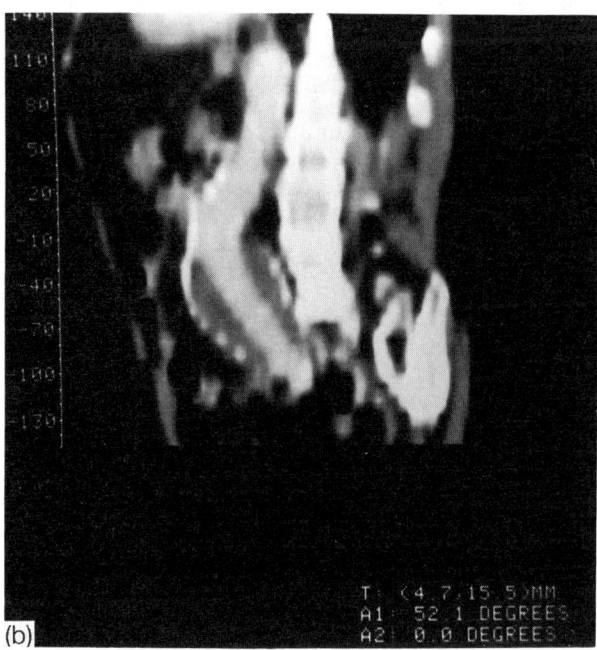

Fig. 4 (a) CT scan in patient with a true, large aneurysm of the abdominal aorta. An outer rim of calcification is well seen. Extensive thrombus formation (arrow) is depicted as a grey zone within which the patent enhanced lumen lies. (b) This is an oblique CT reconstruction of the same patient as shown in Fig. 3. Note the dilated abdominal aorta. Again thrombus is seen surrounding the lumen and calcification forms the outermost border.

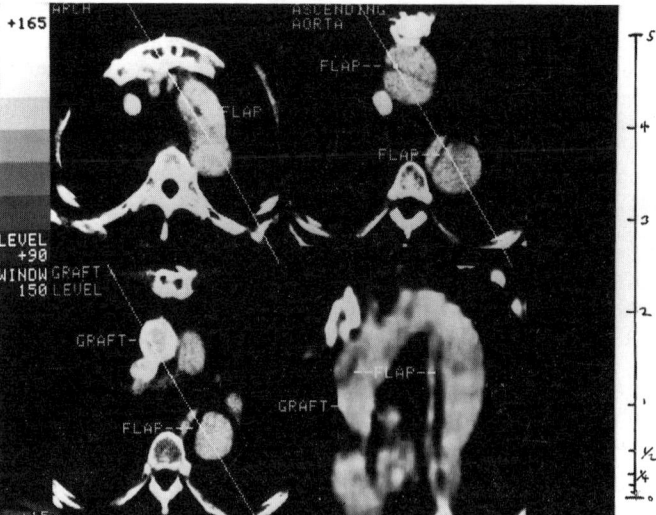

Fig. 5 A CT scan of a patient with an aortic dissection. The upper two panels (contrast-enhanced CT scans) show an intimal flap through the aortic arch and both the ascending and descending aortas. The left lower image is a CT scan through a previously placed Teflon graft in the ascending aorta. The oblique CT reconstruction was created from multilevel cross-sectional images in the plane indicated by the white cursor line selected by the physician. The longitudinal intimal flap is labelled.

region because of the aneurysm. The boundary of the aneurysm is depicted by a ring of calcification within which the thrombus can be seen. The thrombus can be distinguished from the centrally situated lumen, which shows marked contrast enhancement. Figure 4b illustrates a longitudinal oblique reconstruction through this lesion and demonstrates the typical features of a true aneurysm.

Aortic dissection

Dissection of the aorta remains one of the most common catastrophic events affecting the great vessels. The clinical presentation may be acute or chronic. The anatomical site of the tear influences prognosis (page 13.184); hence, the great need is to determine the diagnosis early and to classify the condition as a type A, which affects the ascending aorta, aortic arch or both from a type B dissection which involves only regions of the aorta beyond the left subclavian. The diagnosis may be obvious, but many patients with aortic dissection are not diagnosed early. The definitive diagnostic study has been aortography, particularly for acute situations, but some centres now rely rather on CT as the primary diagnostic modality. CT can demonstrate aortic dissection in a unique cross-sectional manner, as illustrated in Fig. 5. In the figure, the intimal flap separating the two lumens is well seen; CT also allows the selection of any oblique reconstruction plane precisely at right angles to the plane of the dissection (Fig. 5) and can yield the result rapidly, the procedure time being 15–20 min and scan reading, 10–15 min. Conventional angiography is limited by the number of projections possible because of contrast volume load and radiation, even with biplane X-ray systems. Furthermore, it may not demonstrate soft tissue changes, notably haematoma formation. Thus, there may be difficulty in determining the outer boundary of many dissections.

The place of CT in diagnosing acute aortic dissection is still being evaluated, but it has certainly become the method of choice for subacute and chronic dissections. An important consideration is that the false lumen persists in 85 per cent of patients after surgical or medical therapy, and its presence may contribute to recurrence, with extension or rupture of the lesion. Another important aspect in evaluating these patients is to determine the relative blood flow in the aorta and false lumen as well as in vital branches.

graphs. We have found it necessary to use dynamic scanning in the two modes described above in order to assess these lesions adequately. Dynamic CT with bolus injections should be obtained at two or more levels through the aortic arch and root. In addition, a drip infusion with multilevel contiguous scanning is also necessary for reconstructing the whole area of the aorta. Figure 4a illustrates an abdominal aneurysm in a patient in whom cardiac catheterization was attempted from the transfemoral approach, but it was impossible to advance the catheter beyond the mid-abdominal

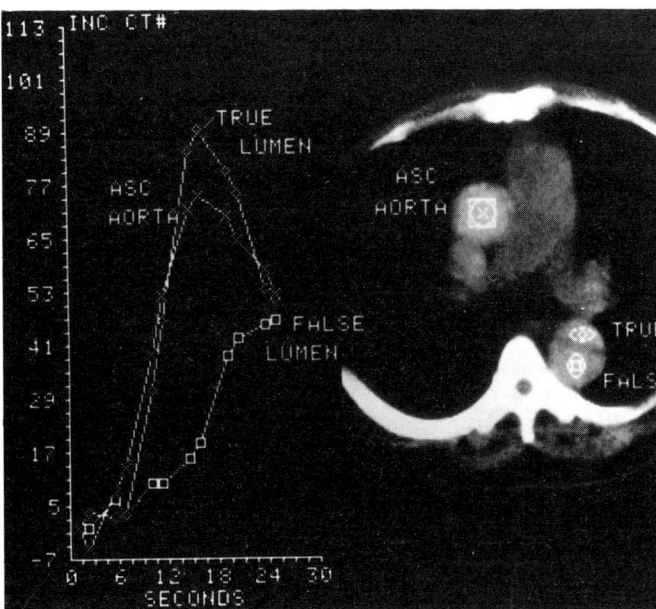

Fig. 6 Graph showing incremental CT number versus time for areas of interest: the ascending aorta (ASC AORTA), the true lumen (TRUE) and the false lumen (FALSE) in the descending aorta. Note the marked delay in peak opacification of the false lumen, suggesting that the communication between the two lumens was distal.

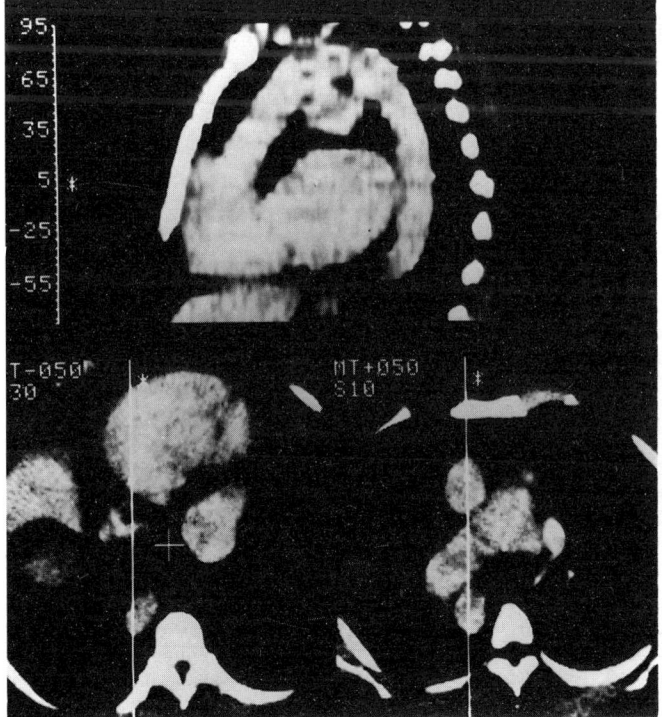

Fig. 7 Transposition of the great vessels. The CT scans show that the aorta is arising from the anterior ventricle, and the aortic arch can be seen in the lateral reconstructed projection image to be abnormally opened in the characteristic manner.

This is not always possible during angiography, but is with CT (Fig. 6).

Aortic malpositions and coarctation

Malpositions of the aorta, occurring either in isolation or in conjunction with a variety of congenital heart lesions (e.g. tetralogy of Fallot and transposition of the great vessels), can also be identified

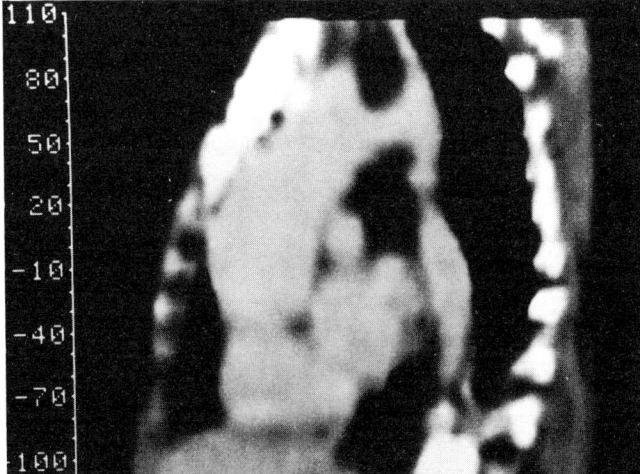

Fig. 8 CT scan illustrating the appearance of coarctation of the aorta. Note that the diameters of the large ascending and small descending aorta are well seen and the relationship of the left subclavian to the site of the coarctation is also demarcated.

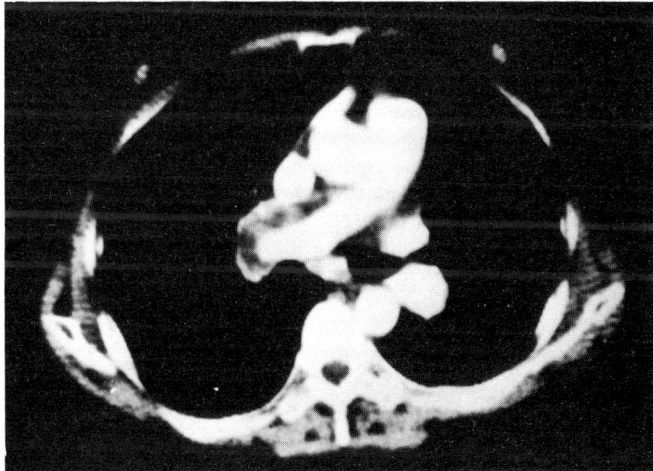

Fig. 9 CT scan through the main pulmonary artery and right main pulmonary artery shows a large non-enhanced filling defect extending eccentrically through the right main pulmonary artery. This proved to be a large pulmonary embolism at surgery.

by CT (Fig. 7). Coarctation (Fig. 8) and pseudocoarctation of the aorta have also been demonstrated by CT. Various other congenital abnormalities, such as persistent left superior vena cava and anomalous pulmonary veins, can be detected; CT is also able to identify the drainage pattern of such structures. Cardiac catheterization in conjunction with angiocardiography, however, remains essential and CT should not yet be regarded as a replacement for it. CT can provide quantitative information besides adequate detailed anatomical diagnosis. The identification of intracardiac shunts and non-invasive measurement of the flow across such lesions is now possible by CT with high speed scanners and is discussed below.

Evaluation of pulmonary arteries and embolic disease

Chest radiography, isotope imaging, and angiography are the present methods used for evaluating the pulmonary vascular system. However, contrast enhanced CT provides anatomical information regarding the size, shape, and position of the main pulmonary artery and its proximal branches. These data may be useful, for example, in pulmonary hypertension. Patients with pulmonary embolism, particularly those with large central lesions, can be readily identified by CT as shown in Fig. 9. Chronic embolism may be associated with severe pulmonary hypertension and in this setting angiography carries a high risk. CT may characterize the extent and location of the thrombus, and is also a safe, useful method for following interval progress especially following surgery.

Acute myocardial infarction

Identification of myocardial ischaemia and has been an attractive prospect since the first CT scanner became available. Laboratory studies have indicated that acute myocardial infarction can be recognized by contrast-enhanced CT. Acute myocardial infarction in patients has also been successfully demonstrated. A vast amount of time and money has been spent during the past two decades in search of a precise method for sizing myocardial infarction. Techniques studied include precordial mapping, measurements of CPK isoenzyme release, nuclear medicine methods, and echocardiography. All have been explored and none are ideal or even adequate for the clinical task. Anterior, septal, and lateral myocardial infarction can be identified by CT in patients, but inferior wall infarcts and small subendocardial ones are not usually visible with present scanners. This is because the scanning plane is often parallel to the posterior wall of the heart. This problem is related to the rigid CT table design and has been overcome in the recently developed cine-CT scanner described below. There are three signs in contrast-enhanced CT images which characterize myocardial infarction. These are a perfusion defect in the infarct zone during the first passage of the contrast agent (Fig. 10); delayed contrast enhancement around the infarct zone, which occurs 10–15 min later after contrast washout elsewhere; and motion abnormalities of the wall. This third finding requires that body scanners be equipped with some form of ECG gating. This capability is available in a few centres; it has merit and will be discussed.

CT of remote infarction and its sequelae

Complications of myocardial infarction may be identified and evaluated by CT. These include thinning of the myocardial wall in the region of the infarct zone, with subsequent compensatory hypertrophy in other regions. Thrombus formation within the left ventricular cavity can be demonstrated by contrast-enhanced CT, and may be difficult to see at angiography. Dilatation or distortion of the left ventricular cavity and aneurysm formation with or without calcification, and isolated or associated mitral and tricuspid valve incompetence can also be shown. The latter may be appreciated with CT by abnormal persistence of contrast in the atria and evidence of dilatation of the atria and cardiac sinus with dynamic (rapid sequential) CT scanning following a bolus injection (0.2 – 0.5 ml/kg body weight) of contrast medium.

Cardiomyopathy

Left ventricular myocardial wall thickness and mass are not easily quantified by any technique. M-mode echocardiography is useful for septal wall thickness and two-dimensional echo is accepted as a reasonably good method for determining total left ventricular mass. All present methods, however, have significant limitations, especially when there is asymmetrical hypertrophy. The need to apply mathematical geometric assumptions is a major limitation for all these techniques. Computed tomography offers a tomographic three-dimensional approach and even without ECG gating, great precision is possible. CT measurements of chamber volumes and mass are independent of chamber orientation (Fig. 11).

Coronary artery bypass graft patency

This was the first cardiac application of CT to gain acceptance. The vast number of operations performed (150 000 annually in the United States alone) and the frequency of recurrent symptoms, notably angina (over 30 per cent of the patients), present a signifi-

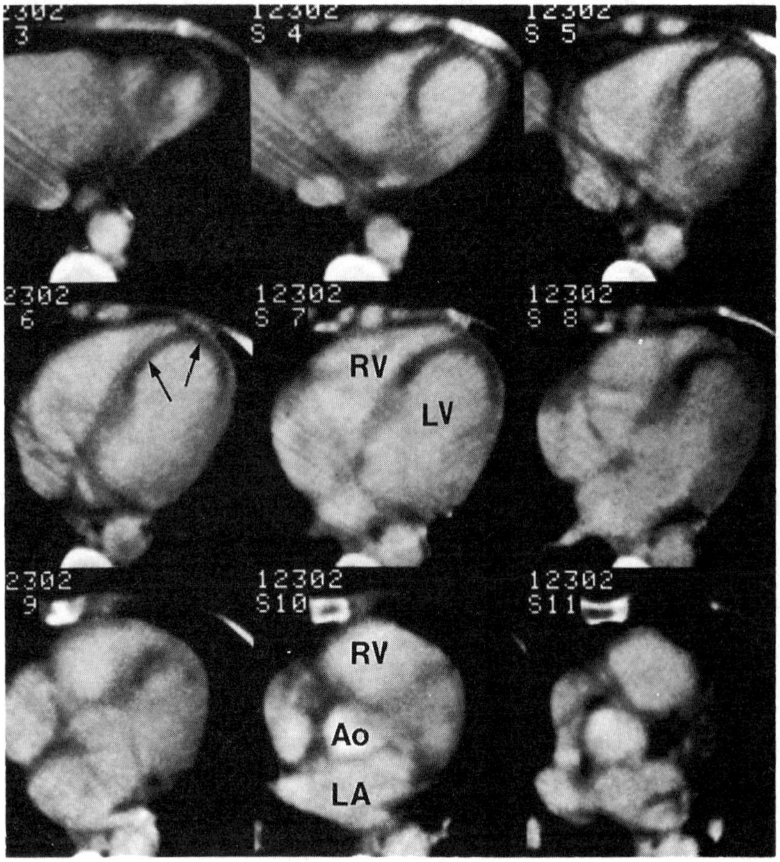

Fig. 10 Acute myocardial infarction. Non-gated CT scan through the ventricles following an intravenous infusion of Conray 400 (1.5 ml/kg body weight) in a patient with an acute (3 day old) anteroseptal myocardial infarction. The infarcted region is depicted as the dark horseshoe-shaped area of myocardium (arrows). The remaining normal myocardium is contrast enhanced, some of which can be seen bordering the infarct. RV = right ventricle, LV = left ventricle, Ao = aorta, and LA = left atrium.

cant diagnostic problem. Selective cardiac catheterization was required to determine graft patency before the introduction of CT. The relatively large size of the vein grafts and their convenient location above the heart where motion is minimal makes them ideal for slow CT diagnostic imaging. The grafts are best seen by giving bolus injections (25 ml) of contrast medium (40 per cent iodine concentration) and using dynamic imaging. Patency is

recognized when there is contrast enhancement of the grafts coincident or just following peak enhancement of the ascending aorta (Fig. 12). The proximal coronary arteries can usually be seen to a variable degree in scans through the left atrium at the aortic root. Dense connective tissue and sometimes calcium may be present in a graft. A diagnosis of patency is still possible in such cases if further contrast enhancement occurs. It is usually necessary to study between two and four levels depending on the number of grafts placed in order to increase the certainty of patency. Furthermore, each graft should be seen adequately on at least two levels. CT is particularly valuable in the early postoperative period. The surrounding fat appears black and allows the contrast-enhanced grafts, which are white on CT images, to stand out prominently. Some respiratory motion may be a concern in acutely postoperative patients, but this should be accepted and does not prevent a good diagnostic study in most cases.

Pitfalls and limitations occur with CT as with all diagnostic techniques. A blind diverticular remnant of an occluded graft is frequently seen during selective angiography. This may mimic a patent graft on a CT examination. Multilevel visualization prevents this error and also identifies the native coronary arteries thereby distinguishing them from vein grafts. One major problem for those not experienced in CT is in appreciating the necessity for a good bolus injection of high iodine-containing contrast agent (40 per cent) as well as a knowledge of the transverse cardiovascular anatomy.

Time–density curves can be generated by the CT scanner from dynamic scan sequences. This is one of the many emerging quantitative methods of CT. The operator defines a region of interest (1 pixel or more) on a CT image using some form of trackball guided cursor. The CT computer is programmed to determine the average density in this region on every scan in that sequence and plots

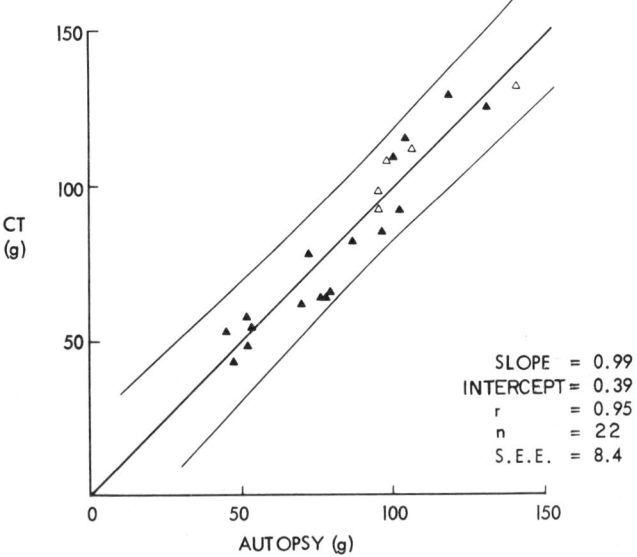

Fig. 11 Relation between autopsy values and computed temography (CT) estimates of left ventricular (LV) mass. Filled triangles, normotensive dogs; open triangles, beagles with left ventricular hypertrophy. The lines on either side of the regression line indicate the 95 per cent confidence limits. (Reproduced from Skioldebrand *et al.*, 1982, with permission.)

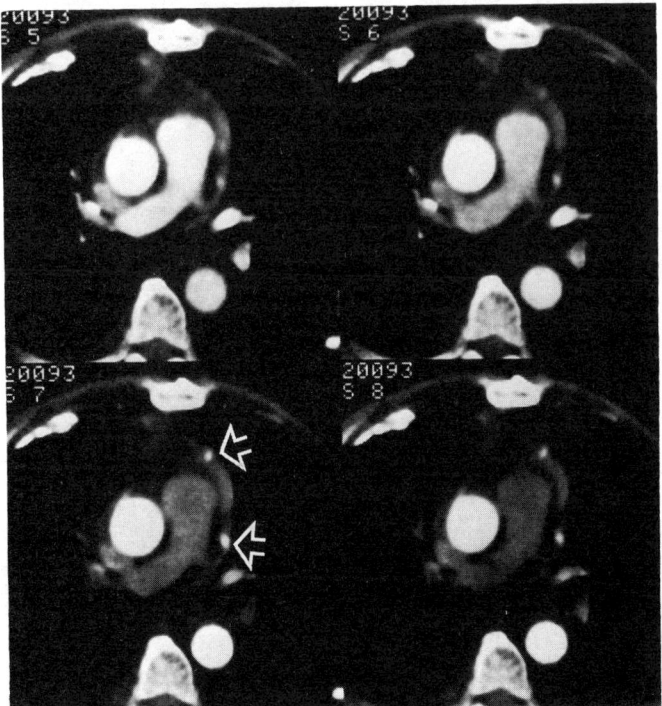

Fig. 12 Four images selected from a dynamic sequence illustrating contrast enhancement of two bypass grafts (arrowed) following enhancement of the ascending and descending aorta. The main trunk and right pulmonary arteries are demonstrated and the bypass grafts are seen to enhance more in images taken later in the series (lower panels, scan numbers 7 and 8) after washout of the pulmonary arteries. The scan exposure time was 1.5 s.

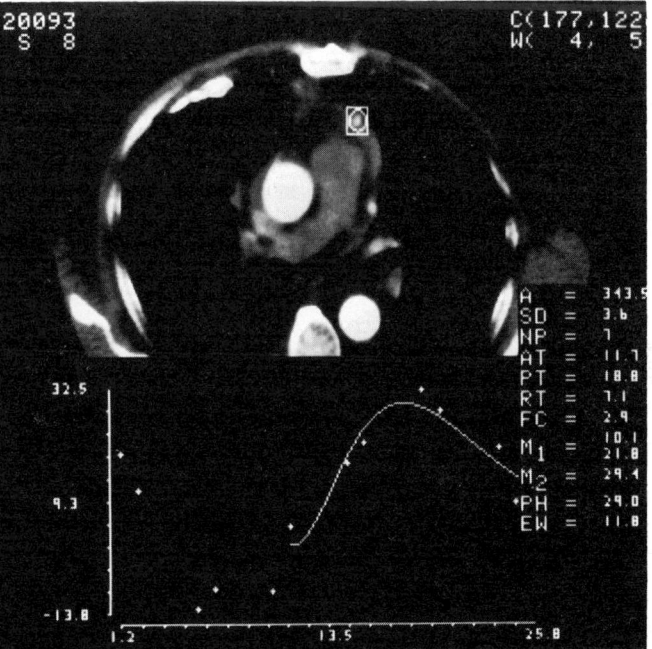

Fig. 13 CT scan from the same dynamic series as Fig. 12. A gamma variate fitted time–density curve has been plotted for the area of interest selected over the more anterior of the two bypass grafts, using an operator-guided trackball cursor, and the curve has been fitted by computer. After performing the fit, the computer calculates various theoretical parameters, such as area under the curve (A), standard deviation of the fit (SD), time of peak (PT), rise time (RT), first moment (M_1), second moment (M_2), and mean width (EW). This approach improves observer confidence in the structure being arterial, by comparison with the curve fitted for the aorta. The area beneath the curve reflects cardiac output. The numbers on the left refer to various characterizations of the curve fit.

a gamma variate curve to these data, which reflects the transit time of contrast agent through that structure, whether this be aorta or bypass graft (Fig. 13). This method has potential to provide information concerning graft flow and may ultimately allow the identification of significant stenotic lesions.

Despite the limitations of whole body CT scanners in terms of their poor temporal resolution of 2–5 s exposure times, CT still remains the best non-invasive method for determining saphenous vein bypass graft patency with a specificity and sensitivity of approximately 95 per cent. Intravenous digital subtraction angiography is not reliable at present and even intra-arterial DSA aortography is prone to false-negative results.

Intracardiac masses

CT compares favourably with two-dimensional echocardiography in accurate diagnosis of left ventricular thrombus and may be as sensitive as echocardiography and probably more specific. Echocardiography appears, however, superior for detecting apical lesions when these are small and mobile. CT is perhaps best used to evaluate patients in whom the echocardiogram is equivocal.

Left atrial thrombus is often a difficult diagnostic problem; the established methods including angiography are insufficiently sensitive. CT provides particularly good anatomical display of this chamber together with the left atrial appendage. Accordingly, a recent study reported a 100 per cent sensitivity and 91 per cent specificity with CT in 28 patients with mitral valve disease for diagnosing left atrial thrombus which was confirmed at the time of open heart surgery. In this same group of patients, sensitivity and specificity was only 60 and 86 per cent for echocardiography and 70 and 88 per cent, respectively, for angiocardiography. If further studies of this type confirm these results CT could become the method of choice in patients suspected of having atrial or indeed, any intracardiac mass lesion.

Cardiac tumours are rare but require differentiation from other intracardiac mass lesions, such as thrombus. CT provides an excellent survey of the chest and mediastinum as well as the heart – all during the same procedure. Thus primary tumours invading the heart walls or tumour thrombus growing within the cardiac chambers or great vessels can be identified by CT. Paracardiac and cardiac masses have been characterized by CT techniques. The value of CT in therapy planning and for interval evaluation of therapy is now established and used routinely for this purpose. Once fast CT scanners become generally available, even mobile tumours, such as atrial myxomas should be visible. Echocardiography is superior to slow CT and remains the preferred modality at present.

Pericardial disease

Echocardiography is established as the most convenient and useful technique for evaluating disease of the pericardium and particularly effusion and haemodynamic effects (page 13.307). Pericardial thickening with constriction is not always diagnosed by echocardiography. Restrictive cardiomyopathy is an important differential diagnosis which may be difficult to identify even at cardiac catheterization. CT offers a non-invasive approach in such patients both as a screening procedure and for definitive diagnosis. The width of the pericardium is normally 2 mm; it is usually greater than 6 mm when constriction is present, and this is readily displayed on cross-sectional CT images. A further helpful CT sign in constriction is the ease with which pericardial calcification can be identified by CT, which allows its precise localization. Figure 14a illustrates this finding. Figure 14b shows the same patient after intravenous infusion of contrast medium. Note the narrowed tubular ventricles, the large atria, and the well-defined atrioventricular groove. These are the classical diagnostic CT signs of constructive pericarditis. CT scanning is greatly underutilized in most hospitals for studying cardiac patients with pericardial problems. CT is also effective in detecting pericardial cystic lesions and other

abnormalities including partial or complete absence of the pericardium.

Congenital heart disease

CT can provide useful diagnostic information in congenital heart disease. The depiction of the cross-sectional anatomy and multiplanar image reconstruction is a powerful diagnostic method. Most cardiologists still rely on established techniques of echocardiography and angiography, primarily because of experience and confidence but also because CT at present cannot yield sufficient cardiac physiological data. However, this is changing with improved CT technology, and it seems likely that fast CT scanning will emerge just as angiocardiography did for routine diagnosis in paediatric medicine as well as in adults with congenital heart lesions. The requirement of contrast medium administration and exposure to ionizing radiation will demand from CT adequate diagnostic information before the technique can become a routine method for clinical practice.

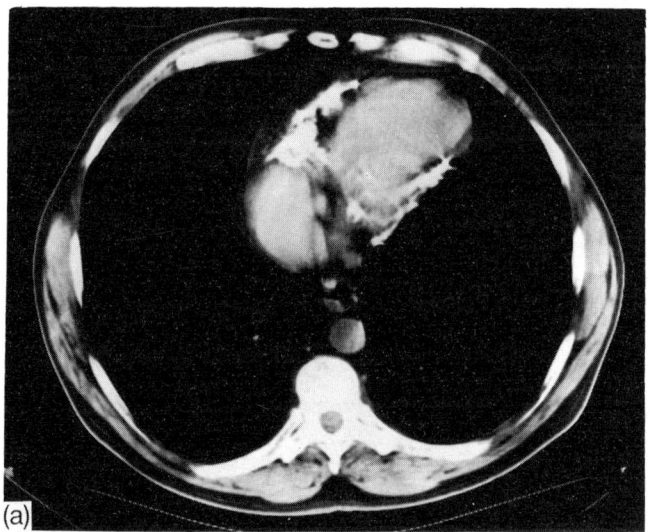

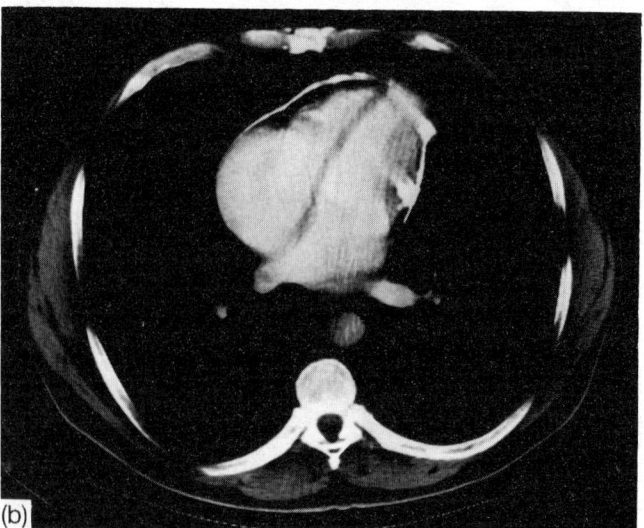

Fig. 14 (a) Dense calcification is seen encasing the pericardium and extending into the atrioventricular groove. (b) Same patient as shown in (a) at another scan level. Calcium is seen circumferentially in the anterior-lateral walls of the greatly thickened pericardium. Contrast enhancement reveals the classical findings of constriction – small compressed tubular ventricles and large atria.

Gated CT

One method of overcoming the limitation of slow CT for analysing cardiac motion is to apply some form of ECG gating. This approach was first attempted in the mid-1970s and has successfully been accomplished with several different CT scanners using either retrospective or prospective gating methods. These techniques allow a gating window of approximately 10 per cent of the cardiac cycle; this is the reciprocal of the number of CT scan revolutions obtained at the same anatomical level. Heat loading on the X-ray tube source is the major limiting technical factor. The need to maintain constant and relatively high blood pool levels of contrast medium is a further requirement and breath holding of 40–50 s or longer is another major clinical disadvantage. Myocardial wall thickening as well as left ventricular cavity dynamics have been analysed using CT images derived from averaged beats obtained by ECG gating. The ability of CT to display both the endocardial and epicardial wall boundaries is a significant advantage over angiography (Fig. 15). CT can, therefore, provide measurement of wall dimensions during different phases of the cardiac cycle. Myocardial wall thickening is known to be a sensitive indicator of ischaemia. CT has the potential to evaluate patients with coronary artery disease and to document the presence and degree of regional ischaemia in terms of reduced wall thickening dynamics. Since standard whole body CT scanners can only scan a single level at a time and gated reconstructions require prolonged breath holding (40 s) during multiple scanner rotations at each level, the contrast medium requirements are rather high for routine clinical applications of this technique.

Role of high-speed CT

Cardiac CT scanning has been used with very favourable results in large numbers of patients in relatively few centres. The limitations of body scanners for cardiac diagnosis include their single slice capability and poor temporal resolution. The early cardiac CT studies with conventional units described above were critical in defining the requirements for successful cardiac CT scanning and are listed in Table 1. Many of these needs were incorporated into the development of the dynamic spatial reconstructor at the Mayo Clinic which was initially designed with 28 X-ray tubes (arranged around the patient) which are synchronously exposed in rapid succession to achieve high-speed scan acquisition. This system pioneered many of the concepts incorporated in fast CT. A more practical approach is that of the cine-CT scanner based upon an electron scanning beam that is magnetically, rather than mechanically, deflected.

Electron beam cine-CT scanner

The problems preventing fast scanning in a conventional body scanner are heat load limitations and the angular momentum of the rotating X-ray tube. The new design replaces the X-ray tube with a magnetically deflected electron beam. The two important advantages are that the ultimate scan speed is limited only by the need to obtain a sufficient number of X-ray photons in a short time and not by mechanical constraints; and secondly, by scanning one or more of the four target rings it is possible to obtain multiple tomographic sections. Technical details of the cine-CT scanner, which produces a very intense beam of electrons in the range of 750 mA, are available in the literature. Figures 16a and b show the cine-CT scanner design and illustrate the two rings of solid-state detectors, which produce two simultaneous 8 mm thick CT scans each time one tungsten target ring is swept by the focused electron beam. The exposure time is currently 50 ms and scans can be obtained at any interval up to 17/s. The scan reconstruction time is presently 10 s. Eight levels can be scanned within 240 ms without the need for table incrementation, although this latter capability is also available. This scanner has a much wider aperture than any conventional CT or magnetic resonance imager, and, in combination with a mobile table, allows patient angulation so that vari-

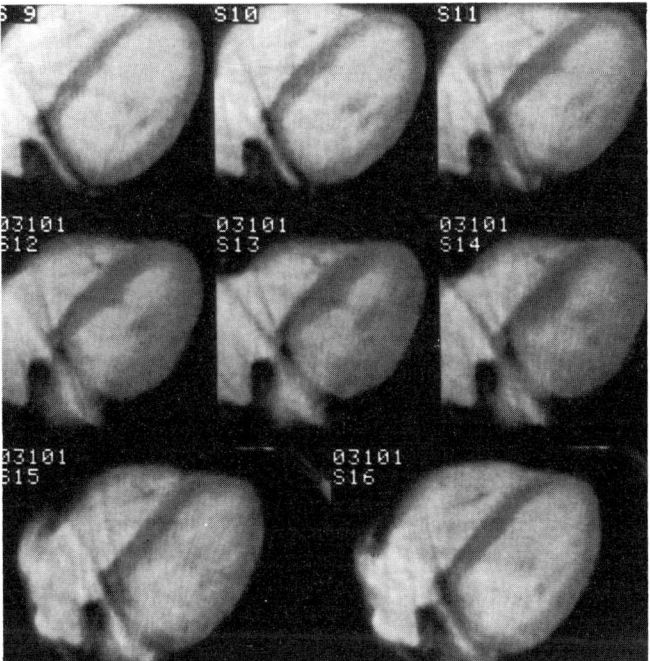

Fig. 15 ECG-gated series of CT scans showing systolic images in the middle row. These reconstructions were obtained by retrospectively gating the CT data to the patients' ECG. Ten scans were obtained at this level and resulted in a gating window of one-tenth of the cardiac cycle, which was approximately 500 ms.

ous cardiac tomographic imaging planes, including the short axis view, can be directly imaged.

Cine-CT scanning techniques

A cine-CT study can be performed rapidly. The first requirement is correct positioning of the patient and accurate localization of the appropriate anatomical scan levels. The left ventricle is usually examined in the short axis plane. This is accomplished by swivelling the table 20° so that the feet are moved to the right with the patient lying supine. Additionally, the table is tilted to elevate the head approximately 15–25°. Electrocardiographic monitoring is used so that the scan exposures can be triggered at selected phases of the cardiac cycle. Localizing scans are then exposed to check the imaging plane and anatomical level and these are reviewed.

Contrast medium administration and scanning options

A flow study is performed first by injecting 0.3 ml/kg body weight of contrast medium at a flow rate of 5 ml/s. A flow controlled injector allows accurate reproducibility and provides greater precision of quantitative analysis. Fifty millisecond scans are obtained at eight contiguous levels, and are all exposed during the same phase of the cardiac cycle, usually systole, on either every heart beat or every second or third beat. Ten scans are usually obtained at each of the eight levels with one 20–25 ml bolus injection in adults (Fig. 17a). There is considerable display flexibility as the images are stored and displayed in the digitized form.

Figure 17b is a geometric on-line magnification of the sixth scan (8.64 s) of the series in Fig. 17a showing the proximal coronary arteries. Figure 18 illustrates a typical scan sequence at one of the eight levels from a dynamic flow-mode cine-CT series. The circulation time is readily obtained from these as each scan is registered in time and anatomical site and displayed on the monitor with each image. This time is used to direct the next phase of a cine-CT study which is the scan acquisition of the movie mode. The flow mode of operation, as will be seen, is also the basis of quantifying vessel, cardiac chamber, and tissue blood flow using gamma variate curve analysis.

The movie mode involves a separate injection of contrast medium with high-speed scanning at the rate of 17 images/s at four, six or eight levels during biventricular contrast enhancement. The scan acquisition period is short, usually between one and four heart beats. The patient is instructed to breath hold in inspiration during the short scanning period.

The scans acquired at 17/s are ECG monitored to ensure that

end-diastole and end-systole are obtained for each level. The cine-CT monitor can display the ECG and indicates the exposure times of each scan on its time base. Usually 8 or 12 levels are scanned to cover the whole ventricular muscle mass and cavities. The CT images are then displayed sequentially as a closed loop movie on the cathode ray oscilloscope for each level. Thcy are also displayed as individual images at various phases of the cardiac cycle.

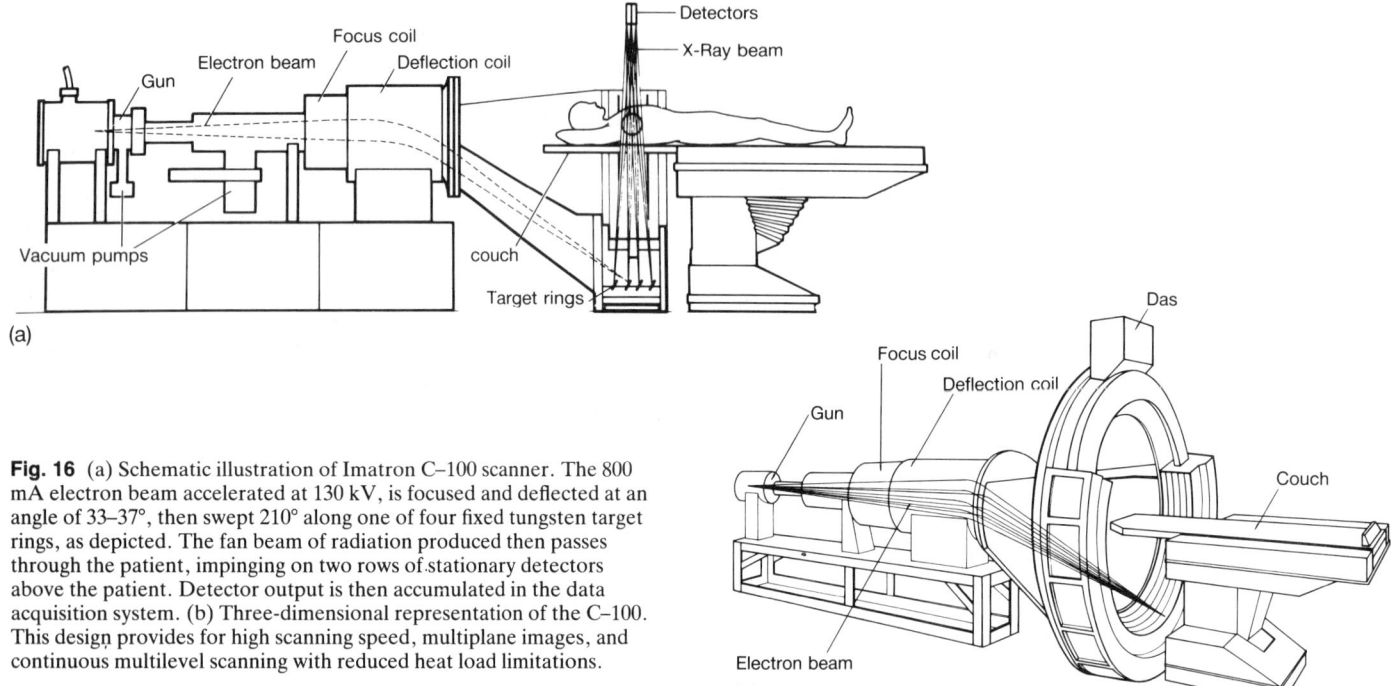

Fig. 16 (a) Schematic illustration of Imatron C–100 scanner. The 800 mA electron beam accelerated at 130 kV, is focused and deflected at an angle of 33–37°, then swept 210° along one of four fixed tungsten target rings, as depicted. The fan beam of radiation produced then passes through the patient, impinging on two rows of stationary detectors above the patient. Detector output is then accumulated in the data acquisition system. (b) Three-dimensional representation of the C–100. This design provides for high scanning speed, multiplane images, and continuous multilevel scanning with reduced heat load limitations.

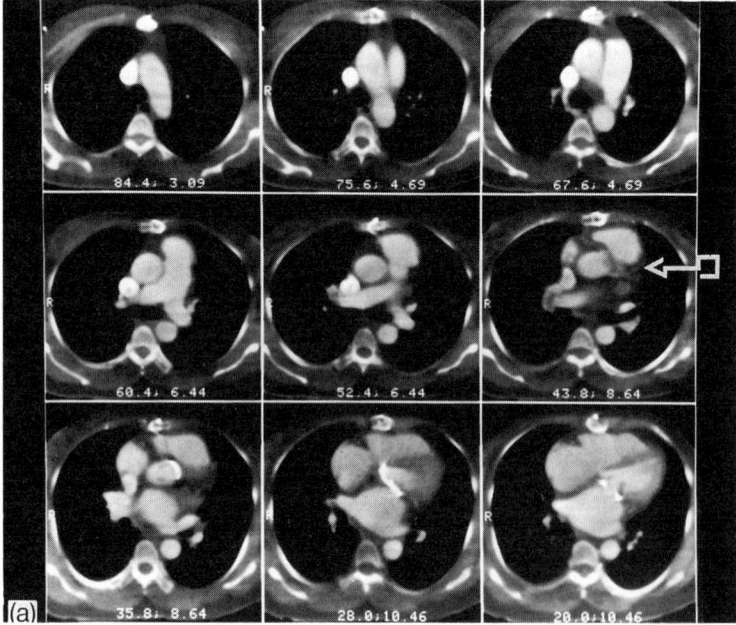
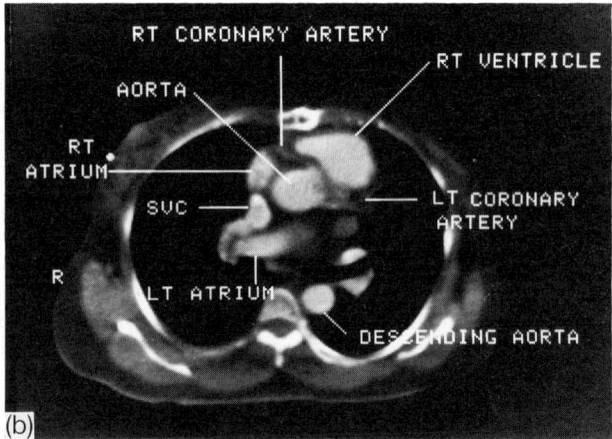

Fig. 17 (a) Illustration of a collection of nine contiguous 8 mm thick scans in a patient with valve prostheses in the mitral and aortic areas. These scans were selected from a dynamic CT flow study at times when both right- and left-sided cardiac structures were contrast enhanced. Note how relatively free from motion streak artifacts these images are despite the dense prostheses. Also, the resolution is adequate for identifying the proximal right and left main coronary arteries and the proximal main branches on the image at 8.64 s (arrow). (b) This image showing the left main, left anterior descending, left circumflex, and main right coronary artery is the same image as the one arrowed in (a). Magnification of this type is possible instantaneously with digitized cine-CT images.

This cinematographic mode demonstrates the changes in cardiac chamber dimensions throughout the cardiac cycle and also enables myocardial wall thickness and thickening to be studied, both qualitatively and quantitatively as shown in Figs 19a and b.

Quantitative cine-CT methods

Left ventricular volumes

The high spatial and density resolution of CT allows the endocardial as well as the epicardial boundaries to be planimetered using a track ball guided cursor and computer-assisted software programs. This technique is illustrated in Fig. 20. The areas of the outlined ventricular cavities are printed on the monitor as each level is planimetered, and are recorded on film using a multiformat camera. The end-diastolic, end-systolic volume, and subsequent global and

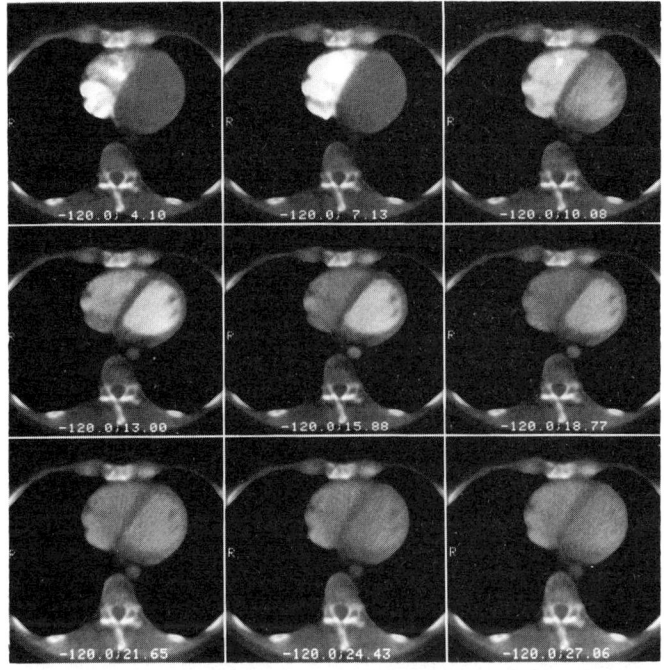

Fig. 18 A sequence of 19, cine-CT 50 ms exposures are shown from the same level illustrating the dynamic or flow-mode using a 20 ml bolus of Conray 400 injected into a peripheral vein. Contrast enhancement occurs progressively from right atrium to right ventricle to left atrium and, finally, the left ventricle and descending thoracic aorta are maximally enhanced. All the CT scans in their sequence were exposed in 50 m/s in diastole using ECG triggering. This ensures good slice registration on the matrix for data analysis.

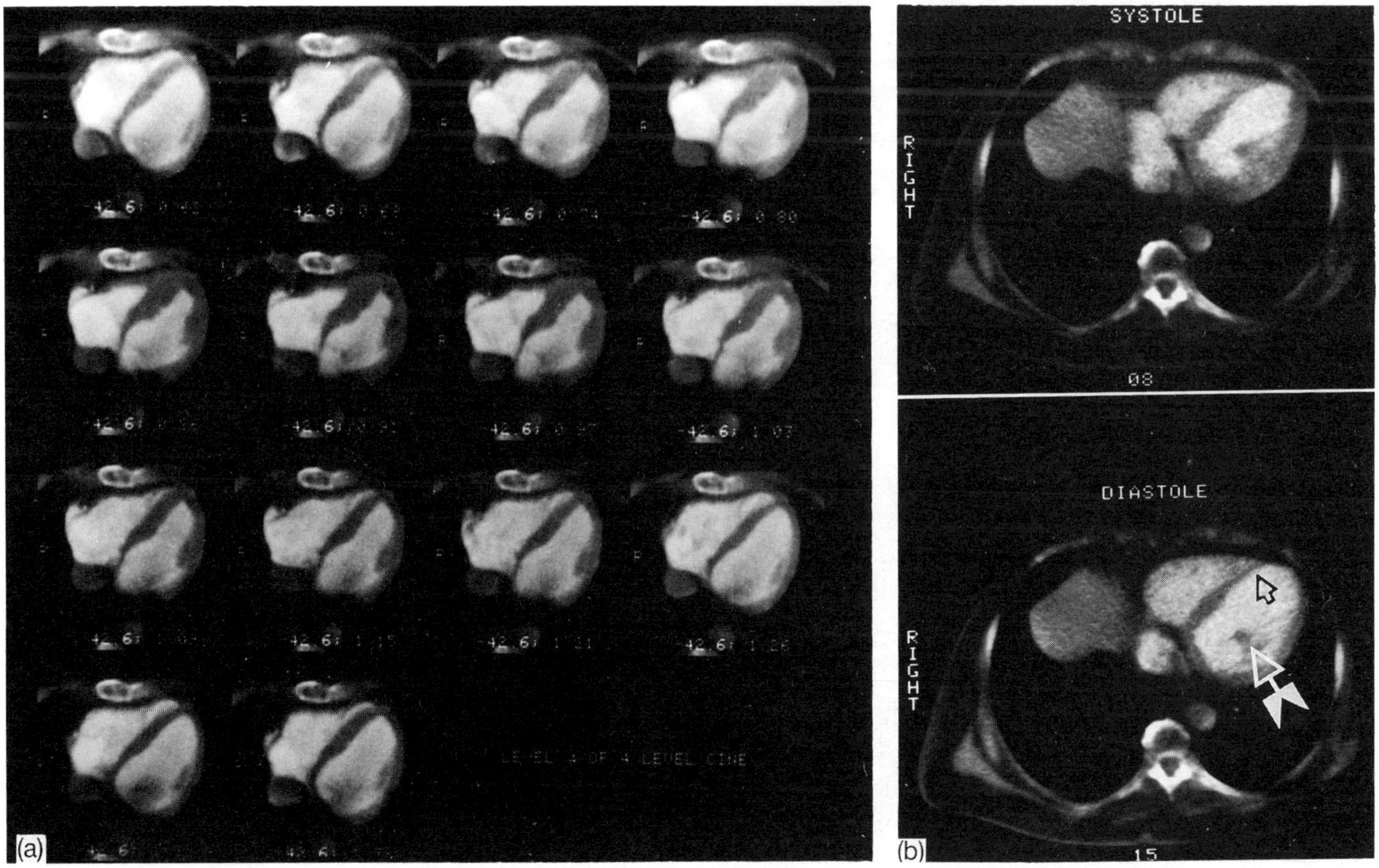

Fig. 19 (a) Illustrates the movie mode of operation of the cine-CT system. Fourteen CT images from a series of contrast-enhanced scans is seen in a patient with a normally contracting left ventricle. Note the various phases of the cardiac cycle depicted. Diastole is represented in the top left panel followed by systolic images in the second row and finally diastole again. All these images were acquired during one heart cycle without the need for any form of ECG gating (averaging). Note how well the myocardial wall boundaries are seen. (b) Systolic and diastolic CT scans from a patient who sustained an old arteroseptal infarction. Note the absence of normal motion as well as myocardial wall thickening in the anterior wall and the anterior portion of the septum, which are markedly thinner than in other regions (black arrow). The right atrium and ventricle are also well defined, and their motion characterized. The right diaphragm and lobe of the liver can be seen adjacent to the heart at this scanning level. The posterior papillary muscle explains the increased density within the left ventricle in this plane (white arrow).

regional ejection fractions are obtained by Simpson's rule. Computed tomography measurement of left and right ventricular volumes has been shown to be independent of chamber orientation unlike angiocardiography and echocardiography which require geometric assumptions in their calculations. Global and regional ejection volume measurements are currently being validated for cine-CT in humans with biplane angiography.

Measurements of left ventricular mass by cine-CT
The ability to define the endocardial and epicardial wall edges accurately and reproducibly by CT techniques has been validated

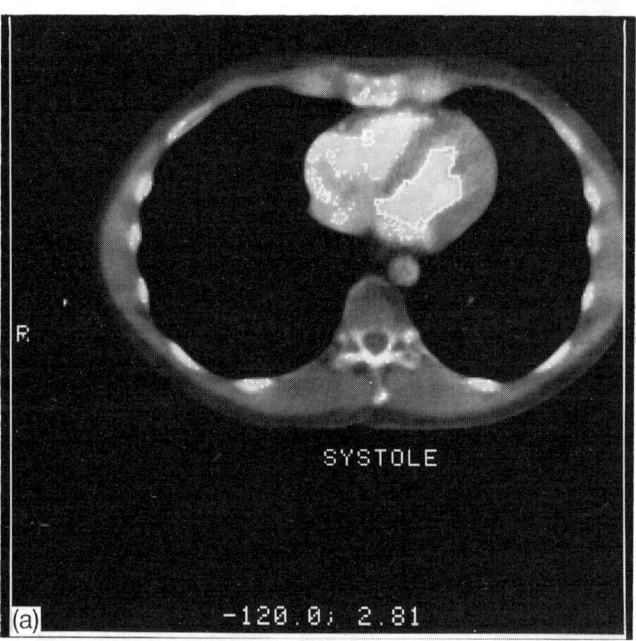

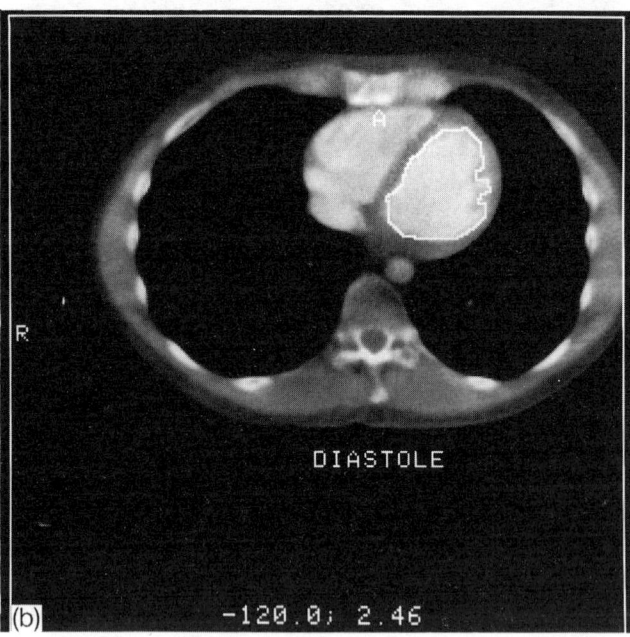

Fig. 20 (a) End-systolic and (b) end-diastolic images from cine acquisition demonstrating calculation of diastolic and systolic left ventricular areas. Endocardial boundary detection was enhanced using a computer density half-contour detection method. Dividing the difference between diastolic and systolic areas by the diastolic area provides the ejection fraction for this 8 mm thick slice. Ventricular volumes are calculated by summation of areas at multiple levels and multiplication by level spacing according to Simpson's rule.

previously for septal wall thickness and myocardial mass in animals. A recent study showed that left ventricular mass in dogs can be measured with cine-CT more precisely than by any other invasive or non-invasive technique. Several centres are performing various validation cine-CT studies of chamber and wall dimensions in humans, and validating their results against other established proven modalities. The tomographic advantages of cine-CT imaging are significant, particularly in conditions in which hypertrophy is asymmetrical as in some types of myopathies (Fig. 21).

The role of cine-CT in myocardial infarction
Until now, the use of slow CT has been limited by the single slice configuration and poor slice registration due to the need for sequential breath holding, as well as multiple injections of contrast medium. The C-100 overcomes these difficulties so that a vast quantity of CT data can be collected with each injection. The effects of ischaemia on wall thinning and contractility can be quantified in humans by cine-CT. In a recent study comprising 24 patients at the University of California, cine-CT provided a reliable assessment of regional wall motion based on left ventricular cavity dynamics (Figs 19a and b). Abnormal contraction patterns by CT correlated in 90 per cent (100/110) of segments with the findings of biplane left ventriculography. It is likely that by adding wall thickening measurements, the cine-CT evaluation CT should be even more sensitive in characterizing ischaemic dysfunction as illustrated in Fig. 21. The sequelae of infarction, namely, thrombus and aneurysm formation, can also be detected and quantified by CT.

Exercise and pharmacological cine-CT stress testing
Wall mechanics have been quantified and validated by cine-CT which can measure wall thickening and thinning during acute ischaemia. Figure 22 illustrates these results. Myocardial wall thickness is measured in this manner at all levels from cardiac apex to base. Supine exercise, using a bicycle ergometer attached to the cine-CT table for exercise stress testing, is presently being evaluated. Interventions with various pharmacological vasodilators

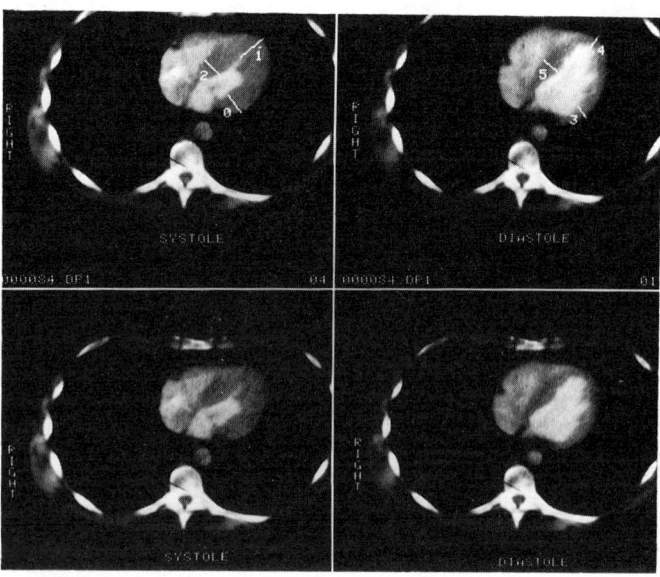

Fig. 21 Systolic and diastolic images are seen in a patient with hypertropic cardiomyopathy. The images in the upper panels are the same as below, but have been analysed to determine regional wall thickness and thickening during the cardiac cycle. Wall thickening is readily appreciated from the movie display and is an excellent index of function. Cine-CT is able to measure the percentage of change with precision. Once the operator defines the points, the computer displays these data numerically on the monitor alongside these images.

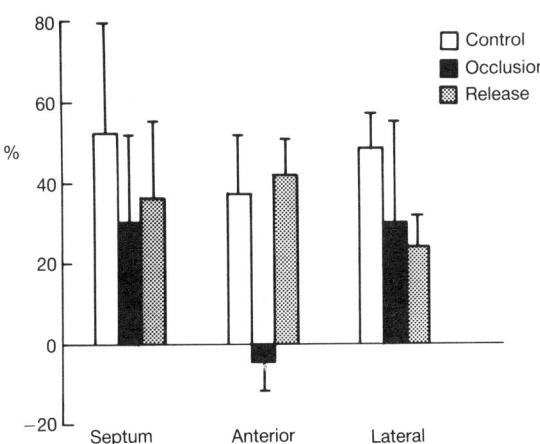

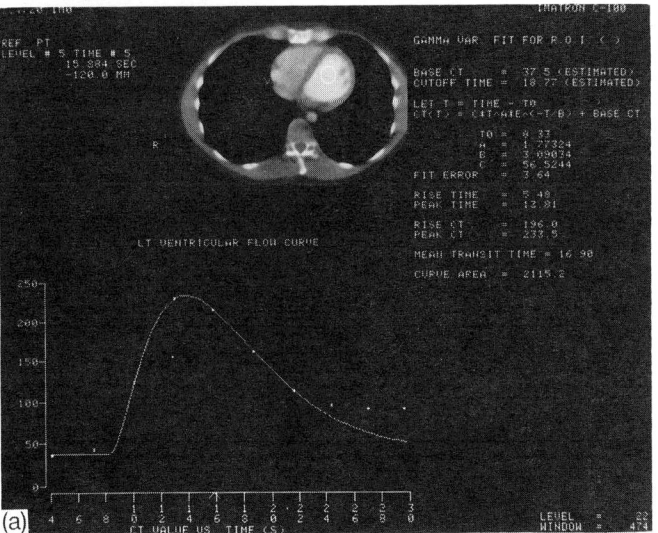

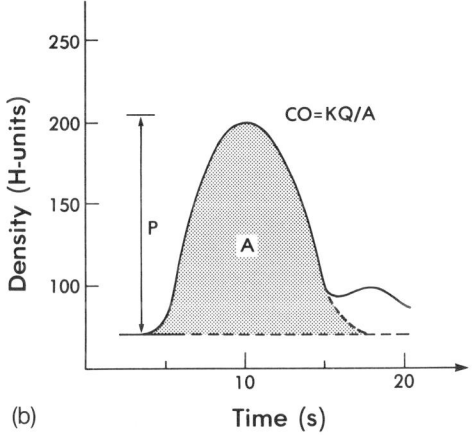

Fig. 22 Graphic representation of end diastolic and end systolic wall measurements in five dogs for the control occlusion and release states of the left anterior descending coronary artery in the septal, anterior, and lateral walls. There is marked decrease in systolic thickness of the anterior wall during acute occlusion of the left anterior descending coronary artery. The other regions show little effect. (Reproduced from Farmer *et al.*, 1985, with permission.)

Fig. 23 (a) Single axial 50 ms image from triggered or flow sequence when contrast bolus is present in left ventricle. Following the placement of a region of interest over left ventricular cavity, computer plots time–mean CT number (density) curve. These points are then fitted to a standard theoretical curve (gamma variate), which corrects for secondary recirculation peak, if present. After performing the fit, the computer calculates various bolus parameters, including the rise time, peak time, and area under the curve, which are simultaneously displayed on the monitor alongside the image. (b) Cardiac output can be determined from area under left ventricular curve (A) is in 23a, if the quantity of iodinated contrast medium injected (Q) is known.

are also being explored with cine-CT to determine whether significant coronary artery disease can be quantified by changes in wall mechanics. These applications are possible because cine-CT provides unique high-speed, high-resolution, cross-sectional imaging during one or more heart cycles.

Coronary artery bypass graft patency by cine-CT

Cine-CT illustrates between two and eight anatomical levels during one bolus injection of contrast agent. This provides greatly improved scan registration during the time of held inspiration and significantly reduces the total volume of contrast medium needed for the study. Furthermore, time–density analysis, as generated by the cine-CT scanner, has the promise of permitting the quantification of graft flow. Internal mammary grafts can also be evaluated. Cine-CT by virtue of multilevel scanning allows not only rapid study, but also enables cine-CT left ventriculography to be performed during the same procedure. Thus, cine-CT should extend our capability for determining graft patency and cardiac function during a single outpatient visit, almost non-invasively.

Measurements of blood flow

No present imaging modality can measure regional myocardial blood flow in absolute terms with any degree of precision. Thallium-201 imaging provides useful but only relative estimates of regional myocardial perfusion. Nearly all our techniques for evaluating ischaemic heart disease are indirect, including coronary arteriography and left ventriculography. Blood flow measurements which are clinically useful may be considered in two groups, blood flow through the cardiac chambers and vessels such as the carotid arteries and coronary bypass grafts and, secondly, and much more difficult, blood flow measurements in tissue.

Cardiac output has been measured and validated by cine-CT. This capability has been assessed in dogs using the gamma variate curve derived from a flow-mode sequence of scans. The area under this curve shown in Figs 23a and b reflects the cardiac output, which is given by the Stewart–Hamilton equation:

$$CO = \frac{X}{c(t)\, \delta\, t}$$

where CO is the cardiac output, X is the quantity of indicator injected into the system and $c(t)$ is the concentration at the sampling site at time t. This concentration is given in terms of density, because a linear relationship exists between indicator (iodine)

concentration and CT numbers over the physiological range. The accuracy of cine-CT has been validated against simultaneous thermodilution measurements of cardiac output and the results, illustrated in Fig. 24, showed excellent correlation ($r = 0.92$) with a mean percentage difference between these techniques of 9.7 per cent over a range of 1.5–6.3 l/min.

Vessel flow can also be characterized using high-speed CT scanning by at least two methods. One approach is to obtain curves, for example, from each carotid artery obtained simultaneously and use the first derivative of this to explore the relationship between slope and arterial occlusive disease. The results are being compared with pre- and postoperative angiographic findings. The carotid arteries are well seen by cine-CT and digital subtraction capability is on-line and helpful in identifying, for example, the vertebral arteries (Table 1).

The second method for measuring flow is to acquire time–density curves at multiple levels for the same bolus injection; hence the peak arrival time can be measured along a vessel. Figure 25 illustrates how the velocity can be calculated for each carotid.

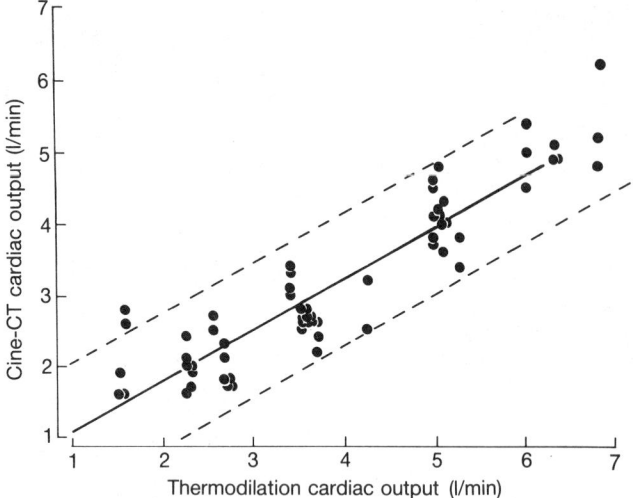

Fig. 24 Demonstration of linear relationship between cine-CT and ther-modilution cardiac outputs. Lease squares regression line is solid; confidence intervals (95 per cent) are broken lines. Solid circles are the individual data prints. Correlation coefficient (r) = 0.92. (Reproduced from Garrett *et al.*, 1985, with permission.)

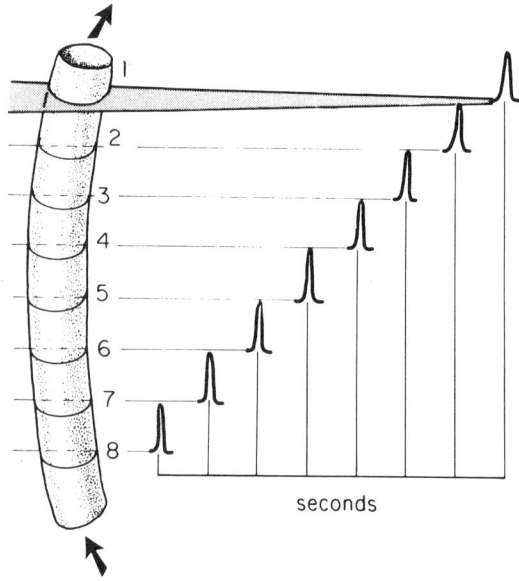

Fig. 25 CT time–density curves generated at eight contiguous levels from a multilevel cine-CT flow sequence during one bolus of contrast medium injected into a peripheral vein. The diagram represents a linear vessel such as the carotid artery. The peak arrival time is given for each flow curve, hence, the velocity profile can be measured in cm/s. Blood flow can be estimated from the velocity if the vessel area is known. This is readily calculated from the many cross-sectional CT images. Bilateral images are acquired for each carotid vessel during the same bolus injection.

Other techniques can also measure velocity, but the cross-sectional images of CT permit the areas of the vessels to be measured simultaneously at each level; hence, the potential for measuring absolute carotid blood flow is apparent. The ability to obtain a bimodal time–density curve over any vascular region involved in left-to-right or right-to-left cardiac shunts provides a measure of the size of the shunt. Absolute myocardial blood flow can be derived by interpreting the relative myocardial time–density curve in concert with the cardiac output, both of which are determined by indicator dilution.

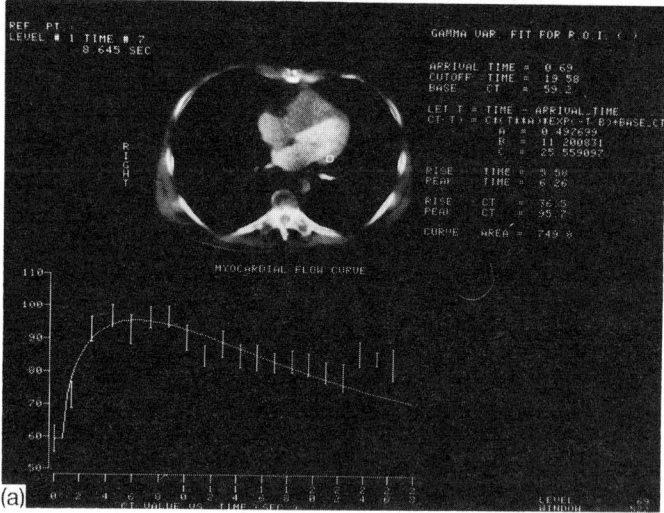

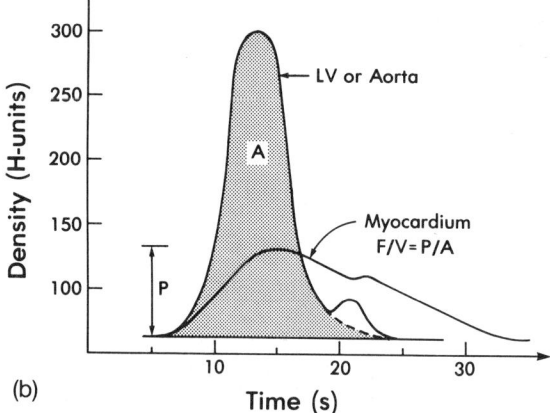

Fig. 26 (a) Myocardial perfusion curve generated over lateral left ventricular wall in a patient with a previous anterior myocardial infarction. Curve analysis provides peak height. Any zone(s) can be analysed around the left ventricular cavity, and at all anatomical levels. (b) Blood flow (F/V) in any myocardial region can be calculated as the ratio of the peak of the time–density curve in that area (P) to the area under the aorta or left ventricle time–density curve (A), which is representative of cardiac output.

For any given contrast injection, as indicated above, measurement of the area under the time–density curves of the aorta and left ventricle is constant and representative of cardiac output. Absolute flow can then be calculated for any myocardial region as the ratio of peak enhancement of the time–density curve in that region to the area under the aortic or ventricular time–density curves (Figs 23a, 26a and b).

This formula assumes that the myocardial contrast washout time is longer than the width of the aortic or ventricular time–density curve. This is true in the myocardium because transit time through the capillary bed is longer than the duration of the systemic venous contrast bolus injection. The theoretical basis which underlies this concept has been discussed in the literature, but the only realistic approach is with three-dimensional imaging techniques which allow accurate sampling. Regional blood flow can be measured by external detectors with a three-dimensional isotope imaging technique. There is, therefore, the realistic prospect of measuring tissue blood flow in humans using high-speed multilevel CT.

Conclusions

The future of direct measurements of flow by cine-CT will depend upon the results of studies now in progress, but the prospect of this

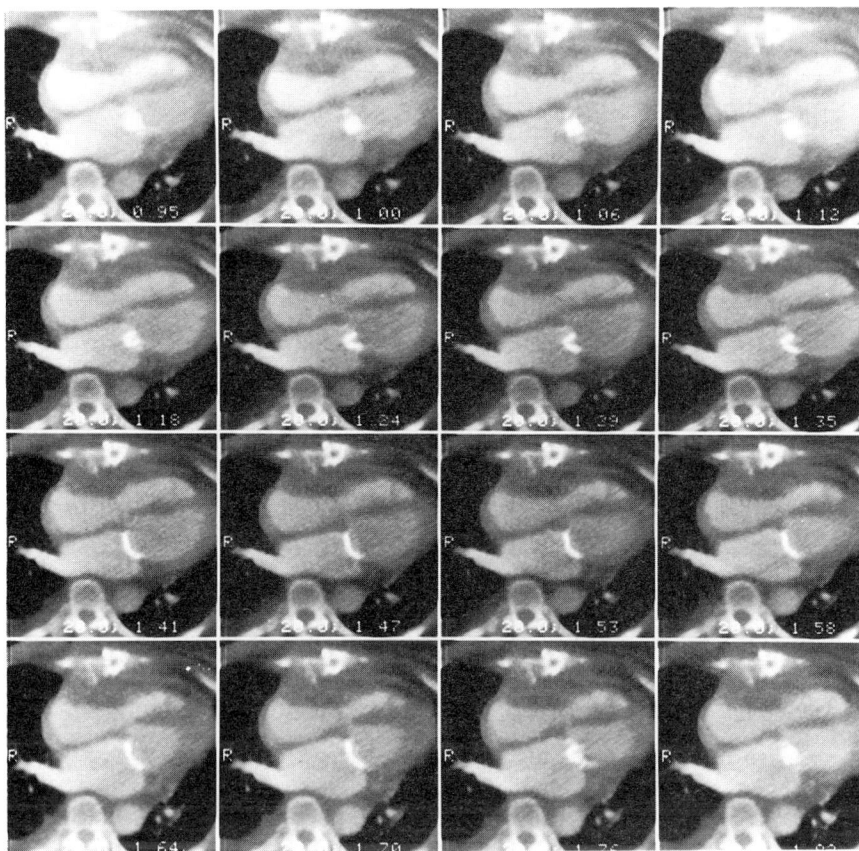

Fig. 27 St Jude mitral prosthesis demonstrated by the movie mode (17 images/s). This is one of four levels scanned simultaneously. The movement and position of the struts which are radio-opaque is well seen. The velocity of their motion can also be estimated. Note that the prosthesis is not obscured by streak artefacts which are a major cause of extensive image degradation with slow conventional CT. The four cardiac chambers are all seen by contrast enhancement; 30 ml or Hypaque 60 was infused into a peripheral vein at 3 ml/s.

new modality for improving the diagnosis and management of patients with coronary artery occlusive disease is exciting. The ability of the high sampling rates for analysing motion creates images which are similar to cineangiography. An example is seen of a prosthetic valve in Fig. 27.

Further validation studies of course are necessary to confirm the capability of cine-CT to provide consistent and quantitative data. Reproducibility studies to verify the precision and specificity of the scanner are in progress. There is, furthermore, every indication that the spatial resolution of cine-CT will be improved and will soon be comparable with state-of-the-art whole body scanners for imaging the body and the brain. The advanced computer software power of the cine-CT system is also likely to extend its applications because of the ease of data extraction for rapid quantitative cardiac CT studies. Image quality is steadily improving and is now almost comparable in the thorax and abdomen to present whole body CT scanners. Improved patient diagnosis can be expected because of the rapid acquisition of images, which allows improved contrast enhancement even while using smaller volumes of contrast medium. This rapidity and improved resolution should significantly increase the number of patients scanned per day compared with conventional CT. It seems likely that high-speed CT electron beam scanners could create a new cardiac and universal imaging modality providing simultaneous anatomical and physiological diagnosis; this prospect, furthermore, could become a clinical reality within the next few years.

References

Boyd, D. P. (1981). Transmission computed tomography. In *Radiology of the skull and brain: technical aspects of computed tomography* (eds T. H. Newton and D. G. Polk), pp. 4357–4371. C. V. Mosby, St Louis, Missouri.

Brasch, R. C., Boyd, D. P. and Gooding, C. A. (1978). Computed tomography scanning in children: comparison of radiation dose and resolving power of commercial CT scanners. *Am. J. Roentgenol.* **131**, 95.

Daniel, W. G., Dohring, W., Stender, H. S. and Lichtlen, P. R. (1983). Value and limitations of computed tomography in assessing aortocoronary bypass graft patency. *Circulation* **67**, 983–987.

Doherty, P. W., Lipton, M. J., Berninger, W. H., Skioldebrand, C. G., Carlsson, E. and Redington, R. W. (1981). Detection and quantitation of myocardial infarction *in vivo* using transmission computed tomography. *Circulation* **63**, 597–606.

Farmer, D. W., Lipton, M. J., Higgins, C. B. *et al.* (1985). *In vivo* assessment of left ventricular wall and chamber dynamics during transient ischemia using cine computed tomography. *Am. J. Cardiol.* **55**, 560–565.

——, ——, Webb, R., Ringertz, H. and Higgins, C. B. (1984). Computed tomography in congenital heart disease. *JCAT* **8**, 677–687.

Garrett, J. S., Lanzer, P., Jaschke, W. *et al.* (1985). Measurement of cardiac output by cine-CT. *Am. J. Cardiol.* **56**, 657–661.

Godwin, J. D., Turley, K., Herfkens, R. J. and Lipton, M. J. (1981). Computed tomography for follow-up of chronic aortic dissections. *Radiology* **139**, 1–660.

Goldstein, J., Lipton, M. J., Schiller, N. B., Ports, T. A. and Brundage, B. H. (1982). Evaluation of intracardiac thrombi with contrast enhanced computed tomography and echocardiography. *Am. J. Cardiol.* **49**, 972 (abstract).

Hounsfield, G. N. (1973). Computerized transverse axial scanning (tomography – Part I. Description of system). *Br. J. Radiol.* **46**, 1016–1022.

Isner, J. M., Carter, B. L., Bankoff, M. S., *et al.* (1983). Differentiation of constrictive pericarditis from restrictive cardiomyopathy by computed tomography imaging. *Am. Heart J.* **105**, 1019–1025.

Kramer, P., Goldstein, J., Herfkens, R., Lipton, M. J. and Brundage, B. H. (1984). Imaging of acute myocardial infarction in man with contrast enhanced computed transmission tomography. *J. Am. Heart Assoc.* **108**, 1514–1523.

Lackner, K. and Thurn, P. (1981). Computed tomography of the heart: ECG-gated and continuous scans. *Radiology* **140**, 413–420.

Lipton, M. J. and Higgins, C. B. (1980). Evaluation of ischemic heart disease by computed transmission tomography. *Radiol. Clin. N. Am.* **18**, 557–576.

—— and —— (1984). Computed tomography. The technique and its use for the evaluation of cardiocirculatory anatomy and function. In *Pediatric cardiac imaging* (eds W. Friedman and C. Higgins), pp. 120–134. W. B. Saunders Company, Philadelphia.

Moncada, R., Baker, M., Salinas, M., *et al.* (1982). Diagnostic role of computed tomography in pericardial heart disease: congenital defects, thickening, neoplasms and effusion. *Am. Heart J.* **103**, 263–282.

Rumberger, J. A., Fiering, A. J., Lipton, M. J., Higgins, C. B. *et al.* (1985). Measurement of myocardial perfusion by ultrafast CT. *J. Am. Coll. Cardiol.* **5**, 500.

Skioldebrand, C. G., Lipton, M. J., Mavroudis, C. and Hayashi, T. T. (1982). Determination of left ventricular mass by computed tomography. *Am. J. Cardiol.* **49**, 63–70.

Thompson, H. H., Starmer, C. F., Whalen R. E. *et al.* (1964). Indicator transit time considered as a gamma variate. *Circ. Res.* **14**, 502–515.

SYMPTOMS OF HEART DISEASE

Dyspnoea

A. GUZ

Dyspnoea (breathlessness in the Greek language) is the sensation of difficult, laboured, uncomfortable breathing. Its presence is signalled by the patient rather than directly observed by the clinician. It presents a formidable clinical problem. Not only does it cause distress and suffering but it results in major socioeconomic consequences by limiting activity. The increase in numbers of survivors of acute cardiopulmonary disorders who are in the chronic phase of their disease means that dyspnoea is becoming more common in clinical conditions that are incurable.

Diseases that give rise to dyspnoea

Diseases may be grouped according to three principal pathophysiological features, although considerable overlap may occur.

(a) Diseases with an increased drive to breathe Disorders in this group include pulmonary embolism, pulmonary oedema, pulmonary fibrosis, and other infiltrations, pneumonia, anaemia, and acidosis; they are all associated with excessive drive to breath. Hypoxia which occurs in many of these diseases adds another drive to breathe. The respiratory frequency is usually increased and the arterial P_{CO_2} is low.

(b) Diseases with an increased hindrance to breathing Disease in this category, causing a decrease in compliance or increase in resistance, including pulmonary infiltrations or congestion, and obstructive disease of the airways.

(c) Diseases associated with a decreased neuromuscular power Diseases in this category include those of the skeleton such as kyphoscoliosis and ankylosing spondylitis, those of the respiratory muscles such as the muscular dystrophies, and those where there is a problem in maintaining neural output to the respiratory muscles as with lesions within the spinal cord including poliomyelitis, polyneuritis, and myasthenia gravis.

It can be seen that with all three pathophysiological groups there is likely to be increased neural output to the muscles of respiration to maintain the required level of ventilation, both at rest and within the neuromuscular mechanisms that are still functioning on exercise.

Patients find that it is extremely difficult to describe the sensation of breathlessness. In general, it is described as not different from normally experienced exercise dyspnoea – with the difference that the sensation is felt at an inappropriately low workload, or at rest. Sometimes, particularly with airway disease, the sensation is described as a tightness in the chest.

Assessment of breathlessness

The time-honoured bedside assessment grades breathlessness according to the activities which are affected (Table 1). Although this method is easily applied, significant changes can occur that are not reflected in the grades.

A 6 or 12 min walking test requires patients to walk as far as

Table 1 Dyspnoea assessment

Grade I	Breathing feels as good as that of others of own age, sex, and build, at work, walking, climbing hills or stairs
Grade II	Able to walk with others of own age, sex, and build on the level; unable to keep up on hills or stairs
Grade III	Unable to keep up on the level, but able to walk about a mile or more at own speed
Grade IV	Unable to walk more than 100 yards on the level without resting because of breathlessness
Grade V	Breathless on talking or undressing or inability to leave house because of breathlessness

they can in their own time and to pause for rest; the distance achieved is the objective measured. Provided that angina, arthritic joint pains or leg muscle fatigue are not limiting factors, such a test can be used as an indirect assessment of dyspnoea. More recently the test has been adapted as a self-paced treadmill walk and this has allowed other relevant physiological parameters to be measured at the same time.

Treadmill or bicycle exercise tests with a standard pattern of increase in workload have also been used to assess dyspnoea. These are very uncomfortable for the seriously dyspnoeic patient and performance in them bears little relation to the problems of daily living. These tests are particularly useful in demonstrating normal or near-normal exercise capacity in some patients with 'psychogenic' breathlessness who complain of hardly being able to walk because they are too breathless.

The 'dyspnoeic index' is not an index of breathlessness. It is the maximum ventilation reached on exercise expressed as a percentage of the maximal breathing capacity achieved voluntarily (or by computation from the forced expiratory volume at 1 s). A high 'dyspnoeic index' has been taken as evidence that the breathlessness is appropriate for the level of exercise achieved; a low value for the index is taken as evidence that the breathlessness is 'inappropriate' for the level of exercise achieved. This index gives no information about the actual sensation of breathlessness during the exercise test.

It is only recently that attempts have been made to estimate directly the intensity of the sensation of breathlessness rather than quantify some objective limitation imposed by this symptom. Over the past two decades a number of workers interested in the genesis of the breathless sensation have employed psychophysical techniques (developed to facilitate sensory measurement) to study the mechanisms of respiratory sensation. These techniques involve subjective assessment of the presence and/or intensity of sensations. The most quantitative of such techniques do, however, depend on establishing a relationship between a sensory stimulus intensity and the perceived sensation. Consequently, considerable attention has been focused on the relationship between actual and perceived changes in respiratory volumes and on the ability of the individuals to identify resistive and elastic loads applied to the respiratory system both in terms of their detection thresholds and magnitude. Moreover, the effect of various experimental interventions (e.g. upper airways anaesthesia) on such relationships is reasonably well documented. Such techniques furnish important information about the neural pathways involved in the perception of respiratory sensations but there is no *a priori* reason for linking these experimentally induced sensory phenomena to that sensory experience commonly referred to as breathlessness. Moreover, these approaches are of limited use for clinically orientated studies in which the efficacy of a putative treatment for the symptom of breathlessness (c.f. pain) is being tested.

In 1969, Aitken reported the use of a 100 mm visual analogue scale in the quantification of sensations experimentally induced by resistive loading. More recently, this technique has been validated (in terms of both reproducibility and sensitivity) for the direct quantification of breathlessness induced by ventilatory stimulation both in normal subjects, and patients with respiratory disease; its use is being increasingly reported in both clinical studies and in those relating to physiological mechanisms underlying this sensation. Normal subjects have been found to show a wide but constant variability in their scaling of breathlessness for equivalent degrees of ventilatory stimulation; this is true irrespective of the type of stimulus. These differences are not explained by the physical characteristics, ventilatory sensitivity or pattern of breathing of the subjects. Relevant sensory information appears to be processed in different but reproducible ways in different subjects; other sensory modalities (for which neurophysiological information is available) have been found to behave in the same way. Judgemental, cognitive, and other non-sensory factors must play an important part in explaining these differences; this is an easily observed phenomenon in any respiratory clinic. A crucial aspect of visual analogue scaling concerns the labelling of the extremes of the scale and the instruments given to the rater (and their understanding of these instructions). For breathlessness, the logical descriptor for the low extreme is 'not at all breathless'. However, two approaches have been described in dealing with the upper limit: terms such as 'extremely breathless' or 'worst imaginable breathlessness' require an assessment relative to a conceived intensity of the sensation, which although ill-defined, would hopefully be somewhat consistent over time in a particular individual; on the other hand, 'anchoring' the scale's upper limit by reference to a level of breathlessness experienced by the subject for a certain level of ventilatory stimulation defines this extreme more rigorously, but is only suitable for short-term studies where the 'standard' can be remembered.

A visual analogue scale could yield 'internal' scaling measurement of breathlessness whereby equal differences in the magnitude of the scaling would represent equal increments of sensation. In practice it seems reasonable to assume that individuals would vary in their ability to make such estimates reliably as well as in their ability to discriminate between differing intensities of the sensation and express these using the scale. For these reasons, the practical use of the scale may well approximate to 'category' or 'ordinal' scaling with the number of categories undefined and varying between subjects. In this respect, the use of overt category scales represents a similar approach although the linking of categories to numbers or semantic statements may introduce subjective bias not associated with an analogue scale. A twelve-point category scale has recently been described for breathlessness, modified from the Borg scale for perceived exertion. Subjective and objective measures during exercise have also been combined in a four-quadrant diagram showing the relationships between a Borg breathlessness scale, ventilation, oxygen comsumption, and an index of increased respiratory muscle work. Scaling of breathlessness is only a useful tool for studying mechanisms and detecting change, if a high level of reproducibility can be obtained. Under carefully controlled conditions, and with reference to objective measures such as ventilation and the stimulus (be it hypercapnia, hypoxia or exercise workload) reasonable reproducibility can be obtained with a visual analogue scale provided the subject is well trained in its use, and instructed in the need to scale a definite dimension of the sensation, such as the intensity of the uncomfortable need to breathe.

Mechanisms of breathlessness

The origin of the sensation of breathlessness remains something of a mystery. Its occurrence in such a wide range of conditions has resulted in a search for a unifying mechanism. In some cases breathlessness is associated with increased ventilation, in others not. A unifying working concept is that in all situations associated with breathlessness, drives to breathe exist which are abnormal, either qualitatively and quantitatively, and which are translated at medullary level into a motor command; this would be the sum of all the nervous traffic to all of the muscles involved in the act of breathing. With a normal respiratory apparatus, an increase in ventilation occurs. With decreased lung compliance or increased lung resistance, and with neuromuscular/skeletal disease affecting the respiratory apparatus, the increased drive to breathe may not produce an increase in ventilation but may nevertheless be associated with breathlessness.

This working concept does not answer the following two basic questions:

(*a*) What combination of receptors need to be activated to give rise to the sensation, and what is their anatomical location?

(*b*) What part of the cerebral cortex is involved in experiencing this sensation?

These questions have never been answered. No investigator has ever described breathlessness experienced during local electrical stimulation of the cortex with the patient conscious. However, this has not been studied in a systematic way, particularly in areas of the orbital cortex of the frontal lobe known to be excited by afferent discharge in the glossopharyngeal and vagus nerves, and also in the sensory cortex between forelimb and hindlimb representations, where phrenic afferents are known to project.

This unifying concept is based on the following evidence:

1. Patients with disease in the medulla (e.g. polioencephalitis, glioma) involving the respiratory 'centre' area, usually do not feel breathless, even though the drives of hypoxia, hypercapnia, lung deflation, are all present; there is no increased motor output to the respiratory muscles, i.e. no ventilatory response. Carbon dioxide added to the inspiratory port of a ventilator maintaining life in such a patient probably causes drowsiness rather than breathlessness, although the opposite view has also been expressed.

2. Afferent drives in the IXth nerve ($P_{O_2}\downarrow$, $P_{CO2}\uparrow$, pH $\downarrow$) and in the Xth nerve (lung collapse, oedema, and microvascular obstruction) do not appear, in themselves, to be felt as breathlessness unless a motor output to the respiratory muscles results. The synchronous discharge of non-myelinated afferents in the alveolar walls of normal humans has been elicited by the injection of the pepper alkaloid capsaicin into the right atrium; there is no ventilatory response, and no breathlessness, but a raw burning sensation in the chest results.

3. Hypoxia, causing a respiratory drive via the cartoid body and the IXth nerve, is a major cause of breathlessness; its correction or prevention usually improves breathlessness.

4. The voluntary control of breathing, presumably originating from the cortex, has a descending pathway to the phrenic and intercostal anterior horn cells that is separate from the descending pathway of the 'automatic' respiratory centre. Voluntary isocapnic hyperventilation is associated with little or no breathlessness in both normals and patients with reduced compliance or high airway resistance. The same ventilation (both in terms of pattern and mechanical work done) achieved during the stimulation of exercise, hypercapnia or hypoxia is accompanied by breathlessness. Thus the activation of respiratory muscle anterior horn cells in the spinal cord in the same manner, by the voluntary pathway as by reflex pathways, has the same results as far as the development of respiratory muscle tension and shortening is concerned, but entirely different results for breathlessness. This must mean that respiratory muscle afferent discharge is unlikely to be relevant to the generation of breathlessness.

5. Patients with complete transections of the spinal cord as high

as C5/6 become breathless with lobar collapse, pulmonary embolus or pneumonia; afferents from the chest wall muscles cannot therefore play a crucial role in the genesis of the sensation.

6. Breathlessness at rest or on exercise is often severe with no evidence of respiratory muscle fatigue. When muscle fatigue is experimentally produced, the accompanying sensation is not that of breathlessness.

7. The removal of abnormal drives to breathe in patients, e.g. correction of hypoxia, carotid body resection, vagal blockade or section, may all improve breathlessness and simultaneously diminish the associated breathing.

Exercise

Breathlessness is brought on or exaggerated by exercise. The mechanisms underlying this can be thought of in terms of extra motor neural output resulting not only from the drive due to exercise but also, in cardiopulmonary disease, from new drives appearing as a result of the development of hypoxia, hypercapnia, metabolic acidosis (IXth nerve), and/or pulmonary venous or arterial hypertension with or without lung oedema (Xth nerve). There is increasing experimental evidence that the intensity of breathlessness grows with the fraction of the maximum respiratory muscle force-generating mechanism utilized in breathing.

Emotional disturbance

The subjective experience of the sensation of breathlessness is dependent on affective factors; the psychosomatic mechanisms are not understood.

Treatment of breathlessness

The best treatment for breathlessness is to cure the cause, e.g. in asthma or anaemia. This is not possible in much chronic cardiopulmonary disease. Careful correction of as many as possible of the pathophysiological features that drive breathing, will improve breathlessness and diminish ventilation. Where this ventilation is excessive no harm results, but there is a danger of worsening respiratory failure where the mechanics of the respiratory bellows is so abnormal that an excessive drive to breathe is required to maintain a normal alveolar ventilation and hence blood gases.

Avoidance of hypoxia, particularly that developing on exercise, is one of the simplest drives to remove, by giving supplementary oxygen via nasal catheters; breathlessness at a given workload is often much reduced. The same drive to breathe can be removed by carotid body resection. Although it is likely that breathlessness improves and exercise tolerance increases, such surgery cannot yet be recommended until proper controlled studies have been done.

Pulmonary denervation has been studied on an experimental basis only; vagus nerves have been anaesthetized or sectioned in the neck. The removal of major drives to breathe, particularly with infiltrative lung disease, has resulted in some striking reductions of both ventilation and breathlessness. Denervated lungs do not have a cough reflex and this should encourage caution before undertaking such a potentially hazardous procedure.

Encouragement of 'adaptation' to the sensation of breathlessness is another approach to treatment. This mechanism, poorly understood, may underlie the benefits of exercise training programmes in patients with chronic obstructive airways disease. Such exercise training may result in improvement of breathlessness even when the training programme is not directed at improving respiratory muscle power.

References

Adams, L., Chronos, N., Lane, R. and Guz, A. (1985). The measurement of breathlessness induced in normal subjects: validity of two scaling techniques. *Clin. Sci.* **69**, 7–16.
—— (1985). The measurement of breathlessness induced in normal subjects: individual differences. *Clin. Sci.* **70**, 131–140.

Aitken, R. C. B., Zeallyey, A. K. and Rosenthal, S. V. (1970). Some psychological and physiological considerations of breathlessness. In *Breathing. Hering-Breuer Centenary Symposium* (ed. R. Porter), pp. 253–273. Churchill Livingstone, London.
Altose, M., Cherniack, N. and Fishman, A. P. (1985). Respiratory sensations and dyspnoea. *J. Appl. Physiol.* **58**, 1051–1055.
Bond, A. and Lader, M. (1974). The use of analogue scales in rating subjective feeling. *Br. J. Med. Psychol.* **47**, 211–218.
Burdon, J. C. W., Juniper, E. F., Killian, K. J., Hargreave, F. E. and Campbell, E. J. M. (1982). The perception of breathlessness in asthma. *Am. Rev. Resp. Dis.* **128**, 825–828.
Burns, B. H. and Howell, J. B. L. (1969). Disproportionately severe breathlessness in chronic bronchitis. *Q. J. Med.* **38**, 277–294.
Cockcroft, A. C. (1985). A self paced treadmill walking test for breathless patients. *Thorax* **40**, 459–464.
Editorial (1986). The enigma of breathlessness. *Lancet* **i**, 891–892.
Killian, K. J. and Campbell, E. J. M. (1983). Dyspnoea and exercise. *Ann. Rev. Physiol.* **45**, 465–479.
—— and Jones, N. L. (1984). The use of exercise testing and other methods in the investigation of dyspnoea. *Clin. Chest Med.* **5**, 99–108.
McGavin, C. R., Artvinli, M., Hase, H. and McHardy, G. J. R. (1978). Dyspnoea, disability and distance walked: comparison of estimates of exercise performance in respiratory disease. *Br. Med. J.* **2**, 241–243.
Plum, F. and Leigh, R. J. (1981). Abnormalities of central mechanisms. In *Regulation of breathing, Part 2, Lung biology in health and disease* (ed. T. F. Hornbeim), pp. 989–1067. Marcel Dekker, New York.
Stark, R. D., Gambles, S. A. and Chatterjee, S. S. (1982). An exercise test to assess clinical dyspnoea: estimation of reproducibility and sensitivity. *Br. J. Dis. Chest.* **76**, 269–278.

Chest pain

W. SOMERVILLE

Pain may originate in the myocardium, pericardium, aorta or pulmonary artery, but myocardial ischaemic pain (angina and the pain of myocardial infarction) outstrips all others in diagnostic importance. It is described fully on page 13.158.

Atypical angina

Atypical angina warrants a comment here. It may present in unusual sites, in the back, jaws, upper arm, forearm, or a finger, spreading to the chest, or in the left side or uncommonly the right side of the chest. It may even be confined to one of these unusual areas and not be felt in the front of the chest at all. Although atypical in site, angina can be suspected or identified from the character of the sensation and its relation to effort and emotion. The entity variously known as *left mammary*, *left breast* or *noncardiac chest pain* is so called because it lacks the essential squeezing, pressing, or tightening quality of ischaemic pain, it is stabbing, pricking or knife-like, and lasts seconds, hours or days. It is usually associated with overbreathing and other anxiety symptoms, especially but not exclusively in women. Left breast (noncardiac) pain may also occur in a person with true angina leading to diagnostic confusion. It often makes its first appearances when angina or infarction is diagnosed in a relation or friend and is particularly common in the early weeks of convalescence after a myocardial infarction. It is an integral part of Da Costa's syndrome (see page 13.80) and often accompanies the systolic click and murmur of prolapsed mitral cusp (although angina may occur here too). It is not caused by coronary atherosclerosis and a normal coronary arteriogram is the rule. It is unlikely to be confused with angina by any physician bearing down on the meticulous details of clinical history. The distinction was elegantly illustrated by Clifford Allbutt: ' . . . surely it is levity to confuse the squalls – *nervose Angstzustände* – of unstable neurotics, mostly women, with the assault of one of the fiercest and most searching afflictions which can fall upon steadfast and resolute men . . . The pain is different, the pulse is different, the panting is different, the behaviour is different, the storm is different, the duration is different, the causes are different, the issue is different . . . '

Table 1 Main distinctions between angina and left breast (non-cardiac) pain

	Angina pectoris	Left breast pain (Da Costa's syndrome, neurocirculatory asthenia)
Site	Central; behind the sternum; across the chest	Left breast
Radiation	Both arms; jaws; back	Left arm
Quality	Constricting; crushing	Prolonged ache; sharp stabs
Duration	2–5 minutes	Seconds or hours
Provocation	During effort; emotion	After effort; fatigue; in bed
Additional symptoms	None	Breathlessness; exhaustion; palpitation; dizziness
ST depression with exercise	Invariable; unaffected by beta-blockade	Sometimes; abolished by beta-blockade
Coronary arteriogram	Abnormal (with rare exceptions)	Normal

The principal points of distinction between angina and left breast pain are summarized in Table 1.

Severe aortic stenosis

This is commonly associated with a classical triad of symptoms, dyspnoea, syncope, and angina. The angina here results from the reduced coronary flow, either by itself or further restricted by coronary arteriosclerosis. Angina occurs only in cases of severe regurgitation.

Aneurysm of the ascending aorta

The pain of *aneurysm of the ascending aorta* is derived from pressure on adjacent structures, particularly rib erosion (pages 13.184 and 13.185).

Dissecting aneurysm

This usually presents with intense chest pain substernal or in the upper back (page 13.191).

Mitral valve prolapse

Mitral valve prolapse, the essential component of the late mitral systolic murmur-click syndrome (Barlow's syndrome, floppy or billowing mitral valve syndrome, see page 13.290) may be responsible for chest pain of different types. A persistent dull ache under the left breast, sometimes with sinus tachycardia or tachyarrhythmias is characteristic. The patient often attributes this to vigorous pounding of the heart. Typical angina may occur and sometimes draws attention to the abnormal mitral valve.

Acute pericarditis

This causes a chest pain sharper than angina, sometimes central, more often left-sided. It lasts for hours, is intensified by breathing, turning in bed, and swallowing, and is lessened by leaning forwards.

Chest pain frequently has a double origin, for example, angina and biliary colic, angina and oesophageal spasm, etc. A common diagnostic pitfall is to identify one component and overlook the other.

Chest pain plays such an important role in angina with 'normal' (or better, 'unobstructed') coronary arteries, and in Da Costa's syndrome, that each of them deserves separate consideration.

Angina with normal coronary arteries

Angina pectoris had been universally accepted as a symptom of transient myocardial ischaemia resulting from coronary atherosclerosis until the mid-1960s. Then, widening experience of coronary arteriography showed that occasionally it could occur with coronary arteries which were free from obstruction or any degree of irregularity of the vessel wall. Confirmatory articles and case reports have proliferated to the extent that a normal coronary arteriogram no longer comes as a surprise in the investigation of angina. The incidence varies from 10 to 30 per cent depending on the accuracy of clinical diagnosis and angiographic interpretation. Evidence of myocardial ischaemia to explain angina despite normal coronary arteries has been readily forthcoming by the demonstration during angina at rest, or after provocation by exercise or pacing, of reduced lactate extraction from arterial blood or lactate production. The ischaemia may or may not be completely reversible, thus explaining the patient-to-patient variation in electrocardiographic findings, thallium scintigraphy, and myocardial biopsy findings.

Associations

Angina is now known to occur in association with a large number of conditions in which the coronary arteries are normal or affected by atherosclerosis so trivial as to be incapable of restricting blood flow. The two commonest are coronary spasm and 'primary' angina (page 13.156). Other suggested mechanisms proliferated in the 1960s and 1970s.

Abnormal oxygen dissociation curve An abnormal oxygen–haemoglobin dissociation curve was recorded in persons with angina and normal coronary arteries whereby the oxygen release from haemoglobin was slow. Certain related factors in the blood have been investigated, including pH (the Bohr effect) and adenosine triphosphate, to explain the slow oxygen release, but the only clue emerging was reduced 2,3-diphosphoglycerate, the principal organic phosphate in red cells.

Hyperventilation Hyperventilation acting via the Bohr effect on the oxyhaemoglobin dissociation curve together with chest wall pain from exaggerated breathing movements, has been cited to explain some instances of chest pain including angina with normal coronary arteries. The clues here are the associated paraesthesiae, palpitation, panic, and dizziness which, with a history of dramatic fighting for breath, point to the hyperventilation syndrome.

Coronary steal Functional circulatory imbalance between different parts of the myocardium whereby blood is shifted from one to the other – 'coronary steal' or *haemometakinesia* – is an attractive proposition in the ischaemic myocardium but unlikely with unobstructed coronary arteries.

Small artery disease Occlusive disease involving small coronary arteries and sparing the larger ones, once a popular hypothesis to explain angina with a normal coronary arteriogram, can no longer be accepted, largely through the advocacy of T. N. James. He doubts the existence of this entity although well aware of non-atherosclerotic conditions especially neuromuscular and musculoskeletal diseases which affect the small arteries only. Recurrent chest pain is common here but should not be confused with angina. Conditions which stenose both small and large coronary arteries are another matter, e.g. diabetes mellitus, amyloid disease, and polyarteritis, when true angina is part of a conventional myocardial perfusion fault.

Systemic sclerosis Polyarteritis and systemic sclerosis present in different forms and angina, myocardial infarction, and sudden cardiac death have been reported in nine such patients. At necropsy, extensive myocardial scarring or necrosis was found in all, but the intramyocardial vessels were normal and unobstructed. A Raynaud-like phenomenon involving histologically normal vessels and producing widespread ischaemia is postulated.

Cardiomyopathy Dyspnoea and angina are the commonest symptoms of hypertrophic cardiomyopathy (idiopathic hypertrophic subaortic stenosis, hypertrophic obstructive cardiomyopathy) (see page 13.221). Small-vessel narrowing may be a part explanation of the angina, for the extramural coronary arteries are widely patent. Disparity between blood supply and oxygen demand by the large muscle mass is an additional factor. Incidentally, a similar supply–demand imbalance has been cited to explain ischaemic electrocardiographic patterns in healthy men undertaking sudden vigorous exercise without a warm-up period.

Oesophageal spasm The pain of hiatus hernia and oesophageal spasm on the one hand, and angina especially angina decubitus on the other, have much in common. Several generations of students at the London Hospital and the National Heart Hospital, London, were taught by Dr William Evans to diagnose oesophageal spasm when recurrent angina-like pain occurred with a normal electrocardiogram; a barium swallow showing terminal oesophageal hold-up or spasm was the decisive test. These views were never widely accepted nor entirely abandoned. Interest in the subject has been re-aroused by Henderson and his co-workers who demonstrated oesophageal spasm by manometric techniques coincidental with angina-like pain provoked by ergometrine injection; they maintain that many instances of 'angina with normal coronary arteries' are in fact oesophageal masquerading as cardiac ischaemia.

Aortic stenosis In severe aortic stenosis with left ventricular hypertrophy (aortic left ventricular gradient of over 50 mm Hg) myocardial oxygen demand may readily exceed supply. The large muscle mass is perfused by coronary arteries compressed by increased ventricular pressures in systole and end-diastole. A further increase by exercise induces angina in over half these patients whether the coronary arteries are diseased or normal. The coronary arteries are more likely to be normal in the younger age groups.

Aortic regurgitation When angina complicates aortic regurgitation normal coronary arteries are found even more frequently. Any of the aetiological types of aortic regurgitation may be responsible, especially syphilitic (with or without coronary ostial stenosis) and rheumatic. The regurgitation is always severe and the peripheral manifestations invariably prominent. The angina is related to low coronary perfusion pressure and the increased demands of the hypertrophied left ventricle. It may be exertional and emotional but the characteristic features peculiar to severe aortic regurgitation whatever the aetiology are occurrence at rest, often at night, prolonged and accompanied by increased heart rate and sweating. The coronary arteries are unobstructed in 80 per cent of cases.

Pulmonary hypertension Patients with primary or acquired pulmonary hypertension and a high pulmonary vascular resistance, whatever the aetiology, may complain of chest discomfort or pain of different types. One of these is angina resulting from low output and inadequate myocardial perfusion, usually triggered off by exertion or any circumstance which increases the heart rate. Most patients are in the first three decades of life when the coronary arteries are open and free from obstruction. Paul Wood made a special study of the Eisenmenger syndrome (pulmonary hypertension with reversed or bidirectional shunt) and documented angina in 20 per cent of patients with pulmonary hypertensive ductus arteriosus, 15 per cent with pulmonary hypertensive atrial septal defect, and 14 per cent with pulmonary hypertensive ventricular septal defect. Although necropsy confirmation was available in only a few, it is certain that these patients had unobstructed coronary arteries. Angina with normal coronary arteries is even more common in primary pulmonary hypertension, occurring in over 20 per cent of cases.

Mitral valve prolapse Mitral valve prolapse, the essential ingredient of the late mitral systolic murmur-click syndrome (Barlow's syndrome, floppy or billowing mitral valve syndrome) may be associated with chest pains of different types. These vary from the discomfort ascribed by the patient to vigorous pounding of the heart, sometimes with sinus tachycardia, rarely with tachyarrhythmias, to a full, long-lasting ache under the left breast. Occasionally angina pectoris is described. Barlow was unaware of this when making his earliest observations in Johannesburg. He suggested that ischaemia of the postero-inferior myocardium resulted from compression of the circumflex artery by the prolapsing posterior mitral leaflet. The commonly seen ST and T changes in II, III, AVF, and V5–6 are more likely to represent localized myocardial ischaemia from abnormal ventricular wall movements as confirmed by ventricular biopsy.

Myocardial bridges Myocardial bridging is a congenital anomaly in which a muscular band constricts or 'milks' the anterior descending artery during systole, normal arterial calibre returning in diastole. Coronary flow, being mainly diastolic, is unlikely to be restricted by this mechanism when the heart rate is below 90. However, when tachycardia occurs for any reason, the constriction can result in angina with ischaemic ECG changes in the anterior leads. It is usually managed effectively by avoiding activity which raises the heart rate to 120 or more and by beta-blockers. Surgical incision of such a band may be considered if it is well-defined arteriographically and the angina is resistant to treatment.

Coronary spasm The concept of coronary spasm, an important feature of Prinzmetal's variant angina, and 'primary' angina has explained to a great extent how angina can occur without a corresponding degree of organic coronary narrowing. Osler in 1910 was well acquainted with the theoretical possibilities of coronary spasm; he invoked it to explain recurrent angina in a man aged 26 years whose coronary arteries at necropsy showed no more than a few atheromatous streaks. The basis of the angina here is myocardial ischaemia, a disparity between myocardial blood demand and supply, identical with angina associated with coronary atherosclerosis. While spasm is the most likely mechanism, and demonstration of spasm in the course of coronary arteriography is now a commonplace event, other possibilities have been broached including an abnormal haemoglobin–oxygen dissociation, already referred to, and atherosclerotic involvement of small vessels not displayed by the coronary arteriogram.

These mechanisms may play a part in some instances but are irrelevant in the majority; coronary spasm is the dominant factor. The demonstration of ischaemia without increased myocardial metabolic demand resulting from spasm of the relevant coronary arteries is attributable to Maseri and his co-workers in Pisa. Maseri coined the term 'primary' angina for this situation, to distinguish it from the classical Heberden's angina. Spasm is responsible in whole for angina with normal coronary arteries and in part for angina with coronary atherosclerosis, hinted at by early writers but put forward more emphatically by Prinzmetal.

Variant or Prinzmetal's angina Prinzmetal and his co-workers claimed that angina at rest with transient ST elevation was the result of sudden increase in smooth muscle tone at or adjacent to a severe stenosis. At first thought to be invariably associated with occlusive coronary lesions, it was subsequently reported with normal or near-normal coronary arteries. Furthermore, ST elevation is not invariable for ST depression has been frequently recorded. This wide variability throws doubt in Prinzmetal's variant angina as a separate clinical entity and supports the concept that different coronary arteries, usually the large epicardial arteries, may be affected by spasm, the artery and site varying from time to time according to unidentified rules. Accordingly, the variability of the direction of ST deviation is readily explicable. Why certain portions of the large coronary arteries, whether intact or the site of atherosclerosis should go into spasm, apparently spontaneously, remains a mystery. Hypotheses are not scarce. A popular one contends that enhanced contractility or spasm is caused by membrane depolarization of cells in the arterial muscular layer resulting from suppressed electrogenic activity of the membrane Na–K pump.

The electrocardiogram

The resting electrocardiogram (ECG) recorded when pain free is usually normal. At one time this was considered to exclude angina as the basis for recurrent chest pain, a view that can no longer be held. Since the normal ECG represents no more than adequate myocardial perfusion at the time the tracing is made, it may be recorded with abnormal coronary arteries allowing adequate resting flow, or with unobstructed coronary arteries which go into spasm from time to time. When spasm and critically reduced flow persist long enough, irreversible ischaemia and even transmural infarction may result. Under these circumstances, an abnormal tracing with QRST changes typical of ischaemia or infarction may be found in a person subsequently shown to have unobstructed coronary arteries by arteriography.

Exercise test

The exercise (stress) test (see page 13.159) sometimes but not invariably clarifies the situation. When a properly conducted exercise test is negative, the chances are high that the coronary arteries are unobstructed.

Can exercise induce spasm in normal coronary arteries? Sympathetic nervous discharge in response to exercise has been well documented and stimulation of alpha-adrenergic receptors is known to produce coronary vasoconstriction. Furthermore, physical exercise has resulted in significant elevation of plasma adrenaline and noradrenaline in persons with normal coronary arteriograms. Arteriographic demonstration of coronary spasm during exercise-induced angina in persons with trivial atheroma would appear to clinch the argument. Exercise can produce coronary spasm when the arteries are the seat of atheroma however mild. False-positive findings, where the ST segments develop ischaemic-like depression although the coronary arteries are unobstructed, can be identified with certainty by repeating the exercise test one hour after 80 mg oxprenolol; a negative result now virtually excludes coronary atherosclerosis.

Provocation test

When coronary arteriography fails to show any obstructive lesion to account for recurrent angina, an attempt to provoke spasm with ergometrine (ergonovine) may be made. All medication is withdrawn for 24 hours and coronary arteriography is performed in the ordinary way. Ergometrine is given by intravenous bolus in three doses, 0.05, 0.10, and 0.25 mg at 3 min intervals. An ECG is taken 1.5 and 3 min after each injection. If ischaemic ST-T changes appear with or without angina, the suspect artery is injected with contrast medium (when the changes appear in leads II, III, and avF, the right coronary is injected; when the chest leads are involved, the left coronary is injected). If spasm has been shown, nitroglycerine is promptly injected into the affected coronary artery or intravenously, the dose being 50–100 µg. A further injection of contrast medium should be made into the affected artery to demonstrate reversal of spasm. The test has many limitations and is seldom essential for diagnosis. Normal coronary arteries show some constriction with ergometrine and the fact that it can induce oesophageal spasm with pain resembling angina and T wave changes without coronary arterial spasm has further reduced its popularity.

Prognosis

The prognosis is good in the absence of any underlying myocardial or metabolic disease. The angina often disappears when the coronary arteries are shown to be normal and the fact is understood by the patient. A population of such patients followed up to seven years after coronary arteriography showed 97 per cent survival compared with 81 per cent survival with minimal stenosis.

Treatment

When the two component parts of this syndrome are confirmed, angina and unobstructed coronary arteries, the first step in management is identification of any factor likely to cause coronary spasm. The commonest is a deep-seated fear of coronary disease, incapacity, and sudden death. Detailed and patient explanation should be given in the presence of the spouse or chosen relative. This should lead on to reassurance emphasizing the good future promised by the unobstructed coronary arteries. This is no time for speculation and guesswork on the doctor's part, for insecurity in diagnosis will be readily pounced on by the alert patient, and the basic fear for survival will be intensified with augmented sympathetic stimulation triggering palpitation and chest sensations of various types. The side effects of excessive drug therapy should be sorted out, particularly the throbbing headache of nitrates, mental dulling, slowing up, bad dreams, muscular pains, bronchospasm, claudication, and depression of beta-blockers, excessive vasodilation of nifedipine, and lethargy of sedation. Patients usually interpret these drug side effects as confirmation of a life-threatening heart disease, thereby prolonging unwarranted invalidism. The reasons for modifying the medication should be confidently and patiently explained.

Stress-producing features of occupation or home-life should be identified and suggestions offered for correcting them. When successful and combined with simple explanation of the injurious effects of smoking on the small arteries throughout the body, the ordinary smoker can invariably be cured and an occasional tobacco addict converted.

These measures are essential when coronary spasm can be indicted. Judiciously chosen drug treatment can often help. The calcium antagonists nifedipine 10 mg twice a day or verapamil 40 mg twice a day, after food, are the most efficient coronary antispasmodics. Beta-blockers may help when anxiety and nervous tachycardia are dominant. To avoid side effects in persons free from organic heart disease, the doses must be smaller than those ordinarily recommended, for example, propranolol 10 mg or oxprenolol 20 mg, two or three times a day. Slow-release or long-acting preparations are usually unsuitable for this purpose.

References

Albutt, C. (1915). Angina pectoris. In *Diseases of the arteries including angina pectoris*, Vol. 2, Section II, Ch. 1.

Barlow, J. B. and Bosman, C. K. (1966). Aneurysmal protrusion of the posterior leaflet of the mitral valve: an auscultatory-electrocardiographic syndrome. *Am. Heart J.* **71**, 166.

Bruschke, A. V. G., Proudfit, W. L. and Sones, F. M. (1973). Clinical course of patients with normal and slightly or moderately abnormal coronary arteriograms: a follow-up study on 500 patients. *Circulation* **47**, 936.

Bulkley, B. H., Klacsman, P. G. and Hutchins, G. M. (1978). Angina pectoris, myocardial infarction, and sudden cardiac death with normal coronary arteries. *Am. Heart J.* **95**, 563.

Cheng, T., Bashour, T., Kelser, G. A., Weiss, L. and Bacos, J. (1973). Variant angina of Prinzmetal with normal coronary arteriograms: a variant of the variant. *Circulation* **47**, 476.

Dart, A. M., Davies, H. A., Lowndes, R. H., Dalal, J., Ruttley, M. and Henderson, A. H. (1980). Oesophageal spasm and angina: diagnostic value of ergometrine (ergonovine) provocation. *Eur. Heart J.* **1**, 91.

Evans, W. (1952). Oesophageal contraction and cardiac pain. *Lancet* ii, 1091.

d'Hemecourt, A. and Detar, R. (1978). Possible physiological basis for locally-induced 'spasm' of large coronary arteries. In *Primary and secondary angina pectoris* (eds A. Maseri, G. A. Klassen and M. Lesch), p. 182. Grune and Stratton, New York.

James, T. N. (1970). The delivery and distribution of coronary collateral circulation. *Chest* **58**, 183.

Kemp, H. G., Elliot, W. C. and Gorlin, R. (1967). The anginal syndrome with normal coronary arteriography. *Trans. Assoc. Am. Phys.* **80**, 59.

Marcomichelakis, J., Donaldson, R., Green, J., Joseph, S. P., Kelly, H. B., Taggart, P. and Somerville, W. (1980). Exercise testing after beta-blockade: improved specificity and predictive value in detecting coronary heart disease. *Br. Heart J.* **43**, 252.

Maseri, A., Severi, S., Chierchia, S., Parodi, V. and Biagini, A. (1978). Characteristics, incidence and pathogenic mechanism of 'primary' angina at rest. In *Primary and secondary angina pectoris* (eds A. Maseri, G. A. Klassen and M. Lesch), p. 265. Grune and Stratton, New York.

Osler, W. (1910). The Lumleian lectures on angina pectoris. *Lancet* **i**, 839.

Prinzmetal, M., Kennamor, R., Merliss, R., Wada, T. and Bor, N. (1959). Angina pectoris. *Am. J Med.* **27**, 375.

Wood, P. (1968). *Diseases of the heart and circulation*, 3rd edn, p. 467. Eyre and Spottiswoode, London.

Da Costa's syndrome

Da Costa's syndrome is a term popularized by Paul Wood as an improvement on effort syndrome, soldier's heart, neurocirculatory asthenia (NCA), and disorderly action of the heart (DAH). These synonyms are all misleading by focusing on one or other feature of the syndrome, not necessarily the most important. They all relate to a disturbance of the autonomic nervous control of the cardiovascular system resulting from intense repetitive emotional stimuli. Fear and anxiety about the safety of the individual or his present or future security are the dominant emotions. The condition proliferates during war when many men are drawn into national service who are unfit for the rigour and discipline of army life. They are soon recognized by their constitutional inability to conform to rules and regulations and to accept responsibility and by their physical incapacity to stand up to routine physical training, cross-country running, gymnastics, and the like. Although passing references to the condition appear in early medical history, the American Civil War provided material for the first detailed clinical description by Jacob M. Da Costa under the appropriate title of 'On irritable heart: a clinical study of a functional cardiac disorder and its consequences'. In the First World War there were 60 000 cases in the British armed forces alone, most of them labelled as malingerers for want of a better diagnosis. None the less they had to be withdrawn from their duties and consequently were numbered as casualties, 44 000 of them eventually receiving pensions. Mackenzie, Lewis, and others studied the condition without discovering a cause beyond exonerating the heart. Wood considered the symptoms in terms of applied physiology. Palpitation resulted from sympathetic nervous stimulation which accelerates the heart rate, raises the blood pressure, and strengthens the heart beat. Dizziness and syncope were perhaps induced by parasympathetic activity which slows the rate, lowers the blood pressure, and weakens the heart beat. The normal person, Wood maintained, is never disturbed by the effects of day-to-day emotions which are too transient and too familiar to cause alarm. Those who seek medical advice have an underlying psychiatric disorder making them excessively sensitive to the circulatory disturbances which in addition are brought on too readily and are persistent rather than transient.

A family history of some kind of emotional instability is present in the majority. In childhood, fears and phobias, stammering, facial tics, nightmares, bed wetting, and fear of the dark attract maternal overprotection. This extends to school life, where kindly matrons and medical officers excuse the timid child from rough games and order extra rest periods. In times of war, they are conscientious objectors or seek out reserved occupations. If conscripted, effort intolerance is the earliest symptom, to be followed sooner or later by the full-blown syndrome. In peacetime, the combination of breathlessness, chest pain, palpitation, dizziness, and exhaustion are to the heart-conscious lay mind, the trademarks of heart disease. It only calls for an ill-informed doctor to attach a label of heart disease or to admit uncertainty by trying out the effects of various cardiac medicines for the conviction of disease to become fixed and the symptoms ineradicable.

Symptoms

The outstanding complaints as described in the patient's words are: (*a*) breathlessness, (*b*) palpitation, (*c*) pain over the heart, (*d*) exhaustion, and (*e*) dizziness. Since these are common features of heart disease, a brief comment on each of them is necessary.

Breathlessness

The term breathlessness in this context means rapid breathing on slight effort, when resting or in bed. Inability to take a deep breath or to 'fill the lungs with air' is invariable. Frequent deep inspirations followed by short expirations are characteristic and are appropriately called 'sighing respiration'.

Palpitation

Palpitation or awareness of forceful rapid beating of the heart is usual with breathlessness. It is brought on by slight effort, often by walking across the room; it occurs also when resting. Relations become at first alarmed and then inured to the patient suddenly breathing rapidly and deeply with all the appearances of mounting distress. Abrupt awakening from sleep with palpitation, breathlessness, and great alarm are characteristic and are often the presenting complaints.

Pain over the heart

Pain over the heart, words used by patients whatever language they speak, may occur with breathlessness and palpitation or by itself. The usual site is inframammary and the customary descriptive terms are a dull ache lasting for hours, stabbing, knife-like, a stitch. Sometimes it is a cramp or constricting, terms alerting the physician to a possible coronary origin, especially when it spreads or shoots down the left arm. It is present at rest or after exercise but sometimes when walking or working with the left arm. It is common in bed, preventing lying on the left side. In isolated dextrocardia, all these sensations affect the right side. The site of the pain is often tender to touch. The cause of the pain is unknown but its origin in the tissues of the chest wall rather than referred is confirmed by Wood's observation that injection of novocaine into the intercostal muscle at the point of greatest intensity provides instant relief, cutaneous or subcutaneous anaesthesia being ineffective.

Exhaustion

Exhaustion is induced by slight effort, persisting during rest and unrelieved by sleep.

Dizziness

Dizziness is usually coupled with overbreathing and elaborated by terms such as 'lightheadedness, about to pass out, a blackout'. Syncope may occur after vigorous overbreathing. Even though unconsciousness may be no more than momentary, the patient in retrospect may claim to have been aware of things for hours.

Headache and sweating are common but not usual presenting symptoms. The headache lasts for hours or is there all the time. It is a pressure on the dome of the skull or the nape of the neck spreading down towards the shoulders. Sweating involves the palms of the hands, axillae, and feet, the emotional sweat areas. Wood pointed out that sweating confined to the palms is emotional; if the backs of the hands are also involved, other causes should be looked for.

The clinical picture of all organic heart disease is coloured by emotion to a greater or less extent, ranging from simple nervous tachycardia to the full-blown Da Costa's syndrome.

Physical signs

Appearance The typical patient has poor physical development, often thin and round-shouldered, and speaks in a timid, apologetic manner. The hands and feet are cold and clammy with coarse finger tremor. Deep sighs punctuate the clinical history and recur, with tachypnoea, during the examination. Tenderness and sometimes hyperaesthesia are present in the left inframammary region. The resting heart rate is over 90, the blood pressure above 150/90, and the pulse jerking in quality. Aortic valve closure is sharp and responsible for the loud second sound. Radiologically, the heart size, shape, and position are normal.

The electrocardiogram may be normal confirming sinus tachycardia. Minor ST depression, 1 mm or less, and low T waves are common when the anxiety element is dominant but are corrected within an hour by a beta-blocker.

Exercise tests are terminated at a low workload by exhaustion, muscular weakness, and overbreathing. Left chest pain is usual but overshadowed by exhaustion and tachypnoea. Sinus tachycardia, disproportionate to the workload is invariable. ST configuration is variable; it is usually normal at the end point but depression of 1mm may develop or persist from the resting state, especially in women. When the test is repeated after a beta-blocker, ST behaviour remains normal in contrast to angina when ST depression persists.

Echocardiogram and radionucleide tests give normal results.

Diagnosis

The combination of breathlessness on trivial effort, palpitation, and chest pain brings the diagnosis to mind. The multiplicity of symptoms disproportionate to the provocative factors is the main clue. The steps necessary to distinguish organic heart disease involving cardiological examination, chest X-ray, and electrocardiograms resting and with exercise may heighten the patient's suspicion of heart disease, and if the physician is not sure of his or her ground, the idea is likely to become fixed.

Left breast pain must be distinguished from angina pectoris especially in an excitable or neurotic patient. The main differential details are set out in tabular form on page 13.76.

Palpitation is often wrongly attributed to paroxysmal tachycardia. When the resting rate is rapid and sweating is a feature, thyrotoxicosis must be excluded. Pulmonary tuberculosis was often diagnosed in earlier days before it became a rarity. Active rheumatic carditis in children may be difficult to differentiate.

Treatment

The two main details in treatment are explanation and reassurance. Quite clearly this approach is impossible until the physician is confident that organic disease in the cardiovascular or other systems is not to blame. Once sure of his ground he should explain, symptom by symptom, how the emotions involved can be responsible while the structure of the heart remains sound. If the physician appreciates the patient's predicament, his fear of disablement or sudden death, he will speak from a position of sympathy and confidence. His equanimity may well be sorely tested. If he gives way to impatience, he will surely fail to drive home his message and the neurosis will be if anything intensified.

Once the patient understands the origin of the symptoms and accepts their harmlessness, improvement may be expected. Progressive daily walking exercises should be part of the regimen and non-aggressive body-building exercises may improve stamina and the sense of well-being. Smoking, alcohol, and sedatives all act in the opposing direction and should be prohibited.

Psychiatric help is seldom necessary for the perceptive physician on his own should be able to identify the origin of the symptoms and signs and to explain them to the patient and the spouse. Medication plays no part, with one possible exception. When palpitation is the dominant symptom, is easily induced by trivial effort, and particularly when sleep is disrupted, small doses of a beta-blocker such as oxprenolol 20 mg or propranolol 10 mg in the morning and before going to bed, will control emotional tachycardia during the periods of adjustment. Higher doses of the order of 120 mg a day should be avoided for they are badly tolerated, increase fatigue, and induce depression.

Prognosis

There is a reasonable chance that treatment will succeed when the personality is adequate and amenable to explanation and reassurance and the condition has lasted no more than a few years. The prognosis is poor when the family history is positive, the domestic environment hostile or unstable, or a motive exists to perpetuate the symptoms for personal advantage. For instance, in wartime, conscripts poorly motivated because of fear or lack of sense of duty will not easily relinquish symptoms which are a sure guarantee of discharge to civilian life. A woman accustomed to the sheltered life of a cardiac invalid is unlikely to take kindly to a diagnosis which will remove her protection from the housewife's chores and responsibilities. A litigant whose case depends on cardiac symptoms dating from a road traffic accident will understandably resist the diagnosis of a normal heart.

References

Da Costa, J. M. (1871). On irritable heart: a clinical study of a form of functional cardiac disorder and its consequences. *Am. J med. Sci.* **61**, 17.

Lewis, T. (1940). *The soldier's heart and the effort syndrome*, 2nd edn. Shaw and Sons, London.

Wood, P. (1941). Da Costa's syndrome (or effort syndrome) *Br. med J.* **i**, 767, 805, 845.

Oedema

J. G. G. LEDINGHAM

1985 marked the bicentenary of William Withering's description of how the dropsy of heart disease might be relieved by the use of extracts of foxglove but the precise explanation of how cardiac oedema arises is still surprisingly incomplete. Heart failure is a difficult term to define, but its clinical features reflect the circulatory adaptations which occur in heart disease to maintain perfusion of brain, heart, and skeletal muscle at the expense of the visceral and skin circulation. How the earliest imperfection in cardiac performance is sensed to set in motion the much better understood efferent effects is a particular difficulty as also is a complete understanding of how the centrally important renal retention of sodium and water is mediated in heart disease.

Starling forces

It is these forces which ultimately determine the rate at which fluid exchanges between the blood volume and the interstitial space. For many years cardiac oedema was attributed, at least in part, to an increase in capillary hydrostatic pressure secondary to the known high central venous pressure of at least some patients with dependent oedema and heart disease. But renal retention of salt and water is known to precede any rise in right atrial and central venous pressure and occurs in high output as well as low output cardiac failure. Nor are there measurements to confirm that any rise in central venous pressure when present makes a *significant* change in capillary hydrostatic pressure on standing. Indeed the explanation for the failure of the feet to accumulate oedema on passive standing in *normal* humans is not yet apparent, although it may depend on regulation of hydrostatic pressure by precapillary arteriolar sphincter as well as on active pumping of interstitial fluid by lymphatic vessels. Whilst a disturbed relationship between capillary hydrostatic pressure, capillary oncotic pressure, interstitial oncotic pressure, interstitial hydrostatic pressure, and/or a change in capillary permeability must be the final mechanism by which interstitial or fluid volume is increased, there has to be retention of sodium and water by the kidney in chronic oedematous states.

Renal retention of salt and water

A reduced capacity to excrete sodium is perhaps the earliest and most sensitive index of some types of cardiac dysfunction. Even when sodium retention and oedema are not evident, an inability to excrete an intravenous or oral sodium load is an invariable feature of all forms of cardiac failure in humans or experimental animals. How does this come about?

Changes in renal haemodynamics

The reduced capacity of the kidney to excrete salt in the earliest stages of impairment of cardiac function is accompanied by a reduction sometimes profound, of total renal blood flow. Glomerular filtration is relatively or absolutely preserved so that there is a substantial increase in filtration fraction. This change alone favours an alteration in glomerulo-tubular balance in that post-glomerular peritubular blood will, as a result of increased ultrafiltration, have a lower hydrostatic and higher oncotic pressure than normal. Sodium in proximal tubular fluid diffuses passively into proximal tubular cells along a concentration gradient. The sites of active transport are on the lateral and basal aspects of the cells where sodium is moved into the corresponding intercellular spaces. A back leak into the tubular lumen then tends to occur by way of the tight junctions between cells which are contiguous with the lateral intercellular spaces. The increase in the physical forces favouring movement of peritubular fluid into peritubular capillaries which results from an increased filtration fraction might then greatly reduce the back leak of sodium through the tight junctions. Such a mechanism is often invoked to account for the increased proximal tubular reabsorption in heart failure (*vide infra*). How important this is, in fact, is difficult to judge. In essential hypertension for instance, the filtration fraction may be equally increased, the total renal blood flow equally reduced, but the capacity of the kidney to excrete a sodium load enhanced rather than blunted.

Redistribution of blood flow

There is some evidence from washout studies using inert gases that the renal blood flow in cardiac failure is not only reduced overall, but is also redistributed away from cortical short loop nephrons to juxta medullary nephrons with much longer loops of Henle and a postulated greater innate capacity to reabsorb salt and water. This mechanism of sodium retention was proposed many years ago. It remains unproven because of the technical difficulties in measuring heterogeneity of blood flow in the kidney in humans and even in experimental animals. There is less enthusiasm for the hypothesis than previously.

Tubular reabsorption of sodium

The glomerular filtration rate is well preserved in mild heart failure at least, and the evidence is overwhelmingly in favour of increased reabsorption of salt and water, relative to the filtered load, as the primary mechanism of fluid retention in cardiac disease.

Proximal tubules

Micropuncture studies in animals in which *acute* administration of noradrenaline or angiotensin II increases filtration fraction also confirm increased proximal tubular reabsorption of sodium. In animals with *chronic* heart failure on the other hand glomerular filtration and tubular sodium reabsorption in superficial nephrons have been found normal.

In humans the increase in free water clearance induced by mannitol infusion in patients with heart failure and the lack of effect of diuretics acting on the distal nephron alone are indications that at least part of the increased tubular reabsorption takes place in the proximal tubule.

Loop of Henle

This is an even more difficult area to study, but the sheer magnitude of the natriuresis which may occur when 'loop' diuretics are given to patients with heart failure has been suggested as evidence of enhanced sodium transport in Henle's loop in cardiac disease.

Distal tubules and collecting ducts

Although quantitatively most of the filtered sodium has been reabsorbed before tubular fluid reaches the distal nephron, recent micropuncture and microperfusion experiments have suggested that the collecting ducts are the site at which critical changes in sodium absorption may occur, very probably in heart failure as well as in states of sodium depletion.

Sensing cardiac malfunction
Afferent mechanisms

A proven mechanism whereby a reduction in cardiac performance triggers the reduction in renal perfusion and salt excretion is yet to be found. The adaptation occurs in both low and high output cardiac failure and is attributed to responses by high and perhaps also low pressure volume receptors in the circulation which may sense absolute or relative changes in distension in relation to flow. Increased interest in the low pressure system has been stimulated by the discovery of the natriuretic factors present in granules in the atria and perhaps released or not by changes in transmural pressure (see page 18.21). These peptides have been shown to be present in plasma in higher concentrations in patients with heart failure than in normal subjects, and the plasma concentration may correlate with both right and left atrial pressures. They possess vasodilatory properties. Their natriuretic effects may be mediated by intrarenal circulatory changes, but the presence of receptors in the renal tubules suggests the possibility also of direct action on tubular sodium transport. Atrial natriuretic peptides tend to increase renal perfusion and to antagonize the vasoconstrictive effects of angiotensin II and noradrenaline. They also inhibit aldosterone and renin secretion, but precisely where they fit into the complex picture of cardiac failure is not not yet known. They are certainly quite separate from the much longer recognized stretch receptors which also lie in the atria and in the pulmonary circulation. Natriuresis and diuresis follows an acute increase in transmural pressure in the atria of dogs, and vice versa. Afferent fibres from these volume receptors travel in the IXth and Xth cranial nerves to the brain stem to modify sympathetic outflow particularly to the kidneys. The presence of similar mechanisms in humans is supported by the natriuretic and diuretic effects of immersion up to the neck in warm water, a manoeuvre which redistributes blood from the periphery to the thoracic capacitance vessels. The paradox about these phenomena is that the experimental observations reflect a natriuretic response to increased atrial pressure, the precise opposite of what occurs in heart failure.

Arterial stretch receptors in the carotid sinus, aortic arch, and juxtaglomerular apparatus are more likely devices to detect deficient filling on the arterial side. Any tendency of the cardiac output to fall, or a reduction in the volume of blood in the arterial tree as would occur in such high output states as arteriovenous fistula could be sensed by these receptors with decreased distension favouring sodium retention and vice versa.

The efferent response
Sympathetic nervous system

Activation of the sympathetic nervous system is well established in heart failure. Adrenergic drive increases cardiac output, and maintains perfusion of brain, heart, and skeletal muscle at the expense of kidney, the visceral circulation, and the skin. It also increases venous tone and reduces the compliance of the capacitance vessels. The effects on the kidney are to reduce renal blood flow while maintaining glomerular filtration, to stimulate renin secretion, and to increase tubular sodium reabsorption directly as well as by these indirect mechanisms.

The renin–angiotensin–aldosterone system

Activation of the renin–angiotensin system has been a prominent feature of experimental models of heart failure. It is also common in progressive cardiac failure in humans and is aggravated by the use of diuretics and a low salt diet. In some stable patients with only mild impairment of cardiac function, plasma renin and aldosterone concentrations may be normal.

Aldosterone

High plasma levels in heart failure relate in part to activation of the renin–angiotensin system and in part to reduced hepatic metabolism secondary to reduced liver blood flow, particularly in the erect posture. The discovery of aldosterone in 1953 seemed likely to provide the answer to sodium retention in oedema states, but the contribution is probably quite small as illustrated by the lack of efficacy of spironolactone given on its own even in very high dosage in restoring sodium balance in any but the mildest of heart diseases.

In normal people administration of mineralocorticoid (aldosterone or desoxycorticosterone) produces only a transient and modest retention of salt and water. Escape with natriuresis occurs after some 3 to 5 days in health, but not in patients with fluid retention. An explanation for this long-standing observation is still lacking.

Hypersecretion of aldosterone would also appear to play little part in the fluid retention of the nephrotic syndrome, an observation which leads to scepticism about its importance in heart failure.

Angiotensin II

Renin secreted by underperfused and adrenergically stimulated juxta medullary cells acts on its substrate within the kidney and in blood to increase production of angiotensin I: some of which results in local effects within the renal circulation (*vide infra*) and some in systemic effects mediated by conversion of angiotensin I to II in the pulmonary circulation.

The *systemic* increase in concentration of angiotensin II has a number of important consequences There are direct pressor effects on vascular smooth muscle, helping to maintain blood pressure and joining with the sympathetic nervous system in increasing renal vascular resistance. The cells of the zona glomerulosa of the adrenal cortex are stimulated to increase secretion of aldosterone. Angiotensin perfusing the area postrema of the brain stem and the circum-ventricular organs of the hypothalamus stimulate increased sympathetic outflow and antidiuretic hormone secretion, respectively. In addition, high plasma levels of angiotensin II augment neuroadrenergic activity in the periperal circulation. All these events will tend to promote fluid retention by inhibiting the renal excretion of both salt and water. Whether angiotensin II stimulates thirst in humans as it does in animals is more debateable (see page 18.18). *Intrarenal* angiotensin I is converted locally to angiotensin II. There is evidence that the local system has at least two important effects. The first is to reduce the ultrafiltration coefficient (Kf) of glomerular capillaries and the surface area available for filtration by stimulating contraction of glomerular mesangial cells. The second is to maintain glomerular filtration at very low perfusion pressures by selectively increasing efferent arteriolar tone. Whether in addition there are direct effects of angiotensin II on renal tubular reabsorption activity is debated. The physiology of the intrarenal renin–angiotensin system is intimately dependent also on intrarenal prostaglandin metabolism.

Prostaglandins

The vascular smooth muscle and endothelial cells of the renal cortex synthesize PGI_2 (prostacyclin) and PGE_2, while thromboxane appears to arise from glomerular mesangial cells. In animal experiments underperfusion of renal tissue results in increased secretion of the vasodilator prostaglandins PGI_2 and PGE_2. Indomethacin

treatment in this situation markedly increases renal vascular resistance and there have been reports of deterioration in patients with heart failure given drugs which inhibit cyclo-oxygenase. Plasma levels of the metabolites of PGI_2 and PGE_2 are also known to be increased in patients with severe chronic heart failure, suggesting an important balance between vasoconstrictive (angiotensin) and vasodilator (PGI_2, PGE_2) hormones within the renal circulation.

In addition to its vasodilator properties, PGE_2 enhances the renal excretion of sodium and attenuates the effects of antidiuretic hormone in mediating water absorption in the collecting ducts.

In practical terms, the ill effects of prescribing indomethacin and like drugs in heart failure are seen largely in those with gross disease and hyponatraemia.

Relationship between intrarenal angiotensin and prostaglandins

Noradrenaline, angiotensin II, and bradykinin are all known to stimulate local release of prostaglandins in the kidney, whilst renin release may itself be mediated in part by local PGI_2, and PGE_2.

Antidiuretic hormone (ADH)

In severe heart failure plasma levels of ADH may reach very high levels despite volume expansion. Hyponatraemia is then commonly present and results from a number of factors (see page 13.100).

Natriuretic hormone(s)

A number of substances, some dialysable, some not, some heat stable, some not, have been extracted from the plasma or urine of volume expanded or uraemic subjects and inhibit sodium transport in toad bladders, frog skin, or renal tubules. These substances, none of which yet has been proven to be a physiologically important natriuretic factor inhibit Na/K ATPase and may react with antidigoxin antibodies. In this they differ fundamentally from the more recently described atrial natriuretic factor (see page 18.32).

Conclusions

Despite ever growing knowledge of the disturbed physiology of heart failure, there remain major uncertainties as to how dysfunction of the left ventricle is sensed, and precisely how renal function is modified towards more or less avid sodium retention.

References

Brod, J. (1972). Pathogenesis of cardiac oedema. *Br. Med. J.* **1**, 222–228.

Cannon, P. J. and Martinez-Maldonado, M. (1983). The pathogenesis of cardiac edema. *Sem. Nephrol.* **3**, 211–224.

Dzau, V. J., Packer, M., Lilly, L. S., Swartz, S. L. , Hollenberg, N. K. and Williams, G. H. (1984). Prostaglandins in severe congestive heart failure. *N. Eng. J. Med.* **310**, 347–352.

Ichikawa, I. and Brenner, B. M. (1984). Glomerular actions of angiotensin II. *Am. J. Med.* **76**, 43–49.

Lancet (1986). Atrial natriuretic peptide. *Lancet* ii, 371–372.

Laragh, J. H. (1985). Atrial natriuretic hormone, the renin–aldosterone axis and blood pressure–electrolyte homeostasis. *N. Engl. J. Med.* **113**, 1330–1340.

Maack, T., Camargo, M. J. F., Kleinert, H. D., Laragh, J. H. and Atlas, S. A. (1985). Atrial natriuretic factor: structure and functional properties. *Kidney Int.* **27**, 607–615.

HEART FAILURE

Heart failure: ventricular disease

D. G. GIBSON

Introduction

Ventricular disease is an important cause of disability and death in patients with coronary artery disease or hypertension, and its presence or absence is a major determinant of the outcome of surgery and postoperative results in patients with valvular or congenital heart disease. It gives rise to characteristic symptoms and physical signs by which it can be recognized clinically, and is treated with a variety of drugs notable for their high incidence of side-effects as well as for their therapeutic potency. Its incidence is high, and increases with age. In the Framingham study, figures of 2 per 1000 in men and 1 per 1000 in women for the age range 45–54 years were found, rising to 8 per 1000 for men and 7 per 1000 for men between 65 and 74 years.

Ventricular structure

Left ventricle

The normal left ventricle is a complex organ, able to transfer energy from the myocardium to the circulation with high mechanical efficiency. A dissection showing some aspects of normal left ventricular anatomy is demonstrated in Fig. 1. The cavity is divided longitudinally into two halves by the anterior cusp of the mitral valve, whose base is in fibrous continuity with the aortic root. The cavity tapers towards the apex, particularly below the insertion of the papillary muscles, where curvature of the inferior wall is reversed, being convex towards the cavity. The inner surface is covered with endocardium and, except on the septal surface, ridges of muscle, trabeculae, from which the two papillary muscles arise. Wall thickness is greatest at the base of the heart, and decreases towards the apex; at the apex itself, myocardium is absent altogether so that endocardium is in direct contact with epicardium. The structure of the left ventricular myocardium is complex. Traditionally, a series of named loops and spirals of muscle are described, but over the last 30 years, these have been shown to

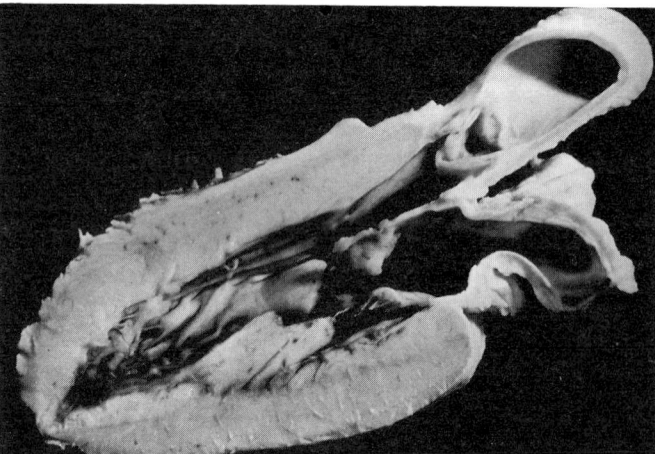

Fig. 1 Normal left ventricular anatomy. The specimen has been sectioned longitudinally. Note the fibrous continuity between the insertion of the anterior cusp of the mitral valve and the posterior border of the aortic root. There is also continuity between the interventricular septum and anterior border of the aorta.

have no clear existence. Rather, myocardium should be thought of as a highly organized and continuously branching structure. The angle the fibres make with the long axis of the ventricle varies. In the mid-wall, particularly towards the base, the fibres are circumferentially arranged, but in the subendocardial and subepicardial regions, they become progressively more oblique, so that those forming the trabeculae and papillary muscles are virtually longitudinal.

Right ventricle

The structure of the right ventricle differs in several respects from that of the left. The pulmonary valve is separated from the tricuspid valve by the muscular infundibulum, a structure that has no counterpart in the left ventricle. This results in the tricuspid and pulmonary valve rings being approximately perpendicular to one another, instead of being almost in the same plane as are the aortic and mitral. The trabeculae of the right ventricle are much coarser than those of the left, and its walls are thinner, since it lacks a well-developed circumferential component.

Pathological changes in ventricular disease

Pathological changes occurring in the heart in patients with ventricular disease are non-specific and, except in rare cases such as acute myocarditis, do not give direct diagnostic information. When coronary artery disease is the underlying cause, the most characteristic finding is fibrosis and degeneration of muscle fibres following local necrosis in the territory of an occluded coronary artery. When overall ventricular function is greatly depressed, generalized fibrosis may be found in the subendocardial region and the bases of the papillary muscles, consisting of nodules up to 1 mm across, with the structure and evolution of larger infarcts. Since its distribution does not correlate with that of any of the major coronary arteries, this fibrosis is probably the result of prolonged subendocardial ischaemia. Exactly similar subendocardial changes are found in patients with congestive cardiomyopathy, when the coronary arteries are normal. In both conditions, left ventricular mass may be moderately increased by up to 150 g. This is due to cavity dilation, since wall thickness remains within normal limits. When the primary abnormality is hypertrophy, the histological picture is virtually the same, whatever the underlying cause. Individual muscle fibre size is increased. The delicate reticular fibrosis normally present between the muscle bundles is greatly accentuated, particularly in patients with clinical evidence of pulmonary congestion. Degeneration of muscle fibres does not occur as in coronary artery disease, but normal myocardial architecture may be replaced by areas of 'fibre disarray', consisting of muscle whorls, often with large bizarre nuclei and fibrosis. These changes are particularly prominent in the myocardium of patients with hypertrophic cardiomyopathy, but may be seen in severe hypertrophy from any cause.

Ventricular function

Many discrete abnormalities of ventricular function can be defined in patients with heart disease, which may be present, either singly or in combination. They may be systolic or diastolic in their timing, and localized or generalized in their distribution. It follows that there is no unique definition of ventricular disease; rather, the problem in the individual patient is to define which of a series of discrete abnormalities is present and to assess the contribution that each makes to overall disability.

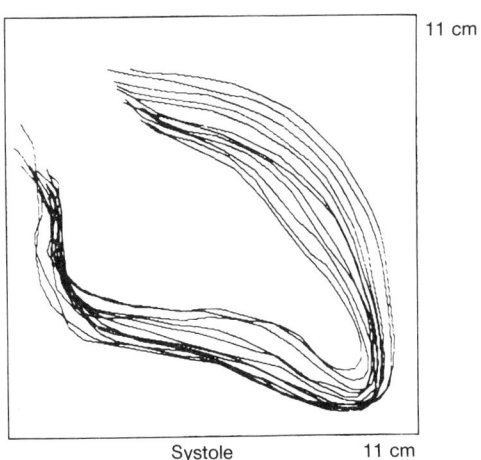

Fig. 2 Normal left ventricular wall motion. The cavity outlines from successive cine frames are shown from the left ventriculogram from a patient with normal left ventricular function.

Left ventricular systolic abnormalities

Systolic abnormalities of left ventricular function can best be defined in terms of wall motion, the term 'wall' here referring to the endocardium, which lies between the myocardium and the blood and which represents the outer border of contrast within the cavity on a cine angiogram.

Normal left ventricle

The normal pattern of left ventricular wall motion is shown in Fig. 2, derived from a left ventricular cine angiogram. The outline of the cavity is shown at 20 ms intervals throughout the period of systole. Inward motion is symmetrical, but not uniform, since its amplitude is greater in the transverse (minor) axis than in the long axis. Normal left ventricular end-diastolic volume is in the range 110–150 ml in the adult, and end-systolic volume is one-third to one-quarter of this so that stroke volume, derived as (end-diastolic volume) − (end-systolic volume), is in the range 80–120 ml. The normal ratio of stroke volume to end-diastolic volume is in the range 55–75 per cent. This ratio, termed ejection fraction, is a sensitive measure of left ventricular systolic pump function. A value of ejection fraction below 50 per cent is good evidence of ventricu-

lar disease. Left ventricular ejection fraction can also be measured by gated radionuclide blood pool scanning, both at rest and on exercise. Ejection fraction normally increases on exercise, since peripheral resistance, and hence resistance to ejection, falls. Except in the elderly, failure of ejection fraction to rise on exercise is evidence of ventricular disease, even if it is within the normal range at rest. Ejection fraction at rest can also be determined by cross-sectional echocardiography. Changes in dimension which parallel those in volume can be recorded with M-mode echocardiography. Shortening fraction is defined as:

$$(Dd - Ds)/Dd \qquad (1)$$

where Dd is end-distolic, and Ds end-systolic dimension. Normal values are within the range 25–40 per cent. The mean rate of reduction of minor axis during ejection, referred to as velocity of circumferential shortening (VCF) is calculated as:

$$(Dd - Ds)/Dd \cdot ET \qquad (2)$$

where ET is left ventricular ejection time. VCF can be determined from echo- or angiograms; normal values are in the range 0.8–1.2/s.

Severe generalized left ventricular disease

The pattern of wall motion in severe, generalized left ventricular disease is shown in Fig. 3a. Though cavity volume is greatly increased, stroke volume is either normal or low, so that ejection fraction is greatly depressed, here to 22 per cent, well below the normal lower limit of 50 per cent. The changed pattern of wall motion is also reflected in the M-mode echocardiogram where measurements of shortening fraction and VCF are both strikingly reduced (Fig. 3b). A large cavity requires wall stress to be increased, and with ventricular dimensions and wall thickness changing little during ejection, this high stress must be maintained throughout systole, rather than falling off as ejection proceeds, as in the normal. This involves a physiological penalty, since myocardial oxygen requirements depend directly on the magnitude of the wall stress and the time over which it is developed.

A dilated left ventricular cavity such as this may occur in the absence of any apparent underlying cause, when it is referred to as congestive or dilated cardiomyopathy. It may represent the end result of a number of disease processes, including myocarditis, coronary artery disease, hypertension, or valve disease. It may also follow administration of drugs such as daunorubicin or long

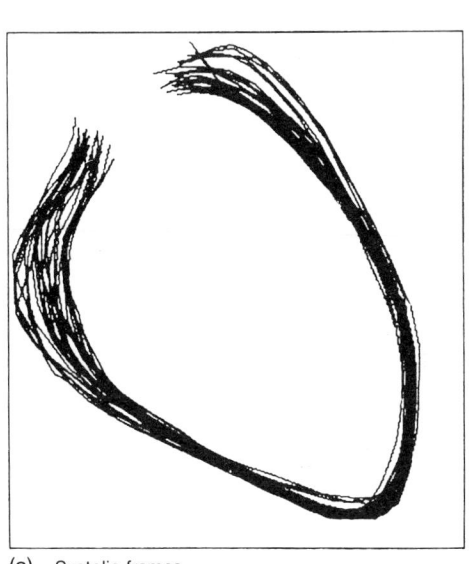

(a) Systolic frames

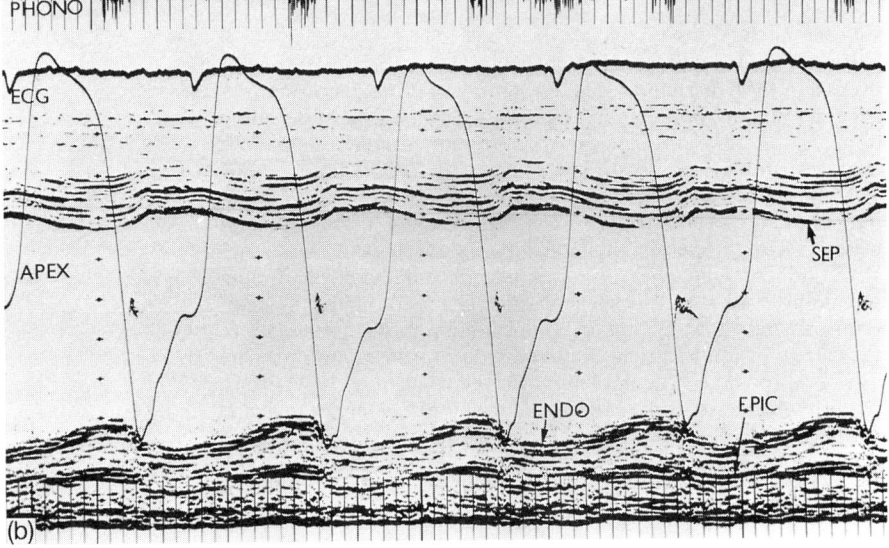

(b)

Fig. 3 (a) Left ventricle wall motion from a patient with severe and generalized left ventricular disease. Note a global reduction in the amplitude of wall movement confirmed in (b) by M-mode echocardiography.

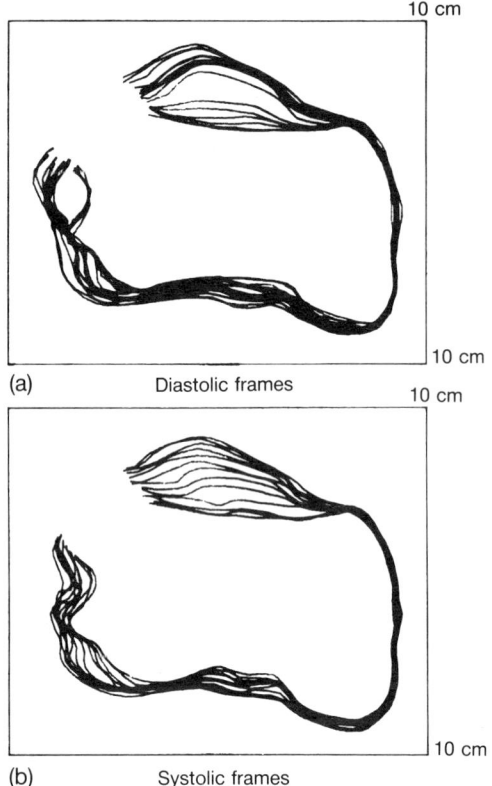

Fig. 4 Left ventricular aneurysm. Note that wall motion is absent at the apex, although its amplitude is normal at the base.

term intake of toxic agents such as ethyl alcohol. In none of these conditions is the exact mechanism of development known, though histological studies show that the muscle fibres are not stretched, since Z band to Z band distances are normal.

The increase in cavity size must thus have occurred by rearrangement of fibres, referred to as slippage, and not by simple distension as would be predicted were it the result of the operation of Starling's law. This is a good example of how chronic abnormalities of ventricular function occurring clinically may bear a superficial resemblance to those induced acutely by drugs or other manoeuvres in experimental animals, although their underlying basis is fundamentally different.

Coronary artery disease
Coronary artery disease is an important cause of left ventricular disease in the West, and leads to a variety of disturbances of ventricular function, both left and right. It may cause generalized dilation of the left ventricular cavity, as described above, but more characteristically, regional abnormalities of wall motion appear, as might be expected when individual coronary arteries are affected. These abnormalities are described in terms of the extent to which the amplitude of endocardial motion is affected. Hypokinesis describes a reduction in amplitude, its direction and timing remaining normal. Akinesis is absence of motion and dyskinesis refers to outward bulging of endocardium throughout systole. Elsewhere in the ventricle the amplitude of wall motion may be increased, possibly to compensate for the reduction elsewhere, a pattern referred to as hyperkinesis. Local replacement of myocardium by scar tissue leads to a contraction pattern of the type shown in Fig. 4, where there is a large akinetic area towards the apex, often described as a ventricular aneurysm. Such aneurysms do not move paradoxically, since scar tissue is almost inextensible at pressures developed by the heart. The wall at the base of the heart moves normally, but in spite of this, ejection fraction is low, and the cavity enlarged. The residual myocardium must thus

develop a higher wall stress than normal, so that overall function is impaired. Dyskinesis occurring after acute myocardial infarction is shown in Fig. 5. The wall moves normally along the anterior wall, but the inferior wall bulges outwards during systole, as the myocardium thins. Overall ejection fraction is normal due to hyperkinesis of the anterior wall.

The timing as well as the amplitude of wall motion may be abnormal in patients with coronary artery disease. In Fig. 6, from a patient with an occluded right coronary artery, the inferior wall is akinetic during systole, but moves inward normally during diastole. The motion of a large segment of the inferior wall is delayed with respect of that of the rest of the ventricle. This interferes with overall function, and greatly reduces mechanical efficiency.

Left ventricular pressure
Abnormalities of pressure are much less specific and sensitive than those of wall motion in diagnosing ventricular disease. The peak rate of rise of left ventricular pressure at the start of systole, peak dP/dt, has been used to assess systolic function. It is measured by differentiating the high-fidelity signal from a catheter-tip manometer inserted into the ventricle. Normal values are in the range 1500–3000 mm Hg/s. Peak dP/dt increases following administration of drugs with a positive inotropic effect, as the rate of myocardial tension development increases, and is reduced by those with a negative inotropic effect. Although low values occur in many types of left ventricular disease, their presence is not diagnostic, since peak dP/dt is also sensitive to changes in ventricular end-diastolic pressure, and is reduced if aortic diastolic pressure is low, as in aortic regurgitation. Asynchronous onset of tension development due to regional left ventricular disease also reduces peak dP/dt. Indices based on peak dP/dt are thus not specific enough to be of diagnostic value in detecting or excluding ventricular disease in individual patients, and are no longer used for this purpose.

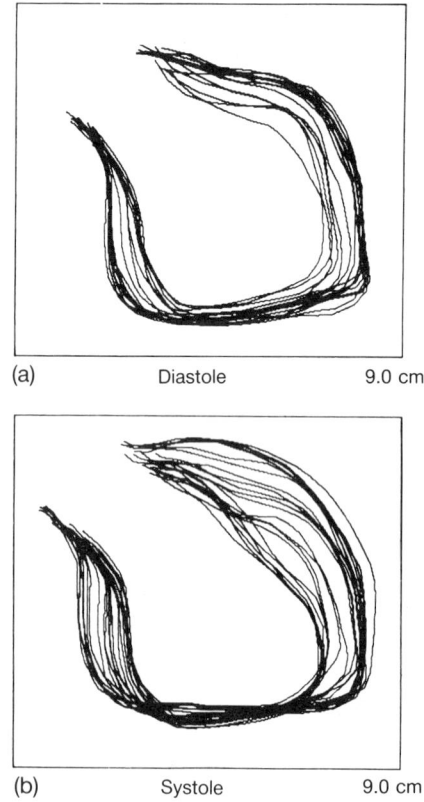

Fig. 5 Left ventricular wall motion in a patient with acute inferior myocardial infarction. Note the outward wall motion during systole along the inferior wall, while movement along the anterior wall is normal.

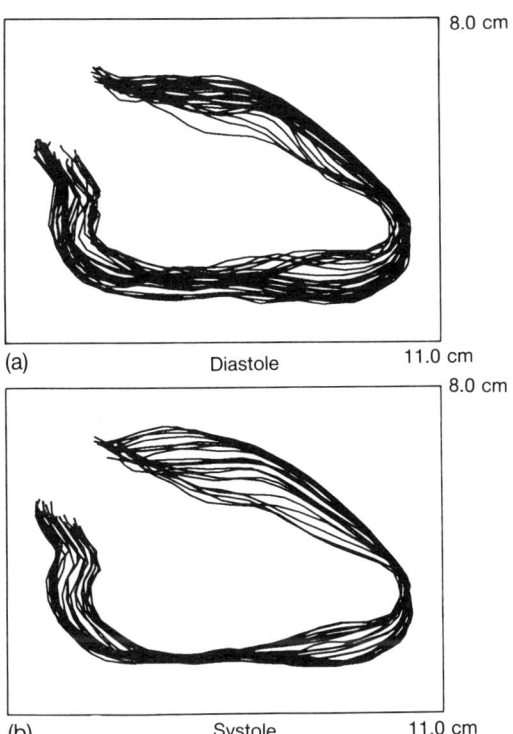

Fig. 6 Inco-ordinate left ventricular wall motion. Note that there appears to have been little wall motion along the inferior wall during systole, but that delayed inward movement in this region occurs in early diastole.

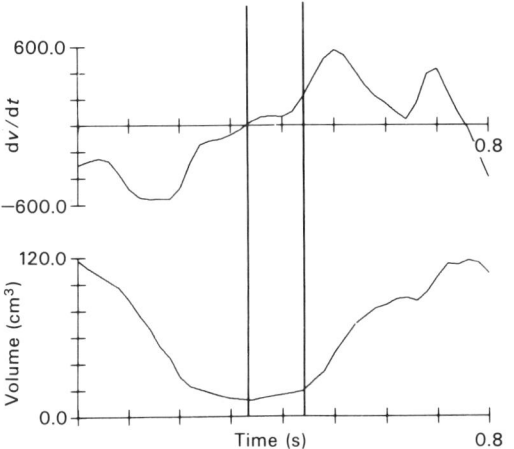

Fig. 7 Left ventricular volume and its rate of change from a normal subject. Note that during diastole, there is an early rapid increase, a mid-diastolic period when it remains virtually constant, and a further late diastolic increase with atrial systole. The vertical lines represent the timing of aortic valve closure and mitral valve opening.

In an attempt to define systolic function more precisely, the possibility of using quantities derived from simultaneous pressure and volume measurements has been investigated. The aim is to find an index of ventricular function which is unaffected by preload or afterload, but which reflects the contractile activity of the myocardium itself. One possible approach has been to investigate pressure–volume relations at end-systole. Experimentally, the end-systolic length of isolated heart muscle depends only on end-systolic tension and contractile state, and is unaffected by the extent of shortening or the end-diastolic length. When extrapolated to the whole heart, this finding suggests that the end-systolic pressure–volume relation might be used in a similar way, to define

contractile state. This method has proved capable of detecting changes due to drugs or other manoeuvres, though whether it is more sensitive than ejection fraction, which also depends on end-systolic volume, in identifying patients with ventricular disease has yet to be determined.

Diastolic function

Abnormalities of ventricular relaxation and filling may be as important as those of systole in limiting exercise tolerance. Left ventricular isovolumic relaxation starts with aortic valve closure, coinciding with A2 on the phonocardiogram, and lasts until mitral valve opening, measured from the M-mode echocardiogram. In normal subjects, its duration is remarkably constant, being 60 ± 10 ms. It may be lengthened in disease, particularly in patients with hypertrophy, when values of up to 200 ms may be seen. Elevation of left atrial pressure has the reverse effect, and at ventricular filling pressures of 30 mm Hg or more, isovolumic relaxation time may be zero or even negative, implying that the mitral valve opens before the aortic valve closes. The duration of isovolumic relaxation time is the result of these two effects so that values from individual patients with ventricular disease show wide scatter.

During isovolumic relaxation, ventricular pressure falls from that in the aorta to that in the left atrium. The rate of pressure decline reflects that of relaxation within the myocardium. It can be quantified as peak negative dP/dt or, if decay is assumed to be exponential, as a time constant. Both these methods show relaxation rate to be reduced in acute ischaemia and ventricular hypertrophy. In chronic ischaemic heart disease, the rate of pressure fall is also reduced, probably because relaxation is asynchronous rather than slow. In such cases, tension persisting in one part of the ventricle while the remainder has relaxed may cause striking local changes in cavity dimension change during isovolumic relaxation at a time when overall volume remains constant.

Ventricular filling

In the normal resting heart, the time available for filling may occupy the greater part of the cardiac cycle, but as rate increases with exertion the length of diastole becomes shorter relative to that of systole. At a heart rate of 160–170 per minute, filling time per beat may drop to less than 100 ms, so that if the normal stroke volume is taken as 100 ml, mean ventricular filling rate must be greater than 1 l/s. It is not surprising, therefore, to find that normal left ventricular filling depends on complex mechanisms and that these become disturbed in disease.

The pattern of left ventricular volume change during diastole is shown in Fig. 7. At rest, filling occurs in three phases. Immediately after mitral valve opening, there is a period of rapid filling, lasting up to 200 ms, when approximately 70 per cent of the stroke volume enters the ventricle. In mid-diastole, or diastasis, volume changes little, and finally, the remaining 30 per cent enters during left atrial systole. These three phases are apparent only at rest. As heart rate increases, diastasis becomes shorter and rapid filling merges into atrial systole. Mechanisms underlying rapid filling become clearer when simultaneous left ventricular pressure changes are considered. Diastolic pressure falls rapidly once the aortic valve closes but only reaches its minimum value 100 ms or more after the mitral valve opens. The greater part of rapid filling thus occurs as ventricular pressure is falling.

During diastasis, left ventricular pressure and volume both remain virtually constant, but in normal subjects, pressure may increase by up to 5mm Hg during atrial systole. It is clear from these interrelations between diastolic pressure and volume, that ventricular filling cannot be considered in terms of a passive elastic structure such as a balloon, since at the time of peak filling, ventricular pressure is falling rather than rising. Normal early diastolic filling has still to be explained in detail, but it seems that the ventricle is deformed at end-systole, with energy stored in its walls as elastic forces. A relaxation starts, the ventricle tends to return to its end-diastolic shape. In the isolated heart, high-fidelity pressure

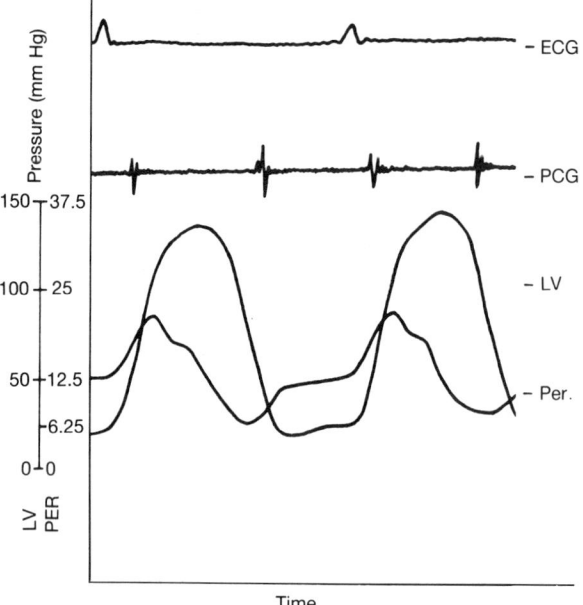

Fig. 8 Measurement of pericardial (Per) and left ventricular (LV) pressure in a patient after open-heart surgery. Note that pericardial pressure is at its lowest early in diastole, but that it rises significantly during the period of left ventricular filling.

measurements show early diastolic pressures to be below atmospheric, compatible with ventricular suction. The complex fibre architecture of the left ventricle would seem ideally adapted to supporting restoring forces of this sort, so that normal early diastolic filling is likely to depend on the integrity of fibre structure.

In normal subjects, peak filling rate, as measured by angiography or gated blood pool scanning, is 500–1000 ml/s or 3–5 end-diastolic volumes/s at rest. On moderate exercise, values approximately double these are seen. Values lower than normal occur, not only in mitral stenosis, but also in left ventricular hypertrophy and coronary artery disease, particularly in the presence of regional abnormalities of systolic function. In cardiomyopathy, major disturbances of relaxation and filling are frequently present, although systolic wall motion is usually normal.

Towards the end of rapid filling, pressure ceases falling, and starts to rise along with volume. It now becomes possible to measure the passive stiffness of the ventricular cavity. Compliance is the slope of the pressure volume curve, being defined as:

$$\Delta P / \Delta V$$

where ΔP and ΔV represent small increments in pressure and volume. As diastole proceeds, so the slope of this curve becomes steeper, meaning that compliance falls as the cavity enlarges. It is thus not possible to derive a single value for the compliance of a ventricle as one would its ejection fraction; the pressure or volume must be also be given at which any estimate of compliance was made, making it difficult to compare results between patients. As an alternative to considering the properties of the cavity as a whole by calculating compliance, the stiffness of the myocardium can be derived. This is somewhat increased in coronary artery disease and hypertension, but the highest values are seen in congestive cardiomyopathy or other conditions where the cavity is enlarged and the ejection fraction low. It is often suggested that there is a direct relation between compliance and filling rate such that stiff ventricles fill slowly. There is no evidence to support this idea. The least compliant ventricles, those with congestive cardiomyopathy, have a normal filling rate, whereas in ventricular hypertrophy, where filling rate is often low, compliance may be virtually normal.

Atrial systole

Approximately 30 per cent of the normal stroke volume normally enters the left ventricle during atrial systole. In left ventricular disease, particularly when early diastolic filling is impaired as in hypertrophy, this component may rise to more than 50 per cent. When compliance is reduced, the increase in ventricular volume during atrial systole will be accompanied by a corresponding increase in the height of the 'a' wave of the ventricular pressure trace, from a normal value of less than 5 mm Hg to 20 mm Hg or more. Left atrial systole increases cavity size and fibre length, and so the force of contraction of the succeeding ventricular systole is enhanced. Increased atrial activity is thus a useful sign of significant left ventricular disease in individual patients.

External influences

Filling of the left ventricle is affected by surrounding structures, including the pericardium and right ventricle. Restriction by the pericardium is well recognized in constriction or tamponade, but there is increasing evidence to suggest that even the normal pericardium may sometimes interfere with filling. This is particularly likely to be the case when the left ventricle is dilated, or after open heart surgery (Fig. 8). Elevated pericardial pressure causes ventricular diastolic pressures to be increased when measured with reference to the sternal angle, although the pressure gradient across the myocardium itself may be normal. Such an increase in pericardial pressure must affect measurements made in all cardiac chambers to an equal extent, and so can be assessed clinically as elevation of the jugular venous pressure. A normal venous pressure makes a pericardial contribution to elevated ventricular filling pressure very unlikely.

In experimental animals, the stiffness of the left ventricle is increased with right ventricular overload. In part, this is due to leftward motion of the interventricular septum, distorting the left ventricular cavity as it fills, and in part to an elevation of pericardial pressure following an increase in right ventricular volume. These effects may underlie the apparent left ventricular disease seen in patients with right ventricular overload. Conversely, left ventricular hypertrophy is frequently associated with a right atrial 'a' wave, again due to increased resistance to filling of the right ventricle. This association was originally described by Bernheim, who ascribed it to the hypertrophied septum bulging into the right ventricular inflow tract.

Left ventricular end-diastolic pressure

Left ventricular end-diastolic pressure (LVEDP) is widely used as an index of diastolic function. It is measured either immediately before (pre-'a') or after (post-'a') atrial systole. Both levels are commonly raised in chronic left ventricular disease, the difference between the two depending on the volume increase of the ventricle and the stiffness of the wall at this time in the cardiac cycle. Normal values of pre-a and post-a end-diastolic pressure are approximately 12 and 15 mm Hg, respectively, but they may rise to over 30 mm Hg in disease. High values may occur with left ventricular cavity dilation or hypertrophy, and are useful, non-specific evidence of disease. They are clinically significant, since in the absence of mitral valve disease, pre-a pressure in the left ventricle is approximately equal to mean left atrial pressure. Values above 25 mm Hg are thus associated with the appearance of Kerley B lines on the chest X-ray, and above 30 mm Hg with the appearance of interstitial pulmonary oedema. Elevated end-diastolic pressure correlates poorly with other manifestations of impaired left ventricular function such as a ejection fraction or inco-ordinate contraction (Fig. 9). End-diastolic pressure clearly depends on end-diastolic volume and wall stiffness, so that an increase in either may cause it to be raised. Simple circulatory overload may lead to a raised end-diastolic pressure by distending an otherwise normal ventricle, while hypovolaemia, induced, for example, by excessive diuretic treatment, may cause end-diastolic pressure to return to normal in spite of severe left ventricular disease. An

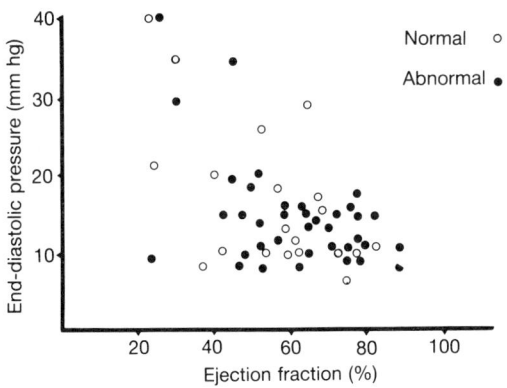

Fig. 9 Relation between end-diastolic pressure and ejection fraction in a group of patients with chronic ischaemic heart disease. Open symbols represent patients in whom contraction pattern is co-ordinate, and closed in whom it is inco-ordinate. Note that even within this single group of patients, there is little relation between these three different aspects of left ventricular disease.

increase in end-diastolic pressure is thus a non-specific marker of disease, and bears no close relation to any single systolic or diastolic abnormality.

Disturbances of cardiac rhythm

Supraventricular or ventricular arrhythmias are common in patients with ventricular disease. Superaventricular arrhythmias include atrial ectopic beats, atrial flutter, and atrial fibrillation, sustained supraventricular tachycardia being much less common. Their exact aetiology is not always clear. In some cases they may be due to the same mechanism as that causing the ventricular disease, as after acute myocardial infarction or in chronic alcoholism. When ventricular disease is chronic and severe, however, they appear to be the direct consequence of high filling pressures and a dilated left or right atrium. Predisposing factors may include an episode of fluid retention or a chest infection. Their clinical consequences vary greatly. Some patients are unaware of any rhythm disturbances at all, while in others, their onset causes severe haemodynamic deterioration. With atrial fibrillation, late diastolic filling due to atrial systole is lost, ventricular rate, particularly at low exercise levels, is much greater than in sinus rhythm, and the cardiac rhythm is irregular. During exercise, the relative increase in ventricular volume with atrial systole is less than at rest so its loss may not be clinically apparent. Diastolic filling time is not always shortened unduly by rapid ventricular rate, since it may be preserved at the expense of abbreviating ejection and isovolumic relaxation times. The haemodynamic effects of atrial fibrillation seem to be greater in patients with hypertrophic disease in whom early diastolic filling is impaired, than in those with simple cavity dilation. If ventricular rate is uncontrolled at rest, treatment with digitalis is required. A therapeutic trial of a small dose of β-blocker may be undertaken when inappropriate tachycardia on exercise seems clinically significant. When the clinical deterioration caused by the onset of atrial fibrillation is severe, and if the patient is not improved by standard treatment, it is reasonable to consider d.c. shock, provided the left atrium is not significantly enlarged. If necessary, sinus rhythm can be maintained with an anti-arrhythmic drug such as quinidine or amiodarone. Disopyramide is contraindicated in patients with cavity dilation, but may be useful with severe hypertrophic disease.

Ventricular arrhythmias play an important part in the clinical picture associated with severe ventricular disease. Isolated ventricular ectopic beats, ventricular tachycardia, either in short salvoes which are clinically inapparent, or in longer symptomatic episodes, and ventricular fibrillation may all be seen. Ventricular arrhythmias are most commonly associated with coronary artery disease. Their incidence is not predictably improved by bypass grafting, and it seems likely that they arise in association with fibrosis, often at the boundary of a ventricular aneurysm. In the absence of coronary artery disease, the commonest clinical association are arrhythmogenic right ventricular dysplasia, and severe generalized left ventricular disease of any sort: hypertrophic or congestive cardiomyopathy, or cavity dilation secondary to valve or other disease. The diagnosis is straightforward if symptomatic attacks of tachycardia develop, but arrhythmias may remain clinically silent, and be detectable only by 24-hour monitoring. If attacks are frequent, sustained, or give rise to symptoms, then treatment is likely to be required. This may involve anti-arrhythmic agents, surgery, or insertion of an automatic implantable cardioverter/defibrillator (see page 13.124).

Right ventricular function

The function of the right ventricle has been studied in very much less detail than that of the left. In the normal subject, it develops a peak pressure of less than 30 mm Hg, and ejects blood into the low resistance pulmonary vascular bed. Pressure changes in the pulmonary artery are delayed with respect to those in the right ventricle, particularly at end-ejection, so that right ventricular pressure has fallen virtually to right atrial level before the incisura is inscribed on the pulmonary artery pressure trace. This delay or 'hang-out' causes the pulmonary valve to close significantly later than the aortic in the normal heart, and explains normal splitting of the second heart sound.

Many aspects of right ventricular function can be described in similar terms to corresponding ones on the left. Right ventricular ejection fraction is normally greater than 50 per cent, and may be reduced in disease. Cavity dilation may be idiopathic, or may result from pressure or volume overload or from coronary artery disease, particularly when the right coronary artery is involved. Right ventricular hypertrophy occurs secondary to pulmonary hypertension or pulmonary stenosis at valve or infundibular level, and is associated with diastolic abnormalities of the type described on the left. In particular, the stiffness of the cavity increases and end-diastolic pressure rises. In such patients, right atrial contraction becomes more prominent, and is associated with a dominant 'a' wave in the jugular venous pulse. As pulmonary artery pressure rises, the dynamics of right ventricular ejection approach those of the left with pulmonary valve closure occurring earlier. The right ventricle differs from the left in a number of respects. It is unique in having an infundibulum, which itself may become hypertrophied, and cause outflow tract obstruction, either as a primary abnormality, or postoperatively in a patient in whom pulmonary valve stenosis has been corrected. A second difference is that atrioventricular valve regurgitation appears to be much commoner on the right side of the heart than the left, and indeed, right ventricular dilation is much the commonest cause of tricuspid regurgitation. Until recently, knowledge of right ventricular function was based only on cardiac catheterization, but it is likely that it will increase rapidly in the next few years with the development of improved methods of study. These include nuclear blood pool or first pass ventriculograms (q.v.) and two-dimensional echocardigraphy with peripheral contrast injection (q.v.), computerized tomographic (CT) scanning or magnetic resonance imaging (q.v.).

Reflex changes occurring in ventricular disease

In intact humans, primary abnormalities of ventricular function are associated with secondary reflex changes which greatly modify the clinical picture. These are complex and poorly understood but appear to involve mechanisms normally maintaining the circulation in the face of changes in blood volume. The most prominent are those whose main effects are to cause peripheral vasoconstriction and renal sodium retention, a response that would be appropriate to hypovolaemia in the normal. The nature of the afferent stimulus is unknown, though it seems to be correlated more closely with a reduction in cardiac output rather than with a low filling pressure. The sympathetic nervous system and the renin–angiotensin axis are both involved, and plasma levels of arginine vasopressin are also elevated. In contrast to these effects, elevation in atrial pressure has been shown experimentally and clinically to be associated with increased levels of atrial natriuretic factor, a peptide of atrial origin, whose main actions are to cause systemic vasodilation, along with an increase in renal blood flow, glomerular filtration rate, and sodium excretion. In patients with severe ventricular disease, the effects of increased sympathetic activity predominate. In the short term, heart rate and force of contraction are increased, as may be seen with the sudden deterioration in left ventricular performance that follows acute myocardial infarction. Here overall pump function is maintained in spite of severe disturbances of regional wall motion. In chronic heart disease, however, myocardial stores of noradrenaline become depleted and sensitivity to beta stimulation reduced so positive inotropic effects become less prominent. Parasympathetic function is less obviously affected, but its overall effect on heart rate is reduced so that the baroreceptor reflexes become less sensitive. The net effect of these reflex changes on the peripheral circulation, is to increase the resistance to ejection and therefore left ventricular afterload. When ventricular disease is severe, this increase in afterload seems inappropriate and deleterious to cardiac function, so that vasodilator therapy has been widely used in an attempt to improve forward flow. These reflex changes also reduce the ability of the cardiovascular system to react to external stimuli, so that patients become more sensitive to minor disturbances, developing pulmonary congestion with chest infections or infusion of small volumes of fluid. Their ability to respond to exercise or postural change is blunted, and their tolerance of surgery greatly reduced. The clinical significance of renin–angiotensin system involvement in these reflex changes has become apparent with the demonstration that angiotensin-converting enzyme inhibitors such as captopril or enalapril are effective in treating patients with severe ventricular disease.

Effect of ventricular disease on exercise capacity

Although cardiovascular function may be normal at rest in patients with heart disease, abnormalities can be unmasked by the stress of exercise. Understanding cardiac function during exercise can thus help to explain the genesis of symptoms seen in many of these patients, as well as forming the basis of a useful means of testing overall cardiac function (q.v.). Exercise may be isometric or dynamic, which have different effects on the cardiovascular system. Isometric exercise, as exemplified by handgrip, consists of a sustained increase in the tension of antagonistic muscle groups without movement. Its main effect is to increase arterial pressure and, to a lesser extent, heart rate. Although cardiac output itself changes little, the increase in arterial pressure causes stroke work and, in particular, left ventricular wall tension to rise. Since systolic wall tension is a major determinant of myocardial oxygen uptake, isometric exercise is a useful experimental method for provoking myocardial ischaemia. However, it may be unfamiliar to the patient, so its effects need not be clearly related to symptoms brought about by everyday activities. For this reason, dynamic exercise, on a bicycle ergometer or a treadmill is more widely used. Patients with possible ischaemic heart disease are best identified with the Bruce protocol (q.v.), in which treadmill rate and slope increase rapidly over a series of 3 min stages. This approach is unsuitable when the aim is to assess exercise tolerance in patients with ventricular disease, and in particular, to detect the relatively small changes brought about by drugs or other interventions. Instead, a lower level is used, and tolerance assessed in terms of exercise duration (Naughton protocol, page 13.159).

Provided neuromuscular or respiratory disease is absent, there is a close and linear relation between exercise capacity and peak oxygen uptake. In normal subjects, peak oxygen uptake is greater than 20 ml/min/m^2. This is reduced in heart disease, a value of 10 ml/min/kg corresponding to severe limitation of exercise tolerance. Normal oxygen uptake depends on ventilation, blood flow, and oxygen extraction. In the absence of severe, primary lung disease, ventilation is not a factor limiting oxygen uptake in patients with heart disease. Similarly, oxygen extraction in the tissues increases with exertion, whether or not heart disease is present. Arteriovenous oxygen difference is approximately 6 vol per cent at a level corresponding to 20 per cent maximum oxygen uptake, rising to 12 vol per cent at peak exercise. Anaerobic metabolism is also related to oxygen uptake in the same way. Venous lactic acid concentration begins to rise, and relative carbon dioxide output increases at approximately 60 per cent maximum oxygen uptake, again whether or not heart disease is present. The factor limiting oxygen uptake in heart disease is therefore reduced forward blood flow.

A number of mechanisms may underlie this reduction in flow during exercise in patients with ventricular disease. These include a small fixed stroke volume, excessive elevation of left ventricular end-diastolic and hence pulmonary capillary pressure causing breathlessness, and failure of the normal positive inotropic response to sympathetic stimulation due to catecholamine depletion. In individual patients with ventricular disease, correlation is virtually non-existent between objectively measured exercise tolerance and a number of indices of resting left ventricular function, including cavity size, ejection time, ejection fraction, and velocity of circumferential fibre shortening. Although other measurements, for example, those of diastolic function, might correlate better with exercise performance, these results must raise the possibility that new disturbances of function appear during exercise that are not apparent at rest. One of these is functional mitral regurgitation, which causes a sharp increase in left atrial pressure. In patients with coronary artery disease, striking abnormalities of regional wall motion and elevation of end-diastolic pressure appear with angina, which a minority of patients may feel as breathlessness. A greater understanding of these additional mechanisms limiting exercise tolerance might form a basis of developing new methods of treatment.

Cardiac function in anaemia

In anaemia, the haemoglobin content, and hence the oxygen carrying capacity of the blood is reduced, so that normal oxygen transport is maintained only with increased flow. This increase in cardiac output is mediated in part by tachycardia, and in part by increased stroke volume associated with a fall in peripheral resistance. Even though peak cardiac output may be normal, peak exercise tolerance is reduced along with haemoglobin content and peak oxygen uptake. The haemodynamic picture at rest in these patients thus resembles that occurring in normal subjects with moderate exercise. Systolic function of both ventricles is usually normal; impairment is uncommon, but when it occurs it is often on the basis of iron overload following multiple transfusions, or possibly to small vessel disease, as seen in sickle cell anaemia. Evidence of overt myocardial ischaemia is unusual except in the presence of obstructive coronary artery disease. Ventricular filling pressures, however, are often moderately increased. This is not evidence of systolic left ventricular disease. In part, this elevation is the result of reduced ventricular compliance, since a small increase in end-diastolic volume due, for example, to increased venous return or to plasma volume expansion secondary to renal sodium retention, will cause the ventricle to work further up the normal passive pressure–volume curve. Any increase in end-diastolic volume will also predispose to pericardial restraint and so to a rise in jugular venous pressure. If fibrosis develops as the result of prolonged and severe anaemia, diastolic stiffness will increase, a process exacerbated by iron overload. Such patients are frequently pronounced to be in 'high output failure'. This is an unsatisfactory term since the primary deficit is in the oxygen capacity of the blood, rather than on the function of the heart, which is well maintained in the absence of intrinsic disease. Its use thus focuses on the homeostatic mechanism maintaining oxygen transport rather than on the primary abnormality.

Effects of heart disease on other organs

Lungs

Pulmonary function may be abnormal in heart disease, since alveolar gas exchange depends on left atrial pressure. Normal left atrial pressure is in the range 7–12 mm Hg. The pulmonary veins are thin-walled and collapsible, so that they are dilated only when the hydrostatic pressure of blood inside them is greater than the surrounding intrathoracic pressure. In the erect position, the point at which collapse occurs is only a few cm above the left atrium. As atrial pressure rises, however, the level to which the veins becomes distended is correspondingly increased, so that they become visible on the PA chest X-ray (page 13.16). Dilation of the upper lobe veins is thus a simple hydrostatic effect, depending on an increase in left atrial pressure, collapsible pulmonary veins and the patient being in the erect posture. In addition, in the erect posture, the hydrostatic pressure of blood is greater in the lower lobes, and indeed, relatively little blood normally flows to the upper zones. When atrial pressure is raised, not only is flow to the upper lobes increased, but that to the lower zones reduced. The mechanism by which this reduction occurs is not fully understood, but it appears to involve active vasoconstriction of the lower lobe arterioles. This causes the characteristic sign on the PA chest X-ray of upper lobe blood diversion (q.v.). When pulmonary capillary pressure reaches 25–30 mm Hg, transudation of fluid into the alveoli occurs, resulting in intra-alveolar oedema if its rate of formation is greater than that at which it is removed by the pulmonary lymphatics. Since the normal oncotic pressure of the plasma proteins is also in the range 25–30 mm Hg, it can be deduced that there is no abnormal increase in pulmonary capillary permeability in heart disease. On the contrary, in patients with long-standing left atrial hypertension, particularly those with mitral valve disease, a number of mechanisms develop which protect against the development of pulmonary oedema. In particular there is thickening of the alveolar membrane, and increased development of the pulmonary lymphatic system to remove transudate.

Pressures in the pulmonary artery are also altered when left atrial pressure rises. Normal mean pulmonary artery pressure is in the range 15–20 mm Hg, so that there is a 10–15 mm Hg pressure drop across the normal pulmonary circulation at rest. When left atrial pressure rises, there is a corresponding rise in pulmonary artery pressure, which may reach 35–40 mm Hg in this way, resulting in passive pulmonary hypertension, without the pulmonary vascular resistance being significantly changed. In active pulmonary hypertension, the resistance also rises, so that the increase in pulmonary artery pressure is much greater, and may reach systemic levels.

Lung function tests are frequently abnormal in heart disease. When left atrial pressure is raised, the lungs become stiffer. Vital capacity and total lung volume both fall with cardiac enlargement, and increase in central blood volume and lung water, and possibly pleural effusions. Peripheral airway resistance rises, due to mucosal oedema and active bronchoconstriction. Reversal of the normal base to apex gradient of blood flow, along with regional inequality in ventilation cause suboptimal gas exchange and ventilation–perfusion mismatch. In particular, the A–a gradient is increased, leading to arterial hypoxaemia, which may be associated with a low P_{CO_2} resulting from hyperventilation. At the same time, DCO is significantly reduced. A number of abnormalities of lung function may thus be found in patients in whom left atrial pressure is raised, which are probably related to the symptom of breathlessness. It must be stressed, however, that these abnormalities are not specific to heart disease, and cannot be used, for example, to assess the relative contributions of heart and lung disease to symptoms in a patient known to have both.

Renal function

Disturbed renal function in patients with heart disease contributes in an important way to the overall clinical picture.

As cardiac output falls, glomerular filtration rate and, in particular, renal blood flow are reduced, and the ratio of the two, filtration fraction, rises. The major abnormality of renal function in heart disease, however, is excessive sodium retention, leading to inappropriate expansion of the volume of extracellular fluid. Possible mechanisms are described in detail elsewhere (page 13.81).

Liver function

Elevation of systemic venous pressure causes hepatic congestion, which causes minor abnormalities of liver function. These include reduced BSP excretion, and slight elevation of enzymes such as SGOT and SGPT. Serum bilirubin is raised, but seldom to more than twice the upper limit of normal, due in part to hepatic dysfunction, and in part to increased intravascular haemolysis causing an unconjugated hyperbilirubinaemia. Although prothrombin time is usually normal or only mildly prolonged, patients may be unusually sensitive to the effects of oral anticoagulants. In general, however, failure of detoxication of drugs in heart disease does not pose problems in practice unless the clinical manifestations are very severe.

After open heart surgery, a characteristic syndrome may appear of severe and prolonged jaundice. This is commonest in patients with long-standing mitral and particularly tricuspid valve disease with hepatic congestion. In such patients, excess blood loss frequently occurs at operation, and the jaundice results directly from the resulting bilirubin load. Serum bilirubin may be considerably raised, approximately half conjugated and half unconjugated. Evidence of hepatocellular failure is not seen, and the jaundice subsides spontaneously. Its occurrence does not affect overall prognosis significantly, and it does not require other than symptomatic treatment.

Ventricular disease and 'heart failure'

Patients with severe ventricular disease are often pronounced to be in 'heart failure', but this term has eluded precise definition. It has been traditional over the past 50 years or so to equate it with the state in which heart fails to meet its 'obligations', or 'to pump blood at a rate commensurate with the requirements of the metabolizing tissues'. These would be excellent definitions if the heart were an organ with a large functional reserve like the bone marrow or the kidney. It would then be possible to speak of a phase in the natural history of ventricular disease when there were no measureable functional consequences, and a later stage, corresponding to 'failure' when circulatory performance was reduced. Unfortunately, this does not apply to the heart, in view of the almost linear relation between oxygen uptake and cardiac output throughout the entire range of performance. The 'requirements of the metabolizing tissues' have never been formally defined. If they include the avoidance of lactic acid accumulation as a result of anaerobic metabolism, then even normal hearts must be said to develop 'failure' with exercise, and to the same extent as those with heart disease. Alternatively, the 'requirements' might be taken as representing the delivery of oxygen to the tissues, again presumably during exercise as well as at rest. If this is so, any condition causing a measureable reduction in peak cardiac output will fulfill the definition of heart failure, whether it is due to ventricular disease, mitral stenosis, pericardial constriction or supraventricular tachycardia. While such a wide definition might be a useful one of 'heart disease' it does not identify what is normally meant by heart failure.

By common usage, heart failure is a clinical diagnosis, and draws attention to a number of similarities between patients with advanced ventricular disease of different types. It refers to some additional but independent developments, late in the stage of the disease, whose effects summate with those of the underlying condition. Its manifestations are similar from patient to patient, and include breathlessness, peripheral oedema, a raised venous pressure, added heart sounds, associated with inappropriate renal sodium retention. Heart failure is usually held to affect the myocardium of one or both ventricles which can be said to 'fail', and to be independent of the underlying condition, so that it is possible to speak of 'heart failure' supervening in a case of valvular disease. Heart failure can be further dissociated from the underlying condition with treatment, so that patients can go 'in' or 'out' of failure. No specific myocardial abnormality has been defined at either a biochemical or physiological level.

Although it has a certain convenience at the clinical level, the drawbacks of setting an undefined term in a position of such importance in the description of a subject should not be underestimated. There are no specific features by which heart failure can be recognized in individual patients, which would allow its presence to be determined independently of additional heart disease. Still less is there any basis for additional qualifying terms such as 'congestive' or 'frank'. As described above, techniques now available demonstrate a wide variety of physiological disturbances in patients pronounced to be in 'failure' on clinical grounds. It is traditionally taught that heart failure is due only to depressed contractility, another undefined entity related indirectly to the maximum velocity of myocardial shortening, which excludes all consideration of diastolic function or inco-ordinate action. Heart failure is an emotive term, and a variety of drugs continue to be proposed for its treatment, particularly in its 'early' stages when it is still 'mild'. Since the effect of a drug depends on the underlying disturbance in the control state, poorly defined criteria are likely to identify patients with a heterogeneous group of functional abnormalities, and thus lead to drugs with useful actions in specific forms of ventricular disease being overlooked. It thus seems preferable to establish the exact diagnosis in each case, in order to understand functional abnormalities more completely, and so treat the patient more effectively. Use of poorly defined terms such as 'heart failure' actively obstructs these aims.

Clinical features of ventricular disease

Symptoms

Limitation of exercise tolerance

Limitation of exercise tolerance is a major manifestation of left or right ventricular disease. In any patient with heart disease, therefore, it is important to establish whether such limitation is present, when the patient's age, sex, background, and habitus are taken into account. Secondly, other causes of limitation, (such as arthritis or neurological disease) must, as far as possible, be excluded. This may not always be possible, for example, when there is evidence to suggest that both heart disease and lung disease are present in the same patient.

Once the presence of limitation of exercise tolerance has been established, its severity should next be determined. This is best done in terms of everyday activities undertaken by the patient. The classification of the New York Heart Association (NYHA) is commonly used for this:

Grade I   Exercise tolerance is uncompromised
Grade II Exercise tolerance is slightly compromised
Grade III Exercise tolerance is moderately compromised
Grade IV Exercise tolerance is severely compromised

This classification is not ideal, since it is largely subjective, and since it contains too few levels, virtually all cardiac patients with significant symptoms falling into Grades III and IV. Unfortunately, it is not always possible to determine the degree of limitation

of exercise tolerance precisely from the history, so that exercise testing may be necessary, particularly for an objective record.

The nature of the symptom or symptoms that limit exercise tolerance must next be established.

1. Breathlessness. This is a common symptom, but unless carefully questioned, patients may describe any sensation associated with limitation of exercise tolerance as breathlessness.

2. Chest pain. This symptom is described in detail elsewhere (page 13.76).

3. Fatigue. Although tiredness is a non-specific symptom occurring in the absence of organic disease, many patients with heart disease describe limitation of exercise tolerance by fatigue, which they clearly differentiate from breathlessness. The symptom is closely related to exertion, and is relieved by rest. It is felt as a heaviness in the limbs, and once it is present, further activity becomes progressively more difficult. It is not uncommonly seen in patients with mixed mitral valve disease and pulmonary hypertension, who are able to differentiate it clearly from the breathlessness present before a previous mitral valvotomy. A low cardiac output, poor peripheral blood flow, and the presence of tricuspid regurgitation predispose to its occurrence; it may be aggravated by β-blocking drugs.

4. Inappropriate tachycardia. Excessive ventricular rate due to atrial fibrillation may severely limit exercise tolerance in the absence of other symptoms. When such patients undergo a formal exercise test, ventricular rate is found to be well controlled at rest, but to rise rapidly at low exercise levels to 150–170 beats/min. This is not prevented by therapeutic digitalization. Often, the patient is unable to describe the sensation associated with inappropriate tachycardia, and may finally decide to call it breathlessness in order to gain the attention of the physician. However, its recognition is important, since it frequently responds specifically to a small dose of a β-blocking drug. Other arrhythmias such as supraventricular or ventricular tachycardia may be precipitated by exertion, but these are rare, and show an inconstant relation to exercise, while the sudden change in heart rate can be elicited by careful history taking.

5. Faintness on exertion. Faintness on exertion due to arterial hypotension is a very important symptom. It results from the combination of a fixed cardiac output and a normal reduction in peripheral resistance. It is commonly seen in aortic stenosis, pulmonary stenosis or hypertrophic cardiomyopathy. It may also occur in coronary artery disease, where it is a sign of severe left ventricular involvement.

6. A significant number of patients with heart disease voluntarily limit their exercise tolerance. This may be on the basis of unpleasant symptoms in the past, or on the advice of their doctor. More difficult to elucidate are cardiac symptoms occurring when the patient knows of the existence of heart disease but does not understand its nature. This state of affairs may lead to anxiety, and so to inappropriate tachycardia on exercise, hyperventilation, or atypical chest pain (pages 13.76 and 13.80). When such symptoms are superimposed on those directly due to the heart disease itself diagnosis may become difficult.

Other evidence of left ventricular disease

1. Orthopnoea is breathlessness that occurs when the patient lies flat, relieved by sitting up. Patients therefore learn to sleep in this position, and the severity of the symptom can be judged from the number of pillows they use. It is strongly suggestive of cardiac rather than lung disease, although this is not invariable, since patients with bronchial asthma also show a preference for sleeping sitting up. A variant of this symptom, also common in patients with left ventricular disease is a dry cough, also relieved by sitting up. Presumably, variation of dyspnoea with posture represents the effects of movement of blood out of the thorax into the systemic vascular bed, and also the deleterious effects of raised pulmonary venous pressure on the lower lobes of the lung in the supine position.

2. Paroxysmal nocturnal dyspnoea. In its most typical form, this is an episode of suffocating breathlessness that wakes the patient at night, relieved by sitting or even standing up, or by making for the window in search of fresh air. Its severity may vary greatly. At its mildest, the patient wakes suddenly with a sense of unease, while at its most severe, it overlaps that seen in acute pulmonary oedema. Common to all is an intense desire to sit up, which gives relief. As with many other symptoms, its physiological basis is not clear. Nocturnal dyspnoea occurs during REM sleep, and may represent the effect of excessive sympathetic activity causing venoconstriction, so that blood moves from the systemic venous system to the pulmonary circulation. If there is associated wheeze, due to bronchospasm, the condition is referred to as cardiac asthma.

3. Acute pulmonary oedema. This is the most severe form of breathlessness. In heart disease, it is due to elevation of the pulmonary venous pressure to levels greater than the oncotic pressure of the plasma proteins, so that fluid leaves the pulmonary capillaries at a rate that cannot be removed by the lymphatics. An attack characteristically begins with a dry cough, and with a feeling of intense breathlessness. The rate and depth of respiration increase, and the patient is forced to sit up gasping for breath, cold, and sweating. The cough becomes productive of pink, frothy sputum, representing intra-alveolar oedema. As free fluid enters the airways, crepitations and evidence of bronchospasm are evident on auscultation over the lung fields. An attack of acute pulmonary oedema may subside spontaneously, or may be a terminal event in spite of treatment.

4. Cheyne–Stokes respiration. Cheyne–Stokes respiration, sometimes seen in patients with chronic pulmonary oedema, consists of alternating periods of apnoea and hyperventilation. It is accompanied by cyclic changes in blood gases, and may represent the effects of interference with normal homeostatic mechanisms by abnormal lung dynamics, loss of sensitivity of the mid-brain centres to hypoxia, and a slow circulation time.

Evidence of right ventricular disease

1. Evidence of systemic venous congestion. Raised systemic venous pressure does not cause symptoms unless it is severe. When it does so, the patient complains of pain in the right upper quadrant of the abdomen, due to distension of the capsule of the liver. It is usually aggravated by exertion, and may even be the factor limiting exercise tolerance. Ascites is also common in patients in whom systemic venous pressure is raised.

2. Underfilling of the left ventricle. Right ventricular disease may manifest itself as a reduction in cardiac output or even cardiogenic shock due to underfilling of the left ventricle. This is particularly likely to occur after acute myocardial infarction, when it may give rise to a clinical picture resembling that due to severe, primary left ventricular disease. The true state of affairs is determined by measuring the left ventricular filling pressure, showing it to be low, rather than high.

Physical signs of ventricular disease

Clinical examination is of considerable value in assessing the presence, nature, and severity of ventricular disease.

Abnormalities of the venous pulse

The venous pulse (pages 13.8 and 13.54) should be carefully examined, since it gives much useful information in assessing right ventricular disease. Its pulsations should be observed in the internal and not the superficial veins. The mean pressure must first be estimated, and expressed in cm above the sternal angle. The posture of the patient is varied so that the entire wave form is adequately displayed. Although the 45° position is usually the most satisfactory, it may be necessary for the patient to sit upright if the pressure is very high. The venous pressure normally falls during inspiration, along with intrathoracic pressure. The reverse pattern, sometimes call venous pulsus paradoxus or Kussmaul's sign,

may occur with pericardial tamponade (q.v.) or with right ventricular disease of any sort. It appears to reflect failure of the ventricle to deal with the transient increase in venous return caused by inspiration. The venous pulse must next be analysed, with particular reference as to whether the main deflection is an 'a' wave or a 'v' wave. An 'a' wave is brief and characteristically 'flicking', preceding the onset of the upstroke of the carotid pulse. It occurs when there is increased resistance to right atrial emptying, and so is seen in tricuspid stenosis, right ventricular hypertrophy or in association with left ventricular hypertrophy (Bernheim 'a' wave). The amplitude of an 'a' wave usually increases with inspiration. A 'v' wave represents the accumulation of blood in the right atrium when the tricuspid valve is closed. The pressure thus rises during ventricular systole, reaching its peak at the time of opening of the tricuspid valve. An increased 'v' wave may result either from a raised right ventricular end-diastolic pressure, or from tricuspid regurgitation, when it is sometimes referred to as a systolic wave. The two descents should also be studied. The 'x' descent occurs after the 'a' wave, and continues throughout ejection, as blood is ejected into the great arteries. The 'y' descent, occurring after the 'v' wave represents early diastolic filling of the right ventricle. An accentuated 'y' descent has a similar significance on the right side of the heart to that of a third sound on the left.

Pulsus alternans

Pulsus alternans describes the condition in which alternate beats in the arterial pulse are weak and strong, occurring with uniform QRS complexes. When the condition is well developed, the difference in amplitude can be detected by palpation. In less obvious cases, it may be necessary to use a sphygmomanometer. Rarely, the difference between the beats is so large that the weak ones do not open the aortic valve, and from the pulse the patient appears to have a bradycardia. In patients with aortic stenosis, pulsus alternans may be detected from alternation of the intensity of the systolic murmur. Pulsus alternans must be distinguished from pulsus bigeminus, which is due to alternate ventricular ectopic beats. In pulsus alternans, the timing of the QRS complexes is regular, but the weak beats may feel slightly delayed, particularly at the radial pulse, because of their slower rate of transmission in the arterial tree. The genesis of pulsus alternans is unknown. All aspects of left ventricular function alternate, including cavity size, contraction velocity, and degree of co-ordination. In spite of this ignorance about its genesis, its recognition is important, since it is a very reliable, though rather uncommon sign of left ventricular disease.

Abnormalities of the apex beat

Left ventricular disease may be accompanied by abnormalities of the apex beat. If cardiac enlargement is severe, the apex is displaced; however, information about overall cardiac enlargement is much better obtained from the PA chest X-ray. More significant is the presence of a sustained apex. In normal subjects, the apex beat moves outwards for the first third of systole only, and thereafter retracts. Failure of this retraction in late systole results in a sustained apex, sometimes described as 'heaving'. It is a non-specific sign, although when present, it requires explanation. It occurs with left ventricular hypertrophy, cavity dilation or left ventricular aneurysm. It may also arise from a right ventricle that is considerably enlarged and palpable at the apex.

Abnormal pulsation may also be felt in the left parasternal region. It may arise from the right ventricle, and be caused by hypertrophy, cavity enlargement or a volume overload such as that caused by a shunt or tricuspid regurgitation. However, it is a non-specific sign, and may be present with severe mitral regurgitation or in coronary artery disease when there are abnormalities of the movement of the anterior left ventricular wall. As with other physical signs, therefore, its significance should not be assessed in isolation, but in conjunction with other clinical evidence.

On occasion, a double apex beat may be palpated. The commonest cause for this is a palpable atrial impulse, which can be felt preceding the main outward movement. Its significance is similar to that of a prominent left atrial sound, although in aortic stenosis or hypertrophic cardiomyopathy, increased left atrial activity is often more easily felt than heard. A double apex may also be due to accentuated outward movement late in ejection, termed a late systolic bulge, associated with a left ventricular aneurysm. Finally, a third heart sound may be so loud as to be palpable, as occurs in severe mitral regurgitation. A double apex beat must not be confused with a palpable first heart sound occurring in rheumatic mitral valve disease (q.v.)

Third heart sound (S3 gallop)
The third heart sound occurs 120–160 ms after the second heart sound. It is usually low pitched, and is best heard with the bell of the stethoscope. Although it is associated in some way with rapid ventricular filling, its exact relation to AV valve motion, blood flow, and ventricular wall motion varies from patient to patient, so that its genesis is still unknown. A third heart sound occurs in a variety of circumstances. It is common in young people, becoming progressively less frequent above the age of 20 years. In patients older than 40 years, it should always be assumed to be abnormal. A third heart sound is the rule in severe non-rheumatic mitral regurgitation (q.v.) and less common, though well documented in rheumatic mitral stenosis. It may also occur in constrictive pericarditis (q.v.), when it is referred to as a muscle knock, and appears to represent sudden cessation of filling. In the absence of these two conditions, a third heart sound implies ventricular disease. It may occur after acute myocardial infarction, or when the left ventricular cavity is dilated and the ejection fraction reduced. It is uncommon in the presence of left ventricular hypertrophy when cavity size is normal and wall thickness increased, possibly because of abnormalities of early relaxation occurring in such patients. Rarely, it may occur in hypertrophic cardiomyopathy, when it carries a poor prognosis. Third heart sounds may also arise from the right ventricle. They can be identified from their increase in intensity during inspiration.

Fourth heart sound (S4 gallop)
A fourth heart sound is due to increased atrial activity. It precedes the first sound, and so may be confused clinically with a split first sound or with the combination of a first heart sound and an ejection click. Since a soft fourth heart sound can frequently be recorded phonocardiographically in patients without significant heart disease, its clinical value has been questioned, However, a clearly audible fourth heart sound is always significant. It can be distinguished from a split first sound or an ejection click by the presence of an unusually soft first sound, with the fourth clearly separate from it. Unlike a third heart sound, a fourth heart sound can occur in left ventricular disease of any sort, a dilated cavity, left ventricular hypertrophy or after acute myocardial infarction. It may also be right sided, when, again, it is accentuated with quiet inspiration. When the underlying cause is treated, the fourth heart sound gets softer, the first sound gets louder, and the interval between the two becomes less.

Summation sound
A summation sound occurs when the third and fourth heart sounds are superimposed, so it requires the presence of ventricular disease and a sinus tachycardia. Once established, a summation sound persists for long periods, so it is often considered a discrete entity.

Abnormalities of the second heart sound
A raised left ventricular end-diastolic pressure is associated with a corresponding elevation of pulmonary artery pressure and an increase in the intensity of the pulmonary component of the second heart sound (P2). If this physical sign is to be elicited, P2 must be correctly identified as the later of the two components,

when splitting is normal. Splitting of the second heart sound may be reversed in left ventricular disease. This may be due directly to left bundle branch block, itself evidence of left ventricular disease, or to prolonged or delayed ejection caused by inco-ordinate wall motion or increased resistance to ejection such as occurs in aortic stenosis or severe hypertension. Reversed splitting may be provoked in a minority of patients wth pre-existing left ventricular disease by β-blocking drugs. In the absence of left bundle branch block, reversed splitting is an uncommon sign of left ventricular disease, but when present, it is a reliable one.

Atrioventricular valve regurgitation
Unlike the semilunar valves, the AV valve cusps are supported by papillary muscles, and their rings, insubstantial structures on their own, are surrounded at the base of the heart by myocardium. Mitral or tricuspid incompetence may thus constitute a significant component of ventricular disease, particularly if cavity dilation occurs. On the left side of the heart, functional mitral regurgitation is frequently attributed to papillary muscle dysfunction, and is associated clinically with a soft pan or late systolic murmur. Unless there is organic disease of the papillary muscle (q.v.), regurgitation is seldom severe, and does not require treatment in its own right. The tricuspid valve is less able to withstand the effects of right ventricular cavity dilation than the mitral valve can those of the left. An elevation of right ventricular cavity size may cause severe tricuspid regurgitation whose presence can be detected from the venous pulse (q.v.). Atricventricular valve regurgitation of this type usually regresses after successful treatment of the underlying ventricular disease and is not often severe enough to require valve surgery.

Basal crepitations
Although basal crepitations may be present in patients with left ventricular disease as a manifestation of early pulmonary oedema, their presence is a non-specific finding, which may occur in otherwise normal individuals, even following deep inspiration or coughing, particularly smokers. This physical sign is easy to elicit, but taken on its own does not constitute evidence of left ventricular disease, unlike the other more specific signs described above.

Manifestations of renal sodium retention
Renal sodium retention results in an increase in the volume of extracellular fluid, and is responsible for many of the clinical features of 'heart failure'.

1. Nocturia. The earliest manifestation of renal sodium retention is frequently nocturia, caused by loss of the normal diurnal rhythm of sodium excretion. In normal subjects, sodium is excreted mainly by day, but if this capacity is impaired by heart disease, it occurs at night when physical activity is low. Nocturia may precede other symptoms of heart disease by several months.

2. Peripheral oedema. Peripheral oedema is a late manifestation of sodium retention, and in order for it to become clinically apparent, there must have been an increase in extracellular fluid of 5–7 litres. Since this is considerably greater than the plasma volume, it is clear that peripheral oedema cannot arise simply from the effects of a raised venous pressure. Its distribution depends on the posture and level of activity of the patient. If the patient is still active by day, then it collects around the ankles, while if the patient is bedridden, then it appears mainly over the sacrum. Its distribution may also be affected by local factors, it is frequently worse over the left than the right ankle, possible because the left internal iliac vein is crossed and partially compressed by the right iliac artery. The more severe the fluid retention, the more extensive the oedema, which may spread to involve the thighs and lumbar region. Cardiac oedema is distinguished from lymphoedema by being pitted (page 13.396), and from that due to venous obstruction by lack of evidence of thrombophlebitis or collaterals. It is similar to that occurring in the nephrotic syn-

drome or hepatic cirrhosis, which is also due to excessive renal sodium retention.

3. Pleural effusion. As sodium retention becomes more severe, fluid is found to collect in the serous cavities. Bilateral pleural effusions appear, which are initially apparent on the PA chest X-ray as blunting of the costophrenic angles, but which may reach volumes of more than a litre. Characteristically, they consist of straw-coloured fluid of low protein content. They can thus be distinguished from those due to pulmonary infarction, which are blood stained, and which may also occur in heart disease.

4. Pericardial effusion. Small pericardial effusions are also common in these patients. They can be detected by echocardiography, or may be found at the time of corrective cardiac surgery. Their volume is of the order of 50–100 ml. They do not give rise to major clinical consequences, although they may contribute to cardiac enlargement demonstrated on PA chest X-ray, and may lead to increasing intrapericardial pressure in patients with severe left ventricular disease. Their resolution is the main cause of the reduction in heart size seen on chest X-ray with diuretic treatment.

5. Ascites. The accumulation of ascites is also a late manifestation of fluid retention. Unlike other manifestations of fluid retention, its development is more closely related to elevation of the venous pressure, and it is particularly common in patients with tricuspid regurgitation or pericardial disease. It is thus often associated with hepatic enlargement and may be perpetuated by protein losing enteropathy (q.v.) associated with high venous pressure.

Investigation of ventricular disease

It is usually possible to establish the presence and nature of ventricular disease using the specialized techniques described elsewhere. However, much useful information can be derived from more simple, routine examinations:

1. Chest X-ray (page 13.16) This is a very helpful investigation.

(*a*) An increase in the transverse diameter of the heart is common in patients with ventricular disease. However, it is not possible to confirm or exclude enlargement of either ventricular cavity from a plain chest X-ray, neither can the presence of hypertrophy be deduced from the configuration of the heart shadow. Severe left ventricular disease may co-exist with a normal heart shadow if cavity size is normal or only moderately increased. It is rare for cardiac enlargement on chest X-ray to be caused by left ventricular hypertrophy alone without any increase in cavity size; when it does so, the increase in wall thickness is usually severe.

(*b*) Selective enlargement of the left atrium on the plain chest X-ray is characteristic of mitral valve disease, but it also occurs in any condition where there is increased resistance to left atrial emptying such as severe left ventricular hypertrophy.

(*c*) Abnormalities of the pulmonary vasculature are amongst the commonest and most significant manifestations of ventricular disease and are described in detail on page 13.18.

(*d*) Though pleural effusion itself is a non-specific finding, the presence of unilateral or bilateral pleural effusions in the presence of pulmonary congestion must raise the possibility of fluid retention.

2. Electrocardiogram There are no specific electrocardiographic abnormalities indicating the presence of ventricular disease. However, it is possible to extract indirect information which may be helpful in individual cases.

(*a*) Evidence of ventricular hypertrophy. Left ventricular hypertrophy may manifest itself as an increase in QRS voltage, or by T wave changes. Both are non-specific. When the sum of the R wave in V5 and the S wave in V2 is more than 35 mm left ventricular hypertrophy is said to be present. However, this criterion is frequently found in normal young men, and may be absent in elderly patients with severe left ventricular hypertrophy. T wave inversion in leads 1, aVf, and V4–6 is a common manifestation of left ventricular hypertrophy in older patients. Its mechanism is unknown, but it appears to relate more closely to diastolic abnormalities than to disturbances of systolic function or the increase in left ventricular mass. Very similar T wave abnormalities may appear in other types of left ventricular disease, especially ischaemic heart disease. Overall, these ECG changes have a sensitivity and specificity only of the order of 70 per cent in predicting the presence of left ventricular hypertrophy. It is thus possible for severe left ventricular hypertrophy to co-exist with an entirely normal ECG.

The cardiographic diagnosis of right ventricular hypertrophy, particularly when due to acquired heart disease, is even more unsatisfactory. The most characteristic ECG feature is a dominant R wave in V1 of amplitude greater than 3 mm, often associated with right axis deviation. This criterion performs even less well than those for left ventricular hypertrophy with specificity and sensitivity of the order of 55 per cent each.

(*b*) Conduction disturbances. The presence of certain conduction disturbances may point to a diagnosis of ventricular disease. Left bundle branch block is very likely to be associated with left ventricular abnormality, while isolated right bundle branch block should be regarded as a normal finding. Increased QRS width due to interventricular conduction delay suggests disease, possibly fibrosis. Left axis deviation is much less specific, and its incidence increases with age. Above the age of 50 years, therefore, it does not require explanation, but below 30 years, left axis deviation may be a pointer to significant left ventricular disease such as cardiomyopathy.

(*c*) Q waves. Q waves are characteristic of coronary artery disease. Their presence correlates poorly with the pattern of coronary artery involvement, but well with left ventricular disease. Q waves in leads 2, 3, and aVf are particularly closely associated with inferior scar tissue. Q waves may also occur in cardiomyopathy, in spite of coronary arteriography being entirely normal. Their genesis in such patients is not well understood. Nevertheless, Q waves are very uncommon in the absence of disease, so that in an individual patient, their presence requires explanation.

(*d*) Left atrial hypertrophy (P mitrale). Evidence of left atrial hypertrophy is present not only in mitral valve disease, but also in patients with left ventricular disease, in whom diastolic abnormalities cause increased resistance to filling. Unlike the other cardiographic abnormalities, evidence of left atrial hypertrophy may vary with the clinical state of the patient.

3. Systolic time intervals See page 13.58.

4. Mechanocardiography See page 13.54.

5. Echocardiography See page 13.34.

6. Nuclear methods See page 13.41.

7. Cardiac catheterization and angiography See page 13.49.

8. Computerized tomographic scanning and magnetic resonance imaging See pages 13.47 and 13.60.

Prognosis of ventricular disease

The prognosis of severe ventricular disease is poor. In the Framingham study, patients pronounced to be in heart failure had an overall survival of 50 per cent at one year, and 30 per cent at two years. That of patients with left ventricular dilation and symptoms corresponding to Grade III or IV of the NYHA is even worse, particularly when due to coronary artery disease. Here, the one-year survival is 35 per cent compared with 65 per cent in those with congestive cardiomyopathy. Once clinical evidence of heart failure has developed, prognosis correlates closely with the severity of indices of left ventricular disease including reduced ejection fraction, high levels of circulating catecholamines, increased peripheral resistance, and low values of stroke work. Death is either from progressive haemodynamic deterioration or occurs suddenly, presumably due to an arrhythmia, in approximately equal numbers of patients.

The same relation between ventricular disease and prognosis can be demonstrated in more homogeneous groups of patients. In those with ischaemic heart disease, ejection fraction is a powerful determinant of survival, regardless of the number of coronary arteries involved or whether or not coronary artery surgery has been performed. In such patients evidence of left ventricular hypertrophy, or increased ventricular ectopic activity, even a single ventricular ectopic beat on a routine ECG, are also independent markers of poor prognosis. In patients with valvular heart disease, both pre-operative and postoperative mortality is affected by the presence of cardiomegaly on chest X-ray, reduced ejection fraction, and the ventricular ectopic beats on ECG. In those with aortic stenosis, the major factors determining poor postoperative survival are left ventricular cavity enlargement, particularly at end-systole, and myocardial fibrosis. The extent of right ventricular disease is the main factor limiting survival after surgery for many types of congenital heart disease. Premature death in association with ventricular disease is thus a major mechanism for the increased mortality associated with cardiovascular disease.

Prevention of ventricular disease

Since the prognosis of ventricular disease is so poor, and since its treatment is so unsatisfactory once it has become clinically apparent, prevention is of major importance. Ventricular disease in a Western population is due mainly to coronary artery disease and hypertension. Methods for the possible prevention of ischaemic heart disease itself are described on page 13.143. Once coronary artery disease has become overt, there are several approaches to reducing the extent of ventricular involvement. In the Beta Blocker Heart Attack Trial (BHAT), there was a reduction in the incidence of myocardial infarction as well as an improvement in survival in treated cases. Both the VA and the Canadian Cooperative Trials of aspirin administration in unstable angina have demonstrated improved survival to be accompanied by reduced incidence of infarction. In the European Coronary Artery Surgery Study, myocardial infarct size in patients with triple vessel disease treated surgically was less than in comparable patients treated medically. Limitation of infarct size at the time of acute myocardial infarction either by pharmacological methods designed to reduce myocardial oxygen requirements or by thrombolysis or acute revascularization would also seem to have the potential of limiting ventricular damage, although this has still to be proved. Prevention of hypertensive heart disease depends on detection and satisfactory long-term treatment of hypertension, and success in this is reflected in the progressive reduction in deaths certified from this cause over the past 20 years. With acquired valvular lesions, ventricular disease occurs when surgery is delayed, or at the time of operation, when myocardial preservation fails. In spite of progress in these two fields, it is chastening to recall that the 10-year survival after mitral valve replacement is only 50 per cent, whatever the initial indication for surgery, and that the main cause of death in these patients is from the effects of left ventricular disease.

Treatment of ventricular disease

Treatment can be considered either from the point of view of improving the very poor prognosis in many of these patients, or of alleviating symptoms, particularly those causing limitation of exercise tolerance.

Improvement of prognosis

There is still little that can be done to improve prognosis once severe ventricular disease is present. There is no evidence to suggest that vasodilator treatment with nitrates or α-adrenergic blocking agents has any effect on prognosis. Combined data from published trials with the angiotensin-converting enzyme (ACE) inhibitors, captopril and enalapril, have suggested some improve-

ment, but a large, controlled trial is required to prove the point. There is no evidence to suggest that drugs with a positive inotropic effect alter prognosis in any way. Beta-blocker administration after acute myocardial infarction improves prognosis over a period of at least two years, both by preventing reinfarction and by reducing the incidence of sudden death. The same may apply to aspirin administration to patients with unstable angina. In those with established angina and either left main stem or triple vessel coronary artery disease, surgical treatment appears to be associated with significantly improved survival compared with medical treatment. Patients with hypertrophic cardiomyopathy in whom ventricular trachycardia has been documented on ambulatory ECG monitoring are at increased risk of sudden death. A recent uncontrolled trial has suggested some reduction with amiodarone administration in doses adequate to suppress episodes of ventricular tachycardia. In spite of progress made in limited areas, the impact of current treatment on the very high mortality of ventricular disease has been small.

Symptomatic treatment of ventricular disease

Specific drugs used in the symptomatic treatment of patients with ventricular disease are described in detail in separate chapters. Nevertheless, there are a number of general principles to be borne in mind in the management of such patients.

1. It is essential than no surgically correctable lesion be overlooked. Such lesions are usually obvious, but on occasion, their clinical manifestations are atypical or silent altogether. This is particularly the case when they co-exist with severe ventricular disease. Well-known examples include silent mitral stenosis, severe calcific aortic stenosis with left ventricular cavity dilation, or acute aortic regurgitation. Malfunction of valvular prostheses, particularly mitral, may also present as severe left ventricular disease with intractible pulmonary oedema. In paraprosthetic mitral regurgitation a systolic murmur is characteristically absent. Such patients, not surprisingly, respond poorly to medical treatment. The appearance of 'heart failure' in a patient with a prosthetic valve should always be taken as evidence of a potential surgical complication. Such patients should be transferred as soon as possible to a cardiac surgical centre where appropriate investigations can be undertaken. After a myocardial infarction, septal rupture causing an acquired VSD may be associated with soft systolic murmur that is similar to that of functional mitral regurgitation. The clinical manifestations of left ventricular aneurysm may be atypical, and its presence should also be questioned in any patient with coronary artery disease and significant pulmonary congestion or cardiac enlargement on chest X-ray. On the right side of the heart, silent pulmonary stenosis in adults may present as isolated right ventricular disease. A silent left-sided lesion such as mitral stenosis may present as severe primary pulmonary hypertension.

2. In many patients, the manifestations of heart disease are aggravated by correctable causes, which should be recognized and eliminated when possible. These are often associated with increased demands on the circulation, and include occult infection, severe anaemia or even pregnancy. In elderly patients, the possibility of thyrotoxicosis should be considered, particularly if atrial fibrillation is present. In a patient with severe heart disease, excessive mental or physical activity may lead to apparent resistance to treatment. In a young patient, vigorous athletic training in the presence of apparently mild heart disease may lead to very significant enlargement of ventricular cavity size. External agents should also be considered, the commonest in western society being alcohol. Treatment with β-adrenergic blocking drugs may also cause clinical deterioration. This is commonest in patients with valvular heart disease, particularly those with atrial fibrillation. In view of the severity of left ventricular disease present in many cases in whom they are administered to treat angina, evidence of deterioration is surprisingly rare. If incipient pulmonary oedema is present, β-blocking drugs, particularly non-selective

ones, may lead to the appearance of breathlessness by aggravating bronchoconstriction.

3. An attempt should be made to identify the type of left ventricular disease present, since this is likely to modify the treatment given. This is usually possible on the basis of the clinical features and non-invasive investigations such as echocardiography or nuclear methods. Thus, in left ventricular hypertrophy, when cavity size and systolic function are normal, and pulmonary congestion due to impaired diastolic function, administration of drugs with a positive inotropic or vasodilator action is likely to be ineffective or dangerous. Additional useful information may be obtained from bedside cardiac catheterization, allowing cardiac output and peripheral resistance to be estimated, and pulmonary wedge pressure, and hence left ventricular end-diastolic pressure to be assessed.

4. The effects of abnormal physiology present in heart disease should be allowed for, both in selecting appropriate drugs, and in following their effects. Unfortunately, many of the clinical pharmacological studies on cardiac drugs have been performed in normal volunteers, where their actions may be quite different from those in disease. A good example is the action of glucagon, an agent proposed for the treatment of patients with severe heart disease. This drug indeed increases cardiac output in normal subjects and those with mild heart disease, but is almost without effect in those in whom ventricular disease is severe. Conversely, the reduction in left ventricular filling pressure caused by nitroprusside causes a striking fall in left ventricular stroke work in normal subjects, but this does not occur in those in whom resting filling pressure and peripheral resistance are high.

Specific measures

1. Reduction in the work of the heart In mild cases this can be brought about by a simple reduction in physical activity, and in more severe ones by admission to hospital for a period of bed-rest. Simple rest frequently induces a diuresis in the absence of any other treatment. If the patient is likely to remain bed-ridden for a significant period, or if there is severe oedema, an anticoagulant such as warfarin or subcutaneous heparin should be given as a prophylactic against peripheral venous thrombosis. One of the main values of vasodilators is to reduce the work of the left ventricle by lowering peripheral arterial resistance, particularly if it is significantly raised initially. Detailed use of these drugs is described on page 13.105. Although acute haemodynamics may improve, administration of nitrates, or α-adrenergic blocking agents over periods of more than a few weeks has not been shown to lead to any sustained improvement in exercise tolerance. The effects of ACE inhibitors are more prolonged.

In very severe cases in whom there is a possibility of substantial improvement either following surgery or by the natural history of the disease, intra-aortic balloon counterpulsation may be considered. This is a specialized procedure, which should be performed in a centre with cardiac surgical facilities available. A balloon-tipped catheter is inserted into the femoral artery and advanced to the descending thoracic aorta. Triggered by the ECG, the balloon is rapidly inflated with 20–40 ml of gas at high pressure during diastole, and deflated during systole. This has the effect of increasing aortic diastolic pressure to higher levels than systolic, and so of improving perfusion of the coronary arteries and other peripheral vascular beds. At the same time, resistance to left ventricular ejection is reduced, when the balloon is deflated during systole, so that left ventricular end-diastolic pressure falls, breathlessness is relieved, possibly with an improvement of coronary, and in particular subendocardial blood flow. This technique leads to a modest increase in cardiac output of around 10 per cent, which may be significant in borderline cases. It is also effective in relieving resistant rest angina and in promoting urine flow.

2. Increase in the output of the heart (*a*) Control of heart rate. If cardiac function is severely impaired, maximum cardiac output occurs when heart rate is between 90 and 120 beats/min. A slow

rate can usually be increased pharmacologically, using atropine (0.6–1.2 mg i.v.), or a catecholamine such as isoprenaline by intravenous infusion at a rate of 1–2 μg/min. If pharmacological means are ineffective, a pacemaker should be used. In patients with severe ventricular disease, a 10–15 per cent increase in cardiac output can be achieved by the use of a physiological pacing system, which takes advantage of the effect of atrial systole on ventricular stroke volume (q.v.). If ventricular rate is rapid due to atrial fibrillation, it should be controlled with a digitalis preparation. Sinus tachycardia in such patients is usually physiological; it should not be regarded as a primary object for treatment, but will fall spontaneously as other means become effective.

(*b*) Cardiotonic drugs. Drugs with a positive inotropic effect are frequently used in the treatment of patients with heart disease. There is still no evidence to suggest that long-term administration of any drug in this class improves prognosis or consistently increases exercise tolerance. This applies to digoxin, and also to amrinone, which has an unacceptably high incidence of side-effects. Drugs with a positive inotropic effect would thus seem to be confined to short-term intravenous use in seriously ill patients, in whom there is some prospect of spontaneous improvement in the underlying disease. The extent to which the beneficial effects of catecholamines such as isoprenaline are due to peripheral vasodilator rather than inotropic actions remains uncertain. A not uncommon clinical problem is the treatment of a low cardiac output state in a patient established on therapeutic doses of a β-blocking drug. Although competitive blockade can theoretically be surmounted by very large doses of agonist, this approach is unsatisfactory in practice. A more reliable alternative is to use drugs whose action is independent of adrenergic mechanisms; glucagon (1–2 mg i.v.), followed by aminophylline (250 mg i.v.) and also by atropine (0.6–1.2 mg i.v.) if heart rate is slow. These drugs can be repeated as often as necessary until the β-blocking drug is metabolized.

3. Treatment of fluid retention This is most conveniently done with diuretics, whose use is dealt with in detail elsewhere (see page 13.98). Their availability has rendered all but mild dietary sodium restriction obsolete as a therapeutic measure. Fluid may also be removed mechanically, especially from the pleural cavity by aspiration, often with considerable relief of breathlessness.

4. Treatment of pulmonary congestion This may be approached in a number of ways. A fall in left atrial pressure may follow use of an arterial vasodilator, or in suitable cases, by a drug with positive inotropic action. As left ventricular function improves, functional mitral regurgitation regresses. Vasodilators acting on the venous side of the circulation, especially nitrates, are invaluable in such patients. Their administration often causes a substantial reduction in left atrial pressure with no significant alteration in forward flow. The same effect may be brought about by venesection. In patients with severe left ventricular hypertrophy, β-blocking drugs or calcium antagonist drugs appear to alter diastolic pressure–volume relations and reduce end-diastolic pressure, although the underlying mechanism of action is unknown. Bronchodilators such as salbutamol 2 mg three or four times daily, or an oral aminophylline preparation may be helpful if symptoms due to bronchoconstriction are prominent. These drugs are also useful when taken last thing at night as a prophylactic against nocturnal dyspnoea.

Treatment of acute pulmonary oedema

Pulmonary oedema represents a severe form of cardiac dyspnoea, so that its treatment lies along similar lines. However, it may present as an acute medical emergency if the attack is severe. The patient should be put into the sitting position. The most effective initial treatment is morphine, 10 mg i.m. or i.v. This not only allays anxiety and pain, if present, but is also a valuable vasodilator. Systemic arterial pressure falls and venodilation occurs, so that blood shifts from the thorax to the systemic vascular bed.

A rapidly acting diuretic should be administered, such as frusemide 20–40 mg i.v., unless the patient is already being intensively treated with diuretics. There is evidence to suggest that frusemide may have effects in addition to being a diuretic, since improvement may precede the onset of a diuresis.

If bronchospasm is a major component, i.v. aminophylline 250 mg over 2–3 min should be given. This drug also has a relaxant effect on vascular smooth muscle, a positive inotropic action independent of the sympathetic nervous system, and reduces sodium reabsorption by the proximal tubule, thereby potentiating diuretic action.

If heart rate is rapid due to atrial fibrillation, it should be controlled by digitalis, as described above. This is likely to be particularly effective in patients with mitral valve disease. Ventricular or supraventricular tachycardia should be promptly treated by d.c. shock in a patient with pulmonary oedema. It may be necessary to intubate the patient first in order for this to be done safely. Appropriate prophylaxis should be given to prevent recurrence of the arrhythmia.

Arterial or venous vasodilators are very valuable in treating and preventing acute pulmonary oedema. In some patients, the excessive sympathetic activity associated with pulmonary oedema may cause severe arterial hypertension, when intravenous infusion of nitroprusside may be particularly effective. If there is a history of repeated episodes, oral or sublingual nitrate can be taken by the patient, in order to abort a major attack. The development of vasodilator drugs has rendered the use of manoeuvres such as rotating tourniquets obsolete.

Intermittent positive pressure respiration may be required if it is not possible to control the attack in any other way. It is recommended in particular, for an exhausted patient in whom P_{O_2} remains low, or, in particular, if a systemic acidosis develops, with evidence of poor peripheral perfusion and low urine flow. The mechanism of its action is not clear. It clearly reduces the work of respiration, and reduces intrathoracic blood volume. It allows blood gases and hence acidosis to be corrected, and so gives time for the haemodynamic state of the patient to stabilize.

Heart transplantation

Increasing expertise with heart transplantation (see page 13.115), and the progressive improvement in its long-term results, now means that this approach can be considered earlier in the natural history of potential recipients. The possibility can then be discussed in good time with patients and relatives, and used to best advantage. Patients should be referred while they are still in good general condition, and before the onset of significant pulmonary vascular disease due to chronic left atrial hypertension or multiple pulmonary emboli.

References

Braunwald, E., Ross, J. and Sonnenblick, E. H. (1967). Mechanisms of contraction in the normal and failing heart. *N. Engl. J. Med.* **227**, 1012.

Bruce, R. A. (1977). Exercise testing for evaluation of ventricular function. *N. Engl. J. Med.* **296**, 671–675.

Denolin, H., Krayenbuehl, H. P., Loogen, F. and Reale, A. (1983). The definition of heart failure. *Eur. J. Cardiol.* **4**, 445–448.

Di Banco, R., Shabetai, R. and Silverman, B. D. (1984). Oral amrinone for the treatment of chronic congestive cardiac failure; results of a multicentre randomized double blind placebo-controlled withdrawal study. *J. Am. Coll. Cardiol.* **4**, 855–866.

Franciosa, J. A., Park, M. and Levine, T. B. (1981). Lack of correlation between exercise capacity and indexes of resting left ventricular performance in heart failure. *Am. J. Cardiol.* **47**, 33–39.

——, Wilen, M., Ziesche, S. and Cohn, J. N. (1983). Survival in man with chronic severe left ventricular failure due either to coronary artery disease of idiopathic dilated cardiomyopathy. *Am. J. Cardiol.* **57**, 831–836.

Grossman, W. and McLaurin, L. P. (1976). Diastolic properties of the left ventricle. *Ann. intern. Med.* **84**, 316–326.

Kammel, W. B. and Feinleib, M. (1972). Natural history of angina pectoris in the Framingham study: prognosis and survival. *Am. J. Cardiol.* **29**, 154–160.

Kaplan, M. M. (1980). Liver dysfunction secondary to hepatic dysfunction. *Pract. Cardiol.* **6**, 39–49.

Noble, M. I. M. (1972). Editorial: problems concerning the application of muscle mechanics to the determination of the contractile state of the heart. *Circulation* **45**, 252.

Rees, P. J. and Clarke, T. L. H. (1979). Paroxysmal nocturnal dyspnoea and periodic respiration. *Lancet* **2**, 1315–1318.

Sagawa, K. (1981). Editorial: The end-systolic pressure–volume relation of the ventricle: definition, modifications and clinical use. *Circulation* **63**, 1223–1227.

Smith, W. (1985). Epidemiology of congestive heart failure. *Am. J. Cardiol.* **55**, A3–8.

Yu, P. N. (1981). Pulmonary edema. *Circulation* **63**, 724.

Treatment

DIURETICS

J. G. G. LEDINGHAM

Why treat cardiac oedema?

The need to treat pulmonary oedema urgently needs no discussion, but there is a place for circumspection in deciding how hard to press treatment in patients retaining fluid other than in the lungs. Massive oedema is unsightly and can be physically inconvenient and sometimes incapacitating. But on occasions physicians substitute a low cardiac output, a feeling of physical exhaustion, and an electrolyte disturbance with renal failure for a relatively mild degree of oedema by overenthusiastic treatment with potent diuretic drugs. There are too cardiac conditions in which removal of fluid from the circulation is quite inappropriate. These include constrictive pericarditis, pericardial tamponade, right ventricular infarction, pulmonary embolism or mitral valve disease when cardiac output is severely compromised.

Conservative measures

The value of bed rest and moderate sodium restriction in the treatment of all forms of fluid retention has been known for years, but these simple approaches have been neglected more than they should have been since the advent of potent diuretics, effective given by mouth. Periods of horizontal rest for an hour or two on working days and for longer periods at weekends may contribute to management surprisingly effectively and are a more physiological way of treating mild cardiac oedema than the use of drugs to inhibit sodium reabsorption in renal tubules. Strict sodium restriction to an intake of less than 20–30 mmol/day is an unpleasant treatment found impractical or unacceptable by most patients, but more modest restriction may reduce the need for drugs and thus reduce risks of toxicity. It is surprising how often house staff report a patient's oedema to be uncontrolled by diuretics when 24-hour urinary sodium excretion exceeds 100 mmol, implying an intake well in excess of that quite generous figure.

Diuretics

When fluid retention is mild but requires relief, one of the benzothiadiazine agents should be the first choice. There has been a tendency since the more potent 'loop' agents became available to prescribe these potentially dangerous drugs unnecessarily. The hazards of extreme hypovolaemia, of aggravating any tendency to urinary retention, and of serious electrolyte disturbance are less with thiazides, agents which inhibit sodium transport in an area just proximal to the distal convoluted tubule. Inhibition at this site, where sodium is reabsorbed without water impairs maximal urinary dilution, but excretion of free water is not completely inhibited since the diluting site in the ascending limb of Henle's loop is not affected. In maximal effective dose the thiazide diuretics are capable of inhibiting reabsorption of some 5 per cent of the filtered load of sodium, quite enough for many patients with cardiac oedema. The dose–response curve of thiazides is a flat one with little difference between small and large doses. Most thiazides affect urinary salt excretion for some 8–10 hours but some, like chlorthalidone, last for as long as 24–36 hours.

Potassium supplements

Because the site of action lies proximal to the area in the distal nephron where potassium is secreted, all thiazide drugs tend to increase urinary potassium losses to a degree dependent on tubular flow rate, the delivery of sodium to the distal nephron, and the extent of secondary aldosteronism present. Chloruresis and potassium loss both tend to produce alkalosis of the extracellular fluid, which, when present, further inhibits renal potassium conservation (see page 18.31). The rate at which potassium may be lost during treatment by thiazide diuretics is, therefore, variable and the need to provide supplements or not equally variable. Arguments as to whether or not they are required are somewhat futile since so much depends on the response of the individual patient and the features of the underlying disease. There is no doubt that severe potassium depletion can be provoked by thiazide treatment, especially perhaps with chlorthalidone, and that such depletion can potentiate cardiotoxic effects of digitalis analogues. When in doubt the wisest course is to prescribe supplements, or to combine treatment with one of the distally acting agents which promote potassium retention. Enteric coated potassium preparations can cause jejunal ulceration and stricture formation. Potassium given as bicarbonate aggravates alkalosis, inhibits renal potassium conservation, and is much less effective than chloride preparations in correcting deficits. Slow-K (Ciba) is probably the preparation of choice, but much can be achieved by advising a high intake of foods naturally rich in potassium content.

Preparations providing thiazide diuretics and potassium in the same tablet are widely available and advertized. They are often prescribed but the amount of potassium incorporated may not suffice to prevent hypokalaemia; separate preparations of diuretic and supplement are preferable since they allow precision and flexibility.

Potassium-sparing diuretics

Spironolactone, amiloride, and triamterene all act on the distal nephron at the site of potassium secretion, promoting a modest increase in sodium excretion but a very significant inhibition of potassium secretion. Spironolactone is a true competitive antagonist of aldosterone, having no effect after bilateral adrenalectomy. Effective doses range from 25 to 400 mg daily and depend on the degree of aldosteronism present. Spironolactone treatment stimulates increased formation of renin, angiotensin, and aldosterone so that dose requirements may increase. Gastrointestinal side-effects of nausea and abdominal discomfort complicate higher dosage and prolonged use of the drug is remarkably commonly complicated by the development of gynaecomastia which may be unilateral or bilateral. The onset of action of spironolactone is delayed for 24–72 hours.

Triamterene and amiloride also act on the distal nephron to inhibit sodium reabsorption and potassium secretion, but are not true antagonists of aldosterone. Triamterene is rather less potent and less well tolerated by patients than amiloride which is perhaps the best of the three distally acting agents for general use. Just as effective in conserving potassium and excreting sodium as spironolactone, it is free of the unpleasant side-effect of gynaecomastia. Effective doses range between 5 and 20 mg daily.

The addition of spironolactone, triamterene, or amiloride to thiazides or 'loop' agents augments sodium excretion and reduces potassium loss, but to a variable degree between patients depending on haemodynamic factors and the activity of the renin–aldosterone system. It is *not* safe to assume potassium homeostasis without regular checks of plasma levels.

Given alone, triamterene, spironolactone, or amiloride are of little value except perhaps in the oedema of liver cirrhosis in which natriuresis needs to be more than usually slowly induced, and

hyperaldosteronism plays a much larger part in aetiology than it does in cardiac or nephrotic oedema.

More resistant oedema

When patients have been shown to be unresponsive to thiazide diuretics combined with amiloride, spironolactone or triamterene, one of the 'loop' agents should be introduced. Frusemide (furosemide), ethacrynic acid, bumetanide, and piretanide all act principally by inhibiting sodium chloride co-transport in the ascending limb of Henle's loop. This is the site in the nephron at which the capacity for sodium reabsorption is difficult to saturate and which is critical to the mechanisms of urinary concentration and dilution. Dilution is achieved here and more distally in the reabsorption of sodium without water. Hypertonicity of the medulla, on which urinary concentration depends, is greatly reduced by inhibition of electrolyte transport at this site. Although they differ structurally, and there is some evidence of additional sites of action in the proximal nephron and perhaps in the second diluting site for frusemide, there is little to choose between ethacrynic acid, bumetanide, and frusemide clinically. All are extremely potent, capable of blocking reabsorption of 25–40 per cent of the sodium filtered at the glomerulus in experimental conditions. All are chloruretic agents and promote a considerably greater excretion of chloride than of sodium. Because they act at a point proximal to the site of potassium secretion which is dependent on tubular flow rates and the rate of delivery of sodium, all tend to increase urinary potassium losses in an amount dependent on the extent of secondary aldosteronism present and the degree of alkalosis induced by chloride deficiency and pre-existing potassium depletion.

These 'loop' diuretic agents are potentially dangerous drugs particularly in the elderly. Their remarkable potency results in a very real risk of extreme hypovolaemia, postural hypotension, circulatory failure, and uraemia when they are given without proper supervision, particularly to patients whose disease would be well controlled by less drastic agents. Weight loss from diuretic therapy should be achieved ideally at a rate not exceeding 1–2 kg/day. Unlike the thiazides which rarely reduce plasma potassium levels below 3 mmol/l, 'loop' agents can reduce potassium to dangerously low levels and a remarkable degree of hypochloraemic hypokalaemic alkalosis can arise over a period of treatment as short as 48 hours.

These caveats apart, the value of 'loop' diuretics properly prescribed and supervized has constituted a major advance in the care of patients whose oedema cannot be controlled by less powerful drugs. Given by mouth, all begin to induce natriuresis and diuresis within one to two hours and have a peak effect at about four hours which is complete at about six hours. The dose response range for oral frusemide extends from 20 to 400 mg or more, of ethacrynic acid from 50 to 200 mg, and for bumetanide from 1 to 8 mg. The relatively short period of action can be used to tailor treatment for individual patients. When the diuretic response is good, patients can take a single dose at a time of day which suits their domestic and work commitments. When oedema is more resistant, divided dosage is more logical and more effective than giving a larger single dose. These diuretics are commonly prescribed in the early morning and at or near noon. A further dose can be given in difficult cases as late as 1700 or 1800 hours, when its effect will be complete before bedtime, and sleep should be undisturbed.

As in the case of thiazides, the natriuretic effects of loop diuretics can be considerably augmented by the addition of spironolactone, amiloride or triamterene. Potassium losses are reduced, but severe hypokalaemia can still complicate combined therapy of this sort. Potassium levels must be checked regularly and supplements given according to need. Again, chloride preparations are mandatory since alkalosis is almost invariable when hypokalaemia complicates treatment by frusemide, bumetanide or ethacrynic acid.

Resistant oedema

A small minority of patients exists in whom sodium restriction, bed rest, and combinations of loop agents, thiazides, and potassium-conserving distal acting drugs fail to control fluid retention. Metolazone may be valuable here especially in patients with renal failure.

The use of drugs which reduce cardiac afterload, of which the angiotensin converting enzyme inhibitors (ACE inhibitors) are the most effective (see page 13.105), may increase cardiac output, renal perfusion, and thus initiate diuresis which once begun tends to continue. Some patients are resistant even to these measures and in extreme cases ACE inhibition may result in an acute fall in glomerular filtration rate, oliguria, and uraemia secondary to inhibition of angiotensin-mediated efferent arteriolar tone. Withdrawal of the ACE inhibitor in such cases restores renal function. In these in whom a feeble cardiac output and poor tissue perfusion is the problem, blood urea and creatinine concentrations will have risen, and there is little or nothing to be gained by any increases in pharmacological onslaught.

In others these warning signs may not be present and in them the possibility of an inadequate absorption of oral diuretics must be considered. Frusemide can be given by intramuscular injection, but more effective and comfortable for the patient is the slow infusion of the drug intravenously by a low volume pump delivering the total 24–hour dose in 100 ml or less of 5 per cent dextrose. Remarkably low doses may be effective given in this way; for instance 40 to 80 mg may induce diuresis when 500 mg given by mouth is ineffective. Patients resistant even to this manoeuvre are rare indeed, and it is doubtful whether the underlying cardiac disorder is worthy of more drastic measures of support, but there are advocates of the use of peritoneal dialysis or haemodiafiltration. Good indications for such an approach must be vanishingly rare.

Complications

Prolonged treatment with loop agents or thiazides induce hyperuricaemia and may cause gout. Hyperglycaemia can be provoked by thiazides particularly and the risk appears greatest in the elderly. The modest hyperlipidaemia associated with thiazides may not be sustained during prolonged treatment, and is of doubtful significance. Hypercalcaemia is increasingly recognized as a consequence of thiazide treatment and should be considered as a possibility before full investigation is begun to seek other causes. Thiazides are also associated with hypersensitivity reactions including photosensitive skin rashes, thrombocytopenia, and acute interstitial nephritis. Hypokalaemia and alkalosis are easily recognized and treated but hyponatraemia presents more of a problem, and hypomagnesaemia has until recently been insufficiently recognized as a problem.

Diuretic-induced hyponatraemia

Cardiac oedema treated by combinations of potent drugs is often accompanied by hyponatraemia of greater or lesser degree. It is, however, never, or almost never, due to sodium depletion, but almost always due to relative water overload.

Mechanism

A number of factors contribute. Increased tubular reabsorption of sodium probably occurs in the proximal tubule in cardiac insufficiency. As a result less sodium and chloride are delivered to the diluting sites where chloride and sodium are reabsorbed without water in the ascending limb of Henle's loop and in the early distal nephron. The capacity of the kidney to excrete free water is thereby decreased. It is decreased further by the use of diuretics which inhibit electrolyte transport at these diluting sites; these include all thiazides, frusemide, ethacrynic acid, bumetanide, and xipamide; indeed all agents except acetazolamide and the relatively weak distal tubular agents. There is good reason therefore why the kidney's ability to excrete a water load is gravely reduced. In addition, patients with heart failure are thirsty. Whether thirst is induced by volume-receptor neurological mechanisms or by increased plasma concentrations of angiotensin II induced by diur-

etics is not known; thirst is clearly inappropriate to both volume and osmotic status. Finally plasma levels of antidiuretic hormone are increased in severe heart failure and this may add its contribution to reduced excretion of free water.

Management

Mild hyponatraemia probably needs no treatment although it can be taken as a sign which indicates a guarded prognosis. More severe hyponatraemia accompanied by constitutional symptoms may require treatment. If diuretic treatment cannot be reduced, the addition of captopril or enalapril may, by improving cardiac performance and renal perfusion, restore normal levels of plasma sodium. Water restriction has been advocated but is rarely tolerated by patients and is not particularly effective.

Demethylchlortetracycline, a drug which in doses of 600–1200 mg induces a degree of nephrogenic diabetes insipidus, has been tried but without great benefit.

Reports that diuretic-associated hyponatraemia may reflect a shift of sodium into cells by inhibition of membrane Na/K ATPase by magnesium depletion draw attention to the importance of magnesium homeostasis in patients treated chronically with diuretics.

Magnesium depletion

Some 15–30 per cent of filtered magnesium is normally reabsorbed in the proximal renal tubule, 50–60 per cent in the ascending limb of Henle's loop, and 5 per cent or so in the distal nephron. Both 'loop' diuretics and thiazides (particularly the former) may on occasion provoke magnesium depletion, especially in subjects whose dietary intake is low, in soft water areas, among alcoholics, and in malabsorptive states. Symptoms and signs are rare but may include depression, muscle weakness, refractory hypokalaemia hypertension, and ventricular or atrial dysrhythmias resistant to treatment. The classical features of magnesium depletion, paraesthesiae, cramp, and tetany associated with accompanying hypocalcaemia are probably never the result of diuretic treatment alone.

In the context of cardiac disease the risks of hypomagnesaemia include supraventricular and ventricular arrhythmias including ventricular tachycardia and fibrillation.

Treatment with magnesium glycerophosphate is quite well accepted in doses of 3–6 g daily providing 12 to 24 hours of magnesium. Other possible preparations include magnesium hydroxide providing approximately 20 mmol in 15 ml but at the risk of diarrhoea and less efficient absorption.

Distal tubular agents (amiloride, spironolactone or triamterene) do not increase urinary magnesium.

Acute pulmonary oedema

Apart from morphine, the most effective agents in the immediate relief of dyspnoea in pulmonary oedema are intravenous injections of 'loop' diuretics, frusemide, ethacrynic acid or bumetanide. There is probably little to choose between the three, but there is most experience with frusemide. Given in a dose of 20–40 mg there is an increase in urinary salt and water excretion within 2 min which reaches a peak at 5–10 min and is complete within 25–35 min unless there is renal retention of the drug secondary to gross impairment of renal function. There is some evidence that the beneficial effects can be contributed to not only by natriuresis and diuresis, but also by falls in left atrial pressure which precede renal effects and may be attributable to dilation of venous capacitance vessels. If ethacrynic acid is given intravenously (50–100 mg) care must be taken to avoid extravasation of the drug into the tissues where it is highly irritant and painful.

References

Davies, D. L. and Wilson, G. M. (1975). Diuretics: mechanisms of action and clinical application. *Drugs* **9**, 176–226.
Dzau, V. J. and Hollenberg, N. K. (1984). Renal response to captopril in severe heart failure; role of furosemide in natriuresis and reversal of hyponatraemia. *Ann. intern. Med.* **100**, 777–782.

Editorial (1986). Atrial natriuretic peptide. *Lancet* **ii**, 371–372.

Seely, J. F. and Dirks, J. H. (1977). Site of action of diuretic drugs. *Kidney Int.* **11**, 1–8.

Sutton, R. A. L. and Dirks, J. H. (1981). Renal handling of calcium, phosphate and magnesium. In *The kidney* (eds B. M. Brenner and F. C. Rector), pp. 551–618. W. B. Saunders, Philadelphia.

Swales, J. D. (1982). Magnesium deficiency and diuretics. *Br. Med. J.* **285**, 1377–1378.

DIGITALIS

J. K. ARONSON

Cardiac glycosides of one sort or another have been used by physicians for thousands of years at various times for the treatment of such conditions as wounds, epilepsy, scrofula, and pulmonary tuberculosis. They were shown to be of value in the treatment of dropsies by William Withering about 200 years ago, and in the treatment of fast atrial fibrillation by Sir James Mackenzie at the beginning of this century.

Nomenclature

Plants of the *Digitalis* species (e.g. *Digitalis purpurea*, *Digitalis lanata*) contain cardiac glycosides, such as digoxin and digitoxin, which are known collectively as 'digitalis'. Other plants contain cardiac glycosides which are chemically related to the digitalis glycosides, and, although it is not strictly correct to do so, by convention these are also included under the heading 'digitalis'. This convention is adopted here and the terms 'digitalis' and 'cardiac glycosides' are used interchangeably.

Clinical pharmacology of digitalis

Pharmaceutical formulations

Digitalis may be given either orally or parenterally. In general, parenteral administration offers no advantage over oral, since glycosides taken by mouth are well and rapidly absorbed. Intravenous administration should be used only in cases of extreme urgency, or when the patient cannot for some reason take oral treatment. The intramuscular route is generally better avoided – absorption is unreliable and the injection may be painful.

Oral formulations

The British National Formulary lists the following oral formulations of digitalis:

Digoxin: tablets (62.5, 125, and 250 μg) and elixir (50 μg/ml)
Digitoxin: tablets (100 μg) and elixir (1 mg/ml)
Lanatoside C: tablets (250 μg)
Medigoxin (beta-methyldigoxin): tablets (100 μg)

Of these, digoxin is the most commonly used, and there are no good reasons to prefer any of the others. Other cardiac glycosides are to be found in other national pharmacopoeias and formularies (e.g. proscillaridin, k-strophanthin, peruvoside), but none has any advantage over digoxin.

Parenteral formulations

The British National Formulary lists the following parenteral formulations:

Digoxin: 250 μg/ml
Deslanoside: 200 μg/ml
Medigoxin: 100 μg/ml
Ouabain: 250 μg/ml

Of these digoxin and ouabain are to be preferred, ouabain having a faster onset and a shorter duration of action.

Pharmacokinetics

The important pharmacokinetic properties of the major cardiac glycosides are listed in Table 1.

Table 1 Important pharmacokinetic properties of the major cardiac glycosides

	Digoxin	Digitoxin	Quabain
Absorption (%)	66 (tablets) 80 (elixir) >90 (elixir in capsules)	>90	<5
Plasma protein binding (%)	25	96	5
Apparent volume of distribution (l/kg)	7.0	0.5	20
Total body clearance (ml/min)	140	3	800
Renal excretion (%)	85	20	50
Hepatic elimination (%)	15	80	50
Biliary excretion (%)	8	20	30
Half-life (normal renal function)	40 h	7 days	20 h
(functionally anephric)	96 h	7 days	60 h

Absorption

Cardiac glycosides are rapidly absorbed after oral administration. Digitoxin is almost completely absorbed, but the extent of absorption of digoxin is dependent on the formulation used: from tablets it is about 66 per cent, from elixir about 80 per cent, and from encapsulated elixir over 90 per cent. There was at one time great variability in the absorption of digoxin from the tablet formulations of different manufacturers, and even between different batches of the same manufacturer. However, because of pharmacopoeial standards for the preparation of tablets, such variability should no longer be a problem. Medigoxin is somewhat better absorbed than digoxin, but early reports that it was more than 90 per cent absorbed were overestimates and the correct figure is about 70–80 per cent. Lanatoside C is itself poorly absorbed, but is partly metabolized to digoxin in the gut; thus the amount of active glycoside entering the circulation after an oral dose of lanatoside C is less than that after an equal dose of digoxin. Ouabain is very poorly absorbed and must therefore be given parenterally.

Distribution

The cardiac glycosides are widely distributed to all the tissues of the body except fat, and therefore have a high apparent volume of distribution of *non-protein-bound* drug in the plasma. However, digitoxin is extensively bound to plasma proteins and that limits the distribution of *total* drug from the circulation into the tissues. The apparent volume of distribution of digoxin is reduced in severe renal failure, and this results in lower loading dose requirements.

Metabolism and excretion

Digitoxin is extensively metabolized to active and inactive glycosides, and this is the major factor contributing to the variability in response. It is excreted to some extent in the bile and subject to enterohepatic recirculation, which can be interrupted by resins such as cholestyramine and colestipol, and by activated charcoal. These agents can therefore be used in the treatment of digitoxin toxicity or self-poisoning.

In contrast, digoxin is 80–90 per cent excreted unchanged via the kidneys in the majority of patients. It is filtered and subject to both passive reabsorption and active secretion. These last two processes on average balance each other, and digoxin renal clearance is therefore approximately equal to creatinine clearance and varies linearly with it. In about 10 per cent of patients, however, digoxin is subject to up to 50 per cent metabolism, probably by gut bacteria before absorption, and this may form the basis of a drug interaction (see below).

Because of its high protein binding and enterohepatic recirculation the half-life of digitoxin is long, about 7 days. It is generally unaffected by renal function, except in the nephrotic syndrome, when loss of protein-bound drug, because of albuminuria, may shorten the half-life to about 5 days. The half-life of digoxin is about 40 hours, and is prolonged in renal failure, being about 96 hours in functionally anephric patients.

The half-life of ouabain is about 20 hours and, since it is 50 per cent excreted unchanged via the kidneys, its half-life is prolonged in renal failure to about 60 hours.

Pharmacodynamics: the relationship to the therapeutic effect

The pharmacological effects of digitalis can be considered at a variety of levels beginning with its effects at the molecular level and progressing to its effects on the whole patient.

At the *molecular* level digitalis has at least three different pharmacological effects. It inhibits the sodium transport enzyme, sodium–potassium adenosine triphosphatase (Na/K ATPase); this is directly responsible for the electrophysiological effects, i.e. the slowing of the heart rate and the arrhythmogenic effects in toxicity. It is also probably indirectly responsible for the positive inotropic effect on the myocardium, via secondary changes in the intracellular disposition of calcium. At very low concentrations digitalis *stimulates* the Na/K ATPase, and in isolation that effect is associated with a small *negative* inotropic effect which is probably of no clinical significance. At similarly low concentrations it may also have a direct effect on the disposition of calcium in myocardial cells, which might in turn result in a positive inotropic effect, but the clinical relevance of this is not known.

At the *tissue* level these actions have a variety of results depending on the tissue involved. In the SA and AV nodes there is prolongation of slow diastolic repolarization and a reduction in automaticity, with a slowing of conduction; these effects are compounded by the direct action of digitalis in stimulating the vagus nerve and in decreasing the response to sympathetic input.

In atrial and ventricular muscle fibres and Purkinje fibres digitalis decreases total action potential duration and increases automaticity. It also stimulates the formation of delayed after-depolarizations, which may contribute to arrhythmias in toxicity. The positive inotropic effect in these fibres occurs because of an increase in the rate of contractility.

Digitalis increases the contractility of vascular smooth muscle by unknown mechanisms, although perhaps due to changes in intracellular calcium disposition secondary to inhibition of Na/K ATPase. It thus tends to increase arterial pressure slightly, but this is of little or no clinical significance.

The major non-cardiac effects of digitalis are exerted on the central nervous system, but the mechanisms at the molecular level are not known. The adverse effects on the eye, at least those involving colour vision, are probably due to inhibition of Na/K ATPase. Digitalis also has direct effects on the gastrointestinal tract, causing diarrhoea and rarely intestinal ischaemia, the mechanisms of which are not known. All of these effects are detailed below under 'Digitalis toxicity'.

Digitalis has a small diuretic effect on the kidney by virtue of inhibition of Na/K ATPase, but its main diuretic effects are due to an increase in renal blood flow, because of increased cardiac output and perhaps because of decreased sympathetic tone.

Clinical uses of digitalis

Indications
Digitalis is indicated for the treatment of cardiac arrhythmias and cardiac failure.

Cardiac arrhythmias
Digitalis is the treatment of choice for atrial fibrillation with a fast ventricular rate, except in a few circumstances. In patients with hyperthyroidism there is a relative resistance to its effects, probably because of alterations in the activity of the Na/K ATPase, and a beta-adrenoceptor antagonist such as propranolol is preferable. Digitalis is contraindicated in patients with accessory conduction pathways, since it slows conduction through the normal conduc-

tion tissues but not through the accessory pathways, thus enhancing the potential for arrhythmias. There is no evidence that digitalis is effective in preventing *paroxysmal* attacks of atrial fibrillation, and other anti-arrhythmic drugs would be preferred for that purpose.

Digitalis is less effective in the treatment of other supraventricular arrhythmias and other drugs should be used as first-line treatment (e.g. in atrial flutter or supraventricular tachycardia). It is better avoided in patients with the sick sinus syndrome, since it may prolong sinus node recovery time and aggravate sinus bradycardia.

Cardiac failure
The recent debate about the usefulness of digitalis in the treatment of cardiac failure has partly been based on misunderstandings about the different issues involved. Those issues may be clarified by considering several discrete questions:

1. Does digitalis exert a positive inotropic effect on the failing heart? There can be little doubt that it does, both during short-term and long-term treatment. One would predict that digitalis would therefore be of value in the treatment of at least some cases of heart failure in the short term. The question of its *usefulness*, as opposed to its *efficacy*, during long-term treatment is discussed below.

2. Does that positive inotropic effect cause an increase in cardiac output with resolution of heart failure? The answer here depends on the cause of the cardiac failure. Digitalis is most likely to be effective in the short-term treatment of cardiac failure with a dilated heart secondary to ischaemic, mitral valvular, hypertensive, and some forms of congenital heart disease. In other circumstances its efficacy is more doubtful.

It is of little value in patients with chronic cor pulmonale or cardiogenic shock, perhaps because of associated hypoxia and acidosis which increase the likelihood of toxicity without altering the therapeutic response. In hyperthyroidism there may also be a decrease in the toxic:therapeutic ratio, and thus a poor response to digitalis.

The efficacy of digitalis after acute myocardial infarction is controversial, but it may increase myocardial oxygen demand, increase vascular resistance, and increase the risk of serious arrhythmias, and is better avoided.

In hypertrophic obstructive cardiomyopathy digitalis is contraindicated because its positive inotropic effects on the left ventricle exacerbate the obstruction to outflow. It is similarly of little value in constrictive pericarditis or tamponade, and there is conflicting evidence of its value in cardiomyopathies.

3. Is the combination of digitalis and diuretics more beneficial than diuretics alone? There is little evidence on which to base an answer to this question. We lack a conclusive comparative study of modern diuretics and digitalis in the treatment of heart failure. Reasonable practice is to use diuretics first. If there is a good clinical response the addition of digitalis is not likely to benefit the patients, but it can be given if the response to diuretics is less than adequate, with a vasodilator as a third line if necessary. Only in patients whose cardiac failure is associated with fast atrial fibrillation is digitalis used as a first choice.

4. If digitalis has been of benefit in the first place does it continue to be of value in the long term? In patients in whom the cause of cardiac failure persists after initial treatment, and in whom there was good indication for using digitalis in the first place, it was tacitly assumed from at least the beginning of this century until recently that long-term digitalis therapy would be of continuing benefit. That may be so in some, although by no means all, patients with chronic atrial fibrillation, but it is not the case in patients with cardiac failure associated with sinus rhythm.

Careful studies of the clinical effects of withdrawing digitalis after long-term therapy, in patients in stable cardiac failure, and in whom plasma digitalis concentrations suggest that they are taking the drug, show that in about two-thirds of cases no clinical deterioration occurs over the subsequent months or even years after withdrawal. In a further one-quarter, although deterioration may be expected following withdrawal, this is likely to respond to appropriate alterations in diuretic therapy. In only about 10 per cent of cases does it seem that long-term digitalis therapy is required. Even in those cases it is not known whether or not vasodilator therapy would be equally effective. There is no clear-cut way in which those 10 per cent can be identified without a trial of withdrawal, although some have suggested that the presence of a third heart sound is a good predictor.

These clinical observations are independent of other observations on the pharmacological and haemodynamic effects of digitalis, which can be demonstrated to be occurring even in patients in whom long-term digitalis therapy seems not to be required. This, therefore, indicates a clear distinction between a persistence of the pharmacodynamic effects of digitalis on the one hand, and the need for its long-term use on the other, since the former does not necessarily indicate the latter.

Should one, therefore, continue digitalis therapy in the long term in the majority of patients in stable cardiac failure? Since it is not possible readily to predict those who will deteriorate following its withdrawal after long-term therapy one practice is as follows: If the plasma digitalis concentration is below the lower end of the recognized therapeutic range (see below) one can assume that the patient does not need the drug and withdraw it – in only a tiny number of patients will worsening of cardiac failure occur. In other cases I continue therapy unless it appears that the risk of toxicity outweighs the risk of deterioration following withdrawal – this is very much a value judgment, but I would include in this category those in whom renal function is steadily deteriorating, and those who have shown themselves to be poor at maintaining potassium balance. If deterioration occurs after withdrawal in such cases I either increase diuretic dosages or add a vasodilator before considering the re-introduction of digitalis, while recognizing that it is not known whether the risks of the adverse effects of long-term diuretic or vasodilator therapy are preferable to those of digitalis.

Dosages

An outline is given here of a regimen for oral administration of digoxin, since the principles are the same for other cardiac glycosides.

Loading dose

It is advisable to start with a loading dose to reduce the delay in onset of effect, and to observe the effects of what appears to be the correct total body load of drug. A suitable total loading dose is 15 μg/kg lean body weight, given in three divided doses at intervals of six hours. This carries a risk of toxicity of about 5 per cent. If evidence of toxicity is seen before the administration of the second or third doses then the loading dose can be curtailed. In patients with renal failure it is better to start with a loading dose of 12 μg/kg. In either case the loading dose can be augmented up to a total of 20 μg/kg if a satisfactory response is thought not to have occurred, but the risk of toxicity then rises to about 10 per cent.

Maintenance

Following the determination of a satisfactory loading dose, the maintenance dose (usually given once daily) can be calculated on the basis of renal function, as assessed by creatinine clearance, measured or estimated. The quick rule of thumb is:

Creatinine clearance	Maintenance dose
100 ml/min	1/3 of loading dose
50 ml/min	1/4 of loading dose
25 ml/min	1/5 of loading dose
10 ml/min	1/6 of loading dose
0 ml/min	1/7 of loading dose

These dosages are based on observations for the most part on elderly patients, and younger patients may require more. Maintenance dosages of digitalis do not need to be altered for patients on chronic dialysis.

When it is not possible to give a loading dose the maintenance dose is based on an intended total body load of 15 μg/kg and varied depending on renal function (e.g. 5 μg/kg if renal function is normal). Since it takes about four half-lives for the drug to accumulate to a steady state it will take between seven days (normal renal function) and two weeks (functionally anephric state) before the maximum effect is achieved without an initial loading dose.

The same principles apply to intravenous therapy but the above dosages should be reduced by a third, based as they are on the assumption of 66 per cent absorption from tablets. When giving any cardiac glycoside intravenously it is best to infuse it over a period of at least 15 min, to reduce the risk of arrhythmias and hypertension.

The corresponding dosages for digitoxin are as follows: loading dose 10 μg/kg; maintenance dose 1.5 μg/kg. Because of its very long half-life maintenance dose therapy with digitoxin without a loading dose takes about four weeks to achieve a maximum effect. Dosages of digitoxin do not need to be altered in renal failure, but may have to be reduced in patients with severe liver impairment.

Factors influencing dosages

There are several factors which may reduce the requirements of digitalis (Table 2). These are of two types: (a) those which increase the amount in the body for a given dose (pharmacokinetic factors), these differ from glycoside to glycoside, as shown in Table 2A; (b) those which increase the response for a given amount of drug in the body (pharmacodynamic factors), these apply equally to all glycosides (Table 2B). Of the former the most important are renal impairment and drug interactions, and of the latter old age and potassium depletion.

Table 2 Factors which may reduce digitalis dosage requirements

A. *Pharmacokinetic factors (increasing the amount of drug in the body without a change in dose)*
Decreased apparent volume of distribution (affecting loading dose)
    Renal failure (digoxin)
    Hypothyroidism (digoxin, digitoxin, ouabain)
Decreased renal clearance
    Renal failure* (digoxin, ouabain, medigoxin)
    Old age (because of reduced renal function)
    Drugs (digoxin): quinidine
                   verapamil
                   spironolactone
                   amiodarone (?mechanism)
Decreased metabolic clearance
    Antibiotics (digoxin)
    Hepatic impairment (digitoxin, medigoxin)
    Withdrawal of hepatic enzyme inducers (digitoxin)

B. *Pharmacodynamic factors (increasing the sensitivity of the tissues without changing the amount of drug in the body)*
Electrolyte and acid–base disturbances
    Potassium depletion*
    Magnesium depletion
    Hypercalcaemia or intravenous calcium administration
    Acidosis and hypoxia
Cardiac disease
    Chronic cor pulmonale
    Cardiogenic shock
    Myocarditis
    Myocardial infarction
Others
    Old age*
    Hypothyroidism

* These are the most important factors to consider.

Digitalis toxicity

The manifestations of digitalis toxicity may be non-cardiac or cardiac. Virtually all the manifestations of toxicity are non-specific, but the concurrence of an ectopic arrhythmia with some form of heart block is particularly suggestive, as is the occurrence of colour vision abnormalities. The risk of digitalis toxicity is still quite high, being up to 29 per cent in patients being admitted to hospital, and up to 16 per cent in outpatients. Mortality rates vary between 4 and 36 per cent, and may be as high as 50 per cent in patients who present with paroxysmal supraventricular tachycardia with block.

Non-cardiac manifestations

The commonest evidence of digitalis toxicity is anorexia, with or without nausea and vomiting. These effects are caused by the actions of digitalis on the brain. Diarrhoea may also occur, and in the elderly may be the only sign of toxicity. Acute intestinal ischaemia has also been reported rarely.

Toxic effects on the nervous system occur more frequently than is generally recognized, and in severe intoxication can occur in up to 65 per cent of patients. The effects include drowsiness, dizziness, acute confusion, bad dreams, restlessness, nervousness, agitation, and rarely seizures. Acute psychoses and delirium may occur, especially in the elderly. Rarely digitalis may cause trigeminal neuralgia.

The toxic effects on the eyes may result in photophobia and blurred vision, and, more commonly (in up to 15 per cent of patients), disturbances of colour vision. Any colour vision disturbance can occur, but the commonest is yellow vision (xanthopsia).

Cardiac manifestations

The cardiac maanifestations of digitalis toxicity are of three kinds: arrhythmias, heart block, and worsening heart failure.

In his review of 726 cases of digitalis toxicity Chung found that the following arrhythmias were the commonest: ventricular extrasystoles (54 per cent), often coupled (25 per cent), and supraventricular tachycardia (33 per cent). Atrioventricular conduction block was also common (42 per cent), whether first degree (14 per cent), second degree (17 per cent), or complete (11 per cent). However, prolongation of the PR interval can occur without other manifestations of digitalis toxicity, and is not reliable evidence of toxicity. Sinus bradycardia is not common (3.4 per cent), and is of poor specificity. Occasionally digoxin toxicity may cause atrial fibrillation (1.7 per cent) or atrial flutter (1.8 per cent). Worsening of heart failure in another series of 148 cases was thought to be a manifestation of digitalis intoxication in 7.5 per cent of cases.

The use of d.c. shock is associated with an increased risk of digitalis-induced arrhythmias. If d.c. shock is necessary in a digitalized patient it is wise to start with low energies (e.g. 10 J), increasing gradually as required. Ideally, where possible, digitalis should be withdrawn 48 hours before elective cardioversion.

Treatment of digitalis toxicity and self-poisoning

It is usually sufficient in uncomplicated cases of digitalis toxicity to withhold the drug and wait. If there is potassium depletion oral potassium chloride should be given. If there are serious arrhythmias intravenous potassium should be used instead, but only life-threatening arrhythmias should be treated with anti-arrhythmic drugs. For ventricular tachyarrhythmias phenytoin is probably the drug of choice, since, unlike other effective anti-arrhythmic drugs, it increases the rate of conduction through the AV node. However, it does depress ventricular automaticity, and it should not be given if there is second- or third-degree heart block. If phenytoin fails then a beta-adrenoceptor antagonist (such as practolol or propranolol) or lignocaine should be used. If there is heart block a temporary transvenous pacemaker should also be inserted. For sinus bradycardia intravenous atropine may be effective, but a pacemaker may be required. In the case of digitoxin the oral administration of activated charcoal, or of cholestyramine or colestipol, may interrupt its enterohepatic recirculation. Antidigitalis antibodies are now available for the rapid reversal of digitalis intoxication, and provide specific therapy.

For the treatment of self-poisoning in an otherwise healthy individual the same principles apply: restoration of potassium, and the administration of anti-arrhythmic drugs as required. However, in these cases the plasma potassium concentration must be carefully monitored, since it may *increase* as a result of extensive inhibition of the Na/K ATPase, and a rising plasma potassium is a poor prognostic sign indicating the urgent need for antibody treatment. In all cases a temporary pacemaker should be inserted as soon as possible, since heart block is the most common cardiac manifestation of digitalis toxicity in a previously healthy heart.

Drug interactions with cardiac glycosides

Pharmacokinetic interactions

Pharmacokinetic interactions with cardiac glycosides affect different glycosides differently, in contrast to pharmacodynamic interactions, which affect all glycosides in the same way.

Absorption

The interruption of the enterohepatic recirculation of digitoxin by activated charcoal and by the resins cholestyramine and colestipol has been mentioned above in the context of the treatment of digitoxin toxicity.

High doses of some antacids decrease the absorption of digoxin when administered concurrently, but these interactions are probably of no clinical significance. Metoclopramide decreases and propantheline increases the systemic availability of digoxin from tablets, but the clinical importance of these interactions is unclear.

Distribution

Quinidine decreases the apparent volume of distribution of digoxin, but this is less important than its effect on the renal excretion of digoxin (see below).

Metabolism

The metabolism of digitoxin by hepatic microsomal enzymes can be induced by drugs such as phenobarbitone, phenytoin, and rifampicin, thus increasing digitoxin dosage requirements.

In the 10 per cent of patients in whom there is extensive metabolism of digoxin by bacteria in the gut before absorption the administration of broad-spectrum antibiotics may reduce the systemic availability of digoxin; the clinical importance of this interaction has not been established.

Renal excretion

The tubular secretion of digoxin is decreased by quinidine (50 per cent), verapamil (40 per cent), and spironolactone (25 per cent), and this leads to reduced dosage requirements of digoxin. Vasodilators may increase digoxin renal excretion by increasing renal blood flow, but the effects, if any, of such interactions on digoxin dosage requirements have not been quantified.

Mechanism unknown

Amiodarone increases plasma digoxin concentrations by an unknown mechanism. It is wise, therefore, to reduce digoxin dosages when amiodarone is also used.

Pharmacodynamic interactions

Drugs which deplete potassium stores will indirectly enhance the actions of cardiac glycosides, without a change in glycoside dose. Of these the most important are diuretics, but other drugs which may be implicated include corticosteroids, amphotericin, and carbenoxolone. A change in potassium disposition may underlie the reported adverse interaction of digitalis with succinylcholine.

Because calcium enchances the actions of digitalis there is an increased risk of cardiac arrhythmias if calcium salts are given intravenously to patients already taking digitalis. This is also thought to be the basis of the reported adverse interaction of digitalis with edrophonium.

Drugs which have pharmacodynamic effects on the heart similar or opposed to those of digitalis will alter the actions of digitalis correspondingly. For example, digitalis enhances left ventricular contractility in patients being given beta-adrenoceptor antagonists, and may be useful in preventing heart failure in those circumstances. There are anecdotal reports of an interaction of digitalis with reserpine, which may be related to alterations in the sympathetic innervation of the heart.

Plasma digitalis concentration measurements

Sensitive radioimmunoassay and enzyme immunoassay techniques are widely available for the measurement of plasma concentrations of digitoxin and of digoxin and related glycosides (e.g. medigoxin), and may be used for four reasons.

1. Monitoring therapy

It is recognized that there is a range of plasma concentrations which is usually associated with a therapeutic response, below which a therapeutic response is unlikely, and above which there is an increased risk of toxicity. For digoxin that range is 0.8–2.0 ng/ml (1.0–2.6 nmol/l) and for digitoxin 20–30 ng/ml (26–39 nmol/l).

It is not usually necessary to check the plasma digitalis concentration during the early stages of therapy. However, if the clinical response is inadequate the finding of a low concentration may help to guide increases in dose, while the use of an alternative treatment is supported by a poor response despite 'adequate' plasma concentrations. During long-term therapy measurement may also be helpful in guiding changes in dosage if renal function starts to deteriorate or if drugs which alter digitalis pharmacokinetics are introduced.

2. Diagnosing digitalis toxicity

If there is a clinical suspicion of digitalis toxicity, a plasma concentration above the recognized therapeutic range tends to confirm it, but toxicity may occur even when plasma concentrations are within the therapeutic range if there is increased sensitivity to digitalis because of any of the factors listed in Table 2B. Of these the most important is potassium depletion, in the presence of which the plasma digitalis concentration cannot be interpreted easily. For this reason the plasma potassium concentration should always be measured before a request for measurement of the plasma digitalis concentration. If there is evidence of potassium depletion digitalis should be withheld until potassium balance is restored.

3. Assessing compliance

The commonest reason for a plasma digitalis concentration below the recognized therapeutic range is poor compliance. But it can also result from pharmacokinetic problems such as impaired absorption or reduced systemic availability, or increased metabolism (e.g. in drug interactions).

4. Determining long-term requirements

The use of the plasma digitalis concentration measurement in determining the need for long-term digitalis therapy is mentioned above under *Clinical uses of digitalis*.

References

Aronson, J. K. (1980). Clinical pharmacokinetics of digoxin. *Clin. Pharmacokin.* 5, 137–149.
—— (1980). Cardiac glycosides and drugs used in dysrhythmias. In *Side effects of drugs annual 5* (eds M. N. G. Dukes and J. Elis), pp. 123–130. Excerpta Medica, Amsterdam.
—— (1983). Clinical pharmacokinetics of cardiac glycosides in patients with renal dysfunction. *Clin. Pharmacokin.* 8, 155–178.
—— (1983). Digitalis intoxication. *Clin. Sci.* 64, 253–258.
—— (1983). Indications for the measurement of plasma digoxin concentrations. *Drugs* 26, 230–242.
—— (1985). An account of the foxglove and its medical uses 1785–1985. (Incorporating a facsimile of William Withering's *An account of the foxglove . . .* , 1785, in an annotated edition.) Oxford University Press, Oxford.
Chung, E. K. (1969). *Digitalis intoxication*. Excerpta Medica, Amsterdam.
Iisalo, E. (1977). Clinical pharmacokinetics of digoxin. *Clin. Pharmacokin.* 2, 1–16.
Noble, D. (1980). Mechanism of action of therapeutic levels of cardiac glycosides. *Cardiovasc. Res.* 14, 495–514.
Perrier, D., Mayersohn, M. and Marcus, F. I. (1977). Clinical pharmacokinetics of digoxin. *Clin. Pharmacokin.* 2, 292–311.
Schwartz, A., Lindenmayer, G. E. and Allen, J. C. (1975). The sodium–potassium adenosine triphosphatase: pharmacological, physiological and biochemical aspects. *Pharmac. Rev.* 27, 3–134.
Smith, T. W. and Haber, E. (1973). Digitalis (review in four parts). *N. Engl. J. Med.* 289, 945, 1010, 1063, 1125.
Symposium (1974). Digoxin bioavailability. *Postgrad. Med. J.* 50 (Suppl. 6), 7–70.

VASODILATORS

K. CHATTERJEE

Vasodilator therapy improves cardiac function and alleviates symptoms of heart failure. It has gained wide acceptance as drug therapy for heart failure. Several parenteral and non-parenteral agents have the potential to be useful in the therapy of heart failure. Knowledge of the principal haemodynamic effects and their relative advantages and disadvantages is essential for appropriate selection of vasodilator drugs in the management of acute or chronic heart failure.

Rationale and mechanisms

Myocardial failure, irrespective of the cause, is frequently associated with reduced cardiac output. Ischaemic heart disease, primary myocardial disease, or an excessive pressure or volume overload (e.g. aortic stenosis, hypertensive heart disease, aortic or mitral regurgitation) may precipitate myocardial failure and consequently decrease contractile function and cardiac output. In response to reduced cardiac output, systemic vascular resistance increases to maintain arterial pressure. The distensibility of the aorta and large arteries (compliance) may decrease in patients with heart failure, which also increases left ventricular ejection impedance. Dilation and increased left ventricular volume are a frequent consequence of myocardial failure; increase in left ventricular volume, however, results in an increase in wall stress or afterload from the Laplace relation. Thus, enhanced systemic vascular resistance, decreased arterial compliance, and increased ventricular wall stress all increase resistance to left ventricular ejection. As an inverse relation exists between left ventricular outflow resistance and its stroke volume, increased resistance to ejection causes a further reduction in cardiac output establishing a vicious cycle (Fig. 1). One of the rationales for vasodilator therapy is to decrease systemic vascular resistance and resistance to left ventricular ejection and an increase in cardiac output, thereby reversing this vicious cycle. The rationale for inotropic therapy is to increase cardiac output by augmenting myocardial contractility.

Increased peripheral venous tone, in heart failure, can also be viewed as a compensatory circulatory adjustment to increased ventricular end-diastolic volume or preload to maintain stroke volume by the Frank–Starling mechanism. An increment in left ventricular volume, however, is usually associated with elevated left ventricular diastolic pressure, which is passively transmitted to the left atrium and pulmonary veins, resulting in pulmonary venous hypertension, the major determinant of symptoms of pulmonary congestion. Many vasodilators reduce intracardiac

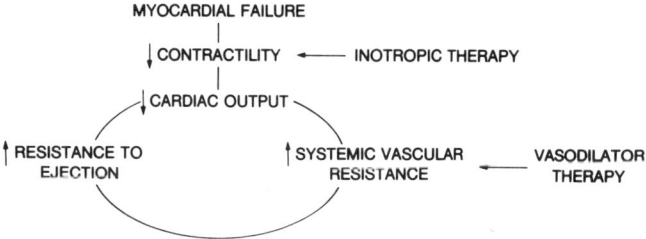

Fig. 1 Myocardial failure is associated with decreased contractility, which decreases cardiac output. Decreased cardiac output may be accompanied by elevated systemic vascular resistance, which increases resistance to left ventricular ejection and causes further reduction in cardiac output, establishing a vicious cycle.

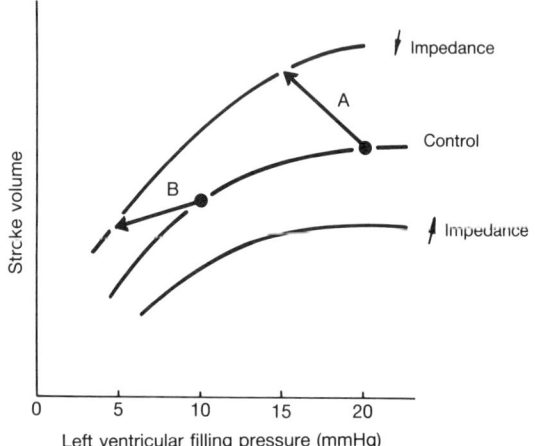

Fig. 2 Left ventricular function curves plotting stroke volume as a function of left ventricular filling pressure. The control curve is in the middle. With a vasodilator drug, there would be a decrease in impedance, which would shift the curve up and to the left. Note that if a patient on the control curve were given a vasodilator with an inital filling pressure of 20 mm Hg, the reduction of filling pressure would be accompanied by an increase in stroke volume (line A). However, if the same patient began at a filling pressure of 10 mm Hg, there would be a decrease in stroke volume (line B). (Reproduced with permission from Parmley and Chatterjee, 1977.)

volume by decreasing peripheral venous tone and venous return to the heart. Decreased systemic and pulmonary venous pressures resulting from small intracardiac volume contribute to the amelioration of symptoms and signs related to systemic and pulmonary venous hypertension. The major objective for the use of venodilators in patients with heart failure is to decrease the venous return to the heart by causing peripheral venous pooling. It needs to be emphasized that when there is increased stroke volume due to concomitant decrease in left ventricular outflow resistance, the net venous return to the heart is still higher than that before vasodilator therapy. An excessive reduction in venous return, however, may cause no increase, or even a decrease, in stroke volume, despite decreased left ventricular ejection impedance (Fig. 2). The net change in stroke volume and cardiac output with a vasodilator is determined largely by the magnitude or reduction of left ventricular volume, which decreases stroke volume and the magnitude of reduction of systemic vascular resistance, which increases stroke volume.

Multiple mechanisms contribute to elevated peripheral vascular tone in patients with heart failure (Table 1). Systemic sympathetic activity is stimulated in many patients and is reflected in increased levels of circulating catecholamines, particularly of noradrenaline (norepinephrine). Although cardiac stores may be depleted, myocardial noradrenaline release is markedly increased in chronic heart failure, indicating enhanced cardiac sympathetic activity.

Alpha adrenergic stimulation, resulting from an activated sympathetic system, promotes peripheral vasoconstriction. The renin–angiotensin–aldosterone system is also activated in heart failure. Plasma renin activity and plasma aldosterone levels may be considerably higher than normal. The precise mechanism for increased plasma renin activity is not known; decreased renal perfusion pressure, enhanced renal sympathetic activity, decreased renal tubular sodium load, and diuretic therapy all may stimulate renin production from the juxtaglomerular apparatus. In the presence of increased plasma renin activity, angiotensin I production increases. In the presence of converting enzyme, increased levels of angiotensin I result in higher levels of angiotensin II, a potent vasoconstrictor. Angiotensin stimulates synthesis and release of aldosterone from the adrenal cortex; aldosterone promotes salt and fluid retention and increases sodium content of the smooth muscles of the vascular bed, which contribute to increased vascular stiffness. Higher plasma levels of vasopressin have also been observed in patients with chronic heart failure, particularly in the presence of markedly depressed left ventricular function. Increased vasopressin levels are observed, despite decreased effective osmolality and hyponatraemia. The significance of higher vasopressin levels in heart failure remains unclear; however, it might contribute to abnormal volume regulation in heart failure (see Table 1).

Classification

Vasodilators potentially useful in the therapy of heart failure can be classified according to their mechanism of action and also according to their principal site of action on the peripheral vascular bed (Table 2). There are a number of vasodilator agents (e.g. hydralazine, nitrates, nitroprusside), which cause direct smooth muscle relaxation of the peripheral vascular bed. Other agents decrease vasoconstrictor tone mediated by the sympathetic adrenergic system. Clonidine decreases peripheral sympathetic outflow by stimulating the alpha-adrenergic receptors located in the central nervous system; on the other hand, drugs like phentolamine or prazosin cause vasodilation by peripheral alpha-adrenergic receptor blockade. Ganglion blocking agents (e.g. trimethaphan or hexamethonium) also cause vasodilation and have been used for the treatment of heart failure. Stimulation of beta-2 adrenergic receptors is associated with peripheral vasodilation, and the pharmacological agents salbutamol and pirbuterol decrease systemic vascular resistance primarily by this mechanism. Inhibition of inward calcium current to the smooth muscles of the peripheral vascular bed is thought to be the primary mechanism by which 'slow channel' (calcium) blocking agents (e.g. nifedipine) cause vasodilation and decrease systemic vascular resistance. Calcium entry blocking agents also attenuate vasoconstriction mediated by alpha-adrenergic stimulation.

There is growing evidence to suggest that, in patients with heart failure, the renin–angiotensin system is stimulated and angiotensin II, the potent vasoactive product of the non-active angiotensin I, plays a significant role in maintaining elevated systemic vascular resistance. Vasodilation and a decrease in systemic vascular resistance can occur from the inhibition or attenuation of the effects of angiotensin II. Saralasin, a competitive antagonist of angiotensin

Table 1 Neurohumoral abnormalities in heart failure

1 Increased systemic sympathetic activity
   Increased circulating catecholamines, particularly noradrenaline (norepinephrine)
2 Increased myocardial noradrenaline release
3 Decreased myocardial noradrenaline stores
4 Decreased myocardial beta receptor density
5 Increased plasma renin activity → increased angiotensin I → increased angiotensin II
6 Increased plasma aldosterone
7 Increased nonosmolal release of vasopressin

Table 2 Mechanism and principal site of action of vasodilators

Vasodilator	Principal mechanism of action	Principal site of action
Nitroglycerin	Direct vascular smooth muscle relaxation	Venous
Nitrates	Direct vascular smooth muscle relaxation	Venous
Molsidomine	Direct vascular smooth muscle relaxation	Venous
Trimethaphan	Ganglion blockade	?Venous
Hydralazine	Direct vascular smooth muscle relaxation	Arteriolar
Endralazine	Direct vascular smooth muscle relaxation	Arteriolar
Minoxidil	Direct vascular smooth muscle relaxation	Arteriolar
Nifedipine	Slow channel (calcium) blockade	Arteriolar, ?venous
Diltiazem	Slow channel (calcium) blockade	Arteriolar, ?venous
Felodipine	Slow channel (calcium) blockade	Arteriolar, ?venous
Phentolamine	Alpha-adrenergic blockade; direct vascular smooth muscle relaxation	Arteriolar, venous
Nitroprusside	Direct vascular smooth muscle relaxation	Arteriolar, venous
Prazosin	Postsynaptic (alpha-1) alpha-adrenergic blockade	Arteriolar, venous
Trimazosin	Postsynaptic (alpha-1) alpha-adrenergic blockade	Arteriolar, venous
Saralasin	Competitive angiotensin II inhibition	Arteriorlar venous
Teprotide	Angiotensin converting enzyme inhibition	Arteriolar, venous
Captopril	Angiotensin converting enzyme inhibition	Arteriolar, venous
Enalapril	Angiotensin converting enzyme inhibition	Arteriolar, venous
Salbutamol	Beta-2 receptor stimulation	Arteriolar, venous
Terbutaline	Beta-2 receptor stimulation	Arteriolar, venous
Pirbuterol	Beta-2 receptor stimulation	Arteriolar, venous
Prostacyclin (PGI_2)	Accumulation of cyclic AMP in vascular smooth muscle	Arteriolar, ?venous
Prostaglandin (PGE)	Accumulation of cyclic AMP in vascular smooth muscle	Arteriolar, ?venous
Clonidine	Centrally mediated inhibition of sympathetic outflow	Arteriolar, venous
Ketanserin	5-hydroxy tryptamine 2 antagonism	Arteriolar, venous

II, and teprotide, captopril and enalapril, which decrease the formation of angiotensin II from angiotensin I by inhibiting the converting enzyme, cause vasodilation by these mechanisms. There is also evidence that prostaglandins are involved in maintaining the peripheral vascular tone. The vasodilators, prostacyclin, and prostaglandin E, appear to cause vasodilation primarily by stimulating the accumulation of cyclic-AMP in the smooth muscles of the vascular bed. Stimulation of serotonergic receptors can potentially increase arteriolar and venous tone. Serotonin antagonism thus can induce vasodilation, the proposed mechanism of action of ketanserin.

Irrespective of the mechanism of action, the major haemodynamic effects of these vasodilator drugs appear to depend on whether they act primarily on arteries or veins. A predominant venodilator (e.g. nitrates) consistently decreases intracardiac volume and systemic and pulmonary venous pressures; an arteriolar dilator, on the other hand, decreases systemic vascular resistance and increases cardiac output. Vasodilators with a balanced effect on arteriolar and venous beds not only decrease systemic vascular resistance and increase cardiac output, but also decrease systemic and pulmonary venous pressures.

The effects of vasodilators on cardiac performance are also dependent on the initial level of left ventricular filling pressure. How the initial level of left ventricular filling pressure can modify the changes in stroke volume is illustrated in Fig. 2. In a patient with heart failure and elevated filling pressure on the control curve, a reduction of aortic impedance will shift the curve upwards. As this portion of the ventricular function curve is relatively flat, an associated decrease in filling pressure will only cause small reduction in stroke volume. The overall result is an upward and leftward shift of the function curve accompanied by an increase in stroke volume (line A). If one begins at a normal or lower filling pressure, a comparable reduction will cause a marked reduction in stroke volume, as this portion of the ventricular function curve is relatively steep. Although the reduction of aortic impedance shifts ventricular function to a new curve (line B), the net result is no change or a decrease in stroke volume. The expected increase in stroke volume due to decreased aortic impedance is more than offset by the reduction in filling pressure. For similar reasons, a marked decrease in filling pressure, below the optimal level during vasodilator therapy may be associated with no change, or even a decrease in stroke volume and cardiac output. In these circumstances, hypotension and reflex tachydardia might be observed.

Haemodynamic effects

The haemodynamic effects of agents which are primarily venodilators (Table 2) are characterized by a marked decrease in right atrial, pulmonary capillary wedge, and pulmonary artery pressures. Left ventricular end-diastolic volume and pressure also decrease consistently. Pulmonary vascular resistance, when elevated secondary to left ventricular failure, tends to decrease. Systemic vascular resistance may not decrease significantly and only a modest increase or no increase in cardiac output or stroke volume is observed. Generally, arterial pressure falls, but only modestly, and in patients with heart failure with elevated left ventricular filling pressure, tachycardia usually does not develop. Nitroglycerin, when administered intravenously, tends to produce more arteriolar dilation than after its sublingual or topical administration with a consequent greater likelihood of a decrease in systemic vascular resistance and increase in cardiac output. The effects of trimethapan, which have been investigated only in a small number of patients, appear to be similar to those of nitroglycerin.

Hydralazine, endralazine, and minoxidil are predominantly arteriolar dilators and cause a significant decrease in systemic vascular resistance and a substantial increase in cardiac output and stroke volume. Nifedipine, diltiazem, felodipine, and prostacyclin also appear to be predominantly arteriolar dilators. These drugs do not cause any appreciable reduction in central venous pressure or pulmonary capillary wedge pressure, because of the lack of significant venodilating effects. Pulmonary vascular resistance tends to fall when it is elevated.

Vasodilator agents such as nitroprusside, with relatively balanced effects on the arteriolar bed and the venous bed, generally decrease systemic vascular resistance and increase cardiac output, and also decrease systemic and pulmonary venous pressure. In the presence of heart failure, as with other vasodilator agents, these drugs do not cause any significant increase in heart rate,

Table 3 Haemodynamic subsets in acute myocardial infarction: therapeutic approach

Subset	Clinical signs	Cadiac index ($1/min/m^2$)	Pulmonary artery wedge pressure (mm Hg)	Therapy
I	No pulmonary congestion No hypoperfusion	>2.2	<18	None required
II	Hypoperfusion No pulmonary congestion	<2.2	<18	Volume expansion
III	No hypoperfusion Pulmonary congestion	>2.2	>18	Diuretics, venodilators
IV	Hypoperfusion Pulmonary congestion	<2.2	>18	In the absence of hypotension: combined arterial and venodilators (inotropes) In the presence of hypotension: vasopressors, inotropes, vasodilators, intraaortic balloon counterpulsation

despite some decrease in arterial pressure. The effects of intravenous salbutamol are generally similar, but tachycardia also develops in most patients. Captopril, enalapril, prazosin, trimazosin, and pirbuterol, having combined arteriolar and venodilating properties, decrease systemic and pulmonary venous pressures and increase cardiac output.

Clinical applications
Vasodilators can be used effectively for the treatment of heart failure in the following clinical circumstances.

1. Pump failure complicating acute myocardial infarction
2. Pump failure due to valvular heart disease
3. Pump failure in postcardiac surgical patients
4. Chronic congestive heart failure
5. Precapillary pulmonary hypertension and primary right ventricular failure

Acute myocardial infarction (page 13.167)
For the treatment of pump failure complicating acute myocardial infarction, it is preferable to use the vasodilator agents with quickly reversible effects. Intravenous preparations of sodium nitroprusside, nitroglycerin, and phentolamine have been used extensively with benefit. Sublingual and topical nitroglycerin and sublingual, oral, and chewable isosorbide dinitrate are also effective. In patients with heart failure associated with elevated left ventricular filling pressure, sodium nitroprusside and phentolamine reduce pulmonary arterial and pulmonary capillary wedge pressures, and increase cardiac output and stroke volume. Systemic and pulmonary vascular resistance decrease, and there is usually a modest decrease in arterial pressure. Nitroprusside usually does not induce tachycardia, despite some fall in arterial pressure. Phentolamine induces tachycardia, irrespective of the initial level of left ventricular filling pressure. The precise mechanism for phentolamine-induced tachycardia remains unclear. In patients without evidence of left ventricular failure, sodium nitroprusside or phentolamine do not improve left ventricular function; although pulmonary capillary wedge pressure decreases, cardiac output and stroke volume may also decrease.

Nitroglycerin and isosorbide dinitrate, irrespective of their mode of administration, produce qualitatively similar haemodynamic responses.

Trimethaphan, a ganglionic blocking agent, has been used only in a limited number of patients, but its effects appear similar to those of nitroglycerin.

Monitoring of cardiovascular function in patients with suspected pump failure allows prompt recognition of sudden change and is necessary to evaluate the response to vasodilator treatment. Mea-

surements of cardiac output and filling pressures provide data by which patients can be categorized into subsets with differing prognosis and appropriate therapy (Table 3). Patients in subset I have no significant haemodynamic impairment and a good prognosis; no intervention is necessary. Patients in subset II improve with volume expansion and vasodilator therapy is not indicated. Most patients with pump failure with acute myocardial infarction fall into subsets III or IV. Patients in whom there is pulmonary congestion, raised left ventricular filling pressure, and maintained cardiac output, without evidence of hypoperfusion, may be treated with diuretics. If adequate reduction of pulmonary venous pressure is not then achieved, vasodilators which predominantly reduce preload (nitroglycerin and other nitrates) can be used. Subset IV patients with decreased cardiac output and elevated left ventricular filling pressure require reduction in both preload and impedance; a vasodilator with balanced effects on arteriolar and venous beds (nitroprusside or phentolamine) is preferable. When pump failure is very severe and associated with marked hypotension, inotropic agents and mechanical assist devices, such as intraaortic balloon counterpulsation, may be required before the addition of vasodilator agents.

One of the aims of treatment is to reduce the extent of myocardial ischaemia and injury. There is controversy about the possible deleterious effects of some of the vasodilators which, because of their potential to cause marked arteriolar dilation, might divert blood flow from ischaemic myocardium to relatively non-ischaemic zones. Venodilators have been reported to increase collateral blood flow to the ischaemic myocardial zones. However, clinical studies have not yet provided any conclusive evidence either for the adverse, or for the beneficial, effects on the extent of myocardial ischaemia with the use of any of the commonly used vasodilators.

One of the potentially hazardous complications of using vasodilators for pump failure complicating myocardial infarction is the development of hypotension. In the presence of myocardial ischaemia or infarction, coronary vascular resistance declines markedly due to the vasodilatory effects of local metabolites. In this circumstance, blood flow to the ischaemic zone is primarily dependent on the perfusion pressure and is likely to fall with a fall in arterial pressure. It is, therefore, essential to avoid significant hypotension. Some broad guidelines for the use of parenteral vasodilators in acute pump failure are listed in Table 4.

Valvular heart disease
In patients with mitral or aortic regurgitation, vasodilator drugs produce haemodynamic and clinical improvement, particularly when heart failure is associated with elevated left ventricular end-diastolic pressure, low cardiac output, and elevated systemic vas-

Table 4 Guidelines for intravenous vasodilator therapy in acute pump failure

1 Determine initial haemodynamics for selection of a vasodilator
2 Start therapy with low initial dose (nitroprusside 15μg/min, phentolamine 0.1 mg/min, nitroglycerin 10μg/min)
3 Gradual increase in infusion rate (every 5–15 min)
4 Monitor changes in blood pressure, heart rate, left ventricular filling pressure, cardiac output, systemic vascular resistance
5 If cardiac output increases, with a decrease in systemic vascular resistance and left ventricular filling pressure, and little change in blood pressure, maintain same infusion rate
6 If blood pressure decreases without change in cardiac output or left ventricular filling pressure, discontinue vasodilator or add inotrope
7 Monitor thiocyanate level during prolonged nitroprusside infusion
8 Substitute non-parenteral vasodilator when chronic therapy is indicated.

Reproduced with permission from Massie and Chatterjee (1979). Vasodilator therapy of pump failure complicating myocardial infarction. Symposium on cardiac emergencies. *Med. Clin. N. Am.* **63**, 25.

cular resistance. An increase in aortic impedance causes worsening mitral or aortic regurgitation; regurgitant volume increases and forward stroke volume increased and cardiac output decline. Conversely, reduction of aortic impedance (analogous to systemic vascular resistance) is associated with decreased regurgitant volume and increased cardiac output. In patients with mitral regurgitation, nitroprusside increases forward stroke volume and cardiac output and decreases pulmonary capillary wedge, right atrial and pulmonary artery pressures. Systemic and pulmonary vascular resistance decrease, with a modest fall in arterial pressure. Heart rate usually does not change. The magnitude of the peak 'v' wave in the pulmonary capillary wedge pressure tracing decreases, suggesting reduction of regurgitant volumes. Analysis of the changes in left ventricular volume during nitroprusside infusion demonstrates reduction of end-diastolic and end-systolic volumes, decreased regurgitant fraction, and increased forward stroke volume and ejection fraction. Left ventricular total stroke volume usually remains unchanged, indicating a redistribution; more blood is ejected forward into the aorta and less backwards to the left atrium. Similar changes are observed in patients with aortic regurgitation, particularly in the presence of low cardiac output and elevated systemic vascular resistance. Increases in forward stroke volume and cardiac output are associated with decreased regurgitant volume, and decreased left ventricular end-diastolic volume and pressure. Prazosin produces similar haemodynamic and clinical responses in patients with mitral and aortic regurgitation, and effects of hydralazine differ only slightly from those of sodium nitroprusside. Forward stroke volume increases with decrease in the regurgitant fraction, but left ventricular end-diastolic volume remains unchanged. As with nitroprusside, the magnitude of the 'v' wave and mean pulmonary capillary wedge pressure, and systemic and pulmonary vascular resistance, decrease. With nitroglycerin, reduction of left ventricular end-diastolic volume is accompanied by decreased left ventricular diastolic and pulmonary venous pressures. Although regurgitant fraction decreases, there is little or no increase in forward stroke volume.

Vasodilators have been used for the treatment of low cardiac output and pulmonary venous hypertension due to aortic and mitral valve stenosis. In patients with mild aortic stenosis, sodium nitroprusside or hydralazine have been shown to increase cardiac output and decrease pulmonary venous pressure. Nitroglycerin relieves angina in patients with aortic stenosis, even without obstructive coronary artery disease, primarily by decreasing myocardial oxygen demand. Nitroglycerin decreases pulmonary venous pressure and relieves the symptoms of pulmonary venous congestion in patients with mitral stenosis. However, tachycardia, hypotension, and a fall in cardiac output can occur because of a marked reduction of left ventricular end-diastolic volume.

Vasodilators, particularly arteriolar dilators, should be used cautiously, if at all, in patients with very severe aortic stenosis. If systemic vascular resistance declines due to peripheral vasodilation, hypotension, and syncope may be precipitated because of the inability to increase cardiac output proportionally in the presence of severe fixed left ventricular outflow obstruction.

Corrective surgery is the preferred treatment for valvular heart disease. Vasodilator therapy is only indicated when surgery is otherwise contraindicated, or needs to be deferred. In patients with acute bacterial endocarditis who develop aortic or mitral regurgitation, vasodilator therapy may be useful to tide over the critical period until infection is controlled. Similarly, in some patients with mitral regurgitation complicating acute myocardial infarction, vasodilators can be used to defer corrective surgery to reduce the operative risk.

Heart failure in postcardiac surgical patients
Vasodilators such as nitroprusside, phentolamine, nitroglycerin, trimethaphan, and hydralazine have been used for the treatment of pump failure complicating cardiac surgery. Monitoring is required to determine the haemodynamic problems of individual patients. When cardiac output is low and systemic vascular resistance is high, an arteriolar dilator is preferable, provided pulmonary venous pressure is not elevated; when pulmonary venous pressure is also raised, a vasodilator with a balanced effect on arteriolar and venous beds is likely to produce a better response.

Primary pulmonary hypertension and right heart failure
Response to a variety of vasodilators has been investigated in patients with primary pulmonary hypertension. Phentolamine, hydralazine, diazoxide calcium antagonists, and angiotensin converting enzyme inhibitors all have been used to decrease pulmonary vascular resistance and pulmonary hypertension. Although an occasional patient may benefit, vasodilator agents, in general, are ineffective in decreasing pulmonary vascular resistance and pulmonary hypertension in far advanced patients. This is particularly true in those who present with evidence of right heart failure in whom pulmonary vascular resistance appears to be fixed. However, a trial of vasodilator therapy is indicated, in view of the extremely poor prognosis. Haemodynamic effects of the different vasodilators should be determined to select the appropriate drug.

Chronic congestive heart failure
For the long-term management of patients with chronic congestive heart failure, a number of oral vasodilators have been investigated and the list of useful drugs in this category is rapidly increasing (Table 5). Although these vasodilators produce qualitatively similar haemodynamic responses, there are significant quantitative differences. Nitroglycerin, isosorbide dinitrate, and pentaerythritol tetranitrate, being predominantly venodilators, decrease systemic and pulmonary venous pressures, but cardiac output may not increase; they are most useful for the relief of signs and symptoms of systemic and pulmonary venous hypertension (dyspnoea on exertion, paroxysmal noctural dyspnoea, orthopnoea, hepatic congestion, and peripheral oedema), but are less effective in the presence of marked peripheral oedema.

Hydralazine, endralazine, and minoxidil cause a marked increase in cardiac output with little or no decrease in pulmonary or systemic venous pressures; they are most useful for the relief of symptoms related to low cardiac output (fatigue, tiredness or lack of energy).

Salbutamol, when given orally, produces effects similar to those of oral hydralazine. There is usually a significant increase in cardiac output with marked reduction in systemic vascular resistance; little or no decrease in pulmonary capillary wedge pressure is observed. With nifedipine, diltiazem, and felodipine, a substantial increase in cardiac output has been noted; a decrease in pulmonary capillary wedge pressure may also occur in some but not all patients.

Prazosin and trimazosin, the postsynaptic alpha-receptor blocking agents, appear to have balanced effects on the arteriolar and venous beds and not only increase cardiac output, but also decrease right atrial and pulmonary capillary wedge pressures. Captopril and enalapril, the orally active angiotensin converting enzyme inhibitors, decrease the level of circulating angiotensin II by preventing its conversion from angiotensin I. They reduce arteriolar tone by attenuating the vasoconstricting effect of angiotensin II; systemic vascular resistance, therefore, decreases with

an increase in cardiac output. There is also a marked decrease of systemic and pulmonary venous pressures due to concomitant venodilation.

Pirbuterol, a beta-2 agonist, also causes a significant increase in cardiac output and reduction of pulmonary capillary wedge pressure, and may be useful for the the long-term treatment of heart failure.

In the majority of patients with chronic congestive heart failure, elevated pulmonary venous pressure, low cardiac output, and

Table 5 The principal haemodynamic effects of non-parenteral vasodilators in chronic heart failure

Vasodilator	Heart rate	Blood pressure	Cardiac output	Systemic vascular resistance	Pulmonary venous pressure	Right atrial pressure	Pulmonary vascular resistance
Nitroglycerin ointment	No change	Slight decrease	No change or slight decrease	No change or slight decrease	Marked decrease	Marked decrease	Decrease
Isosorbide dinitrate	No change	Slight decrease	No change or slight increase	No change or slight decrease	Marked decrease	Marked decrease	Decrease
Hydralazine	No change or slight increase	Slight decrease or no change	Marked increase	Marked decrease	No change or slight decrease	No change	Slight decrease
Endralazine	No change or slight increase	Slight decrease or no change	Marked increase	Marked decrease	No change or slight decrease	No change	Slight decrease
Minoxidil	No change or slight increase	Slight decrease or no change	Marked increase	Marked decrease	No change or slight decrease	No change	Slight decrease
Prazosin	No change or slight decrease	Moderate decrease	Moderate increase	Moderate decrease	Marked decrease	Marked decrease	Decrease
Trimazosin	No change or slight decrease	Moderate decrease	Moderate increase	Moderate decrease	Marked decrease	Marked decrease	Decrease
Captopril	No change or slight decrease	Moderate decrease	Moderate increase	Moderate decrease	Marked decrease	Marked decrease	Decrease
Enalapril	No change or slight decrease	Moderate decrease	Moderate increase	Moderate decrease	Marked decrease	Marked decrease	Decrease
Pirbuterol	Increase or no change	No change or slight decrease	Moderate increase	Moderate decrease	Moderate decrease	Moderate decrease	Slight decrease
Salbutamol	Increase or no change	No change or slight decrease	Moderate increase	Moderate decrease	No change or slight decrease	No change or slight decrease	Slight decrease
Nifedipine	Increase or no change	Decrease or no change	Increase	Decrease	Decrease or no change	Decrease or no change	Decrease
Diltiazem	Increase or no change	Decrease or no change	Increase	Decrease	Decrease or no change	Decrease or no change	Decrease
Felodipine	Increase or no change	Decrease or no change	Increase	Decrease	Decrease or no change	Decrease or no change	Decrease

Table 6 Dose, duration of action, and potential complications of commonly used non-parenteral vasodilators in patients with chronic heart failure

Vasodilator	Usual dose	Duration of action	Potential complications
Topical nitroglycerin	0.5–5 cm every 4 h	Average 4 h	Hypotension, tachycardia
Oral isosorbide dinitrate	20–100 mg every 4 h	Average 4 h	Tolerance, fluid retention
Sublingual isosorbide dinitrate	2.5–10 mg every 2 h	Average 2 h	?exacerbation of angina after sudden withdrawal
Hydralazine	200–400 mg daily in divided doses (twice or three times daily; rarely up to 1200 mg is required)	Average 8–12 h	Headache, tachycardia, hypotension, exacerbation of angina, drug fever, skin rash, nausea, anorexia, abdominal pain, salt and fluid retention, lupus syndrome, polyneuropathy
Minoxidil	10–20 mg twice daily	Average 12 h	Salt and fluid retention, excessive weight gain, hypotension tachycardia, deterioration of renal function, pericardial effusion, excessive hair growth
Prazosin	2–5 mg 4 times daily	Average 6 h	Hypotension (particularly after the first dose), postural hypotension, depression, nausea, anorexia, fluid retention, ?tachyphalaxis
Captopril	6.25–50 mg 3 times daily	Average 8 h	Hypotension, metallic taste, skin rash, drug fever. Nausea, anorexia, ? immune complex membranous glomerulonephritis, leucopenia, renal failure
Enalapril	2.5–10 mg twice daily	Average 12 h	Hypotension, renal failure
Pirbuterol	10–20 mg 3 to 4 times daily	Average 8 h	Tachycardia, arrhythmia, tachyphylaxis
Salbutamol	2.5–25 mg 3 times daily	Average 8 h	Tachycardia, arrhythmia
Nifedipine	10–40 mg 3 to 4 times daily	Average 6 to 8 h	Hypotension, nausea, abdominal pain, constipation, fluid retention
Diltiazem	30–60 mg 3 to 4 times daily	Average 6 to 8 h	Hypotension, nausea, abdominal pain, constipation, fluid retention, skin rash, confusion

increased systemic vascular resistance are the major haemodynamic abnomalities. In these patients, a single vasodilator agent, such as prazosin, trimazosin, captopril, or pirbuterol, can be used to decrease pulmonary venous pressure and to increase cardiac output. Alternatively, an arteriolar dilator like hydralazine, minoxidil, or salbutamol can be combined with a venodilator (nitrates) to achieve the same goal.

Angiotensin coverting enzyme inhibitors (captopril or enalapril) appear to have some advantages over other vasodilators in the therapy of chronic congestive heart failure. These agents decrease aldosterone levels, and sodium and fluid retention, therefore, are infrequent. In contrast, the renin–angiotensin–aldosterone system may be activated during maintenance therapy with direct acting vasodilators, alpha-adrenergic, and calcium entry blocking agents and, frequently, the dose of diuretics needs to be increased. Plasma catecholamine levels tend to decrease with the use of angiotensin converting enzyme inhibitors, whereas, no change or even an increase in catecholamine levels may occur with the use of other types of vasodilators. Myocardial oxygen consumption usually decreases in response to angiotensin converting enzyme inhibitors in patients with ischaemic cardiomyopathy; thus, improved left ventricular function is usually associated with decreased metabolic cost. With the use of other types of vasodilators, no consistent reduction in myocardial oxygen consumption is observed.

The optimal dose range of the vasodilators that is currently available for the treatment of chronic heart failure has not been determined. In general, a larger dose is required for the treatment of heart failure than for hypertension or angina. A low dose should be given to begin with and should be increased gradually to determine tolerance and avoid undesirable side effects. The usual dose, the duration of action, and the important complications of the commonly used oral vasodilators are summarized in Table 6.

References

Ader, R., Chatterjee, K., Ports, T. A. *et al.* (1980). Immediate and sustained hemodynamic and clinical improvement in chronic heart failure by an oral angiontensin converting enzyme inhibitor. *Circulation* **61**, 931–937.

Captopril Multicenter Research Group (1985). A placebo-controlled trial of captopril in refractory chronic congestive heart failure. *Am. Heart J.* **10**, 439–447.

Chatterjee, K. and Parmley, W. W. (1977). The role of vasodilator therapy in heart failure. *Prog. Cardiovasc. Dis.* **19**, 301.

—— and Parmley, W. W. (1980). Vasodilator therapy for chronic heart failure. In *Annual review of pharmacology and toxicology* (eds R. George, R. Ikun and A. Cho), p. 475. Annual Reviews, Palo Alto, California.

—— and Parmley, W. W. (1983). Vasodilator therapy for acute myocardial infarction and congestive heart failure. *J. Am. Coll. Cardiol.* **1**, 133.

Dawson, J. R., Poole-Wilson, P. A. and Sutton, G. (1980). Salbutamol in cardiogenic shock complicating acute myocardial infarction. *Br. Heart. J.* **43**, 523.

Forrester, J. S., Diamond, G., Chatterjee, K. and Swan, H. J. C. (1976). Hemodynamic therapy of myocardial infarction (first of two parts). *N. Engl. J. Med.* **295**, 1356.

Forrester, J. S., Diamond, G., Chatterjee, K. and Swan, H. J. C. (1976). Hemodynamic therapy of myocardial infarction (second of two parts). *N. Engl. J. Med.* **295**, 1404.

Greenberg, B. and Massie, B. M. (1980). Beneficial effects of afterload reduction in patients with congestive heart failure and moderate aortic stenosis. *Circulation* **61**, 1212.

Helfant, R. H., Pine, R., Meister, S. G., Feldman, M. S., Trout, R. G. and Banka, V. S. (1974). Nitroglycerin to unmask reversible asynergy: correlation with post-coronary bypass ventriculography. *Circulation* **50**, 108.

Klugmann, S., Salvi, A. and Camerini, F. (1980). Haemodynamic effects of nifedipine in heart failure. *Br. Heart J.* **43**, 440.

Parmley, W. W. and Chatterjee, K. (1978). Vasodilator therapy. In *Current problems in cardiology* Vol 2 (ed. W. Proctor Harvery), p. 8. Yearbook Medical Publishers, Chicago.

Rouleau, J-L., Warnica, J. W. and Burgess, J. H. (1981). Prazosin and congestive heart failure: short and long term therapy. *Am. J. Med.* **71**, 147.

——, Chatterjee, K., Benge, W. *et al.* (1982). Alteration in left ventricular function and coronary hemodynamics with captopril, hydralazine, and prazosin in chronic ischemic heart failure. A comparative study. *Circulation* **65**, 671.

Stephens, J. D., Banim, S. O. and Spurrell, R. A. J. (1980). Haemodynamic effects of oral salbutamol alone and in combination with sublingual isosorbide dinitrate in patients with severe congestive heart failure. *Br. Heart J.* **43**, 220.

Szczeklik, J., Szczeklik, A. and Nizankowski, R. (1980). Haemodynamic changes induced by prostacyclin in man. *Br. Heart J.* **44**, 254.

CATECHOLAMINES AND THEIR DERIVATIVES

P. FOËX AND A. FISHER

Introduction

The efficiency of the cardiac pump depends upon preload, contractility, and afterload each of which may be influenced by catecholamines and their synthetic derivatives. These agents have been used extensively in the management of acute circulatory failure. However, there is a delicate balance between the therapeutic advantages and disadvantages they produce. This review will mostly deal with their use in the treatment of acute circulatory failure. It must be stressed that the first step in the treatment of acute circulatory failure should always be to ensure that any hypovolaemia is corrected. Once this has been done, the therapeutic approach may include catecholamines, vasodilators, or circulatory assistance using aortic balloon counterpulsation.

Adrenergic receptors

Noradrenaline, adrenaline, and dopamine are naturally occurring catecholamines which, with their structurally related synthetic derivatives, appear to act on at least five types of receptors (Table 1). Originally, Ahlquist postulated the existence of only two types of adrenoceptors which he termed alpha- and beta-receptors, but over the years it has become apparent that both types require subdivision into two subgroups. Alpha-receptors may be either post-synaptic (alpha-1) or presynaptic (alpha-2). Stimulation of the postsynaptic alpha-1 receptors causes peripheral arteriolar con-

Table 1 Cardiovascular effects of adrenergic receptor stimulation

Receptor	Effect
Alpha-1	Peripheral vasoconstriction
	Venoconstriction
Alpha-2	Presynaptic sympathetic inhibition
Beta-1	Positive chronotropy
	Positive inotropy
	Increased a–v conduction
Beta-2	Peripheral vasodilatation
Dopaminergic	Renal vasodilatation
	Mesenteric vasodilatation

striction and venoconstriction. Stimulation of the presynaptic alpha-2 receptors decreases the release of the neurotransmitter. The beta-adrenoceptors are also subdivided into two subgroups. Beta-1 receptors are responsible for most of the cardiac effects while beta-2 receptors are responsible for most of the peripheral effects of beta-adrenergic stimulation. However, beta-2 receptors are also found in the myocardium. In human left ventricular muscle, 85 per cent of the beta-adrenoceptors are beta-1 and 15 per cent are beta-2 receptors. In the human atrial muscle the proportions are, respectively, 75 per cent (beta-1) and 25 per cent (beta-2). Beta-2 receptors play an important role in sinus node function. Finally, specific dopaminergic receptors in the renal, mesenteric, coronary, and cerebral vascular beds are the mediators of dopamine-induced vasodilation. This response is most pronounced in the mesenteric and renal arteriolar territories.

The effects of the catecholamines and of their structurally related derivatives depend upon a basic interaction between the drug and the receptor sites. At the beta-receptors, the result of this interaction is the activation of the enzyme adenylate cyclase in the cell membrane of the target organ or tissues. This, in turn, increases the synthesis of cyclic-AMP (cAMP) in the effector cell and, through the cAMP-dependent protein-kinase, causes the physiological response. At the alpha-1 receptors the interaction between drug and receptor increases the transmembrane flux of ionized calcium and may also modify the turnover of phosphatidylinositol. The natural neurotransmitter at alpha- and beta-receptors is noradrenaline. Beta-1 receptors are equally sensitive to circulating adrenaline and noradrenaline, while beta-2 receptors are more sensitive to adrenaline than noradrenaline. At the dopaminergic receptors, the natural transmitter is dopamine.

The cardiovascular effects of the catecholamines and their derivatives depend upon the type of receptors upon which they act and also upon the state of the circulation at the time they are administered; usually acidosis reduces the efficacy of exogenous catecholamines. Some catecholamines require the release of noradrenaline from sympathetic nerve endings: depletion of noradrenaline stores will decrease their haemodynamic effects. In patients treated with alpha- or beta-receptor antagonists, the effects of catecholamines may differ substantially from those usually observed. More importantly, the efficacy of the catecholamines is a function of two characteristics of the adrenergic receptors which have recently come to light, that is, (a) the state of affinity which is modulated by guanosine nucleotides, and (b) the number of receptors. Hyperthyroidism appears to increase the number of cardiac beta-receptors ('up regulation') while cardiac failure decreases it ('down regulation').

Of the naturally occurring catecholamines and their synthetic derivatives, the most important are noradrenaline, adrenaline, dopamine, isoprenaline, dobutamine, prenalterol, pirbuterol, and salbutamol. The sites of action of these catecholamines are listed in Table 2. From the types of receptors stimulated it is largely possible to predict the effects of these drugs on heart rate, contractility, peripheral vascular resistance, and splanchnic blood flow.

With the exception of salbutamol and of low doses of dopamine that are used to obtain either peripheral or splanchnic and renal

Table 2 Major sites of actions of catecholamines

Drug	Receptors				
	Alpha-1	Alpha-2	Beta-1	Beta-2	Dopaminergic
Noradrenaline	+	+	+	+	
Adrenaline	+	+	+	+	
Isoprenaline			+	+	
Dopamine	+	(+)	+		+
Dobutamine	(+)		+		
Prenalterol			+		
Pirbuterol			+		
Salbutamol				+	

vasodilation, catecholamines are predominantly used to increase the inotropic state of the myocardium. Unless the drug causes vasodilation (e.g. isoprenaline) arterial pressure will increase because of the improved performance of the cardiac pump or because of peripheral vasoconstriction. Catecholamines and their synthetic derivatives have, therefore, been advocated for the treatment of circulatory failure. They are used in the treatment of cardiogenic shock following myocardial infarction, cardiac failure following cardiac surgery, circulatory failure complicating septicaemia, and also to improve cardiac performance during artificial ventilation with positive end-expiratory pressure (PEEP).

Increasing the inotropic state of the myocardium enables the heart to develop more stroke work for a given filling pressure. This beneficial effect cannot be obtained without increasing myocardial oxygen demand. Moreover, stimulation of the beta-1 adrenoceptors causes both inotropic and chronotropic effects. The increase in heart rate that usually accompanies an increase in performance increases myocardial oxygen consumption further. Tachycardia, while increasing oxygen demand, decreases myocardial oxygen supply because it shortens the diastolic filling time of the coronary circulation. Not uncommonly, catecholamine-induced tachycardias are accompanied by the development of arrhythmias that impair the balance between oxygen demand and oxygen supply even more. While the inotropic and chronotropic effects of beta-1 adrenoceptor stimulation are interdependent, the magnitude of tachycardia observed in response to catecholamines is modulated by both baroceptor reflexes and alpha-2 receptor-mediated presynaptic inhibition. At the extremes of the spectrum, noradrenaline causes bradycardia because of arterial hypertension and presynaptic inhibition while isoprenaline causes the largest increases in heart rate because of the reduction of blood pressure that is often associated with its administration. When catecholamines cause an increase in arterial pressure, myocardial oxygen consumption is increased. In the case of a normal coronary circulation, the increased oxygen demand can be met by an increased oxygen supply. Local mechanisms decrease coronary vascular resistance and, therefore, allow coronary blood flow to increase in order to match the increased metabolic requirements. However, in the case of ischaemic heart disease, coronary blood flow and oxygen supply may be critically limited and the increased oxygen demand cannot necessarily be met. Studies of regional myocardial function have shown that wall motion may deteriorate and signs of myocardial ischaemia may develop under the influence of catecholamines. Such considerations would appear to rule out their use in the management of circulatory failure. However, two determinants of coronary blood flow, namely, diastolic arterial pressure and left ventricular end-diastolic pressure are also influenced by inotropic agents. An increase in diastolic arterial pressure accompanied by a reduction of left ventricular diastolic pressure will increase the coronary perfusion pressure gradient and, therefore, coronary blood flow and myocardial oxygen supply; moreover the reduction of left ventricular end-diastolic pressure and volume decreases the oxygen demand. For any therapeutic intervention on the ischaemic heart, it is important to consider its effects on oxygen demand and on oxygen supply. It is useful to remember that the worst offenders of the delicate balance between supply and demand are tachycardia, diastolic hypotension, and left ventricular dilatation.

Haemodynamic profile of the catecholamines

The haemodynamic profile of some of the catecholamines used in clinical practice is summarized in Fig. 1, while the usual doses are listed in Table 3. For most of the catecholamines, administration by continuous infusion is necessary because of their very short duration of action.

Noradrenaline

In the past noradrenaline, the natural neurotransmitter, has been frequently used in the treatment of circulatory failure. Its main

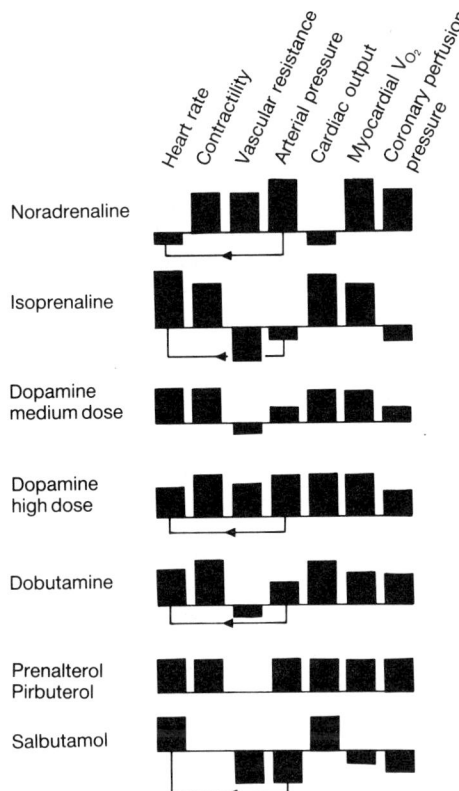

Fig. 1 Haemodynamic profile of selected catecholamines. For each drug, columns above the line indicate an increase and, below the line a decrease of the variable considered. The line joining arterial pressure and heart rate indicates that baroreceptor reflexes may play an important role in the heart rate response.

Table 3 Usual infusion rates of catecholamines

Drug	Infusion rate (µg/kg/min)
Noradrenaline	0.01–0.07
Adrenaline	0.06–0.18
Isoprenaline	0.02–0.18
Dopamine	
Dopaminergic	1–5
Beta-1 effect	5–15
Alpha + beta effects	>15
Dobutamine	2–40
Prenalterol	10–20
Salbutamol	0.2–0.5

haemodynamic effects are alpha-adrenoceptor-mediated arteriolar vasoconstriction and venoconstriction. When venoconstriction predominates, the capillary hydrostatic pressure increases and the intravascular volume decreases. Noradrenaline also stimulates the beta-adrenoceptors increasing the inotropic state of the myocardium. Because of arteriolar vasoconstriction and the positive inotropy, arterial pressure is markedly elevated by noradrenaline but cardiac output usually decreases. The elevation of arterial pressure causes bradycardia, via baroceptor reflexes, in spite of beta-adrenoceptor stimulation. Vasoconstriction predominates in the peripheral vascular beds and is less pronounced in the locally regulated territories, i.e. the coronary and cerebral circulations. Renal, hepatic, and muscle blood flow are all substantially reduced. Prolonged administration of noradrenaline, by reducing peripheral perfusion, may cause or increase tissue acidosis, and may contribute to the development of irreversible shock. The effects of noradrenaline on the myocardium are a combination of increased afterload (alpha-adrenoceptor-mediated vaso-

constriction), increased preload (alpha-mediated venoconstriction) and increased contractility. All these factors contribute to cause large increases in myocardial oxygen consumption. When the coronary arteries are normal, coronary blood flow will increase substantially in response to the increase in oxygen consumption. When the coronary arteries are narrowed, coronary blood flow will still increase because of the increase in aortic diastolic pressure. This may improve myocardial metabolism and myocardial performance. Even in the presence of coronary artery disease, noradrenaline may be useful in the acute phase of resuscitation when the primary goal is to shunt blood away from the skeletal muscle into the cerebral and the coronary circulations. This can be achieved by peripheral vasoconstriction that restores adequate cerebral and coronary perfusion pressures. Outside resuscitation, a rational use for noradrenaline is to increase arterial pressure in septic shock when peripheral vascular resistance may be greatly reduced. Noradrenaline may also be used to prevent hypotension during venodilator therapy with nitroglycerine derivatives. In congestive heart failure, noradrenaline is likely to exert adverse effects. The inotropic response is reduced because of the receptor 'down regulation' while peripheral vasoconstriction is maintained. In this case, elevations of left ventricular end-diastolic pressure are observed, which reduce the coronary perfusion pressure, and worsen the balance between oxygen supply and demand.

Adrenaline

Produced mainly by the adrenal medulla, adrenaline may be administered as an exogenous catecholamine. It acts on the peripheral alpha- and beta-adrenoceptors and also on the cardiac beta-receptors. The increase in myocardial contractility is accompanied by an increase in heart rate, cardiac automaticity, and atrioventricular node conduction. The effect on heart rate differs from that of noradrenaline because adrenaline causes less vasoconstriction and hypertension than noradrenaline. Thus, the direct chronotropic effect (beta-1 adrenoceptor stimulation) is less inhibited by baroceptor reflexes. At low doses, cardiac beta-receptor stimulation is predominant and systemic vascular resistance may decrease, while at high doses alpha-mediated vasoconstriction becomes important. Renal blood flow and glomerular filtration rates are reduced by adrenaline. Coronary vasoconstriction is usually transient and, as metabolic demand increases, coronary blood flow increases because of locally induced vasodilation. However, the development of adrenaline-induced tachycardia and arrhythmias may compromise coronary perfusion and worsen the balance of oxygen supply and demand, thus limiting the value of adrenaline in the treatment of circulatory failure. Because of the marked reduction of renal blood flow and, with prolonged use, the risk of peripheral gangrene, adrenaline is no longer recommended as sole agent for the treatment of circulatory failure, although it is still used in association with other catecholamines.

Isoprenaline

Isoprenaline acts exclusively on the beta-1 and beta-2 adrenoceptors. Its direct effects include marked increases in inotropy, chronotropy, atrioventricular conduction, and automaticity. Peripherally both systemic and pulmonary beta-2 adrenoceptors are stimulated so that diastolic arterial pressure decreases as well as pulmonary vascular resistance. Because of the increase in myocardial performance and the decrease of vascular resistance, large increases in cardiac output are obtained, facilitated by the unbridled chronotropic response. Arterial hypotension causing reflex increases in heart rate contributes to the tachycardia. Moreover, at variance with noradrenaline and dopamine, isoprenaline does not exert any presynaptic effect that could lessen the chronotropic response. Not surprisingly, arrhythmias are frequently observed when isoprenaline is administered, and these constitute a serious disadvantage of the drug. Enhancement of the inotropic and chronotropic state of the myocardium is necessarily accompanied by very substantial increases in myocardial oxygen consumption. In addition, because of the tachycardia and the reduced aortic diastolic pressure, coronary perfusion may be adversely affected and, in the presence of coronary artery disease, signs of myocardial ischaemia may easily develop. Experimentally, isoprenaline has been shown to increase the size of myocardial infarction and to increase the extent of ST segment elevation. Another indication of the imbalance between oxygen demand and oxygen supply is the marked reduction of myocardial lactate extraction caused by isoprenaline.

Because of its adverse effect on the ischaemic myocardium, isoprenaline is not indicated in the treatment of circulatory failure caused by myocardial infarction. Its use after cardiac surgery has declined because of the adverse effect on both myocardial and renal blood flow. However, when circulatory failure is associated with bradycardia, isoprenaline is a useful therapeutic agent that is particularly indicated in the emergency treatment of heart blocks.

Besides its aggravation of myocardial ischaemia, isoprenaline, in common with other catecholamines, may compromise arterial oxygenation in acute respiratory failure by increasing intrapulmonary shunting. One of the mechanisms of this increase in venous admixture is the inhibition of the hypoxic pulmonary vasoconstriction that normally diverts perfusion away from the poorly ventilated areas of the lungs.

Dopamine

The effects of dopamine on the circulation are complex and dose dependent (see Table 3). At low doses, it acts predominantly on specific dopaminergic receptors in the renal and mesenteric vasculature and causes a moderate reduction of diastolic arterial pressure. The major features of the effects of low doses of dopamine are increases in renal blood flow, glomerular filtration, and natriuresis. These effects are mediated by the dopaminergic receptors and are blocked by the butyrophenones, the phenothiazines, and by metoclopramide but not by beta-adrenoceptor antagonists. With higher doses of dopamine, beta-1 adrenoceptor stimulation becomes predominant, myocardial contractility is enhanced, and both cardiac output and arterial pressure increase. The elevation of arterial pressure tends to lessen the chronotropic response to beta-1 receptor stimulation. The tachycardia may also be lessened by the effect of dopamine on the alpha-2 presynaptic receptors. The tendency to arrhythmias is less pronounced with dopamine than with isoprenaline. Enhancement of myocardial performance and elevation of blood pressure are associated with large increases in myocardial oxygen consumption. However, unlike isoprenaline, dopamine tends to increase arterial pressure and to maintain or improve the coronary perfusion pressure. Although the balance between oxygen demand and oxygen supply is unlikely to be as markedly compromised by dopamine as it is by isoprenaline, the risk of increasing myocardial ischaemia still exists. At the highest doses, alpha-adrenoceptor-mediated peripheral vasoconstriction becomes an important determinant of the haemodynamic response to dopamine, and its effects resemble those of noradrenaline. This may be advantageous as the higher diastolic pressure increases coronary perfusion. However, the drawbacks are increased myocardial oxygen demand and reduced peripheral perfusion. Because of its beneficial effects on the renal circulation at low doses and of the lesser risk of arrhythmias, dopamine is extensively used in the treatment of circulatory failure. Dopamine is frequently used in the inotropic support of patients following cardiac surgery; at low and medium doses it has the considerable advantage of improving renal blood flow. Dopamine is effective in the treatment of chronic cardiac failure and may be useful in ischaemic acute renal failure when improving renal blood flow is of major concern.

Dobutamine

By substitution of the isoprenaline molecule it has been possible to obtain a drug exhibiting mostly beta-1 receptor agonist properties. The effects of dobutamine on the beta-2 receptors are considerably smaller than those of isoprenaline; similarly the effects of dobutamine on the alpha-adrenoceptors are much weaker than those of noradrenaline. Dobutamine does not exert any effect on the dopaminergic receptors. One major reason for the development of new synthetic catecholamines is an attempt to dissociate their inotropic and chronotropic properties, because tachycardia has a detrimental effect on the myocardial oxygen balance. Dobutamine, for an equivalent enhancement of the contractile state of the myocardium causes less increase of heart rate than isoprenaline. This may be explained by the lesser effect of dobutamine on the sinoatrial node and by reflex responses. With little or no beta-2-mediated vasodilation and with a modest effect on the alpha-receptors, dobutamine increases arterial pressure; this in turn, via baroceptor reflexes, minimizes the chronotropic response to beta-1 adrenoceptor stimulation. Enhancement of left ventricular performance is reflected by reductions of left ventricular end-diastolic pressure volume which enhance coronary perfusion. However, oxygen demand may still outstrip supply and dobutamine may worsen myocardial ischaemia, particularly in patients in whom it causes tachycardia. Dobutamine is an effective inotropic agent in the treatment of circulatory failure after cardiac surgery and is also very useful for patients with low cardiac output syndromes. When the low output is associated with ischaemic heart disease the combination of a venodilator with dobutamine makes it possible to reduce an abnormally high preload and to augment pump function. This explains why the combination nitroglycerine–dobutamine is fairly widely advocated.

Prenalterol

This selective beta-1 adrenoceptor agonist appears to increase the inotropic state of the myocardium wihout increasing heart rate. Prenalterol increases systolic blood pressure but does not affect diastolic arterial pressure. The less pronounced effect on heart rate may be explained by baroreceptor reflexes elicited by the elevation of arterial pressure. The duration of action of prenalterol is longer than that of the other catecholamines. Its positive inotropy has been demonstrated in patients suffering from myocardial infarction and, provided high doses are administered, it has been successfully used to counteract the effects on the heart of cardioselective beta-adrenergic blockage. While isoprenaline is useful to overcome the effects of non-cardioselective beta-adrenoceptor blockade, prenalterol is the agent of choice to overcome the effects of beta-1 adrenoceptor antagonists. Its place in the treatment of circulatory failure has not been determined yet.

At variance with the other catecholamines prenalterol may be given orally and increases cardiac output in patients with chronic cardiac failure.

Pirbuterol

This sympathomimetic amine exerts more effect on beta-1 than beta-2 receptors, and can be administered orally (20 mg doses). The inotropic effect is combined with arteriolar vasodilatation. Cardiac output and stroke volume are improved while the pulmonary capillary wedge pressure is reduced. Usually pirbuterol does not cause significant tachycardia. The effects of prolonged administration of this drug are not well established but its inotropic efficacy may be compromised by 'down-regulation' of receptors or by the gradual decrease of the number of receptors as cardiac failure worsens.

Salbutamol

Salbutamol is a beta-2 adrenoceptor agonist that has proved of great value in the treatment of bronchial asthma. It shows selectivity for bronchial and vascular smooth muscle beta-adrenoceptors. The major effect of salbutamol on the cardiovascular system is to cause peripheral vasodilation. The reduction of systemic vascular resistance facilitates left ventricular ejection and reduces both systolic left ventricular wall tension and left ventricular end-diastolic volume. The reduction of left ventricular systolic pressure decreases myocardial oxygen demand while the decrease of left ventricular end-diastolic pressure facilitates blood flow to the subendocardium during diastole. Secondary to improved myocardial oxygenation, left ventricular performance may improve. Salbutamol causes increases in heart rate. This may be due to stimulation of the cardiac beta-2 adrenoceptors and to reflexes caused by systolic hypotension. The increase in cardiac output is accompanied by a small increase in myocardial oxygen consumption. However, salbutamol causes more increase in heart rate than other peripheral vasodilators and this limits its usefulness in the treatment circulatory failure associated with ischaemic heart disease. Salbutamol dilates essential and non-essential vascular beds, and is particularly useful when circulatory failure is characterized by protracted vasoconstriction.

References

Bourdarias, J. P., Dubourg, O., Gueret, P., Ferrier, A. and Bardet, J. (1983). Inotropic agents in the treatment of cardiogenic shock. *Pharmacol. Ther.* **22**, 53–79.

Goldberg, L. I. (1977). The pharmacological basis of the clinical use of dopamine. *Proc. R. Soc. Med.* **70**, (suppl. 2), 7–15.

Leier, C. V. and Unverferth, D. V. (1983). Dobutamine. *Ann. Int. Med.* **99**, 490–496.

Mueller, H. D. (1977). Effects of dopamine in haemodynamics and myocardial energetics in man: comparison with effects of isoprenaline and L-noradrenaline. *Resuscitation* **6**, 179–189.

Mueller, H. D., Ayres, S. M., Gianelli, S., Foster Conklin, E. F., Mazzara, J. T. and Grace, W. J. (1972). Effect of isoproterenol, L-norepinephrine and intra-aortic counterpulsation on haemodynamic and myocardial metabolism in shock, following acute myocardial infarction. *Circulation* **45**, 335–351.

Sharma, B. and Goodwin, J. F. (1978). Beneficial effect of salbutamol on cardiac function in severe congestive cardiomyopathy. *Circulation* **58**, 449–460.

Stiles, G. L. and Lefkowitz, R. J. (1984). Cardiac adrenergic receptors. *Ann. Rev. Med.* **35**, 149–164.

Sonnenblick, E. H., Frishman, W. H. and Le Jemtel, T. H. (1979). Dobutamine: a new synthetic cardioactive sympathetic amine. *N. Engl. J. Med.* **300**, 17–22.

CARDIAC TRANSPLANTATION

T. A. H. ENGLISH

Introduction

The first human heart transplant was performed by Christiaan Barnard in 1967. Credit for the subsequent development of cardiac transplantation rests mainly with Dr Shumway and his group at Stanford University in California and it is largely due to their achievements that the last five years has seen an increasing interest in the more general application of transplantation to patients with terminal heart disease. This is illustrated by Fig. 1 which is derived from the register held by the International Society for Heart Transplantation. Latest indications suggest that the number of transplants performed in 1985 will be at least double those for 1984.

During the last few years a number of combined heart and lung transplants have also been performed. These have generally been for conditions associated with severe pulmonary vascular disease such as Eisenmenger's syndrome or primary pulmonary hypertension and, to a lesser extent, for primary lung disorders. The procedure, however, is still in a relatively developmental stage and will not be considered further in this review.

Indications

Cardiac transplantation should be considered for patients in congestive cardiac failure whose prognosis is limited and who continue to deteriorate despite full medical therapy. Usually they will be suffering from irreversible myocardial damage due to ischaemic heart disease or from dilated cardiomyopathy, often of unknown aetiology. Other causes of left ventricular disease such as end-stage valvular heart disease, tumours, sarcoid heart disease, and other rarities are occasionally encountered.

Potential recipients for heart transplantation need careful assessment. This is usually best accomplished by a short stay in the transplant centre after preliminary screening has suggested that the medical criteria for selection will be met. This allows the medical team to review carefully the patient's history, clinical condition, and cardiac investigations, while allowing the patient to become as informed as possible about the probability of duration and quality of survival after transplantation as well as the risks and complications that may be encountered.

Initially it was customary to define age limits of between approximately 15 and 50 years. It is now clear that good results can be obtained in both younger and older patients and therefore the main reason for retaining arbitrary age limits is to act as a filter because demand for the procedure is likely to exceed the necessary resources for many years to come. The pulmonary vascular resistance should not be unduly elevated (more than 6–8 Wood units), as the transplanted normal right ventricle is unable to pump against a high resistance. Active infection is another contraindication, as may be insulin-dependent diabetes. It is desirable for potential recipients to have a stable psychosocial background but it is difficult to deny transplantation on these grounds unless there is a recent history of mental illness.

Selection of cardiac donors

As with potential recipients, criteria for the selection of donor hearts for transplantation are necessary. Because of the prevalence of undetected coronary artery disease in the general popula-

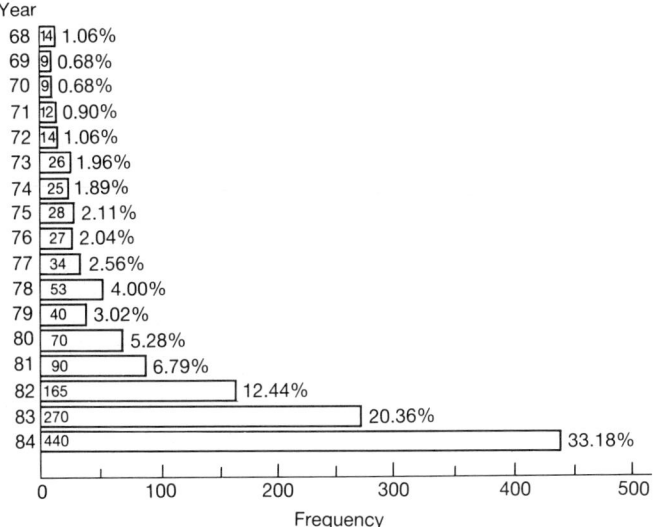

Year	Frequency	%
68	14	1.06%
69	9	0.68%
70	9	0.68%
71	12	0.90%
72	14	1.06%
73	26	1.96%
74	25	1.89%
75	28	2.11%
76	27	2.04%
77	34	2.56%
78	53	4.00%
79	40	3.02%
80	70	5.28%
81	90	6.79%
82	165	12.44%
83	270	20.36%
84	440	33.18%

Fig. 1 Number of transplants performed worldwide (1968–84). (Derived from the Registry of the International Society for Heart Transplantation.)

tion, it is undesirable to accept hearts from donors older than 35 to 40 years. Another reason for using hearts from young donors is evidence from the Stanford group that accelerated graft arteriosclerosis tends to develop more rapidly in recipients with hearts from donors aged more than 35 years.

Most donor hearts come from victims of road traffic accidents or patients with spontaneous intracerebral haemorrhage. Whatever the cause of neurological injury, the diagnosis of brain stem death should be clearly established according to the criteria outlined in the Report of the Royal Medical Colleges and their Faculties (1976). The tests should be repeated on two separate occasions and be performed by two doctors independent of the transplant team, one of whom should have been registered for at least five years. Most offers of cardiac donation arise either because the patient was carrying a donor card, or because the relatives, while agreeing to kidney donation, ask if the heart could not also be used. However, the supply of suitable donor hearts remains a limiting factor and at present about one-quarter of all patients waiting for transplantation die before a heart becomes available. Most hearts are obtained by distant procurement and with present methods of preservation ischaemic periods of up to four hours are well tolerated. Recipients and donors should be matched for size and ABO blood group compatibility. If the recipient has preformed cytotoxic antibodies in the serum, a negative crossmatch with the donor's lymphocytes should be obtained before proceeding to transplantation.

The operation

The operation of orthotopic transplantation involves excising both ventricles and leaving most of the right and left atria, with their respective venous connections, for anastomosis to the donor heart. The pulmonary arterial and aortic connections are completed last. Heterotopic transplantation, which is used infrequently, involves leaving the recipient's heart *in situ* and placing the donor heart in parallel to function as an implanted ventricular assist device.

Standard cardiopulmonary bypass techniques are used for the operation which has a low immediate mortality. Because the donor heart usually provides a normal cardiac output as soon as the operation is completed, most patients recover rapidly from the systemic effects of their pre-operative congestive cardiac failure.

Immunosuppression

As with any organ transplant, permanent immunosuppressive therapy is necessary. This needs to be most intense during the first few months after transplantation when acute rejection is most prevalent.

Until a few years ago, most heart transplant centres used 'conventional' immunotherapy comprising azathioprine and steroids. This was usually supplemented with a postoperative course of antithymocyte globulin, either of rabbit or equine origin. However, since 1982 cyclosporine has formed the basis of most immunosuppressive protocols. The incidence of rejection episodes has been reduced and those that do occur tend to be less acute and more readily reversed. This has resulted in improved probability of survival, fewer serious bacterial infections, and a reduced hospital stay leading to lower costs. Cyclosporine does, however, have several serious side-effects, the most important of which are nephrotoxicity and systemic hypertension. Both tend to be dose related and may compromise long-term graft and patient survival. Present options for dealing with this problem include either converting to conventional immunotherapy after three to six months, or using less cyclosporine by combining it with azathioprine with or without low-dose steroids. A possible future solution is the development of a non-nephrotoxic analogue of cyclosporine.

Postoperative management

After the operation there are two important early and two late complications that face the patient. These are, respectively, rejec-

tion and infection, and the development of accelerated vascular disease in the transplanted donor heart and an increased incidence of malignancy, particularly lymphoma.

Acute rejection tends to be episodic and the earlier it is detected and antirejection therapy instituted, the more likely it is to be reversed. Early rejection tends to be accompanied by oedema of the myocardium and a fall in summated QRS voltages in the ECG and, should this occur, endomyocardial biopsy is indicated. Biopsy is also undertaken if rejection is suspected on other grounds such as general malaise, the development of a third or fourth heart sound, fluid retention, or unexplained atrial arrhythmias. In any event, biopsies are performed at intervals of seven to ten days for the first few months and also to confirm reversal of rejection episodes.

The treatment of acute rejection depends to a certain extent on its timing and severity and whether histological evidence of regression is confirmed or not. Most early rejection episodes respond to intravenous methylprednisolone 1 g daily for three or four days. If particularly severe or recurrent, a course of antithymocyte globulin is added, whereas, if rejection occurs late and is mild, a course of oral prednisolone starting at 1 mg/kg/day and reducing to 0.2 mg/kg/day over two weeks may be all that is necessary.

Infectious episodes are commonest while immunosuppression is at its most intense, i.e. during the first few months or during prolonged treatment of rejection episodes. Bacterial infections are less common since the introduction of cyclosporine but viral and fungal infections, which may be difficult to diagnose and treat, are still an important cause of early morbidity and occasionally mortality. The possibility of donor-transmitted disease also needs to be considered, as may occur if the heart from a donor serologically positive for *Toxoplasma gondii* is transplanted into a serologically negative recipient. Many infections gain entry through the respiratory tract and, if the patient becomes febrile and develops a pulmonary infiltrate, every attempt should be made to identify the infecting organism as quickly as possible. Because of the prevalence of unusual and opportunistic organisms, it is generally best to defer antibiotic therapy until a microbiological diagnosis has been established.

Most patients are ready to leave hospital three to five weeks after transplantation. This interval can be further reduced if appropriate intermediate discharge accommodation is available nearby. After returning home, patients remain initially in close contact with the transplant centre and attend for routine biopsies at three, four, six, and twelve months after transplantation. Gradually, however, the referring physicians assume more and more responsibility for their management. Coronary arteriography is currently undertaken at annual intervals after the second year. This is because some patients develop a progressive coronary occlusive disease in the transplanted donor heart. This is an immunologically mediated lesion which may affect either the large epicardial arteries or the smaller intramyocardial vessels, and, although patients experience no angina because the heart is denervated, it may lead to cardiac failure and the need for retransplantation. Measures for trying to reduce the incidence of this complication include restriction of dietary lipids, regular exercise, and antiplatelet agents in the form of aspirin and dipyridamole. However, this phenomenon is likely to prove the most important determinant of long-term survival after heart transplantation.

As with any group of chronically immunosuppressed patients, there is an increased incidence of malignancy. Of particular interest is the development of lymphomas and lymphoproliferative disorders which may be related to Epstein–Barr virus and which often respond to a combination of intravenous acyclovir and temporarily reduced immunosuppression.

Results

Survival after transplantation is illustrated by experience at Papworth Hospital, where, since 1979, the first 134 patients had 1, 3, and 5 year probabilities of survival of 70, 55, and 51 per cent, respectively. Since cyclosporine was introduced in 1982, the 1 and 3 year survival has risen to 78 and 68 per cent.

Most patients who survive transplantation have excellent cardiac function and this has been documented objectively by left heart catheterization at the time of annual review and by right heart catheterization during rest and exercise. This good cardiac output is reflected subjectively in a much improved quality of life. Evidence for this has been confirmed by a comprehensive independent study of the costs and benefits of cardiac transplantation in the United Kingdom and has led to an increasing demand for the procedure. At present, the main limiting factors to the expansion of clinical cardiac transplantation are financial considerations and the availability of donor organs. With improved immunosuppressive protocols, hospital costs will probably be reduced still further, to the extent that overall costs are likely to be not much more than for a kidney transplant. So far as donors are concerned, there is reason to believe that, with changing public and medical attitudes, many more suitable organs may be offered than are currently made available. Eventually, it is likely that a reliable totally implantable artificial heart will provide an alternative form of heart substitution but at the present stage of technological development the various devices available are suitable only as temporary means of support until transplantation can be undertaken.

References

Barnard, C. N. (1967). A human cardiac transplant: an interim report of a successful operation performed at Groote Schuur Hospital, Cape Town. *S. Afr. Med. J.* **41**, 1271–1274.

Barnard, D. N., Barnard, M. S., Cooper, D. K. C., Churchio, C. A., Hassoulas, J., Novitsky, D. and Wolpowitz, A. (1981). The present status of heterotopic cardiac transplantation. *J. Thoracic Cardiovasc. Surg.* **81**, 433–439.

Bieber, C. P., Jamieson, S. W., Reitz, B. A., Oyer, P. E., Shumway, N. E. and Stinson, E. B. (1981). Complications in long-term survivors of cardiac transplantation. *Transplant. Proc.* **13**, 207–211.

Buxton, M., Acheson, R., Caine, N., Gibson, S. and O'Brien, B. (1985). Costs and benefits of the heart transplant programmes at Harefield and Papworth Hospitals. *Department of Health and Social Services Research Report* No. 12. HMSO, London.

Caves, P. K., Stinson, E. B., Billingham, M. E., Rider, A. K. and Shumway, N. E. (1973). Diagnosis of human cardiac allograft rejection by serial cardiac biopsy. *J. Thoracic Cardiovasc.* **66**, 461–467.

Conference of the Medical Royal Colleges and their Faculties in the United Kingdom (1976). Diagnosis of brain death. *Br. Med. J.* **2**, 1187–1188.

Report from the Council of the British Cardiac Society (1984). Cardiac transplantation in the United Kingdom. *Br. Heart J.* **52**, 679–682.

English, T. A. H., McGregor, C., Wallwork, J. and Cory-Pearce, R. (1982). Aspects of immunosuppression for cardiac transplantation at Papworth Hospital. *Heart Transplant.* **1**, 280–284.

——, Spratt, P., Wallwork, J., Cory-Pearce, R. and Wheeldon, D. (1984). Selection and procurement of hearts for transplantation. *Br. Med. J.* **288**, 1889–1891.

Griepp, R. B., Stinson, E. B. and Bieber, C. P. *et al.* (1977). Control of graft arteriosclerosis in human heart transplant recipients. *Surgery* **81**, 262–269.

Griffith, B. P., Hardesty, R. L., Deeb, G. M., Starzl, T. E. and Bahnson, H. T. (1982). Cardiac transplantation with cyclosporin A and prednisone. *Ann. Surg.* **196**, 324–329.

Krikorian, J. G., Anderson, J. L., Bieber, C. P., Penn, I. and Stinson, E. B. (1978). Malignant neoplasms following cardiac transplantation. *J. Am. Med. Assoc.* **240**, 639–643.

Myers, B. D., Ross, J., Newton, L., Leutscher, J. and Perlroth, M. (1984). Cyclosporine-associated chronic nephropathy. *N. Engl. J. Med.* **311**, 699–704.

Oyer, P. E., Stinson, E. B., Jamieson, S. W., Hunt, S. A., Billingham, M., Bieber, C. P., Reitz, B. A. and Shumway, N. E. (1983). Cyclosporin-A in cardiac allografting: a preliminary experience. *Transplant. Proc.* **15**, 1247–1252.

Pennock, J. K., Oyer, P. E., Reitz, B. A., Jamieson, S. W., Bieber, C. P., Wallwork, J., Stinson, E. B. and Shumway, N. E. (1982). Cardiac transplantation in perspective for the future: survival, complications, rehabilitation and cost. *J. Thoracic Cardiovasc. Surg.* **83**, 168–176.

Ryning, F. W., McLeod, R., Maddox, J. C., Hunt, S. and Remington, J. (1979). Probable transmission of toxoplasma gondii by organ transplantation. *Ann. inter. Med.* **90**, 47–49.

Starzl, T. E., Porter, K. A., Iswatsuki, S., Rosenthal, J. T., Shaw, B. W., Atchison, R. W., Nalesnik, M. A., Ho, M., Griffith, B. P., Hakala, T. R., Hardesty, R. L., Jaffe, R. and Bahnson, H. T. (1984). Reversibility of lymphomas and lymphoproliferative lesions developing under cyclosporin–steroid therapy. *Lancet* 583–587.

Thompson, M. E., Shapiro, A. P., Johnsen, A. M., Reeves, R., Itzkoff, J., Ginchereau, E., Hardesty, R. L., Griffith, B. L., Bahnson, H. T. and McDonald, R. (1983). New onset of hypertension following cardiac transplantation: a preliminary report and analysis. *Transplant. Proc.* **15**, 2573–2577.

Watson, D. C., Reitz, B. A., Baumgartner, W. A., Raney, A. A., Oyer, P. E., Stinson, E. B. and Shumway, N. E. (1979). Distant heart procurement for transplantation. *Surgery* **86**, 56–59.

CARDIAC ARRHYTHMIAS

D. H. BENNETT

An arrhythmia is defined as any cardiac rhythm other than normal sinus rhythm.

Arrhythmias can be divided into disorders of impulse conduction and of impulse formation. Impairment can occur in conduction of either the sinus node impulse to the atria or of the resultant atrial impulse to the ventricles. Disordered impulse formation can be due to an abnormal site of origin and/or rate of impulse discharge.

Only atrial and ventricular activity register on the surface electrocardiogram. The site of impulse formation, sequence of cardiac chamber activation, and functions of the sinus node and the atrioventricular (AV) junction have to be deduced from analysis of atrial and ventricular electrograms.

A single 'rhythm strip' may be inadequate for diagnosis. Scrutiny of several ECG leads recorded during an arrhythmia, preferably simultaneously, may be necessary. For example, atrial activity is often the key to diagnosis but may not be shown clearly in all ECG leads: it is usually best seen in leads II and V_1.

Sinus rhythms

Normal sinus rhythm

Atrial activity begins in the sinus node, which is situated at the junction of the superior vena cava and right atrium, and spreads in an inferior direction. Thus, the atrial electrogram (P wave) is upright in leads orientated towards the inferior surface of the heart (II, AVF) and is inverted in AVR which is orientated towards the superior aspect of the heart. If a P wave does not have these characteristics then it has not arisen from the sinus node (Fig. 1).

Sometimes the P wave is of low amplitude and it is necessary to inspect all leads to establish that there is sinus rhythm.

In adults, normal sinus rhythm is arbitrarily defined as a sinus node rate of 60–100 per minute.

If AV and intraventricular conduction are normal, each P wave will be followed by a ventricular electrogram (QRS complex)

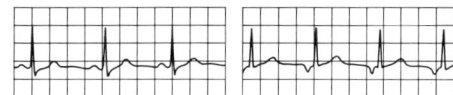

Fig. 1 Lead II during sinus rhythm (on left) and AV junctional rhythm (on right). The P wave is inverted during junctional rhythm.

whose duration is less than 0.08 s after a PR interval of 0.12–0.21 s (Fig. 1). However in some arrhythmias, ventricular activity is dissociated from atrial activity which continues to be initiated by the sinus node. For example, sinus rhythm often coexists with complete AV block.

Sinus bradycardia

This is sinus rhythm at a rate below 60 per minute (Fig. 2). It may be physiological as in athletes or during sleep, or secondary to acute myocardial infarction, sick sinus syndrome, or drugs such as beta-blockers. Non-cardiac disorders, e.g. hypothyroidism, jaundice, and raised intracranial pressure, can also cause sinus bradycardia. The rate may be increased by atropine or pacing but treatment is only indicated when sinus bradycardia causes symptoms.

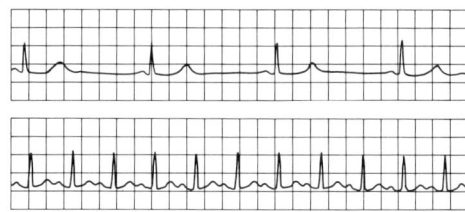

Fig. 2 Sinus bradycardia (above) and sinus tachycardia (below).

Sinus tachycardia

This is defined as sinus rhythm at a rate greater than 100 per minute (Fig. 2). It may be caused by exercise, anxiety, or any disorder which increases sympathetic nervous system activity. Occasionally, sinus tachycardia may be due to a primary disorder of the sinus node (sinus node re-entry).

Sinus tachycardia is usually a physiological response and as such does not require specific treatment. However, if sinus tachycardia is inappropriate, the rate may be slowed by beta-adrenergic blockade.

Sinus arrhythmia

In sinus arrhythmia there are alternating periods of gradual slowing and increasing sinus node rate. The difference between shortest and longest cycle lengths is not greater than 0.16 s. Usually the rate increases with inspiration.

Extrasystoles

The terms extrasystole, ectopic beat, and premature contraction differ in their precise meaning but for practical purposes are equivalent. They refer to an impulse originating from the atria, A V junction (i.e. AV node plus the bundle of His) or ventricles, which arises prematurely in the cardiac cycle (Figs 3–6). Because an extrasystole is premature its coupling interval (i.e. the interval between it and the preceding beat) is shorter than the cycle length of the dominant rhythm. Usually, extrasystoles which arise from the same focus have the same coupling interval and configuration.

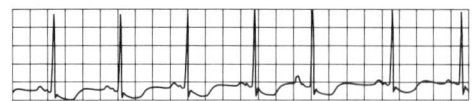

Fig. 3 The fifth beat is an atrial extrasystole, normally conducted to the ventricles.

Atrial extrasystoles

These are recognized by a premature P wave which, because the source and hence direction of atrial activation differ from that during sinus rhythm, will usually be of abnormal shape (Fig. 3). Atrial extrasystoles with a normal P wave configuration are thought to arise from the region of the sinus node.

Most atrial extrasystoles are conducted to the ventricles in the same manner as if the atria had been activated by the sinus node (Fig. 3). However, sometimes atrial extrasystoles, especially those that arise very early in the cardiac cycle, may encounter an AV junction or a bundle branch which has not yet recovered from conduction of the preceding atrial impulse and is, therefore, partially or completely refractory to excitation. Partial and complete refractoriness of the AV junction will result in prolongation of the PR interval and blocked atrial extrasystoles, respectively (Fig. 4). Corresponding impairment of conduction in one or other bundle branch, usually the right bundle, will lead to partial or complete bundle branch block (Fig. 4): this phenomenon of functional bundle branch block is known as 'phasic aberrant intraventricular conduction'. The resultant QRS complex is broad and may be mistaken for a ventricular extrasystole unless a preceding ectopic P wave is identified.

Atrial extrasystoles may be smaller than normal and, because they are premature, may be superimposed on the T wave of the preceding ventricular complex. Often, they are best shown in lead V_1 (Fig. 4).

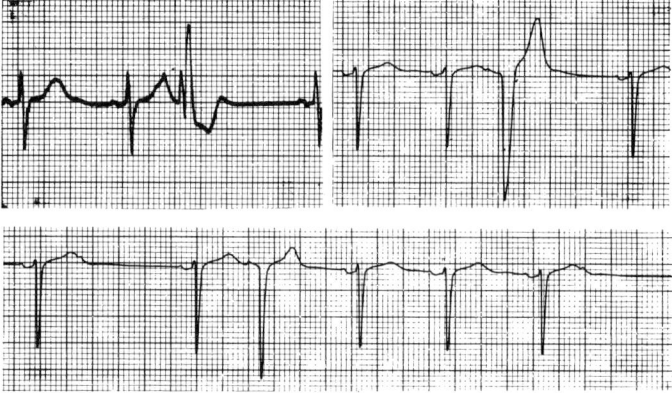

Fig. 4 Three cases of very early atrial extrasystoles, all recorded from lead V_1. The extrasystoles are superimposed on and hence deform the preceding T wave. The upper two examples show phasic aberrant intraventricular conduction of the right and left bundle branches. The lower example shows non-conducted extrasystoles (superimposed on the T waves of the first and sixth complexes) and an extrasystole conducted with partial left bundle branch block (after second ventricular complex).

AV junctional extrasystoles

These used to be termed nodal beats but it is now appreciated that at least part of the AV node is not capable of pacemaker activity and that it is not possible to distinguish between beats of AV nodal and His bundle origin. Hence the more general term 'AV junction'.

AV junctional extrasystoles produce a premature QRS complex similar in configuration to that occurring during sinus rhythm (Fig. 5). The atria as well as ventricles may be activated by the junctional focus, leading to an inverted P wave (i.e. inverted in leads II and AVF) which may precede, follow, or be buried within

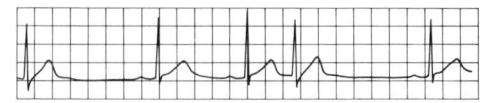

Fig. 5 The fourth beat is a junctional extrasystole.

the QRS complex, depending on the relative speeds of conduction from AV junction to the ventricles and to the atria.

Ventricular extrasystoles

Ventricular extrasystoles are recognized by a premature ventricular complex which is broad (usually > 0.12 s), bizarre in shape and, in contrast to atrial extrasystoles, will clearly not be preceded by a premature P wave (Fig. 6). The abnormal shape and duration of the ventricular complex reflect the abnormal course and consequent slowing of ventricular activation. The abnormal pattern of ventricular activation leads to abnormal recovery and hence ST segment and T wave abnormalities.

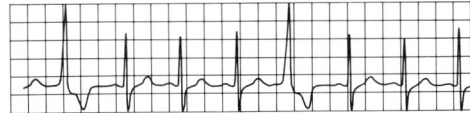

Fig. 6 Unifocal ventricular extrasystoles after first and fourth sinus beats.

Timing of ventricular extrasystoles

Ventricular extrasystoles which occur very early in the cardiac cycle will be superimposed on the T wave of the preceding beat and are called 'R on T' ventricular extrasystoles (Fig. 7). Most episodes of ventricular fibrillation and many episodes of ventricular tachycardia are initiated by R on T extrasystoles though by no means all of this type of extrasystole precipitate an arrhythmia.

Some extrasystoles arise relatively late in the cardiac cycle and may fall, by chance, immediately after a P wave initiated by sinus node activity. These are termed 'end-diastolic' ventricular extrasystoles and should not be confused with atrial extrasystoles with aberrant intraventricular conduction which will, of course, be preceded by a premature rather than normally timed P wave.

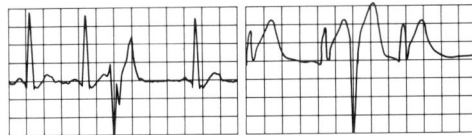

Fig. 7 Two examples of 'R on T' ventricular extrasystoles; one is an interpolated extrasystole (on right).

Compensatory pause

The length of the pause after a ventricular extrasystole depends on whether the extrasystolic impulse is transmitted by the AV junction back to the atria. If there is no retrograde AV conduction, the sinus node will be unaffected and there will be a full compensatory pause, i.e. the lengths of the cycles before and after the extrasystole will equal twice the sinus cycle length (Fig. 6). A full compensatory pause is often regarded as characteristic of a ventricular extrasystole. However, ventricular extrasystoles may be conducted retrogradely to the atria and will thus activate the sinus node. The subsequent sinus node impulse will therefore be discharged earlier than normal and result in an incomplete compensatory pause.

Sometimes there is no pause after a ventricular extrasystole which is referred to as an interpolated beat (Fig. 7).

Frequency of extrasystoles

A number of terms are used to describe the frequency of extrasystoles, particularly when of ventricular origin. When an extrasystole follows each sinus beat, the term bigeminy is applied (Fig. 8), and when there is an extrasystole following every two sinus beats, there is trigeminy. Two ventricular extrasystoles in succession are called a couplet (Fig. 8) and when there are three or more the group is referred to as a salvo or ventricular tachycardia.

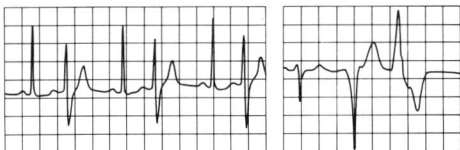

Fig. 8 Ventricular bigemy (on left) and a couplet of ventricular extrasystoles with different foci (on right).

Ventricular parasystole

Ventricular parasystole is an exception to the rule that unifocal ventricular extrasystoles have a constant coupling interval. In parasystole, the ectopic focus discharges regularly, unrelated to and undisturbed by the dominant rhythm. It will activate the ventricles provided they are not refractory due to prior excitation by the dominant pacemaker. Thus, parasystole is characterized by a variable coupling interval, interectopic intervals which are a multiple of a common factor, and because the ventricles may by chance be simultaneously activated by both ectopic and normal pacemakers, by fusion beats (Fig. 9).

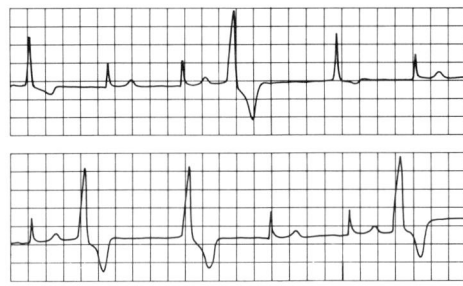

Fig. 9 Ventricular parasystole. The two strips are a continuous recording. Extrasystoles are separated by intervals which are multiples of 1.2 s. The first and fifth ventricular complexes are fusion beats.

Significance and treatment of extrasystoles

Occasional supraventricular and unifocal ventricular extrasystoles can occur in normal hearts and are not necessarily pathological.

Frequent atrial extrasystoles may herald the onset of atrial fibrillation or flutter. In patients with valvar, coronary or myocardial disease, it is advisable to give digoxin so that the ventricular rate may be controlled should these tachycardias arise.

Frequent ventricular extrasystoles during exertion may occur in subjects with normal hearts, but extrasystoles which are frequent at rest or are 'complex' (i.e. multifocal, R on T, or occur in salvoes) are rarely found in the absence of cardiac disease and are associated with an increased cardiovascular mortality. The main concern about ventricular extrasystoles is that they may initiate ventricular tachycardia or fibrillation. In acute myocardial infarction, complex extrasystoles were thought to herald dangerous ventricular arrhythmias but it is now appreciated that they are very common, are not reliable 'warning arrhythmias', and do not usually merit antiarrhythmic therapy. In chronic heart disease, there is a correlation between ventricular dysfunction, which is related to prognosis, and frequency of ventricular extrasystoles. However, recent evidence does suggest that ventricular extrasystoles are an additional and independent risk factor for cardiovascular mortality though there is little data to show that their suppression by drugs will improve prognosis.

Extrasystoles usually cause little or no symptoms but in some patients, even those without structural heart disease, distressing symptoms result from the irregularity in heart rhythm and/or 'thump' caused by increased myocardial contractility with the post-extrasystolic beat. In these patients, therapy may be required for symptomatic rather than prognostic purposes.

Ventricular extrasystoles associated with a bradycardia can

usually be abolished by increasing the heart rate rather than by antiarrhythmic drugs.

Escape beats

Escape beats arise from subsidiary pacemakers when the dominant pacemaker fails to discharge. In contrast to extrasystoles, they are late rather than premature, i.e. the coupling interval is greater than the cycle length of the dominant rhythm (Figs 10 and 11).

Escape beats usually arise from the AV junction though less commonly from the ventricles. The site of origin, like extrasystoles, is determined from their configuration.

Distinction between escape beats and extrasystoles is important because the former should clearly not be suppressed by drugs. If treatment is indicated, it is to increase the heart rate.

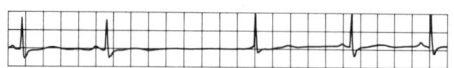

Fig. 10 The third beat is a junctional escape beat resulting from sinus arrest.

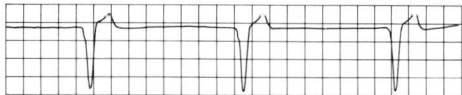

Fig. 11 Three ventricular escape beats resulting from sinus arrest.

Tachycardias of supraventricular origin

Several different tachycardias originate from the atria or AV junction and therefore come under this heading (Table 1). They have one thing in common: because their origin is above the level of the bundle branches, they usually result in narrow ventricular complexes. However, within this group there are major differences in mechanism, ECG characteristics, and treatment. It is, therefore, necessary to specify the type of arrhythmia that one is dealing with and not merely refer to it as a supraventricular tachycardia.

AV re-entrant (paroxysmal supraventricular) tachycardia

This arrhythmia is due to the repeated circulation of an impulse between atria and ventricles (Fig. 12a). It can only occur if there is, in addition to the AV node, a second connection between atria and ventricles. The additional connection is either actually within, but functionally separate from, the AV node or, in the case of the pre-excitation syndromes, is an anatomically distinct pathway between atria and ventricles. The circulating impulse is usually conducted from atria to ventricles by the normal AV junction and then re-enters the atria via the additional connection (Fig. 12b, c). A variety of terms are used to refer to this tachycardia. Some reflect its mechanism, e.g. AV re-entrant, AV junctional re-entrant, and reciprocating AV nodal tachycardia. Others are inappropriate, e.g. atrial tachycardia and junctional tachycardia, because they are also used to refer to tachycardias due to enhanced automaticity (see below).

Table 1 Tachycardias of supraventricular origin

AV re-entrant (paroxysmal supraventricular) tachycardia
Atrial fibrillation
Atrial flutter
Atrial tachycardia
Junctional tachycardia

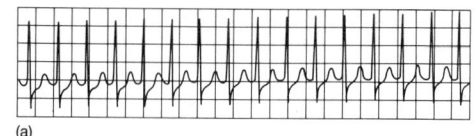

(a)

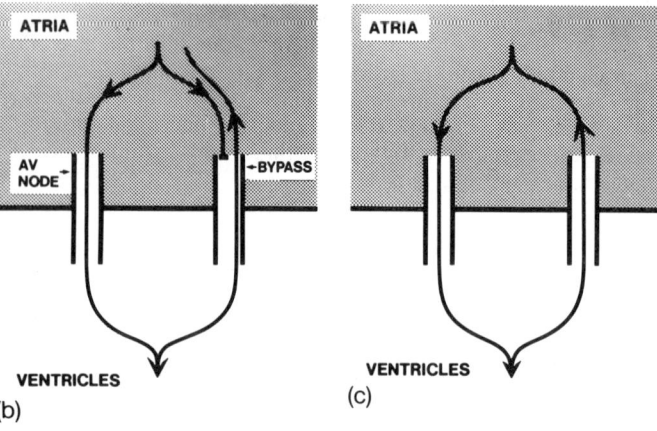

(b)   (c)

Fig. 12 (a) AV re-entrant (paroxysmal supraventricular) tachycardia. (b, c) Initiation of AV re-entrant tachycardia. An atrial extrasystole occurs whilst the bypass tract is still refractory to excitation. The extrasystole is conducted to the ventricles via the AV node by which time the bypass has recovered and can conduct the impulse back to the atria, initiating the re-entrant mechanism.

The basis for AV and other re-entrant tachycardias is the presence of two interconnected pathways which differ in their refractory periods and conduction speeds (some ventricular and atrial arrhythmias are also due to a re-entrant mechanism facilitated by the presence of two functionally dissociated regions within the ventricles or atria, respectively). Tachycardia is initiated when an extrasystole arises at such a time that one pathway is refractory but the other is capable of conduction. The pathway with the shorter refractory period must conduct relatively slowly, allowing the other pathway to recover in sufficient time to perpetuate the circus movement.

ECG characteristics
The tachycardia is regular. In the absence of pre-existing bundle branch block or phasic aberrant intraventricular conduction, the QRS complexes are narrow (Figs 12, 13, and 33).

The rate during tachycardia is usually between 130 and 250 per minute. Assumption of the standing position increases sympathetic tone and consequently the speed of AV nodal conduction with the result that the tachycardia becomes faster.

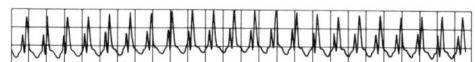

Fig. 13 AV re-entrant tachycardia (lead V$_1$) with phasic aberrant intraventricular conduction causing right bundle branch block.

Since the circulating impulse re-enters the atria after ventricular activation, there will be a 1:1 ratio between atrial and ventricular activity. If the atrial rate exceeds the ventricular rate, whether spontaneously or due to a drug or manoeuvre which slows AV nodal conduction, then the rhythm is atrial tachycardia or flutter.

During sinus rhythm, the ECG is usually normal unless there is ventricular pre-excitation. As in most tachycardias, ST segment and T wave changes can be caused by the AV re-entrant tachycardia and persist for some time after its cessation.

Clinical features
The arrhythmia is common. In most cases the heart is structurally normal, i.e. there is no valve, myocardial or coronary artery disease. Attacks may start in infancy, childhood, or adult life and are often recurrent. The duration and frequency of attacks are vari-

able; they may last for a few minutes or for many hours and may recur several times per day or be separated by many months.

The main symptom is rapid palpitation of abrupt onset. Although the arrhythmia stops suddenly, not all patients are aware of this since sinus tachycardia often follows.

Polyuria may sometimes accompany tachycardia and may relate to release of atrial natriuretic peptide. Faintness, syncope, and chest pain can also occur, particularly with very fast rates. A very prolonged episode of tachycardia may cause heart failure even in a structurally normal heart.

Treatment

Short episodes of tachycardia without distress do not require treatment.

The first approach to termination of the tachycardia is vagal stimulation. By increasing vagal tone, AV node conduction may be slowed and the circuit thereby interrupted. Carotid sinus massage is the best method. Other methods of vagal stimulation include the Valsalva manoeuvre, the 'diving reflex', and eyeball pressure. The latter is painful and not recommended.

If vagal stimulation fails, intravenous verapamil (5–10 mg over 30–60 seconds) will almost certainly terminate the arrhythmia within a couple of minutes. If an adequate dose of verapamil fails, the diagnosis should be reconsidered. If necessary, up to three injections of verapamil can be given in a day. *Verapamil should not be used if the patient has recently received a beta-blocker.* Alternative intravenous drugs include a beta-blocker, disopyramide, amiodarone, and adenosine triphosphate.

If drugs are ineffective or if the clinical circumstances necessitate immediate restoration of sinus rhythm, cardioversion is the simplest approach. Artificial pacing can also be used to terminate the arrhythmia by depolarizing myocardium immediately ahead of the stimulus circulating between atria and ventricles; thereby interrupting the re-entrant mechanism. Simple methods include overdrive right atrial pacing at a rate 20–30 per cent faster than the tachycardia and underdrive right ventricular pacing at 70–100 beats/min. A more sophisticated method is the introduction of a single or couplet of either atrial or ventricular stimuli, whose timing has to be established precisely so that the tachycardia circuit can be interrupted (Fig. 14a). These methods can be employed long-term using a fully implantable pacemaker in patients in whom drugs are ineffective or cannot be tolerated.

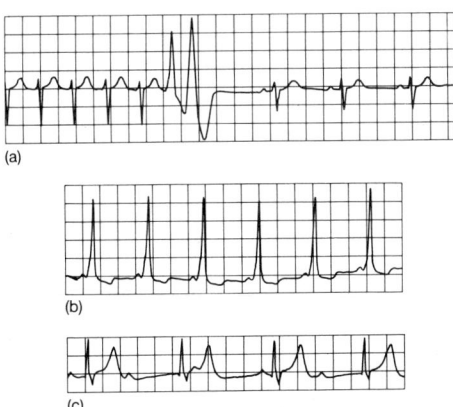

(a)

(b)

(c)

Fig. 14 (a) AV re-entrant tachycardia terminated by a couplet of precisely timed right ventricular stimuli. (b, c) Transvenous ablation in a patient with Wolff–Parkinson–White syndrome due to a septal accessory pathway. Both AV nodal and accessory pathway conduction were interrupted. Upper tracing before, and lower after, the procedure.

Prophylaxis

The patient should be reassured that the tachycardia is distressing rather than dangerous and that it is due to an electrical rather than structural abnormality.

A number of drugs may be of prophylactic value, including beta-blockers (especially sotalol), digoxin, verapamil, disopyramide, and quinidine. Selection of the most effective drug is often a process of trial and error. Amiodarone is likely to be effective in cases where other drugs have failed but should be reserved for refractory cases where the need for tachycardia control outweighs the drug's possible unwanted effects. The patient should keep a record of the number and duration of any attacks so that the effect of therapy can be assessed.

In some patients, both drugs and antitachycardia pacing are ineffective. An alternative is surgical division of one part of the re-entrant circuit: the AV junction or, if accessible, the additional connection. Recently non-surgical ablation of AV conduction has been introduced. This is achieved by passing a high-energy (200–400 joules) direct current shock to the AV junction via a transvenous pacing lead positioned as close to the bundle of His as possible (Fig. 14b, c). In spite of the high energy used, damage is confined to the region of the AV junction and the technique has proved safe. Creation of heart block does necessitate pacemaker implantation. A similar technique has been used in a few patients for ablation of accessory pathways (Fig. 14b, c) and foci of origin of atrial and ventricular tachycardias.

A detailed intracardiac electrophysiological study is required to assess the feasibility of ablation, antitachycardia pacing, and surgery.

Supraventricular tachycardias due to enhanced automaticity

Although the precise mechanisms may be more complex, atrial, tachycardia, flutter, and fibrillation can be considered to be due to enhanced automaticity of atrial ectopic foci. Similarly, junctional tachycardia is due to enhanced automaticity of an AV junctional focus.

Atrial fibrillation

In atrial fibrillation, the atria discharge at a rate between 350 and 600 per minute. Fortunately, the AV node cannot conduct at a sufficient frequency to allow all atrial impulses to reach the ventricles. After an impulse has been conducted to the ventricles, the AV node will be refractory to excitation by other impulses for a short period. Some impulses only partially penetrate the AV node. They will not therefore activate the ventricles but do block or delay succeeding impulses. This process of 'concealed conduction' is responsible for the totally irregular ventricular response characteristic of atrial fibrillation.

Usually the AV node does not allow a ventricular rate in excess of 200 per minute and, when AV node conduction is depressed by drugs or disease, the ventricular response is much slower.

ECG characteristics

The rapid, chaotic atrial activity is reflected by 'f' waves which are irregular in rate and size (Fig. 15). However 'f' waves may not be seen in all leads; usually they are best seen in lead V_1. Clearly, P waves will be absent.

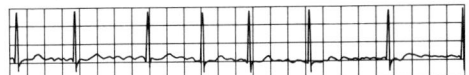

Fig. 15 Atrial fibrillation.

The most important characteristic of atrial fibrillation is the totally irregular ventricular response. Atrial fibrillation, particularly when there is a rapid ventricular rate, is often misdiagnosed because this feature is ignored (Fig. 16). The only circumstance in which there is a regular ventricular rhythm during atrial fibrillation is when there is complete AV block.

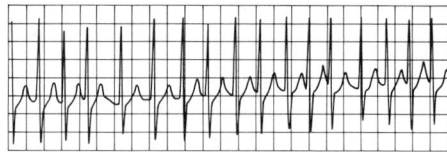

Fig. 16 Atrial fibrillation with a rapid ventricular response. Diagnosis is based on the totally irregular ventricular rhythm.

Sometimes the pattern of atrial activity is so coarse that atrial flutter rather than fibrillation is suspected (Fig. 17). In the latter case, the atrial rate will usually be greater than 350 per minute and the ventricular response will be totally irregular.

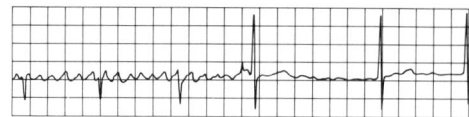

Fig. 17 Atrial fibrillation. Continuous recording as lead changed from V$_1$ to V$_4$, showing how atrial activity can differ in appearance.

Phasic aberrant intraventricular conduction is often seen during atrial fibrillation. It is the result of unequal refractory periods of the bundle branches. An early atrial impulse may reach the ventricles when one bundle branch is still refractory and therefore not capable of conduction whilst the other bundle has recovered and will conduct. The resultant ventricular complex will show bundle branch block. Refractory periods prolong with increasing cycle length. Thus, aberration is usually seen when a beat having a short cycle length follows one with a long cycle length (Fig. 18).

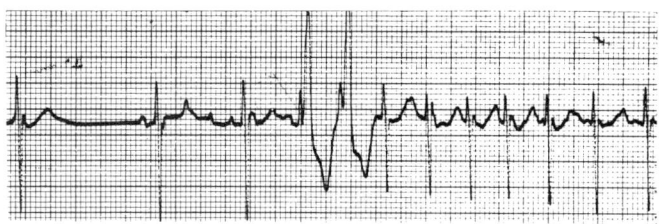

Fig. 18 Atrial fibrillation initiated by an atrial extrasystole superimposed on the T wave of the second ventricular complex (lead V$_1$). There is phasic aberrant intraventricular conduction of the fourth and fifth ventricular beats.

Clinical features

Atrial fibrillation is one of the most common arrhythmias. Causes include rheumatic heart disease, coronary and hypertensive heart disease, thyrotoxicosis, sick sinus syndrome, myopericarditis, dilated and hypertrophic cardiomyopathies, specific heart muscle diseases, constrictive pericarditis, atrial septal defect, alcohol abuse, pulmonary embolism, thoracotomy, and trauma. In a substantial proportion of cases, the arrhythmia is idiopathic and is referred to as 'lone atrial fibrillation'.

Atrial fibrillation may be paroxysmal or persistent. The major determinant of prognosis is the presence or absence of organic heart disease. Paroxysmal lone atrial fibrillation has a normal prognosis.

The arrhythmia results in loss of atrial systole, which may reduce cardiac output and elevate left atrial pressure. During atrial fibrillation, stasis of blood in the left atrium may occur and lead to thrombus formation and systemic embolism. Patients with rheumatic mitral valve disease are at greatest risk whereas embolism is very rare in lone atrial fibrillation. In patients with atrial fibrillation from all causes except mitral valve disease, there is a five-fold increase in the incidence of stroke whereas mitral valve disease increases the incidence seventeen-fold. Several studies

report a high incidence of systemic embolism in atrial fibrillation caused by acute thyrotoxicosis.

Treatment

In most cases, treatment is aimed at controlling the ventricular response to atrial fibrillation by the use of a drug or drugs which depress AV nodal conduction. Although cardioversion will often restore sinus rhythm, there is a high relapse rate, particularly when there is cardiomegaly, marked left atrial enlargement, or when the arrhythmia has been present for a long time. Long-term quinidine, disopyramide, and amiodarone do slightly reduce the relapse rate. When atrial fibrillation has been caused by an acute event, there is a good chance that sinus rhythm will be maintained after cardioversion.

Occasionally, atrial fibrillation with a rapid ventricular response will cause shock or severe heart failure and necessitate immediate cardioversion. When prompt reduction of the ventricular rate is required, digoxin or verapamil can be given intravenously: the latter will work within a couple of minutes. If there is no urgency, control can usually be achieved with oral digoxin. If control is unsatisfactory in spite of apparently adequate digitilization, the addition of verapamil or a beta-blocker will effect control. Occasionally, these measures fail, in which case one may have to resort to amiodarone or even transvenous ablation of the AV junction. In patients with paroxysmal atrial fibrillation, suppression of atrial extrasystoles by quinidine or amiodarone may prevent further attacks.

Anticoagulation to prevent systemic embolism is indicated in cases of rheumatic mitral valve disease and when there is a history of embolism. It should also be considered in the bradycardia–tachycardia syndrome and acute thyrotoxicosis.

Atrial flutter

In atrial flutter, the atria discharge at a rate between 250 and 350 per minute. Usually the atrial rate is close to 300 per minute. Very rarely, the AV node conducts all atrial impulses to the ventricles resulting in a dangerously fast ventricular rate. In most cases, a degree of AV block occurs. In patients with a healthy AV node who are not receiving AV nodal blocking drugs, there is usually 2:1 AV block.

ECG characteristics

The rapid atrial activity is reflected by 'F' waves which are regular. Often, there is no isoelectric line between 'F' waves so that the baseline has a saw-tooth appearance. Although commonly seen, it is not essential for the diagnosis. Some leads show this appearance whilst others, particularly V$_1$, show discrete 'F' waves (Fig. 19).

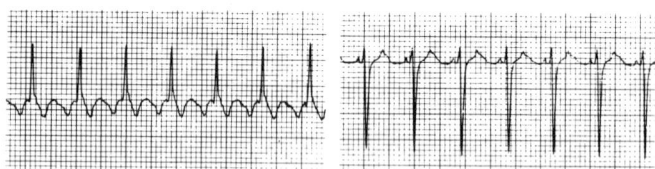

Fig. 19 Atrial flutter with 2:1 AV block. Lead AVF (on left) shows the characteristic saw-tooth baseline whereas lead V$_1$ (on right) shows discrete atrial activity, alternate 'F' waves being superimposed on ventricular T waves.

With a high degree of AV block, atrial flutter is easy to diagnose. However, when there is 2:1 AV block, the rapid ventricular response may conceal atrial activity with the result that the diagnosis is frequently missed, often being mistaken for sinus tachycardia. In 2:1 AV block, the resultant ventricular rate will be approximately 150 per minute. If a patient has this heart rate at rest, atrial flutter should be suspected. Usually, alternate 'F' waves will be superimposed on ventricular T waves and will only be identified by close inspection of the ECG, particularly lead V$_1$. Temporary increase in AV block by carotid sinus massage may aid diagnosis (Fig. 20).

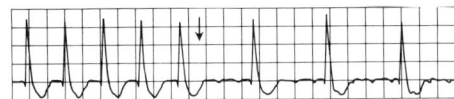

Fig. 20 Atrial flutter with 2:1 AV block. The ventricular rate is slowed by carotid sinus massage (arrow) revealing an atrial rate of 300 per minute.

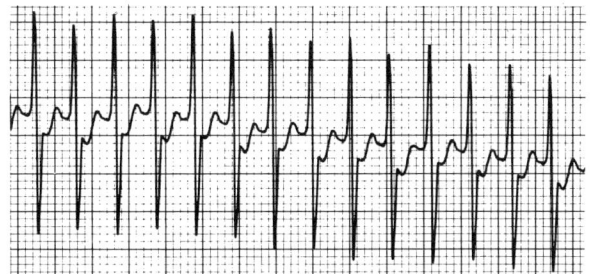

Fig. 21 Atrial flutter with 1:1 AV conduction resulting in a ventricular rate of 300 per minute.

A ventricular rate of 300 per minute suggests atrial flutter with 1:1 AV conduction (Fig. 21).

Causes
Atrial flutter is less common than atrial fibrillation but the causes are the same.

Treatment
It is often difficult to control the ventricular rate during atrial flutter with AV nodal blocking drugs, and a return to sinus rhythm should therefore be sought. Cardioversion is usually successful. An alternative is rapid right atrial pacing for about one minute at a rate 20–30 per cent in excess of the atrial rate. It is important to ensure that pacing stimuli capture the atria; this is usually reflected by a change in ventricular rate. On abrupt cessation of pacing, sinus rhythm will return in approximately one-third of patients. In another one-third, atrial fibrillation will be precipitated but this often reverts to sinus rhythm.

In patients with a rapid ventricular rate, intravenous verapamil can be used to increase the degree of AV block temporarily. In about one-fifth of cases, verapamil will restore sinus rhythm.

Atrial tachycardia
In atrial tachycardia the atrial rate is slower than in atrial flutter, being between 120 and 250 per minute. Usually, there is a degree of AV block though 1:1 AV conduction can occur.

ECG characteristics
Because the atrial rate is slower, there is no saw-tooth baseline appearance (Fig. 22). Like atrial flutter, atrial activity is often best seen in lead V_1. When there is 1:1 conduction, carotid sinus massage will clarify the diagnosis. With fairly high degrees of AV block, because the atrial rate is relatively slow, the rhythm may be misdiagnosed as complete heart block.

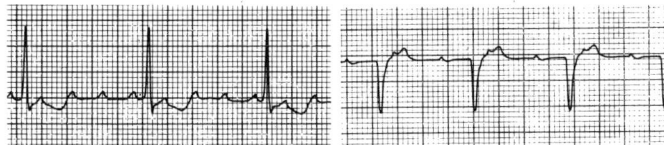

Fig. 22 Two examples of atrial tachycardia with AV block: the atrial rates being 245 (left) and 160 (right) per minute.

Causes
Atrial tachycardia with AV block is commonly due to digoxin toxicity. Although the arrhythmia is often referred to as 'paroxysmal atrial tachycardia with block', the arrhythmia is usually sustained. Other causes include cardiomyopathy, chronic ischaemic heart disease, rheumatic heart disease, and sick sinus syndrome.

Treatment
Digoxin should be stopped if toxicity is suspected. In patients who have not had digoxin this or other AV nodal blocking drugs may be used to control the ventricular rate. A return to sinus rhythm can be affected by cardioversion or rapid atrial pacing.

Junctional tachycardia

ECG characteristics
Usually, the QRS complexes are similar to those of sinus rhythm. The junctional focus may activate both atria and ventricles and thus the QRS complexes may be either preceded by or succeeded by an inverted P wave (Fig. 23). Distinction from the far more commonly occurring AV re-entrant tachycardia may not be possible.

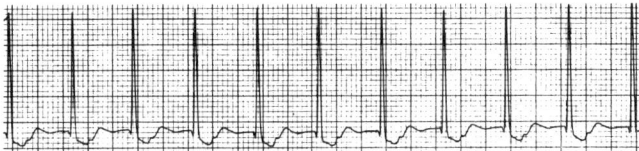

Fig. 23 AV junctional tachycardia due to digoxin toxicity. There is retrograde atrial conduction resulting in a P wave being superimposed on each ST segment.

Causes
Junctional tachycardia may be caused by digoxin toxicity. Most forms of cardiac disease, especially coronary artery disease, can cause the arrhythmia.

Treatment
AV nodal blocking drugs may be effective, depending on the precise site of the arrhythmia focus. Otherwise, a drug which decreases enhanced automaticity, e.g. lignocaine or disopyramide should be used. Where digoxin toxicity is suspected, the drug should be stopped.

Pre-excitation syndromes

In the normal heart, an atrial impulse can only be conducted to the ventricles by the AV node. In the pre-excitation syndromes, there is an additional connection between atria and ventricles. Unlike the AV node, the accessory connection does not delay conduction between atria and ventricles. Thus, an atrial impulse will be transmitted more quickly by the accessory connection and will initate ventricular activation before it has traversed the AV node: hence the term pre-excitation.

Wolff–Parkinson–White syndrome

The syndrome is characterized by a short PR interval, a widened QRS complex due to the presence of a delta wave, and a tendency to paroxysmal tachycardia. It occurs in approximately 1.5 per 1000 of the population.

The syndrome is caused by an accessory connection between atrial and ventricular myocardium. This connection, which is itself ordinary myocardium, is referred to as an accessory AV pathway or bundle of Kent and is congenital in origin. Unlike other pre-excitation syndromes, neither end of the connection is to any part of the specialized conduction system. The bundle of Kent may be situated anywhere in the AV groove.

Sinus rhythm
During sinus rhythm, the atrial impulse is conducted to the ventricles by both the bundle of Kent and the normal AV node. The

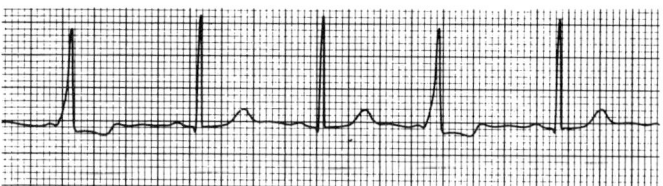

Fig. 24 Intermittent Wolff–Parkinson–White syndrome (first and fourth beats). By comparison with the normal beats, it can be seen how the delta wave both broadens the ventricular complex and shortens the PR interval.

latter pathway conducts more slowly and hence initial ventricular activation is solely due to the bundle of Kent conduction which results in ventricular pre-excitation and thus a shortened PR interval. Because the bundle of Kent is not connected to specialized conducting tissue, early ventricular activation is relatively slow, reflected by slurring of the ventricular complex – the delta wave (Fig. 24). Once the atrial impulse has traversed the AV node, further ventricular activation proceeds normally. During sinus rhythm, therefore, the ventricular complex is a fusion between delta wave and normal QRS complex.

The syndrome is classified into types A and B, depending on the ventricular complex in lead V₁. If predominantly positive, it is type A and if negative type B (Fig. 25). In type A, the bundle of Kent is likely to be on the left side of the heart, and in type B on the right side.

A number of erroneous ECG diagnoses can be made if it is not appreciated that a patient has the Wolff–Parkinson–White syndrome. In type A syndrome, the dominant R wave in lead V₁ can be misinterpreted as right ventricular hypertrophy, right bundle branch block or true posterior infarction. Type B can be mistaken for left bundle branch block. A negative delta wave can be mistaken for a pathological Q wave leading to an inappropriate diagnosis of myocardial infarction (Fig. 25).

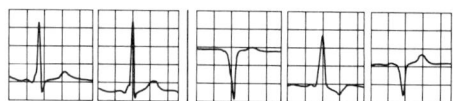

Fig. 25 Wolff–Parkinson–White syndrome. On left, leads V₁ and V₆ from patient with type A syndrome. On right, leads V₁, V₆, and AVF in type B syndrome. The negative delta wave in AVF could be misinterpreted for inferior infarction.

Arrhythmias

Two main arrhythmias can occur: atrial fibrillation and AV re-entrant tachycardia. The former is the less common.

Atrial fibrillation

Ventricular rates during atrial fibrillation are usually faster than in patients without pre-excitation because the bundle of Kent provides an additional route of access to the ventricles and is often capable of very frequent conduction.

Usually, most conducted impulses reach the ventricles via the bundle of Kent and will therefore lead to delta waves. Those impulses reaching the ventricles via the AV node will produce normal QRS complexes. The resultant ECG will, as in all cases of atrial fibrillation, show an irregularly irregular ventricular response (Fig. 26).

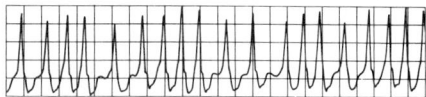

Fig. 26 Rapid ventricular response to atrial fibrillation in Wolff–Parkinson–White syndrome.

The very rapid ventricular response to atrial fibrillation can cause shock and may precipitate ventricular fibrillation. The risk

of ventricular fibrillation is mainly confined to those whose minimum interval between delta waves during atrial fibrillation is less than 250 ms.

AV nodal blocking drugs do not slow conduction in the bundle of Kent and are therefore of no use. Indeed, both digoxin and verapamil can increase the frequency of conduction in the bundle of Kent, leading to a faster ventricular rate, and should be avoided in those patients who are capable of a rapid ventricular response or in patients in whom the ventricular response to atrial fibrillation is not known.

The simplest method of terminating atrial fibrillation is cardioversion. Drugs which impair conduction in the bundle of Kent, such as intravenous disopyramide, sotalol, flecainide, and amiodarone should slow the ventricular rate and will often effect a return to sinus rhythm. These drugs, as well as quinidine, can be used long-term for preventing atrial fibrillation. In patients capable of a very fast ventricular response to atrial fibrillation, rapid atrial pacing can be used to initiate the arrhythmia whilst on oral therapy to ensure the drug does slow the ventricular response.

Surgical division of the bundle of Kent may occasionally be required if drugs are ineffective or cannot be tolerated, especially if the ventricular rate during attacks is dangerously fast.

AV re-entrant tachycardia

The AV junction and bundle of Kent differ in the time that they take to recover after excitation. Usually, the AV junction recovers first. If an atrial extrasystole arises during sinus rhythm when the AV junction has recovered but the bundle of Kent is not yet capable of conduction, the resultant ventricular complex will clearly not have a delta wave. By the time the premature atrial impulse has traversed the AV junction and stimulated the ventricles, the bundle of Kent will have recovered and will be capable of conducting the impulse back to the atria. When the impulse reaches the atria, the AV junction will again be capable of conduction and hence the impulse can circulate repeatedly between atria and ventricles (Fig. 12b, c).

The ECG during re-entrant tachycardia will show regular and narrow ventricular complexes, unless phasic aberrant intraventricular conduction occurs. Unlike atrial fibrillation, there will be no delta waves and thus there will be no clue from the appearance of the ventricular complexes during tachycardia that the patient has the Wolff–Parkinson–White syndrome. However, the timing of atrial activity, if it can be identified, during tachycardia may give a clue as to its mechanism. When the tachycardia is due to dual AV nodal pathways, an inverted P wave immediately follows or is superimposed on the QRS complex. In contrast, in tachycardias due to the Wolff–Parkinson–White syndrome, the P wave occurs half-way between QRS complexes.

Many patients with AV re-entrant tachycardia who have no evidence of pre-excitation during sinus rhythm have been found to have a 'concealed' bundle of Kent when studied by intracardiac electrophysiological testing. A concealed bundle of Kent is only capable of conduction from ventricles to atria. Thus, there will be no delta wave or PR interval shortening but the bundle can transmit impulses in the direction necessary to facilitate re-entrant tachycardia.

Methods for the termination and prevention of AV re-entrant tachycardia are the same whether or not the tachycardia is due to a bundle of Kent (see above).

Lown–Ganong–Levine syndrome

In this pre-excitation syndrome, there is an additional AV connection between atrial myocardium and the bundle of His. Thus, an atrial impulse will reach the ventricles without the normal delay and lead to a short PR interval. Because the tract is connected to the bundle of His, ventricular activation will be normal and there will not, therefore, be a delta wave (Fig. 27). Patients with this syndrome are prone to AV re-entrant tachycardia which should be treated in the usual way.

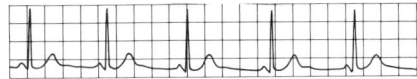

Fig. 27 Lown–Ganong–Levine syndrome. The PR interval is 0.08 s, the QRS complex is normal.

Not all patients with a short PR interval have an AV nodal bypass tract or are prone to paroxysmal tachycardia. Other causes of a short PR interval include a congenitally small AV node and rapid AV nodal conduction due to increased sympathetic activity.

Ventricular tachycardia

Ventricular tachycardia is defined as three or more ventricular extrasystoles in rapid succession. Usually, the rate is between 120 and 250 beats per minute.

ECG characteristics

The ventricular complexes are abnormal in shape and duration (Fig. 28). The duration of the ventricular complex is usually greater than 0.12 s, although occasionally, when the focus is in the proximal intraventricular conducting system, thereby facilitating more rapid ventricular activation, it may be shorter. The rhythm is regular unless there are capture beats (see below).

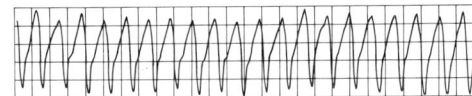

Fig. 28 Ventricular tachycardia with a rate of 235 per minute.

In half of ventricular tachycardias, atrial activity continues to be initiated by the sinus node and, therefore, proceeds independently of ventricular activity. In the other half, the ventricular impulses are conducted via the AV junction to the atria so that they are followed by inverted P waves which are often concealed by the superimposed terminal portion of the ventricular complex (Fig. 29).

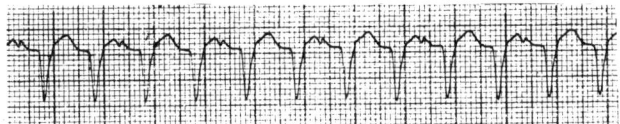

Fig. 29 Ventricular tachycardia. Atrial activity can be clearly seen. In this case, there is, unusually, 2:1 ventriculoatrial conduction.

Identification of independent atrial activity excludes an origin at AV node level or above and is thus an important sign in distinguishing between ventricular tachycardia and supraventricular tachycardia with aberrant intraventricular conduction. There may be direct or only indirect evidence of independent atrial activity.

Direct evidence of independent atrial activity is indicated by P waves inscribed at a slower rate than and dissociated from QRS complexes. Inevitably, some P waves will be concealed by a superimposition of QRS complexes, and not all leads will clearly show atrial activity. Thus, scrutiny of several leads may be necessary.

Indirect evidence of independent atrial activity is indicated by the presence of capture or fusion beats. Capture beats occur when the timing of an atrial impulse during ventricular tachycardia is such that it can be transmitted via the AV junction and activate the ventricles before the next discharge from the ventricular focus. This results in a normal and, therefore, narrower ventricular complex, occurring slightly earlier than the next ventricular extrasystole would be expected (Fig. 30). Fusion beats are caused by a similar process but in this case the ventricles are activated slightly later by the atrial impulse, leading to simultaneous activation of the ventricles by the transmitted atrial impulse and ventricular ectopic focus. The result is a ventricular complex which in appearance is a fusion between a normal QRS complex and ventricular extrasystole (Fig. 30).

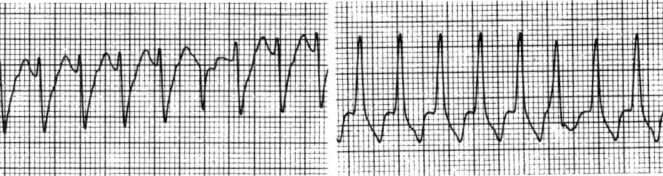

Fig. 30 Ventricular tachycardias. The sixth complex in each example indicates independent atrial activity. There is a capture beat in the case on the left and a fusion beat in the right hand case.

Causes

These include ischaemic heart disease, cardiomyopathy, mitral valve prolapse, digoxin toxicity, and hereditary prolongation of the QT interval.

Clinical features

Ventricular tachycardia can cause shock, cardiac arrest, or progress to ventricular fibrillation. On the other hand, some patients will have minor or even no symptoms. The tachycardia may be sustained or occur in short, self-terminating episodes.

Treatment

Cardioversion is indicated if ventricular tachycardia causes shock or cardiac arrest or if drugs are ineffective or cannot be tolerated.

Lignocaine is the first-line drug. If this fails, mexiletine, tocainide, flecainide and amiodarone are useful second-line drugs. Most antiarrhythmic drugs can, to varying degrees, impair myocardial performance and may therefore cause hypotension or shock. If these complications arise without a return to sinus rhythm, cardioversion should be undertaken quickly because a return to normal rhythm usually improves cardiac output. In general, it is unwise to use more than two drugs before resorting to cardioversion.

Pacing can sometimes be successful in terminating ventricular tachycardia and should be considered when drugs are ineffective, when frequent recurrence necessitates multiple cardioversions or when a pacing wire is already *in situ* for treatment of a conduction disorder. The usual method is rapid ventricular pacing for a few seconds at a rate 10–30 per cent faster than the tachycardia. The arrhythmia is often terminated, although there is a risk of accelerating the tachycardia or of precipitating ventricular fibrillation.

Choice of treatment for the prevention of ventricular tachycardia depends on whether it is likely to recur within a short period of time of its termination, e.g. in acute myocardial infarction or after cardiac surgery. In this case, intravenous lignocaine or, if this has been ineffective, a second-line parenteral antiarrhythmic agent, can be used. Otherwise, an oral agent suitable for ventricular arrhythmias should be used (see below). Occasionally recurrent ventricular tachycardia cannot be prevented by even powerful drugs such as amiodarone. In these patients, there are a number of alternatives. Surgical techniques for the isolation or excision of the arrhythmic focus can be used. However, potential candidates often have very poor ventricular function in which case the risk of surgery is high. Several implantable devices for the termination of ventricular tachyarrhythmias are being evaluated. Tachycardias due to re-entrant mechanisms may be terminated by precisely timed ventricular paced beats but sometimes more dangerous arrhythmias may be precipitated. Furthermore, the electrophysiological characteristics of ventricular tachycardia and hence response to pacing may vary from time to time. Transvenous cardioversion involving the delivery of a 'microshock' can be effective, but microshocks can be painful and there are problems in distinguishing supraventricular from ventricular tachycardia. As with pacing, there is the risk of a microshock leading to a more dangerous arrhythmia. Implantable defibrillators are also being developed. Currently, the devices are bulky and expensive, require thoracotomy for placement of an epicardial electrode, may not reliably recognize ventricular tachycardia or fibrillation, and can provide only a limited number of shocks.

Since ventricular tachycardia can either be dangerous in itself or lead to ventricular fibrillation, it is important to try and ensure that whatever method is employed to control recurrent ventricular tachycardia, it is going to be effective. Therapy should be assessed by ECG monitoring in hospital, and ambulatory electrocardiography. Exercise ECG testing and, in certain situations, intracardiac electrophysiological testing should be also considered.

Idioventricular tachycardia

This is defined as ventricular tachycardia with a rate less than 120 per minute and is also referred to as slow ventricular tachycardia or accelerated idioventricular rhythm (Fig. 31). It is usually seen in acute myocardial infarction. Treatment is unnecessary.

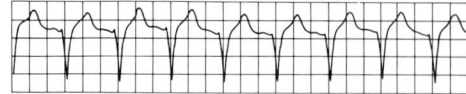

Fig. 31 Idioventricular tachycardia.

Torsade de pointes ventricular tachycardia

This is an atypical ventricular tachycardia characterized by repeated gradual changes in the QRS axis so that complexes appear to twist about the baseline (Fig. 32). *Its recognition is important because it may be aggravated by anti-arrhythmic drugs* and because correction of the underlying cause often terminates the arrhythmia. Causes include the sick sinus syndrome, AV block, hypokalaemia, hereditary QT prolongation syndromes, and drugs such as quinidine, prenylamine, phenothiazines, and tricyclic antidepressants.

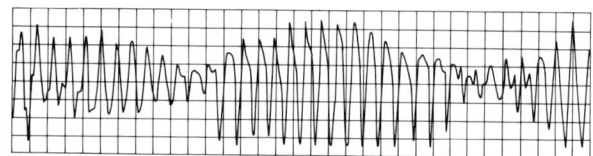

Fig. 32 *Torsade de pointes* ventricular tachycardia.

Hereditary prolongation of the QT interval

There are two conditions in which there is congenital prolongation of the QT interval and a tendency to ventricular tachycardia: the Romano–Ward syndrome and the Jervell and Lange-Nielson syndrome. The former is due to a dominant gene. The latter is due to a recessive gene and is associated with nerve deafness.

Ventricular tachycardia is usually induced by exertion or emotion and often causes syncope. Sudden death can occur, and this may explain why most cases are seen in children or young adults.

The disorders are thought to be an imbalance between left and right sympathetic innervation of the heart. Full beta-blockade is often effective in controlling symptoms. Occasionally, left cervical sympathectomy has been successful.

The QT interval normally shortens with increasing heart rate (partly due to increased catecholamine levels and partly due to the increase in heart rate itself). The QT interval can be corrected for heart rate (QTc) by dividing the measured interval by the square root of the cycle length. The normal QTc is less than 0.42 s.

Distinction between supraventricular and ventricular tachycardias

A tachycardia with narrow ventricular complexes should be assumed to be supraventricular in origin although exceptions to this rule have been demonstrated by His bundle electrocardiography. A tachycardia with broad ventricular complexes is usually ventricular in origin. However, complexes can also be broad during supraventricular tachycardia when bundle branch block has

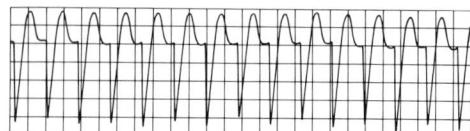

Fig. 33 AV re-entrant tachycardia with left bundle branch block due to phasic aberrant conduction in a patient with Wolff–Parkinson–White syndrome (lead V₁).

been present during sinus rhythm or when phasic aberrant intraventricular conduction (i.e. rate-related bundle branch block) occurs.

Distinction between ventricular tachycardia and supraventricular tachycardia with aberration can be difficult (Fig. 33) but there are some helpful guidelines:

1. If there is direct or indirect evidence of independent atrial activity then a tachycardia arising from above the level of the AV node can be excluded.

2. It is relatively easy to ascertain the origin of a single extrasystole; if the configuration of the extrasystolic ventricular complex is similar to that during tachycardia, a common origin is probable.

3. In patients with coronary artery or myocardial disease, a regular, broad complex tachycardia is almost certain to arise from the ventricles. Atrial fibrillation and flutter may cause aberrant intraventricular conduction but have characteristics whose recognition should prevent confusion with ventricular tachycardia (Fig. 34).

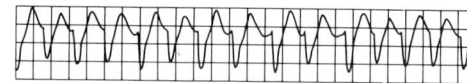

Fig. 34 Left bundle branch block associated with atrial fibrillation. There is the characteristic totally irregular ventricular rhythm.

AV re-entrant tachycardia may also cause bundle branch block but virtually never occurs unless the patient was already prone to the arrhythmia before coronary or myocardial disease was apparent, since these diseases are not going to create the additional AV connection necessary to facilitate this tachycardia.

Two widely quoted guidelines are unreliable. It is said that whereas supraventricular tachycardia is regular, ventricular tachycardia is slightly irregular. In fact, ventricular tachycardia is regular unless there are capture beats and these can cause only minor disturbances to the rhythm. Major haemodynamic disturbance is taken by some to be a sign of ventricular tachycardia. This is incorrect; ventricular tachycardia may cause few or even no symptoms whereas supraventricular tachycardia, particularly when very fast, can cause heart failure or shock. It is surprising how often a regular, broad, complex tachycardia is optimistically diagnosed as being of supraventricular origin in spite of clear evidence to the contrary.

Ventricular fibrillation

This is the rapid, totally inco-ordinate contraction of ventricular myocardial fibres (Fig. 35). It causes circulatory arrest. Occasionally it is a brief event, spontaneously reverting to normal rhythm.

Ventricular fibrillation is usually, but not always, initiated by an 'R on T' ventricular extrasystole. Ninety per cent of deaths caused by myocardial infarction are due to ventricular fibrillation, and this arrhythmia can occur without myocardial infarction in patients with severe coronary disease and may be the first clinical

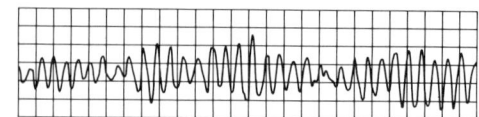

Fig. 35 Ventricular fibrillation.

manifestation of the disease. Other causes include electrocution and severe heart disease of almost any type.

When ventricular fibrillation develops in a heart which was functioning satisfactorily during normal rhythm, it is termed primary fibrillation, whereas if it occurs in the context of cardiac failure or cardiogenic shock, it is termed secondary. Treatment is less likely to be successful in the latter case.

Treatment is discussed below.

Atrioventricular block

AV block is classified into first, second, and third degrees depending on whether conduction of atrial impulses to the ventricles is delayed, intermittently blocked, or completely blocked.

First degree AV block

Conduction of the atrial impulse to the ventricles is delayed, resulting in prolongation of the PR interval (Fig. 36). Usually, delay is at the AV node but rarely it occurs within the atria or bundle of His. First degree AV block may progress to higher degrees of block. In young persons, it may be a benign phenomenon due to high vagal tone.

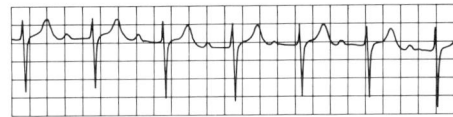

Fig. 36 First degree AV block. PR interval = 0.28 s.

Second degree AV block

In second degree AV block there is intermittent failure of conduction of atrial impulses to the ventricles leading to dropped beats, i.e. P waves not followed by QRS complexes. Second degree block is divided into Mobitz type I (Wenkebach) and Mobitz type II block.

Mobitz type I or Wenkebach AV block

AV conduction is progressively more delayed with each atrial impulse, until there is a complete block, and an atrial impulse fails to be conducted to the ventricles. After the dropped beat, AV conduction recovers and the sequence starts again (Fig. 37). Like first degree AV block, delay usually occurs in the AV node and may be benign due to high vagal tone.

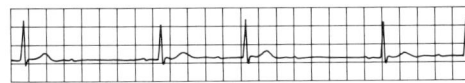

Fig. 37 Mobitz type I (Wenkebach) AV block.

Mobitz type II AV block

Here, there is intermittent failure of conduction of atrial impulses to the ventricles without antecedent progressive lengthening of the PR interval, and thus the PR interval of conducted beats is constant (Fig. 38).

Mobitz type II block is usually due to impaired conduction at a level below the AV node, i.e. within the bundle of His or bundle

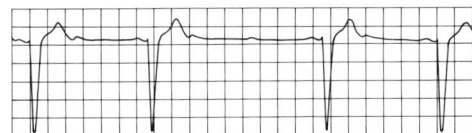

Fig. 38 Mobitz type II AV block. Ratio of AV conduction varies from 2:1 to 3:1.

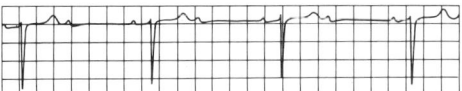

Fig. 39 2:1 AV block.

branches. Block below the AV node is more likely to be associated with Adams–Stokes attacks, slow ventricular rates and sudden death.

The ratio of conducted to non-conducted atrial impulses varies. Commonly, 2:1 AV conduction occurs. A similar pattern may be caused by an extreme form of Wenkebach block so that it is difficult to make prognostic inferences from 2:1 AV block (Fig. 39).

Third degree AV block

Third degree or complete AV block occurs when there is total interruption of the transmission of atrial impulses to the ventricles. It may be due to interrupted conduction at either AV nodal or infranodal level. When the block is within the AV node, subsidiary pacemakers arise in the bundle of His and, unless there is additional bundle branch block, will lead to narrow QRS complexes (Fig. 40). Usually, pacemakers within the bundle of His discharge reliably at a fairly rapid rate. In contrast, in infranodal block, subsidary pacemakers arise in the left or right bundle branches. These pacemakers, which will produce broad ventricular complexes, discharge at slower rates and pacemaker activity is less reliable, so Adams–Stokes attacks are more likely (Fig. 41).

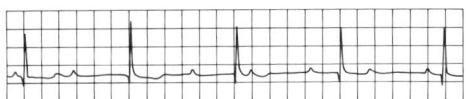

Fig. 40 Complete AV block with narrow ventricular complexes. There is no relation between atrial and the slower ventricular activity.

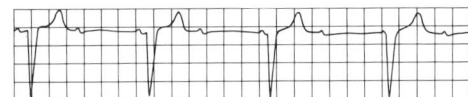

Fig. 41 Complete AV block with broad ventricular complexes.

Occasionally, even during third degree AV block, atrial impulses may be conducted to the ventricles. There is a short period, coinciding with inscription of the latter portion of the T wave, when AV conduction may transiently improve. As a result, atrial impulses falling on this part of the T wave may be followed by a premature ventricular complex. This phenomenon of 'supernormal conduction' should not be confused with extrasystoles (Fig. 43).

Complete AV block can complicate atrial fibrillation and flutter (Fig. 42).

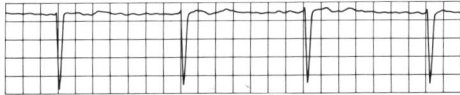

Fig. 42 Complete AV block with atrial fibrillation. The ventricular rhythm is regular.

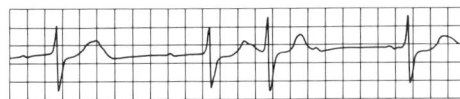

Fig. 43 Complete AV block. The fourth atrial impulse falls during the supernormal phase of AV conduction resulting in the (third) premature ventricular complex.

Table 2 Causes of AV block

Idiopathic fibrosis
Myocardial infarction
Digoxin toxicity
Aortic valve disease
Congenital
Cardiac surgery
Infiltration, e.g. tumour, syphilis, endocarditis
Inflammation, e.g. ankylosing spondylitis, Reiter's syndrome,
      rheumatoid arthritis, scleroderma, sarcoidosis
Rheumatic fever
Dystrophia myotonica
Diphtheria

Causes of AV block

The most common cause is idiopathic fibrosis of the AV junction or bundle branches. This can occur at any age, but it most frequently affects the elderly. Other causes are listed in Table 2. The site of block in inferior myocardial infarction, digoxin toxicity, and congenital block is usually the AV node. In most other situations, block may be nodal or infranodal.

Clinical features of AV block

First degree and Mobitz type I block do not cause symptoms but many progress to higher degrees of block.

In Mobitz II and complete AV block, the resultant low ventricular rate may cause dyspnoea and heart failure. In some patients the ventricular pacemaker may at times discharge very slowly or actually stop, leading to syncope or, if ventricular activity does not quickly return, sudden death (Fig. 44). Ventricular fibrillation and tachycardia arise in some patients as a consequence of the low ventricular rate and may also lead to syncope or death.

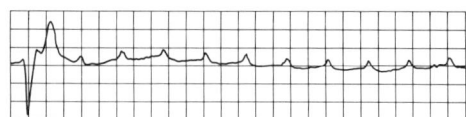

Fig. 44 Ventricular asystole developing during complete AV block.

Recent evidence has shown that in spite of the hitherto good prognosis associated with Mobitz I block, syncope is common and the prognosis in unpaced patients is equally poor for both Mobitz I and Mobitz II AV block. However, Mobitz I block in young people which is transient and often nocturnal is due to high vagal tone and is benign.

Syncope due to transient asystole or ventricular fibrillation is known as an Adams–Stokes attack. It has characteristic features which are of great diagnostic importance because, on the one hand, abnormalities of AV conduction (and also sinus node function) may be intermittent, routine electrocardiography being normal, and on the other hand, in some patients with evidence of disease of the specialized conducting tissues, syncope may be due to unrelated causes such as epilepsy.

In an Adams–Stokes attack, loss of consciousness is abrupt. There is virtually no warning although the patient will sometimes feel that he is going to faint just before actual loss of conciousness. The patient collapses, lying motionless and pale, looking as though he is dead. In a prolonged attack, twitching may develop and progress to a fit. Usually within a minute or two cardiac action resumes, and as consciousness returns there is a flush to the skin. Incontinence does occasionally occur but is not a regular feature as in epilepsy. Unlike epilepsy, recovery is quick.

In some patients, the rhythm disturbance does not last long enough to cause syncope but the patient feels as though he is going to faint (near-syncope) and then recovers. The patient may complain of 'dizziness' but will not experience true vertigo.

Treatment

Cardiac pacing should be considered in all patients with symptomatic AV block and may improve the prognosis of patients with asymptomatic high degrees of block. In patients with syncope, because the next attack may be fatal or cause injury, delay in referral for pacing should be minimal. Artificial pacing is discussed later (see page 13.126).

Even patients with congenital heart block, a relatively benign condition, should be considered for pacing since symptoms can occur and sudden death does occasionally happen.

Bilateral bundle branch disease

Infranodal AV block may be due to a lesion in the bundle of His but is more often caused by disease in both left and right bundle branches. Although the anatomical situation may be more complex, functionally the bundle of His can be considered to divide into three fascicles: the right bundle branch, and the anterior and posterior fascicles of the left bundle branch.

Left anterior fascicular block delays activation of the anterosuperior region of the left ventricle. Initial left ventrical activation will be via the posterior fascicle to the posteroinferior region and will therefore be directed inferiorly, resulting in an initial positive deflection (r wave) in leads III and AVF. Delaycd activation of the anterosuperior region is reflected by left axis deviation of the mean frontal QRS complex (Fig. 45). Conversely, block of the left posterior fascicle results in an initial negative deflection (q wave) in inferior leads and right axis deviation (Fig. 46).

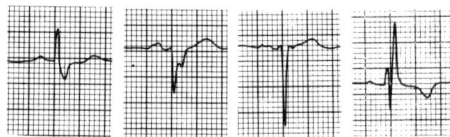

Fig. 45 Bifascicular block: right bundle plus left anterior fascicular block (leads I, II, III and V₁). The latter lesion causes an initial positive vector in inferior leads and left axis deviation which can be quickly diagnosed from a rule of thumb: lead I is predominantly positive and leads II and III predominantly negative.

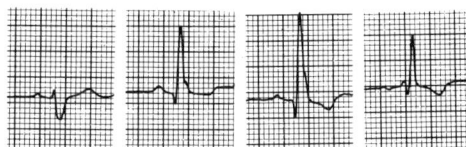

Fig. 46 Bifascicular block: right bundle plus left posterior fascicular block (leads I, II, III and V₁). The latter lesion causes an initial negative vector in inferior leads and right axis deviation: lead I is predominantly negative and both leads II and III predominantly positive.

If conduction is blocked in only two of the three fascicles (bifascicular block), the functioning fascicle will conduct atrial impulses to the ventricles and maintain sinus rhythm. Block in the third fascicle will lead to AV block.

Bifascicular block

The most common pattern of bifascicular block is right bundle branch plus left anterior fascicular block (Fig. 45). The posterior fascicle of the left bundle branch is a stouter structure and has a better blood supply than the anterior fascicle and is therefore less vulnerable.

PR interval prolongation is usually due to impaired AV node conduction, but in the setting of bifascicular block may reflect abnormal conduction in the functioning fascicle.

Trifascicular block

Interrupted conduction in all three fascicles results in complete AV block. In many patients, one of the three fascicles is capable of intermittent conduction so that for part of the time there will be sinus rhythm with evidence of bifascicular block.

The risk of bifascicular progressing to trifascicular block is fairly low. In patients with right bundle and left anterior fascicular block it is in the order of a few per cent per year. The risk is increased when there is right bundle and left posterior fascicular block and when there is alternating right and left bundle branch block.

AV dissociation

AV dissociation occurs when ventricular activity is faster than and independent of atrial activity which continues to be initiated by the sinus node (Fig. 47). Sometimes it is due to enhanced automaticity of a junctional or ventricular pacemaker, often it arises as an escape mechanism during sinus bradycardia.

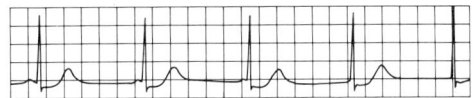

Fig. 47 AV dissociation. The atrial rate is slower than the ventricular rate. The fourth and fifth P waves are concealed by superimposed QRS complexes.

Atrial and ventricular activity are also dissociated during complete AV block. To avoid confusion (e.g. inappropriate pacemaker insertion), the term AV dissociation should be reserved for the former situation, which is due to an abnormality in impulse formation rather than conduction, and in which the atria are slower than the ventricles.

Sick sinus syndrome

The sick sinus syndrome, also referred to as sinoatrial disease, is caused by impairment of either sinus node activity or of conduction of the sinus node impulse to the atria. The result is sinus bradycardia, sinoatrial block, or sinus arrest. In some patients, tachycardias of supraventricular origin may also occur. The term 'bradycardia–tachycardia syndrome' is applied to these patients.

Causes

The most common cause is idiopathic fibrosis of the sinus node. Other causes include ischaemic heart disease, cardiomyopathy, myocarditis, digoxin or quinidine toxicity, and cardiac surgery, especially atrial septal defect repair. Sometimes, antiarrhythmic drugs may precipitate a latent disorder.

Sick sinus syndrome can affect patients of all ages though it is most common in the elderly.

ECG characteristics

Several arrhythmias can occur. They are often intermittent, normal sinus rhythm being present for most of the time. For this reason, ambulatory ECG monitoring is frequently necessary for diagnosis.

Sinus bradycardia

This is a common finding in the sick sinus syndrome.

Sinoatrial block

Sinoatrial block occurs when the sinus node impulse fails to traverse the junction between the node and the atria. Like AV block, sinoatrial block can be classified into first, second, and third degrees. However, only second degree sinoatrial block can be diagnosed from the surface electrocardiogram. Third degree sinoatrial block is indistinguishable from sinus arrest.

In second degree sinoatrial block, there are intermittently dropped P waves, resulting in intervals between P waves which are multiples (often twice) of the cycle length during sinus rhythm (Fig. 48).

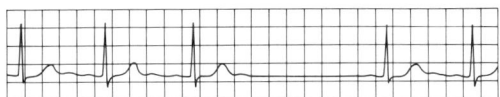

Fig. 48 Second degree sinoatrial block. There is a pause in both atrial and ventricular activity which is twice the sinus node cycle length.

Sinus arrest

Sinus arrest is due to failure of impulse formation by the sinus node. The result is absence of normal P waves (Fig. 49). Unlike second degree sinoatrial block, the pause in normal atrial activity will not be a multiple of the sinus node cycle length.

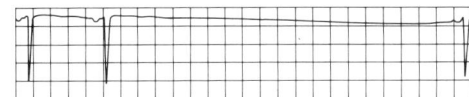

Fig. 49 After two AV junctional beats there is sinus arrest for 4 s which is terminated by a sinus node beat.

Physiological studies have shown that subsidiary pacemakers in the atria, AV junction or ventricles should give rise to an escape rhythm in the absence of sinus node activity. However, in the sick sinus syndrome subsidary pacemakers are often unreliable and sinus arrest may therefore lead to cardiac standstill. Thus, although sinus arrest is attributed to a disorder of sinus node function, where asystole occurs, there is also abnormal automaticity of the more distal specialized conducting system.

Escape beats and rhythms

These arise when, in the presence of sinus bradycardia or arrest, subsidiary pacemakers take over control of the heart rhythm (Figs. 10, 11, 49, and 50). The presence of a junctional or idioventricular rhythm suggests impaired sinus node function.

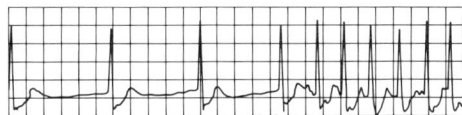

Fig. 50 Bradycardia–tachycardia syndrome. After the fourth beat of a junctional bradycardia, an atrial extrasystole initiates atrial fibrillation.

Atrial ectopic beats

These often occur in the sick sinus syndrome. They may be followed by long pauses because sinus node automaticity is depressed by the ectopic beat.

Bradycardia–tachycardia syndrome

Several tachycardias of supraventricular origin may occur. Paroxysmal atrial fibrillation and flutter are the most common (Fig. 50). Atrial and junctional tachycardia also occur but AV re-entrant tachycardia is not part of this syndrome.

Sinus node automaticity is often depressed by these tachycardias so that termination of the tachycardia leads to a period of sinus bradycardia or arrest. Conversely, tachycardias often arise as an escape rhythm resulting from bradycardia. Thus, tachycardia often alternates with bradycardia.

AV junction disease

Impaired AV conduction is not infrequently found in patients with sick sinus syndrome. In patients with sick sinus syndrome who develop atrial fibrillation, there is often a slow ventricular response even in the absence of AV nodal blocking drugs, suggesting coexistent impaired AV nodal function.

Clinical features

Sinus arrest without an adequate escape rhythm may cause syncope or near-syncope, depending on its duration. Tachycardia often causes palpitation. The frequency of rhythm disturbance is very variable. Some patients will experience symptoms many times per day whereas, in others, symptoms may be separated by intervals of several months. In the bradycardia–tachycardia syndrome there is a high incidence, up to 15 per cent, of systemic embolism.

It should be noted that sinus bradycardia and sinoatrial block during sleep are physiological and are not evidence of sick sinus syndrome if found during the nocturnal hours of a 24 hour ECG tape recording.

Treatment

Drugs rarely prevent sinus bradycardia or arrest and may precipitate tachyarrhythmias. In symptomatic patients, artificial cardiac pacing is necessary to control symptoms.

In the bradycardia–tachycardia syndrome, antiarrhythmic drugs, especially beta-blockers and disopyramide, often worsen sinus node function and thus increase the risk of syncope. It is usually necessary to implant a pacemaker if antiarrhythmic drugs are required.

Atrial rather than ventricular pacing is preferable because it achieves optimal cardiac output, and may prevent systemic emboli and tachyarrhythmias. However atrial pacing is not always possible. In patients where atrial tachyarrhythmias cannot be prevented, the use of anticoagulants to prevent systemic emboli should be considered.

Cardiac arrest

Cardiac arrest is the cessation of an effective cardiac output as a result of a sudden circulatory or respiratory catastrophe. Patients dying from terminal diseases will not benefit from and should not undergo the indignity of cardiopulmonary resuscitation.

Causes include acute myocardial infarction, severe coronary artery disease in the absence of infarction, anoxia, disease confined to the specialized cardiac conducting tissues, electrocution, anaphylaxis, and hyperkalaemia.

Diagnosis

Diagnosis is based on two signs: unconsciousness and absent carotid or femoral artery pulsation. Seconds are vital if a successful outcome is to be achieved, and time should not be wasted in eliciting other signs of cardiac arrest such as dilated pupils, apnoea, and absent heart sounds.

Management

Management is divided into three stages. First, establishment of an artificial circulation, secondly, restoration of spontaneous heart action, and thirdly, aftercare.

Artificial circulation

Once the diagnosis is made, immediate action should be taken. A single blow to the praecordium with the side of a clenched fist may occasionally terminate ventricular tachycardia or fibrillation. If unsuccessful, external cardiac massage and artificial respiration should be instituted immediately.

External cardiac massage The heel of one hand is placed over the sternum (not the precordium) at the junction of its upper two-thirds and lower one-third, and is covered by the other hand. Keeping the arms straight, the sternum should be depressed 3–4 cm at a rate of 60 per minute. Each compression should be sustained so that time spent in compression is equal to that of relaxation.

Cardiac massage increases intrathoracic pressure and thereby propels blood into the arteries. Regurgitation into the venous system is prevented by valves at the superior thoracic inlet and, between chest compressions, the aortic valve remains competent, thus preventing blood flowing back into the heart.

Artificial respiration A clear airway should be ensured by tilting the patient's head backwards, fully extending the neck, and by removing any vomit or foreign material from the pharynx. Mouth-to-mouth respiration should be given by taking a deep breath and, after pinching the patient's nose, blowing forcefully into the mouth, ensuring an airtight seal. The chest should be seen to expand, otherwise respiration is inadequate.

As respiration is given, cardiac massage should be interrupted. When there are two operators, the heart should be massaged five times and then the lungs ventilated once. When there is only one operator, it is best to massage the heart 10 times, then ventilate the lungs twice.

If first attempts at restoration of heart action are unsuccessful, an endotracheal tube should be inserted.

Restoration of spontaneous heart action

The sooner this is achieved the better. Cardiac massage may prevent brain damage for periods of 20 minutes and more. However, the low arterial pressure generated by cardiac massage is insufficient for good coronary artery perfusion, and particularly when there is coronary artery disease, irreversible myocardial damage may result if spontaneous cardiac action is not restored quickly.

Treatment depends on the heart rhythm. The paddles of a modern portable defibrillator also function as sensing electrodes, enabling the heart rhythm to be quickly ascertained.

The electrocardiogram may reveal ventricular fibrillation, ventricular tachycardia, asystole or, very rarely, sinus rhythm. The latter may occur with a very large myocardial infarction, massive pulmonary embolism or cardiac tamponade.

Ventricular fibrillation or tachycardia If there is ventricular fibrillation or tachycardia, the patient should be immediately defibrillated using an initial charge of 200 joules (watt-seconds). If unsuccessful, defibrillation should be repeated at 300–400 joules. Use of the defibrillator is discussed below. If a defibrillator is immediately to hand, no time should be wasted in giving cardiac massage.

If the arrhythmia persists, 100 mg of lignocaine should be given and acidosis should be corrected by 50 ml of 8.4 per cent sodium bicarbonate and then defibrillation repeated. If still unsuccessful, further antiarrhythmic agents such as mexiletine may be tried. Where the amplitude of fibrillation wave is small, 5–10 ml of 1:10 000 adrenaline should be used to coarsen 'fine' fibrillation.

Asystole Resuscitation is often successful when the cause is anoxia or disease of the specialized conducting tissues. In these cases ventilation or the mechanical stimulation of cardiac massage respectively may initiate ventricular activation. On the other hand, asystole due to extensive myocardial damage has a poor prognosis.

When the above measures are ineffective, 10 ml of 10 per cent calcium chloride and 5–10 ml of 1:10 000 adrenaline should be given and acidosis reversed with sodium bicarbonate.

Aftercare

If cardiac arrest was due to ventricular fibrillation or tachycardia, lignocaine or a second-line antiarrhythmic agent should be given to prevent arrhythmias. In patients who have been asystolic, unless there has been readily reversible causes, e.g. anoxia, a temporary pacemaker should be inserted.

If there is impaired consciousness intravenous dexamethasone and frusemide should be given to relieve cerebral oedema. Artificial ventilation may be necessary.

The blood acid-base state should be checked and acidosis reversed by giving 8.4 per cent sodium bicarbonate using the formula:

$$\text{ml required} = \text{body weight (kg)} \times 0.2 \times \text{base deficit}$$

Cardioversion

Cardioversion is the use of an electric shock of high energy and brief duration to terminate a tachyarrhythmia. The shock, which is nowadays direct current, is delivered by two electrodes placed on the chest wall. It depolarizes the myocardium thus interrupting a tachycardia and allowing the sinus node to resume control of the heart rhythm.

Indications

Immediate cardioversion is indicated for the treatment of any tachyarrhythmia which causes cardiac arrest or shock. Elective cardioversion is indicated for the termination of a tachyarrhythmia when anti-arrhythmic therapy is ineffective or contraindicated.

In practice, atrial fibrillation and flutter are the two most common arrhythmias where elective cardioversion is undertaken as a first-line treatment because termination by drugs is likely to be difficult.

Procedure

Facilities for monitoring the ECG and for cardiopulmonary resuscitation must be available. A short-acting anaesthetic or amnesic agent is given, e.g. methohexitone or diazepam. Prior to elective cardioversion, the patient should starve for four to six hours.

The shock is delivered by means of two electrode paddles placed on the chest wall, positioned so that the heart lies between them. Usually, one electrode is placed over the cardiac apex and the other to the right of the upper sternum. Good electrical contact is achieved with the use of electrode jelly applied to the areas beneath the paddles, but not spread right across the chest.

With all arrhythmias except ventricular fibrillation, a synchronizing mechanism is set so that the shock is triggered to coincide with the R or S wave of the electrocardiogram, thus avoiding the ventricular T wave and consequent risk of inducing ventricular fibrillation. The defibrillator is charged to the desired energy level. After ensuring that no one is in contact with the patient or the patient's bed, the charge is released, usually by pressing a button on each defibrillator paddle.

Usually, low energy levels are used initially and if unsuccessful further higher energy shocks are given. The initial energy setting depends on clinical circumstances. For example, atrial flutter usually responds to low energy shocks and 25 joules would be an appropriate initial level. On the other hand, with ventricular fibrillation, it is best to start at 200 joules. With other arrhythmias 50–100 joules are used initially.

With digoxin toxicity, cardioversion may cause dangerous arrhythmias and should only be used as a last resort. Very low levels should be used, starting at 5–10 joules. Cardioversion is safe in the presence of therapeutic levels of digoxin but if there is any doubt, elective cardioversion should be postponed for 24–48 hours after discontinuing the drug.

In patients with atrial fibrillation caused by a condition associated with a high incidence of systemic embolism, e.g. rheumatic mitral valve disease or sick sinus syndrome, the risk of embolism should be avoided by prior anticoagulation for at least two weeks.

Intracardiac electrography

Information derived from this technique, which is also referred to as His bundle electrocardiography, has greatly increased the understanding of conduction defects and tachycardias. In the assessment of the individual patient, the technique has a limited role. Its main uses are for investigating the feasibility of specialized pacing techniques or surgery in patients with tachycardias refractory to drug therapy and in the assessment of the integrity of the sinus node and AV junction in the occasional patient with suspected conduction tissue disease which cannot be confirmed by standard or ambulatory electrocardiography.

Technique

The sequence of cardiac chamber activation, during normal and abnormal rhythms, is studied by recording electrograms from vari-

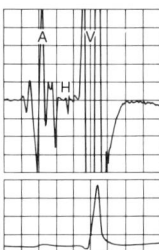

Fig. 51 His bundle electrogram (above) derived by computerized signal averaging technique from surface electrocardiogram (below). His bundle activity (H) can be seen between atrial (A) and ventricular (V) activity. The A–H interval is a measure of conduction time through the AV node, and the H–V interval indicates transmission time through the bundle of His and bundle branches to the ventricles.

ous intracardiac sites using transvenous bipolar electrodes introduced via femoral and antecubital veins, under local anaesthesia.

His bundle activity does not register on the normal surface electrocardiogram, but can be demonstrated using a computerized signal averaging technique (Fig. 51). It can also be recorded from an electrode positioned precisely across the tricuspid valve (Fig. 52). Activity from the low right atrium and interventricular septum is also recorded. The A–H interval indicates the time taken for an atrial impulse to be conducted through the AV node and the H–V interval represents the time taken for transmission through the bundle of His and bundle branches to the ventricles. The latter interval is normally 35–55 ms, any increase indicating impaired conduction.

Activity can also be recorded from the right atrium in the region of the sinus node, left atrium, and ventricles by positioning electrodes in the high right atrium in the coronary sinus (which passes behind the left atrium), and right ventricle respectively. The electrodes can be used to introduce precisely timed single or multiple premature stimuli by means of a programmable pacemaker. Artificial extrasystoles can be used to measure the refractory period of the various portions of the specialized conducting system and to initiate and terminate supraventricular arrhythmias which are caused by re-entry mechanisms.

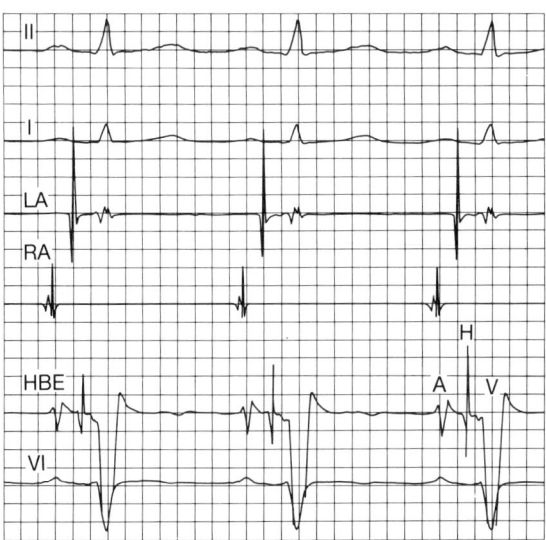

Fig. 52 Simultaneous recordings at 100 mm/s of surface leads II, I and V₁ together with left atrial, right atrial, and His bundle electrograms (LA, RA, and HBE respectively), during sinus rhythm.

Some examples of the uses of intracardiac electrography are shown in Figs 52–56.

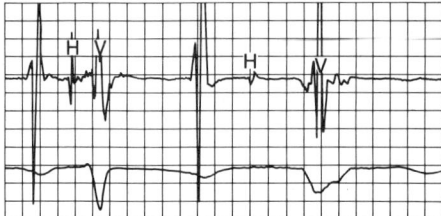

Fig. 53 Simultaneous recordings at 100 mm/s of His bundle (above) and surface (below) electrocardiograms. After the first beat, which is of sinus origin, there is an atrial extrasystole which is conducted with left bundle branch block and an H–V interval of 100 ms, which is twice normal. In the presence of left bundle branch block a prolonged H–V interval suggests impaired conduction in the right bundle branch and in this case confirms the suspicion of conduction tissue disease which could not be demonstrated by repeated surface electrocardiography.

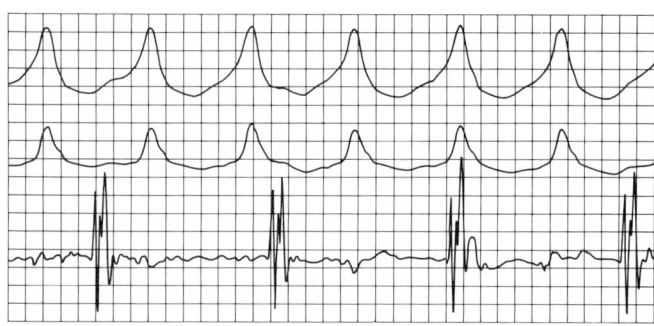

Fig. 54 Simultaneous recordings at 100 mm/s of two surface ECGs (above) and a right atrial electrogram (below). The tachycardia was thought to be supraventricular with phasic aberrant conduction but independent atrial activity points to ventricular tachycardia.

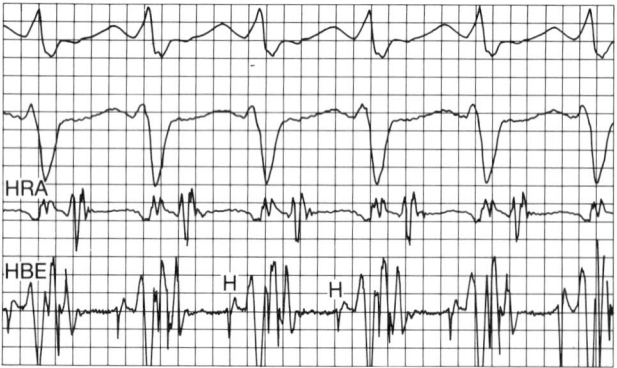

Fig. 55 Simultaneous recordings at 100 mm/s of two surface ECGs (above), a high right atrial electrogram (HRA), and His bundle electrogram (HBE). Each ventricular complex is preceded by His bundle activity (H) indicating supraventricular tachycardia in spite of the broad QRS complexes (110 ms).

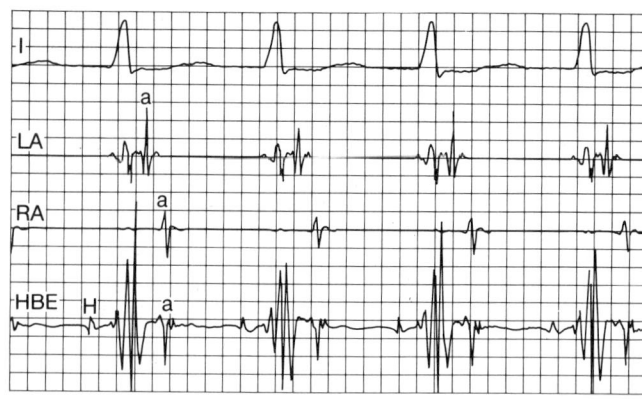

Fig. 56 AV re-entrant tachycardia initiated by a precisely timed premature atrial stimulus, recorded at 100 mm/s. Below lead I, there are left atrial (LA), lateral right atrial (RA), and His bundle (HBE) electrograms. Atrial activity (a) appears in the left atrial electrogram first, indicating that the circulating impulse re-enters the atria via a left-sided bundle of Kent. In this case, the bundle of Kent was concealed, there being no delta wave during sinus rhythm. Had tachycardia been due to dual AV nodal pathways or a right-sided bundle of Kent, atrial activity would be first seen in the His bundle or right atrial electrogram.

Anti-arrhythmic drugs

D. H. BENNETT

This section deals with drugs used to treat arrhythmias. However, drugs are only one form of treatment and in some situations other treatments may be more appropriate (Table 1).

An arrhythmia should not be considered in isolation when deciding how best to treat it. A number of factors may influence the choice of treatment, including the urgency of the situation, the degree of associated circulatory disturbance, the need for short-term or long-term treatment, concurrent administration of other drugs, and the presence of impaired myocardial performance, sinus node dysfunction, or abnormal AV conduction.

Drugs are the mainstay of treatment for arrhythmias but their limitations should be appreciated. First, currently available anti-arrhythmic drugs are of limited efficacy. Second, unwanted effects often occur. The most common are symptoms from the gastrointestinal and central nervous systems, hypotension, heart failure, and impairment of the specialized cardiac conducting tissues. Occassionaly, drugs may be 'pro-arrhythmic' in that they may cause or worsen arrhythmias. Third, with many drugs it can be difficult to maintain therapeutic drug levels. Fourth, though some insight into the mode of action of these drugs has been gained, selection of a drug which is both effective and well tolerated in an individual patient is often a process of trial and error.

Modes of action

The modes of action of anti-arrhythmic drugs can be classified in two ways: according to their effects in the intact heart and according to their effects at cellular level as established by *in vitro* studies. The latter classification is helpful in understanding how drugs work at cellular level but, at least at present, is of limited clinical value.

Table 1 Approaches to treatment of arrhythmias

Anti-arrhythmic drugs
Cardioversion
Artificial pacing
Vagal stimulation (e.g. carotid sinus massage)
Reversal of precipitating factors (e.g. hypokalaemia, digitalis toxicity)
Cardiac surgery

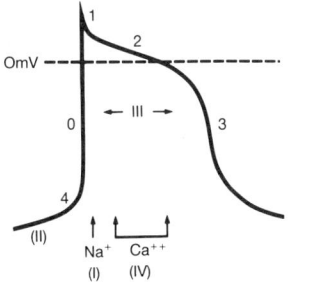

Fig. 1 Diagram of myocardial cell action potential showing its phases 0 to 4, and indicating the modes of action of the antiarrhythmic classes I, II, III, and IV. Na$^+$ and Ca^{2+} indicate the times at which sodium and calcium respectively enter the cell.

Action potential classification

In this classification, drugs are divided into four main classes depending upon their electrophysiological effects at cellular level (Table 2 and Fig. 1).

Class I drugs impede the transport of sodium across the cell membrane during the initiation of cellular activation and thereby reduce the rate of rise of the action potential (phase 0). Many drugs fall into this group. They have been subdivided into classes a, b, and c according to their effect on the duration of the action potential (which is reflected in the surface electrocardiogram by the QT interval): Ia drugs increase the duration, Ib drugs shorten it, and Ic drugs have little effect. The anti-arrhythmic action of Ib drugs is confined to the ventricles whereas Ia and Ic drugs affect both atria and ventricles. Ia and particularly Ic drugs slow intra-ventricular conduction.

Class II drugs interfere with the effects of the sympathetic nervous system on the heart. They do not affect the action potential of most myocardial cells but do reduce the slopes of spontaneous depolarization (phase 4) of cells with pacemaker activity and thus the rate of pacemaker discharge.

Class III drugs prolong the duration of the action potential and hence the length of the refractory period, but do not slow phase 0.

Class IV drugs antagonize the transport of calcium across the cell membrane which follows the inward flux of sodium during cellular activation. Cells in the AV and sinus nodes are particularly susceptible. It should be noted that some calcium antagonists, e.g. nifedipine, do not have an anti-arrhythmic action.

It can be seen from Table 2 that most drugs are in class I, several have more than one class of action, and drugs within class I differ significantly in their clinical effects. Some drugs, e.g. digoxin and adenosine cannot be classified.

Clinical classification

Drugs are divided into three groups according to their main site or sites of action in the intact heart (Fig. 2). The first group consists

Table 2 Examples of action potential classification

	I	II	III	IV
(a)	Quinidine	Beta-blockers	Amiodarone	Verapamil
	Procainamide	Bretylium	Sotalol	Diltiazem
	Disopyramide		Bretylium	
(b)	Lignocaine			
	Mexiletine			
	Tocainide			
	Phenytoin			
	Aprindine			
	Ethmozin			
	Propafenone			
(c)	Flecainide			
	Encainide			
	Lorcainide			

of those whose chief action is to slow conduction in the AV node. These drugs are therefore useful in the treatment of arrhythmias of supraventricular origin but are of little or no use in the treatment of ventricular arrhythmias. In the second group, there are drugs which work mainly in ventricular arrhythmias. The third group comprises drugs which act on the atria, ventricles, and in cases of Wolff–Parkinson–White syndrome, the bundle of Kent. Thus, they may be useful in both supraventricular and ventricular arrhythmias.

Notes on individual drugs

Lignocaine

Lignocaine is the first-line drug for ventricular arrhythmias but is ineffective in arrhythmias of supraventricular origin. The drug is a vasoconstrictor and unlike many other antiarrhythmic agents rarely causes hypotension or heart failure.

Intravenous 100 mg administration over 2 min is usually effective. If not, a further bolus (50–75 mg) should be given after 5 min. Occasional disasters have occurred because of confusion over the several concentrations of lignocaine that are available. For example, 10 cc of 1 per cent lignocaine contains 100 mg of drug.

Lignocaine is often used for short-term prophylaxis of ventricular arrhythmias. Its therapeutic effect is closely related to plasma levels; the therapeutic range is 1.4–6.0 µg/ml. Plasma levels fall rapidly after a bolus injection. Thus it is necessary to give a continuous infusion immediately after the bolus. There is, however, no point in giving a continuous infusion if the bolus has failed to work or, since lignocaine cannot be administered orally, if long-term prophylaxis is required.

It can be difficult to maintain therapeutic levels of lignocaine. With subtherapeutic levels the patient is at risk from arrhythmias, while toxic levels may cause symptoms related to the central nervous system including light headedness, confusion, twitching, paraesthesiae, and epileptic fits. With conventional infusion rates (1–4 mg/min) subtherapeutic levels commonly occur in the first hour or two after the infusion is commenced. A number of regimens have been developed to avoid this problem. These involve the administration of a second bolus 10–15 min after the first and/or giving higher early infusion dosages. However, these regimens may be too complex for routine use and do increase the risk of toxicity.

Lignocaine is metabolized by the liver, and when there is liver disease or hepatic blood flow is reduced by heart failure or by shock, dosages should be halved to avoid toxicity. Hypokalaemia may impair lignocaine's efficacy.

Mexiletine

Mexiletine is similar to lignocaine in its therapeutic and haemodynamic actions but it can be given orally as well as parenterally. There is a narrow margin between therapeutic and toxic effects and symptoms due to toxicity such as nausea, vomiting, confusion, tremor, and ataxia together with bradycardia and hypertension are not uncommon. The therapeutic range of plasma levels is 0.5–2.0 µg/ml.

The oral dose is 200–300 mg eight-hourly. If the patient has not received a prior infusion a loading dose of 400 mg can be given.

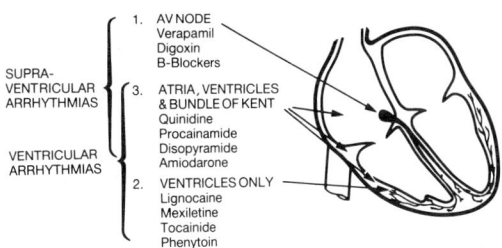

Fig. 2 Clinical classification of antiarrhythmic drugs, showing their principal sites of action.

Up to one-third of patients experience unwanted effects with long-term administration.

Intravenously, the drug is given in a dose of 100–250 mg over 5–10 min, followed by 250 mg over 1 hour and a further 250 mg over 2 hours. The infusion can then be continued at 0.5–1.0 mg/min or oral therapy started.

The drug is mainly metabolized by the liver and doses should be reduced if there is hepatic disease or heart failure. Approximately 10 per cent is excreted unchanged in the urine. Renal excretion is inhibited when urine is alkaline but this is not a problem in practice.

Tocainide

Tocainide is also similar to lignocaine. Like mexiletine it is effective when given either intravenously or orally. Its duration of action is somewhat longer than that of mexiletine, making twice-daily oral administration possible, and intravenous administration is simpler. Forty per cent of the drug is excreted by the kidneys and the dosage should be reduced if there is renal impairment. The therapeutic range of plasma levels is 6–12 μg/ml.

The intravenous dosage is 750 mg over 15 min. The daily oral dosage is 1200 mg. Side-effects include tremor, lightheadedness, confusion, and convulsions. Recent reports of blood dyscrasias associated with tocainide have led to advice that the drug should be restricted to situations where no other is suitable.

Quinidine

Quinidine can be effective in both supraventricular and ventricular arrhythmias. The drug is rarely used parenterally because severe hypotension may result. Orally, its use has been limited because of its reputation for causing dangerous rhythm disturbances, especialy torsade de pointes tachycardia (page 13.126). However, slow-release preparations (e.g. Kinidin Durules) enable therapeutic levels (2.3–5.0 μg/ml) to be maintained with much less risk of toxicity and have the advantage that twice-daily administration (0.5–0.75 g twice daily) is sufficient.

Impaired sinus node and myocardial function are less likely to be worsened by quinidine than by disopyramide or beta-blockers. Because it has a mild anticholinergic action, AV node conduction may be enhanced with a resultant increase in ventricular rate during atrial flutter and fibrillation.

QT interval prolongation occurs with therapeutic doses but lengthening of the QRS complex by more than 25 per cent indicates toxicity. The drug should not be given to patients whose QT interval is already prolonged. Gastrointestinal symptoms are not infrequent. Tinnitus, deafness, thrombocytopenia, and hypotension occasionally occur. Quinidine therapy can elevate digoxin levels and precipitate toxicity. The drug is metabolized by the liver and doses should be reduced if there is hepatic disease.

Procainamide

Procainamide has similar antiarrhythmic properties to those of quinidine. It is not widely used nowadays. It has a short half-life necessitating very frequent dosage when given orally: even with a slow release preparation, eight-hourly administration is necessary. Furthermore, unwanted effects such as systemic lupus syndrome, gastrointestinal symptoms, hypotension, and agranulocytosis make it unsuitable for long-term use. Impaired renal function and a slow acetylator status both reduce procainamide requirements.

N-acetylprocainamide, a metabolite of procainamide, has been shown to have a longer duration of action and not to cause systemic lupus.

Disopyramide

Disopyramide is widely used for both supraventricular and ventricular arrhythmias. However, it is only moderately effective and does have significant unwanted effects.

The intravenous dose is 1.5–2.0 mg/kg up to a maximum of 150 mg, given over no less than 5 min. The injection should be stopped if the arrhythmia is terminated. Therapy can be continued by intravenous infusion at 20–30 mg/hour up to a maximum of 800 mg daily or the patient can be transferred to oral therapy. The oral dose is 300–800 mg daily in three or four divided doses. If necessary a loading dose of 300 mg can be given. The therapeutic range of plasma levels is 2–6 μg/ml.

Given intravenously, the drug is more likely to cause hypotension and heart failure than lignocaine and related drugs and *its use can be disastrous if the recommended minimum period of administration is ignored.*

Orally, the drug's side-effects are mainly related to its anticholinergic (atropine-like) action which often causes a dry mouth, blurred vision, urinary hesitancy or retention, and, by enhancing AV nodal conduction, an increase in the ventricular response to atrial flutter and fibrillation. The drug may precipitate heart failure in patients with impaired myocardial function. It may occasionally induce torsade de pointes tachycardia (page 13.126) and should not be given to patients with QT interval prolongation. Disopyramide may worsen impaired sinus node function and is contraindicated in the sick sinus syndrome. The drug is partially excreted by the kidneys and dosage should be reduced in renal disease.

Flecainide

Flecainide is a potent drug which can be given both orally and parenterally. Its indications include ventricular arrhythmias and pre-excitation syndromes. It has a long half-life of approximately 16 hours. The intravenous dose is 2 mg/kg body weight over not less than 10 min and, because the drug has a significant negative inotropic effect, it should be given more slowly in patients with poor ventricular function. Orally, the dosage is 100–200 mg b.d. After 3–5 days it may be possible to reduce the dose. The therapeutic range of plasma levels is 200–1000 ng/ml

The drug has a narrow therapeutic range and it may be difficult to achieve therapeutic action without unwanted effects. The most common side-effect is visul disturbance, particularly on rotating the head. Lightheadedness and nausea can also occur. The drug can increase the endocardial pacing threshold. Flecainide causes slight prolongation of the QRS complex and hence the QT interval: it does not prolong the JT component of the QT interval as does quinidine and disopyramide. There are a number of reports of the drug causing serious ventricular arrhythmias.

Amiodarone

This drug has several advantages over other drugs. It is highly effective in both supraventricular and ventricular rhythm disorders: even in arrhythmias refractory to other drugs there is a 70 per cent success rate. It has a remarkably long half-life (approximately 28 days) so that the drug need only be given once daily or even less frequently. It does not significantly impair ventricular performance and can be given to patients in heart failure. However, it has important unwanted effects which point to the long-term use of amiodarone being confined to patients with arrhythmias which are dangerous or resistant to other drugs or where the risk of long-term side-effects is not a major consideration because the patient's prognosis is poor, e.g. the elderly and those with severe myocardial damage.

Orally, the drug has a delayed onset of action. It usually takes 3 to 7 days before it takes effect and it may take 50 days to reach its maximal action. When necessary, delay can be minimized by giving large doses, e.g. 1200 mg for 1 or 2 weeks. The dose can then be reduced to 400–600 mg daily. Once it is established that the drug is effective, it is recommended that the dose be progressively reduced until the lowest effective dose is found. Some patients need as little as 200 mg on alternate days. However, in the case of dangerous arrhythmias, it is best not to reduce the dose to less than 400 mg daily.

Intravenous administration will lead to an earlier effect but unlike most drugs an immediate anti-arrhythmic effect rarely occurs: an effect is usually seen within 1–24 hours. The recommended intravenous dosage is 5 mg/kg body weight given over one-half to one hour followed by 15 mg/kg over 24 hours. In an emergency the initial infusion can be given more rapidly – at the risk of marked hypotension. The drug should be given via a central venous line to avoid phlebitis. If this is not possible, frequent change of site of peripheral infusion will usually be sufficient.

The most common long-term unwanted effects are corneal microdeposits and skin photosensitivity. Corneal microdeposits develop in virtually all patients but occular damage does not occur: they disappear if the drug is stopped and are a useful sign of compliance. Skin photosensitivity to UV-A radiation affects over 30 per cent of patients and is the commonest reason for stopping the drug: it may persist for over a year afterwards. Though only a minority experience severe photosensitivity, all patients should be warned about the possibility. Some patients have to avoid prolonged exposure to sunlight (even when shielded by glass) or have to use a barrier cream.

Amiodarone contains iodine and usually causes elevation of both serum thyroxine (T4) and reversed triiodothyronine (T3) with depression of serum T3, the patient remaining euthyroid. However, in a few per cent of patients hypothyroidism (with the usual biochemical changes) or hyperthyroidism (with elevation of both T4 and T3) will develop. Nausea, alopecia, rash, blue-grey skin pigmentation, tremor, and nightmares can occur.

More serious, but uncommon, side-effects include pulmonary fibrosis or alveolitis, neuropathy, myopathy, and hepatitis. These problems are usually but not always associated with high dosage. Pulmonary complications are the most commonly encountered serious unwanted effect and can cause radiological changes similar to those of left heart failure. They usually respond to high doses of corticosteroids.

The drug potentiates both digoxin and anticoagulants. Amiodarone's class III action results in QT prolongation, often with a prominent U wave. There are a few reports of the drug causing *torsade de pointes* tachycardia.

Verapamil

Intravenous verapamil (5–10 mg given over 30–60 s) quickly and effectively slows AV nodal conduction. It is the drug of choice for the termination of paroxysmal (AV re-entrant) supraventricular tachycardia. It will promptly slow the ventricular response to atrial fibrillation and flutter and in a minority of cases, in addition to its action on the AV node, may actually restore sinus rhythm.

Verapamil is less effective given by mouth and because much of each dose is metabolized by the liver, large doses (40–120 mg t.d.s) are required. Oral verapamil is rarely useful alone but is very effective in combination with digoxin in controlling the ventricular response to atrial fibrillation if this cannot be achieved by apparently adequate doses of digoxin alone. Serum digoxin levels are elevated by moderately large doses of verapamil.

Intravenous verapamil is contraindicated if the patient has received an intravenous or oral beta-blocker. Profound bradycardia or hypotension can result and may be fatal. Sometimes, the combination of oral verapamil and a beta-blocker will cause sinus or junctional bradycardia. Because of its depressant effects on the sinus and AV nodes, verapamil is contraindicated in patients with impaired sinus or atrioventricular node function or digoxin toxicity unless a ventricular pacing wire is *in situ*.

Beta-adrenoceptor antagonists

These drugs have antiarrhythmic properties by virtue of their principal action – antagonizing the effects of catecholamines on the heart. They are most effective in arrhythmias caused by increased sympathetic nervous system activity, e.g. those caused by exertion, emotion, thyrotoxicosis, acute myocardial infarction, and the hereditary QT prolongation syndromes.

Beta-blocking drugs slow AV nodal conduction and thus, like verapamil, are useful in arrhythmias of supraventricular origin. However, they are less often successful than verapamil, and, since the latter drug cannot be safely administered once beta-blockers have been given, verapamil is the treatment of choice. Unwanted

bradycardia caused by beta-blockers can usually be reversed by atropine.

Sotalol, in addition to its beta-blocking property, prolongs the duration of the action potential and hence QT interval: it has a significant class III or amiodarone-like action. Unlike other beta-blockers, sotalol has a marked effect upon the refractory periods of atrial and ventricular myocardium and accessory AV pathways. Sotalol is more effective than other beta-blockers for prevention of supraventricular arrhythmias and may possibly be of value for ventricular arrhythmias. There are a few reports of high doses of the drug causing *torsade de pointes* tachycardia, usually in association with other drugs or hypokalaemia. The oral dosage is 160–320 mg daily. Recently, the dextroisomer of sotalol has been shown to have a class III action but insignificant β-blocking properties. D-Sotalol may prove to be clinically useful.

Drug treatment of bradycardia

Artificial cardiac pacing is more effective than drugs in the treatment of bradycardias so that atropine and catecholamines have a limited role.

In patients with symptomatic sinus or junctional bradycardia, particularly in acute myocardial infarction, the anticholinergic action of atropine can quickly restore sinus rhythm. Atropine may also be useful when atrioventricular block is due to impaired atrioventricular node conduction rather than bundle branch disease. In the latter situation, intravenous catecholamines can be useful as a 'first-aid' measure, but pacing is far more effective and safe.

The intravenous dosage of atropine is 0.3–1.0 mg. Tiny doses have been reported to worsen bradycardia and large doses may cause ventricular arrhythmias.

Before the advent of reliable pacemakers, oral catecholamines such as slow-release isoprenaline (Saventrine, 30–120 mg three times daily) were widely used in the treatment of chronic heart block. Nowadays there is little place for these drugs.

References

Barold, S. S. and Friedberg, H. D. (1974). Second degree atrioventricular block. A matter of definition. *Am. J. Cardiol.* **33**, 311–315.

Bennett, D. H. (1985). *Cardiac arrhythmias. Practical notes on interpretation and treatment.* John Wright, Bristol.

Bigger, J. T. (1984). Antiarrhythmic treatment: an overview. *Am. J. Cardiol.* **53**, 8B–16B.

—— et al. (1984). The relationships among ventricular arrhythmias, left ventricular dysfunction, and mortality in the 2 years after myocardial infarction. *Circulation* **69**, 250–258.

Edhag, O. and Swahn, A. (1976). Prognosis of patients with complete heart block or arrhythmic syncope who were not treated with artificial pacemakers. *Acta med. Scand.* **200**, 457–463.

Gallagher, J. J. and Cox, J. L. (1979). Status of surgery for ventricular arrhythmias. *Circulation* **59**, 864–865.

Joy, M. and Bennett, G. (eds) (1984). The First United Kingdom workshop on aviation cardiology: arrhythmias and electrophysiology. *Eur. Heart J.* **5A**, 81–124.

Keefe, D. L. D., Kates, R. E. and Harrison, D. C. (1981). New antiarrhythmic drugs: their place in therapy. *Drugs* **22**, 363–400.

Krikler, D. M. and Curry, P. V. L. (1976). Torsade de pointes, an atypical ventricular tachycardia. *Br. Heart J.* **38**, 117–120.

—— and Goodwin, J. F. (1975). *Cardiac arrhythmias, the modern electrophysiological approach.* W. B. Saunders, London.

Nathan, A. W. et al. (1984). Catheter ablation of atrioventricular conduction. *Lancet* **i**, 1280–1284.

Resnekov, L. (1973). Electroversion. In *Recent advances in cardiology* (ed. J. Hamer), pp. 329–362. Churchill Livingstone, Edinburgh.

Schamroth, L. (1982). *The disorders of cardiac rhythm.* Blackwell Scientific Publications, Oxford.

Vaughan Williams, E. M. (1974). Electrophysiological basis for a rational approach to antidysrhythmic drug therapy. In *Advances in drug research* (eds N. J. Harper and A. B. Simmons). Academic Press, London.

Wellens, H. J. J. (1975). Contribution of cardiac pacing to our understanding of the Wolff-Parkinson–White syndrome. *Br. Heart J.* **37**, 231.

Zipes, D. P. (1985). A consideration of anti-arrhythmic therapy. *Circulation* **72**, 949–956.

PACEMAKERS

R. SUTTON

Pacemakers are employed in the management of bradycardias to maintain the heart rate. The first implant was reported in 1959 and now approximately 200 000 pacemakers are implanted worldwide per year.

Aetiology

The aetiology of bradycardia is most commonly unknown. Histologically the conduction system shows patchy fibrosis occurring in approximately 40 per cent of cases in the United Kingdom. In South America the commonest cause is Chagas' disease. Other causes include coronary artery disease, cardiomyopathy, congenital defects of the conduction system, surgical damage occurring at the time of correction of congenital or valvular defects, calcific aortic valve disease, and drugs such as digitalis.

Presentation

Bradycardias present most frequently with episodes of dizziness (a disturbance of consciousness due to profound fall in blood pressure associated with sudden onset of severe bradycardia or transient asystole), or with complete syncope or a Stokes–Adams attack. Such attacks occur without warning, and may be associated with self-injury. They are usually of short duration and self-limiting, but may be fatal. During the attack, the patient is pale, but if the attack is prolonged, cyanosis ensues with epileptiform seizures. Upon recovery the patient flushes and full consciousness is restored rapidly without amnesia or neurological sequelae. Variations occur in the sick sinus and carotid sinus syndromes with prolonged periods of unconsciousness without a postictal flush and with neurological sequelae rendering diagnosis difficult. Another presentation of bradycardia is with the symptoms and signs of heart failure. In addition to these two presentations the patient may experience palpitation or note his own bradycardia. Severe bradycardia may result in mental confusion or dementia or renal failure due to poor perfusion. It is important to recognize that recurrent falls may be due to transient losses of consciousness; cases may present to orthpaedic or neurological departments. There is no difference in incidence between the sexes and the average age of presentation is 70 years.

Investigation and diagnosis

After clinical examination at which the bradycardia may or may not be present and the effects of low cardiac output may be detected, investigation begins with electrocardiography. Evidence of complete heart block, or Mobitz type II second degree heart block will provide an immediate diagnosis. Blocks at the atrioventricular, or sino-atrial node less commonly lead to symptoms. Frequently sinus rhythm is found but ventricular conduction defects may be present. Trifascicular block raises the strongest likelihood of intermittent episodes of complete heart block. If the electrocardiogram is normal, it is necessary to perform carotid sinus massage on each side separately during rhythm monitoring for 5 s unless the patient has had transient cerebral ischaemic episodes or has a carotid bruit. If more than 3 s of asystole results with reproduction of symptoms, the diagnosis is carotid sinus syndrome. Proof of arrhythmia causing syncope may be obtained by monitoring the cardiac rhythm either as an inpatient or more frequently using ambulatory electrocardiography. If attacks are rare, provocative measures such as exercise stress electrocardiography and electrophysiological testing may be employed. Electrode catheters introduced percutaneously under local anaesthesia into the femoral vein are positioned in the right heart to obtain atrial, ventricular, and His bundle signals. In patients with intermittent heart block the His to ventricular conduction times may be prolonged (normal 35–55 ms). Rapid atrial pacing is used to assess the integrity of the atrioventricular nodal and ventricular conduction and the ability of the sino-atrial node to recover after a period of pacing is delayed in the sick sinus syndrome. None of these electrophysiological tests is absolutely diagnostic and none is performed routinely.

Indications for pacing

Symptoms provide the major indications for permanent cardiac pacing: syncope, dizziness, and heart failure. When complete heart block or Mobitz type II second degree atrioventricular block exist, a pacemaker is advisable even in the absence of symptoms as in these arrhythmias asystole is common and carries a high risk. In other conditions prophylactic pacing is controversial; these include evidence of conduction tissue disease without persistent symptoms following myocardial infarction, cardiac surgery, and in other types of block. Temporary cardiac pacing may be employed in coronary care or postsurgical intensive care units to control transient heart blocks and in the management (together with drugs) of tachyarrhythmias. These conditions do not usually require pacing for longer than 72 hours.

Techniques

The implantation of a pacemaker is a surgical procedure requiring full sterile precautions performed by surgeons or cardiologists usually under local anaesthesia. The central cephalic approached by incision or the subclavian percutaneously are the veins of choice for the lead which consists of a multistrand conductor wire insulated by silicone rubber or polyurethane with an electrode tip usually of platinum alloy and a connector plug at the distal end. The lead is passed with the aid of fluoroscopy and a stiffening stylet in the core of the lead to the right atrium, through the tricuspid valve, and positioned in the apex (anterior) of the right ventricle. Lateral fluoroscopy is useful to confirm the position. Close to the electrode an anchoring device is fitted to the lead which engages the right ventricular trabeculae. The most effective of these is a group of tines which project outwards and backwards from the tip at an angle of 60°. Once the lead is in position tests are made of the signal which the heart will convey to the pacemaker via the lead (electrograms) and the ability of an external pacemaker attached to the lead to pace the heart (threshold testing). If the lead is found satisfactory, it is sutured in the vein or subcutaneous tissues and a subcutaneous pocket over pectoralis major is constructed for the pacemaker which is attached to the lead and implanted (Fig. 1). Prophylactic antibiotics may be used for a few days after surgery. The patient is mobilized on the same day and may be discharged from hospital within a few days. This is a description of an endocardial procedure; an alternative is to place a lead on the epicardial surface of the heart either by an epigastric incision or by thoracotomy which is not done under local anaesthesia and involves a more substantial procedure for the patient. The pacemaker is then usually implanted in the rectus sheath. In young children who will grow rapidly this approach is preferred as a redundant lead can be taken up in the pathway to the heart, though increasingly transvenous approaches are being used for children by means of screw-tipped leads which offer very secure fixation to the endocardium combined with large redundant loops of lead in the venous system.

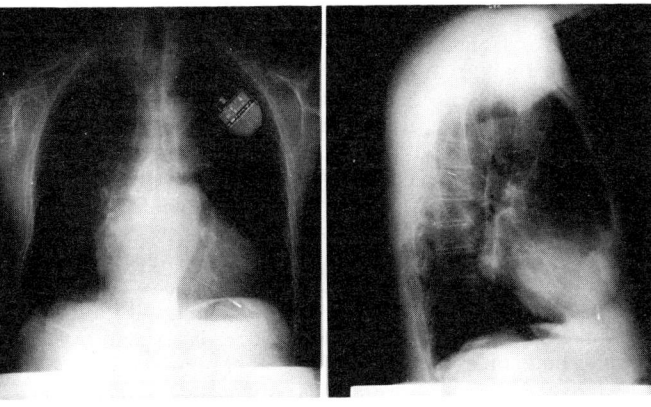

Fig. 1 Chest X-rays. Anteroposterior and lateral projections showing an endocardial pacemaker system with electrode in the right ventricular apex and pacemaker in the subcutaneous tissue over left pectoralis major.

Technology

Pacemakers are manufactured under rigorous conditions of cleanliness and quality assurance. The unit, now weighing approximately 40 g, consists of a battery which is commonly a lithium–iodine cell developed especially for pacemakers. This cell has the advantage of high power to weight and size ratios, predictable discharge behaviour, and long life. Present day cells offer up to 10 years life with low current drain from circuit and electrode. The other major component is the pulse forming circuitry which is now of hybrid type using a silicon chip with the addition of a few discrete components. All pacemakers have a 'sensing' capability where an amplifier picks up spontaneous cardiac activity and uses this to recycle the pacemaker's output. Thus, if the patient returns to normal sinus rhythm, the pacemaker output is inhibited; as soon as the rate of the spontaneous rhythm falls below the set rate of the pacemaker, stimulation of the heart recommences. This is known as demand function (Fig. 2). It can be excluded by placing a magnet over the pacemaker, excluding the sensing amplifier from the circuit, rendering the unit asynchronous or fixed rate. The hybrid circuit is usually sealed hermetically as is the battery and the outer coat of the pacemaker offers another hermetic seal usually being constructed of titanium. There is a feed-through connection to the lead plug which permits electrical connection without loss of hermetic seal. The sealing is necessary to prevent

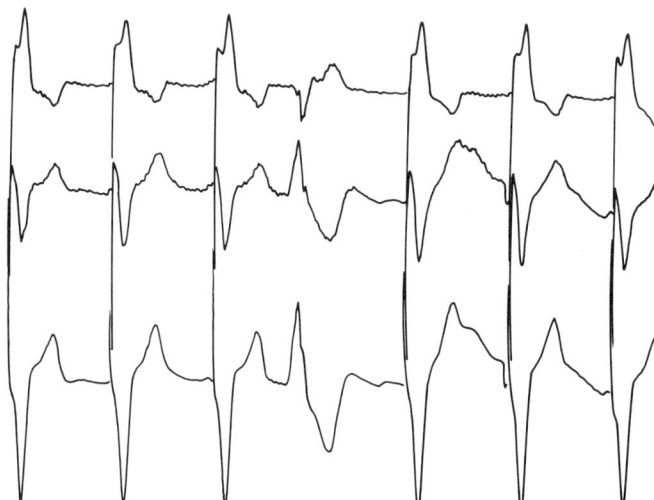

Fig. 2 Electrocardiogram leads V_1, V_2, and V_3 showing ventricular pacing with an extrasystole inhibiting pacemaker's output and recycling it (demand function: see text).

access of body fluids. Part or all of the metal shield may be used as the indifferent pole of the pacemaker system, which has implications for local stimulation and sensing; due to the low current density the pectoralis major is not stimulated. Muscle activity (electromyogram) being 'sensed' as spontaneous cardiac activity is minimized by filtering at the amplifier. An alternative is to use a lead with a second ring electrode close to the tip (bipolar system) and the pacemaker's metal casing then plays no part in the circuit. The bipolar lead has in the past been more vulnerable to fracture. Pacemakers now are often programmable externally. Their rate, output, sensitivity, and refractory periods may be altered transcutaneously by an electromagnetic or radiofrequency programmer allowing more accurate 'tailoring' of the pacemaker to the patient's needs and use of the minimum safe output to prolong battery life.

Pacemaker clinic

Prior to discharge from hospital the pacemaker is checked by electrocardiography (12-lead) for proper capture of the heart with a magnet over the pacemaker if necessary. Chest radiography for lead position is performed as well as electronic analysis of the pulse frequency, stimulus–stimulus interval, and pulse width of the pacemaker's output which should be stable and within milliseconds or in the case of the pulse-width within microseconds of that at implant. Variation may indicate a circuit fault. Programmable pacemakers are checked throughout their range. The patient attends a pacemaker clinic after one month and then at six monthly intervals where a similar protocol is followed together with routine clinical examination including the pacemaker site. Changes in the electronic parameters which are linked to battery voltage can be used to determine an elective pacemaker replacement time well ahead of battery exhaustion. Unexpected changes may indicate circuit or lead faults.

Results

Permanent pacing results in abolition of dizziness and syncope and a marked prolongation in life expectancy in heart block. Improvement in heart failure usually occurs but may need the addition of drugs. Improvement in, or abolition of, symptoms in sick sinus and carotid sinus syndromes is expected but longevity is not influenced. With modern pacemakers and leads, reoperation is rarely necessary until battery exhaustion is imminent.

Complications

Surgical

With proper technique the incidence of infection should be less than 1 per cent. Erosion of the pacemaker through the skin, probably due to pressure necrosis has now been almost eliminated with modern lightweight units. Thrombo-embolism is extremely rare. Local problems such as pain and haematoma are very rarely severe.

Lead

Perforation of heart or venous system is usually benign: proper techniques and modern leads have rendered this rare. If a lead becomes displaced from the endocardium, loss of capture results. This tends to occur in the first few weeks after implant and may be fatal because of sudden cessation of pacing. Modern tined leads have reduced this incidence to less than 2 per cent. Fracture of the wire, insulation, or both may also result in loss of pacing. This occurs rarely and may be anticipated by alterations in the electronic analysis of the pacemaker pulse. Infection may result in endocarditis at the lead tip and, because of the presence of a foreign body, may necessitate the removal of the whole pacemaker system, and the use of temporary endocardial pacing until eradication of the infection when a new permanent endocardial system can be placed or an epicardial system may be preferred. The power required to capture the heart may rise progressively, instead of an early rise followed by stabilization or fall, known as exit block. Its treatment may require a higher pacemaker output or a new lead.

Pacemaker

Premature failure presents either by excessive slowing loss of output or by acceleration (run away). International bodies now collect data on all pacemaker types in order to provide early warnings of pacemaker batch failures, allowing explantation of many before they fail. Runaway protection is now built into all pacemakers. Human error may occur with pacemaker programming; record keeping and checking parameters are essential. Most pacemaker circuit faults occur either as a result of ingress of body fluids or failure of connections between the discrete components and the silicon chip. Hermetic sealing and manufacturer's quality assurance must prevent this as far as is possible. The environment provides most hazards to the pacemaker patient. Electromagnetic interference may arise from many sources, including weapon and theft detectors. Most pacemakers revert to asynchronous mode under these conditions without risk to the patient. Some new software-based highly complex pacemakers may dump their programmes in the face of surgical diathermy. Special care is required in these cases. Halothane and related anaesthetic gases raise the energy required for capture of the heart and should be avoided. Close contact with leaky microwave ovens and working with special apparatus such as arc-welders are contraindicated for pacemaker patients because of possible inappropriate inhibition or acceleration.

Ventricular extrasystoles are not uncommon immediately following lead implant. Competition by the pacemaker with spontaneous rhythm is almost always excluded by the demand function and is further minimized by rate hysteresis where there is a longer interval before the pacemaker takes over than the set pacing interval. Occasionally ventricular pacing may be associated with retrograde atrioventricular conduction. This may be asymptomatic or may cause syncope, by fall in blood pressure, or heart failure. Treatment is by use of an atrioventricular sequential pacemaker with careful programming to avoid an endless loop pacemaker mediated tachycardia.

Developments

Pacemaker application will become more widespread. Pacemakers are making greater use of the silicon chip to become telemetric, now and in the future, self-analysing, and self-programming. Greater account is being taken by pacemaker specialists of circulatory physiology leading to an increasing number of dual chamber pacemakers. These systems have the addition of an endocardial lead in the right atrium, usually in its appendage, and a second amplifier and output stage to allow sensing and pacing in the atria. In addition, a sensed event (P wave) in the atria leads after a suitable delay (PR interval) to ventricular pacing. This function allows a physiological rate response to exertion and emotion, and maintains proper atrioventricular synchrony. When the sinus node function is inadequate other sensors such as respiratory rate and volume, activity and stimulus to T wave interval are being developed to give a physiological rate response to more patients. Pacemakers are being used increasingly for tachycardia control where precisely timed stimuli are employed to interrupt re-entry circuits in conditions such as atrioventricular nodal reciprocating tachycardia, Wolff–Parkinson–White syndrome, and ventricular tachycardia. With the advent of endocardial ablation procedures for arrhythmia control, use of a pacemaker may be needed subsequently where an inadequate escape rhythm results, for example, in His bundle ablation.

References

Davies, M. J. (1971). *The pathology of the conducting tissue of the heart.* Butterworth, London
Elmquist, R. and Senning, A. (1959). An implantable pacemaker for the heart. In *Medical electronics. Proceedings of the Second International Conference in Medical Electronics* (ed. C. N. Smyth), p. 253. Illife, London.
Ginks, W., Siddons, H. and Leatham, A. (1979). Prognosis of patients paced for chronic atrioventricular block. *Br. Heart J.* **41**, 633–636.
Shaw, D. B., Holman, R. R. and Gowers, J. I. (1980). Survival in sinoatrial disorder (sick sinus syndrome). *Br. Med. J.* **21**, 139–142.
Sutton, R., Citron, P. and Perrins, J. (1980). Physiological cardiac pacing. *Pace* **3**, 201–219.
Morley, C. and Sutton, R. (1984). Carotid Sinus Syndrome. *Int. J. Cardiol.* **6**, 287–293.

ATHEROMA: VESSEL WALL AND THROMBOSIS

C. N. CHESTERMAN

Introduction

Occlusive vascular disease due to atherosclerosis and associated thromboembolic phenomena is well recognized as the major cause of mortality and morbidity in developed countries. The disease is a result of the interaction of multiple factors including a genetic predisposition. Although the process is morphologically uniform, there is the fascinating and yet unexplained predilection to affect certain anatomical regions of the arterial tree with greater frequency than others and in a given individual to affect some areas far more severely than others. Thus, the comparative freedom of the arteries of the upper limbs from the atherosclerotic process is notable and tantalizing because it is unexplained. Furthermore, specific risk factors appear to be selectively more important in the development or progression of atherosclerosis at a particular site. Hypertension is particularly associated with the risk of cerebrovascular disease and cigarette smoking with peripheral vascular disease. These factors are discussed further in the sections covering ischaemic heart disease, cerebrovascular disease, and peripheral vascular disease.

The epidemic of atherosclerosis in the twentieth century appears to have peaked in the mid 1960s and the apparent decline in mortality, in particular from ischaemic heart disease, over the past 20 years in the United States, Australia, Finland, Belgium, and other countries (not yet in the United Kingdom) suggests that despite the difficulty in proving formally the effectiveness of modifying 'risk factors', it is likely that such modification has occurred within these populations as a result of public awareness of their possible significance. Other less adequate explanations may be advanced, in particular the improved treatment of clinical events secondary to the disease process.

The occlusion of an artery may be the result of a number of acute events, haemorrhage into an atherosclerotic plaque, embolization of atheromatous or thrombotic material or spasm of a diseased vessel, but in the majority of cases it is caused by thrombosis occurring on an atheromatous and stenosed segment. In each of these instances the situation differs from that pertaining to venous thromboembolism. Common to both, however, are the major factors identified by Virchow in 1856 and which are responsible for

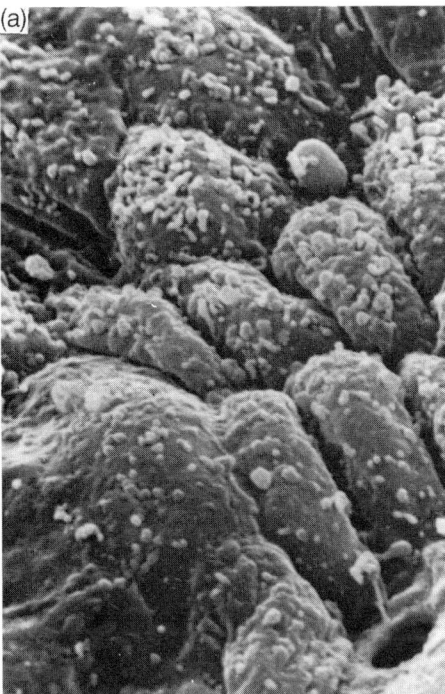

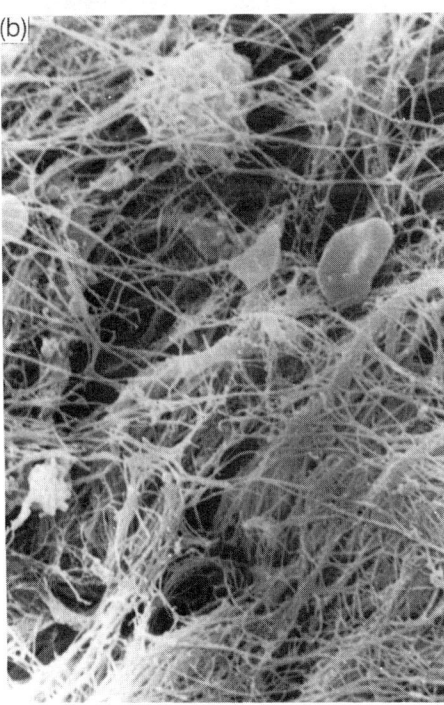

Fig. 1 Scanning electron microscopy of the luminal surface of porcine aorta showing the (a) intact endothelium and (b) subendothelial collagen fibres lying below (× 9600).

modifying the normal haemostatic process so that a thrombus forms. These are to a greater or lesser extent the contributions of altered blood flow, altered blood constituents or an abnormality of the vessel wall.

The vessel wall and blood flow

Circulation of blood depends upon a complicated relationship between components of the blood vessel wall and the flowing blood; this applies obviously to functions such as fluid and solute passage but also with components of haemostasis. The essential requirement is a luminal surface which differs substantially in its

thrombogenic properties from the tissue immediately surrounding it (Fig. 1).

The endothelial lining is formed by a continuous monolayer of cells 25–50 μm long and 10–15 μm wide. The cells overlap to a minor degree. The subendothelium consists of basal membrane, collagen fibrils, proteoglycan rich in carbohydrate, glycosaminoglycans, fibronectin, and elastin. The elastin is continuous with the internal elastic lamina which separates the intima from the underlying media, in arteries consisting mostly of smooth muscle cells arranged in spiral and concentric layers. Externally there is a circumferential condensation of collagen and elastin fibres forming the tunica elastica externa. The adventitia is composed of connective tissue, the fibroblasts being largely oriented longitudinally.

Signals to activate platelets and coagulation proteins remain external to the vessel lumen until there is a breach in the endothelial cell lining and then the sensitivity of the haemostatic system to these signals is very great. Platelets responding to an endothelial breach and adhering to subendothelial tissue, in particular the collagen fibrils are estimated to react within a few milliseconds. In addition, platelet adhesion and subsequent aggregation at the site of laceration of an artery or arteriole takes place despite enormous shear forces compared to those met in the normal circulation. Appreciation of this great susceptibility of platelets to react to an abnormal surface is important when considering the development and the effects of atherosclerosis.

The property of the vessel wall which protects from thrombosis resides in the endothelium. A number of factors have been identified as contributing to this protection including the nature of the membrane glycocalyx; the resulting negative surface charge is probably instrumental in repelling negatively charged platelets. Metabolic characteristics favour the maintenance of circulating platelets in an inactive and non-adherent state. Enzymes in the endothelial membrane rapidly inactivate adenine nucleotides (ADP, ATP) and the cells take up serotonin, thus reducing local concentrations of platelet aggregatory substances. The final product of the endothelial enzymatic degradation of ADP is adenosine which, in itself, is inhibitory to platelet aggregation. The prostaglandin system, commonly a modulater in the interplay between cells, is regarded as important in maintaining the fluidity of blood. Arachidonic acid within the endothelial cell membrane is predominantly catabolized to prostacyclin (PGI_2) a potent inhibitor (by causing elevation of cyclic AMP) of platelet adhesion and aggregation. This highly active metabolite released throughout the extensive area of the endothelial vascular lining has the potential of acting as a circulating anticoagulant and such a proposal was advanced some years ago. The weight of evidence, however, would suggest that circulating prostacyclin levels are too low to have a significant biological effect and this is in part due to the rapidity with which prostacyclin is inactivated in the circulation. Prostacyclin is released in large quantities in response to injury to endothelium and in response to specific coagulation enzymes such as thrombin and vasoactive substances such as bradykinin. Thus its local release is likely to be relevant to limiting thrombosis. Endothelial metabolism of adenine nucleotides and serotonin and the production of prostacyclin all contribute to vasodilation, in itself presumably tending to maintain flow and prevent thrombosis.

Despite the experimental evidence which points to the importance of prostacyclin in the endothelial–platelet interaction, observations in clinical medicine raise some fundamental questions. In conditions in which prostacyclin production is substantially reduced, e.g. in the rare congenital cyclooxygenase deficiency a mild bleeding tendency and no significant predisposition to thrombosis are reported. The parallel deficiency in platelet cyclooxygenase and thus thromboxane A_2 production may provide an explanation for this observation (Fig. 2). However, platelets respond to thrombin and collagen, albeit with reduced sensitivity, in the absence of thromboxane. Similarly, when endothelial prostacyclin production is inhibited by aspirin administration

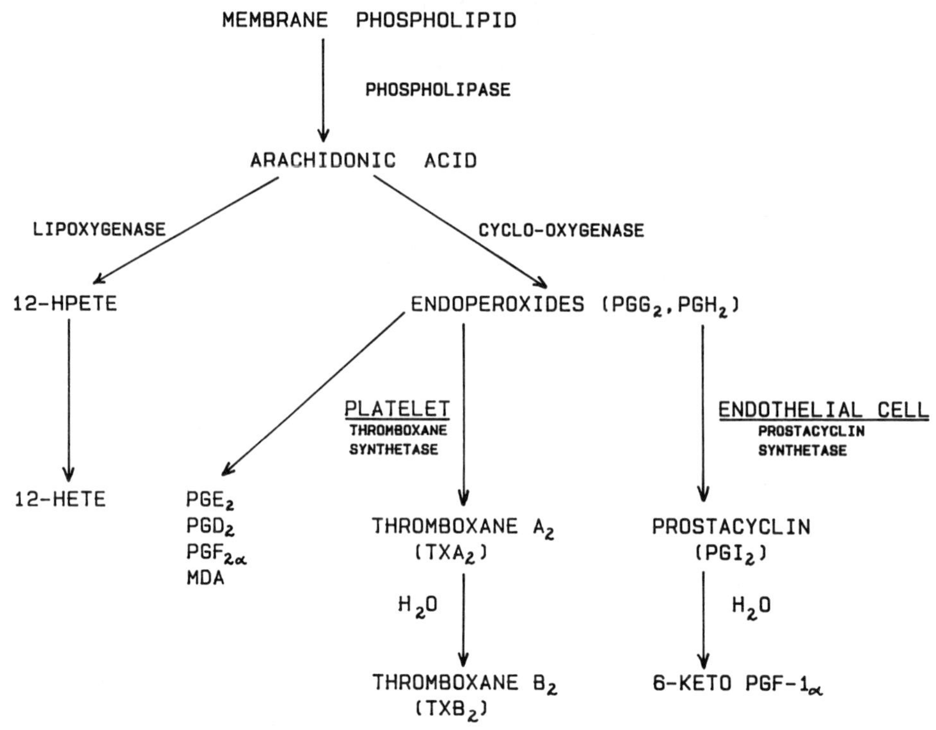

MEMBRANE PHOSPHOLIPID

PHOSPHOLIPASE

Fig. 2 Scheme of arachidonic acid metabolism in the platelet and vascular endothelial cell. Endoperoxides produced by stimulation of platelet cyclooxygenase can be 'shunted' and metabolized by the endothelium to produce prostacyclin.

ARACHIDONIC ACID

LIPOXYGENASE   CYCLO-OXYGENASE

12-HPETE   ENDOPEROXIDES (PGG_2, PGH_2)

PLATELET   ENDOTHELIAL CELL
THROMBOXANE SYNTHETASE   PROSTACYCLIN SYNTHETASE

12-HETE PGE_2 THROMBOXANE A_2 PROSTACYCLIN
         PGD_2 (TXA_2)   (PGI_2)
         $PGF_{2\alpha}$
         MDA H_2O H_2O

THROMBOXANE B_2 6-KETO PGF-1_α
(TXB_2)

(although platelet thromboxane production is also inhibited), thrombosis does not occur.

Vascular endothelium plays a powerful regulatory role in the pathways of blood coagulation. Endothelium synthesizes antithrombin III and binds heparan sulphate and heparin, rapidly inactivating traces of thrombin in the immediate locality. Endothelium is responsible for the production of thrombomodulin, a protein which binds to thrombin and, in doing so, increases by several orders of magnitude the ability of thrombin to activate protein C. This vitamin K-dependent protein then destroys activated factors V and VIII, interrupting the coagulation cascade. Finally, a complex series of endothelial reactions results in the elaboration of plasminogen activator, initiating fibrinolysis and the dissolution of thrombus.

All these processes, integral to maintaining blood fluidity, are presumed to decrease as atherosclerotic disease progresses. Such a decrease may be related to loss of endothelial function as well as to the actual loss of endothelial cells themselves.

Atherosclerosis

Pathology

Atherosclerosis involves the intima of medium and large arteries. The process begins in childhood and the earliest changes observed are areas of diffuse thickening of the musculoelastic intima. As the disease progresses through young adulthood three main lesions are described, namely, the fatty streak, the fibrous plaque, and the complicated lesion. The essential feature of fatty streaks is the accumulation of small numbers of intimal smooth muscle cells surrounded by deposits of lipids. Lipid-laden macrophages are seen very early in experimental models of atherosclerosis. It has been assumed that the fibrous plaque represents a progression from the fatty streak. The question is controversial, however, and because the lipid component in the fatty streak is largely cholesterol oleate in contrast to cholesterol linoleate in the fibrous plaque it may be that the origins of the two lesions are not identical.

The fibrous plaque is composed of lipid-laden smooth muscle cells and macrophages with the deposition of collagen, elastic fibres, and proteoglycan. Further development with calcification, cell necrosis, mural thrombosis, and possibly haemorrhage results in the so-called 'complicated lesion'. The fibrous plaque and to a greater extent the complicated lesion result in luminal narrowing and are associated with subsequent occlusion. Already noted is the predilection for atherosclerotic lesions to occur at specific areas, in particular at the bifurcation of arteries and often with comparatively normal vessel wall between the lesions.

Pathogenesis

Apparently divergent hypotheses regarding the development of atherosclerosis have recently been drawn together in a unified concept by Ross and his colleagues. In the nineteenth century Rokitansky conceived atheroma as an excessive deposition of blood products, in particular fibrin. Virchow described atheroma as an inflammatory process and a 'reactive proliferation'. More recently the proliferation was reported to be due to division of abnormal clones of smooth muscle cells in the vessel wall. Others have regarded atherosclerosis as a degenerative process or even a process due to the progressive accumulation of lipid by 'insudation'.

The unifying concept known as 'response to injury' proposes that atherogenesis involves:

1. Endothelial cell injury
2. The release of factors in the subendothelium which results in the migration of smooth muscle cells through the internal elastic lamina with subsequent proliferation in the intima
3. The synthesis by muscle cells of collagen, elastin, and proteoglycans
4. Intracellular and extracellular lipid accumulation
5. Associated thrombus formation.

Although it was originally suggested that the stimulus to smooth muscle proliferation depended upon a mitogen released from platelets (platelet-derived growth factor) following the endothelial injury, it is likely that this is too simplistic. Growth factors from macrophages, endothelial cells, and smooth muscle cells themselves have similar activity. Thus, atherosclerotic lesions can be induced in experimental animals by producing endothelial dysfunction or by endothelial desquamation and in such models prevented by antiplatelet drugs or by producing thrombocytopenia. In other models, e.g. diet-induced atherosclerosis, endothelial injury is not demonstrable and the earliest abnormalities include the migration of macrophages which can be seen underlying intact

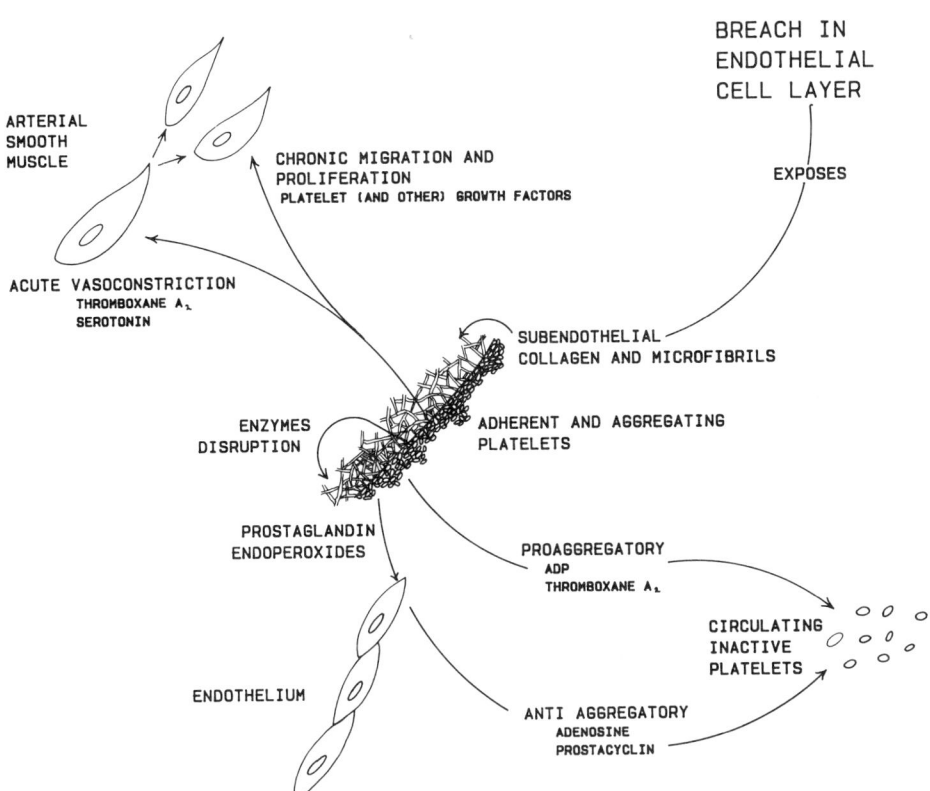

Fig. 3 Main interactions between platelets and the vessel wall maintaining blood fluidity on the one hand and contributing to vessel wall disease on the other when stimulated by endothelial cell injury or loss.

endothelium. In each model, the blood cell, the platelet or macrophage (monocyte derived?) may release the mitogen and provide the stimulus to smooth muscle proliferation.

Endothelial injury

There are many candidates for factors which may injure endothelium, such injury leading to either desquamation, resulting in the exposure of thrombogenic, subendothelial collagen or to impaired cellular function. An example of loss of function short of cell death is demonstrable in cultured endothelial cells. Repeated stimulation of endothelium *in vitro* by thrombin or by mechanical stimuli results in the rapid loss in the ability of the cells to produce prostacyclin. This would favour platelet adhesion, thrombosis, and possibly further vascular injury. Haemodynamic stresses, other forms of mechanical stress and chemical agents may be injurious. At the bifurcations of arteries, endothelial cell turnover is significantly increased, believed to be related to the turbulence of blood flow and both these factors may be related to the tendency of atherosclerosis to develop at these sites preferentially. Platelet microthrombi tend to form at sites of turbulent flow but there is conflicting evidence as to whether wall shear stress or deviation from axially aligned, unidirectional flow is the determining factor. Of chemicals, carbon monoxide toxicity to endothelium has been suggested as an explanation for the higher frequency of atherosclerosis in cigarette smokers. Blood components shown to induce endothelial injury when in excess are homocysteine, the amino acid produced abnormally in hereditary homocystinuria and cholesterol. In both hereditary homocystinuria and congenital hypercholesterolaemia (type II) premature development of atherosclerosis results in vascular occlusions in early adulthood. Other potential injurious agents include immune complexes, viruses, and the products of activated neutrophils. Two problems bedevil interpretation of the significance of these various factors. Firstly there is conflicting evidence regarding the effects of potential endothelial toxins in the laboratory so that, depending on the experimental system, results are not in agreement. Secondly, animal models of atherosclerosis, for obvious reasons require the unnaturally rapid production of lesions and thus involve the use of gross

injury, e.g. the mechanical disruption of endothelium by balloon catheter or the feeding of animals with diets containing massive quantities of cholesterol.

Contributory factors from platelets and coagulation processes to the development of atherosclerosis

Platelet activation and fibrin (thrombus) formation may contribute to the development of atherosclerotic lesions via a number of mechanism which will be briefly outlined. There is little doubt that atherosclerotic plaques contain a significant concentration of fibrin-like material. Fibrin may contribute to cell growth, act as a scaffold for migrating cells and effect the synthesis of connective tissue components by smooth muscle or fibroblasts in the vessel wall. Degradation products of fibrin produced by the fibrinolytic activity of plasmin have similar metabolic capability. Although fibrin is present, particularly as atherosclerotic lesions become established, it is likely that platelets play a more active role in the early proliferative lesion (Fig. 3). Immunologically identifiable platelet-related antigens are found in most fibrous plaques. Further, in experimental animal models of atherosclerosis, platelet-specific proteins rapidly find their way into the intima of the vessel wall. As outlined above, one of the most active proteins released by platelets in this context is the mitogen, platelet-derived growth factor, which has recently been highly purified, characterized, and shown to possess the ability not only to cause smooth muscle cells to proliferate but also to migrate towards the site of release. Platelet-derived growth factor may also effect the biosynthesis of prostaclycin in endothelial cells and the underlying smooth muscle. Other proteins released simultaneously include β-thromboglobulin which has a minor inhibitory effect on prostacyclin production by cultured endothelial cells and a chemotactic effect for mesenchymal cells. Prostaglandin metabolites from platelets, particularly thromboxane A_2 by virtue of its vasoconstricting and platelet aggregating activity, contributes to the progression of thrombosis and the development of atherosclerosis. Another metabolite of arachidonic acid (12-HETE) stimulates migration of aortic smooth muscle cells. Enzymes released from platelets, for example, elastase, may have effects on the basement membrane and aid in disruption of the normal connective tissue stroma.

Experimental observations and pathological findings in human atherosclerosis suggesting the involvement of platelets and coagulation proteins in the development of atherosclerotic vascular disease are supported by clinical and laboratory findings in patients. The problems, however, in assigning a causal role for platelet and coagulation abnormalities in the developmental phases of the disease are legion. As atherosclerosis develops, vessel wall changes are likely to provide a stimulus to platelets to become reactive and to changes in coagulation proteins in the circulation, so that the findings of such abnormalities may reflect secondary phenomena and not primary defects. Nevertheless, it is reasonable to hypothesize that, even if such changes are secondary, they will contribute to atherosclerotic lesion progression or to subsequent thromboembolic phenomena. In patients with established atheroma the results of platelet survival measurements, probably the best index of *in vivo* activation, are somewhat controversial. However, the weight of evidence would favour the existence of subgroups of patients who have shortened platelet survival, elevated plasma levels of platelet release products and increased sensitivity of platelets to aggregating substances. It has been reported that patients with shortened platelet survival have fared less well following coronary artery grafting procedures while platelet abnormalities have been corrected by coronary artery grafting or by antiplatelet drugs in other patients. There is some evidence that the circulating platelets in patients with ischaemic heart disease are larger and functionally more active than in the normal individual. Abnormally high plasma fibrinogen concentration and a reduction in the capacity of the vessel wall to release plasminogen activator (fibrinolytic activity) have been well documented in patients with various forms of atherosclerotic disease.

A further line of investigation has been to seek evidence of platelet or coagulation abnormalities in patients prone to develop vascular disease. Platelets from patients with familial hypercholesterolaemia (type II) are abnormally sensitive to aggregating agents and *in vitro* the acquisition of cholesterol by platelets is associated with increased sensitivity. Diabetes mellitus, particularly in those patients already affected by small vessel disease, is associated with abnormalities in platelet function, elevated plasma fibrinogen levels, reduction in fibrinolytic capacity and significant abnormalities of the factor VIII – von Willebrand factor. The question arises again as to whether these changes, in particular those of fibrinogen and von Willebrand factor, are due to a primary endothelial cell abnormality induced by diabetes rather than to a disturbance in haemostasis. Such a proposition is strengthened by the observation that vascular wall prostacyclin production in vein biopsies from diabetic patients is reduced and experimental diabetes in animals results in deficient prostacyclin synthesis by the vessel wall. Some of the abnormalities described above have been demonstrated in diabetic patients without obvious vascular disease but in whom diabetic control is poor, confusing the issue further.

Perhaps some of the most useful information regarding coagulation factors has been gleaned from the Northwick Park Heart Study, initiated with the object of assessing haemostatic function in ischaemic heart disease. A prospective study of this nature, where observations made on entry to the trial in 1972 have been correlated with the subsequent development of symptoms of ischaemic heart disease, goes part of the way towards assigning a causal role to such abnormalities. Entry plasma concentrations of coagulation factors VII and VIII and fibrinogen were significantly higher in men who subsequently died of cardiovascular causes than in those who have survived. Other coagulation abnormalities and reduced fibrinolytic activity were associated with the subsequent prevalence of ischaemic heart disease but not with cardiovascular death. It should be noted that these coagulation abnormalities appear to be independently important and not associated with other known risk factors.

Plasma lipids in atherosclerosis
(See pages 13.143 and 9.108.)

Reference has already been made to the relationship between plasma lipid levels and development of atherosclerosis. The Framingham study established that hypercholesterolaemia is associated with subsequent risk of development of ischaemic heart disease and this finding has been confirmed in a number of studies. In particular, the absolute level of low-density lipoprotein LDL cholesterol appears to be the most important component and the epidemiological observations are supported by the finding that gelatinous lesions and fibrous plaques in arteries have a high concentration of plasma LDL. The mechanisms by which cholesterol and cholesterol ester accumulate in the vessel wall are unclear but candidates include contributions from uptake by LDL receptor, endothelial damage, and plasma leakage into the artery, binding by fibrin in advanced lesions, enzymatic degradation of LDL with leakage into extracellular spaces, and even the local release of cholesterol by platelets.

The importance of the LDL receptor in the regulation of cholesterol metabolism is illustrated in the condition of familial hypercholesterolaemia (type II). The genetic defect results in a lack of the functional cell surface receptors for LDL, preventing the uptake of lipoprotein from the blood and causing a block in the normal hepatic degradation pathway for very low-density lipoprotein (VLDL). These metabolic alterations are associated with plasma cholesterol levels of six to eight times normal and premature development of atherosclerosis.

Circulating HDL cholesterol reduces the risk of development of vascular disease, again the mechanism being uncertain. HDL may aid the removal of cholesterol from cells by taking up free cholesterol from the plasma membrane thus increasing transport to the liver for catabolism. HDL may also inhibit the cellular uptake of LDL and facilitate the degradation of VLDL. Finally, contributions of cholesterol to the development of atherosclerosis may also be made via additional mechanisms already outlined, by increasing platelet reactivity, by direct injury to the endothelial cell, and by intrinsic mitogenic activity resulting in localized proliferation of smooth muscle cells.

Acute vascular occlusion

Against the background of atherosclerotic disease, ischaemia may be due to increased tissue demand for oxygen, reduced blood flow without occlusion or to acute occlusion. The contribution of blood components may be on the basis of rheological factors, vasoactivity or thromboembolism.

Blood viscosity

Blood viscosity is a significant determinant in occlusive vascular disease. The haematocrit and the plasma fibrinogen level are the two most important factors affecting whole blood viscosity. The viscosity of blood is doubled by a rise in haematocrit from 40 to 50 per cent or an increase in plasma fibrinogen of 1 g/l, at low shear rates. The plasma viscosity in fact correlates closely with plasma fibrinogen. Reference has already been made to the finding of significantly elevated plasma fibrinogen levels in the presence of vascular disease and in diabetics, and also the observation that an elevated plasma fibrinogen concentration is associated with the subsequent development of ischaemic heart disease and cardiovascular death. In the uncommon plasma cell dyscrasias immunoglobulins, particularly IgM paraproteins, may assume greater importance as the cause of increased blood viscosity.

Arterial spasm

Coronary artery and cerebral artery spasm are well documented and either may be superimposed on atherosclerotic or comparatively normal vessels. Spasm of the coronary artery may result in variant angina, severe arrhythmia or acute myocardial infarction. It is possible that platelets stimulated by vessel wall abnormalities account for, or contribute to, coronary spasm in particular by the elaboration of thromboxane A$_2$ a powerful vasoconstrictor. Direct evidence for this link is controversial with plasma levels and coronary sinus levels of platelet products being elevated in some patients studied and not in others. Experiments with anaesthetized animals have shown that intermittent thrombotic occlusions at the site of coronary artery stenosis results in myocardial ischaemia which can be prevented by aspirin or by a thromboxane analogue which inhibits the production and the action of thromboxane. Antiplatelet treatment may improve the outcome in patients with unstable angina but does not appear to influence the variant angina syndrome.

Thrombotic or thromboembolic occlusion

The precise stimuli to thrombotic occlusion or the development of thrombotic material on a diseased atherosclerotic artery are not well defined. The development of critical stenosis with reduction in blood flow, haemorrhage into a plaque, reduction in blood flow for other haemodynamic reasons, and the increase in platelet reactivity due to an increase in circulating catecholamines must all be possible factors. Born has suggested that the initiation of thrombosis may relate to haemodynamic stress. Platelet aggregation is induced at high shear rates and shear stresses that are reached in the presence of a severe stenosis of a vessel. An increase in the viscosity of the blood will also result in an increase in shear stress even though the shear rate remains constant. Direct shear-induced platelet aggregation may occur but also the release of ADP from red cells damaged by shear stress might further contribute to platelet aggregation. Finally, the constitution of the thrombus and whether thrombotic material embolizes or remains adherent are related to the local blood flow and associated shear stresses.

The composition of arterial thrombi differs from the venous. Both appear to originate with a nidus of aggregated platelets. The growth of thrombus in the comparatively sluggish venous system is heavily dependent on fibrin formation with a large erythrocyte and granulocyte component. The development of arterial thrombi depends on the continual acquisition of platelets from the circulation with proportionally less reliance on fibrin and other blood cells. This presumably reflects the effect of flow on the coagulation system and this proposition is supported by *in vitro* experiments.

References

Benditt, E. P. (1977). Implications of the monoclonal character of human atherosclerotic plaques. *Am. J. Path.* **86**, 693–702.
Burch, J. W. and Majerus, P. W. (1979). The role of prostaglandins in platelet function. *Sem. Hemat.* **16**, 196–207.
Fishman, J. A., Ryan, G. B. and Karnovsky, M. J. (1975). Endothelial regeneration in the rat carotid artery and the significance of endothelial denudation in the pathogenesis of myointimal thickening. *Lab. Invest.* **32**, 339–351.
Gerrity, R. G. (1981). The role of the monocyte in atherogenesis. *Am. J. Path.* **103**, 181–190, 191–200.
Harker, L. A. and Ritchie, J. L. (1980). The role of platelets in acute vascular events. *Circulation* **62**, (Suppl. V), v13–18.
Kannel, W. B., Castelli, W. P. and Gordon, T. (1979). Cholesterol in the prediction of atherosclerotic disease: new prospectives based on the Framingham Study. *Ann. int. Med.* **90**, 85–91.
Meade, T. W. (1981). The epidemiology of atheroma and thrombosis. In *Haemostasis and thrombosis* (eds A. L. Bloom and D. P. Thomas), pp. 575–592. Churchill Livingstone, Edinburgh.
Nestel, P. J. (1984). Time to treat cholesterol seriously. *Aust. N.Z. J. Med.* **14**, 198–199.
Niewiarowski, S. and Rao, A. K. (1983). Contribution of thrombogenic factors to the pathogenesis of atherosclerosis. *Prog. Card. Dis.* **26**, 197–222.
Rokitansky, C. (1852). *A manual of pathological anatomy* Vol. 4 (G. E. Day, p. 272. The Sydenham Society, London.
Ross, R. and Glomset, J. A. (1976). The pathogenesis of atherosclerosis. *N. Engl. J. Med.* **295**, 369–377, 420–425.
Virchow, R. (1856). Phlagose und Thrombose in Gefassystem, in *Gesammelte Abhandlungen zur Wissenschaftlichen Medizin*, pp. 458–636 Frankfurt-am-Main, Meidinger Sohn & Co.
Zarins, C. K., Giddens, D. P., Bharadvaj, B. K., Sottiurai, V. S., Mabon, R. F. and Glagov, S. (1983). Carotid bifurcation atherosclerosis. *Circ. Res.* **53**, 502–514.

ISCHAEMIC HEART DISEASE

Epidemiology of ischaemic heart disease

J. I. MANN AND M. G. MARMOT

Of all the chronic diseases, ischaemic heart disease (IHD) has been the object of the most detailed epidemiological study. We now have much information on possible causes of the disease and, with a reasonable degree of precision, can predict its future occurrence; that is, among an apparently healthy adult population we can distinguish those individuals with a high risk from those with a low risk of subsequently developing IHD. The highest risk group has more than 10 times the risk of the lowest risk group. This epidemiological knowledge has provided the basis for efforts to prevent IHD and to reduce its community burden. This chapter reviews the epidemiology and prevention of IHD, beginning with a consideration of the impact of the disease on the population.

Occurrence of ischaemic heart disease

In most industrialized countries IHD is the commonest cause of death. In England and Wales 30 per cent of all deaths among men and 22 per cent of all deaths among women are the result of IHD.

In recent years, in addition to the approximately 156 000 deaths every year in England and Wales, there have been, on average, 115 000 hospital discharges with the diagnosis IHD. It should be stressed that in 60 per cent of all fatal myocardial infarctions, death occurs in the first hour after the attack. Most IHD deaths, therefore, occur too rapidly for treatment to influence the prognosis.

International differences

There are marked international differences in the rate of occurrence of IHD. For example, in one study in seven countries, among men aged 40–59 years initially free of IHD, the annual incidence rate (occurrence of new cases) varied from 15 per 10 000 in Japan to 198 per 10 000 in Finland. Mortality statistics show a similar picture. Table 1 shows that, even among the industrialized countries, mortality rates vary considerably. Some of the variation between countries is undoubtedly due to differences in diagnostic practice and in coding of death certificates, but numerous studies using comparable methods have confirmed that real differences exist in the frequency of disease. In Europe there is almost a threefold difference between France, Italy and Spain, on the one hand, and such countries as Finland and the United Kingdom on the other.

As shown below, these international comparisons have played an important part in the search for causes. The experience of migrants suggests that the variations between countries are likely to be the result chiefly of environmental or behavioural differences. People who have migrated from a low-risk country (e.g.

Table 1 Deaths per 100 000 of the population from ischaemic heart disease in people aged 45–49 in 1977

Country	Males	Females
Finland	296	29
Scotland	229	47
Northern Ireland	223	28
United States of America	193	45
Australia	192	41
England and Wales	188	32
New Zealand	175	64
Canada	175	36
Hungary	166	35
Czechoslovakia	157	21
Norway	137	16
Netherlands	135	23
Israel	111	27
Federal Republic of Germany	110	18
Bulgaria	99	21
Italy	97	15
Sweden	94	16
Romania	74	17
France	59	7
Japan	24	6

Japan) to a high-risk country (e.g. United States of America) tend to have rates of IHD approaching that of the host country.

Time trends

In industrialized countries, IHD emerged as the major cause of death in the twentieth century. This resulted both from a decrease in infectious disease mortality and an increase in the age-specific risk of IHD. The same process is now starting in many developing countries.

The heart disease epidemic appears to have reached its peak, and is even declining in some countries. Figure 1 shows that since 1968 there has been a substantial decrease in IHD mortality in the United States of America and Finland. By contrast, the rate has remained almost unchanged in England and Wales and certain other countries. This change over a short period of time in the United States and Finland encourages us to believe that the disease is preventable, if the causes can be found and modified.

Risk factors

In 1949 Keys suggested that with regard to IHD 'physico-chemical characteristics of the individual should have predictive value'. It was this idea together with the observation in the early 1950s that IHD showed a strikingly different frequency from country to country that stimulated the search for predictive variables (now referred to rather more loosely as risk factors). The term 'risk factors' has come to include not only physicochemical characteristics of the individual, but also aspects of life style such as diet, smoking, and behaviour pattern. From the very beginning it was believed that the discovery of such predictive variables might point the way to preventive efforts even though identification of such variables does not conclusively establish aetiological relationships.

Increasing age, the masculine gender and a family history of premature IHD are three powerful predictors of IHD but will not be considered here in detail because of their irreversibility. It is of considerable interest that most of the potentially reversible risk factors discussed below are predictive of IHD only in relatively young people (usually under the age of 60 years), suggesting that they relate to speed of development of the disease process. The increased risk in association with a family history of premature IHD is explained at least in part by well established genetically determined conditions (e.g. familial hypercholesterolaemia). This is discussed on page 9.108 *et seq.*

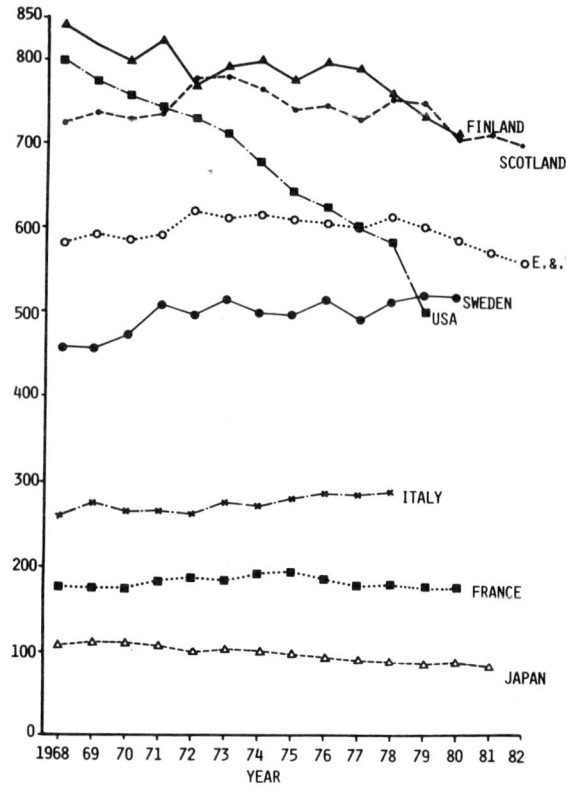

CHD MALES 35–74 – AGE ADJUSTED

Fig. 1 Age-adjusted mortality from ischaemic heart disease in men aged 35–74 in England and Wales and other countries. (Reproduced from Marmot, 1985, Interpretation of trends in coronary heart disease mortality. *Acta med. Scand.* (Suppl.) **701**, 58–65.)

Diet

The evidence provided by epidemiological studies that certain dietary practices may be associated with an increased risk of IHD has been obtained from several different sources:

    1. between-country correlations of IHD rates and food intake
    2. prospective observation of subjects for whom individual diet histories are available
    3. associations between diet (and changes in diet) and various measures of lipid metabolism known to be associated with IHD

Between-country correlations of IHD rates and food intake Most attempts to study dietary determinants of IHD rates have been based on balance sheets of the Food and Agriculture Organization (or, in the United Kingdom, more reliably on household food surveys), and on national mortality statistics before 1970 during which time IHD was increasing (at least in men) in most affluent societies. Positive associations with saturated fat, sucrose, animal protein, and coffee, and negative correlations with flour (and other complex carhohydrates) and vegetables are some of the best described. However, population food consumption data are notoriously unreliable (they are usually derived from local production figures, imports and exports, with no account of quantities not utilized as food), and the accuracy with which mortality is recorded varies from country to country. Consequently, such data do not provide direct evidence concerning aetiology, only clues for further research. Perhaps more interesting are recent studies from the United States of America, the United Kingdom, and Australia, which have examined the downward trend of IHD rates in relation to dietary change. There is certainly some association between the falling IHD rates apparent (particularly in males) in these countries and changes in some nutrients, but in view of the

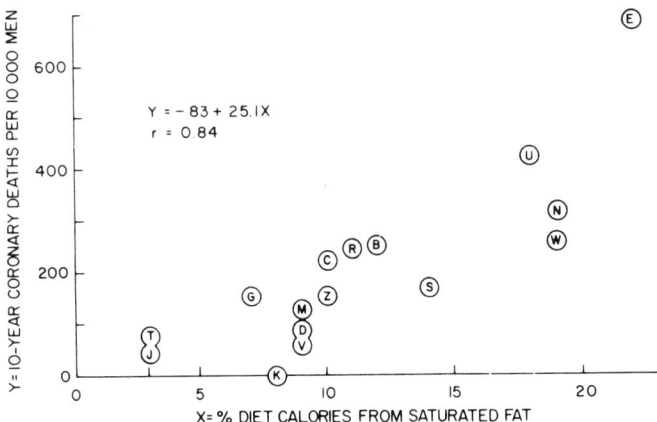

Fig. 2 Ten-year coronary death rates of the cohorts plotted against the percentage of dietary calories supplied by saturated fatty acids.

strong correlations (positive and negative) among different dietary constituents it is difficult to be sure which dietary factor is principally involved or indeed whether dietary change is simply occurring in parallel with some other more important environmental factor (e.g. increasing physical activity or a reduction in cigarette smoking).

Actual food consumption by people in 16 defined cohorts (in seven countries) and 10–year incidence rates of IHD deaths form the rather more reliable basis for the correlations tested by Keys and co-workers. A strong positive correlation was noted between mean (for each cohort) saturated fat intake and fatal IHD incidence ($r=0.84$) (Fig. 2). A weaker association was found with dietary sucrose and a later analysis of the data suggested also a positive relationship with intake of polyunsaturated fat. Protein intake appeared to have no effect on IHD incidence and no data were available concerning dietary fibre.

Prospective observation of subjects for whom diet histories are available In the seven-countries study and some other studies it was not possible to show a relationship between an individual's dietary intake and his subsequent risk of IHD. However, such an association has now been demonstrated in several more recent studies. In one, male bank staff, bus drivers, and bus conductors in London completed at least one seven-day weighed dietary record, and men with a high intake of dietary fibre from cereals had a lower rate of IHD subsequently than the rest. A high energy intake (apparently reflecting physical activity) and, to a lesser extent, the presence of a high ratio of polyunsaturated to saturated fatty acids in the diet were also features of men who subsequently remained free of IHD. In another prospective investigation of employees of the Western Electric Company in Chicago the most striking finding was an inverse association between IHD mortality and consumption of polyunsaturated fat. A positive association was also noted between IHD mortality and dietary cholesterol and with the Keys and Hegsted 'scores' (combined measures of the amount of saturated fat, polyunsaturated fat, and cholesterol in the diet). No association was found between IHD and saturated fat intake considered in isolation. In this study, as in the London study, dietary assessment was carried out very carefully; failure to find similar associations in other prospective studies could be due to insensitivity of their dietary survey techniques.

Diet and lipids Several measures of lipid metabolism described below have been associated with an increased risk of IHD. Of these, only total cholesterol has been convincingly shown to be associated with diet. For example, in the study of Keys and co-workers, mean concentration of cholesterol in the blood was highly correlated ($r=0.87$) with percentage of total calories from saturated fat. In the Western Electric Study changes from one

year to the next in dietary intake of saturated fatty acids and cholesterol were related to changes in serum cholesterol. In the typical western diet about 40 per cent of energy is provided by fat. A substantial cholesterol reduction is achieved when this is reduced to 30 per cent or the ratio of polyunsaturated to saturated fatty acids increases.

The nomadic people of Somalia, Kenya, and Tanzania, whose diets consist mainly of meat, milk, and blood have always aroused particular interest since, despite this diet, they have usually maintained low blood cholesterol levels. It has, however, been pointed out recently that their diet is not in fact habitually high in saturated fat but that intake is subject to much irregularity in food supply on a seasonal basis. There are other apparently conflicting results, but Epstein has pointed out that these seemingly inconsistent findings do not exclude type and amount of dietary fat as major determinants of serum cholesterol levels, provided one concedes that these are not the only factors which determine the distribution of serum cholesterol levels within a population. Another factor which may explain the low cholesterols in East Africa is the fact that fat content and composition of animals varies widely. In Uganda, wild buffalo meat contains one-tenth as much lipid as beef from British cattle, and only 2 per cent of the British beef fatty acids are polyunsaturated as compared with 30 per cent of the meat fatty acids from woodland buffalo. Man's tissue lipids approximate the pattern of his dietary fat intake, and numerous carefully controlled dietary studies have confirmed the cholesterol-lowering effect of polyunsaturated fatty acids.

In addition to the cholesterol-lowering property of polyunsaturated fatty acids, it is conceivable that the findings from the studies carried out in London and Chicago might be explained by another mechanism: certain long chain essential polyunsaturated fatty acids, such as linoleic acid, are reported to reduce the thrombotic tendency of the blood. A significantly lower proportion of linoleic acid is present in the adipose tissue of healthy Scots compared with similar men in Stockholm where IHD rate is one-third lower than in Scotland. Eskimos who have a high intake of eicosapentaenoic acid have prolonged bleeding times, and laboratory studies suggest that a reduced tendency to platelet aggregation may be explained by the effect of these fatty acids on prostaglandin synthesis.

In summary, epidemiological data do give considerable credence to the suggestion that diet is related to IHD, possibly via an effect on both atheroma and thrombosis. Certainly IHD seems to occur very infrequently in communities where the 'western diet' is not consumed, although of course features other than diet characterize such communities. IHD is now being diagnosed with increasing frequency among the black people of East and southern Africa amongst whom the disease was previously regarded as exceptionally uncommon, and it is the more affluent sections of the community who are principally involved. Many have adopted a western life style and made many dietary changes. Further evidence for an aetiological association between diet and IHD is provided by the single factor intervention studies discussed below.

Abnormalities of lipid metabolism

No other blood constituent varies so much between different people as serum cholesterol. From New Guinea to East Finland, the mean serum cholesterol ranges from 2.6 to 7.02 mmol/l (100–270 mg/100 ml) when estimated by the same method in the same age and sex group. Of the *known* risk factors for IHD, total serum cholesterol appears to be the most important determinant of the geographic distribution of the disease. In the seven-countries study median cholesterol values were highly correlated with IHD death rates ($r=0.80$), accounting for 64 per cent of the variance in the IHD death rates amongst the cohorts. Amongst individuals within populations the association is equally strong: in over 20 prospective studies in different countries total serum cholesterol has been shown to be related to the rate of development of IHD, the association being dose-related, occurring in both sexes,

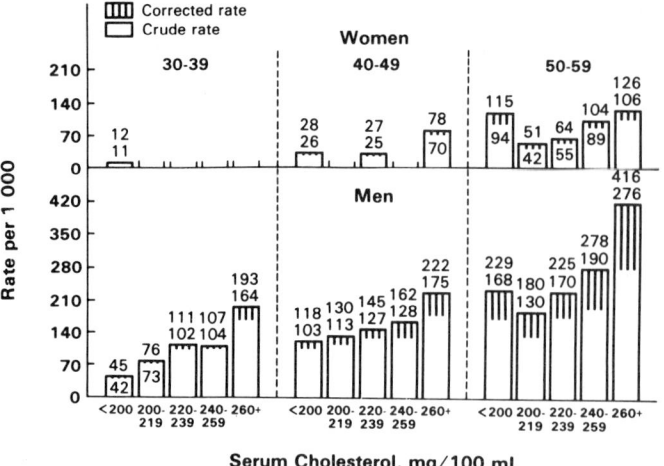

Fig. 3 Twenty-four-year incidence of myocardial infarction, by serum cholesterol levels in the Framingham study.

and being independent of all other measured risk factors. The association in the Framingham study is shown in Fig. 3. Risk of IHD varies over a fivefold range in relation to serum cholesterol levels found in an average American population. There is no discernible critical value: the risk tends to increase throughout the range. Whilst the absolute risk associated with any given cholesterol value varies in different parts of the world, within almost every population sampled the risk is greater in people with higher than with lower values.

The association of total cholesterol with IHD mortality and morbidity appears to derive chiefly, if not entirely, from the low density lipoprotein (LDL) fraction with which it is highly correlated. Low levels of total or LDL cholesterol appear to be associated with an increased risk of non-cardiovascular death (chiefly cancer) but studies in two populations – London and Paris – indicate that this inverse association is confined to deaths in the very early years of follow-up. A low cholesterol may be a metabolic consequence of cancer, present but unsuspected at the time of examination.

Increases in total triglycerides and levels of very low density lipoprotein (VLDL) are usually associated in prospective studies with an increased IHD rate. This increased risk is apparent especially when triglyceride levels are higher than 1.7 mmol/l (150 mg/100 ml), but only two studies (both Scandinavian) have suggested that the association is independent of other measures of lipid metabolism.

Recent interest has centred around the possibility that high density lipoprotein (HDL) may be a protective factor. Where HDL has been measured in prospective studies, low levels do seem to be predictive of subsequent IHD (Table 2), and in communities where IHD is uncommon HDL levels are high. In people over 50 years of age the predictive value of HDL appears to be stronger

Table 2 Levels of high density lipoprotein (HDL) cholesterol and subsequent incidence of ischaemic heart disease in the Framingham Study

HDL cholesterol level (mg/ml)	IHD incidence	Population at risk	Rate/1000
All levels	79	1025	77.1
<25	3	17	176.5
25–34	17	170	100.0
35–44	35	335	104.5
45–54	15	294	51.0
55–64	8	134	59.7
65–74	1	40	25.0
75+	0	35	—

than that of LDL. Below the age of 50 it seems that LDL might be the more important predictor.

Other constitutional factors

Blood pressure Apart from intake of saturated fat and cholesterol levels, blood pressure (both systolic and diastolic) was the only factor measured in the seven-country study which seemed to explain in part the geographic variation in IHD; it appeared to be responsible for about 40 per cent of the variance in the 10-year follow-up of IHD mortality. When considering prospective follow-up of a defined cohort, increased blood pressure has been shown consistently to be associated with a subsequent increase in IHD risk (Fig. 4). It has usually been assumed that a linear relationship exists between blood pressure and subsequent IHD risk, implying the most satisfactory outcome for those with lowest levels of blood pressure. Data from the seven-countries study, however, suggest that the relationship might not be quite so simple, but there is still no suggestion of a cut-off point by which people might be classified as hypertensive or normotensive. The epidemiological data generally indicate that systolic blood pressure is as good a predictor of subsequent IHD as is the diastolic pressure.

Carbohydrate intolerance Prospective studies in affluent societies have shown repeatedly that all manifestations of cardiovascular disease occur more frequently in diabetics than in non-diabetics (Fig. 5). Of particular interest is the fact that diabetic men and women have similar IHD rates, women losing the 'protection' against IHD which is evident in the non-diabetic population. However, observations that diabetics in Africa, East Asia, and Latin America may not experience a similar proneness to atherosclerotic disease raise the question of whether factors other than blood glucose levels are important determinants of the increased risk of atherosclerotic disease in the diabetic. The importance of asymptomatic hyperglycaemia, based on the study of 15 different populations, has recently been reviewed. There is certainly no clear linear trend between carbohydrate intolerance and subsequent development of IHD. There is some evidence of an increased risk in individuals in the top quintiles or deciles of either fasting blood glucose levels or levels one to two hours after a glucose load. It is not conclusively established whether this relationship is an independent one or a consequence of associations between blood glucose and other important risk factors for IHD such as hypertension and hyperlipidaemia which are often associated with carbohydrate intolerance. If not independent, lowering of blood glucose levels without concomitant change in other factors would be unlikely to lower the risk.

Obesity Long-term follow-up data of insured individuals published 30 years ago showed that both men and women rated for overweight developed cardiovascular disease more frequently

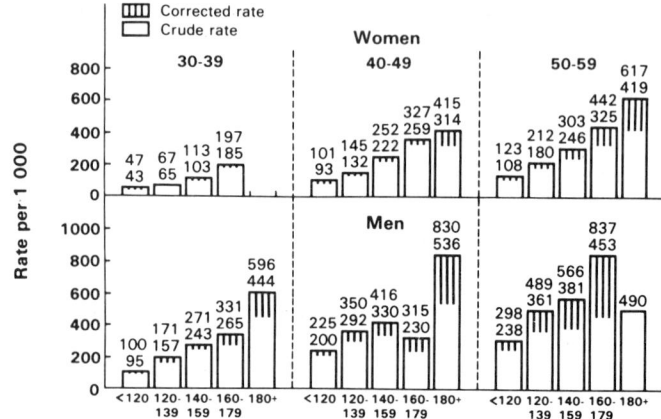

Fig. 4 Twenty-four-year incidence of coronary heart disease, by systolic blood pressure in the Framingham study.

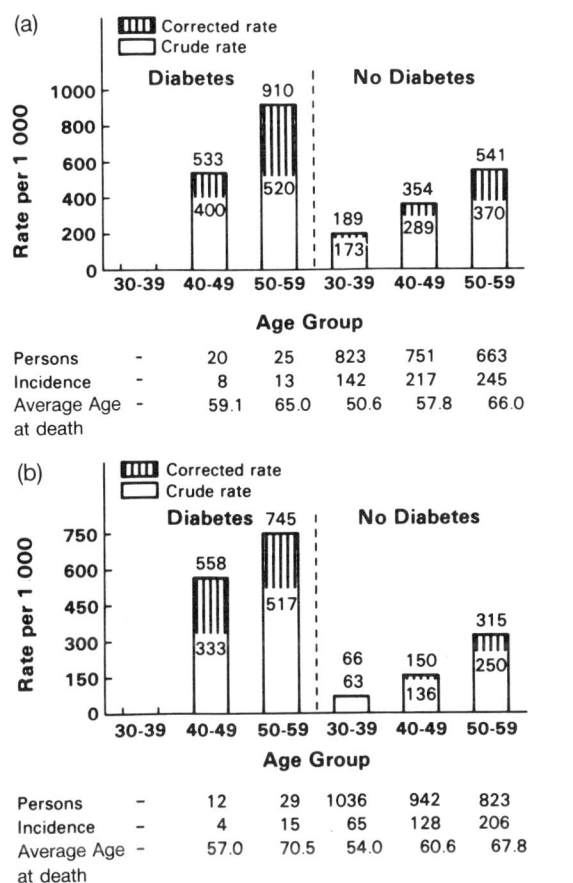

		30-39	40-49	50-59	30-39	40-49	50-59
(a) men	Persons	–	20	25	823	751	663
	Incidence	–	8	13	142	217	245
	Average Age at death	–	59.1	65.0	50.6	57.8	66.0
(b) women	Persons	–	12	29	1036	942	823
	Incidence	–	4	15	65	128	206
	Average Age at death	–	57.0	70.5	54.0	60.6	67.8

Fig. 5 Twenty-four-year incidence of coronary heart disease in subjects with diabetes mellitus, aged 30–59 at entry: (a) men; (b) women.

than the non-obese. Data from at least one prospective study have suggested that this observation is valid and independent of other measured factors. However, there is no indication that obesity explains any of the geographic variations in IHD; moreover, other studies have suggested that if obesity is associated with an increased risk of IHD, it is almost certainly due to an association with other factors such as hypertension. Despite this, the clinical significance of obesity should not be underestimated since reversal may well improve the risk factors which are causally associated with IHD.

Haemostatic factors Almost all epidemiological research into the aetiology of IHD has concentrated on factors which are probably associated with atherogenesis and far less on factors which might primarily increase the risk of thrombosis. The Northwick Park Prospective Heart Study included measures of haemostatic function. Compared with survivors, men who died of cardiovascular disease showed, at recruitment, significantly higher plasma levels of factor VII$_c$ fibrinogen, and factor VIII$_c$. Associations with VIII$_c$ and fibrinogen were at least as strong as that with cholesterol. Fibrinolytic activity was higher in survivors, but the difference was not statistically significant. There were no differences in platelet count or measures of adhesiveness. The data were also examined for any tendency of the three clotting factors to 'cluster' in individual subjects (clustering being defined as concentrations in the top third of the distribution for at least two of the three factors). Clustering was present in 63 per cent of men who died from cardiovascular disease compared with 23 per cent of survivors. Of 367 men with clustering, 4.6 per cent died of cardiovascular disease as compared with less than 1 per cent without clustering. Although the numbers in the study are rather small, the results are certainly compatible with the idea of 'hypercoagulable state' as a major risk

factor for IHD. Recently, data from a prospective study in Sweden have confirmed the importance of fibrinogen as a risk factor.

Physical inactivity
In the seven-countries study physical inactivity did not appear to explain the geographic variation in coronary heart disease (CHD). However, in several prospective studies of defined populations, vigorous exercise at work and in leisure time have been shown to protect against coronary heart disease. Perhaps the most publicized study is that of Morris and his colleagues who asked some 18 000 middle-aged British civil servants (on a Monday morning, without notice) to complete a record of how they had spent each five minutes the previous Friday and Saturday. Men who engaged in vigorous sports, keep fit exercises, and the like had a fatal and non-fatal CHD incidence over the next 8½ years which was about half that of their colleagues who recorded no vigorous exercise (Fig. 6). The effect was noted regardless of age and whether or not other risk factors for CHD were present. Vigorous exercise appeared to reduce the increasing incidence with ageing, so striking in those who did not take vigorous exercise. Vigorous exercise was defined as activity likely to reach peaks of energy expenditure of 31.5 kJ (7.5 kcal) per minute.

To investigate the role of physical activity at work in reducing coronary mortality, some 6000 longshoremen ('dockers') in San Francisco, aged 35–74 years on entry were followed for 22 years or to death or to age 75. Their longshoring experience was compiled in terms of work years according to categories of high, medium and low calorie output. Age-adjusted coronary death rates were 27 per 10 000 work years for the high activity category and 46 and 49 for the medium and low categories respectively. The difference amongst the groups was even more striking with regard to sudden death. Energy expenditure during the type of work defined as 'high output' was in the range of 21.8–31.5 kJ (5.2–7.5 kcal) per minute.

Unfortunately, randomized studies of the effects of vigorous exercise are not feasible. It is difficult to determine whether the observational studies really prove that exercise is beneficial or whether the findings merely reflect a healthier constitution in those who take exercise. There are a substantial number of plausible explanations for a beneficial effect. Physical training is well known to increase the efficiency of cardiac action and to slow the heart. In those who take vigorous exercise a reduced frequency of ectopic beats has been reported. Several other possible 'risk factors' for CHD are favourably influenced by physical activity, including high density lipoproteins, triglycerides, fibrinolytic activity, and obesity. In contemplating possible preventive strategies it should be remembered that epidemiological studies strongly suggest a critical threshold of activity and that near approach to maximal energy output may be more beneficial than overall total output at some lesser intensity of effort.

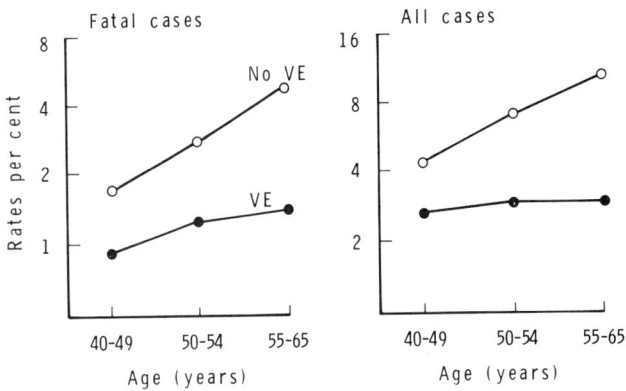

Fig. 6 Rising incidence of coronary heart disease with age in relation to vigorous exercise.

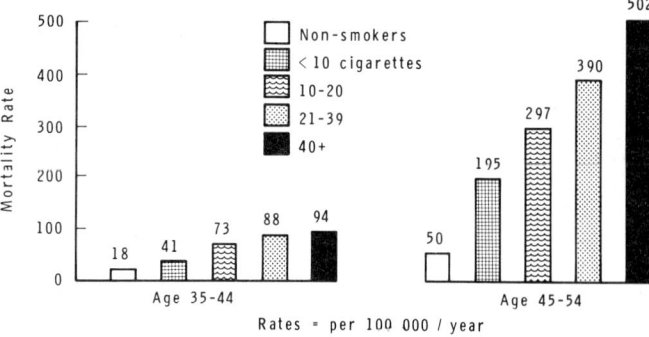

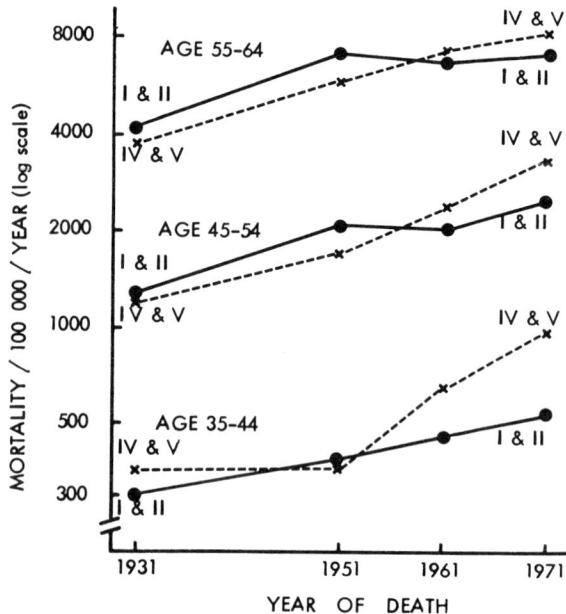

Fig. 7 Mortality rates from ischaemic heart disease in men by number of cigarettes smoked, in two age groups. (From Royal College of Physicians and British Cardiac Society, 1976, Prevention of coronary heart disease. *J. R. Coll. Phycns* **10**, 1–63, by permission.)

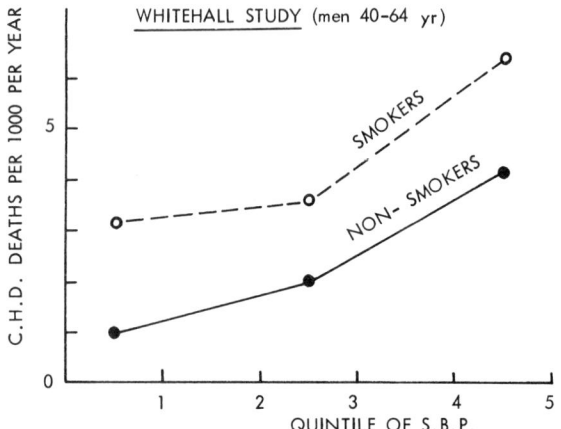

Fig. 8 Smoking is independent of other risk factors (in this case blood pressure) as a cause of IHD. (From Reid, D. D., Hamilton, P. J. S., McCartney, P., *et al.*, 1976, Smoking and other risk factors for coronary heart disease in British civil servants. *Lancet* **ii**, 979–84, by permission.)

Fig. 9 Heart disease mortality (ischaemic, degenerative, and hypertensive) in men in England and Wales according to social class. (Registrar-General's classification based on occupation: I-high V-low.) (From Marmot, M. G., Adelstein, A. M., Robinson, N. and Rose, G. A., 1978, Changing social class distribution of heart disease. *Br. med. J.* **ii**, 1109–12, by permission.)

Smoking

Several longitudinal studies in many countries have shown that people who smoke have a higher incidence of and risk of dying from IHD than non-smokers. Figure 7 reproduces data from one such study. It shows there to be a dose–response relationship: the greater the number of cigarettes smoked, the higher the risk.

In countries where other risk factors are lacking and overall level of IHD is low (e.g. in Japan) smoking appears not to be a risk factor for IHD.

It is not clear how smoking harms the cardiovascular system. Smokers have higher levels of carboxyhaemoglobin than non-smokers. Despite earlier speculation, this is not now generally believed to be the mechanism leading to IHD. Cigarette smoke has been shown to cause endothelial damage, and may affect platelet aggregation. These may be mechanisms in the formation of atherosclerosis and thrombosis, and thus lead to clinical disease. The trend towards filter cigarettes in recent years appears to have made little impact on the risk of cardiovascular disease.

The demonstration of an association between smoking and IHD is not in itself proof that smoking is a cause of the disease. It has been argued that smokers may differ from non-smokers in factors apart from smoking which predisposes them to IHD. The judgement that the smoking–heart disease relationship is causal is strengthened by: (*a*) the consistency of the relationship – it has been demonstrated in many studies in different countries; (*b*) its strength – a risk approximately threefold greater among heavy smokers than among non-smokers; (*c*) its independence of other factors – in the presence of high blood pressure and elevated

plasma cholesterol there is still a higher risk among smokers than among non-smokers (this is shown for smoking and blood pressure in Fig. 8); (*d*) the lower risk of IHD among ex-smokers – the greater the numbers of years as an ex-smoker, the closer the mortality risk to that of a life-time non-smoker; (*e*) the time relationship, for example, in England and Wales over the last 20 years IHD has become more common in working class men than in middle and upper class, and at the same time smoking has decreased in middle and upper class men but not in working class men.

Although people who smoke may indeed be different from those who do not, and those who continue to smoke different from those who give up, the balance of evidence indicates that cigarette smoking is an important cause of IHD.

Psychosocial factors

Socioeconomic In general, IHD is more common in wealthy countries than in poor countries. Paradoxically, in wealthy countries it is the poorer groups who are most at risk. In England and Wales this is a change. In the past, IHD mortality was higher in higher status groups. As shown in Fig. 9, since the 1950s mortality from IHD in working class men has risen more steeply than in middle and upper class men, overtaking the latter by the 1960s. The reasons for the higher rates in lower income groups and for the change are not completely understood. As indicated above, smoking has become relatively more common in working class men and women; they eat somewhat different diets (but not more fat); they tend to be more overweight; they have higher mean blood pressures; they report less leisure time physical activity. It is clear that there are other, as yet unidentified, factors which are also involved. It is of interest that more than one report shows a rise in unemployment to be followed by a rise in IHD mortality.

Psychosocial Many of the great clinicians of history believed that heart disease was related to psychosocial factors. William Harvey ascribed a patient's disease to the fact that he 'was overcome with anger and indignation which he yet communicated to no one'. John Hunter described his own angina pectoris as brought on by 'agitation of the mind . . . principally anxiety or anger'. Hunter reportedly died from an attack which was provoked by a particularly irritating hospital board meeting. Osler enquired after the cause of 'arterial degeneration in the worry and strain of modern life' and described the typical angina patient as the man 'the indicator of whose engine is at full steam ahead'.

These descriptions accord with much current clinical and lay feeling that an acute coronary event or angina pectoris may be precipitated by psychological factors. The difficulty has been to demonstrate this scientifically. Two main approaches have been taken: (a) to identify potentially stressful situations which may increase the risk of IHD; and (b) to identify a particular 'coronary-prone' behaviour pattern.

Stressful situations Much interest has centred on the study of stressful life events. Widowers have a higher mortality from IHD in the six months following bereavement than married men of the same age. There is some other evidence that stressful life events may precipitate myocardial infarction, and studies in Sweden, Israel, and Belgium have produced evidence that stress at work may increase the risk of myocardial infarction and angina pectoris. The Israeli study suggested, in addition, that men who received emotional support were less likely to develop angina as the result of their work problems than men without support.

This leads to the hypothesis that the balance between stressful events and the ability to cope with them determines whether a situation increases the risk of disease.

Coronary-prone behaviour patterns Some of the strongest evidence relating psychosocial characteristics to IHD comes from the studies of 'type A' or 'coronary-prone' behaviour pattern. The type A individual is described as aggressive, striving, ambitious, restless, and excessively concerned with time and deadlines. This pattern of behaviour is particularly common where job stress is reported to be high. In longitudinal studies, type A individuals have greater than twice the risk of developing IHD compared with individuals who do not show this behaviour pattern – type Bs. This increase in risk is independent of the other coronary risk factors described in earlier sections.

It has been shown by coronary angiography and post-mortem studies that type As have a greater average degree of atheroma of the coronary arteries than do type Bs. This suggests the existence of pathological pathways, other than raised lipid levels, which may accelerate atherosclerosis. The possibility that this behaviour pattern may have adverse effects on the cardiovascular system is strengthened by the finding that type A individuals react to stressful situations with greater increases in noradrenaline output than do type Bs.

Much of the work on type A behaviour has come from the United States of America. Initially, European studies affirmed the importance of type A behaviour. More recently, doubt has emerged as to whether this can be generalized to different cultures.

In summary, a wide body of research of varying quality has provided evidence that psychosocial characteristics are causally linked to the development of clinical IHD. The exact nature of this link remains to be elucidated, as does a definition of the type of social environmental situation which may increase the risk of disease. It is not known whether the risk of IHD can be altered by modifying the environment; more evidence is needed on the benefit or otherwise of individual changes in behaviour.

Geographic factors

Climate and season In England and Wales, the mortality from IHD varies with the season. It is consistently higher in winter months. This winter increase may be related to increased spread of infection and/or an increase in pneumonia leading to a greater risk of death in persons already suffering from IHD. It might also be related to ambient temperature itself. Throughout the year there is an inverse association between temperature and IHD – the lower the temperature the higher the mortality.

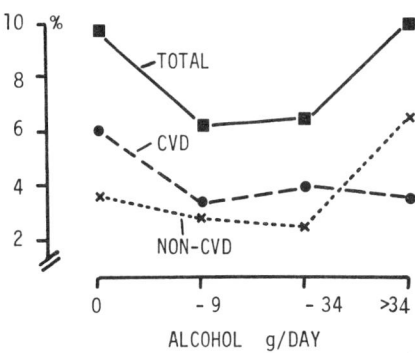

Fig. 10 Ten-year mortality (age-adjusted percentage) all causes, cardiovascular (CVD), and non-cardiovascular (non-CVD) causes according to daily alcohol consumptions (Whitehall study). (From Marmot, M. G., Rose, G., Shipley, M. J. and Thomas, B. J., 1981, Alcohol and mortality: a U-shaped curve. *Lancet* i, 580–83, by permission.)

Data from North America show that there is a rise in IHD deaths after heavy snowfalls. The suggestion has been made that the combination of cold and the unaccustomed physical activity entailed in shovelling snow place an acute burden on the heart.

Support for this association with climatic factors comes from a comparison of IHD mortality rates in different parts of Great Britain. There is a twofold variation in cardiovascular mortality (i.e. IHD, other heart disease and stroke) in Great Britain. The rate is high in Scotland, north-west England, and South Wales, and low in south-east England. The areas with high mortality rates in general have lower average temperatures and more rainy days than the low mortality areas. Although the regional differences in mortality are also negatively correlated with socioeconomic factors and water hardness, there is sufficient variation in all of these factors to disentangle their effects. It has been demonstrated that the negative association between mortality and temperatures is independent of these other factors.

Water hardness Studies in many countries have shown a negative association between water hardness and IHD mortality. The geographic differences in mortality in Great Britain are highly correlated negatively with water hardness: harder water, lower mortality. The association with water hardness is independent of geographic differences in socioeconomic factors and climate.

It is difficult to determine what substance in hard water may be protective, or in soft water may be harmful; for example, water that is hard tends to have a high content of calcium, of carbonate, of nitrate, and of silica. To date there is no evidence that artificial softening of water increases the mortality from heart disease.

Alcohol

Alcoholics and 'heavy' drinkers of alcohol (variously defined) have an excess mortality from IHD. More recently there have been several reports that non-drinkers have a higher mortality from IHD than people who consume a moderate amount of alcohol (up to three drinks per day). Data from one such study are shown in Fig. 10. The consistency of this finding in various studies makes it likely that a moderate intake of alcohol is protective against IHD: it is not other characteristics of the non-drinker which put him at higher risk.

An international study comparing IHD mortality rates showed that the apparently protective effect of alcohol was confined to wine. In particular, in the countries of southern Europe, wine consumption is high and IHD mortality low.

Alcohol intake raises the level of plasma HDL cholesterol. This is a possible mechanism by which alcohol exerts its protective effect. It is also possible that a moderate level of alcohol intake is a successful way of dealing with stress and, thereby, lowering risk. It should be remembered, however, that at higher levels, alcohol consumption is associated with a high risk of dying from non-cardiovascular disease – particularly from cancer.

Possibilities for prevention

Two approaches have been used in studies set up to test the feasibility of preventing premature IHD. The earlier investigations were all aimed at modifying only one factor. These studies, which will be described first, were carried out principally to determine whether the treatment being tested was of benefit in reducing disease frequency. There are several reasons why (with the knowledge of hindsight) these trials could not be expected to produce impressive results. First, the atheromatous process probably starts early in life. Consequently the ideal clinical trial should be started in young people. In fact, very few people under the age of 40 years have been entered into any of the studies and it should not be surprising if such studies fail to demonstrate striking benefit. Secondly, in a disease with multifactorial aetiology it might be expected that modification of only one factor would have little or no effect. Single factor intervention studies can, however, provide useful confirmatory evidence concerning aetiology: modification of a single factor in a randomized study producing reduced frequency of IHD in comparison with the control group is strong evidence that the association between that factor and IHD is causal.

More recently a 'multifactor' approach to prevention has evolved. The approach involves an attempt to modify several risk factors simultaneously, and was initially based on the fact that effects of the factors tend to cumulate. As was shown earlier, a smoker with high blood pressure is at greater risk than a smoker with lower blood pressure. If in addition his plasma cholesterol is high, his risk is increased still further. A pragmatic reason for a multifactor approach in trials of intervention arises from the difficulty in changing one factor at a time. For example, in one study (the United States National Diet Heart Study), 50 per cent of the men who were asked to adhere to a special diet also reduced their cigarette consumption.

Prevention trials may be either primary (carried out in individuals who at the outset have no clinical manifestations of IHD) or secondary (where the subjects already have established disease).

Single factor intervention

Cholesterol reduction by means of diet and drugs Trials of dietary modification aimed at reduction of cholesterol are not truly single factor trials: changes made in one dietary factor inevitably alter another. A decrease in total fat intake, for instance, will either reduce total energy intake or, if the energy level is maintained, require an increase in carbohydrate or protein. A lowering of the percentage contribution from saturated fatty acids will raise the polyunsaturated to saturated ratio whether or not the intake of polyunsaturated fatty acids is increased. Thus all dietary trials are multifactorial within the diet concept.

There have been three studies of *primary* prevention by dietary means. Usually the main feature of the diet has been an increase in the proportion of fat derived from polyunsaturated sources at the expense of saturated fat in order to achieve a ratio of the former to the latter of 1.5 or 2 : 1 rather than 0.3 : 1 which commonly prevails in a typical British or North American diet. Only one (the Los Angeles Veterans Administration Study) has incorporated two essential features of a good clinical trial (random allocation of treatment groups and 'double blind' experimental conditions). This study (with 846 volunteers) showed a significant reduction in atherosclerotic events in the modified diet group compared with the control group and provided evidence that the beneficial effect of the fat-modified diet was via a cholesterol-lowering mechanism (the effect was seen only in those whose cholesterols were high inititally and subsequently fell). Deaths from non-atherosclerotic causes occurred more frequently in the experimental group, thus raising the possibility that such a diet may actually be harmful although the difference between groups was not statistically significant (Table 3). The fact that the participants in this study were

Table 3 Summary tabulation of deaths and atherosclerotic events in the Los Angeles Veterans Administration Study

Category	Number of cases	
	Control	Experimental
Deaths		
Due to acute atherosclerotic event (sole cause)	60	39
Mixed causes, including acute atherosclerotic event	10	9
Due to atherosclerotic complications without acute event	1	2
Mixed causes, including atherosclerotic complication with acute event	10	7
Other causes	71	85
Uncertain causes	25	32
Total	177	174
Atherosclerotic events (fatal and non-fatal)		
Definite myocardial infarction (ECG)	4	9
Definite overt myocardial infarction	47	33
Sudden death	27	18
Total coronary events	78	60
Definite cerebral infarction	25	13
Ruptured aneurysm	5	2
Amputation	5	7
Miscellaneous	6	3

Table 4 Age-adjusted deaths per 1000 person years in the Finnish Mental Hospital Study

	Males		Females	
	Experimental	Control	Experimental	Control
Coronary heart disease	6.6	14.1	5.2	7.9
Cerebrovascular disease	1.7	2.4	2.2	2.0
Other circulatory	3.2	2.5	3.1	2.4
Neoplasms	5.0	4.0	4.1	3.7
Accidents, etc.	2.8	3.5	1.8	1.8
Other causes	15.4	13.0	14.4	11.2
All causes	34.7	39.5	30.8	29.0

relatively old (average 65 years, range 55–89) and followed for only eight years may explain the failure to reflect in the overall mortality the benefit apparent in atherosclerotic deaths.

The other major primary prevention study was started in 1958 in two Finnish mental hospitals (N and K). During the first six years patients in Hospital K continued their usual diet whereas those in Hospital N were fed on an experimental diet rather similar to that used in Los Angeles. After six years the diets used in the two hospitals were reversed. End-points were assessed by physicians unaware of the dietary allocation, but there are major difficulties in the interpretation of this study. The population was, of course, an unusual one. The patients were not the same throughout the 12 years of the study: some were discharged to other institutions and new admissions were added. However, most of the biases would have tended to have produced a negative rather than a positive result. Consequently the reduction in IHD death rates in the experimental as compared with the control periods together with a reduction in overall mortality (at least in men) is of considerable interest (Table 4).

There have been six studies of *secondary* prevention by means of dietary modification. These have shown no consistent trends in terms of outcome, but all have been small (100–450 volunteers) and the final results are therefore subject to a considerable margin of error. The data in Fig. 11, in which confidence limits have been

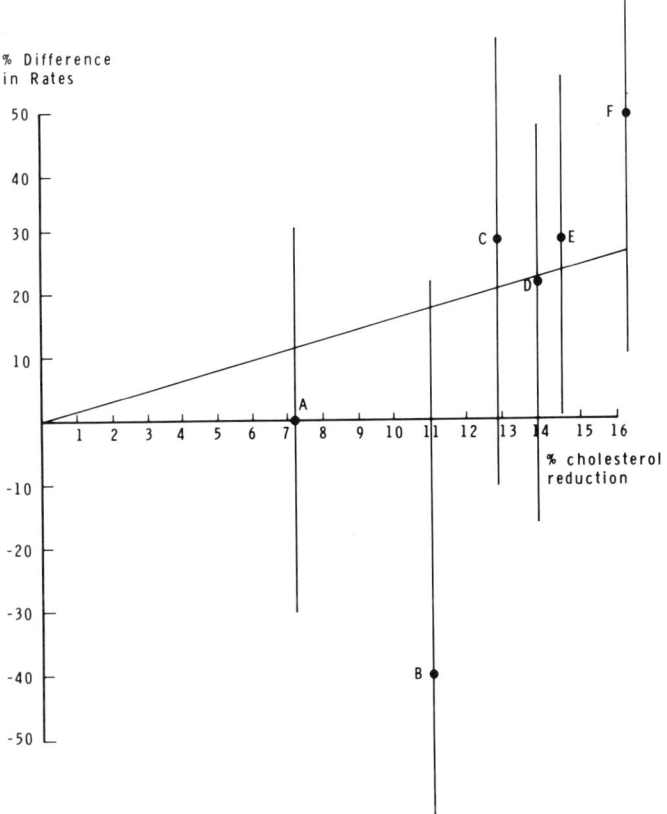

Fig. 11 The percentages of difference in IHD rates (and confidence limits) between experimental and control groups on the randomized dietary studies of primary and secondary prevention.
A= Research Committee to the Medical Research Council (1965). Low-Fat diet in myocardial infarction – a controlled trial. *Lancet* **ii**, 500.
B= Rose, G., Thompson, W. B. and Williams, R. T. (1965). Corn oil in treatment of IHD. *Br. med. J.* **i**, 1531.
C= Dayton, S., Pearce, M. L., Hashimoto, S., Dixon, W. J. and Tomiyasu, U. (1969). A controlled clinical trial of a diet high in unsaturated fat in preventing complications of atherosclerosis. *Circulation* **39** and **40** (suppl. II).
D= Research Committee to the Medical Research Council (1968). Controlled trial of soya-bean oil in myocardial infarction. *Lancet* **ii**, 693.
E= Leren, P. (1970). The Oslo diet-heart study – 11 year report. *Circulation* **42**, 935.
F= Turpeinen, O., Karvonen, M. J., Pekkarinen, M., Miettinen, M., Elosuo, R. and Paavilainen, E. (1979). Dietary prevention of coronary heart disease – the Finnish Mental Hospital Study. *Int. J. Epidemiol.* **8**, 99.

fitted to the results of all the studies (primary and secondary) which have included a control group, are therefore of particular interest. The best regression line is indicated. It is clear that the confidence limits in each case include this line. The relatively small number of subjects in each study have produced the wide confidence intervals and could explain the apparently conflicting findings. Viewing the data in aggregate, however, it is possible to estimate from the graph that, for example, a 10 per cent reduction in cholesterol confers a 15±6 per cent reduction in IHD risk ($p < 0.01$). A similar analysis has been carried out for the randomized studies of cholesterol modification by drugs (Fig. 12). Here a more consistent trend emerges. On the basis of these data a 10 per cent reduction in cholesterol seems to produce a 21±5 per cent reduction in IHD risk. The consistency between the two data sets is remarkable and provides considerable evidence for the aetiological importance of serum cholesterol in IHD.

Undoubtedly the most impressive of the drug trials is the Lipid Research Clinics Coronary Prevention Trial in which cholestyra-

mine and placebo were compared in 3886 men in whom dietary modification failed to reduce cholesterol below 6.9 mmol/l. The cholestyramine-treated group had a 19 per cent lower rate of fatal and non-fatal IHD. The reduction in IHD incidence was proportional to reduction in total and low density lipoprotein cholesterol. Total mortality was also reduced in the cholestyramine-treated group, although the differences were not quite so striking because of a modest, unexplained, increase in deaths due to accidents in the cholestyramine group. The WHO Clofibrate Study showed a beneficial result in terms of non-fatal and all cardiovascular events (in accordance with the cholesterol-lowering effect) but no reduction in fatal IHD in those taking clofibrate. Indeed, mortality from all causes was significantly higher in the clofibrate than the placebo group; the excess mortality increased progressively over time, leading to the suggestion that clofibrate may have long-term toxic affects.

Blood pressure Numerous clinical trials have shown a beneficial effect of treating moderate and severe hypertension, but the benefit has invariably been in terms of stroke. However, two recent studies suggest a reduction also in IHD in association with the treatment of hypertension. The Australian National Blood Pressure Study was a controlled trial of antihypertensive drug treatment

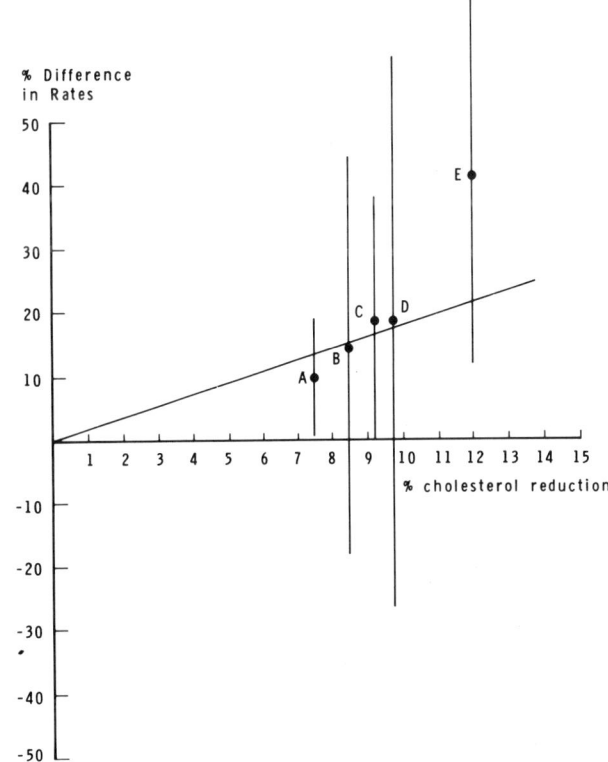

Fig. 12 The percentages of difference in IHD rates (and confidence limits) between experimental and control groups in the randomized studies of primary and secondary prevention drugs.
A= Coronary Drug Project Group (1975). Clofibrate and niacin in coronary heart disease. *J. Am. med. Ass.* **231**, 360.
B= Dewar, H. A. and Oliver, M. F. (1971). Secondary prevention trials using clofibrate. A joint commentary on the Newcastle and Scottish trials. *Br. med. J.* **iv**, 784. [Edinburgh sample.]
C= Committee of Principal Investigators (1978). A co-operative trial in the prevention of ischaemic heart disease using clofibrate. *Br. med. J.* **10**, 1069.
D= Dorr, A. E., Gunderson, K., Schneider, J. C., Spencer, T. W. and Martin, W. B. (1978). Colestipol hydrochloride in hypercholesterolaemic patients. Effect on serum cholesterol and mortality *J. chron. Dis.* **31**, 5.
E= Dewar, H. A. and Oliver, M. F. (1971). Secondary prevention trials using clofibrate. A joint commentary on the Newcastle and Scottish trials. *Br. med. J.* **iv**, 784. [Newcastle sample.]

Table 5 Number of fatal cases in the Australian National Blood Pressure Study

	Intention to treat		On treatment	
	Active	Placebo	Active	Placebo
Ischaemic heart disease	5	11	2	8
Cerebrovascular events	3	6	2	4
Other fatal cases	17	18	5	7

Table 6 Number of deaths by cause, stepped care (SC) and referred care (RC) in the hypertension detection and follow-up programme

Cause of death (ICDA Codes)	Total		With diastolic blood pressures	
	SC	RC	90–104 mmHg	
			SC	RC
All cardiovascular diseases	195	240	122	165
Cerebrovascular diseases (430–438)	29	52	17	31
Myocardial infarction (410)	51	69	30	56
Other ischaemic heart disease (411–413)	80	79	56	51
Hypertensive heart disease (402)	5	7	5	5
Other hypertensive disease (400–401, 403–404)	4	7	2	3
Other cardiovascular diseases (390–458 exclusive of above)	26	26	12	19
All non-cardiovascular diseases	154	179	109	126
Total	349	419	231	291

in men and women aged 30–69 whose diastolic blood pressures were repeatedly 95 mmHg or greater and whose systolic blood pressures were less than 200 mmHg. Eligible subjects were randomized to receive placebo or active treatment (chlorothiazide 500 mg daily initially; methyldopa, propranolol, or pindolol was added if the diuretic alone was inadequate, finally with hydralazine or clonidine if the diastolic blood pressure was still not below 90 mmHg). They were followed for an average of four years; the numbers of trial end-points observed in the various diagnostic categories are given in Table 5. By two methods of analysis fewer cases of fatal IHD occurred in the active than in the placebo group. The numbers, however, were small and the difference just short of statistical significance. The study has shown the possible value of treating what would generally be considered quite mild hypertension and also that treating hypertension even in relatively mild degree may produce a reduction of IHD as well as stroke.

The results of the Hypertension Detection and Follow-up Program in the United States were rather similar. Approximately 160 000 people aged 30–69 were screened. Those considered to require treatment for hypertension were randomized to receive either routine ('referred') medical care or treatment in a 'systematic antihypertension treatment program' ('stepped care'). Five-year mortality from all causes was 17 per cent lower for those receiving specialized treatment, which also achieved consistently better blood pressure results. Table 6 shows that myocardial infarction, as well as other cardiovascular conditions, occurred less frequently in this group.

The results of three major multicentre trials were published in 1985: the MRC trial examined the potential benefit of treating mild hypertension and the relative advantages of diuretics and beta blockers. The European Working Party on Hypertension in the Elderly (EWPHE) recruited patients over the age of 60 years with a diastolic blood pressure at entry of 90–119 mmHg. The third study specifically examined the possible beneficial effects of regimens containing a beta blocker. The MRC and EWPHE studies showed similar reductions in the stroke rate (45 and 52 per

cent, respectively). When considering only fatal strokes the reduction was not statistically significant. With regard to myocardial infarction the MRC study showed almost identical rates in treatment and placebo groups. In the EWPHE study non-fatal myocardial infarctions were not influenced by treatment but there was a significant reduction in fatal myocardial infarction. This suggests a qualitative difference in the elderly heart as a result of which the combination of myocardial infarction and blood pressure is particularly lethal, although there is no indication from either of these studies that treatment modified the hypertensive patients' predisposition to myocardial infarction. The clinical applications of these trials with regard to when and how to treat hypertension have been extensively reviewed (e.g. Treatment of hypertension: the 1985 results. Leading article, *Lancet*, 1985, **2**, 645–647).

Multiple factor intervention

Because of the substantial number of difficulties associated with single factor intervention studies, more recent interest has focused on the 'multiple factor' approach.

Intervention in subgroups A multicentre European trial introduced health education into factories randomly selected from pairs, the non-selected member of the pair serving as a control. The health education included advice on diet, the importance of not smoking, of increased physical activity, of weight reduction and information on hypertension. In addition, men with a mean systolic blood pressure above 160 mmHg were started on hypotensive drug therapy. Only small net reductions in risk factors were achieved and the reduction in overall IHD mortality was only 7.4 per cent. However, support that this represented more than a chance improvement came from analysis of the results from individual centres. The United Kingdom had the worst record of risk factor reduction and showed no evidence of a fall in incidence. Belgium and Italy produced the greatest reduction in risk factors with commensurate changes in incidence; for example, in Belgium, there was a highly significant 24 per cent reduction in IHD.

In the Oslo trial men at high risk of CHD (as a result of smoking or having a cholesterol level in the range of 7.5–9.8 mmol/l) were divided into two groups: half received intensive dietary education and advice to stop smoking; the other half served as a control group. An impressive reduction in total coronary events was observed (31 vs 57 per 1000 over a five-year period) in association with a 13 per cent fall in cholesterol and 65 per cent reduction in tobacco consumption. There has also been a significant improvement in total mortality. Detailed statistical analysis suggests that approximately 60 per cent of the IHD reduction can be attributed to serum cholesterol change and 25 per cent to smoking reduction.

In the light of these relatively encouraging results the findings of the American Multiple Risk Factor Intervention Trial (MRFIT) were rather disappointing. Men at high risk were chosen on the basis of plasma cholesterol and smoking (similar to Oslo) and also of blood pressure. Intervention against these three risk factors for 6 years in the 'special intervention' group produced a reduction in smoking of 50 per cent, in diastolic blood pressure of 10.5 mmHg, and in serum cholesterol of 5 per cent. However, the control group randomized to 'usual care' also showed changes: reduction of smoking of 29 per cent, in diastolic blood pressure of 7.3 mmHg, and in plasma cholesterol of 3 per cent. Clearly a trial which achieves a reduction in plasma cholesterol in the intervention group only 2 per cent greater than the controls cannot be used to show if a reduction in plasma cholesterol will lead to a reduction in IHD incidence. Furthermore over the study period IHD mortality in the United States general population declined by 25 per cent. As a result of this and of the risk factor reductions in controls as well as the intervention group, both groups had lower than predicted mortality and there was no significant difference between the groups.

Perhaps the most interesting aspect of the trial is the fact that when considering only hypercholesterolaemic men or men who smoked (i.e. individuals similar to those participating in the Oslo

Table 7 Total mortality and mortality from cardiovascular disease in men and women aged 30–64 in North Karelia and the control area during 1970–71 and 1976–77 showing average annual age-adjusted rate per 1000 people with 95 per cent confidence limits

	Men		Women	
	North Karelia	Control area	North Karelia	Control area
Total mortality				
1970–71	13.8 ± 0.9	13.6 ± 0.7	4.8 ± 0.5	5.0 ± 0.4
1976–77	11.6 ± 0.8	11.4 ± 0.7	3.9 ± 0.5	3.8 ± 0.4
Difference	2.2 ± 1.1	2.2 ± 1.0	0.9 ± 1.3	1.2 ± 0.6
Mortality from cadiovascular disease				
1970–71	7.7 ± 0.6	7.7 ± 0.6	2.5 ± 0.4	2.5 ± 0.3
1976–77	6.3 ± 0.6	5.8 ± 0.5	1.7 ± 0.3	1.6 ± 0.3
Difference	1.4 ± 0.9	1.9 ± 0.7	0.8 ± 0.5	0.9 ± 0.4

trial) the improvement noted in the special intervention group was comparable with that observed in Oslo. The higher mortality amongst hypertensive men, especially those with ECG abnormalities, has led to the suggestion of adverse effects of the drugs used for treating hypertension. This trial also underlines the near impossibility of achieving an appropriate control group in countries where there is so great an awareness of coronary risk factors and their consequences. It seems most unlikely that further trials will be carried out.

Community approach A different approach has emphasized intervention to change a whole community. One controlled trial, in North Karelia in eastern Finland, assessed the effect of multiple changes (Table 7). As well as health education, there was provision of low fat dairy products and sausages, changed diet in institutions, smoking prohibition in public places and special training of health personnel. These efforts resulted in changes in dietary behaviour and smoking, reduction in blood pressure and a small reduction in plasma cholesterol. There was a reduction in IHD of 18 per cent in North Karelia during the five years of study. This seems unimpressive but the duration of the study so far is probably too short to expect much effect on clinical events. Interpretation of the results is made more difficult by the fact that similar trends were apparent in the control community and, indeed, much of the rest of Finland where, not surprisingly (in view of the high IHD mortality rates), the entire population has changed its behaviour. After 10 years, there is a confirmed decline in IHD mortality in many parts of Finland – possibly greater in North Karelia.

A study of similar design in California successfully produced a reduction in smoking, plasma cholesterol and blood pressure in the experimental as compared with the control areas; however, no change in IHD was detected in this small study. Numbers in the trial are currently being expanded in the hope of producing more data with regard to IHD.

The North Karelia project (like the MRFIT trial) confirms the difficulty of any form of controlled study in a population aware of the high risk of IHD and of measures which might reduce the risk. The approach nevertheless remains a promising one for putting prevention into practice.

Intervention for high risk groups or everyone? There is now reasonable evidence that those at high risk of IHD because of hypercholesterolaemia and smoking will benefit from modification of these risk factors even if the intervention is initiated in middle age. It is not clear whether this applies to those with established clinical IHD nor whether there is an age beyond which a change in life style is no longer of benefit. The trials have not included women, who in general have a lower IHD risk than men. Consensus is gradually emerging concerning the appropriate diet which should be recommended for lowering cholesterol: a reduction in saturated fatty acids, an increase in fibre-rich carbohydrate, and a modest increase in the ratio of polyunsaturated to saturated fatty

acids. The MRFIT trial suggests that consideration must be given to the precise hypotensive agent used, but because of the proven benefit in terms of cerebrovascular disease few would dispute the suggestion that those discovered to have moderate or severe hypertension should be treated. Advice to stop smoking, to modify dietary habits, and a consideration of hypotensive drug therapy (if simple life style modifications have failed) are therefore rapidly becoming part of routine clinical practice when individuals are discovered to be smokers or are found to have raised levels of cholesterol or blood pressure. The role of lipid-lowering drugs is less clear but the Lipid Research Clinic's trial of cholestyramine suggests that some individuals with diet-resistant hyperlipidaemia should be considered as candidates for drug therapy (see page 9.108).

However, concentration only on high risk individuals has two major disadvantages. First, it entails some form of screening or case finding to detect people at high risk. Secondly, it limits the potential benefit of the intervention to the high risk group. For example, the high risk group might be defined – on the basis of smoking habits, blood pressure, and plasma cholesterol levels – as the top 15 per cent of the distribution of these factors in the population. Of the subsequent IHD events in the total population, one would expect that 30 per cent would occur in this high risk group. If, for example, intervention were successful in achieving a 50 per cent reduction in risk in those who participated, this would lead only to a 15 per cent reduction (50 per cent of the 30 per cent of cases which occur in the high risk group) in the rate of IHD in the whole population. In other words, by concentrating efforts only on the 15 per cent of the population at highest risk, nothing would be done to prevent the 70 per cent of cases which occur in the rest of the population not classified as 'high risk'. Clearly, if it were possible to lower the risk level of the whole population, this could have potentially a much greater impact on the population rate of IHD. Many countries with high IHD rates, including the United Kingdom, now have official recommendations suggesting dietary change for the entire population, a view strongly endorsed by a National Institute of Health Consensus Development Conference in December 1984.

Future research

Further intervention trials are unlikely but perhaps equally helpful epidemiological data will be generated from carefully documented information concerning changing incidence of IHD (in countries where IHD is either increasing or decreasing) in relation to measured changes in environmental factors and to changes in risk factor status. Research is also required concerning simple and acceptable means of modifying risk characteristics. There is as yet not even an established method for persuading people to give up smoking, the advantages of which have been established beyond reasonable doubt.

References

Armstrong, B. K., Mann, J. I. and Adelstein, A. M. (1975). Commodity consumption and ischaemic heart disease mortality, with special reference to dietary practices. *J. chronic Dis.* **28**, 455–469.

Carlson, L. A., Bottiger, L. E. and Anfeldt, P. E. (1979). Risk factors for myocardial infarction in the Stockholm Prospective Study. *Acta med. Scand.* **206**, 351–360.

Dawber, T. D. (1980). *The Framingham Study.* Harvard University Press, Cambridge, Mass. and London, England.

Dwyer, J. and Hetzel, B. S. (1980). A comparison of trends of coronary heart disease mortality in Australia, USA and England and Wales with reference to three major risk factors – hypertension, smoking and diet. *Int. J. Epidemiol.* **9**, 65–71.

Epstein, F. H. (1971). Editorial. *Atherosclerosis* **14**, 1–2.

Hjermann, I., Byrne, K. V., Holme, J. *et al.* (1981). Effect of diet and smoking intervention on the incidence of coronary heart disease: report from the Oslo Study Group of randomised trials in healthy men. *Lancet* **ii**, 1303–1309.

Hypertension Detection and Follow-Up Program Cooperative Group (1979). Five year findings of the hypertension detection and follow-up program. *J. Am. Med. Assn* **242**, 2562–2571.

Jenkins, C. D. (1976). Recent evidence supporting psychologic and social risk factors for coronary disease (first of two parts). *N. Engl. J. Med.* **294**, 987–994 and 1033–1038.

Kannell, W. B. and Castelli, W. P. (1979). Is the serum total cholesterol an anachronism? *Lancet* **2**, 950–951.

Keys, A. (1980). *Seven countries.* Harvard University Press, Cambridge, Mass. and London, England.

Lipid Research Clinics Program (1984). The Lipid Research Clinics Coronary Primary Prevention Trial results. I. Reduction in incidence of coronary heart disease. *J. Am. Med. Assn* **251**, 351–364.

Management Committee (1980). The Australian Therapeutic Trial: mild hypertension. *Lancet* **1**, 1261–1267.

Mann, J. I. and Marr, J. W. (1981). Coronary heart disease prevention: trials of diets to control hyperlipidaemia. In *Lipoproteins, atherosclerosis and coronary heart disease.* (ed. N. E. Miller and B. Lewis). Elsevier/North Holland, Biomedical Press, Amsterdam.

Marmot, M. G. (1984). Alcohol and coronary heart disease. *Int. J. Epidemiol.* **13**, 160–167.

Meade, T. W., Chakrabarti, R., Haines, A. P., North, W. R. S. and Stirling, Y. (1980). Haemostatic function and cardiovascular death: early results of a prospective study. *Lancet* **1**, 1050–1054.

Morris, J. N., Marr, J. W. and Clayton, D. G. (1977). Diet and heart: a postscript. *Br. Med. J.* **2**, 1307–1314.

——, Pollard, R., Everitt, M. G. and Chave, S. P. W. (1980). Vigorous exercise in leisure time: protection against coronary heart disease. *Lancet* **ii**, 1207–1210.

Multiple Risk Factor Intervention Trial Research Group (1982). Multiple Risk Factor Intervention Trial. Risk factor changes and mortality results. *J. Am. Med. Assn* **248**, 1465–1477.

Oliver, M. F. (1981). Primary prevention of coronary heart disease: An appraisal of clinical trials of reducing raised plasma cholesterol. In *Lipoproteins, atherosclerosis and coronary heart disease* (eds. N. E. Miller and B. Lewis). Elsevier/North Holland, Biomedical Press, Amsterdam.

Paffenbarger, R. S. and Hale, W. E. (1975). Work activity and coronary heart mortality. *N. Engl. J. Med.* **292**, 545–550.

Pelkonen, R., Nikkila, E. A., Koskinen, S., Plenttinen, K. and Sama, S. (1977). Association of serum lipids and obesity with cardiovascular mortality. *Br. med. J.* **2**, 1185–1187.

Pocock, S. J., Shaper, A. G., Cook, D. G., Packham, R. F., Lacey, R. F., Powell, P. and Russell, P. F. (1980). British Regional Heart Study: geographic variations in cardiovascular mortality, and the role of water quality. *Br. med. J.* **280**, 1243.

Royal College of Physicians of London and British Cardiac Society. (1976). Prevention of coronary heart disease. (Report of a joint working party.) *J. R. Coll. Phycns Lond.* **10**, 1–63.

Shekelle, R. B., Shrycock, A. M., Paul, O., Lepper, M., Stamler, J. *et al.* (1981). Diet, serum cholesterol and death from coronary heart disease: the Western Electric Study. *N. Engl. J. Med.* **304**, 65–70.

Stamler, R. and Stamler, J. (1979). Asymptomatic hyperglycaemic and coronary heart disease. *J. chronic Dis.* **32**, 683–691.

Pathology of ischaemic heart disease

M. J. DAVIES

Acute regional infarction, sudden ischaemic death, and some cases of unstable angina result from thrombosis, in or on, an atheromatous plaque.

Acute myocardial infarction

The controversial role of occlusive thrombi in the pathogenesis of acute infarction has been resolved by clinical angiography. Within four hours of the onset of pain, 87 per cent of cases show the artery supplying the infarct to be occluded. Subsequently this artery may reopen, either spontaneously, or following fibrinolytic therapy. The speed at which flow is restored in some cases suggests that spasm or thrombosis or both processes are responsible for the occlusion. The efficacy of fibrinolysis and the angiographic appearance of filling defects in the lumen during restoration of flow suggest a dominant role for thrombosis. A segment of high-grade stenosis remains, which may diminish in severity over some weeks and can be dilated by angioplasty with relative ease. Coronary thrombosis is thus dynamic, and flow is often restored although, as shown by experimental studies, 20 min of occlusion is sufficient to cause infarction. Autopsy studies show that fatal regional infarction is strongly associated with persistent coronary occlusion in which thrombus has propogated from a proximal nidus over an atheromatous plaque into the more distal normal artery. Radiolabelling studies confirm that the proximal part of the thrombus predates the onset of pain, while the distal tail does not. Reconstruction of the thrombi that are found in fatal infarction, shows that virtually all of them overlie atheromatous plaques which have undergone cracking or fissuring, thus exposing the lipid contents to the blood.

Rare examples of myocardial infarction due solely to spasm are however recorded. Non-regional diffuse forms of myocardial necrosis, in particular circumferential subendocardial necrosis, are caused by factors which produce an overall fall in myocardial perfusion. This may be caused by diffuse stenosis of all three major coronary arteries but also by factors such as hypoxia, elevated left ventricular diastolic pressure, reduced aortic pressure and increased ventricular wall thickness, all of which lead to a fall in subendocardial perfusion irrespective of whether there is structural abnormality of the epicardial coronary arteries. Diffuse subendocardial necrosis may be superimposed on regional infarction in patients with cardiogenic shock and is one form of infarct 'extension'.

Sudden ischaemic death

All pathological studies have emphasized that high-grade chronic stenosis is present in one or more coronary arteries examined after sudden death but only in a minority, comprising up to 30 per cent of subjects, are occlusive thrombi found. Studies in which post-mortem angiography was used, however, have shown over 90 per cent of cases to have atheromatous plaques undergoing fissuring but the overlying intraluminal thrombus is smaller than that found in acute infarction (Fig. 1) and the artery is not totally occluded. Such plaque fissures could cause ventricular fibrillation by a sudden increase in the degree of obstruction due to thrombosis within the plaque or by invoking local arterial spasm. In addition when intraluminal (mural) thrombi are present they can be the source of platelet emboli into the distal myocardium making sudden ischaemic death the cardiac analogue of cerebral transient ischaemic attacks due to platelet emboli from carotid atheroma. The view that the majority of patients who die suddenly from ischaemic heart disease do have an acute and evolving arterial lesion is a considerable change from that expressed in the first edition of this book.

Unstable angina

Clinical angiographic studies show that a high proportion, up to 70 per cent, of patients with progressive recent onset angina have segments of stenosis with ragged outlines, and associated intraluminal filling defects. These appearances are identical to those found in post-mortem angiograms in sudden ischaemic death and are therefore known to indicate plaque fissuring. That unstable plaques undergoing fissuring are the basis of crescendo angina is in accord with the fact that such patients may settle and lose their pain, or develop acute infarction, or die suddenly. As in sudden ischaemic death local arterial spasm may be an additional factor. There is evidence that spasm in arterial segments in which the plaque only involves a quadrant of the wall, leaving a segment of normal medial muscle, may be responsible for the form of unstable angina in which rest pain occurs but in whom the angina is not progressive.

Plaque fissuring

Lipid-rich atheromatous plaques are crescentic shaped masses of free (extracellular) lipid, mainly cholesterol and its esters, encap-

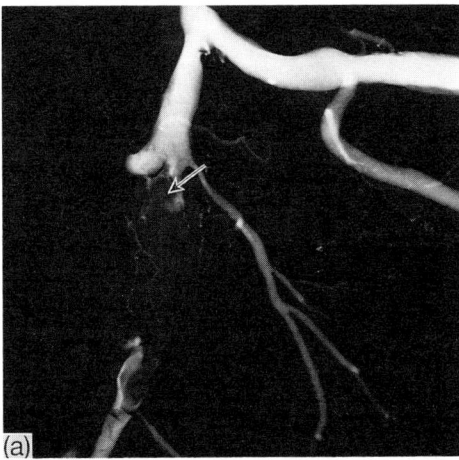
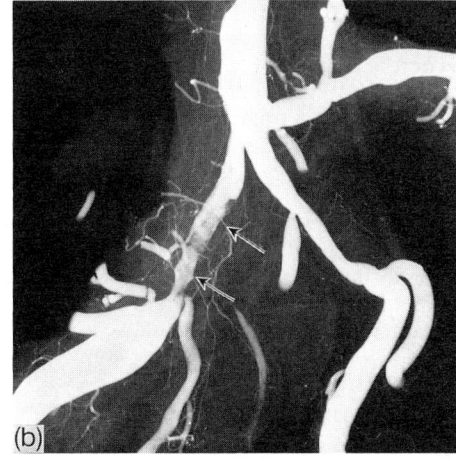

Fig. 1 (a) Post-mortem angiogram in acute anterior infarction. The left anterior descending artery is completely occluded by thrombus (arrow). (b) Post-mortem angiogram in sudden ischaemic death without infarction. The left anterior descending artery shows a stenotic segment (arrows) with an irregular outline and intraluminal thrombi recognized as filling defects but the vessel is patent.

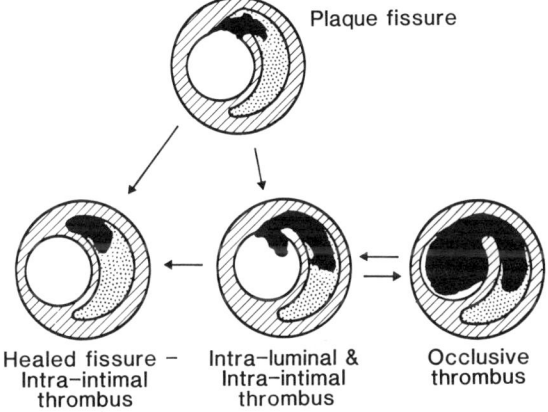

Fig. 2 Diagramatic representation of the events which may follow plaque fissuring as seen in transverse sections. Thrombus is shown as black, the plaque is stippled.

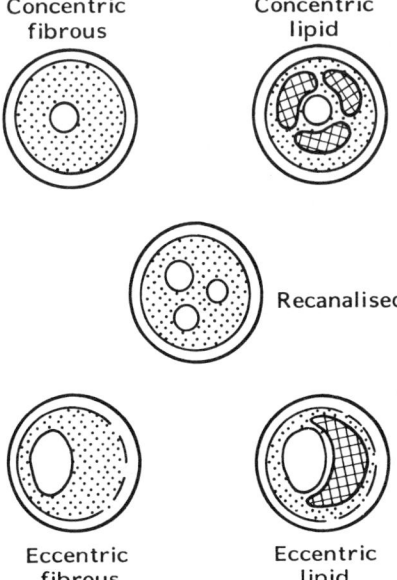

Fig. 3 Diagramatic representations of the various forms of stenosis due to atheroma. Fibrous tissue is stippled, lipid cross-hatched. Opposite eccentric plaques a segment of normal media is retained, although behind the plaque itself medial muscle altrophies. In stenosis due to concentric fibrosis little normal medial muscle remains.

sulated in the intima and separated from the lumen only by a thin cap of fibrous tissue. Breaks (fissures) in the cap allow blood to dissect into the plaque and result in the formation of a platelet-rich thrombus actually within the intima (Fig. 2). The fissure may reseal at this stage leaving a plaque considerably enlarged by virtue of containing a mass of thrombus. Alternatively, thrombus may form within the arterial lumen over the fissure; this thrombus may grow to occlude the lumen and then propagate distally or lyse to allow the plaque to reseal. The process is dynamic, waxing and waning over hours or days before the plaque restabilizes or the artery occludes. Little is known about what invokes plaque fissuring; it could cause, or result from, spasm. A necessary prerequisite, possessed by a minority of plaques only, is a free pool of lipid within the intima.

Stable angina
The vast majority of cases have one or more segments in which atheroma has reduced the lumen diameter by more than 50 per cent (equivalent to 75 per cent stenosis by area if the lumen is circular in shape). The morphological variation in such arterial segments is large.

Up to 60 per cent of patients with stable angina and 85 per cent of those with previous infarction and angina have a segment of artery in which the original lumen is replaced by several smaller channels (Fig. 3) and whose morphology suggests recanalization of a previous occlusive thrombus. Other forms of stenosis are regarded as being formed by the inherent atheromatous process and show a bewildering spectrum of appearances due to different combinations of a number of variables (Fig. 3). The intimal fibrous thickening may be concentric or involve only one quadrant of the artery wall. In the latter case there is a segment of normal arterial wall which may comprise up to 60 per cent of the circumference of the vessel. With concentric intimal disease the lumen is centrally placed, with eccentric disease the lumen is displaced from the central line of the vessel. Any plaque may be predominantly of fibrous tissue or have an even admixture of collagen and histiocyte cells containing lipid, or be lipid rich, that is, have a large pool of extracellular lipid. Most patients have plaques showing all conceivable permutations of these variables, although there is in some cases a preponderance of soft lipid-rich plaques. Calcification develops in the intima at the base of plaques but does not contribute to stenosis directly.

In normal arteries, which have been distended at physiological pressures, the lumen is close to being circular in shape; the internal elastic lamina in the media is smooth implying a state analogus to medial muscle relaxation and not, as illustrated in textbooks, wavy. Over plaques which occupy only a quadrant of the arterial wall the intimal surface is flattened giving a slightly oval-shaped lumen assymetry may be accentuated if spasm occurs in the residual quadrant of normal media. There is good evidence that medial muscle contraction is capable of reducing the circumference of the artery by around 10 per cent which may suffice to invoke symptoms. There is at least a potential for spasm to occur around 20 per cent of stenotic areas present in patients with stable angina.

Angioplasty is used to dilate a range of arterial lesions varying in the amount of lipid, in the physical nature of the stenosis, and in whether or not there is a segment of normal media opposite the plaque. The mechanisms of successful dilation may well differ ranging from extruding lipid into the media, splitting or stretching fibrous plaques, and dilating the normal vessel wall remote from the plaque.

References

Ambrose, J. A., Winters, S. L., Stern, A. *et al.* (1985). Angiographic morphology and the pathogenesis of unstable angina. *Am. Coll. Card.* **5**, 609–617.

Brown, B. G., Bolson, E. L. and Dodge, H. T. (1984). Dynamic mechanisms in human coronary stenosis. *Circulation* **70**, 917–922.

Davies, M. J., Fulton, W. F. M. and Robertson, W. B. (1979). The relation of coronary thrombosis to ischaemic myocardial necrosis. *J. Path.* **127**, 99–109.

—— and Thomas, A. (1984). Thrombosis and acute coronary artery lesions in sudden cardiac ischaemic death. *N. Engl. J. Med.* **310**, 1137–1140.

DeWood, M. A., Spores, J., Notske, R. *et al.* (1980). Prevalence of total coronary occlusion during the early hours of transmural myocardial infarction. *N. Engl. J. Med.* **303**, 897–902.

El-Maraghi, N. R. H. and Sealey, B. J. (1980). Recurrent myocardial infarction in a young man due to coronary arterial spasm demonstrated at autopsy. *Circulation* **61**, 199–207.

—— and Genton, E. (1980). The relevance of platelet and fibrin thromboembolism of the coronary microcirculation with special reference to sudden cardiac death. *Circulation* **62**, 936–944.

Falk, E. (1983). Plaque rupture with severe pre-existing stenosis precipitating coronary thrombosis: characteristics of coronary atherosclerotic plaques underlying fatal occlusive thrombi. *Br. Heart J.* **50**, 127–134.

—— (1985). Unstable angina with fatal outcome: dynamic coronary thrombosis leading to infarction and/or sudden death. *Circulation* **71**, 699–708.

Detection of ischaemic heart disease

R. BALCON

Pathophysiology of cardiac pain

The logical treatment of ischaemic heart disease depends on a good understanding of the pathophysiological mechanisms involved. Important information concerning this continues to accrue with the development of modern technology enabling a fuller study of patients, particularly in conditions of stress during which manifestations of ischaemic heart disease become more obvious. Ischaemia occurs when the myocardium is stressed beyond the limit of its metabolic reserve with maximal coronary vasodilatation and oxygen extraction so that oxygen demand exceeds supply. This thesis was suggested by Burns as long ago as 1809 and has been developed since the early 1920s, supported by a number of clinical and experimental observations. For most of the recent past it was felt that maximum oxygen supply was determined by the level of coronary flow which in turn was fixed by the presence of stenoses in the coronary arteries and that angina pectoris occurred when demand exceeded supply. This theory has been tested in man in the catheter laboratory. Oxygen demand was increased by producing an artificial tachycardia by pacing the right atrium at progressively increasing rates until angina occurred. Demand was assessed by measuring the tension time index (see below). In many patients it was possible by repeating

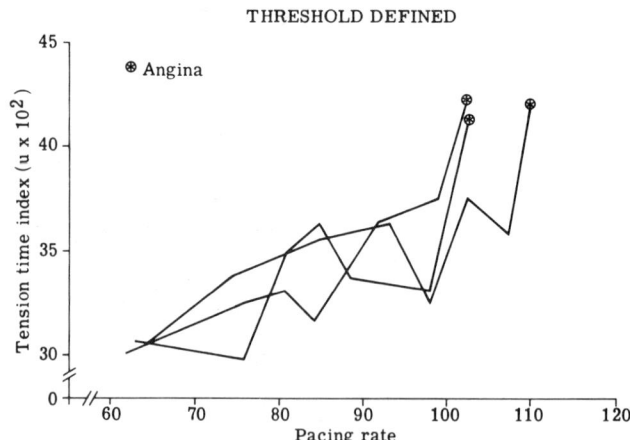

Fig. 1 The three lines show three atrial pacing tests, each terminating in angina. A threshold of myocardial oxygen consumption has been defined above which angina occurs.

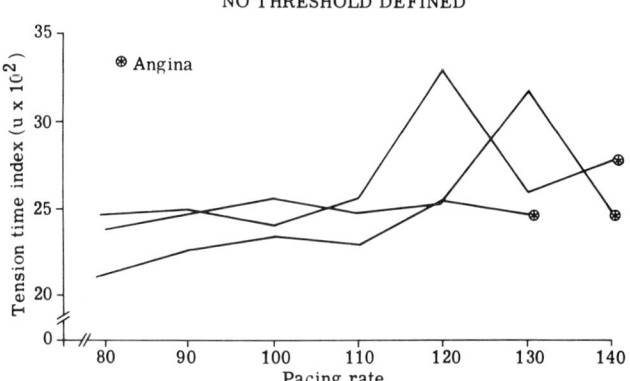

Fig. 2 The three lines shown three atrial pacing tests in one patient. Angina occurs at levels of tension time index previously achieved without pain.

the procedure to define a threshold of demand above which angina occurred (Fig. 1), complying with the theory. In others, however, no such threshold could be found. Figure 2 shows the results in such a patient in whom angina occurred at a tension time index level previously reached without the occurrence of pain.

There are a number of explanations for this latter finding but all require the least modification of the simple hypothesis. Coronary artery spasm was often suggested as a cause of angina but usually rejected because it was thought the heavily diseased vessels would not be capable of it. An early study with exercise testing concluded that the reduction in exercise tolerance after food was reflex in origin and probably due to spasm. Prinzmetal provided good evidence for the implication of coronary artery spasm in his description of a group of patients with intermittent cardiac pain at rest associated with transient electrocardiographic ST segment elevation. Recent work has demonstrated that the simple theory needs to be modified from at least two points of view. First, it has now been clearly demonstrated by angiography that alteration of coronary vasomotor tone does play an important part in atherosclerotic lesions. Indeed, hypersensitivity of the coronary circulation producing localized vasospasm may be the only cause of myocardial ischaemia in some patients (Fig. 3). A considerable body of data has now been published demonstrating that the primary cause of attacks of cardiac pain at rest may be vasospasm. Continuous haemodynamic and electrocardiographic monitoring of such patients has led to the discovery of the second important factor which modifies the simple view of the pathophysiology of angina: that clinical cardiac pain is a relatively late feature in the

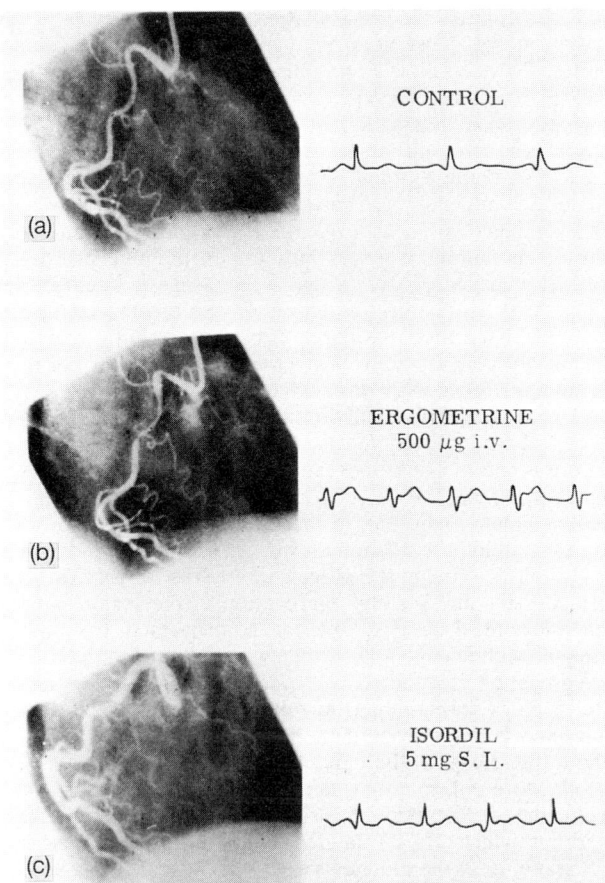

CONTROL

ERGOMETRINE
500 µg i.v.

ISORDIL
5 mg S.L.

Fig. 3 (a) The control right coronary arteriogram and the electrocardiogram which are normal. (b) After ergometrine there is a segment of spasm of the artery associated with electrocardiographic changes and chest pain. (c) The artery after nitroglycerine. It is dilated and the segmental spasm has disappeared.

development of ischaemia. The first changes observed are in the rate of relaxation of the left ventricle, seen as a change in the first derivative of the descending limb of the ventricular pressure curve (dp/dt). This is followed by electrocardiographic changes usually involving ST segment, then an obvious disturbance of haemodynamic variables such as heart rate, systolic blood pressure, and left ventricular end-diastolic pressure. Cardiac pain occurs with these later haemodynamic changes (Fig. 4).

Studies of the left ventricle using both angiographic and isotope techniques have shown that the presence of ischaemia is accompanied by disturbances of function with abnormalities of left ven-

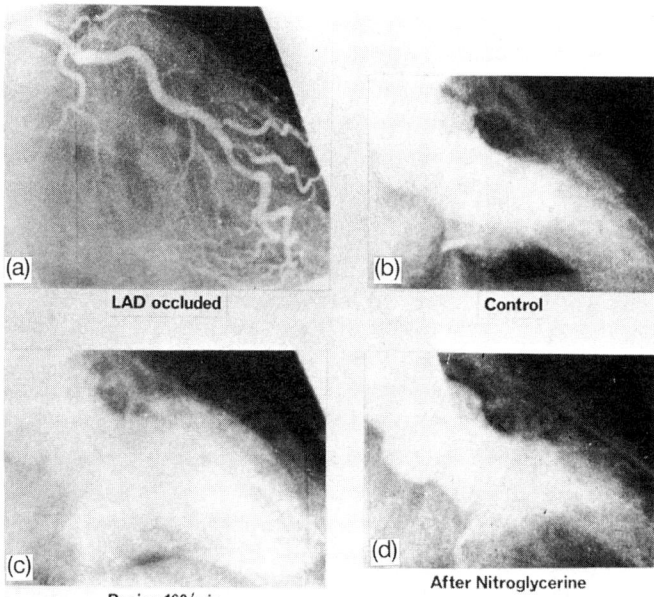

LAD occluded

Control

Pacing 160/min

After Nitroglycerine

Fig. 5 (a) A left coronary arteriogram showing occlusion of the anterior descending branch, only the circumflex branch filing. (b–d) The right anterior oblique left ventricular angiograms are all shown in end-systole and the control shows some disturbance of anterior wall motion. This is greatly increased by pacing to angina and relieved by stopping pacing and giving nitroglycerine.

tricular wall motion developing in the ischaemic regions (Fig. 5). Myocardial ischaemia undoubtedly can be induced in the expected way with primary changes in haemodynamics leading to increased mycardial oxygen demand which cannot be met by supply. This clearly happens on exercise, as mentioned, and can be simulated in the catheter laboratory by pacing. Studies of this kind have helped to elucidate pathophysiological mechanisms. The supply/demand ratio can be evaluated from simultaneously recorded left ventricular and aortic pressures. Left ventricular oxygen demand is determined by the tension in its walls and the state of contractility. The wall tension is a function of intraventricular pressure and volume. It has been shown experimentally, however, that oxygen demand can be approximated from pressure measurements alone. The area under the systolic portion of the left ventricular pressure curve multiplied by the heart rate gives an index (tension time index, TTI) which relates well to the minute myocardial oxygen demand. In a similar fashion, supply can be assessed from the driving pressure for coronary flow – that is, the difference between left ventricular and aortic pressures during diastole. This gives an index known as the diastolic pressure time integral (DPTI)

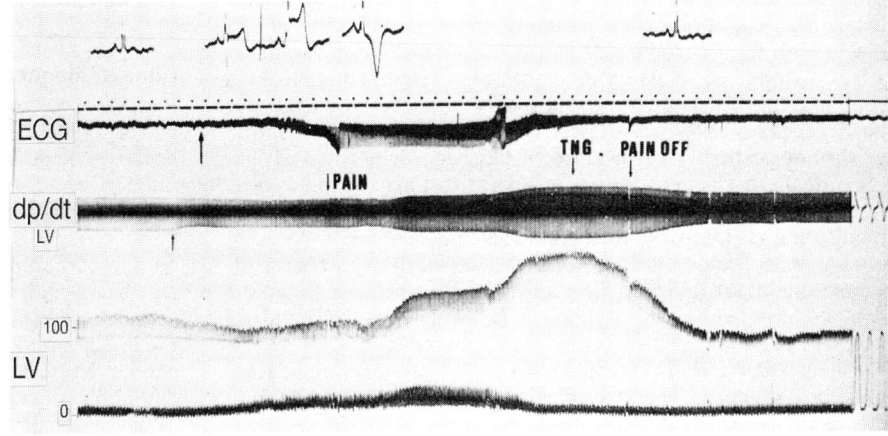

Fig. 4 Continuous recordings of electrocardiogram (ECG), rate of change of left ventricular pressure (Dp/dt LV) and left ventricular pressure (LV) showing the sequence of events in an attack of spontaneous angina at rest. The first to change is dp/dt followed by ECG and left ventricular diastolic pressure; pain occurs last.

ECG

dp/dt
LV

TNG . PAIN OFF

PAIN

100

LV

0

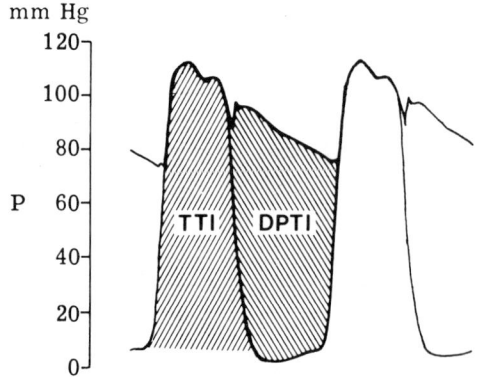

Fig. 6 Left ventricular and aortic pressures showing the method of obtaining myocardial oxygen supply/demand ratio (DPTI/TTI). P = pressure; TTI = tension time index; DPTI = diastolic pressure time integral.

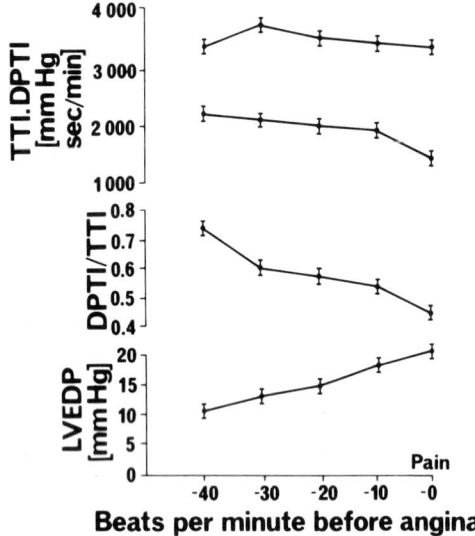

Fig. 7 Lines show mean values for 10 patients with ischaemic heart disease paced to angina. The diastolic pressure time integral (DPTI) falls. Left ventricular end-diastolic pressure (LVEDP) rises, and so the supply/demand ratio (DPTI/TTI) falls progressively and is worst when angina occurs. TTI = tension time index.

(Fig. 6). Studies have shown that the ratio DPTI/TTI is a better indicator of ischaemia than either of these variables alone. Figure 7 shows data from 10 patients with ischaemic heart disease in whom angina was induced by atrial pacing. DPTI has fallen progressively because of the rise in left ventricular end-diastolic pressure; to a lesser extent, TTI has risen leading to a progressive deterioration of the supply/demand ratio, worst at the time of cardiac pain. It is certain now that the supply/demand ratio is adversely affected to a varying degree in different situations by a combination of a reduction of coronary flow caused by the stenoses, changes in left ventricular haemodynamics, and alteration in vasomotor tone. For instance, it has been demonstrated that exertional chest pain as well as attacks at rest may be induced by transient coronary vasospasm. Long-term ambulatory ST segment monitoring has tempered the earlier view that coronary vasospasm is the major cause of most episodes of cardiac pain at rest. Changes in heart rate which would sufficiently increase metabolic demand have been shown to precede many episodes which indeed occurred in patients with more severe coronary disease.

Finally, the role of prostaglandins on the coronary circulation must be considered. The two substances shown to have important effects on the coronary circulation are the prostaglandin endoper-oxidases, thromboxane A_2 (TXA_2) and prostacyclin (PGI_2). These unstable substances have an *in vitro* half-life of a few minutes. Prostacyclin is a coronary vasodilator, and although the effects of thromboxane are less well documented, it has been shown to cause contraction of isolated bovine coronary artery strips. These two substances have opposite effects on platelets, prostacyclin being a potent inhibitor of aggregation and thromboxane A2 inducing aggregation. Platelets activated by contact with a damaged vessel wall release TXA_2 and ADP, and recruitment of circulating platelets into the thrombotic process then occurs (see page 13.138). It has been suggested that adherent platelets may also contribute to vessel wall prostacyclin levels by release of their endoperoxidases. Prostacyclin, in turn, is thought to act as a secondary control mechanism to limit further platelet accumulation. Any vasoconstrictive effect of released TXA_2 produced as a result of platelet adhesion may also be countered by the dilatory effects of locally released prostacyclin.

There is another link between these prostaglandins and ischaemic heart disease. Prostacyclin formation is inhibited by lipid peroxidases which might lead to thrombosis. It has been postulated that excess lipid peroxidation may occur with hyperlipidaemia and that this plays a role in the process of atherosclerosis. This role of prostaglandins and platelet aggregation in the manifestations of ischaemic heart disease is, however, controversial. Even the need for vessel wall damage and contact with collagen to initiate platelet aggregation is doubted by some investigators. For instance, platelet plugs form in plastic tubes when these are damaged. Experimental work in animals has shown that such plugs form without the release of their endoperoxidases and, thus, TXA_2 formation. More information is needed before the exact mechanisms are elucidated. These doubts also make it difficult to evaluate various drugs which affect platelet function. Improvement in our understanding of the platelet–vessel wall interaction is needed to further our knowledge of the mechanisms of the manifestations of ischaemic heart disease and thus make their management more logical.

Other factors, some recognized and some not, might have an important pathogenetic role. Cigarette smoking, for instance, affects platelet stickiness and aggregation, causes vascular endothelial swelling, and vasospasm, and also inhibits fibrinolysis, all of which could lead to reduced coronary flow and myocardial ischaemia.

These advances in our understanding of the pathogenetic mechanisms of angina pectoris have helped to make the management of the problem more logical. They have also made clinical diagnosis more difficult in that the simple view that angina is always related to recognizable precipitating causes and is promptly relieved by their removal and that myocardial infarction can be diagnosed when cardiac pain occurs particularly at rest and is long lasting, is no longer tenable. The studies referred to earlier and others have made it quite clear that prolonged attacks of pain can occur at rest without obvious precipitating cause and need not necessarily indicate that myocardial infarction has occurred.

Clinical diagnosis of angina pectoris

Despite these considerations it is still frequently possible to make an accurate clinical diagnosis of intermittent myocardial ischaemia because the description is so characteristic. Pain which is precipitated by exercise or emotion, especially when there are additional demands for cardiac work because of a recent heavy meal or because of excessive cold or warmth, which occurs in the retrosternal region and radiates to the classic sites of the throat, left arm, and back, and which is described as tight or gripping in nature should be considered cardiac in origin until proved otherwise. If the precipitating cause is exercise, it causes the patient to stop and is relieved promptly by rest. However, in some patients myocardial ischaemia is appreciated in different ways, with mild feelings of aching or discomfort in the retrosternal region or only a difficulty in breathing. The most difficult situation is when it is described as sharp and occurs in the left chest, because it becomes difficult to distinguish this from the common left inframammary pain of no significance (see page 13.76). The site of the pain may vary, there may be no radiation, and the pain may in fact occur in only one of the usual sites of radiation such as the left arm or wrist.

It is possible to compile a list for the differential diagnosis of chest pain. In one study of patients presenting with acute chest pain, 85 diagnoses were eventually made. Such a list, however, is of very little value. From the practical point of view, it is important and often difficult to decide whether the pain is due to myocardial ischaemia or oesophageal dysfunction. For instance, approximately 30 per cent of a group of more than 200 patients whose pain could be induced by acid perfusion of the oesophagus were classified as having angina pectoris using the Rose criteria suggested for field surveys. Oesophageal dysfunction and abnormalities of the thoracic spine probably account for 25–30 per cent of referrals for chest pain, and in a minority of cases the pain is indistinguishable from angina pectoris.

Examination

Myocardial ischaemia is rarely present at rest when the patient is first seen and examination of the cardiovascular system is therefore usually normal. There may, however, be signs of associated factors such as hypertension and its complications. Evidence of hyperlipidaemia may be present with fatty deposits in the classic sites. The presence of arcus senilis and, to a lesser extent, xanthelasmata are, however, unreliable indicators of hyperlipidaemia. Physical signs in the heart are almost always due to the results of left ventricular damage. When this is diffuse, the heart is enlarged and this may be appreciated by palpation although it is much better seen on the chest radiograph. There is often a third heart sound produced by the filling of the ventricle whose compliance is reduced by fibrosis and ischaemia. The damaged ventricle also contracts more slowly than normally, so left ventricular ejection is slower than aortic valve closure later. This may lead to a reversed split or single second heart sound. The findings can be similar with an undamaged ventricle which has a large area of regional ischaemia at the time of examination as judged by the presence of cardiac pain or marked ST segment shift on the electrocardiogram. An aneurysm of the anterior left ventricular wall can often be felt as a diffuse area of sustained forward movement of the precordium, perhaps with the signs of left ventricular dysfunction referred to above. There may be cardiomegaly on the radiograph, often with a distinct bulge on the left heart border. Mitral regurgitation can result from rupture of anterior or posterior papillary muscles which have been involved in infarction. This gives rise to the characteristic pansystolic murmur perhaps heard closer to the sternum, with or without the signs of left ventricular dysfunction. Rupture of the interventricular septum can also occur as a complication of myocardial infarction, and this, too, results in a pansystolic murmur at the left sternal edge. It may be very difficult to distinguish clinically between the two although the chest radiograph may be helpful, showing pulmonary plethora with a ventricular septal defect and pulmonary venous congestion only with mitral regurgitation. The ECG is not usually helpful since both conditions may occur with either anterior or inferior infarction. These two are usually seen as acute complications of infarction and are not found during routine examination of patients with angina pectoris.

Resting electrocardiogram

This is also abnormal when there has been left ventricular damage and may show evidence of previous infarction with Q-waves, failure of R-wave progression across the chest leads, or partial or complete bundle branch block. Persistence of the ST segment elevation of acute infarction often occurs when a left ventricular aneurysm is present.

Fluoroscopy

The chief value of fluoroscopy in current cardiological practice is in the detection of coronary calcification. It is possible to detect calcification with unaided fluoroscopy in 3 per cent of patients with heart disease. Image intensification increases this to 15 per cent over all, and to 54 per cent for patients with ischaemic heart disease. This figure is weighted by the relatively high incidence in older patients. The additional use of fluoroscopy improves the detection rate. 'Ischaemic' electrocardiographic changes are almost nine times more common in asymptomatic men with coronary calcification than in those without calcification. The general correlation between coronary calcification and angiographically demonstrated stenosis is poor, with an overall sensitivity of approximately 65 per cent.

The correlation below the age of 50 years is much better, especially for women in whom it is probably as good as an abnormal electrocardiographic response to exercise. However, the relative rarity of coronary calcification in the younger patients, the need for cine fluoroscopy, and the availability of more definitive diagnostic methods make the search for coronary calcification rather unrewarding. It is more often noticed *en passant* when the cine angiograms are being reviewed, and plays no specific part in the diagnosis. It may affect the management decision in that diffuse calcification is a relative contraindication to aortocoronary bypass surgery. Fluoroscopy has been advocated for the detection of abnormal wall motion in patients with anterior wall left ventricular aneurysms. It is, unfortunately, very unreliable for this and may in fact result in the failure to complete investigations in a patient with a surgically correctable lesion. Kymography is more helpful but is rarely available now.

These diagnostic difficulties and the relative paucity of physical signs make it very important to clarify or strengthen the diagnosis by attempting to demonstrate the occurrence of myocardial ischaemia. The first and most commonly used method for doing this is exercise testing.

Exercise testing: prediction of the presence of disease

ST segment changes Exercise testing has been used for many years in the study of patients with coronary artery disease, although it did not gain great favour until the last decade. In the early years the main emphasis was on the ability to use electrocardiographic ST segment changes to identify patients with coronary artery disease. The main problem has been that some patients with coronary disease have 'negative' tests, and some with normal coronary arteries have 'positive' tests. This has led to the concept of false positive and false negative results. Results depend on the sensitivity of the test (the ability to detect the disease when it is present), on its specificity (the ability to detect coronary artery disease and no other), and on the incidence of the disease in the population under study (Bayes' theorem). They are reasonably good for hospital populations with a high incidence of disease, but relatively poor for population screening where the disease incidence is low. There has also been much discussion about the degree of ST segment depression which should be used in order to define the test as positive. If slight ST segment depression (1 mm or less) is used, the sensitivity of the test is increased but the specificity reduced and the number of false positive results increased. If a greater degree of depression is used, the specificity is improved but the sensitivity reduced. These points are illustrated in Fig. 8 taken from a review of the subject published in 1978. It clearly demonstrates that only a statement of probability about presence of disease can be made, bearing in mind the circumstances of the test and the degree of ST segment change.

R-wave amplitude The amplitude of the R-wave of the electrocardiogram reflects left ventricular volume with change occurring in the same direction so that a decrease in amplitude occurs with a reduction in volume, and an increase with a volume increase. Other factors such as block, electrolyte concentrations and con-

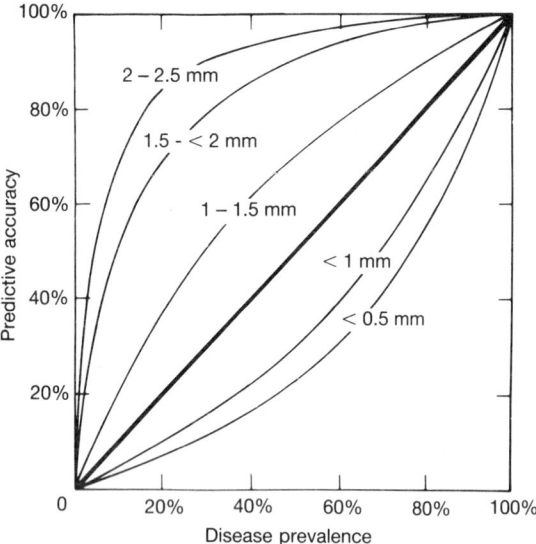

Fig. 8 Relationship between predictive accuracy and disease prevalence according to the degree of ST segment depression (Reproduced by permission of *American Journal of Cardiology*, 1978, **42**, 669.)

ductivity, electrical axis of the heart, and movement of the chest wall and diaphragm also play a part in the changes which occur. The volume of the ventricle increases when part of its wall becomes ischaemic, and this may be detected by a failure of the R-wave amplitude to decrease or increase on exercise which is the normal response. Some workers have shown a good correlation between these changes and the presence of coronary artery disease, and others have not. The changes correlate better if a distinction is made between patients with mild and severe disease, the latter showing positive changes presumably because the degree of ischaemia and thus the increase in ventricular volume is greater. Although the accuracy of the ECG changes during exercise in predicting the presence of coronary artery disease is improved if both ST segment and R-wave changes are considered, the unpredictability of R-wave changes has considerably limited their value and they are little used. The use of multiple electrocardiographic leads, either all 12 standard leads or up to 64 precordial leads, has improved specificity and sensitivity of the ECG changes and is now mandatory. Some workers have used submaximal stress, the test being terminated by reaching a predetermined heart rate – usually 85 per cent of the predicted maximum heart rate adjusted for the patient's age and sex. The predicted maximum is simply derived by subtracting the age from 220 for males or 200 for females. Predictive value is increased when employing maximal tests which are limited by symptoms or potentially dangerous changes such as marked ST segment depression, ventricular dysrrhythmias, or a fall in blood pressure. The risk from maximal tests is greater but still very low. Mortality is about 1 in 20 000 and infarction 1 in 3000.

Prediction of the severity of disease In recent years attention has been directed to other exercise test variables, the maximum workload achieved, the end-point of the test, and the changes in blood pressure and heart rate, in particular to their significance in relation to the severity rather than the presence of coronary artery disease.

Figure 9 shows the correlation between an index of severity of coronary disease and the maximum load achieved during a bicycle ergometer exercise test for more than 500 patients with coronary artery disease. The index is derived from the coronary arteriogram and takes into account the site and severity of all the lesions present. It is expressed as a number ranging from 0 to 100; low numbers indicate severe coronary disease and vice versa. There is

a good general inverse correlation between the severity of disease and the maximum workload achieved.

When patients complaining of exertional angina undergo symptom-limited exercise tests, the symptom which occurs is not always angina. Dyspnoea and exhaustion or fatigue are two other common end-points. If the end-point is angina, however, the patient is more likely to have severe disease. Blood pressure normally rises with exercise, and failure to do so appropriately is another indicator of the severity of both the coronary disease and the left ventricular dysfunction. In summary, severe disease and therefore a less good prognosis is suggested by a low exercise tolerance, a test end-point of angina, a fall or failure to rise of blood pressure, marked ST segment depression on the ECG, and an increased R-wave amplitude.

The most valuable use of exercise testing is in attempting to detect those patients who have severe disease and a poor prognosis and who may therefore be helped by such measures as aorto-coronary bypass surgery. Approximately 80 per cent of patients who have such severe disease can be detected by exercise testing. The problem of how to detect the remaining 20 per cent short of performing coronary arteriography on all patients with suspected disease has not yet been solved.

A new exercise test has been devised which suggests that it substantially solves this problem. The heart rate/ST segment slope (that is, the rate of change of the ST segment with increased heart rate) is measured. This was shown by the group who first reported the test to correlate absolutely with the number of major coronary vessels with at least 75 per cent stenosis. Unfortunately, other workers have not been able to reproduce the results and the test cannot yet be recommended.

Prediction of future coronary events and survival

The prognosis of patients with coronary artery disease is determined to a great extent by the severity of the disease and the degree of left ventricular dysfunction. It is not surprising, therefore, that exercise testing which predicts these also predicts prognosis. In a large five-year study of more than 2000 apparently healthy men the development of clinical coronary events was significantly associated with four variables recorded during a symptom-limited exercise test which they all performed at the outset.

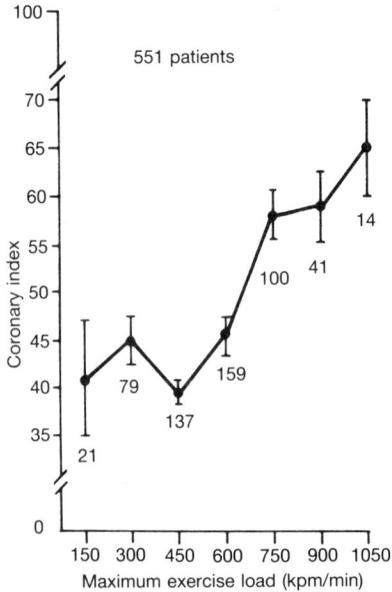

Fig. 9 The graph shows the correlation between severity of coronary disease as judged by the coronary index (see text) and the maximum workload achieved on a bicycle ergometer exercise test. Each point has the standard error and the number of patients. kpm/min = kilopond metres per minute.

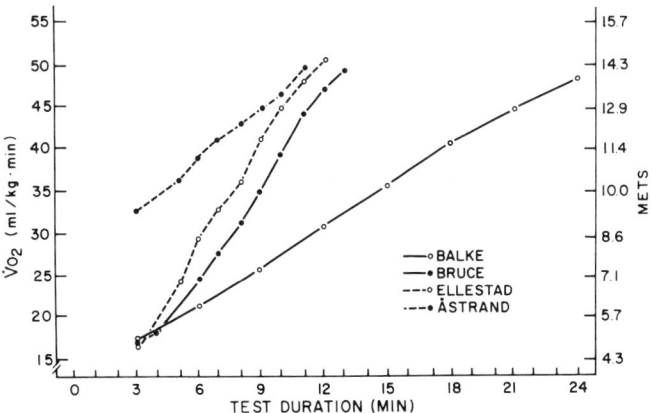

Fig. 10 The rate of change of oxygen uptake and metabolic equivalents for four treadmill exercise test protocols. (Reproduced by permission of *American Heart Journal*, 1976, **92**, 39.)

These were the occurrence of chest pain, a low maximum workload, failure to reach 90 per cent of the predicted maximal heart rate, and 'ischaemic' ST segment depression. This predictive ability of exercise testing applies also to patients wih coronary artery disease.

Method of exercise testing The test has to be maximal to derive from it the type of information referred to above. Bicycle ergometers are often used in Scandinavia and some other European countries and for the new test mentioned above, but the most widespread method is treadmill testing. It has the advantage that patients have only to walk and not cycle (which may be unfamiliar to them). The aim is to achieve maximum oxygen uptake. Most treadmill tests are performed in stages with an increase in inclination and speed of the treadmill at each stage. Figure 10 shows the time course and the relation between maximum oxygen consumption and metabolic equivalents of four commonly used treadmill protocols. Symptom-limited exercise tests such as these should be supervised by a doctor with facilities for cardiac resuscitation.

Twenty-four-hour ECG tape recording The possible occurrence of pain-free episodes of myocardial ischaemia has already been mentioned. Diagnosis can sometimes be facilitated by their demonstration during continuous ambulatory monitoring of the electrocardiogram. It may also help by relating doubful symptoms to definite ST segment changes on the electrocardiogram. Satisfactory recording of the ST segment requires a frequency modulated (FM) tape recorder, preferably recording on two channels simultaneously, to reflect the anterior and inferior left ventricular walls. Analysis of these tapes, usually recorded for at least 24 hours, can be tedious and time consuming but computer methods are being introduced to speed the process. Some recent reports of ST segment changes in 'normals' emphasize the usual need for caution in the interpretation of findings.

Thallium scintigraphy (see page 13.42) Organ perfusion can often be assessed non-invasively by injecting radioactive isotopes and employing appropriately sited external scintillation counters. A scintillation counter employs a sodium iodide crystal which emits a flash of light when struck by a gamma photon. The maximum intensity is at the point of contact, and an array of photomultiplier tubes around the crystal receive varying levels of signals according to the proximity of the scintillation, allowing spatial resolution of the contact. Multicrystal cameras can work faster but their resolution is determined by the size of the individual crystals, which is usually about 1 cm². Systems are being developed which are likely to reduce their size and improve the resolution. Both single and multicrystal cameras are used. This method is more difficult to apply to the heart because of the rapid time course of the changes

which occur. The application of computer processing techniques has, however, made it possible and it was first used for myocardial perfusion studies in 1975.

Thallium–201 is an isotope distributed to the tissues in a way similar to potassium. Although the two substances are subsequently handled differently in the body, the information obtained by following the changes in thallium–201 distributed clinically is useful. It has an actual half-life of 72 hours and biological half-life in myocardium of 7 hours. The duration of exposure to radiation is related to the actual half-life and the rate of excretion; it is longer than required for study, which represents a disadvantage since the patient receives unnecessary radiation. Despite this the whole-body radiation dose is, at worst, in the region of 1 rad and less than 2 rad for organs receiving the highest doses. These levels are compatible with radiation doses which have been in use for medical diagnoses for many years without observable problems. When injected intravenously, thallium is distributed rapidly to the myocardium according to the blood flow, so activity is low in regions of myocardium which are less well perfused. During the next two to four hours the isotope reaches equilibrium in the left ventricular myocardium provided some flow occurs to all regions. Theoretically, therefore, no perfusion would be seen in scarred areas of previous myocardial infarction. If the isotope is injected at a time when areas of the left ventricle have been rendered ischaemic (e.g. by exercise) then defects in perfusion would be detected initially and would disappear later, giving a method of distinguishing between ischaemia and infarction and also of comparing relative perfusion of various regions.

The technique is qualitative and compares perfusion of adjacent areas, relating these to background activity of isotope. In practice, although fixed defects (those which do not change when equilibrium is reached) usually correspond to areas of infarction as judged by angiography, there may be additional ischaemia or ischaemia only. Reversible defects reflect more reliably ischaemia alone. Once again, because the technique is qualitative and makes comparisons between various myocardial regions, it is less valuable in detecting multiple ischaemic areas which may be equally poorly perfused. The problem of overlying areas of left ventricle with varying levels of perfusion and other structures is to a great extent overcome by making counts in multiple projections. Despite these limitations, the technique has been helpful in the evaluation of patients. It may help in the future in detecting non-invasively those patents with severe disease. Its particular use clinically is in doubtful cases where the exercise test result is equivocal. In these circumstances, normal perfusion at peak exercise makes important coronary disease very unlikely. It has, however, been disappointing in helping to decide whether a particular coronary stenosis is causing myocardial ischaemia. It has been helpful in assessing the result of coronary artery surgery.

The test is simple to carry out. The patient performs a standard multistage exercise test, and when the end-point is reached the isotope is administered via a previously inserted intravenous needle. The patient then stands in front of a gamma camera sited over the heart and a standard number of counts are collected in multiple projections, usually left oblique, anterior, and left lateral. The counts are repeated after two to four hours' rest, allowing for equilibration of isotope. The data are computer processed and the result is usually presented as Polaroid colour scintigrams with a colour scale representing varying levels of isotope count.

Non-invasive assessment of left ventricular function

M-mode echocardiography M-mode echocardiography (see page 13.37) is an easily applied non-invasive technique which has proved very useful, especially in the evaluation of valve and congenital heart defects. It is also possible to acquire information about the size and function of the left ventricle in patients with ischaemic heart disease. The technique employs a single ultrasonic piezo-electric crystal used to emit and receive the ultrasound. The wavelength is altered by the different densities of structures through which the ultrasound wave passes. The reflections are converted to an electronic (B-mode) signal displayed on an oscillograph and recorded on moving photographic paper to derive the M-model record. The echo 'window' (i.e. the part of the heart which is accessible to the echo beam without overlying lung) is quite small and only a cross-section of the left ventricle in the region of the mitral valve can be evaluated. The dimensions of this cross-section are increased if the whole ventricle is dilated, and the difference between the end-systolic and end-diastolic dimension is reduced because of the reduced ejection fraction of the ventricle. If the ventricle is dilated and the stroke volume maintained, the ejection fraction is inevitably reduced. Patients with dilated ventricles often have cardiac enlargement on the chest radiograph but this can also be due to localized left ventricular aneurysm. It is extremely important to distinguish between the two situations because the latter is amenable to surgical treatment and has a much better prognosis. In this situation the echo beam misses the aneurysm, but if the remainder of the left ventricle is normal, so is the echocardiogram. It may thus be helpful in distinguishing between the two conditions.

The changes in left ventricular myocardial relaxation which accompany ischaemia have already been mentioned. These may also be detected on the echocardiogram as a reduction in the rate of ventricular filling which can be assessed from the rate of change of the echo dimension. This is accompanied by a prolongation of isovolumic relaxation time, which can be derived from simultaneous echocardiograms used to time the opening of the mitral valve and phonocardiograms to time the closure of the aortic valve. During this period, when both valves are closed, there is no change in volume of the ventricle and relaxation occurs with a change in shape of the ventricle. Computer analysis of the echocardiographic dimensions has also helped to demonstrate that ventricular contraction and relaxation may be inco-ordinate in patients with coronary disease, with regional variations in the state of tension and thickness of the left ventricular wall. Such regional abnormalities may also be detected by two-dimensional echocardiography. This has been developed to widen the area of echo beam. This is currently usually achieved using a multicrystal phased array system with complex technology which enables a field sector of 90 degrees to be viewed. The older oscillating single crystal is still sometimes employed but provides a relatively narrow sector of approximately 30 degrees. A number of different views can be obtained of both the long and short axes of the left ventricle as well as information about ventricular size and regional wall motion. It is even possible to obtain information about the state of the myocardium (i.e. whether normal or fibrotic) from the nature of the echo reflections. The chief limitation of all echo techniques is that good records are not obtainable in all subjects; even when they are, only certain parts of the ventricle can be visualized. Studies during stress, particularly during exercise which exaggerates or produces abnormalities, are not always technically feasible; with increasing experience, however, two-dimensional echocardiography is proving very useful in some patients with ischaemic heart disease. It has particular value in distinguishing between ventricular aneurysm and diffuse myocardial disease, and potentially hazardous invasive investigation can now often be avoided. The two-dimensional method has to a great extent superseded M-mode echocardiography.

Radionuclide angiography Radionuclide techniques (see page 13.41) can also be used to obtain information about left ventricular function. The aim is to keep the isotope in the blood pool rather than in the tissues. Technetium–99m is used. It has a half-life of six hours and can be conventionally made by the decay of molybdenum–99m absorbed on to an alumina column. A generator such as this has a half-life of 67 hours and can be used to produce isotope for a number of days. It is used to label human serum albumin or the patient's own red blood cells. Isotope activity is counted with a gamma camera. Ventricular volume has been shown to correlate

well with count rate, so end-diastolic and end-systolic volumes and the ventricular ejection fraction can be derived from the resulting time–activity curves. Counts can be made during those cardiac cycles when the isotope first passes through the heart (first-pass technique) requiring a rapid-counting multicrystal camera. Alternatively, information is collected from a large number of cardiac cycles over 5–10 minutes and these are 'superimposed' by the computer. The data are then analysed by dividing the cardiac cycle into up to 100 segments or frames by gating the signal. This produces the same type of time–activity curve as the first-pass technique, and average ventricular volumes, ejection fraction and wall motion can all be assessed. Exercise studies are more difficult to perform because of the movement of the precordium during exercise. The ventricle can, however, be stressed by placing the hands in crushed ice. This is a lesser stress than exercise and does not usually produce ST segment change on the electrocardiogram. It does, however, often produce wall motion abnormalities, and, since the same system can be used for thallium scanning, the results of these investigations can be correlated.

Radionuclide techniques therefore give very useful information concerning the presence and effect of lesions in the coronary circulation. They may avoid the necessity of invasive investigation, particularly in patients with symptoms of doubtful origin. They may also be used to observe the effect of various forms of treatment on myocardial perfusion and left ventricular contraction. Their final place is still being evaluated but it seems certain that they will continue to be refined and improved and perhaps play a more important part in the future.

Computed tomographic scanning Computed tomographic scanning is also in the development phase. Computerized radiographic tomography, for instance, has been used widely for diagnosis in many organs. The first-generation apparatus was slow, taking about 20 minutes for each patient since the whole body had to be exposed to the X-ray 'slices'. Data collection for whole body tomography has been reduced to approximately two minutes but this is still much too slow for the heart, which requires information to be collected about 50 times per second to give useful information. Research effort is attempting to solve this problem. A system has been developed using 28 X-ray systems arranged around the patient, exposing rapidly in sequence so that information about the whole 'slice' can be obtained 100 times per second. These data can be analysed and played back dynamically so that the beating heart can be viewed as a whole or in tomographic slices in an infinite number of views.

Blood and myocardium cannot be differentiated from each other, so the cardiac chambers cannot be visualized without the use of radio-opaque medium. This type of apparatus is very expensive and unlikely to come into general use.

Positron emission tomography The use of X-ray tomographic techniques in conjunction with labelling of various metabolic substances with positron-emitting isotopes is being explored. Early results show that the site and size of ischaemic zones can be assessed. The prospects for the future are very exciting, with the possibility of defining the metabolic processes in ischaemia in man non-invasively.

Angiography Selective coronary arteriography was introduced in 1959, and with it for the first time came the ability to demonstrate without speculation the degree and extent of coronary artery disease. It remains the only means for doing this with certainty. This subject is fully discussed elsewhere (see page 13.49). Briefly, however, in the Sones technique the brachial artery is exposed by open dissection and the coronary catheter inserted directly into it and manipulated under fluoroscopic control to the root of the aorta and into both coronary orifices in turn. Ciné film is taken in a number of projections after the injection of 3–8 ml of radio-opaque medium into each coronary artery. Left and right oblique, posteroanterior, and left and possibly right craniocaudal views are often used for the left coronary artery although the last-named projections, which are helpful to separate superimposed branches, are not usually needed for the right coronary artery. The procedure is complete with a left ventriculogram in the right anterior oblique projection and, in some laboratories, a left oblique projection also. The catheter is then removed and the brachial artery repaired. Percutaneous catheterization of a femoral artery using separate preshaped catheters for the two coronary arteries and a third multihole catheter for the left ventriculogram was introduced later but is now the most commonly used method. The injection technique is the same for both.

Provocative tests A number of methods have been used to provoke coronary spasm in the laboratory. The aim of such tests is to demonstrate the cause of angina, especially in patients with apparently normal or mildly diseased coronary arteries. The most commonly used has been the intravenous injection of ergometrine (a smooth muscle constrictor), with subsequent repeat angiography. If the injection induces not only coronary arterial spasm but also the patient's typical pain and ST segment change on the electrocardiogram, it is considered positive. This does not, of course, prove that unprovoked attacks of pain are also caused by coronary spasm but is strong circumstantial evidence that they are. A positive test of this nature occurs in a large proportion of patients with the classic Prinzmetal angina. Variable results, however, occur in other groups of patients in whom the diagnostic problem is more difficult. Coronary spasm may occur alone with pain or ST segment change but not both. Alternatively, pain and/or ST segment change may occur without convincing segmental coronary spasm. The calibre of the whole vessel may be reduced. Finally, ergometrine administration causes haemodynamic changes including elevation of the left ventricular systolic and end-diastolic pressures which adversely affect the myocardial supply/demand ratio and could induce cardiac pain. All of these considerations render interpretation of the results of ergometrine testing difficult, and since the patients in whom it is most likely to be conclusive present the least diagnostic problem its value is doubtful. The test also may cause complications which, very rarely, lead to death and should therefore be performed only with full understanding of the risk, with care, and in circumstances where immediate measures for resuscitation are available.

Digital subtraction angiography Computer techniques are also being applied to angiography. In particular, image enhancement by background subtraction has proved so successful that it is possible to produce high resolution angiograms of non-moving structures such as cerebral and peripheral arteries with intravenous injection, thus greatly reducing the hazards and discomfort of the angiographic procedure. Research is underway to apply these techniques to the heart, so it may be possible in the future to obtain both coronary and left ventricular angiograms without arterial catheters or at least without coronary or left ventricular injection, which would enable the technique to be used much more widely.

Coronary arteriography is a safe procedure when carried out by experienced investigators performing an adequate number of procedures. The investigation is essential before coronary artery surgery is undertaken but there is still controversy concerning indications in other patients. The value of the non-invasive procedures already discussed is still being assessed, so a definite statement which would be accepted universally cannot yet be made. Most cardiologists agree that angiography should be used to exclude coronary disease in the difficult group of patients with chest pain of doubtful origin when the results of exercise testing and radionuclide scanning are equivocal.

The decision is most difficult for patients in whom the clinical diagnosis of angina pectoris is easily made and whose symptoms are well controlled by drug therapy, especially if the patient is young. The problem is to know whether any of these patients should have aortocoronary bypass surgery to improve long-term

survival, and this will be discussed further. If the evolving angiographic techniques fulfill their promise, it is likely that they will be used for all patients with known or suspected coronary disease.

Management of patients with coronary artery disease

Control of 'risk factors'

This subject is discussed fully on page 13.144.

Symptomatic treatment

Principles

Angina pectoris is the chief symptom of coronary disease and the commonest requiring treatment. The principles of medical therapy are to reduce myocardial oxygen consumption and, if possible, to increase myocardial blood supply. As mentioned previously, oxygen consumption is determined in large part by left ventricular wall tension which in turn is related to pressure and volume in the left ventricle. The second important determinant is the contractile state of the left ventricle. This is difficult to define but is reflected in the speed of fibre shortening and, thus, pressure rise. It is exaggerated by inotropic agents such as catecholamines and digoxin, and reduced by various myocardial depressants such as beta-adrenergic blocking agents and calcium antagonists. Heart rate is the final determinant of oxygen consumption since the amount consumed must depend on the number of times events occur in a given period. Drugs which reduce contractility also reduce myocardial oxygen consumption and are therefore useful in the treatment of angina pectoris. Beta-adrenergic blocking agents also reduce heart rate and thus have two possibly beneficial effects on oxygen consumption. However, this must be balanced against the increase in left ventricular volume and wall tension resulting from reduced heart rate; fortunately, this balance is usually in favour of the patient and symptoms are improved. Calcium antagonists also reduce oxygen consumption but have no affect on heart rate. They have additional useful effects in producing peripheral arterial dilatation which reduced systemic and left ventricular pressure and, thereby, myocardial oxygen consumption.

The basis of treatment should be to prevent all attacks of angina, if possible, since any single attack has the potential to proceed to infarction.

Organic nitrates

The group of drugs which have been in use longest for patients with angina pectoris are the organic nitrates, particularly nitroglycerine. The arterial and venous dilatation these drugs produce are both useful (see page 13.105). The venodilatation reduces venous return and left ventricular volume. The arterial dilatation reduces systemic and left ventricular pressure. There is some reflex tachycardia to restore cardiac output but this is not important in the exercising patient.

Nitrates have few important side effects in that they do not have any potentially dangerous effects on left ventricular function. The generalized vasodilatation may produce unpleasant symptoms of flushing and headache, which is the main limitation of their use. Nitrates were thought to be metabolized in the gastrointestinal tract and liver and therefore ineffective when given by mouth; early clinical studies suggested that nitrates did not have a sustained haemodynamic effect when taken orally, but relatively small amounts were used. More recent observations using larger doses both in patients with angina and in those with heart failure have demonstrated sustained haemodynamic and antianginal effects, and the mononitrate metabolites of isosorbide dinitrate have qualitatively similar effects to those of the parent compound. The use of these agents in the management of patients with ischaemic heart disease is now firmly established. Nitrates can also be administered to the skin in the form of ointment; peak effect is late at about six hours, and the duration long. Long-acting oral preparations are now available and these can be used twice daily for background prophylaxis. It is still advisable, however, for patients to use the rapidly acting sublingual or inhalation versions before they undertake physical activity, and, of course, to treat pain which has not been anticipated.

Beta-adrenergic blocking agents

The combination of oral and sublingual nitrates is frequently sufficient to control angina, but, if it is not, a beta-adrenergic blocking agent or calcium antagonist can be added. The first widely used beta-adrenergic blocking agent to be introduced was propranolol. It appeared in the late 1960s and is still one of the most commonly used drugs in the group. The chief observable effect is the bradycardia it produces. A resting heart rate of 55–60 is often used as an index of correct dosage. However, if it is, the drug will appear to be ineffective in a number of patients who then get symptomatic relief with a larger dose. The reduction of the peak heart rate during exercise to approximately 100 per minute has been shown to be a much better index. The variable dose required by different patients has also been well demonstrated. A number of factors may be responsible for this variability but the most important appears to be bioavailability, with as much as 20-fold difference in plasma levels occurring after the same dose has been given to different patients because of differences in elimination of the drug by the liver.

The theoretically most important side effect of propranolol is the induction of heart failure. This has not proved to be an important clinical problem provided the drug is not used in patients who already have indications of important left ventricular dysfunction. The side effects which are most troublesome are related to beta-2 blockade. The beta-2 sites are in bronchial and peripheral arterial smooth muscle, and their blockade can lead to bronchospams and exaggeration of the symptoms of peripheral vascular disease in suceptible subjects. There are also a number of non-specific side effects which may limit its usefulness, such as skin rashes, vivid dreams, gastrointestinal disturbance, fatigue, and, rarely, impotence. The drug is in fact generally tolerated well, side effects occurring in about 5 per cent of patients over all.

Increasing symptoms, myocardial infarction, and death have been observed upon the sudden withdrawal of propranolol. The risk seems to be higher in outpatients than in those in hospital. The exact cause of this phenomenon is not known, but there is some evidence to suggest that it is due to induction by the drug of an increased number of beta receptors of normal affinity. Propranolol is available in a slow release formulation and once-daily administration is possible. This has considerable advantages and greatly increases the likelihood of the patient complying with the regimen.

Many other beta-adrenergic blocking agents have been produced but comparative studies have shown no advantages over propranolol in cardiac effects. Selectivity for beta-1 (cardiac) receptors may be an advantage for some patients who have chest or peripheral vascular disease. Because of the late detection of the dangerous side effects from practolol, there is some reluctance to change from a known safe drug such as propranolol, but atenolol and metoprolol have had considerable clinical exposure without major problems and are probably prescribed more widely now than propranolol.

The combination of beta-adrenergic blocking agents with nitrates has an additive effect and may be synergistic. This combination is the common form of medical therapy for patients with angina at present.

Calcium antagonists

Calcium antagonists inhibit the influx of calcium into the excited myocardial fibre and thus reduce ATP consumption by the contractile system, by reducing the activity of calcium-dependent myofibrillar ATPase (see page 13.3). This leads to a reduction of myocardial oxygen consumption and also has the effect of depress-

ing myocardial contractility. The reduction of oxygen consumption is one reason for the value of calcium antagonists in the treatment of patients with angina. Similar intracellular mechanisms lead to a reduction of tone of vascular smooth muscle and dilatation of coronary arteries and peripheral resistance vessels, two further effects which might lead to a favourable change in the myocardial oxygen supply/demand ratio.

Nifedipine, verapamil and diltiazem are the three calcium antagonist agents which have been widely used in the treatment of angina pectoris. Verapamil is also an antiarrhythmic agent and is more commonly used for that purpose. They have all been shown to have antianginal efficacy.

Nifedipine in particular has been shown to be of value in diminishing attacks of angina in acute and more long-term studies of patients with chronic stable angina. The antianginal effect is about equal to that of beta-adrenergic blocking agents and there is an additive effect if both are used.

Nifedipine and other calcium antagonist agents have proved particularly useful in managing patients in whom coronary artery spasm plays an important aetiological role, especially those with attacks of pain at rest with transient ST segment elevation.

Calcium antagonists need to be given at least 8-hourly. Long-acting preparations are now available but they have not yet been shown to be as effective as the shorter acting varieties. The chief side effects are related to vasodilation rather than to deterioration of left ventricular function although this remains a theoretical hazard. They are often added to other drugs but in some parts of the world are used as a primary agent.

Unstable angina

A number of patients either present with or proceed to a condition described as unstable angina. This is usually defined as angina at rest on minimal exertion either of recent onset or following a period of less severe symptoms. These patients were initially thought to be at very high risk for the develoment of myocardial infarction and were therefore treated as acute medical emergencies. The risk has been defined more clearly now and is not as high as previously thought, but these patients still present an urgent medical problem. They should be treated in hospital, preferably in a cardiac care unit, with bed rest and nitrates usually administered orally and regularly sublingually or intravenously. The presence of recurrent cardiac pain at rest raises the possibility of coronary vasospasm as a contributing mechanism, and for this reason it may be questioned whether beta-adrenergic blocking agents should be used since they could, in theory, aggravate spasm. The point is controversial but in practice it is recognized that the combination of nitrates and beta-adrenergic blocking agents abolish symptoms in the majority of patients. Calcium antagonists should, theoretically, be of most value and there is certainly clinical evidence that they are, so these patients now tend to be treated with 'triple' therapy.

Intra-aortic balloon counterpulsation

Despite intensive medical therapy, a few patients continue to have cardiac pain at rest: and in this situation, two courses are available. The first is to investigate with angiography and proceed to aortocoronary bypass surgery or angioplasty if suitable lesions are found; this will be referred to later. The second is to use intra-aortic balloon counterpulsation with or without subsequent surgery. This technique involves the insertion of a catheter via the femoral artery with an inflatable, finite volume balloon close to its tip. The balloon is placed in the aorta and rapid inflation and deflation are timed by the electrocardiogram. The aim is to inflate the balloon in diastole, thus increasing the perfusion pressure, particularly for the coronary arteries, and so increasing myocardial blood supply. Deflation during systole suddenly reduces resistance to outflow, which reduces left ventricular and aortic pressure and, thus, myocardial oxygen consumption. This method is very effective for the relief of unstable angina. It has the disadvantage of being an inva-

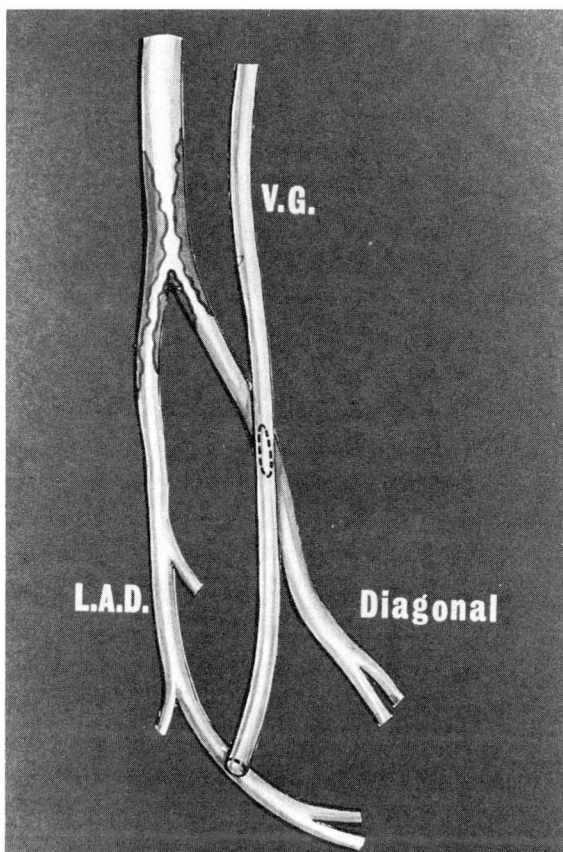

Fig. 11 An atherosclerotic lesion involving the bifurcation of the left anterior descending coronary artery (LAD). A single vein graft (VG) is shown anastomosed side-to-side to the diagonal branch and end-to-end to the anterior descending branch. (Reproduced by permission of Mr J. E. C. Wright).

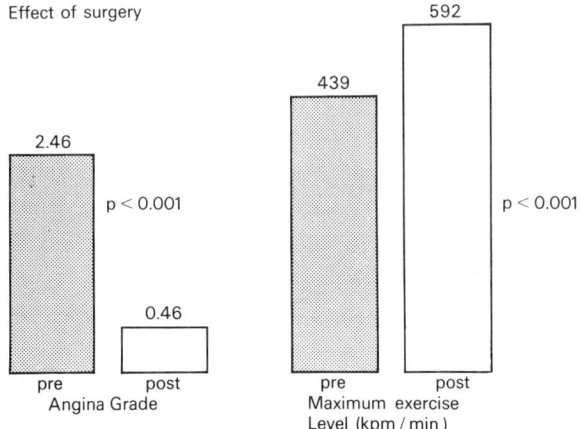

Fig. 12 The two left-hand columns show the change in angina grade and the two right-hand columns the change in maximum exercise load after aortocoronary bypass surgery. kpm/min = kilopond per minute.

sive procedure, the risks of which are mostly related to the insertion of a large catheter into the femoral artery. It is rarely needed now since so many patients respond to medical therapy.

Aortocoronary bypass surgery

Aortocoronary bypass surgery was first introduced in the late 1960s. Since that time a great deal of attention has been paid to the observation of patients who have undergone surgery and prob-

ably more is known about the outcome of this than of any other operation which has ever been performed. Because of this intense study, its place has been reasonably clearly defined although there are still some doubtful areas. The operation consists of bypassing coronary stenoses using vein (usually the long saphenous vein from the leg) and anastomosing it to the aorta and the coronary artery distal to the stenoses. The internal mammary arteries can also be used by dissecting them from the chest wall and anastomosing the distal end to (usually) the anterior descending coronary artery or its diagonal branch. Cardiopulmonary bypass is required but the heart is not opened and so it is not therefore strictly open heart surgery. A number of vein bypasses can be implanted at the same operation and various techniques are available to use a single bypass to deal with two or more stenoses. The commonest of these is to perform a side-to-side anastomosis for the most proximal of the lesions being considered with an end-to-side anastomosis to terminate the graft (Fig. 11). Removal of the atheromatous core by endarterectomy can be performed to facilitate grafting, although the procedure described above often eliminates the need for this; moreover, since endarterectomy may increase the amount of operative myocardial damage because of the inevitable dislocation of side branches, it is not commonly performed.

The postoperative course of these patients is surprisingly uncomplicated compared to that of patients undergoing other forms of cardiac surgery. The additional leg wound gives rise to some increased postoperative morbidity. Operative risk is closely related to the preoperative degree of left ventricular damage and, in its absence, is now less than 1 per cent. The figure rises progressively in patients with serious left ventricular dysfunction. There is particular risk following acute infarction with damage to the intraventricular septum and mitral valve; operative mortality is much increased and may reach prohibitive levels.

The procedure is very effective at relieving angina. It is successful in approximately 85 per cent of patients. Relief of symptoms correlates well with angiographic demonstration that the grafts are patent and perfusing the myocardium well. Physiological studies with exercise and radionuclide techniques also confirm this. Figure 12 shows the effect of surgery on more than 800 patients followed for at least one and up to nine years. Angina is graded 1 to 4, indicating increasing severity. The average grade before surgery was 2.46, and 0.46 after. There was also a demonstrable improvement in exercise tolerance.

Early postoperative studies have shown that the graft patency rate can be expected to be in the region of 95 per cent although, with the passage of time, this figure falls to approximately 70 per cent in five years. The patency rate of internal mammary grafts is rather better than that of vein grafts. However, this progressive slow occlusion of grafts leads to recurrence of symptoms which is also contributed to by progression of the disease in the coronary arteries. Symptoms recur in approximately 8 per cent of susceptible patients every year, although approximately 65 per cent of patients remain symptom-free after five years (Fig. 13). Second and even third operations can be performed, although with more technical difficulties, a higher mortality, and slightly lower success rates.

It is now generally agreed that all patients with severe symptoms despite medical treatment, in whom suitable coronary pathological anatomy and a reasonably preserved left ventricle can be shown, should be treated surgically. Surgical intervention is often suggested earlier, particularly for young patients who wish to lead an active life, either in pursuit of their job or their leisure activities.

Prophylactic drug therapy

Drug treatment may play a part in preventing the progression of coronary disease and myocardial infarction, and sudden death. A number of trials have been performed in order to assess the value of beta-adrenergic blocking agents in this respect, and a summary

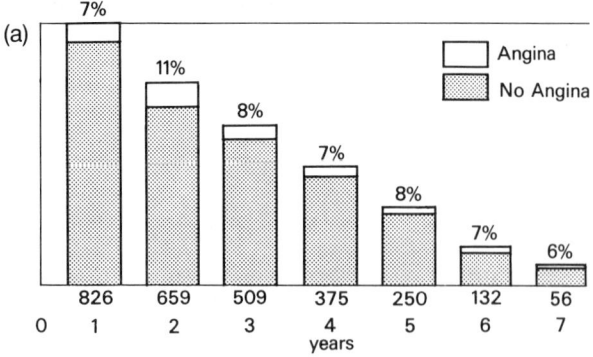

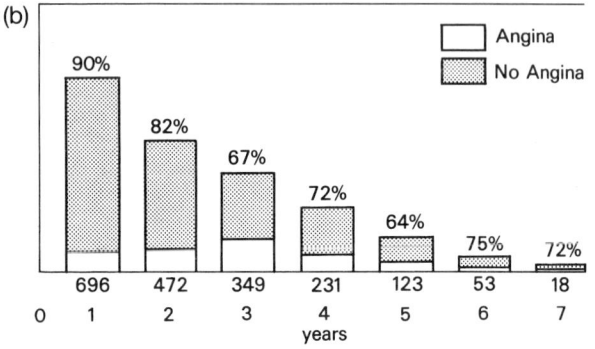

Fig. 13 (a) The rate of recurrence of angina and (b) the percentage of asymptomatic patients. The figure under each column indicates the number of patients.

of the evidence suggests that they do play a part in the prevention of reinfarction and sudden death. The differences in the occurrence of these events reported by these trials have, however, been small and it is not yet accepted practice to give all patients with coronary disease beta-adrenergic blocking agents on this basis alone. This is due at least in part to the possible side effects already mentioned.

A number of other drugs have also been tested. Sulphinpyrazone received considerable attention following a trial of its efficacy which resulted in its widespread use. However, once again, the differences noted were small and no further studies have become available to support the data produced. A combination of dipyridamole and aspirin or either drug alone have effects on platelet function and prostacyclin and thromboxane metabolism which are potentially useful for their prophylactic effects. Clinical trials are in progress which look promising but, once again, their routine use in patients with coronary disease, or indeed in the population in general, is not justified.

Surgery for prophylaxis

For some years there has been controversy as to whether aortocoronary bypass surgery has any prophylactic affect. Early reports suggested that the survival curves for surgically treated patients with severe coronary disease were similar to those with mild coronary artery disease treated medically. There have been three important controlled randomized trials of medical versus surgical treatment, and the results of the first two of these support the initial findings. The latest study (CASS) has not confirmed these findings. The patients studied in this trial, however, were a low risk group since the medically treated patients had only a 1.6 per cent annual mortality rate; it would thus have been very difficult to show any benefit from surgery which itself carries a low but definite mortality. The present position remains in doubt but there is general acceptance that surgery improves the prognosis in the highest risk groups of patients. Figure 14 shows cumulative survival curves for patients taking part in one such trial. The difference in survival for the groups as a whole and for the subset with triple vessel disease is significant at the 1 per cent level. They suggest that patients with severe forms of coronary disease, particularly stenosis of the left main coronary artery or the proximal parts of the three main coronary arteries, have a significantly better survival after surgery. These findings make it extremely important to identify such patients, and this problem has aleady been referred to under the section on coronary arteriography (page 13.162).

Transluminal coronary angioplasty

Angioplasty is a technique for reducing the luminal encroachment of arterial lesions with a balloon catheter passed into the vessel concerned. It was first used for femoral artery obstruction and later adapted for the coronary arteries. It was originally thought to work by 'squashing' the atheromatous plaque and spreading its contents within the arterial wall with subsequent repair of the endothelium. Pathological studies have shown that this is not so and that there is splitting of the plaque and arterial wall involving the intima and the elastic lamina of the media.

Technique

The balloon is non-elastic and is mounted at the tip of a fine catheter with two lumina, one for inflating the balloon and a second at its tip for recording pressure and passage of the catheter over a fine guide wire. The guide is passed through a special guiding cath-

Fig. 14 (a) Cumulative survival curves for all patients and (b) the subset with triple vessel disease from the European Coronary Artery Study Group report. Survival of patients treated surgically is significantly better. M = medical treatment; S = surgical treatment; 3VD = triple vessel disease.

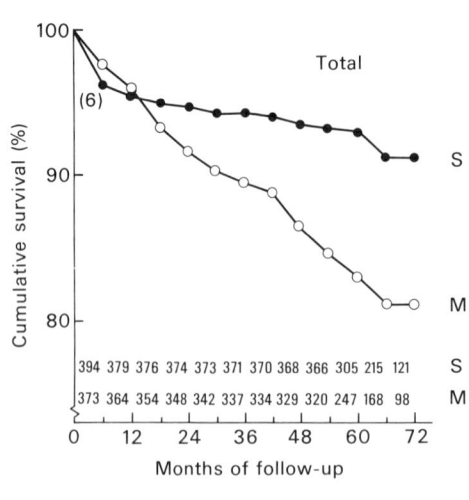

(a)

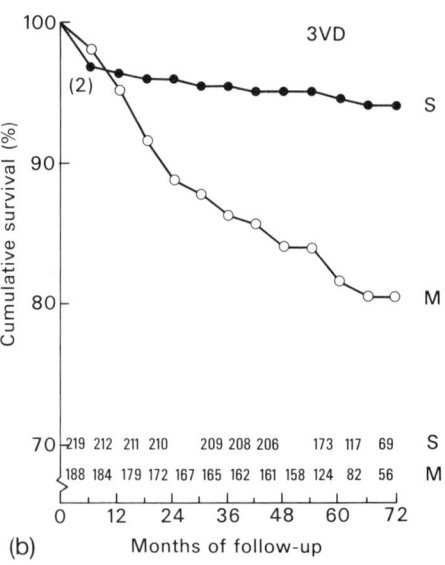

(b)

eter similar to the catheters used to perform coronary arteriography and manoeuvred across the coronary stenosis. The balloon catheter is then passed over the fine guide wire and also positioned across the stenosis. It is then inflated via the second port with a pressure of 4–8 atmospheres, several times for up to 60 seconds each time, until the pressure drop across the stenosis disappears or is maximally reduced.

The procedure would seem likely to produce complications both from the disruption of the arterial wall and the intermittent interruption of coronary flow. These are, however, surprisingly few. The National Heart, Lung and Blood Institute in the United States of America have a registry to record the results of the technique for many centres in both the United States and Europe, and have reported a mortality of 1.3 per cent and myocardial infarction rate of 4.4 per cent in the first 1000 patients studied. Both of these figures were lower for patients with single vessel disease and for those who had not undergone previous aortocoronary bypass surgery.

Primary success was defined as a 20 per cent decrease in degree of coronary stenosis, and this was achieved in 62 per cent of attempts. The result was maintained in 75 per cent of patients in the first months of follow-up. These figures represent the early cases of many centres and therefore include the 'learning curve'. Centres with more experience have better results.

The most suitable patients are those with a single stenosis. These patients have a very good prognosis without surgical intervention, so the only indication for the procedure is failure to control the symptoms with medical treatment – which is a relatively rare problem. Angioplasty is now also being used in some patients with multiple vessel involvement and severe angina, particularly those who cannot be submitted to surgery because of, for instance, lung or cerebrovascular disease. Symptoms may be improved by performing angioplasty on the most severe lesions. The technique is becoming more widespread and the complication rates are falling. With increasing experience and confidence, it will be used more regularly in patients with multivessel disease.

Experimental work is now being carried out on the use of laser catheters to remove coronary atheroma. This would have considerable potential value. The technique has already been attempted successfully in man on a few occasions.

References

Alderman, E. L., Davies, R. O., Crowley, J. J., Lopes, M. G., Brooker, J. Z., Friedman, J. P., Graham, A. F., Matloff, H. and Harrison, D. C. (1979). Dose response effectiveness of propranolol for the treatment of angina pectoris. *Circulation* **51**, 964–975.

Antman, E., Muller, J. and Goldberg, S. (1980). Nifedipine therapy for coronary spasm: experience in 127 patients. *N. Engl. J. Med.* **302**, 1269–1273.

Anturane Reinfarction Trial Research Group (1980). Sulphinpyrazone in the prevention of sudden death after myocardial infarction. *N. Engl. J. Med.* **302**, 250–253.

Bala-Subramanian, V., Lahiri, A., Green, H. L., Stott, F. C. and Raftery, E. B. (1980). Ambulatory ST segment monitoring: problems, pitfalls, solutions and clinical applications. *Br. Heart J.* **44**, 419–425.

Balcon, R. (1980). Prognostic significance of coronary arteriography. *Acta med Port.* suppl. 1, 9–15.

——, and Brooks, N. H. (1984). Correlation of heart rate/ST slope and coronary angiographic findings. *Br. Heart J.* **52**, 304–307.

Baron, D. W., Ilsley, C., Sheiban, I., Poole-Wilson, P. A. and Rickards, A. F. (1980). R-wave amplitude during exercise. Relationship to left ventricular function and coronary artery disease. *Br. Heart J.* **44**, 512–517.

Brooks, N., Warnes, C., Cattell, M., Balcon, R., Honey, M., Layton, C., Sturridge, M. and Wright, J. (1981). Cardiac pain at rest: management and follow-up of 100 consecutive cases. *Br. Heart J.* **45**, 35–41.

Cairns, J. A., Fantus, I. G. and Klassen, G. A. (1976). Unstable angina pectoris. *Am. Heart J.* **92**, 373–386.

Coronary Artery Surgery Study (CASS) principal investigators and their associates. (1983). A randomized trial of coronary artery bypass surgery survival data. *Circulation* **68**, 939–950.

Curry, R. C., Pepine, C. J., Saborn, M. B., Feldman, R. L., Christie, L. G. and Conti, C. R. (1977). Effects of ergometrine in patients with or without coronary disease. *Circulation* **56**, 803–809.

Elamin, M. S., Boyle, R., Kardash, M. M., Smith, D. R., Stoker, J. B., Whitaker, W., Mary, D. A. S. G. and Linden, R. J. (1982). Accurate detection of coronary artery disease by new exercise test. *Br. Heart J.* **48**, 311–320.

Ellestad, M. H., Cooke, B. M. and Greenberg, P. S. (1979). Stress testing: clinical application and predictive capacity. *Prog. cardiovasc. Dis.* **21**, 431–460.

Epstein, S. E. (1978). Value and limitations of electrocardiograph response to exercise in the assessment of patients with coronary artery disease. Controversies in Cardiology II, *Am. J. Cardiol.* **42**, 667–674.

Gruntzig, A. (1981). Percutaneous transluminal angioplasty. Fourth Symposium on Coronary Heart Disease, Frankfurt. Springer-Verlag, Berlin.

Loop, F. D., Proudfit, W. I. and Sheldon, W. C. (1978). Coronary bypass surgery weighed in the balance. *Am. J. Cardiol.* **42**, 154–156.

Lown, B. and de Silva, R. A. (1980). Is coronary arterial spasm a risk factor for coronary artery atherosclerosis? *Am. J. Cardiol.* **45**, 901–903.

Markis, J. E., Gorlin, R., Mills, R. M., Williams, R. A., Schweitzar, P. and Ransil, B. J. (1979). Sustained effect of orally administered isosorbide dinitrate on exercise performance of patients with angina pectoris. *Am. J. Cardiol.* **43**, 265–271.

Maseri, A., Chierchia, A. and Abbate, A. (1980). Pathogenetic mechanisms underlying clinical events associated with atherosclerotic heart disease. *Circulation* **62**, suppl. V, V–3.

Prinzmetal, M., Kennamer, R., Merlis, R., Wada, T. and Bor, N. (1959). A variant form of angina. *Am. J. Med.* **27**, 375–388.

Proudfit, W. L., Brushke, A. V. G. and Sones, F. M. (1978). Natural history of obstructive coronary artery disease: ten year study of 601 non-surgical cases. *Prog. Cardiovasc. Dis.* **21**, 53–78.

Quyyumi, A. A., Wright, C. and Fox, K. (1984). Ambulatory electrocardiographic ST segment changes in healthy volunteers. (1984). *Br. Heart J.* **50**, 460–464.

Russell, D. C. and Balcon, R. (1978). Haemodynamic effects on the myocardial blood-flow supply/oxygen demand ratio in pacing induced angina pectoris. *Cardiovasc. Res.* **12**, 358–363.

Sarnoff, S. J., Braunwald, E., Welch, G. H., Case, R. G., Stainsby, W. N. and Macruz, R. (1958). Hemodynamic determinants of oxygen consumption of the heart with special reference to the tension-time index. *Am. J. Physiol.* **192**, 148–156.

Temple, R. and Pledger, G. W. (1980). The FDAs critique of the Anturane reinfarction trial. *N. Engl. J. Med.* **303**, 1488–1492.

Varnauskas, E. (1982). Long-term results of prospective randomised study of coronary artery bypass surgery in stable angina pectoris. European Coronary Surgery Study Group. *Lancet* **ii**, 1173–1180.

Weintraub, R. M., Aroesty, J. M., Paulin, S., Levine, F. H., Markis, J. E., La Raia, P. J., Cohen, S. I. and Kurland, G. F. (1979). Medically refractory unstable angina pectoris. I. Long-term follow-up of patients undergoing intra-aortic balloon counterpulsation and operation. *Am. J. Cardiol.* **43**, 877–882.

Myocardial infarction

B. L. PENTECOST

Introduction

In the United Kingdom approximately 160 000 deaths occur each year as a result of coronary artery disease. There is considerable regional variation in the incidence of heart attacks; in an urban population of 400 000 people in the Teeside region in Northeast England the incidence of acute myocardial infarction was 4.89 per thousand population per annum between 1972 and 1973. A somewhat lower incidence has been recorded in Oxfordshire, and a substantially higher figure in Edinburgh. There appears to be a genuine increase in the frequency of coronary artery disease from south to north of the United Kingdom, reflected in the two-fold increase in deaths from stroke and ischaemic heart disease in the West of Scotland compared with Southeast England (Fig. 1). The incidence of myocardial infarction varies with both sex and social class. It is three to four times more frequent amongst men than women. The popular concept that coronary artery disease is the scourge of the managerial and professional classes appears to be

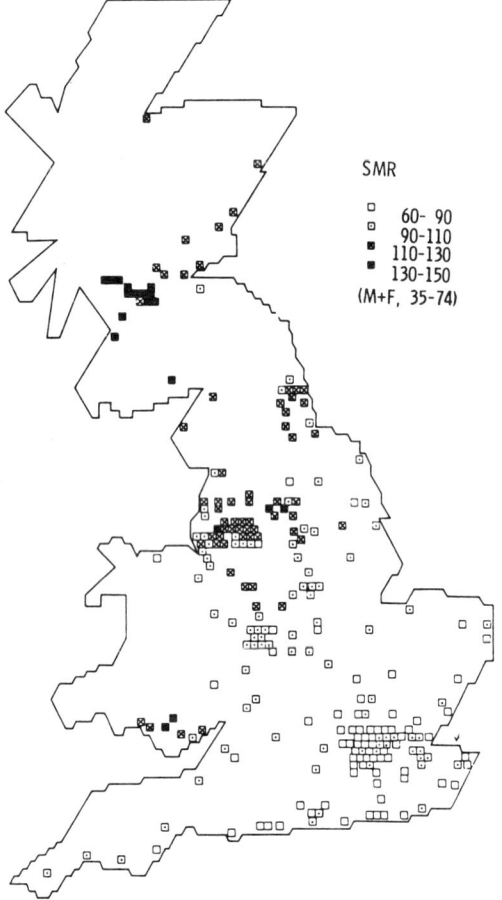

Fig. 1 Standardized mortality ratios (SMR) for cardiovascular disease (excluding rheumatic heart disease) in men and women aged 35–74. A SMR of 100 for a town indicates that its mortality was the same as that for Britain as a whole. (From Pocock *et al.*, 1980, by permission.)

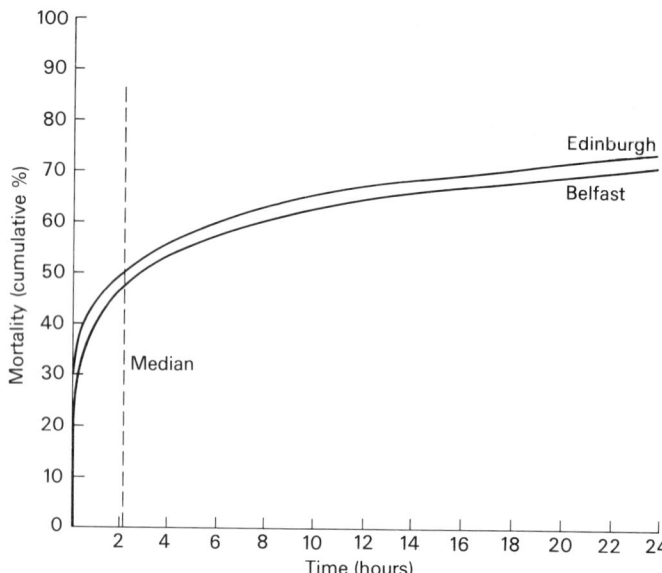

Fig. 2 Cumulative percentage mortality in the first 24 hours after the onset of symptoms of myocardial infarction. Data from Belfast and Edinburgh Studies. (From Fulton *et al.*, 1969, by permission.)

wrong; recent British surveys suggest that myocardial infarction is substantially more common among manual and unskilled workers. This observation is only partly explained in terms of classical risk factors. The relatively high incidence of cigarette smoking among people in social groups 4 and 5 combined with a lower level of recreational physical activity does not completely account for the observed difference.

Approximately 40–50 per cent of patients experiencing a heart attack die within 20 days of the onset. Elderly patients, contrary to popular belief, invariably fare less well than the young and middle aged. Perhaps the most significant statistic concerning myocardial infarction is that half the deaths occur between one and two hours of the onset of symptoms (Fig. 2). Many patients therefore fail to reach medical care, succumbing to potentially correctable ventricular fibrillation. In contrast, a patient surviving long enough to gain admission to hospital is more likely to die as a result of pump failure – intractable left ventricular failure or cardiogenic shock – for which even the best coronary care unit can do relatively little.

Autopsy findings in the two populations are quite different. Arterial occlusion or recent myocardial necrosis cannot often be demonstrated at autopsy among patients dying suddenly, although there is almost invariably evidence of extensive atherosclerosis of the coronary arteries. This contrasts with the classical appearances of myocardial infarction with proximal coronary arterial occlusion found among patients dying several days after the onset of a heart attack.

The problem of sudden death as a result of coronary artery disease underlies two of the most hotly debated issues in clinical man-

agement – the home versus hospital controversy and the place of mobile coronary care units. Some physicians have argued that the problem of sudden death is of such magnitude as to favour mobilizing medical care to minimize delay in reaching patients, and to supplement this process with public education into the symptoms of myocardial infarction and in the technique of cardiorespiratory resuscitation. Others hold that death is frequently so sudden that it defies our ability to deliver skilled medical care in time and that the measures proposed represent a misapplication of scarce medical resources.

Clinical presentation
History

Although acute myocardial infarction may be the first manifestation of coronary artery disease, some 50 per cent of patients admitted to hospital already have a past history of cardiovascular disease. In a survey of 194 patients with myocardial infarction undertaken in Oxford, 44 per cent had a history of angina, 19 per cent previous infarction, and 30 per cent high blood pressure. Among 260 patients recently admitted to hospital in Birmingham within the first six hours of symptoms a similar number provided a history of previous angina or infarction but only 16 per cent were known to be hypertensive. Many patients provide a retrospective history of prodromal fatigue during the preinfarction period but the vague and common nature of this symptom make its significance difficult to evaluate.

Chest or epigastric pain is the presenting symptom in more than 80 per cent of patients. The pain may be recognized as having the same deep pressing, squeezing, or crushing quality as previous angina but it is usually more severe and certainly more persistent. Nitrates, usually so effective in angina, fail to relieve the pain. Occasionally in desperation, patients consume large quantities of nitrates over a short period of time producing hypotension and even syncope. A patient with no previous experience of angina may assume the pain to be indigestion; the frequency of nausea and belching reinforces this belief, with the result that many take dyspepsia remedies before seeking medical attention. Among the Oxford patients two-thirds experienced radiation of the pain to the throat, jaw, arm, and fingers, and sweating was another common feature of the attack. Less frequently myocardial infarction presented as painless dyspnoea or syncope.

Physical examination

The patient's appearance is mainly determined by the severity of pain. This provokes fear and anxiety leading to overactivity of the sympathetic nervous system irrespective of any autonomic imbalance attributable to the process of infarction itself. The clinical picture of a pale, sweating person with a rather thready peripheral pulse and poorly perfused extremities often leads the observer to use the descriptive term 'shock' but this term implies a poor prognosis and should not be used until the beneficial effects of analgesia have been observed.

Findings on physical examination depend upon the extent of myocardial injury. When this is severe, evidence of left ventricular failure is present. Although the patient is orthopnoeic and may show gross radiological changes of left heart failure, physical signs are often sparse. Crepitations over the lung fields may be absent and the jugular venous pressure is usually normal even when left ventricular failure is severe. An atrial or fourth sound is almost invariably present in the acute stages of infarction. When myocardial damage is extensive, a third heart sound is audible, often accompanied by a systolic thrust palpable over the third and fourth left interspaces due to dyskinetic movement of the damaged left ventricular wall. This abnormal praecordial movemen becomes less easily palpable over the succeeding few days except in patients with the most extensive myocardial injury.

Although the patient's blood pressure will almost always fall below previously recorded levels after infarction, this may not be apparent for several hours. The anxiety and fear associated with the illness often mask a fall in pressure for some time and it must never be assumed that maintenance of a normal blood pressure is evidence against infarction. In patients suffering extensive myocardial damage severe systemic hypotension will develop early in the course of the illness.

Fever is usually apparent within 12 hours and is occasionally the first confirmary evidence of infarction appearing before the return of serum enzyme levels from the laboratory. Pyrexia usually settles within four or five days but occasionally persists for a week.

Pericarditis is a sign of extensive infarction which involves the epicardial region of the heart and usually makes its appearance between the second and fourth days. The rub may be persistent and accompanied by further chest pain but is often remarkably transient.

Other physical signs reflect mechanical complications of infarction such as mitral regurgitation or rupture of the interventricular septum and are dealt with in the appropriate sections of this chapter.

Electrocardiography (page 13.21)

Most experienced physicians, although relying heavily on the electrocardiogram for the diagnosis of myocardial infarction, recognize its limitations. The patient who presents with a convincing story of myocardial pain may well have a normal ECG at the time of initial assessment with the classical electrocardiographic appearances of infarction taking some hours to develop. It is doubtful if the ECG is ever totally normal during the infarction process, but many patients experience increasingly frequent and severe angina between attacks of which the electrocardiogram may very well be normal. Indeed the exact time of infarction is often difficult to establish with certainty. The important principle is that the diagnosis of acute myocardial infarction is clinical and the patient should be managed on the basis of the history and the clinician's judgement, irrespective of ECG appearances.

In extensive myocardial infarction involving epicardial tissue, so-called full thickness of Q wave infarction, the initial ECG manifestation is ST elevation – the 'current of injury'. Two processess contribute to this appearance. The dominant mechanism is the diastolic current of injury. During diastole, ischaemic epicardial and subepicardial tissues are incompletely repolarized and therefore electropositive in relation to the completely repolarized surrounding myocardium. This will produce a current flow away from

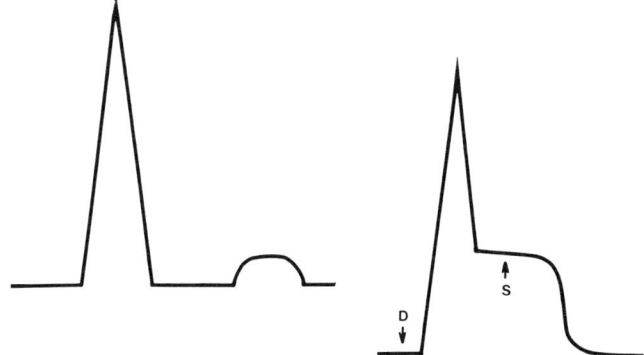

Fig. 3 ST elevation in acute myocardial infarction reflects combined systolic (S) and diastolic (D) current of injury.

the ischaemic tissue resulting in a depressed T Q segment in the signal recorded over the zone of infarction. The systolic current of injury is quantitatively less important. During depolarization, ischaemic tissue is incompletely depolarized with the result that electrical current flows towards the damaged tissue resulting in true ST elevation in the ECG signal (Fig. 3). The elevated ST segment usually describes a curve of upward convexity often matched by reciprocal ST depression in electrodes situated at an angle of 180° (Fig. 4a). Reciprocal ST depression suggests relatively severe myocardial injury and is often associated with occlusive arterial disease remote from the area of infarction. Less frequently the initial electrocardiographic evidence of myocardial infarction consists of an excessive peaking of T waves with some ST elevation, so-called hyperacute infarction (Fig. 5).

The terminal part of the T wave, which is incorporated within the elevated ST segment, often begins to invert below the isoelectric line within the first 24 hours (Fig. 4b). The duration of ST elevation is extremely variable but has usually resolved within one or two weeks. The T wave gradually becomes completely inverted over a period of two or three weeks assuming a symmetrical or 'arrowhead' appearance. T wave inversion usually persists for many months and may even be a permanent feature. It is more common, however, for the T wave to assume a positive or upright appearance in time. Persistent elevation of the ST segments was once regarded as diagnostic of cardiac aneurysm. It is now accepted that such an appearance reflects the presence of an extensive area of akinetic or dyskinetic myocardium as a result of infarction. The distinction is important clinically for it cannot be assumed that persistent ST elevation is evidence of a resectable ventricular aneurysm.

Whereas the current of injury relates to a state of potentially reversible, albeit extensive ischaemic damage, the pathological Q wave is evidence of myocardial destruction. Q wave development within an appropriate clinical setting is diagnostic of myocardial infarction, but it is important to appreciate that Q waves also occur in other pathologies including certain cardiomyopathies and both primary and secondary tumours of the heart. The Q wave phenomenon is often explained in terms of an 'electrical window'. Necrotic myocardium takes no part in the depolarization process and overlying electrodes record activity of underlying and adjacent myocardium. In an extensive infarction involving nearly the whole thickness of myocardium, the surface electrode will record appearances similar to the classical cavity lead avR, i.e. a QS complex or Q wave. A pathological Q wave has a duration of at least 40 ms; this is greater when the Q wave combines with an S wave and durations of 80–100 ms are common. The depth of the pathological Q wave is at least 25 per cent of any accompanying R wave. The development of Q waves is accompanied by a loss of R wave voltage which also reflects reduction of myocardial mass. Both appearances are usually seen within 24 hours of the onset of infarction.

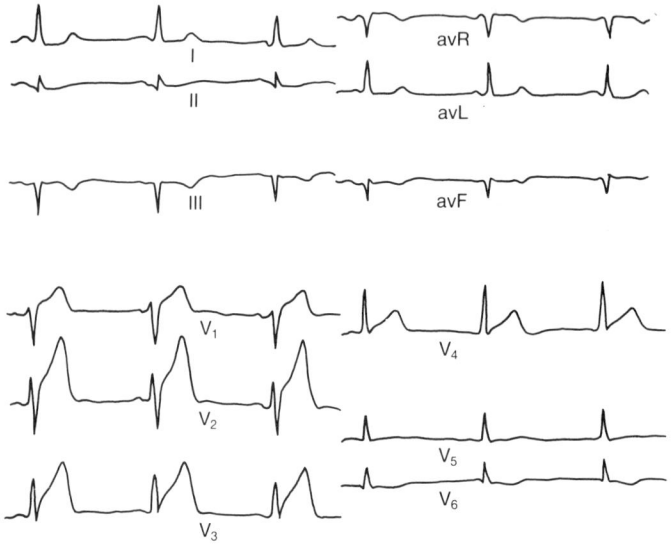

Fig. 5 Hyperacute changes of anterior infarction, ECG shows excessive peaking of T waves V_2 and V_3 with some ST elevation. Patient has previously suffered an inferolateral infarction.

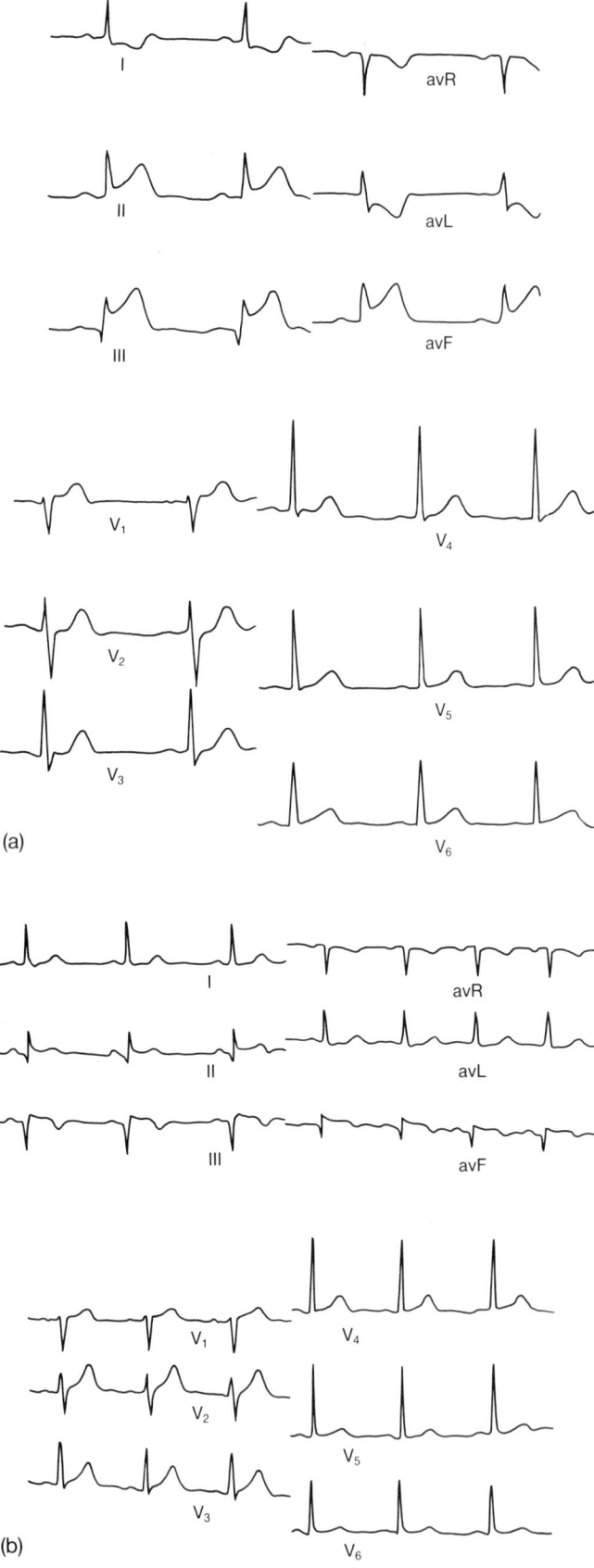

Fig. 4 (a) Acute inferior myocardial infarction. ST elevation in leads II, III, and avF is matched by reciprocal ST depression in I and avL. (b) From the same patient 24 hours later. ST elevation and reciprocal depression are less obvious. T wave inversion developing in III and avF. Pathological Q waves and loss of R wave in II, III, and avF confirm myocardial necrosis.

Q waves were once considered to be permanent features of the electrocardiogram after infarction. This is generally true but with the passage of years the duration of Q waves may become less, only their depth in association with a sloping upstroke to the R wave or notched QRS complex provide clues to the true state of affairs. Another suspicious sign of previous infarction in the anteroseptal region is a progressive reduction in R wave voltage from leads V_1–V_3 rather than the usual increase. It must be said, however, that this appearance is not absolutely diagnostic of previous infarction. Similarly, loss of normal septal Q waves in typically left ventricular leads, 1, avL, and V_5 and V_6 point to previous septal injury, although again various degrees of left bundle branch block may produce similar appearances. Extensive myocardial damage always produces some impairment of conduction and those leads demonstrating the infarction pattern will also show some widening of QRS complexes when compared with preinfarction tracings.

Both right and left bundle branch block may either precede or accompany the development of acute myocardial infarction. In the case of right bundle block there is no interference with intitial septal depolarization so that the formation of pathological Q waves is not obscured (Fig. 6). In left bundle branch block on the other hand the initial electrical forces are not preserved and pathological Q waves do not develop. ST elevation and subsequent T wave changes may, however, still be seen, although the diagnosis of myocardial infarction in the presence of left bundle branch block must often depend upon enzyme studies.

Less extensive myocardial injury may be limited to the subendocardial region of the heart. ECG appearances accepted as compatible with subendocardial infarction are initial ST depression followed by symmetrical inversion of T waves. Other variants encountered are transient ST elevation and subsequent T wave inversion without Q wave formation, as well as isolated T wave changes. These appearances are not specific for the infarction process and require confirmation by enzyme studies.

Electrocardiography provides information on both extent and distribution of myocardial damage and may be analysed to produce a numerical expression of myocardial injury. This ECG score can be used to compare the severity of infarction between different patient populations or as an indication of prognosis. ECG recordings may also be used to provide a dynamic picture of myocardial ischaemia. Multiple electrodes positioned on the praecordium in the pattern of a grid will provide a praecordial map reflecting serial changes in ST segment shift. This technique has

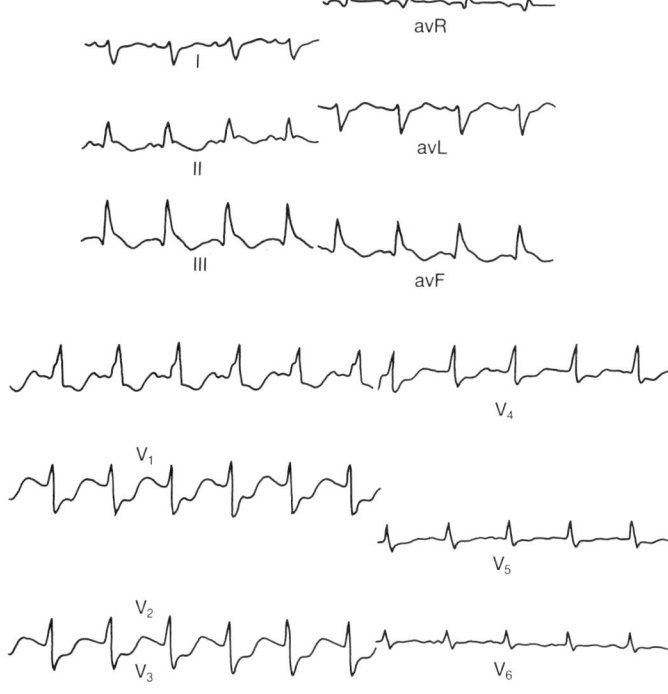

Fig. 6 Right bundle branch block does not obscure the changes of inferior myocardial infarction in this patient. The right axis deviation also suggests the presence of inferior (posterior) hemiblock.

been used as a research tool both to quantify myocardial ischaemia in various circumstances and to demonstrate the effect of therapeutic procedures on ST elevation in acute infarction.

Laboratory investigations

An acute inflammatory response to the presence of dead myocardial tissue results in an elevated neutrophil count and a raised erythrocyte sedimentation rate; both are non-specific findings and of little practical help in diagnosis.

Death of myocardial cells results in the release of intracellular enzymes, the detection of which may help substantiate the diagnosis. Several enzymes have been used in this way. They vary greatly in the time relationships between the episode of infarction and the rise in plasma concentrations as well as in their specifity for myocardial damage. Aspartate transaminase forms part of the routine serum biochemical investigations undertaken in most hospitals and for this reason is the enzyme most frequently used in the diagnosis of myocardial infarction. Elevated serum levels are detectable within 12 to 24 hours of infarction and return to normal approximately 48 to 72 hours later. The enzyme is present in other tissues including liver and lung. Therefore pulmonary infarction will also cause a rise in aspartate transaminase, so too will hepatic congestion as a result of heart failure. The estimation of aspartate transaminase retains a useful role, however, providing the enzyme levels rise to at least twice the upper limit for the individual laboratory and return to normal within two or three days, in which case the test provides good supportive evidence for a diagnosis of myocardial infarction. Lactate dehydrogenase is also released from infarcted myocardium. It has the advantage of a much longer period of elevation for anything up to 10 days after the infarct. It is also contained in other tissues including red cells and lung. The isoenzyme LDH_1, is more specific for heart muscle and this is usually estimated in the form of hydroxybutyrate dehydrogenase. The most specific enzyme for the detection of myocardial injury is the MB isoenzyme of creatine phosphokinase (MB–CPK). MB–CPK serum levels rise within a few hours of infarction and remain elevated for 24 to 48 hours. Unlike creatine phosphokinase it is not released from minor skeletal muscle damage such as

accompanies an intramuscular injection. MB–CPK estimations not only provide a useful diagnostic test but when performed at two-hourly intervals allow the construction of a concentration–time plot, the area of which correlates with the extent of myocardial injury.

The respiratory protein myoglobin is also released from damaged myocardial cells and reaches a peak serum concentration more rapidly than even MB–CPK. It is rapidly excreted through the kidney and serial blood levels often show a series of concentration peaks. This phenomenon may represent a step-wise extension of the infarction but could also reflect reperfusion of necrotic muscle as a result of spontaneous thrombolysis.

Radionuclide imaging (page 13.41)

Several nuclear cardiology techniques have been used both to diagnose myocardial infarction and to evaluate the extent of muscle damage and impairment of left ventricular function. Thallium-201 myocardial perfusion imaging defines the extent of myocardium at risk within four hours of the onset of symptoms and may be used serially to assess the value of such therapeutic interventions as thrombolysis or beta-blockade whereas the 'hotspot' image provided by technetium-99m pyrophosphate may not fully develop for up to 48 hours after infarction, which greatly limits its clinical usefulness. Serial observations of left ventricular function may be achieved by technetium-99m gated blood pool imaging which yields information on both general and regional left ventricular function. To obtain the most comprehensive view of myocardial damage these techniques may each be combined with emission computed tomography and be adapted to provide a limited amount of information via a mobile gamma camera at the bedside.

Differential diagnosis

The clinical diagnosis of myocardial infarction is usually straightforward but occasionally presentation is unusual and confusion with certain other conditions possible.

Aortic dissection

Aortic dissection (page 13.185) presents a considerable challenge to the physician since it is often extremely difficult to differentiate from myocardial infarction. It has become increasingly important in recent years not to miss the diagnosis because the results of early surgical repair of aortic dissection are now encouraging. The severe chest pain accompanying dissection often has a tearing or stabbing quality. Patients frequently describe a radiation of pain along the line of dissection into the interscapular region and sometimes down into the abdomen. The classical sign of absent or diminished femoral pulses occurs so late in the process of dissection as to militate against successful surgical intervention. Careful palpation and auscultation of the subclavian, carotid, and axillary arteries will sometimes provide earlier evidence of dissection in the form of diminished pulsation and arterial bruits. A high-pitched early diastolic murmur of aortic regurgitation may confirm the diagnosis of dissection but it again represents an advanced stage of the process, as does the appearance of a hemiplegia from involvement of the cranial branches of the aortic arch. Dissection of the ascending aorta often tracks back to involve the coronary vessels producing electrocardiographic evidence of infarction. The ECG is thus of limited value in differential diagnosis.

The chest X-ray may show widening of the aortic shadow with medial displacement of intimal calcification towards the lumen. M mode echocardiography of the aortic root will often reveal an intimal 'tag' and demonstrate a double lumen. Computerized tomography has been demonstrated to be particularly useful in diagnosing aortic dissection but it is not available in most district general hospitals. Aortography remains the most certain method of diagnosis but should only be undertaken in a centre where considerable expertise exists. Technically poor aortograms can easily fail to reveal the true state of affairs.

Pulmonary embolus (page 13.355)

This is the classical problem in hospital practice and usually involves a patient who develops chest pain after a period of immobilization due to illness or surgery. Typical presentation results in little difficulty in diagnosis but the description of pain may be vague or unobtainable and the ECG changes can be confusing. Right bundle branch block or T wave inversion over the anteroseptal leads may occur in myocardial infarction or pulmonary embolus; furthermore, hypoxaemia as a result of pulmonary embolism may produce genuine ECG changes of myocardial ischaemia. In addition many enzyme estimations used to diagnose myocardial infarction, including aspartate transaminase and lactate dehydrogenase, are also elevated following pulmonary embolism. Tachypnoea in the absence of radiologically obvious pulmonary oedema is a useful clinical sign of pulmonary embolism. Often the diagnosis must be made on a balance of probabilities. A decision over diagnosis and management must usually be made before the problem can be resolved by such sophisticated techniques as ventilation/perfusion lung scans.

Spontaneous pneumothorax (Section 15)

Uncomplicated spontaneous pneumothorax rarely poses a problem in the differential diagnosis of myocardial infarction but a tension pneumothorax may. I have seen two patients diagnosed initially as cases of cardiogenic shock secondary to myocardial infarction. Right bundle branch block was present in both patients who had presented collapsed, with chest pain and dyspnoea. Physical examination and chest X-ray revealed the correct diagnosis.

Pericarditis (page 13.304)

The pain of pericarditis frequently has a pleuritic component and is often aggravated by changes of posture or swallowing. The ECG changes can be confusing but in pericarditis ST elevation is usually widespread throughout all leads apart from avR. Pericarditis complicating myocardial infarction only accompanies extensive infarcts showing a Q wave formation on the electrocardiogram. In infective pericarditis such Q waves are of course not present.

Oesophageal rupture

The diagnosis of oesophageal rupture should always be considered when severe chest pain and collapse follow a period of violent vomiting. This seems particularly liable to occur when the patient is intoxicated. Pain often radiates through to the back and has a character rather similar to that described for aortic dissection. Occasionally surgical emphysema is present in the supraclavicular region. The classical radiological appearances are those of hydropneumothorax. The level of perforation may be detected by following the passage of some ingested gastrografin.

Prognosis

The overall community mortality after myocardial infarction is approximately 40–50 per cent at one month. The death toll attributable to ventricular fibrillation is at its peak within the first few hours of infarction after which time it is fairly easy to differentiate between patients with a relatively good prognosis and those with poor life expectancy. There is a practical value in the identification of high-risk patients in order to avoid premature discharge from hospital and to provide guidance on the future return to normal physical activity. In addition studies on treatment in the early stages of myocardial infarction should ensure that groups included within any trial are comparable with regard to prognosis at the outset.

Over the years several prognostic indices have been constructed in order to place the matter on a sound statistical basis. Although the intention is to achieve a statistical estimate of prognosis as soon as possible after infarction, in practice several hours must elapse before all data are collected so that the influence of early ventricular fibrillation is past. Essentially all the prognostic indices

have reflected the extent of myocardial damage sustained during the process of infarction. Observations which have been shown to correlate with a relatively poor prognosis have been: *clinical* – tachycardia, oliguria, hypotension, and left ventricular failure; or *electrocardiographic* – Q wave formation and the presence of substantial ST elevation; or *biochemical* – high serum concentrations of cardiac enzymes and a raised blood urea; or *radiological* – appearances of pulmonary venous congestion or pulmonary oedema. All reflect directly or indirectly the extent of myocardial damage and its haemodynamic consequences. Advancing age also has an adverse effect on prognosis, perhaps because infarction tends to be more extensive in the elderly; so too does a history of previous myocardial infarction, hypertension, or diabetes mellitus.

From a practical standpoint it now appears that patients free from left ventricular failure, serious ventricular tachyarrhythmia, and disorders of atrioventicular conduction at 48 hours after admission will probably be fit for hospital discharge at around five to seven days.

Clinical management

General measures

Pain relief Rapid and effective analgesia is the main requirement of most patients in the early stages of myocardial infarction. The opiates, morphine and diamorphine, are most effective for this purpose. When given by slow intravenous injection, either morphine, 10–15 mg, or diamorphine 5–10 mg, result in rapid pain relief. The emetic effects of both drugs result in unwanted circulatory stresses but may be lessened by the routine intravenous administration of cyclizine 50 mg. Among alternative drugs are pethidine, methadone, and pentazocine. Pentazocine has been a source of some concern because a rise in pulmonary artery pressure following its administration has been observed in several studies. This finding has been associated with an elevation of left ventricular end-diastolic pressure in one study, suggesting a negative inotropic effect on the left ventricle. This has not, however, been a uniform observation and a direct effect on pulmonary arterioles has also been postulated. In any event, pentazocine, although an effective analgesic in doses of 30–60 mg intravenously, is probably best avoided because of its tendency to provoke hallucinations.

All the potent analgesics mentioned produce some degree of respiratory depression particularly in the elderly. In the majority of patients this may not be of clinical importance, but in those with severe left ventricular failure or cardiogenic shock, it may impair the patient's ability to correct acid–base imbalance; even so, effective analgesia must never be withheld.

Postural hypotension and bradycardia, very similar to a vasovagal faint, may occur after morphine injection. This is a rare event and unlikely to be seen in hospital but may be provoked by tilting the patient's head up when negotiating a staircase in the process of moving from home to hospital. Correction of the head-up tilt and possibly elevation of the legs is all that is required to correct the situation.

Some patients require a second or third dose of analgesic during the first 24–48 hours of admission, others are particularly anxious and benefit from sedation with a benzodiazepine, e.g. diazepam 2–5 mg thrice daily. The most essential requirement of the patient after analgesia is a sympathetic environment and sensible, informed reassurance from both medical and nursing staff. A major advantage of hospital care is the presence of physicians and nurses familiar with the psychological stresses of this traumatic experience, who are able to explain in simple terms the nature of the illness and provide continual moral support.

Patients with myocardial infarction often present to a medical centre in industry. Such reception areas are frequently staffed by qualified nurses rather than doctors. As a result potent analgesics may not be available; a period of prolonged pain and distress can be avoided by the use of a 50 per cent nitrous oxide/oxygen mixture, which can also be used during transport to hospital. The analgesic effects are rapidly reversed, which allows the patient to provide a history free from the sedative effects of analgesia.

Bed rest The last two decades have seen a progressive reduction in the period of immobilization after myocardial infarction. Prolonged periods of bed rest, with their attendant risks of venous thromboembolism, have given way to early mobilization after two or three days among patients with no major haemodynamic or rhythm disturbances.

Oxygen It is common practice to administer oxygen routinely during the acute stages of myocardial infarction. The appropriate mask has a small dead space and delivers approximately 40 per cent oxygen in inspired air. This practice can be justified on the grounds that a moderate degree of hypoxaemia is commonly encountered either as a result of hypoventilation following opiates or some degree of left ventricular failure. Experimental studies have suggested that routine oxygen therapy might limit the final extent of myocardial damage but the only controlled study undertaken in humans has failed to demonstrate any apparent benefit from routine oxygen administration among patients with no evidence of cardiac failure. It seems reasonable to advise routine oxygen administration during the first few hours of admission, during which time the patient is under the influence of morphine or its derivatives, but to discontinue it thereafter unless there is a specific indication such as the presence of left ventricular failure.

Previous drug therapy Many patients admitted to a coronary care unit will already be receiving beta-blocking agents for angina. If cardiac failure is present, these must be discontinued immediately. If, however, the diagnosis of infarction is in doubt and a state of acute coronary insufficiency is present, then beta-blocking agents should be continued to avoid a potentially harmful increase in myocardial oxygen demand. Among patients with infarction but no signs of failure, there is no clear evidence of benefit from either stopping or continuing beta-blocking drugs. It is the author's practice to discontinue beta-blockade for at least two or three days in the acute stages of infarction but to recommence the drug later during the admission. This is because the majority of patients with angina before infarction do not lose this symptom and continue to require anti-anginal therapy.

Antihypertensive therapy should be discontinued during at least the first few days of admission for there will invariably be a fall in blood pressure. This relatively hypotensive period may persist for several months. Hypertension is likely to return at some future date and such patients require careful follow-up.

Anticoagulation and thrombolysis
Enthusiasm for anticoagulant therapy in the acute stages of infarction faded many years ago. It was originally hoped that anticoagulants might limit the thrombotic process and thereby minimize myocardial damage. In practice the only benefit convincingly demonstrated was a reduction in thromboembolic complications, such as pulmonary embolus. The current practice of early mobilization may well have reduced the risk of this particular complication, but there remain a few patients who for various reasons are immobilized for prolonged periods of and in whom anticoagulant therapy with heparin and warfarin is justifiable. Instead interest has been transferred to the use of thrombolytic enzymes in an attempt to lyse intracoronary thrombus.

Angiography has demonstrated that coronary artery thrombosis is present in nearly 90 per cent of patients investigated within four hours of the onset of infarction, but only 65 per cent after 12 to 24 hours, presumably reflecting spontaneous thrombolysis or the relaxation of arterial spasm. Intra-arterial perfusion of streptokinase results in early reperfusion of the occluded coronary artery in up to 80 per cent of patients. Enthusiasm must however be tempered by the fact that treatment requiring preliminary coronary angiography is unlikely to be available in more than a few highly specialized departments. Interest has therefore been rekindled in the use of intravenous streptokinase. Prolonged infusion with intravenous streptokinase apparently produces a slight reduction in mortality from myocardial infarction, but is not infrequently complicated by troublesome and even fatal haemorrhage. More recently, intravenous infusions of much shorter duration (30–60 min) have been shown to result in recanalization of approximately 60 per cent of occluded arteries with a much lower incidence of bleeding. Intravenous streptokinase also avoids the need for angiography, thereby permitting earlier treatment. It is likely that the problem of avoiding haemorrhage will finally be resolved by the use of tissue type plasminogen activators which have an affinity for plasminogen bound to fibrin, thus limiting their lysing effect to formed thrombus.

The clinical benefits of thrombolysis whether expressed as improved patient survival or preservation of left ventricular function remain to be established. No trial currently available is of sufficient size to resolve this question. It seems highly likely that a delay of more than four hours from onset of symptoms to thrombolysis may result in a reperfused coronary artery without salvage of myocardium but earlier intervention may be of greater therapeutic benefit.

Duration of hospital admission
The duration of inpatient stay has been reduced progressively over recent years. Patients without evidence of left ventricular failure or late ventricular tachycardia or fibrillation, i.e. after the first 12 hours of admission, may be discharged from hospital at approximately one week after admission. The prognosis of such patients is not adversely affected by early discharge, hospital beds are released, and the patient's return to society accelerated. The majority of patients suitable for early discharge are identifiable within 48 hours of admission but all require careful examination and reassessment immediately before leaving hospital.

Arrhythmias and their management (page 13.117)
Contemporary management of acute myocardial infarction has focussed upon the ability to correct ventricular fibrillation and, to a lesser extent, expertise in the management of other arrhythmias including atrial fibrillation and complete atrioventricular block.

Ventricular tachyarrhythmias
Ventricular fibrillation is encountered in approximately 10 per cent of all patients presenting to hospital. The incidence of the arrhythmia is at its peak within the first two hours of the acute illness and any circumstance which facilitates early admission to hospital, including mobile coronary care units or the central position of a city hospital, results in a relatively high incidence of detection of ventricular fibrillation. Ventricular fibrillation occurring in the absence of left ventricular failure or cardiogenic shock is nearly always correctable and a high percentage of patients survive to leave hospital. When the arrhythmia complicates heart failure, successful resuscitation is less frequent. The terms primary and secondary ventricular fibrillation are often used to describe these two sets of circumstances. Classification is usually retrospective and the distinction not always obvious, but the concept retains some practical value as a pointer to the likely outcome of any particular cardiac arrest.

Warning arrhythmia For some years it was considered that the onset of ventricular fibrillation might be predicted by the appearance of premonitory ventricular ectopic activity (Fig. 7). Frequent ventricular premature beats, particularly if repetitive, i.e. occurring in groups of two or three, together with those of multiform or R on T appearance were considered reliable warning of ventricular fibrillation. The importance of this belief lay in the existence of anti-arrhythmic drugs known to suppress such ectopic activity and therefore, by implication, to be capable of preventing the development of ventricular fibrillation. Several studies have now

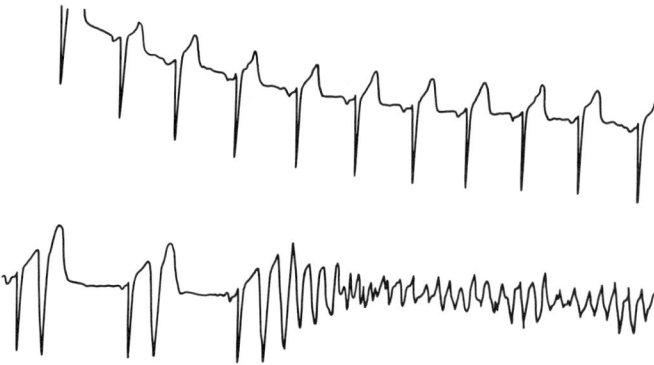

Fig. 7 The upper and lower rhythm traces are a continuous recording of the heart rhythm immediately before the onset of ventricular fibrillation. The lower trace shows ventricular premature beats interrupting the T wave of the preceding sinus beats – R on T appearance – the third ectopic beat appears to provoke ventricular fibrillation.

shown that ventricular fibrillation often develops in the absence of premonitory arrhythmias; furthermore, such warning arrhythmias are seen just as frequently among patients who do not subsequently develop ventricular fibrillation. Thus, both false positive and false negative results abound, so that the concept of warning arrhythmias is largely discredited.

Resuscitation

A natural advantage of the Coronary Care Unit (CCU) is the constant availablity of nursing staff skilled in resuscitation. At the onset of ventricular fibrillation (VF) the optimum management is to remove the patient's pillows so that he or she is supine and to attempt immediate defibrillation. With correct application of electrodes, properly prepared with electrode jelly or pads, a discharge of 100–200 J will restore normal rhythm in the majority of patients.

When there is delay in defibrillation effective cardiorespiratory support is required. The patient must be supported in a supine position on a firm base. The neck is extended and an effective airway secured preferably by endotracheal tube, or at least with an airway and an Ambubag. At the same time external cardiac massage is started. The resuscitator should kneel beside the patient, placing the heel of the left hand on the lower third of the sternum with the right hand on top of the left. Massage can be achieved by the operator rocking backwards and forwards using thigh and pelvic muscles, which is less tiring than an arm action alone. The hands must not slide laterally or inferiorly, which may cause damage to ribs or xiphisternum. The sternum should be depressed 2–3 cm. Effective massage results in a palpable carotid or femoral pulse, previously dialted pupils should return to normal size.

When there has been a delay of more than a few seconds in either detecting or treating cardiac arrest, intravenous sodium bicarbonate is required to correct acidosis and facilitate defibrillation. Sodium bicarbonate 50 mmol i.v. (50 ml of 8.4 per cent solution) is the standard dose which may need to be repeated if the resuscitation procedure is prolonged but repeat injections introduce the problem of a sodium overload for an already damaged myocardium.

Delay in starting effective resuscitation may result in the appearance of a fine ventricular fibrillation on the oscilloscope or even asystole. Fine VF may be coarsened by the use of intravenous adrenalin 0.5 mg, i.e. 0.5 ml of a 1:1000 solution. Adrenalin should not be administered via the bicarbonate infusion. Asystole will sometimes convert to VF with cardiac massage particularly if adrenalin is also given. Atropine 0.6 mg or calcium gluconate (10 ml of 10 per cent solution) may also be used in this situation. VF which gradually deteriorates into asystole in spite of repeated attempts at resuscitation is a desperate situation in which there is

little hope. Cardiac pacing is rarely, if ever, of value in this situation.

Anti-arrhythmic drugs

Attempts to prevent ventricular fibrillation by means of anti-arrhythmic drug therapy have been less successful than is sometimes assumed. Lignocaine has been most comprehensively studied in this context. There is no doubt that lignocaine is effective in suppressing ventricular premature beats but, as already argued, this cannot be accepted as of therapeutic value unless the ectopic activity is so frequent as to be of haemodynamic significance. In the absence of any effective warning of impending ventricular fibrillation any anti-arrhythmic drug would have to be administered routinely to all patients. In one study, 112 patients with acute myocardial infarction were treated with an initial intravenous dose of lignocaine 100 mg followed by continuous infusion of 3 mg/min for 48 hours; no episodes of ventricular fibrillation were encountered. Among a control group of patients receiving no lignocaine, 9 of 111 patients suffered this arrhythmia, but only one succumbed. Although patients were carefully selected to exclude those with evidence of cardiac failure, 15 per cent of the treated group developed troublesome side-effects (mostly paraesthesiae or giddiness and other neurological symptoms) sufficiently severe to require reduction of the infusion rate. The metabolism of lignocaine is critically dependent upon hepatic blood flow and has been shown to be compromised by the presence of cardiac failure complicating infarction. Under these circumstances dangerously high blood levels may be achieved with modest infusion rates. Even in the absence of heart failure steady-state blood levels similar to those recorded among normal subjects are rarely achieved and there is always the danger of lignocaine toxicity when conventional therapeutic dosages are used. Clearance of lignocaine from the circulation under these circumstances is slow so that toxicity is not quickly corrected by discontinuing infusion.

At the present time lignocaine cannot be recommended for administration to all patients with myocardial infarction, particularly when they are treated in well-organized Coronary Care Units. The situation changes somewhat when patients are managed in general medical wards where the level of observation and resuscitative skills may be of a lower order. Even so, in the author's view, there is as yet no anti-arrhythmic prophylaxis regimen of proven value suitable for routine use.

Recurrent ventricular fibrillation

It is in the management of recurrent ventricular fibrillation that the anti-arrhythmic drugs assume greater importance. Intravenous lignocaine is the drug of choice in view of its widespread use and virtual absence of cardiac depressant effects. An infusion should be continued for at least 48 hours of sustained sinus rhythm following multiple episodes of ventricular fibrillation and it is conventional then to prescribe an oral anti-arrhythmic agent, e.g. mexilitine or flecainide. The high incidence of adverse reactions to oral procainamide and the negative inotropic effects and anticholinergic effects of disopyramide make them less suitable for this purpose. Recurrent ventricular fibrillation resistent to therapeutic doses of intravenous lignocaine may often be controlled by amiodarone. Amiodarone has quite different electrophysiological properties to the above-mentioned class I drugs. It prolongs the duration of the action potential and thereby the refractory period, whereas the class I drugs, like lignocaine, procainamide, etc. slow the rate of depolarization with a variable effect on the action potential duration. Although an extremely effective anti-arrhythmic drug and relatively safe in the presence of heart failure when used acutely, there is a high incidence of adverse reactions to long-term administration of amiodarone. A change of therapy to less toxic alternative drugs should therefore be made during the later stages of hospital admission (Table 1).

When ventricular fibrillation occurs repeatedly in spite of appropriate drug therapy, there is a danger that the patient will be

Table 1 Commonly lused anti-arrhythmic drugs in the management of recurrent ventricular tachycardia and fibrillation

Drug	Route	Dose	Effective plasma levels (mg/ml)	Side effects
Lignocaine	i.v.	ID 1 mg/kg infusion 1–3 mg/min	2–5	Circumoral paraesthesiae, giddiness, convulsions, respiratory arrest (most frequent in presence of heart failure)
Procaine amide	i.v.	ID 50 mg/min up to 1 g to control arrhythmia Infusion 2.5 mg/min (oral regime preferred for maintenance)	4–8	Hypotension, flushing, giddiness, heart failure
	Oral	2–4 g/24 h in divided dosage; give every 4 h or use slow release preparation		
Disopyramide	i.v.	ID 2 mg/kg over not less than 5 min–do not give more than 150 mg; infusion 20–30 mg/h	2	Dry mouth, urinary hesitancy and retention, blurred vision, heart failure
	Oral	ID 300 mg Maintenance 400–600/24 h		Note: renal failure or hypokalaemia increase frequency of side effects
Mexiletine	i.v.	ID 25 mg/min up to 100–250 mg Infusion of 250 mg in first hour then 250 mg over second and third hour combined	1–3	Nausea, dizziness, confusion, diplopia, hypotension, myocardial depression
	Continued oral	Infusion 0.5 mg/min ID 600 mg Maintenance 600–800 mg daily		
Amiodarone	i.v.	ID 5 mg/kg over 20–120 min Maximum dose 1.2 g/24 h		Rarely bradycardia/hypotension
	Oral	200–600 mg daily		Corneal deposits, photosensitivity, thyroid dysfunction, neuropathy, pigmentation, pulmonary alveolitis
Flecainide	i.v.	ID 2 mg/kg over 30 min (max 150 mg) then 1.5 mg/kg for 1 h followed by 250 μg/kg/h		Mycardial depression
	Oral	200–400 mg daily		

i.v. = intravenous; ID = initial dose

submitted to increasingly complex multiples of drug combinations in a desperate attempt to prevent further episodes. The negative inotropic effects of these drugs may precipitate cardiac failure and further impair the chances of survival. Overdrive suppression of ventricular tachyarrhythmias is a useful technique on such occasions although not always successful. When episodes of ventricular fibrillation seem to be precipitated by, or are preceded by, bursts of ventricular tachycardia or other complex ventricular ectopic activity, the heart is paced as a rate sufficient to suppress these arrhythmias. Where ventricular fibrillation simply interrupts an otherwise stable sinus rhythm it is the author's practice to pace at around 120 beats/min for at least 24 hours and then slowly to reduce the pacing rate to around 90/min over a period of four to five days. The technique has often been successful in preventing recurrent ventricular fibrillation but has its disadvantages. The price of overdrive pacing is an increased oxygen demand by the injured myocardium, and it might be expected that further chest pain or other evidence of progressive myocardial ischaemia may be provoked. Personal experience suggests that these problems are uncommon.

Ventricular tachycardia
By convention, three or more consecutive ventricular premature beats constitute ventricular tachycardia. In practice two distinct forms of ventricular tachycardia are encountered with very different prognostic significance. Accelerated idioventricular rhythm occurs in around 8 per cent of patients with myocardial infarction and consists of a sequence (usually between 6 and 12 beats) of ventricular premature beats with a rate of between 60 and 120/min (Fig. 8). It often emerges as an escape rhythm during a period of sinus bradycardia and disappears as sinus rate increases. Rarely the heart rate during accelerated idioventricular rhythm may increase sharply, usually doubling, and thereby posing a threat to the patient. In most instances, however, the rhythm appears to be of short duration, benign, and does not require treatment. Ventricular tachycardia with a rate in excess of 150/min tends to occur in

patients with extensive infarction and frequently terminates in ventricular fibrillation. When ventricular tachycardia is sustained, no time should be lost in organizing direct current cardioversion under the influence of a short-acting general anaesthetic. In the few minutes required to set in train these arrangements an injection of intravenous lignocaine 100–120 mg may be made and will quite often convert the arrhythmia to sinus rhythm. Alternatively intravenous diazepam may be slowly administered until the patient is no longer responsive to spoken commands and then cardioversion is undertaken. A prolonged period of inevitable haemodynamic deterioration should not be allowed to pass while ineffectual efforts are made to control the situation with a variety of drug therapies. Even when bouts of ventricular tachycardia are short lived they have a wasteful effect on myocardial oxygen consumption and anti-arrhythmic drug therapy is indicated as with frequent ventricular premature beats (Fig. 9).

Ventricular tachycardia and fibrillation after myocardial infarction occur more frequently among patients with hypokalaemia. In many instances the low serum potassium appears to be an expression of high circulating levels of catecholamines provoked by extensive myocardial injury. It may therefore be that correction of this type of hypokalaemia will fail to reduce the incidence of serious arrhythmias.

The long-term prognosis of patients with ventricular fibrillation depends upon the time at which the arrhythmia occurs with respect to the infarction. Patients resuscitated from ventricular

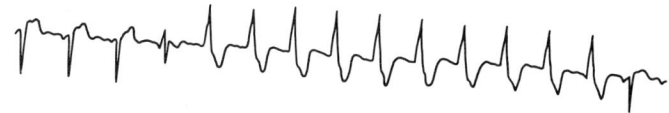

Fig. 8 Accelerated idioventricular rhythm. A 10 beat sequence of this rhythm with a rate of 78 beats/minute interrupts a slightly slower sinus rhythm. The fourth complex is of intermediate appearance between the two QRS shapes and represents a fusion beat.

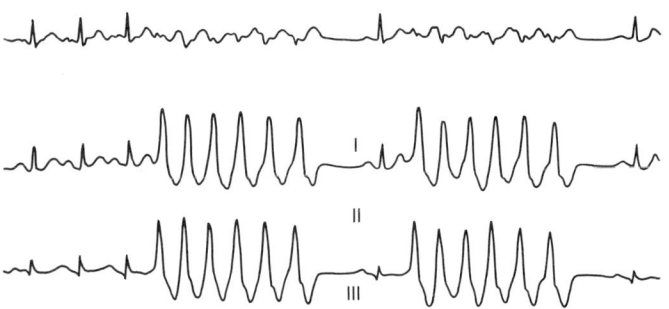

Fig. 9 Short-lived bouts of ventricular tachycardia producing a heart rate of approximately 200/min.

fibrillation within the first four hours of infarction have an excellent long-term prognosis and are usually found to have experienced a relatively minor degree of myocardial injury. Ventricular fibrillation occurring later in the hospital admission is an expression of relatively extensive myocardial damage and carries a less favourable short- and long-term prognosis. It would seem sensible to prescribe an anti-arrhythmic drug free from substantial negative inotropic effects (like flecainide or mexilitine) in such patients for at least six months. There is, however, no firm evidence that such drug regimens actually reduce mortality.

Supraventricular tachycardias

Sinus tachycardia Sinus tachycardia is most commonly an expression of fear or pain in the early stages of infarction; at other times it accompanies left ventricular failure and represents an attempt to maintain adequate cardiac output in the face of a reduced stroke volume. It has been suggested that among patients with anterior infarction a form of sympathetic overdrive may exist, the resulting sinus tachycardia leading to excessive myocardial oxygen consumption, and possibly an extension of myocardial damage. There is some evidence that pharmacological beta-blockade may produce a therapeutic benefit in these circumstances. It must be emphasized, however, that sinus tachycardia is most frequently an essential compensatory response to extensive myocardial damage and that its suppression may be harmful.

Artrial fibrillation This is the commonest atrial tachyarrhythmia encountered among patients with acute myocardial infarction, occurring in approximately 10–15 per cent of all patients admitted to hospital. It is associated with a relatively poor prognosis but this is related to the presence of extensive myocardial damage rather than the haemodynamic consequences of the arrhythmia. Patients suffering atrial fibrillation are relatively elderly and have a higher incidence of radiological changes of left heart failure. Episodes of this arrhythmia are repetitive in more than half the patients involved, which is of importance in clinical management. In a recent Australian study 170 patients from a total of 969 with acute myocardial infarction experienced atrial fibrillation. The mortality at six months was 26 per cent for the whole population studied, those experiencing atrial fibrillation experiencing a significantly higher mortality than those without. The past medical history and localization of infarction bore no relevance to the incidence of the arrhythmia. Ventricular tachyarrhythmias were also commoner among patients with atrial fibrillation but the incidence of cardiogenic shock and atrioventricular block was not. Other workers have reported an association between atrial fibrillation and other atrial arrhythmias, e.g. atrial flutter and paroxysmal atrial tachycardia during the acute stages of infarction.

The management of atrial fibrillation depends mainly upon the resulting ventricular rate. In the majority of patients there is little obvious deterioration in terms of hypotension or dyspnoea and the best policy is to control the ventricular rate by oral digitalis. An initial loading dose of 500 μg of digoxin is advised followed by a further 1 mg in divided dosage over the next 24 hours. Digoxin

will have no immediate effect on ventricular rate which may be slowed by the intravenous administration of either practolol 10–20 mg or verapamil 5–10 mg. These doses may be repeated as required throughout the next 24 to 36 hours. *Verapamil and practolol must not be administered together for fear of producing profound bradycardia or even asystole.*

Among the relatively small number of patients in whom hypotension or dyspnoea follows the onset of atrial fibrillation, cardioversion by direct countershock should be arranged without delay. As with ventricular tachycardia delay will lead to inevitable deterioration in the patient's condition. Occasionally, a patient tolerating atrial fibrillation well initially may subsequently show signs of deterioration. The fear of provoking ventricular fibrillation by direct current cardioversion in the face of previously administered digoxin has been overemphasized. Such patients should not be denied immediate cardioversion. Low energy discharge, 50 J or less, is usually effective and may be less likely to provoke ventricular tachyarrhythmias. I have personally never encountered ventricular fibrillation after such a procedure.

Since atrial fibrillation is frequently repetitive, digitalization should be undertaken among all patients after cardioversion to sinus rhythm.

Bradycardias

Sinus bradycardia Sinus bradycardia is frequently encountered during the first few hours immediately after an inferior myocardial infarction. The bradycardia is usually well tolerated by patients and seldom leads to any complications. There is no justification for increasing the heart rate simply because it falls below the accepted norm. Occasionally, however, bradycardia is associated with hypotension and poor peripheral perfusion of the limbs or, less commonly, the development of frequent ventricular premature beats and short bursts of ventricular tachycardia. The heart rate should then be increased by the use of intravenous atropine. The initial dose should not exceed 300 μg because the administration of atropine occasionally leads to serious tachycardias. If this dose is insufficient to produce a heart rate of between 50 and 60/min, it may safely be repeated during the course of the next 15 min.

Atrioventricular block Approximately 8 per cent of patients admitted to hospital with myocardial infarction develop complete atrioventricular block. Those with inferior infarction usually progress gradually through first degree atrioventricular block (prolonged PR interval) to second degree block of Wenkebach or Mobitz type I variety (Fig. 10). Finally complete atrioventricular block becomes established. The location of block is within the atrioventricular node, therefore the QRS complexes remain nar-

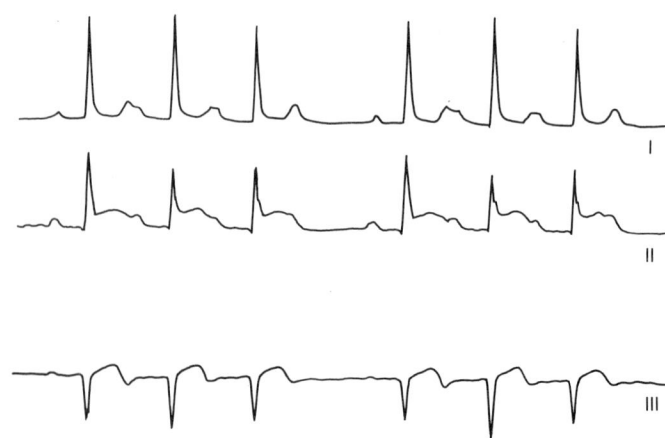

Fig. 10 Patient with an acute inferior myocardial infarction showing Wenckebach phenomenon. There is progressive lengthening of the PR interval until the fourth P wave, which is largely hidden by the previous T wave, is not conducted.

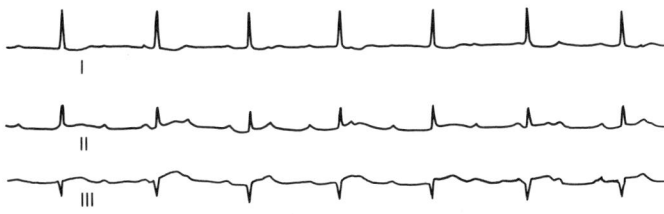

Fig. 11 An ECG from the same patient as shown in Fig. 10 shows development of complete atrioventricular block with a ventricular rate of 43/min.

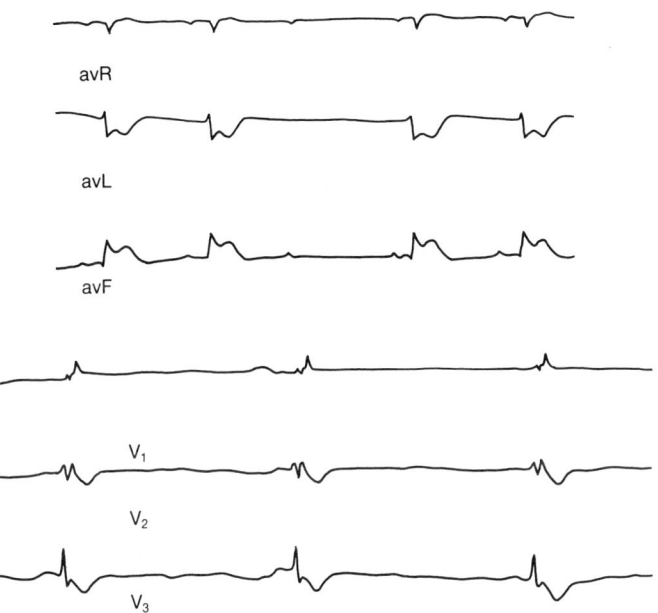

Fig. 12 The upper tracing shows a typical Mobitz type II block; while the same ECG was being recorded complete atrioventricular block developed with a ventricular rate of 22/min. Although this sequence of events is commoner among patients with anterior infarction, in this case the upper trace confirms the presence of an inferior lesion.

row and the escape pacemaker focus distal to the node often results in a ventricular rate of between 45 and 60 beats/min adequate to maintain a satisfactory cardiac output (Fig. 11).

The situation when complete atrioventricular block complicates anterior infarction is very different. The progression through first and second degree block is rarely seen. More often bundle branch block develops, usually right, followed by evidence of bifascicular block, anterior or posterior hemiblock, and finally complete atrioventricular block emerges. Left bundle branch block also represents a form of bifascicular block, i.e. combined anterior and posterior hemiblock, but progresses less frequently to complete atrioventricular block. The prognosis of left bundle branch block is, however, no better than that for other forms of bifascicular block. Occasionally second degree block of the Mobitz type II form is seen before the development of complete block. In Mobitz type II block the QRS complexes are frequently broad and are dropped without preliminary lengthening of the PR interval (Fig. 12). The ventricular rate when complete atrioventricular block complicates anterior infarction is much slower than in the case of inferior infarction, often less than 30 beats/min, and the QRS complexes are broad as a result of the slow intraventricular depolarization. Periods of asystole are common and the profound bradycardia results in severe heart failure as well as the emergence of serious ventricular tachyarrhythmias.

The right coronary artery supplies the atrioventricular node in approximately 85 per cent of people and in a further 5 per cent its

vascular supply arises from a dominant circumflex artery. The clinical picture of inferior myocardial infarction is usually associated with occlusion of one of these two vessels. Patients suffering an inferior infarction may therefore experience disorders of atrioventricular conduction without sustaining extensive myocardial destruction. For an anterior infarction to produce complete atrioventricular block, on the other hand, the amount of myocardium destroyed must be considerable including extensive septal necrosis leading to impairment of conduction through main branches of the His bundle. It is this difference between the extent of myocardial injury which accounts for the remarkably different prognosis between the two clinical situations.

With effective treatment the inpatient mortality among patients with complete atrioventricular block complicating inferior myocardial infarction is around 25 per cent, whereas mortality when the same problem complicates anterior infarction is nearer 50 per cent. Even among survivors the mortality rate over the next six months to one year is extremely high. In all probability this reflects the extent of myocardial injury rather than a recurrence of complete block.

There is no evidence that implantation of a permanent pacemaker reduces long-term mortality among patients with residual bifascicular block after infarction. Indeed problems may be experienced through lack of inhibition of demand pacemakers among patients with extensively damaged ventricular myocardium.

In the case of inferior myocardial infarction it is not always necessary to pace patients with complete atrioventricular block. In those cases where the ventricular rate is adequate, say more than 50/min, and where there is no evidence of heart failure it is safe to observe the patients until normal conduction returns. If the rate should slow further, however, or if signs of left heart failure develop, then pacing should be insititued immediately. In the case of anterior infarction pacing is always required in view of the slow ventricular rate and frequent periods of ventricular standstill. Indeed some physicians advise the insertion of a pacing wire prophylactically with the appearance of right bundle branch block, particularly if this forms part of a bifascicular block pattern, for the subsequent onset of complete block is sudden. The combination of right bundle branch block and posterior hemiblock is particularly likely to proceed to complete atrioventricular block. This is because the posterior fascicle of the left bundle does not share the same vascular supply as the right bundle, whereas the anterior fascicle does. This particular appearance therefore suggests a more widespread vascular occlusion.

Pacing facilities should ideally be available within the Coronary Care Unit, because unnecessary delay while the patient is transferred to another part of the hospital may be fatal. A bipolar pacing electrode is best introduced percutaneously into the subclavian vein from where it is advanced into the right ventricle under fluoroscopic control. The only acceptable location for the tip of the pacing wire is the apex of the ventricle. The proximal leads of the bipolar electrode are connected by a junction box to leads which terminate in a battery powered demand pacing unit. A pacing rate of around 60 to 70 beats/min is usually sufficient. Patients with extensive myocardial injury may deteriorate still further if the damaged ventricles are driven too fast. It is not uncommon to provoke frequent ventricular premature beats or even episodes of ventricular tachycardia or fibrillation while manipulating the electrode wire within the right ventricle. Resuscitation facilities including a defibrillator must always be available. No attempt should be made to suppress ventricular ectopic activity with drug treatment since this will further depress left ventricular contractility.

The subclavian route leaves the patient's arms free for such tasks as washing and feeding but the relatively inexperienced operator may find the approach from a vein situated medially in the antecubital fossa easier to manage. Veins situated in the lateral part of the antecubital fossa drain into the cephalic vein which crosses the clavipectoral fascia on its way to the right atrium. The operator will almost certainly experience difficulty in passing this layer of fascia with the pacing electrode, so laterally situated antecubital veins should be avoided. In those cases where heart block has already developed with periods of ventricular standstill, the presence of other resuscitators performing external cardiac massage and assisted ventilation makes the introduction of the pacing wire by either of the above routes difficult. Under these circumstances puncture of the right femoral vein provides the best approach, allowing the pacing wire to be introduced well away from the area of maximum activity. The wire must be carefully screened up into the right atrium for it frequently enters renal or hepatic veins *en route*. Patients require pacing until normal conduction returns or at least a one-to-one atrioventricular response even though bundle branch block may persist. Very few patients require permanent pacing as a result of persistent complete heart block complicating acute infarction.

Left ventricular dysfunction

With the improved management of cardiac arrhythmias it is the degree of left ventricular dysfunction which often determines the outcome among patients with myocardial infarction and this in turn depends mainly upon the extent of myocardial destruction. The location of myocardial injury is also important. Mitral regurgitation as a result of papillary muscle dysfunction or rupture of the interventricular septum both impose a severe burden upon cardiac function.

Pulmonary oedema

Dyspnoea is the main symptom of left ventricular failure. Clinical examination will reveal the physical signs already discussed earlier, and a chest X-ray demonstrates the extent of pulmonary venous congestion or frank pulmonary oedema.

Treatment should be begun immediately with an intravenously administered diuretic. There is a tendency to overtreat left ventricular failure with excessive amounts of intravenous frusemide or bumetanide which may lead to hypotension as a result of hypovolaemia. Frusemide 40–60 mg intravenously is almost invariably an adequate dose. Diuresis will occur rapidly and there is an accompanying reduction in the severity of dyspnoea long before the radiological appearances of pulmonary oedema disappear. Patients quite often receive excessive diuretics simply because the radiological appearances of left ventricular failure are slow to clear.

Unfortunately the benefits of morphine or diamorphine are sometimes forgotten since the advent of powerful diuretics but they provide the most rapid relief from the distress of dyspnoea. Oxygen is usually administered through a small dead space mask, e.g. MC mask at a flow rate of 4 l/min, thereby providing an inspired oxygen concentration of around 40 per cent.

The place of digitalis in the management of heart failure complicating myocardial infarction remains contentious but many experienced clinicians believe it to be of value even in the absence of atrial fibrillation.

Most patients improve symptomatically on such treatment but some will fail to respond. In this group of patients vasodilator drugs have established a valuable role. The basic principles of vasodilator therapy are dealt with elsewhere (see page 13.105). Ideally haemodynamic monitoring is required for the optimal use of parenteral vasodilator drugs particularly in the presence of severe vasoconstriction when indirect measurement of arterial pressure with a sphygmomanometer is notoriously unreliable. A direct measurement of systemic arterial pressure via an indwelling cannula and an indirect measure of left ventricular filling pressure using a Swan–Ganz balloon catheter in the pulmonary artery provides the optimal conditions for such treatment. Invasive haemodynamic monitoring is not available in many hospitals. There is no need to deny patients in severe pulmonary oedema the benefit of

vasodilator therapy because of imperfect facilities, but the heart rate and arterial pressure must be kept under careful scrutiny.

The drug which has been most extensively studied in the context of severe heart failure complicating myocardial infarction is sodium nitroprusside. Nitroprusside reduces precapillary arteriolar vascular resistance as well as dilating postcapillary capacitance vessels. Among patients with severe left ventricular failure resulting in pulmonary oedema these changes produce an increase in stroke volume, and among hypotensive patients there may be an increase in arterial pressure. Nitroprusside for infusion must be freshly prepared, protected from the light, and administered by an infusion pump, at an initial rate of 10–15 μg/min and the dosage raised by 10 μg increments every 5 or 10 min. The therapeutic effect is most easily studied by measurement of cardiac output by a thermodilution technique, the desired effect being an increase in stroke volume and a fall in left ventricular filling pressure as reflected in the pulmonary arterial wedge pressure.

Systemic hypotension is a potential hazard of vasodilator therapy which is occasionally encountered. It is corrected by stopping the infusion and elevating the patient's legs. Thiocyanate poisoning is only a problem when the infusion is continued for several days when measurement of blood thiocyanate levels are essential. An alternative vasodilator is intravenous isosorbide dinitrate in a dose of 3–12 mg/h.

Cardiogenic shock

When the dominant clinical features of pump failure are systemic hypotension, peripheral vasoconstriction, and oliguria, the term cardiogenic shock is commonly used. The term should be reserved for those patients in whom the clinical picture occurs in the absence of a correctable arrhythmia or unrelieved severe pain. Oliguria and mental confusion are invariably present together with hypoxaemia and a metabolic acidosis. Such patients constitute another form of severe left ventricular dysfunction and also show substantial elevation of left ventricular end-diastolic pressure. Occasionally hypotensive patients are encountered in whom the left ventricular filling pressure is not raised. This situation is nearly always associated with excessive diuretic therapy either during or before the acute illness. Such patients improve when the circulating volume is restored with intravenous fluids.

Although sympathomimetic amines (see page 13.111) have been used to treat cardiogenic shock for several years many experienced clinicians remain sceptical about their value. The problem is that the clinical syndrome is associated with extensive and irreversible myocardial damage so that stimulation of the remaining viable myocardium is short lived and purchased at a cost of rapidly increasing increments of inotropic agent. Even so some patients do experience sustained haemodynamic improvement with inotropic support and maintain their improvement when it is stopped. Such patients presumably reflect those with lesser degrees of myocardial damage but unhappily they have a poor prognosis over the ensuing months.

Dopamine and dobutamine are currently the most widely used sympathomimetic agents in this context. Dopamine at low dosage (2.5 μg/kg/min) results in renal and mesenteric vasodilation mediated through dopaminergic receptors, at higher doses (5–20 μg/kg/min) there is a direct inotropic effect on the myocardium and at higher doses still a pressor effect occurs as a result of alpha adrenergic stimulation of peripheral blood vessels through noradrenalin release. Tachycardia may be a problem which causes excessive myocardial oxygen consumption and the alpha adrenergic effect is also a disadvantage. Dobutamine acts directly on the beta 1 receptors of the heart and is free from any direct or indirect alpha adrenergic effect. Most patients respond to a dose of between 2.5 and 10 μg/kg/min. Dobutamine and dopamine have been used in combination in order to capitalize on the myocardial stimulation of the one and the selective vasodilator of the other drug when both are given in low dosage.

An alternative approach to the problem of cardiogenic shock

has been the introduction of various forms of mechanical assistance for the cirulation. Balloon counter-pulsation has gained widest acceptance. A catheter-mounted balloon is inserted either percutaneously or through a Teflon side-to-end graft into the femoral artery. The catheter is advanced so that the balloon is situated in the distal part of the aortic arch and proximal descending aorta. Inflation and collapse of the balloon is ECG triggered. During ventricular systole the balloon collapses, thereby reducing impedence to left ventricular emptying. In ventricular diastole the balloon inflates thrusting a further 30 ml of blood more peripherally, a feature of considerable functional importance to the coronary circulation which is largely dependent upon diastolic blood flow.

Balloon counter-pulsation appears capable of slightly improving the prognosis among a population of patients with cardiogenic shock. It is difficult to quantify the improvement but perhaps in a population with an expected one month mortality of between 85 and 90 per cent the figure will be reduced to around 70 per cent. The long-term prognosis for such patients, however, remains poor. The technique would appear to be particularly valuable in maintaining life for a week or so in order to permit repair of potentially correctable lesion such as ruptured ventricular septum. The early hope that a fair proportion of patients sustained by counter-pulsation would be found to be suitable for emergency myocardial revascularization has not been realized.

In summary, the treatment of cardiogenic shock remains disappointing as is to be expected in view of its known association with extensive myocardial injury.

Rupture of the interventricular septum

This complication occurs in approximately 0.5 per cent of patients admitted to hospital with acute myocardial infarction. It occurs most commonly between the fourth and sixth day and is usually accompanied by a sudden haemodynamic deterioration. Typically a long systolic murmur is audible over the praecordium, loudest at the lower left sternal edge and frequently accompanied by a palpable thrill. The septum depends mainly upon the anterior descending branch of the left coronary artery for its blood supply. Septal rupture would therefore be expected to complicate anteroseptal infarction most commonly. In fact that incidence of septal rupture is very nearly as high among patients with inferior infarction. This may reflect dependence upon collateral vessels from the posterior descending artery in the presence of severe disease of the anterior descending vessel.

Many cases of ventricular septal rupture escape detection, the patient simply dying in intractable cardiogenic shock or failure. Some patients certainly survive without surgical intervention, one 70-year-old patient of the author's declined surgery after investigations had revealed a definite rupture of the interventricular septum. He remained in reasonably good health for a year and then died following the rapid development of intractable heart failure. Most patients, however, die unless surgical repair can be achieved. The myocardium is easier to handle and repair several weeks after the infarction but patients can seldom sustain an adequate cardiac output to survive this long and intervention must usually be earlier. Recent experience suggests that early repair at around two weeks after infarction results in an acceptable survival rate provided that shock was not present before the onset of septal rupture. Where rupture follows the onset of cardiogenic shock, survival from surgery is rarely if ever achieved and such patients are probably best not submitted to operation.

Mitral regurgitation due to papillary muscle injury

It is difficult to assess the frequency of this complication because it presents a wide spectrum of severity. At one extreme papillary muscle rupture results in a flail mitral valve producing gross pulmonary oedema; alternatively the degree of mitral regurgitation can be trivial as a result of papillary muscle ischaemia and is accompanied by a good long-term prognosis. The posterior papill-ary muscle which derives its blood supply from the posterior descending coronary artery is the more frequently involved. The patient has usually suffered an inferior myocardial infarction. Complete rupture of a papillary muscle is fortunately rare.

The murmur of mitral regurgitation due to papillary muscle injury is very similar in character and distribution to that which accompanies rupture of the ventricular septum. The definitive diagnosis can only be made with certainty by cardiac catheterization. This can be achieved at the bedside without transferring the patient to a catheterization laboratory. A Swan–Ganz balloon catheter can be introduced in the Coronary Care Unit; intravascular pressure and oxygen saturation may then be measured in the pulmonary artery, right ventricle, and right atrium. In rupture of the ventricular septum a clear step-up in oxygen saturation between the right atrium and right ventricle is detected. In the presence of papillary muscle dysfunction and severe mitral regurgitation there will be a prominent 'v' wave recorded in the pulmonary arterial wedge pressure.

Clinical management depends upon the severity of the mitral regurgitation. In patients with a flail mitral valve, surgery presents the only hope of survival. The acute stages of heart failure may be managed by a combination of drug treatment and mechanical assistance using balloon counter-pulsation. This may enable the patient to survive for a sufficient period of time for surgical repair or replacement of the mitral valve to be achieved. Lesser degrees of mitral regurgitation may be managed with drug therapy alone.

The signs of mitral regurgitation may disappear during the convalescent period. In such patients it is likely that improved mechanical performance of left ventricle myocardium occurs compensating for relatively minor ischaemic damage to the papillary muscle.

Cardiac rupture

This condition is substantially commoner than rupture of the ventricular septum and accounts for approximately 10 per cent of all deaths from myocardial infarction in hospital. The free wall of the left ventricle is the usual site of rupture. The underlying pathological process is a dissecting haematoma which pursues a circuitous route through necrotic myocardium to the epicardial surface.

Patients dying from left ventricular rupture are usually men of at least 50–60 years of age who have suffered a transmural infarction. Rupture is relatively rare in the presence of congestive cardiac failure but there appears to be an increased incidence among patients who are hypertensive in the acute phase of infarction. Anticoagulation therapy has been blamed for rupture in the past but this view is no longer held.

Rupture usually occurs within aproximately five to seven days of infarction but may happen as late as three weeks. The patient is usually making an apparent recovery from an extensive infarction at the time. The typical clinical picture is that of chest pain quickly followed by electromechanical dissociation. The heart rhythm as displayed by the ECG monitor shows no change but there is immediate evidence of low cardiac output, often pulses are impalpable within a few seconds of the event. Typical signs of cardiac tamponade may appear but the progression to an undetectable cardiac output is rapid. The ECG then shows agonal slowing of the heart often with disorders of atrioventricular and intraventricular conduction.

In patients in whom the clinical course has been relatively slow, pericardiocentesis followed by successful surgical repair has been recorded. Such an approach is unlikely to be possible in most patients because of the rapid rate of haemodynamic deterioration encountered and the practical difficulties involved in bringing the patient to an appropriate cardiac surgical service.

Systemic embolism The incidence of systemic embolism is difficult to gauge but may be in the region of 2–3 per cent among patients admitted with myocardial infarction. It is usually encountered among patients with full thickness infarcts, the embolus arising from endocardial thrombus which is most frequently located at the apex of the left ventricle. At autopsy the commonest site of major embolism is the cerebral circulation.

Early studies of oral coumarin anticoagulants in myocardial infarction suggested a reduction in the incidence of arterial embolism. For this reason some clinicians continue to use warfarin during the acute phase of infarction but they are in a minority in the United Kingdom.

Pulmonary embolism The current practice of early mobilization has probably reduced the incidence of pulmonary embolus during the last two decades. There is evidence from isotope-labelled fibrinogen studies that thrombus formation in the calf muscles begins on the first day of hospital admission in between one-third to one-half of all patients. The incidence of clinically significant venous thrombosis is of course much less, only thrombus which spreads centrally appears to be associated with embolism. To counter this process heparin would need to be administered from the first few hours of admission. There is interest in the beneficial role of low-dose heparin in the prevention of pulmonary embolism but the majority of physicians appear to restrict the use of anticoagulants to patients experiencing a prolonged period of immobility. Under these circumstances full-dose intravenous heparin therapy is required followed by oral coumarin anticoagulants.

Dressler's syndrome Pericarditis often accompanied by pleurisy and pneumonitis occasionally occurs within one to six weeks of myocardial infarction. When the clinical picture occurs early, it is sometimes difficult to differentiate from the pericarditis directly related to a full thickness infarction.

The pain and fever of Dressler's syndrome frequently settle with aspirin or other non-steroidal anti-inflammaroty drugs but occasionally a short course of oral steroids is required.

Restriction of infarct size

The majority of patients dying in hospital from myocardial infarction do so in pump failure, i.e. intractable left ventricular failure or cardiogenic shock. Both clinical syndromes are associated with the presence of extensive myocardial damage at autopsy. Treatment of pump failure is disappointing and so interest has naturally moved towards the prevention of myocardial necrosis or, expressed another way, the preservation of ischaemic but potentially viable myocardium. The possibility that therapeutic intervention might be of value depends upon two premises. First, it is assumed that following coronary artery occlusion there exists a zone of ischaemic but potentially viable myocardium between the inevitably necrotic muscle, which derived all its blood supply from the occluded vessel, and surrounding tissue which has a totally independent blood supply. Secondly, myocardium must be capable of surviving ischaemia for a sufficient period of time to render intervention feasible and of recovering effective form and function. Experimental studies, involving dog preparations, support the existence of both preconditions. A period of approximately four hours has been shown to exist before irrepairable damage results from ischaemia. Such studies have, however, been undertaken mostly on animals with healthy coronary arteries and a previously non-ischaemic myocardium so that extrapolation of any results to the clinical situation must be made with the utmost caution.

A variety of therapeutic manoeuvres have been demonstrated in animal studies to reduce the final extent of myocardium infarcted. The interventions can be broadly classified into three groups: those calculated to reduce myocardial oxygen demand in order to compensate for impaired blood flow, those which attempt to adjust substrate utilization to the ischaemic state, and finally attempts to improve substrate and oxygen delivery to the marginal ischaemic zone.

Beta-adrenoceptor blocking drugs have been used to reduce myocardial oxygen demand in the management of angina pectoris for several years and are an obvious choice to fulfil the same role

after acute infarctions. Several clinical studies have, however, suggested that beta-blockers given in the acute stage of infarction do not influence survival in the short term. Such observations, are, however, open to the criticism that on many occasions the drugs were not given within the apparently critical three- to six-hour period after coronary artery occlusion when reversal of ischaemic change remains a possibility. It is also possible that death within the short term may be the wrong index by which to judge the results of such an intervention. The quality of long-term survival and the prevalance of such complications as heart failure and the need for diuretics may be more sensitive indices of benefit.

One major study in this field involved the use of intravenous atenolol (5 mg given over 5 min) followed by oral atenolol (100 mg daily) for 10 days. The large population studied were patients admitted within 12 hours of suspected infarction who were not already receiving beta-blockers. Approximately 20–30 per cent were considered suitable for randomization to atenolol or placebo therapy. Among patients in whom the admission ECG had confirmed the presence of infarction, atenolol treated patients had lower MB–CPK release and less R wave loss on the electrocardiogram. Among patients with threatened infarction on admission fewer atenolol than placebo treated patients proceeded to infarction. Although a modest reduction of mortality at 10 days reached statistical significance, the study was conducted on relatively low-risk patients as indicated by the control inpatient mortality of 7 per cent so that this effect was less impressive than the reduction in infarct size. It must be emphasized to those who decide to use acute beta-blockade in myocardial infarction, that the patients in this and similar studies were highly selected in order to exclude all those for whom beta-blockade was likely to be hazardous, e.g. patients who were hypotensive, in heart failure, or with impaired atrioventricular conduction or other forms of bradycardia.

Glucose is theoretically a more appropriate substrate for the ischaemic and therefore hypoxic myocardium than free fatty acids which may indeed exert a toxic effect. The catecholamine release associated with infarction results in antagonism of insulin action and an increase in lipolysis of neutral fat stores. These effects are compounded by the fasting state which accompanies acute illness, resulting in higher circulating levels of free fatty acid which therefore becomes the major substrate for the myocardium. Attempts to improve matters by administering glucose and insulin in association with potassium, to offset the hypokalaemic effects of the combination, have not been successful. Here again, however, most of the studies were undertaken before the critical effects of time on myocardial survival were fully appreciated and long-term follow-up largely neglected.

Routine oxygen therapy has also been shown to result in a reduction of infarct size in an experimental dog preparation but in a study among men with uncomplicated infarction no benefits were demonstrated.

Hyaluronidase has been demonstrated experimentally to increase myocardial survival, presumably through improved diffusion of substrates and metabolites in ischaemic myocardium. Recently, completed controlled trials of both hyaluronidase and one of its purified component enzymes hyaglosidase from the United States and Great Britain have however failed to reveal any significant benefit to patients even when the drugs are administered within a few hours of the onset of myocardial infarction.

Home or hospital?

Reliable and safe resuscitation from ventricular fibrillation dates back to the introduction of direct current defibrillation in the early 1960s. The concept of Coronary Care Units to provide an appropriate level of observation and immediate resuscitation followed naturally. There developed an understandable enthusiasm for the intensive care approach to the problem. It was anticipated that effective treatment would emerge for other major complications of infarction including the pump failure syndrome, and it was

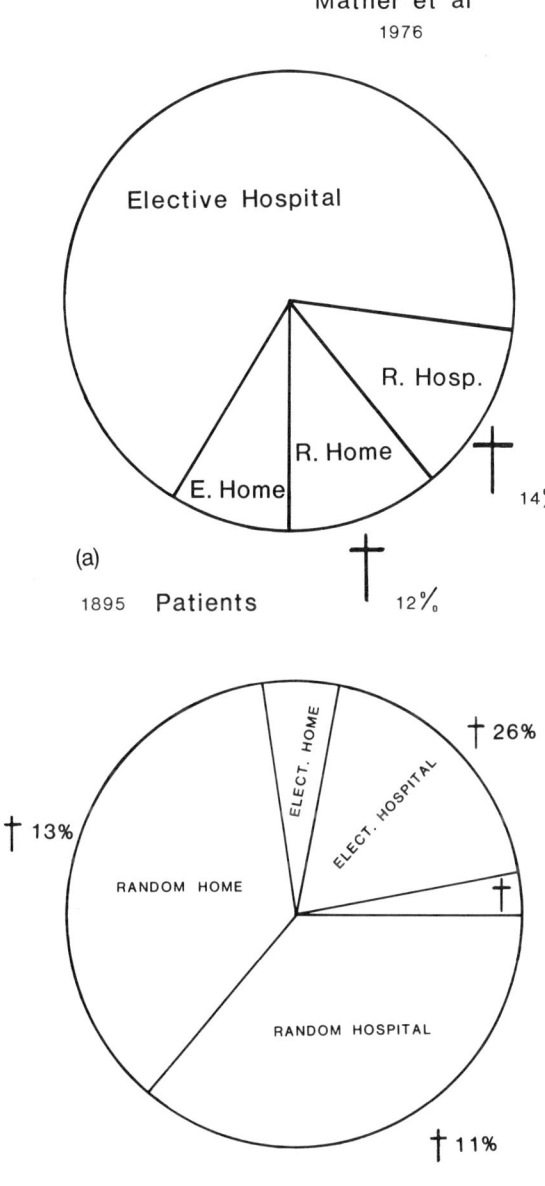

Mather et al
1976

Elective Hospital

R. Hosp.

R. Home

E. Home

14%

(a)

1895　Patients　12%

ELECT. HOME

ELECT. HOSPITAL

26%

13%

RANDOM HOME

RANDOM HOSPITAL

11%

(b)　　363 PATIENTS - OVERALL 6 WEEK MORTALITY 19%

Fig. 13 (a) The West of England study demonstrated that certain patients fared equally well at home as in hospital. Note the relatively small proportion of patients randomized and the low one-month mortality rates. (b) The Nottingham study randomized a greater proportion of patients. The results suggest that low mortality groups can be identified and managed at home, and high risk patients were also identifiable and were admitted to hospital (Hill *et al.*, 1979).

generally assumed that all patients should be admitted to hospital. The first doubts were cast on this philosophy by studies undertaken in the west of England. Approximately 2000 patients with myocardial infarction were assessed at home by their general practitioners and a subgroup randomized to either home or hospital care. No difference could be detected in survival between the two groups. The study was criticized on the grounds that less than a quarter of all patients were randomized and that the more seriously ill had already been admitted to hospital (Fig. 13a). The one-month mortality among randomized patients was in the region of 12 per cent, which in a condition having a mortality closer to 40 or even 50 per cent emphasizes the highly selected nature of the patients studied. In spite of this valid criticism it does

appear that an experienced doctor can identify patients for whom hospital admission offers no advantage over home care. These are patients no longer in pain in whom no rhythm abnormalities or heart failure can be detected. The majority of such patients will be seen several hours after the onset of infarction. In such circumstances home care is probably preferable and certainly cheaper as far as the community is concerned. Supportive evidence for this view has been gathered from studies both in Nottingham (Fig. 13b) and Teeside within the United Kingdom. Many clinicians would, however, argue that these results are only obtained because we are failing to tackle the basic problem of a high mortality within the first few minutes or hours of infarction.

Intensive care provides the ability to correct ventricular fibrillation which is most beneficial during the very earliest stage of the acute illness. It is inevitable, therefore, that studies which are undertaken among patients relatively late in the acute stages of myocardial infarction will demonstrate no benefits from the availability of resuscitative facilities. The problem of delay before patients come under effective medical care was well demonstrated in the Teeside study in which, although 50 per cent of survivors were seen within one hour of the onset of symptoms, only 57 per cent of all patients suffering heart attacks survived long enough to be seen by a doctor. Is it then possible to organize medical care in a way which will reduce significantly the incidence of sudden death? The mobile Coronary Care Unit pioneered in Belfast and adopted with enthusiasm in the USA is one approach. When combined with a programme of public education about the significance of chest pain and the practice of cardiopulmonary resuscitation, the results of prehospital resuscitation are impressive.

The controversy will continue but all studies must be evaluated in the light of what we know of the natural history of myocardial infarction. It seems clear that any impact on the mortality of this condition will depend upon medical assistance, including full resuscitative facilties, reaching the patient early, and this means an increased awareness by patients of the symptoms associated with myocardial infarction. Any studies which assess medical management late in the natural history of the condition are dealing with a highly selected group of patients with a low overall mortality. Such studies are not particularly helpful and tend to avoid the central problem of sudden death and its prevention.

A separate debate exists concerning the justification for CCUs within a hospital service beset by financial difficulties. The question is often asked: 'Could we manage patients equally well in general medical wards?' Many of the studies suggesting an improvement in patient survival as a result of CCU organizations were based on comparisons with earlier inpatient experience, often before effective resuscitation was available. Also the presence of the CCU might well have influenced the admission policy of many general practitioners who might otherwise have kept relatively good risk patients at home. There are no totally satisfactory trials of CCU versus general medical ward care. In one study it was noticeable, however, that resuscitation was attempted less frequently among older patients in a general medical ward than in the CCU. It would be difficult to design an appropriate study now because the CCU is a good training area for resuscitation techniques and therefore the general level of resuscitation is likely to be higher throughout any hospital which possesses a CCU. It follows that any such study would need to compare CCU results with general medical ward care in a hospital with no CCU.

No matter what views are held on the home versus hospital debate there is no doubt that patients will continue to be admitted to hospital if only because they collapse in the city centre or in their place of work. In view of the fact that our principle achievement is defibrillation, and to a lesser extent the management of other arrhythmias, both of which depend for a successful outcome on immediate action it is difficult to believe that the appropriate level of observation and immediate care can be achieved in a general medical ward. The last decade has seen a reduction in the number of nurses and doctors within the hospital during non-office hour periods and this is a further reason for placing high-risk patients within a single area. It is the author's view that in spite of the many limitations of coronary care the CCU retains an important place within the organization of a general hospital.

References

Adgey, A. A. J. (1980). Coronary patient – early treatment? *Br. Heart J.* **44**, 357–360.

Bates, R. J. (1977). Cardiac rupture – challenge in diagnosis and management. *Am. J. Cardiol.* **40**, 429–437.

Campbell, R. W. F. (1980). Placebo controlled study of prophylaxis of ventricular arrhythmias in acute myocardal infarction. *Am. Heart J.* **100**, 995–999.

Chapman, B. L. and Gray, C. H. (1973). Prognostic index for myocardial infarction treated in a coronary care unit. *Br. Heart J.* **35**, 135–141.

Colling, A., Dellipiani, A. W., Donaldson, R. J. and MacCormack, P. (1976). Teeside coronary survey; an epidemiological study of acute attacks of myocardial infarction. *Br. med. J.* **ii**, 1169–1172.

Forfar, J. C., Irving, J. B., Miller, H. C., Kitchen, A. H. and Wheatley, D. J. (1980). The management of ventricular septal rupture following myocardial infarction. *Q. J. Med.* **49**, 205–217.

Fox, A. C., Glassman, E. and Wayne Isom, O. (1978–9). Surgically remediable complication of myocardial infarction. *Prog. cardiovas. Dis.* **21**, 461–484.

Fulton, M., Julian, D. G. and Oliver, M. F. (1969). Sudden death and myocardial infarction. *Circulation* **39**, IV, 182–191.

Gazes, P. C. and Gaddy, J. E. (1979). Bedside management of acute myocardial infarction. *Am. Heart J.* **97**, 782–796.

Hill, J. D., Hampton, J. R. and Mitchel, J. R. A. (1979). Home or hospital for myocardial infarction – who cares? *Am. Heart J.* **98**, 545–547.

Kerr, F. and Donald, K. W. (1974). Analgesia in myocardial infarction. *Br. Heart J.* **36**, 117–121.

Kinlen, L. J. (1973). Incidence and presentation of myocardial infarction in an English community. *Br. Heart J.* **35**, 616–622.

Kuhn, L. A. (1978). Management of shock following acut myocardial infarction. Drug therapy. *Am. Heart J.* **95**, 529–534.

—— (1978). Management of shock following acute myocardial infarction. Mechanical assistance. *Am. Heart J.* **95** 789–795.

Lau, Y. K., Smith, J., Morrison S. L. and Chamberlain, D. A. (1980). Policy for early discharge after acute myocardial infartion. *Br. med. J.* **i**, 1489–1492.

Lie, K. I., Wellens, H. J. J., Downar, E. and Durrer, D. (1975). Observations on patients with primary ventricular fibrillation complicating acute myocardial infarction. *Circulation* **52**, 755–759.

——, ——, Von Capelle, F. J. and Durrer, D. (1974). Lidocaine in the prevention of primary ventricular fibrillation. *N. Engl. J. Med.* **291**, 1324–1326.

Nellen, M., Maurer, B., and Goodwin, J. F. (1973). Value of physical examination in acute myocardial infarction. *Br. Heart J.* **35**, 777–780.

Norris, R. M., Caughey, D. E., Mercer, C. J. and Scott, P. J. (1974). Prognosis after myocardial infarction – six year follow-up. *Br. Heart J.* **36**, 786–790.

Opie, L. H. (1980). Myocardial infarct size. Basic considerations. *Am. Heart J.* **100**, 355–372.

—— (1980). Myocardial infarct size. Comparision of anti-infarct effects of beta blockade, glucose-insulin-potassium, nitrates and hyaluronidase. *Am. Heart J.* **100**, 531–552.

Pantridge, J. F., Adgey, A. A. J., Geddes, J. S. and Webb, S. W. (1975). Dysrrhythmias and autonomatic disturbance in the acute phase of myocardial infarction. In *The acute coronary attack*. Pitman Medical, London.

Pentecost, B. L., De Giovanni, J. V., Lamb, P., Cadigan, P. J., Evemy, K. L. and Flint, E. J. (1981). Reappraisal of lignocaine in management of myocardial infarction. *Br. Heart J.* **45**, 42–47.

Pocock, S. J., Shaper, A. G., Cook, D. G., Packham, R. F., Lacey, R. F., Powell, P. and Russell, P. F. (1980). British Regional Heart Study: geographic variations in cardiovascular mortality, and the rate of water quality. *Br. med. J.* **i**, 1243–1249.

Verstraete, M. (1985). Intravenous administration of a thrombolytic agent is the only realistic therapeutic approach in evolving myocardial infarction. *Eur. Heart J.* **i**, 1243–1249.

Wellens, H. J. J., Bar, F. W., Gorgel, A. P. and Muncharaz, J. F. (1979). Electrical management of early disease with emphasis on the tachycardias. *Am. J. Cardiol.* **41**, 1025–1034.

Yusuf, S., Ramsdale, D., Sleight, P., Rossi, P., Peto, R., Pearson, M., Sterry, H., Furse, L., Motwani, R., Parish, S., Gray, R., Bennett, D. and Bray, C. (1984). Early intravenous atenolol in suspected acute myocardial infarction: Final report of a randomised clinical trial. In *Interventions in the acute phase of myocardial infarction* (eds J. Morganroth and E. Neil Moore), p. 168. Nijhoff Publishing, Amsterdam.

PERIPHERAL ARTERIAL DISEASE

P. J. MORRIS

The increase in the size of the elderly population in developed countries during this century, together with the explosion in cigarette smoking and possibly dietary changes, have led to increased numbers of patients presenting with clinical manifestations of peripheral arterial disease. Coincident with the growth of degenerative arterial disease has been the rapid expansion of arterial surgery as a speciality and in particular of the techniques of reconstructive surgery. Most arterial disease is due to atheromatous degeneration of the arterial wall, and this forms the bulk of the work of peripheral vascular clinics. Embolism, trauma, and vasospastic disorders are important if less common problems. Extracerebral arterial disease and renovascular causes (see page 13.383) of hypertension are discussed elsewhere and will not be dealt with further.

Atherosclerosis

Atherosclerosis is a generalized degenerative disease and is found in all major arteries beyond middle age, and indeed if the fatty streak represents the first stage, then it is widespread even in childhood. The fatty streak is a reversible lesion, which may go on to the next stage of atherosclerosis, the fibrous plaque, which is rarely seen in children, and is unusual before the fourth decade.

Fibrous plaques have a white appearance, are oval in shape, and are covered by endothelium. They are usually seen first in the lower aorta. Some become complicated, with calcification, ulceration, and thrombus formation on the ulcerated surface. It is this complicated lesion which is usually associated with clinical problems, for the enlarging plaques may gradually obstruct the lumen reducing blood flow to a critical level. In contrast to this narrowing of the lumen, destruction of the media by the atheromatous process may lead to dilation of the affected artery rather than occlusion. Although occlusive arterial disease is often considered a different entity to aneurysmal disease because of the different clinical presentation, they both represent different manifestations of the same process.

The distribution of atherosclerosis is peculiarly consistent in that plaques occur in large arteries with a high pressure, and at the bifurcation of arteries, e.g. carotid bifurcation, aorto-iliac bifurcation, or where there is kinking or external pressure on the artery, e.g. adductor canal. At such points flow is disturbed, and the resulting unstable shear stresses may produce endothelial damage as the first stage in the development of atherosclerosis. Although many other factors must be important, this predilection of the lesions for the origin of branches or bifurcations in major arteries,

Table 1 Risk factors for peripheral arterial disease

Smoking of cigarettes	Obesity
Hypertension	Physical inactivity
Diabetes mellitus	Stress
Hypercholesterolaemia	Family history
Hypertriglyceridaemia	

Table 2 The relative risk of intermittent claudication (IC) associated with some of the risk factors in peripheral arterial disease

Risk factor	Relative risk of IC
Systolic pressure $\geq$ 160 mmHg	3.4
Diastolic pressure $\geq$ 90 mmHg	3.2
Serum triglyceride $\uparrow$	2.0
Smoking $\geq$ 15 cigarettes/day	8.8

Adapted from Hughson et al. (1978).

its greater severity in the systemic arterial circulation in comparison to the pulmonary or venous circulation, and its greater severity in large arteries imply an important role in aetiology for haemodynamic or mechanical factors.

Following endothelial damage, which may also be accentuated in experimental models by hypertension, hypercholesterolaemia, high levels of carbon monoxide (comparable to those seen in heavy smokers), and immune complex disease, the normal non-thrombogenic nature of the vessel wall is lost. This property of the vessel wall is probably maintained by the endogenous production of a prostaglandin, which inhibits platelet aggregation. The reparative process is characterized by platelet deposition and lipid infiltration into the area of the injury. This is followed by smooth muscle proliferation in the subendothelial layer of the wall. Collagen may also be produced by the smooth muscle cells, and so the fibrotic plaque has appeared. Further damage may produce a new cycle of plaque growth. Finally, with continuation of the process, calcification and ulceration of the plaque occurs with further thrombus formation on the ulcerated surface. Although the process begins in the intima and subendothelial layer it gradually extends from within out and eventually may extend even in to the adventitia.

Risk factors in peripheral arterial disease
Many risk factors can be identified in peripheral arterial disease, some certain, others less certain (Table 1). These are identical to those implicated in cardiovascular or cerebrovascular disease, but the risk attached to each may be different. For example, hypertension represents a much greater risk for cerebrovascular disease than for cardiovascular or peripheral arterial disease, while smoking is by far the major risk factor in peripheral arterial disease but possibly of minor importance in cerebrovascular disease. As might be expected there is a multiplicative increase in risk in the presence of more than one risk factor.

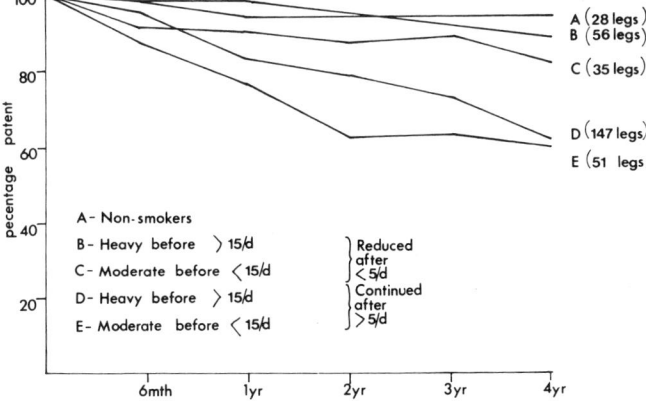

Fig. 1 Accumulative late patency rates for aorto-iliac and femoropopliteal reconstructions based on the pre-operative and post-operative smoking habits. Moderate smokers: 1–15 cigarettes/day; heavy smokers: more than 15 cigarettes/day. After operation smoking was assessed on the basis of smoking less than 5 or more than 5 cigarettes/day. (Reproduced from Myers et al., 1978, Br. J. Surg., with permission on the publishers Butterworth and Co (Publishers)©)

Smoking
This is the major risk factor in peripheral arterial disease (Table 2). Although the mechanism by which it produces atherosclerosis is uncertain it is thought that it is the high level of carbon monoxide (CO) in the form of carboxyhaemaglobin which is responsible for atherosclerosis. Endothelial damage can result from exposure to CO in experimental animals, and prostacyclin production by the endothelium may be depressed, allowing platelet deposition especially in areas at risk for endothelial damage. Of particular relevance to management of patients with peripheral arterial disease are the observations that cessation of smoking will result in less subsequent vascular incidents (e.g. myocardial infarction, stroke, amputation) than occur in those who continue to smoke, and also that the long-term success of arterial reconstruction (as judged by patency rates) is some fourfold greater in patients who give up smoking at the time of surgery than in those who continue to smoke (Fig. 1).

Hypertension
Just as hypertension is an important risk factor in cardiovascular and cerebrovascular disease so it is in the development of peripheral arterial disease. However, once severe occlusive arterial disease is evident, a moderate degree of hypertension may favour increased collateral blood flow around an obstructed artery.

Diabetes mellitus
Patients with diabetes mellitus provide a major part of any vascular clinic's work. Although predominantly presenting with small arteriolar occlusive disease, they are more likely to have occlusive atherosclerosis of major arteries than the normal population. The development of both forms of arterial disease is related to the quality of glucose control, but genetic factors play a role in the development of the small vessel disease.

Hyperlipidaemia
Although hypercholesterolaemia is associated with a greater risk of ischaemic heart disease, there is no clear evidence of its association with peripheral arterial disease, except in patients with familial hypercholesterolaemia. Similarly hypertriglyceridaemia is not clearly established as a risk factor. However, there is one report in a small number of patients that reduction of a high serum cholesterol or triglyceride by diet did cause a regression of atheromatous plaques demonstrated on consecutive femoral angiograms.

Other factors
A number of other factors may be important in the development of peripheral arterial disease (Table 1) but their putative role as risk factors is based in the main on their known role as risk factors in ischaemic heart disease.

Clinical presentation
Acute ischaemia of a limb
The patient with an acutely ischaemic limb presents clinically with a painful, pale, pulseless limb. Most commonly this is due either to acute thrombosis superimposed on an atheromatous stenosis or plaque, or to lodging of an embolus in a major artery to the limb. It should be stressed that there is no difference on clinical examin-

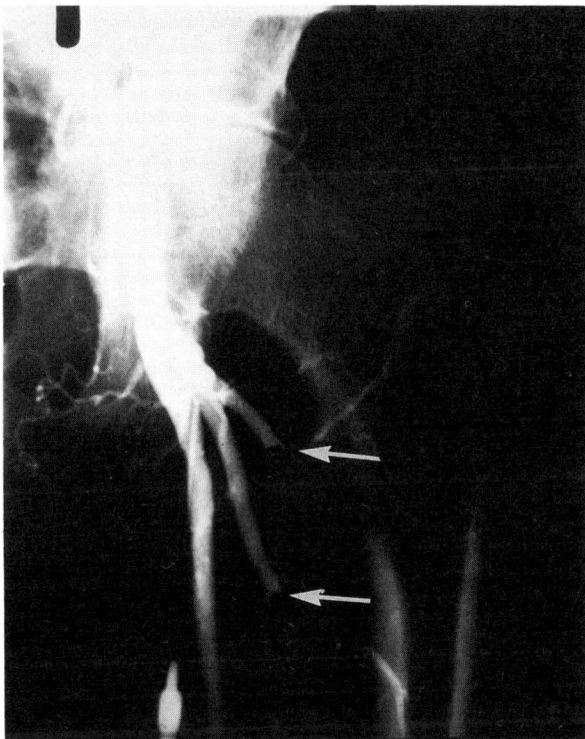

Fig. 2 A femoral angiogram showing the typical appearance of an embolus. On this view two emboli (arrows) are seen in branches of the profunda femoris artery.

ation of the acutely ischaemic limb whatever the cause. A previous history of claudication in the ischaemic limb suggests that it may be due to acute thrombosis, while a history of a previous myocardial infarction, the presence of atrial fibrillation, rheumatic heart disease, or an abdominal aortic aneurysm would favour a diagnosis of embolism. However, only an angiogram will enable an accurate diagnosis of either embolism or thrombosis to be made and the appropriate management instituted (Fig. 2). Arterial trauma, due to road traffic accidents, knife wounds, or gun-shot wounds, are becoming increasingly common, and so too is arterial trauma following the insertion of intra-arterial catheters for diagnosis or therapy. In the presence of ischaemia of a limb following trauma immediate angiography is mandatory. A rare cause of acute ischaemia in the lower limb is phlegmasia cerulea dolens in which massive thrombosis of all the major veins of the limb occurs with gross swelling causing obstruction of the arterial supply.

Chronic ischaemia of a limb

The clinical manifestations of chronic ischaemia range from muscle pain on exercise relieved by rest (intermittent claudication), through rest pain and/or non-healing ulceration, to frank gangrene of the distal part of the limb. Clinical examination will reveal the absence of the appropriate pulses. Although the diagnosis of a severely ischaemic limb is usually quite apparent, that of intermittent claudication may present difficulties. Classically the patient will complain of a cramp-like pain, for example in the calf after walking 100 metres at a constant pace, which disappears within minutes of resting, only to reappear again at the same distance as the patient walks again. Failure of the pain to disappear on resting or its re-appearance at a shorter distance after each rest should draw the attention of the physician to a possible musculoskeletal cause of such symptoms, especially if distal pulses are present on examination. However, it should be remembered that pulses may be present in a limb distal to proximal disease, albeit weaker than the normal side, due to a good collateral flow, but in such cases exercise to the point of claudication will lead to disappearance of the distal pulses. Angiography is performed if reconstructive sur-

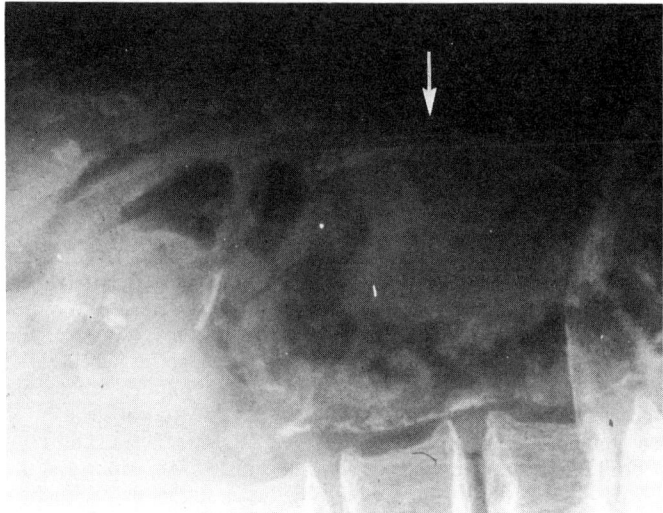

Fig. 3 A lateral plain film of the abdomen in a man found to have a pulsatile mass in his abdomen during an insurance examination, showing a large abdominal aortic aneurysm with calcification in the wall (arrow).

gery is to be considered, but is not used as a diagnostic tool. A variety of conditions may mimic intermittent claudication (and are often grouped together under the heading pseudoclaudication), these including such disorders as spinal stenosis, and arthritis of the knee and hip.

Aneurysms

Abdominal aortic aneurysm This is the commonest aneurysm encountered in clinical practice and may present to the clinician in one of three ways:

1. Ruptured or leaking aneurysm: the patient classically presents with the triad of pain, hypotension, and a pulsatile mass in the abdomen. However, only 50 per cent of patients with a leaking aneurysm will present with all three features. The pain tends to be epigastric radiating through to the back, but may be situated in the loin or even in the testicle. Indeed one of the commonest misdiagnoses is renal colic. A pulsatile mass may be overlooked, especially in the obese patient, if an attempt is not made specifically to feel for a pulsatile mass in a patient with an acute abdomen or shock. In general femoral pulses will be present.

2. Symptomatic or expanding aneurysm: the patient presents with abdominal pain, usually epigastric, or pain in the back of relatively recent onset and is found to have a pulsatile mass on examination. Occasionally the patient may present with ureteric obstruction when a fibrotic inflammatory reaction similar to retroperitoneal fibrosis has occurred around the aneurysm, or an embolus may be shed into the lower limbs causing acute ischaemia.

3. Asymptomatic aneurysm: the patient is found to have a pulsatile mass on examination for some other condition, or a calcified aneurysm is detected on a plain X-ray of the abdomen, again done for some other reason (Fig. 3).

Thoracic aortic aneurysm Although syphilis was the commonest cause of this type of aneurysm, this is no longer the case, the vast majority today being due to atheroma, with a small but significant number resulting from previous trauma. Although the syphilitic aneurysm usually involves the ascending aorta, the atheromatous aneurysm of the thoracic aorta is evenly distributed between the ascending, the arch, and the descending aorta. Most thoracic aorta aneurysms are asymptomatic, and are detected on a chest X-ray performed for some other reason. Very often the first presentation is due to rupture and sudden death. When these aneurysms are symptomatic they are usually large, anterior chest pain being the commonest symptom, but other clinical features due to pressure such as obstruction of the superior vena cava, dysphagia due to

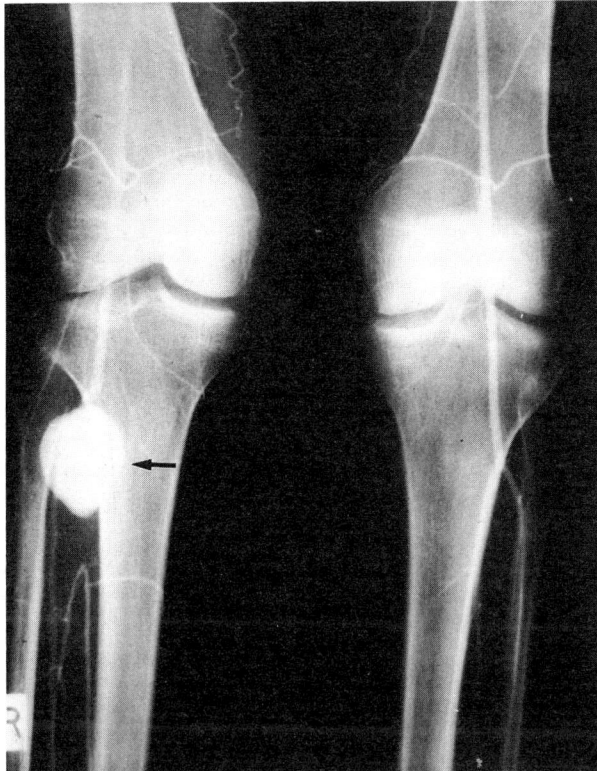

Fig. 4 A mycotic aneurysm (arrow) at the bifurcation of the distal popliteal artery in a young woman with subacute bacterial endocarditis. Other aneurysms were present in the left iliac artery and the right profunda femoris artery.

pressure on the oesophagus, or stridor due to pressure on the trachea, may be present. Aneurysms of the ascending aorta often involve the aortic valve, causing aortic insufficiency, and there may be obstruction of the orifices of the coronary arteries causing myocardial ischaemia.

Dissecting aortic aneurysm The thoracic aorta is the commonest site of dissecting aneurysm, other arteries being involved by extension of the dissection. Dissection is associated with degeneration of the media of the aorta and most patients are hypertensive. In about 50 per cent of cases the dissection starts in the ascending aorta, the next most common site being just distal to the origin of left subclavian artery. The arch of the aorta and the abdominal aorta are uncommon sites of origin. Pain, either substernal or in the upper back, is the most striking presenting feature, often with radiation to the neck or arms. An aortic diastolic murmur or a pericardial friction rub may be heard with a dissection of the ascending aorta, and there may be a significant diminution in the pulse and blood pressure in the right arm. A dissection of the descending thoracic aorta may extend into the abdominal aorta and involve all the major branches of the abdominal aorta, thus being associated with acute renal failure, mesenteric ischaemia, or ischaemia of the lower limbs.

Popliteal aneurysms These are not uncommon and are often associated with aneurysmal disease elsewhere. Although sometimes causing pain due to pressure on surrounding structures, they most commonly present as a pulsatile mass behind the knee or with ischaemia of the distal limb due to thrombosis or embolism.

Other aneurysms Less commonly aneurysms may occur in the iliac, femoral, carotid, splenic, renal, or one of the splanchnic arteries. With the exception of the carotid or femoral artery aneurysm which will usually present as a pulsatile mass, aneurysms elsewhere tend to be asymptomatic until they present as a

major intra-abdominal bleed more often fatal than not. Splenic artery aneurysms are the commonest intra-abdominal aneurysm apart from aortic and iliac artery aneurysms, and are seen more frequently in younger women, in which case there is a marked tendency to rupture during pregnancy. Mycotic aneurysms (better called infected aneurysms) are rare, and usually are seen today as a complication of subacute bacterial endocarditis due to impaction of an infected embolus at a bifurcation or perhaps in the vasa vasorum of the vessel wall (Fig. 4).

Vasospastic disorders
Inappropriate and symptomatic vasoconstriction of the arterioles and arteries of the limbs may be intermittent or persistent. Raynaud's syndrome is the commonest vasospastic disorder. Less common and often not well-defined disorders are acrocyanosis, livedo reticularis, and cold sensitivity following cold injury or trauma.

Raynaud's syndrome Raynaud's syndrome may be defined as intermittent vasospasm of the arterioles of the distal limbs following exposure to cold or emotional stimuli. Classical colour changes are observed, the extremities first becoming pale followed by cyanosis and then redness as the attack passes. This condition may be associated with a variety of underlying disease (Table 3), in which case it is known as Raynaud's phenomenon or secondary Raynaud's syndrome, or on the other hand no underlying condition can be detected, in which case it is known as Raynaud's disease or primary Raynaud's syndrome. True Raynaud's disease occurs mostly in young females, who have intermittent bilateral and symmetrical attacks in the absence of any organic arterial occlusion, and in the absence of severe trophic changes in the fingers or toes. Although upper and lower extremities may be affected, it is most common in the upper limbs.

Patients with Raynaud's phenomenon not only may present with vasospastic features in the hands or feet, but also with other clinical features due to the underlying disease. Trophic changes in the fingers or toes are common. Of all the disorders listed in Table 3, scleroderma is by far the most common. It should be remembered, especially in scleroderma, that the Raynaud's phenomenon may be the presenting clinical feature in many patients, other manifestations of the disease not being evident for several years. Investigations in patients with Raynaud's syndrome will be directed at the possibility of defining an underlying condition, and should include thoracic outlet X-rays, full blood examination, ESR, barium swallow, serum protein electrophoresis, cryoglobulins, cold agglutinins, antinuclear factor, anti-DNA antibody, rheumatoid factor, and perhaps angiography (Fig. 5).

Acrocyanosis This condition virtually only occurs in women and is characterized by cold blue extremities, worse in cold weather but also present in warm weather. The symptoms are not episodic, and all peripheral pulses are present.

Table 3 Underlying disorders which may give rise to Raynaud's phenomenon

1 Collagen diseases
   Scleroderma; lupus erythematosus; rheumatoid arthritis; dermatomyositis
2 Neurogenic lesions
   Thoracic outlet compression; carpal tunnel syndrome; other nervous system diseases
3 Occupational trauma
   Chain saw operators; pneumatic hammer operators; pianists
4 Occlusive arterial disease
   Atherosclerosis; thromboangiitis obliterans; embolism
5 Miscellaneous
   Cryoglobulinaemia; cold agglutinins; macroglobulinaemia; ergot intoxication

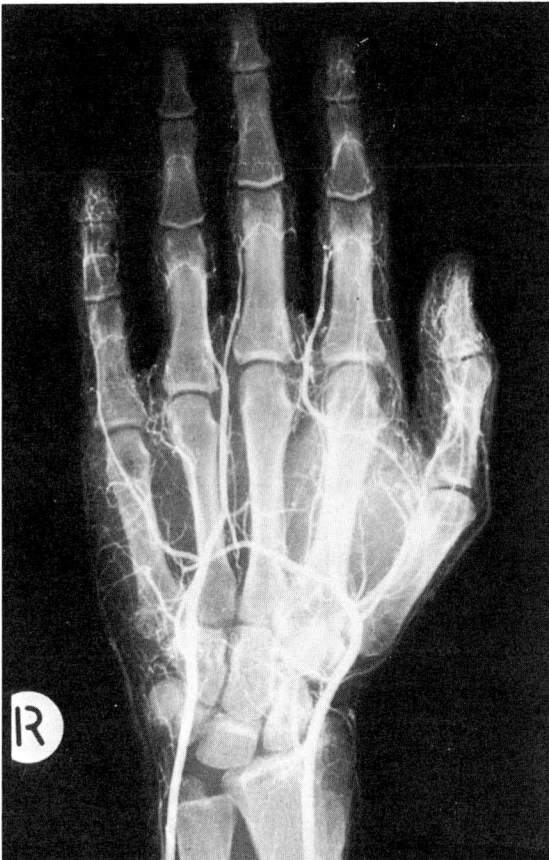

Fig. 5 An arteriogram of the right upper limb in a patient with Raynaud's phenomenon due to scleroderma showing obliteration of most of the digital arteries.

Livedo reticularis This condition is characterized by persistent patchy reddish-blue mottling of the legs (occasionally involving the arms), and tends to be worse in cold weather. It may sometimes be associated with chronic ulceration. It is due to random spasm of cutaneous arterioles, with secondary dilation of capillaries and venules. There may be an underlying vasculitis in some cases.

Cold hypersensitivity following cold exposure or trauma A number of related conditions may be included under this heading, all presumably with a vasospastic aetiology, but following a variety of injuries to the limb or frostbite. Pain is often a prominent feature of the clinical picture, especially when occurring after trauma (when it is usually known as causalgia). The limb is pale and cold, and often shows evidence of disuse atrophy.

Thoracic outlet compression
Compression of any one of the subclavian vein, subclavian artery, or the lower trunk of the brachial plexus, or all three structures, may occur due to a variety of anatomical abnormalities at the thoracic outlet. A cervical rib is perhaps the most easily recognized and so the commonest cause of thoracic outlet compression. But compression of the above structures can occur despite normal anatomy as the structures cross the first rib into the axilla. Patients may present predominantly with neurological symptoms such as pain or paraesthesiae (usually poorly defined rather than with an expected C8-T1 distribution) or vascular symptoms due to either arterial obstruction or venous obstruction. Arterial obstruction may present as a unilateral Raynaud's phenomenon or pallor and pain in the hand when using the arm above the head, or at a later stage with distal emboli to the fingers from a post-stenotic aneurysm. Venous obstruction often presents in the younger person as a spontaneous axillary vein thrombosis (Fig. 6).

Intestinal ischaemia
Acute Generally patients presenting with acute intestinal ischaemia will be elderly, as are most patients with occlusive vascular disease, and will have evidence of generalized atheromatous disease. There may be a possible source of a peripheral arterial embolus, e.g. previous myocardial infarction or atrial fibrillation. However, in addition to arterial thrombosis or embolism, acute intestinal ischaemia may be due to venous thrombosis which is associated with portal hypertension, peritonitis, or a blood dyscrasia. Furthermore, in a significant number of patients with acute intestinal ischaemia, no major arterial or venous obstruction is found at laparatomy or autopsy, the ischaemia being presumed to be due to a low flow state in the bowel wall itself associated with cardiac failure or shock.

The patient presents with an acute abdomen and the features of bowel obstruction, namely colicky abdominal pain, and nausea and vomiting, but associated with tenderness in the early stages, while at a later stage there are all the signs of peritonitis. Diarrhoea is common and is often bloody, especially with acute ischaemia of the large bowel. A peritoneal tap will reveal a serosanguinous aspirate containing leucocytes and at a later stage bacteria. A plain X-ray of the abdomen may show complete absence of gas shadows at an early stage, or fluid levels, sometimes localized to the ischaemic segment of small bowel, while a typical scalloped or finger printing appearance in large bowel may be apparent on barium enema (Fig. 7). However, only an angiogram will confirm an obstruction of a major mesenteric artery with either an embolus or thrombus. Whether this is justified as an investigation of an acute abdomen in patients with possible intestinal ischaemia is debatable. Unless there is obstruction of at least one other major mesenteric artery by atheroma, severe ischaemia of the intestine is unlikely to occur. The mortality associated with acute intestinal ischaemia is high, of the order of 75 per cent, and only early diagnosis offers the patient a chance of survival.

Chronic Patients with chronic intestinal ischaemia present with post-prandial central colicky abdominal pain and weight loss. Usually two of the three main arteries supplying the bowel (coeliac, superior mesenteric, and inferior mesenteric arteries) have to be obstructed for symptoms to result. Angiography with lateral

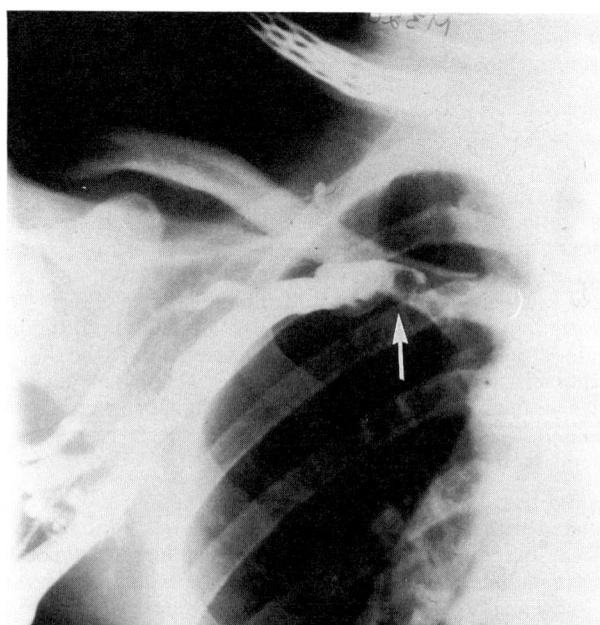

Fig. 6 Axillary venogram in a 25-year-old man with recurrent axillary vein thrombosis and a swollen right arm. Clinical evidence of thoracic outlet compression was evident. At operation the axillary vein was patent but compressed by a fibrous band as it crossed the first rib (arrow). Resection of the first rib relieved the symptoms.

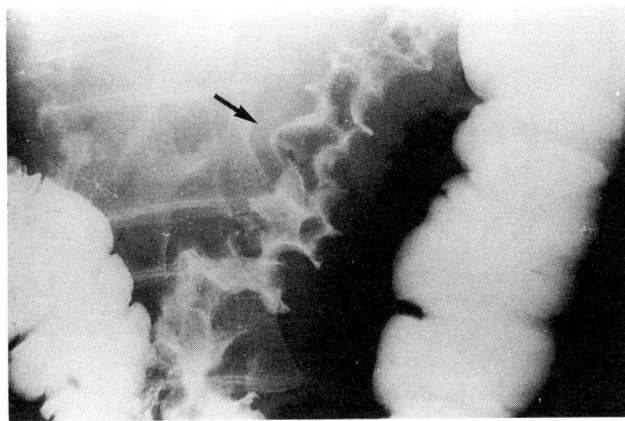

Fig. 7 Barium enema in a 68-year-old man with left-sided abdominal pain and positive occult bloods showing the typical appearance of an ischaemic colitis (arrow).

views will define the vascular lesions but their presence does not necessarily mean that they are responsible for the symptoms.

Compression of the coeliac artery by an unusually low median arcuate ligament of the diaphragm is another postulated cause of chronic intestinal ischaemia, but the existence of this syndrome remains controversial. It is really not known whether chronic mesenteric ischaemia is a frequent cause of symptoms, but probably it is rare. It should also be remembered that the bowel vasculature may be affected by a large number of diseases, e.g. SLE, rheumatoid arthritis, or polyarteritis nodosa, as part of the generalized symptom complex of such disorders.

Investigation of patients with arterial disease

Detection of risk factors

Careful assessment of the blood pressure and a full smoking history are most important, for these are two risk factors that can be corrected. Although this is generally non-rewarding, hypercholesterolaemia and hypertriglyceridaemia should be excluded, especially in the younger patient. Polycythaemia, either vera or secondary, should not be overlooked, but although there is some evidence that hyperfibrinogenaemia with increased viscosity may be associated with peripheral vascular disease, the evidence is not sufficiently strong to warrant this investigation in most patients. Urine examination for glucose and a random blood glucose should be performed routinely to identify diabetes.

Non-invasive assessment of arterial disease

Physiological measurements

It is the physiological dysfunction of arterial obstruction that requires correction rather than the anatomical lesion. Hence efforts are directed at methods which attempt to measure this dysfunction, both qualitatively and quantitatively, of the anatomical lesion recognized by clinical examination and/or arteriography. They also provide a means of following the progress of arterial disease in patients after reconstructive surgery. The tests that are in common use comprise measurements of flow and pressure and analysis of the changes in the flow or pressure patterns.

Peripheral blood flow can be measured relatively accurately and non-invasively by plethysmography, which is available in most vascular laboratories. Radioisotope clearance or distribution provides a semi-invasive method of measuring flow, while at operation flow can be measured by the direct application of an electromagnetic flow meter to the artery in question. However, flow at rest may be normal, and it is only by attempting to increase flow as a result of exercise, arterial occlusion, or by injection of papaverine directly into the artery (all of which produce peripheral vasodilation) that an abnormality may be recognized; for in the presence of arterial obstruction the expected increase in flow does not occur with peripheral vasodilation.

The measurement of pressures in the periphery is the commonest of all the non-invasive techniques used by vascular units as it is simple and reproducible. Generally, pressures are measured by the detection of the return of flow in an artery below a cuff using a Doppler ultrasonic velocity detector, although its sensitivity can be improved with the use of a mercury-in-silastic strain gauge or a photoplethysmograph. Measurement of pressure at the ankle is by far the most useful of the non-invasive measurements of peripheral arterial disease, since these measurements, both before and after exercise, provide an objective assessment of the degree of arterial obstruction. Normally the ankle pressure is expressed as a pressure index which is the ratio of the systolic pressure at the ankle to that in the brachial artery. Normal pressure indices at rest range from 0.9 to 1.2, while those in patients with intermittent claudication range from 0.4 to 0.9, and in patients with rest pain the indices are below 0.4. After exercise or the production of reactive hyperaemia, the pressure and hence the index fall in the presence of arterial obstruction, the rate of recovery giving further information about the degree of ischaemia.

Pressure pulses can only be obtained invasively by intra-arterial catheters or needles, but flow pulses can be obtained not only by electromagnetic flow meters at operation but also non-invasively with an ultrasonic velocity detector. Volume pulses which reflect the arterial wall expansion in response to pressure can be detected with various types of plethysmography.

In most instances the non-invasive techniques described above provide an objective measurement of the clinical assessment of peripheral arterial disease, but in doubtful cases of arterial disease, they can be extremely useful in excluding peripheral arterial disease as a cause of the symptoms.

Transcutaneous oxygen tension can now be measured using polarographic electrodes, and this can provide useful information about the capacity for healing in amputation skin flaps, and so allow the most appropriate level for amputation to be determined.

Imaging techniques

Ultrasound imaging of large arteries, especially the abdominal aorta, has proved invaluable in determining the size of aneurysms, especially as a simple and reproducible method of following patients with small aneurysms where expansion would be an indication for reconstructive surgery. Similarly computer-aided tomographic (CAT) scanning can provide the same information but not as simply.

Radionuclide angiography can be performed by the intravenous injection of ^{99m}Tc pertechnate. It does not produce a clear enough definition for a first-line imaging technique, but it can be a useful way of assessing postoperative graft patency for example. Radioisotopes can also be used for measurements of blood flow by determining the local clearance of ^{133}Xe.

Invasive assessment of arterial disease

Contrast angiography remains the most valuable diagnostic tool for the vascular surgeon, and has not been replaced to any great extent by non-invasive imaging techniques. Direct puncture techniques to inject contrast media have been replaced with retrograde catheter techniques, catheters being inserted via the femoral, axillary, or brachial arteries. The catheter techniques can be performed under local anaesthesia and allow lateral and oblique view to be obtained. Complications of arteriography, comprising thrombosis due to intimal damage and embolism, are uncommon. However, angiograms are unpleasant for the patient, and hence the drive for non-invasive techniques of determining arterial disease.

Digital subtraction angiography is a relatively new development in which contrast is injected intravenously, multiple images of the area in question are stored in a computer in digital form, and as the contrast passes through the area these multiple images are digitally processed, and subtracted from the background leaving the arterial image. The resolution of digital subtraction angiography is inferior to that of a conventional angiogram, but can be enhanced by the intra-arterial injection of contrast. Furthermore, the area that can be shown is relatively restricted without repeated injections of contrast which may reach levels capable of producing renal toxicity. Nevertheless, this technique is proving extremely valuable in certain areas, such as the carotid bifurcation, the renal arteries, abdominal aortic, and peripheral arterial aneurysms, and in the sequential evaluation of known arterial lesions or of reconstructive surgery.

Management of the ischaemic limb

General management

Careful attention must be paid to cleanliness of ischaemic feet or hands so as to avoid infection, and particular care must be given to the cutting of toe nails. In the elderly the nails of ischaemic feet are best trimmed by an assistant or a chiropodist so as to avoid laceration and infection, which may lead to gangrene.

Walking to the point of claudication several times during each day may improve collateral circulation in the patient with intermittent claudication, increasing the walking distance.

Reconstructive surgery and so angiography should not be considered in patients presenting with intermittent claudication until the symptoms have been present for at least three months and continue to interfere markedly with the patient's work or recreation. For it is distinctly possible that the claudication distance first noted by the patient will improve significantly over the succeeding months as collateral circulation develops. Obviously the presence of rest pain and/or gangrene represents an indication for urgent investigation with a view to reconstructive surgery.

Treatment of risk factors

Smoking is by far the most significant risk factor associated with occlusive arterial disease and every effort should be made to stop patients smoking. This edict applies equally well, but for different reasons, to patients with vasospastic disorders. It is just as important to stop patients smoking after reconstructive surgery, for even if patients have smoked for many years, the likelihood of a long-term successful outcome of surgery is fourfold greater in the patient who stops smoking (see Fig. 1). Furthermore, the incidence of other vascular events, e.g. myocardial infarction, is greater in patients with occlusive arterial disease who continue to smoke than in those who stop.

Diabetes must be adequately controlled, and hypertension should be, although hypertension is not such a high risk factor for peripheral arterial disease as it is for cerebrovascular or coronary artery disease. Hypercholesterolaemia and hypertriglyceridaemia probably should be treated, although the evidence that this influences the progress of peripheral arterial disease is sparse and is based mostly on the known association of the various hyperlipidaemias with cardiovascular disease.

Drugs

A variety of vasodilator drugs with different mechanisms of action have been used in the treatment of occlusive arterial disease but with virtually no improvement in any of the clinical features. At this time they have no place in management. Trials of prostaglandin treatment have not been shown to be of value in the ischaemic limb.

Anticoagulants again have no place in the management of occlusive arterial disease. Although during reconstructive surgery, heparin is administered either regionally or systemically before proximal arterial clamps are applied in the course of surgery.

Platelet disaggregators, especially aspirin and/or persantin, are being used more frequently after surgical reconstruction in the expectation of prolonging the patency of bypass grafts, especially distal prosthetic grafts. However, the evidence that these agents do indeed help to maintain patency of peripheral grafts is purely

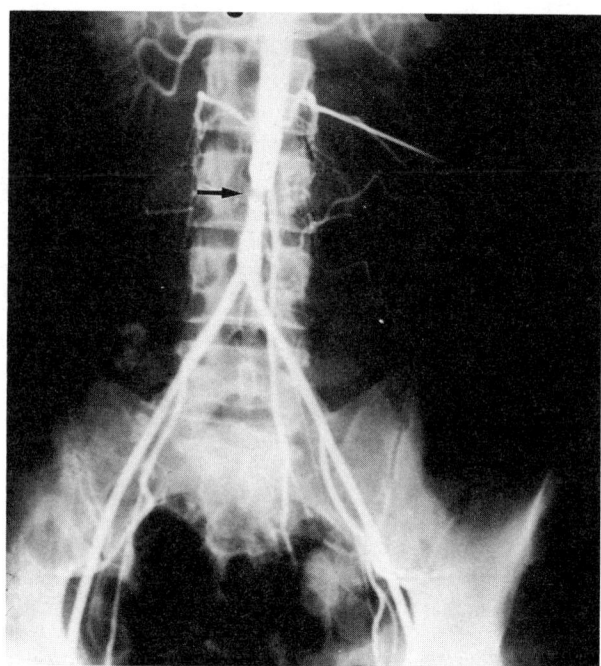

Fig. 8 A translumbar aortogram in a 49-year-old woman with bilateral calf, thigh, and buttock claudication at 100 metres, showing a localized obstruction of the aorta (arrow) with relatively normal vessels above and below. This lesion proved to be eminently suitable for an endarterectomy.

anecdotal at this time, and must await the outcome of current controlled clinical trials.

Reconstructive arterial surgery

Aorto-iliac reconstruction Occlusive disease of the aorto-iliac segment may be treated either by endarterectomy (in which the atheromatous plaque and approximately the inner two-thirds to one-half of the media are removed) or the insertion of a prosthetic graft. Either procedure may give satisfactory results, but endarterectomy is best restricted to relatively localized disease (Fig. 8), a graft being indicated for more extensive disease. Various prosthetic grafts are available but the most satisfactory at this time is a knitted dacron graft. This material best fits the requirements for a prosthetic graft, for it has an adequate porosity to allow ingrowth of fibroblasts to form a false but firmly attached neo-endothelium, it is non-toxic and non-allergenic, it is durable and does not deteriorate, and it is thin-walled and flexible. Usually a bifurcated graft is inserted, the proximal end being anastomosed end-to-end or end-to-side to the aorta above the disease and the two legs of the graft being anastomosed end-to-side to iliac arteries, or just as often to the common femoral arteries below the inguinal ligament. Both procedures give excellent results with patency rates of up to 70 per cent at 10 years being achieved in patients who do not die of cardiovascular or cerebrovascular disease. The long-term patency of bypass grafts is beginning to appear superior to endarterectomy in the aorto-iliac area. Recurrence of disease above or below endarterectomized segments of arteries or a prosthetic graft is common and further surgery for recurrence of symptoms may be required in such cases.

Reconstruction below the inguinal ligament

1. Femoro-popliteal grafts: These are performed for blocks of the superficial femoral artery usually running from the common femoral artery to either the proximal popliteal artery above the knee or the distal popliteal artery below the knee. The ideal graft material is reversed autogenous saphenous vein, and if a suitable vein is not present in the operated leg, the vein is removed from the opposite side. If neither vein is suitable, then it may be poss-

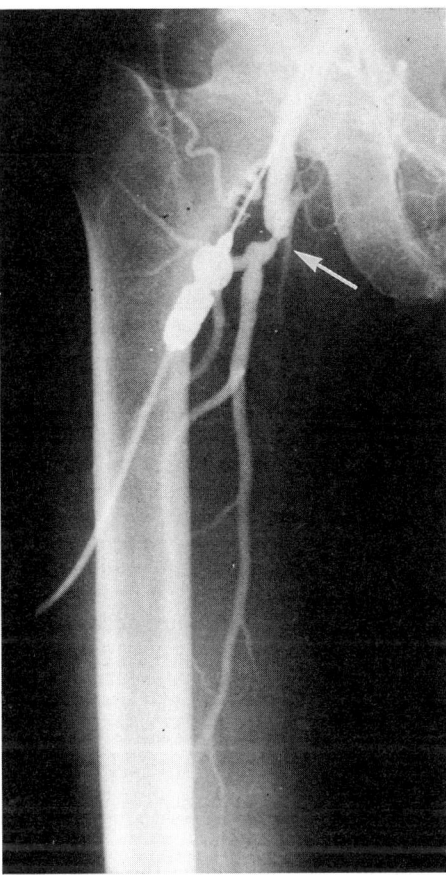

Fig. 9 A femoral angiogram in a 75-year-old man with severe ischaemia of the leg showing a complete block of the superficial femoral artery and a stenosis at the origin of the profunda femoris artery (arrow). As he had severe cardiac disease a profundaplasty was performed under local anaesthetic with relief of the symptoms.

ible to use the cephalic veins from the arm as autogenous vein remains far superior to prosthetic grafts.

Prosthetic grafts below the inguinal ligament have a poor history, new prostheses being introduced with a wave of enthusiasm only to be discarded after several years as the patency rate is shown to fall dramatically after one to two years in comparison to autogenous vein. At the present time three types of prosthetic graft are used below the inguinal ligament: expanded polytetrafluoroethylene (PTFE), glutaraldehyde-tanned umbilical vein supported by a polyester mesh, and double velour knitted dacron. Excellent results are claimed for all three prostheses by their enthusiastic supporters but only time will tell whether such grafts remain patent in the long-term to the same extent that autogenous saphenous veins do.

2. Femoro-tibial grafts. Where no popliteal artery is present but one of the three distal arteries is patent (anterior tibial, posterior tibial, or peroneal), it is possible to use one of these arteries for insertion of a graft arising from the common femoral artery. This type of procedure is only performed for limb salvage, and vein should always be used if possible. The salvage rate in critically ischaemic limbs has been impressive, at least in the short-term.

3. Profundaplasty. When a stenosis at the origin of the profunda femoris artery exists together with a block of the superficial femoral artery, profundaplasty with or without a local endarterectomy may significantly improve the circulation to the limb (Fig. 9). This is a simple procedure which can be performed under local anaesthetic and is ideal as a limb salvage procedure in a poor risk patient. Unfortunately most patients do not have a significant stenosis at the profunda origin.

Extra-anatomical bypass grafts Where aorto-iliac disease exists but the patient is not considered well enough to undergo a major aorto-iliac reconstruction, a prosthetic graft (dacron or PTFE) can be brought subcutaneously from the axillary artery just below the clavicle down to the femoral artery on the same side, with a branch taken off this in the region of the iliac fossa to the opposite femoral artery.

Where one iliac artery only is obstructed, a prosthetic graft can be brought subcutaneously from the femoral artery on the side with a normal flow, just above the pubis, to the common femoral or profunda femoris artery on the obstructed side.

The long-term patency of these extra-anatomical bypass grafts is proving surprisingly good, and as a result they are being used more and more as a first-line reconstructive procedure in the more elderly patient rather than only in patients considered a poor risk for more major reconstructive surgery.

Factors influencing graft patency Numerous factors influence graft patency. The site of the graft is important, for prosthetic grafts have a very high patency rate above the inguinal ligament whereas below the inguinal ligament they are to be avoided in favour of autogenous saphenous vein if at all possible.

Both the inflow and outflow from a graft are important. This is so for all grafts, but especially for grafts below the inguinal ligament.

The continuation of existing risk factors obviously may influence not only the course of the arterial disease but also the patency of reconstructed arteries. None more so than smoking, for continued smoking decreases the likelihood of long-term patency in reconstructed arteries some fourfold. This is the most important factor to be corrected in the patient undergoing reconstructive arterial surgery. However, correction of other risk factors such as hypertension, diabetes, and hyperlipidaemia is just as important because of their prominence also as risk factors in ischaemic heart disease.

Complications of reconstructive surgery Apart from those common to any major surgical procedure, the major complications that are seen after reconstructive arterial surgery are graft thrombosis, which is almost always due either to an unrecognized technical error or poor inflow and outflow, haemorrhage, and infection. Infection in the vicinity of an arterial anastomosis or a prosthetic graft represents one of the most serious complications that can occur in surgery, for it can lead to erosion of anastomoses and life-threatening haemorrhage. In the case of infected prosthetic grafts infection generally can be eradicated only by excising the graft, and replacing it with a new graft generally following an extra-anatomical path well away from the infected site.

Embolectomy Where acute ischaemia of a limb is due to an embolus then the only treatment is embolectomy. With a Fogarty balloon catheter this is a simple procedure and can be performed under local anaesthetic even in the very poor risk patient. Assuming the diagnosis is confirmed by angiography, embolectomy can be performed sometimes as long as four weeks after lodging of an embolus in a distal artery, provided of course that the limb is viable. There is no case for procrastination with anticoagulants in a patient with ischaemia of a limb due to an embolus. This is particularly so in the case of an embolus in the upper limb where it is unusual for the limb to be critically ischaemic and so treatment is often confined to anticoagulation or indeed no treatment is given. However many patients so treated are left with residual claudication in the limb, which can only be prevented by early embolectomy performed under local anaesthetic.

Sympathectomy

In most instances of severe limb ischaemia due to occlusive arterial disease it is the lower limb which is affected. Where reconstruction is not possible, a lumbar sympathectomy may be performed either chemically or by operation. Although chemical sympathectomy by the paravertebral injection of phenol into the vicinity of the sympathetic chain is a simple procedure and can be performed in most poor risk patients, it is not as effective as an operative sympathectomy in which the chain and the second and third ganglia are removed. However, as the results of sympathectomy in patients with severe ischaemia where reconstruction is not possible are not overly impressive, chemical sympathectomy is probably a reasonable approach provided some expertise in the technique is available, and especially in patients considered at high-risk for any surgical procedure.

Percutaneous transluminal angioplasty

This is one of the major developments in recent years in the treatment of occlusive arterial disease, since the development by Gruntzig and Hopff in 1974 of a non-elastomeric double-lumen balloon catheter of polyvinyl chloride that could be expanded to a predetermined size, but no more. The catheter is introduced into the artery by the Seldinger technique and the balloon sited across the stenosis and distended. The actual mechanisms by which dilation is produced is uncertain but it is thought to be due to cracking of the intima and media adjacent to a plaque in an axial direction allowing the media and adventitia to stretch and the lumen, therefore, to dilate as the plaque moves circumferentially. There may also be some crushing of soft atheromatous lesions. Technical improvements in the balloon itself are improving the success rate of dilation.

The indications for this technique are becoming clearer. The lesion par excellence for this treatment is the localized iliac artery lesion, not greater than 2.5 cm long, where over 90 per cent of dilations are immediately successful and two-year patency rates are around 80 per cent. Successful dilation of localized stenoses or occlusions of the superficial femoral artery have been achieved with lesions of less than 10 cm, the immediate success rate being of the order of about 70 per cent. The use of dilation is now being explored for limb salvage in blocks of the superficial femoral artery in patients of high risk for reconstructive surgery. In functional renal artery stenoses percutaneous transluminal angioplasty is becoming the first line of attack for most lesions, with surgery reserved for the failed dilations (page 13.387).

The complication rate for this procedure is small in experienced hands and certainly less than for reconstructive surgery. Complications include distal embolization, significant groin haematomas, thrombosis, false aneurysm, and even death.

Percutaneous transluminal angioplasty has had a significant impact on the management of many patients with occlusive arterial disease and has enlarged the criteria for angiography in the more elderly patient with claudication. However, for the most appropriate use of this technique it is essential that the vascular radiologists and vascular surgeons work closely together in the evaluation of the patient and the selection of the most appropriate treatment for a particular patient.

Amputation

Despite increasing skills in reconstructive surgery for salvage of severely ischaemic limbs, the rate of amputation in hospitals with a specialist vascular unit has not declined, presumably due to the increasing age of the patient population. The level of amputation is dictated both by the limb fitter's requirements for an artificial limb and the likelihood of obtaining primary healing. In occlusive arterial disease there is no place for local amputations of gangrenous toes or even part of the foot, unless of course this is preceded by a successful graft restoring distal circulation. A definitive higher amputation must be performed, and if possible in the case of the lower limb, a below knee amputation should be performed rather than above knee amputation. No satisfactory method exists for determining whether the flaps of a below knee amputation, especially the long posterior flap, have an adequate blood supply to achieve primary healing. Nevertheless with careful technique some 75 per cent of below knee amputations will heal primarily or with a modest delay. This type of amputation allows a much more

effective artificial limb to be fitted in an elderly patient and allows more mobility without an artificial limb.

Rehabilitation of a patient after an amputation is of the greatest importance and must start as soon as the patient recovers from the anaesthetic and continue until the patient is mobile on an artifical limb. This can take many months and is the special task of limb-fitting centres, but the vascular surgeon must pave the way by prior discussions and encouragement as well as providing a suitable stump.

The diabetic foot

The diabetic with peripheral arterial disease not only has small artery disease but is more likely to have large artery disease as well. This possibility must be remembered when an infected or gangrenous toe or foot presents in the diabetic. If large artery disease exists, this should be dealt with on its merits, as reconstruction of an obstructed major artery will improve healing of the distal lesion even in the presence of small vessel disease. The results of reconstructive surgery are no worse in the diabetic than in the non-diabetic patient.

However, having excluded major artery disease, local amputations of gangrenous toes may be performed in the diabetic foot. Healing is slow, but often does occur with care and patience. If infection is present, then the lesion must be laid open extensively with excision of any necrotic tissue or involved tendons. Furthermore the diabetes itself can be difficult to control in the presence of diabetic gangrene, and is best achieved initially with insulin administered on a sliding scale based on four-hourly blood glucose levels (BM stix).

Management of aneurysms
Abdominal aorta

Ruptured This is one of the few true surgical emergencies, and when this diagnosis is made the patient should be taken immediately to the operating room where placement of a clamp on the aorta above the aneurysm should take preference over resuscitation and such procedures as X-rays and the cross-matching of blood. Once the aorta is clamped above the aneurysm resuscitation can begin. The results of surgery for ruptured aneurysm are poor, about 50 per cent of patients surviving at best. Not all patients should be operated on, but the decision not to operate may be difficult. However, as a general guideline patients over 70 years of age who have been hypotensive for over one hour are unlikely to leave hospital alive.

After control of the aneurysm is achieved, the aneurysmal sac is opened, lumbar arteries controlled from within, and either a tube or bifurcated dacron graft laid in the bed of the sac, the proximal end being anastomosed to the neck of the aneurysm and the distal end either to the lower end of the aorta or to the iliac or femoral arteries depending on the extent of the aneurysmal dilation. Usually a woven rather than a knitted graft is used to reduce blood loss on restoring flow to the limbs.

Symptomatic aneurysm In general a symptomatic aneurysm should be operated on whatever its size, for if the symptoms are truly due to the aneurysm then rupture within weeks to months is very likely. However, severe cardiac or respiratory disease is sometimes a contraindication to surgery. In such patients some benefit might be obtained from tacking a sheet of dacron over the aneurysm, with the hope that this will be incorporated in a thick fibrous reaction around the aneurysm, hence preventing further dilation. The surgical procedure of aortic replacement is identical to that described for a ruptured aneurysm and either a knitted or woven graft can be used.

Asymptomatic aneurysm This may provide one of the more difficult management decisions. If the aneurysm is a large one (greater than 6 cm), then there is little doubt that it should be dealt with surgically, for there is good evidence that the likelihood of subsequent rupture of a large asymptomatic aneurysm is high. In the case of the small aneurysm (less than 6 cm), two courses are available. Either the patient is followed regularly and the size of the aneurysm monitored clinically and by ultrasound, or surgery is advised provided that the patient's general health is reasonably sound. In the first instance an increase in size of the aneurysm or the development of symptoms would represent an indication for immediate surgery. The latter course can only be advised provided that a competent vascular surgeon is available and the patient's health is sound. For in the hands of an experienced vascular team, the hospital mortality associated with an elective replacement of an abdominal aortic aneurysm is around 2 per cent. Furthermore, it should be remembered that even patients with a small aneurysm show a decreased survival compared to an age and sex matched population without an aneurysm. This difference is due in part to subsequent rupture of the aneurysm, but also in part to a higher death rate from cardiac and cerebral vascular disease, the aneurysm representing only a marker of the generalized atheromatous disease.

Popliteal artery

Aneurysms of the popliteal artery should always be bypassed or replaced after diagnosis, even though asymptomatic. For if a popliteal aneurysm presents with a severely ischaemic leg due to thrombosis or distal embolization, limb salvage is usually not possible. Either autogenous saphenous vein, dacron, or PTFE can be used as a replacement graft, vein being the most satisfactory.

Thoracic aorta

Rupture of thoracic aortic aneurysms is nearly always followed by sudden death, few cases surviving to reach an operating room, and in these few patients the chances of survival following surgery is remote.

Elective resection of aneurysms of the ascending thoracic aorta or aortic arch present a formidable challenge to the surgeon because of the necessity to interrupt the cerebral circulation. Furthermore, the aortic valve may have to be replaced and coronary arteries reimplanted as part of the replacement of an ascending thoracic aortic aneurysm, while the innominate, left common carotid, and subclavian arteries need to be reimplanted after placement of an aortic arch aneurysm. These procedures are performed under cardiopulmonary bypass together with bypass to the cerebral circulation. In addition deep hypothermia may be employed to reduce cerebral damage.

Elective replacement of descending thoracic aortic aneurysms carries the risk of spinal cord ischaemia and renal ischaemia during the period of clamping of the aorta, and for this reason many surgeons employ extracorporeal bypass to perfuse the lower half of the body while the reconstruction is performed. However, if the anastomosis time can be kept to 30 minutes, then there is probably no need for an extracorporeal circuit.

Woven dacron grafts are used for replacement of thoracic aortic aneurysms to diminish blood loss. Hospital mortality from the procedure is still high, especially in the case of aneurysms of the ascending aorta or arch, and is at least 10 per cent in the most experienced hands.

Dissecting aneurysm

The results of treatment of dissecting aneurysms of the thoracic aorta are poor, and there is no clearly defined plan of management. There are advocates of both surgical and medical treatment, and perhaps a combination of both provides the patient with the best chances of survival. Medical treatment is directed at reducing the blood pressure to normal or below normal levels (the patients inevitably being hypertensive), while surgical treatment is directed at resection of the aorta at the origin of the dissection, closure of the dissection proximally and distally, and replacement of the defect in the aorta by a dacron prosthetic graft. The problems of the surgical technique are the same as for aneurysms of the thoracic aorta.

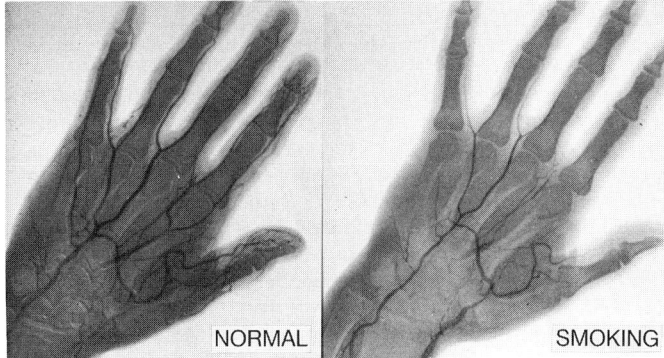

Fig. 10 An angiogram of a hand in a patient with Raynaud's disease before and after smoking half a cigarette showing the induced vasospasm of the small arteries of the hand.

Probably the most appropriate management of the patient with a dissecting aneurysm is firstly to stabilize the blood pressure and then, when the patient's condition is stable, to embark on surgical resection of the dissection in the most favourable circumstances. Mortality will still be high.

Thoraco-abdominal aorta

An aneurysm involving the thoracic as well as the abdominal aorta presents major technical problems as the coeliac, superior mesenteric, and renal arteries arise from the aneurysm. Virtually no patients have survived an emergency resection of such aneurysms, and the mortality of elective resections is still around 30 per cent. The most satisfactory approach is to insert a dacron prosthetic graft from the thoracic aorta to the distal abdominal aorta, followed by implantation of the major intra-abdominal arteries before disconnecting the aneurysm. This inevitably results in prolonged ischaemia of the kidneys and bowel, which is largely responsible for the high mortality.

Other arteries

Aneurysms of other arteries such as the femoral, splenic, and renal arteries should be excised and replaced with a graft if greater than 1.5–2.0 cm in diameter or if symptomatic. For the chances of rupture or other complications, although not really known, are probably higher with these relatively large aneurysms.

Management of vasospastic disorders

General measures

The basis of all treatment initially should be advice on keeping warm and firm encouragement to stop smoking (Fig. 10). Warm clothing (gloves, hats, and boots for the outdoors) and well heated houses are essential. Attention to such measures in the winter months will enable many patients to cope with their symptoms. Emigration to a warmer climate will be of benefit, but is not often a practical solution to the problem. Battery warmed gloves are of value in severe cases.

Drugs

Every vasodilator drug, with their various modes of action, has probably had a trial of treatment in patients with Raynaud's syndrome, sometimes with success but never consistently so. Usually the dosage necessary to produce relief of symptoms in the hands results in unpleasant side-effects. Reserpine is sometimes useful, and some striking claims for benefits of intra-arterial reserpine, at least in the short-term, for patients with severe Raynaud's syndrome have been made. Another approach to severe Raynaud's syndrome which does result in short-term beneficial effect is a guanethidine block, the guanethidine being injected intravenously with a tourniquet on the proximal part of the limb. Plasmapheresis has also been used in some cases with benefit.

Sympathectomy

This remains the most satisfactory treatment but should be reversed for the patient with severe symptoms, despite attention to general measures and drug treatment. Although most patients get an excellent result from sympathectomy in the early months after the operation, relapse of symptoms after six months to two years is common. Relapse occurs in about one-third of patients with Raynaud's disease, and in two-thirds of patients with Raynaud's phenomenon where the operation has been performed usually before the underlying disease has become evident. The results of sympathectomy are poorer once significant trophic changes have occurred in the hands or feet. For usually these are associated with organic changes in the digital arteries, which then play a more prominent role in the clinical features than the vaso-spastic element of the disorder. Thus the decision to perform a sympathectomy should not be delayed too long in patients with severe symptoms.

In the upper limb the sympathetic chain is removed from and including the lower one-third of the stellate ganglion down to the third thoracic ganglion. This may be done either through the root of the neck or through the axilla. A posterior approach is popular in some centres but is cosmetically less attractive than the more commonly used approaches. The procedure is relatively free of complications, the two most distressing being Horner's syndrome if too much of the stellate ganglion is removed, and post-sympath-ectomy neuralgia. The latter begins some 10 days after the procedure and may result in such severe pain that opiates are necessary for relief. Fortunately the neuralgia spontaneously disappears after several weeks.

In the lower limb the second and third lumbar ganglia and intervening chain are excised. The chain is approached retroperitoneally via a small anterior muscle splitting incision in the abdomen. Again the major complication is a post-sympathectomy neuralgia. Failure to ejaculate in the male may rarely follow excision of the second lumbar ganglion, but this is common only if the first lumbar ganglion is excised.

Management of intestinal ischaemia

Acute intestinal ischaemia

Often the patient with acute intestinal ischaemia due to acute thrombosis or embolism presents late and with irreversible ischaemia of part of the small or large bowel, requiring immediate laparotomy and bowel resection. Nevertheless, if some patients are to benefit by embolectomy or reconstruction, then the possibility of this diagnosis must always be borne in mind in the patient with generalized atheromatous disease or a source of embolism who presents with an acute abdomen. Where this possibility exists, the diagnosis can only be established by angiography or less reliably at surgery.

At laparotomy there is usually a need for bowel resection, but if embolectomy or thrombectomy can be performed successfully, it not only reduces the length of bowel that has to be resected but also enhances the healing of the anastomosis. This can be very important, for resection of most of the small bowel will lead to severe malabsorption after operation, often to a degree incompatible with life. If there is the slightest doubt about the viability of any bowel not resected, the abdominal wall should be loosely closed in a single layer and a second laparotomy ('second look') performed after 24 hours. Unfortunately in at least 50 per cent of cases of small and large bowel ischaemia an obvious blockage of a main artery or venous thrombosis is not demonstrable. The ischaemic bowel presumably results from thrombosis of peripheral small vessels in the bowel itself due to a low flow state accompanying some other catastrophe such as a myocardial infarction.

Ischaemia of the large bowel presents with a spectrum of clinical features ranging from mild abdominal pain to frank necrosis of the colon. Obviously the more severe examples will be managed by laparotomy and excision of the ischaemic bowel; preservation of large bowel is not nearly so critical as of small bowel. The less

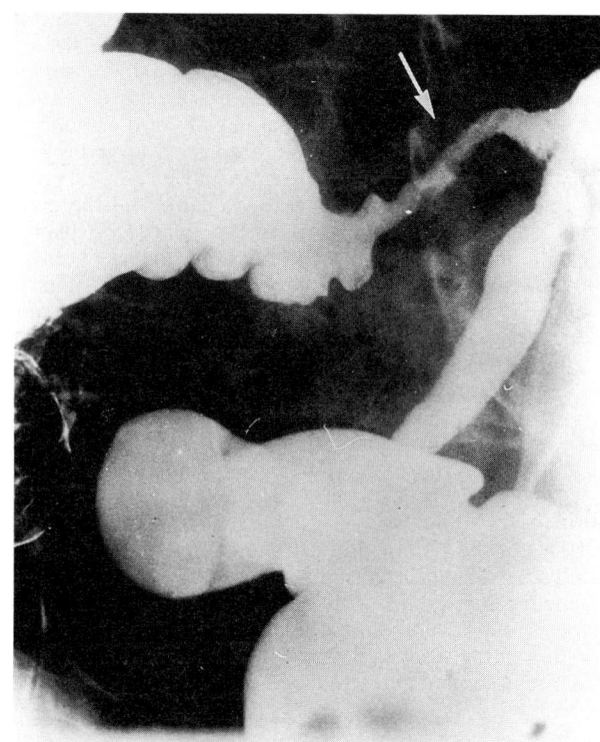

Fig. 11 Barium enema in the same patient shown in Fig. 7, but 11 months later, at which time he presented with large bowel obstruction, showing an ischaemic stenosis of the left transverse colon (arrow).

severe examples can be carefully watched, but with immediate laparotomy if any signs of peritonitis develop. These patients often present months to years later with an ischaemic stenosis and obstruction requiring resection of the stenosed segment (Fig. 11).

Chronic intestinal ischaemia

If this diagnosis can be established, restoration of arterial flow beyond a stenosis can be achieved by a bypass graft from the aorta to the involved mesenteric artery, endarterectomy and patch plasty or transaortic endarterectomy for a lesion at the origin of the artery. In patients in whom a median arcuate ligament syndrome is defined, division of this abnormally low ligament to free completely the coeliac artery will result in cure. The results of reconstruction are excellent if the diagnosis of chronic intestinal ischaemia is correct, but the establishment of this diagnosis is extremely difficult.

Management of thoracic outlet compression

Patients with this syndrome may have demonstrable anatomical abnormalities at the thoracic outlet, but in many no such abnormality can be found. When a clearly defined anatomical abnormality accounts for the clinical features, surgical treatment is indicated with correction of the abnormality, as for instance achieved by excision of a cervical rib. When no apparent abnormality exists, then exercises directed at strengthening the shoulder girdle muscles may be of benefit and should be the first approach to treatment. If no improvement follows, the most appropriate surgical procedure is excision of the first rib which relieves most cases of thoracic outlet compression whatever the cause. This can be done through an axillary approach or an inferior clavicular approach.

If damage to the subclavian artery has occurred as a result of long-standing compression, a post-stenotic aneurysm may be present. As this is a source of emboli, resection of the artery and replacement with a graft is necessary. The most satisfactory approach for such a procedure is a joint approach from above and below the clavicle, without division of the clavicle.

References

Blaisdell, F. W., Steele, M. and Allen, R. E. (1978). Management of acute lower extremity arterial ischaemia due to embolism and thrombosis. *Surgery* 84, 822–831.

Camerini-Davalos, R. A., Bierman, E. L., Redisch, W. and Zilversmit, D. B. (eds) (1976). *Atherogenesis* Vol. 275. New York Academy of Sciences.

Crawford, E. S., Snyder, D. M., Cho, G. C. and Roehm, J. O. (1978). Progress in treatment of thoracoabdominal and abdominal aortic aneurysms involving coeliac superior mesenteric and renal arteries. *Ann. Surg.* 188, 404–422.

Finch, D. R. A., MacDougal, M., Tibbs, D. J. and Morris, P. J. (1980). Amputation for vascular disease: the experience of a peripheral vascular unit. *Br. J. Surg.* 67, 233–237.

Hughson, W. G., Mann, J. I. and Garrod, A. (1978). Intermittent claudication: prevalence and risk factors. *Br. Med. J.* 1, 1379–1381.

Johnston, K. W. (1984). A surgeon's view of peripheral arterial transluminal dilatation. In *Arterial surgery. Clinical Surgery International* Vol. 8 (ed. J. J. Bergan), pp. 147–161. Churchill Livingstone, Edinburgh.

Kannel, W. B., Dawber, T. R., Skinner, J. J., McNamara, P. M. and Shurtleff, D. (1965). Epidemiological aspects of intermittent claudication – the Framingham Study. *Circulation* 32 (Suppl. 2), 121–122.

Loberto, F. W., Johnson, W. C., Corson, J. D. *et al.* (1977). A comparison of the late patency rates of axillo bilateral femoral and axillo unilateral femoral grafts. *Surgery* 81, 33–38.

Maini, B. S. and Mannick, J. A. (1978). Effect of arterial reconstruction on limb salvage: a ten-year appraisal. *Arch. Surg.* 113, 1297–1304.

Marston, A. (1977). *Intestinal ischaemia.* Arnold, London.

Myers, K. A., King, R. B., Scott, D. F., Johnson, N. and Morris, P. J. (1978). The effect of smoking on the late patency of arterial reconstruction in the legs. *Br. J. Surg.* 65, 267–271.

Porter, J. M., Bardana, E. J., Baur, G. M., Wesche, D. H., Andrasch, R. H. and Rosch, J. (1976). The clinical significance of Raynaud's syndrome. *Surgery* 80, 756–762.

Rivers, S. P. and Porter, J. M. (1984). Treatment of Raynaud's syndrome. In *Arterial surgery. Clinical Surgery International* Vol. 8 (ed. J. J. Bergan), p. 185. Churchill Livingstone, Edinburgh.

Roos, D. B. (1979). New concepts of thoracic outlet syndrome that explain etiology, symptoms, diagnosis and treatment. *Vasc. Surg.* 13, 313–333.

Rutherford, R. B. (ed.) (1984). *Vascular surgery* 2nd edn. W. B. Saunders, Philadelphia.

Stephens, W. E. (1979). *Haemodynamics and the blood vessel wall.* C. C. Thomas, Springfield.

Sumner, D. S. (1984). The haemodynamics and pathophysiology of arterial disease. In *Vascular surgery* 2nd edn (ed. R. Rutherford), p. 19. W. B. Saunders, Philadelphia.

Szilagyi, D. E., Rian, R. L., Elliott, J. P. and Smith, R. F. (1972). The coeliac artery compression syndrome: does it exist? *Surgery* 72, 849–862.

——, Smith, R. F., DeRusso, F. J., Elliott, J. P. and Sherrin, F. W. (1966). Contribution of abdominal aortic aneurysmectomy to prolongation of life. *Ann. Surg.* 164, 678–699.

Thompson, J. E. and Garrett, W. V. (1980). Peripheral arterial surgery. *N. Engl. J. Med.* 302, 491–503.

Wald, N. and Howard S. (1975). Smoking, carbon monoxide and arterial disease. *Ann. occup. Hyg.* 18, 1–15.

TAKAYASU'S DISEASE

K. ISHIKAWA

Takayasu's disease was first reported by a Japanese ophthalmologist in 1908. This disease, a chronic inflammatory arteriopathy of unknown cause, occurs in humans the world over but is most frequently diagnosed in Oriental young women. The site of occurrence is the aorta and/or its main branches and the pulmonary artery is often involved. These pathological events lead to occlusive changes in the lumina, often combined with dilation and secondary thrombus formation. Major complications attributed to the disease are Takayasu's retinopathy, secondary hypertension, aortic regurgitation, and aortic or arterial aneurysm. There are geographical variations in the clinical aspects of this disease. The following terms may be identical with what is known today as Takayasu's disease or arteritis entity: Takayasu's arteriopathy, occlusive thromboaortopathy, aortitis syndrome, and non-specific aorto-arteritis.

Aetiology

The cause of Takayasu's disease remains unknown. An autoimmune mechanism may be one factor related to the pathogenesis as partial similarities in clinical systemic symptoms and laboratory findings were noted between this disease in the early phase and systemic lupus erythematosus, and because of response to corticosteroid therapy during the inflammatory active stage. Concerning circulating antibodies against antigens of the arterial wall, however, there have been both positive and negative results. Group A streptococcal infection, association with tuberculosis, hormonal imbalance, ethnic susceptibility, and genetic predisposition have been suggested as pathogenetic factors.

Pathology

The lesions in Takayasu's disease show a panarteritis of the aorta and its main branches and of the pulmonary artery. The lesions of the arterial wall begin with a mesoperiarteritis with subsequent fibrosis and are followed by fibrotic thickening of the adventitia and the vasa vasorum. These lesions lead to an intimal fibrosis,

which progresses usually in marked thickening, often with thrombi. The destruction of the arterial wall leads to both stenotic and ectatic changes of the lumen, especially occlusion. These affected portions are clearly demarcated from the adjacent normal sites and segmental 'skipped' lesions are observed.

Geographical occurrence and variations

Takayasu's disease has a worldwide distribution and the incidence is much higher than previously considered. Geographical and ethnic influences on the incidence of the disease and the general symptoms, age at occurrence, sex distribution, and on the site and morphological changes of arterial lesions have been given attention. Series of over 80 cases have been reported from Japan, the People's Republic of China, India, the USSR, Mexico, and France, where 40 per cent of the patients are immigrants from North Africa.

Classifications

To evaluate the disease status and for a better understanding of the clinical profile in an individual patient, it is pertinent to clarify where the patient belongs in each of varied classifications according to the following three factors: inflammatory activity of the disease as determined by the erythrocyte sedimentation rate (ESR), sites of arterial lesions, and complications attributed to Takayasu's disease.

Inflammatory activity

When the erythrocyte sedimentation rate (ESR, Westergren) is consistently 20 mm/hour or more, in particular over 40 mm/hour, or less than 20 mm/hour, the inflammatory activity may be defined as the active and inactive stage, respectively.

Sites of arterial lesions

According to the location of arterial lesions, the disease is anatomically classified into three types.

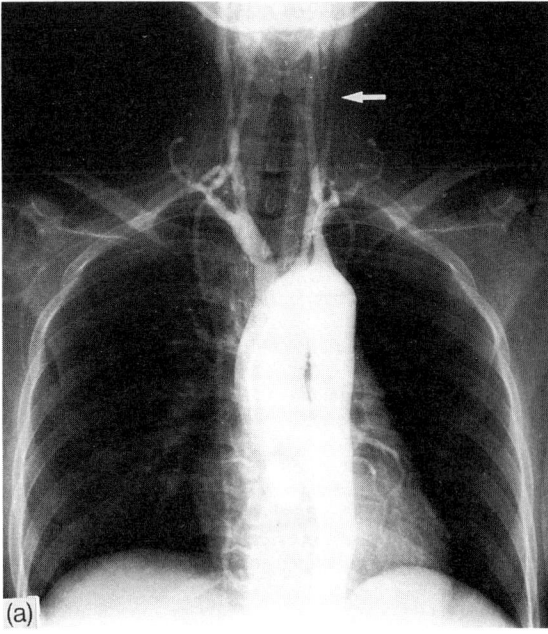

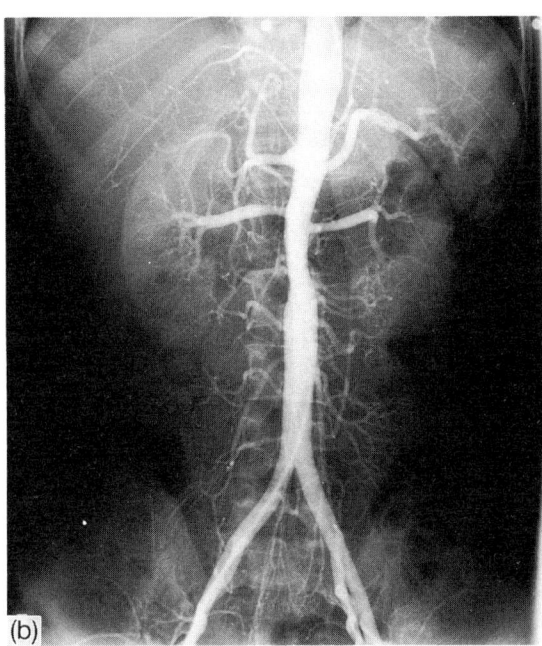

Fig. 1 Aortograms of an 18-year-old Japanese woman with Takayasu's disease in the active stage (ESR, 88 mm/hour), the extensive type, and in group I associated with mild pulmonary arterial involvement. (a) Arch aortogram. Note the segmental narrowing of bilateral common carotid arteries, especially the left distal portion (arrow), but normal appearance of the carotid sinuses. Occlusion or severe narrowing of bilateral subclavian arteries (mid portions). Bilateral vertebral arteries are spared. Mild irregularity of the internal surfaces of the brachiocephalic artery and the thoracic aorta. (b) Abdominal aortogram. Note moderate narrowing of the abdominal aorta (mid portion) and the right renal artery (proximal).

1. The arch type involves the aortic arch and its branches.
2. The descending type involves the descending thoracic and abdominal aorta and its branches.
3. The extensive type which describes the combined arch and descending type (Fig. 1).

Pulmonary arterial involvement is sometimes added in the classification of the disease (Fig. 2).

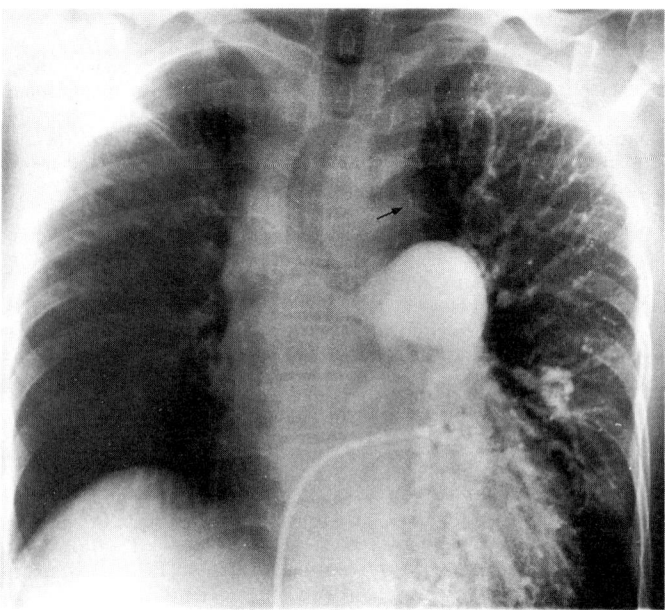

Fig. 2 Pulmonary arteriogram (right ventricular injection) of a 25-year-old Japanese man with Takayasu's disease in the active stage, the extensive type, and in group III. Note occlusion of the right pulmonary artery, no appearance of its branches, and elevation of the ipsilateral diaphragm. Calcification of the aortic knob (arrow). Mild pulmonary hypertension (52/20 mm Hg; mean 30 mm Hg) and moderately increased pulmonary arteriolar resistance (290 dyne s cm^{-5}) were revealed.

Complications
Depending upon the presence and severity of the four complications attributed to the disease, it is classified into four groups (groups I, IIa, IIb, and III).

Group I: uncomplicated Takayasu's disease with or without the involvement of the pulmonary artery (Fig. 1).

Group II: monocomplicated Takayasu's disease; presence of one of the following complications together with uncomplicated Takayasu's disease: (1) Takayasu's retinopathy (Fig. 3); (2) secondary hypertension; (3) aortic regurgitation (Fig. 4); or (4) aortic or arterial aneurysm (Fig. 4). This group is further classified according to the severity of these complications into group IIa (mild or moderate complication) and group IIb (severe complication).

Group III: multicomplicated Takayasu's disease with two or more complications together with uncomplicated Takayasu's disease (Fig. 4).

Clinical features and diagnosis
Takayasu's disease shows protean clinical features and there is a long interval between the onset of symptoms, which begin usually at a young age, and the established diagnosis. At the time of diagnosis, most patients are between the ages of 20 and 40 years. The disease is much more frequent in women. The symptoms and signs may depend on the phase of the disease, the inflammatory activity, the involved site, and major complications.

In general, patients in the early phase are in the active stage and elevated ESR, increased levels of C-reactive protein, increased alpha 2-globulin and gamma globulin values, and slight anaemia are evident. During this phase, most of the patients have general symptoms. The constitutional systemic complaints, which have various grades of severity, are malaise, headache, fever, easy fatigability of the extremities, dizziness, transient visual disturbance, neck pain, mild palpitation and dyspnoea, arthralgia, stiffness of shoulders, and nausea. Syncopal attacks are not

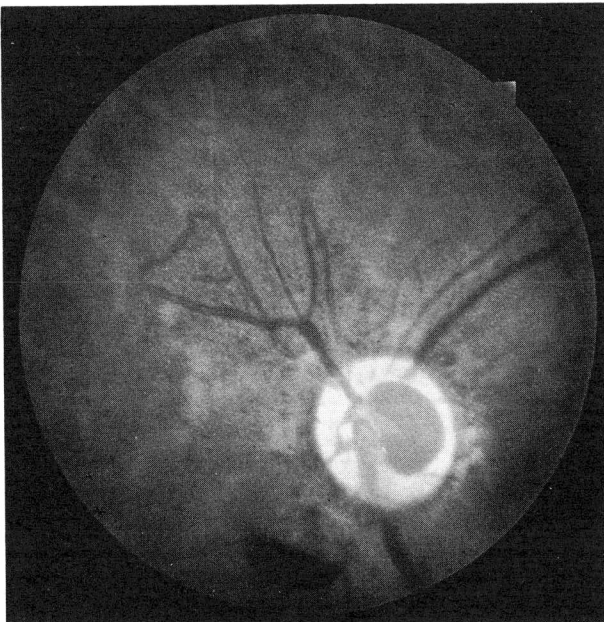

Fig. 3 Fundus photograph of the left eye of a 32-year-old Japanese woman with Takayasu's disease in the suppressed stage of the inflammatory activity, following corticosteroid therapy, and in group III. Note arteriovenous anastomoses (very severe Takayasu's retinopathy) on and around the disc and preretinal hemorrhages. (Reproduced from Ishikawa 1978, Natural history and classification of occlusive thromboaortopathy, Takayasu's disease. *Circulation* **57**, 27, by permission of the American Heart Association, Inc.).

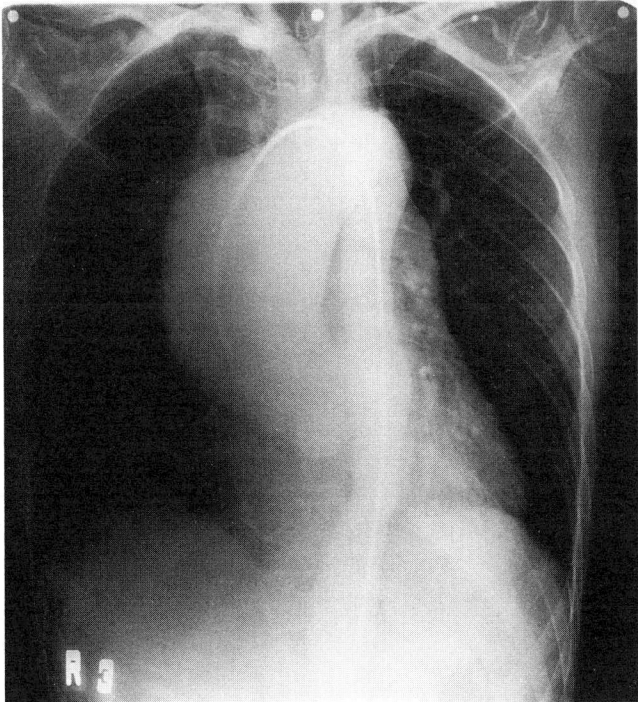

Fig. 4 Thoracic aortogram of a 25-year-old Japanese woman with Takayasu's disease in the active stage, the extensive type, and in group III associated with moderate pulmonary arterial involvement. Note the giant aneurysm of the ascending aorta and mild aortic regurgitation due to annulo-aortic ectasia, and severe irregularity of the internal surface of the entire thoracic aorta. Occlusion or severe narrowing of bilateral subclavian arteries (mid portions).

uncommon in this phase. Haemoptysis occurs rarely. Some patients, however, are asymptomatic and pulselessness, hypertension, or elevated ESR are incidentally detected. The elevated ESR varies in duration with each patient and is generally followed by a gradual return to a normal range.

It is vital for the diagnosis of Takayasu's disease to think of it and to take a careful history as often there are asymptomatic states during some period in the course and a changing pattern of symptoms.

When the grade of narrowing of the involved arteries is advanced in the late phase of the disease, cardiovascular symptoms and signs such as moderate or severe dyspnoea and palpitation on exertion, chest and back pain, recurrent syncopal attacks, intermittent claudication of the arms or legs, pulsus differens or pulselessness, bruits over the affected arteries, and high blood pressure occur. With a careful bedside examination, patients can be broadly classified into one of the three types. It is useful to make a 'pulse–bruit–pressure' diagram which shows the grade of palpability of arterial pulsations, bruits, and tenderness over the affected arteries, and values of blood pressure, including retinal arterial pressure, at various regions. Total aortography, however, is indispensable for the confirmation and differential diagnosis from congenital aortic coarctation at unusual sites, the aortitis of giant cell arteritis, and atherosclerosis alone.

At the time of diagnosis or admission, each of the extensive type, group II, and pulmonary arterial involvement are present in about half the number of patients (Figs. 1, 2, and 4). Coronary arterial lesions are rarely associated with this disease. Plain roentgenograms will often show calcification of the affected aorta and a hyperlucency in the lung area in the occluded pulmonary arterial segments. Pulmonary arteriography or perfusion lung scanning aid diagnosis. Pulmonary hypertension is not rare (Fig. 2). Most patients in the very advanced phase have congestive heart failure or visual disturbances, including blindness.

Treatment and prognosis

Medical

In general, patients with Takayasu's disease in the inflammatory active stage respond well to corticosteroid therapy although this therapy is not completely established for the disease. Not only are complaints reduced but progression of arterial involvement during the active stage of the disease is retarded or prevented. The initial daily dose of corticosteroids is usually 30 to 50 mg of prednisolone, more often the latter, and gradually this is reduced to 10 to 20 mg. It is not uncommon for the drug to be prescribed for these patients for more than four years. Gastric or duodenal ulcer sometimes occur during the treatment.

For symptomatic therapy, digitalis, antihypertensive agents, and antibiotic drugs are often used. All but a few patients in groups I and IIa, especially in the former, are good candidates for medical treatment rather than surgery (Fig. 1).

In a recent large series, from which surgically treated patients were excluded, the ten-year overall survival rate after the diagnosis was established is 89.7 per cent. The ten-year survival rates for patients in groups IIb and III and those in groups I and IIa are 74.2 and 100 per cent, respectively.

The inflammatory activity does not worsen during pregnancy, but various cardiovascular events, including intrapartum cerebral haemorrhage, can occur in the perinatal period in more than half the number of patients. An evaluation of the disease before pregnancy, planning the mode of delivery from both obstetric and non-obstetric indications, and intrapartum and anaesthetic considerations, with special reference to the measurement of blood pressure, are important.

Surgical

Surgical treatments mainly include reconstructive surgery of the aorta and its main branches, endarterectomy, aneurysmectomy, and aortic valve replacement. There are surgical problems specific to the disease. If the inflammation of the arterial wall is active, the possibility of suture failure or aneurysm formation as well as occlusion of the graft is higher than in the case of arterial disease of other causes. It is often difficult to use a calcified aortic wall for the bypass because of the stony hardness of the site.

Surgical results are excellent in some patients who have hypertension secondary to coarctation of the aorta but without significant bilateral lesions of the renal arteries or secondary to narrowing of one renal artery in the inactive stage of the inflammation. However, it is often difficult to decide on surgical indications for patients with Takayasu's disease, as the results of surgical treatments for those in the advanced phase are not always good. In a large series of patients who underwent surgical treatment, 18 patients (27 per cent) died, including 11 (16 per cent) who died at operation, and 7 who died later. Three of the 11 operative deaths were attributed to intracerebral and subarachnoid bleeding after cervical arterial reconstructive surgery. The surgical results seem to depend on the location, extent, severity, and the inflammatory activity of the lesions in the aorta and its main branches.

In general, in patients with this disease who have been selected for surgery, an increased ESR should be lowered by steroid therapy to a normal level (except in emergencies) before surgical treatment. A careful long term follow up is required because of the surgical risks, including an increase of the inflammatory activity after operation. At present, there is no documentation of comparative studies on the long term prognosis for medical and surgical groups of patients with Takayasu's disease.

Among the major factors related to death and severe disability are congestive heart failure, cerebrovascular accidents, and blindness.

References

Deutsch, V., Wexler, L. and Deutsch, H. (1974). Takayasu's arteritis: an angiographic study with remarks on ethnic distribution in Israel. *Am. J. Roentgenol.* **122**, 13–28.

Fiessinger, J. N., Tawfik-Taher, S., Capron, L., Laurian, C., Cormier, J. M., Camilleri, J. P. and Housset, E. (1982). Maladie de Takayasu: critères diagnostiques. *Nouv. Presse Med.* **11**, 583–586.

Gotsman, M. S., Beck, W. and Schrire, V. (1967). Selective angiography in arteritis of the aorta and its major branches. *Radiology* **88**, 232–248.

Ishikawa, K. (1986). Takayasu's disease. In *Extracranial cerebrovascular disease* (ed. F. Robicsek), p. 387. MacMillan, New York.

—— (1978). Natural history and classification of occlusive thromboaortopathy (Takayasu's disease). *Circulation* **57**, 27–35.

—— (1981). Survival and morbidity after diagnosis of occlusive thromboaortopathy (Takayasu's disease). *Am. J. Cardiol.* **47**, 1026–1032.

——, and Matsuura, S. (1982). Occlusive thromboaortopathy (Takayasu's disease) and pregnancy: clinical course and management of 33 pregnancies and deliveries. *Am. J. Cardiol.* **50**, 1293–1300.

——, Uyama, M. and Asayama, K. (1983). Occlusive thromboaortopathy (Takayasu's disease): cervical arterial stenoses, retinal arterial pressure, retinal microaneurysms and prognosis. *Stroke* **14**, 730–735.

Judge, R. D., Currier, R. D., Gracie, W. A. and Figley, M. M. (1962). Takayasu's arteritis and the aortic arch syndrome. *Am. J. Med.* **32**, 379–392.

Kieffer, E. and Natali, J. (1983). Supraaortic trunk lesions in Takayasu's arteritis. In *Cerebrovascular insufficiency* (eds J. J. Bergan and J. S. T. Yao), pp. 395–415. Grune and Stratton, New York.

Kimoto, S. (1979). The history and present status of aortic surgery in Japan: particularly for aortitis syndrome. *J. Cardiovasc. Surg.* **20**, 107–126.

Lande, A. and Rossi, P. (1975). The value of total aortography in the diagnosis of Takayasu's arteritis. *Radiology* **114**, 287–297.

Liu Yu-Qing and Du Jia-Hui (1984). Aorto-arteritis: a collective angiographic experience in 244 cases. *Int. Angio.* **3**, 487–497.

Lupi-Herrera, E., Sánchez-Torres, G., Marcushamer, J., Mispireta, J., Horwitz, S. and Vela, J. E. (1977). Takayasu's arteritis: clinical study of 107 cases. *Am. Heart J.* **93**, 94–103.

Nakao, K., Ikeda, M., Kimata, S., Niitani, H., Miyahara, M., Ishimi, Z., Hashiba, K., Takeda, Y., Ozawa, T., Matsushita, S. and Kuramochi, M. (1967). Takayasu's arteritis: clinical report of eighty-four cases and immunological studies of seven cases. *Circulation* **35**, 1141–1155.

Nasu, T. (1982). Takayasu's truncoarteritis: pulseless disease or aortitis syndrome. *Acta pathol. Jpn* **32** (suppl. 1), 117–131.

Paloheimo, J. A. (1967). Obstructive arteritis of Takayasu's type: clinical, roentgenological and laboratory studies on 36 patients. *Acta med. Scand.* (Suppl.) **468**, 1–45.

Pokrovsky, A. V. and Tsyreshkin, M. D. (1975). Nonspecific aorto-arteritis. *J. Cardiovasc. Surg.* **16**, 181–191.

Sen, P. K., Kinare, S. G., Kelkar, M. D. and Parulkar, G. B. (1973). *Nonspecific aorto-arteritis: a monograph based on a study of 101 cases.* Tata McGraw-Hill, Bombay, New Delhi.

Strachan, R. W. (1964). The natural history of Takayasu's arteriopathy. *Q. J. Med.* **33**, 57–69.

Takayasu, M. (1908). A case with peculiar changes of the central retinal vessels. *Acta soc. ophthal. Jpn* **12**, 554–555 (in Japanese).

Teoh, P. C., Tan, L. K. A., Chia, B. L., Chao, T. C., Tambyah, J. A. and Feng, P. H. (1978). Non-specific aorto-arteritis in Singapore with special reference to hypertension. *Am. Heart J.* **95**, 683–690.

Wong, V. C. W., Wang, R. Y. C. and Tse, T. F. (1983). Pregnancy and Takayasu's arteritis. *Am. J. Med.* **75**, 597–601.

SPECIFIC HEART MUSCLE DISORDERS

C. M. OAKLEY

Definition

The term 'specific' here refers to heart muscle diseases of known cause or associated with disorders of other systems, in contrast to those conditions described on page 13.209. The heart may be involved in many systemic illnesses but disorders of the myocardium caused by systemic or pulmonary hypertension, coronary artery disease, valvular, or congenital anomalies are excluded from this account.

Functional classification (Table 1)

These specific heart muscle disorders may result in weakness of the contractile force of the heart and lead to *dilatation*, may give rise to or simulate *hypertrophy*, or the malfunction may lead to *restriction* of filling. Diaphragmatic weakness in some myopathies may lead to chronic underventilation and *cor pulmonale*. The myocardium is usually diffusely involved but may be focally infil-

trated or damaged. Distinction from a cardiomyopathy is mandatory, as many cases of heart muscle disease can be helped by specific treatment. Endomyocardial biopsy has particular application in these disorders because the histology may be diagnostic.

In most of the specific heart muscle disorders the myocardium shows a generalized reduction in contractile force with failure of ejection, an increase in the residual volume of blood in the ventricles, and consequent progressive dilatation. They thus fall into the same functional category as dilated cardiomyopathy. Myocarditis and sarcoid infiltration may result in *focal damage* to the myocardium, involving mainly the right ventricle in myocarditis or the inflow portion of the left ventricle in sarcoidosis.

In Friedreich's ataxia myocardial hypertrophy is similar to that occurring in hypertrophic cardiomyopathy.

Amyloid infiltration causes a pseudo-hypertrophy and in glycogen storage disease massive accumulation of glycogen swells the

Table 1 Functional classification

	Dilated	
Generalized		Focal
Alcoholic		Myocarditis
Cobalt		Sarcoid
Haemochromatosis		Dermatomyositis
Uraemic		
Phaeochromacytoma		Cor pulmonale
Selenium deficiency (Keshan disease)		Dystrophia myotonica
		Mitochondrial dystrophy
	Non-dilated	
Hypertrophic		Restrictive
Glycogen storage disease		Amyloid
Infants of diabetic mothers		Eosinophilic – Churg–Strauss
Friedreich's ataxia		Neoplastic
		Pseudoxanthoma elasticum
		Carcinoid
		Methysergide

Table 2 Viruses and rickettsiae associated with myocarditis

Viruses	
Enteroviruses	Coxsackie A and B
	Echo viruses
	Polio viruses
Arboviruses	Dengue
	Yellow fever
Influenza	
Herpesviruses	Herpes simplex
	Chickenpox
	Epstein–Barr
	Cytomegalovirus
Mumps	
Rabies	
Rickettsiae	
Chlamydia (psittacosis)	
Coxiella (Q fever)	
Scrub typhus	
Rocky mountain spotted fever	

muscle, reducing the left ventricular cavity size as well as interfering with ejection. Other infiltrations may also cause an increase in wall stiffness which restricts compensatory dilatation.

In carcinoid and methysergide heart disease the impact is on the endocardium, which becomes thickened and scarred with resulting lack of distensibility causing a restrictive picture and involving the heart valves.

The list of causes of myocardial disorder is daunting. Only the more important in which cardiac involvement may be a presenting or dominant feature will be described in detail.

Aetiological classification

Infective

Many viruses have been thought to cause myocarditis but not always with complete proof, and their relationship to chronic myocardial disease and dilated cardiomyopathy is even less clear. The commonest infection is with the Coxsackie group B viruses. Coxsackie group A viruses have also been identified and the emphasis may have been weighted by the ready availability of virological tests for the common group B enteroviruses whereas tests for the group A viruses are inconvenient and expensive. Many enteroviruses, arboviruses and others have been recorded (Table 2). Coxiella (Q fever) may cause either diffuse myocarditis or a focal injury such that it simulates myocardial infarction. Staphylococcal, streptococcal, or diphtheritic toxin may produce an acute reversible depression of myocardial function. Other agents include fungi such as aspergillus, protozoa in Chagas' disease and metazoa in filarial disease such as loa loa.

Metabolic

Important endocrine causes of heart muscle disorder include diabetes and thyroid heart disease (due to either increased or depressed thyroid function), adrenal cortical insufficiency, phaeochromocytoma, and acromegaly.

Storage diseases

The hereditary storage diseases (see page 9.31) include the glycogen storage diseases, Hurler's syndrome, Niemann–Pick disease, Refsum's syndrome, Hand–Schüller–Christian disease, Fabry–Anderson disease, and Morquio–Ullrich disease.

Infiltrations and granulomas

Haemochromatosis, amyloid, and sarcoid heart diseases are the most important of these.

Connective tissue disorders

These include dermatomyositis and systemic sclerosis, systemic lupus erythematosus, polyarteritis nodosa (particularly the Churg–Strauss variant), and rheumatoid arthritis.

Muscular dystrophies and neuromuscular dystrophies

Muscular dystrophies include Duchenne's pseudo-hypertrophic muscular dystrophy, dystrophia myotonica, facioscapulohumeral dystrophy, and the mitochondrial dystrophies. Friedreich's ataxia is a neuromuscular dystrophy with a high incidence of cardiac abnormality.

Sensitivity and toxic reactions

Drugs can cause cardiac damage, especially some of the cytotoxic drugs including particularly the anthracyclines. Others are the antimonials and emetine and the naturally occurring or synthetic sympathomimetic drugs such as isoprenaline. Alcohol and the barbiturates depress myocardial contractile force. Cobalt is a powerful myocardial poison.

Physical agents

Mediastinal irradiation may damage the pericardium, the coronary arteries, and the heart muscle.

Deficiency states

The most important of these is thiamine deficiency, producing beri-beri heart disease, but heart failure is otherwise not caused by starvation. Deficiency of potassium and magnesium can cause myocardial change and arrhythmias. Nutritional deprivation may lead to myocardial atrophy, prolonged QT arrhythmia, and sudden death in anorexia nervosa. Selenium deficiency (Keshan disease) in China causes myocardial failure with dilatation of the heart.

MYOCARDITIS

Myocarditis is an inflammation of the myocyte with or without vasculitis. The myocardium may be damaged in three ways: (a) by direct invasion of the myocyte as in virus myocarditis; (b) by depression of myocardial contraction and of the specialized conducting tissue by bacterial toxins, classically as in diphtheritic myocarditis but rarely also in staphylococcal and streptococcal infections; and (c) by induction of immunopathological processes.

VIRUS MYOCARDITIS

Virus myocarditis is common but the problems of recognition are considerable. Many (perhaps most) cases are missed, particularly when they are mild. Sudden death sometimes reported in the convalescent phase after influenza may be of this cause. By the time the signs of a cardiac disorder are recognized the virus has usually disappeared from pharynx and fauces and the diagnosis has to be made indirectly on antibody titres. The febrile illnesses caused by arboviruses are characterized by myalgia, and this was also the

Table 3 Virological investigation of myocarditis

Throat swab – up to 7 days
Faeces – up to 14 days
Myocardial biopsy
Pericardial fluid
Serological tests – three specimens one week apart

typical feature of Bornholm disease (epidemic pleurodynia or epidemic myalgia) caused by Coxsackie B. It has been pointed out that severe myalgic pain occurring in the course of a virus infection is suggestive of damage to skeletal muscle and hence of possible myocarditis.

Viraemia occurs commonly in virus infections but the heart is only occasionally overtly damaged. Influenza, mumps, and Epstein–Barr viruses probably are also important causes of myocarditis (see Table 2).

Clinical features

The clinical picture of myocarditis is non-specific but fatigue, dyspnoea, palpitation, precordial discomfort, and skeletal myalgia may occur. Examination may reveal tachycardia out of proportion to fever and a third heart sound gallop but at this stage the heart is usually of normal size although congestive features may be seen on the chest radiograph. Conduction defects and arrhythmias may occur and sudden death during influenza outbreaks is well known. Emboli are rare. Electrocardiographic abnormalities are usually transient, with repolarization changes and occasionally conduction defects. If there is associated pericarditis, an underlying myocarditis may be obscured both clinically and on the ECG. It should be suspected when pericarditis is associated with a low output state in the absence of tamponade. When the diagnosis is suspected, cross-sectional echocardiography will confirm it by showing poor contraction of a minimally dilated or normal-sized left ventricle; the changes may be remarkably focal, sometimes involving predominantly the right ventricle. There may be a pericardial effusion even in patients without pericardial pain or a rub.

Live virus probably disappears from the myocardium by six to 10 days (Table 3). A few patients may die at this stage from pump failure, and post-mortem reveals gross myocardial destruction and massive cellular infiltration. Live virus can be recovered. The inflammatory reaction disappears in approximately three weeks. About 75 per cent of patients with clinically overt myocarditis recover fully in a few weeks but sometimes not for up to six months or longer after the illness. Perhaps 10–25 per cent of patients develop progressive heart failure, and if first seen at this stage then they are clinically indistinguishable from patients with dilated cardiomyopathy. This sequence has been reported following dengue fever with myocarditis from Sri Lanka as well as in England following enterovirus infection which is particularly common and lethal in infancy.

Endomyocardial biopsy should be undertaken as soon as the diagnosis is suspected clinically in order to have the best chance of obtaining virus in very early cases or evidence of myocardial destruction or myocytolysis with cellular infiltration in subacute cases (Fig. 1). Later on, sampling errors may become more important and inflammatory infiltrates may be missed.

Treatment

The prospect of preventing progression to chronic heart failure was first encouraged by reports from Stanford that inflammatory infiltrate disappeared after the use of immunosuppressive treatment with steroids and azathioprine only to reappear when this treatment was stopped. The disappearance of inflammatory infiltrates coincided with clinical and functional improvement in the patients. Early excitement and optimism has not been supported in later experience: spontaneous improvement was found to occur in a high proportion of patients presenting with a short history of

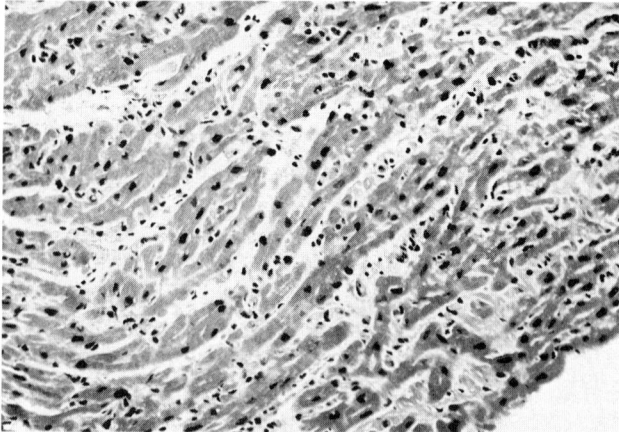

Fig. 1 Photomicrograph of an endomyocardial biopsy from an infant presenting with heart failure. The myocardial fibres are in regular alignment and show evidence of some hypertrophy. The interstitium is widened in which chronic inflammatory cells can be seen. The changes are those of resolving (healing) myocarditis. These features are seen in patients with dilated cardiomyopathy in whom an infectious–immune mechanism is operative. Haematoxylin and eosin × 320. (I am grateful to Dr E. G. J. Olsen for this figure).

symptoms but this improvement did not coincide with biopsy features of myocarditis nor with the use or not of immunosuppressive therapy.

Steroids have been used to treat inflammatory heart disease since the use of cortisone in acute rheumatic fever in which it was not shown to influence the course of the disease. Similarly, cortisone has been used in relapsing pericarditis and the postcardiotomy syndrome when it undoubtedly suppresses the episode although it does not prevent recurrence.

Immunosuppressive treatment should probably be used in patients with a short history, who are very sick, and who have a raised ESR, raised immunoglobulins, and a positive biopsy. Such treatment has not been found to be detrimental even though recent work suggests that virus may still be present in the myocardium by this stage, contrary to previous belief. It is possible, therefore, that Acyclovir or interferon may be helpful at least in early cases. This use of immunosuppressive treatment in acute and subacute myocarditis or in 'acute' dilated cardiomyopathy with a short history should not be applied to patients with chronic dilated cardiomyopathy in whom no evidence of benefit has been shown.

Constrictive pericarditis may develop quite quickly in patients with acute myopericarditis, the venous pressure rising as the heart shadow shrinks on X-ray, and pulmonary congestive changes usually disappear. Such patients usually do very well after pericardiectomy. The absence of any evidence of previous pericarditis in the majority of patients with dilated cardiomyopathy makes it unlikely that in any but a few of these patients is the origin of their disease a previous virus infection, although such an infection may have triggered deterioration of a previously subclinical disease.

There has been interest recently in the chronic illness produced by Epstein–Barr virus, which can cause acute myocarditis. Evidence of this should be sought in patients with chronic ill health and cardiac abnormality following glandular fever.

Features in favour of myocarditis in patients presenting with a clinical picture of dilated cardiomyopathy are:

1. Youth of the patient, with siblings also affected.
2. A short history of acute febrile illness with myalgia at the start.
3. Presentation with only modest cardiac enlargement or with ventricular tachycardia.
4. Raised serum antibody titres to Coxsackie B, mumps, or other viruses.

Table 4 Differential diagnosis of myocardial failure in infancy and childhood

Cardiomyopathies
Endocardial fibroelastosis
Dilated cardiomyopathy
Severe hypertrophic cardiomyopathy with heart failure
The infantile form of cardiomyopathy with histiocytoid change
Restrictive cardiomyopathy with giant atria

Specific heart muscle diseases
Subacute myocarditis
Inherited storage diseases; e.g. Pompe's disease (glycogen storage)
In association with skeletal myopathy, neuromuscular disease or
  polymyositis

Structural heart disease
Anomalous origin of the left coronary artery
Japanese mucocutaneous disease (Kawasaki's disease)

5. Predominant involvement of the right ventricle, sometimes with ventricular tachycardia of right ventricular origin.

6. Focal abnormality seen on ventriculography or on cross-sectional echocardiography.

7. Myocytolysis, fragmentation, and marked cellular infiltration or fibrous tissue replacement seen on biopsy.

8. Hot spots seen on gallium-67 scintigraphy. An increased myocardial uptake of the isotope suggests myocardial inflammation.

Differential diagnosis of myocardial failure in infancy and childhood (Table 4)

Outbreaks of virus infection sometimes occur in maternity and neonatal units after introduction of one of the common enteroviruses by a visitor or staff member. Severe generalized infection in the neonate leads to a severe multisystem illness with lethargy, fever, pharyngitis, acute myocarditis, heart failure, and death, or complete recovery. Such outbreaks are uncommon in developing countries where enteroviruses are more prevalent and therefore newborn children are protected by passively transferred maternal antibodies.

Older children usually produce fever, pharyngitis, and myalgia, sometimes with precordial pain, tachycardia, and dyspnoea. Conduction defects may develop.

Pericarditis is uncommon in young children but produces an acute illness, rarely causing tamponade but sometimes proceeding rapidly to constrictive pericarditis. Chronic heart failure may occur in a few, without intervening pericarditis (Fig. 2). This is sometimes predominantly right ventricular and may be seen also in siblings. Immunosuppressive therapy may be helpful in these cases.

The differential diagnosis includes the infantile form of cardiomyopathy with histiocytoid change. This produces a picture of dilated cardiomyopathy in childhood with a rapidly downhill course and no preceding febrile illness. Characteristic features are seen on biopsy but there is no specific treatment.

Infants surviving endocardial fibroelastosis may go on into a stable asymptomatic disorder in which the left ventricle is chronically dilated but the stroke output and filling pressures may be insufficiently abnormal to generate symptoms. Such patients may survive into adult life or die suddenly from arrhythmia. The diagnosis may be made from recognition of the smooth, highly echo-reflective endocardial lining to the dilated thick-walled left ventricle seen on the short axis view on echocardiography or from the biopsy. Severe hypertrophic cardiomyopathy may present with heart failure but is easily recognized by echo or angiogram as the left ventricle is not dilated and hypertrophy is usually extreme.

Some children may present with heart failure, greatly dilated atria, and a high ventricular filling pressure on the left and the right sides of the heart but without either left ventricular dilatation or hypertrophy and without evidence of endomyocardial fibrosis. The cause of this rare but characteristic picture is unknown.

Congenital anomalies of the coronary arteries should be sought and excluded. Origin of the left coronary artery or a part of it from the pulmonary artery may be missed if not routinely sought during cardiac catheterization and angiocardiography in young patients presenting with left ventricular failure. The ECG sometimes provides a clue but may be non-specific or show only left bundle branch block. Kawasaki's disease (Japanese mucocutaneous disease) (see page 24.1) may permit survival after the acute illness of childhood. Coronary artery involvement with thrombosis, aneurysm formation or narrowing may have given rise to marked left ventricular malfunction or infarction simulating a dilated cardiomyopathy. Kawasaki's disease has been seen in many parts of the world remote from Japan and is not confined to children of Japanese ethnic origin. There may be a place for coronary bypass surgery in rare instances of this condition.

Children with skeletal myopathies are usually all too obviously weak but occasionally milder familial proximal limb girdle myopathies, facioscapulohumeral myopathy, or a mitochondrial dystrophy may be associated with a myocardial disorder at a time when the skeletal myopathy is not readily apparent. Weakness of the diaphragm may cause chronic hypoventilation with pulmonary hypertension and cor pulmonale (Table 5).

Rickettsial myocarditis

Myocarditis commonly complicates infection by chlamydia (psittacosis) causing heart failure and pericarditis (see page 5.355). Fatal

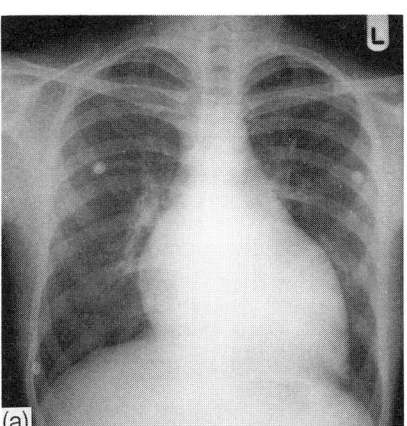
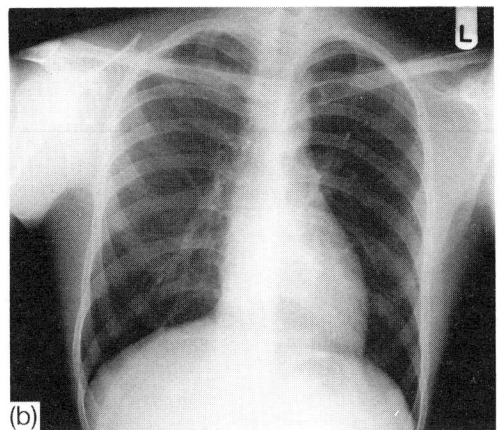
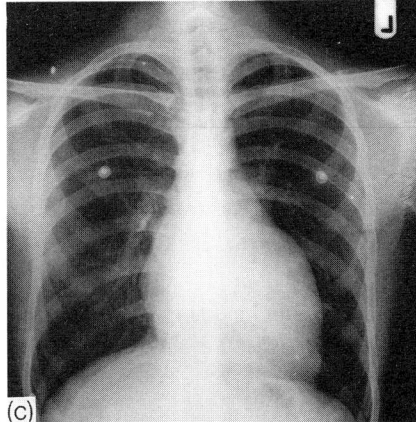

Fig. 2 Sequential chest radiographs from a boy who developed myocarditis with heart failure (*a*) but subsequently improved and became symptom-free with a nearly normal left ventricle (*b*). A year later he again went into heart failure with recurrent ventricular tachycardia which was successfully suppressed with amiodarone (*c*) but the heart remains enlarged.

Table 5 Heredofamilial myopathic, myotonic, and neurological dystrophies in which cardiac disorder may develop

---

Progressive muscular dystrophies
X-linked:
　　Early onset, rapidly progressive (Duchenne)
　　Late onset, slowly progressive (Becker)
Autosomal recessive
Limb girdle (Erb's)
Facioscapulohumeral (Landouzy–Déjérine)
Progressive external ophthalmoplegia (Kearns Sayre)
Mitochondrial

Myotonic
Dystrophia myotonica (myotonia atrophica)

Neurological
Friedreich's ataxia
Hereditary polyneuropathy (Roussy–Lévy)
X-linked humeroperoneal neuromuscular disease
Juvenile spinal muscular atrophy

---

cases show a fibrinous pericarditis with lymphocyte and plasmayte infiltration of the myocardium, interstitial oedema, and subendocardial haemorrhages. Myocarditis is less common in Coxiella (Q fever) infection but a severe focal myocarditis even mimicking acute myocardial infarction has been described. Myocarditis is common in scrub typhus but is rarely severe clinically except in occasional epidemics. The pathology is of a widespread vasculitis involving small vessels.

Bacterial myocarditis
Whereas a virus myocarditis is usually due to direct invasion of the myocyte or to subsequent immunopathology bacterial myocarditis is usually due to bacterial toxin.

Diphtheria
Myocarditis is said to occur in a quarter of cases of diphtheria, and is often fatal. The toxin causes an acute, profound depression of myocardial contraction, often with conduction defects or heart block.

Clinically the signs of cardiac abnormality appear after about a week of illness, with the development of gallop rhythm, heart failure, and elevation of serum cardiac enzymes. Electrocardiographic abnormalities include arrhythmias, bundle branch block, and various grades of atrioventricular block. Repolarization changes are seen. Some patients recover fully, but others show persisting cardiomegaly. The electrocardiographic changes persist longer than the clinical signs.

Treatment should be by the immediate administration of antitoxin with penicillin. If complete atrioventricular block develops, a temporary transvenous pacemaker may be required.

At autopsy the heart muscle is flabby and pale and the chambers are dilated. Microscopy shows fatty infiltration of the myocytes and myocytolysis. An interstitial infiltrate often involves the conducting system in focal areas.

Streptococcus
The cardiac involvement which may follow beta-haemolytic streptococcal infection in predisposed subjects is acute rheumatic fever (see pages 5.168 and 13.277), and this occurs about three weeks after the onset of a streptococcal pharyngitis which has usually been severe and memorable. Direct infection of the heart by the streptococcus is rare at the time of the acute infection but used to be seen when scarlet fever was common. With the modern use of cross-sectional echocardiography we have begun to realize that acute global depression of left ventricular function may be seen during the course of bacterial endocarditis caused by streptococci of the *viridans* group. This is transient and recovers with treatment of the infection. It is presumably caused by bacterial toxin.

Meningococcus
Myocardial involvement is common in meningococcal septicaemia (see page 5.199), with a haemorrhagic myocarditis sometimes associated with intracellular meningococci as well as interstitial myocarditis. Heart failure may be fatal. Purulent pericarditis is common in infancy and may cause rapid tamponade and death.

Spirochaetal infection
Myocarditis may also occur in spirochaetal infections, particularly in Weil's disease (leptospirosis) (see page 5.327).

Protozoal myocarditis (Chagas' disease)
This is discussed on page 13.230.

Heart muscle disease in diabetes
It is well known that the risk of coronary heart disease is increased both in insulin-dependent and in non-insulin-dependent maturity-onset diabetes and that impaired glucose tolerance is frequently discovered in patients with coronary disease (see page 9.51). Diabetics have more atheromatous arterial disease than non-diabetics and they also develop microvascular disease causing diabetic retinopathy, nephropathy, and autonomic and peripheral neuropathy. It is perhaps less well known that they can develop microvascular disease in the heart, and in the Framingham Study it was found that heart failure occurred more frequently than in the non-diabetic population. Microvascular disease is not always easily recognized pathologically and has been the subject of much controversy in the understanding of hypertrophic cardiomyopathy, the heart muscle disease which occurs in Friedreich's ataxia and in syndrome X.

Microvascular disease in the hearts of diabetics was unrecognized for a long time, but, in the young insulin-dependent diabetic, cardiac abnormalities may be found in association with normal extramural coronary arteries. In older diabetics there may be a combination of atheroma and small-vessel disease leading to a reduction of left ventricular function which is excessive for the amount of coronary disease shown on angiography and possibly accounting for the higher mortality of diabetics following coronary bypass surgery compared with non-diabetics.

The small vessels show intimal proliferation and wall thickening with perivascular and interstitial fibrosis. Thickening of the capillary basement membrane has been recognized on electron microscopy, and capillary microaneurysms have been seen in the heart. These cardiac abnormalities usually coexist with microvascular disease in other organ systems.

The recognition of a myocardial microangiopathy was delayed not only because of difficulty in interpreting the pathology but also because the resulting disturbance in function is often subtle and less obvious than, for instance, visual failure resulting from retinal microvascular disease. Until microangiopathy in the heart is advanced the main abnormalities are diastolic with prolongation of the isovolumic relaxation time, resulting in delayed mitral valve opening. In later cases systolic time intervals are also abnormal with prolonged pre-ejection periods and shortened left ventricular ejection time associated with a reduced stroke volume.

Thyroid heart disease
Myxoedema (see page 10.30) is a cause of pericardial effusion, either massive or small, and of heart failure with bradycardia. Subclinical hypothyroidism is common, particularly in the elderly; its correction increases well-being and does not usually intensify anginal symptoms in those with coronary disease.

It is well known that thyrotoxicosis may present with atrial fibrillation and heart failure, and, like hypothyroidism, is not always obvious in older patients. Uncertainty has existed about the cause of heart failure in thyrotoxicosis. It may be attributed to fast ventricular rates in atrial fibrillation which are often poorly controlled by digitalis (see page 13.101). Recent studies have clearly indicated a group of thyrotoxics with depressed left ventricular myocardial function and heart failure which could not be attributed to atrial fibrillation. In them control of the ventricular rate with beta blockers precipitated heart failure whereas in other thyrotoxics administration of beta blockers resulted in an improvement in heart failure which coincided with slowing of the ventricular rate. This indicates that in some patients with thyrotoxicosis cardiac function is depressed and dependent on beta-adrenergic drive. They tend to be older and to have had symptoms of thyrotoxicosis for a long time before diagnosis.

Heart failure in thyrotoxicosis in sinus rhythm is seen occasionally in young people and, like the older ones, they usually have evidence also of proximal skeletal muscle weakness. Both the myocardial failure and the skeletal myopathies improve with correction of the hyperthyroid state.

Rats to whom tri-iodothyroxine (triac) was administered during pregnancy produced offspring showing myocardial hypertrophy. This has been cited as a possible model for hypertrophic cardiomyopathy, but evidence of hypertrophy is minimal in patients with thyrotoxic heart disease and patients with hypertrophic cardiomyopathy are rarely hyperthyroid.

Phaeochromocytoma

Phaeochromocytoma (see page 13.392) may present with recurrent ventricular tachycardia or with normotensive heart failure. It has been associated with marked hypertrophy in the absence of persistent hypertension although probably caused by it. It may then simulate hypertrophic cardiomyopathy. This cause should always be considered in patients with unexplained myocardial syndromes, especially if treatment of heart failure is associated with a rise in blood pressure. Removal of a large phaeochromocytoma was associated with complete resolution of the cardiac abnormality in a 19-year-old boy referred with a diagnosis of probable myocarditis and profound heart failure.

Haemochromatosis and haemosiderosis

Haemochromatosis (see Section 19) is a familial disorder characterized by excessive deposition of iron in many parenchymal tissues. Haemosiderosis develops in association with regular blood transfusion and the iron-loading anaemias.

The heart is dilated and myocardial iron deposits condense in the subepicardium followed by the subendocardium and papillary muscles. The iron deposits are perinuclear but may eventually cover much of the myocyte. Myocardial degeneration and fibrosis develop. The severity of the myocardial dysfunction is proportional to the amount of iron present.

The clinical picture of haemochromatosis is that of a dilated cardiomyopathy in a patient who may have slate grey discoloration of the skin, diabetes mellitus, and gonadal atrophy. The plasma iron level and percentage transferrin saturation are elevated. The ferritin levels are greatly increased in nearly all untreated patients. Occasional younger patients may show none of these features but present with seemingly rather acute heart failure associated with only mild dilatation, high filling pressures, and a restrictive picture of low output failure.

It is possible to mobilize myocardial iron by repeated phlebotomy and to show this on serial endomyocardial biopsy. Improvement in cardiac function can be dramatic in the younger patient with a short history of cardiac symptoms just as it can result in improvement in liver function and the alleviation of diabetes. In older subjects little or no improvement in heart failure may be seen.

Transfusional haemosiderosis may give rise to chronic heart disease. In chronic anaemia it may be difficult to determine whether the chronic anaemia or the associated myocardial haemosiderosis is responsible for the myocardial dysfunction. In these patients, unlike those with familial haemochromatosis, the amount of iron in the heart is roughly proportional to the amount of iron in other organs, and this can be determined easily by liver biopsy.

Chelation of iron by desferrioxamine is useful in thalassaemia and in other anaemias which have to be managed by repeated blood transfusion. This topic is considered in detail in Section 19.

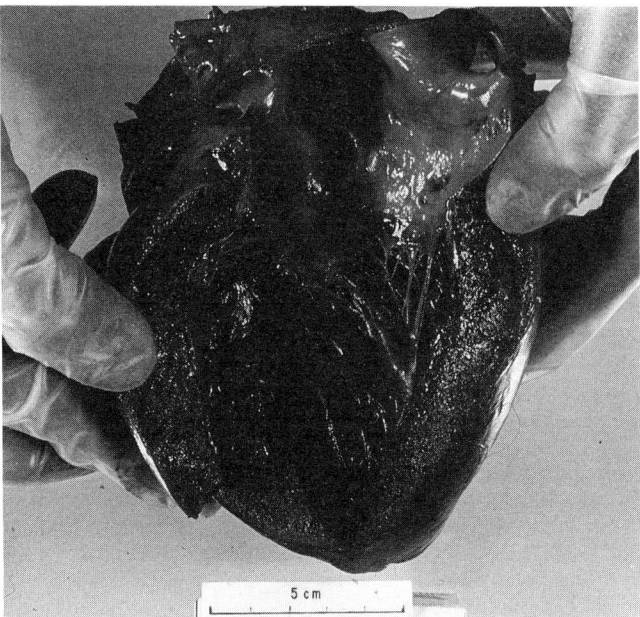

Fig. 3 Cardiac amyloidosis. The muscle is thickened and the cut surface has a 'lardaceous' look. The cavity is not dilated and contains prominent papillary muscles and trabeculae.

AMYLOID HEART DISEASE

Amyloid (see page 9.145) is an abnormal fibrillar protein which can be deposited in almost any organ of the body, although clinical heart disease is not usually recognized until there is extensive cardiac infiltration. Several different types of amyloid fibrils have been distinguished. The amyloid associated with an immunocyte dyscrasia is composed of immunoglobulin light chains whereas in reactive and in familial forms the major protein component varies but is not an immunoglobulin. Senile amyloid is different again. The differing forms of the amyloid fibrils are identified by distinctive light and electron microscopic appearances.

Cardiac involvement is common both in primary amyloid and in amyloidosis associated with multiple myeloma in which it is the commonest cause of death. In reactive amyloidosis clinically significant cardiac involvement is uncommon because the myocardial deposits are typically small and perivascular. In familial amyloidosis (except for the cardiopathic form) the heart is only occasionally overtly involved, and in familial Mediterranean fever death is usually from renal failure but although cardiac involvement is uncommon it can be massive and the cause of heart failure even in the second or third decade. In senile amyloidosis the deposits do not usually result in functional impairment, but occasionally extensive ventricular deposition causes heart failure and may contribute to the susceptibility of the elderly heart to heart failure from seemingly little provocation.

Cardiac amyloidosis is commoner in men than in women, is rare below the age of 40, and is usually seen in the sixth and seventh decades. This contrasts with reactive and familial amyloidosis which affect a younger age group.

Pathology

The heart is overweight but little enlarged, the ventricular wall being thickened but the cavities undilated. The heart may be so firm that its normal shape is retained on the post-mortem table. Its consistency is rubbery and the general appearance of the heart is often not unlike that in hypertrophic cardiomyopathy. The cut surface may have a lardaceous look (Fig. 3). There may be petechiae on the outside of the heart and sometimes a pericardial effusion. Amyloid may be deposited in the valves, which may be thickened.

Table 6 Echocardiographic features of amyloid heart disease

Normal or reduced left ventricular end-diastolic cavity dimension
Normal or increased left ventricular end-systolic dimension
Increased left ventricular wall thickness
Reduced amplitude of left ventricular septal and posterior wall motion
Reduced systolic thickening of left ventricular wall
Increase in thickness of the right ventricular wall
Increase in thickness of the atrial septum
Increase in thickness of valves
Reduced excursion of the mitral valve
Pericardial effusion is frequent
'Granular sparkle' indicating increase in echo-reflectivity of the
  myocardium

In rare cases in which the amyloid is almost confined to the walls of blood vessels the heart may be dilated.

Microscopically, amyloid is found between the myocardial fibres. Extensive deposition in the papillary muscles can lead to clinical mitral or tricuspid regurgitation. Amyloid deposits in the sinoatrial and atrioventricular nodes and the bundle branches explain the frequency of sinoatrial disease, the seemingly excessive sensitivity to digitalis, and the frequency of fascicular blocks on the ECG. Endocardial infiltration is common, sometimes with overlying thrombosis which may lead to embolism. The amyloid material is deposited in and around the walls of the capillaries and small arteries and veins, and may compromise the lumen of arteries, so causing angina. The characteristic staining reactions of primary amyloid are often atypical and the iodine reaction may be negative in the autopsy room. The usual apple green stain with congo red and metachromatic reaction to methyl violet may also be uncharacteristic, and in such cases may lead to the diagnosis being missed even on cardiac biopsy. In such instances electron microscopy reveals the typical fibrillar formation of the amyloid.

Clinical features

Cardiac amyloidosis usually presents with fatigue, shortness of breath or oedema, sometimes with angina, and usually with clinical evidence of heart failure. Involvement of the conducting tissue, low blood pressure, and digitalis intoxication may all contribute to syncope which can be a presenting feature. Sometimes the patient presents with petechiae or haemorrhages into the skin where this is the seat of amyloid infiltration. These are usually periorbital on the face and on the neck and arms (Fig. 4). The tongue can be so enlarged that it leads to dysarthria. The muscles may be weak and, rarely, they may even be enlarged. The lymph nodes are sometimes infiltrated; perineural deposition may lead to a clinical neuropathy and palpable peripheral nerves. Involvement of

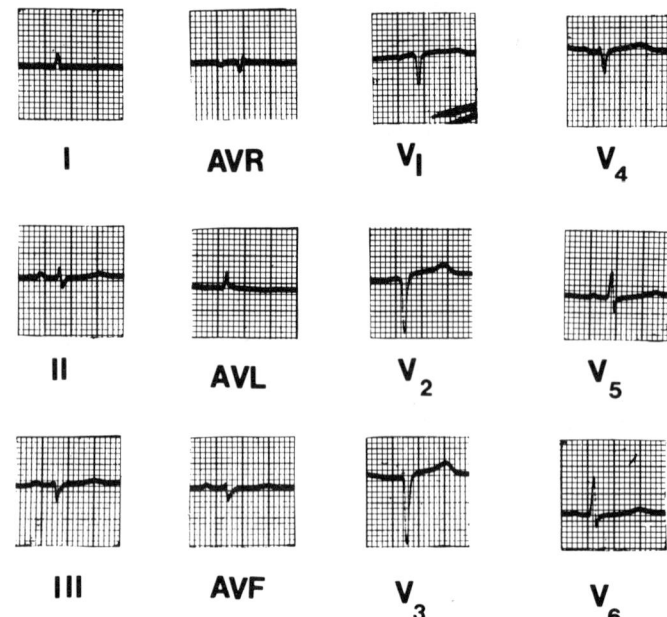

Fig. 5 ECG in amyloid heart disease showing sinus rhythm and extremely low voltage QRS with, in this case, only minor intraventricular conduction defect.

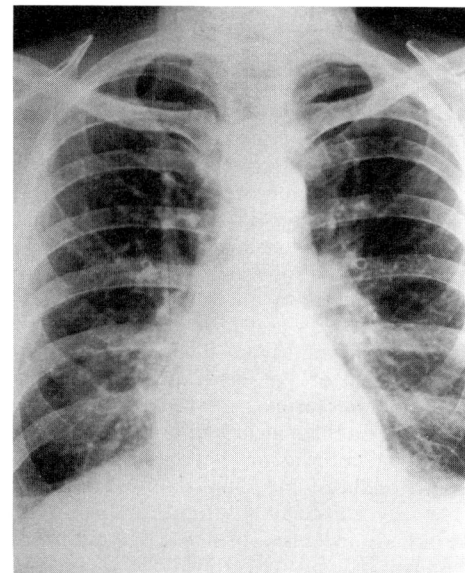

Fig. 6 Chest radiograph in amyloid heart disease. The patient, a man of 64, had been admitted to the coronary care unit with chest pain and suspected myocardial infarction. The heart size is normal but there is gross pulmonary venous congestion.

smooth muscle in the gastrointestinal tract may lead either to constipation or to diarrhoea. The liver is usually enlarged but the spleen is rarely palpable.

The blood pressure is characteristically low and the pulse pressure small. Bradycardia with 2:1 or complete heart block is not uncommon and further reduces an already low cardiac output. The high venous pressure in the neck usually shows a small amplitude pulsation but occasionally a v-wave due to tricuspid regurgitation. The cardiac impulse is quiet or impalpable; typically there are no murmurs and no added sounds although a right ventricular third sound may be heard at the left sternal edge. This tends to disappear if the venous pressure is brought down with diuretics.

These clinical features are explained by the association of systolic and diastolic malfunction without cavity dilatation. This combination determines extremely low stroke output with maximum

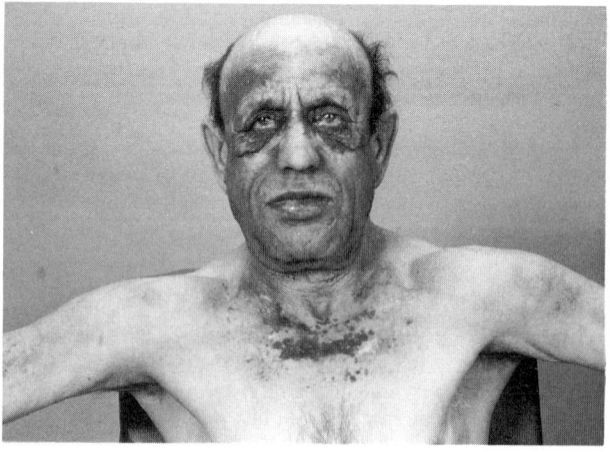

Fig. 4 A 69-year-old man with cardiac amyloidosis. Cutaneous petechiae and enlargement of the lips, tongue, and deltoid muscles were also the result of amyloid infiltration.

minute output achieved only between a very small range of heart rates, tachycardia reducing the stroke volume because of slow filling and bradycardia increasing hypotension because of the small stroke volume. Investigations reflect these haemodynamic abnormalities.

The ECG usually shows strikingly low ventricular voltage and, in the context of the clinical signs, it may be virtually diagnostic (Fig. 5). Q-waves suggesting infarction and atrioventricular and intraventricular conduction defects are common; fascicular blocks may raise the low voltage somewhat. The chest X-ray usually shows a normal or only slightly enlarged heart with pulmonary venous congestion and dilated superior vena cava (Fig. 6). Occasionally the heart shadow is much enlarged because of an associated pericardial effusion.

In the atypical cases with mainly or exclusively intravascular amyloid deposition the clinical and investigational features may be non-specific.

The echocardiographic features also reflect the functional impairment and are usually diagnostic in themselves (Table 6 and Figs 7 and 8). Normal or diminished left ventricular dimensions are associated with reduced amplitude of excursion and great increase in thickness of left and right ventricular walls, sometimes with increased echo reflectivity of the muscle, the so-called 'granular sparkle'. The valve cusps are characteristically thickened but otherwise the valves look normal. There may be a pericardial effusion.

The haemodynamic findings are of greatly increased ventricular filling pressures, usually much higher on the left than on the right side, and there may be moderate pulmonary hypertension (Fig. 9). The early diastolic pressure is raised and left ventricular

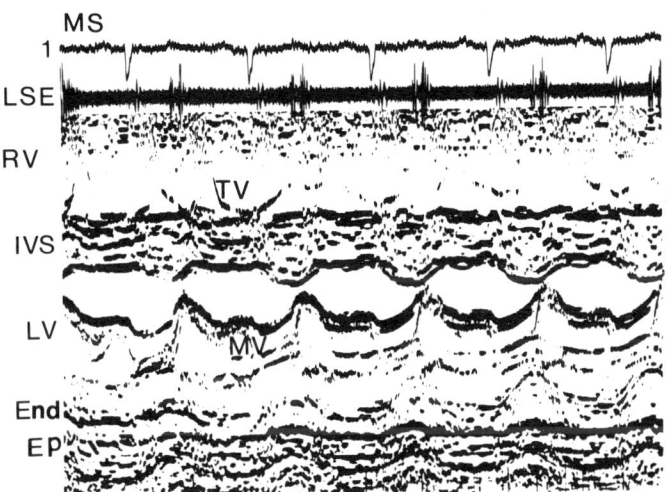

Fig. 7 M-mode echocardiogram in amyloid heart disease showing the features listed in Table 4. From above, ECG (1), phonocardiogram at left sternal edge (LSE) showing widely split second heart sound and no added sounds, thick right ventricle (RV), slightly dilated ventricle showing tricuspid valve (TV), thickened septum (IVS), small left ventricle (LV) with reduced mitral valve excursion (MV), and hypokinetic posterior wall endocardium (End), and epicardium (EP).

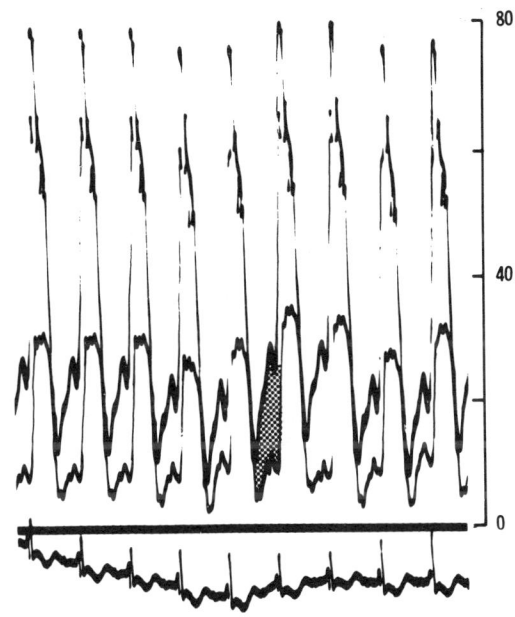

Fig. 9 Simultaneously recorded right and left ventricular pressures (RV and LV) in amyloid heart disease showing that the diastolic pressure in the LV is higher than that in the RV throughout diastole. There was pulmonary hypertension (RV pressure was 60 mmHg) and systemic hypotension (LV pressure under 80 mmHg).

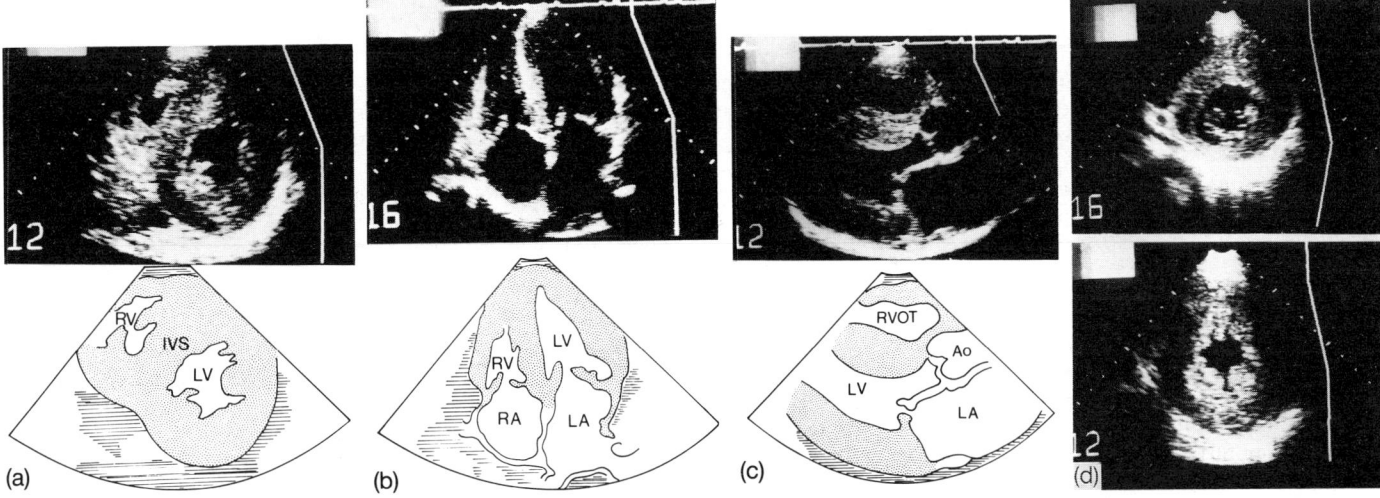

Fig. 8 Cross-sectional echocardiograms in cardiac amyloidosis showing thickened highly echo-reflective walls, small cavities, and thickened valves. (a) Subcostal short axis view of the left and right ventricles. (b) Apical four chamber view. (c) Long axis view. The resemblance to hypertrophic cardiomyopathy (page 13.221) is apparent but the generalized thickening of the valves is seen only in amyloid. (d) Short axis views of the left ventricle: above, at papillary muscle level; below, distal to the papillary muscles. Ao = aorta; IVS = thickened septum; LA = left atrium; LV = left ventricle; RA = right atrium; RV = right ventricle; RVOT = right ventricular outflow tract.

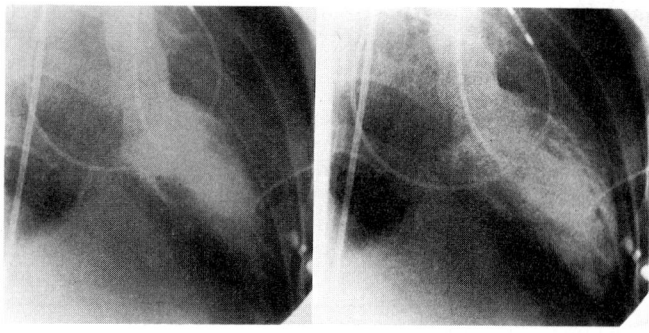

Fig. 10 Left ventricular angiograms from a patient with amyloid heart disease, right agnterior oblique view: systnole on the left, diastole on the right. Note the pacing catheter in the right ventricular outflow tact. The poverty of movement and exaggerated papillary muscles are evident but at first glance the ventriculogram may look normal.

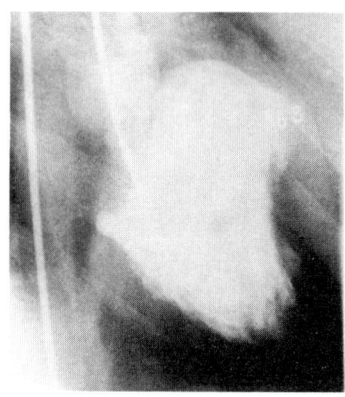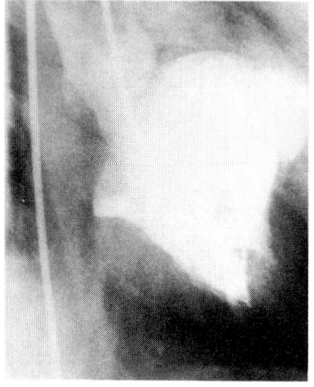

Fig. 11 Left ventricular angiocardiogram in sarcoidosis (right anterior oblique view: diastole on the left, systole on the right) showing gross distortion with proximal dilatation and dyskinesia.

filling continues throughout diastole, so there is no diastolic plateau or square root sign and there is often a considerable a-wave. The features are all unlike constrictive pericarditis, to which there may be a superficial clinical similarity. Systolic function is reduced and a low ejection fraction in the face of a reduced end-diastolic volume accounts for a typically very small stroke volume. During the early stages these volumes may still be normal.

The angiographic appearances are also characteristic and mirror the post-mortem appearance with an undilated left ventricle and marked papillary muscle impressions but no distortion of cavity shape. The trabecular pattern is markedly coarse and gives a shaggy outline (Fig. 10). Systolic emptying is usually depressed but the angiographic appearance may look deceptively normal.

The diagnosis can be confirmed by endomyocardial biopsy. Biopsies of rectum, gingival, or other tissues may be positive but are not invariably so. Because of the frequency of atypical staining reactions, electron microscopic examination is essential.

Treatment

Treatment is ineffective because there is as yet no known way in which to halt the progression of the underlying infiltration. Digitalis should not be used because of the enhanced risk of toxicity and because it does not help if the patient is in sinus rhythm. Diuretics should be used with caution because reduction of the high venous pressure may further reduce forward output but sufficient should be given to relieve uncomfortable oedema. Vasodilators lead to a fall in blood pressure because of inability to augment stroke volume. Patients with bradycardia due to conducting system disease may be helped for a time by implantation of a pacemaker.

While colchicine may result in some removal of the reactive amyloid in familial Mediterranean fever there is no evidence that

any drugs influence the progress of the heart disease in primary amyloidosis or in amyloidosis associated with myeloma. Cardiac transplantation may be contemplated in younger patients who have no evidence of significant amyloid in other vital organs but the time course of the presumably inevitable reappearance of amyloid is still quite unknown.

CARDIAC SARCOIDOSIS

Cardiac involvement is not often recognized clinically in sarcoidosis (see page 5.623) although sarcoid granulomata may be found in the heart in 20–30 per cent of those with the disease at autopsy. Clinical manifestations of cardiac abnormality may even be absent when myocardial involvement is massive. This is because it is focal and contraction of the unaffected part of the ventricle is normal or enhanced. Myocardial sarcoid may result in ventricular arrhythmia, heart block, heart failure, or sudden death. Infiltration of the papillary muscles of the mitral valve resulted in severe mitral regurgitation in one patient, and in another subendothelial deposition in the mitral leaflets caused gross swelling and mitral obstruction. Both of these patients required valve replacement.

The most common presentations are either with ventricular arrhythmias or with heart failure. Ventricular arrhythmias may be associated with normal ventricular function and small granulomata or with massive replacement of myocardium. When this occurs its site typically is in the proximal part of the left ventricle, leading to gross or even aneurysmal dilatation of the proximal ventricle with normal or hyperactive contraction of the apex. This produces an easily recognizable echocardiographic and angiographic picture (Fig. 11). Cardiac biopsy may be negative because of sampling error. There is no effective treatment although steroids are usually given, and there may be no way of knowing whether the disease in the heart is still advancing. Because of the high mortality of cardiac sarcoidosis and the unpredictability of fatal ventricular arrhythmias with this condition, transplantation should be contemplated if there is no important or active disease in the lungs.

ALCOHOL-RELATED HEART DISEASE

Alcohol may cause myocardial damage by three different mechanisms:

1. Associated nutritional defects, particularly of thiamine.
2. Toxic effects due to additives such as cobalt.
3. A direct toxic effect.

Beri-beri heart disease

Beri-beri heart disease may occur in alcoholics but this is a high output failure with rapid heart rate and wide pulse pressure which usually responds completely to thiamine. It is important to consider thiamine deficiency in the alcoholic patient and to give adequate multivitamin B supplementation, but few alcoholics in the United Kingdom are malnourished, vitamin deficient, or derelicts, and many hold down good jobs.

Toxic effects due to additives

The addition of cobalt to beer to stabilize the 'head' led to outbreaks of heart failure among heavy beer drinkers in Canada and Belgium in the 1960s. The 'beer drinker's cardiomyopathy' was seen only in heavy labourers who took most of their daily calories as beer and had associated protein malnutrition. They pursued a rapid downhill course after onset with characteristically widespread myocytolysis seen on microscopy. This disorder is now only of historic interest since discovery of its cause, which was a story of persistent investigation against strenuous opposition from the breweries.

Lead contamination of 'moonshine' has also been implicated in causing a heart disorder in its drinkers.

Direct effects of alcohol

Acute effects

Acute administration of alcohol leads to depression of myocardial contractile force with reduction in left ventricular ejection fraction. This effect is most marked in non-drinkers. Larger doses are required to induce any demonstrable reduction in cardiac function in otherwise fit chronic alcoholics but in chronic alcoholics with a cardiomyopathy an acute challenge with alcohol causes more depression than in non-alcoholics with normal hearts.

The same effects have been shown in experimental animals. A reduction in left ventricular contractile force with dilatation and a fall in stroke output can be measured in conscious chronically instrumented dogs after intravenous infusion of alcohol to blood levels below 150 mg/dl. The intensity of the depression is directly related to blood level and is reversible within 15–30 minutes by haemodialysis. Multiple arrhythmias, ectopic beats, or sustained supraventricular or ventricular tachycardia can also be induced by acute administration and the ECG may develop splintering of the QRS and QT prolongation.

The clinical effects of acute alcohol loading are seen as paroxysmal atrial fibrillation, ventricular ectopic beats, or even ventricular tachycardia. The arrhythmias soon disappear, leaving no other evidence of heart disease, but moderate conduction delays have been seen on high speed high fidelity ECG for up to a week after restoration of sinus rhythm. This 'holiday heart' syndrome is well recognized in countries such as Finland in which heavy drinking is common at weekends, and physicians there are familiar with hospital admission of cases of atrial fibrillation on Mondays.

Binge drinking should always be considered as the possible cause of seemingly 'lone' or recurrent atrial fibrillation in otherwise fit people.

Reduction in systolic and diastolic function of the heart with reduced ejection fraction and increased left ventricular wall stiffness has been shown in non-invasive studies of alcoholic subjects without cardiac symptoms. Invasive studies have shown an abnormal rise in left ventricular filling pressure following afterload stress with angiotensin.

Chronic alcohol-related heart disease

It is uncertain whether alcohol plays a causal or only a precipitating or conditioning role in the development of some cases of dilated cardiomyopathy. Uncertainty concerning the contribution of alcohol to chronic myocardial disease persists because of the impossibility of differentiating between alcohol- and non-alcohol-related cardiomyopathy except by the amount of alcohol said to be consumed.

Arrhythmias in predisposed drinkers have not been shown to presage the development of chronic cardiomyopathy. The difficulties in recognition of alcoholic heart disease are because clinical, laboratory, and pathological findings do not differentiate it from dilated cardiomyopathy. Whilst cardiac biopsies have shown recognizable changes associated with acute infusion of alcohol this does not prove that alcohol causes chronic damage, and nearly all cardiac pathologists agree that they cannot recognize alcoholic from non-alcoholic dilated cardiomyopathy. Some recent claims of increased levels of various enzymes in biopsies from patients with probable alcoholic heart disease compared with non-alcohol-associated dilated cardiomyopathy await confirmation.

Alcohol can cause changes in skeletal muscle, and chronic alcoholics have been shown to develop proximal muscle weakness caused by reduction in the number of type 2 muscle fibres. This is partially reversible after a period of abstinence. Chronic drinkers suffer from the continuous effect of alcohol on the myocardium, and the observation that alcoholic cardiomyopathy improves after abstinence is in keeping with withdrawal of a drug effect. The peak incidence of dilated cardiomyopathy is in middle-aged males who are the group amongst whom chronic heavy alcohol consumption is most common. It has been suggested on no good evidence that 100 g of alcohol per day for ten years is required for the development of alcoholic heart disease but the proportion of such heavy drinkers who develop cardiomyopathy is not known.

Further problems in linking alcohol with chronic heart muscle disease include the observations that heart disease is uncommon in alcoholics with cirrhosis. The teratogenic potential of alcohol is exemplified in the fetal alcohol syndrome but the fetal myocardium has not been shown to be abnormal.

A WHO committee in 1980 admitted that at present one cannot define a causal versus a conditioning role of alcohol and it seems likely that alcohol may be one of several contributory causes of dilated cardiomyopathy in predisposed individuals. We are ignorant both of the frequency of subclinical myocardial malfunction and of its causes. Following apparent recovery from virus myocarditis the myocardium may remain vulnerable if alcohol consumption becomes high in later years. Chronic high alcohol consumption may lead to a state of continued myocardial depression which, although initially reversible through abstinence, eventually becomes progressive once the left ventricle has dilated beyond a certain point.

Complete abstinence from alcohol is mandatory in all patients with dilated cardiomyopathy whether or not it is thought to be of alcoholic origin because, whatever the role played by alcohol, it is certain that alcohol is bad for bad hearts. Cessation of drinking may halt progression in some cases and may even be followed by improvement.

INHERITED STORAGE DISEASES

Fabry's disease

Fabry's disease (see page 9.34) is an X-linked disorder of metabolism characterized by intracellular deposition of a neutral glycolipid in skin, kidney, and myocardium.

The cardiovascular manifestations are variable due to accumulation in myocardium, conducting tissue, mitral valve, and coronary arteries. Renal hypertension may further complicate the clinical picture. Affected subjects are male, and female carriers are usually asymptomatic.

Gaucher's disease

Gaucher's disease (see page 9.33) is a rare disorder of metabolism which results in deposition of cerebrosides in many organs, including the myocardium. This can cause left ventricular systolic and diastolic dysfunction, but clinical evidence of heart involvement is uncommon.

THE HEART IN COLLAGEN VASCULAR DISORDERS

Rheumatoid disease

There is a high incidence of heart disease in rheumatoid arthritis (see page 16.3) which can be classified as:

1. Primary:
   (a) Specific granulomatous;
   (b) Non-specific, e.g. cellular infiltration and fibrosis.
2. Secondary:
   (a) Complicating disease, e.g. amyloid;
   (b) Resulting from rheumatoid involvement of other organs, e.g. the lungs.
3. Pericardial effusion (see page 13.304). Pericardial effusion is very common. While constriction occurs only rarely it is very important as a surgically remediable cause of congestive failure usually occurring in severe active rheumatoid disease.

Systemic lupus erythematosus (SLE)

A key pathological lesion of SLE (see page 16.20) is a diffuse microvasculitis. The heart is commonly involved at autopsy but clinical attention usually is drawn to it only when there is a pericardial rub or effusion, myocardial failure, or murmur due to endocardial involvement. Routine study of SLE patients without overt heart disease using modern non-invasive techniques reveals abnormalities in the majority. Pericarditis is the commonest complication.

The effusion may be clear or blood stained, tamponade may occur or constriction develop. Myocardial abnormalities are very common and are caused by the microangiopathy which may particularly involve the specialized conducting tissue, giving rise to sinoatrial or atrioventricular conduction defects and arrhythmias. Hypertension may compound the myocardial problem. Pulmonary hypertension is not uncommon, especially in patients in whom the 'lupus anticoagulant' can be detected and coronary thrombosis may occur.

The classical Libman–Sacks endocarditis is very rare as a clinical entity but is common at post-mortem examination. It is detectable on echocardiography and may become complicated by infection, which can be occult in steroid-treated patients.

The mitral valve is involved much more often than the aortic, and the wart-like lesions may occur anywhere on the valves. Secondary platelet fibrin aggregates may break off and embolize. Only rarely does marked scarring and deformity develop but mitral stenosis or regurgitation can lead to a need for valve replacement.

Polyarteritis nodosa (PAN)

Involvement of the coronary arteries by PAN (see page 16.28) can cause infarction leading to fibrosis and cardiac failure. Pericarditis can occur with a haemorrhagic and inflammatory exudate. In the Churg–Strauss variant with eosinophilia, endomyocardial disease or even acute myocardial failure may occur.

Scleroderma (diffuse systemic sclerosis)

Involvement of the heart is common, often subclinical but detectable if systolic time intervals are determined and echo measurements are made. Cor pulmonale caused by pulmonary fibrosis, pulmonary hypertension, and systemic hypertension may coexist and can obscure primary involvement, which is caused by coronary intimal sclerosis involving small vessels and consequent diffuse fibrosis. Left ventricular dilatation is progressive and the heart may become very large with all four chambers fibrotic, big, and baggy. Conduction system abnormalities are common.

Myocardial abnormalities and cardiac failure may also occur in Reiter's syndrome (often with aortic regurgitation). Behçet's syndrome, ulcerative colitis, and Whipple's disease.

HEREDOFAMILIAL MYOPATHIC, MYOTONIC, AND NEUROLOGICAL DISORDERS

Cardiac abnormality occurs in the progressive muscular dystrophies, in dystrophia myotonica, and in Freidreich's ataxia (see Table 6). Heart block may occasionally be the presenting problem in patients who are subsequently found to have neuromuscular disorders such as progressive external ophthalmoplegia with pigmentary retinopathy (Kearns–Sayre), dystrophia myotonica, or peroneal muscular atrophy. Others present with conduction system faults plus myocardial disease and are found to have a previously undetected neuromuscular condition such as limb girdle dystrophy. In some patients cardiac complications bring to light their skeletal muscle disease. Rarely, the mothers of patients with Duchenne's X-linked muscular dystrophy have a clinically important dilated cardiomyopathy rather than the more usual abnormalities in the ECG alone. A search should therefore be made for coexisting neuromuscular disease, in young patients who present with conduction system defects or with dilated cardiomyopathy.

Polymyositis

The heart may be involved in polymyositis (see page 16.48) and in dermatomyositis, more commonly in adults than in children, and electrocardiographic abnormality is more common than a clinical heart disorder. Rhythm disturbances and conduction abnormalities occur. Clinical heart failure or mitral regurgitation, probably secondary to papillary muscle involvement, are both rare. Autopsy shows degeneration of elements of the cardiac conducting system and occasionally changes in the myocardium similar to those in skeletal muscle, sometimes with a fibrinous pericarditis.

Friedreich's ataxia

Friedreich's ataxia is a hereditary spinocerebellar degeneration involving the posterior columns and spinocerebellar tracts. It is inherited as an autosomal recessive with onset usually early in the second decade and is relentlessly progressive. It has been estimated that between 10 and 50 per cent of patients show clinical cardiac abnormality and nearly 100 per cent have abnormalities in the electrocardiogram or echocardiogram. There are cardiac abnormalities at necropsy in nearly all, and two-thirds of patients die suddenly. In a few, evidence of heart disease appears before neurological manifestations. More often immobility, kyphoscoliosis, hypoventilation, and chest infections from reduction of intercostal and diaphragmatic muscle power all delay recognition of the cardiac disorder. The earliest sign may be sinus tachycardia but arrhythmia, angina, or the onset of heart failure are the most common presenting features.

At necropsy the heart is found to show left ventricular hypertrophy which is usually concentric even when asymmetrical septal hypertrophy has been documented in life by echo studies. There is hypertrophy of myocardial fibres, interstitial fibrosis, and vagal degeneration.

The clinical features are similar to those of hypertrophic cardiomyopathy but rhythm disturbances are particularly common and the deformed chest and thinness of the subject combine to modify the physical signs. The electrocardiogram usually shows left ventricular hypertrophy and repolarization changes. An echocardiogram may show marked hypertrophy, systolic anterior motion of the mitral valve, and systolic closure of the aortic valve. Left ventricular catheterization shows a raised end-diastolic pressure in the left ventricle and sometimes an outflow tract gradient either at rest or on provocation.

The relationship between the neurological disease and the heart disease remains speculative, the possible common link being an abnormality of the sympathetic nervous system.

Dystrophia myotonica

Dystrophia myotonica (see Section 21) is a progressive multisystem disorder inherited via an autosomal dominant gene whose manifestations are usually delayed until the third or fourth decade. The patients develop a cardiac disorder in about two-thirds of cases. It is recognized more often on the electrocardiogram than clinically, and abnormalities incude sinus bradycardia, tachybrady syndrome, long PR interval, left axis deviation, or left bundle branch block. In addition, there may be repolarization abnormalities or pseudo-infarction pattern. The heart may be enlarged and heart failure may occur, especially if there is an inappropriate bradycardia. Adams–Stokes attacks may develop and a permanent pacemaker may be needed. Diaphragmatic involvement may lead to cor pulmonale from hypoventilation with hypoxaemia, hypercapnoea, pulmonary hypertension, and fluid retention. At necropsy the heart may be enlarged but the myocardium usually appears normal both grossly and under the microscope, although cellular infiltration and interstitial fibrosis have been found with changes in mitochondria and sarcoplasmic reticulum on electron microscopy.

It is thought that the specialized conduction system of the heart is specifically affected in dystrophia myotonica. There is no evidence that the myocardium can manifest myotonia, and in myotonia congenita the heart remains normal. Studies have shown fibrosis of the sinus node and atrioventricular node as well as changes in the bundle of His and bundle branches. It seems, therefore, that the cardiac involvement is a non-myopathic and non-myotonic feature.

Progressive muscular dystrophies

Duchenne's pseudohypertrophic muscular dystrophy (see Section 21) is transmitted by a sex-linked recessive gene from a clinically unaffected mother. Frequent sporadic cases also occur due to new mutations. The onset of symptoms is within the first decade and deterioration is rapid. The muscular dystrophy affects the intercostal muscles and diaphragm. Cardiac abnormalities are an important cause of death but are often masked by scoliosis and frequent chest infections. Death may be sudden or follow progressive heart failure. Electrocardiographic abnormalities are often detected first and the heart size is hard to interpret on a chest X-ray on account of high diaphragms, scoliosis, and a shallow anteroposterior diameter. Sinus tachycardia and arrhythmias are common and the ECG shows a distinctive abnormality specific to the Duchenne disease with tall R-waves in the right chest leads and deep Q-waves in the left precordial leads and limb leads. It is of interest that unaffected female carriers show similar tracings. These changes cannot therefore be explained by thoracic deformity or pulmonary hypertension and there is no hypertrophy of the right ventricle or septum to be found at autopsy. It is thought that the ECG changes reflect a myocardial dystrophy which has a rather constant form. Echocardiography has shown a decrease in posterior left ventricular wall motion which may be in keeping with this theory but, although copious skeletal muscle CPK is released into the plasma, increased concentrations of the cardiac isoenzyme CPK MB are not found.

At necropsy there is sometimes selective scarring in the posterobasal portion of the left ventricle, occasionally extending to the lateral and inferior walls. The small intramural coronary arteries show marked hypertrophy of the media. These changes cannot be held responsible for focal fibrosis since they are generalized.

Other progressive muscular dystrophies

Heart failure may occur in the other progressive muscular dystrophies, including those in which the skeletal muscle dystrophy is mild and only slowly progressive. This has led to the speculation that some cases of apparently isolated dilated cardiomyopathy may be associated with an unrecognized skeletal myopathy.

Cor pulmonale may cause heart failure in muscular dystrophies due to sometimes unrecognized severe diaphragmatic involvement and chronic underventilation. Blood gases should always be checked when heart failure or pulmonary hypertension is seen in a patient with a muscular dystrophy.

Guillain–Barré syndrome

Involvement of intercostal muscles and diaphragm frequently leads to a need for mechanical ventilation. Involvement of autonomic nerves to the heart may be associated with a fixed fast heart rate.

HEART DISEASE CAUSED BY CANCER CHEMOTHERAPY

Cardiac toxicity used to be a rare complication of chemotherapy for neoplastic disease. Vincristine has been associated with the development of myocardial infarction from coronary thrombosis and sometimes causes pulmonary hypertension. Busulphan can cause pulmonary and endocardial fibrosis and some secondary pulmonary hypertension. It was only with the advent of the anthracycline group of drugs that serious cardiac toxicity became a major problem and the limiting factor to the use of these agents.

Adriamycin and daunorubicin are among the most successful agents in the treeatment of some forms of leukaemia, Hodgkin's disease, and solid tumours. Concern about cardiac toxicity has led in some instances to inadequate antitumour treatment whereas other patients have died from cardiac failure induced by these drugs while in complete remission from their disease. The cardiac toxicity is dose dependent, although somewhat unpredictable, and older hearts are much more susceptible. Myocardial dysfunction may occur at two phases of treatment. The first occurs early after the introduction of anthracycline therapy but recovers on temporarily stopping treatment and does not necessarily recur. The second and much more serious type of heart failure relates to cumulative effects of the drug and is refractory to treatment.

When it is severe, survival is short and often under two weeks. In surviving cases cardiac disability may persist.

Cardiac complications are rare in patients receiving less than a cumulative dose of under 500 mg/m^2 body surface area although some instances have been reported. This had led to the suggestion that a combination of anthracycline with other agents such as cyclophosphamide or radiation may have been synergistic in the pathogenesis of cardiac damage.

Pathology

Pathological examination discloses a dilated, pale, and flabby heart, sometimes with mural thrombi. The coronary arteries and valves appear normal. Microscopy reveals a gross reduction in the number of myocytes, degenerative changes in the surviving cells, and fibrosis. Electron microscopy shows reduction in the number of myofibrils, distortion, and breakage of the Z-lines. The mitochondria are distinctly swollen with disrupted cristae containing inclusion bodies. These features have led to the adoption of serial endomyocardial biopsy for the early detection of cardiac damage.

Clinical features

The onset of cardiac failure is usually delayed for between three and six months or even up to three years after the start of treatment but frequently occurs soon after a second course has become necessary because of relapse. The heart failure develops remarkably suddenly, being signalled by sinus tachycardia, fall in blood pressure, dyspnoea, tachypnoea, and gallop rhythm without congestive features. The chest radiograph usually shows little or no cardiac enlargement but some pulmonary venous congestion. Death may be remarkably swift. In the less severely afflicted who survive longer, progressive cardiac dilatation and fluid retention develop. The initial response to diuretics may be good but deterioration usually follows. Early electrocardiographic changes are important, consisting in a fall in voltage only later followed by prolongation of the QRS and repolarization abnormalities. Arrhythmias may occur.

Attempts to recognize the cardiac damage before it has become irreversibly progressive have included measurement of systolic time intervals, serial right heart catheterization, measurement of the cardiac output and pressures, and, most recently, myocardial biopsies. Prolongation of the pre-ejection period/left ventricular ejection time ratio occurs early but often exhibits a threshold phenomenon and therefore is oversensitive. Equally, nuclear changes detected by biopsy antedate clinical disturbance which may never happen, so this also is too sensitive. Attention to QRS voltage on the ECG, to the development of a third heart sound gallop, and to serial echo measurements of left ventricular activity are most useful.

The mechanism of cardiac toxicity is not completely known but is thought to be related to binding of drug to DNA in nuclei and mitochondria. The bound drug is excreted only very slowly from the cell and, since the myocyte cannot reproduce itself, any inhibition of protein synthesis resulting from anthracycline-induced alteration in the DNA template might be very long lasting. Cumulative interference with the processes of normal protein regeneration could explain the delayed onset of toxicity and also the observation that the elderly are most susceptible and children least likely to develop toxicity.

Adriamycin remains one of the best drugs for the treatment of acute myeloblastic leukaemia, and increasing experience with its use has greatly reduced the incidence of serious cardiac toxicity. This has been achieved by wider spacing between individual treatments and careful clinical cardiac examinations. Less cardiotoxic analogues have now been developed.

Irradiation of the heart

The heart may be damaged during radiotherapy to the mediastinum in lymphoma or to the internal mammary nodes in carcinoma of the breast. Although modern techniques have minimized the damage, it still occurs and is seen as acute pericarditis, chronic serous effusions, constrictive pericarditis, right ventricular fibrosis, and occlusion of the anterior descending or right coronary arteries involved in the irradiation fields.

Drug- and toxin-induced endomyocardial fibrosis
Several drugs can cause damage to the endocardium but none causes disease which is identical to endomyocardial fibrosis. Busulphan and methysergide, as well as the anthracycline group of drugs, are known to cause cardiac damage which can involve the endocardium; in long-term survivors of anthracycline and busulphan toxicity, cardiac restriction from endocardial fibrosis may predominate.

Methysergide cardiac toxicity Methysergide damages the valvar endocardium, predominantly of the left side of the heart. It induces mitral regurgitation and stenosis from fleshy swelling and fibrosis of the leaflets together with aortic valve and general endocardial involvement and sometimes mediastinal fibrosis, causing a restrictive syndrome similar to that of constrictive pericarditis.

Carcinoid heart disease In carcinoid heart disease the valves of the right side of the heart are involved predominantly by endocardial fibrosis which may cause tricuspid and pulmonary stenosis. The endocardial fibrosis, although prominent at autopsy, does not usually affect the clinical picture except by valve dysfunction. Mitral valve involvement may occur either from right-to-left shunting of hepatic vasoactive peptides across a patent foramen ovale or even in its absence when pulmonary inactivation of a large hepatic release of peptides is incomplete. Rarely, a lung carcinoid tumour has led to the development of mitral valve disease.

Patients with the carcinoid syndrome used to die in a cachectic state with massive hepatomegaly and there was little indication to consider surgical treatment for valve disease. Caudate lobe compression of the inferior vena cava plus diuretic therapy for the resulting leg oedema together with the inanition led to a low cardiac output state. This minimized the clinical signs, which were further reduced by the jutting ribs of the wasted patients and resultant difficulty in gaining good stethoscopic contact. Now, with effective hepatic embolization of the metastatic liver disease, patients are living longer and better but with more serious heart disease. This may be because the valvar obstruction progresses once it has started or simply because it is more obvious in otherwise well patients. Either way the propriety of cardiac investigation with a view to tricuspid and/or pulmonary valvuloplasty or replacement is not in doubt for patients hampered by cardiac disability and who have a reasonable prognosis otherwise.

Endomyocardial fibrosis in pseudoxanthoma elasticum
The best-known cardiac complication of pseudoxanthoma elasticum (see page 17.33) is coronary artery disease causing angina or infarction at a young age but, rarely, severe endomyocardial fibrosis may occur.

Keshan disease
Keshan disease occurs in a narrow belt from north-west to southeast China in rural areas with poor living conditions. Evidence has now accumulated that the disease is caused by deficiency of selenium. In affected areas the level of selenium in blood and hair is diminished. Young children and women of child-bearing age are most susceptible.

The disease occurs in acute, subacute, chronic, and latent forms. The acute disease often has a fulminating onset with a very high mortality. Hypotension, vomiting, and cardiogenic shock occur. In the chronic disease recurrent or persistent heart failure occurs with dilatation indistinguishable from that in dilated cardiomyopathy. Arrhythmias are common in both acute and chronic forms.

The pathological changes are confined to the heart with myocardial necrosis and replacement fibrosis. Myocytolysis is most prominent in patients who have died from the acute disease whilst fibrosis, most severe in the subendocardial part of the left ventricle, is prominent in the chronic form. The changes resemble those in dilated cardiomyopathy.

Since 1975 oral dietary supplements have been given on a large scale and very few recent cases of the disease have been reported.

Cardiac biopsy
Endomyocardial biopsy of the right or of the left ventricle may be carried out at low risk in young children and adults and, with special techniques, even in young infants. A bronchoscopic bioptome is passed through a long catheter sheath introduced percutaneously into the femoral vein. The left ventricle may be reached either by the trans-septal technique via the femoral vein or retrogradely from the femoral artery.

Biopsies of the right ventricle are probably safer because the right ventricle is trabeculated and the pincer action of the bioptome depends on grabbing a piece of projecting muscle between the jaws. The left ventricle, being smooth, is more likely to be perforated, particularly by the retrograde arterial technique which takes the bioptome towards the apex, whilst the trans-septal technique is more likely to take it to the left ventricular septum. The other hazard of left ventricular biopsy is thromboembolism.

Cardiac biopsy is of use in detecting or confirming the presence of specific heart muscle disease such as amyloid, sarcoid heart disease, or haemochromatosis. It is valuable in the distinction between myocarditis and dilated cardiomyopathy. We have not found it of value in assessing prognosis in dilated cardiomyopathy and have failed to confirm the work of the Düsseldorf school in relating histological and ultrastructural changes to prognosis. So far biochemistry including cell fractionation biochemistry has been disappointing in elucidating the mechanism of development of the myocardial fault in dilated cardiomyopathy but cell fractionation immunological study has had some exciting early results.

References
Abelman, W. H. (1973). Viral myocarditis and its sequelae. *Ann. Rev. Med.* **24**, 145–152.
Bell, E. and Grist, N. R. (1970). Echoviruses, carditis and acute pleurodynia. *Lancet* **1**, 326.
Bengtsson, E. and Lambergr, B. (1966). Five year follow-up study of cases suggestive of acute myocarditis. *Am. Heart J.* **72**, 751–763.
Benson, R. and Smith, J. F. (1956). Cardiac amyloidosis. *Br. Heart J.* **18**, 529–543.
Borer, J. S., Henry, W. L. and Epstein, S. E. (1977). Echocardiographic observations in patients with systemic infiltrative disease involving the heart. *Am. J. Cardiol.* **39**, 184–188.
Brockington, I. F. and Olsen, E. G. J. (1973). Löffler's endocarditis and Davies' endomyocardial fibrosis. *Am. Heart J.* **85**, 308–322.
Bulkley, B. H., Ridolfi, R. L. and Salyer, W. R. (1976). Myocardial lesions of progressive systemic sclerosis. *Circulation* **53**, 283–290.
—— and Roberts, E. C. (1975). The heart in systemic lupus erythematosus and the changes induced in it by corticosteroid therapy. *Am. J. Med.* **58**, 243–264.
Chew, C., Ziady, G. M., Raphael, M. J. and Oakley, C. M. (1975). The functional defect in amyloid heart disease. *Am. J. Cardiol.* **36**, 438–444.
Ferrans, V. J., McAllister H. A. and Halse, W. H. (1976). Infantile cardiomyopathy with histiocytoid change in cardiac muscle cells. *Circulation* **53**, 708–719.
Goodwin, J. F. (ed.) (1985). *Heart muscle disease.* MTP Press, Lancaster.
Greenwood, R. D., Nadas, A. S. and Fyler, D. C. (1976). The clinical course of primary myocardial disease in infants and children. *Am. Heart J.* **92**, 549–560.
Hejmancik, M. R., Wright, J. C., Quint, R. and Jennings, F. (1964). The cardiovascular manifestations of systemic lupus erythematosus. *Am. Heart J.* **68**, 119–130.
Isaacs, H. and Muncke, G. (1975). Idiopathic cardiomyopathy and skeletal muscle abnormality. *Am. Heart J.* **90**, 767–773.
Kawasaki, T., Kosaki, F., Okawa, S., Singematsu, L. and Yanagawa, H. (1974). A new infantile acute febrile mucocutaneous lymph node syndrome (MLNS) prevailing in Japan. *Pediatrics* **54**, 271.
Lebowitz, W. B. (1963). The heart in rheumatoid arthritis (rheumatoid disease). *Ann. intern. Med.* **58**, 102–123.

Letts, A. and Wulff, K. (1976). Myocardiopathy in Duchenne's progressive muscular dystrophy. *Acta paediat. Scand.* **65**, 28–32.

McCue, C. M., Mantakus, M. E., Tingelstad, J. B. and Ruddy, S. (1977). Congenital heart block in newborns of mothers with connective tissue disease. *Circulation* **56**, 82–89.

McDonald, C. D., Burch, G. E. and Walsh, J. J. (1971). Alcoholic cardiomyopathy managed with prolonged bed rest. *Ann. intern. Med.* **74**, 681–691.

McWhorter, J. E. and Carwite, E. (1974). Pericardial disease in scleroderma. *Am. J. Med.* **57**, 566–575.

Mason, J. W., Billingham, M. E. and Ricci, D. R. (1980). Treatment of acute inflammatory myocarditis assessed by endomyocardial biopsy. *Am. J. Cardiol.* **45**, 1037–1044.

Mercier, G. and Patry, G. (1967). Quebec beer drinkers' cardiomyopathy. *Can. Med. Assoc. J.* **97**, 884–928.

O'Connell, J. B., Robinson, J. A., Henkin, R. E. and Gunnar, R. M. (1981). Immunosuppressive therapy in patients with congestive cardiomyopathy and myocardial uptake of gallium-67. *Circulation* **64**, 780–785.

Perloff, J. K., deLeon, A. C. and Doherty, D. (1966). The cardiomyopathy of progressive muscular dystrophy. *Circulation* **33**, 625–648.

Regan, T. J., Ettinger, P. O., Haider, B., Ahmed, S. S., Oldewartel, H. A. and Lyons, M. M. (1977). The role of ethanol in cardiac disease. *Ann. Rev. Med.* **28**, 393–409.

Rubin, E. (1979). Alcoholic myopathy in heart and skeletal muscle. *N. Engl. J. Med.* **301**, 28–33.

Sackner, A., Heinz, E. R. and Steinberg, A. J. (1966). The heart in scleroderma *Am. J. Cardiol.* **17**, 242–259.

Smith, E. R., Sangalang, V. E., Hefferman, L. P., Welch, J. P. and Flemington, C. S. (1977). Hypertrophic cardiomyopathy: the heart disease of Friedreich's ataxia. *Am. Heart J.* **94**, 428–434.

Thoren, C. (1964). Cardiomyopathy in Friedreich's ataxia. *Acta paediat.* **153**, suppl. 1.

THE CARDIOMYOPATHIES

C. M. OAKLEY

Semantics

It is helpful to restrict the term *cardiomyopathy* to heart muscle diseases of unknown cause to emphasize the need to identify the cause, whether it affects the heart alone or is associated with general system disease. When the cause of a cardiomyopathy is identified it becomes a specific heart muscle disorder and is known by this (e.g. sarcoid heart disease) even though the precise aetiology of the disorder may still be obscure.

Disorders of the mycardium caused by systemic or pulmonary hypertension, coronary artery disease, valvular disease, or congential anomalies are therefore excluded.

The cardiomyopathies

Three categories can be identified by their distinctive haemodynamic and pathological characteristics (Fig. 1). The first two are (*a*) *dilated cardiomyopathy* (previously known as congestive cardiomyopathy) in which the malfunction is systolic; and (*b*) *hypertrophic cardiomyopathy* (previously known as idiopathic hypertrophic subaortic stenosis, muscular subaortic stenosis, obstructive cardiomyopathy, asymmetrical hypertrophy or asymmetric septal hypertrophy) in which the malfunction is diastolic. In (*c*) *restrictive cardiomyopathy* the fault is also diastolic and may be myocardial or involve the endocardium. In endomyocardial fibrosis, although the disorder is mainly of the endocardium and involves the atrioventricular valves, the disorder is conventionally regarded as a cardiomyopathy.

Certain disorders do not lend themselves readily to any classification. These include *peripartum* heart disease which may just be dilated cardiomyopathy with a temporal relationship to pregnancy acting as a precipitating factor. Another is *endocardial fibroelastosis* which has a specific pathology but may just be dilated cardiomyopathy with a temporal relationship to infancy.

DILATED CARDIOMYOPATHY

General description

The essential attribute is a reduction in contractile force of the left or right ventricle or both resulting in dilation. The ejection fraction (that proportion of the end-diastolic volume which is ejected at each beat and normally > 0.60 for the left ventricle) is usually profoundly reduced and most patients in whom the condition is recognized have an ejection fraction less than 0.40 with clinical heart failure. Disturbances of ventricular or atrial rhythm are common. Death usually occurs within two or three years of the development of heart failure and is related to the severity of the systolic malfunction and the size of the left ventricle. Death may be sudden, without preceding overt deterioration.

The condition is probably the outcome of a number of different factors operating in a susceptible subject. Previous myocarditis,

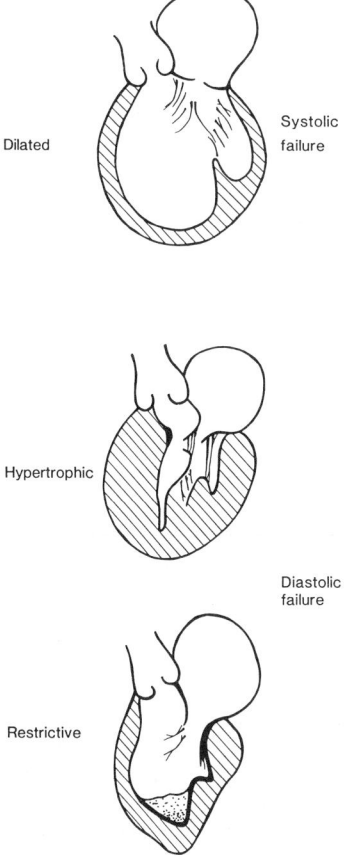

Dilated — Systolic failure

Hypertrophic

Diastolic failure

Restrictive

Fig. 1 The three functionally and pathologically distinct types of cardiomyopathy.

heavy alcohol intake, or hypertension may be important but it is frequently impossible to prove this.

Familial cases are rare; they are usually young and previous myocarditis should always be suspected when they are seen.

Pathology and pathogenesis

The heart is enlarged due to dilatation of the left ventricle and, usually, of all four cardiac chambers, but in some cases only the left ventricle or only the right ventricle is dilated together with its atrium. The weight is increased but the thickness of the left ventricular wall may be normal. The coronary arteries show little or no atheroma even though the disorder is commonest in middle-aged males. When coronary disease is present, distinction has to be made from coronary heart failure; when coronary disease is responsible for left ventricular failure luminal narrowing is usually severe in the major arteries and is associated with focal scarring.

The interior of the left ventricle shows flattening of trabeculae and thrombi in the crevices. The endocardium is usually thickened and patchily opaque but not to the extent seen in endocardial fibroelastosis.

Sometimes the left ventricular wall is greatly thickened; this is especially common in Africa where it gave rise to the term 'idiopathic cardiomegaly' and also a continuing discussion about the contribution of previous hypertension to an eventually normotensive heart failure. Proof of this is sometimes seen when treatment of the heart failure is followed by such improvement in output that sustained hypertension reappears. Modern treatment with afterload reducing agents may obscure this mechanism.

Microscopy shows nuclear changes of hypertrophy but the myocardial fibre diameters are usually normal because of attenuation. Interstitial fibrosis is seen and there may be focal replacement of myocardial fibres but, in contrast to myocarditis, there is usually little or no cellular infiltration. The subendocardium shows an excess of smooth muscle fibres and a variable amount of fibrosis. The small arteries and arterioles are normal. Specific histological changes are absent and the appearances differ very little from those in secondary hypertrophy with failure.

Electron microscopy shows an excess number of mitochondria and abnormal cristae but there are no other special features. Histochemical staining and analysis of subcellular fractions reveal changes in enzymes which are non-specific and secondary to heart failure.

Both humoral and cellular antibodies against myocardial antigens have been reported, as they have in myocarditis. This has been cited as evidence for an immunopathogenesis and causative role of previous myocarditis. The question is controversial. Evidence of previous viral invasion of the heart is usually lacking. Even when high antibody titres are found, the development of a viral myocarditis may have provided the final insult to convert a previously latent cardiomyopathy into one which is clinically overt. Evidence for viral initiation of the disease process has been largely circumstantial and the evidence for dilated cardiomyopathy being a disorder of cellular immunity related to a possibly infective cause has been challenged. Recent immunological studies of subcellular fractions have provided the strongest hints so far of an immunological basis for the disorder.

Incidence and geographic distribution

Dilated cardiomyopathy is common and world wide but the true incidence and geographical distribution are unknown. The reasons are the unknown number of subclinical cases which may exist and inaccurate diagnosis. In Denmark the incidence was estimated at 7 cases per 1 000 000 over all and 23 per 1 000 000 in middle-aged males. This contrasts with an estimated incidence in Malmo, Sweden, of between 50 and 100 cases per 1 000 000 judged clinically and at post-mortem. The big difference in the estimates between two countries with probably a similar population may only partly be accounted for by the exclusion of both alcoholic and early cases from the Danish estimate. The protean symptoms and signs of the condition, particularly in its less advanced forms, together with lack of familiarity with its frequency are responsible for diagnosis often favouring a more fashionable condition. In the West this would usually be coronary artery disease. In developing countries where cardiomyopathies are allegedly more frequent, the explanation may be the rarity of coronary artery disease and the lack of alternative diagnosis apart from hypertensive heart failure from which distinction may be impossible even at autopsy. Mortality figures would not provide a true indication of incidence even if death registration were accurate, as some cases pursue a latent or non-progressive course either indefinitely or until the development of some other cardiac disorders of ageing to which the problem may be attributed. Efforts to detect and treat early cases have been thwarted because mild or even moderate disease is usually asymptomatic. The lack of any simple diagnostic test which can be applied to the recognition of early disease would vitiate a population survey.

Although the disorder appears to be commonest in middle-aged men, the same group in which symptomatic coronary artery disease is most commonly seen, no age is spared. Dilated cardiomyopathy dominantly affecting the right ventricle, seems to be most common in the first two decades when past viral myocarditis may be suspected but often cannot be proved.

Presentation

Presentation is usually with heart failure, arrhythmia, or embolism. Shortness of breath, insidious or sudden and often with cough, may be mistaken for 'virus infection'. Chest pain is mentioned in about 10 per cent of patients. It is usually atypical but may suggest an ischaemic origin.

Any arrhythmia may occur, commonly atrial fibrillation which may precipitate failure, but sometimes supraventricular tachycardia or a ventricular arrhythmia, multiple ectopic beats, or ventricular tachycardia.

Systemic embolism may be the first evidence of the underlying cardiomyopathy. This may occur either in association with the onset of atrial fibrillation or with sinus rhythm. Pulmonary thromboembolism is common at an advanced stage but occasionally determines presentation.

The early symptoms of left ventricular failure may be wrongly ascribed to a chest infection because many of the patients have never previously been ill or indeed a chest infection may complicate pulmonary congestion and be the presenting illness. The development of an arrhythmia or systemic embolism in a previously fit subject should arouse suspicion of an underlying cardiomyopathy. Soft apical systolic murmurs are common due to a dilated left ventricle and mitral regurgitation.

Asymptomatic stage

Asymptomatic patients may be detected during an incidental medical examination because of a mitral regurgitant murmur, clinically evident left ventricular enlargement, or third or fourth heart sounds, an abnormality on the ECG, or cardiac enlargement on the chest radiograph. It is common, however, for such patients to have passed medical examinations without comment within the recent past.

Ejection fraction is depressed in these patients, usually to between 0.40 and 0.50, and echocardiography shows end-diastolic dimensions of between 5.5 and 6.5 cm.

The name 'latent cardiomyopathy' has been given to these patients whose prognosis is unknown. Many show stability during the years of follow-up whilst others show progressive deterioration in left ventricular function either gradually or quite suddenly.

Clinical features

The signs of dilated cardiomyopathy vary from no detectable abnormality to those of severe heart failure.

When the condition is recognized after the first episode of left ventricular failure the rhythm may be regular, perhaps with a

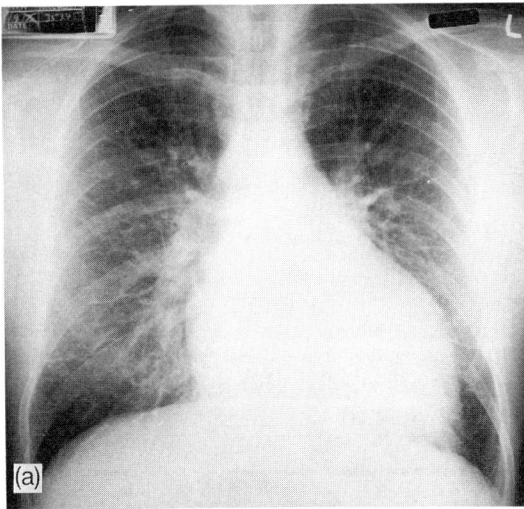

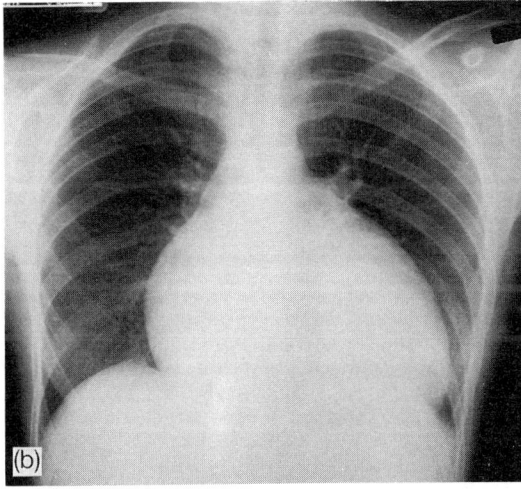

Fig. 2 (a) Typical chest radiograph in dilated cardiomyopathy at time of presentation in left ventricular failure. The left ventricle is greatly dilated and there are marked pulmonary congestive changes. (b) Chest radiograph from a 14-year-old girl with right ventricular cardiomyopathy. The right atrium and right ventricle were massively dilated but the left heart chambers appeared to be normal. The X-ray strongly suggests pericardial effusion but no effusion was present. The lung fields are clear.

slightly raised rate reflecting a reduced stroke, and pulsus alternans may be present. The blood pressure is usually normal but the pulse pressure may be low, with relatively increased diastolic pressure. The venous pressure in the neck is usually raised initially but rapidly falls to normal after a diuretic. The left ventricle is displaced and there may be a palpable fourth or third heart sound gallop. A mitral regurgitant murmur may be heard. There may be crackles at the lung bases.

Response to treatment is usually very rapid; all the abnormal signs may disappear and the patient become asymptomatic but the heart remains enlarged.

In patients who present with a rhythm change or systemic embolus, signs of heart failure may be either absent or ascribable to tachycardia. Evidence of the underlying myocardial fault may need to be sought by special investigation after restoration of sinus rhythm or may appear only during follow-up.

Patients who are detected because of an apical systolic murmur are likely to have left ventricular enlargement disproportionate to the murmur which usually suggests only mild mitral regurgitation.

The ECG abnormalities most commonly found are non-specific and non-focal. They include widening of the QRS, repolarization abnormalities, left or right atrial p-waves, multiple supraventricular or ventricular ectopic beats, a conduction fault such as left anterior hemiblock, or complete left bundle branch block. Low voltage in the standard and limb leads and high voltage in the chest leads is common. Rarely, the ECG is within normal limits at the time of first presentation.

Radiological cardiomegaly may be slight or marked but by the time it is apparent left ventricular malfunction is already considerable (Fig. 2). Usually the left ventricle is the only chamber to be recognizably dilated. Pulmonary congestive changes disappear quickly after the first dose of diuretic.

Differential diagnosis

From structural heart disease

Coronary heart disease Symptoms and signs of left ventricular failure in the absence of a history or focal ECG signs of previous myocardial infarction are more likely to be due to dilated cardiomyopathy than to ischaemic heart disease even if the patient is male and a smoker. A few patients with dilated cardiomyopathy may mention chest pain but this is rarely typical of angina.

Calcific aortic stenosis is a cause of heart failure which is easily overlooked. The murmur may be seemingly insignificant or even absent. A systolic murmur at the base which gets louder (rather than softer) as the patient improves may be caused by underlying aortic stenosis. As such patients need urgent aortic valve replacement, respond poorly to antifailure measures, and may be killed by vasodilator therapy, it is very important to recognize the true diagnosis early. Such valves are nearly always calcified, so fluoroscopy provides easy confirmation and echocardiography enables non-invasive recognition. Patients may survive and benefit from valve replacement even when left ventricular function is initally very poor.

Pericardial effusion may present with breathlessness, failure, and cardiomegaly but in such cases there is pulsus paradoxus, the venous pressure is high, and evidence of left ventricular enlargement and gallop sounds are conspicuously absent. The electrocardiogram is likely to show low voltage in pericardial effusion. Echocardiograms confirm the diagnosis.

Organic mitral valve disease may be suggested if an apical systolic murmur is rather prominent but the left ventricle is dilated more than the left atrium in patients with cardiomyopathy and out of proportion to the evidence of a fault in the mitral valve. Nevertheless, the clinical differentiation occasionally poses difficulty which is not resolved until full investigation has been carried out. The ejection fraction of the left ventricle is rarely less than 50 per cent in patients with organic mitral regurgitation.

From specific heart muscle disease

Some patients give a history of the onset of symptoms following an influenza-like illness and it is in these that the question of postmyocarditic heart failure arises. Often, however, the illness was simply a 'marker' to the patient, the junction between being well and being ill. It is only in a minority of adult patients that the diagnosis of myocarditis can be sustained after serological investigation and myocardial biopsy, and even in these it is not possible to know whether it was a causal or a precipitating factor.

Alcohol is often invoked as a cause for dilated cardiomyopathy. Most adult patients with dilated cardiomyopathy consume alcohol, some immoderately, and its role is always hard to assess (see page 13.205).

The distinction from hypertensive heart failure is often difficult. The diastolic blood pressure is sometimes raised at presentation but rarely to over 100 mgHg. If there is a clear past history of chronic hypertension the diagnosis of hypertensive heart failure is not in doubt even though the blood pressure may have fallen to normal and remained there. Heart failure may get better and hypertension develop in a patient who had been normotensive while in failure and previously regarded as having a dilated cardiomyopathy. There is no clinical or investigative difference between hypertensive heart failure and dilated cardiomyopathy apart from the blood pressure, and this may fall to normal when the hypertensive develops heart failure and not rise to abnormal levels unless left ventricular function improves with treatment. The vasodilator treatment of left ventricular failure and of severe hypertension is, entirely logically, the same for each.

The possibilites of *thyroid dysfunction* or *acromegaly*, a *phaeochromocytoma* which may present with ventricular arrhythmia or left ventricular failure, and *haemochromatosis* need exclusion. The rare *storage diseases* are usually accompanied by an abnormal physical appearance and a family history, and *skeletal myopathies* will not be overlooked.

The *collagen vascular disorders* may present with heart failure; the one most likely to simulate dilated cardiomyopathy and be missed clinically is systemic sclerosis. An unwrinkled face, 'small' mouth, facial telangiectases, tethered skin over face and fingers, and evidence of visceral involvement may be found. *Dermatomyositis*, with or without an underlying malignancy, may also present with heart failure but the involvement of the heart is often patchy such that a patient may present with mitral regurgitation or with focal features suggestive of infarction. The same is true of *sarcoidosis* of the heart, which is often extensive, and presentation with ventricular arrhythmia may mask extensive underlying infiltration with sarcoid granulomata.

Investigation

Investigation has three aims: (*a*) the exclusion of structural heart disease; (*b*) the search for probable causes of myocardial dysfunction (see 'Specific heart muscle disorders', page 13.196); and (*c*) the description and quantification of left and right ventricular function for assessment of the effects of treatment and prognosis as well as for the recognition of occult malfunction in patients presenting with arrhythmia, embolism, or a murmur.

Exclusion of structural heart disease

Coronary heart disease can only be excluded with certainty by coronary angiography. Aortic stenosis is usually recognized by echocardiography but catheterization may be needed for quantification and for coronary angiography before surgery.

General and specific investigations

Full routine biochemistry should always be checked. Immunological investigations including antiheart antibodies, the components of complement, and HLA type may yield clues. Serum iron-binding capacity and ferritin, angiotensin-converting enzyme, serum calcium, and a gallium scan should be considered.

Investigation of left and right ventricular function

Non-invasive investigations Systolic time intervals show decreased left ventricular ejection time and a prolonged pre-ejection period.

M-mode and cross-sectional echocardiography is valuable in both diagnosis and management, and differentiates dilated cardiomyopathy from hypertrophic cardiomyopathy, endomyocardial fibrosis, and amyloid heart disease. It is useful in excluding a large pericardial effusion. The findings are of increased left ventricular dimensions with decrease in systolic contraction which is usually global but may sometimes be asymmetrical (Table 1 and Fig. 3). There may be paradoxical septal movement associated with left bundle branch block. Left ventricular wall thickness is usually normal, even when failure of contractile function is non-uniform, and this usually allows distinction to be made from coronary heart failure in which areas of thinning and of hypertrophy with corresponding akinesia or normal or even increased contraction may be recognized. Movement of the mitral valve is diminished because of low output and occasionally intracardiac thrombi can be seen;

Table 1 Echocardiographic features of dilated cardiomyopathy

Increase in left ventricular cavity dimensions at both end-systole and end-diastole
Reduced excursion of the mitral valve

Cross-sectional echo
Reduced motion of the left ventricular wall which is usually global but may not be perfectly symmetrical
Reduced systolic thickening of the left ventricular wall

M-mode echo
Increased absolute distance of the anterior leaflet of the mitral valve from the septum (>1 cm at *E* point)
Posterior eccentricity of the mitral valve within the left ventricular cavity
Good visualization of the anterior and posterior mitral leaflets in the same plane

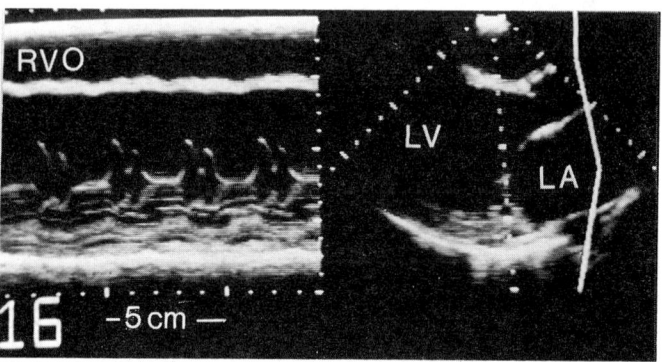

Fig. 3 On the right is a long axis cross-sectional echocardiographic view of the left ventricle in dilated cardiomyopathy showing a greatly increased end-systolic dimension of over 6 cm. The plane of the M-mode beam is shown traversing the tip of the mitral valve and on the left is the M-mode. The features described in Table 1 are seen. LA = left atrium; LV = left ventricle; RVO = right ventricular outflow. The dots are 1 cm apart.

this is unusual, however, as they are commonly small, and big thrombi are much commoner in coronary disease soon after major infarction. Small pericardial effusions are frequent.

Radionuclide blood pool imaging shows the same features. Scans of the right ventricle show it to be of normal size or dilated. Myocardial imaging may show perfusion defects and can be misleading. Positron emission tomography and phosphorus nuclear magnetic resonance imaging may in the future provide clues to the metabolic abnormalities underlying the disorder.

Ambulant ECG recording should be carried out to look for ventricular arrhythmia.

Progress and response to treatment can be assessed serially using M-mode echo with phonocardiogram, apex, and carotid impulse recording for the calculation of both systolic and diastolic time intervals of the left and the right ventricles. Cross-sectional echocardiography is still too insensitive to reveal very small changes in total function. Blood pool scanning allows change in ejection fraction to be measured serially but not absolute volumes.

Serial exercise testing is very important in assessing the initial disability and response to treatment.

Invasive investigations Whenever possible, patients with a suspected dilated cardiomyopathy should be submitted to right and left heart catheterization with selective coronary angiography and both left and right ventricular angiography (Fig. 4). Coronary artery disease may be the cause of the left ventricular failure, and in such patients the left ventricle usually (but not invariably) appears slightly misshapen with recognizable areas of akinesia. Most patients with dilated cardiomyopathy have normal coronary arteries but when coronary artery disease is present it is sometimes hard to be sure whether it is severe enough to account for the cardiac malfunction. In this context it is well to remember that coronary angiograms are usually under-read but that coronary heart failure is rarely seen in the absence of multiple major coronary artery obstructions.

Pervenous endomyocardial biopsy of the right ventricle should be carried out to exclude specific heart muscle disease especially myocarditis. Recent work from Germany has shown that reduced myofibril volume fraction (< 60 per cent) had prognostic significance for both haemodynamic deterioration and death. Patients who improved or stabilized had myofibril volume fractions of more than 60 per cent.

Coronary angiography should not be confined to older patients since anomalous origin of the left coronary artery from the pulmonary artery may present in adult life with non-specific features of left ventricular failure. Neither electrocardiographic changes suggestive of old infarction nor a continuous murmur caused by fistulous flow between the normally arising right and anomalously arising left coronary artery may be in evidence. Other congenital anomalies of the coronary arteries may be found but neither an aberrant circumflex or even the whole left coronary artery arising from the right ostium nor a coronary cameral fistula is usually associated with any significant effect on left ventricular function.

Acquired non-atheromatous coronary artery disease includes coronary thrombosis and/or aneurysm formation in patients who have survived Japanese mucocutaneous disease in their infancy (Kawasaki disease). Coronary thrombosis may also occur in young patients with systemic lupus erythomatosus and in Behçet's syndrome.

Management

General measures include weight reduction when relevant, and alcohol should be forbidden. Other potential myocardial depressants such as tricyclic antidepressants and verapamil should be avoided.

Therapeutic efforts should be directed toward shrinking the left ventricle. Bed rest is helpful in the short term; although it was possible that prolonged bed rest long ago advocated by Birch would prolong life, this will now never be tested as such patients should be considered for cardiac transplantation.

Long-term anticoagulants should be prescribed routinely whether or not sinus rhythm has been lost as they have been shown to be effective in preventing systemic embolism. The risk of venous thromboembolism is also high, as in heart failure whatever the cause.

Modern diuretics leave little place for severe salt restriction, and fluid intake need not be reduced except in advanced low output failure with hyponatraemia or where there is associated renal disease. The introduction of a potassium-sparing diuretic, such as amiloride, early in treatment helps prevent hypokalaemia and is more effective than the use of oral potassium or the later introduction of amiloride when the potassium has already fallen (see page 13.99).

The place of digitalis in the treatment of systolic myocardial failure in sinus rhythm is controversial (see page 13.101). Such patients are easily rendered digitalis toxic because, in contrast to patients in atrial fibrillation, there is no end-point or visible effect. Recognizing this, physicians tend to undertreat even though the inotropic effect of digoxin in acute studies is linear. Ventricular arrhythmias are common in dilated cardiomyopathy and are likely to be increased by pushing digitalis. The effect of hypokalaemia and reduction in dosage required because of interaction with antiarrhythmic drugs such as quinidine, verapamil and amiodarone further reduce enthusiasm for the use of digitalis in the United Kingdom in contrast to the United States. Recent crossover studies have failed to show improvement in left ventricular function or deterioration following withdrawl of chronic use in dilated cardiomyopathy.

Vasodilators are introduced at an early stage, immediately after starting a diuretic (see page 13.105). ACE inhibitors are now acknowledged to be superior to other agents. They have the advantage of inducing both arterial and venous dilatation together with some selectivity so that blood flow to brain and kidney is favoured while on exercise the blood flow to exercising muscles increases though not nearly as much as in health. This is in contrast to patients treated with other vasodilators in whom blood

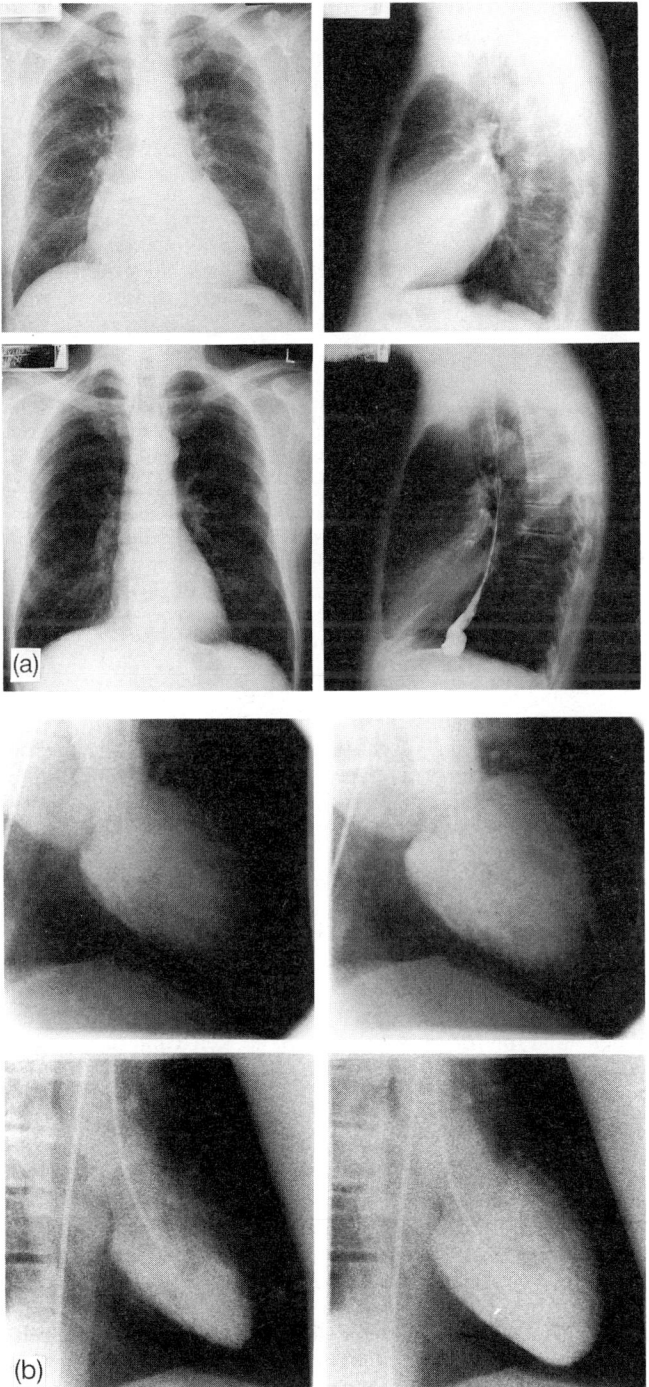

Fig. 4 (a) Matched plain chest radiographs and (b) left ventricular angiograms (right anterior oblique view, systole on the left, diastole on the right) from a patient with severe left ventricular failure; the left ventricle contracts very poorly with a greatly increased residual volume and marked functional mitral regurgitation. The lower lines show the patient two years later when he was off all treatment; the plain film is normal and the angiogram shows that mitral regurgitation has disappeared but the end-systolic volume remains slightly increased.

flow to exercising muscle failed to rise, and accounts for the seemingly paradoxical failure of treatment to improve exercise performance. ACE inhibitors, by antagonizing the increased plasma levels of angiotensin II engendered by heart failure and diuretic treatment, are not only vasodilators but also reduce potassium loss and increased concentrations of vasopressin responsible in part for hyponatraemia in advanced heart failure (see pages 13.100 and 13.94). ACE inhibitors are often associated with a sense of well-being, sometimes almost to the extent of euphoria, another advantage. Either captopril or enalapril may be chosen. Enalapril has the advantage of prolonged action and the side-effects of metallic taste and skin rashes are less common. On the other hand, the first-dose hypotensive effect well recognized with captopril and other vasodilators may be even more severe, delayed, profound, and prolonged after enalapril, suggesting a need to start with very low dosage or even in hospital in patients in whom it is likely that plasma renin and angiotensin levels will be particularly high.

Treatment of arrhythmias is important. Sudden death, embolism, and premature left ventricular decompensation may all result from arrhythmias which may be occult. In the management of atrial fibrillation, a common development in these patients, optimal cardiac function is promoted by a rate which is as nearly regular as possible and which does not become excessive during exercise. Digitalis alone rarely achieves excellent control of atrial fibrillation during exercise but the addition of a beta-blocking drug may improve this if introduced in the manner described for the treatment of heart failure. Amiodarone has been the most successful drug for the regularization of atrial fibrillation and quite frequently promotes the return of sinus rhythm. It has the additional virtue of not having a negative inotropic effect.

In patients with bursts of ventricular tachycardia, multifocal or R on T ventricular ectopic beats, antiarrhythmic drugs should be given. Class I antiarrhythmic drugs should be tried first but if these are unsuccessful amiodarone should be administered. Repeated ambulant ECG tape recordings will be needed.

None of the new inotropic agents (see page 13.111) either synthetic sympathomimetic or bipyridine drugs such as milrinone, has been shown to be useful in the long term or free from serious toxic effects. Any inotrope will be liable to increase metabolic demand and to be arrhythmogenic. In intact man an increase in output will be associated with reflex vasodilatation and it is then impossible to tell whether the beneficial effect was due to primary vasodilatation rather than to an improvement in contractile function. There is a place for short-term use of intravenous agents such as dobutamine in patients who have suffered sudden deterioration, in a bid to salvage them for cardiac transplantation.

The beneficial effect of long-term beta blockade, which was introduced from Sweden in 1975, seems paradoxical particularly when considered in parallel with the use of sympathomimetic inotropes! Metoprolol is started in a very small dose, 12.5 mg twice daily, increasing slowly and gradually under observation to 50 mg twice daily. Only about half of the Swedish patients responded favourably; there was a delay of one month before benefit was seen and deterioration was shown to follow more rapid introduction. Confirmation of the Swedish work was slow to come, but recent German work has confirmed long-term efficacy after an average of six months of treatment and has emphasized that three months may elapse before benefit. The mechanism of the effect is still unknown, but may be to do with release of the denervated failing heart from the ill effects of increased medullary catecholamines, to an improved diastolic length tension relationship, or to the benefits of a slower rate and increased stroke volume. When beta-blocking drugs are given in the catheter laboratory in patients with dilated cardiomyopathy left ventricular function deteriorates acutely and any beneficial effect is seen only with chronic use. Quantification of benefit is elusive because serial studies are necessary and slowing of the heart rate frustrates direct comparison of indices of left ventricular function.

In this difficult situation diuretics and vasodilators should be the first line of treatment. Consideration may then be given to the cautious addition of a beta-blocker, particularly in patients with persistent sinus tachycardia.

Cardiac transplantation (see page 13.115) should be considered in every patient under the age of 60 whose prognosis is probably less than two years. Suitable patients need to have well preserved renal, liver, and pulmonary function without pulmonary emboli or infection, be considered psychologically stable, and have a strong will to survive. The place of cardiac transplantation is now firmly established with survival of over 80 per cent at one year (in the United Kingdom) and greatly improved quality of life as shown in the Buxton report on the Harefield and Papworth patients.

Assessment of benefit from treatment

Patients look for (a) *relief of shortness of breath and oedema*, (b) *improvement in exercise capacity*, and (c) *prolongation of survival*. The first is nearly always easy to achieve with diuretics. Recalcitrant oedema is uncommon in dilated cardiomyopathy and excercise capacity increases but further measurable improvement in exercise performance in severe cases does not often result from the addition of vasodilators unless ACE inhibitors are used. Although the resting cardiac output is often in the low normal range, it fails to rise much on exercise; if the ventricular response to atrial fibrillation is rapid and irregular the output may even fall. Blood flow to exercising muscle does not rise, so the patient quickly gives up because of fatigue and aching muscles. Acid products of anaerobic metabolism cause hyperventilation. Uncontrolled ventricular rates may lead to impaired emptying of the left atrium with a sharp rise in pressure and all of these combine to limit the improvement in performance which one expects in a patient who has lost all external evidence of heart failure.

In mild heart failure great improvement in exercise tolerance comes from the first introduction of a diuretic.

No agents have yet been shown to improve survival after the development of heart failure. In dilated cardiomyopathy as in coronary heart failure the average life span is only about two years after the development of heart failure, although there is a wide scatter and some patients may survive much longer. The impressive improvement in the signs of overt failure which can be achieved has deterred physcians from sending patients forward for transplantation. When these patients die suddenly and 'unexpectedly' this has been related to the presence of potentially life-threatening ventricular arrhythmias detected on ambulant ECG records. In a personal series such arrhythmias were directly linked to left ventricular dimensions and filling pressure. Death, though sudden in terms of how the patient looked clinically, was not 'unexpected' when considered in terms of the size of the left ventricle.

In a study from the Mayo Clinic, 77 per cent of patients were dead within eight years and two-thirds of the deaths occurred within two years of diagnosis. Twenty-three per cent of the patients improved. In our own series of 186 patients, those who survived more than two years after the diagnosis showed a tendency to longer term stability even up to 10 years; adverse predictive features were left ventricular filling pressure(> 23 mmHg) and the dimensions of the left ventricle; end-systolic volume greater than 128 ml/m^2 and end-diastolic volume greater than 173 ml/m^2. In the Mayo Clinic study the adverse features included age over 55 years, cardiothoracic ratio greater than 55 per cent, cardiac index under 3 l/min/m^2 and left ventricular end-diastolic pressure above 20 mmHg. The combination of more than one adverse factor greatly reduced the likelihood of survival beyond three years from the time of diagnosis.

It is hardly surprising that the long-term prognosis is worse in proportion to the severity of the left ventricular malfunction, and this should not be forgotten in planning transplantation. It is true irrespective of how the patient looks clinically.

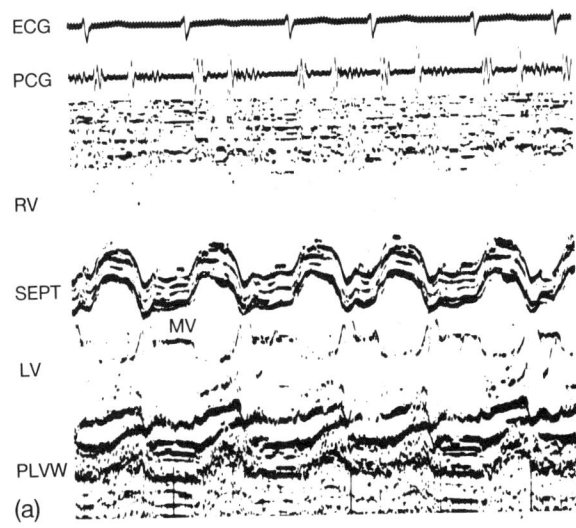

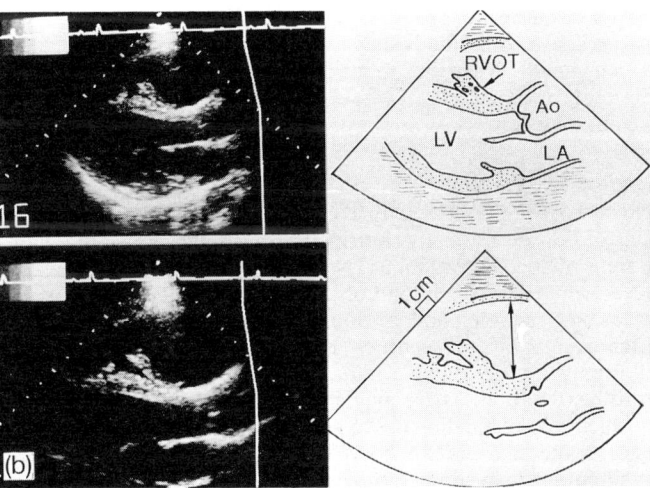

The electrocardiogram gave a clue to a right-sided fault in most of the patients, with T-wave inversion in the right chest leads the commonest feature.

The chest radiograph was sometimes normal in the patients presenting with ventricular tachycardia but in those with heart failure there was marked cardiomegaly (see Fig. 2b).

Cross-sectional echocardiography revealed right ventricular dilation, and when this was marked it was also apparent on M-mode echo (Fig. 5).

Right ventricular angiograms revealed right ventricular dilation (Fig. 6) which tended to be concealed on plain radiographs until it was very marked. The right ventricle showed a normal or reduced trabecular pattern and there was sometimes considerable tricuspid regurgitation. The pulmonary artery pressure was normal but the right ventricular end-diastolic pressure was raised in all.

Endomyocardial biopsy and autopsy usually revealed non-specific findings but five out of 21 patients with this clinical syndrome had evidence of myocarditis and two children were siblings.

Ventricular tachycardia was sometimes hard to treat and three early cases ended fatally. The most commonly effective drug was amiodarone.

Fig. 5 (a) M-mode and (b) cross-sectional echocardiograms in right ventricular cardiomyopathy. Figure 5a shows, from above down, the ECG, phonocardiogram (PCG) with third heart sound, the greatly dilated right ventricular cavity (RV), the ventricular septum (SEPT) which shows paradoxical movement, and the normal-sized left ventricular cavity (LV) containing the mitral valve (MV) and the posterior left ventricular wall (PLVW). Figure 5b shows the long axis end-diastolic view with line drawing on the right. The lower figure is an enlarged view of the right ventricular outflow tract (RVOT) from the same study. It is greatly dilated and measured > 4 cm (arrowed). Ao = aorta; LA = left atrium; LV = left ventricle.

RIGHT VENTRICULAR CARDIOMYOPATHY

Rarely, the right ventricle and right atrium are dilated but the left ventricle appears to be normal or nearly normal on angiography. Such patients comprised only 5 per cent of our cases. They presented either with heart failure or with ventricular arrhythmia which was frequently the sole cause for referral. The severe recurrent ventricular tachycardia typically showed left axis deviation and was found to arise from the right ventricle on electrophysiological testing.

The clinical features varied from a slightly raised venous pressure and right-sided atrial beat or third sound to gross heart failure. The differential diagnosis includes Ebstein's anomaly, right-sided intracardiac tumour, partial Uhl's syndrome, and pericardial effusion.

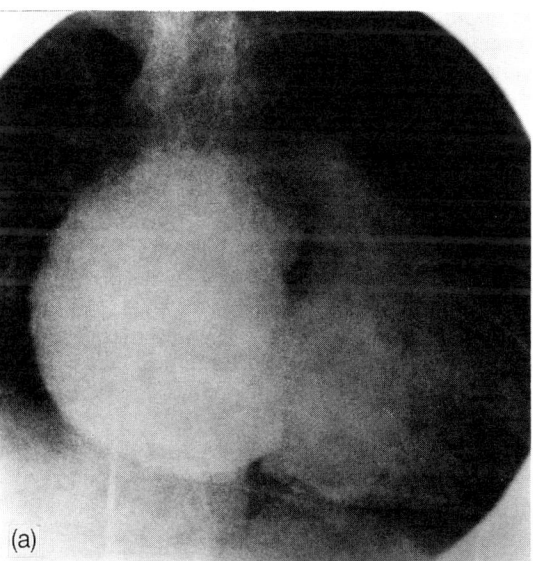

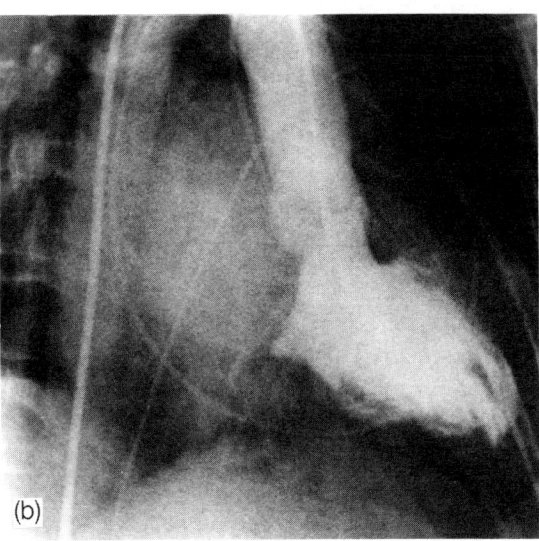

Fig. 6 (a) Right and (b) left ventricular angiograms in right ventricular cardiomyopathy. The right ventricle and right atrium are greatly dilated but the left ventricle is not dilated and contracts normally.

PERIPARTUM HEART FAILURE

The occurrence of unexpected heart failure in the puerperium or late in pregnancy (see page 11.2) has long been recognized, and when a myocardial disorder of mysterious cause presents within three months of childbirth the condition is usually given the purely descriptive label of peripartum heart disease or heart failure. It is still not known whether pregnancy may exert a specific haemodynamic stress on pre-existing but subclinical heart muscle disease analogous to the putative effect of myocarditis or alcohol in precipitating clinical symptoms. Heart failure may develop very suddenly or more gradually with shortness of breath, even acute pulmonary oedema, palpitation, or systemic embolism. Precordial discomfort resembling angina may occasionally occur.

As in dilated cardiomyopathy in the non-pregnant state, the role of hypertension remains ill defined but salt retention, fluid overload, and a rise in blood pressure are probably responsible for the frequency of peripartum heart failure in parts of northern Nigeria where local practice determines that parturient mothers consume a local 'potash' containing large amounts of sodium. The left ventricle appears to be dilated with tachycardia and a third sound gallop, sometimes a mitral systolic murmur, and sometimes also congestive failure. This syndrome among Hausa mothers is almost certainly an 'iatrogenic' high output failure, unrelated to the low output failure of peripartum cardiomyopathy elsewhere and carrying a much better prognosis.

The outcome varies between rapid death, a chronic cardiac disorder, and complete recovery. Recurrence in subsequent pregnancies is usual but not invariable. Autopsy in fatal cases has not contributed to our understanding of the disorder and the clinical appearances, haemodynamic fault, natural history, and myocardial pathology show no clear distinction from dilated cardiomyopathy as it is seen outside pregnancy and in either sex.

It is usually not possible to exclude pre-existing asymptomatic cardiac abnormality, and this is one of the reasons why the causal role of the pregnancy has not been further clarified. Pre-existing hypertension, an immunological disorder related to the pregnancy, and genetic and ethnic factors may all be relevant predisposing agents. Most authors have stressed the problems of multiple rapidly repeated pregnancies in the lowest socioeconomic classes but there are many exceptions. If the stress were largely haemodynamic it would be expected that peripartum heart disease would usually develop in pregnancy but presentation is most commonly linked with lactation, suggesting that the stress may be more nutritional than haemodynamic. In this context it is well known that the normal heart tolerates volume work very easily and heart failure is not known to be precipitated by heavy manual labour in the male, or by athletic activity. It is well known that patients relate the onset of an insidiously developing disease to well remembered landmarks so that in Africa heart failure in young women is related by the patient to pregnancy and in the United Kingdom to previous virus infection.

The treatment is the same as in dilated cardiomyopathy. Lactation should probably be avoided.

ENDOCARDIAL FIBROELASTOSIS

Pathology

Left ventricular dilatation and failure developing in early infancy may be associated with a specific histopathological appearance. Diffuse endocardial thickening covers the internal surface of the left ventricle with a thick white porcelain-like coat and microscopy reveals fibrosis with an excess of elastic fibrils. The left ventricle is both dilated and hypertrophied, and the mitral and aortic valves may be involved with mitral regurgitant and aortic ejection murmurs.

Associations

The condition has traditionally been divided into primary and secondary, and dilated and contracted forms. Although the aetiology is unknown, *primary* endocardial fibroelastosis (EFE) may represent an infantile response to left ventricle dilatation of which the most common cause may be a neonatal or intrauterine myocarditis. The *contracted* form of EFE refers to endocardial thickening and elastosis which frequently accompany serious congenital malfunctions such as aortic atresia and the hypoplastic left heart syndrome. It does not seem helpful to retain the term.

The *dilated* form of EFE may also complicate lesser congenital disorders of the left heart of a type which may cause left ventricular failure in infancy. The main association is with coarctation of the aorta but it is occasionally seen with discrete subaortic stenosis or with aortic valve stenosis.

Although EFE used to be thought invariably fatal (perhaps because an autopsy diagnosis was demanded before the condition could be recognized with certainty), it is well known that many cases survive into adult life. They may then present with dilated cardiomyopathy although there may be a history of heart failure in infancy. Modern techniques allow the thickened endocardium to be identified either by two-dimensional echo or by biopsy. EFE should be suspected in patients of any age if a coarctation is associated with poor left ventricular function.

The condition may occur in sibships without vertical inheritance; this suggests the possibility of an environmental cause or a shared intrauterine infection. A previously noted association with the presence of antibody against mumps is no longer believed to be relevant. It is curious that the incidence of sporadic cases has markedly declined over the last two decades and familial forms are seen more often.

Clinical appearance

Primary EFE presents with congestive heart failure in the first year of life, occasionally shortly after birth but more often at 4–6 months of age. The infant is dyspnoeic and shows hepatomegaly, a raised venous pressure, and often periorbital oedema. He is thin, sweating, irritable, and anxious, with grunting respiration and often cough. The left ventricle is markedly enlarged with a forceful impulse, occasionally a mitral systolic murmur, and usually a third heart sound. There may also be an aortic ejection murmur, in which case distinction has to be made from congenital aortic stenosis as the cause of the heart failure. The pulses, however, are small but jerky in contrast to aortic stenosis with failure in infancy when they may be so small as to be virtually impalpable. The electrocardiogram typically shows extremely high left ventricular voltage with marked repolarization changes and, in the presence of the clinical features, is virtually diagnostic.

Left ventricular angiography reveals a dilated left ventricle with a very smooth interior and there may be mitral regurgitation. The left ventricular diastolic pressure is high and there may be severe pulmonary hypertension.

Treatment

Treatment is traditionally with digoxin and diuretics but vasodilators should also be considered in severe cases. When a child survives the illness of presentation, he very often shows a gradual improvement in the ensuing months and years and may appear to have a normal heart by the age of 5–10 years, but it is not yet known whether such children will add to the numbers of adults developing the clinical picture of dilated cardiomyopathy. Digitalis has a good reputation in EFE and its use has been recommended until years after symptoms and signs have abated. This may be because the drug has been given credit for the survival and improvement of patients in whom this was predestined anyway.

References

Bagger, J. P., Baandrup, U., Rasmussen, K., Moller, M. and Vesterlun, D. (1984). Cardiomyopathy in Western Denmark. *Br. Heart J.* **52**, 327–331.

Bestel, O., Binkarl, F. and Buhler, F. R. (1981). Sustained effectiveness of chronic prazosin therapy in severe chronic congestive heart failure. *Am. Heart J.* **101**, 529–633.

Brockington, I. F. (1971). Postpartum hypertensive heart failure. *Am. J. Cardiol.* **27**, 650–658.

Burch, G. C., Walsh, J. J., Ferrans, V. J. and Hibb, S. R. (1965). Prolonged bed rest in the treatment of the dilated heart. *Circulation* **32**, 852–856.

Cambridge, G., MacArthur, C. G. C., Waterston, A. P., Goodwin, J. F. and Oakley, C. M. (1979). Antibodies to Coxsackie B viruses in congestive cardiomyopathy. *Br. Heart J.* **41**, 692–696.

Colucci, W., Wynne, J., Holman, B. L. and Braunwald, E. (1980). Chronic therapy of heart failure with prazosin: a randomized double-blind trial. *Am. J. Cardiol.* **45**, 337.

Demakis, J. G., Rahimtoola, S. H., Sutton, G. C. *et al.* (1971). Natural course of peripartum cardiomyopathy. *Circulation* **44**, 1053–1061.

Eckstein, R., Mempel, W. and Bolte, H. D. (1982). Reduced suppressor cell activity in congestive cardiomyopathy and myocarditis. *Circulation* **65**, 1224.

Figulla, H. R., Rahlf, G., Nieger, M., Luig, H. and Krenzer, H. (1985). Spontaneous haemodynamic improvement or stabilization and associated biopsy findings in patients with congestive cardiomyopathy. *Circulation* **71**, 1095–1104.

Fitchett, D. H., Sugrue, D. D., McArthur, C. G. and Oakley, C. M. (1984). Right ventricular dilated cardiomyopathy. *Br. Heart J.* **51**, 25–29.

Fuster, V., Gersh, B., Guiliam, E. R., Tajik, A. F., Brandenburg, R. O. and Frye, R. L. (1981). The natural history of dilated cardiomyopathy. *Am. J. Cardiol.* **47**, 525–531.

Goodwin, J. F. (ed.) (1985). *Heart muscle disease.* MTP Press, Lancaster.

Ikram, H. and Fitzpatrick, D. (1981). Double blind trial of chronic oral beta-blockade in congestive cardiomyopathy. *Lancet* **2**, 490–493.

Kühn, H., Breithardt, G., Knierien, H. J., Köhler, E., Lösse, B., Serpel, L. and Loogen, F. (1978). Prognosis and possible presymptomatic manifestations of congestive cardiomyopathy. *Postgrad. Med. J.* **54**, 451.

Massie, B. M., Kramer, B., Slen, E. and Haughon, F. (1981). Vasodilator treatment with isosorbide dinitrate and hydralazine in chronic heart failure. *Br. Heart J.* **45**, 376–384.

Oakley, C. M. (1974). Clinical recognition of the cardiomyopathies. *Circ. Res.* **34/35**, suppl. II, 11.

Olsen, E. G. J. (1979). The pathology of cardiomyopathies. A critical analysis. *Am. Heart J.* **98**, 385.

Packer, M., Medina, N., Yushak, M. and Meller, J. (1983). Hemodynamic pattern of response during long-term captopril therapy for severe chronic heart failure. *Circulation* **64**, 803–812.

Peters, T. J., Wells, G., Oakley, C. M., Brooksby, I. A. B., Jenkins, B. S., Webb Peploe, M. M. and Coltart, D. J. (1977). Enzymatic analysis of endocardinal biopsy specimens from patients with cardiomyopathies. *Br. Heart J.* **39**, 1333.

Pierpoint, G. L., Cohn, J. N. and Franciosa, J. A. (1978). Congestive cardiomyopathy: pathophysiology and response to therapy. *Archs. Intern. Med.* **138**, 1847.

Svedberg, K., Hjalmarson, A., Waagstein, F. and Wallentin, I. (1979). Prolongation of survival in congestive cardiomyopathy by beta receptor blockade. *Lancet* **1**, 1374.

Torp, A. (1978). Incidence of congestive cardiomyopathy. *Postgrad. Med. J.* **54**, 435.

Walsh, J. J., Burch, G. E., Black, W. C., Ferrans, V. S. and Hibbs, R. G. (1965). Idiopathic myocardiopathy of the puerperium (post-partal heart disease). *Circulation* **32**, 19–31.

WHO/ISFC Task Force on the Definition and Classification of Cardiomyopathies (1980). Report. *Br. Heart J.* **44**, 672–673.

RESTRICTIVE CARDIOMYOPATHY

General description

Restrictive cardiomyopathy is characterized by loss of ventricular distensibility and can result from either endocardial or myocardial abnormality. Restriction to diastolic filling may produce signs of heart failure caused by back pressure even though systolic function may be normal.

The commonest cause of a restrictive cardiomyopathy is endomyocardial fibrosis with or without eosinophilia. Löffler's eosinophilic endomyocardial disease and endomyocardial fibrosis were first thought to be different ends of a single spectrum in 1969, and since then abundant evidence has confirmed this. Although endomyocardial fibrosis (EMF) is most common in the tropics and has now been reported from Central and South America, south-east Asia and southern India as well as from equatorial Africa it is also seen in temperate regions including the United Kingdom and the United States of America.

In African EMF an abnormally raised eosinophil count is uncommon but in the United Kingdom patients usually, although not invariably, have a hypereosinophilic syndrome.

In EMF scarring usually affects one or both ventricles and restricts filling. Obliteration of the apices of the ventricles may occur. Involvement of the atrioventricular valves is common but the outflow tracts are spared.

The scarring restricts filling in a way similar to that in constrictive pericarditis except that in EMF the two ventricles may be affected to differing extents and mitral and tricuspid regurgitation are common.

Most patients with restrictive cardiomyopathy have EMF, but a similar diastolic abnormality without atrioventricular valve regurgitation may occasionally result from myocardial fibrosis of unknown cause both in adults and in children in whom 'giant' atrial dilation may develop. Amyloid heart disease is also 'restrictive' but the haemodynamic fault in amyloid is quite different from that in EMF and unique to amyloid heart disease (see Table 5, page 13.201).

THE HYPEREOSINOPHILIC SYNDROME

Cardiac involvement may occur in any disease marked by profound eosinophilia (see page 24.8). The hypereosinophilic syndrome (HES) is defined as an idiopathic eosinophilia of more than 1.5×10^9/l with evidence of tissue injury often involving a number of organs but the main morbidity and mortality are caused by heart disease. Hypereosinophilia may also occur in association with tumours, particularly carcinoma of the bronchus and T-cell lymphomas, in parasitic infections, asthma, the Churg–Strauss variant of polyarteritis nodosa, or in drug reactions. Cardiac involvement may occur in any of these when hypereosinophilia is sustained. HES is not a leukaemia although various forms of leukaemia may enter a hypereosinophilic phase with cardiac and other tissue involvement. There is a heavy male predominance which may be as high as 9:1.

In HES the marrow is full of mature and maturing eosinophils but the circulating eosinophils appear to be hypermature. In patients with cardiac abnormality the eosinophil morphology is almost always strikingly abnormal with a high incidence of vacuolated and degranulated forms. The stimulus to degranulation is unknown.

The relation between eosinophilia and cardiac damage is still unknown (Fig. 7) but it is thought that the strongly positively charged major basic proteins within the eosinophil granules cause tissue injury when released locally into tissues. In patients with HES and no cardiac abnormality the morphology of the circulating eosinophils is usually normal, but if these patients develop morphological abnormalities there is usually cardiac involvement as well.

Although not leukaemic, the hypereosinophilic syndrome pursues a malignant course. British patients with EMF usually also have HES but in African patients with tropical EMF the cardiac damage probably results from previous parastic infection which had produced eosinophilia. It is interesting that Nigerian children admitted to hospital with severe eosinophilia and microfilariasis have been found to have marked cardiac abnormalities. EMF in the tropics is often first seen at the stage of scarring when the cause has gone. EMF in temperate zones is usually not of parasitic origin and the cause, whether a malignancy or HES, is usually still visible. The differences between the two probably relate to the

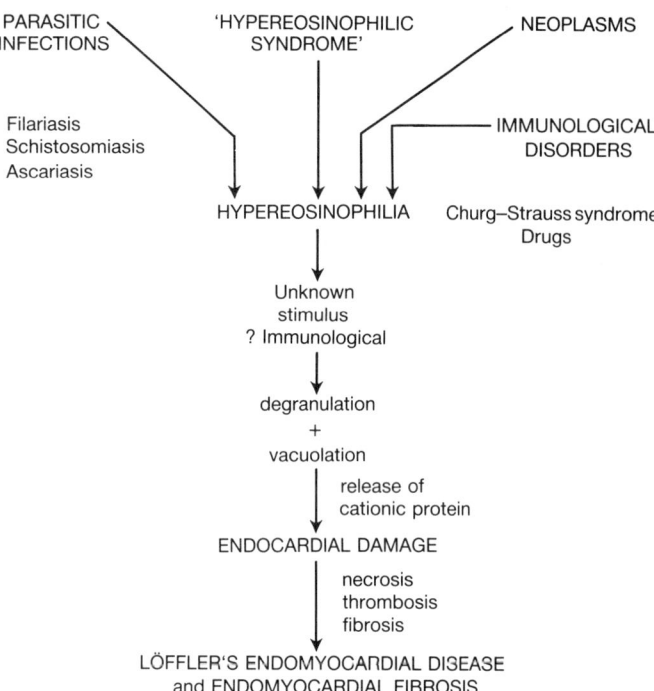

Fig. 7 Eosinophilia and cardiac damage.

severity and acuteness of the initial process. In the tropics a juvenile high parasitic load stimulates a sustained low grade eosinophilia and a long-continued subacute cardiac process which is not severe enough to present until the chronic stage, when eosinophilia may have gone. In cooler climes HES is associated with a higher eosinophilia, with more degranulation, and with more acute and severe cardiac damage which is either rapidly lethal or goes on to EMF with persistence of eosinophilia and progression of cardiac damage until the eosinophilia is suppressed.

In HES multiple organs may be involved in addition to the heart, including the bone marrow, lymph nodes, lungs, and brain. Sometimes there is skin and gastrointestinal involvement. The disease can be seen at any age. The most important clinical features are weight loss, fever, heart failure, and embolism. Less common are skin rash and cough.

Pathology

The cardiac pathology is quite distinctive with dense endocardial fibrosis and overlying thrombosis.

Three stages have been defined: necrotic, thrombotic, and fibrotic. The first is an acute inflammatory reaction with eosinophilic abscesses in the myocardium, particularly in the inner layers. Myocardial necrosis and an arteritis are associated. The endocardium is thickened, often with mural thrombosis. In the second stage the myocardium is infiltrated by eosinophils, and intracavitary thrombi may fill the ventricles. The myocardium is oedematous and the endocardium, including the atrioventricular valves, becomes necrotic. Acute mitral or tricuspid regurgitation may occur or the patient may present with systemic embolism. This stage may mimic a hyperacute rheumatic carditis or the restriction to ventricular filling imposed by massive intracavitary thrombosis may lead to a picture of low output failure with high filling pressures. The diagnosis may be obscure in some patients in whom the hypereosinophilia has regressed spontaneously by the time that the cardiac complications appear. The illness can be devastating and the time from onset of symptoms to death may be anything from days to months.

If the patient survives to the third stage, healing by fibrosis occurs. The arteritis and the cellular infiltrates are no longer seen. The impact of the disease is on the inflow tracts binding down the atrioventricular valves and obliterating the apices of the ventricles but stopping abruptly at the anterior leaflet of the mitral valve on the left side where there is a characteristic rolled edge at the termination of the endocardial fibrosis. The vestibule of the left ventricle and aortic valve are spared. On the right side the infundibulum of the right ventricle and pulmonary valve are also spared; if the sinus of the ventricle is obliterated the infundibulum dilates and takes on some of its function.

Cardiac signs in the acute phase

The patient is ill, febrile, and may simulate acute rheumatic carditis or infective endocarditis. The cardiac signs are variable. The sudden onset of left or congestive heart failure with cardiomegaly and third heart sound gallop is common. Asymmetrical involvement of left and right ventricle may lead to asynchronous third heart sounds. A mitral regurgitant murmur is frequent and systemic embolism is common. Although many patients die rapidly in the acute phase, others survive into the chronic phase, when the cardiac signs are similar to those in 'tropical' EMF except that presentation with gross ascites is uncommon in the West. Most patients have sinus tachycardia, small sharp atrial pulses without pulsus paradoxus, a raised jugular venous pressure often with a systolic regurgitant V-wave, a rather quiet heart with early third heart sound, and often a mitral regurgitant murmur. Tricuspid regurgitant murmurs are rather uncommon even when reflux is massive. The patient may have only signs of mitral regurgitation or only a raised jugular venous pressure.

Investigations

The ESR and C-reactive protein are raised in the acute phase. In cases with hypereosinophilia the disorder is differentiated from classic leukaemia by an absence of immature cells in the blood stream. The marrow, although packed with eosinophils, shows a normal maturation process.

The chest radiograph shows variable cardiomegaly and pulmonary congestion, sometimes with pulmonary infiltration. The electrocardiogram shows non-specific repolarization changes, occasionally with fascicular blocks and sometimes with arrhythmias and voltage changes of left ventricular hypertrophy.

Cross-sectional echocardiography may reveal intracavitary thrombus or bright echoes from the endocardium of the right and left ventricle, cavity obliteration, and valvar involvement (Fig. 8). The left and right atria are enlarged. M-mode echo is less specific but left ventricular and mitral valve motion may be abnormal reflecting the rapid early filling and sudden curtailment of that filling. Outward left ventricular excursion terminates early and is followed by a plateau coincident with the third heart sound (Fig. 9).

The haemodynamic consequences of endomyocardial scarring are restrictive with normal early diastolic pressures and a rapid mid-diastolic rise (square root sign). There may be impairment of systolic function in the acute phase but this is usually normal in the chronic phase. Atrioventricular valve regurgitation may be seen. Catheterization of the left ventricle should be carried out with caution in any phase of the disease because of the risk of dislodging thrombus. Mitral and tricuspid regurgitation may be marked on angiography and both ventricles appear abnormal in shape due to blunting or actual obliteration of the apices of the ventricles (Fig. 10). This may be particularly marked in the right ventricle in which a hypertrophied infundibulum with exaggerated contraction may be seen. In addition, the fibrotic process results in obliteration of the internal architecture of the ventricle such that both appear to be abnormally smooth walled, unless thrombus is present. The appearance of massive intracavity thrombus in the left ventricle may lead to the erroneous diagnosis of a cardiac tumour. In the early acute phase, when left ventricular contraction may be depressed, the shape of the ventricle is far less abnormal (unless it contains thrombus).

Inequality of right and left ventricular end-diastolic pressures at catheterization is an important feature which helps to distinguish cardiac restriction from pericardial constriction, in which the end-diastolic pressures are usually closely similar within the two ventricles.

The diagnosis can be confirmed by endomyocardial biopsy which provides information to help decide whether to treat necro-

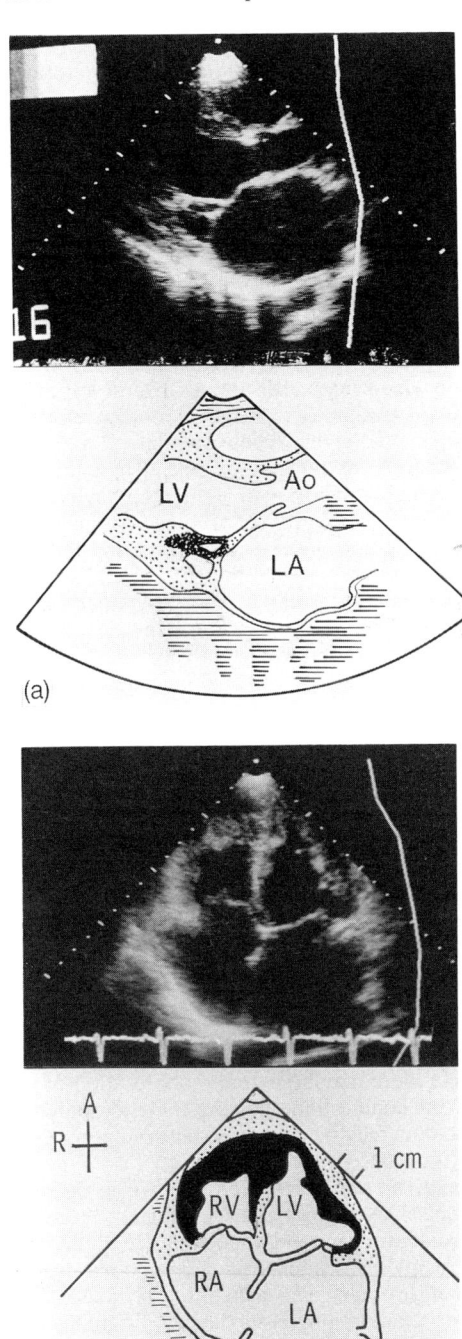

Fig. 8 (a) Systolic long axis cross-sectional echocardiographic appearance in endomyocardial fibrosis. The left atrium is dilated but the left ventricle is of normal size in its outflow portion. An area of bright echoes is seen (darkened on the line drawing underneath) coming from the posterior left ventricular wall and posterior mitral leaflet which are the site of fibrous thickening. (b) Systolic apical four-chamber view. The left atrium is very dilated and the septum bulges towards the right atrium which is also enlarged (the echo fallout in the region of the fossa ovalis does not indicate an atrial septal defect). Both ventricles are small and deformed due to fibrotic obliteration of the apices.

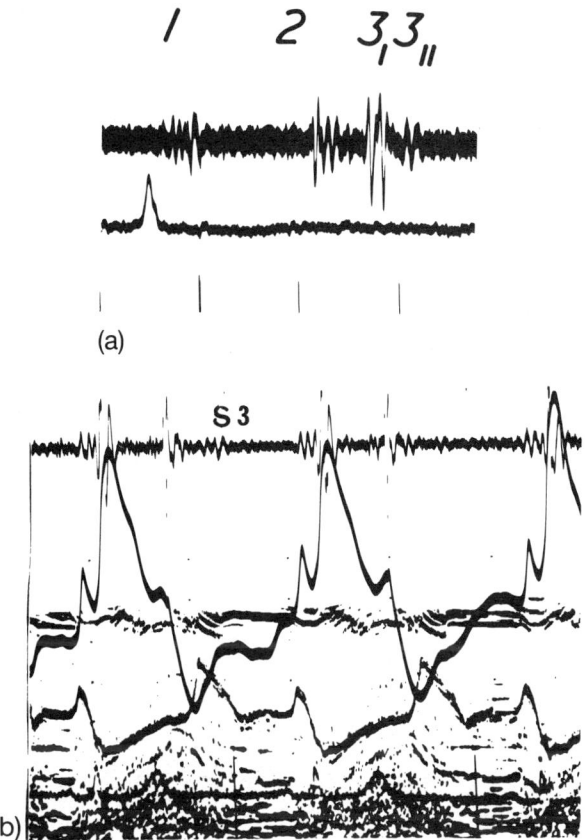

Fig. 9 (a) Phonocardiogram (PCG) in restrictive cardiomyopathy showing asynchronous third heart sounds due to unequal restriction to right and left ventricular filling, and (b) apex impulse with M-mode echo and PCG.

tic or thrombotic disease, which may be susceptible to steroids, as opposed to late fibrotic disease when specific therapy is less important. Biopsy is often abnormal in early cases in the absence of clinical or echo evidence of cardiac involvement. It is important to recognize this possibility when deciding about treatment.

Treatment

The prognosis of HES depends on thromboembolic, cardiovascular, or neurological complications and it is important to lower the eosinophil count as soon as possible. It seems that the use of steroids and cytotoxic drugs has greatly improved the prognosis of these patients. A good response to prednisolone, is most likely in patients with raised serum IgE levels, but the eosinophil count frequently waxes and wanes spontaneously. Steroids may inhibit the mechanisms which cause eosinophil activation or degranulation. They seem to be useful in heart failure caused by acute myocardial necrosis and possibly also in preventing progression to the late fibrotic stage of EMF.

Hydroxyurea reduces eosinophil production and allows steroid dosage to be reduced in patients needing maintenance treatment. The addition of vincristine, given intravenously every two weeks, may result in dramatic reduction of the eosinophil count and an improvement in well being which may be maintained long-term, but bone marrow depression may limit its use.

Thromboembolic problems are common because of endocardial necrosis, and anticoagulants combined with dipyridamole and low-dose (300 mg or less) aspirin are indicated.

The acutely ill hypereosinophilic patient may be temporarily improved (with dramatic falls in eosinophil count) following leukophaeresis and plasma exchange.

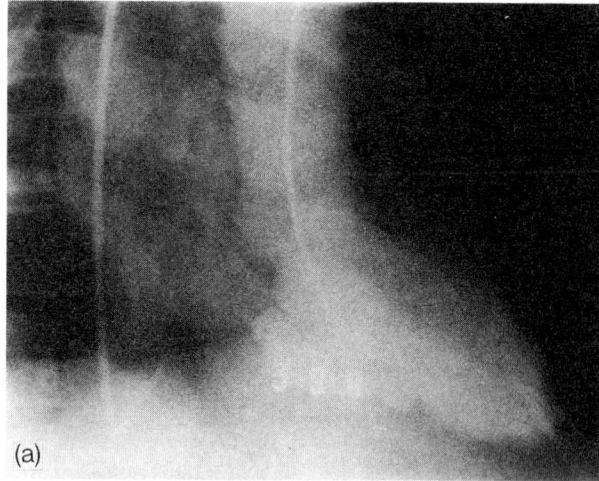

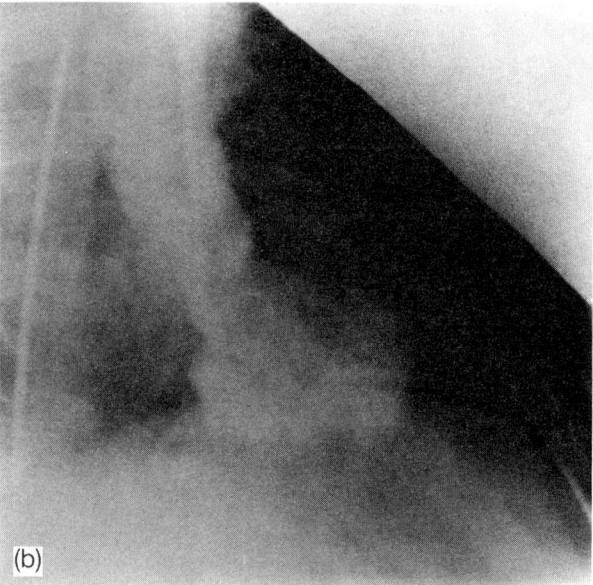

Fig. 10 Left ventricular angiograms in HES showing (a) the normal appearance of the left ventricle at the beginning of the illness when the mitral regurgitation was slight and (b) later on when mitral regurgitation was still slight but the apex appears to have been amputated, the result of cavity obliteration by fibrosis.

'TROPICAL' ENDOMYOCARDIAL FIBROSIS

First described in 1946 from Uganda by Davies and shortly afterwards by Edington from Nigeria, tropical EMF is most frequent from areas 10 degrees north and south of the equator. Although the early descriptions were of very advanced chronic disease, the condition does not seem to differ in its pathology or clinical features from the EMF occurring in non-tropical areas.

Patients in the tropics are younger and tend to come from poor communities with malnutrition and heavy parasite loads (especially filariasis).

African patients tend to present with late fibrotic disease because the population is medically much less supervised and because tropical EMF probably results from a lower grade parasite-induced eosinophilia causing less dramatic and less fatal early illness than the devastating disease of Löffler's original description associated with HES.

The classic appearance of the child with advanced right-sided and often hidden left-sided EMF is with a swollen face and proptosis, tense ascites with everted umbilicus, and stick-thin limbs all caused by a chronically high systemic venous pressure with malnu-

trition accentuated by a protein-losing enteropathy due to the same. Other patients closely simulate rheumatic valvar disease, of which EMF was once thought to be an ethnically determined variation.

Treatment of EMF

Congestive symptoms can be improved by diuretics but overtreatment should be avoided as too great a reduction in ventricular filling pressure may lead to a reduction in cardiac output.

Digoxin is not indicated, as both sinus rhythm and systolic function are usually preserved. A fast heart rate is needed because of the small stroke volume and rapid ventricular filling. Arrhythmias should be sought and ventricular ectopic activity may require specific therapy.

In more than two-thirds of patients both ventricles are involved but in some only the left or only the right ventricle is affected. In patients with severe disease of the right ventricle, left ventricular involvement may be obscured. When mitral regurgitation is severe, valve replacement may be followed by great improvement because the combination of valvar regurgitation with reduced ventricular cavity size causes a disastrous rise in left atrial pressure. So-called decortication (i.e. removal of the endocardium and subendocardial layers) has been popular. It is associated with inevitable replacement of the associated atrioventricular valve and is followed by a great increase in ventricular cavity size because of the development postoperatively of some systolic failure with dilation. This may be associated with a gratifying fall in ventricular diastolic and atrial pressures although the echocardiographic and angiographic appearances of newly impoverished systolic function can be alarming. In general it is preferable to stop at atrioventricular valve replacement, and whenever valvar regurgitation is severe this is usually sufficient. Low profile mechanical valves should be chosen.

Pathology of EMF

The findings are identical in EMF from tropical and from temperate areas, whether or not clinical hypereosinophilia has been present.

The heart is slightly or moderately enlarged and there may be external evidence of obliteration of the right ventricular cavity with retraction and dimpling of its surface. The endocardium may be greatly thickened in the inflow tract and apex of the left ventricle but the thickening stops abruptly at the anterior mitral leaflet where it separates the inflow from the outflow pathways of the left ventricle. The anterior mitral leaflet is rarely affected whereas the posterior leaflet may be bound down in fibrous tissue. In the right ventricle there may be extreme obliteration of the apex and endocardial thickening immobilizing the tricuspid valve leaflets. The infundibulum may be dilated and the pulmonary valve is characteristically normal.

Thrombi may be seen in the ventricles or in the atria although the atria themselves are not usually affected by the disease process. Pericardial effusions and thickening are quite common.

On microscopy the endocardium is characteristically layered with a layer of thrombus over a layer of fibrin and collagen over a very vascular granulation tissue layer containing inflammatory cells and sometimes eosinophils. Calcification and even ossification of the endocardium may occur.

The myocardium may show evidence of hypertrophy or of inflammatory infiltration and the vessels may show some intimal thickening.

References

Andy, J. J., Bishara, F. F. and Soyinka, O. D. (1981). Relation of severe eosinophilia and microfilariasis to chronic African endomyocardial fibrosis. *Br. Heart J.* **45**, 672–680.

Brockington, I. F. and Olsen, E. G. J. (1973). Löffler's endocarditis and Davies' endomyocardial fibrosis. *Am. Heart J.* **85**, 308.

Chew, C. Y. C., Ziady, G. M., Raphael, M. J., Nellen, M. and Oakley, C. M. (1977). Primary restrictive cardiomyopathy. Non-tropical endomyocardial fibrosis and hypereosinophilic heart disease. Br. Heart J. 39, 399–413.

Child, J. S., Levisman, J. A., Abbasi, A. S. and MacAlpin, R. N. (1976). Echocardiographic manifestations of infiltrative cardiomyopathy. A report of seven cases due to amyloid. Chest 70. 726–731.

Chusid, M. J., Dale, D. C., West, B. C. and Wolff, S. M. (1975). The hypereosinophilic syndrome. Medicine (Baltimore) 54, 1–27.

Davies, J. and Spry, C. J. F. (1982). Plasma exchange or leukapheresis in the hypereosinophilic syndrome. Ann. Intern. Med. 96b, 791.

——, ——, Sapsford, R. et al. (1983). Cardiovascular features of eleven patients with eosinophilic endomyocardial disease. Q. J. Med. 52, 23–39.

Davies, J. N. P. (1948). Endocardial fibrosis in Africans. East Afr. Med. J. 25, 10.

—— and Ball, J. D. (1955). The pathology of endomyocardial fibrosis in Uganda. Br. Heart J. 17, 337.

Dubost, C., Maurice, P., Gerbaux, A., Bertrand, E., Rulliere, R., Vial, F., Barrillon, A., Prigent, C., Carpentier, A. and Soyer, R. (1976). The surgical treatment of constrictive fibrous endocarditis. Ann. Surg. 184, 303–307.

Löffler, W. (1936). Endocarditis parietalis fibroplastica mit bluteosinophilie. Schweiz. Med. Wochenschr. 17, 817.

Patel, A. K., D'Arbela, G. and Somers, K. (1977). Endomyocardial fibrosis and eosinophilia. Br. Heart J. 39, 238.

Roberts, W. G., Liegler, D. G. and Cabone, P. P. (1969). Endomyocardial disease and eosinophilia. Am. J. Med. 46, 28.

Schooley, R. T., Parillo, J. E., Wolff, S. M. and Fauci, A. S. (1980). Management of the idiopathic hypereosinophilic syndrome. In The eosinophil in health and disease (eds A. F. Mahmoud and K. F. Austen), pp. 323–339. Grune & Stratton, New York.

HYPERTROPHIC CARDIOMYOPATHY

Hypertrophic cardiomyopathy (HOCM) is an inherited disorder characterized by unexplained, often massive, ventricular hypertrophy, and impaired diastolic function. The hypertrophy may be asymmetrical, involving particularly the upper septum or distal left ventricle. Systolic gradients are common but their significance remains controversial.

Historical

Although almost certainly recognized by earlier cardiac pathologists such as Bernheim and by clinicians such as Osler, HOCM was rediscovered by the pathologist, Donald Teare in 1958. He described asymmetric hypertrophy of the heart in young adults who had died suddenly, including two siblings whose three living siblings were then identified clinically. Round about the same time when Brock was beginning to operate on aortic stenosis, a patient who had presented with severe hypertension but who developed a loud murmur after therapeutic reduction of her blood pressure was found to have a high gradient across the left ventricular outflow tract but at operation only great muscular hypertrophy. Brock's case (published in 1957) is usually cited as the first clinically described case of HOCM. In retrospect, it was a case of severe hypertension with good left ventricular function whose end-systolic volume suddenly diminished as blood pressure was reduced by a ganglion blocking agent. Extensive studies of this exciting new entity followed on both sides of the Atlantic and the disorder was characterized as an inherited disease of seemingly healthy young adults associated with ventricular septal hypertrophy, left ventricular outflow tract obstruction, angina, syncope, and sudden death. It was assumed that the systolic outflow tract gradient indicated obstruction to the outflow of blood and the disease was named 'idiopathic hypertrophic subaortic stenosis' in the United States and 'hypertrophic obstructive cardiomyopathy' in the United Kingdom.

By 1964 Criley had questioned the importance of the left ventricular outflow tract gradient, having demonstrated by cineangiography that the initial outflow of blood from the left ventricle was rapid and that the gradient developed only during mid and late

systole after the left ventricle had contracted down to a normal end-systolic volume and most of the blood had already been ejected. He argued that the gradient was generated by continuing left ventricular contraction after obliteration of the ventricular cavity in late systole and that it was not indicative of true outflow tract obstruction. Criley showed that similar gradients could be induced in animals after inotropic stimulation or haemorrhage. It soon became apparent that only about half of patients with otherwise typical HOCM had outflow tract gradients but the argument continued and indeed still continues in some quarters about the relevance of the gradient in those patients who have one.

With the development of echocardiography came a new and 'echo only' diagnosis known as asymmetric septal hypertrophy or 'ASH' recognized when the width of the septum exceeds that of the posterior left ventricular wall by a ratio greater than 1.3 : 1.

Very quickly a previously rare condition with a bad prognosis became a common condition with a benign prognosis. Although many cases continued to be missed, many more were over diagnosed through M-mode echo, particularly when the echo beam struck the septum normally but travelled obliquely through the wall or when the tricuspid papillary muscle of the septum was included through technical inexactitude.

It was further thought that the bizarre septal histology originally described by Teare was diagnostically specific when in truth these features may be observed to a lesser extent in normal subjects, in secondary hypertrophy, and in congenital heart disease.

Genetic inheritance

Inheritance is usually by an autosomal dominant gene but seemingly sporadic cases also occur. Although some of these may be new mutations, evidence of HOCM is frequently found in family studies of asymptomatic first degree relatives. The inheritance can be likened to that in Marfan's syndrome which is also a disorder for which there is no single diagnostic marker and in which the clinical expression may vary very greatly. Some gene carriers may appear normal and this may account for some of the apparently sporadic cases. In other families the disorder may pursue a persistently malignant course.

HOCM may coexist with certain heredofamilial disorders. These include Noonan's syndrome and lentiginosis. In Friedreich's ataxia the majority of patients die from cardiac causes with greatly hypertrophied hearts (see Section 21).

More difficult is the association of 'too much' or 'asymmetrical' hypertrophy with other causes of hypertrophy. These range from hypertension to aortic stenosis and, particularly, the discrete and tunnel forms of subaortic stenosis. In a disorder such as HOCM which lacks a diagnostic marker it is usually unhelpful to make two diagnoses. A family study has been reported in which congenitally bicuspid aortic valve and HOCM were seen either together or separately; except in such families, it is usually unwise to attribute hypertrophy dually and more important to consider whether the severity of the hypertension or aortic stenosis has been underestimated. It is conceded that some patients with seemingly excessive secondary hypertrophy may have a genetic predisposition to this response or in some cases myocardial hypertrophy may have become asymmetrical because of limitations of blood supply or other factors at cellular level.

Association of HOCM with specific human leucocyte antigens seems likely but the literature is conflicting, probably because of inclusion in most series of hypertensives or of normal subjects with an echo-based diagnosis.

Pathophysiology and pathogenesis

The gross appearance of the typical case of HOCM is very distinctive with massive hypertrophy of the upper ventricular septum and only slight hypertrophy of the free wall of the left ventricle. The disposition of the hypertrophy is widely variable. It may involve only the ventricle distal to the papillary muscles but in many cases these too are markedly enlarged. The right ventricle is usually also hypertrophied, sometimes selectively or the hypertrophy may be concentric in the left or both ventricles.

The heart is overweight due to marked increase in myocardial mass. The ventricular cavities are small but the atria are often dilated and may be hypertrophied, reflecting a high resistance to ventricular filling and sometimes also the effects of atrioventricular valve regurgitation. A fibrous plaque on the left ventricular side of the ventricular septum at the point where the anterior mitral leaflet meets it is typical, and this 'contact lesion' is found both in patients with left ventricular outflow tract gradients and in those without. It is often associated with marked thickening of the anterior mitral valve leaflet, particularly in older patients. In some cases it appears that bunched up chordae rather than the anterior leaflet itself may have met the septum. Turbulence generated during ejection probably determines susceptibility and localization of infective endocarditis in HOCM.

Myocardial fibrosis may be visible and give a 'watered silk' appearance to the cut section, particularly in the upper septum. The myocardial fibre disarray is seen at muscle bundle level, at myocyte level taking the form of 'whorling' with cellular malalignment, and at ultrastructural level with myofibrillar disarray. Despite the lack of specificity the disorganization of myocardial fibre arrangement in the heart appears to be greater in HOCM than in other disorders. This is unhelpful if only a small sample is available and this is why cardiac biopsy is not useful except to exclude other conditions such as amyloid infiltration which may look similar clinically and on echocardiography.

The myocardial cells are thicker, shorter, and more bizarre in shape than in other conditions and the nuclei may appear abnormal. They tend to have a large perinuclear halo of glycogen. These abnormal looking cells are much more common in the septum than in the free wall, particularly in cases with typical asymmetry. Areas of the free wall of the left ventricle often have large areas of ordinary-appearing though hypertrophied cells.

The extramural coronary arteries are usually abnormally large but they are not immune from atheromatous change in older patients. Abnormality of the smaller intramural coronary arteries has been described in the fibrotic areas but may be secondary.

The basic cellular defect is unknown. The disorganization at microscopic level may result from mechanical stresses since it is also seen in other conditions associated with very high systolic pressure. It has been suggested that an abnormal catenoid configuration of the septum, which is genetically determined, could lead to isometric contraction and in turn to cellular disarray. Alternatively, the cellular disarray may be genetically determined and

Table 2 Differential diagnosis of hypertrophic cardiomyopathy

With outflow tract gradient	Without outflow tract gradient
Mitral valve prolapse	Coronary heart disease
Papillary muscle dysfunction	Mitral stenosis
Discrete subaortic stenosis	Left atrial myxoma
Small ventricular septal defect	Constrictive pericarditis
Aortic valve stenosis (in older patients)	Dilated cardiomyopathy
	Athletes

lead to isometric stresses which set up a continuing stimulus to further hypertrophy.

It was early suggested that the condition might result from excessive sympathetic stimulation of the heart due either to overproduction or to abnormal target organ response. This idea initially determined the use of beta-adrenergic blocking drugs in the treatment of the condition but evidence for the concept has weakened over the years.

Clinical evidence for the catecholamine hypothesis is the occasional coexistence of HOCM and phaeochromocytoma, von Recklinghausen's disease and lentiginosis as well as in Noonan's syndrome in which pigmented naevi are also often seen. HOCM in Friedreich's ataxia and in the infants of diabetic mothers can also be linked with increased sympathetic function. In the infants of diabetic mothers noradrenaline secretion is increased in response to exogenous maternal insulin, and these infants often show massive hypertrophy with disproportionate septal thickening which resolves during infancy. Hypertrophy can also be induced in the infants of female rats to which tri-iodothyronine (triac) has been administered during pregnancy. Experimental evidence relates to 'nerve growth factor' which is necessary for the growth of sympathetic neurones, and when administered to pregnant bitches causes an increase in the heart weight of puppies.

Presentation

HOCM may be seen from the neonate to old age. Although presentation is commonly in the second decade, the disorder is most often missed in older patients who are mistakenly thought to have coronary artery disease, mitral prolapse, or aortic stenosis (Table 2). The sex incidence is roughly equal.

The commonest symptom is shortness of breath resulting from a raised left atrial pressure caused by the stiff ventricle and its high diastolic pressure. The tachycardia of exercise makes left atrial emptying even less efficient such that dyspnoea increases and, in addition, the blood pressure may fall due to a fall in stroke

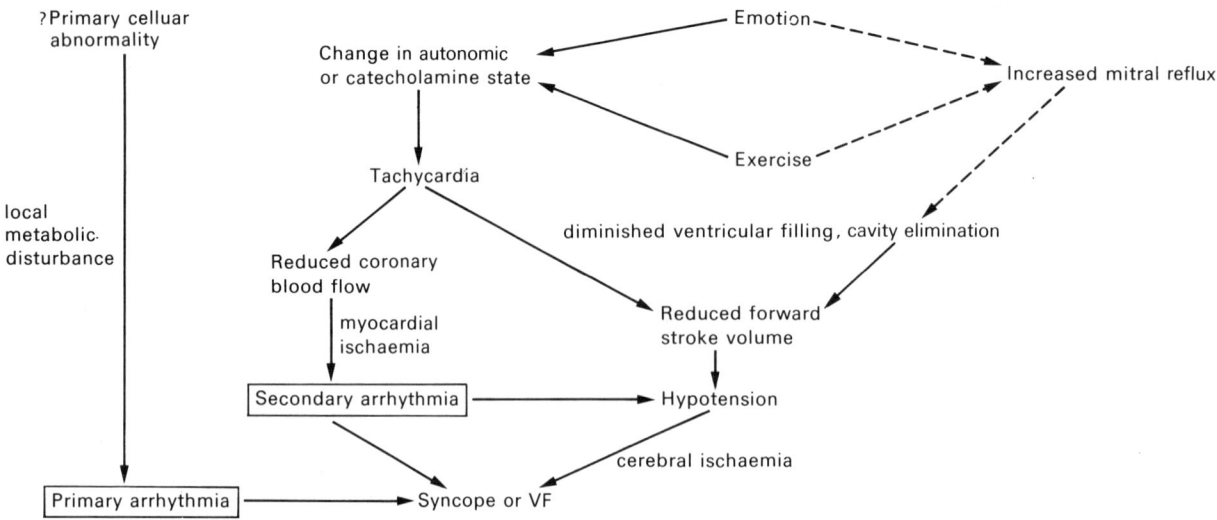

Fig. 11 The mechanisms of syncope and sudden death in hypertrophic cardiomyopathy.

volume, or an arrhythmia may occur due to curtailment of diastolic coronary blood flow. Either may cause syncope (Fig. 11).

Inadequate coronary blood flow may account for angina, which is the second most common symptom, and HOCM should be considered in any young person with typical angina or an older person with a long history of angina of uncertain onset. Older people with HOCM who present with angina of recent onset commonly have coronary artery disease as well.

Arrhythmias are frequent, either occult or causing syncope, palpitation, or dizzy spells. Ambulant ECG monitoring has shown these not to be necessarily tachycardia or bradycardia related. Syncope may also be postural and analogous to the ordinary vasovagal attack except that it may occur with sudden standing rather than from prolonged standing and related to reduced central and left ventricular volume and resultant sudden fall in stroke volume.

Angina in the absence of extramural coronary disease in HOCM has been attributed to narrowing or compression of the intramural coronary arteries or to subendocardial ischaemia related to a high diastolic pressure, increased wall thickness, and myocardial need. Even infarction has been described.

Many cases are asymptomatic. These may be spotted during family studies. In others a murmur or abnormal ECG is found on routine examination and the diagnosis is made by echocardiography.

Elderly patients may present with disabling angina, shortness of breath, or heart failure. Heart failure may develop at any age in patients with severe HOCM; for example, in infancy when left to right shunting may develop across a 'burst' foramen ovale, or in childhood associated with low stroke output and high filling pressure. These features may at first suggest constrictive pericarditis because the heart may still be small. Failure may develop with the onset of atrial fibrillation in patients who have usually had preceding dyspnoea and in old age. Atrial arrhythmias in HOCM seem particularly liable to be complicated by embolism.

Infective endocarditis may occur and the infection can seed from the subaortic and mitral valve area and cause either aortic or mitral regurgitation.

Clinical features

The physical signs are highly variable. In typical cases a positive 'diagnosis of recognition' can be made from the clinical signs alone. In others a firm clinical diagnosis can also be made but by exclusion aided by the ECG and chest radiograph. The most typical signs are those by which the disorder was first recognized and described. The patient is a young adult. The heart rate is regular, the arterial pulses are of normal or seemingly increased volume, and jerky, being rapidly rising and ill sustained. A small dominant a-wave is seen in the venous pulse. The left ventricular impulse is prominent and preceded by a palpable atrial beat giving an anacrotic or double impulse. In some the impulse is a triple shudder, the third element being late systolic following mid-systolic retreat. Such an impulse is diagnostic. Thrills are uncommon but a loud systolic murmur is placed maximally internal to the apex and heard less well in the axilla, at the base, or over the carotid. The murmur is separated from the first heart sound and ceases before the second (Fig. 12). It starts louder and is placed later than the symmetrical murmur of aortic stenosis. Clicks are absent. A soft mid-diastolic inflow murmur may be heard at the apex. There is no opening snap. The atrial beat is usually of too low frequency to be audible but the first heart sound is often mistaken for it because of its separation from the murmur. Third heart sounds are occasionally present but may be right ventricular and heard at the left sternal edge. Evidence of right ventricular enlargement is unusual. Immediate diastolic murmurs are not heard in uncomplicated cases.

Loud murmurs are usually associated with turbulence and with outflow tract gradients but a few patients with loud murmurs have no measurable gradients. Systolic murmurs may be varied by manoeuvres which alter left ventricular size and output (Fig. 13).

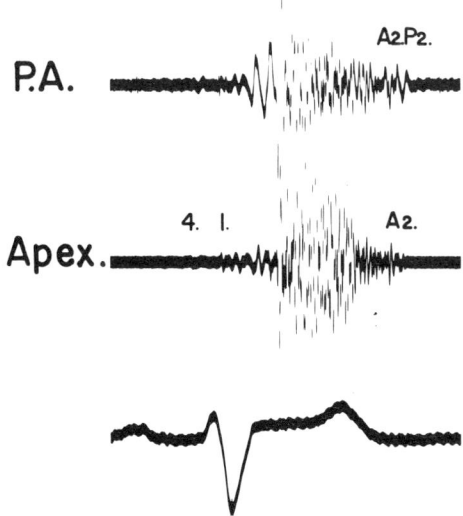

Fig. 12 Phonocardiogram in typical HOCM showing delayed onset asymmetrically shaped crescendo–descrescendo systolic murmur and atrial beat. Pulmonary area (PA) top line and apex underneath.

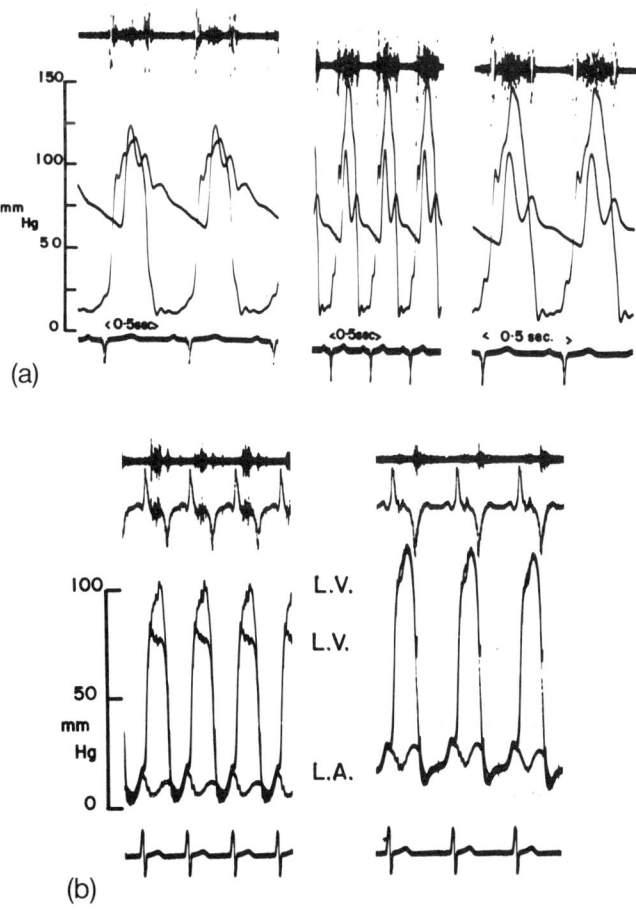

Fig. 13 (a) Simultaneous left ventricular and central aortic pressures with phonocardiograms before and after amyl nitrite inhalation showing development of a gradient and increase in the systolic murmur caused by the drug. (b) Simultaneously recorded left atrial, left ventricular apex and outflow tract pressure, with differentiated ventricular pressure and phonocardiogram above, before and after intravenous phenylephrine 0.3 mg showing abolition both of the subvalvar gradient and of the systolic murmur together with a rise in the left atrial and left ventricular pressures.

A systolic murmur may be abolished by getting the patient to squat suddenly from a standing position or by isometric hand grip exercise. Inhalation of amyl nitrite shrinks the left ventricle and intensifies the murmur. Murmurs may also be provoked during a Valsalva manoeuvre and it may be noticed that murmurs are much louder or appear only in the beat which follows the postectopic pause or after exercise. The second heart sound may be normally or occasionally paradoxically split.

In patients who are murmur-free the palpable atrial beat may reveal the diagnosis and should be sought in the usual way by bringing the apex to maximum prominence; this is usually achieved by getting the patient to turn to the left and hold his breath in expiration or in whatever place in the cycle brings the apex beat into a rib space and onto the finger.

It is not uncommon for the physical signs to have passed for normal on many occasions or even to be 'normal'. This occurs most commonly in big chested middle-aged men.

Athletes

A recent study of sudden death in athletes revealed HOCM in just under half of them. No myocardial fibre disarray could be found in those hearts in which it was sought. This brings to the fore the question whether training can not only develop the subnormal or normal heart to 'supernormal' but may also convert the supernormal heart to an abnormal one with a risk of sudden death. Is the athletic heart syndrome a premorbid condition, and how can it be distinguished from true HOCM?

Adaptation to *isotonic* exercise in athletes includes an increase in left ventricular end-diastolic volume. *Isometric* athletes develop an increase in left ventricular wall thickness which is often more marked in the septum than in the free wall. As most athletes in their training combine both sorts of activity whatever their sport, their hearts usually show a blend of both types of adaptation. Bradycardia, left ventricular hypertrophy with repolarization changes on ECG, and echocardiographic evidence of an increase in wall thickness are found and mirror the clinical findings of high volume pulse, displaced apex beat, ejection systolic murmurs, atrial beats, and third heart sounds. Chest radiographs show cardiothoracic ratios above 50 per cent. Septal hypertrophy with echo 'ASH' has been recorded in more than half of basketball players, and the ratio may reach as high as 2 : 1. 'Muscle-builders' may show grotesque cardiac hypertrophy on echo, particularly those who take anabolic steroids. The implications and reversibility of this hypertrophy are still unknown.

Differentiation from HOCM may be very difficult but two features seem important: (a) the healthy athlete's 'abnormal' ECG becomes normal during exercise, and (b) the end-diastolic left ventricular cavity dimension is increased in athletes whereas it tends to be reduced in HOCM. Both of these criteria still beg the question because the athlete who has developed HOCM, perhaps as a result of his training, must retain an increased stroke volume if he is to be succesful, and hypertrophied hearts, whatever they are called, may have an increased tendency to arrhythmia. HOCM should not be diagnosed in athletes simply because of left ventricular hypertrophy and septal/posterior wall ratio on echo in excess of 1.3 : 1.

Investigation

Electrocardiogram

This is nearly always abnormal in adults but occasionally normal in the young. In children the most common abnormality is voltage evidence of left ventricular hypertrophy, rarely also of right ventricular hypertrophy. In older patients ST and T-wave abnormalities are nearly invariable, suggesting ischaemia, or with steep T-wave inversion simulating previous subendocardial infarction.

In patients who are followed over years the development and progression of abnormality may be seen. There is usually gradually increasing voltage evidence of left ventricular hypertrophy and a progressive tendency for loss of the Q-wave in the left ven-

tricular leads and widening of the QRS. A deep Q-wave may appear in the mid-precordial leads, simulating previous anteroseptal infarction. The T-waves are often upright in leads with abnormal Q-waves and this may help to distinguish HOCM from previous myocardial infarction. The mid-precordial Q-waves have been attributed to a change in the directional activation of the septum, caused either by alteration in its geometry or by fibrosis which has interfered with activation or even rendered it electrically silent so that early posterior forces predominate. Left axis deviation commonly develops and when this is observed the ECG changes meet the criteria for left anterior hemiblock. Complete left or right bundle branch block are uncommon.

Rare patients may show pure right ventricular hypertrophy with right axis deviation and dominant R-waves in the right precordial leads. Such patients may have high right ventricular gradients caused by extensive septal hypertrophy protruding towards the right ventricle during ejection; less often predominant or exclusive involvement of the right ventricle in the hypertrophic process. Left atrial or biatrial P-waves are very common; the P-waves may be more bizarrely tall and wide than in any other disorder, particularly in children with severe disease. In such patients atrial fibrillation commonly develops later and then the characteristic ECG with its left ventricular and left atrial hypertrophy tends to become a non-specifically abnormal ECG which could as well be attributed to any disorder affecting the left ventricle.

A short PR interval has been observed as a common finding in patients with HOCM, particularly in those with evidence of left atrial and left ventricular enlargement when the absence of a preliminary Q-wave in left ventricular leads and a slur on the upstroke of the R-wave may simulate pre-excitation. Although the combination of HOCM with the Wolff–Parkinson–White syndrome has been noted on a number of occasions this may be a chance association of two not uncommon disorders.

Both atrial and ventricular arrhythmias are commonly found on ECG monitoring. These may be of any kind. Treadmill exercise testing may provoke such arrhythmias either during the exercise or during the bradycardia which follows but Holter ambulant ECG recording is more reliable. Ventricular arrhythmias may be predictive of sudden death and because of their frequency it seems sensible to test all patients with HOCM in this way. Exercise testing reveals the extent of disability, which is useful in patients with long-standing symptoms who are used to a disability and may not realize its extent, and for assessing therapy.

Echocardiography (Table 3 and Fig. 16)

Echocardiography is of immense diagnostic value. The cross-sectional technique greatly aids definition of the distribution and severity of the hypertrophy as well as showing the site and mechanism of cavity elimination (see page 13.34).

Using M-mode alone the form of HOCM in which left ventricular hypertrophy is confined to the distal part of the left ventricle may be entirely missed although it is easily recognized by the cross-sectional technique. This was first described from Japan and is a recognizable subset of HOCM characterized by giant inverted

Table 3 The echocardiographic features of HOCM

Cross-sectional echo
Increase in left ventricular wall thickness which may be focal or generalized. Typically most marked in the upper septum, it may be entirely confined to the distal left ventricle and missed on M-mode
Reduced or low normal dimensions of the left ventricle

M-mode
Asymmetrical hypertrophy of the septum compared with the posterior free wall of the left ventricle (ratio >1.3 : 1)
Anterior eccentricity of the mitral valve which 'fills' the left ventricle
Systolic anterior motion ('SAM') of the mitral anterior leaflet on to the septum and delayed onset of diastolic closure
Systolic closure of the aortic valve cusps

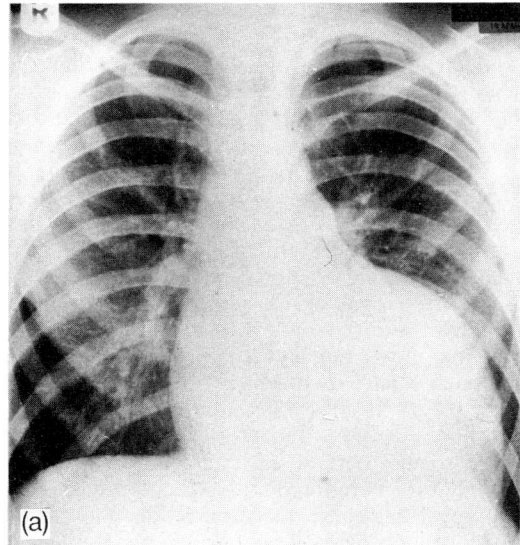

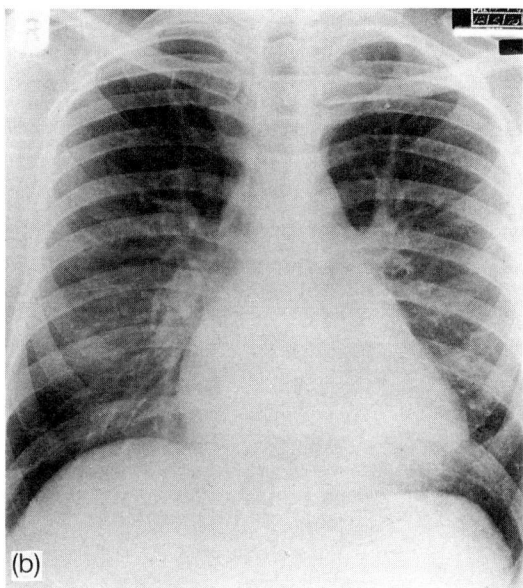

Fig. 14 (a) Chest radiograph showing a markedly prominent left ventricle caused by gross hypertrophy in a boy aged 10 years. (b) Enlarged left atrium (and appendage) with marked pulmonary congestive changes simulating the appearance of rheumatic mitral valve disease from a man aged 41 years with severe HOCM.

T-waves on the ECG and a spade-shaped left ventricle on angiography.

The echo beam in the M-mode should be directed across the ventricular cavity at a level just caudal to the tips of the mitral valve leaflets, which corresponds with the usual area of maximal septal hypertrophy. The cardinal echocardiographic feature of HOCM is an absolute increase in left ventricular wall thickness, particularly of the septum whose thickness may be more than 1.3 times that of the posterior wall ('asymmetric septal hypertrophy'). The width of the cavity is at or below the lower limits of normal both at end-systole and at end-diastole. Systolic anterior movement of the anterior leaflet brings it into apposition with the septum for a varying portion of the rest of systole. In diastole the anterior leaflet shows delayed onset of closure followed by a slow diastolic closure slope. In florid cases the mitral anterior leaflet is on the septum for most of systole after systolic reopening and in early diastole as well. The aortic valve may show systolic closure of the cusps. When well marked these features are diagnostic but no one of the echo features just described is pathognomonic.

Radiography
The cardiothoracic ratio may be normal but the left ventricle is prominent, often with a rather high bulge sometimes even suggestive of aneurysm. The right atrium also may be prominent. In severe cases the lungs show pulmonary venous congestion, and when heart failure develops there may be considerable cardiomegaly but the left ventricle only very rarely becomes dilated (Fig. 14). Valve calcification is not seen in uncomplicated cases. Rarely, the chest X-ray is normal.

Haemodynamics and angiography (Fig. 17)
The cardiac output is usually normal at rest but exercise or emotion-provoked tachycardia is associated with a fall in stroke volume which is sometimes sufficient to cause a fall in blood pressure and syncope. In mild cases the cardiac output may be normal even on exercise. In severe cases the cardiac output is low at rest and falls further with any increment or decrement in heart rate.

Typical cases show a variable gradient between the body of the left ventricle and the vestibule or outflow tract (Fig. 15). This gradient usually occurs at the point where the anterior leaflet of the mitral valve abuts on the ventricular septum during systole. Less often the pressure drop occurs in mid-cavity at the site of apposition of hypertrophied papillary muscles. When the gradient occurs at mitral valve level a catheter introduced trans-septally behind the anterior leaflet enters the high pressure part of the left ventricle with the first beat after entering the ventricle. Artefactual gradients are also easily recorded in HOCM if the catheter tip becomes lodged in a trabecular space because of the small size of the cavity and the greatly hypertrophied muscle. Such artefactual gradients can be recognized because they develop early in systole whereas true gradients are later, the pressure in the left ventricle beginning to rise above the pressure in the left ventricular outflow tract and aorta only after the aortic pressure has reached its peak. The left ventricular pressure shows a characteristic notch at this point (Fig. 16).

Agents which increase contractile force or reduce left ventricular size or both usually increase the gradients which vary cyclically with respiration or change in posture. Changes in the length and intensity of the murmur in such patients reflect these fluctuations and the murmur may be augmented on standing, disappear on

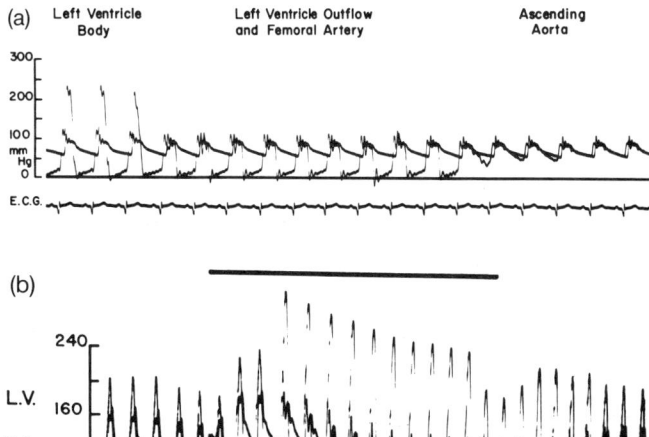

Fig. 15 (a) Simultaneously recorded femoral artery and left ventricular pressures on withdrawal of catheter from the left ventricle showing the subvalvar site of the gradient. (b) Simultaneous left ventricular and brachial artery pressures during a Valsalva manoeuvre showing great increase in systolic pressure difference during the strain period.

squatting, increase during a Valsalva manoeuvre or after amyl nitrite inhalation, or disappear after phenylephrine (see Fig. 13).

A typical feature of HOCM is the phenomenon of post-extra-systolic potentiation wherein the beat following the compensatory pause after a premature beat is associated with an increase in out-flow tract gradient with a higher left ventricular pressure and a lower aortic pressure and pulse pressure than in the regular beats. The post-extrasystolic arterial pulse shows exaggeration of the systolic dip. Careful ciné-angiography studies have shown that in the post-extrasystolic beat there is a fall in forward flow, an increase in mitral regurgitation, and a decrease in end-systolic volume compared with the regular beats. Although an increase in outflow tract gradient also occurs in fixed outflow tract obstruction, both the left ventricular and the aortic pressures rise in the post-extrasystolic beat. The fall in systemic arterial pressure which occurs in HOCM in the post-extrasystolic beat associated with a change in the configuration of the arterial pulse is one of the most specific signs of the disease.

The diastolic pressure in the left ventricle may be elevated throughout diastole, particularly at end-diastole when the a-wave may be very high. The a-wave in the left atrium is augmented although the mean pressure is usually at the upper limit of normal at rest until the advent of heart failure. Despite mitral regurgitation the v-wave rarely exceeds the a-wave in the left atrium except in the post-extrasystolic beat.

Swan–Ganz monitoring of the pulmonary artery and wedge pressures in HOCM during exercise often shows a dramatic rise with tachycardia. This is due to slow left ventricular filling, inad-equate left atrial emptying, and resulting fall in stroke volume which may generate a vicious spiral of increasing rate, diminishing stroke volume, and a fall in blood pressure; either cerebral or myocardial ischaemia may then determine syncope and even death (see Fig. 11). While it is not suggested that patients should ever be exercised to this point, the use of exercise monitoring allows the dose of beta blocker in breathless patients to be adjusted so as to ensure that the heart rate is effectively kept down during exercise in order to avoid the genesis of this potentially fatal vicious spiral. The use of this technique has revealed that syncope in HOCM is not always due to cardiac arrhythmia.

Pressure gradients may also be detected in the right ventricle between the apex and the outflow tract. They are caused by the encroachment of the septum on to the right ventricular cavity. The right ventricular diastolic pressure may be elevated in such patients and the right atrial pressure may show a dominant a-wave.

The left ventricular outflow tract gradients are real but there is no evidence that they are important. Recent studies employing a velocity probe in the aortic root or fractionating the phases of ejection in radionuclide blood pool studies have shown a pattern of ejection in patients with outflow tract gradients similar to those without. Early ejection of blood from the left ventricle is rapid, but later in systole ejection is slow or ceases entirely in patients both with and without gradients. This late curtailment of systolic ejection accounts for mid-systolic closure of the aortic valve leaflets seen on echo. The late deceleration of ejection may be associated with outflow tract turbulence (which is also visible on echo) at mitral valve level, causing a late-onset systolic murmur. Sometimes turbulence occurs during early rapid ejection and gives rise to an early ejection murmur of non-specific type which may tend to mask the more typical late-onset systolic murmur. Another source for a late systolic murmur is mitral regurgitation which

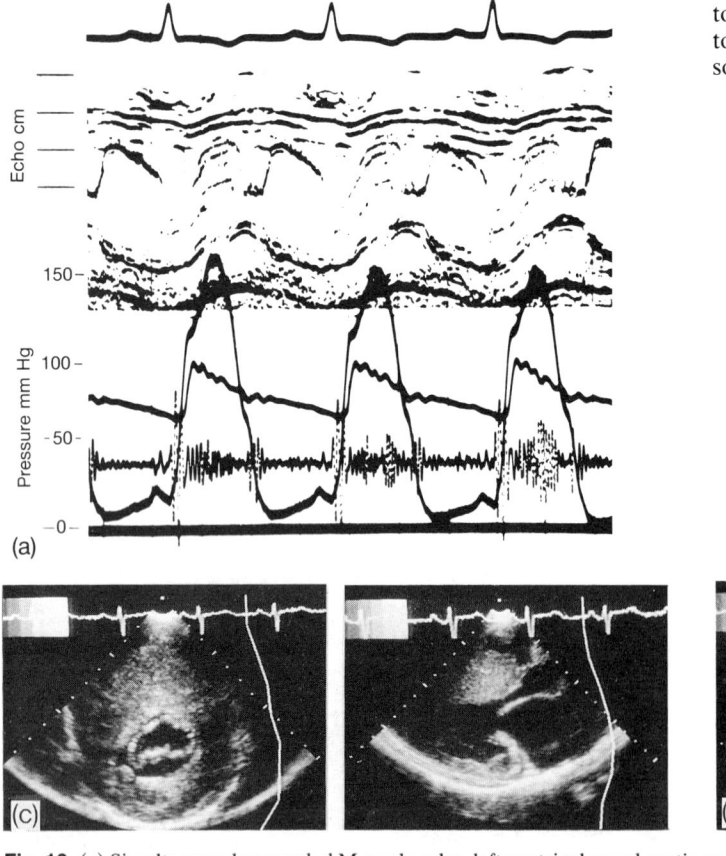

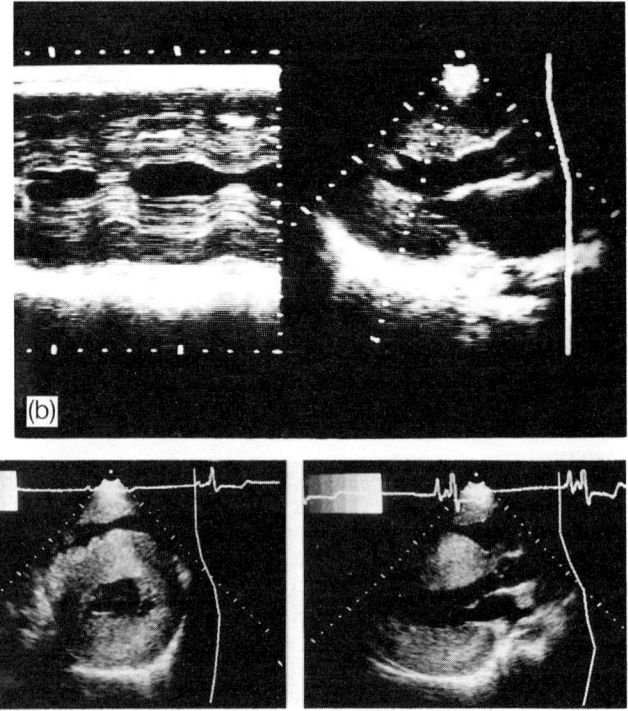

Fig. 16 (a) Simultaneously recorded M-mode echo, left ventricular and aortic pressures and phonocardiogram showing the features listed in Table 3. Note that systolic anterior motion (SAM) coincides with the onset of the gradient. Aortic valve closure is late because of the gradient and mitral valve opening is early because of a raised left atrial pressure, so in this patient the isovolumic relaxation period is greatly shortened. In patients without an outflow gradient and with a normal left atrial pressure this period is usually prolonged. (b) Parasternal long axis view of the left ventricle in HOCM showing the small cavity. On the right the M-mode beam is seen cutting the left ventricle just below the mitral valve, and on the left the M-mode echo shows almost complete elimination of the cavity in systole and a maximum dimension of only 2 cm in diastole. (c and d) Short axis (on the left) and parasternal long axis views of the left ventricle in HOCM showing, in (c), asymmetrical hypertrophy with gross thickening of the septum and normal thickness of the posterior free wall. In (d) the hypertrophy is generalized and symmetrical.

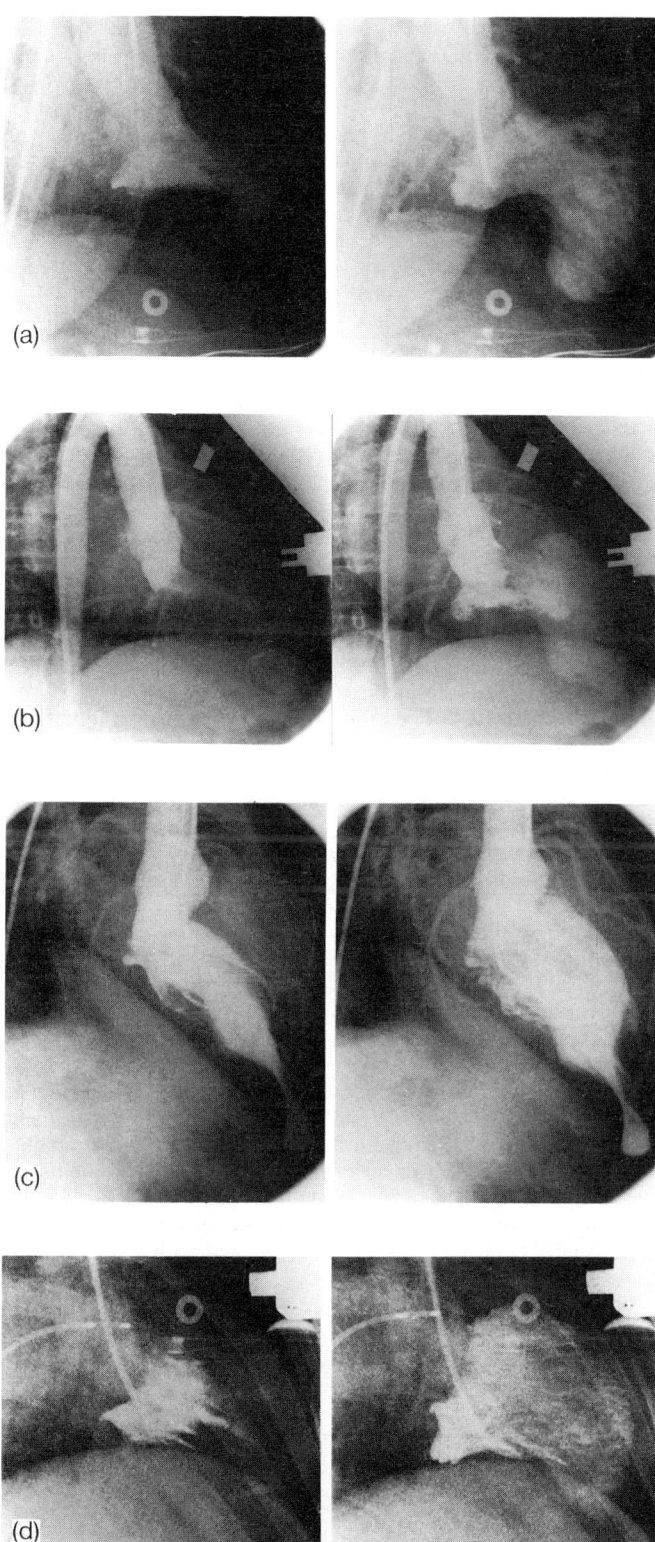

(a)

(b)

(c)

(d)

Fig. 17 Left ventriculograms from four different patients with HOCM illustrating the widely variable appearances (all in right anterior oblique projections with systole on the left and diastole on the right). (a) 'Bent banana' shape with greatly reduced end-systolic volume and huge papillary muscle impression remaining in diastole like the high instep of a misshapen foot. There is some mitral reflux into the left atrium. (b) Greatly elongated and bent cavity with considerable residual contrast in the 'toe' of the left ventricle at end-systole (faintly shown). (c) Multiple muscle indentations into an elongated left ventricular cavity. (d) 'Spade' or turnip-shaped left ventricle in the form of HOCM with hypertrophy confined to the distal part of the left ventricle and giant inverted T-waves on the ECG.

starts when the mitral valve moves anteriorly on to the septum, allowing reflux which is usually small in amount except in post-extrasystolic beats.

Left ventriculography (Fig. 17) shows a typically misshapen chamber, often with a bend in the long axis, and with unusually prominent papillary muscles which may give a 'bent banana' shape to the cavity at the end of ejection. Sometimes a trail of contrast is seen from papillary muscle level to the apex, caused by total obliteration of the cavity at the point of apposition of large papillary muscles. The ventricle resembles a turnip with a long fibre at its tip but has also been called 'spade-shaped'. Occasionally a pool of contrast is left in the extreme apex. Cases with a banana-shaped cavity usually have the most markedly asymmetric hypertrophy with a huge immobile septum and a well contracting and often much less hypertrophied free wall bent around it. The end-systolic volume is reduced in size and often the ventricle appears to empty virtually completely. That there is no single arbiter for the diagnosis of HOCM holds true even for left ventricular angiography and the degree of abnormality varies from minimal to bizarre. Rarely, the angiogram looks normal even in patients with indubitable HOCM by other criteria. Conversely, the left ventricle may appear very misshapen in some older patients with rheumatic mitral stenosis in whom an erroneous diagnosis of HOCM may be made. This becomes particularly difficult since increased rigidity and stenosis of the mitral valve may develop in older patients with HOCM. The diastolic pressure in the left ventricle usually differentiates as well as the presence of an outflow tract gradient which is invariably present in patients with secondary mitral valve changes.

The mitral valve anterior leaflet may be seen in profile in left anterior oblique (LAO) views enhanced by craniocaudal tilt and then the anterior leaflet is seen to bend anteriorly at its junction with the mitral veil giving it a J shape. Reflux into the left atrium takes place posteriorly around it.

A combination of left and right ventriculography carried out simultaneously in this angled LAO projection may allow views of the thickness and configuration of the ventricular septum.

In older patients with HOCM the presenting symptom may be angina; this is often due to acquired atheromatous coronary artery disease, so coronary angiography should always be included in the investigation of patients aged over 40 years.

Management

When HOCM was first recognized, management was designed to relieve the outflow tract gradients by which the disorder was then defined. Since digitalis increases the gradient, this became proscribed, as did isoprenaline and other beta-agonist drugs and nitrates. In recent years more attention has been paid to diastole, slow filling and high diastolic pressures being responsible for tachycardia-related symptoms. When isoprenaline was found to cause an increase in outflow tract gradient and a rise in end-diastolic pressure in the left ventricle, beta-adrenergic blocking drugs were introduced into treatment. These drugs prevent isoprenaline-induced surges in gradient and sometimes reduce the resting gradient although this effect is usually not dramatic. Beta-blocking drugs may also improve the diastolic length tension relationship and result in improvement in the filling characteristics of the left ventricle. More recent studies have suggested that the spectrum of response in HOCM is highly variable, some patients seeming to show improvement in filling and others not. The most constant effect of a beta-blocking drug has been depression of systolic function, shown by a fall in ejection fraction and peak dp/dt with an increase in end-diastolic volume and a variable effect on the end-diastolic pressure.

Undoubtedly the major benefit of beta blockers stems from curtailment of exercise- or emotion-induced tachycardia. Angina is reduced by better maintenance of diastolic coronary blood flow and syncopal attacks are prevented in those instances where they were caused by a drop in blood pressure during sinus tachycardia or during ischaemia-provoked ventricular arrhythmias. Shortness of breath on exertion may also be improved by allowing the left atrium more time to empty. Angina is the symptom which responds best to beta blockers but the overall relief of symptoms in HOCM has been rather disappointing.

Verapamil was introduced for the treatment of HOCM in 1978. The experience of different centres has been inconsistent. It has been found that although outflow tract gradients are reduced when verapamil is given acutely, systolic function is not appreciably altered during 'chronic' use of the drug. Studies of the diastolic function of the left ventricle using blood pool scanning have shown an increased peak filling rate and time to peak filling rate after verapamil compared with before it. Other studies using echocardiography and systolic and diastolic time intervals have shown improved filling characteristics in some patients, but clinical acceptance of verapamil has been disappointing.

Sudden death is the most common way for patients with HOCM to die (see Fig. 11) and it is logical that this be predicted from the detection of ventricular arrhythmias even though these may be asymptomatic. It is our practice to submit all patients with HOCM to an exercise test and ambulant ECG monitoring. If arrhythmias are detected, they should be treated and the efficacy of the treatment tested by repeated exercise and ECG monitoring. Neither propranolol nor verapamil is effective in preventing ventricular arrhythmias in HOCM. Both may slow the rate of atrial arrhythmias but neither prevents them. The drug which has proved to be most effective in arrhythmia prevention has been amiodarone (see page 13.134). This is given in minimal maintenance dose following a loading period. The maintenance dose is judged by repeated ambulant monitoring and is the minimal dose which prevents the arrhythmia. In general, atrial arrhythmias are suppressed in low doses averaging only 200 mg daily but ventricular arrhythmias may need 400 mg or sometimes more than this. Toxic side-effects are usually dose and duration related and are rarely seen in the doses used. Blood levels have little relationship to dosage and are useful ancillary guides. It has been noted that ventricular arrhythmias on Holter recording are uncommon in children, a group in which sudden death is tragically common. This is still unexplained.

When atrial fibrillation first develops in HOCM, the patient very often deteriorates abruptly. This is due more to the irregularity and rapid rate during exercise than to loss of the atrial contribution to left ventricular filling which has become negligible by the time atrial fibrillation develops since the latter is a consequence of atrial overdistension. It is very important, when paroxysmal atrial arrhythmias are first known or suspected, to start the patient on permanent anticoagulant treatment with warfarin because of the high risk of emboli. Atrial fibrillation is rarely well controlled with digoxin alone. Digoxin plus propranolol is better but amiodarone is usually the best, allowing regularization of the rate and often a return of sinus rhythm. Symptomatic benefit from amiodarone is often dramatic even though the drug appears to have no significant haemodynamic effect in HOCM.

Management of pregnancy

Pregnancy and delivery are usually accomplished without difficulty in patients with HOCM (see page 11.12). Because tachycardia, rapid blood loss, and repeated Valsalva maneouvres might be dangerous, elective Caesarean section was practised during our early experience, but after a number of patients had tolerated vaginal delivery it was learned that, as in other heart diseases, Caesarian section was indicated only for obstetric reasons. At first, beta-adrenergic blocking drugs were used routinely throughout pregnancy but pregnant patients with HOCM are now treated according to individual indications.

In a series of 43 pregnancies which went to term, no mothers or babies died. Diuretics were sometimes required for pulmonary congestion and beta blockers for angina. Epidural anaesthesia was considered inadvisable on theoretical grounds. This series was representative of a wide range of the disorder, including patients with very severe disease. Problems in a previous pregnancy did not always recur and deterioration in symptoms could not be predicted by the severity of the outflow tract gradient or by any other feature, although patients whose disease was clinically mild did not develop congestive features requiring diuretic treatment and only two patients showed an increase of angina. It still seems sensible to avoid factors which would increase left ventricular outflow gradients, such as vasodilatation from epidural anaesthesia, hypotension from blood loss, violent expulsive effort, and cardiac stimulant drugs. Oxytocic agents may be given safely. We used to advocate antibiotic prophylaxis against endocarditis but no longer do so for uncomplicated delivery of cardiac patients.

Pregnancy is associated with increased ventricular ectopic activity and it might be argued that pregnant patients with HOCM would be particularly at risk from sudden death and should be protected. Our experience does not support this. A further 58 pregnancies in HOCM patients were not included in the analysis because of insufficient obstetric data but there were no sudden deaths amongst this group. Since recent studies have shown that beta-blocking drugs are ineffective in suppressing clinically important ventricular arrhythmias, rhythm changes in pregnancy should be sought and treated with specific agents whose efficacy is subsequently proven by ambulatory monitoring.

If beta-blockers are given in pregnancy, it is wise to monitor fetal growth particularly carefully, and the heart rate and blood sugar of the neonate should be observed for the first 48 hours after birth since the effect of beta blockers persists considerably longer than would be anticipated from their pharmacological half-life.

Patients rarely ask spontaneously about the eugenic aspects of their disease. In a condition with such a variable outcome it is difficult to advise wisely, although our studies have shown that families tend to run true to form – i.e. that a history of early death from HOCM in a family has predictive value.

Surgical treatment

A number of procedures have been used, of which the most popular is excision of a short length of the hypertrophied upper septum by a transaortic approach. This is the so-called myotomy-myectomy. A more radical approach was to combine the transaortic with a left ventricular approach to resect the lower septum also. The septum has also been approached from the right ventricle. Excision of the mitral valve and replacement with a low profile prosthesis has been advocated for the relief of outflow gradients. All these procedures are usually followed by loss of gradients and some improvements of symptoms. The operative mortality has been high – between 5 and 10 per cent. The indications for surgery have usually been severe symptoms coupled with a high outflow tract gradient.

Surgery may have a role in the treatment of HOCM in the elderly who often have late onset of severe symptoms associated with gross left ventricular hypertrophy and secondary organic changes in the mitral valve. This may be calcified with fixed stenosis and regurgitation consequent upon long-standing distortion of the valve and degenerative changes probably caused by turbulence at the site. Such patients may benefit from mitral valve replacement. Except in these special circumstances, patients with HOCM are better treated medically.

The protagonists of surgical treatment cite a gratifying symptomatic benefit in their patients but even they are unable to prove long-term gain. Postoperative changes in left ventricular function include loss of left ventricular outflow tract gradient, a fall in ejection fraction, an increase in left ventricular end-diastolic volume, and sometimes a fall in left ventricular end-diastolic pressure. The sceptic may regard these as consequences of left ventricular damage caused by difficulties in preservation of the hypertrophied myocardium even by modern cold cardioplegic techniques. Indeed, such changes when marked seem to presage the late development of left ventricular failure seen in at least 25 per cent of the late survivors of operative treatment.

Natural history and the effect of treatment upon prognosis

Retrospective analysis has been carried out at Hammersmith Hospital, London, to assess the prognostic value of clinical, electrocardiographic, and haemodynamic features in 216 patients with HOCM who had been fully investigated and followed for up to 23 years. Of these patients, 49 have died, 24 of them suddenly. The study confirmed clinical folklore: a family history of sudden death, blackouts, or diagnosis in childhood were of ill omen but neither angina, nor shortness of breath, nor palpitation was found to be associated with poor prognosis and no feature in the resting electrocardiogram was of prognostic importance. Very surprisingly, no haemodynamic features nor the amount of hypertrophy were found to help determine prognosis, perhaps because patients with high left atrial pressures had already received diuretics. Neither a resting nor a provocable left ventricular outflow tract gradient proved predictive of early subsequent mortality. This is of particular interest because of a high outflow tract gradient provided the conventional indication for surgical treatment in the past. No clinical, electrocardiographic, echocardiographic, or haemodynamic feature analysed either separately or together revealed any significant difference between the patients who had died and the survivors. It was impossible to assess the effect of propranolol on prognosis because most of our patients had been taking it. Thirty-three patients had undergone myotomy-myectomy and/or mitral valve replacement with nine perioperative deaths. Six of the 24 surgical survivors subsequently died. Surgical treatment may have affected prognosis adversely in a group of patients whose natural outlook should have been no worse than that for the group as a whole. The commonest mode of death in HOCM is sudden and we have shown that this is predicted better from information obtained at the first consultation than by any subsequent laboratory investigation. A minority of patients followed by serial echo have shown progressive wall thinning associated with deterioration in systolic function and increase in diastolic filling pressures without any or only slight increase in left ventricular cavity size.

It can be argued whether or not full invasive investigation is worth doing in HOCM since the combination of clinical features and cross-sectional echocardiography provide the diagnosis and the extended ECG provides the prognosis. Serial cross-sectional echo with Doppler echo will provide much needed information on individual natural history.

Prevention of sudden death

The detection and effective treatment of ventricular arrhythmias comprise the best approach to a reduction of sudden death and improvement in long-term prognosis which has not yet been achieved by any form of medical or surgical treatment. High risk children without demonstrable arrhythmias should probably also be treated.

Summary of management

After HOCM is diagnosed, arrhythmias should first be sought and treated in every patient. If any symptoms remain, these should be treated appropriately either with beta blockers or with verapamil. The precise role of verapamil is not yet defined. The spectrum of haemodynamic abnormality is so wide in HOCM that it may be regarded as composed of many subsets, each with differing pharmacological responses. Until these are identified the approach to symptom relief must be by trial and error.

Surgery is needed only for secondary organic changes in the mitral valve when replacement with a low profile prosthesis may be indicated.

References

Borer, J. S., Bacharach, S. L., Green, M. V., Kent, K. M., Rosing, D. R., Seides, S. F., Morrow, A. G. and Epstein, S. E. (1979). Effect of septal myotomy and myectomy on left ventricular systolic function at rest and during exercise in patients with IHSS. *Circulation* 60, suppl. 1, 82–87.

Braunwald, E., Lambrew, C. T., Rockoff, S. D., Ross, J. and Morrow, A. G. (1964). Idiopathic hypertrophic subaortic stenosis: A description of the disease based upon an analysis of 64 patients. *Circulation* 30, suppl. IV, 3–119.

Brock, R. C. (1957). Functional obstruction of the left ventricle. *Guy's Hosp. Rep.* 160, 221–238.

Criley, J. M. and Siegel, R. J. (1985). A non-obstructive view of hypertrophic cardiomyopathy. In *Heart muscle disease* (ed. J. F. Goodwin), pp. 157–185. MTP Press, Lancaster.

Doi, Y. L., McKenna, W. J., Gehrke, J., Oakley, C. M. and Goodwin, J. F. (1980). M-mode echocardiography in hypertrophic cardiomyopathy; diagnosis criteria and prediction of obstruction. *Am. J. Cardiol.* 45, 1–13.

Emanuel, R. and Withers, R. (1983). Genetics of the cardiomyopathies. *Prog. Cardiol.* 12, 211–223.

Goodwin, J. F. and Oakley, C. M. The cardiomyopathies (editorial). *Br. Heart J.* 34, 545–552.

Henry, W. L., Clark, C. E. and Epstein, S. E. (1973). Asymmetrical septal hypertrophy. *Circulation* 47, 225–233.

Huston, T. P., Puffer, J. C. and Rodney, W. M. (1985). The athletic heart syndrome. *N. Engl. J. Med.* 313, 24–31.

Kaltenbach, M., Hopf, R., Kober, G., Bussman, W. D., Keller, M. and Petersen, Y. (1979). Treatment of hypertrophic obstructive cardiomyopathy with verapamil. *Br. Heart J.* 42, 35–42.

McKenna, W. J. (1983). Arrhythmia and prognosis in hypertrophic cardiomyopathy. *Europ. Heart J.* 4, suppl. F, 225–234.

——, Chetty, S., Oakley, C. M. and Goodwin, J. E. (1980). Arrhythmias in hypertrophic cardiomyopathy exercise and 48 hour ambulatory electrocardiographic assessment with and without beta adrenergic blocking therapy. *Am. J. Cardiol.* 45, 1–5.

——, Deanfield, J. E., Faruqi, A. M., Oakley, C. M. and Goodwin, J. F. (1979). Prognosis and mortality in hypertrophic cardiomyopathy. *Circulation* 60, suppl. II, 154.

Maron, B. J., Koch, J. P., Kent, K. M., Epstein, S. E. and Morrow, A. G. (1980). Results of surgery for idiopathic hypertrophic subaortic stenosis. *J. Cardiovasc. Med.* 5, 145–156.

——, Lipson, L. C., Roberts, W. C., Savage, D. D. and Epstein, S. E. (1978). 'Malignant' hypertrophic cardiomyopathy. Identification of a subgroup of families with unusually frequent premature death. *Am. J. Cardiol.* 41, 1133–1140.

——, Roberts, W. C., Edwards, J. E., McAllister, H. A. Jr, Foley, D. D. and Epstein, S. E. (1978). Sudden death in patients with hypertrophic cardiomyopathy: characterization of 26 patients without functional limitation. *Am. J. Cardiol.* 41, 803–810.

Merrill, W. H., Frier, P. A., Kent, K. M., Epstein, S. E. and Morrow, A. G. (1978). Long-term clinical course and symptomatic status of patients after operation for hypertrophic subaortic stenosis. *Circulation* 57, 1205–13.

Oakley, C. M. (1974). Clinical recognition of the cardiomyopathies. *Circulation* 34/35, suppl. 11, 152–159.

Oakley, G. D. G., McGarry, K., Limb, D. G. and Oakley, C. M. (1979). Management of pregnancy in patients with hypertrophic cardiomyopathy. *Br. Med. J.* 1, 1749–1751.

Olsen, E. G. J. (1983). Anatomic and lightmicroscopic characterization of hypertrophic and non-obstructive cardiomyopathy. *Eur. Heart J.* 4, suppl. F, 1–8.

Pomerance, A. and Davies, M. J. (1975). Pathological features of hypertrophic cardiomyopathy in the elderly. *Br. Heart J.* 37, 305–312.

Sugrue, D. D., McKenna, W. J., Dickie, S. *et al.* (1984). Relation between left ventricular gradient and relative stroke volume ejected in early and late systole in hypertrophic cardiomyopathy. *Br. Heart J.* 52, 602–619.

Swan, D. A., Bell, B., Oakley, C. M. and Goodwin, J. F. (1971) Analysis of symptomatic course and treatment of hypertrophic obstructive cardiomyopathy. *Br. Heart J.* 33, 671–685.

Van Noorden, S., Olsen, E. J. G. and Pearse, A. G. E. (1971). Hypertrophic obstructive cardiomyopathy. A histological, histochemical and ultrastructural study of biopsy material. *Cardiovasc. Res.* 5, 118–131.

CHAGAS' HEART DISEASE

D. S. AMORIM

American trypanosomiasis or Chagas' disease affects a wide variety of human and animal populations throughout the American continent. It is caused by *Trypanosoma cruzi* and transmitted from person to person or from animal to human by a triatomide bug.

Chagas' disease exhibits two basic forms, an acute and a chronic phase, with an intermediate period between the two. In the acute phase the inflammatory actions are intense, and the myocardial fibres are the most important sites of multiplication of the parasite. In the chronic stage of the disease the inflammatory reactions are less intense and not related to the presence of the parasite. Cardiopathy is the most common and serious complication of chronic infection.

The two conditions, acute myocarditis and chronic cardiopathy, have an intimate aetiological relationship. However, from clinical and pathological viewpoints, the acute and chronic phases are almost separate entities.

Infection and disease

Trypanosoma cruzi is a parasite which multiplies mainly in cells of mesodermal or mesenchymal origin. This form of multiplication constitutes a point of fundamental biological importance in the life-cycle of this protozoan and its pathogenic action.

Infections with *T. cruzi* are usually acquired by human beings in the home while asleep at night. Thus far, about 100 species of *Triatoma* (the vectors) have been found on the American continent. It is likely that not all of these species are infected triatomes of the same species.

The acute phase affecting mostly young children in endemic areas is characterized by a febrile illness and the finding of *T. cruzi* in the peripheral blood, decreasing in number as the infection evolves. This stage is very likely associated with cardiac involvement in almost every case. However, it is thought that the acute phase must often pass unrecognized since many adults found to have chronic manifestations of the disease and positive serological tests deny a typical history of a previous acute illness.

If death does not occur in the acute phase, the disease develops into the chronic stage characterized by irregular, extremely low or no parasitaemia. Then the aetiological diagnosis can be made by using more sensitive techniques. Transition from the asymptomatic phase to the stage of chronic visceral involvement is slow (usually 10 to 20 years between the end of the acute phase and the establishment of visceral involvement of chronic infection) and difficult to define clearly.

Although the various manifestations that characterize the chronic stage appear mainly in the cardiovascular system, the disease is responsible for an impressive variety of abnormalities. They include involvement of hollow viscera and interference with homeostatic mechanisms.

Pathology and pathogenesis

In the acute phase, after leaving the blood stream *T. cruzi* become localized in various tissues: the most common are the heart, skeletal muscle, smooth muscle, and connective tissue. They change to the leishmanial (amastigote) forms and multiply by binary fission.

The myocardial fibres are the most important sites of multiplication, although the reasons for preferential selection of the myocardium remain to be determined. Post-mortem examination reveals an acute, severe, diffuse myocarditis with parasites in myocardial cells.

Although inflammatory lesions are sometimes observed in association with ruptured loaded cells, there is no apparent correlation between the location and number of pseudocysts (great swollen cells) and the severity of inflammatory lesions.

In human and animal experimental infections, in addition to myocarditis, inflammation has been seen throughout the conducting system and in the sinus node. Diffuse mononuclear cell infiltration, interstitial oedema, and vascular congestion were revealed in the conducting system of the heart. The amastigote forms were found in all regions of the conducting system.

From systematic investigations in human cases and experimentally or naturally infected animals, damage in the nervous ganglia of the heart has been consistently recorded and is considered an important feature of this disease. The lesions in the nervous cells occur during the acute phase in the vicinity of ruptured pseudocysts, but they are unpredictable in intensity and location.

If in the acute phase of the disease the inflammatory response to *T. cruzi* has been intense, it is less obvious in the chronic stage.

The chief anatomical findings include enlargement of all the cardiac chambers, hypertrophy of the myocardium, an important reduction in the thickness at the apex, mural thrombosis, interstitial fibrosis, some inflammatory foci, and, rarely, persistence of the parasite in the myocardium. In exceptional cases, however, the heart may appear normal in size and shape.

Cardiac biopsies in chronically affected patients are not consistent, and the morphological findings of non-specific focal myocarditis and interstitial fibrosis are indistinguishable from those found in dilated cardiomyopathy.

The histopathological changes revealed by post-mortem examination include focal myocarditis, fibrosis, and myocytolysis. These features usually occur in the absence of demonstrable parasites within myocardial fibres. Focal and diffuse interstitial fibrosis is almost invariably present: its intensity varies between cases and in the same case from one area to another, and predominates in the subendocardium. Fibrosis is conspicuously more severe in the left ventricle, followed in order of frequency by the right ventricle and the right atrium. The interstitial inflammatory reaction may be diffuse or focal, dense and polymorphic: lymphocytes, monocytes, and histiocytes may be present.

Detailed examination of the conducting system in chronic Chagas' heart disease shows extensive and variable changes: atrophy, fibrosis, and fragmentation of specific fibres, chronic inflammation, dilation, tortuosity, and intimal fibrosis of the vasculature. The sinus node may be markedly fibrotic, its specific fibres atrophic, and the sinus main artery frequently altered by thickening.

In the A–V system, distribution of the lesions follow a rather definite pattern: the inferior third of the A–V node, the right half of the main bundle, the right bundle, and the anterior ramification of the left bundle branch. Purkinje fibres are frequently damaged by inflammation and fibrosis.

In chronic chagasic patients, there is significant reduction of the number of nervous cells in the autonomic plexuses of hollow digestive viscera, in the heart, in bronchi, in the spinal cord, and in the cerebellum. These changes are interpreted by many authors to reflect the basic character of the disease in its advanced stage.

An absolute decrease in the number of neuronal cells in ganglia, in the atrial myocardium are consistently observed in chronic Chagas' heart disease, with fibrosis accompanied or not by concomitant inflammation.

An area of thinning of the cardiac wall at the apex is highly characteristic. The diameter of the aneurysm does not usually exceed 5 cm. More than 50 per cent of chronic Chagas' hearts show this unusual alteration; although an overwhelming preponderance are found at the apex of the left ventricle, such lesions may occur at the right apex or both. Mural thrombosis in different stages of organization is very common, within the apical aneurysm but even without aneurysm formation.

A review of necropsy reports shows that apical aneurysm is unrelated to age and heart weight. Those patients dying of chronic disease are more likely to have the lesion, but the mode of death (sudden, or in cardiac failure) appears unrelated to its presence.

Although the pathological findings in Chagas' disease have been described in detail, the exact pathogenesis of cardiopathy as a late complication remains unknown. Inflammatory, immunologic, neurogenic, toxic, and vascular aetiological factors have been proposed. The polymorphism and variable combinations of lesions, the course of the disease, and its variety of clinical manifestations make plausible a complex and multifactorial pathogenesis. Neither direct parasitism nor the inflammatory reaction is the probable mechanism for the recorded lesions in chronic infection. It has been known for a long time that when a parasite pseudocyst ruptures and releases T. cruzi organisms, many of the surrounding uninfected cells are affected by degeneration, necrosis or lysis. The early information was of a hypersensitivity reaction. Later experimental evidence suggested that mammalian cells might share common antigens with T. cruzi so that an antiparasite response could give rise to autoimmune damage to uninfected host cells. Such immunological events would provide an explanation for the widespread destruction of non-parasitic cells in the acute phase of Chagas' disease.

The mechanism through which the neuronal destruction occurs in this disease is uncertain. Neurones are only rarely parasitized in T. cruzi infections and so their destruction is unlikely to be a direct effect of parasite invasion. Some investigators have suggested that neuronal destruction might be produced by a non-specific inflammatory response by a neurotoxin-like substance or by an autoimmune response elicited by parasite antigens that cross-react with host tissue components. In animal models, however, selective adherence of T. cruzi immune lymphocytes to myenteric, parasympathetic ganglion cells, leads to neuronolysis. This can be interpreted as an indication of the high degree of specificity of the destruction of parasympathetic neurons in Chagas' disease. The vast majority of sera (83 per cent) from patients in the chronic phase of Chagas' disease contain antibodies reacting with human neuronal tissue. Intriguingly, although most sera (97 per cent) contain only IgG antibodies, some (7 per cent) contained both IgG and IgM, suggesting that in a high percentage of patients an immune response is associated with neuronal destruction in the acute phase of the disease, but chronic infection and/or the continuous liberation of autoantigen from injured tissue may be the stimulus for the perpetuation of the autoimmune response.

Clinical manifestations and functional disorders
The acute phase
The clinical manifestations of acute Chagas' heart disease do not differ essentially from those caused by acute myocarditis of other aetiologies and are not always conspicuous. In severe cases the symptoms and signs of left and right cardiac failure may develop with dyspnoea, gallop rhythm, cardiac enlargement, and murmurs resulting from dilation of the ventricles. In mild cases detection is less accurate.

Electrocardiographic alterations occur in a relatively large number of patients and are non-specific. Primary T wave changes, low voltage of QRS, prolongation of Q–T interval, and prolongation of the P–R interval are the most common. The appearance of intraventricular block is considered a poor prognostic sign and is apparently caused by severe inflammation and myocardial focal necrosis.

The mortality of the acute phase is about 10 per cent, owing to heart failure or acute meningoencephalitis. If death does not occur in the acute phase, the disease develops into the chronic stage generally without any important symptomatology for a long interval.

The intermediate phase
The expression intermediate phase is open to criticism, because it may be misleading in the sense that it implies inevitable late visceral involvement; but it can be used to indicate the period in which individuals are asymptomatic and apparently healthy in which the only evidence of infection may be a positive serological test. But functional disorders have been shown in some chagasic patients in this intermediate phase. Individuals who are asymptomatic, and have a normal heart size without change in the routine electrocardiogram may develop high risk arrhythmias evident in 24 hour ECG records. Non-invasive nuclear techniques may reveal subnormal increases in ejection fraction or, impaired left ventricular performance can be revealed by echocardiography. The administration of antiarrhythmic drugs probably diminish or prevent serious complications in those patients with 'high risk' arrhythmias.

Screening of an asymptomatic population of chronic chagasic patients is feasible and could include endomyocardial biopsy in addition to non-invasive techniques. What cellular and subcellular evidence is there of changes developing from an 'early' (minor or no symptoms) to an 'established' stage? What are the prognostic implications of, for instance, bundle branch block of immunological abnormalities? Are there demonstrable correlations between morphological and functional disorders and autonomic impairment? All these questions may lead to a better understanding of the physiopathology, and therefore contribute to the treatment of patients. But the relevant investigations have social consequences to the patients. Thousands of otherwise healthy individuals may be abruptly considered unsuitable for their routine work because of minor alterations of uncertain significance revealed by highly sophisticated methods, therefore aggravating their already poor social and economic conditions.

Full assessment of the morbidity due to T. cruzi infection will have to be deferred until solid data of well-planned longitudinal studies are brought to light. Any such attempt must include not only an evaluation of cardiac status, but also the importance of digestive disorders (megaoesophagus and megacolon), features not yet fully investigated.

In one study of morbidity among non-selected patients with positive serology, originating from different areas in a single large country, the prevalence of cardiopathy was nearly 50 per cent and of digestive disorders (megaoesophagus and megacolon) 14 per cent. Both abnormalities were observed in 10 per cent. The proportion of cardiac cases increased progressively between the first and the fifth decades of life, whereas the proportion of digestive cases increased until the seventh decade. A number of studies have shown that nearly half of the cases of chronic Chagas' heart disease are distributed between the ages of 21 and 40 years.

The chronic phase
The clinical manifestations of chronic Chagas' heart disease depend to a large extent on the presence or degree of cardiac failure, on the type of arrhythmia, and on the presence of atrioventricular conduction defects. The most common recognized clinical signs are cardiomegaly, cardiac failure, conduction disturbances, and abnormalities in the repolarization phase of the electrocardiogram. Many cardiac chagasic patients have never had an episode of decompensation; in them the only abnormal findings are alterations in ventricular dynamics revealed by different methods and/or an abnormal electrocardiogram.

Radiological examination is of supplementary value in the assessment of chronic Chagas' heart disease. In general the cardiac silhouette is not distinctive: the size of the heart may vary from normal to enormously dilated, depending upon the degree of myocardial involvement.

Echocardiographic examination reveals abnormal interventricular septum motion, decrease of the left ventricular posterior wall excursion, increase of the systolic and diastolic diameters of the left ventricular cavity, low ejection fraction, and segmental areas of hypokinesia. These are common patterns indistinguishable from those of dilated cardiomyopathy.

Asymptomatic patients

A large number of chronic cardiac chagasic patients are asymptomatic or have only minor symptoms; the cardiac shadow may be normal or only slightly enlarged and the diagnosis of cardiac involvement in them rests upon the demonstration of electrocardiographic abnormalities. Although non-specific, these are valuable in association with epidemiological, serological, and clinical data. Discrepancies in the findings in such patients probably depend on the manner in which groups of cases were selected. Some studies have been epidemiological others were samples of urban populations seeking medical care in hospitals, and still others depended on autopsied cases.

The electrocardiogram shows a great variety of abnormalities, but all forms of arrhythmia and conduction disturbance are common. Two or more alterations are often seen in the same patient. In those in sinus rhythm, right bundle branch block and premature ventricular contractions are by far the most common.

The pattern of right bundle branch block with left axis deviation in this disease has been reported by several authors. The high incidence of right bundle branch block contrasts with the findings of left bundle branch block and has a high diagnostic value in patients under 50 years of age from endemic areas. Although there are discrepancies in relation to the incidence which are difficult to explain, incomplete (first- and second-degree) and complete heart block have also been reported with great frequency.

There is a high incidence of sinus node dysfunction in this disease, which may not be revealed by conventional electrocardiography. Evaluation of sinus node recovery time before and after blockade by atropine can be made by His bundle recordings. In one series, this technique revealed sinus node dysfunction in 5 out of 17 cases. On the other hand, 4 out of 10 patients exhibited a paradoxical response to atropine with a prolongation of the sinus recovery time.

The prognostic value of electrocardiographic changes in chronic Chagas' heart disease has been assessed in a non-selected group of patients followed for nearly two decades. Right bundle branch block, primary ST–T changes, and multifocal ventricular premature beats were significantly more frequent in those who died. Complete atrioventricular block, left bundle branch block, and atrial fibrillation or flutter was also associated with a reduced life-expectancy.

Death in chronic Chagas' heart disease is attributed to myocardial failure, arrhythmias (sudden and unexpected death occurring in many cases), and thromboembolic complications. The level of parasitaemia does not appear to be an aggravating factor, perhaps because of differences in the pathogenicity of various strains of *T. cruzi*.

Autonomic dysfunction

Chagas' disease is a model of spontaneous denervation of the heart, which in the absence of heart failure may be used as an experimental model for the assessment of the autonomic control of cardiac function in humans. In patients with chronic cardiac Chagas' disease, failure of the heart rate to increase after administration of atropine and greatly reduced reflex changes in cardiac rate (tilting from supine to 70° head-up position and from 70° head-up to 30° head-down position, dynamic upright exercise, handgrip isometric exercise, baroreceptor sensitivity during phenylephrine-induced hypertension, and amyl nitrite-induced hypotension) are believed to be functional disorders related to degeneration of the neuronal supply to the sinoatrial region of the heart. Although an impairment in autonomic control appears to exist in patients with chronic cardiac Chagas' disease, there is no demonstrable correlation between this autonomic impairment and the degree of heart dysfunction.

Diagnosis and treatment

The acute phase is characterized by the demonstration of *T. cruzi* in the blood stream, but in chronic cases the diagnostic tests that give best results are those based upon the detection of antibodies dependent on *T. cruzi*. The complement fixation test is valuable because of its sensitivity and specificity; immunofluorescence techniques, xenodiagnosis, and inoculation of laboratory animals are also sensitive indices. Comparative results of complement fixation, immunofluorescence, haemagglutination, and flocculation tests showed relative sensitivity to be 99.2, 99.9, 99.0, and 98.8 per cent, while relative specificity was respectively 99.9, 99.7, 99.6, and 98.3 per cent.

The diagnosis of heart involvement is usually based upon epidemiological profile, conventional physical examination, serum diagnostic tests, and an abnormal electrocardiogram in the absence of any other demonstrable cause. As part of the full cardiological assessment in chronic Chagas' heart disease, however, other noninvasive and invasive techniques are of supplementary value in the detection of early involvement. Two-dimensional echocardiography discloses segmental dyskinesia and apical aneurysm. It may give the first indication of a contractile alteration in an otherwise apparently healthy heart. Radionuclide ventriculography is an alternative way of showing abnormal wall motion and deformity at the apex. Holter monitoring makes it possible to determine the type, number, and severity of arrhythmias, and to assess the effectiveness of antiarrhythmic drugs.

Haemodynamic studies and angiocardiography have been used for the estimation of the size of individual chambers, the extent to which they fill and empty during each cardiac cycle, wall motion, intraventricular thrombosis, and to determine morphological alterations, in particular apical aneurysm of the left ventricle. Electrophysiological studies and endomyocardial biopsy may be of value for early diagnosis and in assessing the effectiveness of proposed therapy.

A characteristic cardiopathy with a positive complement fixation test constitutes a sound basis for the diagnosis of chronic Chagas' heart disease. Chronic Chagas' disease is unlikely in the absence of specific circulating antibodies. In endemic areas, however, because of the prevalence of positive serology, the differential diagnosis between decompensated chronic Chagas' heart disease and dilated cardiomyopathy may be difficult unless the distinctive aneurysm of Chagas' heart disease can be shown in the living patient or at autopsy.

Treatment of chronic Chagas' heart patients is the same as for any other form of cardiomyopathy with comparable clinical manifestations, with the same expectations of symptomatic relief and haemodynamic improvement. There is, however, no evidence that the newer non-glycoside inotropic agents, vasodilator or antiarrhythmic drugs will affect prognosis favourably.

Antiparasitic treatment of Chagas' disease has been attempted since the discovery of the disease. A large number of drugs have been evaluated *in vitro*, in experimental animals, and in humans. None are of proven benefit although some have shown antiparasitic activity of varying degree. Prolonged administration of drugs active on the circulating forms of the parasite should theoretically permit eradication of the infection since continuous destruction of circulating forms should effectively disrupt the life-cycle.

The evaluation of nitrofurane derivatives and nitroimidazole derivatives is based mainly on parasitologic (xenodiagnosis) and serologic criteria (serum diagnostic tests). Both can be rendered negative in the acute phase, but in chronic disease serology remains positive, special treatment can have a considerable effect on parasitaemia, but despite prolonged treatment with more active and less toxic compounds the long-term effect upon the natural history of the disease is unknown.

Public health problems

The transport of *T. cruzi* from natural foci to human dwellings, with the initial establishment or the re-establishment of the domiciliary cycle, may be effected by several mechanisms, including the adaptation of wild insects and the intrusion by humans into natural foci. This is of high practical importance.

Housing transmission of *T. cruzi* infection is a crucial part of the epidemiology. It depends on two major factors: ecological imbalance and poor dwelling conditions in rural areas. Therefore, to a large extent, the disease is related to social development. Study of its control cannot be separated from the study of living conditions of the populations concerned and the risk of infection they run. The persistence of endemic disease is the result primarily of the poor construction of dwellings and the primitive sanitary practices of the populations, which together create conditions favourable for the breeding of triatomes with domestic habits.

It is difficult to obtain reliable and comparable figures of the prevalence of the disease in different areas and of any differences in clinical manifestations, because of the extent of the areas involved, their underdeveloped conditions, and the difficulty in applying suitable serological methods and clinical diagnostic procedures to remote rural areas lacking adequate medical services. In order to obtain a nationwide epidemiological profile based on reliable data, a serological survey was recently carried out under the auspices of the Brazilian government. A total of approximately 1 400 000 samples were collected and analysed by the indirect anti-IgG immunofluorescence test. The prevalence (per 100) varied from 0.31 to 8.8 in different parts of the country. The results from this serological survey were taken as the basis for a national electrocardiographic enquiry. A total of 4982 ECGs were taken in order to evaluate the prevalence of heart disease in individuals with either positive or negative serology for *T. cruzi* infection. Preliminary results reveal that electrocardiographic abnormalities in seropositive individuals were found in a mean of 37.4 per cent (range, 33.3 to 55.6), while in the seronegative subjects it averaged 22.6 per cent (range, 13.0 to 30.0). It is probable that on the American continent nearly 35 million people are exposed to the risk of infection with *T. cruzi*. If the average of the infection rates obtained in the epidemiological surveys carried out in several countries is taken as 20 per cent, it may be calculated that there are at least 7 million people infected with *T. cruzi*.

References

Amorim, D. S., Manço, J. C., Gallo Jr, L. and Marin Neto, J. A. (1982). Chagas' heart disease as an experimental model for studies of cardiac autonomic function in man. *Mayo Clin. Proc.* (Suppl.) **57**, 48–60.

Amorim, D. S. and Olsen, E. G. J. (1982). Assessment of heart neurons in dilated (congestive) cardiomyopathy. *Br. Heart J.* **47**, 11–18.

Andrade, Z. A., Andrade, S. G. and Sadigursky, M. (1984). Damage and healing in the conduction tissue of the heart (an experimental study in dogs infected with *Trypanosoma cruzi*). *J. Pathol.* **143**, 93–101.

Laranja, F. S., Dias, E., Nobrega, G. and Miranda, A. (1956). Chagas' disease: a clinical, epidemiologic and pathologic study. *Circulation* **14**, 1035–1060.

Ribeiro dos Santos, R., Rassi, A. and Köberle, F. (1981). Chagas' disease. *Antibiot. Chemother.* **50**, 115–134.

World Health Organization (1984). *Cardiomyopathies*. Technical Report Series 697, Geneva.

CONGENITAL HEART DISEASE

The anatomy of congenital heart disease

R. H. ANDERSON AND E. A. SHINEBOURNE

The basic anatomy of even the most complex congenital cardiac malformations is not difficult to understand. A simple approach can be made to the naming and origin of the various anomalies. No embryologically derived terms need be used. Nomenclature can be based entirely upon the anatomy as it is observed.

Morphological approach to congenital cardiac malformations

The development of the heart is such that any defect in one segment of the heart can co-exist with any defect in any other. The possibilities for cardiac malformations are therefore enormous. At any time a combination of anomalies may be encountered that has not been seen before. The approach must therefore permit recognition of any combination of lesions that may exist, but must not be so unwieldy that it confuses the understanding of the simpler lesions. The approach which we use enables description of simple lesions and the most complex anomalies: it can be summarized as a *sequential segmental approach*, and is based upon the fact that there are limited numbers of ways in which the cardiac chambers and great arteries can be connected to and related to each other. The important feature of this system is that it requires the establishment, rather than the assumption of a normal basic framework. For example, some very complex malformations such as congenitally corrected transposition produce an apparently normal pattern of circulation. Yet if normality were presumed in these patients, the results of surgical treatment of associated anomalies such as pulmonary stenosis could prove disastrous. The system is designed to simplify the complicated and to make such deterring terminology as 'anatomically corrected malposition' or 'isolated ventricular noninversion' redundant.

The heart can be considered to possess atrial, ventricular, and great arterial segments (Fig. 1). The arrangement of the atrial chambers is the foundation on which to construct the rest of the heart. The way the atria are joined to the ventricles is analysed in terms of the atrioventricular connections, the morphology of the ventricular mass and the relationships of the ventricular chambers. The ventriculo-arterial junction is then examined in exactly the same way. Associated anomalies are then considered in ordered progression, starting at the venous attachments to the atria and working through to malformations of the systemic and pulmonary circulations. These considerations are made in the light of the heart's position within the body described in independent terms.

Atrial position

The arrangement of the atrial chambers is referred to as the atrial arrangement or *situs*. It is usually, but not always, harmonious with the arrangement of the abdominal and thoracic organs, but in difficult cases the arrangement of the atria themselves must be the final arbiter. It is helpful to consider the heart as developing from a five-segment primary heart tube (Fig. 2). The first segment, the sinus venosus, is derived from the venous systems of the embryo and its covering membranes. The second segment is the atrial chamber itself. The third and fourth segments together will form the ventricular loop. Many names have been used to describe these, but the *inlet* and *outlet* components of the loop are simple terms and describe their ultimate role admirably. The final segment is the arterial segment which connects the heart tube to the developing aortic arch systems (Fig. 2). Changes occur concomitantly within these various segments during development, but for

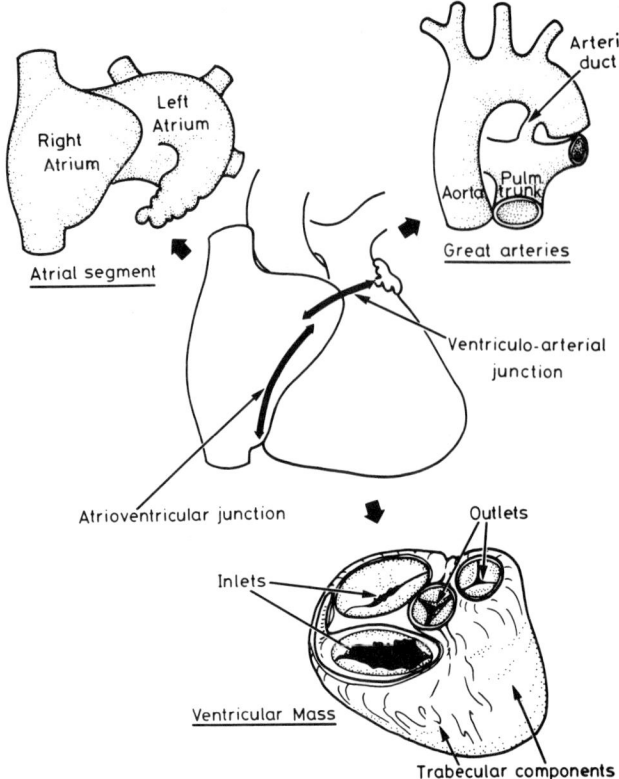

Fig. 1 The segments of the heart and their junctions.

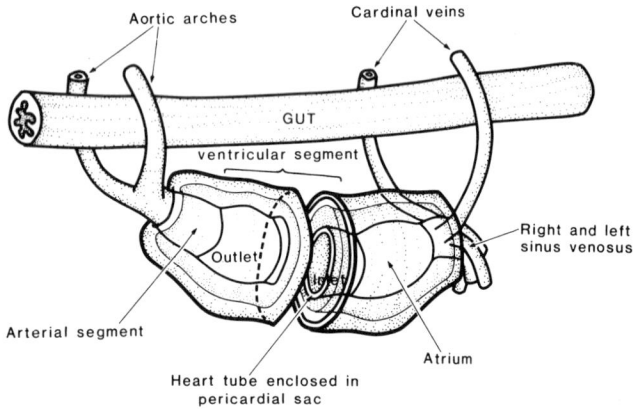

Fig. 2 Artist's representation of the primary heart tube showing its components and venous and arterial connections.

the purposes of description each segment will be considered in the light of its malformations.

Sinus venosus and atrium

The way the sinus venosus and pulmonary veins are incorporated into the atrium determines the atrial arrangement. Initially the sinus venosus is bilaterally symmetrical, receiving three major veins from each side of the embryo (Fig. 3). Normally anastomoses develop in the head and abdomen so that the left-sided venous blood is transferred to the right-sided veins. This, with bilateral atrophy of one set of veins of the original three, results in the sinus venosus being firstly incorporated into the right side of the atrium, and secondly receiving two great veins, the superior and inferior caval veins. The entire left part of the sinus venosus regresses to become the coronary sinus. As the sinus venosus becomes a right-sided structure, the primary pulmonary vein

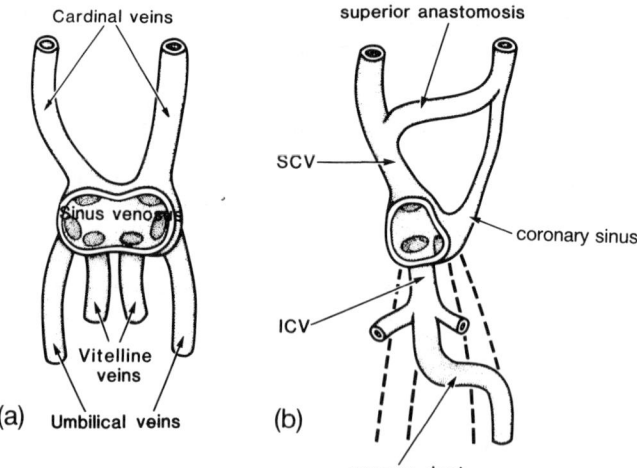

Fig. 3 Diagrams showing the reorientation of the venous connections to the primary heart tube. (a) The initial bilaterally symmetrical arrangement. (b) The arrangement after the development of left-to-right anastomoses.

grows from the left side of the atrium towards the lungs. There it joins with the intrapulmonary venous plexus of which part is reincorporated into the left side of the atrium (Fig. 4). The atrium itself pouches out to form the two atrial appendages, one to either side of the arterial pedicle. Because the right appendage is related to the sinus venosus and the left is not, they have different morphology in their definitive state. The morphologically right atrium has a blunt appendage with a broad junction with the smooth-walled part derived from the sinus venosus, the terminal crest marking the junction (Fig. 5a). The morphologically left atrium has a narrow hooked appendage with a narrow orifice to the smooth pulmonary venous part of the atrium there being no terminal crest (Fig. 5b). The development of usual atrial arrangement (*solitus*) depends on incorporation of the sinus venosus into the right side and of the pulmonary veins into the left side of the atrial chamber.

Should venous anastomoses develop so that the blood drains to the left side of the sinus venosus, the left side will become dominant and the pulmonary vein will grow from the right side of the atrium, giving the mirror-image atrial arrangement (*situs inversus*) (Fig. 6). In both usual and mirror-image arrangements, the sinus venosus and pulmonary veins are lateralized, with a morphologically right atrium to one side and left to the other. Complex malformations occur if lateralization is absent with maldevelopment of both the heart and abdomino-thoracic organs, generally described as visceral heterotaxy, the splenic syndromes, the Ivemark syndrome, etc., names which do nothing to help understand the anomalies. These syndromes represent symmetrical development of the venoatrial segments of the heart to produce *right atrial isomerism* or *left atrial isomerism*. Although these two together are often described as *situs ambiguus*, there is nothing ambiguous about their morphology. The detailed embryology is unknown, but we envisage failure of lateralization of the sinus venosus in right atrial isomerism which would result in both atrial appendages showing right-sided characteristics with bilateral terminal crests (Fig. 7). Because of the central position of the sinus venosus there is no room for development of the pulmonary vein so that anomalous pulmonary venous connection is the rule. Because of isomerism there are bilateral superior caval veins and sinus nodes.

In left atrial isomerism we postulate overdevelopment of the pulmonary veins from both sides of the atrium, squeezing out the sinus venosus. Anomalous systemic venous connection is therefore the rule, particularly drainage of the inferior caval vein via a superior vein (so-called azygos continuation). The atrial appendages are both of the left type and there are no terminal crests (Fig. 8),

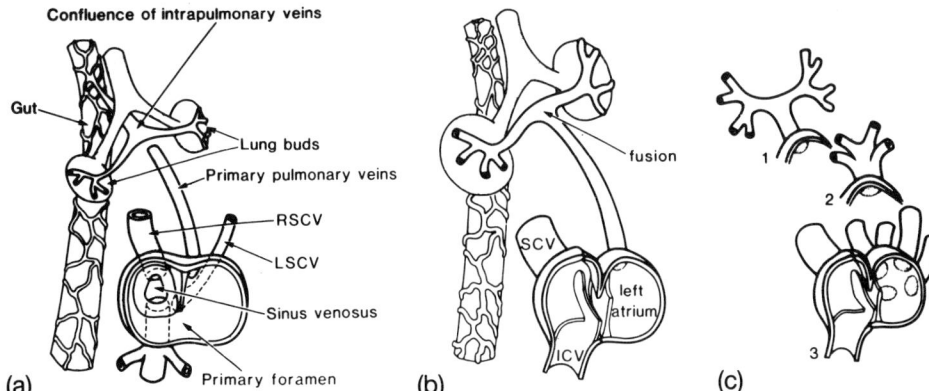

Fig. 4 Diagrammatic representation of the development of the pulmonary veins.

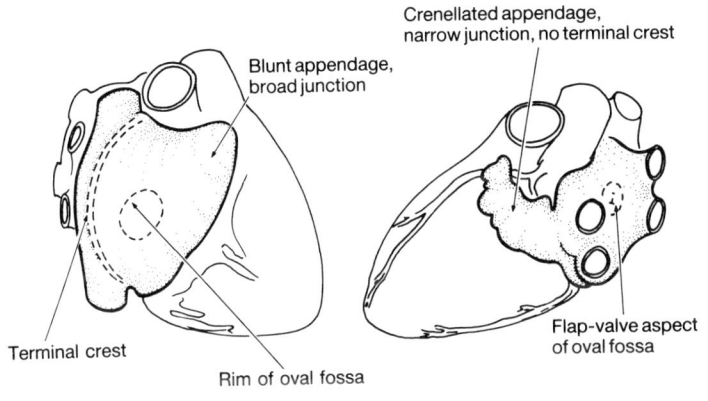

Fig. 5 Drawings showing the differences between the morphologically right atrium and the morphologically left atrium.

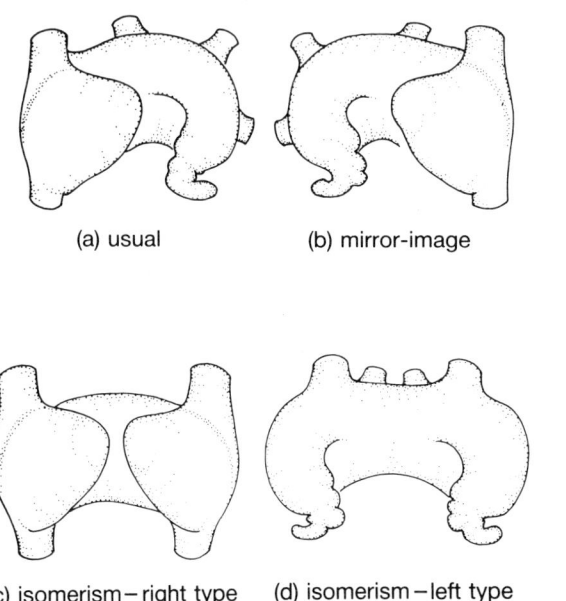

Fig. 6 The four different arrangements of the morphologically right and left atrial chambers which give the different types of atrial arrangement.

but the pulmonary venous connection as expected is bilaterally symmetrical.

When there is atrial isomerism almost always the thoracoabdominal organs also show isomerism. So in right atrial isomerism there are bilateral trilobed lungs with short, eparterial bronchi, and, because the spleen is a left-sided structure, asplenia (Fig. 9a). In left atrial isomerism (Fig. 9b) there are bilateral bilobed lungs with long hyparterial bronchi and multiple spleens (polysplenia).

Atrioventricular junction

Development of the ventricular part of the heart depends on the way the atria have developed, together with the limited ways in which the ventricles connect to them.

Normally the atrioventricular canal is connected initially only to the inlet part of the ventricular loop. When the heart tube has been converted from the straight tube (Fig. 2) to the 'looped' stage, the inlet and outlet parts of the ventricular loop lie more or

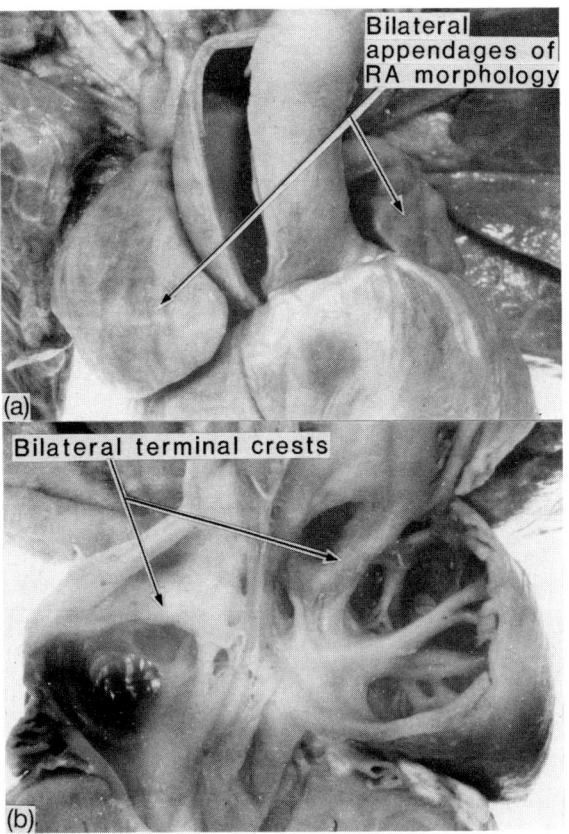

Fig. 7 The bilateral right atrial appendages found in hearts with right atrial isomerism.

less side by side (Fig. 10). Development of the ventricles then depends on the formation of trabecular pouches from both components of the loop. The trabecular pouch which has left ventricular characteristics develops from the inlet part and that with right ventricular characteristics from the outlet part (Fig. 11). By this time, atrial development will have proceeded to the stage at which there are two atrial chambers, be they of lateralized or isomeric

morphology. Whether each atrium establishes a connection to a separate ventricular trabecular component then depends upon development of the inlet component. Normally the heart tube bends so that the outlet part of the loop is closest to the right-sided atrium (d-looping or right-hand looping). Then there is usually growth of the right-sided inlet component so that the right-sided atrium is placed in connection with the trabecular component of right ventricular type (Fig. 12a). This results in a concordant atrioventricular connection when the atria are lateralized, but an ambiguous connection when the atria are isomeric. Rarely the ventricular loop bends so that the outlet part comes closest to the left-sided atrium with resultant junction of the left-sided atrium to the morphologically right ventricle. There is then a discordant atrioventricular connection when there is the usual atrial arrangement (Fig. 12b) but an ambiguous atrioventricular connection when the atria are isomeric.

Diagnosis requires definition of chamber morphology. There are features which always permit differentiation of a right atrial from a left atrial chamber (Fig. 5). It is the morphology of the inlet and trabecular components which enables morphologically right and left ventricles to be distinguished from one another. The right possesses the tricuspid valve in its inlet portion, has a coarse trabecular component, and the extensive septomarginal trabeculation on its septal surface. The left in contrast has the mitral valve in its inlet component, has a fine trabecular component, and a smooth septal surface.

The connections described above presume development of the inlet component to produce an atrioventricular junction in which each atrium is connected to its own ventricular chamber. However, initially both atria are connected to the inlet portion of the ventricular loop which in turn drains to the left ventricular trabecular component. If this arrangement persists, the atria will be connected only to the left ventricle, the right ventricle remaining rudimentary. Alternatively the entire inlet portion can grow to be

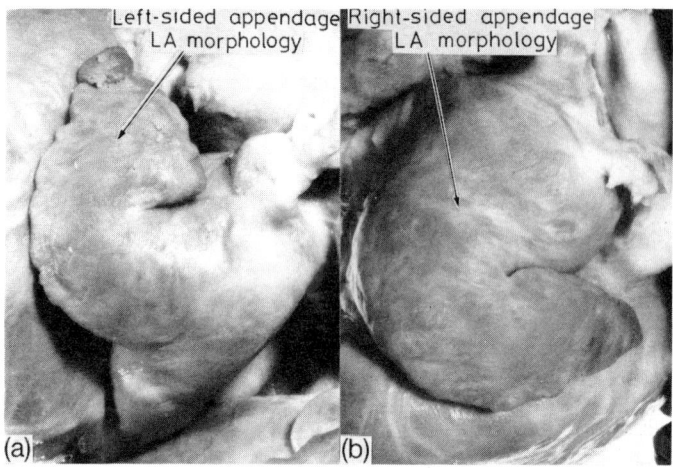

Fig. 8 The bilateral left atrial appendages found in hearts with left atrial isomerism.

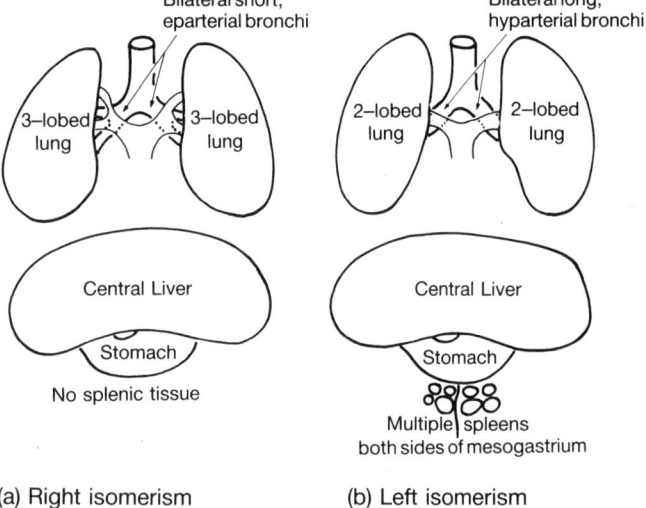

Fig. 9 The arrangement of the thoraco-abdominal viscera usually found (a) with right atrial isomerism and (b) with left atrial isomerism.

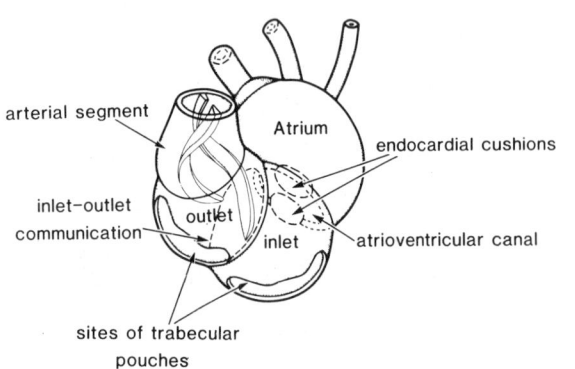

Fig. 10 Diagrammatic representation of the ventricular segment of the primary heart tube after looping has occurred.

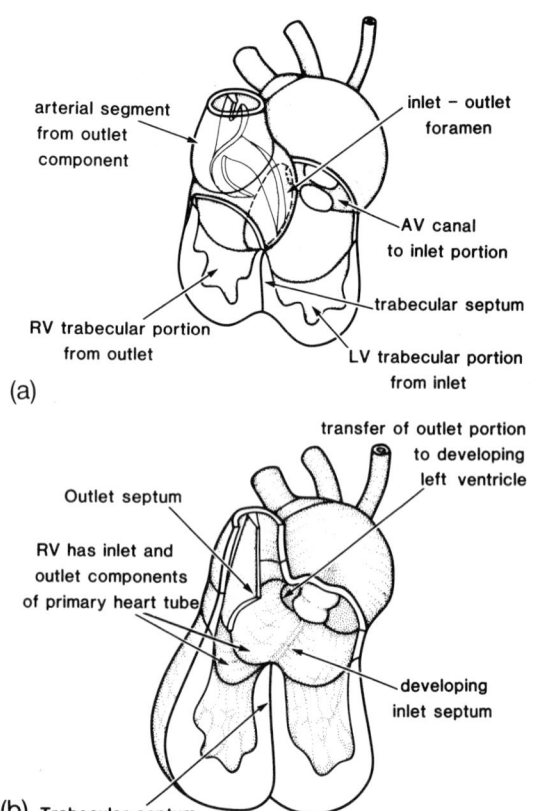

Fig. 11 The subsequent rearrangement of the inlet and outlet portions of the primary heart tube relative to the ventricular trabecular components which pave the way for ventricular septation.

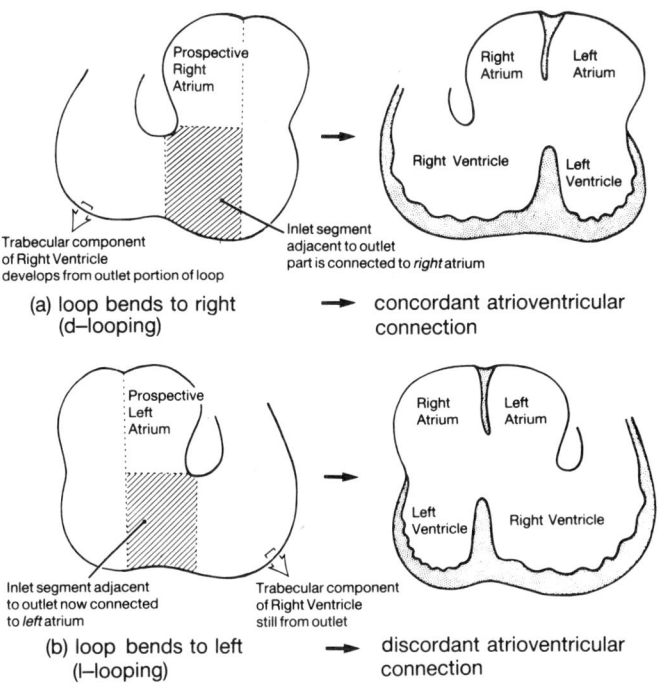

(a) loop bends to right
(d–looping)   →   concordant atrioventricular
                          connection

(b) loop bends to left
(l–looping)   →   discordant atrioventricular
                          connection

Fig. 12 Diagrams showing how bending of the ventricular loop to the right results in atrioventricular concordance whereas leftward looping sets the scene for the development of atrioventricular discordance.

connected to the right ventricle, when the left ventricle will be rudimentary, but still recognizable because of its trabecular component. It is also possible for a common trabecular pouch to grow from the ventricular loop rather than separate right and left ventricular pouches. The atria would then be connected to a solitary ventricle. This is the only situation in which a ventricular chamber will have neither a right nor left ventricular trabecular pattern. Instead it is morphologically indeterminate.

The developments discussed above account for ventricular morphology but not for precise atrioventricular connections which depend on the development of the atrioventricular canal. Usually the atrioventricular canal develops with the inlet portion so that both atria drain through it. When this connection persists the result is a double inlet ventricle of one type or other. It is possible that the atrioventricular canal does not expand. Growth of the atrial septum could then sequestrate either the right-sided or the left-sided atrial chambers from the atrioventricular canal and hence from the ventricular mass with absence of the right or the left atrioventricular connections (see Fig. 13). These arrangements, as with double inlet, can be found when the ventricle receiving the sole connection is of left, right or indeterminate ventricular morphology. Double inlet or absence of one connection can occur with isomeric or lateralized atria (Fig. 14).

Thus there are two basic groups of atrioventricular connections. In the first, each atrium is connected to a separate ventricle with concordant, discordant, or ambiguous atrioventricular connection (Fig. 15a–c). In the second, the atria are connected to only one ventricle to produce double inlet ventricle (Fig. 16a), absent right (Fig. 16b), and absent left (Fig.16c) atrioventricular connections.

The early development of the ventricular loop is largely responsible for determining the ventricular topology by right-hand (d-loop) and left-hand (l-loop) bending of the heart tube. With a right-hand pattern the right ventricle wraps itself round the left so that one's right hand can be applied to the septal surface with the thumb in the inlet and the fingers in the outlet. With a left-hand pattern it is the left which can be applied to the septal surface (Fig. 17). These patterns hold good for concordant, discordant, and ambiguous connections, and when the atria are connected only to a right ventricle. They are of less value when the atria are con-

nected only to a left ventricle and are not applicable when there is a solitary indeterminate ventricle.

Ventriculo-arterial junction
The entire arterial segment of the heart tube is initially positioned above the right ventricular trabecular component. In normal development one sub-arterial outflow tract is transferred to the developing left ventricle so that each ventricle has its own outflow

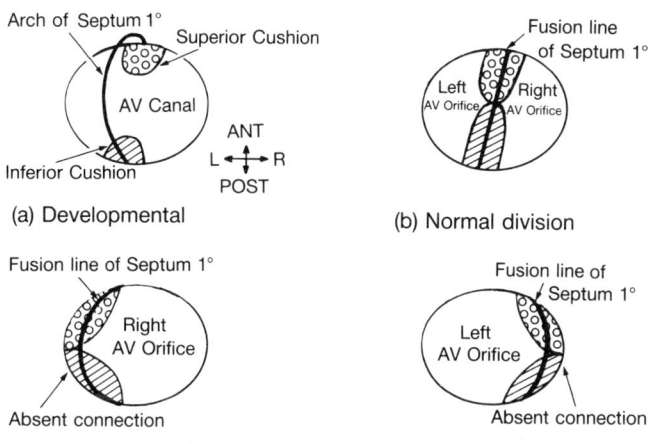

(a) Developmental   (b) Normal division

(c) Absent Left AV Connection   (d) Absent Right AV Connection

Fig. 13 Diagrammatic representation of the way in which division of the atrioventricular canal can produce (b) two atrioventricular orifices, (c) absence of the left atrioventricular (AV) connection, or (d) absence of the right connection.

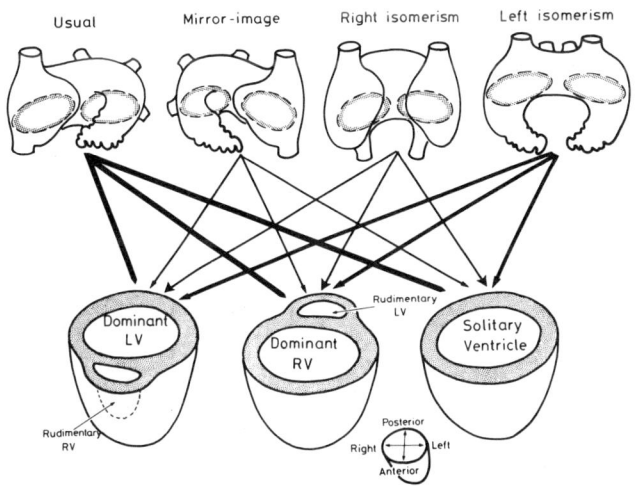

Fig. 14 Diagram showing how double inlet atrioventricular connection can occur with any atrial arrangement and with one of three ventricular morphologies.

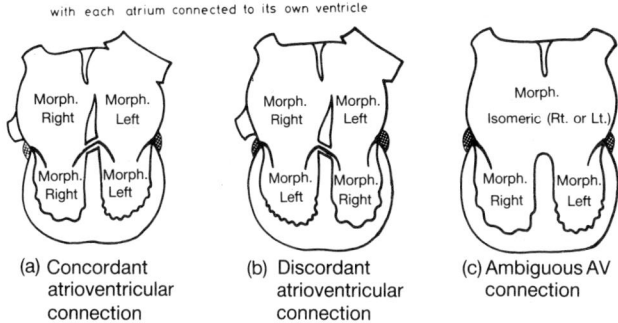

(a) Concordant
atrioventricular
connection

(b) Discordant
atrioventricular
connection

(c) Ambiguous AV
connection

Fig. 15 Diagram showing the three biventricular atrioventricular connections. Options (a) and (b) can occur in either usual or mirror-image atrial arrangements.

tract. The right-sided and posterior component of the outlet segment is transferred to the left ventricular trabecular pouch (Fig.18). Usually the aorta is connected to this outflow portion (concordant ventriculo-arterial connection). Should the pulmonary trunk connect to this part, or if the other part is transferred to the developing left ventricle the aorta remains connected to the morphologically right ventricle and the pulmonary trunk joins the morphologically left ventricle (discordant ventriculo-arterial connection).

Should both arteries retain their initital connection to the right ventricle there will be a double outlet right ventricle, while if both are transferred a double outlet left ventricle results. All of this presupposes septation of the arterial pedicle. If the arterial pedicle is unseptated, there will be a common arterial trunk irrespective of its ventricular connections. Alternatively, if one trunk becomes atretic during development and loses its ventricular connection, there will be a single outlet of the heart with either aortic or pulmonary atresia or very rarely a solitary arterial trunk of unknown nature. The possible connections produced by these mechanisms are summarized in Fig. 19.

Other changes occur in the outlet segment of the heart tube. Potentially both great arteries are supported by a complete ring of outlet musculature, part of which separates the outlets from the inlets, and part forms the anterior wall of the heart. There is also outlet musculature between the subaortic and subpulmonary outflow tracts when the arterial segment is septated. Thus potentially there are complete bilateral muscular outflow tracts (infundibula) which can exist with any connection but are found most frequently with double outlet right ventricle. The possible infundibular morphologies are a bilateral infundibulum; a bilaterally deficient infundibulum; a sub-aortic infundibulum with pulmonary-atrioventricular valvar continuity or a sub-pulmonary infundibulum with aortic-atrioventricular valvar continuity. Arterial relationships are so variable that our practice is simply to describe the position of the aortic valve relative to the pulmonary valve in terms of right/left and anterior/posterior position.

Cardiac position

The segmental possibilities described above are all independent of cardiac position within the chest. If not normally placed, the heart may lie in the middle or to the right and the orientation of its apex is independent of cardiac position.

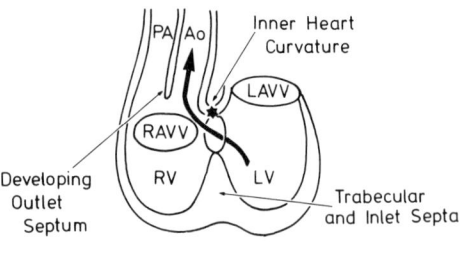

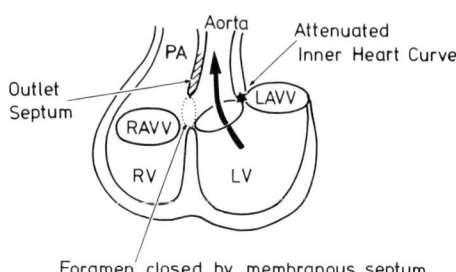

Fig. 18 Diagram showing the way in which the sub-aortic outflow tract is effectively transferred from the right (above) to the left (below) ventricle before the septum is closed by the membranous septum.

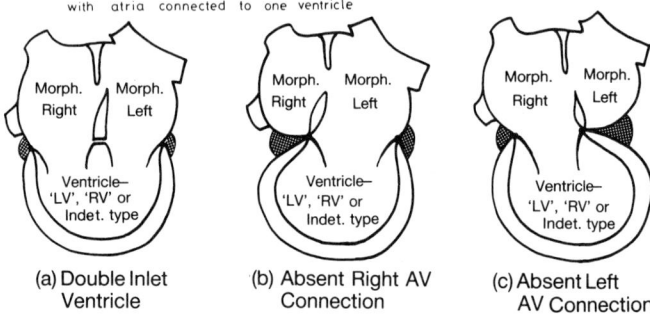

Fig. 16 The options possible in terms of atrioventricular connections when the atria connect to only one chamber in the ventricular mass (univentricular atrioventricular connections).

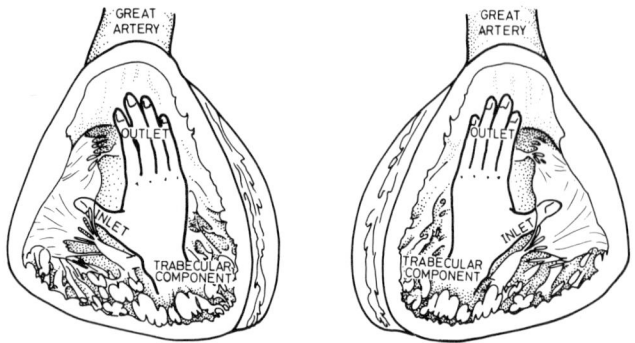

Fig. 17 The different types of ventricular topology which can be interpreted in terms of one's palmar surface applied to the ventricular septum.

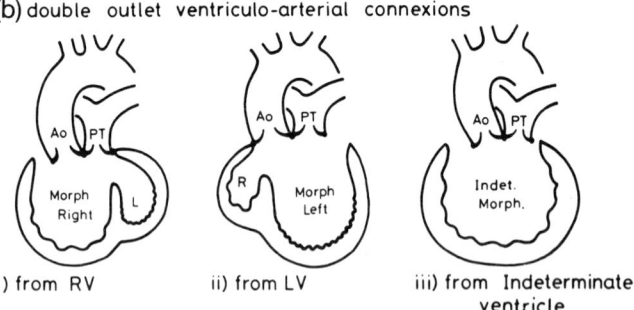

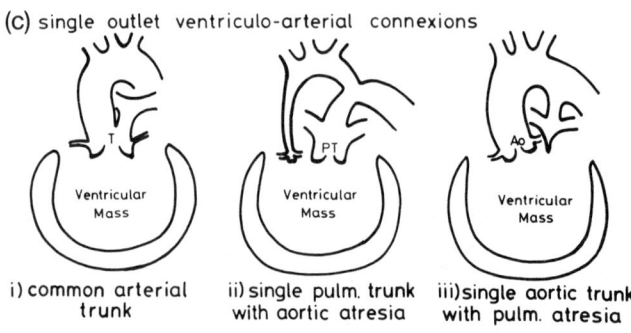

Fig. 19 Diagram showing the different possible ventriculo-arterial connections.

Morphology of specific congenital cardiac malformations

Most lesions are simply holes between the cardiac chambers, anomalies of the valves at the chamber junctions, or anomalous connections of the great veins. Any or all of these anomalies can be found with abnormal chamber combinations and such combinations themselves make up a proportion of congenital anomalies.

Associated anomalies in hearts with normal chamber connections

Anomalous venous connections

Anomalous systemic venous connection Anomalous connections of the systemic veins are rarely of clinical significance. A persistent left superior caval vein is a frequent finding, and it almost always drains via the coronary sinus to the right atrium. This represents persistence of the left sinus venosus. Rarely the 'party wall' between the left atrium and coronary sinus may disappear to a varying degree, leaving a communication between the left superior caval vein and the left atrium. This produces venous desaturation. In its severest form an atrial septal defect remains at the mouth of the coronary sinus and the left superior caval vein drains to the roof of the left atrium. Bilateral superior caval veins draining directly to right- and left-sided atria are much more frequent in atrial isomerism (situs ambiguus). Also frequent in left atrial isomerism is drainage of the inferior caval vein to the atria via the azygos system of veins. When this anomaly occurs in the usual atrial arrangement it produces no symptoms.

Anomalous pulmonary venous connection This produces varying degrees of venous desaturation depending on the number of pulmonary veins connecting anomalously. All combinations are possible, varying from only one part of one lung connecting to a systemic venous site to all the pulmonary veins connecting anomalously. The various sites of anomalous connection (Fig. 20) are to the systemic veins of the thorax (supracardiac connection), to the heart itself either directly or via the coronary sinus (cardiac connection), or to the systemic veins within the abdomen (infracardiac or infradiaphragmatic connection). The calibre of the anomalous connection is important, obstructed connection carrying a much poorer prognosis and being particularly frequent with infradiaphragmatic patterns.

Anomalies of the atrial chambers

Atrial septal defects

The atrial septum is of much smaller dimensions than is first apparent. Much of what appears to be septum consists of infolding of the atrial walls themselves, or is the atrioventricular septum between right atrium and left ventricle. True atrial septal defects must be within the margins of the septum and are therefore limited to interatrial communications in the environs of the oval fossa, although there are several other anomalies which permit interatrial communication.

One part of the septum (the primary septum) grows from the atrial roof between the sinus venosus and the outgrowing primary pulmonary vein (Figs 4 and 21a). It grows down as a crescentic fold and fuses with the endocardial cushions to form the inferior rim of the atrial septum. An interatrial connection is essential during intra-uterine life so, as the lower edge of the primary septum fuses with the cushions, the upper part breaks down to form the secondary foramen (Fig. 21b). The space between the lower edge of the primary septum and the cushions, obliterated during normal development, is the primary foramen. The upper part of the primary septum then forms the flap valve of the oval foramen. If this mechanism is to work properly, the roof of the atrium must become infolded so that the upper edge of the primary septum can abut against the atrial wall. The upper rim of the oval fossa (or the secondary septum) is an infolding of the atrial wall (Fig. 21c).

Normally the higher left than right atrial pressure keeps the oval foramen closed, but in about 25 per cent of normal individuals the flap valve is never anatomically fused to the rim.

A true defect at the site of the oval fossa is almost always due to a deficiency of the flap valve, derived from the primary septum.

This may be because the upper edge of the valve is itself

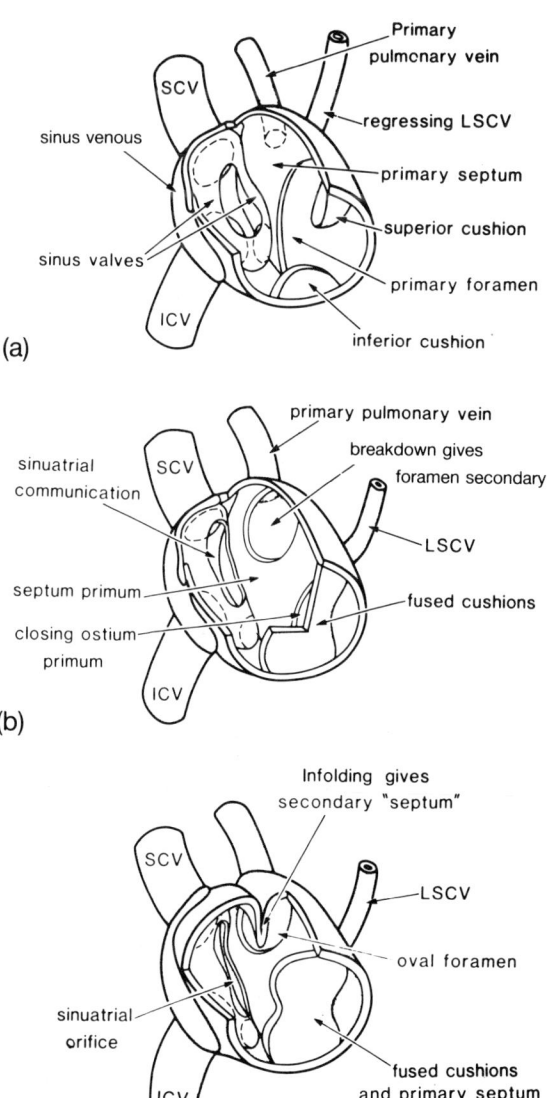

(a)

(b)

(c)

Fig. 21 Drawings showing the stages involved during development of the atrial septum.

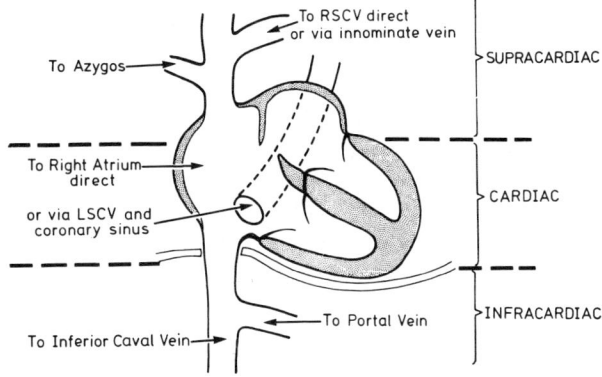

Fig. 20 Diagram showing the possible sites of anomalous connection of the pulmonary veins.

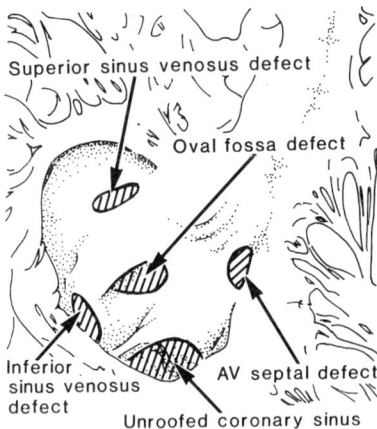

Fig. 22 Diagram showing the different lesions which permit interatrial shunting although not all are within the confines of the normal atrial septum.

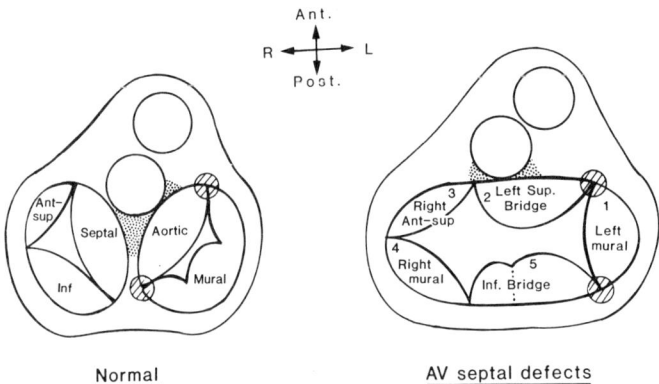

Fig. 23 Diagrams showing the difference between the normal mitral and tricuspid valves and the five leaflet valve which guards the common atrioventricular junction in hearts with atrioventricular septal defects.

deficient or because the flap valve is perforate. A defect due to stretching of the rim can occur but is rare.

The other defects which permit interatrial communications are the so-called sinus venosus defects, the 'ostium primum' atrial septal defect, and a communication at the site of the coronary sinus (Fig. 22). The sinus venosus defect is found in the mouth of one of the great veins, usually the superior caval vein but occasionally the inferior vein. Almost always it is associated with anomalous connection of the right pulmonary veins. The ostium primum defect is found in the region of the atrioventricular septum, and is indeed an atrioventricular septal defect. An interatrial communication at the site of the coronary sinus is rare. It is almost always associated with connection of the left superior caval vein to the roof of the left atrium (unroofed coronary sinus).

Other atrial malformations

Juxtaposition of the atrial appendages occur when both appendages are to the same side of the vascular pedicle. Juxtaposed appendages with the usual atrial arrangement usually lie to the left of the great arteries and are associated with other complex anomalies such as tricuspid atresia or complete transposition. Right juxtaposition is much rarer; it is often associated with an atrial septal defect within the oval fossa.

Division of an atrial chamber is described as cor triatriatum. It can occur in the right atrium due to persistence of the valves of the embryonic sinus venosus. This is associated with complex anomalies, e.g. tricuspid atresia, but can be isolated when it produces stenosis of the right atrioventricular orifice. Occasionally the

dividing membrane may become aneurysmal and rarely may balloon in the right ventricular outflow tract.

Division of the left atrium is more frequent. It can take various forms, and should be differentiated from aneurysmal dilatation of the coronary sinus. Divided left atrium is most usually due to presence of a membrane between the pulmonary venous component of the left atrium and the vestibule. The oval fossa usually is in communication with the vestibular part of the divided atrium which communicates with the left ventricle through a normal mitral valve. It is an important anomaly since it produces pulmonary venous obstruction and has to be distinguished from obstructed total anomalous pulmonary venous connection and various forms of left ventricular inflow obstruction such as mitral stenosis. It is easily recognized echocardiographically and readily dealt with at surgery.

Anomalies of the atrioventricular junction

Atrioventricular septal defects

'Ostium primum' atrial septal defect and 'complete atrioventricular canal' have the same basic morphology, and are best described as atrioventricular septal defects. These anomalies have been presumed to result from various degrees of maldevelopment and malfusion of the atrioventricular endocardial cushions, but there is no positive evidence to support this hypothesis. The major purpose of the cushion is to act as an embryonic 'glue', sticking the centre of the heart together and permitting the process of septation and transfer of the outflow tracts to occur normally around the scaffold provided by the cushions.

Normally the aortic valve achieves a central position between the mitral and tricuspid orifices, the three valves together having a three-leafed clover appearance when viewed from below (Fig. 23). When fusion of the endocardial cushions does not occur, there is a generally 'sprung' appearance of the atrioventricular junction, and the aortic valve does not achieve its normal 'wedge' position. The valvar arrangement in atrioventricular septal defects viewed from above is more like a cottage loaf (Fig. 23). This arrangement is found in both 'ostium primum' defects and 'complete atrioventricular canal' malformations. The difference between the two depends on the morphology of the valve leaflets which guard the 'sprung' junction. The essence of the so-called atrioventricular septal defect is the presence of a common atrioventricular orifice. This common orifice is guarded by a five-leaflet valve (Fig. 23). When the valve leaflets close during diastole there is an interatrial communication between the closed leaflets and the edge of the atrial septum. There is also an extensive interventricular communication between the underside of the valve leaflets and the crest of the ventricular septum (Fig. 24). The difference between this malformation and an 'ostium primum atrial septal defect', a so-called partial atrioventricular septal defect, is that in the latter the valve leaflets common to the right and left ventricles, the bridging leaflets, are fused with each other and also to the crest of the ventricular septum. As a consequence the full extent of the atrioventricular septal defect is between the atrial septum and the valve leaflets, but most is below the level of the atrioventricular junction (Fig. 24). The basic morphology is therefore the same in both defects, including the abnormal left atrioventricular valve (in no way comparable with a normal mitral valve) and the narrowed left ventricular outflow tract. The conduction tissue disposition is also grossly abnormal because of the presence of the atrioventricular septal defect. The morphology explains well the clinical features of these anomalies.

Anomalies of the atrioventricular valves Certain anomalies affect either of the atrioventricular valves, while others have a predilection for the mitral or tricuspid valves respectively. Either valve may be imperforate, more frequently the mitral. An imperforate mitral valve is probably the commonest cause of mitral atresia, but an imperforate tricuspid valve is rarely the cause of tricuspid atresia. This is more usually due to absence of the right atrioventricu-

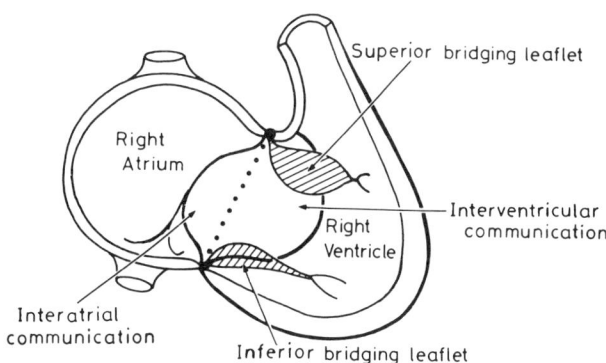

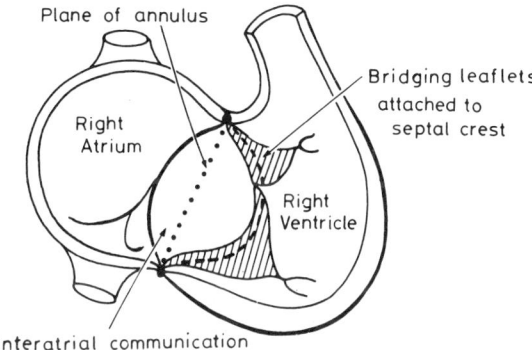

Fig. 24 Diagrams showing the different leaflet arrangements in atrioventricular septal defects with (a) common atrioventricular orifice and (b) separate right and left atrioventricular orifices.

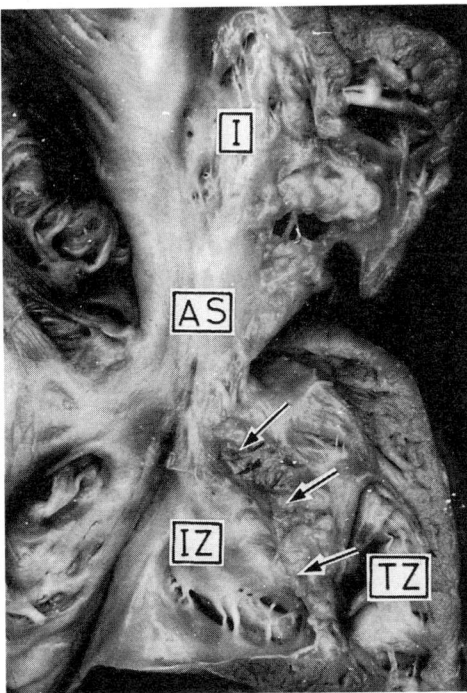

Fig. 25 The opened right atrioventricular junction in a heart exhibiting Ebstein's malformation. IZ shows the septal leaflet of the tricuspid valve plastered down in the inlet zone, and the arrows show how the valve tissue is heaped up at the junction with the trabecular zone (TZ). The inferior leaflet (I) is also dysplastic but the antero-superior leaflet, although dysplastic, is normally positioned.

lar connection. Valve stenosis may be due to various lesions, including valve dysplasia, commissural fusions, etc. A parachute deformity as a cause of stenosis is much more common in the mitral valve, but can occur in the tricuspid valve. The lesions which produce stenosis often additionally produce incompetence. Added to this catalogue should be rare lesions such as a valve arcade, where the papillary musculature extends across beneath the valve leaflet, replacing many of the chords. Valve prolapse is much more important in producing valve incompetence. It is commoner in females and present in up to 2 per cent of the normal population. It is a feature of Marfan's syndrome because of abnormal structure of collagen.

Ebstein's malformation is probably the commonest abnormality of the tricuspid valve. The essence of the anomaly is plastering down of the valve leaflets to the ventricular inlet component so that they are apparently attached more distally in the ventricle than the atrioventricular annulus. The septal and inferior leaflets are most severely affected, while the anterosuperior leaflet becomes a sail-like partition between the ventricular inlet and outlet portions (Fig.25). In its severest form the entire valve is displaced to the ventricular inlet/trabecular junction, and may be imperforate. Ebstein's malformation frequently affects the left-sided tricuspid valve in congenitally corrected transposition. Although exceedingly rare, a similar lesion can affect the morphologically mitral valve.

Anomalies of the ventricular mass

Ventricular hypoplasia

Hypoplasia of the ventricles is most frequently seen in association with atresia of the ventricular outflow tract or else with abnormalities of the atrioventricular valves. Right ventricular hypoplasia is most usually seen with pulmonary atresia and intact ventricular septum while left ventricular hypoplasia is found with aortic atresia. Both anomalies have an exceedingly poor prognosis, and although surgery is improving for pulmonary atresia, few patients with these malformations reach adult life.

In the setting of pulmonary atresia and intact ventricular septum there is a wide spectrum of ventricular size. Rarely the right ventricle is of normal dimensions with a normal tricuspid valve and is separated by an imperforate valve from the pulmonary trunk. More usually the ventricle is hypoplastic. In the least severely affected cases there is global hypoplasia of all three ventricular components with an imperforate pulmonary valve. In the most severely affected the trabecular and outlet components are overgrown, and the ventricular cavity is represented more or less by the hypoplastic inlet portion which usually contains a stenotic miniaturized and dysplastic tricuspid valve. The prognosis is worst in the cases with overgrowth of the ventricular trabecular portion.

In the setting of aortic atresia cases with stenotic or imperforate mitral valves can be distinguished from those with absence of the left atrioventricular connection, but the distinction has little practical significance. In either case the left ventricle has little or no haemodynamic significance, being a slit-like cavity when the left valve is imperforate or a hypoplastic chamber lined with a fibro-elastic layer when there is mitral stenosis. These anomalies together are frequently referred to as the hypoplastic left heart syndrome. Rarely hearts with aortic atresia may have a ventricular septal defect and a more normally sized left ventricle. These are the only cases likely to have a reasonable chance of survival following attempted surgical correction.

Ventricular septal defect

Ventricular septal defect is the commonest congenital cardiac malformation, occurring both as an isolated defect and also as an integral part of anomalies such as double outlet right ventricle and common arterial trunk. A ventricular septal defect is also frequent with other anomalies such as congenitally complete and corrected transposition.

From the stance of the margins, there are three types of defect.

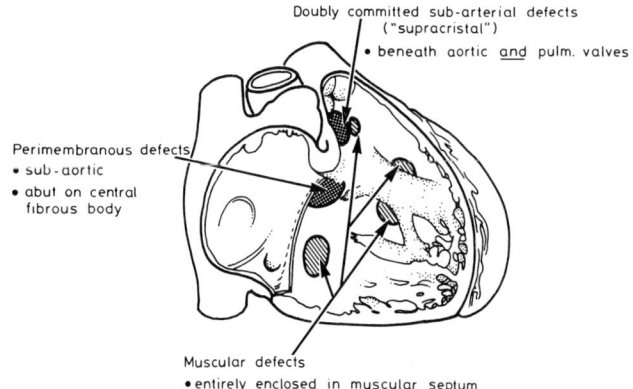

Fig. 26 Diagram showing the morphological features of the different types of ventricular septal defect.

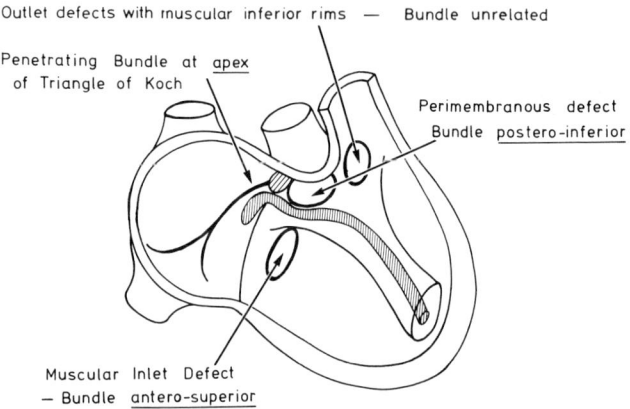

Fig. 27 The relationship of the atrioventricular bundle to various types of ventricular septal defect.

Most are found in the environs of the central fibrous body, whence an area of aortic-mitral-tricuspid valvular continuity forms part of their rim. Incorporated into this fibrous area is the atrioventricular membranous septum, and frequently a remnant of the interventricular membranous septum hangs down as a curtain across the defect from this fibrous zone. The defects are there because of deficiency of the muscular septum around the membranous area, and are designated perimembranous defects (Fig. 26). Much less common are the group whose margins are completely muscular (muscular defects, Fig. 26). The least common is the group of defects which exist because of lack of the outlet part of the ventricular septum. They are therefore beneath both the aortic and pulmonary valves, and indeed are roofed by the conjoint aortic and pulmonary valve rings. This final group may be called doubly committed subarterial defects. Perimembranous and muscular defects can be found opening into the inlet, the trabecular or the outlet components of the right ventricle.

Doubly committed subarterial defects are of necessity between the ventricular outlets but can extend to become perimembranous. Malalignment of the different parts of the ventricular septum can complicate the picture, particularly muscular inlet defects or perimembranous outlet defects.

Increasing knowledge of the site of ventricular septal defects may allow prediction of which will close spontaneously. Of significance in this respect are the size of the defects and their proximity to fibrous structures which may close them off. Small defects are more likely to close than large ones, particularly when in the muscular septum.

Perimembranous defects are likely to close by plastering across them of tricuspid valve tissue or by aneurysmal enlargement of tags derived from the tricuspid valve (so-called aneurism of the membranous septum). Small perimembranous defects opening into the inlet of the right ventricle are most likely to close but any defect with gross malalignment is unlikely to close as are doubly committed subarterial defects. Also of significance is the disposition of the conduction tissues. The atrioventricular bundle is basically postero-inferior to perimembranous defects, antero-superior to muscular inlet defects and unrelated to outlet defects (Fig. 27).

Miscellaneous anomalies of the ventricular mass
Uhl's anomaly is a rare malformation in which the myocardium of the right ventricle is totally deficient so that the chamber becomes a bag with parchment walls. Another malformation is produced by isolated hypolasia of the right ventricle without pulmonary atresia: this is produced by undergrowth of the right ventricular trabecular component. A two-chambered right ventricle results from hypertrophy of the body of the septomarginal or a septoparietal trabeculation. This can occur in varying degree and divides the ventricular trabecular component into inlet and outlet portions. It is frequently associated with tetralogy of Fallot and often with a ventricular septal defect, which may open into either inlet or outlet components of the two-chamber ventricle.

Anomalies of the ventricular outflow tracts
The morphologically right ventricular outflow is a completely muscular stucture, and obstruction can be found at infundibular, valvar or supravalvar levels. Infundibular obstruction is either a sharply defined constriction at the junction of the trabecular and outlet portions or else a long tunnel obstruction of the entire infundibulum. Valve lesions can be due to dysplasia of the valve, particularly in the younger age group, or to commissural fusion of a bifoliate or trifoliate pulmonary valve. The commissures may be so fused to produce a dome shaped valve with a central pin-hole opening. This is also seen particularly in the younger age group and may be similar in its effects to pulmonary atresia. Supravalvar stenosis can affect the pulmonary trunk itself, but is not as frequent as pulmonary artery branch stenosis. Incompetence of the pulmonary valve is of much less significance apart from the particular anomaly when the pulmonary valve is absent. Associated particularly with tetralogy of Fallot, this results in severe dilatation of the pulmonary trunk.

Obstruction of the left ventricular outflow tract can also be found at subvalvar, valvar, and supravalvar levels. Subvalvar obstruction is quite different from that found in the right ventricle because the left ventricular outflow tract is deeply wedged between the mitral and tricuspid valves. It can be divided into fixed and dynamic forms. The most obvious fixed obstruction is a horseshoe shelf-like lesion formed between the septum and the facing leaflet of the mitral valve. When the lesion is more extensive, it can produce a tunnel obstruction of the outflow and is described as such. Other fixed obstructions are produced by anomalous insertion of the atrioventricular valve tension apparatus and herniation of an aneurysm of either the membranous septum or an atrioventricular valve leaflet into the outflow tract. These fixed obstructions can be found either with an intact septum or a ventricular septal defect. When there is a septal defect, a common source of obstruction is malalignment of the outlet septum into the left ventricular outflow tract.

Dynamic obstruction of the outflow tract is due to septal bulging. Although this can be purely haemodynamic, almost always there is dysplasia and hypertrophy of the septal musculature, producing a picture very similar to hypertrophic cardiomyopathy. Indeed, hypertrophic cardiomyopathy itself is a potent source of left ventricular outflow tract obstruction.

Aortic valve stenosis can, like pulmonary stenosis, present in infancy or much later in life. Both can have a congenital basis. When presenting in infancy the valve leaflets are usually thickened and dysplastic and can rarely be repaired to produce a normally functioning valve. Stenosis presenting in later life, if not rheumatic in origin, has its basis in either a bifoliate valve or a trifoliate valve with grossly unequal leaflet sizes. The aortic valve leaflets are rarely of the same size, and it seems that commissural fusion has a predilection to occur between leaflets of particularly disparate size. Supravalvar stenosis is more frequent in the aorta than the pulmonary trunk. It can occur in hour-glass, tubular, or membranous forms. Dilatation and later thickening of the wall of the coronary arteries is also found.

Tetralogy of Fallot

Tetralogy is in essence a malformation of the right ventricular outflow tract. It is the combination of a ventricular septal defect, aortic overriding, pulmonary infundibular stenosis, and right ventricular hypertrophy. The anatomical hallmark is insertion of the septal extension of the outlet septum anterior to the septomarginal trabeculation rather than between its limbs as in the normal heart (Fig. 28). The ventricular septal defect is typically perimembranous but with malalignment of the outlet septum. Rarely the margins may be muscular and when additional absence or hypoplasia of the outlet septum is present the defect will be doubly committed and subarterial. The aortic override can vary between the aortic valve being mostly connected to the left ventricle or mostly connected to the right ventricle. The infundibular obstruction is predominantly due to the anomalous insertion of the septum, but this can be exacerbated by hypertrophy of the septal insertion, the outlet septomarginal trabeculation, or of additional anterior infundibular trabeculations. The right ventricular hypertrophy is a haemodynamic consequence of the other anatomic features. Tetralogy has a particular association with right aortic arch, while a second muscular inlet ventricular septal defect or a common atrioventricular orifice are particularly important but uncommon associated anomalies.

The degree of infundibular obstruction in tetralogy is dependent upon the degree of anterior deviation of the outlet septum. When this is extreme, it produces pulmonary atresia with ventricular septal defect, one form of which is no more than extreme tetralogy of Fallot. This assumes the presence of confluent right and left pulmonary arteries, however small, with the blood reaching the lungs through an arterial duct (ductus arteriosus). In the other main types of pulmonary atresia with ventricular septal defect large systemic collateral arteries supply individual lobes or parts of the lung and the main right and left pulmonary arteries may or may not be present. The precise nature of the pulmonary blood supply and presence or absence of the pulmonary arteries influences both clinical presentation and possibilities for surgical correction.

Anomalies of the great arteries

Aorto-pulmonary window

An aorto-pulmonary window is a communication between the ascending portions of the aorta and the pulmonary trunk. It can be of varying size but is always distinguished from a common arterial trunk because of the presence of separate aortic and pulmonary valves.

Arterial duct (ductus arteriosus)

The arterial duct is the major pathway in the fetus from the ventricular mass to the descending aorta, and represents the left sixth aortic arch. In the fetal circulation the isthmus of the aorta and the right and left pulmonary arteries are all relatively small. After birth there is an almost immediate increase in size of the pulmonary arteries and closure of the duct. The remodelling of the aortic isthmus is a more gradual procedure, but the duct itself is usually effectively closed within two or three days of birth. If the duct remains patent, then persistent patency is the result of an histological abnormality of the ductal wall which distinguishes it from a duct which may be undergoing delayed closure or that commonly found in the premature infant. It is presumably delayed closure that can be stimulated by administration of prostaglandin inhibitors, while these are unlikely to effect closure in a duct with the histological abnormality which favours persistent patency.

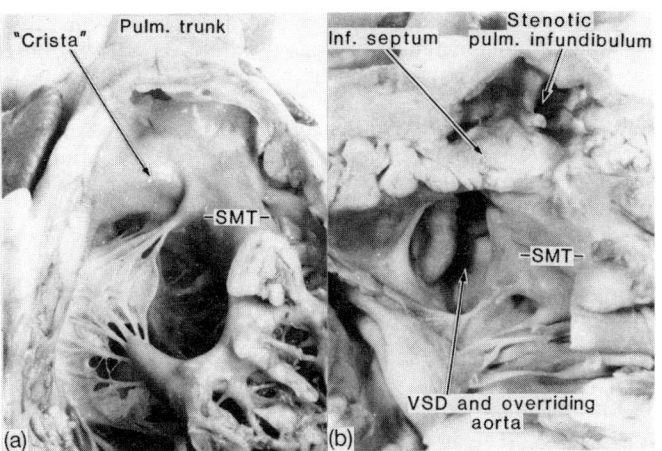

Fig. 28 The basic anatomy of tetralogy of Fallot (b) compared with the normal right ventricular outflow tract (a).

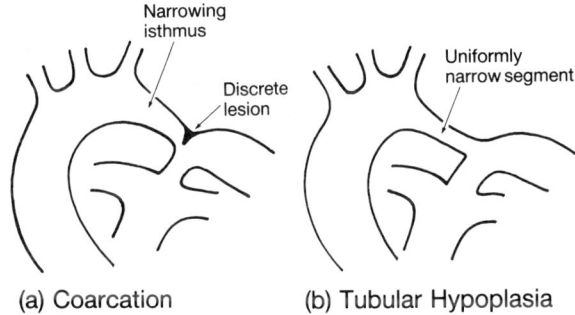

Fig. 29 The difference between (a) discrete coarctation and (b) tubular hypoplasia.

In many malformations a patent or persistent duct is a beneficial finding, and indeed may be the only source of aortic or pulmonary blood flow. This is seen in aortic or pulmonary atresia with or without ventricular septal defect. A patent duct or a ligament is also an integral part of most of the so-called vascular rings (see below).

Anomalies of the aorta and pulmonary trunk

Consideration of numerous types of vascular ring, sling, or 'isolated' arteries is beyond the scope of this book. However, some anomalies of the aortic arches are of particular significance, notably coarctation and interruption of the aortic arch.

Coarctation can take one of two basic forms. It can be an isolated diaphragmatic or curtain lesion within the aortic arch, or it can be a more elongated segment of tubular hypoplasia (Fig. 29). The two forms can co-exist and either can be found with a patent arterial duct. In particular when there is tubular hypoplasia and the duct remains patent there is often an associated intracardiac lesion which has favoured diversion of blood during fetal development away from the aortic pathway and into the pulmonary pathway. Typical lesions are ventricular septal defects with deviation of the outlet septum into the left ventricle, or hearts with univentricular connection to a left ventricle and discordant ventriculoarterial connection and an obstructed ventricular septal defect. In addition to a hypoplastic arch a discrete lesion is also present where the isthmus inserts into the ductal-descending aorta junction. In these cases the coarctation lesion itself is composed of ductal tissue. In contrast, when the duct is closed, coarctation is more frequently an isolated lesion, although in a high proportion of cases there will be a bifoliate aortic valve. The lesion is then formed on the wall of the aorta opposite the ligamental insertion and, when removed, is usually found to be composed of fibrous tissue. Although most usually a discrete coarctation lesion is found at the isthmal junction, pre-ductal or post-ductal lesions can rarely be found. Tubular hypoplasia commonly affects the isthmus, but it may be found in the arch segment between the brachiocephalic and left carotid arteries or between the left carotid and left subclavian arteries. Interruption of the aortic arch probably exemplifies extreme tubular hypoplasia in which the arch becomes atretic, or else disappears completely. It may affect the same segments of the arch, and it too is potentiated by lesions which, during fetal life, divert blood away from the aorta.

Congenital anomalies with abnormal chamber connections

Atrial isomerism

Most patients with congenital heart disease have the usual arrangement of both the atria and the thoraco-abdominal organs and mirror-image arrangements are rare. Patients with neither usual nor mirror-image arrangements have long been known to be harbingers of complex congenital heart disease, and have been grouped together under various terms such as visceral heterotaxy, asplenia, polysplenia, etc. The anatomy is basically that of isomerism rather than lateralization of the organs, and can be recognized by examination of a penetrated chest radiograph. There are two basic groups (see pages 13.234–13.236 and Fig. 9). Right atrial isomerism is almost invariably associated with a bilateral morphologically right or trilobed lung and asplenia. Both atria are of right morphology, probably with bilateral superior caval veins, a common atrium and invariably total anomalous pulmonary venous connection. A common atrioventricular valve is usual and a univentricular atrioventricular connection and pulmonary atresia often co-exist. Most of these patients have a poor prognosis and are seen in infancy.

The heart is more often normal in left atrial isomerism. The lungs are of left morphology and there is usually polysplenia. Both atria are of left morphology, associated often with bilateral superior caval veins, azygos continuation of the inferior caval veins and bilaterally symmetrical drainage of pulmonary veins. The ventricular mass is often normal, but common valves are frequent. Pulmonary stenosis or atresia is not a feature. These patients are much more likely to survive. The condition should always be suspected when azygos continuation of the inferior caval vein is encountered.

Complete transposition

Complete transposition of the great arteries is the combination of concordant atrioventricular and discordant ventriculo-arterial connections. It can exist with a usual or mirror-image atrial arrangement. With usual arrangement the aorta is usually anterior and to the right of the pulmonary trunk, but not sufficiently constantly to warrant use of 'd-transposition' as a synonym for complete transposition. Usually there is a complete subaortic muscular infundibulum and pulmonary-mitral valvar continuity, but infundibular morphology is also variable. The oval foramen is usually probe-patent and initial treatment now consists of rupture of the flap valve of the oval fossa by Rashkind balloon septostomy. Transposition may be complicated by associated lesions such as ventricular septal defect, pulmonary stenosis, patency of the arterial duct, or a combination of these. Exactly the same lesions as produce subaortic stenosis in the normal heart will produce pulmonary stenosis in complete transposition. Other lesions must also be anticipated as a possibility in complete transposition.

Congenitally corrected transposition

Corrected transposition is the combination of discordant atrioventricular and ventriculo-arterial connections and it too can be found in patients with either usual or mirror-image atrial arrangement (Fig. 30). The aortic valve is usually anterior and to the left, but as with the right-sided aorta in complete usual arrangement transposition, not sufficiently constantly to justify the term 'l-transposition'. The hallmark of corrected transposition is malalignment between the atrial septum and the inlet part of the ventricular sep-

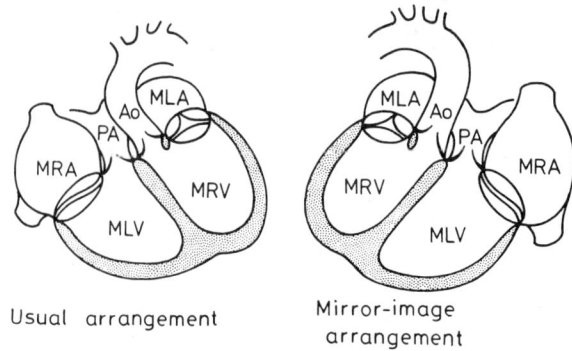

Usual arrangement   Mirror-image arrangement

Discordant atrioventricular and ventriculo-arterial connections

Fig. 30 The chamber combinations which produce congenitally corrected transposition.

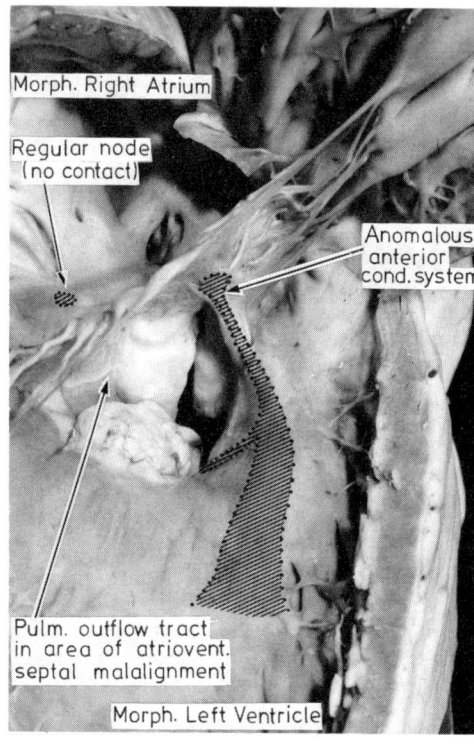

Fig. 31 The malalignment between the atrial and ventricular septa which is the hallmark of congenitally corrected transposition. The position of the conduction tissues has been superimposed on the photograph.

tum (Fig. 31) accounting for the grossly abnormal disposition of the conduction tissues. The regular atrioventricular node in the atrial septum is unable to make contact with the ventricular conduction tissues on the trabecular part of the ventricular system. Instead there is an anomalous anterolateral node in the right atrioventricular orifice which assumes the role of the connecting atrioventricular node. The atrioventricular bundle therefore passes anterolateral to the pulmonary outflow tract from the morphologically left ventricle (Fig. 31). The malalignment also accounts for the frequent association of a ventricular septal defect, pulmonary stenosis, and Ebstein's malformation of the left-sided morphologically tricuspid valve. When there is a ventricular septal defect, the conduction tissues are related to its anterosuperior rim. Pulmonary stenosis may be produced by any of the anomalies which produce left ventricular outflow tract obstruction in the normally connected heart, and aneurysmal tissue tags are particularly common. Heart block of varying severity is frequent because the abnormal disposition of conduction tissue makes it particularly susceptible to fibrotic change.

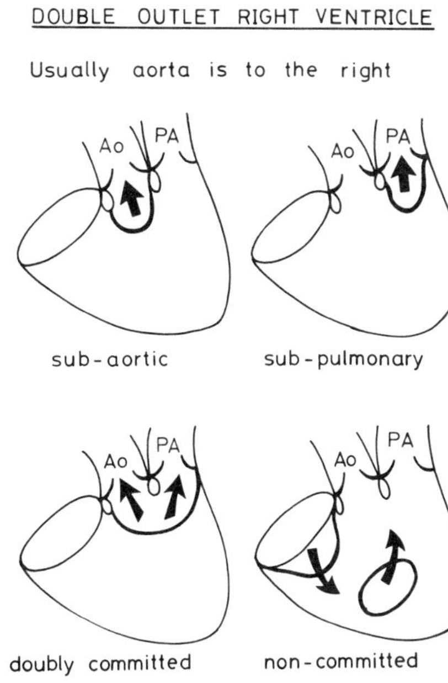

DOUBLE OUTLET RIGHT VENTRICLE

Usually aorta is to the right

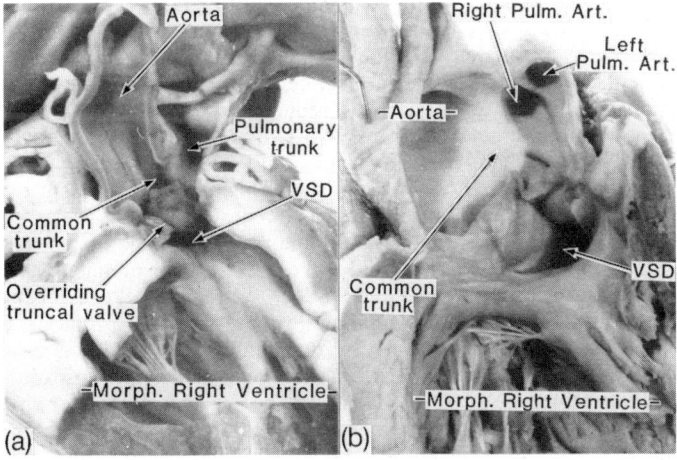

Fig. 32 The positions of the ventricular septal defect in double outlet right ventricle when the aorta is to the right of the pulmonary trunk.

Fig. 33 The morphology of the common arterial trunk as seen from the right ventricle showing (a) the variant with a common pulmonary trunk (type I) and (b) the variant with separate origin of the right and left pulmonary arteries (type II).

Double outlet ventricles

Double outlet right ventricle can exist with any atrioventricular connection. There are many combinations depending on the position of the ventricular septal defect which is almost invariably present, the state of the infundibular morphology, and the interrelationships of the arterial valves. The ventricular septal defect can be subaortic, subpulmonary, doubly committed, or non-committed (Fig. 32), may be perimembranous or have a muscular postero-inferior rim. A bilaterally muscular infundibulum is usual but there may be arterial-atrioventricular valvar continuity. The aortic valve is usually to the right of the pulmonary valve, side by side or anterior but more rarely posterior.

There are two major patterns of double outlet with right-sided aorta. In the first, the ventricular septal defect is in subaortic position and frequently there is pulmonary stenosis. Haemodynamics therefore resemble those of Fallot's tetralogy. In the second group the defect is in subpulmonary position, producing the haemodynamics of complete transposition with ventricular septal defect. Intermediate cases occur because of overriding of the arterial valve.

Double outlet left ventricle is a much rarer finding, which can also exist with any atrioventricular connection but most commonly a concordant one. There is variability in position of the ventricular septal defect or other changes as in double outlet right ventricle. Most usually with a concordant atrioventricular connection the aortic valve is right-sided, the defect is doubly committed, and there is a bilaterally deficient infundibulum.

Common arterial trunk

The common arterial trunk is one of the varieties of single outlet of the heart. The others, single pulmonary trunk with aortic atresia, single aortic trunk with pulmonary atresia, and solitary arterial trunk are only described as such when it is not possible to trace the atretic artery to its communication with a ventricular chamber. There is not likely to be much difficulty in distinguishing a common trunk from the other types of single outlet of the heart. The common trunk is characterized by a single arterial trunk leaving the base of the heart through a common arterial valve and supplying directly the coronary arteries, the aortic arch, and the pulmonary trunk. There may be anomalous origin of one pulmonary artery, or interruption of the aortic arch with the descending aorta supplied by a duct, but the presence of a common valve should permit the common trunk to be readily recognized.

The common trunk can exist with any combination of atria and ventricles, most commonly the normal pattern of the usual atrial arrangement and concordant atrioventricular connection. Usually the trunk is connected to both ventricular chambers, overriding a large subarterial ventricular septal defect, but it can be connected exclusively to either the right or the left ventricle. The subarterial ventricular septal defect most frequently has a muscular postero-inferior rim but can extend to become perimembranous. There is further variability in truncal valve morphology and in aortic and pulmonary arterial anatomy. The truncal valve is trifoliate in the majority of cases, but can be quadrifoliate, bifoliate, or even have five leaflets. The pulmonary arteries can arise from a short common pulmonary trunk (so-called type I), directly from the back of the common trunk (type II), or from either side of the common trunk (type III) (Fig. 33). The aortic arch usually feeds the descending aorta directly, without a duct, but cases are found in which the aortic arch is interrupted and then an arterial duct supplies the descending aorta from the pulmonary component of the common trunk.

Hearts with univentricular atrioventricular connection

The commonest anomalies within this group are the double inlet left ventricle and so-called tricuspid atresia.

Double inlet left ventricle The anomaly, classically described as 'single ventricle', is characterized by connection of both atria to a dominant left ventricle in the presence of an anterior rudimentary right ventricle. The great arteries are usually discordant, so that the aorta arises from the rudimentary right ventricle and the pulmonary trunk from the left ventricle. This type of heart then has further subgroups depending on whether the rudimentary right ventricle and the aorta are left-sided or right-sided. Usually in this anomaly there are two separate atrioventricular valves but there may be a common valve. When there are two valves, one or both may be malformed. Outflow tract obstruction is also common, and obstruction at the ventricular septal defect is associated with coarctation and reduced aortic flow. The prognosis is best when there is a good aortic pathway but sub-pulmonary obstruction, and patients with this combination can survive well into adult life. If surgery is attempted in such patients, then the grossly abnormal conduction tissue must be taken into account, there being an anomalous anterior atrioventricular node as in corrected transposition.

More rarely, double inlet left ventricle can be found with a concordant ventriculo-arterial connection, the pulmonary trunk arising from the rudimentary right ventricle and the aorta from the dominant left ventricle. This combination is known as the 'Holmes

heart' and its clinical presentation is coloured by the high incidence of pulmonary obstruction at the ventricular septal defect. It
therefore presents in a similar manner to tetralogy of Fallot. Other
ventriculo-arterial connections are possible with double inlet left
ventricle but are rare.

Double inlet can also occur to a right ventricle in the presence of
a posterior rudimentary left ventricle. Both great arteries are
usually also connected to the dominant right ventricle so that the
rudimentary left ventricle is no more than a trabecular pouch.

Straddling valves are frequently found with double inlet to
either a right or left ventricle, and a series of anomalies exist in the
presence of straddling valves between hearts with univentricular
and biventricular atrioventricular connections.

Very rarely it is possible to find hearts with double inlet to a solitary ventricle, but a rudimentary second ventricle can usually be
found in these at autopsy, if not during life. These hearts must be
differentiated from those with double inlet to a solitary indeterminate ventricle. Indeterminate ventricles are coarsely trabeculated
and criss-crossed by prominent trabeculations. Of necessity they
can have only double outlet or single outlet as their ventriculo-
arterial connections.

Tricuspid atresia Although very rarely hearts may be found in
which an imperforate valve is responsible for producing tricuspid
atresia, almost always the atresia results from absence of the right
atrioventricular connection. Then the floor of the right atrium is
separated by atrioventricular groove tissue from the ventricular
mass, and the right ventricle lacks an inlet portion, being rudimentary. These also have a univentricular atrioventricular connection.
Most frequently there is a discordant ventriculo-arterial connection, the pulmonary trunk arising from the right ventricle and the
aorta from the dominant left ventricle. Pulmonary stenosis is then
the rule, being produced most usually at the ventricular septal
defect, but sometimes another stenotic area is present between the
trabecular and outlet parts of the right ventricle. Pulmonary atresia can also be found, and sometimes there is no restriction of pulmonary blood flow. A discordant ventriculo-arterial connection
can also be found with tricuspid atresia, and then the aortic flow
from the rudimentary right ventricle is compromised by stenosis of
the ventricular septal defect. This accounts for the frequent
accompaniment of coarctation. Other ventriculo-arterial connections can be found but are rare.

Absence of the right atrioventricular connection can also rarely
be found in hearts with the left atrium connected to right or indeterminate ventricles, and both variants would present as classical
tricuspid atresia. They are, however, very rare.

Absent left atrioventricular connection with the right atrium
connected to a dominant right ventricle may be associated with
aortic atresia and is one of the variants of hypoplastic left heart
syndrome. It can also be found with a patent aorta arising from the
rudimentary left ventricle, or with double outlet from the dominant right ventricle, and then carries a more favourable prognosis.
Absent left atrioventricular connection with patent aortic root is
seen more frequently when the right atrium connects to a dominant left ventricle, the aorta and rudimentary right ventricle being
left-sided. Some refer to this anomaly as 'tricuspid atresia with
corrected transposition', arguing that the absent connection, had
it developed properly, would have become a tricuspid valve. As
with other hearts with absent left connection or imperforate tricuspid valves, there is most frequently obstruction to pulmonary
venous return at the interatrial communication, this being the only
route for pulmonary venous circulation. It is presence or absence
of an obstructive atrial septal defect which determines the clinical
presentation and course.

References

Anderson, R. H. and Becker. A. E. (1980). *Cardiac anatomy – an integrated text and colour atlas*, Gower Medical Publisher, London.

——, Becker, A. E., Lucchese, F. A., Meier, M. A., Rigby, M. L. and
Soto, B. (1983). *Morphology of congenital heart disease*. Castle House
Publications Ltd, Tunbridge Wells.
—— and Shinebourne. E, A. (1978). *Paediatric cardiology 1977*. Churchill
Livingstone, Edinburgh.
Becker, A. E. and Anderson. R. H. (1981). *The pathology of congenital
heart disease*. Butterworth, London.
——, ——, (1983). *Cardiac pathology. An integrated text and colour atlas*.
Churchill Livingstone, Edinburgh, and Gower Medical Publishing, Lon-
don.
Goor, D. A. and Lillehei, C. W. (1975). *Congenital malformations of the
heart. Embryology, anatomy, and operative considerations*. Grune and
Stratton, New York.
Hudson, R. E. B. (1970). *Cardiovascular pathology*, Vol. 3. Arnold,
London.
Okamoto, N. (1980). *Congenital anomalies of the heart. Embryologic mor-
phologic and experimental teratology*. Igaku-Shoin, Tokyo.
Shinebourne, E. A. and Anderson, R. H. (1980). *Current paediatric car-
diology*. Oxford University Press, Oxford.

Congenital heart disease in adults

J. SOMERVILLE

Introduction

Congenital abnormalities of the heart and cardiovascular system
are reported in about 7–12 per 1000 live births. It is doubtful if all
the trivial lesions are recognized in childhood and so the true incidence may be higher. During infancy 50–60 per cent of these
patients need medical and surgical help. In the first decade after
infancy, a further 25–30 per cent require the skills of the cardiac
surgeon to maintain or improve life. Only 10–15 per cent survive
without surgery to adolescence and adult life; these are the 'natural survivors', i.e. those whose natural history permits them to
lead normal lives without surgical treatment.

Many congenital cardiovascular abnormalities which first come
to light in adults have been mild and caused little or no haemodynamic disturbance during childhood. Symptoms develop later in
life because of calcification in valves, progressive myocardial dysfunction, infective endocarditis, or the onset of arrhythmias.
Sometimes more serious lesions cause haemodynamic disorder
and symptoms in the child but he or she survives without treatment because of the development of postnatal adaptive changes in
the heart or pulmonary circulation. Such changes in 'form and
function' may be ultimately destructive, protective or beneficial.

This group of 'natural survivors' whose disease has been modified by time and not by humans is small in comparison to the
increasing numbers of adults and adolescents who have had palliative or direct reparative surgery for congenital cardiac lesions in
childhood and infancy. This larger group of survivors is the product of medical progress in the management of congenital heart
disease. Why do they remain in need of continued medical care?
Many have residual lesions or cardiovascular disease, the result of
the natural evolution of the original lesion; there may be added
iatrogenic problems. Advice is needed from informed physicians
about problems such as pregnancy, genetic risk, the contraceptive
pill, driving capabilities, employment, insurability, adoption, and
jail sentences in relation to their cardiac state and its prognosis.
With increasing success in the surgical treatment of simple and
complex cardiac malformations, the numbers of survivors will
increase. Today's problems are likely to differ from those of 10–15
years hence. Operative treatment has revolutionized the outlook
for patients with congenital heart disease and will achieve more
but the ultimate aim must be to understand the pathogenesis and
prevent congenital heart disease.

Postnatal adaptive changes

The understanding of congenital heart disease in adults requires
knowledge of the adaptive mechanisms which change form and

function of the heart and circulation. The heart at birth is not anatomically or functionally the same as the heart 10, 20 or 50 years later. A congenital structural defect may remain the same or may alter with time and the effects of disordered haemodynamic forces. The heart and blood vessels have few ways of responding to changes of their environment, but profound effects on function may arise from the following postnatal changes.

1. Progressive hypertrophy of abnormally placed muscular bands may lead to obstruction to pulmonary blood flow as in acquired 'infundibular stenosis', bipartite right ventricle, and some forms of subaortic stenosis where there is abnormal muscle placed beneath the aortic valve, particularly when there is discordant ventricular arterial connection.

2. Deposition of endocardial fibrosis/elastic tissue may develop in architecturally abnormal outflows, e.g. fixed subaortic stenosis or fixed infundibular stenosis. These lesions may calcify after 20 years; the same process occurs as a result of endocardial jet lesions which produce no direct haemodynamic upset but provide a site for thrombus formation and infection.

3. Compensatory hypertrophy of ventricular myocardium in response to obstructive and/or regurgitant valvular lesions or increase in peripheral resistance in the pulmonary and systemic circulations may progress with time to fibrosis and irreversible dysfunction.

4. Increasing pulmonary arteriolar disease, by raising pulmonary vascular resistance, may reduce or reverse shunts through associated defects.

5. Spontaneous closure or diminution in size of ventricular septal defect or duct may occur.

6. Valves or outflow tracts may calcify, particularly abnormal semilunar valves or a right ventricular outflow tract which is narrowed. The lesions which have not been severe enough to require surgery before the age of 20 years are prone to calcification later. The most trivial obstruction caused by a bicuspid aortic valve may not declare itself until the seventh or eighth decades as calcific aortic stenosis. Atrioventricular valves also calcify when subjected to pressure loads imposed by distal obstructive lesions. Other factors determine the speed of calcification of congenitally abnormal valves and outflow tracts; these include infection, athletic activity which may increase local trauma, and altered calcium metabolism.

7. Chordae tendinae of malformed, abnormally attached atrioventricular valves and valves subjected to unusual stresses may rupture. This complication usually causes severe regurgitation and tends to occur late in the natural history of complex anomalies such as univentricular hearts, tricuspid atresia, double outflow right ventricle, classic transposition of the great arteries, and even such simple lesions as bicuspid aortic valve stenosis.

8. Aortic valve cusps may prolapse into subarterial ventricular septal defects causing aortic regurgitation and signs of spontaneous diminution or closure of the defect.

9. The term myocardial dysplasia describes a malformation of cardiac muscle in which the functional polarity of cells does not follow the normal tensional alignment; myofibrils and groups of cells are related to each other in a bizarre haphazard criss-cross fashion. The histological pattern itself appears to be non-specific. Areas of dysplasia may change to cause disturbance of ventricular filling or ejection. The amount and site determines the clinical effects. It is extensive in hearts with asymmetrical septal hypertrophy (ASH) which may manifest as hypertrophic obstructive cardiomyopathy, midventricular obstruction, diffuse hypertrophic cardiomyopathy or inflow obstruction of either or both sides of the heart.

Myocardial dysplasia may be found in small areas of normal hearts, particularly in the ventricular septum, but may be more extensive in the myocardium of patients with structural congenital cardiac anomalies. When dysplastic muscle is subjected to pressure strains from distal obstructions which normally lead to hypertrophy (e.g. aortic stenosis, coarctation, pulmonary stenosis) there is a disproportionate increase in its volume which itself may contribute to obstruction to inflow or outflow, disturbance of normal ventricular contractile patterns, and other functional disorders not accounted for by the effects of simple concentric ventricular hypertrophy alone.

The clinical manifestations related to the presence of excessive myocardial dysplasia occur in certain patients with congenital aortic valve stenosis with disproportional septal bulging or late mitral valve prolapse or dysfunction; they may also occur in patients with a small VSD and an inexplicably large left ventricle, in pulmonary valve stenosis, and in ASD with a strange looking left ventricle and mitral regurgitation. These examples show that there is often more disease in the heart than the structural defect alone on which the clinician's attention tends to be focused. The importance for the physician is that congenital heart disease is often congenital cardiovascular disease and as such may manifest some unexpected late cardiac problems.

Changes in cardiac form which develop in response to disordered anatomy and physiology may be beneficial for survival but later the effects are excessive leading to death in childhood, adolescence, or adult life. Changes in form require time to develop and this is the invariable factor which accounts for the differences between hearts in newborns and infants and adolescents or adults.

Morphological changes within the heart and vessels continue in patients who have had extracardiac palliative surgery which prolongs survival, a factor to consider when deciding the timing of more definitive surgery.

In this section only the effects of congenital heart disease in adults and adolescents are emphasized. This selected group of patients does not include all lesions and has special features different from those described in paediatric cardiology textbooks. The vital role of cross-sectional echocardiography in diagnosis and management is discussed elsewhere (see page 13.34).

Classification

The naming and description of congenital cardiac and cardiovascular anomalies have been dealt with in previous chapters (see page 13.233). To present and classify the lesions as they present to the physician is more difficult.

One approach is to classify anomalies of the heart according to the effects on the pulmonary circulation, that is, by dividing conditions into those with increased, decreased or normal pulmonary blood flow. This is unsatisfactory as, with the same basic lesion, it may change during the patient's life, so that the same anatomical defect in the heart could properly be classified in different groups at different points in the evolution of the disease.

Another possibility is to divide lesions which affect primarily the right or left sides of the heart, and leave the septal defects in a special category, separating them from lesions with anomalies of connection. When multiple lesions co-exist it is difficult to decide which is the prime abnormality and the correct categorization.

What is simple and orderly for the medically oriented student may be unacceptable to pathologists, embryologists or surgeons. No classification will suit everyone. For the clinician concerned with congenital heart disease (CHD) what matters is not how did the lesion develop, which has obsessed writers for more than a century, but rather what effects does it produce? The segmental approach to the nomenclature of congenital heart disease has helped indexing and communication, particularly amongst those concerned with complex malformations. It is doubtful if it aids understanding for those who need an introduction to patient management. Recognizing that it is not ideal, lesions are here separated into cyanotic and acyanotic. Like the pulmonary blood flow, this can change but it is an easy starting place as the presence of cyanosis is easily recognized.

Cyanotic congenital heart disease

Central cyanosis is seen when the arterial oxygen saturation is below 85 per cent; lesser degrees of arterial desaturation are not obvious at the bedside. If the presence of central cyanosis is doubtful at rest, exercise or warmth should make it obvious. It is associated with clubbing of the fingers and toes unless arterial desaturation has been established recently. Clubbing of the nails varies from mild heaping up and shininess of the nail beds seen first in the thumbs, to the classic 'drumstick' fingers and toes of severe chronic cyanotic heart disease.

Extracardiac problems are found in adolescents and adults with cyanotic congenital heart disease. These need recognition as they may cause symptoms which are more, or as, troublesome as the symptoms from the basic cardiac defect.

Polycythaemia

In a normally nourished adult with cyanotic CHD who takes and absorbs adequate iron and vitamins, the compensatory polycythaemia is proportional to the systemic arterial desaturation but unusually in excess of the needs, thus causing increased blood viscosity and secondary symptoms. Muzziness, headaches, and 'slowing-up' are described. Venesection, 500–1000 ml, relieves such symptoms. The patient frequently knows when it is time for venesection. The ideal haemoglobin concentration is 17–18 g/dl but in patients in whom concentrations regularly reach levels of 23–25 g/dl it is dangerous to reduce the level acutely to below 20 g/dl. In patients with values exceeding 20 g/dl there is a place for venesection and replacement prior to cardiac or extracardiac surgery to prevent thromboses during or soon after the procedure.

Venesections should be carried out with the patient at rest for a period of hours. The volume removed must be replaced by a volume expander such as dextran or plasma. Dextrose 5 per cent (alone) may be adequate in sporadic venesections of volume less than 500 ml. Never more than 1000 ml of blood should be removed at one period and if this order of venesection is needed, it should be done on two separate occasions separated by at least 24 hours. The common practice of venesection without fluid replacement is dangerous, particularly in patients with the Eisenmenger reaction and should be abandoned. Patients feel weak for five to ten days after excessive venesection, particularly if volume has not been replaced.

Gout

An elevated blood uric acid is common in both sexes perhaps because of increased red cell turnover and associated impaired renal function in adult cyanotic patients. There may be attacks of acute gout in classical sites in males and less commonly females. Wrong diagnosis of this complication is common and patients are often erroneously treated for chronic whitlows, paronychia, or traumatic arthritis. Thiazide diuretics may precipitate the problem but triamterene, spironolactone, and amiloride are free of this complication. Tophi have been reported in men with CHD but not yet in women. Surgical relief of cyanosis prevents polycythaemia and subsequent gout.

Renal problems

The first signs of renal dysfunction are albuminuria and sometimes microscopic haematuria with a few casts. Later creatinine clearance is reduced and oliguria, even anuria, may follow dehydration from any cause. This can be prevented by awareness and provision of adequate fluid intake by mouth and/or intravenously. Diuretics must *not* be given to maintain urine flow until fluid and electrolyte deficits have been adequately replaced. Patients with long-standing polycythaemia and reduced circulating plasma volume are at risk of an acute deterioration in renal function in relation to minor or major surgical procedures. Large doses of contrast media are known to provoke acute renal failure on occasion (see page 18.131) and the risk is probably greater when patients are volume depleted. Hypertonic contrast media increases plasma osmolarity and may thereby cause cerebral or pulmonary oedema in patients with impaired renal function who cannot excrete the osmotic load.

Short periods of intermittent peritoneal or haemodialysis may be needed in some patients with cyanotic CHD, but they readily develop complications such as sepsis, thrombosis or paradoxical emboli which are often fatal. Prevention of oliguria and anuria by early administration of fluid in 'at risk' patients helps prevent serious problems.

Skin sepsis

Adolescents and young adults with cyanotic CHD frequently have serious widespread pustular acne which is more extensive than in the normal adolescent. Spontaneous systemic sepsis from this is unusual but wounds heal poorly with or without acne and stitches should be left in longer than in other patients. Systemic infection following surgery is common in these patients. Non-absorbent suture material or large knots in the subcutaneous layers should be avoided. The responsibility for wound closure should not be left to juniors unaware of such problems.

Attention to skin is vital before surgery and the advice of the dermatologist is useful. Improvement of the arterial oxygen saturation relieves the problem.

Gums

Patients with long-standing polycythaemia and central cyanosis frequently have troublesome bleeding 'spongy' gums. Gingivitis and tooth loss occur prematurely, sometimes hastened by an associated enamel defect. Early and constant attention to dental hygiene is necessary.

Thrombosis and bleeding

Spontaneous venous and less commonly arterial thromboses are a natural consequence of increased viscosity. Their occurrence is reduced by regular venesection and the avoidance of dehydration, prolonged immobilization, and oestrogen contraceptive pills. Low oestrogen preparations have been associated with thromboembolism in patients with haemoglobin levels over 16 g/dl but can be prescribed with minimal risk in the mildly cyanosed with lower haemoglobin levels. Progesterone-only contraceptives have other side-effects and offer incomplete protection (page 11.1).

Any invasive procedure, including venepuncture or intravenous infusion, may precipitate venous thrombosis. This is dangerous because of the risk of paradoxical emboli causing strokes and cerebral abscess. Attacks of spontaneous cortical and cerebral venous thrombosis may mimic the symptoms of cerebral abscess which can be differentiated by brain scan. Haemodilution is the first treatment.

In thrombotic or embolic lesions, anticoagulants may be used provided the patient is in hospital. This has potential danger even though it may prevent further emboli or spreading thrombosis. Control is difficult with frequent haemorrhagic complications which may lead to death, particularly in patients with irreversible pulmonary vascular disease (Eisenmenger reaction). Thus, long-term outpatient anticoagulants are best avoided. If the clinical situation demands anticoagulants, for example, when venous thrombosis is spreading in pulmonary arteries or systemic veins or because of recurrent emboli (uninfected), small intravenous injections of heparin sufficient to prolong the bleeding time slightly above normal and measures to reduce platelet stickiness are recommended. Conventional doses of heparin are contraindicated because of the likely danger of catastrophic haemorrhage. Subcutaneous and intramuscular injections of heparin may cause large haematomas and should be avoided. If bleeding complicates anticoagulation, caution is required in reversing the anticoagulant effects since thrombotic incidents develop readily.

Aspirin and/or dipyridamole are less hazardous and less effective than heparin and can lead to haemorrhage, particularly epistaxis and gastrointestinal. If aspirin is given it should be in the soluble buffered form, administered after meals.

Spontaneous bleeding, except from the gums, is uncommon except after trauma or surgery such as tonsillectomy, tooth extraction, or operations in which vascular adhesions are cut. Cyanotic patients with long-standing severe polycythaemia often have multifactorial clotting defects, sometimes reduced platelet counts, insufficient plasma clotting factors, and defective thromboplastin generation. Assessment of clotting function is needed before any surgery and fresh blood, plasma, and sometimes platelet transfusion should be available.

Relative anaemia
Paradoxically it is possible for cyanotic patients to be relatively 'anaemic' even when the haemoglobin is above 14 g/dl. The haemoglobin concentration may not be high enough for tissue oxygenation when cardiac function is impaired or the red cells may not be the correct size and shape for optimum oxygen transport. In a very cyanosed patient an haemoglobin of 16–17 g/dl may represent important anaemia and if long-standing may cause the heart to be larger than usual or even precipitate unexpected heart failure in sinus rhythm. The blood film may show signs of iron deficiency or macrocytosis but this is often not studied when the haemoglobin is normal, i.e. 14 g/dl or more. Iron, folic acid, or vitamin B$_{12}$ replacement should be given when dietary deficiency has been demonstrated. Anaemia in cyanotic heart disease is uncommon unless there is dietary deficiency, as occurs in patients from developing countries, because of 'food fads', or after gastrectomy or repeated haemorrhages from menorrhagia or gastrointestinal loss. Anaemia is one of the causes of malaise in cyanotic patients and is usually missed when the haemoglobin is above 15 g/dl.

Cerebral abscess
This diagnosis should be considered and excluded in any cyanotic patient with CHD who presents with stroke, new headache, and vomiting, personality change, transient weakness or paraesthesiae, or unexplained low-grade fever and apathy. It may be a lethal complication in adult patients with the Eisenmenger reaction, probably because of circulatory disturbances induced by toxicity, anaesthesia, or secondary haemorrhage.

Pregnancy
Patients with all forms of cyanotic CHD have difficulty in carrying a fetus to term. The major problem is the high incidence of spontaneous abortions between weeks 10 and 14. This may be caused by abnormality in the fetus or its death from hypoxia. Patients with moderate cyanosis (excluding Eisenmenger), i.e. with haemoglobin below 17 g/dl, may carry to term without incident. Such patients need careful obstetric management with rest, short labour, prevention of dehydration to minimize the fall in arterial saturation, immediate attention to sepsis, and to thrombotic or haemorrhagic complications. Pregnancy in patients with the Eisenmenger reaction exceptionally results in a live, normal child. It is a risk to the mother's life, may accelerate deterioration, and should be discouraged, ideally prevented (see page 11.12). Unfortunately, termination carries risks but if done early these are less than the risk of pregnancy.

Contraception
High oestrogen pills are absolutely contraindicated, and there is probably a risk of thrombosis in cyanotics taking low oestrogen preparations but a controlled trial is impossible in view of the relatively small number of patients. Ill effects of contraceptive pills in these patients occur in the first three to six months of administration. Sterilization may be the best solution if pregnancy is contraindicated or unwanted, but even this minor operation has risks in patients with Eisenmenger reaction and should be performed only in optimum circumstances.

Arthritis
Adolescents and adults with chronic cyanotic CHD often complain of painful knees, ankles, and sometimes wrists. The periarti-

cular tissues become thickened with severe long-standing clubbing and cyanotic heart disease. There is usually elevation of the plasma uric acid but the symptoms do not resemble gout and specific antigout treatment is not effective. Only relief of the cardiac condition will improve the joint stiffness but chronic thickening of the ankles and knees will persist in the affected adult.

Tuberculosis and pulmonary problems
It used to be said that patients with a low pulmonary blood flow had a tendency to develop pulmonary tuberculosis. Tuberculosis is a rare disease in the United Kingdom, except amongst immigrants, and so it is not possible to substantiate this concept, but tuberculosis should be excluded when haemoptysis occurs in patients with reduced pulmonary blood flow. A more common cause in cyanotic patients is pulmonary hypertension which commonly develops towards the end of their second decade (see page 13.342).

Causes of cyanosis in congenital heart disease
The haemodynamic disturbances which lead to central cyanosis (systemic arterial desaturation) are:

1. Right to left shunt. The desaturated systemic venous blood can pass from the right side of the heart to the left with defects in the atrial (ASD), ventricular (VSD), or aortopulmonary septa, or a patent foramen ovale (PFO). Normally when a defect is present the shunt is from left to right. Shunt reversal occurs in special circumstances such as: (a) pulmonary vascular disease (Eisenmenger reaction); (b) pulmonary arterial stenosis or banding of the pulmonary artery; (c) pulmonary valve stenosis or atresia; (d) abnormal function of the right ventricle without (a), (b), or (c); (e) tricuspid stenosis/atresia; (f) large Eustachian valve (sometimes called right-sided cor triatriatum) with ASD or PFO.

2. Complete mixing of systemic and pulmonary circulations as in single atrium, univentricular heart, and common trunk. The severity of central cyanosis depends on complications such as the degree of right ventricular obstruction (pulmonary infundibular or valve stenosis) or the degree of pulmonary vascular disease present; the more severe, the lower is the systemic arterial oxygen saturation.

3. Abnormalities of connection: (a) transposition of the great arteries (classic) where right ventricular blood is ejected directly into ascending aorta and left ventricular blood to the pulmonary artery; (b) inferior or superior vena caval drainage to the left atrium or total anomalous systemic venous drainage, a condition most unlikely to be seen in adolescents or adults; and (c) total anomalous pulmonary venous drainage (TAPVD) where some right to left shunt at atrial level is obligatory in order to maintain systemic blood flow.

4. 'Pulmonary' in pulmonary arteriovenous fistula and late after anastomosis of the superior vena cava to the pulmonary artery for treatment of tricuspid atresia (Glenn's operation).

Note that (1), (2), and (3) often co-exist in various combinations. These categories are not intended as a classification of cyanotic heart disease.

Specific disorders

Fallot's tetralogy
This anomaly consists of two basic abnormalities: (a) a large subaortic VSD with cephalad borders formed by aortic valve cusps; and (b) abnormal rotated infundibular bands which can form infundibular stenosis. The pulmonary valve may be mildly stenosed, bicuspid, or normal. Occasionally a suprapulmonary valve stenosis co-exists and may be the major obstruction in Fallot's patients who survive to adult life. Pulmonary artery anatomy is variable. It depends on the size of pulmonary blood flow which in turn relates to severity, form of the obstruction, changes in the

peripheral pulmonary arterioles, and any earlier attempts to improve pulmonary blood flow by 'shunts'. The other two classic features of the 'tetralogy', namely, right ventricular hypertrophy and overriding aorta are secondary to (*a*) and (*b*).

In adults ('natural survivors') the pulmonary arteries are usually well developed although exceptionally survival occurs with hypoplastic pulmonary arteries. Added problems in adults include calcification of the pulmonary valve (after 25 years), aortic regurgitation, and right ventricular failure after 40 years with extensive fibrosis of the myocardium.

Symptoms and presentation

Effort dyspnoea related to hypoxia is common. There may be symptoms from polycythaemia. Rhythm disturbances include atrial fibrillation (after 40 years), supraventricular tachycardia, and spontaneous ventricular ectopics from the right ventricle. Right heart failure is uncommon under the age of 40 years, but may be precipitated by pregnancy, rhythm disturbance, or chronic anaemia from non-cardiac causes. Infective endocarditis occurs and involves the aortic valve with jet lesions on the tricuspid valve from the aortic valve cusp (right coronary) which is contiguous; less frequently the mitral valve becomes involved.

Signs

Clubbing and cyanosis occur in varying degrees depending on the severity of the right ventricular obstruction and age of the patient. Pulses are full and carotid pulsation is prominent. The aortic pulsation may be palpable in the suprasternal notch. 'a' and 'v' waves are easily seen in the jugular venous pulse which may be elevated with rapid 'x' descent if there is right heart failure. The right ventricular impulse is palpable but not the left unless there is an additional lesion such as aortic regurgitation.

The clinical diagnosis of tetralogy of Fallot is characterized by a 'tetralogy' of signs, cyanosis, right ventricular hypertrophy, single second sound (aortic), and pulmonary ejection systolic murmur. Other similar lesions (see variants) share these signs which may be modified by age and severity of the obstruction.

The length and intensity of the ejection systolic murmur is related to the severity of the pulmonary stenosis. The murmur increases or remains unchanged on expiration and is maximal at the second or third left interspace, being conducted to the left and not to the right of the sternum. The milder the stenosis the more the pulmonary flow and the longer and louder is the murmur associated with thrill in mildest cases. The student may meet patients considered to have 'acyanotic Fallot'. This term, used by Wood, refers to the condition of a large subaortic VSD and moderate infundibular stenosis which has allowed a normal or increased pulmonary blood flow initially; cyanosis may appear later or after effort but is not always present at rest. With severe obstruction the murmur is very short and not present in pulmonary atresia. It diminishes with fever, hot weather, and amyl nitrite or any other cause of vasodilation. No murmur arises from the VSD in Fallot because it is large.

Variable added signs include an ejection click from the dilated aorta which is common in Fallot patients over the age of 20 years. There may be a late delayed diastolic murmur (after P₂) when the pulmonary valve is calcified. Aortic regurgitation occurs through the right aortic cusp into the right ventricle causing an immediate diastolic murmur which may be associated with right heart failure and widening of pulse pressure. The venous pressure increases when regurgitation is severe because of reflux into the right as well as the left ventricle. When right heart failure develops, a pansystolic murmur low at the left sternal edge may appear. The left ventricle enlarges if there has been a previous functioning shunt or aortic regurgitation.

Electrocardiographic features of Fallot's tetralogy are: (*a*) right atrial hypertrophy (moderate 3–4 mm P pulmonale); (*b*) right axis deviation; (*c*) right ventricular hypertrophy with mild ST depression or limited T inversion; (*d*) right bundle branch block in

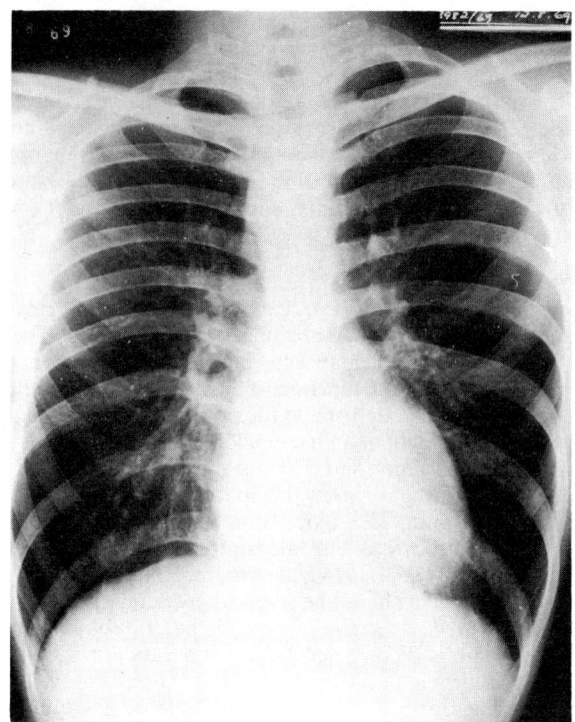

Fig. 1 Chest X-ray from a 25-year-old patient with Fallot's tetralogy showing normal heart size, pulmonary bay, small pulmonary arteries in the hila, and right aortic arch.

older patients with a dilated right ventricle; (*e*) good QR pattern in V₆ in adults but uncommon in children; and (*f*) the P–R interval may be lengthened in patients over the age of 40 years.

The chest X-ray usually shows a normal sized heart but there may be an increase after the age of 40 years, in pregnancy, chronic anaemia, or when there is added aortic regurgitation. There is evidence of right ventricular enlargement with a large ascending aorta and knuckle (Fig. 1); the aortic arch is right-sided in 15 per cent. The pulmonary artery branches are visible, the left usually larger and higher than the right. Pulmonary blood flow is almost normal but may be diminished depending on severity. With very severe obstruction, uncommon in adults, there are small pulmonary arteries with a speckled appearance in the lungs, marked around the bronchi, due to acquired bronchopulmonary collaterals. There is a characteristic pulmonary 'bay' where the main pulmonary artery is normally seen. The infundibular chamber is often prominent and dilated on the left cardiac border. Dilation of the main pulmonary artery is uncommon but may be seen in adults where there has been a raised pulmonary blood flow during infancy. Large (aneurysmal) pulmonary arteries are present when there is an associated 'absent' pulmonary valve. A left-sided superior vena cava is visible in 10–15 per cent.

Haemodynamic changes

Systolic pressures in both right and left ventricles are equal to those in the aorta; right and left atrial pressures are equal unless aortic regurgitation affects one ventricle more than the other. End-diastolic pressures increase after age 35 years and the 'a' wave of the venous pulse is prominent. There is evidence of a right to left shunt at ventricular level and sometimes at atrial level if there is an associated atrial septal defect. Systemic arterial oxygen saturation varies from 70 to 90 per cent depending on the severity of the pulmonary stenosis. The pressure gradient may be present between the pulmonary artery and right ventricular body at infundibular (subvalve), valve, or pulmonary artery level or a combination of these. The main pulmonary artery pressure (PAP) is 10–30 mmHg. Those in whom PAP exceeds 20 mmHg have

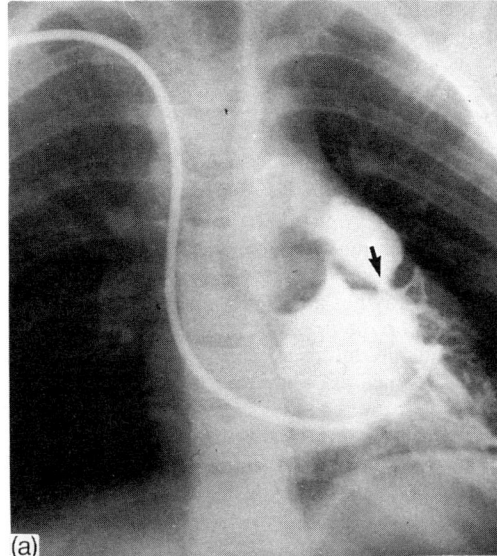

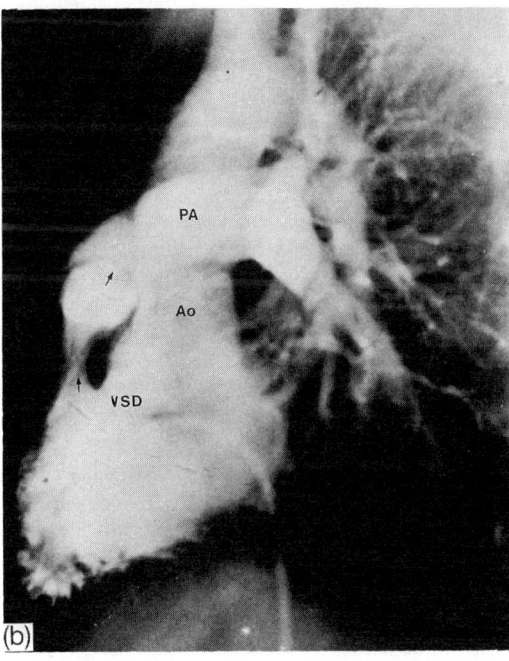

Fig. 2 (a) Anteroposterior view of right ventricular angiogram from a patient with mildly cyanotic Fallot's tetralogy. This shows fixed infundibular stenosis (arrow) beneath a domed pulmonary valve. Medial to this the contrast peaks up beneath the aortic cusps above the large VSD (not seen in this view). (b) Lateral angiogram from a patient with mildly cyanotic Fallot's tetralogy showing infundibular stenosis (lower arrow), domed pulmonary valve (upper arrow), and good-sized pulmonary artery (PA). Ao = aorta; VSD = ventricular septal defect.

usually been through several years without cyanosis at rest and have acquired infundibular obstruction later, having once had a significant left to right shunt. True pulmonary vascular resistance may be elevated despite pulmonary stenosis.

Angiography

Right ventricular angiography shows a large subaortic VSD and right ventricular outflow obstruction (Fig. 2a, b). Aortography shows a dilated aortic root and large tortuous coronary arteries.

Treatment

Complete repair is the ideal treatment, euphemistically referred to as 'total correction'. If the haemoglobin exceeds 21 g/dl and there

is near pulmonary atresia, there may be a place for a preliminary shunt procedure to reduce the red cell mass and the early complications of polycythaemia; in cases so managed, complete repair should be done 6 to 12 months later.

Adults who have not needed or had earlier surgery have good anatomy for primary complete repair. They have more peri-operative complications than children such as sepsis, haemorrhage, renal failure, persistent right heart failure, and prolonged low arterial P_{O_2} which increase morbidity and mortality.

Associated congenital cardiac anomalies

Other common associated congenital cardiovascular abnormalities are (a) left superior vena cava in 15 per cent, (b) right aortic arch in 16 per cent, (c) coronary artery abnormality – a septal branch aberrantly crossing the right ventricular outflow tract is the most important since it may prevent the ideal ventriculotomy and necessitate the use of a valved conduit to bridge the right ventricular obstruction, (d) atrial septal defects (secundum) in 8 per cent (pentalogy of Fallot), (e) aortic valve abnormality, fused or bicuspid in 3 per cent, and (f) additional VSD in muscular septum or other site (5 per cent).

Variants of Fallot which can survive to adolescence or adult life

Absent pulmonary valve

In this curious 'syndrome', the pulmonary valve has failed to form. It usually coincides with subaortic VSDs and acquired infundibular stenosis, thus presenting as atypical Fallot's tetralogy. There are loud ejection systolic and delayed diastolic murmurs (pulmonary regurgitation) at the left sternal edge and aneurysmal dilation of the pulmonary arteries when pulmonary valves are absent. Cyanosis is relatively mild depending on the degree of pulmonary stenosis in the infundibulum and/or main or branch pulmonary artery.

Absence of the body of the 'crista' or interinfundibular VSD

Older patients with Fallot's tetralogy appear with this variant, in which the subaortic VSD encroaches into the outflow tract beneath the pulmonary valve; the rotated septal band of the infundibulum (crista) is absent. The degree of cyanosis depends on the severity of pulmonary valve stenosis; cyanotic attacks do not occur and it is an angiographic diagnosis to be distinguished from double outlet right ventricle. It is important because there are special surgical problems.

Differential diagnosis of Fallot

This depends on distinguishing the condition from pulmonary stenosis and reversed interatrial shunt (closed ventricular septum) and the other lesions with VSD and pulmonary stenosis (PS) whose clinical presentation resembles that of Fallot.

Several lesions have similar physiology and presentation but differ in anatomy. They require accurate diagnosis as their prognosis and management are different from the more straightforward problems of Fallot's tetralogy:

1. One ventricle and PS This is occasionally compatible with longevity: the oldest in my experience was a man aged 69 years without previous palliation who presented in failure with atrial fibrillation.

2. Corrected transposition (atrioventricular discordance, ventricular arterial concordance) with VSD and PS (see page 13.263).

3. Double outlet right ventricle with PS In this, both great arteries arise from the right ventricle and most frequently the ventricular septal defect is subaortic.

4. Transposition of the great arteries (TGA) with VSD and PS (atrioventricular concordance, ventricular arterial discordance) (see page 13.263). When the pulmonary valve stenosis is mild or moderate, these patients may reach adult life.

5. Atrioventricular defect + PS (see page 13.254).

6. Multiple VSDs or VSD, not in Fallot position (diagnosed on biventricular angiography) with infundibular stenosis or pulmonary valve stenosis (PVS). When the VSD is subtricuspid it may close spontaneously or become small so that the patient loses cyanosis and presents as with progressive 'lone' infundibular stenosis.

7. Bipartite right ventricle with VSD In these patients there are anomalous muscle bundles which with time hypertrophy to create a 'low' infundibular stenosis dividing the small cavity of the inflow from the outflow. A VSD may be in any position and when communicating with the right ventricular inflow will be associated with a right to left shunt. However, if it is in the outflow, distal to the obstruction, there may be a left to right shunt or pulmonary hypertension particularly when this appears in adolescents or adults.

Clinical suspicion that the cyanotic patient with pulmonary stenosis does not have straightforward Fallot's tetralogy should arise when:

1. The apex beat is not right ventricular in type; this suggests corrected transposition (atrioventricular discordance) or that only one ventricle is present. The tap of a loud first sound may be felt at the apex when there is one atrioventricular valve.

2. There is a palpable great artery and second sound in the pulmonary area. This occurs when the ascending aorta is anteriorly placed as in true classic transposition (atrioventricular concordance with ventricular arterial discordance) or corrected transposition (atrioventricular and ventricular arterial discordance).

3. The systolic murmur is conducted to the right, rather than the left suggesting that the pulmonary flow is preferentially directed to the right which is characteristic when the pulmonary artery is posterior as in transposition or certain forms of unusual position of the great arteries.

4. There is a giant 'a' wave in the JVP, which can only occur if the right ventricular pressure exceeds systemic indicating that a VSD, if present, is small; or the ventricular septum is intact; or

there is a tricuspid obstruction. It is characteristically found in severe pulmonary valve stenosis with reversed interatrial shunt.

5. There is a combination of severe cyanosis and a long loud systolic murmur which favours the diagnosis of transposition or malposition of the great arteries. In Fallot the more intense the cyanosis, the less the murmur.

6. There is an atypical electrocardiogram for Fallot which may show left axis deviation, a long P–R interval, right or left complete bundle branch block (unless associated with Wolff–Parkinson–White (WPW) syndrome), absent R waves in V_1, V_2, a QR in V_1, and S waves V_1–V_6.

7. The chest X-ray has a narrow pedicle, a great artery making a straight shadow on the upper left mediastinal border to the level of the aortic knuckle due to an abnormally placed anterior aorta (Fig. 3). The presence of pulmonary venous congestion, enlargement of the left atrium or small aortic knuckle signify complications with Fallot or another diagnosis. Any evidence of right or left isomerism (bilateral right or left bronchi) make the diagnosis of Fallot's tetralogy unlikely.

8. There is evidence of a left superior vena cava entering the left atrium.

Clinical diagnosis of other defects (not Fallot) associated with pulmonary stenosis (PS)

Double inlet ventricle with PS (also called single or common ventricle, univentricular heart) There are many forms and combinations of abnormalities (see page 13.265) to account for the varied clinical features. The apex beat feels unusual, i.e. not like a large right ventricle. A strong single first sound is often palpable when there is one voluminous common valve. There is unusual activation in the anterior chest leads of the ECG, either dominant S waves from V_1 to V_6, left ventricular dominance or hypertrophy pattern or less frequently QR complexes in the right chest leads if there is right ventricular or indeterminate morphology of the ventricle. The majority of these hearts have left ventricular morphology. Cross-sectional echocardiography provides useful diagnostic information. The pulmonary stenotic murmur is usually conducted to the right because of the abnormal position of the pulmonary artery.

Corrected transposition ((VSD plus PS) (see page 13.263) is distinguished from Fallot by palpable aortic valve closure (A_2) in the pulmonary area, an unusual electrocardiogram, and chest X-ray which shows a left straight upper border of the mediastinum due to a left anterior ascending aorta.

Double outlet right ventricle plus PS Bedside diagnosis is not possible; two-dimensional echocardiography reveals this anomaly by showing absent aortic/mitral continuity. The clinical signs resemble Fallot but the ECG can show an unusual axis (not right axis deviation). The features are influenced by the site and size of the VSD, the associated anomalies, and the degree of pulmonary stenosis. Restricted VSD, particularly when uncommitted to either great artery, may add signs suggesting aortic stenosis, i.e. carotid thrill and murmur with delay and diminution of A_2.

Transposition of the great arteries (classic form – atrioventricular concordance with ventricular arterial discordance, see page 13.263). The aorta arises from the right ventricle and the pulmonary valve from the anatomical left ventricle. Patients rarely survive to adult life without surgical help but can do so if pulmonary stenosis is mild and associated with a large ventricular septal defect or if there is a large atrial septal defect with an intact ventricular septum. The systolic murmur is long and conducted to the right and associated with severe cyanosis. A_2 is palpable in the pulmonary area and older patients are often erroneously considered to have an Eisenmenger reaction.

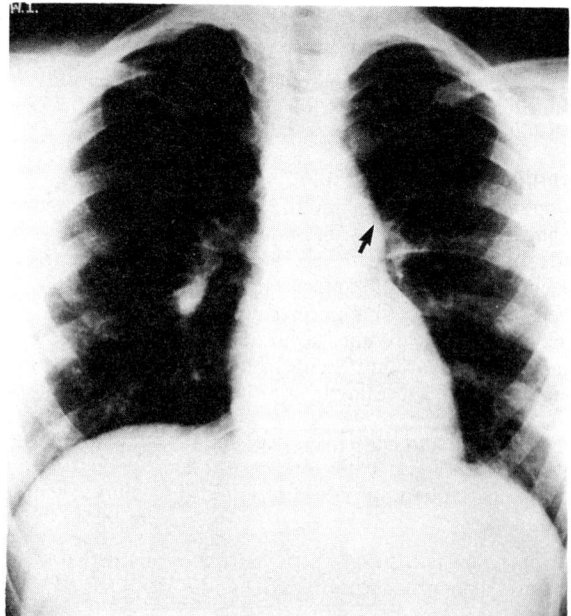

Fig. 3 Chest X-ray from a patient with VSD and pulmonary stenosis and 'corrected transposition' (ventricular inversion). The ascending aorta is anterior and to the left lying on left upper mediastinal border (arrow) making a longer shadow than a prominent pulmonary artery. Physiology is the same as in Fallot's tetralogy.

Atrioventricular defects plus PS Distinguishing features are the ECG with modified left axis deviation ($S_{I, II, III}$ pattern), sometimes an apical pansystolic murmur, and left atrial enlargement.

VSDs in other positions (i.e. not subaortic) with pulmonary valve or infundibular obstruction are diagnosed by echocardiography and angiocardiography. If the VSD is small the physical signs suggest pulmonary stenosis with reversed interatrial shunt.

Fallot's tetralogy after surgery

Patients with Fallot's tetralogy mostly survive because of earlier palliative shunts for hypoxia and cyanotic attacks, or because of radical repair (usually referred to as total correction) with closure of the ventricular septal defect and removal of pulmonary stenosis. Only a few reach adult life without earlier surgery. Occasionally older patients appear with only relief of pulmonary stenosis either because the VSD was left untouched or because it reopened. Such patients have large hearts and are at risk of developing irreversible pulmonary vascular disease.

The aim of systemic to pulmonary artery shunts is to increase pulmonary blood flow which not only results in reduction of cyanosis but also volume load on the left side of the heart leading to enlargement of both left atrium and ventricle. Aortic regurgitation is a usual accompaniment of long-standing shunts in adolescents and should be specifically searched for.

There are various types of shunt, named after the surgeon who designed it:

Blalock–Taussig The subclavian artery is anastomosed to right or left pulmonary artery.

Subclavian autograft A subclavian is joined to a pulmonary artery after transection at its origin and reimplantation lower in the descending aorta in order to prevent upward kinking of the pulmonary artery. Various modifications have been devised by Waterston and Castaneda.

Modified Blalock This technique popularized by de Leval involves the interposition of 'Goretex' tube prosthesis between the subclavian artery and ipsilateral pulmonary artery and has produced good results with less distortion of pulmonary arteries and maintained patency with ideal sized shunts in infants and children. Results appear less satisfactory in adults.

Waterston Through a right thoracotomy a window is made between the ascending aorta and right pulmonary artery, sometimes referred to as Cooley's anastomosis. Although it provides good palliation, particularly in infants, it is associated with problems from kinking of the right pulmonary artery, pulmonary vascular disease on the right, and hypoplasia of vessels centrally and left, overload of the heart, early tamponade, and aneurysm of the right pulmonary artery.

Pott's Through a left posterolateral thoracotomy, an anastomosis is made between the descending aorta and the left pulmonary artery. Although it may initially relieve symptoms, it is a dangerous shunt, tending to be too large, often damaging the left pulmonary artery by kinking or stenotic occlusion, a frequent cause of irreversible pulmonary hypertension and may be difficult to close.

The complications which occur after palliative shunts are:

1. Increasing cyanosis from closure of the shunt or diminution in its size as the patient grows.
2. Acquired atresia of the infundibulum and/or the pulmonary valve.
3. Bronchopulmonary collateral development, particularly when the shunt is poorly or not patent. These vessels may be large, and when present are uncountable and can cause rib notching. There is a risk of major haemorrhage when adhesions are cut in an area where a previous thoracotomy has been performed.
4. 'Subclavian steal'. Sometimes after a bilateral long-standing Blalock operation, the development of collaterals is so extensive that blood is 'stolen' by them from the vertebral artery. The patient may then develop faints on effort or other symptoms of vertebral insufficiency.

5. Cerebral abscess.
6. Infective endocarditis (on aortic valve or shunt), complicated by haemoptysis from aneurysm formation or infection on the shunt.
7. Aortic regurgitation.
8. Biventricular failure.
9. Shortening of arm and smallness of ipsilateral hand after early Blalock *in situ* for over 8–10 years.
10. Residual stenoses or complete obstruction in ipsilateral pulmonary artery.
11. Pulmonary vascular disease (peripheral) related to size, duration *in situ*, and the underlying lesion, i.e. more common in double outlet right ventricle and transposition.

Patients who have had radical repair have dramatic relief of symptoms due to relief of the hypoxia. Residual signs and problems depend on three factors: the completeness of the repair, the residual lesions, and the duration of follow-up. Whether or not late postoperative problems will be different or reduced with earlier 'correction' in infancy remains to be seen.

Clubbing and cyanosis should disappear, but the jugular venous 'a' wave is larger than normal and the right ventricle may remain overactive and even with a palpable bulge if a patch has been used. A systolic ejection murmur is expected, with wide splitting of the second heart sound (related to the complete right bundle branch block in 85–90 per cent) and a diminished but audible pulmonary component preceding a short diastolic rumble of pulmonary regurgitation. Exceptionally, the patient has no murmurs and a normal second sound. The heart on chest X-ray is usually larger than before operation, globular, with a prominence on the left border from the right outflow tract. Lung vascularity may be normal or may increase with a residual VSD or be different in each lung if there is hypoplasia or obstruction in either pulmonary artery; the pulmonary bay fills out by the distended main pulmonary artery. The ECG should show sinus rhythm, variable patterns of right bundle branch block, and variable electrical axis. T inversion may be restricted to V_1 or extend to V_5 and persist. T wave inversion and wide Q waves may be found when there has been prolonged intraoperative ischaemia.

Echocardiography (2DE) is reliable for showing the large subaortic patch closing the VSD, or any detachment, and for delineating the open outflow and increase in size of the pulmonary artery.

Complications after radical repair of Fallot's tetralogy are numerous. They are as follows:

1. Residual VSD may be due to patch detachment or a separate lesion. Large defects produce right heart failure and should not be left without full investigation. Small or moderate VSDs may do no harm except as a site for future endocarditis.
2. Residual pulmonary stenosis, which may be in a main branch at the site of a previous shunt, in the valve, its ring, or infundibular region. It does not increase in severity unless resection of outflow muscle has been inadequate or the patch edge protrudes into the outflow tract.
3. Patent foramen ovale with shunt reversal on effort can occur when the surgeon has not closed the foramen, and right ventricular function is abnormal, or there is associated abnormality of the tricuspid valve.
4. Rhythm disturbances are frequent and include: ventricular ectopic beats which may increase on effort and be a factor in sudden death, paroxysmal ventricular tachycardia, and more rarely complete heart block. This may occur transiently intra- or perioperatively or late, particularly if there has been transient block earlier. Paroxysmal supraventricular tachycardia or atrial fibrillation may develop after 10–20 years. Residual lesions such as important pulmonary stenosis or regurgitation, or residual VSD may predispose but may not be present. Such rhythm disorders may then be related to cannulation, atrial incisions, particularly when transatrial closure of the VSD has been used, or damage to

the sinus node. Nodal tachycardias occur occasionally and usually are related to reoperation for closure of the VSD or more posterior subtricuspid extension of the VSD. Sinus arrest or bradycardias occur unexpectedly and late after repair, probably related to intraoperative damage of the nodes. These problems are less common than in the last decade with improved understanding of the anatomy of the sinus node and its arterial supply.

5. Infective endocarditis. This is uncommon after radical repair but slightly more frequent in patients with shunts that have not been repaired. It occurs with residual VSD, open systemic to pulmonary shunts or on the aortic valve. There is little indication to protect patients after repair of Fallot, unless these residual lesions are present or a prosthetic or biological valve has been used.

6. Right ventricular aneurysm. This occurs at the site of patching of the infundibulum and is uncommon without a raised right ventricular pressure (residual pulmonary stenosis). The aneurysm may increase in the first one to two years and then remains static with calcium deposited in the wall. False aneurysms may occur early. Progressive increase in size with or without elevation of the right ventricular pressure to more than 50 per cent of systemic, requires surgical attention. Rupture is rare unless there is infection or a false aneurysm.

7. Pulmonary hypertension. When a large ventricular septal defect persists and there has been good relief of pulmonary stenosis, the patient develops hyperkinetic pulmonary hypertension which may progress to irreversible pulmonary vascular disease 10–15 years later. Pregnancy can accelerate this process. Such a tragedy should be prevented by early reoperation to the VSD after elevated pulmonary artery pressure and/or a large left to right shunt have been demonstrated by early postoperative catheterization.

8. Pulmonary regurgitation. This has been considered to be a benign complication but, when associated with a persistent VSD or elevated pulmonary artery pressure it can cause chronic right heart failure. Without such complications, when severe, as with some transannular patches or excision of the pulmonary valve cusps, progressive right ventricular dilation occurs over a decade with ultimate right heart failure at the onset of atrial flutter or fibrillation. Pulmonary valve replacement should be advised if cardiomegaly is demonstrated to progress and should be performed before the right ventricle shows signs of failure; the results of later surgery are less good, and the heart remains very dilated and prone to arrhythmias. These late results of pulmonary regurgitation raise doubts about the long-term future of infants who have received patches across the pulmonary annulus.

Table 1 Features which differentiate Fallot from PS with reversed interatrial shunt

	Fallot	PS with reversed interatrial shunt
Squatting	+ (in children)	−
Cyanotic attacks	+ (not present in adults or adolescents)	−
Giant 'a' wave	−	+
P_2 late, audible	Inaudible; A_2 single	±
Long SM to A_2 or later (late crescendo)	±	−
Palpable aorta	Sometimes	−
Extreme RVH, Steep T inv. V_1–V_4	−	+
Right bundle branch block	− (unless over 40 years)	+
P pulmonale > 5 mm	−	+
Right aortic arch	+ (16%)	−
Main PA dilated	− (occasionally when mild)	+
Amyl nitrite ↑ cyanosis; ↓ murmur	+	−

9. Aortic regurgitation. This may be iatrogenic or have been missed prior to the repair as it is common in adolescents and adult Fallot's particularly when shunts have been established over several years. Regurgitation occurs into the right ventricle as well as the left and leads to elevation of the venous pressure with right-sided congestion. Repair may be possible when the lesion is severe or progressive but replacement may be necessary as the aortic ring is so dilated at this stage in Fallot.

10. Myocardial failure. Patients appear in the first decade of follow-up with large or enlarging hearts without a structural lesion to account for this. The presentation is of dilated cardiomyopathy, related to myocardial damage at surgery either with a long ischaemic time or because myocardial protection was inadequate or unsuitable. A line of subendocardial calcification may be visible in the left ventricle in some affected patients. Only general measures for chronic congestive failure are useful; sometimes there is help from removal of a structural cause of failure such as closure of VSD, replacement of regurgitant tricuspid or mitral valves. The risks of reoperation are high. Exceptionally, myocardial damage or dysplasia is present before operation and affects the postoperative course adversely despite adequate surgery.

General state after radical repair of Fallot

Patients with well-repaired lesions mostly live normal lives. They may take the contraceptive pill, go through pregnancy, drive cars provided they have had no syncopal attacks but not hold 'til 70' licences, and have a low risk of infective endocarditis. Preliminary studies from the National Heart Hospital on a selected population show there is at least five times the normal risk for parents, particularly mothers with repaired Fallot's tetralogy, of producing a child with congenital heart disease compared with normals.

Pulmonary valve stenosis with reversed interatrial shunt

The cardinal signs of this and Fallot's tetralogy are similar; both appear in adolescents and adults. If the atrial septal defect is large the heart may not be enlarged but if it is small and the pulmonary stenosis is severe, the heart can be large with extreme right ventricular hypertrophy.

For simplicity, the classical features which differentiate Fallot from PS with reversed interatrial shunt are shown in Table 1.

Pulmonary atresia with ventricular septal defect

The anatomy of the heart resembles Fallot with a large subaortic VSD which may encroach on the outflow tract (unlike Fallot); the right ventricular outflow is blind (atretic) and the infundibular bands may be absent or underdeveloped. The condition is referred to as 'pseudotruncus' as only one artery comes from the heart or extreme Fallot because of the cardiac anatomy. However, the condition of pulmonary atresia plus VSD has specific problems in relation to the pulmonary artery anatomy and systemic supply to the lungs and thus deserves its own name for better understanding and management.

Since both ventricles are connected to the aorta through the large subaortic VSD, the pulmonary flow is dependent entirely on supply from the aorta and/or its branches. There is considerable variation in pulmonary artery development as well as the systemic connections (Fig. 4).

Central arteries may be small (hypoplastic), characteristically taking the form of a 'seagull' on angiography and frequently not supplying all segments of the lung (Fig. 5). This limits the effectiveness of a surgical shunt and prevents 'total correction'. Less frequently and when supplied by a large duct or direct communication of a large systemic collateral artery the pulmonary arteries are large.

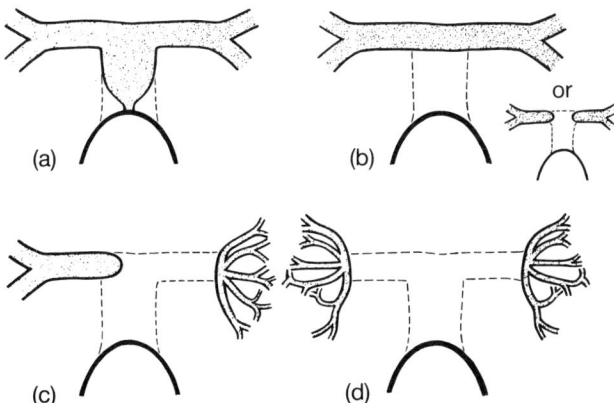

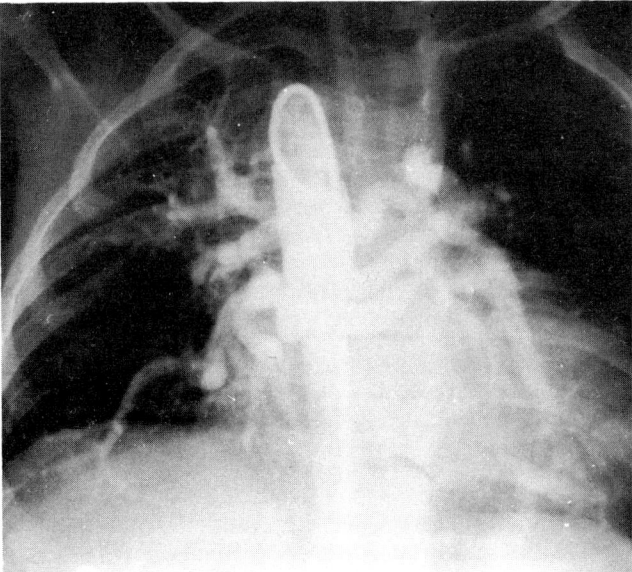

Fig. 4 Types of pulmonary artery development found with pulmonary atresia and VSD. (a) Full set of central pulmonary arteries distal to valve atresia. (b) Right and left central pulmonary arteries without pulmonary trunk. May be confluent or disconnected. (c) One central branch pulmonary artery branching in hilum with absent branch on other side. (d) No central pulmonary arteries.

Fig. 6 Large countable congenital systemic collateral arteries arising from the mid descending thoracic aorta in a patient with complex pulmonary atresia.

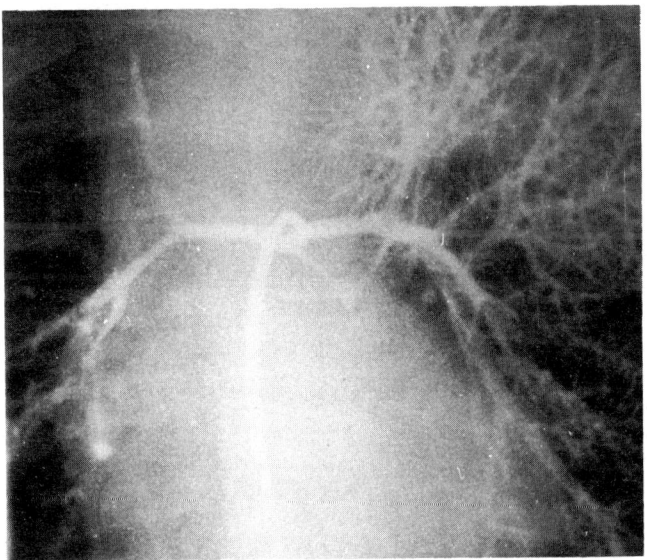

Fig. 5 Hypoplastic pulmonary arteries not supplying all segments of lung on right side from a patient with pulmonary atresia and VSD.

The systemic supply to the pulmonary circulation results from:

(*a*) Duct: if this is the only supply, closure will lead to acute hypoxia as in the neonate. When the duct remains open in adults it may be aneurysmal with associated pulmonary hypertension.

(*b*) Acquired systemic collaterals: these are multiple, uncountable, spidery, thin-walled, arising from mediastinal and intercostal vessels, and take time to develop. They increase after thoracotomy and account for improvement after a shunt has failed or closed. There is increasing evidence that coronary arteries make a contribution in adults and there may be 'steal' from the coronary circulation causing angina which may appear after 20 years in some very cyanotic patients.

Patients with a duct or acquired collaterals usually have well developed central pulmonary vessels which if perfused and made to grow larger may allow radical repair.

(*c*) Congenital systemic collaterals: when present the condition is referred to as 'complex pulmonary atresia'. These patients frequently survive to be adults, particularly if no earlier palliative or reparative surgery has been attempted. The collaterals usually arise from the isthmus, exceptionally from the subclavian, are large, tortuous, countable 1–6, and frequently stenosed at their

origins or as they enter the lung from the hilar (Fig. 6). They take many forms, often bizarre, supply a lobe or segment or whole lung, or connect directly with pulmonary arteries. In 80 per cent of cases central pulmonary arteries are hypoplastic, in 17 per cent they are large, and in 3 per cent they are absent.

One unusual form (1 per cent) is when a single artery arises from the mid-thoracic aorta, supplies all branches to the ipsilateral lung, crosses the mediastinum, and supplies the other lung. Another rare form is a direct coronary artery to main pulmonary artery fistula where there is full development of the central pulmonary arteries.

Right aortic arch occurs in approximately 45 per cent.

Symptoms
In complex pulmonary atresia there may be early cardiac failure and thriving difficulties which improve spontaneously as the pulmonary vascular resistance rises or stenoses on collaterals develop with growth, and cyanosis becomes more marked. Such patients have bulged, deformed chests with intercostal recession from reduced lung compliance. They are dyspnoeic from hypoxia. Haemoptysis may occur in adults or they may present with infective endocarditis on the aortic valve. Severe kyphoscoliosis is a frequent complication. Those without congenital systemic collaterals share the same symptomatology as Fallot but without a history of cyanotic attacks since the right ventricular outflow tract is permanently shut and cannot vary. Adults may appear with atrial fibrillation and right heart failure, contributed to by aortic regurgitaton.

Signs
Pulses are full or collapsing. Cyanosis and clubbing are variable. Carotid pulsation is obvious. The aorta is palpable in the neck or, if right-sided (40 per cent), in the right upper chest. The second heart sound is loud and single (A_2). There are no intracardiac murmurs other than the occasional case with aortic reflux, but an aortic ejection click is constant. Continuous murmurs (inspiratory) from congenital systemic collaterals are audible at the back on either side or in the right or left upper chest. Murmurs are absent when there is one huge collateral without stenoses or when peripheral pulmonary vascular disease is severe as is common in patients who survive beyond 30 years.

Management

Management depends upon the anatomy of the pulmonary arteries and systemic collaterals. In the very blue without congenital systemic collaterals, a shunt is probably the best first step to ensure the development of pulmonary arteries, if present, and to reduce polycythaemia. Adults with complex pulmonary atresia always present a difficult problem and it is often better to do nothing surgically and certainly not any form of repair. Only if a low pressure artery supplying the lung can be found is it worth recommending a shunt procedure. Conservative management of heart failure and polycythaemia is usually the best management. Hypoxic patients who develop any granulomatous lesion in the lung may improve spontaneously with increased pulmonary vascularity although ultimately catastrophic haemoptysis is likely. In patients with severe kyphoscoliosis and hiatus hernia melaena and/or haematemesis can cause death.

Pulmonary atresia after operation

The complications of shunt surgery are the same as in Fallot. However, 'correction' of pulmonary atresia in patients with Fallot type VSD has been made possible by the introduction of cadaver aortic homograft valves by Ross in 1966. Many patients with this treatment have reached adult life. They have similar late problems to Fallot patients but the homograft will require replacement, probably in the second decade. Calcification which starts harmlessly in the graft aortic wall and only later affects the cusps causes stenosis and/or regurgitation. The speed with which this develops depends on how the valve was sterilized (irradiation being disastrously destructive), the residual dynamics, conduit compression, and presence of pulmonary hypertension. The process is quicker in those youngest at the time of surgery.

Late infection of the graft valve in this position is exceptional. Comparative 'valve' survival studies with other biological prostheses have shown the superiority in durability and lack of problems of the homograft in the right ventricular outflow tract. Audibility of pulmonary valve closure (P_2) provides evidence of good pliable valve function and the loss of P_2 shows the cusps are calcified. More problems occur with the dacron conduits used for extension which develop intimal peel obstruction and calcification. Late pulmonary hypertension, right heart failure with pulmonary artery stenoses, and left heart failure from the chronic overload from systemic collaterals are more frequent than after Fallot repair.

Pregnancy is possible and the genetic risk to offspring appear no greater than in Fallot. A normal life and employment are possible.

Pulmonary arterial stenoses

Multiple pulmonary artery branch stenoses occur as part of a generalized congenital arteriopathy (see supra-aortic stenosis, below). A single branch stenosis or multiple stenoses may co-exist with septal defects, a combination which in adults presents with cyanosis and features of pulmonary hypertension. The wrong diagnosis of inoperable Eisenmenger is often made; the correct diagnosis is suggested by the finding of loud, long, widespread systolic murmurs with signs of pulmonary hypertension. The chest X-ray does not show huge central pulmonary arteries or peripheral pruning. The prognosis is better than in Eisenmenger reaction, as the obstruction does not progress in adult life whereas the pulmonary arteriolar disease worsens and increases the right to left shunt in the Eisenmenger syndrome. Such patients may be allowed to have a pregnancy, with careful supervision.

Treatment is usually medical as the disease in the pulmonary arteries may be diffuse, often beyond the hilar vessels and therefore not amenable to surgical relief. Balloon dilation may be helpful and if stenosis is in main pulmonary arteries near the bifurcation, surgical relief may be more successful. Paroxysmal supraventricular arrhythmias are frequent in adults and require

Table 2 Eisenmenger complex: associated defects

Ventricular septal defect (VSD)*
Double outflow right ventricle (DORV)*
A–V canal
Truncus
Aortopulmonary defect
Duct (patent ductus arteriosus)*
Transposition of the great arteries (TGA) with VSD, duct, after shunts, rare with ASD
Double inlet ventricle (single, common, uni) ± mitral atresia*
Tricuspid atresia with large VSD
Atrial septal defect (ASD)
Ostium primum
Common atrium
Hemianomalous pulmonary venous drainage
Total anomalous pulmonary venous drainage (TAPVD)
Pulmonary atresia (complex) with large congenital systemic collaterals

*Rarely associated with coarctation which should NOT be operated on in adolescents/adults in this situation.

control; antifailure measures are needed when right heart failure occurs after the age of 40 years. Patients may have associated systemic hypertension (see supra-aortic stenosis, below) as this is part of diffuse congenital cardiovascular disease in conducting arteries.

Patients with a single branch stenosis and VSD or A–V defect or ASD occur. They show features of pulmonary hypertension with an inspiratory continuous murmur over one side of the chest. The defect may be correctable by opening of the main branch stenosis but much depends on the state of the arterioles in the other lung.

Defects with pulmonary hypertension

Eisenmenger reaction (syndrome)

Wood redefined the Eisenmenger complex as 'pulmonary hypertension at systemic level, due to a high pulmonary vascular resistance with reversed or bidirectional shunt through a large ventricular septal defect'. He pointed out that 'it matters little where the shunt happens to be' and suggested extending the definition of Eisenmenger syndrome to include all other defects associated with such pulmonary hypertension and pulmonary vascular disease. Patients have similar clinical features irrespective of the site of the defect through which the shunt reversal occurs. The syndrome can occur with the defects shown in Table 2.

Certain factors predispose to the establishment of early pulmonary vascular disease. These are associated Down's syndrome, birth at high altitude, associated left-sided lesions such as mitral stenosis or regurgitation, coarctation, multiple chest infections, chronic upper airways obstruction, or perinatal asphyxia. Patients with atrial septal defect acquire pulmonary vascular disease later than in the case of other defects when it usually dates from early infancy or in childhood, below 2 years.

The prognosis is related in part to the site of the defect but also to the way the patient is cared for. Those with an Eisenmenger duct have the best prognosis and survival to the sixth or even seventh decade, although unusual, has been documented.

Symptoms

Dyspnoea is related to the degree of hypoxia. Patients with a duct have 'blue' arterial blood shunted below the left subclavian artery at first and at this stage are not breathless. Symptoms appear when desaturated blood reaches the head, usually in adolescence with the duct; with other defects dyspnoea occurs earlier.

Effort syncope occurs, sometimes early in the disease when hypoxia is not severe. It is a more frequent symptom of primary pulmonary hypertension and is associated with a low fixed cardiac output. Sometimes angina of effort is experienced.

Table 3 Causes of death in Eisenmenger complex

Right heart failure
Sudden
Cerebral abscess
After surgery (cardiac or other)
Haemoptysis
Induction of anaesthesia
Haemorrhage (often anticoagulant-provoked)
Cardiac investigation and angiography
Pregnancy
Infective endocarditis (very rare)

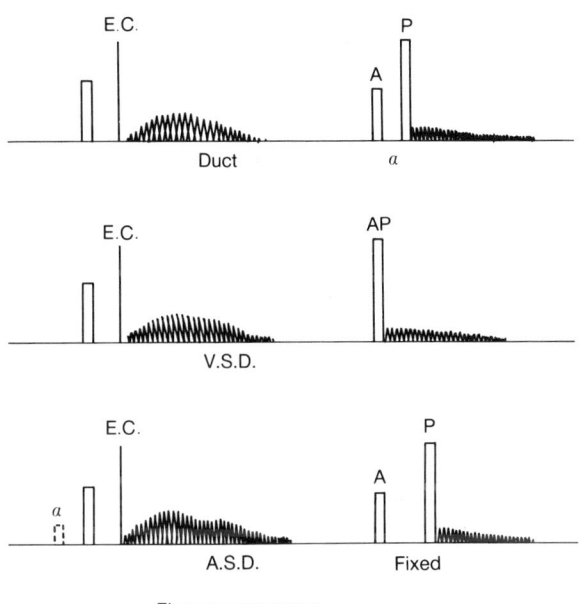

Fig. 7 Physical signs diagram by Dr P. Wood to summarize auscultation in patients with Eisenmenger reaction and defects at different levels. EC = ejection click.

The cardiac reserve is relatively poor so that excess sinus tachycardia with palpitation occurs with exercise, heat, fright, etc. After 35–40 years paroxysmal supraventricular tachycardia is common, particularly with atrial septal defect. The onset of atrial fibrillation produces a rapid downhill course.

There may be massive haemoptysis (pulmonary apoplexy) which is usually terminal when it is associated with rupture of capillaries or occasionally a pulmonary artery itself which may happen after trauma, excitement, or anger. Smaller haemoptyses may occur as the result of infarction and thromboses *in situ*. The incidence of haemoptysis increases with age, starting late in the second decade. Haemoptysis before the age of 15 years in someone with the features of the Eisenmenger reaction should stimulate a search for added left atrial obstruction which can be surgically treated. It is always a sinister symptom and often heralds the end; patients should be rested, venesected, given antibiotics, and sometimes small doses of heparin if there is evidence of pulmonary infarction. If the radiological features persist with fever, a mycetoma may be the cause and antibiotics stopped unless there is good evidence of secondary infection with bacteria.

Right heart failure develops after the age of 40 years in sinus rhythm or precipitated by supraventricular arrhythmias. Digoxin and diuretics may delay the distressing symptoms. The mechanisms by which death occurs are shown in Table 3.

Physical signs

The signs of pulmonary hypertension are uniform (see page 13.346) with right ventricular hypertrophy, pulmonary systolic click, and loud pulmonary valve closure. The patient may not

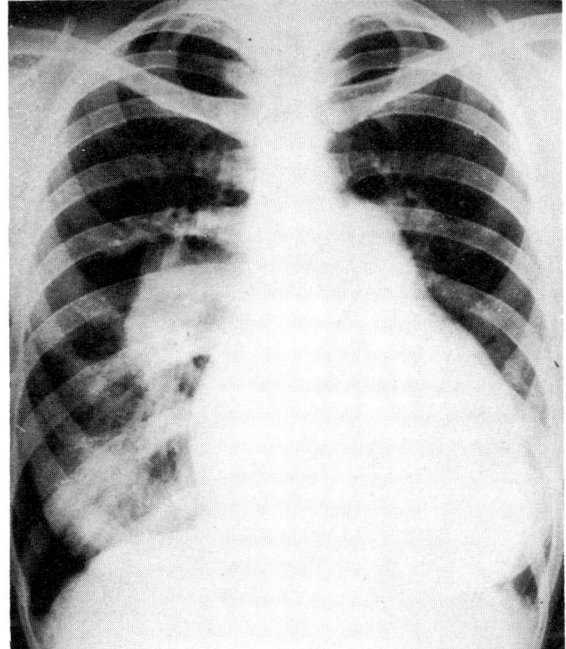

Fig. 8 Chest X-ray from a 35-year-old woman with Eisenmenger ASD showing cardiomegaly, huge central pulmonary arteries with pruned vessels in periphery of lung, and small aortic knuckle.

be cyanosed at rest. With a duct, the toes are clubbed and more cyanosed than the hands – a sign which may be brought out by immersion in warm water; the left hand may be bluer and more clubbed than the right since the origin of the left subclavian is frequently opposite the duct. The behaviour of the second sound reveals the site of the defect, single with VSD or single ventricle, normally split with aortopulmonary shunts, fixed with atrial septal defects (Fig. 7). As the right ventricle fails, fixing of the second sound from delay in P_2 occurs in other defects. Murmurs do not arise from the defects themselves as they are too large to offer any turbulence. However, a pansystolic murmur may appear from tricuspid regurgitation, when the right ventricle fails; this is the probable cause in Eisenmenger's original description.

High-pitched, long inspiratory, immediate diastolic murmur of pulmonary regurgitation is frequent and age related. The most extreme dilation of the main pulmonary artery occurs earliest in patients with a duct in whom a diastolic thrill is palpable with delayed diastolic murmur at the right ventricular apex ('right-sided Austin Flint').

The chest X-ray shows large main pulmonary artery and branches with peripheral pruning. Vessels are large in atrial septal defect and those patients where there was once a large pulmonary blood flow (Fig. 8). When high pulmonary vascular resistance dates from soon after birth the lungs have never carried an increased flow and pulmonary vessels (except for the main pulmonary artery) may be small with lung fields looking oligaemic. In duct and trunk patients the aortic knuckle is prominent. Diagnostic calcification is seen in the duct after 35 years (Fig. 9) and may also appear in atheromatous plaques or thrombus after 40–45 years. When a double inlet ventricle (single) fails, pulmonary venous congestion may appear with the onset of mitral regurgitation. Haemosiderosis with bone formation in the lungs can appear when there is mitral atresia.

The ECG shows varying degrees of right ventricular hypertrophy and axis shift in relation to the lesion and age of the patient.

Differential diagnosis

Patients with the Eisenmenger syndrome must be distinguished from acyanotic Fallot and transposition with pulmonary stenosis.

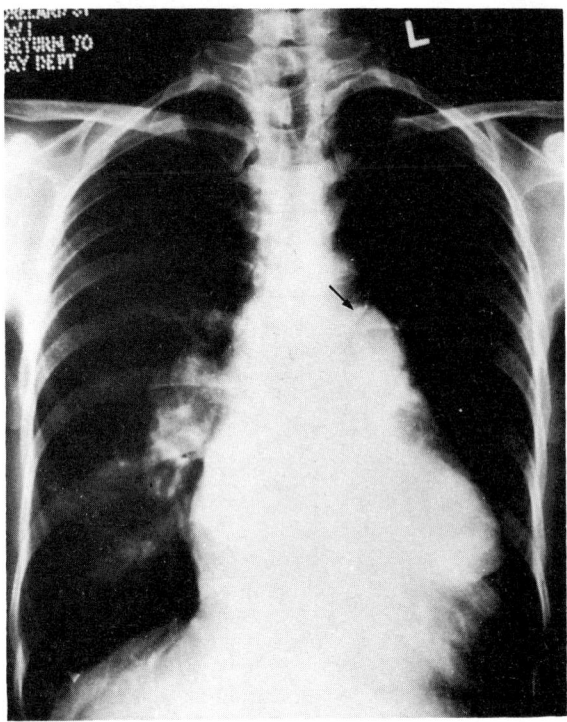

Fig. 9 Penetrated chest PA X-ray showing calcium in large duct (arrow).

A long praecordial systolic murmur suggests either diagnosis and widespread systolic murmurs over the lungs suggest pulmonary arterial stenoses causing the pulmonary hypertension. In the presence of left atrial obstruction with a defect and secondary pulmonary hypertension a delayed diastolic murmur at the apex, P mitrale on the ECG, and an enlarged left atrium with prominent pulmonary venous shadows with haemosiderosis on the chest X-ray, and history of early haemoptysis should raise the suspicion. Abnormal (underdeveloped) right ventricle with reversed interatrial shunt may be confused with Eisenmenger syndrome; large 'a' wave, quiet right ventricle without murmurs and a normal P_2 with normal or small pulmonary arteries on the chest X-ray should make this diagnosis.

Management

The general advice for care of adult patients with cyanotic heart disease must be followed for patients with the Eisenmenger reaction whose circulation readily becomes unbalanced and in whom acute change may lead to death. The systemic and pulmonary artery pressures are the same or the systemic pressure may be lower with atrial septal defect. Any sudden change in volume from vomiting, diarrhoea, haemorrhage or trauma, or a vasovagal episode may lead to death and thus requires urgent expert therapy. Patients should not go to high altitude above 1000 m. Flying is permissible but reduction in effort at the airports is more important than problems in the aeroplane. Oxygen should be available and used at very high altitudes such as in transatlantic and some transcontinental flights together with avoidance of dehydration and alcohol intake. Ordinary driving licences can be issued, provided there is no syncope but should not be asked for 'until 70'. Employment, without insurance, should be encouraged where effort tolerance allows. Appropriate drug management of arrhythmias and heart failure should be instituted when indicated but it is important to remember that all drugs which lower blood pressure should be avoided. Any change in cerebral state, new headaches or transient cerebral signs require urgent investigation to exclude cerebral abscess. Indwelling intravenous lines are a potential source of systemic embolism and even expert nurses require special warning about care with air bubbles etc. The most experienced are some-

times the most vulnerable because they are used to managing necklines or subclavian lines in other patients without complications.

A cerebral embolism may result from a local peripheral vein thrombosis at the catheter site or a cerebral abscess may be the consequence of a minor skin infection. Catheterization and angiography carry the risks of complications and even death in the Eisenmenger patients. Investigative decisions should only be made by the informed senior. Indications are uncertainty of diagnosis by an expert, exclusion of associated treatable left-sided lesions, and controlled trial of possible pulmonary vasodilators. It is important to remember that most vasodilators affect the systemic circulation and that lowering systemic arterial resistance is bad for these patients. However, in early cases without fixed pulmonary arteriolar disease, as occurs in young children, there may be an indication for trial of such therapy. As yet, no drug limited to effects on the pulmonary circulation has been found.

Heart/lung transplantation may offer hope for some of these patients when they become severely disabled with hypoxia but without other organ dysfunction. It is important to ensure that the patient's prognosis and quality of life is not better than that offered by this radical surgical 'solution' before referring the patient.

It is important for the physician to give special advice to patients about pregnancy and contraception. Pregnancy is contraindicated. If conception occurs early termination in hospital with cardiac intensive care should be recommended. If refused, the patient should be in hospital for most of the pregnancy, and early induction of labour or elective caesarian section advised. The progesterone-only contraceptive pill may be used. If unsatisfactory, low oestrogen pills with careful supervision and warnings about side-effects to be reported immediately should be tried. Sterilization may offer a better solution but should only be performed where expert cardiac and anaesthetic care is available as death is a known complication of all anaesthesia and surgery in such patients.

Tricuspid atresia

Adults with this condition have usually had earlier palliative surgery. In this anomaly, the tricuspid valve has not formed (see page 13.240). The systemic blood flows from right atrium to left atrium, left ventricle reaching the pulmonary artery through a 'VSD' leading into a right ventricular outflow when the great arteries are normally related or directly when connected to the left ventricle (with associated transposition or double outlet). Rarely there is associated inversion of the ventricular morphology and so the systemic ventricle has the anatomy of the right ventricle which is usual when there is double outflow with 'tricuspid' or better termed right atrioventricular valve atresia.

The behaviour of the 'VSD', referred to as bulboventricular foramen, mainly controls the clinical picture of tricuspid atresia with normally related great arteries; the presence of pulmonary stenosis is also influential. Most patients have a reduced pulmonary blood flow from reduction in size of VSD ± pulmonary stenosis but if the VSD remains large or there is additional transposition without pulmonary stenosis, pulmonary hypertension with the Eisenmenger reaction will be present in adults. Occasionally patients with tricuspid atresia reach adulthood with the ideal-sized VSD without pulmonary hypertension or previous surgery.

Tricuspid atresia may have the following associations which influence the presentation (all have been seen in adults):

1. Patent foramen ovale (65–75 per cent); atrial septal defect usually secundum, rarely primum defect.

2. Fleshy large Eustachian valve looking like a right-sided cor triatriatum which helps to prevent reflux back to inferior vena cava.

3. Normally related and connected great arteries with or with-

Table 4 Causes of left ventricular hypertrophy and central cyanosis

Tricuspid atresia
Total anomalous systemic venous drainage
Inferior caval drainage to the left atrium
Double inlet ventricle of LV morphology
Pulmonary atresia and intact ventricular septum (with small right
   ventricle)
Occasionally common atrium and A–V canal with pulmonary stenosis
   and/or small tricuspid valve
VSD and tricuspid stenosis
Double outlet right ventricle with tricuspid stenosis (hypoplasia)
RV hypoplasia with atrial septal defect
Absent tricuspid valve and blind right ventricle

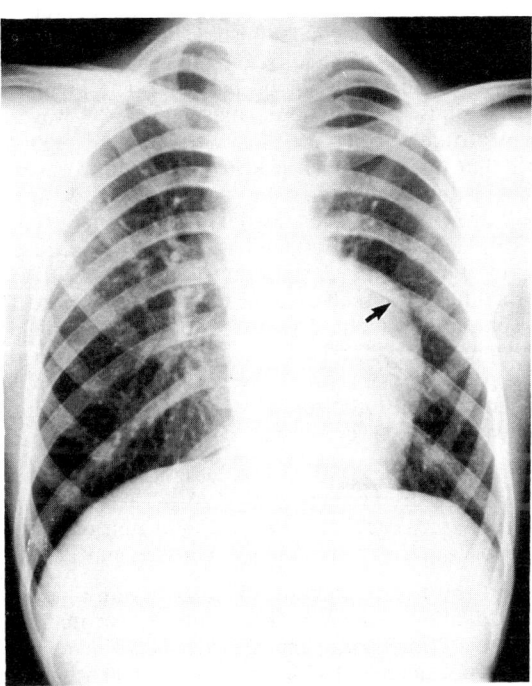

Fig. 10 Chest X-ray from a patient with juxtaposition of the atrial appendages producing characteristic bulge on upper left cardiac border (arrow) from a patient with complex tricuspid atresia.

out pulmonary valve stenosis and less frequently infundibular stenosis.

4. Transposition of the great arteries (TGA – aorta anterior or to left, pulmonary artery posterior) with or without pulmonary valve stenosis. Murmurs are directed to the right chest. The right pulmonary artery is larger than the left. Subaortic stenosis may be acquired when VSD diminishes in size and causes angina and effort syncope.

5. True univentricular heart with or without malposition of great arteries.

6. Ventricular inversion; often with both arteries arising from a systemic ventricle of RV morphology with or without pulmonary valve stenosis, the tricuspid atresia is by definition 'mitral atresia'.

7. Juxtaposition of the atrial appendages; associated with (6) gives a characteristic shadow on chest X-ray (Fig. 10).

8. Mitral 'prolapse' and regurgitation in adults.

Symptoms

Dyspnoea is related to hypoxia or left ventricular failure; the latter accelerated by shunts. Paroxysmal tachycardia, atrial fibrillation, or nodal rhythms occur after 15 years. Haemoptysis may complicate pulmonary hypertension. Ventricular tachycardia may be the cause of fainting in adults – the origin of this unexpected finding awaits evaluation. Angina, effort giddiness, and syncope appear

with progressive obstruction of conduits used in modified Fontan procedure and with associated TGA. Right-sided congestion manifests as a huge liver and ascites and sometimes impending liver failure appears with atrial fibrillation. When such patients present they tend to be erroneously managed as a primary hepatic problem.

Signs (with normally related and connected great arteries)

Besides cyanosis and clubbing a giant 'a' wave is usual and the left ventricle is palpable. There is a variable systolic murmur depending on size of the VSD; if closed and the patient lives on a shunt there may be no systolic murmur. Signs may be modified by earlier palliative procedures. Those with a Glenn anastomosis (superior vena cava to right pulmonary artery) do not have a giant 'a' wave or usual pulsation. When pulmonary resistance is raised the venous pressure is elevated and features of SVC obstruction may appear. An apical pansystolic murmur from mitral regurgitation is common in adults.

The electrocardiogram shows P pulmonale or P mitrale if shunted, normal or left axis deviation and varying degrees of left ventricular hypertrophy, occasional Wolff–Parkinson–White with left bundle branch block (8 per cent). Right ventricular hypertrophy or right axis deviation suggest an additional complication such as TGA, large VSD with pulmonary hypertension, ventricular inversion or wrong diagnosis.

Chest X-ray The right atrium surprisingly may not be prominent because there is no right ventricular inflow, particularly if a Glenn procedure has been done. The left ventricle is large. The pulmonary artery at the hilar and size of peripheral vessels depend on pulmonary flow.

Differential diagnosis

Several other anomalies may present with left ventricular hypertrophy and central cyanosis (Table 4) and must be distinguished from tricuspid atresia.

Treatment

This depends on the disability of the patient and degree of central cyanosis. A systemic–pulmonary artery shunt can be created at relatively low risk, but in adults shunts often thrombose. Right atrial to right ventricular outflow or pulmonary artery anastomosis (Fontan procedure or modifications) using the patient's own pulmonary valve, another biological prostheses or direct right atrial to pulmonary artery anastomosis, succeed if the pulmonary artery pressure is low (below 20 mmHg) and the pulmonary vascular resistance low (below 4 units). This is difficult to calculate correctly: assumptions that the pulmonary arteries are not stenosed and that left ventricular function is adequate may be misleading. When one or more of these criteria are not present, patients are prone to a difficult postoperative period. There is no surgical procedure for those with pulmonary hypertension; only heart–lung transplantation offers hope.

Patients have lived on Glenn anastomoses (SVC to PA) for many years, but after 10–15 years fistulae at capillary level form in the right lung which no longer oxygenates the blood. Shunts, if ideally sized, may last many years but, unfortunately, left ventricular failure develops and may lead to pulmonary hypertension. They may become inadequate often leading to pulmonary artery hypoplasia or stenoses. The late results (i.e. into adult life) of Fontan procedures and modifications performed in early childhood are awaited. Unfortunately, irrespective of what is done, atrial arrhythmias causing congestion and low cardiac output are frequent in tricuspid atresia and associated with an embolic risk. It is vital to maintain sinus rhythm in tricuspid atresia. Attempts to revert atrial fibrillation should be made early with heparin cover and if successful supplemented by an anti-arrhythmic agent such as quinidine but not any drug which diminishes left ventricular function. Heart block may follow the Fontan procedure, and is best managed by epicardial pacing using variable rate devices. Ventricular tachycardia may originate from the abnormal right ventricular outflow or the damaged left ventricle. Amiodarone is probably the most effective agent in this situation as it does not depress left ventricular function in doses adequate to control the arrhythmia. Endocarditis is uncommon except on shunts or the mitral valve in older patients.

Abnormal right ventricle and shunt reversal at atrial level

Ebstein's anomaly

For convenience this is discussed under cyanotic CHD but it is often acyanotic or only mildly so during exercise, rhythm disturbances, fever, or pregnancy. Patients commonly survive to adult life with or without cyanosis.

There are two interrelated basic disturbances: (*a*) the posterior and septal cusps of the tricuspid valve are 'prolonged' into the body of the right ventricle and originate from beneath the true atrioventricular ring, giving the appearance of an 'atrialized' part of the right ventricle; and (*b*) there is abnormal thinning of right ventricular myocardium in the inflow (body) particularly in its anterior part.

The anterior cusp of the tricuspid valve is voluminous, ballooning out to close over the dilated tricuspid ring. Variable degrees of tricuspid regurgitation occur: indeed, the peculiar looking valve may be competent in postnatal life. The right atrium is dilated and thin-walled like the inflow of the right ventricle anteriorly; the right ventricular outflow is mildly hypertrophied. In 80 per cent the foramen ovale is open or defective (ASD), permitting a right-to-left shunt. Other associated abnormalities such as pulmonary atresia or stenosis, VSD, or mitral clefts have been described but such patients are unlikely to survive to adult life. Rheumatic mitral stenosis has been found with Ebstein's anomaly as has non-specific mitral valve prolapse, probably secondary to left ventricular dysfunction which is not uncommon in this condition.

The severity and form of tricuspid valve anomaly and right ventricular dysfunction are most variable. Indeed, there are good reasons to consider this as a primary right ventricular myocardial disease rather than a primary valvular problem which tends to receive all the attention. The right ventricular systolic pressure is low with elevation of end-diastolic pressure; tricuspid regurgitation is usual. It is mild or severe depending on the rhythm, degree of myocardial dysfunction, and age of the patient. In adults in sinus rhythm the right atrial pressure is normal until after the age of 40 years when it may rise. The jugular venous pressure rises considerably with a rhythm change at any age. Left-sided pressures are usually normal and there are no valvular gradients other than an occasional low subaortic gradient when the septum bulges into the small cavity left ventricle and contacts the mitral valve. A right-to-left shunt causing central cyanosis on effort is present at rest in about 65 per cent of patients. The degree of desaturation depends on the degree of right ventricular myocardial dysfunction and the size of the ASD. In most the ASD is not large and the myocardium is the main determinant of this. Left ventricular function may be impaired in adults. Whether this is due to bulging of the dilated right ventricle into the left ventricle (reversed Bernheim) or to an abnormal myocardium is uncertain.

Symptoms

Dyspnoea in relation to hypoxia is usual. Right-sided congestion develops sometimes despite maintained sinus rhythm after 40 years but more often is due to arrhythmias such as paroxysmal supraventricular tachycardia (SVT), atrial fibrillation, nodal rhythm, and complete heart block which are age related but can appear in children or be present at birth. Syncope may occur with SVT because of a fall in an already reduced cardiac output. The

natural history of Ebstein's anomaly is unpredictable and survival to the age of 80 years is possible in those without cyanosis and it can appear an incidental finding at necropsy for other disease. If the patient is severely cyanosed in childhood, survival into adulthood is exceptional without surgical help. In the mildly cyanosed or acyanotic, disability results from rhythm disturbances and subsequent heart failure. Infective endocarditis occurs rarely, and prophylaxis is advisable. Paradoxical emboli from peripheral venous thromboses or atrial fibrillation occur. Haemoptysis is not a feature and if it occurs a search for tuberculosis or another cause should be initiated. Pregnancy is tolerated but rest and increased diuretics are needed to prevent right heart failure.

Signs

The patient is characteristically slender with peripheral cyanosis, cold hands and feet, and a malar flush. Central cyanosis is mild or moderate, rarely severe in adults. Clubbing is variable. Pulses are small with a low to normal blood pressure. The jugular venous pulsation in sinus rhythm shows small flicking 'v' waves as the huge right atrium absorbs the effects of tricuspid regurgitation. Nodal rhythm or heart block lead to huge canon waves. Atrial fibrillation or flutter increases the mean pressure with large 'v' waves, a large pulsating liver, ascites, and oedema. The cardiac apex is displaced to the left and is gentle and diffuse. More obvious pulsation is felt over right ventricular outflow tract.

Abnormalities on auscultation increase on inspiration. The first sound is split, often widely, as is the second with a normal pulmonary component. Atrial and third sounds are present if the P–R interval is prolonged or there is myocardial dysfunction. A short delayed scratchy diastolic with or without a pansystolic murmur are best heard at the lower left sternal edge.

The electrocardiogram shows variable right bundle branch block patterns with low or normal voltage V_1–V_3. The axis may be right or leftward. Wolff–Parkinson–White conduction occurs in 9 per cent. V_5 and V_6 may be normal or QR patterns may be absent.

The chest X-ray usually shows cardiomegaly with right atrial and ventricular dilation, a clear cardiac outline, clear underperfused lungs, and small (low) aortic knuckle (Fig. 11). The main pulmonary artery is not dilated. The heart is occasionally, but rarely, of normal size when the myocardium of the right ventricle is not extensively abnormal and the tricuspid ring not dilated.

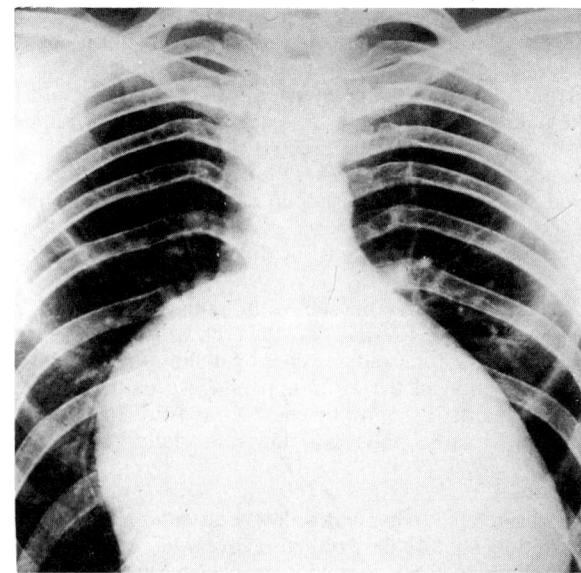

Fig. 11 Typical chest X-ray from a cyanotic 40-year-old with Ebstein's anomaly. Shows gross cardiomegaly mainly from right atrial dilation, clear cardiac outline, and small pulmonary arteries.

Intracavitary electrograms may show characteristic QRS and P wave changes in the lower right atrium. Right atrial angiography shows the huge right atrium and usually opacification of the smaller left atrium with reflux of contrast into the venae and hepatic veins. The tricuspid annulus is visible with separate displacement of the valve cusps in the strangely shaped and abnormally contracting right ventricle. The outflow contracts vigorously.

The left ventricle is bizarrely shaped and sometimes shows abnormal contraction patterns. Similar appearances of the right ventricle and an incompetent tricuspid valve may be seen in Uhl's anomaly and pulmonary stenosis with right heart failure. Dangerous rhythm disorders may occur during catheterization. The diagnosis is well shown by cross-sectional echocardiography.

Management

Rhythm disorders and heart failure respond well to medical treatment. Surgery should only be undertaken when symptoms are severe, from hypoxia, paroxysmal arrhythmias or right-sided congestion or the large heart is shown to be increasing in size. Cardiomegaly alone which may be static for many years is not an indication for surgery.

The aim of surgery in Ebstein's anomaly is to prevent cyanosis by closing the atrial septal defect (or foramen ovale), to restore a competent tricuspid valve by replacement, and to improve right ventricular ejection by plicating the fibrotic anterior portion. Refractory rhythm disorders as part of the Wolff–Parkinson–White anomaly may precipitate the need for surgical help. Attempts should be made to cut the abnormal pathway in these circumstances as well as repairing the basic lesions. Surgery should only be done in experienced centres. The risks are high (15 per cent), but excellent symptomatic benefit can result. Rhythm disturbances including complete heart block and supraventricular tachycardia may persist. Degenerative changes may develop in the tricuspid valve replacement necessitating reoperation.

Differential diagnosis

Ebstein's anomaly in adults must be differentiated from pulmonary stenosis in heart failure, pericardial effusion, Uhl's anomaly (in which all the right ventricle is paper thin), primary right ventricular myocardial diseases such as the rare familial form of progressive fibrosis, and abnormal right ventricle with reversed interatrial shunt.

Echocardiography differentiates pericardial effusion with low voltage on the ECG from Ebstein's anomaly and the other right ventricular diseases. The presence of a significant pulmonary systolic murmur and a dilated main pulmonary artery extending to the left pulmonary artery supports the diagnosis of pulmonary stenosis. Primary right ventricular dilation as in Uhl's or rare myopathies may require angiography and the demonstration of a normally attached tricuspid valve in the correct position. Exceptionally Ebstein's anomaly in adults may appear with a normal-sized heart and no tricuspid regurgitation.

Abnormal right ventricle with reversed interatrial shunt

This unusual condition appears in adolescents and adults. Central cyanosis appears in childhood or even infancy and slowly increases over the years. The right ventricle is described as hypoplastic, underdeveloped, thin, or containing aberrant bands and thickened endocardium. Symptoms are similar to those of Ebstein's anomaly. Signs are also the same but for a large 'a' wave in the JVP, a quiet, usually small, right ventricle, and often normal splitting of first and second sounds. The chest X-ray shows a normal-sized heart with prominent right atrium and normal or diminished lung vascularity. The ECG shows peaked right atrial P waves, a normal axis without right ventricular hypertrophy but left ventricular lead

dominance. An ASD is often seen on echo with bulging of the septum to the left atrium, sometimes a small tricuspid ring or a dilated poorly contracting right ventricle with normal left ventricle and no pulmonary stenosis. Cardiac catheterization confirms normal right-sided pressures. Right ventricular diastolic pressure and 'a' waves are raised and increase further when the patient exercises. Right ventricular angiography confirms the unusual appearance and contraction of the right ventricle. A right-sided 'cor triatriatum' from a large Eustachian valve may be the cause of the problem and is obvious on echocardiography and angiography causing a gradient between right atrium and ventricle.

Management

In those with primary right ventricular pathology and mild symptoms no surgery is necessary. Atrial rhythm disorders should be controlled. If hypoxia or rhythm disorders cause major symptoms, it is justifiable to close the atrial septal defect, thereby preventing cyanosis, thus exchanging cyanosis and dyspnoea for varying degrees of right-sided congestion; it may be difficult to decide when or if this is advisable. If the right ventricular cavity or ejection fraction are below 50 per cent of normal it probably is not. Diuretics given for several months or indefinitely improve symptoms. If there have been rhythm disturbances before operation, they will continue and may even appear for the first time soon after operation. Early surgery is mandatory in the patient with an obstructive Eustachian valve.

Abnormal connections of systemic and pulmonary veins

Inferior vena cava (IVC) to left atrium (LA)

This rare anomaly, when isolated, may manifest for the first time in adolescents and adults. Usually it is found with common atrium or defects associated with isomerism or with inferior vena caval atrial septal defect and its presence is masked by the signs of the septal defect. When isolated, diagnosis is difficult unless considered.

It presents with breathlessness and cyanosis after exercise (legs) or after the first four months of pregnancy. There may be a history of cyanosis persisting after birth and then disappearing after the first two weeks when the pulmonary vascular resistance has fallen to normal.

The signs are of mild to moderate cyanosis, a flat right contour of the normal-sized heart on X-ray and a full left atrium, ventricle, and aortic shadow. P mitrale may be found on the ECG and diagnostic confirmation comes from specific injection of the inferior vena cava. The condition may be iatrogenic after closure of an ASD and should be suspected in any patient who becomes breathless after routine surgical closure of an ASD.

Treatment is by surgical redirection of venous drainage.

Superior vena cava (SVC) to left atrium (LA)

This condition is rarely isolated. It may be associated with common atrium, double outflow right ventricle, coronary sinus ASD with unroofed or absent coronary sinus, and absent right superior vena cava. When isolated, features resemble IVC to LA but cyanosis is only induced by arm movements. Arterial oxygen saturation is 86–90 per cent at rest and cyanosis may not be noted. Surgery is not needed but attention must be given to sepsis in upper limbs, face, and neck once the diagnosis is established.

Total anomalous pulmonary venous drainage (TAPVD)

When all the pulmonary veins drain to the right atrium or a major systemic vein, the right side of the heart and pulmonary circulation become overloaded by the increased pulmonary blood flow. In order to maintain systemic flow an obligatory right-to-left shunt occurs through the atrial septum with and without ASD. Seventy-

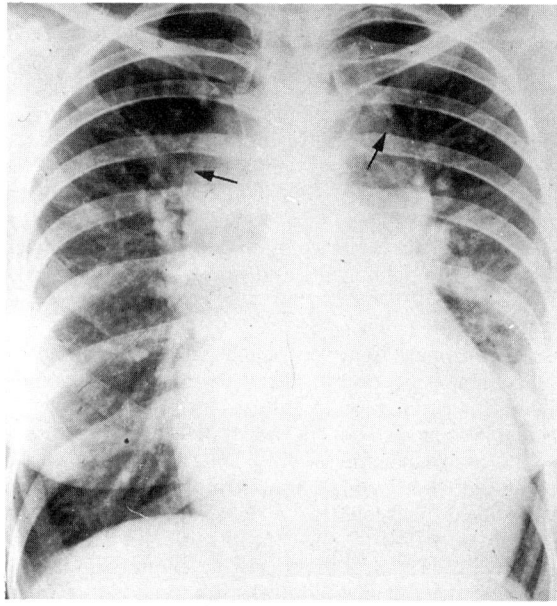

Fig. 12 Chest X-ray from patient with total anomalous pulmonary venous drainage into left ascending vein entering innominate. There is cardiomegaly, pulmonary plethora, and dilation of ascending innominate vein and right superior vena cava (arrows) giving 'snowman' appearance.

five per cent die in the first year; 1–2 per cent may survive to late adolescence or adult life. A good prognosis (i.e. survival to childhood and adult life) is associated with a large atrial septal defect, absence of obstruction in pulmonary venous pathways, drainage to the right atrium or left innominate vein, and normal or only slightly raised pulmonary vascular resistance early.

Late survivors are breathless often with atrial fibrillation, flutter or supraventricular tachycardia. Right heart failure may occur in sinus rhythm and cyanosis and polycythaemia may become severe particularly with the Eisenmenger reaction. The physical signs are those of atrial septal defect with central cyanosis. A continuous murmur – a venous hum – may be heard in the left upper chest, when pulmonary veins drain to the left innominate vein; or over the right chest when veins enter the azygos or right superior vena cava. The murmur is loud when there is mild obstruction at any venous site but such patients rarely survive to adolescence.

The ECG shows P pulmonale, a prolonged or normal P–R interval, right axis deviation, and right ventricular hypertrophy more severe than with ASD; Q waves are absent in V_6 and R waves are small. T inversion extending to V_1–V_4 or V_5 is usual.

When the pulmonary veins enter the right atrium or coronary sinus (exceptional in adults), the chest X-ray looks like that of a large ASD with huge cardiomegaly, dilation of the right atrium and pulmonary arteries with small left atrium and aortic knuckle. When connected to the left innominate, the enlarged upper systemic veins give the cardiac silhouette the appearance of a cottage loaf (or snowman) (Fig. 12).

Diagnosis can be made by echocardiography and catheterization which shows the abnormal channel of pulmonary venous return either after injection of contrast into the pulmonary arteries or into an anomalous pulmonary venous channel. Some elevation of the pulmonary artery pressure is expected and systemic and pulmonary artery saturations are the same or the pulmonary artery exceeds the systemic by 5–7 per cent.

Differential diagnosis is from an unusually large atrial septal defect and cor triatriatum with atrial septal defects. Treatment is operation to anastomose the common pulmonary vein to the left atrium and closure of the ASD provided the pulmonary vascular resistance is not too high. Surgical treatment has produced many adult survivors. The heart may be normal or there may be residual pulmonary hypertension. Atrial arrhythmias occur and nodal rhythm has been found after correction of the coronary sinus drainage type. Although a very serious lesion in infancy, the state of late survivors is excellent provided there is no obstruction at the site of anastomosis to produce pulmonary venous congestion.

Hemianomalous pulmonary venous drainage
This presents as an ASD with slight central cyanosis and often slightly elevated pulmonary vascular resistance (see ASD and cyanosis). Patients are acyanotic at rest. If there is no significant atrial septal defect, the widely split second sound will move freely but not close with respiration. Occasionally the hemianomalous veins enter the IVC/right atrial junction via a confluence of right pulmonary veins which descends to the drainage opening giving the classic 'scimitar' shadow on the chest X-ray (Figs 13a, b). Usually the hemianomalous veins enter the right atrium or left superior vena cava which will appear dilated (like a less rounded snowman shadow).

Partial anomalous pulmonary veins
See ASD, page 13.270.

Anomalies of arterial connection

These anomalies with a basic common pathological feature which distinguishes them from each other include transposition of the great arteries (classic), corrected transposition, corrected malposition, double outlet right ventricle, double outlet left ventricle, and double inlet ventricles (single, uni or common ventricle). They

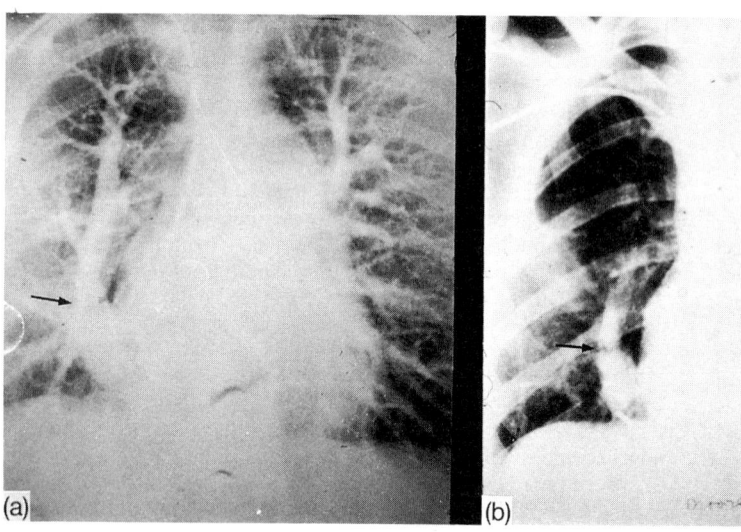

(a)   (b)

Fig. 13 (a, b) Angiogram and chest X-ray from patient with hemianomalous pulmonary veins entering IVC/RA junction. The descending anomalous pulmonary vein is seen as a Scimitar on (b) the chest X-ray and (a) the angiogram (arrows). Left pulmonary veins are draining normally to left atrium.

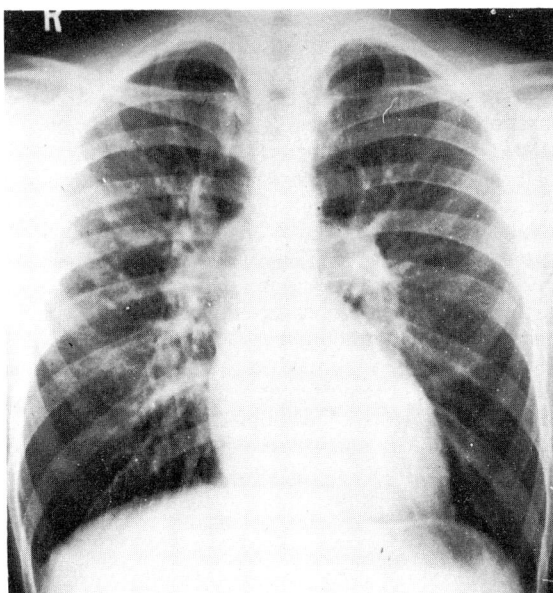

Fig. 14 Chest X-ray from an adult with transposition of the great arteries, VSD, and pulmonary hypertension. It shows narrow vascular pedicle, large branch pulmonary arteries, and 'absent' main pulmonary artery.

uncommonly appear after adolescence unless there has been earlier palliation. Cyanosis is not always evident. Presentation depends on whether pulmonary stenosis or pulmonary hypertension is present.

Classic transposition of the great arteries (TGA) (atrioventricular concordance, ventricular arterial discordance)

Classic transposition describes an anomaly where the right ventricle is connected to the aorta which is usually anterior, but can be in any position and the left ventricle connects to the pulmonary artery which is usually posterior. Adults with TGA sometimes appear without previous surgery but form about 0.5 per cent of patients who have a natural large ASD, pulmonary valve stenosis with VSD, or VSD and ASD and the Eisenmenger reaction. More often they have had childhood palliation with a shunt, banding of the pulmonary artery or more radical therapy with an intra-atrial baffle (Senning, Mustard or Brom modification).

Symptoms include breathlessness from hypoxia, and those of right heart failure after 15–20 years because the right ventricle is often morphologically abnormal as well as hypertrophied and subjected to constant systemic pressure. Abnormally attached tricuspid valve chordae may rupture spontaneously. Infective endocarditis is uncommon but has been seen on tricuspid and mitral valves and the VSD when small. Atrial fibrillation and supraventricular tachycardia occur in the third and fourth decades and there may be troublesome ventricular ectopics.

Signs depend on associated lesions. All patients have clubbing and significant cyanosis. When there is an ASD the ejection murmur is short or absent; the aortic second sound is loud and single in the pulmonary area. The aorta is palpable and there is right ventricular hypertrophy. The heart is usually enlarged with increased flow and pulmonary artery size on the right compared with the left side. Speckly shadows from bronchial-pulmonary collaterals are common in patients with pulmonary stenosis or an ASD. The vascular pedicle is narrow (Fig. 14) or the aorta on the left rises up to the knuckle. The ECG shows right ventricular hypertrophy. The axis is usually right but may be left with certain types of VSD. With VSD and pulmonary stenosis the signs resemble those of Fallot with a long systolic murmur conducted to the right and the aortic sound loud in the pulmonary area. There

may be calcification of the pulmonary valve, visible in the lateral chest X-ray deep in the mediastinum. With VSD or ASD and a patent duct, signs resemble those of Eisenmenger with huge pulmonary arteries and an unusual chest X-ray with an abnormal pedicle.

For diagnosis, patients require right ventricular and left ventricular angiography as a minimum. Efforts should be made to measure pulmonary artery pressure and careful oxygen analysis from all parts of the heart and vessels is vital. The left ventricular pressure is commonly at systemic level or above in adults because of an associated VSD and/or pulmonary stenosis. Sometimes when an ASD is the only mixing site, left ventricular pressure is low. Adult patients can have a spontaneously closed VSD with pulmonary stenosis.

Surgical treatment

Some patients with TGA and ASD may be suitable for intra-atrial baffle (Mustard or Senning procedure) in adult life but this depends on pulmonary vascular resistance. Those with TGA plus VSD plus PVS do well with Rastelli procedure which is closure of the VSD in a way which allows the left ventricle to eject through it into the aorta via the VSD, ligation of the proximal pulmonary artery, and placing a valved conduit between the right ventricle and pulmonary artery distal to the ligature or transection of the pulmonary artery. Those patients with hyperkinetic pulmonary hypertension may be suitable for arterial switch, or a 'palliative switch' in which the VSD is left open. Patients with TGA who survive to adolescence are likely to have a high pulmonary vascular resistance even with pulmonary stenosis.

Since 90 per cent of children born with TGA would die if untreated in the first year of life, survival to adolescence and adulthood usually depends on earlier surgery. Experience of 20 patients who have survived late after intra-atrial baffle shows that complex arrhythmias are common. Right heart failure causing pulmonary oedema is a problem over 20 years and haemoptysis from progressive pulmonary vascular disease occurs. Sudden death may occur despite careful monitoring of rhythm. Several people have lived normal lives in sinus rhythm, and pregnancy has been tolerated and produced a normal child. Late tricuspid regurgitation with and without chordal rupture may result in acute pulmonary oedema. Late results of Rastelli operation have been good, with few arrhythmias. The problems relate to the fate and replacement of the valved conduit between right ventricle and pulmonary artery. There is a danger of bronchial obstruction and pulmonary complications when the conduit is placed on the left of the heart to avoid compression. There are no long-term results in adults of arterial switching yet but aortic (once the pulmonary valve) regurgitation can be expected in some.

Corrected transposition (atrioventricular discordance; ventricular arterial discordance; anterior aorta to the left)

Patients with this basic anomaly often survive into the second decade without surgical treatment. Their survival depends on the associated lesions and the behaviour of the conducting tissue.

The right atrium empties through a bicuspid atrioventricular valve (mitral) into a morphological left ventricle which is connected to a posteromedial pulmonary artery. The left atrium receiving normal pulmonary venous drainage empties through a tricuspid valve, often abnormally formed and placed in a morphological right ventricle which ejects into an anterolateral aorta. Despite the strange anatomy, the circulation flows correctly – hence the name 'corrected' transposition. However, the conducting tissue takes an abnormal course, the coronary pattern is reversed, and the right ventricle and tricuspid valve were not designed to support the systemic circulation indefinitely.

The common associated anomalies are ventricular septal defect with and without pulmonary valve stenosis, subpulmonary

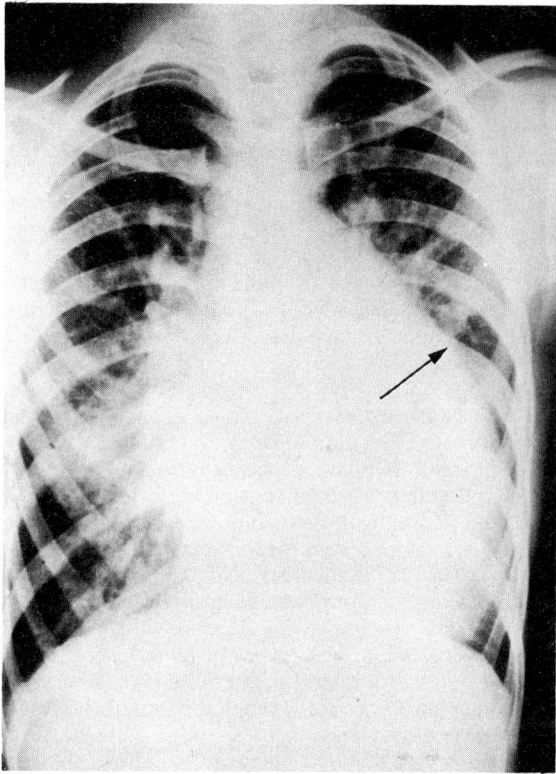

Fig. 15 Chest X-ray from a patient with multiple VSDs, pulmonary hypertension, and corrected transposition showing unusual low bulge on left cardiac border (arrow) from aortic outflow beneath ascending aorta making the straight border up to the aortic knuckle, no obvious dilated main pulmonary artery despite intense pulmonary plethora and cardiomegaly.

obstruction which is not muscular, and Ebstein's anomaly of the left atrioventricular valve causing left atrioventricular valve regurgitation. Aortic stenosis, atrioventricular and atrial septal defect, and left superior vena cava may co-exist. Patients can present as ventricular septal defect with left-to-right shunt and hyperkinetic pulmonary hypertension; when pulmonary stenosis co-exists they look like Fallot; or isolated left atrioventricular valve regurgitation of varying severity; or late onset of left atrioventricular valve regurgitation in fourth decade; or arrhythmias which include sudden complete heart block or sudden death with bizarre supraventricular tachycardias including atrial fibrillation. Complete heart block may date from birth or be acquired at anytime after. The ventricular rate tends to slow with age. Pacemaker implantation may be sufficient to control symptoms, particularly in adults who have well-compensated lesions.

The diagnosis depends on associated defects:

1. With pulmonary stenosis and VSD (resembling Fallot). There is no history of cyanotic attacks since there are no infundibular bands (which are not part of a morphological LV) to constrict the outflow tract. Cyanosis varies according to the severity of the pulmonary stenosis which is usually valvar but occasionally subvalvar caused by fibrous tags or aberrant atrioventricular valve tissue. The feel of the apex beat is non-specific, and arterial pulsation is felt in the pulmonary area due to the anterior aorta. There is a systolic murmur maximal at the lower left sternal edge, A_2 is increased in the pulmonary area, and apical atrioventricular valve regurgitant murmurs are frequent. The ECG shows a prominent QR pattern in II, III, and in V_1, with an rSR in V_6 and aVL. The q wave is absent in the left chest leads even when the systemic ventricle is dilated. The chest X-ray shows a straight left aortic border with the right pulmonary artery higher and larger than the left. The left-sided ventricular outflow tract and aortic sinus may make

a prominence on the left cardiac border in the region of and giving the appearance of a dilated left atrial appendage.

2. With VSD and pulmonary hypertension. The chest X-ray and ECG are unusual for VSD (Fig. 15), with no main pulmonary artery shadow and straight aorta on the left border, and an absent QR pattern of left ventricular overload in V_6.

3. With left atrioventricular regurgitation. Those with a left-sided Ebstein rarely reach adult life but less severe anomalies of the left valve present often with atrial fibrillation, block, or bizarre tachycardia precipitating pulmonary oedema. Diagnosis is made with the usual signs of mitral regurgitation, atypical ECG, and chest X-ray, with evidence of reversed ventricular morphology on two-dimensional echocardiography.

It is possible to have a normal lifespan with corrected transposition without defects or important left atrioventricular valve regurgitation but this is rare as arrhythmias after 40–50 years cause trouble. The systemic ventricle of right morphology fails in the fifth decade and the tricuspid valve develops or increases its regurgitation.

Surgical treatment

It is technically possible to close associated ventricular septal defects and relieve pulmonary stenosis. Relief of pulmonary stenosis may require a valved conduit because access is difficult and there are dangers of producing block or damaging the vulnerable right coronary artery. However, there is a high incidence of problems in relation to malignant arrhythmias, pacing problems for block, and progressive left atrioventricular valve regurgitation after closure of the VSD.

Indications for surgical treatment are severe cyanosis and hypoxia, suprasystemic pressure in the right-sided ventricle, symptomatic hyperkinetic pulmonary hypertension with a large VSD, and severe regurgitation in the left atrioventricular valve which exceptionally will be reparable. Reoperation to replace the regurgitant atrioventricular valve may be needed in the first five years after the first 'corrective' operation. Hence the need for conservative views in management.

Corrected malposition (atrioventricular concordance, ventricular arterial concordance, mitral/aortic discontinuity, anterior aorta)

This curiosity has features of corrected transposition such as the position of the great arteries relative to one another but the morphology of right and left ventricles are not inverted. Subpulmonary and subaortic obstruction are common as is VSD which may close spontaneously, or be large. Basically, the venous blood flows to the right side of the heart and the red blood is in the left heart of correct morphology. Complete heart block is not a special problem but mitral regurgitation may result with resection of subaortic stenosis.

Double outflow right ventricle (DORV)

Both great arteries arise from the right ventricle and left ventricular ejection into the aorta is through the vital ventricular septal defect which can become restrictive thus causing subaortic obstruction. If patients have pulmonary stenosis, they present as Fallot and if not as pulmonary hypertensive ventricular septal defects. Diagnosis is made by echocardiography and angiography showing mitral/aortic discontinuity with the aorta emerging from the right ventricle and pointing anteriorly. The ECG is not diagnostic. If there is subaortic obstruction due to muscle bands or a small VSD, the carotid pulse may be delayed with a thrill and the aortic sound may be delayed and diminished when it should be loud. Left ventricular hypertrophy may be unexpectedly severe. Natural history and management relate to the site of the VSD and the presence or absence of pulmonary stenosis and the competence of atrioventricular valves which may develop chordal rupture in adults. Those with subpulmonary VSD without pulmonary stenosis and uncommitted VSD or atrioventricular canals pose the greatest problems. The easiest to deal with are the most frequent with subaortic stenosis. Those who survive without pulmonary stenosis usually have irreversible pulmonary vascular disease as adults and surgical treatment may be ill advised. Late results of repaired DORV in childhood may be good but there may be problems with aortic regurgitation, subaortic stenosis, ventricular arrhythmias or progressive pulmonary hypertension.

Double inlet ventricle (univentricular, single or common ventricle)

There are many forms and survival depends on the associated anomalies. If pulmonary valve stenosis allows a normal or slightly increased pulmonary blood flow, patients can survive to the fifth to seventh decades finally succumbing to severe heart failure, precipitated by atrial fibrillation. Subpulmonary obstructions usually progress to become atretic and calcified but this may not occur until the second and third decades in a few. Changes in morphology which affect symptoms are acquired subaortic obstruction, subpulmonary stenosis, atrioventricular valve regurgitation, and pulmonary vascular disease.

Treatment is as for tricuspid atresia. Septating the ventricle has produced a few short-term survivors but complete heart block, haemoptysis, and failure have caused problems. It is not known how well are adult survivors.

Univentricular heart with mitral atresia

It is possible to reach adulthood with these anomalies provided the atrial septal defect is large. As well as the features of pulmonary hypertension and univentricular hearts, there are features of pulmonary venous congestion. Massive haemoptysis from capillary rupture occur early and atrial fibrillation in the second/third decade causes rapid deterioration and death.

Pulmonary arteriovenous fistula

Diffuse small or localized large isolated congenital pulmonary arteriovenous aneurysm may occur in the lungs. These patients have varying degrees of central cyanosis and inspiratory continuous murmurs if the fistula is large enough. The condition may be part of Babbington's disease (hereditary telangiectasia). Pulmonary angiography may confirm the diagnosis of single or multiple fistulae in the lung.

Acyanotic congenital heart disease in adults

More patients with acyanotic congenital heart disease than with cyanotic congenital heart disease survive to adult life. Many of the lesions are mild, cause symptoms later, and, when small or modest in size lead to little haemodynamic disturbance.

Right-sided obstructive lesions and other anomalies of the right side of the heart

The main anomalies are: (a) pulmonary valve stenosis; (b) 'lone' infundibular stenosis; (c) bipartite right ventricle; (d) pulmonary artery stenoses; (e) idiopathic dilation of the pulmonary artery; and (f) Ebstein's anomaly (see page 13.260).

Pulmonary valve stenosis (PVS)

Any grade of valve obstruction may be found in adolescents and adults. Severe pulmonary valve stenosis is uncommon in adults unless there has been previous surgery. Patients with 'simple' pulmonary valve stenosis may be cyanosed but more frequently are not.

Table 5 Physical signs in pulmonary valve stenosis (PVS)

	Mild	Moderate	Severe
Pulse	Normal	Normal	Small
JVP	Normal	Dominant 'a' wave on inspiration or exercise	Giant 'a' wave
Apex beat	RV palpable	RV++	RV++
Auscultation	Loud pulmonary ejection click, increases on expiration	Click close to S_1 (absent if valve thick)	No click
	A_2/P_2 interval wide, increases on inspiration	A_2/P_2 interval wider, increases on inspiration	P_2 often very late, soft or not heard
	P_2 audible but late	P_2 audible but late	
	Grade 2 ejection murmur increases on inspiration, maximal 2nd left interspace	Grade 3 murmur + thrill	Loud murmur + thrill – late crescendo over A_2
Other			Mild clubbing (variable) Peripheral cyanosis Malar flush

Anatomy and physiology

The stenosed pulmonary valve may be bicuspid or tricuspid, a pliable dome, or the thick lumpy valve, which is common in patients with Noonan's syndrome or funny faces. After age 35–40 years, the valve calcifies and may become regurgitant. When right ventricular pressures are high (i.e. systemic or suprasystemic), calcification also develops in the tricuspid valve ring, sometimes involving a cusp. The effects of pulmonary valve stenosis are to disturb right ventricular function. Right ventricular hypertrophy occurs when resting right ventricular pressure exceeds 50 mmHg. The actual valve obstruction does not increase after the first decade but increasing infundibular hypertrophy may cause increasing obstruction and the effects on the hypertrophied right ventricle are progressive until fibrosis causes dilation, failure, and tricuspid regurgitation, often worsened or precipitated by atrial flutter and fibrillation.

Symptoms

Fatigue, slight dyspnoea, and effort syncope occur with severe pulmonary valve stenosis. Dyspnoea is more pronounced when there is cyanosis from a reversed intra-atrial shunt on effort. Acyanotic patients are usually symptom-free until the onset of atrial fibrillation or flutter and right heart failure which lead to ascites and peripheral oedema. Adult patients with mild to moderate pulmonary valve stenosis (RV pressures 40–60 mmHg) may appear after age 50 years in right heart failure in sinus rhythm. Infective endocarditis with simple pulmonary valve stenosis is unknown and personal practice is not to use routine prophylaxis.

Signs

The physical signs depend on the severity of the obstruction and the secondary effects on the right ventricular myocardium (Table 5). Pulmonary regurgitation occurs when the valve calcifies. Careful attention to physical signs allows a reliable assessment of severity; cardiac catheterization is often unnecessary.

In right heart failure, the pulse is small and irregular, the JVP high with huge 'v' waves of tricuspid regurgitation, and a third sound increasing on inspiration is obvious. A loud pansystolic murmur difficult to distinguish from the pulmonary ejection murmur may be present at the left lower sternal edge. In such cases, the ejection murmur at the pulmonary area is short.

Electrocardiogram The degree of right ventricular hypertrophy depends on the severity of the obstruction and the length of time it has been present. Minimal changes are right axis deviation, increase in R wave in lead V_1 or splintered S in V_1. More obvious increase in voltage in right chest leads occurs in moderate stenosis with upright T in V_1 and S in V_6. In severe stenosis increased R wave voltage and ST–T wave changes over right ventricular leads are seen. P pulmonale is usual. No true left ventricular complexes are recorded in V_6. QR pattern in V_1 is occasionally seen. With increasing age and/or failure, complete right bundle branch block may develop. In moderate stenosis with progressive cardiac dilation, the T waves become progressively inverted across the right chest leads without increase in voltage of QRS.

Chest X-ray In mild stenosis, the heart is normal in size. Pulmonary blood flow is normal. The main pulmonary artery and left pulmonary artery are dilated. In more severe cases, the heart may be slightly or grossly enlarged. The right atrium is dilated and post-stenotic dilation of the pulmonary artery is present but not as marked as in moderate obstruction. The lung fields appear under-filled with small peripheral vessels (oligaemic) in severe stenosis. The aorta is small, low, and left-sided. Calcification of the pulmonary valve, should be expected after age 35 years, and is best seen on penetrated screening but can be documented by left lateral or anteroposterior views; it appears earlier if the patient is cyanosed and the obstruction is severe.

Differential diagnosis

When stenosis is trivial it may be confused with mild aortic valve stenosis or ASD but pulmonary artery dilation on X-ray and inspiratory murmurs should differentiate PVS from aortic stenosis which do co-exist. To differentiate mild PVS from modest ASD may be difficult and require catheterization in the adult as echocardiography is unreliable. Other causes of a long systolic murmur at the left sternal edge include VSD, infundibular stenosis, subaortic stenosis, and pulmonary artery stenosis.

Severe PVS in failure with right ventricular dilation may be confused with Ebstein, pericardial effusion (no murmurs), or even ventricular septal defect with atrial fibrillation. The appearance of the dilated left pulmonary artery (in comparison to the right) on the X-ray, a late soft P_2, and the 'a' wave if in sinus rhythm should distinguish pulmonary stenosis. It may be difficult to differentiate lone infundibular stenosis without invasive investigation.

Pulmonary valvotomy

The late results of pulmonary valvotomy are excellent; 95 per cent have symptomatic cure. Murmurs persist and pulmonary regurgitation is common. Patients who have had lumpy dysplastic valves are often left with serious pulmonary incompetence, particularly if cusps have been excised. Severe pulmonary regurgitation is not entirely benign long term as it can lead 15–20 years later to progressive right ventricular dilation, frank right ventricular failure with atrial flutter, and fibrillation. Pulmonary valve replacement (with an aortic homograft) has been helpful in a few but the heart diminishes little in size once extreme dilation has occurred – the tricuspid valve may also require surgery as it usually becomes grossly incompetent. This small group of patients requires careful watching – once the heart begins to show acceleration of cardiomegaly, pulmonary valve replacement should be performed before frank failure or atrial fibrillation is established. Provided pulmonary valve and annulus obstruction is relieved, infundibular stenosis should regress. Cyanosis on effort may occur if a patent foramen ovale remains even when PS has been adequately relieved. Endocarditis risks are small so that no prophylaxis is necessary.

When coronary disease with or without hypertension develops in older patients with unrelieved important pulmonary valve stenosis it may take an insidious course to manifest with pulmonary oedema without left ventricular enlargement as it is 'protected' by the pulmonary stenosis. This poses difficulty in management as relief of the pulmonary stenosis will have catastrophic effects on the left ventricle. It may be that only coronary bypass grafting should be done in such unusual circumstances.

There is evidence that in some patients the cardiovascular disease is not limited to the pulmonary valve. There may be associated left ventricular disease which may manifest early as pulmonary oedema and chronic congestion after operation or later as myopathy – hypertrophic or dilated. The concept of more diffuse congenital cardiovascular disease in hearts with congenital structural defects applies to many other conditions besides PVS. It has wide implications for the future of many patients as there may be myocardial, coronary, and aortic abnormalities which are not caused by the obstruction or defect, but which may cause symptoms and signs which cannot be explained by the basic disorder, i.e. pulmonary valve stenosis, on which clinical attention is focused.

'Lone' infundibular stenosis

Anatomy and physiology

Fixed right ventricular outflow tract obstruction below the pulmonary valve is caused by muscle bands which are abnormally placed, at first causing slight obstruction and then slowly hypertrophying in postnatal life; the pulmonary valve may be normal, bicuspid, or minimally stenosed. The infundibular stenosis appears to be the only anomaly in the heart at the time of removal but if a careful search is made there is evidence of a ventricular septal defect (subtricuspid or muscular) which has closed spontaneously earlier leaving only a scar. The speed with which infundibular obstruction develops relates to the stimulus from right ventricular hypertension which initially is determined by the size of the ventricular septal defect, the degree of rotation, and initial size of the bands, and probably the amount of dysplastic muscle present in the abnormal muscle band. Slow enlargement/hypertrophy of bands may cause infundibular obstruction to become critical in the second and third decades. The bands become covered with thickened endocardium. The orifice varies from 1 to 2.5 cm. This anatomical disarrangement is usually associated with a large subaortic VSD, i.e. Fallot's tetralogy and the VSD cannot close spontaneously.

Symptoms and signs

Murmurs have been documented since early childhood. A click never precedes the long pulmonary ejection systolic murmur which is maximal in the third left interspace, conducted into the pulmonary area, and increases on inspiration. P_2 may be heard, delayed, diminished, and heard best in the pulmonary area away from the maximal intensity of the murmur which resembles the murmur of a VSD.

The chest X-ray resembles that of pulmonary stenosis except that both pulmonary arteries are the same size. True oligaemia is rare in adolescents and adults. A prominence on the left border is due to a dilated infundibular chamber. Calcification can occur in the endocardium of the outflow (a vertical linear shadow).

Bipartite right ventricle

This rare form of low infundibular stenosis occurs in adults and raises diagnostic difficulties. Aberrantly placed muscular bands divide the inflow portion of the right ventricle from the outflow and cause obstruction with time to surround a fixed orifice in a muscular partition running from the apex of the right ventricle to the septum. This may be close to the tricuspid valve so that the inflow portion (body) of the right ventricle is small and shallow. If there is a subaortic VSD, it may present as Fallot or it may be missed when associated with an outflow VSD which may be large enough to cause a large pulmonary blood flow and pulmonary hypertension. When present in adults it is usually an isolated abnormality either because a small VSD has closed spontaneously or was not even there.

Symptoms
These include tiredness and slight dyspnoea. Atrial rhythm upsets occur after 40 years.

Signs
The signs suggest a VSD with intense pansystolic murmur at the lower left sternal edge but an 'a' wave is visible and P₂ is delayed. The right ventricle is not obviously enlarged and may not be obviously hypertrophied on the ECG although extensive T inversion in right chest leads suggest abnormality. The presence of left axis deviation makes the diagnosis more difficult. Echocardiography may reveal abnormal bands but is not diagnostic (except in retrospect). Catheterization with angiography is necessary but the high right ventricular pressure cavity may be missed as it is shallow beneath the tricuspid valve. Angiography and careful searching will confirm the diagnosis. Left ventricular angiography should also be performed as there may be a bulging ventricular septum, and aberrantly placed muscle lumps and papillary muscles.

Treatment
Treatment is surgical if there are symptoms and high right ventricular pressure as the lesion progresses to cause myocardial damage and dysfunction. The postoperative results are good; a raised venous pressure may persist.

Differential diagnosis
Other causes of a long, loud systolic murmur at the left sternal edge are:

1. VSD: the murmur is pansystolic and increases on expiration. P₂ is not usually as delayed or diminished and the left ventricle is dominant.

2. Pulmonary valve stenosis: the ejection click, large left pulmonary artery, and more obvious poststenotic dilation distinguish.

3. Subaortic stenosis: there is a soft aortic expiratory diastolic murmur, jerky pulse, a thrill in the suprasternal notch, delayed A₂, and left ventricular dominance.

4. Pulmonary artery stenosis: the long inspiratory murmur is heard higher and is conducted to the lungs.

Idiopathic dilation of the pulmonary artery

This condition has physical signs without symptoms and is compatible with a normal lifespan. In many, perhaps all, it is due to trivial pulmonary valve abnormality – a bicuspid open pulmonary valve – analogous to the floppy bicuspid aortic valve. Since patients do not die as a result of the condition, we do not know if these are constant. Gradients of 5–10 mmHg may be found. Sometimes it is found in patients with stigmata of Marfan's or Ehlers–Danlos and then it is due to pulmonary artery dilation. There is a late pulmonary ejection sound preceding a grade 1 murmur. A₂ and P₂ are normal. Pulmonary diastolic murmurs are frequent and increase on inspiration.

Left-sided obstructive lesions and other anomalies affecting the left side of the heart

The main anomalies are aortic valve stenosis, bicuspid aortic valve, aortic regurgitation, fixed subaortic stenosis, supra-aortic stenosis, coarctation of the aorta, kinked aorta (at isthmus), aorto-left ventricular tunnel, mitral anomalies, and left atrial obstruction.

Aortic valve

Minor congenital abnormality of the aortic valve (bicuspid, slight tricuspid fusion) is said to be the commonest congenital lesion in the cardiovascular system. It is doubtful whether it is more frequent than VSD.

Varying degrees of obstruction occur. Congenital aortic valve stenosis becomes critical around or soon after puberty, occasionally in the third to fourth decades, and thereafter with increasing frequency when calcific aortic stenosis presents maximally in sixth and seventh decades. Isolated calcific aortic stenosis is the result of deposition of calcium on a congenitally abnormal valve. Valve calcification is less in the female and appears later than in males. In patients under 29 years with critical obstruction, the valve remains pliable with flecks of calcium in small myxomatous masses attached to the cusps. Florid calcification under 30 years seems only to occur after previous valvotomy, infection, or with a metabolic upset such as hypercholesterolaemic states or a calcium disorder. The mildly congenitally deformed aortic valve (bicuspid, tricuspid, or rarely quadricuspid) may be regurgitant so that the patient is known to have had an immediate diastolic murmur since childhood.

The physical signs of established aortic valve stenosis depend on severity and pliability. The condition must be differentiated from fixed subaortic stenosis as the management and surgical treatment are different.

In congenital aortic valve stenosis the pathology may not be limited to the aortic valve. Patients may have an unusually thick ventricular septum (perhaps due to excessive myocardial dysplasia), secondary mitral valve dysfunction, and aortic disease with systemic hypertension unmasked after aortic valvotomy or valve replacement.

Fixed subaortic stenosis

This is sometimes referred to as discrete congenital subvalvar obstruction. It is rarely discrete, is probably not congenital (present since birth), but does lie beneath the aortic valve.

The lesion is an accumulation of fibroelastic tissue in the form of a crescent or a complete ring. It may be close to the aortic valve, eccentric, and oblique or 1–2 cm lower. It is never 'membranous' and is attached to a sheet of fibroelastic tissue overlying the bulging and usually excessively hypertrophied ventricular septum. It causes left ventricular outflow obstruction which is mild, moderate or severe, and secondary effects on the aortic valve which develops jet lesions and regurgitation. It may present late in childhood, more commonly in adolescence, and sometimes in an adult. Secondary mitral regurgitation occurs. There is increasing evidence that this is a lesion acquired in postnatal life as the result of some congenital abnormality of the left ventricular outflow tract. Other congenital anomalies of the heart or cardiovascular system occur in 60 per cent, i.e. duct, ventricular septal defect, aortic valve stenosis (bicuspid or tricuspid), and coarctation. There is an interrelationship between fixed subaortic stenosis and obstructive hypertrophic myopathy. In an adult over 30 years with signs of aortic stenosis and no radiological calcification, fixed subaortic stenosis should be the first diagnosis.

Symptoms and presentation
These are as for other forms of aortic stenosis. Left ventricular failure occurs after the age of 40 years. Infective endocarditis on the aortic valve is a risk with signs of severe stenosis, mild regurgitation, and failure.

Signs
Pulses are full and usually slightly jerky. Occasionally small sharp pulses are found when obstruction is severe, close to the aortic valve or the ventricle is failing. There is a prominent 'a' wave in the JVP if the ventricular septum is thick and encroaching on the right ventricular cavity, and a carotid thrill. The apex is left ventri-

cular, powerful, and displaced to the left. There is an ejection systolic murmur, maximal in the third left intercostal space, conducted to the apex and neck. This may be indistinguishable from, and associated with, a pansystolic murmur at the apex. The first sound is normal. There is no ejection sound. The aortic second sound is usually audible but often delayed and splitting, is sometimes difficult to detect or may be reversed. In adults a short immediate diastolic murmur of aortic regurgitation is present.

Chest X-ray shows a left ventricular contour. The aorta appears normal, but a low poststenotic dilation may be seen within the heart shadow. No calcification is evident.

Electrocardiogram There is pure left ventricular hypertrophy without large Q waves in the anterior chest leads; steep ST depression and T inversion are frequent. The axis may be left, normal, and sometimes inexplicably rightwards. Left bundle branch block is common over age 45 years.

Echocardiography M-mode may show premature closure of the aortic valve and a thick abnormal ventricular septum. Cross-sectional echocardiography reveals the shelf protruding beneath the aortic valve. A very thick abnormal ventricular septum is commonly seen and abnormal movement of the mitral cusps are frequent. It may be difficult to differentiate from hypertrophic obstructive myopathy. It is vital to see the actual protruding shelf and not just the thickened septal endocardium. The aortic valve is thickened and opens abnormally with fixed subaortic stenosis.

Investigation
Catheter studies show a subvalvar gradient. Aortography shows minor aortic regurgitation unless there is cusp perforation. Thickened aortic valve cusps open abnormally with concavity outwards but not domed as with valve obstruction. Subvalvar obstruction may be seen as a linear defect, or a small indentation beneath the aortic cusps.

Treatment
The lesion should be resected when diagnosed as it is progressive. All the endocardial thickening attached to the shelf and overlying the ventricular septum must be completely removed by blunt dissection. The condition may reoccur and form 'tunnel' obstruction if resection has been incomplete in childhood or adolescence. Physiologically the left ventricular muscle may behave as in hypertrophic obstructive cardiomyopathy following operation. A picture of congestive myopathy with progressive fibrosis may appear after age 40–50 years.

The aortic valve has a lifetime risk of endocarditis since jet lesions are usual and remain after resection; careful prophylaxis must continue after operation.

The mortality of early resection is low but problems can return. Recurrence of subaortic obstruction is most likely in patients with persistent resting gradients above 25–30 mmHg immediately after operation, in association with a small aortic root, an irregular HOCM-like left ventricle prior to operation, and isoprenaline-stimulated high gradients following operation. Asymptomatic patients with two or more of these features should be watched for electrocardiographic deterioration. Reoperation may be difficult and hazardous as tunnel obstructions present a formidable surgical problem. Total aortic root/valve replacement may be necessary to provide relief of obstruction. Alternatively, the unattractive 'Texas tube' from the apex to the descending aorta has also been used with claimed success but it is doubtful if a good long-term solution will be provided by the addition of this iatrogenic abnormality.

Supra-aortic stenosis
Supra-aortic stenosis describes a narrowing above the aortic valve contiguous with the commissural attachments. It may be mild, appearing as a waist above the sinuses without causing a gradient,

or a severe fibrous constriction above the coronary orifices. When well developed, the aortic cusps hang like a Marlin's nest; the cusps are usually thick and can be regurgitant. Surgical attention is focused on the stenosis and removal is thought to cure the condition. Unfortunately, this is not so as the disease is not localized to the supra-aortic area. The central aorta beyond is grossly abnormal, often seen to be diffusely hypoplastic. Biopsy of the ascending aorta well beyond the supra-aortic narrowing shows constant histological abnormality in the media termed 'higgledy-piggledy', a term to describe disordered, disarrayed musculoelastic fibres of the media. This is most severe in those with obvious aortic hypoplasia where intimal changes may be found even in childhood. The same histological changes in the medial layers occur in those without apparent diffuse narrowing of the aorta and irrespective of whether the supra-aortic stenosis is part of the 'hypercalcaemic' syndrome with its characteristic facies and other features, familial with normal physical features or a sporadic case with none of the known associations. This 'higgledy-piggledy' disorder which extends throughout the major conducting arteries appears in severely affected patients to fade out in the region of the common iliac arteries; at least this was found in the only two patients studied with the familial form. 'Higgledy-piggledy' changes are thus a non-specific result of arterial damage *in utero* from several causes. The actual supra-aortic stenosis is probably the result of more extensive damage at a vulnerable site in the conducting arteries as are the other stenoses at origins of major arteries. These areas may not grow as do the rest of the arteries and so obstruction manifests years or decades later.

Important supra-aortic stenosis has not been found at birth or infancy and so it is doubtful if the lesion itself is congenital. It should, like subaortic stenosis, be regarded as acquired in postnatal life and occurs as part of a congenital arteriopathy. Stenoses occur at other sites, i.e. carotid, innominate, mesenteric, sometimes renal, and peripherally in the pulmonary arteries in about 50 per cent of patients with supra-aortic stenosis. This provides further support for the view that the condition is diffuse.

If supra-aortic stenosis is relieved before growth of the patient has finished, an obstruction may develop distally in the aortic arch or other vessels later. Another association is the degree and form of left ventricular hypertrophy which often co-exists; this appears to be disproportionate to the degree of outflow obstruction and is associated often with severe irregular hypertrophy involving the septum causing cavity obliteration in the left ventricle resembling the appearances of hypertrophic cardiomyopathy. Perhaps the myocardium, particularly the ventricular septum, is abnormally disarrayed (dysplastic) as is the aorta, and when presented with distal obstruction or abnormally inelastic conducting arteries, may hypertrophy erratically and irregularly as in other forms of left ventricular obstruction associated with excess dysplastic muscle. Certainly the conducting arteries in supra-aortic stenosis are thicker and less compliant, thus contributing to the systolic hypertension found in the majority of affected patients. Occasionally the problem complicates other structural congenital heart anomalies such as pulmonary and aortic valve stenosis, duct, or VSD.

Symptoms
When supra-aortic stenosis occurs with the 'hypercalcaemic' facies, a history of early illness in infancy with failure to thrive, repeated infections, and constipation which improve after the first year will be present. Infantile hypercalcaemia may have been detected and treated. Cardiac symptoms are uncommon. Angina occurs late as the coronary arteries are large and well perfused proximal to the obstruction but the walls are often pathologically thick and abnormal. Sometimes a stenosis at the origin of a coronary artery causes angina. Syncope may occur if there is marked septal hypertrophy together with atrial rhythm disturbances in older patients. Fits in adolescence are associated with severe systemic hypertension and carotid or innominate obstruction.

Dyspnoea occurs when the myocardium is grossly hypertro-

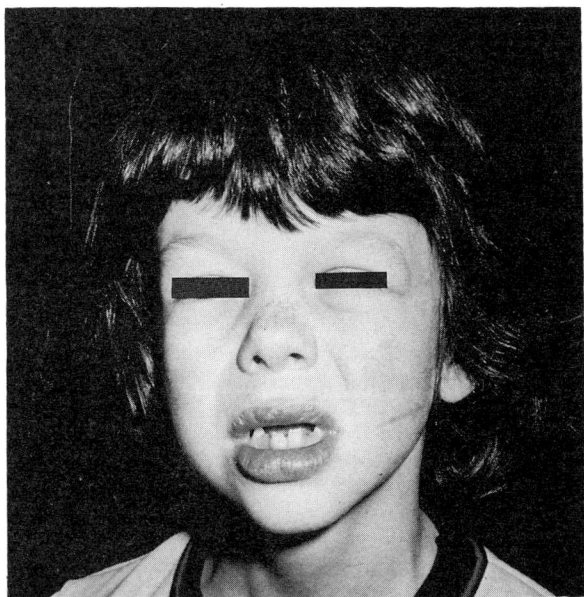

Fig. 16 Classic face associated with supra-aortic stenosis (William's syndrome). Large ridged teeth, prominent jaw, and supraorbital ridges.

phied with secondary mitral regurgitation. Infective endocarditis on the aortic valve is a risk and leads to aortic regurgitation. Prophylaxis is therefore essential. Supraventricular tachycardia may cause problems after age 30 years.

Supra-aortic stenosis is recognized by the following:

1. Signs of aortic stenosis (carotid systolic thrill, left ventricular hypertrophy).
2. Absence of an ejection click in young patients.
3. A murmur maximal at the upper right sternal edge.
4. A clear, loud aortic second sound.
5. Right arm and carotid pulses which are sharp and full unless obstructed at their origin. Left carotid and brachial pulses are usually less sharp. Femoral pulses are normal.
6. Systolic hypertension is common, but not diastolic. If stenosis is severe the systolic hypertension is present only after operation.

In addition there may be other long systolic murmurs in the neck, lungs posteriorly, axilla, or abdomen due to associated arterial stenosis. A specific search for hypertension should be made and care taken to ensure that the true central aortic pressure is being accurately reflected by the peripheral measurements.

If the arteriopathy is part of the 'burnt-out' hypercalcaemic syndrome, the face may be characteristic (Fig. 16) with prominent jaw and supra-orbital ridges, large teeth, mental retardation, and exuberant personality sometimes to the point of manic behaviour. Careful questioning may reveal a story of calcium injections or pills or vitamin D taken during the relevant pregnancy. Familial cases always look normal and siblings and parents should be examined when normal-looking patients present with supra-aortic stenosis.

Electrocardiogram Left ventricular hypertrophy without large Q waves is usual. Severe ST–T wave changes occur exceptionally, usually late, and in association with a HOCM-like ventricle. Right ventricular hypertrophy or right axis deviation co-exist when pulmonary hypertension from pulmonary artery stenosis is present.

The chest X-ray resembles that of aortic stenosis with a small aorta and low knuckle but in milder cases there is high poststenotic dilation of the ascending aorta in adolescents and adults. Lung vascularity may be unusual and dilation of the main pulmonary artery is obvious with pulmonary arterial stenosis.

Investigations

Even when the signs suggest only aortic stenosis, right heart catheterization and pulmonary angiography should be performed as it may reveal pulmonary arterial stenoses. Left ventricular angiography and ascending aortography are mandatory but should include visualization of origin of major vessels which are often cut off in the radiologist's anxiety to 'cone in ' for better definition. Abdominal aortography should be included; unexpected vascular abnormalities are often revealed. Abdominal 'coarctation' may develop particularly in relation to severe associated kyphoscoliosis.

Treatment

If the supra-aortic stenosis causes a gradient over 50–60 mmHg, it should be relieved particularly if there is evidence of abnormal left ventricular and septal hypertrophy. This may be done by 'gusseting'. However, this may disturb aortic valve function and aortic regurgitation may occur and even progress with late cusp avulsion. Systemic (systolic) hypertension is usual after relief of supra-aortic stenosis and is not related to renal arterial stenosis which must be excluded. It may in adults reach levels of 230 mmHg and require therapy. Total aortic root and valve replacement with homograft and reimplantation of coronary arteries may be needed in severe or previously operated patients in order to relieve a diffuse obstruction.

Coarctation of the aorta (page 13.389)

This refers to a narrowing at or proximal to the isthmus but not narrowings in the descending or abdominal aorta which appear to result from acquired disease of the aorta (aortitis), not congenital.

Coarctation is now uncommon in adults as it is diagnosed and treated earlier, but cases may be found at routine examination, with hypertension during pregnancy, with symptoms from aortic valve disease or infective endocarditis.

On exercise or emotion the systolic blood pressure in adult coarctations may rise to levels of 250–300 mmHg and this appears to cause headaches after effort. Leg pains on exertion sometimes occur although if the patient has reached adult life the collateral development is enormous and adequate to prevent claudication.

Back pain may be related to intercostal aneurysms. Angina may come from coronary disease or associated aortic stenosis. Dyspnoea and left ventricular failure occur from coarctation alone in those over 50 years; earlier from added aortic valve disease or in the presence of mitral regurgitation which may be accelerated by the onset of atrial fibrillation. Endocarditis on the aortic or less frequently the mitral valve are risks and cerebral haemorrhage in the young may arise from rupture of associated berry aneurysms. Occasionally infective endocarditis occurs at the coarctation site causing emboli in the legs and toes and false aneurysms.

Signs

Carotid pulses are prominent, but the femorals are diminished or absent. All pulses should be felt as the left subclavian may be involved in the coarctation and therefore diminished and the right be aberrant and arise from below the coarctation. Systolic blood pressure is usually high at rest.

The left ventricle is powerful, and the heart is often enlarged. An apical click from the aortic valve or dilated ascending aorta is usual. A systolic ejection murmur is often heard maximally over the back ($T_{3,4}$) and may be prolonged if it originates in the coarctation: but it is loud in the aortic area and carotids (with thrill) when aortic stenosis is added. An aortic diastolic murmur is frequent in adults. Posterior murmurs are absent in the presence of aortic atresia or interruption.

Collateral vascular development is enormous around the interscapular region, palpable, and visible in the thin person, and best seen with a slanting light on the hunched back. Blood pressure may be normal despite coarctation for a number of reasons, e.g.

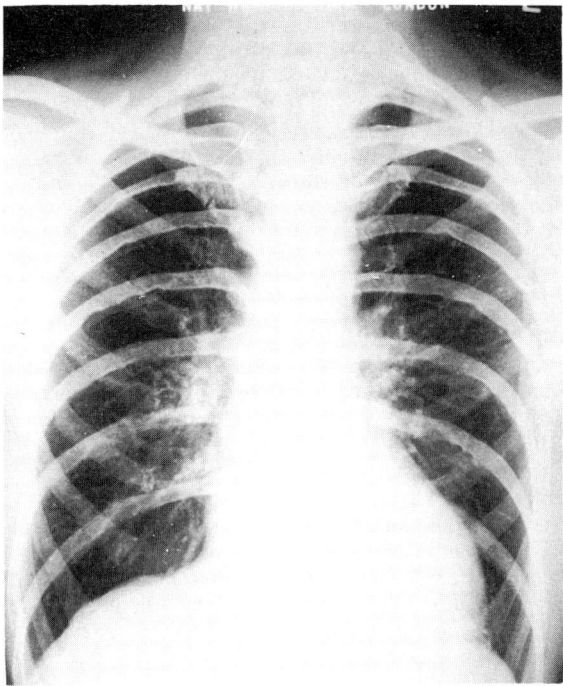

Fig. 17 Chest X-ray from an adult with coarctation of the thoracic aorta showing double (dented) aortic knuckle and bilateral marked rib notching on the under surfaces of the ribs.

severe aortic stenosis, left ventricular failure, aberrant right subclavian artery, stenosed origin of the left subclavian, both subclavians arising below the coarctation, dissection of the aorta, arterial emboli in infective endocarditis on the aortic valve, or after cardiac infarction. However, the femoral pulses are always absent or delayed – this routine feeling for femoral pulses is mandatory in every clinical examination for cardiovascular assessment.

Electrocardiogram The axis is normal. Left anterior hemiblock may develop over 45 years. Varying forms of right bundle branch pattern exist in 7 per cent, the residuum of right ventricular hypertrophy in the neonatal period or spontaneous closure of a ventricular septal defect. Left ventricular hypertrophy with high voltage and usually upright large T waves are to be expected but ST depression and T inversion are unusual unless there is aortic stenosis or regurgitation or both, cardiac infarction, or if the patient is aged over 50 years.

Chest X-ray There is a striking dilation of the ascending aorta and arch, with a double knuckle, and poststenotic dilation of the thoracic aorta (Fig. 17). Intercostal aneurysms may calcify. Lower rib notching suggests a lower coarctation or long segment.

Other features Associated cardiovascular anomalies include a duct (unusual in adolescents/adults), a small VSD, mitral regurgitation, and various abnormalities of the aortic valve. Bicuspid valves not initially stenosed may calcify and become so over the age of 40 years. Others, whether bicuspid or tricuspid, may be stenosed at a earlier age. Floppy or bicuspid valves may cause regurgitation, initially trivial but later significant. Fixed subaortic stenosis develops late, sometimes complicating spontaneous closure of a VSD.

The coronary arteries are abnormal, probably from birth, and hypertension accelerates the development of ischaemic heart disease. Myocardial disease relates not only to hypertension, but large areas of dysplasia, fibrosis, and subendocardial fibrosis which may cause papillary muscle dysfunction and mitral valve prolapse. Berry aneurysms in the cerebral circulation are recognized but rare associations.

Treatment

A coarctation causing elevation of the resting blood pressure should be treated surgically. When blood pressure is normal or only moderately increased, exercise hypertension appears in 95 per cent, which may justify surgical treatment. Over 60 years it is uncertain if removal of the coarctation improves prognosis unless considered necessary prior to treatment of a diseased aortic or mitral valve.

The risks of resecting coarctation in the adult are higher than in the child in view of the aortic changes, aneurysms, severe hypertension, and coronary disease.

Kinked aorta

This minor narrowing of the aortic isthmus looks like a mild coarctation angiographically. Gradients of 0–15 mmHg may be recorded. These are of no haemodynamic significance and require no therapy. In the differential diagnosis from coarctation it should be noted that there is no poststenotic dilation of the thoracic aorta, nor collateral development; femoral pulses are normal and hypertension is not characteristic although patients with kinked aorta may have associated essential hypertension. Associated congenital aortic valve anomalies may require attention.

Aorto-left ventricular 'tunnel' defect

This rare anomaly is a defect, not a tunnel, between the right aortic sinus and left ventricular outflow tract. It presents as serious aortic regurgitation, documented in early childhood. It is characterized by a wide pulse pressure, loud systolic and diastolic murmurs (with thrill) at the left sternal edge, and loud A_2 as the aortic valve cusps are voluminous and pliable. The right aortic sinus is so dilated that it may appear on the chest X-ray as a bulge above the right ventricular outflow; the ascending aorta is hugely dilated as is the left ventricle.

The differential diagnosis is from other causes of gross aortic regurgitation in young people and left coronary artery to left ventricular fistula. Treatment is by operation to close the defect and support the aortic root which is weak. By adolescence, the aortic root is so dilated that the aortic valve remains incompetent and valve replacement may be necessary. The lesion should be treated early in childhood.

Mitral regurgitation (page 13.288)

Minor congenital lesions of the mitral valve such as cleft of the anterior cusp, redundancy of cusp tissue or chordal anomalies may become symptomatic in adults through infective endocarditis, chordal rupture or slow progression of the regurgitation. Diagnosis and treatment is the same as for other forms of mitral regurgitation. When severe the patients present in infancy and childhood.

Left atrial obstruction

When this is of congenital origin, i.e. mitral valve stenosis/cor triatriatum or supramitral valve membrane, the patients do not usually reach adult life without earlier surgical treatment. Occasionally a cor triatriatum with a wide hole in it presents as mitral stenosis in late adolescence. In contrast to mitral stenosis, the left atrial appendage does not enlarge unless there is added valve regurgitation. The echo should make the correct diagnosis.

Communications between systemic and pulmonary circulations, i.e. septal defects

ATRIAL SEPTAL DEFECT

Defects in the atrial septum are often not detected until they cause symptoms in adult life. There are two anatomical groups.

Ostium secundum defects (see page 13.239)

These do not border the atrioventricular valves and are named according to the site in the atrial septum. They may be in the sinus venosus or secundum septum but are grouped together because of clinical similarity.

1. Oval fossa defects (75 per cent) are central, usually about 2 cm in diameter, but exceptionally smaller or much larger.

2. Inferior vena caval defects (7 per cent) are postero-inferior with no posterior rim of septal tissue. Particular problems of this defect are: (*a*) anomalous or pseudo-anomalous drainage of the right pulmonary veins which enter the right atrium close to the midline where the posterior atrial septum is missing; (*b*) a large Eustachian valve which may direct inferior vena caval blood across the defect and cause unexpected cyanosis; and (*c*) the inexperienced surgeon may close the defect and redirect the inferior vena cava to the left atrium resulting in a previously mildly or asymptomatic patient becoming breathless and mildly cyanosed with a small heart and absence of murmurs.

3. Superior vena caval defects (11 per cent) lie at the base of the superior vena cava and are associated with partial anomalous right upper and middle lobe pulmonary veins which enter the SVC and/or RA/SVC junction. The defect itself is usually smaller than other defects and the shunt is contributed to by the anomalous pulmonary veins through which the pulmonary flow is greater than through the normally draining pulmonary veins.

4. Coronary sinus defect. This is a rare ASD in the position of the coronary sinus which is absent or unroofed and sometimes associated with the left SVC entering the left atrium.

5. Other variants (7 per cent) include hemianomalous pulmonary venous drainage with or without ASD, and combinations of categories (1), (2), and (3). The whole atrial septum may be fenestrated.

Physiology

The presence of an interatrial hole permits a left-to-right shunt of blood from left atrium to right atrium once the filling resistance of the right ventricle becomes less than that of the left ventricle after the first weeks of life.

The effects of a long-standing interatrial left-to-right shunt are: (*a*) increased volume load and dilation of the right atrium and right ventricle; (*b*) increased pulmonary blood flow and enlarged pulmonary arteries; (*c*) increase in size of pulmonary veins (not upper lobes only as in left atrial obstruction); and (*d*) reduced flow to the left ventricle and aorta which become smaller than normal with time.

The factors which influence the blood flow across an ASD are: (*a*) compliance of the right ventricle; (*b*) compliance of the left ventricle; (*c*) the size of the defect – least important since most defects are of similar size; and (*d*) atrioventricular valve function. In sinus rhythm the left-to-right flow across the defect is mostly during diastole particularly during atrial systole but when atrial fibrillation occurs the shunt becomes systolic.

Increased flow across the defect is caused by left-sided lesions or by increased systemic resistance. The shunt is decreased by tricuspid valve disease, impaired right ventricular filling (myopathy, hypoplasia, fibrosis, pericardial effusion), by pulmonary stenosis, and pulmonary hypertension. Central cyanosis results from reversal of the shunt.

Symptoms/natural history

Infants are rarely symptomatic with uncomplicated ASD unless early arrhythmias develop as occurs in Holt Oram syndromes and some familial cases with added conducting tissue abnormalities. Symptoms usually develop in adult life, 10–20 per cent in the third decade, a few more in the fourth decade, and the majority over 40 years have complaints. By 50 years, 75 per cent have disability and heart failure, precipitated by atrial fibrillation; dyspnoea, bronchitis, palpitation, cyanosis, and chronic progressive failure continues

Table 6 Causes of central cyanosis in ASD with left to right shunt

Total anomalous pulmonary venous drainage
Hemianomalous pulmonary venous drainage
Cor triatriatum + 2 ASDs
IVC to LA
Huge ASD – common atrium
Abnormal RV, i.e. Ebstein, fibrotic with age
Tricuspid stenosis/regurgitation
Atrial fibrillation
Mild right sided obstructive lesions
Bradycardia

with haemoptysis. Elderly patients over 60 years who remain in sinus rhythm may slip into right heart failure from chronic fibrosis in the stretched ventricle. Paradoxical emboli are rare but do occur particularly with extracardiac surgery or trauma. Pulmonary hypertension occurs in about 8 per cent producing massive cardiac enlargement, cyanosis, and severe failure. It is acquired (see Eisenmenger) in relation to thromboembolism, pregnancy, and life at high altitude. Patients with ASD over 50 years or earlier can acquire ischaemic heart disease and essential hypertension which may precipitate cardiac failure. When atrial fibrillation complicates a small ASD, the ASD may be overlooked as the heart may not be enlarged and the signs are subtle.

Signs

Girls with ASD are said to be slender (gracile habitus). Usually, but not always, the adults are slim. If the defect is large or complicated, a malar flush may be present. Pulses are normal or small if complicated by mitral disease, with moderate to large shunt. Sinus arrhythmia is lost. The venous pulsations are prominent (as in high output states, anaemia, thyrotoxicosis, pregnancy). Central cyanosis can be seen in patients with a left-to-right shunt through an ASD (Table 6).

The right ventricle is overactive and dilated and the left ventricular impulse is usually impalpable. On auscultation the first sound is loud (tricuspid valve closure) and often split, sometimes widely. The second heart sound is widely split in inspiration and expiration. The time interval between $A_2–P_2$ is often fixed to the ear but may widen on inspiration, and not close on expiration when the defect is small or when partial anomalous pulmonary veins contribute more to the shunt than ASD, or in the presence of anomalous caval drainage. The $A_2–P_2$ interval in adults is about 0.06 s. It becomes unusually wide with bradycardia, right ventricular failure, mild pulmonary stenosis, complete right bundle branch block, and severe mitral regurgitation which makes A_2 louder. Delay in A_2, making the split narrower, can occur with left ventricular disease and aortic valve stenosis.

Pulmonary valve closure is loud in adults with ASD irrespective of pulmonary artery pressure. A pulmonary systolic click is usual suggesting pulmonary hypertension which is not necessarily present.

The classic auscultatory features of ASD are shown (Fig. 18). The diastolic murmur is not present in very small defects and in very large hearts with tricuspid regurgitation since the ring is too

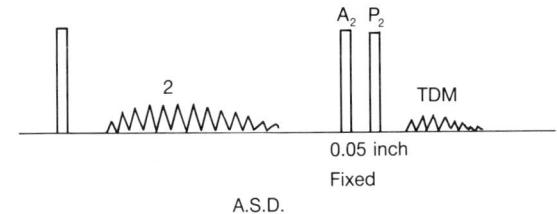

Fig. 18 Auscultation in ASD. TDM = tricuspid diastolic murmur. (Reproduced by courtesy of Dr P. Wood.)

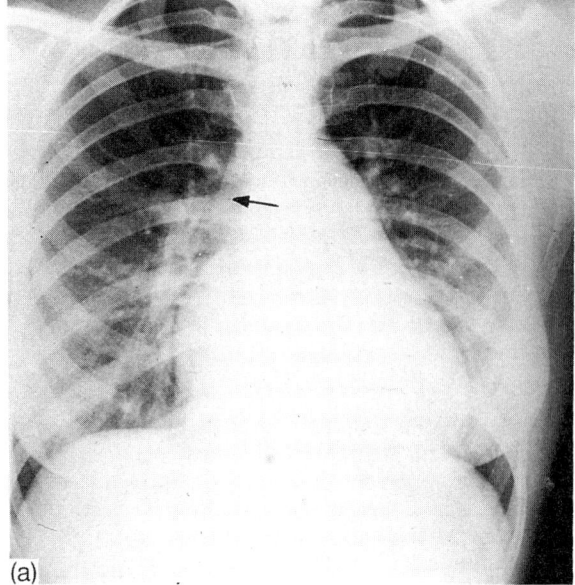

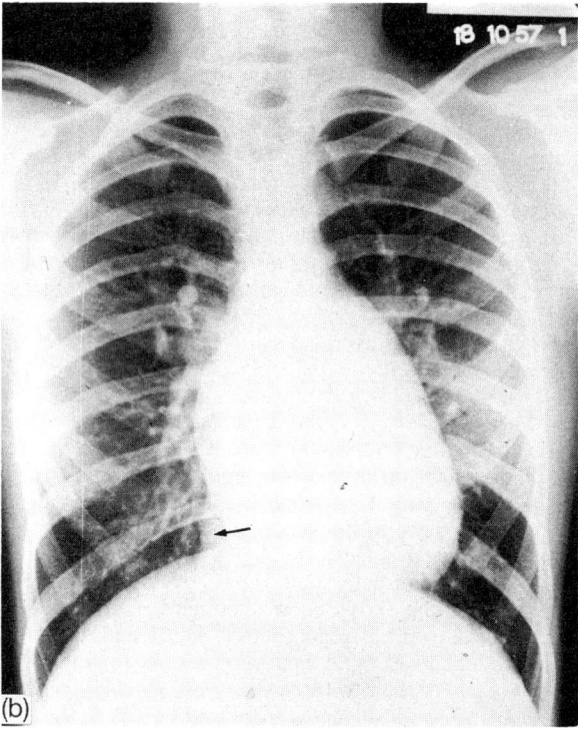

Fig. 19 Chest X-rays from patients with 'secundum' ASD showing cardio-megaly, pulmonary plethora, and small aorta. Special features are: (a) Dilated superior vena cava (arrow) because there is anomalous right upper lobe pulmonary vein entering it in association with SVC defect. (b) Dilation of IVC opposite the uncommon IVC defect.

large to offer any resistance to the torrential flow. A pansystolic murmur occurs in patients in failure from tricuspid regurgitation. Apical murmurs from added mitral valve dysfunction appear frequently with advancing years and a pulmonary diastolic murmur is common over 50 years or in younger patients with pulmonary hypertension.

The chest X-ray of patients in sinus rhythm is typical (Figs. 19a, b). The left atrium is usually normal. The heart size slowly increases over decades with dramatic increase once atrial fibrillation is established. Upper lobe pulmonary veins appear dilated and in the lower lobes, horizontal lines appear like 'Kerley lines',

but thicker and often branching. Shadows of pulmonary infarction *in situ* are frequent. The pulmonary arteries can become aneurys-mal with calcification in atheromatous walls.

The ECG shows right axis deviation, sharp right atrial P waves, slight prolongation of the P–R interval, partial right bundle branch block and absent QR in V_5–V_6. With increasing age there is pro-longation of the P–R interval, an increase in the height of second-ary R.waves (right ventricular hypertension) increasing width of the QRS, and progressive T inversion across RV leads without necessarily increased voltage. Left axis deviation may be present in 7 per cent with secundum defects or may be acquired. P mitrale may develop when the P–R interval is greater than 0.20 s or because of paroxysmal supraventricular rhythm disorder or associ-ated mitral stenosis. Prolongation of the P–R interval above 0.20 s occurs in huge ASDs, in patients over 40 years, sometimes in the Holt Oram syndrome, and occasionally for no obvious reason. Over 40 years pulmonary hypertension (systolic) may develop and increase right ventricular hypertrophy as shown by large R waves in right chest leads.

Cross-sectional echocardiography should show the ASD but sometimes in adults it is difficult to find a clear window to profile the atrial septum. SVC defects are the most difficult to see.

Differential diagnosis

Differential diagnosis of ASD includes particularly mild pulmon-ary stenosis. In elderly patients with cardiomegaly and atrial fibril-lation the condition may mimic cor pulmonale and rheumatic mitral disease or even cardiomyopathy.

Treatment

Atrial septal defects which give rise to physical signs should be closed by operation with few exceptions. These are raised pulmon-ary vascular resistance with severe cyanosis (Eisenmenger), and patients over 65 years with small shunts. The adult over 50 years may present difficulties in assessment as the pulmonary vascular disease may appear more advanced than it is because of the huge pulmonary artery, ejection click, and ringing P_2. Older patients with chronic failure and established atrial fibrillation do benefit but there is a higher morbidity from persistence of recurrent ar-rhythmias, mitral regurgitation, and persistent cardiomegaly.

Patients operated on in the first two decades of life have excel-lent long-term results. They do not suffer from endocarditis unless there are left-sided valve problems. Mitral regurgitation occasion-ally appears. The heart size and electrocardiographic changes regress. The patient may retain an ejection click. Some adults 15–25 years after surgery suffer supraventricular rhythm dis-orders, sometimes nodal bradycardia, and rarely complete block. Whether these are due to surgical trauma or natural history is unknown. Pre-operative rhythm disorders should not prevent physicians referring for surgery the asymptomatic or symptomatic patients because the closure reduces not only the incidence but also the effects of rhythm disturbances. The operation can be con-sidered as 90–95 per cent curative in young patients.

Atrioventricular defects

These account for about 5–10 per cent of all atrial septal defects. These defects with a sickle-shaped cephalad border are in the lower (caudal) part of the atrial septum bounded by the atrioven-tricular valves which are also nearly always anatomically abnor-mal. Other shared anatomical characteristics which enable them to be grouped together are that mitral and tricuspid valves lie at the same level, the outflow of the left ventricle is unusually long and the upper border of the ventricular septum, frequently deficient, is depressed caudally. These features result in abnormal attachment of the mitral valve which gives rise to diagnostic appearances on angiography and echocardiography.

The three major forms are:

1. Ostium primum (75 per cent). The anterior cusp of the mitral

valve is cleft and 20 per cent also have abnormalities of the septal cusp of the tricuspid valve which are probably of no clinical significance. The ventricular septum is functionally intact.

2. Common atrioventricular canal (20 per cent). There are functional atrial and ventricular defects with atrioventricular valve cusps draped like curtains across the defect with and without formation of separate valve rings. Occasionally patients live to adult life with severe pulmonary vascular disease, when anatomy is unusual, e.g. when cusp tissue blocks a VSD or there is mild pulmonary stenosis. There are intermediate anatomical forms of (1) and (2).

3. Common atrium (5 per cent). These patients sometimes reach the third decade. The atrial septum is completely absent or remains as a shallow posterior ridge. The atrioventricular valves and ventricular septum are as in (1) or (2) so that patients present as an ostium primum or common canal with special features. Those who survive the first 10 years usually but not always have a functionally intact ventricular septum. There is frequent association of anomalous drainage of the vena cavae, midline liver, situs ambiguus, and left isomerism. Atrioventricular valves may be normal in rare cases.

Ostium primum defect

The physiology is similar to that of ostium secundum defects. Early pulmonary vascular disease is uncommon unless the defect is large, mitral regurgitation is severe, or there are added lesions such as supramitral valve membrane, coarctation, or duct. Mitral regurgitation increases the left-to-right shunt and in many there is a left ventricular/right atrial shunt through the apex of the cleft. The natural history is worse than in ostium secundum ASD because of the mitral regurgitation and the disturbance of conducting tissue. Behind the posterior edge of the defect is the A–V node and beneath is the bundle of His. Both may become damaged by turbulent flow. Although some patients become symptomatic in childhood and even infancy, the majority reach the second decade. Symptoms come from rhythm disturbances most frequently nodal, complete block, and less frequently and later atrial fibrillation. Infective endocarditis may cause death. Pulmonary vascular disease (Eisenmenger) develops in about 8 per cent. Patients with ostium primum defect can survive to the eighth decade but most die before 30 years. The symptoms are as in other ASDs but with the addition of infective endocarditis and syncope from heart block. Paroxysmal nodal tachycardia and bradycardia may start in adolescence. Signs are also similar to those of secundum patients but with the addition of pansystolic murmur from an incompetent mitral valve in 75 per cent which tends to increase with inspiration. The chest X-ray is also similar but the left atrium is enlarged in 20 per cent.

The striking feature in the ECG which distinguishes ostium primum defects from ostium secundum is the presence of left axis deviation (LAD) in the standard leads associated with an rSR in V_1 and other features typical of ASD (Fig. 20). LAD occurs in 93–97 per cent. When severe right ventricular hypertrophy coexists, the axis may be shifted to the right shoulder and the pattern of ventricular activation may be less easily recognized from the standard leads. Careful scrutiny of the initial direction of the QRS in the frontal plane will provide the clue for there is a qR in lead I and an RS in lead III with a persistent dominant S in lead II. Added right ventricular hypertrophy which shifts the axis towards the right shoulder may be caused by associated pulmonary stenosis, pulmonary hypertension, and coarctation. A normal electrical axis or RAD may occur in unusually small ostium primum defects (2 per cent), in the presence of left bundle branch block, or exceptionally for no obvious reason. Fifty per cent have unusual prolongation of the P–R interval, and P mitrale is common.

Diagnosis

The diagnosis of ostium primum should be made in a patient with the signs of ASD and mitral regurgitation and an ECG showing

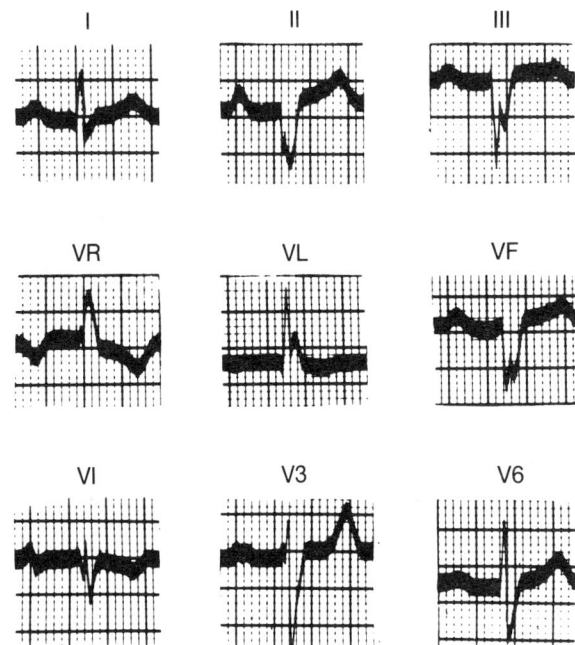

Fig. 20 Typical ECG from patient with ostium primum atrial septal defect (an atrioventricular defect) showing long P–R interval, left axis deviation, and an rSR in V_1.

LAD or abnormal initial activation. Two-dimensional echocardiography shows the lesion clearly as does left ventricular angiography which demonstrates the abnormal outflow and characteristic attachment of the anterior cusp of the mitral valve.

Differential diagnosis

Ostium primum must be differentiated from ostium secundum with LAD, ostium secundum with associated mitral regurgitation, or separate VSD.

Treatment

Closure of ostium primum defects and repair of mitral clefts causing regurgitation is recommended in all patients unless there is advanced pulmonary vascular disease, a small shunt below 1.7:1 (pulmonary to systemic flow) or very abnormal mitral valve anatomy. However, if the patient is symptom-free with evidence of tethered, deficient cusps with palisades of abnormal papillary muscles it is worthwhile delaying to prevent premature valve replacement. Mitral valve replacement in A–V defects has special risks and difficulties because of the long abnormal outflow which may be impinged upon and narrowed by a prosthesis thereby creating subaortic stenosis.

Despite good anatomical 'correction' there may be late problems. Morbidity and mortality are caused by arrhythmias particularly nodal and complete block, and mitral regurgitation which progresses if originally moderate or severe. Endocarditis may develop on mitral valves and rarely subaortic stenosis may progress. There is therefore a need for continued informed supervision of these patients.

Common atrioventricular canal

This is the most severe form of atrioventricular defect with a significant ventricular component of the defect and frequently very abnormal atrioventricular valves or a common valve. Most patients die in infancy or childhood, but survival to adolescence or adult life is possible without prior surgical help when defects are small (5 per cent), in the absence of atrioventricular valve regurgitation (15 per cent), the presence of Eisenmenger reaction (so frequent in Mongols), or moderate pulmonary valve stenosis. Older

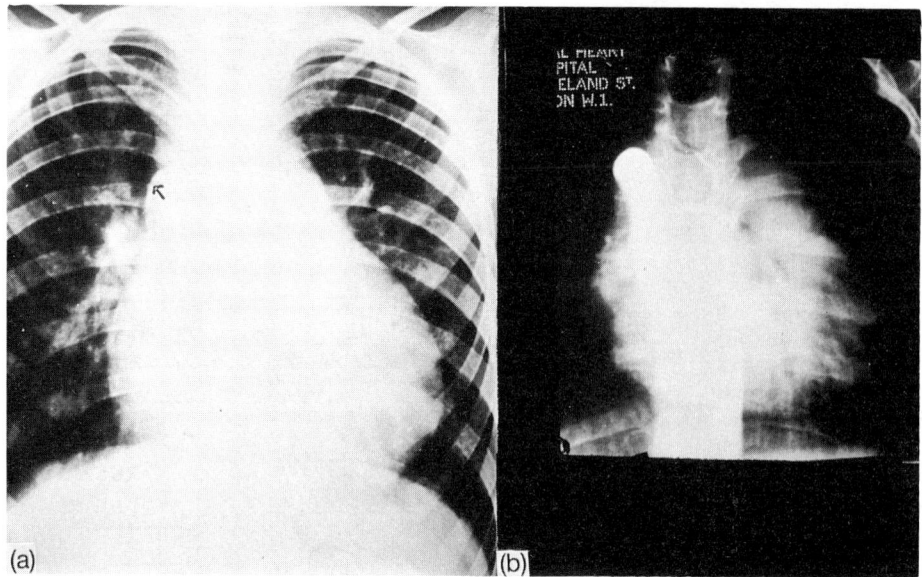

Fig. 21 Chest X-ray and venogram to show dilated azygos vein (arrow) which drains the inferior vena caval blood from a patient with common atrium. IVC ascends on left and crosses the midline to enter azygos.

patients present with cyanosis, rhythm disturbances, haemoptysis, and respiratory infections and cerebral abscess. The physical signs vary according to whether the patient has the Eisenmenger reaction, pulmonary stenosis, or a small defect. The second sound is closely split or single according to the size of the VSD and there may be mitral regurgitation which can be the dominant lesion with a small defect.

The heart is globular on chest X-ray with small aortic knuckle and large pulmonary artery. Radiographic features depend on the size of the shunt and pulmonary blood flow. The left atrium is enlarged unless the atrial component of the defect is large.

The ECG shares typical features with the other atrioventricular defects such as left axis or modified LAD (SI, II, III patterns) and severe right ventricular hypertrophy with a large left-to-right ventricular shunt and large equiphasic complexes in the anterior chest leads with evidence of left ventricular volume overload (QR V_5, V_6) appear (Fig. 20). The P–R interval is prolonged in about 20 per cent.

Diagnosis

Diagnosis is confirmed by echocardiography and angiography. Problems tend to occur in the first 10 years after repair and are similar to those found with repaired ostium primum defect, namely, rhythm disturbances, nodal and complete heart block, symptomatic mitral regurgitation; less frequently stenosis, or chronic haemolysis. Some suffer from progressive pulmonary vascular disease. Dramatic improvement in survival and quality of life is obtained in many survivors.

Common atrium

This is found in 5 per cent of atrioventricular defects. Patients present with signs and symptoms of ostium primum defect or common atrioventricular canal. Only a few survive to the second decade. The diagnosis should be suspected when the patient has the features of A–V defect combined with any one or more of the following: (a) unexpected central cyanosis; (b) situs ambiguus (stomach on right, apex on left or vice versa); (c) abnormal inferior vena caval drainage to the left SVC (via hemiazygos) or right SVC (azygos), or both. The dilated inferior vena cava may be recognized when seen end-on as a coin-shaped shadow in the SVC on the straight X-ray (Fig. 21). The IVC may also drain to the coronary sinus; (d) inverted P waves in standard leads or changing P waves and nodal rhythm; and (e) associated with Ellis van Creveld dwarfism.

The diagnosis is confirmed by cross-sectional echocardiography and angiography.

Surgical treatment

Partitioning of the atrium and repair of the mitral valve with closure of the ventricular septal defect as in other atrioventricular defects is advisable provided pulmonary vascular disease is not severe. Even then, the patient may benefit symptomatically when cyanosis and hypoxic symptoms are abolished. Estimating pulmonary vascular resistance in these patients is difficult in view of the mixing which causes a right-to-left shunt, increased by vena cavae entering to the left of the atrium and causing systemic streaming. Following operation, patients with septated common atrium have more problems with rhythm disorders than do those with other forms of atrioventricular defects. Progressive pulmonary vascular disease appears unexpectedly, particularly with residual mitral regurgitation when the new left atrium is small.

Ventricular septal defect

There is still debate on the nomenclature of VSD which occur at several sites. The natural history is dependent not only on the size of the defect but also the site. A simple classification relating the defect to the contiguous valve – subvalvar – or its site in the muscular septum is used. Defects are thus described as subaortic, subpulmonary, doubly committed subarterial (subpulmonary and subaortic), subtricuspid, and submitral (inlet defects) (Fig. 22). When subaortic they do not close spontaneously as the cephalad border is the aortic valve. In contrast, defects beneath the septal cusp of the tricuspid valve close spontaneously or become small and are the VSDs seen most frequently in adults; small single VSDs also behave like this. Large subaortic or subarterial defects are found in adults manifesting as the Eisenmenger syndrome or mild Fallot. Small subpulmonary or doubly committed subarterial defects in adults present with aortic regurgitation; indeed the prolapsed right aortic cusp may completely close the defect and even cause right ventricular obstruction. Inlet VSD associated with left axis deviation and frequent atrioventricular valve anomalies (subtricuspid and submitral) is rarely found in adults.

VSDs which occur in association with corrected transposition, double outflow right, and left ventricles, tricuspid atresia, and transposition require different classification, as the morphology and landmarks of the right ventricle are different.

Adults and adolescents with VSD appear as follows: (a) small VSD, without elevation of right ventricular pressure and a shunt below 2:1; (b) moderate-sized VSD with slight elevation of RV pressure and infundibular gradient, and shunts between 2 and 2.5:1; and (c) large ventricular septal defect in association with (i) advanced pulmonary vascular disease (Eisenmenger syndrome) or (ii) infundibular and/or mild pulmonary valve stenosis.

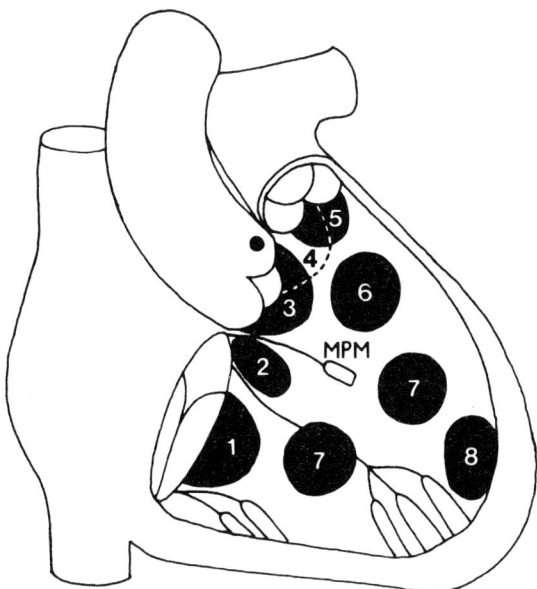

Fig. 22 Diagram to show simple classification of types of VSD as seen from the right ventricle. 1–5, subvalvar; 1, inlet; 2, subtricuspid; 3, subaortic; 4, subarterial doubly committed; 5, subpulmonary; 6–8, muscular; 6, outlet; 7, central; 8, apical; MPM, medial papillary muscle.

Symptoms and signs

These relate to the size of the defect and complications. Problems present with VSD as follows:

1. Infective endocarditis most commonly caused by *Streptococcus viridans* which tends to take an insidious course with low-grade fever, non-specific disability, episodes of unexplained cough diagnosed as 'bronchitis', 'pleurisy', or pneumonitis; the true diagnosis is masked by injudicious use of short courses of antimicrobials handed out in the practitioner's surgery. These symptoms in a previously well patient with a pansystolic murmur demand immediate blood cultures. The vegetations may appear on the tricuspid valve, jet lesions opposite or around the defect, or on the aortic valve and may become large enough to obstruct the outflow tract or tricuspid valve. Cross-sectional echocardiography provides an excellent method for following the size and behaviour of the vegetations. One attack is an indication for surgical closure of the VSD and there is a place for removal of a large vegetation.

2. Atrial fibrillation after age 30 years can precipitate right-sided congestion with tricuspid regurgitation. It may occur spontaneously or in association with pulmonary emboli or lung infections from other causes. Treatment is to convert the patient to sinus rhythm, if possible. It may be worthwhile closing the VSD, however small, as the left ventricular to right atrial shunt can be surprisingly large preventing maintenance of sinus rhythm.

3. Aortic regurgitation may develop with a small VSD (outflow, subarterial) in adult life and progress to embarrass left ventricular function. Reflux can also appear with subaortic VSD although these are less common in adults. It may be acquired as the result of infective endocarditis on an abnormal aortic valve or through prolapse of an aortic cusp – usually the right coronary. The signs of VSD may disappear as the cusp blocks the small defect. There is usually a history of a murmur dating from infancy or childhood. The most common VSDs in adults are beneath the septal cusp of the tricuspid valve already partially closed. In them aortic regurgitation is acquired from spreading infection or primary abnormality of the valve.

The differential diagnosis of VSD with aortic reflux is from causes of a continuous murmur which include ductus, fistulae, ruptured sinus of Valsalva aneurysm, and aortic valve disease. The treatment is surgical and if the aortic regurgitation is due to pro-

lapse, mild or moderate, it should be possible to conserve the aortic valve by repair. If the regurgitation is severe with ring dilation, the valve may have to be replaced to relieve the haemodynamic load on the left ventricle.

4. Aneurysm of the ventricular septum which normally produces no clinical problems. It is an acquired abnormality from spontaneous closure of a VSD beneath the septal cusp of the tricuspid valve which becomes adherent to the margins of the defect and forms an aneurysm which can be identified by two-dimensional echocardiography and left ventricular angiography. Sometimes there is a small hole in it where the defect has not completely closed. There is usually a fibrous reaction around these aneurysms and it is possible for this to invade the conducting tissue causing heart block or a change of electrical axis. If the tricuspid tissue is redundant or voluminous, the aneurysm can enlarge to cause pulmonary stenosis. It does not obstruct the tricuspid valve since it distends in systole.

5. Large left ventricle disproportionate to the expected size for a small VSD. There may be associated electrocardiographic and echocardiographic abnormalities. Either this is a residuum of the effects of a volume overload earlier in life or it is a manifestation of diffuse cardiovascular disease of which the small VSD is one part. Prolapsed mitral cusp may be found in these patients.

6. Spontaneous closure of a VSD which is most common in childhood, but may occur at any age.

Diagnosis of small/moderate VSD

Pulses, venous pressure, and apex beat are normal. There is a pansystolic murmur, moderate or intense and associated with a thrill, maximal at the left sternal edge in the third or fourth interspace, and easily heard at the apex. The murmur is expiratory and occasionally conducted to the right sternal edge. In a very small VSD the murmur may be early systolic or late systolic, opened by a click from the tensing aneurysm of the septum, thus resembling the signs of prolapsed mitral cusp. Sometimes P_2 is slightly delayed if there is associated hypertrophy of the infundibulum or right bundle branch block. With larger VSDs the left ventricle is prominent and overactive and a delayed diastolic murmur is present at the apex.

The chest X-ray can be normal or with prominence of the infundibulum. Pulmonary arteries are normal or slightly enlarged, and the aorta is normal. The left atrium is visible in some with shunts over 2:1 and the left ventricle may be prominent.

The electrocardiogram may be normal. The axis may be leftward or there may be true LAD. A mild form of rSr is frequent in V_1 with features of LV dominance and upright T waves in V_5 and V_6. The addition of aortic regurgitation leads to features of left ventricular overload and even ST–T changes. The presence of pulmonary stenosis may shift the axis to the right and result in right ventricular hypertrophy. Diagnosis is confirmed by two-dimensional echocardiography or left ventricular angiography.

Treatment

Treatment (surgical closure) depends upon symptoms and complications. Without them none is necessary. The prognosis of a small VSD is generally excellent if aortic regurgitation and endocarditis are excluded.

Complications

Many patients have now survived to adult life having had earlier surgical closure of a VSD. Most are symptom-free. However, the following problems have required attention: (*a*) early and late heart block which is rare nowadays; (*b*) ectopics and ventricular tachycardia; (*c*) late sino-atrial problems; (*d*) myocardial damage and dysfunction manifesting as failure which relates to bypass technique or other complications; (*e*) tricuspid and mitral regurgitation, aortic regurgitation; and (*f*) progressive pulmonary hypertension leading to death. This is not as rare as one might hope. There are patients in whom there was pulmonary hypertension before operation but enough left to right shunt to consider and carry out closure of the ventricular septal defect. In them the pulmonary artery pressures may have fallen to 45–60 mmHg at operation, but although resting systolic pressures then settle at 35–50 mmHg much higher figures are reached on exercise so that ultimately vascular disease becomes established and irreversible. Lung biopsy at the time of the operation may give a more accurate idea of the future than the measured PAP at rest. This disastrous and sometimes surprising course can occur after closure of large VSDs but has also been seen after large duct ligation, aortopulmonary window, truncus operation, and Rastelli operation for banded transposition with VSD. If there is doubt about the normality of the pulmonary arterioles, patients should be discouraged from mountaineering, living at high altitude, taking the contraceptive pill, slimming drugs, or indulging in athletics. The question of pregnancy requires careful, informed judgement. Obstetric care must be optimal with expert cardiological and intensive care available at delivery.

Residual VSD despite surgery is common in patients operated on before 1974–75. Patients with residual VSD or left-sided valve lesions should be protected from infective endocarditis.

Sinus of Valsalva aneurysm

Occasionally all three sinuses of Valsalva are aneurysmally dilated but this is usually due to acquired disease. One sinus of Valsalva may be aneurysmal due to deficiency or absence of aortic media and this is congenital. Aneurysmal dilation of a sinus may occur during endocarditis on the aortic valve. The right aortic sinus is most commonly affected. The lesions may be silent or enlarged to cause right ventricular obstruction or affect the conducting tissue causing heart block or left anterior hemiblock. Rupture into the right ventricle or right atrium occurs in men more than women. The patient may complain of a tearing sensation in the chest, becomes rapidly breathless, and soon develops congestive heart failure with hepatomegaly, ascites, and oedema. A loud continuous murmur is heard at the left or right sternal edge. The ECG may show a long P–R interval, right bundle branch block, and mild voltage increase. The chest X-ray shows cardiomegaly and enlargement of the right atrium and right ventricle with mild pulmonary plethora. Sometimes linear calcification of the aortic sinus is seen.

Aortography and right heart catheterization delineate the site and source of the shunt. Surgical closure is urgently required provided infection has been treated or excluded. It may be necessary to operate during active infection. The diagnosis is made from the acute history and finding of continuous murmur to the right or lower left of the sternum and heart failure with a jerky pulse. The condition must be distinguished from other causes of continuous murmur, e.g. dissection of the aorta and aortic regurgitation or other fistulae.

Coronary artery anomalies

Congenital anomalies of the coronary arteries are often symptomless but may cause premature angina, sudden death, or persistent ventricular ectopics or even underlie a cardiomyopathy. A left coronary artery arising from the pulmonary artery may be detected first in adult life but death is common in infancy or later in childhood. It may present with a continuous murmur with evidence of infarction (anterolateral wide Q waves) on the ECG, or with a left ventricular aneurysm in a young person, or mitral regurgitation with infarcted anterolateral wall, or as sudden death.

Treatment is surgical with closure of the fistula and grafting of the left coronary artery into the aorta. It does nothing for previous infarction but may help angina and diminish chances of sudden death.

Single coronary arteries may be discovered in young patients with angina or dilated left ventricle appearing as congestive myopathy.

Coronary artery fistulae may cause a continuous murmur at the left sternal edge and enter the right ventricular outflow, the right atrium, or exceptionally the left ventricle. With long-standing fistulae they may 'steal' from the other coronary arteries and the myocardium causing angina. Calcification may develop in the orifice and in the coronary sinus where the clot may be laid down. Aneurysmal dilation of the vessel and sinus often occur by the time the patient is adult and this may be visible on the chest X-ray. The ECG may show left ventricular volume overload sometimes with anterior ischaemia. The normal resting T waves may invert or flatten on effort.

The fistulae should be closed from within the atrium or ventricle without damaging the normal coronary artery supply. Differential diagnosis is from a duct, if the continuous murmur is at the left sternal edge, other fistulae such as internal mammary, or ruptured sinus which is usually associated with important symptoms and failure. Aortography and selective coronary angiography will make the diagnosis together with oxygen saturation determination in the right heart.

AORTOPULMONARY SHUNTS

Persistent duct (ductus arteriosus)

When the duct remains open into the second decade and thereafter, a left-to-right shunt runs from the isthmus below the aortic knuckle into the top of the bifurcation of the pulmonary arteries. The main pulmonary artery and branches dilate and may cause pulmonary regurgitation, which is common although difficult to separate from the continuous murmur. The pulmonary veins, left atrium, left ventricle, and aorta (ascending and arch) are dilated from accommodating the increased volume of blood. The pulmonary artery systolic pressure may be moderately elevated and the diastolic pressure is low. The levels depend on the age of the patient, size of duct, and where the patient was born, i.e. at sea level or above 3000 m. The pulmonary and systemic pressures may be equal with a balanced or reversed shunt.

Symptoms include breathlessness if there is ventricular dysfunction. Atrial fibrillation may result in heart failure. Infective endocarditis may cause the first symptoms.

Signs

The pulse is jerky and the carotids prominent. The left ventricle is overactive and dilated. The pulmonary artery is often palpable. A continuous murmur, enhanced on expiration, is best heard in the second left intercostal space, loudest near the second heart sound, which is normally split with a loud pulmonary component. A delayed diastolic murmur may be heard at the apex. With large ducts there may be no continuous murmur; instead there is a variable length systolic murmur in the pulmonary area. A pulmonary ejection click is common and the signs of pulmonary regurgitation may be obvious.

The chest X-ray shows cardiomegaly, pulmonary plethora, and large left atrium, pulmonary arteries, and aortic knuckle. Calcium is visible in the duct over 35 years and may be diagnostic when signs are atypical.

The ECG shows left ventricular dominance with large Q waves and increased volume. Occasionally the T waves are flattened or depressed but if inverted may mean added aortic stenosis. The axis is usually normal with exceptional left deviation. Right ventricular hypertrophy only occurs if there is serious pulmonary vascular disease.

The differential diagnosis is from conditions such as VSD with aortic regurgitation, aortic stenosis with regurgitation, or absent pulmonary valve with pulmonary regurgitation. Other diagnoses to consider include aortopulmonary defect, internal mammary or coronary fistulae, pulmonary artery stenosis, pulmonary arteriovenous fistula, and left coronary artery arising from the pulmonary artery.

Treatment

Surgical ligation/section of all ducts which allow a left-to-right shunt is recommended. Although a simple operation with good results, it should be performed by an experienced surgeon; the duct in an adult is treacherous as the tissue may tear or the aorta split.

Aortopulmonary window

This lesion is rare in children and even more uncommon in adults when it is associated with the Eisenmenger reaction. It presents with the same features as a duct but more accentuated because the defect is larger and thus more likely to be associated with pulmonary hypertension and serious pulmonary vascular disease.

The diagnostic problems relate to distinguishing this lesion from a large duct or a large ventricular septal defect. A continuous murmur is exceptional – usually there is a long systolic murmur (not pan) in those with a significant left-to-right shunt and features of pulmonary hypertension; there is often right ventricular hypertrophy.

Common trunk (truncus arteriosus)

Most patients with this lesion die in infancy or early childhood. When seen in adults the condition is complicated by pulmonary vascular disease (Eisenmenger) or rarely by pulmonary artery stenosis.

A single trunk arises from the heart and gives off both pulmonary arteries from the ascending aorta. When the pulmonary arteries arise from descending aorta, the condition is almost always one of pulmonary atresia with a 'blind' atretic right ventricular outflow in front of the aorta. Beneath the common trunk is a large subtruncal VSD and so blood from both ventricles is ejected into the trunk, the amount passing to the pulmonary circulation depending on the pulmonary arteriolar resistance. When pulmonary blood flow predominates, the pulses are full, even collapsing with visible carotids and a palpable enlarged unfolded aorta, particularly obvious when there is a right arch (15 per cent). There is a long systolic murmur, single second sound, sometimes with several components caused by asynchronous closure of 2–5 cusps, together with an immediate diastolic murmur and delayed diastolic apical murmur from increased flow across the mitral valve. There is biventricular hypertrophy and left atrial enlargement together with unusual high, large pulmonary artery branches on chest X-ray. A trace of cyanosis is usual particularly after exercise. The ECG looks like that of VSD. Large QR patterns in V_5-V_6 suggest volume overload of the left ventricle and the possibility of benefit from surgical repair. Diagnosis is confirmed by two-dimensional echocardiography and angiography.

Surgical treatment

Patients with this lesion are probably inoperable by the second decade of life. They have survived because of raised pulmonary vascular resistance. Trunks have been repaired in adolescents with successful late results. Collapsing pulses, little or no cyanosis, a large left ventricle, and pulmonary plethora suggest suitability for operation. The principles of repair are to close the VSD, leaving the trunk connected to the left ventricle, cutting the pulmonary artery origins from the trunk, and joining them to the right ventricle by a valved conduit and closing the hole in the trunk. Late results depend on what conduit had been used and the residual pulmonary vascular disease which may advance.

Hemitrunk

This is a condition where one pulmonary artery arises from the aorta and the other from the right ventricle or is absent. A VSD with pulmonary valve stenosis or atresia may be associated. The physical signs present as a mixture of Fallot and truncus. The chest X-ray shows a marked difference in the perfusion and vascular pattern of the lungs. By the time adult life has been reached irreversible damage to the lung supplied by the pulmonary artery arising from the aorta is likely. If the patient has pulmonary stenosis, it may be worthwhile relieving this or creating a systemic to pulmonary artery shunt on that side. Death from this condition is either from attempted surgery, massive haemoptysis or cerebral abscess.

References

Roberts, W. C. (1979). *Congenital heart disease in adults*. Davis, Philadelphia.

Somerville, J. (1979). Congenital heart disease – changes in form and function. *Br. Heart J.* **41**, 1–22.

Wood, P. (1958). The Eisenmenger syndrome. *Br. med. J.* **2**, 701–709, 755–762.

RHEUMATIC FEVER

J. M. NEUTZE

Rheumatic fever is an illness predominantly of childhood, with major symptoms of arthritis and carditis, a prolonged course and a tendency to recur. It is widely held to be an abnormal immune reaction to an infection with a Group A beta-haemolytic streptococcus. Despite decades of intensive study, the nature of this reaction remains obscure and, in many ways, rheumatic fever is still an enigma. Although the major cause of acquired heart disease in children, rheumatic fever has declined dramatically in the Western world since the 1920s. In underdeveloped countries, it remains a major problem with annual incidence rates of 100–1000 per 100 000 in the childhood age group, compared with fewer than 5 per 100 000 in most Western countries.

Aetiology and pathogenesis

The streptococcus

An association between septic throats and rheumatic fever was noted in the nineteenth century, and in the 1930s there were many reports of outbreaks of rheumatic fever following tonsillitis or scarlet fever in closed communities. With the development of serological tests for streptococcal infections and Lancefield's classification according to the carbohydrate moiety, it became possible to establish the aetiological role of the group A beta-haemolytic streptococcus. Reduction by penicillin treatment of the number of cases of rheumatic fever in epidemics of streptococcal infections, and the near abolition of recurrences with successful penicillin prophylaxis, provide powerful supporting evidence of the role of the streptococcus.

The way in which the streptococcus causes rheumatic fever is still only partly understood. Characteristics of the streptococcus are critical. The organism must be able to attach firmly to pharyngeal cells and produce a brisk antigenic response. Impetigo strains do not cause rheumatic fever. Rheumatic fever has followed infection with many M serotypes, of which there are more than 70, but much more commonly in some (particularly M5) and rarely, if ever, in others (especially M12). The properties of the streptococcus are described in detail on page 5.168.

Streptococci do not persist in cardiac tissues in rheumatic patients. Both the peptidoglycan moiety of the cell wall and Streptolysins O and S have produced cellular damage in experimental situations, but no animal model of rheumatic fever has been developed.

The host reaction
A number of observations have suggested an immune mechanism. The latent period, generally higher antistreptococcal titres in patients who develop rheumatic fever compared with those who do not, and the transient appearance of circulating immune complexes are compatible with such a mechanism. Antiheart antibodies are commonly present in patients with rheumatic fever. It is intriguing that antibodies generated in animals to many streptococcal components cross-react with cardiac tissues. There is also interest in alterations in some lymphocyte responses to streptococcal products in rheumatic patients, raising the possibility of cell-mediated cytotoxic reactions. Much needs to be done before these pieces of the jigsaw can be put together, but an abnormal immune response to infections with certain streptococci remains likely.

Although rheumatic fever is often familial, evidence of a genetic defect is weak. In some communities there is an association with certain racial groups. In Britain, rheumatic fever is much commoner in Asian immigrants, and in New Zealand it is 10 times more common in the Polynesian than in the Caucasian population. Although the suspicion has arisen repeatedly that some races may be intrinsically susceptible to rheumatic fever this has never been substantiated. Crowding, poor housing, poor hygiene, and inadequate medical care all contribute, overcrowding being the predominant factor. Increased rheumatogenicity of streptococci has frequently been demonstrated during epidemics. Possibly heightened rheumatogenicity occurs with repeated upper respiratory infections in crowded communities where there is an undue acceptance of symptoms of infection.

Pathology
The classical histological feature of rheumatic fever is the Aschoff nodule, a perivascular lesion with a central core of necrotic material surrounded by large cells with polymorphous nuclei and basophilic cytoplasm, and an outer layer of lymphocytes. Nodules have a widespread distribution in connective tissues, including those of joints, tendons, and blood vessels. In the heart they are found in myocardial tissue, most valvular lesions consisting of less organized collections of chronic inflammatory cells. The nodules heal by fibrosis, sometimes leading to extensive interstitial myocardial fibrosis.

The mitral valve leaflets become thickened, with impairment of closure exacerbated by ring dilation. Progressive distortion of the leaflets together with shortening and fusion of the subvalvar apparatus may lead to severe regurgitation. Leaflet and chordal fusion may lead to mitral stenosis, the structure of the valve becoming severely distorted by progressive fibrosis and eventually calcification. This process usually progresses slowly over many years, but proceeds rapidly in some children in developing countries. Similar but less severe changes occur in the tricuspid valve in up to 10 per cent of cases. In the aortic valve thickening of the leaflets is also seen, leaflet edges developing a rolled appearance. The dominant lesion is usually aortic regurgitation with relatively minor obstruction.

Clinical features
Rheumatic fever is rare under 4 years of age, most cases occurring in the 6–15 year age group. Some two-thirds of patients give a history of prior sore throat, usually 1–3 weeks before the development of rheumatic symptoms. Although there is considerable variation in the clinical presentation of rheumatic fever, most cases feature migratory polyarthritis, carditis or both. In Western

countries severe carditis has become relatively uncommon, but in developing countries 50 per cent of cases present with carditis which may be fulminating. Presentation may be abrupt with fever and joint pains, or more gradual with a subacute course. In some cases no acute bout is recognized at all, the patient presenting with established rheumatic heart disease.

Arthritis
Arthritis commonly affects larger joints, especially wrists, elbows, knees, and ankles. Hips are affected less often, small joints of the hands and feet rarely, and the spine almost never. Objective signs are usually limited to minor warmth and swelling but pain may be excruciating, especially with pressure or movement. Characteristically one joint will be affected for 2–3 days and then the inflammatory process moves to another region, but often two or more joints are affected simultaneously to some degree. On occasion important symptoms will be restricted to only one joint, sometimes suggesting traumatic or septic arthritis.

Arthralgia without objective signs, may occur in other joints or may be the only feature, symptoms varying from minor discomfort to severe pain. Untreated, joint pains usually settle over 1–4 weeks.

Carditis
This is the most important manifestation of rheumatic fever and the one with permanent sequelae. When carditis occurs in the course of an acute illness featuring fever and arthritis, signs of cardiac involvement are detected in three-quarters of the patients in the first week. In patients with a subacute course, carditis may become manifest later in an illness featuring low grade fever, pallor, and joint aches.

Valvulitis The most common manifestation is the development of mitral regurgitation, consisting initially of a modest apical systolic murmur, but sometimes progressing to a severe leak with an overactive and dilating heart, dyspnoea, and an increasing murmur. Even a minimal leak may be associated with a diastolic murmur, sometimes called a Carey–Coombes murmur, produced by thickening of the valve leaflets. A basal systolic murmur is often present and may be difficult to distinguish from the trivial murmur which occurs in many children with a fever. The appearance of an early diastolic murmur of aortic regurgitation, however trivial, usually clinches the diagnosis of rheumatic fever. Aortic regurgitation may progress rapidly to a severe leak with full and jerky pulses, and an overactive and dilating heart. Major organic involvement of the tricuspid valve is very rare in the acute stage and involvement of the pulmonary valve almost unknown.

Rheumatic myocarditis This further interferes with cardiac function, the left ventricle becoming dilated and contractility impaired. Although some myocardial involvement probably occurs almost universally, severe impairment of left ventricular function is relatively uncommon. Distinguishing the contributions of valvulitis and impaired left ventricular function to cardiac failure may be very difficult but echocardiography, giving a measure of left ventricular contractility, is extremely useful. When pulmonary venous congestion and heart failure develop, severe mitral (and sometimes aortic) regurgitation are usually present with modest reduction in myocardial contractility. Dilation of the mitral valve ring secondary to left ventricular impairment does, however, contribute importantly to the mitral regurgitation.

Pericarditis commonly accompanies myocarditis and should be suspected in the presence of upper abdominal or chest pain. A pericardial rub is quite common with a superficial, scratchy bruit in any part of the cardiac cycle. A moderate pericardial effusion may develop.

A third heart sound is commonly recorded but little weight should be placed on this in the absence of other evidence of carditis. Sinus tachycardia is usual, and supraventricular and ventricular ectopic beats may occur. The P–R interval is frequently prolonged, but clinically important problems with heart block are extremely rare. The Q–T interval is sometimes prolonged.

Carditis is thus diagnosed by the presence of new or changing murmurs, pericarditis or heart failure. Careful monitoring and supervision are required, worsening failure and death being real possibilities in the presence of severe carditis.

Chorea
Sydenham's chorea is an important manifestation. Once present in 50 per cent of patients it is now recognized in fewer than 5 per cent. It has a longer latent period than arthritis or carditis, from 1 to 6 months. It may occur in association with carditis, or as the only rheumatic manifestation – 'pure' chorea. In this case acute phase reactants and streptococcal titres have frequently returned to base line levels. Chorea features jerky, purposeless movements, exaggerated by tension but disappearing in sleep. Choreiform movements lead to clumsiness, grimacing, and unclear speech. In severe cases violent movements and progressive weakness develop. More common is minor clumsiness, sometimes associated with emotional lability. Occult chorea may be diagnosed by testing sustained hand grip. When the patient holds the observer's fingers, minor sudden movements and fluctuations in muscle tension can be detected.

Erythema marginatum and rheumatic nodules
These manifestations are seen much less frequently but may contribute to diagnosis. Erythema marginatum begins as a non-itchy, faint red macule, the erythema spreading outward while the centre returns to normal colour. The margin is often irregular in outline, and adjacent areas may coalesce. The rash usually fades in 24 hours but may recur over a period of months. Carditis is usually present. Although most commonly associated with rheumatic fever, erythema marginatum also occurs in association with acute glomerulonephritis and drug reactions, and occasionally without recognized cause.

Rheumatic nodules usually appear in patients with long-standing carditis. They are firm, painless, 0.5–2 cm in diameter and situated over tendons or bony prominences.

Other associated features
Other features are not specific enough to be diagnostic. Epistaxis is quite common. Abdominal pain is also quite common, particularly at the onset of an attack. Pleural effusions may occur, especially in association with pericardial effusions. 'Rheumatic pneumonia' is described, but frank consolidation is very likely to be due to a concomitant infectious illness. Pulmonary venous congestion may complicate the picture and there are no criteria to distinguish true rheumatic pneumonia.

Diagnosis
Although diagnosis is easy in many cases, a number of factors may cause major problems.

1. There is no single diagnostic test. The diagnosis is made on the basis of the clinical pattern with support from laboratory tests.

2. Many illnesses may mimic the clinical presentation. These include subacute bacterial endocarditis, and viral and other causes of polyarthritis, especially early rheumatoid arthritis. Monoarthritides, including those of septic and traumatic origin, can cause initial confusion. Acute streptococcal infections may be followed by a period of mild fever, lethargy, malaise, and elevated ESR, sometimes lasting several weeks. These reactions may be difficult to distinguish from rheumatic fever but they do not show major rheumatic manifestations and generally have a briefer course. Rheumatic fever rarely settles in less than two months. In fact the average duration of a bout of rheumatic fever is 10–15 weeks, the longer period in patients with carditis.

3. The murmur of a minor congenital cardiac lesion may first be noted during a viral infection. Even in expert hands the distinction

Table 1 Revised Jones criteria for the diagnosis of rheumatic fever

(a) Major criteria	(b) Minor criteria
Carditis	Previous rheumatic fever or
Polyarthritis	rheumatic heart disease
Chorea	Arthralgia (included only in the
Erythema marginatum	absence of frank arthritis)
Subcutaneous nodules	Fever
	Raised erythrocyte sedimentation
	rate, positive test for C-reactive
	protein or leucocytosis
	Electrocardiogram: prolonged
	P–R interval

(c) Evidence of recent group A streptococcal infection
  Raised antibody levels
  Positive throat swab
  Recent scarlet fever

Two major criteria, or one major and two minor criteria, make rheumatic fever very likely if supported by evidence of a preceding streptococcal infection. The absence of the latter should make the diagnosis doubtful, except in situations in which rheumatic fever is first discovered after a long latent period from the antecedent infection (e.g. Sydenham's chorea or low-grade carditis).

of mild congenital aortic stenosis or prolapse of the mitral valve from a rheumatic lesion may be difficult. Echocardiography may establish the presence of a congenital lesion. Changing murmurs and evidence of involvement of both aortic and mitral valves favour rheumatic fever.

4. The features of rheumatic fever may vary according to severity and time of presentation. With early presentation diagnosis may only be possible after a period of observation of clinical progress and laboratory tests. With late presentation some clinical and laboratory abnormalities may have subsided and the clinician may have to be content with a diagnosis of 'probable' rheumatic fever. With a view to providing a basis for diagnosis and minimizing overdiagnosis, Duckett Jones published diagnostic criteria, subsequently modified by the American Heart Association (Table 1).

Laboratory tests
A throat swab should be taken although group A streptococci are isolated in only 15–20 per cent of cases. A blood culture is required to exclude bacterial endocarditis. Mild anaemia and leucocytosis are common.

Acute phase reactants The two most useful acute phase reactants are the ESR and the C-reactive protein which should be measured weekly. The ESR may be depressed by congestive heart failure which tends to increase CRP levels. Later in the illness mild elevation of the ESR may persist after the CRP has returned to normal. It may then be reasonably assumed that residual rheumatic activity is low grade, although the inflammatory process may not have completely subsided.

Streptococcal serology Streptococcal titres should be measured on three occasions at two-weekly intervals. Multiple tests are desirable, usually the streptococcal antistreptolysin O, antiDNAse, and antihyaluronidase. A two-fold rise in titre may be considered diagnostic. Because of the late presentation, titres are usually convalescent and are considered positive when they exceed a given level – 250 for ASO, 320 for antiDNAse, and 300 for antihyaluronidase (see also page 5.168). Using these criteria, positive tests are obtained in over 90 per cent of patients with acute rheumatic fever. The inexpensive streptozyme test is often favoured but shows poor reproducibility and specificity.

Treatment of acute rheumatic fever
Admission to hospital is highly desirable for diagnostic, management, and educational reasons. Following initial blood cultures, a

therapeutic course of penicillin is given, either 1.2 mega benzathine penicillin or 10 days treatment with oral penicillin. Long-term prophylaxis is continued.

Rest

Rest remains the cornerstone of treatment. This recommendation has never been subjected to a controlled trial but is based on clinical observation that symptoms persist and carditis progresses in many patients who are not rested. Patients should remain on bed–chair rest until symptoms subside and acute phase reactants have been normal for two successive weeks. Activity rarely subsides in less than two months even in patients with arthritis alone. In patients with carditis rheumatic activity may persist for a substantially longer period, more than six months in 3–4 per cent. It is likely that earlier mobilization will prove less important in patients who have had arthritis alone and, provided symptoms are settled and the CRP is normal, gradual mobilization may be considered in those with a prolonged course even when the ESR remains mildly elevated. In patients with carditis, however, the period of rest should be strictly maintained. Low-grade activity may continue for many months or even years, leading to progressive valvular and myocardial damage. Once the acute phase reactants have settled, modest restriction of exercise activity is recommended for two weeks only. Measurement of phase reactants is, however, continued, at two-weekly intervals for two months. With this regimen a rebound is unlikely in patients with arthritis alone, but may occur in patients with carditis, rarely requiring a further period of rest.

Anti-inflammatory drugs

Treatment with anti-inflammatory drugs has naturally received intensive study. Joint pains and fever usually settle rapidly with aspirin or steroids. The burning questions are, however, whether either drug has any effect on the duration of the illness or, even more importantly, on the extent of valve damage after the illness. Over 170 papers have failed to show that aspirin has either effect, despite suggestions of benefit in earlier uncontrolled studies.

In a controlled study in the 1960s, Feinstein showed that rheumatic activity was prolonged by the use of steroids, especially if they were used to treat those rebounds in symptoms which occurred as the drug was withdrawn. Although studies without concurrent controls suggested that the extent of valve disease may be reduced by steroid administration, this impression has not been confirmed by controlled studies. A major confounding factor is the fact that patients with minimal carditis during the acute illness rarely show important valvular lesions in the subsequent 5–10 years. A single controlled study by Dorfman with high-dose hydrocortisone showed apparent benefit but contained 30 per cent of patients with minimal carditis. The Cooperative United Kingdom and United States study group, and the United States Combined Rheumatic Fever study group found no benefit from ACTH or prednisone in moderate or high doses. Claims have been made for the efficacy of combined steroids and aspirin but no adequately controlled studies exist. These studies are reviewed in the monograph of Markowitz and Gordis.

One must conclude that, if there is any long-term benefit from suppressive drug therapy, it is so small as to be unmeasurable. Despite this, steroid administration is often recommended for patients with moderate carditis, covering the withdrawal with aspirin because of the rather common rebound in symptoms. Such policies seem to reflect the desire of doctors to administer drugs rather than to allow Nature to effect her cure. Aspirin should be given to control pain, dosage tailored according to need. Prednisone may also be given for this purpose but can usually be reserved for the situation where aggressive carditis appears life-threatening. Steroids sometimes help to arrest progressive heart failure. The required dose of prednisone is usually not more than 40–60 mg daily, and gradual reduction in dosage can usually start within one week. Three points should be noted:

1. Treatment should not be started until the diagnosis is secure.
2. In the situation with deteriorating cardiac output, dilation of the heart, and congestive heart failure, it is often very difficult to assess valve function clinically, but a severe valvular lesion is usually present. Although cardiac surgery carries a somewhat higher risk in this situation, valve replacement may be the only chance of survival. Mortality figures of up to 6 per cent have been quoted for acute rheumatic fever but most cases can be salvaged if care is scrupulous and cardiac surgery is available.
3. Aspirin and prednisone depress acute phase reactants. The bout can not be considered settled until the ESR and CRP have been normal in successive weeks, the first measurement being taken two weeks after stopping suppressive treatment.

Chorea

Treatment of chorea, other than with penicillin prophylaxis, is rarely required and does not influence the duration of symptoms. Bed rest is required only when chorea appears early and phase reactants are still positive, or in the rare case of extreme motor disturbance. For troublesome symptoms phenobarbitone, diazepam (up to 5 mg t.i.d.), or haloperidol (25 mg t.i.d.) are useful.

Recurrence of rheumatic fever and prophylaxis

Recurrence of rheumatic fever

In pre-antibiotic days recurrences of rheumatic fever were recorded in up to 73 per cent of patients. It was subsequently shown that a further streptococcal infection, often with a different strain, preceded each recurrence. The 'rheumatic' patient retains the tendency to develop rheumatic fever with further group A streptococcal infections. The risk of recurrence is highest in the first three years after the first attack, in young patients, and in patients with rheumatic heart disease. Carditis with a recurrence is more common in those patients in whom it was present in the first attack but it may occur in any patient. Recurrent attacks frequently lead to progressive deterioration in valvular and myocardial function. The need for meticulous prophylaxis in all patients is clear.

Prophylaxis

Fortunately the group A streptococcus remains uniquely sensitive to long-term, low-dose penicillin, which may be administered orally or parenterally. Regrettably, non-compliance can reach astonishing levels with oral prophylaxis. In a study in the 1960s Gordis showed that 90 per cent of patients became non-compliant if they had four or more of the following characteristics: female, adolescent, large sibship, not admitted to hospital with acute attack, no activity restriction, unaccompanied to clinic by parents. However conscientious the education programme, a recurrence rate of 30 per cent in five years in susceptible populations must be anticipated, with oral prophylaxis. With rare exceptions, therefore, treatment with benzathine penicillin is recommended. The injection is sometimes painful for 1–2 days but this may be eased somewhat by incorporating a low dose of local anaesthetic with the injection. The minimum treatment period for patients without carditis is often given as five years, or to 18 years of age, but recurrences beyond five years are by no means uncommon. Bland and Jones showed annual recurrence rates of 11 per cent at 5–10 years and 6 per cent at 10–15 years. A minimum treatment period of 10 years is desirable. For patients with established heart disease more prolonged prophylaxis is mandatory and treatment is recommended at least to the age of 45 years. Pressure may rise to change to oral prophylaxis after some years but this is recommended only in particularly reliable patients.

Recommended treatment programme

Benzathine penicillin (with 0.5 ml 2 per cent lignocaine): under 9 years or 27 kg 0.9 megaunits, over 9 years or 27 kg 1.2 megaunits four-weekly. Penicillin VK or penicillin G 250 mg: 2 tablets daily.

Sulphadimidine or sulphadiazine: under 9 years or 27 kg 0.5 g, over 9 years or 27 kg 1.0 g daily.

In a study by Wood in the 1960s percentage annual recurrence rates on these regimens were 0.4 per cent with benzathine penicillin, 5.5 per cent with oral penicillin, and 2.8 per cent with sulphadimidine. Current rates show little change. Blood levels two weeks after benzathine injections are extremely low and higher recurrence rates have recently been reported from some developing countries in patients receiving four-weekly injections. Nevertheless, the recommended routine is four-weekly injections, increasing to three-weekly injections for those with a recurrence. Although peak blood levels are low and unpredictable when oral penicillin is taken after a meal, total absorption is not much changed. It is essential to have a set routine with oral prophylaxis. Often 'first thing in the morning and last thing at night' is best.

The possibility of allergy to penicillin should be borne in mind and adrenalin should be available when giving benzathine penicillin injections. Sulphadimidine or sulphadiazine are satisfactory alternatives for allergic patients. Erythromycin, 250 mg twice daily, is a more expensive alternative.

Bacterial endocarditis

It must be remembered that prophylactic penicillin gives no protection against bacterial endocarditis and, in fact, induces tolerance to penicillin in the viridans streptococci in the buccal cavity. Prophylaxis against endocarditis with dental procedures therefore requires high-dose erythromycin or a combination of a penicillin and an aminoglycoside. In patients with low-grade bacterial endocarditis, blood cultures may not become positive for 3–4 days after the last dose of oral penicillin, or two weeks or more after the last dose of benzathine penicillin.

Prevention of rheumatic fever

Early recognition and treatment of the streptococcal sore throat has been shown to reduce the incidence of rheumatic fever in closed communities and can play an important role, for example, in streptococcal epidemics in schools. Prevention of sporadic cases in a susceptible community is, however, extremely difficult, compounded by the fact that only a minority of patients seek medical care for a streptococcal sore throat. Education about the recognition, complications, and treatment of streptococcal pharyngitis is vital. Systems for taking throat swabs in school and family contacts in cases of acute rheumatic fever are cost effective. Clearly there is a major need in susceptible populations for a co-ordinated programme involving school and community health personnel. The tragedy is that, in the countries where rheumatic fever is the greatest problem, funds are frequently inadequate even to provide long-term penicillin for established cases. Some specific anti-M antisera have been developed but costs of production and the number of antigenic M types constitute formidable problems to a vaccination programme. On the world scene, rheumatic fever is inextricably bound up with socioeconomic factors. Its elimination as a major health factor awaits abolition of poverty, overcrowding, and slum conditions.

References

Ad Hoc Committee of the Council on Rheumatic Fever and Congenital Heart Disease of the American Heart Association (1965) (1984). Jones Criteria (revised) for guidance in the diagnosis of rheumatic fever. Circulation 69, 203A–208A.

Bland, E. F. and Jones, T. D. (1951). Rheumatic fever and rheumatic heart disease: A twenty year report on 1000 patients followed since childhood. Circulation 4, 836–843.

Combined Rheumatic Fever Study Group (1960). A comparison of the effect of prednisone and acetylsalicylic acid on the incidence of residual rheumatic heart disease. N. Engl. J. Med. 262, 895–902.

Combined Rheumatic Fever Study Group (1965). A comparison of short-term, intensive prednisone and acetylsalicylic acid therapy in the treatment of acute rheumatic fever. N. Engl. J. Med. 272, 63–70.

Committee on Rheumatic Fever and Infective Endocarditis of the Council on Cardiovascular Disease in the Young (1984). Prevention of rheumatic fever. Circulation 70, 1118A–1122A.

Dorfman, A., Gross, J. I. E. and Lorinez, A. E. (1961). The treatment of acute rheumatic fever. Pediatrics 27, 692–706.

Feinstein, A. R., Spagnuolo, M. and Gill, F. A. (1961). The rebound phenomenon in acute rheumatic fever. I. Incidence and significance. Yale J. Biol. Med. 33, 259–278.

Gordis, L., Lilienfeld, A. and Rodriquez, R. (1969). Studies in the epidemiology and preventability of rheumatic fever. I. Demographic factors and the incidence of acute attacks. J. Chronic Dis. 21, 645–654.

Markowitz, M. and Gordis, L. (1972). Rheumatic fever 2nd edn. W. B. Saunders, Philadelphia.

Stollerman, G. H. (1975). Rheumatic fever and streptococcal infection. Grune and Stratton, New York.

UK and US Joint Report (1955). The treatment of acute rheumatic fever in children: Cooperative clinical trial of ACTH, cortisone and aspirin. Circulation 11, 343–377.

UK and US Joint Report (1960). The evolution of rheumatic heart disease in children: Five year report of a cooperative clinical trial of ACTH, cortisone and aspirin. Circulation 22, 503–515.

Wood, H. F., Feinstein, A. R., Taranta, A., Epstein, J. A. and Simpson, R. (1964). Rheumatic fever in children and adolescents. III. Comparative effectiveness of three prophylaxis regimens in preventing streptococcal infections and rheumatic recurrences. Ann. Intern. Med. 60 (Suppl. 5), 31–46.

VALVE DISEASE

D. G. GIBSON

Normal mitral valve

Anatomy

The normal mitral valve is a complex structure, consisting of leaflets, annulus, chordae tendineae, and papillary muscles. Its anatomy as studied at autopsy shows an unusual degree of variation between normal subjects. Of the two leaflets, the anterior one is the larger, both from base to margin, and also along its perimeter. It is attached to the root of the aorta and the membranous septum at the base of the heart, and is continuous with the chordae peripherally. It thus passes across the centre of the left ventricular cavity, dividing the inlet from the outlet portion. The posterior cusp is attached to the mitral ring and to the anterior cusp at both commisures. It is continuous with the posterior wall of the left atrium and is divided into three portions by two scallops. The chordae arise from the ventricular margins of both cusps, and are inserted into the heads of the papillary muscles. There are multiple subdivisions in the chordae as they pass from papillary muscles to the cusps, which form an effective secondary pathway, additional to the main one between the cusps, for blood to enter the ventricle. There are two papillary muscles, one anteromedial and the other posterolateral. The former is usually larger and has a more uniform structure than the latter which may be double. Both may have up to six heads, giving rise to chordae. The papillary muscles are continuous with the trabecular and subendocardial layer of the ventricular wall, and both are supplied by a single end-artery. The mitral ring is an insubstantial structure whose function is to support valve cusps only. It is incomplete in the region of the aortic root and the membranous septum. However, it is surrounded by a well-developed circumferential ring of myocardium which supports it, and whose contraction during systole has the effect of significantly reducing the diameter of the valve orifice. Histologically, the normal valve cusp has a dense collagenous core, continuous with the valve ring, the valve fibrosa. This is covered on atrial and ventricular surfaces by a thin layer of loose connective tissue, and finally by endocardium.

Physiology

The normal mitral valve has a cross-sectional area of approximately 5 cm^2 which allows ventricular filling to occur at a peak rate of 500–1000 ml/s, with no measurable pressure gradient across it. Left ventricular filling occurs predominantly during early diastole, the rapid filling phase, and during left atrial systole, with a mid-diastolic period of diastasis when ventricular volume remains virtually constant, and when the mitral valve itself almost closes. As heart rate increases during exercise, diastasis becomes shorter, while the duration of the rapid filling period remains virtually unchanged. At rest, approximately two-thirds of the stroke volume enters during early diastole, and the remaining one-third during left atrial systole. At rapid ventricular rates occurring with peak exercise, left ventricular filling time may fall to less than 100 ms. If stroke volume is taken as being of the order of 100 ml, then mean ventricular filling rate is 1 l/s, which is achieved without measurable pressure gradient across the mitral valve. This gives some idea of the effectiveness of the mechanisms underlying normal ventricular filling.

Mitral stenosis

Aetiology

Chronic rheumatic heart disease is much the commonest cause of mitral stenosis, though a number of other well-defined pathological processes exist. Mitral stenosis may be congenital, when it is frequently associated with other lesions causing obstruction to left ventricular outflow, including aortic or subaortic stenosis, coarctation of the aorta or endocardial fibroelastosis. In such cases, the chordae are usually short, with obliteration of the spaces between them. The leaflets are thick, with rolled edges. The insertion of the papillary muscles may be abnormal, being either directly from the free wall of the ventricle or from the septum. In parachute mitral valve, there is only a single papillary muscle which may be fibrotic, causing interference with normal cusp motion.

Acquired mitral stenosis has been reported in patients with calcified mitral valve ring (q.v.), in infective endocarditis, when bulky vegetations may cause obstruction to flow or to granulomatous infiltration in association with eosinophilia. In nodular rheumatoid arthritis, thickening of the valve cusps has been observed, but true mitral stenosis does not occur. However, in systemic lupus erythematosus, treatment of Libman–Sachs endocarditis with steroids may lead to significant fibrosis, with the development of mitral stenosis. The combination of ostium secundum atrial septal defect and mitral stenosis is frequently referred to as Lutembacher's syndrome, but the mitral stenosis is almost certainly rheumatic, and the association fortuitous.

Rheumatic mitral stenosis

Incidence

The incidence of mitral stenosis varies considerably in different parts of the world, but approximately parallels that of acute rheumatic fever. It is much commoner, and presents earlier, in the Middle East, the Indian subcontinent, and the Far East than in the West. Accurate figures for its incidence are not readily available, but in the West, chronic rheumatic heart disease occurs in less than 5 per 100 000 of the population. In the Third World, values of up to 6 per 1000 are seen in school children.

Pathology

Rheumatic mitral stenosis is due to distortion of the normal mitral valve anatomy with fusion of the commissures. The cusps themselves are thickened, and frequently develop thrombus on their atrial surfaces. The subvalve apparatus may also be affected, with thickening, fusion, and contraction of the chordae tendineae. Finally, the valve cusps or ring may become calcified. The left ventricle is usually normal or small in size in pure mitral stenosis, but occasionally considerable ventricular dilation may occur. The left atrium is characteristically enlarged: its wall may be histologically normal, or there may be evidence of disruption of muscle fibres. Mural thrombosis may be present, most commonly involving the free wall just above the posterior mitral valve cusp (McCallum's patch). In long-standing cases, calcification of the left atrial wall may develop in plaques on its endocardial surface. Changes of pulmonary venous congestion, pulmonary hypertension, and haemosiderosis may develop in the lungs, with dilation and hypertrophy of the right ventricle and functional tricuspid regurgitation.

Pathophysiology

The primary disturbance in mitral stenosis is in left ventricular filling. When the mitral valve area is reduced to approximately 2.5 cm^2, there is a reduction in peak left ventricular filling rate and loss of the normal period of diastasis. This has no functional significance at rest when heart rate is slow and filling period relatively long, but during exercise as the heart rate increases, a pressure gradient develops. If the valve area is smaller, a gradient may be present at rest, with an increase in the mean left atrial pressure. Patients with symptomatic mitral stenosis have a valve area of 0.75–1.25 cm^2. The anatomical site of the stenosis may be either at valve level or below the valve itself, due to fusion of the chordae. Left ventricular cavity size, usually normal in young patients, may be increased in the middle-aged or elderly. This left ventricular disease is an ill-defined entity, but a number of factors may contribute to it, including coronary emboli, distortion of the septum by right ventricular overload, and associated hypertension, itself sometimes secondary to renal emboli. In addition, there is evidence to suggest that the increase in arterial resistance secondary to reduced cardiac output interferes with systolic function, since after successful surgery, cavity size may fall, and the velocity of ejection of blood during systole increases towards normal. Chronic left atrial hypertension causes a corresponding elevation of pulmonary capillary pressure and so to increased transudation of fluid with clinical evidence of pulmonary congestion when it reaches approximately 25 mg Hg.

Further lung disease may result from the development of active pulmonary hypertension, repeated pulmonary emboli or chest infections, haemosiderosis, or even bone formation.

Clinical picture
Symptoms

The symptoms of mitral stenosis usually appear insidiously, and may have been present for several years before the patient seeks medical attention. Their onset may be within 3 or 4 years of the attack of acute rheumatic fever, or be delayed by up to 50 years. Less frequently, the onset is abrupt with an attack of acute pulmonary oedema, systemic embolism, or the onset of atrial fibrillation.

The commonest manifestation of mitral stenosis is a reduction in exercise tolerance. In pure mitral stenosis, the major symptom is usually breathlessness. Less frequently it may be fatigue or a heaviness of the limbs, both clearly related to exercise. Exercise tolerance may also be limited by palpitation due to an inappropriately rapid ventricular rate in a patient with atrial fibrillation. Typical anginal pain may also occur, usually ascribed to previous coronary embolism, but sometimes apparently due to pulmonary hypertension and right ventricular hypertrophy. Late in the disease, nocturnal dyspnoea may be present. Episodes of florid acute pulmonary oedema are less frequent now than appears to have been the case 20 or 30 years ago, due probably to the widespread practice of treating patients with heart disease of whatever severity with powerful diuretics.

Recurrent episodes of chest infection or winter bronchitis are very characteristic. They are associated with cough, purulent sputum, fluid retention, and increased breathlessness. They may precipitate overt pulmonary oedema, and leave a permanent reduction in exercise tolerance after the infection itself has been treated.

Haemoptysis may be caused by chest infection, pulmonary infarction, acute pulmonary oedema, or 'pulmonary apoplexy', the rupture of a small blood vessel within the lung. Massive or recurrent haemoptysis may be the presenting or only symptom of mitral stenosis.

Systemic embolism from the left atrium is common in untreated mitral stenosis, particularly when atrial fibrillation is present. Any organ may be affected, but the commonest sites are cerebral, coronary, splenic, renal, mesenteric, or the arteries of the limbs. Pulmonary emboli may originate in the right atrium as well as the peripheral veins, and cause pulmonary infarction or progressive reduction in exercise tolerance due to an increase in pulmonary vascular resistance.

Fluid and sodium retention is common in untreated mitral stenosis, and manifests itself, initially, by the development of nocturia due to reversal of the normal diurnal rhythm of sodium excretion. Peripheral oedema, ascites, pulmonary oedema, and pleural effusion are clinical evidence of this disturbance when it is severe.

Physical examination

Prolonged low cardiac output may lead to weight loss, peripheral cyanosis, and to the appearance of a malar flush. In pure mitral stenosis, the character of the pulse is normal, although its amplitude may be decreased and the rhythm irregular due to atrial fibrillation. The arterial pulses should always be checked in view of the possibility of previous arterial emboli. The venous pressure is normal unless tricuspid regurgitation is present. An 'a' wave in the venous pulse of a patient with what appears to be pure mitral stenosis should always raise the possibility of additional tricuspid stenosis being present, since it is otherwise unusual even with severe pulmonary hypertension. Palpation of the praecordium at the apex may reveal a palpable first sound, previously called a 'tapping apex', and less frequently, a palpable opening snap. It may also be possible to feel pulmonary valve closure at the base of the heart if severe pulmonary hypertension is present.

A left parasternal heave is usually due to right ventricular hypertrophy caused by pulmonary hypertension, but may also be caused by tricuspid regurgitation, or increased prominence of a normal right ventricle secondary to an enlarged left atrium. In pure mitral stenosis, a sustained apex beat is unusual, but may be seen when the right ventricle is very considerably enlarged or more commonly, because of co-existent left ventricular disease. On auscultation at the apex, the classical findings in pure mitral stenosis are a loud first sound, preceded by a presystolic murmur if the patient is in sinus rhythm, an opening snap, and a mid-diastolic murmur. An early systolic rumble may precede the first sound in some patients with atrial fibrillation, giving a superficial resemblance to a presystolic murmur. It occurs as the valve begins to close at the onset of ventricular systole, the first heart sound occurring only when cusp closure is complete. A loud first heart sound is less specific for rheumatic mitral stenosis than a palpable one, since it may also be caused by a high cardiac output state such as hyperthyroidism. A soft or absent first sound in mitral stenosis strongly suggests that the anterior cusp of the mitral valve is calcified or immobile.

An opening snap is a very characteristic physical sign in mitral stenosis. It is usually loudest at the lower left sternal edge, less commonly the apex or the base, and is likely to be absent if the

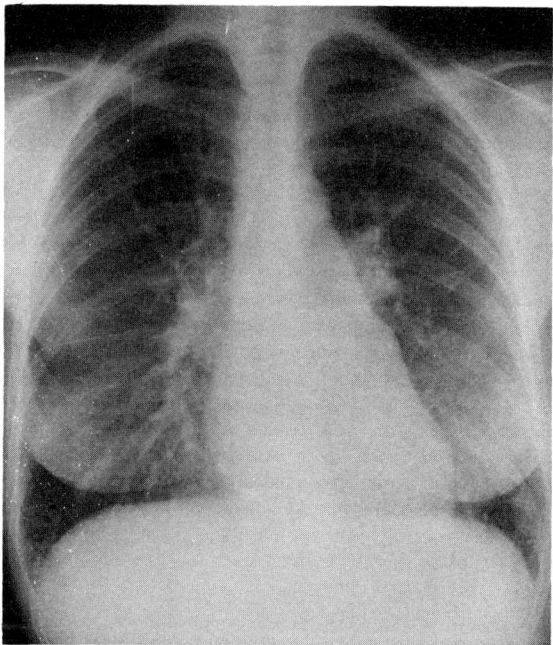

Fig. 1 Chest X-ray from a patient with pure mitral stenosis. Heart size is normal, but the left atrial appendage is enlarged. The upper lobe vessels are dilated and there are Kerley lines at both bases.

valve structure is severely disorganized. The time interval between aortic valve closure and the opening snap becomes shorter as left atrial pressure rises, but this relation is not strong enough to be of value in assessing individual patients, particularly those in atrial fibrillation in whom the interval varies from beat to beat. The mid-diastolic murmur starts after the opening snap, separated from it by appreciable interval. It is low-pitched and persists for a variable period throughout diastole. If the mitral stenosis is mild, the murmur is short, but if the murmur lasts throughout diastole at a normal ventricular rate, then the degree of stenosis is likely to be at least moderately severe. When the rate is rapid due to atrial fibrillation, the murmur may no longer be audible, although in these circumstances, the diagnosis can be suspected from the palpable first sound. However, there exists a group of patients in whom no mid-diastolic murmur is audible even when the heart-rate is controlled, who are referred to as having 'silent' mitral stenosis. These patients frequently have severe pulmonary hypertension, a disorganized valve, and significant involvement of the subvalve apparatus. The exact reason for the absence of the murmur is not clear.

Chest X-ray

The radiological appearances of mitral stenosis are characteristic (Fig. 1). The heart size may be normal or increased, but the most frequent abnormality is enlargement of the left atrium that is selective, i.e. it occurs to a greater extent than that of the heart shadow as a whole. This appears on the penetrated postero-anterior film as a double outline on the right side of the heart shadow, with elevation of the left main bronchus, and enlargement of the left atrial appendix which forms that part of the left heart border just below the main pulmonary artery. Apart from this, the cause of cardiac enlargement is hard to assess radiologically, since it may be due to an increase in size of any of the other three chambers or to the presence of a small pericardial effusion. Mitral valve calcification may be visible on the postero-anterior film just to the left of the spine, on the continuation of the shadow of the left atrium. In the lung fields, the upper lobe veins may be dilated with the patient in the erect position, indicating the presence of a raised left atrial pressure and an increase in the size of the main pulmonary artery reflects the presence of pulmonary hypertension. An

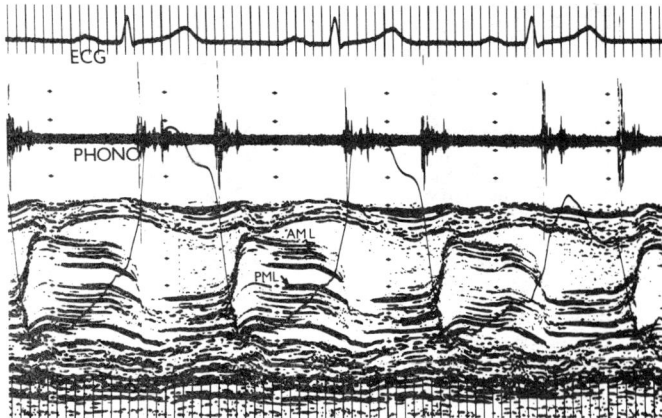

Fig. 2 M-mode echocardiogram from a patient with mitral stenosis. The anterior cusp (AML) is thickened, and its diastolic closure rate is reduced. The posterior leaflet (PML) moves forward during diastole. There is an opening snap on the phonocardiogram, coinciding with maximum forward motion of the anterior cusp.

increase in pulmonary vascular resistance may cause upper lobe blood diversion with a decrease in the prominence of the vessels to the lower zones. When the left atrial pressure reaches approximately 25 mm Hg, evidence of pulmonary oedema may be apparent, with the appearance of lymphatic lines, basal pleural effusions, generalized hazy shadowing, and finally the development of obvious interstitial oedema. Long-standing left atrial hypertension may be associated with pulmonary haemosiderosis, or even bone formation, the latter appearing as dense nodules a few mm in diameter.

Electrocardiogram

The ECG is not very informative in mitral stenosis, but it allows the presence of atrial fibrillation to be confirmed. If the patient is in sinus rhythm, then left atrial hypertrophy is demonstrated by a bifid P wave in lead II and a dominant negative deflection in V1. ECG evidence of right atrial hypertrophy suggests the presence of tricuspid stenosis in addition to mitral stenosis. The electrical axis is usually vertical: right ventricular hypertrophy, if severe, is shown by a dominant R wave in V1.

Echocardiogram

Echocardiography has totally changed the diagnosis and management of patients with mitral valve disease. The characteristic feature of rheumatic mitral valve disease on M-mode echocardiography is a reduction in the mid-diastolic closure rate of the anterior cusp of the mitral valve to less than 50 mm/s for mild mitral stenosis and to 0–20 mm/s for severe involvement (Fig. 2). Cusp fusion is demonstrated by forward, rather than backward movement of the posterior cusp during diastole. Severe fibrosis or calcification of the anterior cusp can be recognized by thickening and a reduction in the amplitude or movement of the echo. The abnormal left ventricular filling pattern can be quantified from left ventricular wall movement, and right ventricular hypertrophy is indicated by posterior displacement of the interventricular septum. On cross-sectional echocardiography, abnormal valve cusp anatomy and restricted motion are apparent on the long axis parasternal view (Fig. 3a), and the valve area can be estimated from the minor axis view (Fig. 3b), provided the cusps are not calcified. It is also possible to assess the degree of subvalve involvement. Occasionally atrial thrombus can be detected (Fig. 4). Continuous wave Doppler can be used to estimate peak mitral transvalvular gradient and mitral valve area (see Figs 8 and 9, page 13.38).

Cardiac catheterization

This investigation is not usually necessary, but may still be required in atypical cases, or when additional coronary artery dis-

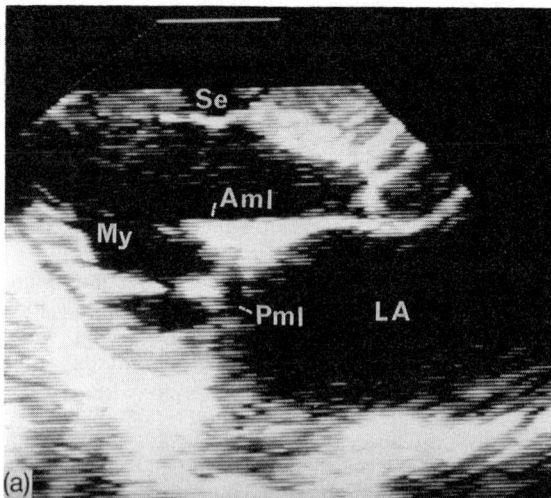

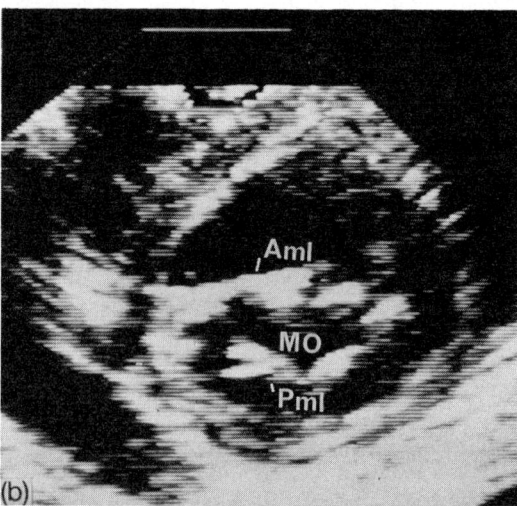

Fig. 3 (a) Two-dimensional echocardiogram from a patient with mitral valve disease, parasternal long axis view taken in mid-diastole. The anterior cusp (Aml) of the mitral valve is thickened, and fails to open normally. LA, left atrium; Se, septum; My, myocardial echoes; whose intensity is increased due to scarring of the subvalve apparatus; Pml, posterior mitral leaflet. (b) Rheumatic mitral valve disease, parasternal minor axis view during mid-diastole, at the level of the mitral valve orifice (MO). Other abbreviations as in (a).

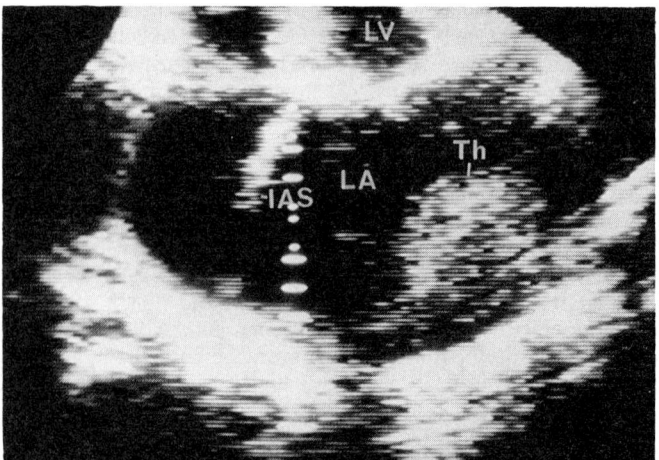

Fig. 4 Left atrial thrombus (Th) in a patient with mitral valve disease. LA, left atrium; LV, left ventricle; IAS, interatrial septum. The left atrium is considerably enlarged.

ease is suspected. The characteristic findings are an increase in left atrial and pulmonary capillary pressure, a diastolic pressure gradient across the mitral valve, and a corresponding increase in pulmonary artery pressure. Cardiac output is usually reduced and pulmonary vascular resistance may be increased. Left ventricular function is normal in the majority of patients, but there may be evidence of left ventricular disease as shown by increased left ventricular end-diastolic pressure and volume and reduced ejection fraction. In a small minority of cases, severe mitral stenosis may be present with no diastolic gradient, indicating that the main abnormality is restriction of ventricular filling rather than obstruction at the valve orifice itself. Unlike echocardiography, cardiac catheterization and angiography give little information about the anatomy of the valve cusps or subvalve apparatus.

Diagnosis

The diagnosis of mitral stenosis is usually straightforward on the basis of history, physical signs, and chest X-ray, and can rapidly be confirmed by echocardiography. When the ventricular rate is rapid, the diastolic murmur may be inaudible, but becomes apparent when the ventricular rate is controlled by digoxin. Cases of silent mitral stenosis may present difficulties, and may mimic primary pulmonary hypertension or left ventricular disease. In such patients, mitral stenosis can often be excluded or confirmed only by echocardiography or direct measurement of left ventricular and left atrial pressures. Mitral stenosis should also be suspected as a source of systemic emboli and as a cause of unexplained atrial fibrillation, particularly in the elderly. In these circumstances, the valve lesion itself may be very mild, so that the usual physical signs may not be present, although the characteristic abnormalities can be demonstrated by echocardiography.

An attempt should be made to quantify the severity of the mitral stenosis as well as diagnosing its presence. Probably the most reliable way in which its clinical significance can be assessed is from the history. The length of the mid-diastolic murmur gives some indication as to the severity of the obstruction, as described above, although it is an unsatisfactory criterion when ventricular rate is increased or the murmur inaudible. Objective measurement of the degree of obstruction at the mitral valve can be obtained from estimates of the diastolic pressure gradient or the mitral valve area obtained from cardiac catheterization, cross-sectional echocardiography or continuous wave Doppler.

Differential diagnosis

Conditions in which an incorrect diagnosis of mitral stenosis may be made

1. Left atrial myxoma (page 13.312). Left atrial myxoma may mimic all the physical signs of mitral stenosis including mid-diastolic and presystolic murmurs, loud first sound, and opening snap ('tumour plop'). It may lead to increasing dyspnoea and systemic embolization, and the length of the history may range from a single acute incident to one of many years' duration. There is often evidence of a systemic illness, and erythrocyte sedimentation rate and plasma proteins are frequently, but not invariably, abnormal. Variable murmurs are often described, but constant ones, or no abnormality at all on auscultation, are equally common. A pressure gradient can usually be demonstrated across the valve if cardiac catheterization is performed, and angiography shows varying degrees of regurgitation. Diagnosis depends on suspicion of the condition, and performing echocardiography, which shows a characteristic mass of echoes behind the mitral valve during diastole, thus allowing left atrial myxoma as a cause of mitral valve disease to be confirmed or excluded. Pulmonary artery or left ventricular angiography are both unsatisfactory, the former being unreliable, and the latter likely to precipitate systemic emboli.

2. Cor triatriatum. This is a rare cause of obstruction to blood flow at left atrial level and may mimic mitral stenosis, particularly in childhood.

3. Pulmonary veno-occlusive disease (page 13.342) may also present as silent mitral stenosis, often with a raised pulmonary wedge but a normal left atrial pressure.

4. Ostium secundum atrial septal defect (page 13.270). Although the differential diagnosis between atrial septal defect and mitral stenosis is usually clear, in occasional cases it may become difficult on clinical grounds because of a loud tricuspid flow murmur, mid-diastolic in timing, preceded by a tricuspid opening snap. With right ventricular enlargement, these signs may be most easily audible at the apex. Pulmonary valve closure is usually, but not always, delayed in atrial septal defect and, in occasional cases, the usual ECG pattern of partial right bundle branch block may be absent. The differential diagnosis can be made by echocardiography. M-mode demonstrates a normal mitral valve and reversed septal motion, and cross-sectional echocardiography will show a negative jet in the right atrium following a peripheral contrast injection.

5. Austin–Flint murmur. In the presence of severe aortic regurgitation, a mid-diastolic murmur may be audible at the apex, although the mitral valve itself is quite normal. This may be accompanied by a loud first sound and a presystolic murmur. On clinical grounds, this murmur can be differentiated from co-existent mitral stenosis by the fact that the first sound is never palpable and an opening snap is never present, but the most satisfactory way of excluding rheumatic involvement of the mitral valve is by echocardiography. This shows a normal diastolic closure rate, often with a high frequency fluttering superimposed on it, reflecting the position of the cusp immediately below the aortic root, and therefore in the regurgitant stream of blood (Fig. 12).

6. There is a small group of patients with aortic regurgitation into a stiff left ventricle in whom end-diastolic pressure may be very high without evidence of systolic dysfunction. These patients may develop atrial fibrillation and pulmonary hypertension so that the clinical picture can mimic that due to combined rheumatic mitral and aortic valve disease.

Conditions in which a correct diagnosis of mitral stenosis may be missed

The diagnosis of mitral stenosis may be missed when the clinical picture mimics other well-known diseases.

1. Primary pulmonary hypertension (page 13.270). In occasional patients with mitral stenosis, the degree of pulmonary hypertension is unusually severe, and apparently out of proportion to the severity of the mitral stenosis. Such cases tend to remain in sinus rhythm throughout the disease, and the mitral murmurs are frequently inaudible since the site of limitation of flow is in the pulmonary circulation rather than at the valve, and since marked right ventricular hypertrophy and enlargement may develop, displacing the left ventricle posteriorly. At cardiac catheterization, the presence of severe pulmonary hypertension may make it impossible to obtain a technically satisfactory wedge pressure. It is essential, therefore, that mitral stenosis is definitively excluded by echocardiography in any patient in whom a diagnosis of primary pulmonary hypertension is considered.

2. Silent mitral stenosis may also present with clinical evidence of pulmonary congestion, so that a diagnosis of heart failure is made without further investigation. Such cases can be suspected clinically, since there is usually no clinical evidence of left ventricular disease, and since ECG shows no evidence of old myocardial infarction or ventricular hypertrophy. The correct diagnosis can be made by echocardiography.

3. In the presence of other valve disease, particularly aortic regurgitation, clinical evidence of mitral stenosis may be suppressed. The correct diagnosis should always be suspected in any patient with what appears to be isolated aortic valve disease who is in atrial fibrillation. Again, the correct diagnosis is made by echocardiography.

Treatment

Medical treatment

1. In patients below the age of 21 years penicillin prophylaxis against further attacks of acute rheumatic fever should be given (see page 13.280).

2. Atrial fibrillation should be treated with a digitalis preparation to control the ventricular rate. Anticoagulant therapy should be given to reduce the risk of systemic embolism to all patients with atrial fibrillation, unless there are very strong contra-indications. It is probably advisable to give this treatment to patients in sinus rhythm with mitral stenosis, particularly the middle-aged and elderly, since the incidence of embolism is not negligible in these patients, and since it is particularly high with the onset of atrial fibrillation. The incidence of embolism is also high when a patient with atrial fibrillation who is not on anticoagulants is admitted to hospital with a rapid heart rate and pulmonary oedema. Intravenous or subcutaneous heparin should be given to such patients until therapeutic anticoagulation with an oral agent is established.

3. Fluid retention associated with mitral stenosis responds well to treatment with diuretics. However, this must be distinguished from radiographic and other changes resulting directly from the raised left atrial pressure, which do not. The raised left atrial pressure is due to blood flow through a fixed resistance so that diuretic treatment could only result in a significant fall if it induced such severe hypovolaemia as to cause a corresponding drop in cardiac output which is clearly undesirable.

4. Chest infections should be treated promptly with appropriate antibiotics. They are often precipitated by fluid retention so that a diuretic should be considered at the same time.

5. In all patients with valvular heart disease, prophylactic antibiotics should be given for all dental manipulations and potentially septic hazards. This should preferably be amoxycillin, 3 g, as a single dose, given three-quarters of an hour before the procedure. If the patient is penicillin sensitive then cephaloridine or erythromycin should be used instead.

Surgical treatment

Mitral stenosis causes mechanical obstruction to the circulation and the most satisfactory treatment is therefore surgical. A number of procedures are available, including mitral valvotomy, open or closed, and mitral valve replacement. The choice of operation depends on the anatomy of the mitral valve determined on the basis of the physical signs and the echocardiogram, the age of the patient, and the surgical resources available. The decision about the first operation is an important one, since it represents the initial stage in a life-time's care of the patient's mitral valve. Closed mitral valvotomy is a relatively simple procedure in terms of the resources that are required, although a satisfactory result presupposes considerable surgical expertise. It is particularly suitable in a young patient, in sinus rhythm, with evidence of a mobile anterior cusp. Open valvotomy requires cardiopulmonary bypass but allows a more complete procedure to be undertaken, and in particular, allows the subvalvular apparatus to be inspected and adherent chordae divided. If the results of valvotomy are found to be unsatisfactory, then it is possible to proceed to valve replacement at the same operation. If the valve cusps are greatly thickened or calcified, then elective mitral valve replacement will be required, using either a mechanical or biological prosthesis. Mechanical prostheses may be of the ball and cage type, such as the Starr–Edwards, or the tilting disc, such as the Bjork–Shiley. All patients with a mechanical valve *in situ* require long-term anticoagulant therapy to prevent systemic emboli. The alternative is a biological valve, usually consisting of an inverted porcine aortic xenograft mounted in a plastic stent. Such a valve has the advantage that anticoagulants are not required if the patient is in sinus rhythm, but the cusps are liable to calcification, perforation or rupture, so that its life is of the order of ten years. These considerations help to determine the type of valve inserted in an individual

patient. For a young woman in sinus rhythm, in whom future pregnancy may be important, a biological valve is to be preferred, since anticoagulant therapy can be avoided. A biological valve may allow anticoagulants to be avoided in the elderly, and should also be considered in those in whom major or repeated thrombotic complications have developed with a mechanical valve, or in those with clearcut contraindications to anticoagulant therapy. A mechanical valve is particularly suitable for other young or middle-aged patients particularly those who are in atrial fibrillation. If the left ventricular cavity is small, then a ball and cage prosthesis should be avoided, and a low profile valve such as a Bjork–Shiley used instead. These considerations should be regarded as no more than guide lines, and the advantages and disadvantages of the different valve substitutes should always be discussed in detail with each patient before surgery. The decision to undertake mitral valve replacement is an important one since resting diastolic pressure gradients and abnormal left ventricular filling can be demonstrated with all currently available prostheses.

It is difficult to lay down hard and fast indications for operation. If the clinical evidence suggests that a closed valvotomy is feasible, then the presence of definite limitation of exercise tolerance is an adequate indication, particularly in a young person. If valve replacement is likely to be required, then symptoms should be more severe. In individual patients, however, the decision is not usually difficult when there has been definite progression of symptoms. It is not often necessary to advise operation in a patient with a normal exercise tolerance, the only exception being repeated systemic emboli unresponsive to anticoagulant treatment. During pregnancy (page 11.12), especially in the middle third, cardiac output increases due to a reduction in peripheral resistance, so that patients with mild mitral stenosis may develop a large pressure gradient and even pulmonary oedema.

Although intended pregnancy might be taken as an indication for valvotomy, a closed operation can be performed quite satisfactorily at any stage. Unless it is due to coronary artery disease, the presence of left ventricular disease is not a contraindication to operation, however severe it may appear to be in terms of increased cavity size or reduced amplitude of wall motion.

Prognosis

In the absence of surgical treatment, mitral stenosis is usually a progressive disease, although the rate is unpredictable. In patients with symptomatic mitral stenosis who refuse operation, 50 per cent survival is of the order of 4–5 years. Unfavourable features include a gradual increase in the severity of the valve disease with disorganization of its structure and superimposed calcification, an increase in pulmonary resistance, and the development of functional tricuspid valve disease, with chronic elevation of the venous pressure leading to cardiac cirrhosis and impaired liver function. Surgical treatment has considerably improved the prognosis, although mitral valvotomy does not prevent progression of the rheumatic process, or reduce the risk of infective endocarditis. It has become apparent that the long-term prognosis of patients in whom mitral valve replacement has been performed is significantly limited, with a 50 per cent survival of approximately 10 years. This applies whatever the original indication for operation. In part these rather disappointing figures reflect valve related complications such as infection or thrombosis, but a major factor limiting survival is the progressive development of left ventricular disease.

Mixed mitral valve disease

Mixed mitral valve disease, the combination of mitral stenosis and mitral regurgitation, is almost invariably rheumatic in origin. In these patients, the mitral regurgitation is not usually severe in terms of the volume load that it imposes on the left ventricle, but it is significant in so far as the increased stroke volume is associated with an increased mitral diastolic pressure gradient, and also because the presence of mitral regurgitation implies a more damaged mitral valve.

Pathology

The pathology of mixed mitral valve disease is similar to that of pure mitral stenosis, except that the disease process has frequently advanced further. The valve cusps are thickened and their edges everted so that the mitral valve orifice becomes fixed. The chordae tendineae are frequently shortened and thickened and the valve apparatus may become calcified. In addition, the patient may well have had a previous mitral valvotomy which led to symptomatic improvement for a number of years but which did not alter the progress of the disease.

Clinical picture

Symptoms

As with pure mitral stenosis, the main complaint is of progressive reduction in exercise tolerance, although dyspnoea is frequently less prominent than fatigue or palpitations on exertion. Exacerbation of symptoms may result from chest infection or fluid retention, and systemic embolism remains a possibility.

Physical examination

Patients are usually in atrial fibrillation. The pulse character is normal unless additional aortic valve disease is present. The venous pressure may be raised due to a raised right ventricular end-diastolic pressure, to tricuspid valve disease, or to obstruction to right heart filling due to massive enlargement of the left atrium. On palpation of the praecordium, a left parasternal heave is often present whose mechanism is the same as in patients with pure mitral stenosis. The first sound is not usually palpable and a sustained apex beat suggests the presence of additional aortic disease or impaired left ventricular function, since rheumatic mitral regurgitation is rarely severe enough to cause clinical evidence of left ventricular hypertrophy.

On auscultation the first heart sound is soft, reflecting the presence of thickening or calcification of the anterior cusp, rather than the degree of mitral regurgitation, as was once held, and the opening snap either soft or absent. Mitral regurgitation causes a pan systolic murmur which is loudest towards the axilla, reflecting fibrosis and retraction of the posterior cusp. The mid-diastolic murmur is not usually full length, but may be loud, or even palpable, due to the increased left ventricular stroke volume. Ankle oedema or even ascites may be evidence of fluid retention, although these are unusual in the absence of tricuspid regurgitation.

Chest X-ray

This shows an enlarged heart with selective enlargement of the left atrium. In mixed mitral valve disease, the left atrium may be very large indeed with a volume of up to 3 litres ('giant left atrium') (Fig. 5). There may be calcification in the wall of the left atrium as well as in the mitral valve cusps. The lung fields show similar changes to those of pure mitral stenosis.

Electrocardiogram

This confirms atrial fibrillation and may show voltage changes of left ventricular hypertrophy, particularly deep S waves in the anterior leads rather than large R waves in V5 and 6. Since the patient is likely to be taking digitalis, it is not usually possible to comment on the T wave changes.

Echocardiogram

A reduced diastolic closure rate with anterior movement of the posterior cusp during diastole confirms the presence of rheumatic mitral valve disease. The cusp itself is usually thickened and amplitude of its movement reduced (Fig. 2). Left ventricular cavity size may be increased due to valvular regurgitation or

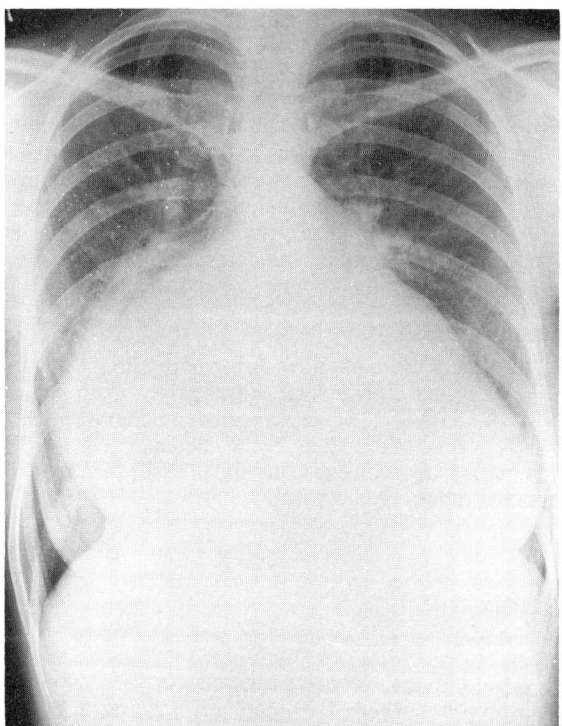

Fig. 5 Chest X-ray from a patient with mixed mitral valve disease, showing gross cardiac enlargement, due mainly to dilation of the left atrium.

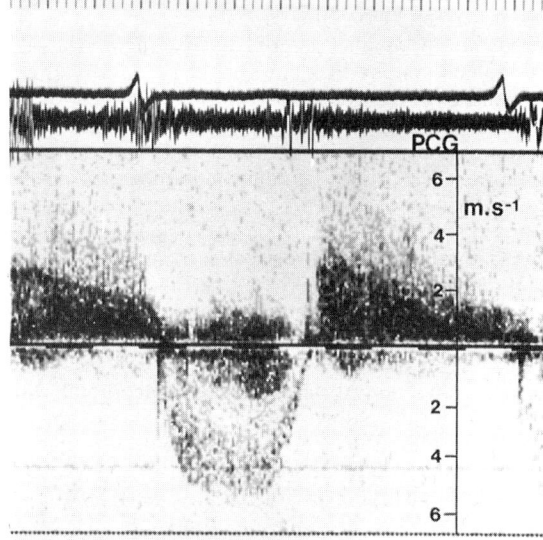

Fig. 6 Doppler cardiogram from a patient with mixed mitral valve disease, showing mitral regurgitation as a downward deflection during systole, and forward flow through the mitral orifice during diastole as an upward deflection. Peak diastolic velocity is increased due to mitral obstruction. (Gain increased for optimal recording of systolic flow velocity.)

additional left ventricular disease. The diastolic gradient across the mitral valve can be estimated with continuous wave Doppler, which can also be used to detect regurgitation flow into the left atrium (Fig. 6).

Diagnosis

This is not usually in doubt. The severity of the overall lesion is best determined from the symptoms. Attempts to determine the relative importance of the stenosis and regurgitation are unhelpful, since the two lesions are qualitatively different, so there is no way of comparing them, and since as has been pointed out, the mitral regurgitation is seldom severe. It is much more important to establish the presence or absence of other valvular lesions, particularly of the aortic valve. A giant left atrium, although producing a striking X-ray appearance, is not necessarily evidence that the disease is scvere, and its presence may actually improve the prognosis by damping the oscillations of the left atrial pressure. Similarly, the presence and severity of the pulmonary hypertension is not of major importance in determining the severity of the symptoms, or in assessing the timing or risk of operation.

Treatment
This is on exactly the same lines as for pure mitral stenosis. Surgery will almost certainly involve mitral valve replacement with a prosthesis or a biological valve. In a small number of cases, repair of the valve can be undertaken, but in rheumatic, as distinct from non-rheumatic mitral valve disease, the place of such conservative procedures is rather limited.

Mitral regurgitation

Aetiology
Unlike mitral stenosis, which is nearly always due to chronic rheumatic heart disease, there are a number of causes of pure mitral regurgitation (Table 1). The commonest of these is the floppy mitral valve. This condition has been described in the literature under a number of names, based either on its pathology or on its clinical features. Thus it has been referred to as mucinous or myxomatous degeneration, or as a ballooning or billowing mitral valve. As described below, it is probably responsible for a significant proportion of patients described as having mitral valve prolapse, or the mid-systolic click late systolic murmur syndrome.

Floppy mitral valve, which is relatively common above the age of 50 years, is a non-inflammatory process which may affect either cusp, partially or completely. The most striking abnormality is an increase in cusp area, causing folding and upward doming into the left atrium during systole. The chordae may become elongated, tortuous, and thinned, predisposing to chordal rupture. The elongated chordae can undergo fibrosis, as can the cusps, leading to an erroneous diagnosis of chronic rheumatic involvement. Ulceration of the cusps may also occur, predisposing to thrombosis on their surface, and also to infective endocarditis. The ring circumference may be normal or increased. The papillary muscles are normal. Histologically, the central valve fibrosa is abnormal with large areas in which fibrous tissue is either absent altogether, or where the collagen bundles are fragmented, coiled or disrupted, lying in pools of abnormal acid mucopolysaccharide. Over the atrial surface of the cusp, a dense layer of laminated collagen forms. There is no evidence of vascularization or of inflammatory cells in the absence of secondary infective endocarditis.

The cause of sporadic cases of floppy mitral valve is unknown. However, similar appearances may accompany Marfan's syndrome, thoracic deformities such as straight back or depressed sternum, pseudoxanthoma elasticum, Ehlers–Danos syndrome, and osteogenesis imperfecta. An association with thyrotoxicosis has also been reported. The incidence of the sporadic condition tends to rise with age, and individual case histories suggest that it may be a benign and very chronic process.

Infective endocarditis is an important cause of mitral regurgitation, which may affect the valve directly or be secondary to an infection on the aortic valve. Vegetations developing on the cusps vary from small nodules along the line of apposition to large, friable masses up to 10 mm or more in diameter which are especially common when the organism is a fungus. Cusp perforation is characteristic of staphylococcal infection. Lesions on the anterior cusp of the mitral valve may occur in association with aortic endo-

Table 1 Common causes of pure mitral regurgitation

Structures affected	Anatomical fault	Pathogenesis
Valve cusps	Congenital cleft	Primum atrial septal defect
	Redundant cusp	Marfan's syndrome 'Floppy valve'
	Perforation	Infective endocarditis
	Distortion and scarring	Rheumatic fever
	Iatrogenic	
Chordae tendineae	Redundant chordae	'Floppy valve' Marfan's syndrome
	Ruptured chordae	'Floppy valve' Marfan's syndrome Infective endocarditis Rheumatic
	Chordal shortening	Rheumatic Endomyocardial fibrosis
Papillary muscle	Dysfunction	Ischaemic heart disease Cardiomyopathy
	Prolapsing mitral valve cusp	Various
	Rupture	Acute myocardial infarction
Valve ring	Dilation	Severe left ventricular disease
	Calcification	Various

carditis, usually involving the right coronary cusp. These 'jet lesions' may appear as localized perforations or as aneurysms and may be severe enough to require mitral valve replacement in affected patients. Rarely, the vegetations may be large enough to cause mitral valve obstruction: much more commonly, the haemodynamic disturbance is of pure regurgitation. Infective endocarditis may also involve the chordae, particularly in patients with floppy mitral valve. It may occur on an otherwise normal valve, particularly in the old or debilitated, but more commonly the valve is abnormal due to minor congenital abnormality, previous rheumatic involvement, floppy mitral valve, hypertrophic cardiomyopathy, or calcification of the mitral valve ring.

Pathophysiology of mitral regurgitation
Pure mitral regurgitation is associated with a large increase in left ventricular output. The pressure in the left atrium is lower than that in the aorta, and the resistance to left ventricular ejection is reduced, so the stroke volume may be up to three times normal. Ejection begins almost immediately after the start of left ventricular contraction, and at the time of aortic valve opening, up to one-quarter of the stroke volume may already have entered the left atrium. The relative forward and backward flows depend on the relative resistances in the two directions, which has therapeutic significance in the treatment of severe mitral regurgitation. At the end of ejection, left ventricular filling begins early since the phase of isovolumic relaxation is very short. Left ventricular end-diastolic cavity size is not greatly increased, particularly when the history is short, but end-systolic size is considerably smaller than normal due to the low resistance to ejection. Left ventricular output is also maintained by the short period of relaxation before filling starts and by a sinus tachycardia which is almost invariably present in significant non-rheumatic mitral regurgitation.

Clinical picture
The clinical picture of pure mitral regurgitation is very variable, depending on the underlying pathology, the severity of the regurgitation and presence or absence of additional left ventricular disease. These clinical patterns will be described separately, recognizing that they overlap so the relation between the clinical picture and the underlying aetiology is not an invariable one.

Ruptured chordae tendineae

Ruptured chorda is often associated with severe mitral regurgitation. Though the onset of symptoms is usually gradual, in a minority of cases it may be so sudden that patients are able to describe exactly what they were doing at the time of their onset. In these latter cases, symptoms are most severe at the start, and tend to improve over the next few weeks, as left ventricular function adapts to the volume load, although even in this more compensated phase, severe limitation of exercise tolerance by breathlessness or fatigue may persist. On enquiry into the past history, a murmur has not infrequently been heard, often many years previously, and described as 'innocent' or 'benign'. The most severe cases may present in intractable pulmonary oedema and require immediate intermittent positive pressure respiration. On the other hand, when the regurgitation is only moderately severe, it is remarkably well tolerated for many years with minimal symptoms.

Clinical examination

Patients are usually in sinus rhythm until late in the course of the disease if the mitral regurgitation is non-rheumatic. Sinus tachycardia is frequent when regurgitation is severe, and the pulse 'jerky', implying that its amplitude is normal although the upstroke is rapid. The venous pressure is normal unless severe pulmonary hypertension is present. The praecordial impulse at the apex is prominent and sustained, and may be double due to a palpable third sound. A systolic thrill may also be present. A left parasternal heave is frequently apparent in severe mitral regurgitation, and usually reflects the presence of a large and expansile left atrium or of left ventricular disease, rather than right ventricular hypertrophy. The first sound is not palpable. On auscultation, the first sound is normal or reduced in intensity and the most prominent features are a loud pan systolic murmur and a third heart sound. The third sound may be rather more high-pitched than that associated with left ventricular disease, and may be confused with the second, thus leading to the murmur being mistimed. This mistake can be avoided by knowing that confusion can exist thus starting auscultation at the base of the heart where the second sound can be appreciated, and 'inching' the stethos-cope towards the apex, when the second sound can be heard to bury itself in the murmur and the third sound appear. If the mitral regurgitation is very severe, then left atrial and left ventricular pressures may equalize before the end of systole, so that the murmur stops early and, in occasional cases presenting with acute pulmonary oedema and shock, the mitral valve is effectively absent, and there is no murmur at all. Unlike rheumatic mitral regurgitation, the position at which the amplitude of the murmur appears maximal is variable, and may be at the apex, down the left sternal edge, at the back, to the left of the spine, or even on the top of the head.

Chest X-ray

The radiographic picture reflects the haemodynamic disturbance. Most characteristically, overall heart size is normal or only moderately enlarged, with selective enlargement of the left atrium, although not to the same extent as in rheumatic mitral valve disease (Fig. 7). The pulmonary vasculature reflects the presence of an increase in mean left atrial pressure. A chest X-ray taken soon after the onset of severe mitral regurgitation may show the characteristic picture of pulmonary oedema with a normal-sized heart. If the condition is severe and long-standing, considerable cardiac enlargement may develop due to co-existent left ventricular disease.

Electrocardiogram

The ECG usually shows sinus rhythm with only moderate left ventricular hypertrophy. There may, in addition, be evidence of left atrial hypertrophy. Frequent ventricular ectopic beats are characteristic of mild or moderate mitral regurgitation.

Echocardiogram

On the M-mode, the mitral valve echo may be abnormal, showing prolapse, with cusp remnants visible in the left atrium during systole. The left ventricular end-diastolic dimension is increased and end-systolic dimension reduced, compatible with a large stroke volume and normal left ventricular function. A rheumatic aetiology is excluded by a normal or increased diastolic closure rate. Cross-sectional echocardiography confirms the presence of very active left ventricular wall motion. It is also possible to get a clearer view of the extent of systolic cusp prolapse into the left atrium. The extent of the jet within the left ventricle can be determined by pulsed Doppler, or displayed directly by colour flow mapping. The velocity of the regurgitant jet as measured by continuous wave Doppler (Fig. 8) depends on the systolic pressure difference between left atrium and left ventricle and not the severity of retrograde flow; it can thus be used to give some idea of the height of the left atrial 'v' wave if left ventricular systolic pressure is known.

Cardiac catheterization

The haemodynamic disturbance is usually clear on clinical and non-invasive grounds, so that cardiac catheterization is only required to confirm or exclude coronary artery disease. The usual findings are increased right heart pressures, with 'v' waves in the pulmonary capillary pressure of up to 60 or 70 mm Hg. Left ventricular angiography demonstrates the presence of mitral regurgitation by reflux of contrast back into the left atrium from a left ventricular cavity that is normal or only moderately increased in size.

Papillary muscle dysfunction

Mitral regurgitation associated with primary left ventricular disease is usually referred to as papillary muscle dysfunction. Normal mitral closure depends on the integrity of the myocardium as well as that of the valve apparatus itself. In part, the position of the cusps is maintained during systole by contraction of the papillary muscles as the left ventricular cavity gets smaller. This mechanism may be disturbed in a number of ways. The papillary muscles themselves may be affected by ischaemic or other left ventricular

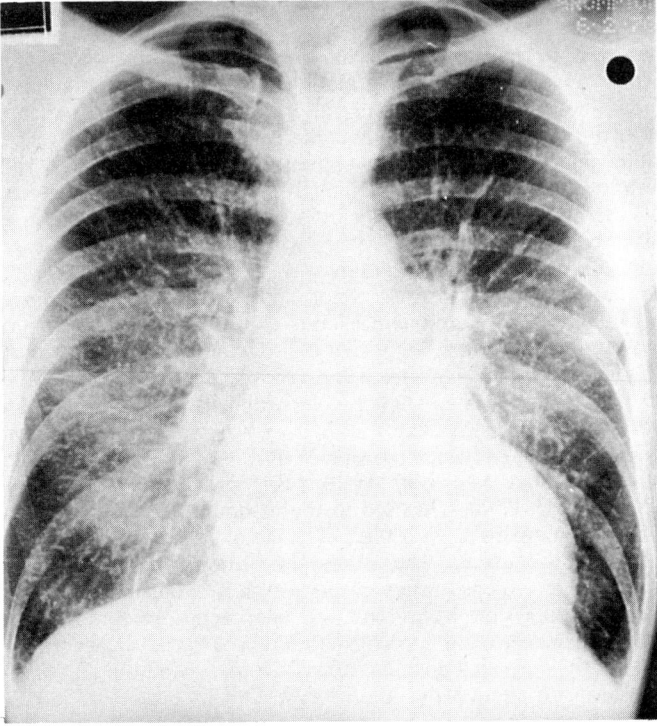

Fig. 7 Chest X-ray showing acute pulmonary oedema due to acute mitral regurgitation resulting from ruptured chordae tendineae.

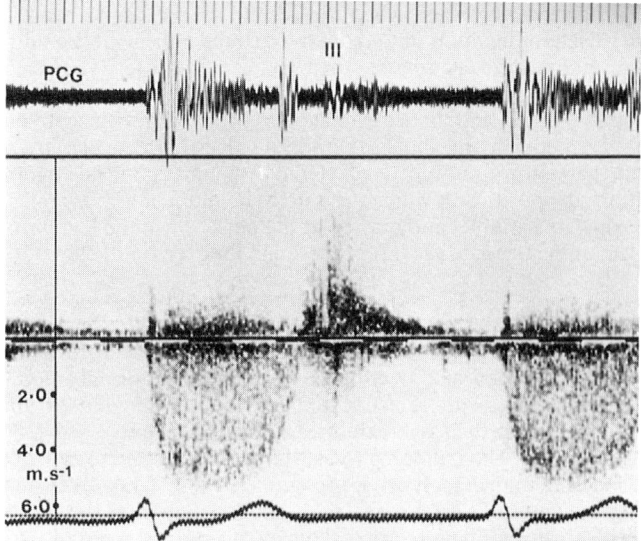

Fig. 8 Doppler cardiogram from a patient with pure mitral regurgitation, showing regurgitant flow as a downward deflection during systole. Diastolic flow velocity pattern is normal, with peak velocity coinciding with the third heart sound (III) on the phonocardiogram (PCG).

disease, leading to ischaemia or fibrosis, so that their ability to contract is impaired. If left ventricular cavity size is greatly increased, then the relation between wall movement and papillary muscle shortening may be abnormal. In hypertrophic cardiomyopathy, the greatly hypertrophied papillary muscles and abnormal cavity shape may contribute to the characteristic forward movement of the whole mitral valve apparatus during systole, which is associated with a gradient between the left ventricular cavity and the aorta as well as significant mitral regurgitation. Finally, the mitral ring itself is supported in systole by circumferentially arranged myocardium at the base of the heart. The mitral regurgitation itself occurring as the result of papillary muscle dysfunction is not usually severe, the only exception being after acute myocardial infarction. The clinical picture is thus dominated by the left ventricular disease. The presence of mitral regurgitation is demonstrated by either a late or a pan systolic murmur, which often varies in its intensity and timing from day to day, and which becomes softer with successful treatment of the underlying condition. In addition, there is evidence of left ventricular disease or congestive cardiomyopathy.

Echocardiography is informative, when it demonstrates a large cavity with poor wall movement, quite different from the picture seen in severe mitral regurgitation. If the underlying cause is hypertrophic cardiomyopathy, echocardiography allows the pathognomonic features of this condition to be demonstrated.

Cardiac catheterization confirms the presence of a raised left atrial pressure, secondary to a corresponding elevation of the left ventricular and end-diastolic pressure. Left ventricular angiography shows a dilated and poorly functioning left ventricle with reflux of contrast into the left atrium. It tends to accumulate here due to poor forward flow, thus leading to overestimation of the amount of regurgitation.

Ruptured papillary muscle

This is an unusual complication of acute myocardial infarction, causing a relatively sudden deterioration in the patient's clinical condition. Complete rupture of a papillary muscle may occur, or only a single head may be involved. Complete rupture usually occurs 2 to 5 days after the infarct, and is rarely associated with survival for more than 24 or 48 hours, death being due to cardiogenic shock and pulmonary oedema. A pan systolic murmur may be audible at the apex. Partial rupture, i.e. loss of one of the

heads, occurs rather later after the infarct, and like complete rupture, causes a striking deterioration in clinical state, along with the development of a pan systolic murmur. However, more prolonged survival is possible. The posteromedial papillary muscle is involved more frequently than the anterolateral, by both partial and complete rupture. When complete rupture occurs, death usually occurs before definitive treatment can be undertaken, but partial rupture can potentially be recognized by cross-sectional echocardiography and treated by early mitral valve replacement, once the haemodynamic state has been stabilized. The prognosis, however, is significantly worse than that after chordal rupture due to the almost invariable additional presence of severe left ventricular disease.

Dilated mitral valve ring

Dilation of the mitral valve ring is an uncommon cause of mitral regurgitation. It may well be the basis of some cases described as having 'papillary muscle dysfunction'. However, in younger patients, a clinical picture indistinguishable from that due to a floppy mitral valve may be found at surgery to have resulted from considerable dilation of the mitral ring with no evidence of any abnormality of the valve cusps or subvalve apparatus. Such patients usually come from areas where chronic rheumatic heart disease is endemic, and in addition, minor degrees of cusp fusion may be found at operation. A minority of such patients have severe left ventricular disease, presenting a clinical picture similar to that of congestive cardiomyopathy. Mitral ring dilation may complicate long-standing left ventricular enlargement, particularly that secondary to chronic aortic regurgitation. It is also a feature of mitral regurgitation due to chronic rheumatic heart disease. It is not possible to diagnose its presence with any degree of certainty preoperatively. If the regurgitation it causes is haemodynamically significant, mitral valve replacement or repair is indicated in the same way as with ruptured chorda.

Mitral prolapse

Prolapse of the mitral valve cusps into the left atrial cavity during systole is a non-specific finding that may occur in many different types of mitral valve disease, trivial or severe. Such prolapse can be documented in a number of ways, the most satisfactory being direct inspection at the time of operation. Alternatively, it may be detected by left ventricular angiography or echocardiography. Unfortunately, these various methods are not in complete agreement about the presence of mitral prolapse in individual patients. In ostium secundum atrial septal defect, for example, left ventricular angiography frequently shows evidence of mitral prolapse, although the valve is usually quite normal to inspection at the time of operation. Similarly, echocardiography and angiography may disagree, particularly in patients with coronary artery disease, when only the former method shows mitral prolapse to be present. The ability to demonstrate abnormalities of mitral valve movement by echocardiography has led to considerable interest in prolapse, and, unfortunately, to not a little confusion. Two M-mode echocardiographic patterns of valve movement have been demonstrated, late systolic and holosystolic prolapse. In the former, cusp position is normal for the first half to two-thirds of systole, but then a sudden posterior movement of one or both cusps occurs, often accompanied by a mid-systolic click and late systolic murmur (Fig. 9). This finding has led to the assumption that mitral prolapse is synonymous with the syndrome of mid-systolic click and late systolic murmur. The other echocardiographic pattern is of holosystolic prolapse, when cusp position is abnormally posterior throughout systole. On cross-sectional echocardiography, the diagnostic criterion of mitral prolapse is backward displacement of part of the cusp to a position at least 2 mm behind the line of the valve ring, taken as the line of cusp attachment. Systolic cusp apposition along the commisures is normal, unless severe mitral regurgitation is present, when one cusp moves backward into the left atrium becoming completely separated from the other. Mitral

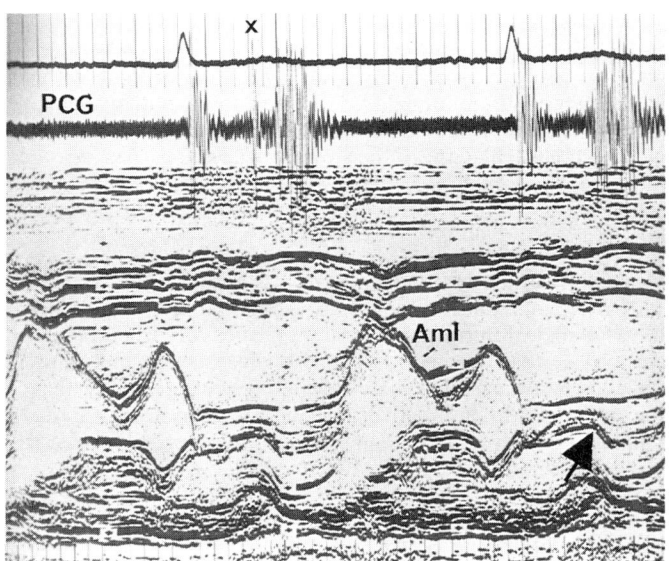

Fig. 9 Mitral valve prolapse, M-mode echocardiogram. Mid-systolic prolapse occurs, marked by the arrow. This is associated with a mid-systolic click (x) and late systolic murmur on the phonocardiogram (PCG).

prolapse as demonstrated by echocardiography, does not represent a single disease entity. In some instances, the echocardiographic diagnosis may be erroneous, the appearance of off-axis echoes from the normal mitral valve apparatus being confused with that of mitral prolapse. Since cusp and chordal redundancy are found in a significant proportion of normal subjects at autopsy, the suspicion must arise that many of the patients in whom minor degrees of prolapse are demonstrated are not, in fact, abnormal at all. Thus, M-mode findings of mitral prolapse have been described as occurring in up to 21 per cent of a series of apparently healthy females of college age, strongly suggesting that the criteria for normality have been inappropriately set. Nevertheless, it does appear that a significant number of patients do have some abnormality of the mitral valve, particularly those in whom phonocardiographic or cross-sectional echocardiographic features are present. This may be a floppy mitral valve with a minor degree of mitral regurgitation. In others, it may be early cardiomyopathy. Whatever their exact anatomical basis, these clinical and echocardiographic findings appear to have a number of clinical associations.

(a) Non-rheumatic mitral valve disease, with evidence of mitral prolapse, predisposes to infective endocarditis, particularly when due to a minor degree of cusp or chordal redundancy. Thus, all patients in whom minor mitral valve abnormalities are suspected should have prophylactic antibiotic for dental manipulations and other potentially septic hazards.

(b) Young people with evidence of mitral prolapse have a significantly increased risk of cerebral embolism. This again appears to result from non-bacterial thrombotic vegetations due to cusp ulceration. This complication is unusual, and the risk does not justify treating all patients with evidence of mitral prolapse with long-term anticoagulants.

(c) A minority of patients develop chest pain. This may be characteristic of angina pectoris, or more commonly, it is 'atypical'. It may be accompanied by T wave changes on the ECG, affecting particularly the inferior leads. Left ventriculography may show abnormalities of regional wall motion, particularly affecting the inferior wall. Coronary arteriography is normal, in typical cases showing neither fixed disease nor spasm. The genesis of the pain remains obscure, and in a significant number of cases it may well have no organic basis, simply being the result of anxiety in a patient in whom a diagnosis of organic heart disease has been made.

(d) Ventricular ectopic beats, again a normal finding, are said

to be commoner in this condition. In very occasional cases, recurrent ventricular arrhythmias may occur, which may be life-threatening. The majority of such patients are female, aged 20–60 years. Approximately half have a history of syncopal or presyncopal episodes. A late systolic murmur is common, but a mid-systolic click is unusual. The resting ECG almost invariably shows T wave abnormalities and ectopic beats. Left ventriculography, when it is performed, characteristically demonstrates severe mitral prolapse. The autopsy appearances are those of floppy mitral valve. However, in the absence of severe left ventricular hypertrophy, mitral valve abnormalities are a very unusual case of sudden death in the general population.

Mitral prolapse should not therefore be regarded as a single disease entity, but a non-specific finding. The echocardiographic evidence should be reviewed in detail before the diagnosis is made, and M-mode findings should not be accepted in isolation unless they are supported by phonocardiography or cross-sectional echocardiography. Mitral regurgitation, when present, and other associated abnormalities should be treated on their own merits.

Endomyocardial fibrosis (EMF) and eosinophilic endomyocardial disease

These two diseases are both characterized by fibrosis of the endocardium and underlying myocardium. EMF (page 13.261) occurs in equatorial regions in Africa and South America, and in South India, where it is a common cause of heart disease, particularly in the lower socioeconomic groups. Eosinophilic endomyocardial disease (page 13.217) is a rare condition, occurring in temperate regions and apparently representing the effects of direct injury to the heart by eosinophils. In both conditions, atrioventricular valve regurgitation occurs due to fibrosis and shortening of the papillary muscles, and in both the effect of the increased volume load on diastolic pressures is accentuated by subendocardial fibrosis which restricts ventricular filling. Intracavity thrombus and pericardial effusion may also occur. The dominant effect of EMF is on the right side of the heart, while that of eosinophilic endomyocardial disease is mainly on the left. Both are potentially treatable operatively with mitral or tricuspid valve replacement and subendocardial resection of fibrous tissue.

Mitral ring calcification

Heavy calcification of the base of the heart, frequently referred to as 'mitral ring calcification' is a disease of the elderly. It is commoner in females, and its incidence is increased in the presence of left ventricular hypertrophy. The calcification itself is found in the base of the posterior cusp of the mitral valve, in the central fibrous body spreading to the upper part of the interventricular septum and the anterior cusp of the mitral valve. The condition may coexist with calcific aortic stenosis. In spite of the common name for the condition, calcification is not found in the mitral ring itself, which in any case is an insubstantial structure. It usually causes no symptoms, and is detected incidentally either from a systolic murmur or, when more extensive, from calcification in the region of the mitral valve on chest X-ray. However, it is not a totally benign condition, since it is associated with a number of clinically significant complications. The cusp abnormality is a potential source of cerebral emboli, and the incidence of transient ischaemic attacks in such patients is increased. It is also a focus for infective endocarditis. Approximately half the patients with significant mitral ring calcification have abnormalities of conduction, including high-grade atrioventricular block, sinus node disease or left bundle branch block. Abnormalities of mitral cusp motion are common, and may cause mitral regurgitation severe enough to require valve replacement. In rare cases, calcification may narrow the valve orifice enough to cause clinically significant mitral stenosis, with diastolic gradients of up to 20 mm Hg.

The diagnosis is best made by echocardiography, which shows the anatomical distribution of the calcification at the base of the heart. The extent of interference with mitral valve function can be judged qualitatively by the extent of cusp movement, and quantified more precisely from continuous wave Doppler. The presence of left ventricular hypertrophy should always be sought. This may be severe, and even show the characteristics of hypertrophic cardiomyopathy. If mitral valve disease is severe, cardiac catheterization may be considered necessary.

In the absence of complications, no treatment is required other than prophylaxis against infective endocarditis. Complications are treated on their own merits.

Diagnosis of mitral regurgitation
The diagnosis of mitral regurgitation itself is usually straightforward on the basis of the physical signs. It should always be borne in mind that mitral regurgitation, unlike mitral stenosis, has a number of causes, and may be secondary to other disease, particularly of the left ventricle. The physical signs may be atypical when the regurgitation is severe, since the pressures in left atrium and left ventricle may equalize during systole, so that the murmur becomes shorter, or absent altogether if the mitral valve is destroyed. Such patients may present with cardiogenic shock of sudden and unexplained onset with a chest X-ray showing pulmonary oedema and a normal-sized heart. Echocardiography demonstrates very active left ventricular wall movement, providing that the poor peripheral blood flow is due to valvular regurgitation rather than left ventricular disease. In addition, it may show abnormal mobility of one or both mitral valve cusps. In patients who present with more typical signs, the main diagnostic problem is to decide the relative contributions of the valvular regurgitation and left ventricular disease to the overall clinical state. This may be difficult and even after echocardiography and cardiac catheterization, the final decision may not be clearcut particularly in longstanding cases.

Differential diagnosis
Ventricular septal defect (VSD)
A congenital VSD may persist into adult life and cause a pan systolic murmur maximal at the lower left sternal edge (maladie de Roger). However, such a VSD is invariably small, with no haemodynamic consequences and thus does not cause cardiac enlargement, limitation of exercise tolerance or abnormality on the chest X-ray. Acquired VSD, due to septal perforation, may present as a pan systolic murmur developing in the first few days or weeks after a myocardial infarction. Unlike the small congenital VSD described above, its presence may be associated with a large left-to-right shunt. In addition, it is situated in the muscular, rather than in the membranous septum, so that the physical signs to which it gives rise are significantly different. The differential diagnosis from mitral regurgitation is an important one since either condition may require surgical treatment. This distinction cannot be made clinically or on the basis of the chest X-ray or ECG. The presence of a VSD can be diagnosed at the bedside from a simple right heart catheter, by demonstrating a left-to-right shunt at right ventricular level. It may be possible to see the abnormality itself with two-dimensional echocardiography, from either an apical or a subcostal view. Either may show a defect in the muscular septum, with impaired movement of its apical segment. The diagnosis can be confirmed by demonstrating a negative jet in the right ventricle following a peripheral contrast injection. Definitive preoperative diagnosis requires left ventricular contrast angiography, since as well as the VSD, there is frequently a ventricular aneurysm or a significant area of hypokinesis, and, in addition, significant mitral regurgitation may be present. In individual patients, the main problems are to decide the relative contribution of valvular regurgitation and left ventricular disease to overall clinical state, and on the optimal timing of operation. These may be difficult, and, even after full investigation, the final decision may not be clearcut.

Aortic valve disease
The ejection systolic murmur of aortic valve disease is frequently audible at the apex, where it may be louder than at the base, and have a slightly different quality. However, this is not an adequate basis for diagnosing additional mitral regurgitation and it is essential to establish that the timing of the murmur is pan systolic, either from its relation to the second heart sound, or in aortic regurgitation, from its relation to the start of the early diastolic murmur.

Tricuspid regurgitation
The pan systolic murmur of tricuspid regurgitation may be mistaken for that of mitral regurgitation, particularly when the right ventricle is greatly enlarged. The presence of tricuspid regurgitation can be suspected from an elevated venous pressure with systolic waves, and confirmed using contrast echocardiography or Doppler. In severe mitral regurgitation, however, additional tricuspid regurgitation may be present and the distinction between the two becomes academic.

Hypertrophic cardiomyopathy
Patients with hypertrophic cardiomyopathy frequently present with a systolic murmur, maximal down the left sternal edge, whose characteristics, on auscultation, appear half way between ejection and a pan systolic murmur. A proportion of such cases do, in fact, have significant mitral regurgitation, but, in a minority, the murmur appears to emanate from the left ventricular outflow tract, and is associated with a significant pressure difference between the left ventricular cavity and the aortic root. The diagnosis can readily be made by echocardiography, the M-mode technique showing systolic anterior motion of the anterior cusp of the mitral valve.

Prognosis
The prognosis of mild or moderately severe, primary mitral regurgitation is excellent, with 20–30 year survival being well documented. The main risk factor in such patients is the development of infective endocarditis, or chordal rupture, both of which lead to a sudden increase in the severity of the regurgitation. When the regurgitation is severe enough to cause significant symptoms and cardiac enlargement, the prognosis becomes much more limited, 50 per cent survival in such cases being of the order of 2–3 years. The prognosis in secondary mitral regurgitation depends on that of the underlying condition. If this is left ventricular disease, the overall outlook is likely to be poor.

Treatment
Mild mitral regurgitation is well tolerated and does not require treatment apart from prophylactic antibiotics for all dental manipulations and potentially septic hazards. Such patients should be followed up at annual intervals, since mitral regurgitation, particularly when due to degenerative disease, may be progressive. When mitral regurgitation is due to papillary muscle dysfunction, treatment is that of the underlying condition which usually means administration of digitalis, diuretic, and vasodilator. If the patient has hypertrophic cardiomyopathy, however, then treatment with a β-adrenergic blocking drug or a calcium antagonist may be more appropriate.

Severe mitral regurgitation, which causes significant symptoms in spite of medical treatment, is best managed by mitral valve surgery. This will involve either mitral valve replacement, or in suitable cases, mitral valve repair. Repair is most satisfactory when regurgitation is due to rupture of the chordae normally supporting the middle third of the posterior cusp. The operation consists of approximating the two outer scallops, and has proved a very satisfactory one. When chordal rupture or redundancy affects the anterior cusp, repair is not usually feasible, and replacement is normally undertaken. After acute chordal rupture, it is frequently possible to treat the patients medically with rest, digitalis, and

Table 2 Types of valuvar aortic stenosis

Valvular
    Congenital
    Calcified bicuspid valve
    Rheumatic
    'Senile' (calcified tricuspid valve)
    Infective endocarditis (rare)
    Hyperlipidaemia (rare)
Fixed subaortic stenosis
Supravalvular

diuretics for several weeks, while the left ventricle compensates for the increased volume load, often with considerable clinical improvement, so that surgery becomes a less hazardous procedure than an emergency operation in the acute stage would have been.

Very severe mitral regurgitation may require emergency treatment on account of intractible pulmonary oedema or a low output state. Such pulmonary oedema is best treated by intermittent positive pressure respiration. The most effective means of managing a low cardiac output state associated with mitral regurgitation is not to administer cardiotonic drugs, such as digoxin or isoprenaline, but to give a vasodilator. This reduces the peripheral resistance, and thus increases the volume of blood entering the aorta at the expense of that going back into the left atrium. Sodium nitroprusside, by continuous intravenous infusion, at a dose of 20–200 μg/min as a 0.01 per cent solution is the agent most frequently used. This requires that arterial pressure, and preferably pulmonary wedge pressure and cardiac output, are measured at frequent intervals in order to control the infusion rate. If these facilities are not available, then intravenous salbutamol at a rate of 10 μg/min can be used, when such monitoring is unnecessary. Vasodilators, with or without intermittent positive pressure respiration, may make it possible for the cardiac state to be stabilized long enough to allow the underlying diagnosis to be confirmed and cardiac surgery arranged.

Vasodilators are also very effective in patients with papillary muscle dysfunction associated with severe left ventricular disease where their use may lead to a temporary, but nevertheless, useful symptomatic improvement.

Aortic stenosis

Aortic stenosis represents a fixed obstruction to left ventricular ejection at the level of the valve cusps. Significant fixed obstruction to the left ventricular outflow tract may also develop immediately above the sinuses, when it is referred to as supravalvar aortic stenosis, or below the valve, within the left ventricular cavity, referred to as subaortic stenosis.

Aetiology

Types of aortic stenosis are summarized in Table 2.

Aortic valve stenosis is an important cause of cardiac disability, and though commonest in elderly males, it may present at any time of life. Congenital aortic stenosis, due to a valve with only a single commissure is most frequent in infancy or childhood. A much more common abnormality, the congenital bicuspid valve, consisting of two approximately equal-sized cusps, may be detected as an incidental finding early in life, but not give rise to significant haemodynamic abnormality unless it becomes calcified or involved by infective endocarditis. Rheumatic aortic stenosis develops as the result of commissural fusion in a tricuspid valve and may subsequently become calcified. Senile or degenerative aortic stenosis results from deposition of calcium in a bicuspid valve in the absence of any inflammatory process. Very rarely, vegetations in infective endocarditis, or lipid deposits occurring in

hyperlipidaemia may be bulky enough to cause a significant left ventricular outflow tract obstruction.

Pathophysiology

The presence of aortic stenosis leads to the development of a pressure gradient between the left ventricular cavity and the aorta, which in symptomatic cases, may be greater than 50–70 mm Hg at rest, and reach over 200 mm Hg on exertion. The resistance is a fixed one, and thus differs from the increased peripheral vascular resistance of systemic hypertension, which falls during exercise. As a result of the increase in stroke work, left ventricular hypertrophy develops, with the thickness of the wall increasing although the cavity size is normal or even reduced. This hypertrophy causes an increase in the diastolic stiffness of the cavity so that end-diastolic pressure may rise causing pulmonary vascular congestion. Increased left ventricular wall thickness also predisposes to ventricular arrhythmias. Late in the disease, when left ventricular involvement is severe, the cavity becomes dilated and more spherical in shape. In the majority of cases, calcification is confined to the aortic valve, but in a minority it may spread to involve either cusp of the mitral valve or the atrioventricular node, and thus give rise to a prolonged P–R interval or even to complete heart block. Finally, aortic stenosis is most common in a population of patients in whom the incidence of ischaemic heart disease is high, so that obstructive coronary artery disease may contribute, coincidentally, to the development of symptoms or impairment of left ventricular function.

Clinical picture

Symptoms

The three characteristic clinical features of aortic stenosis are breathlessness, chest pain, and syncope. Breathlessness in aortic stenosis is frequently associated with an elevated left ventricular end-diastolic pressure and it occurs at first on exercise, but later at rest. A common mode of presentation is with an attack of pulmonary oedema precipitated by some unusual exertion. Paroxysmal nocturnal dyspnoea is common in late stages of the disease. The length of the history of breathlessness from its onset until it becomes severe is usually only of the order of 1–2 years, and thus considerably shorter than that of mitral stenosis. Angina occurring in aortic stenosis is clinically indistinguishable from that due to ischaemic heart disease, and indeed, in many cases this is the underlying cause. However, typical anginal pain can occur in aortic stenosis in patients in whom the large and medium-sized coronary arteries are normal. The mechanism for this is uncertain; its presence is associated with an abnormal pattern of coronary flow, and in particular with reduction in its peak velocity which characteristically occurs early in diastole. In the absence of obstructive coronary artery disease, angina in such patients is associated with prolonged left ventricular relaxation and slow filling, characteristic of hypertrophy. Syncope in aortic stenosis probably reflects a number of different types of disturbance. In some patients, it is clearly related to exertion and appears to be due to hypotension resulting from the combination of exercise-induced vasodilation and a limited cardiac output. In others, it results from transient complete atrioventricular block due to involvement of the atrioventricular node by calcification, from short periods of ventricular fibrillation or tachycardia, or from carotid sinus hypersensitivity. Exactly similar mechanisms may underlie the greatly increased incidence of sudden death in these patients.

Clinical examination

The physical signs of aortic stenosis are very characteristic. The carotid pulse is slow rising with a reduced amplitude and an early notch on the upstroke, followed by a thrill. The venous pressure is usually normal until late in the disease, but a small 'a' wave is frequently present. This is not necessarily due to pulmonary hypertension, but appears to be related in some way to the presence of left ventricular hypertrophy causing increased resistance to right ventricular filling (Bernheim 'a' wave). The apex beat is sustained and is often double, due to the presence of an additional left atrial impulse. On auscultation, the first sound is normal or reduced, and may be preceded by a fourth heart sound, although this is often difficult to hear even when an atrial impulse is palpable. The second sound is single when the valve is calcified, due to lack of the aortic component. In younger patients with mobile aortic valve cusps, aortic valve closure may be audible, but delayed, so that splitting of the second sound is reversed. When left ventricular disease is severe, pulmonary valve closure is accentuated. The characteristic ejection systolic murmur is maximal at the base of the heart, and is also audible over the right common carotid artery. It may seem longer than the ejection systolic murmur of, for example, anaemia or thyrotoxicosis due to prolongation of ventricular systole and delay in aortic valve closure. An additional short, soft early diastolic murmur is nearly always present, although this does not imply haemodynamically significant aortic regurgitation.

Chest X-ray

Heart size is normal in uncomplicated aortic stenosis. If it is increased, the underlying cause is likely to be unsuspected aortic regurgitation, left ventricular cavity dilation, or very severe left ventricular hypertrophy, when the cavity may be normal in size but the myocardium up to 50 mm in thickness. Increased left ventricular filling pressure may cause left atrial hypertension and thus dilation of the upper lobe vessels as well as selective enlargement of the left atrium in the absence of organic mitral valve disease. The aortic root is nearly always dilated and the aortic valve calcified in older patients which is best seen on the lateral chest X-ray or with screening.

Electrocardiogram

ECG characteristically shows changes of left ventricular hypertrophy, although it may be entirely normal, even in the presence of severe aortic stenosis. Left atrial hypertrophy is shown by a bifid P wave in lead II or a dominant negative deflection in V1. Conduction disturbances include left anterior hemiblock, left bundle branch block, prolonged P–R interval, or complete heart block. Poor progression of R waves across the chest leads is common, and appears to be evidence of septal hypertrophy rather than anterior myocardial infarction.

Echocardiogram

If the aortic valve is calcified, disruption of the normal anatomy can be demonstrated by M-mode, but in younger patients, it may appear entirely normal, even when severe aortic stenosis is present. Cross-sectional echocardiography is very useful for demon-

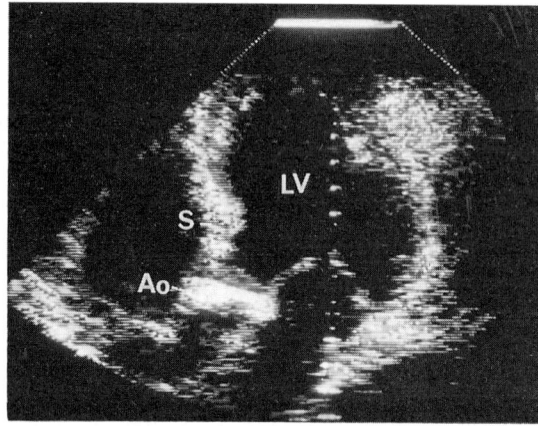

Fig. 10 Aortic stenosis, two-dimensional echocardiogram from apical four-chamber view, showing left ventricle (LV) and heavily calcified aortic valve (Ao). Se, septum.

strating abnormalities in the left ventricular outflow tract (Fig. 10). Thickening and reduced mobility of the valve cusps can nearly always be demonstrated. In young patients with a bicuspid valve, doming of the cusps during systole can be seen, while in older patients, a calcified aortic valve appears as an immobile mass. Echocardiography is also of value in studying left ventricular anatomy and function. Hypertrophy can be assessed as an increase in the thickness of the posterior wall and the septum. Abnormal diastolic properties of the ventricle are associated with a reduction in the diastolic closure rate of the mitral valve, although the cusp echo itself is normal, and the posterior cusp moves in a posterior direction during diastole, in contrast to rheumatic mitral stenosis. The hypertrophy itself may be concentric, or may involve the septum to a much greater extent than the posterior wall, resembling the pattern seen in hypertrophic cardiomyopathy. The papillary muscles are also likely to be hypertrophied, with apical cavity obliteration. The peak gradient across the valve during ejection can be reliably estimated using continuous wave Doppler.

Cardiac catheterization

The aortic systolic gradient can be measured directly at cardiac catheterization (Fig. 11). In uncomplicated cases it is usually greater than 60 mm Hg, but may be lower in the presence of severe left ventricular disease, when stroke volume is reduced. Left ventricular end-diastolic and mean left atrial pressures may be raised, associated with a corresponding increase in right heart pressures. Angiography allows left ventricular cavity size to be assessed, and additional aortic regurgitation can be detected from an aortic root injection. Co-existent coronary artery disease can be diagnosed by coronary arteriography.

Diagnosis

A complete diagnosis of aortic stenosis depends not only on establishing the anatomical abnormality, but also its severity and the degree of associated left ventricular disease. Mild aortic stenosis is associated with a normal carotid pulse and a short systolic murmur which stops well before the second sound, reflecting the fact that a pressure gradient is present between the left ventricular cavity and the aorta only during the first part of systole. In addition, both components of the second heart sound are audible and splitting is normal. If mild aortic stenosis is due to a bicuspid valve, then an ejection click and a short early diastolic murmur may also be present. Severe aortic stenosis associated with advanced left ventricular disease may cause atypical physical signs, with a carotid pulse of small amplitude, but normal upstroke, but apart from this, significant aortic stenosis should not be diagnosed unless the upstroke of the carotid pulse is modified. The presence of left ventricular hypertrophy can be diagnosed from the apical impulse which is characteristically sustained, although not necessarily displaced, since the heart size is normal. A double impulse due to a palpable left atrial contraction is further evidence of left ventricular hypertrophy, and its presence correlates with reduced diastolic distensibility. A raised left ventricular end-diastolic pressure can be deduced from accentuation of pulmonary valve closure, which forms the only component of the audible second sound. The severity of left ventricular disease does not necessarily parallel that of aortic stenosis, and it is not uncommon to see mild aortic stenosis in association with severe left ventricular disease.

Differential diagnosis

1. Hypertrophic cardiomyopathy (see page 13.221). Patients with hypertrophic cardiomyopathy may also have a history of dyspnoea, chest pain, and syncopal attacks, which may be very similar to that associated with valvular aortic stenosis, although its duration may be longer. On physical examination the carotid pulse is normal or jerky, rather than slow rising, and the systolic murmur, when present, tends to be louder down the left sternal edge, or even at the apex rather than at the base of the heart and

over the carotid arteries. The definitive diagnosis is made by echo-cardiography or left ventricular angiography, which shows obliteration of the apical part of the left ventricular cavity at end-systole.

In some patients with valvular aortic stenosis, left ventricular hypertrophy may be unusually severe, and come to resemble that seen in hypertrophic cardiomyopathy.

2. Fixed subaortic stenosis (see page 13.267). This condition characteristically presents in children and young adults who are asymptomatic, but in whom a systolic murmur is found at routine examination. The physical signs differ from those of aortic valve stenosis in the same age group in that an ejection click is absent, and a short early diastolic murmur usually present. As with valvular aortic stenosis, there is clinical and cardiographic evidence of left ventricular disease which may be very severe. Cross-sectional echocardiography demonstrates the site of obstruction to left ventricular outflow, and is capable of distinguishing between a discrete membrane or a more extensive tunnel stenosis. M-mode echocardiography may show mid-systolic closure of the aortic valve, which is not specific to this condition, but is none the less rather suggestive of its presence. The gradient can be estimated by continuous wave Doppler. Definite confirmation of the diagnosis can also be made by left ventricular angiography which demonstrates the presence of a small chamber immediately under the aortic valve.

3. Congestive cardiomyopathy (see page 13.209). Patients with advanced aortic stenosis may occasionally present with severe breathlessness, a large heart on X-ray, a small volume pulse with a normal upstroke, a third heart sound, and pan systolic murmur due to papillary muscle dysfunction. This clinical picture represents one possible outcome of patients with untreated aortic stenosis. The diagnosis can be suspected from the presence of calcification in the aortic valve on lateral chest X-ray and can be confirmed by demonstration of a gradient across the valve of 30–40 mm Hg at cardiac catheterization. If the clinical state can be improved by medical management, then the typical physical signs of aortic stenosis may reappear.

4. Heart block. Patients with aortic stenosis may develop complete heart block and, with the slow heart-rate and corresponding increase in stroke volume, the slow-rising pulse may not be apparent, so that the condition can mimic uncomplicated complete heart block. The combination should be suspected when the systolic blood pressure is low or normal, since it is raised in uncomplicated heart block with a slow ventricular rate. The true diagnosis becomes apparent when ventricular pacing is instituted.

Prognosis

Mild or moderately severe aortic stenosis without evidence of left ventricular disease is well tolerated. By contrast, severe aortic stenosis with symptoms of left ventricular disease has a poor prognosis, with a 50 per cent survival of less than two years. These patients are at risk from sudden death as well as acute pulmonary oedema.

Treatment

Medical treatment has little to offer in aortic stenosis, since in mild cases, it is unnecessary and in severe ones ineffective. However, it is essential that all patients with aortic stenosis, of whatever severity, have prophylactic antibiotic for any potentially septic hazard. Patients with severe left ventricular disease and fluid retention will benefit from a period of bed-rest and treatment with a diuretic before operation is contemplated, but it must be remembered that the primary abnormality is a mechanical one, which cannot be significantly modified by altering renal sodium handling by diuretic agents. Prolonged treatment of such patients with large doses of powerful diuretics merely induces potassium depletion with a corresponding increase in the risk of postoperative rhythm disturbances.

Severe aortic stenosis is a surgical condition, and aortic valve replacement in such patients is an extremely effective operation. In uncomplicated cases, it can be carried out with low mortality and morbidity, and thus should be considered in all patients in whom the disease causes significant symptoms. It is likely to relieve breathlessness, angina, or syncope, whether due to ischaemic heart disease or to the aortic stenosis itself. If coronary artery disease is also present, saphenous bypass grafting is usually performed at the same operation. In general only one or two coronary arteries are grafted, and there is still no evidence of either symptomatic or prognostic benefit from this additional procedure. The combined operation implies that all patients should be studied with coronary arteriography pre-operatively, and increases the length of the operation itself. Patients with severe aortic stenosis and advanced left ventricular disease should always be urgently considered for valve replacement however bad their clinical condition. Although the risks of operation are naturally higher, the striking improvement in symptomatic state in many survivors compared with the uniformly poor prognosis untreated makes the operation well worthwhile. At the other extreme is the patient who is asymptomatic, but who is found to have a systolic murmur and evidence of significant aortic stenosis at routine examination. Although a decision will clearly be influenced by local surgical facilities and the preferences of the patient, it should be remembered that such patients show an increased incidence of sudden death, and also that, if they are followed up, they almost invariably develop symptoms within 1 or 2 years. The choice between a biological and a mechanical valve must also be made. Since patients with aortic stenosis are likely to be in sinus rhythm, using a biological valve will allow anticoagulants to be dispensed with which may be an advantage in elderly patients who commonly come to surgery. On the other hand, in the aortic position, the performance of mechanical valves over the years has been very satisfactory, lasting 15 or 20 years. In a young patient, with no contraindication to anticoagulant therapy, therefore, there is much to be said for a mechanical valve, at least until the problem of long-term survival of biological valves is clarified.

Aortic stenosis and incompetence

Aetiology

The combination of aortic stenosis and regurgitation usually results from chronic rheumatic heart disease, but may also be caused by infective endocarditis on a previously stenotic valve. As with mixed mitral valve disease, the additional regurgitation may not be severe enough to constitute a significant volume load on the left ventricle, but nevertheless, causes significant alterations to the pathophysiology. This may be due to the increased stroke volume causing a corresponding increase in the pressure gradient across the valve, although the orifice itself is not greatly narrowed. A more significant factor is that if left ventricular cavity size is normal and its wall thickness due to hypertrophy, then it is relatively indistensible during diastole. A moderate increase in stroke volume will thus result in a disproportionate increase in end-diastolic pressure and, therefore, in mean left atrial pressure. It is clear that this is due solely to altered diastolic properties of the ventricle, although the resulting pulmonary congestion is frequently said to be evidence of 'heart failure'.

Clinical picture

The clinical features of mixed aortic valve disease do not differ significantly from those of pure aortic stenosis, except that breathlessness is usually the most prominent symptom. On examination, those cases who are uncomplicated remain in sinus rhythm until late in the disease, and atrial fibrillation suggests the presence of additional rheumatic mitral valve disease. A subgroup of patients, in whom the mitral valve is normal, however, should be recognized in whom left ventricular end-diastolic pressure is greatly raised, and who resemble those with rheumatic mitral valve dis-

Table 3 Causes of aortic regurgitation

Cusp
  Distortion
    Rheumatic
    Rheumatoid
  Perforation
    Infective endocarditis
    Traumatic
Ring
  Dilation
    Dissecting aneurysm
    Marfan's syndrome
    Syphilis
    Ankylosing spondylitis
    Reiter's syndrome, ulcerative colitis
Loss of support
  Associated ventricular septal defect

ease by developing atrial fibrillation, selective left atrial enlargement, and severe pulmonary hypertension. The character of the carotid pulse is modified in mixed aortic valve disease, being bisferiens, implying the presence of a notch half way up the upstroke. As in pure aortic stenosis, left ventricular hypertrophy is shown by a sustained apical impulse, with or without a palpable left atrial contraction. The diagnosis is confirmed by the presence of aortic systolic and diastolic murmurs, maximal down the left sternal edge. If the patient is in atrial fibrillation, evidence of additional rheumatic mitral valve disease should be sought, with particular reference to a palpable first heart sound, an opening snap, and a mid-diastolic murmur. Chest X-ray shows moderate cardiac enlargement and, in older patients, evidence of aortic valve calcification. Selective enlargement of the left atrium suggests the presence of additional mitral valve disease. ECG confirms left ventricular hypertrophy. Echocardiography can be used to measure left ventricular cavity size and thus to gain some idea of the severity of the regurgitation from the stroke volume. The technique can also be used to confirm or exclude the presence of rheumatic mitral valve disease.

Diagnosis and treatment

Differential diagnosis from pure aortic stenosis or regurgitation is largely academic. In particular, any attempt to assess the relative importance of stenosis and regurgitation is misplaced since the treatment of the condition is surgical, with aortic valve replacement, the same criteria being applied as described in the previous section.

Aortic regurgitation

Aortic regurgitation is an important form of valvular heart disease, and may result from a number of pathological mechanisms which are summarized in Table 3.

Pathology

Chronic rheumatic involvement leads to the characteristic appearance of a tricuspid valve whose cusps are thickened, with rolled edges, and whose commissures are fused. There may be superimposed calcification or thrombosis. The vegetations of infective endocarditis may lead to cusp destruction or perforation and frequently spread to involve the sinus of Valsalva, the atrio-ventricular node and the interventricular septum, where abcess formation may occur. Organisms may also be carried to the anterior cusp of the mitral valve, where they cause 'jet lesions'.

Isolated dilation of the aortic root is now the commonest cause of significant aortic regurgitation in the Western World and is associated with normal cusps, which fail to appose completely during diastole. This can also result from a 'flask-shaped' aneurysm of the ascending aorta, often seen in Marfan's syndrome, or isolated medionecrosis. Syphilitic aortitis causes dilation of the valve ring, with aneurysm formation of the ascending aorta and involvement of the coronary ostia. Dilation of the ring may also occur in association with connective tissue diseases such as ankylosing spondylitis, rheumatoid arthritis, Reiter's syndrome, or relapsing polychondritis. Dissecting aneurysm involving the aortic root may separate the cusps from the valve ring; and the presence of a high ventricular septal defect or Fallot's tetralogy may leave the cusps unsupported from below. Systemic hypertension aggravates the extent of regurgitant flow whatever the severity of the valve lesion, and severe aortic regurgitation itself is frequently accompanied by systolic hypertension. However, there is no definite evidence to suggest that hypertension alone causes clinically significant aortic regurgitation.

Pathophysiology

Aortic regurgitation is associated with an increase in left ventricular stroke volume with a corresponding increase in left ventricular cavity size. Wall thickness is within normal limits, but left ventricular mass is increased. In moderately severe aortic regurgitation, the stroke volume is twice normal, and when it is severe, up to three or even four times normal. The characteristics of ejection are altered in that the end-diastolic pressure in the aorta is low, so that the resistance to ejection of blood by the left ventricle is reduced. This, together with the large stroke volume, explains the characteristic rapid upstroke and large volume pulse. Additional peripheral vasodilation may be present which also contributes to the large stroke volume. In long standing cases, left ventricular cavity size increases out of proportion to the stroke volume, with loss of the normal myocardial architecture, so that the cavity becomes more spherical in shape, and ejection fraction falls. The walls become stiffer, so that end-diastolic pressure rises and pulmonary congestion develops.

Clinical picture

Patients with aortic regurgitation remain asymptomatic for many years. When symptoms develop, they are commonly those of left ventricular disease, with breathlessness the most prominent one. This usually occurs on exercise, but the presenting symptom may be nocturnal dyspnoea, or an attack of acute pulmonary oedema precipitated by severe exertion. Chest pain may also be a prominent symptom resulting from reduced coronary perfusion pressure during diastole, co-existent coronary artery disease, or ostial involvement in syphilitic aortitis. A rather similar retrosternal pain, aggravated by exertion, may develop in patients with aneurysms of the ascending aorta in whom the coronary arteries are normal, which seems to originate from the aortic root itself. Aortic dissection may also cause severe central chest pain.

The physical signs of aortic regurgitation are characteristic. The carotid pulse has a large amplitude and a rapid upstroke, and is described as 'collapsing'. A notch may be palpable towards the end of the upstroke, whose presence is compatible with the diagnosis of pure aortic regurgitation, and does not imply the presence of significant aortic stenosis. This latter diagnosis is also excluded by the presence of visible arterial pulsation in the neck (Corrigan's sign). It is also useful to elict a waterhammer pulse (a waterhammer was a Victorian toy consisting of an evacuated glass tube containing water, which moved from one end to the other with a bump when it was tipped) by elevating the forearm and feeling its knocking quality with the palm of the hand through the muscles. Other physical signs which depend on an increase in stroke volume and peripheral vasodilation, which include capillary pulsation, visible in the nail beds, and de Musset's sign, nodding of the head in time with the heart beat are now largely of historical interest. Of greater practical importance is Durosiez' sign, which is elicited by compression of the femoral artery and listening proximally with the stethoscope for a diastolic murmur. A positive test implies retrograde flow in the femoral artery due to aortic regurgitation of at least moderate severity. It may remain positive in patients in whom severe left ventricular disease prevents the development of the other peripheral signs of aortic regurgitation.

The peripheral pulses should always be checked to exclude coarctation of the aorta. The venous pressure is normal until late in the course of the disease, although the venous pulse may show a Bernheim 'a' wave. The left ventricular impulse is sustained indicating the presence of hypertrophy: a palpable 'a' wave is much less common than in aortic stenosis, and when present often denotes additional left ventricular disease. On auscultation, the characteristic finding is an early diastolic murmur, maximal down the left sternal edge: less commonly, it is loudest at the apex or even in the left axilla (the Cole–Cecil murmur). An ejection systolic murmur is nearly always present, reflecting the presence of a large stroke volume, and not necessarily due to additional stenosis. Aortic valve closure is not usually audible, but pulmonary hypertension is due to a raised left atrial pressure. At the apex, a third heart sound may be present, if the left ventricular cavity is dilated, but more commonly, a mid-diastolic murmur may be audible, indistinguishable from that of mitral stenosis (Austin–Flint murmur). This may continue throughout diastole, and be associated with presystolic accentuation and even a loud first heart sound, though the last is never palpable. In addition, there may be a mitral pan systolic murmur due to dilation of the valve ring.

These classical signs of aortic regurgitation may be modified in a number of circumstances. If infective endocarditis has caused cusp perforation, then the early diastolic murmur may have a high-pitched musical quality, a so-called 'seagull murmur'. In the presence of severe left ventricular disease, or less commonly, of rheumatic mitral stenosis, the collapsing pulse, and other evidence of aortic regurgitation may be lost, although the aortic diastolic murmur persists. It is worth noting, however, that Durosiez' sign frequently remains positive in these circumstances if the regurgitation is moderate or severe. Of particular importance is the recognition of severe aortic regurgitation of rapid onset, usually due to infective endocarditis affecting the aortic valve. The patient presents with a low cardiac output state, normal or reduced pulse volume, sinus tachycardia, and on auscultation the main abnormality a loud, low pitched early diastolic bruit resembling a third sound, which appears to represent rapid left ventricular filling from the aorta. A short early diastolic murmur is sometimes audible, and Durosiez' sign is positive.

Chest X-ray

Significant aortic regurgitation is always accompanied by cardiac enlargement on chest X-ray. The aortic root is usually dilated, but the aortic valve not necessarily calcified. The pulmonary vasculature remains normal until severe left ventricular disease develops (Fig. 11).

Electrocardiogram

This usually shows left ventricular hypertrophy on voltage and T wave criteria, with left atrial enlargement. Left bundle branch block may develop, and indicates the presence of left ventricular disease. A long P–R interval in association with aortic regurgitation is very suggestive evidence of disease of the aortic root.

Echocardiogram

Left ventricular cavity size can be measured by echocardiography and stroke volume estimated. Rheumatic mitral valve disease can be excluded if the cusp echo is thin and posterior movement of the posterior cusp demonstrated during diastole. In chronic isolated aortic regurgitation, a characteristic high frequency fluttering motion is superimposed on the anterior cusp echo during diastole, probably due to its position in the regurgitant stream of blood immediately below the aortic root (Fig. 12). Less commonly, similar movement can be seen superimposed on the septal echo. In infective endocarditis, vegetations can be identified on the aortic valve cusps, which replace the usual slender aortic cusp echoes. In

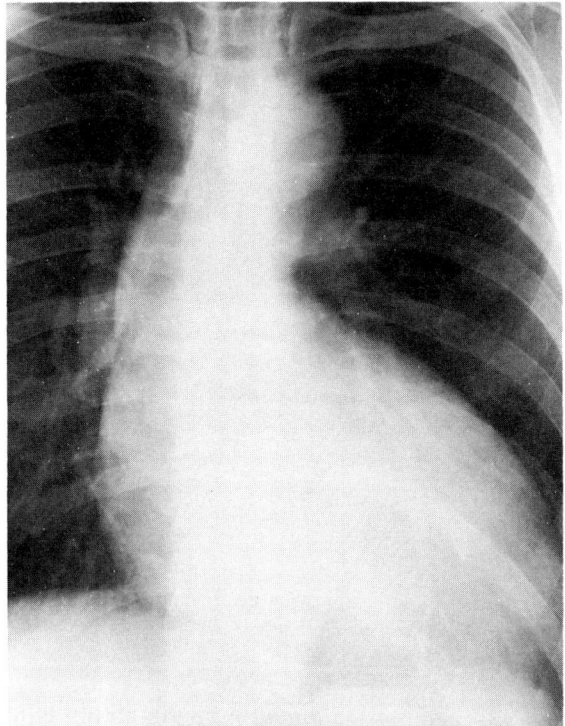

Fig. 11 Chest X-ray from a patient with chronic aortic regurgitation showing cardiac enlargement and dilation of the ascending aorta.

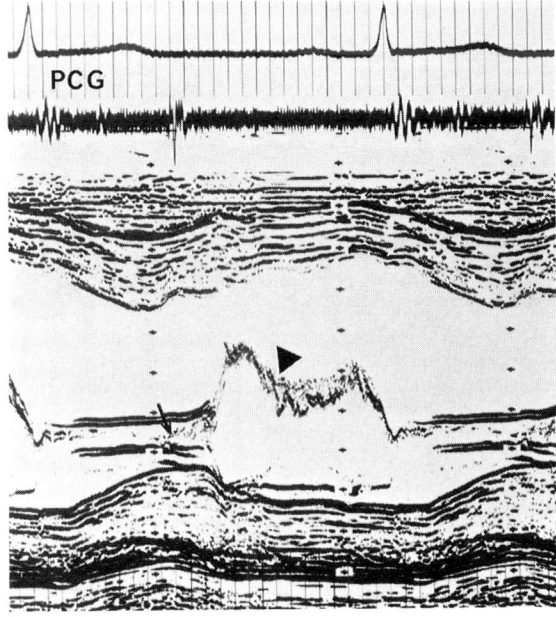

Fig. 12 Chronic aortic regurgitation, M-mode echocardiogram, showing 'flutter' on the anterior cusp of the mitral valve, marked by the arrow. PCG, phonocardiogram.

acute aortic regurgitation, mitral valve movement is very abnormal, showing premature closure (Fig. 13). This results from severe regurgitation into a relatively non-compliant left ventricular cavity causing the pressure to rise, and thus leading to mitral valve closure in mid-diastole. Its presence implies that left ventricular and aortic diastolic pressures are equal, so that the coronary perfusion pressure is zero. A less common echocardiographic manifestation of the same phenomenon is premature opening of the aortic valve cusps before the onset of ejection (Fig. 14). Cross-

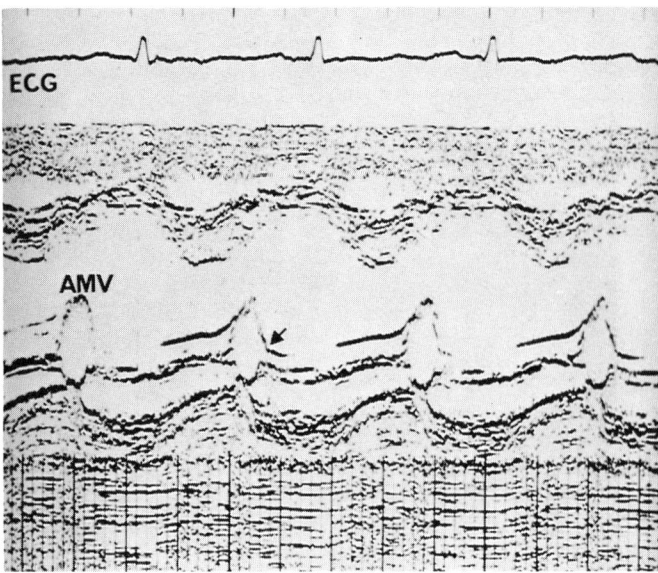

Fig. 13 M-mode echocardiogram showing premature mitral valve closure (arrow) in a patient with acute aortic regurgitation due to infective endocarditis.

and the state of the left ventricle assessed. The presence or absence of symptoms is an unsatisfactory way of assessing the severity of either the regurgitation or the left ventricular disease. Patients with severe regurgitation may remain asymptomatic with a normal or near normal subjective exercise tolerance in spite of a high end-diastolic pressure and even of pulmonary oedema on the chest X-ray. In addition, patients with no more than moderate disease and normal left ventricular function may develop non-specific symptoms. To some extent these problems can be circumvented by exercise testing. In uncomplicated cases, the severity can be judged more satisfactorily from the carotid pulse and from the heart size on chest X-ray, but direct measurement of left ventricular cavity size and stroke volume by echocardiography or angiography is a more reliable method. Left ventricular disease can be suspected clinically from accentuated pulmonary valve closure, and from chest X-ray by the presence of pulmonary vascular congestion and inappropriate cardiac enlargement, but again, left ventricular function is most satisfactorily assessed by echocardiography or angiocardiography. The clinical picture of chronic aortic regurgitation is significantly modified by co-existent mitral stenosis. In some patients, the mitral stenosis dominates the clinical picture. There is a reduction in forward stroke volume and the peripheral evidence of aortic regurgitation is muted, with reduction in pulse volume and in its collapsing quality. The severity of

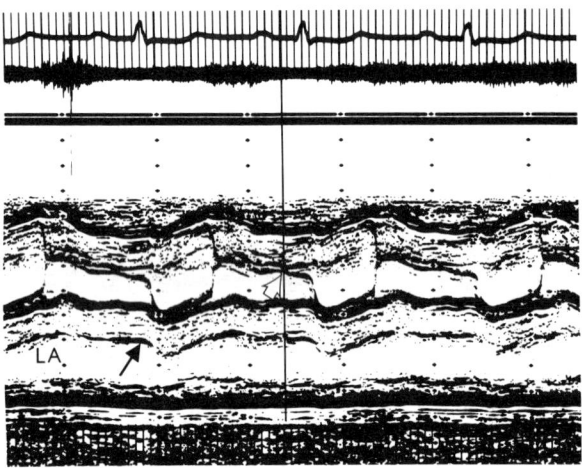

Fig. 14 M-mode echocardiogram showing premature aortic valve opening (arrow), preceding the onset of the QRS complex of the ECG in a patient with acute aortic regurgitation due to infective endocarditis. The double echo of the posterior aortic wall was due to an abscess (arrow), separating it from the left atrium (LA).

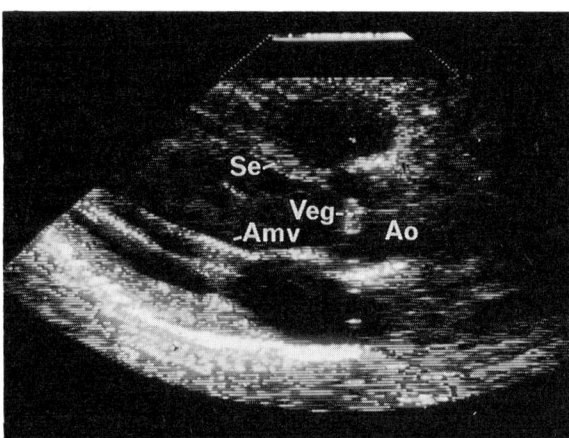

Fig. 15 Two-dimensional echocardiogram, parasternal long axis view, of a patient with aortic endocarditis, showing vegetation (Veg) on aortic valve. Amv, anterior mitral valve cusp; Se, septum; Ao, aortic root.

sectional echocardiography enables the aortic root to be observed in greater detail. Dilation or dissection can frequently be detected, and in patients with infective endocarditis, vegetations can be demonstrated (Fig. 15), and abcesses involving the structures around the aorta may be observed (Fig. 16). The presence of a regurgitant jet in the aortic root or the left ventricular outflow tract can also be detected by Doppler cardiography.

Cardiac catheterization
Left ventricular pressures are normal until late in the disease. Rheumatic mitral valve disease can be excluded by lack of a diastolic gradient between the left atrium and the left ventricle. Aortography allows the diagnosis of aortic regurgitation to be confirmed by filling of the left ventricle, and also allows disease of the aortic root to be confirmed or excluded.

Diagnosis
As with aortic stenosis, it is not enough to establish the presence of aortic regurgitation; the severity of the lesion must be estimated

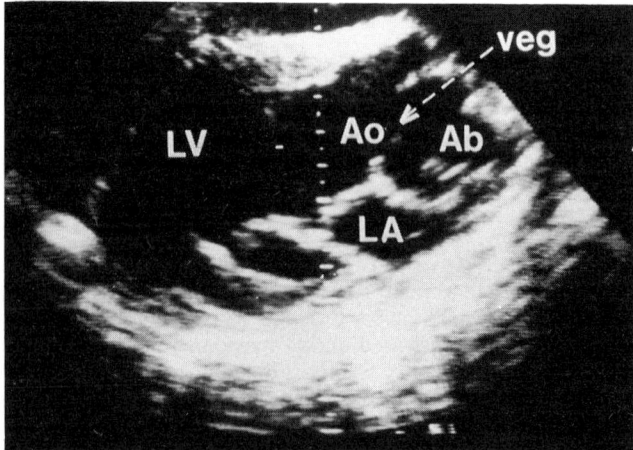

Fig. 16 Parasternal long axis view of aortic root (Ao) showing an abscess cavity (Ab) containing a vegetation (Veg), bulging into the left atrium (LA). LV, left ventricle.

the regurgitant flow may thus be underestimated. If it is left uncorrected when the mitral stenosis is treated, the clinical picture of severe aortic regurgitation will appear after operation. Alternatively, aortic regurgitation may dominate the picture, with the mitral stenosis going unnoticed, or the apical diastolic rumble misinterpreted as an Austin–Flint murmur. Provided the correct diagnosis is made, such cases do well after double valve surgery, even if there is cavity dilation, since the mitral stenosis appears to have a protective effect on left ventricular function. The diagnosis of acute aortic regurgitation may present difficulties when the classical physical signs are modified, although the condition should be suspected in any patient with severe systemic infection, low cardiac output state, and a normal or slightly collapsing pulse, with pulmonary congestion on chest X-ray. Echocardiography is a particularly valuable means of making a definite diagnosis non-invasively, demonstrating aortic vegetations, a large stroke volume, and premature mitral valve closure. Angiography should be avoided unless other methods of making the diagnosis are not available, due to the depressant effect of contrast medium on cardiac function.

It is also important to confirm or exclude other valve disease. Co-existent aortic stenosis is often diagnosed on the basis of an ejection systolic murmur, but this does not constitute adequate evidence, and in order to confirm its presence clinically, a bisferiens pulse should be present. Additional rheumatic mitral stenosis is best confirmed or excluded by echocardiography, although the presence of atrial fibrillation, a palpable first sound, or an opening snap makes its presence very likely on clinical grounds. Mitral regurgitation leads to an additional pan systolic murmur at the apex, which may sound continuous with the early diastolic murmur across the second sound. It usually results from dilation of the valve ring in the absence of organic mitral valve disease, and thus indicates the presence of considerable left ventricular enlargement.

Although it is usually unnecessary to establish the exact aetiology of the aortic regurgitation, syphilis should be excluded, since the possibility of ostial stenosis modifies the technique used at coronary arteriography. It is also important to investigate the possibility of disease of the aortic root. This should be suspected if there is a history of chest pain that is not clearly anginal in nature, and also from excessive dilation of the ascending aorta on chest X-ray or a long P–R interval on ECG. The most satisfactory investigation is an aortogram or a CT scan although it is often possible to obtain excellent visualization of the aortic root by cross-sectional echocardiography.

Differential diagnosis

In the presence of severe pulmonary hypertension, dilation of the pulmonary artery may occur with the development of functional pulmonary incompetence which gives rise to a soft early diastolic murmur (Graham–Steell murmur), but no evidence of abnormality of the carotid pulse. Difficulty in diagnosis usually arises when the patient has pulmonary hypertensive mitral valve disease, and an early diastolic murmur. In these circumstances, aortic regurgitation may not necessarily cause an abnormal carotid pulse. In many cases, the differential diagnosis can only be made by aortography or by pulsed Doppler, but on clinical grounds, pulmonary incompetence is more likely when there is other evidence of severe pulmonary hypertension, and in particular, when chest X-ray shows the main pulmonary artery to be greatly dilated. Pulmonary incompetence may be diagnosed by echocardiography if regurgitant flow is demonstrated in the right ventricular outflow tract after a peripheral contrast injection.

Aortic regurgitation should also be distinguished from other causes of aortic run-off, which include persistent ductus arteriosus, ruptured sinus of Valsalva aneurysm or coronary arteriovenous fistula. These all cause an increase in pulse pressure, and a continuous murmur down the left sternal edge, which may be confused with the combination of aortic regurgitation and mitral regurgitation. Additional abnormalities which may give rise to confusion are the combination of aortic regurgitation and a ventricular septal defect, and finally, the rare anomaly of aortic left ventricular tunnel, in which the haemodynamic disturbance is identical to that of aortic regurgitation. If these abnormalities are suspected, then cardiac catheterization, and biplane aortograms are essential, though even after full investigation, the exact diagnosis may still be in doubt.

Prognosis and treatment

Mild or moderately severe aortic regurgitation is well tolerated and requires no treatment other than prophylactic antibiotic to prevent infective endocarditis. In young patients, excessive athletic activity should be discouraged, since this may provoke considerable cavity dilation. Severe aortic regurgitation is treated by aortic valve replacement. If the patient has symptoms due to aortic regurgitation, the decision as to timing of the operation is not difficult. There remains, however, a group of patients with disease of intermediate severity in whom there is no clear indication for operation. They are usually asymptomatic, or if they have symptoms, these are non-specific and not clearly related to the presence of valve or left ventricular disease. Clearly, it is desirable to avoid premature valve replacement in such patients, exposing them unnecessarily to the morbidity and risk of surgery as well as to the problems associated with a prosthetic valve. At the same time, it is very important to operate before irreversible left ventricular disease develops. Unfortunately and in spite of much investigation, the uncertainties in assessing prognosis in this group of patients remain very wide. However, a number of guidelines for determining the timing of surgery can be recognized. Subjective exercise testing is unreliable, but a significant reduction in exercise tolerance in a standard treadmill test is a useful pointer towards operation. Normal performance, however, does not exclude severe disease. Valve replacement in an asymptomatic patient may also be indicated if left ventricular cavity size is greatly increased or if the regurgitation very severe. Attempts to identify specific measures of cavity size, such as an end-systolic dimension of 5.5 cm on M-mode echocardiography have proved unsatisfactory. Indications for operation include an enlarging heart on X-ray or echocardiography, provided the increase is greater than the uncertainty associated with the method of measurement; this is a 1 cm increase in heart size on chest X-ray, or a 5 mm increase in transverse dimension on M-mode echo. A history of infective endocarditis or the appearance of evidence of diastolic left ventricular disease are also relative indications. The quality of local surgical facilities, the preferences of the patient, as well as difficulties in communication or travelling must all be taken into account. If it is decided not to operate, it is essential that any patient with significant disease is kept under regular review, with at least annual, and preferably six monthly chest X-rays, since severe left ventricular disease may become apparent over a period as short as 1–2 years, even in the absence of significant symptoms.

Acute aortic regurgitation is a surgical emergency. It is nearly always due to infective endocarditis, so an attempt should be made to isolate an organism and to start antibiotic therapy preoperatively. One of the most useful criteria for emergency aortic valve replacement has proved to be the presence of premature mitral valve closure on the M-mode echocardiogram. When emergency surgical facilities are not available, the haemodynamic state can sometimes be stabilized with vasodilator treatment as with severe mitral regurgitation. However, the patient should be transferred as soon as possible to a centre capable of performing open heart surgery, so that operation can be performed if progress is not maintained. Delaying operation so that a prolonged course of antibiotics can be given is strongly contraindicated in such patients, since the valve is rarely sterilized, and further deterioration in left ventricular function inevitably occurs.

Acquired tricuspid valve disease

Tricuspid stenosis

Although functional tricuspid stenosis may occur with a large flow through the right heart such as occurs in an atrial septal defect, organic tricuspid stenosis is almost invariably due to chronic rheumatic heart disease. Rheumatic tricuspid stenosis always co-exists with mitral valve disease, although its incidence is about one-tenth of the latter. The two conditions are similar both with respect to their pathology and to the functional disturbance that they cause. The valve cusps become thickened, and the commissures fused, so that the cross-sectional area of the orifice is reduced. Involvement of the subvalvar apparatus, however, is uncommon. The primary functional abnormality is obstruction to right ventricular filling associated with a diastolic pressure gradient across the valve. In clinically severe tricuspid stenosis, however, this gradient is smaller than it would be with mitral stenosis, and is usually within the range 3–10 mm Hg. This causes a corresponding increase in right atrial pressure, which leads to fluid retention, manifesting itself as ascites and peripheral oedema.

Clinical picture

The problem is to recognize the presence of additional tricuspid stenosis in a patient known to have mitral and possibly also, aortic valve disease. This is not always possible on clinical grounds, but a number of indications may be sought. There are no specific findings in the history. If the patient is in sinus rhythm, then tricuspid stenosis is frequently associated with an 'a' wave in the venous pulse and with evidence of right atrial hypertrophy on ECG. These findings are unusual in the presence of pulmonary hypertension and mitral stenosis alone. The venous pulse may also be abnormal in patients in either sinus rhythm or atrial fibrillation in that the 'y' descent is slow. This may be difficult to recognize clinically, but may be suspected when the rate of fall of the venous pulse is less than its rate of rise. On auscultation, a separate tricuspid mid-diastolic murmur may be audible. This is similar in timing to a mitral one, but it is higher in pitch, resembling an aortic diastolic murmur in this respect. It is maximal down the left sternal edge or in the epigastrium. A tricuspid opening snap may also be present; it is later than a mitral one and its timing with respect to pulmonary valve closure varies with respiration. It may be possible to document separate mitral and tricuspid opening snaps phonocardiographically in the same patient.

Chest X-ray may be suggestive, since right atrial enlargement frequently causes dilation of the heart shadow to the right of the midline. These appearances, however, are non-specific, and may be present with functional tricuspid regurgitation, or even a giant left atrium. Echocardiography can be used to give a specific diagnosis. Cross-sectional echocardiography shows doming of the tricuspid valve into the right ventricle during systole, in the apical four chamber view (Fig. 17). A pressure gradient as low as 1 mm Hg will manifest itself as an increased blood flow velocity across the valve, which can be quantified by continuous wave Doppler, and the effective valve area estimated as for mitral stenosis. Cardiac catheterization will often demonstrate a diastolic pressure gradient across the tricuspid valve, but if cardiac output is low, severe stenosis may co-exist with no measurable gradient. Right atrial angiography can also be used to demonstrate tricuspid doming with a central orifice through which the dye passes. It may also demonstrate, in very rare cases, a right atrial tumour as the cause of the tricuspid stenosis. It is nevertheless true that an appreciable number of cases of organic tricuspid stenosis reach operation without a definite diagnosis having been made, and in the majority of these, its presence is detected at surgery by direct palpation of the valve cusps. Previously undiagnosed tricuspid stenosis may be unmasked by successful mitral valve surgery, which allows cardiac output to increase, causing a corresponding increase in the tricuspid diastolic pressure gradient. This leads to severe postoperative

Table 4 Causes of tricuspid regurgitation

Organic
Rheumatic
Infective endocarditis
Ebstein's anomaly
Atrioventricular canal
Carcinoid syndrome
Endomyocardial fibrosis
Prolapsing cusp
Functional

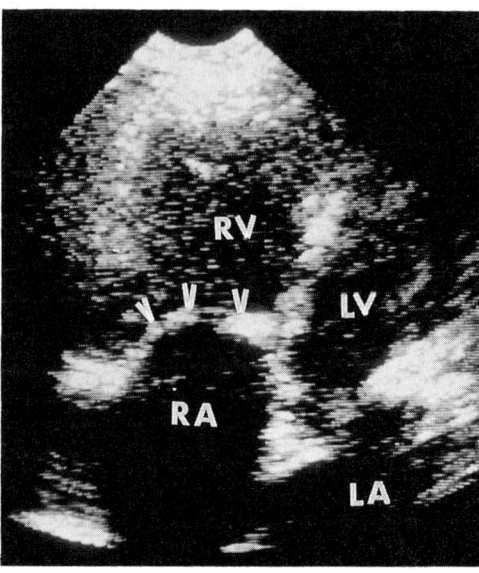

Fig. 17 Rheumatic tricuspid stenosis, apical four-chamber view showing doming and thickening of the tricuspid valve during diastole (arrows). LA, left atrium; LV, left ventricle; RA, right atrium; RV, right ventricle.

ascites and oedema in a patient thought to have had a satisfactory operation, and may lead to difficulties in diagnosis unless this possibility is considered.

Treatment

Fluid retention should be treated with moderate doses of diuretic but prolonged administration of inappropriately large doses merely leads to potassium depletion. Definitive treatment is surgical consisting of either valvotomy or tricuspid repair, at the time that the other valve lesions are dealt with. Tricuspid valve replacement is avoided whenever possible, in view of the physiological significance on the right side of the heart of the diastolic pressure gradient across all normally functioning prostheses. An additional procedure on the tricuspid valve increases the operative risk of mitral valve surgery due to the greater postoperative incidence of jaundice and arrhythmias.

Tricuspid regurgitation

As with mitral regurgitation, a number of different pathological processes may cause tricuspid regurgitation, which are indicated in Table 4.

Tricuspid regurgitation is frequently functional, occurring in association with dilation of the right ventricular cavity. It is particularly common in patients with pulmonary hypertensive mitral valve disease, but may also occur with primary pulmonary hypertension, or in the terminal stages of many types of congenital heart disease, particularly those with a significant left-to-right shunt. The tricuspid valve is appreciably more liable to develop functional regurgitation than the mitral valve.

Organic tricuspid regurgitation may be congenital, as an isolated abnormality, or associated with an abnormal displacement of the valve towards the apex of the right ventricle (Ebstein's anomaly, see page 13.260). A cleft tricuspid valve may also occur in ostium primum atrial septal defect (see page 13.270). Acquired, organic tricuspid regurgitation may be rheumatic in origin, or result from infective endocarditis of a previously normal valve, which occurs particularly commonly in drug addicts. Right-sided endomyocardial fibrosis causes progressive obliteration of the right ventricular cavity with distortion of the tricuspid subvalvular apparatus. The carcinoid syndrome is also associated with severe tricuspid regurgitation, and similar findings may occur after methysergide therapy. The tricuspid valve may show mid-systolic prolapse in a manner exactly similar to that of the mitral valve.

Clinical picture

The clinical features of tricuspid regurgitation are those of severe and chronic elevation of the venous pressure, often in association with disease on the left side of the heart. The symptoms are nonspecific, although, when tricuspid regurgitation supervenes in a patient with mitral stenosis, it is often associated with an increase in the prominence of fatigue as a factor limiting exercise tolerance instead of breathlessness. Symptoms may also be related to the development of oedema or ascites: hepatic enlargement may be associated with nausea, and upper abdominal or epigastric pain frequently aggravated by exercise. The main physical sign of tricuspid regurgitation is a raised venous pressure with a prominent systolic wave, which is almost a *sine qua non* for the diagnosis. The mean venous pressure may be very high, greater than 15 cm, with pulsations visible in the retinal vessels or palpable in the femoral veins. The high venous pressure is also responsible for the protein-losing enteropathy that sometimes occurs in the same way as with constrictive pericarditis (page 13.309). In approximately two-thirds of patients, there is associated systolic expansile pulsation of the liver which may be considerably enlarged and tender. In long-standing cases, however, hepatic fibrosis develops so that this is no longer evident. Hepatic dysfunction may also be associated with mild jaundice, which with increased skin pigmentation, gives these patients a very characteristic appearance. In approximately one-third of cases, a tricuspid pan systolic murmur is present, which is audible down the left sternal edge. Although it is said to increase in intensity during inspiration, this may be difficult to demonstrate in individual patients, so that it may be indistinguishable from that of functional mitral regurgitation. The findings on chest X-ray depend mainly on other cardiac disease present, but, as with tricuspid stenosis, there may be well marked dilation of the heart shadow towards the right. ECG may show right atrial hypertrophy in isolated tricuspid regurgitation if the patient remains in sinus rhythm, but otherwise dominated by the other cardiac disease present. It is possible to make a definitive diagnosis by two-dimensional echocardiography by demonstrating the appearance of contrast in the inferior vena cava after injection into peripheral vein. Tricuspid regurgitation can readily be detected by continuous wave or pulsed Doppler, but these techniques have the disadvantage, from the clinical point of view, that their sensitivity is very high, so that minor and haemodynamically insignificant regurgitation may give rise to a very prominent flow signal. In addition, the difference between right atrial and right ventricular systolic pressures can be estimated from the peak retrograde blood velocity. Right ventricular cavity size is usually increased and septal movement reversed due to right-sided volume overload. Cardiac catheterization confirms the presence of high right atrial pressures with a prominent systolic wave.

Treatment

Medical treatment with bed-rest, diuretics, and vasodilators may allow right ventricular cavity size to decrease and thus restore competence to the tricuspid valve. Isolated tricuspid incompetence, unless very severe, or accompanied by right ventricular disease, is well tolerated, and does not require surgery unless there is

right-to-left shunting through a patent foramen ovale causing severe cyanosis or polycythaemia. When tricuspid regurgitation occurs in association with rheumatic heart disease involving the left side of the heart, it frequently subsides spontaneously after the latter has been dealt with surgically, although there is a case for routine tricuspid valve plication or repair to prevent tricuspid regurgitation developing in the immediate postoperative period in patients with severe pulmonary hypertension. If the tricuspid valve is badly damaged and the symptoms of fluid retention, chronic venous hypertension or reduced exercise tolerance severe, tricuspid valve replacement can be considered. This is often a high-risk procedure, and a prosthesis that is satisfactory in the mitral position must be regarded as causing at least moderately severe tricuspid stenosis when it is used to replace the tricuspid valve. For this reason, conservative operations are performed on the tricuspid valve, whenever possible.

Carcinoid heart disease

A characteristic form of heart disease develops in patients with metastatic carcinoid disease affecting predominantly the right heart, with thickening of the tricuspid and pulmonary valves and enlargement of the right ventricular cavity. The left side of the heart is rarely involved, unless a septal defect is present. Microscopically, the thickening is due to deposits of fibrous tissue, but there is no evidence of inflammation. Not all patients with carcinoid disease develop cardiac manifestations, but when they are present they may progress, even after removal of the tumour (see Section 12).

Clinical picture

Patients may demonstrate the well-recognized manifestations of the carcinoid syndrome of flushing, telangiectasia, bronchoconstriction, and intestinal hypermotility. The venous pressure is raised, due partly to tricuspid valve disease and partly to right ventricular disease, and it is these manifestations which dominate the clinical picture from the cardiac point of view.

Chest X-ray shows cardiac enlargement. ECG findings are non-specific but include low-voltage QRS complexes and evidence of right ventricular hypertrophy. Echocardiogram may show very considerable enlargement of the right ventricular cavity, often to a degree unusual in acquired heart disease. Tricuspid regurgitation, if present, can be demonstrated by echocardiography. Since the underlying carcinoid disease may progress slowly, the tricuspid regurgitation may be worth treating in its own right by repair or replacement. Treatment of the carcinoid disease itself may be by surgical excision of the tumour, if this is possible, by cytotoxic agents (e.g. cyclophosphamide) or by serotonin antagonists (e.g. methysergide).

Acquired pulmonary valve disease

Acquired pulmonary valve disease is unusual. The commonest form is that associated with severe pulmonary hypertension and dilation of the pulmonary valve ring, causing mild regurgitation. This commonly occurs in association with pulmonary hypertensive mitral valve disease, causing a soft early diastolic murmur (the Graham–Steell murmur), but an identical picture may be present with severe pulmonary hypertension from any cause. Although the murmur itself is early diastolic in timing, there is no associated abnormality of the carotid pulse as would be expected in aortic regurgitation. Nevertheless, the differential diagnosis on clinical grounds may be difficult when the mitral valve disease is severe. However, it may be possible to demonstrate retrograde flow in the right ventricular outflow tract following a peripheral contrast injection. Aortic regurgitation can be confirmed or excluded by an aortogram.

Rheumatic pulmonary regurgitation is extremely rare, although an increase has been reported in populations exposed to considerable altitudes, but even when present, it contributes little to over-all disability. Pulmonary regurgitation may also form part of the carcinoid syndrome, or be iatrogenic, following pulmonary valvotomy for pulmonary stenosis. It is associated with short early diastolic murmur, and may contribute to the elevated venous pressure that may persist for a variable period after pulmonary valvotomy. It is of no clinical consequence and requires no specific treatment.

Management of patients with valve prostheses

Valve replacement has been a major advance in the treatment of patients with valvular heart disease. Large numbers of patients have been treated in this way over the past 25 years since the operation was introduced with very significant improvement in their quality of life. Valve prostheses may be mechanical or biological. Mechanical prostheses inserted over the last 10 years are likely to be either the ball and cage type, of which the commonest example is the Starr–Edwards one, or the tilting disc. The former has the advantage of a 25 year follow-up, with remarkable reliability. The latter has a larger effective orifice area in relation to the size of the ring. Further developments in this direction include the more recently introduced St Jude Medical valve. Biological prostheses consist of a plastic stent on which cusps made from some biological material are mounted. The cusps may be derived from porcine aortic valve or pericardium. Minor differences in performance exist between these various valve substitutes, but these are of little clinical significance. All fall short of their natural counterpart in performance *in vivo*. Under resting conditions, pressure differences are present across mitral prostheses, which range from 4–5 mm Hg for the Starr–Edwards to 2–4 mm Hg for the Bjork–Shiley and porcine bioprostheses. In addition, all have a rigid mitral ring which interferes with ventricular function. Systolic gradients across aortic prostheses are in the range 10 to 25 mm Hg at rest, increasing on exercise. The main factors guiding choice of one or other of them is the durability of the prosthesis and the likely incidence of thrombotic complications. Unfortunately it has become clear that in spite of the great improvement in outlook, patients with valvular prostheses are at significantly increased risk of cardiac complications and death in comparison with matched normal controls. Present operative mortality is in the region of 3–5 per cent for single valve replacement and approximately 10 per cent for double valve replacement. Long-term survival studies have shown that 10-year survival after single valve replacement is approximately 50–55 per cent, and after double valve replacement 35–45 per cent. For reoperation, mortality is higher, the exact figure depending on the circumstances in which surgery is performed.

Late complications of valve replacement

1. Thromboembolism

This is a major complication associated with all mechanical prostheses. Long-term anticoagulant therapy with a drug of the warfarin type is thus essential in all patients in whom these prostheses have been inserted, and even with satisfactory control an incidence of significant events, including transient weakness, dysphasia or visual disturbances of 1–2 per cent per annum can be expected. At the same time, anticoagulant therapy itself is associated with haemorrhagic complications severe enough to require admission to hospital with an incidence of approximately 1 per cent per annum. In a small minority of patients, emboli are much more frequent in spite of good anticoagulant control. Initially such cases should be given an antiplatelet agent such as dipyridamole, and the anticoagulant dose adjusted accordingly. The possibility of some other cause for the neurological manifestations must always be considered, such as cerebrovascular disease. However, frequent embolization may be associated with thrombosis of the prosthesis, and if it cannot be suppressed medically, reoperation and replacement with a biological prosthesis may be necessary. In

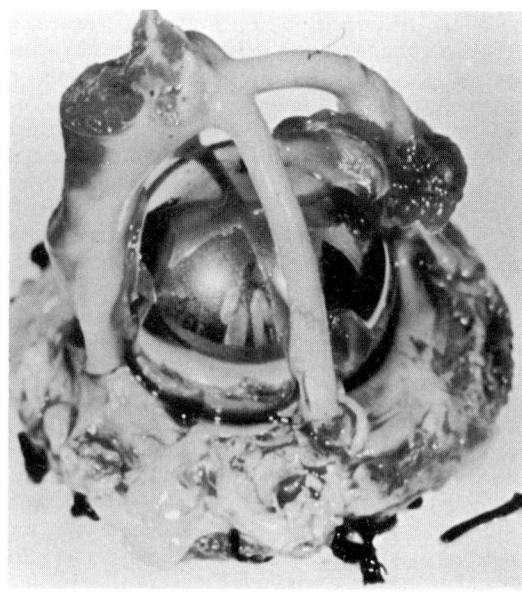

Fig. 18 Thrombosed Starr–Edwards prosthesis, removed at emergency operation.

such cases, the diagnosis of multiple cerebral emboli must be established beyond all question, since the operative mortality of reoperation is significantly greater than for a first operation. The incidence of thromboembolic complications is lower with biological prostheses, so that long-term anticoagulant therapy can be dispensed with in patients in sinus rhythm after aortic or mitral valve replacement: however, many surgeons recommend a short course of 2–3 months in such patients while suture lines become endothelialised. Patients with atrial fibrillation and mitral valve replacement will require standard long-term anticoagulant therapy. In developing countries, mitral replacement in particular may have to be performed in children under the age of 15 years, in whom biological valves are unsuitable. The use of a mechanical prosthesis might seem appropriate, but facilities for regular prothrombin estimations are not available, while uncontrolled administration of standard doses of warfarin are associated with unacceptable risk of haemorrhage. This therapeutic dilemma is, at present, unsolved, although the use of small doses of warfarin, e.g. 2 mg daily, without anticoagulant control has been advocated. It would seem that clinical trials in this area would be justified.

2. Limited prosthetic function

In a minority of patients, however, valve replacement may give rise to severe haemodynamic disturbances, so that in extreme cases, the condition of the patient may be worse after the operation than before. This usually arises when the valve ring or the ventricular cavity is very small so that it proved necessary to insert a correspondingly small prosthesis. A small mitral prosthesis may cause a resting diastolic pressure difference as high as 20 mm Hg and a small aortic prosthesis a systolic gradient of up to 50 mm Hg. A second, related problem is the insertion of a prosthesis particularly of the ball and cage type that is too large for the ventricle. In the mitral position, the cage may impinge on the septum and obstruct the left ventricular outflow tract causing subaortic stenosis, while in the aortic position, obstruction may develop between the ball and the aorta. Normally, such complications are avoided by the use of a low profile prosthesis, such as a Bjork–Shiley. They are sometimes referred to by the sonorous description of 'valve prosthesis–patient mismatch'.

3. Infection

Patients with prostheses, mechanical or biological, are at greatly increased risk of infective endocarditis. The infecting organism may have been introduced at the time of operation, when it usually manifests itself within two months of surgery. Later infections are blood borne. It is thus essential that all patients receive full antibiotic prophylaxis for dental manipulations and other potentially septic hazards in a course lasting for at least 48 hours, rather than in the single dose currently recommended for routine dental prophylaxis. Infective endocarditis is a very serious complication, and rarely responds to antibiotic therapy alone. A second valve replacement is nearly always required, often in a seriously ill patient in whom the valve ring may be infected and friable.

4. Prosthetic dysfunction

This is an important cause of morbidity in patients who have undergone valve replacement. There may be structural damage to the prosthesis itself, which is uncommon in mechanical valves, though occasional batches may undergo strut fracture due to metal fatigue. It is much commoner with biological prostheses, when cusps may become calcified, perforated, or detached. Calcification of porcine bioprostheses regularly occurs within 1–2 years in children under the age of 15 years. Mechanical prostheses are subject to thrombosis. This may take two forms. Deterioration in function may be insidious over a period of several months or years due to ingrowth of organized clot (pannus) usually from the atrial side (Fig. 19). This may be associated with an increased incidence of emboli in spite of adequate anticoagulant therapy. Alternatively, the prosthesis may clot acutely; this is particularly likely to occur with the Bjork–Shiley prosthesis in the mitral position, and represents a surgical emergency. It can often be recognized clinically, the patient presenting with pulmonary oedema or in a low output state, and the closing click of the prosthesis no longer audible. Operation is required as soon as possible, since marked deterioration may occur within hours. If the condition of the patient is so poor as to preclude anaesthesia, intravenous streptokinase should be given, at a dose of 500 000 u stat, followed by 100 000 units hourly, though the risk of systemic embolism is appreciable. Such treatment may be associated with improvement within a few hours; the streptokinase is then neutralized, and surgery undertaken. Finally, paraprosthetic regurgitation may develop. In the aortic position, this may have been present since the original operation, and its presence is associated with heavy calcification of the original valve extending into the valve ring. Its sudden appearance always raises the possibility of infection of the prosthesis. Mitral paraprosthetic regurgitation usually results from part of the circumference tearing away from the valve ring. Again, infection should always be considered, but regurgitation is well documented in its absence.

Management of prosthetic dysfunction

Stenosis or regurgitation associated with a prosthesis does not have the same physical signs as the corresponding lesion of the native valve. In general, it presents as deterioration in cardiac state, whose progress may be acute or chronic. The patient complains of reduced exercise tolerance, followed by orthopnoea. On examination, the venous pressure is raised, the liver enlarged, and chest X-ray shows further cardiac enlargement and the development of pulmonary congestion. When a mitral prosthesis is involved, there are characteristically no murmurs, other than those of tricuspid regurgitation; an aortic systolic murmur may be present, but its intensity and timing differs little from that of a normally functioning prosthesis. The clinical picture may thus be indistinguishable from that of ventricular disease or 'heart failure'. It is essential, therefore, that the possibility of a prosthesis-related complication is considered in all such patients. This requires echocardiography, Doppler, and possibly cardiac catheterization by an experienced operator. All patients presenting in this way should thus be referred to a unit where these investigations can be performed, and emergency surgery, if necessary, can be undertaken.

Haemolysis

All mechanical prostheses are associated with increased intravascular haemolysis. This rarely gives rise to clinical problems when the prosthesis is functioning normally, and anaemia does not occur. The extent of haemolysis can be estimated from a peripheral blood film, which shows fragmented forms, from depression or absence of serum haptoglobin, and from an increase in LDH levels. Haemolysis may become significant with a normally functioning prosthesis when the patient has a compensated haemolytic state of some different aetiology, such as congenital spherocytosis or thalassaemia minor. In these circumstances, there is a risk of the extent of haemolysis becoming severe. Mild paraprosthetic regurgitation whose severity is insufficient to give rise to any haemodynamic complications may cause clinically significant haemolysis. In such cases, it may be undesirable to expose the patient to the risk of reoperation, particularly if the original valve leak was due to some predictable cause such as calcification of the valve bed, and so likely to recur. Provided that haemolysis is not severe, such cases can usually be treated medically on maintenance therapy with iron and folic acid. A requirement for transfusion, however, is a strong indication for reoperation.

Left ventricular disease

This is now a major cause of morbidity and mortality after valve replacement. There is no single cause. In many patients, severe left ventricular disease was present preoperatively, and though some improvement frequently occurs with correction of the valve disease, function never returns to normal. Operation itself causes additional damage. Methods of preservation of myocardium during the period of cardiopulmonary bypass have improved very considerably over the last five to ten years with the general introduction of cold cardioplegia, but before then ischaemic arrest and particularly coronary perfusion appear to have been associated with myocardial damage which may take several years to become manifest. Postoperatively, the presence of a prosthesis may interfere with ventricular function. This is particularly the case if there is any disparity in size with the site at which it is inserted. A rigid mitral ring invariably leads to abnormal function. Coronary emboli may arise from the prosthesis. Many patients are of an age to have additional coronary artery disease; there is no evidence to suppose that routine bypass grafting at operation affects the development of ventricular disease.

Left ventricular disease after valve replacement presents its usual clinical features. There is progressive limitation of exercise tolerance and breathlessness due to reduction in cardiac output and pulmonary congestion. Venous pressure becomes raised, and the earliest clinical evidence may relate to right rather than left ventricular disease, with elevated venous pressure, fluid retention, and hepatic congestion. Auscultatory signs may be modified, and in particular third and fourth heart sounds are not audible in patients with mechanical mitral prostheses. Chest X-ray shows an increase in heart size and pulmonary congestion. ECG may show Q waves, but their absence is of no significance. The differential diagnosis of ventricular disease after valve replacement is thus with prosthetic dysfunction, and it is essential that a comprehensive diagnosis is established in any patient who fails to progress, or whose improvement after operation is not maintained. Echocardiography has proved of great value in such patients, since it allows the very active left ventricular wall motion that accompanies a paraprosthetic leak to be distinguished from the dilated cavity and poor shortening fraction that usually accompanies left ventricular disease. Continuous wave Doppler can be used to detect significant gradients across biological valves. However, unless the diagnosis is clear from non-invasive investigation cardiac catheterization is required to settle the diagnosis beyond doubt. The prognosis once clinically apparent left ventricular disease has developed is poor, usually being of the order of 1–2 years, so it is essential that no remediable cause is overlooked.

Follow-up of patients after valve replacement

It is clear, therefore, that after valve replacement, patients require regular follow-up. This must be for life, and after recovery from the operation itself, should be at least at six monthly intervals, with regular chest X-ray and ECG. It is also very helpful if echocardiography can be performed early so that a baseline can be established to detect any deterioration, Dental prophylaxis is essential. Deteriorations must be detected early, and investigated in detail so that life-threatening complications are not missed, and essential treatment implemented early when it has the greatest chance of success. Only in this way will the maximum benefits of valve replacement surgery be realized.

References

Ball, C. J. D., Williams, A. W. and Davies, J. N. P. (1954). Endomyocardial fibrosis. *Lancet* i, 1049.

Barnett, H. J. M., Boughner, D. R., Taylor, D. W., Cooper, P. E., Kostuk, W. J. and Nichol, P. M. (1984). Further evidence relating mitral valve prolapse to cerebral ischemic events. *N. Engl. J. Med.* **302**, 139–144.

Borer, J. S., Bacherach, S. L., Green, M. V., Kent, K. M., Henry, W. L., Rosing, D. R., Seides, S. F., Johnston, G. S. and Epstein, S. E. (1978). Exercise-induced left ventricular dysfunction in symptomatic and asymptomatic patients with aortic regurgitation: assessment with radionuclide cineangiography. *Am. J. Cardiol.* **42**, 351–357.

Bulkley, B. H. and Roberts, W. C. (1976). The heart in systemic lupus erythematosus, and change induced in it by corticosteroid therapy. *Am. J. Med.* **58**, 243–264.

Davies, M. J., Moore, B. P. and Braimbridge, M. C. (1978). The floppy mitral valve. Study of incidence, pathology, and complications in surgical, necropsy and forensic material. *Br. Heart J.* **40**, 468–481.

Fauci, A. S., Harley, J. B., Roberts, W. C., Ferrans, V. J., Gralnick, H. R., Bjornson, B. H. (1982). The idiopathic hypereosinophilic syndrome. Clinical pathophysiologic and therapeutic considerations. *Ann. intern. Med.* **97**, 78–92.

Fenoglio, J. J., McAllister, H. A., DeCastro, C. M., Dvavia, J. E. and Cheitlin, M. D. (1977). Congenital bicuspid valve after age 20. *Am. J. Cardiol.* **39**, 164–169.

Fowler, N. and van der Bel-Kahn, J. M. (1979). Indications for surgical replacement of the mitral valve with particular reference to common and uncommon causes of mitral regurgitation. *Am. J. Cardiol.* **44**, 157.

Fulkerson, P. K., Beaver, B. M., Auseon, J. C. and Graber, H. L. (1979). Calcification of the mitral annulus. Etiology, clinical associations and therapy. *Am. J. Med.* **66**, 967–977.

Goldschlager, N., Pfeifer, J., Cohn, K., Popper, R. and Selzer, A. (1973). The natural history of aortic regurgitation. A clinical and haemodynamic study. *Am. J. Med.* **54**, 577–588.

Hammer, W. J., Roberts, W. C. and DeLeon, A. C. (1978). Mitral stenosis secondary of combined 'massive' mitral anular calcific deposits and small hypertrophied left ventricles. *Am. J. Med.* **64**, 371–376.

Jeresaty, R. M. (1976). Sudden death in the mitral prolapse click syndrome. *Am. J. Cardiol.* **37**, 317–318.

Leatham, A. and Brigden, W. (1980). Mild mitral regurgitation and the mitral prolapse fiasco. *Am. Heart J.* **99**, 659–664.

Linch, D. C., Gillmer, D. J., Whimster, W. F. and Keates, J. R. W. (1980). Rheumatoid aortic valve prolapse requiring emergency aortic valve replacement. *Br. Heart J.* **43**, 237–240.

Oakley, C. M. and Olsen, E. G. J. (1977). Editorial. Eosinophilia and the heart. *Br. Heart J.* **39**, 233–237.

Procacci, P. M., Savran, S. V. and Schreiter, S. L. (1976). Prevalence of clinical mitral prolapse in 1169 young women. *N. Engl. J. Med.* **294**, 1086.

Rahimtoola, S. H. (1983). Valvular Heart Disease: a perspective. *J. Am. Coll. Cardiol.* **1**, 199–215.

Roberts, W. C. (1970). The congenitally bicuspid aortic valve. *Am. J. Cardiol.* **26**, 72–83.

——, Hehoe, J. A., Carpenter, D. F. and Golden, A. (1968). Cardiac valvular lesions in rheumatoid arthritis. *Arch. intern. Med.* **122**, 141–146.

Ross Jr, J. (1981). Left ventricular function and the timing of surgical treatment in valvular heart disease. *Ann. intern. Med.* **94**, 498–504.

Ruckman, R. N. and van Praagh, R. (1978). Anatomic types of congenital mitral stenosis: report of autopsy cases with consideration of diagnosis and surgical implications. *Am. J. Cardiol.* **42**, 592–601.

Selzer, A. and Cohn, K. E. (1972). Natural history of mitral stenosis: a review. *Circulation* **45**, 878–890.

Smith, H. J., Neutze, J. M., Roche, A. H. G., Agnew, T. M. and Barratt-Boyes, B. G. (1976). The natural history of rheumatic aortic regurgitation and the indications for surgery. *Br. Heart J.* **38**, 147–154.

Smith, N., McAnulty, J. H. and Rahimtoola, S. H. (1978). Severe aortic stenosis with impaired left ventricular function and clinical heart failure: results of valve replacement. *Circulation* **58**, 255–264.

Vaughton, K. C., Walker, D. R. and Sturridge, M. F. (1979). Mitral valve replacement for endocarditis caused by Libman Sachs endocarditis. *Br. Heart J.* **41**, 730–733.

Vijayaraghavan, G., Cherian, G., Krishnaswami, S. and Sukumar, I. P. (1977). Left ventricular endomyocardial fibrosis in India. *Br. Heart J.* **39**, 563–568.

——, ——, ——, —— and John, S. (1977). Rheumatic aortic stenosis in young patients presenting as combined aortic and mitral stenosis. *Br. Heart J.* **39**, 294–298.

Vlodaver, Z. and Edwards, J. E. (1977). Rupture of ventricular septum or papillary muscle complicating myocardial infarction. *Circulation* **55**, 815–822.

Waller, B. F., Morrow, A. G., Maron, B. J., Del Negro, A. A., Kent, K. M., McGrath, F. J., Wallace, R. B., McIntosh, C. L. and Roberts, W. C. Etiology of clinically isolated, severe, chronic pure mitral regurgitation: analysis of 97 patients over 30 years of age having mitral valve replacement. *Am. Heart J.* **104**, 276–288.

Wood, P. (1954). An appreciation of mitral stenosis. Part 1. Clinical features. *Br. Med. J.* **1**, 1051–1063.

—— (1954). An appreciation of mitral stenosis. Part II. Investigations and results. *Br. Med. J.* **1**, 1113–1124.

—— and Gibson, R. V. (1955). Diagnosis of tricuspid stenosis. *Br. Heart J.* **17**, 552.

PERICARDIAL DISEASE

D. G. GIBSON

Anatomy of the pericardium

The normal pericardium is a double structure, consisting of fibrous and serous components. The fibrous pericardium is a thick, unyielding membrane which protects the heart from surrounding organs, fusing with the central tendon of the diaphragm below, and with the great vessels above, 1–2 cm beyond their origins. The serous pericardium, in which the heart is invaginated, itself has two layers, a parietal layer which lines the fibrous pericardium, and a visceral layer, sometimes called the epicardium, which covers the surface of the heart and origins of the great vessels. The pericardial cavity is thus a potential space normally containing only a few millilitres of fluid, but with a capacity of up to 600 ml, which may be further increased in pericardial disease.

Physiology of the pericardium

The normal pericardium is not essential to life, since the pericardial space is commonly obliterated after open heart surgery, and since both layers may be removed in patients with constrictive pericarditis with no apparent ill effect. Pericardial pressure has not been directly measured in normal humans, although there is evidence to suggest that its mean value may be up to 5 mm Hg negative to atmospheric. In animals, it increases during isovolumic contraction, and falls to its lowest point during early relaxation and filling. It is probable that the presence of the normal pericardium limits the stroke volume during exercise, and thus prevents inappropriate distension of ventricular myocardium. In disease, the pericardium may restrict ventricular filling. In part, this simply reflects an increase in the pressure in the pericardial space, and in part direct restraint by surrounding structures. Both have the effect of increasing myocardial surface pressure, i.e. the force per unit area acting perpendicular to the epicardium. Whether restraint by the normal pericardium is of clinical significance remains to be determined, but its influence has been invoked as a mechanism limiting filling when the left ventricular cavity is dilated. It is also possible that elevation of pericardial pressure may be a mechanism by which enlargement of one ventricle causes an increase in diastolic pressure in the other.

Congenital anomalies of the pericardium

Congenital abnormalities of the pericardium are uncommon, with an incidence of approximately 1–2 per 10 000 autopsies. Congenital absence of the pericardium may be partial or complete. A partial defect involving the left side of the pericardium is about four times as common as the complete form. Either type may be associated with additional cardiac anomalies in about one-third of cases, including atrial septal defect, Fallot's tetralogy or sequestrated pulmonary segments. Clinical features include non-specific chest pain and sinus bradycardia, and the ECG shows right axis deviation. The chest X-ray is characteristic, demonstrating a shift of the heart to the left, with prominence of the pulmonary artery. Heart size is increased, and the lower border of the heart shadow may be ill-defined. Echocardiography shows increased right ventricular size and reversed septal motion, as occurs in atrial septal defect. If the defect of the pericardium is partial, the atrial appendix may herniate through it, and even strangulate, leading to a clinical picture suggesting acute pericarditis. If the defect is larger, the left ventricle may herniate and undergo torsion. Alternatively, lung may become trapped within the pericardial space. These complications are treated surgically by enlargement of the defect.

Pericardial cysts

Pericardial cysts are rare. They have a variety of embryological origins, and may be continuous with the pericardium or separate from it. They do not usually cause symptoms and are discovered at routine chest X-ray, when they present as mediastinal masses. A computerized tomographic (CT) scan may give some indication of their nature, but the exact diagnosis is usually established only when they are removed surgically.

Mulibrey nanism

Mulibrey (MUscle, LIver, BRain, EYe) nanism is an autosomal recessive, characterized by growth failure, a triangular face often with hydrocephaloid skull, hypotonia, peculiar voice, large liver, and yellowish dots and pigment dispersion in the optic fundi. The majority of cases have pericardial constriction due to congenital thickening of the pericardium, and this may be responsible for many of the clinical features. Histologically, the pericardium shows simple fibrous thickening. Considerable improvement may result from pericardiectomy.

Pericardial disease

Diseases of the pericardium may be considered from two points of view. The first is aetiological, since in common with other serous membranes, the pericardium is affected by a number of disease processes. The second is in terms of the physiological and clinical disturbances that they produce. There is no fixed relation between the two, so that an account will be given first of different diseases affecting the pericardium, and then of the three main syndromes of acute pericarditis, pericardial tamponade, and pericardial constriction.

Table 1 Diseases affecting the pericardium

Acute idiopathic pericarditis
Infections
  Viral
  Bacterial (including TB)
  Toxoplasmosis, amoebiasis
  Histoplasmosis, actinomycosis
  Nocardiosis
  Echinococcal
Other inflammatory
  Postcardiotomy
  Dressler's syndrome
In association with other systemic disease
  Connective tissue disorders (systemic lupus erythematosus, rheumatoid, rheumatic fever, scleroderma, polyarteritis nodosa, giant-cell arteritis)
  Uraemia
  Hypothyroidism
Neoplastic
  Primary or secondary
Physical agents
  Radiation, blunt trauma
Haemorrhage
  Trauma, aortic dissection
  Anticoagulant therapy
Drug-induced
Chylopericardium

Aetiology

Diseases affecting the pericardium are summarized in Table 1.

Acute idiopathic pericarditis is a disease occurring characteristically in young adults. Prospective studies have strongly suggested a viral aetiology in approximately half, the commonest agent being Coxsackie B. When the outbreak occurs as an epidemic, approximately equal numbers of those affected show manifestations of pericarditis and myocarditis. The most characteristic clinical feature is chest pain, but flu-like symptoms, palpitation, orchitis, skin rash, encephalitis, and radiographic evidence of pleural effusion or pneumonitis have been reported. The condition is usually self-limiting, but in a small minority of cases may progress to constriction. The virus may be identified serologically from paired specimens taken two weeks apart, or recovered from throat or rectal swabs.

Pyogenic bacterial infection of the pericardium is much more unusual, but may be due to blood-borne infection of a previously sterile effusion or by direct extension from the lungs or pleural space. The organisms most commonly involved are staphylococci, pneumococci or streptococci. Bacterial infection of the pericardium is not usually an isolated event, but occurs more commonly in a patient with overwhelming disease elsewhere, or one in whom the response to infection is suppressed, either therapeutically or as the result of disease.

Tuberculous infection is an important cause of pericardial disease particularly in the Third World. It may take the form of acute pericarditis, pericardial effusion, or pericardial constriction. Acute pericarditis appears to be a 'primary' response, and so is an exudative lesion whose basis is allergic. Chronic pericardial effusion and pericardial constriction both reflect granulomatous disease, often with fibrosis and calcification in the late stages. Both parietal and visceral layers of the pericardium may be affected, so that spread of disease to the myocardium follows. In the first instance, treatment is with antituberculous drugs. The place of corticosteroids is undetermined. Drainage of the effusion or surgical relief of chronic constriction may also be required.

Fungal pericarditis is much less common, but infection with actinomycosis, coccidioidomycosis, and histoplasmosis have all been reported, the last leading to pericardial constriction and calcification. Pericardial calcification due to hydatid disease is increasingly recognized in areas where the disease is endemic, and may require surgical treatment if cardiac compression occurs.

Myocardial infarction Evidence of acute pericarditis may be found in up to 15 per cent patients in the first 24 to 72 hours after acute myocardial infarction. This may take the form of a friction rub, implying that the infarction was a transmural one. It seldom gives rise to symptoms other than dull retrosternal pain, which may be differentiated from that due to the myocardial infarction itself by its variation with respiration. Not surprisingly, patients who develop evidence of pericarditis have more extensive ST changes and a slightly higher risk of arrhythmic complications. Echocardiography may demonstrate a small pericardial effusion. The effusion itself seldom requires treatment, although anticoagulant therapy is contraindicated as long as the rub persists.

Pericardial involvement is an important component of the post-cardiotomy syndrome. This is an acute febrile illness occurring within 6 to 9 months of cardiac surgery. The onset is sudden, with pleural or praecordial pain associated with a pyrexia of up to 40 °C. The chest X-ray may show enlargement of the heart shadow or pleural effusions. The ECG is unchanged. The condition is usually self-limiting, but may recur. Diagnosis is by exclusion, particularly of infective endocarditis or cytomegalic inclusion disease resulting from transfusion. Treatment is with aspirin or indomethacin. Rarely, a large pericardial effusion may develop, requiring aspiration or even surgical drainage. Dresler's syndrome is a related condition, occurring two weeks to several months after myocardial infarction in 3–4 per cent of cases. It also presents as as self-limiting febrile illness, accompanied by pericardial or pleural pain, and by pneumonitis in more severe cases. Like the postcardiotomy syndrome, it responds to aspirin or indomethacin.

A small pericardial effusion is present in virtually all cases of acute rheumatic fever, and may be associated with epicardial inflammation. Less commonly, it may be large enough to cause cardiac enlargement on chest X-ray, and so to suggest the presence of myocardial disease. It may be associated with the clinical features of acute pericarditis, and constriction has been recorded in a small number of cases. Healing is virtually complete, although rheumatic pericarditis may be responsible for adhesions found at the time of cardiac surgery in patients with chronic valvular heart disease. Diagnosis of effusion is best made by echocardiography, and the condition must be distinguished from rheumatic myocarditis or severe valve disease.

Pericardial involvement is well recognized in patients with rheumatoid arthritis, particularly in males with subcutaneous nodules and positive serology. Transient pericardial pain, symptomatic pericardial effusion or pericardial constriction may all occur. Pericardial involvement is also common in systemic lupus erythematosus, whether spontaneous or precipitated by drugs such as procainamide or hydrallazine. Pericardial pain, asymptomatic effusion or chronic constriction have all been reported. Massive pericardial effusion may also occur in scleroderma, polyarteritis nodosa, and giant cell arteritis.

Pericardial involvement is common in untreated chronic renal failure. It usually presents with pericardial pain and a rub, which may both subside with the development of a pericardial effusion. The commonest manifestation is fibrinous pericarditis associated with a haemorrhagic pericardial effusion due to capillary bleeding. Tamponade may develop due either to liquid blood or clots. Collagenous thickening of the pericardium is much less common, but may give rise to constriction. Either of these complications may require surgical relief. The incidence of pericardial complications has been greatly reduced by adequate treatment of renal failure by dialysis or renal transplantation.

Pericardial effusion may be present in patients with untreated hypothyroidism, leading to moderate enlargement of the heart shadow on chest X-ray (Fig. 1), although clinically silent. The effusion itself has a high cholesterol content which may produce an unusual secondary pericarditis with cholesterol deposits which

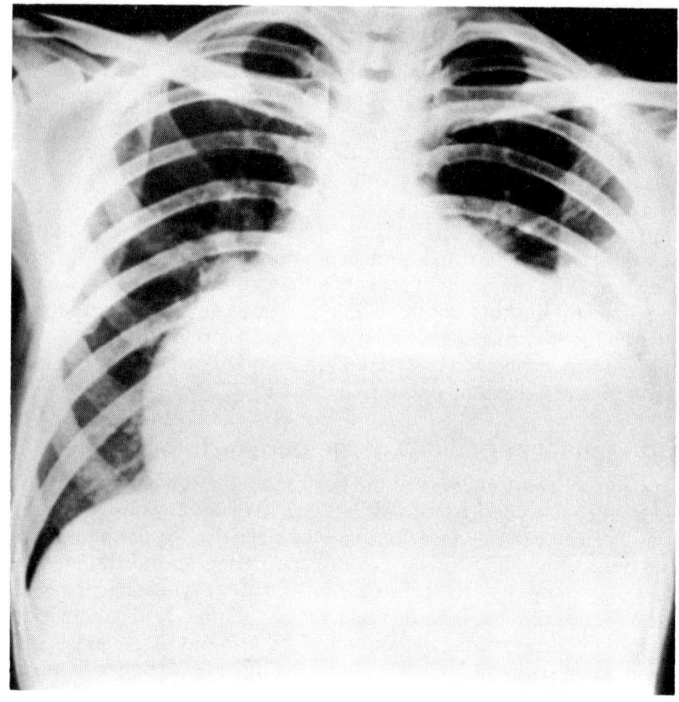

Fig. 1 PA chest X-ray of a patient with a large pericardial effusion. The heart shadow is greatly enlarged and globular in configuration. The lung fields are normal.

have a 'gold paint' appearance. The pericardial effusion does not require treatment in its own right, and subsides when replacement therapy is given.

Malignant involvement of the pericardium may be due to primary tumours, the commonest being mesothelioma or sarcoma, but much more commonly it is metastatic, or due to lymphomatous involvement of the pericardium. Clinical manifestations include recurrent supraventricular arrhythmias or atrial fibrillation as well as pericardial tamponade or constriction. On aspiration, the fluid is usually heavily blood stained. Positive diagnosis is best made by open biopsy, and at the same time a window is left into the pleural space to prevent recurrence.

Pericarditis may be caused by radiation at a dose of more than 4000 rad (40 Gy) to the mediastinum. It is usually asymptomatic, and a rub is unusual, but transient cardiac enlargement and minor ECG changes may occur. Small amounts of pericardial fluid can be demonstrated by echocardiography. However, in a minority of cases, a significant pericardial effusion may develop. This may occur up to two years after the end of the course of radiotherapy and may be severe enough to require surgical treatment for tamponade. At operation, the pericardium is found to be thickened by fibrosis with dense adhesions. This clinical picture must be distinguished from a recurrence of the original malignancy. In a small minority of patients, pericardial constriction may occur up to 40 years after the radiation.

Haemorrhage into the pericardium is an important cause of tamponade. It may occur with aortic dissection involving the ascending aorta. If the leak is large, it will cause pericardial tamponade with hypotension and death, but small volumes of blood frequently accompany aortic dissection. They can be detected by echocardiography, and may be responsible for ST-T wave changes on ECG. Pericardial haemorrage may also result directly from trauma, blunt injury as well as stab wounds, and after open heart surgery. It may be induced by anticoagulant administration, or may follow invasive procedures such as direct left ventricular puncture or pacemaker insertion. Symptoms may occur at the time of bleeding, or may be delayed by 2–3 weeks, possibly due to autolysis of blood clots causing an increase in the volume of fluid in the pericardial space. Delayed tamponade produces a characteristic syndrome of elevation of venous pressure, fluid retention, and a low cardiac output which may be mistaken for myocardial disease. Haemorrhage into the pericardium from any cause may lead to delayed pericardial constriction. This may be the basis of constriction occurring in a small number of patients up to 10 years after open heart surgery.

Clinical syndromes associated with pericardial disease

Acute pericarditis

Clinical findings

There are three main components to the clinical syndrome of acute pericarditis: chest pain, pericardial rub, and ECG changes. The pain is usually retrosternal, continuous, and sharp or 'raw' in character. It is frequently aggravated by sudden movements or deep inspiration, and it is sensitive to position, being relieved by sitting up. Less commonly, it may resemble angina pectoris, or may be mild, resembling 'non-cardiac' pain. If it is associated with dyspnoea, it is usually because inspiration is painful, so that the patient adopts an unfamiliar pattern of breathing. The onset of the pain is usually sudden, but in the acute idiopathic form, may have been preceded by several days' malaise or other non-specific symptoms.

On examination, the main abnormality is the presence of a pericardial rub, which may be audible in any position over the praecordium. In patients with sinus rhythm, the rub has two components in each cardiac cycle, corresponding to atrial and ventricular systole. Rubs are frequently evanescent, and may be sensitive to posture. They are often louder in inspiration, particularly if the patient experiences an increase in pain at this time. Irregularity of the pulse, due to supraventricular arrhythmia is also common with acute pericarditis, particularly when due to renal failure, or immediately following operation. Supraventricular ectopic beats, atrial flutter, and atrial fibrillation are all seen.

The third clinical feature of the syndrome of acute pericarditis is an abnormal ECG. Symmetrical elevation of the ST segments occurs in over 90 per cent of patients. Early in the illness, the T waves are upright, but over the next two to three weeks, they become inverted. These T wave changes are variable in their incidence, direction and extent, probably dependent on the distribution and degree of more permanent epicardial injury. They usually regress completely over a few weeks, but a minority of cases are left with minor, non-specific abnormalities, only to be detected many years later at a routine ECG.

Chest X-ray

Chest X-ray is usually uninformative. It may show cardiac enlargement, but it is not possible to tell whether this is due to pericardial fluid, an increase in left ventricular wall thickness or enlargement of one or more cardiac chambers.

Echocardiography

Echocardiography is the method of choice for detecting pericardial effusion. On the M-mode, pericardial fluid is demonstrated as an echo-free space between the epicardial and parietal pericardium, posterior to the left ventricle, but not extending behind the left atrium, where there is no potential pericardial space (Fig. 2). The distance between the two echoes bears an approximate relation to the quantity of fluid present, and as little as 50 ml can be detected under favourable circumstances. The thickness of the pericardium itself can also be estimated. Two-dimensional echocardiography gives more anatomical information about the distribution of fluid, and may be particularly helpful if the effusion is loculated (Fig. 3). In addition, pericardial adhesions can frequently be demonstrated.

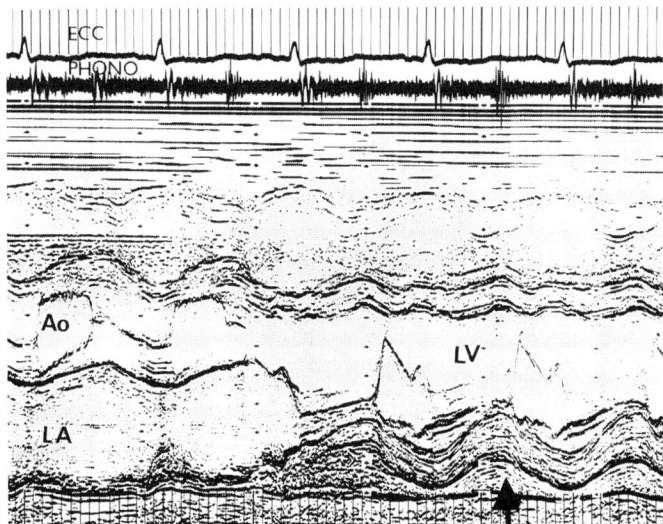

Fig. 2 M-mode echocardiographic sweep from left atrium to left ventricle. A pericardial effusion is present posterior to the left ventricle (LV), marked by an arrow. The effusion does not extend to the level of the left atrium (LA). Ao = aortic root.

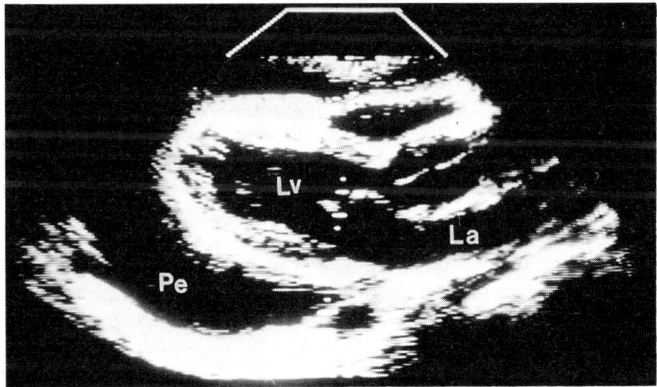

Fig. 3 Two-dimensional echocardiogram, parasternal long axis view, showing a large pericardial effusion (Pe) posterior to the left ventricle (LV). LA = left atrium.

Cardiac catheterization

This investigation is not usually required unless echocardiography is impossible technically, or when the primary disturbance is pericardial thickening. The most satisfactory technique is to inject contrast in the right atrium, and follow it through the pulmonary circulation to the left side of the heart. Abnormal pericardial thickening can be demonstrated as an increase in the distance between the right atrial cavity and the right heart border, and also between the left ventricular cavity and the left heart border, the outer margin of the myocardium being identified by the position of the coronary arteries.

Diagnosis

This is usually straightforward, although it is possible that either the late systolic murmur of mitral prolapse (qv) or the systolic 'scratch' of Ebstein's anomaly (qv) might be mistaken for a pericardial rub. An underlying cause should always be considered when a diagnosis of acute pericarditis is made. In addition, evidence of co-existent myocarditis must be sought, including a third or fourth heart sound, dilated upper lobe vessels on chest X-ray, and enlargement of the left ventricular cavity with a reduction in the amplitude of wall motion on echocardiography.

Treatment

Idiopathic acute pericarditis is usually self-limiting, requiring symptomatic treatment only. In view of the possibility of additional myocarditis, the patient should be rested until the pain has subsided. Pericarditis due to Dressler's syndrome or the post-cardiotomy syndrome is likely to respond to aspirin or indomethacin. When symptoms are very severe, or when repeated drainage of the pericardial effusion is necessary, steroids may be indicated, provided a specific infection has been excluded as a cause. Supraventricular arrhythmias are likely to respond to a therapeutic dose of digitalis or a β-blocking drug; d.c. shock is not recommended, since reversion to the original rhythm nearly always occurs while the pericarditis is still active even if it was initially successful. Pericarditis is often part of a generalized disease which should be treated appropriately.

Pericardial tamponade

Pericardial tamponade is a complication of pericardial effusion, in which the pericardial pressure is high enough to interfere with ventricular filling. The volume of fluid required to cause cardiac compression varies considerably. If the fluid has collected slowly, 1–2 litres may be present, but if it has collected rapidly or if the pericardium is rigid, very much smaller volumes may lead to cardiac tamponade.

When pericardial pressure is raised, a number of mechanisms maintain cardiac output. Right and left atrial pressures rise to maintain a normal transmural pressure across the ventricular walls at end-diastole. A sinus tachycardia is present, since such ventricular filling as occurs, does so in early diastole. This means that stroke volume is small and fixed, and an adequate cardiac output depends on heart rate. Finally, peripheral vascular resistance increases, so that arterial pressure is maintained in spite of a reduction in flow.

Patients with pericardial tamponade, therefore, present with clinical evidence of a low cardiac output. The skin is cold and sweaty, the pulse volume small, and urine flow reduced. A sinus tachycardia is usually present, although systolic arterial pressure may be above 100 mm Hg. Of particular importance is the physical sign of 'pulsus paradoxus', meaning a reduction in arterial pressure and pulse pressure with inspiration. This is very characteristic of tamponade, and when present implies severe embarrassment of the circulation, so that its recognition is essential. Normally, there is a slight reduction in arterial pressure during inspiration as the intrathoracic pressure drops which is accentuated in patients with increased airways resistance. Arterial pulsus paradoxus is thus an accentuation of the normal response rather than being paradoxical in any way. What is abnormal is the extent to which the arterial pressure falls. In early cases, this is 10–15 mm Hg; 10 mm Hg being taken as the upper limit of normal unless the patient has bronchospasm. In more severe cases, the reduction in arterial pressure can readily be palpated at the radial artery, and in patients with severe circulatory embarrassment, it may disappear altogether during inspiration. The mechanism of pulsus paradoxus is still uncertain, though a number of mechanisms are involved. Direct measurement of pericardial pressure shows it to rise during inspiration, probably due to distortion of the almost spherical cavity by downward movement of the diaphragm. This increase is accompanied by a concomitant rise in right atrial and central venous pressure, originally described by Kussmaul. However, on the left side of the heart, pulmonary venous pressure fails to rise appropriately, falling below that in the pericardium, so that there is a striking drop in left ventricular filling and hence stroke volume. At the same time, the amplitude of septal motion with respiration is greatly increased, so that on inspiration, right ventricular volume is maintained only at the expense of almost complete obliteration of the left ventricular cavity. During expiration, the reverse is seen. The normal inspiratory increase in systemic venous return is thus only maintained by

interfering with filling of the left ventricle from the pulmonary veins.

Abnormal right atrial filling in pericardial tamponade is reflected in abnormalities of the systemic venous pulse. The pressure is always considerably raised, and, indeed, if it is less than 10 cm above the sternal angle, tamponade is unlikely. In severe cases, it is more than 20 cm, so that it may be difficult to see the top, even with the patient sitting up. If a central venous pressure line is in place, then a further increase can be observed with inspiration (Kussmaul's sign). Both 'a' and 'v' waves are visible, although their amplitude is small, reflecting elevation of the mean venous pressure. Abnormalities of the venous pressure should be regarded as suggestive only, and not diagnostic of tamponade.

The precordial impulse is not usually palpable, and the heart sounds are quiet. Of particular significance is the absence of added sounds whose presence would be expected if the cardiac state were a manifestation of myocardial disease. A pericardial rub does not exclude a large effusion, with tamponade.

Chest X-ray

A large, globular heart is characteristic of pericardial effusion (Fig. 1), though similar appearances may be seen in congestive cardiomyopathy. Of much greater significance is the absence of pulmonary congestion, which again would be expected if myocardial disease were the main abnormality. Pulmonary oedema is most unusual in uncomplicated cardiac tamponade.

Electrocardiography

This demonstrates sinus tachycardia, often with low voltage QRS complexes, but with no Q waves or conduction disturbance that might suggest myocardial disease. If the effusion is large, then electrical alternans may be present, when the QRS complexes of alternate beats show different morphology, resulting from the heart swinging to and fro in a large, and therefore usually malignant, pericardial effusion.

Echocardiography

The is a most important investigation since it allows rapid and unequivocal diagnosis of the presence of pericardial fluid. The diagnosis of tamponade itself is a physiological one, and cannot be made by echocardiography, but its presence can be suspected from an increase in the amplitude of septal motion with respiration, associated with diastolic collapse of the right ventricule on expiration, and also with a low amplitude of left ventricular wall motion. If electrical alternans is present, then the echocardiogram confirms the rotatory motion of the heart within the pericardial space.

Cardiac catheterization

This investigation is not usually necessary, and certainly should not be undertaken routinely, since it may well delay essential treatment. However, it may be required in cases where the physiological disturbance is not clear-cut. Right heart catheterization shows considerable elevation of the mean right atrial pressure, with superimposed 'a' and 'v' waves. Right ventricular pressures are increased throughout diastole. Pulmonary artery pressure may be slightly raised, but diastolic pressures throughout the heart, in right atrium, right ventricle, and left ventricle all tend to equalize at a value of approximately 20–25 mm Hg. Angiography demonstrates an increase in the thickening of the pericardial space. The left ventricle may be distorted and its cavity almost obliterated at end-systole.

Differential diagnosis

The main step in the differential diagnosis of pericardial tamponade is to consider the possibility in a patient presenting with a low cardiac output state. The condition must thus be distinguished from hypotension due to left ventricular disease, massive pulmonary embolism, hypovolaemia or overwhelming sepsis. Hypovolaemia is ruled out by the very high venous pressure, while absence of added sounds and radiographic evidence of pulmonary venous congestion make severe left ventricular disease rather unlikely. Massive pulmonary embolism is usually accompanied by characteristic ECG abnormalities, and by a loud third heart sound audible down the left sternal edge, but can only be definitively excluded by pulmonary angiography or a ventilation perfusion scan. Features of cardiac tamponade may complicate other conditions, such as severe left ventricular disease, when there may be a significant increase in pericardial pressure. Strong evidence of a primary diagnosis of tamponade, however, is arterial pulsus paradoxus, particularly when palpable at the wrist, and electrical alternans on the ECG. If the echocardiogram shows, in addition, the presence of a significant pericardial effusion, then the diagnosis can be taken as established.

Treatment

Pericardial tamponade requires emergency treatment by pericardial aspiration if it is associated with arterial hypotension or marked arterial paradox. Aspiration should be performed in an area where resuscitation facilities are available, and the ECG should be monitored throughout. It is helpful to perform an echocardiogram just before the aspiration is undertaken, to determine the safest spot to insert the needle, and to get some idea of the best direction in which to aim it. Ring transducers have been designed to allow echocardiography to be performed throughout the aspiration; if available, these are useful, but are not essential. The subcostal or the apical route may be used. For the former, the local anaesthetic needle is inserted under the xiphisternum, just to the left of the mid-line, and directed cranially, and a little towards the left. The pericardium is thick in this region, and there is often a 'give' as the needle passes through. The alternative approach is from the apex, just inside the area of cardiac dullness, directing the needle towards the right shoulder. This latter approach has the disadvantage that one of the terminal branches of the left anterior descending coronary artery may be traumatized. On entering the pericardial space by either route, straw coloured fluid may be withdrawn, thus confirming the diagnosis. A larger needle, or preferably a polythene cannula is then inserted, and up to 500 ml removed. If the effusion is larger than this, continuous drainage is advisable. Many pericardial effusions, particularly those due to malignant disease, are heavily blood stained, and may appear indistinguishable from blood when they are withdrawn. They can be differentiated from blood obtained from puncture of a chamber by their colour, since the haemoglobin in them is desaturated, and by their failure to clot, since blood that has been in the pericardial space for any time has become defibrinated. If necessary, the haematocrit of the fluid can be determined and compared with that of blood taken simultaneously.

Pericardial aspiration relieves the acute emergency, but it is also necessary to diagnose the underlying cause, and to prevent recurrence. The most satisfactory way of managing such patients is to undertake open biopsy through a limited thoracotomy. This allows an adequate specimen of tissue to be obtained for histology under direct vision, and drainage to the pericardial space to be assured by making a window to the pleural cavity. It is also possible to deal with a loculated effusion or to remove blood clots whose presence may cause tamponade. If the diagnosis is not in doubt, or if surgical treatment is undesirable, a plastic intravenous catheter is left *in situ*, and attached to an underwater drain, with suction applied.

Pericardial constriction

Pericardial constriction is the haemodynamic disturbance due to restriction of ventricular filling by thickening of the pericardium. In many cases, there may also be myocardial atrophy and fibrosis of the subepicardial layer of the ventricular wall. Constriction is nearly always due to generalized thickening of the pericardium, but in rare cases the process may be concentrated in the region of the atrioventricular grooves. Calcification may be present, either in plaques, or forming a continuous shell around the heart.

Pathophysiology

Pericardial constriction prevents cardiac filling in late diastole. Early diastolic pressure is normal in the ventricles, but since the pericardium is indistensible, a normal or reduced stroke volume causes a striking increase in filling pressure. This abnormality of ventricular filling is reflected in the venous pulse, and also in the left atrial pressure trace, since both sides of the heart are usually affected symmetrically. Diastolic pressures in both ventricles are raised to an equal extent, a haemodynamic finding that is of diagnostic significance. Ventricular diastolic pressures remain equal during interventions such as deep inspiration or catecholamine infusion. Ventricular volume increases rapidly during early diastole, but 100–150 ms after mitral valve opening stops abruptly, due to limitation by the non-compliant pericardium. The venous pulse is also abnormal during systole with accentuation of the normal dip during ejection. In well-developed cases, the increase in mean venous pressure may be considerable, causing hepatic enlargement, ascites, and peripheral oedema. Constriction has the effect of limiting stroke volume, so that cardiac output is maintained by a rapid heart rate. Sinus tachycardia is therefore common, although in long-standing cases, atrial fibrillation is frequently present.

Clinical findings

The clinical picture is dominated by obstruction to right ventricular filling. In well-developed cases, the venous pressure is greatly raised, up to 20 cm above the sternal angle, showing abrupt early systolic and 'y' descents. The former is present, whether or not the patient is in atrial fibrillation, since it depends on ventricular ejection rather than atrial systole for its genesis. The prominent 'y' descent represents the drop in venous pressure from a very high value just before the start of right ventricular filling towards a normal early diastolic value (Fig. 4). The venous pulse thus reflects the difference between the haemodynamic disturbance of constriction, and that of tamponade, when filling pressure is high throughout diastole. The precordial impulse is not usually palpable, and on auscultation the heart sounds are soft. In addition, a prominent early diastolic sound is frequently present, described as a 'pericardial knock', which is rather earlier, and of higher pitch than the usual third heart sound (Fig. 4b). Its timing corresponds to that of the abrupt end of rapid filling. The liver is enlarged, and in patients with long-standing disease, there may be jaundice, and other evidence of hepatic dysfunction. Ascites may be very prominent, and may even be the presenting symptom. Peripheral oedema may also be present.

Chest X-ray

The heart shadow may be enlarged due to pericardial thickening but the lung fields are clear. In cases presenting in the West, an important finding is calcification of the pericardium, which may be present either as multiple plaques or more frequently, as a rim covering the right ventricular and diaphragmatic surfaces of the heart (Fig. 5). In a minority of cases, the chest X-ray may be entirely normal.

Electrocardiography

The ECG may show a number of non-specific findings including atrial fibrillation, low voltage QRS complexes, T wave flattening or, less commonly, right ventricular hypertrophy. There are no diagnostic features.

Echocardiogram

This may indicate the presence of pericardial fluid or thickening, but is frequently unhelpful. The abnormal pattern of left ventricular filling may be reflected in the lack of increase in left ventricular transverse dimension during the later part of diastole, but this is a non-specific finding.

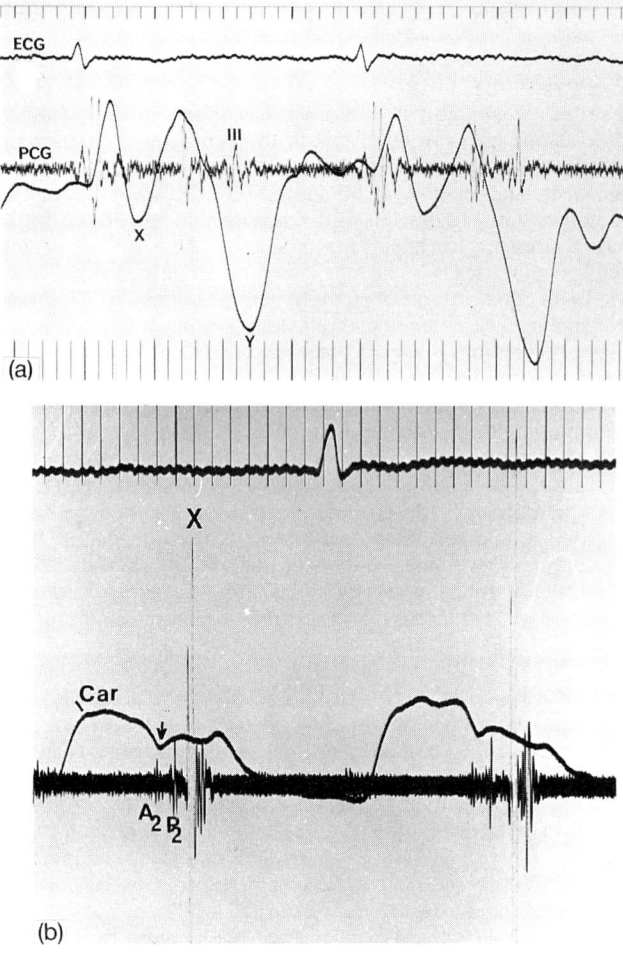

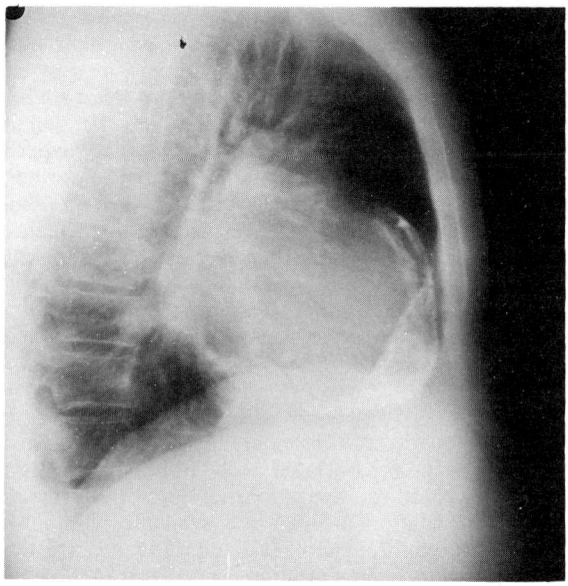

Fig. 5 Lateral chest X-ray showing distribution of pericardial calcification in a patient with pericardial constriction.

Fig. 4 (a) Phonocardiogram and indirect jugular venous record from a patient with constrictive pericarditis and atrial fibrillation. Early systolic (x) and diastolic (y) descents are present, together with a third heart sound (III). (b) Phonocardiogram and indirect carotid pulse from a patient with constrictive pericarditis, showing a ventricular knock (x). This is high pitched, and earlier than the third heart sound shown in (a). A2 on the phonocardiogram just precedes the dicrotic notch of the carotid pulse (marked by arrow), and this is followed by pulmonary valve closure (P2).

Cardiac catheterization

Cardiac catheterization confirms the presence of considerable elevation of left and right atrial pressures, which may be approximately equal to one another, provided the constriction is uniform. Superimposed left and right ventricular traces show identical diastolic pressures. Right atrial angiography demonstrates the presence of pericardial thickening.

Alternative clinical presentations

A number of less common clinical presentations have been described.

1. Localized constriction may lead to atypical features. Thus, compression of the outflow tract of the right ventricle may cause subpulmonary stenosis, with a significant pressure gradient between the right ventricular cavity and the pulmonary artery. Alternatively, the atrioventricular groove may be involved, causing functional mitral or tricuspid stenosis, with diastolic murmurs. In occasional cases, a band of calcification surrounding the heart has been described . Such cases are very unusual.

2. Elevation of systemic venous pressure may lead to a protein-losing enteropathy, causing hypoproteinaemia, and thus aggravating ascites and peripheral oedema. Biopsy may demonstrate lymphangectasia, and small bowel X-ray shows diffuse thickening of jejunal and ileal folds with flocculation and segmentation of barium. In addition, selective loss of T lymphocytes may occur, leading to impaired cell-mediated immunity.

3. Nephrotic syndrome, which regresses after correction of constriction, has been documented. Renal biopsy shows focal or diffuse glomerular thickening without hypercellularity. Renal vein thrombosis may occur, probably as a secondary, rather than a primary phenomenon.

4. Occult constrictive pericardial disease. This atypical form of the disease has been described in which resting filling pressures are normal, but where characteristic haemodynamic changes can be induced by rapid volume infusion. Patients present with non-specific limitation of exercise tolerance. Chest X-ray is either normal or shows border-line cardiomegaly, and ECG non-specific T wave changes. There is frequently a history of acute pericarditis. At operation, the pericardium is found to be thickened.

5. The combination of hepatomegaly, ascites, and jaundice may mimic primary liver disease.

Differential diagnosis

1. Malignant disease. The clinical picture of weight loss, hepatomegaly, and ascites may suggest the presence of malignant disease, particularly if the elevated venous pressure is mistaken for superior caval obstruction. This diagnosis can be excluded by observation of the characteristic wave form.

2. Myocardial disease. It may be very difficult to distinguish constrictive pericarditis from myocardial disease. One reason for this is that both conditions may co-exist, so that it is necessary not only to distinguish them, but also to assess the extent to which either or both are contributing to a raised venous pressure and impairment of cardiac function. This is not always possible clinically, but a number of indications exist: the more prominent pericardial component, the earlier the timing of the early diastolic sound with respect to A2, and the higher its pitch. Conversely, pulmonary congestion on chest X-ray, or an ECG showing conduction disturbances, left ventricular hypertrophy or Q waves suggests that myocardial involvement is likely to be present. When constriction is the main disturbance, then the characteristics of ventricular ejection are normal, while with myocardial disease, the pre-ejection period may be prolonged, and ejection time shortened. In addition, the response to treatment is rather different. The venous pressure drops with effective diurectic therapy in nearly all patients with myocardial disease, while it remains raised

in those with constriction. It may be extremely difficult to separate the two conditions when myocardial disease is due, not to depressed systolic function, but to infiltration of the ventricle with fibrous tissue or amyloid, leading to the clinical picture of restrictive myocarditis. In these circumstances, the dynamics of ventricular filling may be identical with those in constrictive pericarditis, and if the patient has significant symptoms, an exploratory operation, with pericardial and myocardial biopsy followed by pericardial strip, is entirely justified.

3. Other causes of obstruction to right ventricular inflow. The most important of these is tricuspid stenosis (see page 13.300), or in very rare cases, by a right atrial tumour. Tricuspid regurgitation is usually secondary to pulmonary hypertension, but if due to endomyocardial fibrosis (page 13.216) it may mimic pericardial constriction.

4. Right ventricular infarction. Right ventricular infarction is a not common manifestation of coronary artery disease. It is usually associated with inferior Q waves on the ECG, reflecting disease of the right coronary artery. The venous pressure may be considerably raised, and the right ventricular cavity dilated. Since the distensibility of the right ventricle is reduced, the venous pulse may resemble that of constriction. The diagnosis should be considered in patients with known coronary artery disease, particularly in the presence of inferior Q waves on ECG. It can be confirmed non-invasively by the demonstration of a large and poorly functioning right ventricle, either by blood pool scanning or by two-dimensional echocardiography. At cardiac catheterization, right ventricular filling pressure is raised disproportionately to any increase in pulmonary artery pressure, and, in addition, there are usually significant differences between right- and left-sided diastolic pressures.

Treatment

At first sight it would seem that tachycardia, a raised venous pressure, peripheral oedema, and ascites could be treated medically. However, it must be emphasized that these clinical features all result from the high filling pressure that is essential to maintain an adequate cardiac output, and that their 'correction' with diuretics is not only useless, but dangerous. This is particularly the case with paracentesis, which may cause an abrupt reduction in filling pressure and the development of hypovolaemic shock. It is usual to assume a tuberculous aetiology, though this becomes increasingly unlikely in the West. Antituberculous chemotherapy is thus started before operation but continued postoperatively only if the diagnosis is confirmed by histology and culture.

Treatment of chronic constrictive pericarditis is surgical, and operation should be recommended in all patients in whom there is significant limitation of exercise tolerance or evidence of fluid retention that cannot be controlled by a moderate dose of diuretic. It is necessary to remove the thickened pericardium from the anterior and inferior surfaces of the heart, and from the atrioventricular sulci. The operation may be a long and difficult one since, in long-standing cases, disease may not be confined to the pericardium itself, but may have spread deep into the muscle of the right ventricle. It is usually possible to perform the operation without cardiopulmonary bypass, but in difficult cases, its use may help in freeing the ventricles more completely than would have been the case without it. In many patients, the venous pressure remains considerably raised following operation, even to the same level as before. However, with digitalis and diuretic treatment it gradually falls over the succeeding weeks and months, with corresponding improvement in the clinical condition of the patient.

Other manifestations of pericardial disease

1. Postoperative pericardial tamponade. A modified type of pericardial tamponade may occur due to the presence of clots within the pericardium. This is commonest after cardiac surgery, but may also be seen in uraemia or with cardiac trauma. It is due to localized blood clots within the pericardium, particularly posterior to the left atrium. Clinically, it presents with a drop in the rate of urine flow, a reduction in skin temperature, and finally, with the development of hypotension and a low cardiac output. The atrial pressures may be normal or raised, and, unlike typical pericardial tamponade, are not necessarily equal. Arterial and venous pulsus paradoxus do not occur. Chest X-ray and ECG show no specific abnormality, although it is important to rule out myocardial infarction as a cause of impaired cardiac function. The condition is suspected in a patient who has bled rather heavily after operation, and is diagnosed and treated by reopening the chest and removing the blood clots. In a small minority of patients, a localized pericardial collection may obstruct right ventricular inflow, presenting with raised venous pressure and fluid retention. The possibility of postoperative heart failure or residual tricuspid valve disease may be raised. The correct diagnosis is made by two-dimensional echocardiography, which demonstrates compression of the right atrium by a loculated effusion. Treatment is by drainage.

2. Tuberculous pericardial constriction in the Third World runs a very different course from that seen in the West. It occurs early in the disease, and may be the presenting feature, or may supervene when an effusion has been drained. Patients present with sinus tachycardia rather than atrial fibrillation, very high venous pressure with ascites, and weight loss. The venous pressure does not show the characteristic pattern of deep early systolic and 'Y' descents. A third heart sound is present in about half. Chest X-ray shows a normal sized heart, but characteristically a 'shaggy' heart border. There is no pericardial calcification. ECG shows sinus tachycardia and non-specific T wave changes only. Two-dimensional echocardiography is very helpful, demonstrating separation of the two pericardial surfaces by amorphous echoes, which can be shown to arise from fibrocaseous material. There may also be small, loculated effusions. The amplitude of ventricular wall motion is reduced. Treatment is initially medical with antituberculous chemotherapy. During the subacute phase, the response to operation is poor, particularly if echocardiography demonstrates fibrocaseous material in the pericardial space. Surgery is indicated if deterioration continues for more than 6 weeks after starting chemotherapy, or if clinically significant fluid retention continues once the infection has been eradicated.

3. Effusive–constrictive or subacute pericarditis. This entity combines features of pericardial constriction and tamponade. There is constriction caused by thickening of the visceral pericardium, with effusion outside this, often loculated. Not only does it occur with tuberculosis, as described above, but has also been recorded in association with malignant disease, uraemia, after blunt chest trauma, in rheumatoid arthritis, and after pyogenic infection of the pericardium. It usually progresses to more typical features of pericardial constriction within a year. Clinical features include a large heart shadow, a 'shaggy' left border, and a raised venous pressure. Patients usually remain in sinus rhythm. As might be expected, the clinical course is variable, and treatment depends on the aetiology. However, if the venous pressure is greatly raised, surgical exploration may be considered, though the risks of operation in the presence of active infection are increased.

References

Baldwin, J. J. and Edwards, J. E. (1976). Uremic pericarditis as a cause of tamponade. *Circulation* **53**, 896–901.

Bush, C. A., Stang, J. M., Wolley, C. F. and Kilman, J. W. (1977). Occult constrictive pericardial disease. Diagnosis by rapid volume expansion and correction by pericardectomy. *Circulation* **56**, 924–930.

Caird, R., Conway, N. and McMillan, I. K. R. (1973). Purulent pericarditis followed by early constriction in young adults. *Br. Heart J.* **35**, 201–203.

Carty, J. E., Deverall, P. B. and Losowsky, M. S. (1975). Retrosternal pain, widespread T wave inversion and collapse of left lower lobe with effusion. Strangulated atrial appendix. *Br. Heart J.* **37**, 98–100.

Chesler, E., Mitha, A. S. and Matisonn, R. E. (1976). The ECG of constrictive pericarditis: pattern resembling right ventricular hypertrophy. *Am. Heart J.* **91**, 420–424.

Dressler, W. (1959). The post-myocardial infarction syndrome. A report of 44 cases. *Archs intern. Med.* **103**, 28–37.

Friedman, A., Sahn, D. J. and Haber, K.(1979). Two-dimensional echocardiography and B-mode ultrasonography for the diagnosis of loculated pericardial effusion. *Circulation* **60**, 1644–1649.

Hancock, E. W. (1971). Subacute effusive constrictive pericarditis. *Circulation* **43**, 183–192.

Heilbrun, A., Kittle, C. F. and Dunn, M. (1963). Surgical management of echinococcal cysts of the pericardium. *Circulation* **27**, 219–226.

Hirschman, J. V. (1978). Pericardial constriction. *Am. Heart J.* **96**, 110–122.

Kahn, A. H. (1975) Pericarditis of myocardial infarction. *Am. Heart J.* **90**, 788–794.

Lorell, B., Leinbach, R. C., Pohost, G. M., Gold, H. K., Dinsmore, R. E., Hutter, A. M., Pastore, J. O. and Desanctis, R. W. (1978). Right ventricular infarction: clinical diagnosis and differentiation from pericardial tamponade and pericardial constriction. *Am. J. Cardiol,* **43**, 465–471.

Martin, R. G., Ruckdeschel, J. C., Chang, P., Byhardt, R., Bouchard, R. J. and Wernick, P. H. (1975). Radiation induced pericarditis. *Am. J. Cardiol.* **35**, 217–220.

Mounsey, P. (1955). Annular constrictive pericarditis. *Br. Heart J.* **21**, 325–334.

Nelson, D. L., Blaese, R. M., Strober, W., Bruce, R. M. and Waldman, T. A. (1975). Constrictive pericarditis, intestinal lymphangectasia and reversible immunologic deficiency. *J. Pediat.* **86**, 548–557.

Perheentupa, J., Autio, S., Leisti, S., Raitta, C. and Tuuteri, L. (1973). Mulibrey nanism, an autosomal recessive syndrome with pericardial constriction. *Lancet* **ii**, 351–355.

Peterson, V. P. and Hastrup, J. (1963). Protein losing enteropathy in constrictive pericarditis. *Acta med. scand.* **173**, 401–411.

Pitt, A., Cutforth, R. H., Bender, H. W., Humphreys, J. O., Sterling, G. R., Criley, J. M. and Ross, R. S. (1971). Intrapericardial cyst formation in constrictive pericarditis simulating tricuspid stenosis. *Circulation* **40**, 219–225.

Robertson, R. and Arnold, C. T. (1965). Acute constrictive pericarditis. *J. thorac. cardiovasc. surg.* **49**, 91–100.

Schrire, V. (1967). Pericarditis (with particular reference to tuberculous pericarditis). *Aust. Ann. Med.* **16**, 41–51.

Shabetai, R. (1970). Symposium on pericardial disease. *Am. J. Cardiol.* **26**, 445–455.

Smith, W. G. (1970). Coxsackie B pericarditis in adults. *Am. Heart J.* **80**, 34–46.

Spodick, D. H. (1974). ECG in acute pericarditis. *Am. J. Cardiol.* **40**, 470–474.

Tubbs, O. S. and Yacoub, M. H. (1968) Congenital pericardial defects. *Thorax* **23**, 598–607.

Voelkel, A. G., Peietro, A., Folland, D., Fisher, M. L. and Parisi, A. F. (1978). Echocardiographic features of constrictive pericarditis. *Circulation* **58**, 871–875.

Wood, P. (1961). Chronic constrictive pericarditis. *Am. J. Cardiol.* **7**, 48–61.

LEFT ATRIAL MYXOMA

T. A. TRAILL

Tumours of the heart are rare. At least 80 per cent are secondary deposits involving the pericardium, or occasionally the myocardium. Cardiac myxoma, typically a large pedunculated lump of amorphous material occupying the left atrium, is the most common primary neoplasm, and since this lesion is today readily diagnosed and treated, it is also the most important. Estimates of the prevalence of such a rare condition are necessarily approximate and range from 1–5 per 10 000 in autopsy series, or 2 per 100 000 in the general population, with a sex ratio of 2:1 women predominating. As a cause of left atrial obstruction, myxomas are 200–400 times less common than mitral stenosis. The majority of patients are between 30 and 60 years, but there are reports of tumours occurring in infants and in the elderly. The aetiology is obscure. Six instances of familial occurrence have been recorded, some of these involving successive generations as well as siblings, but most cases are sporadic. Rare examples have been reported of myxomata occurring in both the heart and other organs, including breast and skin, but besides this there are no known associations with other diseases.

Pathology

Cardiac myxomas are invariably benign. Local invasion is unknown and metastatic growth is exceptional, despite the lesions' situation in the blood stream. Recurrence after removal is usually due to incomplete excision of the base, but is attributable in some cases to multicentric growth, just as are the 30 or so reported cases of multiple tumours occurring within a single heart.

Myxomas are usually polypoid masses arising from a stalk, ranging in size from 3 cm to as much as 10 cm or more, with a smooth or lobulated surface and gelatinous consistency. They are frequently covered with more or less adherent thrombus. More than 75 per cent occur within the left atrium, with the base of the pedicle arising from the fossa ovalis or its rim. Occasionally they arise from the base of the mitral valve leaflets, from the posterior part of the left atrium, within the right atrium or, rarely, the ventricles. Left atrial tumours, being freely mobile, descend into the mitral orifice during ventricular filling, and may thus acquire an indentation on the circumference corresponding to the atrioventricular valve ring.

The histology is that of a loosely woven sparsely cellular connective tissue tumour, with very infrequent mitotic figures. Several cell types are identifiable including undifferentiated stellate and polygonal cells, as well as smaller numbers of fibroblasts, smooth muscle and endothelial cells. Among these are found macrophages and plasma cells. Rarely other mesodermal tissues may be found, including bone. It is suggested that all of these are differentiated from a primitive multipotential mesenchymal cell, and that the predilection of these tumours for the atrial septum reflects the incidence of such cells in the subendothelium of this region. The abundant myxoid stroma contains large amounts of an acid mucopolysaccharide similar to chondroitin C as well as glycoprotein and variable numbers of collagen and elastic fibres.

Clinical features

Presentation

Although the present wide availability of echocardiography has made the laboratory diagnosis of atrial myxoma quite straightforward, it remains true that the prerequisite for recognizing this rare lesion is to include it in the differential diagnosis of patients presenting with symptoms and signs of much more common conditions. Three patterns of presentation may be distinguished, which reflect the main pathophysiological effects of the tumour.

Left atrial obstruction In about 50 per cent of cases, the history and physical examination suggest mitral stenosis, with left ventricular inflow obstruction as the chief pathophysiological change.

Thus the presenting symptoms include progressive breathlessness, orthopnea, paroxysmal nocturnal dyspnea, fluid retention, and atrial arrhythmias. Examination suggests rheumatic heart disease, and before the routine use of ultrasound, a few such patients were referred for mitral valvotomy and the lesion was first diagnosed at surgery.

Systemic embolism Systemic emboli occur in about 40 per cent of patients and are frequently the first manifestation of disease. In contrast to mitral stenosis such emboli often occur while patients are in sinus rhythm. They may be sizeable, for example, large enough to occlude the aortic bifurcation, and besides thrombus they frequently contain tumour material, so that histological examination may be diagnostic. Thus, when systemic emboli are removed from patients they should always be sent to the pathology laboratory. When emboli occur in young people, patients in sinus rhythm or where there is no obvious source, even in the absence of abnormal cardiological signs, patients should be referred for echocardiography.

Constitutional effects In about a quarter of patients constitutional effects of the neoplasm predominate. These include fever, weight loss which is more conspicuous than in mitral stenosis and often occurs without severe left atrial obstruction, Raynaud's phenomenon, finger clubbing, both of which are rare, a raised erythrocyte sedimentation rate, which is present in about 60 per cent of patients, and abnormal serum proteins with elevated immunoglobulin levels. These changes are usually attributed to abnormal proteins secreted by the tumour, although the nature of these has not been determined. Other haematological abnormalities include anaemia, which may be due to mechanical haemolysis, polycythaemia, associated particularly with right atrial tumours, leucocytosis, and thrombocytopaenia. Such constitutional changes may lead to an initial diagnosis of infective endocarditis in patients who have heart murmurs, or to the suspicion of collagen vascular disease or occult cancer.

Physical signs

In many patients specific cardiovascular signs of myxoma are inconspicuous or absent. In others they vary from a prominent first heart sound to obvious changes similar to those of mitral valve disease. These include apical systolic murmurs, somewhat more common than diastolic rumbles, and occasionally signs of pulmonary hypertension with accentuated pulmonary closure and elevated jugular pressure. Many patients have an audible 'tumour plop' in early diastole, analogous to a mitral opening snap. On combined echocardiographic and phonocardiographic recordings this is seen to coincide with the end of the tumour's downward movement into the ventricle, usually a short time after mitral valve opening; similarly the accentuated first heart sound occurs at the end of the early systolic movement of the mass into the atrium, and may be identified graphically as a notch on the upstroke of the apexcardiogram. A rare but specific feature of the condition is variation of the auscultatory findings with change in posture.

Investigations

The chest X-ray and electrocardiogram do not help to distinguish myxoma from mitral valve disease. Left atrial enlargement is common but seldom marked and signs of pulmonary venous hypertension are infrequent. Calcification within the tumour is rarely demonstrable.

Echocardiography

While the first account of left atrial myxoma diagnosed during life was not until 1951, it is now exceptional for the diagnosis to be made first at autopsy. This is chiefly attributable to the wide availability of echocardiography which has proved itself both reliable and specific for recognizing these tumours. The characteristic pattern of left atrial myxoma is easily recognized, and it is no accident that the echocardiographic appearance of these lesions was among

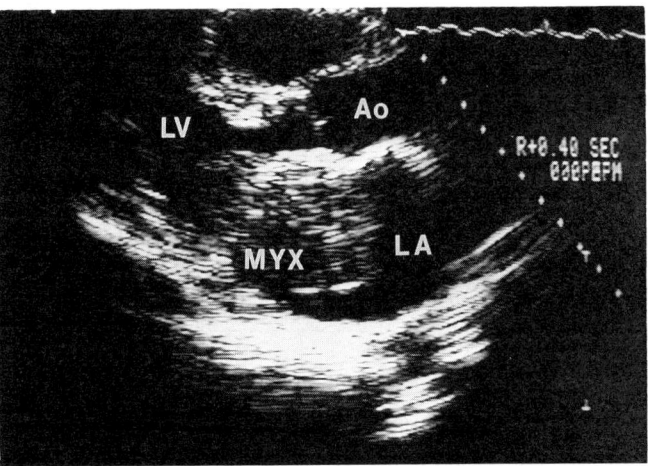

Fig. 1 Two-dimensional echocardiogram showing a long-axis section through the left heart. The myxoma (MYX) lies at the mitral orifice. LA, left atrium. LV, left ventricle; Ao, aorta.

the first clinical reports by ultrasonographers, in 1957. Figure 1 illustrates a typical echocardiogram from a patient with left atrial myxoma. This long axis section shows the characteristic dense mass of echoes from the tumour lying at the mitral valve orifice. The cross-sectional technique demonstrates the mobility of the mass as it flops to and fro within the atrium, restrained only by its peduncle. This pattern of motion also makes for easy diagnosis when only the M-mode technique is available. When the beam is swept from the inlet portion of the left ventricle up to traverse the left atrium, the tumour mass is demonstrated at the mitral orifice in diastole, and in the left atrium during systole. Differential diagnosis is from left atrial ball thrombus, a lesion which is today probably even rarer than myxoma. Since in either case surgical exploration is required, distinguishing these lesions is academic. Smaller left atrial masses may be papillary fibroadenomas or infective vegetations due to endocarditis. These can usually be distinguished by their clinical context.

Cardiac catheterization

In almost all cases, the echocardiographic appearance is sufficiently characteristic to obviate the need for further studies. Angiography may rarely be ordered for clarification or confirmation. Contrast studies are performed in the left ventricle, when sufficient mitral regurgitation may allow recognition of the tumour as a mobile filling defect within the left atrium, or by follow through injection of dye into the pulmonary artery. Transseptal catheterization of the left atrium is contraindicated.

Treatment and prognosis

Atrial myxoma is treated by urgent surgical removal with its pedicle. This has been performed successfully, on cardiopulmonary bypass, since 1954. Early figures for operative mortality reflect the high risk of all heart surgery at that time. Currently the operation may be performed safely with a low risk comparable to that of surgery for rheumatic mitral valve disease. It is important to ensure complete removal of the base, and it is recommended that full thickness excision be performed, with repair of the defect in the atrial septum, if necessary with a patch.

Functional results of surgery are good. Some patients are left with mitral regurgitation but this is seldom severe. However, even with histological confirmation of full excision of the tumour base, a significant number of recurrences occur, in as many as 5 per cent of patients followed for five years. It is therefore necessary to perform regular postoperative echocardiography even in the asymptomatic majority of patients.

References

Ferrans, V. J. and Roberts, W. C. (1973). Structural features of cardiac myxomas: Histology, histochemistry and electron microscopy. *Human Path.* **4**, 111–146.

Prichard, R. W. (1951). Tumors of the heart: Review of the subject and report of one hundred and fifty cases. *Arch. Pathol.* **51**, 98–123.

St John Sutton, M. G., Mercier, L.-.A., Giuliani, E. R. and Lie, J. T. (1980). Atrial myxomas: A review of clinical experience in 40 patients. *Mayo Clin. Proc.* **55**, 371–382.

INFECTIVE ENDOCARDITIS

B. GRIBBIN

Introduction

Infective endocarditis is a condition characterized by a microbiological inflammation of the endocardial lining of the heart chambers, great vessels, or valves. Traditionally the disease has been classified as bacterial or fungal and acute or subacute, and although the latter distinction is far from absolute there is an advantage in retaining it because of the very different mode of presentation at the two ends of the disease spectrum.

Acute infective endocarditis is caused by a virulent pyogenic organism such as *Staphylococcus aureus* or *Streptococcus pneumoniae* and leads to rapid tissue destruction often in the absence of pre-existing heart disease, with both local and metastatic abscess formation. Patients present early, cardiac failure is common, and mortality remains high with death supervening in days or a few weeks despite intensive medical and surgical treatment. Early recognition and treatment is of the utmost importance if patients are to survive.

Subacute infective endocarditis, often caused by viridans-type streptococci presents as chronic ill health of weeks or even months duration. The patient usually has underlying acquired valvular or congenital heart disease, and the prognosis is good provided that the condition is recognized and adequate treatment is given before further tissue damage leads to haemodynamic deterioration and heart failure.

The importance of adequate antibiotic treatment tailored to the organism involved cannot be overemphasized and makes it advisable to classify infective endocarditis not only in the clinical context, as acute or subacute, but also in terms of the organism. The usefulness of this approach is underlined when one considers that the same organism may produce different forms of the disease; for example, *S. aureus* infection may run a subacute course and conversely viridans-type streptococci may produce severe tissue damage and early death.

Although the number of patients at risk in the community must be large, infective endocarditis is uncommon with a prevalence of approximately 1000 cases each year in England and Wales. The pattern of the disease has changed considerably since antibiotics were introduced over 40 years ago. From being a disease mainly of young adults, the mean age of those afflicted is now in the fifties and the fall in the incidence of chronic rheumatic heart disease which is commoner in women, has meant that there is now a preponderance of males with the aortic valve most often affected and valve prolapse the commonest underlying mitral abnormality. In addition endocarditis has emerged as a serious complication of valve surgery and intravenous drug abuse.

Microbiology

Attention has already been drawn to the fact that virulent organisms such as *Staphylococcus aureus* and *Streptococcus pneumoniae* may, if favoured by circumstances, cause endocarditis. Organisms which colonize the skin and the mucous membranes of the upper respiratory tract, lower bowel, and genitourinary system may also gain access to the circulation and it is clear from animal work as well as clinical studies that these commensal organisms can cause infective endocarditis. This is more likely to occur when certain factors conspire to overwhelm the normally effective defence mechanisms of the body. For example, instrumentation of the mouth and upper respiratory tract, lower bowel, bladder or urethra may result in a large number of resident organisms entering the blood stream at the same time. Sustained bacteraemia may also result from skin infections at the site of intravenous cannulation or arteriovenous shunts in haemodialysis patients. The effect which this may have is influenced by the presence of underlying heart disease and especially prosthetic heart valves, and whether or not the effectiveness of the host defence mechanisms has been compromised by disease or by drugs such as corticosteroids and other immunosuppressive agents. In the majority of patients, however, the portal of entry cannot be readily ascertained and in many more an alleged dental origin is based on circumstantial evidence only.

Streptococci

In the preantibiotic era approximately 90 per cent of subacute endocarditis was caused by streptococci of the viridans type. Now the incidence is 35 to 50 per cent of all cases although greater in subacute infections. The commonest organisms are *Streptococcus mitior*, *Streptococcus mutans* and *Streptococcus sanguis*. As the proportion due to viridans infections has fallen so there has been an increase in the number of microaerophilic and Lancefield group D streptococcal cases reported. The former produce a subacute illness like that of viridans and respond similarly to treatment but require anaerobic culture. Group D streptococcal infection is often caused by *Streptococcus bovis* which tends to produce a subacute illness and is highly sensitive to penicillin. It may be mistaken in the laboratory for *Streptococcus faecalis*, another group D organism, which can gain entry from the gastrointestinal or genitourinary tract and can lead to an acute or subacute illness, usually in the elderly. This organism and the related but much less common *Streptococcus faecium* are intrinsically more resistant to penicillin but have in addition the ability to acquire new mechanisms of antibiotic resistance. Combination treatment with high-dose penicillin or ampicillin plus an aminoglycoside is usually required. Group A beta-haemolytic streptococci are now a rare cause of endocarditis, perhaps because penicillin is prescribed promptly for throat infections.

Staphylococci

Staphylococcus aureus causes about 20 per cent of all cases of infective endocarditis but more than 50 per cent of the acute form. In approximately half of these a predisposing heart lesion is not recognized and the portal of entry may be a localized abscess or furuncle, although contaminated entry sites for intravenous cannulae are another largely avoidable source. Frequent skin infections and an increased carrier state can also explain the predisposition of 'mainline' heroin addicts to staphylococcal endocarditis which then usually involves the right heart. Left heart involvement leads to a rapidly progressive illness with abscess formation in the heart and elsewhere and with an overall mortality of about 30 per cent. The lethal nature of this infection and the frequent paucity of abnormal cardiac signs at presentation makes it advisable to consider a prolonged course of antibiotics for any patient in whom *Staphylococcus aureus* is found in more than one blood culture. This is especially true if there is underlying valve disease or a delay in starting treatment. Most strains of *Staphylococcus aureus* (particularly hospital strains) produce an enzyme which splits the β-lactam ring of penicillin and so confers resistance to the drug. Resistance to other antibiotics also occurs and this together with the fact that it may be impossible to achieve an adequate antibacterial effect within abscesses has resulted in a move towards earlier surgical intervention.

Staphylococcus epidermidis is an ubiquitous skin commensal and when isolated in blood cultures is often considered to be a contaminant. However, the diagnosis of endocarditis can be made when persistently positive blood cultures occur in the context of the appropriate clinical setting, usually an illness of many weeks to months duration with evidence of valvular disease. This organism has assumed greater importance over the past few years because it is now the commonest cause of prosthetic valve infection, occurring early or late after surgery and it is also being isolated more frequently from 'mainline' drug addicts. Despite a low level of virulence it can be extremely difficult to eradicate and relapse may occur when antibiotics are stopped.

Gram-negative bacteria

It is of interest that whereas Gram-negative bacteraemia and septicaemia are commonly encountered, endocarditis caused by these organisms remains unusual. However, they do cause endocarditis in drug addicts who usually have no pre-existing heart disease, and in prosthetic valve recipients, accounting for up to 20 per cent of infections occurring early after surgery. The prolonged use of broad-spectrum antibiotics may predispose to this form of infection and numerous organisms have been implicated. Some, such as *Bacteroides* species, *Haemophilus* species, and *Cardiobacterium hominis* gain entry from the mouth or upper respiratory tract. Others such as *Escherichia coli* and *Proteus* species are more likely to occur after urinary tract infections, and *Serratia marcescens*, *Enterobacter* species, and *Pseudomonas* species after heart surgery. There is great variability in the clinical presentation which may be acute or subacute, but despite the ability of Gram-negative organisms to secrete endotoxin the picture of septic shock is unusual. Typically bulky vegetations occur and blood cultures are positive although anaerobic cultures may be necessary and some organisms grow slowly and require special culture techniques.

Unusual organisms

Acute endocarditis caused by *Streptococcus pneumoniae* is rare perhaps because treatment for pneumococcal pneumonia is usually prompt and effective. However, it may occur in the absence of clinically evident lung disease and has a high mortality often with extensive abscess formation in the heart. It may also co-exist with pneumococcal meningitis and it has been reported that type 12 *Streptococcus pneumoniae* is more likely to cause widespread infection by virtue of the fact that haematogenous spread from the lung is common.

Q-fever endocarditis is typically a chronic illness caused by *Coxiella burneti* which is transmitted to humans by respiratory secretions or inhalation of infected dust. Its importance lies in the need to consider it in any case of fever and heart disease with negative blood cultures, especially if there is a history of occupational exposure to cattle or sheep. An increase in or a greatly elevated titre of complement-fixing antibody is diagnostic and long-term treatment with tetracycline may be necessary.

Chlamydia psittaci is another rare cause in which a history of exposure to birds is expected and the complement fixation test should be positive.

Yeasts and fungi are usually opportunistic invaders in patients given cytotoxic drugs, corticosteroids, or protracted courses of antibiotics and so may lead to secondary infection of the heart in patients already being treated for bacterial endocarditis. Fungal endocarditis in drug addicts is most often due to *Candida parapsilosis* whereas *Candida albicans* is one of the main causes of prosthetic valve infection, very likely gaining entry at the time of heart surgery. In general *Candida* and *Aspergillus* species are most commonly involved but many others have been reported. Typically, large friable vegetations are produced and the diagnosis may be made only after histological study and culturing of emboli removed surgically. Diagnosis is not always easy and although *Candida* may be grown from the blood in about 75 per cent of cases, infection accompanied by severe valve destruction can occur without positive blood cultures and without a change in the agglutinin titre to *Candida*. The precipitin test may be more sensitive and its value in prosthetic valve endocarditis enhanced if a routine preoperative measurement is available for comparison. *Aspergillus* is rarely cultured from the blood even in cases with disseminated infection and large intracardiac vegetations.

Finally, it is worth bearing in mind that antibiotics such as penicillin which inhibit bacterial cell wall synthesis may occasionally be responsible for persistence of partly damaged organisms with deficient cell walls. These protoplasts may survive and be resistant to further penicillin treatment and yet reform when the antibiotic is stopped. Special culture techniques are necessary to isolate these forms which can be killed by the addition of an aminoglycoside. Their place in the aetiology of infective endocarditis is uncertain.

Pathology

Underlying heart disease

In the United Kingdom underlying heart disease will not previously have been detected in some 40 per cent of patients with infective endocarditis. Of the others the sort of contributing heart disease has changed considerably over the past three decades. At the beginning of this period (and still in certain parts of the world) chronic rheumatic heart disease accounted for 80–90 per cent of cases in adults with the mitral valve most commonly involved, but now the proportion due to this is less than half. This reduction has followed a decline in the incidence of acute rheumatic fever and also perhaps a greater awareness of non-rheumatic causes of valvular disease, for example, mitral valve prolapse and age-related degenerative changes, particularly of the aortic valve, but also affecting the annulus of the mitral. The aortic valve is now the commonest site for infective endocarditis. Infection may also develop on the mural endocardium in the region of a myocardial infarction or ventricular aneurysm.

Congenital heart disease (page 13.233) is present in most children with endocarditis and in approximately 10 per cent of adults. The risk of infection increases over the second decade of life and again substantially over the age of 20 years. Most of the common congenital abnormalities predispose to infection although it only occurs in patients with atrial septal defects if there is an associated mitral valve abnormality, and involvement of a stenotic pulmonary valve is also very uncommon. A ventricular septal defect is an important predisposing state with the risk of contracting endocarditis by the age of 30 years estimated at 9.7 per cent with a lifelong risk of about 12 to 13 per cent. This risk is increased further if there is associated aortic reflux. Early surgery has virtually abolished persistent ductus arteriosus, once commonly associated with endocarditis, as a site of infection and made it much less likely with ventricular septal defects, tetralogy of Fallot, and coarctation of the aorta. This is not the case, however, for aortic stenosis in which the risk may actually increase after valvotomy perhaps because a measure of aortic reflux is frequently produced. Cyanotic congenital heart disease in one form or another is still the commonest underlying abnormality in children with endocarditis and those who survive palliative or corrective surgery for the more complex abnormalities such as tetralogy of Fallot, pulmonary atresia, and tricuspid atresia now represent a new population at risk, not only by virtue of their continuing survival but also because of residual defects and the presence of prosthetic materials used in repair procedures. For example, there is a considerable risk of endocarditis in patients with tetralogy of Fallot or other cyanotic conditions treated by an aortopulmonary shunt, and to a lesser extent also in those who receive a valved conduit used to link the right atrium or right ventricle with the pulmonary arteries.

The presence of any foreign material in the heart increases the risk of infective endocarditis although this is much more for prosthetic heart valves than pacemaker electrodes and patches used to close intracardiac defects.

Pathogenesis

In studying the pathogenesis of endocarditis attempts have been made to discover why some forms of heart disease are more susceptible to infection than others, how a blood-borne micro-organism manages to colonize the lining of the heart, and why some forms of micro-organism seem to be more adept at this than others.

The vegetation is the initial lesion and is composed of platelets, fibrin, macrophages, and organisms. Observation has shown these to be more common on the left side of the heart and on the free margins of incompetent valves, particularly on the atrial aspect in mitral reflux and the ventricular side in aortic reflux. They are also found on the right side of the ventricular septum in ventricular septal defects and distal to the constriction in coarctation of the aorta. In order to explain the localization of these excrescences Rodbard showed that when an aerosol containing bacteria was blown through a narrowing in an agar tube, most organisms settled immediately distal to the constriction. He then postulated that the ideal haemodynamic conditions for producing infective endocarditis consist of a high-pressure source forcing blood through a narrow orifice into a low-pressure chamber. Furthermore, if a defect allows a high velocity of blood to pass through it, as, for example, would be the case in valvular reflux, small ventricular septal defect or persistent ductus arteriosus, then endothelial damage occurs, not only at the site at which organisms would be expected to settle but also where the jet of blood impinges on the wall of the low-pressure chamber. The latter explains why satellite lesions may form on the left atrial wall in mitral reflux, on chordae tendineae in aortic reflux, and on the tricuspid valve and free right ventricular wall in ventricular septal defect. Also low-pressure haemodynamic forces such as exist in mitral stenosis, large ventricular septal defects and atrial septal defects are unlikely to result in endocarditis.

Endothelial abrasion caused by turbulence is followed by deposition of platelets with or without fibrin, which then builds up to form a small sterile vegetation, so called non-bacterial thrombotic endocarditis. The stage having been set, blood-borne organisms may then adhere to the vegetations and provoke further deposition of platelets, fibrin, and macrophages (Fig. 1). It seems that the capacity for different organisms to colonize sterile vegetations varies considerably, perhaps because some adhere more readily or because others are lysed in the circulation by antibody and complement. The chance of sticking to a small vegetation may be increased by the clumping of bacteria brought about by agglutinating antibodies although this concept is controversial. Animal studies have shown that virulent organisms such as *Staphylococcus aureus* can stick directly to undamaged endothelium and can also stimulate platelet aggregation. As the vegetation grows, organisms become incorporated and to some extent protected from defence mechanisms by layers of fibrin, and those in the depths of the vegetation may enter a resting phase with a very low metabolic rate. Valve tissue under the vegetation shows a variable amount of damage with attempts at healing and ingrowth of capillaries in subacute and necrosis in acute cases. The subsequent course of infected vegetations is variable. Some, especially in fungal endo-

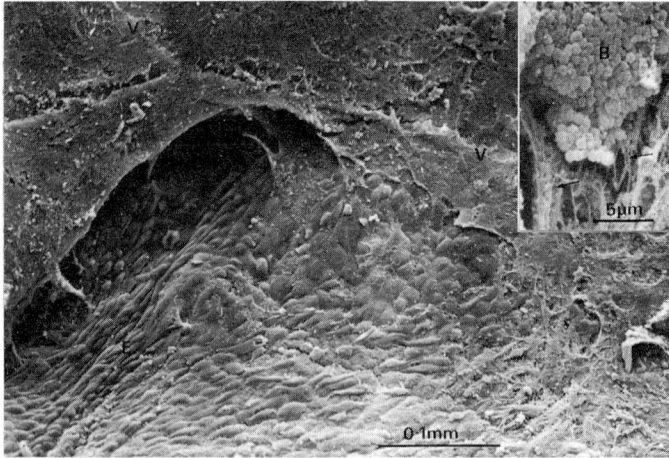

Fig. 1 Scanning electron micrograph of a leaflet of a human aortic valve showing the normal surface covered by endothelial cells (E) adjacent to an area with a large vegetation (V). Inset: detail of the surface of the vegetation showing a group of bacteria (B) surrounded by strands of fibrin (arrows). (Micrograph courtesy of D. J. P. Ferguson.)

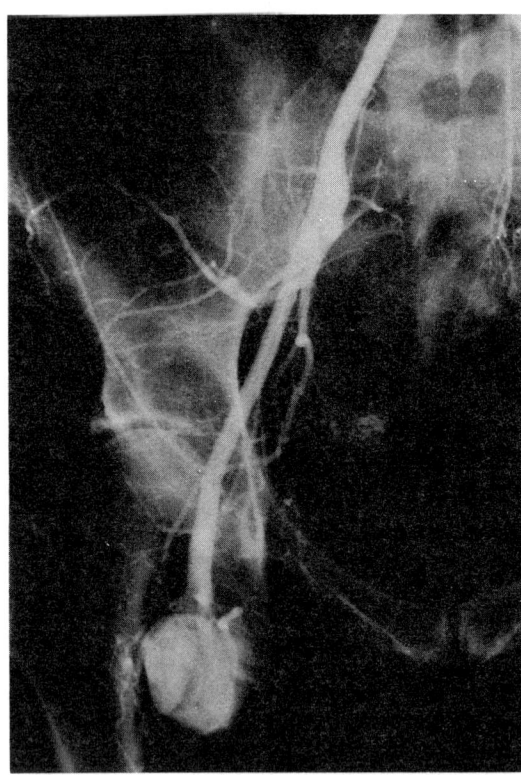

Fig. 2 A mycotic aneurysm of the right femoral artery.

carditis, become very large but even in bacterial cases their size may be sufficient to obstruct a valve orifice. In some, erosive rather than proliferative lesions are prominent leading to perforation of cusps and necrosis with abscess formation burrowing from the valve into adjacent tissue. More commonly found around the aortic valve, this process can damage the conducting pathways of the heart and weaken the aortic root, resulting in perforation and shunting of blood from the aorta to the pericardial space, the right atrium, or other adjacent chamber. Multiple myocardial abscesses resulting either from direct spread or septic embolization are another complication and evidence of myocarditis can be found in the great majority of patients studied at autopsy. With adequate treatment healing of vegetations may occur. They shrink, become endothelialized and organized from the base, and at subsequent surgery may be recognized as small fibrotic and calcified nodules on the valve.

Pericarditis can follow direct spread of infection from a valve ring abscess or myocardial abscess and can also occur as a complication of coronary embolism and myocardial infarction. In addition sterile pericarditis can occur presumably as an immunological phenomenon but this is uncommon.

Systemic emboli are a major threat and occur more commonly than can be detected clinically although all too often a patient may develop the disabling features of a cerebral or coronary embolus. In ventricular septal defect and other forms of right-sided endocarditis emboli pass into the pulmonary circulation and present clinically as pneumonia or as a pulmonary infarction. The incidence of embolism is related to the presence of vegetations detected by echocardiography and has been reported in 30 to 40 per cent of this group. Microemboli too are thought to be common and may be one of the causes of the peripheral stigmata of the condition such as Osler's nodes and the small petechial haemorrhages found in the skin and mucous membranes. They may also be responsible for an inflammatory myocarditis, the effect of which on overall cardiac function is usually difficult to judge. Mycotic aneurysms are localized arterial dilations caused by embolization of infected vegetations. In small peripheral arteries impaction of such an embolus may be enough to weaken the adjacent wall structure but in larger vessels the initial injury can be best explained by microembolization of the vasa vasorum followed by inflammatory change in the wall, destruction of wall elements, and dilation. Even if all infection is then eradicated, progressive dilation may still occur by mechanical means because, as the diameter of the artery increases so the tension stretching the wall rises and eventually this may lead to rupture (Fig. 2).

Immunology

In infective endocarditis the persistent bacteraemia provides an exceptional challenge to antibody production by B lymphocytes and plasma cells and such is their response in some cases that it contributes to the pathogenesis of the condition. Levels of antibody specifically directed against the invading organism are increased but in addition there is a generalized hypergammaglobulinaemia which is most apparent in patients whose illness has gone untreated for six weeks or longer. This exaggerated increase in immunoglobulin explains the presence of rheumatoid factors, including antibodies directed against specific antibacterial antibodies (antiglobulins), false positive antibody test for syphilis (VDRL), cryoglobulins, and antinuclear antibodies. Of the other autoantibodies present, antiheart antibodies reflect antigen release from damaged myocardial cells.

Tissue damage can result from the combination of excess circulating antigen and antibody into immune complexes which may pass through capillary walls and be deposited in subendothelial tissues. In some instances these complexes may form in situ but in either case complement factors are then activated and acute inflammatory injury ensues. It remains controversial whether some of the peripheral manifestations of infective endocarditis are due solely to immune complex deposition. Roth spots in the fundi, Osler's nodes, and petechial haemorrhages may have different or more than one cause, including immune complex deposition, microembolization, and increased capillary permeability. Rarely vasculitic skin lesions may occur with areas of haemorrhage and necrosis and these too are likely to be manifestations of immune complex deposition. Infective endocarditis may also be complicated by renal disease (page 18.42). Infarction is caused by embolism but immune complex deposition is known to cause the two other renal manifestations of the condition, focal glomerulonephritis, and diffuse proliferative glomerulonephritis. Renal biopsies have shown changes of glomerulonephritis in the majority of patients studied, although many with mild histological changes have no detectable abnormality of the urine or of renal function.

As a rule improvement follows antibiotic treatment but rarely inflammatory changes progress and lead to irreversible renal failure and then immunofluorescent studies show deposition of immunoglobulins and complement factors in the capillary walls of the glomerulus, along the basement membrane and in the mesangium. Destruction of glomeruli is thought to result from the opsonic activity of complement which leads to polymorphonuclear leucocyte infiltration and the release of enzymes which then injure vascular endothelium and the basement membrane.

Symptoms and signs of infective endocarditis

Attention has already been drawn to the two ends of a wide spectrum of clinical presentation with the rapid onset of severe symptoms in the acute variety and chronic ill health of a non-specific nature in subacute cases. However, as most of the peripheral stigmata of endocarditis are now less common and heart murmurs may be absent, missed or at least considered unremarkable, an atypical presentation can cause diagnostic difficulties. For example, a patient may come under care initially with neurological or psychiatric disability or perhaps following sudden loss of vision due to a central retinal artery occlusion. If one is aware of these diverse manifestations of endocarditis, the correct diagnosis should be considered and the relevant investigations done. Usually, however, the clinical features are characteristic of the condition with fever, marked constitutional symptoms, and evidence of heart disease.

Fever

This occurs at some time or another in nearly all patients and in most it is prominent and associated with sweats, chills, and occasionally rigors. The fever itself is often low grade in the subacute variety falling to normal some time during a 24-hour period but spikes over 40 °C may occur. Elderly patients, those in congestive cardiac failure, and those in renal failure may have a blunted pyrexial response but even in them an elevated temperature can usually be recorded on several occasions.

Constitutional symptoms

These consist of malaise with body aches and pains and are often summed up as 'flu-like'. In some, anorexia and weight loss are prominent and in others exhaustion. Aching joints and muscles and low back pain are common, headaches and arthritis less so and rarely severe. The low back pain may be disabling and if so may be the main presenting feature.

Cardiac abnormalities

At the time of presentation most patients with subacute endocarditis do not complain of newly acquired symptoms of heart disease. Of course, if endocarditis complicates a cardiac abnormality severe enough in its own right to cause effort dyspnoea or anginal chest pain, then the infection with its concomitant fever and anaemia is likely to cause further deterioration. However, cardiac failure is the most sinister complication and the commonest cause of death. The development of any symptoms or signs of decompensation should alert the physician to the possibility of acute aortic or mitral reflux or to an acute myocardial infarction caused by a coronary artery embolus.

Heart murmurs are detected in nearly all patients with subacute infection and in the majority of acute ones although careful auscultation will often be required to make a diagnosis of mild aortic reflux in those thought to be free of valve disease. Some day-to-day variation in the intensity of murmurs is not uncommon and the importance of changing murmurs in infective endocarditis lies in the detection of progressive valve damage, for example, a louder and longer early diastolic murmur suggesting greater aortic reflux, or in the same patient a new blowing systolic murmur at the apex suggesting secondary involvement of the mitral valve. Care should be taken to elicit confirmatory signs elsewhere such as tachycardia, cardiac enlargement, or an increase in pulse pressure. A pericardial friction rub, if heard, implies an extension of infection from a valve ring abscess.

Extracardiac manifestations

Peripheral stigmata Of these only petechial haemorrhages and splenomegaly are relatively common. Neither is specific for endocarditis but the former may be detected on the trunk, limbs, and mucous membranes. Particular care should be taken when examining the eyes because small conjunctival haemorrhages are more significant than isolated splinter haemorrhages which are found often under the fingernails of unselected hospital patients. Similar or slightly larger haemorrhages may be found in the fundi and some with central pale areas have come to be called Roth spots although different from the large exudates originally described by Roth in patients with septicaemia. Osler's nodes are circumscribed, indurated, red, tender lesions which occur most frequently in the pulps of the fingers and toes but may also be found in the thenar and hypothenar eminences and on the sides of the fingers. Often their appearance is preceded by the sudden or insidious onset of a burning discomfort, although in some patients this may be no more than a sensation of heightened sensitivity. They may be multiple and usually disappear after a few days. Janeway lesions are rare and are described as transient, non-tender, macular patches on the palms of the hands or soles of the feet and occasionally the fingers and toes. Clubbing of the fingers is usually seen in patients with long-standing disease. Splenomegaly is variable, and although most likely to be prominent in those with a chronic illness, it may not be detected in patients with infection of considerable duration and yet be obvious in someone presenting with a two-week history.

Renal abnormalities The pathogenesis of renal disease in endocarditis has been described. Renal infarction may present with loin pain and haematuria. Glomerulonephritis is seldom severe enough to cause symptoms of end-stage renal failure but more often function may be compromised sufficiently to justify close monitoring of potentially nephrotoxic drugs such as gentamicin. The urine may be normal even in patients who have histological evidence of glomerulonephritis but haematuria and proteinuria are not uncommon. These renal abnormalities usually disappear with effective antibiotic treatment. Rarely a progressive rise in serum creatinine with haematuria and proteinuria can be caused by an acute interstitial nephritis caused by penicillin or other antimicrobials in which case the fever persists and a skin rash is usual (page 18.132).

Neurological abnormalities These are common and may well be the mode of presentation, especially in the elderly. As in any severe infection a fluctuating confusional state with short-term memory impairment, disorientation, and behavioural changes may be prominent and yet is reversible with adequate antibacterial treatment. Presumably these changes are related to brain cell damage, either through interference with normal metabolism or by more direct damage from microemboli or vasculitis. Cerebral emboli, mainly in the distribution of the middle cerebral artery, have been reported to occur in 17 per cent of endocarditis cases and can lead to hemiplegia, sensory loss, and other focal abnormalities. Similar features may follow rupture of a mycotic aneurysm which tragically may occur up to two years after apparent cure of the infection. Most of these are in the territory of the middle cerebral artery and rupture leads to subarachnoid haemorrhage or intraventricular haemorrhage. In some cases aneurysm rupture may be preceded by a clinically evident embolus to the same vascular territory.

Meningo-encephalitis occurs and characteristically produces headache and neck stiffness. The cerebrospinal fluid is usually sterile but may show an increase in white cells and if associated with acute endocarditis, especially when *Staphylococcus aureus* is involved, purulent meningitis may be demonstrated with the organism grown from the spinal fluid. Multiple cerebral abscesses

are then the rule whereas a single large collection of pus is more typically a complication of endocarditis in children with cyanotic congenital heart disease. Pneumococcal endocarditis is perhaps the variety most likely to be associated with a purulent meningo-encephalitis.

Investigations

Blood culture

This is the single most important investigation and should be carried out as soon as possible in any patient suspected of having endocarditis. Correct aseptic skin preparation and a no-touch technique should be used and normally three blood samples are taken over a 24-hour period. Patients suspected of having acute endocarditis should be started on antibiotics after two or three samples are taken over an hour. Conversely it may be best to continue culturing for a few days in less acute cases particularly when the patient has already had a short course of antibiotic treatment or if initial cultures are negative at 48 hours. Serial sampling can also be a useful way of determining the relevance of an organism such as *Staphylococcus epidermidis* which could be a skin contaminant if found in only one or two samples. Although the magnitude of bacteraemia in endocarditis is small it does tend to be persistent and so it is not surprising that blood cultures are positive in about 90 per cent of cases and in nearly all of these the organism will be grown from the first sample.

Negative blood cultures occur in 10 per cent of cases. They are said to be more common in patients with congestive cardiac failure and in those with renal complications, the explanation of which may be that if the patient has survived a low-grade disorder without adequate treatment for months, a high level of antibodies and other natural bactericidal factors might then sterilize the blood, although organisms persist in vegetations. Such a patient would be expected to develop immune complex renal disease and cardiac failure.

Patients with right-sided endocarditis may develop positive cultures only after seeding of the lung by infected pulmonary emboli. Some negative results can be explained by poor culture techniques or by previous antibiotic treatment, although even under the latter circumstance organisms usually can be grown from the blood. Furthermore, it is not always realized that some organisms, for example, Gram-negative bacilli, may require several weeks to grow in culture and advice should be sought about special culture techniques for anaerobes, microaerophilic organisms, nutritionally variant streptococci, cell-wall deficient organisms, and fungi. *Coxiella burneti* which causes Q-fever endocarditis should always be considered in culture-negative cases and appropriate serological testing may make the diagnosis. If prior antibiotic treatment is ruled out then most cases of apparent culture negative endocarditis are probably caused by Gram-negative bacilli, in which case large vegetations may be seen on echocardiography, or nutritionally variant streptococci.

Blood tests

There is no set pattern of changes in infective endocarditis. The haemoglobin concentration is likely to be well maintained in acute cases whereas in subacute infections values below 10.5 g/dl occur in about half. The anaemia is normochromic and normocytic and is probably due to marrow suppression although haemolysis occasionally plays a part. The white cell count is variable, perhaps as high as 20 000–30 000/mm^3 (predominantly polymorphonuclear leucocytes) and yet in both acute and subacute cases the count may be normal or even slightly depressed, although a shift to the left is usual. The erythrocyte sedimentation rate too is variable and ranges from normal values of 20 mm/hour to over 100 mm/hour.

In subacute cases the concentrations of immunoglobulins rise. The presence of autoantibodies can be inferred from a positive VDRL test and a high titre of rheumatoid factors. Circulating immune complexes can be detected and in many the level seems to correlate directly with the duration of illness, the presence of extracardiac manifestations such as glomerulonephritis or skin changes, and inversely with serum complement values. In most hospitals it is not possible to measure immune complexes but total or selective serum complement values are more readily available and can provide confirmatory evidence of endocarditis and particularly of immune complex disease. Furthermore, because effective treatment is followed by a fall in immune complex levels and a rise in serum complement, with reversal of these changes in cases of relapse, their assay may prove useful as a way of determining disease activity. Complement consumption may of course be offset by increased production, allowing normal levels in patients with active disease. Serial measurement of C-reactive protein is also helpful.

Serological tests are useful in several instances. Q-fever endocarditis can be diagnosed by a rising or elevated titre of antibodies to *Coxiella burneti* phase one and phase two antigens. Likewise the agent causing psittacosis, a rare cause of endocarditis, can be identified by a high titre of complement fixing antibody. The place of serological tests in the diagnosis of fungal endocarditis will be discussed below.

Electrocardiogram

The electrocardiogram should always be recorded early in the course of the illness because it adds to the information about the nature of the underlying heart disease, and serial records can show changes which imply extension of infection, myocardial damage, and haemodynamic deterioration. For example, prolongation of the P–R interval in cases of aortic valve endocarditis signifies likely extension of the infection from the aortic ring into the conducting tissue at the top of the intraventricular septum and a similar suspicion can be raised if left bundle branch block develops. Prominent supraventricular or ventricular arrhythmias may be the only indication of an extravalvular abscess or myocarditis. Changes of acute myocardial infarction may provide an explanation for sudden clinical deterioration and marked ST segment depression in someone with acute aortic reflux indicates poor subendocardial perfusion and unlikely survival with medical treatment alone.

Echocardiography

This plays an important role in the investigation of patients with endocarditis (see page 13.34). It rapidly provides serial records of chamber dimensions and ventricular function as well as detecting evidence of pre-existing rheumatic or degenerative valve disease. By displaying premature closure of the mitral valve leaflets it can strongly support the diagnosis of acute aortic reflux (Fig. 3) and because of its ability to show vegetations it can support a clinical suspicion of endocarditis when blood cultures are negative and

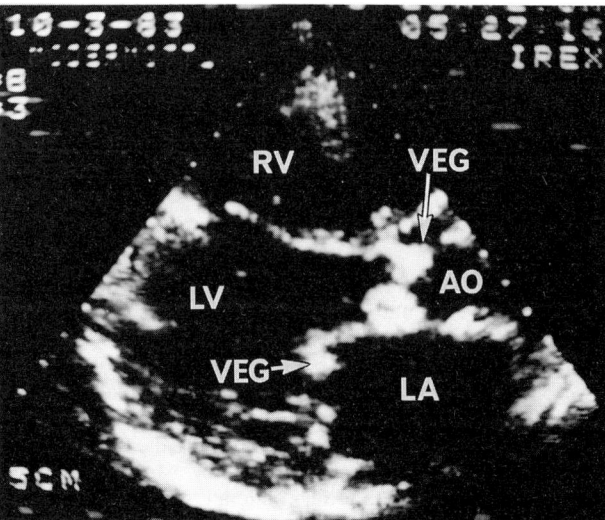

Fig. 4 Two-dimensional echocardiogram showing vegetations (veg) on the aortic valve and the anterior leaflet of the mitral valve. LA, left atrium; AO, aorta; RV, right ventricle; LV, left ventricle.

confirm particular valve involvement in others. Early reports using the M-mode technique describe vegetations as shaggy, irregular, mobile echoes, not restricting valve motion. Two-dimensional echocardiography is more sensitive (Fig. 4) and vegetations of only 2–3 mm can be visualized although it may not be easy to distinguish these from eccentric thickening of aortic cusps or the thick echoes seen in some cases of mitral valve prolapse. Most studies have shown that vegetations, certainly those greater than 1 cm in size, are associated with embolic complications and an increased mortality. Large vegetations, for example, those clearly seen by the M-mode technique carry a substantial risk and should influence any decision being made about surgical treatment. Echocardiography is useful also in demonstrating other complications of endocarditis such as pericardial effusion and perivalvular abscesses. It is less helpful in the patient with a mechanical prosthetic valve because of the echoes created by the prosthesis itself although valve dehiscence may be seen. With regard to porcine valves, large vegetations should be evident but thickening of valve leaflets reported in endocarditis, also occurs as an age-related degenerative change.

Special clinical problems

Aortic root infection

Cardiac failure developing during endocarditis usually has its basis in severe and progressive valve damage with the aortic valve most often involved. Under these circumstances acute aortic reflux is likely to be present, and if in addition there is electrocardiographic evidence of prolonged atrioventricular conduction or a pericardial friction rub is heard then extravalvular extension of infection and an aortic ring abscess is a strong possibility. If this is indeed present, then the subsequent course is likely to be one of sudden catastrophic cardiac failure brought about by further aortic valve damage, rupture of a sinus of Valsalva aneurysm or by secondary involvement of the mitral valve with leaflet perforation or rupture of chordae tendineae. Alternatively a failing myocardium may be unable to sustain such a heavy haemodynamic load in the face of a reduced diastolic coronary perfusion pressure and inflammatory changes. This state may be prevented in some patients if acute or progressive aortic reflux is diagnosed early enough, effective antibiotic treatment is started without unnecessary delay, and if it is realized that surgery often offers the best chance of survival. Early diagnosis rests on an awareness that the physical signs of acute aortic reflux may be misleading and quite different from those found in the more familiar situation of chronic reflux. In acute

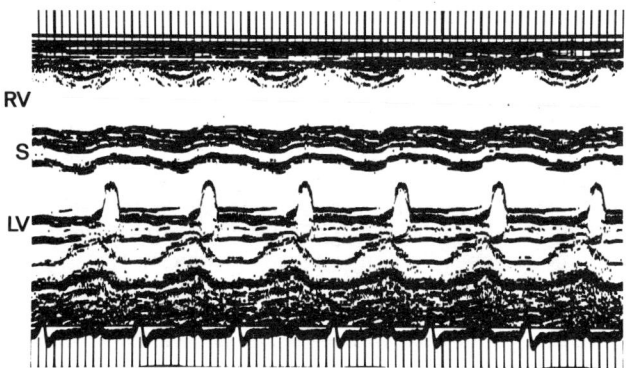

Fig. 3 Echocardiogram from a patient with acute aortic reflux showing that the mitral valve is open only during the early part of diastole. The electrocardiogram shows first degree atrioventricular block which can also lead to early closure of the mitral valve leaflets, RV, right ventricle; S, interventricular septum; LV, left ventricle.

aortic reflux of more than moderate severity a normal left ventricular cavity suddenly receives a large volume in diastole so that left ventricular pressure increases abruptly from early diastole, to such an extent that it exceeds left atrial pressure and premature closure of the mitral valve occurs (Fig. 3). Stroke volume hardly changes and cardiac output is maintained by an increase in heart rate. Observation of such a patient therefore will reveal a tachycardia, a prominent but normally positioned apex beat, and a low systolic and diastolic blood pressure with perhaps some increase in pulse pressure. However the peripheral pulses may not be collapsing in character. On auscultation the first sound is soft or absent, depending on the prematurity of mitral valve closure and the early diastolic murmur may be difficult to hear and limited to the very beginning of diastole. A low pitched diastolic Austin–Flint murmur represents mitral flow passing through the valve as it is being forced shut by the high left ventricular pressure. If the mitral valve is also infected and mitral reflux is present, then the protection afforded to the pulmonary circulation by early closure of the mitral valve is lost and pulmonary oedema may be uncontrollable. The combination of the clinical features of an aortic root abscess with valve reflux and moderately severe cardiac failure is an indication for surgery. An attempt is then made to replace the valve and excise as much necrotic and infected tissue as possible. The results of surgery are largely determined by preoperative left ventricular function and are likely to be better in those patients referred before the onset of severe cardiac failure.

Infective endocarditis in children and the elderly
Endocarditis in children is uncommon and in most instances the presentation is similar to that in adults, although in infancy it is usually one of generalized sepsis, underlying heart disease is infrequent, and mortality is high. The majority of older children have congenital heart disease, most commonly tetralogy of Fallot, ventricular septal defect or a bicuspid aortic valve. A number of reports have drawn attention to a recent increase in the incidence of *Staphylococcus aureus* endocarditis often associated with cardiac surgery or wound sepsis after general surgery. Peripheral stigmata such as Osler's nodes and petechial haemorrhages are less common than in adults and severe constitutional symptoms with joint pains and splenomegaly more common. Right-sided endocarditis complicating tetralogy of Fallot or ventricular septal defect may present with pneumonia, pleuritic chest pain, and haemoptysis although with both these conditions the aortic valve may also be involved with a subsequent risk of systemic emboli. Unfortunately children with cyanotic congenital heart disease seem to have more dental caries and periodontal disease than other children of similar age.

In the elderly the clinical presentation is often atypical and it may be the relatives who seek advice because the patient has become confused, disorientated, and lethargic. Fever may not be evident and the physical signs unimpressive with perhaps a systolic murmur thought to be due to aortic sclerosis, although careful scrutiny may detect haemorrhages in the conjunctivae, the fundi, or the mucous membranes of the mouth. This form of presentation is commoner in men who may give a history of previous urinary tract instrumentation.

Prosthetic valve endocarditis
The risk of this postoperative complication has fallen over the years and in reported series is now about 2 per cent with the first few months being the main danger period although the patient remains vulnerable. The Mayo clinic experience indicates that this form of endocarditis accounts for 16 per cent of all cases treated in a cardiac referral centre.

The condition has been classified as early or late onset varieties with the dividing line at two months after surgery. When infection occurs early, one assumes that organisms have gained entry during the perioperative period, perhaps from contaminated cardiopulmonary bypass equipment, from wound infection or from intra-

venous or intra-arterial cannulation sites. *Staphylococcus epidermidis* is the commonest organism isolated and approximately half of early cases can be attributed to this and *Staphylococcus aureus*, with Gram-negative bacilli and *Candida* spp. causing most of the remainder. The microbiological profile of late onset prosthetic valve endocarditis is similar to that of native valve involvement with streptococci assuming the predominant role. In either case the disease tends to produce necrosis of the valve annulus which leads to separation of the sewing ring and the development of a periprosthetic leak. Abscesses may track into adjacent myocardium particularly if staphylococci are involved. Less common and mainly affecting the mitral valve is functional stenosis caused by ingrowth of vegetations which obstruct the valve orifice and the free movement of the disc or poppet. Porcine valves are as susceptible to infection as mechanical ones with retraction and perforation of leaflets another cause of valve reflux. The clinical picture may be one of persisting postoperative fever although in time valve malfunction will be recognized, for example, by an early diastolic murmur caused by an aortic periprosthetic leak. Mitral prosthetic valve malfunction may be less easily detected and the advent of cardiac failure or a systemic embolus may be the first clue.

Three other causes of persisting or recurrent postoperative fever should be borne in mind. The first is residual infection in the lung, urinary tract or healing wounds. The second is the postperfusion syndrome in which fever occurs from two to eight weeks postoperatively and is associated with 'flu-like' symptoms, splenomegaly, and a lymphocytosis with atypical lymphocytes. A virus infection transmitted from transfused blood is thought to be responsible and the cytomegalovirus antibody titre may be raised. Recovery is usually uneventful over a two-week period. The third condition is the postpericardiotomy syndrome which can occur from one week to two months postoperatively and consists of fever, pericardial, and pleuritic pain often with effusions, and a high erythrocyte sedimentation rate. This responds to anti-inflammatory drugs but may recur.

The mortality of early prosthetic valve endocarditis is high although there may have been a decline in recent years from over 70 per cent to 41 per cent. No doubt this reflects the increasing use of further surgery which should be carefully considered in all patients other than those with highly sensitive organisms, who are free of heart failure, and in whom valve malfunction is apparently absent.

Prevention is extremely important and consists of clearing septic foci preoperatively, performing routine checks for contamination of equipment, and removing all intravascular cannulae and bladder drainage tubes as soon as possible. Prophylactic antibiotics are widely used to cover the perioperative period.

The clinical presentation of late onset prosthetic valve endocarditis is similar to that of native valve infection although systemic emboli appear to be more common and the importance of taking blood cultures from any patient with a prosthetic valve and unexplained fever cannot be overemphasized. Confirmation of valve malfunction can be provided by radiological screening to detect abnormal movement of the valve constituents, cardiac ultrasound, and cardiac catheterization. The mortality of late prosthetic valve endocarditis is now about 21 per cent and prevention is directed towards giving appropriate parenteral antibiotics for any manipulation or instrumentation likely to give rise to a bacteraemia. This is also recommended for any infection in which a bacterial cause can be assumed or proved. The details of antibiotic treatment for prosthetic valve endocarditis are described below but one further therapeutic requirement may be anticoagulation. Evidence favours the view that the risks of stopping routine anticoagulation are greater than those of continuing this form of treatment.

Infective endocarditis in dialysis patients
In one large study of 1014 patients with chronic renal failure treated with haemodialysis and followed over a 12 year period,

only four patients with infective endocarditis were diagnosed (0.35 per cent) although 9.5 per cent had an episode of bacteraemia. Other studies have estimated the incidence to be much higher. The source of infection is usually the access site with external arteriovenous cannulae proving more of a risk than arteriovenous fistulae and *Staphylococcus aureus* is by far the most common organism involved. Diagnosis may be delayed because the clinical features which might alert a physician to the possibility of endocarditis are not uncommon in the dialysis population as a whole: febrile episodes, heart murmurs, and anaemia.

Infective endocarditis in drug addicts

In many parts of the world this is a growing problem, with some hospitals in the United States reporting the illicit use of intravenous heroin as the commonest predisposing factor in cases of endocarditis. Typically the patient is a young male addict without previously recognized heart disease and with a relatively short history of illness. It is perhaps not surprising that the narcotic solution prepared and injected under unhygienic conditions should carry the risk of infection but adulterants also play a part. Less than 10 per cent of the powder used to make up the solution may be pure heroin, the remainder comprising bulk powder such as starch or lactose. The intermittent injection of these contaminants can lead to right heart endothelial damage which may predispose to subsequent infection with bacteria or fungi. The commonest organism involved is *Staphylococcus aureus* (62 per cent) which in most cases gains entry from septic skin spots and superficial phlebitis. Streptococci, mainly group D organisms, make up about 20 per cent of cases and *Pseudomonas aeruginosa* about 5 per cent. Fungal endocarditis occurs more often in the addict population with *Candida parapsilosis* the organism most commonly isolated. Double and even multiple infections are also commoner in addicts than in the general population.

The tricuspid valve is the one most often involved and the clinical presentation owes much to the shedding of emboli into the pulmonary circulation. Thus fever, dyspnoea, cough, haemoptysis, and pleuritic chest pain make up the typical features, with *Staphylococcus aureus* infections also complicated by the formation of microabscesses in several body tissues. Although examination may provide clear evidence of tricuspid valve disease, this is not always the case and abnormal physical signs in the heart may be few, particularly if the patient presents early. The venous pressure is likely to be elevated but the absence of a large 'V' wave should not rule out the possibility of tricuspid reflux. A soft short systolic murmur perhaps increasing with inspiration may be present at the lower left sternal edge and in more florid cases the systolic murmur may be pansystolic and accompanied by a short mid-diastolic noise giving a to and fro quality. However, because of the inconstancy of these localizing signs, one should always consider right-sided endocarditis in mainline addicts who present with pneumonia. Staphylococcal infection of the tricuspid valve has a good prognosis if adequately treated with antibiotics, but pseudomonas or candida infections may only be controlled after surgical excision of the valve. The presentation of left-sided endocarditis in addicts is usually acute with rapid valve damage and early development of heart failure. Under such circumstances valve replacement may be required and the risks of surgery are no greater than in non-addicts although long-term survival may be threatened by the patient's unwillingness to comply with medical advice.

Management of infective endocarditis

General principles

The purpose of treatment is to sterilize infected cardiac tissue and by so doing limit the extent of damage and prevent life-threatening complications such as systemic emboli and cardiac failure. In most instances adequate antibiotic treatment is all that is required but in selected cases, usually patients in cardiac failure, surgery has an important role to play sometimes early in the hospital course. In order to devise a rational plan of management which

may cover a period of four to six weeks, it is important to have accurate identification of the organism involved and to know its sensitivity to various antimicrobials. To some extent the course of the illness can be predicted if, in addition, the nature and severity of the underlying heart disease is known. This exercise can be useful in deciding upon the degree of surveillance required for individual patients and in particular whether complications such as acute valvular damage are likely. An attempt also should be made to find the source of infection, because this too may require treatment, an obvious example being a periapical dental abscess which would require drainage.

The principles of antibacterial treatment have been laid down as a result of experimental work in animals and clinical experience in humans. In general the consensus is that bactericidal drugs should be used in preference to bacteriostatic, that parenteral treatment is indicated and that bolus intravenous injections are preferable and possibly more effective than intravenous infusions or intramuscular administration. If in-dwelling intravenous needles are used, they should be changed every two days or at the first sign of local inflammation. An intravenous cannula should only be used if it can be inserted under strict aseptic conditions, usually in the subclavian vein and with further manipulation limited to a part of the cannula proximal to the site of skin entry which itself should be protected with antifungal and bactericidal spray or cream. If these precautions are not observed, there is a risk of secondary infection.

Sensitivity should be judged by laboratory testing in which the organism is added to culture media containing measured amounts of antimicrobial. The minimum concentration required to inhibit growth (MIC) is determined and subculture then allows measurement of the minimum bactericidal concentration (MBC). The range of antimicrobials used in this way depends on the nature of the organism and resistant bacteria should be tested against multiple agents, singly and in combination, so that synergy can be detected. Further, adequate bactericidal activity should be demonstrated by checking the effect of serial dilutions of the patient's serum against a standard inoculum of the organism, using blood drawn immediately before a dose. If possible this test should be carried out in all patients shortly after starting treatment and the bactericidal effect should be apparent at a dilution of one in eight or greater. If such an effect is present in higher dilutions, this is not a reason to reduce the administered dose, because it is likely that *in vitro* tests underestimate the blood levels required to sterilize vegetations and there can be a poor correlation between the serum antibacterial effect and clinical outcome. The duration of treatment is determined by several factors but is usually weeks. Those patients with staphylococcal infection, a prosthetic heart valve, or a delay in diagnosis will require six weeks treatment, and fungal endocarditis often has to be treated for considerably longer.

Antimicrobial treatment

The drug doses recommended below are for adult patients.

Streptococcus viridans

In general this group is highly sensitive to penicillin but there is a degree of variability in this and as accurate identification and antibiotic sensitivity testing may be delayed, it is best to start treatment with benzylpenicillin 7.2 g (12 megaunits) daily given intravenously in six 4-hourly doses, combined with gentamicin in a dose of 1 mg/kg eight hourly which provides a synergistic effect. When penicillin sensitivity is confirmed the gentamicin can be stopped although it is my policy to take advantage of *in vitro* synergism by continuing gentamicin at the low dose of 40 mg twice daily for two weeks and then benzylpenicillin alone for a further two-week period. The same treatment is advocated for *Streptococcus bovis* infections.

In patients with penicillin allergy treatment should be started with vancomycin 1 g intravenously over 60 min every 12 hours plus gentamicin 80 mg twelve hourly. Blood levels of vancomycin and gentamicin should be monitored frequently and consideration should be given to the possibility of treating with vancomycin alone.

Group D streptococci

These organisms are much less sensitive to penicillin and although large doses of benzylpenicillin in combination with gentamicin are usually effective, sensitivity to ampicillin or amoxycillin is often better and the recommended treatment is ampillicin 8 to 12 g/day given six hourly plus gentamicin 3 mg/kg/day. Treatment with both drugs should continue for six weeks. The concentration of gentamicin in the plasma must be checked at intervals. Satisfactory peak levels lie between 5 and 10 mg/l and if toxicity is to be avoided, trough levels should be less than 1.5 mg/l. In patients allergic to penicillin there is no clearly defined and tested second line drug, but the cephalosporins have proved unsatisfactory and should not be used. The best drug is probably vancomycin 1 g intravenously given slowly twelve hourly in combination with gentamicin, but one should remember that both drugs can be nephrotoxic and ototoxic.

Streptococcus pneumoniae

Pneumococcal infective endocarditis is rare. It runs an acute course and is particularly likely to form abscesses. Surgery may be required at some point but medical treatment comprises benzylpenicillin 9.6–12 g/day (16–20 megaunits) alone or in combination with low dose gentamicin (40 mg bd). Benzylpenicillin should be given in a dose of 14.4 g (24 megaunits) daily in patients who have coexistent purulent meningoencephalitis. Treatment should be continued for four weeks.

Staphylococcus aureus

This infection should always be suspected in the clinical context of acute endocarditis. Several blood cultures can be drawn over an hour and then antibiotic treatment should be started without further delay. *In vitro* and animal experimental studies have demonstrated improved killing with combined penicillin and gentamicin treatment and despite lack of clinical confirmation, combination treatment is usually recommended. Because most strains of *Staphylococcus aureus* involved in infective endocarditis produce penicillinase it is advisable to start treatment with flucloxacillin 2 g four hourly given by the intravenous route and accompanied by gentamicin 3 mg/kg/day in divided doses and benzylpenicillin 7.2 g (12 megaunits) daily. As soon as antibiotic sensitivity is known either the penicillin or the flucloxacillin can be withdrawn and dosage adjusted if necessary. Prolonged treatment is usually necessary and a six-week course prescribed but if serum bactericidal activity is satisfactory, the risk of ototoxicity makes it advisable to stop the gentamicin after two weeks or even earlier in the elderly or in those with poor renal function. In this regard, netilmicin is claimed to be less toxic than gentamicin.

In patients allergic to the penicillins, vancomycin with or without rifampicin in a dose of 600–900 mg daily, eight hourly or gentamicin should be given. Unfortunately medical treatment is often unsuccessful and mortality remains high with some patients being saved by surgical intervention.

Staphylococcus epidermidis

This organism tends to produce a subacute illness which is difficult to cure. Antibiotic resistance is common and even when a prolonged course is given of two drugs shown to be bactericidal *in vitro*, relapse may still occur after discontinuation of the treatment. Flucloxacillin and gentamicin are often given or vancomycin with or without rifampicin are other possibilities but it has to be stressed that the choice is determined by laboratory testing, and treatment should be continued for weeks. Most patients with this form of prosthetic valve endocarditis require surgery.

Gram-negative bacillary infection

These infections are uncommon but tend to occur in the elderly, in patients with prosthetic heart valves, in drug addicts, and in those with compromised defence mechanisms. It may be difficult to achieve adequate blood levels of antibiotics which are bactericidal for the organism when tested in the laboratory, and combination treatment should be used with surgical removal of the infected valve often necessary. *Pseudomonas aeruginosa* infection should be treated with pipericillin up to 16 g daily or ticarcillin 20 g/day plus tobramycin 3–5 mg/kg/day for four weeks. The newer cephalosporins such as cefsulodin and ceftazidime may prove satisfactory alternatives. *Haemophilus* species infection may respond to ampicillin in high doses (12–18 g/day) plus gentamicin or to cefotaxime which has the reputation of being very effective in cases of *Haemophilus influenzae* infection. *Escherichia coli* is the commonest cause of Gram-negative bacteraemia but infective endocarditis is rare. Ampicillin and tobramycin should be given for four weeks if laboratory tests confirm sensitivity of the organism to this combination. Indole-negative *Proteus* strains tend to be sensitive to ampicillin and this should be used with gentamicin. Indole-positive strains are more likely to be resistant to antibiotics and the choice must be made on the basis of sensitivity testing in the laboratory with a measure of effectiveness confirmed by demonstrating bactericidal activity in the patient's serum.

Most strains of *Klebsiella* are sensitive to the cephalosporins and *Serratia marcescens* should be treated with cefotaxime plus gentamicin. *Salmonella* species infection may respond to ampicillin and gentamicin with chloramphenicol an alternative. *Enterobacter* infection too may be treated with ampicillin and an aminoglycoside but this is another group in which laboratory testing is the main guide to therapy.

Fungal infection

This poses considerable therapeutic difficulties. The chances of cure with medical treatment alone are extremely small and even combined medical and surgical treatment is often unsuccessful. However, it is standard practice in some centres to recommend surgical removal of the infected valve followed by eight weeks of antifungal treatment. When only the tricuspid valve is involved excision may be quite well tolerated and valve replacement can be postponed until completion of a six to eight week course of medical treatment. It may be that in most patients complete eradication of the organism is impossible and one can hope only to inhibit growth. Certainly late relapse of fungal endocarditis, sometimes years after completion of treatment, suggests that long-term inhibition is possible. Amphotericin B, a fungicidal drug, given in doses of up to 1.5 mg/kg/day for six to eight weeks should be used, although it is extremely toxic and immediate side effects are prominent. For that reason regimens have been devised, one of which is to give 0.25 mg/kg intravenously on the first day with an increase of 0.25 mg/kg/day each day until 1 mg/kg is being given. 5-Fluorocytosine can be given orally and may be fungicidal for some strains of *Candida* and fungistatic for others. It is best to give this with amphotericin B and then it can be continued alone for some months after the six-week course of combined therapy. The dose of 5-fluorocytosine is 100–200 mg/kg/day in four divided doses given orally.

Unusual forms of infective endocarditis

Q-fever endocarditis can be treated effectively with tetracycline 2 g/day alone or in combination with co-trimoxazole (320 mg trimethoprim and 1600 mg sulphamethoxazole daily). Prolonged treatment is required and should be continued until sustained clinical improvement is associated with a fall in phase 1 antibody titres to *Coxiella burneti*. Prolonged therapy with tetracycline is also required for psittacosis infection.

Treatment in patients with negative blood cultures

It has already been stressed that in the clinical context of acute endocarditis, antibiotic treatment directed against *Staphylococcus aureus* should be started without delay. In those patients with a subacute presentation and negative blood cultures the possibility of a different diagnosis should be considered. Left atrial myxoma, acute rheumatic fever, collagen vascular disease, recurrent pulmonary emboli, and marantic endocarditis can all mimic infective endocarditis. It is often appropriate to await initial blood culture results, but the clinician may decide to start antibiotic treatment before these alternative diagnoses can be excluded and before laboratory results are available. If so, treatment should be directed against streptococcal infection including group D streptococcal strains. Thus benzylpenicillin 12 g (20 megaunits) daily plus gentamicin 3 mg/kg/day should be started or alternatively amoxycillin 6 g daily in divided doses plus gentamicin. In patients with a prosthetic valve initial treatment should cover possible staphylococcal infection.

Side effects of drugs
Hypersensitivity reactions can complicate treatment with virtually all the antibacterial drugs used in infective endocarditis. This is particularly the case for all forms of penicillin which on occasions may cause an illness which mimics endocarditis itself with persistent fever, aches, and pains, elevated erythrocyte sedimentation rate, and interstitial nephritis with red cells and protein in the urine. When penicillin is given in very large doses it may also cause convulsions although this is unlikely to be a problem when doses of less than 18 g/day (30 megaunits) are given to adult patients with normal renal function. The aminoglycosides are ototoxic and nephrotoxic and plasma levels should be checked in all patients but notice should also be taken of the total dose of gentamicin administered because there is some evidence that this too may influence toxicity. Vancomycin can cause cochlear damage and again blood levels are required if the drug is to be given for more than two days.

Surgical treatment of infective endocarditis
The surgical approach to the treatment of infective endocarditis began in 1940 when ligation of an infected persistent ductus arteriosus led to a cure. Because most deaths from endocarditis occur as a result of cardiac failure, itself a complication of aortic or mitral valve damage, it seems logical to attribute a prominent role to surgery in its management. However, suturing a prosthetic valve into a potentially infected site seems to go against basic surgical tenets and for that reason only those patients in gross cardiac failure were at first considered suitable. These were patients with an expected mortality with medical treatment alone of up to 89 per cent and yet this was reduced to approximately 23 per cent by combined medical and surgical treatment. Moreover it was found that the risk of developing infection of the prosthetic valve was low at 4 per cent, even when surgery was carried out before completion of the antibiotic course.

Postoperative survival has been shown to be largely determined by the degree of preoperative left ventricular failure and so it seems evident that an attempt must be made to recognize patients who may deteriorate rapidly. These include patients with *Staphylococcus aureus* or pneumococcal endocarditis characterized by rapid tissue destruction, patients with evidence of aortic root infection, and those with changing heart murmurs indicating further valve damage. The presence of obvious valvular vegetations visualized by echocardiography is not by itself an indication for surgical referral but complications appear commoner in this group with a 30 per cent incidence of major emboli and cardiac failure reported. It is clear that any patient with progressive cardiac failure should be referred early for a surgical opinion and even those with mild to moderate failure on medical treatment are best served by referral to a cardiac centre where surgery can be carried out if necessary.

Surgery followed by antibiotic treatment may also be required in order to eradicate persisting infection often with *Staphylococcus epidermidis* or Gram-negative organisms, and combined surgical and medical treatment offers the best chance of cure in fungal endocarditis. Early onset prosthetic valve endocarditis is often caused by *Staphylococcus epidermidis*, *Staphylococcus aureus*, Gram-negative organisms or fungi, and for that reason surgery may be required either because of persisting infection or valve malfunction. Endocarditis occurring more than three months after valve replacement is more likely to be cured by medical treatment alone but close supervision is required to detect early evidence of dehiscence or mechanical derangement of the prosthesis.

Response to treatment and prognosis
The patient's sense of well being usually returns within a few days of starting effective antibiotic treatment. The fever settles within four or five days unless sustained by extravalvular abscess formation or drug hypersensitivity. With *Staphylococcus aureus* infection the elevated white cell count should fall rapidly although with all forms of infection the erythrocyte sedimentation rate may take weeks to return to normal as may the anaemia and the serological abnormalities. The C-reactive protein concentrations will fall more quickly (page 9.157). Peripheral stigmata such as petechial haemorrhages can also occur during the first week or two of treatment and splenic enlargement may take months to resolve.

Prognosis
Prognosis is influenced by many variables. It is worse in cases of prosthetic valve endocarditis and in the elderly and if diagnosis and treatment have been much delayed so that valve damage, cardiac failure, and cerebral and coronary emboli are more likely to have complicated matters. Major emboli, usually to the brain, can occur even after completion of antibiotic treatment and late rupture of a mycotic aneurysm can tragically maim a patient who has apparently made a complete recovery. Overall mortality is quoted at about 30 per cent but there is some evidence that this is an overestimation and a survey of endocarditis in the British Isles during 1981 and 1982 gives a mortality of 30 per cent for staphylococcal infections, 14 per cent for bowel organisms and 6 per cent when sensitive streptococci are involved. Fungal infection carries a worse prognosis which is improved by combined medical and surgical treatment. Of the survivors who achieve bacteriological cure, 20 per cent may have some incapacity caused by complications and some of them will require late valve replacement for cardiac failure. Patients discharged from hospital without major complications have a long-term prognosis similar to that expected in someone of the same age and with the same underlying heart disease.

Prevention of infective endocarditis
Many diagnostic and therapeutic procedures involving minor tissue trauma or the spillage of blood can produce bacteraemia, and under these circumstances susceptible patients must be at risk of developing infective endocarditis. However, when one considers the large number of patients having dental and other procedures, about 5 per cent of whom are susceptible, the risk must be small. For that reason it has not been possible to prove that antibiotic prophylaxis in humans prevents infective endocarditis. However despite this constraint it has been generally accepted that prophylactic antibiotics should be used because experimental work in an animal model has shown that endocarditis can be prevented by prior administration of antibiotics. Furthermore, circumstantial evidence is available from clinical studies linking the onset of infective endocarditis with previous dental and other forms of instrumentation although the relative importance of the former has been debated. A recent British survey found that 14 per cent of endocarditis cases had undergone dental treatment within three months of the start of the illness although in another 7 per cent poor dental hygiene was incriminated. Under these circumstances *Streptococcus viridans* species are the commonest organisms isolated and it seems sensible to offer antibiotic prophylaxis directed against streptococci to susceptible patients having any dental pro-

Table 1 Antibiotic treatment for the prophylaxis of infective endocarditis

	Standard risk			High risk*
Dental treatment	Amoxycillin 3 g orally 1 hour before. Can be given twice within the same month	Penicillin allergy: erythromycin 1.5 g orally 90 min before and 500 mg orally six hours later	Amoxycillin 1 g and gentamicin 120 mg intramuscularly 15 min before the procedure followed by 500 mg amoxycillin orally six hours later	Penicillin allergy: vancomycin 1 g given over 60 min followed by gentamicin 120 mg given intravenously
Dental treatment†, upper respiratory tract surgery— under general anaesthesia	Amoxycillin 1 g intramuscularly before induction and 500 mg orally six hours later. Can be given twice within the same month.	Penicillin allergy; vancomycin 1 g over 60 min followed by gentamicin 120 mg given intravenously before induction		As above
Genitourinary, gastrointestinal tract investigations or surgery	Amoxycillin 1 g and gentamicin 120 mg intramuscularly immediately before induction and 500 mg amoxycillin given six hours later	Penicillin allergy: vancomycin 1 g over 60 min followed by gentamicin 120 mg given intravenously		As above

*High-risk patients are those with prosthetic heart valves and those who have a previous history of endocarditis. The dose of oral amoxycillin in children should be half of the adult dose for those less than 10 years and a quarter for those under the age of 5 years. The dose of intramuscular amoxycillin is half of the adult dose for those under 10 years. The dose of vancomycin for children is 20 mg/kg bodyweight and that for gentamicin is 2 mg/kg body weight. Intramuscular injections of amoxycillin should be given in 2.5 ml of 1 per cent lignocaine.

†An alternative to parenteral administration is 3 g amoxycillin orally four hours before anaesthesia and a further 3 g as soon as possible after the operation.

cedure which causes gingival bleeding. Instrumentation and surgery of the alimentary and genitourinary tracts are also potential sources of heavy bacteraemia involving group D streptococci and Gram-negative organisms, the former being more likely to cause endocarditis.

A vexed question is how to detect patients at risk. Almost 50 per cent of cases have no recognized pre-existing cardiac abnormality and so any kind of selective prophylaxis will not be offered to this group. Patients with known valvular or congenital heart disease should have antibiotic cover as should those with a past history of rheumatic fever and those with a heart murmur, unless judged to be normal. Mitral valve prolapse is associated with an increased risk but it remains controversial whether this extremely common condition should be covered, at least in the absence of mitral reflux. This should be decided on an individual basis, but in all, emphasizing the potential benefits of good dental care. Increased susceptibility seems to occur in patients who are immunosuppressed, diabetic patients, and those who abuse alcohol. The risk of infective endocarditis is certainly greater in patients with prosthetic valves and in those with a previous history of endocarditis and in them parenteral antibiotic cover should be given for any procedure which could conceivably cause a bacteraemia. This includes uncomplicated childbirth which is otherwise not an indication for prophylactic treatment.

The drugs chosen must take into account the likely dominant organism gaining entry from a particular site, the nature of the underlying heart disorder, any history from the patient of hypersensitivity to antibiotics, and also the circumstances under which the drug will be given. Dental treatment is the most common indication for prophylaxis and any recommendation should take into consideration the fact that combination antibiotic treatment given parenterally is difficult to implement and has proved impracticable in dental practice. The recommendations made by the British Society for Antimicrobial Chemotherapy should be followed and are presented in Table 1. It was thought unnecessary to offer antibiotic prophylaxis to standard risk patients having minor obstetric and gynaecological procedures, gastrointestinal endoscopy or barium enema studies. High-risk patients such as those with prosthetic heart valves should be covered as should patients having surgery or instrumentation of the genitourinary tract.

References

Bayliss, R., Clarke, C., Oakley, C. M., Somerville, W. and Whitfield, A. G. W. (1983). The teeth and infective endocarditis. *Br. Heart J.* **50**, 506–512.

—— and Young, S. E. J. (1983). The microbiology and pathogenesis of infective endocarditis. *Br. Heart J.* **50**, 513–519.

Cates, J. E. and Christie, R. V. (1951). Subacute bacterial endocarditis: a review of 442 patients treated in 14 centres appointed by the Penicillin Trials Committee of the Medical Research Council. *Q. J. Med.* **20**, 93–130.

Cherubin, C. E. and Neu, H. C. (1971). Infective endocarditis at the Presbyterian Hospital in New York City from 1938–67. *Am. J. Med.* **51**, 83–96.

Report of a Working Party of the British Society for Antimicrobial Chemotherapy (1982). The antibiotic prophylaxis of infective endocarditis. *Lancet* **ii**, 1323–1326.

Report of a Working Party of the British Society for Antimicrobial Chemotherapy (1985). Antibiotic treatment of streptococcal and staphylococcal endocarditis. *Lancet* **ii**, 815–817.

CARDIOVASCULAR SYPHILIS

B. GRIBBIN

Introduction

Cardiovascular syphilis is no longer a prominent cause of heart disease, and even in specialized cardiac units it is now a rarity. Natural history studies have shown that about 12 per cent of untreated syphilitic patients will eventually develop cardiovascular complications. Although gummata can occur in the pericardium, myocardium, and endocardium, and have been implicated in patients presenting with Stokes–Adams attacks caused by involvement of the atrioventricular node or the bundle of His, the characteristic lesion is an aortitis. This follows spirochaetal infection of the aortic wall and leads to an endarteritis and periarteritis of the aortic vasa vasorum, initially in the adventitia and subsequently in the media. Lymphocytes and plasma cells surround these small feeding vessels and obliterative changes result in the loss of medial smooth muscle and elastic fibres, occasionally with frank necrosis and eventually with fibrous tissue replacement. This causes scarring of the aortic wall and weakening of its structure. Macroscopically the intima becomes thickened in a gelatinous patchy fashion and fibrosis produces an irregular linear thickening which has been termed the tree-bark appearance. Intimal scarring may involve the ostia of the coronary arteries which are susceptible to further narrowing by accelerated and superimposed atheroma. The ascending aorta is involved in about half of all cases, the arch is next in frequency, and the descending aorta in only 10 per cent with changes virtually limited to that part of the vessel lying above the renal arteries. As the aortic wall structure weakens so dilation occurs resulting in aneurysm formation, which in turn leads to further dilation with the risk of rupture. The major branches of the aorta may also be affected, especially the innominate artery. Enlargement of the aortic root and separation of the cusp commissures causes aortic reflux, and although thickening and retraction of the leading edges of the cusps also occurs, this is thought to be a secondary change due to abnormal turbulence rather than a consequence of direct syphilitic involvement of cusp tissues.

Clinical features

Because cardiovascular syphilis may take up to 40 years after primary infection to become apparent, most patients are middle-aged or elderly, with men more often affected. Patients with aortitis can present in four main ways: asymptomatic aortitis, aneurysm formation, aortic reflux, and lastly as the result of coronary artery ostial stenosis. The latter three are not mutually exclusive and aortic reflux plus ostial stenosis may co-exsist with aneurysm formation.

Aortitis in asymptomatic patients is usually diagnosed as the result of radiographic findings of a dilated ascending aorta with calcification in the wall (Fig. 1). Aortic calcification is common particularly in the elderly and hypertensive population but then it is virtually limited to the aortic knuckle and descending aorta. When visible in the ascending aorta, syphilitic aortitis should come to mind and supporting evidence such as mild aortic reflux may be noted. Serology is likely to be positive.

Aortic aneuryms tend to be saccular rather than fusiform and occur most commonly in the ascending aorta, also in the arch, and with increasing rarity down the descending aorta. This is in contrast to atherosclerotic aneurysms which tend to involve the distal aorta below the renal arteries. The clinical features vary depending on the site of the aneurysm, its size, and whether or not compression and even erosion of adjacent structures occurs. A large aneurysm may cause no symptoms but pain can be a prominent

feature, often sustained and boring in nature, influenced by position, and exacerbated by impending rupture. With ascending aortic aneurysms pain is felt in the upper chest wall to the right of the

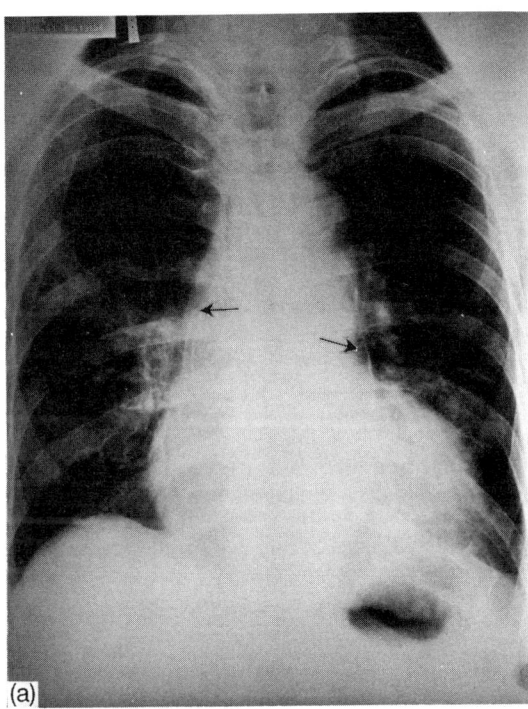

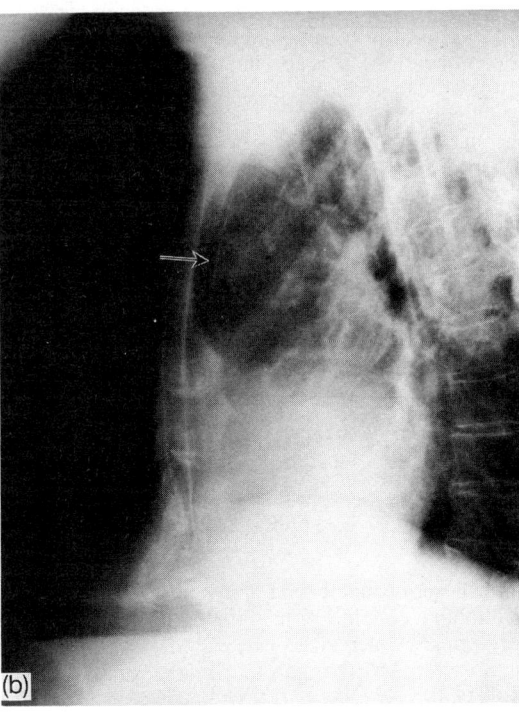

Fig. 1 PA and lateral radiographs showing evidence of syphilitic aortitis. A line of calcium (arrowed) is visible in the wall of the dilated ascending aorta.

sternum and with large aneurysms a bulge may appear at this site and erosion of ribs and even sternum may be apparent on radiographs. Aneurysms of the arch produce pain over the upper sternum and occasionally in the throat and there may be visible arterial pulsation in the root of the neck with tracheal deviation. Pressure on upper mediastinal structures can produce superior vena cava obstruction, dysphagia, stridor, and a tracheal tug. Involvement of the upper descending aorta causes pain between the scapulae or to the left of the spine, and there is a risk of hoarseness from pressure on the left recurrent laryngeal nerve and complications arising from compression of the left main bronchus. Rupture can occur into the bronchus, into the left pulmonary artery or the left pleural space, and erosion of vertebrae may result in chronic and debilitating pain.

Syphilitic aortic reflux may have a number of features to help distinguish it from the more usual varieties. Radiographic or clinical evidence of aneurysmal dilation of the ascending aorta is one, and explains the fact that the early diastolic murmur may be heard best at the right rather than the more usual left sternal edge position. Furthermore, an ejection click may be audible and probably occurs as a result of sudden distension of the dilated aortic root by the large stroke volume. However, these auscultatory signs are not entirely specific and may be found in patients with annuloaortic ectasia, now a more common condition characterized by a flask-like dilation of the proximal ascending aorta. Even severe aortic reflux may be well tolerated for many years, but eventually the volume overload of the left ventricle is likely to lead to cardiac failure which then carries a poor prognosis without surgical intervention.

Coronary ostial stenosis is not restricted to cases of syphilitic aortitis and may occur as a variant of the more usual atheromatous coronary artery disease. It presents as angina, the true nature of which may be missed unless a thin line of calcification is noted in the ascending aorta or there is other evidence of syphilitic disease in the cardiovascular system or elsewhere. Myocardial infarction may occur as a further complication.

Diagnosis
The diagnosis of cardiovascular syphilis is usually made by detecting a positive serum antibody test in a patient who may give a history of past syphilitic infection, and who has evidence of aortitis or one of its complications. It is also important to note that 10–25 per cent of patients with cardiovascular syphillis have central nervous system involvement.

Non-specific antibody tests such as the Venereal Diseases Research Laboratory (VDRL) test may be negative in cardiovas-cular syphilis, but specific tests such as the fluorescent treponemal antibody absorption test (FTA-ABS) remain positive, even after treatment.

Treatment
If patients with cardiovascular syphilis have not received effective antibiotic treatment in the past, they should receive a course of penicillin, given as procaine penicillin 1.5 g (900 000 units) intramuscularly daily for 10 days. Benzathine penicillin given as 4 g (2.4 megaunits) intramuscularly is less satisfactory but useful if only one clinic visit is likely. Patients known to be allergic to penicillin can be treated with tetracycline 500 mg orally four times daily for 30 days. If the VDRL test is positive then effective treatment should result in a fall in titre over a 1–2 year period. In all cases the cerebrospinal fluid should be examined and if antibody tests are found to be positive, then further cerebrospinal fluid examination should be performed to demonstrate a similar fall in titre. Although it is generally accepted that antibiotic treatment is indicated, there is no evidence that the severity of aortitis is in any way altered, and in fact there has been concern that provocation of a Jarisch–Herxheimer reaction might lead to inflammatory swelling of the aortic wall with the risk of rupture or further critical narrowing of ostial stenosis. However, large number of patients with cardiovascular syphilis have been given penicillin without untoward effects and whereas the Jarisch–Herxheimer reaction can rarely occur, it has never been shown to cause life-threatening changes in the aortic wall.

Surgery may be required to deal with the complications of aortitis. Symptoms of ischaemic heart disease caused by severe ostial stenosis have been successfully relieved by endarterectomy of the coronary orifices, and also by aorto-coronary saphenous vein bypass grafting. Aortic valve replacement has been carried out for severe aortic reflux. Saccular aneurysms have been excised and scarred aortic tissue replaced by grafts. Indications for the latter form of surgery are based on the need to relieve pain, to prevent rupture, the risk of which is considerable when the aneurysm reaches 6 to 7 cm in diameter, and the need to decompress adjacent organs such as the left main bronchus, pulmonary artery or oesophagus.

References
Heggtveit, H.A. (1964). Syphilitic aortitis. A clinicopathologic autopsy study of 100 cases, 1950 to 1960. *Circulation* **29**, 346–355.
Rimsa, A. and Griffith, G.C. (1957). Trends in cardiovascular syphilis. *Ann. intern. Med.* **46**, 915–924.

THE PULMONARY CIRCULATION

The pulmonary circulation in health and disease

J. S. PRICHARD AND G. de J. LEE

Introduction
This chapter describes the broad design and functional behaviour of the pulmonary circulation in the healthy lung as well as the common responses which take place within it as a result of perturbations imposed upon the organ by diseases, often entirely unrelated aetiologically.

The chapter is intended to be read in conjunction with those that follow relating to cor pulmonale, pulmonary hypertension, pulmonary oedema, and pulmonary embolism, to help the general reader to spot the precise malfunctions reponsible for the clinical manifestations of the above conditions, on which to base rational therapy, prognosis, and differential diagnosis.

The role of the pulmonary circulation
The whole of the cardiac output is delivered to the lungs for gas exchange which must be accomplished equally efficiently over wide ranges of blood flow and ventilation.

This requirement imposes three major constraints on the pulmonary circulation. The first is that the passage time for individual red blood cells through the alveolar capillaries must be long enough for complete oxygen exchange to take place by diffusion. The second constraint is that any increase in blood flow through the capillaries must be achieved without any great increase in intracapillary hydrostatic pressure. Thirdly, regional blood flow must be regulated to match local variations in regional ventilation.

The flux of water from capillaries into the tissues of organs depends upon the balance of forces between the organ's capillaries and the tissues surrounding them. In the case of the lung, if the hydrostatic pressure within the capillaries were to exceed the plasma oncotic pressure it would perturb the equilibrium regulating the diffusion of water and solute across the alveolar capillary membrane. Normally this prevents fluid movement into the lung interstitium other than for nutritive purposes, in spite of unrestricted diffusion of respiratory gases.

In disease, various adaptive mechanisms operate to protect the lung from early alveolar flooding manifest as pulmonary oedema. Other mechanisms also allow redistribution of both blood flow and ventilation away from local areas of disease to more normal areas of the lung.

The alveolar–capillary microenvironment also conceals many important metabolic, immune, and barrier functions which together protect the lung as a gas exchanging organ. Capillary sieving, proteolysis, and phagocytosis remove cellular and proteinaceous debris deposited in the lungs from the systemic venous system, as in venous thromboembolism.

The cells of the lung microcirculation, particularly endothelial cells, interstitial macrophages, and mast cells, provide an immense variety of metabolic, humoral, autocoidal, and immunological functions whose individual actions are becoming increasingly understood, but whose modes of corporate action have still hardly been studied. The lung metabolizes endogenous steroids; its endothelial cells manufacture the necessary enzyme to convert angiotensin I to angiotensin II, as well as inactivating bradykinin and other vasoactive amines. The tight epithelial junctions of the alveolar walls with their sentinel alveolar macrophages, reinforced by tissue macrophages in the same alveoli, are strategically placed to resist microbial invasion of the body through the airways.

From time to time, various perturbations disturb the normally protective cellular, autocoidal, humoral, and immune responses of the lung, particularly in association with haemorrhagic shock, severe body trauma, and septicaemia. Under such circumstances, complex and still poorly understood, cascade reactions take place which involve the activation of complement, local granulocyte aggregation, release of kinins and arachidonic acid metabolites, platelet activating factor, and many other cellular mediators including their contained combat enzymes, particularly proteases and free oxygen radicals. This inappropriate inflammatory reponse leads to massive microvascular lung injury with ensuing catastrophic proteinaceous pulmonary oedema. It is here that the main thrust of lung research is currently being applied.

Morphology

The structure of the pulmonary vasculature differs markedly from that of the systemic vessels. The difference applies throughout the system to include the large and small pulmonary arteries and veins, whose media are poorly developed compared with comparable vessels in the systemic circulation.

The lungs also possess two blood supplies, the bronchial circulation and the pulmonary circulation.

The bronchial circulation

This circulation normally contributes less than 10 per cent of the total blood flow to the lungs. Its function is largely nutritive to the walls of bronchi, larger pulmonary vessels, interstitium, and interstitial pleura. It has an important characteristic, relevant in disease. It possesses a dormant precapillary component which anastomoses with the pulmonary arterioles. This enlarges in conditions leading to cyanosis from ineffective alveolar blood–gas exchange, such as in chronic lung disease and congenital heart disease with right-to-left shunts. Under such circumstances the bronchial circulation may contribute a large fraction of the total blood flow to the alveoli, effectively becoming a reperfusion system to boost gas exchange.

There is a further beneficial effect from the increased precapillary bronchopulmonary anastomosis in localized chronic lung disease. The bronchial arterial pressure, being at systemic level and thus above pulmonary arterial pressure, tends to deflect pulmonary arterial blood flow away from the diseased areas to more normally ventilated areas, thus helping ventilation/perfusion relationships to remain as normal as possible.

The pulmonary arterial and venous systems

Compared with similar vessels in the systemic circulation, the pulmonary arteries are thin-walled with relatively wide lumina (Fig. 1). The pulmonary trunk is about half as thick as the aorta. Both it and the large pulmonary arteries exceeding 1000 μm in diameter are normally very distensible. Their media contain few smooth muscle fibres and consist mainly of elastic fibrils, collagen, and an acid mucopolysaccaride ground substance attached via a basement membrane to the intima composed of endothelial cells.

The larger muscular pulmonary arteries possess both an internal and external elastic lamina in contrast to the pulmonary veins, which only have an internal elastic lamina. Below about 100 μm the muscle fibres within the artery become discontinuous and finally disappear at the level of the pulmonary arterioles. These have a single internal elastic lamina resting upon a basement membrane applied to the intima of the vessel composed of endothelial cells. Their scanty adventitia consists of collagen interspersed with elastic fibres.

The appearance of the pulmonary venules is virtually indistinguishable from that of the arterioles. Commencing near the bronchioles, they pass into the connective tissue septa between secondary lobules to become pulmonary veins which lie separated from the bronchi. Their media consists of irregularly arranged circular and oblique smooth muscle fibres, interspersed with collagen.

The large extraparenchymal pulmonary veins which lie external to the lung in the loose areolar tissue of the mediastinum and which connect the lung to the left atrium are largely composed of collagen with some elastic fibres. In contradistinction to the large pulmonary arteries they are virtually indistensible but readily collapsible.

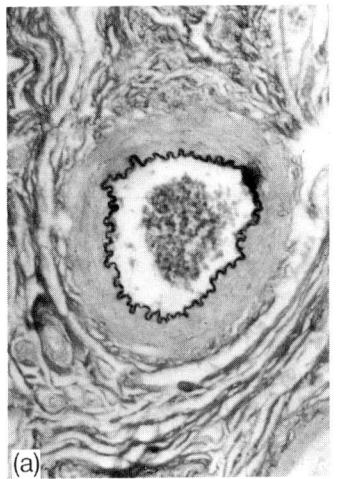 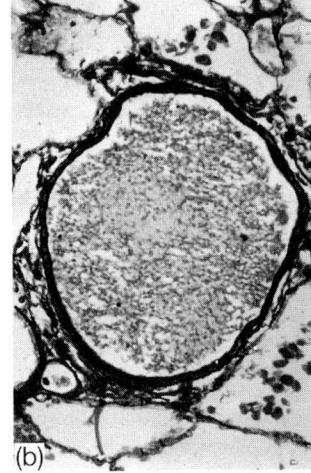

Fig. 1 Comparison of (a) a systemic (prostate) and (b) a pulmonary artery. The pulmonary artery is a thin-walled vessel with a limited capacity for vasomotion. (Photomicrograph kindly given by Professor D. Heath.)

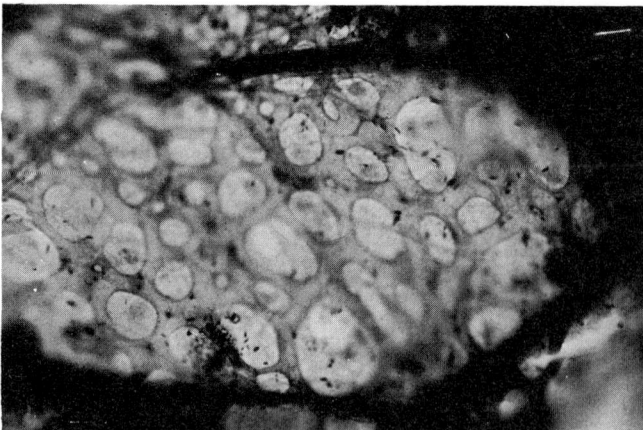

Fig. 2 Lung capillaries. The pulmonary capillaries are arranged as a meshwork around the alveoli.

The pulmonary capillaries

The human lung contains approximately 300×10^6 alveoli each surrounded by a mesh of capillaries so short that they resemble a fenestrated 'sheet' through which blood is transported as a fine film (Fig. 2). Erythrocytes need only remain within the capillaries for 0.03 s for gas exchange, so despite an estimated 70 m² area for alveolar capillary gas exchange, the lung capillary volume is as little as 150–200 ml. The capillary volume nicely accommodates the maximal stroke volume delivered to it by the right ventricle. Most of the capillary bed comprises the alveolar capillary sheet. It is therefore susceptible to alveolar gas pressure. However, some capillaries are located at the angles of the alveoli in the deformable extra-alveolar connective tissues joining contiguous alveoli. These vessels are not directly susceptible to alveolar pressure and remain patent even when alveolar gas pressure exceeds capillary hydrostatic pressure.

The tissue and fluid layers which lie between the gas-filled lumen of the alveolus and the blood-filled capillary constitute the alveolar–capillary blood–gas barrier. Since both the alveolus and the capillary are supported by connective tissue, their epithelia are separated in many places. However, in other regions the vascular endothelium and alveolar epithelium are so closely juxtaposed that the two basement membranes fuse and no connective tissue is interposed. The geometric mean thickness of the barrier is approximately 0.5 μm, which offers little resistance to gas exchange for diffusion (Fig. 3). Despite the delicacy of the lung microcirculation, electron microscopy also reveals its deeper complexity, whose components also provide the non-respiratory metabolic and protective functions briefly mentioned above.

The lung lymphatics

The lymphatic capillaries are relatively large, blindly ending vessels formed from a thin irregular endothelium with a poorly developed basement membrane. The individual cells are only weakly attached to each other by feebly developed adhesions and often adjacent cells may be separated by gaps as large as 1–10 μm.

Lymphatic vessels are not present in alveolar walls but begin at the level of the respiratory bronchioles. Thus any fluid which enters the alveolar interstitium is first contained within its collagen matrix. The matrix gel then acts as a wick connecting the alveolar interstitium to the lymphatics which then run centrally to the hila, coalescing as they do so. One group forms the right lymphatic duct. Another group unites to form the tracheobronchial duct which joins the thoracic duct just before it enters the venous system. A third group of posterior mediastinal lymphatics run through the caudal mediastinal node also to join the thoracic duct.

Drainage of fluid by the lymphatics is continuous but can be

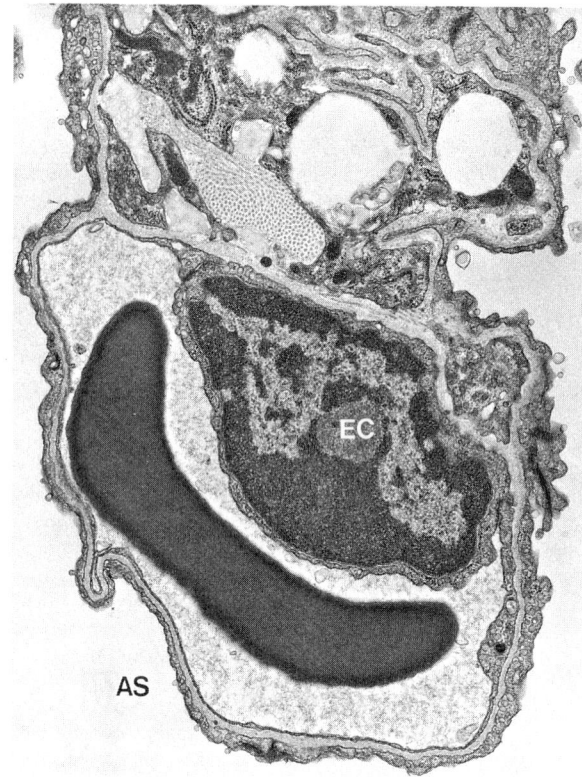

Fig. 3 The pulmonary microcirculation and blood–gas barrier. EC, endothelial cell; AS, alveolar space. (Reproduced by courtesy of Dr E. Schneeberger.)

enchanced by three factors. First, the basement membrane is attached by fibres to the surrounding connective tissues so that any tissue swelling opens and holds patent the vessels. Secondly, lymphatic vessels in the lungs, like those elsewhere, are actively pulsatile. This pulsatility, together with endolymphatic valves, forms an active pumping system. Third, lung movements, working in conjunction with the endolymphatic valves, form a second pumping system analogous to the muscle pump in the systemic lymphatic system. Normally total lung lymph flow is less than 10 ml/hour, but in diseases leading to increased transcapillary water filtration lymph flow may increase several fold, as in chronic venous pulmonary hypertension of mitral stenosis.

Nerve supply of the pulmonary blood vessels

The pulmonary arterial and venous systems of the lung are liberally supplied by both the sympathetic and parasympathetic nervous systems. Afferent and efferent fibres are present in both systems. In spite of this, the normal lung circulation has low inherent reflex vasomotor activity. Even in diseases leading to pulmonary hypertension associated with medial hypertrophy of the muscular pulmonary vessels, therapeutic attempts to reduce pulmonary vascular resistance using pharmaceuticals to block reflex vasomotor activity are very disappointing.

Pressures, volumes, and resistance in the pulmonary circulation

The pulmonary circulation receives the entire output from the right ventricle. In the adult this ranges from 5 to 8 l/min at rest up to 25–30 l/min during exercise. Despite the large blood flow, the system operates at a low pressure of approximately one-fifth that of the systemic pressure because the pulmonary vascular resistance is itself low (Table 1).

Table 1 The pulmonary circulation: representative normal adult values

Intrapulmonary blood volume	900 ml
Pulmonary capillary blood volume	100–200 ml
Pulmonary artery pressure	25/15 mmHg
Pulmonary capillary pressure*	7 mmHg
Pulmonary vascular resistance	20–120 dyne s cm^{-5}
Pulmonary venous pressure	5 mmHg

* Calculated value for the mid-point of the upright lung.

The longitudinal distribution of pressure within the pulmonary circulation differs considerably from that of the systemic bed, where the arterioles are the major resistance vessels. No such situation exists in the lungs where resistance is fairly evenly distributed. Probably about 40–50 per cent of total resistance lies in the arteries and arterioles, with further 30 and 20 per cent contributions from capillaries and veins, respectively. This distribution of resistance suggests a fairly even pressure drop throughout the system. Calculations give a mean capillary pressure of about 7 mmHg at the mid-point of the upright lung.

The amount of blood in the pulmonary circulation is important because variations in its volume may influence venous return to the left heart, efficiency of gas exchange, and the mechanical behaviour of the lungs. Furthermore, the vertical distribution of the volume of blood in the upright lung is responsible for characteristic radiological appearances in health and disease. The normal pulmonary blood volume between the pulmonary valve and left atrium is approximately 900 ml, of which only 150–200 ml are in the gas-exchanging lung capillaries. However, the distensibility of the pulmonary circulation and its reserve unperfused capacity in the upright position is such that the central blood volume may increase by as much as 500 ml when changing from the upright to the lying position. This may be of little consequence in health, but when the pulmonary vascular pressures become elevated by subclinical or overt heart failure, the shift may cause further pressure rise and precipitate pulmonary oedema.

When upright, the distribution of blood volume in the lung increases vertically from apex to base. This parallels the regional distribution of blood flow, which shows an eight-fold increase from top to bottom of the lungs (see below). Ventilation is also heterogeneous, increasing from top to bottom of the lungs, but less steeply than does blood flow. Both the distribution of ventilation and of blood flow are partly determined by the anchorage of the blood vessels at the hilum as well as gravitational effects. Because of gravity, lower regions are relatively compressed by the weight of lung above them. In the upright position, vessel diameters increase from the top to the bottom of the lung as a result of gravitional increase in hydrostatic pressure unopposed by any baroregulatory mechanism.

The obstacle to blood flow presented by the pulmonary circulation is usually quantified as the pulmonary vascular resistance. Resistance is a concept derived from the rheology of laminar, non-pulsatile fluid flow in tubes of invariant dimension. Use of this term in the pulmonary circulation is a gross simplification, but useful practically. The calculation of vascular impedance is a more correct theoretical approach, but its greater complexity limits its usefulness.

Pulmonary vascular resistance is calculated as the pressure drop between the pulmonary artery and left atrium, divided by the blood flow.

$$R = (Ppa–Pla) / \dot{Q}$$

where Ppa is the mean pulmonary artery pressure, Pla is the mean left atrial pressure, $\dot{Q}$ is pulmonary blood flow and R is the pulmonary vascular resistance. Normal values for pulmonary resistance in humans at rest are 0.1–0.15 torr/ml/s. When expressed in cgs units, these results should be multiplied by 1328, giving values of 130–200 dyne s cm^{-5}.

Regulation of the pulmonary circulation

Because the lung blood vessels are so frugally supplied with smooth muscle in their walls, pulmonary arterial resistance to blood flow is low and vasomotor reflex vasomotion is capable of playing only a subsidiary role in the regulation of blood pressure and flow into and out of the lung capillary bed for gas exchange. Variations in blood flow to the lung capillaries are thus largely dominated by *passive* responses consequent upon changes in lung morphology due to respiration; by changes imposed by haemodynamic events taking place in the left atrium; by changes in the systemic circulation occurring either because of systemic baroreceptor or humoral activity there; or due to the effects of variations in venous return to the heart during respiration, exercise or as a result of changes in posture. Figure 4 lists these interrelationships in diagrammatic form. It also indicates the *active* vasomotor responses which take place. An excellent review of these has been written by Barer (1980).

Virtually all vasomotor activity, other than the weak reflex activity mentioned, is chemically mediated. This includes vasoconstriction from hypoxia and hypercapnia as well as from local humoral effects of catecholamines, serotonin, other kinins, histamine, cyclo-oxygenase products of arachidonic acid metabolism etc. Although the effects of these humoral mediators have been demonstrated experimentally, they are not shown in Fig. 4 because the homeostatic roles of most of them are still unclear.

Much the most important factor producing local peripheral arterial vasoconstriction in the environs of the lung capillaries is a combination of hypoxia and hypercapnia. This has obvious teleological importance; for example, the redistribution of blood flow away from locally diseased areas of the lung to more normal areas for gas exchange as in centrilobular emphysema or lobar pneumonia. The peripheral pulmonary arteries and venules appear more sensitive to chemically induced vasomotion than to reflex effects, while the larger conducting radicals of the pulmonary arterial system appear to respond more to reflex stimulation than to hypoxia or catecholamines. This has relevance in the selection of agents to reduce pulmonary resistance in the relief of pulmonary hypertension.

There is growing evidence to suggest that hypoxia and release of vasoactive amines exert their effects not only upon the myofibrils of the arterioles and venules but also on actin and myosin components of the myofibroblasts present in the alveolar interstitium at the corners of alveoli. Active motility of this kind could provide a local autoregulatory mechanism for adjusting ventilation/perfusion ratios at alveolar level.

Hypoxic vasoconstriction is thought to be caused in three ways: first by direct excitatory action through depression of mitochondrial phosphorylation leading to shifts in cytosolic metabolite concentrations, membrane depolarization, calcium influx, and contraction; second, by chemical mediators released by hypoxia from extravascular lung tissue, e.g. mast cells, neuroepithelial bodies or autonomic nerve endings; finally, hypoxia may reduce the endothelial content of endothelium derived relaxant factor (EDRF) leading to reduction in small vessel calibre. These concepts have obvious implications for possible future pharmacological management of cor pulmonale.

Regional pressure–flow relationships in the pulmonary circulation

The behaviour of the pulmonary arterial and alveolar–capillary systems

Because the normal pulmonary arterial system offers such low resistance to blood flow and has so little reflex vasoregulatory

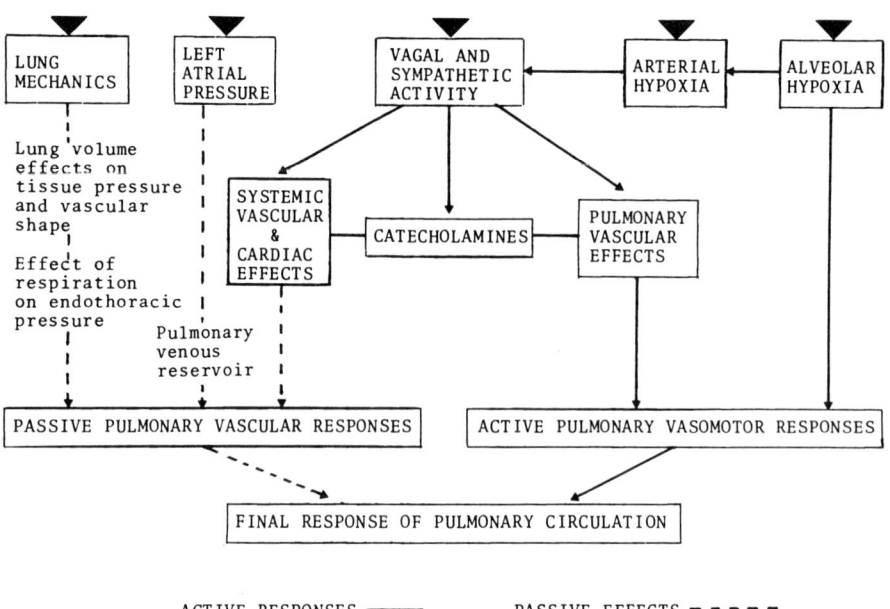

ACTIVE RESPONSES ———   PASSIVE EFFECTS – – – – –

Fig. 4 The regulation of the pulmonary circulation.

capability, it would not be surprising if pressure–flow relationships within the pulmonary circulation were regulated largely by physical means and that the pulsatile ejection of blood by the right ventricle generated pulsatile blood flow throughout the system.

Three interdependent physiological features of the pulmonary circulation were discovered in the late 1950s and early 1960s which support this. First, Cournand and colleagues found that the rise in pulmonary blood flow with exercise was not accompanied by a similar rise in mean pulmonary artery pressure because the pulmonary vascular resistance fell as cardiac output increased. Second, Bannister and Torrance, using the isolated perfused lung, and West and Dollery, using radioactive gases in human studies, demonstrated that there was a marked gradient of perfusion from top to bottom of the resting upright lung. Flow per unit volume of lung was eight times greater at the base of the lung than at the extreme apex, which was barely perfused at all. Third, Lee and Du Bois discovered that blood flow through the lung capillaries remained pulsatile throughout the cardiac cycle. Not only is capillary blood flow pulsatile but so also is the exchange of the respiratory gases, although in the case of carbon dioxide release the pulsatility is less marked because of its high tissue solubility (Fig. 5).

The three phenomena have a common mechanism which depends upon the pulmonary microvessels behaving as a vertical stack of 'Starling resistors' within the lung (Fig. 6). A Starling resistor is a thin-walled collapsible tube through which fluid flows and which is surrounded by a pressure reservoir. In the lung, the pressure reservoir equates with the alveoli. The collapsible tubes are the capillaries whose arteriolar inflow and venular outflow pressures will be the products of the pulmonary artery and left atrial hydrostatic pressures combined with the gravitational pressures within them occasioned by the height of each capillary system above or below the cardiac origin of the pulmonary artery and left atrium, respectively.

The vertical height of the human lung is approximately 30 cm. Normally pressure rises to approximately 30 cmH$_2$O only during the peak of systole. Thus, at the very top of the lung in normal erect humans (West: zone 1) the reservoir pressure (alveolar pressure) will be atmospheric but its vascular inflow pressure will only approach that level for a brief period during systole. Venular outflow pressure in zone 1 will be subatmospheric throughout the cardiac cycle because the normal left atrial pressure rarely exceeds

12–15 cmH$_2$O. Thus, under resting conditions in zone 1, there is little or no blood flow through the lung capillaries except during part of systole.

Further down the lung (West: zone 2) arterial pressure will be greater than alveolar pressure (which is again atmospheric), but alveolar pressure will still be greater than venous pressure. Under these conditions flow is determined by the difference between alveolar and arterial pressure and not by the arterial to venous pressure difference. Since the mean vascular pressures increase progressively down the zone while the alveolar pressure remains constant, there is a steady increase in perfused capillary volume as well as total blood flow down zone 2.

In zone 3, both the arterial and the venous pressures are greater than alveolar pressure and each is augmented by the same gravitational amount as the zone is descended. In zone 3 all capillary

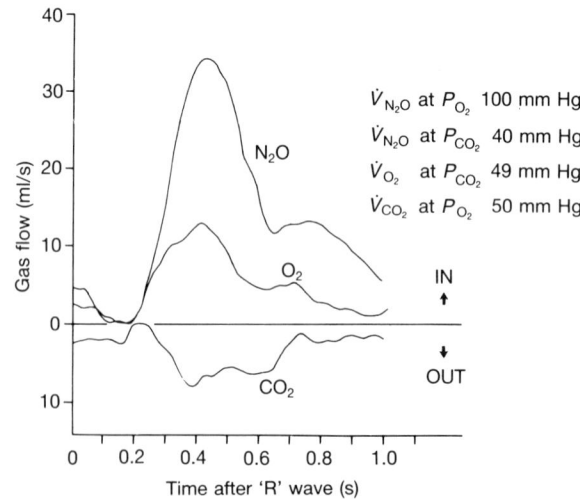

Fig. 5 The effect of pulsatile lung capillary blood flow upon oxygen and carbon dioxide exchange. Pulmonary capillary blood flow, estimated from the rate of N$_2$O uptake, is compared with the rate of flow of O$_2$ into and CO$_2$ out of the lungs, measured by the body plethysmograph method. (Reproduced from Bosman *et al.*, 1965, *Clin. Sci.* **28**, 295, with permission.)

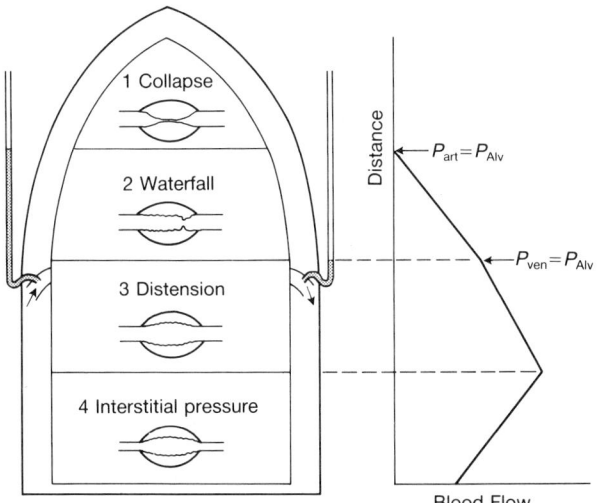

Fig. 6 The upright human lung as a vertically stacked pile of 'Starling resistors'. In zone 1 there is no blood flow (except through 'angular' vessels, see text) because alveolar pressure is greater than both arterial and venous pressure. In zone 2 arterial pressure is greater than alveolar pressure which in turn exceeds venous pressure. Here flow is determined by the arterial–alveolar pressure difference and increases progressively as the lung is descended. In zone 3 both arterial and venous pressures are greater than alveolar pressure so flow is determined by arterial–venous pressure difference. This is constant and independent of height, so it cannot account for the increasing flow observed which may be due to increasing calibre of the vessels as pressure within them increases. There is some doubt about the existence of zone 4 in normal individuals. In this zone, it is postulated that flow may be restricted by perivascular cuffing.

systems are recruited for perfusion because their intracapillary hydrostatic pressure exceeds alveolar pressure. The rate of blood flow through the region depends on the mean arteriovenous pressure difference, modulated in a pulsatile fashion throughout the cardiac cycle as a result of the pressure events taking place simultaneously in the right ventricle and left atrium, respectively. A small increase both in regional perfusion volume and flow occurs with descent through the zone, probably because of a gravitational increase in overall hydrostatic pressure in vessels below the heart which in turn causes their distension, thereby lowering resistance to flow.

There is probably a fourth zone (zone 4) at the extreme base of the lungs where regional blood flow may diminish despite the continued rise in intravascular pressure. There has been controversy about this, but the implication is that the alveolar interstitium in the lowermost areas is subject to greater hydrostatic transcapillary fluid transfer than elsewhere. The resulting reduction in interstitial distensibility could increase capillary resistance in the region. In diseases leading to pulmonary venous hypertension, for example, mitral stenosis, this could have some homeostatic benefit for gas exchange, for the further rise in pulmonary venous pressure will also increase interstitial fluid content at the lung bases. This will occur before overt pulmonary oedema is recognized clinically. The consequent increase in local vascular resistance will further impair blood flow to the bases, leading to its redistribution to the upper zones of the lung.

The gravitational relationships between regional intracapillary and alveolar gas pressure described above have two important homeostatic effects when blood flow increases during exercise. They help both to regulate pulmonary vascular pressure and maintain optimal blood gas exchange. The pulmonary artery pressure will tend to rise as blood flow increases with exercise. This will lead progressively to more and more vertical recruitment of the pulmonary capillary bed from base to apex, accompanied by increasing evenness of blood flow distribution throughout the

lung. With sufficient increase in blood flow, all alveolar–capillary units will be recruited. Alveolar–capillary recruitment thus allows a progressive reduction in pulmonary vascular resistance to take place as blood flow increases. As a result, both the pulmonary arterial and microvascular pressures rise much less than would have been the case if the system had maintained a fixed volume. However, once all alveolar–capillary systems have been recruited, further increase in pulmonary blood flow will be accompanied by a linearly related rise in pulmonary arterial pressure.

Alveolar–capillary recruitment also increases the capillary surface area, so diffusing capacity increases. Moreover, optimal kinetics for gas exchange are preserved for, despite the overall increase in blood flow through the capillary bed as a whole, the recruitment of successive alveolar–capillary units ensures that red cell velocity through individual units remains remarkably constant.

Pulmonary capillary blood flow, the nature of its pulsatility

The physical behaviour of the pulmonary arterial and alveolar–capillary systems together determine the pulsatile nature of lung capillary blood flow. During peak ejection by the right ventricle, the systolic input pressure from the pulmonary artery to the capillaries will temporarily exceed the alveolar gas pressure in all lung zones. As a result, capillaries from the bottom to the top of the lungs will accommodate flowing blood. When diastole ensues, the pulmonary arterial pressure and blood flow velocity both begin to fall, so blood flow will first cease in the uppermost alveolar capillary systems as the input pressure from the pulmonary artery to the capillaries drops below alveolar gas pressure in that zone. Only in the more dependent parts of the lung where both pulmonary arterial and venous pressures exceed alveolar gas pressure will the capillaries continue to conduct at a rate determined by the arteriovenous pressure difference between them. Thus, during each cardiac cycle, a tidal rise and fall of distributed blood flow takes place up and down the lungs during systole and diastole, respectively.

Pulsatile capillary blood flow is jealously preserved even in diseases leading to pulmonary arterial hypertension of whatever cause. This is surprising, for a rise in pulmonary arteriolar resistance from the peripheral vascular changes taking place in these diseases might have been expected to damp out such pulsation. However, it has been shown that when the pulmonary arterial resistance (R) rises, there is a reciprocal fall in compliance (C) proximal to the site of increased resistance. As a result, the time constant of the arterial system as a whole remains constant ($R \times C = kt$) so that lung capillary flow pulsatility is largely unaffected.

The role of the pulmonary veins

The pulmonary venous system is also designed to protect the autonomy of lung capillary blood flow free from pressure perturbations from the left atrium, despite the absence of valves in the pulmonary veins. Lung capillary blood flow remains normally pulsatile even when large pressure transients are generated in the left atrium, for example, from cannon waves in complete heart block.

When blood flow is measured in the large pulmonary veins outside the lungs near the left atrium it is found to be pulsatile, but its pattern is different from that in the capillaries. Its wave form is virtually a mirror image of left atrial pressure events. But, under experimental conditions when pulmonary vein flow is isolated from the left atrium, its wave form still resembles the capillary flow pulse. These observations might suggest that some component of the pulmonary venous system is highly compliant so it absorbs left atrial pressure waves and prevents them from reaching the lung capillaries. However, human post-mortem studies reveal that the pulmonary veins are largely indistensible and therefore non-compliant. Instead, it has been found that the large extraparenchymal pulmonary veins, lying in the loose areolar tissue of the mediastinum before their entry into the left atrium, are highly collapsible structures whose cross-sectional dimensions are

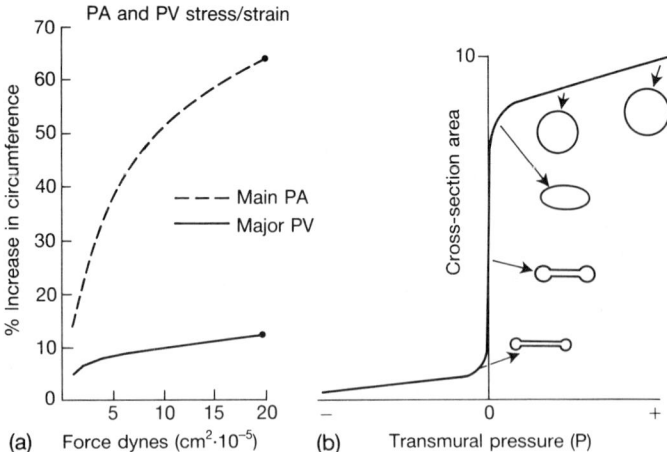

Fig. 7 (a) Stress–strain relationships obtained from circumferential strips of human pulmonary artery and pulmonary vein, post-mortem. The pulmonary artery is highly distensible. The pulmonary vein is virtually inelastic. (Reproduced from Banks *et al.*, 1974, *Thorax*, with permission.) (b) Schematic diagram showing how the extraparenchymal pulmonary veins behave as collapsible tubes whose cross-sectional dimensions change over a narrow range of transmural pressure.

capable of changing from a cylindrical, fully filled state to one of complete collapse and emptiness over a narrow transmural pressure range (Fig. 7). Their combined volume, when full, is about the same as one stroke volume of the heart.

The extraparenchymal pulmonary veins thus provide a variable volume reservoir which decouples venous outflow from the lungs from left atrial events. At normal left atrial pressures, during ventricular systole, the veins collapse as they empty into the left atrium. As left atrial pressure rises, particularly during the 'a' and 'v' waves, the veins refill and their cross-sectional dimensions become circular once more (Fig. 8). These events take place from 0 to 16 mmHg transmural pressure. Thereafter the veins are capable of distending slightly.

Thus, the extraparenchymal pulmonary veins of the lungs, though indistensible, alter their shape and volume cyclically during each heart beat with very little change in their transmural pressure. This effectively prevents pressure pulsations from the left atrium from reaching the lung capillaries so that lung capillary outflow remains largely independent of downstream pressure, even with moderate elevation in mean left atrial pressure from left-sided heart disease. Moreover, since the aggregate volume of the large pulmonary veins is similar to the stroke volume of the heart, they also act as a reservoir which supplies a relatively constant inflow to the left atrium, despite beat-to-beat changes in right ventricular stroke output.

Within the lungs themselves, the behaviour of the veins connecting the capillary bed to the large extraparenchymal pulmonary veins remains obscure. However, their histology suggests that they have relatively little distensibility so they probably add little further protection to capillary outflow.

Transvascular fluid dynamics

The homeostatic role of pulsatile blood flow in the capillaries

The preceding sections have outlined how the pulmonary arterial, capillary, and venous systems together normally regulate lung capillary blood flow for optimal gas exchange with minimal fluid transudation.

In general, these same mechanisms also operate in diseases known to be associated with most forms of pulmonary vascular hypertension. They have been listed in Table 2. Both the arterial and venous systems appear to impart a largely autonomous fluid

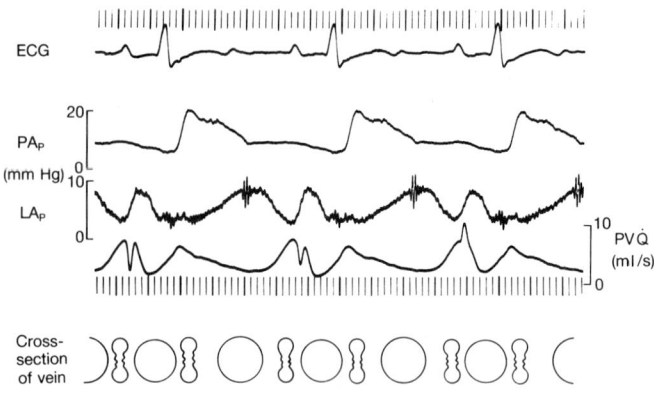

Fig. 8 The pulmonary veins. The relationship between pulmonary artery pressure (PA_p), left atrial pressure (LA_p), pulmonary venous flow ($PV\dot{Q}$) and pulmonary venous distension in the dog. Note that left atrial pressure events dominate $PV\dot{Q}$: when LA_p is high $PV\dot{Q}$ is low and when LA_p is high $PV\dot{Q}$ is low. The pulmonary veins are distended at high LA_p and collapsed at low LA_p. (Reproduced from Rajagopalan *et al.*, 1979, *Cardiovasc. Res.* **13**, 684, with permission.)

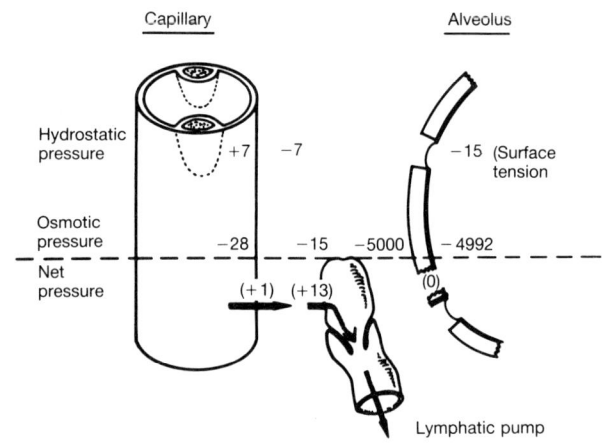

Fig. 9 Pressures causing fluid movement between lung water compartments. Pressures are expressed as mmHg. (Reproduced from Prichard, 1982, *Edema of the lung*. Charles C. Thomas, Springfield, Illinois, with permission.)

dynamic status upon the capillary gas exchange units of the lung which, together, form a gravity dependent, variable volume vascular bed designed to be largely independent of active vasomotor control.

Fluid exchange between the intravascular and interstitial compartments is determined by the balance of forces first described by Starling in 1896. The pressure for outward water filtration from the capillary results from the sum of its own hydrostatic pressure and the subatmospheric interstitial tissue pressure. This is almost, but not quite, balanced by the reabsorption pressure caused by the gradient of colloid osmotic pressure between interstitial fluid and plasma. The small net excess results in a flux from capillary to interstitium, which is removed as lymph by the lymphatics, pumping against an interstitial pressure which is normally subatmospheric and estimated to be in the order of −7 mm Hg (Fig. 9).

To operate the system, the capillaries must be freely permeable to water and small ions but must present a significant barrier to plasma proteins, which generate oncotic pressure. Physiological studies show that this is so, and electron microscopy demonstrates that the capillary endothelial cells are joined by discontinuous adhesions giving small aqueous pathways of macromolecular dimension, joining intravascular and interstitial spaces.

Table 2 Factors affecting lung capillary blood flow

Physical factors		
Pulmonary arteries	Compliance × resistance = $K(t)$	Stabilize capillary inflow conditions over wide pulmonary arterial pressure range
Alveolar–capillary relationships Steady flow ⎫ conditions Pulsatile flow ⎭	'Waterfall effect' Gravity-dependent zones with added 'tidal' effects	Hydrostatic capillary recruitment which regulates pulmonary arterial pressure and allows optimal capillary gas exchange
Pulmonary veins Intraparenchymal veins Large extraparenchymal veins	Behaviour still obscure Indistensible but collapsible Combined capacity equivalent to right ventricular stroke volume	Lung capillaries 'decoupled' from left atrium Pulsatile capillary flow preserved 'Venous reservoir' provided for left heart
Chemical and reflex responses		
Hypoxia Hypercapnia	Local action	Powerful peripheral pulmonary arterial vasoconstriction Less active on large pulmonary arteries Vein behaviour not fully elucidated
pH	Reflex action	Weak peripheral pulmonary arterial constriction More powerful constriction of larger pulmonary arteries Vein behaviour still obscure
Vasoactive amines		
Hydrostatic, oncotic and autocoidal factors	Alterations in capillary permeability	Mechanisms not yet elucidated

The negative interstitial hydrostatic pressure results from the chemical nature of the glycoproteins which make up most of the interstitial space. These giant molecules, more than 10^6 dalton in weight, contain large numbers of mucopolysaccharide chains, each of about 50 000 dalton, bound to a central core of protein and hyaluronic acid. The side-chains are all strongly anionic and mutually repulsive. This mutual repulsion is translated into a hydraulic force by chemical interaction between water and the macromolecular side-chains so that the whole of the interstitial space may be likened to a sponge avid to imbibe water under conditions of deranged fluid balance.

The colloid osmotic pressure (oncotic pressure) of the interstitial fluid is high partly due to the transcapillary leak of plasma proteins and partly due to the influence of what has been termed the interstitial 'exclusion volume' for water. Analysis of interstitial fluid shows that its protein concentration is only about half what should be expected from oncotic pressure estimations. This discrepancy can be explained if 50 per cent of the interstitial water has had protein 'excluded' from it because that water is entrapped within the confines of the mucopolysaccharide gel, whose interstices are too small to allow macromolecules, such as albumin, to enter.

Efficient gas exchange depends upon the alveolar–capillary interstitium being capable of disposing of water without widening the blood–gas barrier through interstitial swelling should capillary pressure rise. Five mechanisms enable this:

1. Macromolecular sieving. Increasing transcapillary hydrostatic pressure increases water flux but not protein permeability. Consequently, the ratio of water to protein flux increases and the interstitial fluid oncotic pressure falls.

2. Increased water entry into the interstitium produces a *relative* diminution of the 'excluded' volume. So a larger proportion of the interstitial water will be available to macromolecules, which will further reduce the interstitial oncotic pressure.

3. The increased interstitial water content raises the interstitial hydrostatic pressure, which therefore becomes less negative.

4. Lymph flow increases in response to the increase in transcapillary water flux.

5. Pulsatile capillary blood flow probably has a vital role in reducing transcapillary water flux during normal exercise as well as in disease.

Why is it that the lungs so jealously guard capillary blood flow pulsatility even in disease? Figure 10 shows that only in systole does

the capillary hydrostatic pressure temporarily exceed the hydrostatic–osmotic equilibrium between capillary lumen and the alveolar interstitium. So, in systole, the net balance of forces temporarily facilitates fluid flux outwards from capillary lumen to interstitium. However, during diastole the intracapillary hydrostatic pressure will fall below the plasma osmotic pressure so the net flux of water will be reversed towards the capillary lumen again.

At rest, the diastolic period of each cardiac cycle is longer than its systolic period so the tendency will be to maintain the alveolar–capillary interstitium in a dry state. With exercise, capillary recruitment has some limiting effect upon the rise in pulmonary capillary pressure, but heart rate also increases and so the diastolic period of the cardiac cycle becomes shorter and shorter. This results in the development of a net outward flux of water from capillary to interstitium. Though small in total volume, the alveolar interstitial gel is avid for water as already explained. As the

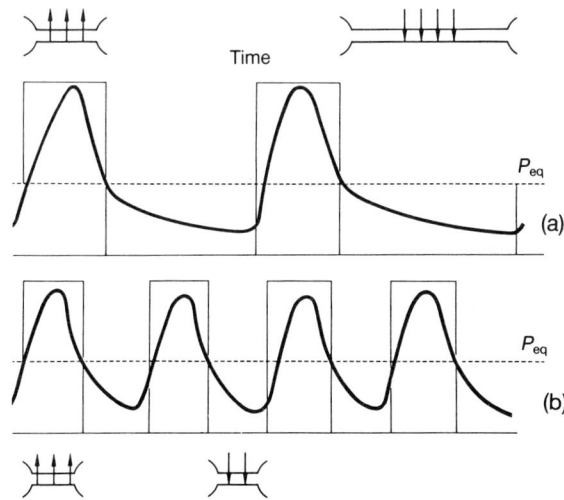

Fig. 10 Schematic diagram to show the movement of fluid in relation to capillary hydrostatic pressure. Only during systole does transcapillary hydrostatic pressure exceed the transcapillary hydrostatic–osmotic equilibrium (P_{eq}) and net flux is from capillary lumen to the interstitium. In diastole, the net forces are towards the lumen. At rest (a), when diastole is longer than systole, the interstitium tends to be 'dry' but during exercise (b), when diastole is short, the interstitium becomes charged with fluid.

interstitium becomes charged with water the alveolar walls become turgid and less compliant. Strategically located within the interstitium at the corners of the alveoli are afferent vagal nerve endings, termed J receptors. These respond maximally when lung interstitial compliance is reduced. They excite breathlessness.

As a result of the breathlessness, the individual stops exercising, the heart rate returns to normal, the duration of the diastolic period of the cardiac cycle once more exceeds that of the systolic period, fluid present in the alveolar interstitium returns to the capillaries, interstitium compliance returns to its resting state, and the sensation of breathlessness disappears. Normally the breathlessness of exercise occurs long before alveolar flooding takes place, though extreme exercise beyond the point of endurance can lead to acute pulmonary oedema, particularly at altitude.

The preservation of capillary pulsatility in diseases leading to pulmonary venous hypertension, such as mitral stenosis or left ventricular dysfunction, imparts protection over and above that possible if steady flow conditions existed. For example, with mean pulmonary venous pressure elevated to a level approaching plasma osmotic pressure (approximately 30 mm Hg), *provided* the heart rate is within normal limits, there will still be a considerable period during diastole when the pulmonary venous and capillary hydrostatic pressures fall below the osmotic equilibrium level. Consequently, good therapeutic control of heart rate is an important requirement when managing patients liable to hydrostatic pulmonary oedema.

Diseases leading to pulmonary arterial hypertension do so as a result of medial hypertrophy in the peripheral arteries and arterioles leading to increased peripheral arterial resistance to blood flow into the capillaries. This effectively down-regulates their mean hydrostatic pressure towards osmotic pressure level, or even lower. Details of these diseases will be found in subsequent chapters. However, as already explained, the concomitant reduction in pulmonary arterial compliance which accompanies the increased peripheral arterial resistance in such circumstances, effectively preserves pressure and flow pulsatility into the capillaries even at mean pulmonary artery pressure levels as high as 70 mmHg, with the protective advantages regarding fluid homeostasis already described in the case of pulmonary venous hypertension.

Finally, the major site of fluid input to the lung interstitial space, the pulmonary capillary bed, is some distance from the terminal lymphatics in the peribronchial connective tissue. Water passage from the alveolar interstitium to the origins of the lymphatics is accomplished by a gradient of tissue pressure which results from differing properties of the connective tissues. In the alveolar septa the tissue is 'tight' so that pressure rises rapidly with increasing hydration. In the peribronchial regions the tissue is 'loose' and is able to swell with little increase in tissue pressure. This functional differentiation between the perialveolar and peribronchial connective tissue is a further provision defending the integrity of the alveolar–capillary apparatus for gas exchange, for when lung oedema first begins to develop it does so preferentially in the loose connective tissue surrounding the bronchi remote from the gas exchanging areas.

References

Barer, G. W. (1980). Active control of the pulmonary circulation. In *Pulmonary circulation in health and disease* (eds G. Cumming and G. Bonsignore), p. 81. Plenum Press, New York.
Cudkowicz, L. (1968). *The human bronchial circulation in health and disease*. Williams and Wilkins, Baltimore.
Harris, P. and Heath, D. (1977). *The human pulmonary circulation*. Churchill Livingstone, Edinburgh.
Hughes, J. B., Glazier, J. B., Maloney, J. E. and West, J. B. (1968). Effect of lung volume on the distribution of pulmonary blood flow in man. *Resp. Physiol.* **4**, 58.
Jacobs, E. R. (1983). Mediators of septic lung injury. *Med. Clin. N. Am.* **67**, 701.
Lee, G. de J. (1983). The pulmonary circulation in health and disease. In *Scientific foundations of cardiology* (eds P. Sleight and J. V. Jones). Heinemann, London.
McMurty, I. F., Stanbrook, H. G. and Rounds, S. (1982). The mechanism of hypoxic vasoconstriction: a working hypothesis. In *Oxygen transport to human tissues* (eds J. A. Loeppky and M. L. Riedesel), p. 79. Elsevier North Holland, Amsterdam.
Paintal, A. S. (1977). The nature and effect of sensory inputs into the respiratory centres. *Fed. Proc.* **36**, 2428.
Prichard, J. S. (1982). *Edema of the lung*. Charles C. Thomas, Springfield, Illinois.
Rajagopalan, B., Bertram, C. D., Stallard, T. and Lee, G. de J. (1979). Blood flow in pulmonary veins III: simultaneous measurements of their dimensions, intravascular pressure and flow. *Cardiovasc. Res.* **13**, 684.
Reuben, S. R. (1971). Compliance of the human pulmonary arterial system in disease. *Circ. Res.* **29**, 40.
Riley, R. L., Himmelstein, A., Motley, J. L., Weiner, H. M. and Cournand, A. (1948). Studies of pulmonary circulation at rest and during exercise in normal individuals and in patients with chronic pulmonary disease. *Am. J. Physiol.* **152**, 372.
Ryan, J. W. and Ryan, U.S. (1977). Pulmonary endothelial cells. *Fed. Proc.* **36**, 2683.
Said, S. I. (1973). The lung in relation to vasoactive hormones. *Fed. Proc.* **32**, 1972.
Said, S. I. (1974). Endocrine role of the lung in disease. *Am. J. Med.* **57**, 453.
Vane, J. R. (1969). The release and fate of vasoactive hormones in the circulation. *Br. J. Pharmacol.* **35**, 209.

Pulmonary oedema

J. S. PRICHARD AND G. de J. LEE

Acute fulminant pulmonary oedema is a terrifying but fortunately uncommon event when the patient literally suffocates in his own body fluids. Much more commonly, the clinician is called to treat pulmonary oedema in its less acute form, as breathlessness disturbs the patient long before serious alveolar flooding has begun.

Because pulmonary oedema is so common a manifestation of left-sided heart disease and since its relief by diuretics is so effective, there is a temptation to forget other causes. It is therefore prudent to make the diagnosis of hydrostatic pulmonary oedema of cardiac origin only when other manifestations of heart disease are also present and to consider wider causal possibilities in all other circumstances despite apparent relief from diuretics.

Pulmonary oedema has many possible causes and these frequently occur in combination. Only by careful analysis of the pathophysiological data, inferred first from meticulous clinical assessment, will the contributing factors be identified.

Before proceeding with this chapter, the reader is encouraged to read the chapter on pulmonary circulation in health and disease (page 13.326) where many of the homeostatic mechanisms which protect the lung from oedema are described.

The nature and origin of pulmonary oedema

The continuous movement of water and solute from the lung capillaries into the interstitium is regulated by the differential permeability of its endothelium to water, small ions and protein as well as by changes in the balance between the hydrostatic and osmotic forces across its membrane (Fig. 1a, b). The relationship is that of the Starling hypothesis and this suggests that perturbation of any of four factors, alone or in combination, could lead to oedema (Fig. 2). These are hydrostatic pressure, colloid osmotic (oncotic) pressure, endothelial permeability, and lymphatic drainage. Abnormalities in the first three will cause oedema by increased water filtration into the interstitial space, while the last will diminish drainage.

Experimentally, the development of pulmonary oedema may be characterized by the relationship between tissue water and micro-

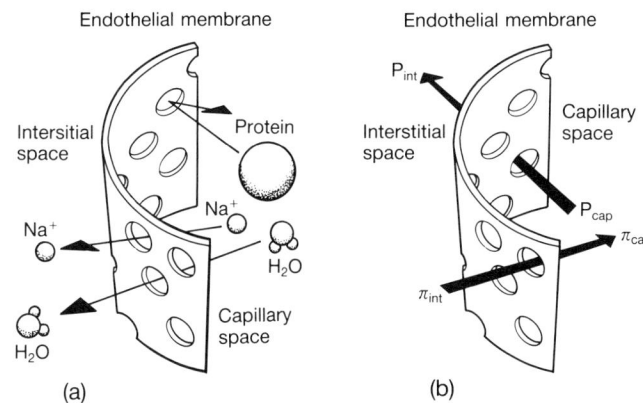

Fig. 1 (a) The lung endothelial membrane is permeable to water and electrolytes, but less permeable to macromolecules. (b) The Starling equation: $\bar{Q}_f = K\,(P_{cap} - P_{int}) - K\sigma\,(\pi_{cap} - \pi_{int})$ where $\bar{Q}_f$ is the net fluid filtration rate, K is the filtration coefficient, σ is the reflection coefficient, $(P_{cap} - P_{int})$ is the hydrostatic pressure gradient from the capillary lumen to interstitial space, and $(\pi_{cap} - \pi_{int})$ is the oncotic pressure difference across the capillary membrane.

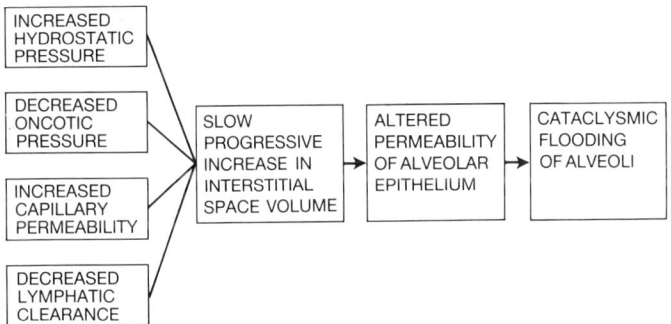

Fig. 2 The initiation of pulmonary oedema and the sequence of development.

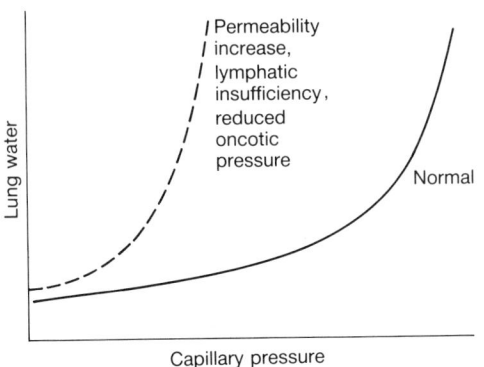

Fig. 3 Lung water content and capillary pressure. In the normal lung tissue, the water content does not begin to increase until capillary pressure is approximately 30 mmHg. Where colloid osmotic pressure (e.g. plasma protein concentration) is reduced, endothelial permeability is increased or the lymphatic pump is impaired, the whole curve is shifted to the left. (Reproduced from Prichard, 1982, *Edema of the lung.* Charles C. Thomas, Springfield, Illinois, with permission.)

vascular hydrostatic pressure (Fig. 3). The water content of the normal lung rises very little until transcapillary hydrostatic pressure exceeds 25–30 mmHg. Thereafter, the rise is rapid. The pressure–volume curve is shifted leftwards if the plasma oncotic

pressure is reduced, if endothelial permeability increases or if lymphatic drainage is impaired. Figure 3 illustrates the interactions between these factors as, at low and normal capillary pressures, reduction in either oncotic pressure or lymphatic clearance do not cause oedema readily, but at higher hydrostatic pressures their adverse effects are much more dramatic.

A striking feature of normal lung is that the pulmonary capillary pressure can rise as high as 30 mmHg before any significant accumulation of water takes place. This is due to a 'safety factor' which is multifactorial (see page 13.129). Its most important components are the preservation of pulsatile capillary blood flow and the drainage potential of the lymphatic system. In response to faster transcapillary water flux, the lymphatics can increase their flow some ten times above normal before becoming overwhelmed. The situation in which transcapillary and lymph fluxes can increase with relatively little change in tissue water content emphasizes that pulmonary oedema is a dynamic phenomenon. Tissue and alveolar flooding represent the end stage, reached when lymphatic drainage capacity is exceeded. Only then does fluid accumulation begin, at first slowly in the interstitial space, then rapidly when alveolar flooding begins.

The sequence of oedema accumulation

At functional residual capacity the total lung volume is approximately 3.5 litres, about 75 per cent of which is gas filled. The remainder consists of water and solids, of which about half is blood. The circulating blood volume is between 750 and 900 ml. The interstitial tissues contain about 250 ml of water, with a similar amount in the cells.

When fluid first starts to accumulate in the interstitial tissues, it does so around the blood vessels and airways because the peribronchial connective tissue is loosely structured and swells easily without any great change in tissue pressure initially. When this perivascular 'sump' has filled and become turgid, interstitial swelling will spread to the alveolar walls, impairing gas diffusion. Finally, after a phase of progressive alveolar wall thickening, fluid begins to accumulate in the alveoli themselves. This final phase begins when interstitial water has already increased some 30 per cent (Fig. 4).

At first, fluid in the alveoli is confined to the alveolar angles. Subsequently, complete flooding of individual alveoli takes place. A striking microscopic feature is the way in which alveoli are either completely filled with fluid or else have only minimal accumulation in the angles. There are no half-filled alveoli.

Flooding is a 'quantal' event so that flooded alveoli are scattered at random through the affected area. During this process, although the volume of each alveolus is smaller when fluid filled than when air filled, atelectasis is uncommon and air is rarely trapped.

The quantal nature of alveolar flooding arises from the interaction of surface and tissue forces upon the alveolar walls (Fig. 5). The immediate precipitating factor is an increase in epithelial permeability caused by swelling of the alveolar walls distorting the epithelial cellular junctions, normally some 20 times less permeable than those of the capillary endothelium. As a result, the dimensions of the alveoli become unstable because the normal relationship between alveolar pressure and volume reverses as they fill with fluid (phase 2, Fig. 5). There are two reasons for this. The first is related to the role of surfactant. Surfactant, a lipoprotein secreted by type 2 alveolar cells, normally assists the alveoli to remain gas filled by lowering the surface tension of their moist walls, which would otherwise lead to their collapse. The surface tension lowering effect of surfactant is directly proportional to the surface area of the liquid film it covers. As fluid fills the alveolus, its gas–liquid surface area is reduced and its surfactant is diluted so that surface tension within the alveolus is transformed into a constant inward force acting upon the wall independent of its surface area.

The second factor leading to alveolar instability results from the

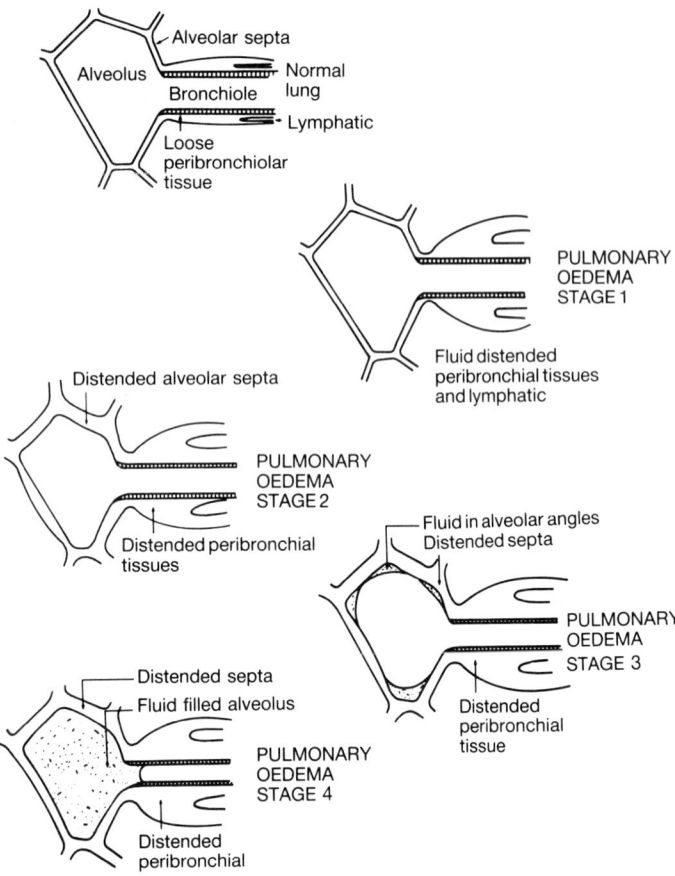

Fig. 4 Stages in the development of pulmonary oedema. Stage 1 – peribronchial swelling; stage 2 – distended alveolar septa; stage 3 – limited accumulation of fluid in alveolar angles; stage 4 – alveolar flooding. (Reproduced from Prichard, 1982, *Edema of the lung.* Charles C. Thomas, Springfield, Illinois, with permission.)

PRESSURE-VOLUME RELATIONSHIPS FOR THE ALVEOLAR UNIT

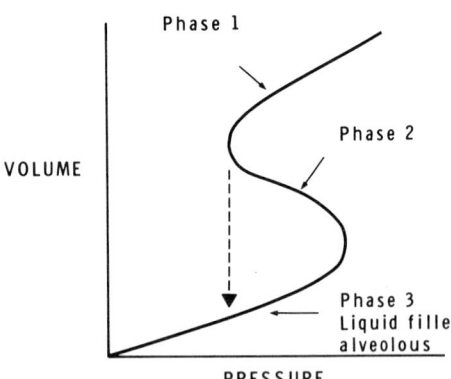

Fig. 5 Pressure–volume relationships in the alveolus. Phase 1 represents the normal alveolus lined by surfactant. Tissue elasticity, osmotic balance, and the presence of surfactant combine to produce a direct, mechanically stable relationship between pressure and volume. Phase 2 represents the situation in which alveolar permeability has increased. Any influx of fluid into the alveolus decreases the overall surface area. At these lower dimensions, surfactant is inoperative and surface tension is independent of area. The relationship between volume and pressure is that of an air bubble in liquid ($P = 2T/R$) and unstable. The air volume therefore shrinks as air is expelled until phase 3 is reached. Here the remaining air is a 'bleb' at the bronchiolar orifice.

oedematous thickening of the alveolar walls, which leads to widening of their epithelial cell junctions. This damage facilitates water movement, without increasing transepithelial osmotic pressure or tissue distortion. Because elastic and osmotic forces can now play little part in epithelial fluid homeostasis, the overall relationship between air volume and pressure within the alveoli becomes similar to gas bubbles in liquid, where gas pressure is inversely related to volume ($P = 2T/R$, where P is the luminal pressure within the alveolus, R its radius, and T its wall surface tension, now constant). This unstable situation, which helps to drag fluid into the alveoli, only ceases when the alveoli are fully flooded.

Hydrostatic pulmonary oedema

Any increase in capillary hydrostatic pressure whether from cardiac failure, fluid overload or pulmonary venous occlusion, augments the rate of water flux into the interstitium. At first, tissue water increases very little because molecular sieving, increased tissue pressure, and decreased macromolecular exclusion all help to limit the amount of transendothelial flow, provided the lymphatic pump keeps pace (page 13.328). However, once the capacity of the lymphatic pump is exceeded, interstitial oedema starts to form with fluid which contains little protein. The fluid first begins to collect in the lower parts of the lung, because hydrostatic pressures are greatest there. The increased microvascular resistance so produced leads to the characteristic redistribution of blood flow away from the lung bases to higher regions, as in mitral stenosis.

Pulmonary oedema and reduced plasma oncotic pressure

Reduction in plasma oncotic pressure increases fluid transudation into the lung interstitium, which may lead to pulmonary oedema at lower hydrostatic pressures than would otherwise be expected. This factor is frequently overlooked in clinical practice where it may be important, particularly in the intensive care ward where prodigal use of crystalloids, particularly when overall fluid balance may be difficult to assess clinically, can lead to sudden pulmonary oedema.

The role of the lung lymphatics

The lung lymphatic system provides the lung with its most important 'safety factor' against oedema. It can normally increase its clearance rate at least ten-fold before being overwhelmed. In chronic pulmonary venous hypertension, as in mitral stenosis, even larger lymph flows are possible because of lymphatic hypertrophy. The activity of the lymphatics is a key feature in determining the onset and severity of hydrostatic oedema. So, without lymphatic hypertrophy, acute elevations of pulmonary vascular pressure will produce acute life-threatening pulmonary oedema at levels which, in chronic states, cause little distress and are recognizable clinically by the characteristic radiological changes of lymphatic hypertrophy (Kerley B lines).

High-permeability pulmonary oedema

Endothelial damage from a variety of mechanical, chemical, and inflammatory perturbations also produces pulmonary oedema by increasing water flux into the interstitium. But, unlike hydrostatic oedema, there is also a transcapillary leak of protein. This has three serious consequences. First, the oncotic pressure of the interstitial fluid increases so that one of the major mechanisms for limiting the progress of oedema becomes unavailable. Second, much of the protein which enters the interstitium and alveoli is fibrinogen which coagulates. Initially, fibrinolysis by plasminogen limits damage from interstitial coagulation, but this defence is soon exhausted and clearance of the coagulum ceases. Third, the fibrin coagulum impairs lymphatic drainage. It also stimulates interstitial fibrosis. The late effects of this process may be chronic cyanosis from impaired oxygen diffusion from alveolar–capillary block due to chronic alveolar interstitial fibrosis.

Routine methods of diagnosing high-permeability lung oedema are limited so that additional experimental approaches have been devised, some of which are now evolving into clinical practice. Studies of pulmonary lymph, obtained by cannulation, micro-aspirates of interstitial fluid, and measurement of alveolar fluid contents have all shown high concentrations of plasma proteins in pulmonary oedema due to increased capillary permeability. Radiolabelled markers, notably serum albumin and transferrin, injected intravenously, and subsequently counted over the lungs over a period of time are being used increasingly to obtain direct estimates of lung capillary permeability from measurements of the rate of the rate of rise in local radioactivity due to the flux of the marker from capillary lumen to interstitial tissue (Fig. 6). It is also possible to make non-invasive measurements of transcapillary transfer kinetics of γ-emitting radiolabelled macromolecules, notably albumin and transferrin, using external counting equipment placed over the chest.

A large number of causes of high permeability pulmonary oedema are now known (Table 1). They appear to fall into two main groups: those in which lung damage is caused directly from trauma or inhalation of toxic substances and those in which damage appears to be the result of inappropriate activation of the normal defence mechanisms of the lungs, producing an inflammatory response as if to microbial invasion via the alveoli.

The inflammatory process, when appropriately mounted against an aerosol of invading organisms such as the pneumococcus, produces a cascade of reactions which involves their phagocytosis by macrophages and granulocytes, and subsequent destruction by activated proteases and free oxygen radicals. Complement and immune proteins are rapidly mobilized from the circulation to the site of invasion via the alveolar endothelial cell junctions whose permeability is greatly augmented. All the above reactions are controlled and modulated by autocoids released by the alveolar macrophages and endothelial cells. These include thromboxane, the prostaglandins and prostacyclin, leucotrienes B4, C4, and D4,

Table 1 Causes of pulmonary oedema

Disorders of ultrafiltration in the lungs
Excessive capillary pressure
  Venous hypertension
    Left ventricular failure
    Mitral stenosis
    Cardiomyopathies
    Loculated and/or constricting pericarditis
    Left atrial myxoma
    Thrombus in left atrium
    Pulmonary venous thromboses
    Cor triatriatum

  Pulmonary capillary hypertension, normal venous pressure
    Hypoxia
    Increased plasma volume
    Exposure to high G
    Altitude

  Acute pulmonary arterial hypertension
    Hyperkinetic states
    Packing pulmonary emboli
    Collagen diseases (rare)
    Idiopathic pulmonary hypertension
    Drugs (aminorex fumarate)
    Secondary to reflex systemic vasoconstriction
    Secondary to release of catecholamines

Reduced plasma colloid osmotic pressure
  Reduced plasma protein concentration
    Overhydration
    Nephrotic syndrome
    Hepatic failure
    Malabsorption
    Protein-losing enteropathy
    Malnutrition

Disorders of capillary permeability
  Humoral release
    Catecholamines, histamine, bradykinin, serotonin, arachidonic acid
     metabolites

  Inflammatory and immune responses of obscure cause
    Following hypovolaemic shock, closed body trauma, septicaemias,
     etc.

  Direct chemical action
    Hypoxia, O_2 poisoning, smoke, chemical fumes – NH_4, SO_2,
     paraquat etc.

  ? Reflex
    Postictal, acute hydrocephalus

Failure of lymph clearance
  Lymphatic obstruction
    Mediastinal obstruction
    Carcinomatous lymphatic infiltration
    Prolonged inadequate positive pressure ventilation

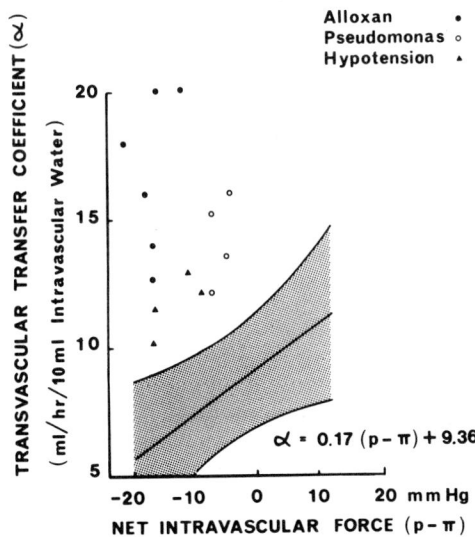

Fig. 6 Experimental demonstration of increased pulmonary endothelial permeability to serum albumin in dog lung using ^{123}I-albumin *in vivo*. Note that the transvascular transfer coefficient for albumin is affected by the net intravascular pressure. This is because the latter determines water movement and this in turn partially entrains albumin by solvent drag. However, following the administration of an endothelial toxin (alloxan), Gram-negative bacteria or a period of hypotension, the transvascular transfer coefficient increases markedly and lies well outside the 95 per cent confidence limits for the normal values. (Reproduced from Prichard, *et al. Clin. Sci.* **59**, 105, with permission.)

platelet-activating factor, fibroblast stimulating factor, interleukin 1, and many others.

Detailed understanding of how the inflammatory cascade works is exciting intense research because its inappropriate activation leads to catastrophic high-permeability pulmonary oedema. Thus, from time to time, the acute inflammatory response is set in motion by a number of apparently unrelated clinical events such as severe closed body trauma, acute hypovolaemic circulatory failure or septicaemia, particularly when associated with Gram-negative organisms. This leads to acute life-threatening respiratory failure because of massive high permeability pulmonary oedema from acute endothelial injury, usually unassociated with any change in transcapillary hydrostatic pressure. The condition is referred to clinically as the adult respiratory distress syndrome (ARDS) (see page 15.161 and 14.12 *et seq.*).

Although the various disorders which precipitate the syndrome are common, ARDS develops relatively infrequently and is remarkably unpredictable. An important early step in its initiation appears to be granulocyte aggregation in the lung capillaries, activated by complement.

Sheep with chronically implanted lung lymph fistulae have been used to model ARDS experimentally. Intravenous infusion of *Escherichia coli* endotoxin activates the alternative pathway of complement, leads to aggregation of granulocytes in the lung, and initiates an immediate rise in lung lymph flow associated with a transient rise in pulmonary artery pressure, almost certainly produced by local release of thromboxane. Later, despite the subsequent return of pulmonary arterial pressure towards normal, the high lymph flow persists, but now becomes proteinaceous at a time when $PGF1_\alpha$ and leucotriene B4 may be detected in the arterial blood leaving the lungs. Increased capillary permeability is responsible for the phase of proteinaceous lymph flow. However, this is *not* an invariable response to endotoxin challenge despite the fact that granulocyte aggregation occurs in every case. Moreover, the response does not occur if the animal has previously been rendered agranulocytic.

In humans, there is a correlation between circulating C5a and the severity of ARDS and examination of bronchoalveolar lavage fluid (BALF) obtained from patients with ARDS reveals the presence of large numbers of degranulated leucocytes. The fluid also has a high protein content, unlike normal BALF which contains very little protein and a cell count composed almost entirely of alveolar macrophages.

A critical question is how the granulocytes themselves become activated to release free oxygen radicals and proteases, once induced to aggregate and adhere to capillary endothelium through the action of complement. One factor which may amplify initial endothelial damage comes from the effects of local ischaemia. Oxygen-starved cells lose high-energy phosphates so that intracellular ATP falls and the cation pumps can no longer keep calcium out of the cytosol. The calcium influx activates a calcium-dependent protease in the cytosol, which leads to the proteolytic conversion of normally innocuous xanthine dehydrogenase to xanthine oxidase. This leads to the release of highly destructive free oxygen radicals, particularly from granulocytes and macrophages.

A second link between permeability oedema and the inflammatory cascade relates to the role of arachidonic acid metabolites, whose various vasodilator prostaglandins and leucotrienes also increase vascular permeability. Their effects are augmented by the presence of activated C5a complement, as also are the actions of bradykinin and histamine.

No general view yet unifies understanding of what first initiates endothelial response to the various toxic substances which may associate to cause high permeability oedema. A link in common might be provided by the existence of a permeability receptor controlling endothelial pore size and junctional integrity, responsive to mediators released from locally activated macrophages, mast cells, and granulocytes as well as to damage by peroxidation. This could explain not only mechanisms based upon C5a complement activation but also account for the action of endothelial toxins such as alloxan and ANTU, which have been studied extensively experimentally.

The agents of endothelial damage so far discussed have all been blood-borne. However, lung damage also results from inhaled and aspirated substances which first effect the alveolar epithelium (Table 1). The damage may be from noxious gases or, as in 'aspiration pneumonia' and drowning, from inhaled liquids. Aspiration of stomach contents causes severe damage to the blood–gas barrier even when the aspirate is not markedly acidic. In seawater drowning, it is assumed that hypertonicity is sufficient in itself to cause epithelial damage, but the lung injury from freshwater inhalation is more obscure, for up to 72 hours after resuscitation 'secondary drowning' may occur, leading to acute respiratory failure due to the rapid filling of the lungs with fluid having a high protein content.

Table 2 The multifactorial nature of pulmonary oedema

	Hydrostatic pressure	Oncotic pressure	Endothelial permeability	Lymphatic drainage
Shock lung (ARDS)	(From treatment)	+	+	(+)
Hepatic failure		+	+	
Renal failure	+	(+)	+	
Neurogenic	+		+	
Fluid overload	+	+		
Pulmonary emboli	+		+	
Myocardial infarction	+	(+)	(+)	
Carcinomatosis		(+)		+
High altitude	+		(+)	(+)

Clinical considerations

Table 1 lists the main causes of pulmonary oedema, classified according to the predominant pathophysiological mechanisms. The clinician should never forget that more than one cause may be operating in case one remediable factor may be neglected at the expense of another. Moreover, if the multifactorial nature of pulmonary oedema is not continuously borne in mind, therapy itself can become positively harmful. For example, following a period of traumatic hypotension with possible occult pulmonary endothelial injury, overvigorous blood transfusion may be the very factor which accelerates the clinical manifestations of ARDS. The pulmonary oedema which may develop as a result of some clinical disorders may almost invariably have a multifactorial basis. Some examples of these are set out in Table 2.

Descriptions of the clinical manifestations and management of the commoner diseases listed in Table 1 are to be found in other chapters. But from time to time some of the less obvious causes of pulmonary oedema need careful exclusion. Some of these are mentioned below.

Loculated constrictive pericarditis is not uncommon in patients with chronic renal failure undergoing regular dialysis. When it embarrasses predominantly left ventricular function, pulmonary oedema may ensue. Echocardiography is helpful in excluding the condition, which may be difficult to recognize clinically as the usual signs of pericardial tamponade may be missing other than a low cardiac output state, tachycardia, and hypotension. Often located posteriorly, the usually bloodstained fluid is difficult to aspirate percutaneously. Fortunately open drainage is rarely necessary, for strict attention to fluid regulation during dialysis usually leads to resolution.

Pulmonary venous thrombosis is comparatively rare, but should always be considered in cases of obscure pulmonary oedema. It may be idiopathic or present as a subsidiary manifestation in such conditions as polyarteritis nodosa, systemic lupus erythematosus or occult neoplastic disease. Commoner in women, who are often middle aged, increasing lassitude, and breathlessness, sometimes with low grade fever are the presenting symptoms. Ultimately gross effort dyspnoea and pulmonary oedema, usually with pleural effusions, develop. The signs of pulmonary hypertension are present, but diagnostic proof of its venous origin is difficult. At cardiac catheterization, difficulty in obtaining a clear pulmonary artery wedge pressure tracing associated with a normal left atrial pressure, measured directly by the transseptal route, should alert suspicion. Pulmonary artery angiography should demonstrate poor segmental drainage in the regions affected by thrombosis. Open lung biopsy will confirm the diagnosis but is dangerous, so it should only be undertaken when there is real fear of missing an alternative cause of the oedema. Prognosis is bad, usually less than a year from diagnosis. Treatment is palliative with diuretics and long-term anticoagulants to prevent extension.

Left atrial myxoma, ball thrombus of the left atrium and cor triatriatum are all rare causes of pulmonary oedema from pulmonary venous hypertension. They must not be missed as all are remediable by surgery. Their clinical presentation may be very similar to that of pulmonary venous thrombosis, for often the characteristic episodic mitral diastolic murmurs that occur with left atrial myxoma and ball thrombus are not heard. All three conditions also enter into the differential diagnosis of tight mitral stenosis. Two-dimensional echocardiography helps diagnose them all.

Pulmonary arterial hypertension At first sight, pulmonary oedema secondary to pulmonary arterial hypertension would seem to be unlikely since the raised pressure is usually associated with marked peripheral arteriolar disease at precapillary level. This should protect the capillaries from high pressures, but high output states with secondary hypertension can be associated with pulmonary oedema, especially following exercise. This is usually avoided because acute exertional breathlessness is such a prominent symptom of the underlying condition.

Pulmonary arterial thromboembolism may occasionally lead to pulmonary oedema. Experimentally, two hypotheses are advanced: local overperfusion by diversion of blood flow away from occluded sites; and humoral alteration of permeability, for the oedema fluid is often protein rich. The clotting cascade could be involved as prior heparinization prevents experimental oedema developing. Clinically, pulmonary oedema is often associated with small haemoptyses particularly in patients suffering showers of small emboli which pack distal to the precapillary bronchopulmonary anastomosis. Post-mortem studies suggest that microvascular hypertension and hyperperfusion in the neighbourhood of patchily infarcted lung is responsible for the oedema. Invariably initial symptoms are insiduous, with increasing unexplained breathlessness and right heart failure, sometimes with mild jaundice from associated breakdown of haemoglobin in the infarcted tissue. A search for associated occult neoplastic disease is wise. Initial heparin therapy, followed by long-term anticoagulants for at least three months is generally recommended.

High altitude oedema It has long been known that some apparently normal people who ascend rapidly to high altitudes experience acute pulmonary oedema. The condition is a particular instance of oedema due to severe hypoxia. It develops in a minority of individuals who have an exaggerated pulmonary artery pressor response to hypoxia and who develop pulmonary hypertension at high altitude. The oedema could result from fluid leakage due to high pressure within the microvessels or, alternatively, heterogeneous vasoconstriction with consequent extreme hyperperfusion of those areas less vasoconstricted. A further contribution may arise from the release of vasoactive amines and their action upon contractile filaments within endothelial cells leading to separation of their junctions. In addition to standard management involving rest, oxygen therapy, and diuretics, suggestions that hypoxic vasoconstriction is due to abnormal calcium entry into the endothelial cells has prompted the trial of calcium-blocking agents such as verapamil and nifedipine. Their usefulness is unproven.

Pulmonary oedema following acute intracranial lesions A large variety of intracranial lesions may occasionally be associated with pulmonary oedema. Damage to the nucleus of the tractus solitarius and the hypothalamus probably initiates the intense systemic sympathetic vasoconstriction and catecholamine release necessary to shift sufficient blood to the pulmonary circulation to cause acute distensive pulmonary hypertension, reaching 410/210 mm Hg in one recorded case. This leads to hydrostatic pulmonary oedema and, if sufficiently severe, damage also to the endothelium leading to less easily resolved oedema from permeability change.

Expansion pulmonary oedema Pulmonary oedema after apparently successful aspiration of a pleural effusion or with expansion of a collapsed lung was first observed as long ago as 1875. The incidence is rare but may be reduced by ensuring that negative pressures in the pleural space during re-expansion do not exceed 10 cm H_2O, that no more than 1.5 litres of pleural fluid are aspirated at any one time and that the procedure is stopped if cough develops. The mechanism is uncertain. Permeability change is unlikely, but loss of surfactant during collapse may play a key role during re-expansion.

Disorders of capillary permeability The reader is referred to page 15.161 describing the adult respiratory distress syndrome. Many of the conditions associated with this florid disorder can also be associated with less dramatic degrees of pulmonary oedema. It is a good rule always to consider the possibility that a permeability abnormality might exist as an associated cause in all cases of pulmonary oedema. The history can be particularly helpful, particularly with regard to possible infections such as mild influenza, possible reactions to drugs or occupational chemicals. The possibility of oxygen toxicity should be borne in mind in patients in intensive care, though prolonged ventilation with mixtures containing less than 65 per cent oxygen are usually safe.

The resolution of pulmonary oedema

Hydrostatic and oncotic pulmonary oedema can resolve rapidly once the cause is removed, but this is rarely the case when increased permeability is the problem. Slow resolution is then the rule, leaving some permanent damage, manifest either by a reduced oxygen diffusing capacity or more serious manifestations of alveolar fibrosis.

Resolution of hydrostatic oedema occurs when the capillary pressure returns to normal allowing osmotic and lymphatic removal of fluid from the tissues, but the mechanism removing fluid from the alveoli is less well understood. A considerable amount of fluid is removed by coughing and ciliary drainage, but little is known regarding final clearance and restoration of normal alveolar epithelial integrity.

In permeability oedema, fluid clearance is less efficient because fibrin entering the interstitium soon forms a coagulum. The protein stimulates local fibromyocytes to differentiate to fibroblasts. Alveolar fibrosis is the end result in severe cases. Nothing is known about the process of endothelial repair. Epithelial cell replacement is by transdifferentiation from type II pneumocytes.

Pulmonary function in oedema of the lung

The oedematous lung shows a mixture of restrictive and obstructive defects, although the former dominates. The restrictive component arises from decreased lung compliance, due predominantly to vascular congestion, and to a lesser extent interstitial oedema and dilution of surfactant.

Sometimes increased airflow resistance may cause rhonchi and a reduction in forced expiratory volume per second (FEV_1), but usually it is difficult to detect clinically because it predominantly occurs in small airways which contribute relatively little to overall resistance. Lung compliance may fall by as much as 75 per cent in severe pulmonary oedema. The resistive and obstructive defects together increase the work of breathing so that breathlessness and tachypnoea become a prominent feature, due partly to the stimulation of the alveolar 'J' receptors of the vagus.

Tachypnoea and ventilation perfusion mismatch lead to hypoxia with hypocapnia. But in about 20 per cent of severe cases, carbon dioxide retention with respiratory acidosis occurs without the presence of chronic airway disease. A number of mechanisms have been proposed. They include uncontrolled oxygen administration accompanied by low central carbon dioxide sensitivity, respiratory muscle fatigue, and severe ventilation perfusion imbalance. Although hypoxia is the rule it may occur surprisingly late, partly because oedema first accumulates away from the alveoli and partly because increased vascular resistance in the oedematous areas redirects perfusion to better ventilated areas.

The hypoxia and hypercapnia are usually accompanied by mild metabolic acidosis but occasionally the base deficit may exceed

15 mEq/l. Frank metabolic acidosis is most likely in patients with severe oedema, who already have carbon dioxide retention, severe heart failure with peripheral circulatory failure or other organ system failures such as uraemia.

The diagnosis of pulmonary oedema

The diagnosis of pulmonary oedema is by clinical observation and the chest X-ray. Nuclear techniques can now detect changes in both lung capillary endothelial and epithelial permeability, while simple protein analysis of bronchoalveolar lavage fluid also helps detect capillary epithelial damage.

The earliest symptom of pulmonary oedema is inappropriate breathlessness. Dyspnoea will tend to occur more or less acutely at first, often following exercise. Later there is paroxysmal nocturnal dyspnoea because of postural and hydrostatic factors. Only then are the signs of diminished breath sounds at the bases and fine lung crepitations likely to be found. Serial vital capacity measurements are useful, correlating inversely with the severity of oedema. The effectiveness of therapy can be assessed by plotting improvement in serial vital capacity measurements.

The chest X-ray, lung water distribution, and pulmonary oedema

The most sensitive and easily available tool for spotting early pulmonary oedema is the posteroanterior chest radiograph (Figs 7 and 8). *Pre-oedema* is the earliest sign reflected by the vascular changes seen on the X-ray, which become distended and engorged, with redistribution to the upper zones. *Interstitial oedema* follows and is characterized by a number of changes:

1. *Septal lines, perilobular lines, and rosettes* all represent engorged lymphatics. Septal lines were first identified by Kerley. *Type A* are ragged, unbranched, and run towards the hilum. *Type B* are short, sharp, horizontal, and seen in the costophrenic angles. *C lines* are fine, interlacing, and seen most easily in the central and perihilar regions. Perilobular lines and rosettes are found on close inspection in about 3 per cent of X-rays. They probably represent the lymphatics encircling the respiratory acini. There is a tendency for pulmonary oedema of rapid onset to be associated more with the early appearance of A and C lines. Also these are commoner in pulmonary oedema from increased endothelial permeability, so are helpful clues to ARDS. Type B lines are most often seen in oedema from chronic pulmonary venous hypertension. Indeed, there is excellent correlation between the density of Kerley B lines and left atrial pressure in mitral stenosis. The lines are rarely seen below a left atrial pressure of 13.5 mm Hg, are commonly found in the region of 22 mm Hg and are invariably present when the left atrial pressure exceeds 30 mm Hg.

2. *Visible interlobar and accessory lung fissures.*

3. *Perivascular and peribronchial cuffs* contribute to the homogeneous circular shadows formed by the already distended blood vessels and also give ring shadows round bronchi, seen close to the hilum.

4. *Micronoduli* consist of small round densities < 3 mm due to fluid accumulating round small blood vessels.

5. *Blurring and hazing of the hilar regions* represent the beginning of true interstitial oedema.

6. *Diffuse clouding* due to increased lung density represents the final phase of interstitial oedema.

Alveolar oedema appears as patchy and 'fluffy' loss of translucency either around the hila in a 'butterfly' or 'batswing' pattern or predominantly in the lower zones. Pleural effusions may develop and there is a loss of lung volume.

The detection of breakdown in lung capillary permeability

It is now possible to obtain quantitative estimates of permeability non-invasively. A marker is injected intravenously with subsequent measurement of radioactivity in serial blood samples and at the surface of the chest. In the lung, a gradual rise in counts

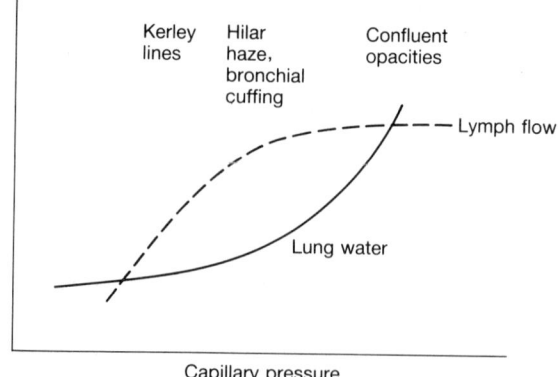

Fig. 7 Radiological signs and pulmonary pathophysiology. Kerley lines are a particularly useful radiological sign as they occur at a stage where lymph flow and transinterstitial water flow have both increased but where appreciable tissue swelling has not yet appeared. (Reproduced from Prichard, 1982, *Edema of the lung*. Charles C. Thomas, Springfield, Illinois, with permission.)

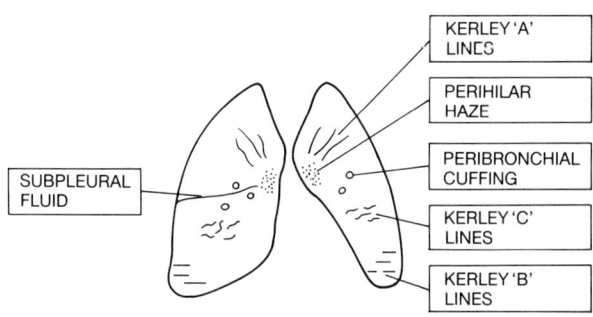

Fig. 8 Characteristic radiological appearances in interstitial oedema (see text). (Reproduced from Prichard, 1982, *Edema of the lung*. Charles C. Thomas, Springfield, Illinois, with permission.)

takes place, due to the marker leaving the plasma compartment to enter the interstitium. The rate of rise of radioactivity in the chest relative to that in the blood provides an estimate of capillary permeability. The faster the rise in chest counts, the greater will have been the permeability of the capillaries of the underlying lung. Using a non-diffusible marker, such as indium-labelled red cells, and a freely diffusible marker, such as radioactive sodium iodide, one may also measure lung blood and interstitial fluid volumes.

Figure 9 shows how the methods have been applied in patients with pulmonary oedema to find out whether changes in hydrostatic pressure or lung capillary permeability were responsible for the increased interstitial fluid volumes present, compared with a normal group. The figures in brackets represent pulmonary artery precapillary wedge pressures, obtained by Swan–Ganz catheterization. The severity of the lung oedema, represented by the interstitial volume, was similar in both the cardiac group of patients and those with pulmonary oedema from ARDS. In cardiac oedema, the rate constant for the transfer of albumin from plasma to interstitium (K_p) was within normal limits, the oedema being caused by raised transcapillary pressure. In ARDS the lung oedema was due solely to increase in capillary permeability (K_p).

Bronchial toilet in the intensive care ward often involves the aspiration of secretions from the peripheral airways of the lung by fibreoptic bronchoscopy. Changes in capillary epithelial permeability may be assessed from sizing analysis of the proteins present in the aspirate. Generally the protein content is low in cardiac oedema, but in permeability oedemas the protein content of alveolar fluid may approach that of plasma itself.

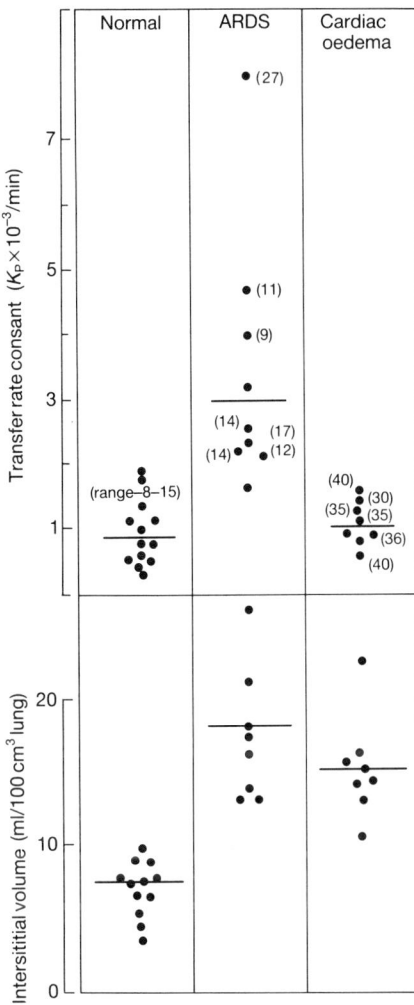

Fig. 9 Lung interstitial fluid volume and pulmonary capillary permeability, expressed as the transcapillary transfer rate constant for albumin (K_p). A comparison between normal subjects, patients with cardiac pulmonary oedema and patients suffering from high permeability pulmonary oedema from ARDS. (Figures in brackets show pulmonary capillary wedge pressure, mmHg.) (Reproduced from Lee, Kanazawa and Hussein, data submitted for publication 1985. Figure by permission of authors.)

Treatment of pulmonary oedema

Since pulmonary oedema may result from increased microvascular pressure, decreased plasma colloid oncotic pressure, increased microvascular permeability or impaired lymphatic drainage, treatment of each form should ideally include measures specific for the major pathophysiological cause; but, with the exception of reduction of elevated hydrostatic pressure, these are rarely particularly effective and the clinician has to rely on general supportive measures combined with meticulous fluid balance and monitoring of oncotic pressure.

Hydrostatic pulmonary oedema

The commonest causes are acute or chronic left-sided heart disease. The patient is most comfortable in the 'trunk up, legs down' position to help pool blood in the dependent parts of the systemic circulation. Thigh cuffs inflated to occlude venous return can act in the form of a bloodless phlebotomy. Dyspnoea should be relieved with morphine. This drug has important vasodilator effects on the systemic venous system thus helping reduce venous filling pressure to the heart, performing a 'pharmacological phlebotomy' by shifting blood from the lesser to the major circulation. Particularly in severe heart failure with cardiogenic shock, morphine is best

administered slowly intravenously in a moderate dilution volume to help deliver it to the effective circulation. Morphine sulphate, 10 mg, diluted in 20 ml saline, given at a rate of 1 mg/min until the patient is tranquil, brings relief, free of risk from respiratory depression.

A bolus dose of 100 mg frusemide, or 40–80 mg ethacrynic acid, administered intravenously should be given. These act both by 'pharmacological phlebotomy' and by diuresis. If the patient is in extremis or heavily sedated it is wise to catheterize the bladder, since rapid diuresis leading to acute bladder distension may induce intense reflex systemic vasoconstriction and disaster.

Hypoxia is relieved with a standard face mask or nasal prongs delivering oxygen at relatively high flow rates, up to 10 l/min. This provides an inspired oxygen concentration of about 60 per cent. If the patient's arterial oxygen tension continues to fall, and/or hypercapnia develops, tracheal intubation and intermittent positive pressure ventilation will be needed.

The use of inotropic drugs (page 13.111) and vasodilator therapy (page 13.105) also play their part for patients with severe pulmonary oedema due to left ventricular dysfunction (page 13.85).

The use of digoxin needs thought. If the patient is already receiving the drug, it may be best to stop it to avoid toxicity, particularly if large amounts of diuretic are being given. But if the cardiac failure is associated with fast atrial fibrillation or other tachyarrythmias, it will be harder to relieve the pulmonary oedema without good heart rate control.

For rapid effect, intravenous amiodarone, given in a loading dose of 300 mg over half an hour, followed by a maintenance infusion of 150–300 mg six hourly via a catheter advanced to the vena cava, is probably more effective and less hazardous than digitalis.

The patient who becomes refractory to digoxin and diuretics often progresses to a state in which a low cardiac output and borderline low blood pressure, oliguria, and intense peripheral vasoconstriction combine with persisting pulmonary oedema. In such a state, reduction in left ventricular afterload by means of vasodilators has a place, the use of angiotensin-converting enzyme inhibitors being particularly effective. Any further improvement in left ventricular function demands the use of inotropic agents such as dopamine, which require facilities for careful haemodynamic monitoring.

Manipulation of osmotic and oncotic pressures

A reduction in plasma oncotic pressure may play some part in pulmonary oedema, as in crystalloid fluid overload, hepatic failure or nephrotic syndrome. In the case of fluid overload, the most appropriate therapy is the use of diuretics, for these not only reduce the extracellular and blood volumes but also return plasma oncotic pressure towards normal.

Diuretics are also an appropriate approach in the rare cases where pulmonary oedema complicates hypoalbuminaemic states. The use of salt-free albumin and plasma concentrate is often disappointing and may even be counterproductive when the condition is also associated with permeability damage as in ARDS.

Management of high-permeability pulmonary oedema

General principles of management relate to attempts to block the inappropriate inflammatory cascade usually responsible for the condition.

There is experimental evidence that *prior* administration of glucocorticoids to animals given lipopolysaccharide to trigger complement activated lung injury reduces its severity, but there is little clinical evidence that steroids can benefit pulmonary oedema once endothelial damage has begun. However, there is some logic in their use, for evidence is now very strong that granulocytes aggregate in the lungs of patients with ARDS as a result of complement activation. Steroids can not only reduce their aggregation but also diminish free radical production. Until a conclusive answer is produced, clinicians will continue to use steroids in large doses despite the absence of adequate supportive clinical data.

The supplementary calcium and xanthine oxidase dependent cell-destructive mechanism leading to the release of oxygen free radicals within granulocytes and macrophages may be suppressed by phosphodiesterase inhibitors, allopurinol, and calcium-blocking drugs. These are being studied experimentally, but no conclusions are yet available. Similarly, the use of allopurinol or nifedipine is of unproven benefit. The injection of superoxide dismutase and catalase is accompanied by a number of practical problems which limit their clinical use. An injectable specific inhibitor of the NADPH oxidase responsible for neutrophil-generated oxygen free radicals would be a powerful tool if it could be developed.

Inhibition of the metabolic pathways of arachidonic acid by non-steroidal anti-inflammatory substances and by aspirin are undergoing therapeutic trials. No evidence of their effectiveness clinically is yet available. At present therefore the only treatment available is to limit transcapillary fluid flux by meticulous attention both to plasma oncotic pressure regulation and to reduce pulmonary transcapillary pressure through diuretic therapy. Diuretic therapy is often limited by hypovolaemia, particularly in patients undergoing positive pressure ventilation. Another problem is that severe respiratory failure in high-permeability lung oedema may require prolonged high concentration oxygen therapy, itself a risk because of oxygen toxicity.

Positive pressure ventilation

At first sight, it would seem attractive to increase alveolar gas pressure in cases of severe hydrostatic pulmonary oedema, not least to avoid alveolar collapse. Positive pressure ventilation can be effective in severe pulmonary oedema uncontrolled by other measures. Its efficacy in promoting gas exchange may be augmented by applying positive end expiratory pressure, but there is little evidence that this reduces the extent of the lung oedema.

References

Aberman, A. and Fulop, M. (1972). The metabolic and respiratory acidosis of acute pulmonary oedema. *Ann. intern. Med.* **76**, 173.

Albert, R. K. (1985). Least PEEP: Primum non nocere. *Chest* **87**, 2–4.

Anonymous (1986). Adult respiratory distress syndrome. *Lancet* i, 301–303.

Brigham, K. L. and Meyrick, B. (1984). Interaction of granulocytes with the lungs. *Circ. Res.* **54**, 623–635.

—— and —— (1986). Endotoxin and lung injury. *Am. Rev. Resp. Dis.* **133**, 913–927.

Cohen, A. B. (1983). Proteases and anti-proteases in the lung. *Am. Rev. Resp. Dis.* **127**, S2–S27.

Gorin, A. B., Kohler, J. and De Nardo, G. (1980). Non-invasive measurement of pulmonary transvascular protein flux in normal man. *J. Clin. Invest.* **66**, 869.

Guyton, A. O. and Lindsey, A. W. (1959). Effect of elevated left atrial pressure and decreased plasma protein concentration upon the development of pulmonary oedema. *Circ. Res.* **7**, 649.

Hocking, W. G. and Golde, D. W. (1979). The pulmonary alveolar macrophage. *N. Engl. J. Med.* **301**, 580–587, 639–645.

Kapanci, Y. and Elemer, G. (1981). Permeability pathways of alveolar capillary membrane during pulmonary oedema. *Eur. Heart J.* **2**, Suppl. a, 125.

Kerley, P. (1962). Cardiac failure. In *A textbook of X-ray diagnosis* Vol. 2 (eds S. C. Shank and P. Kerley), pp. 97–107.

Nicholson, D. P. (1983). Corticosteroids in the treatment of septic shock and the adult respiratory distress syndrome. *Med. Clin. N. Am.* **67**.

Pistolesi, M. and Giuntini, C. (1978). Assessment of extravascular lung water. *Radiol. Clin. N. Am.* **16**, 551.

Prichard, J. S. (1982). *Edema of the lung.* Charles C. Thomas, Springfield, Illinois.

Schneeberger, E. E. (1976). Ultrastructural basis of alveolar capillary permeability to protein. In *Lung liquids* (eds R. Porter and M. O'Connor), pp. 3–21. Excerpta Medica, Amsterdam (Ciba Foundation Symposium 38).

Staub, N. C. (1980). The pathogenesis of pulmonary edema. *Prog. Cardiovasc. Dis.* **23**, 53.

Sugarman, H. J. *et al.* (1982). Gamma scintigraphic analysis of albumin flux in patients with adult respiratory distress syndrome. *Am. Rev. Resp. Dis.* **125**, 279.

Taylor, A. E. and Drake, R. E. (1978). Fluid and protein movement across the pulmonary microcirculation. In *Lung water and solute exchange* (ed. N. L. Staub). Dekker, New York.

Vismara, L. A., Leaman, D. M. and Zellis, R. (1976). The effect of morphine on venous tone in patients with acute pulmonary edema. *Circulation* **54**, 335.

Pulmonary hypertension

G. de J. LEE

Introduction

Unlike systemic hypertension, where a specific cause for the raised arterial pressure is found only in a minority of cases, the development of increased pulmonary arterial pressure (pulmonary hypertension) is the commonest response of the lung blood vessels to diseases of all kinds. So, although primary or idiopathic pulmonary hypertension occurs, it is rare; its diagnosis is made by exclusion.

This chapter will consider pulmonary hypertension arising from causes other than lung disease, which is covered separately on page 13.350 on cor pulmonale.

Just as in systemic hypertension, the definition of pulmonary hypertension depends entirely upon what limits are put on normality. Table 1 shows normal values for intracardiac pressures and for derived pulmonary and systemic haemodynamic indices. Both the pulmonary artery pressure and resistance are approximately five times lower than in systemic circulation. As one ages, the resting cardiac output tends to fall and there is a general rise both in systemic and pulmonary arterial pressure.

Pulmonary hypertension may be said to exist when the systolic pulmonary artery pressure exceeds 30 mmHg or a mean arterial pressure of 20 mmHg.

Physical considerations

The simplest conceptual model linking vascular resistance to blood flow and pressure within the pulmonary and systemic arterial systems is to consider the analogy of Ohm's law for electrical circuits in which $I = E/R$ where I = current, equivalent to flow (Q); E = voltage, equivalent to pressure (P); and R = resistance.

Thus in the human circulation we may write: $Q = P/R$. Conductance (C), the reciprocal of resistance, describes the ability of the fluid conducting system to accept flow at a given pressure difference across the system, expressed as ml/s/mmHg ($C = 1/R$).

Resistance to blood flow depends upon a number of factors, including the physical characteristics of the vascular bed, blood viscosity, and whether blood flow is laminar or turbulent. Below a certain critical velocity, blood flow is laminar and stable, with individual fluid laminae sliding over one another within the vessel. Blood ejected into the aorta and pulmonary artery from the cardiac ventricles has an initial flat velocity profile across the diameter of the vessel. This becomes parabolic over a linear distance down the vessel equivalent to approximately twenty times its initial diameter. This is due to friction from the vessel walls.

Poiseuille's Law defines these relationships for a Newtonian fluid within rigid tubes:

$$Q = \frac{(P_1 - P_2)\, r^4}{8\, \eta\, L} \qquad (1)$$

where Q = flow rate, $P_1 - P_2$ = the pressure difference between the entry and exit points, r = radius, η = viscosity, and L = the length between the entry and exit points.

If either the length of the tube or the viscosity of the fluid were to double, flow velocity would be halved. If, on the other hand, flow velocity stayed constant then the pressure gradient would

Table 1A Normal intracardiac, systemic and pulmonary haemodynamic values

	Maximum normal pressures		
	Systolic (mm Hg)	Diastolic (mm Hg)	Mean (mm Hg)
Right atrium	'a' 7 'v' 5	'x' 3 'y' 3	5
Right ventricle	25	End diastolic pressure pre 'a' wave post 'a' wave	3 7
Pulmonary artery	25	15	18
Left atrium (direct or via PA wedge)	'a' 12 'v' 10	'x' 7 'y' 7	10
Left ventricle	100–120	End diastolic pressure pre 'a' wave post 'a' wave	7 12
Aorta	100–120	60–80	80–107

After Sokolow and McIlroy (1982).

Table 1B Derived haemodynamic values

Index	Normal range
Cardiac Index (CI) $= \dfrac{\text{Cardiac output}}{\text{Body surface area (m}^2)}$	2.8–4.2 l/m^2
Stroke vol. index (SV1) $= \dfrac{\text{SV}}{\text{BSA}}$	40–70 ml/m^2
Stroke work index (SWI) $= \text{SV} \times (\overline{\text{SAP}} - \overline{\text{PAW}}) \times 0.0136$	40–80 gm/m^2
Systemic vascular resistance (SVR) $= \dfrac{80\,(\overline{\text{SAP}} - \overline{\text{RA}})}{\text{CO}}$	770–1500 dyne/s/cm^{5*}
Pulmonary vascular resistance (PVR) $= \dfrac{80\,\overline{\text{PA}} - \overline{\text{PAW}})}{\text{CO}}$	20–120 dyne/s/cm^{5*}

After Sokolow and McIlroy (1982).
* Divide by 80 to obtain mmHg/l/min.
CO = Cardiac output l/min.
BSA = Body surface area (m^2).
$\overline{\text{SAP}}, \overline{\text{RA}}, \overline{\text{PA}}, \overline{\text{PAW}}$ = mean arterial, right arterial, pulmonary arterial, and pulmonary artery wedge pressures, respectively (mm Hg).
SV = stroke volume (CO/heart rate) in ml.

double. If the tube radius were to double then fluid velocity would increase sixteen-fold, hence the physiological effectiveness of small diameter changes in the peripheral arterial system in blood flow regulation.

If the calibre and length of the tube as well as the fluid viscosity remain constant, resistance is found to be directly proportional to both fluid viscosity and tube length but inversely proportional to the fourth power of its radius.

The geometric components and viscosity can be measured in the circulation to provide a constant; so, for practical purposes, the relationship between pressure flow, and resistance can be simplified to:

$$Q = \frac{P_1 - P_2}{R} \text{ and } R = \frac{P_1 - P_2}{Q} \qquad (2)$$

Because blood vessels are not rigid, these relationships are non-linear, so that if the pressure difference between inflow and outflow sites is increased linearly, flow increases exponentially as a result of vascular distension. This will be accompanied by a reciprocal fall in vascular resistance.

When fluid flow exceeds a certain velocity, its laminar profile becomes disturbed and turbulence ensues. This is characterized by unpredictable random fluctuations in motion of elements within the fluid continuum, which cannot be predicted in detail. As a result there is a great increase in both wall friction and resistance to blood flow.

Turbulent blood flow occurs most readily in large diameter vessels, at high fluid velocities and when blood viscosity is low. Turbulence can be predicted from the Reynolds number (Re) given by:

$$Re = \frac{V\,D\,\varrho}{\eta} \qquad (3)$$

where D = diameter, V = velocity, ϱ = fluid density, and η = fluid viscosity. The Reynolds number for blood is normally less than 1000. Turbulence develops at Reynolds numbers over 3000. In areas of turbulence, the necessary applied pressure difference to maintain flow will need to increase with the square of the mean linear velocity ($P = kV^2$). This imposes obvious extra demands upon ventricular function in valvular disease. The downstream effect of exceeding the critical Reynolds number in the face of a constant driving pressure difference is that the loss of kinetic energy from the resulting turbulence leads to a *decrease* in flow. This will obviously affect the blood flow adversely through diseased vessels.

Since both pressure and flow is repetitive and pulsatile, they can be subjected to harmonic (Fourier) analysis to obtain dynamic information of the hydraulic input impedance (Z) of the arterial system. This is a complex ratio of pressure and flow at the site of inputs to the system, i.e. at the root of the aorta or pulmonary artery. Studies of impedance spectra yield important information to the bioengineer and physiologist on the dynamic factors regulating total fluid energy supply and consumption between the ventricular pump and the periphery. Their interest to clinicians is largely theoretical.

The mechanisms responsible for pulmonary hypertension

The principle stimuli evoking a response in the pulmonary arterioles are (a) alveolar hypoxia, for example, from high altitude or chronic lung disease; (b) pulmonary venous hypertension, as in mitral stenosis; and (c) vascular distension due to high blood flow as in large congenital left-to-right intracardiac shunts.

In all cases the main site of reaction is the smooth muscle of the pulmonary arterioles. All the stimuli mentioned cause arteriolar vasoconstriction that is at first functional, spasmodic, and reversible (except in the case of congenital shunts). With time, the vasoconstriction stimulates organic smooth muscle hypertrophy, which ultimately becomes irreversible and complicated by secondary reactive and degenerative changes.

The age at which the patient is first exposed to these stimuli as well as their duration, determines the ultimate response of the pulmonary vascular system. Stimuli present from birth cause the severest and least reversible changes. All the above stimuli interact. For example, a combination of hypoxia from high altitude combined with pulmonary venous hypertension from mitral valve disease will lead to accelerated pulmonary hypertension. Moreover, once the pulmonary vasculature has become damaged peripherally, local complications further accelerate the process and pulmonary hypertension will tend to increase, as local thromboses and emboli tend to occur which further contribute to pulmonary vascular obstruction.

Tissue destruction by chronic lung disease will further decrease the normal capacity of the pulmonary circulation to accommodate changes in lung blood flow. Thus, the principle mechanism causing chronic hypertension in chronic lung disease is loss of lung tissue, caused by a combination of inflammation, fibrosis, and atrophy. Clinical manifestations of cor pulmonale from chronic lung disease will not be recognizable until approximately seven-eighths of the pulmonary circulation has been destroyed. Alveolar hypoxia in chronic lung disease, potentiated by hypercapnoea and respiratory acidosis, imposes an additional reversible element of resistance which overloads the right heart, especially during acute respiratory infections.

The vascular pathology in hypertensive pulmonary vascular disease

Pulmonary hypertension produces changes in the large pulmonary arteries so that they begin to resemble the structure of the aorta. Atheroma, normally rare in the pulmonary artery, is also common. It is an indication of long-standing pulmonary hypertension.

The muscular pulmonary arteries and arterioles, veins and venules all develop changes in their walls in response to a number of different perturbations all leading to pulmonary hypertension. There are five pathological groups of arterial change: (1) Changes following long term hypoxia; (2) changes from venous outflow obstruction; (3) changes from chronic thromboembolic obstruction; (4) vasoactive or plexogenic arteriopathy; and (5) necrotizing arteritis.

1. Changes following long-term hypoxia Chronic hypoxia from any cause stimulates the formation of smooth muscle bundles arranged longitudinally within the intima and media of the muscular pulmonary arteries extending proximally. Muscularization of the arterioles between internal and external elastic laminae also occurs. In addition there will be destructive loss of lung parenchyma if chronic obstructive lung disease is present. Details about

the reversibility of the vascular changes in hypoxic pulmonary hypertension may be found on page 13.350 on cor pulmonale.

2. Changes resulting from pulmonary venous outflow obstruction Intimal fibrosis will also take place in the pulmonary veins when they are submitted to high transmural pressures from any cause. The changes are non-specific; for example, they are found in hyperdynamic pulmonary hypertension, as in atrial septal defect, as well as in obstructive venous hypertension from mitral stenosis. The specific changes of venous pulmonary hypertension are found in the media of the veins which respond by hypertrophy and condensation of the smooth muscle. The arterial changes which accompany venous hypertension usually only develop to the stage of medial hypertrophy and intimal fibrosis represented by grade 3 in Table 2. This is important clinically because it indicates that even if severe pulmonary hypertension develops in mitral stenosis it is virtually always reversible following surgical relief of the stenosis. This may well be the reason that plexogenic arteriopathy does not develop secondary to pulmonary venous hypertension; for plexogenic arteriopathy only develops in the severest forms of vasoactive and hyperdynamic pulmonary hypertension.

3. Changes due to chronic microvascular obstruction from recurrent thromboembolism Gradual occlusion of the peripheral pulmonary arterial bed may occur occultly from recurrent multiple small pulmonary emboli which build up to occlude the peripheral radicals of the pulmonary arterial system, become organized by inflammatory cells, fibrose and often partially recanalize. The muscular pulmonary arteries proximal to the occlusions show intimal fibrosis and medial hypertrophy. The larger proximal arteries become distended and atheromatous. Survival is usually short, death being due to right heart failure. This may explain why plexogenic arteriopathy is not usually a feature of the pathology of thromboembolic pulmonary hypertension.

4. 'Vasoactive or plexogenic arteriopathy' develops as the result of vasoconstrictive and hypertrophic changes in the muscular pulmonary arteries and arterioles from a variety of stimuli. In particular it is found in response to increased microvascular distension caused by increased transmural pressures resulting from persistently elevated pulmonary blood flows from birth, associated with large left-to-right intracardiac shunts. For reasons not yet understood, identical pathological changes are also found in pulmonary hypertension sometimes associated with liver cirrhosis and portal vein thrombosis, in so-called 'primary' pulmonary hypertension and in dietary pulmonary hypertension.

The persistently increased pulmonary blood flow of even large left-to-right shunts may be accommodated initially with little rise in mean pulmonary arterial pressure at rest. But further increase in cardiac output with exercise can only be accomplished by increasing the driving pressure through the vascular bed which has already reached the limit of its distensibility due to the presence of the shunt. Thus, over the years, progressive changes in the structure of the pulmonary arterioles and arteries take place in response to the rise in pulmonary artery pressure imposed by such high flows.

Heath and Edwards (1958) have defined six grades of change in the muscular pulmonary arteries and arterioles in vasoactive pulmonary hypertension. The morphological changes which occur are summarized in Table 2.

In large congenital shunts with pulmonary hypertension, the earliest grade of vascular changes represent a persistence of the fetal characteristics of the pulmonary circulation. In the large arteries elastic fibres continue to predominate. Within the muscular pulmonary arteries and arterioles, the changes associated with high blood flow rates from birth continue as a gradual increase in thickness of the muscular media, sandwiched between distinct internal and external elastic laminae. These changes largely protect the vascular structures distal to the site of increase resistance at arteriolar level, so that the veins are largely unaffected.

Table 2 Pathological changes in hypertensive pulmonary vascular disease leading to 'plexogenic pulmonary arteriopathy'

	Grade of hypertensive pulmonary vascular disease					
	1	2	3	4	5	6
Type of intimal reaction	← None →					
		←————————— Cellular —————————→				
			←——— Fibrous and fibroelastic ———→			
				←——— 'Plexiform lesion' ———→		
State of media of arteries and arterioles	←——————————— Hypertrophied ———————————→					
			←——— Some generalized dilation ———→			
				←——— Local 'dilation lesions' ——→		
					←——— PH* ———→	
						←— NA† —→

Taken from Harris and Heath (1977) Table 16.1.
* Pulmonary haemosiderosis associated with distended, thin-walled arterial vessels throughout the lung.
† Necrotizing arteritis.

All the subsequent pathological changes (Grades 2–6) are thought by Harris and Heath to represent the secondary pathological effects of the pulmonary hypertension itself.

If the intramural vascular tone maintained by the contractile fibres of the media remains persistently severe, than patchy death of medial cells takes place, allowing fibrinogen to penetrate the vessel walls from the bloodstream. The presence of fibrin in the walls of the pulmonary arterioles stimulates local myofibroblasts to form 'onion-skin' proliferations of concentrically arranged collagen and elastin lamellae. The medial and intimal hyperplasia which results leads to local and vascular obstructions as well as patches of fibrinoid necrosis.

The process leads on to the formation of a number of different 'dilation lesions', shown diagramatically in Fig. 1. Heath distinguishes three main types:

(a) Vein-like branches of hypertrophied muscular pulmonary arteries These usually emerge from parent arteries proximal to a point of obstruction from any cause. For instance, they can be found in pulmonary vascular obstruction from Bilharzia. The new vessels act as collateral channels to supply the alveolar capillaries.

(b) Angiomatoid lesions These are very rare and have only been seen in pulmonary hypertension associated with ventricular septal defects. They arise in small pulmonary arteries just proximal to points of fibrotic occlusion.

(c) Plexiform lesions These consist of complex distensions of the smallest pulmonary arteries to form thin walled sacs with connections to the alveolar capillaries. Endothelial proliferation and thrombosis often occur within them. The site of their development in relation to local areas of microvascular occlusion raises the question that precapillary anastomoses with bronchial arterioles could be implicated. Heath considers this to be unlikely.

Only a small proportion of patients with congenital left-to-right cardiac shunts go on to develop severe pulmonary vascular disease with plexiform lesions. Once the stage of concentric-laminar intimal proliferation, plexiform, and other dilation lesions has developed, the obstructive process has become so advanced that pulmonary vascular resistance rises rapidly, producing the clinical and radiological associations of a low cardiac output, reversal of the intracardiac shunt with cyanosis, and increased peripheral vascular radiotranslucency.

As already mentioned above plexiform pulmonary arteriopathy is also found in the rare combination of pulmonary hypertension associated with liver cirrhosis and some cases of hepatic portal vein thrombosis. In both conditions release of vasodilator substances from the liver may be responsible, for hepatic failure is often terminally associated with a high cardiac output state.

Plexiform lesions do not occur in pulmonary hypertension secondary to obstruction to pulmonary venous outflow as in mitral stenosis, nor in pulmonary thromboembolic disease.

Because plexogenic pulmonary arteriopathy is also a common terminal finding in patients dying from 'primary' pulmonary hypertension, the elucidation of the pathogenic stimulus leading to the formation of the lesions could be important for diagnostic and therapeutic reasons.

5. Necrotizing arteritis occurs very rarely. It is found only in most extreme cases of pulmonary hypertension from any cause.

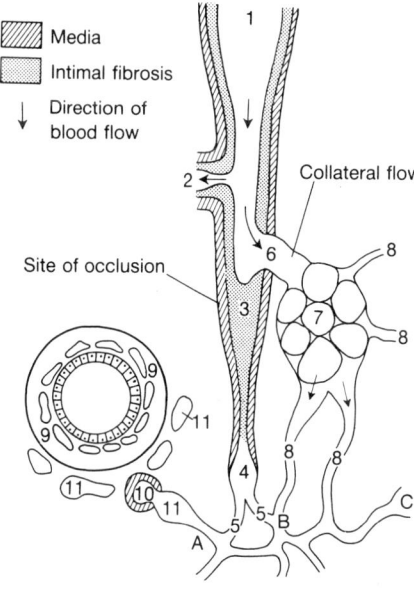

Fig. 1 Diagram to show the origin and probable connections of small, thin-walled blood vessels in the lung in grade 5 hypertensive pulmonary vascular disease. 1 = Dilated muscular pulmonary artery with thin media and intimal fibrosis: this is part of the generalized dilation proximal to the site of vascular occlusion. 2 = Hypertrophied muscular pulmonary artery arising as a side branch of 1 with heaped-up intimal fibrous tissue at the site of origin. 3 = Terminal muscular pulmonary artery totally occluded by fibrous tissue: the media may be thick, as shown, or abnormally thin. 4 = Terminal dilated pulmonary arteriole. 5 = Capillaries in alveolar walls arising from pulmonary arteriole. 6 = Dilated, thin-walled, vein-like branch of hypertrophied parent muscular pulmonary artery. 7 = Localized 'dilation lesion': an angiomatoid lesion is shown. 8 = Capillaries in alveolar walls arising from dilation lesions. 9 = Dilated thin-walled vessel in sub-mucosa of small bronchus. 10 = Small bronchial artery in fibrous coat of small bronchus giving rise to thin-walled branches shown as 11. A = Broncho-pulmonary anastomosis at capillary level. B = Anastomosis between capillaries arising from parent muscular pulmonary artery and from 'dilation lesions'. C = Possible anastomosis between thin-walled vessels derived from pulmonary artery and those derived from pulmonary vein. (Reproduced by permission from Harris and Heath, 1977, *The human pulmonary circulation*. Churchill Livingstone, Edinburgh.)

The changes in the pulmonary circulation are equivalent to the changes found in the systemic circulation in malignant hypertension. The muscular pulmonary arteries show acute fibrinoid necrosis. The necrotic muscle induces an inflammatory invasion by polymorphonuclear leukocytes with a few eosinophils. Granulation tissue replaces the whole vessel with ultimate fibrotic obliteration of the vessel, sometimes with infiltration by new capillaries.

Clinical features of pulmonary hypertension

Because pulmonary hypertension so rarely occurs as an independent entity, symptoms and signs relating to the causal disease predominate in the milder cases. As the severity of the pulmonary hypertension increases it modifies, and ultimately dominates the usual clinical signs of the causative disease. Thus in severe pulmonary hypertensive disease from mitral stenosis, cardiac output is greatly reduced and the usual mitral diastolic murmur may disappear because diastolic flow velocity through the valve may be so low that turbulent flow never develops (the low Reynolds number is maintained). In congenital heart disease, left-to-right shunt flows will become lower and lower as right and left heart pressures equalize as a result of the pulmonary hypertension. Thus, the usual diastolic flow murmur heard in atrial septal defect may disappear; in ventricular septal defects pansystolic left-to-right shunt murmurs will tend to shorten and become quieter, while in persistent patent ductus arteriosus the continuous murmur will disappear.

Intense fatigue, breathlessness even at rest, and faintness on exertion, often culminating in syncope, are all features of severe pulmonary hypertension.

Chest pain resembling angina of effort may arise as a result of the high right ventricular workload and reduced coronary blood flow associated with the low output capability of the right ventricle, overloaded by the pulmonary hypertension. A small volume pulse, peripheral vasoconstriction, cool extremities, and peripheral cyanosis all reflect the low cardiac output state.

Haemoptysis with episodes of pleural pain suggests recurrent pulmonary embolism. Haemoptyses without pain occur in severe pulmonary venous hypertension and also in the late stages of plexogenic arteriopathy.

Central cyanosis is not a feature of pulmonary hypertension, unless associated with reversal of a previous left-to-right intracardiac shunt. However, if a patient presents with dyspnoea at rest, central cyanosis, and clinical signs of pulmonary hypertension, but no evidence of an intracardiac shunt, then occult recurrent pulmonary embolism is a likely diagnosis. Support for this can be acquired quite simply from arterial blood gas analysis; for if both a low PO_2 *and* low PCO_2 is found, serious ventilation perfusion mismatch exists.

The severity of pulmonary hypertension, particularly venous pulmonary hypertension can be assessed clinically quite accurately if simple clinico-physiological principles are followed. Thus the physician first examining a patient with breathlessness from mitral stenosis can be fairly sure of significant pulmonary venous hypertension if basal lung crepitations can be heard under stable resting conditions. Evidence of increased pulmonary venous and transcapillary hydrostatic pressures is also obtained from the chest X-ray if redistribution of the venous vascular shadows from the base to apex is found, particularly if also associated with the presence of Kerley B lines.

Significant pulmonary arterial hypertension is present if the pulmonary arterial component of the second heart sound is accentuated. The high diastolic pressure due to severe pulmonary arterial hypertension will lead to forceful closure of the pulmonary valve with an accentuated, often palpable, pulmonary closure sound which may be audible at the apex. A further auscultatory clue to the pulmonary arterial hypertension can be obtained from the relationship between the aortic and pulmonary components of the second heart sound during expiration. The closer the pulmonary second sound approaches the aortic component, the higher the pulmonary artery pressure is likely to be, provided right bundle branch block is not present.

Plainly, long-standing pulmonary hypertension will lead to right ventricular hypertrophy, an increasingly palpable right ventricular heave and the presence of an increasingly prominent right atrial 'a' wave transmitted to the neck veins because of the increased force of the right atrial systolic contraction needed to overcome the elevated end-diastolic right ventricular pressure of an increasingly embarrassed right ventricle. Atrial fibrillation will develop at some stage, but is often quite a late manifestation.

A right ventricular third heart sound, often with an (atrial) fourth sound superimposed, leads to a summation gallop being heard. The pulmonary valve may become incompetent in severe pulmonary hypertension, leading to the presence of a basal diastolic murmur which may become louder on inspiration. An early pulmonary systolic ejection sound or even a short murmur may be heard when there is significant dilation of the main pulmonary trunk. This may sometimes be confused with the presence of a soft systolic murmur, increasing during inspiration, due to the development of tricuspid valve incompetence, verified by the presence of a right ventricular 'v' wave visible in the jugular venous pulse.

Investigations in pulmonary hypertension

The chest X-ray
(See page 13.16). This commonly shows little overall cardiac enlargement until heart failure supervenes, or unless the causative condition itself is responsible for specific chamber enlargement. Enlargement of the main pulmonary trunk is usual but variable. It causes a prominent convexity of the upper left mediastinum between the aortic knuckle and the upper left border of the heart (left ventricle and left atrial appendage). The left and right main pulmonary arteries and their proximal branches are also enlarged. In contrast, in severe pulmonary hypertension, the peripheral pulmonary arteries appear to have been pruned so that they are much narrower than normal. This leads to increased radiological translucency peripherally.

The size of the peripheral pulmonary arteries also helps the clinican decide whether or not there is a high pulmonary blood flow. Thus, patients with large septal defects and hyperdynamic pulmonary hypertension show plethoric lung fields with engorged peripheral vessels, whereas patients who are developing a low output state from pulmonary hypertension associated with severe vascular changes will show conspicuous peripheral vascular pruning, as in congenital septal defects with the Eisenmenger syndrome (see page 13.256) or in 'primary' pulmonary hypertension.

The appearance of the lung fields will also give clues to the association of pulmonary hypertension with primary lung disease, such as emphysema; with areas of increased density from fibrosis; or areas of increased translucency from pulmonary embolism.

The electrocardiogram
This shows the pattern of right ventricular hypertrophy (page 13.25) with right axis deviation (more than $+ 120°$) in the limb leads, dominant R and T inversion in the right precordial leads, and a dominant S wave in the left precordial leads. Right atrial enlargement is shown by tall, often peaked P waves in right precordial leads and in the inferior leads.

The pattern may be modified when pulmonary venous hypertension is also present from mitral stenosis, for the associated dilation and hypertrophy of the left atrium will lead to the development of bifid P waves and a negative terminal deflection in lead V_1.

If both left and right ventricular hypertrophy is present, as in large ventricular septal defects with pulmonary hypertension, then tall R waves will be found in the left precordial leads with large biphasic RS complexes in the mid-precordial leads, indicating biventricular hypertrophy. In cor pulmonale the electrocardiograph is a remarkably insensitive aid in the diagnosis of right ventricular hypertrophy from pulmonary hypertension. The increased residual lung volume of emphysema associated with chronic obstructive lung disease leads to diaphragmatic depression with the result that the heart tends to hang vertically and rotate clockwise. This may be recognized by inversion of both the right and left unipolar limb leads associated with deep S waves in both.

Right bundle branch block is common. In pulmonary hypertension from congenital atrial septal defects, it will be present from birth. In septum secundum defects the terminal portion of the QRS complex will be orientated anteriorly (producing an rsR′ in V_1) and rightward (producing a permanent S wave in lead 1). Left axis deviation in a young patient with a right ventricular conduction defect, pulmonary hypertension, and a tendency to cyanosis with exercise suggests the presence of an ostium primum atrial septal defect.

The echocardiograph
This has two useful roles. The first, and less important, assists in assessing the severity of the pulmonary hypertension. The pulmonary valve echo tends to show a reduced 'a' wave excursion, an increased 'b' to 'c' slope, a prolonged right ventricular pre-ejection period and a mid-systolic notch. However echocardiographic visualization of the pulmonary valve is notoriously difficult and the findings, when obtained, show poor correlation with the severity of the pulmonary hypertension. Assessment of right ventricular cavity size and right ventricular wall thickness is also somewhat unreliable because it is often difficult to obtain clear chamber definition. This is because of interference from overlying lung tissue, particularly in patients with emphysema.

The second, major, use of echocardiography is in finding the underlying cause of the pulmonary hypertension. Thus in venous pulmonary hypertension, it helps to verify the presence and severity of mitral stenosis and to exclude rarer conditions such as left atrial myxoma and cor triatriatum. In hyperdynamic pulmonary hypertension particularly when used with contrast enhancement, echocardiography is a remarkably precise non-invasive tool for localizing and defining the size of intracardiac septal defects.

Cardiac catheterization
Catheterization enables one to quantify the severity of pulmonary hypertension, to relate this to pulmonary blood flow, to calculate pulmonary vascular resistance, and to obtain direct evidence of pulmonary venous and left atrial pressures. These measurements combined with pulmonary angiography, which has the risk of precipitating acute right heart failure or ventricular fibrillation from sudden pump overload from the injectate, may be essential if accurate diagnosis is needed in difficult cases of unexplained severe pulmonary hypertension.

Arterial blood gas analysis
The usefulness of arterial blood gas analysis in differential diagnosis of intracardiac shunts and in detecting ventilation–perfusion abnormalities has already been mentioned. The analyses should be undertaken both at rest and under exercise. *Regional* localization of ventilation–perfusion abnormalities in pulmonary embolism or lung infarction is made using inhaled and injected radioactive markers, combined with gamma scintigraphy. The information should be used only as confirmatory evidence and *not* depended upon as a reliable diagnostic tool.

Lung biopsy
Biopsy has an important but restricted place in the diagnosis of otherwise unexplained pulmonary hypertension. The use of the fibreoptic bronchoscope allows transbronchial biopsy specimens to be obtained. These are unsatisfactory for tissue diagnostic purposes in cases of obscure pulmonary hypertension. Open biopsy, from several different sites is needed for accuracy. This inevitably imposes risks to patients who have often already reached the limit of their cardiorespiratory reserve. Lung biopsy should therefore be reserved only for those cases where there is deep doubt about the aetiology of the pulmonary hypertension associated with

Table 3 Aetiological diagnosis in pulmonary hypertension

1 Conditions leading to pulmonary venous hypertension
  (a) *Chronic left ventricular failure* from any cause
  (b) *Left atrial outflow obstruction*
      Mitral valve disease
      Obstructive cardiomyopathy
      Constricting pericarditis
      Left atrial myxoma
      Left atrial thrombus or tumours
      Cor triatriatum
  (c) *Pulmonary venous occlusive disease*
      Idiopathic pulmonary venous thrombosis or venous thrombosis secondary to neoplastic disease
2 Conditions leading to pulmonary arterial hypertension
  (a) *Viscous, obstructive and obliterative causes*
      Polycythaemia rubra vera. Sickle cell disease.
      Emphysema, chronic obstructive lung disease
      recurrent thromboembolism. Tumour emboli
  (b) *Reactive vascular responses*
      Sarcoidosis. Systemic sclerosis and CRST disease.
      Goodpasture's syndrome
      Polyarteritis nodosa
      Fibrosing interstitial alveolitis
      Bilharziasis, filariasis, eosinophil granuloma
      Aminorex fumarate and adulterated rapeseed oil ingestion
  (c) *Vasoconstrictive causes*
      Chronic hypoxia
      Raynaud's phenomenon of the lung in systemic sclerosis
      Hepatic cirrhosis. Hepatic portal vein thrombosis
      Serotonin release from carcinoid syndrome
      Eisenmenger response to large left-to right shunts from birth
      'Primary' pulmonary hypertension
  (d) *Hyperdynamic causes*
      Chronic hypoxia, CO_2 retention and acidosis
      Anaemia
      Left to right heart shunts
      Chronic arteriovenous fistulae
      Paget's disease
      Thyrotoxicosis
      Liver failure
      Beri-beri

serious apprehension that a remediable cause is being missed, such as sarcoidosis or polyarteritis nodosa or recurrent pulmonary embolism. Even here it could be argued that a therapeutic trial of drugs such as steroids or immunosuppressants combined with oral coagulants is a less hazardous course to follow.

The aetiological diagnosis of pulmonary hypertension
Usually, even in severe pulmonary hypertension leading to right heart failure, the clinician will have little difficulty in linking the condition to appropriate underlying causal factors if he or she is methodical. Table 3 attempts this by means of a pathophysiological approach. The reader is referred to appropriate chapters for full accounts of the diseases listed.

Conditions leading to pulmonary venous hypertension
Disorders of left ventricular function
Chronic left ventricular strain from severe *systemic hypertension, or aortic valve disease* will ultimately lead to the left ventricular failure, venous hypertension and pulmonary oedema. The manifestations and management of pulmonary oedema are considered on page 13.334.

Ischaemic heart disease and the broad group of *congestive cardiomyopathies* will also present with symptoms and signs of left ventricular failure with or without a history of effort angina. Clinical, radiological, and echocardiographic evidence of left heart hypertrophy and chamber dilation will be found. A gallop rhythm and third heart sound will be present. The electrocardiograph may show changes of ischaemia at rest. An electrocardiograph following maximum tolerable exercise should be undertaken where ischaemic heart disease is suspected without typical findings.

Acute regional constriction of the left ventricle by an acute *pericardial effusion*, particularly in patients with chronic renal failure maintained on dialysis therapy, may develop a low cardiac output state with pulmonary oedema. The effusion is readily detected by echocardiography. Aspiration of the fluid percutaneously is difficult. In severe cases, open drainage will be needed, but often moderate doses of prednisone produce resorption. *Constricting pericarditis* will present with similar, but less acute, symptoms and signs. When unexplained pulmonary oedema occurs without left heart enlargement and without infection as a basis, consider *obstructive left ventricular cardiomyopathy*. This is usually associated with a collapsing pulse and a late systolic murmur best heard to the left of the sternum. Echocardiography confirms its presence. Obstructive cardiomyopathy having been excluded, proceed to consider other causes of left atrial and pulmonary venous obstruction.

Left atrial outflow obstruction

Mitral stenosis is the commonest cause and difficulties in recognizing it in severe pulmonary venous and arterial hypertension with low cardiac output have already been mentioned. The echocardiograph enables the diagnosis to be confirmed and other left atrial obstructive lesions excluded, such as *left atrial myxoma*, ball thrombi in the left atrium, tumours, and *cor triatriatum* (see also page 13.334).

Pulmonary veno-occlusive disease is extremely difficult to diagnose. It is thought to be rare, but this may be due to failure of recognition. The clinical features are the same as those in patients with severe 'primary' pulmonary hypertension, though often complicated by the presence of pulmonary oedema and pleural effusions. Proof of diagnosis may be difficult. Cardiac catheterization reveals an elevated pulmonary artery pressure. Difficulty in obtaining a clearly transmitted left atrial pressure wave form from a pulmonary artery wedge pressure tracing should alert suspicion. The left atrial pressure measured directly by the trans-septal route will be normal, thus excluding tight mitral stenosis and other left atrial disorders. Pulmonary artery angiography shows regions of poor perfusion where the thromboses are present. Open lung biopsy shows occlusion of individual veins by organized thrombus, fibrosis, and some recanalization. Engorged hyperplastic lymphatics are found in profusion. The aetiology of venous thrombo-occlusive disease is not known but it may sometimes occur as a subsidiary manifestation of polyarteritis nodosa, other connective tissue disorders or occult neoplastic disease. Prognosis is poor. Treatment is palliative with diuretics and long-term anticoagulants.

Conditions leading to pulmonary arterial hypertension independent of venous hypertension

By far the commonest cause of pulmonary arterial hypertension is *chronic obstructive lung disease* associated with hypoxia, often acutely exacerbated by acute respiratory infections (see page 13.350).

Recurrent systemic venous thromboembolism is the next most common cause of pulmonary arterial hypertension. Recurrent attacks of breathlessness, often with pleuritic pain and haemoptysis, with or without manifestations of leg vein thrombosis, suggest the diagnosis. But insidious onset of the more protean symptoms of pulmonary hypertension, namely, unexplained breathlessness, fatigue, signs of right ventricular overload, and a low cardiac output state are equally common. *These are the presenting symptoms of all unexplained cases of pulmonary hypertension.* Aetiological diagnosis is by exclusion, the term 'primary' pulmonary hypertension being confined to those cases where no

aetiological factor can be found. For further information on chronic thromboembolic pulmonary hypertension refer to page 13.355.

Pulmonary hypertension from large intracardiac shunts has been discussed elsewhere in this chapter. When severe pulmonary hypertension has reached the stage of plexogenic arteriopathy, haemoptyses are not infrequent. By this stage a low cardiac output state will have developed as well, with balance or reversal of the intracardiac shunt so that central cyanosis will be a guiding sign to the underlying congenital heart lesion.

Polycythaemia, by increasing blood viscosity, will exacerbate pulmonary hypertension in the cyanotic stages of previously hyperdynamic congenital heart disease as well as in *cor pulmonale* and in *polycythaemia rubra vera*. The polycythaemia also increases the risks of further deterioration from intravascular thrombosis. A therapeutic compromise has to be reached between the need to maintain compensatory augmentation to oxygen transport capacity and the wish to reduce viscous resistance to pulmonary blood flow. Regular venesection to maintain the haemoglobin level in the region of 17 g per cent appears helpful in reducing right ventricular load. Long-term oral anticoagulants are also advisable.

Tropical disease and pulmonary arterial hypertension

Severe *sickle cell disease* particularly in the young, may be associated with sequestration crises. Red cell sequestration in the lungs, with resulting increased viscosity, vascular stasis, and even complete blockage of the microvasculature may occur leading to local areas of infarction and acute pulmonary hypertension. Recurrent episodes can lead to microvascular destruction, fibrosis, and chronic hypertensive changes.

Pulmonary arterial hypertension from tropical parasitic infestations excite complex partially immune inflammatory responses with the formation of granulomata in the lungs as in Bilharziasis from *Schistosoma mansoni* but less commonly from *Schistosoma japonica* infestation. The early symptoms are allergic with attacks of asthma with sputum and mild fever. Slowly severe pulmonary hypertension develops, leading to chronic right heart failure within a few years. There is also liver involvement with cirrhotic change and ascites.

Particularly in the Far East, *filariasis* and *tropical eosinophilia* associated with helminth infestations other than filariasis produce both an allergic and granulomatous response to the larvae, with scattered lesions in the lung substance, liver, and sometimes the lymph glands. Again, attacks of asthma, often with purulent blood streaked sputum, are the presenting symptoms. Gradually the insidious symptoms of fatigue and breathlessness herald the development of pulmonary hypertension. A careful history should alert the clinician to the possibility of tropical parasitic exposure, particularly if associated with a high eosinophil percentage in the differential white count.

Virtually all other causes of pulmonary arterial hypertension listed in Table 3 present insidiously and their differentiation from one another and from unexplained 'primary' *pulmonary hypertension* nearly always present difficulty. The remainder of this chapter will therefore consider them together with the latter condition.

Unexplained or 'primary' pulmonary hypertension

Few aetiological clues are obtained from the history, with the rare exceptions of pulmonary hypertension associated with recent dietary disasters, such as the European 'epidemic' of pulmonary hypertension in the mid 1960s due to the slimming agent 'aminorex fumarate' and the Spanish outbreak in 1981 from the *ingestion of adulterated rape seed oil* for cooking.

These two examples illustrate the importance of a meticulous history in the search for causes, including enquiry into drug usage. For example. the chemical structure of aminorex fumarate was found to be closely related to that of adrenaline and amphetamine. Some herbals are suspect, particularly those containing pyrrolizidine alkaloids. Experimental animals fed foliage and seeds of the species Crotalaria and Senecio develop pulmonary hypertension from muscularization of their pulmonary arterioles with necrotizing arteritis. The common ragwort, Senecio jacobaea, contains such alkaloids. It can be bought from any health store.

Pulmonary hypertension complicating *cirrhosis of the liver and portal venous hypertension* is possibly more likely to occur in patients treated surgically with portocaval shunts. Vasoactive substances released from the failing liver have been suggested as a cause, but without evidence.

Pulmonary hypertension may be a complicating manifestation of an increasing spectrum of *autoimmune* diseases affecting the lung. The list given in Table 3 is by no means complete, for instance, pulmonary interstitial disease and pulmonary hypertension may occur in *rheumatoid arthritis* and in association with an increasing number of connective tissue disorders, in *Goodpasture's syndrome*, *polyarteritis nodosa*, and *fibrosing alveolitis*. Pulmonary hypertension may also occasionally develop as a late sequel post-partum, following the complication of *amniotic fluid embolism*.

'Primary' pulmonary hypertension is likely to become a diminishing clinical entity as knowledge increases. It occurs at all ages, but particularly in younger adults. In adults the condition is four times commoner in women than in men, though in children the sexes are involved in roughly equal numbers. The disease is occasionally familial, occurring in siblings or in parent and child.

The symptoms and signs are those of severe pulmonary hypertension of whatever cause and have been described in previous sections.

The course, prognosis, and management of pulmonary hypertension

Mild and moderate degrees of pulmonary hypertension are usually asymptomatic and there may be few abnormal signs. Primary pulmonary hypertension is commonly far advanced before it is recognized, for the symptoms of fatigue and weight loss are so protean that the clinician fails to recognize the condition till overt symptoms of cardiorespiratory embarrassment develop. Deterioration is rapid. Most patients whose mean pulmonary artery pressure at rest is greater than 6 kPa (50 mmHg) are dead within five years. Treatment is palliative and, at best, delays the relentless course of the disease with progressive right heart failure. Death may be sudden from lethal cardiac arrhythmias or from pulmonary embolism.

Long-term anticoagulants are therefore logical to use, but care must be exercised because of deteriorating liver function from congestive heart failure. Diuretics assist in the control of systemic oedema. The patient's breathlessness, of reflex origin and rarely associated with cyanosis, is not particularly relieved by oxygen, though its effect in relieving vasoconstriction has theoretical sense. Palliative relief of breathlessness at rest, particularly to assist sleep at night in terminal cases, may require opiates.

Vasodilator drugs given intravenously have been shown to produce temporary reduction in pulmonary vascular resistance (e.g. prostacycline, diazoxide, phentolamine). Long-term administration of oral agents such as hydralazine in increasing doses three to four times a day to a limit compatible with reasonable maintenance of the systemic arterial pressure, is reported to be effective in some cases. An equal number of reports can be found contradicting this finding. The use of calcium-inhibiting agents, particularly nifedipine in oral doses of 20 mg thrice daily, is also currently fashionable for primary pulmonary hypertension.

Selecting patients with pulmonary hypertension who are most likely to respond beneficially to long-term oral vasodilators is best achieved at the time of diagnostic cardiac catheterization by testing whether or not there is an acute vasodilator response to oxygen breathing and to intravenous challenge with phentolamine 5 mg intravenously, given slowly over 10 min.

Once pulmonary hypertension has reached the stage of having

developed vascular occlusive changes with fibrosis and microvascular necrosis, vasodilator drug therapy of any kind is likely to be largely ineffective. The best hope depends on very early diagnosis, in turn dependent on constant awareness that protean symptoms of weariness, weight loss, and periods of unexplained malaise could possibly be associated with one or other of the occult causes of vasoactive or reactive pulmonary arterial hypertension. If spotted early, the granulopathies in particular may well respond to appropriate medication, assisted by vasodilator drugs used when early vasoactive vascular pathology still predominates.

Prophylactic long-term oral anticoagulant treatment to prevent superadded intrapulmonary microvascular thromboses from imposing further deterioration is particulary important.

Experience of combined heart–lung transplantation is as yet small, but in some selected patients has had limited success.

References

Asherson, R. A., Mackworth-Young, C. G., Boey, M. L. *et al.* (1983). Pulmonary hypertension in systemic lupus erythematosus. *Br. med. J.* **287**, 1024–1025.

Camerini, F., Alberti, E., Klugman, S. *et al.* (1980). Primary pulmonary hypertension effects of nifedipine. *Br. Heart J.* **44**, 352–356.

Cohen, M. L. and Kronzon, I., (1981). Adverse hemodynamic effects of phentolamine in primary pulmonary hypertension. *Ann. int. Med.* **95**, 591–592.

Collins, F. S. and Orringer, E. P. (1982). Pulmonary hypertension and cor pulmonale in the sickle hemoglobinopathies. *Am. J. Med.* **73**, 814–821.

Cotter, L. (1984). Vasodilator treatment of primary pulmonary hypertension. *Adv. exp. med. Biol.* **164**, 359–368.

Douglas, J. G., Munro, J. F., Kitchin, A. H. *et al.* (1981). Pulmonary hypertension and fenfuramine. *Br. med. J.* **283**, 881–883.

Fahey, P. H., Utell, M. J., Condemi, J. J., Green, R. and Hyde, R. W. (1984). Raynaud's phenomenon of the lung. *Am. J. Med.* **76**, 263–269.

Fishman, A. P. and Pietra, G. G. (1980). Primary pulmonary hypertension. *Ann. Rev. Med.* **31**, 421–431.

Gessner, U. (1972). Vascular input impedance. In *Cardiovascular fluid dynamics* Vol. 1 (ed. D. H. Bergel) pp. 315–349. Academic Press, London, New York.

Gurtner, H. P. (1979). Pulmonary hypertension, 'plexogenic pulmonary arteriopathy' and the appetite depressant drug aminorex: post or propter? *Bull. Physiopathol. Respir. (Nancy)* **15**, 897–923.

Harris, P. and Heath, D. (1977). *The human pulmonary circulation*. Churchill-Livingstone, Edinburgh.

Kennedy, T. P., Michael, J. R., Huang, C-K. *et al.* (1984). Nifedipine inhibits hypoxic pulmonary vasoconstriction during rest in patients with chronic obstructive pulmonary disease: a controlled double-blind study. *Am. Rev. Resp. Dis.* **129**, 544–551.

Klinke, W. P. (1980). Treatment of primary pulmonary hypertension. *Am. Heart J.* **100**, 587–588.

Lockhart, A., and Reeves, J. T. (1984). Plexogenic pulmonary hypertension of unknown origin. What's new? *Clin. Sci.* **67**, 1–5.

Lupi-Herreran, E., Sandoval, J., Seoane, M. and Bialostozky, D. (1982). The role of hydralazine therapy for pulmonary arterial hypertension of unknown cause. *Circulation* **65**, 645–650.

—— E., Seone, M. and Verdejo, A. (1984). Hemodynamic effect of hydralazine in advanced, stable chronic obstructive pulmonary disease with cor pulmonale. Immediate and short-term evaluation at rest and during exercise. *Chest* **85**, 156–163.

Noriega, A. R., Gomez-Reino, J., Lopez-Encuentra, A. *et al.* (1982). Toxic epidemic syndrome. Spain 1981. *Lancet* **ii**, 697–702.

Person, B. and Procter, R. J. (1979). Primary pulmonary hypertension response to indomethazine, terbutaline and isoproterenol. *Chest* **76**, 601–603.

Poderoso, J. J., Biancolini, C. A., Del Bosco, C. G. *et al.* (1983). Captopril versus hydralazine in primary pulmonary hypertension. *J. Clin. Pharmacol.* **23**, 563–566.

Rabinovitch, M., Keane, J. F., Norwood, W. I., Castaneda, A. R. and Reid, L. (1984). Vasculature structure in lung tissue obtained at biopsy correlated with pulmonary haemodynamic findings after repair of congenital heart defects. *Circulation* **69**, 655–667.

Rich, S., Martinez, J., Lamb, W. and Rosen, K. M. (1982). Captopril as treatment for patients with pulmonary hypertension. *Br. Heart. J.* **48**, 272–277.

Rose, A. G. (1983). Pulmonary veno-occlusive disease due to bleomycin therapy for lymphoma. *S. Afr. Med. J.* **64**, 636–638.

Ruskin, J. M. and Hutter, A. M., Jr (1979). Primary pulmonary hypertension treated with oral phentolamine. *Ann. Int. Med.* **90**, 772–774.

Sokolow, M and McIlroy, M. B. (1982). *Clinical cardiology.* Lange, Los Altos.

Tsoue, E., Waldhorn, R. E., Kerwin, D. M., Katz, S. and Patterson, J. A., (1984). Pulmonary veno-occlusive disease in pregnancy. *Obs. Gyn.* **64**, 281–284.

Ungerer, R. G., Tashkih, D. P., Furst, D. *et al.* (1983). Prevalence and clinical correlates of pulmonary arterial hypertension in progressive systemic sclerosis. *Am. J. Med.* **75**, 65–74.

Cor pulmonale

J. S. PRICHARD

Introduction

The term cor pulmonale denotes right heart failure associated with a wide variety of diseases of the lung parenchyma, airways, thoracic cage, and respiratory control mechanisms, The association has been recognized since the middle of the nineteenth century and a variety of expressions such as 'pulmonary heart disease', 'emphysema heart', and 'black cardiacs' has been used. However, from the time of the introduction of the term cor pulmonale in the 1950s, there have been attempts to emphasize hypertrophy of the right ventricle rather than actual cardiac failure, as in the WHO definition of 1961 which was 'hypertrophy of the right ventricle resulting from diseases affecting the function and/or structure of the lung, except where these pulmonary alterations are the result of diseases that primarily affect the left side of the heart'. The definition makes no reference to occlusive pulmonary vascular diseases and although these have been included in cor pulmonale by some authors, they will not be discussed here.

The view adopted here is that right heart hypertrophy and eventual failure are consequences of a high afterload produced by pulmonary hypertension and that the hypertension is itself a result of physiological and anatomical changes in the lung caused by the primary disease. It is necessary to distinguish between

(*a*) *Pulmonary arterial hypertension* which is the initiating event and which creates the high afterload against which the ventricle must work.

(*b*) Subsequent *hypertrophy of the right ventricle* – cor pulmonale – which is adaptive to the pulmonale hypertension and allows normal cardiac output and filling pressure despite the raised afterload.

(*c*) Eventual *right heart failure* which occurs when the hypertrophied ventricle is no longer able to compensate for the hypertension and venous pressure becomes elevated.

Throughout discussion of cor pulmonale a continuing problem is the use of the term 'right heart failure'. 'Cardiac failure' is a term usually used to denote an inappropriate relationship between venous filling pressure and output which, in cardiac disease, arises from intrinsic damage to the heart. In cor pulmonale, on the other hand, there is no evidence of intrinsic abnormality of the heart; the problem is increased right ventricular afterload and there may even be sufficient functional reserve for the cardiac output to increase in response to hypoxia and exercise (see also page 13.326).

Pathological changes

The lungs

Cor pulmonale may be secondary to many diseases (Table 1) and the features of one or more of these will therefore be present. In the diseases of the parenchyma and airways, marked pulmonary pathology may be seen but where the problems are those of the thoracic cage, of neuromuscular disease or of the respiratory control mechanisms, lung damage may be very slight. However, a

Table 1 Diseases associated with cor pulmonale

Diseases of the lung parenchyma and intrathoracic airways
  Chronic obstructive lung disease
  Asthma (severe, recurrent or chronic)
  Bronchiectasis (including cystic fibrosis)
  Pulmonary interstitial fibrosing and granulomatous diseases

*Occlusive pulmonary vascular disease**
  Multiple pulmonary emboli
  Schistosomiasis
  Filariasis, tropical eosinophilia
  Sickle cell disease

Disorders of the thoracic cage
  Kyphosis (particularly when deformity angle >100°)
  Scoliosis (particularly when deformity angle >120°)
  Thoracoplasty
  Pleural fibrosis

Neuromuscular disease
  Poliomyelitis
  Myasthenia gravis
  Amyotrophic lateral sclerosis
  Myopathies and muscular dystrophy

Disturbance of respiratory control
  Idiopathic hypoventilation syndrome
  Obesity–hypoventilation syndrome
  Cerebrovascular disease

*Obstruction of extrathoracic airways**
  Tonsils and adenoids in children

* These causes of cor pulmonale are not discussed in this chapter.

common pattern of abnormalities of the smaller pulmonary blood vessels can be found wherever cor pulmonale has developed. This comprises the development of longitudinal muscle in the intima of pulmonary arterioles and muscular pulmonary arteries, the formation of a distinct media of circular muscle in the pulmonary arterioles and medial hypertrophy in the muscular pulmonary arteries. Of these, muscularization of the arterioles appears to be the lesion most closely associated with the development of pulmonary hypertension and right ventricular hypertrophy. These changes were first and most clearly identified in chronic obstructive airflow disease but have been noted in all conditions characterized by chronic hypoxia including kyphoscoliosis, the obesity hypoventilation syndrome, and persistent residence at high altitudes.

The right ventricle

Right ventricular hypertrophy is the hallmark of cor pulmonale but its extent varies greatly. Increases in weight range from slightly above normal (60 g) to as high as 200 g whilst the ratio of left ventricular weight (plus septum) to that of the right ventricle may fall below 2.5 and the right ventricular wall thickness may become greater than 0.5 cm. These figures and ratios are only approximate for, particularly in the case of the ventricular weight ratio, the pattern may be totally obscured by other co-existing disease, such as hypertension or ischaemic vascular disease, which may affect the left heart.

The left heart

A number of studies have shown that the left ventricle becomes hypertrophied in patients with cor pulmonale even where there is no atheromatous, hypertensive or valvular disease. This may be a response to hypoxia and/or erythrocytosis.

The carotid body

In chronic hypoxia, the carotid body becomes enlarged as a result of an increased number of chief cells. The clinical significance of this hypertrophy is not known.

The pathogenesis of cor pulmonale

As the majority of cases of cor pulmonale occur in chronic obstructive lung disease, the view was put forward by Budd in

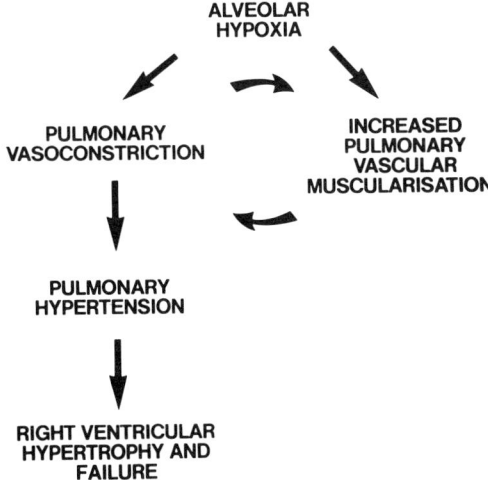

Fig. 1 Pathogenesis of oedema in cor pulmonale.

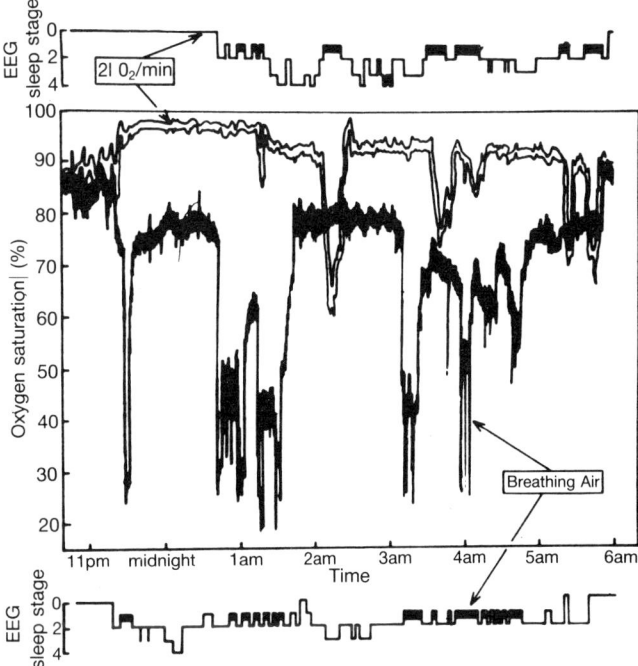

Fig. 2 Oxygen saturation measured by ear oximeter and EEG sleep stage throughout the night in a 'blue-boater' when breathing 2 l O$_2$/min through nasal prongs (above) and when breathing air (below). (Reproduced from Douglas *et al.*, 1979, Transient hypoxaemia during sleep in chronic bronchitis and emphysema. *Lancet* i, 1, with permission. Illustration kindly provided by Professor Flenley.)

1840 that emphysematous destruction of lung parenchyma led to obstruction of pulmonary blood flow because of anatomical reduction of the pulmonary capillary bed. This view held until the 1960s although it was never able to take into account the dynamic nature of changes in pulmonary artery pressures and it produced no explanation for cor pulmonale in diseases where severe lung damage was not a feature. Finally, when methods of quantification of lung pathology became available, it was found that there was no correlation between degree of emphysema or internal lung area or any other index of parenchymal damage and right ventricular hypertrophy.

Evidence now suggests that hypoxia is the initiating event common to all forms of cor pulmonale (Fig. 1). This leads to pulmonary vasoconstriction which causes pulmonary hypertension and increased afterload. Thereafter, hypertrophy and subsequent failure follow. The following evidence supports this hypothesis:

1. Experimentally induced pulmonary hypertension in animals leads rapidly to right ventricular hypertrophy.

2. The inhalation of a gas mixture with a reduced oxygen content so that arterial oxygen tension falls below 7 kPa raises the pulmonary vascular resistance in isolated perfused lungs, in experimental animals, in 60–70 per cent of normal subjects, and patients with lung disease. This phenomenon of *pulmonary hypoxic vasoconstriction*, first clearly described by von Euler and Lillestrand in 1948, differentiates the pulmonary from the systemic circulation. The response arises within lung tissue and is independent of perfusing fluids and the autonomic nervous system. One or more chemical mediators is probably involved since isolated pulmonary artery strips constrict in response to hypoxia only if some lung parenchyma remains adherent. It has been suggested that intrapulmonary chemoceptors must exist to mediate the reaction and, although these have not been identified, circumstantial evidence suggests that an unidentified autocoid released from mast cells may be the proximal cause of vasoconstriction.

3. Patients with *established* cor pulmonale are inevitably hypoxaemic and there is a reasonable correlation between the degree of hypoxaemia and that of ventricular hypertrophy.

4. Long-standing hypoxia causes significant changes in the structure of pulmonary blood vessels so that these become muscularized and more capable of sustained vasomotor activity. This phenomenon, by increasing the muscularity and vasomoticity of the pulmonary circulation, could provide the mechanism by which pulmonary hypertension becomes progressively more severe and self-sustaining.

5. Long-term relief of hypoxia will cause some lowering of even a chronically raised pulmonary vascular resistance.

The problem in accepting this otherwise logical chain of events has

always been the fact that, early in cor pulmonale when right ventricular enlargement can be documented, the pulmonary vascular resistance is often not raised except during periods of exacerbation. Also, right heart hypertrophy may be present before many attacks of decompensation and episodes of pulmonary hypertension have occurred. Observations upon arterial oxygen saturation during sleep provide an hypothesis which seems able to explain the missing link. The studies involve continuous measurement of arterial oxygen saturation in patients with respiratory disease by the use of an ear oximeter (Fig. 2). Oxygen saturation is not stable even during day time but at night, large and rapid changes occur. Episodes of desaturation are particularly likely during periods of rapid eye movement (REM) sleep and, in turn, these are associated with elevated pulmonary arterial pressure and vascular resistance. Not only is each episode of desaturation accompanied by a period of pulmonary hypertension but a stepwise progression of pulmonary artery pressure takes place with each successive episode. It is tempting to see in these periods of pulmonary hypertension the link between lung disease and right ventricular hypertrophy.

Hypoxia, whether from alveolar hypoventilation, ventilation/perfusion imbalance or reduced environmental oxygen is thus the common cause of pulmonary vasoconstriction and cor pulmonale. However, other factors can play a part. Erythrocytosis may be present as a response to hypoxia and, where the haematocrit exceeds 0.55, increased resistance to flow and red cell clumping can become significant. Where pulmonary arteritis is present, as in some collagenoses, this may in itself be a factor increasing pulmonary vascular resistance and, in the CRST variant of systemic sclerosis, myxomatous change in the small and medium-sized pulmonary arteries may have a similar pathophysiological effect. In chronic obstructive lung disease, high expiratory intra-alveolar pressure may be an additional factor and, although not the primary cause, physical destruction of the vascular bed may also contribute. In advanced obstructed airways disease, fewer than 20 per cent of the capillaries and small vessels remain and this reduction may explain the extreme pressure changes which result from small increases in cardiac output.

Clinical features

Natural history

Cor pulmonale occurs in patients in whom there is a long-standing history of hypoxia from disease of the lung parenchyma, airways, thoracic cage or respiratory control mechanisms (Table 1). None is invariably associated with the condition which only develops in the more severe cases in which hypoxia is prominent.

The natural history of the condition consists first of a period in which right ventricular hypertrophy and strain are developing but frank right ventricular failure has not yet occurred. Subsequently, the first attack of right heart decompensation appears and is frequently triggered by an episode of pulmonary infection. The age at which the signs and symptoms first appear is determined largely by the underlying primary pathology and may stretch from adolescence to old age. Similarly, the period of hypoxia and pulmonary arterial hypertension which precedes the onset of cor pulmonale may also vary very greatly from months to years. The right heart failure is usually treated satisfactorily at first but relapses occur with increasing frequency and with less response to treatment until eventually death results. Little is known of the mode or mechanism of death except that it most frequently occurs during a period of heart failure unresponsive to treatment.

In the Western World, the commonest cause is undoubtedly chronic obstructive lung disease (COAD) but even in this disorder fewer than 50 per cent of patients will ever develop right heart hypertrophy and failure. These are usually men presenting in their late 50s and, as might be expected, the disease is commoner amongst the hypoxic 'blue bloaters' than amongst the emphysematous 'pink puffers'. Overall, the incidence of cor pulmonale is largely determined by the prevalence of chronic obstructive lung disease and is commonest where smoking is widely practised and air pollution heavy. In British industrial cities, 30–40 per cent of clinical heart failure a decade ago, arose from this cause whilst comparative figures from Delhi in India were 15 per cent and for the USA only 6–7 per cent. In the 1960s and 1970s between 50 and 60 per cent of patients with COAD and cor pulmonale died within three years of the onset of cardiac failure but most authors are agreed that survival now is probably somewhat longer.

Clinical signs

Apart from the primary disease, the clinical signs are associated with:

(a) Pulmonary hypertension
(b) Right ventricular hypertrophy
(c) Right heart failure

These three constitute a chronological sequence but since the phases merge imperceptibly into each other, no attempt will be made to describe them in order.

In the thorax, the enlarged right ventricle may produce a sternal heave (unless masked by deformity or distortion of the chest wall) while cardiac pulsations may also be felt in the epigastrium. The heart beat may be rapid or irregular for arrhythmias may develop (see below). An emphasis to the pulmonary component of the second heart sound, a pulmonary valvular click and (unless bundle branch block is present) shortening of the interval between the components of the second heart sound all denote pulmonary hypertension. Frequently, when frank right heart failure is present, the systolic murmur of tricuspid incompetence can be heard and a right ventricular third heart sound develops. More rarely, the diastolic murmur of pulmonary incompetence may occur.

Outside the thorax no signs are present until the right heart begins to fail. Then, the central venous pressure becomes raised. It is usually visible as an elevated jugular venous pressure in the neck and if tricuspid incompetence has developed a v-wave can be

Table 2 ECG changes in cor pulmonale

Right axis deviation of mean QRS vector
R/S ratio in V1 >1
R/S ratio in V6 <1
S1, Q3 or S1, S2, S3 patterns
Clockwise rotation
P Pulmonale (increased P wave amplitude in II, III, aV1)
Isoelectric P wave in I or right axis deviation of P vector

Notes
1. The presence of chronic obstructive lung disease and deformity of the chest wall and thoracic cage may confuse ECG interpretation considerably.
2. Arrhythmia and conduction defects are not included.

seen. An enlarged and often tender liver becomes palpable and in the presence of tricuspid incompetence may be pulsatile. Oedema commonly forms in the legs and/or sacrum but appears later in the non-hypercapnic than in the hypercapnic forms of cor pulmonale. Ascites and pleural effusion are relatively rare. Hepatic dysfunction may result but, acutely, this is usually only detectable biochemically. If the heart failure persists, hepatomegaly, cardiac cirrhosis, and splenomegaly may eventually result. In extreme and chronic cases persistently elevated venous pressure may lead to renal dysfunction, proteinuria, and, rarely, nephrotic syndrome.

Routine investigations

Blood gas oxygen tensions are usually in the range 6–7 kPa or lower: arterial carbon dioxide tensions are more variable. If the primary disease is associated with alveolar hypoventilation, hypercapnia is present with carbon dioxide tensions raised to between 8 and 9 kPa (or higher). On the other hand the interstitial lung diseases are associated with hyperventilation and carbon dioxide tensions are below normal. Haematocrit is frequently raised, often above 55 per cent.

Radiological appearances are often dominated by the primary pathology and, particularly where emphysema is present, diaphragmatic descent and increased thoracic diameters may obscure cardiomegaly. When the right ventricle becomes detectable, the left cardiac border is displaced laterally but the apex gives the appearance of pointing upward. In the lateral view, the upward displacement of the right atrium gives an increased density in the upper anterior part of the heart shadow. The central pulmonary arteries are prominent and it has been suggested that, on the standard AP radiograph a diameter of >16 mm for the right pulmonary artery and >19 mm for the left pulmonary artery may be diagnostic of pulmonary hypertension. The more peripheral vessels show rapid tapering. If frank right ventricular failure is present, the superior venacaval and azygos vein shadows may be enlarged.

ECG changes arise from hypertrophy of the right ventricle (particularly the crista supraventricularis) and dilation of the right atrium. The basic changes are set out in Table 2 (see page 13.24) but may often be partially masked by the primary disease. Thus, where obstructive lung disease is present, the diaphragm is depressed, the AP diameter of the chest increased, and the electrical conductivity of the lungs changed. The heart becomes more vertical and rotated left so that the right atrium and right ventricle lie more anteriorly while the apex is more posterior. These features affect the ECG by causing clockwise rotation, low QRS voltage, and, occasionally, large Q or QS waves in the inferior and/or mid-praecordial leads reminiscent of healed myocardial infarction. Similarly, in diseases associated with deformity of the chest wall and thorax, problems arise from alterations in the anatomical position of the heart. Over the spectrum of cor pulmonale, correlation of ECG changes with autopsy proven right ventricular hypertrophy (particularly in the presence of chronic obstructive airways disease) is closest with a frontal plane mean QRS axis between 90° and 180°. Although this produces a high degree of diagnostic accuracy a large number of cases would be missed if this were the only criterion used and assessment of each ECG by reference to a number of features is necessary. Usually about 20 per cent of patients show p-pulmonale (a p-wave >2 mm in standard lead II) whilst between 70 and 80 per cent have a pattern of right ventricular strain or hypertrophy (with a dominant R in V1 or V3 and/or a dominant R in aVr and a dominant S in V5).

Rhythm and conduction disturbances may also be detected. The former are mainly supraventricular and paroxysmal atrial tachycardia, nodal rhythms, and wandering pacemakers are not infrequently seen. Right bundle branch block is the commonest conduction defect.

Pulmonary haemodynamics are assessed by cardiac catheterization (see Table 3). In the early phases changes may be minimal and the pulmonary artery pressure may rise only during exertion or exacerbations. Radionuclide studies, including thallium-201 imaging and first pass angiocardiography may be used to assess right ventricular size and function at an early stage but are not in routine use. Echocardiography may also assist but its application is frequently frustrated by emphysema.

Sleep studies involving continuous transcutaneous oximetry can help in studying patients who have mild hypoxia whilst awake but in whom there is doubt about the cause of pulmonary hypertension.

Body fluids, fluid compartments, and renal function The presence of oedema suggests that total body water and exchangeable sodium have increased. These changes have been observed frequently and may result from decreased renal blood flow, increased renin–aldosterone secretion and the consequent reduced water and electrolyte clearances which usually precede frank cor pulmonale.

However, sodium and water retention may not be the only cause of oedema for in some cases, although body weight falls as expected during treatment it frequently returns to the pretreatment levels in convalescence without reappearance of oedema. Two interrelated factors may be responsible. Firstly, much of the oedema may be due to a shift of fluid from the intracellular to the extracellular fluid, possibly exacerbated by the need for extracellular buffering where hypercapnia is present. The increase in weight during convalescence may then be due to increased synthesis of body tissue, a suggestion which is supported by a severe decrease in total body potassium observed during acute attacks.

The differential diagnosis of cor pulmonale

In many patients, right heart failure, hypoxia, and respiratory disease co-exist. The question then arises, 'Is this cor pulmonale?' To answer may be difficult for respiratory diseases are common and the non-respiratory causes of pulmonary hypertension all lead to secondary hypoxia. The differential diagnosis usually consists of:

1. Cor pulmonale itself
2. Pulmonary hypertension from unrecognized left heart failure or pulmonary veno-occlusive disease

3. Pulmonary arterial occlusive disease from emboli
4. Primary pulmonary hypertension

The diagnosis of cor pulmonale requires demonstration (a) that the respiratory disease is sufficiently severe to generate the necessary degree of hypoxia; (b) that no other cause of pulmonary hypertension is present.

In the first instance, the severity of respiratory disease will be evaluated clinically but detailed pulmonary function tests and blood gas measurements will also be needed. For cor pulmonale, the degree of hypoxia required is <65 mmHg (8.7 kPa), but this is only a very rough guide as the vasoconstrictive response to hypoxia is very variable. Furthermore, the recent recognition of the various sleep apnoea syndromes suggests that studies of oxygen tension during sleep may be necessary to establish the diagnosis in patients where waking oxygen tensions are only mildly lowered.

In the elimination of cardiac causes of pulmonary hypertension, left heart failure can usually be identified by clinical examination but mitral stenosis and shunts may present problems which require echocardiography, radionuclide studies or catheterization for their solution. In perplexing cases, measurement of wedge pressure may be particularly valuable as a normal study eliminates both left heart failure and pulmonary veno-occlusive disease.

Large pulmonary emboli may frequently be identified by a clinical history aided by ventilation/perfusion scanning and, if necessary, pulmonary angiography. On the other hand, insidious, recurrent small emboli may be extraordinarily difficult to diagnose. If the diagnosis is considered, a search for a source should be made and pulmonary angiography performed. However, it may be impossible to identify small emboli even by angiography, particularly where the pulmonary circulation is already damaged by some other process such as emphysema.

The diagnosis of primary hypertension can only be made when all other causes have been eliminated and, in the case of differentiation from multiple emboli, this may be all but impossible.

Treatment of cor pulmonale

The object of treatment of cor pulmonale is reduction of the workload of the right ventricle by lowering of pulmonary vascular resistance and pulmonary arterial pressure. To this end success depends upon:

1. Treatment of the primary disease to relieve respiratory failure
2. Use of supplemental oxygen to reduce hypoxia and pulmonary vascular resistance
3. Reduction of oedema by use of diuretics and fluid restriction

More controversial are:

4. Venesection
5. Use of digoxin to obtain an inotropic effect on the right ventricle
6. Reduction of pulmonary artery pressure by pulmonary vasodilators

Table 3 Pressure and flows in the pulmonary circulation in cor pulmonale

	Normal individual	Phase I pulmonary hypertension	Phase II right ventricular hypertrophy	Phase III frank cardiac failure
Pulmonary artery pressure (mmHg)	18–20	30–40	40–50	40–50
Pulmonary wedge pressure (mmHg)	6–8	6–8	6–8	6–8
Right ventricular end Diastolic pressure (mmHg)	4	4	8–10	14–16
Cardiac output (l/min)	6	6	6	6 (variable)

As yet incompletely evaluated is:

7. Diminution of intrapulmonary ventilation–perfusion imbalance by use of almitrine bismesylate.

Treatment of primary disease

The condition most commonly responsible for cor pulmonale is chronic obstructive lung disease and the episodes of frank heart failure commonly appear during infective exacerbations. At this time, there is an acute deterioration of pulmonary function, an increase in ventilation–perfusion imbalance and heightened hypoxia. Therefore, the more rapidly and effectively the infective exacerbation can be overcome the less the strain on the right heart. The essentials of treatment are a combination of physiotherapy and appropriate antibiotics.

Also, chronic obstructive lung disease (whether or not a result of underlying asthma) may be associated with reversible airways obstruction. In these cases, whether by use of steroids or bronchodilators, the relief of airways obstruction will reduce the work of breathing, will reduce intra-alveolar pressures, and will aid the clearance of lung secretions and infection. Irrespective of the bronchodilator used, however, the immediate result of bronchodilation will be increased hypoxia due to increased ventilation – perfusion imbalance and it is essential that supplemental oxygen should also be given.

The same principles apply to treatment of bronchiectasis but other lung conditions causing cor pulmonale are more difficult to treat. In the fibrosing diseases and pneumoconioses there is an increased tendency to pulmonary infections which should be treated promptly. Otherwise the mainstay of treatment is supplemental oxygen. Deformation of the spine and chest wall have been treated surgically but the effects upon pulmonary function and pulmonary vascular physiology have been disappointing. In the hypoventilation syndromes various artificial methods for sustaining ventilation have been attempted and include extrathoracic cuirasses and phrenic nerve pacemakers. Patients with obesity-hypoventilation syndrome frequently improve greatly after weight reduction and, for all these groups, sublingual medroxyprogesterone or protriptyline may be a suitable respiratory stimulant.

Supplemental oxygen

Hypoxia is a feature of all the diseases which lead to cor pulmonale and it is therefore reasonable to consider whether the provision of supplemental oxygen might not prevent the development of the condition or alleviate its consequences.

Supplemental oxygen has been used in the treatment of acute exacerbations of chronic obstructive airways disease since the development of controlled titrated administration by Campbell and his colleagues in the early 1960s. The oxygen is used to maintain cerebral function, to reduce pulmonary artery pressure, and to aid the resolution of oedema.

For long-term treatment recent results suggest that oxygen given in low dose (2 1/min) or low concentration (24 per cent) for long daily periods over a number of months or years has a beneficial effect. In a number of trials, it has been shown that mortality, morbidity, and frequency of hospital admissions are reduced for patients with advanced disease and also that pulmonary artery pressure and haematocrit may be reduced (Fig. 3). The oxygen must be breathed continuously for at least 12–15 hours each day; continuous use for 24 hours has a greater benefit than for the shorter period; patients with hypercapnia may benefit most; in men, although morbidity may be reduced by 50 per cent after 3–4 years there is a lag of about 18 months before benefits become apparent; in women, the effects are more dramatic and immediate.

The results of these trials may have considerable consequences when the very high incidence of chronic obstructive disease and the relatively high cost of providing continuous oxygen are considered. At present, oxygen may be provided by one of three methods: compressed gas, oxygen concentrator or liquid oxygen

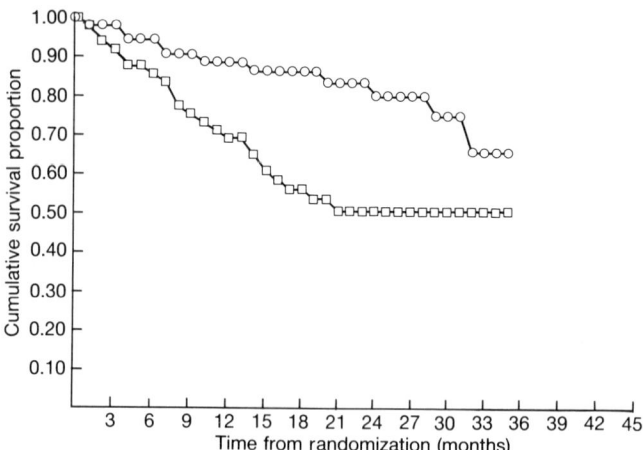

Fig. 3 Overall mortality of patients with chronic obstructive lung disease treated with continuous (O) or nocturnal only (□) oxygen therapy. Mean pulmonary vascular resistance in the nocturnal therapy group was 330 dyne/s cm⁵ and in the continuous group 333 dyne/s cm⁵. (From Nocturnal Oxygen Therapy Trial Group, 1980, *Ann. intern. Med.* **93**, 391, by permission.)

systems. All are expensive either in respect of the initial apparatus or in terms of continual resupply.

Diuretics

In cardiac failure, by the time frank oedema has developed, the accumulation of fluid and increased central venous pressure are no longer adaptive responses to increased afterload. The use of diuretics reduces oedema, improves peripheral circulation, allows improved ventricular contractile efficiency by reducing intravascular volume and may also improve gas exchange in the lung if pulmonary extravascular water has increased.

Usually, powerful loop diuretics such as frusemide are used. There is no evidence that any one diuretic is more effective than others but in resistant cases combinations may be necessary. The addition of spironalactone is logical in view of the raised aldosterone levels. Finally, fluid restriction to 1000–1500 ml/day may be tried.

There is an important relationship between oxygen treatment and diuretic therapy. It has frequently been observed that the administration of oxygen alone will improve cardiac failure and diuresis occurs. Consequently, the dose of diuretic is less when supplemental oxygen is being given. Also, once the acute exacerbation which led to the frank heart failure has been satisfactorily treated, pulmonary vascular resistance and diuretic requirement may both fall. Where this happens, failure to reduce the dose of diuretic can lead to hypovolaemia, hypotension, and prerenal failure.

A final complication of diuretic therapy may be metabolic alkalosis in the presence of potassium deficiency. This is a particular problem in chronic obstructive airways disease for the alkalosis may reduce yet further the CO_2 sensitivity of the medullary centres. To avoid this, potassium chloride supplements should be given or potassium sparing diuretics (such as spironalactone or triamterene) added.

Venesection

The increase in haematrocrit in chronic hypoxia is initially an adaptive response to reduced oxygen saturation. As the haematrocrit rises progressively above 50 per cent, blood viscosity increases significantly and this increase, together with thrombosis and sludging in the pulmonary circulation, adds to right ventricular strain. Thus the disadvantages of the increased red cell mass begin to outweigh the advantages of the increased oxygen-carrying capacity and venesection has been advocated. Haemodynamic studies have shown that optimal benefit is obtained by reduction of haematocrits above 60 per cent to values in the mid or low 50s and that this should be achieved by exchange transfusion with low molecular weight dextran solutions.

Digoxin

It is doubtful if digoxin is therapeutically effective in cor pulmonale unless atrial fibrillation needs to be controlled. In the absence of fibrillation, evidence that its administration improves pulmonary haemodynamics or right ventricular performance is lacking. On the other hand, it is certainly known that in hypoxia and potassium depletion, digoxin is potentially liable to cause cardiac arrhythmias.

Pulmonary vasodilators

The use of these drugs which include acetylcholine, hydralazine, calcium entry blockers and angiotension converting enzyme inhibitors has not yet been assessed although the success of afterload reduction in left heart failure would suggest that they might have a role.

Almitrine bismesylate

This reduces ventilation–perfusion imbalance in the diseased lung, possibly by action on intrapulmonary chemoreceptors. It has been shown to improve arterial oxygenation in patients with severe COAD but its role in cor pulmonale remains doubtful as it may induce pulmonary hypertension.

References

Alpert, J. S. (1979). Pulmonary hypertension and cardiac function in chronic obstructive pulmonary disease. *Chest* **75**, 651–652.
Barer, G. R. (1980). Active control of the pulmonary circulation. In *Pulmonary circulation in health and disease* (eds G. Cumming and G. Bonsignore), p. 81. Plenum Press, New York.
Block, A. J., Boyser, P. G. and Wynne, J. W. (1979). The origins of cor pulmonale. *Chest*, **75**, 109–116.
Fishman, A. P. (1980). Cor pulmonale: general aspects. In *Pulmonary diseases and disorders* (ed. A. P. Fishman), pp. 397–409. McGraw-Hill, New York.
Heath, D., Brewer, D. and Hicken, P. (1968). *Cor pulmonale in emphysema*. Charles C. Thomas, Illinois.
Howard, P. and Suggett, A. (1983). In *Scientific foundations of cardiology* (eds P. Sleight and J. V. Jones), pp. 323–332. Heinemann, London. don.
Matthay, R. A., Schwarz, M. I., Ellis, J. H. *et al.* (1981). Pulmonary hypertension in chronic obstructive pulmonary disease: determination by chest radiography. *Invest. Rad.* **16**, 95–100.
Matthay, R. A., Bergen, H. J., Davies, R. A. *et al.* (1980). Right and left ventricular exercise performance in chronic obstructive pulmonary disease: radionuclide assessment. *Ann. intern. Med.* **93**, 234–239.
Medical Research Council Working Party (1981). Longterm domiciliary oxygen therapy in chronic cor pulmonale complicating chronic bronchitis and emphysema. *Lancet* **i**, 681–686.
Nocturnal Oxygen Therapy Trial Group (1980). Continuous nocturnal oxygen therapy in hypoxaemic chronic obstructive lung disease. *Ann. intern. Med.* **93**, 391–398.
Stretton, T. B. (1985). Provision of long-term oxygen therapy. *Thorax* **40**, 805–801.
Stuart-Harris, C. H. and Hanley, T. (1957). *Chronic bronchitis, emphysema and cor pulmonale*. John Wright, Bristol.
Symposium (1972). Myocardial function in chronic pulmonary disease. *Bull. Physiol–Pathol. Resp.* **8**, 1395.
Thenot, A. (1983). Almitrine bismesylate: facts, deductions and therapeutic perspectives. *Eur. J. Resp. Dis.* (Suppl. 126) **64**, 331–332.

Pulmonary embolism

G. A. H. MILLER

Other than rare causes such as fat embolism, amniotic fluid embolism, and embolism by neoplastic cells and parasites, the vast majority of pulmonary emboli are due to dislodgement of venous thrombi and their impaction in the pulmonary circulation. Venous thrombosis is very common. Factors responsible can be classified conveniently under three headings: stasis, damage to vessel wall, and an alteration in the coagulability of the blood (Virchow's triad). Although the mode of action of these factors in causing venous thrombosis is not fully elucidated, one or more of these three factors is usually present when venous thrombosis has occurred. Thus deep venous thrombosis is common when there has been prolonged bed rest or compression of the leg or pelvic veins. Deep venous thrombosis occurs during and after surgery – particularly abdominal or pelvic surgery; it occurs during pregnancy, in women taking oestrogen-containing oral contraceptives, and following trauma – particularly trauma to the lower limbs. The situations which predispose to deep vein thrombosis are also those which predispose to pulmonary embolism. It is important that in about 50 per cent of cases of deep vein thrombosis there are no symptoms or signs pertaining to the lower limbs. The occurrence of pulmonary embolism may be the first evidence of extensive deep vein thrombosis.

The true incidence of pulmonary embolism is unknown and estimates of its frequency vary depending on the basis for the diagnosis – clinical, post-mortem, or following investigation. Although frequently missed or misdiagnosed, pulmonary embolism is common and its incidence may be increasing. It has been estimated to cause some 21 000 deaths each year in the United Kingdom. Although it is not known how many patients have massive pulmonary embolism it is known that of those who die of massive embolism some two-thirds are dead within two hours of the onset of symptoms. Since it takes time to organize specific treatment and time for such treatment to take effect, it follows that a significant reduction in mortality will only be achieved by adequate prevention. It has been shown that prevention is possible, for example, by the use of low dose subcutaneous heparin before, during, and after surgery. It has also been shown that certain patients are at increased risk of developing deep vein thrombosis and pulmonary embolism. Such patients include those over the age of 50, those who are undergoing abdominal or pelvic surgery, and those who have had previous episode of thrombosis or embolism. Heparin prophylaxis need not, therefore, be given to all patients but should be given to high-risk patients at times of increased risk, for example, before surgery.

Clinical syndromes

Pulmonary embolism due to blood clot can present in a number of ways depending on the volume of embolic material and the duration of the disease. There are therefore not one but several clinical syndromes (see Table 1).

Acute minor embolism

This occurs when a small amount of blood clot impacts in a small, distal pulmonary artery. It is probable that in the majority of instances minor pulmonary embolism is silent but symptoms and signs occur when there is a pleural involvement and 'pulmonary infarction'. When this happens there is pleuritic pain and haemoptysis, a pleural rub, and fine crepitations may be heard. The term 'pulmonary infarction', though clinically useful, has caused confusion since the lung possesses a dual blood supply (bronchial and pulmonary arteries), and infarction with necrosis can probably only occur in an abnormal lung with defects of one or other arterial supply. Nonetheless the syndrome commonly occurs in patients with previously normal lung; there is exudation of fluid and cells into alveolar spaces but necrosis does not occur. This exudate may be detected as a shadow on the chest X-ray. Such 'infarct shadows' appear rapidly (within 24 hours) and usually resolve completely within a few days although they may leave a linear scar.

Since at least half of the pulmonary arterial tree has to be obstructed before there is a detectable rise in pulmonary arterial pressure, it follows that there is *no* haemodynamic disturbance in minor pulmonary embolism. Symptoms and signs are confined to those of 'pulmonary infarction' and specific treatment is not required.

Table 1 Clinical syndromes of pulmonary embolism

Clinical syndrome	Symptoms	Signs	P_a systolic pressure	Treatment
Acute minor pulmonary embolism	Pleurisy/haemoptysis (or none)	Pleural rub crepitations (or none)	Normal	None needed (heparin for DVT)
Acute massive pulmonary embolism	'Collapse'/syncope Acute onset dyspnoea Chest pain	RV failure V/Q disturbance Shock	41 mmHg ± 1.2	Embolectomy or streptokinase
Subacute massive pulmonary embolism	Gradual onset dyspnoea (days or weeks) Pleurisy/haemoptysis Painful swollen leg (DVT)	RV failure V/Q disturbance Shock	54 mmHg ± 5.0	Embolectomy or streptokinase
Chronic thrombo-embolic pulmonary hypertension	Gradual onset dyspnoea Effort syncope	Pulmonary hypertension	85.2 mmHg ± 5.7	None effective

Acute massive pulmonary embolism

This occurs when the volume of embolic material is sufficient to obstruct 50 per cent or more of the pulmonary arterial tree. Thus, in this condition there *is* a haemodynamic disturbance which may be profound. The consequences of this haemodynamic disturbance dominate the presentation. Since most or all the embolic material may impact in central pulmonary arteries, pleural involvement is not an essential part of the syndrome, and pleuritic pain and haemoptysis are present in less than a third of patients with massive pulmonary embolism. When such symptoms are present they frequently antedate the onset of massive embolism and are due to minor premonitory emboli occurring before dislodgement of the massive embolus.

The haemodynamic disturbance of massive embolism may be categorized under three headings:

1. Acute right ventricular failure
2. Acute disturbance of pulmonary ventilation and perfusion
3. Acute reduction of cardiac output

Acute right ventricular failure The result of sudden obstruction to right ventricular outflow is to cause acute dilatation of the right ventricle. Right ventricular filling pressure (end-diastolic pressure) rises with consequent elevation of central venous pressure. The normal, thin-walled, right ventricle is poorly adapted to generate a high pressure and when acutely stressed is unable to generate a pressure much in excess of 50 mmHg. Thus, signs of pulmonary hypertension or right ventricular hypertrophy are absent. In particular pulmonary valve closure is not loud; indeed pulmonary valve closure is usually inaudible during the first 24 hours following embolism. The result of delayed right ventricular ejection and a low stroke output with early aortic valve closure is to cause wide splitting of the second heart sound, and this is the usual finding after 24 hours have elapsed.

Right ventricular failure is detected clinically both by a raised central venous pressure and by the appearance of an added sound in diastole ('gallop rhythm') best heard at the left sternal edge. This added sound is probably a 'summation gallop' – that is to say fusion between a third heart sound (filling sound) due to the high end-diastolic pressure and a fourth heart sound due to forceful atrial contraction which 'fuse' as a result of the sinus tachycardia which is almost always present. It is observed that the gallop rhythm may be absent when (*a*) there is pre-existing atrial fibrillation (loss of fourth heart sound), or (*b*) when, after 24 hours, the right ventricular filling pressure has fallen (loss of third heart sound).

A symptom which may be ascribed to right ventricular failure and dilatation is central chest pain indistinguishable from angina pectoris. This symptom is present in about one-third of patients with massive embolism and is of importance since its presence in a shocked patient may lead to an erroneous diagnosis of myocardial infarction. In myocardial infarction with shock, however, there is *left* ventricular failure and pulmonary venous hypertension result-

ing in orthopnoea – the patient prefers to sit up. In massive pulmonary embolism the patient prefers to lie flat and may lose consciousness if sat up. There are two probable reasons for this. Firstly, when there is severe hypotension, cerebral blood flow may be critically reduced in the upright position. Secondly, the failing right ventricle is critically dependent on a high filling pressure (Starling effect) and this in turn depends on venous return which is maximal in the supine position.

Acute disturbance of pulmonary ventilation and perfusion This, the second of the three haemodynamic consequences of massive pulmonary embolism, is an obvious result of obstruction to pulmonary flow, though the mechanisms responsible for the observed symptoms and signs are not fully understood. The chief symptom to be included under this heading is the sudden onset of acute dyspnoea. The signs observed are that there is tachypnoea and that the patient is hyperventilating. Some degree of arterial desaturation is present in virtually all cases though cyanosis is clinically detectable in only two-thirds of patients. Arterial saturation averages 85 per cent and the combination of arterial desaturation and hyperventilation leads to the characteristic finding of a low arterial P_{O_2} (average 50 mmHg) and a low arterial P_{CO_2} (average 35 mmHg). The mechanism responsible for this arterial desaturation is not fully understood. In a proportion of cases it may be due to right-to-left shunting across a patent foramen ovale. In other patients it is probable that there is atelectasis of affected zones; perfusion of these zones is not totally absent and this perfusion of non-aerated lung results in a shunt-like effect and arterial desaturation.

The obstruction to pulmonary flow and the resulting increase in pulmonary artery pressure can probably be explained as a simple mechanical effect of the embolic material. An alternative explanation which has been proposed is that there is an additional vasoconstrictive effect which may be mediated by serotonin released by interaction between platelets and emboli. Although there is no direct evidence for such an effect in man, this postulated serotonin effect is the basis for some of the treatments which have been proposed (see below).

Acute reduction in cardiac output This, the third of the triad of haemodynamic consequences of massive pulmonary embolism, is the result of obstruction to right ventricular ouput. Pulmonary venous return to the left heart falls and cardiac output falls abruptly. This sudden fall in cardiac output is undoubtedly responsible for the commonest presenting symptom of massive pulmonary embolism – 'collapse'. This may take the form of a brief episode of syncope resulting from reduced cerebral flow or may be so severe a fall in output that the patient dies within seconds or minutes of the onset of embolism. The low output is responsible for signs of shock – a low or unrecordable arterial pressure with a sinus tachycardia and small volume, sharp upstroke, pulse. The periphery is constricted and cerebration may be impaired and urine flow low or absent. *The diagnosis of massive pulmonary*

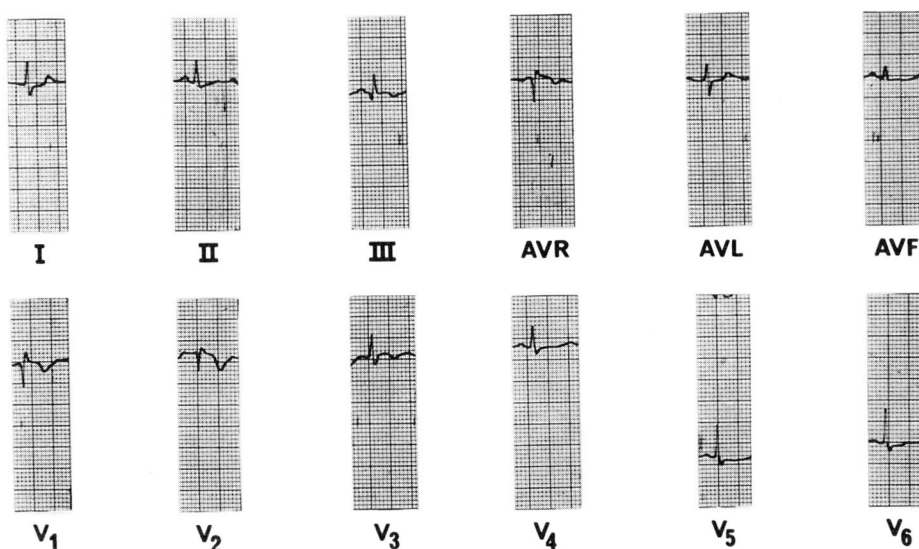

I   II   III   AVR   AVL   AVF

V₁   V₂   V₃   V₄   V₅   V₆

Fig. 1 Acute massive pulmonary embolism. Electrocardiogram, showing the most commonly found pattern of electrocardiographic abnormalities. There is an S wave in lead 1, a Q wave in lead 3 with T wave inversion in lead 3 and there is T wave inversion in the anterior chest leads, leads V_1–V_3.

embolism is made when the signs of right ventricular failure are detected in a shocked patient who is acutely short of breath.

The symptoms and signs of massive pulmonary embolism and their physiological basis are summarized in Table 1.

Aids to diagnosis
Useful (and simple) aids to diagnosis are: (*a*) the ECG; (*b*) the plain chest X-ray; and (*c*) arterial blood gases (already discussed above).

The electrocardiogram
The classical electrocardiographic abnormalities associated with acute massive pulmonary embolism reflect abnormalities of right ventricular depolarization (the QRS complex) and repolarization (the T wave). The most commonly seen electrocardiographic pattern consists of: an S wave in lead 1; a Q wave in lead 3; and T wave inversion in lead 3 with or without T wave inversion over the right ventricle (leads V_1 to V_3 or V_4). This pattern is conveniently remembered as the S_1, Q_3, T_3 pattern (Fig. 1). Other commonly seen abnomalities include partial or complete right bundle branch block. One or other of these abnormalities are seen in 85 per cent of patients with proven acute massive pulmonary embolism. It is important to remember that massive pulmonary embolism can exist without any ECG abnormality in 15 per cent of cases. On rare occasions there may be left-sided ECG abnormalities (e.g. ST-T wave changes over the left ventricular leads V_4–V_6). It is possible that such changes occur in patients with co-existing occult coronary artery disease. The electrocardiographic changes may be evanescent and this could explain the occasional finding of a normal ECG.

The plain chest X-ray (Fig. 2)
This is of considerable help in the diagnosis of massive pulmonary embolism. The result of impaired perfusion of affected areas of lung is to cause a reduction in the radiologically visible pulmonary markings in affected zones – patchy oligaemia. This abnormality can nearly always be detected by the trained eye and may be the only radiological abnormality present. Other radiological abnormalities which may be present can be classified under two headings: (*a*) those which reflect abnormalities of pulmonary artery perfusion; and (*b*) those which reflect loss of lung volume – usually due to prior pulmonary 'infarction'. In the first category is the so-called 'plump' or 'pear-shaped' hilar shadow due to abrupt cut-off of a slightly dilated pulmonary artery at the site of occlusion by an embolus. This is most easily seen at the right hilum as the left is obscured by the heart shadow. Although there may be slight

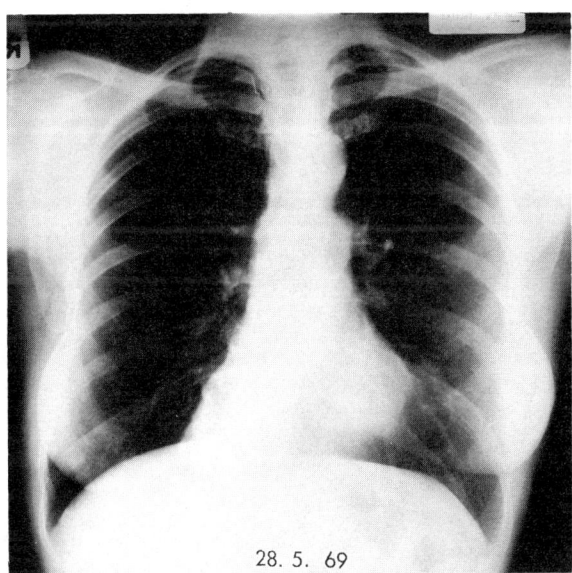

28. 5. 69

Fig. 2 Acute massive pulmonary emboslism. Plain chest X-ray showing oligaemia – reduced pulmonary vascular markings – affecting both lung fields. Heart size is normal and the pulmonary artery is not dilated.

enlargement of the pulmonary arteries, obvious enlargement of the main pulmonary artery does not occur – nor is it to be expected since this is a sign of pulmonary hypertension, and pulmonary artery pressure is not greatly elevated in patients without previous cardiorespiratory disease. Included in the second category are such radiological abnormalities as 'infarct shadows' (which are seldom wedge-shaped) and elevation of one or other dome of the diaphragm.

Investigation
Pulmonary embolism may be confirmed or excluded by two techniques: (*a*) pulmonary arteriography, or (*b*) scintillation scanning. The advantage of cardiac catheterization and pulmonary arteriography is that it establishes (or excludes) the diagnosis beyond doubt. Emboli are seen as filling defects within the contrast-filled pulmonary arteries, and the severity and distribution of embolism can be accurately determined (Fig. 3). To some extent pulmonary angiography helps to determine the age of emboli since recent emboli bulge into the contrast-filled pulmonary artery giving a convex filling defect. Later on (days or weeks) gradual lysis of

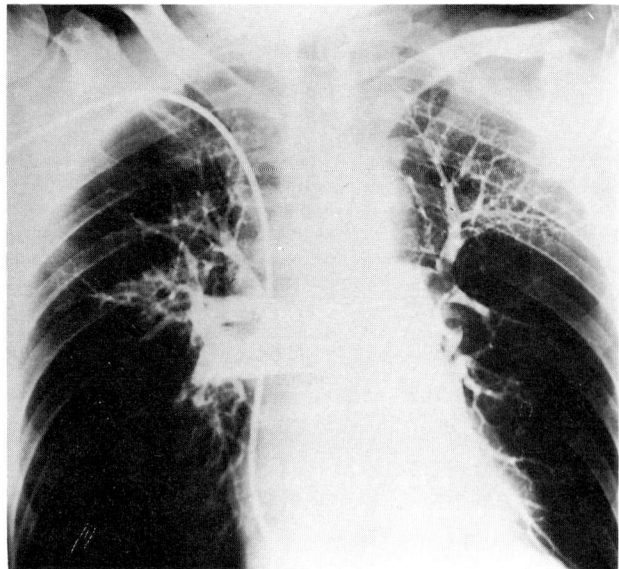

Fig. 3 Acute massive pulmonary embolism. Pulmonary arteriogram; radio-opaque contrast has been injected into the main pulmonary artery via a catheter introduced from the right arm. Pulmonary perfusion is grossly diminished in all but the left upper zone. Recent emboli are seen as filling defects within the left pulmonary artery and causing an abrupt 'cut-off' of the right lower lobe pulmonary artery.

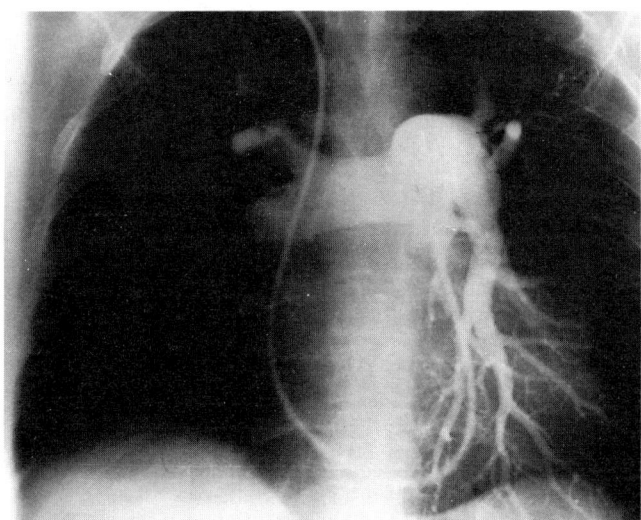

Fig. 4 Chronic thrombo-embolic pulmonary hypertension. Pulmonary arteriogram; the presence of severe pulmonary hypertension is indicated by the considerable dilatation of the main and right and left pulmonary arteries. Filling defects are not seen and the right pulmonary artery terminates in a convex fashion where naturally occurring thrombolysis has partially removed obstructing embolism. In recent embolism the embolic material would have been seen as a filling defect bulging into the contrast-filled right pulmonary artery. The thrombo-embolic nature of the disease is assumed from the asymmetrical involvement with sparing of the left lower lobe pulmonary artery. Compare with Fig. 3.

emboli and their contraction leads to the appearance of a concave filling defect or an abrupt 'cut-off' of a pulmonary artery.

The disadvantage of pulmonary arteriography is that it can only be performed by experienced personnel and requires a catheterization laboratory. In experienced hands there is little if any risk, and the diagnosis can be established without the need for the patient's co-operation.

Scintillation scanning for pulmonary embolism may be by using an isotopically labelled substance injected into a peripheral vein – 'perfusion scanning'. Alternatively, this may be combined with the inhalation of an isotopically labelled gas – ventilation/perfusion scanning. While a normal perfusion scan excludes massive pulmonary embolism, false positive results can occur though these are usually associated with an abnormal chest X-ray. The addition of a ventilation scan improves the specificity of lung scanning in the diagnosis of pulmonary embolism. Such combined ventilation and perfusion scans will show perfusion defects unaccompanied by defects of ventilation – a finding specific for pulmonary embolism.

Subacute massive pulmonary embolism

This clinical syndrome is of importance since it can cause problems of diagnosis and management. Patients with this condition are suffering from massive or sub-massive embolism but have a history extending for days or weeks. Whereas in acute massive embolism the dominant symptom is syncope and acute onset dyspnoea, patients with subacute embolism frequently give a history suggestive of deep venous thrombosis (e.g. a painful swollen leg) together with episodes of pleuritic pain and haemoptysis and of gradually increasing breathlessness without syncope. At cardiac catheterization such patients are found to have significantly higher pulmonary artery pressures than are found in acute massive embolism (see Table 1), suggesting that the longer duration has allowed the right ventricle to generate a higher pressure in response to a similar degree of obstruction to pulmonary flow. With this exception other findings are similar to those in acute massive embolism.

Chronic thrombo-embolic pulmonary hypertension

The fourth clinical syndrome resulting from pulmonary thrombo-embolism is fortunately rare since the prognosis is grave and treatment is ineffective. The thrombo-embolic origin of the condition is often speculative since the pathological findings may be non-specific and a history of deep vein thrombosis and pulmonary embolism is frequently lacking. The diagnosis is made when asymetric occlusions of pulmonary arteries are demonstrated in a patient with severe pulmonary hypertension. Such patients present with a history of increasing breathlessness and, often, of effort syncope. Abnormal physical signs are confined to those of pulmonary hypertension and are often overlooked until the terminal stages of the disease.

The haemodynamic disturbance is of severe obstuction to pulmonary flow with very great elevation of pulmonary artery pressure. The degree of obstruction may be no greater than in acute massive embolism, but the considerable higher pulmonary arterial pressure (Table 1) indicates that considerable right ventricular hypertrophy has taken place with time so that the thick-walled hypertrophied ventricle can now generate a higher output and much higher pressures than can the non-hypertrophied ventricle. The physical signs and investigative findings reflect this severe pulmonary hypertension. Thus, pulmonary valve closure is loud but is physiologically split (moves with respiration) allowing distinction from pulmonary hypertension which has developed in response to a long-standing left-to-right shunt. The electrocardiogram shows the changes of right ventricular hypertrophy rather than the 'strain' pattern of acute embolism. The plain chest X-ray shows the same patchy oligaemia but there is marked enlargement of the main pulmonary artery reflecting the high pressure in the pulmonary circulation. Pulmonary arteriography demonstrates these enlarged pulmonary arteries and shows asymmetric occlusions of pulmonary vessels characteristic of thrombo-embolism. However, filling defects are no longer seen (Fig. 4).

Differential diagnosis

Acute minor pulmonary embolism

From other causes of pleuritic pain and haemoptysis, e.g. pneumonia.

Acute and subacute massive pulmonary embolism

From other causes of 'collapse' and shock. The condition most often misdiagnosed as massive pulmonary embolism is septicaemic shock. Patients suffering from septicaemia may have collapsed some days after an operation thus suggesting pulmonary embolism. They are dyspnoeic and peripherally cyanosed. The central venous pressure is not raised, however, and this should distinguish such patients from those with massive embolism. Other conditions which may be misdiagnosed as pulmonary embolism include myocardial infarction and concealed haemorrhage. An important source of diagnostic difficulty occurs when *minor* embolism occurs in a patient who is breathless or shocked from another cause. Thus the diagnosis of pulmonary embolism becomes difficult when there is co-existing cardiorespiratory disease. In such cases the haemodynamic disturbance is due to the underlying disease but the sudden onset of pleuritic pain due to superadded minor embolism may suggest that the whole illness is due to massive embolism.

Chronic thrombo-embolic pulmonary hypertension

The differential diagnosis is from other causes of pulmonary hypertension. When this is secondary to pulmonary venous hypertension (e.g. mitral stenosis), this should be clear from the differing X-ray appearances. Primary, or idiopathic, pulmonary hypertension has an identical haemodynamic disturbance and is only distinguished by the symmetrical and uniform reduction in pulmonary vascularity seen in primary pulmonary hypertension.

Management

In minor pulmonary embolism no treatment is required other than the relief of symptoms, since there is no haemodynamic disturbance and the condition usually resolves without sequelae. The occurrence of embolism should alert the physician to the presence of deep venous thrombosis and the possibility of further, perhaps fatal, embolism. Since minor embolism is very common, it is impossible to investigate all cases (e.g. by venography) but anticoagulant treatment is a wise precaution.

The management of acute massive pulmonary embolism can be summarized under three headings:

1. Immediate resuscitation
2. Definitive treatment
3. Aftercare

Resuscitation

The objects are: (*a*) to reverse the metabolic effects of a cardiac arrest should it have occurred; (*b*) to minimize the hypoxaemia; (*c*) to preserve right ventricular function; and (*d*) to reduce the severity of obstruction to pulmonary flow. The effects of (*c*) and (*d*) will be to improve cardiac output and tissue perfusion but there may be a place for the administration of vasopressors (e.g. metaraminol) in addition. (*a*) and (*b*) above are achieved by the intravenous administrations of sodium bicarbonate and by giving oxygen by mask or endotracheal tube. Right ventricular function is critically dependent on a high filling pressure so that the importance of preserving venous return cannot be overemphasized. It is for this reason that patients with massive embolism prefer to lie flat since venous return is maximal in the supine position. No drugs should be given which might cause vasodilatation and operations on the inferior vena cava play no part in the management of the acute phase of massive pulmonary embolism. Some patients with massive, but not imminently lethal, pulmonary embolism have been shown to be improved by administration of 500 ml of Dextran 70, a plasma expander.

Ideally resuscitation should reduce the degree of obstruction to pulmonary flow although it is uncertain to what extent this can be achieved immediately. It is possible that some of the increased resistance to pulmonary flow may be due to serotonin-mediated vasoconstriction which can be reversed by intravenous heparin in high doses. While no direct evidence exists for such a mechanism in man the immediate administration of 15 000 units of heparin intravenously will not prejudice subsequent treatment and may be beneficial. External cardiac massage may cause some onward propulsion of emboli so that they cause a lesser obstructive effect in relation to the increasing area of the pulmonary vascular bed. External massage is, in any case, likely to be used in a collapsed patient although in pulmonary embolism the left ventricle does not need support – the usual reason for cardiac massage.

Other resuscitative measures which have been advocated include the 'immediate' institution of femoro-femoral (partial) cardiopulmonary bypass, the removal of the embolus by a special suction catheter advanced from the femoral vein, the intrapulmonary infusion of urokinase, and emergency pulmonary embolectomy using inflow occlusion (modified Trendellenberg

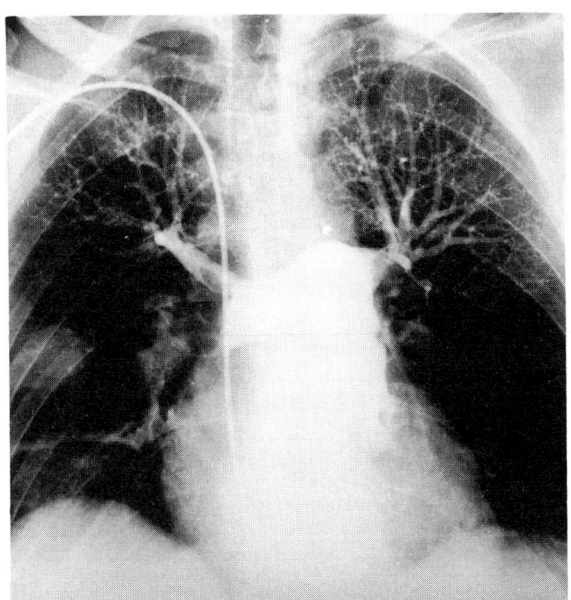 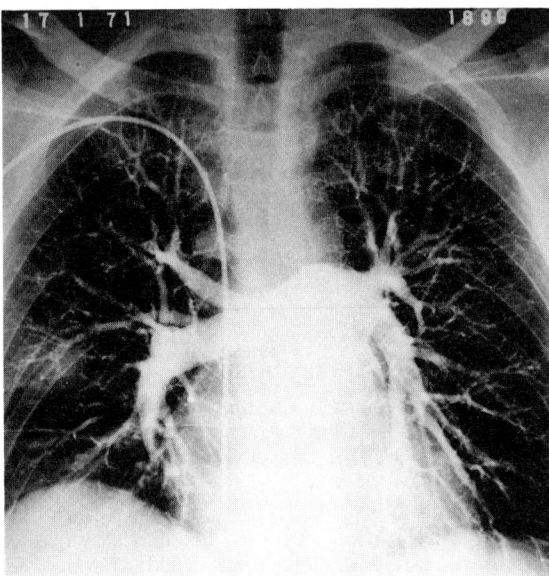

Figs 5 and 6 Acute massive pulmonary embolism. Treatment by enhanced thrombolysis – streptokinase. Fig. 5 shows the pulmonary arteriogram obtained on admission with typical features of acute massive pulmonary embolism. Streptokinase was infused for 72 hours and pulmonary arteriogram shown in Fig. 6 then obtained. There is almost complete lysis of all emboli. Had treatment been with heparin there would have been very little change at this time. An 'infarct shadow' is seen in the right mid-zone.

operation) instead of total cardiopulmonary bypass. Such techniques clearly merge into definitive treatment, discussed below.

Definitive treatment
It is essential that the diagnosis be established beyond doubt before definitive treatment is started – pulmonary embolectomy, for example, carried out on a patient shocked from a cause other than massive embolism is unlikely to result in survival. Thus the first step is to perform pulmonary arteriography (or lung scanning) without delay.

Three types of treatment are available: (*a*) anticoagulants – heparin; (*b*) thrombolytic drugs – streptokinase or urokinase (Figs 5 and 6); and (*c*) pulmonary embolectomy on cardiopulmonary bypass.

Heparin has no thrombolytic effect and where this is the only treatment used recovery will be delayed and dependent on naturally occurring thrombolysis. Heparin alone should only be used for embolism of relatively minor severity. Where there is massive embolism and shock, thrombolytic drugs or pulmonary embolectomy should be employed and are probably equally effective. Streptokinase can be given in a standard dosage of 250 000 units in the first hour followed by a maintenance infusion of 100 000 units/hour for 24 hours. Steroid cover can be given to prevent the occasional sensitivity reaction. Thrombolytic agents are contra-indicated where there is an increased risk of haemorrhage. Accepted contra-indications include:

Major surgery within the preceding five days or total hip replacement within the preceding ten days.

Active bleeding lesions of the gastrointestinal or genitourinary tract.

Carotid or translumbar aortic puncture within the preceding four weeks.

A history of cerebrovascular accident.

Severe renal or hepatic insufficiency.

Hypertension.

Pregnancy, lactation, and a period of ten days or less postpartum.

When thrombolytic therapy is contra-indicated, the patient should be transferred to a unit where emergency embolectomy can be performed on cardiopulmonary bypass. Pulmonary embolectomy can also be life-saving in the occasional patient who deteriorates despite thrombolytic therapy or who is suffering from such massive embolism that it seems unlikely that thrombolysis will exert its effect soon enough to prevent death. In patients with massive embolism and shock who have survived long enough for definitive treatment to be given (streptokinase or embolectomy) the mortality should not be more than 25 per cent. Most of the deaths which occur despite such treatment are due to brain or other organ damage occurring at the time of the initial cardiac arrest and resuscitation.

Natural history and aftercare
Recurrent embolism and chronic thrombo-embolic pulmonary hypertension are rare complications of energetically treated pulmonary embolism, whatever the treatment used. Patients should be maintained on anticoagulants for at least three months. Patients who have had one episode of deep vein thrombosis/pulmonary embolism are at increased risk of further thrombo-embolic episodes when exposed to situations in which thrombosis might occur (surgery, bed rest, etc.). Anticoagulant cover should be given to such patients whenever they are exposed to such further risk. Where thromb-embolism has resulted from the use of oestrogen-containing oral contraceptives, another contraceptive method should be used.

There are a very few patients who continue to have repeated pulmonary emboli despite good anticoagulant control or who, for some reason, cannot be maintained on anticoagulants. Such patients are at risk of developing thrombo-embolic pulmonary hypertension and in them there may be a place for inserting a 'filter' in the inferior vena cava. Various operations and devices have been developed for this purpose but are not without complications and do not provide complete protection against recurrent embolism. In the author's view such procedures, though frequently performed are rarely, if ever, indicated.

Many patients who have had a pulmonary embolus for no obvious reason subsequently develop neoplastic disease which was unsuspected at the time of embolism. An attempt shoud be made to discover occult neoplasia in such cases.

In summary, most, if not all, patients who survive acute or subacute embolism will eventually recover normal or nearly normal pulmonary and cardiac function. Recurrent embolism and thrombo-embolic pulmonary hypertension are very rare complications.

References
Miller, G. A. H. (1981). Pulmonary embolism and infarction. In *Scientific foundations of respiratory medicine* (eds J. G. Scadding, G. Cumming and W. M. Thurlbeck), pp. 698–711. Heinemann, London.
British Medical Journal (1980). Consensus Development. Thrombolytic therapy in treatment. Summary of an N.I.H. Consensus Conference. *Br. med. J.* **280**, 1585.

HYPERTENSION

Essential hypertension

P. SLEIGHT

The size and nature of the problem
Some impression of the enormous importance of hypertension as a cause of death can be gleaned from the fact that in one painstaking prospective study (Framingham, Massachusetts) 37 per cent of men and 51 per cent of women who died of cardiovascular disease had been noted previously to have had an arterial pressure over 140/90 mm Hg on at least three occasions. The mortality of such subjects was more than double those with normal arterial pressure. This study was of a random sample of the population, not just hospital patients or those who consulted a physician. The bulk of the deaths occurred with no warning. A similar increase in risk has been calculated from life insurance data (Fig. 1).

Death due to hypertension is sometimes directly related to the bursting effect of a very high pressure on arteries. These deaths, due to cerebral haemorrhage or dissecting aneurysm, and those due to heart failure from the increased pressure work of the left ventricle are particularly associated with the relatively small number of people with very high pressures, say over 180 mm Hg systolic. They are important because they are almost entirely preventable by treatment as may also be deaths and morbidity from cerebral thrombosis. But the great majority of deaths attributable to hypertension are caused by coronary artery disease. The bulk of these occur at much less spectacular pressures, around 140–160 mm Hg systolic, and are not so readily controlled by treatment of hypertension (Fig. 2).

There is at present great controversy about the evidence for and against drug treatment of this type of mild hypertension, with systolic pressures in the region of 140–160 mm Hg and diastolic pressures in the region of 90–100 mm Hg.

The reports of the Medical Research Council (MRC) mild

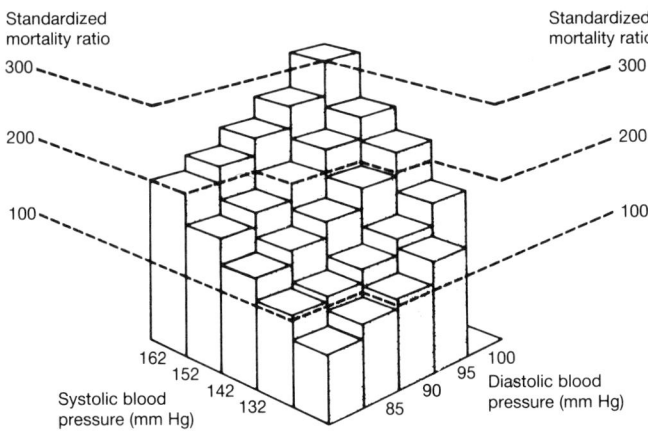

Fig. 1 Life insurance data linking risk and levels of arterial pressure, standardized to average risk (= 100). (Data from MRC Working Party, 1977, *Br. med. J.*, with permission.)

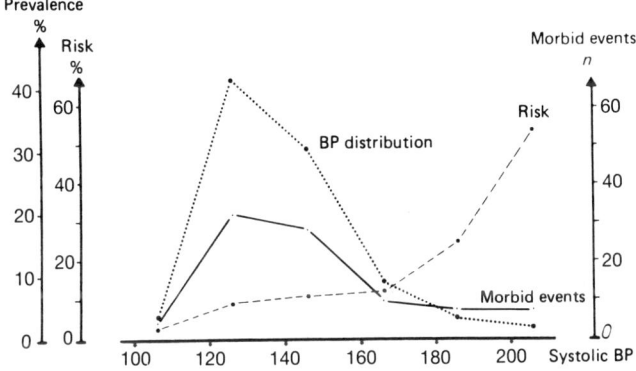

Fig. 2 Number of morbid events (solid line), risk (dashed line), and BP distribution (dotted line) in a 13.5 year follow-up of 865 males aged 50 years at entry to the Gothenberg study. Note that the bulk of the morbid events occurs at lowish levels of hypertension. (Reproduced from Wilhelmsen, 1979, *Clin. Sci.* **57**, 455s–458s, with permission.)

hypertension trial, the International Primary Prevention Study in Hypertension (IPPSH), and the European trial of treatment of elderly patients will be discussed later (see page 13.371), but the overall impression is that treatment of mildly raised blood pressure in patients without other risk factors for vascular disease and particularly in women may cause side-effects which outweigh rather marginal benefits.

The adverse effects of cigarette smoking are far more important than the benefits of drug therapy in mild hypertension. Changes in lifestyle, e.g. reduction in cigarette smoking, weight, and fat intake, and increase in exercise, may have much to offer.

Definition
The definition of high blood pressure depends entirely upon what arbitrary limits are put on normality, for there is no dividing line between normal and abnormal. In practice 'normal' values will be different for each group dealt with, whether young or old, pregnant or non-pregnant. The level of arterial pressure in a defined population is a continuously distributed variable in the same way as serum cholesterol or urea. The consequences of the actual level of pressure in a given person will depend not only on the measured level but also upon certain 'risk' factors such as age, race, gender, glucose tolerance, cholesterol, and smoking habits. Hypertension is thus not a disease or abnormality in the same sense as gout, nephritis or pneumonia. The disease processes associated with high arterial pressure are the consequences of the damage caused to the heart or to the arterial wall by a given level of pressure.

A further difficulty concerns the actual measurement of blood

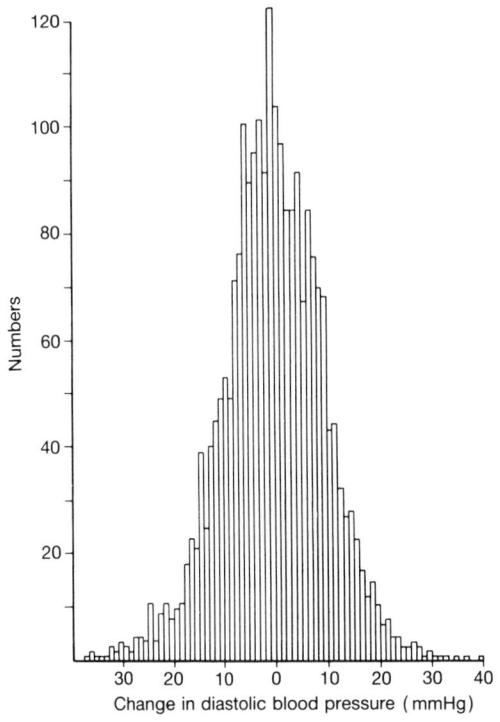

Fig. 3 Frequency distribution of the change in diastolic blood pressure in 2289 of the 3001 subjects at rescreening one year after the initial survey. (Reproduced from Hawthorn, Greaves and Beevers, 1974, *Br. med. J.* **iii**, 60, with permission.)

pressure. The defence or alerting reaction of the subject to the examiner can cause a spurious reading. For this reason it is usual to measure the pressure on several occasions and to allow the subject time to become familiar with the surroundings, which should be as free from tension as possible (see below). When pressures are measured repeatedly in a population, it will be found that although the mean levels on separate occasions are usually closely similar, there is frequently individual variation which may be as great as 30 mm Hg (Fig. 3); indeed 'within subject' variation can be as much as 50 per cent of 'between subject' differences.

Thus, if one took the common arbitrary upper limit for 'normal' as 140/90 mm Hg, a subject classified as hypertensive on one occasion might be normal on the next or vice versa. For this reason it is wise (unless the pressure is dangerously high) to forego labelling a person as abnormal until two or three readings at least have been obtained on separate occasions spread over a few weeks. If only one reading is taken then about one-third of the United Kingdom population will have a diastolic blood pressure more than 90 mm Hg; if six readings are taken the frequency drops to about 5 per cent. A practical and proven strategy is to take three separate readings over 3–4 weeks, unless the earlier readings, coupled with other physical findings (e.g. retinal haemorrhages or lesser evidence of end organ damage) dictate immediate treatment.

Systolic or diastolic pressure?
Despite the fact that nearly all advice on treatment is based on diastolic pressure, the evidence on prognosis from two large studies (Framingham and Whitehall) suggests that the systolic pressure is a better predictor and, since its range is greater, it is probably a better discriminator. It is certainly easier to measure, particularly with automatic devices. Future studies should pay more attention to it.

The next problem, whether to define a level as abnormal or not, is usually solved by reference to the degree of risk attached to that level. It has been suggested that a level carrying a morbidity two to three times that of the general population should be regarded as

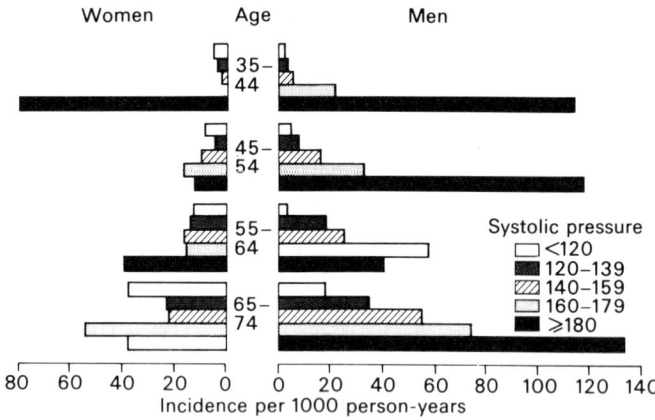

Fig. 4 Incidence of all cardiovascular–renal deaths, myocardial infarctions, angina pectoris, and cerebrovascular accidents according to systolic pressure, age, and sex in Rhondda Fach and the Vale of Glamorgan, 1971. (Reproduced from Miall and Chinn, 1974, *Br. med. J.* **iii**, 600, with permission.)

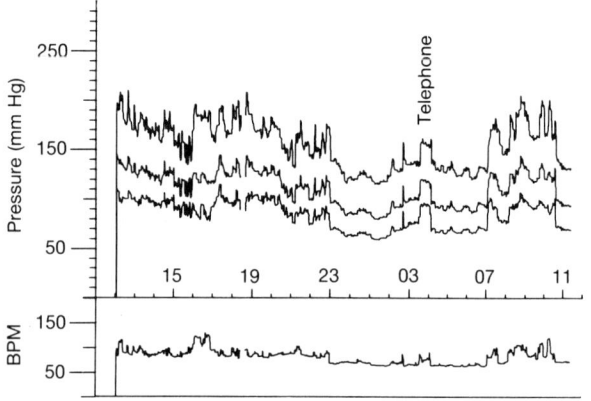

Fig. 5 Computerized printout of means of every 2 min over 24 hours for blood pressure (systolic, diastolic, and mean), and heart rate, from intra-arterial ambulatory monitoring.

abnormal. This is essentially a practical definition of hypertension. From population studies such as those carried out in Framingham, Massachusetts, and the Medical Research Council studies in South Wales, we now have quite good data on the relative risks or morbidity for levels of both systolic and diastolic pressures separately related to other risk factors such as age and sex (Fig. 4).

Labile hypertension
Because of the arbitrary division between normal and abnormal (often taken as 140/90 for the general population), it sometimes happens that an individual finds himself normal on one reading and abnormal on another. Such findings have given rise to the term 'labile' hypertension. I believe this to be an artefact. A continuous record of intra-arterial pressure over 24 hours in anyone, whether clearly hypertensive, or clearly normal, shows enormous variability over the day and night (Fig. 5). The variability of arterial pressure (defined as the standard deviation from the mean) rises in proportion to the individual's resting pressure level. There is no clear evidence for any other form of lability.

The defence reaction
If life expectancy is related to blood pressure, the line shows a continuous rise in longevity as resting blood pressure falls and this is true within quite 'normal' levels of pressure. Notwithstanding the very great power of casual or 'office' blood pressures to predict future risk it is becoming increasingly evident that an even better prediction is achieved by ambulatory blood pressure recording. It

is very important to be sure of our measurements before an individual is sentenced to long-term treatment.

Long-term intra-arterial measurements of blood pressure in untreated hypertensive subjects at home and work, away from hospitals and doctors, have been performed. When the waking intra-arterial records were compared with the average of several conventional cuff readings, the intra-arterial measures in about one-third of the subjects were much lower and fell within the normal range (Fig. 6). This 'pseudo' hypertension from cuff measurements was much more common in those who were free of any ECG or ocular manifestations of hypertension. It seems clear, therefore, that there are many people who, as a result of a well-developed 'defence' or alerting reaction, masquerade as hypertensives. It may be possible to identify this important group less invasively by the use of home blood pressure measurement by the subject or spouse. These measurements of home blood pressure show good correlation with intra-arterial measurements.

The error from the defence reaction seems to be a particularly important problem in subjects with 'borderline' hypertension. Since the publication of the HDFP trial US physicians are being urged to treat subjects with diastolic blood pressures in the range of 90–95 mm Hg and certainly in the range of 95–100 mm Hg. Yet it is with just such levels that the greatest discrepancies between casual and ambulatory blood pressures are found. Left ventricular hypertrophy correlates best with blood pressures recorded at work.

Equally important, ambulatory blood pressure recording with reliable automatic devices seems to reduce or abolish the defence reaction, so that the fall in cuff blood pressure seen with placebo tablets is not seen with 24 hour records. It is possible using this technique to distinguish effects of treatment on blood pressure which may be lost by inherent 'noise' from cuff measurements.

Despite all this there is no current 'gold standard' for ambulatory recording, since most of the data relating prognosis to blood pressure comes from office cuff measurement. We need to establish a similar large body of knowledge relating ambulatory blood pressure to prognosis.

Measurement techniques
Since blood pressure is measured in the arm by an indirect method, errors in technique may be very important. Particular attention should be paid to:

1. Making sure the subject is at ease, either lying or sitting, in order to reduce muscle tension.

2. The cuff around the arm should be at the level of the heart.

3. The position of the arm may influence the apparent pressure irrespective of the hydrostatic level with respect to the heart. The

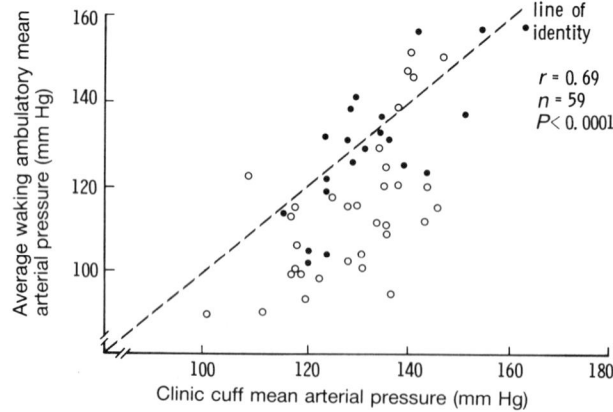

Fig. 6 Comparison of waking intra-arterial versus cuff mean arterial blood pressures (open circles, patients with no LV hypertrophy or fundus changes). This suggests that a high proportion of patients have artefactually high blood pressure readings on conventional cuff measurement. (Reproduced from Floras *et al.*, 1981, *Lancet*, with permission.)

best measure seems to be obtained in a seated subject with the forearm supported horizontally and with the cuff at heart level.

4. The cuff should be of sufficient size to be able to occlude the brachial artery effectively. The size of cuff must be selected for differing limb sizes. A rough guide is that the width of cuff should be about half the arm circumference. In practice a cuff width of 2.5 cm is suitable for newborn infants, with 5, 8, and 12 cm cuffs available for 3–12 year olds. The length of the bladder is frequently rather short (35–42 cm is ideal) and for adult arms with the usual 23 cm bladder it is necessary to take care to place this over the artery on the medial aspect of the arm. Thigh cuffs (17.5 cm × 35 cm bladder) should be used on the arm of obese subjects. It is equally important that the cuff should be neatly and smoothly applied to obviate herniation of the bladder.

5. The mercury column should be lowered at a rate of approximately 2–3 mm/s.

6. There is still considerable debate as to what should be defined as the diastolic pressure, namely, the change from loud to 'muffling' (4th phase) or the disappearance of sound (5th phase) as used in the United States and epidemiological studies. There have been relatively few careful comparisons of intra-arterial and cuff measurements but those studies which have been made suggest that cuff methods give systolic measures which are about 5 mm too low and that both 4th and 5th phases overestimate diastolic pressure. The 5th phase (disappearance) is therefore preferable.

7. One of the commonest sources of error is caused by observer 'digit preference' for readings ending with 0 or 5 and usually 0 or 5 below the true reading. This can be eliminated by the use of a special sphygmomanometer in which the scale or zero are randomly altered and a correction added later (Hawksley muddled zero manometer). Such a manometer is recommended for any clinical trial or for epidemiological measurements. Electronic or otherwise automated methods have many problems, particularly in the measurement of diastolic pressure. Of the many current models the Remler device seems to be the best validated. Of the cheaper digital electronic devices the one manufactured by Takeda Medical, Japan, gives adequate accuracy. Newer devices will be available shortly to monitor beat-to-beat finger blood pressure accurately for a limited time (30–60 min).

8. It is also important to consider other environmental factors such as room temperature, noise, alcohol, caffeine, and recent cigarette smoking (see below).

Aetiology and classification of hypertension
Even after thorough investigation, a specific cause for a raised arterial pressure is found only in some 5 per cent of cases. When no such case can be found hypertension is designated essential or primary, and the term 'secondary' is used to classify those patients in whom a renal, endocrine or other rare abnormality can be found.

Benign and malignant hypertension
Among all cases of hypertension a small proportion can be recognized in which the level of pressure has risen suddenly. In some of these, the physical force of the rise in pressure changes the nature of the disease and its prognosis from a slowly progressive form (misnamed 'benign') to an accelerated form which is truly named malignant since, untreated, the majority of subjects will die within 6–12 months. The cause of this transition appears to relate to sudden loss of the ability of arterioles to resist the raised arterial pressure with consequent insudation of plasma and fibrin into the vessel wall, an associated abrupt rise in peripheral resistance, and fall in tissue perfusion particularly in kidney and brain. The pathological hallmark of this change is a hyalinization of the arterioles – the so-called 'fibrinoid' necrosis. The clinical and pathological features will be discussed below.

Secondary hypertension
The causes and their investigation and management are described on page 13.382. The question of how hard to look for these causes involves a fine and often personal appreciation of the costs (both financial and the morbidity from invasive investigation) and the benefits. In general most physicians are less obsessional in their search in older subjects, particularly women; when there is a family history of hypertension; when the levels of pressure are relatively mild; when the pressure responds well to simple treatment; and when there is no evidence or sudden recent change of the malignant phase.

Essential hypertension
This is a diagnosis of exclusion. Despite careful and energetic search for a primary cause, a diagnosis of essential hypertension is made in 95 per cent of hypertensive subjects. For this reason many patients undergo only minimal investigation (urinalysis and estimation of urea and electrolytes). In the United Kingdom epidemiological surveys have shown that perhaps only 2–3 per cent of patients are referred to a hospital, the majority being supervised by their general practitioner.

There is considerable doubt about the cost-effectiveness of screening patients with high blood pressure for a primary cause. For example, intravenous pyelography is not free from risk, it is uncomfortable, and the therapeutic and diagnostic yield is minimal; many surveys have confirmed this and most physicians now carry out initial pyelography only when the subject is below 40 years old or there is a suspicion of renal disease in the history or on examination. There is a better case for more aggressive investigations if the patient's hypertension is difficult to control with drugs or there is a sudden deterioration after prior good control. Whether to proceed directly to angiography or whether first to do pyelography will depend on the clinical cicumstances.

Aetiology
There is general agreement with the view that the cause of essential hypertension is multifactorial. Some of the factors involved will be considered below.

Family history and genetic background
A family history of raised blood pressure is common. Platt proposed a single dominant gene as a result of his study of the blood pressures of relatives of subjects with hypertension. Pickering was able to refute this theory pointing out that the hypothesis was based on a fallacy arising from the statistical unreliability of the relatively small numbers in Platt's survey. Pickering proposed a multiple genetic influence on arterial pressure and no data have been collected since which negate this concept. The ease with which some Japanese strains of rats can be selectively bred for hypertension suggests that the number of genes involved need not necessarily be large (see below).

Population studies have shown a greater correlation of blood pressure between siblings than that between parents and their children. Twins show greater concordance than spouses, suggesting that genetic factors are more important than environment (see below, under salt intake). Some idea of the power of the genetic influence can be obtained from population studies which show that close relatives of a subject whose blood pressure is 50 mm Hg above the population mean will themselves have pressures 14 mm Hg above the mean.

'Tracking' of blood pressures
There is some evidence that the blood pressure trends of an individual are determined very soon after birth, but it is not possible at present to be sure of this since 'tracking' studies of infants' blood pressures do not show very strong correlations with pressures taken a few years later. Longitudinal studies of arterial pressure have shown that older subjects in the top or bottom 10 per cent of their group, with regard to arterial pressure, stay in the same percentile for many years. Those whose pressure is at the upper end of the range as young adults may be destined to become the hypertensives of the future. There is much debate and few facts as to the

reasons for this. Some recent surveys show that height and body weight are important predictors of pressure and involve skeletal age and growth hormone levels. Nevertheless such 'tracking' from childhood only accounts for some 30–50 per cent of the variation in adult blood pressure, and, in general, early measures of pressure have not been very predictive of future risk. Arguments continue about the relative importance of genetic influences and those of the common family environment, for instance, diet and salt intake among other factors.

Salt intake

The influence of sodium intake upon arterial pressure is another area of controversy. One of the biggest problems is the inability of single 24-hour collections of urine to reflect sodium intake accurately. Those who believe that a high salt intake is an important cause of hypertension point out that there is a strong correlation between the average salt intake of different populations and the incidence of high blood pressure and cardiovascular complications, such as stroke, which accompany hypertension. For example, in Japan the fish diet (containing much salt) is associated with an above average incidence of hypertension. Primitive populations in Amazonia or Africa have a sodium intake of less than 10 mmol/day; they do not develop hypertension, nor does blood pressure rise with age. These correlations are at first sight highly persuasive. However, many other variables such as body weight, nutrition, cultural factors, and other dietary factors (e.g. percentage of polyunsaturated fatty acids) tend to confound the issue.

Opponents of the salt theory point out that within populations there is little or no evidence that an individual's arterial pressure is closely correlated with sodium intake (or excretion, which is easier to measure). Studies of spouses with similar salt intake have not shown any striking influence of intake on arterial pressure. There has been some epidemiological evidence from a Gothenburg study of 50-year-old men that there is a weak *negative* correlation between arterial pressure and sodium excretion. The same has been found in Scotland, and the carefully executed National Health and Nutrition Survey in the United States (NHANES-I) found no correlation between blood pressure and salt intake in a representative sample of the population.

There is no doubt that *extreme* dietary restriction of salt (to less than 10 mmol/day) will reduce arterial pressure, but such extreme restriction would be quite unacceptable as a public health measure. The argument at present is whether a moderate reduction to say less than 80 mmol/day is worthwhile. We do not have adequate information on which to judge this issue. In general the trials have been of short duration on selected subjects, with poor and often inadequately frequent measures of blood pressure, with insufficient control of confounding variables such as environmental temperature, and other dietary changes associated with reduced salt intake. Above all, too few subjects have been studied.

An important part of the argument concerns the mechanism(s) by which excess salt might raise pressure. De Wardener has postulated a defect in the renal excretion of sodium in hypertensives which might lead to an increase in a circulating natriuretic hormone. He and his colleagues have found evidence for such a substance (disputed by others) which they believe may favour hypertension by its postulated effect on cation transport in arteriolar smooth muscle.

These intriguing studies have now been complemented by work on cation fluxes in red and white cells. The findings between investigating groups are not all mutually compatible but do strongly suggest that subjects with essential (but not secondary) hypertension have a genetically determined defect in cell membrane transport which leads to an increase in intracellular sodium. The same defect can be detected in normotensive relatives of hypertensive subjects, and it has been suggested that this, in the presence of a high salt intake, might eventually lead to changes in cell physiology which could cause hypertension. There is some evi-

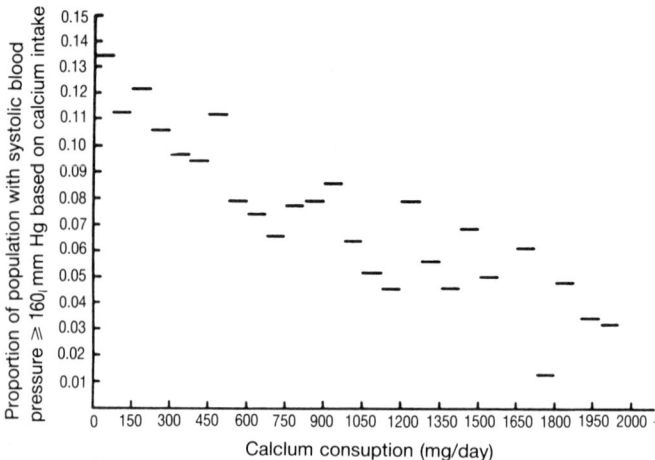

Fig. 7 Risk of hypertension (systolic blood pressure 160 mm Hg) for a subject in the NHANES I, 1971–74, (10 419 people) based on his or her peer group (adjusted for age, race, and sex), and dietary calcium intake. (Reproduced from McCarron *et al.*, 1984, with permission.)

dence that increased intracellular sodium may be paralleled by increased intracellular calcium. If such a defect were present in arterial smooth muscle, it would be a plausible explanation for increased arteriolar tone. However, there are several recent studies which raise doubts and the matter remains unresolved.

It has been argued that, to be effective, sodium restriction should be applied in the crucial early months of life. Again there is now some evidence of a small significant effect of such restriction on pressure but there remains the possibility that sodium restriction at this age might carry some hazard such as increased risk of severe hypovolaemia in the face of any stress caused by gastro-enteritis or blood loss.

Although much has been made of animal models such as the Dahl strain of salt-sensitive rat, it is now clear that these salt-sensitive animals are also sensitive to many other environmental factors, such as noise, and not only to salt intake. It is also possible to breed animals whose pressures rise with salt restriction.

Some well-controlled studies have shown a fall in arterial pressure with moderate sodium restriction; others have failed to do so, among subjects with mild hypertension or among children of parents whose arterial pressure was known to be in the upper third of the blood pressure distribution. A large international study (INTERSALT) is now under way.

Potassium and magnesium supplementation

Some studies have suggested that increased dietary potassium may lower arterial pressure, but again the evidence is conflicting and the best designed investigations have not supported this approach. The suggestion that magnesium depletion, whether caused by diuretic therapy or otherwise, might also provoke a rise in arterial pressure reversed by magnesium supplements is also controversial.

Dietary calcium

McCarron and his colleagues have postulated that there may be abnormalities of calcium metabolism involved in the pathogenesis of essential hypertension. The US dietary survey (NHANES-I) showed a striking correlation between low calcium intake and high systolic arterial pressure (Fig. 7). Low dietary calcium appeared to be the most consistent dietary predictor of hypertension. They calculated that a person consuming less than 300 mg/day of calcium had an 11–14 per cent risk of hypertension; a diet containing 1200 mg/day had an associated risk of 3–6 per cent. It is likely that there are important interactions between calcium and other dietary constituents so that the relationships and mechanisms may not be simple. There is certainly no generally agreed relationship between dietary calcium and arterial pressure. There is rather more evidence now for an abnormality of calcium metabolism either within cells or across their membranes. Support comes from measurement of intracellular calcium in platelets and other cells, and perhaps most persuasively from the studies of Robinson and colleagues in London. They found that the forearm vascular resistance of hypertensive subjects was reduced more by the calcium channel blocking agent verapamil infused into the brachial artery, than by nitroprusside infusion; the reverse was found in normotensive subjects suggesting a functional difference in the role of calcium in the control of arterial smooth muscle tone in hypertensives.

Environmental lead exposure

Earlier associations between raised blood lead concentrations and hypertension suggested that the apparent positive correlation might have been associated with a confounding parallel increase in alcohol consumption. Cigarette smoking also raises blood lead levels. More recently the second US nutrition survey of 20 322 persons (NHANES-II) found a direct relationship between lead blood levels and both systolic and diastolic blood pressures, particularly in young men and women (21–55 years). It was thought possible that the relationship might operate via a lower serum calcium, since both ions follow similar metabolic pathways. Although these results could have very wide public health implications and might (via the petrol engine) provide reasons for urban/rural differences in blood pressure, we should still be cautious. The regression coefficients found in NHANES-II were very low, so that blood lead might only account for a very small proportion of the variability of pressure of the population. Studies in the United Kingdom do not confirm an association between blood lead and blood pressure. Studies of industries with great exposure to lead show no high prevalence of hypertension related to blood lead levels.

Conclusions

The recent studies of the relation between sodium, calcium, and lead intake and blood pressure have raised more questions than they have answered. We are not at the stage where one can advocate mass policies for populations; the evidence for dietary sodium restriction is at best suggestive.

Other environmental factors

Alcohol

Because of the well-recognized skin vasodilation caused by alcohol we tend to overlook the evidence that its general effect is vasoconstriction, particularly in muscle beds. It is now clear that even moderate alcohol intake raises blood pressure. In one important study, the well known fall in blood pressure on admission to hospital was shown to result at least in part from alcohol withdrawal. When subjects supplemented the hospital diet with 3 pints of beer/day blood pressure did not fall! Several population studies have shown a strong positive correlation between chronic alcohol intake and blood pressure; the relation is independent of any concomitant weight gain. When patients remain hypertensive despite drug therapy one should always try to discover whether there is a hidden alcohol problem. It has been estimated that a 1 mm fall in blood pressure results from 100 ml reduction in ethanol/week.

Vegetarian and polyunsaturated fat diets

Well-controlled studies have shown that a Vegan diet, or a diet high in polyunsaturated fatty acids, may lower blood pressure by about 5 mm Hg. These diets are not generally acceptable to the population at large so it is important to determine which are the active ingredients of such changes.

Noise

Studies of noisy environments, such as airport communities or heavy industry, have shown that raised environmental noise levels can raise blood pressure.

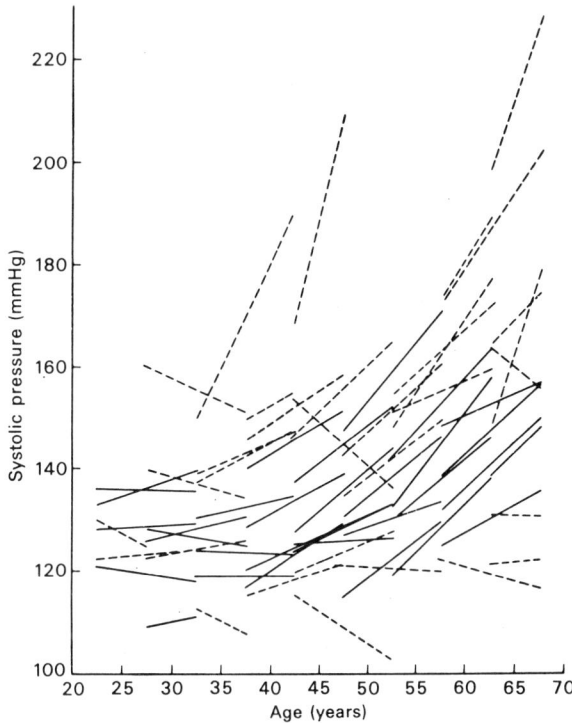

Fig. 8 Trends of mean systolic pressure for males followed up for 10 years in Rhondda Fach and the Vale of Glamorgan. Solid line, groups with 10 or more subjects; dotted line, groups with less than 10 subjects. (Reproduced from Miall and Chinn, 1973, *Clin. Sci. mol. Med.* **45**, 23S, with permission.)

Age changes

In western nations, blood pressure usually rises with age. In males this happens steadily, but in females there is very little rise until after the menopause. Surveys of the population of the Rhonda Fach have confirmed this trend (Fig. 8). Although the figure suggests that the rise accelerated with age, the data fit equally well a linear as opposed to an exponential relation, i.e. they do not therefore provide evidence for or against the operation of a vicious circle. The cause of the rise in arterial pressure with age is not clear. Plasma renin declines with age, whereas catecholamines rise with age. It seems probable that the age-related rise in arterial pressure is secondary to structural thickening and degenerative changes in arteries and arterioles. Blood pressure does not necessarily always rise with age, e.g. in the natives of New Guinea and in many other remote populations.

Environmental temperature

Until the very large MRC trial (about 17 000 subjects) of mild hypertension it was not generally realized that there is about 3–7 mm Hg difference in systolic blood pressure between winter and summer in the United Kingdom for about 20 °C temperature difference. The lower figure applies to young and the upper to older subjects.

Coffee and cigarettes

Drinking coffee (200 mg caffeine) elevates blood pressure by about 10/8 mm Hg for 1–2 hours. Cigarette smoking causes a shorter term rise in pressure but the combination of cigarettes and coffee produces a greater and more lasting effect which is still present at 2.5 hours. Overall most studies of the longer term effects of cigarette smoking show a lower blood pressure in smokers, but this appears to be largely related to weight. Malignant hypertension is more common in cigarette smokers than nonsmokers. These studies emphasize that it is important to consider cigarette and caffeine intake when measuring blood pressure.

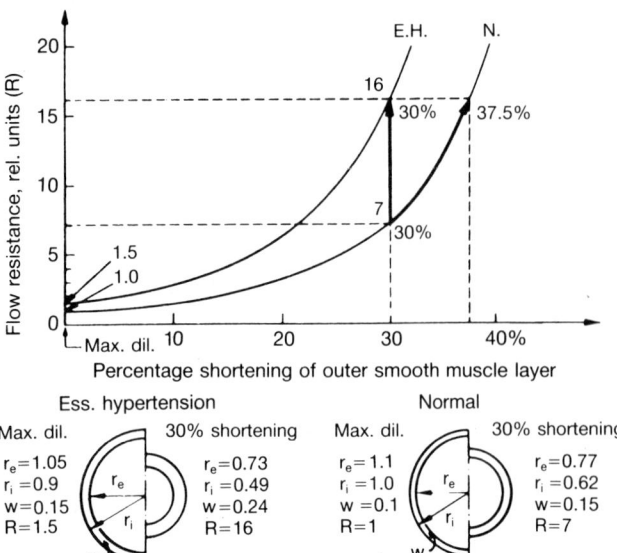

Fig. 9 Showing the large change in resistance (and hence arterial pressure) which follows from the same percentage shortening of arteriolar smooth muscle, when one vessel (hypertension, E.H.) has a slightly thicker wall than the normal vessel (N). r_e, external radius; r_i, internal radius; w, wall thickness; nominal resistance units, R. (Reproduced from Sivertsson, 1970, after Folkow *et al.*, *Acta physiol. Scand.*, Suppl. 342, with permission.)

Structural changes in small arteries

Folkow has emphasized the important role of adaptive changes in the vessel walls, particularly in the arterioles. In experimental animals these changes develop in a matter of days, and regress if the hypertension is reversed.

Figure 9 shows how relatively small changes in the wall thickness of these narrow vessels can have quite profound changes on the resistance to flow and hence the arterial pressure. The same degree of smooth muscle shortening will result in a much greater increase in flow resistance in the thicker hypertensive vessel. Looked at in another way, this means that a high resistance can be obtained in response to fewer sympathetic nerve impulses or lower concentrations of humoral agents such as angiotensin or circulating catecholamines. Normal levels of urinary or blood catechols or of angiotensin do not therefore exclude these agents as being important in the genesis of hypertension, since normal levels may lead to inappropriately high vascular resistance in these adapted arterioles.

Recent work in humans confirms that left ventricular hypertrophy is reversible by hypotensive treatment, and suggests that vascular changes may also be reversible.

The sympathetic nervous system

Many of the drugs used to control hypertension act via the autonomic nervous system. The recent development of more precise methods of analysis of catecholamines in the blood and urine has promoted a revival of interest in the role of the sympathetic nerves in essential hypertension. At present the question cannot be resolved since the evidence is conflicting; there is, however, a bias towards a positive role.

Some of the conflicting evidence may be the result of patient selection. Another problem is that estimation of either urine or plasma catecholamines at best give a shadowy indication of the activity of the sympathetic system. Figure 20 (page 13.379) gives a much simplified scheme of noradrenaline release from the nerve terminal. Most of the catechols released are reabsorbed into the nerve terminal and perhaps less than 5 per cent are taken up by the blood and then excreted in the urine. Despite this large re-uptake of noradrenaline, recent studies have shown good correla-

tion between direct measurement of muscle sympathetic nerve activity in humans and plasma catecholamines.

There is considerable overlap between plasma noradrenaline levels in hypertensive compared with normotensive subjects, with no clear increase in the hypertensive group. Some evidence suggests a relation between arterial pressure and plasma noradrenaline in younger subjects and normals but none in older hypertensives. It is clear that the sensitivity of β-adrenoreceptors is reduced in older subjects; there is less evidence for a suggested reduction in α-receptor sensitivity in older subjects.

At one time it was suggested that the β-2 positive feedback loop seen in Fig. 20 might be important in the genesis of hypertension. The hypothesis was that environmentally induced rises in plasma adrenaline might result in re-uptake of more adrenaline into the storage vesicles, which was then available for release with noradrenaline in response to a nerve impulse to stimulate β-2 presynaptic release of further catechols. Critical evidence for this mechanism of amplification is missing and recent work casts doubt upon its validity.

Important peptides such as neuropeptide Y may be released by autonomic nerves and interact with catecholamine release. Neuropeptide Y is a potent vasoconstrictor. The newer work on this and the powerful vasodilator, calcitonin gene-related peptide add to the complexity of elucidating the relationship between blood pressure and simple indices of adrenergic function.

The activity of the sympathetic nervous system is increased in many forms of experimental hypertension, such as that caused by renal artery stenosis or by DOCA-salt/administration, but the mechanism by which the sympathetic system is excited in hypertension is unclear, whether by reduced afferent inhibitory input (e.g. from arterial baroreceptors) or from cortical or hypothalamic modulation of the baroreflex arc, or from a reduction of cortical control of sympathetic neurones which are independent of the circulatory reflexes.

Recordings from human sympathetic nerves have been made by placing microelectrodes in the peripheral nerves of conscious people. These have shown the great influence of environmental stimuli of apparently the most trivial nature on the short-term control of sympathetic outflow. The influence of mental arithmetic in producing significant rises in blood pressure is also well established. It has been suggested that constant repetition of such alerting stimuli might lead to labile and then sustained hypertension.

Neurogenic hypertension

Animal models of neurogenic hypertension caused by cutting the so-called 'buffer' nerves (carotid sinus and aortic baroreceptors) differs from essential hypertension in several respects. First, the pressure is extremely variable; secondly, there is a disproportionate tachycardia; thirdly, the pressure may return to normal at night; and, fourthly, the degree of arteriolar and cardiac hypertrophy is less marked. In clinical medicine the hypertension that most resembles this pattern is that associated with cerebral tumours and with other pathology in the brain stem.

Baroreflex sensitivity in hypertension

There is a marked diminution in baroreflex sensitivity with increasing age and with increasing levels of resting mean arterial pressure. Figure 10 shows that in any age group the subject's resting arterial pressure is closely related to the baroreflex sensitivity. Is the loss of reflex control the cause of the hypertension or is it merely that the baroreceptors are damaged by hypertension? We do not know the answer to this question but both mechanisms may be operative to produce a vicious circle. The carotid sinuses are one of the most common sites in the body for the development of atheroma. Whatever the cause of hypertension in a given case, ineffective baroreceptors probably contribute to impaired homeostasis of arterial pressure (Fig. 11).

Post-mortem study of the carotid sinus has shown a very gross increase in wall thickness with age: this change is very apparent

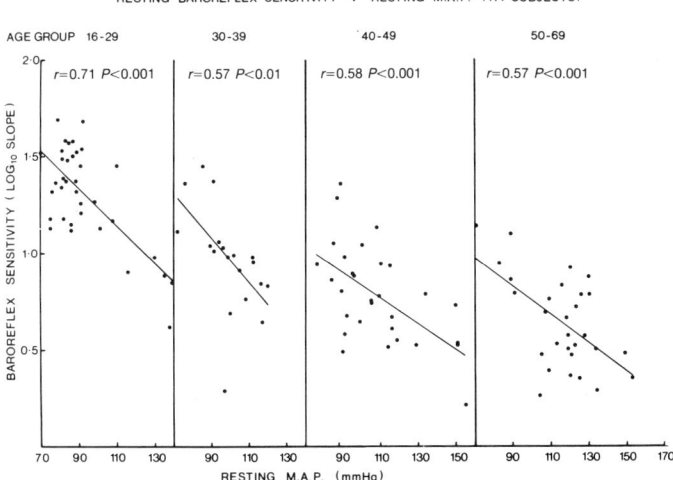

RESTING BAROREFLEX SENSITIVITY V RESTING M.A.P. (114 SUBJECTS)

Fig. 10 Resting log baroreflex sensitivity in 114 subjects classified according to age and resting mean arterial pressure. The reflex control of heart rate becomes increasingly poor with higher arterial pressure and with advancing age. The method used gives a numerical value to the degree of bradycardia which reflexly results from a provoked rise in arterial pressure caused by a pressor agent such as phenylephrine.

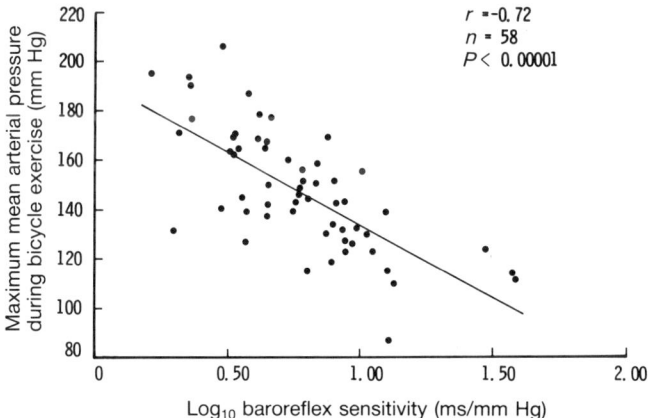

Fig. 11 Relationship between maximum mean intra-arterial pressure reached during bicycle exercise and the logarithm of the baroreflex sensitivity in 58 subjects. (Reproduced from Floras, 1981, *Neural regulation of blood pressure in hypertension*, D. Phil. thesis, University of Oxford, with permission.)

even at the age of 25 years. Guyton has questioned whether the baroreceptors have any long-term influence on blood pressure. Others disagree with this viewpoint, particularly since there is much animal data indicating that either lesions of the afferent input to the CNS or interruption of the reflex arc in the medulla can lead to severe and sustained high blood pressure.

The role of the central nervous system and psychological factors
Some spontaneously hypertensive rats (SHR) have an abnormal nervous reaction to environmental stimuli. They show sharper and more sustained rises in arterial pressure when their cages are disturbed than do normotensive controls. There is evidence too of a greater sympathetic discharge in these animals.

Do these animal studies implicate the CNS in the genesis of high blood pressure in humans? Pickering has stated that factors acting through the mind are among those most difficult to evaluate. Early work attempted to find some psychological abnormality or personality type in subjects with hypertension. None has shown any influence of psychotic illness on raising arterial pressure, nor has there been any increased incidence of anxiety neurosis among

hypertensives. Indeed, randomized population studies both in the United Kingdom and Sweden have demonstrated that subjects with high blood pressure complain less than matched normal controls. Whether this is a true well-being or whether it represents a tendency to 'bottle things up' and be a non-complainer is not clear. One hypothesis (Wolff) states that hypertension results from suppressed emotion. Crude but gross intervention, such as frontal leucotomy, has no clear-cut influence on arterial pressure.

Although there is a clear relation between mental or emotional stress and a temporary rise in blood pressure, there is no evidence that this leads to a sustained rise. This cannot be construed as evidence against a relation between the mind and arterial pressure, since adequately controlled studies would be almost impossible to carry out. What constitutes a stress to one subject would not necessarily do so for another.

A recent study from Glasgow has suggested that a community of schizophrenics leading an institutional life had a slower than expected increased in blood pressure with age. This finding reinforces the feeling that environmental factors may have a substantial influence on blood pressure.

Influences of biofeedback or transcendental meditation
Because of the association of hypertension with western society and its absence in certain less-developed cultures, attempts have been made to lower arterial pressure by meditation or mental relaxation. There is now evidence that biofeedback can reduce pressure. There have been several well-controlled studies. The subject is given information about the level of arterial pressure and asked to try to raise or lower this pressure. Several groups have now reported successful use of biofeedback in the voluntary control of heart rates or blood pressure. Although these studies have been of great scientific interest, it is disappointing that for the most part the changes produced have been very small, of the order of a few mm Hg only. Nor do we have any evidence that the technique can be used by the subject when not given any instrumental feedback. The techniques need dedication and time. They do not seem likely to be adopted widely.

The role of the kidney in essential hypertension
Few would disagree with Guyton that the kidney is of great importance in the determination of arterial pressure. His thesis states that if the arterial pressure rises the kidney excretes more salt and water until it again reaches equilibrium at the original arterial pressure. A decreased renal mass will need a higher arterial pressure to excrete the obligatory salt and water load imposed by the dietary intake. The level of the blood pressure at this equilibrium point could of course be altered by changes in the tone of the glomerular arterioles, as well as by a reduction in renal mass. Since this arteriolar tone is influenced by arterial and cardiac receptors, the renal and neural schools of high blood pressure could, in theory, be reconciled.

Powerful evidence for the role of the kidney has been gathered from elegant experiments in rats, which have shown that the high blood pressure of selectively bred, spontaneoulsy hypertensive rats can be lowered by transplanting the kidneys of normotensive rats and vice versa (Fig. 12). Transplanting the kidneys of the Japanese SHR also leads to hypertension. These experiments are not totally convincing since, particularly in the SHR, the kidney which is transplanted may have been subject to some structural change which resulted from the donor animals' blood pressure. In humans there is some evidence that hypertension may regress after transplantation of a kidney from a normotensive donor and vice versa.

Natriuretic hormone
De Wardener has long advocated the existence of a circulating natriuretic hormone and has more recently argued that such a hormone, by inhibiting sodium transport in cells other than renal tubules, might lead to changes in arterioles favouring increased sensitivity to vasconstrictive stimuli (see page 13.364).

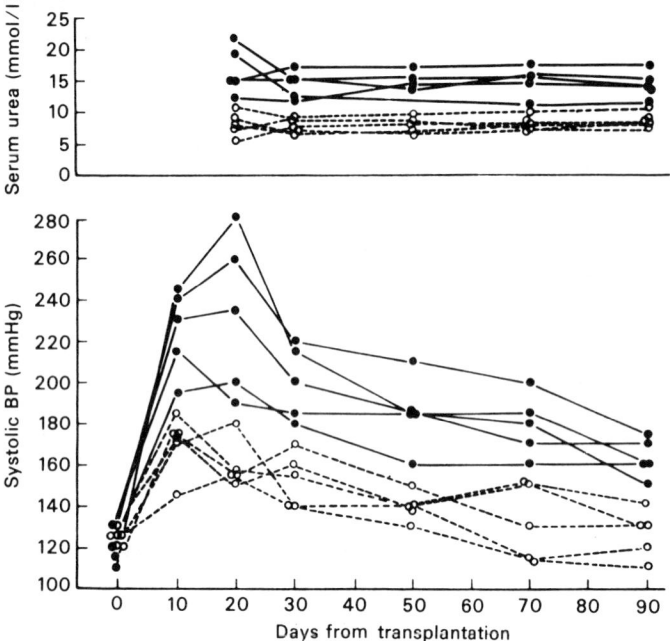

Fig. 12 Systolic blood pressure (BP) and serum urea of young normotensive recipient rats after transplantation of kidney from young normotensive (open circles) and hypertensive (filled circles) rats (prehypertensive stage). (Reproduced from Bianchi *et al.*, 1974, *Clin. Sci.* **47**, 435, with permission.)

Atrial natriuretic peptide

This has no effect on membrane Na–K–ATPase and is not in contention as the de Wardener natriuretic hormone. It is a powerful vasodilator, resembling nitroprusside in its action which is mediated by cyclic GMP. It also antagonizes the vasoconstrictive effects of noradrenaline and angiotensin II, and inhibits both renin and aldosterone secretion. There are preliminary reports of raised levels in untreated essential hypertension, a finding compatible with, but not diagnostic of, a compensatory response either to raised pressure itself or the hypothetical reduced renal capacity for salt excretion.

Antidiuretic hormone (arginine vasopressin)

In the last few years there has been renewed interest in the role of vasopressin blood pressure control. Levels of vasopressin are elevated in malignant hypertension and in several experimental models. The hypertensive action of vasopressin seems particularly potent, and at physiological concentrations if the baroreflexes are impaired; but overall evidence is against an important role for ADH in human hypertension.

Physical fitness and blood pressure

Several anecdotal as well as controlled studies have confirmed that blood pressure is lowered acutely by exercise. The effect is substantial, about 10–12 mm Hg, and lasts for a few hours. It also appears likely from studies of more prolonged exercise that increased physical fitness (such as obtained by 20–30 min of moderate exercise 4–5 times a week) is accompanied by significant lowering of blood pressure (by about 7–10 mm Hg).

Pathology

The pathology of essential hypertension represents the combination of adaptive and degenerative changes in the heart and circulation.

Adaptive changes

The heart in essential hypertension may at first appear normal both on clinical examination and investigation by X-ray, ECG, or echocardiography. With time there is a gradual hypertrophy of the left ventricle. The individual cardiac cells increase in size and probably in number. There is a very close linear relationship between the weight of the heart and the subject's arterial pressure. This phenomenon, seen in humans, can be reproduced experimentally. Lowering of arterial pressure by treatment can result in a regression of the hypertrophy, but different drugs reducing pressure to the same extent may result in different degrees of regression of hypertrophy. Cardiac hypertrophy may result from sympathetic stimulation to the heart, as the final common path, whatever the original stimulus. The failure of vasodilator drugs to induce regression as readily as antisympathetic agents supports this, but the question remains open.

Adaptive changes to 'work hypertrophy' are also seen in the arterial tree, particularly in the small arteries and arterioles. There is thickening of the muscular media (see Fig. 9) and intima with important consequences since in these small vessels a minor increase in wall thickness has quite large effects on peripheral resistance. These adaptive structural changes allow the circulation to sustain a higher arterial pressure without the metabolic 'expense' of increased catecholamine drive. They may be part of the reason why removal of the cause of secondary hypertension does not always result in a complete lowering of arterial pressure to normal.

These adaptive changes in heart and arterial tree correlate better with direct or ambulatory estimates of arterial pressure than with casual ('office') pressures (see Fig. 6).

Degenerative changes

The adaptive changes described above may be gradually progressive over many years. Eventually degenerative lesions develop in both heart and arteries and lead to the lethal consequences of hypertension. Three changes impair the performance of the heart: first, the larger muscle fibres increase the volume of tissue between capillaries and thus the vascular supply becomes more tenuous; secondly, the increased left ventricular thickness increases the pressure gradient from epicardium to endocardium rendering the inner third of the muscle relatively ischaemic; thirdly, the coronary vessels develop atheromatous lesions which aggravate development of ischaemic fibrosis in the heart or even provoke myocardial infarction. The consequence is the development of hypertensive heart failure – one of the common terminations of the patient with hypertension.

Equally important are the generalized degenerative arterial lesions. The mechanisms of these are not fully understood but appear to be due to several factors. The high arterial pressure leads to a greater rate of filtration of plasma through the arterial wall. Certain lipoprotein fractions are preferentially retained in the vessel wall so leading to degenerative lesions which are not peculiar to hypertension; but there is no doubt that high pressure accelerates their development. The predilection for certain sites in the vascular tree may be related to differing shear forces causing damage to vascular endothelium at sites such as arterial junctions, particularly carotid and iliac, where turbulence is common.

The consequence of medial and intimal hypertrophy is most important in the kidney and brain. Thickening of the renal interlobular and arcuate vessels results from medial hypertrophy, elastic reduplication, and intimal proliferation. Afferent arterioles and some glomeruli become hyalinized with associated tubular atrophy and interstitial fibrosis. Some impairment of renal function is common but significant renal failure is uncommon unless the malignant phase supervenes. Similar pathological changes occur in mesenteric vessels but are uncommon in muscular arteries.

Ross Russell has emphasized the importance of the Charcot-Bouchard aneurysm and the frequently associated 'lacunae' (dilation of small arteries in the brain) in the genesis of haemorrhagic stroke. These small micro-aneurysms must be clearly distinguished from the saccular or 'berry' aneurysm seen on angiography. They occur in older people in close association with hypertension and are overlooked at post-mortem unless a careful search is made. They are most common in the region of the thalamus and white matter surrounding the corpus striatum. They are up to 1 mm in size and are probably a major cause of cerebral haemorrhage. Histologically there is a local absence of smooth muscle in the vessel. The wall of the micro-aneurysm consists of collagen and some remnants of elastica with a variable amount of fatty hyaline material.

Thrombotic stroke does not arise from these Charcot-Bouchard lesions but from arteriosclerosis of larger vessels, commonly the middle cerebral or the carotid vessels in the neck. These arteriosclerotic lesions of the larger supplying arteries to the brain are also the source of emboli of platelets ('white bodies'), which have been seen impacting in the retina of patients with transient ischaemic attacks. There they may break up after which the neurological function (in this case vision) is restored.

The pathology of hypertensive retinopathy

Arteriosclerotic change
It is important to realize that increased light relex, increased tortuosity, and arteriovenous nipping are signs which may reflect either hypertension, arteriosclerosis or both.

Hypertensive change
There are changes more specific to hypertension. At very high arterial pressures there may be irregularity of the calibre of the arterioles such that there is an appearance of local constriction followed by dilation. The dilated regions are then the abnormal ones with dilation representing breakdown of the autoregulatory constriction in response to a rise in transmural pressure (the normal response is some times called the Bayliss effect). At an earlier and more benign stage, the whole arteriolar bed may be constricted and the normal ratio of vein to artery, 3:2, increased. This diminution in calibre is not absolutely specific to hypertension; it may occur if the retinal arterial pressure is diminished by upstream arterial narrowing or occlusion.

'Cotton wool' exudates are due to ischaemia resulting in increased axonal transport in normal neurones near a micro-infarct. Fluorescein angiography in some instances demonstrates blockage of the arteriole just proximal to the 'spot', and absent capillary filling. The lesions may be exactly reproduced by microsphere emboli in the experimental animal. Final breakdown of the vessel leads to flame-shaped haemorrhages (the shape determined by the parallel nerve fibres) or deeper 'blot' haemorrhages. 'Cotton wool' spots and haemorrhages of hypertensive origin are stigmata of the malignant phase and underlying fibrinoid necrosis. Both can resolve in a few weeks if arterial pressure is lowered effectively.

Elschnig spots, small, round and three to four times the diameter of a major retinal artery, are choroidal infarcts, rarely seen now except in the retinopathy associated with pre-eclampsia, where the pressure rise is often acute and the vessels little protected by gradual hypertrophy. They are best seen on fluorescein angiography.

All of these exudative lesions may develop when arterial damage occurs from other causes in the absence of hypertension. Common causes are severe anaemia of rapid onset and uraemia, but also include hypoxia, collagen disease with arteritis (e.g. systemic lupus erythematosus) and subacute bacterial endocarditis.

Papilloedema, or swelling of the optic disc is also a marker of malignant hypertension and may be present with or without haemorrhages or exudates. The mechanism of its development is not clearly understood. It may be due to general brain oedema secondary to breakdown of autoregulation of flow in the face of very high pressure. It is not always associated with raised intracranial pressure but is probably related to a slowing down of slow axonal transport in the optic nerve. Nerve function is usually well preserved.

Papilloedema is also seen in raised intracranial pressure from, for example, a cerebral tumour. Cerebral tumour or raised intracranial pressure from any cause may lead to secondary hypertension (Cushing's reflex). The exact mechanism is obscure but is possibly related to sympathetic discharge caused by ischaemia of vital medullary centres. It can thus be seen then that occasionally we may be faced with a therapeutic dilemma. Is the patient who presents with stupor, hypertension, and papilloedema suffering from hypertensive encephalopathy or is the hypertension secondary to the high intracranial pressure of a space-occupying lesion in the skull? Here it is important to search for evidence of prior hypertension, e.g. clinical left ventricular hypertrophy on the ECG, but this may be absent (see below). A computer-aided tomographic (CAT) scan may be helpful.

In a subject with hypertension these retinal changes are not usually seen unless the diastolic arterial pressure is more than 125 mmHg (or has risen very rapidly) and usually considerably higher. The diagnosis of a hypertensive retinopathy with haemorrhage and papilloedema, constitutes a medical emergency. Immediate steps should be taken to lower the arterial pressure gently. The patient should not wait for the next outpatient clinic.

Fibrinoid necrosis: the malignant stage
Essential hypertension has been divided into benign and malignant phases although the former is often far from benign. The damage caused depends largely on the duration of the raised pressure and other factors which may impair the ability of the circulation to withstand pressure. If the pressure is very high or the rate of rise has been abrupt, an accelerated phase may supervene with very rapid deterioration in the health of the patient (the so-called malignant change) with the patient dying within 6–12 months unless treated. Formerly there was great speculation about the cause of this change. The hallmark of the phase is the appearance of a pink staining material in the wall of the resistance vessels (small arteries and arterioles) resembling fibrin (so-called fibrinoid necrosis). This change, which leads to a severe reduction in the lumen of the vessel, is responsible for the rapid development of micro-infarcts in retina and kidney. It can occur in any form of hypertension from whatever cause, provided the pressure is high enough, or rises sufficiently rapidly.

Experimental studies of animals made severely hypertensive by a number of differing methods, in which a colloidal carbon marker has been injected into the circulation at the time when the animal was developing the malignant phase, have shown that these very high pressures breach the vascular endothelium. Plasma constituents (and carbon) enter the vessel wall and rapidly damage the muscle cells of the media, with deposition of material giving the staining reaction for fibrin. The wall swelling may occlude the vessel. Examination of arterioles of the gut has shown alternating segments of 'constriction' and dilation. It is the dilated segments that are damaged and show fibrinoid change. These lesions have been shown to be reversible in animals and presumably in humans since treatment of the malignant phase is compatible with prolonged survival thereafter, as shown by Pickering and his colleagues.

Echocardiographic studies in subjects with malignant hypertension have shown little evidence of left ventricular hypertrophy. This suggests that in many cases the course to malignant hypertension has been of short duration.

Hypertensive encephalopathy
The patient who presents with hypertension and coma may, with treatment, make a full and often surprising recovery without evidence of stroke or focal damage. This picture, which is always seen following fits associated with high blood pressure, is sometimes called hypertensive encephalopathy. The pathology underlying this condition has been the subject of much controversy. Port-mortem reports are, almost by definition, rare. Oedema, scattered haemorrhages, and small infarcts of the brain have all been seen. Classic experimental studies by Byrom, with obser-

vations of both the retina and the surface vessels of the brain through a transparent window, suggested that the clinical picture was caused by the lesion of segmental vascular constriction, with capillary stasis and oedema as described above. More recent observations implicate a 'breakthrough' of cerebral autoregulation, with vascular and tissue damage both related to overperfusion and physical damage to vessel walls, which is maximal in the dilated areas.

Clinical picture

Hypertension is a condition with at first no symptoms. Despite the popular opinion that headaches are a common symptom of high arterial pressure, properly controlled studies of an unselected population have shown that this is not so. Hospital and general practitioner studies are biased because a patient complaining of headache is more likely to have the blood pressure measured. Only one symptom has been shown to be more common among hypertensive subjects than normotensive controls. This is dyspnoea, presumably due to a combination of a higher pulmonary venous pressure secondary to increased left ventricular stiffness, plus some cases of true left ventricular failure as a result of hypertensive left ventricular disease. Subjects with very high blood pressure in the malignant phase do suffer from severe headache. This is characteristically worse in the morning and may be present on waking. Such patients form but a small proportion of the whole and there are so many other more trivial causes of headache that the symptom overall has little diagnostic value.

The surprising feature of studies of symptoms of high blood pressure is that people with high arterial pressure have less than others.

Once the degenerative consequences of hypertension have begun, symptoms may be due to failure of the heart (dyspnoea, orthopnoea, nocturia, frank left ventricular or congestive heart failure), the coronary circulation (angina or infarction), the cerebral circulation (stroke, severe headache, visual deterioration, or hypersensative encephalopathy), or the kidney (uraemia, anaemia, fatigue, vomiting or oedema).

Physiology of the circulation in hypertension

The only striking abnormality of the circulation in uncomplicated hypertension is the rise in the calculated peripheral arterial resistance. The consequence is that the normal variability in arterial pressure is exaggerated. This is evident in 24-hour recordings of intra-arterial blood pressure obtained in subjects carrying out their normal work and sleeping at home. It is clear that the arterial system can tolerate very large rises in blood pressure which occur during everyday events. For instance, during coitus in normotensive subjects arterial pressures may double and heart rates reach 140/min.

Signs

The changes in the arterioles of the fundus have been described above under the section on Pathology (see page 13.369).

The pulse feels forcible and is more difficult to compress in diastole. A powerful left ventricle may be felt, particularly if the patient is turned to the left. There may be an aortic ejection click and an apical or aortic systolic ejection murmur caused by turbulence secondary to aortic dilation. Sometimes this is enough to cause aortic incompetence, but this is very uncommon and always raises the question of aortic dissection (see below).

Course and prognosis

Essential hypertension is a disease with an extremely variable prognosis. Some of the reasons for this are understood and will be discussed below. The outcome in any subject is probably determined by the interplay of the actual level of arterial pressure and the duration for which it is raised, causing wear and tear on vessels which are variably resistant to this stress. Largely as a result of the careful studies done in Framingham, over the last 20 years, a

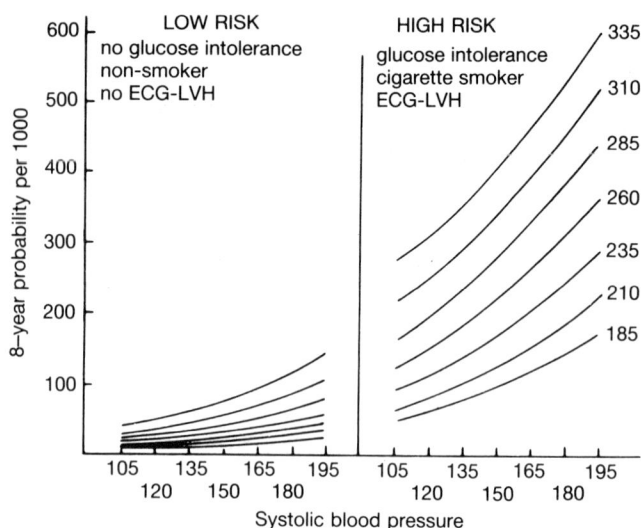

Fig. 13 Risk of cardiovascular disease according to systolic blood pressure and serum cholesterol value in otherwise high and low risk subjects: 35-year-old men. (Framingham Study, 18-year follow-up.) (Reproduced from Kannel and Dawber, 1974, *Br. J. hosp. Med.* **7**, 508, with permission.)

reasonably clear picture of the quantitative aspects of these 'risk factors' have been found in the middle-aged American.

Prognosis depends on the height of the arterial pressure

There is a clear correlation between arterial pressure and risk of death. Thus a subject with a systolic arterial pressure of 100 mm Hg will be less at risk than one with 120 mm Hg. A person with a systolic arterial pressure of 170 mm Hg will have about twice the mortality risk of the person whose pressure is 120 mm Hg.

Other factors (see below) may contribute to increase the risk.

Influences which accentuate the risk

As one might expect, the wear and tear on vessels may be accentuated by other conditions concomitant with hypertension. The most striking of these are:

1. Gender. It is well known that women withstand raised arterial pressure better than men, particularly before the menopause, when the risk of death or morbidity is about half that of men.
2. Abnormal blood lipids. At the same arterial pressure, a serum cholesterol of 8.64 mmol/l will carry a five-fold risk of cardiovascular disease, compared with a cholesterol of 4.77 mmol/l. The ratio of high to low density lipoprotein (preferably > 20 per cent) may slightly improve the estimate of risk, and some recent studies suggest that the apolipoprotein values may be a better guide still.
3. Cigarette smoking.
4. ECG evidence of left ventricular hypertrophy.
5. Glucose intolerance.
6. Obesity. This is a complex and unresolved area since obesity is frequently associated with raised serum lipids. On the other hand, the difficulties in measuring blood pressure accurately in the obese may lead to an overestimate of arterial pressure and hence a better prognosis than might have been expected.

The importance of associated risk factors

Figure 13 shows that the risk of morbidity or death at any level of arterial pressure will vary many times, depending on the presence of one or more of other adverse factors such as cholesterol, cigarette smoking, and diabetes. The decision on whether to treat an individual patient depends on an assessment of the balance of the risk factors against the side-effects of treatment; it depends, therefore, not only on arterial pressure, but also the other factors which act as 'multipliers' in the risk equation. For this reason, it is more logical to treat men rather than women at borderline levels of arterial pressure, as clearly shown by the MRC trial of mild hypertension, where women fared best on placebo (see below).

Morbidity from hypertension

The increase in morbidity with increase in arterial pressure is more striking for stroke and heart failure than for coronary or peripheral artery disease. However, in terms of impact on the community, there are about three to five times more cases of coronary disease than stroke, particularly in younger age groups. In Framingham, for instance, the annual incidence of stroke was 66 per 10 000 and coronary heart disease 306 per 10 000 in men with hypertension. The bulk of these deaths occur in subjects with relatively modest degrees of hypertension (see Fig. 2).

Treatment

The high prevalence of hypertension in western populations and the serious consequences of pressure upon the heart, brain, and kidneys as a result of arterial degeneration have been summarized above.

If treatment were free of side-effects, particularly since it is demonstrably effective in reducing dramatically the ravages of stroke and heart failure (and probably to some degree of coronary disease), it would be justifiable to offer treatment to the very large number of subjects with only minor elevations of pressure. Furthermore, since hypertension is usually an entirely symptom-free condition until the subjects suffer a stroke or myocardial infarction, there is a case for screening the population as a whole. The difficulty with this approach is that antihypertensive drugs are far from free of side-effects so acceptability of treatment is restricted at least in some patients.

The effects of treatment on morbidity

The Veterans' Administration studies have provided the best data on the effects of antihypertensive drugs on long-term prognosis. Their first trial of therapy for more severe hypertension (diastolic pressure greater than 115 mm Hg) was ended early because of the adverse morbidity and mortality in the control group. A second trial was then mounted for patients with diastolic pressures from 90 to 115 mm Hg. This too showed a highly significant improvement in the treated group, where morbidity was only one-third of that of the control group assessed over five years. However, the greatest benefit was in the 110–115 mm Hg group and there was considerable doubt about the benefits of treating the 90–110 mm Hg diastolic level. Furthermore, the Veterans' Administration patients were highly selected for both their adherence to a drug regimen and were remarkable for evidence of hypertensive vascular disease. It seems likely that the comparable levels for general practitioner or outpatient attenders in the United Kingdom would be 100–125 mm Hg diastolic, particularly since morbid events in the control group in the Veterans' Administration study occurred in about 55 per cent over five years – an unexpectedly high rate.

Recent trials of treatment of mild hypertension

The Australian blood pressure trial compared the effect of active versus placebo treatment in about 3500 men and women with mild hypertension, aged 30–69 years, free of any signs of cardiovascular disease, and followed for four years. There was a two-thirds reduction in cardiovascular mortality in the treated group, mainly due to stroke reduction. There was also a non-significant reduction in the incidence of ischaemic heart disease. The initial blood pressures in the patients who experienced symptoms of ischaemic heart disease were not different from those who did not. No differences in trial end points were seen between treated and placebo patients with pressures < 95 diastolic. About half the placebo patients' blood pressures fell below 90 mm Hg by 3 years.

The US HDFP trial The US hypertension detection and follow-up programme (HDFP) was a community study of about 11 000

people who were randomized either to obsessional clinic care or routine care by their private physicians. The latter were equally effective in the treatment of severe hypertension but less so with mild hypertension. This was understandable since at that time it was not at all clear whether it was worthwhile treating patients with diastolic blood pressure in the range 90–105 mm Hg. The trial showed that mortality was 20 per cent lower in this milder category, when treated in the clinic, with particular benefit among Blacks.

The HDFP trial is the only large study to suggest that treatment of subjects with diastolic pressures in the range 90–95 mm Hg was clearly beneficial. Because of the enormous financial and public health implications of this recommendation and the absence of any confirmatory evidence from the other studies it is important to realize that the design of this HDFP study has aroused considerable controversy, both within and outside the United States. It has been difficult to be sure whether the differences in mortality between the 'usual' and 'special' care groups are due to more careful control of blood pressure or to better general health care.

During 1985 three other important studies reported their main results.

The IPPPSH trial The International Prospective Primary Prevention Study in Hypertension (IPPPSH) randomized about 6400 men and women aged 40–64 years and with diastolic blood pressures of 100–125 mm Hg to receive treatment starting with oxprenolol or placebo, followed by supplementary drugs in order to reduce diastolic blood pressure to 95 mm Hg or less. Event rates were clearly related to blood pressures achieved on treatment, rather than index pressures (Fig. 14). Diuretics were used as supplementary therapy in 67 per cent of the oxprenolol group and 82 per cent of the 'placebo' group. Overall there were no significant differences between the two types of treatment. As in the MRC trial (below) there was a suggestion that the β-blocker regime was better for non-smokers. Smokers had twice the cardiac and cerebrovascular complications of non-smokers. Smoking or not was a much more important determinant of prognosis than differences in control of arterial pressure.

MRC mild hypertension trial This very large study (over 17 000 patients, 85 000 patient years of treatment) randomized men and women aged 35–64 years with phase V diastolic blood pressures of 90–109 mm Hg to placebo, propranolol 240 mg or bendrofluazide 10 mg/day (perhaps a large dose). The trial was largely conducted on a general practice (and middle-class) population. It showed a significant reduction in strokes of 1.4/1000 patient years for those on active treatment versus 2.6/1000 patient years for those on

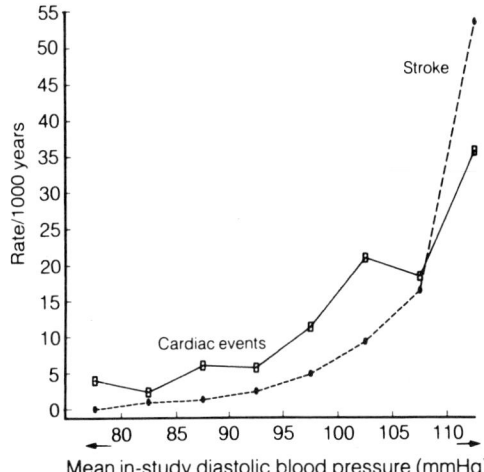

Fig. 14 Cardiac events and stroke rates per 1000 patient years of treatment in the IPPPSH trial related to diastolic blood pressure during the trial. (Reproduced from IPPPSH Collaborative Group, with permission.)

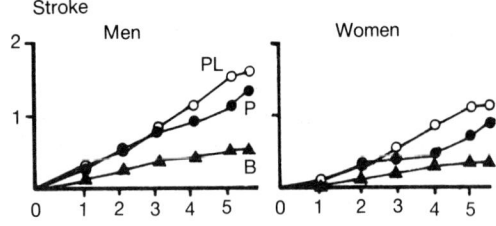

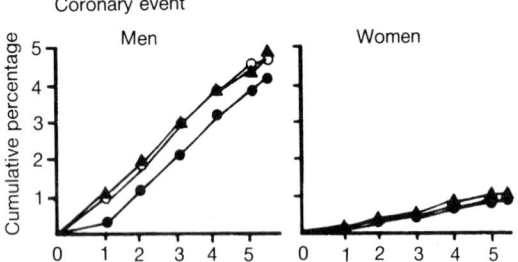

Fig. 15 Cumulative percentage of people with terminating events (stroke, coronary event) by sex and by randomized treatment, in the MRC mild hypertension trial (triangle, bendrofluazide 10 mg daily; closed circles, propranolol, up to 240 mg daily; open circles, placebo). (Reproduced from MRC Working Party, 1985, *Br. Med. J.* **291**, 97–104, with permission.)

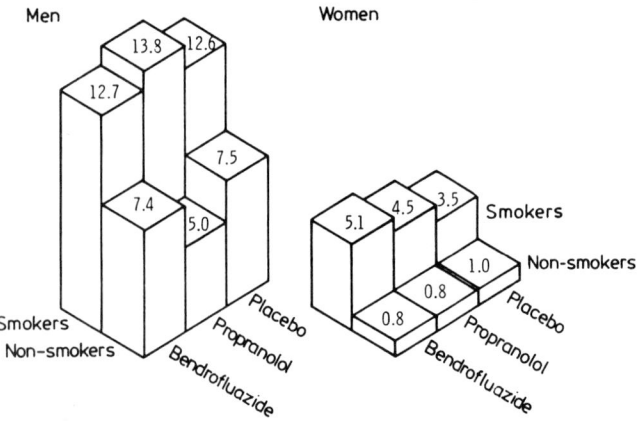

Fig. 16 Incidence of coronary events per 1000 person years of observation according to randomized treatment regimen and cigarette smoking status at entry to MRC trial. (Reproduced from MRC Working Party, 1985, *Br. Med. J.* **291**, 97–104, with permission.)

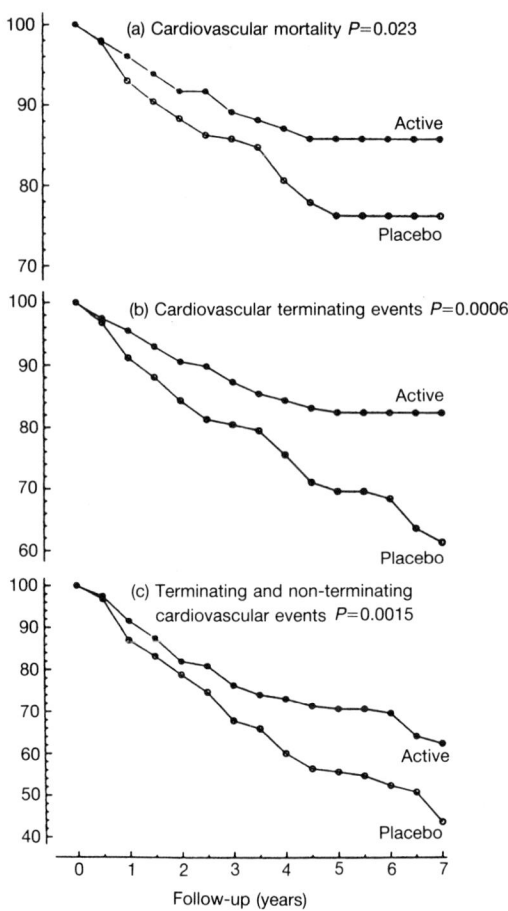

Fig. 17 Cumulative percentage of survivors without events calculated by the life table method for the patients on randomized treatment in the European trial of treatment of high blood pressure in the elderly. (Reproduced from Amery *et al.*, 1985, with permission.)

observation only (P = <0.01), but no significant reduction in ischaemic cardiac events (5.2 versus 5.5/1000 patient years, Fig. 15).

Post hoc analysis showed significantly less benefit for women and for smokers on propranolol. Coronary events were less frequent in non-smokers on propranolol (Fig. 16).

Males were more likely to drop out of thiazide treatment (because of impotence) and females from the propranolol group (because of cold extremities). About 25 per cent of the actively treated patients withdrew because of side-effects.

Despite favourable results in some categories, there was no overall reduction in mortality from all causes. Even for stroke, 850 patients had to be treated for 1 year to prevent one stroke. More than 95 per cent of the control group were free of complications over the 5-year follow-up.

The elderly (over 60 years, EWPHE) The European trial of treatment of high blood pressure in the elderly (EWPHE) randomized 840 patients aged over 60 years (diastolic BP 90–119) to hydrochlorothiazide plus triamterine (plus methyldopa if necessary) or

placebo treatment. Overall, there was a non-significant 9 per cent reduction in total mortality with active treatment. In the double blind analysis, cardiovascular mortality was reduced by 38 per cent and myocardial infarction by 60 per cent (Fig. 17). This trial was difficult to mount and sustain, but was of considerable importance as it was the first serious attempt to quantify benefit in the elderly. Those with lower levels of blood pressure appeared to benefit as much as those in the higher ranges. The findings on coronary mortality in particular are strikingly in contrast to the other recent trials in younger subjects. It may be that the largely clinic- and hospital-based population in the EWHPE trial represents a more severely hypertensive population.

What do the recent trials tell us?

It is disappointing that in several trials there was no significant reduction in mortality from all causes. There was generally a reduction in specific cardiovascular causes, particularly stroke, which was reduced more by thiazides, especially in women.

A very large number of people have to face the inconvenience, risks, and side-effects of treatment to save one life. A possible explanation for rather borderline results of therapy on all cause mortality in mild hypertension is that the number of disease-related end points may be rather small compared with non-hypertension-related deaths such as neoplasm, accidents etc. In other words, over the relatively short 3–5 year term possible in a clinical trial the 'noise' drowns out the cause-specific reductions in mortality. The failure to reduce coronary mortality may be due to the weak power of short-term trials to discern a small but perhaps worthwhile reduction in a disease with such a long incubation period, or it may be that there are balancing harmful effects of treatment such as a lowered coronary perfusion pressure and/or adverse metabolic effects on serum lipids and electrolytes.

Side-effects
Not surprisingly the side-effects of diuretic and β-blocker treatments are different. Men particularly complained of impotence and loss of libido on diuretic treatment, which was also associated with more feelings of anxiety, dizziness, and cramps, and also metabolic effects such as gout and glucose intolerance. Breathlessness, lethargy and (in women) cold extremities caused withdrawal from β-blocking agents.

More interest has focussed on the possible long-term effects of both thiazide diuretics and β-blockers on serum lipids. There is not a large effect of β-blockers on total cholesterol but HDL cholesterol falls; there is also a rise in triglycerides. These adverse changes are greatest with non-selective β-blockers, less with selective β-blockers and small or non-existent with strong ISA (pindolol). The effects with diuretics are rather more worrying with rises in total and LDL cholesterol, which appear to persist.

The MRC and IPPPSH trials give no support to the theory that thiazide diuretics may be more dangerous than β-blockers except perhaps in non-smoking males.

Smoking and hypertension
The trials *do* show that the difference in mortality between smokers (risk about double) and non-smokers is far greater than the difference between alternative drug regimes or between any active and placebo treatment.

The *post hoc* analysis of both the MRC and IPPPSH trials showed that male *non-smokers* had about a 50 per cent (IPPPSH) or 30 per cent (MRC) reduction in coronary mortality with β-blockade whereas there was no reduction (MRC) or possibly excess coronary mortality (IPPPSH) with predominantly diuretic-based treatment. *Smokers* showed no reduction in coronary mortality by either treatment compared with placebo in the MRC trial. The IPPPSH trial had no true placebo group. Since this unexpected interaction was found by 'data dredging' one has to be cautious about accepting conventional levels of significance; but that it has been seen in both these large trials does add weight to the finding. What then might be the underlying mechanism?

Both oxprenolol and propranolol are fat soluble, interfere with the liver P_{450} enzyme system, and are non-selective. The lack of benefit with these non-selective drugs in smokers might be attributable to blockade of vasodilator $β_2$-receptors in peripheral vasculature which would combat the rise in catecholamines and blood pressure evident during smoking. Indeed the rise in blood pressure during smoking is less with cardioselective β-blockers (atenolol, betaxolol, metoprolol, acebutolol) than with non-selective agents. It is possible therefore that smokers might derive benefit from cardioselective β-blocking agents but this is speculation.

In the light of these difficulties a WHO/International Society of Hypertension working group has offered draft guidelines for the evaluation and treatment of the 10–20 per cent of adults who have borderline hypertension (Fig. 18).

Non-drug treatment of mild hypertension
There is a correlation between obesity and hypertension in cross-sectional studies and many (but not all) studies suggest that weight reduction also reduces arterial pressure however modestly, probably independently of dietary salt. Dietary restriction, particularly of carbohydrate, may have its effects by reducing sympathetic nerve output, probably by a central mechanism. A lowered intake of fat, alcohol, and weight reduction, increased physical exercise, and above all abstinence from cigarette smoking are of paramount importance and are particularly useful to implement in the weeks or months when the level of blood pressure is being assessed by multiple readings, or home or ambulatory measurements.

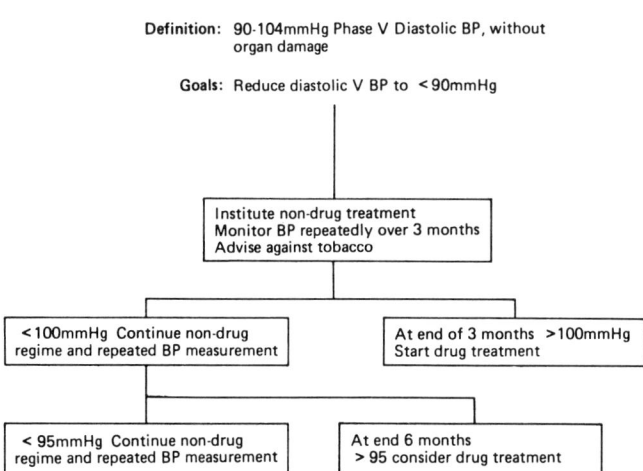

Fig. 18 Draft guidelines for treatment of mild hypertension (1986). (Reproduced from Konigstein WHO/ISH Workshop, December 1985.)

Screening for hypertension
The justification for screening programmes for hypertension is that the disorder is symptomless, common, and, at higher levels of pressure at least, is worth treating.

The rule of halves An important facet to the effectiveness of a screening programme is the education of individual doctors. Screening programmes have revealed a group of hidden hypertensives equal in number to those already known to the practitioner. Moreover, the blood pressure control of half of the previously known cases is unsatisfactory. Thus, of the whole population at risk, only about 25 per cent will be receiving effective treatment (i.e. diastolic pressure below 100 mm Hg). Furthermore, death rates in men from hypertension are greater than in women, but it is women who receive treatment much more frequently than men.

Method of screening
In the United Kingdom the best and most economical method is to take the blood pressure of all persons making contact wih their general practitioner. Studies in South Wales have shown that this can be done very effectively by the practice nurse; 95 per cent of one practice was screened during a two-year period. In a Scottish general practice 61 per cent of males and 69 per cent of females contacted their general practice clinic in one year; by three years, the figures had risen to 84 and 87 per cent, respectively. Thus no special effort or screening 'drive' has to be made.

Specific therapy
My own personal prejudices and general strategy are outlined below together with the properties of individual drugs. It is best to master a few of these and stick to them, and wise to change prescribing habits slowly and only after an adequate controlled trial has shown clear advantages in change.

General strategy Attention to the patient's lifestyle may be important in a few cases but in general it is very difficult to change. Nevertheless, it is proper to try to dissuade people from smoking and to tackle the difficult task of losing weight, if obese, and of not gaining weight if they are of normal weight. It is important to emphasize the importance of future surveillance. Too many people with previously known mild hypertension present later with stroke or malignant hypertension, having had no intervening measurement of blood pressure.

Mental relaxation can be urged more easily than achieved. Sometimes regular graded exercise will cause a simultaneous feeling of well-being. The value of regular exercise in lowering arterial pressure is not proven, but recent evidence is encouraging, particularly as pressure reduction is accompanied by other favourable changes.

Mild or moderate benign essential hypertension

After establishing (see page 13.362) that the raised pressure appears to be a sustained finding during an initial surveillance period of at least three to six weeks and sometimes months, and at least three to four readings, drug therapy may be commenced. This initial period can be used to control weight and advise on diet and lifestyle. If the patient is below 40 years of age and there is no family history of hypertension, screening tests for a surgically curable cause can be carried out (see page 13.382).

For the initial drug, the choice lies between a thiazide diuretic and a β-blocker. The choice can be varied depending on several factors. For women, a diuretic might well be the first choice. For men in whom there are no contraindications, a cardioselective β-blocker is my first choice. All β-blocking agents seem almost equally effective in lowering pressure but a longer acting agent has some advantages in terms of compliance. A water-soluble agent is not metabolized in the liver and is less likely to penetrate brain lipids. The former property is the most useful since people vary greatly in the rate at which they metabolize the fat-soluble β-blockers in the liver. This means that the lipid-soluble drugs, e.g. propranolol, metroprolol, timolol, oxprenolol, may show great intcrindividual variability in plasma levels for the same dose. In practice this means that the dose must be titrated (tedious) and that about 10 per cent of patients (who are slow metabolizers) may be over dosed. At present, atenolol is my own personal preference. Beta-blockers with intrinsic sympathetic activity appear less desirable in the presence of ischaemic heart disease. The combination of angina and hypertension is best treated with a β-blocker; while a β-blocker alone is best for patients with tachycardia and when mild sedation would seem appropriate. Beta-blockade may be more effective in patients with a raised plasma renin level but this investigation will not be available in the majority of cases.

When heart failure is present a diuretic is clearly the first choice. If oedema is present then it is usual to add potassium or use a potassium-sparing diuretic. Unlike the situation with heart failure, it does not appear necessary to supplement with extra potassium in patients with hypertension but without oedema unless they are receiving digoxin when a low serum potassium might predispose to arrhythmia. Some physicians, however, favour amiloride, which does have a potassium-sparing effect, as does spironolactone; the latter has more troublesome side-effects, particularly gynaecomastia.

Studies in the United Kingdom, United States, Sweden, and Norway, of long-term (two to three years) β-blockade following myocardial infarction, have demonstrated a significant lowering of sudden death (presumably from arrhythmia) in people treated with a β-blocker compared with a placebo. Since many subjects with hypertension have overt or hidden coronary disease, β-blockers might have an important advantage over thiazides. The case is supported by the now known beneficial effects of intravenous atenolol given at the onset of myocardial infarction. However, neither the MRC nor the IPPPSH trial gave real support for any significant advantage of β-blockers in the primary prevention of myocardial infarction.

If arrhythmia complicates hypertension, and particularly if β-blocking agents are contraindicated (e.g. bronchospasm or peripheral vascular disease) a calcium channel blocking agent has advantages. Verapamil in a dose of 40–120 mg tds is best for arrhythmia. Nifedipine or diltiazem have less anti-arrhythmic properties but may be very useful where peripheral vasodilation is wanted, e.g. peripheral vascular disease.

Where a single agent is ineffective it is preferable to change drugs or to add a second agent rather than increase the dose of the first agent further. The current choice to add to an initial β-blocker lies between a diuretic and nifedipine (see below), depending on the factors discussed above. Nifedipine alone may sometimes cause a reflex tachycardia (particularly troublesome if angina is also present). The combination of delayed release nifedipine and a β-blocker is particularly effective in combating the tachycardia and cold extremities from the respective drugs used singly. In the past it has been the standard 'step care' regime to use first a diuretic or a β-blocker and then combine both if the first treatment is inadequate. A recent interesting study questions this strategy. It was found that the same patient rarely responded equally to a β-blocker or a thiazide used singly. The better strategy was to *exchange* one for the other and only use the combination if the exchange failed. Furthermore, the combination was often ineffective. This underlines the modern tendency to use more logical second-line treatment, e.g. nifedipine with β-blocker or ACE inhibitor with diuretics. Another possible second or third strategy is to add a vasodilator such as hydralazine or prazosin. Most vasodilator agents given alone may lead to a troublesome reflex tachycardia and so are best used in combination with a β-blocker.

Triple therapy (β-blocker, diuretic, and nifedipine or vasodilator) will be effective in 90–95 per cent of patients. In those who are resistant, or suffer undue side-effects, the addition of a centrally acting agent, such as α-methyldopa may be effective but its main side-effect – fatigue – can be troublesome. There is also considerable loss in libido.

Clonidine, although an effective and interesting hypotensive agent, causes marked sedation. Like methyldopa (which leads to the formation of α-methyl noradrenaline), it is an α-adrenoceptor-stimulating drug. It appears to act by facilitation of the baroreflex arc by a central nervous action on interneurones in the medulla. It also may have a peripheral effect on the reactivity of arterial smooth muscle. It is recommended in subjects who have a combination of hypertension and migraine, since it has been shown to be useful in relieving migraine headache. It is also useful in patients who experience diarrhoea on methyldopa. The principal risk of prescribing clonidine is the so-called 'overshoot' phenomenon. This refers to the severe rise in arterial pressure when clonidine is stopped suddenly. Within hours, the patient experiences an autonomic 'storm' with tachycardia, sweating, intense anxiety, and severe hypertension. Its incidence is difficult to quantify. Some physicians report that they have never seen a case. Where care is taken to record pressures carefully, it seems to be quite common, and sometimes very alarming rises are seen. It is not seen after a short course or a single dose. Its mechanism is not understood. The rapidity and potential severity of its onset makes one reserve this drug for patients with migraine or in whom the earlier drugs have failed, and then only with careful explanation to the patient of the need to avoid sudden withdrawal.

Calcium channel blocking agents have a valuable and growing place in treatment. Unlike the β-blockers they appear individually to be quite different in their actions, so that some are more specific for veins compared with arteries and others more effective on the heart.

Another drug useful for severe and resistant hypertension is the potent vasodilator minoxidil, which may be particularly effective in patients with renal hypertension. However, it has considerable toxicity, leading to excess hair growth and oedema; the former is usually severe enough to bar its use in women.

Combined α- and β-blockade

A combination of α- and β-blockade is theoretically attractive, but may result in undue postural hypotension. Labetalol, has α- and β-blocking properties combined in the same compound. Although the α-blocking potency is relatively mild labetalol appears to be significantly better in hypotensive potency than a β-blocker alone, and although postural and exercise hypotension occur with this drug they have not been too much of a problem so far.

Emergency treatment of malignant hypertension

When reducing arterial pressure from very high levels particularly when there is evidence of fibrinoid necrosis the aim should be a smooth reduction over some hours. There is good evidence that very sudden reduction in pressure may lead to neurological damage in the so-called 'watershed' areas of the brain at the boundary between large supplying vessels such as the middle cerebral and posterior cerebral arteries.

Parenteral treatment is no longer considered necessary, unless there is coincident left ventricular failure, dissecting aneurysm, hypertensive encephalopathy or eclampsia. If these complicating factors are present, diazoxide given in repeated 50 mg boluses reduces pressure rapidly. A useful alternative is hydralazine 5–20 mg by slow intravenous injection or intramuscularly. Both drugs may cause a troublesome reflex tachycardia which can be suppressed by a concomitant β-adrenergic blockade. This problem is well obviated by the use of bolus doses or infusions of labetalol. Recent evidence suggests that oral or more rapidly acting sublingual nifedipine may be particularly effective in inducing a smooth and relatively rapid fall in arterial pressure with minimal risk of inducing cerebral ischaemia or infarction.

Although malignant hypertension is still a medical emergency, bed rest in hospital, together with conventional oral therapy with a β-blocker and diuretic will usually lower pressure within a few hours and to an acceptable degree.

Hypertension in pregnancy
See pages 11.4–11.8.

Does cerebrovascular disease contraindicate therapy?
For many years it was believed that cerebral blood flow might be compromised if arterial pressure was lowered, since a high perfusion pressure may be necessary to perfuse an occluded or stenosed vessel. However, controlled studies have shown that survival is greater if arterial pressure is lowered in stroke survivors. This is probably due to prevention of further cerebral haemorrhage, prevention of further arterial degeneration, and to the great intrinsic capacity of the cerebral circulation to autoregulate flow.

There remains a problem in the management of *acute* stroke, often accompanied by very high arterial pressures, and without certainty as to whether hypertension is an acute consequence of stroke or vice versa. It is reasonable to advise in this situation a conservative approach. The risks are to leave a high pressure untreated with possible consequent further hypertensive damage to the brain, or to lower pressure too far and induce focal neurological damage due to hypoperfusion or infarction. Most physicians would settle for an arterial pressure around 160/100 in this difficult situation.

The treatment of the uraemic patient
Renal failure can affect the drug therapy of hypertension in several ways. First, lowering arterial pressure may, by lowering renal perfusion pressure, exacerbate the renal failure. In practice, this does not commonly occur except in the management of malignant hypertension. Secondly, the presence of a high circulating renin may antagonize the action of hypotensive agents and render them ineffective. Some patients with terminal renal failure and malignant hypertension have been almost impossible to control with regard to blood pressure, even on ultrafiltration haemodialysis. Nephrectomy, by removing the source of renin, was once used to reverse this process. This drastic step may now be averted by use of minoxidil and the newer agents such as angiotension-converting enzyme inhibitors or nifedipine combined with better control of salt and water balance. Thirdly, drugs excreted by the kidney may accumulate and cause toxic effects (such as paralytic ileus in the case of ganglion blocking agents) or very severe hypotension.

An ideal drug in renal failure might be one which preserves or even increases renal blood flow. Hydralazine was once in vogue and is effective combined with a β-blocking agent to reduce tachycardia. More effective now are the angiotensin-converting enzyme inhibitors, but both captopril and enalapril are renally excreted

and should be given only in very small doses to patients in renal failure, or who are taking high doses of diuretics. In such reduced doses both drugs are effective and safe. Effective control of blood pressure may lead to a rise in GFR in some patients in whom hypertension (usually in the malignant phase) is the cause of renal failure. In most cases renal failure progresses despite good control, but it is probable that uncontrolled hypertension accelerates the rate of loss of renal function in all patients with renal failure.

Should we ignore high blood pressure in the elderly?
Most physicians are less aggressive in treating elderly subjects, particularly women, in whom a raised pressure is found casually. The results of the EWPHE trial (see above) give support for active treatment in the elderly. Unfortunately, elderly subjects with stiff vessels are more prone to side-effects of drugs, particularly postural hypotension. It is reasonable to give a trial of therapy to see how well it is tolerated; if bad side-effects occur treatment can be abandoned unless hypertension is severe with good evidence of end organ damage.

Do we stop treatment before anaesthesia?
Drug therapy of hypertension was at one time discontinued before surgery and anaesthesia, in order to allow an intact autonomic nervous system to respond to such crises as bleeding and to obviate interaction with drugs given by the anaesthetist. This is no longer acceptable since patients with uncontrolled hypertension experienced more dangerous surges of arterial pressure than treated patients, particularly during anaesthetic induction. Arrhythmias and ischaemic ST depression are also significantly more frequent and severe in the untreated. The anaesthetist is able to use control of blood volume by transfusion to combat undue hypotension. Many of the drugs, particularly β-blockers, are competitive in nature and can therefore be reversed, if necessary by increasing doses of agonist. It is important to note that seemingly very large doses of catecholamines may be needed. A possible exception is that some cardiac surgeons prefer to withdraw β-blockade at least two days pre-operatively in order, perhaps, to reduce the risk of low cardiac output postoperatively. This has not been examined systematically and carries obvious risks in those with ischaemic heart disease.

Drug interaction
Mono-amine oxidase inhibitors will antagonize all drugs which aim to reduce sympathetic discharge; more specifically, tricyclic antidepressive drugs compete with guanethidine and bethanidine and reduce the degree of block produced by these drugs of the re-uptake of noradrenaline by the nerve ending, thus directly antagonizing the sympathetic blocking agents. Indomethacin and other non-steroidal anti-inflammatory agents interact with several hypotensive agents, rendering them less effective, although this interaction may only be temporary and unimportant in the long term.

Is poor control better than no control?
The Veterans' Administration and another more recent study have shown that poor treatment is significantly better than no treatment at all.

Specific drugs
Diuretics
The thiazide diuretics and the closely related phthalimidine (chlorthalidone) diuretics are extremely valuable hypotensive agents, particularly since they have the effect of increasing the hypotensive effects of other drugs, whatever their mechanism of action. It does not matter greatly which thiazide is used, although chlorthalidone is favoured by some because of its longer duration of action. The choice should be dictated by price and familiarity. Tables 1 and 2 list the hypotensive agents more commonly used in the Oxford hospitals, together with the local cost per week.

Table 1 Principal hypotensive drugs and National Health Service costs (1986) (excluding many useful fixed combinations)

Drug	Usual daily dose (mg)	Tablet size (mg)	Approximate NHS* cost/week (pence)	Proprietary names	Advantages (A) Disadvantages (D)
Thiazides/natriuretics					A: cheap (thiazides), no sedation, well tolerated D: K depletion, gout, diabetes, rashes, agranulocytosis
Amiloride	5–10	5	13–26	Midamor	A: cheap, less metabolic effects than thiazides, K sparing
Chlorothiazide	500–1000	500	13–26	Saluric	
Hydrochlorothiazide	25–100	25, 50	10–20	Hydrosaluric, Diurema, Esidrex	
Hydroflumethiazide	25–50	50	6–12	Hydrenox	
Bendrofluazide	2.5–5	2.5, 5	2–4	Aprinox, Centyl, Berkozide, Urizide, Neonaclex	
Methylchlothiazide	2.5–5	5	14	Enduron	
Cyclopenthiazide	0.25–0.5	0.5	6–12	Navidrex	
Polythiazide	1–4	1	19–39	Nephril	
Chlorthalidone	25–50	50, 100	10–20	Hygroton	A: longer acting (24 hours plus)
Indapamide	2.5	2.5	140	Natrilix	A: rapid onset, long acting
Spironolactone	50–200	25, 50, 100	99–198	Aldactone, Spiroctan, Laralactone, Diatensec, Spiretic	A: K sparing D gynaecomastia
Xipamide	20–40	20	68–136	Diurexan	
Piretanide	6–12	6	59–118	Arelix	
Loop diuretics					
Frusemide	40–80	40	13–26	Lasix, Dryptal Fruselic Frusid	A: useful in high dose in renal failure D: shorter fiercer action
Bumetamide	1–5	1, 5	35–130	Burinex	
Vasodilators					
Hydralazine	75–200	25, 50	30–80	Apresoline	A: useful in renal failure D: reflex tachycardia, SLE in high dose (200 mg/day or less in slow acetylators), flushes, nausea
Prazosin	4–20	0.5, 1, 2, 5	97–436	Hypovase	A: less reflex tachycardia D: 'first dose' hypotension, dry mouth
Diazoxide	30–300 i.v.		270/dose of 300 mg	Eudemine	A: rapid action, within 1–2 min D: nausea, tachycardia, diabetes
Minoxidil	10–50	2.5, 5, 10	177–889	Loniten	A: useful in resistant cases D: Na retention, hypertrichosis, tachycardia
Indoramin	50–200	25, 50	177–709	Baratol	
CNS active drugs					
Methyldopa	500–2000	125, 250, 500	41–111	Aldomet, Medomet, Dopamet	A: safe in pregnancy, cheap D: sedation, loss of libido, diarrhoea, positive Coombs' test
Clonidine	0.1–1.2	0.1, 0.3	104–418	Catapres	A: migraine, diarrhoea D: overshoot–hypertension on stopping
Adrenergic blockers					
Guanethidine	20–50	10, 25	16–32	Ismelin	A: longer action (24 hours) D: postural hypotension, diarrhoea, impotence, dry mouth
Bethanidine	30–200	10, 50	136–817	Esbatal, Bendogen	D: shorter action (4 hours)
Calcium-blocking agents					
Verapamil	120–260	40, 80, 120	95–280	Cordilox	A: useful in asthmatics, anti-arrhythmic D: constipation
Nifedipine	30–60	5, 10, 20 (retard)	256–511	Adalat	A: peripheral vasodilation D: flushing, headaches
Lidoflazine	360	120	242	Clinium	A: coronary vasodilation
Diltiazem	180–360	60	350–700	Tildiem	D: tinnitus, headaches
Angiotensin converting enzyme inhibitors					
Captopril	25–150	25, 50, 100	460–1540	Capoten	A: some bradycardia despite hypotension D: side-effects on bone marrow in high dose, occasional rash, taste disturbance
Enalapril	10–40	5, 10, 20	259–519	Innovace	A: less rash and taste problems and longer acting than captopril D: first dose hypotension and renal failure more prolonged than captopril

* NHS cost is intended only as a rough guide; it is the usual MIMS retail price at December 1985, not allowing for special discounts.

Table 2 Beta-adrenoceptor-blocking agents

Drug	Daily dose (mg)	Tablet size (mg)	Approximate NHS cost/week (pence)	Proprietary names	ISA	MSA	Cardio-selective (81)	Lipo-philic	Per cent protein bound	Approximate plasma half-life (h) (oral)	Urine recovery per cent of oral dose	Per cent of drug excreted unchanged	Slow release preparation available	Combined with diuretic available
Non-selective β-blockers														
D: bronchospasm, heart failure, cold hands, fatigue, dreams, masks hypoglycaemia in insulin-dependent diabetics														
A: in angina or arrythmias, lowers plasma renin in low dosage, reduces sudden death														
Alprenolol (not available in UK)	200–800	40, 80		Aptin	+	+	0	++	85	2–3	90	41	Yes	
Nadolol	80–240	40, 80	188–566	Corgard	0	0	0	0	30	15–37	25	95		
Oxprenolol	160–320	20, 40, 80, 160 (SR)	91–273	Trasicor	+	+	0	+	80	2	75–95	5	Yes	Yes
Pindolol	10–45	5, 15	149–447	Visken	+	0	0	+	57†	3–4	95	40		Yes
Propranolol	160–320	10, 40, 80, 160, 80 & 160 (SR)	57–115	Inderal (plus other generic preparations)	0	+	0	++	95	3–4	96	4	Yes	Yes
Sotalol	160–600	40, 80, 160, 200	82–290	Beta-cardone, Sotacor	0	0	0	0	54†	5–15	75+	95+		Yes
Timolol	10–30	10	61–184	Blocadren, Betim	0	0	0	+	10	5–6	66	25		Yes
Cardioselective β-blockers														
A: less brochospasm and similar advantages to non-selective, above														
Acebutolol	400–800	100, 200, 400	197–394	Sectral	+	+	+	0	30–40	1–2–11* (*metabolite)	38	56		
Atenolol	50–200	50, 100	43–174	Tenormin	0	0	+	0	25–30	6–15	80–90	90		Yes
Metoprolol	200–400	50, 100, 200 (SR)	61–245	Betaloc, Lopressor	0	Weak ±	+	+	12	3–4	95	5	Yes	Yes
Practolol		No oral preparation		Eraldin i.v.	+	0	+	0	32†	No oral preparation	95	5		
Betaxolol	20–40	20	192–385	Kerlone	0	±	+	+	?	16–20	?	?		
Combined α- and β-blockade														
Labetolol	200–800	100, 200, 400	84–336	Trandate	0	0	0	0(+)	50	4	60	5		

ISA = intrinsic sympathetic activity, MSA = membrane stabilizing activity, HSA = human serum albumin.
* Costs will vary quite widely, depending on hospital contracts.
† HSA values only.
With acknowledgements to Miss Jenny Dorey, Pharmacist, John Radcliffe Hospital, Oxford.

The mode of action of diuretics is probably two-fold: an initial decrease in blood volume and cardiac output is followed over months by a poorly understood fall in peripheral resistance and gradual return of the blood volume towards normal. The fall in peripheral resistance may be due to a direct effect on smooth muscle, although it is difficult to explain why this takes some weeks to appear; alternatively an autoregulatory adjustment in smooth muscle tone may occur in response to the diminution in organ flow consequent upon the initial fall in cardiac output. There is some new evidence linking the thiazides to alterations in prostaglandin metabolism in the vessel wall.

The suggestion that smooth muscle relaxation is related to a diminished salt and water content of the vessel wall is rendered less likely since the related compound diazoxide also relaxes smooth muscle, but with simultaneous salt and water retention.

The thiazides are cheap but suffer the long-term disadvantages of hypokalaemia, hyperglycaemia, and hyperuricaemia. Since there is a frequent association of hypertension and hyperuricaemia, the development of clinical gout is not rare in subjects on thiazide diuretics. Hyperglycaemia is not usually troublesome, but frank diabetes may appear in some subjects who had initially normal glucose tolerance when thiazides are given continuously for some years. We are also now more concerned with the possible ill-effect of magnesium depletion induced by those agents in relation to cardiac arrhythmias.

Is potassium supplementation required?
The long-term results of minor depletion of whole body potassium are not known. Weakness and muscle cramps occur in more severe depletion and cardiac arrhythmias are more common in patients receiving digitalis and thiazides in combination.

Studies of whole body potassium suggest that potassium supplementation is not necessary in patients who do not have oedema and who are not receiving digitalis. Severe (greater than 30 per cent) depletion of total body potassium is unusual with a serum concentration over 3.5 mmol/1. A check of serum potassium after some weeks of treatment and intermittently thereafter is sensible.

Dosage
Thiazides have the advantage of a flat dose–response relationship. If the lowest dose is not effective, there is little further effect on arterial pressure from doubling it, but metabolic ill-effects are likely to be aggravated. Evidence suggests that 2.5 mg bendrofluazide or equivalently small doses of other thiazides are effective. There is also an increasing tendency to prescribe potassium-sparing compounds such as amiloride or spironolactone. Both have been shown to be as effective as thiazides but without associated ill-effects on potassium, uric acid or magnesium metabolism.

Adrenergic-blocking drugs
Alpha-receptors are mainly distributed in vascular smooth muscle where noradrenaline acts to cause vasoconstriction and an α_1 effect. Alpha$_2$-receptors are usually presynaptic and act to limit the release of further noradrenaline when this is present in the synaptic cleft.

Beta-receptors are also divided into two subgroups. Beta$_1$-receptors predominate in the heart (where both noradrenaline and adrenaline have positive inotropic and chronotropic effects), and β_2-receptors in the bronchi and vascular smooth muscle cause relaxation (mediated mainly by adrenaline).

Blocking agents have been developed for all these receptors. Figure 19 classifies the main groups of β-blockers acting on cardiac and vascular receptors and gives examples of drugs in each category. The original β-blocking agents were non-selective, blocking both β_1 and β_2 effects. Inevitable side-effects were of vasoconstriction and bronchial narrowing which can be so dangerous in asthmatic subjects (see below). Selective β-blockade drugs are at best only relatively selective so that they too may promote dangerous bronchoconstriction in susceptible patients.

Partial agonist activity (PAA)
Whether intrinsic sympathomimetic activity has any therapeutic value is open to considerable doubt and controversy. It is theoretically possible that some such activity might prevent too slow a heart rate at rest, or perhaps diminish the tendency to bronchospasm, whilst still effectively blocking higher levels of sympathetic activity. There is no good evidence to support this possibility.

Membrane stabilizing effect
The presence or absence of a membrane stabilizing or local anaesthetic action is not thought to be of any significance at clinical dose levels. At very high doses this 'quinidine-like' effect may cause myocardial depression.

Cardioselectivity
The selective or β_1-blocking agents may, on rare occasions, be given successfully to patients with asthmatic tendencies. However, cardioselectivity is only relative and extreme caution should be taken in prescribing these drugs to asthmatics; *they should be given, if at all, under immediate medical supervision* with β-adrenoreceptor agonists and resuscitation equipment available.

Another theoretical advantage of selectivity is the relative lack of blockade of peripheral arterial β_2-receptors, so that one might expect less trouble from claudication and Raynaud-like symptoms from the use of selective agents. In practice, no such advantage is evident, but β_1-receptor-blocking drugs are less likely to block mobilization of glucose and are therefore preferable in patients

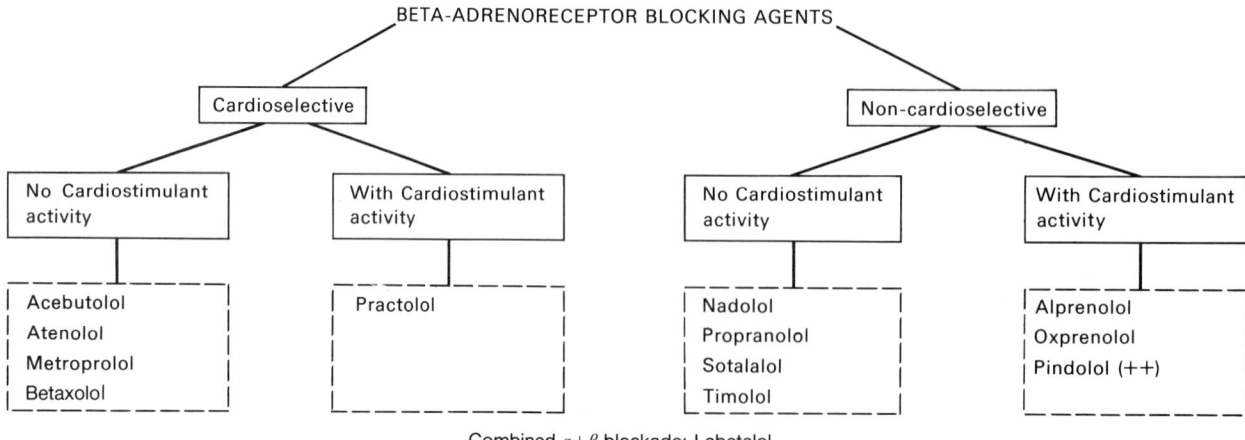

Combined $\alpha+\beta$ blockade: Labetalol

Fig. 19 A classification of β-adrenoceptor-blocking drugs.

such as treated diabetics liable to hypoglycaemia. All in all there is a good case for using a cardioselective β-blocker as first choice, since they appear clinically to be just as effective as non-selective blockers in lowering arterial pressure.

Liver metabolism
When a drug is substantially and rapidly metabolized by the liver (e.g. propranolol), oral treatment is more complicated since a variable amount of the effective drug may be lost on the first pass through the liver. If the subsequent metabolites still have β-adrenoreceptor-blocking properties, this effect is mitigated, but this is not always the case. The practical result is that it is necessary to titrate the dose in every individual. Some of the newer agents (e.g. atenolol) do not have this snag and they are therefore easier to prescribe and one may only have one step in titration (usually to double the initial dose).

Central nervous system penetration
The earlier β-blockers, such as propranolol and oxprenolol, are lipid-soluble and easily penetrate brain tissue. They are therefore more likely to give rise to troublesome CNS side-effects such as drowsiness and excessive dreams. Atenolol and nadolol are water-soluble and do not have this effect, although they can still reach areas of the brain (e.g. the area postrema in the medulla) where there is no blood–brain barrier.

Pharmacokinetics
The half-life of the differing agents varies from 2 to 3 hours to over 24 hours. At present nadolol has the longest half-life; this drug, betaxolol, and atenolol can therefore be given once daily. Single doses of short-acting β-blockers do not give effective cover over the whole day and night, unless they are specially formulated as slow-release preparations. Slow-release metoprolol and propranolol are effective.

Mode of action
Although propranolol has been in clinical use now for over 15 years, we still do not understand all its actions. A strange dissociation in time between immediate effect on heart rate and the delayed (days or weeks) effect on blood pressure were noticed in early work with propanolol but this delay is not such a feature of the newer β-blockers with which an effect may be seen with the initial dose. A reduction of cardiac output is unlikely to be the whole story since drugs with high intrinsic sympathetic activity still lower arterial pressure, while cardiac output at rest appears normal. Another possibility is by way of effects on synaptic neurotransmission.

The mode of release of noradrenaline from a nerve terminal is much more complex than originally thought. A simplified diagram outlining the feedback control loops for catecholamine release is shown in Fig. 20. We now know that the sympathetic varicosities where noradrenaline is stored are also acted upon by a very large number of other peptides, such as angiotensin, neuropeptide Y, and many others. It may be that an important action of β-blockers lies in the blockade of the positive feedback loop mediated by a presynaptic β-receptor. A similar action may be important in the central nervous system since it is believed that β-blockers, like the α-adrenergic drugs clonidine and α-methyldopa, may have important central effects on sympathetic nervous tone. Certainly these three agents induce drowsiness and sedation as a common side-effect. Vivid dreams are also a frequent consequence of β-blockade.

High renin is not a necessary prerequisite for the hypotensive action of β-blockers. However, it is true to say that renin-dependent hypertension does respond well to these drugs. In this connection it may be relevant that β-blockers have now been shown to interfere with the peripheral potentiation of noradrenaline by angiotensin, locally in the vessel wall.

Toxic effects
Side-effects of β-blockade are uncommon and rarely serious and are listed in Table 1. Fatigue and sedation are the most common and often wear off with time.

Dosage
Although the half-life of many of the drugs is of the order of 6 hours, it is usually quite satisfactory to dose twice daily for hypertension for many drugs, and once daily for several others (atenolol, nadolol, or slow-release preparations). The dose should be gradually increased every few days until a satisfactory pressure is reached or until no further fall occurs.

Vasodilators
A particular factor leading to a revival of interest in vasodilators in general was the development of the β-blocking agents, which very effectively control the reflex tachycardia and renin release which may accompany their use. Because of the risk of induced systemic lupus erythematosus, particularly in slow acetylators, hydralazine, even in low dosage is less used now than it was only a few years ago. Calcium antagonists and ACE inhibitors are increasingly prescribed in its place.

Hydralazine
Hydralazine dilates arterioles and reduces peripheral resistance, cardiac output, and renal blood flow increase. Caution should be exercised in subjects with coronary disease, since a rise in cardiac work may aggravate ischaemia. For hypertensive emergencies, 5–20 mg intravenously will usually lower blood pressure effectively in 15–20 min, but this is rarely necessary and may be dangerous.

Prazosin
Prazosin blocks α_1-receptors. It is a useful drug, but caution is necessary since the first dose is sometimes associated with a large postural fall in pressure so that syncope has occurred. It is recommended that this can be eliminated if the first dose is: (a) small (0.5–1 mg) and (b) given at night on going to bed. It is not a persistent effect and further doses may be increased without problems.

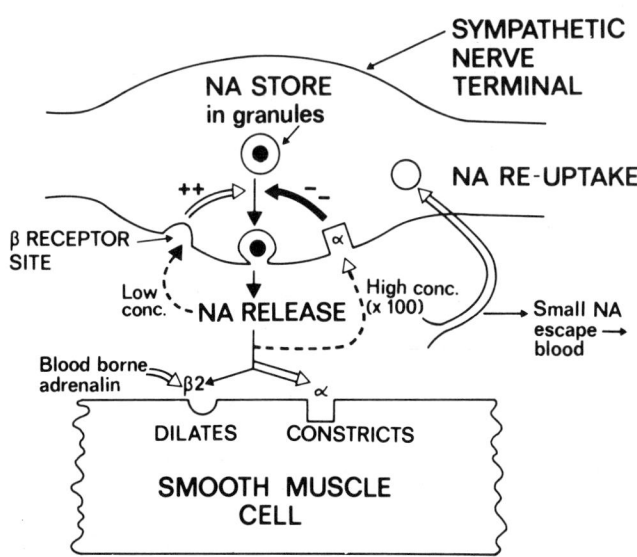

Fig. 20 Simplified diagram of noradrenaline (NA) release from a sympathetic nerve terminal, to show the feedback loops (dotted lines) which control the rate of release. Initial low concentrations increase the rate of release, but at concentrations about 100 times greater, the release is inhibited by the presynaptic α-receptor. We now know that several similar feedback loops, involving angiotensin, acetylcholine, serotonin, and prostaglandins exert similar fine control of noradrenaline release. (After Langer, 1976, *Clin. Sci. mol. Med.* **51**, Suppl. 3, 4235, with permission.)

Minoxidil

This is a very powerful vasodilator particularly useful in end-stage renal failure. It does have severe side-effects (hirsutism and fluid retention) and its long-term place is limited. Dosages range from 2 mg daily to 15 or even 20 mg twice daily.

Diazoxide

Diazoxide was at one time popular for parenteral treatment of hypertensive emergencies. It has also been used for chronic oral treatment but resultant hyperglycaemia and gastrointestinal side-effects have made it of largely historic interest.

Sympathetic blocking agents

Bethanidine and guanethidine are rarely used now. They differ principally in the longer duration of action of the latter. These drugs and debrisoquine act by depleting the catecholamine stores in nerve endings. When given intravenously this initial depletion can lead to a rise in blood pressure mediated by catecholamine release. Guanethidine is taken up by the same pathway that is responsible for the re-uptake of noradrenaline by nerve endings and apparently displaces noradrenaline from these stores. The side-effects of the drugs are mainly postural and exercise hypotension, diarrhoea, and failure of ejaculation. For these reasons, they are scarcely used in initial treatment but may be necessary for subjects refractory to other therapy. The combination of methyldopa and a sympathetic blocking agent has an additive hypotensive effect. The initial starting dose of guanethidine is usually 10 mg daily; because of its long duration of action it is wise to increase the dose slowly, at intervals of one week.

Alpha-adrenergic blocking agents

Phentolamine and dibenyline are used in the pre- and peroperative management of phaeochromocytomas (page 13.395). They may also be useful in those now rare cases in which the patient has become refractory to such agents as guanethidine because of medical sympathetic denervation of the vessel walls; the smooth muscle in these cases may become hypersensitive to small amounts of circulating catechols. Small doses of an α-blocker can reverse this and restore responsiveness. Postural hypotension is to be expected from use of these agents.

Angiotensin converting enzyme (ACE) inhibitors

These drugs are effective in all grades of hypertension and are growing in reputation and usage. Inhibition of the formation of angiotensin II and a delayed antisympathetic effect are both important mechanisms of action. The contributions from reduced catabolism of bradykinin or a postulated reduction of vasopressin release are probably less certain.

Captopril

Most experience has been gained with the orally active drug captopril. This is relatively short acting but can be used twice daily in hypertension. Its action begins within 30 min and peaks at 1–2 hours. It contains SH bonds which may or may not be responsible for the now uncommon side-effects of rash and alterations in taste. Used in moderate dosage (below 75 mg/day) it has been very well tolerated. Indeed the well-being experienced by the patient on ACE inhibition is such a striking feature that it was suspected that it might be exerting a direct effect on mood, but systematic mood alteration has not been found in clinical trials. In mild hypertension side-effects are found in about 3 per cent of subjects; this compares very well with the 10–20 per cent of complaints with either diuretics or β-blockers. Side-effects encountered when the drug was introduced at excessive dosage were more serious so that ACE inhibitors are not yet in widespread use as first-line drugs in mild hypertension.

Care must be taken to avoid undue hypotension and/or renal failure in patients with high angiotensin levels, e.g. in bilateral renal artery stenosis (listen for renal bruits), or more commonly in the patient who has been vigorously treated with diuretics. It is best to withdraw these drugs and then begin captopril with a small (6.25 mg or less) initial dose. If severe hypotension does not occur in the next 2–3 hours it is then safe to increase the dose over the next few days from say 12.5 mg bd to 75 mg bd at maximum. It is often useful and indeed necessary to add a diuretic at this stage. It is best to avoid potassium-sparing diuretics and use thiazides alone with no potassium supplementation.

Enalapril

This is the first of the rivals to captopril. It does not contain SH bonds and may therefore have less side-effects, but this is not yet proven. It is a pro-drug and is slower in onset and longer in action than captopril. If a hypotensive reaction does occur it may therefore be more troublesome. The initial recommended dose of 10 mg is now thought to be too high and it is safer to begin with say 2.5 mg, again preferably after 2–3 days without diuretics. The usual maintenance dose is 10–40 mg daily. Very rarely hypersensitivity may lead to angioneurotic oedema with any ACE inhibitor. Although enalapril may be more convenient to use in the long-term (because of its longer duration of action), the delay in onset of effect (and side-effects) means that it should be started only very cautiously outside hospital.

Calcium channel-blocking agents

Three drugs are currently available on the United Kingdom market, verapamil, nifedipine, and diltiazem. Unlike the β-blockers, where differences in action depend on ancillary and pharmacokinetic considerations, there are considerable differences in tissue specificity between the calcium blockers.

Verapamil

Verapamil (dose 40–120 mg 8 hourly) is quite useful as monotherapy, especially in patients with contraindications to β-blockade. It causes modest vasodilation but its action on the SA node and conducting tissue aborts any reflex tachycardia. This action is also useful in patients who exhibit arrhythmia or angina in addition to hypertension. In high dosage it may cause constipation, sometimes amenable to an increase in dietary fibre.

Nifedipine

Nifedipine (10–30 mg bd or tds), particularly in the twice daily retard (20 mg) preparation, is now frequently used with a β-blocker as second-line therapy. It causes more peripheral vasodilation than verapamil and may thus provoke a reflex tachycardia when used alone. It sometimes causes peripheral oedema (not due to heart failure, but probably to dilator effects on the arteriolar precapillary sphincter) and headache is common.

Diltiazem

Diltiazem (60–120 mg tds) is not currently licensed for hypertension, but is for angina. It appears to be somewhere between nifedipine and verapamil, with perhaps more coronary and less peripheral vasodilation. It has more effect on conduction than nifedipine. Both verapamil and diltiazem should be avoided if there is any conduction problem.

Drugs acting on the central nervous system

Methyldopa

Methyldopa is a drug whose predominant action is thought to be central. It is 100 times more active if given into the cerebral ventricles, compared with systemic administration. Its hypotensive action can also be abolished by intracerebral injection of dopa decarboxylase inhibitors or α-adrenergic-blocking agents such as phentolamine.

Since the peripheral sympathetic nervous control is relatively unchanged qualitatively, the incidence of postural hypotension is small. For this reason it was a major advance over the sympathetic- and ganglion-blocking agents, and therefore gained widespread acceptance which it still enjoys. Because of the side-effects of sedation and depression it is presently losing ground to other agents. Although a positive antiglobulin (Coombs') test develops in over 20 per cent of patients on long-term therapy, frank haemolytic anaemia is rare.

Clonidine

This drug, which also has α-adrenergic properties, was first developed as a nasal decongestant.

It has proved active in the CNS in extremely small doses. The systemic daily dose in humans is also small: 100 μg three times daily. It appears to potentiate the baroreflex arc, possibly by stimulation of an interneurone with an adrenergic synapse; this resetting appears to be a principal mechanism of its hypotensive action. The drug may, in addition, have primary peripheral actions which reduce the reactivity of vascular smooth muscle to both constrictor and dilator agents – a possible factor in its use in migraine.

The intravenous form of the drug (150–300 μg) lowers blood pressure in 15–20 min and also causes considerable drowsiness. There is some evidence that further increase in dosage may have less hypotensive effect, possibly due to the direct α-adrenergic constrictor action on vascular smooth muscle.

The principal side-effects – sedation and dry mouth – appear to be central in origin. Its clinical use is limited because of the potential dangers of the large overshoot in arterial pressure which occurs when the drug is abruptly stopped after chronic administration.

Newer drugs

Ketanserin

This is a relatively specific antagonist of 5HT-2 receptors but with some α_1-adrenergic-blocking properties, which have caused some argument as to its mode of action in lowering arterial pressure. It has been speculated that serotonin may regulate the vasoconstrictor effects of noradrenaline and angiotensin, so it remains possible than an antiserotonin mechanism is involved in its hypotensive action.

It may be used as monotherapy and it has been claimed to be particularly effective in the elderly. Side-effects are not negligible and consist mainly of mild headache or fullness in the head.

Piretanide

This is a new diuretic, said to spare potassium and also to have vasodilator properties.

Indoramin

Indoramin is an α_1-adrenergic blocking drug which has recently been re-introduced as a vasodilator which is less likely to cause reflex tachycardia than, for instance, hydralazine. It is also claimed to have a lignocaine-like antiarrhythmic action. It causes some sedation and may also cause failure of ejaculation (dose 25–100 mg bd).

Conclusions

Physicians are today besieged by an army of salesmen eager to promote their particular hypotensive drugs. A condition as widespread and potentially dangerous as hypertension is big business. The wise physician will select patients for treatment with care; he will bear in mind his duty to minimize the adverse effects of what, for the patient, is a life-sentence; he will be very aware of the possibility of falsely high readings from anxiety and the defence reaction; he will particularly restrict his own therapeutic armoury to a few drugs which he knows well; above all, he will resist the temptation to change the drug treatment of a patient who is satisfactorily controlled, even if the therapy might look a little old-fashioned to his colleagues. The MRC trial has re-emphasized the very low risks posed by mild hypertension for many; it is important that the risks of treatment are known to be less!

Treatment which is life-long demands (except in the case of malignant hypertension, which is a true medical emergency demanding instant treatment) a firm diagnosis based on successive readings over three to four weeks, or even longer. Once begun, treatment should not be stopped lightly; all of us have seen patients presenting with stroke after another doctor – finding a normal blood pressure – has told the unfortunate patient that there is no need to take therapy. If treatment is stopped, it is gross negligence not to follow that patient for one to two years, and preferably indefinitely at two or three year intervals.

The treatment of hypertension by specific and increasingly sophisticated drugs represents one of the great successes of the pharmaceutical industry over the last 20 years, and accounts in great part for the encouraging fall in mortality from this common disorder (Fig. 21).

References

Amery, A., Birkenhager, W., Brixko, P. *et al.* (1985). Mortality and morbidity results from the European Working Party on high blood pressure in the elderly trial. *Lancet* i, 1349–1354.

Armitage, P. and Rose, G. A. (1966). The variability of measurements of casual blood pressure. *Clin. Sci.* **30**, 325.

Beilin, L. J. and Arkwright, P. D. (1983). Alcohol and hypertension. In *Handbook of hypertension* Vol. 1 (ed. J. I. S. Robertson), pp. 44–63. Elsevier, Amsterdam.

Boon, N. A. and Aronson, J. K. (1985). Dietary salt and hypertension. Treatment and prevention. *Br. med. J.* **290**, 949–950.

——, Harper, C., Aronson, J. K. and Grahame-Smith, D. G. (1985). Cation transport functions *in vitro* in patients with untreated essential hypertension: a comparison of erythrocytes and leucocytes. *Clin. Sci.* **68**, 511–551.

Brennan, P. J., Greenberg, G., Miall, W. E. and Thompson, S. G. (1982). Seasonal variation in arterial blood pressure. *Br. med. J.* **285**, 919–923.

Brown, J. J., Lever, A. F., Robertson, J. I. S. and Semple, P. F. (1984). Should dietary sodium be reduced? The sceptics position. *Q. J. Med.* **53**, 427–437.

Brunner, H. R., Waeber, B. and Nussberger, J. (1985). Blood pressure recording in the ambulatory patient and evaluation of cardiovascular risk. *Clin. Sci.* **68**, 485–488.

Chaine, G. J. and Kohner, E. M. (1982). Hypertensive retinopathy. In *Hypertension* (eds P. Sleight and E. D. Freis), pp. 92–116. Butterworth, London.

Conceicao, S., Ward, M. D. and Kerr, D. N. S. (1976). Defects in sphygomomanometers, an important source or error in blood pressure recordings. *Br. med J.* **1**, 886.

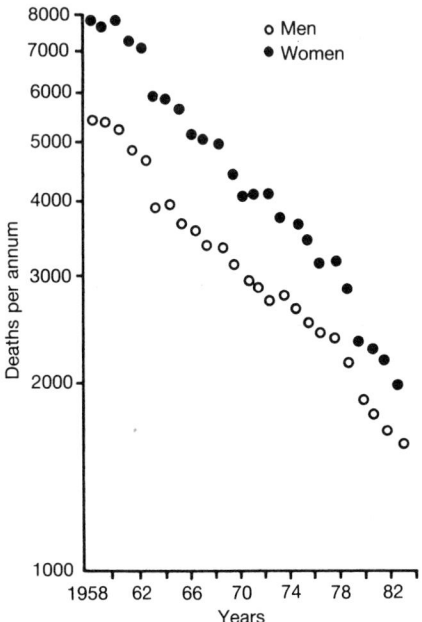

Fig. 21 Mortality from hypertensive heart disease in England and Wales since 1958. (Source: Code 402 from the Registrar General's annual reports.) (Reproduced from Dollery and Corr, 1985, *Br. Heart J.* **54**, 234, with permission.)

Curtis, J. J., Luke, R. G., Dustan, H. P. *et al.* (1983). Remission of essential hypertension after renal transplantation. *N. Engl. J. Med.* **809**, 1009–1015.

Davies, M. H. (1971). Is high blood pressure a psychosomatic disorder? *J. chron. Dis.* **24**, 239.

Goldstein, D. S. (1983). Plasma catecholamines and essential hypertension. An analytical review. *Hypertension* **5**, 86–99.

Graham, D. I. (1975). Ischaemic brain damage of cerebral perfusion failure type after treatment of severe hypertension. *Br. med. J.* **4**, 739.

Guyton, A. C., Coleman, T. G., Cowley, A. W., Manning, R. D., Norman, R. A. and Ferguson, J. D. (1974). A systems analysis approach to understanding long-range arterial blood pressure control and hypertension. *Circulation Res.* **35**, 159.

Harlan, W. R., Landis, J. R., Schmouder, R. L., Goldstein, N. G. and Harlan, L. C. (1985). Blood lead and blood pressure. Relationship in the adolescent and adult US population. *J. Am. Med. Assoc.* **253**, 530–534.

Henry, J. P., Stephens, P. M. and Santisteben, G. A. (1975). A model of psychosocial hypertension showing reversibility and progression of cardiovascular complications. *Circulation Res.* **36**, 156.

Hypertension detection and follow-up Programme Co-operative Group (1979). Five year finding II. Mortality by race, age and sex. *J. Am. Med. Assoc.* **242**, 2572–2577.

—— (1979). Five year findings I. Reduction in mortality. *J. Am. Med. Assoc.* **242**, 2562–2571.

—— (1982). The effect of treatment on mortality in 'mild' hypertension. *N. Engl. J. Med.* **307**, 976–980.

IPPPSH Collaborative Group (1985). Cardiovascular risk and risk factors in a randomised trial of treatment based on the betablocker oxprenolol. *J. Hypertension* **3**, 379–392.

Kannel, W. B. and Dawber, T. R. (1974). Hypertension as an ingredient of a cardiovascular risk profile. *Br. J. hosp. Med.* **7**, 508.

Ledingham, J. G. G. (1983). Management of hypertensive crises. *Hypertension* Suppl. III **5**, 114–119.

Lichtenstein, M. J., Shipley, M. J. and Rose, G. (1985). Systolic and diastolic blood pressures as predictors of coronary heart disease mortality in the Whitehall study. *Br. med. J.* **291**, 243–245.

Lund-Johansen, P. (1982). Haemodynamics of hypertension with and without treatment. In *Hypertension* (eds P. Sleight and E. D. Freis), pp. 173–182. Butterworth, London.

MacMahon, S. W., Macdonald, G. J., Bernstein, L., Andrews, G. and Blacket, R. B. (1985). A randomized controlled trial of weight reduction and metoprolol in the treatment of hypertension in young overweight patients. *Clin. Exp. Pharm. Phys.* **12**, 267–271.

Management Committee (1980). The Australian therapeutic trial in mild hypertension. *Lancet* **i**, 1261–1267.

—— (1982). Untreated mild hypertension. *Lancet* **i**, 185–191.

Masterton, G., Main, C. J., Lever, A. F. and Lever, R. S. (1981). Lower blood pressure in psychiatric inpatients. *Br. Heart J.* **45**, 442.

Medical Research Council Working Party (1983). Ventricular extrasystoles during thiazide treatment: substudy of MRC mild hypertension trial. *Br. med. J.* **287**, 1249–1253.

—— (1985). MRC trial of treatment of mild hypertension: principal results. *Br. med. J.* **291**, 97–104.

Miall, W. E. and Chinn, S. (1973). Blood pressure and aging: results of a 15–17 year follow-up study in South Wales. *Clin. Sci. mol. Med.* **45**, 235.

—— (1974). Screening for hypertension: some epidemiological observations. *Br. med. J.* **3**, 595.

Murphy, M. B., Scriven, A. J. I. and Dollery, C. T. (1983). Role of nifedipine in treatment of hypertension. *Br. med J.* **287**, 257–259.

Nichols, M. G. (1984). Reduction of dietary sodium in Western Society: Benefit or risk? *Hypertension* **6**, 795–801.

Nielsen, P. E. (1981). Physiological and methodological aspects of blood pressure measurement in normotensive and hypertensive subjects (ed. P. E. Neilsen). *Acta med. scand.* **670** (Suppl.), 1–104.

—— and Janniche, H. (1974). The accuracy of ausculatory measurement of arm blood pressure in very obese subjects. *Acta. med. scand.* **195**, 403.

Omvik, P. and Lund-Johansen, P. (1984). Combined captopril and hydrochlorothiazide therapy in severe hypertension: long-term haemodynamic changes at rest and during exercise. *J. Hypertension* **2**, 73–80.

Patel, C., Marmot, M. G., Terry, D. J., Carruthers, M., Hunt, B. and Patel, M. (1985). Trial of relaxation in reducing coronary risk: four year follow up. *Br. med. J.* **290**, 1103–1106.

Perloff, D., Sokolow, W. and Cowan, R. (1983). The prognostic value of ambulatory blood pressure. *J. Am. Med. Assoc.* **249**, 2793–2798.

Pickering, T. G. and Harshfield, G. (1985). What is the role or ambulatory blood pressure monitoring in the management of hypertensive patients? *Hypertension* **7**, 171–177.

Pocock, S. J., Shaper, A. G., Ashby, D., Delves, T. and Whitehead, T. P. (1984). Blood lead concentration, blood pressure and renal function. *Br. med. J.* **289**, 872–874.

Poston, L., Sewell, R. B., Wilkinson, S. P., Richardson, P. J. Williams, R., Clarkson, E. M., MacGregor, G. A. and de Wardener, H. E. (1981). Evidence for the circulating sodium transport inhibitor in essential hypertension. *Br. med. J.* **1**, 847.

Potter, J. F. and Beevers, D. G. (1984). Pressor effect of alcohol in hypertension. *Lancet* **i**, 119–121.

Prys-Roberts, C., Meloche, R. and Foëx, R. (1971). Studies of anaesthesia in relation to hypertension. *Br. J. Anaesth.* **43**, 122.

Robinson, B. F. (1984). Altered calcium handling as a primary cause of hypertension. *J. Hypertension* **2**, 453–460.

Ross Russell, R. W. (1975). How does blood pressure cause stroke? *Lancet* **iv**, 1283.

Sivertsson, R. (1970). The haemodynamic importance of structural vascular changes in essential hypertension. *Acta. physiol. scand.* Suppl. 343.

Sleight, P. (1985). Differences between casual and 24-h blood pressures. *J. Hypertension* **3** (Suppl. 2), S19–23.

—— (1985) Editorial. Ambulatory monitoring of blood pressure. *Hypertension* **7**, 163–164.

—— (ed.) (1980). *Arterial baroreceptors and hypertension.* Oxford University Press, Oxford.

Taguchi, J. and Freis, E. D. (1974). Partial reduction of blood pressure and prevention of complications in hypertension. *N. Engl. J. Med.* **291**, 329.

Thomas, J. P. and Thomson, W. H. (1983). Comparison of thiazides and amiloride in treatment of moderate hypertension. *Br. med. J.* **286**, 2015.

Tudor Hart J. (1970). Semi-continuous screening of a whole community for hypertension. *Lancet* **iii**, 223.

Veterans' Administration Co-operative Study (1970). Effects of treatment on morbidity in hypertension – results in patients with a diastolic blood pressure averaging 90 through 114 mm Hg. *J. Am. Med. Assoc.* **213**, 1143.

Weber, M. A. and Drayer, J. I. M. (1984). Single-agent and combination therapy of essential hypertension. *Am. Heart J.* **108**, 311.

Webster, J., Newnham, D., Petrie, J. C. and Lovell, H. G. (1984). Influence of arm position on measurement of blood pressure *Br. med. J.* **288**, 1574–1575.

Weidmann, P., Uehlinger, D. E. and Gerber, A. (1984). Antihypertensive treatment and serum lipoproteins. *J. Hypertension* **3**, 297–306.

Secondary hypertension

J. G. G. LEDINGHAM

Introduction

If on repeated measurement a patient's blood pressure is thought to be high enough to justify treatment by antihypertensive drugs, the question arises as to how far investigation should be taken before such treatment begins. Although primary causes of hypertension which can be reversed by treatment are rare, the finding of such a cause may spare the patient from a lifetime of taking drugs. Perhaps equally important, an underlying disease may be uncovered which needs treatment in its own right, e.g. diabetes mellitus, obstructive uropathy, analgesic kidney damage, collagen vascular disease, or endocrine disease. There may be a lead in the history or clinical examination (Table 1). Most commonly, such is not the case. How far should investigation then go in the frequently encountered problem of the patient with moderate hypertension, most likely to be 'essential' in origin? Most would agree that the simple approach outline in Table 2 is adequate, with other investigations reserved for the patient in whom essential hypertension is unlikely, or who fails to respond to, or perhaps co-operate with, drug treatment (Table 3).

Causes

The many possible causes of hypertension are listed in Table 4. Most are extremely rare. Precise figures are hard to come by.

Table 1 Features suggesting secondary hypertension in the clinical examination

History	Examination
Known renal disease	Femoral pulses delayed
Thirst, polyuria, nocturia	Palpable kidney(s)
Dysuria	Enlarged bladder
Haematuria	Uraemic features
Loin pain, colic	Oedema
Stones, gravel	Abdominal bruits
Abdominal trauma	Features of Cushing's or acromegaly
Analgesic consumption	Cafe au lait patches
Oral contraceptives	Neurofibromata
Other drugs (see Table 4)	Orthostatic hypotension*

* May occur in untreated phaeochromocytoma.

Table 2 First-line investigations in hypertension

Urine	Reagent strips for protein, blood, sugar
	Microscopy for casts and cells
	Culture
Blood	Haemoglobin, ESR
	Urea, uric acid
	Creatinine, fasting sugar
	Electrolytes, fasting lipids
Radiology	Chest X-ray
ECG	For left ventricular hypertrophy*
Echocardiography	For left ventricular wall thickness

* 30 per cent of patients in the Framingham study with left ventricular hypertrophy died in five years.

Table 3 Features suggesting need for further investigation

Clinical features suggesting a primary cause
Abnormalities of urea, creatinine, potassium in plasma
Proteinuria, haematuria, glycosuria
Hypertension under 30 years of age
Malignant hypertension
Uncontrolled hypertension

Table 5 Frequency of various diagnoses in hypertensive patients

Diagnosis	Percentage of group
Essential	90
Oral contraceptive induced	4
Renovascular disease	3
Chronic renal disease	2
Primary aldosteronism	0.4

From Ferguson (1975). *Ann. intern. Med.* **82**, 761–756, by permission.

Much depends on the selection of cases referred to individual centres, less to the extent to which the physician is prepared to take investigation. Analysis of series of unselected patients suggests a frequency of secondary hypertension of only some 10 per cent. Data from East Lansing are shown as an example (Table 5). In other series, phaeochromocytoma, Cushing's syndrome, and coarctation of the aorta feature, but each amounts to less than 0.5 per cent of the total. Other causes are even more uusual.

Despite the rarity of secondary hypertension, there are a number of conditions in which appropriate treatment may cure hypertension. These are sought after particularly eagerly; they include vascular disease, unilateral renal parenchymal disease, hypertension related to the oral contraceptive, Cushing's syndrome, coarctation of the aorta, phaeochromocytoma, primary aldosteronism (adenoma), renin-secreting tumours, liquorice addiction, and treatment by carbenoxolone sodium or sympathomimetic appetite suppressants or nasal sprays. A high alcohol intake may aggravate underlying hypertension or even act as a primary cause in some cases (see page 13.365).

Renal vascular diseases

The frequency of renal vascular diseases as a cause of hypertension is difficult to assess, partly because so many publications come from specialized centres, partly because the diagnosis may be missed in less specialized centres, and partly because of a difficulty in definition. Since extensive narrowing of the renal arteries by atheroma or fibrous dysplasia may occur in subjects with a

Table 4 Causes of secondary hypertension

Unilateral renal diseases	Bilateral renal diseases	Adrenal disorders	Drug associated	Other
Renal artery:	Glomerulonephritides	Primary aldosteronism	Oral contraceptive	Coarctation of aorta
stenosis	Interstitial nephritis	Cushing's syndrome	Corticosteroids	Pre-eclampsia
atheroma	Pyelonephritis	Phaeochromocytoma	Carbenoxolone sodium	Acute intermittent
fibrous dysplasia	Polycystic disease	DOC excess	Liquorice addiction	porphyria
trauma	Analgesic kidney	Corticosterone excess	Sympathomimetics	Acute lead poisoning
Pyelonephritis	Systemic sclerosis	Congenital adrenal	Monoamine oxidase	CNS disorders:
Obstructive nephropathy	Other collagen vascular	hyperplasia	inhibitors	raised intracranial
Vesico-ureteric reflux	diseases	Glucocorticoid-remediable	Application of skin	tension
Dysplasia	Thrombotic	hypertension	mineralocorticoid	tetanus
Ask-Upmark kidney	thrombocytopenic	Extrarenal renin secreting	ointment	poliomyelitis
Trauma	purpura	tumours		? Acromegaly
Tumour (including renin-	Post-partum renal failure	11β-hydroxysteroid		Alcohol addiction
secreting)	Haemolytic–uraemic	dehydrogenase		
Tuberculosis	syndromes	deficiency		
Cyst	Obstructive uropathy			
Irradiation	Vesico-ureteric reflux			
	Dysplasia			
	Gout			
	Diabetes mellitus			
	Amyloidosis			
	Tuberculosis			
	Irradiation			
	Chronic renal failure (any			
	cause)			

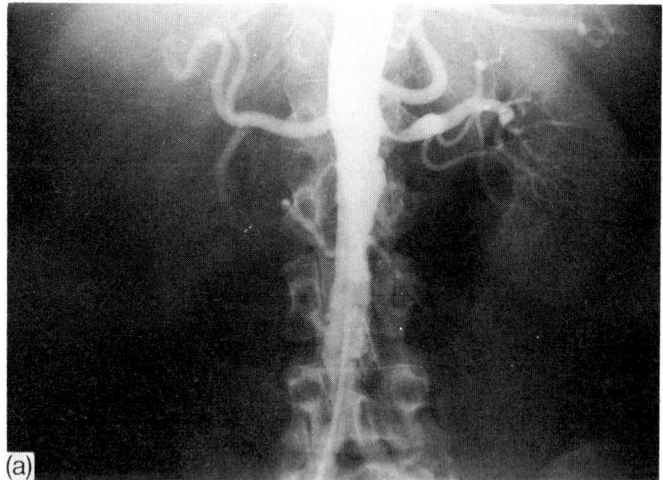

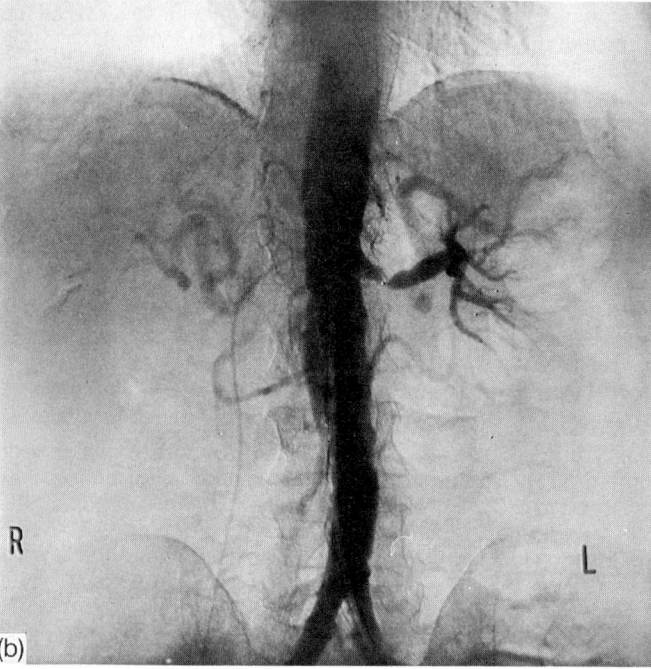

Fig. 1 (a) Aortography in a patient with atheromatous renal vascular disease; the right renal artery is totally occluded, the left tightly stenosed at its origin. Splenic and hepatic vessels are healthy, but there is extensive atheroma in the aorta. (b) Another patient with extensive atheroma, an occluded right renal artery and tight stenosis on the left.

normal arterial pressure and since atheromatous lesions may arise *de novo* in the renal arteries of patients with essential hypertension, one can only be sure of the diagnosis retrospectively if hypertension has been cured by surgery. Even then there is a dilemma, since it is likely, if not certain, that surgical correction of a long-standing arterial lesion, the original cause of hypertension, may fail if there are secondary vascular changes, particularly in the contralateral kidney. With these reservations, it is probable that only some 3–5 per cent of all hypertensive patients owe their arterial pressure to renal disease. The most common lesion is atheroma.

Atheromatous renal vascular disease
Atheromatous lesions tend to occur at or near the junctions of the renal arteries with the aorta. They are found principally in middle-aged patients, rather more in men than in women, but especially in cigarette smokers of either sex. The renal arterial lesion is only one facet of a generalized disease. Patients with atheromatous

lesions of the renal arteries often suffer also from angina, intermittent claudication, and transient ischaemic attacks or stroke because of atheroma in other major vessels (Fig. 1). These lesions contribute to the remarkably poor prognosis in this group of patients, whether treated medically or by renovascular surgery. For this reason many physicians will not search for this condition with particular diligence.

Fibrous dysplasia
This term describes a number of different conditions affecting the intima, media, and adventitia of renal and other arteries. The commonest manifestation is medial fibroplasia with mural aneurysms. In contrast to atheroma, the lesions occur predominantly in the distal two-thirds of the renal arteries, often extending into the intrarenal branches. The typical radiological appearances, which resemble a 'string of beads' (Fig. 2) represent alternating areas of stenosis from medial fibrosis and of aneurysmal dilations in areas deficient in the internal elastic lamina and muscle. In some patients with fibromuscular hyperplasia a single smooth tight stenosis may be the angiographic appearance, closely resembling an atheromatous lesion. In such a case the absence of extrarenal atheroma would suggest the possibility of hyperplasia but the diagnosis depends ultimately on histology.

The classical lesions of fibromuscular hyperplasia may affect one or both renal arteries and may be found also in the carotoid, coeliac axis, mesenteric, and iliac vessels, although morbid consequences of involvement of extrarenal vessels is unusual. All forms of fibrous dysplasia may progress, but medial fibroplasia does so less than the other less common varieties. The disorder occurs much more commonly in women than in men; although a disease of the young (third and fourth decades predominantly), it may be diagnosed for the first time in patients aged 50 years or more.

The response to reconstructive surgery or balloon angioplasty is generally excellent and the long-term prognosis much better than for atheromatous renal vascular disease.

Other renal vascular lesions
Arteritis, aneurysm, arteriovenous fistula, embolism, or intimal trauma of the renal arteries may cause hypertension which is also associated on occasion with lesions from cyst or tumour distorting the arterial blood supply to the kidney.

When to investigate potential renal vascular disease
Investigations to identify patients with renal arterial lesions should only be undertaken if there is good reason to suppose that surgical reconstruction, balloon angioplasty or uninephrectomy is likely to produce a better result than medical treatment. The 'routine screening' intravenous urogram (IVU) has no part in proper management. Antihypertensive drugs have improved greatly in range, effectiveness, and acceptability to patients, but so have surgical techniques, and balloon angioplasty has added another possible approach to treatment of renovascular disease. Judgement of whether or not to consider surgery or angioplasty can only be made with confidence from a proper trial of medical versus surgical and/or angioplastic treatment, among a large number of properly randomized patients. No such trial has taken place. The uncontrolled Mayo Clinic experience reported in 1974 suggested a better prognosis for surgically treated patients. While this conclusion, although widely quoted, is at best debatable, particularly as antihypertensive treatment has since improved in efficacy and acceptability, most are agreed that fibrous dysplastic lesions are best treated surgically or by angioplasty whenever these approaches are technically feasible.

The physician denied the results of a good controlled trial should even so have a clear idea of what surgery or angioplasty can offer, *before* submitting the patient to the relevant tests. Table 6 gives the results of surgery in several large series reported since 1965. The outcome has not changed significantly over 20 years, apart from Kaufman's experience in Los Angeles which shows

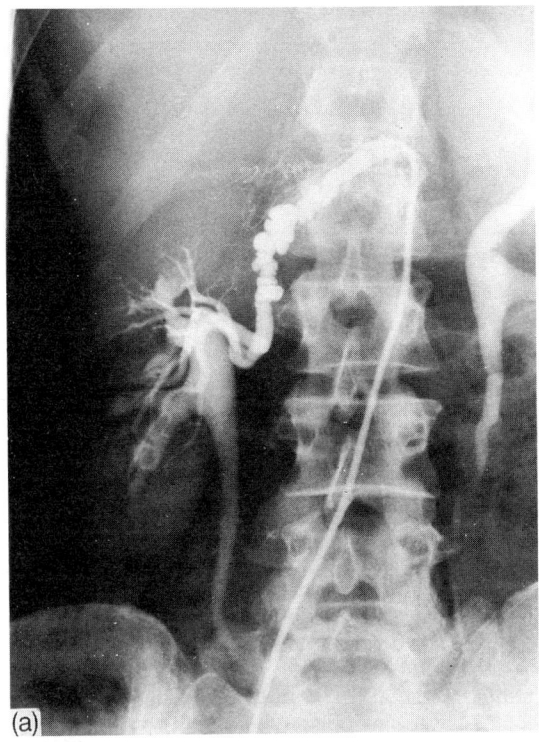

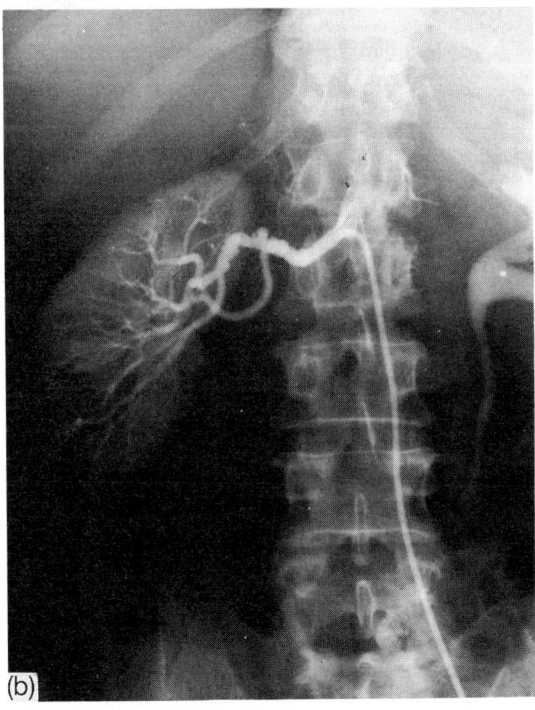

Fig. 2 Selective right renal angiography in two patients with hypertension due to fibromuscular hyperplasia.

what can be achieved by a highly skilled and experienced team. Renal vascular surgery should be undertaken only in specialized centres; there is no place for the occasional operation. Even if this precept is followed, overall expectation of cure by surgery is unlikely to be more than 50 per cent, but this figure, representing as it does a wide variety of cases, obscures the good results to be expected in fibromuscular disease.

It is still too early to be sure about the response to balloon angioplasty but results would appear to approximate closely to those of reconstructive surgery (see later).

No clinical features reliably distinguish renal vascular disease from essential hypertension. Pointers include a known onset of high arterial pressure in patients unusually young or unusually old for essential hypertension, the presence of abdominal bruits, malignant hypertension or hypertension particularly resistant to drug treatment; but none of these are of more than marginal value.

A reasonable set of criteria on which to base the decision to investigate are:

Hypertension in the young Although essential hypertension appears to be more common in the young than was once believed, severe hypertension under the age of 30 years merits full investigation for a primary cause. The presence of an abdominal or loin bruit in this age group is particularly suggestive of fibrous dysplastic disease.

Drug-resistant hypertension When the whole range and combination of antihypertensive drugs either fail to control arterial pressure, or do so only at the cost of unacceptable side-affects, a full search for a surgically remediable cause should be made.

Trauma Sudden onset of a raised arterial pressure following injury which might have involved the renal areas suggests a lesion of the kidneys or renal artery potentially reversible by prompt vascular surgery or nephrectomy.

Renovascular renal failure Atheromatous renal vascular disease is all too often bilateral with complete occlusion of one renal artery and severe stenosis of the other side a not uncommon finding (see Fig. 1).

Renal function is then compromised and may deteriorate further and suddenly with any increase in vascular obstruction. In this situation, reconstructive surgery or balloon angioplasty on one or both sides may prove surprisingly effective, not only in restoring renal function but also in improving arterial pressure. Renovascular renal failure occurs most commonly in middle-aged male patients who have smoked and in whom there is evidence of generalized atheroma. Hypertension is often of long-standing and associated with evidence of mild renal dysfunction. A sudden onset of renal failure, often accompanied by worsening hypertension are indications of further impairment of renal perfusion, which should be investigated by renal angiography.

Malignant hypertension The malignant phase is more common in patients with renal hypertension than in those without a detectable primary cause. It is taken by most physicians as an indication to investigate for renal vascular disease.

Table 6 Results of surgery (reconstruction or nephrectomy) in apparent renovascular hypertension 1965–83

Reference	Number of patients	Cured (%)	Improved (%)	Failed (%)	Early postoperative deaths (%)
Meltzer (1965)	297	42	30	28	8
Morris *et al.* (1966)	432	41	40	12	7
Hunt *et al.* (1974)	100	51	27	6	16
Maxwell (1975)	502	51	15	28	6
Kaufman (1979)	142	80	15	3	2
MacKay *et al.* (1983)	39	54	31	15	0

The hyponatraemic hypertensive syndrome The rare combination of severe hypertension with hyponatraemia, hypokalaemia, polyuria, polydipsia, and weight loss is associated with gross increases in activity of the renin–aldosterone system and is usually a manifestation of tight unilateral renal artery stenosis, although a very similar syndrome can also occur in patients with chronic renal failure treated by intermittent haemodialysis.

How to investigate renal vascular disease

Rapid-sequence urography

The physiological basis of the detection of a renal vascular lesion by intravenous urography depends on the delay in the rate at which dye reaches the tubules and the enhanced tubular reabsorption of salt and water which occur in an ischaemic kidney, resulting in an increased concentration of the dye and lesser urine volume on the side of the lesion. A rapid sequence of pictures at 1, 2, 3, 4, 5, 15, and 30 min should be taken in every case. Features indicating vascular disease include focal atrophy in lesions of branches of renal vessels, decreased renal size (disparity of more than 1.5 cm in length), delay in the first appearance of a nephrogram, increased density of the pyelogram, and lesser distension of the renal pelvis and calyces all on the side of the lesion. The most reliable signs are the disparity in size and delay in the appearance of the dye. In experienced hands, this technique detects some 80 per cent of patients in whom later angiography shows unilateral disease. It is much less accurate if disease is bilateral or segmental. Accuracy also depends on the degree of stenosis present. Complete occlusion is detected in 95 per cent of cases, but if the obstruction occludes less than 50 per cent of the lumen, only some 20 per cent of cases are picked up. The IVU is of no value in predicting prognosis after surgery.

Isotope renography

The original renographic techniques using ^{131}I hippuran gave a high incidence of false-positive results in patients subsequently proven to have essential hypertension. Gamma cameras linked to computers detecting ^{123}I isotopes provide blood background subtraction and much improved imaging. These developments allow measurement of total and divided renal blood flow and glomerular filtration rates, giving more accurate data about the blood supply and function of individual kidneys.

Where facilities are available, a combination of radionuclide imaging and rapid sequence urography provide the best screening tests for renal arterial lesions. Again, the demonstration of a lesion cannot predict the blood pressure response to its removal.

Renal angiography

Angiograms serve to identify and detect renal arterial lesions but do not assess their functional significance. Good pictures should be obtained of the aorta and its branches including the iliac vessels as well as the renal vasculature. Selective renal angiograms, while providing excellent pictures of the distal renal vessels, may miss proximal stenosis and do not provide the surgeon with sufficient information about the rest of the local vascular tree. Renal angiography is not without complication. Mortality may be as high as 0.1 per cent and local pain and haemorrhage are occasional problems. Transient renal failure may be provoked by any procedure in which radiocontrast media are injected intravenously (see page 18.131). Intravenous administration with digital angiography is an advance in this respect.

Divided renal function tests

Tests of the function of individual kidneys by selective ureteric catheterization are usually uncomfortable for the patient and are often accompanied by haematuria, renal colic, and on occasion, by a period of oliguria or anuria. There is no evidence that they predict the outcome of surgery; few units still use this technique.

Table 7 Renal vein renin ratios in predicting outcome of surgery

Number of patients	Ratio increased (over 1.6:1)		Ratio not increased	
	Improved	Not improved	Improved	Not improved
412	267	19	64	62

Data from several series.

Renin–angiotensin system

1. Renin in peripheral blood Renin activity or concentration in peripheral venous plasma is raised in only some 50 per cent of patients in whom surgery returns arterial pressure to normal.

2. Renal vein renin Comparison of the renin activity in blood taken from the two renal veins simultaneously is a more sensitive index of the outcome of subsequent surgery, as shown in Table 7, but false-positive and false-negative results are evident in published series. Their true incidence may be higher in unreported series and a number of recent publications have suggested the test to have no predictive value. Certainly many patients in whom the ratio of concentrations between the stenosed and intact sides is less than the traditional 1.6 to 1 are helped or even cured by reconstructive surgery or angioplasty. Particular problems arise when the disease is bilateral or segmental, when there is difficulty in placing the catheter in the renal veins or when samples are diluted by caval or gonadal blood. The test is therefore not to be taken as an absolute criterion but only as one of a number of important factors to be considered in making the decision of whether or not to proceed to reconstructive techniques or nephrectomy. In one series of 126 patients, surgery was successful in about half the patients in whom the renal vein renin ratios were less than 1.6 to 1.

Stimulation of renin release by dietary sodium restriction or the use of drugs such as hydralazine, frusemide or converting enzyme inhibition increases the differential values of renin activity on the two sides but these manoeuvres have not been shown to provide a substantially better prediction of the outcome of surgery. Nor is the failure to suppress renin release by the contralateral kidney an absolute indication that surgery or angioplasty will fail.

3. Antagonists of the renin–angiotensin system These are of three kinds. Competitive inhibitors of angiotensin II such as saralasin have some agonistic effects and must be given parenterally. They are therefore of limited usefulness. Angiotensin-converting enzyme inhibitors (ACE inhibitors) such as captopril or enalapril are free of agonistic effects and are active given by mouth. They are not *specific* inhibitors however, and while they prevent conversion of angiotensin I to II they also inhibit catabolism of bradykinin. True renin inhibitors have now been developed but are not generally available; their usefulness in diagnosis and in prediction of the outcome of surgery is not yet known.

Saralasin and ACE inhibitors both reduce arterial pressure *acutely* in patients with renovascular disease in broad proportions to the pretreatment activity of the renin–angiotensin system. Both also cause a fall in arterial pressure in salt-depleted normal subjects. No sound evidence exists that the *acute* blood pressure response to these agents can predict the outcome of surgery or angioplasty. In contrast, the *long-term* response to treatment with captopril or enalapril has been shown to have predictive value and may prove to be more valuable in this respect than measurement of renal vein renin ratios. Caution is required in applying such a test because of the ill effects of ACE inhibition on renal function on those rare occasions when stenosis is tight in a single functioning kidney or in bilateral disease. Where renal perfusion is grossly reduced, glomerular filtration pressure is dependent on efferent arteriolar tone, increased in this situation by local production of angiotensin II, which is prevented by ACE inhibition. Loss of glomerular filtration rate with substantial acute rises in blood urea and creatinine concentrations may therefore complicate ACE inhibition treatment in the few patients at risk. Renal dysfunction is reversible when ACE inhibition is stopped, but there is a risk, probably very small, of renovascular occlusion complicating the phase of ACE inhibition, particularly if this is continued despite substantial loss of renal function. In unilateral tight renal artery stenosis, overall renal function remains unchanged, but sometimes this finding obscures a considerable deterioration in the affected kidney, compensated by the performance of the contralateral organ.

Selection of patients for surgery or angioplasty

Since no single investigation or combination of factors distinguishes patients in whom surgery or angioplasty will succeed from those in whom they will fail, decisions must be made on imprecise grounds. Features which favour a surgical or radiological approach include youth, the presence of fibromuscular disease, the absence of widespread atheroma, a renal vein renin ratio exceeding 1.6 to 1, a good long-term (6–8 weeks) response to ACE-inhibiting drugs, a failure to respond to other antihypertensive drugs, an acute loss of renal function and above all the appearance of a lesion(s) which looks amenable to surgical or angioplasty reconstruction.

Surgical treatment

The removal of a kidney or part of a kidney in the hope of curing hypertension should be avoided whenever possible. Loss of functioning nephrons without cure of hypertension is not good treatment of a disease whose natural history includes impairment of renal function. Only when the damaged kidney contributes little or nothing to renal function is uninephrectomy acceptable. Whenever possible reconstructive techniques should be used, preserving or improving renal function as well as offering the chance of amelioration or cure of hypertension. A number of methods are in current use: (*a*) saphenous vein bypass, (*b*) arterial autograft bypass, (*c*) dacron graft bypass, (*d*) resection and reanastomosis, (*e*) autotransplantation to iliac fossa, (*f*) 'bench' surgery, (*g*) splenorenal bypass, and (*h*) endarterectomy.

Percutaneous transluminal angioplasty

This technique, which has been in use since 1978, is reported to be an effective and safe method of treating renal vascular stenoses without open surgery. The procedure involves catheterization of the involved artery by the Seldinger technique (Fig. 3). A guide line is then used to traverse the stenosis. The balloon dilation catheter is then appropriately placed and inflated for half to one minute at pressures from 75 to 90 PSL. Access to renal vessels can be via femoral or axillary arteries depending on the site of stenosis and ease of entry. Dilation by balloon results not from compressing the plaque as was thought initially, but by splitting and fracture of the plaque involving intima and media.

Long-term results of balloon angioplasty have been variably reported, but cure, improvement, and failure appear to be achieved at rates not greatly different from those achieved by surgery. Again patients in whom renal vein renin concentrations are increased, and those with fibromuscular hyperplasia do best.

The site of the stenotic lesion is important, the least good results being achieved in those in whom the stenosis involves the aorta and ostium of the renal artery.

Complications of the procedure occur in some 6 to 15 per cent of patients. The most serious are of dissection of the renal artery with partial infarction of the kidney, or rupture of the balloon, which can then embolize to kidney or other vessels. Transient renal failure perhaps due to injection of contrast has also been reported.

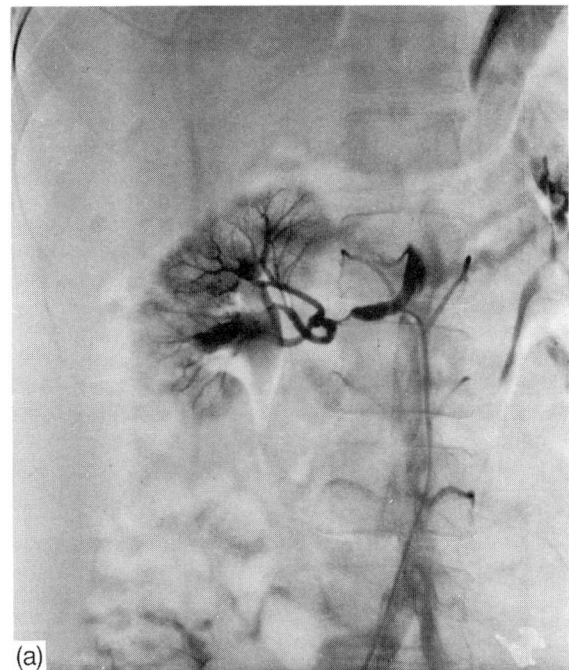

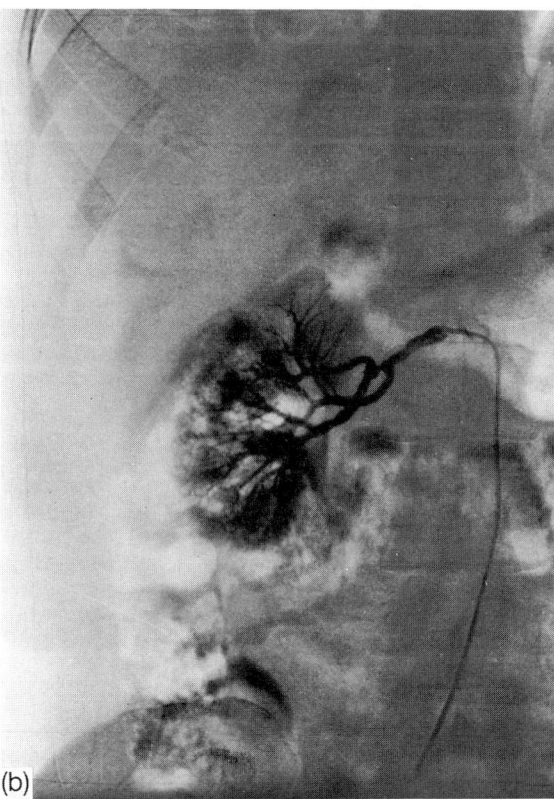

Fig. 3 Selective right renal angiograms illustrating (a) a lengthy stenosis due to fibromuscular hyperplasia in a 19-year-old girl, and (b) the appearance after successful transluminal angioplasty. (Reproduced by permission of Dr E. W. L. Fletcher.)

Unilateral renal parenchymal disease

Pyelonephritic scarring or dysplasia of a single kidney are probably the commonest forms of unilateral parenchymal renal disease in which nephrectomy is an option in treatment. Since the first successful operation in 1937 opinions have been divided about the role of surgery in such cases. A more conservative approach than taken in renovascular disease is proper, since operation leads to loss of renal tissue in every case. Published data are considerably fewer than in the case of renal vascular disease. Surgical results are probably less good than after nephrectomy for renovascular disease with cure to be expected in perhaps 30 per cent of patients, but with improvement in control in a rather large number. Surgery specifically designed to relieve hypertension should only be undertaken when the affected kidney contributes little or nothing to renal function or when blood pressure is uncontrolled despite maximal tolerated doses of combinations of antihypertensive drugs, including minoxidil, captopril or enalapril and nifedipine.

Although there have been claims that measurement of renal vein renin activity is of value in predicting blood pressure response to surgery for renal parenchymal disease, the evidence is thin and inconsistent. Nor would it be wise to proceed on the assumption that the blood pressure response to antagonists of the renin–angiotensin system (such as saralasin or ACE inhibitors) has useful predictive value.

References

Bengtsson, U., Bergentz, S-E. and Norbäck, B. (1974). Surgical treatment of renal artery stenosis with impending uraemia. *Clin. Nephrol.* **2**, 222–229.

Dean, R. H. and Foster, J. H. (1977). Surgical management of renovascular hypertension in older patients. *Med. Clins. N. Am.* **61**, 643–653.

Ferguson, R. K. (1975). Cost and yield of the hypertensive evaluation: experience of a community based referral clinic. *Ann. intern. Med.* **82**, 761–765.

Dustan, H. P. (1984). Renovascular hypertension and azotemia. *N. Engl. J. Med.* **311**, 1114–1115.

Horvath, J. S., Baxter, C. R., Sherbon, K., Smee, I., Roche, J., Ultrer, J. B. and Tiller, D. J. (1977). An analysis of errors found in renal vein sampling for plasma renin activity. *Kid. Int.* **11**, 136–138.

Horvath, J. S., Waugh, R. C., Tiller, D. J. and Duggin, G. G. (1982). The detection of renovascular hypertension: A study of 490 patients by angiography. *Q. J. Med.* **51**, 139–146.

Hunt, J. C., Sheps, S. G., Harrison, E. G., Strong, C. S. and Bernatz, P. E. (1984). Renal and renovascular hypertension: a reasoned approach to diagnosis and management. *Arch. intern. Med.* **133**, 988–999.

Kaufman, J. J. (1979). Renovascular hypertension: the UCLA experience. *J. Urol.* **121**, 139–144.

Levine, D. C. (1984). Percutaneous transluminal angioplasty of the renal arteries. *J. Am. Med. Ass.* **251**, 759–763.

MacKay, A., Boyle, P., Brown, J. J., Cumming, A. M., Forrest, H., Graham, A. G., Lever, A. F., Robertson, J. I. S. and Semple, P. F. (1983). The decision on surgery in renal artery stenosis. *Q. J. Med.* **52**, 363–381.

Maxwell, M. H. (1975). Cooperative study of renovascular hypertension: current status. *Kid. Int.* **8**, Suppl. 5, S153–S160.

Meltzer, J. I. (1965). Recent advances in hypertension. *Am. J. Med.* **39**, 616–645.

Morris, G. C., DeBakey, M. E., Crawford, E. S., Cooley, D. A. and Zanger, L. C. C. (1966). Late results of surgical treatment for renovascular hypertension. *Surg. Gyn. Obs.* **122**, 1255–1261.

Siampoulos, K., Sellars, L., Mishra, S. C., Essenhigh, D. M., Robson, V. and Wilkinson, R. (1983). Experience in the management of hypertension with unilateral chronic pyelonephritis: Results of nephrectomy in selected patients. *Q. J. Med.* **52**, 349–362.

Sos, T. A., Pickering, T. G., Sinderman, K., Saddekri, S., Case, D. B., Silane, M. F., Vaughan, E. D. and Laragh, J. H. (1983). Percutaneous transluminal renal angioplasty in renovascular hypertension due to atheroma or fibromuscular hyperplasia. *N. Engl. J. Med.* **309**, 274–279.

Youngberg, S. P., Sheps, S. G. and Strong, C. G. (1977). Fibromuscular disease of the renal arteries. *Med. Clin. N. Am.* **61**, 623–641.

Weinberger, M. H. (1985). Renovascular hypertension: Introduction: questions, current knowledge and clinical implications. *Am. J. Kid. Dis.* **5**, A85–A92.

Hypertension in chronic renal disease

Chronic renal diseases are the most common cause of secondary hypertension. Figures from renal units show that glomerulonephritis in its various forms is the commonest condition to bring the patient to regular dialysis or transplant surgery, with chronic pyelonephritis, reflux nephropathy, polycystic disease, and analgesic-

abuse kidney the other major causes. The mechanism(s) by which these diseases cause an elevation of arterial pressure are quite uncertain. One of the difficulties in finding an explanation is the common observation that hypertension is a feature of only *some* patients with those disorders. A patient with any form of renal disease may have a normal arterial pressure for many months or years and then suddenly develop hypertension without any apparent change in renal function. If there is a progressive diminution of glomerular filtration rate, hypertension becomes more common and more severe, with a prevalence at end-stage renal failure (from any cause) of about 90 per cent. Sodium and water retention are usual in advanced renal failure. Control of blood pressure in these patients by ultrafiltration haemodialysis and sodium restriction can usually be achieved, and this supports the concept of 'volume-dependent' hypertension in at least some patients. In others (much rarer) blood pressure fails to fall in response to these measures; body fluid volumes may be frankly low and plasma renin very high. Some such patients have been submitted to bilateral nephrectomy with cure of hypertension, but such desperate measures are almost never needed now.

Good control of arterial pressure in patients with chronic renal failure is an important part of their management, not only to prevent cardiovascular complications, but also to preserve the diseased kidney from nephrosclerosis and the ravages of malignant hypertension.

Hypertension in acute glomerulonephritis

The clinical syndrome of acute nephritis comprises proteinuria, haematuria, the passing of red cell casts, oliguria, impairment of glomerular filtration, hypertension, and mild oedema. In the now rare condition of poststreptococcal acute nephritis, hypertension is usually transient but may be severe enough to reach the malignant phase. Acute nephritis may present with pulmonary oedema, or with the neurological manifestations of hypertensive encephalopathy rather than the more widely recognized features of smoky urine and oedema. The persistence or otherwise of hypertension in any acute glomerular disease depends on the evolution of the disease in the kidney. In most people's experience the vast majority of patients with acute poststreptococcal nephritis make a complete recovery with a fall to normal levels of arterial pressure, but Baldwin has challenged this view, suggesting that prolonged follow-up of patients who had earlier shown evidence of complete recovery reveals an unexpectedly high number with hypertension and renal failure. Results from a later series from South Australia support more traditional views on prognosis and only four of 57 patients developed persistent hypertension, mild in each case.

The mechanisms by which arterial pressure is increased in the various acute nephritic syndromes are not completely resolved. The retention of sodium and water, together perhaps with renin activity in plasma inappropriately high have been invoked, but the evidence is not conclusive.

Renin-secreting tumours

Benign haemangiopericytomas in the kidney may contain cells resembling those of the juxtaglomerular apparatus. Plasma renin (from the tumour), angiotensin II, and aldosterone are increased with resultant hypokalaemic alkalosis. Hypertension tends to be severe and affects mostly young people of either sex. The tumours are usually small and are easily missed on angiography. Diagnosis of this very rare condition may require a demonstration of high renin activity in the renal vein blood of the affected kidney. The response to surgical removal of the tumour is excellent.

A similar syndrome may result from hypersecretion of renin from Wilm's tumours, from renal carcinoma or from extrarenal tissues such as pancreatic, pulmonary, hepatic or Fallopian tube carcinoma. The total renin produced by these rare tumours has been found to contain an unusually high proportion of inactive (big) as compared to active renin.

References

Baruch, D., Corvol, P., Alhenc-Gelas, F., Dutloux, M-A., Guyenne, T. T., Gaux, J-C., Raynaud, A., Brisset, J. M., Duclos, J-M. and Menard, J. (1984). Diagnosis and treatment of renin-secreting tumours. *Hypertension* **6**, 760–766.

Brod, J., Bahlmann, J., Cachovan, M. and Pretschner, P. (1983). Development of hypertension in renal disease. *Clin. Sci.* **64**, 141–152.

Brown, J. J., Fraser, R., Lever, A. F., Morton, J. J., Robertson, J. I. S., Tree, M., Bell, P. R. F., Davidson, J. K. and Ruthven, I. S. (1973). Hypertension and secondary hyperaldosteronism with a renin-secreting juxtaglomerular cell tumour. *Lancet* **ii**, 1228–1232.

Conn, J. W. (1977). Primary reninism. In *Hypertension* (eds J. Genest, E. Koiw and O. Kuchel), pp. 840. McGraw-Hill, New York.

Corvol, P. (1984). Tumour-dependent hypertension. *Hypertension* **6**, 593–596.

Ganguly, A., Gribble, J., Tune, B., Kempson, R. L. and Luetscher, J. A. (1973). Renin-secreting Wilm's tumour with severe hypertension. *Ann. intern. Med.* **79**, 835–837.

Ledingham, J. M. (1971). Blood pressure regulation in renal failure. *J. R. Coll. Phycns London* **5**, 103–134.

The oral contraceptive and hypertension

Hypertension caused by the oral contraceptive pill is one of the commoner forms of secondary hypertension. Although the rise in pressure is usually mild, rare patients develop severe hypertension and the malignant phase, reversed by withdrawal of oral contraceptives, has been described. The increased risk of stroke among women taking oral contraceptives appears to be independent of changes in arterial pressure.

Hypertension has been reported to occur in as many as 15 per cent of women taking combined oestrogen–progestogen preparations, or in as few as 1 or 2 per cent. A recent estimate is that arterial pressure increases above 140/90 mm Hg in between 2 and 5 per cent of women followed over 5 years. The true prevalence of hypertension among pill takers must depend on the selection of patients observed, how long they are followed, and criteria for diagnosing 'hypertension'.

Weir and colleagues have compared the blood pressures of 325 women taking combined oestrogen–progestogen preparations with a group of control women using cervical diaphragms or intrauterine devices. There were significant increases in both systolic and diastolic pressure in the pill takers, but not in the control group. The rise in pressure occurred in most cases within two years, but in some women blood pressure continued to rise progressively over five years. Eight women (4 per cent of those at risk) developed increases in systolic pressure exceeding 25 mm Hg, with the largest individual rise being 41 mm Hg. Diastolic pressures rose 34 and 24 mm Hg, respectively, in two women to reach figures of 94 and 98 mm Hg. No correlation was found in this study between change in blood pressure and dose of oestrogen or progestogen, past history of pre-eclampsia, family history of hypertension, change in weight, cigarette smoking or social class.

The mechanism by which oral contraceptives increase blood pressure is unknown. Changes occur in various components of the renin-angiotensin system but to the same degree in women whose blood pressure rises and in others in whom it does not. Sodium and water retention is associated with oestrogen treatment but again not selectively in those who become hypertensive. This is an important point since it has become common practice to prescribe low oestrogen compounds or preparations containing progestogen alone to those women whose blood pressure has increased on the standard drug.

That this might not be sound practice was suggested by the study of the Royal College of General Practitioners which showed the lowest rates of 'hypertension' in women taking the higher doses of oestrogen, while the highest rates were recorded in those taking preparations with the highest progestogen content. But hypertension in this study was imprecisely diagnosed, and other work would suggest that the risk of hypertension is less on the 30 μg oestrogen combined preparation and much less among women taking progestogen alone, although even this sort of oral contraceptive can cause an increase in arterial pressure in women in whom the combined preparation has been associated with hypertension.

In most patients with oral contraceptive-induced hypertension withdrawal of the drug corrects blood pressure within three months although a longer period (up to 18 months) may be needed in a few cases. It follows that patients should be advised to stop oral contraceptives for at least 18 months if there is a suspicion that hypertension has been pill induced. Whether or not women with established hypertension should be denied oral contraception is less easy to decide. Most doctors would at least discourage patients in this category since both elevated arterial pressure and regular consumption of oral contraceptives carry an increased risk of coronary artery and cerebrovascular disease.

References

Blumenstein, B. A., Douglas, M. B. and Hall, W. D. (1980). Blood pressure changes and oral contraceptive use; a study of 2676 black women in the South Eastern United States. *Am. J. Epidemiol.* **112**, 539–552.

Hall, W. D., Douglas, M. B., Blumenstein, B. A. and Hatcher, R. A. (1980). Blood pressure and oral progestational agents: A prospective study of 119 black women. *Am. J. Obs. Gyn.* **136**, 344–348.

Laragh, J. H. (1976). Oral contraceptive-induced hypertension: nine years later. *Am. J. Obs. Gyn.* **126**, 141–147.

Roberts, J. M. (1981). Oestrogens and hypertension. *Clin. Endocrinol. Metab.* **10**, 489–512.

Weinberger, M. H. and Weir, R. J. (1983). Oral contraceptives and hypertension. In *Handbook of hypertension*, Vol. 2 (eds W. H. Birkenhager and J. L. Reid), pp. 196–207. Elsevier, Amsterdam.

Weir, R. J., Briggs, E., Mack, A., Naismith, L., Taylor, L. and Wilson, E. (1974). Blood pressure in women taking oral contraception. *Br. Med. J.* **1**, 533–535.

Coarctation of the aorta

Coarctation of the aorta (see page 13.269) is usually diagnosed in childhood but it may be missed and present with hypertension in later life, often refractory to treatment. The disorder is commoner in males by a ratio of 4:1, and may be associated with other congenital abnormalities such as Turner's syndrome, patent ductus arteriosus, septal defects, mitral valve lesions, septal hypertrophy, and a bicuspid aortic valve. Preductal infantile coarctation (a narrowing between the origins of the left carotid or subclavian arteries and the ductus) does not allow survival to adult life without correction. The adult form of the disease is associated with narrowing in the region of the ductus lower down the aorta. In this condition blood is carried to the distal aorta by enormously enlarged collateral vessels; transverse cervical, transverse scapular, intercostal, internal mammary, and superior epigastric arteries. In adults the disease presents with hypertension much aggravated by exercise and usually associated with a systolic murmur best heard along the left heart border. It is diagnosed by feeling femoral and radial pulses simultaneously; the femoral may be absent, but is more commonly delayed compared with the radial. Enlarged collateral vessels are most easily seen by observing the patient from behind, when an oblique beam of light directed to the back may show arterial pulsation around the scapulae. Symptoms are not particularly specific, but fatigue in the legs during exertion may occur.

The diagnosis of coarctation is confirmed by aortography or computerized tomographic (CT) scanning which will demonstrate the position and length of the narrowed segment. Treatment is by surgical excision and is best undertaken under the age of 5 years. Untreated patients, though they may survive well into adult life are at risk of bacterial endocarditis as well as of the cardiovascular complications of uncontrolled hypertension.

The arterial pressure after surgery is improved but is not often restored completely to normal compared to age- and sex-matched populations. A paradoxical rise of arterial pressure may occur in the first 24 hours after surgery, perhaps due to baroreceptor-induced increased sympathetic activity, detectable by an increase in urinary catecholamines and plasma noradrenaline.

The mechanisms of hypertension in coarctation is disputed. It may be due to the mechanical effects of aortic obstruction, to changes in the activity of the renin–angiotensin system, a resetting of the baroreceptors, or all of these things.

References

Cheitlin, M. D. (1977). Coarctation of the aorta. *Med. Clin. N. Am.* **61**, 655–673.
de Leeuw, P.W. and Birkenhager, W. H. (1983). Coarctation of the aorta. In *Handbook of Hypertension*, Vol. 2 (eds W. H. Birkenhager and J. L. Reid), pp. 1–17. Elsevier, Amsterdam.
Sellors, T. H. and Hobsley, M. (1963). Coarctation of aorta: effect of operation on blood pressure. *Lancet* **i**, 1387–1391.

Cushing's syndrome

Cushing's syndrome (see page 10.69 *et seq.*) is caused by an increased secretion of hydrocortisone by the adrenal cortex and is mimicked closely by prolonged treatment with cortisone and its pharmacological analogues, used to treat a variety of diseases. Pituitary-dependent disease is most common. More rarely there is a primary abnormality of the adrenals – adenoma or carcinoma. ACTH-like peptides may also be secreted by certain tumours of non-endocrine tissues (particularly oat-cell carcinoma of the bronchus) but when this occurs the clinical features of Cushing's syndrome, including hypertension, are often absent. Modest hypertension is common (some 70–80 per cent of patients) in Cushing's syndrome and in a few cases it may be severe or even in the malignant phase. Welbourne, in a large series was unable to find any correlation between the severity of the biochemical changes in his patients and the arterial pressure. Nor is it certain that cortisol itself induces the hypertension. Cardiovascular disease is a common cause of death in Cushing's syndrome.

The response of the blood pressure to adrenalectomy or pituitary surgery has not been a subject of careful study by endocrinologists, but in most patients pressures fall after surgery. The responses in some may be delayed and incomplete.

The mechanism(s) by which cortisol may increase arterial pressure are still uncertain. They do not appear to depend on sodium retention. Hypotheses concerning altered vascular reactivity, the renin–angiotensin system or the sympathetic nervous system are unproven.

References

Krakoff, L. R. and Elyovich, F. (1981). Cushing's syndrome and exogenous glucocorticoid hypertension. *Clin. Endocrinol. Metab.* **10**, 479–488.
O'Neal, L. W., Kissane, J. M. and Hartroft, P. M. (1970). The kidney in endocrine hypertension. *Arch. Surg.* **100**, 498–505.
Ross, E. J., Marshall-Jones, P. and Friedman, M. (1966). Cushing's syndrome: diagnostic criteria. *Q. J. Med.* **35**, 149–192.
Welbourne, R. B., Montgomery, D. A. D. and Kennedy, T. C. (1971). The natural history of treated Cushing's syndrome. *Br. J. Surg.* **58**, 1.

Primary aldosteronism (Conn's syndrome)

This term is no longer sufficiently specific to indicate a single disorder, but embraces the entities of *aldosterone producing adenoma* or *carcinoma*, *idiopathic hyperaldosteronism*, and *glucocorticoid remediable hyperaldosteronism*. Each of these is associated with excessive and *relatively* autonomous production of aldosterone, and together the three conditions account for less than 1 per cent of all patients with hypertension. Adrenal hyperplasia with or without nodules is found in most cases of idiopathic hyperaldosteronism, but the glands may on occasion appear normal macroscopically and microscopically.

The increase in arterial pressure which occurs in these rare disorders may be directly attributable to sodium retention and volume expansion but the failure of bilateral adrenalectomy to restore normotension in idiopathic hyperaldosteronism gives reason for doubt. It is also possible that mineralocorticoids produce changes in the responsiveness of resistance vessels to pressor stimuli by a mechanism independent of sodium retention.

The cause of bilateral hyperplasia is not known in either idiopathic hyperaldosteronism or glucocorticoid remediable hyperaldosteronism. Renin activity is suppressed, plasma potassium low, and ACTH concentrations are not increased. The possibility of 'tertiary' hyperaldosteronism with the original stimulus renin, later suppressed by autonomous adrenal hyperplasia has been suggested but no proven example exists. It is also possible that idiopathic adrenal hyperplasia is part of the spectrum of essential hypertension and closely related to the 30 per cent of patients with that diagnosis in whom plasma renin activity is reduced ('low-renin essential hypertension').

Another explanation put forward is that hyperplasia in idiopathic aldosteronism is secondary to overproduction of 'aldosterone-stimulating factor', a glycoprotein of molecular weight 26 000 Dalton, which has been isolated from human urine, plasma, and pituitary tissue. Reports of high plasma and urinary concentrations of this substance in idiopathic hyperaldosteronism support this concept, but how its output is regulated and what changes occur in adenomatous aldosteronism are not yet known.

All these conditions present with hypertension associated with a tendency to hypokalaemia and renin suppression. Some 60 per cent of such cases are caused by adenoma, and 40 per cent by hyperplasia. Glucocorticoid remediable hypertension forms only a tiny proportion of the latter.

Presenting features

Clinical suspicion of the diagnosis of primary aldosteronism (whether caused by adenoma or hyperplasia) is most often raised by hypokalaemia with alkalosis. Hypokalaemia is common enough in hypertensive patients and in the majority the cause will be diuretic treatment or hyperaldosteronism secondary to hypersecretion of renin, the consequence of renal disease or severe essential hypertension; other causes to be considered are Cushing's syndrome or hypokalaemia secondary to liquorice addiction or treatment by carbenoxolone sodium as well as renin-secreting tumours and congenital adrenal hyperplasia (see below). Reliance on hypokalaemia or even hypokalaemia and suppression of plasma renin activity will result in a proportion of these cases being missed. Whilst in most patients with adenoma hypokalaemia is persistent, it may be intermittent or even absent. The frequency of normokalaemic aldosteronism is difficult to define, but reported figures range from 10 per cent of cases (Glasgow) to 25 per cent (Cleveland). Both of these are referral centres with a known interest in the syndrome. It is probable that in unselected populations normokalaemic primary aldosteronism is sufficiently rare to ignore for practical purposes. Specific symptoms of primary aldosteronism are uncommon and relate to severe hypokalaemia. Thirst and polyuria arise because of the effects of hypokalaemia on urinary concentration (see page 18.23). Associated symptoms include muscle weakness, which may amount to paralysis, cramps, paraesthesiae, and tetany. Most of the early reports emphasized the benign nature of the hypertension of primary aldosteronism, but in recent years it has become apparent that hypertensive vascular disease is often severe and the accelerated phase has been described.

Diagnosis

The diagnosis of primary aldosteronism whether due to adenoma, carcinoma, idiopathic aldosteronism or glucocorticoid remediable hyperaldosteronism is made by demonstration of an hypokalaemic alkalosis with increased aldosterone secretion, unsuppressed by a high salt intake, and suppression of plasma renin activity which fails to rise in response to the erect posture or sodium depletion. Plasma sodium concentrations tend to be at or slightly above the upper limit of the normal range in contrast to the hyponatraemia of secondary hyperaldosteronism.

A number of approaches to the important differentiation between adenoma and hyperplasia have been made. Patients with adenoma tend to have more severe biochemical changes, with higher aldosterone secretion and lower renin activity and potassium concentrations. Quadric analysis, multiple logistic analysis, and linear discriminant analysis have been used to distinguish, but these methods are difficult to apply outside specialist units. The most valuable methods to distinguish are by trial of dexamethasone treatment, by assessment of diurnal and postural changes in plasma aldosterone, and by bilateral adrenal vein catheterization.

Glucocorticoid remediable hyperaldosteronism

In a small minority of patients presenting with hypertension, hypokalaemia, hyperaldosteronism, and suppressed renin activity, treatment with glucocorticoid (usually dexamethasone 2 mg daily) reverses all of these abnormalities in some 2 to 3 weeks. A feature which may be useful in diagnosis is that there is often a remarkable fall in plasma aldosterone concentration between a sample taken when supine at 8.00 a.m. and one taken after 4 hours of being up and about at 12.00 noon. This fall of aldosterone on standing suggests an adrenal more under the control of ACTH than of angiotensin II. Indeed it has been suggested that the excess aldosterone production in this syndrome comes from zona fasciculata rather than zona glomerulosa cells, or that the number or responsiveness of ACTH receptors in the adrenal have been enhanced. The true explanation is unknown.

Diurnal and postural changes in diagnosis

There is evidence to suggest that aldosterone secreting adenomas (like the hyperplasia of glucocorticoid remediable hypertension) are more sensitive to control by ACTH than by angiotensin II while in idiopathic hyperaldosteronism the reverse is true. These concepts form the basis of the use of diurnal and postural changes in plasma aldosterone in diagnosis. Blood is taken at 8.00 a.m. before the patient has got up, and again at 12.00 noon after 4 hours of ordinary activity. A rise of plasma aldosterone in the erect sample suggests a postural response to angiotensin II and is seen in normal subjects, and in idiopathic hyperaldosteronism. No change or a fall are typical of an adrenal adenoma, but also of glucocorticoid responsive hyperaldosteronism and of an even rarer entity, 11-β-hydroxysteroid dehydrogenase deficiency (*vide infra*). This is a useful screening test but results can on occasion be difficult to interpret or misleading. Accuracy can be enhanced by volume expansion for three days before the test is performed, by prescribing a sodium intake of 250–300 mmol/day supplemented with fludrocortisone 0.5 mg daily.

Adenoma versus hyperplasia: other methods

Adrenal venography fails to detect the smallest tumours and may result in rupture of the vein or occasionally infarction of the adrenal. The best approach is undoubtedly adrenal vein catheterization with measurements of aldosterone concentrations in relation to cortisol in the adrenal veins on either side. In patients with hyperplasia similar concentrations are found on the two sides, but in adenoma cases the concentration is increased on the side of the lesion and suppressed on the other side.

Adrenal vein catheterization, which is technically difficult and sometimes impossible, is not always necessary. Large tumours are rare (most measure 10–40 mm across) in primary aldosteronism but when present can be detected by arteriography, ultrasound or computerized tomography. These techniques give no information about function in the adenomas which they may demonstrate. More useful is radionuclide imaging by labelled cholesterol scintiscans (Fig. 4a, b), undertaken during treatment by dexamethasone. This approach does provide information about secretory function on the two sides and will detect all but the smallest (less

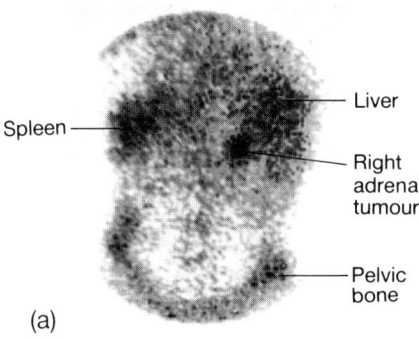

(a)

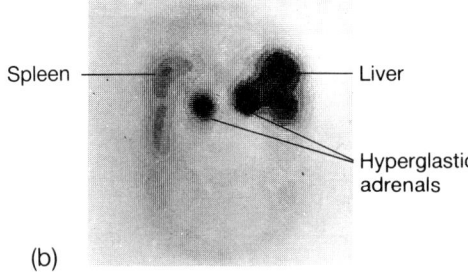

(b)

Fig. 4 (a) Adrenal scintiscan in a patient with a 2 cm diameter right-sided aldosteronoma. Gamma camera picture on the second day after intravenous scintadren. Dexamethasone 2 mg six hourly was begun 48 hours previously. (b) Scintiscan as in (a) but indicating bilateral adrenal hyperplasia. (Reproduced by permission of Dr B. Shepstone.)

than 5 mm) of adenomas. If both scintiscans and adrenal vein catheterization fail, a case can be made for a surgical examination on both sides and removal of any detected adenoma. Hyperplastic glands should not be removed.

Treatment

Glucocorticoid remediable hypertension

This is diagnosed by the response to 2–3 weeks treatment with dexamethasone 2 mg daily. A smaller dose may then suffice to control the disease without undue Cushingoid complications. When this is not possible, spironolactone or amiloride can be used in conjunction with dexamethasone or alone.

Idiopathic hyperaldosteronism

Treatment of this condition should be medical and not surgical. Spironolactone (200–400 mg/day) corrects the electrolyte abnormalities and usually improves control of arterial pressure. Amiloride (20–70 mg/day) is as effective and induces fewer side-effects in high dosage. Other antihypertensive drugs may be required to obtain acceptable control of arterial pressure.

Aldosterone secreting adenoma

Surgical removal of adenomas results in cure of hypertension in 50–60 per cent of cases and correction of hypokalaemia in every case. Transient mineralocorticoid deficiency may develop postoperatively and is best treated by parenteral DOCA or oral 9-α-fluorohydrocortisone. Preoperative treatment for 4 to 6 weeks by amiloride or spironolactone (see above) corrects electrolyte disturbances and lowers arterial pressure. It may also predict the long-term response to surgery; good control within four weeks of such medical treatment indicates good postoperative blood pressure control, and vice versa.

References

Beevers, D. G., Brown, J. J., Ferris, J. B., Fraser, R., Lever, A. F., Robertson, J. I. S. and Tree, M. (1976). Renal abnormalities and vascular complications in primary aldosteronism. Evidence on tertiary aldosteronism. *Q. J. Med.* **45**, 401–410.

Biglieri, E. G. (1984). The pituitary and idiopathic hyperaldosteronism. *N. Engl. J. Med.* **311**, 120–121.

Davies, D. L., Beevers, D. G., Brown, J. J., Cumming, A. M., Fraser, R., Lever, A. F., Mason, P. A., Morton, J. J., Robertson, J. I. S., Titterington, M. and Tree, M. (1979). Aldosterone and its stimuli in normal and hypertensive man: are essential hypertension and primary aldosteronism without tumour the same condition? *J. Endocrinol.* **81**, 79p–91p.

Ferris, J. B., Brown, J. J., Fraser, R., Lever, A. F. and Robertson, J. I. S. (1983). Primary aldosterone excess. Conn's syndrome and similar disorders. In *Handbook of hypertension*, Vol. 2, *Clinical aspects of secondary hypertension* (ed. J. I. S. Robertson), pp. 132–161. Elsevier, Amsterdam.

Ganguly, A. (1982). New insights and questions about glucocorticoid-suppressible hyperaldosteronism. *Am. J. Med.* **72**, 851–854.

Hogan, M. J., McRae, J., Schamberlan, M. and Biglieri, E. G. (1976). Location of aldosterone-producing adenomas with ^{131}I-19-iodocholesterol. *N. Engl. J. Med.* **294**, 410–414.

McAreavy, D., Brown, J. J., Cumming, A. M. M. *et al.* (1981). Pre-operative localisation of aldosterone-secreting adenomas. *Clin. Endocrinol.* **15**, 593–606.

Streeten, D. M. P., Tomycz, N. and Anderson, G. H. (1979). Reliability of screening methods for the diagnosis of primary aldosteronism. *Am. J. Med.* **67**, 403–413.

Swales, J. D. (1983). Primary hyperaldosteronism: How hard should we look? *Br. Med. J.* **287**, 702–703.

Vaughan, N. J. A., Jowett, T. P., Slater, J. D. H., Wiggins, R. C., Lightman, S. L., Ma, J. T. C. and Payne, N. N. (1981). The diagnosis of primary aldosteronism. *Lancet* **i**, 120–125.

Inborn errors of corticosteroid synthesis and metabolism

11-β-hydroxysteroid dehydrogenase deficiency

Hypertension and hypokalaemia, but with suppression of both aldosterone and renin, suggest the presence of a non-aldosterone mineralocorticoid. In a number of children this pattern has been described with the additional feature that the hypertension, far from being improved by hydrocortisone treatment, is aggravated. An impaired catabolism of hydrocortisone can be shown, with prolonged plasma half-life. Spironolactone and amiloride correct hypokalaemia and reduce arterial pressure in these rare patients.

Congenital adrenal hyperplasia

The various conditions comprising congenital adrenal hyperplasia are discussed on pages 10.69–10.83. Among these, deficiency of 11-β-hydroxylase and 17-α-hydroxylase cause hypertension with hypokalaemia. In both conditions renin activity in plasma is suppressed by an overproduction of deoxycorticosterone as a result of the biochemical defects in normal steroid synthesis. Aldosterone secretion is reduced or normal.

11-β-hydroxylase deficiency presents in infancy or early childhood with virilization in both sexes. Deficiency of 11-β-hydroxylase prevents normal production of cortisol and of aldosterone. Adrenal androgen synthetic pathways are intact. Reduced cortisol production results in high plasma concentrations of ACTH which stimulates overproduction of androgens, and increased secretion of DOC and 11-deoxycortisol (compound S).

17-α-hydroxylase deficiency leads to abnormalities in both adrenal and gonadal steroid synthesis in both sexes. Impaired cortisol production stimulates increased ACTH secretion, but biochemical pathways for aldosterone production are intact. High levels of both DOC and aldosterone are to be expected, but although plasma levels of DOC, corticosterone, and 18-hydroxycorticosterone are high, aldosterone production is low. This unexpected finding may result from suppression of renin and angiotensin because of volume expansion, but an associated enzymatic defect inhibiting conversion of 18-hydroxycorticosterone to aldosterone has also been suggested. An eunuchoid body build and deficiency of secondary sexual characteristics with pseudohermaphroditism in the male and primary amenorrhoea in the female reflect gonadal

dysfunction. Diagnosis in this condition may be delayed until adult age. Diagnostic biochemical features include increased production rates of DOC, corticosterone, 18-hydroxyprogesterone and deficiency of pregnantriol, 17-hydroxyprogesterone, cortisol, and 11-deoxycortisol. Low levels of testosterone or oestrogens are associated with an increase in plasma FSH and LH.

References

Bricaire, H., Luton, J. P., Laudat, P., Legrand, J. C., Turpin, G., Corvol, P. and Lemmer, M. (1972) A new male pseudohermaphroditism associated with hypertension due to a block in 17-α-hydroxylation. *J. Clin. Endocrinol. Metab.* **35**, 67–72.

Eberlein, W. R. and Bongiovanni, A. M. (1956). Plasma and urinary corticoids in hypertensive form of congenital adrenal hyperplasia. *J. Biol. Chem.* **223**, 85–94.

Gabrilove, J. L., Sharma, D. C. and Dorfman, R. I. (1965). Adrenocortical 11β-hydroxylase deficiency and virilism first manifest in an adult. *N. Engl. J. Med.* **272**, 1189–1194.

New. M. I. and Seaman, M. P. (1970). Secretion rates of cortisol and aldosterone precursors in various forms of congenital adrenal hyperplasia. *J. Clin. Endocrinol. Metab.* **30**, 361–371.

Oberfeld, S. E., Levine, L. S., Carey, R. M., Greig, F., Ulick, S. and New, M. I. (1983). Metabolic and blood pressure responses to hydrocortisone in the syndrome of apparent mineralocorticoid excess. *J. Clin. Endocrinol. Metab.* **56**, 332–339.

Liquorice and carbenoxolone sodium

Large quantities of liquorice eaten regularly may cause hypertension, hypokalaemia, and alkalosis. Plasma renin activity and plasma aldosterone are both suppressed by the mineralocorticoid effects of glycyrrhetinic acid contained in liquorice. The same features are present in patients on chronic treatment with carbenoxolone sodium given for peptic ulcer. Glycyrrhetinic acid is again responsible for mineralocorticoid effects. Hypertension and hypokalaemic alkalosis are both reversed on stopping the offending agents, but may take several days or even weeks to do so.

Deoxycorticosterone and corticosterone excess

There have been examples of hypertension and hypokalaemia, reversed by spironolactone and apparently caused by isolated overproduction of DOC. Carcinoma of the adrenal with hypertension, hypokalaemia, and oedema can also be associated with overproduction of corticosterone.

References

Brown, J. J., Fraser, R., Love, D. R., Ferris, J. B., Lever, A. F., Robertson, J. I. S. and Wilson, A. (1972). Apparently isolated excess deoxycorticosterone in hypertension. *Lancet* **ii**, 243–247.

Conn, J. W., Rovner, D. R. and Cohen, E. L. (1968). Liquorice-induced pseudoaldosteronism. *J. Am. Med. Ass.* **205**, 492–496.

Cumming, A. M. M., Boddy, K., Brown, J. J. *et al.* (1980). Severe hypokalaemia with paralysis induced by small doses of liquorice. *Postgrad. Med. J.* **56**, 526–529.

Phaeochromocytoma

A tumour secreting catecholamines is the cause of hypertension in perhaps 0.5–1.0 per cent of patients with high blood pressure. Phaeochromocytomas arise in chromaffin cells of neuro-ectodermal origin. They may, therefore, be found anywhere in the sympatho-adrenal system from the neck down to the bifurcation of the aorta or lower in the pelvis and on occasion in the urinary bladder. Tumours of extra-adrenal origin are sometimes referred to as paraganglionomas.

The occurrence of phaeochromocytomas in families is well recognized. These familial tumours nearly always arise from the adrenal medulla, and both adrenals are involved in 70 per cent of cases. Other abnormalities are associated in some families, and may arise less commonly in sporadic cases as well.

Associated disorders in familial cases

Sipple's syndrome consists of adrenal phaeochromocytoma (bilateral in 70 per cent) and medullary carcinoma of the thyroid; many patients harbour a parathyroid adenoma or hyperplasia as well. This familial disorder, also designated multiple endocrine neoplasia (MEN) type II or type IIa is inherited in an autosomal Mendelian dominant pattern, but sporadic cases have also been described. The thyroid tumours arise from the 'C' cells which synthesize calcitonin. They may also produce prostaglandins, serotonin, and ACTH. Plasma concentrations of calcitonin are not always raised, but may increase pathologically in response to an infusion of pentagastrin, calcium or glucagon. Diarrhoea may occur, perhaps related to overproduction of prostaglandins or serotonin. ACTH from the thyroid or the phaeochromocytoma itself may on occasion cause Cushing's syndrome.

Familial phaeochromocytomas with medullary thyroid carcinoma are also associated with neuromata in the mucosa of the lips, tongue, conjunctivi, and eyelids, and sometimes in the mucosal, submucosal, muscular or serosal layers of the walls of the gut. This latter condition of intestinal ganglioneuromatosis may cause diarrhoea or constipation and dilation of the colon which may be misdiagnosed as congenital megacolon. The body habitus of some of these patients resembles Marfan's syndrome with long extremities, poor muscular development, dorsal kyphosis, pectus excavatum, and pes cavus; neither lens dislocation nor aortic disease have been described.

This constellation of abnormalities has been variously designated multiple endocrine neoplasia (MEN) type IIb or type III (Fig. 5). MEN type I affects the anterior pituitary parathyroid, and adrenal glands as well as pancreatic islets with adenomatous, carcinomatous or hyperplastic change. Carcinoid tumours may be associated, but not phaeochromocytoma. Among patients presenting with medullary carcinoma of the thyroid, some 3 per cent can be shown to have an associated phaeochromocytoma.

Neurofibromatosis (von Recklinghausen's disease) occurs in 5 per cent of patients with phaeochromocytoma and may be associated with familial or sporadic cases. Looked at the other way around, phaeochromocytomas are found in only some 1 per cent of patients presenting with neurofibromatosis. A recent report has associated phaeochromocytoma, neurofibromatosis, and duodenal carcinoid.

The von Hippel–Lindau syndrome of angiomatous change in the retinal vessels and cerebellar haemangioblastoma has been linked with phaeochromocytoma but the association is remarkably rare. Tuberose sclerosis (see page 24.10) and neurofibromatosis may co-exist, but not with phaeochromocytoma, at least to date. Astrocytomas and cystic tumours of the cerebellum may be associated with phaeochromocytomas but may also produce fluctuating hypertension and suggestive symptoms in the absence of a tumour secreting catecholamines.

Pathology

Ninety per cent of phaeochromocytomas arise in the adrenal medulla and 99 per cent are found within the abdomen or pelvis. The commonest extra-adrenal site apears to be the organ of Zuckerkandl, adjacent to the bifurcation of the aorta. Phaeochromocytomas in the chest are mostly found in the paravertebral region; the very rare chromaffin tumours arising in cervical ganglia, including glomus jugulare tumours, are mostly chemically inert but have been known to secrete catecholamines, and in others there may be an associated phaeochromocytoma in the mediastinum.

Adrenal phaeochromocytomas vary in size from a few millimetres across to very large vascular and often cystic masses weighing as much as 3 kg. They are bilateral in some 10 per cent of cases and more commonly when the condition is familial. The diagnosis of malignancy is not possible by histological examination; it depends rather on clinical or macroscopic pathological demonstration of invasion and metastasis, usually to liver, lung or bone. Some 10 per cent of adrenal phaeochromocytomas are malignant, and malignancy is more likely in familial cases. The suggestion that the oversecretion of adrenaline as well as noradrenaline is an indication of an adrenal rather than an extra-adrenal lesion is not always true; extra-adrenal phaeochromocytomas can synthesize adrenaline on occasion. Tumours contain variable amounts (from 0.08 to 50 mg/g) of catecholamines depending on storage and turnover. Noradrenaline usually predominates, but a tumour containing 99 per cent adrenaline has been described, and in others dopamine has been present in large amounts. There are no biochemical features which reliably distinguish benign from malignant tumours, although a very high secretion of dopamine is suggestive of malignancy.

Clinical features

In autopsy series, up to one-third of phaeochromocytomas have been shown to be undiagnosed in life. In these, the tumours have usually been the cause of sudden death caused by massive outpouring of catecholamines in association with such events as anaesthesia, surgery, parturition or trauma.

There have been a number of case reports of phaeochromocytomas presenting to the surgeon with abdominal pain, circulatory failure, and shock due to infarction of the tumours. This diagnosis is easily missed and in reported cases death has occurred in the course of anaesthesia or surgery for an apparently surgical cause of an 'acute abdomen'. Similarly, hypertension in pregnancy is easily attributed to pre-eclampsia; on occasion the cause is a phaeochromocytoma which, if not accurately diagnosed, is likely to prove fatal during labour or at Caesarian section.

Tumours causing hypertension occur at any age from infancy to old age, but are most commonly diagnosed between the ages of 20 and 50 years. Hypertension is sustained in some 50 per cent of adults with the disease, but in most of the remainder blood pressure is normal between paroxysmal attacks. Whether hypertension is sustained or not, episodic acute rises in pressure are common. The usual pattern is of an increase in both systolic and diastolic pressures in attacks, but in patients in whom the major product of the tumour is adrenaline there may be a rise in systolic pressure and pulse rate with a normal or frankly low diastolic pressure (in one case a figure of 230/40 was recorded). It is in this rare group of patients that hypotension may develop, often closely following a hypertensive episode. Rare cases have also been described of consistently normal arterial pressure despite the presence of a functioning tumour.

A number of classical symptoms are commonly described in paroxysms of hypertension caused by secretion of catecholamines by the tumours. These are listed in rough order of frequency in

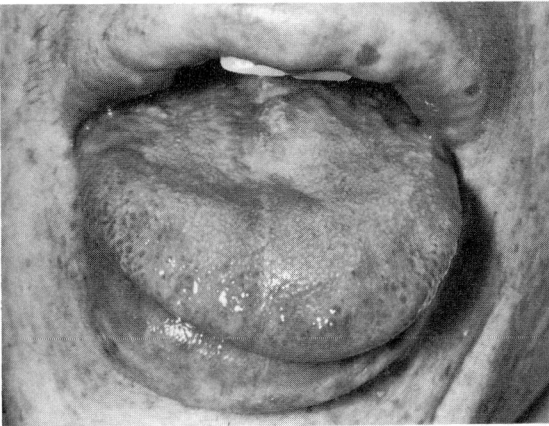

Fig. 5 Multiple endocrine neoplasia type 2B (sometimes called type 3) and phaeochromocytoma. Note skin pigmentation and multiple mucosal neuromata.

Table 8 Common symptoms of phaeochromocytoma

Symptom	Percentage affected	
	Paroxysmal	Persistent
Headache	92	72
Sweating	65	69
Palpitation	73	51
Anxiety, fear	60	28
Tremor	51	26
Pain in chest, abdomen	48	28
Nausea ± vomiting	43	26
Prostration	38	15
Severe weight loss	14	15

Adapted from Manger and Gifford (1977).

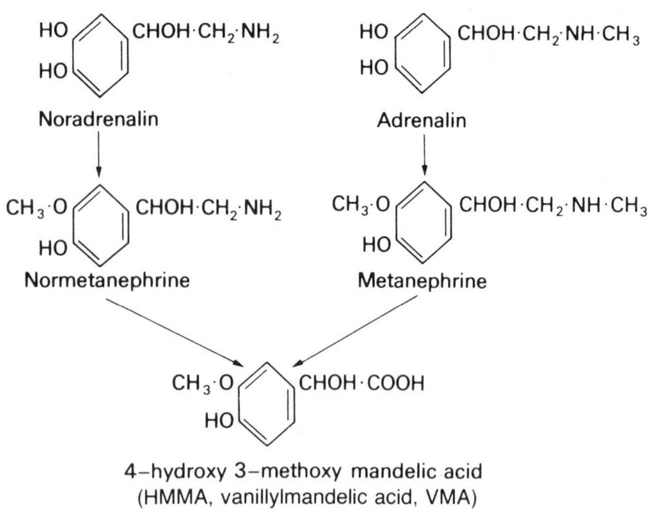

Fig. 6 The degradation of adrenaline and noradrenaline to 4-hydroxy, 3-methoxymandelic acid.

Table 8. Severe, usually pounding headache, sudden in onset, is the commonest of these and sweating, palpitation, apprehension, and tremor are often prominent. A variety of precipitating factors have been described. Most have in common an alteration in physical pressure on the tumour; bending, straining at stool, lying in a particular position, or the wearing of a tight girdle may provoke attacks when the tumour is abdominal. Swallowing has been recorded to induce attacks in a tumour lying adjacent to the oesophagus and they may be associated with micturition in cases of phaeochromocytoma of the bladder. Other relatively frequent triggers are exercise, anxiety, and laughter. In many patients paroxysmal attacks are associated with an ashen pallor, chiefly of the face and upper body; sometimes the skin is mottled and a cyanotic purple flush may succeed pallor. Attacks may occur several times in a day or more rarely, but in most cases symptoms arise at least once a week. They are usually relatively short-lived lasting in most cases between 15 min and 1 hour. After an attack, patients describe a sense of overwhelming exhaustion and weakness with a tendency for muscles to ache.

Physical signs suggesting the diagnosis are rare. Tumours may be large enough to be felt in the abdomen. *Cafe au lait* patches or neurofibromata in an hypertensive patient should suggest the diagnosis. Postural hypotension may be found in as many as 70 per cent of untreated patients with a phaeochromocytoma. This phenomenon, once attributed to volume depletion induced by a long-standing vasoconstriction and venoconstriction is now thought to arise because of a blunting of the orthostatic autonomic reflexes by chronic oversecretion of catecholamines. A paradoxical rise in blood pressure after treatment by β-adrenergic blocking drugs or postganglionic sympatholytic agents may occur in patients with phaeochromocytoma.

A careful examination of the thyroid for signs of medullary carcinoma is important, particularly in patients in whom there is a family history of phaeochromocytoma. The urine should be examined for glucose which can be demonstrated at the time of an attack in some 30 per cent of patients.

Differential diagnosis
A number of conditions may give rise to symptoms suggestive of phaeochromocytoma. Chief amongst these are anxiety states, hyperventilation, thyrotoxicosis, recurrent hypoglycaemia, and in some patients, recurrent episodes of angina. Severe pain from ischaemic heart disease may be accompanied by an increase in plasma and urinary catecholamines and with appropriate symptoms. Cerebral tumours have been reported as rare associations with phaeochromocytoma but may also mimic that condition particularly when they arise in the posterior fossa when systemic hypertension and headache may coincide with a mild rise in plasma and urinary catecholamines.

Another cause of phaeochromocytoma-like symptoms and signs is alcohol withdrawal after heavy drinking.

Investigation
A firm diagnosis of phaeochromocytoma depends on the demonstration of overproduction of catecholamines reflected by biochemical assays in urine or blood or both. Since no measurement, done on one occasion only, completely excludes the diagnosis, the length to which investigation should be taken depends on the index of suspicion that a phaeochromocytoma may be present. In the context of hypertension, signs of the malignant phase, resistance to treatment, a paradoxical blood pressure response to β-adrenergic blockade, and a postural fall in arterial pressure without other explanation can be taken as firm indications as well as more classical symptoms suggestive of paroxysmal secretion of catecholamines.

Urine
For many years, assays of noradrenaline and adrenaline, or of their metabolites normetadrenaline, metadrenaline, and vanillylmandelic acid (VMA) in 24-hour urine samples have been the mainstay of diagnosis (Fig. 6).

These are relatively simple assays, but which is the best to perform in a given case varies depending on the relative activities of catechol-*o*-methyltransferase (in synthesis) and monoamine oxidase (in catabolism) in the tumour as well as on storage and urinary excretion rates. Table 9 shows representative figures for normal ranges, but these will differ between laboratories using different assay methods.

Analysis of the contributions to total excretion by noradrenaline or adrenaline and their meta-derivatives is not of significant value in determining the site of tumour, despite suggestions that the

Table 9 Approximate* normal ranges in urine and plasma of catecholamines and their metabolites

Measurements	Normal range
24-hour urine excretion of:	
VMA	< 35 µmol (7 mg)
Metadrenaline	< 2 µmol (0.4 mg)
Normetadrenaline	< 4.5 µmol (0.9 mg)
Total metanephrins	< 5.0 µmol (1 mg)
Noradrenaline	< 0.5 µmol (100 µg)
Adrenaline	< 0.1 µmol (20 µg)
Plasma concentrations	
Adrenaline	< 1.5 nmol/l
Noradrenaline	< 10 nmol/l

* True normal ranges vary between laboratories and methods.

presence of adrenaline in excess may indicate an adrenal rather than extra-adrenal phaeochromocytoma. Large amounts of dopa and dopamine have been taken to suggest malignancy but examples have been described in which this pattern of excretion was associated with benign tumours.

In patients in whom the clinical evidence points strongly to phaeochromocytoma, repeated assays may be necessary. These should include both VMA and the metadrenalines, the latter probably the more reliable index. In one series VMA excretion in patients with proven tumours was normal on a single occasion in 25 per cent of cases and in another the 24-hour urine VMA was falsely negative in 25 of 43 patients. Assay of the metadrenalines misses fewer cases and when in doubt it is best to assay VMA, the meta products, and urinary free catecholamines. Catechols and their metabolites are unstable products; urine must be kept cool and below pH 3.5 in the 24-hour collections. Care must be taken to ensure complete collection. The excretory products of a number of substances may affect urinary assay. These include methyldopa, monoamine oxidase inhibitors, phenothiazines, and an excessive intake of bananas, coffee, tea, and chocolate. Plasma and urinary levels may be much increased on withdrawal of clonidine.

In patients with paroxysmal hypersecretion of catechols, diagnosis may be difficult to confirm biochemically and may require repeated testing, particularly of urine collected immediately after symptomatic attacks.

Plasma

Techniques of radioenzymatic or high-performance liquid chromatography (HPLC) assay of noradrenaline and adrenaline in plasma are now established and are becoming more generally available. Opinion is divided about the relative merits of plasma and urinary assays of catechols in the diagnosis of phaeochromocytoma. Some suggest that plasma noradrenaline assays in particular are to be preferred in a difficult case. Others disagree and point out the potentially greater value of urinary assays when hypersecretion is intermittent. Further experience is required in a larger number of patients. In the meantime, suspicious cases in which one assay technique does not confirm should be reinvestigated by all available methods.

The greatest care should be taken to be sure that blood samples for catechol assays are taken from patients at rest and through an indwelling needle or catheter which has been inserted some 30–60 min before sampling to avoid the effects of discomfort and stress.

Suppression tests

Pentolinium test

This is based on the hypothesis that a ganglion-blocking drug will inhibit release of catecholamines from adrenergic nerves and normal adrenal medulla, while leaving unchanged autonomous secretion by a tumour which lacks a preganglionic nerve supply. Plasma noradrenaline and adrenaline are measured before and 10 and 20 min after 2.5 mg of pentolinium given intravenously. A fall in both catecholamines is expected in normal subjects but a failure of adrenaline concentrations (in particular) to fall suggests a phaeochromocytoma. The originators of this test report only three false-positives and no false-negatives in a series of 50 patients, but others have not found it so helpful and pentolinium is not available everywhere.

Clonidine

This centrally acting α-adrenergic agonist might be expected to reduce plasma levels of noradrenaline secreted from nerve endings but not from phaeochromocytomas. In this test plasma is taken before and at 1, 2 and 3 hours after 300 μg of clonidine given by mouth. Failure of plasma noradrenaline plus adrenaline (measured by catechol-o-methyltransferase) to fall below 2.95 nmol/l (500 pg/ml) suggests the presence of a tumour.

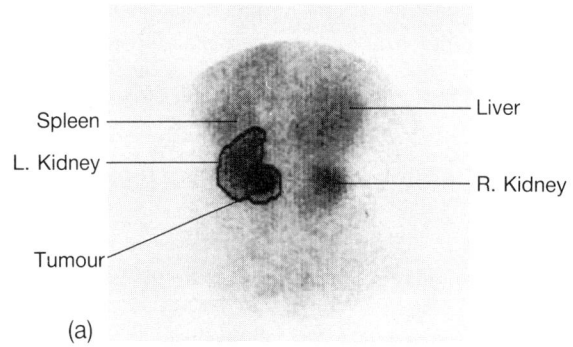

(a)

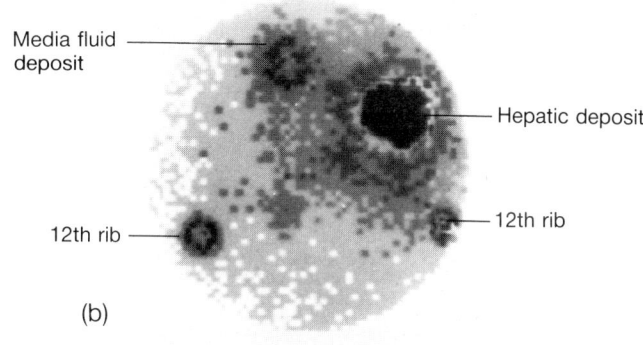

(b)

Fig. 7 (a) MIBG scan and superimposed ^{99}Tm DMSA renal scintiscan to show phaeochromocytoma near the lower pole of the left kidney. (b) MIBG scan showing secondary deposits of phaeochromocytoma in the right lobe of the liver and mediastinum.

Localization

Where computerized tomography (CT scanning) is available, this has become the method of choice for locating phaeochromocytomas, and is reported to detect tumours as small as 1 cm in diameter. Another sophisticated method is scintigraphy using ^{131}I meta-iodobenzylguanidine (MIBG) which is selectively taken up by adrenergic cells (Fig. 7a). Scintigraphy may detect tumours missed by CT scanning, is capable of indicating an adrenergic origin in unidentified tumours, and may be particularly useful in locating metastatic spread in malignant cases (Fig. 7b).

These techniques are not available in all parts of the world. Ultrasound may be useful. Longer established procedures include intravenous urography and angiography. Both these can provoke catechol secretion by the tumour resulting in dangerous and on occasion fatal hypertensive crises. It is essential, therefore, to begin treatment with α- and β-blockade for several days before any radiological investigation involving the injection of contrast material or selective venous sampling. Phenoxybenzamine should be given in a dose sufficient to eliminate hypertensive surges and to lower arterial pressure to normal or near normal levels. Dose requirements range from 10 to 30 mg three times daily and on rare occasions a dose is as high as 60 mg three times daily. Beta-adrenergic blockade, given to prevent cardiac arrhythmias, should be withheld until α-blockade has been established; β-blockers given alone are likely to raise arterial pressure in the presence of a phaeochromocytoma. Dose requirements are usually small, not more than 40 mg three times daily of propranolol. Labetalol has been advocated and used successfully, but has more β- than α-blocking properties which should render it less suitable than individually adjusted doses of phenoxybenzamine and propranolol.

Venous sampling

Catheterization of the inferior vena cava or superior vena cava with sequential sampling for noradrenaline and adrenaline concentrations may be used to localize tumours not found by simpler techniques, particularly when multiple tumours are suspected. Plasma concentrations vary very rapidly and may increase markedly in response to distress and pain, so that results must be interpreted with caution. Concentrations in samples from adrenal veins depend on adrenal blood flow which may be low in normal subjects and very high from vascular tumours. A useful approach to this problem is to apply a correction factor based on measurement of cortisol concentration.

Treatment

Surgery is the treatment of choice and is curative in some 75 per cent of cases. In those in whom arterial pressure does not fall substantially, persistence of hypertensive vascular changes or co-existence of essential hypertension may be responsible, but it is essential to check by urine and blood assays that tumour removal has been complete.

The surgical removal of a phaeochromocytoma is a hazardous procedure which should be undertaken only by a team of surgeons and anaesthetist experienced in the management of cardiovascular crises which are likely to occur during and immediately after surgery. The patient should come to operation fully α- and β-blocked. Arterial pressure and heart rate and rhythm should be monitored throughout induction of anaesthesia and surgery. Solutions of phentolamine, isoprenaline, noradrenaline, and practolol should be prepared and ready to use. Whole blood and plasma volume-expanding solutions such as purified protein fraction should also be to hand. Operative mortality in the best hands is about 3 per cent.

Malignant and inoperative cases

When surgical removal is not feasible or has been incomplete, medical management can be remarkably successful. Alpha-methyl-*p*-tyrosine (Alpha-MT) inhibits the hydroxylation of tyrosine to dopa and therefore reduces synthesis of both noradrenaline and adrenaline. This drug controls arterial pressure and symptoms, but at the expense of undesirable gastrointestinal and neurological side-effects and impairment of renal function in some cases. Phenoxybenzamine is to be preferred and is effective in total daily doses of 40–80 mg. Most patients with diagnosed treated malignant phaeochromocytoma survive several years; tumours are slow-growing and death is usually caused by cardiovascular complications.

References

Allison, D. J., Brown, M. J., Jones, D. H. and Timmis, J. B. (1983). Role of venous sampling in locating a phaeochromocytoma. *Br. Med. J.* **286**, 1122–1124.

Bravo, E. L. and Gifford, R. W. (1984). Pheochromocytoma: diagnosis, location and management. *N. Engl. J. Med* **311**, 1298–1303.

Goldfien, A. (1981). Phaeochromocytoma. *Clin. Endocrinol. Metab.* **10**, 607–630.

Jones, D. H., Reid, J. L., Hamilton, C. A., Allison, D. J., Wellbourn, R. B. and Dollery, C. T. (1980). The biochemical diagnosis, localisation, and follow-up of phaeochromocytoma: the role of plasma and urinary catecholamines. *Q. J. Med.* **49**, 341–361.

Kieser, H. R., Beaven, M. A., Doppman, J., Wells, S. and Buja, L. M. (1973). Sipple's syndrome: medullary thyroid carcinoma, pheochromocytoma and parathyroid disease. *Ann. intern. Med.* **78**, 561–579.

Lancet (1984). Iodobenzylguanidine for location and treatment of phaeochromocytoma. *Lancet* **ii**, 905–907.

Manger, W. M. and Gifford, R. W. (1977). *Phaeochromocytoma*. Springer-Verlag, New York.

—— and —— (1982). Hypertension secondary to pheochromocytoma. *Bull. NY Acad. Med.* **58**, 139–158.

Swenson, S. J., Brown, M. L., Sheps, S. G., Sizemore, G. W. and Van Heerden, J. A. (1985). Use of ^{131}I-MIBG scintigraphy in line evaluation of suspected phaeochromocytoma. *Mayo Clin. Proc.* **60**, 299–304.

Winkler, H. and Smith, A. D. (1972). Phaeochromocytoma and other catecholamine-producing tumours. In *Handbook of experimental pharmacology. New Series* Vol. 23 (eds H. Blaschko and E. Muscholl), p. 900, Springer-Verlag, Berlin.

Lymphoedema

J. G. G. LEDINGHAM

Introduction

On occasion, local oedema can be caused predominantly by inadequacy of lymphatic drainage of extracellular fluid. Such inadequacy may be related to hypoplasia of lymphatic vessels or to structural change related to trauma, surgery, inflammation, fibrosis or neoplasm.

Anatomical considerations

Lymphatic vessels permeate the extracellular spaces of the body. The smallest of them, lymphatic capillaries, are thin-walled, blind-ended structures found especially around collecting venules. They are lined by a thin layer of endothelial cells, with a discontinuous basement membrane. Anchoring filaments, attached laterally, probably mediate the size of intercellular clefts. Vesicles within endothelial cells probably undertake pinocytosis, for instance, of proteins which are taken up by the lymphatic system. Numbers of lymphatic capillaries join to form the collecting lymphatics of larger dimension, lined also by a single layer of endothelium, but with a continuous basement membrane, a layer of smooth muscle cells, and valves retarding retrograde flow. Collecting lymphatics themselves merge to form larger vessels which tend to aggregate along veins. The largest lymphatic trunks ultimately join the thoracic duct which itself empties into the junction of the internal jugular and subclavian veins in the thorax.

Normal physiology

Interstitial fluid is derived from net filtration across capillary membranes dependent on the forces described by Starling in 1896. These are the intracapillary hydrostatic pressure opposing that of the interstitial fluid and the plasma and tissue fluid colloid oncotic pressures. The formation of interstitial fluid is determined by these forces and by the coefficient of ultrafiltration of the relevant capillary wall. Capillary filtration pressure on the arteriolar side is regulated by the precapillary arteriolar sphincter as well as by gravitational forces, whereas on the venous side there is no such sphincter to 'protect' from high venous pressures. On passive standing therefore, arterial and venous pressures in the legs increase in parallel, so that the arteriovenous gradient is not altered; but absolute hydrostatic pressure increases according to the vertical distance of the capillary in question below the heart. The capillary pressure in the feet on quiet standing has been measured and reaches some 125 cm H_2O. The normal plasma oncotic pressure is some 33 cm H_2O. Not surprisingly, therefore, the volume of the feet increases rapidly over some 2–3 min on quiet standing, and after 10–15 min swelling continues steadily at a rate of some 20–30 ml/hour. The mechanisms preventing more rapid capillary transudation and therefore oedema in such a situation are three-fold. Much the most important is precapillary vasoconstriction, which attenuates the rise in capillary hydrostatic pressure and may, by reducing the area of functional perfused capillaries, reduce the coefficient of ultrafiltration. Extreme ultrafiltration of the much reduced blood flow results in only modest changes in hydrostatic and oncotic pressure in the extracellular fluid but a marked increase in intracapillary oncotic pressure. Venous blood draining a foot passively dependent for some 30–40 min may contain protein to a concentration of over 9 gm/l with a haematocrit as high as 52 per cent at a time when the haematocrit of the forearm venous blood is at 42 per cent. This rise in oncotic pressure, mediated in part by reduced flow, is critical to the limitation of the rate of formation of tissue fluid.

Increased rates of formation of tissue fluid are known to occur in dependent limbs when heating or other vasodilatory influences relax precapillary arteriolar tone, when there is fluid overload, and when venous pressure is increased by obstruction. Rates are decreased by vasoconstriction, particularly when there is a deficit of blood volume.

Colloid osmotic pressure depends not only on protein concentration but also on charge and ionic strength. On quiet standing colloid osmotic pressure may rise from around 33 to 60 cm H_2O in 30–40 min. Such an increase allows local plasma oncotic pressure to balance the increased hydrostatic pressure with resultant filtration equilibrium.

A change in interstitial tissue fluid pressure postulated at one time to be an important factor in limiting tissue fluid formation is no longer considered so. Some tissue fluid is reabsorbed at the venous end of the capillaries but the remainder by the lymphatic system.

Lymphatic flow

Lymphatic valves resemble functionally those of the venous system. Local fluid accumulation results in considerable dilation of the lymphatic vessels, at least in part mediated by the physical action of the attached fibrils such that distension of the extracellular fluid space pulls on the walls to increase the lumen. Although tissue fluid formation is increased in dependent limbs there is no corresponding increase in lymphatic flow in the absence of muscular activity. Passive or active exercise does however augment lymphatic flow very considerably. The passage of lymph within the thorax into the subclavian veins is considerably influenced by intrathoracic pressure with a marked increase observed to accompany hyperventilation.

Protein in lymph

Capillaries leak protein, most of which is returned to the circulation by way of lymphatic uptake and transport while little or none is reabsorbed by way of the vascular capillaries.

Lymphatic oedema

Congenital lymphatic hypoplasia may induce local oedema from earliest infancy. Familial oedema, coming on at any age or in either sex but mostly at puberty and in girls, is also due to lymphatic hypoplasia as can be demonstrated by lymphangiography.

Structural damage to the lymphatic systems sufficient to cause local oedema, may be the consequence of neoplastic infiltration, of scarring from trauma or irradiation, or of chronic lymphangitis from such infective agents as *Wucheria bancrofti*, lymphogranuloma venereum or recurrent streptococcal infection.

The swelling of lymphatic oedema is initially painless, pits readily, and subsides at night. With time, however, fibrosis develops in the interstitial tissues of the affected limb such that the oedema resolves much less easily with posture and becomes 'brawny' (firm and non-pitting). The skin itself may become considerably thickened and pigmented. Indolent ulcers tend to develop at sites of pressure. The skin of a chronically oedematous area is abnormally susceptible to bacterial infection.

Lymphatic oedema fluid contains a higher concentration of protein than is the case with oedema of cardiac, renal or hepatic origin.

Treatment

Treatment is very unsatisfactory. The affected part should be elevated above the heart whenever possible and at other times supported externally by firm elastic bandaging or appropriate elastic hosiery, applied after a period of postural drainage. Devices designed to massage the affected part through the night or at other times of rest can be helpful. Prevention of skin sepsis or prompt treatment of it are important in their own right and to prevent further lymphatic insufficiency.

References

Kinmonth, J. B. and Taylor, G. W. (1954). The lymphatic circulation in lymphoedema. *Ann. Surg.* **139**, 125–136.

Michel, C. C. (1979). Fluid movement through capillary walls. In *Handbook of physiology; the cardiovascular system* Vol. IV, 2nd edn, pp. 375–409. American Physiological Society, Washington.

Mortimer, P. and Regrand, C. (1986). Lymphostatic disorders. *Br. Med. J.* **293**, 347–348.

GEOGRAPHIC VARIATION IN HEART DISEASE

Africa

E.H.O. PARRY

The rich diversity of geography and climate, of people and culture, and of health and disease, thrust themselves upon any student of medicine in Africa. Inevitably those who read about Africa think primarily of its tropical subSaharan belt: the countries of the Mediterranean littoral and of the more temperate Maghreb are considered less, on account of a differing climate and people; but in terms of the delivery of health care these countries share the problems of all African countries.

The draw of the cities and the neglect of agriculture in many countries has led to a diminished food supply per head of population. Urban migrants often live wretchedly in shanty town squalor, so that both they and their children are far worse off than they were in their rural villages. Water supply, disposal of all wastes, heavy pressure on urban clinics, and appalling overcrowding, all promote the spread of microbial disease. In addition, there is growing evidence that the rush to the cities is bringing an increase in cardiovascular disease, notably in the rise of blood pressure in urban migrants and in the urbanized African. Sadly the hope of Health for All by the Year 2000, including its cardiovascular component, seems now to be little more than a mirage. Although it is dwarfed by the pressing problems of nutrition and gastrointestinal

infections in infants, cardiovascular disease is still important and will become more important in its demands on health care services. This is not a happy picture.

Clinical methods and investigations

While so little is known about the epidemiology of cardiovascular disease, every patient is a potential source of new and valuable information. The problem can be expressed thus – why should this patient from this place fall ill with this cardiac disease at this time? Social, geographical, and seasonal factors can all be important in the genesis of cardiac failure in the African patient. Such basic data are the first priority in investigation and should ideally be complemented by further planned field studies. For example, the percentage of rheumatic heart among cardiac patients was compared in Francophone countries in Maghreb (43.8 per cent), Sahel (21.3 per cent), and rain forest (17.8 per cent). Why the differences? Where are other similar studies?

The clinical history can be very misleading if ideas borrowed from the medicine of the industrialized societies are introduced. A visiting research team at an African teaching centre, with a questionnaire designed in New York, concluded that over 50 per cent of the patients had ischaemic heart disease. This was because the question about chest pain was interpreted by the patients as the discomfort due to breathlessness. This sort of difficulty will continue unless trained doctors work in their own home area where they are familiar with the idioms and ideas prevalent among the local people, or until physicians begin to see health and disease in the context of a people's culture.

The physical signs are frequently far advanced and it is common to see patients in left ventricular failure with pulsus alternans, and severe pulmonary oedema; those with hypertensive disease with advanced retinopathy or renal failure; those with mitral valvular disease with significant pulmonary hypertension; and many patients with the signs and effects, in addition, of anaemia and hypoproteinaemia. A mastery of physical signs is very important as signs alone are so often the rock on which the working diagnosis is built.

The investigations of cardiovascular disease are now so complex in the industrial society that the gap between what is possible there and what is feasible in the Third World countries of Africa has grown so much that it is unbridgeable. However, a good P-A radiograph of the chest, perhaps a 12-lead electrocardiogram, and basic tests to define a sign such as pallor or jaundice, provide the essentials in most patients. A blood film will reveal whether there are many neutrophils or eosinophils, which is highly relevant in acute pyogenic infection and in possible cases of early endomyocardial fibrosis (EMF). Where they are available, advanced techniques are exceedingly helpful for precise anatomical diagnosis: for example, angiocardiography was elegantly used at Ibadan to define the distorted ventricles in EMF, idiopathic tropical aortitis, and annular subvalvular aneurysm of the left ventricle; and immune complexes were identified in Zaria in patients who had meningococcal pericarditis. But the advances in Africa in the years ahead will depend on tests for the diagnosis of early disease and in the definition of mechanisms of disease, such as the eosinophilia in EMF, and on planned epidemiological and preventive studies.

The pattern of cardiovascular disease
Differences from those in the industrialized countries
The outstanding differences are the absence of significant occlusive vascular disease due to atheroma, and the frequent cardiac sequelae of infection. Far less important is the presence of certain distinctive syndromes such as EMF.

There is growing evidence, however, that ischaemic heart disease is increasing in established residents in every African city. For example, at the Baragwanath Hospital in Johannesburg, it accounted for 0.9 per cent of deaths due to cardiovascular disease in 1959, whereas in 1976 the percentage had risen to 11.7 per cent. The same story, but not as great an increase, is repeated for many other places. Why should this be? Epidemiological data are scanty, but urban Africans are heavier, have a higher blood pressure, plasma cholesterol, and proportion of fat in their diet than rural people, and tend to smoke and take little physical exercise. Yet, despite all these risk factors in settled urban people, clinical coronary artery disease is uncommon; the reasons for this have not yet been explained. In contrast, ischaemic heart disease is exceptionally rare (or unknown) in a patient who lives in a rural area and who eats subsistence staple foods, works on the farm most days, and does not smoke. Similarly, venous thrombo-embolism, though rare, is apparently increasing too; it is seen relatively often in some cities in Senegal, Sudan, and Uganda. Could this also be part of the change of the pattern of disease with urbanization?

The heart and infections
In children, *Staphylococcus aureus* pneumonia after measles may lead to septicaemia, with infective endocarditis or pyogenic pericarditis. Rheumatic heart disease, often with established mitral stenosis, is common in children below the age of 10 years. But the Duckett–Jones criteria for acute rheumatic carditis have to be reviewed and revised if used in Africa: nodules, chorea, and erythema marginatum are extremely uncommon.

Infection by nephritogenic streptococci of the skin of children is very common and may appear in epidemics. Acute glomerulonephritis may be overt or occult: this renal damage could reasonably explain why there is much hypertension in young adults. But no longitudinal studies are available. Streptococcal pyoderma which may also complicate scabies, is a problem of poverty, overcrowding, and a bad supply of water.

In adults, an acute myocarditis during an infection may make difficult the management of a patient with meningococcaemia, typhoid, typhus, sleeping sickness, relapsing fever, and possibly some viral infections. Pulmonary oedema during an intravenous infusion may be the first evidence that the heart is affected, unless an unexplained tachycardia or a gallop rhythm have been detected and myocardial damage has been invoked as their cause.

In areas where *Schistosoma mansoni* is endemic and transmission is high, notably Egypt and Sudan, cor pulmonale due to a peri-oval obliterative arteritis is familiar; by contrast, in wet and forested areas heavy hookworm loads produce a severe iron deficiency and anaemic cardiac failure. Tuberculosis has many possible effects: destructive lung disease with hypoxic cor pulmonale, kyphoscoliotic heart disease due to Pott's disease of the spine, and constrictive pericarditis; ventricular aneurysms have been associated with, but not proven to be due to, tuberculosis also. In some countries tuberculosis is the commonest cause of cor pulmonale.

Infective endocarditis, when it complicates staphylococcal and pneumococcal infections, may be missed during life because signs of the primary infection, for example, pyomyositis or a confusional state or a metastatic abscess, or post-partum pelvic infection, dominate the clinical picture.

The problem of cardiomyopathy
Apart from infections in adults a major and significant conundrum is cardiomyopathy. It commonly accounts for at least 20 per cent of all cardiovascular admissions in adults, and may be impossible to distinguish, if a distinction is valid, from hypertensive heart failure which also accounts for about 20 per cent in most countries. Alcohol is certainly important in its genesis in certain areas but there is increasing evidence that hypertension, untreated and not complicated by ischaemic heart disease, is the basis of many cases. First, the disease appears in the same age groups as hypertensive cardiac disease; second, patients previously known to be hypertensive, have normal blood pressures when they are admitted with their dilated cardiomyopathy; third, the blood pressure may rise to 'hypertensive' levels in some patients as the myocardium regains its tone with effective treatment: finally, the aortic arch diameter in cardiomyopathy patients is only a little less than the diameter in patients with hypertension, and is much greater than normotensive controls.

What then is this cardiomyopathy? Are we seeing the effect of sustained afterload on a left ventricle free from associated coronary disease? Or are we merely attaching an elegant word of Greek derivation to a syndrome of cardiac failure without obvious cause. A syndrome, not a disease entity, in which a major factor may be incriminated – in most patients hypertension, in some alcohol, and in a few, perhaps a former viral infection.

Workers at Ibadan have emphasized that cardiac failure in patients with cardiomyopathy is more common if the patients are anaemic, hypoproteinaemic or poor. The picture of a man of about 40 years, with a large heart, mitral incompetence, a third heart sound, and gross systemic and pulmonary congestion is so familiar, and can be so easily treated, at least initially, that the unsolved problems of its pathogenesis are easily forgotten in the press of busy work.

Pericardial disease
Rapid constriction and early signs of obstruction to right-sided inflow are characteristic in the pyogenic pericarditis caused by *Streptococcus pneumoniae* or *Staphylococcus aureus*. In an adult with pyomyositis, or a child after measles, the diagnosis may be

very difficult, but an enlarging tender liver and distant heart sounds are helpful signs; a chest radiograph may be of little help because an opacity due to lower lobe consolidation obliterates one border of the heart. Early pericardiectomy with appropriate antibiotics is now judged the most reliable treatment.

Pericardial tuberculosis is reported in many patients; it is conspicuously common in Swaziland. It has often advanced to severe constriction, with irreversible hepatic fibrosis, by the time the patient is seen first. As health care improves, cases are defined earlier, during the phase of acute pericardial effusion, when antituberculosis chemotherapy with or without surgery offers hope of complete cure.

Endomyocardial fibrosis (EMF)

Even though the new term eosinophilic endomyocardial disease embraces EMF and Loeffler's endocarditis, and the eosinophil has been incriminated as the cause of the cardiac damage, many problems are still unsolved in tropical Africa. Why is the EMF syndrome rare in the drier regions of Africa? Why is it more prevalent in Rwandans in Kampala than in the indigenous Baganda? What causes the disease to become 'burnt out'? Can the early phase be identified and arrested? The diagnosis of the established disease – a varying combination of signs of cardiac constriction, and atrioventricular valvular incompetence of the left or right or both ventricles – is not difficult although lone mitral incompetence may be very difficult to distinguish from rheumatic mitral incompetence. The primary challenge is the early stage of the disease: its recognition, mechanism, control, and ultimately its prevention.

Peripartum cardiac failure

In mothers in Northern Nigeria, this syndrome is a beautiful example of the relationship between culture, environment, and disease in Africa. The traditional beliefs of the mothers make them protect themselves against cold after delivery and so the nursing mother lies on a heated, and often very hot, bed for at least 40 days; she also takes a sodium-rich lake salt in order to make her breast milk flow. The sodium and heat loads, aggravated by the very hot weather particularly just before the rainy season starts, contribute to cardiac failure. Some mothers recover quickly from their hypervolaemic high output state: others develop an irreversibly dilated heart. Hypertension may also be a factor in the pathogenesis of the syndrome in some women.

Treatment

By far the most important problems are the management of cardiac failure and the effects of hypertension in the adult; and of cardiac disease due to infection in children.

Successful long-term management of the patient with cardiac failure may not succeed because:

1. The patient does not understand the need to take drugs continuously, as he thinks of treatment as one large dose at the beginning and no more.

2. A continuous supply of drugs is not available because communications between the rural centre and headquarters are bad, or because the national budget is so small *per capita* that money cannot be spared for cardiac drugs.

3. The patient lives far away from the referral centre: there are no resources, nor is there the interest, to bring him or her back to a specialist clinic, or to visit at home if the patient does not attend the centre for follow up. Unless money is given, the cost of a journey by public transport may well be a significant slice from a subsistence income so that the patient just cannot attend.

Because money is short, every member of the health team has to come to terms with the fact that every patient cannot be treated with the drugs which are prescribed so effortlessly by physicians in richer countries. Again, because health care is given primarily by members of the health team with little knowledge of cardiac drugs, and even less opportunity to keep informed about new remedies, it is essential for specialist physicians to prescribe as simply as possible, so that all drugs used in chronic health care can be understood and handled by those with no more than auxiliary training. Ideally, drugs should be given once per day so that the pattern of life of the patient is not upset and there is little to remember.

Cardiac surgery has a low priority and it would be very difficult for a minister of health to justify the opening of a cardiac surgical unit (except for political prestige) until primary care, and maternal and child health clinics are fully established throughout the country. Happily there are skilful general surgeons who have successfully handled the surgery of pyogenic pericarditis and closed mitral valvotomy, which are the major common problems for which surgery is practicable.

Prevention of cardiovascular disease

Although it seems inevitable that coronary disease and the complications of hypertension will become more common as urbanization accelerates, the pressing need now is to prevent the major infections associated with cardiovascular disease. Streptococcal infections of the throat and skin prevail where people are crowded and denied a good water supply; the pyogenic respiratory and thus pericardial complications of measles can only develop where severe measles is not prevented in a good child health programme; and tuberculosis will not disappear until a comprehensive antituberculosis programme succeeds. More optimistically, schistosomal cor pulmonale may recede now that oxamniquine and praziquantel are available to treat *S. mansoni*.

Programmes already attempted afford little cheer. In a study in Soweto, Johannesburg, only 17 per cent of children who had been in hospital with rheumatic heart disease were attending for follow up until a programme of secondary prevention was established. In this, health visitors worked through the local health clinics and with an academic department of community health. Yet, even with such a team, only 38 per cent were being seen at follow up at 8 months.

In Zaria, Northern Nigeria, only the tenacity of a full-time social worker enabled us to follow up, at a referral cardiac clinic, a cohort of women with peripartum cardiac failure: it was effective but expensive.

Successful prevention will depend on comprehensive primary care; good liaison between rural clinics and larger referral centres; positive interest and commitment by hospital oriented physicians; and, most daunting of all, an attack across a broad front on the indifference which accepts, but does not attempt to alleviate, the deprivation and disadvantage which are the hallmark of all too many people in rural and urban Africa today.

The future

It will become increasingly difficult to justify very expensive investigative and surgical cardiac units in much of Africa until a basic health service is widely enjoyed. But much can still be learned if clinical data are carefully collected, prolonged follow up is established, and the epidemiology of disease is patiently plotted. For many years, precise and accurate definition of cardiac signs will be more important than advanced investigative ventures in the majority of patients, and the relief of symptoms by a few manageable and cheap drugs will remain the aim of treatment.

References

Andy, J. J., Bishara, F. F. and Soyinka, O. O. (1981). Relation of severe eosinophilia and microfilariasis to chronic African endomyocardial fibrosis. *Br. Heart J.* **45**, 672–680.

Davidson, N. Mc. D. and Parry, E. H. O. (1978). Peripartum cardiac failure. *Q. J. Med. N. S.* **47**, 431–461.

Edgington, M. E. and Gear, J. S. S. (1982). Rheumatic heart disease in Soweto – a programme for secondary prevention. *S. Afr. med. J.* **62**, 523–525.

Falase, A. O., Ayeni, O., Sekoni, G. A. and Odia, O. J. (1983). Heart failure in Nigerian hypertensives. *Afr. J. Med. med. Sci.* **12**, 7–15.

Isaacson, C. (1977). The changing pattern of heart disease in South African Blacks. *S. Afr. med. J.* **52**, 793–798.

Jaiyesimi, F. (1982). Acquired heart disease in Nigerian children: an illustration of the influence of socio-economic factors in disease pattern. *J. trop. Paed.* **28**, 223–229.

Mabogunje, O. A., Adesanya, C. O., Khwaja, M. S., Lawrie, J. H. and Edington, G. M. (1981). Surgical management of pericarditis in Zaria, Nigeria. *Thorax* **36**, 590–595.

Latin America

M. RIGATTO

For descriptive purposes Latin America has been considered as the American continent south of the United States. The Pan American Health Organization divides Latin America into four areas: Temperate South America, Tropical South America, Continental Middle America, and Caribbean Middle America. Brazil (41 per cent of the Latin America area) has approximately one-third of its population (from São Paulo to the south) in Temperate South America. Nevertheless in the statistical data used in this chapter all Brazil is included in Tropical South America.

Temperate South America

Temperate South America had 41 million inhabitants in 1980. The so-called South Cone of Latin America – Argentina, Chile, and Uruguay – has a profile of cardiovascular diseases similar to those of North America or Western Europe. Diseases of the heart lead mortality statistics accounting for 24.5 per cent of all deaths. Cerebrovascular disease stands in third place with 9.6 per cent of the total. Together, they account for more than twice the percentage of the second leading cause of death from malignant neoplasms (16.9 per cent) in 1979.

A number of factors may account for the similarities of disease pattern with the West. The life span is long, 69.5 years in Uruguay, 69.2 in Argentina, 65.7 in Chile, in 1980, with 4 per cent of the population above 65 years of age; a reasonable income *per capita* (US$ 1859 in 1980); a high literacy rate, 94 per cent in Uruguay and Argentina, 88 per cent in Chile; a dominant urban population, 82.2 per cent in 1980; a slowly growing population, 1.27 per cent in 1980–85, the slowest in Latin America; a population of heavy smokers, 50 to 60 per cent of the adults; a high average caloric intake, 3358 calories *per capita* in Argentina, 2927 in Uruguay, 2644 in Chile; a high prevalence of elevated systemic arterial pressure, from 10 to 20 per cent of the adult population, according to different studies. Only Chagas' disease, common in the north of Argentina, makes a dissounding note.

Tropical South America

Tropical South America had 204 million inhabitants in 1980. The disease pattern is different. Infectious diseases are the leading causes of death. Among cardiovascular disorders Chagas' cardio-myopathy is particularly prevalent in the centre and northeast of Brazil and in Venezuela. Cor pulmonale due to schistosomiasis is also found in this area of Brazil and in Surinam. The disease of Monge (cor pulmonale due to altitude) is found among the numerous inhabitants of the top of the Andes, particularly in Peru and Bolivia.

In contrast to Temperate South America, in the tropical zones malaria, Chagas' disease, leishmaniasis, schistomiasis, plague, dengue, yellow fever are endemic. There is undernutrition with an average intake of 2049 cal *per capita* in Bolivia to 2436 in Venezuela (1975–77); *per capita* income is low (US$ 1504 in 1980); literacy rates are also low ranging from 63 per cent in Bolivia to 82 per cent in Venezuela (1976); the lifespan is less, e.g. 61.3 years in the period 1975–80. Only 1.7 per cent of the population is above 65 years of age. The urban population is smaller (65 per cent). These are important causes and/or consequences of a less advantageous

health profile. The prevalence of high blood pressure and smoking habits in adults are apparently not different from those of southern areas of the continent. But their effects are minimized by the shorter lifespan.

Middle America

In Middle America these two broad patterns of disease are again discernible. Continental Middle America (93 million inhabitants in 1980) extends to the north the same health problems as in Tropical South America; while Caribbean Middle America (31 million inhabitants in 1980) has higher health standards and approaches the pattern described for Temperate South America.

This geographical outline is only valid in its broad perspective. In all Latin America there are areas which depart significantly from the dominant regional profile. An example is Costa Rica whose health standards are unusually high for Continental Middle America. Another is Trinidad and Tobago whose population (1 190 000 inhabitants, in 1981) has an unusually high incidence of several chronic diseases: diabetes mellitus, hypertensive disease, ischaemic heart disease, and cerebrovascular disease.

Epidemiological data on *congenital heart disease* are scanty. Apparently its incidence in Latin America is not different from that of other parts of the world. No regional differences have been described.

Acute rheumatic fever is rather uniformly widespread in Latin America. According to data from the late seventies, the age-adjusted death rate per 100 000 population varies between 0.1 and 0.3 in most countries except Ecuador with 0.7 and Barbados with 0.8 who have the highest rates. The age-adjusted death rate per 100 000 population for chronic rheumatic heart disease varies between 1.0 and 3.5 in most countries except Chile with 3.8, and Trinidad and Tobago, with 5.0, who have reported higher rates. As a reference point, the rates for the United States and Canada, at the same date were, respectively, 0.1 and 0.0 for acute rheumatic fever, and 2.5 and 2.7 for chronic rheumatic heart disease.

From a historical and regional viewpoint, the heart conditions more closely linked to Latin America are *Chagas' disease* and *chronic cor pulmonale*. Chagas' disease was fully characterized and established as an entity, in Brazil, by Carlos Chagas, in 1909. It is discussed on page 13.230. The concept of cor pulmonale as a syndrome was first advanced and documented by the Argentinian School of Medicine. Two peculiar types of chronic cor pulmonale have been described in South America: that due to hypoventilation at altitude, described by Monge, in Peru, and that due to lung involvement by the ova of *Schistosoma mansoni*, described in Brazil.

Chronic cor pulmonale was first described under the title of 'the black cardiac' by Ayerza in Buenos Aires during a student lecture in 1901. He referred to patients with chronic lung disease who presented, at an advanced stage of their clinical course, with heart failure characterized by severe cyanosis, dyspnoea, oedema, and, at autopsy, pulmonary disease and marked right ventricular hypertrophy. The vivid expression 'black cardiac' was probably justified by the summation of central (lung disease) and peripheral (circulatory failure) causes of cyanosis.

Ayerza did not publish his lecture but a few of his disciples did under the title 'Ayerza's disease'. In 1909, Marty emphasized the importance, recognized by Ayerza, of chronic lung disease as the origin of right ventricular overload. But Elizalde and Arrillaga, in 1920, impressed by the finding of spirochaetes in the lungs of some patients, adopted the designation 'pulmonary arteritis', giving chronic lung disease second place as a cause for the disturbance. For a decade the world medical literature, particularly European, tended to consider the disease of Ayerza as a disorder of the pulmonary artery. In the early thirties, studies from Argentina re-established the pathophysiological basis of Ayerza's disease as due to severe alveolar hypoventilation leading to the clinical picture of polycythaemia, cyanosis, and right ventricular overload.

From 1925 to 1929, Monge, from the University of Lima, characterized the 'disease of the Andes' or the 'erythraemias of altitude', now designated as chronic mountain sickness, 'chronic *soroche*', or 'Monge's disease'. The clinical picture is seen in people living at high altitude, usually above 3000 metres, who lose acclimatization to environmental hypoxia. It is characterized by alveolar hypoventilation leading to hypercapnia and to an exacerbation of the hypoxaemia, the polycythaemia and pulmonary hypertension normally prevalent in these individuals. In due course, these disturbances lead to right ventricular overload and to neuropsychiatric manifestations. Overt right ventricular failure may be seen in advanced cases. The patients improve with bloodletting and/or, oxygen administration. Recovery, in days or weeks, is the rule after the patient has been moved to sea level. As yet it is not fully understood why some people, born and living at altitude or born at sea level but living for many years at altitude, should suddenly lose their established acclimatization to the hypoxic environment.

Besides describing medicinal features of the disorder, Monge recognized the secondary nature of the polycythaemia and distinguished it from polycythaemia rubra vera.

In 1922, Harrop documented a reduction in the pulmonary diffusion capacity of these patients. In 1960, Hurtado attributed the hypoventilation to a reduction in the sensitivity of the respiratory centre to carbon dioxide. In 1966, Severinghaus, attributed hypoventilation to a reduced sensitivity of the peripheral chemoreceptors to hypoxia and in 1969, Stella demonstrated a significant increase in size of the carotid body in altitude dwellers. The present concept is of cor pulmonale secondary to the alveolar hypoventilation.

Indeed patients with known causes of alveolar hypoventilation, as bronchitis, emphysema, obesity, kyphoscoliosis, or with diffusion problems, as diffuse interstitial fibrosis, sarcoidosis, silicosis, may, at altitude, develop a clinical picture similar to Monge's disease. The designations 'secondary chronic mountain sickness' and 'Monge's syndrome' have been proposed for these cases.

An intriguing observation relevant to the understanding of the pathophysiology of Monge's disease is the fact that Himalayan dwellers, living at altitudes equivalent to those in the Andes, do not present any disease comparable to it. Humidity and the mining activities in the Andes have been put forward to explain the difference.

Chronic cor pulmonale due to *Schistosoma mansoni* involvement of the pulmonary circulation has been described in Brazil where there are 8 to 10 million people infected by this parasite, also present in other South and Middle America countries. The mechanical blockade of pulmonary vessels by the ova of the parasites and the intravascular and perivascular reactions to them, leading to granulomatous formation and, eventually, to interstitial fibrosis, have been considered the cause of the increased pulmonary vascular resistance. It is estimated that two-thirds of the persons infected with *Schistosoma mansoni* have lung involvement by the parasite, but only 1 per cent show clinical changes attributable to it. In some patients lung involvement leads not to a clinical picture of cor pulmonale but to cyanosis and finger clubbing without elevated pulmonary arterial pressure. In such cases the development of venoarterial shunts has been described.

Conclusions

In broad perspective cardiovascular diseases are tending to become increasingly important causes of death in Latin America. From 1970 to 1979 total deaths due to diseases of the heart increased from 21.4 to 24.5 per cent in Temperate South America, from 6.5 to 12.7 per cent in Tropical South America, from 6.2 to 9.6 per cent in Continental Middle America, and from 18.7 to 23.2 per cent in the Caribbean. On the other hand, the percentage of total deaths due to cerebrovascular disease increased from 8.7 to 9.6 per cent in Temperate South America, from 2.5 to 4.9 per cent in Tropical South America, from 2.3 to 2.8 per cent in Continental

Middle America, and from 8.4 to 9.2 per cent in the Caribbean. In Tropical South America diseases of the heart moved from third to first place in the rank order of leading causes of death. Cerebrovascular disease moved from ninth to seventh place in Continental Middle America and from tenth to seventh place in Tropical South America. Possible reasons for these trends are the increasing lifespan (58.7 years in Latin America as a whole in 1965–70, to 62.5 years in 1975–80), and, particularly among women, an increasing prevalence of smoking and an increasing use of hormonal contraceptive pills.

Significant public health efforts against Chagas' disease, schistosomiasis, and streptococcal pharyngitis, may reduce the relative importance of these entities as a cause of cardiovascular disease. Six countries which reported comparative death rates for chronic rheumatic heart disease in the mid-seventies showed, on average, a 40 per cent reduction in these rates by 1980.

Public campaigns mainly inspired by medical associations are increasing consciousness of the risks of smoking, lack of exercise and high blood pressure. The Pan American Health Organization has been a powerful ally in this endeavour.

References

Andrade, L. A., Paronetto, F. and Popper, H. (1961). Immunocytochemical studies in schistosomiasis. *Am. J. Path.* **39**, 589–598.

Cavalcanti, I. de L., Thompson, G., Souza, N. and Barbosa, F. S. (1962). Pulmonary hypertension in schistosomiasis. *Br. Heart J.* **24**, 363–371.

Faria, J. L. de, Barbas Fº, J. V., Fujioka, T., Lion, M. F., Andrade e Silva, V. and Décourt, L. V. (1959). Pulmonary schistosomotic arteriovenous fistula producing a new cyanotic syndrome in Manson's schistosomiasis. *Am. Heart J.* **58**, 556–567.

Pan American Health Organization (1982). *Health conditions in the Americas 1977–1980*. Washington, DC.

Porter, R. and Knight, J. (1971). *High altitude physiology: cardiac and respiratory aspects*. CIBA Foundation Symposium. Churchill Livingstone, Edinburgh.

Taquini, A. C. (1954). *El corazon pulmonar*. Ateneo, Buenos Aires.

Southeast Asia

S. HATHIRAT

Published epidemiologic studies of cardiovascular diseases in Southeast Asia are scarce. A few show increasing morbidity and mortality from these diseases during the past 30 years. Cardiovascular events now rank second or third among the leading causes of death; a substantial upsurge from the sixth or seventh position of 20–30 years ago. However, it is still not the number one killer as in western countries, particularly North America and Europe.

The changing pattern and the cause

The increases in cardiovascular morbidity and mortality in Southeast Asia are due mainly to coronary heart disease, and, to a much lesser extent, to cardiomyopathy or miscellaneous cardiac problems, such as idiopathic cardiac arrhythmias, aortic disease (including Takayasu arteritis), cardiac tumours, and unclassified cardiac problems. However, rheumatic heart disease is on the decline. These trends are similar to those in China, but different from those in Japan or western countries. In the latter, coronary mortality has decreased since the late 1960s. There are no significant changes in the incidences and/or mortality rates for congenital, infectious, hypertensive, pulmonary, nutritional, or metabolic heart diseases.

The possible causes of these changing patterns will be discussed. An interesting finding is the higher cardiovascular mortality of the Australasian Aborigines as compared to the White inhabitants. This has been related to various socio-environmental effects including socio-cultural change and imposed migration into a reserve far distant from their homeland.

Ischaemic heart disease

This disease was rarely seen 20–30 years ago except in elderly diabetic and hypertensive patients particularly those with high administrative responsibility. During the past 10–20 years, it has presented itself in all strata of the population over 30 years of age, and certainly more in populations at high risk.

The increase in prevalence and mortality of this disease probably reflects the change of life style which has become more and more westernized. Diets have become richer in proteins and fats, technology has led to sedentary habits, and the rapid influx of western culture and materialist civilization has led to socio-economic stress. The way of life in Southeast Asia is changing so that the old and simple ways are being replaced by a more materialistic and selfish environment.

Rheumatic heart disease

The decline in prevalence of this disorder over the past 10–20 years probably reflects a decrease in incidence due to the improvement in housing and living standards as a result of improved economics, and to a much lesser extent, the use of penicillin in the eradication and treatment of streptococcal infections.

In recent years, rheumatic heart disease has become very rare in Singapore children. In two recent surveys in Thailand this disease was found in none of the children under the age of 15 years in a rural community, and in only three confirmed and six possible cases out of 31 040 Bangkok school children (a prevalence of 0.1 and 0.2 per 1000, respectively).

The decline in the mortality rate of this disease may be attributed to the decreased incidence and the improved medical and surgical treatment.

Congenital heart diseases

These diseases occur in about 6–8 per 1000 live births, a rate which is quite similar to that of developed countries. The lack of change in incidence in Southeast Asia does not reflect improving premarriage examination and counselling, antenatal care, and/or rubella vaccination because preventable congenital heart diseases like congenital rubella syndrome and Down's anomaly are present in only 5 per cent of the Southeast Asian patients, a figure which is about half of that reported in the West.

More awareness, better diagnostic and therapeutic techniques including surgical correction, and improved nursing care have reduced the mortality rate of this group of disorders.

Infectious heart disease

Better antibiotics and improved penicillin prophylaxis during dental and surgical procedures in congenital and valvular heart diseases have reduced the incidence and mortality rates of some kinds of infectious endocarditis. However, these improvements have been counterbalanced by infective disease associated with increasing intravascular and intracardiac instrumentation and intravenous heroin addiction.

In addition, a decrease in pyogenic and tuberculous myopericarditis has also been countered by an increase in viral and other non-bacterial myopericarditis.

Hypertensive heart disease

The insignificant change in prevalence and mortality from hypertension probably reflects a balance between an increase in its incidence and a decrease in morbid events as a result of earlier diagnosis and better antihypertensive treatment.

Pulmonary heart disease

Acute cor pulmonale or pulmonary thromboembolism is a rare entity in this area. Chronic cor pulmonale due to massive pulmonary destruction from tuberculosis, pneumonias, and bronchiectasis has decreased due to earlier diagnosis and better treatment of these pulmonary infections, but an increase in chronic cor pulmonale due to chronic obstructive pulmonary disease from increased air pollution and cigarette smoking has counterbalanced the above decline.

Nutritional and metabolic heart disease

The prevalence and mortality rates of nutritional heart disease, particularly cardiac beriberi and anaemic heart failure, have decreased substantially during the past 10 years due to better nutrition and treatment of hookworm. Coincidentally there has been a trend towards an increased incidence or recognition of such disorders as thyrotoxic and myxoedematous heart disease.

Miscellaneous cardiac diseases

The increase in the prevalence of these disorders may be attributed to the discovery of more cardiac problems and their inclusion into the International Classification of Disease (ICD 9 and 10), and to more awareness and better diagnostic techniques including transcatheter endomyocardial biopsy.

Clinical features, investigation, and treatment

Ischaemic heart disease

The presenting features are similar to those of western populations. Presentation in young women is usually associated with systemic lupus erythematosus or Takayasu arteritis which may be controlled by immunosuppressive therapy. Those due to coronary atherosclerosis are investigated and treated as they are in the developed countries with increasing coronary bypass graft surgery and thrombolytic therapy.

The trends towards investigation and treatment of coronary heart disease with the most recent advances in technology and drugs impose serious burdens to the health care system and the socio-economics of Asian countries. Sadly, there is a reluctance to take preventive measures against the new life-style which has probably precipitated the upsurge of this disease and the current approach is increasingly complicated by anxiety symptoms and a variety of iatrogenic problems.

Rheumatic heart disease

The presenting features, investigation, and treatment are similar to those of developed countries. For those requiring surgery, closed heart surgery can be carried out in several hospitals, and open heart surgery in a few big units. Rheumatic valvular surgery still ranks second in cardiac surgery in Southeast Asia in contrast to the situation in western countries, particularly the United States.

Congenital heart disease

The types, clinical features, investigation, and treatment of these diseases, are also similar to those of the developed countries. Ventricular septal defect and Tetralogy of Fallot including its variants are commonest. With the decline of rheumatic heart disease together with better diagnostic, anaesthetic, and surgical techniques, congenital heart surgery has now become the leading cardiac surgery in this area. Almost all correctable congenital cardiac lesions can be treated.

Infectious heart disease

Streptococcal organisms particularly *streptococcus viridans* still remain the major organisms in infective endocarditis, but endocarditis in heroin addiction in this area is mainly due to staphylococcal and, less often, polymicrobial infection. The difficulty in treating endocarditis in heroin addiction is well known, particularly the resistance to treatment. Relapse or reinfection usually occurs within a year due to the return of addiction.

The clinical features, investigation, and treatment of infective endocarditis, myocarditis, and pericarditis are similar to those of the developed countries. Resection of infected valves is occasionally performed for uncontrollable infection or intractable heart failure with good results except in those with heroin addiction.

Non-bacterial, particularly viral, myocarditis, still remain a diagnostic and therapeutic challenge because of inadequate diagnostic and therapeutic techniques.

Hypertensive heart disease

The types and causes of hypertension are similar to those in the West except that renal artery stenosis is due mainly to Takayasu arteritis, rather than atherosclerosis or fibromuscular dysplasia which are the major causes in the West.

In the early or active phase of Takayasu arteritis (page 13.193) with elevated erythrocyte sedimentation rate, migraine-like symptoms, erythema nodosum, palpable bruit, and/or aneurysmal pulsation of large arteries complicated by renovascular hypertension, prolonged use of corticosteroids will alleviate the symptoms and return the patient to normal life with or without the reduction of arterial pressure. In cases of severe and resistant renovascular hypertension, the use of captopril may help in control. Surgical correction of the obstructive lesion or removal of a destroyed kidney are occasionally successful in controlling hypertension.

Pulmonary heart disease

Acute cor pulmonale is rare in this area because pulmonary thromboembolism is seldom seen except in occasional obstetric or gynaecological patients or others with multiple fractures. This is probably due to the rarity of deep vein thrombosis in the Southeast Asian population except those of western descent. Acute pulmonary thromboembolism is successfully treated medically in almost all cases except occasional cases of massive amniotic fluid embolism complicated by diffuse bleeding, and of multiple open fractures complicated by septicaemia.

The clinical features, investigation, and treatment of chronic cor pulmonale are similar to those of the West.

Nutritional and metabolic heart disease

Anaemic heart failure in this area is usually due to intestinal parasites (particularly hookworm) or to thalassaemia. Prolonged and gradual blood loss may lead to haemocrit values of less than 10 per cent. Such profound anaemia results in cardiomegaly and congestive heart failure, which respond well to packed red cell transfusion, diuretics, and iron supplement in cases of iron deficiency.

Cardiac beriberi In children, cardiac beriberi is usually seen in infants less than 6 months old, born and breast-fed by malnourished mothers with glove-stocking hypoesthaesia or hyperesthaesia and pedal oedema. Usually following an upper respiratory tract infection, the child becomes restless, dyspnoeic, and swollen over the abdomen and feet. Clinical features include a rapid pulse, voice hoarseness, hepatosplenomegaly, and later circulatory shock. The response to thiamine is dramatic.

In adults, cardiac beriberi occurs most commonly in young muscular men without evidences of malnutrition or of known heart diseases, a picture very different from that in the West. Physical examination and pretreatment chest roentgenogram and electrocardiogram do not usually help in the diagnosis. Therefore, when acute congestive heart failure follows strenuous physical work, a febrile episode, or an alcoholic binge in such a man, 100 mg of thiamine hydrochloride should be given intravenously without digitalis or diuretic. A dramatic clinical improvement within a few hours followed by massive diuresis, will confirm the diagnosis. Erythrocyte transketolase activity and other laboratory tests may

be misleading and usually delay the diagnosis and treatment. Serial chest films will show the rapid resolution of pulmonary congestion and regression of cardiac size after thiamine treatment. Serial electrocardiograms will show a marked reduction of heart rate, disappearance of right axis deviation, increased QRS voltage, and giant T inversion in right precordial leads within 2–3 days of treatment, when the patient is already well. The post-treatment giant T inversion may lead those who are not familiar with this entity to mistakenly diagnose acute anterior subendocardial infarction or acute pulmonary embolism.

Thyrotoxic and myxoedematous heart failure The clinical features, investigation, and treatment of these disorders do not differ from those in the West.

The prospect

Although the causes of the changing prevalence of various cardiovascular diseases in Southeast Asia are mainly speculative, there is little doubt that the changes are real and substantial.

The establishment of universal community-based morbidity registries which would greatly improve the quality of data is a particularly important priority for developing countries whose national resources are limited. The trend towards increasingly expensive investigation and treatment of cardiovascular diseases without adequate primary or secondary prevention threatens to bankrupt these countries.

References

Guzman, S. V. and Yason, J. V. (1979). Cardiovascular community control programme in the Philippines. In *Report of a WHO meeting on comprehensive cardiovascular community control programmes*, Alberta, November 1978, pp. 38–42. World Health Organization, Geneva.

Hathirat, S. and Jumbala, B. (1975). Giant T inversion in cardiac beriberi. *J. Med. Assoc. Thai.* **58**, 636–641.

——, (1978). Modern medicine in Thailand to-day: problem and treatment. *J. Med. Assoc. Thai.* **61**, suppl. 3, 17–24.

Lochaya, S., Watthana-Kasetr, S., Suvachittanont, O., Triyanond, K., Pongpanich, B., Sudhas Na Ayudhya, P., Hathirat, S., Na Ranong, V. and Srivorapangpan, R. (1983). Prevalence of heart diseases in school-age children in Bangkok. *J. Med. Assoc. Thai.* **66**, 789–798.

Panichewa, S. and Hathirat, S. (1982). Fulminant cardiac beriberi with severe acidosis. *J. Med. Assoc. Thai.* **65**, 566–569.

Piza, Z. and Uemura, K. (1982). Trends of mortality from ischaemic heart disease and other cardiovascular diseases in 27 countries, 1968–1977. *Wld Hlth Stat. Q.* **35**, 11–47.

Reed, D. M. and Feinlab, M. (1983). Changing patterns of cardiovascular diseases in the Pacific Basin: report of an international workshop. *J. Community Hlth* **8**, 182–205.

Sindhvananda, K. (1981). Incidence and epidemiology of cardiovascular disease in Thailand. In *Cardiovascular disease* (eds S. Lochaya, B. Pongpanich and P. Sakornphant), pp. 6–10. Bangkok Medical Publisher, Bangkok.

Trigger, D. S., Anderson, C., Lincoln, R. A. and Matis, C. E. (1983). Mortality rates in 14 Queensland Aboriginal reserve community. Association with 10 socio-environmental variables. *Med. J. Aust.* **1**, 361–365.

Wu, Y. K., Wu, Z. S. and Yao, C. H. (1983). Epidemiologic studies of cardiovascular diseases in China. *Chin. Med. J.* **96**, 201–205.

Yip, W. C. L., Tay, J. S. H. and Tan, N. C. (1982). Congenital heart disease in Singapore – present problems and future perspective. *Singapore Med. J.* **23**, 133–139.

SECTION 14
INTENSIVE CARE

INTENSIVE CARE

R. D. BRADLEY

Intensive care does not exist as a medical speciality. It is a form imposed upon present day medicine by what is technically possible on the one hand and economic necessity on the other. The account which follows attempts to add comments upon disease from the very special point of view of its management within an intensive care unit. The experience upon which the comments rest was gained from over 15 000 patients in a single unit with very diverse commitments encompassing coronary care, pacemaking, post-operative cardiac surgical care, the dialysis of patients with circulatory problems, head injuries, respiratory failure, circulatory failure, diabetes with serious metabolic disturbance, intoxications, and major trauma including burns.

The general philosophy of the unit has been to provide the space, equipment, and staff necessary for the performance of *medical* as opposed to *surgical* operations not possible in a normal ward.

The practical management of the patients has to be a blend of the expertise of the permanent staff of the unit, with that of the physicians and surgeons under whose care the patients were initially admitted to the hospital. Success depends not only upon special competence of the unit staff with the very sick, but also their ability to communicate and co-operate with the entire hospital staff.

At best, the special competence with the very sick is not merely confidence born of familiarity, but the ability to clarify situations which are often very muddled. This depends partly upon techniques for the investigation of patients who may well be deemed too sick to be investigated. A few measurements in such situations are worth a deal of conjecture.

There is a logical difficulty in the management of some very sick patients, which is not widely appreciated. The dilemma which faces the physician is that on the one hand diagnosis must come before treatment, and on the other that the physical signs upon which the diagnosis depends tend to disappear as the patient approaches death. A grossly hypotensive patient with an intestinal perforation may have few abnormal abdominal physical signs; partial restoration of the patient's circulation with a volume expander will restore the abdominal physical signs.

The solution to this seeming impasse depends upon arriving at a diagnosis in stages, each stage allowing some supportive manoeuvre which will not obscure the diagnosis.

Major acute derangements of the circulation

The word *shock* is commonly used to describe all major acute circulatory disturbances. The term has the value of brevity but little else to recommend it. It is imprecise, cannot be measured, and is applied to circulatory states which differ profoundly when analysed. The gravest disadvantage of the idea of shock as a physiological entity is the pervasive quest for some form of treatment which might be universally applicable.

The human circulation may deteriorate to the point of death in many different ways. Reversal of the process of deterioration can only be undertaken in a logical fashion if the diagnosis is known and the adjustments most likely to produce optimum performance of the circulation under those circumstances are understood.

The ensuing account describes in broad terms how the diagnosis may be pursued, and the circulatory manipulations appropriate to most acute circulatory disorders, based upon their abnormal physiology.

A systematic approach to patients with *major acute circulatory disturbances* of an unknown nature is outlined in Figs 1 and 2. Most of the measures and the order in which they are undertaken require no further comment. The early elimination of the possibility that the patient has a tension pneumothorax is required because the condition does not belong in either of the main groupings in the subsequent system of diagnosis. There is usually little difficulty in the diagnosis of a tension pneumothorax providing its existence is considered. It should be remembered that a relatively shallow pneumothorax, in the presence of emphysema, is potentially lethal and extremely difficult to diagnose from the physical signs, or the chest X-ray. With any life-threatening pneumothorax the venous pressure will appear raised.

The central venous pressure

It will be seen that assessment of the venous pressure occupies a critical position in the diagnostic scheme, and this should be measured with a catheter advanced to lie within the thorax. Introduction of the catheter through the internal jugular vein has the advantage that its position does not require radiographic confirmation. The subclavian approach carries a small risk of producing a pneumothorax.

Pressures within the circulation must be measured relative to some fixed point. The sternal angle is convenient and does not pose the uncertainties of mid-chest if the patient is unable to lie flat. It is to the sternal angle that all the figures quoted in this Section are related. The range of normal venous pressures may be from +3 to −5 cm of water.

It is possible in practice to divide patients suffering from major acute circulatory derangements into a group with central venous pressures above +1 cm and a group below −3 cm. Should a patient present with an obvious profound circulatory disturbance and a filling pressure lying between the limits described above, dual pathology is the likely explanation. Acute myocardial infarction and diabetic ketoacidosis are a relatively common combination and serve as a reminder that it is possible to have heart failure without a raised venous pressure.

Once the height of the venous pressure is known, a decision has to be made in the light of the patient's condition, for if this is deteriorating, there is now information upon which to base logical first-stage supportive therapy without risk of concealing the diagnosis.

In the high filling pressure group, the rapid provision of support requires the administration of an inotropic agent which preferably should not raise systemic resistance: dopamine in doses up to 6 μg/kg/min supplemented by dobutamine, if greater dosage is required. If this regimen fails to restore a urine output of 0.5 ml/kg/hour, or if the arterial systolic pressure remains below 80 mm Hg, adrenaline should be added, and the dose adjusted to between 0.01 and 0.4 μg/kg/min to produce acceptable levels of blood pressure and perfusion. If the initial level of systolic arterial pressure is less than 60 mm Hg, it is likely that adrenaline will be required. In the presence of sepsis, doses as high as 2 μg/kg/min may stabilize the circulation. In cases where the heart rate is slow, the inotropic agent of choice is isoprenaline in a dose of 0.007 to 0.07 μg/kg/min.

Should supportive intervention be required at this juncture in the low filling pressure group, blood should be taken for haematology (Hb, or haematocrit, white cell count, platelet count, blood grouping, and serum for possible cross matching), and chemistry (electrolytes, urea, sugar, and plasma proteins). Only then should the filling pressure of the right heart be restored toward normal with a plasma expander. If a normal right atrial pressure fails to produce an adequate circulation there must also be something amiss with the heart, and an inotropic agent should be administered in addition to the plasma expander.

Low venous pressure group (−3 cm or below)
Further logical separation of patients in this diagnostic group is not usually a matter of great difficulty, and depends, as is indicated in Fig. 2, on clinical observation of the state of the peripheral circulation and the haematocrit.

Low venous pressure – low venous tone group
If the cause of the fall in venous pressure is a drop in venous tone, as may occur in barbiturate and opiate intoxication, certain brain stem lesions, and in some patients with septicaemia, then the limb veins will appear to be of normal calibre or even dilated, and the limbs will be of normal temperature or warmer than normal.

These patients may retain a moderate cardiac output with arterial pressures as low as 50 to 60 mm Hg because the systemic resistance is also low. They may even produce urine normally when hypotensive. The general circulatory treatment, as opposed to specific treatment aimed at the cause, should be to raise the central venous pressure toward normal with a plasma expander. Restoration of a normal venous pressure in these patients will only partially restore the arterial pressure, because of the low systemic vascular resistance. Attempts to raise the arterial pressure to normal by raising the venous pressure to high positive values are a common iatrogenic cause of pulmonary oedema.

Low venous pressure – high venous tone group
If oligaemia is the cause of a low venous pressure, the normal vascular reflexes will produce venoconstriction and cold extremities. If the haematocrit or haemoglobin is normal, the probable cause is acute haemorrhage. Should the haematocrit be high, renal or gastrointestinal loss of fluid, electrolyes, and plasma proteins should be sought. Common causes of gastrointestinal loss of this nature are gastrointestinal perforations, peritonitis, pancreatitis, dysentery, toxic megacolon, and septicaemia. The loss may be into the lumen of the gut, the peritoneal cavity or both. Renal losses on this scale occur in diabetic ketoacidosis, the polyuric phase of acute tabular necrosis, and certain 'salt-losing' chronic renal disorders (Section 18). The diagnostic scheme just described will, of course, break down should chronically severely anaemic patients, in becoming oligaemic by loss of salt and water, raise their low haematocrit to normal. Although the diagnosis of acute haemorrhage will be incorrect, the conclusion that the oligaemia should be treated initially with whole blood remains true.

Ideally oligaemia should be treated by the replacement of whatever fluid has been lost. This may have to be modified by considerations such as the changes in blood viscosity which occur with oligaemia, and the changes in the circulation which may have occurred during the period of oligaemia.

Blood viscosity changes
As blood flow rate falls, viscosity rises disproportionately, and as the haematocrit increases, viscosity rises exponentially. Also after injury it has been shown that red cell dispersion is abnormal for at least three days, perhaps because of an increase in fibrinogen levels. All of these changes increase the chance of intravascular sludging. Moderate haemodilution is probably of advantage in countering these changes. There is evidence that tissue oxygen requirements may be met by an increase in perfusion associated with the lowering of the haematocrit. The theoretical optimum level of haematocrit in the presence of poor flows may be as low as 30 per cent.

Much has been made of the microcirculatory effects of low molecular weight dextrans although their capacity to make any measurable difference to blood fluidity, beyond that due to dilution, has been difficult to demonstrate in the concentrations obtained clinically. These solutions are hyperosmolar and will transfer fluid from other compartments into the circulation.

Volume and rate of circulatory fluid replacement in oligaemia
It might be thought that the volume of the replacement should equal the volume which has been lost from the circulation, and although this is probably ultimately true, it is not a particularly helpful concept. The volume which has been lost is not usually known, and although the remaining circulating volume can be estimated with isotopic techniques, replacements based upon measurements of volume in this way may cause serious circulatory problems. The reason for this apparent anomaly is the variability in the capacity of the vascular bed. There are few more powerfully constrictive influences upon the systemic capacity vessels than oligaemia. The events which occur in that part of the circulation during haemorrhage and transfusion can be illustrated diagrammatically. In Fig. 3, the central venous pressure is plotted on the ordinate, and the change of volume of blood in the systemic

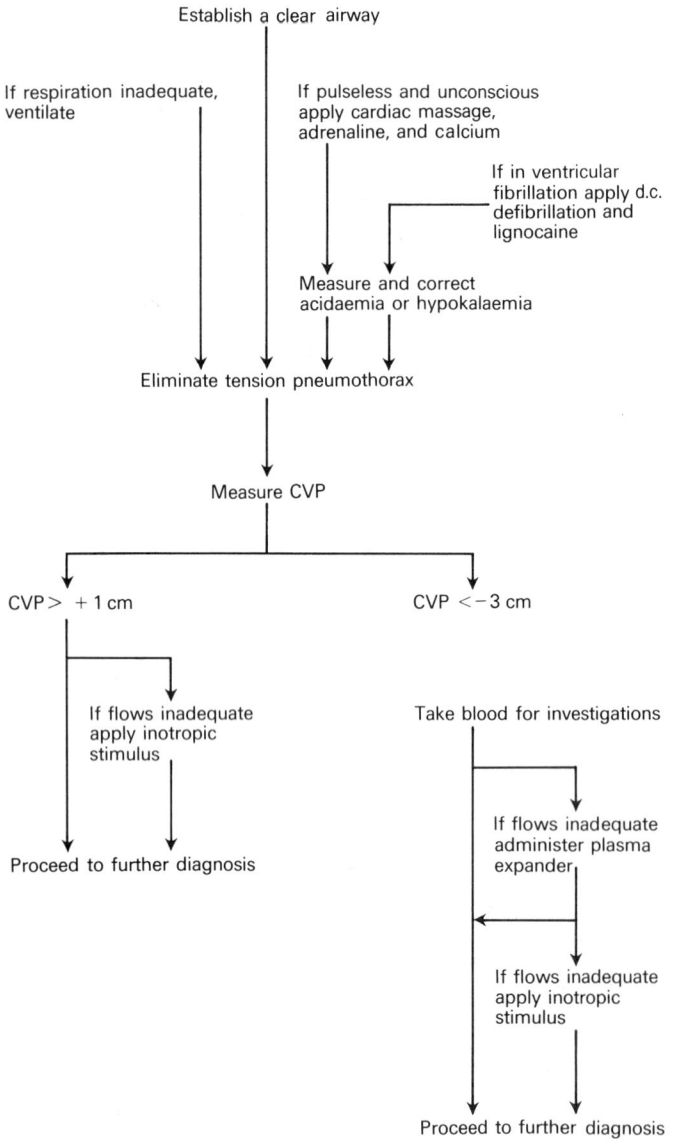

Fig. 1. A systematic approach to patients with acute circulatory disturbances: see text.

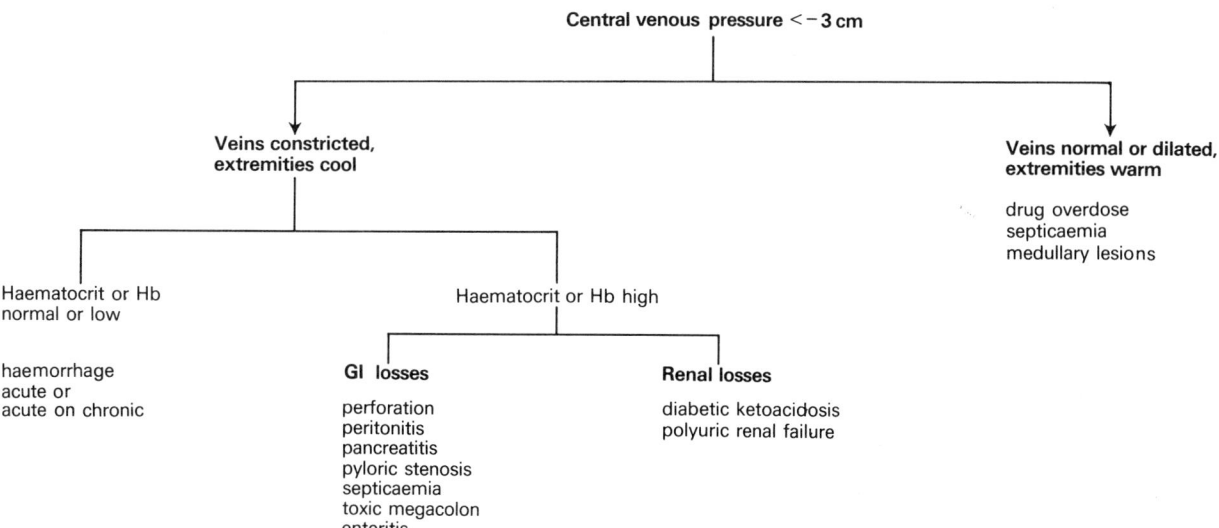

Fig. 2. The approach to patients with circulatory insufficiency where the central venous pressure is low: see text.

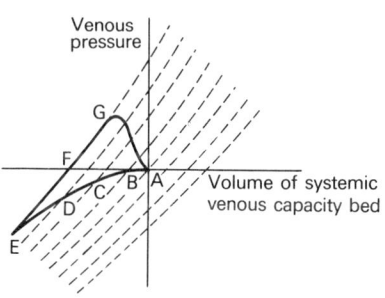

Fig. 3. As blood is removed from the circulation, the venous pressure falls little initially, but later more steeply, as the patient proceeds to lines of greater venous tone. With retransfusion the patient should follow the path EDCBA; return via EFGA may produce pulmonary oedema.

venous capacity vessels on the abscissa. Each broken line represents a line of constant venous tone (an isophleb) ranging from maximum on the left to diminished venous tone on the right. During haemorrhage, volume is lost from the venous bed, but initially the drop in venous pressure is very small as the veins constrict upon the shrinking volume; the changes are described by the line A, B, C, D, E in Fig. 3. Only latterly is there a sharp fall in the venous pressure and with it the cardiac output and arterial pressure.

In ideal circumstances during transfusion the opposite path is retraced. Events may not follow this simple course. A low cardiac output, coldness, pain, apprehension, and possibly acidaemia and hypoxia may all cause the venous system to remain tightly constricted. If the venous system remains constricted in the face of transfusion, the patient may take the path E, F, G in Fig. 3, and the venous pressure may rise to undesirably high levels before the volume of blood which was lost from the system has been replaced. The fact that the heart must generate its own blood supply causes a circulatory disturbance of a compound nature. Oligaemia and low filling pressures cause a normal heart to produce a reduced cardiac output. If these changes are gross and sustained, the impairment of coronary flow will add the complication of a failing heart with an impaired ability to generate work at any given filling pressure. Recognition of this compound disturbance depends upon the observation that restoration of the venous pressure to normal levels fails to restore the peripheral circulation.

Resolution depends upon the correction of acidaemia or hypoxia, and the administration of an inotropic stimulus. Plainly inotropic drugs given during a period of coronary underperfusion may produce myocardial damage. The damage will be reduced by breaking out of this circulatory disturbance with the minimum of delay.

High venous pressure group (+1 cm or above)
The diagnosis of patients with profound circulatory disturbance in the high venous pressure group is commonly achieved by clinical examination and inspection of the ECG and chest X-ray. In the event that it is not possible to make the diagnosis in this way or if the diagnosis requires substantiation because of the nature of the treatment to be undertaken, left and right heart catheterization and angiography are possible at the bedside within the unit. Ready availability of these facilities not only provides a lower threshold to investigation, but also allows measurements to continue to be made over a longer time course than would be possible in a catheter laboratory.

Immediate supportive measures
The immediate supportive measures available in this group are the correction of any acidaemia or hypoxia, positive pressure ventilation, and inotropic stimulation.

It has been shown that if all other variables are held constant the contractility of an isolated papillary muscle preparation varies linearly with change in pH. The correction of severe degrees of acidaemia is mandatory and because the relation referred to is linear, the aim should be a normal pH. The sodium load which this implies may require subsequent treatment.

The requirement to minimize hypoxia in the presence of a seriously impaired circulation needs no comment. The value of positive pressure ventilation in low cardiac output states has long been recognized intuitively, but there is now substantial experimental evidence, both animal and human, that circulatory performance and survival rates are both improved if the energy required for the performance of ventilation is supplied by a machine.

Diagnosis, pathological physiology, and management of patients in the high venous pressure group
The notes which follow about the conditions in this group are peculiar to the management of these problems in an intensive care unit, but the principles can be applied without elaborate facilities for measurement.

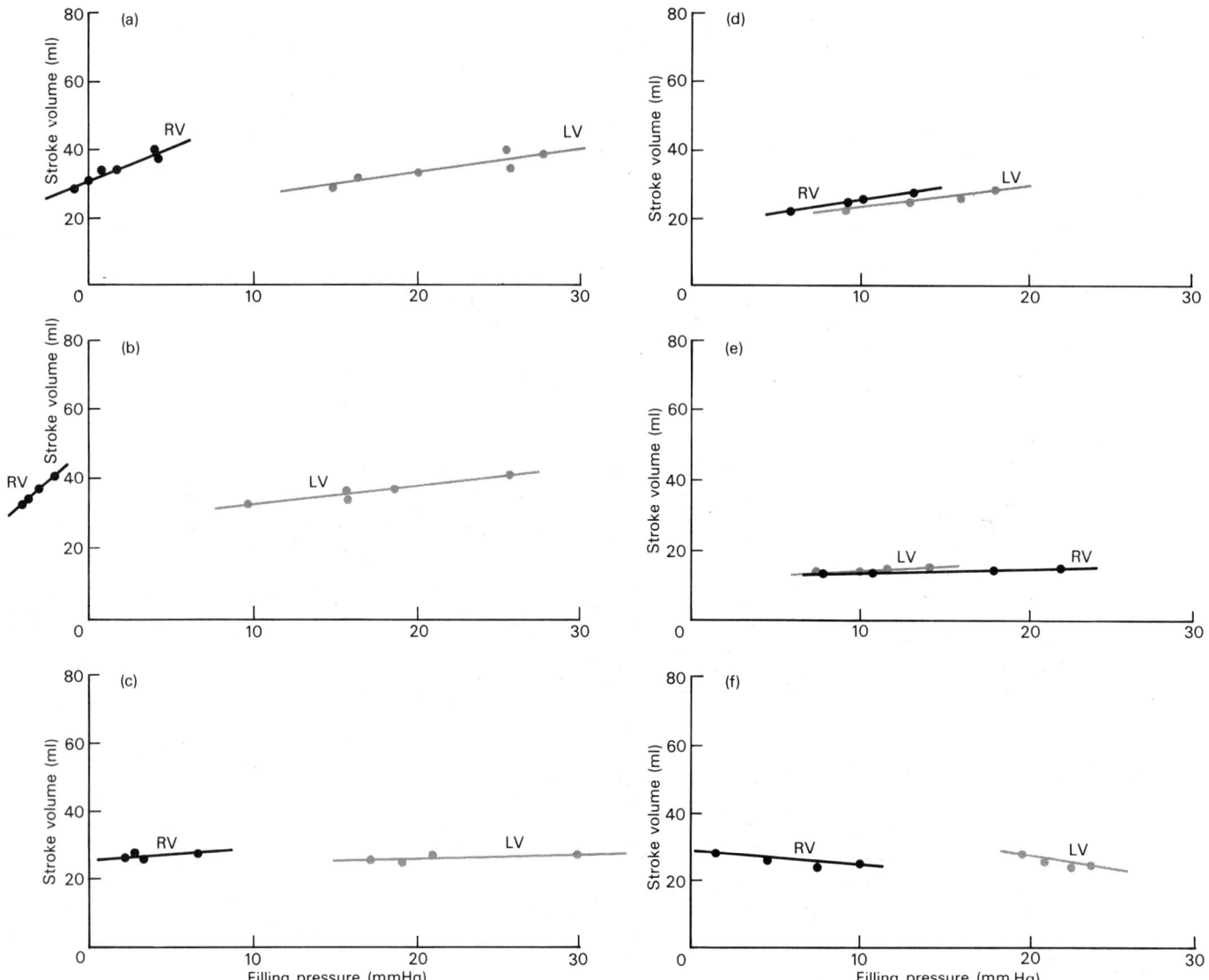

Fig. 4 (a–c) Equations of stroke volume in acute anterior myocardial infarction showing wide separation of the equations and consequent susceptibility to pulmonary oedema. (d, e) From cases of acute inferior infarction. The relation between left and right atrial pressures preserves the patient from pulmonary oedema, and reduction of the right atrial pressure will only diminish the stroke volume. (f) Inferior infarction complicated by inferior papillary dysfunction, and mitral regurgitation producing separation of the equations similar to that seen in anterior infarction.

Acute myocardial infarction

The management of dysrhythmias and heart block are dealt with elsewhere in this book (Section 13). The complications of acute myocardial infarction requiring consideration here are pulmonary oedema and impairment of the cardiac output.

Diagnosis In the great majority of cases this follows from the history and the ECG, and later confirmation is provided by an appropriate rise in enzymes.

Pathological physiology (i) The venous tone is high, and the compliance of the venous system can be measured by observing right atrial pressure (RAP) change in relation to rapid removal of volume from the circulation. In acute myocardial infarction measurements of compliance made in this way vary from 50 ml/mm Hg change in RAP to 150 ml/mm Hg: the least values relate in general to patients with lower values of cardiac output.

(ii) The relation between the filling pressure of the two sides of the heart and the flows generated is illustrated in Fig. 4. The equations of stroke volume versus filling pressure in the first three cases (a), (b), and (c) are of the pattern most commonly seen in acute

anterior or lateral myocardial infarction. The wide separation of the equations occurs because although both ventricles are damaged, the left ventricle is affected disproportionately.

Failure of a ventricle, or an increase in the resistance against which it ejects, will move its equation downward and to the right, and inotropic stimulation or a reduction in the resistance faced by the ventricle, will move its equation upward and to the left, making the gradient steeper. For these reasons worsening left ventricular performance or an increase in systemic vascular resistance separates the equations of the right and left heart, and conversely worsening right ventricular function or an increase in pulmonary vascular resistance approximates the equations.

Most commonly in acute inferior or diaphragmatic myocardial infarction both ventricles are involved with the emphasis on right ventricular damage. This results in close approximation of the left- and right-sided equations, as shown in the examples in Fig. 4d and e.

The equations shown in Fig. 4f are from a case of inferior myocardial infarction with papillary muscle dysfunction resulting in acute mitral regurgitation.

(iii) Systemic vascular resistance is the difference between mean arterial pressure and mean right atrial pressure in mm Hg divided by the cardiac output in l/min. In a normal person this gives a value of 18 units [(90–0)/5]. In cases of acute infarction this is raised to values from normal to as high as 60 units.

Pulmonary vascular resistance is the difference between mean pulmonary artery pressure and mean left atrial pressure in mm Hg divided by the cardiac output in l/min. In a normal person this gives a value close to 1 unit [(10–5)/5]. In acute myocardial infarction, the pulmonary vascular resistance may be less than normal where the left atrial pressure is high and the volume of blood in the pulmonary circuit increased. In some patients with acute infarction, who have been treated with beta blockade, the pulmonary resistance may be grossly increased to 10 or 12 units. (In the measurement of pulmonary vascular resistance it is sometimes acceptable to use pulmonary wedge pressure or left ventricular end diastolic pressure instead of the left atrial pressure).

Management In any case of heart failure there are two entirely separate issues to be considered: impairment of the cardiac output and pulmonary oedema. It is important to consider them separately, for measures which improve one may make the other worse.

Pulmonary oedema Pulmonary oedema is potentially lethal and must be treated or death will ensue from failure of ventilation due to enormous increases in the work of breathing and failure of gas exchange.

The formation of pulmonary oedema occurs as pulmonary capillary pressure rises above a critical value. The critical value is approximately $0.57 \times$ the plasma albumin level in g/l. The rate at which the oedema forms is proportional to the amount by which this value is exceeded. Once formed the rate at which pulmonary oedema will reabsorb is related principally to the amount by which the pulmonary capillary pressure is reduced below the critical value, and also partly to the level of pressure in the subclavian veins; this is because the lymphatic drainage of the lungs is into the innominate and subclavian veins.

As pulmonary capillary pressure rises, breathlessness may occur before levels which will produce oedema are reached. As the pressure rises the lung vessels become increasingly turgid due to a transfer of blood from the systemic to the pulmonary system. This causes the lungs to become stiffer and in most, but not all patients, produces the sensation of breathlessness.

The pulmonary capillary and left atrial pressure are likely to rise to levels which will engender pulmonary oedema when the pattern of damage to the heart causes wide divergence of the equations of ventricular function Fig. 4a, b, c, and f. In the example shown in Fig. 4b the disproportionate damage to the left ventricle is so extreme that negative values of right atrial pressure correspond to left atrial pressures productive of pulmonary oedema.

If the equations are close together as is commonly the case in uncomplicated inferior or diaphragmatic myocardial infarction (Fig. 4d and e) pulmonary oedema will not appear even at remarkably high right atrial pressures.

The reversal of pulmonary oedema requires that the pulmonary capillary and left atrial pressures be reduced below the critical pressure (24 mm Hg if the albumin level is 42 g/l) by a sufficient margin to produce a useful rate of reabsorption. The ratio of slopes of the equations for the left and right heart determine the degree of reduction in right atrial pressure necessary to produce the required fall in left atrial pressure. In acute anterior infarction the ratio of slopes varies from the normal 2:1 to ratios as high as 8:1. A fall in left atrial pressure of 10 mm Hg will be brought about by reducing the right atrial pressure between 1 and 5 mm Hg depending upon the ratio in the individual case.

The reduction in circulating volume needed to depress the right atrial pressure depends largely upon the systemic venous tone which is raised, and as was stated, the compliance of the system is such that removal of between 50 and 150 ml of volume are required for each mm Hg fall in right atrial pressure.

Water is distributed between the plasma space and the extracellular space in a ratio dependent upon the concentration of the plasma proteins. If the protein concentration is normal, reduction of the circulating space by 100 ml implies a removal of about 450 ml from the combined plasma and extracellular spaces.

Although the pathological physiology of anterior and lateral myocardial infarction makes the complication of pulmonary oedema likely to occur, it also makes it very senstive to treatment by the removal of relatively small volumes of salt and water, for the reasons given above.

Treatment of pulmonary oedema by removal of volume from the circulation inevitably causes a reduction in cardiac output which in its turn may be as threatening as the original pulmonary oedema. The reduction in cardiac output occurs because the ventricles generate less work as their filling pressures are reduced and because the removal of volume from the circulation increases the resistance of the systemic and pulmonary circulations. The treatment of pulmonary oedema by infusion of a sodium nitroprusside solution does not carry this penalty. The diminution in venous tone which it produces reduces right and left atrial pressures and ventricular stroke work, but this is offset by a fall in systemic and pulmonary resistance and a modest increase in heart rate. The penalty is a lower arterial pressure and diminished coronary perfusion pressure; a consequent increased mortality has been demonstrated. Positive pressure ventilation and the sedation which accompanies it produce similar circulatory changes to those of sodium nitroprusside with the reservation that the changes in pulmonary vascular resistance are variable and difficult to interpret. This approach to treatment has considerable advantage in the presence of a marginal cardiac output; the greatly increased work of ventilation no longer has to be provided by the patient. Patients with papillary muscle dysfunction (Fig. 4f) may be responsive to any measure which reduces left ventricular volume. The negative sloping equations of stroke volume in response to a diminution in atrial pressures seen in this case as a result of removal of volume from the circulation, are only explicable either as errors of measurement, or that each of the points obtained must lie on a separate equation with a positive slope, which increases as volume is removed.

Positive pressure ventilation and sedation have certainly proved very effective in relieving the acute mitral regurgitation in these patients. The physical signs change with dramatic speed, the left atrial pressure falls and the stroke volume equations move together again into the configuration most commonly seen in diaphragmatic myocardial infarction. Provided that the papillary muscle does not rupture, these patients can be weaned from the ventilator as their infarct matures, using vasodilators to continue the afterload reduction. It is important that they be kept relatively well sedated at the time of removal from the ventilator, in contrast to normal practice. If the papillary muscle ruptures it is sometimes possible to contain the pulmonary oedema with positive pressure ventilation, sedation, and vasodilators. If these manoeuvres fail, the afterload reduction can be augmented by balloon counterpulsation. The aim is to support the patient for long enough from the time of infarction for surgical replacement of the mitral valve to be possible.

Impairment of cardiac output There are five approaches to increasing a cardiac output critically impaired by myocardial infarction.

Firstly, the heart rate can be increased with atropine or with atrial pacing; the latter is more easily controlled and can be continued over many days. In practice it is found that in badly failing hearts, with relatively flat performance equations, cardiac output rises linearly with heart rate up to rates just over 100/min, but diminishes at higher rates. Myocardial oxygen consumption is very closely related to the proportion of time spent in systole, and therefore to rate.

Secondly, the cardiac output can be increased by raising the

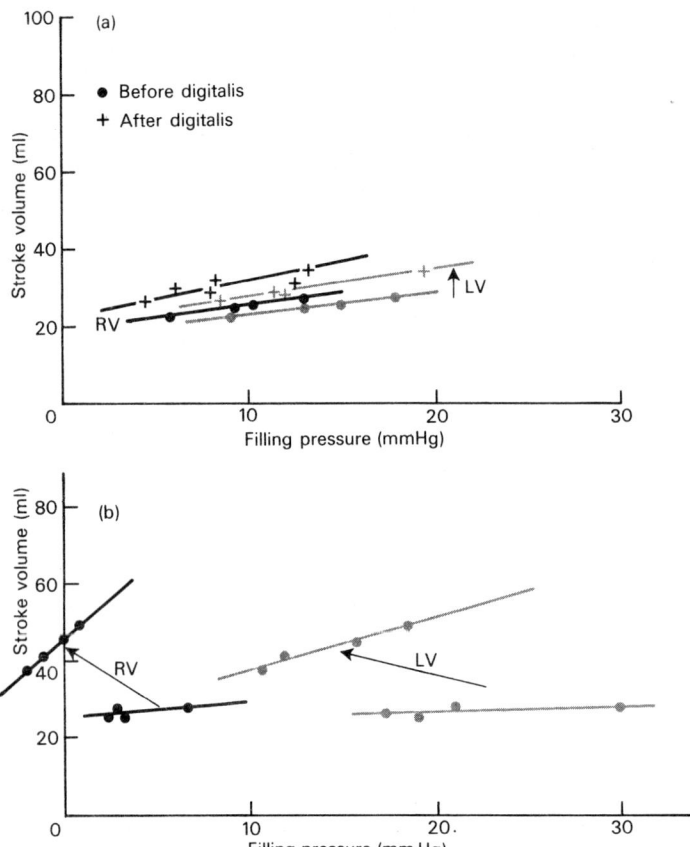

Fig. 5. (a) The effect of digitalization contrasted with (b) stimulation with isoprenaline in patients with acute myocardial infarction. Isoprenaline produces a greater shift of the equations upward and to the left.

filling pressures of the two sides of the heart. This is of least value when most needed, because the equations relating filling pressure to stroke volume become flatter as the damage to the ventricles increases. In the worst cases, the gain is negligible. This manoeuvre produces the most strikingly beneficial results in those whose hearts still have useful positive sloping equations, but whose cardiac outputs have been reduced to grossly inadequate levels with diuretics. The case of inferior myocardial infarction illustrated in Fig. 5a has a cardiac output of 1.9 l/min at a right atrial pressure of 6 mm Hg, rising to 2.4 l/min at a right atrial pressure of 13 mm Hg. This very high level of right atrial pressure is tolerable because the corresponding left-sided filling pressure is 18 mm Hg. The configuration of the left- and right-sided equations most commonly associated with acute inferior myocardial infarction protects them from pulmonary oedema. *If there is no pulmonary oedema treatment of a high venous pressure with diuretics is harmful because it will reduce the cardiac output.* If the filling pressures of the left and right heart are raised with a plasma expander, the expansion of the systemic and pulmonary beds will also reduce their resistance. In the case of the overdiuresed small volume circulation this is a very important effect.

Thirdly, an inotropic stimulus may be given which will increase the work generated by the ventricles at any given filling pressure. Examples of agents which have this action are calcium, adrenaline, isoprenaline, dopamine, dobutamine, and digoxin (Section 13). Some of these agents are more powerful than others; Fig. 5 illustrates the relative effects of digoxin and isoprenaline. It is a general truth that the worse the performance of the heart, the less its response to any inotropic agent; this is shown in Fig. 6 and relates to the fact that with increasing damage there is less surviving muscle to respond. Acidaemia and hyperkalaemia impair the

response to these agents, which all have the disadvantage that they are likely to increase the extent of an existing infarction by increasing myocardial oxygen demand.

There are some patients who, following infarction have sufficient potentially viable myocardium to survive, but whose cardiac output and coronary perfusion are temporarily reduced to levels which will not allow that survival. This often follows an acute dysrhythmia which has either reverted spontaneously or with treatment. Inotropic agents are the only rapidly effective method of breaking out of this circle, which exists because the heart must generate its own blood supply. The inotropic agents undoubtedly cause damage, but without them the patient will not survive.

At the other extreme there are patients with insufficient heart muscle to permit survival however they are treated. Between these two groups, there is an area of present uncertainty where the use of inotropic agents may, in spite of their known harmful effects, prevent patients entering a cycle from which they cannot escape because of inadequate perfusion.

Fourthly, cardiac output can be increased by diminishing the resistance of the pulmonary and systemic circuits. It should be remembered that the physiological concept of increasing flows by diminishing the ventricular afterload assumes that the filling pressure of the ventricle is kept constant. If vasodilators such as sodium nitroprusside are used to increase flows in contradistinction to the control of pulmonary oedema, it should be remembered that they are also venodilators, and a plasma expander will be required to maintain the right and left atrial pressures; this combined therapy minimizes the drop in coronary perfusion pressure. As already pointed out a volume expander will enhance the reduction of systemic and pulmonary resistance, this effect is especially marked if the resistance values are very high or where the circulating volume is small.

Sodium nitroprusside and the longer term orally administered drug prazosin both markedly reduce myocardial oxygen consumption, and are particularly valuable in the presence of a dilated left ventricle, their hypotensive effect being then less marked.

Fifthly, cardiac output may be increased by counterpulsation with an intra-aortic balloon. This technique might be grouped with agents operating by reduction of afterload. Like those agents it produces a marked drop in myocardial oxygen consumption, but in addition some of the energy required to drive blood around the systemic circulation is derived from the filling of the balloon. The physiological changes produced by counterpulsation both in the internal and external economy of the heart are all beneficial pro-

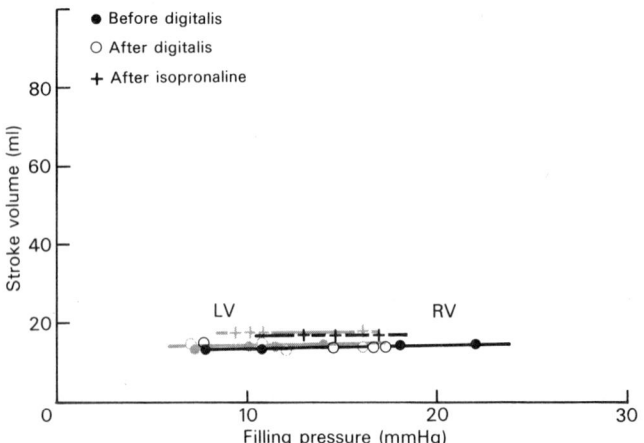

Fig. 6. With extreme impairment of function the stroke volume equations (●) are flat, so that stroke volume cannot be increased by adjustment of the filling pressures. Digitalization (○) produces no change, and isoprenaline (+) a very modest elevation of the equations.

ducing an increase of cardiac output of the order of 0.5 l/min at a considerably lower myocardial oxygen consumption. Yet the application of the technique in the field of acute myocardial infarction has been of limited value.

Experience has shown that the majority of patients suffering acute infarction *who are unable to survive without counterpulsation* cannot be weaned from its support. Moreover those few with massive myocardial damage who have been supported and weaned from counterpulsation have a very limited prognosis (Section 13).

There are two relatively rare complications of acute myocardial infarction in which balloon counterpulsation is of value in supporting the patient until surgical treatment can be undertaken. These are papillary muscle rupture already considered in this section, and rupture of the interventricular septum. Counterpulsation is effective in reducing the run-off into the left atrium or the right ventricle, and increasing the proportion of left ventricular ejection which goes to the aorta.

Massive acute pulmonary embolism

(See Section 13.)

Many patients die with pulmonary emboli present in their lungs, but relatively few die due to pulmonary embolism. The incidence of life threatening embolism is relatively small.

Diagnosis

The diagnosis of pulmonary embolism can only be made with certainty by pulmonary angiography. Isotopic scanning techniques may be suggestive of the diagnosis but do not offer the degree of certainty necessary before embolectomy can be undertaken.

Pulmonary angiography can be accomplished very rapidly at the bedside using a portable image intensifier and a video recording system. Examples of angiograms obtained in this manner are shown in Fig. 7. Catheterization of the pulmonary artery through a sheath placed in the internal jugular vein by Seldinger's technique has the advantage of ease of manipulation of the catheter to the pulmonary artery, compared to the more conventional approach through the femoral vein, which may harbour a further clot.

Pathological physiology of acute massive pulmonary embolism

(i) The venous tone is very greatly raised probably as a response to the gross impairment of cardiac output. The compliance of the system may be as little as 30 ml volume change/mm Hg·change in the right atrial pressure.

(ii) The relation between the filling pressure of the two sides of the heart and the flows generated is illustrated in Fig. 8. A considerably raised pulmonary vascular resistance and a reduction in right ventricular stroke work in relation to filling pressure, conspire to move the right ventricular equation relating stroke volume to filling pressure so far downward and to the right from its normal position, that it moves through the left ventricular equation and comes to lie upon its far side. This has consequences of the greatest importance.

The depression of right ventricular stroke work is related to an acute change in ventricular diameter which interferes with the generation of tension in the wall of the ventricle in a manner which might be expected from the application of Laplace's law.

(iii) The pulmonary vascular resistance in the presence of an acute life-threatening pulmonary embolus is usually in the range 12 to 16 units. Higher values up to 25 units can be sustained with chronic packed pulmonary emboli because the right ventricle is hypertrophied.

The systemic vascular resistance is raised to values between 25 and 50 units with the result that the systemic arterial pressure is better preserved than the cardiac output. The fact that the blood pressure may be only moderately reduced should not militate

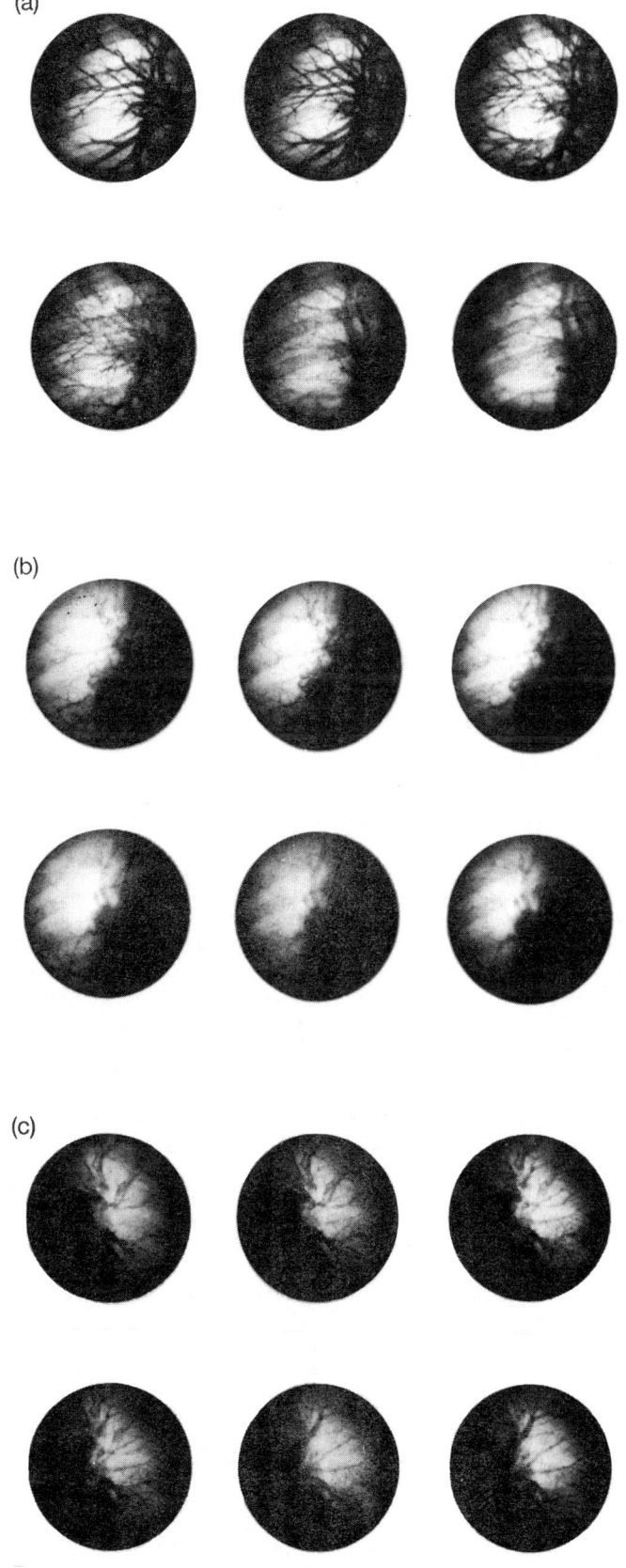

Fig. 7. Frames from bedside pulmonary angiograms using portable image intensifier (Siemens Siremobil 2) and video-recorder (International Video Recorders). (a) A near-normal right lung. (b) The right lung of the patient showing near-complete obstruction. (c) Left lung of same patient showing considerable obstruction with pulmonary emboli.

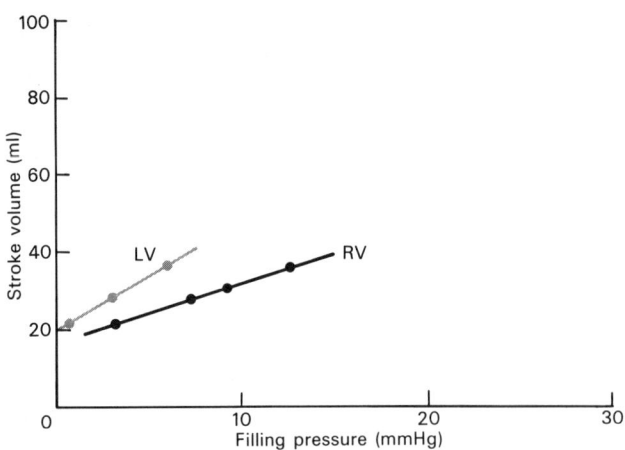

Fig. 8. The equations of stroke volume in acute pulmonary embolism are laterally transposed.

against the diagnosis nor should it be allowed to engender a false sense of security.

The doubling of systemic resistance is a reflex response probably triggered by the very considerable impairment of cardiac output. There is some evidence that the increase in pulmonary resistance to values over ten times normal is in part reflexly engendered, and not entirely related to obstruction of the vessels by emboli.

Management

Patients with acute pulmonary embolism in whom the right atrial pressure is found to be in excess of 15 mm Hg are in an unstable circulatory state which can only be controlled with sufficient rapidity by pulmonary embolectomy. Providing that cardiopulmonary bypass can be instituted before cardiac arrest occurs, there is a very good chance of success.

The threat to life in massive pulmonary embolism depends upon the reduction of cardiac output which follows obstruction of the pulmonary circulation, and the circulation can be manipulated to diminish the degree of obstruction without surgical removal of the embolus. The essence of this manipulation is the expansion of the remaining pulmonary vascular bed with a volume expander such as plasma. This manoeuvre will reduce considerably the very high pulmonary vascular resistance which is the central problem. Two effects are involved: the raising of the right atrial pressure from 3 to values of 12 or 15 mm Hg increases the work output of the right heart (See Fig. 9), and, more importantly, distribution of some of the administered plasma into the pulmonary circulation reduces the pulmonary vascular resistance by as much as one half. As will be seen from Fig. 8 the elevation of right atrial pressure produces a considerable increase in cardiac output without the production of pulmonary oedema because the left atrial pressure is very much lower than the right. Oedema may appear subsequently when flow is restored, in that part of the pulmonary circulation which was obstructed. This is probably due to damage to the basement membrane, for it occurs at low pulmonary capillary pressures.

The administration of inotropic agents will increase the work output of the heart and improve flows. Their use increases the importance of minimizing hypoxaemia and acidaemia. Digitalization is a valuable insurance against the appearance of atrial flutter or fibrillation, which are common in pulmonary embolism.

Volume expansion, inotropic stimulation, and oxygen may be sufficient to stabilize the patient's circulation whilst the natural process of thrombolysis takes place. Where there is no risk of provoking haemorrhage the thrombolytic process can be accelerated with streptokinase or urokinase.

Equally important in the management of these patients is the

avoidance of measures having the opposite physiological effects. Sedation, diuretics, haemorrhage, the induction of anaesthesia, vena caval ligation, and the administration of contrast material during angiography may all precipitate the patient's death by reducing the right atrial pressure. The sequence of events is as follows: the fall in right atrial pressure decreases the stroke volume pumped into the lungs, the matching fall in stroke volume from the left heart only occurs when there has been a net transfer of blood out of the pulmonary circulation, causing the left atrial pressure to fall. The loss of volume from the pulmonary bed causes a further sharp rise in its resistance which with the diminished right ventricular stroke work still further reduces the right ventricular output. Unless this chain of events is interrupted it must end in circulatory arrest. The changes can be prevented by maintaining the right atrial pressure with volume expanders and the stimulation of venous tone with alpha agonists such as phenylephrine. For similar reasons it is important to avoid drugs which have a negative inotropic effect including those which reduce the patient's own catechol secretion.

The measures described above do not detract from the need for heparinization and venous ligation to diminish the chances of further embolization.

Cardiac tamponade

(See also Section 13.)

The critical physiological disturbance which appears with tamponade is impairment of cardiac output by interference with the filling of the heart.

Diagnosis

The clinical physical signs of restlessness, oliguria, breathlessness, and hypotension stem from the diminished cardiac output. The systolic descent in the venous pressure is due to a fall in pressure in the pericardial sac at the time of ventricular ejection. Pulsus paradoxus, which is not paradoxical but an exaggeration of a normal phenomenon, when it appears in tamponade, is principally due to failure of transmission of the intrathoracic pressure swings to the left atrium. During inspiration the fall in intrathoracic pressure is transmitted to the pulmonary veins; if this fall is not also transmitted to the left atrium it will produce a diminution in the effective filling pressure of the left heart, and a fall in arterial pressure. The absence of pulsus paradoxus does not exclude the presence of tamponade, neither does the presence of a pericardial rub exclude a large pericardial effusion.

Echocardiographic confirmation of a pericardial effusion, although usually correct, is not always so, whereas a right atrial angiogram is a definitive investigation if the patient has a large

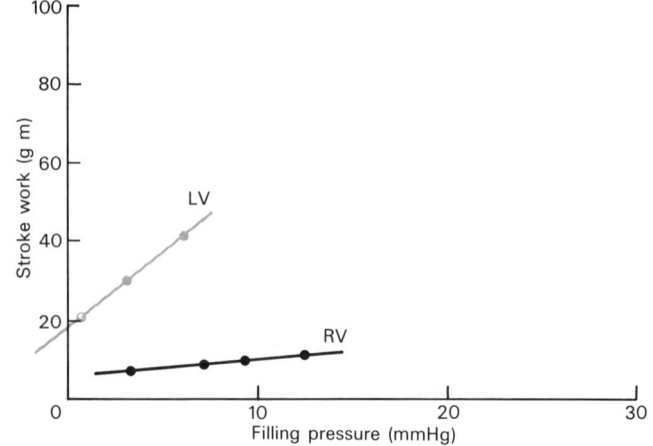

Fig. 9. The equations of stroke work in acute pulmonary embolism.

(a)

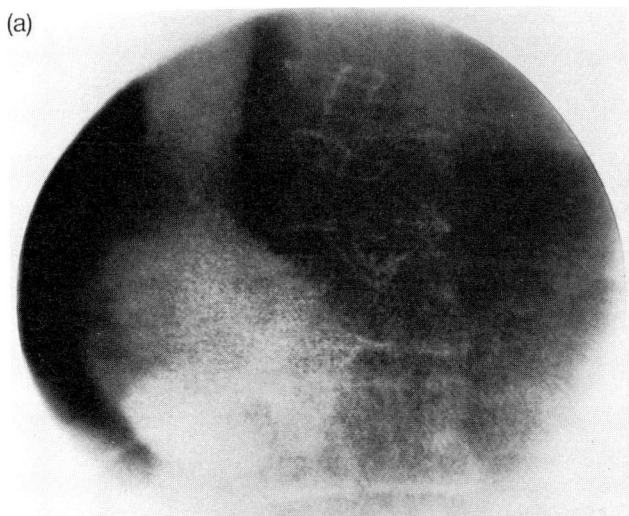

(b)

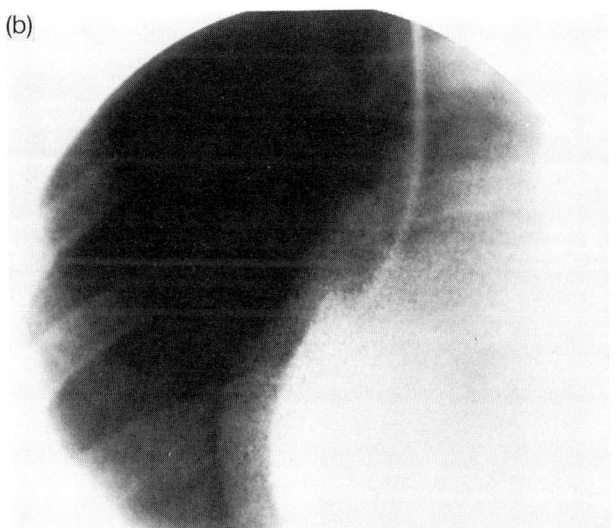

Fig. 10. Right atrial angiograms from (a) a normal and (b) a case of tamponade.

enough pericardial volume to produce tamponade. Figure 10 compares a normal with a case of tamponade.

Pathological physiology
The venous tone is high. The equations of function of the left and right heart move together and eventually are coincident as tamponade worsens, and the systemic vascular resistance is high.

Management
Until the effusion is drained cardiac output can only be sustained by maintaining high right and left atrial pressures. In the limiting case these may both be as high as 15 mm Hg.

The safety of the procedure of tapping the pericardium has been much enchanced by not attempting to drain the fluid through the needle with which the puncture is made, but by replacing the needle with a soft catheter over a Seldinger guide wire. The catheter should have multiple side holes, and it is possible by the use of dilators and sleeves in conjunction with the Seldinger guide wire to introduce a drain of appreciable size.

If because of clotting it is impossible to remove the pericardial fluid in the above manner, or if it is probable that an actively bleeding vessel requires to be controlled, a surgical approach is necessary.

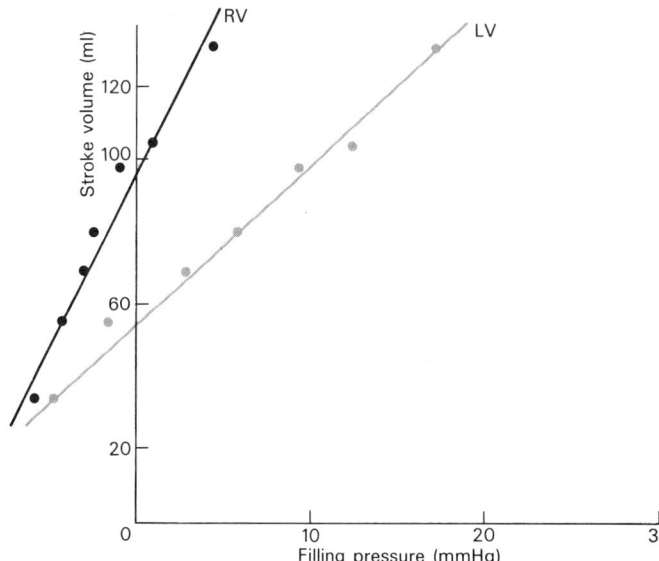

Fig. 11. Equations of stroke volume in relation to filling pressure for the left and right heart of a patient with a normal heart.

Overtransfusion
(See also Section 19.)

The critical lesion which appears in overtransfusion is the appearance of pulmonary oedema. The diagnosis depends principally upon the realization that sufficient fluid may have been administered.

Pathological physiology
Initially the circulation may be characterized as follows:–

(a) The venous tone is low and the compliance of the system may be as great as 300 to 350 ml volume change/mm Hg right atrial pressure change. The venous pressure is moderately raised in spite of this because of the very large circulating volume.

(b) The equations of function of the two sides of the heart are normal (Fig. 11) and the cardiac output greatly raised in response to the raised filling pressures.

(c) The pulmonary and systemic vascular resistance are reduced.

(d) The rate at which pulmonary oedema appears in the lungs is proportional to the amount by which the critical pulmonary capillary pressure has been exceeded. The critical pulmonary capillary pressure is related to albumin concentration ($0.57 \times$ plasma albumin in g/l), which may well have been greatly reduced, depending upon the nature of the transfusional insult.

If the pulmonary oedema is allowed to accumulate unchecked, this pattern changes so that the venous tone rises, driving the right atrial pressure to values as high as 25 mm Hg, and the equations of function of both sides of the heart move towards those of extreme failure (Fig. 12) and the cardiac output dwindles from its previous elevated levels to grossly impaired values.

Management
In the initial phase described, the pulmonary oedema will probably be brought under control by lowering the left atrial pressure by 12 mm Hg. The relative slopes of the equations of a normal heart imply that this will be achieved by a fall of half this magnitude in the right atrial pressure. The compliance of the system is such that this will entail removal of approximately 2 litres from the circulation. If the distribution of fluid between the circulation and extracellular space were normal this would necessitate the removal of as much as 6 or 7 litres of fluid from the combined spaces. A diuresis of this size takes time to accomplish, and for this reason if the situation is threatening, rapid control can be obtained by removing 1.5 to 2 litres of blood from the circulation.

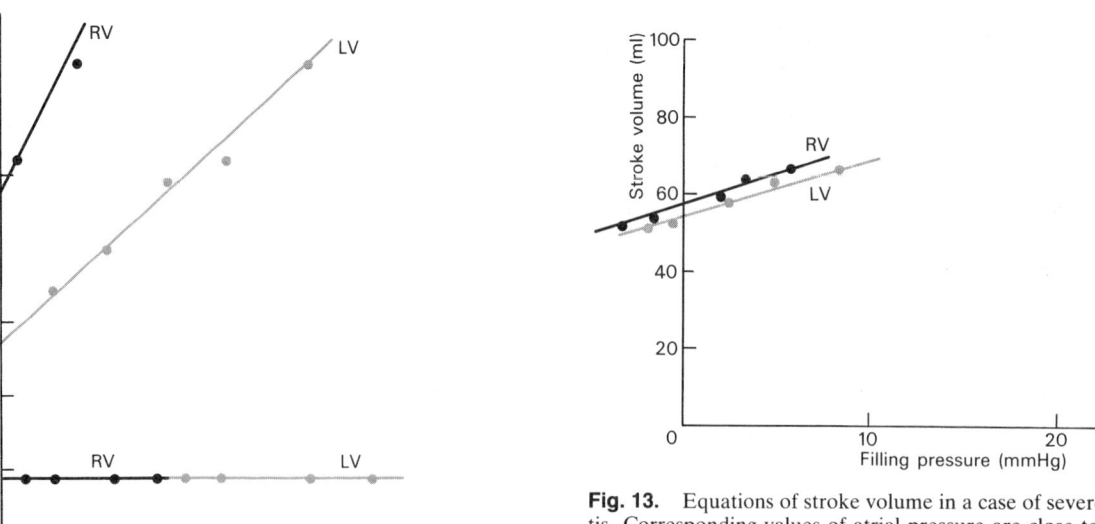

Fig. 12. Stroke volume equations of a case of extreme pump failure compared with those of a normal.

This can be stored in order that the red cells and albumin can be returned to the patient as the matter is brought in hand by diuresis. The volume and nature of the fluid to be removed and its distribution between the body compartments will vary with the nature of the infused fluid which caused the problem.

If the insult has reached the physiological stage at which the right atrial pressure is inordinately high, the patient should be ventilated, inotropic agents infused, and the left-sided filling pressure (pulmonary wedge pressure or left ventricular end diastolic pressure) controlled by circulatory volume adjustment at a level which will allow the slow reabsorption of the pulmonary oedema.

The circulatory failure associated with obstructive airways disease

(See also Section 15.)

The term cor pulmonale is not used because this may be taken to include pulmonary embolism which creates a different pattern of physiological disturbance.

The critical lesion in asthma and chronic bronchitis is obstruction of the airways and adjustment of the circulation should be directed toward relief of the obstruction.

Diagnosis

The diagnosis is made from the obvious physical signs of obstructive airways disease in the presence of a raised arterial carbon dioxide tension and lowered arterial oxygen tension, whilst the patient is breathing air.

Pathological physiology

Patients in a stable circulatory state with obstructive airways disease show the following features:

(*a*) The venous tone is very much less raised than in severe pulmonary embolism, the compliance of the system being of the order 150 ml volume change/mm Hg change in right atrial pressure. The raised venous pressure is principally due to water and salt retention. This contrast with acute pulmonary embolism may relate to the passage of sufficient time to allow the water retention to occur.

(*b*) The important features of the performance of the heart in obstructive airway disease are illustrated by the equations in Figs 13 and 14. In contrast to pulmonary embolism the cardiac output generated is normal or raised depending upon filling pressure. The equations of stroke volume of the right and left heart are

Fig. 13. Equations of stroke volume in a case of severe chronic bronchitis. Corresponding values of atrial pressure are close together due to the coincidence of a raised pulmonary vascular resistance (PVR 4 units) and a low systemic resistance (SVR 15 units), in the presence of normal stroke work equations (Fig. 14) for both sides of the heart. The important difference between this patient and cases of pulmonary embolism is the very much higher values of stroke volume.

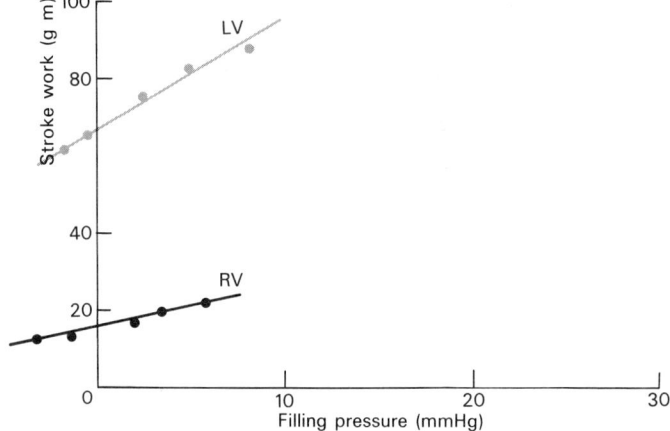

Fig. 14. The stroke work equations for both left and right heart of the patient with severe chronic bronchitis.

moved into close apposition. That of the right heart is moved to the right by the combined influences of a raised pulmonary vascular resistance and right ventricular dilation and that of the left heart is moved to the left by a lower than normal systemic vascular resistance. The consequences of these changes are a relatively good cardiac output and immunity from pulmonary oedema over a wide range of filling pressures.

(*c*) The pulmonary vascular resistance is moderately elevated to values of the order four to eight times normal, and the systemic resistance reduced (14 to 16 units), perhaps due to hypercapnia.

The above circulatory state may be destabilized by a number of events which are probably most commonly precipitated by extremes of hypoxaemia. The obvious signal that the patient has entered this unstable state and is likely to die within a few hours is coldness of the limbs. The physiological nature of this change is that terminally the patient's heart is failing and its equations of performance are falling.

Management

In the stable state described above, the optimal conditions are achieved by reducing the patient's atrial pressures to values around zero. Although cardiac output will be less at these values than at the naturally occurring values of between 5 and 10 mm Hg, circulatory flows are not the major problem, and the airway obstruction, which is critical, is improved by reducing the atrial pressures. The improvement in airway resistance may be due to a reduction of the pressure in the system into which the lymphatics from the bronchial mucosa drain.

The relative compliance of the venous system, and the distribution of the retained salt and water imply that a relatively large diuresis is required – 3.5 litres to lower the right atrial pressure by 7 mm Hg.

The avoidance of treating such patients with high concentrations of oxygen in the inspired air in order to preserve their ventilatory drive has been greatly stressed. It is no less important to avoid the extremes of hypoxaemia which by raising pulmonary vascular resistance and depressing ventricular function are likely to induce the unstable circulatory state discussed above. Once the patient enters this cycle of depression of cardiac function evidenced by coldness of the limbs, reversal of the trend can only be induced by positive pressure ventilation and inotropic stimulation. The decision to adopt such measures must depend upon judgements of the degree of reversability of the patient's airways disease.

The artificial ventilation of patients with airway obstruction of this degree presents special difficulties essentially because any further rise in functional residual capacity of the lungs produces a sharp rise in pulmonary vascular resistance. This will be discussed in the section of this chapter dealing with positive pressure ventilation (page 14.12).

Septicaemia and the circulation

The most important feature of circulatory derangement due to sepsis is the intense variability of the nature of the disturbances produced, not only between different patients but often in the same patient as a function of time. Therapy that is at one moment beneficial may become harmful, and logical treatment can only be applied upon a background of continuing analysis of the circulation.

Diagnosis

The diagnosis should be suggested by the occurrence of hypotension in the presence of any infective process (see Section 5).

Pathological physiology

(a) The venous pressure is determined by the interaction of the venous tone and the volume contained within the circulation, and in the presence of sepsis the venous tone may be abnormally high or low, the compliance of the system may be as little as 50 ml or as great at 350 ml volume change/mm Hg change in right atrial pressure. Similarly the circulating volume may be disturbed in either direction. Oligaemia may be produced by the loss of fluid containing albumin into the peritoneal cavity or distended loops of bowel. Oliguric renal failure and overgenerous intravenous therapy are common causes of an opposite volume change.

(b) The heart may be normal or may fail in the sense that it produces less work from both ventricles in relation to their filling pressure. A normal ventricle will show a moderate diminution in stroke work in response to afterload reduction, but the impairment of stroke work seen in many of the patients with sepsis has been massive. In contrast others with sepsis in whom the systemic vascular resistance has been reduced to one-third of normal have retained normal stroke work equations. It seems reasonable to conclude that in some the heart muscle is affected, and in others not. This assessment is the only arbiter of heart failure in these circumstances; the significance of the venous pressure is often in doubt because of the many influences described.

(c) The systemic vascular resistance may be as low as 2 units or

may be considerably raised, and the pulmonary vascular resistance may be altered in either direction.

The venous tone and systemic vascular resistance do usually vary in the same direction, and when both are raised in association with depressed ventricular stroke work, produce all the accepted physical signs of heart failure: a high venous pressure, deficient cardiac output, and sometimes a high enough left atrial pressure to generate pulmonary oedema.

The fact that the heart is failing may be obscured where deficient ventricular function is associated with a low venous tone and systemic vascular resistance, because the venous pressure is not raised and the cardiac output may be as high as 10 or 12 l/min. These relatively high flows are generated by a defective heart because the resistance to flow may be as little as one-tenth of normal.

(d) Pulmonary oedema may occur in sepsis because of a raised left atrial and pulmonary capillary pressure, or because of damage to the capillary basement membrane in which case the oedema appears at normal pulmonary capillary pressures and has a protein content approximating to that of the plasma. Very commonly pulmonary oedema is iatrogenic stemming from unavailing attempts to restore the arterial blood pressure to normal in the face of a grossly reduced systemic vascular resistance.

(e) Perhaps the most bizarre of all the unpredictable changes observable in the presence of sepsis is the breakdown of the normal distribution of blood flow to individual organs.

Aortography of a patient with sepsis showed the vessels of the coeliac axis and the renal arteries to be so constricted that they did not fill with contrast medium in spite of a seemingly more than adequate cardiac output of 7 l/min. The patient was anuric at the time of the investigation, and at post-mortem all the vessels in question appeared normally patent. These focal abnormalities of distribution of flow can be observed to change very much with time, and are perhaps responsible for the generation of severe degrees of metabolic acidosis which appear in sepsis in the presence of more than adequate values of cardiac output.

(f) Any of these changes may be further compounded by the appearance of a consumptive coagulopathy.

Management
(See also Section 5.)

The one therapeutic manoeuvre of unequivocal value is the administration of appropriate antibiotics in adequate dosage *without delay*. Delay is important because of the rate at which bacteria multiply; it may be much reduced if a stock of blood culture medium is readily available.

Life-threatening septicaemia may be due to a single organism as is commonly the case with pneumococcal, meningococcal, streptococcal, and staphylococcal infections. If these are strongly suspected or proven, treatment with a single appropriate antibiotic is allowable. This is not the case with septicaemias secondary to intestinal perforations where although blood cultures may yield a single organism, there are likely to be multiple organisms, and contamination of the circulation is likely to be continued. It is illogical to accept that failure to grow an organism excludes its presence; anaerobic organisms were the cause of septicaemia before techniques were available for their culture.

In the absence of a clear indication that a single organism is involved, broad-spectrum antibiotic cover is required and should only be changed if an insensitive organism is grown. Negative blood cultures are not a logical reason for changing or stopping antibiotic therapy in a patient with the circulatory hallmarks of sepsis; rather they are an indication of some measure of control being achieved with the existing therapy.

Oligaemia due to loss of protein-containing fluid from the circulation is best treated with plasma, and the heart failure which is very commonly present in severe sepsis, but unrecognized clinically because the venous pressure may not be raised for the reasons already discussed, is best treated with inotropic agents.

Adjustments of the right- and left-sided filling pressures to produce optimal flows without risk of pulmonary oedema should be made for both oligaemia and heart failure.

In the presence of severe hypotension due to sepsis it is impossible to tell clinically whether the systemic vascular resistance is high or low, the matter can only be analysed by invasive measurement. When the resistance is below 7 units the distribution of perfusion is very severely deranged and infusions of alpha-agonists such as noradrenaline can be used to raise the resistance and paradoxically may restore urine flow and warmth to cold limbs. If the systemic resistance is raised by these means to values between 10 and 15, the heart continues to enjoy the benefits of afterload reduction.

In those cases where the systemic vascular resistance is found to be raised, a sodium nitroprusside infusion affords an easily controllable degree of dilation. Most commonly these patients also have depressed myocardial function, in which case dobutamine offers both a positive inotropic effect and systemic vasodilation, and low-dose dopamine may have the additional benefit of increasing renal blood flow.

Corticosteroids in high dosage have been said to improve the distribution of bloodflow, and to stabilize damaged capillary endothelia, reducing leakage of plasma from the vascular compartment. *A large multicentre, double blind, randomized trial, soon to be published, shows steroids to be of no benefit, and to be associated with a higher mortality in patients with the syndrome of severe circulatory derangement due to sepsis. Provided that the atrial pressures are controlled, steroids have no effect on cardiac output, systemic vascular resistance or arterial pressure. The present balance of evidence suggests that steroids should not be used in this condition.*

Acute dissections of the thoracic aorta

The important possible circulatory consequences of aortic dissection are obstruction of any of the branches of the aorta, aortic regurgitation, and haemorrhage into the pleural or pericardial space; the latter may result in cardiac tamponade.

Diagnosis

The history of a sudden agonizing pain in the chest or abdomen may be associated with symptoms or signs relating to obstruction of any of the aortic branches. The chest X-ray may show a widened mediastinal shadow or pleural effusion, but definitive diagnosis depends upon aortic angiography which is possible with relatively little disturbance to a well-sedated patient, as a bedside manoeuvre. Catheterization of the true aortic lumen may entail the use of unusual approach sites such as the axillary arteries, and confirmation that the catheter lies in the true aortic lumen depends upon retrograde passage across the aortic valve to the left ventricle (Fig. 15).

Pathological physiology

The angular shearing forces which act to extend an existing fault or tear in the aortic lining are related to the wavelength of the harmonics which go to make up the pressure pulse propagated along the aorta by the heart. The shorter the tear and the greater the length of the pulse wave the less likely it becomes that the tear will extend.

Management

Medical treatment is directed toward control of the hypertension that is so often an antecedent factor in the causation of aortic dissection, and the attenuation of the pulse wave by interference with the rate of ventricular ejection by beta blockade. The trials of medical treatment suggest that the systolic arterial pressure should be reduced to 100 mm Hg provided the patient continues to pass more than 30 ml urine per hour.

Intense beta blockade with propranolol and hypotensive agents

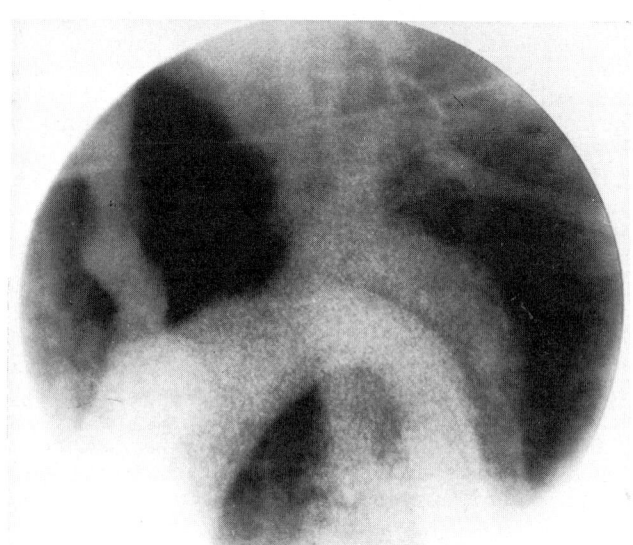

Fig. 15. Aortic angiogram of an acute aortic dissection obtained with portable equipment at the bedside.

which are effective in the recumbent posture provoke water and salt retention which in turn may make control of the hypertension more difficult. Minoxidil may achieve control when other agents fail but is particularly prone to produce fluid retention. Physical considerations suggest that depression of the rate of ventricular ejection is the most important factor.

A recent trial of medical and surgical treatment demonstrated that for dissections originating in the ascending aorta, surgical treatment had a considerable advantage. For aortic dissections originating in the region of the left subclavian artery medical and surgical treatment offered a very similar mortality. Failure of perfusion of a major organ or limb is always an indication for a surgical approach.

Positive pressure ventilation

Positive pressure ventilation has been in use in the treatment of ventilatory failure for 25 years. The effectiveness of the technique increased very considerably when valves which allow the pressure in the system to be maintained at a level above atmospheric throughout the ventilatory cycle became available.

The mechanical arrangements of ventilators differ; those that are volume cycled inflate the lungs by the volume selected, whereas pressure cycled ventilators achieve a tidal volume which is the resultant of the compliance of the patient's lungs and chest wall on the one hand and the pressure to which the ventilator is set to inflate them on the other.

Both types of ventilator, and various subdivisions within each group can be manipulated by the physician to achieve the same end in terms of the amount of ventilation delivered and the manner of its delivery. The matching of the pattern of ventilation delivered, and the disturbance of the patient's pulmonary physiology, is therefore largely independent of the type of ventilator which is used.

Indications for mechanical ventilation

The indications for the employment of positive pressure ventilation embrace all those conditions which may cause ventilatory failure. Delay in its institution commonly adds the problems of renal failure and cerebral oedema because widespread damage has usually occurred before ventilatory failure causes cardiac arrest.

The headings under which the indications for positive pressure ventilation may conveniently be considered are respiratory, circulatory, neurological, and musculoskeletal, posttraumatic and postoperative.

Respiratory indications

Patients suffering from pneumonia, pulmonary oedema, asthma, chronic bronchitis, pulmonary fibrosis or massive atelectasis can almost always be prevented from dying from ventilatory failure by the use of a mechanical ventilator. Patients with pneumonia may still die due to the toxic effects of the infection on other organs, but inability to maintain ventilation at a level which will sustain life is most unusual with modern ventilators suitably adjusted to match the patient's disease.

The judgement that the patient's condition has deteriorated to a level which justifies mechanical ventilation is complex. It depends not only upon the observation that, with appropriate measures short of positive pressure ventilation, the patient is unable to ventilate the arterial blood adequately and that there is a worsening trend in the arterial blood gas tensions; equally important is the observation that the patient's own respiratory efforts are inducing a state of increasing physical exhaustion which is likely to be irreversible. Implicit within the judgement of the level of exhaustion which can be tolerated, is an appreciation of the patient's general state of fitness and the adequacy of systems other than the patient's lungs. The physician must also consider the reversibility or otherwise of the patient's underlying condition, before embarking upon treatment which may be viewed as the medical equivalent of a surgical operation. Broadly this will depend upon an estimate of the proportion of the pulmonary disorder which is reversible.

Circulatory indications

The value of positive pressure ventilation in low cardiac output states has long been recognized, but Macklem's group have now provided substantial experimental evidence that circulatory performance and survival rates are both improved if the energy required for the performance of ventilation is supplied from an external source. For these reasons a cardiac output of less than 2 l/min in a 70 kg patient or a cardiac index of less than 1.2 l/m²/min is of itself an indication for mechanical ventilatory support. The sharp increase in the ventilatory workload occasioned by pulmonary oedema, in addition to its interference with pulmonary gas exchange, make this condition particularly susceptible to treatment with positive pressure ventilation when it cannot be contained sufficiently rapidly by manipulation of the circulation.

Neurological and musculoskeletal indications

Weakness of the respiratory muscles occasioned by acute infective polyneuritis, poliomyelitis, myasthenia gravis, or rarely multiple sclerosis may be sufficiently severe to make ventilatory assistance necessary. In general such assistance will be required when the patient's vital capacity falls below 1 litre because the patient will then be incapable of generating a cough of sufficient force to maintain a clear airway. The possibility that any of these conditions may be complicated by bulbar weakness may dictate that the ventilatory assistance is provided as positive pressure ventilation via an endotracheal tube. Where it is clear that there is no bulbar weakness and that this will not appear, ventilatory support may be provided by other techniques more appropriate to chronic weakness such as tank ventilators, cuirasses, or rocking beds.

Following traumatic head injuries and in cases of brain damage secondary to asphyxiation or periods of cardiac arrest, an initial period of partial neurological recovery is not infrequently followed by neurological death due to cerebral oedema. There is evidence that the occurrence of this cerebral oedema may be prevented by hyperventilation. Reduction of the arterial carbon dioxide tension to values between 25 and 30 mm Hg (3.3 and 4.0 kPa) acts by reducing cerebral blood flow to control the development of the oedema. Ideally, ventilation undertaken for these

reasons should be monitored by extradural measurement of intracranial pressure, since premature withdrawal of the treatment may be followed by overwhelming cerebral oedema which is irreversible by the time that signs of upper midbrain compression appear.

Respiratory depression of a central nature due either to drug overdose or the action of anaesthetic agents may necessitate a period of mechanical ventilation.

Underventilation due to kyphoscoliotic deformities may require treatment with a mechanical ventilator but the results are poor unless undertaken to deal with an acute episode of ventilatory insufficiency precipitated by a potentially reversible pulmonary infection, or to provide support during a postoperative period when the patient's ventilatory capacity is further reduced temporarily.

Posttraumatic and postoperative indications

Patients who have sustained traumatic chest injuries may be best treated with a period of positive pressure ventilation, either because a segment of the chest wall is moving paradoxically secondary to fracture of the rib cage at more than one point on its circumference, or as an adjunct to the management of pain, or in the treatment of respiratory failure due to contusion of the lung.

An uncontrolled flail segment of the chest wall is inevitably complicated by collapse and consolidation of the underlying segment of lung and also impairs ventilatory capacity by its paradoxical movement. These complications can be prevented either by wiring the rib fractures, or by positive pressure ventilation. Pain can be controlled either by epidural anaesthesia or by sedation and positive pressure ventilation, which is the obvious treatment of choice where the three problems of paradoxical movement, lung contusion, and pain co-exist. The chest wall usually becomes stable and the pain occasioned by the patient's own respiratory effort becomes tolerable within a period of ten days.

Following cardiac operations for the circulatory reasons already discussed, and following abdominal operations where for some reason the abdomen remains either distended or acutely painful, an elective period of positive pressure ventilation is an effective means of avoiding pulmonary complications.

Extensive burns involving the chest wall may impose a remarkable degree of restriction upon the chest wall which is best treated by escharotomies and positive pressure ventilation.

Technical considerations involved in the institution of positive pressure ventilation

Endotracheal intubation

Positive pressure ventilation requires intubation of the trachea by either the oral or nasal route or through a tracheostomy. The details of technique are all directed toward the minimization of laryngeal and tracheal damage.

A tube diameter of 9.5 mm in an adult male and 8.5 mm in a female patient leaves a small space between tube and trachea which can be sealed by minimal inflation of the cuff. The cuff should be inflated until the leak, audible with a stethoscope over the trachea, just disappears. Tracheal damage is occasioned by the use of tubes of small diameter because high cuff pressures are then necessary to produce an air seal.

Oral endotracheal tubes are preferred because although nasal endotracheal tubes may be marginally less uncomfortable for the patient, the fact that smaller tubes have to be used because of the diameter of the nasal airspace increases the likelihood of tracheal damage, and also makes aspiration of the airway with catheters more difficult.

The factors which increase the chance of laryngeal abrasion from an endotracheal tube are the shape of the female larynx, oedema of the head and neck, and of greatest importance, movement of the tube relative to the patient, due to restlessness, hiccoughing, or respiratory efforts. Where all these factors are reduced to a minimum an oral endotracheal tube can be used for a maximum of two weeks. Except in children, a longer period of ventilation requires the formation of a tracheostomy.

Plastic tubes should be used in preference to rubber because they produce less tissue reaction. The length of the tube should be adjusted before insertion so that the connector at the proximal end of the tube buttresses the tube as it lies between the patient's teeth to prevent severence or compression of the tube. The distal end of the tube must lie well above the carina. Inadvertent intubation of the right main bronchus is manifested by diminished movement of the left chest. The correct positioning of the tube should be confirmed radiologically after insertion.

In small children nasotracheal tubes are preferred to oral because the most important consideration is stability of the tube. Stability is difficult to ensure because the distance between the larynx and carina is small, and the tolerance between an ideally placed tube half way between these points and inadvertent extubation is correspondingly small. These problems are best countered by anchorage of a nasal tube to a wire frame secured to the child's forehead with adhesive pads.

The nasal endotracheal tubes used for small children are non-cuffed and the tube diameter selected is such that there is a modest leak of a half to one litre of gas per minute between the tube and the trachea. The leak is compensated for by augmentation of the minute volume and forms a non-traumatic cushion between the tube and trachea. The tube should be changed to the other nostril at least each week or more frequently if it becomes part obstructed with inspisated secretions, but this arrangement can be used for long-term ventilation if necessary. Tracheostomy should be avoided in small children.

Matching the ventilator settings with the patient's disease

The matching of the ventilator to the patient's physiological disturbance is made at a number of levels.

The first approximation With the notable exception of patients suffering from obstructive airways disease, the minute volume is adjusted to bring the arterial carbon dioxide tension to a level between 30 and 35 mm Hg (4 and 4.7 kPa). This mild degree of overventilation increases the patient's tolerance of the ventilator by diminishing the ventilatory drive. In an adult the minute volume required to achieve this is likely to lie between 6 l/min if the patient has normal lung function and 22 l/min with extremes of pulmonary disorder. An estimate is made of the patient's degree of disturbance, and the ventilator adjusted to deliver a minute volume related proportionately to this estimate of dysfunction. The oxygen concentration of the inspired gas is adjusted with the aim of producing an arterial oxygen tension between 100 and 150 mm Hg (13 and 20 kPa). The desired end is achieved by a process of successive approximation by measurement of the arterial blood gases and adjustment of the ventilator.

Oxygen toxicity Inspired oxygen concentrations in excess of 75 per cent are undesirable since they engender pathological changes in the lung. Animals ventilated with 100 per cent oxygen show changes in the alveolar basement membrane after 10 hours and after two days there is an intense fibroblastic reaction in the lungs. Inspired oxygen concentrations in excess of 75 per cent are therefore only acceptable for a very short period where the arterial oxygen tension is below 50 mm Hg (6.6 kPa) in spite of mechanical ventilation.

Detailed matching of disease and ventilator Patients requiring ventilation who have normal lungs, pneumonia, pulmonary oedema, or atelectasis are best ventilated at a slow rate, with an inspiratory time as great as 30 per cent of the respiratory cycle and with a pause in full inspiration. Theoretically an inspiratory pause allows redistribution of gas from overventilated to underventilated alveoli. In practice it is difficult to demonstrate that the introduction of a pause makes any measureable difference to the efficiency

of ventilation. Its practical importance is that it allows the pressure within the airway to be measured under conditions of no gas flow.

In an adult a respiratory rate of 15/min is more efficient than more rapid rates. In children a suitable rate is determined, once the required minute volume is known, by holding the minute volume constant and varying the rate until the observed excursion of the child's chest wall seems appropriate to its size.

Patients in this respiratory group all benefit very considerably from being ventilated with an end expiratory pressure raised above atmospheric pressure unless cardiac output is severely impaired. The application of a positive end expiratory pressure (PEEP) has been an important advance in the technique of mechanical ventilation. PEEP valves allow gas to escape freely from the airway during expiration down to a selected pressure between 0 and 20 cm H_2O. Their closure at a pressure above atmospheric has the effect of inflating the lungs to a greater functional residual capacity (FRC) over the course of a few breaths. Once equilibrium is re-established between the inspired and expired gas volume, the patient continues to be ventilated with the original values of tidal and minute volume, but with the lungs held inflated to a larger FRC, so that their volume in inspiration and in expiration are both increased by the same amount.

Experimental evidence suggests that the optimum value of PEEP, from both respiratory and circulatory points of view, is that end expiratory pressure at which the compliance of the lungs is greatest. This can be determined by measuring the excursions in airway pressure occurring between end expiration and the inspiratory pause. The ideal value of PEEP is that at which the pressure swings are the minimum for the same applied tidal volume.

PEEP is contraindicated in low cardiac output states for the reason that it further lowers the cardiac output, and in obstructive airways disease, where its application worsens lung compliance and raises the pulmonary vascular resistance.

The pattern of mechanical ventilation required by patients with severe asthma or major obstructive airways disease for any other reason, is unlike that for any other disease. In essence it entails deliberate underventilation, avoidance of any measure which might further increase the already large FRC and, in the case of acute asthma, intense humidification.

The inception of positive pressure ventilation unless correctly managed can prove lethal in these patients. The lungs should be oxygenated from a face mask and an isoprenaline infusion started before anaesthesia is induced for the placement of an endotracheal tube. The patient should then be intubated under general anaesthesia and underventilated with a gas mixture containing 75 per cent oxygen. No attempt should be made to reduce the arterial carbon dioxide tension from the high levels that it will have attained in such patients before they are subjected to ventilation. Ventilation of an adult with 6 l/min in such circumstances may well correspond with an arterial carbon dioxide tension of 70 mm Hg (9.3 kPa) or more. An increase in minute volume will produce an increase in both FRC and pulmonary vascular resistance, with a deleterious effect upon the circulation. If the patient's deterioration before ventilation was rapid, the respiratory acidosis will not have been offset by the retention of bicarbonate, and this should be administered to bring the arterial pH toward normal.

The underventilation and consequent high arterial carbon dioxide tension make it necessary to continue the anaesthesia and muscle relaxation.

A slow ventilatory rate and an inspiratory phase as short as 5 per cent of the cycle allow greater time for expiration. An inspiratory pause theoretically allows redistribution of gas from overventilated to underventilated alveoli, but makes little demonstrable difference to the efficiency of ventilation.

A positive end expiratory pressure is absolutely contraindicated in patients whose disease has already raised their FRC beyond the point at which the compliance of their lungs improves. In the severe asthmatic PEEP constitutes a threat to life by increasing the pulmonary vascular resistance.

The use of an expiratory choke to limit the rate of emptying of the lungs has been advocated to prevent premature closure of small airways so allowing more complete alveolar emptying. The pattern of emptying is converted from an exponential to a linear form. The improvement in the arterial gases so obtained is usually modest, and the benefit is probably outweighed by the potentially very dangerous threat posed by minor maladjustment of this control, limiting the expiratory rate sufficiently to cause an increase in FRC.

Humidification and warming of the air delivered to the patient is important whatever the nature of the disease which has occasioned treatment by mechanical ventilation. In the case of acute asthma, the eventual dislodgement of viscid bronchiolar casts, which intense humidification produces after about 10 hours, is central to successful treatment. As the airways are cleared of this material, the pulmonary abnormalities diminish, allowing the alveolar ventilation to be increased.

Patients with restrictive abnormalities either of the lungs or chest wall, as may occur in fibrosing alveolitis or kyphoscoliosis, require modification of the ventilatory pattern in the sense of a smaller tidal volume and higher respiratory rate. The optimal rate can be found in each case by measurement of the arterial blood gases whilst the minute volume is held constant and the respiratory rate raised. A fall in the optimal rate will be found where it has been possible to reverse a fibrotic change.

Where ventilation has been undertaken with the object of reducing or preventing cerebral oedema, it might be expected that PEEP would have the effect of raising intracranial pressure by transmission of the raised intrathoracic pressure to the theca through the rich plexus of veins around the vertebral bodies within the thorax. Direct measurement of the intracranial pressure in a very limited number of cases suggests that this may not be so.

Management of the ventilated patient

Once patient and machine have been matched according to the nature of the disease process, there are details of management which relate to all ventilated patients.

The effect of gravity is paramount and the optimum drainage of secretions from the airway is achieved with the patient lying horizontal, and alternating from side to side so that a coronal plane through the chest is truly vertical. This ideal may be rendered impossible by multiple injuries or may require to be sacrificed in some degree by the greater importance of nursing a patient threatened with cerebral oedema in a steeply head up position. Similarly where the greatest threat to life is circulatory instability, patients must remain flat on their backs.

Aspiration of the airway is necessary with a frequency related to the amount of the secretions. This should be carried out with catheters as aseptically and atraumatically as possible.

Atelectasis can usefully be treated by manual inflation of the chest with an anaesthetic bag. A series of hyperinflations of the lungs are followed by sudden disconnection of the endotracheal tube simulating a cough, followed by aspiration of the airway. This process should not be employed indiscriminately and is contraindicated in the presence of a precarious circulation and in severe obstructive airway disease.

Restlessness in a ventilated patient should never pass unheeded, and makes the measurement of the arterial blood gases obligatory. The commonest cause is underventilation, the basis for which should be determined and the ventilation increased. Circulatory inadequacy may be manifested by restlessness without any demonstrable change in the respiratory status, and the deterioration of any ventilated patient must always suggest the possible occurrence of a pneumothorax. It is almost always possible to continue ventilating a patient despite the presence of a pneumothorax, but an adequate chest drain must be inserted.

The requirement of patients with oral endotracheal tubes for sedation is immensely variable and must be adjusted to the individual. Restlessness in spite of adequate ventilation and sedation is an indication for either curarization or early conversion to a tracheostomy.

Weaning from the ventilator

A period of mechanical ventilation may either be terminated abruptly or by gradual transfer of the ventilatory workload from machine to patient. In either case the factors which govern the possibility of the patient's independence of the ventilator fall under three headings: the adequacy of pulmonary function, the likely work cost of spontaneous ventilation, and the patient's capacity to sustain such a workload.

The simplest measure of adequacy of pulmonary function, which is available in any ventilated patient, is the relation of the minute volume and inspired oxygen concentration, supplied through the ventilator, to the arterial blood gas tensions which they engender. An arterial carbon dioxide tension between 30 and 35 mm Hg (4.0 and 4.7 kPa) in response to a minute volume of 6 l is likely to be associated with substantially normal lungs. If the minute volume required to produce this level of alveolar ventilation is in excess of 12 l for a 70 kg patient, who has been ventilated, it is unlikely that the patients' own ventilatory efforts will sustain them other than briefly. Between these limits there is a spectrum of respiratory dysfunction which may be compatible with a reversion to spontaneous ventilation, necessitating a judgement of the balance between the implied workload, and the patient's competence to undertake this.

Patients whose pulmonary pathology is best treated with a positive end expiratory pressure during mechanical ventilation should *not* be weaned from positive pressure as a prelude to weaning from the ventilator. The very considerable benefits of PEEP are best maintained in order that the lungs are in the best possible condition at the moment of separation from the ventilator.

An estimate of the likely workload is provided by the size of the minute volume and of the pressure swings in the airway generated by the conjunction of patient and ventilator. Although neither value may remain unchanged once the patient is divorced from the ventilator, both are good indicators.

Estimation of the patient's ability to support the workload requires examination of the cardiovascular system, the nervous system, and the abdomen.

Withdrawal of ventilatory support in the presence of a cardiac output which is less than half the normal resting value is likely to lead to further circulatory deterioration. An elevated left atrial pressure or any residual pulmonary oedema will increase the work of breathing by stiffening the lungs. A pulmonary vascular resistance greater than 10 units is a contraindication to the removal of ventilatory support for at least 48 hours after cardiopulmonary operations, and for longer periods if the pulmonary vascular resistance is higher. Premature removal of support probably causes death by provoking a sharp rise in pulmonary vascular resistance, which is not reversed by reventilation. If this is the mechanism, infusion of acetyl choline into the pulmonary artery might be effective where reventilation fails.

Lungs which have been flooded with pulmonary oedema as a result of insults to the capillary basement membrane, rather than for hydraulic reasons, require to be ventilated for a minimum of 6 days following the insult. Premature cessation of ventilation results in extensive atelectasis. It seems possible that the surfactant mechanism is destroyed and requires time to regenerate. The pulmonary oedema in such cases has the same appearance as the patient's plasma and the same albumin concentration.

Central nervous depression whether organic or metabolic in origin, and, most important, the integrity of the patient's brain stem and spinal cord function, together with any damage to the phrenic and intercostal nerves, may all make adequate spontaneous ventilation impossible. Wasting and weakness of the respiratory muscles have the same effect, and in this context the atrophy of the muscles which results from prolonged periods of artificial ventilation is of particular importance. The sensory nervous system is also involved, in as much as pain is commonly a transcending respiratory depressant.

Abdominal distension and tenderness interfere with diaphragmatic movement and are of especial relevance to the patient's ability to cough. A vital capacity of at least 1 litre and the apposition of the vocal cords are necessary for the production of an effective cough, without which an initially adequate ventilatory capacity is likely to deteriorate.

Whilst any of these circulatory neuromuscular or abdominal considerations may offer a clear contraindication to the discontinuation of mechanical ventilation, the requirement for fine judgement in cases of doubt is obviated by allowing the patient to breathe a high flow of a suitable gas mixture from an anaesthetic bag, whilst still intubated. This manoeuvre will very quickly make any deficiencies of drive or neurological integrity obvious from the movements of the chest wall and the movements of the diaphragms inferred from those of the abdomen. It also allows a judgement to be made of the likelihood that the patient will become unduly exhausted. The deficiencies of this trial are the increased airway resistance presented by the endotracheal tube and the intolerance of the tube, which some patients show after the withdrawal of sedation. A brief trial of this nature also leaves in doubt the patient's longer term independence of the ventilator.

The problems of sedation are to some extent overcome by the replacement of all other forms of sedation with nitrous oxide for a period of hours to allow excretion of the other agents. The effects of nitrous oxide wear off very rapidly allowing a brief time for the trial assessment and a decision, if all seems well, to remove the endotracheal tube. Nitrous oxide is not suitable for long-term sedation because of bone marrow changes and after 24 hours neutropenia.

Careful observation of the patient in the first hours after the removal of ventilatory support will confirm or confound the decision. The most important indications for reventilation are those of respiratory distress, a rising respiratory and pulse rate, and the appearance of such effort being required as can only end in increasing exhaustion. From the circulatory point of view the most favourable response is a fall in right atrial pressure and a small rise in arterial pressure. A rise in both venous and arterial pressure suggests that apprehension or pain require treatment with mild sedation or analgesia. A rise in right atrial pressure, a fall in arterial pressure, a diminished hourly urine output and cooling limbs suggest that ventilatory support should be restored.

Evidence of underventilation in the sense of a rising carbon dioxide tension is not of itself an indication for reventilation unless it is extreme (over 65 mm Hg or 8.6 kPa), or unless it is due to weakness rather than the unwanted persistence of sedation, for which small doses of respiratory stimulants are effective.

If exhaustion is evident, the patient should be restored to the ventilator before serious derangement of the arterial blood gases occurs. For this reason these measurements are of less importance than is commonly believed in the solution of this problem.

Laryngeal obstruction following removal of an endotracheal tube is suggested by the appearance of wheeze which is predominantly inspiratory rather than expiratory, and not associated with overinflation of the chest. This may well respond to intravenous hydrocortisone. If this is not effective, it is necessary to pass through the intermediate steps of reintubation and conversion to a tracheotomy. The breathing of helium mixtures is not of value, because the gas flow through the restriction breaks down and becomes turbulent rather than laminar.

The weaning of the tracheostomized patient from the ventilator presents few of these problems, because the tube is tolerated without sedation and should be left in place until the process is successfully completed.

Because a tracheostomy makes it possible to separate the patient from the ventilator intermittently for gradually increasing periods of time, if necessary over the course of many days, this is

the method of choice where the respiratory muscles have been subject to wasting. Most chronic bronchitics can only be weaned from a ventilator in this manner, when the oedema of the airway and the infective process in their lungs has been reduced to the absolute minimum. Tracheostomy in these patients has the added advantage of allowing continued aspiration of the airway.

Underventilation of chronic bronchitic patients prior to their removal from the ventilator decreases rather than increases their ventilatory drive in accord with changes in intrathecal pH, and is not of value. The inspired oxygen concentration should of course be limited during weaning, in contradistinction to the requirements at the initial inception of ventilation in such patients.

Tracheostomies are best closed allowing them to shrink down around uncuffed metal tubes which are daily decreased in size. A flap valve allows the patient to talk and provide a more effective cough than is possible with no occlusion. When sufficient shrinkage has occurred, the tube can be replaced with an occlusive dressing.

Haemodialysis in the presence of circulatory disorder

The abnormalities of the circulation which commonly lead to serious circulatory difficulties during haemodialysis are the combination of an incompliant venous capacity bed, and a heart which is failing in the sense of a limited ability to generate useful work in relation to its filling pressure.

The volume of water normally excreted over a 24 hour period is removed during haemodialysis in perhaps as little as 4 hours. This allows time for movement of fluid between the extracellular space and the circulation such that the loss from the circulation is a moderate proportion of the total loss. In the presence of an incompliant venous system with a high tone, the diminution in right atrial pressure resulting from any given volume loss is multiplied by a factor which may be as great as 10. If this larger change in right atrial pressure impinges upon a heart with impaired equations of performance, the resulting fall in cardiac output, although modest because of the reduced slopes of the equations, is from a low to an insupportable level, and is likely to occasion further renal damage. Haemodialysis undertaken under these conditions is best supervised with continuous monitoring of the right atrial and arterial pressures.

The fall in cardiac output can be mitigated by the administration of inotropic drugs during the dialysis, and the fall in venous pressure by expansion of the circulation and maintenance of a high central venous pressure.

The even removal of water throughout the 24 hours which is possible with peritoneal dialysis represents a great advantage where these circulatory difficulties exist. The risk of peritoneal infection with conventional peritoneal dialysis, continued for longer periods of time, has made this method undesirable in the presence of prosthetic heart valves. Methods evolved for continuous ambulatory peritoneal dialysis offer the promise of a system which is minimally disturbing to the circulation and acceptably less likely to produce infection.

Arteriovenous haemofiltration, which uses the pressure gradient between the patient's arterial and venous system to drive blood through a capillary haemofilter has the same considerable advantage that it can be used to remove fluid from the circulation evenly and continuously. An ultrafiltrate is removed from the patient through the capillary haemofilter and is discarded. The volume removed is replace with an artificial fluid and the rate of this replacement in relation to the rate at which ultrafiltrate is removed from the patient determines the net rate of fluid removal. Although originally developed for the removal of water, sodium, and potassium, the filtration rates obtained are usually high enough to compensate in some measure also for renal failure, since the average rate of removal and replacement of 8 ml/min corresponds to a similar glomerular filtration rate.

Fig. 16. Pupillary responses associated with various lesions: **1**, Optic nerve. **2**, Optic tract. **3**, Midbrain pretectum. **4**, Midbrain oculomotor nuclei. **5**, Emerging third nerve fibres in midbrain. (Reproduced with permission from Plum and Posner, *The diagnosis of stupor and coma.* F. A. Davis.)

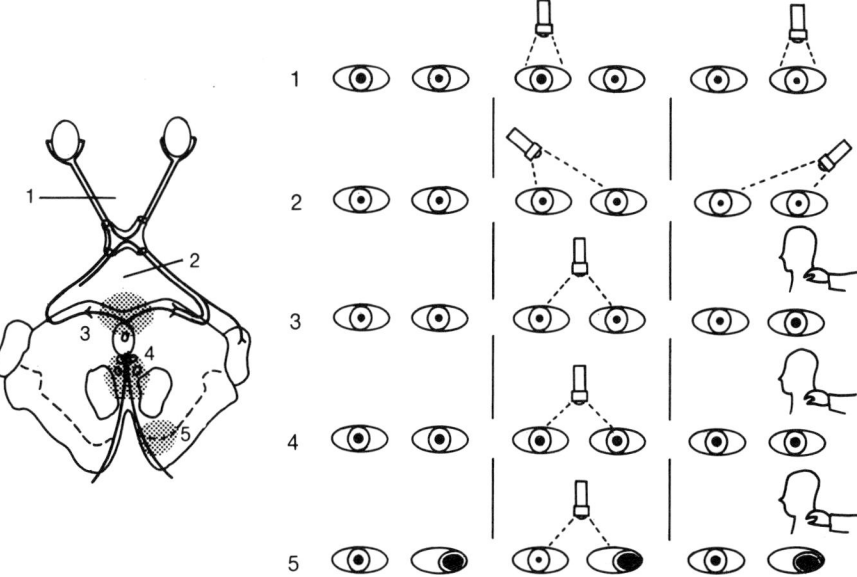

Diagnosis and management of the unconscious patient

Much of the substance of this section is taken from the work of Posner and Plum, whose contribution to this topic marked such an advance in the neurological assessment of the unconscious patient. The eventual management of such a patient will vary according to the diagnosis, but the need for a clear airway, adequacy of both ventilation and circulation, and the elimination of hypoglycaemia transcend all else, if the patient is not to be exposed to further needless brain damage.

The first approximation to the diagnosis depends upon the history and physical signs. The patient's inability to give any history must not preclude enquiry being made of relatives or witnesses concerning the mode of onset of the coma.

Any injury to the head, the appearance of either blood or CSF in the auditory meati, or nose, or bleeding into the orbits, or the presence of meningism are of obvious significance. The neurological assessment of the unconscious patient depends upon observation of the patient's responses to a relatively small number of manoeuvres some of which are not applicable to a conscious patient. There follows a relatively detailed account of these manoeuvres and the information they may yield.

Brainstem function

Consciousness probably depends upon interaction between the reticular formation in the midbrain and pons and hemispheric structures, and may be interfered with by damage to any of these areas. In the case of the hemispheres the damage must be bilateral to produce loss of consciousness.

The brain stem is accessible to moderately detailed examination even in the absence of consciousness. This assessment depends upon:

1. The pupillary responses.
2. Abnormalities of resting gaze of the eyes.
3. Observation of eye movements induced by stimulation of the patient's vestibular apparatus, either in response to movement of the head or by caloric stimulation.
4. The corneal reflexes.
5. The presence of a jaw jerk.
6. The ability of the patient to swallow and gag.
7. The pattern of any spontaneous respiratory movements that may be present.
8. The ciliospinal reflex.

As will be seen when they are considered in detail, these responses may be interfered with by depression of brain stem function or damage to the cranial nerves. In practice it is not usually difficult to discern where the problem lies.

The pupils

(See also Section 21.)

The localization of lesions to the optic nerve, optic tract, and either the pretectal or oculomotor nuclear region of the midbrain is most succinctly summarized by the diagram in Fig. 16 taken from Posner and Plum.

Tectal midbrain lesions produce midposition (4 mm) or widened (5 to 6 mm) pupils which are unreactive to light, but which may spontaneously fluctuate in size (hippus) and dilate in response to a painful stimulus to the skin of the neck (ciliospinal reflex). Lesions of the oculomotor nuclear region of the midbrain interrupt both sympathetic and parasympathetic supply to the eye producing midposition pupils, which do not react to any stimuli and are often non-circular in outline and slightly unequal in size. Pontine lesions produce bilaterally small pupils. Lateral medullary lesions produce a Horner's syndrome, but do not interfere with the response to light. Third nerve lesions produce pupillary dilation and if the lesion is complete are accompanied by an oculomotor palsy producing downward and outward gaze of the affected eye.

Fixed dilated pupils following a cardiac arrest may be due to cerebral damage but the pupils will also dilate in response to adrenaline and atropine, and although in these circumstances they may still respond to light, it is often difficult to detect the response. Since intense sympathetic stimulation and the administration of these drugs are common accompaniments of a cardiac arrest it is wise to be guarded about the significance of such pupils following an arrest.

Metabolic depression of the brain stem produces even depression of all the brain stem functions with the important exception that the pupillary light response is preserved.

Eye movements and disorders of gaze

The resting position of the eyes, and their response to movement of the head or caloric stimulation of the vestibular apparatus, are potentially more revealing than any other bedside observation that may be made about an unconscious patient.

Most conjugate gaze disorders in comatose patients are the

result of destructive lesions because compression and metabolic disturbances affect the supranuclear oculomotor pathways symmetrically. Conjugate deviation of the eyes away from the side of a hemiplegic arm and leg has the same significance as a hemianopic field defect toward the arm and leg; the lesion is hemispheric. Conjugate deviation of the eyes toward the paralysed arm and leg may occur in the early irritative stages of a hemispheric lesion, but is otherwise the result of a lateral pontine lesion.

Disconjugate lateral deviation of both eyes may be the result of a nuclear lesion in the midbrain; if this is the cause, the pupils will not react to light. Metabolic depression can produce a similar deviation, but the pupils react and stimulation of the patient commonly causes the eyes to assume a central position.

The oculocephalic responses are elicited by holding the eyelids open and rotating the patient's head rapidly to one or other side, *and then holding the head still*. (This should be done with a light touch, and the response to flexion may only be tested when it is clear that there is no question of a neck injury). If the patient is unconscious the eyes will initially be 'left behind', but will subsequently 'catch up' with the movement of the skull, and come to occupy their original resting position in relation to the skull. The movements so elicited are called 'Dolls-Head eye movements'. These movements will only occur if the overriding influences controlling eye movement from the hemispheres are suppressed, and the oculomotor and vestibular components and the connections between them in the brain stem are still functioning.

The caloric responses are elicited, provided that the tympanic membrane is intact, by slow irrigation of the auditory canal with at least 50 ml of ice-cold water. The patient's head should be positioned 45°, head up, with the eyelids held open. In an unconscious patient with an intact brain stem both eyes will deviate toward the irrigated ear. In a patient feigning loss of consciousness the manoeuvre is extremely unpleasant and will produce nystagmus with the slow component toward the irrigated side and possibly vomiting. If the vestibular and oculomotor components or the connections between them in the brain stem are non-functioning as a result of either a focal lesion or severe generalized metabolic depression, the eyes will not move in relation to the skull.

In metabolic and drug-induced coma the oculocephalic and caloric responses are present at first because of the removal of the overriding hemispheric influences, but disappear later as brain stem function is depressed. Caloric stimulation provides a much stronger stimulus than head turning and may therefore still produce a response when the Dolls-Head eye movements have already been lost.

Both manoeuvres will demonstrate a sixth nerve palsy by absence of lateral movement of the affected eye and make the oculomotor consequences of a third nerve palsy very obvious since the affected eye remains turned laterally and downward whilst the other moves in relation to the skull. Failure of either eye to move to the nasal side of the midline is evidence of an internuclear lesion in the brain stem. The presence of Dolls-Head eye movements is good evidence that the patient is unconscious except in the presence of blindness or lesions affecting the connections between the motor eyefields on the frontal cortex and the oculomotor nuclei. These exceptions may seem to render this test of unconsciousness of little value, but in practice patients who have Dolls-Head eye movements for these reasons are usually obviously conscious.

The transition from unconsciousness to consciousness is usually heralded by the appearance of small quick conjugate movements of the eyes interspersed within the Dolls-Head movements. Oddly these rapid movements which represent the beginnings of the ability to fixate always precede the reappearance of any response to menace.

Relatively rapid jerking movements of both eyes commonly occur during grand-mal seizures. Retraction nystagmus due to the simultaneous contraction of all the extraocular muscles is associated with mesencephalic lesions, and caudal pontine lesions produce a repetitive and very distinctive rapid downward movement of the eyes followed by a slow upward return to the mid-position. This phenomenon is known as ocular bobbing and is very specific to lesions in this area.

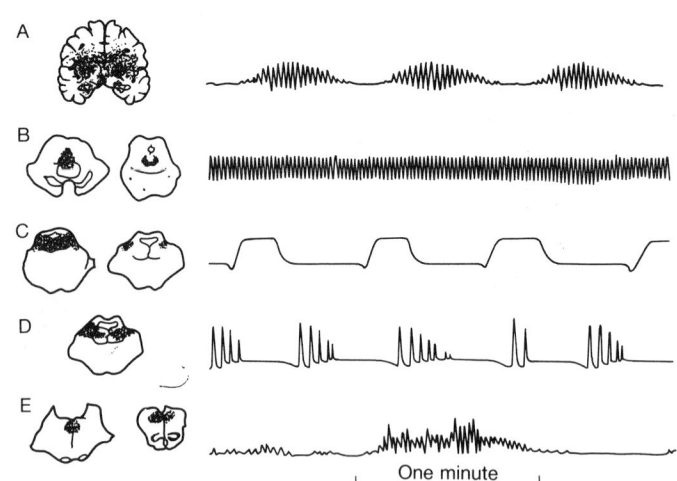

Fig. 17. Abnormal respiratory patterns associated with pathological lesions (shaded areas) at various levels of the brain. Tracings by chest-abdomen pneumograph, inspiration reads up. (A) Cheyne-Stokes respiration. (B) Central neurogenic hyperventilation. (C) Apneusis. (D) Cluster breathing. (E) Ataxic breathing. (Reproduced with permission from Plum and Posner, *The diagnosis of stupor and coma*. F. A. Davis.)

The jaw jerk and corneal responses
The presence of an abnormally brisk jaw jerk signals a bilateral upper motor neurone lesion above the motor nucleus of the Vth cranial nerve, and always suggests the possibility of a pseudobulbar palsy. The corneal reflexes test the integrity of the Vth and VIIth cranial nerves and a small pontine section of the brain stem and will be depressed with bilateral hemispheric damage.

Swallowing and the cough reflex
The total reliability of the swallowing mechanism should always be mistrusted in any unconscious patient. Overflow of saliva from the patient's mouth is simple evidence of an inability to swallow, but the fact that the patient does not cough when fluid is instilled into the mouth is no guarantee of the continence of the swallowing mechanism unless the cough reflex has been demonstrated to be intact by laryngeal stimulation with a suction catheter.

Any patient who cannot guard their airway should ideally be positioned on their side, slightly head down and without a pillow, so that one corner of the mouth is at a lower level than any other part of the upper airway. This requirement may well conflict with the need to position the patient steeply head up to limit the generation of cerebral oedema. Should this conflict arise, it is a clear indication for the placement of a cuffed endotracheal tube to isolate the airway from the pharynx.

The respiratory pattern
Distortions of the normal respiratory pattern may assist in the localization of the neurological disturbance. The characteristic patterns associated with lesions at various levels are illustrated in Fig. 17.

The respiratory patterns in Fig. 17a and d are both examples of *Cheyne Stokes breathing*. In Fig. 17d, where the lesion is at the junction of pons and medulla, Cheyne Stokes breathing will occur in the presence of a normal lung to brain circulation time of approximately 8 s, and a respiratory cycle length of 16 s measured from apnoea to apnoea. In this case the periodic respiration appears because the mechanism which turns ventilation on and off is damaged, analogous to a sticky thermostat switch. In long-cycle Cheyne Stokes breathing, where the respiratory cycle length may be from 30 to 200 s, the essential lesion is *not* neurological, but a prolonged lung to brain circulation time, occasioned either by a diminished cardiac output or an expanded central blood volume or commonly both. The system exhibits periodicity in this case because blood which has been relatively hyper- or hypoventilated in the lungs takes an abnormally long time (always half the respiratory cycle length) to reach the brain stem and exert its moderating influence. This form of Cheyne Stokes respiration is frequently revealed by the administration of opiates which probably act in the same non-specific way as the deep-seated hemispheric lesions in Fig. 17a, by removing hemispheric influences which otherwise conceal the abnormal respiratory pattern.

Abnormal hyperventilation (Fig. 17b) may be associated with focal, usually destructive lesions in the midbrain and pons, and an apneustic respiratory pattern (Fig. 17c) with similar lesions in the pons (see also Section 21). The apneustic pattern always betokens a neurological lesion, but hyperventilation is only rarely due to focal brain stem damage and the diagnosis is only tenable in the presence of other evidence of midbrain or pontine damage, and in the absence of a metabolic cause.

Ataxic irregular patterns of respiration (Fig. 17e) shading into apnoea are associated with medullary depression occurring for any reason.

Frequently it is necessary to inspect the respiratory pattern of a patient who is already being ventilated. To prevent hypoxia during the period that the patient is left to his or her own respiratory devices, the lungs should be washed out with 100 per cent oxygen from an anaesthetic bag. Whilst the patient remains apnoeic the arterial carbon dioxide tension will rise at a rate of approximately 2 mm Hg/min, and the spontaneous respiratory pattern may not emerge until the carbon dioxide level has risen considerably, but with the preoxygenation described, this should be possible without hypoxaemia.

The ciliospinal reflex

The ciliospinal reflex is a homolateral pupillary dilation evoked by pinching the skin of the neck. It probably depends upon both active sympathetic stimulation, and inhibition of the parasympathetic outflow from the Edinger–Westphal nucleus. It is enhanced by depression of hemispheric function, but its principal significance is to indicate that there are functioning long tracts passing through the entire length of the brain stem.

The motor responses of the limbs

The cerebral hemispheres are more sensitive to hypoxia, malperfusion, and metabolic depression than the brain stem. In an unconscious patient, if the brain stem can be shown to be intact to the system of testing already described, then the responses of the limbs to noxious stimuli can be used as a test of hemispheric and spinal cord function. The noxious stimulus may be applied as pressure in the region of the stylomastoid foramena, supraorbital pressure, tracheal suction, vigorous cutaneous stimulation over the sternum or pressure applied to the nail beds. The responses of the limbs are graded as in the Glasgow Coma Scale (Section 21) from, at best, an attempt to remove the stimulus, to localization of the site of stimulation, to flexion and external rotation of the arms coupled with extension, internal rotation, and plantar flexion of the legs (decorticate rigidity), to extension and internal rotation of the arms with hyperpronation of the hands and powerful extension of the legs (decerebrate rigidity) and finally, at worst, a failure to produce any movement of either arm or leg.

These responses clearly involve the sensory elements of the nervous system as well as the motor and require that the long tracts in both brain stem and spinal cord are intact. Decerebrate rigidity is associated experimentally with brain stem disorders and commonly appears with damage at this level, but it is also seen in the absence of other brain stem signs with widespread hemispheric damage such as occurs following hypoxia where the anatomical changes have been confined to hemispheres.

The motor responses together with the limb reflexes and the plantar responses may make it possible to determine that one hemisphere is disproportionately affected suggesting a focal lesion.

There are two clinical syndromes associated with expanding supratentorial mass lesions which must be recognized. Symmetrical supratentorial expansion interferes with the midbrain structures from above downwards. Initially it produces bilaterally unresponsive mid-position pupils, and loss of upward gaze of the eyes in response to head flexion followed by loss of the lateral component of the Dolls Head eye movements. Usually if the signs have progressed to the stage of loss of the lateral eye movements, the damage is irretrievable, and will be followed in order by signs of pontine and hind brain destruction. Asymmetrical supratentorial expansion (the *uncal syndrome*) produces progressive dilation of the pupil on the same side as the lesion, followed by an oculomotor palsy as the third nerve is progressively stretched by herniation of the uncal portion of the temporal lobe downwards between the edge of the tentorium and the midbrain. This is followed by dilation of the other pupil to the mid-position and loss of the Dolls' Head eye movements due to midbrain compression or sometimes wide dilation of the other pupil perhaps due to stretching of the other third nerve as a result of the further distortion of the midbrain.

The ocular fundus

Subhyaloid haemorrhages tend to be associated with either subarachnoid or intracerebral haemorrhage, and obvious diabetic changes may establish that the patient has long-standing diabetes. Perhaps the most important fact of which the physician should be aware is that patients presenting with acute coma and who have raised intracranial pressure very rarely have papilloedema. In patients who succumb as a result of overwhelming cerebral oedema, angiography reveals total obstruction of the cerebral circulation probably due to compression of the cerebral capillaries, but the circulation through the retinal vessels is preserved, consonant with the observation that these patients do not have papilloedema.

Investigations

The techniques of examination which have been described are all possible in an unconscious patient and an intelligent analysis of the patient's responses should make it possible to determine whether the patient has a focal or generalized disturbance affecting the brain stem or hemispheres, and whether the disturbance is progressing for better or worse and at what rate.

If the patient is unconscious and has focal signs, the most useful investigation is likely to be a computerized tomography (CT) scan. If a CT scan is not available decisions about further investigation in this group of patients will depend upon the direction and rate of change of the signs. If there is improvement, it is reasonable to delay angiography, but if there is deterioration at a rate which allows it, angiography should be undertaken seeking a treatable space-occupying lesion. If deterioration is rapid the patient should be transferred directly to theatre for exploratory burr holes if there is any possibility that the signs are due to an extradural haematoma.

If the patient is unconscious and does not have focal signs, but has meningism, a lumbar puncture should be performed seeking evidence of subarachnoid haemorrhage or meningitis. If the history is very strongly suggestive of subarachnoid haemorrhage and CT scanning facilities are readily available, a scan is the preferred investigation, as it is thought that lumbar puncture may further destabilize patients with subarachnoid haemorrhage. It should be borne in mind that some patients with meningitis especially those who are very ill may not have menigism, so that other signs of infection in combination with unconsciousness are an indication for lumbar puncture. The prognosis of those with meningitis who are unconscious before the institution of treatment is so bad that the outcome may not be influenced by diagnosis or treatment.

The remaining group of patients who are unconscious, and who have neither focal signs nor meningism, are likely to be suffering from generalized brain contusion, anoxic damage, the postictal stage following a fit, metabolic coma, or drug intoxication. The metabolic causes of coma, hepatic or renal failure, carbon dioxide narcosis, and hyperglycaemia are usually very obvious on other clinical grounds, and hypoglycaemia should always be tested for at a very early stage in the examination of any unconscious patient. The metabolic cause which is sometimes missed is that due to porphyria. Drug intoxication can only be proved by appropriate chemical testing and most laboratories require guidance as to the drugs they should be seeking. There are, in the United Kingdom, a number of poisons centres from whom advice may be sought. Intoxication due to carbon monoxide may be missed; its neurological manifestations in the acute phase are identical to those of hypoxia, and the half-time for its clearance from the blood is 250 min if the patient is breathing air, and is reduced to 50 min if the patient breathes 100 per cent oxygen. There may therefore be little of the gas remaining in the blood, by the time that its presence is sought.

Management of the unconscious patient

It is inappropriate to detail here the treatment of space-occupying lesions, subarachnoid haemorrhage, meningitis, and the various causes of metabolic coma and intoxications considered in the section on investigation. It is the general aspects of management, and those appropriate to an intensive care unit, which will be considered.

Immediate measures

The clearance and maintenance of the airway takes precedence over all else. How this is achieved depends upon the setting in which the patient is first seen and what apparatus is to hand. Gravity is always available and it may be sufficient to position the patient on his or her side with no pillow under the head so that one corner of the mouth is the lowest part of the upper airway. It is important to avoid flexion of the neck until cervical injury has been excluded.

In the early management of an unconscious patient in hospital, the placement of a cuffed endotracheal tube has so many advantages that it is perhaps easier to separate those patients who may be safely managed without this intervention; essentially those who can be demonstrated to cough in response to laryngeal stimulation, and who will swallow without coughing if a small quantity of water is instilled into the mouth. Such patients will usually be sufficiently reactive that they will not tolerate endotracheal intubation. The important advantages of intubation are the ability to clear the major airways and protect them from any further obstruction or soiling, especially if gastric lavage is necessary. Also there is freedom to position the patient optimally in response to either neurological or circulatory requirements, and the option that the patient may be ventilated mechanically. If there be any doubt as to the adequacy of spontaneous ventilation, the patient must be ventilated. The practical disadvantage of intubation is that it may be necessary to use anaesthetic agents or muscle relaxants which will obscure the trend of neurological events. Agents with the briefest duration of action should be used, ideally perhaps only suxamethonium chloride.

The autoregulatory nature of the cerebral circulation tends to preserve the perfusion of the brain against circulatory inadequacy, but any such state must be dealt with appropriately. Similarly, cerebral metabolism must be protected by the treatment of hypo- or hyperglycaemia.

When the integrity of the CSF compartment has been breached, usually because of a fracture of the base of the skull, it is normal practice to give soluble sulphonamides and penicillin. Microbiological advice suggests that the sulphonamides are unlikely to be active against the organisms likely to cause meningitis, and that the value of such prophylaxis is very doubtful.

Measures for the control of intracranial pressure

After damage to the brain, from whatever cause, it is common to observe a trend of improvement in the function of the nervous system followed, usually after a period of between 10 and 72 hours by a rapid and often catastrophic deterioration. Given that an expanding intracranial haematoma has been excluded in the manner outlined in the section on investigation, this deterioration follows a rise in intracranial pressure and an increase in intracranial water. CT scanning suggests that the water is distributed both intravascularly and as oedema fluid. The view has been expressed that once damage of a certain severity has occurred the outcome is inevitable and that the excess intracranial water is not instrumental in the destruction of the brain, but the fact that the patient's nervous system may improve to function at levels approaching normal consciousness after the insult and yet be overwhelmed subsequently is very persuasive evidence to the contrary. The angiographic evidence suggests that the increase in fluid obstructs the cerebral circulation by compression at capillary level and that the intracranial venous system and the retinal circulation are not obstructed, explaining the absence of papilloedema in the presence of gross rises in measured intracranial pressure.

If the inferences drawn from the above observations are correct, it becomes very important to limit the rise in intracranial pressure by every possible means. It is neither possible nor desirable to measure the intracranial pressure of every unconscious patient, but where it is known that there has been a profound cerebral insult and there is evidence of a good initial recovery, there is a strong case for such monitoring. The pressure may be measured intradurally or extradurally; both approaches are effective in that they warn of a rise in intracranial pressure although they may not yield the same values. The intradural system, because of the risks of infection, can only be used for 48 hours which in many cases is too brief a period. Experience with monitoring in selected cases has demonstrated that the single most effective measure for the reduction of intracranial pressure is to position the patient as steeply head up as possible, in the sitting position. This may compromise the ideal management of the lungs or circulation, but may have to take precedence. Intracranial pressure measurement also offers a solution to the dilemma that, on the one hand, it would be beneficial to sedate the patient whose restlessness will drive the intracranial pressure up still further, yet on the other, the sedation will obscure changes in the neurological signs. Pressure measurement gives much earlier warning of change which requires intervention than the signs of midbrain compression, which only appear when the damage to the brain stem is near to irreversible.

Experimental evidence suggests that dexamethasone is only effective in the limitation of cerebral oedema if it is administered before the cerebral damage occurs, but it is currently accepted practice to use both dexamethasone and hyperventilation to an arterial carbon dioxide tension of between 25 and 30 mm Hg in an attempt to limit cerebral oedema formation. Perhaps the best evidence that these measures may be effective comes from the observation that cessation of either may produce a sharp rise in intracranial pressure in some patients for as long as 10 days after the initial cerebral insult, and that their reintroduction returns the pressure to its original level. In this study both interventions could eventually be stopped without a rise in the intracranial pressure.

Both osmotic and renal tubular diuretics can be used effectively in the control of intracranial pressure. Mannitol as a bolus is very effective if used as a temporary measure to allow time for surgical intervention, but has the disadvantage that after about four hours it causes the intracranial pressure to rise. This problem can be circumvented by continuous infusion, but if a sustained effect is required it is probably simpler to use frusemide. It must be remembered that, although a low right atrial pressure and a strongly negative water balance will reduce oedema formation wherever it is occurring, diuresis must not be taken to the point at which the circulation is jeopardized.

Two further measures aimed at reducing brain damage may conveniently be considered at this point, although they operate by reducing cerebral metabolism rather than by acting directly on oedema formation, i.e. the administration of barbiturates in high dosage and cooling of the patient to 31 °C. Although both are effective in reducing cerebral metabolism, the most recent evidence from three controlled trials failed to show any advantage for the use of barbiturates after head injury, or anoxic brain damage. The use of corticosteroids following traumatic head injury tested by comparison of predicted outcome between centres also failed to show any difference.

References

Aubier, M., Trippenbach, T. and Roussos, C. (1981). Respiratory muscle fatigue during cardiogenic shock. *J. Appl. Physiol. Respirat. Environ. Exercise Physiol.* **51**, 499–508.

Barber, R. E., Lee, J. and Hamilton, W. K. (1970). Oxygen toxicity in man: a prospective study in patients with irreversible brain damage. *N. Engl. J. Med.* **283**, 1478–1484.

Bell, J. A., Bradley, R. D., Jenkins, B. S. and Spencer, G. T. (1974). Six years of multidisciplinary intensive care. *Br. Med. J.* **ii**, 483–488.

Bradley, R. D. (1973). Shock. In *Recent advances in surgery* (ed. S. Selwyn Taylor), pp. 275–296. Churchill Livingstone, Edinburgh and London.

—— (1977). *Studies in acute heart failure.* Edward Arnold, London.

—— (1978). Intensive care. In *Progress in clinical medicine* (eds A. R. Horler and J. B. Foster), pp. 303–319. Churchill Livingstone, Edinburgh.

——, Jenkins, B. S. and Branthwaite, M. A. (1970). The influence of atrial pressure on cardiac performance following myocardial infarction complicated by shock. *Circulation* **42**, 827–837.

Branthwaite, M. A. (1980). *Artificial ventilation for pulmonary disease.* Pitman, London.

Braunwald, E., Covell, J. W., Maroko, P. R. and Ross, J. Jr (1969). Effects of drugs and of counterpulsation on myocardial oxygen consumption. Observations on the ischaemic heart. *Circulation* **40**, Suppl. 4, 220–228.

Burn, J. M. B. (1970). Design and staffing of an intensive care unit. *Lancet* **i**, 1040–1043.

Chamberlain, D. A., Leinbach, R. C., Vassaux, C. E., Kastor, J. A., De Sanctis, R. W. and Sanders, C. A. (1970). Sequential atrioventricular pacing in heart block complicating acute myocardial infarction. *N. Engl. J. Med.* **282**, 577–582.

Chatterjee, K., Parmley, W. W., Ganz, W., Forrester, J., Walinsky, P., Crexells, C. and Swan, H. J. C. (1973). Haemodynamic and metabolic responses to vasodilator therapy in acute myocardial infarction. *Circulation* **28**, 1183–1193.

Cohn, J. N., Guiha, N. H., Broder, M. I. and Limas, C. J. (1974). Right ventricular infarction, clinical and haemodynamic features. *Am. J. Cardiol.* **33**, 209–214.

Cournand, A., Motley, H. L., Werko, L. and Richards, D. W. (1948). Physiological studies of the effects of intermittent positive pressure breathing on cardiac output in man. *Am. J. Physiol.* **152**, 162–174.

Guyton, A. C. and Lindsey, A. W. (1959). Effect of elevated left atrial pressure and decreased plasma protein concentration on the development of pulmonary oedema. *Circ. Res.* **7**, 649–657.

Guyton, A. C. (1963). *Circulatory physiology: cardiac output and its regulation.* pp. 380–383. W. B. Saunders, Philadelphia.

Macklem, P. T. and Roussos, C. S. (1977). Respiratory muscle fatigue. A cause of respiratory failure? *Clin. Sci.* **53**, 419–422.

Miller, G. A. H., Sutton, G. C., Kerr, I. H., Gibson, R. V. and Honey, M. (1971). Comparison of streptokinase and heparin in the treatment of isolated acute massive pulmonary embolism. *Br. Med. J.* **ii**, 681–684.

Mueller, H., Ayres, S. M., Gianelli, S., Conklin, E. F., Mazzara, J. T. and Grace, W. J. (1972). Effect of isoproterenol, L-norepinephrine and intra-aortic counterpulsation of haemodynamics and myocardial metabolism in shock following acute myocardial infarction. *Circulation* **45**, 335–352.

Pontoppidan, H., Geffin, B. and Lowenstein, E. (1972). Acute respiratory failure in the adult: *N. Engl. J. Med.* **287**, 690–698, 743–752, 799–806.

Replogle, R. L., Meiselman, H. J. and Merrill, E. W. (1967). Clinical implications of blood rheology studies. *Circulation* **36**, 148.

Urokinase Pulmonary Embolism Trial (1973). A national co-operative study. *Circulation* Suppl. 2.

Wheat, M. W. and Palmer, R. F. (1968). Dissecting aneurysms of the aorta: present status of drug versus surgical therapy. *Progr. Cardiovasc. Dis.* **11**, 198–210.

Yatsu, F. M. (1986). Cardiopulmonary–cerebral resuscitation. *N. Engl. J. Med.* **314**, 440–441.

SECTION 15
RESPIRATORY DISORDERS

AN INTRODUCTORY REVIEW

J. CROFTON

The function of the respiratory tract in mediating gas exchange exposes it to an atmosphere containing a wide variety of damaging fumes and particles, and the perfusion of the lungs by the whole of the cardiac output exposes them to micro-organisms, clots, and chemicals carried by the blood stream. It is therefore not surprising that respiratory diseases bulk large in medicine and have major economic implications. An overview of their prevalence, mortality, causes, and social importance forms the subject matter of this introduction.

The importance of respiratory diseases

Prevalence

In general practice in Britain consultation and episode rates for respiratory diseases are higher than for any other disease grouping, about 250 consultations per 1000 population per year. A survey of 1000 families in Newcastle found that respiratory disease was the commonest health problem in children under 5 years, constituting half of all illnesses. In adults, general practice consultation for upper respiratory tract infection is much less than in children but chronic bronchitis and asthma each account for 30–40 consultations per 1000 population per year and form an important proportion of the general practitioner's work.

Today it is most unusual for a general practitioner to pick up a case of tuberculosis, yet in the mid 19th century this was the single commonest cause of death in Britain. The attack rate was very high and the mortality rate about 50 per cent. Improving social conditions led to a steady decrease in these rates, briefly interrupted by the two world wars and accelerated, some 30 years ago, by the introduction of modern chemotherapy and BCG. It is now a relatively minor problem in Britain despite residual higher rates in some immigrant groups. But in the world as a whole the picture is much grimmer. There has been no decrease in prevalence in most countries in the Third World. Indeed, as their populations have greatly increased and their attack rates have failed to fall, there is probably more tuberculosis in the world now than there was 30 years ago.

The impact of environmental air pollution on the lungs is exemplified in occupational respiratory diseases. Coalworkers' pneumoconiosis, stone and haematite miners' pneumoconiosis, silicosis, stannosis, and many others have been long recognized and, at least in Britain, steps have been taken to prevent them by controlling dust and monitoring exposure. In 1950 more than 4000 cases were notified each year. In 1982 a ten-fold reduction had been achieved, to 467 new diagnoses of coalworkers' pneumoconiosis and 96 new pneumoconiosis diagnoses in other industries.

There has been much concern in recent years about asbestos risks, previously underestimated. Diffuse pulmonary fibrosis (asbestosis) is serious enough but recent concern is due to evidence that asbestosis strongly predisposes to lung cancer, greatly enhancing the carcinogenic effect of tobacco smoking. The public has been further alarmed by the association of even relatively minor exposure to certain types of asbestos dust with the development, usually after a very long interval, of pleural mesothelioma. In contrast to the development of lung cancer in asbestosis this form of malignant disease is unrelated to tobacco smoking. Numerically, asbestos-related diseases are not of great importance in the United Kingdom, but world-wide there are pockets of very high incidence such as in Canada, South Africa, and the USSR,

regions where there is both mining of asbestos and manufacture of products from it.

Byssinosis has been a recognized hazard in the cotton, jute, and hemp industries for centuries. It gives rise to wheeze and breathlessness, but is a disease not yet completely understood. The importance of fumes and dusts in causing occupational asthma has only recently been appreciated. It has now become a statutorily certifiable disease in Britain, and in certain other countries.

The inhalation of dusts containing organic materials can give rise to an allergic alveolitis. The naming of the first discovered of these as 'Farmers' Lung', after the occupational group in whom it is most prevalent, has led to the proliferation of a rash of picturesque names for other similar disorders described in many different parts of the world – paprika-pickers' lung, maple bark strippers' lung, budgerigar fanciers' lung, etc. etc.

Mortality

The mortality from respiratory disease varies strikingly with age and to some extent with sex. Current statistics from England and Wales are given in Figs 1 and 2. It will be noted that lower respira-

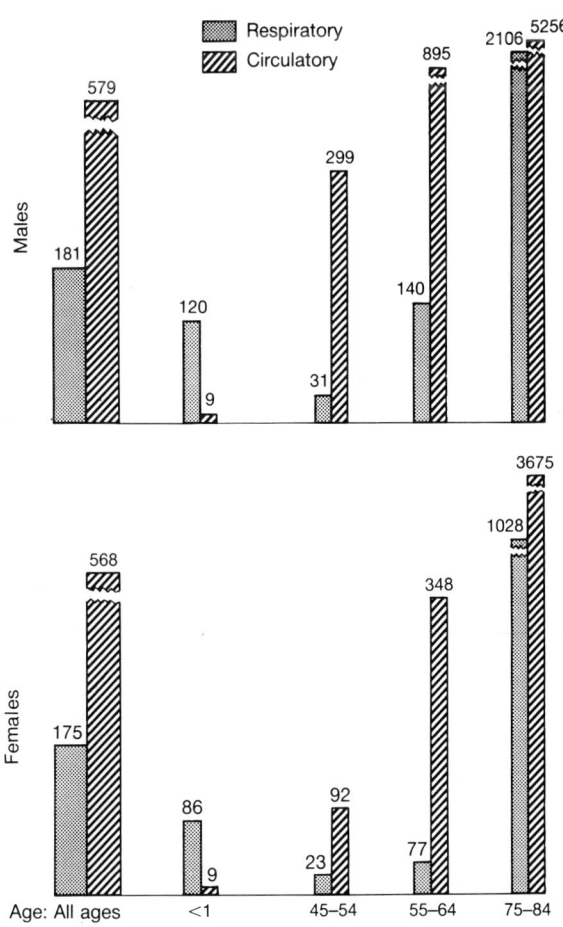

Fig. 1 Mortality per 100 000 population from diseases of the respiratory (ICD 460–519) and circulatory (ICD 390–459) systems at selected ages in England and Wales in 1982. *Source*: Registrar General's Report, Office of Population Censuses and Surveys.

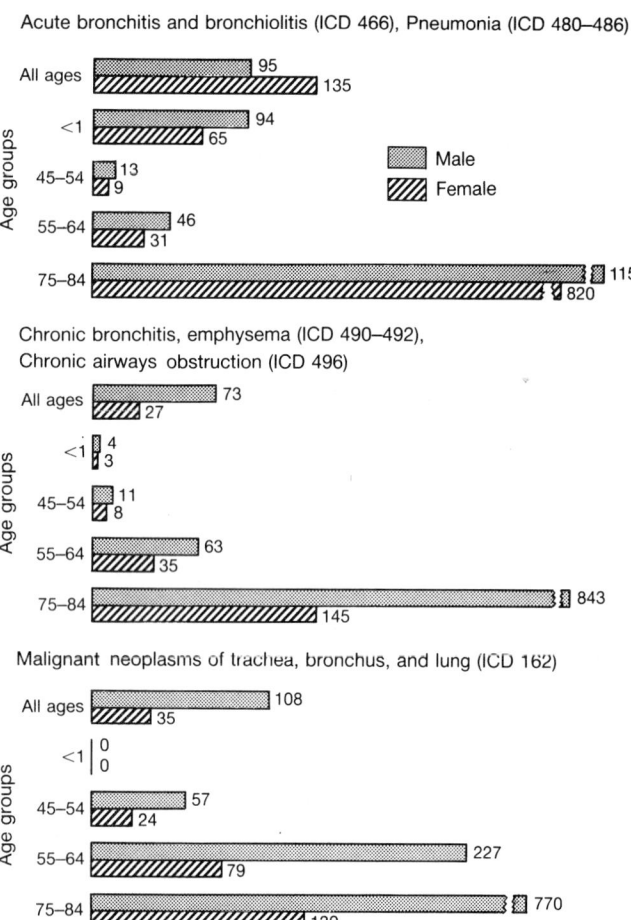

Fig. 2 Mortality rates per 100 000 population from the main groups of respiratory diseases at selected ages, and by sex, in England and Wales in 1982. *Source*: as Fig 1. The higher mortality rate from respiratory infections for females at 'All ages', in contrast to their lower rates than males in the specific age-groups, is due to the much larger numbers of women surviving into old age with its higher respiratory mortality.

tory tract infections make a major contribution in infancy and in old age, with malignant neoplasms of trachea, bronchus, and lung, and the diseases of airway obstruction, more important in middle age: a much higher mortality from respiratory than from circulatory diseases occurs in infancy, but there is a dramatic reversal of this in middle age when the rate for cardiovascular disease, mainly ischaemic, becomes much higher than the rate for respiratory disease.

There is still a possibility for improvement, through earlier diagnosis and better treatment, in infant respiratory mortality. There may also be some scope for improvement in the pneumonia of old age, though the diagnosis on death certificates in the old often lacks precision and the scope may be less than might at first glance appear. But a high proportion of the deaths from lung cancer and from chronic bronchitis and emphysema are theoretically preventable if tobacco smoking was to be effectively controlled.

International comparisons

International comparisons of respiratory mortality are difficult, as few Third World countries have accurate statistics. In many countries in Africa, South and Central America, and Asia infant mortality rates are 30 or more times higher than in North America or Europe. In most of these countries about a third of these deaths are due to respiratory infection. Figure 3 shows comparisons between some developed and developing countries for mortality from respiratory infections. Malnutrition, poor housing, and inadequate treatment probably contribute to the differences.

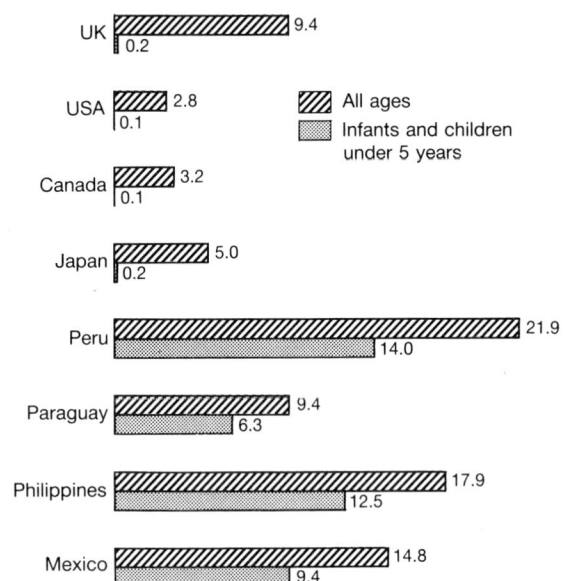

Fig. 3 Mortality from acute respiratory infections as a percentage of deaths from all causes in selected countries (for available years 1973–78). *Source*: Chrétien *et al.* (1984).

There are considerable international variations too in mortality from chronic bronchitis, emphysema, and chronic obstructive lung disease. Although these differences probably to a large extent reflect different smoking habits, other factors may also play a part. Industrial and domestic atmospheric pollution was formerly important in Britain and in certain other countries but has now been greatly reduced. In many Third World countries, though factory chimneys are rarities, domestic smoke may act synergistically with tobacco smoke. Increasing industrialization bringing atmospheric pollution unfortunately often goes hand in hand with increasing affluence and tobacco smoking and, unless the Third World countries read the message so evident in Western mortality statistics, they too will reap a bitter harvest of chronic lung disease. In addition there is suggestive, if not yet conclusive, evidence that inadequately treated respiratory infections in childhood may leave a residuum which contributes to chronic bronchitis and bronchiectasis in adult life.

On the whole the mortality rates for lung cancer also reflect differences in smoking patterns between countries, and between the sexes in those countries, though there are certain anomalies. For instance, the rates in females in Hong Kong and northwest India are higher than might be expected from their smoking habits and in these areas it seems likely that there may be some other factor operating.

Sadly, in morbidity and mortality from smoking-related diseases, the countries of the British Isles show a grim primacy which represents for them by far their greatest challenge to preventive medicine. Equally sadly, the smoking epidemic which has caused so much havoc in industrialized countries is now beginning to affect the non-industrialized nations so that, just as they are emerging from the burden of ill-health from malnutrition and infection, they will be struck down by an epidemic of chronic obstructive lung disease, ischaemic heart disease, and lung cancer.

Causative factors in respiratory disease

Infection

Much of the mortality due to lower respiratory infection is due to bacterial pneumonia. The single most important causative organism both in Britain and elsewhere is *Streptococcus pneumoniae*, and this despite the fact that it is potentially susceptible to many antibiotics. Pneumonia acquired in hospital may be due to a wide range of organisms and is often more difficult to treat. Although so far there is no widely available specific chemotherapy for viral infections, these are less often fatal. If agents are developed which are specific for particular viruses rapid diagnosis will become much more important. In many developing countries pulmonary tuberculosis remains a major challenge. Curative chemotherapy is now a reality and techniques have been developed which should make prevention feasible, but the scale and cost of the undertaking are formidable.

Tobacco smoking

Tobacco smoking is the major cause of lung cancer, chronic bronchitis, and chronic obstructive lung disease which, together with ischaemic heart disease, are responsible for a high proportion of the mortality in the later years of working life (Figs 1 and 2), both in Britain and in most other industrialized countries. Tobacco smoking by pregnant mothers affects the unborn child, by parents makes infants more liable to lower respiratory tract infections, and by married men increases their wife's risk of lung cancer.

It is not surprising, therefore, that smoking is accepted as the most important preventable cause of death in Britain. Unfortunately there are considerable counter pressures from the powerful tobacco industry so that, though much has been done, much more could be done. Stemming from the second (1971) of a series of reports on the subject by the Royal College of Physicians of London, the establishment of a campaigning body, Action on Smoking and Health (ASH), has done much to rouse public opinion and has obtained steadily increasing support from professional organizations. Government financed health education bodies devote more than a quarter of their resources to the problem.

Educational programmes are becoming more enthusiastic, especially since research has begun to evolve techniques which are demonstrably effective in children. The media have taken a major interest in the subject and have been increasingly supportive. With a majority of the population in England and Wales now non-smokers (Fig. 4) peer-pressure is beginning to have its effect, resulting in mounting action to decrease smoking in public places and on public transport. Health considerations have led to the raising of taxation on cigarettes which has been repeatedly shown to decrease consumption. Unfortunately advertizing and tobacco-industry sponsorship of sport and cultural events, which may have a major influence on the young, have not yet been adequately controlled. Although it is often difficult to demonstrate the specific effect of any one measure (apart from a sharp increase in tobacco duty) there has clearly been a cumulative effect from all these activities. It has been calculated that in Britain one million people give up smoking every year.

The decreases in smoking outlined above, together with the decrease in the tar content in cigarettes and the increasing use of cigarette filters, are now beginning to have an effect on mortality. In Britain death rates from lung cancer in males in early middle age have dropped, in some age groups, by as much as 50 per cent, though at the moment this is largely compensated by increased rates in older cohorts. Unfortunately the rates in women, who started smoking later and have only recently begun to give up, are still rising sharply. There has been a substantial decrease in death rates from chronic bronchitis/emphysema in males, though the decrease in atmospheric pollution (see below) has probably also made a contribution.

Atmospheric pollution

Only a little over 30 years ago Britain probably had the most polluted atmosphere in the world. The great London smog of 1952, with 4000 excess deaths within a few days, alarmed the public and led both to intensive research and to government action. As a result of the subsequent *Clean Air Acts* smoke pollution has fallen by 90–95 per cent. Research at the beginning of this campaign showed the very important effect of atmospheric pollution, together with tobacco smoking, in causing death in patients with

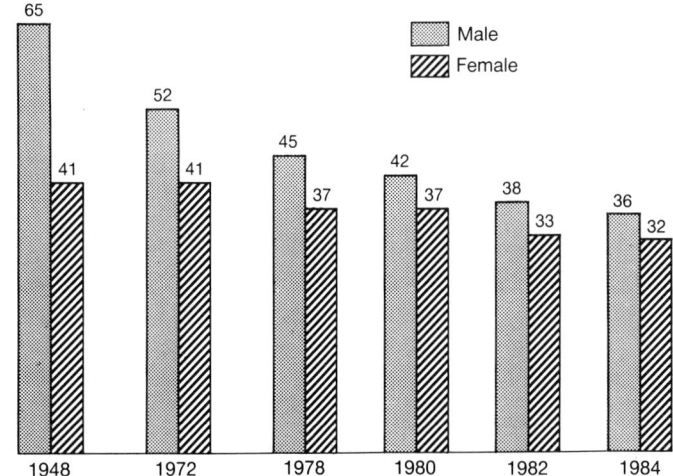

Fig. 4 Percentage adult smokers in Great Britain 1948–82. Figures for 1948 include Northern Ireland; those for Great Britain alone not separately available: *Source*: Capell (1978). Remaining figures from General Household Survey. *Source*: OPCS Monitor GHS 8.

chronic bronchitis. The aetiological contribution of pollution to lung cancer has been much less easy to demonstrate. In consequence it is difficult to determine with certainty whether smoke reduction is one of the factors responsible for the decrease in mortality in younger males.

Immunological aspects of respiratory disease

The great advances currently being made in immunology have important implications for respiratory disease. Impairment of the immune defences by disease, tobacco smoking, alcohol, or medication predisposes to respiratory infection and makes that infection more difficult to treat. There is increasing evidence that the mobilization of the immune system by known, or so far unknown, agents may have adverse effects, resulting in either functional abnormality, as in asthma, or in tissue damage, as in cryptogenic diffuse fibrosing alveolitis. The identification of immunoglobulin E as an important component of the immediate reaction to an allergen led to massive research on the immunological aspects of asthma. This interest has now extended to more long-term reactions, which are probably more important in the clinical disease and in the pathogenesis of chronic asthma. So far we have glimpses of only part of the picture, but progess is rapid and the pathogenesis of asthma may become much clearer in a few years.

Conclusions

Respiratory diseases are clearly of great importance, not only to the public health but also to the economy. They afflict, at least to a minor degree, virtually everyone in the population. Their prevention, particularly the prevention of smoking-related diseases, provides the major challenge to preventive medicine both in Britain and in many other countries. Their diagnosis and treatment is relevant to almost every branch of clinical medicine. The following sections review in greater detail this immense and challenging field.

References

Bulla, A. and Hitze, K. L. (1978). Acute respiratory infection; a review. *Bull. Wld Hlth Org.* **56**, 481–498.

Capell, P. J. (1978). Trends in cigarette smoking in the United Kingdom. *Hlth Bull. (Edin.)* **36**, 286–294.

Chrétien, J., Holland, W., Macklem, P., Murray, J. and Woolcock, A. (1984). Acute respiratory infections in children: a global public health problem. *N. Engl. J. Med.* **310**, 982–984.

Crofton, J. and Douglas, A. (1981). *Respiratory diseases* 3rd edn. Blackwell Scientific Publications, Oxford.

Fry, J., White, R. and Whitfield, M. (1984). *Respiratory disorders*. Churchill Livingstone, London.

Leowski, J. (1984). *Acute respiratory infections – the magnitude of the problem*. A report from the Tuberculosis and Respiratory Infections Unit, Division of Communicable Diseases, World Health Organisation, given at XIth International Conference for Tropical Medicine and Malaria. Calgary, Canada.

Royal College of Physicians (1970). *Air pollution and health*. Pitman, London.

Royal College of Physicians (1983). *Health or smoking?* Pitman, London.

World Health Organization (1980). *Viral respiratory diseases. Report of a WHO Scientific Group*. Technical Report Series 642. World Health Organization, Geneva.

THE STRUCTURE OF THE LUNG AND ITS INVESTIGATION

Pulmonary anatomy

M. S. DUNNILL

The structure of the lungs is adapted to the functions of gas transport in airways, gas mixing in the acini and gas transfer from air to blood across the alveolar-capillary membrane.

Airways in the conducting zone

Trachea

The tracheobronchial tree in man consists of an irregularly branching dichotomous system of tubes. It begins with the trachea which is 10 cm in length but only half is in the thorax. In cross-section the trachea is shaped like a D, the straight portion lying posteriorly and having a wall lacking cartilage and composed largely of smooth muscle and connective tissue. The curved portion is anterior and contains the cartilaginous rings which are more accurately described as horse-shoe shaped. There are approximately 20 of these cartilages which prevent total collapse of the airway when it is subject to positive transmural pressure although narrowing may be present due to invagination of the posterior wall.

Bronchi and bronchioles

The trachea divides into right and left main bronchi which have the same general shape in cross-section as the trachea and are extrapulmonary. Within the lung the bronchi divide in a dichotomous manner. Apparent trichotomous branching is caused by extremely short branches. It is an important general rule that in intrapulmonary bronchi two daughter airways have a greater cross-sectional area than the parent airway. They also have a much more irregular arrangement of cartilage than in the trachea and main bronchi. In transverse section up to four cartilaginous plates can often be seen in larger airways and these are placed circumferentially in the bronchial wall. As the bronchi become smaller, cartilage decreases in quantity and tends to be found mainly at points of bifurcation.

In the right lung, which has three lobes, the main bronchus divides into an upper and lower lobe branch and the latter gives off a branch to the middle lobe. In the left lung, which has two lobes, the main bronchus divides into upper and lower lobe branches. Division of these five bronchi occurs into named segmental bronchi which supply the bronchopulmonary segments of the lung (Table 1). These are separate distinct units, originally described by the Guy's Hospital surgeon Brock, and are of importance because they can be surgically removed without excision of the entire lobe.

Further dichotomous branching takes place in the bronchi until bronchioles are formed. These are defined as airways without cartilage and mucous glands in their walls, and they divide in a similar manner until the terminal bronchiole is reached. Distal to terminal bronchioles airways contain alveoli in their walls and are termed respiratory bronchioles. The terminal bronchioles supply the respiratory unit of the lung known as the acinus. The total number of generations, that is of branching, varies in different parts of the lung but it is estimated that there are approximately 25 000 terminal bronchioles.

Histology of airways in the conducting zone

The airways are lined by a pseudostratified columnar ciliated epithelium containing a variety of cell types. In the trachea and larger bronchi this epithelium is several layers thick but becomes greatly thinned towards the periphery of the lung and is only one cell thick at the level of the terminal bronchiole.

Basal cells are situated immediately adjacent to the basement membrane and are small, pyramidal in shape, and have a high nuclear cytoplasmic ratio. When overlying ciliated cells are damaged, it is these which proliferate and differentiate to replace them.

Feyrter cells, also known as K cells, are interspersed with basal cells and are also present in the bronchial glands. They form part of the APUD (amine precursor uptake decarboxylation) system being allied to Kultschitzsky cells of the small intestine. They are maximal in number in smaller bronchi. Electron microscopy reveals characteristic intracytoplasmic bodies approximately 100 nm diameter composed of a central electron-dense core surrounded by a translucent halo and bounded by a membrane. These are known as dense core vesicles. It is thought that they have an endocrine function and there is some evidence they they have chemoreceptor properties as they have been shown to degranulate under hypoxic conditions. These cells have dendritic type cytoplasmic processes which extend through the mucous membrane towards the luminal surface. The bronchial carcinoid tumour and probably the oat-cell carcinoma are both derived from the Feyrter cell. The dense core vesicles found in these tumour cells are the site of abnormal hormone production often associated with these neoplasms.

Intermediate cells lie on basal cells and have an elongated shape. They are thought to develop into columnar cells.

Table 1 Segmental bronchi: named bronchopulmonary segments

Right upper lobe	Left upper lobe
Apical	Apico-posterior
Posterior	Anterior
Anterior	
Right middle lobe	Lingula
Lateral	Superior
Medial	Inferior
Right lower lobe	Left lower lobe
Apical	Apical
Anterior basal	Anterior basal
Lateral basal	Lateral basal
Posterior basal	Posterior basal
Medial basal or cardiac	

Ciliated cells are found in respiratory mucosa from the level of the trachea to the terminal bronchiole. They play a vital part in pulmonary defence as the mucociliary escalator constitutes the major method whereby particles are removed from the respiratory tract. They are the most frequent cell in the trachea and main bronchi. The nucleus occupies a basal position. The cytoplasm contains mitochondria near the apex and lysosomes are often prominent. Yet their most important feature is seen on the luminal aspect of the cell surface where cilia are to be found together with microvilli. There are approximately 200 cilia to each cell and individually they measure 6 μm in length and 0.3 μm in diameter. Cross-sections of cilia reveal a constant arrangement of two central longitudinal microtubules enclosed in a sheath which is itself surrounded by a matrix containing nine double microtubules. This is often referred to as the nine plus two structure. One of each of the pair of tubules found in the outer units is slightly larger than the other and is notable for possessing a short diverging projection made up of the protein dynein and usually referred to as the dynein arm. These structures are involved in ciliary motility and are missing or deformed in conditions of ciliary immotility such as Kartagener's syndrome. Ciliary fibres continue into the outer portion of the cell cytoplasm, become triplet in form, and are associated with a densely staining structure near the apex of the cell known as the basal body from which further fibres pass into the cytoplasm. The exact functional significance of this complex structural arrangement is not understood, but it has been suggested that the peripheral microtubules are concerned with contraction, deriving their energy from adenosine triphosphate, and the central fibres have a co-ordinating function.

Goblet cells are much less common than ciliated cells in normal respiratory mucosa. They have a basally placed nucleus and prominent Golgi apparatus. Ribosomes and granular endoplasmic reticulum in the cell cytoplasm synthesize the protein component of mucus which is combined with the carbohydrate component in the Golgi zone. Small mucinogen droplets are formed which gradually increase in size, coalesce to form a large vacuole, move towards the apex of the cell, and are finally expelled from the cell surface by exocytosis. The precise appearance of the cell depends upon the stage of the cycle of mucus production at which the cell is observed.

Clara cells are most numerous in bronchioles where they appear singly or in groups of two or three. Their surface projects further into the lumen of the airway than adjacent ciliated cells. This characteristic allows their presence to be suspected in light microscope sections but certain identification requires electron microscopy. There are numerous mitochondria and plentiful smooth endoplasmic reticulum is found near the luminal surface together with many small electron-dense granules. The function of these cells has been the subject of considerable argument but it is highly probable that they are concerned with secretion of a surfactant-like substance. Certainly this cytoplasm is rich in lipoprotein and oxidative enzymes.

Distribution of cells in the airways

In the trachea and large bronchi the pseudostratified columnar epithelium is several layers thick. Towards the periphery the epithelium becomes gradually thinner so that in pre-terminal bronchioles there are only one or two cell layers, goblet cells are not found, and Clara cells are plentiful. In terminal bronchioles ciliated cells are still present although they are cuboidal in shape but generally they are absent in the respiratory bronchioles.

Bronchial glands

These form an important feature of the bronchial wall and are responsible for the major portion of secretion entering the bronchial lumen. They are seromucinous in type but in addition to serous and mucous cells contain, in their collecting ducts, myoepithelial cells and ciliated cells. These ducts pass through the bronchial mucosa to open into the bronchial lumen. The glands are situated between mucosa and cartilage as well as between and deep to cartilage. The mucous component of these glands increases greatly in chronic bronchitis. Serous cells have small electron-dense granules in their cytoplasm and secrete lysozyme and neutral glycoprotein. Ultrastructurally mucous cells are similar to goblet cells and secrete acid glycoprotein. The cells found in collecting ducts include occasional Feyrter type cells similar to those in surface bronchial epithelium.

IgA-containing plasma cells may be prominent in the interstitial tissues of these glands and the conversion of this immunoglobin to its dimeric form with addition of the J and secretory components takes place here.

Submucosa

The submucosa contains loose fibrous connective tissue as well as smooth muscle. There are fairly numerous thin-walled vessels which in inflammatory or allergic states dilate and exhibit increased permeability with resulting oedema. This submucosal oedema may contribute to airways obstruction in small bronchi due not only to swelling of the submucosa but also to transudation of oedema fluid into the bronchial lumen.

Bronchial smooth muscle

In the main bronchi as in the trachea smooth muscle lies posteriorly being attached to the two ends of the horse-shoe shaped cartilages. In intrapulmonary bronchi muscle is present in the submucosa and although it may appear discontinuous in histological sections, it is in fact a spiral or helical structure with two components, one turning to the right and the other to the left. At varying points this muscle has connections to the perichondrium formed by bands of collagen and reticulin. The proportion of muscle in the bronchial wall is greater in smaller than larger airways reaching a maximum in terminal bronchioles.

The importance of smooth muscle in producing resistance to air flow in man is debated. In asthma where airway resistance is markedly raised bronchial muscle is certainly greatly increased in volume. In normal lungs the small airways account for only a minor proportion of total airway resistance, but in chronic bronchitis and emphysema peripheral airway resistance increases very greatly though it seems this is accounted for more by peribronchial fibrosis than by contraction of hypertrophied smooth muscle.

Respiratory zone

The acinus

The pleural surface of the lung has a mosaic appearance due to septa composed of thin strands of collagenous tissue surrounding veins and lymphatics. These septa, which can be seen very clearly in adult town dwellers' lungs because of carbon deposition in lymphatics, outline secondary lobules of the lung described by Miller. It would be convenient if these constituted the main respiratory unit, that is if each lobule was supplied by a terminal bronchiole. Unfortunately this is not so and each secondary lobule contains between two and five terminal bronchioles. The important unit of the respiratory zone of the lung is the *acinus* and this is defined as that portion of the lung distal to the terminal bronchiole. In man there are approximately 25 000 acini. They tend to be pyramidal in shape with the terminal bronchiole and muscular pulmonary artery entering at the apex. The dichotomous branching process extends beyond the terminal bronchiole which then divides into two respiratory bronchioles concerned not only with conduction of gas to and from more distal portions of the acinus but also with gas exchange in alveoli that arise from portions of their walls. There are usually two or three orders of respiratory bronchioles which finally divide into alveolar ducts which are entirely surrounded by alveoli and from which alveolar sacs and terminal alveoli arise.

Alveoli

These vary somewhat in shape and size. Those in upper zones of lung are larger than those at the base. The shape of the alveolus has been likened to a truncated cone superimposed on a cone but it varies considerably with respiration. The maximum alveolar diameter lies between 200 and 250 μm. Their walls contain numerous capillaries and a little connective tissue and are shared between adjacent alveoli.

Alveolar cells

The alveolus has a continuous cellular lining composed mainly of two types of cell. Type I pneumocytes have greatly attenuated cytoplasm which covers by far the greater portion of the alveolar surface. In the cytoplasm there are few mitochondria and little in the way of endoplasmic reticulum. The cells are joined one to another and to type II pneumocytes by tight junctions. Type I pneumocytes provide a major part of the barrier to gas exchange but the enormous surface area of the cell renders it particularly liable to damage by inhaled noxious agents. Hyaline membranes seen in the neonatal distress syndrome and in adults following inhalation of toxic materials or ingestion of substances such as paraquat, are largely formed from necrotic cellular material derived from type I pneumocytes together with exudate from alveolar capillaries.

Type II pneumocytes are cuboidal in shape and although probably more numerous than type I pneumocytes occupy little of the surface of the alveolus. They have blunt microvilli on their luminal aspect and their cytoplasm contains, in addition to numerous mitochondria and much endoplasmic reticulum, characteristic vacuoles with lamellated osmiophilic bodies. These can sometimes be seen discharging their contents onto the alveolar surface. The material discharged is pulmonary surfactant. Although in routine histological sections type I alveolar epithelium appears to be in direct contact with air, *in vivo* there is a layer of surfactant present over the entire surface. Using special perfusion fixation techniques this can be demonstrated under the electron microscope as an extra-cellular osmiophilic layer.

In addition to secretion of surfactant type II pneumocytes have another important function in that they are the progenitor of type I cells. If the latter undergo necrosis, which happens readily if they are exposed to pulmonary poisons, type II cells proliferate giving rise to the appearance of cuboidal cells lining alveoli which is so frequently encountered in histological sections in 'interstitial' lung disease. Provided the noxious stimulus is removed they may differentiate into type I pneumocytes and restore the alveolar lining.

Another cell, the type III pneumocyte, sometimes referred to as a brush cell because of prominent regular microvilli on its luminal border, has been described. It is found in alveoli and sometimes in airways. Its function is not fully understood but it is thought to be concerned with chemoreception or to be connected with fluid absorption.

The alveolar wall contains a network of intercommunicating capillaries. In gaps between capillaries are small quantities of connective tissue and occasional interalveolar communications known as pores of Kohn. Alveolar endothelial cells contain numerous caveolae which have small 'diaphragms'. The membranes lining these caveolae contain enzymes engaged in metabolism of angiotensin I and bradykinin. The interstitial tissues contain at least two types of cell, one of which has myofilaments and because of its juxtaposition to the pulmonary capillaries is considered to have some control over their diameter. The other cell is a macrophage.

Alveolar macrophages form a very important part of the pulmonary defence mechanism. They are bone marrow derived but there is evidence that some may proliferate in the interstitial tissues of the alveolar walls before entering the alveolar spaces. Following ingestion of foreign particles or bacteria macrophages migrate to the level of the respiratory bronchiole where they either enter lymphatics or join the mucociliary escalator. Bacterial clearance from the lung is dependent on alveolar macrophages and may be depressed by such divergent factors as virus infection, intoxication with ethanol, cold, hypoxia, and starvation. Of great importance is the inhibitory effect of cigarette smoke on macrophage activity. It results in release of enzymes such as collagenase and elastase which may cause permanent damage to lung parenchyma and are of considerable consequence in the pathogenesis of emphysema.

Lung growth

At birth the lung has its full complement of non-alveolar airways, that is airways proximal to the terminal bronchiole, and the process of bronchial branching is complete. This is not true of the alveoli. The precise number of alveoli present at birth is disputed but it is probably in the region of 20 to 40×10^6 whereas adult lungs have at least 300×10^6 and maybe more. It is probable that the full complement of alveoli is present by the age of eight years. Disorders of post-natal growth may well be of importance in certain rare forms of 'congenital' emphysema.

The alveolar surface area in the adult is usually quoted as being of the order of 70–80 m^2. In the neonate it is approximately 3 m^2. This considerable increase takes place by addition of new alveoli in early childhood but thereafter occurs as a result of increase in size of existing alveoli. Figures given for alveolar surface area must not be regarded as 'absolute' as they are based on light microscope measurements. The estimate will increase the higher the magnification as finer and more subtle undulations of the alveolar surface are revealed. Yet values obtained by light microscopy are of great help in comparative studies allowing one to assess the considerable reduction of surface area that takes place in destructive disorders of the pulmonary parenchyma such as emphysema.

Regeneration of bronchial epithelium

A remarkable property of bronchial mucosa is its power to regenerate following the shedding of columnar epithelium, which often takes place in acute bacterial or viral infections and as a consequence of transudation of fluid across the basement membrane in submucosal oedema. The ciliated columnar epithelial cells, intermediate cells, and goblets are desquamated together with some basal cells but many of the latter remain to proliferate and replace the lost mucosa. At first the new lining consists of a simple stratified squamous type epithelium which, after approximately three weeks, differentiates into a columnar ciliated form. This phenomenon is of clinical importance as during the period of regeneration when the airways are lined by non-ciliated epithelium one of the main defence mechanisms of the lung is defective and secondary infection is liable to occur. Ciliary function may not return to normal even when cilia can be seen on microscopy, as initially atypical compound forms are found with a deranged microtubular structure.

Pulmonary circulation

Pulmonary arteries

Pulmonary arterial structure is adapted to functional requirements of a low pressure system. Pulmonary arteries provide low resistance for transmission of total cardiac output. Gravity rather than constriction of muscular vessels plays an important role in directing flow to different portions of the pulmonary vascular bed.

The pulmonary trunk in the fetus, where there is pulmonary hypertension, and in the neonate has a similar structure to that of the aorta with a media composed of numerous parallel elastic laminae enclosing smooth muscle fibres and a little acid sulphated mucopolysaccharide. There is a clearly defined internal elastic lamina and a thin intima. During the first few months of life, following the fall in pulmonary artery pressure at birth, the media involutes to adopt an 'adult' form. The greatest change is seen in the arrangement of elastic laminae which instead of exhibiting a regular parallel pattern become scanty, short, widely spaced, and irregular in shape often having clubbed ends. The remaining part of the media is composed of connective tissue containing plentiful ground substance and irregularly orientated smooth muscle fibres. The importance of these changes lies in the observation that in children and adults dying with severe pulmonary hypertension the pulmonary trunk shows only atheroma provided the hypertension has been acquired during life. On the other hand, if it has been present since birth, the media has a fetal or aortic configuration of elastic tissue.

Elastic or conducting pulmonary arteries extend from the pulmonary trunk to vessels with an external diameter of approximately 1 mm. They lie adjacent to the bronchi and bronchioles, roughly follow the same branching pattern, and are enclosed in a common connective tissue sheath. Their structure reflects their function, namely conducting blood rather than influencing direction of blood flow. The media of these vessels provides their characteristic feature with concentric parallel elastic laminae. Near the hilum there may be up to 20 such laminae but at the periphery in smaller vessels only three or four are found. Smooth muscle cells lie between the elastic fibres. The intima is composed of a layer of endothelium together with a thin layer of fibrous connective tissue which lies on the clearly defined internal elastic lamina.

Muscular pulmonary arteries, which also accompany airways and are found at the level of the terminal and first order respiratory bronchioles, range from approximately 1000 μm to 100 μm in external diameter and have a media defined by internal and external elastic laminae. They show a striking quantitative difference from the thick-walled systemic muscular arteries in that in transverse sections the thickness of the media accounts for less than 10 per cent of the total diameter of the vessel. In pulmonary hypertension a considerable increase in medial thickness, often accompanied by intimal fibrosis, is found.

Pulmonary arterioles are defined as vessels less than 100 μm external diameter. They have exceedingly thin walls composed of endothelium and a single elastic lamina which sometimes splits to enclose a single spirally wound smooth muscle fibre.

Pulmonary capillaries are adapted to the process of gas exchange between blood and air in alveoli without leakage of red cells into the alveolar space. The vessels are of small diameter, thus following the Laplace law, have low tension in their walls, and are perfused at low pressure. If pulmonary capillary pressure was higher, the wall would have to be thicker in order to prevent leakage of red cells and this would seriously impair gas exchange. Pulmonary capillaries are arranged in an intercommunicating network in the alveolar wall. Their endothelial cells possess thin attentuated cytoplasm lying on a thin basement membrane which is mostly fused with that on which the alveolar epithelial cells lie. Narrow slits can be seen between one endothelial cell and the next and thus the major resistance to fluid flow through the alveolar wall is provided by the epithelial cells and their tight junctions.

Pulmonary venous system
Pulmonary venules are indistinguishable from pulmonary arterioles but they drain into veins situated in the interlobular septa. These veins pass to the apex of the secondary lobules where they join airways and pulmonary arteries. The walls of pulmonary veins are made up of collagen, acid mucopolysaccharide, elastic fibres, and irregularly arranged smooth muscle. There is often no clear demarcation between media and adventitia but there is often a somewhat indistinct line of elastic tissue separating the thin intima from the media.

Bronchial arteries
The bronchial arterial system arises directly from the aorta and provides the lung with the systemic arterial supply which is particularly valuable in supplying oxygen and nutrition to the upper zones which are not well perfused by the low pressure pulmonary circulation. These vessels have the structure of systemic muscular arteries with a thick muscular media and follow airways throughout the lung. They communicate with the pulmonary arteries at capillary level in the bronchial submucosa. In inflammatory bronchial diseases, notably saccular bronchiectasis, these communications may enlarge considerably to form true bronchopulmonary arterial anastomoses. Many bronchial carcinomas gain their blood supply almost exclusively from the bronchial circulation.

Lymphatics
Lymphatics are not found at the level of peripheral alveoli. Most authorities consider they commence at the level of the respiratory bronchiole and then follow airways to the hilum of the lung. They are joined by a second system which has its origin in the pleura and in the interlobular septa. They are formed of endothelium with very little surrounding connective tissue. Valves are present ensuring flow towards the hilum. Small aggregates of lymphoid tissue are found within the lung usually situated adjacent to bronchial bifurcations and larger nodes are present at the hilum.

Nerve supply
The precise innervation of the lung is ill understood. It receives both efferent and afferent fibres via the vagus nerve. It is thought that efferent fibres are responsible for constriction of bronchial smooth muscle. Stimulation of vagal efferent fibres in experimental animals also results in increased secretion from bronchial seromucinous glands and dilatation of pulmonary arterioles. Non-adrenergic inhibitory nerve fibres have recently been demonstrated but the importance of this system in man needs to be elucidated. Nerve endings can be seen in between the cells of the respiratory mucosa in large airways and these are derived from vagal afferent fibres and are concerned with the cough reflex. Afferent fibres are also derived from stretch receptors in both airways and alveoli. Nerve endings have been described in close relation to type I pneumocytes in alveoli and these are thought to be afferent and related to J receptors. It is also possible that nerve endings which have been seen in close relation to type II pneumocytes may be concerned with nervous control of surfactant secretion. The lung receives no sympathetic nerve supply.

References
Dunnill, M. S. (1982). *Pulmonary pathology*, Churchill Livingstone, Edinburgh.

Reid, L. (1967). *The pathology of emphysema*. Lloyd Luke, London.

Scadding, J. G., Cumming, G., and Thurlbeck, W. M. (1981). *Respiratory medicine*. Heinemann, London.

Thurlbeck, W. M. (1978). *The lung, structure function and disease*. Williams and Wilkins, Baltimore.

Weibel, E. R. (1963). *Morphometry of the human lung*. Springer Verlag, Berlin.

Diagnostic bronchoscopy and tissue biopsy

M. F. MUERS

Diagnostic bronchoscopy and tissue biopsy are an integral part of the investigation of respiratory disease, but should be regarded as complementary to, rather than substitutes for, simpler diagnostic tests.

Bronchoscopy (Table 1)
Bronchial abnormalities may present in many ways, some of which do not immediately suggest endobronchial disease, as, for example, recurrent infections or breathlessness with a normal chest radiograph. Diagnosis at bronchoscopy is not confined to visible lesions; the simultaneous use of flexible sampling instruments and fluoroscopy allows biopsy of distal bronchi or lung parenchyma.

Rigid bronchoscopy is usually performed under general anaesthesia, and oxygen Venturi ventilation. Bronchoscopy using the flexible bronchofibrescope is performed using sedation and topical anaesthesia. The bronchoscope is usually passed transnasally, but may be passed transorally alone or via an endotracheal tube. Standard fibrescopes cannot be used in small children. Using the rigid

Table 1 Indications for bronchoscopy

Diagnosis
  Suspected malignancy
  Unexplained haemoptysis
  Unexplained localized or diffuse radiographic opacity
  Unexplained respiratory symptoms
  For bronchoscopic bronchogram
  For microbiological sampling
Therapy
  Removal of secretions, foreign body
  Endobronchial surgery
  Laser treatment of malignancy

bronchoscope with appropriate telescopes, the bronchial tree can be inspected as far as the proximal portions of the segmental bronchi. About 70 per cent of bronchogenic neoplasms are therefore within the field of view of both instruments. In practice, the flexibility of the fibrescope is of greatest advantage when examining segments of the upper lobes, or the apical segments of the lower lobes. If they are carefully performed, both methods should be regarded as safe.

The survey of British practice during 1983 revealed a complication rate of 0.12 per cent and a mortality rate of 0.04 per cent from 40 000 bronchoscopic procedures, 96 per cent of which were performed using the fibreoptic bronchoscope. The major cause of morbidity in this series was the problem of respiratory depression due to inappropriate sedation.

In addition to visual evidence of luminal endobronchial or extrabronchial lesions, tissue samples can be obtained at bronchoscopy for histological, cytological, microbiological, and immunological examination. Bronchial wall biopsies are obtained by forceps, and other samples which can be taken include brush biopsies, catheter suction specimens, needle aspirates, bronchial secretion aspirates, and limited bronchial saline lavages. The technique of transbronchial biopsy is used to sample parenchymal lung tissue (Fig. 1). Forceps are advanced peripherally under fluoroscopic control, and tissue is sampled within a centimetre or two of the pleural surface. Multiple specimens can be obtained.

Bronchoscopic bronchograms
Bronchographic contrast medium can be injected either directly through the suction channel of a fibreoptic bronchoscope, or through a narrow catheter, and selective (segmental or lobar) bronchograms, or full unilateral or bilateral bronchograms of good quality can be obtained. This is a useful complementary investigation when endobronchial appearances are normal, and the problem under investigation is, for example, haemoptysis, or a chronic productive cough with a normal chest radiograph or persistent unexplained lobar or segmental shadowing. In these circumstances, and particularly in patients over 40 years of age, a selective bronchogram may reveal unsuspected bronchiectasis, or, less commonly, stricture, as, for example, due to endobronchial sarcoidosis, or tumour.

Percutaneous needle biopsy
Needle aspiration of the lung was first used by Leyden in 1883 to diagnose pneumonia and in recent years has been used increasingly to sample peripheral lesions where malignancy is suspected. Under screening control, a needle is advanced perpendicular to the chest wall and during suspended respiration guided into the target lesion at a premeasured depth below the pleura. Tissue aspirated through a fine needle (e.g. spinal needle, tumour needle, or Rotex needle) is suitable for cytological or microbiological examination, but cannot give information about lung architecture. For this purpose either a wider bore cutting needle, e.g. Vim Silverman or Tru-cut, or the more elaborate trephine drill are used.

The use of these techniques and that of open lung biopsy is discussed in the four following sections.

Diagnosis of localized lung lesions
The most important differential diagnosis is carcinoma, and if simpler investigations are inconclusive it is usually appropriate to proceed to bronchoscopy if tissue diagnosis is required. At bronchoscopy, the sensitivity of catheter sampling, brush biopsy, and tissue biopsy are about 80 per cent for visible lesions. The few published studies show that about a 10–15 per cent increase in diagnostic sensitivity results from the combination of cytological and histological sampling, compared with histological sampling alone. There is now ample evidence that the sensitivity of both saline lavage and postbronchoscopy sputum tests is inferior.

Biopsy of peripheral (non-visible) lesions through the bronchoscope is less successful than for proximal lesions, and the diagnostic sensitivity is only about 50 per cent. It is as low as 30 per cent for lesions less than 2 cm in diameter. Because of this, a percutaneous needle biopsy under single or biplane fluoroscopic control is probably a better method. The most widely used and safest technique is fine needle aspiration. A diagnostic accuracy of about 80 per cent should be expected, and this will be progressively higher with larger and more peripheral lesions. However, this method offers only a 60 per cent accuracy in the cell-typing of tumours, and offers only limited information about benign lesions. Carefully performed cutting needle biopsies, again under screening control, have a comparable success rate, but the likelihood of a large pneumothorax is greater (perhaps 1–5 per cent). Haemorrhage needing treatment is recorded in 0.5 per cent and is especially likely when lesions more than 8 cm from the pleural surface are sampled. Because these histological specimens provide better information in non-malignant lesions, it seems rational in the author's opinion, to prefer the aspiration method as a routine, but to advise cutting needle biopsy if a benign lesion is suspected and must be biopsied, or if an accurate neoplastic cell type is imperative. Strict attention to the detail of biopsy technique is advised in order to reduce the risk of complications.

Diagnosis of diffuse parenchymal lung disease
General
The role of tissue biopsy in the diagnosis and management of patients with diffuse lung disease is one of the most perplexing problems in thoracic medicine. Published series do not give adequate answers to the questions of when and how the lung

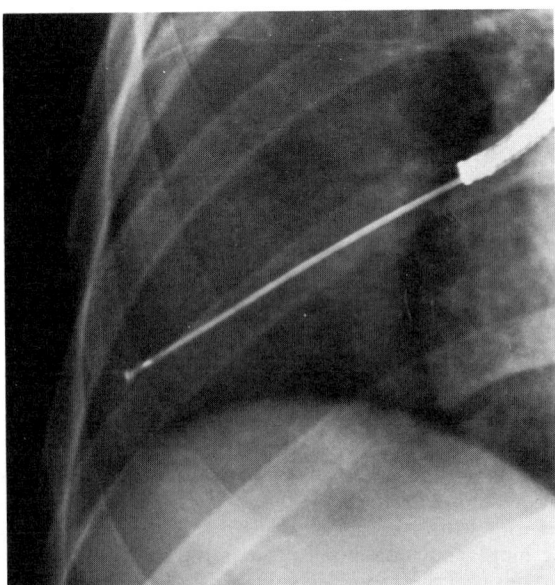

Fig. 1 Transbronchial lung biopsy through the fibreoptic bronchoscope. The flexible forceps can be seen sampling peripheral lung tissue in the right lower lobe. The bronchoscope has been wedged in a lobar bronchus. *Diagnosis*: Miliary tuberculosis in a renal transplant patient.

should be biopsied, since there are unquantifiable biases of patient selection, and it is often uncertain how the achievement of precise tissue diagnoses has benefited patients or altered the management of their condition. Furthermore, even with adequate tissue sampling, a proportion of all reported series have shown non-specific interstitial changes which are impossible to classify nosologically with present histological techniques.

Practical points are as follows: first, biopsy should not be considered until simpler non-invasive procedures have been exhausted. Secondly, biopsy should not be considered if a tissue diagnosis will not result in any change of treatment, or will not allow a more accurate prognosis to be made, for example, if a patient has a well-established non-progressive alveolar fibrosis. Thirdly, biopsy should be performed by experienced operators, or under their immediate supervision, and the safest techniques should be preferred. Fourthly, biopsy should not be performed if the occurrence of a complication, especially a pneumothorax, in the presence of reduced respiratory reserve will endanger the patient.

Technique

Needle aspiration is unsuitable. Drill biopsy and cutting needle biopsy have comparable specimen success rates (90 per cent) diagnostic yield rates (70–80 per cent) and complication rates (20–50 per cent for pneumothoraces, and 5–15 per cent for haemorrhage). Specimens obtained by the trephine are larger. Multiple transbronchial biopsies provide acinar tissue in 90 per cent of cases and diagnostically useful specimens are obtained in about 80 per cent of most series. Fewer complications are reported than with percutaneous techniques (pneumothoraces in 2.1 per cent and haemorrhage in 0.5 per cent of 3400 patients reported in the British 1983 series). The disadvantage of these biopsies is their small size (1–2 μm^3) and crush artefact. Open lung biopsy by the limited thoracotomy method introduced by Klassen (1949) remains the final arbiter in difficult cases. Pneumothoraces needing intubation occur in about 4 per cent of cases and are the major complication.

A rational approach to biopsy depends upon an assessment of the likely diagnosis after clinical and non-invasive evaluation. Transbronchial biopsy should be suitable if the diagnosis is likely to be widespread granulomata (e.g. sarcoidosis or allergic alveolitis), diffuse malignancy (lymphangitis or alveolar cell carcinoma), diffuse infection (e.g. disseminated tuberculosis or pneumocystis) or if the diagnosis may be the rarer conditions of alveolar proteinosis, or idiopathic pulmonary haemosiderosis.

If the likely diagnosis is a fibrosing alveolitis on the other hand, then the situation is more complex. If all that is required is a confirmation of interstitial alveolar fibrosis, and the exclusion of, for example, malignancy or granulomata, then transbronchial biopsies may suffice, although the proportion of negative (unsatisfactory) specimens may be high. If a more detailed histological assessment is required, then an experienced operator may choose a drill or cutting needle biopsy, but otherwise the physician should advise an open biopsy.

For other cases, the author would advise a transbronchial biopsy, and proceed to an open biopsy if no diagnosis was achieved. However, if the provisional diagnosis is of vasculitis, then an open biopsy alone is recommended.

Broncho alveolar lavage

This technique is a routine investigation in some centres, and is complementary to biopsy. At bronchoscopy, aliquots of 50 ml saline are injected in to a single basal segment until an aspirate volume of 150 ml is retrieved. This contains a harvest of free lung cells (pulmonary alveolar macrophages and leucocytes) and after cyto-centrifugation, absolute yields and differential cell counts as well as functional studies can be made.

Lavage in normal non-smoking subjects shows a preponderance of macrophages (more than 90 per cent) with 7 per cent of the cells

being lymphocytes. Their numbers are markedly increased in smokers. It has been shown that characteristic distribution profiles occur in active sarcoidosis (increase in lymphocytes) and cryptogenic fibrosing alveolitis (increase in polymorphs). However, although a characteristic cell profile may complement a clinical diagnosis, or even assist diagnosis in the presence of an inadequate biopsy, most centres will still rely on histology for diagnosis in the majority of cases.

Tuberculosis

Recent studies have shown that fibreoptic bronchoscopy can accelerate the diagnosis in cases of suspected tuberculosis with negative sputum smears. Fifty three of 134 such patients (40 per cent) from three series have had positive microscopical examination of bronchial brushings or transbronchial biopsies. A further 36 per cent yielded specimens which were positive on culture. Therefore bronchial brushings and transbronchial biopsies may effect a rapid diagnosis if this is needed, and will provide useful additional material especially if sputum specimens are inadequate or are unobtainable.

Pulmonary lesions in the immunocompromised patient

Since one of the major differential diagnoses is infection, it is important to obtain multiple specimens such as brushings, aspirates, and biopsies, both for specialized microscopy and for culture. Fibreoptic bronchoscopy is therefore the preferred method, and several series have shown a diagnostic yield above 70 per cent.

The technique of intensive cytological examination of limited, segmental lavage specimens (three 20 ml samples) appears to be particularly useful in transplant patients. However, success in achieving a diagnosis in this way depends critically on the co-operation of an experienced cytopathologist.

Patients of this type may need pretreatment with fresh frozen plasma and platelets. Sheathed brushes and sterile catheters have been shown to avoid the problem of specimen contamination by irrelevant upper respiratory tract flora. Failure to diagnose is probably best rectified by open lung biopsy even in these high-risk patients. Several centres have reported the use of bronchoscopic techniques to diagnose pulmonary shadowing in patients with AIDS, particularly because many of these patients have pneumocystis pneumonia. Careful attention has to be paid in these patients however to the problem of decontamination of the instruments and infection of operating personnel. Percutaneous needle aspiration, despite a possibly lower yield, may be considered an expedient alternative.

Pleural biopsy

As pleural disease is usually accompanied by effusion, needle aspiration is the first choice for diagnosis. Fluid is sent for microbiological, cytological, and biochemical analysis. This should be followed on the same occasion, in nearly all instances, by pleural biopsy. The latter has a reputation for being difficult and unrewarding. This is because the use of the usual instrument, the Abram's punch, needs practice, and because too few samples are taken. It is often impossible to be sure that pleura has been obtained, and it has been shown that multiple biopsies at the same site increase the diagnostic yield to 70 per cent for malignant effusions and 85 per cent for tuberculous effusions. Thoracoscopy and biopsy under direct vision may be needed in difficult cases.

Surgical biopsy

Mediastinoscopy requires a general anaesthetic and is a rigid tube inspection of the mediastinum via an anterior cervical incision. It is used to obtain specimens from mediastinal nodes, particularly on the right side, as well as from other lesions such as thymic tumours. For the former it is probably safer and more satisfactory than perbronchial needle biopsy through the rigid bronchoscope, and for the latter it is the only available method apart from anterior mediastinotomy or open thoracotomy.

Occasionally biopsies of palpably enlarged supraclavicular nodes are taken for diagnosis of intrathoracic disease. Likely causes are secondary malignancy, sarcoidosis, tuberculosis, or lymphoma.

Therapeutic bronchoscopy

The rigid bronchoscope is a superior instrument in nearly every instance, and may be used for the removal of secretions, or foreign bodies, and for endobronchial surgery such as polypectomy.

In the intensive care unit on the other hand, flexible fibrescopes are preferred for patients on IPPV. Bronchial lavage and the removal of secretions using the wider bore endoscopes may be life-saving. The problem of parenchymal tissue sampling from patients on IPPV and PEEP is a daunting one, but successful transbronchial biopsies without the development of large pneumothoraces or lung cysts at the biopsy site have been reported.

In the last five years, techniques have been developed for the treatment of haemorrhage and bronchial obstruction due to carcinoma by high energy laser photocoagulation via a flexible fibreoptic probe passed down the instrument channel of a flexible bronchoscope. At present the indications for this treatment are limited, and the technique is available at only a few centres. However, it does offer possible palliative treatment to patients in whom additional radiotherapy may not be possible, and repeated treatments can be undertaken under local or general anaesthesia.

References

Brutinel, W. M., Cortese, D. A. and McDougall, J. C. (1984). Bronchoscopic phototherapy with the neodymium – YAG laser. *Chest* **86**, 158–159.
Editorial (1983). Fibreoptic bronchoscopy and sputum-negative tuberculosis. *Lancet* i, 337–338.
Flower, C. D. R. and Verney, G. I. (1979). Percutaneous needle biopsy of thoracic lesions – an evaluation of 300 biopsies. *Clin. Radiol.* **30**, 215–218.
Flower, C. D. R. and Schneerson, J. M. (1984). Bronchography via the fibreoptic bronchoscope. *Thorax* **39**, 260–263.
Harrison, B. D. W., Thorpe, R. S., Kitchener, P. G., McCann, B. G. and Pilling, J. R. (1984). Percutaneous trucut lung biopsy in the diagnosis of localized pulmonary lesions. *Thorax* **39**. 493–499.
Mitchell, D. M. and Collins, J. V. (1980). Fibreoptic bronchoscopy. In *Recent advances in respiratory medicine* (ed. D. C. Flenley), pp. 91–104. Churchill Livingstone, Edinburgh.
Scadding, J. G. (1970). Lung biopsy in the diagnosis of diffuse lung disease. *Br. Med. J.* **2**, 557–564.
Simpson, F. G., Arnold, A. G., Bellfield, P. W., Muers, M. F. and Cooke, N. J. (1986). Postal survey of medical bronchoscopies in the United Kingdom. *Thorax* (in press).
——, ——, ——, —— and —— (1986). Postal survey of bronchoscopic practice by physicians in the United Kingdom. *Thorax* **41**, 311–317.
Steel, S. J. and Winstanley, D. P. (1969). Trephine biopsy of the lung and pleura. *Thorax* **24**, 576–584.
Stradling, P. (1976). *Diagnostic bronchoscopy* 3rd edn. Churchill Livingstone, Edinburgh.
Zavala, D. C. and Hunninghake, G. W. (1983). Lung lavage. In *Recent advances in respiratory medicine* (eds D. C. Flenley and T. L. Petty), pp. 21–33. Churchill Livingstone, Edinburgh.

Radiology

F. W. WRIGHT

The cornerstone of radiological investigation of the chest is plain chest radiography, using inhaled air as the main contrast medium. The radiographs should be taken in maximum inspiration and have as much of the thorax displayed as possible. This comment may seem superfluous but it is surprising how many (posteroanterior) views do not show the area behind the heart, the mediastinum, the larger air passages, or all of the lung bases. The domes of the diaphragm are not straight but curved and lesions may be concealed behind them. A virtue of high kV (150–200) as opposed to low kV (60–90) X-rays is that with high kV the radiographs show these areas well, although they will, at first sight, tend to look rather greyer than normal.

Various other radiological techniques (Table 1) can be used to investigate particular aspects of thoracic structural abnormalities and to a smaller extent pulmonary function, but each is subsidiary to a proper interpretation of the plain radiograph.

The recognition of normal from abnormal in the chest radiograph depends, as elsewhere, on a knowledge of normal anatomy and of the likely findings in relation to disease processes. The scheme which follows is designed to help pick out the salient features which may be found in any of the organs on the chest radiograph. Most observers will take a quick look at a chest radiograph before scrutinizing the various structures in detail. It is important for students and doctors to have a system to which they adhere, but the order in which they look at each feature is less important than keeping to a scheme and hence not forgetting important features and signs.

General points

It is essential in radiology as with other medical procedures, to remember that radiographs are taken of patients. Note the name of the patient, particularly for what it reveals about sex and nationality. Also note the approximate age of the patient (older patients tend to have an enlarged heart, emphysema, calcification in the bronchi, costal cartilages, or coronary arteries, etc.). Whilst most patients having chest radiographs will have the salient clinical details furnished on a request form, these may not be known to the student. In any case, it is very useful to be able to examine chest radiographs critically as an academic exercise, before knowing the clinical details, and to have a second look after knowing these.

Checklist

The following is suggested but more detailed discussion follows. Scan the PA and lateral chest radiographs (Fig. 1) for:

1. Real or apparent increased transradiancy of one lung: (*a*) apparent due to *absent breast* or rotation; and (*b*) real due to Mac-

Table 1 Radiological methods of examining the chest

Plain films: PA and lateral, including expiration view (especially for inhaled foreign body)

Fluoroscopy: diaphragmatic movement, mediastinal movement, obstructive emphysema (especially in children with foreign bodies) position of lesions prior to tomography, etc.

Bucky views (using moving grid) for ribs and spine

Tomograms
   AP
   Lateral
   Inclined frontal and transverse axial ⎫ Not available in all
   Computer ('body scan' or CT) ⎭ hospitals

'Lung scans' or isotope scintigrams: ventilation and perfusion studies made with a gamma camera

Bronchograms: frequently superseded now by tomograms for the demonstration of tumours (the soft tissue component is much better shown on tomograms), but still important for the assessment of bronchiectasis

Radiologically assisted biopsy: percutaneous or transbronchial

Pneumothorax

Pneumomediastinum

Pneumoperitoneum

Ultrasound for diagnosis of pleural fluid collections, peripheral cysts adjacent to chest wall and the localization of these prior to drainage

Note that lordotic or apical views are now rarely taken as tomograms show apical lesions more clearly

leod's syndrome, massive embolism, unilateral emphysema, pneumothorax, etc.

2. The position of the trachea and major bronchi: distortion may be due to external pressure, as from mediastinal masses, the pull of collapsed or fibrotic lung tissue, or displacement from a contralateral pneumothorax or pleural effusion.

3. Diminished lung size, abnormal position of fissures, or crowding of the ribs signifying collapse or fibrosis.

4. Abnormality of the vascular shadows at the hilum or in the lung fields.

5. Intrapulmonary consolidation, nodules, or masses.

6. Shadows in the costophrenic angles, under the lungs, or extending up the chest wall, especially posteriorly and laterally due to pleural fluid.

7. Abnormalities in the shape or blurring of the outline of the cardiac shadow.

8. Diaphragmatic abnormality caused by phrenic nerve palsy,

lung collapse, or pushed up by enlarged liver. Normally the right side is 1.5–2 cm higher than the left, but normal variants are common. Beware of spurious elevation due to 'subpulmonary' effusions, or trans-diaphragmatic herniae, which may contain bowel (e.g. stomach or bowel) or colon (Morgagni and Bochdalek herniae).

9. Abnormal mediastinal shadows such as a dilated oesophagus or hiatus hernia.

10. Lesions of bone especially secondary deposits (lytic or sclerotic), in the spine, or ribs. Lytic deposits particularly with bronchus, kidney, bowel, myeloma, or thyroid. Sclerotic or mixed deposits with reticulosis, breast or prostate (especially after treatment), also rarely with other tumours such as villous papilloma of rectum, medulloblastoma, etc. Note evidence of previous thoracotomy shown by a deformed rib, or sternal suture wires, notching of the ribs caused by coarctation of the aorta, Paget's disease, fibrous dysplasia, renal rickets or neurofibromata, deformed ribs due to hyperparathyroidism, etc.

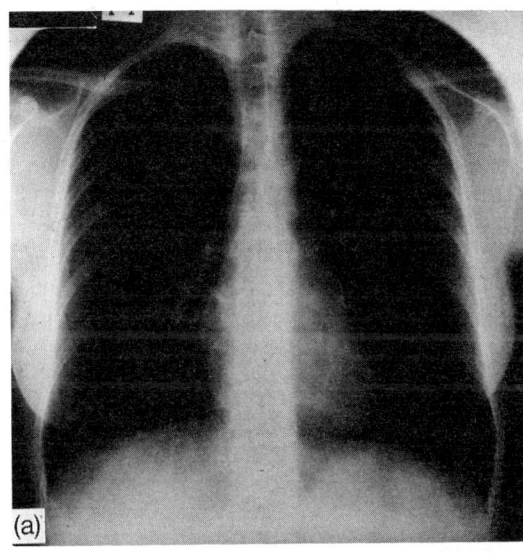

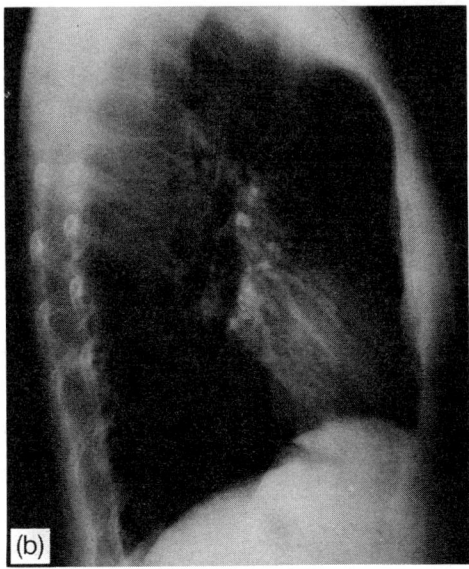

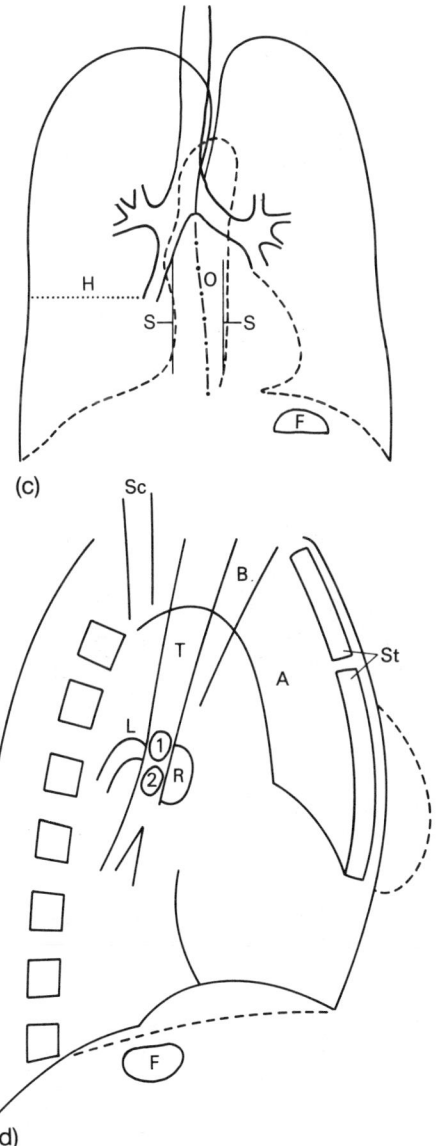

Fig. 1 (a, b) Normal PA and lateral chest radiographs of a young adult female taken at 150 kV. The breast shadows do not obscure the underlying lung and trachea, and hilar structures are well demonstrated. On the lateral view note the increased density (white) due to muscles in the posterior part of the axillae and the relative translucency (black) anteriorly and above the heart and also inferiorly behind the heart and over the lower dorsal spine. (c) Diagram of PA view showing the larger air passages, the paraoesophageal line (O), and the descending aorta. F = fundus of the stomach; H = horizontal fissure; S = paraspinal lines. (d) Some important features on lateral chest radiograph. T = trachea; B = shadow due to bronchocephalic vessels; Sc = scapulae; St = sternum; R, L = right and left pulmonary arteries; A = aorta; 1,2 = ring shadows superimposed on trachea due to right and left upper lobe bronchi respectively.

The plain postero-anterior view

Most frontal views are taken postero-anterior (PA) with 2 m or more tube–film distance; the author uses 3 m, 150 kV, and an air gap between the patient and the cassette. Portable or chair examinations may often be done anteroposterior with shortened tube–film distance and with geometric projectional enlargement of the heart.

The trachea, carina, and main bronchi should be visible through the upper and middle mediastinal shadows. The trachea is not usually straight and is commonly a little over to the right of the midline at the thoracic inlet. It may be compressed or deviated by a goitre in the neck or displaced with lung collapse especially of a lung or upper lobe. Commonly in the elderly it is somewhat too long and becomes tortuous. A similar situation occurs with bilateral upper lobe fibrosis. The right main bronchus is shorter and more horizontal than the left. On the right the intermediate bronchus descends almost vertically to branch into the right middle and lower lobes (see Figs 1, 2, 9, and 11). The carina should be seen through the heart shadow and normally has an angle of about 70°, but may be widened due to subcarinal node enlargement or left atrial enlargement as with mitral stenosis. Usually the lobar bronchi can be made out, but smaller branches are commonly not seen except on tomograms. Bronchial wall thickening is, however, seen in fibrocystic disease, chronic bronchitis, and bronchiectasis.

Blood vessels are usually visible as far as the outer third of the lungs, but may be seen right out to the periphery in congestion or with other causes of pulmonary plethora. Pulmonary artery enlargement may occur in both hila, as with emphysema or cor pulmonale, or be unilateral if the blood supply to the contralateral lung is impaired. The number of vessels on either side should be roughly equal – if not, suspect a collapsed lobe or a previous lobectomy, the 'fan sign' (Fig. 3). It is important to note that the position of the pulmonary arteries is different from the pulmonary veins and these are easily recognized with a little practice (see Fig. 4).

Note the position of the horizontal fissure which is seen on about 60 per cent of PA chest views. It normally runs laterally at the level of the anterior end of the right fourth rib. With collapse its position may be altered, being elevated with upper lobe collapse or depressed with middle or lower lobe collapse (Fig. 5).

The cardiac and diaphragmatic outlines are entirely dependent on air-filled lung being adjacent to them. When fluid is present in the pleura or if the adjacent lung is opaque, i.e. collapsed or consolidated, then these outlines may be obscured or lost. This is known as the *silhouette sign* (an Americanism, positive when the silhouette is lost). Thus loss of the right lower cardiac outline implies that the middle lobe is opaque or on the left of the lingula. Note that a collapsed and opaque lower lobe will lie behind the heart shadow and not affect its outline.

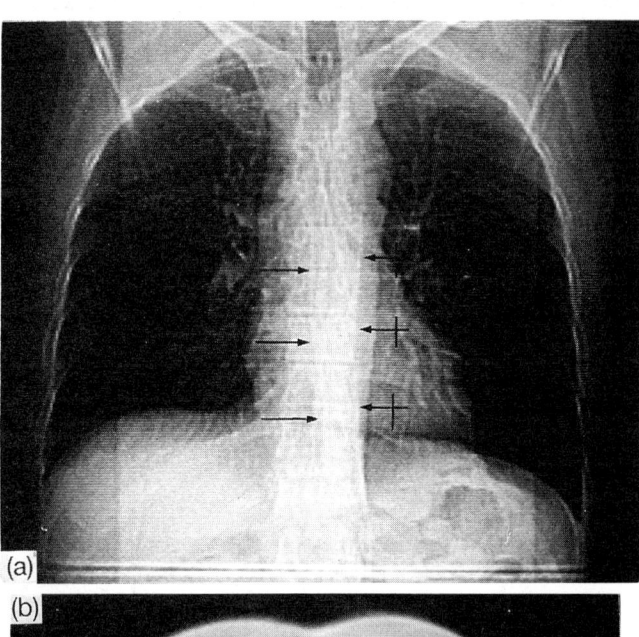

(a)

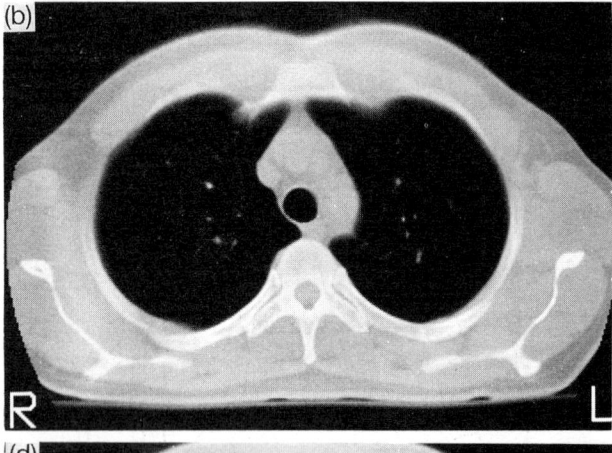

(b)

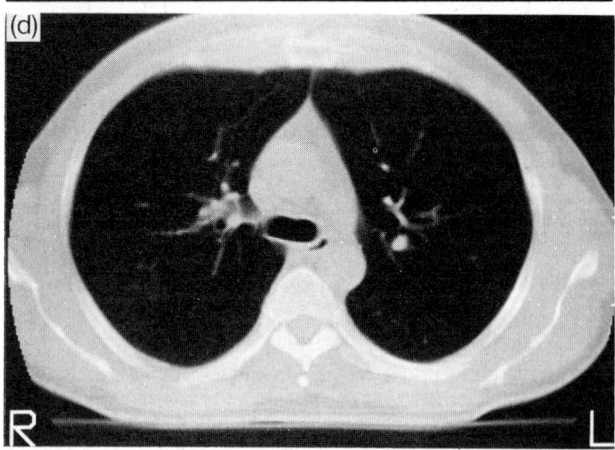

(d)

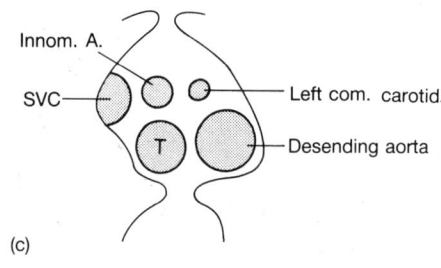

(c)

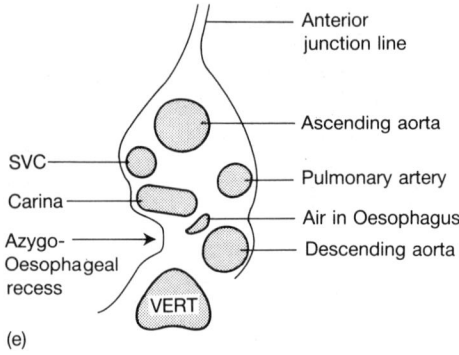

(e)

Fig. 2 (a) AP view of author's chest using 'scout view' on CT apparatus showing the anatomy extremely well. Note the paraoesophageal (→) and left paraspinal (⊢) lines. The left cardiac outline is 'stepped' due to cardiac pulsations during the traverse through the narrow X-ray beam. (b, c) Cross-sectional view of the author's chest just below the level of the aortic arch. (d, e) Cross-sectional view of the author's chest at the level of carina.

With well 'penetrated' or high kV views, not only should one see collapsed lower lobes more readily, a dilated oesophagus (Fig. 6) or hiatus hernia (Fig. 7), retro-cardiac masses, etc. but also the normal anatomy. The descending aorta normally descends on the left side of the posterior mediastinum. It may be tor-

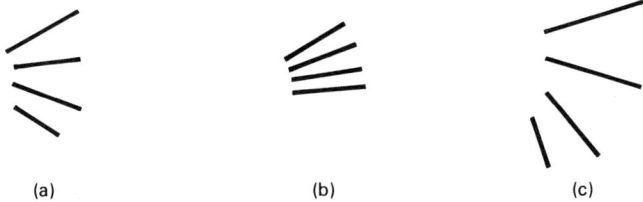

Fig. 3 The 'fan sign': (a) normal; (b) vessels 'crowded', i.e. reduced volume; (c) vessels splayed apart due to previous lobectomy or lobar collapse, which may not be readily apparent. There is compensatory over-expansion of the rest of the lung and only half the normal number of vessels is seen in a given area. (Adapted from Wright, 1973, by permission.)

tuous in the elderly. Dilation may be uniform or more localized as with an aneurysm. Dissecting aneurysms may 'leak' causing mediastinal swelling, and a blood-stained or serous 'sympathetic' left pleural effusion. On well penetrated views a line following the oesophagus may be seen – the paraoesophageal line (Fig. 1c). A second line defines the left border of the descending aorta. Paraspinal, and junctional lines between the two lungs (especially in the upper mediastinum) may also be seen (Fig. 2a). These lines may also be lost with opacity of the adjacent lung, and they are commonly displaced by masses arising in the adjacent mediastinum. Note also that the medial borders of the lungs are not straight from front to back and that they are moulded by the mediastinal structures. Thus superiorly the most medial part of the right upper lobe commonly passes to the left of the mid-line in front of the spine whilst anteriorly in front of the heart the two upper lobes are only separated by a thin septum (see Fig. 2b).

The azygos vein is usually seen above the right main bronchus, but may lie within an accessory fissure in the right upper lobe, when it forms an 'azygos lobe' (see Fig. 25). It is dilated in heart

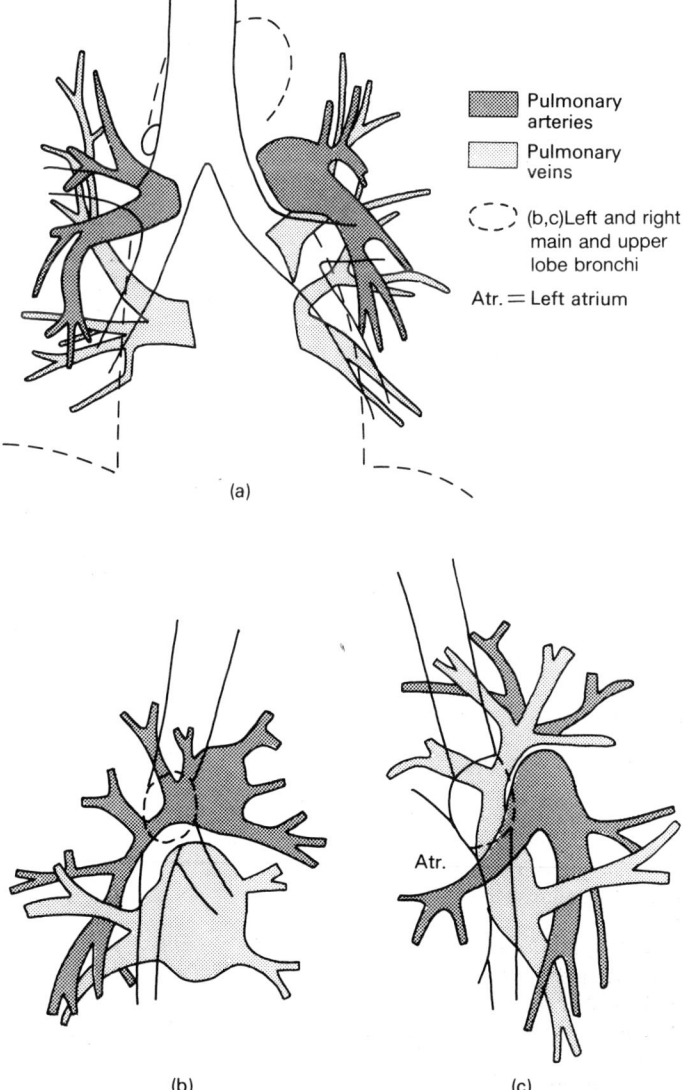

Pulmonary arteries

Pulmonary veins

(b,c)Left and right main and upper lobe bronchi

Atr. = Left atrium

Fig. 4 Positions of the larger pulmonary vessels: (a) PA view; (b) right lateral view; (c) left lateral view. Normally on the lateral view the shadows from the two sides are superimposed but they are shown separately here to clarify the anatomy. Note that the left interlobar pulmonary artery lies posterior to the carina whilst that on the right lies anterior – an important point when considering mass lesions. (Adapted from Wright, 1973, by permission.)

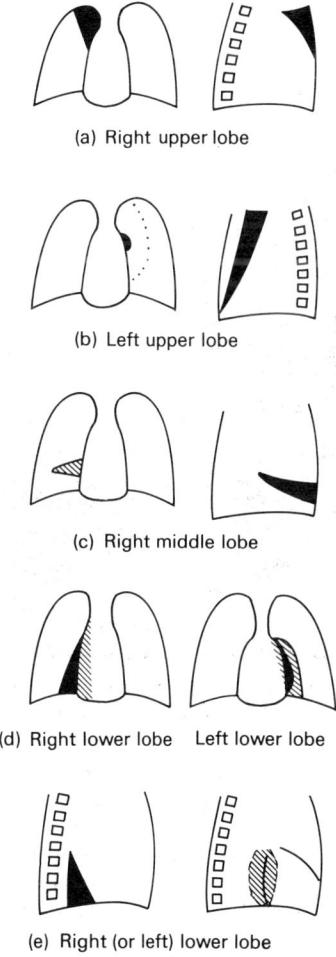

(a) Right upper lobe

(b) Left upper lobe

(c) Right middle lobe

(d) Right lower lobe   Left lower lobe

(e) Right (or left) lower lobe

Fig. 5 Patterns of lobar collapse. Note with left lobe collapse how the right upper lobe herniates to the left in front of the collapsed left upper lobe; the silhouette sign with right middle lobe or lingular collapse (loss of the adjacent cardiac outline); and that a right middle lobe collapse may not be seen as an opaque shadow on the PA view – as it may not be tangential to the X-ray beam – to show this a lordotic view used to be done, but a lateral view is better. A collapsed lower lobe is largely seen behind the corresponding side of the mediastinum which will also tend to be displaced to this side. On lateral views a collapsed lower lobe may not be obvious and will show as increased density over the lower dorsal spine and loss of the posterior part of the diaphragmatic outline on the affected side. (Adapted from Wright, 1973, by permission.)

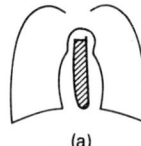 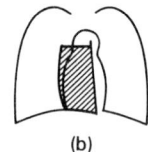

(a)   (b)

Fig. 6 Achalasia. Note in (a) the mildly dilated oesophagus with air/fluid level behind the cardiac shadow, and in (b) the hugely dilated oesophagus has extended to the right of the cardiac border to produce a double shadow. No fundal gas in the stomach.

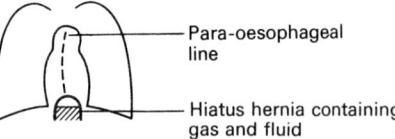

Para-oesophageal line

Hiatus hernia containing gas and fluid

Fig. 7 Hiatus hernia behind the heart. Note the absence of the normal fundal gas bubble below the left side of the diaphragm, with both achalasia and hiatus hernia.

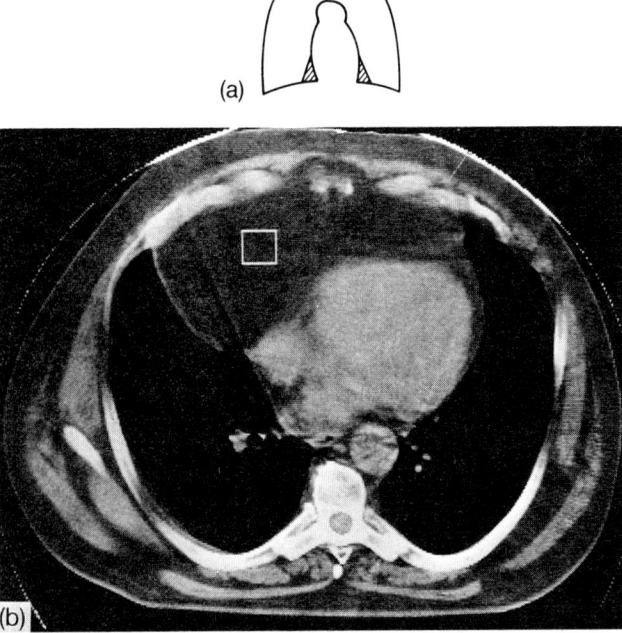

Fig. 8 (a) Pericardial fat pads. (b) Large mass of fat in front of the heart – small rectangular box gives density reading of minus 125 Hounsfield units.

failure, superior vena caval obstruction, pregnancy, etc., and in normal people tends to be larger on views taken with the patient lying down compared with those in the erect position. As shown in Fig. 23 there are lymph nodes (the 'azygos nodes') present alongside it which may become enlarged and sometimes give rise to confusion. These nodes may particularly be enlarged with neoplasms of the right upper lobe.

Note the position of the gastric air bubble and splenic flexure and any alteration in the position of these. They may be displaced with an enlarged liver or spleen. With a subpulmonary effusion the apparent thickness of the left side of the diaphragm may be increased due to fluid under the lung. In achalasia gas may be trapped in the dilated oesophagus by fluid in the lower oesophagus with the patient erect; the oesophagus may also be considerably dilated, and since it lies in the posterior mediastinum behind the heart, its border may be seen through the heart or even to its right giving an apparent 'double shadow' to the right side of the heart. If no gas is seen in the stomach below the diaphragm, consider an hiatus hernia or achalasia (Figs 6 and 7).

Triangular masses at either of the lower aspects of the heart may be due to fat, especially in obese patients. These are very common and are termed 'fat pads' (Fig. 8).

The diaphragm may be paralysed on either side by a phrenic palsy. It may also be elevated on the right side by an enlarged liver. Minor eventrations or a lobulated appearance are common but may also be due to masses below the diaphragm. Apparent abnormalities of the diaphragm may be due to trans-diaphragmatic herniae such as a Morgagni hernia which occurs between the sternal and costal origins of the diaphragm. Through this opening the liver, omentum, or bowel (especially colon) may herniate and with the last colonic gas shadows may be seen in the thorax. A posterior deficiency in the diaphragm may give rise to a Bochdalek hernia. Interposition of the colon may also occur in front of and above the liver; this is a feature which is common in children and the elderly, sometimes known as the Béclère or Chilaiditidi syndrome.

Chest deformity such as a depressed sternum ('pectus excavatum') may cause the heart to be displaced to the left and apparently to be enlarged; often the area of the right middle lobe appears abnormal, with spuriously added vascular shadows; the anterior ends of the ribs are more vertical than normal; a lateral view is confirmatory. 'Pectus carinatum' (or pigeon chest deformity) with an anteriorly bowed sternum may be a congenital anomaly or be associated with asthma. Chest deformities due to severe kyphosis or scoliosis or a combination of both may cause considerable difficulty in interpretation.

A point always to be considered on a PA view is whether an apparent hilar mass is really hilar, or whether it overlies the hilum, either anteriorly or in the apex of a lower lobe. Such will usually be readily apparent on a lateral view, but may often be deduced from the PA, as the mass will be superimposed over the normal hilar anatomy.

The lateral radiograph

Commonly the diseased side is placed closer to the cassette, but with a 2 m or more tube-film distance, this is really immaterial. Note particularly:

1. The position of the trachea.

2. The spines of the scapulae which usually appear as dense lines about 10° to the vertical over the upper part of the lungs, but behind the position of the trachea. They must not be confused with other structures.

3. The normally air-filled lung which occupies the space in the upper anterior (retro-sternal) part of the chest. When opaque this area may be opacified by enlarged nodes (within the thymus), a thymic mass, or goitre (note that one-third of intra-thoracic goitres become displaced to lie behind the trachea).

4. The normally darker and more translucent area over the lower dorsal vertebrae as compared with the lighter and more opaque area over the upper dorsal spine, due to the thickness of the shoulders and associated muscles. When this picture is reversed think of a lower lobar collapse or pleural fluid.

5. Displacement of the oblique and horizontal fissures may indicate collapse or fibrosis. For patterns of lobar collapse see Fig. 5.

6. The hilar shadows are different on the two sides (see Fig. 4). Note that the left pulmonary artery lies *posterior* to the trachea and carina, whilst the right pulmonary artery lies *anterior*. This means that any mass lying anteriorly in the left hilum or posteriorly on the right cannot be a vascular mass, and is most likely to be due to enlarged nodes.

7. Ring shadows of the main and upper lobe bronchi (Fig. 4a).

8. The two domes of the diaphragm can usually be seen as separate shadows, the right normally higher than the left and as in the PA view the stomach and/or the splenic flexure may be seen under the left dome. Occasionally the hepatic flexure passes up under the right dome (see under PA view). Part of one dome may be obscured by pleural fluid or unaerated lung (the 'silhouette sign').

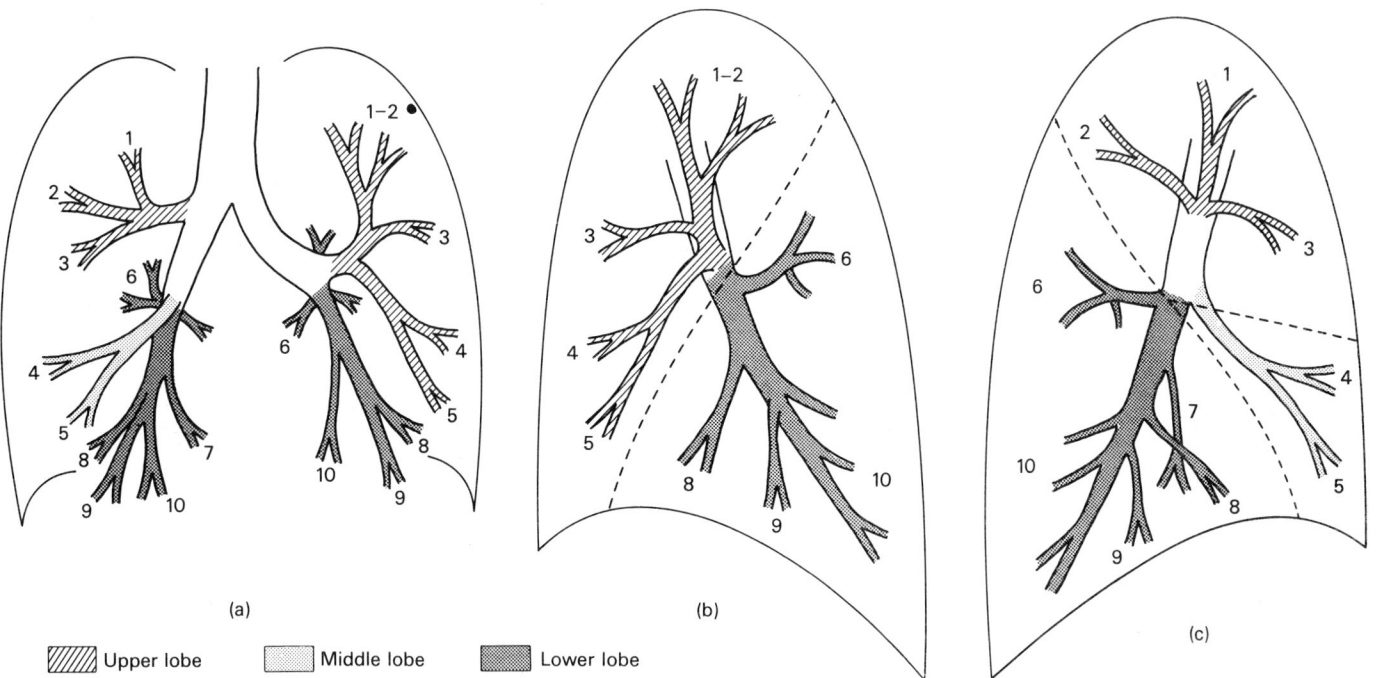

(Adapted from Wright, 1973, by permission, and from Pallardy and Remy, 1970. *Illustrations of radiological anatomy*. Kodak Pathé, by courtesy of CERR, Paris.)

Fig. 9 Bronchial anatomy: diagram of lobar and segmental anatomy. Note: the 'intermediate bronchus' is the common bronchial stem, below the origin of the upper left lobe bronchus, which passes to the right middle and lower lobes.

Right	Left
	Upper lobe
1 Apical	1 2 } Apico-posterior
2 Posterior	3 Anterior
3 Anterior	4 Superior lingula
	5 Inferior lingula
	Middle lobe
4 Lateral	4 Superior lingula
5 Medial	5 Inferior lingula

Right	Left
	Lower lobe
6 Apical	6 Apical
7 Medial basal (cardiac)	8 Anterior basal
8 Anterior basal	9 Lateral basal
9 Lateral basal	10 Posterior basal
10 Posterior basal	

Legend: Upper lobe / Middle lobe / Lower lobe

Bronchial anatomy and disease

A diagram of bronchial anatomy is shown in Fig. 9. As already mentioned, the larger bronchi may be seen on plain radiographs, but bronchial detail is best seen on tomograms or bronchograms. Deformities due to tumour, infection, or bronchiectasis may be demonstrated. With tumours both intrinsic and extrinsic masses may be present. Extrinsic masses may displace or compress bronchi, whilst intrinsic tumours may give rise to an endobronchial mass or an irregular or 'rat-tailed' stenosis (Fig. 11).

The advantage of tomography over bronchography, for the demonstration of tumours, is that soft tissue shadows as well as bronchial deformities are readily demonstrated. For central lesions involving the hilar and mediastinal areas, the author has used a horizontal X-ray beam and a circular blurring motion (on a transverse axial tomograph – both the patient and the cassette rotate) to give an 'inclined frontal tomogram', parallel to the tracheo-bronchial tree (Figs 10a–c). For peripheral lung lesions a longitudinal tomographic movement is employed. With lateral tomograms the patient is always in the erect position to avoid mediastinal distortion which occurs if he is laid on his side. With the advent of CT, this is now used to show the extent of lung tumours and their spread through the lung to the hilum and mediastinum (Fig. 11).

In *bronchiectasis* the bronchi become distorted and dilated, often with destruction and obliteration of their smaller branches. In gross disease the dilated bronchial sacs may be seen on plain radiographs, filled with air and/or fluid, but in lesser cases they are demonstrated better by a bronchogram. For this a contrast medium (usually oil-based, as it is much less of an irritant than water-soluble media) is introduced either through a needle inserted into the trachea via the crico-thyroid membrane or through a translaryngeal catheter directly into a bronchus.

Collapse, consolidation, and other effects of bronchial obstruction

Lobar collapse is commonly produced by an endobronchial obstructive lesion, but can also be caused by a long-standing loss of volume as in bronchiectasis. (The term 'atelectasis' should be avoided as it is not synonymous with collapse, and properly refers to congenital collapse, i.e. a part of the lung which has never been expanded.) Collapse is not the only effect of bronchial obstruction. Before this happens one may see obstructive emphysema on a chest radiograph taken in expiration (Fig. 12). Consolidation distal to an obstruction may also occur, as may breakdown or abscess formation. The cause of an obstruction may be demonstrated by tomography, e.g. a tumour, or may be inferred from the patient's history, e.g. a foreign body in a child, or a mucous plug in an asthmatic, postoperative or sick patient. A view in expiration is particularly important with a non-opaque inhaled foreign body since the diameter of the bronchial wall will be less in expiration and hence the obstruction greater. An expiration view is also often used to accentuate the size of a pneumothorax. However, most pneumothoraces that are clinically important are readily seen on inspiration views. Diagnosis is particularly important if the patient is shortly to travel by air (at a lower atmospheric pressure) when the pneumothorax will then be much larger.

A very useful guide to distinguish between collapse, due to bronchial obstruction, and consolidation is to note the '*air bron-*

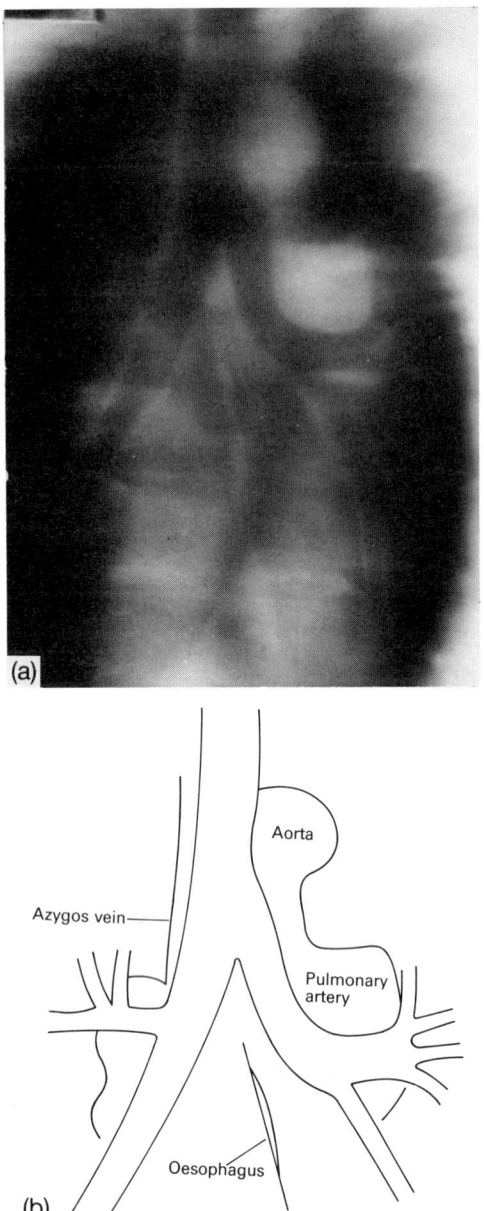

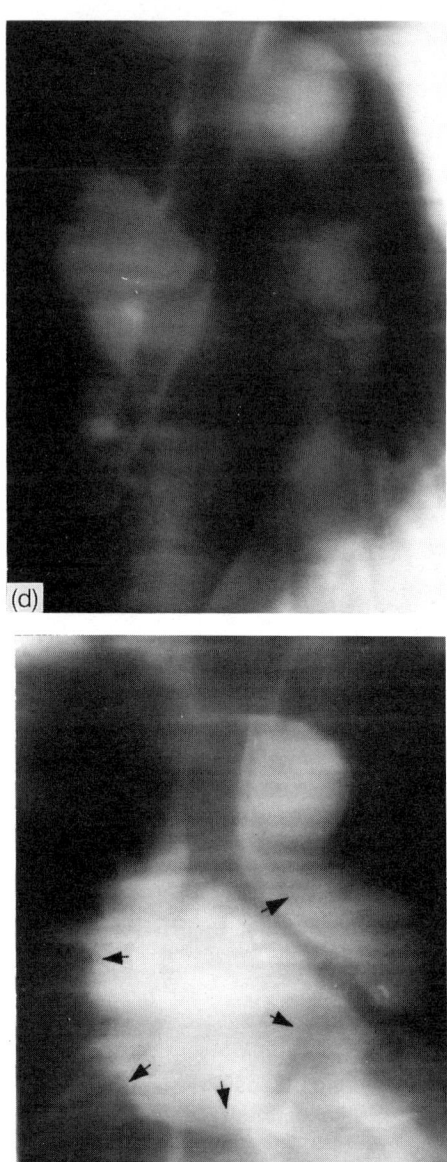

Fig. 10 (a, b) Normal tracheobronchial tree with subcarinal anatomy (shown by inclined frontal tomography). (c) Huge subcarinal nodes in a patient with bronchial carcinoma. The right hilar nodes are also enlarged. Note the severe compression of the main bronchi and old calcification within the nodes due to past tuberculous infection. The patient had severe stridor on the slightest exercise. (Reproduced from Wright, 1973, by permission.) (d) Endobronchial mass in the intermediate bronchus with a larger extrabronchial mass, lobulated in its outline.

chogram' which occurs with consolidation (Fig. 13a). With collapse the bronchi are often fluid-filled because of the obstruction and as the lung is opaque there is no contrast difference between them.

Fluid-filled bronchi or mucocoeles may be seen distal to blocked segmental bronchi, due to air passing from one segment to another by 'collateral air drift', through the *inter-alveolar pores of Kohn* (Fig. 13b). These mucocoeles are particularly seen with slowly growing endobronchial tumours – adenomas and some malignant tumours, but may also occur proximal to mucous plugs, e.g. in aspergillosis.

The collateral air pathway also accounts for some 'sequestrated segments' being aerated. In this uncommon condition the alveolar parts of the affected segment develop normally from mesenchymal elements but the segmental bronchi fail grow into them. This usually occurs at the lung base and may be complicated by repeated infections and abscess formation.

Bronchial anatomy and collateral air drift also have to be con-

sidered in the distribution and extent of other pathological processes, particularly pneumonia. In 'lobar pneumonia' consolidation usually stops at the pleural border of the lobe and one suspects that its spread occurs mainly through the tissue planes and the interalveolar connections. In bronchopneumonia on the other hand, transbronchial spread of infection gives a more patchy and widespread distribution of disease, whether it be spread from a breaking down tuberculous focus, from other bacterial or virus infection, or from inhaled gastric contents. The concept of a 'bronchial embolus' is also important when considering the causation of a lung abscess (Brock, 1954).

Pulmonary nodules and masses

Tiny multiple nodules

These are seen because multiple tiny opacities augment one another, and a few may not be seen at all.

A scheme of differential diagnosis is given in Table 2.

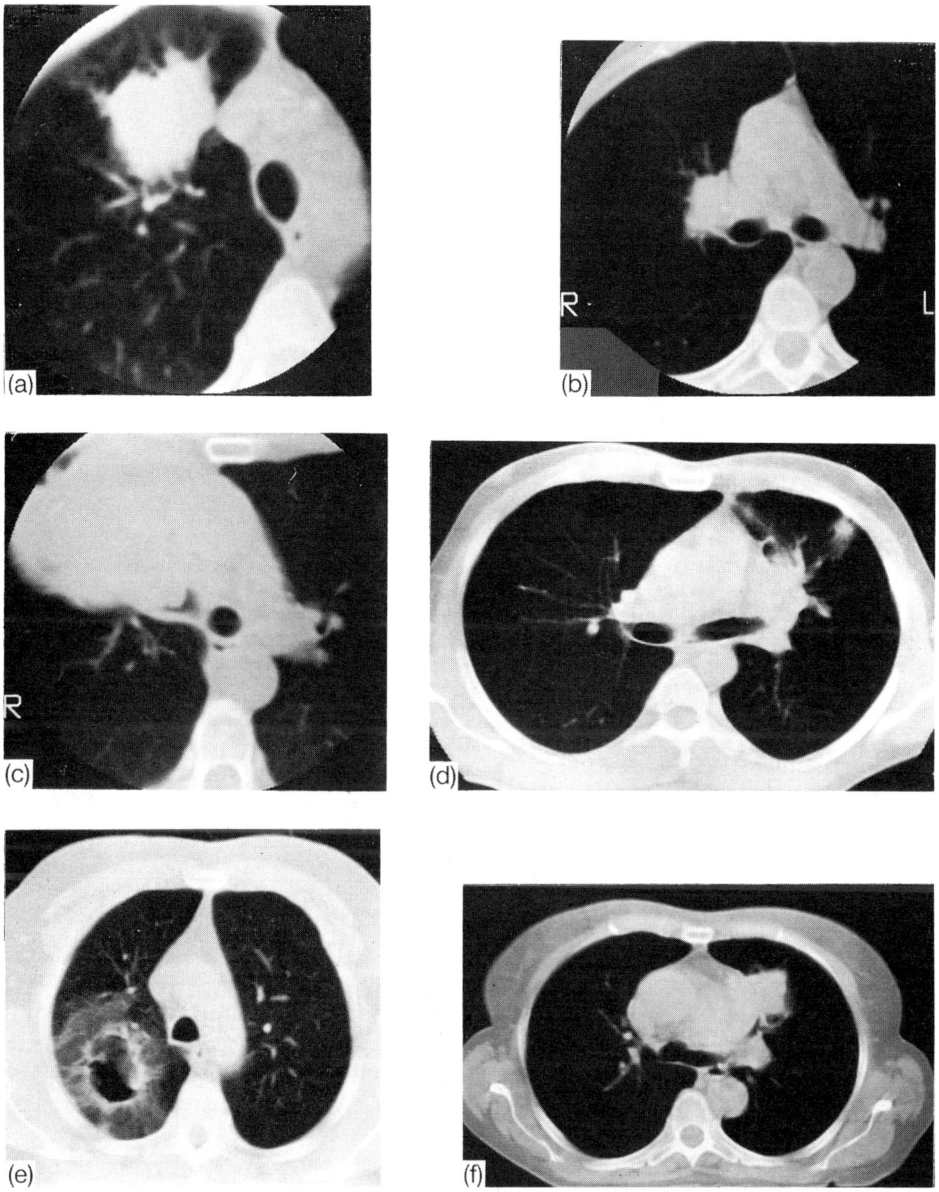

Fig. 11 (a, b) Irregular tumour in RUL with right hilar node enlargement. (c) Endo-bronchial tumour in RVL bronchus with collapsed RUL. (d) Mass at origin of LUL bronchus, with enlarged L hilar nodes. (e) Breaking down tumour in right lung with fine spread of tumour outwards into the adjacent lung – the 'corona maligna'. (f) Tumour in LUL extending into thymic fat and involving the left phrenic nerve.

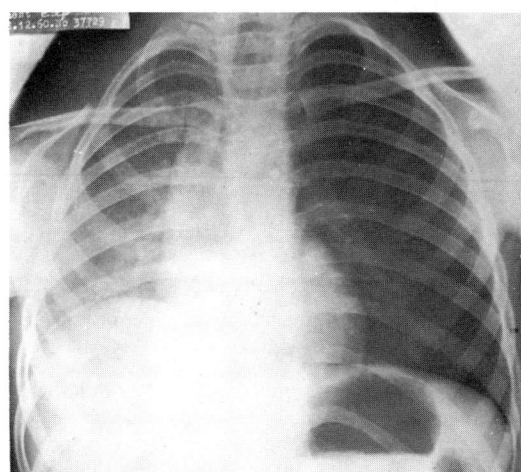

Fig. 12 Obstructive emphysema of the left lung in a small child due to an inhaled apple core. Radiograph taken in *expiration* – the left lung cannot deflate. (The inspiratory radiograph appeared normal). (Reproduced from Wright, 1973, by permission.)

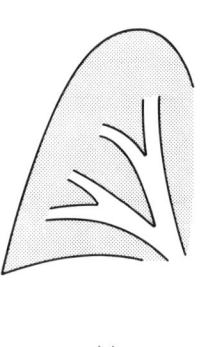
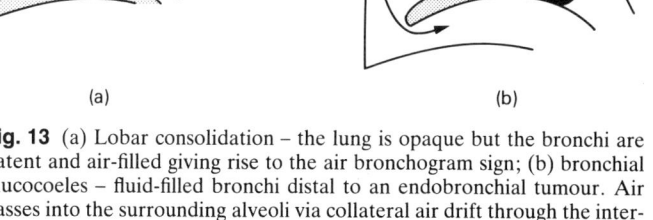

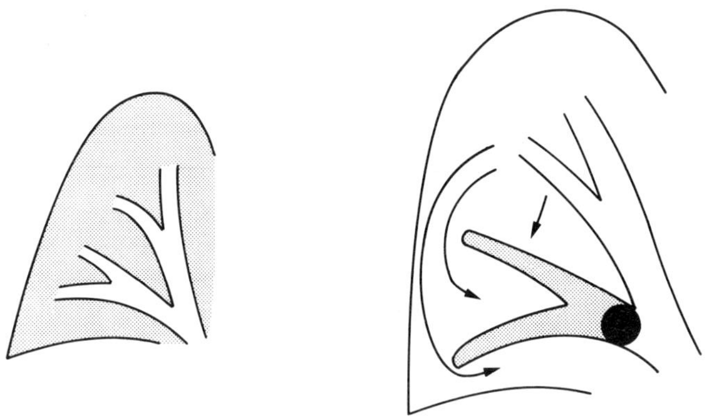

Fig. 13 (a) Lobar consolidation – the lung is opaque but the bronchi are patent and air-filled giving rise to the air bronchogram sign; (b) bronchial mucocoeles – fluid-filled bronchi distal to an endobronchial tumour. Air passes into the surrounding alveoli via collateral air drift through the inter-alveolar pores of Kohn, and interbronchiolar canals of Lambert.

Table 2 Tiny multiple nodules

Micronodules (under 1 mm)
  Pneumoconiosis, stage 1–2; coal miners; fettlers; quarry workers, etc.
  Inhaled metal, Fe: haematite workers; knife and lens polishers using rouge (ferric oxide)
Miliary (1–2 mm) nodules
  Tuberculosis
  Sarcoid
  Miliary carcinoma
  Acute alveolitis or bronchiolitis: infection or allergic
  Acute chickenpox pneumonia: especially in adolescents or adults
If calcified
  Previous chickenpox pneumonia
  Histoplasmosis
  Microlithiasis pulmonale in mitral stenosis
  Rarely, 'stony lung' disease
3–4 mm nodules
  Sarcoid
  Secondary deposits
  Bronchopneumonia
  Bronchopneumonic tuberculosis

Transient patchy shadows or nodules of varying size may also be due to allergic causes (e.g. inhaled foreign protein as in bird fancier's lung, or injected protein as antihaemophilic globulin).

In considering the differential diagnosis of tiny nodules, note that tuberculosis tends to affect the upper two-thirds of both lungs, sarcoidosis tends to affect the middle two-thirds, that pneumoconiosis will often spare the apices (because of bullae there), and that when all parts of the lungs are affected one should think of miliary carcinomatosis.

Larger nodules or masses
A scheme of differential diagnosis, according to the various radiographic appearances is given in diagrammatic form in Fig. 14.

Naturally the age of the patient, contact with tuberculosis, and clinical history or occupation will make certain causes more likely. For example, a primary lung tumour is more common in patients over 40, who have been smokers, whilst younger patients are more likely to have tuberculosis or hamartomas. Secondary deposits are more likely to be seen in patients who have had primary tumours and patients with coal miners' pneumoconiosis are most likely to have masses due to progressive massive fibrosis (PMF).

Calcification is almost never seen *in vivo* in primary lung tumours, but is not uncommon in tuberculomas or hamartomas (usually non-malignant masses of cartilage, bone, fat, and muscle). This last commonly gives a 'popcorn' appearance. Rarely calcification is seen in secondary deposits particularly from osteogenic sarcomas.

Adenomas most commonly occur in young adult females and may have both an endobronchial and a larger surrounding mass. The slowly growing endobronchial component may lead to mucocoeles and bronchiectasis in the obstructed area of the lung. Adenomas tend to grow slowly and are usually regarded as benign, but occasionally metastasize.

Fibrotic nodules may not only be due to PMF, but also to scars from pulmonary embolism, rheumatoid disease (the necrobiotic nodule, often referred to as Caplan's syndrome when it occurs in coal miners) or varieties of granulomatous disease.

Other points about lung tumours
Bronchial tumours tend to present on chest radiographs as either 'central' or 'peripheral'. Peripheral tumours are commonly nodular (see above) but may break down and cavitate. Central tumours which develop in the larger bronchi are often advanced at the time of diagnosis. Both types may have considerable hilar or mediastinal nodal spread or more distal metastases. Some apparently central tumours may, however, be metastatic from peripheral tumours since lymphatic vessels not only pass to the bronchopul-

Radiological appearance	Differential diagnosis
Small round focus	Carcinoma / Tuberculoma / Adenoma / Hamartoma / Metastasis especially if multiple / Rare causes such as rheumatoid nodule, polyarteritis, or infarct
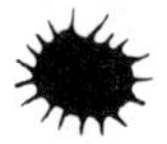 Spiculation or scalloping	Carcinoma / Tuberculoma
Notching or umbilication	Carcinoma / Adenoma / Hamartoma
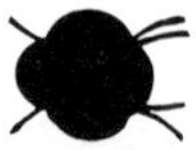 Vessels entering or radiating vessels	Carcinoma, arterio-venous malformation
Satellite sign	Carcinoma
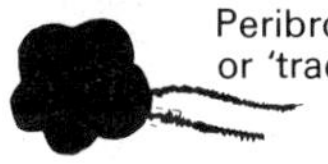 Peribronchial infiltration or 'track to hilum'	Carcinoma / Infection
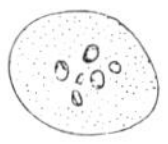 Mass with calcification	Tuberculoma / Adenoma / Hamartoma ('popcorn' calcification) / Metastasis (bone sarcoma) / Carcinoma unlikely unless old tuberculosis focus incorporated in tumour
Large round mass	Carcinoma / Bronchogenic cyst / Hydatid cyst / Secondary deposit (e.g. from sarcoma) / Adenoma
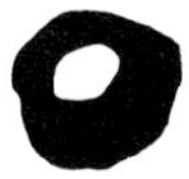 Mass with cavity, often eccentric	Carcinoma / Infarct (especially if infected) / Fungus infection (may contain a fungus ball or mycetoma) / Rarely metastasis (squamous primary or rapidly growing tumour e.g. sarcoma) / Lung abscess (if acute)
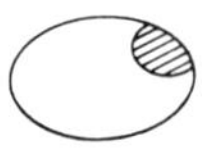 Thin-walled cavity (may have nodule on its inner wall)	Emphysematous bulla / Tuberculosis / Bronchial carcinoma (very occasionally), perhaps due to check valve mechanism as also occurs in staphylococcal pneumonia

Fig. 14 Diagrammatic differential diagnosis of peripheral lung masses.

monary nodes but also anastomose with the lymphatic vessels in the walls of the larger bronchi.

Bronchial tumours may spread to the pleural surface of a lobe, and may be limited by this for a while until adhesions form or spread into the pleura takes place. When extension occurs into the chest wall, much pain is caused, and bone erosion may also be seen (note that a tuberculous abscess is usually painless). With a tumour in the apex of the upper lobe there may be destruction of the upper ribs and adjacent dorsal spine, the Pancoast tumour (Fig. 15) with involvement of the lower part of the brachial plexus and the cervical sympathetic chain. Blood-stream spread may also occur into ribs and spine and also produce pulmonary metastases (lung to lung).

The bronchiolar or alveolar cell carcinoma is a relatively uncommon type of lung tumour which may start as a small nodule, an area of consolidation, spread to nodes or give a miliary type of

Table 3 Position of lung lesions as a help to differential diagnosis

Apex (i.e. the part of the lung above the clavicle)
  Bullae
  Tuberculosis
  Aspergillosis
  Neoplasm—especially Pancoast tumour with rib erosion
Mid zones
  Consolidation due to pneumonia
  Fibrosis due to sarcoid (look also for nodal enlargement)
Bases
  Chronic disease with collapse and small (0.3–1.5 cm) cavities:
    bronchiectasis
  Consolidation: pneumonia or embolism
  Collapse: inhaled FB, food, etc.
  Fibrosis: fibrosing alveolitis
  Tiny cavities or honeycombing (0.2–0.4 cm): scleroderma
  Linear basal collapse; often with horizontal (or sometimes vertical)
    lines of collapse, not uncommon in women who wear tight corsets
    and of little significance; may also occur with other conditions
    producing poor diaphragmatic movement and in some cases of
    pulmonary embolism

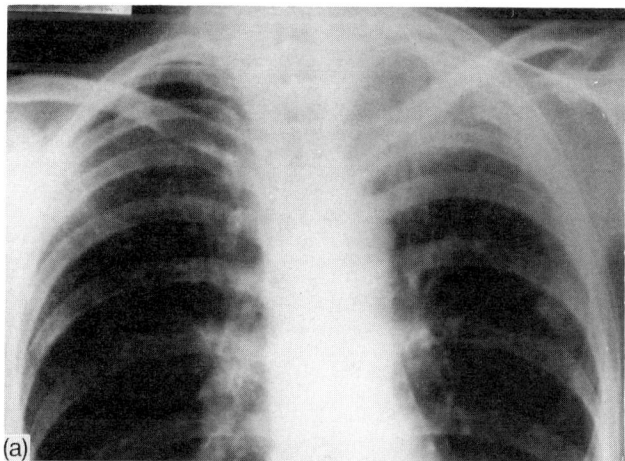

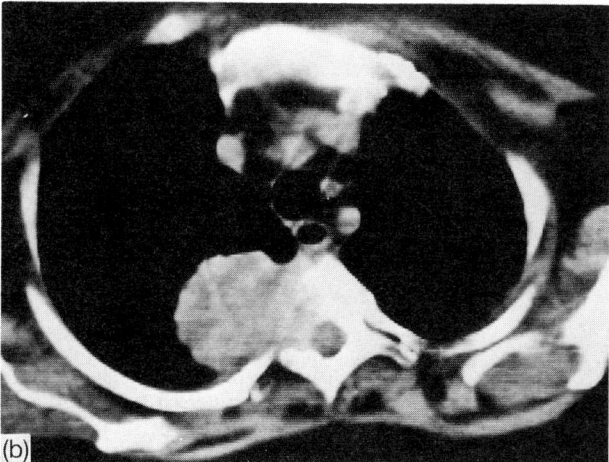

Fig. 15 (a) Pancoast tumour of left apex. Note the eroded left third and fourth ribs. (b) CT of Pancoast tumour eroding an upper dorsal vertebra.

appearance. Not uncommonly it appears to spread through the bronchi to give rise to multiple lesions resembling bronchopneumonia (airborne spread). Bone metastases may be sclerotic. Tracheal tumours, also rare, are best shown on tomograms, and should be suspected if a patient has a central stridor.

Hypertrophic pulmonary osteoarthropathy may accompany finger and toe clubbing particularly with primary lung and pleural tumours (most commonly bronchial and bronchiolar neoplasms), but may also be seen with an empyema. The radiological features of this are periosteal reactions along the lower shafts of the radius and ulna, femora, tibiae, and fibulae, and along the shafts of the metacarpals and metatarsals.

The solitary pulmonary nodule

This radiographic abnormality raises problems in diagnosis because, if due to a primary pulmonary neoplasm which has not metastasized, then it falls into the small group likely to do well with surgery, and if not then an unnecessary thoracotomy will be carried out.

Pointers to a malignant diagnosis are age (over 45 years), male sex, heavy smoking history, a mass more than 2 cm in diameter with an ill defined spiculated margin or lobulated shape, and no calcification. Pulmonary metastatic deposits especially from renal tumours can be solitary and round. Benign lesions which may cause solitary round lesions are tuberculomas (and in appropriate parts of the world similar lesions due to other granulomatous infections such as histoplasmosis), hydatid cysts, pulmonary infarcts, or benign tumours (for a detailed list see Table 4).

Cavitating lung lesions

Any lung lesion which becomes infected or outgrows its blood supply may cavitate, but certain features may suggest the underlying cause (Fig. 16):

1. Bullae are the commonest cavities (see below).

2. Pneumonia with lung abscess, appears as an area of lung consolidation with a cavity. The aetiology is discussed elsewhere (see page 15.103). In staphylococcal pneumonia cavitation may be real and due to lung breakdown, or be appparent and due to pneumatocoeles or bullae, as a result of bronchial distortion and air trapping.

3. Tuberculosis is suggested by multiple cavities and lung infiltration especially in the upper lobes or apices of lower lobes. There may also be an associated chronic lesion containing calcification.

4. Neoplasm. Commonly primary lung tumour masses break down to give an eccentric irregular cavity within the mass. (They may also cause a more distal lung abscess.) Those which seem to break down most often are squamous tumours, which commonly

Table 4 The solitary pulmonary nodule: common causes

Cause	Frequency (%)
Carcinoma of bronchus (including pulmono-pulmonary metastasis)	80
Other lung tumours: malignant and potentially malignant (carcinoid, hamartoma, neurological tumours) Metastasis from extra-thoracic primary (breast, kidney, gut, uterus, gonads)	10
Granulomatous lesions (tuberculous, fungal) Circumscribed pneumonia Pulmonary infarcts Wegener's granuloma Rheumatoid nodule Hydatid cyst Lipoid pneumonia Arteriovenous fistula Fibrotic nodule (progressive massive fibrosis)	10

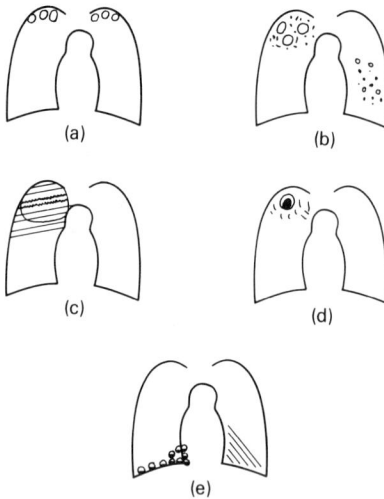

Fig. 16 Some apical and basal lung lesions: (a) apical bullae; (b) tuberculosis – note mutifocal infiltration and cavities and bronchopneumonic spread to contralateral lung; (c) plombage – note the adjacent rib resection; (d) thick-walled cavity containing a mass (aspergilloma) with old tuberculous scarring present; (e) basal bronchiectasis (shown by partially fluid-filled cavities or thickened dilated bronchi).

produce a thick-walled cavity having an *irregular* inner border. Secondary tumours may also occasionally cavitate particularly those which are rapidly growing (e.g. sarcoma or poorly differentiated tumour) or those of squamous origin (e.g. from throat, cervix, etc.). Rapidly growing or cavitating neoplasms which lie towards the periphery of the lung may also give rise to a spontaneous pneumothorax.

5. A pulmonary infarct may cavitate especially if infected as in drug addicts, diabetics or patients undergoing haemodialysis treatment with an infected shunt. These may be multiple.

6. Cavitating pneumoconiotic nodules are suggested if there are other smaller nodules and pulmonary fibrosis.

7. Rheumatoid and other necrobiotic or granulomatous nodules may also cavitate.

8. Fungus infections in which the cavities may contain a mycetoma or fungus ball (aspergilloma).

Basal cavities, often containing fluid, are commonly due to bronchiectasis. A 'honeycomb' lung appearance may be due to a collagen disease such as scleroderma, histiocytosis or adenoma sebaceum and may present with a secondary pneumothorax (see page 15.54).

Bullae and emphysema (see also page 15.84)
Thin-walled bullae though usually readily seen on plain radiographs, are better demonstrated on tomograms. They may occur anywhere, but are most commonly seen at the apices. They seem to result from lung atrophy, either physiological (at the apices) or in relation to a disease process. Such cavities may become large, forming pneumatocoeles which compress the remaining lung tissue to cause severe respiratory distress. Bullae may also become infected and contain fluid levels.

Emphysema can be difficult to diagnose on plain chest radiographs. It is not synonymous with the overdistension which occurs in asthma, and may be present with normal or only slightly overinflated lungs especially in emphysema of the centrilobular type. One should look for signs of lung destruction – smaller and fewer than normal pulmonary vessels, fibrosis, and bullae which may occupy part or even a whole lung. A lung perfusion scan may give a lacework pattern, i.e. a lung 'full of holes'.

Pulmonary fibrosis
Pulmonary fibrosis may be localized or more general giving a fine or coarse pattern in the lungs with severe scarring, bullous forma-

tion, or superadded cor pulmonale in severe cases. The fibrosis may be localized or generalized. Fibrosis causes not only lines of scarring in the lungs, but also loss of volume in the affected parts (unless these are re-expanded by bullae), and a loss of definition or indistinct outlines of the heart and diaphragm (Fig. 17).

Fibrotic shadows may be difficult to discern, especially if they are fine or diffuse. They may be present in association with nodules, e.g. in sarcoid or pneumoconiosis. Sometimes the terms 'reticular' or 'reticulonodular' are used in relation to fibrosis or fibrosis and nodules. The problem in using these terms is that they often seem to confuse and this author prefers to avoid them. A network pattern of blood vessels and alveoli is present in all normal lungs, and the recognition of an altered pattern is of paramount importance. This recognition can only readily be achieved with practice, but the observer should always try to note whether the fine vessel pattern is normal, accentuated (as in pulmonary plethora), reduced (as with emphysema), whether there are fine nodules superimposed, fibrosis, engorged septal lines (as with congestion) or cavities of whatever size from very small to quite large.

On an underexposed radiograph, or one with poor inspiration, the fine peripheral vascular shadows will sometimes appear as small 'nodules' or a 'network', yet if closely studied each will be seen to be continuous with a small vessel. The nodules in this case are vessels seen 'end on'. Normally no vessels are visible in the outermost 1–2 cm of lung. 'Nodular' and 'fibrotic' shadows are in addition to these.

In the various forms of fibrosing alveolitis (see page 15.123) the thickening of the alveolar walls causes a diffuse fine fibrosis, particularly at the lung bases (Fig. 17d).

In scleroderma, not only may there be fibrosis, but breakdown of alveolar walls may form small honeycomb-like cavities. Fibrosis leads to loss of distinct outlines to the diaphragm and heart, elevation of hila, bullous formation, and often a small volume chest. (Note that patients with fibrosing alveolitis commonly have basal crepitations on auscultation, whereas those with fibrosis due to sarcoidosis, pneumoconiosis etc. do not.)

In considering the differential diagnosis of pulmonary fibrosis look also for signs of:

1. Previous tuberculosis often with calcified lung foci and calcified hilar mediastinal nodes.

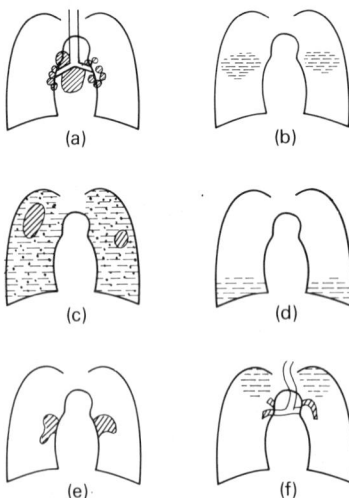

Fig. 17 Sarcoidosis, pulmonary fibrosis, and cor pulmonale; (a) bilateral hilar, subcarinal, and azygos node enlargement: sarcoidosis; (b) mid-zone fibrosis: sarcoidosis; (c) diffuse fine fibrosis, small nodules, and larger nodules due to coalescence (PMF): pneumoconiosis; (d) fine fibrosis starting at lung bases: fibrosing alveolitis. A similar picture but with added tiny cystic changes (honeycombing) may be seen with scleroderma; (e) cor pulmonale: enlargement of interlobar pulmonary arteries bilaterally; (f) elevated hila, tortuous trachea, and bilateral upper lobe fibrosis due to past tuberculosis.

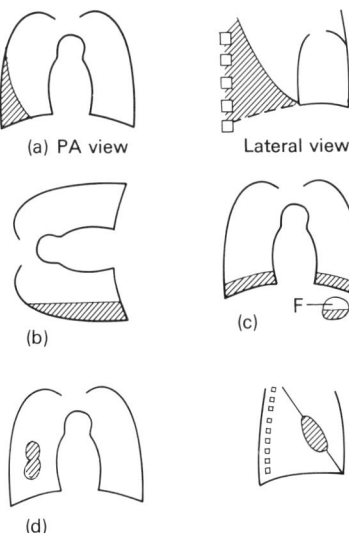

Fig. 18 Some patterns seen with pleural effusions; (a) free fluid lying mainly postero-laterally in the right pleural cavity; (b) decubitus view (patient lying on right side) with horizontal X-ray beam; the fluid has moved under the effect of gravity; (c) subpulmonary effusions: note the apparent extra thickness of the left side of the diaphragm, i.e. between the stomach gas and the lung. On the right side such fluid may not be so readily apparent unless gas is present in the peritoneal cavity; (d) loculated fluid in oblique fissure.

2. Nodal enlargement, occasionally with calcification (sarcoidosis)
3. Coalescing or nodular shadows (pneumoconiosis)
4. Pleural plaques and/or calcification above the diaphragm (asbestosis)
5. Pleural effusions and/or thickening (rheumatoid arthritis)

Localized fibrosis can be the result of previous pneumonia, infarct, or other lung diseases. Previous radiotherapy treatment will often give rise to sharply delineated areas of fibrosis which do not correspond to the normal anatomical landmarks in the lungs, but take up the shape of the treatment fields. Such may be seen at the lung apex in a patient who has had treatment to the nodes for cancer of the breast, alongside the mediastinum after 'mantle' treatment for reticulosis, or in the area of a treated lung neoplasm.

Pleural effusions

Small pleural effusions commonly give rise to an opacity in the costophrenic angle. As they become larger the fluid rises around the lung and commonly fills the posterolateral aspect of the pleural cavity to give an opacity bounded by a curved line concave towards the hilum. The fluid also tracks around the lung (unless a hydro-pneumothorax is present), producing opacity medially and as a thin line over the upper lobe to the apex. Sometimes it becomes localized and collects in the oblique fissures (the 'vanishing tumour' which frequently clears in a few days), over the apex of the lower lobe, at the base posteriorly or beneath the lung as a subpulmonary effusion. This last gives a spurious appearance of a thickened dome of the diaphragm. On the left side detection of a subpulmonary effusion is aided by noting the position of the stomach gas bubble – on the right it may be more difficult unless there is gas in the peritoneal cavity.

Freely moving fluid can be demonstrated by the use of a *decubitus* view, with the patient lying on his side and a horizontal X-ray beam. The patterns of pleural effusions are shown in Fig. 18.

The type of pleural fluid cannot be determined by radiography but may sometimes be inferred, e.g. empyema after pneumonia, blood or chyle after trauma, etc.

Ultrasound

Normally the air-filled lung prevents ultrasound examination of thoracic structures, except for the heart. However, when there is pleural fluid, including pus or empyema (and also with a superficial cyst) there is then a very good 'window' for the linear array or spinning types of probes of real-time ultrasound apparatus. It is then a very easy matter to confirm the presence of fluid or masses, if these are adjacent to the chest wall. Adhesions and debris within the fluid may also be visualized. The examination is best carried out with the patient sitting or standing, and is more accurate in this respect than CT.

The method is very valuable for the localization of the fluid prior to drainage or biopsy.

Ultrasound may also be used to assess pericardial effusions, or via the normal 'window' of the liver to assess the right side of the diaphragm, its movement, overlying or underlying fluid, pus etc., e.g. in a subphrenic abscess.

Pleural and chest wall masses

Masses may be due to primary or secondary tumours or may be encysted fluid or pus. Secondary tumours in the ribs may cause destruction (often with a soft tissue mass) or sclerosis, but such destruction is also seen with direct extension into the chest wall, e.g. the Pancoast tumour (Fig. 15), and may also be seen with a metastatic abscess, e.g. in tuberculosis with a 'cold' abscess in the chest wall. Secondary pleural tumours are more common than primary i.e. mesothelioma but both usually give a coarse nodular outline to the affected pleural cavity (Fig. 19a). Primary pleural tumours may be benign, e.g. fibroma giving a well oulined mass. Both this and a mesothelioma may be accompanied by a pleural effusion. Note also apparent pleural masses – plombage (sponges, leucite balls, etc.) which used to be inserted to collapse the upper part of a lung and help to heal tuberculosis, in preference to the more disfiguring operation of thoracoplasty.

In order to determine whether a mass is pleural, in the lung, chest wall, or mediastinum occasionally fluid may be replaced by air (artificial pneumothorax) to partially collapse the lung and show the abnormality more clearly. Intraperitoneal gas may also be useful in showing clearly the under aspect of the diaphragm, e.g. with a subpulmonary effusion or to show a diaphragmatic tumour.

Pleural calcification

Calcification in the pleura may signify a previous empyema, often tuberculous if the patient has had artificial pneumothorax treatment – often with gross pleural thickening as well. Chronic fibrous pleurisy which can follow other causes of empyema or result from haemothorax may also calcify. Asbestosis (see page 15.113) causes pleural plaques especially anterolaterally, in the interlobar fissures, and over the diaphragm where their calcification looks similar to 'icing sugar on cake' (Fig. 19b). If not visible on plain radiographs or ordinary tomograms, these plaques are readily shown by computerized tomography. Pulmonary fibrosis, pleural and lung neoplasms are also complications of asbestosis. Occasionally a benign 'whorled nodule' is produced (Fig. 19c).

Pulmonary circulation

Not only is it important to study the pulmonary vessels when considering the possibility of collapse, mass or nodular lesions, but changes in them must also be noted with other diseases.

Pulmonary embolism

When a large part of the lung has its blood supply shut off by embolism, then the vessels in that part of the lung will be less distended and less visible. This occurs before infarction supervenes, when there will then appear an opaque, and often wedge-shaped shadow with its point towards the hilum, followed often by pleural reaction or fluid. Sometimes there is collapse of the affected part of the lung. With larger emboli, the main pulmonary artery

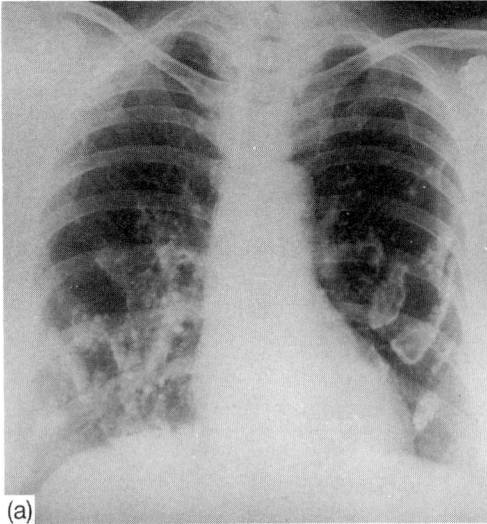

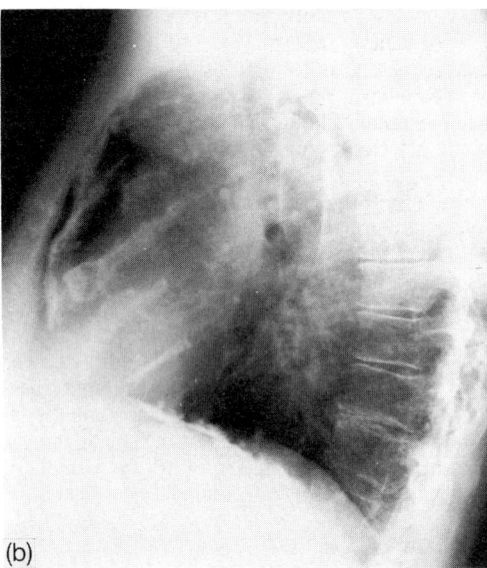

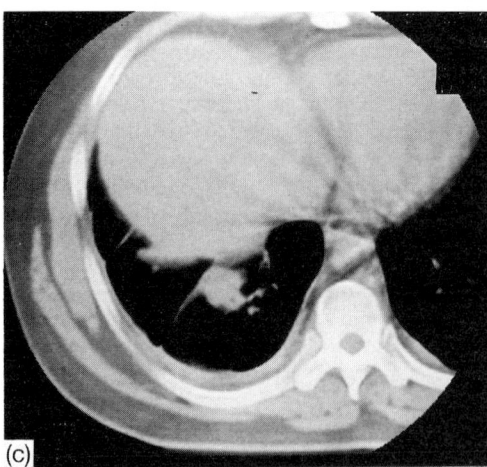

Fig. 19 (a, b) Calcified pleural opaques including 'sugar icing' on the diaphragm (asbestosis). This woman suffered from asbestosis as a result of washing her husband's clothes (it may also give rise to diffuse fibrosis, pleural or pulmonary tumours). (c) Pleural plaques, pleural thickening in fissure and 'whorled nodule' secondary to asbestosis.

shadow may become enlarged due to the more distal obstruction and diversion of blood will occur to the unblocked portions of the pulmonary circulation.

The most convenient way of demonstrating a pulmonary circulation defect is with an isotope study, in which labelled particles (50–100 μm) are injected intravenously. $^{99}Tc^m$ (half-life six hours) is most commonly used. However, not all perfusion defects are due to emboli and some are due to localized emphysema which may not be apparent on the plain radiographs. Other transient defects may be secondary to small areas of collapse secondary to mucous plugs in asthma. The best time to do the examination is in the acute stage, and in most centres a ventilation study using ^{133}Xe or $^{81}Kr^m$ as a gas is also carried out but labelled inhaled particles may also be used. Typically in the case of pneumonia, ventilation will be reduced but perfusion will be normal in the affected area, while for embolism ventilation will be normal and perfusion reduced (Fig. 20).

However, not all cases are as clear cut as this, particularly if they are not examined at the start of the illness. In the later stages of pneumonia (especially staphylococcal) there will also be a perfusion deficit. Likewise, when there is localized emphysema or consolidation supervenes on embolism, ventilation in the diseased area will be impaired.

Because of the problems in trying to distinguish between the areas of embolism and emphysema (in the absence of consolidation), it may be helpful to consider the ventilation and perfusion mismatch as a ratio.

V/P>1   Wasted (i.e. too much) ventilation is nearly always due to a vascular lesion, e.g. embolism.

V/P<1   Wasted perfusion is usually due to airways disease.

Note also that emboli and infarcts tend to resolve either spontaneously or with treatment so that a follow-up lung scan in a few days' time, will usually show improvement.

Pulmonary plethora
Too much blood in the pulmonary vessels (arteries and veins), is usually due to cardiac failure, but may also be caused by polycythaemia or a left-to-right shunt.

Cor pulmonale
Cor pulmonale tends to give large main (hilar) pulmonary arteries and peripheral narrowing.

Pulmonary congestion
This may be due to a variety of causes, e.g. local noxious agent (e.g. infection), allergy to drugs, heart failure (or overtransfusion, etc.), or lymphatic blockage. Radiological signs are:

1. Fullness of pulmonary veins, and upper lobe blood diversion (see below).

2. Interstitial oedema is shown by septal engorgement. Pulmonary septa are connective tissue planes containing lymph vessels and are normally invisible. When thickened, they give rise to lines (Fig. 21) on chest radiographs. Kerley's A lines radiate from the hila especially in the upper and mid zones and do not reach the lung edge, whilst B lines are horizontal, about 2 cm in length and are best seen at the periphery of the lung bases. C lines are short lines radiating at different angles to give a network pattern. B lines are commonly seen in patients with chronic cardiac failure (e.g. mitral stenosis). These and A lines may also be found in acute cardiac failure (e.g. myocardial infarction) and are very prominent in lymphangitis carcinomatosa. C lines are commonly present in dust diseases. Obliquely running D lines have since been described mainly in the middle lobe and lingula.

3. Concomitant pleural effusions.

Alteration in size of one pulmonary artery relative to the other
This will happen if the blood flow to one lung is severely impaired, e.g. with fibrosis, unilateral transradiant lung (Macleod syndrome,

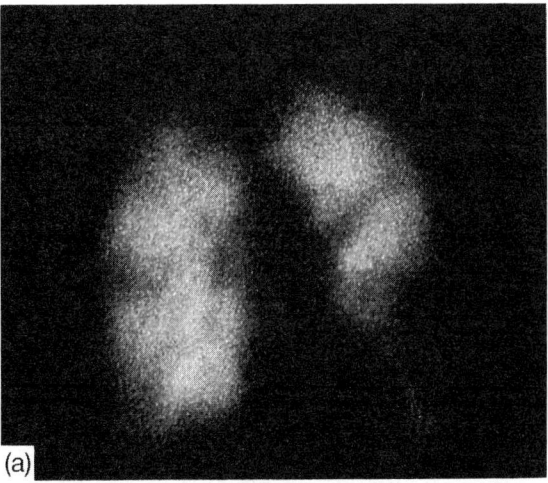

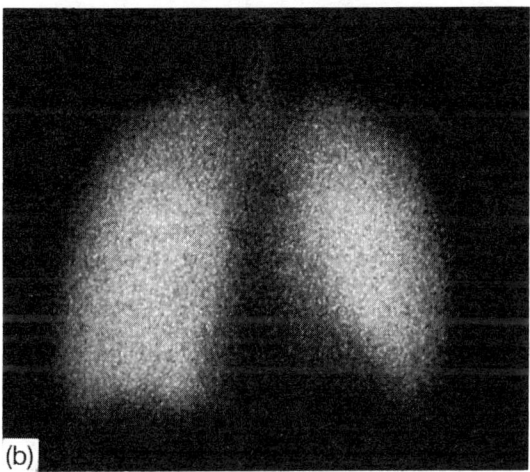

Fig. 20 Lung scan: (a) perfusion study using $^{99}Tc^m$-labelled albumen showing large defect at left base and smaller defects elsewhere in both lungs; (b) ventilation study, using $^{81}Kr^m$, showing normal appearance.

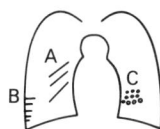

Fig. 21 Kerley's lines. Note 'C' lines give a fine network pattern. ('D' lines similar to 'A' and 'B' lines are especially seen in the right middle lobe and lingula overlying the shadow of the heart on the lateral view.)

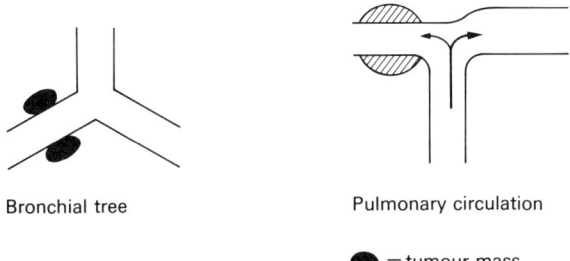

Bronchial tree   Pulmonary circulation

● = tumour mass

Fig. 22 The paradoxical hilar enlargement sign – the contralateral main pulmonary artery is enlarged because of diminished blood flow through the artery on the other side. Not only may this occur with a tumour (Oeser *et al.*) but also with other causes of unilateral diminished pulmonary perfusion, e.g. acutely in pulmonary embolism, chronically in Macleod's syndrome, or unilateral pulmonary scarring or fibrosis. (Reproduced from Wright, 1973, by permission.)

see page 15.66), pulmonary embolism blocking the blood supply to one lung, or sometimes with a bronchial neoplasm involving or stimulating a narrowing of one pulmonary artery. In the latter instance dilation of the contralateral artery will give rise to the *paradoxical hilar enlargement sign* (Fig. 22) and on occasion such has been diagnosed as the primary neoplasm, when it lies on the opposite side.

Blood diversion

One also has to consider blood diversion not only in a contralateral direction but also vertically. With our upright posture the apices of the lungs are rather poorly perfused, which is one reason for the development of apical bullae. Diversion of blood from lower to upper lobes occurs with increased pulmonary venous pressure (mitral stenosis or congestive cardiac failure), basal emphysema, or embolism. A decreased perfusion of the upper lobes with increase in the lower lobes occurs in upper lobe emphysema or embolism. In mitral stenosis obliterative basal vascular changes may take place.

Intrathoracic lymph nodes

It is important to know the approximate positions of the hilar and mediastinal lymph nodes and the pattern of lymph drainage through them. Lymph, draining from the cisterna chyli in the abdomen, passes up through the thoracic duct in front of the dorsal spine to the left subclavian vein. Usually mediastinal nodes do not fill on pedal lymphography, but may occasionally do so. Drainage from the mediastinal nodes occurs into both the thoracic and accessory thoracic ducts. Drainage from the right and left lungs is shown in Fig. 23. In particular, one should note how spread of tumours can take place into the contralateral side of the mediastinum, the position of the azygos nodes, the large group of subcarinal nodes (sometimes referred to as the 'sump', see Fig. 10b), and the nodes around the aortic arch on the left, involvement of which can often result in left recurrent laryngeal palsy. The right recurrent laryngeal nerve turns around the subclavian artery, not the aortic arch (unless this is right sided): it may sometimes become involved by a right apical (or Pancoast type) of lung tumour.

Nodes should, if possible, be differentiated from vessels on plain radiographs or tomograms, by their nodularity, by overlapping the vessels, and in difficult cases by opacifying the vessels with contrast medium at angiography or during computerized tomography.

In *sarcoidosis* nodal enlargement is particularly seen in the bronchopulmonary (hilar nodes), the azygos region, and the *subcarinal* nodes. These latter are usually the largest. They are often poorly seen on plain films or conventional tomograms but are readily seen on those taken with high kV and on inclined frontal (or rotational) tomograms. Usually the disease is symmetrical on either side of the chest. Nodal enlargement may occur without lung infiltration, and may be accompanied by erythema nodosum. In most patients nodal enlargement will resolve spontaneously, but rarely the nodes remain enlarged or may calcify. Pleural effusions are almost *never* seen in sarcoidosis unless complicated by some other disease, e.g. tuberculosis.

With *reticulosis* (especially Hodgkin's disease) nodal enlargement tends to be asymmetrical. Enlargement of anterior mediastinal or thymic nodes is common and may be massive.

Finally one must not forget tuberculosis as a cause of lymph node enlargement particularly in primary tuberculosis in children. The typical Ghon focus (Fig. 24) with a small peripheral lesion and central node enlargement is well known, and nodes may sometimes be very large and extend up to the mediastinum. Nodal enlargement seems to be particularly dangerous in the lower right hilum where pressure may cause collapse of the right middle lobe, in the right hilum causing obstructive emphysema and in the right upper mediastinum adjacent to the superior vena cava which seems particularly prone to lead to miliary tuberculosis.

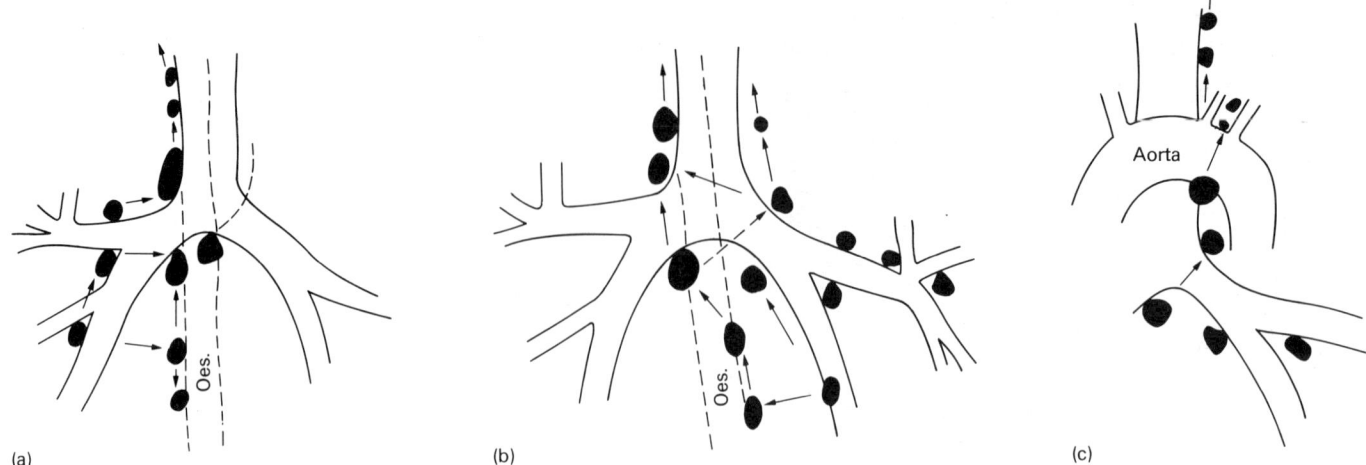

Fig. 23 Diagram of hilar and mediastinal lymph nodes: (a) nodes draining the right lung, and (b) and (c) the left lung. Note how the lymph flow and hence spread of tumour cells may take place to the contralateral side, also the large group of subcarinal nodes, and those around the aortic arch, involvement of which by tumours commonly leads to a left recurrent laryngeal nerve palsy. (Reproduced from Wright, 1973, by permission.)

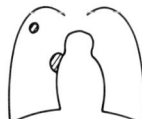

Fig. 24 Ghon focus in primary tuberculosis – peripheral focus in lung and enlargement of hilar lymph nodes.

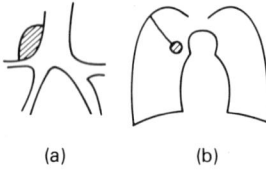

Fig. 25 (a) Enlarged azygos node (diagram of tomogram); (b) the azygos vein may sometimes pass through the right upper lobe in an 'azygos fissure'.

Azygos node enlargement may be seen with tuberculosis, sarcoidosis, and tumours. It is often readily distinguished from distension of the azygos vein by being (a) very large, (b) associated with other lymphadenopathy, and (c) distended with the patient supine and much smaller when sitting or standing (Fig. 25).

In Eastern peoples, tuberculous lymph node enlargement may be massive and may be associated with mediastinal abscesses or metastatic bone lesions, e.g. in ribs. Negroid peoples may exhibit rounded lung infiltrates in sarcoidosis or tuberculosis resembling metastases.

References

Armstrong, P. and Wastie, M. L. (1981). *X-ray diagnosis*. Blackwell Scientific Publications, Oxford.

Brock, R. C. (1954). *The anatomy of the bronchial tree*, 2nd edn, Oxford University Press, London.

Felson, B. (1973). *Fundamentals of chest roentgenology*. W. B. Saunders, Philadelphia.

—— and Felson, H. (1950). Localisation of intrathoracic lesions by means of the PA roentgenogram: the silhouette sign. *Radiology* **55**, 363.

Fraser, R. G. and Paré, J. A. P. (1970). *Diagnosis of diseases of the chest*. W. B. Saunders, Philadelphia.

——, —— (1977). *Organ physiology: structure and function of the lung with emphasis on roentgenology*, 2nd edn. W. B. Saunders, Philadelphia.

Kerley, P. (1933). Radiology in heart disease. *Br. med. J.* **ii**, *v*, 594.

—— (1951). In *Textbook of X-ray diagnosis*, by British Authors vol. 2, (eds S. C. Shanks and P. Kerley). Lewis, London. (See also 3rd edn, 1962).

Kohn, H. N. (1983). Zur histologie der indurirenden fibrösen pneumonie. *Münchener Medicinische Wochenschrift* 42–45.

Kreel, L., Slavin, G., Herbert, A. and Sardin, B. (1975). Intralobar septal oedema: D lines. *Clin. Radiol.* **26**, 209.

Lillington, J. T. and Jampolis, R. N. (1977). *A diagnostic approach to chest disease*. Williams and Wilkins, New York.

Nagaishi, C. (1972). *Functional anatomy and histology of the lung*. University Park Press, Baltimore.

Oeser, H., Ernst, H. and Gerstenberg, E. (1969). Das 'paradoxe hiluszeichen' beim zentralen bronchuskarzinom. *Fortschritte auf dem Gebiete der röntgenstrahlen*. **110**, 205.

Pillardy, G. and Remy, J. (1970). *Diagram of bronchial anatomy*. Kodak Pathé and Cercle d'Études et des Recherches Radiologiques, Paris.

Pancoast, H. K. (1932). Superior pulmonary sulcus tumours (tumours, characterised by pain, Horner's syndrome, destruction of bone and atrophy of hand muscles). *J. Am. med. Assoc.* **99**, 1391.

Paul, L. W. and Juhl, J. H. (1972). *The essentials of roentgen interpretation*. Harper and Row.

Pierce, J. W. and Grainger, R. G. (1975). In *Textbook of radiology* (eds D. Sutton and R. G. Grainger). Churchill Livingstone, Edinburgh.

Simon, G. (1978). *Principles of chest X-ray diagnosis*. Butterworth, London.

Wright, F. W. (1973). *The radiological diagnosis of lung and mediastinal tumours*. Butterworth, London (2nd edn in preparation).

THE FUNCTION OF THE LUNG AND ITS INVESTIGATION

N. B. PRIDE

The primary function of the lungs is to act as a gas exchanger supplying oxygen to the tissues and removing the carbon dioxide produced by cellular respiration. Though the exchange of gases between the alveoli and pulmonary capillary blood is achieved by passive transport, the efficiency of the lungs as a gas exchanger depends on many active processes, ranging from the workings of the ventilatory pump to the production of the surfactant lining layer of the alveoli which reduces the pressures needed to expand the lungs.

Measurement of arterial blood O_2 and CO_2 at rest and during exercise provides the ultimate tests of whether the lungs are performing adequately as a gas exchanger. Obvious abnormality of blood gases at rest is usually only found with relatively advanced lung disease and may not be present when there are considerable abnormalities in other aspects of lung function.

The plan of this section is first to review the most important aspects of normal lung function, indicating briefly the abnormalities which may be found in disease; then to detail the ways in which these different aspects of function may be tested in clinical practice. The functional changes produced by individual diseases are dealt with in the sections specifically dealing with these diseases.

Pulmonary physiopathology

Ventilatory pump, lung, and airway mechanics

In normal subjects resting tidal ventilation (about 5–6 l/min) is only a small proportion of the maximum ventilatory capacity, which is greater than 100 1/min. Even on strenuous, sustained exercise, ventilation does not usually increase above about 80 1/min. But in many lung diseases impairment of the ventilatory capacity becomes the dominant factor limiting exercise tolerance, while abnormalities in the mechanical properties of the lung greatly impair the efficiency of pulmonary gas exchange and predispose to the eventual development of respiratory failure.

Respiratory muscles

Ventilation of the lungs is produced by the action of the inspiratory muscles in expanding the chest cage and lowering pressure on the pleural surface of the lungs leading to their expansion. In normal subjects at rest the diaphragm is probably responsible for most of inspiration, acting primarily by its downward piston action, but also by its insertional action on the lower ribs, leading to their elevation and outward expansion. Some inspiratory muscle activity continues through the first part of expiration which 'brakes' the recoil of the lungs and slows expiratory flow. The later part of expiration is usually passive allowing the lungs to return to the neutral position of the respiratory system.

When ventilation increases (as on exercise), diaphragmatic and intercostal muscle activity increases in inspiration and accessory muscles such as the sternomastoids, are recruited; postinspiratory activity of inspiratory muscles is reduced and may be replaced by increasing activity of expiratory intercostal and abdominal muscles. In addition, there are co-ordinated actions of muscles of the upper airway which, on inspiration, widen the alae nasi, pharynx, and larynx, and prevent the passive narrowing of these structures which would otherwise result from the negative airway pressures developed during vigorous inspiration.

The contractile properties of the respiratory muscles are similar to those of other skeletal muscles, though there are suggestions that the respiratory muscles may be less prone to fatigue. The optimum length of the diaphragm for generating tension is at lung volumes around or below the normal resting breathing position and its ability to develop tension decreases considerably at larger lung volumes. Many clinical problems with the respiratory muscles are a consequence of their working at a mechanical disadvantage. Examples are diseases distorting the rib cage, such as kyphoscoliosis, and airflow obstruction where increase in end-tidal lung volume shortens the initial length of all inspiratory muscles and often flattens the domes of the diaphragm so that its contraction then narrows rather than widens the lower rib cage (Hoover's sign). Because in most respiratory diseases increased pressures are required to expand the lungs while hypoxaemia and loss of muscle bulk may further reduce muscle performance, there has been much recent speculation as to whether chronic fatigue of ventilatory muscles ('pump failure') contributes to ventilatory failure. Though such chronic fatigue probably occurs in neurological or muscle diseases its occurrence in patients with chronic airflow obstruction remains uncertain; however, most clinicians accept that acute inspiratory muscle fatigue sometimes plays an important role in severe asthma.

Lung volumes and distensibility

The elasticity of the lungs causes them to collapse to a very small volume when no expanding force is applied. In contrast, the chest wall has a large resting or 'neutral' volume. Thus the end-tidal volume is the volume at which the tendency of the chest wall to recoil outwards exactly balances the tendency of the lungs to collapse inwards. When the respiratory muscles are relaxed (as at the end of a tidal expiration or under anaesthesia) the volume of the lungs (functional residual capacity, FRC) in a normal subject is in the range 2–3 litres which is about half the lung volume during a full inspiration (total lung capacity, TLC) (Fig. 1). At the resting breathing position with respiratory muscles relaxed, pleural surface pressure is about -5 cmH$_2$0 (-0.5 kPa) (referred to atmospheric pressure). Inspiratory muscle activity reduces this pressure to -8 or -9 cmH$_2$0 (-0.8 or -0.9 kPa) during quiet tidal breathing. In normal lungs about 80 per cent of the tidal change in inspiratory pressure is dissipated in overcoming forces attributable to the elasticity of the lungs and only 20 per cent in overcoming airflow resistance.

The elastic properties of the lungs represent the combination of tissue elasticity and the surface properties of the alveoli. The surfactant layer lining the alveoli, produced by type II alveolar cells,

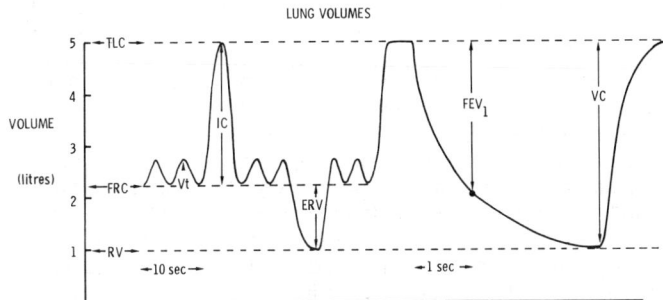

Fig. 1 Static and dynamic lung volumes indicated as a record of tidal breathing against time, followed by expiratory and inspiratory forced vital capacity manoeuvres for which the time scale has been expanded. TLC, total lung capacity; FRC, functional residual capacity; RV, residual volume; FEV, forced expiratory volume in 1 s; IC, inspiratory capacity; Vt, tidal volume; ERV, expiratory reserve volume; VC, vital capacity.

greatly reduces surface forces. The increase in lung volume produced by a given increase in lung distending pressure declines as the lungs are expanded towards TLC. Increase in lung volume also shortens the inspiratory muscles and impairs their ability to reduce pleural surface pressure so that expansion of the lungs is limited at the volume (TLC) at which their recoil pressure (the difference between alveolar and pleural pressure) is exactly balanced by the most negative pleural pressure that can be generated by the inspiratory muscles. In young normal subjects, pleural surface pressure at TLC is about -30 cmH$_2$O (-3 kPa).

A reduced TLC ('restrictive lung disease') is found either when the lungs have low compliance and cannot be expanded normally above their resting volume, or when inadequate expanding forces are applied to the lungs. In lung fibrosis reduced compliance can be due to loss of functioning peripheral lung units rather than thickening of the alveolar wall and interstitium of surviving ventilated units. A similar mechanism probably applies when there is fluid filling of the alveoli in pneumonia or pulmonary oedema. Absence of the surfactant lining layer has been shown to be a definite cause of reduced compliance only in the lungs of premature infants with respiratory distress syndrome of the new-born. But surfactant production is inevitably affected in other severe lung diseases which damage type II alveolar cells and are responsible for the adult respiratory distress syndrome. A thick cortical rim of fibrotic pleura may prevent a normal lung expanding. Weakness of the inspiratory muscles leads to inadequate expanding forces on the surface of the lungs and a reduced TLC. Uncoupling of the lung from the chest wall due to air or fluid in the pleural cavity also increases pleural pressure and reduces resting and maximum lung volumes.

An increase in TLC in adult life occurs when the lungs are easily distended and have low recoil pressure and is only found in emphysema. An increase in end-tidal volume (FRC) is however found in most patients with intrapulmonary airflow obstruction whether or not they have emphysema. This hyperinflation is probably sustained by continued activity of the inspiratory muscles through expiration.

Airway mechanics

In addition to the pressures required to distend the lungs pressure is dissipated in overcoming the resistance to air flow in the branching system of the airways. The resistance of the normal tracheobronchial tree is very low (1–2 cm H$_2$O/1/s or 0.1–0.2 kPa/1/s) so that during quiet tidal breathing alveolar pressures only fluctuate about ± 1 cmH$_2$O (± 0.1 kPa) around atmospheric pressure. Airways expand as lung volume is increased and are 30 to 40 per cent larger in calibre at full inspiration (TLC) than at full expiration (residual volume, RV). Although airway distensibility does not make a significant contribution to the distensibility of the lungs as a whole, the increase in airway calibre as the lungs are inflated results in a significant decrease in airflow resistance, so that airway narrowing can be partially overcome by breathing at a larger lung volume. The calibre of the airways at any lung volume is under the control of the autonomic nervous system. Most normal subjects have some bronchomotor tone mediated by vagal efferent nerves. This tone can be removed by β-adrenoceptor agonists or atropine, reducing airflow resistance by about 30 per cent. The role of the sympatho-adrenal system in controlling airway tone is less clear; in humans, sympathetic nerves may not directly innervate bronchial muscle, though they probably modulate the activity of the vagal ganglia in the airway wall. The many adrenoceptors in normal bronchial muscle probably respond to circulating catecholamines rather than to sympathetic nerve stimulation.

Airway tone shows a circadian rhythm which is greatest at about 4.00 hours and least in mid-afternoon. Tone can be briefly increased by many inhaled stimuli, such as cold air, inert dust, cigarette smoke, and sulphur dioxide, and other air pollutants. These stimuli act on irritant or cough receptors situated immediately under the airway epithelium which trigger reflex broncho-

constriction; both afferent and efferent nervous pathways run in the vagus nerve. There is a wide range of airway responsiveness to exogenous stimuli in healthy, asymptomatic subjects and reactivity is increased for some weeks after respiratory tract infections and for a shorter period after exposure to environmental pollutants. The airway hyperreactivity found in asthma is an exaggeration of this normal response, one effect of which is to increase the amplitude of the circadian rhythm in airway calibre; as timing is unchanged this leads to the characteristic early morning worsening of symptoms.

Airways are kept patent for gas flow by their clearance mechanisms. The nose traps large particles (such as pollen); if it is bypassed and foreign material is inhaled and impacts on the airway wall, cough is reflexly stimulated by firing of irritant receptors, which are concentrated in the larynx, trachea, and major airways. The glottis is closed, the bronchi constrict, and there is a rise in intrathoracic (pleural and alveolar) and airway pressure; with sudden opening of the glottis there is an explosive decompression of airway pressure, leading to rapid narrowing of central airways and a burst of high velocity gas flow through them. The shearing action of cough is only likely to be effective in the central airways. In more peripheral airways, the mucus carpet carried towards the glottis by the beating of the cilia is the effective mechanism for removing secretions and smaller foreign bodies. Apart from forming a depository for small particles, airway secretions moisten and smooth the airway wall and so may have a role in reducing the frictional component of airflow resistance. Impaired cough is found with gross expiratory muscle weakness. Mucociliary transport is impaired in patients with immotile cilia and in some chronic lung diseases. The extent to which other clearance mechanisms can compensate for this impairment is uncertain, but impaired transport can be found in healthy, asymptomatic subjects.

Another important role of the airways, particularly the upper airway and nasal passages, is to condition the inspired and expired air. Under normal ambient conditions at rest, heating and humidification of inspired air to body temperature and 100 per cent saturation with water vapour is achieved by the time it reaches the carina. When the volume of inspired air is large, cold, and dry and the nose is bypassed (as occurs with strenuous exercise on cold, wintry mornings) or when tracheostomy or endotracheal intubation is performed, conditioning of inspired air may not be complete until it has penetrated further into the lungs. However, because the total mucosal surface area available for air conditioning rapidly increases as the periphery of the lung is approached, it is unlikely that alveolar temperature ever deviates from core body temperature. Central airway cooling and water loss during strenuous exercise is believed to be the immediate stimulus provoking the bronchoconstriction that occurs after strenuous exercise in many asthmatic subjects, but it is not clear precisely how this triggers the generalized airway narrowing as changes in central airway temperature on exercise are similar in asthmatic and normal subjects.

Total airflow resistance is the sum of the resistance of a complex branching system with 20 or more generations of airways arranged in series and with many parallel pathways in the more peripheral airway generations. Because each succeeding airway generation from trachea out to the periphery is smaller in size, the resistance offered by each individual *airway* of successive generations increases. However, the effect of the diminished calibre of each individual airway is far outweighed by the increase in the total number of airways in each generation which results in the total cross-sectional area available for gas flow at any fixed distance from the trachea increasing dramatically as the alveoli are approached (Fig. 2). Because the velocity of gas flow depends on the ratio of bulk flow to cross-sectional area, convective flow of gas is at a maximum in the trachea and central airways and slows progressively towards the periphery, so that in the terminal airways gas flow occurs solely by diffusion. As a consequence, at

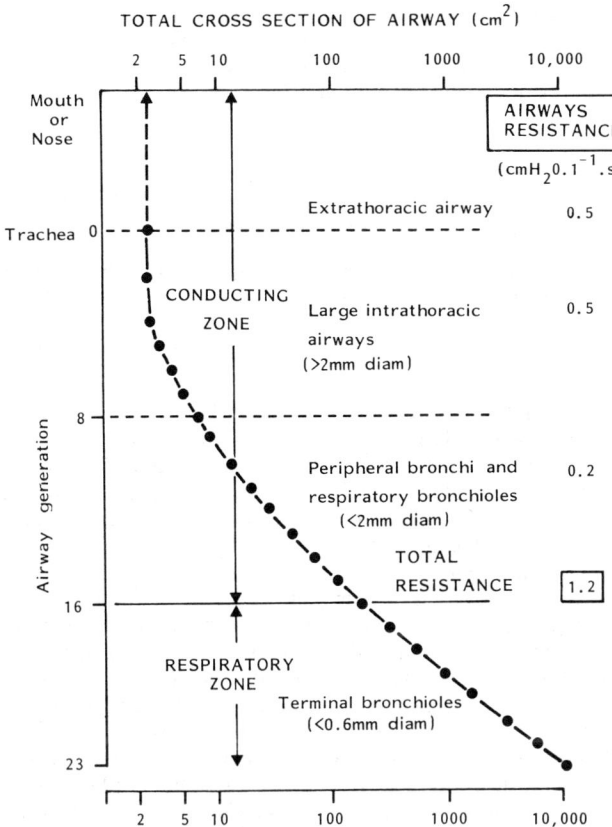

Fig. 2 Relationship between airway generation (trachea = 0), total cross-section of airways in a given generation, and airways resistance in a normal subject breathing at mid-lung volume. Over 80 per cent of the total resistance is in the extrathoracic airway and larger intrathoracic airways (generations 0–8), and the remainder in peripheral conducting airways (generations 8–16 ≃ airway diameters 2.0–0.6 mm). There is no significant resistive pressure drop in the terminal bronchioles which have an enormous total cross-sectional area. If the subject breathes via the nose the extrathoracic contribution to resistance may be even greater. (Based on anatomical data of Weibel, 1963, with permission.)

FRC in healthy subjects only about 20 per cent of the total airways resistance is due to airways of 2 mm diameter or less (Fig. 2). Breathing through the nose assists particle removal and the conditioning of inspired air, but increases airflow resistance. This may account for the switch to mouth breathing that occurs when ventilation is greatly increased on exercise.

During quiet breathing, the subatmospheric pleural pressure throughout the breathing cycle slightly distends the airways. With vigorous expiratory efforts, as in a cough, central airways are dramatically compressed by the positive pleural pressures which may exceed +100 cmH₂0 (+ 10 kPa). Complete airway closure does not occur because the positive pleural pressure not only compresses the central airways (which increases resistance) but also increases the driving pressure for expiratory flow, alveolar pressure. Above a certain minimum expiratory pressure, these two tendencies precisely counterbalance each other so that at any given lung volume, flow reaches a maximum plateau value which remains constant with further increases in pressure. The compressed central airways act as the flow-limiting mechanism and the plateau value of maximum expiratory flow provides the physiological basis for the widely used tests of forced expiration and their relative independence from the precise expiratory pressure applied.

Many lung diseases diminish the calibre of the airways, increasing airflow resistance and reducing maximum expiratory flow. Airway narrowing may result from disease of the airway wall or lumen (as in asthma or the obstructive bronchiolitis of smokers) or from loss of the normal forces distending the airways (as occurs with the alveolar destruction of emphysema). When narrowing of the intrapulmonary airways is present, dynamic narrowing of the central airways and flow limitation occurs on expiration at unusually low flows and pleural pressures, so that reductions in maximum flow and increases in airflow resistance characteristically are much greater on expiration than on inspiration. In contrast, if the site of airway narrowing is in the extrathoracic airways, changes in inspiratory flow and resistance may predominate and, if severe, are associated with inspiratory stridor.

The site of intrapulmonary airway narrowing has been particularly studied in smokers with varying combinations of irreversible airway disease and emphysema (chronic obstructive pulmonary disease). Pathological studies suggest that the usual site of fixed disease of the airway wall and lumen leading to increased resistance is in the small peripheral airways of less than 2–3 mm diameter. Because these airways account for only a small proportion of normal airflow resistance, considerable disease can develop insidiously in this 'quiet zone' of the lung before obvious increases in total airflow resistance and reductions in maximum expiratory flow are found. The site of airway narrowing in asthma is much less certain, both because it probably varies from patient to patient (and probably within a patient as asthma varies), and because physiological studies cannot be backed up by appropriate pathological evidence.

Pulmonary gas exchange

At rest an average tidal inspiration adds 350–500 ml of fresh air to the initial lung volume of about 3 litres. The inspired air filling the conducting airways at the end of inspiration makes no contribution to pulmonary gas exchange and is exhaled unchanged at the start of the subsequent expiration. In the normal subject the volume of these conducting airways is about 120–150 ml (anatomical dead space) so that only about two-thirds of each breath mixes completely with alveolar gas.

The fall in partial pressure of oxygen as it is transported from ambient air to the tissues via a perfectly homogenous lung is shown schematically in Fig. 3. Tissue hypoxaemia can arise from a decrease in ambient P_{O_2} or abnormal gradients at any of the subsequent stages. However, diffuse lung disease characteristically leads to inhomogeneity of mechanical and gas exchange properties of the lungs. Uneven ventilation leads to widespread differences in local alveolar and end-capillary P_{O_2}; the resulting ventilation/perfusion imbalance is the commonest cause of arterial hypoxaemia in lung disease.

Alveolar P_{O_2} and P_{CO_2}
The value of P_{O_2} in alveolar gas can be estimated from the simplified form of the alveolar gas equation:

$$\text{Alveolar } P_{O_2} = \text{Inspired } P_{O_2} - (\text{Alveolar } P_{CO_2}/R)$$

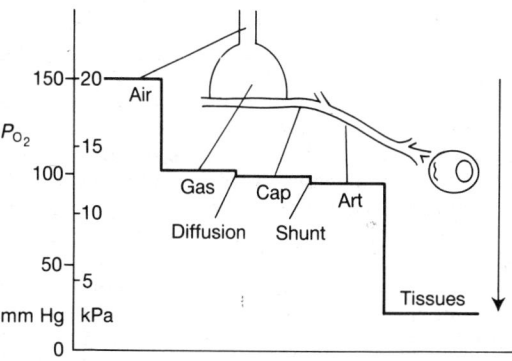

Fig. 3 Scheme of fall in P_{O_2} between ambient air and tissues, assuming a perfectly homogenous lung. (Modified from West, 1977, *Ventilation/blood flow and gas exchange*, 3rd edn. Blackwell Scientific Publications, Oxford, with permission.)

where R is the respiratory exchange ratio, which is normally about 0.8. Alveolar P_{CO_2} is assumed to be the same as arterial P_{CO_2}.

When air is breathed at sea level the inspired P_{O_2} in tracheal gas is 150 mmHg (20 kPa), so that with a normal arterial P_{CO_2} of 40 mmHg (5.3 kPa), alveolar P_{O_2} is 100 mmHg (13.3 kPa).

If the lungs function as perfect gas exchangers, arterial P_{O_2} equals alveolar P_{O_2}. Any inefficiency results in arterial P_{O_2} being less than alveolar P_{O_2}.

Mechanisms of a low arterial P_{O_2}

Arterial P_{O_2} is reduced if alveolar P_{O_2} is reduced or if there is an abnormal difference between alveolar and arterial P_{O_2}.

Alveolar P_{O_2} is reduced when there is a low inspired P_{O_2}, as at altitude, or when alveolar ventilation is inadequate. For a given carbon dioxide production alveolar ventilation is inversely related to mean alveolar P_{CO_2}. Thus with a reduction in total and alveolar ventilation, alveolar and arterial P_{CO_2} rise and (if air is breathed) alveolar P_{O_2} falls. Arterial hypoxaemia solely due to reduced ventilation and a low alveolar P_{O_2}, with the lungs functioning normally as a gas exchanger, occurs with extrapulmonary disease, for instance, when the central drive to breathing is depressed by drugs, anaesthesia, or neurological disease, when respiratory muscle movement is impaired in neuromuscular disorders or when the upper airway is acutely obstructed.

Arterial P_{O_2} is slightly less than alveolar P_{O_2} in normal lungs. Three physiological mechanisms may contribute to the normal alveolar-arterial P_{O_2} difference: (a) diffusion defect (defined as a difference between alveolar P_{O_2} and the P_{O_2} in end-capillary blood as it leaves contact with alveolar gas); (b) ventilation-perfusion imbalance (in which pulmonary capillary blood P_{O_2} fully equilibrates with local alveolar P_{O_2} but there are local differences in alveolar and pulmonary venous P_{O_2}); and (c) shunt (where some mixed venous blood escapes contact with alveolar gas). The same mechanisms are responsible for the much larger alveolar-arterial P_{O_2} differences found in many forms of lung disease.

Diffusion across the alveolar–capillary membrane Transport of oxygen and carbon dioxide across the alveolar-capillary membrane occurs by passive diffusion. Pulmonary arterial blood entering the proximal end of the capillary has a P_{O_2} of about 40 mmHg (5.3 kPa) compared to an average P_{O_2} of 100 mmHg (13.3 kPa) on the alveolar side of the alveolar-capillary membrane. Oxygen therefore moves rapidly from the alveoli into the blood, increasing its P_{O_2} and oxygen saturation and reducing the gradient in P_{O_2} between alveolar gas and capillary blood. At rest it probably takes about 0.25 s for alveolar gas and capillary blood to come into complete diffusion equilibrium; as blood normally remains about 0.75 s in contact with alveolar gas on each transit through the lungs, there is no measurable difference between alveolar and end-capillary P_{O_2} and there are considerable reserves of diffusion capacity. These reserves are stressed by strenuous exercise or a low inspired P_{O_2}. Diffusion limitation probably only occurs in normal lungs when these stresses are combined and strenuous exercise is performed at considerable altitude, as for instance when attempting to climb Mount Everest without added oxygen.

In disease there are several mechanisms by which diffusion limitation could become a cause of arterial hypoxaemia, particularly during exercise. The most familiar is widespread thickening of the alveolar wall, which increases the distance for gas to diffuse into capillary blood producing 'alveolar-capillary' block. This has been suggested as a mechanism of hypoxaemia in fibrosing alveolitis, asbestosis, and similar conditions. However, in areas of gross alveolar damage, local ventilation is more reduced than blood flow and hypoxaemia due to ventilation//perfusion imbalance appears to be quantitatively more important than a diffusion defect. Another cause of diffusion limitation in disease is a reduced total area of alveolar-capillary membrane, as occurs with the breakdown of alveolar walls in emphysema. A loss of accessible alveolar-capillary membrane also occurs with fluid filling of the alveoli (pulmonary oedema, extensive pneumonia), following extensive lung resections, and indeed with extensive fibrosis. In abnormal lungs, diffusion limitation may be confined to certain areas of the lung which have a large blood flow (and short pulmonary capillary transit times for red blood cells) and a low ventilation (reducing local alveolar P_{O_2}), while in other areas no difference between alveolar and end-capillary P_{O_2} occurs. Diffusion limitation is generally now accepted as a much less important cause of hypoxaemia in lung disease than ventilation/perfusion imbalance.

Ventilation/perfusion imbalance Pulmonary gas exchange would be most efficient if in every acinus there was a uniform ratio of alveolar ventilation to pulmonary capillary blood flow close to 1.0. In practice a whole range of ventilation/perfusion ($\dot{V}/\dot{Q}$) ratios is found even in normal lungs.

1. Regional differences due to gravity. In the normal lung the distribution of ventilation and perfusion (and of $\dot{V}/\dot{Q}$ ratios) is not uniform because of regional differences due to the effects of gravity. In the normal upright lung blood flow (per unit of lung volume) at rest is much greater at the base than at the apex of the lung. In the supine or lateral decubitus position the dependent part of the lung again has greater blood flow.

There is also a gravitational gradient of ventilation (again assessed per unit of lung volume) which in the normal upright lung results in more ventilation of the bases than of the apices of the lungs, but the gradient is less marked than that for blood flow. The differences in ventilation occur because the distending pressure on the lung (the difference between alveolar and pleural pressure), and hence regional lung volume, is smaller in the dependent areas of the lung. This is due to a gravitational gradient of pleural pressure, which is about 6 cmH₂O (0.6 kPa) higher (less subatmospheric) at the base than at the apex in the upright position. Because the compliance of lung units is greater at small volume than at large, if a uniform change in inspiratory pleural pressure is applied the increase in volume is greater at the base than at the apex of the lung. This distribution of ventilation can be reversed at small lung volume below FRC in sitting normal subjects when the distending pressure in the dependent areas of the lung may be so low that airway closure occurs and basal ventilation is then decreased. In the supine position, where FRC is reduced, dependent zones may have closed airways throughout a tidal breath and this may be an important cause of hypoxaemia when there is a low FRC as during anaesthesia and in some subjects with obesity.

Because the gravitational gradient of perfusion is greater than that of ventilation, there is a five-fold variation in $\dot{V}/\dot{Q}$ ratios down the normal upright lung and, according to calculations by West, alveolar P_{O_2} may vary from over 130 mmHg (17 kPa) at the apex to about 90 mmHg (12 kPa) at the bases. Hence there is no single value of alveolar P_{O_2} even in the normal lung. The value of alveolar P_{O_2} derived by the alveolar gas equation is a notional *ideal* alveolar P_{O_2} which would occur in the absence of any inequality of $\dot{V}/\dot{Q}$ ratios. In each region of the lung, blood leaving the alveoli normally comes into equilibrium with alveolar P_{O_2} (and P_{CO_2}), and so apical pulmonary venous blood has a P_{O_2} of 130 mmHg and basal blood a P_{O_2} of 90 mmHg. The P_{O_2} in mixed systemic arterial blood lies between these two values, the precise value depending on the quantities of blood at each P_{O_2} which are mixed in transit through the left side of the heart. Despite the apparently important regional differences in $\dot{V}/\dot{Q}$ ratios in the normal lung, these have surprisingly little effect on arterial P_{O_2} which is only about 4 mmHg (0.5 kPa) below ideal alveolar P_{O_2} in young, normal subjects.

2. Differences within a lung region. In disease, inequalities of $\dot{V}/\dot{Q}$ ratios are much more pronounced and are more important within a region than between regions. Whereas in the normal upright lung the lowest $\dot{V}/\dot{Q}$ ratio at the bases may be 0.6, in disease it is common to have $\dot{V}/\dot{Q}$ ratios of 0.1 or less, chiefly because of reduced ventilation but also because loss of pulmonary capillaries in other areas may increase blood flow through surviving per-

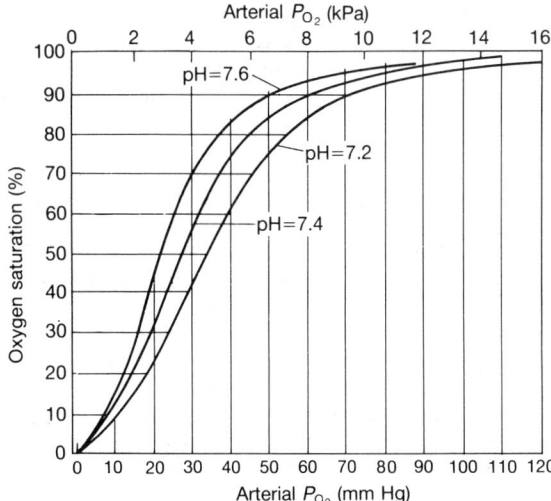

Fig. 4 The relationship between arterial P_{O_2} and percentage oxygen saturation of haemoglobin at three different levels of arterial pH. Apart from a more acid pH, increases in P_{CO_2}, temperature or 2–3 DPG also cause shifts of the curve to the right.

fused areas. Units of low $\dot{V}/\dot{Q}$ ratio which are well perfused play the dominant part in causing arterial hypoxaemia in lung disease. The hypoxaemia occurs because of the shape of the O_2 dissociation curve (Fig. 4). Blood leaving units with a high $\dot{V}/\dot{Q}$ ratio does not contain much more oxygen than blood leaving alveoli with a normal $\dot{V}/\dot{Q}$ ratio, and so high $\dot{V}/\dot{Q}$ units cannot compensate for the low oxygen content of blood leaving low $\dot{V}/\dot{Q}$ units. The final mixed arterial P_{O_2} depends on the respective oxygen contents (not P_{O_2}) of the blood leaving low and high $\dot{V}/\dot{Q}$ units. An abnormal spread of $\dot{V}/\dot{Q}$ ratios also adversely affects CO_2 exchange. But because the CO_2 dissociation curve is nearly linear, blood leaving units with a high $\dot{V}/\dot{Q}$ ratio has a low P_{CO_2} and, provided there is some increase in total ventilation to compensate for the inefficiency of gas exchange, it is possible to keep arterial P_{CO_2} normal. The differing effects of $\dot{V}/\dot{Q}$ imbalance on arterial P_{O_2} and P_{CO_2} therefore occur because the inefficiency of CO_2 exchange (but not O_2 uptake) can be compensated for by a relatively small increase in total ventilation.

By far the most important cause of arterial hypoxaemia in lung disease is $\dot{V}/\dot{Q}$ imbalance due to intraregional inequalities of ventilation which are not precisely balanced by corresponding changes in perfusion. Most diseases of the intrapulmonary airways and of the alveoli are unevenly distributed, with increases in resistance and/or reductions in compliance of affected areas. The consequence is that a high proportion of the tidal volume goes to the most normal parts of the lung, which are relatively overventilated in relation to their blood flow. In the poorly ventilated areas of the lungs, there is usually some reduction in local blood flow but this is not sufficient to prevent the development of abnormally low $\dot{V}/\dot{Q}$ ratios. The reduction in local blood flow sometimes occurs because the pathological process affecting alveoli or peripheral airways also narrows or obliterates blood vessels (as in emphysema and fibrosing alveolitis); this accounts for many apparently 'matched' defects on regional ventilation and perfusion scans. Hypoxic pulmonary vasoconstriction is probably less important in adjusting local blood flow. Thus $\dot{V}/\dot{Q}$ imbalance may be just as severe in acute asthma, where the pulmonary vessels are normal, as in emphysema, where there is a tendency for vessel destruction to occur in overinflated areas which are poorly ventilated.

When the primary pathological abnormality is in the pulmonary vessels, as in pulmonary embolism without infarction, ventilation is well maintained in the areas of reduced blood flow and $\dot{V}/\dot{Q}$ ratios are high in these areas. High $\dot{V}/\dot{Q}$ areas reduce the efficiency of CO_2 excretion but cannot account for the hypoxaemia often

found in acute, severe pulmonary embolism. One possible mechanism for this hypoxaemia is that, in maintaining cardiac output, regions with unoccluded pulmonary vessels have increases in blood flow without accompanying increases in ventilation, so that $\dot{V}/\dot{Q}$ ratios in the unaffected areas are reduced. Because alterations in $\dot{V}/\dot{Q}$ ratios in diseased areas are often accompanied by complementary changes in $\dot{V}/\dot{Q}$ ratios in unaffected areas of the lung, an increased spread of $\dot{V}/\dot{Q}$ ratios (rather than isolated evidence of either high or low $\dot{V}/\dot{Q}$ areas) is the characteristic finding in disease.

Shunt When pulmonary blood flow continues to lung units which are totally unventilated, the $\dot{V}/\dot{Q}$ ratio is zero and blood with mixed venous values of O_2 content will be added to the systemic arterial blood increasing the difference between ideal alveolar P_{O_2} and arterial P_{O_2}. (An identical effect will be found with a right-to-left intracardiac shunt). Shunt through the lungs is negligible in normal lungs. In lung disease an increased shunt is particularly associated with conditions with massive consolidation (alveolar oedema, 'shock' lung, etc.); large increases in shunt are not found in intrapulmonary airway obstruction, even when there is considerable airway occlusion as in asthma, suggesting that some ventilation reaches alveoli beyond occluded airways by collateral pathways. Increasing inspired O_2 improves arterial hypoxaemia satisfactorily if it is due to low $\dot{V}/\dot{Q}$ ratios but has only a small effect when hypoxaemia is due to a large shunt.

Relation between arterial P_{O_2}, O_2 saturation, and tissue oxygenation

The vast majority of oxygen in the blood is carried as oxyhaemoglobin. At a normal P_{O_2} of 85 mmHg (11.3 kPa) or more, percentage saturation (oxygenation) of haemoglobin is close to 100 per cent (Fig. 4) so giving normal subjects higher inspired O_2 to breathe has little effect on O_2 saturation while small reductions in P_{O_2} have little deleterious effect. But below a P_{O_2} of about 60 mmHg (8.0 kPa) small falls in arterial P_{O_2} are associated with large falls in O_2 saturation.

The O_2 content of the blood at a given P_{O_2} will be reduced if there is a reduction in available haem binding sites (anaemia, occupation by carboxyhaemoglobin) or a shift to the right of the O_2 dissociation curve with increase in P_{50} (P_{O_2} at which 50 per cent of haemoglobin is oxyhaemoglobin). The difference between arterial P_{O_2} and tissue P_{O_2} inevitably depends on cardiac output and local blood flow. It is therefore impossible to stipulate a 'safe' level of arterial P_{O_2} for all circumstances. Patients with long-standing chronic hypoxaemia and a good cardiac output can tolerate remarkably low levels of arterial P_{O_2} which would cause unconsciousness if suddenly applied to a normal subject. Markers of inadequate tissue oxygenation are crude; a rise in blood lactate at rest indicates a gross defect.

Respiratory control of acid–base balance

Carbon dioxide entering red blood cells reacts with water to form carbonic acid, most of which dissociates to form hydrogen and bicarbonate ions;

$$CO_2 + H_2O \rightleftharpoons H_2CO_3 \rightleftharpoons H^+ + HCO_3^-$$

The CO_2 produced by cellular respiration is by far the largest source of production of hydrogen ions in the body so the lungs play a major role in controlling blood pH. The amount of CO_2 in the blood can be rapidly regulated by the lungs but adjustment of HCO_3^-, which is regulated by the kidneys, is much slower. The arterial pH depends on the dissociation constant of carbonic acid (which can be represented as a constant, 6.1) and the balance between the two routes of excretion, as indicated by the classical Henderson–Hasselbach equation:

$$\text{Arterial pH} = 6.1 + \log_{10}(HCO_3^-/0.03\ P_{CO_2}\ \text{mmHg*})$$
$$\text{*In SI units } 0.225\ P_{CO_2}\ \text{kPa}$$

When there is chronic elevation of P_{CO_2} (more than 48 hours), there is usually an associated rise in HCO_3^- so that the pH may return to within the normal range (7.36–7.44). Thus measuring pH as well as P_{CO_2} in hypercapnic respiratory failure helps to decide whether a rise in arterial P_{CO_2} is acute or not.

(A comprehensive account of acid–base homeostasis is given on page 9.164).

Pulmonary circulation

The major function of the pulmonary circulation is to deliver blood in a thin sheet to the alveolar–capillary membrane for gas exchange. This is achieved with a low mean pulmonary artery pressure, which is only about 15 mmHg (2 kPa) at rest, so allowing gravitational differences in vascular pressure to have large effects on the distribution of pulmonary blood flow. In keeping with this low pressure, the walls of normal pulmonary arteries and arterioles contain little muscle and resistance to blood flow is distributed relatively evenly between arteries, capillaries, and veins. In the upright posture blood flow is very low at the lung apices in the resting normal subject and increases progressively down the lung at least until near the bases. The distribution of flow becomes more even during exercise. In upper regions of the lung, though pulmonary arterial pressure exceeds alveolar pressure, alveolar pressure may be greater than pulmonary venous pressure and then the effective driving pressure for local blood flow is the difference between local arterial and alveolar pressures; in dependent parts of the lung the conventional difference between pulmonary arterial and venous pressure is the effective driving pressure for flow.

In normal lungs the balance between transvascular hydrostatic pressures, tending to filter fluid out of the small blood vessels, and transvascular osmotic forces which tend to retain fluid in the microcirculation, results in a very small net outflow of fluid which is drained through the interstitium and then via lymph vessels running in the connective tissue sheaths around larger vessels and airways. When the capacity of this drainage system is exceeded, fluid accumulates in the interstitial space around arteries and subsequently in the alveoli. Increases in pulmonary capillary pressure or increases in permeability of the vascular endothelium predispose to pulmonary oedema.

Pulmonary arterioles constrict and arterial pressure rises in response to overall alveolar hypoxia, as occurs on going to altitude. The extent of this vasoconstriction is quite variable between individuals. An acid pH increases the vasoconstrictor effect of hypoxia. With prolonged alveolar hypoxia, pulmonary artery muscle hypertrophies. Local alveolar hypoxia also causes some local pulmonary vasoconstriction, which will tend to divert blood away from such hypoxic areas.

Apart from the major function of pulmonary gas exchange, the smaller pulmonary blood vessels act as a filter of emboli and the large area of vascular endothelium plays an important and selective role in the metabolism of a variety of circulating vasoactive (and often bronchoactive) substances. The best known is the conversion of angiotensin I to angiotensin II by angiotensin-converting enzyme on the luminal surface, but the endothelium is also involved in the inactivation or removal of circulating bradykinin, serotonin, and noradrenaline and some prostaglandins while some forms of pulmonary vasodilation are dependent on relaxing factors produced by the endothelium.

Primary disorders of the pulmonary circulation without involvement of the lungs or heart may cause narrowing of the arterioles ('primary' pulmonary hypertension), endothelial damage, and increased capillary permeability (believed to be the underlying abnormality leading to the 'acute respiratory distress syndrome') or, rarely, pulmonary veno-occlusive disease.

Local occlusions of the pulmonary arterial tree are much commoner and are usually due to thrombotic emboli, but occasionally to pulmonary vasculitis. The characteristic physiological abnormality is areas of high $\dot{V}/\dot{Q}$ ratio but, surprisingly, hypoxaemia is common in acute pulmonary embolism in the absence of obvious infarction. Three mechanisms have been suggested.

First, if there are many parallel pathways occluded or having a high vascular resistance, a large proportion of the pulmonary blood flow may pass through surviving low resistance pathways which traverse alveoli with normal ventilation, so that the $\dot{V}/\dot{Q}$ ratios in these lung units are low. Secondly, in association with a high pulmonary vascular resistance, cardiac output may fall, so that P_{O_2} of mixed venous blood falls and therefore the effect on arterial blood of low $\dot{V}/\dot{Q}$ units will increase. Thirdly, the rise in pulmonary arterial pressure may occasionally open up shunt pathways, increasing the proportion of the pulmonary blood flow evading contact with alveolar gas.

Increases in pulmonary artery pressure (at first on exercise, but with more advanced disease also at rest) are found in many chronic pulmonary diseases, particularly in patients with chronic airflow obstruction, but also when there is severe reduction in lung volumes. In most hypoxaemic patients with pulmonary hypertension there is structural damage to the lungs and it is impossible to apportion the roles of loss of vessels, muscular hypertrophy in the arterioles, vasoconstrictor responses to hypoxia, and increased haematocrit to the increase in pressure. Giving oxygen usually only results in a small acute drop in pulmonary artery pressure, though treatment over many weeks with oxygen through much of the 24 hours can lead to larger reductions in pressure – probably by inducing regression of hypertrophy of arteriolar muscle. The role of hypoxia (and the acid pH produced by episodes of hypercapnia), however, is clear in the chronic pulmonary hypertension found in patients with normal lungs who have chronic hypoxaemia due to abnormal control of ventilation, as occurs in the obesity–hypoventilation ('Pickwickian') syndrome.

Reductions in local pulmonary blood flow are frequently found in areas of gross lung disease; often these may be due to the pathological changes involving both alveoli and pulmonary vessels (emphysema, advanced lung fibrosis), but they are also found in asthma. Because of the associated changes in structure and local expansion of the lung, it is difficult to quantify the role of local pulmonary vasoconstriction in response to alveolar hypoxia, but compensation by this mechanism appears to be rather small in lung disease.

Control of ventilation

The control of the respiratory muscles is complex because a voluntary control system has been superimposed on an automatic control system. The automatic control system, situated in the brain stem, is concerned primarily with O_2, CO_2 and acid–base homeostasis. When metabolic requirements are modest, this automatic system can be over-ridden by the voluntary control system, which arises in the cerebral cortex, and the ventilatory system can be used for other activities such as talking, coughing, and singing. In ordinary waking life, breathing is characterized by its disorderliness. Because of this strong behavioural component, there is great difficulty in studying control in humans, except under extreme metabolic stress which over-rides the voluntary system (heavy exercise, breathing hypoxic or hypercapnic mixtures), or during sleep or anaesthesia. Even putting in a mouthpiece and wearing a nose clip increases ventilation.

Nevertheless, in all the differing physiological conditions imposed by changes in mechanical load (nose or mouth breathing, supine or standing posture) or metabolic load (vigorous exercise may increase O_2 consumption and CO_2 output 10-fold), neurological output in normal man is adjusted to maintain arterial P_{O_2} and P_{CO_2} overall within rather narrow limits. The regulation of neurological output from the central pool of neurones controlling respiratory muscles in the pons and medulla is influenced by the degree of respiratory stimulation by the reticular activating system (which is dependent on the state of wakefulness) and three main sensor systems, apart from the 'over-ride' provided by behavioural influences from higher centres. These are (a) the peripheral chemoreceptors in the carotid and aortic bodies; (b) the central chemoreceptors on or beneath the ventral surface of the medulla; and (c) mechanoreceptors in the larger airways and lung parenchyma.

A low arterial P_{O_2}, high arterial P_{CO_2}, or acid pH all stimulate ventilation, although it is difficult to dissociate the effects of P_{CO_2} and pH. The effects of hypoxaemia are mediated via the peripheral chemoreceptors, while an increased P_{CO_2} acts mainly to stimulate central chemoreceptors with a much smaller effect on peripheral chemoreceptors. The role of mechanoreceptors is more difficult to define but probably they are particularly important in determining the pattern and timing of breathing.

Abnormal patterns of ventilation with grossly irregular, periodic (Cheyne–Stokes) or very fast or slow breathing may be found in acute (and rarely in chronic) disease of the central nervous system.

During sleep a distinctive pattern of recurrent obstruction of the oropharynx leading to transient hypoxaemia may be found in grossly obese patients and some non-obese subjects with abnormalities of the upper airway. This appears to be due to a disproportionate reduction in activation of the genioglossus and other pharyngeal muscles compared with the thoracic cage muscles during sleep; in some subjects daytime hypoxaemia and hypercapnia develop together with reduction of the ventilatory responses to oxygen and carbon dioxide (obesity–hypoventilation or 'Pickwickian' syndrome). These episodes of apnoea are associated with continued breathing efforts against the obstructed airways; in addition 'central' apnoea with cessation of respiratory efforts may be found during sleep. (For further discussion see page 15.158).

In lung disease the characteristic change in breathing is an increase in total minute ventilation, leading to a low arterial P_{CO_2} and an alkaline pH though often arterial P_{O_2} remains below normal. However, the increased ventilation is not removed when inspired oxygen is increased so as to bring arterial P_{O_2} to above normal values; the implication is that the increased ventilation is not due to chemical factors but that stimulation of mechanoreceptors (especially the J-receptors in the lung parenchyma) is involved. Depression of the central drive to breathe with reduced minute ventilation occurs after drugs or anaesthesia but in the absence of these factors is usually not a feature of chronic lung disease, even when there is a raised P_{CO_2}. Most patients with hypercapnic respiratory failure have a slightly increased minute ventilation and the raised P_{CO_2} reflects the gross inefficiency of the lung as a gas exchanger. Bizarre breathing patterns with gross irregularities and sighs suggest a psychogenic cause.

Lung function testing

Simple tests of ventilatory capacity and arterial blood gases measure the mechanical characteristics of the ventilatory pump and the adequacy of pulmonary gas exchange. Carbon monoxide transfer indicates the gas exchange capacity of the lungs, which may be reduced when blood gases remain normal. The pulmonary circulation is relatively inaccessible to simple techniques.

Tests of ventilatory mechanics
Minute ventilation
Until recently measuring ventilation at rest has played only a small part in clinical assessment, except in the intensive care unit. This is because methods that require breathing via a mouth-piece with the nose clipped are not well tolerated by breathless patients, always add some dead space, and generally increase minute ventilation. Newer, less obtrusive methods, in which pneumographs or magnetometers are used to measure expansion of rib cage and abdomen, have shown that minute ventilation in healthy subjects at rest is less than previously believed – commonly about 5–6 1/min. Methods which monitor chest wall expansion are influenced by postural changes and, even with careful calibration, it is difficult to achieve an accuracy better than ±10 per cent, but they are particularly valuable for detecting irregularities in pattern of breathing, as during sleep.

Increased ventilation (often with a disproportionate increase in frequency) is found in many lung diseases and in various metabolic disorders (renal failure, diabetes mellitus, aspirin poisoning). Reduced total ventilation is much less common and is usually due to sedative drugs or neuromuscular disease. In most patients with chronic irreversible airflow obstruction, minute ventilation is slightly above normal values, even in episodes of acute respiratory failure.

Static lung volumes
See Fig. 1.

Vital capacity (VC) is the volume expired from full inflation (TLC) to full expiration (residual volume, RV) and can be measured by a spirometer or by integrating expired flow at the mouth. A reduction in vital capacity can occur with a reduction in TLC (as in lung fibrosis or inspiratory muscle weakness) or an increase in RV (as occurs in emphysema, asthma, and other forms of intrapulmonary airway disease) and therefore, on its own, provides non-specific information.

Functional residual capacity (FRC) and total lung capacity (TLC)
In normal lungs there is a close relation between the resting breathing volume (FRC), the fully expanded volume of the lung (TLC), and vital capacity. This relationship is lost in disease, where a small vital capacity may be associated with either decreased or enlarged FRC and TLC.

FRC can be measured either by gas dilution or by whole body plethysmography. In the gas dilution methods a known volume and concentration of a foreign, relatively insoluble gas (usually helium) is allowed to mix with resident intrapulmonary gas the volume of which is measured from the difference between the initial and final concentration of marker gas. In normal lungs a single breath test provides a reasonable estimate of lung volume, but multi-breath methods lasting more than five minutes may be required to achieve mixing in patients with intrapulmonary airway obstruction. In the whole body plethysmograph method the subject makes panting efforts against a closed shutter while seated in a large, air-tight chamber. As mass movement of gas is prevented, changes in alveolar volume during this manoeuvre are due to compression and rarefaction of alveolar gas. Once change in alveolar volume and pressure are known the alveolar volume can be calculated using Boyle's law. The volume inspired during a maximum inspiration or expiration from FRC can then be measured with a spirometer to derive TLC or RV. The plethysmographic method often gives higher values than the gas dilution method for FRC in severe intrapulmonary airway disease. Some of this difference occurs because plethysmography measures intrathoracic gas which is hardly in communication with the airway (bullae and other very poorly ventilated areas). An accurate estimate of thoracic volume can also be obtained from planimetry of standard postero-anterior and lateral chest radiographs taken at full inflation. Corrections have to be made for tissue and vascular volumes of the lungs so as to estimate gas volume.

Measuring TLC and FRC is useful to elucidate the cause of a reduction in vital capacity. Intrapulmonary airway disease consistently leads to a rise in RV and FRC, while TLC is either normal or, in some subjects with emphysema, increased. When TLC is increased, the accompanying increase in RV is almost always greater, so that there is still a decreased vital capacity. Reductions in vital capacity in lung fibrosis, respiratory muscle weakness, and chest wall deformity are accompanied by decreases in TLC and FRC.

Tests of forced expiration and inspiration
Tests of forced expiration were originally introduced empirically as a simple method for estimating maximum ventilatory performance. The volume expired in the first second of a forced expiration commenced from TLC (forced expiratory volume in one second, FEV_1) (Fig. 1) was found to relate well to the maximum voluntary ventilation that could be sustained over 15 s both in subjects with normal lungs and in the presence of many lung diseases.

The physiological basis of these tests is complex and depends on the development of plateaux of expiratory flow at any particular lung volume once a certain minimum expiratory pressure is achieved. Provided flow plateau conditions are achieved, the values obtained do not depend on the pressures applied but only on the mechanical characteristics of the lungs and airways. In contrast, tests of forced inspiration are much more dependent on the applied inspiratory pressures. Both forced expiration and inspiration may be analysed as change in volume versus time (by spirometry) (Fig. 1), or as change in instantaneous flow rate (usually measured by a pneumotachograph) versus change in lung volume (maximum flow–volume curve). Standard spirometric measurements are the FEV_1 and the vital capacity; the latter may be obtained from the forced expiration (forced vital capacity, FVC) or from a separate, slower full expiration. In airway disease FVC may be considerably less than the slow VC. Normally FEV_1 is more than 70 per cent of the VC. Two patterns of spirometric abnormality can be distinguished – 'obstructive' in which, although there is usually some reduction in FVC, FEV_1 is reduced even more so that FEV_1/FVC ratio is low, and 'restrictive' in which a small FVC is associated with normal or even accelerated emptying on forced expiration and a normal or increased FEV_1/FVC ratio. The maximum flow–volume curve (Fig. 5) shows that normally on expiration flow rapidly rises to a peak value and then declines in an approximately linear fashion. Peak expiratory flow (PEF) can also be measured simply with the Wright peak flow meter. The most effort-dependent part of expiration is close to full inflation and therefore in measuring PEF the subject must take a full inspiration and make a rapid and forceful start to the subsequent full expiration. Provided subject co-operation is obtained and gross expiratory muscle weakness is not present, a reduction in maximum expiratory flow usually indicates intrinsic airway disease or reduction in lung recoil. For clinical assessment of ventilatory function, FEV_1 and VC (or FVC) are usually adequate, although these tests will not pick up mild airway disease. In asthma the value of PEF is closely related to the value of FEV_1, and because PEF can be measured by simple meters which can be used by patients in the home or at work, this measurement is particularly useful for identifying asthmatic episodes and their response to treatment. The maximum flow–volume curve cannot be used to distinguish different mechanisms of intrapulmonary airway narrowing, but a distinctive curve is found when obstruction is extrathoracic (Fig. 5).

Airways resistance

Airways resistance is the ratio of driving pressure (difference between alveolar and mouth pressures) to instantaneous gas flow. Alveolar pressure can be obtained non-invasively with a body plethysmograph or derived from oesophageal pressure obtained via a balloon-catheter system. Although resistance is measured during resting breathing, its precise value varies according to the lung volume at which it is measured, the phase of respiration (inspiration or expiration), the size of the laryngeal aperture, and the flow rate. Consequently the measurement is more suitable for research, particularly into airway pharmacology, than for clinical assessment.

Lung recoil pressure and compliance

Lung recoil pressure is the difference between alveolar and pleural pressure. Pleural pressure is estimated from the pressure measured by a balloon-tipped catheter placed in mid-oesophagus. The relation between lung recoil pressure and volume is obtained by interrupting inspiration and expiration during vital capacity manoeuvres when mouth pressure will equal alveolar pressure. The change in volume for unit change in recoil pressure is the static lung compliance. Analysis of lung recoil and compliance helps in examining mechanisms of airflow obstruction and also in determining whether a reduction in TLC is due to extrapulmonary (when there is a low recoil pressure at TLC) or intrapulmonary

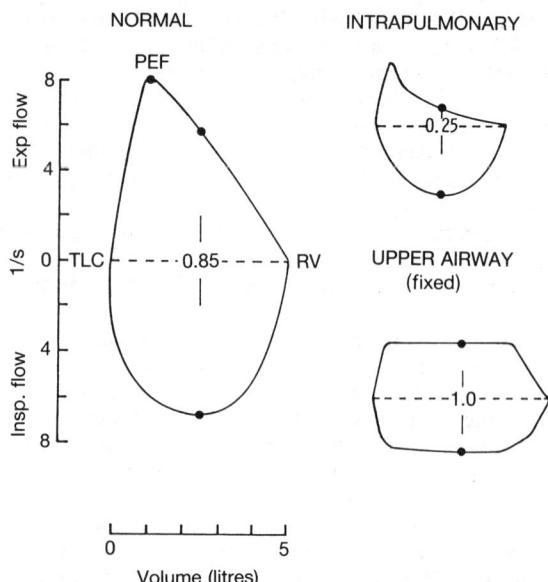

Fig. 5 Characteristic maximum flow–volume curves for a normal subject (left) and for a patient with intrapulmonary airflow obstruction (upper right) and with obstruction of the upper (extrathoracic) airway (lower right). In intrapulmonary airways narrowing, maximum expiratory flow is reduced more than maximum inspiratory flow but in upper airway obstruction the reduction in inspiratory flow is equal to (or sometimes greater than) reduction in expiratory flow. Solid dots on the curves indicate values of maximum expiratory and inspiratory flow at 50 per cent vital capacity and the ratio of these flows is shown on the zero flow line of each curve (horizontal dashed line).

(when there is a high recoil pressure at TLC and low compliance) causes. A low recoil pressure and a high static compliance is found in emphysema. Lung compliance measured during ordinary or accelerated tidal breathing reflects the effects of airway disease as well as the static elastic properties of the lung. The effective dynamic compliance of the lungs is reduced below static compliance when there is peripheral airway narrowing. Airway pressure during an end-inspiratory pause is often used to assess compliance in patients on assisted ventilation in the intensive care unit; this indicates the total compliance of lungs and chest wall which is normally about half that of the lungs alone.

Tests to define the site and mechanism of airflow obstruction

An increased airways resistance or reduced maximum expiratory flow is produced by primary disease at any site along the tracheobronchial tree or may be secondary to a loss of airway distension as occurs in emphysema.

The role of loss of airway distending forces can be assessed by relating maximum expiratory flow or resistance to the corresponding lung recoil pressure, rather than to lung volume. If airway obstruction is extrathoracic, distinctive maximum flow-volume curves may be obtained (Fig. 5). Due to the serial distribution of airway geometry, values of PEF and airways resistance reflect mainly the dimensions of large airways in normal subjects, but this cannot be assumed to apply in airway disease which inevitably distorts the serial distribution of airway dimensions. Comparing measurements of resistance or maximum expiratory flow breathing air and an 80 per cent helium, 20 per cent O_2 mixture gives some information on the serial site of narrowing, improvement on helium–oxygen being present when airway narrowing is central and absent when it is in peripheral airways. An immediate improvement in airway function after bronchodilators is assumed to be due to reduction in bronchial muscle contraction.

Tests to detect minor peripheral airway disease

Minor changes in the peripheral airways, which commonly develop in smokers, cannot be detected by standard spirometric tests or by measuring airways resistance, but lead to reduced maximum flow in the last 25 per cent of FVC, a fall in dynamic lung compliance as respiratory frequency is increased, and an abnormal single breath N_2 test (see below). Once airway disease becomes sufficiently advanced to lead to changes in standard spirometry these additional tests provide little further information.

Airway reactivity

In subjects with asthma there is an increased tendency for airways narrowing to occur in response to a whole range of stimuli (e.g. exercise, hyperventilation, breathing cold air, hypo- or hyperosmolar aerosols, or constrictor drugs such as histamine or cholinergic agonists). This reactivity may be quantified using an incremental dose–response technique. Most commonly histamine or methacholine are used as the stimulus and the dose increased until a 20 per cent fall in FEV_1 is produced. Airway reactivity is often increased in smokers with chronic airflow obstruction.

Mucociliary clearance

Mucociliary clearance is assessed by inhaling radionuclide labelled microspheres and following their clearance from the airways after impaction.

Respiratory muscle function

The most popular test, introduced by Hutchinson in the mid-19th century, is to measure mouth pressure when voluntary maximum inspiratory or expiratory efforts are made against a closed valve. Properly performed, this indicates the overall strength of inspiratory or expiratory muscles. Bilateral paralysis of the diaphragm can be suspected if there is orthopnoea and paradoxical inspiratory indrawing of the abdominal wall (especially in the supine position). The pressure developed across the diaphragm during maximum inspiratory efforts can be measured by placing balloon-catheters in the oesophagus and stomach. A reduction in vital capacity in the sitting position is often found in respiratory muscle weakness: a further fall of 25 per cent or more in VC on adopting the supine position is said to be characteristic of diaphragmatic weakness. Serial measurements of peak expiratory flow or vital capacity may be useful in monitoring conditions where muscle strength varies rapidly, e.g. myasthenia gravis.

Work of breathing

If there is any abnormality of lung or airway mechanics, the inspiratory muscles have to produce larger pressures to maintain a normal minute ventilation. Because of the associated inefficiency of pulmonary gas exchange, in many patients with lung disease minute ventilation at rest is increased. If there is a raised FRC with hyperinflation of the chest wall, the inspiratory muscles work at a mechanical disadvantage and expend more energy to generate a given inspiratory pleural pressure. All these mechanisms stress the inspiratory muscles and increase their oxygen consumption. In normal subjects the oxygen consumption of the respiratory muscles is very small even during exercise, but, with disease, particularly airflow obstruction, they may account for a significant proportion of the total oxygen consumption.

The mechanical work of breathing can be calculated from changes in oesophageal pressure and volume during tidal breathing, but the oxygen consumption of the respiratory muscles can only be measured in the research laboratory.

Tests of pulmonary gas exchange
Distribution and mixing of inspired gas

Inequalities of ventilation and inefficient gas mixing may be either between regions or within regions. The topographical distribution of ventilation can be examined by placing counters over the chest wall and detecting the distribution of inhaled radionuclides such as ^{133}Xe or $^{81}Kr^m$. The lung volume at which airways begin to close (closing volume) can be measured by asking the subject to inhale a small quantity of a foreign gas (argon, helium, or ^{133}Xe have all been used) at the beginning of an inspiration from RV. Because of

basal airway closure this foreign gas is preferentially distributed to the lung apices. During the subsequent expiration an abrupt rise in concentration of the foreign gas at the lips indicates that gas is now coming preferentially from the apices due to closure of airways at the bases. Closing volume in the upright position is well below FRC in young non-smokers but rises with age when it may occur within the tidal breathing range. Increases in closing volume occur in many smokers at an early stage in the development of airway disease.

In normal subjects much of the inequality in ventilation is on a regional basis. In most diseases of the lung, however, inequalities within a region are of greater importance than inter-regional differences. This applies even in diseases like asthma and emphysema, where obvious inequalities of ventilation are easily demonstrated by radioactive gas methods. These inequalities may be detected by tests which follow gas mixing by sampling expired air at the mouth. A simple single breath test measures the expired nitrogen concentration at the mouth after a preceding vital capacity breath of 100 per cent O_2. The rate of rise of expired N_2 over the middle part of the expiration indicates the unevenness of ventilation; towards the end of the breath there may be a sharp rise in N_2 concentration which corresponds to closing volume. Other techniques are based on the rate of equilibration when helium is washed in or nitrogen washed out of the lung to measure FRC and on the difference between the volume measured by a single breath test using a foreign gas and that obtained from multibreath techniques or body plethysmography.

Transfer factor for carbon monoxide

The transfer of carbon monoxide across the alveolar–capillary membrane and into combination with haemoglobin within the red blood corpuscle mimics the uptake of oxygen. In normal lungs this transfer can be used to define a true diffusing capacity of the lungs, which depends on the diffusivity of the gas and the available area and thickness of the alveolar–capillary membrane. The usual technique is to inhale a full breath of a gas mixture containing a very low carbon monoxide concentration and to measure the gas transferred during 10 s breathholding at TLC. The physiological significance of this measurement in lung disease is less clear cut as carbon monoxide transfer is then affected by inhomogeneities of ventilation, blood flow, and indeed diffusing capacity as much as by a true loss of area or increase in thickness of the membrane. Values are also reduced if there is anaemia, but correction can be made for haemoglobin level. In lung disease the test provides a simple, non-invasive indicator of the ability of the lungs to transfer gas into the blood. Values of carbon monoxide transfer are reduced (particularly when expressed per unit lung volume, transfer coefficient) in emphysema and in infiltrative and fibrotic diseases but are well preserved in asthma. By measuring carbon monoxide transfer at two or more levels of alveolar P_{O_2}, it is possible to obtain separate values for transfer across the alveolar–capillary membrane and transfer into the haemoglobin within the red blood corpuscle and so derive pulmonary capillary blood volume. The technique is difficult to apply when there is significant lung disease but is useful in investigating abnormalities of the pulmonary circulation. Serial measurements of carbon monoxide transfer can also be used to monitor the number of haemoglobin binding sites (intra- and extra-vascular) accessible in the lungs in intrapulmonary haemorrhage.

Assessment of arterial hypoxaemia and hypercapnia

Usually P_{O_2} and P_{CO_2} are measured on direct arterial samples. There are various less invasive ways of obtaining almost as good information. Instead of taking arterial blood, capillary blood can be sampled from the vasodilated ear, and P_{O_2} and P_{CO_2} measured with electrodes needing microsamples. Instead of measuring P_{O_2}, O_2 saturation can be continuously measured with an ear oximeter. This is particularly useful for studying transitory hypoxaemia as may occur during sleep. Arterial P_{CO_2} can be estimated by measuring mixed venous P_{CO_2} with a simple rebreathing technique. Finally sensors which measure P_{O_2} and P_{CO_2} in the warmed, vasodilated skin are being developed.

Arterial P_{O_2} values can only be fully assessed if the inspired P_{O_2} and arterial P_{CO_2} are known; a rough check on the alveolar-arterial P_{O_2} difference can then be made from the alveolar air equation (see page 15.27), assuming $R = 0.8$. For accurate measurement of this difference, a simultaneous collection of all expired air is made for several minutes and its volume, O_2, and CO_2 content measured. If arterial hypoxaemia is due to a low alveolar P_{O_2} (with reduced total ventilation), the alveolar–arterial P_{O_2} difference is normal; if hypoxaemia is due to a diffusion defect, $\dot{V}/\dot{Q}$ imbalance or shunt, the alveolar–arterial P_{O_2} difference is widened. Although this difference is a useful index of the efficiency of pulmonary gas exchange, it is dependent on inspired O_2 concentration, the difference widening as inspired O_2 is increased. However, with a changing inspired O_2 the arterial P_{O_2}/alveolar P_{O_2} ratio should remain approximately constant if the efficiency of pulmonary gas exchange remains the same.

Most evidence suggests that (at least at rest) diffusion limitation is not important in the hypoxaemia of lung disease, so resting alveolar–arterial P_{O_2} difference can be assumed to be due to either shunt ($\dot{V}/\dot{Q}$ ratio $= 0$) or to ventilation/perfusion imbalance chiefly due to units with very low $\dot{V}/\dot{Q}$ ratios. The contribution of these low $\dot{V}/\dot{Q}$ units to hypoxaemia can be expressed by calculating the proportions of pulmonary blood flow which would have to completely bypass ventilated lung (i.e. $\dot{V}/\dot{Q} = 0$) and so act as *venous admixture* to mixed arterial blood to produce the same alveolar–arterial difference. This calculation includes both areas of shunt and of low $\dot{V}/\dot{Q}$ ratio. Attempts to distinguish shunt from low $\dot{V}/\dot{Q}$ areas by measuring the alveolar–arterial P_{O_2} difference while breathing 100 per cent O_2 are unreliable because the high inspired O_2 leads to loss of volume in low $\dot{V}/\dot{Q}$ units and their conversion to unventilated units.

Whereas units with low $\dot{V}/\dot{Q}$ ratios chiefly cause hypoxaemia, units with high $\dot{V}/\dot{Q}$ ratios have most effect on the efficiency of carbon dioxide elimination. The effect of these units can be expressed by an analogous calculation of the proportion of the tidal breath (V_t) which would have to act as dead space (V_d) completely avoiding contact with pulmonary blood ($\dot{V}/\dot{Q} = \infty$) to produce the same effect on the efficiency of CO_2 elimination:

$$V_d/V_1 = (\text{Arterial } P_{O_2} - \text{mixed expired } P_{CO_2})/\text{Arterial } P_{CO_2}$$

This equation derives the physiological dead space (V_d), which at rest is normally 30 per cent or less of the tidal volume but may rise up to 50–60 per cent in lung disease. This calculation includes the inspired gas which only penetrates as far as the conducting airways and is subsequently expired (anatomical or series dead space). The difference between anatomical and physiological dead space is sometimes called alveolar (or parallel) dead space.

These calculations simulate the effects of an enormous range of $\dot{V}/\dot{Q}$ ratios in disease by a three compartment model of the lung, with zero, normal, and infinite $\dot{V}/\dot{Q}$ ratios. A research method using an infusion of fluid containing six inert gases, enables a much more complete distribution of $\dot{V}/\dot{Q}$ ratios to be simulated. This analysis distinguishes between shunt and low $\dot{V}/\dot{Q}$ units and can be used to predict values of arterial P_{O_2}. If actual values of arterial P_{O_2} are lower than predicted from the extent of shunt and $\dot{V}/\dot{Q}$ imbalance, the implication is that a diffusion defect is also present.

The regional distribution of overall $\dot{V}/\dot{Q}$ ratios can be estimated from sequential measurements of regional ventilation, perfusion, and lung volume using appropriate radionuclides. This is chiefly useful for studying the physiology of normal lungs, as in disease considerable inhomogeneity of $\dot{V}/\dot{Q}$ ratios occurs within the fields covered by the counters.

Arterial P_{CO_2} is determined by the relation between metabolic CO_2 production and alveolar ventilation. Conventionally alveolar ventilation is calculated from the difference between total ventilation and the dead space ventilation, so alveolar ventilation (1/min)

$= \text{total ventilation} \times [1 - (V_d/V_t)]$. This calculation defines alveolar ventilation as the volume of gas leaving the alveoli each minute which has a P_{CO_2} equal to arterial P_{CO_2}. As the mixed alveolar P_{CO_2} is much lower than arterial P_{CO_2} in the presence of $\dot{V}/\dot{Q}$ inequality, alveolar ventilation so defined is always lower than the true volume of gas leaving the alveoli per minute and the terms alveolar hypoventilation and hyperventilation merely indicate that the arterial P_{CO_2} is above and below normal respectively.

A raised arterial P_{CO_2} is found if mixed alveolar P_{CO_2} is increased (as occurs when total ventilation is reduced below metabolic needs) and may be found if arterial P_{CO_2} is higher than mixed alveolar P_{CO_2} (as occurs with $\dot{V}/\dot{Q}$ imbalance). If the efficiency of CO_2 excretion is decreased by $\dot{V}/\dot{Q}$ imbalance and the V_d/V_t ratio is increased, a normal arterial P_{CO_2} often can be maintained by an increase in total ventilation. The pattern of breathing also has an influence as the V_d/V_t ratio will be higher with small than with large tidal volumes. Patients with airflow obstruction and a raised P_{CO_2} tend to breathe with a small tidal volume.

Pulmonary circulation

Non-invasive assessment remains a problem as hyperinflation of the lungs often obscures clinical and electrocardiographic signs, radiological clues to the presence of increases in pulmonary vascular pressure are imprecise, and the radionuclide methods used for assessing left ventricular function are less accurate for assessing the right ventricle. Pulmonary capillary blood volume can be estimated from measurements of carbon monoxide transfer at two or more different levels of alveolar P_{O_2}, but the measured volumes are surprisingly small. Direct measurements of pulmonary vascular pressures therefore are still used for assessing the response to drugs, oxygen or exercise. It is useful to measure arterial P_{O_2} during studies of pulmonary vasodilator drugs as these may worsen the $\dot{V}/\dot{Q}$ balance by preferentially dilating vessels supplying low $\dot{V}/\dot{Q}$ areas, which may be sites of hypoxic vasoconstriction.

Detecting small increases in extravascular lung water before frank alveolar oedema appears is also difficult. None of the research methods developed have proved to be both simple and accurate. Comparisons with the research methods have, however, shown that abnormalities in the chest radiograph appear with a surprisingly small increase in extravascular water.

The only widely used test of the pulmonary circulation is the assessment of the regional distribution of pulmonary blood flow after venous injection of radiolabelled microspheres, to detect pulmonary embolism. Pulmonary embolism also leads to an increase in minute ventilation, physiological dead space and Vd/Vt ratio, and a reduction in arterial P_{O_2}. In the presence of significant lung disease similar changes may occur in pulmonary function and local perfusion defects can only be interpreted as evidence of embolism if there are no 'matched' defects in the ventilation scan.

Control of ventilation

The ventilatory response to hypoxia or hypercapnia can be studied by steady-state or rebreathing methods. These techniques are most useful when lung mechanics are normal as in studies of the effects of drugs or anaesthesia in normal subjects or of unusual patients with abnormal central control of breathing. Impaired responses to hypoxia and hypercapnia are found in many patients with chronic airflow obstruction, but when there are abnormalities of ventilatory mechanics, a given neurological output inevitably results in less ventilation than in a normal subject. A better idea of neurological output may be obtained by measuring oesophageal pressure throughout the breath or mouth pressure during a transitory 0.1 s occlusion at the start of a breath. Recent studies with these techniques have generally reduced the role of decreased central drive and emphasized the role of impairment of respiratory muscle and lung mechanics in reducing the ventilatory response in such patients.

Exercise capacity

Breathlessness on exercise is one of the major symptoms of lung disease, and exercise tests play an important part in quantifying effort intolerance, investigating its cause, and monitoring progress and response to treatment. They are also used for confirming a diagnosis of exercise-induced asthma and ischaemic heart disease.

Despite a great amount of research the mechanisms responsible for increasing ventilation in parallel with the increase in metabolic load and O_2 consumption are still not well understood. An increased ventilation in relation to O_2 consumption is found at high work loads in normal subjects when blood lactate begins to rise. In lung disease increased ventilation is particularly found with fibrosing alveolitis and primary pulmonary hypertension; some of this increase may be due to stimulation of peripheral chemoreceptors by a fall in arterial P_{O_2} during exercise, but mechanoreceptor stimulation has also been implicated as increasing inspired O_2 does not restore exercise ventilation to normal values.

In chronic airflow obstruction and fibrosing alveolitis, exercise tolerance appears to be limited by the impaired ventilatory capacity.

Quantitative exercise tests usually involve either a treadmill or a bicycle ergometer. Many clinical problems can be investigated by a simple progressive work load test on a bicycle ergometer measuring ventilation, heart rate, electrocardiogram, and O_2 consumption. This will often indicate whether exercise is limited by the cardiac response or by ventilation and give an objective measurement of maximum O_2 consumption. More elaborate measurements including arterial blood gases and cardiac output may occasionally be required. Simple step tests and the distance walked on the flat in 6 or 12 minutes can be used to assess progress in patients with more severe disability.

Physiological variation in lung function

Body size, sex, and ethnic differences

Lung size is generally related to body size and particularly to height. Height is used to predict expected values of TLC and the subdivisions of lung volume, FEV_1, and PEF, and carbon monoxide transfer factor. The difference in lung function between men and women partly reflects differences in body size but, at a given height, TLC is about 20 per cent greater in men than women. Similarly there are ethnic differences, apart from those explained by height, lung volumes being about 15 per cent larger in Caucasians than in Asians.

Growth and ageing

Lung function is fully developed by about 18 to 20 years and probably remains constant (at least in non-smokers) until about 30 years old. After this age, many aspects of lung function slowly deteriorate even when there is no exposure to tobacco or environmental pollution. Thus FEV_1 and VC, CO transfer factor, and exercise capacity all fall with increasing age. Forced lung emptying slows and because FEV_1 falls more than VC, FEV_1/VC also drops. Loss of lung recoil leads to increase in FRC and RV with age, while increased $\dot{V}/\dot{Q}$ imbalance leads to a larger difference between alveolar and arterial P_{O_2} and a fall in arterial P_{O_2}. Aspects of lung function that do not change with increasing age are TLC, arterial P_{CO_2}, and pH and airways resistance.

Posture, sleep, and diurnal variation

A number of physiological factors potentially impair lung function at night in healthy subjects. End-tidal lung volume (FRC) is lower in the supine position than when sitting or standing; in older subjects this may lead to airway narrowing and even closure of airways in dependent regions of the lungs and to a reduction in arterial P_{O_2}. Ventilation becomes more dependent on the diaphragm and total intrapulmonary blood volume increases. During sleep, total ventilation falls and there is a small fall in arterial P_{O_2}

and a rise in arterial P_{CO_2}. There may also be a disproportionate reduction in the inspiratory activation of tongue, palatal, and pharyngeal muscles, leading to partial obstruction of the airway and snoring. Finally, the circadian rhythm of airway tone peaks in the early hours of the morning.

In patients with cardiopulmonary disease many of these effects may be amplified and account for the frequency of problems with breathing and oxygenation at night. Thus in subjects with daytime hypoxaemia due to $\dot{V}/\dot{Q}$ imbalance, the usual small fall in ventilation and arterial P_{O_2} when asleep causes much larger falls in oxygen saturation and delivery to the tissues. In some obese men, the mechanisms normally responsible for snoring may be exaggerated, particularly after alcohol, leading to repeated episodes of complete obstruction of the airway and hypoxaemia at night. In patients with active asthma, the amplitude of the circadian rhythm in airway function is greatly increased compared to normal subjects, leading to the common symptom of wheezing in the early hours of the morning.

Environment, smoking, and pollution

The most obvious environmental factor is altitude which reduces inspired and arterial P_{O_2}; ventilation is stimulated so that arterial P_{CO_2} is also reduced (see page 6.99). Smoking has both immediate and long-term effects. The carbon monoxide in the blood occupies up to 10 per cent of the haemoglobin-binding sites which would otherwise be used to carry oxygen. Some compensation is achieved by an increase in red cell mass in smokers. Inhalation of cigarette smoke also produces immediate increases in airflow resistance and minute ventilation. Regular cigarette smokers show deterioration in many aspects of lung function – notably in FEV_1 and other tests of maximum expiratory flow, tests of unevenness of ventilation, and carbon monoxide transfer factor. Subtle differences in lung function between smokers and non-smokers can be detected in subjects in their twenties; though these changes are sometimes reversible in the early years of smoking, in middle age and beyond they usually persist indefinitely after quitting smoking. In Westernized countries, the effects of smoking on lung function are now quantitatively more important than general environmental pollution. This may not be the case in some Third World countries, for instance, in societies where domestic cooking and heating fuels generate extremely polluted air in confined living quarters.

References

Cotes, J. E. (1979). *Lung function* 4th edn. Blackwell Scientific Publications, Oxford.

Douglas, N. J. (1984). Control of breathing during sleep. *Clin. Sci.* 67, 465–471.

Exercise testing in the dyspneic patient (1984). *Am. Rev. Resp. Dis.* 129 (suppl), S1–S100.

Forster, R. E. and Ogilvie, C. M. (1983). The single breath carbon monoxide transfer test 25 years on: a reappraisal. *Thorax* 38, 1–9.

Gibson, G. J. (1984). *Clinical tests of respiratory function*. MacMillan, London.

Green, M. and Moxham, J. (1985). The respiratory muscles. *Clin. Sci.* 68, 1–10.

Milic-Emili, J. (1982). Recent advances in clinical assessment of control of breathing. *Lung* 160, 1–17.

Pride, N. B. (1983). Physiology. In *Asthma* 2nd edn (eds T. J. H. Clark and S. Godfrey), pp. 12–56. Chapman and Hall, London.

Remmers, J. E. (1984). Obstructive sleep apnea. A common disorder exacerbated by alcohol. *Am. Rev. Resp. Dis.* 130, 153–155.

Snashall, P. D. (1980). Pulmonary oedema. *Br. J. Dis. Chest* 74, 2–22.

West, J. B. (1977). Ventilation-perfusion relationships. *Am. Rev. Resp. Dis.* 116, 919–943.

—— (1985). *Respiratory physiology – the essentials* 3d edn. Blackwell Scientific Publications, Oxford.

THE RESPONSES OF THE LUNG TO INHALED PARTICLES

M. E. TURNER-WARWICK

General introduction

The airways and acinar gas exchanging parts of the lungs are exposed to a wide range of materials contaminating the air we breathe. The lung presents a surface area of around 500 m^2 to some 7000 litres of air every 24 hours. Several systems have been evolved to defend and protect various parts of the lungs from the types of particles liable to reach them. When these defences are overwhelmed, a variety of inflammatory responses develop which recruit additional biological processes to aid degradation or expulsion of the inhaled noxious agent. These processes, however, often result at the same time in considerable tissue damage to the lungs of the host, which not only compromizes the normal physiological functions of the lung in the acute phase but may, as a result of healing and formation of scar tissue, lead to permanent and sometimes progressive fibrotic damage in the long term.

In this chapter, we therefore have to consider the normal clearance mechanisms from the lungs of particles of various types and sizes, as well as the various diseases which result from their deposition.

Deposition of particles

The ways in which aerosolized particles leave the atmosphere and settle onto various parts of the respiratory tract depend in part on their size (and to a lesser extent their shape) and in part on factors relating to the anatomical structure of the dividing system of airways. Inertial impaction is the main mechanism for large particle deposition (particles from a few microns to about 100 μm). Gravitational sedimentation is the major mechanism for particles of around 0.5–50 μm. Deposition by diffusion or Brownian movement accounts for deposition of only very small particles. The site of deposition of particles of different sizes will depend on the many physical factors mentioned. In general, the hairs of the nasal mucosa trap the majority of particles over 20 μm and up to 50 per cent of those down to a diameter of 5 μm. Even on mouth breathing, particles of 10 μm and over settle almost completely in the trachea. Particles of 1–2 μm are of optimal size to be deposited in the alveoli. Particles of less than 1 μm fail to settle out on the airways and are exhaled, unless they reach, and are deposited in, the alveoli.

Many recent studies using isotope-tagged particles have shown that the penetration of particles of standard size into the lungs depends upon breathing patterns (size of breath and frequency of breathing). The deposition is particularly modified by diseases of the airways, more central deposition being found in smokers and those with chronic inflammatory changes in the bronchi.

Normal defence mechanisms of the lung

A summary of the range of defence systems of the lungs is set out in Table 1. These can be divided conveniently into non-specific systems, in other words, general systems not 'purpose made' against individual antigens, and specific humoral and cellular mechanisms developing after 'priming' of the host against a particular agent. The non-specific mechanisms can be further divided into those which can be regarded as 'physical' defences of the lung and those involving humoral and cellular mechanisms. The specific defences may also be discussed under the headings of humoral and cellular responses. These have to be considered both in terms of those developing locally in the lungs (requiring special sampling techniques to study them) and those developing systemically as a result of agents reaching the reticuloendothelial system of the body (reflections of which may often be obtained from samples of circulating blood).

Clearance of particles

Particles settling on the surface of larger airways may trigger irritant receptors present near the surface of the bronchial mucosa to stimulate a forcible expulsive manoeuvre, namely, cough. The cough reflex can be triggered by stimulation of afferent fibres in the larynx, trachea, and major bronchi.

Particles settling on the mucociliary blanket of the bronchial mucosa are wafted centrally by the co-ordinated action of the cilial escalator (Fig. 1). Much is now known about the factors determining normal cilial action. In particular, their microstructure (described on page 15.6) is crucial to normal function. Under certain (probably genetically determined) circumstances the dynein arms of cilial microtubules are defective leading to immotile or inco-ordinated cilial action and this results in bronchial infections and perhaps subsequent bronchial wall damage. A typical example of this situation is found in Kartagener's syndrome.

Cilial function is also modulated by many external factors and now that techniques are available to study cilial action *in vitro*, detailed information on factors modulating co-ordinated cilial performance is accumulating rapidly. Certain serum factors appear to slow or arrest cilial action and further definition of these may help explain some aspects of the pathogenesis of chronic obstructive airways disease. Factors from certain bacteria especially *pseudomonas aeruginosa* have now been identified which slow cilial action. A serum factor present in patients with cystic fibrosis which can arrest cilial action has been recognized for a number of years.

Study of inhaled agents capable of altering cilial action has only just begun but of particular interest is the fact that extracts of cigarette smoke have been shown to reduce cilial beat frequency.

Table 1 A summary of the range of defence systems of the lung

Non-specific (i.e. general systems not directed against specific antigens)

Physical	(a) Reflex expulsion of particles by cough
	(b) Mucociliary clearance in the upper and lower respiratory tracts
	(c) Lining materials – mucus, surfactant
Humoral	(a) Antimicrobial agents – lysozyme, interferon, lactoferrin
	(b) Complement
	(c) Natural antibodies
Cellular	(a) Macrophages in airways, alveoli, and interstitium
	(b) Polymorphonuclear granulocytes; perhaps eosinophils
	(c) Other mononuclear cells – 'killer' cells

Specific

Humoral	(a) Local sIgA in central airways
	(b) Local mainly IgG in peripheral airways
	(c) IgG and IgM antibodies reaching lungs from the systemic circulation
Cellular	(a) Specifically sensitized lymphocytes derived from BALT*, intrapulmonary, and hilar lymphoid tissue (T and B cells)
	(b) Specifically sensitized lymphocytes originating from the reticuloendothelial system generally

*Bronchial associated lymphoid tissue.

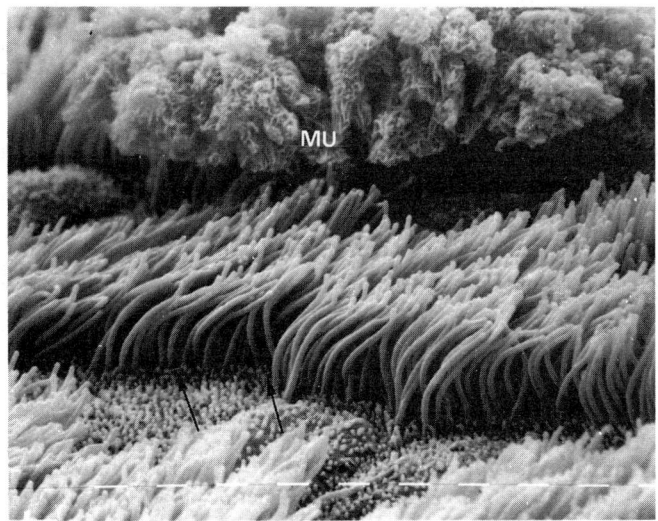

Fig. 1 Scanning electron micrograph to demonstrate a field of tracheal cilia. Their wave form is partially preserved and mucus (MU) is moved only by their tips. Microvilli are numerous between the cilia (arrows) and while shorter are also present on the non-ciliated cells (foreground). Glutaraldehyde and osmium tetroxide: uranyl acetate and lead citrate. × 6000. (Reproduced by courtesy of Drs P. K. Jeffery and T. Brain.)

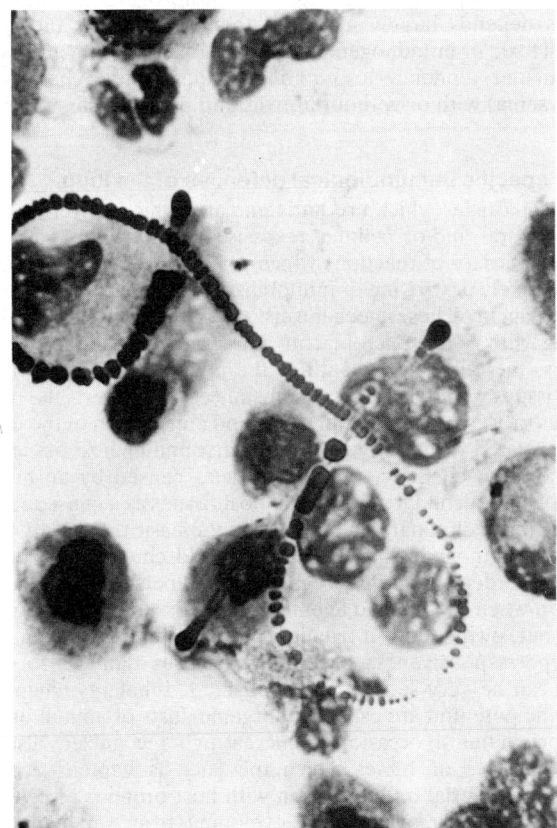

Fig. 2 Lung lavage cytocentrifuge preparation showing alveolar macrophages clustered around an asbestos fibre.

Cilial epithelium in humans can be found as far distally as the terminal bronchioles. When particles settle more distally in the lungs they have to be cleared by other mechanisms.

Macrophages

Particles settling in the acinar parts of the lung are mainly cleared by alveolar macrophages. How effectively a particle is taken up

into a macrophage depends upon its size and shape – some particles such as asbestos fibres may, through their shape, be difficult to phagocytose and several macrophages may be seen 'co-operating' in an attempt to clear such agents (Fig. 2).

The effectiveness of phagocytosis varies with the state of the macrophages at the time and many factors can modulate their phagocytic ability. These include their age, their state of 'activation', the presence of factors enhancing phagocytosis such as opsonins, and factors reducing it such as cigarette smoke. Where particles are toxic to macrophages (e.g. silica) this will tend to impair effective uptake of particles further.

Alveolar macrophages containing their phagocytosed burden travel or are wafted from the alveoli towards the terminal bronchioles, here to reach the mucociliary escalator. In view of these facts it is not surprising to find that there is a 'watershed' in clearance of particles just distal to the terminal bronchiole where the macrophage clearance system meets clearance by cilial action. This fact may be one reason why this area of the lung is particularly vulnerable to noxious particles and is the region where initial deposition can be of particular importance in relation to local tissue damage (Fig. 3).

Alveolar macrophages with their contained burden also migrate into the interstitium of the lung, penetrating the lymphatics and so reaching peripheral lung lymphoid tissue or the hilar nodes. Dense deposits of particles such as carbon can be seen etching these pathways in the lungs of coal miners. Eggshell calcification of hilar nodes in silica workers are a consequence of silica reaching the nodes by these routes (Fig. 4). The linear 'Kerley' lines seen on the chest radiograph of those exposed to coal dust are a further clinical example of the increased lymphatic load of particle clearance. These examples show how an understanding of basic defence mechanisms of the lung may be reflected in everyday clinical observations.

Local non-specific humoral antimicrobial agents

A number of antigen non-specific substances with antimicrobial properties are found in bronchoalveolar secretions. *Lysozymes* identified and studied by Inoue and his colleagues have the properties of proteolytic enzymes, acting either directly or, sometimes, in concert with complement and secretory IgA, to immobilize and destroy micro-organisms within the bronchial lumen. *Interferon* has been identified in local lung secretions as well as in the serum and tissue spaces and appears, amongst its many properties, to reduce virus colonization of cells. *Lactoferrin* is an iron-binding protein formed within bronchial serous glands and

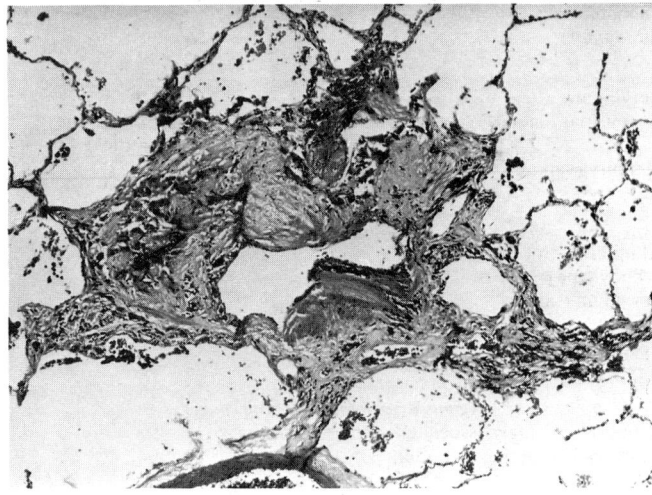

Fig. 3 Peribronchiolar fibrosis with embedded asbestos bodies demonstrating the burden of dust deposition at the watershed between the alveoli and the cilial escalator of the airways.

has bacteriostatic properties due to its ability to compete for iron with micro-organisms. The quantitative changes in these substances during disease have not been studied in much detail but are clearly of potential importance. There is, for example, some evidence that in diseases where mucus glands hypertrophy, levels of lactoferrin in the secretions fall.

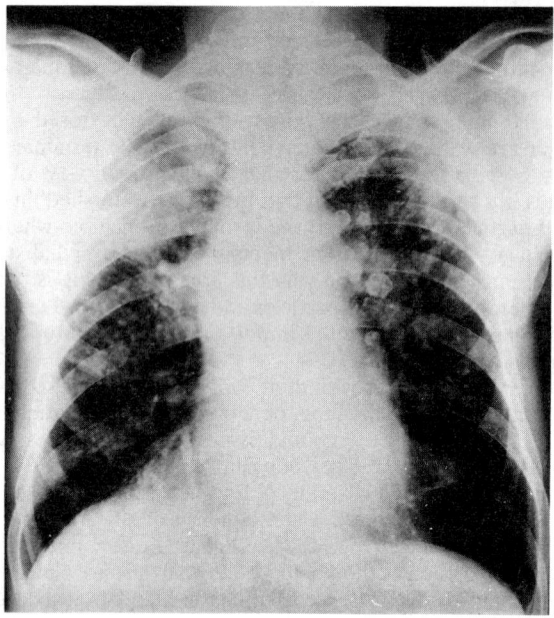

Fig. 4 Chest radiograph of a slate worker exposed to silica, demonstrating 'eggshell' calcification in the hilar lymph nodes. (Reproduced by courtesy of Professor P. Elmes.)

Table 2 Inorganic dusts of occupational importance causing radiographic abnormalities

Metals	Non-metals
Non-fibrogenic	
Antimony	Carbon (in moderate amounts)
Barium	
Cerium (and rare earth elements)	
Chromite	
Iron	
Tin	
Titanium	
Zirconium	
Fibrogenic	
Beryllium	Asbestos
Cobalt (hard metal)	Carbon (in large quantities)
Mercury (vapour)	Kaolin (??)
	Silica
Granuloma-forming	
Aluminium (foreign body type)	Talc (foreign body type)
Beryllium (sarcoid type)	
Cobalt (foreign body type)	
Agents associated with lung cancer	
Asbestos – strongly associated with asbestosis	
Alpha-radiation, e.g. Uranium	
Thorium	
Haematite	
Fluorspar	
Chloroethers – coal volatiles (? benzpyrene)	

Complement is a normal component of serum and broncho-alveolar secretions. When 'activated', it plays an important role in normal defence, not only by its direct cytotoxic effect on membranes of cells, but also as an opsonin, acting on the cell membrane of phagocytic cells, so facilitating ingestion of particles of all sorts. A number of agents are known to activate complement *in vitro* by the pathway which is independent of specific antibody; these agents include bacterial endotoxins, components of bacterial cell walls such as lipopolysaccharide, aggregated immunoglobulin, endotoxins, and an increasing number of organic materials, e.g. *Micropolyspora faeni* as well as inorganic particles including silica and asbestos (see page 4.57). If this activity can be demonstrated in human lungs *in vivo*, local lung complement could play an important role in defence in the absence of antibodies. Its well-defined role in association with complement-fixing specific antibodies is, of course, a separate issue and will be discussed below.

The non-specific mechanisms of lung defence summarized so far are important in the clearance of all types of particles including those which are biologically inert (i.e. neither toxic to tissues nor antigenically active) as well as those which initiate biological tissue reactions. They are, of course, the only systems of importance in the clearance of biologically inert particles. When the inhaled dust load from such inert particles is very heavy, clearance is incomplete, and this can result in a very abnormal chest radiograph without any clinical or physiological evidence of damage to the structure of the lungs. The basis for classifying various types of inorganic dust pneumoconioses into non-fibrogenic and fibrogenic groups depends largely upon whether the agent is biologically active (toxic or immunogenic) or not (Table 2). Some agents have a particular tendency also to induce destructive changes (i.e. emphysema) with or without fibrosis and this is discussed on page 15.43.

Local specific immunological defences of the lung

Inhaled particles which are antigenic and which therefore stimulate humoral and/or cellular responses in the lungs generate a complex variety of reactions which may be protective to the host by effectively destroying or immobilizing the potentially damaging inhaled agent. These mechanisms are particularly important for dealing with living microbial invaders and, under ideal circumstances, the outcome is death of the invader without damage to host tissues. Under most circumstances, however, the advantageous processes resulting in death and elimination of the invader are associated with some damage to surrounding host tissues. The balance between direct injury to tissues caused by an invading microbe and secondary damage to host tissues as a consequence of its attempt to eliminate the invader, is the basic dichotomy underlying the pathogenesis of much acute and chronic lung disease. Those disorders commonly regarded as 'hypersensitivity diseases' develop when the inhaled agent has little tissue injuring potential *per se* but, owing to its antigenic potential and to the immunological hyperresponsiveness of the host causes damage to tissues which can be very serious and even fatal. Inhalants having such antigenic potential are especially organic dusts of animal or vegetable origin but on occasion, as increasingly recognized, also inorganic particles or fumes which may act as haptens acquiring antigenic potential on interaction with host proteins or cell membranes. Occupational asthma developing from small molecular weight inorganic materials such as isocyanates, platinum salts, and phthalic anhydride are probably examples in this category.

Antigen is first taken into macrophages and there is now evidence that alveolar macophages are Ia receptor site positive indicating cell activation and act as antigen presenting cells initiating lymphocyte immune responses through interleukin-1 production. Macrophage/lymphocyte interaction stimulates proliferation and differentiation of T as well as B cells and thus permits cell-mediated as well as antibody responses. Subsets of T cells acting as helper or suppressor cells modulate the response.

It is important to recognize that these humoral and cellular events may develop locally in the airways and acinar parts of the lung, or may be stimulated in lymphoid tissue at distant sites, in which case differentiated cells or their products reach the lung through the pulmonary and bronchial circulations. Recent studies emphasize the substantial capacity of the lung to develop *local* immunological reactivity which is not necessarily reflected in serum or cell samples obtained from peripheral blood. For this reason it is becoming increasingly important to obtain samples for study directly from the lung; this is now possible using broncho-alveolar lavage. Further, studies, both in experimental animals and in humans in which antigen is introduced either by inhalation via the airways or systemically by parenteral injection, emphasize the distinctive types of immunological response which occur depending upon the route of administration. Agents introduced directly into the lung tend to stimulate formation of *local* antibody and sensitized cells; such antibodies can be demonstrated in only small amounts in samples from systemic blood. The converse is the case following parenteral administration of antigen.

Local antibody

The predominant immunoglobulin in bronchial secretions is IgA in dimer form (sIgA). This is secreted from plasma cells located around the central airways in the lamina propria of the bronchial mucosa and especially around the bronchial mucus and serous glands. Immunoglobulin is secreted in dimer form linked through the Fc portions of the molecule via a 'J' chain. In transit across or through the bronchial epithelial cells, an additional protein becomes attached to the dimer – the secretory piece. The molecular size of IgA in bronchial secretions is thus greater than that found in the serum, mainly 11s in secretions and mainly 7s in serum. Secretory IgA and serum IgG also have different biological properties. Secretory IgA appears to be more resistant than serum IgG to the action of proteolytic enzymes and its special function may be to block bacterial and viral adherence to mucosal surfaces, thus preventing colonization of epithelium by microbes and their penetration into the body.

The formation of specific local IgA has been demonstrated as a result of intranasal inoculation of virus to inhaled bacterial antigens and to inhaled allergens.

In view of all of these observations, there is presumptive evidence that sIgA is important in the defence of the lungs. However, there is still much discussion on the role of IgA (both local and systemic) in normal host defence. The argument arises because there are a number of healthy individuals in whom there is an almost complete absence of IgA in the circulation and local secretions. In these individuals, other defence systems presumably deputize. On the other hand, studies on patients with a predisposition to repeated lung infections show that the commonest immunological abnormality is a partial IgA deficiency. Thus Cole and his colleagues showed that a partial or complete IgA deficiency was present in 83 of 218 (38 per cent) patients with recurrent chest infections. Whether the IgA deficiency *per se* is responsible or is a marker for some associated immunological defect has not yet been clarified. Subtypes of IgA have now been identified and study of these may elucidate further defects of protective immunity in the respiratory tract.

IgE immunoglobulin is also secreted locally from plasma cells in the tonsils and central airways. These immunoglobulin secreting cells are present in all individuals but are especially prominent in atopic subjects. Studies using inhaled antigens in atopic subjects have demonstrated relatively more specific local IgE antibody production and less specific IgA compared with normal controls. The relationship of the local production of IgE antibody to normal host defence is a hotly debated and unresolved subject. There is some evidence that IgE immunoglobulin-secreting cells become established in relatively or transiently IgA-deficient individuals. Whether IgE has survived phylogenetically as an amplification response, when the local IgA defences are overwhelmed, is an attractive but quite unproven possibility. Others contend that IgE

plays no useful protective role in normals, but becomes important in the development of hypersensitivity responses in individuals with a genetically determined predisposition to form this type of antibody in response to antigenic stimulation (see pages 15.41 and 15.76). If IgE is a wholly undesirable characteristic with regard to health and the lungs, it is perhaps surprising that this immunological system has survived through the evolution of humans. An alternative explanation involving its role in protection against helminth infections has been postulated but is outside the context of the present chapter.

IgG-secreting plasma cells increase relative to those containing IgA in more distal airways and the humoral responses nearer to the acinar parts of the lung therefore change. Challenge studies have been performed to identify the origin of IgG in broncho-alveolar secretions. The results suggest that part of the specific IgG appears to be generated locally and part is derived from systemic responses. Specific IgG antibody has many mechanisms of action in normal defence (see page 4.49), but a particularly important role in the lung appears to be its opsonizing function, facilitating phagocytosis of particles by macrophages and polymorphonuclear granulocytes. Thus, in the lung, the interdependence of specific humoral and non-specific phagocytic cell performance becomes crucial to normal host defences.

Local cellular defence

There is increasing evidence that inhaled antigen may sensitize T lymphocytes locally. Further stimulation of these cells results in secretion of lymphokines, not only expanding specific lymphocyte populations through interleukin-2 but also by a number of important actions in the inflammatory response. For example, lymphokines increase vascular permeability, as well as showing chemotactic properties for polymorphonuclear leucocytes, eosinophils, and particularly monocytes.

The intensity of local cellular immunological responses in a wide variety of acute and especially chronic lung disease is often reflected in the light microscopy appearances of lung biopsy specimens. Lymphocytic infiltrates are often prominent and collections of lymphocytes containing germinal centres reflect their potential for local immunoglobulin production. Proof of local antibody formation can be obtained both by immunofluorescent and immunochemical studies using monoclonal antibodies on lung biopsy specimens which demonstrate plasma cells and immunoglobulin production within germinal centres. Culture of lymphocyte populations separated from lung lavage samples can be used to demonstrate their capacity to secrete antibody *in vitro*. Lung lavage samples have shown large numbers of active T lymphocytes in certain disorders, especially hypersensitivity pneumonitis and sarcoidosis, when the same cells cannot be demonstrated in peripheral blood samples. Interestingly these two conditions are characterized by different subtypes of T cells; predominantly T 'helper' cells in sarcoidosis and T 'suppresser' cells in hypersensitivity pneumonitis. The full explanation for this difference is not yet known.

Biological responses in the lungs to inhaled particles

Having dealt briefly with normal defence mechanisms in the lung, the range of biological responses to inhaled particles must now be reviewed since these form the basis of the many different types of tissue injury underlying the clinical patterns of the diseases we observe. Whilst many of the well-studied biological responses to inhaled antigens can be considered under the heading of immunological reactions, it is important to note that there is increasing evidence of biological effects resulting from the inhalation of various types of particle which have not been included within the *conventional* scope of immunology, but which are now being incorporated under that heading. Some of these are listed in Table 3. Further, it must also be noted that immunological responses can often be detected using *in vitro* tests from samples taken from

Table 3 Some biological responses to inhaled particles

Responses	Examples of agents	Consequences
None	Inert particles, e.g. iron, barium, tin, etc.	Abnormal radiograph with physiological or clinical abnormality
Toxic to macrophages	Silica and asbestos	Fibrogenic response, e.g. silicosis, asbestosis
Activation of macrophages	Asbestos, beryllium (low dose), silica	Liberation of a variety of proteolytic enzymes and possible fibrogenic factors
Adsorption of proteins	Silica and asbestos	May reduce toxicity of agent to cells; may stimulate antiprotein antibodies, e.g. rheumatoid factor
Immunological stimulation of specific antibodies and sensitized T cells	Microbial agents Organic dust Beryllium	Inflammatory reactions, e.g. pneumonia, hypersensitivity pneumonitis
Alternative pathway of complement activation	*M. faeni* Silica, asbestos	*In vivo* effects uncertain
Neoplasia	Chromium Uranium	Lung cancer

Table 4 Some consequences of 'activation' of macrophages

Synthesis and release of lysosomal enzymes	Local tissue damage
Synthesis and release of neutral proteases including collagenase and elastase	Breakdown of type I and III collagen and elastin. Splitting of C5 with formation of chemotactic factors for neutrophils and eosinophils
Release of chemotactic factor especially for neutrophils	Increased local accumulation of neutrophils
Synthesis and release of complement components and enzymes cleaving such components	Generation of complement fragments augmenting inflammatory responses
Release of fibroblast stimulating factor and fibronectin	Increasing fibroblast production of collagen
Synthesis and release of plasminogen activating factor	Influencing local coagulation and fibrogenesis
Synthesis and release of prostaglandins	Capable of modulating lymphokine mediated reactions with up or down regulation of inflammatory response

Macrophage toxicity

In vitro studies using particles of silica have demonstrated their capacity to be ingested by, and then to kill, phagocytosing macrophages. Similar effects have now been seen with appropriate doses of asbestos fibres. The lethal effects of these dusts on alveolar macrophages *in vivo* can be seen in dusted experimental animals

and in lung lavage samples from humans following occupational exposure. Electron microscopic preparations of the cell pellets obtained from lavage samples reveals these changes most readily.

In spite of these observations, it has been difficult to demonstrate an overall defect in phagocytosis. This is presumably due to the recruitment of new populations of macrophages from circulating monocytes which rapidly replace the defunct cells. For this reason (in addition to others such as the multiplicity of defence mechanisms in the lung), a general susceptibility to infections is not usually observed in those with silicosis or asbestosis. The frequency of tuberculosis in silicosis may, however, be due to a defective degradation of this particular bacillus for which macrophage-dependent defences may be especially important.

'Activation' of macrophages

In suitable doses, a wide range of materials can stimulate the alveolar macrophage causing a general increase in the biological functions of the cell. For this change the word 'activation' has been widely applied. It is, however, important to appreciate that an agent may not stimulate all macrophage functions equally. For instance, while phagocytosis (e.g. uptake of latex particles) may be increased in some instances, stimulation of secretory products (e.g. secretion of proteolytic enzymes) may predominate under other circumstances. Indeed, there is some evidence that macrophages may adapt into a predominantly phagocytic phase depending on the stimulus and conditions. Under other circumstances, phagocytosis and secretion are linked. For example, small doses of silica (below toxicity level) have been shown to stimulate lysosomal enzyme secretion without cell death and asbestos fibres have the same effect. A wide range of other agents causing granuloma formation have been shown by Allison and his colleagues to have the same property. These include microbial agents such as *Mycobacterium tuberculosis* and *M. faeni*. Metals such as beryllium, and, of particular interest, preformed immune complexes of various types, also cause changes in the macrophage characteristic of 'activation'.

The consequences of macrophage 'activation' not only include changes in the micromorphology of the cell itself with increased ruffling of the cell membrane shown on scanning electron microscopy, and increased spreading of the cell on glass, but also an increase in secretion of a range of substances influencing, in their turn, inflammation in neighbouring host tissues. Some of these effects are listed in Table 4.

The interaction of a variety of agents with macrophages has been emphasized because it illustrates a rapidly expanding field of

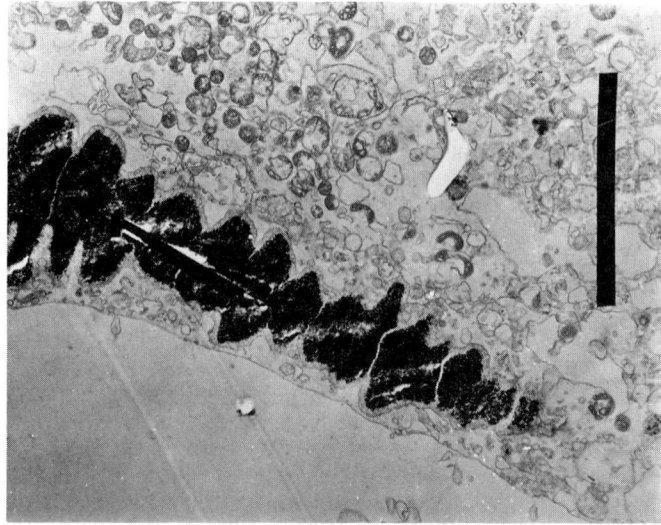

Fig. 5 Electron micrograph showing an asbestos fibre coated with host-derived iron-containing protein.

knowledge about the pathogenesis of inflammatory responses to inhaled antigens in the lungs which are not mediated by factors typically regarded as within the scope of immunological responses.

Adsorption of proteins

Some inorganic particles such as silica and asbestos adsorb host-derived proteins onto their surface (Fig. 5). In some instances, (e.g. asbestos bodies) these may protect the host, rendering the particle less susceptible to ingestion by macrophages and the various adverse biological consequences discussed above. On the other hand, adsorption of proteins onto the surface of particles may modulate the antigenicity of such proteins and stimulate auto-antibody production or other immunological responses to them. A possible source for the altered immunoglobulin, which stimulates the production of rheumatoid factor in inorganic dust pneumoconiosis may, at least in part, be the adsorption of body protein onto particle surfaces.

Complement activation

An ever-extending range of agents capable of triggering the cascade of complement activation *in vitro*, without the intervention of specific antibody, is now recognized. In the context of this chapter, such agents include endotoxins, *M. faeni*, silica, and asbestos. The consquences of such 'activation' is an amplification of the local inflammatory response. No doubt the list of agents capable of acting in this way will extend rapidly now that *in vitro* techniques have been developed and are reasonably simple. As Allison has pointed out, it is of some interest that at least *in vitro* the macrophage itself contains all the components to promote the alternative pathway of complement activation; the cell can produce not only C3 and factor B but also some initiating factors such as proteases (e.g. cathepsins). Thus, under certain circumstances, it is at least theoretically possible that activity within the macrophage itself can perpetuate the generation of activated complement with its tissue-damaging consequences. If this can be confirmed *in vivo*, it would have a bearing on the pathogenesis of progressive inflammatory changes in the lung which no longer appear to be dependent on the presence of the initial inhaled trigger.

Immunological responses to inhaled agents

The majority of inhaled organic particles, both living and non-living, stimulate antibody production which can be identified in the circulation and (in those instances in which it has been sought) also in lung lavage supernatants. When the host is exposed to antigen for the first time, specific antigen is generated first of all with IgM and IgG somewhat later. This sequence has been exploited in an attempt, for example to identify in a clinical context active tuberculosis by detecting the presence of IgM antibodies in the circulation. Currently diagnostic antibody tests have not yet been completely validated but major studies are underway and such a test may become satisfactory for clinical use in the near future.

As emphasized earlier, the development of such circulating antibodies following inhalation exposure does not necessarily mean that any local lung disease of clinical relevance has developed. For example, titres of circulating antibody to influenza virus increase following droplet infection, but in the majority of cases there is no accompanying pulmonary disease. Circulating precipitating antibodies are frequently found following inhalation of non-living organic dusts (e.g. avian protein or extracts of *M. faeni*) in exposed but clinically healthy individuals. Even where circulating antibodies are found in association with lung disease this alone is not proof of their participation in pathogenesis. For example, antibodies to *Haemophilus influenzae* are frequently found in patients with chronic bronchitis in which this bacteria is frequently isolated. However, the fact that titres of antibody do not appear to fluctuate with exacerbations of disease suggests that the presence of antibodies reflects more the presence of bacterial antigen rather than necessarily its damaging consequences.

Although the presence of circulating antibody under some circumstances may be no more than an epiphenomenon, its detection may, of course, have very considerable practical diagnostic value. For example, the detection of antibodies to *Pneumocystis carinii* has proved a valuable diagnostic procedure in elucidating the nature of certain opportunist infections in immunologically compromised individuals especially when isolation of the organism itself may, on occasion, prove difficult. The diagnostic value of serological techniques demonstrating a rising titre of antibody in association with acute disease is, of course, a useful diagnostic procedure irrespective of the role of the antibody in pathogenesis. The identification of specific antibody in the circulation may also be diagnostically useful where the particular antibody is rarely found in normal individuals. Thus its detection may at least help to identify an agent which may be responsible for the disease irrespective of the mechanism of pathogenesis. Such identification is especially useful in individuals with appropriate clinical features.

The value of detecting circulating sensitized lymphocytes as a diagnostic indicator of disease has not been explored extensively, but some reports suggest that in avian protein hypersensitivity pneumonitis there is a closer association between pulmonary symptoms and sensitized lymphocytes in the peripheral blood than with the presence of circulating antibodies. However, other workers have found evidence of peripheral blood lymphocyte sensitization in apparently healthy exposed individuals. Lymphocyte sensitization to beryllium has been demonstrated to be closely associated with lung involvement.

As noted earlier in this chapter, the immunological responses most closely relating to pathogenesis are more likely to be found in the lung itself and the rapid advances coming from the study of lung lavage and lung extracts are confirming this view. Indeed, the cell profile obtained from lung lavage samples is often quite distinct from that found in the blood. For instance, in avian protein hypersensitivity, the predominant inflammatory cell is the T lymphocyte and many are found in the 'activated' state. Evidence of specific sensitization of lymphocytes isolated from lung lavage samples has been demonstrated in some individuals when none could be demonstrated using circulating lymphocytes. Herein lies the probable explanation of the conflicting reports regarding lymphocyte sensitization from blood derived samples.

A very well-recognized example of the importance of local antibody in the development of lung disease due to inhaled antigens is the classic example of the immediate IgE-mediated reaction in some asthmatic patients. The cellular basis of this reaction in relation to cytophilic IgE antibody on the mast cell membrane leading to the liberation of histamine, SRS.A (now identified as leukotrienes C4 and D4), neutrophil chemotactic factor, and many other inflammatory mediators, following stimulation with the appropriate antigen, has been discussed in a separate section of this book (Section 4). In the context of this chapter, it is of interest to note that certain common allergens in the United Kingdom (e.g. housedust mite excreta and pollen grains) both have a similar, large particle size (around 10–20 μm) which results in proximal deposition in the nose and central airways sites which are similar to the major distribution of IgE plasma cells in the airways.

Special examples of IgE-mediated asthma are found in some occupational asthmas. These individuals are exposed to agents not normally present in the environment and the development of sensitization and lung disease has been followed in a number of instances in newly exposed populations. For example, of those exposed to various salts of platinum, the first to be affected are atopic individuals whether or not they have suffered previously from asthma. On more prolonged exposure, non-atopic workers are eventually sensitized. IgE antibodies have been found in the circulation of these workers and immediate prick tests have been demonstrated using platinum salts appropriately linked to sepharose particles. Antigen challenge studies confirm the association between antigen and development of symptoms. Thus, occupational asthmas produce an elegant model in which to follow the evolution of specific IgE antibody, its potential development in various subpopulations of exposed individuals, and its role in pathogenesis.

If antigen/antibody interaction occurs predominantly at very central sites in the airways, another explanation has to be sought for the widespread narrowing of airways throughout the bronchial tree and the extensive inflammatory changes seen at autopsy in asthmatic patients. Part of the extensive airways narrowing may depend on histamine-stimulated reflex narrowing of airways over a much wider area than the original immunological stimulus. However, the explanation of the widespread eosinophilic inflammatory reaction is much more difficult. One obvious possibility is that much of the pathogenesis of asthma depends on non-immunological events and is not related to antigen stimulation or IgE antibody, but very little is known about the nature of these alternative mechanisms. It is likely that they may be particularly important in non-atopic 'intrinsic' asthmatic patients where IgE appears to be less important. The role of the neutrophil in asthma is now attracting much attention, especially in relation to 'late' asthmatic reactions. It should not, however, be forgotten that in chronic asthma, histology shows a predominance of mononuclear cells surrounding airways, and their role has so far hardly been studied at all.

In summary, a wide variety of immunological responses may be observed in relation to inhaled living and non-living organic and inorganic materials. Some of these indicate the presence of antigen only, others reflect previous exposure to antigen and represent markers or mediators of protective immunity, responsible for the lessening of clinically important tissue responses (e.g. protective antibodies to influenza or *M. tuberculosis*). Others are directly involved in tissue damaging immunological reactions and are intimately connected with pathogenesis of the clinical disease.

The role of the three major categories of response discussed above (i.e. IgG antibody, cell-mediated, and IgE-associated responses) in the development of different clinical patterns of asthma which can be observed is not so far clear.

Neoplasia

Certain inhaled agents including cigarette smoke, chromates, and uranium are closely associated with an increased incidence of carcinomas, but not necessarily with other pulmonary disease (Table 2). The mechanism of induction of these neoplastic changes is not known in any detail but may depend as much on the influence of these agents on the various immunological responses controlling neoplastic cell proliferation as on causing the direct mutation of cells.

In other instances, such as occur in asbestos workers, there is an increased incidence of lung cancer especially in those in whom a fibrogenetic inflammatory response has already developed (i.e. in those with asbestosis). Further, cigarette smoking has a powerful associated influence on the development of cancer in these particular patients. Thus, the development of neoplastic change in some instances is interdependent upon other external and/or internal factors.

Other aspects of pathogenesis and inhaled particles

The foregoing discussion has been confined to the analysis of biological components triggered by the inhalation of various types of particles. It is also important to summarize the various fields of study particularly relating to the *pathogenesis* of lesions which develop in the lung.

Immune complexes in the lung

Exposure to an inhaled antigen in an individual previously 'primed' either to microbial or non-living organic agents is an exceedingly common situation. The opportunity for immune complexes to form locally is obviously great and the clinical relevance of this must be discussed. The consequences of such antigen/anti-

body interaction depends upon the relative amounts of antigen and antibody involved (i.e. complex formation in antibody or antigen excess, or in equivalence), the overall amount of complex formed and its size. The latter depends not only on quantitative factors, but also on other things such as affinity of antibody and whether complement is or is not involved. A detailed discussion of these many variables is outside the context of the present chapter but a brief outline can be given.

Complexes in antibody excess rapidly precipitate and are taken up by phagocytic cells which are degraded by the intracellular mechanisms already outlined (page 15.41) with the consequent protection of the host from the invader. In antigen excess, complexes may solubilize. Whether such soluble complexes reach the circulation from the air spaces is not precisely known but the fact that circulating immune complexes have been detected in patients with hypersensitivity pneumonitis suggests that this may occur; its frequency has to be worked out.

Complexes forming in equivalence, at least under experimental circumstances, may form local granulomas (see below).

Where inhaled antigen reacts in the lungs with large amounts of circulating antibody a florid tissue-damaging Arthus reaction may result. Examples of this may include fulminating measles pneumonia in previously immunized children, respiratory syncytial virus pneumonia in infants with high circulating maternal antibody, and possibly some cases of florid chicken pox pneumonia occurring in adults. The influence at a cellular level of local complexes may also be important. *In vitro* studies have shown that immune complexes activate macrophages inducing the sequence of events discussed on page 15.40. Immune complexes may also occupy C3b or Fc receptor sites on a range of inflammatory cells with these membrane receptors (e.g. macrophages, neutrophils, eosinophils, B cells, and T helper and suppressor cells), and by blocking these sites diminish further responses of the cell to subsequent challenge. For example, the normal antibody dependent cytotoxicity killing potential of some lymphocytes may be reduced in this way, and important lymphocyte/macrophage interactions may also be diminished. Some impaired handling of microbial or other noxious agents may in part be due to blocking of membrane sites by immune complexes. This sequence of events might be important in clinical circumstances such as bronchiectasis or cystic fibrosis where circulating immune complexes are readily demonstrated (page 15.101). It must be recognized that at the present time technical methods available for demonstrating immune complexes are numerous and of varying sensitivity. In addition to this, they demonstrate different components of the complex (in some instances a complement component, in others an antibody component) and results in the clinical context will therefore vary, depending upon the techniques used. It should also be appreciated that the detection of circulating complexes is not synonymous with tissue damage; further, even the identification of complexes deposited in tissues cannot be necessarily equated with local damage. For instance, immune complexes may be detected in biopsies from normal skin sites of patients with systemic lupus erythematosus (SLE). Thus the same critical arguments summarized in relation to the role of circulating antibodies in pathogenesis must also be applied when immune complexes are considered.

Granuloma formation

The characteristic pathology in the lungs following the inhalation of certain types of particles is the formation of epithelioid granulomas. These are especially typical following inhalation of a variety of organic dusts and of beryllium.

There are several hypotheses to explain the formation of these particular lesions. While the final answer is not yet known, it is probable that, like fibrogenesis (see below), several different mechanisms are involved under different circumstances. A few of these can be summarized:

1. Spector and Heesom showed that the intravenous injection of preformed immune complexes in equivalence resulted in granu-

loma formation in the lungs. Thus, under special circumstances, granuloma formation may be induced by immune complexes alone.

2. Much more commonly, however, granulomas are associated with antigens which particularly sensitize lymphocytes, for example, *M. tuberculosis*, beryllium, and avian proteins. Lymphokines secreted from T cells are known to inhibit macrophage migration and to contain a chemotactic factor for monocytes. These together could explain the local accumulation of tissue histiocytes and epithelioid cells.

3. Allison has noted that those agents characteristically associated with granuloma formation in the lungs are those which 'activate' macrophages, and macrophages have also been purported to secrete a chemotactic factor recruiting monocytes. Under these circumstances the stimulus to granuloma formation could be independent of immune complexes and sensitized lymphocytes.

4. Granulomas under some conditions appear to form in the neighbourhood of persisting undegradable foreign material (e.g. foreign body granulomas). They also occur under other circumstances where, for immunological reasons, there may be defective clearance of agents (e.g. granulomas seen in some immune deficiency states).

Thus, persistence of a non-degradable agent in tissues may be a potent stimulus for granuloma formation.

Granuloma formation in hypersensitivity pneumonitis

In the subacute stage of this disorder, and independent of the particular antigen, granuloma formation is a characteristic histological finding. The mechanism for this is not clearly established but some observations can be made. Both in experimental models and in humans, immunofluorescent studies have only rarely demonstrated deposition of immune complexes in or around granulomatous lesions. Positive fluorescence has occasionally been reported in human biopsies but the distribution of this is not located in the granulomas.

So far, systematic assessment of 'activation' of alveolar macrophages in lung lavage has not been reported in any detail and deserves further study.

M. faeni has been shown to activate complement by the alternative pathway and complement fragments, especially C3b which can activate macrophages without participation of antibody. Allison has shown that *M. faeni* activates macrophages directly *in vitro*. Thus, macrophage activation may well be increased by mechanisms which are independent of immune complex formation.

Granulomas in hypersensitivity pneumonitis frequently show intracellular accumulation of foreign material and the persistence of such material may also be important.

Lymphocyte sensitization in peripheral blood and in lung lavage samples has now been observed in cases with hypersensitivity pneumonitis, beryllium disease, and tuberculosis. In all three conditions the predominant cell type in bronchoalveolar samples is the T lymphocyte. A lymphocyte-dependent mechanism is therefore likely to hold a central place in the development of granulomas in these disorders.

In conclusion, it appears that on the basis of current observation it is probable that several different mechanisms may play a part in granuloma formation even in a single individual exposed to a single inhaled agent. Thus, the arguments in favour of any one hypothesis exclusive of another may turn out to be a false philosophy.

A further clinical problem in hypersensitivity pneumonitis is why some individuals progress from the development of granulomas to irreversible fibrosing destruction of the lung and others do not. Part of the explanation is likely to depend on the dose of antigen and the frequency of exposure which together determine the severity of the acute inflammatory changes. Other factors such as those controlling the dynamics of collagen formation may well also be important and this area is now being actively explored.

Fibrogenesis

The clear distinction which exists clinically between those inhaled agents which induce lung fibrosis and those which do not probably reflects an important difference in the handling by the lung of these two groups of particles (see Table 2).

One of many unresolved problems is why some early and acute lesions tend to progress to fibrosis and why others do not. Where certain types of cell death occur without loss of architectural integrity of the lung, cell regeneration, particularly type II pneumocytes spreading to replace destroyed type I pneumocytes, may restore the lung to normal without the development of fibrosis (e.g. normal resolution of lobar pneumonia). Where the early lesions are associated with destruction of lung architecture then healing is by organization and scar formation. Persistence of the inflammatory response (for whatever reason) also plays a major part in stimulating fibroblastic proliferation. This response may depend particularly upon fibroblast stimulating factors and fibronectin derived from activated macrophages. A potential factor in lung stroma destruction would appear to be tissue-damaging proteases liberated from phagocytic cells. On this basis, Allison proposed a two-stage theory of fibrogenesis. Particles toxic to macrophages are first taken up into these cells by phagocytosis; silica-induced damage to the plasma membrane, for instance, allows permeation of lysosomal enzymes into the macrophage cytoplasm with cell death and a consequent discharge of tissue damaging acid hydrolases into the surrounding tissues. Moreover, liberation of neutral proteases including collagenases and elastase results in disruption of collagen and elastin in alveolar stroma. Macrophages also liberate a small molecular weight fibrogenic factor which increases protein uptake by fibroblasts and increases secretion of collagen (i.e. fibroblast growth factor). The two-stage theory proposed by Allison is in line with early *in vitro* experiments reported by Hepplestone and Styles and more recent ones using nucleopore chambers inserted intraperitoneally into mice reported by Bateman and colleagues. The general hypothesis of soluble fibrogenic factors secreted from activated macrophages is supported by the fact that phagocytosis of particles which do not activate or are not toxic to macrophages (e.g. latex or carbon) fail to induce fibrosis.

Destruction of collagen by collagenases may generate collagen fragments which are themselves antigenic. Kravis and colleagues have demonstrated lymphocyte sensitization to type I collagen in fibrosing lung disease in humans and such a reaction could lead to further local tissue destruction, in turn stimulating further fibroblastic proliferation. Thus, once fibroblastic proliferation has been stimulated, circuits may develop allowing for persistence of the fibrosing response which is no longer dependent upon the local primary agent. Controlling mechanisms in fibrogenesis therefore become very important but so far little is known about these. Collagenase activity is counterbalanced by collagenase inhibitors and there is preliminary evidence from protease kinetic studies that the properties of different types of inhibitors change in patients with different types of fibrosing lung disorders. Whether these changes are primary or secondary effects is at present unclear.

The fibroblast is also able to control the amount of collagen leaving the cell by rapid degradation of newly synthesized procollagen within the cell itself. The intracellular and extracellular events involved in the dynamics and control of collagen degradation, formation, and modelling, are complex and are difficult to study in humans, and at present are not understood in detail. However, it is important to recognize that the process of fibrosis in the lungs is a dynamic one and it should no longer be viewed necessarily as end-stage immutable scarring. This view is further supported by immunofluorescence and biochemical studies designed to identify different types of collagen during tissue repair. Type III collagen increases in the early stages of tissue repair and has a greater susceptibility to proteolytic action, and may be remodelled or even totally reabsorbed spontaneously or in response to treatment. On the other hand, type I collagen appears to be less reversible.

Other experiments suggest that some agents are able to stimulate fibroblasts directly without the intermediate step of macrophage phagocytosis. Several groups of workers have suggested that asbestos fibres have this potential while coal, glass, and quartz do not.

A third mechanism of fibrogenesis is suggested by studies showing that antigenic stimulation of sensitized lymphocytes results in the release of lymphokines which will stimulate fibroblasts directly.

In conclusion, when considering the pathogenesis of lung disease relating to inhaled particles, not only must the interaction of humoral and cellular responses be considered in the more acute stages but the subsequent events leading to the formation, deposition, and control of collagen must also be considered.

The interaction of effects of inhaled particles in relation to altered host factors

So far, this chapter has considered particularly the effects of various inhaled particles on previously healthy and normal individuals. There are many situations where inhaled microbes or non-living particles have exaggerated or unusual effects because the 'soil' is abnormal. In some instances, the mechanism for this unusual susceptibility has been postulated. For example, in patients with α_1-antitrypsin deficiency the additional deleterious influence of smoking on the development of destructive emphysema may be due to smoking-induced accumulation of neutrophils or macrophages in the lung and the associated uncontrolled release of proteases from these cells. The explanation for the apparent synergism between the carcinogenic influence of asbestos or uranium and cigarette smoking, although well-established epidemiologically, is unknown in terms of cell events.

The influence of microbial inhalants on the immunologically compromised host is well recognized and different types of microbial invaders tend to predominate in different types of deficiency. For example, those with various types of B cell deficiencies tend to develop recurrent but rapidly resolving bacterial infections while those with T cell deficiencies tend to be more susceptible to tuberculosis, viral, fungal infections, and to *Pneumocystis carinii*. Those with generalized depression due to immunosuppressant drugs are also susceptible to inhaled microbes which are uncommon pathogens under normal circumstances, e.g. Nocardia, Candida, etc.

Under some circumstances, host factors may alter the typical pathology induced by an inhaled particle. For example, in coal workers with rheumatoid arthritis or circulating rheumatoid factor, the inhalation of coal dust is more likely to induce large nodules not dissimilar in histological appearance to those of rheumatoid nodules, i.e. Caplan's syndrome. However, the exact explanation at a cellular level of this altered tissue response remains quite unknown. These few examples emphasize a fact which is a central issue to this chapter. Namely, that the lung responses to inhaled agents show a wide spectrum of changes in the pulmonary tissue which is substantially modulated by the varied capacity of host cells to react.

Effects of cigarette smoke on the lungs

As Government health warnings correctly state, cigarette smoke is the commonest, and in epidemiological terms, the most seriously damaging of all inhaled particles in humans. Extensive studies have now been carried out, both regarding the clinical syndromes relating to adverse effects of cigarette smoke and on the cellular events forming the underlying pathogenic basis for these lesions. Cigarette smoke, quite apart from being most unpleasant to those who do not smoke, can be shown to have an adverse effect on vir-

Table 5 Effects of cigarette smoke on lung tissue and host defences*

	Effects
Bronchi	
Ciliated epithelium	Depression of cilial action
	Destruction of ciliated epithelium
	Reduced regeneration
Mucus gland hypertrophy	Hypersecretion
	Interference with cilial action
Bronchial muscle irritability	Increased susceptibility to microbial infection, e.g. chronic bronchitis, obliterative bronchiolitis
Epithelium	Carcinogenesis
Acini	
Surfactant	Diminished surface tension
Alveolar walls	Destruction with development of emphysema
	Effects on type I and type II cells
Immune systems	
Local sIgA	Sputum levels increased
Alveolar macrophages	Morphological changes
	Increased lysozymal content
	Increased numbers of macrophages
	Diminished opsonization of microbes
	Diminished killing
	Increased pigment (kaolinite)
Lymphocytes	Diminished Ab formation
	Diminished natural cytoxicity
	Impaired local T cell transformation
	Diminished activated T cells at 37 °C
	Diminished PHA and Coconavalin A responses
Neutrophils	Increased in lavage fluid
Supernatants of lavage	Decreased α_1-antitrypsin
IgE	Induction of type I responses to tobacco products with potential asthma
Co-factor	
Cancer	Asbestos
	Uranium
Emphysema	α_1-antitrypsin deficiency
Asthma	Irreversible airflow obstruction
Coal	'Protective' from pneumoconiosis
	Hypersensitivity pneumonitis

*Some of the numerous effects which have been reported.

tually every defence mechanism in the lung. Some of the evidence for this statement is summarized in Table 5.

In view of the profound effects of tobacco smoke on so many cells in the lung, and the prevalence of the smoking habit throughout the world population, the additional influence of smoking has to be sought and analysed in every study concerning any lung disease – in many, additive detrimental effects have already been demonstrated.

Conclusion

This chapter has attempted to outline some of the varied and complex responses occurring in the lung following inhalation of various materials. In spite of the complexities of the subject, a great deal is now known about the interaction of components at a cellular level and factors which influence these. It is necessary to analyse and describe these individually. However, in humans, during life, it is important to emphasize that many of the different processes described will be occurring simultaneously. It is important to remember that a single agent may induce varied patterns of lung disease in different individuals, either because of different circumstances of exposure (e.g. dose and duration) or because of the varied host response. This may be a characteristic of the individual; it may be dependent on genetic factors or a response dependent upon previous priming by an external agent.

Throughout this chapter an attempt has been made to cite samples in lung disease where individual events have been well demonstrated, rather than to attempt a systematic review of each of the huge number of different inhaled particles to which the lung can be exposed. The latter approach would not only be unduly cumbersome, but at the present time there are too many gaps in our knowledge for it to be a useful exercise.

Lastly, throughout this chapter there has been repeated reference to tissue-damaging events which develop in the lung in the trail of particle damage, which may then set up persisting circuits of inflammation which are no longer dependent on the presence of the primary agent. It is the control of these secondary circuits which may prove to be of particular importance in determining chronic inflammation in the lung. The implication of this understanding for clinicians is that identification and intervention at an early stage of lung disease has to be our goal and in clinical terms this implies early case finding and preventive medicine in its widest sense.

References

Allison, A. C. (1977). Mechanisms of macrophage damage in relation to the pathogenesis of some lung diseases. Respiratory defence mechanism, Part II. In *Lung biology and health in disease* (eds J. D. Brain, D. F. Proctor and L. Reid), Ch. 26. Marcel Dekker, New York.

Bateman, E., Emerson, R. and Cole, P. J. (1981). Mechanisms of fibrogenesis. Ch. 11. In *Lung biology in health and disease* (eds H. Weill and M. Turner-Warwick). Marcel Dekker, New York.

Bienenstock, J. (1984). *Immunology of the lung and upper respiratory tract.* McGraw Hill, New York.

Cole, P. J. (1980). Recurrent bronchial infections and bronchiectasis. In *Advanced medicine* Vol. 16, Royal College of Physicians of London (ed. A. J. Bellingham), pp. 59–72. Pitman Medical, London.

Hunninghake, G. W., Gadek, J. E., Kawanami, O., Ferrans, V. J. and Crystal, R. G. (1979). Inflammatory and immune processes in the human lung in health and disease: evaluation by bronchoalveolar lavage. *Am. J. Path.* **97**, pp. 149.

Newman Taylor, A. J. (1980). Occupational asthmas. *Thorax* **35**, pp. 241.

Johnson, K. J., Chapman, W. E. and Ward, P. A. (1979). Lung immunopathology: a review. *Am. J. Path.* **95**, pp. 793.

Reynold, H. Y. and Newball, H. H. (1976). Milieu of the human respiratory tract. Immunologic infectious reactions in the lung. *Lung biology in health and disease* Vol. 1 (eds C. H. Kirkpatrick and H. Y. Reynolds). Marcel Dekker, New York.

Turner-Warwick, M. (1978). Defence mechanisms. *Immunology of the lung* Ch. 5. Edward Arnold, London.

THE CLINICAL PRESENTATION OF CHEST DISEASES

D. J. LANE

The presenting symptoms of chest diseases are few, but the structural and functional disturbances which these symptoms reflect are numerous, and the underlying disease entities are very many. It is a useful starting point to consider the symptoms of lower respiratory tract disease under just three headings: cough, breathlessness, and chest pain.

Cough may or may not produce sputum. Patients occasionally report the expectoration of sputum while denying that they have cough. This seems to be a socially determined separation of the act of 'clearing the throat' to expell sputum from a non-productive cough which, perhaps because it appears to have no purpose, is regarded as more sinister. Breathlessness is itself a complex symptom. Wheezing and stridor, audible accompaniments to the act of breathing, are rarely reported without breathlessness and so will be considered with it. Discussion of the third member of the triad, chest pain, will include mention of chest tightness.

In the analysis of symptoms it is important to recognize and differentiate between the pathology or disordered physiology likely to be responsible for the symptoms, and the clinical diagnoses associated with that symptom. The investigation of mechanism, though superficially of little clinical relevance, can be the key to symptomatic treatment, creating opportunities for relief when the underlying condition is untreatable. Knowledge of the clinical significance of symptoms is largely empirical but forms the essential diagnostic base of clinical medicine. Thus research into the mechanisms of, for example, breathlessness will continue to be a proper concern of clinicians as long as disabling and irreversible conditions such as chronic airways obstruction exist. In contrast, knowing the mechanism of dyspnoea in pleural effusion is unimportant besides knowing how to relieve the dyspnoea by draining the effusion, and being able to diagnose the clinical condition causing it.

Cough

Coughing is a defensive reflex designed to clear and protect the lower respiratory tract. The act of coughing is essentially a forced expiratory effort against a transitorily closed glottis which then opens allowing a sudden expulsion of air from the lungs. Except perhaps when the cough arises from laryngeal irritation, there is an initial deep inspiration which presumably allows the respiratory muscles to act to greater mechanical advantage. This could however, draw the offending material deeper into the bronchial tree. The pressure which builds up behind the closed glottis can reach as much as 40 kPa and, if often repeated in a sequence of coughs, can seriously impede venous filling of the heart. The consequent drop in cardiac output is responsible for the well described 'cough syncope'.

The cough reflex can be initiated by the stimulation of irritant receptors in the larynx, trachea, and major bronchi. These receptors respond to mechanical irritation by intraluminal material such as mucus, dust, or foreign bodies, and to chemical irritation by fumes and toxic gases such as sulphur dioxide. Mechanical events within the thorax, such as sudden and large changes in airway calibre or lung collapse, can also stimulate cough receptors. The afferent fibres run in the branches of the superior laryngeal nerve and the vagus to the medulla, where the resultant efferent activity of virtually the whole of the respiratory musculature is co-ordinated. The explosive action of the respiratory muscles produces laryngeal air velocities which can approach the speed of sound and is accompanied by laryngeal and bronchial constriction, mucus secretion, and a transient systemic hypertension.

The clinical description of cough relies on its sound, its timing, and whether or not there is expectoration. A dry cough with an irritative hacking quality, short and often repeated, is heard in inflammatory conditions of the pharynx, in tracheobronchitis, and in early pneumonia. With laryngitis the sound is harsh and hoarse ('croup'). The long inspiratory sound that gives whooping cough its name is also produced by tracheal and laryngeal inflammation. Abductor paralysis of the vocal cords creates a cough that is prolonged and lowing like the sound of cattle, and hence described as 'bovine'. The usual cause is pressure on the left recurrent laryngeal nerve by lesions in the thorax: carcinoma of the bronchus, or oesophagus, enlarged (usually neoplastic) hilar nodes, or, now very rarely, aortic aneurysm. If similar lesions press on the trachea but spare the nerve, the cough has a hard metallic quality described as 'brassy'. Unilateral abductor palsy of the larynx does not affect the voice and even with additional adductor palsy the voice often remains good. Complete paralysis of both cords gives aphonia and a weak ineffectual cough. Weakness of the thoracic muscles as in polyneuritis or the muscular dystrophies will lessen the expulsive force in coughing, as will the general weakness of prostration, toxaemia, or the deeper states of unconsciousness. Cough may be suppressed when there is severe thoracic or upper abdominal pain.

A cough may fail to produce expectoration because there is nothing to produce, because the secretions are swallowed, as is almost universal in children, because of weakness as outlined above or because the secretions are too viscid. In the latter three instances the sound quality of the cough differs from that of a dry cough in the sense that secretions can be heard moving in the major airways. This type of cough and the cough productive of sputum may be described as 'moist' or 'loose'.

Certain aspects to the timing of coughing may give useful diagnostic clues. A cough that awakens in the small hours of the night suggests asthma: wheezing need not be evident. Cough with expectoration on arising in the morning is characteristic of chronic bronchitis, though may also be reported by the asthmatic. A bout of coughing after food or when lying down after food, points to oesophageal, pharyngeal or neuromuscular disease causing aspiration into the lungs. Changes of posture can also set off coughing in the bronchiectatic: the free expectoration of sputum at any time of day is common in these patients. A dry cough which persists over many weeks can signify a neoplasm, but a non-productive barking cough that has lasted years is more likely to be a nervous habit often perpetuated by psychogenic factors.

Phlegm, the secretions of the lower respiratory tract, is admixed with nasal and pharyngeal secretions as well as saliva to give expectorated sputum. It has been very difficult to study the natural secretions of the healthy tracheobronchial tree in man for only about 100 ml is produced daily and most of this is swallowed. In disease the quantity of secretions is often sufficient to swamp contamination in the upper respiratory tract, so that valid observations can be made, but in clinical medicine, no less than in research, it is important to obtain expectorated material that has actually come from the lungs.

Mucus is visco-elastic. Its viscosity or stickiness influences the effect of forces applied to it in coughing. Initially it resists flow and then as increasing force is applied it becomes more and more liquid, returning to its original state when flow stops, rather like a dripless paint. The elasticity of sputum appears to alter with the rate of application of stress to it, and may be important in relation to the rate of beating of the bronchial epithelial cilia. Intrabronchial mucus appears to exist in two layers, one of low viscosity and high elasticity touching the cilia, and above this a more viscous layer which, in disease, carries globules of mucus.

Though airway mucus is 95 per cent water it derives its distinctive physical characteristics from its glycoprotein content. Two components in these glycoproteins, sialic acid and sulphate, enable airway mucus to be chemically analysed and identified *in situ* in histological sections. At least four glycoproteins have been identified in human bronchial mucus and are found to be produced in various combinations from different mucuous cell types. Serous fluid is produced from other cells in the bronchial glands, and with water, lipids and proteins makes up a transudate component of sputum that can be separated from the glycoproteins. Although bronchial secretions do not show diagnostically distinctive changes in disease, there is, for example, a shift towards greater glycoprotein production in chronic bronchitis, and greater transudate formation in asthma. In infection both components increase and the breakdown of leucocytes and of bronchial mucus increases the DNA content of sputum, making it less viscid. The accumulated

debris of cells and micro-organisms imparts a yellow colour to infected sputum and the subsequent action of verdoperoxidase derived from leucocytes gives a green colour.

The distinction between infected and non-infected sputum is one of the most obvious descriptive features of sputum that is relevant in clinical medicine. Non-infected mucoid sputum is variously described as clear, white, or jelly-like. Exceptionally viscid mucoid sputum is sometimes seen in asthma, and the patient may report seeing pellets of even branching plugs of mucus that are presumed to be casts of small bronchi. In bronchopulmonary aspergillosis similar pellets or casts have a dark brown colour. In city dwellers and those in dusty occupations mucoid sputum can be various shades of grey. Coal miners may produce jet black sputum (melanoptysis) if an area of fibrosis breaks down and is expectorated.

In most lower respiratory tract infections pus is admixed with mucus to produce mucopurulent sputum. Pure pus can be expectorated from a lung abscess or from stagnant bronchiectactic cavities. An offensive smell to the sputum, especially in these last two conditions, often comes from infection with anaerobic organisms. A rarely seen but distinctive brown discoloration ('anchovy sauce') comes from the pus from an amoebic lung abscess (usually secondary to hepatic amoebiasis).

Patients rightly regard the presence of blood in the sputum as of sinister significance. Despite this in most series a definite cause for haemoptysis is only found in about half of the cases. In the assessment of haemoptysis it is important to establish first that the blood stained material has come from the chest and not from the gastrointestinal tract. Some patients find this difficult. Accompanying features of an appropriate disease are usually present, but it is worth remembering that in haemoptysis there is usually froth due to admixed air, and the blood is bright red, not dark brown. Gastric contents should be acid, bronchial alkaline. Another trap for the unwary is contamination with blood from the nose or upper respiratory tract.

It is unwise to attribute haemoptysis simply to 'bronchitis' or infection. In bronchiectasis, however, haemoptysis not uncommonly mixes with mucopurulent sputum. In the early stages of pneumococcal pneumonia a 'rusty' staining of mucoid sputum is quite characteristic. In tuberculosis, frank blood in otherwise mucoid sputum is well recognized. Sudden haemoptysis is a hallmark of pulmonary embolism with infarction. In bronchial neoplasia there may be streaking of the sputum, often daily, with blood or more substantial bleeding with clots. Recurrent blood staining of the sputum is seen in idiopathic pulmonary haemosiderosis and also, though usually over a shorter time span, in Goodpasture's syndrome, both uncommon conditions. Cardiac conditions associated with blood in the sputum are pulmonary oedema, with its pink frothy sputum and mitral stenosis. The recurrent haemoptyses of the latter condition are infrequently seen today. In a general context, it may be necessary to consider thoracic trauma, endometriosis, or a blood coagulation disorder as causes of haemoptysis.

In the investigation of haemoptysis the chest radiograph will often indicate a likely diagnosis, for example an apical tuberculous infiltrate or a neoplastic hilar mass, but this must be backed up by appropriate microbiological or cytological examination of the sputum. Old, presumably healed and calcified tuberculous lesions may be a sufficient cause for haemoptysis simply due to local bronchiectasis though reactivation and invasion by mycetoma must be considered. Bronchiectasis and pulmonary infarction may, on the other hand, not be evident on a plain radiograph. Both should give a suggestive history. A bronchogram is seldom required to diagnose (as opposed to manage) bronchiectasis, but ventilation/perfusion scanning is of great value in diagnosing pulmonary embolism. If examination of the sputum and radiology, plain or specialized, yields no obvious cause for the haemoptysis then bronchoscopy needs to be considered. After a single haemoptysis in a young person, this can be deferred for a month. If then there has been no recurrence and radiology is normal, no further action need be taken. A recurrence of haemoptysis or a single episode in an older person, especially a smoker, are indications for early bronchoscopy, not omitting a careful look at the pharynx and larynx on the way. Selective bronchography through the bronchoscope may be useful in delineating areas of unsuspected bronchiectasis.

Apart from its appearance the only other macroscopic attribute to sputum is its quantity. Excessively large quantities of sputum are found in bronchiectasis especially where this is widespread, as in cystic fibrosis and in the rare alveolar cell carcinoma where large quantities of watery mucus may occasionally be produced. The amount of sputum in both chronic bronchitis and in asthma is very variable but can, in individuals, be excessive. Briefly pulmonary oedema leads to the production of a large quantity of frothy sputum.

Expectorated sputum should be subjected to microscopic and microbiological investigation as appropriate. Microscopy will, in a haemotoxylin-eosin preparation, yield evidence of infection in terms of pus cells, or allergy in terms of eosinophils. Gram staining may give useful immediate clues to an infecting organism and acid–alcohol fast bacilli will point to mycobacterial infection, almost invariably tuberculosis. Special stains are required if fungi are suspected. Culture requirements vary and can only be anticipated by the microbiologist if he is given appropriate clinical information. This is especially true if anaerobic infection is suspected: anaerobes do not survive long in air and sputum suspected of containing them must be transported in an oxygen-free environment. The frequent disappointment expressed over the results of the routine microbiological examination of sputum often arise because the technique is regarded as routine. Sampling, transportation, and preparation must be done quickly but with care: some respiratory pathogens survive poorly, others do not stain with conventional stains, and most fail to grow when antibiotic therapy has been given even though infection is still evident. The cytological examination of sputum for malignant cells can only be done by an expert, but in skilled hands it is invaluable and time saving.

The investigation of a patient with cough very often reveals a recognizable condition responsible for the cough. This may well be treatable, even if the only appropriate advice is to stop smoking. If the condition is not treatable, or if no cause can be found, symptomatic measures need to be considered. Two lines of approach are open: to suppress the cough or, accepting the cough as inevitable, to make expectoration easier.

All cough suppressants in common use act centrally. Most are opiate derivatives. Codeine and pholcodeine have a weak antitussive action but made into a sweet syrup seem to have a soothing effect. Methadone and the stronger opiates are more powerful in suppressing cough but they depress respiration and cause constipation as well. In terminal bronchial carcinoma they are invaluable. Attempts to suppress cough by a peripheral action on bronchial afferent receptors have not been conspicuously successful. Inhaled local anaesthetic may be helpful, and its effect on cough may long outlast its anaesthetic action: it may perhaps break a vicious cycle in which cough leads to throat irritation and hence further stimulus to coughing. Drugs which act on the production of bronchial mucus will lessen cough if their purpose is the expectoration of that mucus. Atropine is used to this end preoperatively, but rarely in disease. Corticosteroids can diminish mucus production in alveolar cell carcinoma and in asthma. In the latter condition disodium cromoglycate will act likewise.

Water is said to be the most effective expectorant. Certainly dehydration causes a drying of the bronchial secretions. But there are a multitude of agents which it is claimed will increase sputum quantity or accelerate its expectoration. The volatile oils such as menthol probably act as direct irritants. The inorganic salts such as potassium iodide probably have to cause vomiting if they are going to assist expectoration. The movement of particles up the mucociliary escalator of the bronchial tree has been charted using radio-

isotope techniques and shown to increase under the influence of ingested guiaphenesin (present in several 'cough medicines') and inhaled beta-adrenergic agonists, 2-mercapto-ethane sulphonate and hypertonic (1.2M) saline.

Attempts to decrease the viscosity of sputum using mucolytic agents have been clinically disappointing despite definite in vitro evidence of activity. These strictures apply to both bromhexine and orally administered cysteine derivatives. Inhaled acetyl-cysteine works more convincingly as a mucolytic but has the great disadvantage of inducing bronchoconstriction.

Most patients with haemoptysis require no more than treatment appropriate to their underlying condition, but occasionally haemoptysis is massive and life-threatening. The recorded mortality of 50 per cent with haemoptysis of 200 ml or more includes patients with initially poor respiratory reserve, as well as those who asphyxiate. At bronchoscopy it may be difficult to locate the source of bleeding but local endoscopic measures may be applicable: topical adrenaline application, balloon tamponade, and cold saline lavage. An open surgical approach (lobectomy or pneumonectomy) carries a mortality of up to one third and if operative intervention is contemplated bronchial arteriography should be considered. The source of bleeding is from the bronchial arteries so that embolization of the appropriate bronchial artery has been successfully used to control massive haemoptysis in a high proportion of actively bleeding patients. Its effect is, however, temporary.

Breathlessness

This major symptom of pulmonary, cardiovascular, and other systemic diseases suffers much because it is so frequently referred to by physicians as dyspnoea. Whilst patients sometimes do speak of difficulty in breathing, they more frequently use the terms 'breathlessness', 'short of breath', 'out of breath', or even more colloquially 'puffed'. It is usually only on direct questioning that specific features or associations of breathlessness, such as the effect of position, reveal clues that are likely to be useful clinically. Despite the often quoted statement of Comroe that dyspnoea is not tachypnoea, hyperpnoea, or hyperventilation, but difficult, laboured, or uncomfortable breathing, patients are quite unaware of these fine distinctions. Rapid breathing, the necessary increase of breathing in response to metabolic demands, and ventilation in excess of metabolic requirements are all at times described by patients as breathlessness. Just what degree or quality of awareness of respiratory movement deserves to be called breathlessness is probably indefinable: awareness undoubtedly varies from patient to patient and even within the same subject from time to time. The implication of most terms used by patients to describe this type of pulmonary sensation is, however, that in some way the performance of the respiratory apparatus ('breath-') is not meeting ('-less') a demand placed on it.

Any attempt to understand breathlessness from the standpoint of disordered physiology must start with a brief description of the appropriate features of the performance of the respiratory apparatus. The respiratory muscles are supplied by motor nerve fibres from cervical and thoracic anterior horn cells, from C3 to T12. Like all other anterior horn cells, the respiratory motor nerve cells are served by pyramidal fibres from the motor cortex in the precentral gyrus. Directives from the cortex enable respiratory movement to be modulated to serve such functions as talking, singing, holding the breath, voluntary hyperventilation, and the performance of lung function tests. This pathway will also be responsible for the conscious, and perhaps unconscious, transmission of anxiety or a calming influence on respiratory performance. But, to an extent that is unparalleled in other mammalian skeletal muscle, the respiratory motor neurones are under dual control, the second component being the motor output from the brainstem respiratory centres responsible for involuntary or automatic respiratory movement. This is the movement necessary to satisfy metabolic requirements for oxygen supply and CO_2 removal.

For the purposes of understanding breathlessness, respiratory centre activity, explained in more detail on page 15.30, may be seen as under the influence of chemical and neurogenic stimuli. The chemical stimuli of hypoxia and acidaemia are of relevance to the breathlessness of high altitude and diabetic coma. This is not to say that the hyperventilation induced by these means is the sole cause of breathlessness, but to deny that it plays a part is quixotic. The general traffic of neurogenic stimuli impinging on the reticular formation from all sources maintains a certain level of activity in the medullary respiratory neurones irrespective of more specific stimuli. The modest quietening of this activity in sleep is associated with a small drop in minute ventilation, and the dramatic curtailment of spinal ascending information that sometimes occurs following high spinal tractotomy (usually for intractable pain) can completely abolish automatic medullary respiratory activity. There is no clear-cut association between increased reticular formation activity causing hyperventilation and states of breathlessness, but the increase in ventilation at the very onset of exercise is thought to be neurogenic in origin possibly quite specifically originating from the exercising muscles.

Through the vagus nerve, the respiratory centre receives information from the lungs. This originates in bronchial epithelial irritant receptors, intraluminal stretch receptors, and interstitial J receptors within the alveolar and capillary network (see page 15.7). Stimulation of all these receptors will produce reflex effects amongst which, for example, tachypnoea might easily make up a component of breathlessness in an appropriate setting. Whether the afferent information travelling up the vagus itself reaches the sensorium, or whether it merely modulates some other afferent pathway, is not clear. Afferent information that undoubtedly reaches consciousness is that concerning the rate and degree of thoracic cage movement, and, quite accurately, a sense of lung volume (degree of lung inflation/deflation). This information presumably comes from joint, tendon, and muscle receptors in the chest wall, and for sense of movement (of air) perhaps also from the oropharyngeal mucosa. It seems evident that information from these latter sources is part of natural and healthy sensation: it also seems likely that the same channels will signal increased rate or depth of movement which if excessive (in some way fairly specifically for that individual) will be described as breathlessness. In exercise the description 'breathless' often comes at the point where the smooth linear relation between ventilation and oxygen consumption is disturbed. Ventilation becomes excessive for metabolic requirements. How this becomes described as a shortness or loss of breath is not at present clear.

Two 'unnatural' respiratory sensations that can only be inadequately mimicked in an healthy individual are those associated with abnormal lung mechanics (as for example in airways narrowing) and muscle paralysis. An obvious parallel for the first is breathing through an external resistance. This technique has been widely used by those investigating dyspnoea. The useful finding that may have some bearing on the clinical situation is that in resistance breathing the ability to detect an increased load depends, not on the absolute magnitude of the load, but on the ratio of that load to the basal, i.e. pre-existing, loading of the system. Thus a given absolute increase in airways resistance will be much more obvious to an individual with near normal airways function than to one already suffering a considerable increase in resistance due to airways narrowing. The sensations of those few normal individuals who have undergone muscle paralysis (usually curarization) for experimental purposes, include phrases such as 'choking' and 'I would give anything to be able to take one deep breath'. These are similar to the reported symptoms of patients with paralytic diseases affecting the respiratory muscles. The element of inadequate performance is stressed. Whether this sensation can be at all simulated by the voluntary withholding of respiratory movement, as in breathholding, is very doubtful. This much studied experimental

model undoubtedly gives sensations most of which probably arise from the diaphragm twitching ineffectually. It is difficult to see where this fits into a clinical setting.

If any common thread can be drawn between these examples, it is at the level of an interaction between the drive to breathing and achievement; a drive in excess of what is metabolically needed or cerebrally tolerable; or a drive that fails to achieve because of poor performance or mechanical loading of the respiratory system. The neurophysiological implications of this hypothesis are that there should be monitoring systems for both drive and performance. It is obviously feasible for the brain to assess and in some way sum the various drives to breathing but tentative suggestions have also been made that there may be a monitoring system for motor output. The muscle spindle has been proposed as the likely detector of achievement but several objections exist to this proposal, not least that in the diaphragm, the most important muscle of respiration, there are relatively few muscle spindles.

When it comes to the application of these principles to disease, some parallels are obvious but an example from one common condition—acute bronchial asthma—will illustrate that the situation is not straightforward and is frequently multifactorial. In acute asthma there may be excessive drive from bronchial irritant receptors, and there is often cortical drive expressing itself in anxiety, even panic, as well as hyperventilation. There is clearly poor performance on account of the increased resistance of narrowed airways but, in addition, it seems likely that the respiratory muscles will act at a mechanical disadvantage on account of lung hyperinflation.

Whilst bearing these neurophysiological points in mind when it comes to devising symptomatic measures for the relief of breathlessness, the clinician must still largely rely on an empirical approach to the analysis of this symptom. Such an analysis will rely on four characteristics of breathlessness; its quality, its timing, its severity, and the circumstances which precipitate or relieve it.

Qualities in breathlessness are difficult to define. Most patients can go no further than saying that they are 'short of breath'. The asthmatic will generally recognize the quality of wheeze and, contrary to the physiologists opinion, usually finds it more difficult to breathe in than out. An asthmatic who develops more persistent breathlessness between attacks often recognizes this as 'different from my asthma'. A sense of suffocation is a feature of massive pleural effusions and of pulmonary oedema. Phrases such as 'I can't fill my lungs properly', 'I need to take a big breath' suggest the possibility of psychogenic breathlessness, but muscle weakness must be carefully excluded.

Timing is of the greatest value in separating out conditions likely to be associated with breathlessness. There are five categories. Breathlessness may be of dramatic onset (over minutes), acute onset (over hours), subacute (over weeks), or chronic (over months or years), or it may be intermittent. Table 1 gives a guide to conditions falling into these categories. The sub-divisions are not rigid. Asthma again provides an example. About half of all acute attacks of asthma build up in less than 24 hours: but some asthmatics slowly deteriorate over a week or so and, occasionally when there are anaphylactoid features perhaps with laryngeal spasm as well, the asthmatic can be transformed from an asymptomatic state to desperate breathlessness and unconsciousness within 15 minutes. Asthma is also, of course, intermittent though some patients have chronic exertional breathlessness as well. Likewise left ventricular failure, though usually developing over hours, may be dramatic in, for example, aortic valve rupture or more persistent in long-standing hypertension. The pattern of breathlessness in certain disorders depends on the stage of the disease and the structural or functional changes it causes. Thus in early sarcoidosis diffuse infiltration of the lungs can cause the quite rapid development of breathlessness over several days or a week or so; on the other hand the late fibrotic stage of sarcoid will be associated with relentlessly progressive breathlessness as pulmonary reserve diminishes. Breathlessness in a condition such as

Table 1 Conditions causing breathlessness classified by rate of onset

1 Dramatically sudden: over minutes
  Pneumothorax
  Pulmonary embolism
  Pulmonary oedema
2 Acute: over hours
  Pneumonia
  Acute pulmonary infiltrations, e.g. allergic alveolitis
  Asthma
  Left ventricular failure
3 Sub-acute: over days
  Pleural effusion
  Bronchogenic carcinoma
  Sub-acute pulmonary infiltrations, e.g. sarcoidosis
4 Chronic: over months or years
  Chronic airflow obstruction
  Diffuse fibrosing conditions
  Chronic non-pulmonary causes, e.g. anaemia, hyperthyroidism
5 Intermittent: episodic breathlessness
  Asthma
  Left ventricular failure

Table 2 The MRC breathlessness scale

1 Troubled by shortness of breath when hurrying on level ground or walking up a slight hill
2 Short of breath walking with other people of own age on level ground
3 Have to stop for breath when walking at own pace on level ground

Table 3 A classification of acute breathlessness by grade of severity (based on the Jones index)

Grade I	Able to do housework or job with difficulty
Grade IIa	Confined to chair/bed but able to get up with moderate difficulty
Grade IIb	Confined to chair/bed and only able to get up with great difficulty
Grade III	Totally confined to a chair or bed
Grade IV	Moribund

carcinoma of the lung will be determined by the pattern of structural change: whether there is, for example, bronchial stenosis, collapse, or pleural effusion.

The severity of breathlessness is gauged traditionally on scales relating to activity. Two such scales one from the Medical Research Council chronic bronchitis questionnaire and the other the Jones index for acute asthma are shown in Tables 2 and 3. Many other scales have been devised. All have two faults. The first is that there is a temptation to suppose that the grading system with which you are familiar is universally known; it is not and thus it is usually preferable to stick to a description of the amount of exercise limitation. Secondly no scale suggests a convention for dealing with variable breathlessness. Very few patients have a consistent level of severity of breathlessness, but any attempt to introduce a range of severity will have to be accompanied by some assessment of the time extent of each grade, an almost impossible task.

The circumstances under which breathlessness is experienced can give important diagnostic clues. Only psychogenic breathlessness bears no relation to exertion or is experienced only at rest, though many patients with organic diseases are breathless at rest as well as on exertion: this is an expression of the severity of their breathlessness. Breathlessness made worse by lying flat (orthopnoea) is characteristic of left ventricular failure, as is nocturnal awakening with suffocating breathlessness and frothy sputum production (paroxysmal nocturnal dyspnoea). These patients are relieved by sitting or standing up. The asthmatic can also awaken in the small hours of the night with breathlessness accompanied by coughing and wheezing, or these symptoms may be delayed until

the normal awakening hours. Any sputum produced under these circumstances is likely to be sticky and mucoid in the asthmatic. Post-exertional breathlessness and the immediate triggering of an episode of wheezing breathlessness by non-specific irritants (dust and fumes) or specifically allergic stimuli (pollen, animal danders, etc.) also characterize the asthmatic. In occupational asthmas breathlessness will bear a temporal and circumstantial relation to the working environment. In byssinosis the first day at work is characteristically troublesome (Monday morning tightness). Patients with Type III hypersensitivity reactions (e.g. bronchopulmonary aspergillosis, page 15.81, or extrinsic allergic alveolitis, page 15.119) will notice breathlessness four to six hours after exposure. An intercurrent respiratory tract infection will worsen breathlessness in patients with any form of diffuse airway or parenchymatous lung disease.

Spontaneous improvement occurs in most breathless patients with rest or the removal of trigger factors, the post-exertional breathlessness of the asthmatic being an important though temporary exception. Patients with pulmonary hypertension even with severe exertional breathlessness, improve dramatically quickly immediately they sit down.

Breathlessness as an isolated symptom is likely to be due to diffuse parenchymal lung disease such as emphysema or diffuse fibrosis, to pulmonary hypertension or to extrathoracic conditions.

In the investigation of the breathless patient, the clinical history may immediately suggest a likely cause. Beyond this the two most helpful pointers are simple lung function tests and chest radiology. Spirometric testing will define three groups; normal, an obstructive pattern, and a restrictive pattern (see page 15.32). The chest radiograph will be of most value in furthering the diagnosis in conditions giving a restrictive pattern. The further investigation of the patient with airflow obstruction is dealt with on pages 15.80 and 15.87.

Breathlessness in a patient with normal spirometric testing and a clear chest radiograph presents special problems. Four categories should be considered. Is there intermittent disease? Are the tests being used too crude to pick up significant abnormalities? Is there extrathoracic disease? Is this psychogenic breathlessness?

Many asthmatics reviewed in a clinic will have normal lung function. The value of serial recordings of lung function over several days in these patients cannot be over emphasized. Conditions affecting the heart and pulmonary circulation may also be intermittent but more often the problem is that conventional tests of lung function do not seem to demonstrate significant abnormalities when there is quite considerable dyspnoea. Tests for muscle power and the integrity of the pulmonary vascular bed are required to diagnose early neuromuscular conditions weakening respiratory movement and the easily missed pulmonary hypertension. The hyperventilation of acidosis as in uraemia or diabetic coma is not often described by patients as breathlessness and is otherwise easily diagnosed. Hyperthyroidism and anaemia should however not be forgotten as causes of breathlessness. It is said that 60 per cent of patients with a Hb of less than 8 g/dl will have this symptom.

Psychogenic breathlessness is a diagnosis by exclusion though there may be clues in the history and examination. The quality of the breathlessness has been described above. The sighing and irregular breathing will be readily noticeable to a keen observer. Associated complaints directly related to the hyperventilation are paraesthesiae in the hands and, perhaps, feet, tetany, dizziness, and collapse. Apparently non-specific features such as fatigue, insomnia, muscle weakness, or vague chest pains may all be part of the syndrome. Depression and anxiety may both be aspects of the underlying psychiatric state. By definition, in pure psychogenic breathlessness, the chest radiograph and lung function are normal. But some patients may develop breathlessness because they have been told that they have 'a shadow on the lung', or through anxiety exhibit a degree of breathlessness disproportionate to a mild functional abnormality. The latter patients tend to have an obsessional personality or may be looking for compensation for supposed 'lung damage' due to injury or to their occupation. The obverse of this situation, the patient with a severe lung function abnormality, usually airflow obstruction, who is little distressed by breathlessness, is discussed on page 15.86.

The relief of breathlessness is best achieved by treating the underlying condition. This may mean the removal of 'mass' lesions (pneumothorax, pleural effusion) or the treatment of pneumonia or alveolitis. Airflow obstruction can only be excluded with measurement and useful reversibility often exists. Loss of muscle power is occasionally treatable as in myasthenia gravis or may recover spontaneously. An approach to breathlessness through these channels must not be neglected even when the underlying condition is untreatable (pleural effusion in carcinoma of the bronchus, or a reversible steroid responsive component in a patient with chronic airflow obstruction).

The symptomatic treatment of breathlessness is far from satisfactory. It may be usefully considered along the lines of disordered physiology. An excessive drive may be dampened, for example, oxygen for the hypoxic. A direct approach to the vagal afferent system has met with little success: local anaesthetic to the airways gives a short-lived effect and may itself be irritant. In a select few with intense breathlessness due to diffuse infiltrative disease, vagotomy in the thorax has given some relief. Psychogenic breathlessness may be helped with beta-blockers (but asthma must be excluded with absolute certainty). The opiate sedatives are a traditional remedy but can, of course, dangerously depress respiration: there has been a sad failure to find opiate derivatives with a more selective action on breathlessness. Diazepam and promethazine have given subjective relief to some patients disabled by breathlessness from severe emphysema. The use of rehabilitation measures is considered on page 15.88. Induced hypothyroidism is a measure which has been employed to reduce oxygen demands in the severely breathless.

Chest pain

The greater part of the lower respiratory tract is insensitive to pain. Most parenchymal lung disorders proceed to an advanced state without pain. The parietal pleura on the other hand is exquisitely sensitive to painful stimuli and unpleasant sensations can arise from the tracheo-bronchial tree.

Typical pleural pain has a sharp stabbing and knife-like character and is accentuated by movement. Hence it is aggravated by respiration and coughing so leading to rapid shallow breathing and a suppressed cough. That it is less obvious during expiration than inspiration is one reason for now believing that the pain is not due to friction between the two roughened inflamed surfaces. The pain is more likely to be due to stretching of the inflamed pleura. The afferent pain fibres pass up the intercostal nerves save for those from the central portion of the diaphragm which run in the phrenic nerve to the cervical cord (C3/4). Central diaphragmatic pleurisy is thus referred to the lateral side of the neck and shoulder tip: indeed local anaesthesia to the shoulder trigger area can relieve diaphragmatic pleurisy. The outer portions of the diaphragm are served by intercostal nerves (T7–12) causing referred pain to be felt in the lower thorax, lumbar region, and upper abdomen.

Most conditions giving rise to pleuritic pain are acute and inflammatory in origin: either infective when there is usually associated pneumonia (pleurisy is especially common in pneumococcal pneumonia) or infarctive as in pulmonary embolism. Rather less frequently the immunologically based pleurisies (as in systemic lupus erythematosus or rheumatoid disease) give pain. Recurrent pleurisy at the same site should suggest bronchiectasis and at different sites broncho-pulmonary aspergillosis.

If pleurisy progresses to pleural effusion, the sharp pain largely disappears, to be replaced by a dull and more constant ache or heaviness, quantitatively roughly proportional to the amount of fluid. Pleural fibrotic disease is rarely painful but pleural neoplasia frequently is. The severity and quality of pain depends on the degree of pleural inflammation and the extent of the tumour especially outside the chest. A superior sulcus tumour of bronchial origin (Pancoast) infiltrating the brachial plexus gives very severe and persistent pain in the distribution of C8 T1 and T2.

Chest wall pain can mimic pleurisy and conditions in the chest wall provide its most important differentials. Pain due to strain or tearing of thoracic muscles can be quite sharp and since it may be caused by coughing, and may cause shallow respiration, it can easily be confused with pleurisy. There is however always local tenderness over the affected muscle and none of the ancillary investigations for pleurisy (see page 15.55) prove positive. Patients with persistent cough or distressing breathlessness due especially to asthma may complain of muscular pain around the lower rib cage.

Epidemic myalgia or Bornholm disease (see page 5.99) is a bothersome manifestation of Coxsackie B infection giving fever and recurrent muscle pain. If the intercostal muscles are involved (pleurodynia) the associated breathlessness and tachypnoea can exactly mimic pleurisy. So can the pre-eruptive stage of thoracic herpes zoster which gives a stabbing pain in the distribution of the affected nerve. Costal cartilage pain is generally not inflammatory. In Tietze's disease there is a painful protuberance of one or more costal cartilages probably due to asymmetrical growth of the rib cage. Osteoarthritis and dislocation of the costosternal joints can give chronic pain. Rib fractures rarely present diagnostic problems: cough fracture in osteo-porotic bone should be remembered. Most primary chest wall tumours are not painful, but the more common metastatic disease of bone frequently is, and may be symptomatic before radiological change is evident.

Perhaps the commonest chest pain of all is left inframammary pain. This is a transitory sharp but quite severe pain, felt over the apex of the heart at rest or on mild activity. It lasts up to a few minutes and may cause a catching of the breath or shallow breathing. Its cause is unknown but it seems totally benign.

Sensations arising from the tracheobronchial tree are less easy to characterize as painful though some are exceedingly unpleasant. Instrumentation of the trachea causes pain referred to the anterior chest wall. This is usually abolished by vagotomy and is most likely to be perceived from irritant receptor discharge. Tracheal inflammation, as in infective tracheobronchitis or following the inhalation of toxic vapours, causes a raw painful sensation retrosternally. It is difficult to say how much or how often sensations arising from the main airways are describable as pain. There is often a component of what is described by the patient as tightness. This sensation is a common complaint of patients with generalized airflow obstruction, though it is probably naive to think that the sensation is a direct appreciation of airways narrowing. Further complicating the interpretation of sensation in these conditions is the almost universal association with coughing which of itself if persistent can lead to soreness in the upper airways and trachea.

Finally the mediastinal structures of the thorax are responsible for a multitude of pains the majority of which are dealt with elsewhere in the sections on cardiology and gastrointestinal disease. Myocardial ischaemia, pericarditis, pulmonary embolism, aneurysm, oesophagitis, and referred abdominal pain will all need to be considered in the differential diagnosis of central chest pain. Most have distinctive features that will rarely lead to confusion with the few central pulmonary lesions likely to give mediastinal pain. Besides pain due to inflammatory conditions of the trachea, only neoplasia is a common culprit. A central bronchial carcinoma or hilar nodes associated with it can be responsible for a deep dull aching pain in the centre of the chest. In the early stages of sarcoidosis with hilar lymph adenopathy and in lymphoma a similar pain may occasionally be recorded.

Other pulmonary symptoms

Patients or their relatives on their behalf may complain of noisy breathing, generally using the word wheeze. A harsh inspiratory wheezing sound arising from obstruction in the larynx or major airways is termed stridor. There may be accompanying hoarseness or features of intrathoracic disease. Wheeze is the externally audible counterpart of the rhonchi heard with the stethoscope in asthma and obstructive bronchitis. It is always accompanied by breathlessness and is a term frequently used by asthmatic patients to describe their respiratory distress.

When airflow obstruction is suspected, specific enquiries should be made for the features of bronchial irritability. In response to changes in atmospheric conditions (especially temperature), or to the inhalation of dusts, fumes, or vapours, the patient with irritable bronchi will respond with a variety of symptoms: cough, tightness in the chest, wheeze, or breathlessness.

Patients may rarely complain that they are cyanosed or have finger clubbing: these are more often elicited as physical signs (see below).

General history in the patient with pulmonary disease

A full history is essential emphasizing the following features: (a) the cardiovascular system for features which might indicate cardiac disease as a cause or aggravating factor in breathlessness; (b) the legs for fluid retention (ankle oedema) as a result of lung disease or any suggestion of deep venous thrombosis; (c) the upper respiratory tract for infective or allergic disorders; (d) the skin for a history of eczema or urticaria; (e) the locomotor system or elsewhere for the features of rheumatoid or collagen-vascular disease; (f) the nervous system for the effects of respiratory failure or neuromuscular disease that might impair ventilatory control; and (g) many systems for pointers to metastatic spread or the non-metastatic manifestations of malignant disease.

The past history may reveal atopy or other allergic disease, tuberculosis or other serious infective disease especially in childhood. It is always worth asking about previous chest radiographs which may be obtainable for comparison.

Note must be made of smoking history for its influence as an aetiological factor and alcoholism because of its effects on antibacterial defences. Steroid and immunosuppressive therapy will also depress defences and a detailed drug history is essential because of the wide variety of toxic effects on the lungs which are now recognized (see page 15.141).

A complete occupational and environmental history is of the utmost importance. Whilst the mining industries will be obvious, many other occupations which create dusts of both inorganic and organic materials are now recognized as presenting hazards to the chest (see page 15.116). Certain working environments may lead to exposure to organisms likely to cause pulmonary infection: *Chlamydia psittaci* from contact with domestic or wild birds: *Coxiella burnetti* in slaughterhouses and amongst cattle; tuberculosis through working with immigrants or vagrants.

Finally certain disorders have a familial predisposition. These include asthma and other atopic diseases (see page 15.75), cystic fibrosis (see page 15.101), Kartagener's syndrome (see page 15.100), familial fibrocystic pulmonary dysplasia (a form of fibrosing alveolitis, see page 15.123), pulmonary lymphangio-myomatosis (see page 15.136), and alveolar microlithiasis (see page 15.140). A family or personal contact history of tuberculosis should be noted as should any record of previous tuberculin testing or BCG.

Physical signs in pulmonary disease
Extrathoracic signs
Whilst a full physical examination can reveal several features relevant to the diagnosis and management of pulmonary disease, such as lymphadenopathy, arthropathy, or skin lesions, there are two physical signs of special importance that require description; cyanosis and clubbing.

Cyanosis is the blue discoloration imparted to the nail beds, lips, and tongue by hypoxaemic blood. Peripheral cyanosis due to a sluggish peripheral circulation as in cold weather will leave the tongue still pink, whereas in central cyanosis the tongue will be blue and the peripheries blue yet often warm. The oft repeated statement that it requires 5 g of reduced haemoglobin before cyanosis can be detected is false. A saturation of 87 per cent (2.6 g of reduced Hb) is readily detectable. Cyanosis is less marked in severe anaemia and more obvious in polycythaemia. The curious phenomenon of orthocyanosis (due to hypoxia occurring only in the upright position) is generally associated with pulmonary arteriovenous malformations.

Clubbing of the fingers Loss of the natural angle between the nail and the nail bed in a properly manicured finger, and a boggy fluctuation of the nail bed are cardinal signs of clubbing. An increased curvature to the nail and enlargement of the end of the finger develop later. The toes may also be affected. The differential diagnosis of clubbing of the fingers includes many extrathoracic conditions but, as far as the lungs are concerned, three categories deserve consideration: (a) suppurative disease especially bronchiectasis of long standing and also, acutely, lung abscess and empyema, but not uncomplicated bronchitis; (b) fibrosing alveolitis and asbestosis, but rarely other diffuse fibrotic diseases; and (c) malignant disease especially carcinoma of the bronchus but also pleural malignancy. If finger clubbing is associated with hypertrophic pulmonary ostoarthropathy (HPOA), a painful osteitis of the distal ends of the long bones of the lower arms and legs, then there is associated malignancy in 95 per cent of cases.

There is no totally satisfactory explanation for clubbing and HPOA. Pathologically there is abnormal vascularity and new bone formation in the peripheries, and evidence for abnormal bronchopulmonary anastomoses in the lungs. The latter may be under vagal control since vagotomy has sometimes abolished clubbing in lung cancer patients. These intrathoracic channels may allow through to the systemic circulation substances normally detoxified by the lungs which could be responsible for the peripheral changes. There is evidence to support a role for reduced ferritin in this respect.

Inspection of the chest
The pattern of breathing and the configuration of the chest must be observed. The normal respiratory rate when the subject believes himself to be unobserved is around 10–14 per minute. Higher rates than this are commonly recorded in the healthy but a rate above 20 per minute is abnormal. Pneumonia, many interstitial lung disorders, and abnormal drives to breathing including anxiety will increase rate. If the chest is free to move, tidal volume will increase also, but this is not the case with restrictive disease or painful conditions of the thoracic cage or upper abdomen. An abrupt stop to inspiration when there is pain can be seen. The frequency of deep sighs, normally 8 to 10 per hour in quiet breathing, is greatly increased in psychogenic breathlessness when there may be a quite irregular breathing pattern including phases of rapid breaths or relative apnoea. A regular alternation of apnoeic periods of 5 to 30 or more seconds with a period of increasing and then decreasing ventilation characterizes Cheyne–Stokes respiration. This and several other irregular breathing patterns are usually associated with brainstem or cerebral lesions.

In observing respiratory movement particular attention must be paid to expansion. Poor movement of the chest on one side only always indicates pathology on that side. Generally poor expansion is seen in the hyperinflated chest of the patient with severe airflow obstruction and in the fixed thoracic cage of advanced ankylosing spondylitis. In airflow obstruction two other features may be observed: an indrawing of intercostal spaces during inspiration (reflecting the negative intrapleural pressure necessary to draw air into the lungs), and abnormal movement over the lower chest. Normally the lower chest moves outwards during inspiration. In gross hyperinflation the diaphragm is flat and its contraction merely causes the lower thoracic cage to move inwards. In the same patients the anterior abdominal wall may move inwards during inspiration instead of outwards. This asynchrony of movement carries a poor prognosis.

The configuration of the body as a whole – weight loss or obesity – will be relevant in both reflecting and contributing towards respiratory disorders. Abnormalities of the shape of the chest are well recognized. An increased anteroposterior diameter to give the 'barrel-chest' is as often a sign of the kyphosis that accompanies senile osteoporosis as it is the hyperinflation of emphysema and chronic airflow obstruction. Pectus carinatum (pigeon chest), an outward protuberance of the sternum may reflect severe attacks of asthma in childhood when it may be accompanied by bilateral indrawing of the anterior portions of the lower ribs (Harrison's sulci): it is now rarely due to rickets. The opposite, pectus excavatum (depressed sternum) is a congenital anomaly (see page 15.61). Scoliosis of skeletal origin is of importance because of the severe impairment of respiratory movement it causes and can lead to respiratory failure (see page 15.168). Localized collapse and fibrosis may draw in the adjacent rib cage (which will also move poorly) and, if severe, unilateral fibrosis of the whole lung can cause a scoliosis with its curvature towards the affected lung.

Palpation of the chest

This is used to confirm the observed patterns of chest expansion, and to identify the position of the trachea and apex beat. The trachea should be localized in the suprasternal notch with the index finger. With the patient looking directly forwards, any deviation of the trachea from the mid-line should be assessed using a combination of touch and vision. As with the trachea, the position of the apex beat can reflect pressure against or traction on mediastinal structures, but due consideration must be given to displacement of the apex beat due to intrinsic cardiac disease.

The detection of the transmission of vocal sounds by the placing of the palm of the hand on the chest (vocal fremitus) should be abandoned in favour of vocal resonance (listening with the stethoscope for voice sounds) except for simultaneous comparison of the two sides of the chest.

Percussion of the chest

In properly performed percussion the examiner listens for the pitch and loudness of the percussed note and both listens and feels for the post-percussive vibrations which gives the note its resonance. The sides of the chest must be compared from identical sites. A dull note lacks resonance and is higher in pitch and softer than a normal percussion note: it signifies the presence of solid tissue or fluid underneath the percussed area. A hyperresonant note has these qualities reversed, is more difficult to detect, and occurs over hyperinflated lung or an air filled space.

Auscultation of the chest

Three types of sound can be heard coming from the lung: breath sounds, adventitious sounds, and voice sounds. Normal breath sounds are better termed just this, rather than 'vesicular'. They are certainly not generated in the vesicles or alveoli of the lung where air flow is too low, but probably reflect turbulent flow in major bronchi. The pattern and intensity of breath sounds reflects regional ventilation. Thus in the normal upright lung at the apex breath sounds are loudest in early inspiration and at the bases in mid-inspiration. Breath sounds are quietened over areas of atelectasis. During expiration normal breath sounds rapidly fade out probably due to decreasing air flow rate. Bronchial breathing is heard over airless lung as in consolidation, atelectasis, or dense fibrosis. There is some resemblance to the sounds heard over the normal trachea, but, by comparison with normal breath sounds, bronchial breathing is higher in pitch and more blowing in quality. It does not have to be loud. Bronchial breath sounds are classically heard throughout both inspiration and expiration. Very quiet

breath sounds are heard over hyperinflated lungs as in emphysema or when breath sounds are prevented from reaching the chest wall by a layer of air or fluid (pneumothorax, pleural effusion).

The terminology of adventitious sounds is confused. This arises because whereas Laennec originally used the term *râles* (rattle) to embrace all added sounds, Latham in 1876, introducing the classification dry and moist sounds, applies *râles* exclusively to the former and *rhonchi* to the latter. The established convention in the United Kingdom is to drop *râle* altogether and to call interrupted non-musical sounds crepitations, and continuous musical sounds rhonchi. The move to replace crepitations with the term crackles and rhonchi with wheezes has not gained universal acceptance. Crepitations (or crackles) may be coarse or moist when they are probably due to the movement of sputum in large airways, or fine when they may be created by small airways snapping open as pressures equalize in a distal lung compartment. Coarse early inspiratory and expiratory crepitations are often heard in respiratory tract infection, especially in patients with chronic obstructive lung disease, whilst fine late inspiratory crepitations are characteristic of pulmonary oedema and fibrosing alveolitis. Occasionally a single mid- to late inspiratory 'squawk' is heard in patients with a variety of pulmonary fibroses.

Rhonchi (or wheezes) signify obstruction in airways. A sound of single pitch (monophonic) in inspiration and/or expiration that cannot be altered by coughing to shift mucus, signifies localized obstruction in a major airway. Several sounds of varying pitch (polyphonic) heard randomly in inspiration and expiration are typical of the widespread airways obstruction of asthma and chronic obstructive bronchitis. A polyphonic wheeze on forced expiration signifies diffuse airflow obstruction and can be a useful sign when tidal breathing is free of rhonchi.

The only other added sound, a pleural rub, is a superficial grating noise heard over an area of pleurisy (see below).

Voice sounds (a long sound such as 'ninety-nine' is favoured) are transmitted by normal lung but not by air space or fluid, and pass through solid lung with undue clarity, even allowing whispered sounds to be heard (whispering pectoriloquy). Certain physical characteristics of solid lung allow low frequency sounds to be filtered out leaving a sound of bleating or nasal quality (aegophony): this is especially noticeable over the top of a pleural effusion (see page 15.55).

Common presentations in respiratory disease

The ways in which a patient with pulmonary disease presents to the clinician are threefold; with one or more of the symptoms of respiratory disease already described; with a radiological abnormality; or with extrapulmonary symptoms that are due to or part of a syndrome that includes pulmonary disease.

Presentation with cough, breathlessness, or chest pain as sole or predominant symptom has been discussed. By combining symptoms with physical signs and radiology, certain well defined syndromes can be recognized: (*a*) the syndrome of respiratory tract infection with its subgroups recurrent infections and the slowly resolving pneumonia; these are discussed below and further referred to on page 15.91; (*b*) the syndrome of airways obstruction considered on page 15.84; (*c*) the syndrome characterized by a presentation with chest pain and breathlessness of which pneumothorax and pleural effusion are described in this section; and (*d*) the syndromes of solid lung, consolidation, and atelectasis which are also described below.

Occasionally radiological abnormalities may be the presenting feature of respiratory disease rather than a part of the assessment of a patient with respiratory symptoms. Two appearances which are especially likely to be picked up on routine or coincidental chest radiology are the solitary pulmonary nodule (page 15.16) and diffuse widespread radiological change (page 15.117).

Finally acute and chronic respiratory failure (see page 15.167), sleep apnoea (see page 15.156), cor pulmonale (see page 13.350), and secondary polycythaemia (see page 19.155) produce non-pulmonary symptoms but are of primary importance as manifestations of lung disease, and many generalized disorders (especially collagen-vascular diseases and malignancy) may have pulmonary disease as part of their clinical presentation.

The syndromes of respiratory tract infection

Respiratory tract infection is suggested by a combination of features pointing to infection *per se* together with others localizing infection to a site in the respiratory tract. Systemic upset, malaise, fever, and sweating are present if the infection causes toxaemia, a likely accompaniment to deep parenchymal infection of the lung as in pneumonia (and with some upper respiratory tract infections) but less commonly seen with uncomplicated bronchial infection. Mucopurulent sputum production whilst inevitable with bronchial infection may be absent, especially in the early stages of pneumonia and when infection is loculated in the lung or pleural space. The site of infection may be localized by the symptom of pain, soreness in the throat in pharyngitis, a retrosternal rawness in tracheitis and pleuritic pain with pneumonia, and by physical and radiological signs details of which are given elsewhere in this chapter and on page 15.71. The frequently expressed disappointment with physical signs which appear negligible in relation to extensive radiological shadowing is only partly due to undue reliance being placed on radiology at the expense of clinical skills in examination. To give the classical signs of consolidation an extensive alveolar exudate is required. Very often pneumonia is patchy or to a significant extent interstitial. Crepitations without other abnormality may be the only localizing feature on clinical examination.

In chronic respiratory tract infection, systemic features take the form of weight loss, fatigue, and anorexia often with low grade or recurrent fever. Physical signs in the chest are variable depending on the site of infection, often being minimal with tuberculosis: in bronchiectasis the crepitations are usually coarse and have been described as 'leathery'. Clubbing may occasionally be seen subacutely (developing over a few weeks) in lung abscess and empyema, and is a characteristic feature of bronchiectasis.

A combination of symptoms, signs, and radiology can define a series of syndromes of respiratory tract infection as listed in Table 4. Some are obvious on symptoms alone, others are only revealed radiologically. Further details of these syndromes are found elsewhere in this textbook.

An integral part of the clinical assessment of the patient with respiratory tract infection is an attempt to predict the causative organism from clues given in the history, the physical signs, and the radiographic appearances.

Specific historical clues can be knowledge of a prevailing epidemic of infection in the area e.g. influenza, or circumstantial clues such as contact with birds to give psittacosis. A history of contact by the patient with other individuals who might also have respiratory tract infection may provide useful aetiological clues, the technique of contact tracing being most extensively applied in the search for a source of infection or for transmission of tuberculosis (see page 5.289).

Micro-organisms which invade the lungs are not always inhaled from the environment. Some, especially pneumococci and

Haemophilus influenzae, reside in a relatively saprophytic way in the airways of those with some abnormality in local pulmonary defence mechanisms. These organisms can certainly be cultured from the bronchi of otherwise healthy chronic smokers and their clearance is impaired, particularly when there is associated airflow obstruction. Similar problems arise in those with asthma, bronchiectasis, and fibrosing alveolitis. A relatively minor, usually viral, infection can upset the balance between host defences and these resident organisms which then become locally invasive. Other internal sources of organisms which can cause lower respiratory tract infection are the oropharynx and oesophagus, both by aspiration, the abdomen by transdiaphragmatic spread from hepatic or subphrenic abscess, and also the skin and venous cannulae.

The soil into which an infecting organism is sown plays an important part in determining not only the extent of the infection, but also the type of organism likely to gain hold. The important distinction between a primary pneumonia – that occurring in a previously healthy individual – and a secondary pneumonia in which some predisposing feature influences the development of the infection, is considered in more detail on page 15.93. Inborn or acquired abnormalities of antibacterial defences as well as iatrogenic immunosuppression necessary to the management of patients with organ transplants and those receiving chemotherapy for malignant and other disorders, produce the most dramatic examples of exotic and rampant infection. Suppression of antibacterial defences is also seen to a great or lesser extent in a wide variety of diseases, for example, in the congested lungs of those with heart failure and in those with systemic lupus erythematosus or rheumatoid disease. In cystic fibrosis staphylococci and, at times, psuedomonas reside in the bronchiectatic cavities and can invade lung tissue. In diabetes there is an association with tuberculosis. The alcoholic is prone to pneumococcal and to severe gram-negative bacterial pneumonias, and the drug addict to metastatic streptococcal lung abscesses. Extreme non-specific insults, exposure to cold, malnutrition, prematurity, and debility in the elderly all increase the likelihood of serious chest infections.

Whilst consideration of the above points from the clinical history can give important clues, the physical examination of the patient is relatively unrewarding in terms of identifying the type of infecting organism. *Herpes labialis* is very suggestive of pneumococcal infection and a general examination may reveal potential sources of endogenous infection. Features of septicaemia and toxaemia merely point in a general way to serious acute bacterial rather than viral infection. Confusion and other pointers to cerebral dysfunction can accompany pneumococcal and legionella infection.

Investigations that point to a specific infection rather than suggesting infection *per se* (e.g. leucocytosis) include the presence of cold agglutinins for mycoplasma infection, hypokalaemia for legionella, and deranged liver function tests in pneumococcal septicaemia. However, abnormalities such as the latter may just reflect underlying disease and so are unreliable.

Though clues such as those described above may suggest a particular infection, it is fundamental to the proper management of respiratory tract infections that attempts are made to establish a precise microbiological diagnosis. Material from the respiratory tract is most readily obtained from expectorated sputum. This will, however, be unreliable if the invading organism can be an oropharyngeal contaminant, and unrewarding if antibiotics have already been given. If pulmonary parenchymal infection with organisms that can be found in the mouth is suspected, or if the patient can produce no sputum even with the aid of physiotherapy, then there are three possible approaches. These are (*a*) transtracheal aspiration through the cricothyroid membrane with or without the injection of a few ml of normal saline; (*b*) fibre-optic bronchoscopy (see page 15.9), though even here care has to be taken to avoid oropharyngeal contamination; and (*c*) percutaneous lung aspiration with a fine bore needle. Though each technique carries certain inconveniences and complications, the use of .

Table 4 Syndromes of respiratory tract infection

Upper respiratory tract	Lower respiratory tract
Coryza	Acute tracheitis
Acute pharyngitis/tonsilitis	Acute bronchitis
Quinsy	Acute bronchiolitis
Acute epiglotitis	Pneumonitis
Acute laryngitis	Pneumonia
	Lung abscess
	Pleurisy
	Empyema

these invasive methods should probably be more widely used in the investigation of serious pneumonic chest infections. Any pleural fluid present should be aspirated and cultured, and blood culture should never be neglected.

Non-bacterial infections may be diagnosed from serological evidence as discussed elsewhere under specific infections, and indirect evidence of present or past infection may be obtained by appropriate cutaneous sensitivity tests.

Chest pain with breathlessness

Pulmonary syndromes characterized by chest pain and breathlessness with absent or minimal cough, mostly involve the pleura; pneumothorax, pleural effusion, and early pneumonia. Pulmonary embolism (see page 13.355) and myocardial infarction (see page 13.167) both dealt with elsewhere, enter into the differential diagnosis.

Pneumothorax

A leak of air into the pleural space produces an immediate sensation which may be so slight as to be described as a twinge or discomfort, or such a severe sharp tearing pain that the patient fears imminent death. Occasionally central chest pain radiating to the neck mimics a myocardial infarction. Persisting pain after this usually has a pleuritic quality and may be especially noticeable when the lung has almost reinflated.

Breathlessness may be noticed only as a modest limitation in exercise tolerance, but is commonly marked, initially as a sudden tachypnoea concurrent with the pain. Even a modest pneumothorax in a patient with pre-existing lung disease can cause a sharp increase in breathlessness.

The physical signs of air in the pleural cavity are hyper-resonance with silence. The decreased or absent movement of the affected side of the chest gives the first clue. The percussion note is hyper-resonant, but many find this aberration more difficult to detect than dullness. Breath sounds are quiet, or in a large pneumothorax absent, apart from the distant muffled sounds of the other lung. A clicking sound may be heard synchronously with the heart beat in left-sided pneumothorax (Hamman's sign). At times any sounds transmitted through the air-filled cavity can have a metallic quality. This is the basis of the coin or bell test in which sounds produced on one side of the chest by tapping one coin with another, are listened for on the other side: the test may be equally well done with finger percussion.

A plain postero-anterior chest radiograph is mandatory whenever a pneumothorax is suspected. Air rises, so that the upper lobe is the first to collapse. The extent of the pneumothorax is determined by identifying the line of the visceral pleura. Interestingly with a small pneumothorax, because blood flow in the lung reflexly decreases with collapse, the density of lung tissue is little altered. Only with a large pneumothorax does the collapsed lung appear as a dense clump of tissue close to the hilum and lower mediastinum. A lateral view is only required if the air seems to be loculated: the lateral decubitus view may show up a small pneumothorax. So will an expiration film. This view, though frequently requested, is seldom necessary unless a small pneumothorax is likely to be important clinically because of serious pre-existing chest disease. The important radiographic differential diagnoses are a large emphysematous bulla, obstructive emphysema, and congenital unilateral emphysema.

Additional features which must be sought on physical examination and radiology are those which signify the type of pneumothorax, point to complications, or reveal evidence of causative pathology.

Clinical progress depends on the size and extent of the tear and of any underlying pathology. A small tear often seals when the lung collapses. With no further leak, the pneumothorax is described as closed and there is gradual clinical recovery. Alternatively, especially in association with pre-existing pathology, there is a persistent leak (an 'open' pneumothorax) creating a bronchopleural fistula. The lung remains deflated with persistent symptoms and recovery is impossible without intervention. The most critical situation clinically is the development of a valve mechanism, the tear opening during inspiration but flapping closed during expiration. Pressure builds up in the pleural space, giving a tension pneumothorax. There is suffocating dyspnoea and extreme anxiety. The mediastinal structures move away from the affected side and eventually there is cardiovascular collapse: a medical emergency.

Other dangerous complications of pneumothorax are bilateral pneumothorax, rapidly fatal if not recognized, and haemopneumothorax due to the tearing of a blood vessel in an adhesion, or to any form of trauma. Haemopneumothorax is rare, occurring in not more than 5 per cent of all pneumothoraces. A sudden cardiovascular collapse ('haemorrhagic shock') in a patient with pneumothorax should suggest this complication if tension pneumothorax has been excluded. Fluid in a pneumothorax cavity is detectable clinically by basal dullness which shifts with the patient's position, a succussion splash, and a horizontal line outlining the opaque fluid on the chest radiograph. Besides blood the fluid may be serous (hydropneumothorax) or purulent (pyopneumothorax). Previously seen in pyogenic and tuberculous infection these complications are now more likely to signify underlying neoplasia.

Air escaping through into the tissues of the chest wall, neck and sometimes beyond is recognizable clinically by the swelling it causes, and the crinkling sensation given on palpation. This subcutaneous emphysema appears as linear translucent streaks on the chest radiograph. The latter may also reveal mediastinal emphysema.

Most pneumothoraces are spontaneous. The alternatives are artificial and traumatic. Artificial pneumothorax, once in common use as an aid to the healing of tuberculous cavities, is now used only for specialized pleural radiology or thoracoscopy. Thoracic wall trauma can be associated with pneumothorax following penetrating injury, fractured ribs, or ruptured bronchus. Pneumothorax is an inevitable accompaniment to thoracotomy, and an accidental complication of pleural or lung biopsy, or large vein cannulation.

Spontaneous pneumothorax can itself be divided into two categories. In the one, sometimes known as benign pneumothorax or pneumothorax simplex, there is clinically inapparent or unimportant lung disease. In the other the pneumothorax is symptomatic of a large variety of often serious pulmonary disorders.

Benign pneumothorax occurs chiefly in young men aged 20–40 years with an incidence averaging about 10 per 100 000 population per year. Male to female sex ratio is 5 to 6 to 1 and affected individuals are often tall and asthenic. The underlying lesion is usually a small apical bulla or bleb perhaps situated in an area of minor fibrosis, sometimes suggesting a congenital malformation of a few distal lobules. Whilst it is often commented that sudden movement or the lifting of heavy objects induces pneumothorax in these individuals, there is no clear proof of this.

Pneumothorax may be symptomatic of localized or generalized intrapulmonary disease. The emphasis given previously to tuberculosis as a cause is quite unplaced now. Primary (bronchial or oesophageal) neoplasms or metastatic deposits are more likely candidates for a pneumothorax caused by localized disease. Subpleural deposits from sarcomas and metastatic abscesses, especially staphylococcal, feature here. But the majority of symptomatic pneumothoraces are related to diffuse disease, predominantly emphysema and asthma. A sudden symptomatic deterioration into more severe breathlessness or the unexplained onset of respiratory failure in this type of patient should suggest pneumothorax. Diffuse fibrotic pulmonary disease especially when this leads to honey-combing can be complicated by pneumothorax. The list is long and includes fibrosing alveolitis (see page 15.123), sarcoid (see page 5.623), and certain pneumoconioses (see page 15.109), as well as rarities such as Hand–Schuller–Christian disease, neurofibromatosis, lymphangio-myomatosis, and tuberous sclerosis. A curiosity is the occurrence of a usually left-sided pneumothorax in women at the time of the menstrual cycle (catamenial pneumothorax). The underlying pathology seems to be endometriosis. Generalized disorders of connective tissue such as Marfan's syndrome and Ehlers–Danlos syndrome are associated with an increased incidence of pneumothorax.

Various considerations determine what action is taken. A pneumothorax that occupies less than 20 per cent of the unilateral thoracic area, occurring in an asymptomatic young patient in a sedentary occupation, can safely be left to seal itself. Most of these will disappear within six weeks. Symptoms, complications, underlying disease, or a need to get back to full activity will all swing the decision towards drainage. In uncomplicated pneumothorax simple aspiration of the air using an intravenous cannula syringe and three-way tap is often sufficient and can be repeated. However, the standard procedure is to insert under local anaesthesia, an Argyl or Malecot catheter in the 4th or 5th intercostal space in the axilla or in the 2nd intercostal space anteriorly (Fig. 1). The underwater seal, though it slightly limits mobility, is usually preferable to mechanical one-way valves which quite easily become clogged with secretions. Posturing or occasionally a second drain may help clear a persistent pocket of air. The value of suction is much debated. It does seem to assist reinflation in some instances, but it is unlikely that any pump in current use can cope with the flow likely through a bronchopleural fistula. Too rapid reinflation can lead to unilateral pulmonary oedema in the affected lung. If the air in the pleural space can be replaced by oxygen in the early stages, its absorption after the tear has healed will probably be quicker, but this artifice is seldom employed.

Tension pneumothorax is a medical emergency and demands the urgent insertion through the anterior chest of whatever needle or cannula is immediately to hand. After the hiss of escaping air has died down and the cardiovascular state recovered, formal tube drainage can be instituted.

Tube drainage is continued till all bubbling of air has ceased for 24–48 hours. Ensuring that this is not due to a blocked tube, the tube is then clamped. Radiographic check is made to ensure the lung remains inflated. The tube can then be removed.

Recurrence of pneumothorax is not infrequent; 1 in 6 to 9 if

treated by tube drainage and up to 1 in 3 if there has been no intervention. At the second tube drainage an attempt may be made to excite a pleural reaction. When they were available, red rubber tubes used for drainage served this purpose: modern plastics are too inert. The patient's own blood, tetracycline, iodized talc, and mepacrine have all been used with varying success rates and varying discomfort to the patient, though the latter can be avoided with prior intrapleural local anaesthesia.

A third pneumothorax on one side or a persistent pneumothorax after two to three weeks tube drainage generally calls for thoracic surgery. The pleural surface may be abraided with gauze swabs (pleuradesis) or inflamed with silver nitrate (very painful), or the parietal pleura may be removed over the thoracic wall (pleurectomy). An emphysematous bleb can be undersewn or a diseased segment resected. Recurrence rate after pleurectomy is near zero.

Pleurisy and pleural effusion

The sharp stabbing pain of classical pleurisy (see page 15.50) is readily recognized. In pleural effusion this pain is absent and a slowly developing pleural effusion may be painless throughout until it causes local discomfort by virtue of its size. An acute pleurisy will engender respiratory distress by the pain it causes with respiratory movement, and there is some breathlessness with all but the smallest effusions. A very large effusion produces a suffocating breathlessness.

The clinical recognition of a pleural effusion depends on the combination of dullness to percussion with quiet breath sounds. The affected side moves poorly if at all but is not collapsed inwards. In effusions of sufficient size, the apex beat is displaced away from the affected side. Percussion note is classically dull. Provided the fluid is free to move in the pleural cavity, the area of dullness is determined by gravitational forces and not, as in lobar consolidation, delineated by anatomical boundaries. It requires a fine ear to pick up Ellis' S-shaped line: a slightly higher level of dullness in the axilla when the patient is in the sitting position. Large effusions which displace mediastinal contents may produce an area of dullness at the opposite base close to the mid-line (Grocco's sign). Breath sounds are quiet but often have a bronchial character. This is especially so over the upper border of the effusion beneath which there will nearly always be compressed and rather solid lung, but if there is underlying consolidation bronchial breathing may be more widespread over the effusion. Likewise there may be an area of aegophony: it is instructive to listen for the quality of voice sounds as the stethoscope is moved progressively down the thorax. From normal sounds above the effusion there follows aegophony over the edge of the effusion and then a gradual loss of sounds further down to the base where the effusion is deepest. The diagnostic added sound of pleurisy is the pleural rub, a superficial grating or rasping sound synchronous with late inspiration and early expiration, best heard at the bases and rarely at the apices. A soft friction rub may be mistaken for crepitations but is not altered by coughing: it can be made louder by pressure with the stethoscope. Inflammation of the pleura close to the heart can give a friction rub that synchronizes with the heart beat but it will cease if the breath is held.

The distribution of these signs will not follow a classic pattern if the effusion is loculated, and if fluid is only present in the fissures none of these signs will be found. Any underlying disease whether responsible itself for the effusion (pneumonia, neoplasm) or not, may contribute to the observed signs, so confusing the diagnostic criteria. The not uncommon occurrence of bilateral effusions must be remembered.

The normal pleural space contains a very little fluid: most estimates state about 5 ml each side and certainly no more than 20 ml. It has the electrolyte composition of interstitial fluid and a low protein content. There is evidence that it is formed by the parietal pleura and absorbed by the visceral pleura. There is probably a continual flux of fluid through the pleural space with its exact

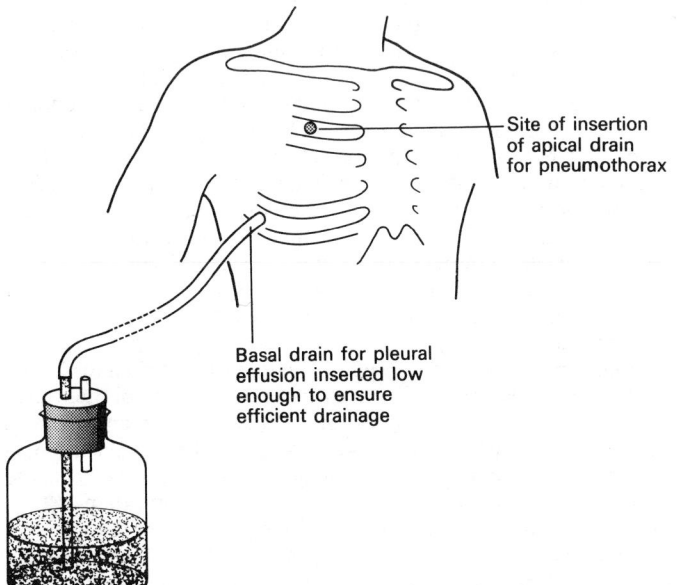

Site of insertion of apical drain for pneumothorax

Basal drain for pleural effusion inserted low enough to ensure efficient drainage

Fig. 1 Standard drainage sites for pneumothorax and pleural effusion with illustration of underwater seal device.

amount depending on hydrostatic and osmotic forces and lymphatic drainage. Thus an accumulation of fluid can form if these forces are upset, haemodynamically as in heart failure or osmotically in hypoalbuminaemic states such as the nephrotic syndrome or malnutrition. Impaired lymphatic drainage due to developmental, traumatic, or neoplastic abnormalities of major lymph vessels especially the thoracic duct will lead to fluid accumulation in the pleural space. But the majority of pleural effusions are related to increased capillary permeability in response to inflammation (both infective and other), to ischaemia (as in pulmonary infarction), and to neoplastic infiltration.

The diagnostic approach to the pleural effusion is three-pronged. The clinical findings will give some clues. Radiology will define the extent and localization of the fluid, and may point to other pulmonary and sometimes extrapulmonary disease which may be responsible. Thirdly the fluid itself must be examined cytologically, microbiologically, and biochemically.

In analysing pleural effusions it is useful to think clinically of categories of causative condition because the presentation of disease is as likely to be with general features of the disorder as with those directly attributable to the effusion. Thus malaise and fever will point to an infective aetiology, cardiac symptoms or oedema to a pleural transudate, and arthropathy to collagen-vascular disease. Trauma and abdominal conditions should give distinctive symptoms and signs, and malignancy whether primarily intrathoracic or metastatic from elsewhere will inevitably make itself known at some stage.

Radiology both of the thorax and elsewhere will help confirm many of these clinical pointers. If a pleural effusion is discovered without any radiological clues, then it is likely to be due to tuberculosis (see page 5.289), mesothelioma (see page 15.157), small deposits of other intrathoracic malignancies, or to Meig's syndrome. This rare syndrome occurs in women and consists of pleural effusion (usually right-sided, less often left or bilateral) in association with a pelvic tumour. The latter is usually ovarian and frequently benign (ovarian fibroma, thecoma, etc.) or less frequently adenocarcinoma. The fluid is usually a transudate and the mechanism of its formation is disputed. Removal of the pelvic tumour in Meig's syndrome leads to resolution of the hydrothorax.

Bilateral pleural effusions suggest initially the formation of transudates from an extrathoracic cause. Pleural effusions are commonly found in heart failure and the nephrotic syndrome and less frequently in acute glomerulonephritis, uraemia, hepatic cirrhosis, and myxoedema, and in all these examples the fluid may be bilateral. There is, however, a predilection for the right side which may alone be involved. In some instances an actual gap in the diaphragm has been demonstrated. It has been said that the appearance of a left-sided effusion alone in a patient with heart failure should prompt a search for an alternative cause, for example, pulmonary infarction. If heart size is normal in a patient with bilateral effusions, then almost half will be due to malignancy, usually metastatic cancer (from breast or an intra-abdominal primary) or lymphoma. Pleural effusion is a not infrequent finding in lymphoma and leukaemia: a variable proportion appear to be due to lymphatic blockage from enlarged hilar and mediastinal nodes, but venous obstruction, direct infiltration of the pleura, and infection also account for some cases.

Pleural fluid may appear to the naked eye clear and of a variable yellow or straw colour, cloudy or frankly purulent (empyema), blood stained (haemothorax), or opalescent (chylothorax). Sufficient fluid may be removed for diagnostic purposes using a 20 or 30 ml syringe and a 21 gauge needle. All necessary investigations can be carried out on this volume except specific gravity (SG). This physical characteristic has been used to distinguish between transudates and exudates using the figure of 1.016 as the dividing line. Yet up to 30 per cent of pleural transudates associated with heart failure have been shown to have an SG of greater than this, and as many exudates a lower figure.

The distinction between a transudate and an exudate is often obvious on simple clinical grounds but when this fails and important management decisions rest on an answer to this question, other tests may help. The discriminative power of the fluid protein content, using a dividing line of 30 g/litre leads to a lower misclassification rate than SG, though still around 10 per cent. An improved discrimination can be achieved by considering also the pleural fluid lactic dehydrogenase (LDH) level. A figure of in excess of 200 IU or a pleural fluid to serum LDH ratio of greater than 0.6 points to an exudate.

The cytological findings in pleural fluid in benign effusions are rarely absolutely diagnostic but are of greater value in malignant disease. A light cell content of chiefly mesothelial cell derived from the pleural lining, and macrophages (a mixture of phagocytic cells from various sources) characterizes a transudate. Mesothelial cells showing histological signs of activity are present in most exudates but can predominate (more than 70 per cent) in pulmonary infarct effusion, and are very scarce in tuberculous effusions and empyema. Macrophages are found to a variable extent in all effusions. Well preserved neutrophil polymorphonuclear leucocytes are frequent in sterile inflammatory effusions and predominate in infected effusions showing degenerate forms in empyema pus. The exception to this pattern is tuberculosis, where, although in the very early stages there may be a neutrophil excess, very quickly lymphocytes come to predominate constituting 80–100 per cent of all cells examined. Such a high lymphocyte count is only rarely encountered in chronic infections of other origins but may sometimes be seen in malignant (especially lymphomatous) effusions where, however, accompanying mesothelial cells are likely. A high eosinophil count in pleural fluid always raises expectations of a specific diagnosis. This hope is unfounded. In two-thirds of instances where eosinophils make up more than 20 per cent of the cells, air or blood has been allowed into the pleural cavity (spontaneous pneumothorax, trauma, surgery, etc.) and in a miscellaneous remainder pulmonary infarct and malignancy figure more than any 'allergic' disorder.

Malignant cells are found in pleural fluid when there is invasion of the pleural cavity by growth. In any series of cases with effusion and malignant disease, lymphatic block will be responsible for fluid formation in some. The reported positivity rate for the cytological diagnosis of malignancy in pleural fluid of around 60 per cent therefore represents a reasonable though by no means totally satisfactory situation. Malignant cells are only reliably recognized by an experienced cytologist. They tend to be of large size with a high nuclear to cytoplasmic ratio showing a uniformity of appearance, mitoses, and a tendency to clump. It is often possible to designate their cell type or even suggest an extrapulmonary origin.

Culture of pleural fluid is, like that of sputum, often disappointing. This, more than anything, is likely to be due to examining the fluid at a late stage after antibiotics have already been given. Failure to culture for anaerobes is again a fault. *Mycobacterium tuberculosis* is very rarely cultured from a tuberculous effusion. Despite this, most infective effusions and empyemas (see page 15.104) will be due to bacteria rather than other organisms. *Mycoplasma pneumoniae* can occasionally give a pleural effusion, viruses almost never do and of the parasites only *Entamoeba histolytica* features at all frequently.

Other characteristics in pleural fluid can be of diagnostic and even of prognostic help. An acid pleural effusion (pH less than 7.10) carries a risk of progression to loculation or empyema in parapneumonic effusions. A low pH may also be recorded in tuberculous effusions whereas malignant effusions (which can also be lymphocytic) are more likely to have a pH greater than 7.40. A low pleural fluid glucose (less than 30 mg/100 ml) in the face of a normal blood glucose strongly suggests rheumatoid disease being present in three-quarters of effusions associated with this condition. However, low fluid glucose has also been recorded in tuberculosis, malignancy, and empyema. The left-sided pleural effusion that can be associated with pancreatitis almost invariably has a high amylase content. Adenosine deaminase activity is high in tuberculous effusions (greater than 30 IU/l) and apparently in no others, and lysozyme is raised in chronic infection (tuberculosis, empyema) but these tests are rarely applied in routine clinical practice.

Tests on pleural fluid in rheumatoid arthritis and systemic lupus erythematosus have sometimes given a positive rheumatoid factor or antinuclear factor, or low complement levels but results have not been consistent.

Blood in pleural fluid is not uncommon. Setting aside accidental haemorrhage during pleural aspiration, a count of less than 10 000 red blood cells/ml is not diagnostic but counts above 100 000 cells/ml are only seen in malignancy, pulmonary infarction and trauma.

The therapeutic aspiration of a pleural effusion should be done under generous local anaesthesia. The patient should be seated leaning slightly forwards and with the head and arms comfortably supported. The needle must be of sufficient bore to allow fluid of any consistency (including pus) to be aspirated easily. If a pleural biopsy is required (as it almost always is at a first therapeutic tap), then the Abrams needle should be used for aspiration as well as biopsy (see page 15.9). A syringe of at least 50 ml size saves time and effort.

The indications for continuous tube drainage are empyema and malignant effusion. In empyema open drainage may be used with antibiotic or antiseptic instillation. Several techniques recommended for the treatment of malignant effusions require open drainage to empty the pleural space as much as possible both before and after the instillation of cytotoxic or sclerosing solutions.

Empyema. This is the presence of pus in the pleural space. The fluid is frequently loculated. The aetiology and management of empyema is discussed on page 15.104.

Chylothorax. Subdiaphragmatic and left-sided thoracic lymph drains up the thoracic duct. Damage to or disease of the thoracic duct in the thorax leads to the leakage of lymph into the pleural space, a chylothorax. The fluid is white and contains fat.

The clinical features are those of a rapidly developing pleural effusion. Though there may be a latent period of about a week and rarely longer before sufficient fluid accumulates to make itself obvious, after aspiration rapid reaccumulation is the rule. Vital nutrients are removed in the aspirated pleural fluid and weight loss and malnutrition are dangers.

The condition is rare. Various traumatic causes are described: hyperextension of the spine, blunt injury to the thoracic cage, the strain of severe coughing or vomiting, and rarely knife or gun shot wounds. The thoracic duct may be unwittingly severed in upper thoracic surgery. The commonest non-traumatic cause of chylothorax is intrathoracic malignancy involving the thoracic duct or subclavian artery. Benign lymph node or vascular conditions including congenital malformations and filarial infestation may lead to chylothorax, and it has been described in more than a third of patients with lymphangiomyomatosis (see page 15.136).

A true chylothorax in which lymph accumulates in the thoracic cavity is to be distinguished from other milky white effusions. The transformation of degenerating cells into cholesterol (pseudochylous) or fat globules (chyliform) is seen in fluid collections of long standing of many origins, but especially in tuberculous and malignant effusions.

Chronic pleural thickening. After haemothorax and empyema (especially that due to tuberculosis) the pleura may heal by fibrosis producing a plaque of tissue up to 2 cm in thickness and occasionally encasing the whole lung. In severe cases there is dras-

tic reduction in lung volume with impairment of lung function. Considerable restoration of function can follow decortication.

Bilateral pleural thickening is rarely seen after uraemia but is a consistent feature of asbestosis. The latter and other pleural conditions associated with exposure to asbestos are dealt with elsewhere (asbestosis, page 15.113; pleural plaques and mesothelioma, page 15.157).

Consolidation and atelectasis

These two syndromes depend for their detection on physical signs supported by radiological findings. The symptoms which cause these patients to present vary widely with the causative condition. Consolidation and atelectasis are not traditionally considered together but whilst there are certain instances where there is either pure consolidation or pure atelectasis very often there is a mixture of the two.

Consolidation refers to an airless state of the lung due to the filling of the alveolar space with exudate or cellular material. The bronchi remain patent and the overall size of the lobe or segment is unaltered. The physical signs of consolidation are reduced movement over the affected area of lung with a dull percussion note and bronchial breathing. The dulling of the percussion note is not as marked as that in pleural effusion. The bronchial breathing is most marked over the deepest parts of the consolidation and may be quite harsh in quality: it can be associated with aegophony and whispering pectoriloquy. Yet in other instances of indisputable consolidation, bronchial breathing is never heard, often because the relevant bronchus is blocked. In lobar consolidation the physical signs delineate the surface markings of the affected lobe.

Atelectasis refers to an airless state of the lung due to the collapse of distal bronchi and alveoli beyond a site of bronchial obstruction. The volume of the affected lobe or segment therefore shrinks and surrounding lung is pulled on to fill the void (compensatory emphysema). The physical signs of atelectasis are reduced movement over the affected area of lung with a dull percussion note and quiet or absent breath sounds. Vocal resonance will be impaired. The trachea will be deviated towards a collapsed upper lobe, and the apex beat towards a collapsed lower lobe. With complete atelectasis of a lobe the collapsed lung shrinks right up against the mediastinal structures giving minimal physical signs on the surface of the thoracic cage and so making the lesion very difficult to detect clinically.

The combination of consolidation with atelectasis occurs when there is mucus impaction in a bronchus draining a pneumonic lobe or segment, where enlarged lymph nodes at the hilum press on a draining bronchus, or when infection builds up behind a bronchial obstruction. Though many instances of the latter will be malignant, benign lesions – endobronchial sarcoidosis, amyloidosis, adenomas, and especially in the young, foreign bodies – must never be forgotten.

Further confusion is injected into the interpretation of physical signs when a pleural effusion complicates pneumonia or a malignant mass. Radiology, can help sort out these cases.

References

Forgacs, P. (1977). *Lung sounds*. Ballière Tindall, London.
Lane, D. J. (ed.) (1976). *Tutorials in post-graduate medicine*, Vol. 5. *Respiratory disease*, Heinemann, London.
Scadding, J. G. and Cumming, G. (1981). *Scientific foundations of respiratory medicine*. Heinemann, London.

STRUCTURAL DISORDERS OF THE THORACIC CAGE AND LUNGS

C. OGILVIE

This section deals with structural faults in the thoracic cage and lungs. For convenience, these will be described under anatomical headings although their clinical importance relates more to functional disorder than to structural distortion.

The spinal column

Our main concern here is with thoracic spinal disorders which disturb respiratory function. Other diseases of the spine and neuromuscular causes for respiratory failure are dealt with elsewhere. Abnormalities of the vertebral column directly impair respiration if they interfere with the mechanical action of the ribs and diaphragm or prevent full expansion of the lungs. Scoliosis and ankylosing spondylitis have these effects but kyphosis alone has little clinical impact on respiration and will not be considered further here.

Scoliosis

Aetiology

Scoliosis is a lateral curvature of the vertebral column, sometimes accompanied by a backward curvature (kyphoscoliosis) or by rotation. Scoliosis may be functional or structural.

Functional scoliosis is reversible, the curvature being abolished by forward flexion of the spine. It may result from faulty posture

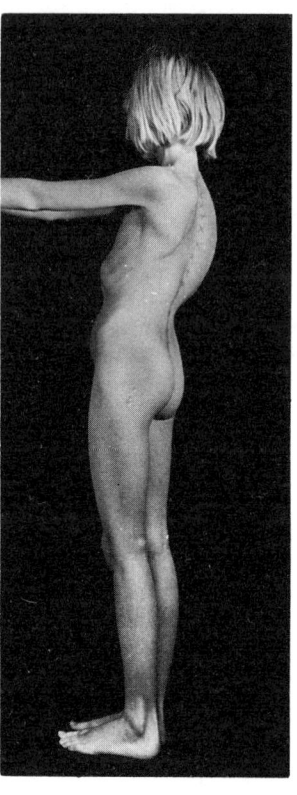

Fig. 2 Thoracic scoliosis: the ribs are prominent on the convex side of the curvature posteriorly and the concave side anteriorly (see also Fig. 1).

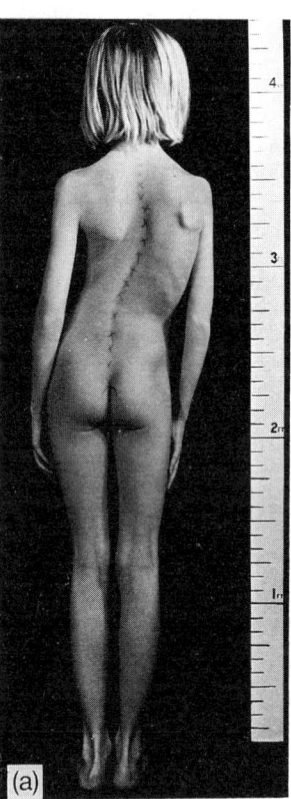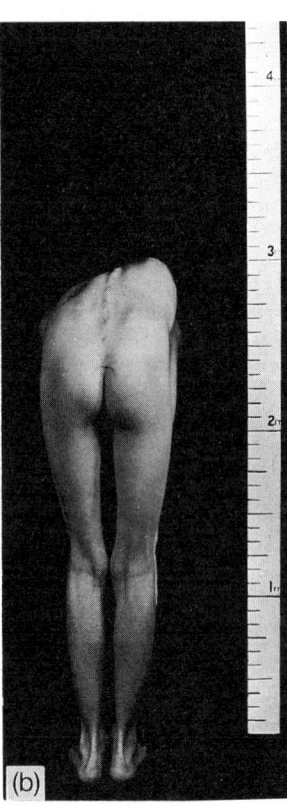

Fig. 1 (a) Mid-thoracic scoliosis in an eleven-year-old girl. (b) On forward bending, the curvature persists with a rib hump (not a kyphus) on the convex side.

as, for example, when there is inequality of leg length. There is no structural abnormality of the vertebrae, the curvature is not progressive, and there are no respiratory symptoms.

Structural scoliosis is irreversible and not abolished by forward flexion of the spine (Fig. 1). There may be rotation and wedging or other deformities of the affected vertebrae and the condition can progress to respiratory or cardiac failure in middle life. Congenital vertebral anomalies account for about 15 per cent of these cases and a further 15 per cent are due to or associated with neuromuscular disorders: poliomyelitis, muscular dystrophy, or congenital conditions such as neurofibromatosis, syringomyelia, and Friedreich's ataxia. Structural scoliosis occasionally results from surgical or other trauma to one side of the chest, gross pulmonary fibrosis, metabolic bone disease or vertebral tumours.

In about two-thirds of all patients presenting with scoliosis, the aetiology is not apparent but the clinical picture is sufficiently consistent to suggest some common pathogenetic factors. Unless otherwise stated, the account which follows applies especially to this so-called idiopathic form of the disease.

Clinical features

The idiopathic type of scoliosis develops during the period of spinal growth and may present at any time from infancy to adolescence. It is commonest in girls from 10 to 15 years of age and is often noticed first by the mother when helping her child to choose a dress or at a routine school medical examination. At this stage, there are usually no symptoms other than those arising from the emotional reaction to physical deformity; dyspnoea in particular is more often due to unrelated causes such as asthma or anaemia from menstrual loss than to the scoliosis.

The scoliosis is most commonly mid-thoracic in site with the convexity of the curve towards the right side. This sideways curvature is usually accompanied by rotation of the spine so that the ribs are more prominent posteriorly on the convex side of the curvature and anteriorly on the concave side (Fig. 2). The shoulder tends to be lower on the concave side and the waist indented. The prominence of the ribs and scapula on the convex side, which persists when the patient bends forward (Fig. 1), simulates a kyphosis but idiopathic scoliosis is in fact rarely associated with kyphosis and the commonly used term 'kyphoscoliosis' is a misnomer.

With severe deformity, breathing tends to be rapid, shallow, and predominantly abdominal. Chest expansion may be unequal and incoordinate and, in some cases, there is paradoxical recession of one hemithorax giving a side-to-side or 'curtain' movement of the chest as a whole. There may be accessory respiratory activity of the neck and shoulder muscles. Breath sounds are unevenly distributed and usually less intense on the concave side. Inspiratory basal crackles, which tend to disappear with deep breathing, probably result from expiratory closure of peripheral airways because of shallow breathing at low lung volume. Cyanosis, jugular venous engorgement, oedema, and other signs of cardiac or respiratory failure may complicate idiopathic scoliosis in middle life but, in childhood or adolescence, these signs suggest either a severe congenital scoliosis, associated perhaps with a cardiac anomaly, or a scoliosis of paralytic origin.

The physical examination of a scoliotic patient must include a careful search for possible causes as well as for the effects of the scoliosis. Neuromuscular disorders and congenital cardiac, neural, and urinary tract anomalies should be sought in every case.

Assessment

Radiographic and laboratory investigations may be required to determine the cause and prognosis of the scoliosis, to discover if symptoms such as dyspnoea are due to the scoliosis or to unrelated causes, to exclude associated congenital defects, and to decide whether treatment is needed, and, if so, whether the patient would tolerate surgery.

Radiography

Spinal radiography will reveal any congenital malformation of the vertebrae and will also show the level, severity, and configuration of the curvature. In general, high curves with an angle greater than about 60° are likely to result in cardiorespiratory failure in adult life.

Chest radiographs are needed to help rule out congenital cardiac defects and to ensure that there is no pulmonary cause for dyspnoea. A film should be taken with the patient rotated until the spines at the apex of the curvature are centrally placed (i.e. facing the X-ray source). The heart is then displayed in its conventional postero-anterior perspective and the lung on the convex side of the curve is no longer hidden by the shadow of the spine.

Screening of the diaphragm to exclude paralysis is essential in every case. Paradoxical movement on sniffing suggests a neuromuscular cause for the scoliosis and may also account for unexplained effort dyspnoea or orthopnoea.

Other radiographic techniques may be needed to detect associated congenital anomalies of the skeleton, the cardiovascular system (angiography), or urinary tract (intravenous pyelography).

Cardiography

The chief difficulty in the cardiographic investigation of a scoliotic subject is the change of heart position in relation to the usual anatomical landmarks. In general, however, the sternum overlies the heart so that precordial electrodes may still be sited in relation to the sternum as in conventional practice. Electrocardiographic abnormalities arising from alteration in cardiac position cause a variability in the distribution of the mean QRS vector (giving either left or right axis deviation) and, in children especially, a high QRS voltage in precordial leads due to abnormal proximity of the heart to the chest wall. Because of the frequency of QRST changes due to right axis deviation in scoliotic subjects, a tall P wave (over 3 mm) in standard leads 2 and 3 is probably the most reliable electrocardiographic sign of pulmonary arterial hypertension complicating the scoliosis.

Respiratory function

The chief physiological signs of thoracic scoliosis are reduction in lung volume and hypoxia. The distribution of inspired gas is usually normal and the diffusion coefficient (diffusion per unit lung volume) higher than normal so that hypoxia has been attributed to impaired alveolar ventilation from rapid shallow breathing, collapse of peripheral alveolar units due to the restricted expansion of the lungs, and mismatching of ventilation and perfusion. On exercise, the maximum oxygen uptake is limited by ventilatory factors and the oxygen cost of breathing is abnormally high; the arterial oxygen tension falls and the pulmonary arterial pressure rises. Hypoxic constriction of pulmonary arterioles is the principal though not the sole cause of pulmonary arterial hypertension and right ventricular failure; compression of the pulmonary capillary bed may be an additional factor. Hypoxia is accompanied by hypercapnia when ventilation is severely impaired.

The mechanical action at the costovertebral joints is disturbed, but the compliance of the lungs and the thoracic cage is normal at least in young patients with scoliosis. Conventional spirometric tests for airflow obstruction are normal but airways resistance may be increased as a result of reduction in lung volume; premature closure of the smaller peripheral airways during expiration may also contribute to the ventilatory defect.

Regional lung function studies have disclosed no consistent differences between the function of the lungs on the convex and concave side of the curvature but inequality in size of the two lungs – the lung on the concave side of the curvature being smaller – may contribute to the mechanical inefficiency of ventilation. In severe cases, however, the normal gradient of increasing perfusion from apex to base in the erect posture may be abolished due to loss of lung height.

Physiological tests help to determine the severity and prognosis of thoracic scoliosis and fitness for surgical procedures; they can also provide an objective assessment of response to surgery. The tests of greatest practical value are those available in most general hospitals: spirometry, blood gases, and a simple exercise test.

Interpretation of physiological tests, especially spirometry, is made difficult by the fact that most formulae for the prediction of normal values are based on age and height. Because scoliosis causes loss of height, most workers now use formulae based on other variables such as arm-span, tibial length, 'uncoiled' height, or weight. Unfortunately, none of these methods is reliable in all circumstances.

Management

Scoliosis can develop insidiously and progress rapidly in childhood or adolescence. The first step in management is therefore the early recognition by school screening programmes of the 2 or 3 per cent of children who develop this deformity. It is difficult to predict which of these cases are likely to deteriorate and progress to cardiac and respiratory failure in adult life. Decision to treat must therefore depend upon regular review and accurate measurement – with the help of radiographs and clinical photographs – of the angle of the curvature.

The orthopaedic treatment of an increasing curvature is outside the scope of this book. It is sufficient here to say that, in the early stages, conservative measures involving the use of a brace (e.g. the Milwaukee brace), traction, and other forms of physiotherapy are usually tried. Later, surgical fusion of the spine along with a prosthetic splint (e.g. the Harrington rod) may be needed. Cosmetic procedures such as excision of the rib hump and overlying scapula sometimes help to diminish the deformity. Spinal surgery may possibly prevent cardiac and respiratory complications but cannot be expected to relieve them. These are indeed a contra-indication to surgery and call for medical management as described on page 15.169.

Ankylosing spondylitis

(See also page 16.11.) This is an inflammatory arthritis which chiefly affects the axial skeleton of young men; it may be associated with non-articular lesions including iritis, pulmonary fibrosis, and aortic reflux. The respiratory complications of the disease result from involvement of the costovertebral joints, fibrotic changes in the upper parts of the lungs or, more rarely, left ventricular failure due to aortic disease.

Pathophysiology

The inflammatory process usually starts in the sacroiliac joints and only later spreads upwards to involve the thoracic spine. Ankylosis of the costovertebral joints prevents full expansion of the thorax and reduces chest wall compliance. At first, the vital capacity is preserved by greater excursion of the diaphragm but later it falls and the residual volume increases but there is usually no evidence of airflow obstruction. Changes in the relative proportions of costal and diaphragmatic movement alter the normal relationship of ventilation to perfusion, mainly by reducing apical ventilation; there may also be some redistribution of mechanical stresses on the lung. The kyphosis has little impact on pulmonary function but extreme degress of cervicothoracic kyphosis can disturb the swallowing mechanism, constrict the trachea, and make tracheal intubation difficult or impossible.

The pathogenesis of pulmonary disease in ankylosing spondylitis remains obscure. Patchy inflammatory lesions appear in the upper parts of the lung and progress to confluent areas of dense consolidation with fibrosis, cavitation, bronchiectasis, and bulla formation. The cavities are sometimes huge and are commonly invaded by fungi, especially aspergillus fumigatus, to form a mycetoma. There is no histological evidence of a granulomatous or vasculitic process nor of a tuberculous or other specific infective cause. The apical predominance of the lesions may reflect the altered distribution of ventilation and the mechanical stresses imposed by increased excursion of the diaphragm.

Clinical features

Ankylosing spondylitis rarely causes dyspnoea. In the early stage of the disease, the patients are usually otherwise healthy young men with arthritis confined to the sacroiliac joints. As the disease progresses to involve the thoracic spine, the patients may have already abandoned vigorous exercise because of either increasing age or disability from arthritis in the joints lower down. As in the case of scoliosis, dyspnoea should not be attributed to restriction of the thoracic cage, even when the vital capacity is greatly reduced, until all other possible causes have been excluded. Arthritis in the intervertebral or costovertebral joints may give rise to pain related to breathing and this may simulate pleuritic pain. There is some evidence that patients with ankylosing spondylitis are more prone to respiratory infection, perhaps because of the impaired mechanics of coughing, and certainly the reduced ventilatory reserve puts them at greater risk of respiratory difficulties following bronchopulmonary infection, chest trauma, or surgery. Cough, profuse purulent sputum, and haemoptysis – sometimes life-threatening – are the principal symptoms of the apical pulmonary lesions.

Clinical examination of the chest may reveal a dorsal kyphosis and diminished chest expansion with a corresponding increase in abdominal excursion. Signs of fibrosis, consolidation, or cavitation may be evident at the apices. An aortic diastolic murmur and a left ventricular thrust should be carefully sought, especially in patients complaining of dyspnoea.

Investigation

The chest radiograph is helpful to demonstrate the characteristic bilateral apical cavitating lesions although tomography may be needed to show up a mycetoma. Left ventricular enlargement may be seen in patients with aortic valve disease and the classical 'bamboo' spine should be apparent in the lateral radiograph. Relevant laboratory investigations include lung function tests, vital capacity especially, to measure the degree of thoracic involvement, the ESR to assess activity of the disease, aspergillus precipitins in cases of suspected mycetoma, sputum culture for fungi and other secondary invaders, and HLA status to help confirm the diagnosis (the great majority are HLA-27).

Management

The management of ankylosing spondylitis is dealt with elsewhere (see page 16.14). There is no specific treatment for the thoracic complications of the disease except for secondary infection (see treatment of fungal diseases, page 15.81). In particular, there is no evidence to show that mobilizing the thoracic cage by rib osteotomy improves dyspnoea or prevents pulmonary complications. The general principles of management, including prophylactic measures and pre-operative assessment, are similar to those applicable to other restrictive conditions of the thoracic cage.

The ribs

Disease of the ribs may present as a chance radiological finding (e.g. congenital anomalies), a localized swelling (e.g. tumour or infection), pain interfering with breathing (e.g. fractures), or as one part of a widespread neoplastic or metabolic disorder.

Congenital abnormalities

Congenital anomalies of the ribs are often evident in chest radiographs. The commonest are bifid, fused, or extra ribs. Except for occasional cases of cervical rib (prolonged transverse process of C7), these are usually symptomless. Congenital vascular anomalies may cause rib erosions, notably the notching of the lower borders of the upper ribs in cases of aortic co-arctation (see page 13.269).

Primary tumours and local infections

Primary tumours and local infections of ribs are relatively rare but should be considered when a patient presents with a localized rib swelling. Of the former, solitary myeloma, chondroma, and osteochondroma (the last two sometimes undergoing sarcomatous changes) are the most frequent and treatment is by surgical excision. Fibrous dysplasia and eosinophilic granuloma are rare non-neoplastic causes of localized rib swelling.

Osteomyelitis of the ribs, often staphylococcal, can occur in children and as a complication of draining an empyema; tuberculosis, typhoid, and actinomycosis are rarer causes of rib infection. Treatment consists of antibiotics followed if necessary by surgical drainage or excision.

Abnormalities of the costal cartilages

These include (a) costochondritis, in which there is pain, swelling, and tenderness over the upper costal cartilages; and (b) abnormal motility of the chondrosternal joints giving rise to painful clicking on inspiration or movements of the trunk. Costochondritis may respond to local infiltration with hydrocortisone. An abnormally mobile cartilage may have to be excised if pain cannot be relieved by analgesia or local anaesthesia.

Fracture

This is the commonest acquired lesion of the ribs. It is important because it can cause severe pain and impair respiration and also because it may be the first sign of more generalized disease (see below).

The immediate cause of a rib fracture is trauma but this may be so slight as to be unrecognized by the patient. Gross direct trauma, as in a road accident or a fall against furniture, leads to multiple rib fractures and severe pain. In these cases, the relationship to injury is clear unless there was impairment of consciousness by alcohol or head injury. Fractures may also arise from indirect trauma such as coughing or carrying heavy shoulder burdens. These stress fractures usually occur in the axillary area of only one or two ribs and disability is correspondingly less. Fractures from carrying heavy burdens tend to involve upper ribs and cough fractures the lower ribs. Cough fracture has been attributed to the contrary motions of the upper and lower rib cage during violent expiratory effort: the upper rib cage is moved inwards by expiratory muscle contraction while the lower rib cage is forced outwards by raised intra-abdominal pressure. Local pain and relationship to trauma is least evident in the case of pathological fractures associated with neoplastic or metabolic bone disease; the rib fracture may only come to light in a routine radiograph and is usually overshadowed by other manifestations of the disease.

Symptoms

The chief symptoms and signs of rib fracture are pain on inspiration or coughing and local tenderness. Pain may also be elicited by exerting inward pressure on the rib cage with both hands spread out in the axilla ('springing'). Multiple rib fractures, especially when associated with sternal fracture, may lead to a 'flail' chest with paradoxical movements, the thoracic cage being drawn inwards during inspiration. Pain induces rapid shallow breathing which, in combination with paradox, can cause hypoxia and hypercapnia from ventilatory failure especially in bronchitic patients. Fractures due to direct trauma may be associated with laceration of the lung from rib displacement resulting in haemoptysis or haemopneumothorax. The radiograph is helpful in demonstrating the fractures, to show whether they are recent (no callus formation), and to exclude underlying bone disease and haemopneumothorax.

Management

The management of rib fracture without ventilatory failure consists of pain relief. If simple analgesics are not effective, opiates such as pethidine 50 or 100 mg may be given to patients without a previous history of respiratory disease. Infiltration of the site of the fracture with a local anaesthetic may be helpful in some cases. Ventilatory failure (hypoxia and hypercapnia) due to a flail chest or pre-existing chronic bronchitis is an indication for tracheal intubation and intermittent positive pressure ventilation if it cannot be relieved by bronchodilators and physiotherapy to remove retained secretions.

Metastatic and metabolic bone disease

(See also Section 17.) This may first present with a pathological rib fracture or with lytic or sclerotic rib changes in a routine chest radiograph. Tenderness and swelling at the site of the lesion may be detected.

The commoner neoplastic causes are carcinoma of the lung, breast, or kidney, and myelomatosis. These usually produce osteolytic lesions; osteosclerosis suggests a primary in the prostate.

Osteoporosis with or without pathological fractures is often evident in a radiograph of the ribs; the commoner types are the osteoporosis of post-menopausal women and that due to corticosteroid therapy. Various disorders of calcium metabolism such as hyperparathyroidism can also present with radiographic changes in the ribs.

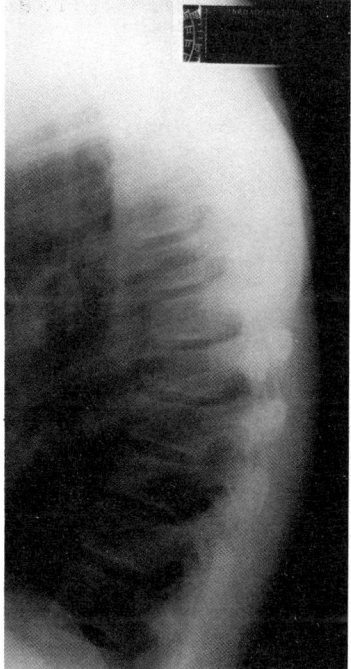

Fig. 3 Wire suture in fractured sternum.

The sternum

The chief abnormalities of the sternum are fracture and deformity.

Fracture of the sternum

This may result from steering wheel injury or from a surgical approach to the heart by median sternotomy. Sternal fracture can lead to ventilatory failure from instability of the chest wall (see under rib fractures above). Suturing of the fracture is a routine after sternotomy and may also be needed in traumatic cases (Fig. 3).

Sternal deformity

Deformities of the sternum are either congenital or acquired during childhood. They are rarely of more than cosmetic importance.

Funnel chest (pectus excavatum) (Fig. 4)

This consists of a depression of the sternum and inward curving of the costal cartilages associated with fibrous replacement of the anterior part of the diaphragm. It is a relatively common deformity, occurring in 2–3 per cent of children. Minor defects of both respiratory and cardiac function have been recorded: these include abnormally increased work of breathing and reduced cardiac stroke volume during vigorous exertion. The deformity occasionally causes dyspnoea but does not predispose to cardiac or respiratory failure in later life. Radiographic displacement of the heart to the left and rotational changes in the electrocardiogram may be wrongly interpreted as evidence of heart disease. Surgical elevation of the sternum is sometimes justified for cosmetic reasons.

Pigeon chest (pectus carinatum) (Fig. 5)

A pigeon deformity of the chest results from undue prominence of the sternum with lateral flattening of the chest wall. When the deformity is asymmetrical, the forward bulge consists of the anterior ends of the ribs rather than sternum. The deformity does not of itself give rise to cardiac or respiratory symptoms but may be a marker of underlying disease. For example symmetrical anterior

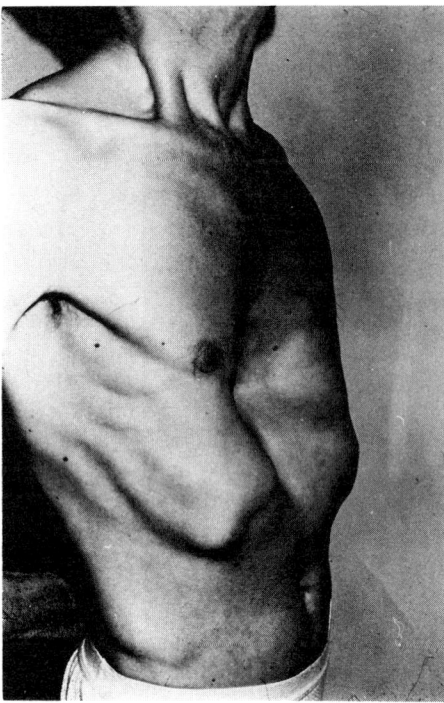

Fig. 4 Pectus excavatum (funnel sternum). (From Ogilvie, C. (1980). *Symptoms and signs in clinical medicine*. John Wright, Bristol, by permission.)

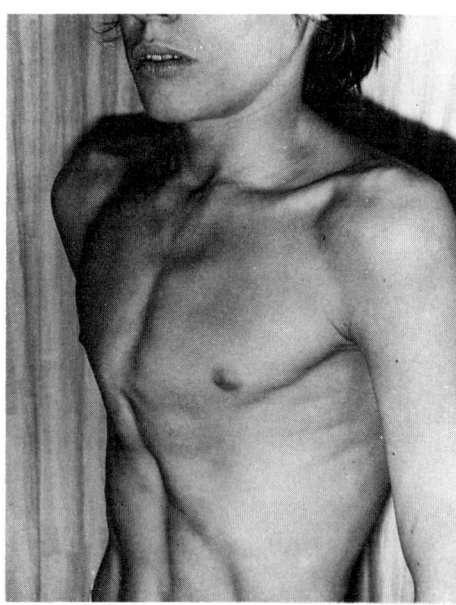

Fig. 5 Pectus carinatum (pigeon chest). A 15-year-old boy troubled with asthma throughout childhood but symptom-free now (Reproduced from Ogilvie, 1980, *Symptoms and signs in clinical medicine*. John Wright, Bristol, by permission.)

prominence of the chest is sometimes found in patients who had asthma during childhood. This has been attributed to airflow obstruction causing inspiratory retraction of the ribs, an effect more likely to occur in poorly nourished rachitic children. Asymmetrical prominence of the anterior chest wall occurs in scoliosis (see page 15.58) and in various congenital syndromes (e.g. Marfan's syndrome), some of which may be associated with heart disease.

The diaphragm

Paralysis

Causes
The commoner causes of diaphragmatic paralysis are listed in Table 1. Unilateral paralysis is most often due to involvement of the phrenic nerve in the thorax by a bronchial carcinoma. Bilateral paralysis usually results from a peripheral neuropathy or myopathy.

Clinical features
Paralysis of the diaphragm should always be considered as a possible cause for otherwise unexplained dyspnoea on effort. Orthopnoea due to abnormal ascent of abdominal viscera into the thorax in the supine position may be wrongly attributed to cardiac causes. Gastric distension and flatulence may occur when the left hemi-diaphragm is paralysed. Nocturnal hypoventilation in cases of bilateral paralysis gives rise to disturbed sleep and morning headaches.

Breath sounds are diminished over the lung base on the affected side. Because the paralysed diaphragm assumes a resting expiratory posture, the basal percussion note will be dull in right-sided paralysis due to elevation of the liver. When the left side is paralysed, the gas-filled stomach gives a tympanitic note and borborygmi may be abnormally audible over the base of the left lung. Paradoxical (i.e. inward) movement of the abdominal wall during inspiration may be observed in the supine position, especially in patients with bilateral paralysis.

Diagnosis
The diagnosis of diaphragmatic paralysis may be established and its effects measured by radiographic and physiological methods.

Radiography
Postero-anterior and lateral chest radiographs usually show elevation of the diaphragm but this is not always evident especially in bilateral paralysis. Displacement of the heart toward the opposite side may be mistaken for cardiac enlargement. Plate atelectases, presumably due to compression and inadequate ventilation of the lung base, are not uncommon and such cases have been mistakenly diagnosed as pulmonary embolism (Fig. 6). The diagnosis of phrenic paralysis is established by demonstrating paradoxical movement on fluoroscopic screening. This is not always apparent in the upright posture because the downward drag of the abdominal viscera may prevent the paradoxical upward movement of the diaphragm on inspiration; screening should therefore include examination in the supine posture. Paradoxical movement may not be present on normal breathing and is best elicited by a short sudden inspiration (i.e. sniffing). A hilar mass may be seen in patients with a neoplastic cause for phrenic paralysis but, when this is not so, the radiographic investigation should include hilar tomograms and radiographs of the cervical spine.

Table 1 Causes of phrenic paralysis

Site of lesion	Cause
Anterior horn cell (C3–5)	Poliomyelitis
	Motor neurone disease
	Syringomyelia
Nerve roots (C3–5)	Cervical spondylosis
	Herpes zoster
Brachial plexus	Trauma: falls on shoulder or head; surgical
Phrenic nerve	Tumour: bronchial carcinoma
	Peripheral neuropathy
	Surgery
Diaphragm muscle	Myopathy

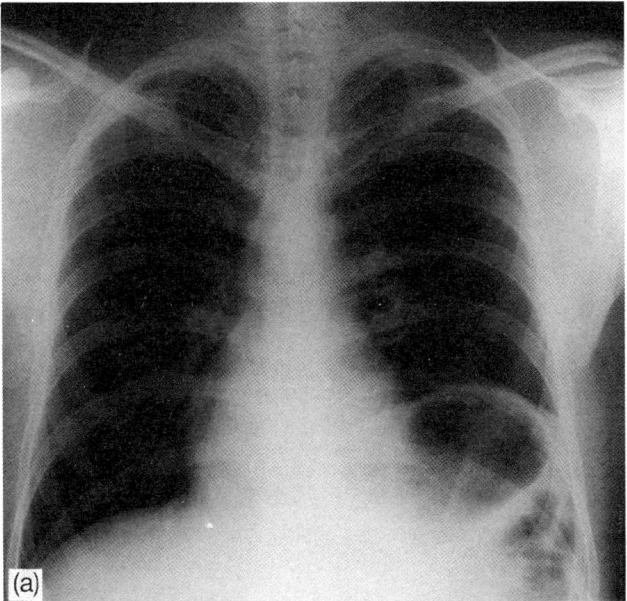

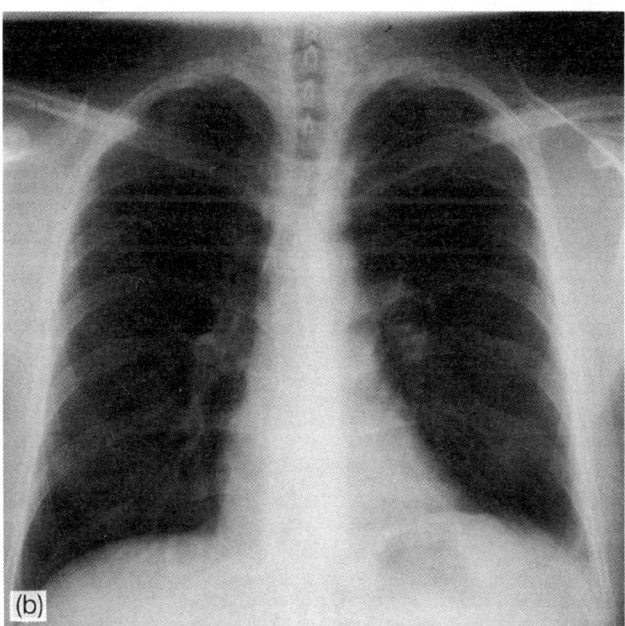

Fig. 6 Paralysed left diaphragm before and after surgical plication.

Physiological measurements

When phrenic paralysis is suspected, standard lung function tests should be carried out in the supine as well as the upright posture. The vital capacity is reduced in the upright posture but falls further on lying down from 10–20 per cent in unilateral paralysis to 50 per cent in bilateral paralysis (in normal subjects, the fall is less than 5 per cent). The forced expiratory volume in one second (FEV_1) is usually normal but the maximum voluntary ventilation, which reflects inspiratory as well as expiratory effort, is reduced to below the value predicted from the FEV_1. Hypoxia and hypercapnia may occur in the supine posture especially in patients with bilateral paralysis. Regional lung function studies show impaired basal ventilation on the affected side. In cases of bilateral paralysis, the dependent lung when the patient lies on one side has less ventilation but more perfusion than the upper lung with resulting hypoxia. The lung is less compliant than normal, possibly due to widespread atelectases (see above). The most reliable way to recognize and measure diaphragmatic paresis is by recording

transdiaphragmatic pressure from simultaneous measurements of gastric and oesophageal pressures; a relatively low intragastric pressure during inspiration suggests phrenic paresis. The contribution of the intercostal muscles and diaphragm to inspiration can also be measured by less invasive techniques using either magnetometers or light stripes projected on to the torso. Recent physiological studies have shown that fatigue of a normally innervated diaphragm may simulate phrenic paralysis and contribute to ventilatory failure.

Management

Neoplastic invasion of the right phrenic nerve, or of the left phrenic nerve above the hilum, is an indication of inoperability. Phrenic paralysis due to a peripheral neuropathy may respond to treatment of the neuropathy. Some traumatic cases recover spontaneously over a period of months but recovery is unpredictable and uninfluenced by treatment. Patients with orthopnoea or symptoms of nocturnal hypoventilation should be advised to sleep in the upright posture. Lowering and fixation of the diaphragm by surgical plication may improve the vital capacity, abolish paradox and prevent orthopnoea (Fig. 6).

Eventration

Eventration is a condition characterized by fibrous replacement of the diaphragm of unknown cause but possibly congenital in origin. It is usually left sided but eventration of the anterior part of the right diaphragm may occur. (Fig. 7). The clinical features and management are similar to those described under diaphragmatic paralysis except that no neurological cause is ever apparent. Eventration is relatively common in infancy when it may be a cause of respiratory distress requiring urgent treatment by plication of the diaphragm.

Hernia

Gastric herniation through the oesophageal hiatus is the commonest form of diaphragmatic hernia (see Section 12).

Herniation may rarely occur through the foramina of Morgagni and Bochdalek. In the former, abdominal contents pass anteriorly between the costal and sternal insertions of the diaphragm

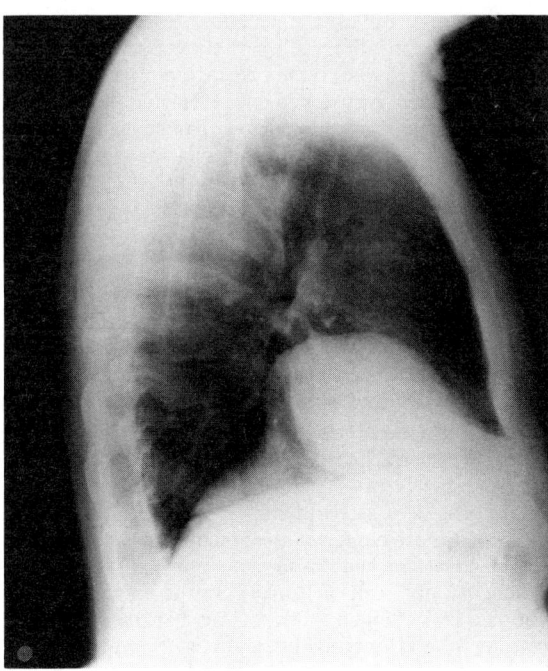

Fig. 7 Right lateral chest radiograph showing eventration of the anterior part of right diaphragm.

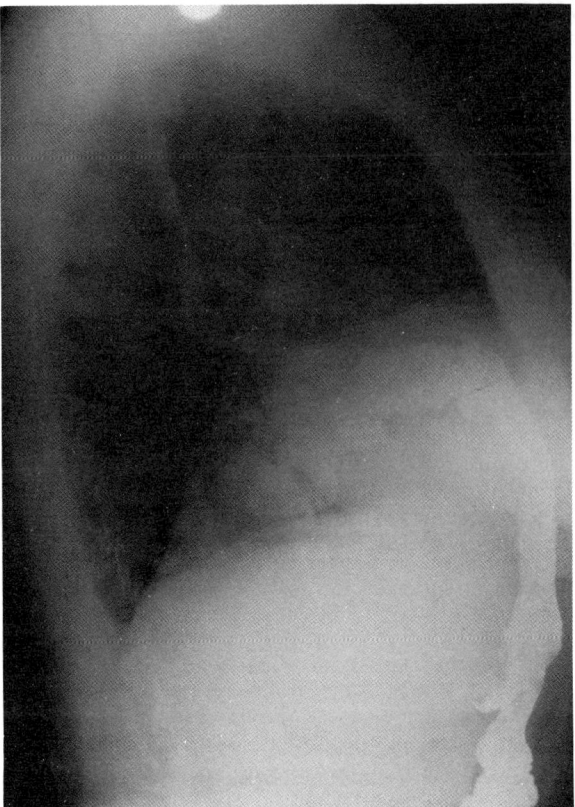

Fig. 8 Barium enema showing large bowel within a hernia through the foramina of Morgagni (right lateral chest radiograph).

(Fig. 8). In the latter, herniation occurs through the pleuroperitoneal hiatus and may give rise to respiratory distress in infancy.

Traumatic diaphragmatic hernia follows rupture of the diaphragm but actual herniation of abdominal viscera into the thoracic cavity may not occur for months or even years after the original injury. The diagnosis should be suspected when a patient who has recovered from severe chest trauma later presents with respiratory symptoms. The chest radiograph may show pockets of air, sometimes with fluid levels, due to the presence of bowel or stomach in the thorax. This may be mistaken for a loculated pneumothorax or lung abscesses but the correct diagnosis can be established by barium meal and enema. Rupture of the liver through the right diaphragm can simulate a raised diaphragm but the two can usually be distinguished by fluoroscopy and an isotope liver scan.

The trachea

Tracheal stenosis

Causes

The commonest causes for tracheal narrowing are compression by malignant lymph-nodes and other mediastinal tumours, or a primary tumour in the tracheal wall. Non-neoplastic causes include congenital atresia, fibrotic stricture secondary to trauma or to granulomatous processes (sarcoid, tuberculous or Wegener's), and amyloidosis. Of these benign causes, the most frequent is the stricture which follows tracheal intubation. This may occur at the site of the tracheostomy itself or it may result from pressure necrosis by the inflated cuff of an endotracheal tube or the distal end of the tracheostomy tube. This type of stricture is becoming less common with the methods and materials now used for tracheostomy. Sarcoidosis rarely produces a tracheal stricture but is an important cause of multiple bronchial stenoses.

Clinical features'

The principal symptom of tracheal stenosis is wheezing dyspnoea. At first, this may be evident only on effort but later occurs at rest, especially in bed at night. There may also be recurrent bronchial infections distal to the obstruction. These symptoms are easily confused with those of asthma and chronic bronchitis.

Stridor is the chief sign of tracheal stenosis but may not be apparent during normal breathing. It is best heard after exercise or during hyperventilation through the open mouth. With the stethoscope, a fixed wheeze is audible over the trachea becoming fainter over the lungs. When the stenosis affects the portion of the trachea within the thorax, the sound tends to be louder in expiration because the trachea is subject to intrathoracic expiratory pressure; the converse holds true for narrowing of the extrathoracic trachea. These differences, and also the distinction between main airway narrowing and diffuse distal airways narrowing (as in asthma and emphysema) may be demonstrated by flow–volume curves (see Fig. 2). With extreme degrees of tracheal narrowing, violent ineffectual respiratory effort, cyanosis, and sudden death may result when a relatively minor additional insult, such as a mucus plug or inhaled food, occludes the narrowed trachea completely.

A plain postero-anterior chest radiograph, if well penetrated, may show tracheal narrowing but this can be defined more clearly by tomography (Fig. 9). The diagnosis is confirmed by bronchoscopy using both the rigid and fibreoptic instruments. The former allows assessment of tracheal mobility (fixation suggests mediastinal malignancy as the cause of the stenosis) and the latter is more suitable for passing through the tracheal stenosis to exclude associated bronchial stenoses. When there is extreme narrowing of the trachea, no attempt should be made to obtain a biopsy because the resulting oedema or haemorrhage may cause asphyxia. Flow–volume curves, as already mentioned, help to determine the level of the airway obstruction and are of practical value when for any reason bronchoscopy is not feasible.

Treatment

Tracheal stenosis associated with an acute granulomatous condition such as sarcoidosis or Wegener's granuloma may improve

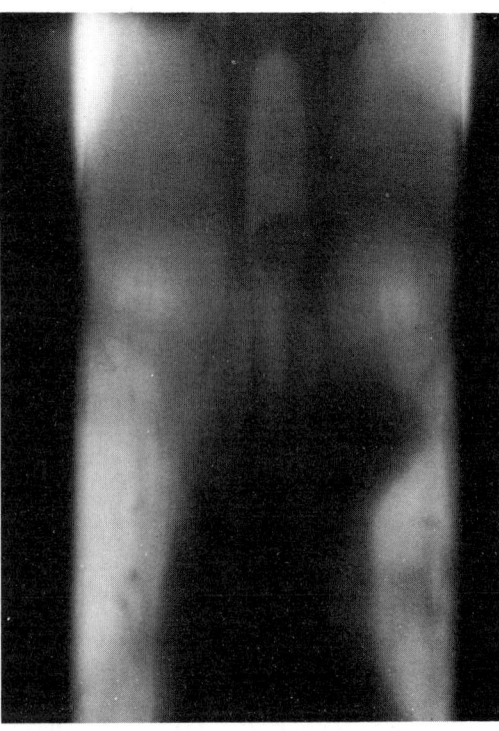

Fig. 9 Tomogram showing narrowing of the trachea by a chondroma.

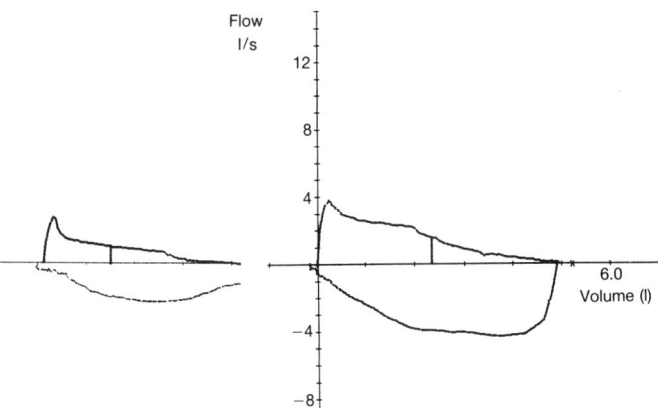

Fig. 10 Flow volume loop before and after bougie dilatation of bronchial strictures due to sarcoidosis.

with corticosteroids. Fibrous stricture may be treated by bougie dilatation (Fig. 10) but, if the patient's condition permits, surgical resection with end-to-end anastomosis is the treatment of choice.

Tracheo- and bronchopathia osteoplastica

This is a rare disease of unknown cause mainly affecting elderly men and characterized by cartilaginous and calcific nodules projecting into the trachea and main bronchi; these nodules are evident in tomograms and at bronchoscopy. They arise from between the normal cartilage rings and are commonest in the lower two-thirds of the trachea. The disease may present with clinical features of bronchial obstruction but is more often a chance radiographic or necropsy finding.

Tracheobronchomegaly

A rare congenital disease of children and young adults in which there is abnormal widening of the trachea and major bronchi with laxity of the cartilaginous rings due to atrophy of the elastic and muscular tissue. The result is a rasping ineffectual cough, difficulty in expectoration, and dyspnoea because of the increased collapsibility of the airways. There is a tendency to recurrent respiratory infection. Radiography shows the airways dilatation and on bronchoscopy the airways appear to have an irregular surface. A marked exaggeration of the normal calibre change between inspiration and expiration can easily be seen.

Relapsing polychondritis

This rare systemic disease affects cartilage in a variety of anatomical sites. Inflammation and destruction of cartilage occurs with the release of chondroitin sulphate. Narrowing of major airways results; this may be relatively fixed, or variable, due to increased flaccidity resulting from the loss of cartilaginous support.

Tracheomalacia

This condition is usually a developmental defect characterized by weakness of the tracheal walls due to a deficiency of cartilage. Although pathologically it is distinct from relapsing polychondritis and does not affect other cartilaginous structures, the respiratory symptoms are similar.

It is important to recognize that apposition of the extrathoracic tracheal walls in inspiration or of the intrathoracic walls in expiration does not necessarily indicate tracheomalacia. The former may result from forceful inspiration when there is upper airway obstruction and the latter from forceful expiration in cases of asthma or emphysema.

The bronchi and vessels

Congenital bronchial anomalies

Variations in bronchial segmental anatomy

These are common but of little clinical importance except in the interpretation of bronchoscopic or bronchographic appearances and the planning of resectional surgery.

Bronchogenic cyst

This is the result of duplication of the primitive foregut from which the trachea, bronchi, and oesophagus are derived. It occurs most often in the region of the tracheal bifurcation. The cyst has a thin wall which may contain any of the elements found in normal bronchial wall. In the absence of infective complications, it is filled with clear fluid and does not communicate with the lumen of the bronchial tree. Bronchogenic cyst is usually a chance finding in a chest radiograph where it appears as a smooth rounded opacity lying posteriorly in the superior or middle mediastinum. A large cyst may rarely compress the trachea, main bronchi, or oesophagus to cause dyspnoea and feeding difficulties in children. An infected cyst can rupture into the bronchus and cause symptoms suggestive of bronchiectasis or lung abscess; in these cases a fluid level may be seen in the radiograph. Surgical excision is necessary only for those cysts causing symptoms but may be the only way of proving the nature of the radiographic opacity.

Congenital cystic bronchiectasis

Bronchiectasis may arise from congenital causes such as immunoglobulin deficiency or an abnormal mucociliary mechanism as in fibrocystic disease and Kartagener's syndrome. It may also develop when a bronchus fails to communicate with the main bronchial tree as in congenital bronchial atresia and sequestration of the lung (see below). True congenital cystic malformation of the bronchi is probably very rare.

Congenital vascular anomalies

See page 13.233 for those of cardiac rather than pulmonary significance.

Aberrant vessels

Variations in the number and origin of pulmonary vessels, especially the bronchial arteries and pulmonary veins, are frequent but unobtrusive, coming to light only on angiography or at thoracotomy. Aberrant extrapulmonary vessels are more likely to present a diagnostic or therapeutic problem relating to the lungs. Three will be mentioned: right-sided aorta, azygos lobe, and bronchopulmonary sequestration.

Right-sided or double aortic arch may be mistaken in the chest radiograph for a mass in the right upper mediastinum but the diagnosis can be established by screening for pulsation and by arch aortography. The aberrant aorta or its branches may compress the oesophagus to cause dysphagia or the right main bronchus to produce dyspnoea, stridor, or a localized wheeze; in these cases, surgery may be needed.

Azygos 'lobe' is caused by the azygos vein looping over the medial part of the right upper lobe which is then partially separated from the remainder of the lobe by an infolding of pleura. This pleural fold is seen in the chest radiograph as a thin line curving out from the mediastinum with the oval shadow of the azygos vein at its lower end. This is a relatively common but harmless anomaly.

Bronchopulmonary sequestration refers to an area of lung supplied by an aberrant artery arising from the aorta or one of its branches and drained by a pulmonary vein; the bronchi are usually dilated or cystic but do not communicate freely with the rest of the bronchial tree. The sequestration may be intralobular (usually the posterior basal segment of the lower) or extralobular (usually between the diaphragm and lower lobe) and is rather commoner

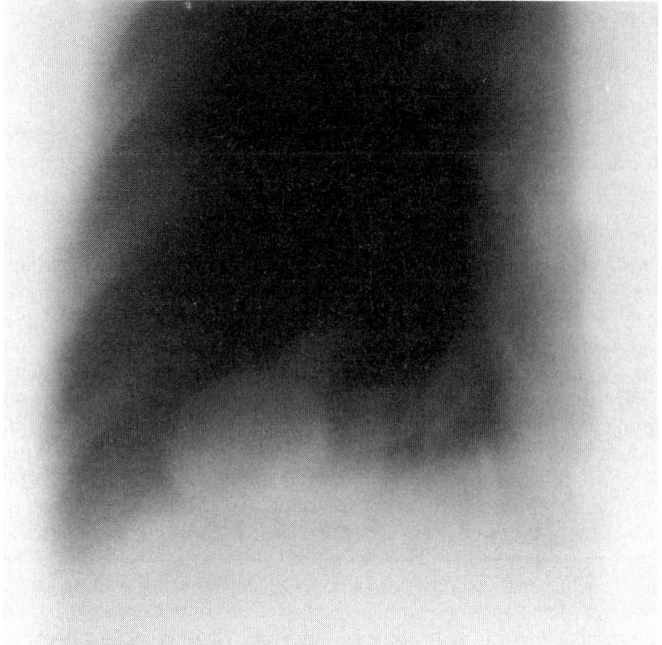

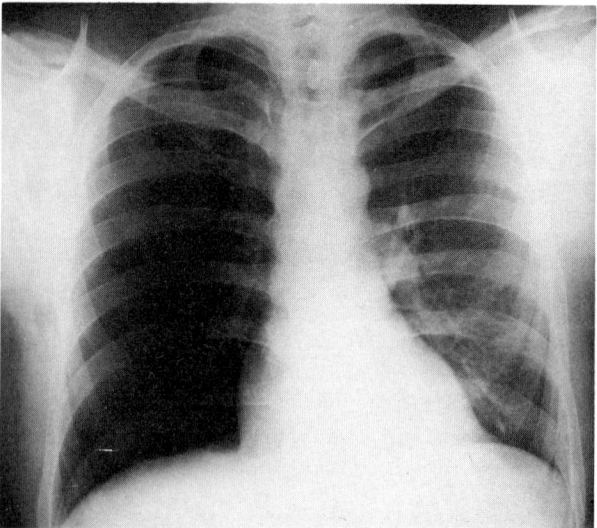

Fig. 12 Macleod's syndrome: note hypertransradiant right lung with diminished hilar and peripheral vascular shadows and central mediastinum.

Fig. 11 Tomogram of the right lower lobe showing a congenital arteriovenous fistula with large feeding vessel.

on the left than the right side; congenital diaphragmatic herniae are present in nearly half the cases of extralobular sequestration. In the chest radiograph, a sequestrated lobe may show as a rounded basal opacity resembling a tumour or as a cystic area with or without a fluid level. The diagnosis is established by retrograde aortography to display the aberrant blood supply. About a third of all cases present with symptoms during the first decade of life, usually recurrent infections with abscess formation, and in these surgical excision of the sequestrated lobe is indicated. Urgent surgery may also be needed to deal with haemoptysis when this is of systemic arterial origin.

Congenital arteriovenous fistula

This rare malformation arises as a persistence of the fetal precapillary communication between pulmonary artery and vein. There may be multiple fistulae and about half the cases are associated with hereditary haemorrhagic telangiectasia. Blood flowing direct from artery to vein bypasses the pulmonary capillary bed and thus causes a shunt hypoxia. A large shunt leads to cyanosis, polycythaemia, finger clubbing, and an overlying murmur heard best in maximal inspiration. Cerebral symptoms may result from polycythaemia, paradoxical embolus or an associated intracranial vascular malformation. Epistaxis and other features of haemorrhagic telangiectasia may occur in the patient or other members of the family and there can be massive haemoptysis. Some cases first present with an abnormality in a routine chest radiograph (Fig. 11). This consists of a rounded or lobular opacity usually in the lower zone and the main feeding vessel may be seen entering the lesion from the hilum; calcification can occur but pulsation is rarely detectable. The size of the lesion decreases with a Valsalva manoeuvre. The diagnosis is confirmed and multiple lesions excluded by pulmonary angiography. Treatment is by surgical excision but this may not be feasible if the lesions are too numerous.

Unilateral hypertransradiancy: Macleod's syndrome

Macleod's syndrome has been attributed to an obliterative bronchiolitis, probably of virus origin, occurring during early childhood. This leads to alveolar overinflation but, because the original damage occurred during the period of lung growth, the affected

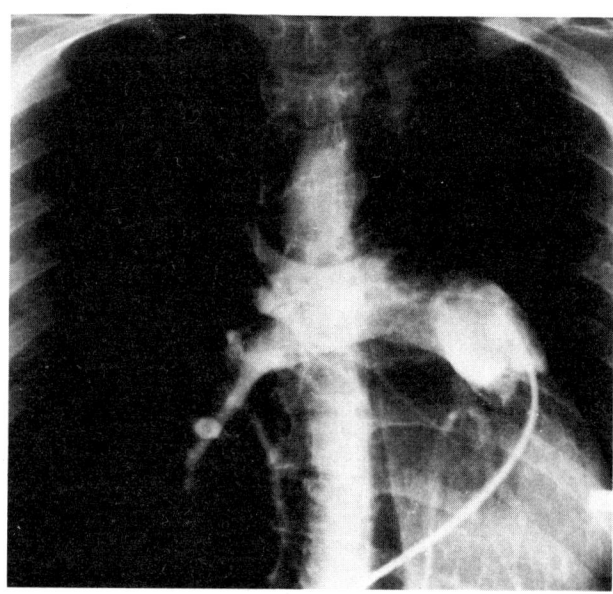

Fig. 13 Pulmonary arteriogram showing congenital absence of the left pulmonary artery.

lung becomes hypoplastic with fewer alveoli and a smaller pulmonary artery than on the normal side.

There is sometimes a history of acute respiratory infections during childhood. In adult life, this tendency may continue and a few patients develop chronic bronchitis with persistent cough, sputum, and dyspnoea, but Macleod's syndrome is more often a chance radiographic finding in a symptomless subject. In a few cases, there are reduced expansion and breath sounds with a normal or increased percussion note on the affected side.

The chest radiograph shows increased transradiancy of the whole or part of one lung with diminished hilar and peripheral vascular shadows (Fig. 12). The mediastinum is central or displaced towards the affected lung but may shift towards the opposite side on expiration because of air trapping. Peripheral dilatation and 'pruning' of the bronchial tree with irregularity of calibre may be evident on bronchography. The spirometric pattern is usually mildly obstructive and lung function studies show that both ventilation and perfusion of the affected lung are reduced.

Table 2 Causes of unilateral hypertransradiancy. This list includes the final diagnosis in patients originally referred to the author as possible cases of Macleod's syndrome

Technical	Poorly centred film
Chest wall	Scoliosis
	Absent pectoral muscle
	Mastectomy
	Contralateral lipoma
Pleura	Pneumothorax
	Contralateral thickening
Pulmonary artery	Congenital absence
	Embolic occlusion
Airways	Obstructive overinflation
	Macleod's syndrome
Lung parenchyma	Compensatory overinflation
	Bullous emphysema

The differential diagnosis of Macleod's syndrome calls for the exclusion of other causes of hypertransradiant lung (see Table 2). Most of the causes listed in Table 2 can be identified by clinical examination or by postero-anterior, lateral, and expiratory chest radiographs. Bronchoscopy may be needed to exclude obstructive causes for overinflation, bronchography to rule out overinflation secondary to a contracted segment or lobe, and pulmonary angiography to exclude occlusion or congenital absence of one pulmonary artery (Fig. 13).

Management involves the treatment of secondary infections in the abnormal lung but these are rarely severe or frequent enough to justify pneumonectomy.

References

Arborelius, M., Lilza, B. and Senyk, J. (1975). Regional and total lung function studies in patients with hemidiaphragmatic paralysis. *Respiration* 32, 253.
Baxter, J. D. and Dunbar, J. S. (1963). Tracheomalacia. *Ann. Otol.* 72, 1012.
Borgeskov, S. and Raahave, D. (1971). Long term results after operative correction of funnel chest. *Thorax* 26, 74.
British Medical Journal (1973). Bronchial cysts. *Br. med. J.* 2, 501.
Castile, R. G., Staats, B. A. and Westbrook, P. R. (1982). Symptomatic pectus deformities of the chest. *Am. Rev. resp. Dis.* 126, 564–568.
Davies, D. (1972). Ankylosing spondylitis and lung fibrosis. *Q. J. Med.* 41, 395.
Editorial (1971). Lobar obliterative bronchiolitis (Macleod's syndrome) *Br. med. J.* 3, 264.
Guest, J. L. and Anderson, J. N. (1977). Tracheobronchomegaly. *J. Am. Med. Assn.* 238, 1754.
Harley, H. R. S. (1971). Laryngotracheal obstruction complicating tracheostomy or endotracheal intubation with assisted respiration: a critical review. *Thorax* 26, 493.
International symposium on the diaphragm (1979). *Am. Rev. res. Dis.* 119, no. 2, part 2 suppl.
Jones, R. S., Kennedy, J. D., Hasham, F., Owen R. and Taylor, J. F. (1981). Mechanical inefficiency of the thoracic cage in scoliosis. *Thorax* 36, 456–461.
Landing, B. H. (1979). Congenital malformations and genetic disorders of the respiratory tract (larynx, trachea, bronchi and lungs). *Am. Rev. resp. Dis.* 120, 151–185.
Macklem, P. T. (1981). Normal and abnormal function of the diaphragm. *Thorax* 36, 161–163.
Martin, C. J. (1974). Tracheobronchopathia osteochondroplastica. *Arch. Otolaryngol.* 100, 290–293.
Newsom Davies, J., Goldman, M., Loh, L. and Casson, M. (1976). Diaphragm function and alveolar hypoventilation. *Q. J. Med.* 45, 87.
Rademaker, M., Redmond, A. D. and Barber, P. V. (1983). Stress fracture of the first rib. *Thorax* 38, 312–313.
Roaf, R. (1980). Spinal deformities, 2nd edn. Pitman Medical, London.
Savic, B., Birtel, F. J., Tholen, W., Funke, H. D. and Knoche, R. (1979). Lung sequestration: report of seven cases and review of 540 published cases. *Thorax* 34, 96.
Sluiter-Eringa, H., Orie, N. G. M. and Sluiter, H. J. (1969). Pulmonary arteriovenous fistula: diagnosis and prognosis in uncomplainant patients. *Am. Rev. res. Dis.* 100, 177.
Wright, C. D., Williams, J. G., Ogilvie, C. M. and Donnelly, R. J. (1985). Results of diaphragmatic olication for unilateral diaphragmatic paralysis. *J. Thorac. Cariovasc. Surg.* 90, 195–198.
Zorab, P. A. and Siegler, D. (eds) (1979). *Scoliosis 1979.* Academic Press, New York.

THE UPPER RESPIRATORY TRACT

The pharynx

W. S. LUND

Anatomy and physiology

The pharynx consists of a roughly funnel-shaped fibromuscular tube extending from the base of the skull to approximately the level of the VIth cervical vertebra. It is divisible into three zones which lie behind the nose, mouth, and larynx, respectively, viz, the naso-, oro-, and hypopharynx.

The pyriform fossae recesses which lie on either side of the larynx, are often termed 'the lateral food channels' and it is down these that a bolus of food passes during the second stage of deglutition.

The internal division of the superior laryngeal nerve, a branch of the Xth cranial nerve (sensory supply to the upper half of the larynx) runs beneath the mucous membrane of its floor.

The muscular coat of the pharynx is comprised mainly of three paired voluntary muscles, the superior, middle, and inferior constrictors. The lower half of the inferior constrictor (the cricopharyngeal muscle) with its fellow on the opposite side forms an important sphincter which prevents air from being sucked into the oesophagus during inspiration, and conversely protects the pharynx.

Posteriorly the pharynx is separated from the cervical vertebrae by the retropharyngeal space which contains lymph-nodes. The tonsils and adenoids lie in the pharynx and are part of Waldeyer's ring of subepithelial lymphoid tissue encircling the upper end of the alimentary and respiratory tracts. The adenoids lie between the roof and posterior wall of the nasopharynx. Lower down on each side of 'the ring' are the palatine tonsils. The bottom of the ring is completed by the lingual tonsils on the upper surface of the base of the tongue.

Waldeyer's ring possesses only efferent lymph vessels. The adenoids drain into the upper deep cervical nodes. The tonsils send vessels initially to the tonsillar node which is situated a finger's breadth below and behind the angle of the jaw. The remainder of the pharynx drains to the deep cervical nodes.

The nerve supply to the pharynx is chiefly from the pharyngeal plexus which is formed by branches of the IXth and Xth cranial nerves. Both of these nerves have branches going to the ear which explains why painful lesions in the upper air and food passages can frequently cause earache.

Deglutition

Food is carried to the stomach after mastication by a series of co-ordinated movements of the muscles of the mouth, pharynx, and oesophagus.

The first stage is voluntary and involves passing the bolus backwards into the oropharynx. The next pharyngeal stage is reflex and carries the bolus downwards through the cricopharyngeal sphincter and into the oesophagus by means of peristalsis affected by the constrictors. The emptying of the pharynx is helped by gravity in the vertical position and a thrust downwards by the back of the tongue, at the same time the nasopharynx is closed off by the soft palate, and the larynx shut. The epiglottis is swept backwards to cover the laryngeal inlet like a lid. It divides the bolus into two streams which pass laterally down into each pyriform fossa only to join behind the arytenoids in the midline and thus through into the opening of the oesophagus.

DISEASES OF THE PHARYNX

Conditions affecting the pharynx will be considered under the following headings:

1. Pharyngitis.
2. Enlargement and inflammation of the tonsils and adenoids.
3. Neoplasia.
4. Miscellaneous.
5. Lump in the throat.

Important features in the history of throat trouble

The duration of symptoms and their relationship to swallowing, both food and saliva, is essential. A direct enquiry as to whether a change of diet has been made because of the throat trouble is helpful in deciding on severity. Some idea of the level or site to which the patient refers the symptom is important with particular reference to its constancy and whether it is unilateral or generalized. Information about associated complaints such as hoarseness and earache must be sought, remembering to ask about gastro-oesophageal symptoms which can occasionally produce a referred pharyngeal clinical picture.

Serious disease should be suspected in the presence of

1. Unilateral symptoms.
2. Constant site.
3. Worsening with swallowing.
4. Localized pain.
5. Referred otalgia.
6. Voice change.
7. A hard lump in the neck.

Always examine the head and neck for a primary growth since 60 per cent of cervical metastases arise from a tumour in the upper alimentary and respiratory tracts. A biopsy of the lump must not be done until this examination has been carried out along with checking other nodal areas and excluding an enlarged liver and spleen. Remember 'hidden sites' of a tumour, namely, nasopharynx, tonsil, back of tongue, and valleculae.

Pharyngitis

Inflammation of the pharynx is frequently limited to the oropharynx, but all three parts may be involved, together or separately.

Acute pharyngitis

The cause in 90 per cent of cases is viral with haemolytic streptococci accounting for more serious infections. *Streptococcus pneumoniae* and *Haemophilus influenzae* are also incriminated especially as secondary invaders.

Symptoms vary from a slight sore throat lasting for only a few days with minimal malaise and mild pyrexia to intense throat symptoms with toxaemia and fever. The patient may have difficulty in swallowing even his saliva with the palate and uvula oedematous causing irritation. The disease often goes in epidemics.

The pharynx is uniformly injected and red with the lateral pharyngeal bands particularly affected. The lymphoid follicles on the posterior pharyngeal wall and the lingular tonsils are frequently hypertrophied with slough and exudate on them. The tonsils will present a similar appearance. The upper deep cervical nodes bilaterally are enlarged and tender. Referred earache is not uncommon.

Complications include laryngeal oedema, Ludwig's angina (cellulitis of the surroundings of the submandibular salivary glands), and a cervical abscess.

When exudate is present diphtheria, Vincent's angina ('trench mouth' caused by a Gram-negative fusiform *Bacillus spirillium*), and moniliasis must be excluded. The prodromal manifestations of the examthemata should be remembered and blood dyscrasias excluded by haematological investigation. However, the most important entity to be differentiated is acute tonsillitis. In children it is often difficult to make the correct diagnosis, but acute pharyngitis is a generalized condition affecting the whole of the oropharynx, whereas acute tonsillitis is a localized infection. The former is frequently preceded by head cold and occurs in epidemics whereas tonsillitis starts abruptly without any warning.

Gonococcal pharyngitis should also be remembered as an uncommon entity.

Management

Culture of a throat swab may eventually establish the diagnosis, but treatment must rely on clinical judgement. The white cell count may help differentiate between a viral and a bacterial infection.

In the milder cases resolution occurs on simple conservative therapy, but in the more severe cases penicillin is essential.

Oropharyngeal candidiasis

Known also as moniliasis or 'thrush', this is an infection with the yeast-like organism *Candida albicans*. There are white patches on the fauces, palate, gums, and tongue, which usually cause minimal discomfort. The condition is rare except in patients receiving therapy which influences local oropharyngeal defences, e.g. broad-spectrum antibiotics, cytotoxics, radiotherapy, and especially corticosteroids, both systemic and local (viz, inhaled steroids used in the treatment of asthma).

Chronic non-specific infection

This is a common condition predisposed to by excessive mouth breathing or overindulgence in tobacco and alcohol and exposure to dry and dusty atmospheres. Some patients appear to have an unduly sensitive throat with possibly a vasomotor type of pharyngeal mucosa producing constant irritation and hawking up of phlegm.

Chronic pharyngo-oesophagitis: Paterson Brown–Kelly or Plummer–Vinson syndrome

This is a rare condition characterized by submucosal inflammation, classically in the postcricoid region producing a web or concentric stenosis, but also occurring at any level in the oesophagus.

The clinical picture of upper alimentary tract dysphagia in a middle-aged woman with iron deficiency anaemia is characteristic and there is often associated koilonychia, with other stigmata, e.g. atrophic glossitis.

The importance of recognizing the condition apart from it being a sign of severe anaemia, is that it is a premalignant entity.

Chronic specific infections, such as syphilis and tuberculosis are now very rare.

Enlargement and inflammation of the tonsils and adenoids.

Acute tonsillitis

The tonsils being covered by the mucous membrane common to the oropharynx will become inflamed as part of a generalized pharyngitis. An accurate record of true tonsillitis is all important in making a subsequent decision about surgery.

Acute tonsillitis is predominantly a disease of childhood, with the peak incidence in the fifth and sixth years of life, but it also occurs in adolescence and early adulthood, often as a periodic exacerbation of chronic tonsillitis.

Viruses, especially adenoviruses are commonly the initial infecting organism. However, secondary bacterial invasion occurs frequently with the haemolytic streptococcus having a particular predilection for the tonsils.

Symptoms and signs

The infection is heralded by a dry throat, malaise, slight fever, and thirst. Once fully developed sore throat exacerbated by swallowing is the predominant symptom with headache and general malaise.

In the young child acute tonsillitis may present atypically as pyrexia of unknown origin, earache, cervical lymphadenopathy or abdominal pain.

The tonsils are swollen, red, and spotted with purulent exudate or in severe cases a purulent 'false' membrane. The tonsil nodes on both sides of the neck are enlarged and tender.

Scarlet fever, Vincent's angina, diphtheria, granulocytopaenia, and leukaemia, enter into the differential diagnosis and the anginose form of glandular fever deserves special mention. However, it usually affects an older age group and is associated with more extensive lymphadenopathy.

Treatment

In mild cases fluids and analgesics are sufficient. In severe cases it is wise to assume that the infection is due to a streptococcus against which penicillin remains the most universally effective agent.

Complications

Local suppuration can occur in the peritonsillar space (quinsy), parapharyngeal compartment or in the cervical nodes. Some children have a susceptibility to acute otitis media after tonsillitis.

Quinsy

This is an infection of the potential space between the tonsil and superior constrictor muscle. Cellulitis occurs initially, quickly followed by pus with abscess formation.

Pain is very severe, unilateral, and maximal behind the angle of the jaw radiating to the ear. Trismus makes it difficult to look into the mouth. The oedematous uvula is displaced across the midline to the opposite side, and the tonsil downwards and medially to occlude the oropharyngeal isthmus. Cervical nodes on the affected side are large and tender.

Urgent treatment in hospital is required to prevent oedema of the supraglottis and aspiration of pus. Penicillin is essential and surgical incision through the mucosa at the maximal point of swelling gives immediate relief if an abscess is unequivocally present.

Systemic complications of acute tonsillitis, namely, rheumatic fever, acute glomuleronephritis, chorea, and subacute bacterial endocarditis are seen principally in association with group A beta streptococcal infection, but fortunately have been rare since the advent of antibiotics.

Chronic tonsillitis

Chronic tonsillitis is usually a complication of acute tonsillitis, but may also become established more insidiously. In severe cases attacks of acute tonsillitis may occur once every six weeks or so with the throat feeling constantly sore and uncomfortable inbetween attacks. They are most frequently seen in childhood, although chronic tonsillitis is by no means uncommon in teenagers and young adults.

The clinical picture may occur in relation to tonsils of varying shape, size, and appearance, with combined elements of infection in the crypts, fibrosis or hypertrophy. In the adult the important differential diagnosis of unilateral enlargement of the tonsils is malignancy. Lymphosarcoma is particularly prone to declare itself in this way.

There is no medical treatment that will eradicate chronic tonsillitis. Radical enucleation of the tonsils is the only certain cure.

The size of the tonsils is usually unrelated to the frequency and severity of acute infections in them, but occasionally their physical size along with large adenoids can lead to the so-called dangerous 'sleep apnoea' syndrome (see page 15.158).

Adenoids

The adenoids frequently become enlarged and chronically infected. Simple hypertrophy is physiological between the ages of 3 and 7 years. Excessive enlargement relative to that of the nasopharyngeal space leads to nasal and Eustachian tube obstruction.

Nasal obstruction causes chronic mouth breathing, difficulty in eating, and a toneless 'nasal' voice. Blockage of the Eustachian tube predisposes to secretory otitis media or glue ear. A sterile collection of fluid, often thick and mucoid, collects in the tympanic cavity producing severe conductive deafness.

Glue ear is one of the commonest diseases causing deafness in children.

Inflammation of the adenoids is evident as a postnasal drip with an irritating cough and recurrent acute otitis media. Cervical adenitis may be found involving the upper deep cervical and the posterior triangle nodes.

Surgery of the tonsils and adenoids

Tonsils

Great care has to be taken in evaluating the patient with a tonsillar problem. The importance of the history must be stressed as appearance is often misleading. The ENT surgeon, therefore, is very dependent upon the general practitioner and his assessment of the problem.

Indications for surgical treatment of tonsils are:

1. Four unequivocal attacks of tonsillitis in the preceding 12 months, except in a child who starts getting tonsillitis only on going to school. The tendency to allow children to 'grow out' of the trouble should be avoided. The operation with efficient medical and nursing care is virtually uncomplicated (mortality 0.008 per cent of all operations 1979/83, Registrar General's figures). In about 15 per cent of children physiological atrophy of Waldeyer's ring of lymphoid tissue does not occur at 7 to 8 years so that tonsillitis can continue into the teens and even beyond.

The only practical alternative to surgery is prolonged antibiotic therapy over a period of several months. This is only effective in 50 per cent of cases but is definitely preferable to surgery in the very small child.

2. Peritonsillar abscess is rare but when accompanied by preceding attacks of acute tonsillitis surgery is required.

3. Persistently enlarged cervical nodes with a history of chronic tonsillitis.

4. Gross hyperplasia of the tonsils giving rise to symptoms of chronic upper airway obstruction with the sleep apnoea syndrome (page 15.158).

5. Histological examination in rare cases of suspected neoplasm.

Adenoids

Indications for adenoidectomy are:

1. Persistent mouth breathing with a toneless nasal voice. Excessive and persistent snoring and chronic nasal discharge, though it should be remembered that adenoidal atrophy occurs in virtually 100 per cent of children by the age of 10 years.

2. Recurrent attacks of otitis media and conductive deafness due to secretory otitis media.

For glue ear, myringotomy and aspiration of the middle ear under the operating microscope will also be required to restore normal hearing. A ventilation tube (grommet) is usually inserted, remaining *in situ* for several months, acting as an artificial Eustachian tube.

3. If the problem is just a tonsillar one, most surgeons will couple the operation with removal of adenoids. If it is 'just adenoids', a decision has to be made about taking out the tonsils as well. The incidence of all complications, although small, with the combined operation, is twice that of the adenoids alone. However, the chances of subsequently needing to do a tonsillectomy after an adenoidectomy is 1 in 8 below 5 years of age and 1 in 16 above this age.

Neoplasms

Benign tumours are very rare. Juvenile angiofibroma of the nasopharynx deserves mention. It produces nasal obstruction, unilateral conductive deafness, and recurrent severe epistaxes. A squamous cell papilloma can be found as a sessile or pedunculated mass arising from anywhere on the pharyngeal wall.

Malignant tumours of many histological types are seen, but by far the most frequent is squamous cell carcinoma. In the nasopharynx it has an interesting racial distribution, common in the Cantonese population, accounting in Hong Kong for 30 per cent of all deaths from carcinoma compared with 0.5 per cent in most other countries.

Squamous cell carcinoma of the oropharynx is rare before the age of 50 years. Men are five times more commonly affected than women. Tobacco smoking or chewing is a causal factor. Another primary growth in the upper alimentary or respiratory tract is found in about 10 per cent of cases.

In the hypopharynx half the squamous cell carcinomas arise in the pyriform fossa: the postcricoid space is also an important site in women.

Lympho-epithelioma is an unusual tumour found in sites of subepithelial lymphoid tissue in the pharynx. It presents in the younger age group with a tendency to early and widespread metastases, but it is very sensitive to radiotherapy. It is almost certainly a carcinoma surrounded by masses of lymphocytes.

Clinical features

Metastatic cervical lymph-node enlargement is often the presenting sign of pharyngeal carcinoma.

Local symptoms of primary nasopharyngeal tumour are nasal obstruction and deafness due to involvement of the Eustachian tube. Pain in the distribution of the Vth cranial nerve can be an early symptom. Involvement of other cranial nerves occurs late in the disease by extension into the middle cranial fossa and retro-orbital and antral spaces.

Carcinoma of the oropharynx causes enlargement of the ipsilateral tonsil with persistent unilateral sore throat made worse by swallowing. Referred earache is common and occasionally spitting of blood from an ulcerative lesion. Some cases of tonsillar carcinoma have been mistaken for a quinsy, the latter being extremely rare over 50 years of age.

With carcinoma in the pyriform fossa at first there may be no more than a 'catch' in the throat, or a slight sticking of food. The patient frequently points accurately to the pyriform fossa at the level of the thyroid. Pain on swallowing occurs later with referred earache a frequent complaint. Hoarseness indicates an extension into the larynx, or involvement of the recurrent laryngeal nerve. A metastatic lump in the neck is often an early symptom.

Postcricoid carcinoma may complicate the Plummer–Vinson syndrome. Malignant change should be suspected when dysphagia worsens, with localized pain or referred otalgia.

Treatment

Radiotherapy is the usual primary type of treatment, reserving surgical excision for residual or recurrent disease and metastatic cervical nodes.

Prognosis is poor. Only one-third survive 5 years even with very early localized disease and no lymph-node involvement. Early diagnosis is therefore essential. Postcricoid carcinoma carries a particularly poor prognosis. A combination of radiotherapy and elective radical surgery (pharyngo-laryngo-oesophagectomy) provides the best chance of a cure.

Miscellaneous

This includes general diseases, dermatological conditions, neural dysfunctions, and foreign bodies.

Feeling of a lump in the throat

This is a very common complaint. The lump is usually referred to either cricoid or suprasternal notch level. The history is all important, in particular the relationship of the symptom to swallowing of food, and saliva ('quilting'). If only present with quilting and indeed if made better or absent with a normal swallow the condition is seldom anything serious.

Once a neoplasm has been excluded the aetiology is either local or distant. Under local causes cricopharyngeal spasm (or failure of the sphincter to relax), posterior pharyngeal pouch, pharyngeal paralysis or postcricoid web, and globus hystericus should be considered. Spasm is by far the commonest cause, cine radiography being of enormous value in assessing the patient. Globus hystericus should only be diagnosed as a last resort and is comparatively rare.

Distant causes include lesions of the gastro-oesophageal junction level, e.g. reflux, hiatus hernia, carcinoma, which reflexly produce symptoms in the pharynx. It is most important to assess the lower end of the oesophagus to exclude the disease at this site once the pharynx and cervical oesophagus have proved normal.

The larynx

W. S. LUND

Anatomy and physiology

The larynx consists of the signet ring-like cricoid cartilage and the V-shaped thyroid cartilage. Within this framework are the paired arytenoid cartilages and the epiglottis, a curved and leaf-shaped structure.

The intrinsic muscles of the larynx are all inserted into the muscular process of the arytenoid and all of them except one, the posterior crico-arytenoid, are adductors of the vocal cord. The muscles are supplied by the recurrent laryngeal nerve, (derived from the vagus nerve), the only exception being the cricothyroid muscle (a tensor of the vocal cords) which is innervated by the external laryngeal nerve.

The muscles of the larynx have three functions: (1) to open the glottis, allowing the passage of air, (2) to close the glottis and vestibule (the interval between the true and false cords), denying entry of food during swallowing, and (3) to regulate the tension of the vocal cords for speaking.

Laryngeal pathology

The majority of laryngeal lesions give rise to voice change. It is mandatory, therefore, that any patient complaining of an alteration in the voice must have the larynx inspected within one month of the onset of symptoms. If this rule is obeyed an early diagnosis can be made, greatly improving the prognosis with regard to treatment.

Laryngeal pathology may be classified under the usual headings. Congenital lesions are of considerable importance in surgical practice, but need not be discussed here. Attention will be focused on inflammatory, neoplastic, and some miscellaneous conditions.

Laryngitis

Four types of inflammation require mention:

(a) Acute simple laryngitis
(b) Acute epiglottitis
(c) Acute laryngo-tracheo-bronchitis
(d) Chronic non-specific laryngitis (tuberculosis, etc. are now rare, but should be remembered in atypical cases).

Acute simple laryngitis

Children are prone to this condition because immunity against infection is still being acquired. The submucosa of the child's larynx is particularly loose and laryngeal spasm occurs especially easily. In the adult, smoking predisposes to acute laryngitis as part of a generalized upper respiratory tract infection.

Symptoms and signs in the child are croupy cough, huskiness, and the very frightening feature of nocturnal stridor. Hoarseness predominates in the adult.

The diagnosis is usually straightforward and treatment (humidification, sedation, and possibly antibiotics) effective. The voice must be rested. When stridor is present the differential diagnosis is widened to include acute epiglottitis, laryngo-tracheo-bronchitis, and possibly a foreign body.

Acute epiglottitis

This is a rare entity, but since it can be a lethal disease of terrifying swiftness, it is essential that every practitioner is able to recognize it, the condition being caused by the *Haemophilus influenzae* type B organism.

Clinical features

The peak incidence lies between 2 and 3 years, but older children and adults can be affected.

Inflammation is maximal above the vocal cords where the epiglottis can swell up to ten times its normal size. Sudden airway obstruction develops with barely any warning typically within a few hours in a previously healthy child. The classic triad is sore throat, followed by dysphagia and dyspnoea.

Cough is usually slight or absent. Fever may reach 41° C with toxaemia and prostration. The child sits up, drooling saliva and the chin thrust forward. There are enlarged nodes in the neck. The face is ashen, pinched with anxiety and wide-eyed with fear. Difficulty in breathing is entirely inspiratory with accompanying stridor. Hypoxaemia leads to irritability followed by somnolence and coma.

Management

No attempt should be made to view the epiglottis by depressing the tongue as this will precipitate acute asphyxia. Clinical suspicion demands urgent admission to hospital.

Immediate relief of the airway obstruction is mandatory by means of either nasotracheal intubation, tracheostomy or preferably bronchoscopy. There is rarely time for radiology.

Along with safeguarding the airway, humidification is supplied by ultrasonic mist, oxygen is given as well as ampicillin intravenously (chloramphenicol is an alternative). Corticosteroids may be used to control oedema after an airway has been established. Extubation is usually possible after 1 to 4 days. Prompt action and immediate hospitalization on the slightest suspicion can now render this deadly disease harmless.

Acute laryngo-tracheo-bronchitis

The peak incidence of this condition is in children aged between 6 months and 3 years when it often complicates measles, scarlet fever, whooping cough or chicken pox. Various organisms have been isolated, the majority being para-influenza viruses with secondary bacterial invaders.

Clinical features

There is a preceding history of upper respiratory tract infection followed by the onset of a characteristic croupy cough likened to 'the bark of a seal'. Hoarseness is often present with stridor being biphasic instead of wholly inspiratory as in acute epiglottitis. Indurated swelling of the subglottic structures with resulting purulent sputum obstructs the main airway. Respiration is rapid and difficult: the child may find it easier lying down. After hours of struggling the child becomes fatigued and can slip into respiratory failure.

Management

Laryngo-tracheo-bronchitis is a deadly disease. Humidification and nebulized mucolytics are the basic management, together with sedation and tracheobronchial toilet as necessary with a nasotracheal tube, or tracheostomy. Antibiotics are useful if bacterial secondary invasion occurs.

Chronic non-specific laryngitis

This condition is most frequently seen in middle-aged men and is due to a condition of faulty use of the voice, chronic infection of the upper respiratory tract, and exposure to pollution, especially cigarette smoke. Hoarseness is the overriding symptom, intermittent at first, and then persistent.

Treatment is difficult. Vocal rest and elimination of the irritating factors, especially smoking, are essential. Squamous metaplasia and keratosis may require endoscopic removal with histological investigation being important.

Neoplasms and cysts of the larynx

Benign tumours

Simple laryngeal tumours are not uncommon. The great majority of cordal benign 'tumours' are not neoplastic (e.g. vocal nodules seen in professional voice users). Of true benign neoplasms the commonest is the papilloma. Diagnosis can usually be made by simple inspection, though confirmation by histological examination must be sought. In recent years the laser has proved a very useful method for removing these growths.

Malignant tumours

Cancer of the larynx accounts for about 2 per cent of all malignant disease. The most frequent type is the squamous cell carcinoma, generally well differentiated, with the glottic region being the commonest site. Direct extension can occur either upwards or downwards. There are practically no lymph vessels in the true vocal cord so there is very little tendency for involvement of the neck nodes. This feature combined with the early onset of symptoms makes the prognosis more favourable than for carcinoma anywhere else in the body. Lymphatics increase in the supraglottic region with a greater tendency for tumours at this site to give rise to cervicall lymphadenopathy.

Clinical features

Hoarseness beginning without obvious cause is the main early symptom of malignant disease of the larynx. A persistent, continuous huskiness unrelieved by simple treatment in a middle-aged or elderly patient should suggest immediate referral for an indirect laryngoscopy. Other symptoms such as dyspnoea, cough, referred earache, dysphagia, and bleeding occur late in the natural history of the disease.

Unfortunately, practically any other disease affecting the larynx may exhibit symptoms compatible with malignancy. Examination of the neck for metastases and radiological examination with special reference to lateral and PA plain films of the larynx will help. A chest radiograph is obligatory.

Treatment

Essentially, this consists of either surgery, radiotherapy or a combination of both. Early diagnosis is of supreme importance as modern irradiation techniques in localized glottic cancer give a 5-year survival rate of the order of 90 per cent with preservation of the larynx. When cervical metastases are present a radical neck dissection is required, worsening the prognosis.

Miscellaneous conditions of the larynx

Subglottic stenosis

The condition is not uncommon and can cause a severe, harsh, barking, biphasic stridor and dyspnoea. A congenital form is due to considerable thickening of the anterior arch and lateral parts of the cricoid. The acquired type (usually in adults) is associated with granulation tissue over the vocal processes of the arytenoids and is due to prolonged intubation.

Paralysis of the vocal cord

The course of the recurrent laryngeal nerves determines the presentation. The right nerve comes off the vagus in the root of the neck, but the left arises intrathoracically at the hilum of the left lung where it winds around the arch of the aorta. Both nerves then ascend in the tracheo-oesophageal sulcus being intimately related to the posterior surface of the thyroid lobe before entering the larynx. By virtue of its longer course the left recurrent nerve is affected twice as often as the right.

In a complete paralysis the affected cord lies in the paramedian position producing a gap at the level of the glottis. The normal cord being unable to hyperadduct across the midline to meet the fixed one, produces a breathy whispery voice lacking in strength. This is quite unlike the true hoarseness of lesions such as carcinoma of the cords.

Cord paralysis may be produced by a lesion either in the vagus itself (see Table 1) or in one of the recurrent nerves. In relation to the latter on both sides various types of thyroid pathology are relevant with intrathoracic lesions such as enlarged hilar glands, carcinoma of the bronchus, selectively affecting only the left nerve.

In a case of vocal cord paralysis where no aetiology is determined it is assumed that some type of neuritis has affected the recurrent nerve.

An injection of Teflon paste into the paralysed cord to increase its bulk can produce a significant improvement in those cases where speech therapy has been unsuccessful.

Dysphonia

The larynx, like any other muscular organ, is prone to misuse, abuse, and strain, producing changes in the character and quality of the voice. This is particularly so in professional voice users, such as singers, actors, teachers. The history will usually establish the diagnosis, but it is essential that the larynx is examined to exclude any more serious pathology.

One particular 'voice-production problem', functional aphonia,

Table 1 Lesions of the vagus nerve causing cord paralysis

1. Lesions in the CNS
   (*a*) Supranuclear lesions; rare, must be very large
   (*b*) Brain stem nuclear lesions: denote involvement of the nucleus ambiguus; e.g. bulbar palsies
2. Posterior cranial fossa: e.g. meningitis, acoustic tumours
3. Jugular foramen: e.g. skull fractures, tumours
4. Neck: injuries, neoplasms, enlarged nodes

is most frequently seen in young women. The voice is suddenly reduced to a whisper for no apparent reason. A bilateral adductor paralysis is noted, the vocal cords remaining widely apart on attempted phonation. However, cough is normal when the glottis may be seen to close efficiently.

The nose and sinuses

W. S. LUND

Anatomy (Fig. 1a, b)

The nasal cavities which are separated by a cartilaginous and bony septum have three downwardly curved shelves, the conchae (or tubinates), projecting from their side walls. These overhang three anteroposteriorly running passages, the meatuses. Opening into the inferior meatus is the nasolachrymal duct, while the orifices of virtually all the sinuses open into the middle meatus.

The mucous membrane covering the inferior and middle conchae contain large venous sinuses, and are covered by ciliated columnar epithelium. The uppermost part of the medial and lateral walls is the olfactory area supplied by the olfactory nerves which pass through the thin cribriform plate.

The paired ethmoidal labyrinths, each containing a variable number of air cells, lie under the cribriform plate lateral to the superior and middle conchae. The orbits lie immediately lateral to each ethmoidal labyrinth. The maxillary antra are below the orbits, three of four upper teeth being closely related to them. The frontal sinuses which vary enormously in size (and indeed may be entirely absent) open into the nose via a duct which runs through the anterior ethmoidal air cells.

Physiology

Nasal function can be considered under three headings.

1. Respiration.
2. Protection.
3. Smell.

Respiration

The normal pattern of nasal respiration is established from birth and it has been known for infants to asphyxiate when unable to breathe through the nose. Mouth breathing is learnt by about six months of age.

Inspiratory and expiratory air currents pursue a well-recognized curved pathway through the nose which may be interfered with by a deviated nasal septum, polyps, enlarged turbinates, etc.

Protection

The lower respiratory tract is in part protected by the nasal functions of purification, warming, and moistening of the inspired air. Purification is affected by the vibrissae at the front of the nose. The cilia move the mucus 'blanket' which contains lysozymes backward into the pharynx. Warming is established by the rich vascular arrangements of the nasal mucosa with the inspired air being almost completely saturated in the nose. The ciliary mechanism is extremely important and may be damaged by drying, e.g. excessive central heating and factors producing nasal obstruction, certain drugs such as local decongestants that are not isotonic and cause rebound congestion, and excessive heat or cold.

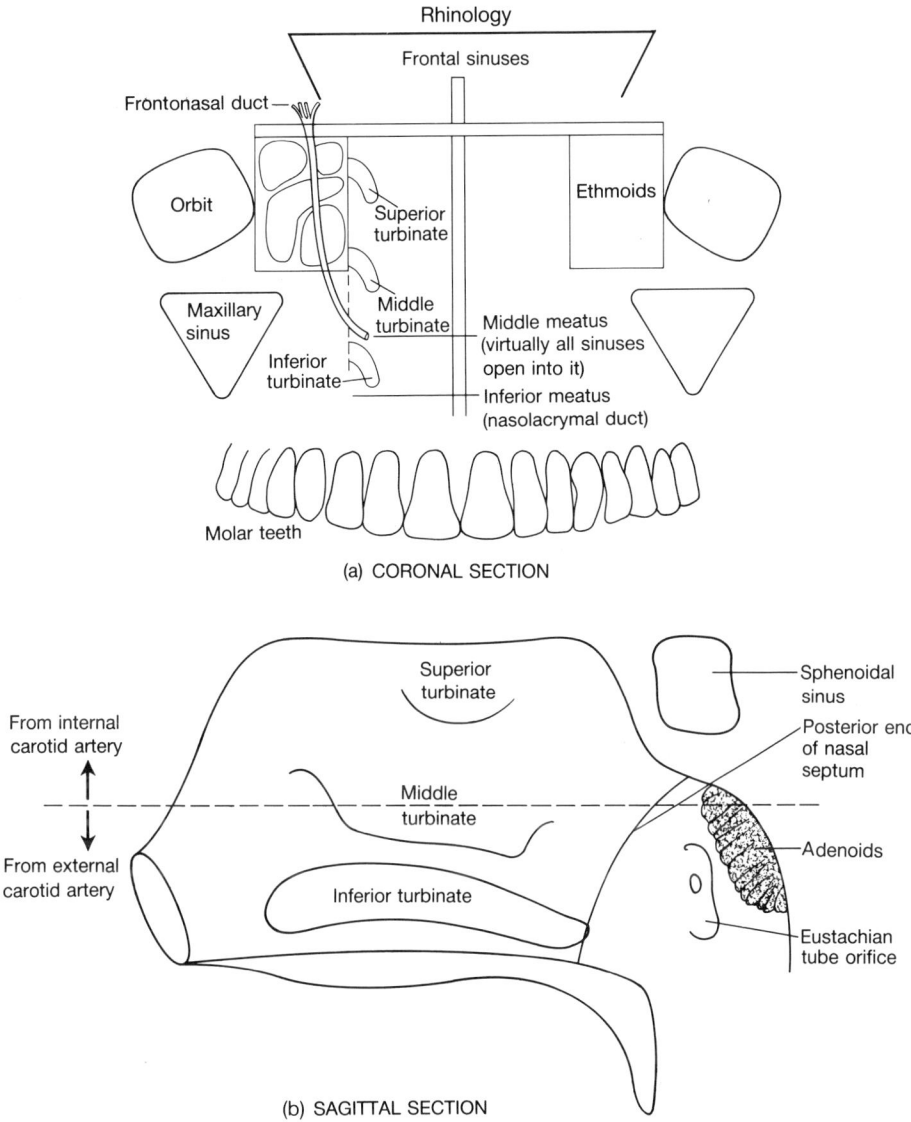

Fig. 1 (a, b) Anatomy of the nose and sinuses.

Smell

The odour of a substance is probably related to the shape of its molecules. Olfaction is closely associated with taste as flavours are largely perceived through the olfactory apparatus. The olfactory mucosa possesses three types of cell, namely, the olfactory cell with a central axon passing through the cribriform plate, supporting cell, and basal cell.

Rhinology

The history is important with certain well-recognized symptoms suggesting particular clinical conditions.

(a) A *watery* rhinorrhoea, sneezing, and alternating nasal obstruction indicate an allergic and/or vasomotor rhinitis.

(b) *Purulent* rhinorrhoea, a postnasal drip (with frontal headache) suggest sinusitis.

(c) Nasal obstruction may be *unilateral* or *bilateral*. When unilateral the diagnosis lies between a deviated nasal septum, sinusitis or a tumour. Bilateral obstruction occurs with allergic/vasomotor rhinitis and polyps.

(d) Bleeding (epistaxis) is usually due to trauma or hypertension, occasionally a bleeding disorder and rarely a tumour.

(e) Loss of sense of smell (anosmia) can be related to almost any condition.

The danger signs in rhinology are shown in Table 1.

Rhinitis

This is a common condition characterized by variable nasal obstruction, watery rhinorrhoea, sneezing, and reduction of smell.

Infective rhinitis is initially viral, but secondary bacterial

Table 1 Danger signs in rhinology

Tumour is suggested by

1 Serosanguinous discharge
2 Swelling of the cheek
3 Unilateral nasal polyp
4 Unilateral nasal symptoms in an adult

Especially if associated with

5 An enlarged node in the neck
6 Lower cranial nerve palsies
7 Closed swollen eye in a child or young adult
8 Swollen upper eyelid and headache

invasion occurs quickly. Allergic rhinitis may be difficult to distinguish from early infective rhinitis. It can be seasonal as exemplified by hay fever or perennial due to the house dust mite, dog hair, cat fur, etc.

Vasomotor rhinitis is a frequently encountered entity caused by 'parasympathetic overdrive', and made worse by pollution, central heating, cigarettes, alcohol, stress, etc.

Management

A careful history is essential. The degree of the problem and severity of symptoms must be assessed accurately to avoid overtreatment. Special investigations may include skin tests for an allergic state and sinus X-rays to exclude secondary infection.

When obvious infection is present antimicrobials, e.g. penicillin with or without metronidazole, may be required, together with a local decongestant (Otrivine – Xylometazoline or 1 per cent ephedrine in normal saline) and an inhalant (steam, Vic or Karvol). Use of the former must be limited to a two-week course to avoid the rebound phenomenon and the development of 'rhinitis medicamentosa'.

In allergic rhinitis, desensitization is of value for seasonal pollen hay fever. Avoidance of specific allergens should be recommended if practical. Cromoglycate (Rynacrom) is helpful as a prophylaxis, along with antihistamines to control sneezing and rhinorrhoea, but of greatest value are the topical corticosteroids, beclomethazone diproprionate (Beconase), budesonide (Rhinocort), and flunisolide (Syntaris). These have proved of enormous value in reducing mucosal sensitivity. To be effective a two month course is required. Rebound does not occur, side-effects are nonexistent, and the preparation can be repeated at regular intervals.

Surgical reduction in size of the inferior turbinates can be carried out if nasal obstruction is the principal complaint due to gross swelling of the mucosa.

Nasal polyps

This condition frequently accompanies allergic/vasomotor rhinitis and complicates sinusitis. The polyps have a grey 'peeled grape' appearance and arise from the oedematous mucosa of the ethmoid air cells. They are invariably *bilateral* and appear in the middle meatus. Diagnosis is made on inspection with treatment by intranasal surgical excision, followed by topical steroids.

Sinusitis

The maxillary antrum is the most commonly affected; the frontal and ethmoidal sinuses more rarely though more seriously and usually secondary to maxillary disease.

Maxillary sinusitis

In acute sinusitis the infection is mixed bacterial, secondary to a viral rhino-sinusitis, or more rarely apical/peridontal tooth disease. Eighty per cent of chronic cases are predisposed to by allergic/vasomotor rhinitis.

Considerable malaise accompanies acute sinusitis with mucopurulent rhinorrhoea, nasal obstruction, facial pain/frontal headache with or without upper toothache. Tenderness may be present over the affected sinus and on tapping the upper teeth. The nasal mucosa is swollen and pus may be seen in the middle meatus. A swollen cheek does *not* occur in uncomplicated maxillary sinusitis. In the acute form it is usually due to dental disease, and in the chronic form to an antral tumour.

Radiographs show mucosal thickening in the maxillary sinus, an appearance, however, which can occur in uninfected vasomotor rhinitis. A completely opaque antrum, i.e. a 'white-out', or a fluid level is however pathognomonic of infection.

Treatment consists of antibiotics, a local decongestant, and humidification. If resolution does not occur then an antral washout will be required, and failing this an intranasal antrostomy. Irreversible chronic disease needs a Caldwell Luc with total removal of the infected sinus lining.

Complications

Acute frontal sinusitis

Pus and swelling in the middle meatus obstructs the frontonasal duct, poor drainage results with secondary infection of the frontal sinus. Primary frontal sinusitis can follow jumping into water with an upper respiratory tract infection and this can produce pus under tension, an *empyema* of the sinus. It is a dangerous condition since it occurs in a closed bony cavity with a long duct; infection can spread to the orbit and anterior cranial fossa.

The clinical picture is one of severe pain over the eye with marked constitutional upset. Swelling of the upper eyelid is frequently present. Percussion of the affected sinus exacerbates the pain. The condition demands hospitalization with intravenous antibiotics. If there is no improvement after 24 hours the sinus should be trephined through its floor.

Acute ethmoiditis

This occurs typically in children and young adults. There is a swollen, closed eye with the danger of peri-orbital abscess, orbital cellulitis, and blindness. Admission to hospital is essential.

Nasal obstruction

This very frequent symptom when it occurs alone and is constant, suggests a deviated nasal septum or polyps (bilateral). When it occurs alone and is variable, vasomotor rhinitis is the likely cause and if accompanied by watery rhinorrhoea, then rhinitis. If accompanied by mucopurulent rhinorrohoea think of sinusitis and if the discharge is serosanguinous and unilateral then it may be a tumour.

Severe crusting and bleeding with nasal obstruction point to an intranasal granuloma.

Upper repiratory tract granulomas

Sarcoidosis Involvement of the upper respiratory tract occurs in about 1:20 of patients with sarcoidosis. As with the disease as a whole the male:female rate is 1:2. The spectrum of other sarcoid lesions seen in this subgroup is wide but not strikingly different from sarcoid overall, though there is a strong association with skin lesions especially lupus pernio. However, two-thirds of these patients have no symptoms elsewhere at presentation.

The nasal mucosa is most often involved. Sarcoid lesions here cause nasal discharge and obstruction. Inspection reveals a granular erythematous mucosa with crusting. Nasal perforation is an uncommon complication. Punctate areas of destruction may be seen on nasal radiographs due to bone involvment.

Less commonly there may be sarcoid deposits in the larynx and pharynx leading to hoarseness and obstruction.

Steroids are helpful but not often sufficient if only given topically.

Wegener's granulomatosis This condition is described elsewhere (page 15.133). The nasal granulomas which occur as part of a full Wegener's syndrome may occasionally occur alone (lethal midline granuloma). The clinical features of bilateral nasal crusting and serosanguinous discharge are not specific. Septal perforation and destructive lesions of the nasal and sinus bones are seen more often than in sarcoid. Regrettably histology does not confirm the diagnosis, but other investigations, e.g. ESR, CXR, MSU etc. are essential.

When part of a generalized Wegener's granulomatosis, treatment is with systemic steroids and immunosuppressive agents. Localized midline granuloma can respond well to radiotherapy.

Fractured nose

It is important to check for a septal haematoma and other associated facial fractures. X-rays are unhelpful, but may be necessary for medico-legal reasons.

Nose bleeds (epistaxis)

Eighty per cent of nose bleeds arise from Little's area on the front of the septum. They occur in young patients and are easy to stop. Twenty per cent come from further back, usually in the elderly patient and need a postnasal pack on admission to hospital.

Aetiology The vast majority are spontaneous (or due to minor trauma), but it is important to remember anticoagulants, thrombocytopaenia, clotting disorders, and tumours. Hypertensive patients probably do not bleed more often, but the bleeding is more severe when they do.

Management This must be considered under two headings.

1. General. An attempt should be made to assess blood loss and the patient's cardiovascular state. If there is any degree of 'shock' then admit to hospital immediately, especially in the elderly. Blood should be cross-matched and given as necessary.

2. Local. The nose must be examined with a head-light in order to try to identify the source of the bleeding. Clots should be blown of sucked out and a 10 per cent cocaine spray (with or without 25 per cent cocaine paste) applied to the nasal cavity which is then inspected carefully.

If the bleeding is anterior then the vessel can be cauterized with silver nitrate or trichloracetic acid once the nose is dry. If the bleeding is posterior, packing is required with a Simpson balloon (an inflatable finger cot); admission to hospital is required.

Acknowledgement
We would like to acknowledge the help of Mr M. P. Rothera, Clinical Lecturer, the Department of Otolaryngology, the Radcliffe Infirmary, Oxford, in the planning of this chapter on the nose and sinuses.

DISORDERS OF THE AIRWAYS

Asthma

A. J. WOOLCOCK

The problem of definition

Asthma is a disease of the airways. Since 1952 it has been defined as widespread narrowing of the airways which changes its severity over short periods of time either spontaneously or under treatment. This definition gives no indication of the nature of the disease or, indeed, if a specific disease, identifiable as asthma, exists. It is not a suitable definition for epidemiological studies or for studies involving interventions on precisely defined groups of patients. Lack of a more precise definition reflects our poor understanding of the cause of asthma.

It is now recognized that asthmatics with current symptoms have bronchial hyperresponsiveness (BHR). This is defined as narrowing of the airways in response to a wide variety of provoking agents which have little or no effect in normal subjects. The degree of BHR can be accurately and reproducibly measured with an inhalation test using histamine or methacholine. However, asthma cannot be defined solely as the presence of BHR to inhaled histamine or methacholine because patients with other airway diseases, including chronic airflow limitation, have airways which are hyperresponsive to these agents.

Definition

In this chapter, asthma is defined as bronchial hyperresponsiveness together with intermittent symptoms of wheezing, chest tightness or cough. Symptoms in the last 12 months distinguish 'current' from 'past' asthma. Bronchial hyperresponsiveness is defined as a 20 per cent fall in the 1 s forced expiratory volume (PD20FEV1) in response to a provoking dose of histamine or methacholine of less than 8 μmol.

There are individuals who have asthmatic symptoms only in the pollen season or on exposure to occupational agents. Many of these people do not have BHR to histamine and methacholine and do not have symptoms induced by stimuli other than pollen or occupational agents. They are better defined as having either seasonal allergic or occupational asthma, and appear to be different from the group with asthma as defined above, except during times of exposure to these agents.

Epidemiology

Prevalence of asthma

Accurate figures for the prevalence of asthma in different populations are not available because of the lack of an agreed definition and because it is now well known that asthma is underdiagnosed in some populations. However, there does appear to be a wide variation between populations. It is common in Australia and New Zealand where the cumulative prevalence has been shown to be as high as 12 per cent in some groups of children. The prevalence is lower in Europe and in the United States and extremely low in most developing countries, particularly in village communities. In Western countries it is more common in children than in adults and it is more frequent in boys than in girls.

Prevalence of BHR

To date there have been few studies of the prevalence of bronchial responsiveness in different communities. Figure 1 shows the results of studies in children and adults in Australia. In both age groups, the distribution of increased responsiveness was continuous. Many people with mild and intermediate levels of BHR had no symptoms and many were non-atopic (as defined by skin prick tests). Approximately 18 per cent of children and 14 per cent of

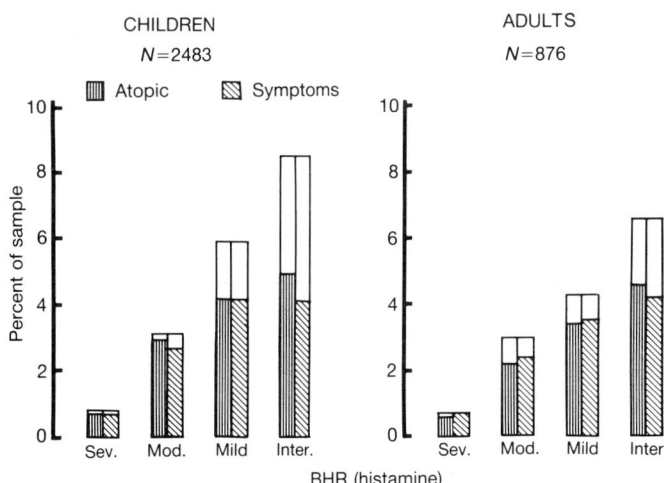

Fig. 1 Prevalence of bronchial hyperresponsiveness (BHR) in a sample of Australian children (aged 8–10 years) and adults. The degree of BHR shown here as severe, moderate, mild, and intermediate, is defined in Fig. 3. The proportion who were atopic and had symptoms consistent with asthma are also shown. The prevalence of severe and moderate degrees of BHR was similar in the two age groups but there were more children with mild and intermediate degrees of BHR, and a greater percentage of these children were nonatopic and without symptoms.

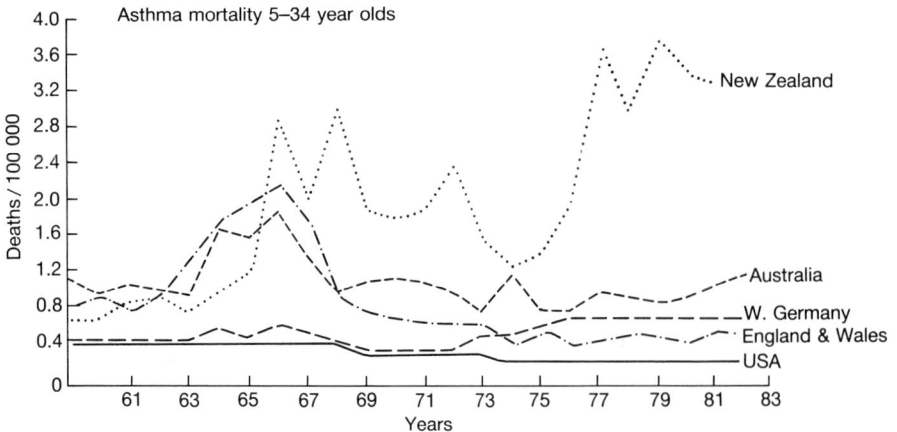

Fig. 2 Death rates for 5–34 year olds in several countries between 1959 and 1980. There was an increase in the 1960s in several countries and a recent increase in New Zealand persists. (This figure is redrawn from data published by Jackson *et al.*, 1982, *Br. med. J.* **285**, 771–774.)

adults had BHR. The cumulative prevalence of asthma, as defined above and shown by the sloped hatching, was 12 per cent in children and 8.5 per cent in adults.

Mortality

Before this century, reliable observers stated that asthma was not a fatal disease. Now it is recognized that asthma mortality can be as high as 3 per 100 000 per year in some countries. The highest rates are in New Zealand followed by Australia, England, European countries, and then North America. There was a rise in death rates in some countries in the 1960s but now the rates are steady in most countries with the exception of New Zealand, where there has been an increase in recent years. Recent mortality figures from several countries for those aged 5 to 34 years (where the diagnosis is likely to be accurate) are shown in Fig. 2. Retrospective analyses have shown that most deaths occur outside hospital and result from underestimation by the physician and/or the patient of the severity of the disease.

Natural history

The abnormality appears to wax and wane with time. It commonly starts in childhood and then improves spontaneously in early adult life. It can also occur for the first time in middle age. However, there is evidence that many adults with so-called newly diagnosed asthma had the disease in childhood. There is some controversy as to the age at which asthma can first be diagnosed because the bronchial smooth muscle is not well developed in the first year of life. It is generally agreed that although a child who wheezes before the age of 2 years may well have asthma, it is not possible to be certain about the diagnosis before this age.

There is increasing evidence that children with mild asthma, as assessed by frequency and severity of attacks or by measurements of BHR, are more likely to become symptom free and perhaps reach normal levels of BHR after adolescence. On the other hand, when the BHR is severe, the abnormality seems to be irreversible and the child continues to have asthma. Early age of onset and the presence of severe infantile eczema also carry a poor prognosis. Chronic asthma in adult life can lead to irreversible airways obstruction but how much of this is due to inadequate treatment is not known. There is no evidence that asthma leads to emphysema.

Aetiology

The cause of asthma is unknown. There is an abnormality in the control of the airway lumen and particularly in the control of bronchial smooth muscle (BSM) which permits the airways to narrow excessively in response to a wide variety of stimuli which have little or no effect on the airways of normal people. The nature of this abnormality is discussed further below. It is probably acquired and, once present, a variety of provoking stimuli including exercise, airway drying, infections, allergens, sulphur dioxide, and emotional upsets can trigger attacks. If the BHR is severe, only small amounts of a provoking stimulus are needed to produce an

attack and the patient is liable to have symptoms continuously unless treatment is given. If the BHR is mild, much stronger provoking stimuli are needed to cause airway narrowing and attacks are less frequent. Atopy, acute respiratory infections in childhood, and genetic factors are thought to be associated with asthma.

Atopy

The association between asthma and atopy is so strong that in some countries asthma is regarded as primarily an allergic disease and asthmatics are treated by allergists with a view to reducing the degree of allergy present. The majority of young asthmatics are atopic. Circulating IgE antibodies to common aeroallergens can be demonstrated by either radioimmunoabsorbent tests (RAST) or simple skin prick tests which are equally reliable. Recent epidemiological studies have shown that up to 40 per cent of some adult populations are atopic, as judged by skin tests, but the current prevalence of asthma is closer to 5 per cent. Thus, not all atopic people have asthma. Equally many asthmatics do not have any evidence of atopy (Fig. 1). There is no evidence that allergic mechanisms are responsible for the initial onset of BHR although there is good evidence that allergic asthmatic subjects become worse, with increased BHR and more symptoms, after exposure to allergens and are improved when isolated from allergen exposure.

In the laboratory, inhalation of allergens in the asthmatic may cause an immediate or a late airway response and often the responses differ not only in time course (Fig. 3) but also in mechanism (Table 1). Late reactions probably involve inflammatory cells which enter in response to chemotactic factors released during the initial reaction. Late, more than immediate, reactions appear to alter existing levels of BHR.

It seems likely that seasonal allergic asthmatics have an antibody–antigen reaction in the airways on inhaling the allergen, with

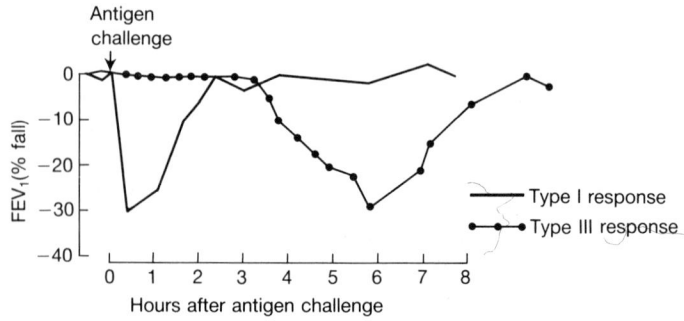

Fig. 3 Changes in FEV$_1$ after an antigen challenge showing a 'type 1' or early response and a 'type 3' or late response. Usually, both responses occur in reponse to allergen but isolated early or late responses sometimes occur.

Table 1 Differences between early and late reactions to allergen challenge

	Early	Late
Time of onset	10 min	4–8 hours
Duration	30–60 min	24–36 hours
Prevented by	(a) β_2 agonist aerosols	(a) Prevention of early
	(b) Sodium cromoglycate	reaction
		(b) Corticosteroids
Reversed with β_2-agonists	Easily	With difficulty
Probable mechanisms	Bronchial SM contraction ± oedema	Inflammation with cellular infiltration

release of sufficient mediators to narrow the airways and to cause symptoms. On recovery, if no further exposure occurs, the airways behave normally. This group of atopic subjects, although exposed to allergens does not appear to develop the underlying abnormality of BHR which characterizes other asthma sufferers (see below). Thus, although there is a close association between atopy and asthma they are not identical and the nature of this association requires clarification.

Childhood infections

There is now good evidence in developed countries that asthma is common in children who have had severe viral infection before the age of 2 years. The role of infections later in childhood is not so well established. There is much anecdotal evidence that infections can precipitate asthma for the first time in adults. There seems to be good evidence that viral (and perhaps bacterial) infections alter the response of lymphocytes and neutrophils to β-adrenergic stimulation, even in normal subjects. If this occurs in a patient with asthma, it may well precipitate an attack. The mechanism by which infection induces BHR, if indeed it does, is unknown.

Genetic factors

The role of genetic factors in the development of asthma is far from clear. It is commonly said that there is a genetic component to asthma but the association is much stronger for atopy than for asthma. In fact, studies in twins do not show a strong genetic component to BHR. Although in some animal studies there is suggestion of a genetic factor operating to determine BHR, studies of relatives of people with BHR have given conflicting results. At present it is far from proven that induction of BHR requires a genetic factor.

Autonomic nervous system (ANS) in asthma

Beta-adrenergic system

It is generally agreed that there is no direct sympathetic nerve supply to the bronchial smooth muscle in humans. However, endogenous and exogenous catecholamines have a strong influence on BSM tone via the β_2-adrenoceptors found throughout the length of the bronchial tree. When stimulated they cause relaxation of the cells via adenyl cyclase and cyclic AMP.

In asthma there is some evidence for altered function of the β_2-adrenoceptors in the airways. However, there have been no systematic studies of the number of β_2-receptors along the length of the bronchial tree in asthmatic airways. In normal and atopic subjects down regulation of the β_2-receptors on BSM occurs with long-term use of adrenergic drugs but there is no evidence that this occurs in patients with asthma. Normal people cannot be made to have BHR with β-blockers and it does not seem that BHR in asthma is simply the result of abnormal β_2-receptors. A number of other cells in the airways including mast cells, leukocytes, basophils, and epithelial cells have β-receptors. Studies using white cells indicate that β_2-receptor function can be decreased for a time after administration of adrenergic drugs, after allergen exposure, and after upper respiratory tract infections, but there is no evi-

dence that there is an abnormality of β-adrenergic functions of the white cells in asthmatics outside these circumstances.

Cholinergic system

There is a good cholinergic nerve supply to the airway smooth muscle which extends throughout the airways. There are cholinergic receptors on the BSM which can be blocked by atropine and related drugs. There is no evidence that the structure, numbers or functions of these receptors are altered in asthma although the afferent side of the reflex may have increased activity due to changes in the sensitivity of the sensory nerve endings. It has been suggested that BHR is due to an exaggerated activity of the parasympathetic pathways because all asthmatics have exaggerated responses to cholinergic agonists (methacholine, carbachol, acetylcholine) and that muscarinic antagonists are effective bronchodilators. However, there are many arguments against this idea. Firstly, asthmatics have exaggerated responses to a large number of chemical agents (see below), secondly, cholinergic antagonists are relatively poor bronchodilators compared with β_2-agonists and thirdly, many studies have shown that they have slight (or at the best variable) effects in protecting against provocation of attacks. By comparison, β_2-agonists are vastly superior prophylactic drugs. There is indirect evidence for cholinergic receptors on human mast cells and basophils but no evidence that they function abnormally in patients with asthma. Overall, present evidence suggests that cholinergic innervation and receptors in the lung are normal in asthma and that the cholinergic reflex is extremely active in many unstable asthmatics contributing to the smooth muscle contraction and perhaps to mucus secretion.

Alpha-adrenergic system

There is now little doubt that there are α-receptors in the human airways. They respond to circulating noradrenaline and cause bronchial smooth muscle contraction. These effects are difficult to show in vivo in normal subjects even when the β-receptors are blocked. However, in asthmatics there is good evidence that α stimulation causes airway narrowing. There is also some evidence that α stimulation causes increased release of mediators from mast cells.

Overall function of the ANS in asthma

There is some evidence for minor abnormalities in the ANS function of the blood vessels of the skin and of the pupil. However, overall, asthmatics do not suffer from severe abnormalities of autonomic function and patients with stable asthma probably have little demonstrable abnormality of the autonomic nervous system. If any abnormality exists it appears to be an overdependence of the airways on β_2-adrenergic stimulation and an increased responsiveness to α-adrenergic stimulation.

Cellular function in asthma

Bronchial smooth muscle cell

There is evidence for histamine, prostaglandin, and leukotriene receptors in addition to the β_2-adrenergic, cholinergic, and α-receptors on the BSM cell. The function of all these receptors in the maintenance of normal BSM tone is unknown. In spite of a great deal of work with these mediators, there is no evidence that the number or the sensitivity of any of their receptors is abnormal in patients with asthma or that they cause or contribute to BHR.

In subjects with severe asthma who die of the disease, the BSM is hyperplastic and hypertrophied. However, no other structural or ultrastructural abnormality of the BSM has been described. The function of the BSM is thought to be abnormal because of the severe and rapid narrowing of airways which occurs during spontaneous and induced attacks. There is some evidence that muscle excised from patients with asthma contracts normally in an organ bath.

If all bronchial smooth muscle cells shortened maximally in vivo (20 per cent of their resting length) the airways would close. This probably occurs only rarely but it seems likely that BSM cells of asthmatics are able to shorten more than those of normal subjects. Thus, the abnormality appears to be in the control of the BSM cells in the living airway.

Mast cells

In human lungs there are mast cells along the length of the airways. Many are in the mucosa close to the epithelium and some are in the lumen. The normal function of the mast cells is largely unknown although they appear to be an inflammatory cell with modified lysosomal 'packages' in their granules.

Direct evidence that the lung mast cells are abnormal in asthma is not available. There is some evidence that they are increased in number in lavage fluid and that they more easily release mediators than the mast cells of normal subjects. However, most of the studies have been done on allergic asthmatics and it is not clear if these differences are simply due to the allergic state.

It is tempting to speculate that in the allergic person, low level and constant mediator release from mast cells over a period of time is the cause of the underlying bronchial hyperresponsiveness but there is no published evidence for this apart from observations which show that exposure to allergens increases, while withdrawal from exposure decreases pre-existing levels of BHR.

Mediators

The role of mediators in controlling BSM tone and in the inflammatory process in normal subjects is largely unknown. In asthma there is much speculation about their role in producing BHR but little evidence. On the other hand, their role in producing attacks in individual patients is becoming clearer. The mediators from human lung mast cells include histamine, heparin, prostaglandin D2, leukotrienes, and proteoglycans.

There is no evidence that the nature of mediators released from mast cells is altered in asthma although there is some evidence for greater amounts. The products of arachadonic acid metabolism can be influenced by drugs and perhaps by diet so that it is possible that the amounts of prostaglandins and leukotrienes released may vary between and within different patients. In the presence of BHR very small amounts of mediator can cause airway narrowing while the chemotatic mediators probably play a role in late reactions and chronic asthma. There is no evidence that mediator release itself causes asthma to develop.

Epithelial cells

These may prove to be most important in asthma. At present it is known that they produce two mediators, 5 Hete and leukotriene B4, as well as an inhibitory substance. Epithelial cells are frequently shed in asthma even when the disease is clinically quiescent. Increased permeability of the epithelium has been much discussed as the cause of BHR but there is no convincing evidence to support this theory.

Inflammatory cells

The pathology of asthma is characterized by the infiltration of the airways by eosinophils and other inflammatory cells which migrate in response to chemotactic factors released by mast cells, macrophages, and lymphocytes. Eosinophils contain a substance, major basic protein, which damages the airway and is responsible for the large amorphous, pink masses in the mucus and submucosa seen in patients who have died with asthma.

Neutrophils also infiltrate the airways in acute attacks of asthma. However, their role is unclear. In an animal model, mild degrees of increased BR can be induced with ozone yet if these animals are depleted of neutrophils this does not occur.

Mucus secreting cells

In asthma, goblet cell metaplasia is common, probably a response to mediator release, and there is hypertrophy of the mucous glands. Cholinergic stimulation increases secretion of mucus while β-adrenergic stimulation seems to have little effect except to reduce viscosity. It is not known if the mucous glands and secretions are functionally abnormal in asthma even though plugging with thick mucus is almost invariable in patients who die with severe asthma and mucous plugs are known to exist in small airways even in the symptom-free state. Some asthmatics have excess mucus secretion during attacks whilst others do not.

Vascular endothelial cells

Oedema of the airways is commonly listed as one of the causes of obstruction of the airways in asthma. Oedema of the bronchial wall will occur if there is a leak of protein followed by fluid from the microvasculature. This leak probably occurs through venules. Using the hampster cheek pouch model, it is known that venular endothelial cells contract in response to many of the mediators which contract BSM in vitro leaving a gap through which a leak occurs. This contraction can be prevented by β_2-agonists and theophylline. Very little is known about the control of vascular endothelial cells in the human airway in health or in asthma.

Pathology

The macroscopic findings in the lungs of people who have died during a crisis of asthma are well described. The characteristic features are overinflated lungs which do not deflate when the thorax is opened, widespread plugging of airways with thick mucus, but no evidence of emphysematous changes. The airway walls can be seen to be thickened and there is sometimes evidence of bronchiectasis in the upper lobes.

Histologically, desquamation of the epithelium, hypertrophy of the smooth muscle, thickening of the basement membrane, and infiltration with eosinophils are the findings which characterize the pathology of asthma. Other features which are not unique to asthma include inflammatory cell infiltration, hyperplasia of the mucous glands, and goblet cell metaplasia. Of particular interest is the shedding of the epithelium which is a feature of the asthmatic airway even in the absence of a crisis. The cause of this shedding is unknown but may be the result of the severe oedema caused by protein leak which, in turn, is produced by mediators acting on the microvasculature.

Little is known about the pathology of the airways in the symptom-free state apart from evidence for residual mucous plugs in the small airways. Recent studies of mucosal biopsies have shown that the epithelial cells are severely deranged even in the well asthmatic.

Nature of bronchial hyperresponsiveness in asthma

Within the population there is a continuum between normal and increased bronchial responsiveness (BR). Figure 1 shows the distribution of BHR in adults and in children in a study using histamine, but others have used methacholine and hyperventilation with cold air to show a similiar distribution. From extensive clinical studies it is known that patients with asthma are unlikely to experience symptoms when the PD20FEV1 to histamine or methacholine is greater than 8 μmol. For this reason, this level is chosen to describe BHR. It must be recognized that this cut off point is arbitrary. Occasionally subjects with more severe levels of BHR can be asymptomatic while others with well-documented symptoms have lesser levels of BHR. Furthermore, the test is reproducible only to one doubling dose of the inhaled bronchoconstrictor and varies with a number of factors.

Figure 4 shows typical dose–response curves to inhaled histamine, methacholine, and methoxamine (an α agonist) in an asthmatic and in a normal subject. Patients with asthma have similar responses to histamine and methacholine while normal subjects are more sensitive to histamine. Furthermore, the dose–response curves of normal subjects reach a plateau while those of the asthmatic do not, even after a 60 per cent fall in the FEV_1. This suggests that in vivo, the airway smooth muscle of subjects with asthma is able to contract to a greater degree than that in normal subjects perhaps because the asthmatic subject lacks an inhibitory

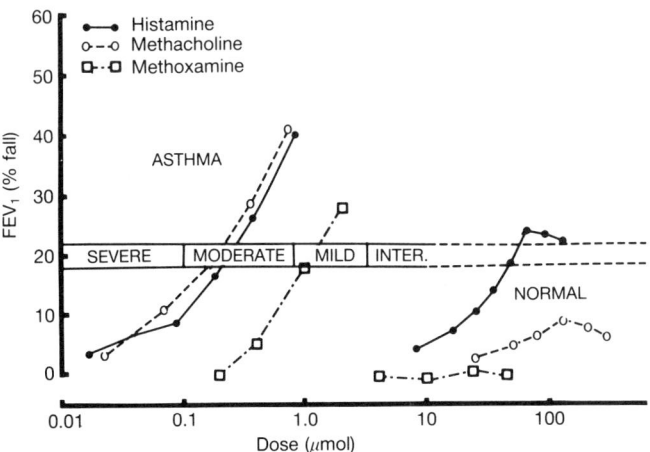

Fig. 4 Dose–response curves to inhaled histamine, methacholine, and methoxamine (an α-agonist) obtained from a patient with moderately severe asthma and from a normal subject. The asthmatic curves to histamine and methacholine were similar and did not plateau and there was a response to methoxamine, whereas the normal subject was more sensitive to histamine than to methacholine, the curves reached a plateau and there was no response to methoxamine.

mechanism. The figure also shows the ranges for severe, moderate, mild, and intermediate levels of BHR defined on the basis of large numbers of clinic patients. Most people with intermediate levels of BHR do not have symptoms.

There are innumerable studies of increased 'bronchial reactivity' in patients with a variety of diseases, in normal subjects after respiratory infections and following exposure to ozone, and in animal models. The airway responses to histamine and methacholine can be shown to increase after many different insults, especially when a very sensitive indicator such as airway resistance or conductance is used to measure the response and no deep inspiration is taken. This increased response does not mean that the animal, the normal subject or the patient has acquired the abnormality which is basic to asthma. The BHR of asthma has certain characteristics, some of which are listed in Table 2. Further definition of these characteristics may lead to better definitions of asthma.

From time to time people are described as having symptoms of asthma who do not have a response to histamine or methacholine when they are well. Some of them undoubtedly have seasonal allergic asthma as defined above and some have occupational asthma. Others are non-allergic and can be demonstrated to improve slowly after an attack. It may well be that there exists another form of airways disease characterized by airway narrowing which improves with treatment (i.e. is reversible) but is not the same disease as asthma. This suggests that, as with allergen exposure, it is possible, in some circumstances which are not understood, to have mediator release sufficient to narrow the airways in the absence of BHR. If a person has normal responses to histamine, methacholine, and cold air hyperventilation challenges it is difficult to make a diagnosis of asthma at that particular time.

Table 2 Characteristics of BHR in asthmatic and normal subjects

	Asthma	Normal
Response to histamine (H) and methacholine (M)		
(a) PD20FEV1 (μmol)	< 8.0	> 20
(b) Shape of curve	No plateau	Plateau
(c) Relative sensitivity to H and M	H = M	H > M
Effect of a big breath on dose response curve	None or shifts to left	Shifts to right
Response to cold air hyperventilation	Yes	No
Response to α agonist	Yes	No

Table 3 Factors known to produce airway narrowing in patients with asthma

Inhaled	Non-inhaled
Aeroallergens	Exercise
House dust mites	Emotional stress
Pollens	Respiratory infections
Animal danders	
Fungal spores	
Stuffings (kapok, feathers)	
Osmotic stimuli	Ingested substances
Nebulized hypertonic saline	Aspirin
Nebulized hypotonic saline	Alcohol
Sulphur dioxide	Nuts, shellfish, fruits
Surface of beverages	Beta-blockers
Air pollution	
Mediators	
Histamine	
Acetylcholine (methacholine etc.)	
Prostaglandins D_2 and F_{2a}	
Leukotriene C_4	
Adenosine	

Factors known to provoke attacks of asthma

Table 3 lists factors known to provoke airway narrowing in asthmatic subjects.

Allergens

These are probably the most widely studied experimental and natural provoking substances. However, many things remain unknown about their role in causing symptoms in normal life outside the experimental laboratory. How do they penetrate to the airways? What is the role of the nose in protecting the airways? Do they usually cause late reactions? Why do not all atopic people have asthma?

Some aeroallergens are confined by locality and season – birch pollen in the Scandinavian spring, grass pollen in the British early summer and ragweed pollen in North America in late summer. With pollen allergens associated allergic symptoms in the eyes and nose are common but not universal and frequently occur without asthma. Other aeroallergens, such as the house dust mite, are more widespread being found in many parts of the world and favouring the warm humid conditions in bedding. Allergens from animals include not only skin scales (dander) but also particles of hair and proteins derived from saliva and urine.

Exercise and osmotic stimuli

Attacks of asthma can be produced by exercise. Whilst subjects with a wide variety of pulmonary and cardiac disorders will complain of breathlessness during exercise, this recovers with rest. Only in the asthmatic does wheezing breathlessness come on after exercise. Typically there is a fall of over 20 per cent in spirometric indices of lung function (FEV$_1$ or PEF) which is maximal 5–10 min after the end of exercise and recovers over a time course of 30–60 min. The response is most likely to be produced by sustained exercise over 6–8 min and is 'dose related' in the sense of being greater, the higher the exercise ventilation achieved. After exercise-induced asthma there is a refractory period of 2–4 hours during which repeat exercise produces a much smaller effect. Exercise-induced asthma is worse in a dry cold environment and can be prevented by breathing moist air during exercise. Simple hyperventilation with cold dry air without exercise, and the inhalation of nebulized non-isotonic solutions (water or hypertonic saline) will also produce airways narrowing. It now seems likely that all these effects can be explained either in terms of heat loss across the bronchial mucosa or by alterations in osmolality. The mechanism whereby these changes induce the airway narrowing is not known. Mediator release has been shown to be present in some studies but not proven as the cause.

It appears that most people with asthma and BHR to histamine and to methacholine react to exercise and 'osmotic' stimuli. There is no evidence that exercise-induced asthma exists in isolation from other forms of provocation even though individual subjects may give a history that exercise is the major or perhaps sole provoking agent experienced in daily activity.

Infections

It is well recognized that viral infections commonly cause attacks of asthma. However, there have been very few studies of either BHR or lung function serially in asthmatics with documented viral infections. Secondary bacterial infection is widely held to occur and to perpetuate the inflammatory reactions which give rise to prolonged airways narrowing. Though this may be the case in some chronic asthmatics and in those who smoke cigarettes (and so have a resident bronchial bacterial flora) many patients diagnosed as having asthma repeatedly induced by infections, respond to treatment designed to prevent allergic reactions and not to antimicrobial therapy.

Sulphur dioxide

It is not usually appreciated that this gas, in concentrations as low as 2 ppm, can cause severe narrowing of asthmatic airways and probably all patients with asthma react to it. Its importance lies in the fact that levels of SO_2 in the air can exceed this concentration due to air pollution and at the surface of beverages which use SO_2-producing products as preservatives. It is commonly thought it acts via irritant airway receptors, but this is not true.

Others

There are many substances for which there is documented evidence for asthma provocation. These include some foods and drugs, emotional factors, and non-specific trigger factors such as strong smells and cigarette smoke.

Thus the asthmatic is at risk from a large number of potential provoking agents and exposure to them will cause airway narrowing, depending on the dose and on the degree of BHR present. It is this ability to respond to a wide range of provoking substances that characterizes the true asthmatic from subjects with seasonal allergic, occupational, and food-induced asthma.

Clinical manifestations

The symptoms and physical findings in asthma vary with age, the severity and duration of the disease, the amount and nature of treatment, and with the presence of complications. Many asthmatics have only occasional attacks of mild wheezing often in response to known trigger mechanisms and otherwise live perfectly normal lives. Indeed this is the aim of modern treatment. In most Westernized communities asthma starts for the first time in the first decade of life and may be troublesome for a variable number of years. Virtually nothing is known about the factors which initiate or terminate a spell of asthmatic symptoms within the lifetime of a given asthmatic. Two clinical patterns of asthma cause more concern – the acute severe attack, and chronic or persistent asthma.

Acute severe asthma

A typical attack in a young patient with uncomplicated asthma is not difficult to diagnose. It often begins with an irritating cough. The patient complains of difficulty with breathing, especially during inspiration, and may interpret this difficulty as tightness in the chest, or as wheezing. Breathlessness alone, without the other symptoms, is rare. Symptoms of asthma can come on very rapidly sometimes transforming the patient from apparent normality to a state of severe disability within less than 30 min. Around 40 per cent of severe attacks build up in less than 24 hours. When acute severe asthma develops over a longer time spell the prodromal phase is characterized by nocturnal awakening with cough or wheezing breathlessness, increasing exertional breathlessness during the day, and a failure of bronchodilator therapy to produce effective relief.

Clinical examination during an attack usually reveals a distressed patient with hyperinflation of the chest, rapid breathing, and widespread rhonchi (wheezes). In mild attacks and during very severe attacks, rhonchi may not be present. Since they may also be heard in patients with other diseases, rhonchi should not be relied upon for making the diagnosis or for estimating the severity of the attack. A tachycardia greater than 120 min and pulsus parodoxus greater than 15mm/Hg are useful indicators of severe asthma. Exhaustion, cyanosis, and a low blood pressure are signs of serious import indicating cardiorespiratory failure.

Chronic asthma

The chronic asthmatic usually gives a history of multiple acute attacks, but occasionally the disease develops insidiously and the patient presents with severe airway obstruction and gives a history of increasing breathlessness on effort. Other clinical manifestations of chronic asthma include the emotional effects of long-term illness, irreversible airways obstruction, and the side-effects of corticosteroid therapy.

Function of the lungs

The mainstay of assessment both during attacks and in the interval period is measurement of expiratory flow rate either with a spirometer which records timed forced expiratory volumes or with a peak flow meter to record peak expiratory flow rates. When the patient is well, the best values for expiratory flow should be recorded and used as a guide to severity of attacks and amount of prophylactic treatment needed. Serial twice-daily readings are an invaluable guide to progress and the effects of treatment. There have been a number of attempts to measure aspects of respiratory and cardiovascular function during acute attacks of asthma and to compute an index of severity. Apart from indices of airways function the most reliable guide to the severity of the attack is the blood gas tensions and these assume even greater importance if the patient is too distressed to record a forced expiration. Analysis of the cause of death of patients both in and out of hospital in recent years has consistently shown that the patient and/or the physician was unaware of the severity of the situation because the status of the patient had been inadequetely assessed.

Patients with severe asthma usually have some degree of airway obstruction and hyperinflation even when symptom free. The cause of the hyperinflation is thought to be continued action of the inspiratory muscle during expiration. The diffusing capacity is usually normal and is useful for distinguishing asthma from emphysema.

Differential diagnosis

In the acute attack in a young person, there are few other diseases from which to distinguish asthma. However, in the young child wheezing can be caused by bronchiolitis and by foreign bodies in the airways. In the adult with chronic asthma, particularly when the symptoms are slowly progressive, the disease must be distinguished from chronic left heart failure and from chronic obstructive lung disease. Occasionally pulmonary eosinophilia (Churg–Strauss syndrome, page 15.133), pulmonary emboli, and the carcinoid syndrome can present as asthma.

Complications

The complications to be aware of in the acute attack are pneumothorax or pneumomediastinum and airway plugging leading to death in respiratory failure. In the chronic asthmatic, complications include the development of irreversible airways obstruction, the side-effects of corticosteroids, bronchopulmonary aspergillosis (sometimes with bronchiectasis), and, in a few patients, eventually cor pulmonale.

Complicated forms of asthma
Occupational asthma

Occupational asthma has been defined above. The subjects do not need to be atopic and with some substances a very high percentage

Table 4 Sensitizing agents in occupational asthma

Material	Industrial exposure
Plicatic acid	Wood milling, carpentry
Platinum salts	Platinum refining
Isocyanates	Paints, varnishes, plastic industry, insulation, packaging, coatings for wires in electronics
Epoxy resins	Hardening agents in plastics and adhesives
Colophony fumes	Resin from pine trees used in solders and hot melt glues
Proteolytic enzymes	Biological detergents
Insects or animals	Laboratory workers
Flour and grain	Milling and baking

of the work force may be affected. The definition depends on establishing airway narrowing to a substance found at the work place (or other special environment). Since the substance may cause only 'late' responses with symptoms at night, a careful history is needed. It is important to differentiate non-specific irritability of the airways in dusty situations and true asthma with exacerbations at the workplace from exclusively occupational asthma. The best means of treatment is to cease all exposure to the chemical involved.

Substances which cause occupational asthma include wood dust, of which western red cedar is the most common (the substance implicated is plicatic acid), isocyanates and proteins from laboratory animals, and many others (see Table 4).

Bronchopulmonary aspergillosis
When asthma is associated with transient lung infiltrates and eosinophilia, it is likely that the cause is the fungus *Aspergillus fumigatus*. Its presence in the airways acts as a potent allergen though it does not invade the bronchial walls or lung tissue. The condition is confirmed by finding circulating precipitins and positive skin prick tests to *A. fumigatus*. Clinically the patient may have dyspnoea, pleuritic chest pain in attacks, and typically coughs up tenacious plugs of brown mucus. Attacks of asthma do not always accompany these episodes. Repeated attacks can lead to a characteristic proximal bronchiectasis. The treatment is with oral corticosteroids in high dose for several days. This almost invariably controls the episode and the chest radiograph returns to normal. Relapses are common and may not be prevented by inhaled corticosteroids.

Aspirin sensitive asthma
Approximately 3 per cent of adult asthmatics are sensitive to aspirin. Ingestion of small amounts causes severe attacks with both immediate and late responses. Many of these patients have late onset asthma and some have nasal polyps. The treatment is avoidance although patients have been desensitized by daily ingestion of the drug starting with extremely small amounts. Some of these asthmatics show cross reactions with tartrazine, benzoic acid, and other azo dyes and food preservatives whilst yet others respond to one or more of these substances but not to aspirin. To confuse the issue further the very occasional patient seems to get bronchodilation with aspirin.

Treatment
Aims of treatment
Patients with severe asthma are at risk of death in an attack, at risk of developing irreversible airways disease, and at risk from the side-effects of corticosteroids. Until a cure is known, treatment should be planned with the aim of protecting the patient from these risks. This can be achieved by decreasing BHR to a level where provoked attacks rarely, if ever, occur and by maintaining normal lung function without producing serious side-effects due to long-term corticosteroid use.

Acute attacks
The majority of asthmatics have mild asthma and most of their acute wheezy episodes can be reversed by β_2-agonists given as an

aerosol. The actions, modes of use, and complications of these drugs are described below. The underlying abnormality in asthma is manifested as a relative overdependence on β_2-stimulation so these drugs are of primary importance.

In severe acute attacks the dose of bronchodilator that can be given by a metered dose aerosol is insufficient (namely, 0.1 mg per inhalation of salbutamol or 0.25 mg for terbutaline). The larger doses which can be delivered using a nebulizer (2.5 to 10 mg of either salbutamol or terbutaline) are frequently indicated. With the widespread use of nebulizers, the intravenous route is rarely necessary now for β_2-stimulant therapy in acute asthma though some will still use it for infusion of a xanthine, e.g. aminophylline. Whilst some very severe acute attacks will respond to β_2-stimulants alone it is wise to give corticosteroids as well as 100 to 300 mg of hydrocortisone hemisuccinate even though the onset of action may not be apparent for several hours. There have been few controlled trials of these drugs alone and in combination in severe acute asthma but, with adequate supportive therapy most patients now recover, even from very severe attacks.

Prophylactic and long-term treatment
It is becoming increasingly clear that the most important aspect of treatment is prophylaxis and the prevention of attacks. If the patient has been documented with lung function and measurements of BHR to have mild asthma, treatment can be given just for symptoms but patients with more severe disease require prophylactic treatment. Effective prophylactic treatment requires cooperation between doctor and patient. The doctor must be willing to set aside time to explain about the illness, its treatment, and possible complications. The patient must be willing to continue treatment regularly even when the asthma seems quiescent and to measure lung function frequently as a guide to the amount of medication required.

Figure 5 shows the changes in dose–response curves to histamine in a patient treated for 4, 6 and 7 months with a prophylactic regimen of a β_2-adrenergic aerosol, inhaled beclomethasone diproprionate, and sodium cromoglycate taken regularly, four times a day. The drugs needed to keep severe asthmatics symptom-free, with normal lung function and with gradually lessening degrees of BHR vary, but inhaled corticosteroids are extremely important and some patients require oral steroids for short periods of time.

The long-term benefits of prophylactic treatment have not yet been evaluated. However, it is clear that with regular prophylactic treatment, the level of BHR can be reduced, lung function kept close to normal, and almost all attacks avoided, even in the most

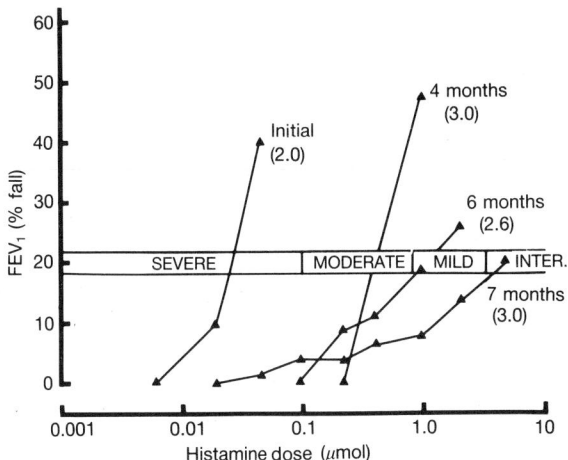

Fig. 5 Dose-response curves to histamine from a patient with severe asthma treated for 7 months with prophylactic therapy with three drugs inhaled four times per day. Each response was recorded 6 hours after any therapy had been taken.

severe asthmatic. Hopefully it will also be shown to lessen the risk of irreversible changes in airway function.

Drugs used to treat asthma

Asthma therapy is best administered by aerosol. The local high dose of the drugs lessens systemic side-effects and, in the case of β_2-adrenergic drugs prophylactic effects against all forms of provocation (allergens, exercise, SO_2, mediators) are only obtained when the drug is given as an aerosol.

Beta-2-adrenoceptor agonists

The effectiveness of these drugs, both for treatment and preventing asthma attacks, has led to their widespread use. Most of the abnormalities which have been documented in asthma can be corrected, partially or fully, by the administration of these drugs. Their known actions include relaxation of contracted BSM cells, prevention of contraction of BSM cells by various stimuli in a dose-related manner, increased clearance of mucus, decreased viscosity of mucus, decreased release of mediators from cells near epithelial surfaces, and prevention of leaking by the microvascular system with mediators. Regrettably for all of these actions the effects are short-lived, having disappeared by 4–6 hours.

In spite of their ability to both reverse and prevent attacks and to alter the life styles of most asthmatics, there has been a reluctance in many countries to use these aerosols, probably from a misapprehension that they cause dangerous side-effects. Some tremor and mild tachycardia occur but they rarely inconvenience the patient. The other concern has been that they may produce tolerance. Although this has been demonstrated experimentally in normal subjects, it has not been shown in asthmatics. Beta-2-adrenergic aerosols have been taken by some patients with chronic asthma for almost 25 years. They continue to respond and have not developed side-effects.

The main problem with all inhaled therapy is effective delivery. Not all patients find the metered dose aerosol easy to use even with careful instruction. Small children, the elderly, and the infirm may never master the technique. Alternative delivery devices using dry powder and spacer devices (even nebulizers) help but in some oral therapy is the only alternative.

Corticosteroids

Corticosteroids have revolutionized the treatment of asthma. Their mode of action is unknown but probably rests largely on their ability to reduce the number of inflammatory cells in the airways. The introduction of steroids for the aerosol route has led to a reduction in dose required and thus in the side-effects. After almost 15 years of use these drugs are proving to have few major side-effects and it is now recognized that inhaled steroids are the treatment of choice when corticosteroids are indicated for more than two weeks. The dose needed is that required to achieve the aims of treatment as stated above.

Candidiasis of the pharynx is the commonest side-effect. It can be treated without stopping the drug and appears to be a local problem only. Aphonia which is not related to the candidiasis, and may be a myopathy of the laryngeal muscles, also occurs and limits the use of the drug in a few patients.

Sodium cromoglycate

This drug, originally developed for its antiallergic properties, is well documented to protect against provoked attacks by allergens, exercise, and sulphur dioxide. It is a pure prophylactic agent having no immediate bronchodilator activity. Initially it was regarded as a drug which stabilizes mast cells but recently doubt has been cast on its exact mode of action. It certainly seems to act as though it is preventing release of mediators but it clearly has other actions. For the best results it must be given regularly and in sufficient doses to prevent attacks. It is remarkable for the paucity of side-effects.

Numerous attempts have been made to find a clinically useful oral 'antiallergic', modelling research on the supposed properties of cromoglycate. Whilst many drugs have been produced few have received widespread support. Ketotifen has antihistaminic properties as well as some antiallergic activity but its performance clinically has been disappointing partly because of sedative side-effects in adults.

Anticholinergic drugs

This group of drugs includes atropine and the synthetic atropine-like drug, ipratropium bromide, which appears to have the bronchodilating properties of atropine without its side-effects. They are less effective bronchodilators than the sympathomimetic amines and work in some asthmatics more than in others. Effectiveness has to be assessed in the individual patient allowing an adequate time for the maximum response which may be more than 30 min.

Non-drug treatment of asthma

Allergists treat patients with asthma with injections of substances to which they are sensitive. There is evidence that symptoms improve and the amount of treatment needed lessens with time. However, in the best placebo controlled trials, the long-term aims of treatment have not been stated and neither the duration of improvement nor the long-term changes in BHR have been studied.

It is possible that the future of asthma treatment lies in this direction but at present it should only be used as first-line treatment for mild asthma which responds readily to inhaled bronchodilators. There seems little doubt that desensitization is both effective and important for subjects with allergies to insect stings but these patients usually do not have asthma as a major problem. It is of interest that aspirin intolerance can be treated with long-term desensitization using small doses.

Removal of aeroallergens from the environment is often difficult. Where a specific animal dander is implicated there is usually no problem. Pollens can be avoided to a limited degree by staying away from offending countryside at the appropriate time of the year. Cutting back the load of house dust mite allergens is much more difficult. Really rigorous control does help clinically and also reduces BHR, but for most asthmatic families the demands are too arduous and time consuming. There is some hope that specific pesticides may kill off the mites in bedding.

Beverages containing SO_2, certain alcoholic drinks, and aspirin have long been recognized to cause attacks of asthma and it is well recognized that other substances in the diet may be unrecognized causes of deterioration in asthma. The prevalence of diet-related asthma is unknown but one study showed that 10 per cent of children with chronic perennial asthma responded to treatment with an elimination diet. There is growing interest in the fatty acid and tryptophan content of the diets of asthmatics and it may well be that diet modification will play an important role in the long-term management of the severe asthmatic in the future.

References

Anderson, S. D. (1983). Current concepts of exercise induced asthma. *Allergy* **38**, 289.

Barnes, P., Fitzgerald, G., Brown, M. and Dollery, C. (1980). Nocturnal asthma and changes in circulating epinephrine, histamine and cortisol. *N. Engl. J. Med.* **303**, 263.

Brown, P. J., Greville, H. W. and Finucane, K. E. (1984). Asthma and irreversible airflow obstruction. *Thorax* **39**, 136.

Chan-Yeung, M., Lam, S. and Koener, S. (1982). Clinical features and natural history of occupational asthma due to western red cedar (Thuja plicata). *Am. J. Med.* **72**, 411.

Clarke, T. J. H. and Godfrey, S. (eds) (1983). *Asthma*. Chapman and Hall, London.

Hargreave, F. E. and Woolcock, A. J. (eds) (1985). *Bronchial hyperresponsiveness: methods of measurement*. Astra Pharmaceuticals, Ontario.

Paterson, J. M., Woolcock, A. J. and Shenfield, G. (1979). Bronchodilator drugs. State of the art. *Am. Rev. Resp. Dis.* **120**, 1149.

Townley, R. G., Ryo, U. Y., Koltkin, B. M. and Kay, B. (1975). Bronchial sensitivity to methacholine in current and former asthmatic and rhinitic patients and control subjects. *J. Allergy Clin. Immun.* **56**, 429.

Trembath, P. W. (1980). Corticosteroids in asthma: inhaled or oral. *Drugs* **20**, 81.

Weiss, E. B., Segal, M. S. and Stein, M. (eds) (1984). *Bronchial asthma. Mechanisms and therapeutics* 2nd edn. Little, Brown and Co., Boston.

Chronic bronchitis, emphysema, and chronic obstructive airway disease

M. K. BENSON

Introduction

Over the past 25 years there have been many attempts to clarify the terminology and definitions applied to the above conditions. None has been entirely successful and confusion still exists. Clinically there are two main components to these disorders: mucus hypersecretion with cough and excess sputum production and breathlessness consequent upon impaired respiratory function. Although these often co-exist, either may occur in isolation. Further difficulties arise with the realization that impaired lung function can itself involve at least two pathological processes: airways disease and emphysema. Again these frequently occur together and whilst the pathologist may distinguish between the two, clinically they are impossible to separate.

Definitions

Chronic bronchitis is defined *clinically* as a condition characterized by chronic or recurrent cough with excess sputum production occurring in the absence of any other pathology.

Emphysema is defined *pathologically* as a condition characterized by enlargement of air spaces distal to the terminal bronchiole accompanied by destruction of their walls.

The terms chronic obstructive airway disease (COAD), chronic obstructive pulmonary disease (COPD), and chronic obstructive lung disease (COLD) are used synonymously and have been introduced to include all patients who have irreversible and usually progressive airflow limitation resulting from a combination of airway disease and emphysema.

In this chapter these conditions will be considered under two main clinical entities, those of mucus hypersecretion (chronic bronchitis) and airway obstruction (COAD).

Chronic bronchitis

The airways of normal individuals are constantly exposed to a variety of inhaled irritants. They are protected by a lining of mucus, secreted by bronchial glands, which traps particulate matter and is removed by the co-ordinated beating of the ciliary escalator. Coughing is a normal physiological response which aids removal of inhaled particulate matter or excess sputum.

The normal response to inflammation or irritation is increased mucus production which is then expectorated. Continued irritation leads to chronic mucus hypersecretion which is the hallmark of simple chronic bronchitis.

Epidemiology

Chronic bronchitis has tended to be regarded as 'the British disease'. Prevalence figures vary considerably and vary with definition, with the age group studied, and with smoking habits and industrialization. Figures tend to be higher in industrialized countries, although in recent years high prevalence rates have emerged from countries such as India, Malaysia, and Papua New Guinea.

The major problem with many epidemiological studies is the variation in definition with respect to 'chronic bronchitis'. In Britain a general practitioner survey conducted in the early 1960s concentrated on the age group 40–65 years and yielded a prevalence of 8 per cent in men and 3 per cent in women. However, the diagnostic criteria used in this study included cough, mucus production, and breathlessness due to airway obstruction and it is likely to underestimate the prevalence of simple mucus hypersecretion which is undoubtedly more common than airway obstruction.

The morbidity due to chronic bronchitis is mainly the result of increased susceptibility to acute infections. In Britain it represents the largest single cause of loss of work accounting for 31 000 000 lost working days in 1973–74. Infections tend to be more common in the autumn and winter months.

High mortality rates are not the consequence of uncomplicated chronic bronchitis, but are associated with impaired lung function. There are wide international variations with particularly high rates in the United Kingdom. Some of the differences may reflect diagnostic habits, but in Britain high tobacco consumption and atmospheric pollution have both made significant contributions. Now that both are decreasing, this is being reflected in the fall in mortality.

In virtually all countries, prevalence rates are considerably higher for males than females with ratios of approximately 5:1. Differences in mortality due to urbanization have been very apparent in the past but in the United Kingdom death rates are now similar in urban and rural areas; a consequence of measures to control air pollution. There is a steady increase in mortality with descending socio-economic class. Much of the difference can be accounted for by differences in smoking habits, although other environmental factors undoubtedly contribute.

Pathology

The pathological hallmark of chronic bronchitis is the increased numbers of goblet cells within the bronchial mucosa and the hypertrophy of the mucous glands. Such changes were first quantified by Reid who compared the thickness of the gland layer to the thickness of the bronchial wall (the Reid Index). An alternative approach has been a point counting method employed by Dunnill and colleagues to estimate the percentage volume of the bronchial wall occupied by mucus glands. An increase in gland mass is found in 'normal smokers' as well as patients with a history of mucus hypersecretion, although there is no clear division between normal and abnormal. Two other features are notable by their absence. Unlike changes seen in patients with asthma, an increase in the smooth muscle within the bronchial wall is not a feature of chronic bronchitis. A cellular inflammatory infiltrate is also absent, except in patients dying with an acute infective exacerbation.

Pathophysiology

The development of mucus hypersecretion can be regarded as an enhancement of the normal physiological response to inhaled irritants brought about by continued exposure. The main consequence of excess mucus production is, paradoxically, impairment of normal clearance mechanisms. This can be demonstrated *in vivo* by measuring the rate of removal of inhaled radiolabelled particles. In patients with chronic bronchitis, time for clearance is prolonged when compared with normal individuals. This is partly because the normal ciliary clearance mechanism is unable to cope with the increased volume of mucus, which tends to pool in lobar and segmental bronchi until expectorated as sputum. In addition changes in the composition of mucus have been demonstrated with an increased ratio of sulphated to sialic acid mucin in the bronchial mucus of smokers. The extent to which rheological changes in the mucus impair clearance remains a matter of debate. To compound these changes, ciliary function is also impaired by the direct depressant effect of cigarette smoke and eventually squamous metaplasia also occurs with damage to and replacement of the normal ciliated epithelium.

Impaired clearance mechanisms result in an increased susceptibility to acute respiratory infections. Bacteria gaining access from the upper respiratory tract are not cleared effectively and clinical infection results with an acute inflammatory infiltrate and expectoration of purulent sputum.

Clinical features

Many individuals with simple chronic bronchitis (mucus hypersecretion without airway obstruction) only present to their doctors during an acute infective exacerbation and regard their cough as an inevitable consequence of their smoking habit – 'a smokers cough'. Coughing usually produces mucoid sputum especially on waking and expectoration is often initiated by the first cigarette of the day. Symptoms tend to be worse during winter months when there is an increased likelihood of developing acute infective exacerbations often associated with an upper respiratory tract infection. Sputum changes from grey or mucoid to yellow or purulent. In the majority of patients, the illness is mild but may be accompanied by fever and constitutional symptoms. Occasionally broncho-pneumonia may result. In patients with underlying lung damage and airway obstruction the consequences may be more serious (*vide infra*).

Examination is usually unremarkable, although the patient may have a rattly cough. If available sputum should be inspected as part of the examination.

Differential diagnosis

Chronic bronchitis is, by definition, a diagnosis based on exclusion of other pathologies. In non-smokers presenting with chronic cough, a specific cause can often be identified. In smokers, or those exposed to industrial dusts or fumes, the situation is more difficult. It is however dangerous to apply the label 'chronic bronchitis' without considering other possibilities, especially when the patient feels that there has been a change in his usual cough. The following possibilities should be considered.

Chronic sinusitis with post-nasal drip This can usually be diagnosed on a careful history supplemented by radiology of the nasal sinuses.

Bronchiectasis (page 15.100) There may be a history of previous lung damage. The cough is often productive of moderate or large amounts of purulent sputum.

Bronchial neoplasm (page 15.147) Like chronic bronchitis, this is smoking-related, and the two conditions may co-exist. Haemoptysis is a sinister symptom and should not be attributed to bronchitis alone. A chest radiograph is usually abnormal, although when small endobronchial lesions are present there may be no radiological abnormality.

Asthma (page 15.80) Although episodic wheeze and breathlessness are the cardinal features of asthma, occasionally a cough, especially at night may be the presenting feature.

Aspiration A cough, especially one which occurs on lying down, may be a feature of aspiration of regurgitated gastric contents occurring in patients with a hiatus hernia or oesophageal reflux. It may also be associated with pseudo bulbar palsy.

Chronic pulmonary infections Of these pulmonary tuberculosis remains the most important. A chest radiograph is invariably abnormal.

Treatment

Mucus hypersecretion is a direct consequence of continued mucosal irritation. If the irritant stimulus, whether it be cigarette smoke or atmospheric pollution, is removed, the symptoms of cough and sputum production resolve over a period of weeks even in patients with long-established disease.

Drug treatment is of no real value. Expectorants tend to act as bronchial irritants, either by their direct action or via vagal reflexes. Thus whilst they encourage expectoration, they also result in further mucus production. The best expectorant is the first cigarette of the day: it is not however a treatment to be recommended.

Drugs such as bromhexine and carbocisteine are marketed as mucolytics for use in chronic bronchitis. Although laboratory studies have demonstrated reduced sputum viscosity as a result of their use, the majority of clinical studies have shown no subjective or objective benefit and routine use of these drugs is not recommended.

Acute infective exacerbations are usually due to *Haemophilus influenzae* and *Streptococcus pneumoniae*. The majority of cases respond to oral ampicillin, co-trimoxazole or erythromycin (see page 15.92).

Chronic obstructive airway disease

Pathology

Patients with chronic obstructive airway disease may have a combination of emphysema and airway narrowing. Only the pathologist can differentiate between the two.

Emphysema has been defined by Thurlbeck as an abnormal permanent increase in size of the respiratory portion of the lung beyond the terminal bronchiole, accompanied by destructive changes. Classification is based on the portion of the lung involved, the two main types being centrilobular emphysema, in which destruction is localized to the respiratory bronchioles and acini at the centre of each lobule and pan acinar emphysema which involves the majority of the alveolar tissue of the acinus but tends to spare the respiratory bronchioles. If the disease is extensive, large areas may coalesce to form thin-walled cysts or bullae.

In centrilobular emphysema, the macroscopic appearance is characterized by abnormal air spaces occupying the central portion of the lobule, but surrounded by normal lung tissue. The upper zones are more frequently affected than the lower zones. Histologically the respiratory bronchioles that supply emphysematous areas are usually the foci of chronic inflammation and scarring. The functional importance of centrilobular emphysema is difficult to quantify, since it is invariably associated with airway disease, both of which may contribute to the clinical picture.

Because of its more generalized nature, *pan acinar emphysema* may be clinically recognizable. The main macroscopic features are the generalized hyperinflation and gross enlargement of air spaces within the acinus. Peripheral bullae are often present and the lower zones are predominantly affected. The normal architecture is totally disorganized and this is best seen histologically, the affected lung being devoid of normal alveoli, which are replaced by thin-walled sacs of varying size.

Airway disease The pathological changes found in patients with chronic mucus hypersecretion have already been described. Whilst it might be assumed that glandular hypertrophy and excess mucus within the bronchial tree leads to airway obstruction, epidemiological studies have suggested that the two processes are not directly connected. Some patients undoubtedly develop changes in the smaller more peripheral airways. Hogg and his colleagues first drew attention to 'small airways disease' affecting airways less than 2 mm in diameter. In pathological terms, disease is not limited to this section of the bronchial tree but their small initial diameter makes individual airways more susceptible to narrowing, obliteration, and total destruction.

Pathogenesis

The development of both emphysema and airway disease may depend on exposure to a variety of external factors together with an intrinsic susceptibility. Of extrinsic factors, epidemiological studies have focussed attention on smoking, atmospheric pollution, and infection.

Cigarette smoking

Cigarette smoking is associated with an increased mortality from chronic bronchitis and emphysema. In a survey of medical practitioners conducted by Doll and Peto, the death rates from chronic bronchitis were significantly higher in cigarette smokers than in non-smokers and increased with the amount smoked. The causal relationship can also be inferred by the fall in mortality which accompanied an overall decrease in smoking habits among doctors occurring at a time when smoking in the general population was increasing. Subsequent prospective studies in the United Kingdom, Canada, and the United States have all shown an accelerated annual rate of decline of lung function in smokers.

The natural history is illustrated in Fig. 1. In non-smokers there is a gradual decline in lung function with respect to age, the fall in FEV_1 being about 35 ml/annum. Smokers tend to have a more rapid rate of decline with those destined to develop disabling airway obstruction losing function at rates exceeding 90 ml/year. These changes can be detected by periodic screening but it is only when the FEV_1 falls to less than 50 per cent predicted that symptoms become apparent. Any subsequent small loss in function will have a much greater impact on the degree of exercise limitation. Ex-smokers have decreased morbidity and lower annual fall in the FEV_1 when compared with those who continue to smoke.

The ways in which cigarette smoke can affect airway function are summarized on page 15.44. However, despite the overwhelming epidemiological and experimental evidence linking smoking and chronic obstructive airway disease, only a minority of smokers develop disabling disease. Whether these individuals have an intrinsic susceptibility remains the subject of debate.

Atmospheric pollution

Atmospheric pollution has in the past been an important aetiological factor in the pathogenesis of chronic bronchitis and emphysema. This has been shown by the correlations in both prevalence and mortality rates with the degree of urbanization and increased atmospheric pollution. However, in Britain, the effects of air pollution are now disappearing. As a result of the *Clean Air Acts* and changes in domestic heating, smoke emission has fallen dramatically. This decrease in pollution has contributed to the decline in morbidity and mortality from chronic bronchitis and emphysema although it is difficult to dissociate this effect from that of a decrease in smoking habits.

Studies in other industrialized societies have confirmed the relationship between atmospheric pollution and bronchitis, although a Swedish study concluded that smoking was a far more important factor. In developing countries, domestic smoke may contribute

towards bronchitic symptoms although it is likely that with the rapid increase in tobacco consumption, mortality rates will also increase.

Infection

There is some evidence from prospective studies of a correlation between respiratory tract infections in childhood and chronic respiratory symptoms in adult life. It has been suggested that childhood infections lead to an increased susceptibility to subsequent extrinsic factors such as cigarette smoking. However, the relationship need not be a causal one, since there may simply be a common factor, such as a genetic predisposition which increases susceptibility to infections and pollutants.

In patients with established disease, infective exacerbations undoubtedly have at least a temporary effect in worsening lung function. Some studies have shown a correlation between permanent loss of respiratory reserve and frequency of exacerbations. However long term studies in the United Kingdom by Fletcher and colleagues and in Canada by Bates have shown that loss of function occurs independently of respiratory infections.

Intrinsic factors

The best documented example of a constitutional abnormality which predisposes towards the development of chronic obstructive lung disease is the relation between emphysema and α_1-antitrypsin deficiency. Alpha$_1$-antitrypsin is a serum protein capable of inhibiting several types of proteolytic enzymes. Smokers have been shown to have increased amounts of elastase and protease in alveolar neutrophils and macrophages and these observations have led to the hypothesis that emphysema is caused by the unrestricted action of proteolytic enzymes.

At present some 30 co-dominant protease inhibitor (Pi) genotypes have been indentified which determine the level of circulating antitrypsin. The most common allele in all populations tested is PiM and the resulting phenotype (MM) results in normal levels of antitrypsin. PiZ was the first variant to be recognized in the Pi system and in the homozygous state (phenotype ZZ), which occurs in approximately 1 in 5000 of the United Kingdom population, α_1-antitrypsin levels are virtually non-existent. This can be detected on serum electrophoresis by the absence of the α_1 globulin band. Individuals with this deficiency are prone to develop severe basal emphysema at a relatively young age especially if they are smokers. Screening of the families of patients with this deficiency may be of value in that affected individuals should be strongly counselled not to smoke and to try and avoid exposure to industrial pollutants. It must be stressed that the majority of patients with emphysema are not deficient in α_1-antitrypsin and in them the pathogenesis of their lung destruction remains uncertain.

The role of other possible constitutional factors remains speculative. Dutch investigators have suggested that patients who develop airway obstruction have an increased reactivity or sensitivity to cigarette smoke. There is, however, no direct evidence to support this hypothesis and a specific allergy to smoke has not been demonstrated.

Pathophysiology

Although airway disease and emphysema are separate pathological processes affecting different areas of the respiratory apparatus, both result in airway narrowing and consequent limitation of airflow within the bronchial tree. Areas of the lung become poorly ventilated with resultant ventilation perfusion mismatching. When disease is extensive, respiratory failure is an inevitable result.

Airway size normally varies with lung volume. This variation is a direct result of elastic forces operating on the walls of the bronchi, the lung elastic recoil. Airways increase in size during inspiration and become smaller near to residual volume when closure of certain airways may occur. In emphysema the main physiological abnormality is a loss of elastic recoil. This has several physiological consequences. Firstly, it permits the expansion of the lung to

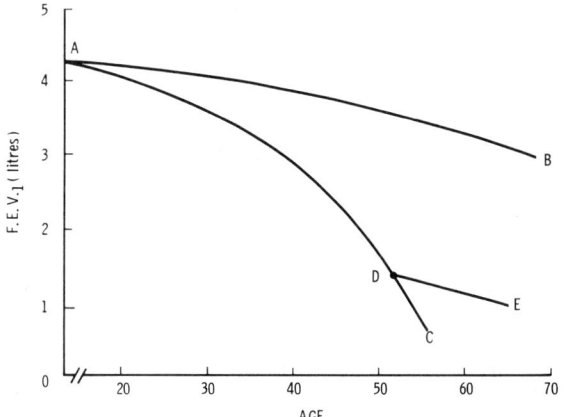

Fig. 1 Diagrammatic representation of decline in lung function with respect to age. Line AB represents a normal individual. The line AC represents the development of disease in a smoker, clinical presentation occurring at point D. The DE represents the rate of change if the patient stops smoking.

a greater degree than normal and thus total lung capacity is increased. Secondly, during expiration, the loss of recoil results in earlier closure of airways, air trapping, and a marked increase in residual volume. Thirdly, the main driving pressure resulting in expiratory flow is the elastic recoil of the lung. Since flow rates are directly proportional to the driving pressure as recoil is lost so expiratory flow rates diminish. Finally there is a loss of normal surface area for alveolar gas exchange and a reduction in transfer factor for carbon monoxide.

Mention has already been made of the pathological changes occurring in the small peripheral airways. Resistance to airflow is the sum of a series of resistances forming a branching pattern. At each airway generation or division, individual bronchi are small but the total cross-sectional area rapidly increases because of the large number of individual bronchi. These smaller peripheral airways are, because of their size, more susceptible to total occlusion or obliteration, but the physiological consequences only become apparent when there is extensive disease. The physiological result of pure airway narrowing will have certain features in common with pure emphysema. Airway resistance will be increased, maximal expiratory flow rates will be reduced and air trapping will occur resulting in an increase in residual volume. Areas of ventilation perfusion mismatching are more likely to occur with consequent respiratory failure.

One further factor which has received relatively little attention but which may contribute significantly to expiratory flow limitation, is the dynamic compression of larger airways which may occur during forced expiration. This is difficult to demonstrate pathologically but is frequently seen bronchoscopically when the posterior wall of the trachea invaginates and complete occlusion may result. This observation may explain why some patients have a higher expiratory flow rate during a relaxed expiratory manoeuvre than during a forced manoeuvre.

Clinical features

Patients with airflow limitation present with a history of breathlessness and a reduced exercise tolerance. Since the symptoms usually develop insidiously, many patients regard the exercise limitation as part of the normal ageing process until it reaches a stage where it interferes with everyday activity. Often the patient will date his or her symptoms from an acute infective illness although careful questioning will reveal that exercise has been limited for some longer period of time. As the disease progresses, exercise becomes more limited so that the patient may have difficulty in undertaking tasks such as dressing, washing or even talking. Stimulation of irritant receptors lining the bronchial mucosa irritates a reflex response resulting in mucus secretion, cough, and bronchoconstriction.

Physical signs

In patients with mild or moderate disease there may be no abnormal signs. Tachypnoea will become evident on exercise but the respiratory rate may be normal at rest. In patients with severe disease expiration is prolonged, often with pursed lips breathing and inspiration is consequently shortened. Increased inspiratory effort is evidenced by the use of accessory muscles and there is frequently intercostal recession. In order to give the muscles of the upper thorax greater mechanical advantage, the patient often leans forward slightly, resting on outstretched arms. The chest is hyperinflated with poor expansion, low diaphragm, and reduced cardiac and hepatic dullness. A tracheal tug, whereby the trachea descends on inspiration, is also evidence of hyperinflation. Breath sounds are often reduced in intensity, an observation which has been correlated with the severity of the airways obstruction. Coarse inspiratory rhonchi are a variable feature usually attributed to excess mucus in relatively large airways.

Chronic respiratory failure is an inevitable consequence of end-stage obstructive airway disease. Some patients present with severe breathlessness early in the course of their disease, although

arterial blood gas analysis reveals only modest abnormalities with a slightly reduced P_{O_2} and normal P_{CO_2}. These 'pink puffers' contrast markedly with the 'blue bloaters' who appear less incapacitated but who bear the hallmarks of severe respiratory failure. These ends of a clinical spectrum were at one time felt to represent patients with pure emphysema (pink puffers) or pure chronic bronchitis (blue bloaters). In fact clinicopathological studies do not support this neat division. It may be that differences relate more to the severity of the underlying disease although there may also be differences in the sensitivity of the respiratory centre.

Hypoxaemia is manifest by central cyanosis, best detected in the lips and tongue. This is usually obvious when the partial pressure of oxygen falls below about 8 kPa. At very low levels (less than 4 kPa) agitation, confusion, and impaired consciousness may result. Chronic hypoxia may result in a compensatory or secondary polycythaemia. The polycythaemic patient will have a weather-beaten, dusky complexion resulting from a combination of cyanosis and a raised haematocrit. Cor pulmonale (page 13.350) frequently occurs in patients who are chronically hypoxic. Pulmonary hypertension develops with evidence of right ventricular hypertrophy, an elevated jugular venous pressure, hepatic congestion, and peripheral oedema, signs which may account for the bloated appearance. Hypercapnia may be less easy to recognize clinically. An elevated P_{CO_2} is a vasodilator resulting in warm peripheries and a bounding pulse. Headaches, especially early morning, are due to dilation of cerebral vessels and occasionally papilloedema occurs. In severe hypercapnia, CO_2 narcosis with drowsiness and eventual coma occurs. This may be precipitated by the use of sedatives, hypnotics or alcohol. A coarse flapping tremor is a further feature of severe hypercapnia although the mechanism of this is uncertain.

Acute complications

Patients with established airway obstruction and chronic respiratory failure are susceptible to relatively minor additional pulmonary insults which result in a further limitation in exercise tolerance and worsening respiratory failure. In such circumstances there are a number of possible contributory causes.

Acute respiratory infections

As in patients with uncomplicated chronic bronchitis, those with chronic airflow obstruction are also more prone to develop acute infective exacerbations. The most common infecting organisms are again *Haemophilus influenzae* and *Streptococcus pneumoniae*. Such infections obviously assume more importance in patients with limited respiratory reserve. The patient may be pyrexial and sputum volume will usually be increased in amount and will appear purulent. Auscultation of the chest may reveal coarse rhonchi and a few scattered crepitations especially when there is associated broncho-pneumonia.

Left ventricular failure

Whilst right heart failure is a feature of cor pulmonale, it should not in itself result in impaired gas exchange. Left ventricular failure will result in increasing dyspnoea. The mechanism whereby left heart failure occurs in patients with chronic respiratory failure is uncertain, although it may in part be a consequence of the hypoxia. There may be signs of left ventricular strain with third and fourth heart sounds, but it may be difficult on clinical grounds to separate worsening due to patchy broncho-pneumonia from that due to left heart failure. Even with the aid of a chest radiograph the differentiation can be difficult.

Pneumothorax

Rupture of a bulla on the pleural surface may occur, especially in patients with emphysema, resulting in a pneumothorax. Because the chest is already hyperinflated and hyperresonant, this may be difficult to detect clinically. Any patient with rapidly worsening dyspnoea should be X-rayed to exclude this possibility.

Pulmonary emboli or thromboses

These are often present on autopsy in patients with chronic airway disease and may account for a sudden clinical deterioration. Confirmation of the diagnosis in life can be particularly difficult since the electrocardiograph, pulmonary perfusion scan, and even angiogram are likely to be abnormal because of the underlying airways disease.

Differential diagnosis

The differential diagnosis to be considered in a patient presenting with breathlessness as the main symptom is considered elsewhere (page 15.47). Identification of airway obstruction as a major factor is relatively easy using simple tests of forced expiration. Spirometry with measurements of the forced expiratory volume in 1 s (FEV_1) and the forced vital capacity (FVC) provides objective physiological evidence and can be used as a guide to treatment. The peak expiratory flow rate is less reliable since it is more dependent on muscular effort and will be reduced in patients with restrictive as well as obstructive lung disease.

Having established the presence of airway obstruction, the differential diagnosis will usually lie between chronic obstructive airway disease and asthma. Less common causes include large airway obstruction (page 15.90), obliterative bronchiolitis (page 15.89), and occasionally left ventricular failure. The latter condition should be easy to detect on clinical and radiological grounds.

The clinical differentiation between COAD and asthma depends mainly on the spontaneous variability or the reversibility of the airway obstruction following treatment. Diagnostic procedures which have been developed to try and separate these two conditions have included the regular measurements of peak flow to assess spontaneous variability, bronchodilator response to inhaled β-sympathomimetics, therapeutic response to systemic steroids, and measurements of bronchial hyperreactivity in respect to constrictor stimuli. The major difficulty encountered when using this classification is the lack of a distinct boundary between 'reversible' and 'irreversible' disease. Even patients with apparently irreversible airway obstruction will show a small reduction in airway resistance following inhaled bronchodilators.

Investigations

The investigations are aimed at establishing the type and severity of the disease and in detecting associated complications.

Radiology

The plain posterior–anterior radiograph may show little abnormality even in patients with severe disease. The most common finding is hyperinflated lung fields with low flat diaphragms and an apparently elongated cardiac shadow. In patients with pulmonary hypertension the proximal part of the pulmonary arteries will be enlarged. Emphysema is difficult to diagnose reliably from the chest radiograph except when severe. The peripheral vessels will be thin or reduced in number. Bullae may be associated with generalized emphysema, but can also occur in isolation. They can be recognized by their fine margin around an avascular air space.

Patients with a history of repeated acute infections may have radiographs which show patchy fibrotic changes, presumably as the consequence of their repeated infections. Cardiac enlargement may be seen although it is difficult to distinguish between enlargement of left and right ventricular chambers.

Pulmonary function tests

The most useful tests are those of forced expiration, and include the FEV_1, FVC, and peak expiratory flow rate. In general patients whose symptoms are due to airway obstruction will have an FEV_1 reduced to approximately 50 per cent of the predicted value (often 1.5 l or less). In patients with severe disease the figure may be much lower. As a practical point, at least three measurements should be performed and further measurements made if the curves do not superimpose. The vital capacity should be measured both as part of a forced manoeuvre, but also during a gentle expiration. In patients with emphysema, the slow vital capacity may be significantly greater than that obtained during a forced expiration. In assessing any patient with airway obstruction, these measurements should be made before and after the use of an inhaled sympathomimetic bronchodilator. It may also be useful to see what additional benefit can be obtained by an anticholinergic drug. It is generally impractical to assess all patients with regular peak flow measurements, steroid trials or measure their bronchial reactivity. The decision to undertake these will depend on the clinical situation and the response to inhaled bronchodilators. Whilst asthma may occur in individuals who smoke, irreversible disease rarely occurs in non-smokers, and any non-smoker presenting with severe airway obstruction should be regarded as having asthma until proved otherwise.

Other measurements of lung mechanics include the measurement of residual volume and total lung capacity, recordings of airway resistance using the whole body plethysmograph, and the measurement of lung compliance. Whilst these tests may give some clues as to the underlying pathophysiology, they are rarely of any clinical use in everyday practice. Arterial blood gas measurements are usually necessary in any patient who is ill enough to be admitted to hospital. In addition, their measurement as an outpatient can provide a useful basis for deciding of the appropriateness or otherwise of domiciliary oxygen therapy.

One further assessment of global function can be made by recording exercise capability. The simplest method is to use the 12 min walking test, in which the distance walked during this period of time is measured. The result of the test is very susceptible to a learning process on repeated testing but with care may show improvement when conventional spirometry is unchanged after therapeutic intervention.

Blood tests

Secondary polycythaemia may develop and is usually related to the degree of chronic hypoxia. A raised white cell count suggests the presence of infection and a blood eosinophilia should alert the clinician to the possibility of asthma. Biochemistry is usually normal apart from a raised serum bicarbonate in patients with carbon dioxide retention.

Sputum examination

Culture of purulent sputum is likely to reveal either *H. influenzae* or *Strep. pneumoniae*. Sputum eosinophilia, as with blood eosinophilia, raises the possibility of a reversible component to the airway disease.

The electrocardiogram

In cor pulmonale there is evidence of right ventricular and right atrial strain. The P-wave is taller and more pointed than normal especially in lead 2 (a P-pulmonale). Right ventricular strain and hypertrophy occur with a dominant R-wave in leads V 1–3 and inverted T-waves. A right bundle block is the commonest conduction defect.

Treatment

The potential for significant improvement is limited in patients with severe irreversible airway disease, particularly when associated with emphysema. In view of this, preventative aspects must assume great importance. In patients with established disease management involves those measures which can be employed in the long-term and the additional action which is necessary in an acute exacerbation.

Prevention

The main aetiological factors where action is possible are in reducing atmospheric pollution and in stopping cigarette smoking. In the United Kingdom the levels of atmospheric pollutants have fallen dramatically with the implementation of smokeless zones and with alternative methods of fuel combustion. Action with respect to smoking has been much less evident, although there has been a steady fall in cigarette consumption particularly in social classes 1 and 2. In addition to increased public awareness of the hazards of smoking, it will need an alteration in social attitudes, combined with fiscal and legislative measures, e.g. a prohibition of all forms of cigarette promotion. A few countries have taken effective action, and there is increasing acceptance of smoking-free areas in public places. However, the aggressive promotion of cigarettes in developing countries will undoubtedly produce an increase in smoking-related diseases currently prevalent in Western society. Screening of smokers for the detection of early disease is technically possible using relatively simple spirometric methods. Whether such a policy is appropriate is debatable since it assumes that the patient will stop smoking when there is early disease and does not take into account the possible development of other smoking-related illnesses.

Long-term management of established disease

In patients with established disease it is difficult to strike a balance between therapeutic nihilism and the overenthusiastic use of a variety of measures which at best will be of marginal benefit. The most important single measure is to prevent further deterioration by persuading patients to stop smoking. Although this will not lead to a marked improvement in lung function, continuation will lead to further deterioration in respiratory reserve. Stopping smoking is often easiest during an acute exacerbation when motivation is greatest. Additional support from aids such as substitute cigarettes, nicotine chewing-gum or hypnotherapy may offer temporary benefit although at the end of one year's follow-up, all methods have a high relapse rate.

Those patients most severely affected will need advice and support in modifying their life-styles. Relatively simple aids such as the provision of a wheelchair may permit greater mobility. The ability to continue work will depend to a large extent on the patient's occupation. The problem is obviously greater in those patients with heavy manual jobs, and it is in social classes 4 and 5 that there is an increased prevalence in the disease.

Drug treatment

Although a variety of drugs are used in patients with chronic airway obstruction, the majority are of dubious value. They can be divided into those which improve lung function and those which may simply relieve symptoms.

Bronchodilators will produce the much smaller objective improvement in lung function than that seen in patients with asthma. However, even a small improvement may be of value in patients with severe airflow limitation, and continued use is justified if the patient derives symptomatic benefit. Inhalation of a sympathomimetic agent, e.g. salbutamol, or an anticholinergic, e.g. ipratropium bromide, can produce some improvement and a combination has been shown to produce slightly greater bronchodilation than either agent alone. Usually these are given via a metered dose pressurized inhaler, the standard dose being between 2 and 4 puffs, four hourly. Higher doses of either of these drugs can be delivered from a nebulizer, whereby a compressed gas flow can result in dispersal of a liquid into droplets. The small particles are carried out of the nebulizer suspended in air. Patients with severe disease may prefer this form of treatment, although it is often difficult to demonstrate significant physiological changes. The placebo effect which results from the use of a mechanical aid may be appreciated; against this has to be balanced the cost of purchasing a nebulizer.

Oral methylxanthines are widely used in patients with chronic obstructive airway disease. Theoretically they result in some bronchodilation and may also have effects on the respiratory centre, respiratory muscles, and as a diuretic. However, the majority of clinical trials have demonstrated no subjective or objective benefit and this together with their side-effects should mitigate against routine use.

Corticosteroids are known to be effective in the management of asthma. The response to steroids in patients with apparently stable chronic airflow limitation cannot be predicted reliably, but occasionally this form of treatment is unexpectedly beneficial. Long-term steroid treatment should only be instituted after a therapeutic trial, taking into account both subjective and objective changes. Such a trial is indicated in any non-smoker with significant airway obstruction, as well as in any patient who despite apparently irreversible airways obstruction has some features suggestive of asthma. These include an increase in the FEV_1 after a bronchodilator (20 per cent improvement is an arbitrary figure), objective evidence of spontaneous variability and blood or sputum eosinophilia. The usual regimen is prednisone 30 mg daily for a period of two weeks, administered when the patient is in a stable clinical state rather than during an acute exacerbation. If the patient has shown no response the prednisone can be stopped. If there is a significant improvement the oral steroids can be tailed down, whilst inhaled steroids are substituted.

Patients who fall into the pink puffing category are severely limited by their dyspnoea. Symptomatic relief can be obtained by the judicious use of respiratory depressants, such as diazepam, or opiates. It must be stressed that such treatment should only be taken after careful evaluation and blood gas analysis since the same drug may result in fatal carbon dioxide narcosis in patients who have a reduced respiratory drive.

Antibiotics are indicated for acute infective exacerbations. Early treatment is important and it is often sensible for the patient to have a reserve supply of antibiotics with instructions to commence treatment if sputum becomes purulent. The value of long-term maintenance antibiotics is debatable and the results of studies in the 1960s showed no convincing benefit.

In patients with right heart failure complicating severe lung disease, diuretic treatment is effective in controlling peripheral oedema in the majority of patients. Cardiac glycosides are of little value. In patients with intractable failure bed rest and additional inspired oxygen may be beneficial.

Physical therapy

A variety of non-pharmacological measures have been tried to relieve the symptoms of breathlessness, to improve exercise tolerance, and to assist the patients feeling of well-being. Measures include exercise training, physiotherapy aimed at improving functional aspects of respiratory muscles, assisted ventilation, and the use of domiciliary oxygen. Assessment of the value of some of these measures is difficult since there is likely to be a strong placebo element. Indeed simply adopting a positive approach may in itself improve the patient's morale and influence the therapeutic response.

Exercise training

A variety of training methods have been used with training periods lasting from 4 weeks to 12 months. The most economical programmes are those in which the patient is asked to do simple exercises, such as walking for a fixed time or stair climbing, which they can perform in their own homes. Regular assessment at clinic visits is an important component. Results vary but modest increases in exercise capacity have been reported with a diminution in the sensation of breathlessness and generally increased confidence. The physiological basis for any improvement is poorly understood but may be due to enhanced haemodynamic efficiency and oxygen utilization.

Specific chest physiotherapy is aimed at enhancing mucus clearance, modifying abnormalities of the breathing pattern, and training of respiratory muscles. Therapeutic measures such as postural drainage are of no value in the majority of patients except perhaps during acute infective exacerbations.

The value of breathing exercises is difficult to establish. A change to low frequency breathing may improve gas exchange. However, many patients intuitively adopt a pattern of respiration which is most comfortable. This includes pursed lip breathing, a slow relaxed expiratory phase, and a posture which gives maximal mechanical advantage to the accessory muscles.

Respiratory muscle training attempts to increase the power of respiratory muscles and reduce fatiguability. Recent measures have involved short periods of breathing through an inspiratory resistance. There are conflicting results as to the value of this form of training although gas exchange is undoubtedly impaired whilst the resistance is imposed.

Intermittent positive pressure breathing has been used to assist ventilation and to deliver bronchodilator aerosols. There is considerable debate about the long-term value. Any benefit is likely to be marginal and the practical and financial limitations mitigate against its routine use.

Respiratory failure

The management of acute respiratory failure and the indications for long-term domiciliary oxygen in patients who are chronically hypoxic are discussed elsewhere (page 15.169).

Related clinical syndromes

Bullous emphysema

A bulla is defined as a thin-walled emphysematous space greater than 1 cm in diameter. Bullae may arise either in association with generalized disease or occur in isolation. Spontaneous rupture of what would normally be small insignificant bullae is the most likely cause of a spontaneous pneumothorax.

Large bullae, which can easily be seen on a chest radiograph, represent areas in which there has been greater destruction of lung tissue with coalescence of several smaller bullae. Occasionally these may occur in association with a ball valve obstruction of a larger bronchus. Under these conditions the bulla enlarges and compresses the surrounding lung. Giant cysts tend to form in those areas of the lung more prone to other forms of emphysema, especially in the lung apices.

Clinical features

A moderate sized bulla occurring in isolation will not give rise to any symptoms but may be seen on routine chest radiograph. Breathlessness is the main symptom when there is general emphysema or when the cyst is so large as to impair the function of one lung. Patients would usually be smokers and symptoms develop insidiously. A more acute presentation will occur if there is an associated pneumothorax.

On examination the chest is likely to be hyperinflated with reduced movement of the affected lung. Breath sounds will be reduced or absent.

Investigations

Large bullae are usually seen radiologically as localized, thin-walled, well-demarquated areas of avascularity. If there is marked compression of surrounding lung this is obviously due to the crowding together of normal vascular markings. When bullae are in association with generalized emphysema, comparison of inspiratory and expiratory films reveals little change in volume. By contrast a localized bulla will remain inflated whilst the remaining normal lung becomes virtually airless. Assessing the extent to which the bulla is compressing normal lung is important since it may determine the value of surgical resection. A plain PA radiograph is usually insufficient to assess this and traditionally angiography or bronchography is used to demonstrate crowding together of normal vessels or bronchi. However, these procedures have to some extent been superseded with the advent of computerized tomography.

The degree to which respiratory function is impaired will depend on the size of the bulla and the extent to which there is generalized emphysema. Where there is a solitary large bulla,

residual volume will be increased, but there is usually no evidence of generalized airway obstruction and spirometry may be normal. The value for total lung capacity will depend on the method of measurement. Helium dilution will underestimate the true lung volume because of poor ventilation of the bulla. Body plethysmography will give a more accurate figure and the difference between the two values may give an estimate of the size of the bulla.

When there is more generalized disease, lung function is more severely affected. Residual volume and total capacity are often increased and there is evidence of airways obstruction.

Treatment

There is no drug therapy which is likely to improve lung function significantly in patients with emphysema. Bronchodilators may minimally improve airway function. The main therapeutic decision is whether surgery is likely to offer any benefit. The best results are obtained when there is a single large bulla compressing otherwise normal lung. Surgical removal or decompression results in expansion of the compressed lung and an improvement in lung function. Beneficial results are less likely if there is generalized disease and in patients with severely impaired lung function, surgery carries a high risk.

Unilateral lung radiolucency (MacLeod's syndrome)

This syndrome is one which derives from radiographic appearances. MacLeod described several patients whose chest radiograph showed unilateral hypertransradiency with a small pulmonary artery and poorly developed vascular branches. Bronchographically there is irregular dilation of the larger bronchi. Pathologically the affected lung is often reduced in size and when removed from the chest does not deflate. There is often evidence of patchy obstruction or obliteration of smaller bronchi. MacLeod suggested that the appearances result from damage in childhood, probably resulting from an infective bronchiolitis.

Clinical features

The majority of patients are asymptomatic. A few may complain of exercise-related breathlessness and occasionally there may be a history of repeated respiratory tract infections. Usually there is no recollection of what might be regarded as the initiating infective episode.

On examination there is reduced movement of the infected hemithorax with diminished air entry.

In functional terms there is sometimes evidence of airway obstruction with a modest increase in residual volumes. Isotope ventilation and perfusion scanning demonstrates reduced ventilation and blood flow to the affected lung. Radiologically it may occasionally be difficult to distinguish this condition from generalized emphysema in which there is asymmetry between the two lungs. Compenstory emphysema in association with a collapsed lobe should be obvious by the presence of the collapsed lobe and by the reduced number of the vessels.

There is no specific treatment indicated for this condition and the prognosis is good.

Bronchiolitis obliterans

Bronchiolitis obliterans is essentially a pathological diagnosis whereby bronchioles become obstructed by organizing exudate, granulation tissue, and fibrosis. It may be the end result of a variety of initiating stimuli. It can follow exposure to poisonous gases such as oxides of nitrogen or chlorine. There has been a few instances in which it is associated with a respiratory tract infection possibly due to an adenovirus. In addition, a variant may be associated with rheumatoid arthritis.

Clinical features

The history is usually relatively short and the main symptoms are cough, productive of mucoid sputum, and breathlessness.

Occasionally chest pain or haemoptysis may be associated. On examination there may be scattered inspiratory crackles. Radiographic features may vary and three main patterns of disease have been observed. Alveolar opacities are most common and represent varying degrees of collapse or consolidation at a subsegmental level. Nodular shadows of varying sizes have also been recorded and occasionally there is evidence of hyperinflation. Respiratory function is also variable, some patients showing a restrictive defect, others showing more evidence of airway obstruction. There is no response to bronchodilators and although steroids are frequently used there is no clearly documented evidence of benefit. The prognosis is poor and the disease usually progresses over a period of weeks or months.

Diseases of the trachea

Disorders primarily affecting the trachea are relatively uncommon although, since they often present with symptoms of cough, breathlessness, and wheeze, they may be mistaken for bronchitis or asthma. Tracheal narrowing or obstruction is the end result of a number of pathological processes and the mode of presentation will vary with the rapidity of onset and severity of the obstruction.

Acute tracheal obstruction

This is most common in infants and young children because of the small calibre of the trachea. Infective causes predominate and acute laryngotracheo bronchitis is usually due to parainfluenza or respiratory syncitial virus infections. The cause of respiratory distress is usually apparent from the history with symptoms of malaise, cough, fever, and sore throat. The presence of serious airway narrowing is evidenced by the respiratory distress, tachypnoea, harsh inspiratory stridor, and marked intercostal recession and indrawing of the lower ribs.

Foreign bodies

Obstruction of the air passages by foreign bodies is again most frequent in infants and young children. The objects most frequently aspirated are peanuts, sweets, coins, and plastic toys. The consequences of an inhaled foreign body will depend on its size. Total occlusion of the airway will rapidly result in death from asphyxiation. Smaller objects impacting more peripherally may present at a later stage with a history of cough and recurrent chest infections. In an emergency the foreign body may be dislodged from the upper airway using the using the Heimlich manoeuvre whereby sudden abdominal compression results in a rapid exhalation.

Chronic tracheal obstruction

In contrast to acute tracheal obstruction where the cause is usually obvious, chronic tracheal obstruction is frequently misdiagnosed as being due to asthma or bronchitis. Although the clinical features will vary to some extent with the underlying cause, breathlessness and cough occur most frequently. Stridor is a useful diagnostic sign sometimes present at rest or becoming apparent during exercise. Its timing is usually during inspiration but may also be during expiration. Intercostal recession occurs when there is severe obstruction and high negative intrapleural pressures are needed to generate inspiratory flow.

Aetiology

There are a variety of conditions which may affect the upper airway and result in obstruction. In general there are three different mechanisms: intraluminal obstruction, extrinsic compression, and abnormalities of the tracheal wall resulting in increased collapsibility of the trachea.

Tracheal tumours are undoubtedly the commonest cause of intraluminal narrowing or obstruction. Compared with the larynx and bronchi, the trachea is a rare site of primary cancer although frequently tumour can spread from more distal sites in the bronchial tree. The commonest primary cancer of the trachea is a squamous cell carcinoma. Adenoid cystic carcinomas (cylindromas) are slightly less common. Patients with tracheal neoplasms are often treated for asthma for some time before the correct diagnosis is made.

Tracheal stenosis may occasionally be congenital, but most commonly occurs as a complication of intubation or tracheostomy. Stenosis after a tracheostomy may occur at the stoma or at the level of the inflatable cuff. The most susceptible portion of the trachea is where the mucosa overlies rigid cartilaginous rings and pressure of the cuff results in necrosis, ulceration, and subsequent fibrosis. New endotracheal tubes which have a large volume, low pressure cuff are less likely to cause tracheal damage.

The causes of extrinsic compression of the trachea are usually more obvious and include malignant lymph nodes, thymic tumours, thyroid enlargements, and aortic aneurysms.

Investigation

The diagnosis of a tracheal obstruction is relatively easy once the diagnosis is suspected. Clues may be obtained from physiological tests or from radiology but the diagnosis is usually confirmed by direct inspection at bronchoscopy.

Physiologically tracheal narrowing will result in reduced airflow in or out of the lungs. A fixed stenotic segment will result in low inspiratory and expiratory flow rates. The expiratory spirogram will appear as a straight line (Fig. 2). If cartilaginous support of the trachea is absent, the intrathoracic segment will be compressed during expiration. The extrathoracic segment will collapse on inspiration.

Tracheal narrowing is frequently missed on the plain radiograph. Thoracic inlet view and tracheal tomograms are likely to yield more information.

Treatment will depend on the underlying cause of the obstruction.

Primary diseases of the trachea

There are a number of rare conditions which affect the tracheal wall and cartilaginous supports. These include tracheomalacia, tracheobronchomegaly, tracheopathia osteoplastica, and relapsing polychondritis. Each of these will briefly be considered.

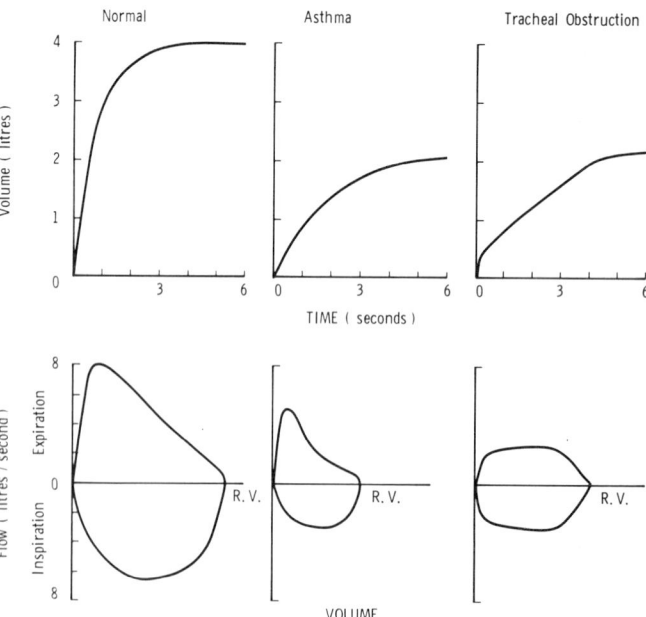

Fig. 2 Representative flow volume curves and spirometry in normal subject, patient with asthma, and patient with tracheal stenosis. Note the reduced peak flow and constant maximal expiratory flow rate seen spirometrically as a straight line.

Tracheomalacia

This condition is characterized by a weakness of the supporting cartilage within the tracheal wall. In some patients it is a developmental defect and may be associated with other congenital abnormalities such as a cleft palate. Acquired forms may follow tracheostomy and also occur in patients with severe chronic obstructive airway disease. The abnormal flaccidity of the tracheal wall has two main consequences. The cough mechanism is impaired resulting in retention of mucus and recurrent infections. In addition symptoms include wheezing and shortness of breath occurring as a result of the premature collapse of major airways during expiration. The dynamic changes in calibre of the trachea occurring during respiration can be visualized bronchoscopically or demonstrated by cine-radiography.

Tracheobronchomegaly

This rare disease is characterized by an unusual increase in diameter of the trachea and main bronchi. It is probably congenital and has been associated with Ehlers–Danlos syndrome. Pathologically there is atrophy of the connective tissues of the trachea and main bronchi. Cough is ineffective and as a result respiratory tract infections and bronchiectasis are associated features. The condition is obvious on tracheobronchogram.

Tracheopathia osteoplastica

This condition is characterized by the development of nodules or spicules of cartilage and bone projecting into the lumen of trachea and bronchi. It is exceedingly rare and occurs almost exclusively in middle-aged and elderly men. The patient is frequently asymptomatic although a dry cough may be a presenting feature. The majority of cases have only been diagnosed at autopsy. A few patients have been diagnosed on the basis of the bronchoscopic appearances. A plain radiograph is usually normal but tomography of the trachea will reveal the projecting spicules.

Relapsing polychondritis

This unusual and interesting systemic disease affects cartilage in a variety of anatomical sites. Information and destruction of cartilage occurs with the release of chondroitin sulphate. The sites most commonly affected are the pinna, nasal septum, larnyx, and trachea. More rarely the aortic valve may be affected. Respiratory involvement is the most serious complication and may result in death from airway obstruction and complicating pneumonia. Corticosteroid drugs in higher doses may help in the acute phases but the disease often progresses despite their use.

References

Bjartveit, K. (1978). The Norwegian Tobacco Act. *World Smoking Hlth* 3, 29–31.

Dolan, D. L., Lemmon, G. V. and Teitelbaum, S. T. (1966). Relapsing polychondritis. *Am. J. Med.* 41, 285–299.

Doll, R. and Peto, R. (1976). Mortality in relation to smoking: 30 years observations on male British Doctors. *Br. Med. J.* 2, 1525–1536.

Flenley, D. C. and Warren, P. M. (1980). Chronic bronchitis and emphysema. In *Recent advances in respiratory medicine*, No. 2 (ed. D. C. Flenley), p. 206. Churchill Livingstone, Edinburgh.

Fletcher, C., Peto, R., Tinker, C. and Speizer, F. E. (1976). *The natural history of chronic bronchitis and emphysema.* Oxford University Press, Oxford.

—— and Pride, N. B. (1984). Definition of emphysema, chronic bronchitis, asthma and airflow obstruction: 25 years on from the CIBA symposium. *Thorax* 39, 81–85.

Geddes, D. M., Corrin, B., Brewerton, D. A., Davies, R. J. and Turner-Warwick, M. (1977). Progressive airway obliteration in adults and its association with rheumatoid disease. *Q. J. Med.* 46, 427–444.

Gosink, B. B., Friedman, P. J. and Liebow, A. A. (1973). Bronchiolitis obliterans: roentgenological-pathological correlation. *Am. J. Roent.* 117, 816–832.

Hogg, J. C., Macklem, P. T. and Thurlbeck, W. M. (1968). Site and nature of airway obstruction in chronic obstructive lung disease. *N. Engl. J. Med.* 278, 1355–1360.

Hugh-Jones, P. and Whimster, W. (1978). The aetiology and management of disabling emphysema. *Am. Rev. Resp. Dis.* 117, 343–378.

King, K., Mandaw, B. and Kamen, J. M. (1975). Tracheal tube cuffs and tracheal dilation. *Chest* 67, 458.

Macklem, P. T. (1972). Obstruction in small airways – a challenge to medicine. *Am. J. Med.* 52, 721–728.

Macleod, W. M. (1954). Abnormal transradiency of one lung. *Thorax* 9, 147–153.

May, J. R. (1972). *The chemotherapy of chronic bronchitis and allied disorders* 2nd edn. Hodder and Stoughton, London.

Miller, R. D. and Hyatt, R. E. (1969). Obstructing lesions of the larynx and trachea. Clinical and physiological characteristics. *Mayo Clin. Proc.* 44, 145–161.

Orie, N. G. M., Sluiter, H. T., De Vries, K., Tammeling, C. J. and Witkop, J. (1961). The host factor in bronchitis. In *Bronchitis. Proceedings of the international symposium on bronchitis at Gronigen, the Netherlands* (eds N. G. M. Orie and H. J. Sluiter), pp. 43–51. Royal Vangorcum Assen.

Petty, T. L. (ed.) (1978). *Chronic obstructive pulmonary disease.* Marcel Dekker, New York.

Pride, N. B., Barter, C. E. and Hugh-Jones, P. (1973). The ventilation of bullae and the effect of their removal on thoracic gas volumes and tests of overall pulmonary function. *Am. Rev. Resp. Dis.* 107, 83–98.

Woolcock, A. J. (1980). The pathogenesis of chronic obstructive lung disease with particular reference to the small airway hypothesis. In *Recent advances in respiratory medicine*, No. 2. (ed. D. C. Flenley), p. 45. Churchill Livingstone, Edinburgh.

CHEST INFECTIONS

Acute infections of the lower respiratory tract

J. T. MACFARLANE

Introduction

Infections of the respiratory tract are one of the commonest illnesses to affect humans, whether healthy or debilitated by other disease.

This section discusses lower respiratory tract infections, adopting a practical and clinical approach. Further details of specific pathogens and individual syndromes can be found in other parts of the textbook.

Bronchial infections

Acute tracheo-bronchitis in previously healthy people

This is so common that few think it unusual to have at least one attack each year. It is usually caused by virus infection including adenovirus, influenza virus, Respiratory Syncytial virus (especially in infants and the elderly), and enteroviruses (particularly Coxsackie A21). Atypical infections with *Mycoplasma pneumoniae* and *Chlamydia psittaci* sometimes present as acute bronchitis in young adults.

Symptoms include a dry, tickly cough and retrosternal soreness. Mucoid sputum may be produced. Associated upper respiratory tract symptoms are common. The patient does not look ill and the chest is clear. Investigations are not normally required: the white blood count will be normal and chest radiograph clear. Sometimes the virus can be cultured from a nasopharyngeal swab.

Treatment is symptomatic and antibiotics are not needed. Compound cough mixtures may be helpful at night, largely due to their sedative properties.

Acute bronchitis in those with pre-existing chronic bronchitis

Presentation

Chronic bronchitis is characterized by persistent production of excess bronchial mucus. Those affected by this syndrome are liable to suffer repeated acute exacerbations characterized by an increase in sputum purulence and worsening cough that lasts for 48 hours or more. In addition, there may be general malaise, a mild fever, increased breathlessness, increased sputum volume or thickness, and increased difficulty in expectoration. Such exacerbations are more common in the winter months.

Aetiology

Identifying the supposed role of acute bronchial infection in such exacerbations can be difficult. Over three-quarters of patients with stable chronic bronchitis have *H. influenzae* present in their sputum and in a third *S. pneumoniae* is also found. Therefore the culture of these pathogens during an exacerbation is not necessarily informative. Long-term studies of patients with chronic bronchitis suggest that although the incidence of positive sputum cultures for *H. influenzae* and *S. pneumoniae* does not rise during exacerbations, the actual numbers of bacteria (particularly pneumococci) do increase. Regarding non-bacterial causes, viruses have been associated with 40–60 per cent of acute exacerbations particularly in winter months, and the reported incidence of *M. pneumoniae* infection (proven on serological testing) is 1–8 per cent. Mycoplasma colonize the lower respiratory tract in chronic bronchitis in a higher proportion, but their role in acute exacerbations is unclear.

Clinical features

These reflect both the infection itself and the associated underlying lung disease. Sputum is usually mucopurulent and produced in greater quantities, though not necessarily with greater ease, than in the stable bronchitic state. Scattered, coarse crepitations may be heard on auscultation, particularly at the bases, with a variable accompaniment of wheezes. Radiographically the chest is usually clear, though some peribronchial thickening and infiltration may be noted. Dyspnoea and disturbance of lung function will be determined by the degree of pre-existing obstructive airways disease.

Management of acute exacerbation

Because *H. influenzae* and *S. pneumoniae* are found with such regularity in sputum from these patients, routine sputum culture is unnecessary during an exacerbation unless the patient is seriously ill or the presentation unusual. Antibiotics appear to hasten recovery. The choice of antibiotic is not crucial provided it is effective against the two common pathogens. Studies have shown equally good response with ampicillin, amoxycillin, co-trimoxazole, and erythromycin. Tetracycline previously widely used in this setting, is less popular now because of side-effects and because of increasing bacterial resistance, particularly amongst common strains of *H. influenzae* but also some *S. pneumoniae*.

Treatment is given for 7–10 days or until the patient improves and sputum purulence resolves. Patients with severe chronic bronchitis may also require treatment for airflow obstruction and for respiratory and cardiac failure during an exacerbation (page 15.168).

Prophylactic measures

The place of measures to prevent acute exacerbations in patients with chronic bronchitis is not clear. Antibiotic prophylaxis with such agents as daily tetracycline or weekly long-acting sulfametopyrazine has been shown to be helpful but only in patients with frequent (six or more per year) exacerbations. Regular *N*-acetylcysteine appears to reduce the rate of winter exacerbations in people with chronic simple bronchitis. An influenza vaccination in the autumn is helpful.

Acute bronchial infections and asthma

Adults with asthma frequently date the start of their condition from an attack of acute bronchitis. Acute infective bronchitis, particularly due to viral infection, can lead to a state of airways hyperreactivity. This explains the persistence of cough and wheeze for several weeks after an acute bronchitic illness. In certain susceptible people this appears to initiate the development of true asthma.

It is very important to identify such patients as the treatment and prognosis of asthma is so different from that of a simple infective bronchitis. Persisting cough and wheeze, particularly at night, together with a reduced peak expiratory flow rate all point to the development of asthma. All too often such patients receive repeated and inappropriate courses of antibiotics, whereas they really need bronchodilators or even corticosteroids.

In patients with established asthma, bacterial infections are an unusual cause of acute exacerbations and antibiotics have little place in the routine management of acute asthma. Similarly viral infections have been implicated in only 10–20 per cent of acute exacerbations.

Bacterial superinfection following acute viral bronchitis

A viral bronchitic illness may be complicated by bacterial superinfection. This is of more clinical importance when a pneumonic illness develops and is therefore considered later in this chapter (page 15.93).

Pneumonia

History

Pneumonia has been recognized for many centuries. 'Peripneumonia' was described by Hippocrates in the 4th century BC. The erroneous concepts of anatomy and physiology which prevailed up to the last century hampered any real understanding of the nature of pneumonia, though it was regarded as some sort of inflammation of the lung. Treatment included leeches, cupping, and stupes applied to the chest, and emetics, tonics, and purges, to draw the inflammation away from the chest. Vigorous blood letting was popular, particularly in Britain.

In 1834 Laennec paved the way for our modern understanding of lobar pneumonia by describing the three stages of consolidation that are still recognized today. Pathologically these include a first state of engorgement: the lung when cut, is wet, oedematous, and congested. In the second stage of red hepatization, the lung is dry, red, friable, and solid like liver. Thirdly, grey hepatization occurs with softening of the cut lung and exudation of yellow purulent fluid which denotes resolution. Laennec also perfected the use of the stethoscope and described the crepitous rattle (crepitation) as a pathognomonic sign of the first stage of peripneumonia. Red hepatization was heralded by the development of bronchial breathing, and resolution by the return of crepitations (rhonchus crepitous redux).

Towards the end of the 19th century the cause of pneumonia became a matter of hot debate with some expounding atmospheric conditions as the cause and others infection. It was Friedländer, between 1881 and 1884, who first found bacteria in the lungs of fatal cases of pneumonia using the staining techniques of his colleague Gram, and Fraenkel who, in 1884, first isolated an organism which he called 'pneumoniemikroccus' (pneumococcus) from a 30-year-old man dying of pneumonia. The identification of the pneumococcus rapidly led to a realization of its importance as a cause of pneumonia and to the production of specific antisera for treatment. By the early 20th century microbiologists had become expert and quick at typing and isolating pneumococci as a guide to specific serum therapy.

With the discovery of penicillin and other antibiotics, the problem of pneumonia seemed to be conquered and interest in the condition waned. It was however recognized that there was a group of pneumonias, which did not behave like lobar pneumococcal pneumonia, in that they were generally not severe and did not respond to penicillin. These 'atypical' pneumonias were subsequently identified as being caused by *Chlamydia psittaci* (psittacosis), *Coxiella burneti* (Q fever), and *Mycoplasma pneumoniae* (Eaton's agent).

The next major event in the history of pneumonia was the first outbreak of Legionnaires' disease in 1976. The immense interest generated by this discovery sparked off an awareness that pneumonia of all types was still a common cause of morbidity and mortality, even in the days of readily available antibiotics.

The continuing importance of pneumonia

Pneumonia remains a common cause of hospital admission. Over 12 000 adults between 12 and 79 years of age were admitted to hospitals in England and Wales with primary pneumonia in 1980. Pneumonia still has a significant mortality. The death rate in England and Wales for males of all ages between 1968 and 1972 was around 80 per 100 000 population and about half that for women. The figure for males in the United States was 34 per 100 000 and 141 per 100 000 for Mexico. The figures are considerably higher in patients over 65 years of age. Pneumonia (with influenza) ranks fifth among causes of death in the United States. In developing countries, pneumonia is one of the commonest causes of hospital admission in both children and adults (see page 15.171).

Classification of pneumonia

The traditional divisions of pneumonia are by radiological appearance or microbiological cause. Neither are of much practical help to the clinician. The radiological description of pneumonia as lobar, lobular, segmental, and bronchopneumonia does not help in either diagnosis or management. Similarly, grouping under aetiology presupposes that the clinician knows the cause of the pneumonia when the patient first presents – a theoretically ideal but, in practice, very unusual situation.

A useful, practical classification of the types of pneumonia includes reference to the clinical circumstances under which the pneumonia is acquired and to the clinical background of the particular patient. Thus pneumonia may be acquired in the *community* or in *hospital* (nosocomial) and may be *primary*, that is, occurring in a previously healthy individual or *secondary*, that is, developing in an individual in whom some recognizable predisposing factors operate.

This section will consider community acquired pneumonias, most of which are primary, and certain secondary pneumonias such as those occurring in an influenza epidemic, pneumonia in patients with chronic obstructive lung disease, and pneumonia in the very young and the elderly. Nosocomial pneumonia, which invariably is secondary to some pre-existing disease or abnormality in antimicrobial defences, is also discussed.

Pneumonia in the immunocompromised patient is a special example of secondary pneumonia that is of increasing importance. This complex problem is dealt with on page 15.106.

Recurrent pneumonia This describes three or more separate attacks of pneumonia in the same patient (see page 15.99).

Pneumonia acquired in certain specific parts of the world can be due to unusual infections peculiar to particular geographical areas. Aspects of these infections are described on pages 15.171 and 15.173.

Community-acquired pneumonia

Introduction

This continues to be a common cause of acute hospital admission. There are few studies of the incidence in the community of patients not requiring hospitalization, but studies in a large group health practice in Seattle suggested an annual rate of 10–15 cases per 1000 population (all ages). Only 16 per cent of cases required hospital admission. Community studies in Nottingham suggest that a General Practitioner will see about 8–10 cases of pneumonia each year, in adults between 16 and 79 years, and will manage three-quarters of them at home. Those with pneumonia only constitute about 6 per cent of all the patients that they treat for respiratory infections with antibiotics. In Britain, 25 million prescriptions for antibiotics are written each year for new episodes of respiratory illness (all ages). Therefore, a substantial number of patients are being treated for pneumonia in the community. Pneumonia is commoner in the winter months. It has been suggested that winter air of low humidity dries the nasopharyngeal mucosa and impairs local defences.

Aetiology

Before the introduction of antibiotics, the predominance of pneumococcal infection as a cause of pneumonia emerged very clearly. Reports on over 14 000 cases of lobar pneumonia by Cecil in 1927 and Heffron in 1939 found pneumococcal infection in over 95 per cent. After the discovery of antibiotics and their subsequent widespread use, the pattern appeared to change. Recent hospital studies of adults admitted from the community with pneumonia in the United Kingdom have produced widely varying results (Table 1), depending on where, how, and when the study was performed.

Antibiotics given before admission to hospital reduce the ability to culture common pathogens from sputum, blood, and body fluids, and this is one reason for disappointing microbiological results. In some studies no pathogen has been identified in up to half of the cases. Pneumococcal infection may still be the cause in many of these undiagnosed cases because pneumococcal antigen can be detected by countercurrent immunoelectrophoresis in up to three-quarters of cases. The detection of bacterial antigen is much less affected by prior antibiotics or delay in specimen collection (see page 5.188). Some viral and atypical pneumonias are also underdiagnosed because both acute and follow-up serological samples are needed to identify such infections.

The main conclusions from British studies is that community-acquired pneumonia is caused by a limited number of organisms. *S. pneumoniae* is the principal pathogen. Other bacteria are uncommon but include *H. influenzae* and *S. aureus* (particularly in association with influenza virus infection). In some areas legionella pneumonia must be considered. Although *H. influenzae* is usually seen in those with chronic lung disease, it can sometimes be a primary pathogen in previously fit adults. Infections with the Gram-negative coccal bacteria, *Neisseria meningitidis* group Y and *Branhamella catarrhalis* have been reported infrequently but Gram-negative bacillary infections are very unusual. Viral and atypical pneumonias, particularly *M. pneumoniae* infection, form a sizeable group. Viral infections are usually associated with superadded bacterial pneumonia. These conclusions have important implications for deciding on antibiotic treatment.

In contrast, community-acquired pneumonia in the United States is reported to be much more frequently due to Gram-negative and staphylococcal infection than in Britain. This is probably because debilitated patients, alcoholics, and drug abusers form a larger proportion of patients with pneumonia in studies from centres in North America.

The causes of community-acquired pneumonia not requiring

Table 1 Causes of adult community-acquired pneumonia found in recent British hospital-based studies

Type of pneumonia (several mixed infections)	Multicentre study (British Thoracic Society, 1985) ($n = 453$) (%)	London study (McNabb et al., 1984) ($n = 80$) (%)	Nottingham study (Macfarlane et al., 1982) ($n = 127$) (%)	Bristol study (White et al., 1981) ($n = 210$) (%)
Streptococcus pneumoniae	34*	50*	76*	11.5
Legionella species	2	1.2	15	1.5
Staphylococcus aureus	1	3.7	2.4	4
Haemophilus influenzae	6	6	3	2
Mycobacterium tuberculosis	0	2.5	1	0
Other bacteria	3	3.7	0.8	2
Mycoplasma pneumoniae	18†	0	2.4	14†
Psittacosis/Q fever	4	0	6.3	4.5
Viral	8	6.2	8.6	15
No pathogens identified	33	36	3	52

* Pneumococcal infection also diagnosed by detection of pneumococcal antigen.

† One or more mycoplasma epidemics during study period.

hospital admission have not been studied extensively. Surveys from Plymouth, England, Sweden, and Seattle, North America, found mycoplasma pneumonia in 15–20 per cent of cases and viral infection in only 5–7 per cent. Legionella pneumonia was found in 1 per cent of cases in Seattle. A community study in Nottingham has helped to clarify the role of bacteria in this situation. Pathogens were identified in 53 per cent of 236 adults with pneumonia including *S. pneumoniae* in 78 (33 per cent), *H. influenzae* in 24 (10 per cent), tuberculosis in 3, *S. aureus* in 2, and *L. pneumophila* in 1. In addition, viruses were found in 30 cases and atypical pneumonia in 6. This pattern is very similar to hospital-based studies.

Clinical features

It is usually not possible to identify the cause of a pneumonia from the history and signs on presentation. The time of year may be of some help in indicating the cause. Influenza is usually seen in epidemics in February and March and Respiratory Syncytial virus in December to February, whereas legionella pneumonia is commoner in the summer months. Mycoplasma infection has definite 3–4 year periodicity throughout the world and suspicion will be heightened during an epidemic, the last one being in 1982–83.

Symptoms

Males are affected more commonly than females by a ratio of 2–3 to 1. General symptoms include those of any febrile illness, malaise, anorexia, sweating, aches and pains, and headache. There may be a preceding history of upper respiratory tract symptoms, particularly with viral and mycoplasma infections. Respiratory symptoms are variable but classically include cough, sputum, and dyspnoea, pleural pain, and, less commonly, haemoptysis (Table 2).

Sputum is usually mucoid, scanty or absent early on in the illness, particularly with legionella and atypical pneumonias. Purulent sputum develops later.

Non-respiratory symptoms sometimes dominate the picture and mask the diagnosis. Lower lobe pneumonia may present with abdominal pain, rigidity, and ileus, and should be excluded in anyone with an 'acute' abdomen. Marked confusion may also be seen in patients with any severe pneumonia and it is a feature of legionella pneumonia in less seriously ill patients. Meningitis, hypoxia, and metabolic upset must also be considered in the confused patient. Severe headache, cerebellar dysfunction, memory loss, and myalgia also occur with legionella pneumonia. Vomiting and diarrhoea are prominent in some cases, though they may be the result of initial antibiotic therapy.

Enquiry should be made about recent contact with pet birds or fowl at home or work (possible psittacosis), contact with farm animals (for Q fever), recent foreign travel or stays in large hotels or hospitals (for legionella pneumonia) or contact with others with pneumonia, influenza or chicken pox.

Table 2 Symptoms in 127 consecutive adults with community-acquired pneumonia

Symptom	Percentage
Fever	86
Headache	55
Muscle aches	44
Nausea/vomiting	48
Diarrhoea	24
Sore throat	19
Dyspnoea	67
Pleural pain	62
Cough	92
New sputum production	54
Haemoptysis	15

Source: Macfarlane, unpublished data.

The duration of symptoms before hospital presentation varies with the severity of the illness, but is usually 3–7 days. Ten to 14 days are not unusual with atypical pneumonia, especially mycoplasma infection. Pneumococcal pneumonia may present abruptly with fever, rigors, cough, and pleural pain. Adults with influenza or chicken pox who develop lower respiratory symptoms may deteriorate quickly and should be assessed and treated as a matter of urgency.

Physical signs

The patient usually looks flushed and unwell with tachypnoea and a tachycardia. High temperatures (greater than 39.5 °C) and rigors occur in young people, especially with pneumococcal and legionella pneumonia. Elderly or debilitated patients may have little or no rise in temperature, the main sign being a raised respiratory rate. Herpes labialis is a feature of pneumococcal infection, being found in a third of cases. Examination of the chest may show reduced movement of the affected side particularly if pleural pain is prominent and the patient may splint that side by shallow breathing and hand holding. Classic signs of lobar consolidation are uncommon and bronchial breathing occurs in less than one-third of cases; inspiratory crepitations are the commonest focal sign. A pleural rub may be heard even in the absence of pleural pain. On occasions, chest examination appears normal and the extent of radiographic shadowing comes as a surprise.

Signs outside the chest may be found. Upper abdominal tenderness and confusion are not uncommon in more severely ill patients. A rash is unusual with community-acquired pneumonias, but it has been reported with mycoplasma and psittacosis pneumonia. Usually any rash is secondary to antibiotic therapy.

It is important to emphasize that respiratory symptoms and signs may not be elicited even in the presence of extensive pneumonia. This is particularly the case in the very young, elderly or debilitated patient and the diagnosis may be missed without a chest radiograph.

Investigations

General

The total white cell count is over 15.0×10^6/dl in the majority of patients with bacterial pneumonia, with the differential showing a neutrophilia (Table 3). However, in legionella pneumonia the total white cell count is usually not above 15.0×10^6/dl and sometimes there is a lymphopenia. In patients with uncomplicated atypical or viral pneumonia a near normal white cell count is usual. A low white cell count can be found in the very ill and is a poor prognostic sign. Marked red cell agglutination on the blood film should suggest the presence of cold agglutinins which are raised in over 50 per cent of cases with mycoplasma pneumonia. Cold agglutinin titres are normally measured in the laboratory but a screening test can be useful at the bedside. A few drops of fresh blood are mixed with the same volume of sodium citrate (as found in a standard prothrombin tube) and this is left in the fridge for 2–3 min to reach about 4 °C. Coarse agglutination of the blood, seen as the cooled tube is rotated, is usually associated with cold agglutinin titres of greater than 1:64.

Abnormal liver function tests are common and may be found in a third of patients with pneumococcal pneumonia and half with legionella pneumonia. Raised blood urea and creatinine, hyponatraemia, hypoalbuminaemia, proteinuria and haematuria can be seen with any severe pneumonia. Marked hypoalbuminaemia can develop quickly, probably due to a combination of sequestration of plasma protein into the lung and generalized increased vascular permeability from toxaemia. Patients ill enough to require hospital admission will often be hypoxic, and sometimes acidotic. Hypercapnia denotes the onset of ventilatory failure. Signs of multisystem involvement are less usual with atypical pneumonias.

Specific

Many patients with mild pneumonia, treated successfully in the community, will not need any investigations, except for a chest radiograph after clinical recovery to confirm resolution. For patients who are ill enough to require hospital treatment, the aim is to identify the cause of the pneumonia as soon as possible. Blood, any pleural fluid, and, if possible, sputum, should be collected for culture before antibiotics are started, because a single dose can interfere with the culture of common pathogens such as *S. pneumoniae* and *H. influenzae*.

Gram staining of sputum (and pleural fluid) sometimes gives a quick and accurate indication of the pathogen, if predominant numbers of one pathogen are seen in a good sputum specimen. Although the specificity of the Gram stain is high, the sensitivity is

Table 3 Initial total white cell count ($\times 10^6$/dl) in 268 patients with different types of community-acquired pneumonia

	10.0 or less	11–15	More than 15
Pneumococcal ($n = 93$)	15%	32%	53%
Legionella ($n = 78$)	53%	36%	11%
Mycoplasma ($n = 85$)	61%	28%	11%
Psittacosis ($n = 12$)	58%	42%	0%

Source: Macfarlane, unpublished data.

low. Predominant numbers of Gram-positive diplococci on Gram stains are only seen in 10–20 per cent of patients with pneumococcal pneumonia. If more than ten squamous epithelial cells are seen in each low-powered field, the specimen is probably of oropharyngeal origin and is of little use. Because the bacterial flora of sputum represents a mixture of organisms from the lower respiratory tract and those acquired during passage through the mouth, isolation of a pathogen may not reflect what is occurring in the lung itself. The specificity of the culture may be improved by washing or diluting the sputum. Even then sputum culture is a relatively insensitive method of diagnosis for bacterial pneumonia. Less than half of patients with untreated bacteraemic pneumococcal pneumonia have pneumococci isolated from their sputum. Isolation of a pathogen from blood or pleural fluid culture provides certain evidence of its importance.

The commonest practical problem is that over half of the patients have received an antibiotic before hospital admission and this greatly reduces the usefulness of Gram stains and culture of secretions and body fluids. The detection of bacterial antigen can partially overcome this problem and is particularly helpful in pneumococcal infection (see page 5.188).

The diagnosis of non-pneumococcal bacterial pneumonia raises similar problems to those encountered with pneumococcal pneumonia. Potential pathogens like staphylococci, meningococci, and streptococci can be part of the normal respiratory flora. *H. influenzae* can be cultured in mucoid sputum in over half of patients with chronic bronchitis. Over a quarter of hospitalized patients may carry Gram-negative organisms in their upper respiratory tract, particularly if they are receiving broad-spectrum antibiotics. There are no tests available for detecting antigens from these other bacteria and serological testing for bacterial precipitating antibodies is of no value in diagnosing acute infections.

The major limitation of diagnostic virology is the length of time required for isolating and identifying a particular virus. The direct fluorescent antibody staining technique for detecting viral antigens in respiratory secretions has been useful in the rapid diagnosis of Respiratory Syncytial virus bronchiolitis in children, but is not widely used for other viruses. Of the organisms causing 'atypical' pneumonia, only *M. pneumoniae* can be grown with any ease, though even here growth may take several weeks despite using a specifal diphasic medium.

To diagnose viral and atypical pneumonias by serological methods, blood should be collected early in the illness and again 10–14 days later or during convalescence. A four-fold or greater change in specific antibody titre is accepted as evidence of recent infection. Unfortunately the result often arrives too late to influence the management of the patient. A single sample taken late in the illness showing a high titre does not distinguish between a recent or past infection. The detection of a raised specific IgM antibody by the indirect fluorescent antibody test can overcome this problem, and is also used for the early detection of *M. pneumoniae* infection.

The majority of cases of legionella pneumonia are diagnosed serologically by repeat indirect fluorescent antibody testing. Only about 10–15 per cent are identified in the acute phase of the illness by culture of the organism or by direct fluorescent antibody staining of organisms in lower respiratory secretions or lung biopsy material. About a third of cases will have detectable antibody levels (titres ≥ 16) on admission and this may be a pointer to the diagnosis in populations with a low background of seropositivity, such as in Britain.

Invasive techniques for investigating pneumonia

Two problems inhibit further advances in sputum diagnosis. Contamination of sputum by oropharyngeal organisms has already been mentioned. In addition about a quarter to a third of patients with pneumonia cannot produce sputum for testing. Various invasive techniques have therefore been developed to overcome these problems. They are usually reserved for patients with severe infection. Close liaison between the clinicians and the microbiologist is essential at this stage so the correct specimens are collected in the optimum manner, and transported rapidly to the laboratory where they are processed immediately.

Transtracheal aspiration This technique, first described by Pecora in 1963, is widely used in North America and Europe. A needle is inserted through the cricothyroid membrane and a sterile catheter is passed through it towards the carina. Uncontaminated lower respiratory secretions can then be aspirated. Small quantities of sterile saline are sometimes injected first to obtain a better sample. The technique is useful for diagnosing anaerobic infection. Although local neck emphysema and haemoptysis are not uncommon, significant side-effects such as large bleeds and mediastinal emphysema are rare. Occasional deaths are reported usually in patients with bleeding disorders. Often a saline injection with a small gauge needle and syringe through the cricothyroid membrane (without recourse to catheters etc.) will be enough to produce a deep cough specimen of respiratory secretions and this is a simple and safe technique.

Percutaneous lung aspiration This technique was first used in 1920 to follow the clearance of pneumococci from the lungs of patients with lobar pneumonia. More recently it has been used extensively to investigate pneumonia in children in whom sputum is often not available and tracheal aspiration is difficult. The small samples of 'lung juice' obtained can be examined by Gram stain, culture, direct fluorescent antibody staining (e.g. for *L. pneumophila*), and countercurrent immunoelectrophoresis for bacterial antigen. Pneumothorax can occur in up to 10 per cent but the need for drainage is unusual; significant haemoptysis is rare. The use of slim 25 gauge needles reduces any risk of complications and the technique can be performed at the bedside if necessary. It is contraindicated in patients having assisted ventilation.

Bronchoscopy Fibreoptic bronchoscopy will provide bronchial secretions, bronchoalveolar lavage fluid, and transbronchial biopsies from specified areas of the lung. Some contamination of equipment by passage through the nasopharynx is inevitable. Protected catheters partially overcome this problem. Bronchoscopy is rarely needed for patients with community-acquired pneumonia, except to exclude a bronchial obstruction, but is increasingly used for investigating pneumonia in the immunocompromised patient. A high diagnostic yield is reported from bronchoalveolar lavage and protected catheter brush specimens in patients with lung infections and AIDS. Local anaesthetics, such as lignocaine, are bacteriostatic and may impair the culture of pathogens from bronchoscopic specimens.

Open lung biopsy This is most effective biopsy method for diagnosing the cause of both infective and non-infective lung shadowing. A specific diagnosis can be made in over three-quarters of cases. It is rarely used for investigating community-acquired pneumonia but has an important part to play in the management of pneumonia in the immunocompromised host (see page 15.106).

Radiographic features

The initial radiographic pattern is not particularly helpful in differentiating types of community-acquired pneumonia. Homogeneous lobar or segmental shadows are commoner than patchy shadows in bacterial pneumonia, but they are also seen in over half the patients with atypical pneumonia. Multilobe involvement is common with severe infection. The lower lobes are most often affected in all types of pneumonia. Pleural effusions are seen in about a quarter of all cases and more will be revealed be lateral decubitus films. Although some degree of pulmonary collapse should raise the possiblity of an endobronchial obstruction (e.g. tumour, foreign body, mucus plug), it occurs in a quarter of otherwise uncomplicated cases of community-acquired pneumonia. Hilar lymphadenopathy is seen with mycoplasma pneumonia and occasionally in psittacosis. Lung cavitation is unusual except with staphylococcal and pneumococcal serotype 3 pneumonia or in immunosuppressed patients. An intense inflammatory and exudative response may produce a swollen lobe with a displaced interlobar fissure. This is said to be a feature of klebsiella pneumonia but is also seen with other severe infections.

The rate of radiographic resolution can be surprisingly slow, and lags considerably behind clinical recovery. It is related to the cause of the pneumonia, the age of the patient, and the presence of any underlying chronic lung disease (Fig. 1). Atypical pneumonias clear quickly. Radiographs return to normal by 2 months in the majority following mycoplasma pneumonia. At the other extreme, radiographs may not clear for several months after legionella and bacteraemic pneumococcal pneumonia.

Differential diagnosis

When there is a classic history of fever, malaise, sweats, cough, discoloured sputum, pleural pain, and dyspnoea, together with the clinical and radiographic signs of lung consolidation, a diagnosis of pneumonia is usually obvious. The commonest diagnostic confusion is with pulmonary infarction or atypical pulmonary oedema. A source of pulmonary emboli or evidence of valvular disease or cardiac failure should be sought by physical examination. On occasions the distinction is very difficult and treatment may have to be given for more than one condition until the true diagnosis becomes clearer. Less common conditions that enter the differential diagnosis include acute alveolitis, pulmonary eosinophilia, bronchoalveolar lung tumours, and more chronic lung conditions. Subdiaphragmatic conditions such as subphrenic or hepatic abscess or acute pancreatitis may present like lower lobe pneumonia often with an accompanying pleural effusion.

Secondary pneumonias acquired in the community

Some circumstances require careful consideration in the context of community-acquired pneumonias because of their influence on clinical presentation, likely pathogens, and antimicrobial therapy. These include the occurrence of pneumonia during an influenza epidemic, pneumonia in patients with pre-existing chronic bronchitis and chronic obstructive airways disease, and pneumonia at extremes of age.

Bacterial pneumonia with influenza

Since influenza virus A was first isolated in 1933, a link between viral and subsequent bacterial infection has been recognized. Secondary bacterial pneumonia with *S. pneumoniae*, *S. aureus* or

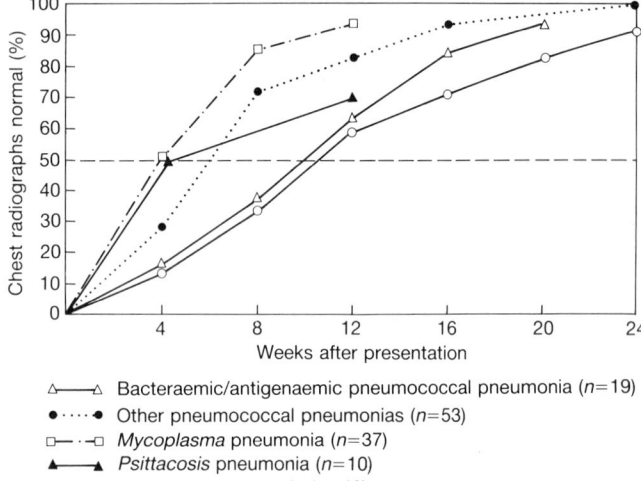

Fig. 1 Rate of radiographic clearance for different types of adult community-acquired pneumonia. (Adapted from Macfarlane *et al.*, 1984, *Thorax* **36**, 566–570, with permission of the editor of *Thorax*).

H. influenzae is now the most common pulmonary complication of influenza. Rarely the influenza virus itself causes pneumonia (see page 5.57).

The pattern of bacterial infection varies. Necropsy studies have shown that the principal bacterial pathogen during the 1918–19 influenza epidemic was *H. influenzae*, whereas during 1957 it was *S. aureus*, and in 1969–70, *S. pneumoniae*.

There are several reasons why viral infection may promote explosive bacterial superinfection. There is increased susceptibility of the respiratory tract to bacterial colonization which is most evident about a week after the onset of the viral infection. The ciliated epithelium of the bronchial tree is destroyed by virus invasion and therefore mucociliary clearance is reduced. There also appears to be suppression of the activity of the alveolar macrophages and reduction in lysozyme activity – other essential features of the lung defences.

Usually the patient experiences the typical symptoms of influenza, starts to improve, and then 3–10 days later suddenly deteriorates with rigors, chest pain, dyspnoea, and cough with discoloured or blood-stained sputum. In approximately a third of cases, the pulmonary symptoms blend with the influenza. Pregnant women and those with chronic cardiac or respiratory diseases are particularly at risk. Influenza virus and staphylococcal infections are often a lethal combination.

Complications vary with the nature of the bacterial organism (see infectious diseases section) but overall prognosis is not good. The mortality of postinfluenza bacterial pneumonia remains high at 20–25 per cent even in young previously well people.

Bacterial pneumonia in patients with pre-existing chronic obstructive lung disease

It is not easy without a chest radiograph to determine whether parenchymal lung infection is present in the chronic bronchitic or emphysematous patient suffering an acute infective exacerbation. Symptoms will resemble those described above for the acute bronchitic infection though the addition of pleuritic chest pain suggests pneumonia as does a generally rather sick patient.

Radiographic features are less likely to be a classic lobar consolidation than to reveal patchy segmental or subsegmental infiltrates scattered throughout the lung fields. An apical distribution will need to be distinguished from tuberculosis and a basal distribution may suggest aspiration which occasionally can be a predisposing factor. Peribronchial infiltrates are common. If there is much emphysematous bulla formation inflammatory changes in surrounding lung may form a halo around cystic areas and occasionally a cyst may partially fill with infected fluid.

Whilst *S. pneumoniae* and *H. influenzae* will still be important organisms in these pneumonic consolidations, consideration will also have to be given to the possible presence of aspirated anaerobic organisms and staphylococci.

Community-acquired pneumonia in childhood and old age

Whilst pneumococcal pneumonia is still the commonest pneumonia in infants and children, staphylococcal pneumonia is important in the first year of life (especially the first 3 months) and at all ages non-bacterial infections feature more importantly than in the adult. Pneumonia may occasionally be seen as a complication of the viral childhood exanthems such a varicella, measles, and rubella. *H. influenzae* B infection, a major cause of upper respiratory tract infection in infancy and early childhood, also occasionally gives segmental infiltrates or lobar consolidation.

In the elderly a much higher percentage of patients have non-pneumococcal bacterial pneumonia. Pathogens reported in geriatric patients hospitalized with community-acquired pneumonia have included Gram-negative bacilli in 6–37 per cent of cases, *H. influenzae* in up to 20 per cent, *S. aureus* in 2–10 per cent, and anaerobic infections in a proportion. The increased incidence of Gram-negative pneumonias is also seen in patients transferred from nursing homes. The occurrence of these pathogens in community-acquired bacterial pneumonias in the elderly cannot entirely be explained by previous antibiotic exposure and the suggestion is that ageing antibacterial defences allow this wider range of organisms access to the lungs and fail to prevent the development of pneumonias. Aspiration of oropharyngeal contents in debilitated patients also plays a part.

Management of community-acquired pneumonias

General measures

Patients with acute pneumonia should be in bed. Fever and pleuritic pain can often be relieved by regular aspirin or indomethacin. Adequate hydration is essential. For patients managed at home, the severity of the illness and the need for hospital admission should be assessed regularly (see prognostic factors on page 15.98). On occasions this will be influenced by psychological and social factors. Pneumonia developing in someone with influenza or chicken pox is particularly worrying. Patients with severe pneumonia should be admitted urgently to a hospital which has facilities for assisted ventilation. For patients ill enough to be in hospital, correction of hypoxia is very important. An arterial oxygen tension of 6.5 kPa or less or a rising arterial carbon dioxide is an indication of severe pneumonia and assisted ventilation may well be required for advancing respiratory failure. This can be life-saving and should be started early. Therefore patients with severe pneumonia are best managed on an intensive care unit or similar high dependency area where they can be carefully monitored. Although the outlook of patients with pneumococcal and staphylococcal pneumonia who require assisted ventilation is poor, those with Legionnaires' disease, atypical pneumonia, and varicella pneumonia have a recovery rate of over 50 per cent. Chest physiotherapy and postural drainage are rarely helpful in the acute stage and may exhaust a toxic and ill patient. When there is increased sputum production during recovery, physiotherapy can be useful. In patients with severe infection and in whom recovery is slow and prolonged, adequate enteral or parenteral nutrition is important.

Specific measures

Antibiotics

The cause of the pneumonia is not usually known when the patient is first seen and therefore lists of pathogens matched to ideal antibiotics are of little help. In practice, a 'best guess' antibiotic choice has to be made, depending on the type of patient, severity of infection, and any aetiological clues from the clinical picture.

Mild or moderate pneumonia In most patients with mild pneumonia the most likely infecting agent is the pneumococcus or, less commonly, the other few pathogens already described. The choice lies therefore between a penicillin and erythromycin. Although penicillin is highly effective against the pneumococcus, the poor absorption of oral penicillin V and the inconvenience of injections of penicillin G usually mean that a well-absorbed, broad-spectrum agent such as ampicillin or amoxycillin is chosen. Erythromycin is particularly appropriate during times of mycoplasma epidemics, although gastrointestinal intolerance can be a problem. Tetracycline though helpful for atypical organisms is often no longer effective for the pneumococcus.

In those with pre-existing chronic lung disease an antibiotic which is also effective against *H. influenzae* is required. Ampicillin and amoxycillin will fit the bill. Co-trimoxazole and chloramphenicol are other alternatives. Oral cephalosporins are rarely of much value.

Severe pneumonia The physician needs to be on the alert for any signs of deterioration (see prognostic factors below). Severe pneumonia, even in previously fit people, can evolve rapidly and the mortality remains high in spite of apparently effective antibiotics. Antibiotics should be given as soon as samples have been taken for culture. By far the commonest cause of the community-acquired pneumonia is still pneumococcal infection and any anti-biotic choice must provide effective cover against it. Penicillin-resistant pneumococci are a significant problem in only a few countries so far. Other possible causes of severe community-acquired pneumonia include the atypical infections, *H. influenzae* (especially in those with chronic lung disease) and *Legionella pneumophila*. High doses of intravenous penicillin (1–2 megaunits 6-hourly) and erythromycin (as erythromycin lactobionate 600–1000 mg 6-hourly) together provide good initial cover for all these pathogens. Ampicillin (500–1000 mg 6-hourly) should replace penicillin for patients with a history of chronic lung disease such as chronic bronchitis when an haemophilus infection may be more likely. The incidence of ampicillin-resistant haemophilus species in Britain is about 14 per cent. In areas of the world where the resistance rate is higher, a cephalosporin could be used instead. Patients allergic to penicillins can be given erythromycin alone in high doses or combined with a cephalosporin. Phlebitis at the cannula site with intravenous erythromycin can be reduced by a slow dilute infusion. During a period of influenza, or where there is a chance of secondary staphylococcal pneumonia, fluclox-acillin should be used as well. The antibiotics are adjusted appro-priately as soon as investigations identify a specific pathogen.

Duration of antibiotic therapy

Patients with uncomplicated pneumonia are usually treated with antibiotics for 7–10 days. This may be unnecessarily long in some cases. Studies in Africa have shown equally good results when treating pneumonia for 1, 3, and 7 days. The duration of therapy for those with more severe pneumonia is judged on clinical response. In the presence of lung cavitation, treatment may be needed for 3 or 4 weeks.

Failure to improve

The majority of patients will improve quickly within a few days after starting treatment. If recovery is unsatisfactory the causes shown in Table 4 should be considered.

Intrathoracic complications

Pleural effusions are the commonest intrathoracic complication and a sample should be aspirated to exclude an empyema. Usually

Table 4 Factors to consider when a patient with pneumonia is responding poorly to initial therapy

Factors	Action
Improvement expected too soon	Continue – review again (improvement slow in elderly and debilitated)
Diagnosis of pneumonia wrong (?pulmonary infarction/oedema)	Review history, examination, and data
Organism resistant to antibiotic/ unexpected organism involved	Review history. ?travel abroad. ?avian contact
	Review microbiological data
	Consider alternative or invasive investigations
Complicating pulmonary disease (e.g. bronchial obstruction, bronchiectasis)	Review chest radiograph; consider bronchoscopy
Local intrathoracic complications (e.g. empyema, lung abscess)	Repeat chest radiograph Aspirate any pleural fluid
Secondary complications (e.g. deep venous thrombosis, intravenous cannula infection)	Detailed clinical examination
Metastatic infective complication (e.g. arthritis, endocarditis, meningitis)	Detailed clinical examination
General factors (e.g. dehydration, hypoxia)	Treat appropriately
Allergic reaction to antibiotic (usually after several days therapy)	Take allergic history; look for rash; consider stopping/changing antibiotic

these effusions are clear, straw-coloured, sympathetic exudates with a high protein content and sparse neutrophils, and are sterile. The fluid can be tested for bacterial antigen. Empyemas occur in up to 5 per cent of pneumonias, although the incidence is higher with some patients such as *S. aureus* and streptococci or if post-mortem findings are included (see page 15.104).

Following a severe pneumonia, some degree of pulmonary fibrosis may occur with a resulting restrictive lung defect. Persist-ent intrapulmonary streaky opacities may be seen on the chest radiograph. Abnormalities in lung function and tracheobronchial clearance have been reported many months after apparent recov-ery from mycoplasma pneumonia.

Prognostic factors

Prognosis is related to the pathogen, the host and the interplay between the two. A positive blood culture is a bad prognostic sign in bacterial pneumonias, the mortality of bacteraemic pneumococ-cal pneumonia being 25–33 per cent compared to 5 per cent for non-bacteraemic cases. Pulmonary infections with *S. aureus*, *H. influenzae* or Gram-negative bacilli carry a poor prognosis. On the other hand patients with atypical pneumonia generally do well. The mortality of community-acquired legionella pneumonia is 5–15 per cent.

Mortality and morbidity rise with increasing age of the patient and the presence of co-existing chronic illness (such as cardiac or respiratory disease or diabetes). Other factors indicative of a poor prognosis for bacterial pneumonias include confusion and delir-ium, tachypnoea (of 30 breaths per minute or more), hypotension (diastolic pressure of 60 mm Hg or less), new cardiac arrhythmias, a low total white cell count (5.0/dl or less), abnormal renal func-tion (blood urea of 7 mmol/litre or more), hypoalbuminaemia (less than 25 g/litre) and severe hypoxia (PaO_2 less than 8 kPa breathing air). Multilobe involvement on the initial chest radio-graph and subsequent spread of the shadows in spite of treatment are worrying features.

Nosocomial pneumonia

Introduction

This is a new episode of pneumonia developing more than 48 hours after a patient has entered hospital for whatever reason. The infection is usually identified by the development of fever, purulent respiratory secretions, elevated white cell count, and a new pulmonary infiltrate on the chest radiograph. Nosocomial respiratory infections have been estimated to occur in 0.5–5 per cent of hospitalized patients and to rank third behind urinary infections and wound infections in the frequency of hospital-acquired infections.

Pathogenesis

The infection usually arrives from aspiration of nasopharyngeal contents, inhalation of bacteria from contaminated equipment or rarely by haematogenous spread.

Some aspiration of nasopharyngeal secretions is common even in healthy people, particularly during sleep. The normal lung copes easily with this, both because the bacteria are relatively non-pathogenic and because the local pulmonary defences are working normally. However, colonization of the nasopharynx with Gram-negative bacilli occurs in 30–40 per cent in hospitalized patients. The frequency can be even higher in patients receiving broad-spectrum antibiotics or those who are seriously ill. These bacilli arise by the direct contamination of the nasopharynx from the hos-pital environment.

Patients who are ill, bed-bound, have impaired consciousness from their illness or from drugs, or who have neurological disease will be more likely to aspirate such pathogens. Reduced ability to clear bronchial secretions after a general anaesthetic and impaired coughing after thoracic or abdominal surgery are further risk factors and occasionally impaired general antimicrobial defences contribute to the development of these infections.

The risk of postoperative pneumonia is associated with increasing age, smoking habit, obesity, the presence of chronic illness, long preoperative stay, prolonged anaesthesia, and thoracic and upper abdominal operations.

Inhalation of bacteria from contaminated respiratory equipment such as ventilators, nebulizers, intubation equipment, humidifiers, and nasogastric tubes is a particular problem in respiratory and intensive care use. Spread of pathogens via the hands of the personnel must be remembered. The presence of malignancy and the prior use of antibiotics, steroids or cytotoxic drugs increase the risk of nosocomial pneumonia.

Pneumonia caused by haematogenous spread of infection from a distant site is uncommon but may arise after intra-abdominal infection or as a result of infected pulmonary emboli. Intravenous cannulae left *in situ* for long periods are a potential source of blood stream infection.

Pathogens implicated

The spectrum of pathogens encountered in nosocomial pneumonia is much wider and more varied than that for community-acquired pneumonia. Gram-negative bacilli comprise about half of all isolates and Gram-positive bacteria, of which *S. aureus* is the commonest, less than a quarter. Specific circumstances may make one particular infection more likely. Respiratory equipment and aerosol units harbour pseudomonas, and klebsiella; the presence of bowel or urinary tract infection favours *E. coli* and proteus-type organisms; *Serratia marcescens* can survive in certain disinfectant fluids; and any situation which encourages aspiration from the oropharynx can produce a pneumonia due to klebsiella, pseudomonas or a whole range of anaerobes including Gram-negative bacilli of bacteroides and fusobacterium species, Gram-positive cocci, and various Gram-positive clostridial species. The potential list of pathogens causing nosocomial pneumonia in the immuno-compromised host is even more varied (see page 15.107). Outbreaks of nosocomial legionella infection have been caused by colonization of hospital heating and water systems. Mists generated by contaminated cooling towers and ward showers have also been implicated. Debilitated and immunosuppressed patients are most at risk.

Diagnosis

The diagnosis of a pneumonia is not usually difficult providing the patient is carefully examined. Sometimes the diagnosis will only be suspected after a chest radiograph is performed in a patient who has deteriorated for no obvious cause.

Identifying the pathogen is more difficult. Colonization of the oropharynx by a variety of hospital-acquired pathogens means that sputum examination is generally unhelpful. If blood, sputum or pleural fluid cultures are negative, invasive techniques may be required to obtain lower respiratory secretions (see above). Serological tests for legionella infection should be considered.

Treatment

Because of the variety of potential pathogens, it is advisable to use wide spectrum or combination antibiotics as initial therapy, pending the results of tests. These may include a wide spectrum third generation cephalosoprin such as cefotaxime with or without an aminoglycoside such as gentamicin. If there is a high probability of pseudomonas infection an appropriate penicillin derivative such as azlocillin or ticarcillin may be used instead of a cephalosporin. For suspected anaerobic infection, penicillin, metronidazole or clindamycin will have advantages. Physiotherapy aids the clearance of infected secretions and used postoperatively may help to prevent nosocomial pneumonia. In spite of therapy, the mortality is high ranging from 25 to 50 per cent and in survivors there is a considerable prolongation of hospital stay.

Prevention

The frequency of nosocomial respiratory infection may be reduced by such measures as prevention of smoking pre-operatively, early postoperative mobilization, hospital staff hygiene, scrupulous care of respiratory equipment, and infection control in high risk areas such as intensive care units.

Recurrent pneumonia

In patients with a history of three or more episodes of pneumonia, several possibilities need to be considered.

Localized respiratory disease

Recurrent pneumonia in the same part of the lung raises the possibility of a bronchial or pulmonary abnormality. Localized bronchiectasis or bronchial obstruction are the commonest reasons. Obstruction may be intraluminal (e.g. foreign body), intramural (e.g. bronchial stenosis, adenoma or carcinoma) or due to compression from outside (e.g. by lymph-nodes). Intrapulmonary sequestration may present as recurrent basal pneumonia. This is a development abnormality where a portion of the lung has an arterial supply from the systemic circulation and little or no normal bronchial architecture. The disorder may be discovered by chance on a radiograph or because of recurrent infection in early adult life.

Generalized respiratory disease

When pneumonia recurs in different sites, a more generalized disorder is likely. The commonest is chronic obstructive lung disease, perhaps with some bronchiectasis. Rarely the problem is one of impaired pulmonary defences as in the immotile cilia syndrome. Chronic sinusitis can lead to recurrent lower respiratory infections due to aspiration of infected material.

Non-respiratory problem

Aspiration of pharyngeal or oesophageal contents may be caused by neuromuscular conditions such as muscular dystrophy, motor neurone disease, multiple sclerosis, strokes or disorders of oesophageal motility in achalasia and scleroderma. Rarely pharyngeal diverticulae, tracheo-oesophageal fistula or gastro-oesophageal reflux can be implicated.

Alcoholics, drug abusers, and epileptics are liable to recurrent pneumonia during episodes of depressed consciousness.

Immune deficiency states are an uncommon cause of recurrent pneumonia but their recognition is important because of the availability of replacement therapy in antibody-deficient syndromes.

Prevention of pneumonia

Better housing and working conditions and better health of the community have contributed greatly to the reduced incidence of community-acquired pneumonia.

Vaccination has been helpful in specific instances and may have a greater role to play. Postmeasles pneumonia, a common occurrence in children in developing countries, can be reduced by a measles vaccination campaign and pertussis immunization reduces the frequency of respiratory complications of whooping cough. Pneumococcal vaccination has been shown to be effective in reducing serious pneumococcal pneumonia. It can be considered in patients who are particularly liable to severe pneumococcal infection, such as those with chronic respiratory and cardiac disease, sickle cell disease, and in those due to have a planned splenectomy. Influenza vaccination in the autumn gives some protection to patients who are debilitated and in whom an attack of influenza or its complications could be serious.

References

British Thoracic Society Research Committee (1985). Multicentre study of community acquired pneumonia. *Thorax* **40**, 693–694.

Fekety, F.R., Caldwell, J., Gump, D., Johnson, J. E., Maxson, W., Mulholland, J. and Thoburn, R. (1971). Bacteria, viruses and mycoplasmas in acute pneumonia in adults. *Am. Rev. Resp. Dis.* **104**, 499–507.

Gump, D. W., Phillips, C. A., Forsyth, B. R., McIntosh, K., Lamborn, K. R. and Stouch, W. H. (1976). Role of infection in chronic bronchitis. *Am. Rev. Resp. Dis.* **113**, 465–474.

Knight, V. (1973). *Viral and mycoplasmal infections of the respiratory tract.* Lea and Febiger, Philadelphia.

Levison, M. E. (1984). *The pneumonias. Clinical approaches to infectious diseases of the lower respiratory tract.* John Wright, PSG Inc., Boston.

Macfarlane, J. T., Finch, R. G., Ward, M. J. and Macrae, A. D. (1982). Hospital study of adult community acquired pneumonia. *Lancet* **ii**, 255–258.

Macfarlane, J. T., Miller, A. C., Smith, W. H. R., Morris, A. H. and Rose, D. H. (1984). Comparative radiographic features of community acquired Legionnaires' disease, pneumococcal pneumonia, mycoplasma pneumonia and psittacosis. *Thorax* **39**, 28–33.

McNabb, W. R., Shanson, D. C., Williams, T. D. M. and Lant, A. F. (1984). Adult community acquired pneumonia in central London. *J. R. Soc. Med.* **77**, 550–555.

Putnam, J. S. and Tuazon, C. (1980). Symposium on infectious lung diseases. *Med. Clin. N. Am.* **64**, 317–576.

Reynolds, H. Y. (1981). Respiratory infections. *Clin. Chest Med.* **2**, 1–168.

Verghese, A. and Berk, S. L. (1983). Bacterial pneumonia in the elderly. *Medicine* **62**, 271–285.

White, R. J., Blainey, A. D., Harrison, K. J. and Clarke, S. K. R. (1981). Causes of pneumonia presenting to a district general hospital. *Thorax* **36**, 566–570.

The suppurative lung diseases

J. M. HOPKIN

Bronchiectasis lung abscess, and empyema are not diseases of the past in developed countries and are an important source of morbidity and mortality in the Third World. Late or missed diagnosis and undertreatment are common.

Bronchiectasis

Bronchiectasis, defined as permanent and abnormal dilation of the bronchi and generally accompanied by suppurative inflammation, is the end result of a diverse group of pathologies (Table 1) Bronchial health and defence rests dominantly on the normal action of the mucociliary escalator, though other elements including immunoglobulin function, clearly make important contributions. Mucociliary clearance may be impaired by local obstruction, ciliary abnormality or excessive or unusual mucus production, all of which will predispose to secondary infection. Infection itself, producing inflammatory change and excess mucus, may lead to obstruction especially in childhood when bronchial calibre is small.

Bronchiectasis develops from the combined destructive action of bronchial obstruction and bronchial infection with inflam-

Table 1 Underlying cause of bronchiectasis

(*a*) Postpneumonic
  Measles, pertussis, tuberculosis, other pneumonias
(*b*) Mechanical bronchial obstruction
  Foreign body, carcinoma, nodal compression
(*c*) Immunologic disease
  Allergic bronchopulmonary aspergillosis
(*d*) Gamma globulin deficiencies
  Congenital and acquired
(*e*) The immotile cilia syndrome
(*f*) Cystic fibrosis
(*g*) Neuropathic disorders
  The Riley–Day syndrome, Chagas' disease
(*h*) Idiopathic

mation, when these are protracted. In general, it is the medium-sized bronchi (generations 4–9) that are involved and the distribution clearly depends upon the underlying disorders. The resulting bronchiectasis may take a cylindrical, saccular or cystic form, and different morphologies can occur in the same patient. Bronchiectatic saccules have thin fibrotic walls with loss of cartilage and may frequently be blind ending. There is inflammatory change with extensive submucosal lymphocyte and plasma cell infiltration, which can be exuberant enough at focal points to produce pseudopolyps. The pseudostratified columnar epithelium is hypertrophied with focal areas of squamous metaplasia. One notable feature is the presence of dilated thin-walled blood vessels in the submucosa which are often the site of bronchopulmonary anastomoses. The surrounding lung will show varying degrees of fibrosis and inflammatory change.

The classic circumstance for the development of *postinfective bronchiectasis* has been severe respiratory infection in childhood in the prevaccination and preantibiotic era, particularly with measles and pertussis. Secondary infection leads to blockage of bronchi with secretions and debris with consequent collapse especially in the lower lobes. Weakening of the bronchial wall by inflammatory change, distention by secretions, and retraction by transmitted negative intrapleural pressure via the collapsed lung, all contribute to permanent dilation and damage of the bronchus.

Bronchiectasis results from *tuberculous infection* following extensive upper lobe postprimary disease or by compression of the long middle lobe bronchus on the right by hilar lymphadenopathy associated with primary disease.

Other *obstructive causes* include foreign bodies, bronchial neoplasms, and allergic bronchopulmonary aspergillosis where, on a background of asthma, protracted plugging of a bronchus associated with intense immunological inflammation results in secondary collapse and infection.

Various *hypogammaglobulinaemic* states have been associated with the development of chronic bronchial sepsis with or without morphological bronchiectasis and these include X-linked hypogammaglobulinaemia, late onset primary hypogammaglobulinaemia, hypogammaglobulinaemia associated with thymoma, hypogammaglobulinaemia resulting from lymphoproliferative disease (especially chronic lymphatic leukaemia), IgA deficiency, and selective IgG deficiencies (especially IgG2). Selective IgA deficiency generally involves both circulating and secretory levels, the former being the stronger predictor of risk of infection which may take the form of repeated acute infections or of chronic bronchial sepsis. There is also evidence that functional deficiencies may produce the same result and here normal circulating gammaglobulin levels are accompanied by an inability to mount measured responses to tetanus toxoid or polyvalent pneumococcal vaccines. Recognition of these hypogammaglobulinanaemic syndromes (with the exception of IgA deficiency) is important because bronchial sepsis may be greatly helped by replacement therapy.

Abnormal ciliary action can certainly result in chronic bronchial sepsis and bronchiectasis. *Kartagener* first described his *syndrome* of situs inversus, chronic sinusitis, bronchiectasis, and infertility 40 years ago. In the 1970s it was shown that both the respiratory cilia and the sperm from such patients are abnormal. The tail of the sperm and the cilia share a common ciliary motor or axoneme consisting of 9 microtubular doublets encircling two central microtubules (Fig. 1). The outer doublets have two rows of short trajections, the dynein arms and a radial spoke each A variety of structural abnormalities, seen on electromicroscopy, including the absence of one or both rows of the dynein arms, spoke or spokeheads are associated with little or no ciliary movement or measured tracheobronchial mucociliary clearance. These heterogeneous abnormalities give a clinical disorder with an incidence of approximately 1 in 20 000, where inheritance seems to be autosomal recessive and where it is assumed that one or another axonemal protein is absent. The syndromes result in bronchiectasis, sinusitis, and frequently salpingitis and otitis media. Situs inversus

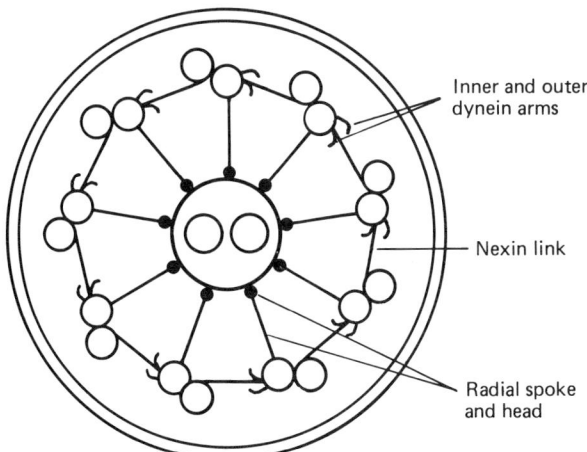

Inner and outer
dynein arms

Nexin link

Radial spoke
and head

Fig. 1 Schematic cross-section of the mid portion of a cilium showing nine outer pairs and one central pair of microtubules and their connections. (Reproduced by courtesy of Dr B. A. Afzelius.)

seen in approximately half the patients with the immotile cilia syndrome and associated with the orginal Kartagener's syndrome, is thought to result from impaired organ rotation following ciliary abnormality. The shared abnormality in the sperm leads to infertility.

Cystic fibrosis is becoming increasingly prevalent as a cause of chronic bronchiectasis since the advent of antibiotics has prolonged the lives of those with the disorder. It is the commonest lethal autosomal recessive disorder in Britain with an incidence of 1 in 2000 births with a carrier frequency of 1 in 22. The disorder is characterized by affection of exocrine glandular function and a high sweat sodium concentration. In those that survive the childhood complications of meconium ileus and intussusception, the disease is increasingly dominated by its respiratory manifestations. Significant pancreatic disease with malabsorption remains in 85 per cent or more although this seems to wane with time. The meconium ileus equivalent with small intestinal obstruction in older children and adults can be fatal. Other manifestations are liver and biliary problems and secondary endocrine failure giving diabetes mellitus. Despite a welter of research, the basic abnormality is as yet unidentified. It seems likely that disturbance of exocrine function in the lungs and pancreas follows difficulties in the clearance of increased amounts of mucus of low water content (but normal viscosity). It is possible that recent observations on defective chloride ion transport in the sweat glands and bronchial epithelium of individuals with cystic fibrosis may be important and relevant to the water content of secretions. The most exciting development has been the localization of the cystic fibrosis gene locus to the mid portion of the long arm of chromosome 7 by the use of restriction fragment length polymorphisms in genetic linkage studies. This should lead fairly quickly to the identification of very closely linked polymorphic markers that could be successfully used in antenatal diagnosis and lead in the longer term, by increasingly sophisticated gene walking techniques, to the identification of the cystic fibrosis gene itself and its protein product.

In the *Riley–Day syndrome* (a rare autosomal recessive condition found in Jewish people) and Chagas' disease, it appears that autonomic disturbance leads to major hypersecretion of mucus and secondary bronchial obstruction and suppuration.

In some individuals, no underlying cause is apparent but there is some evidence that one subgroup comprises individuals with hypergammaglobulinaemia, positive autoantibodies and co-existing inflammatory disease in other tissues such as thyroiditis, ulcerative colitis, and rheumatoid disease.

Clinical manifestations and diagnosis

The clinical features of bronchiectasis will vary with the cause and extent of the disease. Some postinfective cases with only small seg-

ments of disease may be entirely asymptomatic or develop purulent sputum only after coryzal illnesses. Posttuberculous upper lobe disease may be similarly asymptomatic, perhaps because of natural gravitational drainage of secretions. Either may declare itself with haemoptysis, which is a frequent complication of all forms of bronchiectasis.

At the other end of the spectrum of clinical severity, individuals with extensive postinfective bronchiectasis present a classical clinical picture with moderate to large amounts (500 ml/24 hour) of deeply purulent sputum on a daily basis over a number of years, punctuated by episodes of self-limiting haemoptyses or by 'exacerbations' which may be accompanied by pleuritic pain. Recurring pleurisy at one site over a number of years is particularly characteristic of bronchiectasis. Extensive disease, completely untreated, results in disabling and progressive ventilatory disturbance leading to cor pulmonale accompanied potentially by other complications such as lung abscess, empyema, brain abscess, and amyloid. Curiously, some individuals with fairly extensive chronic disease seem unaware of any disturbance, presumably swallow a good deal of sputum, and present late with some worsening of symptoms, or some complication, particularly haemoptysis. However, in most forms of bronchiectasis symptoms can be traced to childhood.

In *cystic fibrosis*, the disease is extensive, progressive, and severe, although there is accruing evidence of milder forms presenting in middle adult life and these may represent true genetic variants. In the *immotile cilia syndrome*, whilst disease and symptoms are very significant, reasonable longevity may be expected with adequate medical care.

In the great majority of patients with extensive bronchiectasis, sinusitis and nasal disease are present, producing purulent discharge and occasionally leading to nasal polyposis. This may simply result from a shared defect in mucociliary clearance within the nose or from extension of infection from the lungs. Again in patients with extensive disease, significant airflow obstruction may be present and there is good evidence that a reversible component susceptible to simple bronchodilators, can occur. This reversible airflow obstruction, however, does not seem necessarily related to the high incidence of skin test reactivity to common allergens found in individuals with bronchiectasis especially those with cystic fibrosis. This seems to be a secondary phenomenon for these individuals rarely suffer from asthma, hay fever or eczema.

Physical signs may be absent in mild cases but in extensive disease the characteristic findings are of fixed coarse crepitations over the affected segment, variable finger clubbing, halitosis, and signs of generalized airflow obstruction with hyperinflation and prolonged expiration with wheezes. An occasional patient's 'white or cream' sputum can be floridly purulent on direct inspection and this simple action is therefore important. Halitosis and offensive fetid sputum implies anaerobic infection, but this is now more rare since courses of many simple antibiotics will tend to clear such organisms.

There is increasing evidence, particularly when special culture media are used, that *Haemophilus influenzae* is the most important organism in sustaining continued infection and inflammation. In cystic fibrosis, *Staphylococcus aureus* is important in childhood but eventually in this disease, persistent infection with *Pseudomonas aeruginosa* is almost universal. The plain chest radiograph is abnormal in the great majority of cases; although the quoted figures of greater than 90 per cent abnormality depend on retrospective viewing of films once the diagnosis is established. The abnormalities include increased markings, patchy consolidation, collapse with a crowding of markings (which may be difficult to visualize in the left lower lobe behind the heart), and direct evidence of dilated bronchi in the form of tubular, finger or ring shadows of circular hair lines of 1–2 cm in diameter which may have fluid levels (Fig. 2). In cystic fibrosis, the changes are dominantly in the mid and upper zones with nodules and streaks in addition to hyperinflation. The formal demonstration of bron-

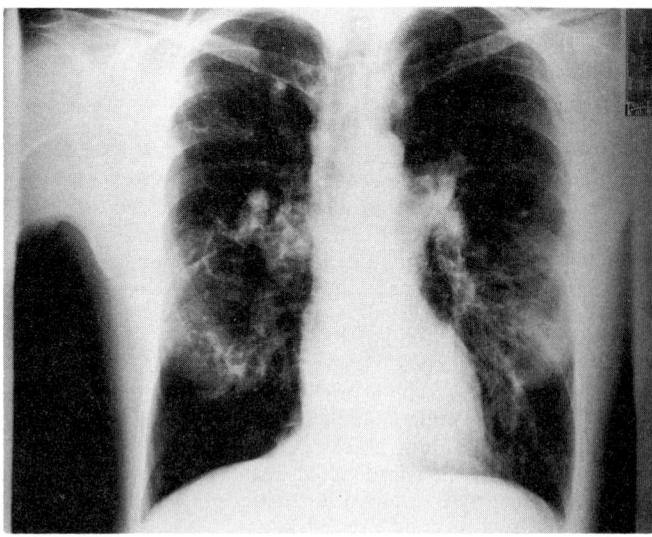

Fig. 2 Chest radiograph of a 40-year-old man with postinfective cystic bronchiectasis showing typical ring shadows.

chiectasis in life depends upon bronchography, when the features are dilated bronchi, abruptly blind ending bronchi, and bronchial filling defects due to excessive secretion. Bronchograms do however carry some morbidity, should be performed after postural drainage and perhaps a course of antibiotics, and require anaesthesia in children.

In many patients bronchograms are not required as the clinical diagnosis – often with support from the plain chest radiograph – is beyond reasonable doubt. If however surgery is contemplated for local disease, then bronchography is crucial to assess the distribution of disease accurately. Recently bronchography has been performed using aqueous propyliodone as a contrast medium via the fibreoptic bronchoscope. This allows for direct inspection to exclude local obstruction, for siting a source of bleeding, and the performance of less traumatic regional bronchography.

Once a diagnosis is established, then an attempt to assess the underlying cause is important in determining further management.

Local disease, suggested on physical examination or chest radiograph, implies that the underlying process has been childhood pneumonia, or obstruction. *Allergic bronchopulmonary aspergillosis* will be supported by a preceding history of asthma, the demonstration of positive prick tests and the presence of precipitins to *Aspergillus fumigatus*. Measurement of *immunoglobulins* and their subsets is relatively simple. *Kartagener's syndrome* will be suggested by situs inversus and the absence of frontal sinuses. A simple nasal saccharin test with measurement of the time taken to taste provides a sensitive, but non-specific test for mucociliary clearance. Although sepsis can result in some secondary depression of ciliary activity, tissue obtained from brush nasal biopsy viewed on light microscopy shows absent ciliary activity in the *immotile cilia syndrome* and electron micrography shows consistent structural ciliary defects. *Cystic fibrosis* may be suggested by other exocrine glandular abnormalities, but especially pancreatic disease. The measurement of sweat sodium by the pilocarpine iontophoresis method should be diagnostic (including in adults when two sweat sodium results of greater than 90 mmol/l or two values between 70 and 90 not suppressable by 9-fludrocortisone are obtained).

Management

Management aims are the control of symptoms and, if possible, disease progress by medical means, the encouragement of the patient to sustain as normal and active a life as possible, and the occasional cure by surgery.

Many patients with mild disease require no more than courses of an antibiotic during spells of active bronchial infection. For more significant disease where larger volumes of infected sputum are constantly present, some aid beyond coughing may be required to clear secretions from dependent bronchi. Postural drainage, positioning the affected segment(s) uppermost, performed on rising and before retiring is particularly helpful aided by gentle percussion of the chest and by forced expiratory manoeuvres. Many patients are happy to continue with this regimen although others may find it tedious enough to use it only at the time of colds or exacerbations when it may be required frequently through the day. In many patients, bronchodilators such as inhaled salbutamol will help airflow obstruction. General advice on avoiding smoking and taking exercise is important, as is reassurance about the generally self-limiting nature of recurrent haemoptysis.

The role of antibiotics is not clearly resolved. There is little doubt that they help during spells of increased sputum volume and purulence with or without haemoptysis but the value of long-term suppressive treatment is uncertain. A British Medical Research Council placebo-controlled study in the 1950s showed that tetracycline 500 mg q.d.s. on 2 days a week over a year significantly reduced the volume and purulence of sputum and the number of days in bed and lost from work. The benefits were however not dramatic and the authors recommended this treatment only for the very severely affected. More recently, it has been shown that the achievement of high antibiotic levels in sputum by an oral regimen of amoxycillin 3 g b.d. can have major effects on sputum purulence in a significant proportion of patients. This has raised the unanswered question whether such treatment used long-term would favourably influence the progression of the disease without hazard.

Currently, many physicians restrict antibiotics to 7–14 day courses for episodes of worsening of symptoms often following coryzal illnesses. Ideally, such treatment should be based on the result of sputum culture, using special media. In fact, *Haemophilus influenzae* seems to be the most important organism and, in practice, courses of antibiotics such as ampicillin, amoxycillin, tetracycline or co-trimoxazole are used successfully without recourse to culture on each occasion.

Surgical treatment may be highly successful in the few patients with significant symptoms not responding to medical treatment in whom disease is bronchographically demonstrated to be localized. It seems that young patients in particular may expect a good outcome. Surgery may be contemplated in more extensive disease when there is direct bronchoscopic evidence of repeated troublesome bleeding from one site but as with any other form of pulmonary resection a critical assessment of overall lung function is crucial.

In *hypogammaglobulinaemia* replacement therapy prepared from pooled plasma may have an important protective role. In *allergic bronchopulmonary aspergillosis* vigorous treatment of episodes of local plugging with oral steroids should prevent the development of bronchiectasis and modern antifungal therapy may offer some further hope in future.

Cystic fibrosis presents special problems in management and such patients may require collaborative or special unit care. Bronchopulmonary infection with staphylococci will specifically require the addition of an antibiotic such as cloxacillin. Persistent infection with pseudomonas poses special difficulties but evidence is available that for patients in steady decline requiring repeated admissions, then vigorous intravenous therapy with a suitable penicillin (e.g. piperacillin) or cephalosporin (e.g. ceftazidime) combined with an aminoglycoside may be successfully followed by medium- to long-term daily inhaled treatment with carbenicillin and gentamicin. In a proportion of patients this has led to marked recovery of pulmonary function and well-being. The development of orally active antipseudomonal drugs such as ciprofloxacin may also prove to be useful in this respect. Pancreatic malabsorption and meconium ileus require appropriate management (see page 12.143). Families will require expert genetic counselling. The risk of a further sib being affected is of course 1 in 4. In individuals with cystic fibrosis, only the females are fertile and all their children will be carriers: the risk of producing an affected infant is 1 in 44 [half times the chance of the spouse being coincidentally a carrier (1/22)]. The detection of low levels of intestinal alkaline phosphatase in amniotic fluid, a phenomenon secondary to meconium ileus in the fetus, has offered one method of attempting antenatal diagnosis. When performed in special centres and for high risk (1 in 4) pregnancies the sensitivity seems to be 90 per cent with a false-positive rate of 6 per cent.

Prevention

Prevention of postpneumonic disease depends on good nutrition, successful immunization against measles, pertussis, and tuberculosis, and vigorous treatment of lower respiratory tract infection in childhood. Increasingly accurate gene analysis should lead fairly shortly to accurate antenatal diagnosis in cystic fibrosis.

Lung abscess

The term lung abscess is applied to infections resulting in suppurative inflammation with necrosis of lung seen typically as a cavitating, usually rounded pneumonic opacity on the chest radiograph. The underlying causes of such a lesion are listed in Table 2.

The commonest cause for the development of lung abscess is *aspiration* of debris or fluid, with bacterial contamination. Oropharyngeal secretions may contain up to 10^8 anaerobes/ml even in health with higher concentrations being present in the presence of oropharyngeal sepsis. Most normal individuals aspirate to some small extent during sleep but this is cleared by the mucociliary escalator and perhaps coughing. These defences can be particularly overwhelmed during spells of impaired consciousness, for example, after general anaesthesia, in alcoholism, and drug overdosage, in epilepsy, or following a cerebrovascular accident. It is notable that the incidence of lung abscess has significantly diminished following increased standards of anaesthesia and postoperative care. Other risk factors for the development of lung abscess are excessive volumes of aspirate as may occur in oesophageal disease or heavily infected aspirate as in oropharyngeal sepsis or periodontal disease. The dominant organisms are anaerobes, including fusiforms, bacteroides species, and anaerobic cocci. In hospital, colonization of the mouth and upper airways by Gram-negative bacteria and staphylococci may make these organisms important.

Aspiration of infected material results in a severe purulent reaction in the alveoli with necrosis of lung which may be exacerbated by partial obstruction of the bronchus by debris. Progression across interlobar fissures and into the pleural space to produce a secondary empyema are both possible. The cavity of the abscess is composed of debris, pus cells, and organisms with a wall of granulation tissue with fibrosis. Nearby pulmonary arteries may show marked intimal fibrosis. Aspiration lung abscesses occur at typical sites influenced by gravity and bronchial geometry. Most form in the right lung which continues in a more direct line from the trachea than the left. Aspiration in the supine position leads to disease in the apical segment of the lower lobe or posterior segment of the upper lobe, in the lateral position to disease in the axillary subsegments of the posterior and anterior segments of the upper lobe and in the upright position, as in dental manipulation, to disease in the right lower lobe.

Bronchial obstruction leading to infection of retained sputum with no means of escape is an increasingly common cause of lung abscess in Britain, bronchial carcinoma being the chief cause of the obstruction. Foreign body is an important cause in childhood. More rarely one or more lung abscesses may result form *vascular embolization of infected material* to the lung as in septicaemias of diverse origin, in right-sided endocarditis, infected intravenous cannulae, and 'mainline' drug abuse. Extension of a *subphrenic abscess or hepatic amoebic abscess* may lead to a secondary abscess formation in the right lower lobe. Some organisms can produce necrosis of the lung as a complication of severe pneumonia without significant aspiration or obstruction. *Staphylococcus aureus* and *Klebsiella pneumoniae* are particularly liable to do this, although pneumococcus type 3 may rarely do so.

Clinical features

The illness generally begins as a pneumonitis with associated shivers, fever, cough, and pleuritic chest pain. At some stage, not usually earlier than a week, the abscess discharges into a bronchus resulting in cough producing large amounts of blood stained frankly purulent sputum. Other than the general constitutional signs of an infective process, there may be no decisive physical signs beyond a local area of crepitations, progressing rarely at that site to the so-called 'amphoric' breathing, and the development of finger clubbing. Empyema ensues in up to 20–30 per cent in some series.

A more chronic course is well recognized where less severe symptoms progress over weeks or months, a course which may be punctuated with brief improvements following courses of antibiotics, when the diagnosis has not been suspected.

When one or more lung abscesses are secondary to a bacteraemic or septicaemic illness, the clinical picture may be dominated by the features of the latter.

Diagnosis

Lung abscess should be considered in the differential diagnosis of any severe acute or chronic and relapsing respiratory infection, particularly when there has been a lapse of consciousness, or when oesophageal disease or oropharyngeal sepsis are present. Chest radiographs taken early after an aspirational event may show non-cavitating pneumonitis but the microbiological implications are the same, suggesting primarily anaerobic infection with Gram-negative organisms and staphylococci as other possibilities.

In the context of an illness where purulent sputum or general features such as fever imply infection, the diagnosis of abscess is suggested by the radiological appearances of a rather rounded pneumonic opacity typically with a cavity, in which a fluid level may be seen. The presence of an abscess in the apical segment of the lower lobe or the posterior segment of the upper lobe should raise the possibility of aspiration (Fig. 3). At sites away from these then the possibility of an accompanying obstructing bronchial carcinoma becomes more likely, particularly with advancing age in a cigarette smoker. A lung abscess in the right lower zone raises the possibility of spread from a contiguous subphrenic or hepatic abscess. Multiple abscesses suggest a blood-borne source of infection.

The differential diagnosis for a solitary cavitated lesion (other than suppurative bacterial infection) includes tuberculosis and fungal infections such as actinomycosis, histoplasmosis, coccidiomycosis, a cavitating squamous cell carcinoma, a non-infected pulmonary infarct, and Wegener's granulomatosis. Many of these possibilities may be discounted on clinical grounds and, if not, by reasonably simple further investigation.

Blood cultures should be taken. Sputum should be examined by

Table 2 Underlying causes of lung abscess

1 Aspiration
 Altered consciousness, oesophageal disease, oropharyngeal sepsis
2 Bronchial obstruction
 Carcinoma of the bronchus, foreign body
3 Vascular embolism of infected material
 Bacteraemias and septicaemias of diverse origin
4 Direct spread of contiguous suppuration
 Subphrenic or hepatic abscess
5 As part of pneumonia
 Usually with particular organisms, e.g. staphylococcus, klebsiella

microscopy and culture for bacteria, including tuberculosis, and fungi though it may not be a suitable sample for study of anaerobes due to contamination during expectoration through the mouth unless a deep sample collected cleanly at physiotherapy with rapid transport to the laboratory is used. In this respect fibreoptic bronchoscopy may be particularly useful in providing deep specimens for accurate microbiological assessment. Bronchoscopy is also useful in excluding obstruction by a foreign body or carcinoma and in clearing debris from the affected bronchus as an aid to postural drainage of the abscess. If available, quantitative gas–liquid chromatography studies on sputum for volatile fatty acids from anaerobes may also be useful as a strongly positive chromatogram suggests real anaerobic infection rather than oral contamination.

Management

The single most important aspect of treatment is effective antimicrobial therapy. As has been emphasized, the most important organisms in aspirational disease are generally anaerobes and therefore unless aerobic Gram-negative organisms or staphylococci are recovered, treatment should be based on benzylpenicillin, 2–3 megaunits q.d.s. initially, changing to oral therapy once there has been clinical improvement and resolution of fever. Treatment in general should be continued for 4–6 weeks. When there are laboratory or clinical doubts about the sensitivity of the anaerobe to penicillin, then addition of metronidazole is appropriate. Postural drainage with vigorous percussion will aid the clearance of pus. Ultimately recovery will be seen in 70–80 per cent.

If there is failure to resolve, a repeat bronchoscopy allowing the clearance of the relevant bronchus and a reassessment of malignant and other microbiological possibilities is useful before considering surgical resection. The presence of a carcinoma will require definitive management in its own right and an accompanying distal abscess is not a contraindication to surgery. The presence of an obstructing carcinoma makes abscess resolution by medical means less likely and so encourages surgical intervention although this will be a complex decision depending on the general state of the patient and the staging of the tumour.

In single or multiple lung abscesses secondary to bacteraemia or septicaemia, the antibiotic of choice should be ultimately dictated by blood culture results but in practice will begin with a combination of antibiotics given parenterally to cover a broad spectrum of bacteria.

Prevention

Prevention of aspirational disease depends upon the awareness of the pulmonary risks of oropharyngeal sepsis, oesophageal disease, and uncontrolled altered levels of consciousness.

Empyema

The term empyema is given to a purulent pleural effusion. The excess of white cells present is an expression of viable organisms continuing to initiate the chemotaxis of white cells and therefore denotes active intrapleural infection. Empyema usually follows a *pulmonary infection* in the form of pneumonia, lung abscess or bronchiectasis, but may occur after *septicaemia*, *thoracic surgery* or *penetrating chest wounds* or following *transdiaphragmatic extension* from a *subphrenic or hepatic abscess*. *Tuberculous empyema* once a complication of advanced pulmonary disease and of artificial pneumothorax is now becoming rare in developed countries (see page 5.289). Lowered resistance to infection, multifactorial in origin, in *rheumatoid disease* results in an increased risk of empyema.

Infection in the pleural space results in the production of an inflammatory exudate with varying numbers of pus cells and, depending on the organism involved, the production of fibrinous adhesions between visceral and parietal pleura which may result in loculation of the fluid. The presence of a bronchopleural fistula will result in a pyopneumothorax. Failure to resolve rapidly results in the sequential deposition of layers of fibrin with trapped cellular debris on both pleural surfaces, but particularly the parietal. Progressive fibrosis leads to markedly impaired pulmonary expansion and chest wall deformity.

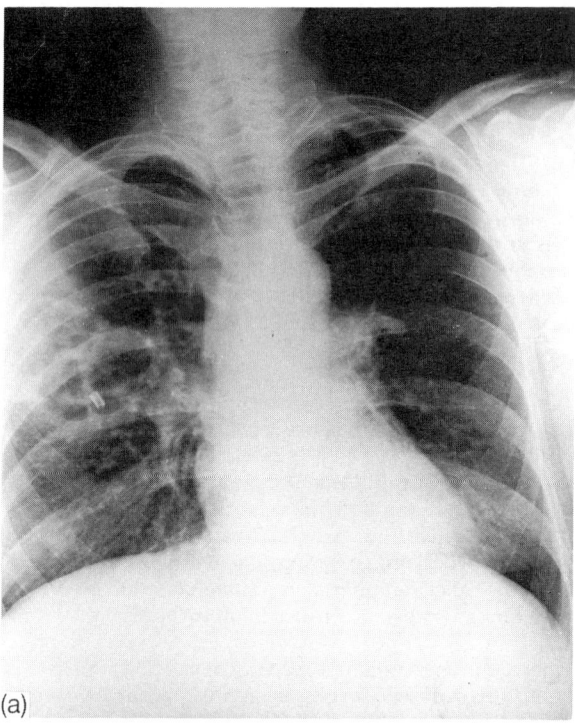

(a)

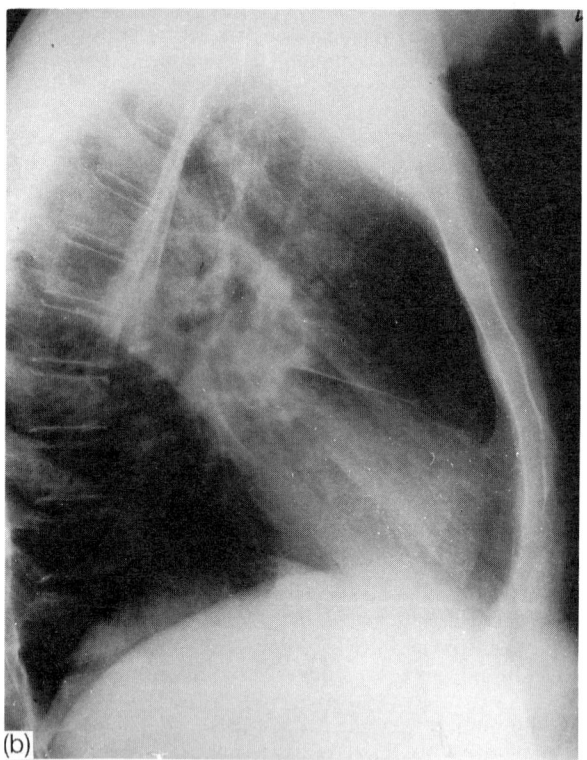

(b)

Fig. 3 Chest radiographs (PA and R lateral) of a 50-year-old man with treated acute myeloid leukaemia, cough, and unremitting fever, showing an abscess in the right upper lobe. Specimens taken at bronchoscopy showed numerous Gram-negative rods found to be the anaerobe *Bacteroides bivius* on culture. An excellent clinical and radiological outcome followed treatment with metronidazole.

The organisms implicated will depend on the underlying cause of the empyema. Following simple pneumonia, a single organism may dominate, whereas mixed growths are common in other disease. Pneumococcal empyema has become distinctly less common since the advent of antibiotics. Following extension from a subphrenic abscess, faecal organisms are likely to be present. Spread from an hepatic abscess may be due to amoebic disease (see page 5.466). Rarely, an aspergilloma of the pleural space, following years after surgery or artificial pneumothorax for tuberculosis or following spontaneous pneumothorax or pneumonectomy, may produce an empyema. Overall, the organisms most frequently found to be responsible have been anaerobes, staphylococci, and Gram-negative organisms.

Clinical features and diagnosis

Empyema is most commonly seen as an acute disorder complicating the course of pneumonia and generally presents as failure of this pneumonia to resolve or as a recurrence of symptoms and signs some days after an apparent recovery. Clinical features include malaise with shivers and pleuritic pain. Fever and leucocytosis may be found and careful examination of the chest usually shows an area of stony dullness.

Chronic empyema usually results from failure to diagnose or treat adequately an acute empyema but may arise from chronic infection as in tuberculosis or actinomycosis, or form an underlying carcinoma or chronic pulmonary sepsis. More rarely chronic empyema may result from the retention of an intrapleural foreign body following surgery or trauma. The features of chronic empyema are continuing malaise, pain , and occasionally purulent sputum, with progression to the development of normochromic anaemia, weight loss, finger clubbing, and chest wall deformity.

The chest radiograph will confirm the presence of an effusion, usually posteriorly and in chronic disease there is typically crowding of the ribs associated with a dense pleural opacity (Fig. 4). The presence of a fluid level implies a leak of air from a previous pleural aspiration, a bronchopleural fistula or, more rarely, the presence of gas-forming organisms (e.g. after trauma when *Clostridium welchii* may be involved). The development of a bronchopleural fistula often leads to the patient's being aware of a foul odour on coughing or to the expectoration of large amounts of purulent sputum. The diagnosis of empyema is confirmed by the demonstration of purulent fluid of varying degrees on pleural aspiration – a wide-bore needle being required to ensure extraction of thick pus.

In acute empyema complicating pneumonia, the fluid aspirated needs careful microscopy and culture for aerobic and anaerobic bacteria, and in chronic empyema, these methods, together with studies for tuberculosis and actinomycosis are needed. In tuberculous empyema, the organism is usually visible on Z-N staining of the pus and pleural biopsy is not required, in contrast to non-purulent tuberculous effusions. Foul-smelling fluid suggests anaerobic infection and all specimens, irrespective of odour, should be taken to the laboratory rapidly in a syringe from which air bubbles have been expressed. Methods such as countercurrent immunoelectrophoresis for pneumococcal antigen and gas–liquid chromatography for volatile fatty acids from anaerobes may be helpful, particularly if antibiotics have already been used. In amoebic disease, microscopy of temporary wet mounts of pleural fluid or sputum may identify the trophozoites. Close collaboration with the microbiologist is crucial for the production of meaningful results. Pleural fluid cytology may be helpful in excluding malignancy, but otherwise bronchoscopy will be required in unexplained disease or when there is clinical suspicion. Bronchograms may be needed to exclude bronchiectasis. An ultrasound examination may help the precise localization of a loculated empyema and help exclude the presence of a predisposing subphrenic or hepatic abscess.

Management

The principles of treatment are obliteration of the empyema space and eradication of infection. In the first instance, therefore, treatment consists of evacuation of purulent fluid and administration of an antibiotic. Thin fluid may be removed by repeated aspiration but more success is likely, especially with thick pus, by the insertion of one or more large indwelling intercostal tubes with drainage to an underwater seal until the effluent is non-purulent. The choice of antibiotic to be used systemically will be influenced by

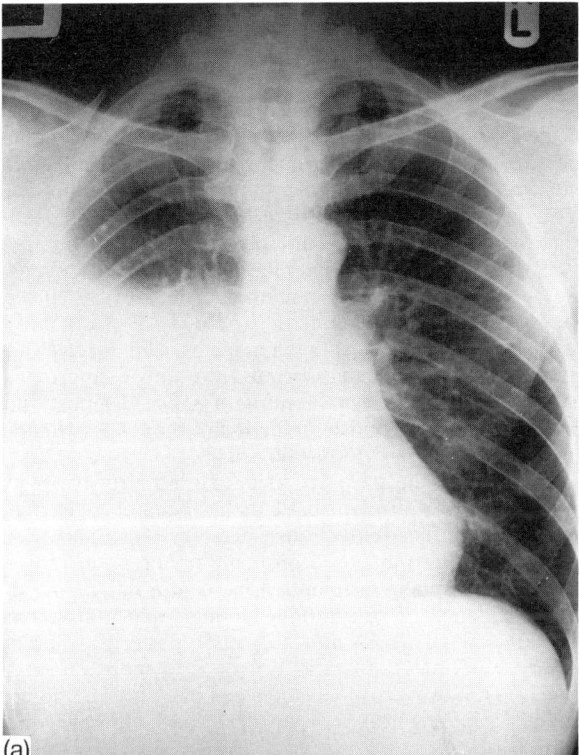

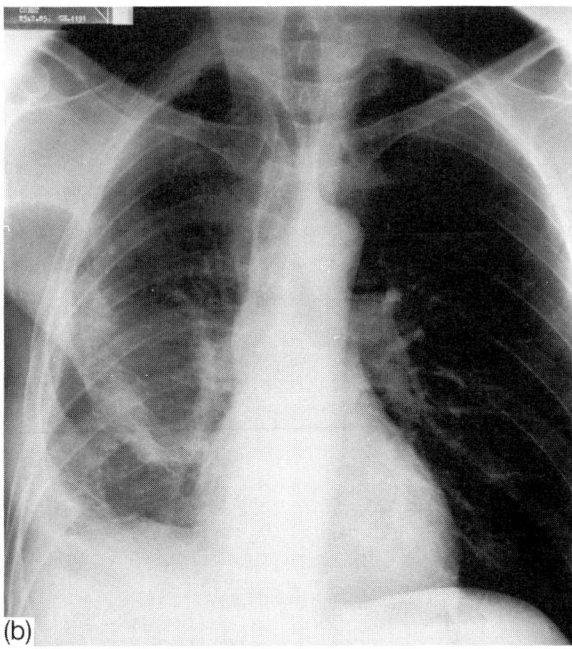

Fig. 4 Chest radiographs, before and after treatment of a 51-year-old man with a chronic empyema and associated glomerulonephritis with renal impairment and the nephrotic syndrome. Microbiology on the pleural pus produced a growth of the Gram-negative *Morganella morgani*. Successful treatment of the empyema with surgery and appropriate systemic antibiotics also led to complete resolution of the renal lesion.

the clinical circumstances and the knowledge that anaerobes, staphylococci, and Gram-negatives are commonly implicated, but ideally should be guided by the microbiological findings. After clinical improvement, and full expansion of the lung and resolution of fever have occurred, antibiotics should probably be continued for some 2–3 weeks. The rare fungal empyema should respond to drainage and intrapleural institution of amphotericin.

Not uncommonly, an empyema may fail to resolve because of unextractable thick pus, extensive loculation, the development of bronchopleural fistula or the presence of gross fibrin and debris deposition on the pleura. Under these circumstances, surgery for the clearance of the pleural space and decortication of the lung or closure of a bronchopleural fistula is essential. The results of surgical treatment are good and failure to achieve adequate drainage by aspiration or indwelling tube should lead to prompt consultation with a thoracic surgeon. It is probably wise to continue appropriate antibiotic treatment for 2–3 weeks following successful surgery.

References

Afzelius, B. A. (1976). A human syndrome caused by immotile cilia. *Science* **193**, 317–319.

Bartlett, J. G. and Finegold, S. M. (1974). Anaerobic infections of the lung and pleural space. *Am. Rev. Res. Dis.* **110**, 56–77.

Brock, R. C. (1952). *Lung abscess*. Oxford University Press, Oxford.

Cochrane, G. M. (1985). Chronic bronchial sepsis and progressive lung damage. *Br. Med. J.* **290**, 1026–1027.

Crofton, J. W. and Douglas A. C. (1981). *Respiratory diseases* 3rd edn. Blackwell Scientific Publications, Oxford.

Delikaris, P. G., Conlan, A. A. Abramor E., Hurnitz, S. S. and Studi, R. (1984). Empyema thoracis – a prospective study on 73 patients. *S. Afr. Med. J.* **65**, 47–49.

Editorial (1985). Prenatal diagnosis in cystic fibrosis. *Lancet* **i**, 1199.

Hodson, M. E., Norman, A. P. and Batten, J. C. (1983). *Cystic fibrosis* Bailliere Tindall, London.

Knowlton, R. G. *et al.* (1985). A polymorphic DNA marker linked to cystic fibrosis is located on chromosome 7. *Nature* **318**, 380–382.

Medical Research Council (1957). Prolonged antibiotic treatment of severe bronchiectasis. *Br. Med. J.* **2**, 255–259.

Quinton, P. M. (1983). Chloride impermeability in cystic fibrosis. *Nature* **301**, 421–422.

Wainwright, B. J. *et al.* (1985). Localisation of cystic fibrosis locus to human chromosome 7 cen-q 22. *Nature* **318**, 384–385.

Pulmonary infection in the immunocompromised host

C. H. FANTA AND J. E. PENNINGTON

Introduction

The lung is among the most frequent target organs for infectious complications in immunocompromised hosts. Furthermore, the mortality for pulmonary infection in immunocompromised patients is high, often exceeding 50 per cent. In one report, the occurrence of lung infiltrate and fever among neutropenic patients with haematologic malignant diseases was associated with 62 per cent mortality, while a group of similar patients also with fever and neutropenia, but without lung infiltrates, had only a 9 per cent episode-related mortality. Thus, fever and a new lung infiltrate in the immunocompromised host pose an urgent clinical problem, demanding prompt diagnosis and specific treatment.

Unfortunately, the usual diagnostic methods for evaluation of pneumonia are less useful in immunocompromised patients. A decision whether to use invasive techniques to determine the exact aetiology of the pneumonia or else to use empirically chosen therapy must be made. On the one hand, the broad range of aetiologies and appropriate therapies confound empirical choices; on the other hand, debilitating illness may make invasive procedures

such as lung biopsy hazardous. The choice between the two approaches must rest on knowldege both of the various pulmonary diseases seen in this setting and their patterns of presentation and also of the yield and risks of available diagnostic procedures. In this chapter, discussion will focus on the most severely immunocompromised patient groups. These include patients with haematologic neoplasias, patients rendered neutropenic by chemotherapy, organ transplant recipients, and the recently described group with acquired immunodeficiency syndrome (AIDS).

Incidence

The precise attack rate of pneumonia among various groups of immunocompromised hosts is uncertain. However, all agree that the incidence of pneumonia is highest among patients with haematologic malignancies, bone marrow transplant recipients, and patients with AIDS. For example, in patients with lymphoma who are receiving intensive chemotherapy, the lung is the most common site of serious infections, and deaths from infection are most often associated with pneumonia. Patients with acute leukaemia in relapse suffer an episode of pneumonia once every 60 days of patient risk. Interstitial pneumonias occur in as many as 55 per cent of bone marrow transplant recipients who survive 30 days posttransplantation, with an associated mortality of approximately 60 per cent. Finally, among patients with AIDS, the most frequent cause of death is opportunistic infection of the lungs (usually with *Pneumocystis carinii* or cytomegalovirus).

In recent years, the intensity of immunosuppressive regimens employed in renal transplant patients has been decreased. While this has clearly reduced infectious (including pulmonary) complications, pneumonia remains a problem among renal (and other solid organ) transplant recipients. One centre has reported a 24 per cent incidence of pneumonia among renal graft recipients between 1966 and 1978. A mortality of 50 per cent, often due to pulmonary superinfections, was noted. In a more recent series (1977 to 1979), however, the incidence of pneumonia among renal transplant recipients was 12 per cent, and all survived their infection.

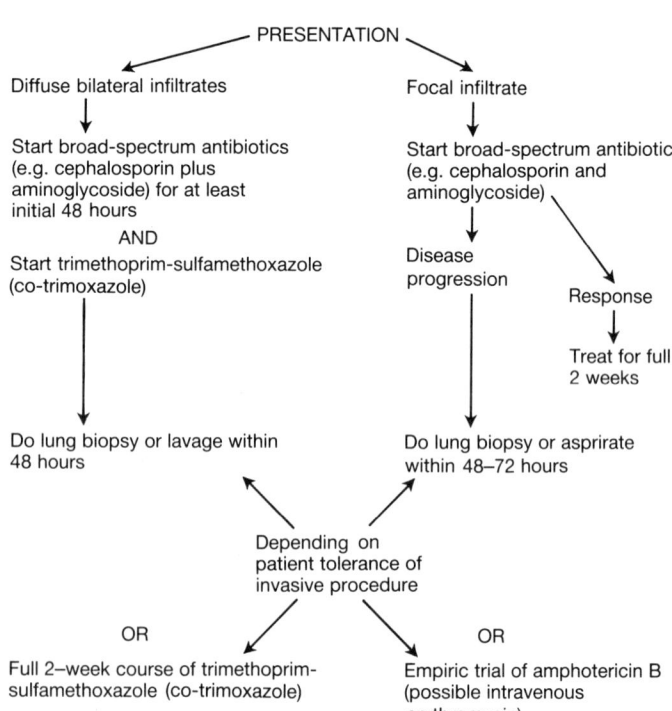

Fig. 1 Management scheme for fever and pulmonary infiltrates in the immunocompromised host.

Table 1 Common aetiologies for pneumonia in immunocompromised patients

Aetiology	Usual underlying conditions	Usual diagnostic methods	Treatment
Bacteria			
Gram-negative bacilli (examples: *Klebsiella*, *Escherichia coli*, *Pseudomonas*)	Haematologic neoplasia with neutropenia	Blood culture, sputum culture, empiric ('response' to antibiotics)	Cephalosporins or ticarcillin, plus an aminoglycoside
Staphylococcus	Haematologic neoplasia	Same	Semisynthetic penicillin or cephalosporins
Pneumococcus	Transplants (especially bone marrow) and splenectomy	Sputum or blood culture	Penicillin
Nocardia	Transplants, lymphoma, AIDS	Invasive procedures (rarely, sputum examination)	Sulphonamides or co-trimoxazole
Legionella	Transplants, corticosteroid therapy, lymphoma, AIDS	Indirect fluorescent antibody titre, direct fluorescent antibody preparation, charcoal–yeast extract media culture	Erythromycin alone or with rifampin
M. tuberculosis	Transplants, AIDS	Sputum culture, lung biopsy	INH, rifampin, ethambutol
M. avium intracellulare	AIDS	Sputum or blood culture, lung biopsy	Ansamycin, clofazimine (unpredictable sensitivities for other drugs)
Fungus			
Aspergillus, *Phycomycetes*	Neutropenia, transplants	Lung aspirate or biopsy	Amphotericin B
Cryptococcus	Transplants, lymphoma, AIDS	Lung aspirate or biopsy, spinal fluid examination, serum latex agglutination test	Amphotericin B plus 5-fluorocytosine
Parasite			
Pneumocystis carinii	Transplants, corticosteroid therapy, AIDS	Lung biopsy or aspirate	Co-trimoxazole
Toxoplasma gondii	Transplants	Lung biopsy, serology	Pyrimethamine plus sulphadiazine
Strongyloides	High-dose corticosteroids	Sputum and stool examination or duodenal aspirates	Thiabendazole
Virus			
Cytomegalovirus	Transplants, lymphoma, AIDS	Lung biopsy, serology and culture	None proven to be effective
Varicella-zoster virus	Hodgkin's disease, renal and bone marrow transplant	Clinical appearance, lesion cultures	Acyclovir
Herpes simplex	Bone marrow transplant	Lung biopsy and culture	Acyclovir

Table 2 Non-infectious causes of fever and pulmonary infiltrates in immunocompromised patients

Tumour	Drug reaction
Radiation pneumonitis	Bleomycin
Pulmonary haemorrhage	Cyclophosphamide
Pulmonary infarction	Busulfan (after very long periods
Leukoagglutinin reaction	of treatment)
Non-specific interstitial pneumonitis	Methotrexate
	Bis-chloroethylnitrosourea
	(BCNU)
	Cyclohexylnitrosourea (CCNU)
	Mitomycin
	Chlorambucil
	Melphalan
	Procarbazine

Aetiologies

Numerous reviews have stressed the large number of potential aetiologic agents which may cause pneumonia in the immunocompromised host. Table 1 provides a list of the most common opportunistic infectious agents causing pneumonia in immunocompromised patients, and also describes the diagnostic and therapeutic approaches most likely to be successful for each. It should be kept in mind that there are also a number of non-infectious causes of fever and lung infiltrates in this patient population (Table 2).

Clinical approach

The development of pneumonia in an immunocompromised patient should be considered a clinical emergency. Thus, early and specific therapy should be instituted. Even if an invasive diagnostic procedure is to be used, it is likely that, on clinical grounds, empirically chosen antimicrobial agents will be given quite soon after presentation. In choosing empiric antimicrobial agents, consideration of the underlying type of immune defect (Table 3), and the radiographic pattern of pulmonary infiltrate at the time of clinical presentation (Table 4), may be useful. Also, the tempo of pneumonia development may suggest certain aetiologies over others. For example, bacterial pneumonias progress rapidly (one or two days), while fungal and protozoan pneumonias are less fulminant (several days, to a week or more). Viral pneumonias are usually not fulminant, but on occasion may develop quite rapidly.

After consideration of all facets of the clinical presentation, a strategy for clinical management can be developed. Figure 1 provides basic management strategies which may be employed for diffuse and focal pneumonias in immunocompromised hosts. It should be emphasized that this is a general scheme, and that each patient must be considered in the light of the specific risk factors noted in Table 3 and the tempo of disease progression.

Invasive diagnostic procedures

If it is decided that an invasive diagnostic procedure will be employed, several choices of technique are available. These include percutaneous needle aspiration, fibreoptic bronchoscopy (biopsy and/or lavage), and open lung biopsy. Percutaneous cutting-needle biopsies are hazardous and are rarely performed in these patients. The relative yields of the most common techniques, their associated risks of complications, and commonly recognized indications for their use are listed in Table 5. In general, the more morbid procedure of lung biopsy via thoracotomy is preferred when: (a) the most likely aetiology for the pulmonary infiltrate is a non-infectious process; (b) the

Table 3 Association between immune defect and aetiologies for pneumonia

Immune defect	Usual aetiologies
Granulocytopenia	Gram-negative rods (examples: *Escherichia coli*, *Klebsiella*, *Pseudomonas*)
	Staphylococcus aureus
	Aspergillus
	Mucor
Cell-mediated immune deficiency	Herpes-group viral agents (example: cytomegalovirus)
	Pneumocystis carinii
	Nocardia
	Cryptococcus
	Legionella
	Mycobacterium
	Aspergillus
Hypogammaglobulinemia or splenectomy	*Pneumococcus*
	Hemophilus influenzae

Table 4 Causes of focal and diffuse pulmonary infiltrates in immunocompromised patients

Focal infiltrate	Diffuse infiltrate
Gram-negative rods	Cytomegalovirus (and other Herpes group agents)
Staphylococcus aureus	
Aspergillus	*Pneumocystis carinii*
Malignancy	Drug reaction
Nonspecific interstitial pneumonitis	Non-specific interstitial pneumonitis
Cryptococcus	Bacteria (uncommon)
Nocardia	*Aspergillus* (advanced)
Mucor	*Cryptococcus* (uncommon)
Pneumocystis carinii (uncommon)	Malignancy
Tuberculosis	Radiation pneumonitis (uncommon)
Legionella pneumophila (or other *Legionella*-like organisms)	Leucoagglutinin reaction
Radiation pneumonitis	

Table 5 Invasive diagnostic techniques for immunocompromised patients with pneumonia

Procedure	Specimens provided	Yield	Complications	Comments
Percutaneous needle aspiration	Fluid aspirate; sometimes a small core of tissue	For localized pulmonary infections = 70–80%	Pneumothorax requiring evacuation (10%); hemoptysis (2–5%); empyema (rare)	Particularly useful for peripheral nodules or cavitary infiltrates
Fibreoptic bronchoscopy	Bronchial washings, bronchial brushings, transbronchial lung biopsy (approximately 1.0–1.5 mm in diameter); bronchoalveolar lavage	Overall yield = 40–50%. In certain infections (e.g. pneumocystis), the yield exceeds 90%	Hemoptysis (5%); pneumothorax requiring evacuation (5%)	Particularly useful for focal or diffuse infiltrates suspected of being infectious in aetiology
Open lung biopsy	Lung tissue (approximately 2–4 cm in size)	Approximately 90%	Delayed pneumothorax; wound complication; prolonged ventilator dependence	Necessary to establish diagnosis based on histopathology, such as radiation pneumonitis, drug-induced lung disease, or 'non specific interstitial pneumonitis'

Table 6 Staining and cultivation techniques recommended for specimens obtained by invasive techniques

| Potential aetiologic agent | Staining techniques | | Culture techniques | |
	Fresh material	Fixed tisue	Medium	Period of incubation (time to preliminary identification)
Legionella sp.	Direct immunofluorescent antibody	Dieterle, acid-fast (*L. micadadei*)	Charcoal yeast extract	3–5 days, sometimes up to 10 days
Nocardia	Modified acid-fast, gram	Modified acid-fast, gram	Sabouraud	Minimum of 5 days, up to 4 weeks
Cryptococcus	India ink	H & E, PAS, MSS, mucicarmine	Sabouraud	4–7 days, occasionally up to 4–6 weeks
Aspergillus	Potassium hydroxide	H & E, PAS, MSS	Blood agar, Sabouraud	1–2 weeks
Mucor (*Phycomyces*)	Potassium hydroxide	H & E, MSS	Sabouraud	1–2 weeks
Mycobacterium sp.	Acid-fast (Ziehl–Neelson, Kinyoun)	Acid-fast stains	Lowenstein–Jensen	Up to 4–6 weeks
Pneumocystis	MSS	MSS	—	—
Cytomegalovirus	Tzanck preparation, *in situ* DNA hybridization, immunofluorescence (monoclonal antibodies)	H & E, *in situ* DNA hybridization	Cell culture (fibroblasts)	2–10 days when inoculum high, up to 6 weeks

H & E, haematoxylin and eosin; MSS, methenamine silver stain; PAS, periodic acid–Schiff.

rapid progression of disease toward respiratory failure dictates a need for immediate definitive diagnosis; (c) bleeding tendency, hypoxaemia, or an unco-operative patient contraindicates other procedures; and (d) a non-diagnostic result (including 'non-specific interstitial pneumonitis') has been obtained by other methods. Recently, the technique of bronchoalveolar lavage via the fibreoptic bronchoscope has proved highly effective in recovering organisms in immunocompromised patients with pulmonary infections. This technique has been particularly useful in diagnosing *Pneumocystis carinii* in patients with AIDS. A few centres have also reported success using pleuroscopically guided lung biopsy in patients with diffuse lung infiltrates. The diagnostic yield of any invasive procedure will be greatly enhanced by a close collaboration with pathology and microbiology laboratory services. Some of the special culture and staining techniques commonly used to identify potential pathogens are detailed in Table 6.

Prevention

A major advance in the care of immunocompromised patients has been the identification of measures effective in preventing certain pulmonary infections. Foremost among these is low-dose oral co-trimoxazole (i.e. one double-strength tablet once or twice daily). Its routine use has virtually eliminated pneumocystis pneumonia among renal and bone marrow transplant recipients, and has caused a dramatic decline in the incidence of nocardia infections among heart transplant patients. Mycobacterial disease can be avoided by isoniazid chemoprophylaxis administered to tuberculin-positive patients facing a period of prolonged immunosuppression. Pneumococcal vaccine provides important prophylaxis for high-risk populations, particularly patients who have undergone splenectomy. In the near future, cytomegalovirus pneumonia may also be preventable by prophylactic administration of immune serum globulin, recombinant interferons, or attenuated live vaccine.

References

Fanta, C. H. and Pennington, J. E. (1983). Pneumonia in the immuno-compromised host. In *Respiratory infections: diagnosis and management* (ed. J. E. Pennington), pp. 171–185. Raven Press, New York.

Murray, J. F., Felton, C. P., Garay, S. M., Gottlieb, M. S., Hopewell, P. C., Stover, D. E. and Teirstein, A. S. (1984). Pulmonary complications of the acquired immunodeficiency syndrome. Report of a National Heart, Lung, and Blood Institute workshop. *N. Engl. J. Med.* **310**, 1682–1688.

Ramsey, P. G., Rubin, R. H., Tolkoff-Rubin, N. E., Cosimi, A. B., Russell, P. S. and Greene, R. (1980). The renal transplant patient with fever and pulmonary infiltrates: etiology, clinical manifestations, and management. *Medicine* **59**, 206–222.

Stover, D. E., Zaman, M. B., Hajdu, S. I., Lange, M., Gold, J. and Armstrong, D. (1984). Bronchoalveolar lavage in the diagnosis of diffuse pulmonary infiltrates in the immunosuppressed host. *Ann. intern Med.* **101**, 1–7.

Williams, D. M., Krick, J. A. and Remington, J. S. (1976). Pulmonary infection in the compromised host. Part I. *Am. Rev. Respir. Dis.* **114**, 359–394.

——, —— and —— (1976). Pulmonary infection in the compromised host. Part II. *Am. Rev. Respir. Dis.* **114**, 593–627.

PNEUMOCONIOSES*

A. SEATON

Most lung diseases are caused or provoked at least in part by the inhalation of harmful material. A wide range of lung conditions, including lung cancer (asbestos, α-radiation, chloromethyl ethers, nickel), pneumonia (legionnaire's disease in hospitals), asthma (flour, isocyanates, epoxy resins), allergic alveolitis (farmer's lung, maltworker's lung), and toxic pneumonitis (silo-filler's disease, chlorine poisoning, cadmium poisoning) may occur as a result of workplace exposure. When exposure to mineral dust in the workplace results in a diffuse, usually fibrotic reaction in the acinar parts of the lung, the condition is generally called a pneumoconiosis.

Although mines have been recognized to be unhealthy places since Roman times, the distinction between tuberculosis and a specific effect of dust in the causation of respiratory disease was not made until the mid-nineteenth century. By this time silicosis, often complicated by tuberculosis, was widespread amongst metal miners, tunnellers, potters, and cutlers. During the same period the industrial revolution stimulated the need for coal and the production of this fuel resulted in increasing numbers of sufferers from coalworker's pneumoconiosis. This in turn was not distinguished from silicosis until the late 1940s and in some countries even today the two conditions are referred to by the one name.

In Britain today and generally through Western Europe and the United States, dust control in the mines and decline of the traditional industries with a silica hazard has resulted in a sharp reduction in the numbers of workers suffering from these two diseases, though less perfect preventive measures in other countries, and especially in the development of these industries in the Third World, will ensure that humans will continue to suffer respiratory illness from working in mines. At the same time, the rise of the asbestos and chemical industries has added new problems for society in weighing the benefits of the product against the cost in terms of human morbidity. Fortunately, these problems are all potentially soluble by the application of preventive measures and these will be emphasized in the sections that follow.

Coalworker's pneumoconiosis

Coalworker's pneumoconiosis is a disease of the lungs caused by inhalation of coalmine dust, a complex mixture of coal, kaolin, mica, silica, and other minerals. It remains the most prevalent of the pneumoconioses in Britain, though improved dust control in the coal mines combined with a reduction in the labour force has reduced the numbers of men with the condition considerably over the last two decades. The importance of coal as a source of energy and as a chemical feedstock for the future ensures that man will be required to produce it after stocks of oil have declined and vigilance will have to be maintained to prevent increasing demand from being attended by increasing dust exposure of the workforce.

Aetiology and pathology

The pathogenicity of coal dust depends on several factors, not all of which are completely understood. It is, of course, essential, if lung damage is to occur, for the dust to be inhalable to acinar level within the lung. Thus the particles must have the appropriate aerodynamic characteristics, essentially making them equivalent to a sphere of unit density between 7 and 0.5 μm in diameter. Once inhaled, the particles must be able to overcome the lung's defences. Some, containing a high proportion of quartz (crystalline silicon dioxide), are toxic to macrophages and cause their disruption after phagocytosis. Such particles seem to be cleared predominantly to the lymph nodes where they remain and set up a

* See also page 6.147.

fibrotic reaction that ultimately destroys the node. Some, however, remain in the peribronchiolar and perivascular parts of the acinus, where whorled fibrosis occurs leading to the typical silicotic nodule. The mechanisms of fibrogenesis are not fully understood but damage to macrophages by quartz has been shown to result in stimulation of fibroblasts to produce collagen through the action of an uncharacterized fibrogenic factor. Most coal dust, however, contains relatively little quartz and yet such high carbon dust is often most harmful in epidemiological terms. For example, in anthracite mines in South Wales in the United Kingdom and in Pennsylvania in the United States the dust is almost pure carbon and yet the pneumoconiosis rates have traditionally been the highest in the country. Such dust is often not particularly toxic to macrophages so some other explanation of its harmfulness to miners needs to be sought. One clue to this may be that anthracite miners have relatively more dust in their lungs than other miners, suggesting that excessive exposures and/or impaired clearance may be factors. Certainly there is a well-demonstrated dose–response relationship between exposure to coalmine dust and risk of pneumoconiosis.

The matter of pathogenesis is further complicated by the observation that some mines with high quartz levels have much lower risks of pneumoconiosis than other pits with similar levels of quartz. This is probably explained by the presence of other minerals in the dust, some of which can react with the surface of the quartz crystal and thus alter its toxicity, and such an effect has been demonstrated *in vitro*.

In conclusion, the pathogenicity of coalmine dust depends primarily on the amount of respirable dust that is inhaled to acinar level. Thereafter its effects are dictated by its composition (high carbon and high quartz dusts, in different ways, being particularly dangerous) and by the presence or absence of other minerals that may interfere with the activity of any quartz present. Finally, the factor of individual susceptibility must play some part, though no genetic markers of this have so far been identified.

Pathologically, coalworker's pneumoconiosis is characterized by the presence of multiple centriacinar and interlobular foci of dust, inflammatory cells, macrophages, and reticulin or collagen, the coal macule (Fig. 1). In miners exposed to relatively high proportions of quartz, the lesions come more to resemble the silicotic nodule. The presence of small discrete nodules is known as simple pneumoconiosis, and when sufficient numbers of these lesions are present they become visible on a radiograph. Complicated pneumoconiosis, or progressive massive fibrosis (PMF), is present by definition when one or more of these lesions is more than 1 cm in diameter (Fig. 2). This occurs either by aggregation together of several, usually collagenous, smaller nodules or by a more diffuse

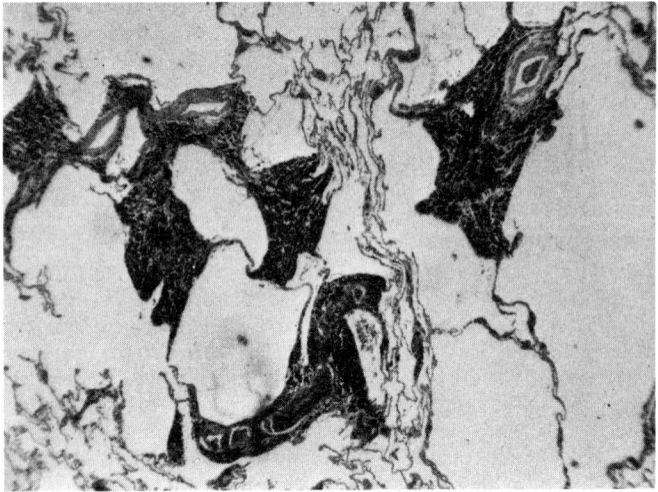

Fig. 1 Simple coal macules, showing accumulation of dust and macrophages around centre of lobule with some associated emphysema.

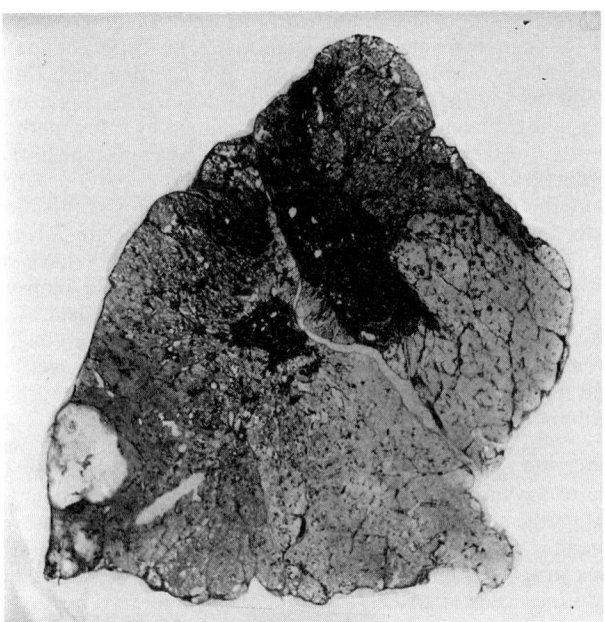

Fig. 2 Whole lung section of a coalminer whose radiograph is seen in Fig. 4, showing progressive massive fibrosis.

accumulation of dust associated with dead cells and ischaemic necrosis of lung tissue. The former, less common, mechanism occurs especially in relation to relatively high quartz exposures while the latter seems more frequent with exposure to high carbon dusts. With either type, or with intermediate types, there is a tendency for the lesions to grow and to be associated with surrounding bullous emphysema, ultimately being responsible for destruction of large volumes of the lung.

The aetiology of PMF is not wholly understood. It is more common in the upper lung zones and in taller men, suggesting an important relationship to lung clearance mechanisms. High carbon or high quartz dusts are particularly liable to cause PMF and the higher the dust exposure, the greater a person's risk. Tuberculous infection is no longer an important factor, though it may well have been in the past. The rheumatoid diathesis seems to be responsible for initiating a particular type of PMF (Caplan's syndrome) in very occasional cases, but this is not an important factor overall.

Clinical features

Simple coalworker's pneumoconiosis causes no symptoms or physical signs. This fact is of considerable importance, as symptoms of respiratory disease in a miner with this condition are due to some other cause, such as bronchitis, heart failure or asthma, which may be treatable. In keeping with this, the simple form of the disease is not associated with any important physiological abnormality. Radiological progression or regression of simple pneumoconiosis occurs only very rarely after dust exposure ceases, apparent regression sometimes being associated with the development of emphysema.

The danger associated with simple pneumoconiosis is that it predisposes to PMF. The risk of PMF is directly related to the profusion of simple pneumoconiosis on the radiograph. It may occur during working life or appear for the first time after (often many years after) dust exposure ceases. It may even occur when there is no apparent simple pneumoconiosis on the radiograph. In general PMF progresses and causes a mixture of restriction of lung volumes and, due to associated emphysema, airways obstruction. Ultimately it may lead to cor pulmonale and death. However, the rate of progression is very variable. In general, the earlier PMF develops in a person's life, the more rapidly progressive and thus the greater a threat to health it is.

The patient with PMF may complain of shortness of breath and symptoms of cor pulmonale. An unusual, but pathognomonic, symptom is the expectoration of the black contents of a cavitated lesion, melanoptysis. Finger clubbing is not a feature and its presence suggests other disease. Abnormal signs in the chest, if present, relate to the presence of bullae, though sometimes lobar collapse can occur.

Coalworker's pneumoconiosis is not associated with an increased risk of tuberculosis or lung cancer, though obviously these diseases can occur in coalminers and should be suspected if haemoptysis, finger clubbing or rapid progression of radiological changes occur. The association between pneumoconiosis and emphysema has been controversial, but there is now clear evidence of a parallel association between dust exposure and two effects – pneumoconiosis and airways disease. The more dust a miner has been exposed to, the greater his risks of pneumoconiosis on the one hand and productive cough, reduction in FEV_1, and presence of centriacinar emphysema on the other. Of course the latter risks are also related to cigarette smoking, and the effect of dust exposure seems to be additional.

The radiological lesions in simple pneumoconiosis are predominantly rounded opacities between 1 and 5 mm in diameter, though small irregular and linear opacities and Kerley B lines are frequently present also. The round opacities tend to be more profuse in the upper and mid zones whereas the irregular lesions predominate in the lower (Fig. 3). Progressive massive fibrosis almost always starts in an upper zone, gradually increasing in size until it may occupy up to a third of the lung. Such lesions are frequently multiple. They are often shaped like short fat sausages, their outer border curved with the chest wall and separated from the pleura by bullous emphysema (Fig. 4). Calcification is not a feature of coalworker's pneumoconiosis, but cavitation of massive fibrosis may occur. Caplan's syndrome is the name given to the combination of rheumatoid disease and several round nodules (usually between 1 and 5 cm in diameter) in the lungs of a coalminer. The lesions have a rheumatoid histology and rarely cause any serious pulmonary impairment. They may cavitate and occasionally coalesce to produce massive fibrosis. The radiological features of coalworkers' and other pneumoconioses are best described in terms of a set of standard films produced by the International Labour Organization. Use of these standards is mandatory for any epidemiological studies of pneumoconiosis.

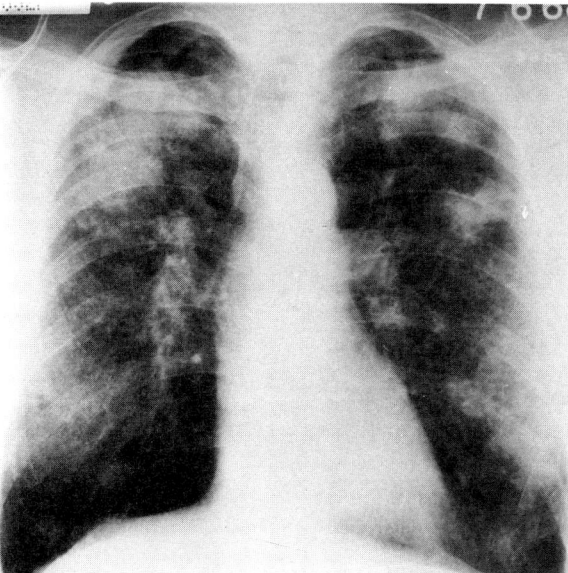

Fig. 4 Chest radiograph of a coalminer showing progressive massive fibrosis in the upper zones, associated with some bullous emphysema and small round shadows throughout both lungs.

Prevention and management

Epidemiological work has shown a dose–response relationship between the total weight of respirable coal dust to which miners have been exposed and their risks of developing simple pneumoconiosis. This has allowed a standard to be set for coalmine dust levels which is resulting in a fall in the prevalence of the disease in British coalmines. Its success depends on regular monitoring of the respirable dust by a gravimetric sampler, constant attention to dust suppression by ventilation and the use of water at points of dust production, and regular radiography of the workforce. Massive fibrosis is prevented at present by preventing men from getting simple pneumoconiosis, though studies are under way which will provide evidence on a dose–response relationship between PMF and dust exposure and which may lead to the development of a new dust standard. The present British standard is 7 mg/m³, measured in the air returning from the coal face.

If a man develops simple pneumoconiosis late in his career, no action normally needs to be taken, apart from (in the United Kingdom) advising him to apply to the Pneumoconiosis Panel via the Department of Health and Social Security for assessment of disablement and possible benefit payments. A younger man, with several years of further dust exposure ahead, should be advised to work in an area of approved low dust conditions. This advice will be given in Britain by the Medical Service of the National Coal Board. Men with more than the earliest stages of simple pneumoconiosis are eligible for certification by the British Pneumoconiosis Panel. Currently about 400 new cases are certified annually, compared to about 2000 in 1960, and 4000 in 1950.

Silicosis

Silicosis is the fibrotic disease of the lungs due to inhalation of crystalline silicon dioxide. Such a disease has been recognized in metal miners and masons since ancient times but assumed particular importance in the cutlery and pottery trades in the 19th century. Silicosis may affect anyone involved in quarrying or carving, mining or tunnelling, grinding or sandblasting, if the dust generated contains silica. In Britain the traditional trades that caused the disease, pottery and cutlery, flint knapping, sandblasting, tin and iron mining, and slate quarrying, have either introduced safe substitute materials or have declined, so true silicosis is now quite rare. Sporadic cases still occur, usually in the production of slate

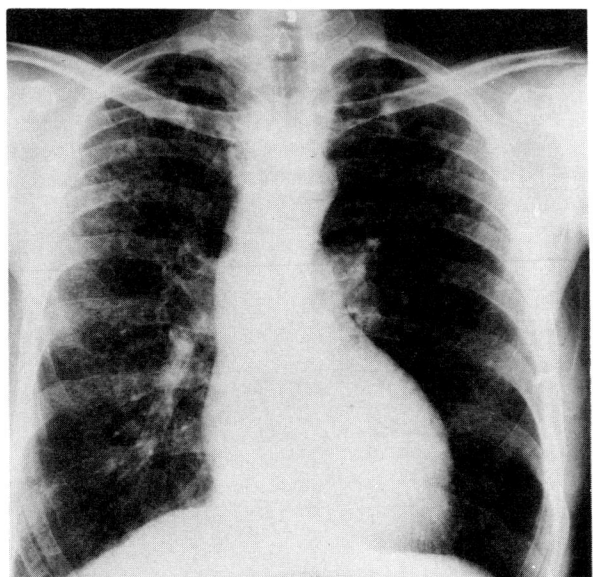

Fig. 3 Radiograph of a coalminer showing small round lesions of simple pneumoconiosis. Note irregular shadows at bases also.

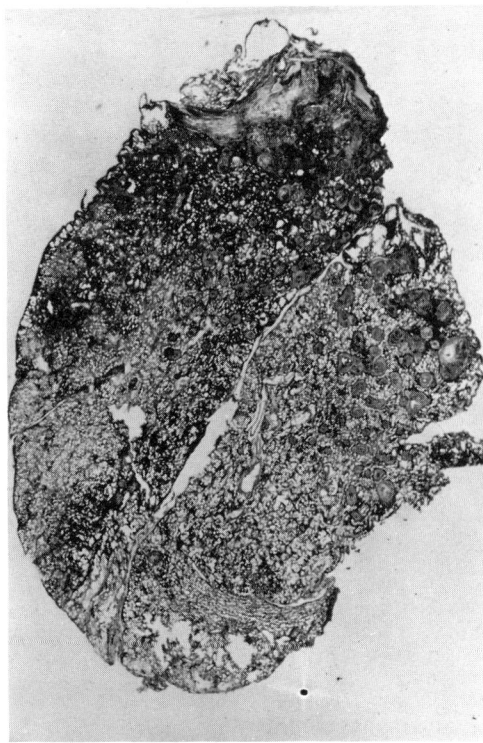

Fig. 5 Whole lung section from a coalminer whose work had predominantly been in hard rock, showing silicotic nodules in upper parts of upper and lower lobes.

or granite, amongst miners cutting through rock and in fettlers in foundries.

Aetiology and pathology

Crystalline silica is present in the earth's crust usually as quartz, though other forms such as crystobalite and tridymite occur occasionally. All are extremely toxic to macrophages. Inhaled particles small enough to reach the alveoli and respiratory bronchioles are engulfed by macrophages and would in normal circumstances be carried up the airways to the mucociliary escalator or via the interstitial lymphatics to the pulmonary and hilar nodes. These clearance mechanisms fail when overloaded with silica, the macrophages being killed and liberating their enzymes, and the silica initiating a fibrous reaction typically around the respiratory bronchiole or in the lymph-nodes. A very heavy overload of silica causes a more acute reaction with damage also to type 2 pneumocytes and consequent exudation of surfactant-containing fluid into the alveoli giving an appearance of pulmonary oedema.

The macroscopic inspection of silicotic lungs shows fibrous pleural adhesions, enlarged lymph-nodes that contain fibrotic, often calcified, nodules, and grey nodules throughout the lung. These nodules vary from a few mm to several cm in diameter and are more profuse in the upper zones (Fig. 5). They may be calcified and they have a typical whorled appearance when cut across (Fig. 6). The largest lesions consist of many such whorled nodules that have become confluent and this massive fibrosis may, as in coalworker's pneumoconiosis, undergo ischaemic necrosis and cavitate. Under the microscope the silicotic nodule is seen to consist of concentric layers of collagen surrounded by a zone of doubly refractile silica particles, macrophages, and fibroblasts. The nodule may contain the remnants of the respiratory bronchiole and arteriole, which become destroyed by fibrosis.

Acute silicosis appears macroscopically like pulmonary oedema. Under the microscope, the alveoli are filled with eosinophilic fluid and the alveolar walls contain plasma cells, lymphocytes, fibroblasts, and silica.

Clinical features

Silicosis presents a spectrum of clinical appearances, depending on the circumstances in which it is contracted. The most severe, acute silicosis, may be acquired from a relatively brief but very heavy exposure such as occurs in sandblasting without respiratory protection. Such patients become intensely breathless and die within months. The radiograph shows appearances resembling pulmonary oedema. Less heavy exposure causes progressively less dramatic symptoms, ranging from a progressive upper lobe fibrosis with slowly increasing exertional dyspnoea over several years (accelerated silicosis), to radiographic nodular change similar to coalworker's pneumoconiosis unassociated with any symptoms or physical signs. The latter type of silicosis is the most common and is usually associated with exposure to dust containing 10 to 30 per cent silica over a prolonged period. Simple nodular silicosis differs from coalworker's pneumoconiosis in that the lesions tend to be large (3–5 mm) and that it is progressive even after dust exposure ceases. Lesions both increase in size and become more profuse. Moreover, extensive simple silicosis may be associated with some

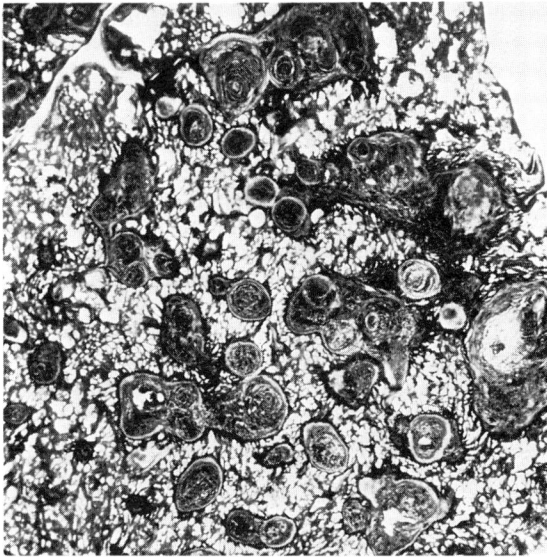

Fig. 6 Silicotic nodules, showing typical whorled appearance.

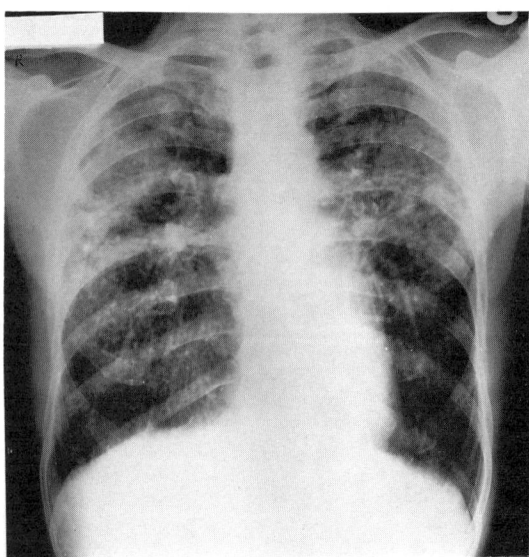

Fig. 7 Radiograph of slate miner, showing extensive simple silicosis in upper and mid zones with early progressive massive fibrosis and eggshell calcification of hilar nodes.

restriction of lung volumes, though it is not complicated, again unlike coalworker's pneumoconiosis, by emphysema. Accelerated silicosis and PMF cause lung restriction and lead to cor pulmonale and cardiorespiratory failure.

Apart from evidence of cardiac failure or distortion of lung architecture by extreme degrees of massive fibrosis, physical signs are not prominent in silicosis. Clubbing and crackles are not usually present. The diagnosis depends on a history of silica exposure and the radiographic features. The most characteristic of these are nodules between 3 and 5 mm in diameter, predominantly in the upper zones, and eggshell calcification in the hilar nodes (Fig. 7). This latter is a pathognomonic feature, only occurring otherwise, very rarely, in sarcoidosis. All forms of silicosis are liable to be complicated by tuberculosis, nowadays in Britain usually due to reactivation of a quiescent lesion.

Other mycobacterial diseases (*Mycobacterium kansasii* and *avium-intracellulare*) also occur more frequently than would be expected in silicotics. The epidemiological evidence of a relationship between silicosis and lung cancer has so far been inconclusive. There does not seem to be a strong link and there may well be none. Pneumothorax is an occasional complication of silicosis, as it is of any disease associated with diffuse lung fibrosis.

Subjects with silicosis, especially of the accelerated type, seem to be at increased risk of the development of autoantibodies and of rheumatoid disease, scleroderma, and systemic lupus erythematosus; these conditions have been described in about 10 per cent of some series of silicotics. Focal glomerulonephritis has also been described in acute silicosis; whether this is a direct toxic effect or due to autoantibodies is not known.

Prevention and management

There is surprisingly little evidence on which to base a hygiene standard for crystalline silica. The current threshold limit value in Britain for respirable silica is 0.1 mg/m^3. Any industry, except coalmining, in which airborne silica may be a hazard, is obliged to keep levels below this figure, by appropriate ventilation, extraction, and other dust suppression measures. In coalmining, for historic reasons, quartz exposures are controlled by total dust levels rather than the silica component of the dust. If higher levels are inevitable, the worker should wear appropriate respiratory protection though this must be regarded as a second-best and potentially risky procedure. Once a worker has developed the disease, he should be prevented from working with silica again. The only medical management necessary is regular sputum examination for tubercle bacilli, as tuberculosis accelerates the lung damage but responds normally to modern chemotherapy. Such examinations in Britain are often arranged by the Pneumoconiosis Panels, to whom the man should apply for industrial injuries benefit.

Asbestosis

Asbestosis is pulmonary fibrosis caused by exposure to fibres of asbestos. It was originally described in the 1900s and its importance as an occupational disease was recognized by epidemiological studies in the 1930s. However, in the first century A.D. Pliny recorded that the weavers of wicks for the lamps of the vestal virgins wore masks for respiratory protection, so some recognition of its hazards goes back to antiquity.

Asbestos is mined principally in Canada, South Africa, and the USSR. It is a generic term for a group of fibrous silicates, the most important being chrysotile (white), crocidolite (blue), and amosite (brown). Chrysotile has a serpentine configuration and breaks up into microfibrils while the other types are straight and less liable to longitudinal fracture (Fig. 8). All types are resistant to physical and chemical destruction which gives them their commercial value in fireproofing, insulation, reinforcement of cement, weaving into cloth, bonding in brake linings, and so on. The asbestos is obtained by crushing the rock to release the fibres which are then carded and transported in non-porous bags to the user industry.

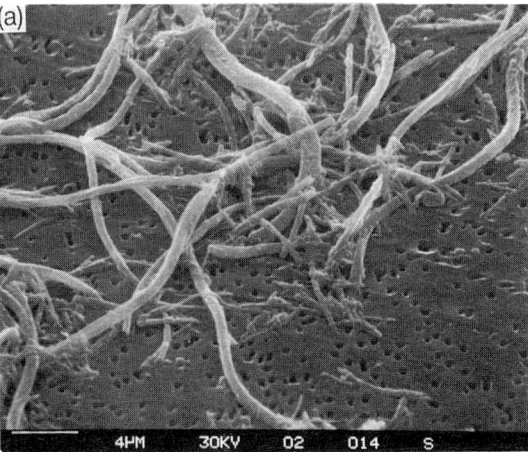

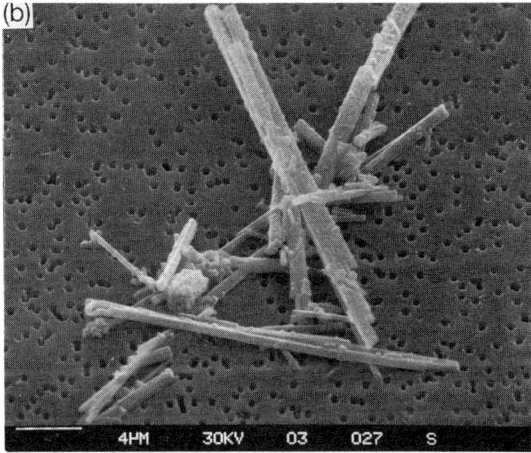

Fig. 8 Scanning electron micrographs of (*a*) chrysotile and (*b*) amosite on Millipore filters. Note curly configuration and microfibrils of chrysotile. Scale bar: 4 μm.

It is important to know that asbestos causes several separate pleuropulmonary lesions. All types of asbestos cause pleural plaques, asbestosis, and lung carcinoma, and risks of the last two are related to the amount of asbestos inhaled. Crocidolite and amosite cause mesothelioma in humans and this disease, though probably also dose-related requires smaller and less prolonged exposure to cause it. Chrysotile, like the other types of asbestos, causes mesothelioma when injected intrapleurally into rats but has only rarely been shown to be associated with mesothelioma in exposed human populations, in spite of being the most commonly used fibre commercially. Further details of mesothelioma can be found in the section on neoplastic disorders (page 15.157).

Aetiology and pathology

It seems likely that the harmful asbestos fibres are those less than 3 μm in transverse diameter and greater than 10 μm in length, that is, those sufficiently narrow to be inhaled to the alveolated part of the lung yet too long to be dealt with adequately by macrophages. All types of asbestos are equally toxic to macrophages *in vitro* and all can cause fibrosis and carcinoma when inhaled by rats. Moreover, injection of any asbestos type (and indeed many fibrous non-asbestos minerals) into the peritoneum of rats causes mesothelioma in a high proportion of cases. It seems likely that the absence of clear human epidemiological evidence linking chrysotile with mesothelioma is related to its curly configuration, which reduces the number of fibres penetrating deep into the lung, and its propensity to break up into minute short fibrils that can eventually be removed from the lung by the action of macrophages. The fibrogenicity of asbestos is probably related, as with coal and

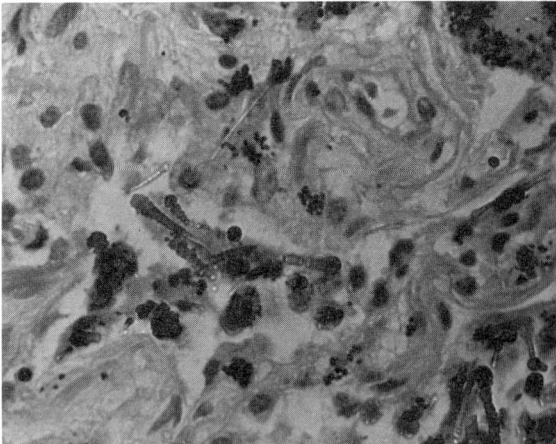

Fig. 9 Histological appearance of asbestosis, with interstitial fibrosis, asbestos bodies, and several uncoated fibres.

silica, to the destruction of macrophages which are unable to cope with fibres much longer than themselves and the liberation of substances that activate fibroblasts to produce collagen.

The macroscopic appearance of an asbestotic lung is of grey fibrosis, progressing to honeycombing, and predominant in the lower zones. Yellow, shiny parietal pleural plaques are also usually present though these frequently occur also in the absence of pulmonary fibrosis. Under the microscope, the appearances are of interstitial fibrosis with minimal cellular infiltrate or desquamation of type 2 pneumocytes. Larger asbestos fibres may be seen coated with a protein–ferritin complex, the asbestos or ferruginous bodies, while smaller fibres remain uncoated but may still just be visible with the light microscope (Fig. 9). However, for every fibre visible by light microscopy, several hundred uncoated fine fibres can always be found on electron microscopy. Pleural plaques have the appearance of basket-weave collagen, and fibres are almost never seen within them.

Clinical features

Asbestosis occurs in people exposed regularly to airborne asbestos at their workplace and not as a result of occasional exposure. It is more likely to be seen in trades involving the application or removal of asbestos in lagging and insulation than in asbestos mining, preparation or weaving where control of fibre levels is nowadays more careful.

The symptoms of asbestosis are shortness of breath, initially on exertion, and dry cough. Physical signs, repetitive end-inspiratory basal crackles and finger clubbing, commonly precede symptoms. The disease is usually progressive, the speed of progression probably being related to the dose of asbestos to which the lungs have been subjected, and results in increasing disability and death from cardiorespiratory failure. Forty to fifty per cent of smokers with asbestosis die of bronchial carcinoma and there is evidence of a multiplicative increase in risk with these two causes. There is no increased risk of tuberculosis in asbestosis.

The radiological appearances of asbestosis are identical to those of cryptogenic pulmonary fibrosis, that is predominantly basal irregular linear shadowing progressing to honeycombing (Fig. 10). The presence of pleural plaques, which frequently calcify, is an indication of asbestos exposure and may help in the differential diagnosis (Fig. 11). In advanced asbestosis the pulmonary fibrosis obscures the cardiac borders, giving a shaggy appearance. As with other pneumoconioses, the radiological appearances are best described by comparison with International Labour Organization standard films.

Asbestosis causes a restrictive pattern of lung function, with reduced volumes and transfer factor. These measurements are the most suitable for screening for the disease and for following its

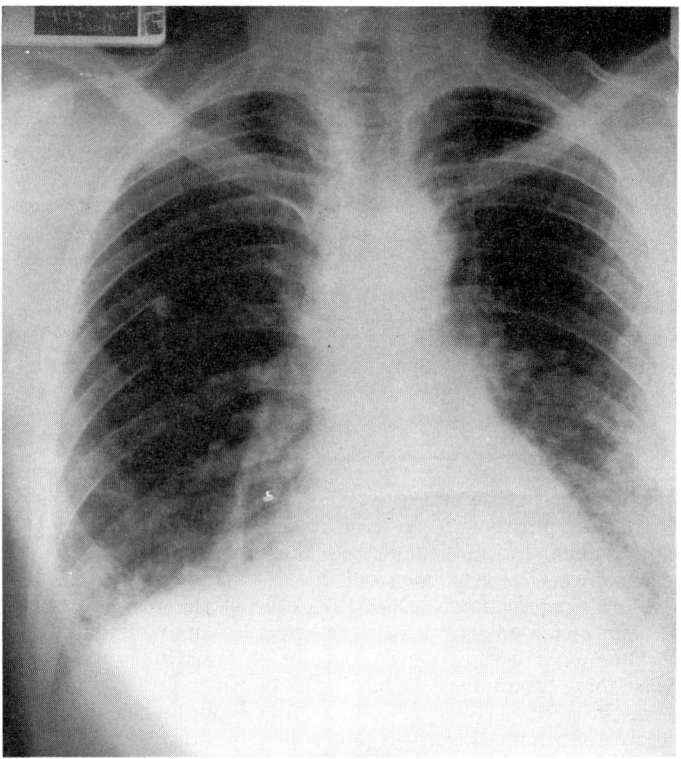

Fig. 10 Radiograph of lagger with asbestosis. Note irregular basal and mid zone fibrosis.

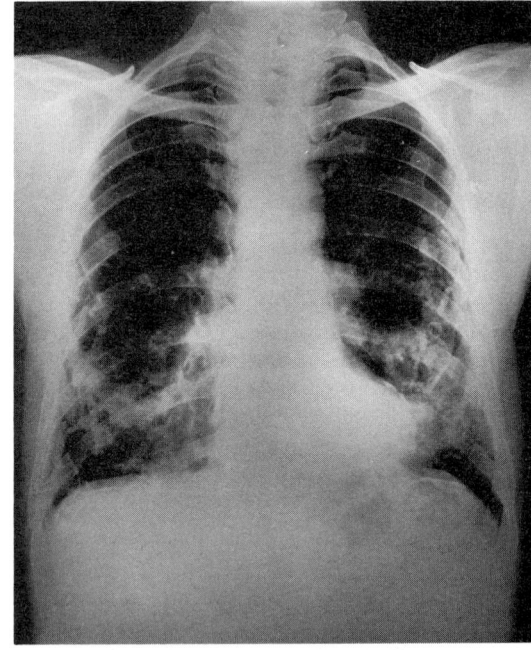

Fig. 11 Radiograph of lagger showing extensive calcified pleural plaques.

progress. Pulmonary compliance is also reduced in relation to the extent of the fibrosis and in the later stages arterial oxygen desaturation occurs.

Pleural plaques cause no symptoms and are usually a coincidental finding on routine chest radiography. A more diffuse form of pleural thickening, which can cause breathlessness and restricted lung volumes, occurs infrequently and rarest of all is benign asbestos pleural effusion. This develops within the first two decades after exposure as a transient haemorrhagic effusion and is diagnosed by the exclusion of infective and malignant causes. It is important to appreciate that there is no evidence that any of these benign disorders predisposes to pleural mesothelioma.

Prevention and management
The prevention of asbestosis, as of other pneumoconioses, depends on reduction of the exposure of individuals to fibre levels that have been shown to be insufficient to cause the disease in a lifetime of exposure. The determination of such a level should ideally be based on epidemiological evidence of the dose–response relationship. Unfortunately, the difficulties of making sensible and reproducible measurements of airborne fibres and the unreliability of such measurements when made, as well as the uncertainties attached to the early diagnosis of asbestosis, have prevented the formulation of really reliable evidence on which to base a standard. The present British standard for chrysotile of 0.5 respirable fibre per ml has been based on work that suggests such levels would, breathed over a working lifetime, result in asbestosis in fewer than 1 per cent of those exposed. More strict standards apply to exposure to crocidolite, which is no longer imported into Britain, and to amosite. Work on standardization of counting and the epidemiology of exposure to fibres is currently taking place in order to increase confidence in exposure standards. Furthermore, many industries are introducing other fibrous or crystalline minerals where possible in place of asbestos. Such new materials may entail hazards in themselves and it is important that they should be subjected to the same scrutiny as asbestos both by toxicity testing and epidemiological studies.

Regular medical and radiological examination of asbestos workers is essential to early detection of asbestosis and there is some evidence that removal of the worker from exposure at this stage is associated with slower progression. Workers should also be advised not to smoke in view of the interaction between cigarettes and asbestos in causing lung cancer. Once the disease is suspected, the British worker should apply to the Pneumoconiosis Panel for assessment for industrial injuries benefit. Currently about 80 asbestotics are certified each year.

Risks of asbestos-related disease in the non-occupationally exposed population
Much anxiety has been engendered amongst the general public by media interest in asbestos, and doctors may find themselves being asked about, for example, the risks to children of asbestos wall panelling in houses or asbestos inserts in ironing boards. In general it can be stated that asbestosis only occurs in people working regularly for years with asbestos. This included, however, at least in the past, wives washing dusty clothes of asbestos workers and people working near asbestos workers or living alongside dusty asbestos factories. Occasional or incidental exposure to asbestos can be dismissed as a significant cause of asbestosis. Lung cancer risks, similarly, seem to be significantly increased only with the doses of asbestos that lead to asbestosis, and individuals who don't smoke and who only have asbestos fittings in their houses can be reassured that their risks of this disease are negligible. Finally, the risk of mesothelioma is again dose-related, although it is well established that a sufficient dose of crocidolite or amosite can be inhaled in a period of intense exposure to the material of as short as six months. Of the 400 or so cases occurring in Britain each year, almost all give a history of having worked with asbestos and have large numbers of fibres in their lungs. Small and occasional exposures to amosite or crocidolite are highly unlikely to entail an important risk, but if significant exposures are thought to be occurring in the domestic or general environment, steps should be taken to eliminate them.

Other silicate pneumoconioses
Several silicates apart from asbestos are of commercial importance and some of these have been shown to cause pneumoconiosis. Talc, hydrated magnesium silicate, is mined as soapstone in the United States, China, and the Pyrenees. It is milled and has many uses including cosmetics, the rubber industry, paints, ceramics, and pharmaceuticals. Kaolin, hydrated aluminium silicate, is quarried in Southwestern England, Georgia in the United States, Japan, Egypt, Germany, and Czechoslovakia. It is used mainly in ceramics, paper, and paint manufacture and in pharmaceuticals. Fuller's earth, calcium montmorillonite, is an absorbent clay quarried in England, the United States and Germany. It was used originally in fulling or removing grease from wool and now in oil refining and bonding foundry moulds. Mica is a complex aluminium silicate, occurring in two forms, muscovite and phlogopite. The former is mined in the United States and India and used in fire-resistant windows and manufacture of paper and paint. Phlogopite, mined in Canada, is used in the electrical industry because of its resistance to heat and electricity.

Two widely used silicate materials are not established as causes of pulmonary disease: cement and vitreous fibres. Though cement exposure has occasionally been reported to be associated with pneumoconiosis, the evidence for this is flimsy. It is often mixed with asbestos and asbestosis may occur in the production of this material. Artificial vitreous fibres (glass wool and rock wool) have not so far been shown to cause pulmonary fibrosis or neoplasia in humans exposed to them, though mesothelioma has been produced by intraperitoneal injection in rats. It is possible that commercial production of finer fibres of these materials might be hazardous and vigilance is required in these industries as the need for safer substitutes for asbestos increases.

Talc pneumoconiosis
Talc is commonly contaminated with tremolite, a non-commercially exploited form of asbestos, and silica and it has been difficult to disentangle the effects of these components. The disease appears clinically to resemble asbestosis, with finger clubbing and basal crackles, though radiological descriptions emphasize lesions predominantly in the mid zones with nodular as well as reticular components. Massive fibrosis has been described.

Talc has been shown to be associated with pulmonary disease in a number of other circumstances. Bronchoconstriction may occur in children exposed to high concentrations and drug takers may get granulomatous reactions in the lungs either by intravenous injection or inhalation of ground-up tablets. The widespread use of talc for producing pleurodesis has fortunately not been shown to be associated with the later development of mesothelioma, probably because the grades of talc used have not been contaminated with tremolite.

Kaolin pneumoconiosis
Kaolin causes a pneumoconiosis similar to coalworkers' pneumoconiosis with small discrete nodular lesions initially and a tendency to produce massive fibrosis. It has been described in workers involved in drying and milling processes in the production of china clay; kaolin may also be the component of the dust responsible for pneumoconiosis in the now defunct Scottish shale extraction industry. There is no evidence linking kaolin pneumoconiosis with carcinoma or tuberculosis.

Fuller's earth pneumoconiosis
This condition has been described in workers extracting the material. It seems to be a benign nodular pneumoconiosis similar in pathological and radiological appearances to coalworker's pneumoconiosis, though progressive massive fibrosis has not been described.

Mica pneumoconiosis
A few reports of radiological change in those exposed to ground mica have been recorded, but there is no recent publication describing pathological or clinical features.

Fibrous erionite

Exposure to this fibrous hydrated aluminium silicate occurs in certain areas of Turkey and probably elsewhere in the Middle East. The populations of several villages have been exposed for many generations as they use local erionite rock as stucco and whitewash in their homes. Pleural plaques, pulmonary fibrosis, and both lung cancer and mesothelioma are endemic in these villages. Fortunately fibrous erionite has no general commercial use, but this episode illustrates the potential dangers of inhaling fine fibrous material, whether asbestos or some other mineral.

Berylliosis

Beryllium is a metal that is used in the nuclear industry and in the production of X-ray tubes. It was used in ceramics, metallic alloys, and fluorescent lights until its toxicity was recognized and it was replaced by other materials. It is mined as the ore mostly in South America and extracted by chemical processes.

Beryllium is highly toxic when inhaled, though it may also cause granulomatous ulcers on contact with the skin. Inhalation of high concentrations causes an acute pneumonitis and tracheobronchitis, which may be fatal. Chronic berylliosis, which may occur as a sequel to acute exposure, usually follows more prolonged exposure to lower levels. It is not common in Britain, no more than about 50 cases having been diagnosed, but has been recorded much more frequently in the United States. Reported cases have occurred in workers with beryllium and in wives exposed to dust from their husbands' clothes, and in people living near the factories.

The patient with chronic berylliosis presents with cough and shortness of breath. The features mimic those of sarcoidosis; bilateral pulmonary mottling with upper lobe fibrosis is the usual radiographic feature initially, bilateral hilar lymphadenopathy being less common. The disease progresses typically to diffuse fibrosis (Fig. 12), but the rate of progression is very variable. The functional lesion is a restrictive pattern with low transfer factor. The progress of the disease can usually be controlled with corticosteroid therapy but this needs to be continued indefinitely in most cases.

The pathological lesion is identical to that of sarcoidosis, with non-caseating granulomas and varying amounts of interstitial fibrosis (Fig. 13). The diagnosis is made on the basis of history of exposure, compatible clinical and histological features, and a negative Kveim test. A skin patch test is inadvisable as it can cause sensitization.

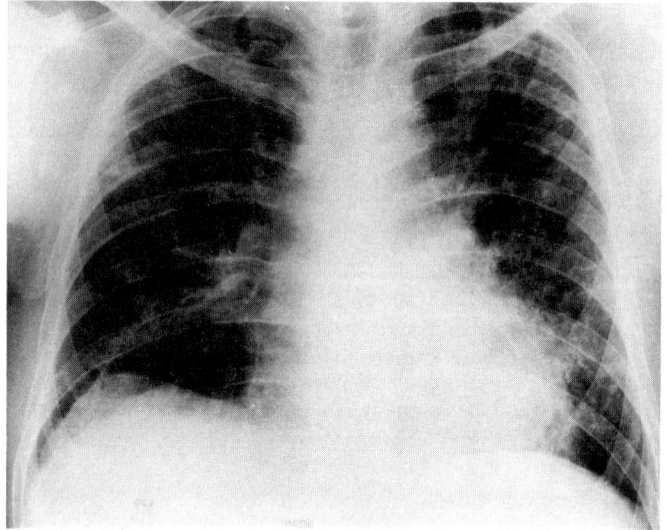

Fig. 12 Radiograph of beryllium refinery worker showing diffuse fibrosis of berylliosis.

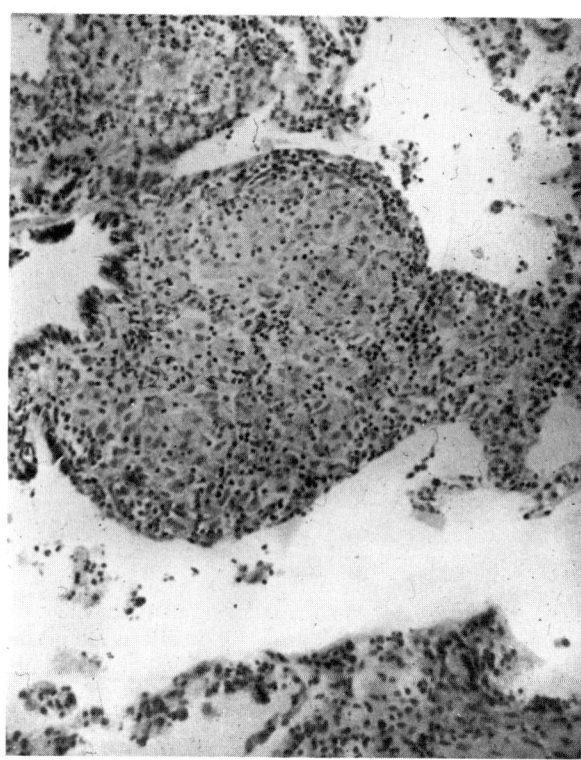

Fig. 13 Photomicrograph of a lung from a man with berylliosis, showing granuloma indistinguishable from that found in sarcoidosis.

Berylliosis is prevented by keeping exposures below the threshold limit value ($2 \ \mu g/m^3$), though as it is a hypersensitivity disease even this will not prevent all cases. Proper respiratory protection should be provided in the event of spills where acute berylliosis could occur.

Other pneumoconioses

Many other pneumoconioses have been described, though most are of very limited prevalence and are relatively benign. Haematite lung, occurring in iron ore miners, used to be seen in Britain in Cumbria. This is a fibrotic reaction to a mixed dust containing silica and iron. Radiographically it resembles silicosis and pathologically only differs from it in that the lungs are coloured red. However, there is an increased risk of lung cancer in the disease, probably related to radiation in the mines. Closely related to haematite lung is siderosis, a benign pneumoconiosis occurring in welders and other workers in iron foundries. Complicated pneumoconiosis rarely occurs. The radiological lesions often regress after exposure ceases. Barium processing and tin refining may be associated with the development of dramatic radiological nodular shadowing, baritosis, and stannosis, respectively. These are completely benign conditions, the radiological appearances reflecting the collection of radio-opaque dust in macrophages. Pneumoconiosis associated with a diffuse fibrotic reaction in the lungs has been described in work with aluminium oxide (Shaver's disease) and tungsten carbide (hard metal disease). A pneumoconiosis resembling that in coalminers has been described in workers with graphite and other forms of carbon, and in shale miners. A benign pneumoconiosis, consisting of simple accumulations of dust and macrophages with minimal nodular radiological shadowing has been described in workers producing polyvinyl chloride.

References

Henderson, V. L. and Enterline, P. E. (1979). Asbestos exposure: factors associated with excess cancer and respiratory disease mortality. *Ann. NY. Acad. Sci.* **330**, 117–126.

Hurley, J. F., Burns, J., Copland, L., Dodgson, J. and Jacobsen, M. (1982). Coalworkers' simple pneumoconiosis and exposure to dust at 10 British coalmines. *Br. J. Industr. Med.* **39**, 120–127.

International Labour Organization (1980). *Guidelines for the use of ILO International classification of radiographs of pneumoconioses.* ILO, Geneva. *(Occupational Safety and Health Series no. 22 (rev. 80)).*

Liddell, D. (1981). Asbestos and public health. *Thorax* **36**, 241–244.

Morgan, W. K. C. and Seaton, A. (1984). *Occupational lung diseases* 2nd edn. W. B. Saunders Ltd, Philadelphia.

Peto, J. (1979). Dose–response relationships for asbestos-related disease: implications for hygiene standards. Part 2. Mortality. *Ann. NY. Acad. Sci.* **330**, 195–203.

Ruckley, V. A., Gould, S. J., Chapman, S., Davis, J. M. G., Douglas, A. N., Fernie, J., Jacobsen, M. and Lamb, D. (1984). Emphysema and dust exposure in a group of coalworkers. *Am. Rev. Resp. Dis.* **129**, 528–532.

Seaton, A. (1983). Coal and the lung. *Thorax* **32**, 241–243.

Seaton, A., Dick, J. A., Dogson, J. and Jacobsen, M. (1981). Quartz and pneumoconiosis in coalminers. *Lancet* **ii**, 1272–1275.

Ziskind, M., Jones, R. N. and Weill, H. (1976). State of the art: silicosis. *Am. Rev. Resp. Dis.* **113**, 643–665.

ALVEOLAR AND INTERSTITIAL DISEASES

The clinical evaluation of alveolar and interstitial lung disease

M. E. TURNER-WARWICK

Introduction

The evaluation of so-called interstitial disease of the lungs poses one of the most challenging and exciting problems in respiratory medicine. The problem is challenging because of the huge number of theoretical possibilities, ranging from the relatively common to the horrendously rare. Perversely some of the most uncommon are treatable, and may occur in quite young individuals. For these reasons however uncommon, they should never be missed. The subject is exciting because there is almost always an answer. The objective is to arrive at a certain diagnosis which often involves considerable sleuthwork, with the minimum inconvenience to the patients.

This introductory chapter will describe with unrepentant personal bias a practical approach to the diagnosis and evaluation of a patient presenting with radiographic bilateral widespread shadowing. The chapter will *not* include discussion on more localized unilateral shadows. It will however be recognized that not all bilateral shadowing affects all parts of the lung uniformly. A radiographic starting point is practical because this is often the first certain indication that the patient has indeed a widespread alveolar and/or interstitial problem.

The clinical history

The first fact to establish is the probable duration of disease. Many patients present with breathlessness and its duration and speed of deterioration are important. Most acute diseases will be identified fairly readily although chronic interstitial disease may be very slow in its development and remain subclinical even for years. Direct questioning is usually needed to establish whether previous chest radiographs have been taken; if so they must be seen and reports alone are inadequate.

A full occupational history is critical because job descriptions alone may not indicate the full range of exposure. For example, rivetters in shipbuilding programmes during the Second World War were often exposed to as much asbestos as the laggers themselves. An intelligent occupational history entails knowledge of the materials which do and do not cause interstitial disease and the type of symptoms that these patients may experience. Hobbies are equally important and are sometimes deliberately withheld from the doctor. Pigeon breeders, for example, are liable to considerable financial loss if they have to sell their birds; the budgerigar in the sitting room is 'part of the furniture' and may not be recognized as a possible culprit by the patients.

Other points in the personal history have recently become important with the recognition of AIDS amongst special groups especially homosexuals. They often present with pneumocystis pneumonia.

A history of medications is important. A wide variety of unrelated drugs may cause acute or chronic interstitial lung disease (page 15.143). The lung disease may be a complication of the systemic disorder for which the drug is being used or be due to the drug itself (e.g. gold in rheumatoid arthritis). Some drugs are used over very long periods for an entirely separate complaint and are easily overlooked even on direct questioning (e.g. nitrofurantoin in the treatment of chronic urinary infections). Lung disease associated with cytotoxic drugs may be a complication of the underlying malignant disease (e.g. lymphomatous infiltrates of the lung), may be a toxic effect of the drug (e.g. bleomycin lung) or are often due to an opportunist infection consequent upon the cytotoxic drug treatment (e.g. pneumocystis pneumonia). Clearly treatment in each of these situations is completely different. Other specific symptoms may be important. Most interstitial lung disease is associated with very little sputum although some patients have an irritating dry cough. A patient with extensive bilateral shadowing (often maximal towards the bases) with widespread crepitations on auscultation and finger clubbing may at first sight appear to have cryptogenic fibrosing alveolitis but if much sputum is present it may be an alveolar cell carcinoma (if mucoid) or widespread bronchiectasis (if purulent).

Small persisting haemoptyses are often ignored especially when long standing but immediately suggest the possibility of pulmonary haemosiderosis.

The points highlighted above do no more then illustrate the range of history which may immediately give an important indication of the most likely diagnosis. More details will be given in the specific chapters that follow.

The physical signs

If the patient has persisting widespread radiographic shadows and finger clubbing without cough or sputum the shortlist of possibilities narrows very considerably (cryptogenic fibrosing alveolitis and asbestosis being high on the list). While many patients with widespread alveolar wall fibrosis or inflammatory infiltrates have basal fine crepitations, patients with granulomatous disease or disseminated tumours usually have no added sounds. Physical signs in other systems (e.g. suggestive of connective tissue or heart disease) can be of even greater help than physical signs in the lungs themselves.

The chest radiograph

This will be described in full detail in the individual sections which follow but analysis of the type of shadow, nodular (i.e. 'regular' in the International Labour Organization (ILO) classification) reticular (i.e. 'irregular' in the ILO classification) or confluent (i.e. alveolar filling), their distribution in the upper, middle or lower zones or their peripheral or more central distribution can be of great importance in setting diagnostic likelihoods. The additional appearances of honeycombing suggestive of alveolar wall destruction or linear shadows with upper zone contraction commonly seen in 'fibrotic' sarcoidosis or hypersensitivity pneumonitis can also be very helpful. A finely tuned interpretation of the radiograph in the context of the history and physical signs will often provide a high index of suspicion to the most likely diagnoses or at least a short list of possibilities.

Lung function tests

As a diagnostic tool conventional lung function tests can be relatively disappointing. Their real value is in following the progress of patients either during treatment or before treatment is started.

Many patients with interstitial disease show a reduction of lung volumes (i.e. the so-called restrictive defect) and this may or may not be accompanied by a reduction in the transfer factor for carbon monoxide (DLCO), reflecting perhaps the extent of compromize of the pulmonary capillary bed.

The tests are of relatively little diagnostic value except when they are in substantial discord with other features (e.g. showing a severe obstructive defect in a non-smoker in a patient with widespread shadows). The tests are also very variable in individual patients with known persisting sarcoidosis many of whom have entirely normal lung function tests. Evidence of airflow limitation in patients with widespread radiographic shadows may be due to a bronchiolar component of the primary pathology, may be attributable to cigarette smoking or to co-existing destructive emphysema or of course to coincidental asthma.

Computerized tomography

The introduction of high-class, high-resolution computerized tomography can be very useful in defining the distribution of lesions, in defining parenchymal lesions in the presence of pleural disease and in distinguishing lower zone shadows due to blood diversion (e.g. upper zone emphysema) from real interstitial disease. A study of patients in the prone as well as the supine position is particularly useful in distinguishing interstitial disease from blood diversion.

The next step

Having collated the history, chest radiograph, physical signs, and the lung function tests in that order of importance, the experienced physician is likely to be in a position to decide on the most probable diagnosis or at least a very small shortlist of the most likely. The wise physician will always remember that with such a wide range of outside possibilities he or she may well be wrong! The next step is to decide, under the full clinical circumstances, how important it is to make a definite diagnosis at all. For example, in an elderly patient with few symptoms and a known abnormal radiograph over several years, especially if there are additional disorders such as ischaemic heart disease, it may be wise to investigate no further.

However, the more acute the onset and the younger the patient the more it is, in the author's view, essential to obtain a definite diagnosis at the outset. This is so for several reasons. Rare treatable conditions often masquerade as common ones (e.g. alveolar proteinosis is often diagnosed as sarcoidosis). The prognosis of diseases differs widely. The indications for, and the nature of, treatments can also differ widely. In some (e.g. cryptogenic fibrosing alveolitis) there is growing evidence that treatment at an early cellular stage, often when symptoms are minimal, offers the best chance of response and control of this otherwise progressive and potentially lethal disease.

Having decided that there are not overriding reasons for allowing a diagnosis to remain unproven (and in the author's view this is the way round the question should be presented) the next step is to decide which is the least traumatic and most certain way of making a firm diagnosis. Many specific investigations

may obviously be appropriate including detection of organic dust precipitins in the blood or the detection of neoplastic cells in the sputum. Thereafter two more invasive procedures should be considered.

Bronchoalveolar lavage

This simple procedure performed through the fibreoptic bronchoscope passed under a local anaesthetic allows samples of cells to be washed from the alveolar spaces. It may be diagnostic or it may provide substantial support for a diagnosis indicating fairly strongly the next most appropriate diagnostic step.

Pathognomonic appearances

Provided the samples are prepared in the correct way lavage can provide a virtually certain diagnosis in certain rare conditions like pulmonary haemosiderosis (Pearl's stain for iron-laden macrophages), alveolar proteinosis (the macroscopic appearance of the supernatant or electron microscopic appearances of laminated proteinaceous material), and eosinophilic granuloma (Langerhans cells with typical inclusions on electron microscopy). It may yield important information about infections, especially opportunist infection (e.g. fungi, acid-fast bacilli or *Pneumocystis carinii*).

Other cell appearances may be highly suggestive of inorganic dust exposure (e.g. asbestos bodies in large numbers, talc crystals or the giant cells so typical of hard metal exposure).

The differential inflammatory cell profile although not pathognomonic may point strongly to the most likely cause. A very high lymphocyte count suggests hypersensitivity pneumonitis, although of course it is occasionally seen in other conditions. A moderately raised lymphocyte count favouring sarcoidosis rather than cryptogenic fibrosing alveolitis, and a raised neutrophil and/or eosinophil count in the absence of inorganic material is more in keeping with cryptogenic fibrosing alveolitis.

This very brief description of the diagnostic value of lavage can often suggest whether a mucosal biopsy or a transbronchial biopsy is likely to confirm the diagnosis or whether it is probable that an open biopsy with its more adequate sample is likely to be necessary.

The choice of biopsy

Where there is a strong chance of sarcoidosis a mucosal biopsy which can be done at the same time as the lung lavage will often show a granuloma. Where this fails and granulomatous disease is suspected a small lung sample provides highly characteristic pathology (e.g. a well-formed granuloma) and is all that is necessary; under these circumstances a transbronchial biopsy is likely to provide adequate material.

Where a less specific pathology is likely and particularly where the stage of disease is important for establishing the likelihood of response to treatment, then a larger (and uncrushed) sample obtained by open biopsy gives the maximum chance of making a certain diagnosis and giving some indication about the chances of therapeutic response.

Biopsy before or after treatment?

All too often patients are treated blindly sometimes with an inadequate dose of steroids and when they fail to respond or indeed have deteriorated further, they are referred for a second opinion regarding the diagnosis. At this stage biopsy or lavage may carry a greater risk. Some are only referred when they are very sick indeed and may have been allowed to slip into an irreversible stage. There is good evidence that open biopsy in patients on corticosteroids has a higher complication rate. The author's view is that the correct time for histological confirmation of disease is before treatment, not afterwards.

Clearly the question of the need for biopsy and the preferred method is a very contentious one, but the scheme outlined above has over the years brought to light otherwise overlooked treatable conditions. Furthermore, it has provided a much more secure basis for frank discussion with patients about their chances of response and prognosis, and about selection of drugs (which themselves have considerable toxicity), in a field where otherwise there remains a great deal of uncertainty. There is still much to be learnt and with more information the recommendations set out here may well need to be modified or radically changed. Currently it appears to have much to commend it.

Evaluation of patients under treatment

Even when meticulous systemic investigation and diagnosis has been made, all too often, treatment is monitored quite inadequately. Meticulous comparison of the whole series of radiographs (not just the two consecutive ones) together with plotted trends of lung function tests, together with other parameters where relevant (e.g. decrease in precipitins or lavage lymphocytes after removal of antigen), are essential. This is so because trends of change can be quite slow. The general objective is to use medication to restore optimally the measurements available (usually the chest radiograph and lung function tests) as well as to improve symptoms and then to titrate drug doses to the lowest which maintain optimal improvement. Where suppressive rather than curative treatment is the aim, carefully planned follow up against titrated doses of drugs would seem to be a more logical approach than arbitrary courses of random doses for arbitrary periods of time which pay no regard to the activity and natural history of the disease in that individual.

Against this background of principles, the details of management of individual cases may be considered.

Extrinsic allergic alveolitis

D. J. HENDRICK

Historical background

Farmer's lung is often regarded as the prototype of the bronchiolar/alveolar disorders that result from hypersensitivity to inhaled organic dusts. They are known collectively by the term extrinsic allergic alveolitis (EAA), though it is recognized that the underlying inflammatory response occurs diffusely throughout the gas exchanging tissues and is not confined to the alveoli. For this reason many prefer the term hypersensitivity pneumonitis. These alveolar disorders were not clearly distinguished from asthma until 1932 when Campbell published his celebrated report describing three affected English farm workers. The appellation farmer's lung was suggested later in 1944. The disease was nonetheless recognized in Iceland in the 19th century, and probably contributed to the occupational ailments of grain workers so graphically described by Ramazzini in the 18th century.

Part of the eminence of farmer's lung itself stems from its industrial importance, and part from its historical role in the understanding of EAA. Its relation to the inhalation of dust from mouldy hay, straw or grain had been recognized from the outset, but it was not until 1961 when Pepys and colleagues demonstrated the presence of precipitins to antigens of mouldy hay in patients suffering from the disease that the idea of an allergic aetiology gained general acceptance. These and other investigators showed that the main sources of antigen were contaminating thermophilic actinomycetes, particularly *Micropolyspora faeni* and *Thermoactinomyces vulgaris*. These thermophilic microbes (they are actually bacteria not fungi) colonize fermenting damp vegetable produce as it heats up. When it eventually dries, a respirable dust laden with antigenic microbial spores is released. Symptoms are consequently most common during winters following wet summer harvests, when hay or grain is used for feeding stock.

For deposition of the dust to occur predominantly in the gas exchanging tissues, particle size must be largely confined to the range 0.5–5μm. This encompasses the diameters of many antigenic

bacterial and fungal spores and a large number of microbial species are now recognized causes of EAA. In addition, the disease has been noted to follow exposure to a variety of antigens derived from animal, vegetable, and even chemical sources, both in the workplace and in the home.

Clinical features

Acute form

The acute form of EAA is the most easily recognized because symptoms are often quickly distressing and incapacitating, and have a high degree of specificity. Following a sensitizing period of exposure which may vary from weeks to years, the affected subject experiences repeated episodes of an influenza-like illness accompanied by cough and undue breathlessness some hours (usually 3–9) after commencing exposure to the relevant organic dust. The systemic 'flu'-like symptoms generally dominate those that are essentially respiratory in nature, and the subject complains most of malaise, fever, chills, widespread aches and pains (particularly headache), anorexia, and tiredness. He is unlikely to exercise himself and may well put himself to bed. He may therefore be unaware of undue shortness of breath, though he is likely to develop a dry cough without wheeze and some difficulty taking deep, satisfying breaths. Occasionally there is an asthmatic response in addition to that in the gas exchanging tissues and wheezing becomes a further feature.

Affected subjects soon learn to associate symptoms with the causative environment, despite the delay in onset after exposure begins. Recognition is particularly easy for groups such as farmers, malt workers, and pigeon fanciers for whom these risks are likely to be well known because colleagues have already become affected. In some cases, however, there may be a tendency to deny such a relationship for fear of compromising the ability to pursue livelihood or hobby, and the clinical history may appear much less convincing than it should.

The severity and duration of symptoms depend on exposure dose. With low levels of acute exposure, symptoms are mild and persist for a few hours only. When occupation is responsible, the affected worker may feel unwell only at home during the evening or night, and be fully recovered by the following morning. Severe responses from particularly heavy exposures may, however, require several days or even weeks for complete resolution.

In exceptionally severe cases, life-threatening respiratory failure may develop and emergency admission to hospital becomes necessary. Death is not unknown. Respiratory distress at rest with fever and gravity-dependent crackles comprise the major physical signs, breathing being fast but shallow. Clubbing is rarely seen, especially in the acute form of the disease. Hypoxia is typically accompanied by hypocapnia, and the chest radiograph shows a diffuse alveolar filling pattern. Spontaneous recovery can be expected to begin within 12 to 24 hours, and can be speeded up with corticosteroids. Supplemental oxygen will be required in the interim, and in rare cases there may be a brief need for mechanical ventilatory support.

Most subjects recover fully from each acute exacerbation, and if the cause is recognized and further exposure avoided, there is little risk of persisting pulmonary dysfunction. It is not always realistic to expect affected individuals to avoid further exposure, however, especially among farming communities, and there is some risk that continuing exposure and repeated acute exacerbations will eventually be associated with permanent impairment of lung function. In practice, a greater risk lies with continual low levels of exposure, which are insufficient to provoke clinically recognizable acute responses but may nevertheless lead to the chronic form of the disease.

Chronic form

In some subjects, EAA expresses itself in a much less dramatic though potentially more serious way. There is a slowly increasing loss of exercise tolerance due to shortness of breath but no systemic upset apart from an occasional prominent loss of weight. This is the result of diffuse pulmonary fibrosis which has often been progressing for years before the affected subject seeks advice. The slower the progression, the longer the delay, and the greater the degree of permanent fibrotic damage. Eventually hypoxia and pulmonary hypertension may supervene, and the right heart fails. There are no acute exacerbations, and each day and each month are much like any other. The clinical features are similar to those of other varieties of pulmonary fibrosis, and it may prove extremely difficult to distinguish this form of EAA from cryptogenic fibrosing alveolitis, sarcoidosis or other slowly progressive forms of pulmonary fibrosis.

The chronic form of EAA is typically seen in the subject who keeps a single budgerigar (known as a parakeet in the United States) in the home. The level of antigenic exposure to avian dust is comparatively trivial (compared to the farm worker forking bales of heavily contaminated hay in a poorly ventilated barn) but it is encountered almost continuously, especially if the affected subject is a housewife or elderly pensioner confined largely to the home. The different exposure patterns are mainly responsible for the distinct forms of EAA, though differences in host responsiveness probably exert an additional influence. There may consequently be considerable variability in clinical features among individuals affected by the same source of antigenic exposure.

Intermediate forms
The fact that the acute form of EAA can be produced by provocation tests in subjects with the chronic form of the disease emphasizes the major role that dose exerts in determining the clinical nature of the response that occurs. It is therefore possible for acute exacerbations to occur in subjects manifesting predominantly the chronic form of the disease, and for a limited degree of recovery to follow cessation of exposure. Depending on exposure dose and host responsiveness a variety of intermediate forms will be recognized, and some subjects will experience different patterns of response at different times. In general, however, the indi-

Table 1 Agents reported to cause extrinsic allergic alveolitis

Agent	Source	Disease
Microorganisms		
Alternaria	Paper mill wood pulp	Wood pulp worker's lung
Aspergillus clavatus	Whisky maltings	Malt worker's lung
Aspergillus fumigatus	Vegetable compost	
Aspergillus versicolor	Dog bedding (straw)	Dog house disease
Aureobasidium pullulans	Redwood	Sequoiosis
Bacillus subtilis	Domestic wood	
Cephalosporium	Sewage	Sewage worker's lung
?Cryptococcus neoformans/	Japanese summer air	Summer type hypersensitivity
?Trichosporon cutaneum		pneumonitis
Cryptostroma corticale	Maple	Maple bark stripper's lung
Graphium	Redwood	Sequoiosis
Lycoperdon	Puffballs	Lycoperdonosis
Merulius lacrymans (dry rot)	Domestic wood	
Mucor stolonifer	Paprika	Paprika splitter's lung
Penicillium casei	Cheese	Cheese washer's lung
Penicillium chrysogenum/cyclopium	Domestic wood	
Penicillium frequentens	Cork	Suberosis
Saccharomonospora viridis	Logging plant	
Sporobolomyces	Horse barn straw	
Streptomyces albus	Soil/peat	
Thermophilic actinomycetes	Hay, straw, grain	Farmer's lung
(Micropolyspora faeni,	Mushroom compost	Mushroom worker's lung
T. sacchari/vulgaris)	Bagasse	Bagassosis
Miscellaneous ?bacteria/?fungi/	Air conditioners,	Humidifier lung
?amoebae/?nematode debris	humidifiers, tap water	Sauna taker's lung
Animals		
Arthropods (Wheat weevil–	Grain dust	
Sitophilus granarius)		
Birds	?Bloom/?excreta	Bird fancier's lung
Fish	Fish meal	Fish meal worker's lung
Mammals		
Pituitary (cattle, pig)	Pituitary extracts	Pituitary snuff taker's lung
Hair	Fur	Furrier's lung
Urine (rodents)	Urinary protein	Rodent handler's lung
Vegetation		
Wood (Ramin–Gonystylus bacanus)	Wood dust	Wood worker's lung
Chemicals		
Bordeaux mixture (fungicide)	Vineyards	Vineyard sprayer's lung
Cobalt dissolved in coolants	Tungsten carbide grinding	
Diphenyl methane diisocyanate	Plastics industry	
Formaldehyde*	Laboratory	
Pauli's reagent	Laboratory	
Pyrethrum	Insecticide spray	
Hexamethylene diisocyanate	Plastics industry	
Toluene diisocyanate	Plastics industry	
Trimellitic anhydride	Plastics industry	

* One subject, possibly toxic not allergic response.

vidual affected by the chronic form of EAA should be satisfied if no further progression occurs, because in some cases fibrotic damage continues despite cessation of exposure.

Causative agents

Table 1 lists the various agents reported to cause EAA. Most are micro-organisms that are found contaminating a variety of vegetable products. Although those associated with the most celebrated disorders, farmer's lung, mushroom worker's lung, and bagassosis, are usually thermophilic, the majority are not. Even with mouldy hay and farmer's lung there is evidence that non-thermophilic organisms (e.g. *Aspergillus* spp) may occasionally be involved. Some microbial contamination may occur during growth of the vegetable host, but most of the antigenic load is usually acquired after harvest. Prolonged storage under damp conditions therefore increases the risk of EAA substantially, while drying to reduce the water content below 30 per cent greatly lessens the risks.

Inevitably there are situations where contamination arises with a number of different microbes and affected subjects show antibodies to several of them. Unless time-consuming provocation tests are carried out with extracts of the individual microbial species, it is not possible to identify a single responsible agent. It is conceivable that several could be relevant in these circumstances. This is a characteristic feature with contaminated humidifiers and air conditioners, and a great variety of bacteria, fungi, protozoa (amoebae), and metazoa (nematode debris) have been suggested as possible causes of humidifier lung.

Humidifier lung is also distinguished by the presentation of antigen in soluble rather than particulate form, and by the comparative rarity of radiographic abnormalities. The latter may depend on the former, though radiographic abnormalities are not uncommon when thermophilic organisms are involved and they are not unknown in their absence. Perhaps a more important feature of humidifier lung is the rapidly increasing frequency with which it is being recognized in both the workplace and the home. It may become the most common cause of EAA in developed countries, especially those of North America where prevalences of 15–52 per cent have been suggested in populations from contaminated offices. In Britain, bird fancier's lung may be more prevalent at present, simply because of the great popularity of keeping budgerigars and pigeons. Budgerigars are kept in some 12 per cent of British homes, and 0.5–7.5 per cent of the population involved are likely to have EAA as a consequence, albeit mildly in most cases. Pigeon keeping is 40 times less common, and the measured prevalence of pigeon fancier's lung has been a good deal more varied (0–21 per cent). This may reflect both true differences between groups of pigeon breeders as exposure levels vary according to number of birds, duration of exposure, loft ventilation, cleaning habits, etc. and artefactual differences arising as a result of selection bias and the notorious lack of compliance shown by pigeon fanciers in epidemiological studies. The responsible avian antigen and its precise source has yet to be identified, but bloom from the feathers containing saliva and secretory IgA is currently favoured over dust emanating from dried droppings.

The prevalence of farmer's lung rarely exceeds 10 per cent, even in areas of high rainfall, and where modern farming methods are used prevalence rates as low as 2–3 per cent have been observed. The farming population at risk represents a mere 1–2 per cent of the population at large, though there are marked regional variations. Even smaller populations are employed making whisky from germinating barley (maltings), raising mushrooms on a variety of antigenic composts, or handling bagasse (the fibrous stem that remains when sugar is extracted from sugar cane); but within some of these populations EAA was a common problem until excessive exposure levels were controlled. EAA associated with animals other than birds is extremely uncommon as is the case with the few chemicals currently reported to induce alveolitis. These two further groups of causative agents together with a few uncontaminated vegetable dusts nevertheless emphasize the wide range of working and domestic environments that may lead to EAA.

Mechanisms

The presumption that complexes of antigen and complement-activating antibodies (type III, Arthus hypersensitivity) are primarily responsible for EAA is now largely discarded. The evidence for deposition of immune complexes is not convincing, and neither IgG nor IgM antibodies are uniformly demonstrated in the sera of affected subjects unless sensitive detection techniques such as the enzyme-linked immunosorbent assay or radioimmunoassays are used. More importantly these antibodies are frequently found in subjects who are similarly exposed but clinically unaffected, irrespective of the method of detection. Furthermore, vasculitis, a cardinal feature of the experimental Arthus reaction, is not characteristically present, the acute inflammatory reaction being lymphocytic/mononuclear rather than polymorphonuclear. Lung tissue is most commonly examined during subacute phases of the disease, at which time a non-caseating granulomatous response suggesting type IV cell-mediated hypersensitivity is the usual finding, coupled with oedema and thickening of the alveolar walls, monocytic infiltration, and the presence of giant cells and epithelioid cells.

It could be argued that these histological appearances merely represent a healing reaction, but the finding of an acute T lymphocyte response in fluid obtained at bronchoalveolar lavage strongly supports the current consensus that cell-mediated hypersensitivity plays the dominant role in EAA. This is not to say other mechanisms play no role, nor that all inflammatory diseases of the gas exchanging tissues induced by organic dusts share a common mechanism. Indeed, the onset of symptoms within a few hours of exposure coupled with polymorphonuclear leucocytosis in peripheral blood does favour the participation of an additional (perhaps priming) immunological or toxic process. Components of a number of organic dusts associated with EAA are known to activate complement by the alternative pathway and this, with or without type III hypersensitivity, could prove to be relevant.

In fact, bronchoalveolar lavage in similarly exposed subjects has shown excess numbers of T lymphocytes whether they were clinically affected or not, though the proportions of T cell subpopulations may vary according to disease activity and the circumstances of exposure. In an intriguing study of an animal model of EAA, monkeys which developed characteristic reactions to inhalation challenge showed a helper T cell lymphocytosis (T4 cells with monoclonal T cell antisera) in bronchoalveolar fluid and a deficiency of suppressor (T8) cells, compared to the monkeys giving no clinical reaction who showed responses with both T4 and T8 cells. When the non-reactors were challenged again after low doses of body irradiation had impaired suppressor but not helper cell function, characteristic reactions were noted. These observations suggest that a relative impairment of suppressor cell function is fundamental to the development of EAA – a situation which has close parallels with sarcoidosis. It is interesting that lymphopenia in peripheral blood is a typical feature of acute exacerbations of the disease, the T lymphocytes migrating from blood to lungs within hours of the provoking exposure. It is small wonder that studies of systemic and local immune responses have given discordant results, and it is clear that continuing research should address both aspects of the immune response.

The systemic 'flu'-like symptoms that are so characteristic of the acute form of EAA are indistinguishable from grain fever in grain workers, 'Monday fever' in cotton workers, and humidifier fever in subjects exposed to microbially contaminated humidifiers. In these three situations, the febrile disorder is not characteristically associated with alveolar inflammation, raising the possibility that its occurrence with the acute form of EAA is an independent phenomenon, not an integral part of EAA itself. In favour of this hypothesis has been the finding of high levels of endotoxin from

Gram-negative bacteria (which are known to provoke these symptoms) in grain dust, cotton dust, contaminated humidifiers, and many of the 'mouldy' vegetable dusts that cause EAA. Not all inducers of EAA are contaminated with endotoxin, however, and so this hypothesis is not entirely satisfactory. In particular, inhalation provocation tests with uncontaminated bird serum in subjects with bird fancier's lung reproduce both alveolar and 'flu'-like responses, even in those who have the chronic form of the disease. The 'flu'-like response evidently is an integral feature of the acute form of EAA but it is relatively non-specific and can occur in many other situations.

EAA occurs in families only sporadically, and no association with HLA phenotypes has been demonstrated. It is therefore unlikely that genetic predisposition plays a major role in its development. It has been suggested that an acute inflammatory episode (from viral infection or the inhalation of microbial toxins or chemicals) may be necessary to disrupt the normal equilibrium of mucosal and local immunological defences, and thereby permit antigen to be presented in a fashion that leads to hypersensitivity. Smoking evidently does not provide such a disruptive effect, since smokers show reduced antibody responses and possibly have a lesser prevalence of EAA than non-smokers. The smoker without antibodies is, however, particularly liable to find his respiratory symptoms attributed to other diseases, and so this negative association between EAA and smoking may have been exaggerated.

Diagnosis
Establishing a diagnosis of EAA involves three areas of investigation: the lungs, the exposure, and the evidence of hypersensitivity.

Pulmonary investigations
In many cases EAA is first suspected after the presence of a diffuse alveolitis or progressive pulmonary fibrosis is known. With the acute form of the disease the chest radiograph will commonly show no abnormality unless symptoms are moderately severe. With the latter, there is a widespread alveolar filling pattern, particularly in the lower and mid-zones. This may resolve within a mere 24–48 hours once exposure has ceased. In more subacute forms, irregular small opacities are seen within the same distribution, simulating asbestosis. These may persist for several weeks despite cessation of exposure, and if exposure continues honeycombing may develop. By contrast, it is the upper zones that are predominantly affected by the irreversible fibrotic process that characterizes the chronic form of EAA. This may simulate sarcoidosis or even tuberculosis, and may lead to considerable shrinkage and distortion. In practice, the radiographic appearances vary considerably from patient to patient, and correlate poorly with clinical disease.

Lung function studies show impaired carbon monoxide gas transfer with a restrictive ventilatory defect though residual volume is characteristically increased suggesting air trapping as a result of bronchiolar involvement. Occasionally there is obstruction of the large airways also. Compliance is decreased and the arterial blood shows hypoxia (particularly on exercise) with hypocapnia.

Biopsy may be helpful in distinguishing EAA from cryptogenic fibrosing alveolitis (CFA) and other non-granulomatous alveolitides but is not commonly needed. The evolving technique of bronchoalveolar lavage may prove to be more helpful. EAA, like sarcoidosis, is associated with a T lymphocyte response in the alveolar fluid (lymphocytes represent > 10–20 per cent of recovered cells) whereas CFA characteristically produces a polymorphonuclear leucocyte response.

Exposure investigations
In many cases the history alone provides the evidence of relevant exposure. An independent account of the exposures involved can be invaluable. Ideally, industrial hygiene measurements are made so that respirable agents can be accurately identified and quanti-

fied. These are sophisticated investigations, mostly indicated when EAA is first suspected in an environment not previously associated with the disease, particularly in industries where many individuals may be at risk and where modification of the plant and its respirable environment may be a costly matter.

Immunological investigations
Laboratory demonstration of an IgG antibody response to the inducing organic dust is the most widely used method of 'confirming' hypersensitivity, but this has proved to be unsatisfactory as has the use of skin tests. Although affected subjects tend to have higher antibody levels than unaffected but exposed colleagues, most investigators have found the antibody response to correlate more closely with exposure than with disease. Tests for type IV hypersensitivity have been even more unsatisfactory. In practice the absence of a precipitin response is extremely uncommon in subjects eventually proved to have EAA, providing they are non-smokers.

When diagnosis remains in doubt, some form of inhalation challenge test may be considered necessary. The simplest method involves close supervision of experimental periods spent away from the suspected environment with similar periods of continuing exposure. The acute form of the disease is likely to be recognized in this way, though the procedure can be time-consuming and there may be practical problems of compliance. When a definitive diagnosis is particularly important formal laboratory-based provocation tests can be used. These employ a variety of techniques from nebulizing soluble extracts to recreating natural environmental exposures in an exposure chamber. Positive reactions are uncomfortable, and if excessive doses are administered they can be hazardous. Tests of this nature should consequently be restricted to centres with special experience.

Management
Of the individual
Management centres on reducing further exposure to the offending agent to a minimum. There is no place for desensitization. Ideally, the affected individual changes the relevant working or domestic environment completely, but this may mean a profound loss in income or great expense and is often unrealistic. Nor is it fully justified on purely medical grounds since continued exposure does not lead inevitably to progressive disease. A recent 15-year follow-up survey of farm workers presenting with the acute form of farmer's lung showed that while the majority continued to live on farms only a minority developed pulmonary fibrosis or impairment of carbon monoxide gas transfer.

The affected individual who continues to work in the occupation responsible for the disease can often reduce exposure substantially by changing the pattern of his particular duties. An alternative is the use of industrial respirators, which filter out 98–99 per cent of respirable dust from the ambient air. They are especially valuable when exposures are intermittent and comparatively brief. Whatever course is followed, continuing exposure should be accompanied by regular medical surveillance. If there is no progression, it is reasonable for reduced levels of exposure to continue.

When there is progressive disease, exposure should cease. This may involve a loss of earnings, and may entitle the affected worker to compensation. In Britain, industrial injuries legislation provides limited compensation from central government for both disability and loss of earnings for EAA of occupational origin. Acceptance of such compensation no longer debars the recipient from seeking redress in the civil courts, which is the primary mechanism of compensation in many countries. Rarely, the individual with progressive disease will refuse to change his occupation or hobby and the physician must weigh the possible advantages of long-term steroid therapy against the well-known risks.

Of the environment
Once EAA is recognized in one individual, the environment concerned should be assessed for the risk it poses to others. In many

circumstances this will be well known already, and exposure levels will be within the range considered acceptable.

When EAA arises in unfamiliar circumstances there may be a need not only to identify the causative agent but to survey the population at risk by questionnaire and serological investigations.

Modifications can always be made to the environment to lessen the level of exposure, but their extent will be limited by expense and must be justified by need. Dry storage and adequate ventilation are the two most important factors when vegetable produce is involved, and in some farming areas there is benefit in drying produce artificially after harvest. When ventilation and humidification systems are themselves responsible for EAA, major mechanical alterations may be necessary and the methods of humidification and temperature control changed. The crucial need is to reduce the ease with which airborne microbes are able to proliferate in stagnant collections of water. The need for rapid air changes coupled with close control of humidity and temperature poses formidable problems. The use of recirculated filtered air is the most economical, but effective filters are expensive and can become contaminated themselves, increasing rather than decreasing the load of respirable microbial antigens. The use of heat exchangers minimizes the cost of temperature control if contaminated exhaust air is not recirculated but does not conserve water.

References

Banaszak, E. F., Thiede, W. H. and Fink, J. N. (1970). Hypersensitivity pneumonia due to contamination of an air conditioner. *N. Engl. J. Med.* **283**, 271–276.

Braun, S. R., doPico, G. A., Tsiatis, A., *et al.* (1979). Farmer's lung disease: long term clinical and physiologic outcome. *Am. Rev. Resp. Dis.* **119**, 185–191.

Hendrick, D. J., Faux, J. A. and Marshall, R. (1978). Budgerigar fancier's lung: the commonest variety of allergic alveolitis in Britain. *Br. Med. J.* **2**, 81–84.

——, Marshall, R., Faux, J. A. and Krall, J. M. (1980). Positive 'alveolar' responses to antigen inhalation provocation tests: their validity and recognition. *Thorax* **35**, 415–427.

Leatherman, J. W., Michael, A. F., Schwarz, B. A. and Hoidal, J. R. (1984). Lung T cells in hypersensitivity pneumonitis. *Ann. intern. Med.* **100**, 390–392.

Morgan, D. C., Smyth, J. T., Lister, R. W. and Pethybridge, R. J. (1973). Chest symptoms and farmer's lung: a community survey. *Br. J. indust. Med.* **30**, 259–265.

Pepys, J., Jenkins, P. A., Festenstein, G. N., Lacey, M. E., Gregory, P. H. and Skinner, F. A. (1963). Farmer's lung. Thermophilic actinomycetes as a source of 'farmer's lung hay' antigens. *Lancet* **2**, 607–611.

Peterson, L. B., Thrall, R. S., Moore, V. L., Stevens, O. and Abramoff, P. (1977). An animal model of hypersensitivity pneumonitis in the rabbit. Induction of cellular hypersensitivity to inhaled antigens using Carageenan and BCG. *Am. Rev. Resp. Dis.* **116**, 1007–1012.

Cryptogenic fibrosing alveolitis

I. W. B. GRANT

This form of alveolar and interstitial lung disease, to which the term idiopathic pulmonary fibrosis (IPF) is applied in the American literature, differs from other types of fibrosing alveolitis (or interstitial fibrosis) in that it has no extrapulmonary manifestations, as with the multisystem connective tissue disorders, nor any identifiable cause, such as a pulmonary allergic reaction to an external agent, radiotherapy or drug sensitivity. Histologically, it is in most cases readily distinguishable from the 'secondary' forms of interstitial fibrosis seen in pulmonary asbestosis, sarcoidosis, and idiopathic pulmonary haemosiderosis, because the characteristic features of these primary diseases can usually be recognized even when the fibrosis has reached a fairly advanced stage. The pathologists may have problems, however, in deciding whether fibrosing alveolitis is the end-stage of chronic extrinisic allergic alveolitis ('hypersensitivity pneumonitis' in American parlance),

or is caused by radiotherapy or drug reactions. Such possibilities must always be excluded by a carefully taken clinical history before any case of fibrosing alveolitis is labelled as 'cryptogenic' from the histological appearances.

These observations may seem to suggest that cryptogenic fibrosing alveolitis is a diagnosis which can be made only by a process of elimination. In fact, the condition can be recognized clinically with a fair measure of confidence in patients with progressive exertional dyspnoea without wheeze who present with gross digital clubbing, persistent bilateral auscultatory crackles, a radiographic picture of shrunken lungs with diffuse reticulonodular shadowing, and physiological evidence of restrictive lung disease. In most such patients lung biopsy will merely confirm the diagnosis, but occasionally it will reveal some other form of diffuse pulmonary disease not suspected from the history or from the results of non-invasive investigations.

Historical background and terminology

Cryptogenic fibrosing alveolitis was first reported by Hamman and Rich in 1944 under the title 'Acute diffuse interstitial fibrosis of the lungs'. Their four patients all had a rapidly progressive form of the disease terminating fatally within six months, but it has subsequently been recognized that most cases pursue a much more chronic course, some surviving for several years without treatment. The term 'fibrosing alveolitis' was introduced by Scadding in 1964, 'cryptogenic' being added later to exclude cases with identifiable aetiological factors. This term was soon accepted in the United Kingdom as an appropriate description of a disease in which the alveolar walls are thickened by pleomorphic cellular exudate and fibrosis, and the alveolar spaces contain variable numbers of macrophages and desquamated pneumocytes. It was recognized that the predominance of each element in this histological pattern could vary from case to case, and even from one site to another in the same lung, but most British pathologists believed that these differences were not inconsistent with the concept of a single disease entity. Liebow *et al.* (1965), however, separately identified those cases in which the most prominent feature was the proliferation of alveolar macrophages and shedding of pneumocytes into the alveolar spaces, and coined the term 'desquamative interstitial pneumonia' to describe them. Liebow and Carrington (1969) then devised an extended classification of what they called 'interstitial pneumonia', which included undifferentiated interstitial pneumonia (UIP), desquamative interstitial pneumonia (DIP), undifferentiated interstitial pneumonia with bronchiolitis obliterans (BIP), lymphocytic interstitial pneumonia (LIP), and giant cell interstitial pneumonia (GIP). Yenokida and Crystal (1985), however, took issue with this classification by expressing the view, previously held by most British pathologists, that the first three are all forms of IPF, i.e. cryptogenic fibrosing alveolitis, each perhaps representing a different response to whatever has caused the alveolitis, whereas LIP and GIP are not morphological variants of that disease but manifestions of some unrelated immunological disorder. Although that view is widely accepted, there may be grounds for subdividing cryptogenic fibrosing alveolitis (IPF) into 'mural' (UIP) and 'desquamative' (DIP) types, if one or other of these histological patterns predominates, since this distinction may have some bearing on the nature of the radiographic abnormalities and perhaps on the response to corticosteriod therapy.

Theories of causation

Because of the histological similarity between the pulmonary lesions in cryptogenic fibrosing alveolitis and those observed in some multisystem connective tissue disorders, it is possible that all forms of fibrosing alveolitis have an immunological basis, involving some kind of autoimmune process. Support for that hypothesis is provided by the fairly frequent finding of organ non-specific auto-antibodies in the blood and the good response in some cases to the administration of corticosteroids, but it is disputed by some authorities mainly on the grounds that lung auto-antibodies have not been detected in the serum. Immune complexes, containing IgG and complement C3 have, however, been demonstrated in lung biopsy specimens, and it has been suggested (Yenokida and Crystal, 1985) that these may be generated as a result of an abnormal immune response to some extrinisic agent, such as a virus. Although the mechanism of immune complex formation in the lung remains obscure, their presence would appear to be the main factor in initiating a sequence of events which damages the connective tissue in the alveolar septa and the alveolar pneumocytes. These events probably include interaction of the immune complexes with macrophages, which are then stimulated to produce neutrophil chemotactic factor. The resultant accumulation and destruction of neutrophils may then release cytotoxic oxidases and proteases which are finally responsible for the alveolitis. The interstitial fibrosis may either be a reparative reaction to tissue damage caused by the alveolitis or an independent process resulting from the release from activated macrophages of substances which either act as chemoattractants to fibroblasts or stimulate their proliferation and increase their capacity to produce collagen. The pathogenesis of pulmonary fibrosis is discussed in more detail on page 15.43.

Pathology

In cryptogenic fibrosing alveolitis the lungs at autopsy are small, firm, and rubbery, having lost their normal spongy texture, and advanced interstitial fibrosis often produces the histological pattern of 'honeycomb lung' (see page 15.135). Biopsy earlier in the course of the disease, however, shows more specific changes at various stages of evolution. The alveolar septa are thickened by oedema, cellular exudate, and fibrosis, the degree of each depending on whether the alveolitis is acute or chronic, on the stage of the disease at which the biospy material is obtained, and on the site from which the biopsy is taken. The cellular exudate consists mainly of lymphocytes and macrophages but significant numbers of neutrophils and a few eosinophils are present in the more acute forms of disease. The exudate and fibroblastic proliferation may be so exuberant, particularly in acute cases, as to cause the cell-packed alveolar septa to herniate into the air spaces, some of which may be almost completely obliterated. The changes in the alveolar epithelium consist of the shedding of normal pneumocytes into the air spaces and their replacement by cuboidal epithelial cells. In the 'desquamative' form of the disease numbers of macrophages and neutrophils migrate into many of the air spaces, and when added to the debris of pneumocytes, may mimic an inflammatory intra-alveolar exudate. A hyaline membrane may be present within some alveoli.

About 10 per cent of patients with cryptogenic fibrosing alveolitis develop lung cancer. This figure is significantly in excess of the expected incidence, and cannot be accounted for by differences in age, sex, and smoking habits. The higher incidence of lung cancer has been noted in all forms of fibrosing alveolitis. The various histological types of tumour occur in the same proportions as in patients without that disease.

Clinical features

Cryptogenic fibrosing alveolitis is an uncommon disease, with a prevalence of only 2–3 per 100 000. It generally affects adults between the ages of 40 and 70 years, but occasionally occurs in younger subjects, including children.

The presenting symptom is usually breathlessness on exertion, although some patients may also complain of tiredness. The rate at which the dyspnoea increases in severity varies considerably from one patient to another. The acute form of the disease described by Hamman and Rich is relatively rare. In most cases the respiratory disability increases steadily over a timespan of 1 to 3 years, but in a few, particularly older, subjects it may remain almost static for even longer periods.

Most patients have a dry cough, often quite severe, from the start, and in the later stages of the disease bacterial infection becomes an increasingly frequent complication. In the vast majority of patients (about 90 per cent) a marked degree of digital clubbing develops at an early stage, and numerous coarse inspiratory crackles, with end-inspiratory high-pitched rhonchi, are audible on auscultation, chiefly over the lower lobes. In advanced cases bronchial breath sounds may be heard over areas of confluent fibrosis.

Pneumothorax is a complication of the late fibrotic stage. Type I respiratory failure eventually supervenes, and although this is usually accompanied by pulmonary hypertension, most patitents succumb from severe hypoxaemia before they develop right ventricular failure and peripheral oedema.

Radiological abnormalities

1. In most cases, particularly the more acute, the volume of the lung fields is symmetrically reduced, as shown by the abnormally high position of the diaphragm.
2. There is a combination of reticular, nodular, and striate shadowing throughout both lung fields. This is seldom completely uniform in distribution, usually being more conspicuous in the lower lobes. It has been suggested that the nodular type of shadowing is associated with the desquamative form of the disease, and the reticular and striate types with the mural form.

Pulmonary function tests

1. In all cases there is a restrictive ventilatory defect, with proportionate reductions in the forced expiratory volume in 1 s (FEV_1) and vital capacity (VC). The latter, being a rough index of lung compliance, is the more useful of these two measurements for the assessment of improvement or deterioration.
2. The carbon monoxide transfer factor (Tl_{CO}) is reduced, and falls steadily as the disease progresses.
3. In the early stages the partial pressure of oxygen in arterial blood (PaO_2) may be subnormal only on exercise, but in advanced cases the alveolar–arterial oxygen tension gradient is markedly increased, and the patient becomes severely hypoxaemic at rest. At this stage hyperventilation increases the degree of respiratory distress, and the partial pressure of carbon dioxide in arterial blood ($PaCO_2$) may fall to 4 kPa or less.

Other investigations
Blood
The haemoglobin level is seldom elevated, even in patients with chronic hypoxaemia, who might be expected to become polycythaemic. Anaemia is also uncommon except in the presence of chronic bacterial infection in damaged lung tissue, which is a frequent late complication. The total and differential white cell counts are usually normal, but the erythrocyte sedimentation rate is always moderately raised. The serum globulin is increased, chiefly the IgG fraction, but serum complement levels are usually normal. In 10–12 per cent of cases tests for antinuclear and/or rheumatoid factors are positive.

Bronchoalveolar lavage
The diagnostic value of this procedure in cryptogenic fibrosis alveolitis has not yet been fully established, but it is beginning to produce interesting and encouraging results. The total yield of cells is very much higher than in normal subjects, and these are predominately macrophages and neutrophils, with eosinophils in some cases. Biochemical studies, still in an early stage of development, may later increase the scope of this investigation.

Scintigraphic lung scanning
The ^{67}Ga scan is abnormal in 60–70 per cent of patients with cryptogenic fibrosing alveolitis. This probably reflects the number of activated macrophages, and possibly also neutrophils, in the alveolar walls and spaces, and thus the 'activity' of the alveolitis.

Since its results lack specificity, it is more useful for monitoring progress than as a diagnostic procedure.

Lung biospy

A firm diagnosis of fibrosing alveolitis can usually be made by lung biopsy, although other considerations, previously mentioned, must be taken into account before it is deemed 'cryptogenic'. Since the tiny and probably unrepresentative specimens obtained by transbronchial or percutaneous biopsy seldom provide the pathologist with sufficient tissue for accurate histological interpretation, open biopsy by thoracotomy is without question the only certain means of achieving this objective, two or three specimens being taken from where there are different degrees of visible or palpable abnormality in the lung. Thoracotomy is not devoid of risk, particularly in hypoxaemic patients, and a decision to advise open lung biopsy must, as Professor Turner-Warwick has emphasized in the Introduction to this Section, balance any such risk against that of failure to make a secure histological diagnosis. In patients with suspected cryptogenic fibrosing alveolitis who are under the age of 70 years and are reasonably fit in terms of general health and respiratory function, there is a strong case for lung biopsy, since it provides the physician with information which is essential for correct treatment and rational patient management.

Treatment and progress

The administration of an oral corticosteroid, such as prednisolone, is followed by complete relief of symptoms and objective evidence of improvement in only 15–20 per cent of cases, but in a further 30 per cent there may be some degree of subjective improvement, although this is often only temporary. A good response is observed more frequently in younger patients with acute forms of the disease where cellular infiltration in the alveolar septa is more conspicuous than fibrosis in lung biopsies. There is also some evidence, not yet fully substantiated, that the response to corticosteroids is more favourable when 'desquamative' features dominate the histological picture.

A high dose of prednisolone (60 mg/day) should be given initially, and after a few weeks this should be reduced cautiously to a maintenance level of 10–15 mg/day. Adjustments in this dose may be indicated from time to time and these should be governed by regular assessment (every 2–3 months) of the radiographic appearances and of trends in the VC, PaO_2, $PaCO_2$, and Tl_{co}. If facilities are available, serial ^{67}Ga lung scans may also be of value in monitoring the response to treatment, but repeated bronchoalveolar lavage, although potentially useful, will be declined by most patients, and is clearly not essential. The sudden withdrawal of treatment or too rapid a reduction in dosage may precipitate an acute relapse of the disease.

Older patients with a long history, in whom alveolar septal fibrosis is the dominant histological feature, seldom respond to corticosteroid therapy, but they tend to deteriorate more slowly.

If prednisolone in high dosage produces unacceptable side-effects, it can be partially or completely replaced by azathioprine or cyclophosphamide, but treatment with these drugs alone seems to have no specific advantages.

In the later stages of the disease oxygen will be required to correct hypoxaemia, but dyspnoea may become so distressing that it can be relieved only by opiates, which in these circumstances should not be withheld.

References

Hamman, L. and Rich, A. R. (1944). Acute diffuse interstitial fibrosis of the lungs. *Bull. John Hopkins Hosp.* **74**, 177–204.

Liebow, A. A. and Carrington, C. B. (1969). The interstitial pneumonias. In *Frontiers of pulmonary radiology* (eds M. Simon, E. J. Potchen and M. Le May), pp. 102–141. Grune and Stratton, New York.

——, Steer, A. and Billingsley, J. G. (1965). Desquamative interstitial pneumonia. *Am. J. Med.* **39**, 369–404.

Turner-Warwick, M. (1978). Interstitial pneumonias and fibrosing alveolitis. *Immunology of the lung*, pp. 216–248. Edward Arnold, London.

——, Burrows, B. and Johnson, A. (1980). Cryptogenic fibrosing alveolitis: clinical features and their influence on survivial. *Thorax* **35**, 171–180.

——, ——, ——, (1980). Cryptogenic fibrosing alveolitis: response to corticosteroid treatment and its effect on survival. *Thorax* **35**, 593–599.

Scadding, J. G. (1964). Fibrosing alveolitis (correspondence). *Br. Med. J.* **2**, 686.

Yenokida, G. G. and Crystal, R. G. (1985). Idiopathic pulmonary fibrosis and the 'interstitial pneumonias'. *Current perspectives in the immunology of respiratory diseases*' (eds E. J. Goetzl and A. B. Kay), pp. 128–147. Churchill Livingstone, Edinburgh.

Radiation alveolitis

I. W. B. GRANT

This iatrogenic form of alveolitis, which may follow the exposure of lung tissue to ionizing radiation (X-rays) in therapeutic dosage, has histological similarities to cryptogenic fibrosing alveolitis although, in the earlier stages at least, the changes in the alveolar epithelium and the migration of macrophages into the air spaces are usually more conspicuous than the cellular exudate and fibrosis in the alveolar septa.

Factors influencing the development and extent of the pulmonary changes

Severe radiation alveolitis was once a fairly common complication of 'wide-field' irradiation of the whole thorax in diseases such as lymphoma and multiple secondary deposits in the lungs from testicular or thyroid tumours, but this form of radiotherapy has now been abandoned. Irradiation of extrapulmonary structures such as breast, mediastinum, oesophagus, and spine employs techniques which reduce to a minimum the dose of X-rays absorbed by lung tissue and ensure that it affects only small volumes of lung, but occasionally, for reasons unknown, radiation alveolitis develops outside the treatment field. In these circumstances, and also when a bronchial carcinoma is irradiated, the degree and extent of the pulmonary damage may be sufficient to cause impairment of respiratory function in addition to abnormal radiographic shadowing. In general, the severity of radiation alveolitis is dose-related but it may be aggravated by the administration, before or after radiotherapy, of cytotoxic drugs such as Adriamycin or by pulmonary bacterial infection.

Course of the disease

Mild radiation alveolitis following, for example, radiotherapy for breast carcinoma is usually asymptomatic unless the patient has pre-existing impairment of pulmonary function, and is recognized only if the chest is X-rayed. In more severe cases the patient complains of exertional dyspnoea 3 to 6 weeks after the end of the course of radiotherapy. At this stage, there is thickening of the alveolar septa by oedema and chronic inflammatory cells, and also enlargement and desquamation of alveolar epithelial cells, the second feature usually predominating. Without treatment the respiratory disability may become rapidly more severe, and cause death from hypoxaemia, but in some cases there is gradual spontaneous improvement after a few weeks. In either event, fibroblasts begin to replace the inflammatory cells in the alveolar septa, and the end result in patients who survive is interstitial fibrosis (radiation fibrosis) of varying degree and extent.

The pathogenesis of radiation alveolitis is not fully understood, but it may be an immunological reaction to alveolar cells rendered antigenic by the effects of ionizing radiation.

Clinical and other findings in severe cases

1. The patient is dyspnoeic at rest or on mild exertion, and central cyanosis will often be present. Because of the sudden decrease in lung compliance, some patients exhibit 'door-stop breathing', in

which there is an abrupt halt to every inspiration. Coarse inspiratory crackles are audible over the affected regions of the lung.

2. The chest radiograph in the early stages shows dense patchy shadowing mainly confined to the irradiated areas of lung, but in some cases extending beyond the margins of the treatment field. Later, the shadowing assumes a more fibrotic pattern, in some cases conforming fairly sharply to the irradiated area but in others extending more widely and involving both lungs.

3. If the radiation alveolitis is localized, there may be only minor disturbances of pulmonary function, but when it is extensive and progressive, the VC falls sharply, with a proportionate decrease in FEV_1 and reductions in total lung capacity and $T1_{CO}$. Continued deterioration leads to the development of type I respiratory failure, with severe hypoxaemia caused by ventilation–perfusion imbalance and hypocapnia induced by hyperventilation.

Treatment and prognosis

Patients with localized radiation alveolitis recover without treatment, but there is often residual pulmonary fibrosis. Those with severe dyspnoea and extensive pulmonary shadowing in the acute phase should always be treated with prednisolone, starting with a dose of 60 mg/day. The response varies considerably from case to case. In some patients there is dramatic improvement, but in others, the treatment appears to be of little or no value. Even in those who respond well initially relapse is apt to follow a premature reduction in the dose of prednisolone, which should usually be maintained in these cases at a level of about 20 mg/day for up to 3 months.

References

Douglas, A. C. (1959). Treatment of radiation pneumonitis with prednisolone. *Br. J. Dis. Chest.* **53**, 346–355.

Whitfield, A. G. W., Bond, W. H. and Kunkler, P. B. (1963). Radiation damage to thoracic tissues. *Thorax* **18**, 371–380.

Pulmonary manifestations of connective tissue disorders

D. M. GEDDES

The lungs, being chiefly made up of blood vessels and connective tissue, are vulnerable to involvement by all the connective tissue disorders. Not only may the lungs be affected in a number of different ways, but also the pleura and chest wall may be sites of disease. While pulmonary involvement is often mild and clinically unimportant, occasionally the lung is the main organ involved and in some disorders the lesions can be fatal. The spectrum of pulmonary complications of these disorders is summarized in Table 1. Fuller descriptions of the connective tissue diseases appear elsewhere in this textbook and this section will concentrate exclusively on the pulmonary features of these disorders.

Systemic lupus erythematosus (SLE)

Incidence

The reported incidence of pulmonary involvement in SLE varies widely. Whilst figures up to 70 per cent emerge from autopsy studies, significant clinical lung disease, though undoubtedly common, may only be found in 30 per cent. Spontaneous and drug-induced SLE are similar in this respect.

Pathogenesis

There are four main mechanisms of pulmonary damage:

1. Direct effect of SLE on lung tissue. The relative importance of immune complex damage as opposed to cell-mediated tissue antigen directed auto-aggression is unclear but there is evidence to suggest both operate.

2. Indirect effect of SLE on the lung secondary to involvement of another organ system, e.g. thrombocytopenia contributing to pulmonary haemorrhage; uraemic pulmonary oedema.

3. Infection. The patient with SLE is predisposed to infection both as a result of the disease itself and on account of the drugs used to treat it.

4. Drug toxicity.

Clinical patterns

The clinical manifestations of SLE in the pulmonary system vary widely and symptoms such as cough, with or without mucoid or mucopurulent sputum, dyspnoea, and pleuritic pain are by no means specific. Haemoptysis is rare but can be massive. Fever is either associated with early onset acute disease or with superimposed infection in more chronic disease.

Pleuropericarditis

This is common and presents with pleuritic pain and breathlessness often with fever. Chest radiographs show pleural effusions, usually bilateral and small, but sometimes unilateral and occasionally massive: there may in addition be evidence of pericarditis or pericardial effusion. The pleural fluid contains more than 30 g/l protein with normal sugar and predominant lymphocytes: LE cells may be seen and ANF is often high, while complement activity is low. Though the findings are often non-specific pleural aspiration and biopsy should be done to exclude infection.

Spontaneous resolution is not infrequent but persisting or relapsing disease responds well to corticosteroids. Although a few

Table 1 Pulmonary involvement in connective tissue diseases

	Airways	Alveoli	Pleura	Thoracic cage
Systemic lupus erythematosus	—	Pneumonia Lupus pneumonitis Atelectasis Pulmonary oedema Fibrosing alveolitis	Pleurisy Effusions	High diaphragms (vanishing lung)
Rheumatoid arthritis	Bronchiectasis Obliterative bronchiolitis	Pneumonia Fibrosing alveolitis Nodules	Effusion	—
Systemic sclerosis	Bronchiectasis	Aspiration pneumonia Fibrosing alveolitis	Effusion	Scleroderma of chest wall
Dermatomyositis	Neoplasm	Aspiration pneumonia Fibrosing alveolitis	—	Myositis of respiratory muscles
Ankylosing spondylitis	—	Upper zone fibrosis	—	Fusion of costovertebral joints

patients experience frequent relapses and some have progressive multisystem disease, the prognosis in this form of SLE is usually good.

Atelectasis

This is a radiographic diagnosis which may be made in isolation on a routine film but more commonly is seen in association with pleurisy (above), pneumonia or diaphragmatic disease (below). The usual mechanism is poor respiratory excursion secondary to pain or poor diaphragmatic movement. Surfactant abnormalities or pulmonary venous involvement have also been suggested as mechanisms but on inadequate evidence. Typically there are bilateral basal linear shadows 1–4 cm in length, so-called 'plate atelectasis'. Sometimes the lines extend from diaphragm to hilum crossing segmental boundaries when their pathogenesis is more obscure.

No specific investigations or treatment are required although corticosteroids may be needed for the associated pleurisy or pneumonia.

Lupus pneumonitis

The clinical picture is of pneumonia or pulmonary infarction with fever, cough, and rapid respiration, and a reduction in arterial P_{O_2}. The consolidation is usually basal, often bilateral and occasionally associated with pleural fluid.

The diagnosis can only be made presumptively. Infection and haemorrhage may be excluded by bronchoscopic lavage and empirical antibiotic therapy. Lung biopsy can be considered but carries an appreciable risk in these patients. Lupus pneumonitis responds to corticosteroids and immunosuppressive treatment.

High diaphragms (Fig. 1)

A few patients develop diaphragmatic elevation in the absence of any lung or pleural disease. There is progressive breathlessness usually without other symptoms or abnormal clinical findings. The probable cause is a diaphragmatic myopathy although the evidence for this is incomplete and subclinical lung or pleural inflammation may sometimes contribute. The lung volumes are low and the diaphragm cannot generate normal pressures. Lung compliance appears appropriate for the low volume. No treatment has been shown to influence the progression of this disorder.

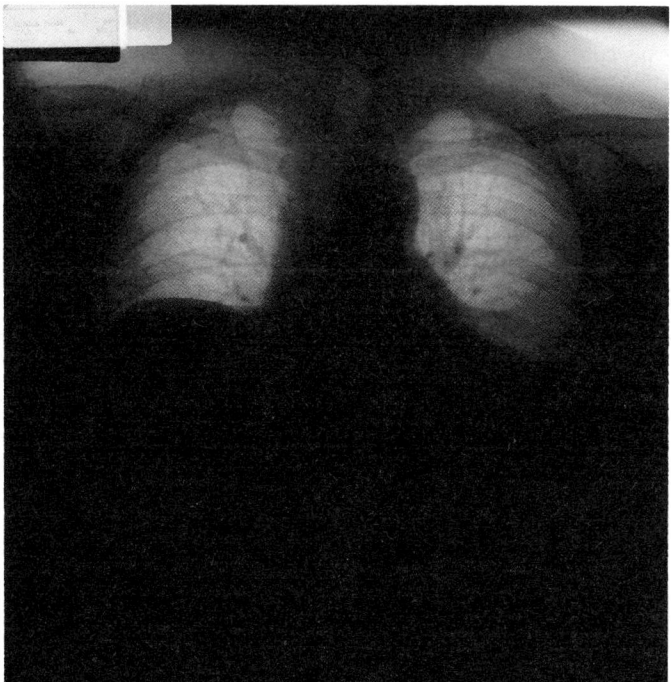

Fig. 1 High diaphragms in a patient with SLE causing the 'vanishing lung' syndrome.

Fibrosing alveolitis

This is rare in SLE in spite of high levels of circulating immune complexes and the occasional demonstration of immune complex deposition with complement activation in the pulmonary capillaries. Some degree of fibrosis may also follow lupus pneumonitis, and cyclophosphamide therapy is occasionally implicated. There is diffuse lower zone radiographic shadowing with crackles and occasionally clubbing. Response to corticosteroids and immunosuppressive drugs is unpredictable.

Rheumatoid disease

Incidence

Pulmonary involvement in rheumatoid disease is seldom very important clinically. However, subclinical involvement is frequent. Minor abnormalities of lung function have been reported in 20–40 per cent of patients and amyloid deposits in the pulmonary vasculature are common. Lung disorders in rheumatoid disease occur more frequently in men than women. This probably reflects smoking habits since smoking is an additional risk factor either by increasing pulmonary capillary permeability or by initiating an inflammatory response. Patients with severe seropositive nodular rheumatoid disease are those most likely to develop pulmonary complications.

Clinical patterns

Pleural effusion

This is the commonest form of pulmonary involvement occurring in 2–8 per cent of cases and may precede the development of overt arthritis. The effusions are usually asymptomatic, unilateral, small, and tend to organize rather than progress. Only rarely is an effusion massive and recurrent. The features of the fluid are similar to those of synovial fluid in rheumatoid joints and it is likely that the same pathological processes affect both serous membranes resulting in an inflammatory exudate. The protein is > 30 g/l with a low sugar and high lactate dehydrogenase. There is often a characteristic cytological picture of degenerating polymorphs, amorphous extracellular material, and epithelioid cells (which may be multinucleate). Rheumatoid factor is present in the fluid, often in high titres.

Pleural aspiration and biopsy should be performed to exclude infection and malignancy. Empyema is a surprisingly common complication of rheumatoid disease. Treatment of uncomplicated rheumatoid pleural effusion is seldom needed but persistent accumulations of fluid may need repeated aspiration. Chemical pleurodesis is occasionally required.

Fibrosing alveolitis

Though this occurs in less than 1 per cent of patients with rheumatoid disease, because of the frequency of the disease, fibrosing alveolitis is more likely to be seen in association with rheumatoid than with any of the other connective tissue disorders. Immune complex deposits have been reported to occur in the pulmonary vessels and may initiate the alveolitis which progresses slowly to fibrosis. The clinical picture of breathlessness, dry cough, basal crackles, and sometimes clubbing is identical to cryptogenic pulmonary fibrosis although the clinical course is often more benign. A tissue diagnosis is not usually required and treatment seldom has any striking effect. A trial of corticosteroids possibly with immunosuppressive drugs should be considered for severe or progressive disease but should be stopped if the chest radiograph or lung function tests do not improve.

Pulmonary nodules

These have the same histology and presumably the same aetiology as subcutaneous rheumatoid nodules with which they are frequently associated. They can be single or multiple, small or large (up to 7 cm in diameter), and tend to be situated peripherally in the lung. They may grow or occasionally disappear, and not infrequently cavitate. Rarely rheumatoid nodules calcify, erode a rib or break down to cause a pleural effusion or bronchopleural fistula.

The clinical problem is to exclude malignancy or infection at an early stage. If the nodules are multiple, unchanging, and causing no symptoms they can be observed. A new solitary nodule, especially if it is growing or has cavitated, may need a thoracotomy for precise diagnosis. No treatment is required once the diagnosis is made.

Rheumatoid nodules in the lung are sometimes seen in coal miners in association with an often mild simple pneumoconiosis (Caplan's syndrome). They develop more rapidly than progressive massive fibrosis and often occur in crops. Apart from coal dust deposited in them, they are indistinguishable from other rheumatoid lung nodules histologically and clinically behave in the same way.

Obliterative bronchiolitis
This complication is very rare but can be fatal. The small airways are narrowed by chronic inflammation which obliterates the lumen. Autoimmune inflammation, a persistent severe viral infection, and penicillamine have all been suggested as causal factors.

Breathlessness develops quite rapidly, usually without a history of viral infection and may stabilize or progress to respiratory failure. Widespread inspiratory crackles and an occasional midinspiratory squeak can be heard over the lung fields but the chest radiograph is normal. Lung function tests show fixed small airways obstruction. Corticosteroids and possibly immunosuppressive drugs should be given to try to prevent obliteration and to suppress active inflammation but there is little evidence of benefit.

Bronchopulmonary sepsis
Some patients with rheumatoid disease develop frequent and severe chest infections. There are many factors involved and these include general debility, poor nutrition, and relative immunosuppression both from the rheumatoid disease itself and its treatment, difficulty in coughing and expectorating secondary to painful arthritis, and possibly diminished local host defences secondary to an associated sicca syndrome. The bronchiectasis which develops can be difficult to treat because the arthritis makes physiotherapy painful.

Drug toxicity
Some of the drugs used in rheumatoid disease have specific pulmonary side-effects. These include pulmonary eosinophilia (aspirin), acute alveolitis (penicillamine), and progressive lung fibrosis (gold) (see page 15.143).

Systemic sclerosis
Lung involvement in this disorder is evident in 90 per cent of patients at autopsy or on lung function testing, though few have clinically important symptoms or abnormal chest radiographs. The disease is commoner in women and in late middle age. Four facets of the disease affect the pulmonary system.

Recurrent bacterial infection
Aspiration pneumonia secondary to oesophageal disease contributes to lower lobe fibrosis and bronchiectasis.

Fibrosing alveolitis
This is manifest radiographically as basal reticular or reticulonodular infiltration perhaps with cyst formation and is due to a combination of systemic sclerosis affecting the lung connective tissue together with the effects of organizing aspiration pneumonias. There is progressive loss of lung volume and the fibrosis causes increasing breathlessness which is largely uninfluenced by treatment.

Pulmonary hypertension
This produces breathlessness with relatively normal lung fields on chest radiograph. The proximal pulmonary vasculature may be

fibrosed but may also be overreactive as shown by an increase in pulmonary artery pressure on cooling the skin. There are no reports of treatment of this complication, though some vasodilators are known to affect the pulmonary circulation.

Scleroderma of the chest wall
Occasionally chest expansion is limited by rigid skin.

Dermatomyositis
Dermatomyositis and polymyositis both cause muscle pain and weakness and this has implications for the respiratory system if it involves thoracic cage or oropharyngeal muscles.

Respiratory muscle involvement
Myositis of the diaphragm and intercostal muscles results in breathlessness and small lung volumes with basal atelectasis.

Aspiration pneumonia
This occurs as a result of pharyngeal and laryngeal myositis. In combination with thoracic muscle involvement it can lead to an end-stage picture of respiratory failure.

Fibrosing alveolitis
This is relatively rare, has no specific features, and responds poorly to treatment.

Neoplasm
Malignancy of the lung or elsewhere can occur with dermatomyositis and may then be the underlying cause of the disorder.

Sjögren's syndrome
This chronic autoimmune disorder usually affects middle-aged women and is characterized by keratoconjunctivitis sicca, xerostomia, and, in about half the cases, evidence of a systemic connective tissue disorder. Pulmonary involvement is not common and seldom important clinically. The bronchial mucosal glands can be involved and this presumably alters pulmonary secretions. However, there is no evidence that this impairs mucociliary clearance. Fibrosing alveolitis, transient pulmonary infiltrates, and recurrent infections are other reported features, and can occur independently of any underlying connective tissue disorder.

Ankylosing spondylitis
This condition with its male predominance and early occurrence (third decade) involves the lungs in two ways.

Reduced rib movement
Restricted chest expansion is due to fusion of the costovertebral joints. While this can cause breathlessness, functional impairment is usually mild.

Upper zone fibrosis
This is usually bilateral with slow progression from apical pleural fibrosis to interstitial fibrosis with cavitation. The chest radiograph resembles that seen in fibrotic tuberculosis but infecting organisms cannot usually be found. Various species of atypical mycobacteria are occasionally isolated and should be treated appropriately. Aspergillomas may develop in the cavities but need not be treated unless haemoptysis is life-threatening. Removal at thoracotomy is then necessary but there is a considerable postoperative morbidity in these patients.

Mixed connective tissue disease
This disorder with a mixture of clinical features of systemic sclerosis, SLE, polymyositis, and rheumatoid disease seldom presents with pulmonary features though functionally and radiographically more than three-quarters will have some abnormality. Late in the disease significant pulmonary hypertension is the chief feature. Fibrosing alveolitis is a rare complication but a few patients have been reported with unusually rapid progression of the fibrosis.

References

Fairfax, A. J., Haslam, P. L., Pavia, P. *et. al.* (1981). Pulmonary disorders associated with Sjögren's syndrome. *Q. J. Med.* **199**, 279–295.

Frazier, A. R. and Miller, R. D. (1974). Interstitial pneumonitis in association with polymyositis and dermatomyositis. *Chest* **65**, 403–407.

Geddes, D. M., Corrin, B., Brewerton, D. A. *et al.* (1977). Progressive airway obliteration in adults and its association with rheumatoid disease. *Q. J. Med.* **46**, 427–449.

Gibson, G. L., Edmonds, J. P. and Hughes, G. R. V. (1977). Diaphragm function and lung involvement in SLE. *Am. J. Med.* **63**, 926.

Haupt, H. M., Moore, G. W. and Hutchins, G. M. (1981). The lung in SLE. *Am. J. Med.* **71**, 791–798.

Hunninghake, G. W. and Fauce, A. S. (1979). Pulmonary involvement in collagen vascular disease. *Am. Rev. Resp. Dis.* **119**, 471–503.

Scadding, J. G. (1969). The lungs in rheumatoid arthritis. *Proc. R. Soc. Med.* **62**, 227–238.

Sullivan, W. D., Hurst, D. J., Harman, C. E. *et al.* (1984). A prospective evaluation emphasising pulmonary involvement in patients with mixed connective tissue disease. *Medicine (Balt.)* **63**, 92–107.

Pulmonary haemorrhage disorders

D. M. GEDDES

A range of different disorders can cause recurrent bleeding from the pulmonary capillaries producing the clinical triad of haemoptysis, diffuse alveolar opacities on the chest radiograph, and anaemia. These conditions can be classified as follows

1. Chronic pulmonary venous congestion. Mitral stenosis, left ventricular failure, pulmonary veno-occlusive disease (see Section 13).
2. Goodpasture's syndrome
3. Idiopathic pulmonary haemosiderosis
4. Pulmonary vasculitis usually associated with connective tissue disorders, e.g. SLE
5. Bleeding disorders (see page 19.211).

Goodpasture's syndrome (see page 18.43)

Goodpasture originally described a man who died with pulmonary haemorrhage and glomerulonephritis. The syndrome is now usually considered as a triad of these two features together with the demonstration of antibodies to glomerular basement membrane.

Pathology and pathogenesis

Although there is sometimes a history of a recent viral infection or hydrocarbon inhalation, the initiating event is unknown but presumably involves the unmasking of a previously hidden antigen. Antibodies to one or more basement membrane antigens circulate and deposit in the kidneys to produce a glomerulonephritis and in the lungs to damage vessel walls and allow bleeding. Immunofluorescence shows a linear deposition of antibody along the basement membrane with additional complement deposition in some 60 per cent. Presumably the lungs share the same basement membrane antigen as the kidneys since a more generalized deposition of antibody along other vascular basement membranes has not been observed (though there is binding of antibody to choroid plexus). The vast majority of patients are smokers: it is thought that smoking initiates some degree of pulmonary damage or inflammation which allows bleeding to occur. This implies that antibasement membrane antibody deposition in the lung may occur more commonly but remain clinically silent.

Histologically the lungs show red cellls in the alveoli following acute bleeding and later there are haemosiderin-laden macrophages. The glomeruli show focal proliferative and necrotizing glomerulonephritis usually with crescent formation. There is no vasculitis in the pulmonary or other systemic blood vessels. Electron microscopy shows swelling and defects in the basement membrane but no immune complexes.

Clinical features

The syndrome predominantly affects young male smokers who present with cough, breathlessness, and haemoptysis. Pulmonary symptoms usually come first with haemoptysis heading the list. Renal disease may be missed at this stage because it is only evident as proteinuria or microscopic haematuria. Within a few days or weeks renal involvement becomes clinically obvious and may progress rapidly to renal failure. The haemoptysis is intermittent and ranges from occasional streaks to massive fatal bleeding. Systemic symptoms of fever, joint pains or weight loss are unusual.

The chest radiograph shows patchy shadows due to intra-alveolar blood. These shadows may be single or multiple or occur diffusely throughout both lung fields (Fig. 1). The shadows resolve over the course of two weeks unless there is further bleeding. At the time of bleeding there may be arterial hypoxaemia, reduced lung volumes, but increased carbon monoxide gas transfer as the inspired carbon monoxide is taken up by the blood within the lungs. This test can be used to monitor the progress of the pulmonary bleeding. Haemosiderin-laden macrophages are found in the sputum. Prolonged severe bleeding leads to an iron-deficiency anaemia. Renal function may be normal initially and then deteriorates over days to weeks.

The diagnosis is confirmed by demonstrating circulating antibasement membrane antibodies (present in 90 per cent) or by demonstrating linear immunofluorescence on renal biopsy. The antibasement membrane antibody titre does not correlate well with clinical progress.

Treatment

The main treatment is plasma exchange which must be started early before there is irreversible renal damage and continued until antibasement membrane antibodies are absent. Steroids and immunosuppressant drugs may be helpful temporarily to control the pulmonary haemorrhage but probably have only a secondary role in controlling the renal disease. Nephrectomy may be required for uncontrollable pulmonary haemorrhage or for irreversible renal failure. Transplantation can be successful but must be delayed until after the disappearance of antibasement membrane antibody.

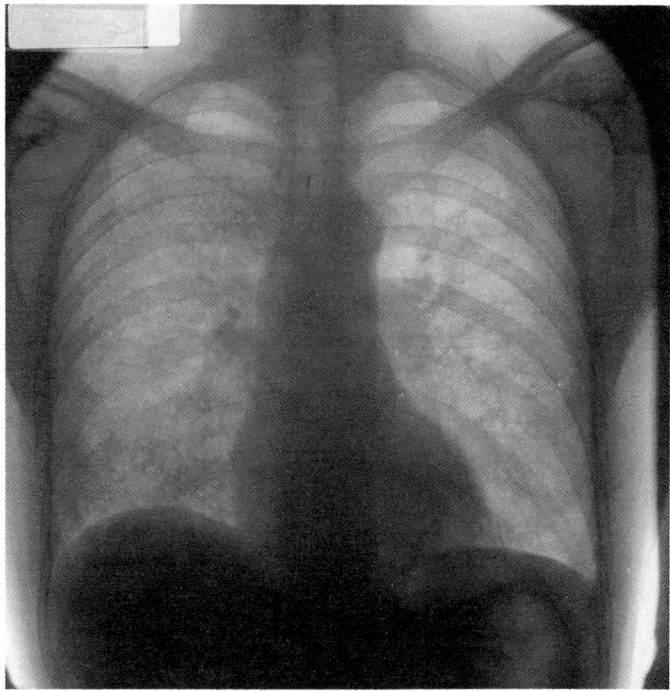

Fig. 1 Intra-alveolar haemorrhage in a patient with Goodpasture's syndrome.

Prognosis

The outlook from Goodpasture's syndrome has improved dramatically in recent years partly as a result of plasma exchange and partly because milder degrees of the syndrome are being recognized. With adequate treatment the majority of patients can now be expected to survive.

Idiopathic pulmonary haemosiderosis

Introduction

This is a rare disorder of children and young adults in which there is recurrent bleeding into the lungs. The extravasated blood is taken up by macrophages which become loaded with haemosiderin, and repeated bleeding may cause an iron-deficiency anaemia. Blood in the alveoli is in some way fibrogenic and diffuse pulmonary fibrosis eventually develops. Other conditions which cause recurrent alveolar bleeding such as mitral stenosis and chronic severe left ventricular failure can result in identical pathological changes.

Pathology and pathogenesis

The cause of idiopathic pulmonary haemosiderosis is unknown. Immune complexes are not found in the serum or pulmonary capillaries, there is no evidence of antibasement membrane antibody and the electron microscopic appearance of the basement membrane shows no consistent abnormality. Serum IgA is elevated in over half the cases and there have been reports of associations with rheumatoid arthritis, cow's milk antibodies, and gasoline products. Coeliac disease is another association and this subgroup shows a high incidence of HLA B8 antigen. However, none of these is a consistent finding and they do not shed light on the cause of the disorder. Histologically the lungs show intra-alveolar blood and normal alveolar walls in the acute stage, and intra-alveolar haemosiderin-laden macrophages and non-specific interstitial fibrosis in chronic disease.

Clinical features

Idiopathic pulmonary haemosiderosis presents either as recurrent acute pulmonary bleeding or as progressive breathlessness with diffuse radiographic changes. The acute bleeds are more common in childhood and may be life-threatening. Physical examination is unhelpful and the chest radiograph shows very variable alveolar shadowing due to blood. These shadows clear completely over 1–3 weeks. Repeated bleeds may cause severe iron-deficiency anaemia which itself gives rise to symptoms and eventually a large bleed can be fatal. The more chronic form chiefly occurs in adults when progressive breathlessness and iron-deficiency anaemia are the main features. Haemoptysis in the chronic form is usually of small volume and occasional. Systemic symptoms are rare. Some patients with the more indolent disease eventually die of acute massive bleeding but slow progression to diffuse pulmonary fibrosis with honeycombing is more usual. The chest radiograph shows widespread fine discrete nodules with subsequent contraction due to the fibrosis. Lung function tests show progressive loss of volumes with reduction of gas transfer: an obstructive defect occurs occasionally and this is unexplained.

Treatment

The treatment is supportive during the acute bleeding and artificial ventilation is occasionally required. The role of corticosteroids, cytotoxic drugs, and plasma exchange in limiting acute or chronic bleeding is unclear. They should be tried when the disease is progressing but there is no good evidence of benefit. Chelating agents to remove pulmonary iron and so limit fibrosis have been suggested but are also unproved. Occasional patients appear to recover spontaneously with or without a degree of permanent pulmonary damage.

Other causes of alveolar haemorrhage

Alveolar haemorrhage occurs in a variety of other disorders which are considered elsewhere in this textbook. Though the haemorrhage can be equally as dramatic as in Goodpasture's syndrome or as persistent as in idiopathic pulmonary haemosiderosis (IPH), it is generally overshadowed by other features of the disease in question. A list will provide a differential diagnosis and a means of cross referencing.

Systemic lupus erythematosus In this disease alveolar haemorrhage is a rare but serious lung manifestation characterized by massive intra-alveolar bleeding without evidence of pulmonary vasculitis: 70 per cent of cases in a series of 23 were fatal.

Systemic vasculitides particularly those with prominent necrosis, may present with alveolar haemorrhage though this complication is unusual in the better characterized syndromes such as Wegener's granulomatosis.

Rapidly progressive glomerulonephritis whether immune complex-mediated or not may be accompanied by alveolar haemorrhage. Indeed in half of immunofluorescent negative cases haemoptysis and pulmonary infiltrates have been recorded, though the pattern of the pulmonary disease is often mild.

Alveolar haemorrhage has been reported to result from various exogenous agents such as D-penicillamine, lymphangiography contrast media, and trimellitic anhydride fumes or powder.

References

Leatherman, J. W., Davies, S. F. and Hoidal, J. R. (1984). Alveolar haemorrhage syndromes: diffuse microvascular lung haemorrhage in immune and idiopathic disorders. *Medicine (Balt.)* **63**, 343–361.
Peters, D. K., Rees, A. J., Lockwood, C. M. and Pusey, C. D. (1982). Treatment and prognosis of anti-basement membrane antibody mediated nephritis. *Transp. Proc.* **14**, 513–521.
Soergel, K. H. and Sommers, S. C. (1962). Idiopathic pulmonary haemosiderosis and related syndromes. *Am. J. Med.* **32**, 499–511.
Teague, C. A., Doak, P. B., Simpson, I. J. *et al.* (1978). Goodpastures Syndrome: an analysis of 29 cases. *Kidney Int.* **13**, 492–504.

Pulmonary eosinophilia

D. J. LANE

Introduction

The finding of a significant peripheral blood eosinophilia excites the imagination and interest of clinicians when seen in association with evident disease in some organ or system. Various different syndromes have thus been defined and attempts made to classify each in the context of other similar disorders. Perhaps nowhere has this led to such a profusion of confusing terminology and classification as in the context of pulmonary disease. 1952 was a seminal year in this field seeing the publication in the United Kingdom of Crofton's classification of the 'pulmonary eosinophilias' and in the United States of Reeder and Goodrich's introduction of the term the 'PIE syndrome' – pulmonary infiltration with eosinophilia. At that stage many cases had no defined aetiology. Subsequently a whole variety of specific causes has been identified, but the later attempt by Citro and colleagues in 1973 to separate those cases with a defined cause from those without seems meaningless and unnecessary since the actual clinical presentation can be the same whether a cause has been defined or not.

Classification

An overview of the various classifications based on clinical features rather than aetiology suggests that these conditions should be broadly divided into three categories (see Table 1 for variations in terminology).

Table 1 Classification of the pulmonary eosinophilias

Pulmonary eosinophilia with alveolar exudate without airways
  involvement
  Simple pulmonary eosinophilia: Loeffler's syndrome
  Prolonged pulmonary eosinophilia: eosinophilic pneumonia
Pulmonary eosinophilia with alveolar exudate and airways disease
  Asthma
  Allergic bronchopulmonary aspergillosis
  Tropical eosinophilia
Pulmonary eosinophilia with angiitis and granulomatosis
  Allergic granulomatosis: Churg–Strauss syndrome
  (Polyarteritis nodosa)
  Wegener's granulomatosis
  Bronchocentric granulomatosis

1. Pulmonary infiltrations due to an eosinophilic alveolar exudate without airways involvement. This category includes the acute syndrome described by Loeffler in 1932 and renamed by Crofton as simple pulmonary eosinophilia, as well as the more chronic cases variously called prolonged pulmonary eosinophilia (Crofton) and eosinophilic pneumonia.

2. Pulmonary infiltration with eosinophilia but including a component of airways obstruction, as well as parenchymal lung disease. Allergic bronchopulmonary aspergillosis and tropical eosinophilia are classic examples in this group.

3. Pulmonary infiltrations with eosinophilia and with or without airways involvement but with evidence of a systemic disorder which may be predominantly vascular or granulomatous in pathology: polyarteritis nodosa, allergic granulomatosis, and the hypereosinophilic syndrome fall into this category.

Other conditions in which peripheral eosinophilia is part of a well-defined disease which may include pulmonary involvement as part of its clinical presentation are generally excluded from consideration under these headings, e.g. hydatid disease, Hodgkin's disease.

Loeffler's syndrome (simple pulmonary eosinophilia)

Clinical features
The essential features of the syndrome are transitory, migratory pulmonary shadows with modest peripheral eosinophilia seen in patients with a mild self-limiting illness. Some cases are truly asymptomatic, being discovered incidentally. Most have a cough, sometimes with oddly yellowish sputum and containing an abundance of eosinophils, and a few have general malaise and a mild fever. The pulmonary shadows are fan-shaped areas of consolidation, often peripheral, sometimes rather nodular, which last a few days only and appear haphazardly in various lobes, seldom following a truly segmental pattern, in some cases being single, in others multiple.

Laboratory findings
Though autopsy studies have rarely been performed except by chance (this being a benign self-limiting disease), the histology of these consolidations seems to consist, as might be expected, just of alveolar consolidation with an eosinophil-filled exudate. The peripheral eosinophilia is obvious but rarely gross: a differential of more than 20 per cent in a modestly raised total white cell count is unusual, and more often it will be 10–20 per cent of eosinophils and total white cell count that is at the high end of the normal range.

Pathogenesis
Patients who develop Loeffler's syndrome are often atopic and may have other manifestations of an atopic diathesis such as angio-oedema. The defined causes of the syndrome all suggest an allergic reaction, and are many and various. Two broad groups with a third miscellaneous collection emerge from analysis of the literature. From the first described cases a reaction to parasites has featured as a recognizable aetiology. The list is long including *Ascaris lumbricoides* (and occasionally *Ascaris suum*), *Ankylostoma*, *Trichuris*, *Trichinella*, *Taenia*, and *Strongyloides*. Drugs form a second important category, Loeffler's syndrome being well described after administration of para-amino salicyclic acid, aspirin, sulphonamides, penicillin, and imipramine. It may also be seen with nitrofurantoin though this more often gives a diffuse reticular nodular alveolar exudate (see page 15.143), toxic smoke, and lymphangiography contrast medium. A significant minority of cases of Loeffler's syndrome remains unexplained.

Treatment
Treatment is that of the causal agent if indicated. The syndrome itself resolves spontaneously and is never fatal. Avoidance of the precipitating agent, if defined, is advised.

Eosinophilic pneumonia and prolonged pulmonary eosinophilia

In several respects, particularly the association of pulmonary infiltrates with peripheral eosinophilia and in the wide range of defined causes, this syndrome is similar to simple pulmonary eosinophilia. Indeed the differences may lie entirely in degree and duration rather than anything fundamental. The division in terms of duration at one month is arbitrary but often about right clinically.

Clinical features
Prolonged pulmonary eosinophilia may last several months. It is associated with more severe clinical symptoms than simple pulmonary eosinophilia. Fever, often high and swinging, is usual, weight loss may occur and a range of associated systemic features have been described: focal, skin and hepatic necrosis, hepatosplenomegaly, and atopic manifestations such as rhinitis, sinusitis, and angio-oedema. The pulmonary disease is usually extensive causing dyspnoea and hypoxia with signs of consolidation on clinical examination. Radiologically the shadows may be pneumonic (hence the term eosinophilic pneumonia): the solid and confluent peripheral consolidations earn these cases the description 'the negative photographic image of pulmonary oedema'. They last several days or a week or so, though also like the shadows of Loeffler's syndrome, vary in site during the course of the illness. Eosinophilic pleural effusion has been recorded.

Pathology
Pathologically there are macrophages, lymphocytes, and polymorphs in the alveolar exudate together with the eosinophils and in some cases evidence of angiitis or even granuloma formation making these cases shade into the more sinister disorders of allergic or Wegener's granulomatosis. The white cell count is usually more than 10 000 and eosinophils more than 10 per cent with records existing of 70 per cent eosinophils in very high total counts (up to 100 000).

Management
Causes and hence treatment cover the same range as that described for simple pulmonary eosinophilia but often no cause is evident. These cryptogenic cases respond dramatically to corticosteroid therapy which is usually required for 6-12 months and occasionally for longer.

Pulmonary eosinophilia with bronchial involvement
Introduction
Some degree of eosinophilia is common in straightforward bronchial asthma. Counts of above 0.4×10^9 are considered a helpful

diagnostic pointer in this condition. Figures greater than about 1.0×10^9 however suggest that a specific cause should be sought. Two syndromes stand out. The first is exemplified by allergic bronchopulmonary aspergillosis and consists of asthma, fleeting pulmonary infiltrates with a tendency to mucus impaction, and bronchial wall damage which leads to proximal bronchiectasis. In the United Kingdom and probably most other westernized countries *Aspergillus* sensitivity accounts for more than 90 per cent of patients presenting with this syndrome. Rarely other agents included in the list given for Loeffler's syndrome and fungal species such as *Candida* can cause the same syndrome, whilst other cases remain cryptogenic. Further details of allergic bronchopulmonary aspergillosis are given on page 15.81. The second syndrome in this category is tropical eosinophilia.

Tropical eosinophilia

This term was coined by Weingarten in 1943 for a condition seen in the tropics and characterized by asthmatic airways obstruction, parenchymal lung damage, and a marked peripheral eosinophilia. The early noted beneficial response of these patients to arsenicals suggested a parasitic aetiology.

Incidence

The disease is endemic in the Indian subcontinent especially in the northwest as well as in Malaysia, Indonesia, and also parts of Africa and South America. In Singapore it is noted that the disease is confined to Indians, sparing the Chinese population.

Clinical features

Clincally, the typical presentation is with a persistent dry cough especially at night. Dyspneoa quickly follows with typically asthmatic nocturnal exacerbations. Non-asthmatic features are a tendency to fever and haemoptysis. Wheeze predominates on auscultation but there may also be crepitations. The latter reflect the diffuse parenchymal component of the disease which gives the typical radiological appearance of bilateral mottling which may in places become confluent. In the later stages of the disease, if untreated, persistent dyspnoea reflects irreversible airways obstruction and pulmonary fibrosis, and there can be terminal respiratory failure and cor pulmonale. Lung function tests, as expected, show a mixed obstructive and restrictive defect. The peripheral white cell count is usually elevated, often very high and there will be at least 20 per cent of eosinophils and often a much higher proportion.

Pathogenesis

The aetiology of this syndrome is now satisfactorily worked out. There is no reasonable doubt that microfilarii are the cause, most often *Wucherichii bancrofti*. The pathological lesions, focal granulomata in an infiltrate of eosinophils, neutrophils, polymorphs, and macrophages do not contain recognizable microfilia. Nor are the filaria found in the blood stream in relation to obvious exacerbations of the pulmonary eosinophilia. These facets of the pathology have hindered confirmation of the aetiology but are not surprising since the condition represents an allergic response to the worm or part of it. Complement-fixation tests are often positive but the most reliable diagnostic test appears to be a direct immunofluorescent technique developed in recent years using a papain digest which must include the cuticle of the worm and exclude other blood products.

Prognosis and treatment

A good prognosis is possible if the condition is recognized and treated early with diethyl carbamazine in a daily dose of 6–8 mg/kg body weight orally, given for a week, though occasionally longer courses may be necessary.

References

Citro, L. A., Gordon, M. E. and Miller, N. T. (1973). Eosinophilic lung disease (or how to slice PIE). *Am. J. Roent.* **117**, 787.

Crofton, J. W., Livingstone, J. L., Oswald, N. C. and Roberts, A. I. M. (1952). Pulmonary eosinophilia. *Thorax* **7**, 1.

Epstein, D. M., Tuormina, V., Gefter, W. B. and Miller, W. T. (1981). The hypereosinophilic syndrome. *Radiology* **140**, 59.

Middleton, W. G., Paterson, J. C., Grant, I. W. B. and Douglas, A. C. (1977). Asthmatic pulmonary eosinophilia. A review of 65 cases. *Br. J. Dis. Chest* **71**, 115.

Pearson, D. J. and Rosenow, E. C. III (1978). Chronic eosinophilic pneumonia (Carringtons): a follow up study. *Mayo Clin. Proc.* **53**, 73.

Udwadia, F. E. (1979). *Progress in respiratory research*, Vol. 7 *Pulmonary eosinophilia*. Karger, Basel.

Pulmonary vasculitis and granulomatosis

D. J. LANE AND D. M. GEDDES

Introduction

Though various forms of systemic vasculitis were well described in the 19th century, notably by Schonlein and by Kussmaul, syndromes which include a prominent pulmonary component were not well defined before about 1930. Klinger noted an association of pulmonary lesions with polyarteritis in 1931 and this was followed in 1939 by Wegener's description of the granulomatous vasculitis that bears his name. Churg and Strauss put allergic granulomatosis on the map in 1951 and the now classic paper by Leibow in 1973 divided the pulmonary granulomas into five on morphologic grounds.

Classification

Classification of these disorders is not however satisfactory. Grouping based on morphology does not necessarily tally with clearcut clinical syndromes, and features of one clinical entity seem to merge imperceptibly in individual patients with features of another. The reasons for this are complex, partly explained by our lack of knowledge about aetiology, partly by the wide variation in the size and distribution of vessels involved (and so a variable clinical picture), and partly by the failure to find laboratory tests that can help distinguish one condition from the next.

Broadly speaking the vasculitides can be divided into three categories as shown in Table 1. The granulomatous vasculitides in which the lungs are prominent sites of pathology form the subject matter of this section. The hypersensitivity vasculitides in which the lungs are occasionally involved as part of a systemic disease are dealt with at various places in the textbook and the pulmonary vascular and granulomatous manifestations of the connective tis-

Table 1

The granulomatous vasculitides
    Allergic granulomatosis and angiitis
    Classic Wegener's granulomatosis
    Limited Wegener's granulomatosis
    Lymphomatoid granulomatosis
    Necrotizing sarcoidal granulomatosis
    Bronchocentric granulomatosis
Hypersensitivity vasculitis
    Anaphylactoid purpura
    Mixed cryoglobulinaemia
    Vasculitis associated with malignancy, infection, drugs
Pulmonary vasculitis with connective tissue diseases (page 15.126)
    Rheumatoid disease
    Systemic lupus erythematosus
    Systemic sclerosis
    Dermato-polymyositis
    Mixed connective tissue disease

sue disorders are described elsewhere in this section of the book (page 15.126).

Pathogenesis

Much has been surmised but little is definitely known about the aetiology of these disorders. A genetic predisposition seems unlikely despite known HLA associations with certain connective tissue disorders. If the conditions are acquired there seems no pattern of consistent association with external agents. There are specific examples of associations between polyarteritis nodosa and either drug therapy (e.g. sulphonamides) or infections (specifically hepatitis B), but these associations do not appear to extend to the granulomatous manifestations of vasculitic lesions listed save for one, bronchocentric granulomatosis. This disorder is linked with *Aspergillus fumigatus* infection but in fact it differs significantly from most of the other disorders to be considered in lacking vasculitis and systemic manifestations. Immune mechanisms for vascular injury seem possible since immunoglobulins and complement fragments can be demonstrated in vessel walls but where the process is initiated or why it chooses blood vessels is unknown.

Churg–Strauss syndrome: allergic granulomatosis

In 1951 Churg and Strauss described a group of young adults with a history of asthma who developed evidence of systemic vasculitis in association with a marked peripheral eosinophilia. Subsequently other cases have been described though the condition is not common (English literature by Lenham *et al.*, 1984; 154 cases) and both before and since it seems likely that other examples of the condition have been described as polyarteritis nodosa, eosinophilic pneumonia or Loeffler's syndrome.

Clinical features

The sex ratio shows a slight preponderance of males and the age of diagnosis is usually late in the fourth decade. Preceding this there will have been a history of rhinitis and then asthma though the onset of these is usually in early adult life rather than in childhood. Peripheral eosinophilia then becomes marked and there may be eosinophilic infiltrates in various organs especially the lungs. It is the appearance of vasculitis in the mid to late 30s that alerts the physician to the true diagnosis. The overall clinical course can be acute and rapidly fatal with heart failure but is more usually sub-acute and relapsing.

The diagnostic triad is therefore asthma, eosinophilia, and vasculitis. Pulmonary infiltrates that accompany the asthma are patchy and transient, not especially favouring any lobe or zone: hilar lymphadenopathy, pleural effusion, and both fine small and large (non-cavitating) nodules are described in some cases. The eosinophilia is greater than 1.5×10^9/l unless reduced by therapy, and so greater than that seen in conventional atopic asthma but less than that found in the hypereosinophilic syndrome. Vascular lesions affect the body widely. A mononeuritis multiplex is perhaps the commonest being seen in two-thirds of patients: other neurological abnormalities are infrequent, perhaps an optic neuritis or rarely involvement of other cranial nerves. Abdominal pain is a frequent complaint reflecting vascular lesions in the bowel which resemble those in eosinophilic gastroenteritis in causing mass lesions with the potential for intestinal obstruction, and also ulceration leading to haemorrhagic diarrhoea. Vasculitis of the skin vessels gives a variety of maculopapular, urticarial or purpuric rashes and there may also be subcutaneous granulomatous nodules. Whilst a focal segmental glomerulonephritis may occur this is not common and rarely dominates the clinical outcome by causing fatal renal failure. The upper respiratory tract features usually remain simply 'allergic' in type with coryza congestion and polyposis rather than vasculitic or granulomatous lesions.

Laboratory findings

There is little help from investigations, apart from the eosinophilia, in either making the diagnosis or understanding the aetiology. A normochromic, normocytic anaemia is not uncommon and the ESR is usually high. Skin prick tests are often positive for common environmental allergens reflecting the atopic status, as does the elevated IgE. Other immunological tests are disappointing: rheumatoid factor, C_3, and IgG are inconsistently abnormal. A family history of atopic or allergic disease is relatively infrequently recorded (20 per cent).

Eosinophils dominate the histological picture with a dense infiltrate of these cells in almost all lesions together with foci or eosinophilic necrotic material and Charcot–Leyden crystals. Immunocytochemical studies reveal the presence of large amounts of potentially toxic compounds secreted by the activated eosinophils. Of these both eosinophil cationic protein and eosinophil protein-X can be shown to be toxic to cardiac muscle and other cells. It seems likely that these products may be responsible for the development of the damaging lesions of this syndrome. Necrotizing vasculitis can usually be demonstrated in vessels in and around the lesions, but granulomas have been found in less than half of the cases examined at autopsy.

Pathogenesis

These findings suggest no special aetiology and the disorder may just represent an unusual progression of allergic disease in a subset of predisposed atopic individuals. There is a disturbing report of six atopic patients who developed a systemic vasculitis after hyposensitization treatment.

Treatment

One fortunate aspect of the disease is that steroids are almost universally successful, transforming a previously poor prognosis into one in which death is now uncommon. Cytotoxics are rarely needed. Hypertension can be a problem especially since steroid therapy may need to be maintained for months or years.

Wegener's granulomatosis

The classic triad of upper respiratory tract and lower respiratory tract granulomas combined with a necrotizing focal glomerulonephritis make this syndrome the best known and most easily identified of the pulmonary granulomatous vasculitides. Involvement of two of the three sites is said to be sufficient to make the diagnosis but lack of the glomerulonephritis makes the disease less than 'classical': alternatively there may be vasculitic lesions elsewhere.

Clinical features

The disease can strike at any age though it is commonest in the fifth decade. There is probably some predominance in men. Pulmonary involvement can be heralded by cough, haemoptysis, and some chest pain, but often the radiology seems out of all proportion to the symptoms and paucity of physical signs, and can be the only manifestation of pulmonary involvement in a patient who presents with renal disease. The chest radiograph can show a kaleidoscope of changing pulmonary opacities which frequently cavitate but may regress spontaneously. Nodules reach up to 9 cm in size and are usually multiple and bilateral. Other pulmonary features include more widespread 'pneumonic' or reticulonodular shadows, bronchial obstruction leading to atelectasis and pleural involvement giving effusion, pneumothorax, and even bronchopleural fistula. Lymphadenopathy is uncommon.

In the upper respiratory tract granulomas in the nose may produce little more than coryza with epistaxis and some nasal crusting, but extensive destruction is possible leading to nasal septal perforation and saddle nose, or there may be ulcerative lesions of the sinuses, palate or pharynx.

The third component of the classical disease is an acute

glomerulonephritis, often asymptomatic, sometimes acute and fulminating (and occasionally accompanied by such pulmonary haemorrhage that Goodpasture's syndrome is suggested). Hypertension is rare.

Beyond these features there is often malaise, fever, and arthralgia. Vasculitic lesions can affect the skin (papular, vesicular or bullous), the nervous system (uveitis, orbital pseudo tumour, peripheral neuropathy), the cardiovascular system (pericarditis and coronary arteritis), and infrequently elsewhere. There may be a normochromic, normocytic anaemia with an elevated ESR. Rheumatoid factor, ANF, and smooth muscle antibodies are occasionally positive and serum IgA may be raised.

Pathology

The pathological lesions are granulomatous nodules built up from lymphocytes, plasma cells, and histiocytes. Giant cells form and the centre of the nodule is frequently necrotic. Within the nodules and at a distance from them there is a necrotic vasculitis affecting both arteries and veins. Pulmonary nodules usually show this characteristic histology whereas nasal granulomas are often less specific in appearance, largely due to local superinfection. The renal lesion is a focal necrotizing glomerulonephritis with frequent crescent formation similar to that seen in Goodpasture's syndrome or the Henoch–Schonlein syndrome. There is no distinctive pattern of immunofluorescence.

Prognosis and treatment

Prognosis though variable is generally poor if the condition is untreated. Death in about five months from renal failure is the quoted figure. However, occasional cases seem to survive untreated much longer (on the basis of a retrospective diagnosis) and the prognosis overall has been transformed by cyclophosphamide therapy, 1 to 2 mg/kg body weight/day continued for at least a year. Corticosteroids are often added certainly for an initial phase but may not be necessary. A remission rate of over 90 per cent is now to be expected.

Limited Wegener's granulomatosis

In this variant of the disease, pulmonary granulomas are the only consistent manifestation. Their histology and radiographic appearance are as in the classic disease. The condition may be diagnosed when a nodule is removed on suspicion of malignancy. There is no glomerulonephritis and nodules outside the lungs are uncommon and not associated with a damaging vasculitis. They have been recorded most often subcutaneously, but also in the kidneys. The disease evolves slowly, and may even stabilize or regress without treatment. Response to corticosteroid therapy is recorded.

Necrotizing sarcoid granulomatosis

Liebow included this amongst the five pulmonary granulomas which he delineated in 1973. It is uncommon, less than 100 cases having been described to date. A wide age range of adults has been affected and females seem more prone to the disorder than males. Presentation is usually with non-specific respiratory complaints such as cough or chest pain, though a quarter are asymptomatic. In all instances chest radiology is striking showing usually multiple nodules which may be down to miliary in size and are frequently confluent. They are especially seen in the lower zones and do not cavitate. Hilar nodes may be seen on the chest radiograph and are often found pathologically.

Neither a systemic vasculitis nor a glomerulonephritis are part of the clinical picture but the only extrapulmonary feature recorded that resembles sarcoidosis is uveitis, and this is very rare.

Pathology

Histologically the nodules are sarcoid-like, epithelioid giant cell granulomas differing from the better known disease in that they

quite frequently show necrosis and also a vasculitis. There is cellular infiltration with lymphocytes, histiocytes, and plasma cells of the walls of both arteries and veins leading to vessel destruction and local infarction.

Prognosis and treatment

Prognosis is good. Survivals of a decade or more are quite common. Surgical removal often seems to result in cure and in cases not subjected to thoracotomy, steroids with or without cytotoxics give good remission, the occasional relapse responding equally well.

Bronchocentric granulomatosis

This is essentially a morphologic diagnosis of a condition which lacks clearcut clinical, radiological or immunological features, though there is increasing support for the concept that it represents an unusual but specific bronchial reaction to a sustained inflammatory insult and that this insult most often comes from fungi of the *Aspergillus* species.

Clinical features

Originally described by Liebow in 1973 in his paper on the pulmonary granulomas there is little evidence now to link this with conditions such as Wegener's granulomatosis. It most commonly presents as localized pulmonary shadowing in a patient with persistent cough and dyspnoea. The dyspnoea has the characteristics of asthma in about half of the cases, often the younger patients. Those with asthma usually have a high peripheral eosinophil count. Radiographically an isolated mass or alveolar infiltrate confined to one lobe is the usual picture so that it is not surprising that many of these patients are diagnosed histologically after thoracotomy. Changes are more commonly seen in the upper lobes and other radiological presentations are multiple nodules or infiltrates or even a diffuse alveolar infiltrate. Pleural involvement, cavitation, and hilar lymphadenopathy are rare. The disease has no extrapulmonary manifestations, though there are case reports of an association with rheumatoid arthritis.

Pathology

Histologically the lesions consist of necrotizing granulomas centred on an airway and surrounded by collapsed, consolidated lung. Microscopically epithelioid cells are arranged radially to form granulomas. The bronchial lumen is filled with inspissated mucus which together with the ulcerated bronchial wall and the peribronchial tissues is infiltrated by eosinophils and eosinophilic masses. Though there may be chondritis and destruction of cartilage, there is no arteritis.

Aetiology

In 1975 Katzenstein described the finding of *Aspergillus fumigatus* spores in the bronchi of some of these patients. Positive prick tests, raised *Aspergillus* IgE and IgG have subsequently been variably reported in these patients especially those with asthma, making the condition in most respects identical to allergic bronchopulmonary aspergillosis. Even in patients without asthma, eosinophilia or positive *Aspergillus* serology, some workers have claimed that laminated clusters of fungal elements and eosinophils can be found on careful histological staining. Others take the view that the lesions represent a tissue reaction that results from prolonged inflammation due to a variety of insults even though *Aspergillus* species may be the commonest amongst these.

Management

Treatment is often inadvertently by surgical resection at a thoracotomy carried out for supposed bronchial malignancy. However, if the condition is suspected in life corticosteroids will clear the consolidation, even though repeated courses may be needed. Residual damage leading to bronchiectasis is recorded but on the whole prognosis is good. No studies of antifungal agents have been reported but ketoconazole would be worth a trial.

Other forms of pulmonary vasculitis

The lungs may be involved to a limited degree in the hypersensitivity vasculitides such as anaphylactoid (Henoch–Schonlein) purpura or essential mixed cryoglobulinaemia. Besides the cutaneous lesions, the hepatosplenomegaly, and other systemic features, the patchy pneumonitis usually revealed only on the chest radiograph, is unimpressive. Likewise in the vasculitides associated with malignancy, infection or drugs, any pulmonary involvement is minor.

In two other vasculitic disorders, perhaps related, a systemic vasculitis may be associated with pulmonary artery aneurysms. These are Behçet's syndrome and the Hughes–Stovin syndrome.

Behçet's syndrome

Haemoptysis, infiltrates on the chest radiograph, which may cavitate, and fibrosis, focal or generalized, have all been reported. These are probably all manifestations of a pulmonary vasculitis, but sometimes occur in association with vena caval thrombosis, in which instance pulmonary emboli are a likely contributing cause. The lung manifestations may precede the systemic disease by some years, during which time the diagnosis is obscure (see also page 24.13).

Hughes–Stovin syndrome

Pulmonary artery aneurysms, unusual in Behçet's syndrome, are the hallmark of this rare and peculiar disorder characterized clinically by haemoptysis from rupture of the aneurysms. Histologically the lesions are an eosinophil angiitis. There may be an accompanying glomerulonephritis.

References

Churg, A., Carrington, C. B. and Gupta, R. (1979). Necrotizing sarcoid granulomatosis. *Chest* **76**, 406–413.

Fauci, A. S., Haynes, B. F., Katz, P. and Wolff, S. M. (1983). Wegener's granulomatosis: prospective clinical and therapeutic experience with 85 patients for 21 years. *Ann. intern. Med.* **98**, 76–85.

Israel, H. L., Patchefsky, A. S. and Saldana, J. J. (1977). Wegener's granulomatosis, lymphomatoid granulomatosis and benign lymphocytic angiitis and granulomatosis of lung: recognition and treatment. *Ann. intern. Med.* **87**, 691–699.

Lanham, J. G., Elkom, K. B., Pusey, C. D. and Hughes, G. R. (1984). Systemic vasculitis with asthma and eosinophilia: a clinical approach to the Churg–Strauss syndrome. *Medicine (Balt.)* **63**, 65–81.

Liebow, A. A. (1973). Pulmonary angiitis and granulomatosis. *Am. Rev. Resp. Dis.* **108**, 1–18.

Other granulomas and related disorders

For sarcoidosis see page 5.623.

Histiocytosis-X (eosinophilic granuloma of lungs)

This is a somewhat diverse group of three conditions in which the lungs are infiltrated by abnormal histiocytes. Since the aetiology and pathogenesis are unknown it is unclear whether they represent a spectrum of a single disorder or distinct entities which happen to share some pathological features. The extrapulmonary clinical features are summarized in Table 2.

Pathology and pathogenesis

The lungs are infiltrated by morphologically distinct histiocytes called histiocytosis-X cells. Histiocytosis-X cells resemble macrophages with indented nuclei. The cytoplasm is pale and eosinophilic and contains PAS-negative granules called X-bodies. These are rod or racquet-shaped inclusions which are seen in the periphery of the cell sometimes contiguous with the plasma mem-

Table 2 Histiocytosis X

Disease	Age	Extrapulmonary manifestations	Prognosis
Letterer-Siwe	Infants	Hepatosplenomegaly Anaemia purpura	Poor
Hand Schuller Christian	Children Young adults	Skull deposits Diabetes insipidus	Variable
Eosinophilic granuloma	Adults	Lytic bone deposits Long bones, pelvis, skull	Slow progression, occasional remission

brane. Electron microscopy reveals a pentalaminar structure with occasional formation of intercellular junction complexes. Histiocytosis-X cells are associated in the tissues with variable numbers of eosinophils and sometimes lymphocytes, fibroblasts, and giant cells. In places these come together to form granulomas. Nodular clusters of cells collect around blood vessels giving the appearance of a vasculitis and sometimes around small airways to cause an obliterative bronchiolitis. There is some extension into the alveolar walls as in fibrosing alveolitis. Fibrosis develops in association with this cellular infiltrate and in later stages the fibrosis is the dominant feature progressing to a relatively acellular honeycomb lung.

The pathogenesis is unknown. The X-bodies are somewhat suggestive of virus structures but there is no other evidence to support an infectious cause. On the other hand histiocytosis-X cells resemble Langerhan's cells of the skin which have an immune function. Some minor alterations of immunity have been reported in histiocytosis-X such as circulating immune complexes and altered T cell function, but these are likely to be epiphenomena.

Clinical features

The more aggressive childhood disorders (Letterer–Siwe, Hand–Schuller–Christian disease) present with progressive breathlessness, general malaise, weight loss, and sometimes anaemia or purpura. Diabetes insipidus is associated with infiltration of the base of the skull. The pulmonary infiltration usually progresses with increasing breathlessness to pulmonary hypertension and terminal right heart failure. Recurrent spontaneous pneumothoraces are common and may be intractable or fatal. The childhood diseases progress to death within a few months or years.

The more indolent adult disease (eosinophilic granuloma) is usually confined to the lung and is not part of a multisystem disease, but it may be found on routine chest radiograph in the course of the investigation of a lytic bone lesion. Sex distribution slightly favours males. Symptoms consist of dyspnoea, cough perhaps with sputum and chest pain, though up to one-fifth are asymptomatic. One-third have fever, malaise or weight loss. A high proportion of patients (80 per cent or more) are, or have been, smokers. Physical examination is often relatively normal: crackles occur only in the later stages and clubbing is rare. The chest radiograph shows diffuse bilateral reticulonodular shadowing with no specific features. This progresses to honeycombing with cystic air spaces which are predominantly peripheral and in the upper zones (Fig. 1). Pneumothorax may occur. Lung function is normal initially but eventually lung volumes and carbon monoxide gas transfer are reduced. A minority of patients have obstructive spirometry presumably due to peribronchial disease. There is no good parallel between symptoms, radiographic change, and lung function, each of which may change independently of the others.

Transbronchial biopsies may be diagnostic but more usually show non-specific changes. Open lung biopsy provides definitive histology but is seldom necessary and may be hazardous in the later stages when lung cysts have developed. A bone scan is better than a skeletal radiographic survey in assessing bone involvement.

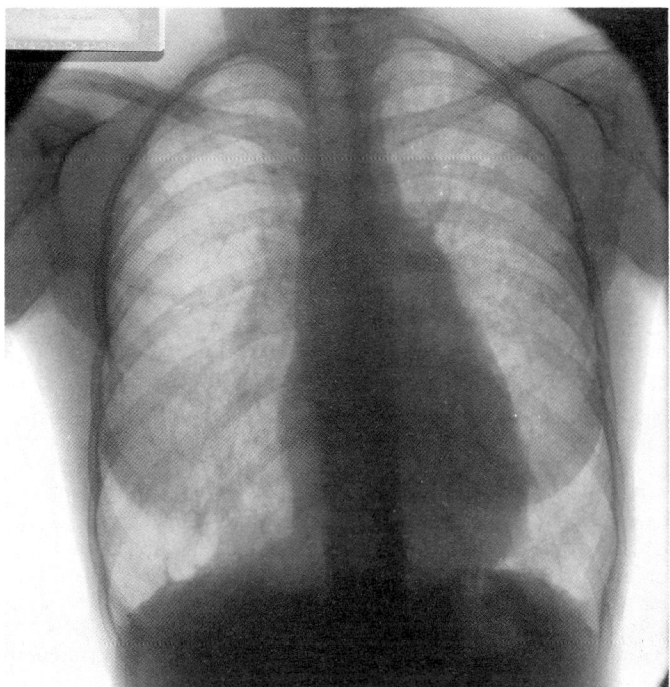

Fig. 1 Chest radiograph of a patient with eosinophilic granuloma of lung showing granulomas and fibrosis with bulla formation.

Prognosis

Most cases progress slowly over many years but sometimes spontaneous regression is seen. Unfavourable features are extremes of age, multisystem disease, extensive cyst formation with pneumothoraces, and reduced diffusing capacity. Histological findings do not predict outcome.

Treatment

Mild stable disease can be left untreated but progressive disease may be influenced by corticosteroids or cytotoxic drugs. The true value of this treatment is difficult to assess since spontaneous remissions are quite common and no controlled trials have been performed. More usually the disease progresses in spite of therapy. The bone lesions can be treated by radiotherapy or curettage.

Lymphangiomyomatosis (lymphangioleiomyomatosis)

This rare condition occurs almost exclusively in women of reproductive age. There is proliferation of immature smooth muscle throughout the peribronchial, perivascular, and perilymphatic regions of the lung and often more widespread infiltration of extrapulmonary lymph-nodes and lymphatics. The histological appearances are somewhat similar to tuberous sclerosis but a family history is lacking and the natural history of the two conditions is different.

The presenting features are breathlessness together with diffuse shadowing of the chest radiograph. There are fine reticulonodular infiltrates affecting the lung fields uniformly often in association with increased lung volumes. Chylous pleural effusions are quite common due to lymphatic obstruction, and pneumothorax or haemoptysis are frequent complications. Lung function tests show a mixed obstructive and restrictive pattern with considerable reduction of diffusing capacity. The diagnosis is made on lung biopsy although the clinical picture can be almost diagnostic especially when chylous effusions are present with interstitial lung disease.

Treatment with progesterone or tamoxifen has been successful in a few cases, while androgens and ovarian ablation have not. Chemical pleurodesis may be required for recurrent chylous effusions.

Tuberous sclerosis

This is a hamartomatous proliferation of various tissues which manifests itself as some combination of mental retardation, fits, adenoma sebaceum, retinal phakomas, periunqual fibromas, and renal tumours. The lungs are involved in about 1 per cent of cases. The condition is inherited with an autosomal dominant pattern of inheritance, but sporadic cases also occur.

Lung disease presents with progressive breathlessness and an abnormal chest radiograph although some patients are identified on routine testing. Complications include pneumothorax and occasionally haemoptysis. There is progressive pulmonary fibrosis with honeycombing and eventually cor pulmonale and death within about 5 years of the onset of pulmonary symptoms. No treatment has been shown to be effective.

Neurofibromatosis

Pulmonary involvement in neurofibromatosis is rare and may take many different forms. These include neurogenic tumours arising within the thorax and involving mediastinal and intercostal nerves or intrathoracic meningocoeles. The lungs are occasionally affected by non-specific fibrosis when the presenting features are breathlessness with diffuse lower zone shadowing on chest radiograph, restrictive spirometry, and reduced diffusing capacity. The pathological changes are indistinguishable from other forms of lung fibrosis. Occasionally there are co-existing upper zone bullae and while these may simply be due to traction on the lung from the lower zone fibrosis they are an unusual finding and may therefore be a reflection of the underlying disorder of connective tissue.

References

Carrington, C. G., Cugell, D. W., Gaensler, E. A. *et al.* (1977). Lymphangioleiomyomatosis: physiologic–pathologic–radiologic correlations. *Am. Rev. Resp. Dis.* **116**, 977–995.

Colby, T. V. and Lombard, C. (1983). Histiocytosis-X in the lung. *Human Path.* **14**, 847–856.

Dwyer, J. M., Hickie, J. B. and Garvan, J. (1971). Pulmonary tuberose sclerosis. *Q. J. Med.* **40**, 115–121.

Friedman, P. J., Liebow, A. A. and Sokoloff, J. (1981). Eosinophilic granuloma of lung. *Medicine (Balt.)* **60**, 385–396.

Massaro, D., Katz, S., Matthews, M. J. and Higgins, G. (1975). Von Recklinghausen's neurofibromatosis associated with cystic lung disease. *Am. J. Med.* **38**, 233–240.

LYMPHOCYTIC INFILTRATION OF THE LUNG

D. M. GEDDES

The classification of disorders of the lung characterized by lymphocytic infiltration is evolving and is not yet satisfactory. The patient usually presents with a systemic illness which includes fever, malaise, and weight loss together with an abnormal chest radiograph. Occasionally the abnormal radiograph is the only finding. The diagnosis is made on lung biopsy which shows lymphocytic infiltration as the dominant feature amongst a variety of other findings. In view of the wide spectrum of clinical and pathological features attempts have been made to classify such patients into distinct diagnostic categories. There is, however, considerable overlap and the features also change with time, a proportion progressing to lymphomas. Some lymphocytic infiltrates do in fact appear to represent an early stage of lymphoma confined to the lung. The term 'pseudo lymphoma' was coined by Saltzstein in 1963 for lung tumours containing relatively mature lymphocytes in a mixture of other cells with some germinal centres and no lymph-node involvement. A predominance of poorly differentiated lymphocytes, lymph-node enlargment, and pleural seeding implies more aggressive lymphomatous behaviour. Five disorders of the lung characterized by lymphocytic infiltration will be considered here. Further details of lymphoma in the lung are found in Section 19.

Lymphocytic interstitial pneumonitis

Introduction

This occurs in isolation or as a complication of a systemic disorder such as systemic lupus erythematosus (SLE) or Sjögren's syndrome. There have also been occasional reports of an association with chronic active hepatitis, myasthenia gravis, and pernicious anaemia. The alveolar walls are infiltrated by mature lymphocytes, plasma cells, and immunoblasts. Germinal foci occasionally occur but lymph-nodes are not involved. However, a proportion of cases progress to lymphocytic lymphoma.

Clinical features

Breathlessness accompanies extensive infiltration and systemic symptoms of fever, weight loss, and arthralgia are common. If the condition progresses to lymphoma then systemic symptoms become more pronounced and lymphadenopathy develops. Other patients progress slowly to pulmonary fibrosis with the development of lower zone crackles and clubbing.

The chest radiograph initially shows lower zone infiltration similar to fibrosing alveolitis. This may progress to generalized fibrosis or, when lymphoma develops, more homogeneous lung shadowing with lymphadenopathy. Protein electrophoresis is often abnormal with a polyclonal or monoclonal increase in gammaglobulin, however, about 10 per cent have hypogammaglobulinaemia. Malignant transformation is more common in association with Sjögren's syndrome particularly when there is a monoclonal band. It has therefore been suggested that regular measurements of serum protein may identify malignant change early.

Treatment

Treatment with corticosteroids or cytotoxic drugs can lead to improvement. Different therapies have not been evaluated. A proportion of patients die from infectious complications, some develop lymphoma with a variable course and others progress to end-stage pulmonary fibrosis.

Plasma cell interstitial pneumonitis

This is very similar to lymphocytic interstitial pneumonitis except that plasma cells predominate in the pulmonary infiltrate. Progression is into multiple myeloma or Waldenstrom's macroglobulinaemia.

Benign lymphocytic angiitis

This is a relatively benign condition presenting clinically with one or more pulmonary nodules on a chest radiograph usually taken in a patient with a mild non-specific illness. The nodules represent a localized angiitis around small pulmonary arteries. Histologically there is an infiltrate of lymphocytes, plasma cells, and histiocytes usually without necrosis. Spontaneous resolution is well recorded though the occasional evolution into lymphomatoid granulomatosis suggests that some cases are less benign.

Immunoblastic lymphadenopathy (angio-immunoblastic lymphadenopathy)

The lungs are occasionally involved in this generalized disorder of lymph-nodes. There is proliferation of B-lymphocytes with involvement of lymph-nodes, liver, and spleen, skin, and sometimes lung. A wide range of different drugs have been implicated as a cause in individual cases. There is usually anaemia, polyclonal hypergammaglobulinaemia, and often peripheral eosinophilia. The Coomb's test may be positive. The chest radiograph shows alveolar infiltrates in about 15 per cent of cases, pleural effusion in 10 per cent and thoracic lymphadenopathy in about 40 per cent. The diagnosis is established on lymph-node biopsy but lung biopsy may be required to exclude opportunistic infection. Corticosteroids are the mainstay of treatment but cytotoxic therapy may be needed for progressive disease. While some patients progress rapidly to death within a few months of diagnosis from either opportunistic infection or immunoblastoma many have relatively indolent disease with only a little progression over many years.

Lymphomatoid granulomatosis (see also page 19.185)

This disease, first described by Liebow in 1972 is a widespread granulomatous disorder pathologically characterized by destructive lymphoreticular infiltrates based around small arteries and with its clinical features dominantly pulmonary, neurological, and cutaneous.

Clinical findings

Most patients are between 30 and 50 years of age although occasional cases appear in childhood or old age. There is a slight male preponderance. Presenting features are either non-specific – fever, malaise, and weight loss, or refer to the organs involved. For the lungs this is usually cough, perhaps dyspnoea, and sometimes haemoptysis. Radiographically the appearances are of fleeting areas of patchy consolidation especially peripherally and at the bases: cavitation can occur. In the nervous system a variety of centrally or peripherally placed lesions can cause hemiparesis, ataxia, blindness, paraesthesiae or lower motor neurone paralyses. Skin lesions are variable but often consist or widespread erythematous maculopapular nodules which may ulcerate. Many other organs such as the heart, liver, adrenals, pancreas, and prostate may be involved, but whilst the kidneys deserve inclusion, clinical evidence of renal disease is unusual, in contrast to its importance in Wegener's granulomatosis. Likewise though the features histologically are hard to distinguish from malignant disorders of the lymphoreticular system, the lymph-nodes, spleen, and bone marrow are rarely involved unless the disorder is manifesting, late in its course, truly lymphomatous transformation.

Pathology and pathogenesis

Laboratory findings are non-specific and unhelpful. Tests for auto-antibodies or immune complexes have not proved useful either in aiding diagnosis or in understanding the aetiology of lymphomatoid granulomatosis. The histological features are of a heavy infiltrate of atypical lymphoreticular cells with plasmacytoid features, rather sparse granuloma formation, and an angiitis of small and medium-sized arteries which leads to infarction and a coagulative necrosis. Whilst the variegated nature of the infiltrate, the presence of angiitis in areas distant from parenchymal involvement, and the sparing of lymphatic tissues are pointers against this being a primary malignant disorder, there is a strong feeling that lymphomatoid granulomatosis is a form of lymphoma.

Prognosis and treatment

There is little doubt that a proportion (variously given as between 13 and 47 per cent) will develop a malignant lymphoma and die from this complication. The types of lymphoma recorded are immunoblastic sarcoma, T cell, and diffuse large or mixed cell lymphomas. An alternative hypothesis suggests that the disorder is an acquired abnormality of lymphocyte function in a susceptible host.

Whilst the occasional patient seems to achieve a spontaneous recovery, death rates up to 90 per cent have been recorded. In a small prospective study this depressing outlook was improved to a rate of 53 per cent by the combined uses of prednisolone and cyclophosphamide. If remission is achieved the long-term outlook looks good with several patients being able to stop therapy. If no remission occurs, malignant lymphoma refractory to further treatment seems to be the rule.

References

Katzenstein, A. L., Carrington, C. R. B. and Liebow, A. A. (1979). Lymphomatoid granulomatosis: a clinico-pathological study of 152 cases. *Cancer* **43**, 360–373.

Kradin, R. L. and Mark, E. J. (1983). Benign lymphoid disorders of the lung. *Human Pathol.* **14**, 857.

Vath, R. R., Alexander, C. B. and Fulmer, J. D. (1982). The lymphocytic infiltrative lung diseases. *Clin. Chest Med.* **3**, 619–634.

MISCELLANEOUS DISORDERS

B. J. HENDRICK

Pulmonary alveolar proteinosis

First described in 1958, pulmonary alveolar proteinosis (PAP) has proved to be a rare but interesting disorder that exerts its primary effects in the alveolar spaces. Over a period ranging from months to years, these become filled with an amorphous, largely cell-free, lipoproteinaceous material which is not readily expectorated. There are two major consequences. Depending on the number of alveoli involved, ventilatory function becomes restricted, the lungs become stiff, and shunting occurs at the alveolar capillary level causing hypoxia and in some cases death from respiratory failure. In many cases, however, extensive involvement does not occur, there being little or no progression, or even spontaneous remission. The second major consequence, and a not uncommon cause of death, is secondary infection. The responsible organisms are generally those that are associated with intracellular infection and impaired T lymphocyte function, *Nocardia* being particularly prominent.

Clinical features

Males appear to be affected more commonly than females, but all age groups may be involved. The cause in most cases is unknown, though an apparently identical (though relentlessly progressive) disorder can arise within months of massive exposure to respirable mineral dust, especially silica, both in the unfortunate worker exposed negligently without adequate respiratory protection and in experimental animal models. A few reports describe affected sibships, and some associate PAP with haematological malignancies, the use of cytotoxic agents, or immunodeficiency disorders. The secreted material is rich in protein and phospholipid, and stains strongly with periodic acid–Schiff (PAS) reagent and eosin. It also contains myeloid bodies which are probably derived from lamellar bodies of surfactant-producing type II pneumocytes. It is likely that the secretions themselves are chiefly the product of these cells, but it is unclear whether their accumulation results from excessive or abnormal production, or from impaired resorption by the type II pneumocytes or the alveolar macrophages. In most cases the PAS stain is taken up uniformly, as is peroxidase-labelled immunoglobulin raised against the apoprotein of surfactant. In others, particularly those associated with haematological or immunological disorders, uptake is heterogeneous, and it has been suggested that fundamentally different processes underlie this 'secondary' form of PAP. The vulnerability to infection with 'opportunistic' organisms coupled with the *in vitro* demonstration of a number of abnormalities of macrophage function incriminates the macrophage more than the pneumocyte in this respect. It has been shown, however, that ingestion of the material may itself cause impairment of phagocytic function in macrophages harvested from normal control animals.

The affected subject usually presents with progressive shortness of breath due to the disease itself or with a pneumonic illness due to superimposed infection. Occasionally, the disease is first recognized from the appearances of an incidental chest radiograph. Cough is common and may be productive, particularly if there is infection. Low-grade fever, haemoptysis, and pleuritic pain occur infrequently, though some authors report an initial febrile incident. There may be crackles and clubbing in advanced stages, and fever becomes characteristic when infection supervenes. When *Nocardia* is not responsible for this, *Aspergillus, Candida, Cryptococcus,* cytomegalovirus, *Histoplasma, Mucor,* mycobacteria, *Pneumocystis,* and viruses are the most common culprits.

Diagnosis

The chest radiograph characteristically shows an alveolar filling pattern, which radiates from the hila and simulates pulmonary oedema. There is no associated evidence of heart failure, however, and the appearances may be somewhat patchy and asymmetrical. Diffuse pulmonary fibrosis is rare, unless provoked by complicating infection, though a micronodular infiltration is occasionally seen. Hilar lymphadenopathy is characteristically absent. Pneumonia or aspiration may be suspected initially, but the cough produces little or no sputum, and no organisms are isolated if the disease remains uncomplicated. The key to diagnosis rests with the demonstration that the alveolar secretions are strongly PAS positive but contain no organisms and no excessive cellular response. Indeed the macrophages appear to be deficient in numbers as well as function. Occasionally the sputum provides diagnostic material, identification of lamellar bodies or their debris by electron microscopy being particularly useful. More commonly bronchoalveolar lavage or lung biopsy is required.

Management

In perhaps a third of cases, no appreciable disability develops and the disease remits spontaneously or fails to progress. The choice of treatment, when necessary, is strictly limited. Corticosteroids are of no value and may increase the risk of infection. Prolonged periods of inhalation therapy with expectorants (potassium iodide) or proteolytic enzymes (trypsin) have been claimed to offer some benefit, but have caused frequent irritative responses in the airways. The most effective measure has been physical removal of the secretions by alveolar lavage. This is usually performed under general anaesthesia using a double lumen endotracheal tube, one lung being repeatedly lavaged with a total of 20–40 litres of warm buffered saline (often with heparin and acetyl cysteine), the other being mechanically ventilated. When severe respiratory failure has already supervened despite ventilatory support, cardiopulmonary bypass has been used successfully to maintain gas exchange during the lavage procedure. An alternative is sequential lobar lavage using a fibreoptic bronchoscope and cuffed catheter. Further lavage is usually necessary every few weeks or months but the activity of the disease may lessen and the frequency of this need diminish. Sometimes there is fatal progression with a prominent loss of weight despite repeated lavage.

A considerable threat to life comes from complicating infection, and this should be quickly recognized and treated. An accelerated clinical course together with the development of fever, increased (and productive) cough, malaise, evidence of systemic infection, and the radiographic demonstration of cavitation or pleural effusion all provide pointers to its development. Blood cultures together with smear and culture studies of sputum may identify the organism or organisms responsible, but often bronchoscopy with brushings and diagnostic lavage is needed. Sometimes a biopsy procedure is considered necessary, particularly when the underlying presence of alveolar proteinosis is not clearly established. When 'opportunistic' organisms are involved, the eradication of infection may prove to be difficult, perhaps reflecting the underlying impairment of macrophage function.

References

Claypool, W. D., Rogers, R. M. and Matuschak, G. M. (1984). Update on the clinical diagnosis, management, and pathogenesis of pulmonary alveolar proteinosis (phospholipidosis). *Chest* **85**, 550–558.

Freedman, A. P., Pelias, A., Johnston, R. F., Goel, I. P., Hakki, H. I., Oslick, T. and Shinnick, J. P. (1981). Alveolar proteinosis lung lavage using partial cardiopulmonary bypass. *Thorax* **36**, 543–554.

Rosen, S. H., Castleman, B. and Liebow, A. A. (1958). Pulmonary alveolar proteinosis. *N. Engl. J. Med.* **258**, 1123–1142.

Singh, G., Katyal, S. L., Bedrossian, C. W. M. and Rogers, R. M. (1983). Pulmonary alveolar proteinosis. Staining for surfactant apoprotein in alveolar proteinosis and in conditions simulating it. *Chest* **83**, 82–86.

Pulmonary amyloidosis

Recent advances in understanding the complex mechanisms responsible for amyloidosis have led to a modified method of classification. The proteinaceous material (it is not in fact related to starch) that gives the characteristic staining appearance with Congo Red is composed of a fibrillar polypeptide and a non-fibrillar glycoprotein. They produce a unique β-pleated structure that is deposited progressively and widely in the body's organs, eventually interfering with their function. The glycoprotein (amyloid P or AP protein) comprises a mere 10 per cent of amyloid tissue. It is derived from a parent serum protein (SAP) and is common to all types of amyloid tissue. The fibrillar protein on the other hand is of two distinct types.

The type seen with 'primary' amyloidosis and amyloidosis associated with myeloma is derived essentially from immunoglobulin light chains or their N-terminal fragments, and is known as AL protein. It is the product of a plasma cell clone (though

Table 1 Classification of pulmonary amyloidosis

Systemic amyloidosis
    Amyloidosis with lymphocyte or plasma cell dyscrasia (primary)
    Systemic reactive amyloidosis (secondary)
    Familial amyloidosis
Localized amyloidosis

macrophages may contribute under monocyte influence), and monoclonal immunoglobulin (M-component) may sometimes be detected in the serum as may Bence-Jones protein in the urine. The type seen with 'secondary' amyloidosis and most of the familial forms of amyloidosis (AA protein) is derived from an acute phase serum component (SAA), presumably by proteolytic cleavage. The chronic inflammatory diseases associated with persistently raised levels of SAA (and C reactive protein) are indeed those that are most commonly associated with secondary amyloidosis, but only a small minority of affected subjects show evidence of complicating amyloidosis. This implies there is in these subjects some derangement of the SAA degrading process or the SAA protein itself.

The differing patterns of organ dysfunction associated with these two types of amyloidosis remain unexplained, but much overlap evidently occurs and it seems likely that both proteins become deposited widely as the disease progresses. It also remains unclear why deposition is a systemic process in some cases but local in others. This is a more crucial matter to the clinician and is central to the proposed new classification (Table 1).

Pulmonary involvement

The lungs are not commonly the major target organ in amyloidosis, but may become infiltrated with both types of amyloid protein. Rarely, hilar or mediastinal lymph-nodes are involved as well. When systemic amyloidosis is associated with AL protein, the kidneys and heart bear the brunt of the damage, though the lungs are said to be involved in the majority of cases. With systemic reactive amyloidosis, the lungs are involved only in a minority of cases. When pulmonary involvement is symptomatic, the disease is often localized and is usually due to deposition of the light chain-derived protein. Its effects depend on the site of deposition. The following varieties, in descending order of epidemiological importance, are the most clearly recognized:

1. Tracheobronchial. Discrete and usually multiple masses of amyloid protein enlarge in the walls of the airways or the peribronchial tissues causing cough, obstruction, and sometimes bleeding. The obstructed airways may lead to wheeze, stridor, breathlessness, atelectasis, and infection, and may eventually give rise to bronchiectasis. When a single lesion is involved it may simulate the effects of a bronchial adenoma, appearing as a polypoid mass on endoscopic inspection.

2. Parenchymal nodule(s). Discrete nodules or masses, which may be single or multiple, are seen within the lung parenchyma on the chest radiograph. They rarely cause symptoms or disrupt lung function and may eventually calcify, cavitate or even ossify. They are likely to simulate bronchial neoplasms and so become resected.

3. Alveolar-interstitial. Amyloid tissue is deposited diffusely throughout the alveolar walls and interstitium of the lung. There is progressive breathlessness and dry cough. Scattered crackles are characteristic and there may be pleural effusions. Eventually respiratory failure supervenes as ventilation becomes increasingly restricted and gas transfer impaired.

Diagnosis

The diagnosis rests essentially on the demonstration of amyloid tissue in an affected organ. When the protein is derived from plasma cells or lymphocytes, it may be possible to demonstrate light chains in the urine or M-component in the serum, and a plasma cell or lymphocyte dyscrasia may be clinically evident. When systemic reactive amyloidosis is the diagnosis, a provoking chronic inflammatory disease should be obvious, and high levels of SAA and C reactive protein will be present in the serum. Histochemical studies in the laboratory should, in any event, identify the specific biochemical nature of the protein obtained at biopsy.

Management

Treatment of the systemic disease associated with AL protein is usually unrewarding. There is an inexorable accumulation of amyloid tissue in the affected organs, and death occurs within 1–2 years. Survival is even shorter when myelomatosis is present. There is some point in trying cytotoxic agents such as melphalan since responders are encountered sporadically, but these agents are not often helpful. Corticosteroids may actually worsen deposition of protein in the kidneys. Ultimately, organ transplantation may become the only hope of survival, and when renal failure is the only immediate threat to life, this is often carried out.

The outcome of systemic reactive amyloidosis is dependent on the accompanying inflammatory disease. If this can be controlled, the deposition of amyloid tissue may be halted. It may also be halted or lessened by the use of colchicine, which interferes with the metabolism of SAA. Systemic reactive amyloidosis is nevertheless a serious disorder and usually ends fatally within a few years.

A current experimental approach, which may prove to be of benefit to both types of amyloidosis, is the use of dimethylsulphoxide. This denatures amyloid tissue, and has been shown to produce urinary excretion of amyloid-like material. Its place in the management of human disease is yet to be established, however.

With the local forms of the disease of whatever aetiology, the outlook is a good deal brighter. Progression may be slow, and the disease may become quiescent. The tracheobronchial deposits can sometimes be resected or depleted piecemeal endoscopically, but there is some risk of serious bleeding from this. Parenchymal nodules in the lung rarely need to be removed provided their histological nature is not in doubt. The diffuse alveolar-interstitial form of pulmonary amyloidosis tends to be relentlessly progressive, irrespective of whether the disease is confined to the lungs, and shows little response to therapy.

References

Buxbaum, J. N., Hurley, M. E., Chuba, J. and Spiro, T. (1979). Amyloidosis of the AL type. Clinical, morphologic and biochemical aspects of the response to therapy with alkylating agents and prednisone. *Am. J. Med.* **67**, 867–878.

Glenner, G. G. (1980). Amyloid deposists and amyloidosis: the β fibrilloses. *N. Engl. J. Med.* **302**, 1283–1292, 1333–1343.

Ravid, M., Robson, M. and Keder, I. (1977). Prolonged colchicine treatment in four patients with amyloidosis. *Ann. Intern. Med.* **87**, 568–570.

Rubinow, A., Celli, B. R., Cohen, A. S., Rigden, B. G. and Brody, J. S. (1978). Localized amyloidosis of the lower respiratory tract. *Am. Rev. Resp. Dis.* **118**, 603–611.

Thompson, P. J. and Citron, K. M. (1983). Amyloid of the lower respiratory tract. *Thorax* **38**, 84–87.

Pulmonary alveolar microlithiasis

This is a very rare disorder which is remarkable for a number of unusual if not unique features. Tiny (0.2–3 mm) calcified concretions are formed progressively in the alveolar spaces which produce a striking and truly unique appearance on the chest radiograph. As profusion (but not size) increases the lung fields become diffusely and densely opaque, there being a mere haziness initially when profusion is yet mild. At this stage the lower zones only appear to be affected, simply because they represent a greater volume of lung tissue on the two-dimensional radiograph. Almost invariably the affected subject is symptom free when an

initial film is taken for incidental reasons, and there may be wonder that this can be possible when the radiograph is grossly abnormal. Measurement of lung function during this asymptomatic stage, however, reveals little or no abnormality, and the affected subject may remain well for many years. In most cases there is slow progression and eventually exercise limitation, dry cough, occasional haemoptysis, respiratory failure, and cor pulmonale supervene, the lungs becoming stiff, ventilation restricted, and gas transfer impaired. Survival of 10–20 years is characteristic. At death, extensive areas of the chest radiograph show a 'white-out' appearance due to the considerable accumulation of calcium, the lungs are difficult to cut, and they sink in water.

At present there are few clues to the cause of this curious disorder and there is no effective means of therapy – features that are themselves unusual at a time of rapid advance in medical science. No abnormality of calcium metabolism has been demonstrated, but a disproportionate number of cases occur in siblings which points to a genetic rather than environmental basis. This is supported by the reported deaths of two newborn infants from the disease. It is nonetheless possible that environmental factors operated during pregnancy, and no clearcut pattern of Mendelian inheritance has been described. The disease usually presents in middle age, but the whole age spectrum may be involved and both sexes are equally represented. Physical signs are conspicuous by their absence for most of its long course, though crackles, clubbing, and signs of respiratory failure are observed in its final stages. The radiographic appearances are specific making biopsy an unnecessary diagnostic procedure.

References

O'Neill, R. P., Cohn, J. E. and Pellegrino, E. D. (1967). Pulmonary alveolar microlithiasis – a familial study. *Ann. Intern. Med.* **67**, 957–967.

Viswanathan, R. (1962). Pulmonary alveolar microlithiasis. *Thorax* **17**, 251–256.

Lipoid (lipid) pneumonia

Exogenous

When mineral or vegetable lipids are aspirated into the alveoli of the lungs, they usually prove to be relatively inert but difficult to remove. Lung lipases have little effect, and the macrophages are slow to transport the free or emulsified material into the lymphatics. The result is a chronic low-grade inflammatory response that may lead to secondary infection and/or local fibrosis. It is known as lipoid pneumonia. Some animal lipids may, however, be degraded by lung lipases to release more irritating fatty acids. In these circumstances a brisk pneumonitis may occur.

Such aspiration is not common in the population at large, but is seen not infrequently within certain subgroups. Most affected are the elderly who are accustomed to use paraffin nasal drops and aperients. A portion of the nasal dose is likely to enter the trachea, as may part of the ingested dose if the subject then reclines in bed or has difficulty swallowing. It is not irritating to the tracheal mucosa, and so coughing is rarely excited. The reluctant child forced to swallow cod liver oil is said to have undergone similar risks, while in wartime shipwrecked sailors have occasionally aspirated diesel oil. Less unwilling inhalers of mineral oil and vaseline have been the blackfat tobacco smokers of Guyana, who obtain a more satisfying smoke by mixing these additives to native tobacco leaf. A distinctive picture of progressive and often fatal pulmonary fibrosis complicates this habit in some 20 per cent of blackfat users, but has not been observed among non-smokers. In more recent times, lipoid pneumonia has been recognized in workers exposed to oil mists and burning fats.

The inflammatory response may give no symptoms, the subject presenting by chance with an abnormal chest radiograph, or may lead to productive cough with low grade fever. Often there is a cyclical course with intermittent symptoms. Repeated aspiration may lead to fibrotic shrinkage of the affected segment or segments, or to persistent consolidation. Either may closely simulate bronchial carcinoma, and many resections have been carried out for this reason. When more substantial quantities are aspirated the radiographic abnormalities are necessarily more diffuse, and when dependent segments are involved the true nature of the disorder is more obvious.

The key to diagnosis lies with the demonstration of lipid material within the sputum or its macrophages. If lung tissue is resected or undergoes biopsy, there may be fibrosis, evidence of chronic inflammation, and foreign body granulomata/giant cells in addition to lipid material retained within alveoli and macrophages. An innovative use of computerized tomography has recently identified excess deposits of lipid in lipoid pneumonia from its X-ray absorption characteristics, a technique which could offer a valuable alternative to biopsy or alveolar lavage in the diagnosis of 'atypical pneumonias'. The key to management lies with identifying the misuse (or abuse) of lipid/paraffin, and in persuading the misuser to adopt alternative habits. During episodes of secondary bacterial infection, there is an obvious role for antibiotics.

Endogenous

Unfortunately the body may itself produce an excess of lipid (chiefly cholesterol) within the lungs at sites of chronic inflammation, though this is not a common phenomenon. This lipid will also be ingested by macrophages and may be recovered in the sputum. Sputum macrophages laden with lipid are not therefore pathognomonic of aspiration from an exogenous source, though chemical tests can distinguish the two varieties. Endogenous lipid is most commonly deposited when chronic inflammation accompanies bronchiectasis, bronchial carcinoma or some other cause of persisting localized bronchial obstruction, and appears to depend on cigarette smoking. The radiological appearances are of a persisting pneumonia, which may also stimulate resection for fear a carcinoma is present.

References

Corrin, B. and Soliman, S. S. (1978). Cholesterol in the lungs of heavy smokers. *Thorax* 33, 565–568.

Miller, G. J., Ashcroft, M. T., Beadnell, H. M. S. G., Wagner, J. C. and Pepys, J. (1971). The lipoid pneumonia of blackfat tobacco smokers in Guyana. *Q. J. Med.* 40, 457–470.

Oldenburger, D., Maurer, W. J., Beltaos, E. and Magnin, G. E. (1972). Inhalation lipid pneumonia from burning fats. *J. Am. Med. Assoc.* 222, 1288–1289.

Wheeler, P. S., Stitik, F. P, Hutchins, G. M. Klinefelter, H. F. and Siegelman, S. S. (1981). Diagnosis of lipoid pneumonia by computed tomography. *J. Am. Med. Assoc.* 245, 65–66.

Lipid storage disease

Gaucher's disease and Niemann–Pick disease are characterized by hereditary inborn inabilities to degrade the body's production of, respectively, glucocerebroside and sphingomyelin. The metabolic defects lie with deficiency (or absence) of the appropriate catabolic enzymes. Each disease is manifested in various forms, usually in Ashkenazi Jews, indicating that a number of distinct genetic abnormalities occur. The effect of these deficiencies is a steady accumulation of the two endogenous lipids within the histiocytes of many organs, particularly those of the liver, spleen, bones, and lymph-nodes. In some forms, central nervous system involvement is characteristic and dominates the clinical picture. The lungs may become infiltrated in both disorders, uncommonly in Gaucher's disease but commonly in the classical acute neuronopathic variety of Niemann–Pick disease.

The interstitial space and the alveolar walls are primarily affected, and the chest radiograph shows a diffuse reticulonodular pattern representing focal accumulation of lipid-laden histiocytes. Pulmonary involvement is rarely symptomatic, however, and is usually of little concern compared with other affected organs. As a result the pulmonary disease is rarely the subject of diagnostic enquiry, the derangement of lipid storage having been recognized already. The excess accumulation of glucocerebroside within histiocytes of affected organs produces a characteristic appearance and the cell can be recognized diagnostically as the Gaucher cell. Accumulation may also occur within the ribs, and the chest radiograph may show characteristic lytic lesions in addition to evidence of a diffuse micronodular infiltration. The equivalent 'foam cells' of Niemann–Pick disease are similarly diagnostic, but bone destruction does not seem to occur, possibly because death from neurological disruption occurs at an early age (2–4 years).

No definitive therapy is available for either disease, but with Gaucher's disease the chronic non-neuronopathic varieties are generally associated with survival into adult life. Occasionally, the pulmonary vasculature may become infiltrated, emboli of Gaucher cells from bone marrow may impact in the pulmonary arterial tree, or deposits may develop directly in the pulmonary capillaries. Pulmonary hypertension may then lead to death from respiratory failure.

References

Jackson, D. C. and Simon, G. (1965). Unusual bone and lung changes in a case of Gaucher's disease. *Br. J. Radiol.* 38, 698–700.

Smith, R. R. L., Hutchins, G. M., Sack, G. H. and Ridolfi, R. L. (1978). Unusual cardiac, renal and pulmonary involvement in Gaucher's disease. *Am. J. Med.* 65, 352–360.

Wolson, A. H. (1975). Pulmonary findings in Gaucher's disease. *Am. J. Roentgenol.* 123, 712–715.

DRUG-INDUCED LUNG DISEASE

G. J. GIBSON

Deleterious effects of drugs on the lungs and airways are an increasing problem and often a source of diagnostic confusion. Adverse reactions to some well-established drugs were identified several decades ago, e.g. exacerbation of asthma after ingestion of aspirin was described in 1910 and the toxic alveolitis produced by gold salts in 1945. A rapidly expanding pharmacopoeia has produced many further problems and widened the spectrum of drug-induced respiratory disease. This review will be limited to direct effects of drugs in usual therapeutic doses on the airways, alveoli, pulmonary vasculature, and mediastinal structures. Indirect

effects, such as the predisposition to opportunistic lung infection resulting from cytotoxic agents or the worsening of respiratory failure after sedatives, are excluded as are the consequences of overdosage or inadequate control of dosage (e.g. pulmonary haemorrhage with anticoagulants).

Airway reactions

Airways obstruction induced by drugs usually presents as an exacerbation of pre-existing asthma, rather than *de novo* development of respiratory disease. Exceptions occur with certain agents

Table 1 Drugs which may produce or exacerbate asthma.

Pharmacological effects		Cholinergic agents e.g. carbachol pilocarpine
		Cholinesterase inhibitors e.g. pyridostigmine
		Prostaglandin $F_2\alpha$
		Histamine release e.g. curare derivatives
		β sympathetic antagonists
Idiosyncratic effects	Oral:	Analgesics and anti-inflammatory agents
		Aspirin
		Indomethacin
		Mefenamic acid
		Flufenamic acid
		Phenylbutazone
		Fenoprofen
		Ibuprofen
		Diclofenac
		Naproxen
		Paracetamol
		Tartrazine-containing preparations
		Carbamazepine
	Parenteral:	Penicillin
		Iron-dextran complex
		Aminophylline
		Hydrocortisone
		N-acetyl cysteine
	Inhaled:	Ampicillin
		Benzyl penicillin
		Cephalosporins
		α-methyl dopa
		Cimetidine
		Piperazine
		Psyllium
		Pancreatic extract
		Pituitary snuff
		Ipratropium bromide (hypotonic solution)

which on repeated inhalation are capable of sensitizing a previously healthy individual and these present a particular problem in the pharmaceutical industry (see below).

The relevant drugs may conveniently be divided into those which produce a more or less predictable effect, related to their pharmacological properties, and secondly those which produce airways obstruction due to an idiosyncratic effect (Table 1).

Pharmacological effects

Cholinergic drugs such as carbachol given systemically occasionally produce bronchoconstriction and in very sensitive asthmatic patients exacerbations have even occurred after use of pilocarpine eye drops. An inhaled anticholinergic agent would seem a logical approach to this problem and has been shown to be effective in reversing occasional untoward effects of cholinesterase inhibitors in asthmatic patients with myasthenia gravis.

The bronchoconstrictor prostaglandin, $F_2\alpha$, if used to induce abortion, may be hazardous in asthmatic patients. Bronchoconstriction after thiopentone, opiates, and muscle relaxants (tubocurarine, suxamethonium, and pancuronium) is probably due to their capacity to release histamine.

A more common problem is worsening of airways obstruction by β-adrenergic antagonist drugs. Although these have been increasingly refined to select agents with the least β_2 antagonism, thus minimizing effects on the airways, none is completely specific for β_1-receptors. The degree of selectivity varies, with propranolol the least, and practolol probably the most, selective agent used so far; unfortunately practolol causes its own distinctive side-effects (see below) and is no longer available for long-term use. Of the currently marketed β-blockers, atenolol and metoprolol seem to have the least adverse effects on airway function but many patients with asthma will show a reduction in FEV_1 or peak flow

on therapeutic doses of these agents and considerable caution is necessary. The problem of β-blockers in patients with clearcut asthma is relatively straightforward but the situation with chronic airways obstruction is less clear. Adverse reactions in such patients are less common and usually less severe, and many patients who develop symptoms with worsening airways obstructon after use of β-blockers are subsequently recognized as 'latent asthmatics'.

Idiosyncratic reactions

In their most dramatic form these present as acute anaphylaxis and among the causative agents penicillin and intravenously administered iron dextran are noteworthy. N-acetyl cysteine given intravenously in severe paracetamol poisoning has recently been shown to produce exacerbations of asthma and caution is necessary in asthmatic patients.

The drugs producing idiosyncratic reactions most frequently are the analgesics and although aspirin-induced asthma has long been recognized, its mechanism remains uncertain. Most patients who are sensitive to aspirin react also to other analgesics with widely differing chemical structures (Table 1) making an immunological reaction unlikely. All the anti-inflammatory agents incriminated are inhibitors of prostaglandin synthesis via the cyclo-oxygenase pathway and it is presumed that their adverse effects are mediated in this way, perhaps with diversion of arachidonic acid metabolism to the production of bronchoconstrictor leukotrienes, but the exact mechanism and why only a proportion of asthmatics are affected is not clear. Deaths have been reported with aspirin and indomethacin. Of the commonly used analgesics, paracetamol seems to be the least likely to provoke a significant response, although occasional adverse reactions are well documented. An interesting feature which has recently come to light is that under carefully controlled conditions most aspirin-sensitive asthmatics can be made tolerant to further aspirin by ingesting graded doses over a couple of days. This state of tolerance can then be maintained by daily treatment with aspirin but sensitivity returns within a few days of discontinuing regular treatment.

Many patients with analgesic-induced asthma are also sensitive to the azo dye tartrazine, a commonly used colouring agent in medications (especially those coloured yellow, orange, or red), and also in foodstuffs. Usually reactions to tartrazine are not as severe as with aspirin but, since tartrazine is an approved food and drug additive, its presence is usually not declared and the extent of the problems it may cause is not clear. If tolerance to tartrazine can develop in a similar way to aspirin tolerance the majority of the populations in advanced societies may be chemically desensitized to its effects because of the ubiquitous presence of tartrazine in processed, canned, and packeted foods, Ironically tartrazine was in the past present in some medications used to treat asthma! Many drug manufacturers are currently removing tartrazine from their formulations but at the time of writing it still lurks in such apparently innocent generic formulations as linctus codeine BP.

The potential exacerbation of asthma by drugs used to treat it presents a particularly acute dilemma as a drug effect may be difficult to dissociate from spontaneous deterioration. Apart from potential problems related to tartrazine there are well-documented cases of worsening asthma after both intravenous aminophylline and hydrocortisone; the latter may be particularly a problem in asthmatic patients with analgesic sensitivity. Recently it became apparent that some patients with markedly hyperreactive airways reacted adversely to the anticholinergic agent ipratropium bromide when nebulized in a hypotonic solution. The preparation has now been changed so that the solution is isotonic and this will hopefully remove the problem. Bronchodilator and other drugs formulated as a dry powder sometimes have an irritant effect, as also may the propellants used in pressurized aerosols.

Asthmatic reactions have been reported following the inhalation of several drugs, usually during the manufacturing process (Table 1). The affected patients are usually non-atopic with no history of respiratory disease prior to exposure; on challenge testing the asthma is often of the 'late' type and the condition appears likely to be a specific immunological response, with a good prognosis if the subject is removed from the offending drug. Inhalation of organic substances of animal or vegetable origin may also produce sensitization, usually in atopic individuals; these include extracts of the weed psyllium used as an osmotic laxative, pancreatic extract used to treat cystic fibrosis, and pituitary snuff.

Alveolar reactions

There is no generally accepted classification of alveolar reactions, which range from acute pulmonary oedema or the adult respiratory distress syndrome at one extreme to an insidiously developing pulmonary fibrosis at the other. The reactions are conveniently considered under three main headings (Table 2). Of the drugs which may produce acute pulmonary oedema, hydrochlorothiazide and salicylates are the commonest; in the case of the former there is good evidence that the oedema is non-cardiogenic, and it appears to be an occasional idiosyncratic reaction not shared by other thiazide drugs. In the case of salicylates there is a more clear relationship to dose, with reactions usually seen in frank overdose (as also occurs with opiates), but occasionally in chronic ingesters with high serum levels. Problems related to isoxsuprine have occurred with its use as a tocolytic agent and other drugs, including sympathetic stimulants and corticosteroids also used to arrest premature labour, have been less commonly implicated.

Several drugs produce widespread alveolar damage ('pneumonitis' or 'alveolitis') which may or may not be followed by fibrosis (Table 2). Patients may present acutely with cough, fever, shortness of breath, and occasionally systemic upset. Alternatively slowly progressive fibrosis may present with gradually worsening dyspnoea and widespread shadowing on the chest radiograph. The mechanism(s) of such reactions are generally uncertain but in some cases, including bleomycin, carmustine, amiodarone, and nitrofurantoin there is evidence of a relationship to dose or duration of treatment. Recent evidence in the cases of nitrofurantoin and bleomycin has suggested mechanisms involving the production of toxic oxygen radicals in the lungs, perhaps providing a link with the known pulmonary toxicity of oxygen itself and with the synergistic adverse effects of high oxygen concentrations and some cytotoxic agents.

The anti-arrhythmic agent amiodarone has caused problems in many countries over the last 5 years. The literature to date includes more than 50 patients with pulmonary reactions associated with this drug, of whom approximately one-third have died. Since most of the patients have serious cardiac disease, a common problem of differential diagnosis is the distinction from cardiogenic pulmonary oedema. Histologically the lungs show thickening and fibrosis of alveolar walls usually with a mild inflammatory reaction; the alveolar spaces show abundant 'foamy' macrophages due to accumulation of phospholipid within lysosomes. This characteristic appearance of the macrophages is not necessarily accompanied by other evidence of pulmonary toxicity and is also found in other tissues of patients being treated with the drug.

Cytotoxic and immunosuppressive drugs represent an increasing problem and the majority have been reported to cause pulmonary complications. Bleomycin causes the most frequent problems, followed by busulphan and methotrexate. Cyclophosphamide and azathioprine, which, because of their rôles in non-malignant disease, are perhaps the most widely used agents in this group of drugs, produce adverse pulmonary reactions only rarely. In most cases it is not clear whether the effects are due to direct toxicity or to hypersensitivity. With bleomycin, however, there is evidence of a dose relationship: cumulative doses of less than 150 mg are unlikely to cause serious reactions, whereas death due to respiratory failure consequent upon severe fibrosis has occurred in about 10 per cent of patients receiving more than 500 mg. The recorded frequency of adverse reactions varies with the means by which they are detected; for example, on clinical and functional criteria fibrosis occurs in 5–10 per cent of patients treated with busulphan but pathological and cytological evidence suggests lung toxicity in a much higher proportion. The frequency of overt lung involvement may also be related to length of survival as determined by the primary disease. With busulphan the average interval between starting treatment and the appearance of toxic effects can be as long as four years and in some cases the lung changes appear to progress after the drug has been discontinued. Other factors which may increase the toxicity of a given drug include advanced age of the patient and synergistic effects with other drugs, with radiation to the lung, or with subsequent inhalation of high oxygen concentrations.

Histologically most cytotoxic drugs produce evidence of diffuse alveolar damage with destruction of lining cells, formation of hyaline membranes, and a variable inflammatory infiltrate and degree of fibrosis. Fibrosis is particularly common with busulphan and bleomycin and rare with methotrexate. With methotrexate and procarbazine (and very occasionally with bleomycin) there may be blood and tissue eosinophilia and correspondingly a good therapeutic response to steroids. The possibility of cytotoxic drug-induced malignancy in the lungs has been suggested and there are cases of alveolar cell carcinoma recorded in patients with fibrosis induced by busulphan, but since this association is recognized with diffuse fibrosis of any cause, a direct aetiological relationship is doubtful.

Eosinophilic reactions in the lung include conditions which would be classified as Loeffler's syndrome, simple or prolonged pulmonary eosinophilia, and eosinophilic pneumonia. Tissue eosinophilia may be a more consistent feature than peripheral blood eosinophilia. Sulphonamides are the drugs most frequently reported as causes of pulmonary eosinophilia, and reactions have even occurred to a vaginal cream containing sulphonamide; sulphonamide sensitivity may also explain some of the reactions to sulphasalazine and to chlorpropamide which is chemically related. The pulmonary eosinophilia recorded with aspirin appears to be separate from aspirin-induced asthma. Nitrofurantoin may produce an acute eosinophilic reaction in addition to the more insidious fibrosis described above. The rôles of gold salts and

Table 2 Alveolar reactions

Acute pulmonary oedema/ARDS
    Hydrochlorothiazide
    Salicylates
    Isoxsuprine
    Naloxone

Diffuse lung injury (alveolitis) and/or fibrosis
    Oxygen
    Hexamethonium
    Nitrofurantoin
    Amiodarone
    Cytotoxic agents

	Bleomycin	Melphalan
	Mitomycin C	Cyclophosphamide
	BCNU (carmustine)	Cytosine arabinoside
	CCNU (lomustine)	6 mercapto purine
	Busulphan	Azathioprine
	Chlorambucil	
Eosinophilic reactions	Sulphonamides	Nitrofurantoin* (acute
	Penicillins	reaction)
	Tetracycline	Methotrexate*
	Aspirin	Procarbazine*
	Naproxen	Gold salts*
	Sulphasalazine	Penicillamine*
	Chlorpropamide	
	Chlorpromazine	
	Imipramine	
	Carbamazepine	
	Phenytoin	

* Eosinophilia not consistent.

penicillamine in this type of reaction have been a matter of some debate but the evidence suggests that either may occasionally provoke a reaction. However, the suggestion that drugs may be responsible for many of the cases of fibrosing alveolitis associated with rheumatoid arthritis seems unlikely. Penicillamine has also been incriminated in two other types of adverse pulmonary reaction: firstly, Goodpasture's syndrome with pulmonary haemorrhage when used in high doses in treatment of Wilson's disease and, secondly, obliterative bronchiolitis, an unusual form of airways obstruction which is seen occasionally in patients with rheumatoid arthritis. The evidence against penicillamine in the latter case is not conclusive.

The clinical severity of eosinophilic reactions is very variable ranging from a transient and asymptomatic radiological opacity to a severe illness with dyspnoea, cough, fever, and hypoxaemia due to widespread eosinophilic pneumonia. Concomitant asthma has been noted in particular with carbamazepine, but is not otherwise a common feature. The chest radiograph shows fluffy opacities frequently with a peripheral or predominantly upper lobe distribution. The reactions are often accompanied by a diffuse maculopapular skin eruption. The prognosis is usually good: the changes often subside spontaneously on withdrawal of the drug or in more severely ill patients there is usually a dramatic improvement on instituting treatment with corticosteroids. Although repeated exposure to the offending agent will continue to produce reactions, the severity of these may progressively decrease.

Two reports of pulmonary eosinophilia occurring in asthmatic patients treated by inhaled corticosteroids probably resulted from the unmasking of an eosinophilic pneumonia as oral steroids were reduced and there is no good evidence of any cause and effect relationship.

Pulmonary vascular reactions

Pulmonary thromboembolism related to use of the contraceptive pill is well established; its incidence correlates with the oestrogen content and has been reduced since introduction of low oestrogen preparations.

Of great theoretical interest was the statistical association between pulmonary hypertension and the use of the anorectic agent aminorex in Switzerland, Germany, and Austria. Since the drug was withdrawn the epidemic of pulmonary hypertension has subsided and no similar rise was seen in countries which did not introduce this agent. Occasional cases of pulmonary hypertension have been reported in patients taking various amphetamine-like agents and in a recent report two patients had been treated with fenfluramine. Although the evidence against other anorectic agents is not conclusive, experience with aminorex indicates the need for a careful drug history from all patients with unexplained 'primary' pulmonary hypertension. Two patients with pulmonary hypertension who were taking the now obsolete antidiabetic agent phenformin have also been reported and a reduction of pulmonary vascular resistance was documented after withdrawal of the drug; it was suggested that pulmonary hypertension in these patients might have resulted either from lactate production or from an α sympathetic stimulating effect of phenformin.

Analgesics given during labour have been implicated in the development of pulmonary hypertension in the newborn; drugs such as aspirin, indomethacin, and naproxen delay premature labour but may also by their inhibitory effects on prostaglandin synthesis cause constriction of the ductus arteriosus *in utero* leading to postnatal pulmonary hypertension and respiratory distress.

Pleura and mediastinum

Hilar and mediastinal adenopathy are occasionally seen as part of the generalized lymphadenopathy produced by the anticonvulsant phenytoin and mediastinal lipomatosis has been reported in patients on large doses of steroids.

Drugs which have been associated with pleural reactions (fluid or thickening) are shown in Table 3. Numerous agents have been

Table 3 Drugs associated with pleural reactions

Drug-induced lupus syndrome	Procainamide
	Hydralazine etc.
Oculo-muco-cutaneous syndrome	Practolol
Isolated	Methysergide
	Dantrolene
	Methotrexate
	Bromocriptine

reported to produce a systemic lupus (SLE)-like syndrome (see page 16.20). The anti-arrhythmic procainamide is the one most often implicated but others include gold, hydralazine, isoniazid, penicillamine, and sulphonamides. Although the main target structure both in the lupus syndrome and with methysergide is the pleura, there may be some fibrosis of adjacent areas of lung.

A more recently recognized problem concerns the selective β-sympathetic antagonist practolol. This produces a characteristic 'oculomucocutaneous' syndrome; although patients with the latter have high titres of antinuclear factor, LE cells are not usually found, and the syndrome differs from lupus in that ocular symptoms are not usually a feature of drug-induced SLE. In many patients pleural effusions and subsequent pleural thickening have been reported in association with the characteristic corneal ulceration, discoid rash, and fibrinous peritonitis. Patients with practolol-induced pleurisy sometimes develop effusions months or years after discontinuing the drug and a careful drug history is therefore necessary from patients with unexplained pleural effusions or thickening. The chronic changes have in some cases led to significant respiratory disability. As with procainamide and methysergide, pulmonary involvement has been reported in some patients but the predominant abnormality is related to the pleural surface. Other β-sympathetic antagonists, in particular acebutolol, have been reported as occasionally causing an alveolar or pleural reaction but it seems unlikely that other β-blockers cause the full-blown and severe 'practolol syndrome'.

The drug methysergide used for the treatment of the carcinoid syndrome and occasionally for migraine may induce mediastinal or pleural fibrosis with or without retroperitoneal fibrosis. Improvement follows early withdrawal of the drug. Methotrexate has been associated with pleurisy, independent of its alveolar effects, and the smooth muscle relaxant dantrolene, which is used for relief of spasticity, has been reported to produce an unusual type of pleurisy with effusion in which fluid and blood eosinophilia are prominent. There is no evidence of any parenchymal abnormality and although the changes gradually resolve on withdrawing the drug, some residual pleural fibrosis may remain.

Complications of radiological procedures

Lipoid pneumonia may follow bronchography with oily media. This is an oleogranulomatous reaction which may lead to fibrosis and sometimes to a localized mass simulating a neoplasm. Similar reactions can follow aspiration into the lungs of oily medicine (laxatives).

Lymphangiographic media which drain through the thoracic duct and so into the venous circulation, enter and can impact in the pulmonary circulation. This is often symptomless but may cause dyspnoea and cough with the expectoration of fat globules or haemoptysis. The chest radiograph shows a fine stippling and occasional deaths have been recorded.

References

Brewis, R. A. L. (1981). Respiratory disorders. In *Textbook of adverse drug reactions* (ed. D. M. Davies), pp. 154–187. Oxford University Press, Oxford.

Ginsberg, S. J. and Comis, R. L. (1982). The pulmonary toxicity of antineoplastic agents. *Sem. Oncol.* **9**, 34–51.

Van Arsdel, P. P. (1984). Aspirin idiosyncracy and tolerance. *J. All. Clin. Immunol.* **73**, 430–443.

TUMOURS OF THE LUNG, MEDIASTINUM, AND PLEURA

N. W. HORNE AND S. G. SPIRO

Carcinoma of the bronchus

In most technically advanced countries lung cancer is acknowledged to be the most important cancer in men and to be rapidly approaching the same position in women. For example, the tumour currently causes about 35 000 deaths annually in England and Wales. There has been a downturn recently in younger men and the death rate in men is now stabilizing but in women it continues to rise and will continue to do so if current trends are maintained. So long as smoking remains popular the mortality rate is likely to fall only very slowly.

Whereas there has been a significant improvement in survival in diseases such as Hodgkin's disease, and to a lesser degree, leukaemia and cancer of the kidney and larynx, there has really been no improvement in the survival rate from lung cancer. Between 17 and 20 per cent survive for one year after registration, but only 6 to 8 per cent are alive five years later, compared with over 50 per cent for breast and cervical cancer.

Despite the very poor prognosis of lung cancer it is very important that each patient with this disease be carefully assessed as much can be done to ameliorate the suffering of many patients and some can be cured of the disease. However, in palliative treatment the withholding of technological advances in investigation and therapy requires as much skill and judgement and compassion as their employment.

Aetiological factors

Tobacco

The increase in mortality from lung cancer in every country appeared to coincide with the increase in tobacco usage, particularly cigarette smoking, after what seemed to be an appropriate latent interval. Early retrospective studies showed that there were, amongst patients with carcinoma of the bronchus, many fewer non-smokers and many more heavy smokers than among the controls, and that there was a degree of association between the amount smoked and the risk of lung cancer. Prospective studies amongst which the long-term study of British doctors is particularly informative, confirmed the increased risk of death from lung cancer from any tobacco use but most specifically from usage of cigarettes, there being a strong dose–response relationship with the number of cigarettes smoked. This is illustrated in Table 1. The most important variable in smoking intensity is the

number of cigarettes smoked but other variables include the depth of inhalation, number of puffs, butt length, use of a filter, and the type of tobacco smoked. Further evidence of a causal relationship became apparent in a further study which documented the reduction in risk following cessation of smoking: after cessation of smoking for 15 years the ratio of rates compared to non-smokers fell from 15.8 : 1 to 2 : 1 or if expressed in a different way fell to 11 per cent of that pertaining to continuing smokers. Wide differences in smoking habits are now seen between social classes with 49 per cent of unskilled manual workers smoking, compared with only 17 per cent of professional workers. However, during the last ten years the number of adult men smoking in England and Wales has fallen from 51 to 36 per cent, and from 41 to 32 per cent in adult women (OPCS General Household Survey). The effect of the lower tar-containing cigarettes has just had time to become established, and could be responsible for declining death rates in young men. Passive smoking (the inhalation of other people's smoke by non-smokers) has recently become an emotive issue, and appears to increase the risk of lung cancer in the non-smoking wives of heavy smokers about 1.5 times.

Occupation

A number of different factors have now been identified as being associated with lung cancer: subjects who develop this disease as a result of their occupation represent a small but important group. The association of *asbestos* with lung cancer is now firmly established, various studies identifying a risk factor of 4.9 to 7.3 times those who are not specifically exposed to asbestos. There is a much greater risk for the asbestos industry worker if he smokes cigarettes, one study identifying the risk at 93 times that in non-smokers not exposed to asbestos. In Norway it has become illegal to employ a smoker in an asbestos-related job. Exposure to *radioactive isotopes*, mainly radon daughters, occurs among various groups of miners particularly those involved in the mining of pitchblende and uranium; *polycyclic aromatic hydrocarbons* are believed to be responsible for the increased risk in workers in the gas and coke ovens and in foundry workers; *nickel* refining, *chromate* manufacture, and *arsenical* industrial workers are also exposed to a higher risk of lung cancer. The amount of lung cancer caused by occupational exposure may well have been underestimated in the past.

Air pollution

The decline in male mortality is occurring earlier than would be expected from changes in smoking habits. The high mortality figures in the United Kingdom and Germany compared to, for example, France and Italy seem likely to be in part due to heavy industry and coal burning. Analysis by county in the United States shows an association between lung cancer deaths and counties with chemical, petroleum, ship building, and paper industries. Legislation for cleaner air has caused both environmental and occupational pollution to fall dramatically in the past 30 years, and this has preceded changes in smoking habits.

There is a high incidence of lung cancer among women in Hong Kong. This has been shown to be associated not only with cigarette smoking but with the habitual use of the kerosene stove in small and poorly ventilated kitchen rooms.

Pathology and pathogenesis

A detailed understanding of the natural history, pathology, and pathogenesis of bronchial carcinoma is becoming more and more important as the assessment, management, and prognosis of the

Table 1 Death rate from lung cancer in males by smoking habits when last asked (British Doctor's Study)

Tobacco use category	Death rate (age standardized per 100 000)
Non-smokers	10
Ex-smokers	43
Continuing smokers	
Any tobacco	104
Pipe and/or cigar only	58
Mixed	82
Cigarette smokers only	140
Number smoked per day	
1–14	78
15–24	127
25 or more	251

Table 2 Classification of epithelial tumours of the lung (based on revised WHO classification)

	Frequency (%)		Frequency (%)
Main			
Epidermoid carcinoma (squamous cell)	35	Adenocarcinoma Acinar Papillary Bronchiolar alveolar	21
Small cell carcinoma Oatcell Fusiform Others	24	Large cell carcinoma With stratification With mucin-production Giant cell Clear cell	19
Less common Tumours showing mixed differentiation		Bronchial gland Adenoid cystic Muco-epidermoid Others	
Carcinoid tumours			
	Carcinoma *in situ*		

disease depends largely upon the cell type and the presence or absence of metastases at the time of presentation. It has been estimated that about seven-eighths of a tumour's life will have passed when it is diagnosed and that the vast majority, and perhaps all tumours, will be disseminated at this time.

The World Health Organization orientated classification of lung cancer according to cell type and the approximate distribution of each type as a percentage of all lung cancers is shown in Table 2. The four main histological types of bronchial carcinoma are epidermoid (squamous) cell, small (oat) cell anaplastic, adenocarcinoma, and large cell carcinoma. Tumours which have matured sufficiently to form readily identifiable markers, keratin and gland formation, for example, appear to have a less aggressive nature.

Epidermoid (squamous) carcinomas seem to arise most commonly in segmental and subsegmental bronchi in response to repetitive carcinogenic stimuli or inflammation and irritation. The mucosal lining is most susceptible to injury at the bifurcation of bronchial structures. Dysplasia is followed by carcinoma *in situ* when the entire thickness of the mucosa may be replaced by proliferating neoplastic cells. These changes may be strictly localized or multicentric. Tumour infiltration follows loss of the basal membrane. The precise origins of small cell carcinomas remain an enigma and those of adenocarcinomas are not precisely defined. The latter may arise from the mucosal lining or from the submucosal bronchial mucous glands. A significant number of lung tumours arise in the periphery of the lung, perhaps three-quarters of adenocarcinomas and large cell anaplastic malignancies, one-third of epidermoid and one-fifth of small cell carcinomas. Epidermoid has a relatively slow growth rate (volume doubling time 90 days) and the lowest incidence of distant haematogenous metastasis; small cell tumours grow rapidly (volume doubling time 30 days) and there is very early dissemination by both haematogenous and lymphatic routes, metastasis being present in more than 90 per cent of patients at the time of diagnosis. Adenocarcinomas and anaplastic large cell tumours occupy an intermediate position.

Epidermoid (squamous) carcinoma These tumours, commonly referred to as 'squamous cell', are composed predominantly of flattened to polygonal-shaped neoplastic cells that tend to stratify, form intercellular bridges, and elaborate keratin. About 60 per cent present as obstructive lesions in lobar and main stem bronchi. The tumours tend to be bulky and to produce intraluminar granular or polypoid masses. As a result distal pneumonia and abscess formation is common and cavitation is seen in about 10 per cent. The cells are usually well differentiated, but in some cases differentiation is poor and the appearances are those of predominantly anaplastic cells, frequently arranged in the classical pattern of stratifying sheets.

Small (oat) cell anaplastic carcinoma is now recognized as a pathologically and clinically distinct form of lung cancer. Small cell lung cancer may originate from the amine precursor uptake and decarboxylation (APUD) series of cells. The tumour is composed of neoplastic cells with dark oval to round spindled nuclei and scanty indistinct cytoplasm arranged in ribbons, nests, and sheets. The cells tend to crush easily on biopsy and extensive areas may be necrotic. This type of tumour presents as a proximal lesion in 75 per cent of cases and may arise anywhere in the tracheobronchial tree and rapidly invade vessels and lymph-nodes, disseminating widely even before symptoms arise from the primary tumour. Extensive advanced disease exists in more than half the patients on presentation. The tumours often have a glossy reddish appearance and may stenose the bronchial lumen circumferentially for several centimetres. The cells secrete hormones which give rise to characteristic clinical syndromes in 10 per cent of cases.

Adenocarcinoma This tumour forms acinar or granular structures, having prominent papillary processes, and may be mucin-provoking. About 70 per cent appear to originate peripherally in the lung and are frequently fairly circumscribed: in about 10 per cent the initial presentation is a pleural effusion. If related to bronchi they tend to cuff and stenose the lumen. They occasionally arise in old tuberculous scars.

Large cell These tumours, which have been described as a 'wastepaper' category, include all tumours that show no evidence of maturation or differentiation. They are composed of pleomorphic cells with variable enlarged nuclei, prominent nucleoli, and nuclear inclusions, and abundant cytoplasm: they are mucin-producing in many instances. The tumours tend to be bulky and are often necrotic; they are frequently peripheral, they invade locally, and disseminate widely, about half the patients having disseminated disease on presentation. Though they are highly malignant and undifferentiated the cure rate after surgery is surprisingly high, but radiotherapy is ineffective in controlling the disease. Large cell carcinoma is a smoking-related disease in over 90 per cent of patients.

Bronchioloalveolar carcinoma There has been considerable controversy as to whether this tumour, which has the least association with tobacco intake, arises from alveolar or bronchial epithelium, but derivation from the alveolar type II cell has been suggested. The tumour tends to spread as cuboidal or columnar 'epithelium' along the lining of the alveoli, with single or multiple rows of cells and often papillary formation. There is production of a large amount of mucus in 20 per cent of cases and it is believed that malignant cells shed into the mucus may carry over into relevant anatomical sites in the contralateral lung. Some authorities however believe the tumour to be multicentric in origin, and diffuse nodular lesions are to be found on radiographic examination in some patients. Invasion of neighbouring tissue and lymph-nodes and blood stream metastases are less common than in other cell types. There is some resemblance to metastases from adenocarcinomas emanating from other organs and this sometimes leads to confusion. The form often called malignant pulmonary adenomatosis tends to grow along alveolar septa as a framework, and it may be difficult to distinguish it from metastatic tumour from colon, breast, and pancreas.

Carcinoid tumours are described on pages 15.156 and 12.59.

Carcinoma in situ Many investigators have suggested that cells undergoing malignant change do not necessarily invade the lungs at the onset of this biological mutation, but continue to exist at a particular location (cancer *in situ*). Exfoliated cancer cells sloughed from such a location may be seen fortuitously by the cytologist : even more rarely such a site may be biopsied at bronchoscopy.

Clinical features

The clinical abnormalities associated with lung cancer vary considerably. In about 5 per cent of patients the initial presentation is a radiographic abnormality found on routine examination and unassociated with symptoms: on the other hand patients may present with extremely advanced disease from which death rapidly occurs.

The clinical features may be due to local development of the tumour in the lung, including bronchial obstruction; invasion of contiguous structures in the thorax and mediastinum; metastasis through blood or lymph vessels; and endocrine, metabolic, and neurological syndromes.

Cough is the most common initial presenting symptom. Because cough is a symptom of so many respiratory disorders, the possibility of tumour may be overlooked or other cause attributed to it, particularly in smokers who may have had chronic bronchitis for many years. Patients who have a persistent cough should have a chest radiograph, particularly if they are 40 years or over and are smokers. A change in the cough habit is significant and also requires investigation. If the trachea or main bronchi are involved the cough may be brassy in character and may be accompanied by wheezing or stridor. If cough is manifestly ineffective involvement of the recurrent laryngeal nerve should be suspected.

Sputum Expectoration of sputum may be due to spread of the tumour itself or to infection occurring distal to bronchial obstruction. In the early stages of the disease the sputum is often grey and viscid; it is usually purulent in the presence of infection distal to a tumour and in cavitated tumours. The increasing value of sputum cytology in diagnosis is described below.

Haemoptysis which occurs as a sole presenting symptom in about 5 per cent, and at some stage in the disease in 50 per cent of patients, is a symptom not easily ignored by patient or physician. The degree varies from streaking of the sputum with blood to significant amounts, but massive haemoptysis is rare except as a terminal event. The most significant description given by patients is that of coughing up blood every morning for several days in succession. The introduction of the flexible bronchoscope has led to readier investigation of patients with haemoptysis and this is to be commended.

Wheeze may be observed in a few patients, localized persistent wheeze even after coughing being a significant observation associated with bronchial obstruction.

Stridor is a feature which is ill-recognized and often confused with wheeze. It is due to narrowing of the glottis, trachea or major bronchi and is best heard after the patient coughs and then breathes in deeply with the mouth open.

Dyspnoea is a presenting symptom only in a small number of patients. As the disease progresses, dyspnoea is inevitable, being proportionate to the amount of lung involvement, including collapse of the lung due to endobronchial disease causing airway narrowing or obstruction. Progressive breathlessness is also a salient feature of malignant pleural and, rarely, pericardial effusion, of superior vena caval obstruction and of lymphangitis carcinomatosis.

Chest discomfort is a common symptom occurring in up to 40 per cent of patients at diagnosis. The discomfort is often of an ill-defined nature and may be described in terms of intermittent aching somewhere in the chest. Definite pleural pain may occur in the presence of infection but invasion of the pleura by tumour may well be painless. Invasion of ribs or vertebrae however causes continuous gnawing pain locally. A tumour in the superior pulmonary sulcus (Pancoast) causes progressive constant pain in the shoulder, upper anterior chest or interscapular region, soon spreading to the arm once the brachial plexus is invaded. Other symptoms of this type of tumour include weakness and atrophy of the muscles of the hand, Horner's syndrome, hoarseness, and spinal cord compression at levels D1 and D2.

Lack of energy and, more particularly, *loss of interest* in normal pursuits is a symptom of great importance; a sensation of vague ill-health occurs commonly.

Fever, chills, and night sweats may occur due to chest infection but fever may very rarely be present in rapidly progressive tumours without evidence of infection, especially if there are hepatic metastases.

Invasion of adjacent intrathoracic structures
This gives rise to certain specific clinical features.

Involvement of the last cervical and first thoracic segment of the sympathetic trunk by cancer produces *Horner's syndrome* manifested by a drooping eyelid, sunken eyeball, narrow palpebral fissure, contracted pupil, and lack of thermal sweating on the affected side. Malignant infiltration of the recurrent laryngeal nerve – almost always the left branch due to its course adjacent to the left hilum – gives rise to *vocal chord paralysis*. The right recurrent laryngeal nerve is rarely affected in the base of the neck. Recurrent aspiration pneumonias may follow vocal chord paralysis. Extension of the tumour with invasion or compression of the superior vena cava with secondary thrombosis results in the characteristic features of *superior vena caval obstruction* – awareness of tightness of the collar, fullness of the head, and suffusion of the face especially after bending down, blackouts, breathlessness, engorgement of veins with a downward venous flow in the neck, the upper half of the thorax and arms, oedema of the face often being observed.

Dysphagia is due to compression of the oesophagus from without due to tumour masses and only rarely to direct invasion. *Cardiac* metastases usually occur late in the disease and are manifested clinically by tachycardia, arrhythmias, pericardial effusion, breathlessness, and cardiac failure. Invasion of the *phrenic nerve* results in elevation of the hemidiaphragm which is seen to move paradoxically on fluoroscopic examination.

The clinical features associated with involvement of the *ribs, spine,* and *pleura* are described elsewhere. Very rarely bronchogenic carcinoma causes *spontaneous pneumothorax*. It must not be forgotten that spread of tumour to the other lung may occur or that double primaries may co-exist.

Metastatic lesions
Metastatic lesions from lung cancer may occur in any organ of the body and produce symptoms which form the presenting complaint.

Metastases to *nodes*, particularly those in the scalene area, which are usually the first nodes involved which can be palpated clinically, are frequent and should be sought for with great care, the best position for examination being from behind the patient seated relaxed in a chair. The side affected usually corresponds with the side of the lung lesion, the exception being that tumours from the left lower lobe may metastasize to the nodes in the right scalene area. Involvement of the nodes in the floor of the supraclavicular fossa is equally common.

Bony metastases are common particularly in small cell tumours and occur predominantly in the ribs, vertebrae, humeri, and femora. Early involvement may be detected by a rise in alkaline phosphatase of bony origin, isotope scanning or biopsy. Conventional skeletal surveys are often unhelpful and occasionally misleading. *Liver secondaries* are common and may be silent although a rise in liver enzymes and particularly alkaline phosphatase of liver origin may be an early sign. Isotope liver scans and ultrasound may detect involvement in a liver which is not clinically enlarged but as the metastases develop the liver becomes grossly enlarged with an irregular outline. Friction rubs may sometimes be heard over a grossly involved liver. Metastases to *brain* may account for the presenting symptom in lung cancer in 4 per cent of patients and may be encountered at some time in the illness in 30 per cent. The symptoms simulate those of any expanding brain tumour. The *kidneys* and *adrenals* are involved in 15–20 per cent of patients, rarely producing symptoms. The *skin* should be examined for the presence of the typical slightly bluish umbilicated lesions of tumour spread. Subcutaneous metastases may be found in almost any site.

Endocrine and metabolic manifestations

It is becoming more apparent that many hitherto unexplained and often unusual manifestations of malignant disease are the result of endocrine and metabolic manifestations of the cancer itself. Cancer cells appear to be able to synthesize polypeptides that mimic virtually all the hormones produced by conventional endocrine organs: hence the term 'ectopic hormones'. From time to time the clinical features resulting from ectopic hormone secretion precede those of the pulmonary tumour emphasizing the importance of a high index of suspicion in such circumstances. Unfortunately, in current practice, there is no ectopic hormone measurement which can be used for effective screening purposes. Numerous examples have now been cited of multiple hormonal abnormalities with associated clinical syndromes in the same patient.

Syndrome of inappropriate secretion of antidiuretic hormone (SIADH) The continued secretion of vasopressin (antidiuretic hormone, ADH), in an amount in excess of the body's needs leads to overhydration in both the intracellular and extracellular compartments. The cerebral oedema resulting from water intoxication causes drowsiness, lethargy, irritability, mental confusion and disorientation, fits, and coma being the most profound features. Peripheral oedema is remarkably rare. The patient is usually asymptomatic unless the sodium falls below 120 mEq/litre and the hyponatraemia is dilutional in type with a low serum osmolality. Urine osmolality usually exceeds 300 mosmol/kg. This syndrome is most commonly associated with small cell lesions and may be obvious in 10 per cent of cases and in many more if they are studied closely, and also occurs in some cases of pleural mesothelioma. Restriction of fluid to a daily intake of 700–1000 ml may redress the hyponatraemia while demethylchlortetracycline (demeclocycline) 600–1200 mg daily is often highly effective. Azotaemia may occur as a result of increased urea production and a mild drug-induced nephrotoxicity so that adjustment of dosage may be necessary. Infusion of hypertonic saline is hazardous often precipitating cardiac failure or cerebral oedema.

Ectopic ACTH syndrome Secretion of an adrenocorticotrophic substance by a small cell carcinoma or bronchial carcinoid leads to bilateral adrenal hyperplasia and to secretion of large amounts of cortisol. The onset of symptoms may be so acute that death may occur within a few weeks and the typical features of Cushing's syndrome such as cutaneous striae and the characteristic distribution of body fat do not have time to develop. Chief clinical features are thirst and polyuria, oedema, pigmentation, and hypokalaemia. Hypertension and profound myopathy may also be present. Serum cortisol is elevated: the level is not suppressed by dexamethasone, loss of the diurnal rhythm of cortisol level occurs, and hypokalaemic alkalosis may be present, the plasma potassium often being below 3.0 mmol/litre and bicarbonate more than 30 mmol/litre. Drugs which block adrenocortical steroid biosynthesis may produce partial and reversible medical adrenalectomy and metyrapone in doses from 250 mg thrice daily to 1 g four times daily may cause disappearance of symptoms; an excellent quality of life can be achieved thereby for several months. Obviously removal of the tumour, if practicable, is of value as is chemotherapy as the latter will deal with ectopic sources of hormone as well as hormone secreted by the primary tumour. Reappearance of symptoms usually heralds tumour recurrence.

Hypercalcaemia This feature may be associated with ectopic secretion of parathormone by squamous cell cancers but it must be remembered that it is more commonly due directly to the presence of multiple bone metastases. The primary tumour may also produce a cyclic AMP-stimulating factor or a prostaglandin causing hypercalcaemia. Its presence is unlikely to be recognized symptomatically unless the serum calcium exceeds 12 mg/100 ml: levels of 20 mg/100 ml are sometimes encountered. The main clinical features are nausea, vomiting, abdominal pain, and constipation; polyuria, thirst, and dehydration; muscular weakness and psychosis and drowsiness and eventually coma. The calcium level drops dramatically within 48 hours if the tumour is removed and also falls after radiotherapy or chemotherapy. The associated dehydration requires replacement of 5 litres of fluid intravenously in 24 hours. Corticosteroids are effective in about half the cases, using 400 mg of hydrocortisone and 100 mg prednisolone in 24 hours initially. Other treatments which are sometimes effective are calcitonin 200–400 units 8-hourly, mithramycin 10–15 μg/kg by infusion over 4 hours on alternate days, aspirin 2–4 g/day and indomethacin 50–100 mg/day.

Gynaecomastia Swelling of the breasts which may be painful occurs mainly in the subareolar area, and there may be atrophy of the testes. The association is chiefly with large cell carcinomas. Increased gonadatrophin production is the cause.

Hyperthyroidism occurs rarely but neither goitre nor eye signs are prominent features. *Spontaneous hypoglycaemia*, the *masculinizing syndrome* in young women and *hyperglycaemia* are very rarely encountered. Pigmentation associated with α- and β-melanocyte stimulating hormone may occur. The *carcinoid syndromes* are described on page 12.59.

Neuromyopathies The term carcinomatous neuropathy is used to describe those abnormalities of the central nervous system, the peripheral nerves, the muscles, and the autonomic nervous system occurring in association with malignancy. These disorders may be subdivided as follows: myopathies (polymyositis, myasthenia, and dermatomyositis) and neuropathies (sensory and mixed sensorimotor, encephalopathy, and myelopathy). Toxic, infective, nutritional, and autoimmune causes have been suggested but none fully substantiated. Neuromyopathies respond variably following treatment of the primary tumour by surgery, radiotherapy or chemotherapy. Most neuromyopathies are not tumour cell type specific except for the Lambert–Eaton syndrome seen occasionally in small cell lung cancer patients, often preceding the appearance of a tumour by up to 15 months. It is characterized by proximal muscle weakness, depressed tendon reflexes often returning following repetitive exercise, autonomic features, and difficulty with swallowing. There may be an autoimmune aetiology for this condition which is currently treated with prednisolone and 3,4-amidopyridine, 10–20 mg q.i.d.

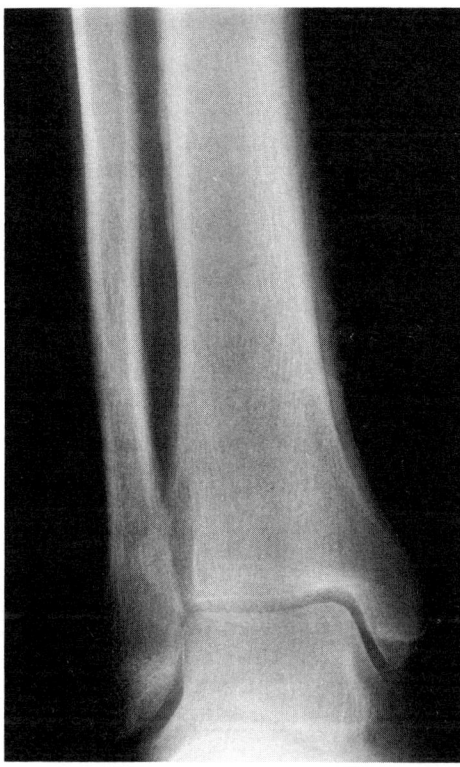

Fig. 1 Hypertrophic pulmonary osteoarthropathy. Note the periosteal reaction resembling elm bark affecting the long bones mainly in the regions of the ankles (and wrists).

Finger clubbing and hypertrophic pulmonary osteoarthropathy

Finger clubbing accompanies a variety of intrathoracic disorders. Gross clubbing is readily recognizable: its early presence may best be demonstrated by the ability to rock the nail on its abnormally spongy bed. Clubbing of the toes is usually present also. Its incidence in lung cancer has been variously reported as being between 10 and 30 per cent. Clubbing may disappear after resection of tumour. The precise mechanism for the development of clubbing has not yet been determined.

Hypertrophic pulmonary osteoarthropathy (HPOA), which may be preceded by finger clubbing alone, consists of periostitis, arthropathy, and usually gross finger clubbing. It is most commonly associated with lung tumours but is also very common in pleural tumours, preceding the diagnosis of tumour in about one-third of patients. It is much commoner in peripheral lesions and in squamous tumours.

The long bones of the extremities are affected by a periosteal reaction resembling elm bark, the changes being symmetrical and affecting mainly ankles and wrists, the knees and elbows being involved less commonly. Synovial thickening and joint effusions are rare. The typical radiographic appearances are shown in Fig. 1. The affected areas are hot and painful and sometimes oedematous. In severe cases walking becomes impracticable. The facial features are sometimes thickened and gynaecomastia is present in 10 per cent of cases. Removal of the tumour is followed by immediate regression of HPOA, but symptoms recur if there is regrowth of the tumour. Vagotomy alone is sometimes effective supporting the theory of vagal mediation of increased blood flow as an aetiological factor in HPOA.

Miscellaneous The *haematological* effects of lung cancer are normally non-specific and normocytic normochromic anaemia is the most common form. More rarely leukaemoid reactions and polycythaemia are observed. *Venous thrombosis* and thrombophlebitis

Table 3 Definitions for staging bronchogenic carcinoma (American Joint Committee on Cancer Staging 1973)

TO	No evidence of primary tumour
TX	Tumour proven by the presence of malignant cells in bronchopulmonary secretions but not visualized roentgenographically or bronchoscopically, or any tumour that cannot be assessed
TIS	Carcinoma *in situ*
T1	A tumour that is 3.0 cm or less in greatest diameter, surrounded by lung or visceral pleura, and without evidence of invasion proximal to a lobar bronchus at bronchoscopy
T2	A tumour more than 3.0 cm in greatest diameter, or a tumour of any size that either invades the visceral pleura or has associated atelectasis or obstructive penumonitis extending to the hilar region. At bronchoscopy, the proximal extent of demonstrable tumour must be within a lobar bronchus or at least 2.0 cm distal to the carina. Any associated atelectasis or obstructive pneumonitis must involve less than an entire lung, and there must be no pleural effusion
T3	A tumour of any size with direct extension into an adjacent structure such as the parietal pleura or chest wall, the diaphragm, or the mediastinum and its contents, or a tumour demonstrable bronchoscopically to involve a main bronchus less than 2.0 cm distal to the carina; or any tumour associated with atelectasis or obstructive pneumonitis of an entire lung or pleural effusion
NO	No demonstrable metastasis to regional lymph-nodes
N1	Metastasis to lymph-nodes in the peribronchial or the ipsilateral hilar region, or both, including direct extension
N2	Metastasis to lymph-nodes in the mediastinum
MO	No (known) distant metastasis
M1	Distant metastasis such as in scalene cervical, or contralateral hilar lymph-nodes, brain, bones, liver, or contralateral lung

Summary staging

Stage I		*Stage III*	
(operable)	T1 NO MO	(inoperable)	T3 any N or M
	T1 N1 MO		N2 any T or M
	T2 NO MO		M1 any T or N
Stage II	T2 N1 MO		
(operable)			

due to hypercoagulability are common complications of malignancy and may precede the detection of the underlying cancer, recurrent migratory phlebitis resistant to anticoagulation being an ominous feature. Marantic *endocarditis* is extremely rare as are *skin lesions* such as acanthosis nigricans, dermatomyositis, hypertrichosis languinosa, and erythema gyratum repens. The *nephrotic syndrome* is also rarely encountered.

Staging and investigations

The sophistication of investigations applied to make the diagnosis and the assessment of lung cancer will vary according to the stage of presentation, cell type, age, and general condition of the patient.

The very rapid doubling time of small cell lung cancer (SCLC) causes it to disseminate rapidly and widely and at diagnosis is very rarely considered operable. However, the slower doubling times for squamous and adenocarcinomas, together with the relatively lesser tendency for squamous cell cancers to disseminate makes surgery the best option whenever possible for the non-small cell lung cancers (NSCLC). A precise anatomical staging classification was only applied to lung cancer in 1973 and immediately demonstrated that the prognosis of NSCLC depended heavily on the extent (or stage) of the disease. The introduction of the TNM staging system (T describing the primary tumour, N the extent of regional lymph node involvement, and M the absence or presence of metastases, see Table 3) encouraged an orderly assessment of investigations and selection of cases for surgery.

The following investigations form the basis for the diagnosis and staging of patients with lung cancer.

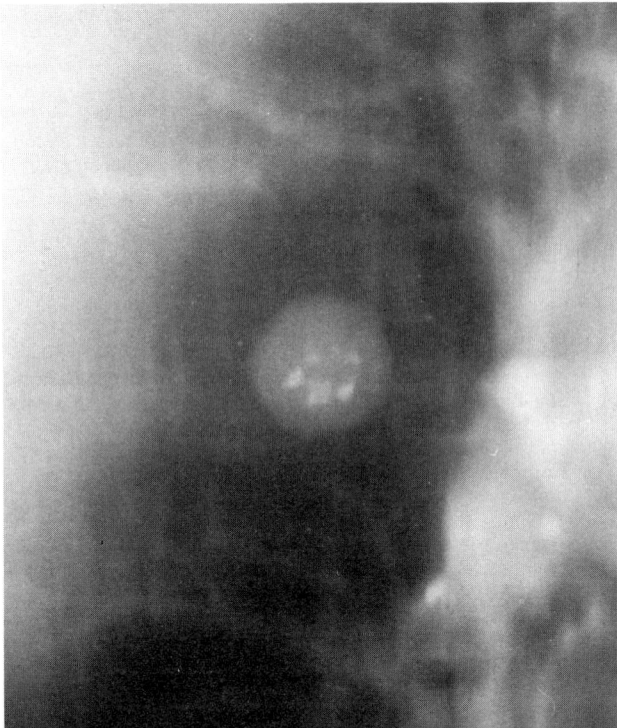

Fig. 2 Tomographic cuts only rarely contribute to the precision of diagnosis in solitary pulmonary nodules. The calcification in this lesion is however pathognomic of a chondroma: this was confirmed at thoracotomy.

Intrathoracic investigations

Radiological assessment

The value of the chest radiograph in the diagnosis and management of pulmonary neoplasm needs no emphasis. Good radiological accomplishments – the quality of radiographic technique and the experience of the observer – enhance the accuracy of diagnosis and the assessment of progress. There is however an inherent inability of the radiological method alone to go all the way in making a precise diagnosis, the so-called 'coin' lesion being a good example. No initial examination is complete without a lateral film. Fluoroscopy is a useful step with observation of diaphragmatic movement and opacification of the oesophagus by barium in order to detect diaphragmatic paralysis and displacement of the oesophagus by tumour or nodes. A lordotic view sometimes gives additional information by demonstrating a lesion in the medial segment of the middle lobe as well as in regions hidden behind the sternal end of the clavicles and the first ribs. Coned views of the ribs may help where rib invasion is suspected clinically. It is on completion of these investigations that a discussion between clinician and radiologist is invaluable. The decision can then be made as to whether tomography or, very rarely, bronchography would give useful additional information. One or two selected tomographic cuts, for example, may suffice to define cavitation or calcification (Fig. 2). The place of needle biopsy under fluoroscopic control and of radio-isotope imaging, ultrasound, and computerized tomographic (CT) scanning is described below. Radiographic examination of the skull and skeletal surveys may be required in the search for metastasis.

The finding of a normal radiograph of the chest does not exclude bronchial carcinoma as, from time to time, patients presenting with haemoptysis and a normal chest radiograph are found to have a central tumour on bronchoscopy. The rounded or ovoid shadow of a peripheral tumour is described in greater detail below: these are sometimes cavitated (Fig. 3a, b). The common appearance of a tumour arising from the main central airways (70 per cent of all cases) is enlargement of one or other hilum: even

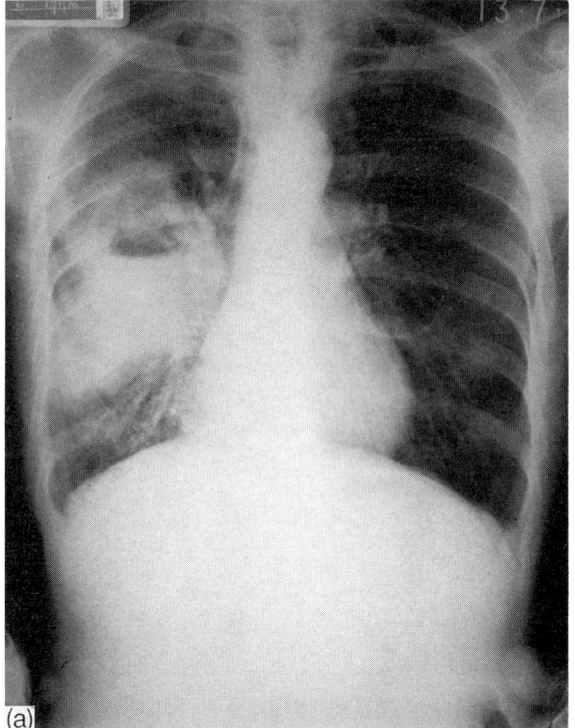

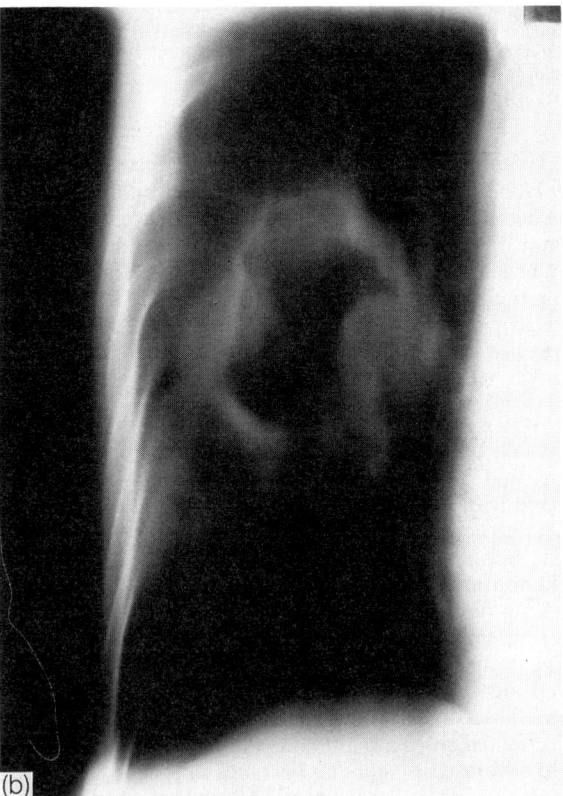

Fig. 3 (a, b) Squamous peripheral tumours tend to cavitate to reveal typical polypoid protuberances on the cavity wall.

experienced observers have difficulty sometimes in determining whether a hilar shadow is enlarged or not and if there is any suspicion, investigation by bronchoscopy and tomography should be pursued. Consolidation and collapse distal to the tumour may have occurred by the time the patient presents, the tumour itself often being obscured in the process. One of the pitfalls is to misinterpret progressive collapse in serial films as 'clearing' of the opacity. Other radiographic appearances which may confuse the diagnosis are inflammatory-like infiltrates in oat cell and adeno-carcinoma (Fig. 4) and apically located masses or so-called super-ior sulcus tumours (Pancoast) which may be misdiagnosed as pleural caps.

The mediastinum may be widened by enlarged nodes. Involve-ment of the phrenic nerve may lead to elevation of the hemidiaph-ragm which becomes paralysed and moves paradoxically on sniffing. Tumour spreading to the pleura causes effusion, but such an abnormality may be secondary to infection beyond obstruction caused by a central tumour. The ribs and spine should be carefully examined for the presence of metastasis. Spread of tumour from mediastinal nodes peripherally along the lymphatics gives the appearance characteristic of lymphangitis carcinomatosa, bilateral hilar enlargement with streaky shadows fanning out into the lung fields on either side. Rarely, localized obstructive emphysema may be observed.

Bronchoscopy
This procedure which is described in detail on page 15.7, is fre-quently the definitive diagnostic method in lung cancer. Like many procedures that depend on close accurate and rapid obser-vation, experience is the most important ingredient in endoscopic interpretation. Tissue removed at bronchoscopy is an essential means of establishing the diagnosis and cell type before embarking on a programme of further staging and treatment. The amount of material biopsied is generally smaller with the fibreoptic instru-ment and this can occasionally cause problems in specificity of cell type with NSCLC, but only rarely with SCLC. The extent of visualization and sites within reach of the biopsy forceps is much greater with the flexible than with the rigid bronchoscope particu-larly in the upper lobes. The rigid instrument is often preferred if the presence of an adenoma is suspected, and is preferred by some in the assessment of central lesions as with this instrument the resistance produced by extrabronchial masses can be sensed more easily: others claim that mobility can be as readily gauged throughout the flexible instrument during respiration and cough-ing. Modern techniques of brushing or washing material from smaller bronchial segments augment the positive yield. When cancer cells are found without a radiologically visible lesion, one is looking for very subtle changes in the mucous membranes particu-larly at carinae and such areas should be biopsied, the site of the

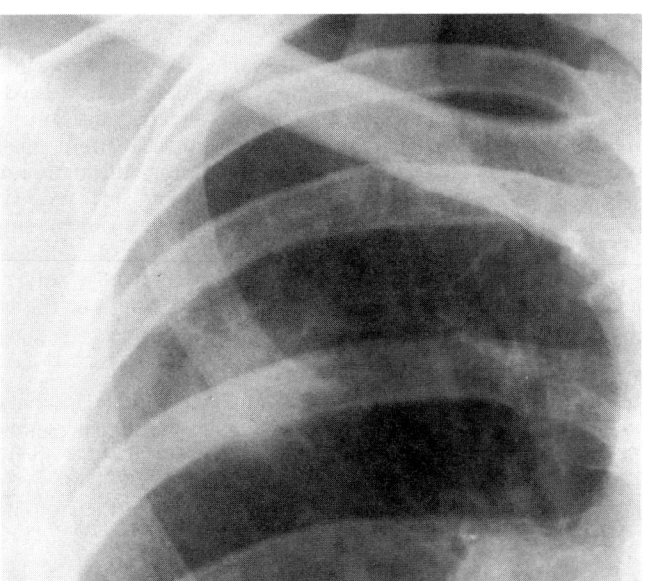

Fig. 4 Small areas of indefinite opacity provisionally diagnosed as inflam-matory. Confirmed as adenocarcinoma on sputum cytology and sub-sequently by lymph-node biopsy.

specimen being very carefully labelled. Rarely the nasopharynx is the source of such cells. Bronchoscopic examination also yields valuable information regarding suitability for surgical resection. Resection is regarded as unsuitable if the main carina is recog-nized as being invaded, or unequivocally broad with splaying of the main bronchi and immobility on respiration, where there is involvement of the trachea unless it be limited to the right lateral wall or tumour found to involve main bronchus within 1.5 cm on the left side. Histological confirmation is now obtainable in 85–90 per cent of bronchoscopically visible lesions.

Transbronchial biopsy
Transbronchial biopsy via the fibreoptic bronchoscope is useful in the diagnosis of circumscribed lesions beyond the range of direct vision or of more diffuse lesions such as may be seen in adenocar-cinoma and bronchoalveolar cell carcinoma. It is advisable to manoeuvre the placement of the biopsy forceps under fluoro-scopic control. A positive yield of 60–70 per cent has been obtained in circumscribed lesions, greatest in those over 4 cm in diameter. Pneumothorax follows the procedure in about 5 per cent and important haemorrhage in 1–2 per cent almost always in the presence of haemorrhagic diathesis. Fatalities are extremely rare.

Percutaneous needle biopsy
This may be carried out either by a Vim-Silverman, Menghini or Trucut needle in large lesions close to the pleura, by aspiration needle biopsy. Concentration of the tiny fragments which are sometimes obtained into a larger mass increases the positive yield. The procedure should be done under fluoroscopic control and should be avoided in patients with poor respiratory function or with bleeding diathesis. Positive yields as high as 90 per cent have been reported, the yield depending upon meticulous technique and the competence of the pathologist. However, the method remains the least satisfactory for cell type specificity being most inaccurate for NSCLC. It is a useful diagnostic method in patients in whom exploratory thoracotomy may be hazardous or to try to determine whether a solid mass is a primary, secondary or benign tumour. Pneumothorax occurs in about 25 per cent of patients, some 5 per cent requiring intubation. Slight haemoptysis may fol-low the procedure.

Sputum cytology
Cytological examination of sputum is a very useful non-invasive step in the diagnosis of malignant pulmonary disease. A high degree of competence in the cytologist to whom specimens are submitted is of inestimable value.

The patient should be encouraged to cough deeply and to raise sputum from the deeper parts of the chest because material for examination, if it is to be of value, must come from the lower res-piratory tract. Skilled physiotherapists can give considerable assistance in obtaining satisfactory material: a warm aerosol may help. The yield increases according to the number of specimens examined and three consecutive morning specimens should be submitted in the first instance. Rapid transport to the laboratory is important as delay in preparation leads to overgrowth of organ-isms and to loss of histological definition. In the hands of an expert cytologist receiving good quality specimens, 80 per cent positivity can now be obtained, the yield being greater from larger tumours in major segmental bronchi, for such exfoliate well. False-posi-tives are rare in competent hands.

Thoracoscopy
With the advent of more recently introduced diagnostic tech-niques, the indications for thoracoscopy have declined. Visualiza-tion of the parietal and visceral pleura has an important part to play in the diagnosis of effusions and in pleural tumours as biopsy of lesions can be carried out under direct vision, absence of pleural tumour being important in decisions about resectability of a lung tumour. Thoracoscopy is inadvisable in the absence of effusion or

pneumothorax and is unsatisfactory in the presence of empyema or gross haemothorax. However, in otherwise operable tumours with a pleural effusion that is not blood stained and without positive cytology or pleural biopsy – thoracoscopy may be a useful next step in determining operability.

Computed axial tomography

Thoracic CT scanning has been a useful advance in the staging of lung cancer. It will identify the site, size, and extension of the tumour far more clearly than conventional radiology. It identifies mediastinal lymphadenopathy frequently when the PA and lateral chest radiographs and also tomography fail to show any abnormality. Mediastinal lymphadenopathy on CT scanning is arbitrarily taken to be pathological by most centres if the glands are greater than 1.5 cm in diameter. However, previous infective conditions such as tuberculosis and reactive hyperplasia to the tumour can cause appearances identical to that of malignant enlargement. Thus positive CT scans of the mediastinum may be falsely positive in up to 50 per cent of cases, although this figure is now less with the newer more rapid scanning time machines. Mediastinal lymphnode biopsy (mediastinoscopy) must therefore be performed to confirm an abnormal finding. A normal CT scan for mediastinal lymph-node enlargement or for direct mediastinal invasion by the primary tumour is sufficiently reliable to exclude the necessity for mediastinal biopsy prior to thoracotomy.

Extrathoracic investigations

In general the ability to identify small metastatic deposits is as unsatisfactory for lung carcinomas as for other solid tumours. The available techniques are relatively crude and this in part explains the high extrathoracic relapse rate following so called 'curative' resections for NSCLC. In patients with no symptoms other than those caused by their primary tumour, if there is no clinical evidence of neurological, hepatic or bony disease and normal biochemistry then radio-isotope scans of brain, liver, and bones will be unhelpful. Brain scans have a high accuracy in detailing cerebral metastases in patients with neurological symptoms. In patients with a palpable liver and/or abnormal liver function tests a liver scan or ultrasound should be performed. Bone scans have a high false-positive rate due to Paget's disease, active arthritis, healing fractures, renal disease, and hyperparathyroidism. However, in patients with bone pain, local tenderness or non-specific symptoms of weight loss or malaise, a bone scan should be requested.

In patients with SCLC bone marrow aspiration is often performed and a single sample can be positive in up to 40 per cent of subjects. In apparently operable cases of NSCLC the incidence of tumour in the marrow is too small to justify the procedure as a routine. *Biopsy* of enlarged lymph-nodes and skin metastases should be carried out whenever indicated. If an isolated hepatic or bony lesion identified with isotope or CT scanning appears the only contraindication to surgery, this should be biopsied under radiological control.

It is important to evaluate *lung function*. Simple spirometry is usually adequate but it may be necessary to evaluate exercise capability in a more sophisticated manner in some patients particularly if surgery is to be undertaken. The ability to climb one flight of stairs without breathlessness has been claimed to be a very good indication of fitness for resection.

The staging investigations for NSCLC are summarized in Fig. 5. The final procedure prethoracotomy is the assessment of the mediastinum. If CT scanning is available this may, if normal, allow the surgeon to proceed directly to thoracotomy. If abnormal or no CT scan is available mediastinal exploration should first be performed.

Routine cervical mediastinoscopy in patients who otherwise appear radiologically operable on conventional films and tomography, will yield mediastinal lymph-node involvement in 10–15 per cent of all cases considered for surgery. To this should be added

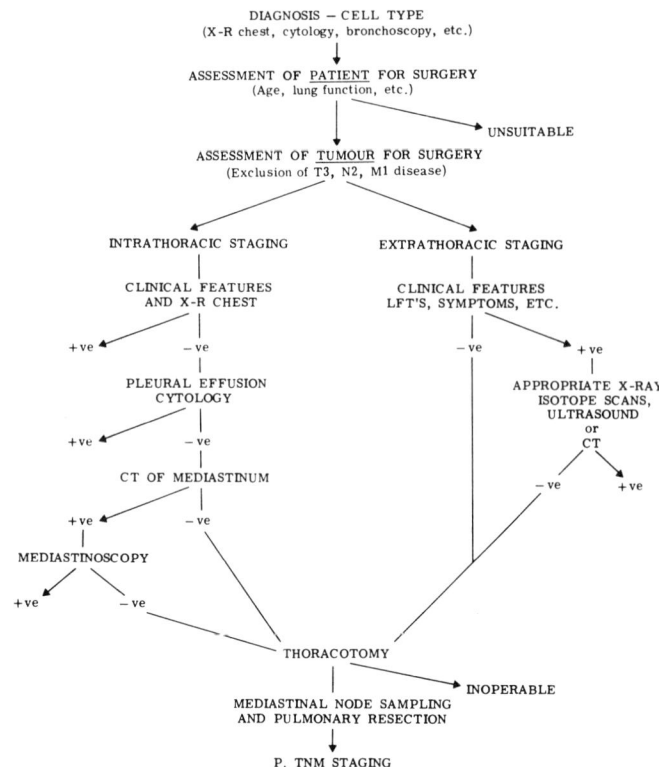

Fig. 5 Preoperative staging of non-small cell lung cancer. +ve, positive; −ve, negative; CT, computed tomography, pTNM staging, i.e. postsurgical pathological staging. (Reproduced from Spiro and Goldstraw, 1984, The staging of lung cancer. *Thorax* **39**, 401–407, by permission.)

the value of left anterior mediastinotomy, an approach through the bed of the second left costal cartilage to inspect glands draining tumours from the left upper lobe. The mediastinum may be involved in up to 50 per cent of patients with a peripheral poorly differentiated tumour, and in a much greater percentage of centrally occurring lesions although many of them will have an abnormal mediastinum on routine chest radiograph.

Treatment

In 1903 Osler wrote: 'The practice of medicine is an art, not a trade; a calling, not a business; a calling in which your heart will be exercized equally with your head.' The philosophy he expressed is appropriate to the management of bronchial carcinoma 80 years later for crucial decisions in management often have to be made on more than one occasion in the patient's lifetime the alternative lying between aggressive and supportive treatment, and wise decisions cannot be made unless full information is available from careful and skilful investigation and assessment. In the following paragraphs the three main modalities of treatment – surgery, radiotherapy, and chemotherapy – are described and their application in various clinical situations discussed.

Surgery

Surgery remains the single modality most likely to be curative in NSCLC. In SCLC the very occasional patient, usually presenting with a peripheral tumour, who after extensive staging investigations remains operable is occasionally cured. These patients are rare but nevertheless have a 5-year survival rate in the region of 30–40 per cent.

Prior to surgery the patient should have been carefully staged (Fig. 5) and his chances of long-term survival will be greatly influenced by this. All patients with stage III disease should be rejected for thoracotomy, but those with stage I and II disease resected. In general patients with squamous cell carcinomas have

Table 4 Ranges for survival according to pre-operative staging in non small cell lung cancer (pooled data)

Stage	Per cent survival	
	3 years	5 years
T1 N0	60–75	42–75
T2 N0	25–54	20–45
T1 N1	35	30
T2 N1	20–40	10–35
T1 N2		0–20*
T2 N2		0–10*

* Small selected series of operated patients with mediastinal disease.

Table 5 Contraindications to surgical treatment

Absolute	
General clinical state	Serious cardiac disease, poor respiratory function
Metastasis	
Distant	Lymph-nodes, liver, bone, brain, etc.
Intrathoracic	Involvement of recurrent laryngeal nerve, sympathetic trunk or phrenic nerve, superior vena cava, trachea, oesophagus, pericardium, heart
Chest-wall	Pleura, rib, medial to angle
Bronchoscopic appearances	Widened fixed main carina, tumour within 1.5 cm of origin of left mainstem bronchus
On mediastinoscopy	Diagnosis of small cell, involvement of subaortic, carinal or paratracheal nodes

Relative		
Advanced age	Poor physical state	Superior sulcus tumour (Pancoast)

a higher 5- and 10-year survival rate than adeno and large cell carcinomas and the more differentiated the tumour the better the prognosis. Table 4 summarizes survival data at 3 and 5 years for pre-operatively staged NSCLC. Clearly small peripheral lesions with no nodal disease fare best (up to 75 per cent 5-year survival in some series), but the survival rate decreases both with size of tumour and presence of hilar node involvement.

In all, approximately 20 per cent of patients who present with NSCLC eventually come to thoracotomy. Most of the others are excluded almost immediately because of clinically evident metastatic disease, radiological or bronchoscopic evidence of inoperability, too advanced an age to withstand surgery, significant associated other illnesses or inadequate lung function. Of those having a 'curative' resection the 5-year overall survival rate remains approximately 25 per cent and at 10 years 16–18 per cent. Death from local or distant recurrence of the tumour is equally probable, highlighting the inadequacies of current staging techniques. However, the careful application of the TNM system and the advent of more sophisticated scanning equipment may further improve selection.

The major contraindications to resection are summarized in Table 5. Cardiac and respiratory complications are the most common source of postoperative morbidity and mortality and it is essential that the reserve capacity of heart and lungs be evaluated. Patients in the high risk cardiac complication category are those who have sustained myocardial infarction in the preceding three months, or who have uncontrolled arrhythmias. A history of angina of itself does not contraindicate surgery: the ultimate in sophisticated surgery is simultaneous tumour resection and coronary bypass!

Pulmonary function evaluation must always be made prior to consideration for resection. The simplest test for assessing pulmonary function is the FEV_1 and FVC. Pneumonectomy should probably not be undertaken if the patient cannot achieve an FEV_1 of more than 1.2 litres, bearing in mind that patients who have co-existent chronic obstructive airflow disease may not sustain the current value in exacerbations. In the middle range of ventilatory capacity the risk of resection is a matter of judgement based on the estimate of maximum tolerable resection and assessment of the functional integrity of the non-tumour bearing lung. Combination of pulmonary function tests, including the 12-min walking test, and regional function studies using xenon-133 may be used in patients with borderline function. Clinical judgement, however, is the ultimate factor in the determination of operability. As lung cancer is such a serious disease consideration may have to be given from time to time to carrying out resection in patients whose physical performance defies the results of pulmonary function tests.

Only very rarely is there an indication for palliative surgery and resection should not be considered in the presence of intra-thoracic or distant metastasis. There are diametrically opposite views as to whether operation should be undertaken in Pancoast tumours.

Advanced age is not an absolute contraindication to surgery. Patients over 70 years of age appear to tolerate pneumonectomy badly, but in good risk patients in this age group, consideration should be given to surgery if it seems probable that tumour removal will be achieved by lobectomy. Patients in very poor general condition usually withstand surgery badly.

Even in the best of hands the perioperative mortality for pneumonectomy may reach 10 per cent, and this increases with the age of the patient. The mortality for lobectomy is always much lower, 1–4 per cent.

Radiotherapy

Patients who are excluded from surgery by reason of adverse prognostic factors, advanced stage of tumour or other coincidental disease constitute the largest group treated with radiotherapy. Although the usual goal of radiotherapy will be palliative, there will be a small group of patients in whom more aggressive therapy will be used in the hope of cure or at least long-term survival, particularly in those who have refused surgery. Radiotherapy for lung cancer is limited by the comparative radiosensitivity of three critical normal tissues likely to be included in the radiation beam: normal lung, spinal cord, and heart each of which has a critical tolerance dose. Increased radiation dose leads to greater killing of tumour cells but may produce unwanted normal cell damage. Radiation dose must be expressed not only in terms of total dose but also numbers of fractions and overall time. There is no clear evidence for an optimum radiation dose but doses of 5000 to 6000 rad in 5 to 6 weeks are appropriate; higher doses will be associated with unacceptable morbidity.

The role of radiotherapy

Curative It seems that about 5 per cent of patients with localized disease of non-small cell type will be cured by appropriate doses of radiotherapy. For such tumours the comparable figure for surgery is 30 per cent and therefore radiotherapy in such a group should be reserved for patients who refuse surgery or are unfit for other medical reasons. Its role in small cell cancer is described below. Radical radiotherapy is inappropriate in the presence of extrathoracic metastasis, in bilateral lesions, tumour mass greater than 6 cm diameter, severely impaired pulmonary function, and poor general physical state. Advanced age is not, of itself, a contraindication.

Palliative Many patients with inoperable lung cancer are given radiotherapy at some stage of the disease. It is of particular value in the relief of local skeletal pain, e.g. in ribs or vertebrae, and in severe recurrent haemoptysis. Relief of bronchial obstruction to reduce the risk of distal pneumonia may be obtained. Superior vena caval obstruction is also relieved. Whole brain irradiation is sometimes used for relief of symptoms associated with cerebral metastases and is often combined with dexamethasone.

Preoperative radiotherapy The value of radiotherapy given 4–8 weeks before operation remains a matter of debate. Although some series have suggested improved survival the large randomized series conducted by the National Cancer Institute (NCI) and the Veterans Administration in the United States failed to substantiate this and there was some excess morbidity in the group treated with adjuvant preoperative radiotherapy in the NCI study.

Postoperative radiotherapy The role of localized radiotherapy after operation also remains unclear though few would deny its application where there has been complete resection of the tumour except at the bronchial stump margin or at the chest wall which is really an extension of the primary tumour mass.

Complications The main complications are dysphagia occurring commonly in the third week of treatment and radiation pneumonitis which should be rare and may develop about four weeks after the end of treatment though it may be delayed for as long as 12 weeks.

The full potential of radiotherapy may not yet have been realized. The value of high linear energy techniques, or radiosensitizers such as mizonidazole and of radiotherapy plus hyperthermia are being evaluated at present, as is the technique of the interstitial implantation of radioactive isotopes (iodine-125) planted at thoracotomy.

Chemotherapy

Non-small cell lung cancer Despite many cytotoxic drugs showing modest activity against these tumours there is no good evidence that they prolong survival in inoperable patients. There have been hundreds of studies of single agent and combination regimens but very few controlled studies. Response rates (i.e. reduction in tumour volume by at least 50 per cent) of up to 30 per cent have been commonly reported but owing to lack of control data, non-comparative data, or using historical controls as the comparison, there is no convincing evidence that chemotherapy prolongs survival for these cell types. Newer agents such as etoposide, ifosfamide, and cisplatin are currently being evaluated but until a significant survival advantage is shown, the use of cytotoxic agents in the treatment of NSCLC is not recommended outside clinical trials.

Small cell lung cancer This cell type has been separated from the other types of lung cancer because of its very different biological and clinical features. It has an explosive growth pattern so that the TNM staging classification makes no impact on prognosis or survival, almost certainly because careful staging puts most patients into the inoperable category and because small metastases remain undetected for a few months. Simple staging has however some prognostic impact and those staged to have limited disease – tumour confined to one hemithorax and the ipsilateral supraclavicular fossa – fare better than those with extensive disease, causing involvement of any site outside the hemithorax. The natural history of untreated SCLC is about three and a half months for limited disease and 1.8 months for extensive disease.

Small cell lung cancer is much more sensitive to cytotoxic chemotherapy than the NSCL tumours with a much higher response rate for several cytotoxic drugs (see Table 6). Although the administration of single agents resulted in response in terms of tumour shrinkage there was no noticeable improvement in median survival until the cytotoxic drugs were used in combination. In the late 1970s there was a very rapid improvement in median survival using three and four drug combinations but responses have subsequently reached a plateau. Nevertheless with modern combination cytotoxic treatment given, usually on an outpatient basis every three weeks, the median survival for limited disease has been extended to 14–18 months, and for extensive disease to 9–12 months. Most combinations include cyclophosphamide, doxorubicin, etoposide, vincristine or methotrexate. All these regimens have side-effects. Most patients will experience some nausea and

Table 6 Response rates of small cell lung cancer to cytotoxic drugs used as single agents

Drug	Responding (%)
Methotrexate	39
Vincristine	33
Cyclophosphamide	31
Etoposide	30
Doxorubicin	25
Procarbazine	25
Cisplatin	13

vomiting; alopecia is practically universal. Care has to be taken to ensure bone marrow recovery before the next course is given and safe lower limits of total white cell and platelet counts have been achieved. Anaemia is treated by transfusion as necessary. Life-threatening septicaemia can occur in 1–4 per cent of patients but treatment-related deaths are uncommon.

Much effort has been applied during the last 5 years to improving the median and long-term survival of patients with small cell lung cancer. In general those patients in whom further progress is to be made are those who present with limited disease and a high performance status. Extensive disease patients tend to have a universally bad prognosis and very few survive beyond two years. However, it seems that single metastatic sites such as bone and bone marrow are not as sinister as the brain or the liver and therefore the occasional extensive disease patient does extremely well with chemotherapy but in general the treatment offered to those with extensive disease tends to be palliative. Studies assessing the quality of life in all patients presenting with SCLC have noted that over 70 per cent of patients have important symptoms such as weight loss, malaise, bone pain, dyspnoea, and haemoptysis.

The majority of these patients will have extensive disease. Reassessment of symptoms after three months of chemotherapy has shown relief of these symptoms in 60–70 per cent of sufferers, making chemotherapy worthwhile with the benefits of chemotherapy in terms of symptom relief far outweighing the potential side-effects.

Intensifying the dosage or the frequency of administration of the cytotoxic agents has been thoroughly assessed without striking benefit on median survival data. Smaller advantages are occasionally seen but these have to be balanced by the increased toxicity resulting from this more aggressive approach. Attempts to overcome or delay the emergence of cell resistance to chemotherapy have involved alternating combinations of drugs, but these more complicated regimens have not been rewarding either.

The optimal duration of treatment in terms of achieving the best possible median survival is not known as the early studies continue to treat completely responding patients for a year following the response and the partial responders (< 50 per cent reduction in tumour mass) until relapse. However, recent studies of six months of chemotherapy have shown no disadvantage in terms of median survival and this is an important area for further research.

The role of radiotherapy in small cell lung cancer has recently been clarified. Whilst the cell type is extremely sensitive to radiotherapy and the addition of radiotherapy to the primary tumour site and mediastinum will usually decrease the relapse rate at the primary site, its addition to combination chemotherapy has shown no advantage for median survival in patients with either limited or extensive disease. Whilst this is disappointing and reflects the failure of chemotherapy to control the distant disease it has a major practical impact on management and transferring patients to regional centres for mediastinal irradiation appears unnecessary.

The role of radiotherapy in patients presenting with superior vena caval obstruction has also recently been studied. Approximately 10 per cent of patients with SCLC present with superior vena caval obstruction and are usually regarded as a radiothera-

Table 7 Complete responses and survival in small cell carcinoma

Therapy	Number of patients	Complete responses (%)	Median survival (months)	One year survival (%)	Long term survival (%)	
					LD*	ED*
Placebo	55	0	2.5	5		
Radiotherapy	235	—	6.0	20	<5	
Cyclophosphamide	363	1.1	5.0	18	0	0
Eight other active single drugs	468	2.7	5.5	15		
Combination chemotherapy (two, three, and four drugs)	1201	15.0	8.5	25		
Combination chemotherapy (three and four drugs)	452	23.0	9.0	40	5–10	1–3
Combination chemotherapy plus radiotherapy	984	31.0	11.0	47	8–15	2

Adapted from Spiro (1979). Carcinoma of the bronchus. *Medicine*, 3rd Service, p. 1206, with permission.
* LD, limited disease; ED, extensive disease.

peutic emergency. However, these patients respond as well as other types of presentation of SCLC and should be given chemotherapy. The objective and subjective response is the same as for radiotherapy given as an isolated treatment, and the median survival following chemotherapy is better than for radiotherapy alone and in fact is identical to that of other presentations of SCLC.

An important role for radiotherapy in SCLC is prophylactic cerebral irradiation (PCI). The incidence of relapse in the brain in SCLC is up to 40 per cent during life and the likelihood increases with prolonged duration of survival. Although PCI does not in itself affect median survival (due to its rarely being an isolated site of relapse) it both delays and decreases the incidence of cerebral metastases which if allowed to occur are a major source of debility, often condemning the patient to spend the remainder of his or her life in hospital. The current policy is to offer PCI to those patients who enter a complete response following chemotherapy, i.e. after three months or so of treatment. The usual dose is 2000–3000 rad given over 5 to 10 days.

Data is now accumulating on the long-term survival of patients with SCLC treated with chemotherapy with or without additional irradiation. There are hardly any long-term (> 2 years) survivors in extensive disease patients. In those presenting with limited disease about 8–15 per cent of patients are alive at two years (Table 7). It appears that most of these have had both PCI and mediastinal irradiation in addition to chemotherapy but as yet no controlled data is available to ascertain whether radiotherapy, although not improving the median survival for all limited disease patients, may be a factor in achieving long-term survival.

Unfortunately not all patients alive at 2 years are disease free and about 25 per cent will still relapse with small cell lung cancer up to 6 years following treatment. A few patients will develop second neoplasms. Furthermore, of those apparently cured up to 40 per cent develop a 'CNS syndrome' of memory loss, confusion, and ataxia which makes them unable to return to their previous occupations. Whether this is due to the chemotherapy, PCI or both, or the malignant disease itself is not yet clear.

Adjuvant immunotherapy
The belief that there may be a spontaneous immunological response to lung cancer is supported by the occasional regression of histologically proven tumours and the variable rate of progression of similar histological types of tumour in different patients.

A large percentage of patients with lung cancer show evidence of immunosuppression demonstrable by impaired reactions of

delayed cutaneous hypersensitivity and impaired ability of lymphocytes to undergo transformation *in vitro* upon stimulation with various antigens and mitogens. Immunotherapy in lung cancer is based on the following premises: there is a host defence mechanism against tumours which is largely immunological in nature, that depression of this mechanism allows growth and spread of the tumour, and that correction of this immunosuppression would impair growth of the tumour. Removal of a large burden of tumour by resection seems to influence the host–tumour relationship in some way, perhaps by allowing the host's immune system respite to recover sufficiently to destroy the microscopic foci of tumour cells scattered throughout the body: often, unhappily, this is too great a residual burden.

The three most widely used non-specific immunopotentiator drugs are BCG, *Corynebacterium parvum*, and levamisole, these agents causing a general stimulation of all cells concerned with the immunological response in the hope that some of the activated immunocompetent cells will attack tumour cells as a result. However, all studies with these agents, administered in a variety of ways have shown no effect on inhibiting either local or disseminated disease recurrence rates nor hence survival.

General management
There are certain complications which require specific measures to alleviate symptoms.

Patients who seem likely to survive for 6 months or more and who have *vocal chord paralysis* find considerable help in morale from the operation of Teflon injection into the affected chord which restores voice production in a high percentage of cases. Occurrence of upper airway obstruction causing *stridor*, or obstruction of the lower major airways is usually initially treated in NSCLC patients with radiotherapy. Should this complication recur or be unsuitable for radiotherapy it could be suitable for laser photocoagulation administered either via the fibreoptic bronchoscope or under general anaesthetic via a rigid instrument. Laser therapy for carcinoma of the bronchus is still a new and developing field but seems most suitable as a palliative treatment in central tumours occluding large airways. There are technical limitations to its application via the flexible bronchoscope but with the rigid instrument removal of considerable quantities of tumour can be achieved in a single treatment session.

Superior vena caval obstruction in non-small cell lung cancer or relapsed small cell cancer should be treated by radiotherapy under steroid cover.

Infection distal to tumour requires antibiotic therapy and, where appropriate, oxygen therapy and bronchodilators. *Severe recurrent haemoptysis* may be controlled by radiotherapy or chemotherapy.

Malignant pleural effusion recurs after aspiration unless the pleural space is obliterated. Chemical pleurodesis can be induced by a number of agents by intrapleural instillation or by the more invasive procedures of talc pleurodesis or pleurectomy. Intrapleural tetracycline is most commonly used but bleomycin or radioactive colloidal gold also give successful pleurodesis in 50–70 per cent of patients. Recent studies with intrapleural bleomycin (105 mg) and *Corynebacterium parvum* (7 mg) have demonstrated a very high success rate with very few side-effects.

Skeletal pain, if localized, responds well to irradiation: bone involvement in SCLC is common and often responds well to chemotherapy. The general management of pain is discussed in Sections 21 and 28. It should not be forgotten that the expertize of neurosurgical pain control can be extremely valuable.

Metastasis from hormone-dependent tumours may respond well to specific treatment such as radioactive iodine or non-specific treatment as already described. Dexamethasone 4–16 mg orally daily may control the symptoms of brain metastasis and if so this should be consolidated with radiotherapy to prevent severe steroid-induced myopathy. Prednisolone 20 mg orally daily is often used for improving the sense of well-being as are blood transfusion or hyperalimentation.

Terminal care is described in Section 28, but it cannot be emphasized too much how important is the combined support to the patient and the family given by the family doctor, the nursing organizations, and the hospital team. The service given by hospitals to the community should not be merely diagnostic and therapeutic but should include terminal care facilities for those patients in whom such is thought appropriate.

Prevention

Lung cancer is an almost totally preventable disease and is very largely due to smoking, and particularly the smoking of cigarettes. The strategy of any preventive measures must be based on the observations that lung cancer is extremely rare in non-smokers (the exception being adenocarcinoma of the bronchus in Chinese women in Singapore and Hong Kong), the absence of a threshold limit below which no effect is produced though the risk increases proportionately to the amount smoked, the benefit from stopping smoking is evident within five years and the risk for an ex-smoker at any given time after stopping is determined by the length of time he had smoked before he stopped. Strenuous efforts must thus be made to persuade people not to start smoking, to establish more effective methods of enabling people to stop smoking and to promote further research into effective methods of health education. The promotion of low tar, low nicotine, low carbon monoxide cigarettes, now capable of production, may have made a small contribution to prevention, but low tar cigarettes are not a substitute for giving up smoking. Penal taxation by governments may also help.

The identification of occupational hazards and appropriate measures to safeguard the health of employees are clearly important preventive measures, even although the number at risk is very small.

Prospective lung cancer screening programmes in males 45 years and older and who smoke at least 20 cigarettes per day have been carried out on an experimental basis using both chest radiographs and pooled three-day sputum analysis every four months. They are unlikely to form the basis of standard practice as there is yet no evidence that early detection is translated into increased cure rate.

Carcinoid tumours

The slow-growing intrabronchial lesions previously grouped under the heading of bronchial adenoma have now been reclassified into bronchial carcinoids, adenoid cystic tumours, and muco-epidermoid tumours. They are not related to cigarette smoking, and tend to be diagnosed at a younger age than carcinoma of the bronchus. True bronchial adenomas derived from bronchial glands are rare. These tumours were once thought to be benign but they are potentially and often frankly malignant being capable not only of destructive local growth but also of metastasis to regional lymphnodes in about one-third of patients and in about 10 per cent to distant organs especially liver and brain. They are occasionally located in the trachea.

The most common symptoms are cough, haemoptysis, and recurrent pneumonia though not infrequently the lesion is discovered on routine radiographic examination before symptoms develop. Carcinoids may produce the classical symptom pattern of intermittent cyanotic flushings, intestinal cramps and diarrhoea, bronchoconstriction, and cardiovascular lesions only in a few cases particularly when there are liver secondaries. The radiological appearances are those of a solitary nodule or pulmonary collapse or obstructive hyperinflation. As the majority of the tumours occur in main stem or the proximal portions of lobar bronchi, bronchoscopy is usually the definitive diagnostic measure. The tumour appears as a white or pink polypid or lobulated mass, the bronchial mucosa appearing to be intact: biopsy may be followed by brisk haemoptysis.

Surgical resection is the treatment of choice: the tumour is relatively resistant to deep X-ray therapy. In the absence of regional spread or distant metastases, 5-year survival prospects are excellent but if there is involvement of regional nodes, survival rates fall to 70 per cent. Some aggressive carcinoid tumours carry a much worse prognosis. The mechanism and the management of the general symptoms of the carcinoid syndrome are described on page 12.59.

Mediastinal tumours (cysts and new growths)

Most mediastinal tumours and cysts are discovered by routine radiographic examination: a few declare themselves because they have spread to affect neighbouring structures, e.g. neural tumours, or have become infected, e.g. teratomas. Malignant change, pressure symptoms, and infection occur sufficiently frequently in many of the tumours to warrant surgical removal at the time of discovery unless there are clear contraindications to operation such as advanced age, severely impaired respiratory or cardiac function, or clear indication of a primary tumour elsewhere in the body. There are certain limited investigations which may help in differential diagnosis: examination of peripheral blood and bone marrow if lymphoma is suspected, barium swallow in foregut reduplication, and radioactive iodine administration to detect heterotopic thyroid tissue.

By convention, tumours of the trachea, oesophagus and heart are excluded in a classification of tumours of the mediastinum. The anatomical site of the lesion often gives the best lead to diagnosis (Fig. 6). The commonest tumour of the mediastinum is secondary carcinoma most frequently from bronchogenic carcinoma. Lymphomatous lesions are usually due to Hodgkin's disease or to non-Hodgkin's lymphoma and are described in Section 19. In a 10-year period during which 3000 patients with bronchial carcinoma were treated, Le Roux recorded a total of 105 patients with mediastinal cysts and tumours. Of these 30 were neural tumours, 21 teratomas, 20 pericardial cysts, 17 cysts and tumours of thymic origin, 14 foregut reduplications, and only 3 heterotopic mediastinal thyroids.

Neural tumours are the commonest and always lie posteriorly in the paravertebral gutter. They arise from the sympathetic trunk or

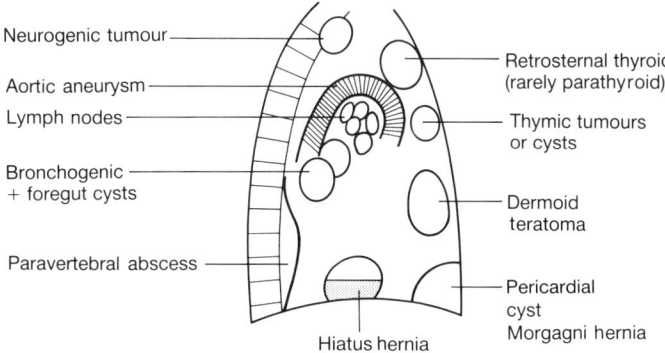

Fig. 6 Common mediastinal tumours (cysts and new growths).

from one or more intercostal nerves, several histological types being described: neurilemmoma, neurofibroma, neurosarcoma, ganglioneuroma, and malignant neuroblastoma. Symptoms are uncommon but incarceration in the thoracic inlet may give rise to pressure effects such as Horner's syndrome, splaying and erosion of ribs, and, if they are large, oesophageal displacement. Occasionally neural tumours extend in dumbbell fashion into the spinal canal and a neurofibroma is sometimes associated with von Recklinghausen's disease. They appear radiologically as ovoid opacities of smooth outline and uniform density frequently flattened against the posterior chest wall. Loss of outline and irregularity may indicate malignancy.

Teratomas are derived from all three germinal layers and are composed of tissues foreign to the organ in which the tumour is found: if they contain a predominance of ectodermal elements they are called dermoid cysts. They are almost always situated anteriorly. The serum chorionic gonodotrophin and α-feto-protein levels are often elevated in this condition and are diagnostic. Symptoms of breathlessness, stridor or substernal pain may arise from pressure and if they become infected they may give rise to symptoms of recurrent respiratory infection, greasy material, and rarely hair being expectorated. If they are large, the ribs may bulge outwards and a pulmonary systolic murmur may be found. The opacity is well defined and may have a rind of calcium: teeth may be clearly seen on occasion.

Parapericardial or pleuropericardial cysts are thin-walled and often called 'springwater' cysts from their content of clear liquid. They are found in the anterior cardiophrenic angle – the right more than the left and there seem to be no complications. The herniation of extraperitoneal fat or a peritoneal-lined hernia through the right foramen of Morgagni most commonly simulate these cysts.

Thymic tumours and cysts present in one of three ways: with myasthenia gravis with a symptomless opacity found at routine radiography, or with evidence of a malignant mediastinal tumour which has produced superior vena caval obstruction, pleural or pericardial effusion or phrenic paralysis. Their pathological classification is fraught with difficulty. The radiographic appearance is of an anterior mediastinal shadow extending downwards in front of the pericardium: if large they may have a bilateral presentation and extend to the level of the diaphragm. Loss of hairline definition suggests malignancy. Thymic tumours should be resected irrespective of the presence of myasthenia gravis.

Mediastinal thyroids are usually a retrosternal extension of a goitre though there may occasionally be true heterotopic thyroid tissue anywhere in the anterior mediastinum. Rarely, dyspnoea, stridor, and dysphagia are present: vocal chord paralysis and obstruction of great veins may also occur and there may be haemorrhage into the mass. Scanning with radioactive iodine is of value in diagnosis but not all heterotopic thyroids take up the isotope. Radiologically the mass lies in the upper mediastinum and is

more prominent on one side (usually the right) than the other: the trachea is displaced and may be narrowed. Calcification is occasionally present.

Foregut duplications and cysts are congenital anomalies and are sometimes given distinct names based on their anatomical position or their lining, e.g. bronchogenic gastrogenous or enterogenous cyst. One type of developmental error occurring in the first few weeks of life 'the split notochord syndrome' results in the formation of a cyst lying posteriorly and associated with vertebral abnormalities. The second type occurs at about the sixth week and gives rise to a true duplication. The cysts are commonly found at the tracheobronchial junction mainly on the right side, and may be intra- or extraluminal. Malignant change does not occur but infection, haemorrhage or rupture may cause dramatic symptoms.

Rare tumours such as lipoma or liposarcoma, fibroma or fibrosarcoma, haemangioma, chondroma, hydatid cyst, and cystic hygroma may arise anywhere in the mediastinum.

The other conditions which enter into the differential diagnosis are aneurysm of the aorta, lymph-node enlargement from whatever cause, hernias, meningoceles, and mediastinal abscess.

Tumours of the pleura

The commonest tumour of the pleura is a metastasis from a primary carcinoma of the lung, effusions from such tumours usually being unilateral. Metastatic spread may also occur from other primary sites such as breast, stomach, pancreas or uterus: in such cases the effusion is occasionally bilateral. Pleural malignancy with effusion also occurs in lymphomas, including Hodgkin's disease, and lymphosarcoma. The differential diagnosis of pleural effusion is discussed on page 15.55.

Pleural fibroma

This tumour may be a chance finding on routine radiography. It is a localized tumour, well-encapsulated, and sometimes pedunculated, and may be as large as a grapefruit. The histological appearance varies from acellular tissue with masses of collagen to highly cellular, anaplastic sarcoma-like cells. Hypertrophic pulmonary osteoarthropathy and clubbing of the fingers are commonly present. Dull chest pain may occur. Pleural fibromas should be removed surgically as some behave as slowly growing malignant tumours.

Pleural mesothelioma

The association of mesothelioma with exposure to asbestos (page 15.1) is now accepted and has been established in up to 90 per cent of cases in various series. The male:female ratio is about 3:1 and most cases occur in the 40–60 year old age group.

In diffuse mesothelioma small granular flakes of tumour spread to form diffuse sheets of thick, rubbery, yellowish-grey tissue which encase the lung and infiltrate the cortex. Local extension into the pericardium and through the diaphragm occurs, and there is spread to mediastinal nodes in about half the cases: distant metastases are surprisingly common at autopsy (50–70 per cent) though less frequently obvious clinically. A number of different pathological types are described: tubulopapillary, sarcomatous, undifferentiated polygonal, and mixed.

The onset of the disease is often insidious, dull chest pain, breathlessness, and asthenia being commonest, cough, weight loss, and fever being less frequent, haemoptysis being rare. Encroachment on mediastinal structures may cause vocal chord paralysis or Horner's syndrome. Massive pleural effusion is the characteristic radiographic feature. It is very difficult to make the diagnosis by pleural cytology and tumour tends to grow along the needle track after paracentesis or along the scar of a thoracotomy incision. A history of exposure to asbestos should make one suspect the presence of this tumour especially if severe pain is present in the absence of rib destruction.

The disease is highly malignant and the average survival after diagnosis is 8 to 10 months. The management is that of malignant pleural effusion (page 15.156). The reported response to chemotherapy or immunotherapy is not encouraging except in a few early cases. The effects of pleurectomy and radiotherapy are equally discouraging.

References

Arnold, A. M. and Williams, C. J. (1979). Small cell lung cancer: a curable disease? *Br. J. Dis. Chest* **73**, 327–348.

Coombs, R. C., Ellison, M. L. and Neville, A. M. (1978). Biochemical markers in bronchogenic carcinoma. *Br. J. Dis. Chest* **72**, 263–287.

Crofton, J. W. and Douglas, A. C. (1981). *Respiratory diseases*. Blackwell Scientific Publications, Oxford.

Geddes, D. M. (1979). The natural history of lung cancer: a review based on rates of tumour growth. *Br. J. Dis. Chest.* **73**, 1–17.

Greco, F. D. and Oldham, R. K. (1979). Current concepts in cancer; small cell lung cancer. *N. Engl. J. Med.* **301**, 355–358.

Morstyn, G., Ihde, D. C., Lichter, A. S., Bunn, P. A., Carney, D. N., Glatstein, E. and Minna J. D. (1984). Small cell lung cancer 1973–1983: Early progress and recent obstacles. *Int. J. Rad. Oncol. Biol. Phys.* **10**, 515–539.

Spiro, S. G. and Goldstraw P. (1984). The staging of lung cancer. *Thorax* **39**, 401–407.

Staging of lung cancer (1979). American Joint Committee for Cancer Staging and End-Results Reporting: Task Force in Lung Cancer.

SLEEP-RELATED DISORDERS OF BREATHING

J. R. STRADLING

This chapter covers a relatively new field, the disorders that result from abnormalities of breathing during sleep. The most dramatic is the obstructive sleep apnoea syndrome, a condition characterized by recurrent hypoxaemia and arousal, due to obstruction of the pharyngeal airway during sleep with consequent excessive daytime sleepiness. However, there are other conditions where marked nocturnal hypoxaemia and central apnoea can occur with or without symptoms during wakefulness. Understanding of these conditions, as well as details of their prevalence and morbidity, is far from complete. Some of them undoubtedly lead to morbidity and mortality and thus it is important to be aware of their existence. To understand how a problem with breathing can arise during sleep, and not be apparent during wakefulness, it is necessary to discuss some of the normal changes in the physiology of respiration occurring during the different phases of sleep.

Normal physiology of breathing during sleep (Table 1)

Sleep can be divided into two basic phases: non-rapid eye movement (non-REM) and rapid eye movement (REM) sleep. Non-REM sleep has progressive depths (numbered 1 to 4) and is characterized by increasing amplitude and decreasing frequency of the electroencephalographic (EEG) waves. Stages 3 and 4 are also called slow wave sleep (SWS). REM sleep has an EEG pattern similar to that in the awake state and is associated with intermittent synchronous, binocular rapid eye movements. The tone in postural muscles is suppressed and the body becomes limp with occasional bursts of phasic muscular activity. It is this phase of sleep during which we dream.

During drowsiness, as the subject drifts in and out of the early stages of non-REM sleep, breathing can be periodic (waxing and waning) and irregular. Short periods of complete apnoea are normal during this stage and are common in the elderly. As SWS develops the breathing becomes very regular and the overall drive to the respiratory muscles is reduced leading to a small rise in $PaCO_2$ and fall in PaO_2. Sensitivity to induced hypoxaemia and hypercapnia is a little reduced compared to wakefulness, but the brain stem seems to be controlling breathing and all the classical respiratory drives are operative. It is probably more appropriate to view this change the other way round and to think of wakefulness as adding an extra cortical drive to the classical brain stem ones.

During REM sleep the breathing becomes less regular than during SWS, particularly during the bursts of phasic muscular activity referred to above. The muscles having a postural function (that REM sleep inhibits) include intercostal, laryngeal, pharyngeal, and tongue; all of which also have a respiratory function, particularly during inspiration. This loss of function leads to the pharynx becoming a relatively unsupported floppy tube and predominant abdominal (diaphragm) breathing.

Also during REM sleep there is some evidence that the ventilatory drives from classical stimuli (hypercapnia, hypoxaemia, Herring–Breuer, airway irritants) are reduced or can be intermit-

tently suppressed. This sort of experimentation is difficult and species differences exist. However, in humans, the response to progressive hypoxia and hypercapnia is reduced. Perhaps of more importance is that the arousal responses to all these stimuli are suppressed in REM sleep. Thus more severe disturbances of gas exchange are tolerated before arousal and corrective measures are taken. Only the response to complete airway occlusion is actually faster during REM than non-REM sleep. It seems likely that during REM sleep breathing can again be overridden by cortical activity, as it is whilst awake; whereas during non-REM sleep only classic drives via the brain stem are present.

Thus breathing during sleep, and particularly REM sleep, is different to wakefulness and this accounts for the development of problems perhaps only during one or other of the sleep stages.

Obstructive sleep apnoea

In 1877 Broadbent of St Mary's Hospital in London was one of the first to recognize that a patient of his snored heavily and had obstructed inspiration repeatedly throughout sleep. Gastaut, Tassinari, and Duron in 1965 were the first to document recurrent upper airways obstruction during sleep in an obese, sleepy patient though an association between obesity and respiratory failure was recognized by Osler who first used the term Pickwickian for such patients.

Table 1 Sleep and breathing

	Non-rapid eye movement sleep	Rapid eye movement sleep
Electroencephalogram (EEG)	Progressively slower and higher amplitude	Similar to the awake pattern
Eye movements	Initially slow and pendular, then none	Bursts of rapid, binocular movements
Breathing	Initially periodic, then regular. Mainly ribcage and a little less than during wakefulness	Irregular and further reduced. Mainly abdominal (diaphragm) breathing
Factors controlling breathing	Brain stem and classical stimuli although reduced compared to wakefulness	Cortical overriding and reduced responses to classical stimuli
Postural muscle tone, e.g. in pharynx	A little reduced	Very much reduced
Arousal response	Small changes in PaO_2 and $PaCO_2$ are enough to arouse	Large changes in PaO_2 and $PaCO_2$ are needed to arouse

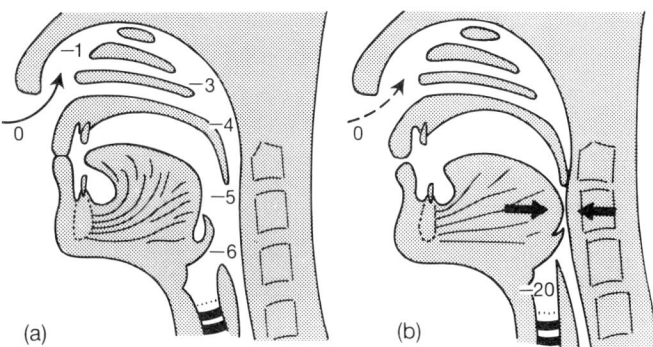

Fig. 1 Saggital section through head. (a) Normal situation during inspiration. As air is inhaled there is a pressure drop across structures offering a resistance (e.g. turbinates) and thus a negative pressure exists in the pharynx behind the tongue. Pressures in cm H_2O. (b) In obstructive sleep apnoea this negative pressure sucks in and collapses the pharynx preventing inspiration.

The main symptoms of this condition are hypersomnolence, heavy snoring, and restless sleep. They are often not appreciated by the patient but will be reported by the spouse. They may develop over many years and have been preceded by loud snoring alone, which should be regarded as a 'forme fruste' of this condition. Other symptoms include poor concentration, morning headaches, and impotence. Hypersomnolence often develops at a time when the body weight is increasing indicating that loud snoring has developed into recurrent obstruction. An observant spouse will also have noticed that there are apnoeic pauses between snoring and sometimes violent movements in association with the apnoea. As the condition progresses the hypersomnolence leads to a deterioration in personality and intellect. Redundancy, divorce, and recurrent car accidents may follow. Occasionally nocturnal enuresis occurs in adults. This symptom is found more frequently in children with this condition who may also be mistakenly regarded as retarded because of inability to concentrate at school.

The genesis of these symptoms is related to the changes in ventilatory drive and postural muscle tone during sleep described above. It seems that during inspiration some tone is required in the pharyngeal muscles to keep the pharynx open, if this drops below a critical level then the walls can simply collapse together and produce apnoea (Fig. 1). This may only occur during REM sleep but in most patients, with sufficient sleep disruption to cause daytime hypersomnolence, apnoeas occur in both REM and SWS. In order to overcome this obstruction the patient with obstructive sleep apnoea has to arouse (partially or completely) in response to the asphyxia. This arousal increases the drive to the muscles in the pharynx and the walls are pulled apart, usually with loud snorting and snoring noises. The patient may then hyperventilate enough to stop producing any respiratory efforts for a short while (central apnoea). As the patient drifts into deeper sleep again the narrowing pharynx vibrates with each inspiration and this gives rise to loud snoring. The pharynx then collapses again and the cycle is repeated over and over again with partial or complete arousal each time (Fig. 2). The periodicity of this cycle varies between 30 and 120 s in different individuals. This form of obstruction may be responsible for some cot deaths.

Recurrent nocturnal hypoxaemia and hypercapnia as a result of obstructive sleep apnoea may eventually carry over into the day with resetting of PaO_2 and $PaCO_2$ levels. Cyanosis, polycythaemia, and ankle oedema become obvious and if untreated the patient dies either suddenly at night or more slowly in respiratory failure. This final stage of diurnal respiratory failure seems to occur almost exclusively in patients with associated lung conditions such as asthma or chronic airways obstruction. Thus in a patient presenting with cor pulmonale, but only mild to moderate airways obstruction, obstructive sleep apnoea should be considered as a possible additional diagnosis. The reported cases of sudden nocturnal death in obstructive sleep apnoea have largely been in patients who also had chronic airways obstruction.

On physical examination most patients with this problem appear normal apart from a very high incidence of obesity. Recent evidence suggests though that even patients who appear normal probably have a small pharyngeal lumen such that the normal further reduction during sleep is critical. This is likely to be the primary problem rather than a subtle abnormality of upper airway control only present during sleep. Certainly no such abnormality has been demonstrated awake. However, there are correctable features worth looking for in perhaps a third of cases that are known to precipitate, or aggravate, obstructive sleep apnoea. These can be broadly divided into three:

1. Conditions that lead to encroachment upon the pharynx and reduce the lumen, thus making collapse and obstruction easier; for example, obesity, acromegaly, small jaw, mucopolysaccharidoses, superior vena caval obstruction, enlarged tonsils, and probably myxoedema.

2. Conditions that produce nasal or nasopharyngeal obstruction and thus accentuate the negative pressure in the pharynx during inspiration, e.g. a previously broken nose or congenitally deviated septum, rhinitis (allergic or infective), enlarged adenoids, and nasal valve obstruction.

3. Drugs that depress respiration such as alcohol, sedatives, and strong analgesics. These agents seem to reduce preferentially the drive to the upper airway muscles thus accentuating the col-

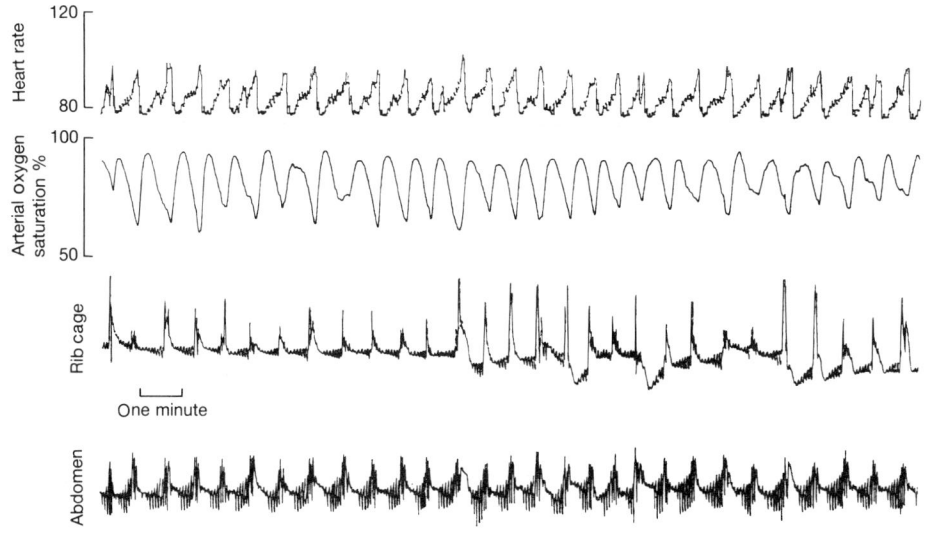

Fig. 2 Sleep tracing from a patient with obstructive sleep apnoea. Note the phasic pattern of the ribcage and abdominal movements: the cycle of very little movement, frustrated movements, and the deep unobstructed inspiration repeated every 40 s. The level of oxygen in the arterial blood seen by the ear with an ear lobe oximeter lags about 10 s behind representing the lung-to-ear circulation time. The instantaneous heart rate mirrors the arterial saturation. This pattern persisted throughout the night.

lapse, as well as inhibiting arousal and thus lengthening the apnoeas.

Rare forms of sleep apnoea occur in the Shy–Drager syndrome and can follow damage to the larynx by, for example, rheumatoid arthritis. In these cases it is the larynx that obstructs during sleep rather than the pharynx.

Investigation of these patients should include an upper airway examination for the features mentioned above, a screen for the predisposing conditions, and a sleep study. The parameters that need monitoring during a period of sleep are disputed. The overnight recording of multiple signals including EEG, EMG, eye movements, nasal and oral air flow, chest and abdominal movement, ear oximetry, ECG, and oesophageal pressure (polysomnography) is regarded as essential in some centres. For clinical purposes this is not so and the absence of such expensive equipment should not prevent the diagnosis being made. Ear oximetry and observation should be adequate to make the diagnosis. The obstructive apnoea leads to paradoxical movements of the chest and indrawing of neck soft tissues. These movements and the struggling appropriate for an asphyxiating person are unforgettable. One useful screening test is to ask the patient's spouse to record the characteristic and continuous snore–silence–snore pattern at home. A second useful screening test is 24-hour ECG monitoring. If the replay system is programmed to plot R–R interval then cyclical changes with a periodicity of 40 to 80 s, in time with the apnoeas, are often noted. A new oximeter that continuously records oxygen saturation from a non-invasive finger probe is available. It can be used in the patient's home and may become the best screening test in future. If these screening tests are normal then persisting hypersomnolence should be investigated with a full sleep study which may reveal other problems such as nocturnal myoclonus. In this condition repeated movements of the leg(s) produce recurrent arousals with consequent sleep deprivation: the patient may not be aware of these movements.

Treatment of obstructive sleep apnoea can be difficult. The level of therapeutic intervention has to be determined by the degree of disability from hypersomnolence and respiratory failure. Correction of predisposing conditions, such as stopping alcohol or sedatives, weight loss, or surgery to straighten a deviated septum and remove enlarged tonsils, is always worth trying first. Tracheostomy (bypassing the obstruction) is absolutely successful but attended by its own problems. However, in serious cases it is life-saving and can be closed later if other treatments can be instituted. In North America, uvulo-palato-pharyngoplasty has achieved some success, an operation involving the removal of all the redundant tissue from the pharynx. However, its value has not been adequately proven and cannot be recommended as a routine procedure at present. Surgery in these obese patients is hazardous and not to be undertaken lightly. The tricyclic antidepressants have a small place but probably only help in the milder cases.

The most ingenious and successful recent development has been the use of continuous nasal positive airway pressure delivered via a nasal mask (or sealed nasal canulae) during sleep. These systems raise the pressure in the pharynx by about 5 to 15 cm H_2O and hold open or 'splint' the airway. The patient breathes a normal minute volume but at a higher airway pressure. The air is humidified and warmed by the nose as usual. This treatment is totally effective except in a small minority who cannot tolerate the nasal mask. Commercial systems are becoming available.

Successful treatment of pure obstructive sleep apnoea can lead to correction of any daytime hypercapnia indicating that it is the nocturnal apnoea itself that leads to persisting respiratory failure.

The true incidence of this disorder is unknown. One centre in North America has seen over 1000 cases but no interested unit in England has seen more than 40 cases. The condition is much commoner in men. Population surveys are difficult but one estimate from Israel puts the overall incidence at 1 per cent of the male working population though not all of these would complain of symptoms. The main problems in estimating incidence are in selecting a random sample of subjects who are not influenced in their decision to volunteer for sleep studies by having relevant symptoms. Second, there exists a continuum between non-snorers, heavy snorers, and obstructive sleep apnoea. The point at which apnoeas at night become responsible for minor symptoms of hypersomnolence is difficult to determine and may vary from one individual to another and with age. One study on people over 65 years found more than 30 per cent had more than five apnoeas (more than 10 s each) per hour. Symptomatically there was no difference between these subjects and non-apnoeic controls. Other studies have found a correlation between overnight hypoxaemia and increases in morning confusion in patients with Alzheimer's dementia. A recent study on healthy and apparently asymptomatic subjects, over 65 years, showed 9/24 with more than 8 arousals per hour associated with breathing irregularities. Two of these subjects had previously unrecognized hypersomnolence on subsequent formal testing. More work is required to determine at what point abnormalities of breathing during sleep lead to daytime symptoms. The current limit for normality (five apnoeas, of more than 10 s each per hour) is too low. The third problem is in detecting and quantifying hypersomnolence. Many people regard daytime naps and a degree of sleepiness as normal, particularly as they grow older. There is no reliable and simple way to measure sleepiness for epidemiological purposes. At present narcolepsy is probably the commonest misdiagnosis although nocturnal myoclonus is the third major cause of daytime hypersomnolence.

Sleep hypoventilation and central apnoea

Sleep hypoventilation and central sleep apnoea should probably be considered together since they are different only in degree. Normal people hypoventilate at night with consequent small rises in $PaCO_2$ and falls in PaO_2. Short periods of apnoea due to temporary loss of drive are also normal (called 'central' as opposed to 'obstructive' apnoea). These can occur during both stages 1 and 2 non-REM and REM sleep. At sea level normal people have nearly fully saturated haemoglobin on the flat part of the dissociation curve and these small falls in PaO_2 are unimportant. However, if a patient has a daytime PaO_2 on the steep part of the dissociation curve then easily measurable falls in oxygen saturation will occur. This extra hypoxaemia may be instrumental in hastening the long-term effects of hypoxaemia but is normally unavoidable and largely depends on the starting level of PaO_2.

In patients with chronic airways obstruction, cystic fibrosis, kyphoscoliosis, and asthma, nocturnal hypoxaemia can be considerable but to what extent it contributes to the overall respiratory failure is not clear. The degree of hypoventilation in these conditions is probably considerably more than that in normal subjects during REM sleep. Because such patients depend on intercostal and accessory muscles of respiration to a greater extent than normal people, it is likely that the REM sleep inhibition of these muscles is more serious to overall ventilation. In patients with bilateral diaphragm paralysis, totally dependent on intercostal and accessory muscles of respiration, the REM sleep-associated hypoventilation and even apnoea is profound. Although bilateral diaphragm paralysis usually occurs as part of a general neuromuscular condition in some cases (such as in acid-maltase deficiency) it is an early or isolated finding and leads to respiratory failure before general weakness is apparent. This rare condition is one of the causes of 'central' sleep apnoea since the patient appears to simply stop breathing at times during the night.

Another cause of central sleep apnoea is absent or reduced hypoxic and hypercapnic drives. These can be impaired by exposure to recurrent hypoxia and hypercapnia but more commonly by brain stem lesions. Occasionally, they are congenitally deficient. During wakefulness a person with impaired hypoxic and hypercapnic drives has a stimulus to breath from the cortex and reticular activating system (the 'awake' drive referred to earlier). On falling asleep this drive is lost and the person stops breathing, the so-called 'Ondine's curse'. During REM sleep the cortical activity may produce respiratory activity again. These patients may present with hypersomnolence from sleep disruption but more usually in severe respiratory failure.

Recently, some cases of hypersomnolence and central sleep apnoea have been recognized as variants of obstructive sleep apnoea. It seems that when the pharynx collapses, rather than struggling to inspire, a reflex cessation of drive to breath occurs. This occurs particularly if the subject is lying supine. There is often snoring and the clinical presentation, consequences, and therapy are similar to classical obstructive sleep apnoea.

Thus central sleep apnoea can be due to a variety of underlying conditions and is not a diagnosis in itself. Once discovered, and felt to be symptomatic, further investigations are required to elucidate the cause.

Treatment for central sleep apnoea or hypoventilation is required if respiratory failure carries over into waking hours with hypoxaemia and hypercapnia. Whether idiopathic and symptomless central apnoea with only nocturnal hypoxaemia requires treatment is disputed. At present the most successful management of these patients is assisted overnight ventilation with external devices such as a cuirasse, or a rocking bed. The cuirasse ventilator is like the old 'iron lung' but consists of a small shell, fitting around the patient, connected to an intermittent vacuum pump that draws out the chest wall. A rocking bed simply pushes the diaphragm up and down by gravity. These therapies are of proven benefit even when only used overnight for the ventilatory failure of bilateral diaphragm paralysis, kyphoscoliosis, old extensive thoracoplasty, and some neuromuscular disorders. They are even being tried in patients with chronic hypoxic lung disease. If the central apnoea is truly central, and the phrenic nerve and diaphragm are still intact, then phrenic nerve pacing is possible. All these procedures can sometimes actually precipitate obstructive apnoea since the patient's own respiratory drive is suppressed so that during the induced inspiration the pharynx is not being activated and can collapse.

Overnight ventilation therapy usually improves any daytime hypercapnia and hypoxaemia sometimes to normal. This may result from preventing the nocturnal deterioration in blood gases and thus 'resetting' the respiratory control mechanisms to normal; or possibly by relieving any fatigue of the respiratory muscles that are working under adverse conditions, such as in kyphoscoliosis. Benefit may result simply from resting the muscles so allowing them to deliver the pump action demanded by the respiratory centre during the day. Studies are underway to define the place of overnight ventilation in a variety of conditions causing respiratory failure.

The scope of a sleep disorders clinic

In North America many hospitals have sleep investigation units but these are as yet a rarity in the United Kingdom. A sleep disorders clinic will be asked to see a variety of problems other than those related to abnormalities of breathing described above. In a survey of 8000 such referrals over 5 years from several centres in North America, and one in Italy, three main groups of disorders were being diagnosed. These diagnoses were made after sleep monitoring, deemed to be necessary in 80 per cent of the original referrals. (1) Insomnia accounted for 30 per cent, mainly from psychiatric causes. (2) Hypersomnolence accounted for 45 per cent, mainly due to sleep apnoea, narcolepsy, and nocturnal myoclonus. (3) Parasomnias or dysfunctions associated with sleep accounted for 20 per cent. This group consisted of gastro-oesophageal reflux, fits, sleep-walking, and symptoms of choking or difficult breathing for which no cause could be found.

Overall less than 20 per cent of patients in such a broad referral category will have a primary disorder of nocturnal breathing; hypersomnolence as a referral symptom increases this figure to 40 per cent.

References
Guilleminault, C., Tilkian, A. and Dement, W. C. (1976). The sleep apnoea syndromes. *Ann. Rev. Med.* **27**, 465–484.
Phillipson, E. A. (1978). Control of breathing during sleep. *Am. Rev. Resp. Dis.* **118**, 909–939.
Saunders, N. A. and Sullivan, C. E. (1984). Sleep and Breathing. In *Lung biology in health and disease* Vol. 21. Marcel Dekker, New York.
Stradling, J. R. (1986). Controversies in sleep-related breathing disorders. *Lung* **164**, 17–31.
—— and Phillipson, E. A. (1986). Breathing disorders during sleep. *Q. J. Med.* **58**, 3–18.

ADULT RESPIRATORY DISTRESS SYNDROME

A. FISHER AND P. FOËX

Introduction

The term adult respiratory distress syndrome (ARDS) is used to describe an acute, life-threatening respiratory failure which occurs in subjects with previously healthy lungs without primary left ventricular failure. It is associated with a large and ever-increasing number of unrelated clinical disorders, yet has uniform physiological, radiological, and pathological features. The present title was introduced by Ashbough in 1967 because of the morphological similarities to the neonatal respiratory distress syndrome and has replaced the many synonyms used in the past. The title is sometimes criticized for obscuring reference to specific aetiological causes which might influence management.

Although major trauma, acute hypovolaemia, Gram-negative septicaemia, and overwhelming microbial pulmonary infections are the most frequent precursors of ARDS, the inclusion of all non-cardiogenic disorders causing respiratory failure produces a prodigious list of associated disorders (Table 1). An inciting event can be assigned in about 80 per cent of cases of ARDS and often this is non-pulmonary.

Incidence

It is difficult to record accurately the incidence of a poorly defined disorder but the Division of Lung Disease Task Force estimated that 150 000 cases occurred annually in the United States, an incidence of 0.6/1000 population. Patients with ARDS account for about 5 per cent of admissions to intensive therapy units. The incidence appears to be increasing due to more effective resuscitation and intensive care of the critically ill. A recent prospective epidemiological study of 34 872 patients admitted to three university hospitals in the United States revealed the overall incidence of ARDS to be 0.25 per cent of hospital admissions.

Clinical presentation

Since ARDS follows a variety of direct and indirect lung insults, its development varies in time and intensity but the morphological and symptomatic changes that occur have led to the recognition of a sequential progression of events.

Table 1 Disorders associated with ARDS

1	Hypovolaemic shock			
2	Infection	(a) Pulmonary (microbial, fungal, pneumocystis, malaria)		
		(b) Extrapulmonary (septicaemia)		
3	Trauma	(a) Thoracic		
		(b) Extrathoracic		
4	Embolism	(a) Fat		
		(b) Amniotic fluid		
		(c) Cellular aggregates		
5	Inhalation	(a) Gas	(i) irritant (e.g. nitric oxide, smoke)	
			(ii) Non-irritant (e.g. oxygen)	
		(b) Liquid	(i) Gastric juice	
			(ii) Fresh and salt water	
6	Haematological	(a) Disseminated intravascular coagulopathy		
		(b) Massive blood transfusion		
7	Metabolic	(a) Diabetic ketosis		
		(b) Uraemia		
8	Neurogenic	(a) Cerebral oedema		
		(b) Intracranial haemorrhage		
9	Drugs	Including heroin, aspirin, propoxyphene, barbiturates		
10	Others	(a) Pancreatitis		
		(b) High altitude		

Phase 1

This is the period of initial resuscitation, with repletion of hypovolaemia. Excessive use of bicarbonate, loss of chloride in gastric contents, and oxidation of citrate in transfused blood may produce a metabolic alkalosis aggravated by a respiratory component following hyperventilation in response to pain. Unless there has been direct pulmonary damage, the lungs are dry on ausculation and the chest radiograph is clear.

Phase 2

This is a deceptive period of 24–72 hours' duration when the patient is haemodynamically stable with no obvious respiratory distress except mild tachypnoea. Serial blood gas analysis at this time, however, might reveal subclinical hypoxaemia due to intrapulmonary shunting.

Phase 3

During this period, the hypoxaemia worsens with an increasing intrapulmonary shunt. The patient becomes clinically cyanosed and dyspnoeic. The chest compliance falls demanding higher inflation pressures. The chest radiograph may reveal the classical picture of widespread bilateral intra-alveolar and interstitial infiltrates, which become progressively more confluent though sparing the costophrenic angles and apices. Increasing hypoxaemia produces disturbed cerebral and renal function and, unless management reverses the course of the disease, the final phase is entered.

Phase 4

Refractory hypoxaemia develops with increasing pulmonary hypertension and right ventricular dysfunction. Hypercapnia and hypoperfusion contribute to a mixed respiratory and metabolic acidosis and multiorgan failure follows. Sepsis and renal failure frequently occur in this terminal phase.

Pathology

Despite the heterogeneity of initiating conditions leading to ARDS, there is homogeneity of the morphological changes found in the lung at autopsy. Macroscopically it may be heavy, red, and liver-like or light, grey, and fibrous, depending on whether the disease has been of short or long duration. Microscopically two phases can be distinguished:

Acute exudative phase

Interstitial oedema is accompanied by damage to and necrosis of capillary endothelial and alveolar type I epithelial cells. Fibrin and

platelet thrombi develop in the capillaries and there is adherence of leucocytes to areas denuded of endothelium. Later, the oedema becomes perivascular, peribronchial, and intra-alveolar in distribution and accompanied by focal alveolar haemorrhages. The damaged type I alveolar cells together with fibrin and other plasma proteins constitute the characteristic hyaline membrane which lines the alveoli, alveolar ducts, and some respiratory bronchioles.

Chronic proliferative phase

There is regeneration of the capillary endothelium and alveolar epithelium accompanied by interstitial infiltration by lymphocytes, fibroblasts, and deposition of collagen which may proceed to fibrosis. The damaged type I alveolar cells are replaced by more granular type II alveolar cells often cuboidal in shape producing a hyperplastic appearance with a thickening of the air–blood interface. The alveolar lining of surfactant, normally produced by these cells is absent.

Pathogenesis

A finding in all patients with ARDS, whether the initiating cause is mediated by the blood stream or the airways, is an increase in total lung water caused by a disturbance in the normal fluid flux between the intravascular and extravascular compartments in the lung. The factors governing the normal distribution of lung water are expressed in the Starling equation:

$$F = K\,(P_{\mathrm{cap}} - P_{\mathrm{is}}) - \Theta\,(\Pi_{\mathrm{cap}} - \Pi_{\mathrm{is}})$$

where F is net filtration rate, K is the filtration coefficient, P_{cap} and P_{is} are the capillary and interstitial hydrostatic pressures, π_{cap} and π_{is} are the capillary and plasma protein osmotic pressures, and θ is the protein reflection coefficient. Normally the outward transcapillary hydrostatic pressure difference slightly exceeds the inward transcapillary protein osmotic pressure difference, producing a continuous flow of water and solutes. In ARDS, interstitial lung water increases, exceeding the capacity of the lymphatic drainage, producing intra-alveolar pulmonary oedema and intrapulmonary shunting of venous blood.

Plasma protein osmotic pressure

In trauma and acute illness, there is a reduction in plasma protein concentration and osmotic pressure which may be further reduced by crystalloid infusion. It cannot be assumed that interstitial protein osmotic pressure remains steady and evidence suggests an interstitial loss of osmotically active material occurring as the plasma protein osmotic pressure falls, preserving the transcapillary gradient. Reductions in plasma protein concentration, however, do lower the threshold at which pulmonary capillary hydrostatic changes become significant.

Lymph drainage

The normal lymph drainage is only 25–30 ml/hour but this can increase 20-fold in response to relatively small changes in interstitial pressure from fluid accumulation. High intrathoracic pressures during IPPV or high levels of PEEP may impair this function but they are unlikely to play a primary role in the genesis of interstitial oedema in ARDS.

Pulmonary capillary permeability and hydrostatic pressure

Although stress-evoked stimulation of the sympathetic nervous system in the critically ill will produce pulmonary venoconstriction and pulmonary hypertension, emphasis is moving away from neurohumoral mechanisms in the pathogenesis of ARDS. There is convincing evidence that increased pulmonary vascular permeability with increased postcapillary resistance is largely responsible for the increase in lung water. Fluid obtained from the airways of patients with ARDS has a higher protein content than that from normal subjects or patients with cardiogenic pulmonary oedema. In animal experiments, lymph collected from chronically implanted fistulae increases both in amount and protein content

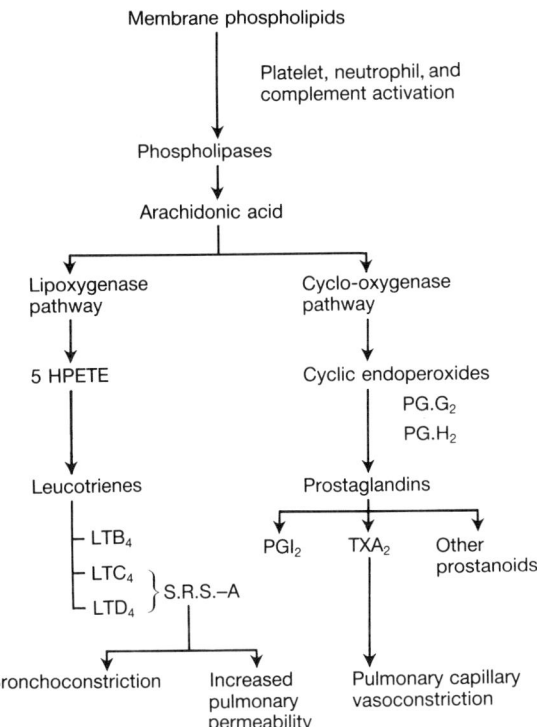

Fig. 1 Pathogenesis of ARDS: arachidonic acid metabolism.

following endotoxin-induced shock. Using radioisotope-labelled tracers such as ^{123}I-albumin or ^{99m}Tc-albumin a transmicrovascular flux of protein can be demonstrated indicating increased endothelial permeability. The cause of this increased permeability has been the focus of much research and speculation.

Neutrophils and complement activation

There is mounting evidence suggesting that the neutrophil plays a key role in the pathogenesis of ARDS. In sheep there is a neutropenia within 60 min of endotoxin infusion correlating with the subsequent hypoxaemia. The high flow and high protein content of lymph following the endotoxin injection can be attenuated by previously rendering the animal neutropenic. In humans, radiolabelled neutrophils can be seen by lung scan to sequester in the lungs of patients with ARDS with increased numbers demonstrable in bronchoalveolar lavages (BAL). The mechanism by which neutrophils microembolize in the pulmonary circulation probably involves the alternative pathway activation of complement with the release of neutrophil-aggregating components, particularly C5a. In experimental animals embolization of the pulmonary microcirculation and a pulmonary capillary leak can be induced by infusion of activated complement. In humans, clinical causes of ARDS such as endotoxaemia, trauma, and pulmonary infection are also known to activate the complement cascade and elevated levels of C5a have been claimed as a useful predictor for the development of ARDS in the critically ill. The neutrophil is well equipped to induce injury in the lung. Intracellular granules can release proteinases such as elastase, collagenase, and cathepsins which, by degrading structural components such as elastin, collagen, basement membranes, and fibronectin, can lead to disorganization of the interstitium and damage to capillary endothelial and alveolar epithelial cells. Proteinases may also cleave fibrinogen, the Hageman factor, complement, and the other plasma proteins producing further embolization by blood constituents such as platelets, mast cells, fibrin, and fibrinogen degradation products, often demonstrable by balloon-occluded segmental pulmonary angiography. Their presence is enhanced by deficiency of opsonic fibronectin impairing the phagocytic function of the reticuloendothelial system. Histamine, platelet activated factor, serotonin,

bradykinin, and other vasoactive substances may be released by these embolized blood products, contributing to the permeability and hydrostatic pressure changes in the pulmonary microcirculation. The activated neutrophils may also be responsible for oxidant damage to the lung by the excessive generation of highly toxic oxygen radical molecules. The free radical superoxide (0^-_2) can participate in several chemical reactions yielding hydrogen peroxide (H_2O_2) and the extremely cytotoxic hydroxyl radical (OH^-). These molecules are normally used in a protective role against bacteria but, by overwhelming the antioxidant defence mechanisms, such as superoxide dismutase, they act in an aggressive manner destroying intracellular enzyme systems and cell wall structure of both the pulmonary capillary endothelial and alveolar epithelial cells. The toxic oxygen radical molecules can do further damage, inactivating enzyme inhibitors such as α_1-antitrypsin, thus encouraging proteinase activity.

Arachidonic acid metabolism

The lung is an important organ in arachidonic acid metabolism producing metabolites with a remarkable spectrum of biological activity. There is increasing evidence that these metabolites might be involved in the pathogenesis of ARDS. They are released from cell membrane phospholipids, not only by activated neutrophils, but also by mast cells, platelets, and complement-dependent mechanisms. Two functionally active groups of substances, the prostaglandins (PG) and the leukotrienes (LT), are produced by separate metabolic pathways (Fig. 1).

Oxidative metabolism of arachidonic acid by the cyclo-oxygenase pathway sequentially produces two cyclic endoperoxides (PGG_2 and PGH_2). These intermediate prostaglandins are rapidly converted by specific enzymes into diverse vasoactive products, the most important being thromboxane A_2 (TXA_2), an intense pulmonary vasoconstrictor and platelet aggregator, and prostacyclin (PGI_2) an anti-aggregator and pulmonary vasodilator substance. A disturbance in the normal metabolic balance in favour of TXA_2 could result in pulmonary capillary hypertension by postcapillary vasoconstriction and mechanical obstruction by microaggregates. Increased prostacyclin production may increase intrapulmonary shunting by preventing the normal hypoxic pulmonary vasoconstriction. In experimental animals it has been found that pretreatment with cyclo-oxygenase inhibitors such as indomethacin or meclofenamate can abolish endotoxin-induced pulmonary hypertension, although the increased pulmonary vascular permeability is unchanged.

The alternative lipoxygenase pathway of arachidonic acid metabolism produces several groups of metabolites depending on the source of the lipoxygenase enzyme. Neutrophils possess the enzyme responsible for producing 5-hydroperoxyeicosa tetranoic acid (5, H.PETE) which is the precursor of a family of active substances known as leukotrienes. Leukotriene B_4 is a potent neutrophil chemotaxin while leukotrienes C_4 and D_4 are the main constituents of the slow reacting substance of anaphylaxis (SRS-A) which, in the lung, can produce bronchoconstriction, microvascular vasoconstriction and increased capillary permeability. The pathogenesis of ARDS is thus extremely complex and involves interrelated immune, coagulation, and biochemical responses which, although producing similar end-stage manifestations, probably employ differing pathways, depending on the specific aetiology. A simplified sequence of the mechanisms involved is shown in Fig. 2.

Physiological features

Abnormalities of pulmonary function correlate well with the pathological changes described.

Reduced compliance and lung volume

The stiffness of the lung is determined directly by the tissue elasticity and alveolar surface tension and indirectly by the lung volume. In ARDS altered surfactant production and function result in alveolar instability and diffuse microatelectasis. All lung

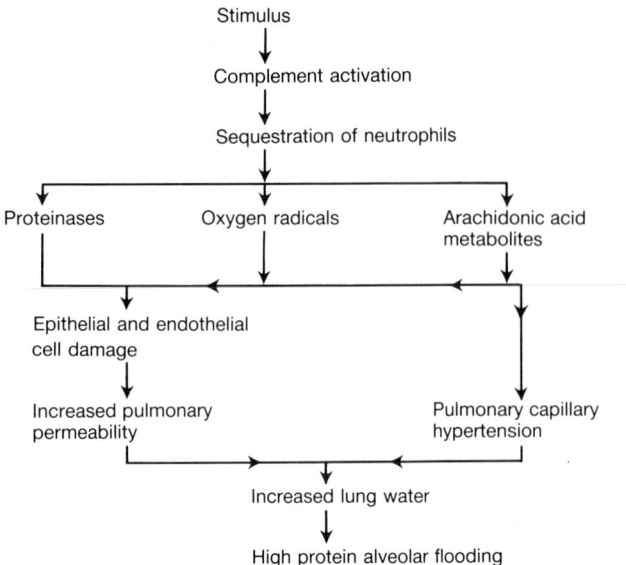

Fig. 2 A summary of the pathogenesis of ARDS.

Table 2 Criteria for diagnosis of ARDS

Characteristic chest radiograph
Hypoxaemia
Reduced lung compliance
Pulmonary hypertension (>30/15 mm Hg)
Normal PCWP (<15 mm Hg)
High protein pulmonary oedema

Table 3 Management of ARDS

Oxygenation	(a) Uptake
	(b) Delivery
	(c) Demand
	(d) Toxicity
Pulmonary haemodynamics	(a) Vasoconstriction
	(b) Microembolization
	(c) Increased permeability
Fluid balance	(a) Crystalloid
	(b) Colloid
Prophylactic management	(a) Steroids
	(b) Antibiotics
	(c) Nutrition

volumes are reduced. Physiologically, the most important is the functional residual capacity (FRC) which, if greatly reduced, produces small airway closure during expiration, with air trapping in the distal alveoli. Subsequent absorption atelectasis produces more reduction in lung compliance and further impairs gas exchange.

Alterations in gas exchange

The most sinister feature of ARDS is an inability to maintain arterial oxygen tensions without toxic levels of inspired oxygen concentration (FiO$_2$). Three mechanisms operate in producing this hypoxaemia:

(a) Perfusion of underventilated alveoli ($\dot{V}_A/\dot{Q}$ mismatch) The fluid accumulation in the lung progresses from an interstitial to a peribronchial distribution before alveolar flooding occurs. Narrowing of the small airways results in a large number of alveoli, particularly in the dependent lung zones, having a reduced but finite $\dot{V}/\dot{Q}$ ratio.

(b) Perfusion of non-ventilated alveoli (true shunt) The normal physiological shunt (3–5 per cent of the cardiac output) is produced by small intrapulmonary A–V anastomoses, together with the bronchial and Thebesian circulations. In ARDS the intrapulmonary shunt can increase to 60–70 per cent of cardiac output, partly by a few direct A–V anastomoses opening up but mainly by perfusion of non-ventilated alveoli.

(c) Impaired diffusion In addition to thickening of the alveolar capillary septum, there is a reduced capillary blood volume with decreased transit time. The relative contributions of these three mechanisms are variable and not easily assessed. If true shunt rather than $\dot{V}/\dot{Q}$ mismatch was the main contributor, increasing FiO$_2$ would not alter the shunt, whereas theoretically it would lessen the contribution made by the alveoli with a low but finite $\dot{V}/\dot{Q}$ ratio. In practice, however, increasing FiO$_2$ has a variable effect on the shunt, not only in different patients, but also in the same patient, during different phases of the disease. The usual response to increasing FiO$_2$ is an increase in intrapulmonary shunt, an active response which may be found in patients with ARDS either throughout the disease or at different times during evolution of the disease. This active response is associated with a more favourable prognosis than a fixed shunt uninfluenced by increasing FiO$_2$.

Increased work of breathing

In spontaneously breathing patients, an increase in the dead space/tidal volume (VD/VT) ratio may seen particularly with microembolization of the pulmonary capillaries. Increased effort required to keep the arterial carbon dioxide tension normal and reduced lung compliance can lead to respiratory failure unless respiration is mechanically assisted.

Diagnosis and management

ARDS is a clinical diagnosis, the criteria for which are listed in Table 2. Tachypnoea, hypoxaemia, and a similar chest radiograph make the differentiation from cardiogenic pulmonary oedema difficult. ARDS should, however, be suspected if acute respiratory failure (PaO_2<6.7 kPa breathing 60 per cent oxygen) occurs in association with a recognized precipitating cause and if the circulation is hyperdynamic with normal or slightly raised pulmonary capillary wedge and central venous pressures. Blood gas analysis may often reveal hypoxaemia due to intrapulmonary shunting before the classical radiological appearance of ARDS develops.

Early recognition with appropriate pharmacological and supportive therapy favourably influences the prognosis, but, unfortunately, no simple laboratory test or bedside measurement accurately predicts the onset of this condition. The indices of pulmonary gas exchange and pulmonary compliance are not sufficiently sensitive to detect early interstitial oedema, becoming abnormal only when alveolar oedema occurs. Changes in lung volumes, particularly FRC, do occur earlier but are not applicable to bedside monitoring. Non-invasive methods of measuring lung water and permeability changes may prove to be useful in screening patients but perhaps the most useful method of identifying incipient acute respiratory failure is by C5a assays, high levels of which have been positively associated with the onset of ARDS.

The aim in the management of ARDS is to support all body systems until the integrity of the alveolar capillary membrane is restored and, although the correction of tissue hypoxia is the cornerstone, other supportive measures listed in Table 3 are also of utmost importance.

Oxygenation

Oxygen uptake

(a) Intermittent positive-pressure ventilation (IPPV) If the arterial oxygen tension cannot be maintained above 6.5 kPa with an FiO$_2$ of 0.5 in the spontaneously breathing patient, intubation and ventilatory support are indicated. A volume preset ventilator delivering a large tidal volume (10–15 ml/kg) with a slow inspiratory phase and prolonged expiratory pause produces the most efficient gas exchange. If hypoxaemia persists, other manoeuvres, designed to increase FRC and improve oxygenation are indicated.

(b) Positive end expiratory pressure (PEEP) Recent evidence suggests that pulmonary extravascular water is either unchanged or increased. The beneficial effects are produced by an increase in FRC and a decrease in intrapulmonary shunting derived by recruitment of lung units previously unavailable for gas exchange. The compliance of the lung may also be improved by an increase in the lung volume and surfactant conservation. Its benefits are limited, however, by cardiac output changes and the dangers of barotrauma such as pneumothorax, pneumomediastinum, and surgical emphysema. Although modest levels of PEEP (5–10 cm H_2O) are unlikely to reduce cardiac output more precise information can be obtained by thermodilution cardiac output measurements. Alternatively, the assessment of mixed venous oxygen content ($C_{\bar{v}}O_2$) can be used; assuming an unchanged oxygen consumption, a fall in $C_{\bar{v}}O_2$ would indicate a reduced cardiac output. Very high levels of PEEP (up to 30 cm H_2O) have been advocated, the cardiac output being maintained by volume loading and inotropic support, but the obvious dangers impose limitations on its use. More conventionally a level of PEEP is selected which is compatible with an unchanged cardiac output or an unchanged static lung compliance.

(c) Asynchronous independent lung ventilation (AILV) This technique employs a double lumen endobronchial tube, each limb of which is connected to a separate ventilator thus allowing optimum respiratory function to be obtained from each lung independently, by varying ventilatory indices and inspired oxygen concentrations. Although the concept of AILV is attractive, in practice it demands a high degree of nursing care to preserve accurate tube placement and the duration is limited by the risk of trauma to the bronchial tree.

(d) High frequency ventilation (HFV) The traditional concepts of alveolar ventilation and dead space have been questioned by satisfactory gas exchange occurring at ventilatory 'frequencies' up to 40 Hz. HFV can be divided into high-frequency jet ventilation and high-frequency oscillation depending on the speed of ventilation and the apparatus. The physical principles involved in explaining the efficacy of this mode of ventilation invoke the enhancement of convection and the accelerated diffusion of gas molecules. Ventilators, with negligible compressible volumes are required and these, by delivering pulses of oxygen-enriched air, achieve efficient alveolar ventilation and gas exchange with low transpulmonary pressures and reflex inhibition of spontaneous respiration. The advantages are, therefore, adequate blood gas exchange with lessened risk of barotrauma and minimal effects on pulmonary and systemic circulations. In clinical practice, humidification is difficult and its role in the management of ARDS has yet to be fully assessed.

(e) Membrane oxygenation The technical and physiological advances made in extracorporeal oxygenation during open heart surgery led to the hope that, by using a similar technique with a membrane oxygenator, the lungs of patients with ARDS would have time to recover while oxygenation and perfusion of vital organs was maintained. Initial enthusiasm was tempered, however, by the disappointing results of a randomized prospective multicentre trial in the United States. More attention has recently been paid to a modification of this technique using a large area membrane lung with low extracorporeal blood flows (1–1.5 l/min) to remove carbon dioxide. A low ventilatory rate (3/min) prevents atelectasis and oxygenation is maintained by using a carinal catheter delivering 300 ml oxygen/min. The low intra-alveolar tensions, low ventilatory rates, and low inflation pressures avoid the adverse iatrogenic effects of conventional IPPV. Although initial results of this technique in the management of ARDS are encouraging, further experience is required before a final assessment can be made.

Oxygen delivery
The amount of oxygen available to the tissues is a direct function of arterial oxygen content, cardiac output, and the position of the oxyhaemoglobin dissociation curve. In ARDS hypoxaemia reduces the arterial oxygen content and cardiac output may be lowered by hypovolaemia or by PEEP. Adequate filling of the vascular compartment is necessary and inotropic support may be required to restore an effective cardiac output. The interdependence of biventricular function must be remembered. Right ventricular failure secondary to increased pulmonary vascular resistance impairs left ventricular forward flow and may also produce left ventricular compression by a leftward shift of the interventricular septum. In such instances the pharmacological reduction of the excessive pulmonary vascular resistance might be considered. Anaemia should be corrected by transfusion of filtered fresh blood. Metabolic and respiratory alkalosis producing a leftward shift of the oxyhaemoglobin dissociation curve with reduced oxygen availability should be avoided.

Oxygen demand
High oxygen requirements may be reduced by heavy sedation and, when indicated, muscle relaxation. Although hypothermia (30 °C) increases the amount of oxygen dissolved in the blood and reduces the oxygen demand, there is no firm evidence that it improves the prognosis in ARDS; oxygen availability is reduced by the leftward shift of the oxyhaemoglobin dissociation curve, thus lessening the benefits of hypothermia.

Oxygen toxicity
The devastating effect of oxygen on the lung was described by Lorraine Smith as early as 1899, but it was not until 1967 that evidence appeared correlating histological changes of both early and late ARDS with high inspired oxygen concentrations. Experimental evidence suggests that the elevated alveolar oxygen concentration, not the arterial oxygen tension, is responsible for the toxicity. The mechanism involves the reduction of molecular oxygen to highly reactive and potentially cytotoxic radicals which overwhelm the antioxidant defence enzymes causing intracellular enzyme damage and loss of membrane integrity.

The severity of oxygen toxicity is dependent on both the FiO_2 and the duration of exposure. It is also influenced by biochemically induced tolerance, previous lung disease, and the age and weight of the patient. The variability of a patient's susceptibility does not allow a safe inspired oxygen concentration to be predicted accurately. From a practical point of view, it is believed that an FiO_2 of < 0.5 can be safely administered for prolonged periods, whereas an FiO_2 of > 0.8 can produce deleterious effects in the lung within 48 hours. On occasions, however, it is impossible to maintain adequate oxygenation unless potentially toxic inspired oxygen concentrations are used. In these circumstances the full range of therapeutic manoeuvres should be employed in an attempt to lower the FiO_2. The use of free radical scavengers such as superoxide dismutase enzymes has yet to be shown clinically to be effective in preventing oxygen toxicity.

Pulmonary haemodynamics
There is no therapy in current use which will improve $\dot{V}/\dot{Q}$ mismatch by changes in pulmonary haemodynamics. Infusions of vasodilator drugs such as glyceryl trinitrate, sodium nitroprusside or prostacyclin all non-selectively reverse vasoconstriction throughout the whole pulmonary vascular bed reducing the pulmonary artery pressure but at the expense of systemic arterial oxygenation. Pulmonary hypertension in ARDS may also be caused by microembolization of the pulmonary circulation by particulate blood products. It is possible that this embolization is enhanced by plasma fibronectin deficiency which can be corrected by cryoprecipitate infusions, but neither the use of anticoagulants nor the infusion of streptokinase has been shown to be useful or safe. The use of pharmacological preparations in the management of the permeability defect of the microcirculation has not yet been established. Cyclo-oxygenase inhibitors such as the non-steroidal, anti-

inflammatory drugs, can reduce the pulmonary hypertension but without abatement of the increased permeability. Similarly specific antivasoactive drugs such as the antihistamines have proved ineffective while lipoxygenase inhibitors are not yet in clinical use. The role of steroids is discussed later.

Fluid balance

There is still debate about the effects of crystalloid and colloid infusions on the flux of water and solutes across the pulmonary endothelium when there is increased permeability as in ARDS. There is general agreement that the initial therapeutic goal must be the restoration of circulating blood volume but the dilemma as to which type of fluid to use exists because it is not known at what stage the pulmonary capillary leak occurs, nor if it is a sudden or gradual event. Some studies have demonstrated that colloid infusion, by increasing plasma protein osmotic pressure, reduces extravascular lung water accumulation, while other authorities maintain that colloid infusions extravasate into the interstitium, abolishing the transcapillary protein osmotic pressure difference. Certainly when the capillary leak is established, even large molecules pass into the interstitium and the protein content of the alveolar fluid can approach that of plasma. It is probable that in early ARDS colloid infusions do not augment the pulmonary transcapillary flux of proteins provided the microvascular hydrostatic pressure does not rise significantly. Thus careful monitoring of systemic and pulmonary perfusion pressures is critical and the use of a flow-directed balloon catheter essential. By maintaining a pulmonary capillary wedge pressure (PCWP) between 8 and 12 mm Hg a guide to the rate and volume of infused fluid can be obtained while sequential measurements of plasma protein osmotic pressure and haematocrit enable the type of infused fluid to be more precisely selected. It must be remembered that high levels of PEEP may overestimate the PCWP and central venous pressure measurements. Relative or absolute fluid overload should be managed by diuretic therapy, although more recently it has been suggested that ultrafiltration is a more efficient method of treating pulmonary oedema.

Prophylactic management

(a) Steroids The use of high-dose corticosteroid therapy in the prevention and management of ARDS remains controversial. A recent comprehensive review of the literature (Nicholson, 1983), however, suggests that their early use is indicated and Table 4 lists possible actions in ARDS. The most convincing evidence of their beneficial effect is the prevention of complement activation and neutrophil sequestration in the lung when given early in endotoxin-induced ARDS in animals. Until prospective clinical trials in humans prove to the contrary, high-dose corticosteroids (30 mg/kg 6 hourly for 48 hours) are indicated if started early in the disease process.

(b) Antibiotics The role of infection in the aetiology and prognosis of ARDS cannot be overemphasized. It is estimated that 85 per cent of patients with established ARDS have an infective focus, either intra- or extrapulmonary. Strict aseptic suctioning techniques must be used and the sterility of ventilators ensured. Intensive efforts must be made to identify the micro-organism and appropriate antibiotics started. The changing bacterial pattern in patients on ventilators can be followed by taking daily specimens of tracheobronchial secretions. When no organism can be iso-

Table 4 Action of steroids in ARDS

Stabilization of cellular and lysomal membranes
Inhibition of platelet aggregation
Inhibition of neutrophil response to activated complement
Improvement of reticuloendothelial system function
Inhibition of cell arachidonic acid release
Increase in cardiac output
Increase in plasma 2–3 DPG
Lowering of total peripheral resistance
Mild cardiac inotropic action

lated, the decision to start a prophylactic broad-spectrum antibiotic regimen must be determined by the clinical state of the patient.

(c) Parenteral nutrition Patients with ARDS invariably suffer nutritional depletion which, if uncorrected, leads to muscle weakness, particularly of the respiratory muscles, and lessened cellular mediated immunity predisposing to infection. Hyperalimentation or parenteral feeding must, therefore, be started early in the management of patients.

Outcome

The mortality of ARDS has changed little during the last ten years and, in spite of therapeutic innovations, is more than 50 per cent, rising to more than 80 per cent when accompanied by renal failure. Although improvement in lung function can occur for up to six months approximately 40 per cent of survivors of ARDS have abnormal pulmonary function on follow-up. Reduced vital capacity and ventilatory restriction are the most common defects but, in general, the quality of life of the survivors justifies their demanding and expensive care.

References

Ashbaugh, D. G., Bigelow, D. B., Petty, T. L. and Levine, B. E. (1967). Acute respiratory distress in adults. *Lancet* **ii**, 319–321.

Bone, R. C. (1980). Treatment of severe hypoxemia due to the adult respiratory distress syndrome. *Arch. intern. Med.* **139**, 347–350.

Brigham, K. L. and Meyrick, B. (1986). Endotoxin and lung injury. *Am. Rev. Resp. Dis.* **133**, 913–927.

Gaitononi, L., Agostoni, A., Presenti, A. *et al.* (1980). Treatment of acute respiratory failure with low-frequency positive-pressure ventilation and extracorporeal removal of CO_2. *Lancet* **ii**, 292–294.

Hammerschidt, D. E., Weaver, L. J., Hudson, L. D., Craddock, P. R. and Jacob, H. S. (1980). Association of complement activation and elevated plasma C5a with adult respiratory distress syndrome. Pathophysiological relevance and possible prognostic value. *Lancet* **i**, 947–949.

Lee, F. and Massard, D. (1979). The lung and oxygen toxicity. *Arch. intern. Med.* **139**, 347–350.

Nicholson, D. P. (1983). Corticosteroids in the treatment of septic shock and the adult respiratory distress syndrome. *Med. Clin. N. Am.* **67**, 717–723.

Pontoppidan, H., Wilson, R. S., Rie, M. A. and Schneider, R. C. (1977). Respiratory intensive care. *Anesthesiology* **17**, 96–116.

Sibbald, W. J., Anderson, R. L. and Holliday, R. L. (1979). Pathogenesis of pulmonary edema associated with the adult respiratory distress syndrome. *CMA.J.* **120**, 445–450.

Sjöstrand, U. (1980). High-frequency positive-pressure ventilation (HFPPV): A review. *Crit. Care Med.* **8**, 345–364.

Staub, N. C. (1980). The pathogenesis of pulmonary edema. *Prog. cardiovasc. Dis.* **XXIII**, 53–80.

RESPIRATORY FAILURE AND THE MANAGEMENT OF SEVERE RESPIRATORY DISABILITY

J. B. L. HOWELL

While deteriorating lung function may cause increasing disability through limitation of exercise capacity, breathlessness, cough, sputum, etc. the ultimate danger to the survival of the patient is disturbance of gas exchange – 'respiratory failure'.

The functional capacity of the lungs is such that considerable reduction is possible before gas exchange is impaired. Increased hindrance to breathing is overcome by increased ventilatory drive, V/Q mismatching may be compensated by regulation of local vascular and airway resistance, and small reductions from normal in P_{O_2} have little effect on arterial O_2 saturation. However, a stage may be reached when no further compensation is possible and significant deviations from normality occur. This stage is termed 'respiratory failure', and once reached even a small further deterioration will cause rapid worsening of arterial blood gases. Operationally, respiratory failure is usually defined as being present when the P_{O_2} is less than 8 kPa and the P_{CO_2} is greater than 6.5 kPa.

Types of respiratory failure

Although blood gas abnormalities occur in combination, a disturbance of oxygenation can occur separately from failure of CO_2 elimination. The term 'oxygenation failure' is sometimes used to describe reduction in P_{O_2} in contrast to 'ventilatory failure' which is indicated by a raised P_{CO_2}.

Oxygenation failure (type I respiratory failure)

Whereas small deviations in arterial P_{CO_2} from normal values are always of clinical significance, quite large reductions in P_{O_2} from the normal values of 12–13 kPa to about 8 kPa cause only small changes in oxygen saturation, and hence have little impact on tissue oxygenation or clinical condition. Below this level oxygen saturation falls rapidly. It would be of little value therefore to refer to small reductions in arterial P_{O_2} as respiratory (or oxygenation) failure; the term is reserved for reduction below 8 kPa (at normal barometric pressure).

As an isolated abnormality this is not uncommon occurring against a background of chronic lung disease, such as pulmonary fibrosis, bronchiectasis, or chronic obstructive lung disease. Alternatively, 'oxygenation' failure may occur with pulmonary congestion due to left ventricular failure or with pulmonary pathology leading to V/Q mismatching, e.g. pulmonary embolism, pneumonia, arteriovenous communications. With acute inflammatory episodes superimposed upon chronic bronchitis and airflow obstruction, there may be associated ventilatory failure (see below).

Ventilatory failure (type II respiratory failure)

Except when due to failure of central neurological control, even small changes in the P_{CO_2} are resisted by the powerful response of the ventilatory control apparatus (see page 15.30). Although the range of normal CO_2 responsiveness is wide, the power of this mechanism can be great: on average the respiratory muscles approximately double their power (work rate) above the resting level for every 0.13 kPa rise in P_{CO_2}.

Thus, any reduction in alveolar ventilation, as, for example, when resistance to breathing is increased in a severe asthmatic attack, will recruit increased respiratory muscle drive and will limit the elevation of P_{CO_2}. Elevation of P_{CO_2} by more than say 6.5 kPa or above implies either mechanical loading of extreme severity or impairment of CO_2 sensitivity or a combination of both.

Elevation in P_{CO_2} may also occur secondary to metabolic alkalosis, e.g. due to persistent vomiting, but here it represents a change in threshold and not impairment of responsiveness to further changes in P_{CO_2}.

Whilst the division into oxygenation and ventilatory failure is important in understanding mechanisms, of more immediate value in determining management is the division into acute and chronic respiratory failure.

Acute respiratory failure

Acute respiratory failure may occur with failure of any component of the respiratory apparatus from brain to lungs. Causes include interference with the neuromuscular apparatus (e.g. sedative drugs, central neurological lesions, poliomyelitis, polyneuropathy, polymyositis), acutely compromised mechanics of the chest (e.g. stove-in chest, bilateral pneumothorax), and severe airflow obstruction.

The commonest situation in which acute respiratory failure occurs is an acute episode of worsening airflow obstruction in a patient with chronic bronchitis and emphysema especially if respiratory failure is present or has occurred previously. Acute respiratory failure in these patients may also occur postoperatively or when sedative or narcotic drugs have been injudiciously administered.

Essentials of management in patients with chronic airflow obstruction

When confronted with such a patient two questions require an immediate answer so that urgent measures may be instituted as required: (a) does the patient require immediate oxygen therapy; and (b) can he raise his bronchial secretions?

Need for O_2 therapy

The immediate danger is tissue hypoxia. Surprisingly low levels of arterial oxygen can usually be tolerated because the associated hypercapnia leads to vasodilation and a good cardiac output ensures sufficient 'oxygen flow' to the tissues. Arterial P_{O_2} levels as low as 2.5 kPa have been recorded without evidence of gross tissue hypoxia in the form of lactic acidosis. However, cerebral function is often temporarily impaired and raised serum γ GTP and AST concentrations indicate hypoxic damage to hepatic cells. Such a patient is clearly in a perilous situation and survival is dependent upon a good cardiac output being maintained.

Because it is not always possible to judge whether circulatory failure is imminent, it is prudent to induce a modest improvement in arterial oxygenation, without seriously reducing the hypoxic ventilatory drive. This may be achieved by controlled oxygen administration (e.g. by Ventimask, or other devices, delivering about 24 per cent O_2), which initially will raise the alveolar P_{O_2} by about 2.7 kPa and the arterial P_{O_2} somewhat less depending upon V/Q relationships in the lungs. Even this degree of amelioration of hypoxaemia may reduce ventilatory drive significantly and should be monitored by serial measurements of arterial (or mixed venous) P_{CO_2} at appropriate intervals depending on the clinical situation and facilities available. If 24 per cent O_2 is well tolerated, the patient may be given a higher concentration, e.g. 28 per cent, but it must be remembered that underventilation may develop gradually over many hours.

If on the other hand, the patient is ashen, sweating, with cold extremities, and feeble pulse, hypoxia has already impaired cardiac output and the patient is in urgent need of oxygen in high concentration, and this should be administered without delaying for any further assessment – the situation is critical.

When CO_2 sensitivity is unimpaired, e.g. as in most patients with asthma, oxygen may be administered freely with the aim of raising arterial P_{O_2} above 8 kPa. It is most unlikely that sufficiently high inspired O_2 concentrations can be achieved with face masks currently in use or that it will be administered for long enough to produce oxygen toxicity, usually only a danger when oxygen is used with artificial ventilation.

While correction of dangerous hypoxaemia is the first essential, attention also needs to be given to the cause of the respiratory failure, which is increased V/Q mismatching due to increased secretions and worsening of airflow obstruction. There is a need therefore to raise secretions and to improve airways obstruction.

Removal of secretions

This may achieve dramatic improvement both in oxygenation and alveolar ventilation and must be vigorously pursued. If the patient is sufficiently alert and co-operative, he or she should be encouraged to raise secretions by coughing but should be allowed to rest and recover breath and strength after each attempt. Ideally, the efforts should be directed by experienced staff, chest physiotherapists and trained nurses usually being the most effective. A positive pressure demand ventilator, such as the Bird ventilator, may permit more effective coughing to be achieved but often patients will not tolerate the face mask or mouthpiece. If patients are not able to co-operate because of drowsiness associated with the hypercapnia, hypoxaemia, and exhaustion, they may be aroused sufficiently to co-operate for a few minutes by intravenous analeptics, e.g. nikethamide 2 ml intravenously combined with aminophylline 250 mg intravenously (useful both as a bronchodilator and possibly as a respiratory stimulant). The patient's general condition may improve rapidly and induce false optimism. The physician must recognize that objective measures of pulmonary mechanics may have changed only slightly and that continued vigilance and therapy may have to be continued intensively for 48 hours or longer in many cases. Judgement is needed, therefore, on the compromise between the need for continuing physiotherapy and the need for rest and unsedated sleep.

Bronchodilators

An immediate effect on airways narrowing can be achieved to a limited extent with nebulized bronchodilators. Objective response in these patients to β_2-agonists is often disappointing even using up to 5 mg of inhaled salbutamol or terbutaline. There may be greater benefit from ipratropium bromide (0.5 mg), and if so this can be repeated 4 hourly. Continued use of aminophylline by slow intravenous infusion (0·5 mg/kg body weight/hour) should be monitored with blood level measurements to ensure both that the therapeutic range is achieved (10–20 μg/ml) and that toxic levels above this range are avoided.

If the patient is unable to cough effectively, despite improved oxygenation and modest bronchodilatation achieved with these conservative measures, a period of artificial ventilation with intensive bronchial toilet via endotracheal intubation may be needed. While some patients may be able to maintain adequate bronchial toilet after a single bronchoscopy, the majority require a period of intubation for 48 hours or longer. Provided the patients are not grossly overventilated, and this is unlikely if a patient-triggered ventilator (e.g. Bird) is employed, difficulty in weaning off the ventilator is rarely a problem. As a general guideline, those patients who previously had a good level of activity and were not in chronic respiratory failure, fare better with IPPV, than the long-term house-bound respiratory cripple. When these essential decisions have been made, other aspects of the treatment need to be considered.

Antibiotics

Most infections will respond to amoxycillin or ampicillin 500 mg four times daily or to co-trimoxazole 2 tablets twice daily. In some individuals, previous experience or the results of sputum cultures may indicate the need for additional or alternative antibiotics (e.g. gentamicin, flucloxacillin, cefotaxime).

Diuretics

In patients with pre-existing chronic respiratory failure, sodium retention producing a degree of pulmonary oedema is common. Intravenous or oral diuretic therapy (e.g. frusemide 40–120 mg) may improve ventilatory and gas exchanging function.

Digitalis

The value of digitalis is not proven in this situation and as it may induce dangerous arrhythmias in hypoxic and acidaemic states, it is probably best avoided unless an arrhythmia, e.g. atrial fibrillation, is already present.

Corticosteroids

If the patient has been receiving long-term corticosteroid therapy, an increase in dosage may be required. Hydrocortisone 100 mg six-hourly intramuscularly or intravenously should be sufficient.

When there has beeen no previous corticosteroid therapy, its use in the hope of reducing bronchospasm will need to be considered. In most cases no harm will follow such treatment, but it is well recognized that a period of severe respiratory failure may be followed by gastrointestinal bleeding and corticosteroid therapy might be expected to increase this tendency. Therefore, if a patient is progressing satisfactorily, steroids should not be given. They should be reserved for the patient who remains very ill or in whom improvement is not maintained and for any in whom an underlying allergic disorder of the bronchi is suspected.

Respiratory stimulants

The acute use of a single injection of a respiratory stimulant has been mentioned. Controversy exists over the value of repeated injections or continuous infusion of respiratory stimulants. The argument is over the relative contributions of hypoventilation and of V/Q mismatching to the observed blood gas abnormalities. Almost certainly both operate to different degrees in different patients. Absolute hypoventilation is difficult to measure with certainty if no antecedent values are available: but an obtunded patient with slow, irregular breathing and a rapidly rising P_{CO_2} especially on oxygen therapy, presents a clear clinical indication for a trial of a respiratory stimulant. On the other hand if the patient is already fighting for breath further respiratory stimulation could be harmful by leading to the metabolic production of more CO_2 than the inefficient lungs can eliminate. Two drugs deserve consideration. Doxapram, a central respiratory stimulant in high dosage, predominantly acts on the peripheral chemoreceptors in the conventional continuous i.v. infusion dose of 0.5–3 mg/min. Overdose can lead to epileptiform seizures but the margin of safety is wider than with earlier drugs in this class. Almitrine is a potential alternative. It also acts on the peripheral chemoreceptors and may as well influence V/Q matching in the lungs. It is still an experimental drug not yet widely available in all countries.

Acute respiratory failure in other settings such as thoracic cage trauma or acute neuromuscular disease is considered elsewhere. In general when the prognosis is good but the likely period of ventilatory failure prolonged or unpredictable, artificial ventilation is used with less restraint than in patients with long-standing, severe, chronic obstructive lung disease.

Chronic respiratory failure

This may occur rarely with normal lungs and rib-cage, e.g. primary alveolar hypoventilation, Pickwickian syndrome, or following bulbar poliomyelitis; it may also occur with gross structural abnormalities of the thorax, e.g. kyphoscoliosis, post-thoracoplasty. However, the commonest cause of chronic respiratory failure is chronic airflow obstruction in the presence of impaired CO_2 responsiveness when the clinical picture is generally that of a 'blue 'bloater' (see page 15.86). It is now recognized that sleep apnoea may occur in many of these patients and sometimes play an important part in generating the clinical syndrome (see page 15.158).

Respiratory failure with chronic airflow obstruction

There is usually a long history of increasing dyspnoea on exertion associated with chronic productive cough and a tendency to repeated winter bronchitis. Oedema of the feet and ankles may occur before the breathlessness becomes extreme, unlike the patient with the 'pink and puffing' presentation. When the severity of symptoms has become evident, the situation is likely to be complex and there are many components to be assessed in planning therapy.

The clinical approach to assessment

A careful history ensures that the patient recognizes the physician's interest in the condition and that the physician appreciates not only the nature of the patient's disability, but also any anxieties about its likely progressions and probable misconceptions about its nature. The assessment will include recognition of exacerbating factors and especially the possibility that an allergic component may be present even when severe irreversible airflow obstruction exists. This is suggested whenever the symptoms associated with bronchial hyperreactivity are present, namely, prolonged morning chest tightness, attacks of nocturnal dyspnoea, or evidence of marked bronchial 'irritability', i.e. breathlessness or wheezing in response to inhaled atmospheric irritants such as cold air, smoke, fumes.

The severity of airflow obstruction should be assessed clinically and measured using simple spirometry, and any disproportion between these and the severity of the disability noted. This may lead to recognition of associated disorders such as heart failure, pulmonary embolism, asthma or bronchial neoplasm, or to psychological factors including anxiety and depression. However, it is important to recognize that the correlation between severity of disability and indices of airflow obstruction, e.g. FEV_1 and PEFR, is often poor, and one cannot conclude that discrepancies necessarily indicate psychological abnormalities or co-existing disease. For example, gross overinflation of the lungs places the respiratory muscles at varying degrees of mechanical disadvantage as may be seen when in-drawing of the lower thoracic cage occurs during inspiration. This would not be reflected in FEV_1 measurements but is likely to generate dyspnoea.

Respiratory failure can only be reliably recognized by blood gas measurements: though cyanosis certainly indicates hypoxaemia even this is deceptive in the presence of anaemia or polycythaemia, and the clinical features of CO_2 retention are known to be unreliable.

Evidence of the major complications of chronic respiratory failure – cor pulmonale (see page 13.350) mental impairment, and secondary polycythaemia – will be noted on clinical and routine laboratory testing.

When a full assessment has defined the nature of the disability, the severity of the disorder, the patient's psychological reaction to its consequences, and a proper rapport between patients and doctor has been established, the management of the patient can be planned rationally.

Management of severe disability associated with chronic respiratory failure

1. Ensure that the severity of the airflow obstruction is minimized by the avoidance of inhaled irritants, especially smoking, and careful attention to the therapeutic approaches detailed on page 15.168, namely:

   (a) Treatment of infections
   (b) Aerosol bronchodilator therapy
   (c) A therapeutic trial of 'anti-allergic' therapy
   (d) Mucolytic therapy (page 15.84).

Table 1 Guidelines for long-term oxygen therapy (minimum 15 hours a day and 2l/min)

---

1 Absolute indications: patients with stable chronic obstructive airways disease having
   $FEV_1 < 1.5$ litres
   $FVC < 2.0$ litres
   $PaO_2 < 7.3$ kPa
   $PaCO_2 > 6.0$ kPa
2 Other patients with chronic obstructive lung disease having similar spirometry and hypoxaemia but *no* hypercapnia may benefit
3 Palliative use: patients with severe hypoxaemia but usually without hypercapnia due to advanced pulmonary fibrosis and other lung infiltrations
4 Other conditions. Great care should be exercised in giving long-term oxygen therapy to hypoxic, hypercapnic patients in whom abnormalities of ventilatory control are a primary cause (e.g. obesity, kyphoscoliosis, muscle diseases)

---

2. Improve gas exchange by:

(a) Diuretics to diminish pulmonary oedema if present.

(b) Oxygen therapy. There are three main ways in which oxygen can be used in the chronic situation. First, a supply at home enables the patient to use oxygen for short periods before and to aid recovery from a bout of exercise. Second, oxygen supplementation may be provided during exercise from a portable supply, either a small lightweight cylinder of compressed gas or, less commonly available, liquid oxygen. Many patients who would benefit are not prepared to accept the embarrassment of wearing a mask or nasal cannulae in public and it is important therefore to assess its effectiveness and acceptability before and at intervals after embarking on this costly approach. The third way in which oxygen may be used is 'continuously' which in practice should be for more than 15 hours each day. In multicentre trials in the United Kingdom and the United States improved survival and well-being have been demonstrated in chronically hypoxic patients, especially those who have had an episode of cor pulmonale, though the criteria for selection differed in the two major trials. Against these benefits has to be set the inconvenience of being tied to the end of an oxygen delivery system for long hours on end. In the present state of knowledge, consideration for long-term oxygen therapy should probably be restricted to patients with severe chronic airflow obstruction ($FEV_1 < 1.5$ l) marked hypoxaemia ($PaO_2 < 7.3$ kPa or 55 mmHg), pulmonary hypertension, and polycythaemia (see Table 1). Such long-term oxygen therapy requires ten or more of the conventional oxygen cylinders each week. The development of oxygen concentrators for use in the home has improved the feasibility and reduced the running costs of this approach, but further studies are needed to evaluate more fully the benefit in terms of quality of life as well as increased survival.

(c) Venesection. This is a controversial topic but there is general agreement that with marked elevation of the haematocrit, venesection to bring the haematocrit below 55 per cent should be undertaken especially in patients with intractable high elevation of the jugular pressure.

(d) Intermittent positive pressure breathing (IPPB). There is no evidence that periods of assisted breathing with a patient-demand positive pressure ventilator is of long-term benefit for patients with respiratory failure associated with airflow obstruction but it may provide comfort during an acute exacerbation and a more effective route of administration of bronchodilator drugs. There is however a risk that some patients may become dependent upon this assistance and diminish their mobility and independence even more. But for patients with neurological and musculoskeletal disorders with relatively normal lungs there is benefit to be gained. In some of these cases, a cuirasse-type ventilator, used at night, may be of even greater benefit.

(e) Carbonic anhydrase inhibitors e.g. acetazolamide (Diamox) 250 mg twice daily, dichlorphenamide (Daranide) 50 mg twice daily. The role of these drugs is limited but they are worth a therapeutic trial especially when a patient remains oedematous with a high P_{CO_2} and a high bicarbonate concentration. A short course may induce a diuresis and may improve sleep apnoea, but long-term administration is not required.

(f) Surgery. Removal of isolated, large emphysematous cysts ('disappearing lung syndrome') may result in a dramatic improvement in gas exchange which is often maintained. Removal or plication of emphysematous bullae in generalized emphysema rarely induces benefit of lasting duration. The immediate postoperative risks, e.g. bronchopleural fistula, are high. Permanent tracheotomy (fenestration) has been performed in some patients. It provides access to the trachea for removal of secretions and this may be helpful in some patients who are particularly troubled in this way. Though it reduces anatomical dead space it does not, in practice, appear to improve alveolar ventilation. Unless the tracheotomy is performed in such a way that the patient normally breathes through the oronasopharynx, complications with lack of humidification and with speaking may outweigh any benefit. This procedure is very rarely performed and few have much experience of it.

3. The place of physiotherapy and 'breathing exercises' is controversial. Proponents claim to be able to train patients to modify their breathing patterns and the use of different respiratory muscles to aid ventilation, but objective evidence that this can be maintained during exercise is scant. Nevertheless, many patients claim symptomatic benefit and should not be denied this approach because our understanding of its mechanism is unclear (see also page 15.88).

4. Prevention and management of acute exacerbations. Advice about minimizing chances of infection may be needed, but by the time the disease is advanced patients are often well aware of this. Prophylactic influenza vaccination is often of value and should be given a trial. A detailed knowledge by the doctor of the illness and its effects over a prolonged period of time will enable a rational decision to be made whether to resuscitate vigorously in an episode of acute respiratory failure, or whether to accept that the end of the road has been reached.

5. Psychiatric reactions. Anxiety and depression are common in chronic disability, and may require treatment in their own right. But in addition they may be associated with increased ventilatory drives and hyperventilation, either episodically at rest, or on exertion, in either case leading to distressing dyspnoea. The ability to increase alveolar ventilation is limited by the mechanical state of the chest and the usual features of hypocapnia may therefore be less prominent, but should be suspected whenever symptoms are disproportionately severe and accompanied by lightheadedness or dizziness and paraesthesia. A short period of voluntary overbreathing may reproduce these symptoms and confirm their mechanism. Hyperventilation is most likely to occur in those with meticulous, perfectionist, obsessional personalities, and may be associated with factors such as bereavement, resentment, and illness. Fear about the nature of an illness is common in association with chronic disability and the severe and often bizarre symptoms of hyperventilation lead to even greater apprehension and a vicious circle is established. A convincing explanation of the nature of hyperventilation is not only reassuring but may reduce or even remove the tendency for it to occur. It is necessary to treat depression effectively, tricyclic antidepressants usually being sufficient. Low doses of benzodiazepines, e.g. diazepam 2–4 mg as required up to thrice daily, are sometimes helpful if ventilatory drives seem excessive; however, care is needed with both these forms of treatment not to worsen ventilatory failure, especially at night.

6. Explanation and reassurance. While it is by no means universal, many patients appreciate an explanation, in reassuring terms, of their disorder. A simple account of expiratory flow limitation may assure them that it is not lack of determination that prevents them from undertaking greater physical exercise. Many have feelings of guilt and self-reproach and often attempt the impossible through their mistaken concepts of their disorder. Some have great fear of 'emphysema', a term that carries connotations as bad as, if not worse than, cancer for some. The term is best avoided unless some reassuring explanations can accompany it.

Although it may be difficult to achieve, patients should be encouraged to remain as physically fit as possible, taking regular exercise within their capabilities, avoiding being overweight, taking alcohol to excess and, of course, smoking.

It is a great reassurance to many to be able to start treatment of incipient or established bronchial infections on their own initiative, from a stock of antibiotics at home without reference to a doctor.

Finally, being able to talk to someone about their problems, anxieties, the effect of the disorder upon their domestic and social life, and sometimes their prognosis is a comfort to many patients and is a most important role of the doctor. Alone, patients may be unable to adjust to their limited, often precarious existence but the knowledge that their doctor is understanding and interested may delay the time when enjoyment of living is lost.

The social isolation of the respiratory cripple can be made more tolerable by home visits from health visitors and day care facilities in chest units. Easy parking facilities, financial allowances, and wheel chairs should be considered to assist the mobility of the respiratory cripple.

References

Anthonisen, N. R. (1982). Hypoxaemia and oxygen therapy. *Am. Rev. Resp. Dis.* **126**, 729–733.

Hodgkin, J. E. (ed.) (1979). *Chronic obstructive pulmonary diseases: current concepts in diagnosis and comprehensive care.* American College of Chest Physicians, Park Ridge Illinois.

Nocturnal Oxygen Therapy Trial Group. (1980). Continuous or nocturnal oxygen therapy in hypoxemic chronic obstructive lung disease. *Ann. intern. Med.* **93**, 391–398.

Petty, I. L. (ed.) (1982). *Intensive and rehabilitative care: a practical approach to the management of acute and chronic respiratory failure* 3rd edn. Lea and Febiger, Philadelphia.

Report of the Medical Research Council Working Party. (1981). Long-term domiciliary oxygen therapy in chronic hypoxic, cor pulmonale, complicating chronic bronchitis and emphysema. *Lancet* **i**. 681–685.

Warren, P. M., Flenley, D. C., Millar, J. S. and Avery, A. (1980). Respiratory failure revisited: acute exacerbations of chronic bronchitis between 1961–68 and 1970–76. *Lancet* **i**, 467–471.

GEOGRAPHIC VARIATION IN RESPIRATORY DISEASE

Africa

B. TEKLU

Introduction

Respiratory diseases are one of the commonest and most serious causes of morbidity and mortality globally. This is especially true of Africa. Tuberculosis which is associated with low socio-economic status is widespread throughout Africa while lung cancer, a scourge of the affluent and industrialized societies, is very rare. The three commonest respiratory diseases in Africa are acute respiratory infection (ARI), tuberculosis, and bronchial asthma. Because of limited diagnostic facilities several respiratory diseases remain undiagnosed in many African countries.

Acute respiratory infection

The World Health Organization (WHO) reported in 1972 that ARI was one of the commonest causes of morbidity and mortality worldwide. The average annual mortality for 88 countries in the world was 55/100 000 population but for the nine African countries reported, the mortality rate was twice this. Deaths occurred mostly in infants, small children, and the elderly. ARI accounted for 6.3 per cent of all causes of death, and 75 per cent of these respiratory deaths were due to pneumonia.

Pneumonia

About two-thirds of all pneumonias are caused by *Streptococcus pneumoniae*. Other less commonly isolated organisms from pneumonias include *Haemophilus influenzae*, *Staphylococcus pyogenes* and *Klebsiella pneumoniae*. Although infrequently diagnosed because of lack of facilities mycoplasma pneumonia occurs in young adults, especially among military recruits. It is usually mistaken for pneumococcal pneumonia and fails to respond to penicillin. However, when tetracycline or erythromycin is administered the response is fairly prompt. Three per cent of all pneumonias are due to Klebsiella, and in contrast to the developed countries, it occurs in previously healthy young male Africans but with the typical radiographic picture.

Pneumonia occur most frequently in the dry season in Nigeria and just before and at the beginning of the rainy season (May–June) in Ethiopia.

In six Black African countries, pneumonias were the commonest respiratory disease requiring medical admission. Admittedly, admission criteria vary a great deal from one country to the other. This in turn influences mortality rates which vary between 1.3 per cent in South Africa and 17 per cent in Kenya and Ethiopia. The majority of those who die have underlying complicating diseases like diabetes and cirrhosis. The overall mortality rate of pneumonias before the advent of antibiotics was 19 per cent in Kenya in contrast to 46 per cent in the USA.

Clinically, pneumonia presents with the classical symptoms of fever, rigors, chest pain, cough, and rusty sputum. However, several patients present with only one or two of these symptoms. In addition, some may present with non-respiratory symptoms like diarrhoea, muscle tenderness, and enlarged liver and jaundice. Pneumonias must be differentiated from amoebic liver abscess and typhoid fever.

The simplest and cheapest way to confirm the diagnosis is by Gram-stain of sputum. The presence of many polymorphonuclear leucocytes and predominant Gram-positive diplococci is typical of pneumococcal pneumonia. Radiographs are very useful when available. Cultures of lung aspirate, pleural fluid, and blood could be diagnostic when positive.

Only those seriously ill, with complications or a serious underlying disease, need be admitted to hospital. The rest can be treated as outpatients with one injection of long-acting penicillin to be followed by oral penicillin or ampicillin for 5 to 7 days. This eliminates the cost of hospitalization and avoids patients returning for daily injections.

A survey of pneumonia from Zambia in 1984 found that only about 10 per cent of patients failed to respond to penicillin and that an aminoglycoside was often effective in these cases. Most of the deaths occurred in this group even though overall mortality was commendably low at 4.2 per cent. Age over 65 years, absence of fever or leucocytosis, hypotension, and multiple lobe involvement were unfavourable features.

Complications include lung abscess, empyema, sterile pleural effusion, pericarditis, endocarditis, and meningitis. The commonest complication encountered in Nigeria was jaundice which was attributed to both hepatocellular damage and haemolysis from glucose-6-phosphate dehydrogenase (G6PD) deficiency.

Lung abscess

This is a not uncommon condition in the African and the clinical presentations are no different from those seen in developed countries, except that factors like alcoholism and poor dental hygiene that predispose to aspiration and lung abscess are infrequently encountered.

In South Africa the organisms most frequently isolated were the aerobic oropharyngeal flora and very infrequently anaerobes. In Tunisia, the organisms isolated were in most cases staphylococci, streptococci, pneumococci, klebsiella, and enterobacter. Ninety-four per cent of the cases have single cavities in upper lobes or in the apical segments of the lower lobes. The majority do well on high-dose intravenous penicillin over 4–6 weeks but about one-fifth of patients require either surgical drainage, lobectomy or pneumonectomy.

Bronchiectasis

This is one of the common suppurative diseases of the lungs in the tropics. In most reported series from Africa, bronchiectasis is the fourth leading respiratory disease requiring hospitalization. The aetiology and clinical presentations are very similar to those in the West. Most cases give a childhood history of pneumonia, measles or whooping cough. Cystic fibrosis is, however, not reported from Africa.

Croup (epiglotitis and laryngotracheitis)

This condition in its most serious form is caused by *Haemophilus influenzae* type B and occurs most frequently in children and young adults. The clinical picture starts as an upper respiratory infection and patients gradually develop stridor, brassy cough, and breathlessness. In some cases it may even progress to asphyxiation and sudden death.

Chronic respiratory infection

Pulmonary tuberculosis

This is the most serious chronic respiratory disease facing Africa today. The aetiology is *Mycobacterium tuberculosis* in almost all cases, although there are few cases of *M. bovis* and atypical mycobacteria isolated. *Mycobacterium africanum* involves the lungs and is indigenous to Central and West Africa. Its biological behaviour falls between *M. tuberculosis* and *M. bovis*.

Although reporting is incomplete and inaccurate the WHO figures for 1977 show a prevalence of as high as 475/100 000 population in Botswana with an annual mortality rate of up to 70/100 000 population both in Botswana and Djibouti. It is estimated that two-thirds of smear-positive tuberculosis cases remain undetected. The defaulter rate is in the range 50 to 70 per cent. Lack of staff and money compounded by inefficient organization and management mean that tuberculosis control will remain virtually unattainable over the coming several decades in most countries of Africa.

Case finding and treatment is the cornerstone of tuberculosis control anywhere. With all the prevailing constraints touched upon, tuberculosis control should have a very pragmatic approach in Africa:

1. In education of the public, mass media is essential, and community participation in the control of tuberculosis mandatory.

2. Case finding and treatment should concentrate on smear-positive cases which are the major sources of further infection.

3. Competent microscopists should be trained and simple microscopes like that of MacArthur be readily available in remote areas. Even if there is no electricity, daylight can be used.

4. The standard treatment regimen for the poorer African countries should be isoniazid and thiacetazone for 12–18 months provided the side-effects of the latter are not high and serious. This regimen should be supplemented with streptomycin for the initial two months. For the few resistant and relapse cases rifampicin, pyrazinamide, and ethambutol should be available. Fully supervised twice weekly therapy with streptomycin and isoniazid after a 2-month intensive therapy with streptomycin, isoniazid, and thiacetazone should be encouraged.

5. Most patients should be treated on an ambulatory basis except those critically ill or with serious complicating underlying disease. All tuberculosis control should be integrated into the general health programme, and hospitals must accept tuberculosis patients. Tuberculosis sanatoria are expensive and unnecessary, their creation should discouraged, and those already in existence should be closed gradually.

6. BCG vaccination should be continued as part of the Extended Programme of Immunization (EPI) in spite of the evidence from South India that BCG gave no protection against tuberculosis. Even though this was a well-controlled prospective study, the negative results could be explained on the basis of high infection rate, non-specific sensitization, and other epidemiological factors in the community. Furthermore, the study did not include children.

7. Unnecessary activities like mass miniature radiography (MMR) or active case-finding using village elders should be discouraged. These are very expensive exercises with too low a yield.

8. Last but not least, governments should have a definite commitment to the control of tuberculosis.

Fungal infection (see page 5.447)

Deep fungal infections occur in Africa. *Histoplasma capsulatum* has been identified in South Africa, Zaire, Zimbabwe, and Gabon. But African histoplasmosis which is caused by *Histoplasma duboisii* has been reported mostly from Nigeria and also from other West and Central African countries, Senegal, Ghana, Cameroon, Ivory Coast, and Zaire. It affects mostly skin, bones, lymph-nodes, and other viscera, and only occasionally the lungs. The disease occurs in those who visit bat infested caves. Cryptococcosis is a ubiquitous infection especially in the compromised host, in leukaemias, lymphomas, and Hodgkin's disease. Actinomycosis is infrequently encountered but aspergillosis is seen in asthmatics and chronic bronchitics.

Bronchial asthma

This disease has gained importance recently in many parts of Africa. Unfortunately there are no reliable population-based statistics on the prevalence of this disease. However, from hospital data, bronchial asthma is one of the commonest respiratory problems in Africa outstripped only by pneumonias and tuberculosis. Bronchial asthma constitutes 1–3 per cent of all medical admissions. In Nairobi, Kenya, 2.6 per cent of emergency room visits were for asthma. In Addis Ababa asthma comprised 3 per cent of all medical admissions and 1 per cent of emergency room visits. Sixty per cent of the cases occur in the last one-third of the rainy season and immediately following the rains.

Bronchial asthma occurs mostly in adults but other atopic disease is extremely rare. There is a family history of asthma in 20 per cent of cases. In many parts of Africa it is more common in the higher socio-economic groups while the opposite is true in other parts of Africa. That intestinal infestation with round worms plays a role in the pathogenesis of asthma is unsubstantiated. Serum IgE levels are often lower in asthmatics than in controls. It is possible that the increased IgE levels in the controls secondary to heavy intestinal helminthiasis may act as a non-specific blocking immunoglobulin giving protection against asthma. The prick skin tests show that the commonest allergy is to house dust mites. With regard to management, cost becomes a critical factor and selective β_2-adrenergic drugs in any form, steroid aerosols, and the chromones are too expensive. Therefore, one has to be content with simple and cheap drugs like ephedrine, theophylline, and prednisolone.

Other respiratory diseases in Africa

Lung cancer

This neoplasm is being reported increasingly in the African continent. The more affluent the society, the higher the incidence of lung cancer. Again hospital experience reveals that there is a small but definite increase in lung cancer cases over recent years in Black African countries which has become a source of concern lately. This increase may partly be attributed to the improvement in diagnostic facilities and increasing awareness of the disease amongst physicians. The cases reported from large general hospitals (teaching hospitals) do not exceed 5 per cent. This is true of Ethiopia, Uganda, Kenya, Tanzania, and Zambia while the corresponding figure for Tunisia was six-fold higher. But as cigarette smoking is increasing in epidemic proportions in Africa its full impact will be felt several years hence. As serious antismoking campaigns are launched in the West and smoking is on the decline, at least in some countries, cigarette manufacturers are now concentrating their efforts on the Third World. Cigarette advertizing is unscrupulous and virtually uncontrolled in Africa and as a result it is paying the advertizer a dividend. It is sad to discover that the same brand of cigarette sold to Africa has a much higher content of tar and nicotine than that sold in Europe or North America, thus making cigarette consumption in Africa potentially more lethal.

Chronic bronchitis and emphysema

This is not such a major problem as in the developed countries. Again with increasing smoking it will become a major health problem in Africa as already evident in the more affluent African countries.

Parasitic diseases

The lung is affected in a variety of ways by various intestinal and extra-intestinal parasites. Details of these diseases are given elsewhere in this book.

Of the Protozoan diseases, amoebiasis is seen in which liver abscess can rupture into the diaphragm and result in pleural effusion.

The migration of larvae of ascaris, hookworm, and strongyloides through the lungs produces respiratory symptoms of cough, copious amounts of sputum with generalized malaise, and itching. There is a high eosinophilia and with the chest radiograph showing diffuse mottling or fluffy infiltrates; this is an example of Loeffler's syndrome.

The lodgement of eggs of *Schistosomiasis mansoni* and *Haema-*

tobium in the pulmonary arterioles and capillaries causes pulmonary hypertension and fibrosis. The end-stage is chronic cor pulmonale. This clinical entity is most common in Egypt.

Hydatid disease is endemic throughout Africa but more common in North and South Africa. The patient presents with cough, sputum production, and haemoptysis without constitutional symptoms. In several cases it is an incidental radiographic finding.

Paragonimiasis Typically this is a disease of the Far East but several cases occur in West Africa especially the Cameroon where raw or poorly cooked crab and crayfish are consumed. Classically the patient develops cough, sputum production, haemoptysis, and constitutional symptoms. The chest radiograph may show an infiltrate in the lungs that may later progress to fibrosis and calcifications. The diagnosis is confirmed by identifying the typical egg in the sputum.

Occupational lung diseases

In general, Africa is not an industrialized continent and hence occupational lung diseases are not a major health concern in most African countries. Silicosis and other pneumoconioses, however, are encountered amongst workers in the large goldmines of South Africa and Zimbabwe, and in the copper mines of Zambia. Some small-scale local industries can also be a hazard to the lungs. For example, in Nigeria, stone cutting to prepare domestic grindstones has been associated with extensive silicosis. Grindstones are widely used in both East and West Africa to grind grains and vegetables at home. The stones are cut from open sandstone quarries and the grinding surfaces are carefully chiselled with primitive tools to make them smooth. The whole process is dusty; and worse still, the cutting and finishing of these grindstones takes place in deep pits that are poorly ventilated. These professional stone cutters present with classical signs and symptoms of silicosis with the typical radiographic findings.

Byssinosis is fairly common in Egypt and Tanzania. Occupational asthma due to wood, vegetable, and grain dusts may be common although documentation is lacking. Small-scale industries that are ubiquitous in many African countries have little legislation about waste disposal and protection of employees and the environment.

Chronic cor pulmonale

The commonest cause of this entity is almost exclusively tuberculosis in the less developed countries of Africa while in the more affluent countries, chronic bronchitis is the major cause.

Miscellaneous diseases affecting the lung

Sarcoidosis is very rare in Africans, in contrast to Black Americans in the United States, providing evidence that environment is one important factor in the causation of the disease. Only a few mild cases have been reported from Ethiopia, an average of 1–2 per year in a large teaching hospital. Fewer cases were reported from West Africa (Ghana, Nigeria and Senegal).

Microlithiasis A case report has appeared in the literature from Tunisia. Legionnaire's disease, histiocytosis X, and some other exotic diseases of the lung have not yet been identified in the African continent.

The practice of respiratory medicine in Africa is both gratifying and challenging to keen young physicians. It is gratifying because the majority of the respiratory diseases are treatable and potentially curable, challenging because there are several yet unidentified diseases, a fertile ground for clinical investigation using simple clinical tools and basic laboratory facilities.

References

Bulla, A. (1981). Worldwide review of reported tuberculosis morbidity and mortality. *Bull. Intern. Union Against Tuberculosis* **56**, 111–118.
—— and Hitze, K. L. (1978). Acute respiratory infections – a review. *Bull. Wld Hlth Org.* **56**, 481–498.
Clark, B. M. and Greenwood, B. M. (1968). Pulmonary lesions in African Histoplasmosis. *J. Trop. Med. Hyg.* **71**, 4–10.
Cockshott, W. P. and Lucas, A. O. (1964). *Histoplasmosis duboissi. Q. J. Med.* **33**, 223–238.
Fox, W. (1964). Realistic chemotherapeutic policies for tuberculosis in the developing countries. *Br. Med. J.* **1**, 135–142.
Teklu, B. (1980). Patterns of respiratory diseases in a general hospital in Addis Ababa. *Ethiop. Med. J.* **18**, 135–143.
—— (1983). Primary pulmonary neoplasms in Ethiopians. *E. Afr. Med. J.* **60**, 374–379.
Warrell, D. A. (1975). Respiratory tract infections in the tropics. *Practitioner* **215**, 740–746.
Warrell, D. A., Fawcett, I. W., Harrison, B. D. W., Aganah, A. J., Iby, J. O., Pope, H. M. and Maberley, D. J. (1975). Bronchial asthma in the Nigerian Savanna. *Q. J. Med.* **44**, 325–347.
——, Harrison, B. D. W., Fawcett, I. W., Mohammed, Y., Mohammed, W. S., Pope, H. M. and Watkins, B. J. (1975). Silicosis among grindstone cutters in the north of Nigeria. *Thorax* **30**, 389–398.

Latin America

M. RIGATTO

The Pan American Health Organization acknowledges four regions in Latin America: Temperate South America, Tropical South America, Continental Middle America, and Caribbean Middle America. For descriptive purposes, Latin America is taken as America south of the United States.

Brazil with its vast size (41 per cent of Latin America) and large population (33 per cent of Latin America) has part of its territory in Temperate South America (Sao Paulo and south of it: one-third of Brazilian population) and part in Tropical South America. It has the largest population both in Temperate and Tropical South America. In the statistical data available and used in this chapter Brazil is included as a whole, in Tropical South America.

A strong general characteristic of Latin America is its young population. In 1980, 15.4 per cent of the population were below 5 years of age, in contrast to 7.2 per cent in North America. On the other hand, only 4.1 per cent were above 65 years of age, in contrast to 11.0 per cent in North America. Sixty-one per cent of the Latin American population are below 25 years of age.

A consequence of this age distribution is the predominant importance of respiratory diseases affecting infants, children, and adolescents. On this basis, acute respiratory infections stand out as the most important respiratory diseases in Latin America. They exceed all others both in incidence and lethality.

Acute respiratory tract infections

Among acute respiratory infections influenza and pneumonia are the most important though upper respiratory infections usually of viral aetiology are the most common. In developed countries most serious lower respiratory tract infections in children appear also to be viral, but in developing countries, as in most of Latin America, bacterial pneumonias, mainly due to *Streptococcus pneumoniae*, play an important role in child mortality. Pneumonias due to respiratory syncytial virus may also cause death in infants.

Influenza and pneumonia

In 22 countries of Latin America, at all ages, these conditions led, in 1979, to an age-adjusted death rate of 55.5/100 000 population, approximately six times the rate for either tuberculosis (9.7 in 29 countries) or lung cancer (8.9 in 29 countries). They ranked as the leading cause of death in Continental Middle America, as the second in Tropical South America, as the fifth in the Caribbean, and as the sixth in Temperate South America. This order runs parallel with the percentage of the population constituted by children under 5 years of age in each of these regions – 16.7, 15.8, 12.6, and 10.4 per cent, respectively, and with the illiteracy rate – 21.3, 21.7, 12.7, and 6.6 per cent, respectively. *Per capita* gross domestic product and the caloric intake *per capita* are highest in Temperate South America where mortality and the other indices are lowest.

Childhood mortality

In children whooping cough and the pulmonary complications of measles add significantly to the burden of respiratory infections in Latin America. Overall considering data from 11 countries, respiratory infections, excluding tuberculosis, accounted for 22.5 per cent of all deaths of children under the age of 1 year and for 20.4 per cent of deaths of children 1 to 4 years of age. They stand as the most important cause of infant mortality (excluding perinatal deaths) and as the second most important cause of child mortality. In 1980, in 17 countries, for children under 1 year, the death rate per 100 000 population for influenza and pneumonia was 874. In that same year, in North America, that rate was 46. Again for children under 1 year of age, the age-specific death rate per 100 000 population for whooping cough was 46.2 in Latin America and 1.4 in North America; for measles, during the seventies, it was 64.2 in Latin America and 0.2 in North America. For children 1 to 4 years of age, the rates are smaller but still impressive: for influenza and pneumonia, in the same 17 countries, 158; for whooping cough, 11.5; for measles, 44.8.

Tuberculosis

Once the leading killer, tuberculosis does not figure any more among the ten most important causes of death in Latin America. From 1969 to 1979 mortality rates for tuberculosis per 100 000 population dropped from 18.3 to 9.4 in Temperate South America, from 21.7 to 13.4 in Tropical South America, from 18.1 to 12.1 in Continental Middle America, and from 7.0 to 4.4 in the Caribbean. In this same decade, the drop in North America was from 2.7 to 1.3.

Chemotherapy, improved health conditions, and BCG vaccination are responsible for the progress achieved. Nevertheless, it is pertinent to consider that the incidence of tuberculosis has dropped, on average, no more than 5 per cent per year, far from the 14 per cent achieved by some developed countries. The use of BCG, while still only partial, is growing. From 1977 to 1980 the number of countries adopting it rose from 18 to 26. On average, 50 per cent of the children under 1 year were vaccinated in these countries.

The drop in mortality has made morbidity data a better index for tuberculosis. Countries with a sufficient level of diagnosis and notification, like Argentina, Brazil, Chile, Colombia, Costa Rica, Cuba, Uruguay, and Venezuela have already adopted it. In Latin America, as a whole, in 1980, 216 000 new cases were registered. It is believed that underregistration is of the order of 30 per cent, so that 280 000 new cases would be a better estimate. The countries with the highest rates of reported cases per 100 000 population are Bolivia (224), Haiti (165), Peru (137), French Guyana (101), Paraguay (96) and Colombia (82). The rate for South America is 69, for Middle America 29, and for North America 12.

Smoking related respiratory diseases

Lung cancer, bronchitis, and emphysema, the smoking-related diseases, have not yet reached in Latin America the importance they already have in developed countries. Nevertheless, while all other important respiratory diseases are being significantly reduced, they show a definite tendency to increase in both the morbidity and mortality statistical tables. The large and effective antismoking campaigns in action in developed countries have pushed the tobacco industry's interests towards the developing countries. With a market free of restrictions on propaganda, sales to minors, and high tar/high nicotine brands, the tobacco industry is planting in Latin America its most macabre harvest. Around 50 per cent of the adult population smoke. The prevalence among women is smaller but is rapidly growing.

Lung cancer

Lung cancer is the tumour with the fastest growing incidence in Latin America. In males, in most countries, it shares first place with cancer of the stomach, having a definite lead in Argentina and Cuba. Among females it is already very common in Cuba. Data from nine countries of Latin America, around 1979, yielded an age-adjusted death rate per 100 000 population of 11.4 for males and 3.2 for females. In Argentina it is 25.3 for males and 3.3 for females. In Cuba it is 20.6 for males and 7.1 for females. At this same time, in North America, the rate for males was 30.5 and for females 8.9.

Bronchitis and emphysema

In spite of being more notorious for morbidity than for mortality, these are among the ten leading causes of death in Middle America and Tropical South America. They are rapidly becoming one of the most frequent diagnoses in the intensive care units of the continent. For prolonged absenteeism from work they lead too, thus becoming among the most costly diseases of the community. Their age-adjusted death rate per 100 000 population in Latin America, in 1978, was 13.9; in Temperate South America 16.6; in Tropical South America 12.1; in Continental Middle America 18.1; and in the Caribbean 5.7.

Other disorders of the airways

Bronchial asthma

In Latin America asthma has as variable a prevalence as it has in other parts of the world. Epidemiological studies in Barbados (1973), Cuba (1974), Puerto Rico (1976), Chile (1981), Argentina (1982), and Brazil (1984) have yielded a prevalence of asthmatic children of 1.1, 9.7, 5.4, 2.9, and 6.7 per cent, respectively. Different criteria to define the condition and its prevalence make comparisons difficult.

Mucoviscidosis

This has been detected in several parts of Latin America, almost in every place it has been searched for. Nevertheless there is a feeling that it is much less frequent than, for instance, in the United States. The high percentage of non-White races in Latin America may have a bearing on this.

Two respiratory entities which have a more peculiar connotation to Latin America are paracoccidioidomycosis and the respiratory problems of adaptation to altitude.

Paracoccidioidomycosis (page 5.447)

This infective disease, less properly called South American Blastomycosis, is caused by a fungus, the *Paracoccidioidis brasiliensis*, described by Lutz, in Brazil, in 1908. Both men and women may be infected but the progressive disease is almost exclusive to males between 20 and 60 years of age, with a preponderance in the White race. Contrary to what was previously thought, the disease is not contracted through the skin or mucosae but by inhalation. A primary nodule in the lung has been described. The disease closely mimics pulmonary tuberculosis. The lungs are the most common site of infection but the skin and mucosae are also frequently affected. The disease is limited to Latin America but widely distributed through it. The countries with greatest incidence are Brazil, Venezuela, and Colombia, in South America, and Guatemala, in Middle America. Infected individuals may be detected through a skin reaction to paracoccidioidin. For treatment, sulphonamides are suppressive and amphotericin B is curative. Ketoconazole is showing promising results.

Respiratory disorders of high altitudes (page 6.101)

South America, along the Andes, has a large human population living at high altitude. The adaptation of humans to altitude is complex and if inadequate may end in respiratory failure.

Acute mountain sickness (page 6.101)

This is a condition affecting lowlanders 6 to 90 hours after rapid ascent to altitude. The symptomatology includes lethargy, insomnia, headache, nausea, vomiting, and dyspnoea. In more severe cases, cyanosis, crepitations in the lungs, papilloedema and other signs of cerebral oedema may be found. The cause is unknown. Fluid retention may play a role and preventive treatment with diuretics is apparently useful.

High altitude pulmonary oedema may be seen in high altitude dwellers 9 to 36 hours after return from a few weeks at sea level. This is not left ventricular failure. Pressure in the pulmonary artery may be three to four times greater than usual but the wedge pressure is normal. Right ventricular failure may ensue. The condition benefits from oxygen administration and recedes with return of the patient to sea level. In fatal cases pulmonary congestion, intravascular thromboses, and perivascular haemorrhages around dilated arterioles and capillaries are usually found. Hyaline membranes in the alveolar spaces may also be present. The important muscularization of the pulmonary arterioles and the blunting of the hypoxic respiratory drive, which occurs in natives or longliving dwellers at altitude, have been considered as bases for the phenomenon. A very marked vasoconstriction, induced by the environmental hypoxia, would lead to extreme pulmonary hypertension, in some cases with pressure levels above systemic, and transarterial leakage.

Chronic mountain sickness (page 6.105)

This was first described by Monge, in publications from 1925 to 1929. In the local idiom it is called soroche. It is a progressive loss of acclimatization, for unknown reasons, in natives born and living at altitude throughout their lives or in highlanders born at sea level but for many years living at altitude and fully acclimatized to it. The condition is more common in young males. It is characterized by headache, dizziness, easy fatigability, paraesthesia, somnolence, and decreasing mental activity. In advanced cases right ventricular failure may be present. Cyanosis and finger clubbing are outstanding. Laboratory examinations show a very low oxygen arterial saturation (< 70 per cent) and polycythaemia, with haematocrits and haemoglobin as high as 80 per cent and 25 g/dl, respectively. The heart is enlarged but radiographically the lung fields are clear. The ECG shows right ventricular strain. Apparently in Monge's disease there is a magnification of the changes peculiar to the normal adaptation to altitude: polycythaemia, increased pulmonary artery pressure, ventilatory hyposensitivity to hypoxia. The patient improves with oxygen administration and recovers, in days or weeks, on descent to lower altitudes. Normalization of pulmonary artery pressure takes longer.

Public health and respiratory disease in Latin America

The respiratory health of Latin America is improving. The acute respiratory infections are considered the first priority by local health authorities and by the Pan American Health Organization. Vaccination, prophylactic use of antibiotics for bacterial complications of viral infections in high risk populations, and the steady development of health resources have been the major tools at work. Raising standards of living, improving nutrition and housing conditions, avoiding overcrowding particularly in cold weather, are important but more difficult goals to achieve.

In 1980, approximately 50 per cent of children of 30 countries under 1 year of age received a first dose of triple (DPT) vaccine and 30 per cent the third dose. One-third of them, in 20 countries, were vaccinated against measles.

These measures, despite the fact that they are incompletely applied, led to encouraging results. The age-adjusted death rate for influenza and pneumonia per 100 000 population in children under 1 year of age, in 17 countries, dropped from 1410 in 1970, to 874 in 1979, and for whooping cough, from 123 to 46. These achievements were decisive contributions to the 60 per cent reduction in infant mortality registered in Latin America from 1950 to 1980 (119 deaths per 1000 living births, in 1950, against 44 per 1000 in 1980), and for the even more impressive decline in mortality for children 1 to 4 years of age (from 14.8 per 1000 in 1950, to 4.4 per 1000 in 1980 – a 70 per cent drop).

Tuberculosis has deserved priority, for decades, from public health authorities. The progress obtained has been substantial. In the perspective of the Pan American Health Organization, in spite of the expected large increase in population, the number of new cases diagnosed per year is likely to drop from 280 000 in 1980 to about 100 000 in 1990.

The battle against smoking is a different one. The economic interests involved in the smoking issue make governmental authorities poor allies in this kind of war. Nevertheless, national anti-smoking campaigns promoted by community forces, and led by medical associations, are underway in most countries. The national leaders of these campaigns have joined forces and, since January 1984, with the support of the International Union Against Cancer (UICC), Latin America has become the first continent to recruit all its countries on to a Coordinating Committee dedicated to controlling the tobacco epidemic. Up to now the creation of a public awareness that 'smoking is harmful to health' has been the main achievement. Several laws, particularly at municipal and provincial level, have been enacted restricting propaganda and prohibiting smoking in public places like schools, hospitals, and magazine stores. In Brazil, a steady decline in the number of cigarettes sold per year has been observed: from 143 billion cigarettes in 1980 to 129 billion in 1983. In October 1984 the Pan American Health Organization officially joined the antismoking campaign in Latin America. With this sort of collaborative endeavour some hope exists that the inevitable epidemic of smoking-related diseases may yet be contained.

References

Londero, A. T. (1972). The lung in paracoccidioidomycosis. In *Paracoccidioidomycosis*. Proceedings of the First Pan American Symposium, pp. 109–117. Pan American Health Organization, Washington, DC.

Pan American Health Organization (1982). *Health conditions in the Americas 1977–1980*. Scientific Publication no. 427. Washington, DC.

Porter, R. and Knight, J. (1971). *High altitude physiology*. CIBA Foundation Symposium. Churchill Livingstone, Edinburgh.

Monge, C. (1929). *Les erythrémies de l'altitude*. Masson, Paris.

Southeast Asia

S. BOVORNKITTI

Southeast Asia comprises Brunei, Burma, Indonesia, Kampuchea, Laos, Malaysia, the Philippines, Singapore, Thailand, and Vietnam. Besides their geographical proximity and their predominantly tropical climate, the countries of this region share several similarities. For example, most are developing countries with rural communities accounting for about 80 per cent of the total population; such people earn their living from agriculture or forestry, although this generalization does not apply to Singapore, which has developed rapidly during the past two decades to become more industrialized than the others. Nonetheless, a population profile of all these nations would reveal a highly diversified people, according to their respective racial, cultural, educational, and economic backgrounds.

With this as a backdrop, it is obvious that some notable infectious diseases (namely, melioidosis, amoebiasis, filariasis, malaria, paragonimiasis, gnathostomiasis, strongyloidiasis, leptospirosis, and tuberculosis), which are more prevalent in Southeast Asia than in other geographical zones of the world, would be related to the following environmental characteristics:

1. Tropical climate. This together with the underdeveloped

nature of the affected areas provides an ideal environment for the causative organisms, specific vectors, and intermediate hosts of certain infectious diseases.

2. Cultural habits. These inadvertently favour exposure of the local inhabitants to diseases and preserve carriers.

3. Economic and educational status. Lack of knowledge about diseases and lack of money to eliminate the causes or to treat the sick people in some of the countries further enhance the persistence of infection.

The geographical and cultural factors, likewise, produce some variation in the types of disease prevalent among the different countries of the region. On the other hand, certain disorders that are prevalent in the West are virtually absent or rarely seen in Southeast Asia. Included in this category are coccidioidomycosis, blastomycosis, nontuberculous mycobacteriosis, sarcoidosis, and a number of interstitial lung diseases.

Parasitic infections of the lung

Pleuro-pulmonary amoebiasis (page 5.466)
Hepatic amoebiasis occurs as a serious complication of amoebic dysentery. One of the natural courses of the amoebic liver abscess is to rupture into the right hemithorax producing empyema thoracis or hepato-bronchial fistula.

Diagnosis of pleuro-pulmonary amoebiasis is established by the characteristic reddish brown, the so-called anchovy sauce-like aspirate, either from the liver or the pleural cavity, or expectorate from the lung, all of which fluids are bacteria-free but often contain amoeba trophozoites. Serology, scanning, and sonography techniques have now greatly simplified diagnosis; a negative serology test provides strong evidence against the diagnosis.

For treatment, metronidazole is currently the drug of choice. Drainage of the pleural cavity must be done in every case.

Tropical eosinophilia
This is an occult filarial infection occurring as a result of an alteration in host immunity to the parasite and is manifested by persistent hypereosinophilia and pulmonary symptoms resembling an asthmatic attack. Lymph-nodes, liver, and spleen may be enlarged.

Chest radiographic findings may vary from those that look normal to those with ground-glass and miliary appearance or small areas of consolidation. IgE levels are high and ESR is raised. Microfilaria are not found in the blood but their remnants (Meyer–Kouwenaar bodies) may be revealed in the lungs, liver, lymph-nodes or spleen, and the filarial complement fixation test is positive.

Treatment with diethylcarbamazine relieves symptoms and results in a decrease in the blood eosinophil count and the titre of the serology test.

In Southeast Asia filariasis is caused by infections with *Wuchereria bancrofti*, *Brugia malayi*, and *B. timori*. Transmission of infection is established by mosquitoes of Culex, Anopheles and Mansonia species which act as vector and intermediate host.

The high incidence of tropical eosinophilia among Indians both in their own country and overseas is noteworthy and may suggest a genetic predisposition in certain racial groups.

Malaria (page 5.474)
This still poses a major public health problem in most Southeast Asian countries. The disease is generally limited to rural communities in or near forested areas, mountains, and foothills, especially in newly opened land settlements or semiforested areas.

Respiratory signs and symptoms, which occur in 3–10 per cent of patients with acute falciparum malaria present a clinical spectrum that varies from mild upper respiratory tract complaints to fatal pulmonary oedema. In most cases, pulmonary oedema becomes manifest during hospitalization and is unresponsive to vigorous therapy. Patients do not have overt evidence of conges-

tive heart failure, fluid retention or peripheral circulatory collapse before the onset of the pulmonary episode. Microscopic findings include severe congestion of pulmonary capillaries, thickened alveolar septa, diffuse pulmonary oedema, focal hyaline-membrane formation, and scattered areas of intra-alveolar haemorrhage.

Treatment for severe cases of falciparum malaria with pulmonary complication requires intensive medical care together with prompt intravenous institution of quinine hydrochloride (600 mg in 300 ml normal saline), repeated 8 hourly for 7 days. Oral route administration (650 mg t.d.s.) is reserved for recuperating or milder cases. Oral tetracycline (250 mg q.d.s. for 7 days) is supplemented when the critical period is over.

Paragonimiasis (page 5.586)
The lung flukes *Paragonimus westermani*, *P. heterotremus*, and *P. skjabini* are endemic in much of Southeast Asia with cases reported in the lower central part of Thailand, the Philippines, and southern Vietnam.

Infection is acquired by eating raw or uncooked crayfish or land crabs infected with the larval stage of the worms.

Many persons infected with Paragonimus are symptom-free; others have symptoms of chronic bronchitis or bronchiectasis. Chronic cough, which is worse in the morning and productive of tenacious brown or rusty sputum, is the most common presentation. Haemoptysis is irregular and seldom severe. Most patients remain in good health despite a long history of the disease. Physical findings are non-specific and often normal. There may be eosinophilia in the sputum or blood. Chest radiographs are normal at some stage in approximately one-fifth of the patients. The most common findings are patchy infiltrates and radiolucencies in the mid-lung fields. Pleural thickening and effusion may be seen.

The diagnosis is based on the patients' geographic origin and relative well-being as well as whether the chronic cough has persisted for a very long period. Ova can be detected on unstained sputum smear. Serological tests such as countercurrent immunoelectrophoresis have proved useful.

Bithionol (a dose of 30–50 mg/kg orally on alternative days for a total of 10–15 doses) or praziquantel (a dose of 25 mg/kg orally thrice a day) are the treatments of choice.

Human gnathostomiasis (page 5.558)
This is a disease caused by the larva or immature stage of *Gnathostoma spinigerum*, a nematode parasite found in feline and canine stomachs. Humans acquire the infection by eating the uncooked flesh of second intermediate hosts (i.e. fish, frogs, snakes, lizards, chickens, ducks, rats, and mongooses), and sometimes by applying the flesh as a poultice.

The clinical manifestations are caused by the wandering of the worm through almost any tissue except bone, giving the characteristic intermittent migratory swellings in the skin and less commonly in internal organs such as the lungs. The parasite has been seen expectorated from patients with eosinophilic pneumonitis, or following symptoms indicating irritation of the upper respiratory tract. Eosinophilic pleural effusion and hydropneumothorax have occasionally been encountered.

Diagnosis is suggested by clinical characteristics, and geographical and dietary history. The presence of blood eosinophilia is supportive and the identification of the worm is confirmative. An immunoenzyme test for IgG antibody against the antigen from an extract of the third-stage larva showing a titre of 1:1600 is indicative, while a titre of 1:400 is only suggestive.

Treatment is curative by surgical removal of the parasite; but in practice only supportive, symptomatic, and anti-inflammatory treatments are normally carried out. Metronidazole at a dose of 400 mg orally thrice daily for three weeks has been claimed to reduce the recurrence rate, the duration of swelling and the eosinophil count in the blood.

Strongyloidiasis

In heavy infections by *Strongyloides stercoralis*, wheezing, coughing, breathlessness, and sometimes haemoptysis may occur during the stage of larval migration through the lungs, and such infections are usually associated with gastrointestinal symptoms and blood eosinophilia. Larvae have been identified in sputum or bronchial aspirate from heavily infected patients. A severe and sometimes fatal form of infection has occurred in immunosuppressed patients who die because of massive alveolar haemorrhage.

Thiabendazole and mebendazole are both effective against adult worms, although neither kills migrating larvae. Therefore, all patients should receive further courses of treatment two and four weeks after the first one.

Bacterial infections

Melioidosis (page 5.245)

Melioidosis is an infectious disease caused by a Gram-negative bacillus, *Pseudomonas pseudomallei*, which is found as a saprophyte widespread in the soil of the tropical areas of Southeast Asia such as Northeastern Thailand and the Malay Peninsula. Bacterial growth requires reasonably high temperatures (range 18–42 °C; best at 37 °C), high humidity, and frequent rainfall to allow stagnant pools and muddy water-courses to accumulate. During the dry season, the organisms live in the relatively moist clay layers of the soil; in cleared areas, the top soil inhibits the growth of the organisms during dry periods. In the rainy season, the organisms rise to the surface with the watertable. It is at this time that infection occurs most frequently through the contamination of cuts and sores with *Ps. pseudomallei*. Transmission of infection by the respiratory route occurs as the organisms on the soil surface become airborne during periods of strong wind. Venereal transmission has been documented, but direct transmission from person to person by other routes has never been reported.

Subclinical disease is quite common among people who live in the endemic areas of Southeast Asia. The frequency of serologically positive asymptomatic individuals varies from 6 to 29 per cent among people native to the region. Reactivation of latent melioidosis occurs during periods of altered body defense mechanisms following burns, diabetic ketoacidosis, steroid therapy or acute infectious diseases leading to the highly fatal septicaemic type of disease. The more usual clinical forms are a relatively mild pneumonia and chronic pulmonary cavitation mimicking pulmonary tuberculosis.

The diagnosis is established by culturing *Ps. pseudomallei* from the sputum or bronchial aspirate and/or positive serological tests.

Specific treatment for melioidosis includes administration of effective antimicrobial drugs, i.e. co-trimoxazole, tetracycline, kanamycin, chloramphenicol, and novobiocin, singly or in combination. Surgical treatment is mandatory for the removal of localized lesions in some deep organs.

Leptospirosis (page 5.327)

Pulmonary involvement (mostly haemorrhage) occurs frequently in leptospirosis. It is manifested by a dry cough, occasionally with blood-stained sputum. There may be crepitations on physical examination. A variety of patterns shown by chest radiographs includes small patchy lesions, confluent infiltration or even consolidation. The lesions are prevalent in the periphery of the lung.

Treatment with penicillin (streptomycin, tetracycline, and erythromycin as alternatives) should be given within four to seven days of the onset of the disease.

Pulmonary tuberculosis

This remains the leading respiratory disease in Southeast Asian countries. Despite the considerable advances achieved in recent years in the management and control of tuberculosis, the incidence has declined only slowly during the past 15 years. Persistence of infection and disease have mainly been attributed to poor resources, drug resistance, and default from treatment. The developing countries are handicapped by a shortage of staff and other resources in the medical and public health services. Ideally sputum-positive cases should be treated as early as possible and with a highly effective regimen to cut short the spread of infection to non-infected persons. A high prevalence of initial drug resistance becomes an obstacle to the implementation of the two-drug combination regimens; triple-drug regimens elevate the cost of treatment and the defaulter rate. Eighty per cent of the population in the region are agricultural workers and their earnings are seasonal. This financial problem together with the nature of their occupation and the difficulty of completing the course of treatment causes a high rate of default.

All the aforementioned factors ultimately lead to ineffective eradication of infectivity and prevention of relapses; hence the inability to eliminate the disease from the countries in the region.

References

Bovornkitti, S. and Tandhanand, S. (1959). A case of spontaneous pneumothorax complicating gnathostomiasis. *Dis. Chest* **35**, 328.
—— (1981). Sarcoidosis in Asia. In *Sarcoidosis* (ed. Japan Medical Research Foundation), p. 339. University of Tokyo Press, Tokyo.
——, Jaroonvesma, N., Klinvimol, T. and Dhepchatri, A. (1976). Intrathoracic complications of amoebiasis. *Siriraj Hosp. Gaz.* **28**, 1229.
Kangsadal, P. and Bovornkitti, S. (1960). A case of gnathostomiasis with spontaneous hydropneumothorax. *J. trop. Med. Hyg.* **63**, 67.
Maranetra, N. and Bovornkitti, S. (1983). Respiratory disorders in Southeast Asia: viewpoint from Thailand. *Med. Prog.* (*special issue*), 117.
Marks, S. M., Holland, S. and Gelfand, M. (1977). Malarial lung: report of a case from Africa successfully treated with intermittent positive pressure ventilation. *Am. J. trop. Med. Hyg.* **26**, 179.
Sitprija, V. (1983). Leptospirosis. In *Oxford Textbook of Medicine* Vol. 1, 1st edn (eds D. J. Weatherall, J. G. G. Ledingham, and D. A. Warrell), p. 5.297. Oxford University Press, Oxford.
Strauss, J. M., Groves, M. G., Mariappan, M. and Ellison, D. W. (1969). Melioidosis in Malaysia. II. Distribution of *Pseudomonas pseudomallei* in soil and surface water. *Am. J. trop. Med. Hyg.* **18**, 698.
Viranuvatti, V., Bovornkitti, S. and Prijyanonda, B. (1966). Early diagnosis of intrathoracic involvement of amebiasis by intrahepatic instillation of radio-opaque material. *Am. J. Proctol.* **17**, 507.

SECTION 16
RHEUMATOLOGY AND CONNECTIVE TISSUE DISORDERS

IMMUNOPATHOLOGY OF RHEUMATOID ARTHRITIS

G. S. PANAYI AND H. M. CHAPEL

Despite its name, rheumatoid arthritis is a systemic disease with extra-articular manifestations present in most if not all patients. For this reason it is more logical to call it *rheumatoid disease*. The immunopathological description of rheumatoid disease must therefore attempt to explain its extra-articular as well as its articular features. The evidence for disordered immune function is convincing and includes serological evidence (hypergammaglobulinaemia, the presence of rheumatoid factors), cellular evidence (splenomegaly, lymphadenopathy, accumulation of lymphocytes, and macrophages in the inflamed synovial membrane), and its association with HLA-DR antigens. However, since the cause of rheumatoid disease (RD) is still unknown, it is not clear what triggers these abnormal immunopathological events. Naturally where there is ignorance speculation is rife. From experimental models in animals two main hypotheses have been proposed which may not necessarily be mutually exclusive. The first proposes that RD is caused by infectious agents such as bacteria, mycoplasma or viruses. This has led to several studies to implicate various organisms in the pathogenesis of human RD; there is some evidence that Epstein–Barr virus, proteus mirabilis, and more recently parvovirus may be involved in a proportion of patients. The second proposes that the disease is the expression of disordered immunity leading to an autoimmune attack on the body's own constituents. The current favourite is autoimmunity to immunoglobulin G, which would explain the production of rheumatoid factors. Autoimmune features may be triggered by infection by a variety of organisms, thus making the search for a single aetiological agent unproductive. The most striking feature of human and mouse studies is that the development of chronic persistent arthritis in animals is exquisitely dependent on genetic factors. Thus mycoplasma arthritis can be induced easily in one strain of mice while another is totally resistant. Hence the genetic basis of RD may be the proper starting point at which to look at causative factors.

Genetic factors

Classical genetic studies of the distribution of RD in families in mono- and dizygotic twins showed that there was a small but definite contribution of genetic factors to the disease. In recent years our understanding of these genetic factors has undergone a revolutionary change since the discovery of an association between RD and alloantigens of the major histocompatibility complex. Family studies have shown that the susceptibility gene is not linked to HLA; thus this is a true association. The human genes for the major histocompatibility complex (MHC) are present on the short arm of the sixth chromosome (Fig. 1). Three major classes of gene products are associated with the MHC; the human leucocyte antigens (HLA) (page 4.15) represent classes I and II. The association between HLA and RD involves the class II antigens.

Investigations have shown that 70 per cent of patients with rheumatoid arthritis possess HLA-DR4 and calculations indicate that an individual with this HLA antigen is six to twelve times more likely to develop the disease than one who is negative. It is worth noting that within the MHC (Fig. 1) there are genes which control the expression of some of the complement components (C2, C4, and factor B) and since complement is so intimately involved in the genesis of immune-mediated inflammation, such genes may also be involved in the development of rheumatoid disease, though there is no evidence to support this at present.

What does the association of HLA-DR4 with rheumatoid imply about the immunopathogenesis of the disease? It is possible that this HLA antigen is a marker for genes which regulate either the development of autoimmunity to such self-components as IgG or an abnormal host response to an environmental agent. It is worth noting that although some 25 per cent of Caucasians are HLA-DR4 positive only some 5 per cent at the most of such populations have rheumatoid, so that clearly other factors are involved in causing the disease. Furthermore, 30–40 per cent of patients with RA are negative for DR4, depending on the population studied. In some ethnic groups, an association with DR1 and RA has been shown. This has raised the question as to whether or not there is a very precise epitope in class II antigens which permit susceptibility to RA. Recent studies with monoclonal antibodies to class II MHC antigens suggest that there is. The mechanism by which this epitope determines disease susceptibility remains a matter of speculation; does it act as a receptor for the aetiological agent, is it responsible for poor T4 cell-macrophage interaction and failure to remove this agent or does its alteration by an invading organism lead to altered self-antigen and autoimmunity?

Immunological features

Serological

Immunological abnormalities in the serum of patients consist of an hypergammaglobulinaemia, especially of immunoglobulins G and M, and the presence of rheumatoid factors. Rheumatoid factors are autoantibodies of IgG, IgA, and IgM classes directed against immunoglobulin G as the autoantigen. Only M rheumatoid factors can be measured routinely by agglutination reactions (sensitized sheep red blood cell test). There are also increased immunoglobulin and rheumatoid factor concentrations in synovial fluid, much of which is synthesized locally in the joint. There are a variety of other autoantibodies found in RD including antinuclear factors, anticollagen, and antikeratin antibodies but these are not thought to be important immunopathogenically.

What is the evidence that rheumatoid factors are of importance in the immunopathogenesis of rheumatoid? First, high titres of rheumatoid factors, both G and M, correlate closely with the presence of very severe erosive joint disease, nodules, vasculitis (including vasculitic-mediated complications such as neuropathy), and interstitial pulmonary fibrosis. Secondly, rheumatoid factors, and especially of the immunoglobulin G class, can associate to form immune complexes which have been detected in the synovial membrane, synovial fluid, serum, skin, nodules, and around blood vessels. These

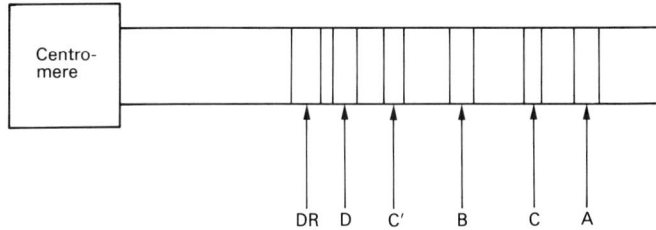

Fig. 1 The structure of the human major histocompatibility complex which is present on the short arm of chromosome 6. The HLA alleles are designated as A, B, C, D, and DR. The region containing alleles coding for the complement components C2, C4, and factor B is designated by <u>C</u>′.

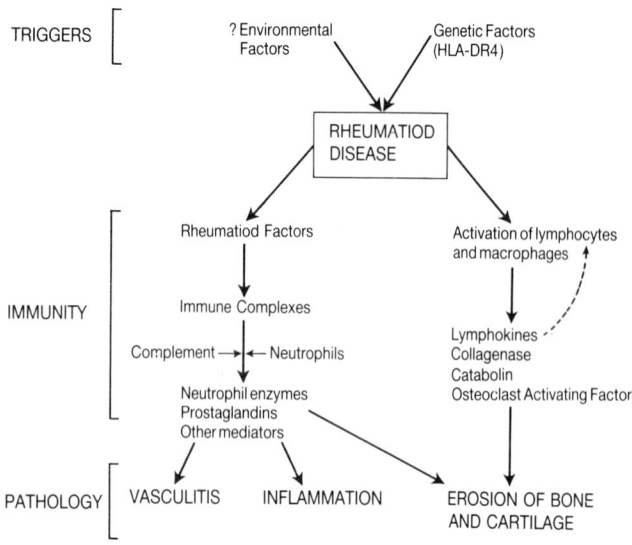

TRIGGERS

? Environmental Factors

Genetic Factors (HLA-DR4)

RHEUMATIOD DISEASE

IMMUNITY

Rheumatiod Factors

Activation of lymphocytes and macrophages

Immune Complexes

Complement → ← Neutrophils

Lymphokines
Collagenase
Catabolin
Osteoclast Activating Factor

Neutrophil enzymes
Prostaglandins
Other mediators

PATHOLOGY

VASCULITIS   INFLAMMATION   EROSION OF BONE AND CARTILAGE

Fig. 2 A schematic representation of the major events thought to be involved in the immunopathogenesis of rheumatoid arthritis.

immune complexes are thought to mediate pathogenicity because they can be phagocytosed by neutrophils, monocytes, and macrophages with the release of a variety of inflammatory mediators, including prostaglandins, and hydrolytic, proteolytic, and other degradative enzymes. In addition, immune complexes containing rheumatoid factors can activate the complement cascade which generates inflammatory and chemotactic substances, such as C3A and C5A, with further accumulation of inflammatory cells. The evidence for complement activation is convincing and can usually be shown directly in inflammatory fluids from the joint and pleura by the presence of C3 breakdown products. It is unusual, however, to show direct complement consumption in the serum, though this may occur in the severe systemic vasculitis of RD. A convincing immunopathological pathway can be constructed involving the production of rheumatoid factors, their self-association into immune complexes, and activation of the complement cascade leading to joint inflammation, and, because of the common link of vasculitis, to many of the extra-articular features as well (Fig. 2).

Cellular

Despite all the current interest in immunology concerning the role of helper and suppressor thymus-dependent (T) lymphocytes in the aetiopathogenesis of autoimmune disease, no convincing disturbances in the numbers or functions of circulating lymphocytes have as yet been demonstrated in RD. The distinct cellular abnormality consists of the accumulation of large numbers of plasma cells in bone marrow, thymus, lymph-nodes, spleen, and the rheumatoid factors. Indeed the inflamed rheumatoid synovium produces as much immunoglobulin, mainly as rheumatoid factors, on a weight-to-weight basis, as the spleen from an immunized animal. Thus the cellular basis for production of rheumatoid factors is well established although we are still ignorant of the factors which switch on this process.

Immunoglobulins and rheumatoid factors are products of plasma cells which are the differentiated progeny of stimulated bone marrow derived (B) lymphocytes. T lymphocytes are also activated, the evidence for which includes the finding of lymphokines in synovial fluids and their production by rheumatoid synovial explants cultured *in vitro*. Lymphokines have a variety of biological properties including the ability to activate other T cells, act as helper factors for B cell differentiation, stimulate macrophages, and to stimulate fibroblasts to produce collagen. The latter may be of importance in bringing about the eventual fibrosis seen in a 'burnt-out' synovial

membrane and perhaps in the development of interstitial pulmonary fibrosis. Activated macrophages produce prostaglandins and other inflammatory mediators, enzymes, in particular collagenase which degrades synovial and articular cartilage collagen, and osteoclast activating factor which, as its name implies, activates osteoclasts to erode bone synergistically with released prostaglandins. Macrophages may also be responsible for the production and release of catabolin, a protein which diffuses through the articular cartilage inhibiting the synthetic activity of chondrocytes and stimulating them to release enzymes capable of degrading the cartilage. This pathway is potentially a very destructive one as the chondrocytes, from within the cartilage itself, would be reinforcing those damaging events acting on the cartilage from without (Fig. 2).

Pathological features

The pathological features of rheumatoid are to be found in the synovial membrane, lymph-nodes, blood vessels involved with vasculitis, and nodules, although none of these features are pathognomic with the exception of the nodules.

In the rheumatoid synovial membrane there is a marked increase in the number of macrophages both in the synovial lining cell layer (type A cells) and in the subsynovial tissues. These macrophage-like cells have at least four functions in the immunopathology of the disease. These are: phagocytosis of immune complexes, release of degradative enzymes, release of accessory factors stimulating T lymphocytes and fibroblasts, and in antigen presentation. The lymphocytes infiltrating the synovial membrane are predominantly of the T cell population and in particular of the helper class. In functional terms therefore the synovial membrane has macrophages which can present antigen to T helper lymphocytes which in turn help B cells to differentiate into immunoglobulin producing plasma cells. The particular mechanisms which lead the inflamed synovium at the joint margin to invade bone and cartilage are not known at present.

Rheumatoid nodules begin as areas of vasculitic involvement in skin subject to excessive pressure such as the extensor surface of the forearm. Indeed the role of local factors in the expression and development of disease have received little attention. Thus, in addition to areas of local high pressure determining the development of nodules, it has long been known that disease in the dominant hand can be more severe than that in the non-dominant and development of paralysis in a limb can lead to significant improvement in pre-existing rheumatoid disease. Whether these effects are due to changes in blood flow and hence the quantity of immune complexes capable of being deposited in that area or the release of antigen(s) due to joint movement is not known. In blood vessels involved with vasculitis, immunoglobulins and complement can be demonstrated by immunofluorescence. Subsequently inflammatory cells can enter and damage the vessels. In nodules, the characteristically palisaded tissue macrophages (histiocytes) surround the central area of hyaline necrosis. Around the histiocytes are scattered lymphocytes and the occasional plasma cell. Whether nodules are 'autonomous' immunologically functioning tissue, like the rheumatoid synovium, still awaits investigation.

References

Fox, R. I., Lotz, M., Rhodes, G. and Vaughan, J. H. (1985). Epstein–Barr virus in RA. *Clin. Rheum. Dis.* **11**, 665–688.

Lee, S. H., Matsuyama, T., Logalbo, P., Silver, J. and Winchester, R. J. (1985). Ia antigens and susceptibility to RA. *Clin. Rheum. Dis.* **11**, 645–664.

White, D. G., Mortimer, P. P., Blake, D. R., Woolf, A. D., Cohen, B. J. and Bacon, P. A. (1985). Human parvovirus arthropathy. *Lancet* i 419–421.

Youinou, P., Le Goff, P., Saout, J., Courtois, B., Shipley, M. and Lydyard, P. M. (1985). Activation of T lymphocytes in blood and joints of patients with RA. *Rev. Rheum.* **52**, 473–477.

Young, C. L., Adamson, R. III, Vaughan, J. H. and Fox, R. I. (1984). Immunohistologic characterisation of synovial membrane lymphocytes in rheumatoid arthritis. *Arth. Rheum.* **27**, 32–39.

CLINICAL FEATURES OF RHEUMATOID ARTHRITIS

M. I. V. JAYSON AND D. M. GRENNAN

Introduction

Rheumatoid arthritis was the term introduced by Sir Alfred Baring Garrod in 1859 to describe a chronic inflammatory disease of peripheral joints which he distinguished from acute rheumatic fever and gout. It is now defined as a chronic or subacute, systemic inflammatory disorder principally involving the joints with a peripheral symmetrical inflammatory non-suppurative arthritis. The disease pursues a long course with exacerbations and remissions. It is likely that the disorder presently known as rheumatoid arthritis consists of several different disease entities and the splitting of rheumatoid arthritis into subgroups may occur in the future. The term 'rheumatoid disease' is often used to emphasize the systemic features and multisystem complications which occur in many patients.

The antiquity of rheumatoid arthritis is of possible aetiological as well as historic interest. There is a lack of palaeopathologic evidence on examination of skeletal remains for the existence of rheumatoid arthritis prior to the eighteenth century, although suggestive descriptions of the disease have been found in writings in Sanscrit in the second century AD and from authors in Asia Minor in first, second, and tenth centuries AD. This is in contrast to other forms of arthritis such as gout and ankylosing spondylitis which have frequently been identified. This suggests that rheumatoid arthritis has only appeared relatively recently but the evidence remains uncertain.

Prevalence and incidence

Modern population studies utilize the criteria of the American Medical Association and classify patients as having classical, definite, probable or possible disease. In Britain definite and classical disease occurs in 0.5 per cent of adult males and 1.8 per cent of females. This figure increases with age to reach a peak of 2 per cent of males and 5 per cent of females over the age of 64 years. In addition there are many patients with less severe but probable forms of rheumatoid arthritis who do not meet the diagnostic criteria for definite or classical disease. The disease frequency is constant throughout Europe and does not vary significantly with latitude. The prevalence appears less in primitive populations but this may well be due to a much shorter life-span. Studies in Africa have shown a higher prevalence in urban than in rural negroes of the same background. It is possible that diet or other factors associated with urban life may predispose to the disorder.

Established rheumatoid arthritis is commoner in females than in males, the sex ratio being between 2:1 to 3:1. The predisposition for females appears less in patients with early disease and in those in whom it starts over 60 years. The more equal sex ratio in early disease may be because the condition is nearly as common in men but is more likely to remit spontaneously, or perhaps because men with mild symptoms are more likely than their female counterparts to seek medical advice. No age group is exempt but the peak incidence occurs between 35 and 55 years in women and 40 to 60 years in men. The contraceptive pill may protect against the development of the disease. The onset is more common in winter. This might be due to lowering of the pain threshold in cold weather increasing the chances of arthritis being noticed, or to cold precipitating the onset of vasculitic phenomena.

Familial aggregation

There is an increased incidence of the disease in relatives of affected patients. This familial aggregation is most marked in severe forms of rheumatoid disease. Tissue typing studies have shown a significant association between the histocompatibility antigen DR4 and seropositive rheumatoid arthritis.

Disease onset

Rheumatoid arthritis may develop in an acute, subacute or insidious fashion. The onset is very sudden over the course of a day in between 10 and 20 per cent of patients and may be associated with systemic illness and fever. It develops insidiously in 50 to 70 per cent of patients and this pattern may be associated with a worse prognosis. Many patients describe prodromal symptoms such as aches and pains and stiffness before the definite onset of the disease. In some there are apparent precipitating factors such as joint trauma or intercurrent systemic viral infections but whether they are relevant or merely co-incidental is not established.

Articular features

Rheumatoid arthritis is typically a symmetrical peripheral polyarthritis most commonly involving the proximal interphalangeal and metacarpophalangeal joints of the hands, the wrists, metatarsophalangeal (MTP) joints, ankles, knees, and cervical spine. The shoulders, elbows, and hips are less commonly involved. Any synovial joint in the body may be affected particularly in the more severe forms of the disease. A distinction must be made between the active inflammation and synovitis of early rheumatoid arthritis and the secondary destructive changes found in later disease. Actively inflamed joints are stiff and painful particularly on movement and on examination they are tender, warm, and swollen. Similar inflammation commonly affects the synovium lining tendon sheaths in the wrists, hands, and elsewhere. Muscle wasting may appear early in the course of the disease and appears due to reflex inhibition particularly in the presence of large articular effusions as well as in the later destructive stages of the arthritis. While the disease is active the patients are usually most stiff in the early morning on wakening and may take several hours to loosen up. The patients complain of stiffening (or gelling) with inactivity during the day. As the disease progresses cartilage, bone, and ligament damage become increasingly pronounced to produce the typical deformities seen in long-standing destructive rheumatoid arthritis. Secondary osteoarthritic changes may follow in damaged joints.

The progression of radiological change in rheumatoid arthritis is:

(a) Soft tissue swelling produced by synovial hypertrophy and joint effusions.
(b) Periarticular bone osteoporosis.
(c) Loss of joint space secondary to cartilage erosion.
(d) Bone erosions and deformities.

Hands and wrists

Rheumatoid arthritis produces classical and readily recognizable changes in the hands. In early disease there may be spindling of the fingers due to synovial hypertrophy and effusions in the interphalangeal joints. Similar soft tissue swellings occur in the metacarpophalangeal joints and wrists (Fig. 1). Diffuse swelling and stiffness of the fingers together with triggering of the fingers may appear as a result of tenosynovitis in the flexor tendon sheaths.

Similar flexor-tenosynovitis at the wrist can compress the median nerve and produce the carpal tunnel syndrome. The characteristic symptoms are pain and paraesthesiae in the hand and fingers often spreading proximally even as far as the side of the neck. The symptoms are worse at night, often waking the patient, and are relieved by shaking the hand and flexing and straightening the fingers. The little finger is usually pain free but may be involved if the superficial branch of the ulnar nerve is also compressed at the wrist. Wasting of the thenar eminence and sensory loss in the median nerve distribution are present in more severe forms of the disease. Tinel's sign may be positive and nerve conduction tests will confirm the diagnosis. The symptoms of a carpal tunnel syndrome may be the presenting features of rheumatoid arthritis.

Tenosynovitis of the extensor tendons at the wrist is common. Extensor tendon rupture with 'dropped fingers' can occur at a surprisingly early stage of the arthritis.

Persisting synovitis, weakening of the joint capsule, muscle wasting, tendon ruptures, and destruction of the articular surfaces lead to characteristic rheumatoid hand deformities (Figs. 2 and 3). These include ulnar deviation at metacarpophalangeal (MCP) joints, swan neck deformity with hyperextension at the proximal interphalangeal and flexion at the distal interphalangeal joints, Boutonniere (buttonhole deformity) at the proximal interphalangeal joints, and the Z-thumb deformity.

The mechanisms producing these deformities are complex. Factors leading to ulnar deviation are:

(*a*) In the normal grip, the fingers move into ulnar deviation.

(*b*) The joint capsules of the MCP joints are weaker on the radial than the ulnar sides.

(*c*) Weakening of the radial sides of the joint capsule and the radial insertions of the interossei by inflammation.

(*d*) The volar supports of the flexor tendon sheath are weakened by inflammation allowing the tendons to bow-string ulnarwards during gripping.

(*e*) Ulnar displacement of the extensor tendons in early deviation makes them slip off the dorsal surfaces of the MCP joints to lie between them and then they exacerbate the development of ulnar deviation by acting as a bow-string.

The swan-neck deformity is probably caused by palmar subluxation of the proximal phalanges at the MCP joints with intrinsic muscle contracture and tethering of the lateral extensor slips at the proximal interphalangeal joints to produce hyperextension. At the distal interphalangeal joint the flexion deformity is produced by the pulling effect of the now overstretched profundus tendon working against weakened or ruptured terminal extensor tendons. In the Boutonniere deformity, chronic synovitis of the proximal interphalangeal joint stretches or ruptures the central dorsal slip of the extensor tendon allowing the joint to protrude between the two lateral slips of the extensor tendons.

Prolonged synovitis at the wrist can contribute to the poor grip of the rheumatoid hand. Chronic inflammation in the inferior

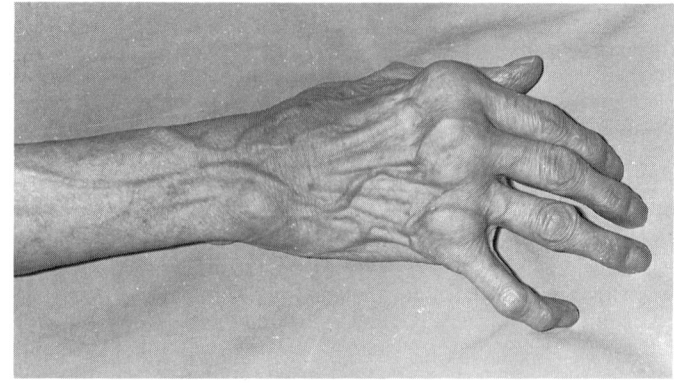

Fig. 2 Rheumatoid hand deformity with ulnar deviation at the MCP joints and muscle wasting.

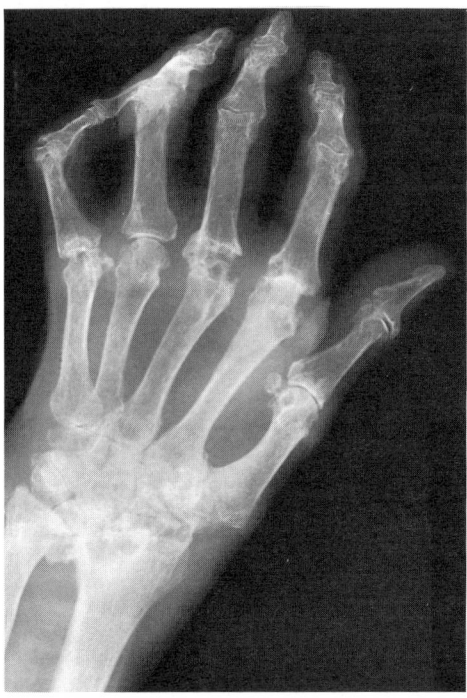

Fig. 3 Radiograph of advanced rheumatoid arthritis of the hands showing erosions and extensive destructive changes.

radio-ulnar joint may destroy the triangular disc and allow the distal end of the ulna to sublux dorsally. Abrasion by this caput ulnae together with inflammatory tenosynovitis may rupture the extensor tendons particularly to the ring and little fingers.

Feet and ankles

Involvement of the feet and ankles is common but often neglected. Radiological abnormalities occur in the MTP joints in most patients, although only half of these have clinical problems. Active synovitis in the MTP joints can produce pain and tenderness best elicited by lateral squeezing of the joints. The synovial swelling of active disease together with destruction of the ligament between the metatarsal heads may broaden the forefoot and separate the toes to produce the 'daylight' sign. The typical forefoot deformity of rheumatoid arthritis is dorsal subluxation of the proximal phalanges and the distal displacement of the fibro-fatty cushion normally on the plantar surface of the MTP joints so the patient walks on the unprotected metatarsal heads. Callosities form in the soles and are usually most obvious under the second and the third metatarsal heads where weight bearing is carried out

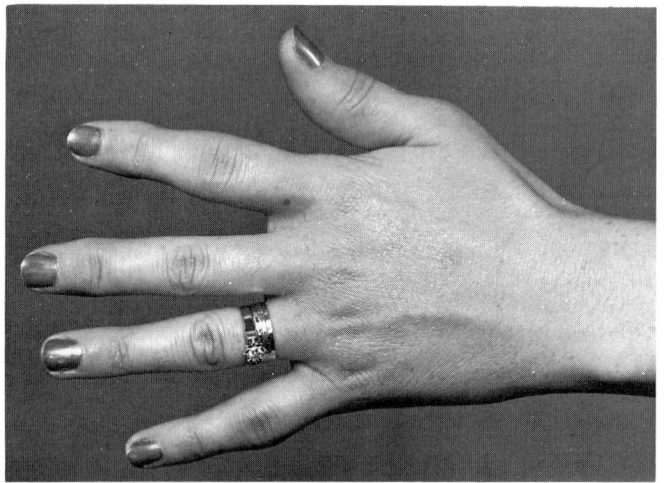

Fig. 1 Early rheumatoid arthritis of the hands.

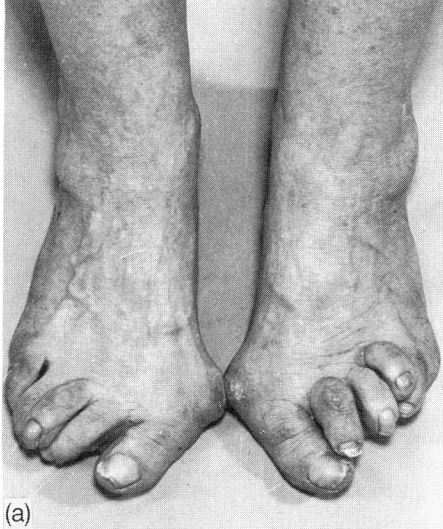

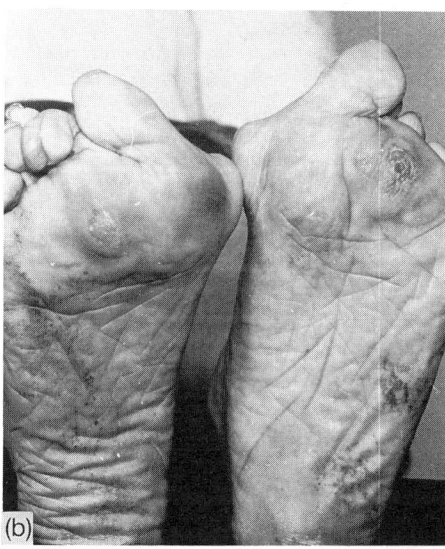

Fig. 4 (a) Dorsal view of rheumatoid feet showing hallux valgus, overriding toes, and pes plano-valgus deformities. (b) Plantar-view of rheumatoid feet showing callosities under subluxed metatarsophalangeal joints.

(Fig. 4b). Not surprisingly, patients with these deformities complain of 'walking on stones'. Callosities may also develop on the dorsal surfaces on the toes because of rubbing on the shoe uppers. A wide variety of deformities of toes may develop. Hallux valgus deformity is common in rheumatoid arthritis (Fig. 4a) but of course frequently occurs in patients who do not suffer from this disease.

Rheumatoid synovitis may develop in the subtaloid and midtarsal joints and be demonstrated by direct pressure and passive movements of the joints. Chronic arthritis in this region can lead to the pes plano-valgus deformity (Fig. 4a). Synovitis can develop in the Achilles bursa and erosions develop on the posterior surface of the calcaneum. Subcutaneous nodules can develop in the heel pads and occasionally cause discomfort on standing. Synovial hypertrophy sometimes develops in the peroneal tendon sheaths laterally and around the flexor tendon sheaths medially. The latter can compress nerves producing the tarsal tunnel syndrome which is analogous to the carpal tunnel syndrome in the upper limb.

Knees
A large synovial effusion in the knee may produce reflex inhibition of quadriceps contraction and rapidly lead to muscle wasting. The

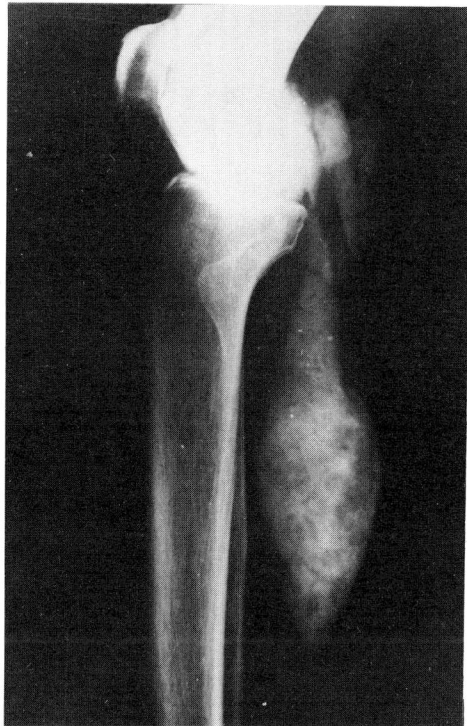

Fig. 5 Arthrogram of knee to show a popliteal (Baker's) cyst which extends into the calf.

effusion may be obvious with distension of the supra-patella pouch and the joint margins. The synovial space may communicate posteriorly with a Baker's cyst in the popliteal fossa which can extend down the calf (Fig. 5). The communication is valve-like allowing fluid to be pumped from the knee to the cyst but not easily to return. In early disease, before significant capsular fibrosis has developed, the joint may rupture posteriorly. Rheumatoid synovial fluid is extremely irritant producing pain and swelling in the calf and the symptoms are frequently misdiagnosed as due to a deep venous thrombosis. The correct diagnosis can usually be made from the history of a prior swelling of the knee which decreased at the time of the sudden onset of pain in the popliteal space and calf. The diagnosis is confirmed by an arthrogram. Treatment involves reduction of the amount of fluid in the joint by aspiration and local steroid injection together with bed rest. Occasionally acute joint rupture and deep vein thrombosis may co-exist in the same leg. Anticoagulants should only be given in rheumatoid patients for venogram proven calf vein thromboses to avoid the risk of haemorrhage into the joint space and soft tissues.

Chronic inflammation of the knee may damage the cruciate ligaments producing antero-posterior instability or medial and lateral ligament weakness with medial and lateral instability. In advanced rheumatoid damage in the knee, fixed flexion with inability to flex the knee properly and valgus or varus deformities together with instability and reduced range of further flexion make walking and other physical activities difficult and painful.

Elbows and shoulders
Inflamed olecranon bursae and rheumatoid nodules around the elbows are common but true arthritis affecting the elbows is less frequent. Severe destructive changes can occur leading to fixed flexion deformity, loss of further flexion, and instability making use of the forearm difficult. A particular problem can be that of getting the hand to the face and mouth for washing and feeding. Pain in the shoulder can be referred from the neck or be due to involvement of the acromio-clavicular joint, subacromial bursa, rotator cuff, and bicipital tendon as well as the gleno-humeral

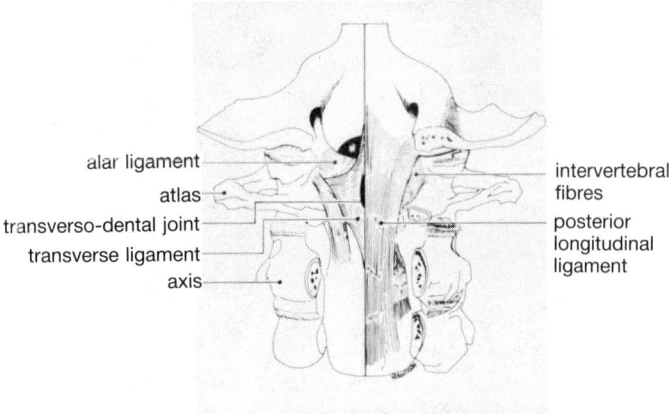

Fig. 6 Stylized sketch of ligaments of upper cervical spine. (Reproduced from Bunton *et al.*, 1978, *Br. J. Rheum.* **51**, 963, by permission of the Editor.)

joint. The shoulders must always be examined carefully as knowledge of the precise source of the symptoms will dictate management.

Cervical spine

Rheumatoid involvement of the neck is found in radiographs of up to 80 per cent of patients but fortunately is often asymptomatic. In a few patients it causes severe neurological damage or even death. The common radiological findings are osteoporosis, apophyseal joint erosions, erosion of the vertebral end plates, loss of disc space, and subluxation at the atlanto-axial and lower cervical disc levels.

Atlanto-axial subluxation occurs in around 25 per cent of rheumatoid patients seen in hospital but only about a quarter of these will have symptoms or signs of neurological damage. In the normal cervical spine the odontoid peg is kept in close apposition to the back of the anterior arch of the atlas by a network of ligaments including the posterior longitudinal ligament, the transverse ligament of the atlas which is part of the cruciate ligament, the apical ligament of the odontoid process, and the alar ligaments (Fig. 6). Destruction of this network of ligaments allows the odontoid peg to move posteriorly during cervical flexion with risk of compressing the cervical cord. On lateral X-ray of the neck in flexion the distance between the odontoid peg and posterior border of the anterior arch of the atlas increases to more than 3 mm (Fig. 7).

Less commonly lateral or vertical subluxation of the atlanto-axial joint occurs. All forms of atlanto-axial subluxation are commonest in patients with the worst peripheral joint disease. Symptoms suggesting atlanto-axial disease include high cervical pain made worse by neck movements and which may radiate to occipital, temporal or retro-orbital areas. Some patients complain of a 'clunk' on nodding their heads or develop peculiar postures of the neck.

Atlanto-axial disease is important because of the danger of compression of the spinal cord or vertebral vessels with shooting pains in the arms and legs, limb weakness, and sphincter disturbances. In severe cases complete quadriplegia or even sudden death may occur. The interpretation of weakness is difficult in the patient with widespread rheumatoid disease and the presence of increased muscle tone and reflexes in the lower limbs may be the only signs of early neurological damage. Patients are at special risk during general anaesthesia when the normal protective reflexes are lost so that *any rheumatoid patient about to have a general anaesthetic should always have the neck X-rayed in flexion and extension and the anaethetist warned if there is any instability*.

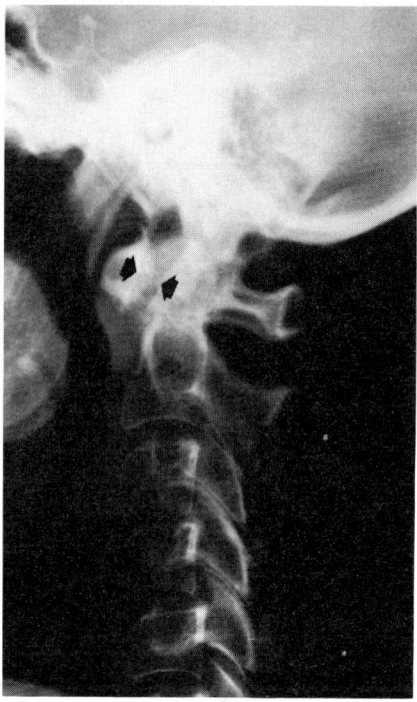

Fig. 7 Lateral X-ray of cervical spine in flexion showing anterior subluxation of atlas on axis. Arrows indicate the gap between anterior arch of the atlas and the ondontoid peg.

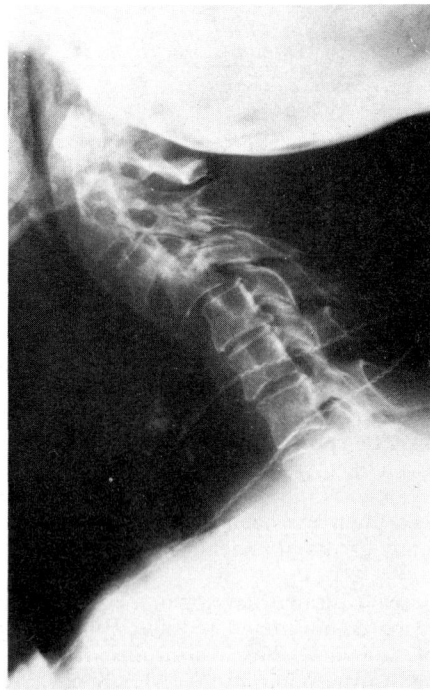

Fig. 8 Lateral X-ray of cervical spine showing gross subluxation of C2 on C3 and C3 on C4.

Subluxation of the cervical vertebrae may also appear at levels below the atlanto-axial region and be associated with neurological abnormalities (Fig. 8).

Rheumatoid cervical subluxation with severe pain or neurological involvement may be treated initially by immobilizing the neck in a cervical collar or skull traction in bed. Severe pain or neurolo-

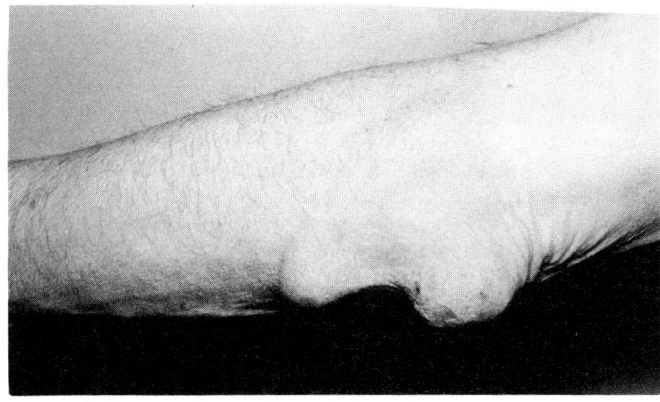

Fig. 9 Rheumatoid nodules and olecanon bursitis.

gical damage unresponsive to rest, or showing progression of the physical signs, may require surgical decompression and fixation.

Other joints

The rheumatoid process can involve all synovial joints. In contrast with the sero-negative arthritides the hips are often spared. In the lumbar spine the apophyseal joints may be affected producing back pain and this can lead to a lumbar scoliosis and changes in the intervertebral discs. Hoarseness and pain on swallowing may be due to synovitis of the crico-arytenoid joints.

Temporo-mandibular involvement produces pain on chewing.

Extra-articular features

General

There is a rough correlation between the severity of joint disease and the likelihood of extra-articular manifestations. Particularly in the elderly but also in some other patients initial features such as fever, weight loss, lassitude, and anaemia may be out of proportion to the arthritis. It is essential to distinguish systemic illness due to the rheumatoid disease process from that due to a supervening infection or intercurrent neoplasm. There is a slightly increased risk of developing a reticulosis. In some this could be related to immunosuppressive therapy.

Nodules

Together with rheumatoid hand deformities, subcutaneous nodules form the hallmark of seropositive rheumatoid disease. The nodules are discrete, firm, non-tender subcutaneous swellings, and are larger and more constant than the smaller nodules of rheumatic fever. They occur particularly in areas subjected to mechanical stress and are found in about 20 per cent of patients. The commonest site for rheumatoid nodules is the extensor aspect of the forearm and over the olecranon (Fig. 9). Repeated minor trauma through resting on the forearms is believed responsible. Over the sacrum nodules may ulcerate and become infected and can lead to severe bed sores. Rheumatoid nodules occur elsewhere such as in flexor tendons, the sclera, and within the aortic valve, myocardium, larynx, and vocal cords.

Histological examination shows a central zone of fibrinoid necrosis surrounded by a palisade of fibroblasts and chronic inflammatory cells. The exact pathogenesis of the nodule is uncertain but it is thought to be due to deposition of antigen–antibody complexes.

Vasculitis

Inflammation of blood vessels can produce the more serious systemic features of the disease and underlie many of the other extra-articular complications. All sizes of blood vessels may be involved and the vascular changes vary from a bland intimal hyperplasia to inflammatory pan-arteritis or pan-phlebitis sometimes associated with extensive vessel wall necrosis. When this latter change affects medium-sized arteries it may be histologically indistinguishable

from polyarteritis nodosa. The clinical spectrum of rheumatoid vasculitis ranges from often asymptomatic nail-fold and splinter infarcts to life-threatening disease with visceral infarction and neuropathy. Rheumatoid vasculitis may cause cutaneous ulceration and gangrene of the digits. Pulmonary hypertension has been described in association with vasculitis of the pulmonary artery.

Rheumatoid vasculitis more often develops in patients with severe destructive forms of arthritis, nodules, and other extra-articular features. It is thought to be due to immune complex deposition in the vessel wall and various studies have demonstrated circulating immune complexes, cryoglobulinaemia, and high titres of circulating IgM and IgG rheumatoid factors and of antinuclear antibodies. Systemic corticosteroid therapy or a sudden change in steroid dosage is sometimes blamed for precipitating vasculitis but this is uncertain as it is those patients with the worst forms of arthritis who are at the greatest risk of both developing vasculitis and receiving corticosteroids.

Pulmonary

Pleurisy and pleural effusion These are the commonest forms of rheumatoid pulmonary disease and often precede frank synovitis. Analysis of the pleural fluid from a rheumatoid effusion typically shows a sterile fluid with lymphocytosis, an elevated protein, low sugar content, reduced complement C3 levels, ragocytes (macrophages with IgM containing inclusions), and containing antinuclear antibodies and IgM rheumatoid factor. These abnormalities are not seen in all rheumatoid pleural effusions but may help in the differentiation from other causes. A pleural biopsy often only reveals non-specific chronic inflammatory infiltration but occasionally may demonstrate rheumatoid pathology.

Interstitial fibrosis Diffuse interstitial pulmonary fibrosis or fibrosing alveolitis may complicate rheumatoid arthritis and is identical with the less common cryptogenic form. As in the idiopathic condition there is finger clubbing, progressive dyspnoea, coarse basal crepitations, and widespread pulmonary shadowing on radiographs. The prognosis is poor with most patients dying within about five years. The results of treatment with corticosteroids have been disappointing but occasional patients respond to azathioprine or cyclophosphamide.

In contrast to the low frequency of symptomatic interstitial disease, asymptomatic interstitial involvement shown by lung function tests in the absence of radiological changes is not uncommon in rheumatoid disease and other connective tissue disorders such as systemic lupus erythematosus (SLE).

Pulmonary nodules Rheumatoid nodules may occur in the lungs of rheumatoid patients. Their main significance lies in the difficulty in differentiating them from other causes of pulmonary shadows. Their size varies from a few mm to 4 cm in diameter and occasionally they may cavitate to form necrobiotic nodules and cause haemoptysis.

In Caplan's syndrome, intrapulmonary nodules and massive fibrosis occur in the lungs of workers with rheumatoid arthritis exposed to various forms of inorganic dust (silica, asbestos, etc.). The original description by Caplan was in coal miners with rheumatoid arthritis. It has since been found that seropositivity for IgM rheumatoid factor even in the absence of clinical evidence of rheumatoid arthritis predisposes the lungs to develop these changes in response to exposure to dust.

Obstructive bronchitis and bronchiolitis Rheumatoid patients have an increased frequency of airways obstruction irrespective of smoking history. In addition there is a more severe form of obstructive airways disease associated with rapidly progressive and usually fatal obliterative bronchiolitis in the absence of chronic bronchitis and emphysema. Fortunately this seems very rare. It may be associated with penicillamine therapy.

Both the obstructive airways disease and the interstitial fibrosis of rheumatoid disease are associated with the inheritance of certain phenotypes producing reduced (but not absent) α_1 antitrypsin levels. This may be of pathogenic significance as α_1 antitrypsin inhibits a wide range of proteolytic enzymes and a similar association has been found between α_1 antitrypsin deficiency and pulmonary emphysema (page 9.44).

Cardiovascular

Pericarditis is common but frequently missed. Echocardiography suggests that a pericardial effusion may be present in 55 per cent of patients with nodular disease and in 15 per cent with non-nodular rheumatoid arthritis. Rarely life-threatening disease may occur with constrictive pericarditis or cardiac tamponade.

Non-specific valvulitis has been described in up to 30 per cent of autopsies of rheumatoid patients but specific granulomata occur much less commonly. Clinical evidence of valvular heart disease in rheumatoid patients has in the past been ascribed to other causes such as previous rheumatic fever. Rheumatoid valvulitis usually affects the aortic and more rarely the mitral valves. Generally the abnormalities have no functional significance but occasionally they produce incompetence.

Non-specific inflammatory changes and rheumatoid granulomata may be found in the myocardium of rheumatoid patients. Rarely coronary arteritis and conduction defects occur.

Haematological

Anaemia (page 19.66 *et seq.*) Anaemia is common and roughly correlates with disease activity and the ESR. The anaemia of rheumatoid disease is similar to that of other forms of chronic inflammation and is usually normocytic and normochromic but sometimes hypochromic and less commonly microcytic. This anaemia is characterized by normal or increased body iron stores in which the iron is thought to be sequestered in the reticuloendothelial system in a form which is unavailable for haemopoiesis. This is probably a non-specific consequence of chronic inflammation. In addition rheumatoid patients have an increased blood volume and some haemodilution. There is a degree of ineffective erythropoiesis and red cell survival is reduced. This haemolytic element is mild. More severe haemolysis is usually due to drug hypertensivity.

The principal practical problem is to differentiate iron-deficiency anaemia produced by gastrointestinal bleeding from the anaemia of chronic disease. This bleeding is largely a consequence of drug therapy but there is also an increased risk of peptic ulceration in rheumatoid arthritis irrespective of treatment. Not uncommonly this iron-deficiency anaemia co-exists with that associated with rheumatoid arthritis itself. In the anaemia of rheumatoid disease, the serum iron is low, total iron binding capacity normal or low (in contrast to the elevated total iron capacity in iron-deficiency anaemia), serum ferritin elevated, and bone marrow examination shows increased stainable iron within reticuloendothelial cells and a reduced number of sideroblasts. The absence of an elevated serum ferritin level in anaemic rheumatoid patients suggest there is a low iron store and a need for supplementary iron.

A megaloblastic anaemia is uncommon in rheumatoid patients but may be more frequent than in age-matched controls. Serum folate levels are reduced but red cell folate levels are usually normal or only slightly low.

The usual anaemia of rheumatoid disease does not respond to iron, folate or vitamin B_{12} therapy. Its severity reflects the activity of the arthritis and as the disease comes under control the haemoglobin level will usually improve.

Felty's syndrome This syndrome descibes the association between rheumatoid arthritis, splenomegaly and leucopenia. Other features which may occur include a normocytic, normochromic anaemia, thrombocytopenia, lymphadenopathy, cutaneous pigmentation, persistent skin ulceration, and weight loss. The leucopenia may be profound with less than 800 white cells/mm³ although more commonly the white cell count lies between 800 and 2500/mm³. The differential count shows a neutropenia which

often fluctuates spontaneously. The main hazard is recurrent infections although in some patients the neutropenia may not produce clinical problems. Felty's syndrome is usually found in patients with severe, nodular erosive disease, and other extra-articular features. Although neutropenia can precede arthritis, it is more likely that some other cause for neutropenia is present in patients with minimal joint problems. Patients with Felty's syndrome often have high titres of IgM rheumatoid factor and antinuclear antibodies. The commonest bone marrow changes are granulocyte maturation arrest which may disappear after splenectomy.

The pathogenesis of Felty's syndrome is uncertain. Most evidence suggests that the splenomegaly is responsible for the neutropenia although it is uncertain whether this is due to increased peripheral pooling, depression of granulopoiesis by a splenic humoral factor or autoimmune neutrophil destruction and phagocytosis by the spleen.

Treatment of Felty's syndrome is only indicated if it causes recurrent infections, severe anaemia due to hypersplenism, persistent cutaneous ulceration or thrombocytopenic bleeding. Treatment with corticosteroids produces inconsistent results and may make the infections worse. Splenectomy produces an increase in the white cell count and usually reduces the risk of infection. However, even though the white cell count rises, some patients continue to develop infections and some have even died within a few weeks of operation from overwhelming septicaemia. Lithium carbonate and testosterone have been used to correct the neutropenia of Felty's syndrome with variable success.

Thrombocytosis An increase in the platelet count occurs and correlates roughly with the articular disease activity and ESR. Investigations show that there is an increase in the formation and turnover of platelets in the blood.

Eosinophilia Eosinophilia develops in a minority of patients with active rheumatoid disease. More commonly it is found in patients with drug hypersensitivity reactions.

Other The commonest cause of haematological abnormality other than anaemia in rheumatoid arthritis is drug toxicity. Leucopenia, thrombocytopenia, eosinophilia, and less commonly haemolytic anaemia may all develop as adverse reactions.

SJÖGREN'S SYNDROME

Sjögren's syndrome (page 16.41) is the association of keratoconjunctivitis sicca (KCS) and/or xerostomia with rheumatoid arthritis or other connective tissue disease such as systemic lupus erythematosus. The lack of tear and salivary secretions which characterize the condition are caused initially by lymphocytic infiltration of the salivary and lacrimal glands progressing in more severe forms of the disease to generalized fibrosis and complete destruction of acinar tissue. Secretions from other epithelial surfaces may be affected so that patients can develop dysphagia, recurrent otitis media, chronic respiratory disease, dyspareunia, and dryness of the skin.

In KCS both the mucus and watery content of tears may be affected. Patients complain of grittiness and irritation of the eyes and of photophobia. In the early stages of the disease inadequate coating by mucus of the endothelium of the conjunctiva and cornea causes formation of dry patches and keratinization of the conjunctiva. Later, thick adherent strands of mucus form and are associated with filamentary keratitis. With the lack of the bacteriostatic lysoszymes in tears, secondary bacterial infection is common.

Dryness and stickiness of the eyes is worse on waking with difficulty in opening the eyes. Schirmer's tear test using a length of sterile filter paper hooked over the lower lid, is a rough guide to the presence of subnormal tear formation. Wetting of the filter paper less than 15 mm over 5 min is considered subnormal. The Schirmer tear test may be repeated using 10 per cent ammonia to stimulate tear secretion and confirm reduced tear flow. Slit lamp examination will show the abnormal tear film and mucus strands and instillation of Rose Bengal dye will show up the mucus strands.

The oral features of Sjögren's syndrome are due to involvement of the parotid, submandibular, and buccal glands. The absence of saliva produces dryness of the mouth and dysphagia which can be extreme and lead to weight loss. There may be recurrent parotid gland swelling and dental caries because of poor oral hygiene.

Simple atrophy of the lacrimal and salivary glands occurs in the elderly and labial gland biopsy is useful for identifying Sjögren's syndrome. The changes in these readily accessible minor glands mimic those in the parotid glands. Symptomatic Sjögren's syndrome is found in about 15 per cent of rheumatoid patients seen in hospital but many more have asymptomatic histological abnormalities. Other tests which have been used include measurement of salivary flow rate after cannulation of the parotid ducts, radioisotope scanning, and sialography.

Sjögren's syndrome in rheumatoid patients is found particularly in those with severe forms of the disease and extra-articular features. Other disorders described in association with Sjögren's syndrome include autoimmune thyroid disease, pernicious anaemia, renal tubular acidosis, glomerulonephritis, Raynaud's phenomenon, and high incidence of adverse drug reactions particularly to antibiotics and gold therapy. Patients with Sjögren's syndrome also have an increased risk of developing lymphomas particularly if treated with radiotherapy or immunosuppressive drugs.

Although the oral and ophthalmological features of Sjögren's syndrome associated with rheumatoid arthritis are similar to those in the sicca syndrome unassociated with connective tissue disease, there are certain immunological and genetic differences between the two. The sicca syndrome is associated with histocompatibility antigen HLA DR3 while rheumatoid arthritis both alone and with Sjögren's syndrome is associated with HLA DR4.

The ophthalmic symptoms are relieved by artificial tears such as hydroxymethylcellulose drops and some patients require topical antibiotics for secondary bacterial infections. In a few patients with more severe forms of KCS, coagulation of the nasolacrimal duct may be required. The oral manifestations of the disease are treated symptomatically and good oral hygiene and dental care is essential in view of the risk of caries.

Other ocular features
Scleritis
Scleritis is a deep inflammation of the sclera to be distinguished from the more superficial and relatively innocuous episcleritis. Pathological examination of the areas of scleritis will show typical rheumatoid inflammation. Scleritis is less frequent than Sjögren's syndrome in association with rheumatoid arthritis and is commonest in patients with vasculitis and other systemic disease complications.

The symptoms of scleritis vary from minimal or none to excruciating pain. The appearance is of diffuse or nodular inflammation but in necrotizing scleritis, the involved dead area is white. Perforation may occur through this and lead to loss of the eye. The complications of scleritis include perforation of the sclera (scleromalacia perforans; Fig. 10), uveitis, glaucoma and cataracts. When scleritis heals, the sclera becomes translucent and the blue/black underlying choroid can be seen. Despite appearances the translucent sclera is not thinned. It is not scleral translucency but rather necrotizing scleritis that may lead to scleromalacia perforans.

The treatment of scleritis is with local steroid drops and anti-inflammatory drugs in the first instance or with systemic steroids and immunosuppressives for more severe disease.

Episcleritis
Episcleritis may occur in association with scleritis but on its own is a mild self-limiting disease. It is doubtful whether episcleritis has any special association with rheumatoid arthritis.

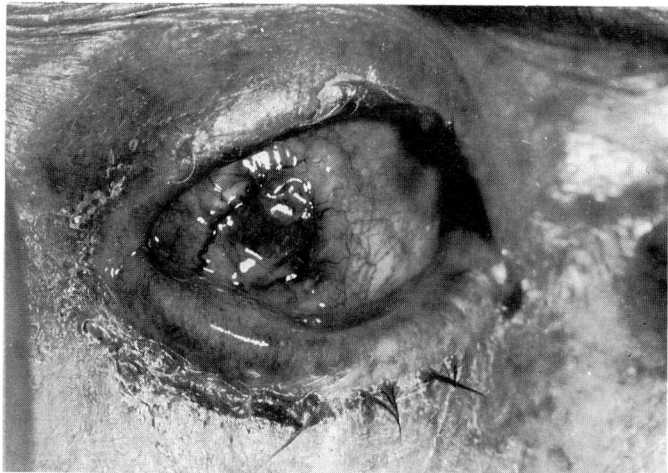
Fig. 10 Scleromalacia perforans.

Corneal involvement
Keratolysis (corneal melting) and limbal guttering are rare but formidable ocular complications which can lead to corneal perforation. They may be due to vasculitis of the circumcorneal vessels.

Neuromuscular
Peripheral neuropathy
Rheumatoid peripheral neuropathies fall into two main groups – a mild, mainly sensory neuropathy and a severe sensorimotor neuropathy often of the mononeuritis multiplex type. The milder neuropathy often presents as a symmetrical glove and stocking hypoaesthesia and paraesthesiae with only minor weakness. This type of neuropathy is common in women and occurs in mild as well as severe disease. Electromyographic tests may show slowing of motor or sensory conduction. The severe sensorimotor neuropathy is commoner in men and develops in association with destructive nodular rheumatoid disease, widespread vasculitis, and high titres of IgM rheumatoid factors. The mortality in these patients is high. The motor signs are predominant, often start suddenly, and are accompanied by mild sensory symptoms. Electromyography usually shows denervation of muscle. Rheumatoid neuropathies are thought to be produced by vasculitis of the vasa nervorum. Biopsy of the sural nerve in both types of neuropathy also shows both axonal and segmental demyelination.

Entrapment neuropathy
Nerve entrapment syndromes are easily treated and should be distinguished from the neuropathies described above. They include median nerve compression at wrist (carpal tunnel syndrome), posterior tibial nerve of the ankle (tarsal tunnel syndrome), and ulnar nerve compression at the elbow.

Cervical myelopathy
The neurological complications of atlanto-axial and subaxial subluxation have already been described (page 16.6). The neurological complications of cervical spine disease can occasionally present as peripheral sensory loss and mimic a peripheral neuropathy.

Muscular disease
Muscle atrophy in rheumatoid patients is usually attributed to reflex inhibition and disuse because of articular inflammation. Occasionally muscle atrophy and tenderness appear out of proportion to the joint disease and biopsies show inflammatory changes in the muscle. Some patients have rheumatoid arthritis–polymyositis overlap syndromes. Muscle weakness can be due to drug therapy. Drug-induced myopathy is most often due to corticosteroids but can also result from chloroquine. Penicillamine can cause a myasthenic syndrome.

Renal

Mild impairment of renal function is not uncommon. On renal biopsy the commonest histological abnormality is interstitial nephritis and this may be due to either pyelonephritis or drug toxicity. Hypercellularity of the glomerular tuft and glomerulonephritis may occur in patients with systemic disease but is uncommon and may reflect an overlap syndrome with SLE. Renal amyloid may cause proteinurea and renal failure and will be considered separately.

Antirheumatic drug therapy is an important cause of renal disease in patients with arthritis. Analgesic nephropathy (pages 18.67 and 18.108) with renal papillary necrosis may present with haematuria, renal colic, hypertension, chronic renal failure or recurrent urinary tract infections. Phenacetin was formerly regarded as the main culprit but is now excluded from antirheumatic drugs. Aspirin alone may cause analgesic nephropathy but in view of the large amounts consumed it seems that this is uncommon. Prostaglandin synthetase inhibitors such as the propionic acid derivatives and other anti-inflammatory drugs may produce a variety of renal problems. Both gold and penicillamine can induce an immune complex glomerulonephritis and penicillamine a form of Goodpasture's syndrome (page 18.36).

Hepatic

Hepatosplenomegaly occurs in about 11 per cent of rheumatoid patients. Asymptomatic minor elevations of serum alkaline phosphatase and impaired bromsulphthalein excretion are common particularly in those with Sjögren's syndrome. Liver biopsies are often normal or show non-specific fatty change, Kuppfer cell hyperplasia, or mild lymphocytic infiltration of the portal tracts. Amyloidosis is less common but a more serious cause of hepatic enlargement. Various drugs including salicylates, phenylbutazone, and some propionic acid derivatives may produce hepatotoxicity.

Other

Generalized lymphadenopathy may occur in rheumatoid patients and in particular those with Felty's syndrome. If biopsied, the glands show nodular hyperplasia.

Peripheral oedema can be troublesome in some rheumatoid patients. There are many causes including anaemia, hypoalbuminaemia, stasis in immobile patients, chronic joint rupture, venous and lymphatic obstruction by cysts, lymphatic obstruction by fibrin or lymphangitis, and increased capillary permeability.

Periarticular osteoporosis is a consequence of joint inflammation. It may be mediated by the release of prostaglandins or an osteoclast activating factor. Generalized osteoporosis is common in patients with more severe arthritis. It is due to a variable combination of the severity of the disease, loss of mobility, the effects of drugs, and in particular corticosteroids and an inadequate diet.

Clinical course and prognosis

The clinical course of rheumatoid arthritis is very variable. The type of patient seen in hospital has more active disease pursuing a long course of exacerbations and remissions but only a minority develop severe progressive destructive disease. In one ten-year follow up study of rheumatoid patients admitted to hospital, 20 per cent were functionally normal, 41 per cent had some restriction of daily living, 27 per cent marked restriction of daily living but only 11 per cent were severely disabled. In contrast, in the community many patients with very mild rheumatoid disease are never referred to hospital. The identification of prognostic factors is important in planning management to avoid overtreating patients with mild non-destructive disease and to pick out those patients with a poor prognosis for a more active treatment programme. Factors which suggest a poor prognosis include: (a) failure to respond to non-steroidal anti-inflammatory drugs, (b) early development of radiological erosions, (c) poor functional capacity early in the disease course, (d) the presence of extra-articular features such as anaemia, nodules, scleritis, vasculitis etc., (e) a persistently raised ESR, (f) high serum titres of IgM rheumatoid factor or antinuclear factor, (g) histocompatibility antigen DR4. HLA DR3 may indicate patients at risk of side effects from gold or penicillamine.

Although the life-span of patients with rheumatoid arthritis is slightly reduced, in general the causes of death are similar to those of the population at large.

Complications

Septic arthritis

This is a serious and frequently fatal complication and is seen particularly in patients with severe debilitating nodular disease who are receiving steroids. There may be a preceding history of an infected lesion such as an ingrowing toenail, boil or an ulcerating nodule. Rarely infection is introduced by an intra-articular injection. Septic arthritis may present as a hot painful joint which is disproportionally inflamed compared with the arthritis elsewhere. This may be followed by fever and rigors. However, particularly in the more debilitated patients, this complication may present as just general ill health or even a generalized disease flare. Fever and leucocytosis may be absent. The diagnosis is made by culture of blood and synovial fluid which should be undertaken whenever the complication is suspected. *Staphylococcus aureus* is the commonest organism but occasionally streptococci, pseudomonas, and Gram-negative bacteria can be responsible.

Amyloidosis

Evidence of amyloid deposition is found in about 10 per cent of rectal biopsies from rheumatoid patients. Amyloid can produce hepatosplenomegaly, proteinuria, cardiac failure, malabsorption or gastrointestinal haemorrhage. The diagnosis is based upon rectal, gingival or if appropriate renal biopsy. Although no therapy is of proven value there are anecdotal reports that immunosuppressive drugs such as chlorambucil can help.

Differential diagnosis

Diagnosis of established classical rheumatoid disease with symmetrical arthritis in a typical distribution, nodules, and positive tests for rheumatoid factor is not difficult. However, at an earlier stage the disease may be confused with other conditions.

Seronegative spondyarthropathies

Ankylosing spondylitis, psoriasis, Reiter's syndrome, Crohn's disease, and ulcerative colitis may be associated with a peripheral arthritis. Factors which suggest this group of conditions include asymmetry of the arthritis, involvement of predominantly medium and large joints, sacro-iliitis or spondylitis, distal interphalangeal joints involvement, urethritis, mouth ulcers, iritis, colitis, family history of a seronegative arthropathy or related disorder, and persistent negative serological tests for rheumatoid factor in a patient with established disease.

Systemic lupus erythematosus (SLE)

In SLE the peripheral arthritis is ususally mild and non-erosive. Recurrent arthritis can lead to ulnar deviation of the fingers or a reversible swan-neck deformity due to involvement of the periarticular structure and is one cause of Jaccoud's syndrome. Less commonly patients with SLE develop erosive arthritis. Features suggestive of SLE in a patient with polyarthritis include facial rash, photosensitivity, skin ulceration, serositis, nephritis, CNS involvement, and positive tests for antinuclear factor combined with a negative or low titre rheumatoid factor.

Primary osteoarthritis

The bony swellings around the terminal and proximal interphalangeal and first metacarpophalangeal joints of primary generalized osteoarthritis are easily distinguished from rheumatoid changes even though there may be an inflammatory component in osteoarthritis. As both rheumatoid and osteoarthritis are common it is not surprising that the two conditions may co-exist.

Gout

The clinical history, distribution of arthritis, and presence of tophi usually makes the diagnosis obvious. Occasionally tophaceous deposits over the elbow may be confused with rheumatoid nodules. The diagnosis is confirmed by the presence of urate crystals in synovial fluid and tophi and the measurement of the serum uric acid.

Acute benign polyarthritis

Acute polyarthritis follows certain viral infections such as rubella or rubella vaccination and may be confused with early rheumatoid arthritis. These forms of arthritis remit completely without residual damage. A careful history together with viral studies will usually distinguish them.

Juvenile chronic arthritis

Arthritis in childhood, often known as Still's disease, includes a miscellany of conditions grouped together under the term juvenile chronic arthritis (JCA). This may be defined as arthritis commencing below the age of 16 years with an inflammatory arthritis affecting four or more joints over at least a three-month period or in fewer joints with a synovial biopsy confirming appearances similar to those of adult rheumatoid arthritis. Other causes of joint disease are excluded by careful examination of follow-up over a year. Many children with JCA will eventually develop adult forms of polyarthritis such as rheumatoid arthritis, ankylosing spondylitis, psoriatic arthritis, and various forms of connective tissue disease such as SLE. Often it is difficult to classify the disease type and only gradual evolution over the years allows its characterization within an appropriate group. The principal types of JCA are:

Systemic

There is a high swinging fever worst in the afternoon and usually associated with a macular rash, lymphadenopathy, splenomegaly, hepatomegaly, pleurisy, and pericarditis. The polyarthritis may be surprisingly mild and usually resolves but about a quarter of patients develop very severe progressive arthritis.

A similar problem can develop in adults with a swinging pyrexia, macular rash, visceral inflammation, and a relatively mild polyarthritis. This is known as Adult Onset Still's Disease.

Polyarticular rheumatoid factor negative

This type is commonest in young girls although any age group may be affected. Any joint may be involved and there may be similar but milder systemic features.

Pauci-articular

This is defined as arthritis affecting three or less and often only one joint. There are two separate types.

The first most commonly occurs in girls under 5 years and affects large joints such as the knee. Extra-articular features are rare except for chronic iridocyclitis which occurs in up to 50 per cent of patients. Those developing this complication usually have developed antinuclear antibodies. Regular examination of the eyes with a slit lamp (preferably by an ophthalmologist) is mandatory in all children with JCA but particularly in this group because of the high risk and because children of this young age may not complain if they develop ocular problems.

The second form affects older boys, commonly affects large joints of the lower limbs and may be complicated by sacroiliitis, spinal involvement, and acute iridocyclitis. They possess the tissue type HLA B27. Ths is a form of juvenile ankylosing spondylitis.

Juvenile rheumatoid arthritis

This is rheumatoid arthritis occurring in a child and is associated with positive tests for rheumatoid factor. The prognosis for these children is worse than for other forms of JCA.

References

Ansell, B. M. (1982). *Rheumatic diseases in childhood*. Butterworth Scientific, London.
Calin, A. (1983). *Diagnosis and management of rheumatoid arthritis*. Addison-Wesley, Menlo Park, California.
Gardner, D. L. (1972). *The pathology of rheumatoid arthritis*. Edward Arnold, London.
Lawrence, J. S. (1977). *Rheumatism in populations*. Heinemann, London.

SERONEGATIVE ARTHRITIDES

A. HARVEY AND V. WRIGHT

Introduction

The term seronegative arthritides is applied to a group of arthritides with specific characteristics, chief of which are a consistent absence of rheumatoid factors in the serum, a tendency to axial skeletal involvement, and a strong clinical and genetic association with ankylosing spondylitis. The association with ankylosing spondylitis has resulted in the adoption of the more accurate term seronegative spondarthritides to describe the group. This helps distinguish them from seronegative rheumatoid arthritis and other arthritides such as gout and osteoarthritis, which, though seronegative for rheumatoid factors, do not have an association with ankylosing spondylitis. The diseases which qualify for inclusion in the seronegative spondarthritis group are: (*a*) ankylosing spondylitis, (*b*) psoriatic arthritis, (*c*) reactive arthritis (including Reiter's disease and dysenteric arthritis), (*d*) enteropathic arthritis (associated with ulcerative colitis, Crohn's disease, Whipple's disease, and intestinal bypass for morbid obesity), and (*e*) Behcet's syndrome. Each of these conditions will now be considered in turn.

Ankylosing spondylitis

Definition and prevalence

Ankylosing spondylitis is an inflammatory arthritis of the spine which by definition involves the sacro-iliac joints and is sometimes associated with an asymmetrical peripheral arthritis. Ocular, cardiac, and pulmonary extra-articular manifestations of the disease are also well recognized. It predominantly affects young males and the first symptoms usually occur before the age of 30 years, the peak being in the late teens and early twenties. It is rare for the symptoms to develop after the age of 45 years. The overall mean prevalence of the disease in Western populations is approximately 0.1 per cent. A higher prevalence is seen in Haida Indians, but it is less common in Negroes than Caucasians.

Aetiology

The exact aetiology of ankylosing spondylitis is still unknown. The familial nature of ankylosing spondylitis has been stressed for many years, and a genetic basis for this has been provided by the discovery that between 88 and 96 per cent of patients with ankylosing spondylitis carry the tissue type antigen HLA B27 (compared with between 4 per cent and 8 per cent of the normal population). Ankylosing spondylitis occurs in only about 1 per cent of patients who carry HLA B27 and it is postulated that environmental factors, specifically carriage of gastrointestinal or genitourinary micro-organisms, act as triggering factors in individuals rendered genetically susceptible by cell surface expression of the HLA B27 coded polypeptides. In support of this hypothesis, excretion of Klebsiella bacterial species in the stools has been associated with clinical activation of peripheral arthritis and iritis in some studies, but not with spondylitis activity, although other evidence is conflicting. Immunological evidence of Klebsiella infection has also been associated with active disease, and *in vitro* evidence of immunological cross-reactivity between Klebsiella bacterial wall antigens and the HLA B27 coded polypeptides has been demonstrated in some, but not all, studies. Immunoglobulin A (IgA) concentrations are usually elevated in ankylosing spondylitis. Recent demonstration of increase in salivary secretory IgA has provided additional evidence of activation of mucosal defences within the gastrointestinal tract, although other work suggests this is merely a manifestation of active disease.

An alternative theory is that it is a locus distinct from, but closely associated with, the HLA B27 locus, which acts as a predisposing factor. The demonstration that HLA B27 positive relatives of ankylosing spondylitis patients have a 5–16-fold increased risk of developing ankylosing spondylitis compared with unrelated B27 positive individuals supports this hypothesis.

Why the axial skeleton is predominantly involved is still not understood. The spread of an infective agent from the pelvic organs via the pelvic and paraspinal lymphatics to the spine has been suggested, but there is no direct evidence for this. Although such a theory might explain spinal involvement, it still leaves unexplained the extraspinal features of the disease, such as peripheral arthritis and iritis.

Pathology

The brunt of the inflammatory process seen in ankylosing spondylitis is borne at the sites of attachment of ligaments, tendons, and joint capsules to bone. Such a site is known as an enthesis and the resultant damage an enthesopathy. This comprises a focus of chronic inflammatory cells, adjacent bony erosion, and later features of healing by fibrosis and new bone formation. The common sites for this pathology are the annulus fibrosus of the intervertebral discs leading to the characteristic syndesmophyte formation seen on X-ray (Fig. 1), the iliac crests, the ischial tuberosities, greater trochanters, calcaneae, and patellae. A similar pathology is seen in the sacro-iliac joints. The process starts in the lower third of both joints, and leads initially to bony erosion of the joint margins, and then secondary ossification and ankylosis which ultimately involves the whole joint. The peripheral synovitis is similar histologically to that of rheumatoid arthritis, but in general leads to less cartilage destruction. This may be related to the relative paucity of IgM-producing plasma cells and absence of rheumatoid factor in ankylosing spondylitis. However, the hip joints can be severely damaged and may become ankylosed.

Clinical features

A gradual onset of low back pain often with bilateral sciatic radiation as far as the knees, worse on waking and eased by exercise, occurring in a young male is the classical presentation of the disease. Several episodes of such pain may have been experienced before the patient is persuaded to see his practitioner, the symptoms often being regarded by the patient as non-specific muscular strain or 'lumbago'. Low back pain is an extremely common complaint, but care in taking a history will usually establish bilaterality of symptoms and a definite 'stiffening up' at rest, unlike the symptoms of disc disease or apophyseal joint damage, which are eased by rest. As the spine becomes progressively involved pain will be experienced at higher levels and pain around the rib cage, exacerbated by deep breathing and coughing, heralds the involvement of the costovertebral joints. This is sometimes an early feature of the disease and can masquerade as pleurisy. Cervical spine involvement usually occurs later in the disease, and results in pain and a grating sensation on movement. The spinal involvement can stop at any stage and only a small proportion of patients go on to total spinal ankylosis.

A peripheral arthritis occurs in up to 30 per cent of patients, in 10–20 per cent of whom it may precede the onset of back symptoms. It usually affects the hips and the knees and can occur as an acute monoarthritis. The wrists and shoulders may also be involved, but the small joints of the hands and feet are only rarely affected. The asymmetry of the peripheral arthritis is a useful diagnostic aid and helps distinguish the disease from rheumatoid arthritis. Swelling, pain, and tenderness of the sternoclavicular, manubriosternal, and costochondral joints are frequently experi-

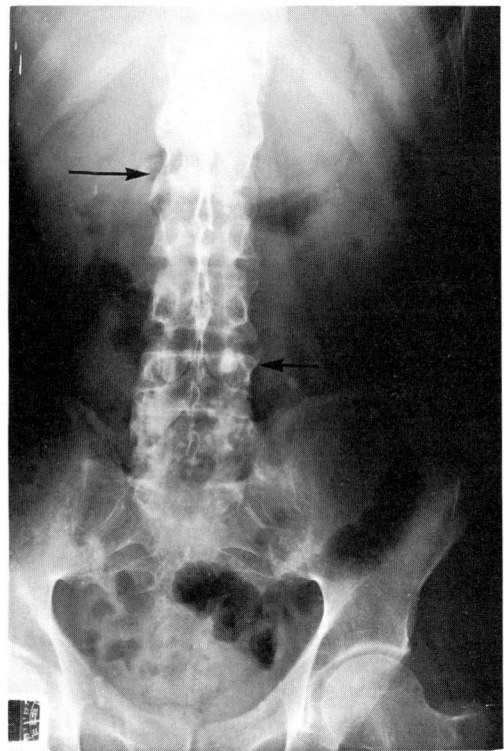

Fig. 1 Lumbar spine X-ray of a patient with ankylosing spondylitis showing syndesmophyte formation (arrows) in the lumbar spine and fused sacro-iliac joints. Note the more advanced state of syndesmophytes at the thoracolumbar junction; in some regions bony bridging has occurred (T12-L1, L1-L2).

enced during exacerbation of the disease. The pubic symphysis may also be similarly affected. Other peripheral musculoskeletal symptoms not directly involving joints also occur. Plantar fasciitis resulting in severe heel pain can be a presenting symptom. Achilles tendinitis and tenderness over the iliac crests, ischial tuberosities, and greater trochanters may also be found. In fact, any point of ligamentous attachment to bone may be the site of tenderness and pain.

In the early stages of the disease, examination may reveal bilateral sacro-iliac tenderness and pain over the sacro-iliac joints on springing the pelvis. This latter manoeuvre can be achieved either by firm downward pressure over both anterior superior iliac spines with the patient supine, or by even pressure over the sacrum with the patient prone. Loss of the normal lumbar lordosis is an early sign of vertebral involvement and results in the flattening of the lumbar curve on forward flexion. Loss or diminution of lateral flexion of the lumbar spine occurs early but forward flexion may be apparently well preserved. Careful examination will reveal that most of this flexion is achieved at the hip joint and not in the spine itself. The interspinous distances of the lumbar vertebrae remain fixed on forward flexion as the disease advances and the vertebrae become ankylosed. A careful survey of the peripheral joints must also be made and signs of synovitis, hip involvement, and tenderness over any enthesis such as the calcaneae, greater trochanters, and ischial tuberosities should be noted. In advanced disease the classical poker spine with marked thoracic kyphosis leading to the 'question mark posture' makes diagnosis easy. The abdomen bulges forwards and diaphragmatic breathing becomes marked as the costovertebral articulations becomes fixed. Chest expansion is restricted relatively early in the disease and is one of the more important objective clinical measurements. Systemic manifestations such as fever and weight loss may occur especially during severe exacerbations. Very occasionally, patients present with total spinal ankylosis and deny any history of back trouble.

Complications

Iritis

Non-granulomatous anterior uveitis occurs in approximately 20 per cent of patients with ankylosing spondylitis. It may be the presenting feature of the disease and has an association with the peripheral arthropathy, though not with the severity of the spondylitis. Iritis can be a troublesome complication and lead to much distress for the patient. Prompt treatment with steroid eye drops is mandatory if the secondary complications of posterior and anterior synechiae with the risk of glaucoma are to be avoided.

Cardiovascular disease

A non-specific aortitis resembling syphilitic aortitis is seen in approximately 4 per cent of patients with ankylosing spondylitis of at least 15 years duration. It results in lone aortic incompetence which can be of such severity as to warrant valve replacement. The arch of the aorta may also be involved, leading to aneurysmal dilation. Involvement of the conducting system may rarely cause bradyarrhythmia or complete atrioventricular block. Cardiomyopathy and pericarditis have also been described.

Neurological complications

These are a direct result of the spinal pathology in ankylosing spondylitis. Spinal cord damage may result from traumatic fractures of the rigid cervical spine and spinal fractures can occur at other levels. Surprisingly, cases of atlantoaxial subluxation occurring spontaneously have been described. The risk of tetraplegia is high in these patients. Lesions of the cauda equina can also occur with pathological evidence of an inflammatory arachnoiditis, and sacral root pain due to the involvement of the nerve roots as they run over the sacro-iliac joint can give rise to classical sciatica. An association between ankylosing spondylitis and multiple sclerosis has been reported anecdotally.

Pulmonary complications

Pulmonary function tests usually show a mild restrictive abnormality of ventilation, but in general lung function remains remarkably well preserved despite severe restriction of thoracic cage movement. Ventilatory capacity is preserved by increased diaphragmatic excursion. The only parenchymal lung involvement in ankylosing spondylitis is rare and takes the form of apical fibrosis, cavitation, and occasionally calcification leading to radiological diagnostic confusion with pulmonary tuberculosis. Patients can present with cough, increased dyspnoea, and even haemoptysis. The cavities may become secondarily infected with aspergillus and the formation of mycetomas may occur.

Amyloidosis

Secondary amyloidosis is well recognized in long-standing ankylosing spondylitis and in one autopsy series 6 per cent of spondylitic patients died of uraemia from this complication.

Investigations

Radiology

This is the most important investigation in ankylosing spondylitis. A definite diagnosis cannot be made in the absence of radiological evidence of bilateral sacro-iliitis. The earliest sign of this is a loss of definition of the lower joint margins followed by erosive changes and juxta-articular sclerosis extending to the whole of the joint. Eventually complete ankylosis occurs, but occasionally the old joint line can still be seen as a 'ghost' and in this event ankylosis may be missed unless the radiograph is carefully scrutinized. Changes at the sacro-iliac joint are usually the earliest radiological signs of the disease. In early sacro-iliitis, where radiography may be equivocal, quantitative scintigraphy and computerized tomography (CT scan) have both been reported to improve resolution. As the disease extends up the spine, features such as squaring of the lumbar vertebral bodies, calcification of the annulus fibrosus resulting in syndesmophyte formation, calcification of the interspi-

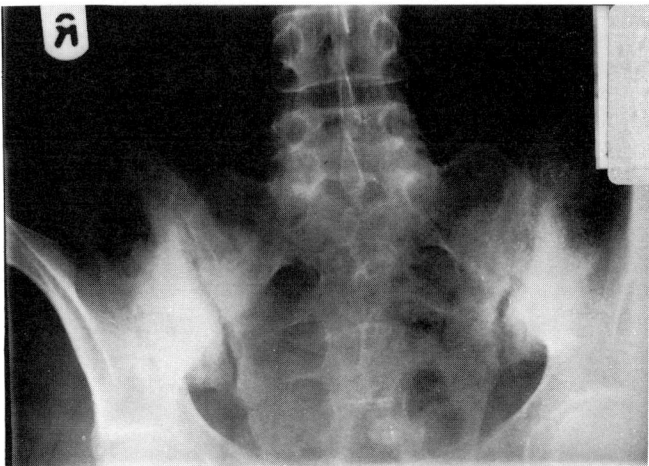

Fig. 2 Bilateral sacro-iliitis in a female patient with ankylosing spondylitis. Sclerosis of the sacro-iliac joint margins is well shown. Erosive changes are also seen especially on the left.

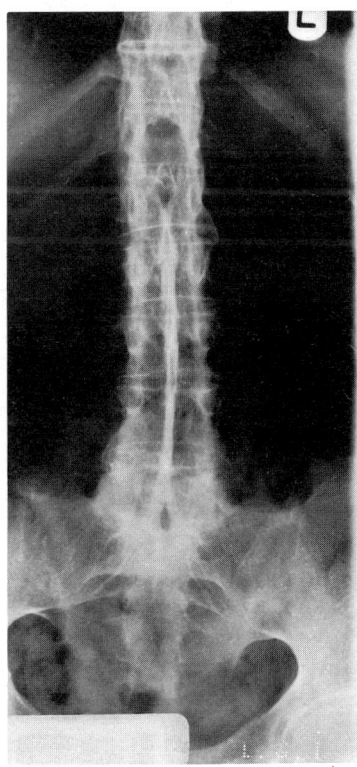

Fig. 3 Advanced changes of ankylosing spondylitis showing calcification in the interspinous ligament (known as the 'dagger sign'), ankylosis of the lumbar vertebrae, and the sacro-iliac joints.

nous ligaments, and sclerosis and ankylosis of the apophyseal joints are seen (Figs 1–4). Total spinal involvement with ankylosis results in the classical radiological appearance of the bamboo spine.

Erosions of the ischial tuberosities often accompanied by soft tissue calcification, also seen around the iliac crests and greater trochanters, are frequent radiological associations with the changes seen in the spine (Fig. 5). Erosions, sclerosis, and ankylosis of the pubic symphysis are also common. Of the peripheral joints the hip is by far the most comonly affected radiologically. Initially cartilage loss is seen as a narrowing of the radiological

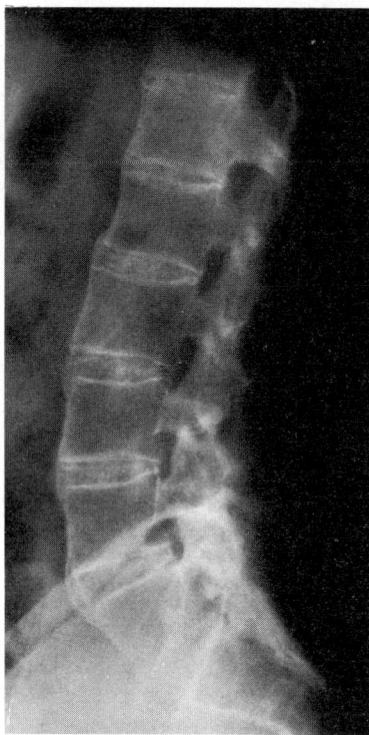

Fig. 4 The 'bamboo' spine of ankylosing spondylitis. This patient had had active disease for over 15 years resulting in total spinal ankylosis. Note fusion of posterior facet joints and intervertebral disc calcification which is sometimes seen in long-standing disease.

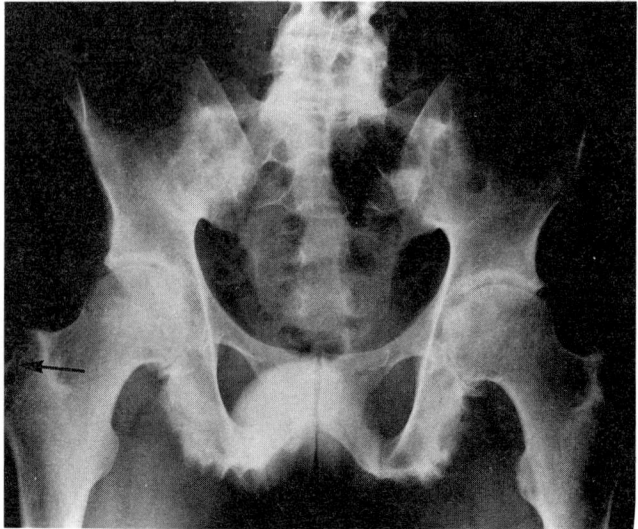

Fig. 5 Pelvic X-ray of a patient with ankylosing spondylitis showing fusion of the sacro-iliac joints and marked erosion and periosteal new bone formation around the ischial tuberosities. Similar though less severe changes are seen in the right greater trochanter (arrow).

joint space and is followed by bony erosion, sclerosis, and finally ankylosis in advanced cases.

Laboratory tests

The ESR is raised during exacerbations of the disease, particularly in the early phases. However, this finding is by no means invariable and the ESR is a relatively poor guide to the activity of the disease. Plasma viscosity, C-reactive protein, and alpha-2 globulin show a closer correlation with disease activity, particularly for peripheral arthritis and iritis, reflecting the systemic acute phase response. Elevation of immunoglobulin A is characteristic of active disease in ankylosing spondylitis, except when peripheral arthritis predominates, when IgG elevation is more likely, as in rheumatoid arthritis. Rheumatoid factors are absent from the blood and the sheep cell agglutination and latex tests are negative. Circulating immune complexes are not present in the serum, and although complement metabolism is increased, serum complement levels are normal or elevated. Some patients with long-standing disease run a low-grade normochromic normocytic anaemia and a leucocytosis is occasionally seen in acute attacks. Recent reports of elevation in alkaline phosphatase and gamma glutamyl transpeptidase during disease flares remain to be confirmed. HLA typing shows the presence of B27 in 96 per cent of patients with ankylosing spondylitis, but the test should not be used routinely as a diagnostic aid in view of the fact that only a small percentage of the total population with B27 develop the disease (see Aetiology).

Treatment

The main aims of treatment are to reduce pain and stiffness and to prevent deformity. A combination of non-steroidal anti-inflammatory drugs with a vigorous home exercise programme to maintain normal spinal posture is usually sufficient. Oral corticosteroids are effective anti-inflammatory drugs, but should be avoided because of the necessity for chronic administration and its associated side-effects. Short-term benefit may be gained from pulsed methyl prednisolone which has both early anti-inflammatory and late immunosuppressive actions. Long-acting anti-rheumatoid drugs, such as myocrysin and D-penicillamine, have no proven effect on either axial or peripheral arthritis in ankylosing spondylitis. Severe destructive peripheral arthritis may respond to immunosuppressive drugs such as azathioprine. Radiotherapy of the axial skeleton is no longer used because of the high incidence of late leukaemia, but local joint irradiation may still have a place in severe peripheral oligoarthritis.

Prognosis

Uncomplicated ankylosing spondylitis does not alter life expectancy but can impinge on the quality of life, though with judicious use of anti-inflammatory drugs and active physiotherapy this can be kept to a minimum in the majority of patients who usually continue in full, gainful employment all their working life. The pattern of involvement at 10 years' disease duration has been shown to predict long-term morbidity, and early development of hip involvement, peripheral joint involvement, and iritis are associated with poor long-term functional status. A minority suffer a particularly aggressive form of the disease which can result in total spinal ankylosis in two or three years and little can be done to prevent this. However, even in these patients, emphasis on posture and physiotherapy can reduce the likelihood of gross spinal deformity that can result without proper supervision. Amyloidosis and cardiac involvement in long-standing disease carry a definite, though small, mortality.

Psoriatic arthritis

Definition and prevalence

This is an inflammatory, seronegative arthritis occurring in patients with psoriasis. It has several distinct clinical patterns, one of which also involves the spine and may be indistinguishable from ankylosing spondylitis. Approximately 7 per cent of patients with psoriasis develop arthritis, suggesting an overall population prevalence of 0.1 per cent. The sex incidence is to some extent determined by the type of psoriatic arthritis. Thus there is a male predominance in the distal type whereas females predominate in the other types.

Aetiology

As in ankylosing spondylitis, there is strong evidence of inherited factors playing a key role in the aetiology of psoriatic arthritis.

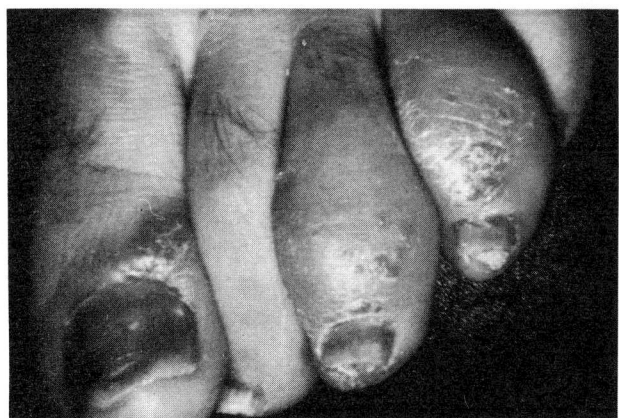

Fig. 6 Psoriatic arthritis involving the toes. Note 'sausage-shaped' swelling of the digits indicating a dactylitis. There is a nail dystrophy and psoriatic skin lesions are also seen.

Psoriatic arthritis is 50 times more common in the families of patients than it is in the normal population. Studies of HLA types have been performed in patients with psoriatic arthritis and in addition to the types associated with uncomplicated psoriasis (A1, B13, B17, and CW6), an increase in B27, DR4, and DR7 has been reported in separate studies. HLA B27 has specifically been associated with psoriatic spondylitis and with distal interphalangeal joint disease, and DR4 has been associated with the rheumatoid pattern of joint involvement (see below). Infection, trauma, and neurotrophic effects have been implicated as additional factors precipitating the arthritis. It is interesting that a minority of patients present with arthritis before developing psoriasis.

Pathology
Chronic inflammatory changes in the synovium with villous hypertrophy and often marked fibrosis but without pannus formation are the non-specific characteristics of psoriatic arthritis. Rheumatoid granulomata are not seen but erosive cartilage damage and bone destruction may be marked. Periostitis, particularly of the shafts of the phalanges contributing to the uniformly tender sausage-shaped digits (dactylitis) is often seen (Fig. 6). Juxta-articular osteoporosis as found in rheumatoid arthritis is not a feature, but bony ankylosis of peripheral joints occurs more commonly than in rheumatoid arthritis.

Clinical features
Five clinical subgroups of psoriatic arthritis are generally recognized:

1. Predominant involvement of the distal interphalangeal joints, often in an asymmetrical fashion (Fig. 7) and associated with a dactylitis.
2. Severe deforming arthritis sometimes showing widespread ankylosis or having the clinical appearance of an arthritis mutilans (Fig. 8) (uncommon).
3. Arthritis that is clinically indistinguishable from rheumatoid disease but which follows a more benign course.
4. Oligo- (or mono-) arthritis distributed in an asymmetrical fashion affecting any synovial joint (this is the commonest form of psoriatic arthritis). Enthesopathy, including achilles tendonitis and plantar fasciitis, may be a prominent feature in this subgroup.
5. Ankylosing spondylitis occurring either on its own or in association with any of the above groups. This accounts for approximately 5 per cent of all types of psoriatic arthritis.

In the majority of patients, skin lesions antedate the onset of the arthritis, though in a few patients the reverse is true. Arthritis is found 10 times more commonly in patients with severe skin involvement than in those with mild involvement. One should always make a careful search for psoriatic plaques in the scalp,

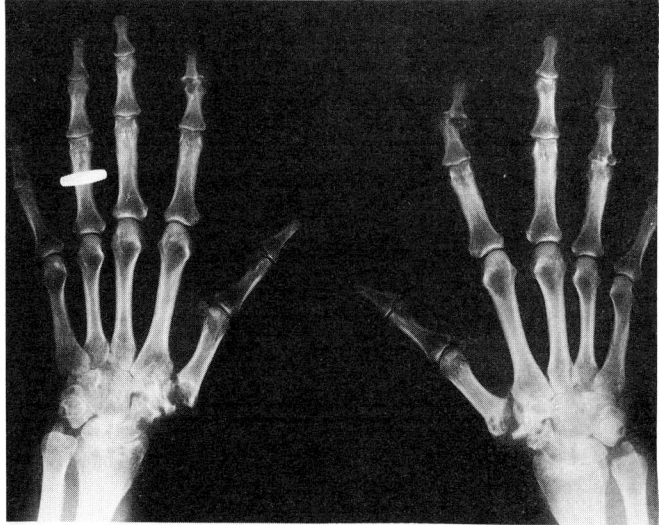

Fig. 7 Typical radiological appearance of psoriatic arthritis of the hands. Distal interphalangeal joint involvement is prominent in the index fingers but changes are also seen in the proximal interphalangeal joint of the right ring finger demonstrating the asymmetrical distribution of the arthritis. The metacarpophalangeal joints and the ulnar styloids, a common site of erosive change in rheumatoid disease, have been spared. Both carpi however show advanced erosive changes.

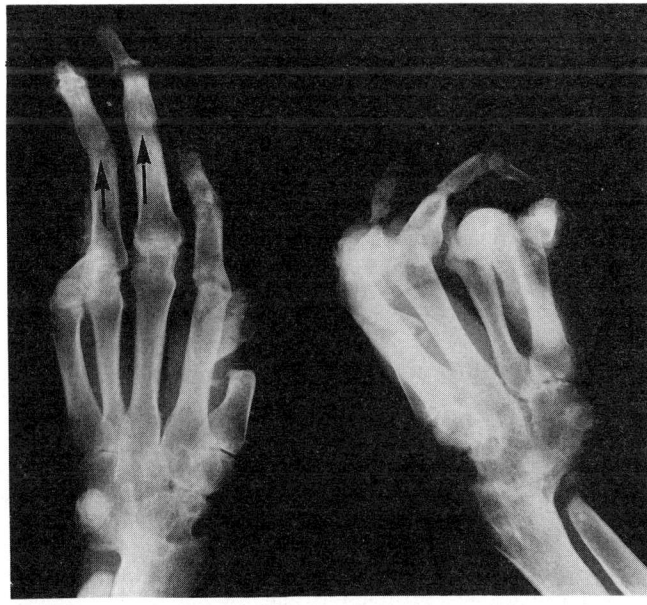

Fig. 8 X-ray of the hands of a patient with psoriatic arthritis of the mutilans type. Several interphalangeal joints are fused (arrows) as are both carpi. Note advanced bony destruction with typical 'whittled' bone ends.

behind the ears, in the umbilicus, and in the natal cleft as well as at the more usual sites, as occasionally severe arthritis is seen with minimal skin involvement. Only rarely is there a strict temporal relationship between exacerbations of psoriasis and of the arthritis. In the arthritis mutilans type the psoriasis tends to be extensive and long-standing, making a double misery for the patient. The mutilating type also has a relationship with pustular psoriasis of the palms and soles. Interestingly psoriatic nail changes such as pitting, ridging, hyperkeratosis, and onycholysis are more frequently seen at the onset of the arthritis than are the skin lesions (Fig. 9). Sometimes there is a curious juxtaposition of a psoriatic nail and an affected distal joint. Overall 81 per cent of patients with psoriatic arthritis have nail changes compared with 32 per

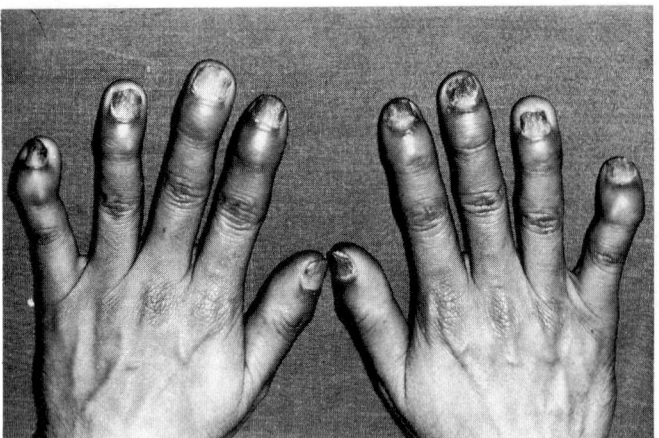

Fig. 9 Psoriatic arthritis of the 'distal' type showing involvement of the distal interphalangeal joints and the associated nail dystrophy.

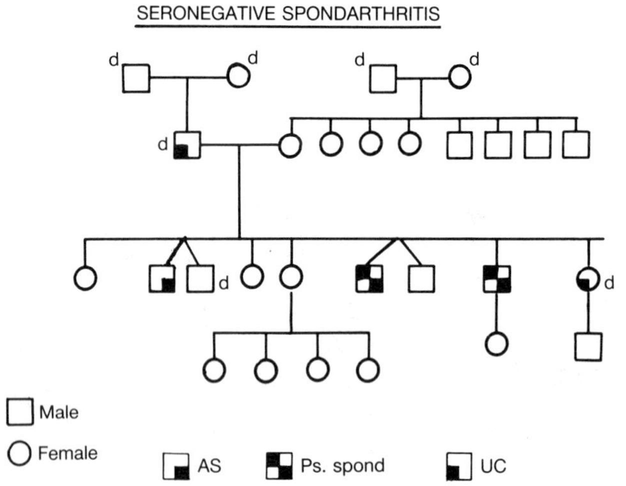

SERONEGATIVE SPONDARTHRITIS

☐ Male
◯ Female
◲ AS   ◆ Ps. spond   ◪ UC

Fig. 10 Family tree to show an aggregation of ankylosing spondylitis, psoriatic spondylitis, and spondylitis with ulcerative colitis. (Reproduced from, 1971, *Proc. R. Soc. Med.* **64**, 663.)

cent of patients with a similar distribution of uncomplicated psoriasis.

The association of psoriasis and ankylosing spondylitis has been recognized for over 20 years, and there is familial evidence showing aggregation of sacro-iliitis and spondylitis in blood relatives of patients with psoriatic arthritis (Fig. 10). Sacro-iliitis alone without spondylitis is also seen and asymmetrical spinal involvement sometimes only affects the cervical spine.

Asymmetrical seronegative arthropathies other than psoriatic arthritis occurring in patients with concomitant psoriasis can sometimes cause diagnostic difficulty. Gout, either of the monarticular or polyarticular variety, can simulate psoriatic arthritis both clinically and radiologically. The finding of crystals of sodium urate in the synovial fluid will prove the diagnosis of gout. Moderately elevated serum uric acid levels are sometimes seen in patients with severe psoriasis and this finding alone should not exclude a diagnosis of psoriatic arthritis, though markedly elevated levels make gouty arthritis a stronger possibility. Osteoarthritis of the erosive variety affecting the distal and proximal interphalangeal joints can sometimes be indistinguisable from psoriatic arthritis. Inflamed Heberden's nodes can add to the diagnostic confusion, but careful radiological assessment usually resolves the difficulties. Extra-articular features are rare in psoriatic arthritis. Ocular involvement, including conjunctivitis, iritis,

scleritis, and keratoconjunctivitis sicca, is the most common extra-articular feature. Spondylitic heart disease predominantly affecting the aortic valve is occasionally seen and in these patients the skin lesions are usually pustular. Amyloidosis also occurs. Subcutaneous nodules are not a feature.

Investigations
Radiology
Although an important investigation in psoriatic arthritis, radiology can sometimes confuse the diagnosis. Many of the changes are indistinguishable from rheumatoid arthritis, but the following features should be noted: (*a*) asymmetry of joint involvement with emphasis on erosive changes in the distal interphalangeal joints and a relative sparing of the metacarpophalangeal joints, (*b*) periosteal thickening particularly in the phalanges, (*c*) 'whittling' of bone ends leading to the 'pencil-in-cup' appearance of the distal interphalangeal joints, (*d*) joint ankylosis, not usually seen in rheumatoid disease (see Fig. 8), and (*e*) spinal involvement with sacro-iliitis, fusion of the sacro-iliac joints, ligamentous calcification, sometimes leading to the classical bamboo spine of ankylosing spondylitis. A rare type of paravertebral ossification in the lumbar and thoracic areas may occur at some distance from the vertebral body.

Laboratory findings
The ESR is elevated in acute phases of the arthritis. A mild normochromic anaemia is not uncommon in long-standing disease. Hyperuricaemia is said to be a frequent finding in psoriasis and is common in patients with more extensive skin involvement. It shows no correlation with the arthritis. Elevated gamma and alpha-2 globulins have been reported in psoriatic arthritis as have other immunoglobulin abnormalities, particularly elevated IgA levels, but these findings are inconsistent. Rheumatoid and antinuclear factors are absent from the blood but are occasionally found in synovial fluid. Synovial fluid complement levels, as in all seronegative arthritides, are either mildly elevated or normal. Synovial fluid cell counts can be very high in the acute psoriatic joint with a polymorphonuclear preponderance, but in general the counts are lower than those seen in active rheumatoid synovitis. Synovial biopsy is not helpful. Determination of histocompatability antigens is not a useful diagnostic test in psoriatic arthritis for reasons already outlined.

Prognosis and treatment
Fortunately, the arthritis mutilans type of psoriatic arthritis is rare and when present is often confined to the hands, although occasionally it can be generalized and such a patient with numerous ankylosed joints presents a pathetic sight. Few patients run such an aggressive course, and in the majority the outlook is good, with joint changes confined to the distal interphalangeal joints or a few other joints. Spinal involvement is extremely variable, although total ankylosis is the exception rather than the rule. The general principles of management with non-steroidal, anti-inflammatory drugs and physical therapy apply to psoriatic arthritis. For aggressive joint disease, methotrexate, either orally or intramuscularly, has been shown to be of benefit if simpler methods fail, although liver toxicity may preclude its prolonged use in some patients. Recently the vitamin A derivative, etretinate, has been shown to benefit the arthritis as well as the skin lesions in psoriatic patients.

Reactive arthritis
Introduction
This term refers to the development of an inflammatory synovitis associated with (and apparently resulting from) infection with micro-organisms at a site distant from the joint, and without evidence for synovial invasion by micro-organisms. In the context of seronegative spondarthropathies, Reiter's disease, arthritis associated with bacterial enteritis and with acne are all reactive arthri-

tides, although other conditions such as rheumatic fever and the polysynovitis resulting from several viral infections including rubella, are also reactive arthritides but without features otherwise associated with the seronegative spondarthropathies.

Reiter's disease

Definition and prevalence

Reiter's disease comprises a triad of symptoms: (a) seronegative polyarthritis affecting the lower limbs predominantly, (b) conjunctivitis, and (c) non-specific urethritis. Two types are generally recognized, genital, usually following promiscuous sexual exposure and intestinal, usually following an attack of bacillary dysentery. It is now increasingly accepted that not all cases exhibit this classical triad and the most consistent features are non-specific inflammation of the lower urogenital tract and a recurrent polyarthritis. Overall prevalence figures are not available but about 2 per cent of patients with non-specific non-gonococcal urethritis attending clinics for sexually acquired diseases in the United Kingdom develop Reiter's disease. The frequency of the disease following dysentery was 0.24 per cent of 150 000 cases of dysentery in one large study but considerable geographical variation exists. The population frequency reflects the prevalence of the HLA B27 antigen, with one or two exceptions. The majority of cases occur between the ages of 16 and 35 years and the male to female ratio is approximately 20:1. The male preponderance may be exaggerated in view of the fact that urethritis often goes undetected in females. The apparent rarity in children reflects the rarity of sexually acquired infection, but postdysenteric disease occurs.

Aetiology

The current aetiological concept of Reiter's disease is that of a primary infective agent inciting a specific host response in genetically predisposed individuals. There seems little doubt that the disease follows an infection of the bowel or lower genitourinary tract. In the intestinal form various infective agents have been implicated, chief amongst which are shigella, salmonella, and yersinia, but in some cases no specific causative organisms can be isolated. A non-specific polyarthritis without associated urethritis and conjunctivitis is sometimes seen after gastroenteritis caused by salmonella or yersinia. This reactive arthritis may be a *forme fruste* of Reiter's disease and is discussed below. Both types show a high correlation with carriage of tissue type B27. In the venereal form of the disease, attention has been focused on the chlamydia group of organisms and mycoplasma/ureaplasma. The organisms can be isolated from carefully taken urethral and cervical smears in patients with non-specific urethritis. They have also been isolated from the synovium, urethra, and conjunctiva of some patients with Reiter's disease. In addition, antibodies to chlamydia have been found in high titre in some patients with sexually acquired reactive arthritis, and synovial fluid lymphocyte responses to antigenic preparations of ureaplasma, chlamydia, and enteric bacteria have been shown to differ between patients with sexually acquired and enteric acquired reactive arthritis, and from patients with rheumatoid arthritis. There is little information on the familial aspects of the disease but an inherited tendency to develop the disease has been suspected for a long time. In a family study in the United Kingdom an increased prevalence of sacro-iliitis, spondylitis, and psoriasis was found in relatives of patients with Reiter's disease. In addition to this epidemiological evidence, tissue typing of patients with Reiter's disease reveals a frequency of between 63 and 90 per cent of B27. In terms of risk factors, a B27 positive male runs a 20 per cent risk of developing the disease following an attack of dysentery.

Pathology

There are no specific pathological lesions unique to Reiter's disease. The synovial histology is generally indistinguishable from that of rheumatoid synovitis. The histology of keratoderma blenorrhagica (see below) is indistinguishable from pustular psoriasis.

Clinical features

The symptom triad of acute arthritis, conjunctivitis, and non-specific urethritis occurring between one and four weeks after sexual exposure or an attack of dysentery in a young man is the classical presentation of Reiter's disease. The arthritis is commonly a monoarthritis, usually of the knee, but any synovial joint can be involved. The disease may not present with the classical triad and a physician should always be alert to the possibility of Reiter's disease in any young man with an acute non-traumatic monoarthritis. It is usually self-limiting and may be transitory, lasting no more than two or three days. Occasionally the synovitis can be extremely acute with tense effusions and knee joint rupture. Multiple joints can be involved asymmetrically and the acute stage can develop into one of chronic relapsing destructive arthritis particularly of the knees and forefeet. Flare-ups in the arthritis are not necessarily associated with further episodes of infection. The spine may also be involved in about 20 per cent of cases. Sacro-iliitis, sometimes asymmetrical, is the most common finding, but spondylitis extending up the spine, although usually confined to the lumbar region, is also seen. This results in ligamentous calcification and a stiff back. The fully developed bamboo spine of ankylosing spondylitis is rarely seen.

Tendinitis and fasciitis, particularly of the Achilles tendon and plantar fascia, can be extremely troublesome and interfere markedly with the patient's general mobility. Periostitis gives rise to tenderness of the shafts of the phalanges and contributes to sausage-shaped digits similar to those seen in psoriatic arthritis.

Ocular lesions

Conjunctivitis is usually mild and may escape the patient's notice. It is sometimes associated with a sterile discharge which subsides in one to four weeks. More severe cases are occasionally seen which progress to episcleritis, keratitis, and corneal ulceration. Anterior uveitis may also occur. Less than one in ten patients have this early in the course of the disease, but it may affect as many as 30 per cent of patients with recurring arthritis. When sacro-iliitis is present, nearly half the patients develop uveitis. Other ocular complications, such as intra-ocular haemorrhage or retrobulbar neuritis, occur rarely.

Urethritis

A history of a clear urethral discharge accompanied by minimal dysuria can be obtained from the majority of patients with sexually acquired Reiter's disease, provided it is sought diligently. The discharge is sterile on routine culture. Occasionally symptoms may be severe and accompanied by acute haemorrhagic cystitis and prostatitis. Mild prostatitis is determined by the finding of 10 or more leucocytes per high-powered field in the fluid obtained after prostatic massage and is an invariable finding in Reiter's disease. Care, however, must be exercised in the interpretation of this finding as approximately 29 per cent of normal males will be deemed to have prostatitis on these grounds. Urethritis is also a common finding in the dysenteric form of the disease.

Mucocutaneous lesions

Keratoderma blenorrhagica is the characteristic skin lesion of the disease. It is usually confined to the palms and the soles and manifests itself as brown macules initially. The lesions progress to pustules and become scaly, closely resembling those of pustular psoriasis (Fig. 11). It can spread to involve the trunk and the scalp but rarely involves the face. Nails may also be affected with a dystrophy resembling that of psoriasis, but nail pitting does not occur, and this has been suggested as a useful differentiating feature. Subungual hyperkeratosis can be severe and lead to the shedding of the nails. Circinate balanitis and painless shallow buccal ulce-

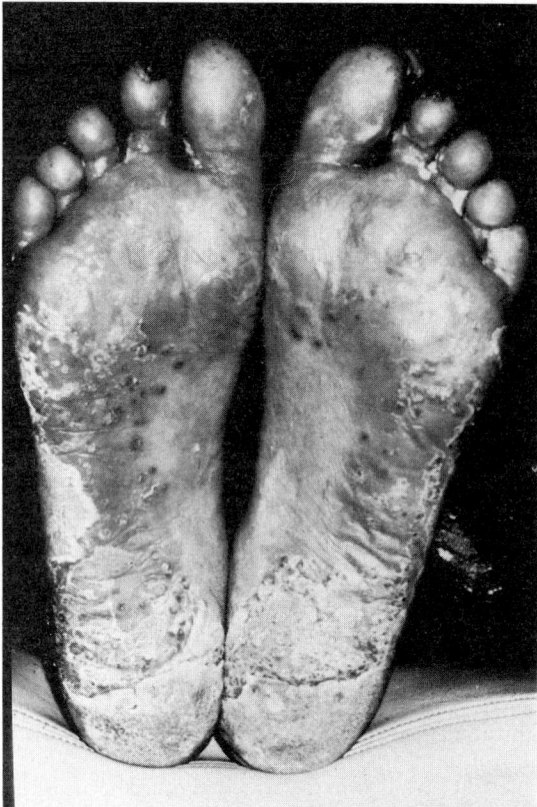

Fig. 11 Keratoderma blenorrhagica on the soles of a patient with Reiter's disease.

ration are also characteristic of the disease, and are often over-looked.

Other clinical manifestations

Many patients run a low-grade fever at the onset of the disease but occasionally systemic upset may be more severe with high fever and weight loss. Reports in children suggest a much greater prominence of systemic features of fever, lymphadenopathy, spleno-megaly, and also pleuritis. Cardiac involvement is well recognized. Pericarditis, myocarditis, aortitis indistinguishable from that seen in ankylosing spondylitis, and conduction defects have all been reported. Pleurisy and transient pulmonary infiltrates are occasionally seen. Amyloidosis is a rare complication. Neurological complications occur in about 1 per cent of the patients and include peripheral neuropathy, transient hemiplegia, and meningoencephalitis.

Investigations

Radiology

In the early stages of the disease, the X-ray changes are limited to soft tissue swelling around affected joints. If the disease progresses, cartilage loss with ultimately bony erosion may be seen particularly in the knees and feet. Patients with sacro-iliitis will usually develop changes in the sacro-iliac joints similar to those seen in ankylosing spondylitis. Ligamentous calcification and facet joint ankylosis are usually not as marked as that seen in ankylosing spondylitis and syndesmophyte formation is often asymmetrical as in psoriatic arthritis. Calcaneal spurs in Reiter's disease are said to have a different radiological texture to those in ankylosing spondylitis, being more ebullient and fluffy.

Laboratory tests

The ESR is considerably elevated during the acute phases of the disease, and in common with other spondarthritides the ESR can remain elevated for long periods after the acute phase has settled.

Polymorphonuclear leucocytosis, sometimes marked, is also found during exacerbations. Patients often develop a mild hypoch-romic or normochromic anaemia.

Serum proteins are usually normal but a moderate rise in gamma globulins is often detected. Rheumatoid factors are not found in the serum in any greater frequency than in the normal population. In one study B27 was found in up to 75 per cent of patients with Reiter's disease, contrasted with 9 per cent in uncomplicated non-specific urethritis, and in 6 per cent of controls. Synovial fluid analysis reveals a typical acute inflammatory fluid having a high polymorphonuclear leucocyte count but sterile on culture. The demonstration of excess polymorphs in a urethal smear may provide important supportive evidence for the diagnosis, and Gram stain should be undertaken to rule out gonorrhoea which may present similarly.

Prognosis and treatment

In the majority of patients the disease is manifested initially by a transient monoarthritis associated with conjunctivitis and urethritis, and is usually self-limiting. A large proportion (between 34 and 38 per cent) will suffer recurrent or sustained disease activity, and between 11 and 15 per cent will suffer functional limitation sufficient to prevent employment. This minority of patients, usually those with a more severe initial attack and associated with mucocutaneous manifestations of the disease, such as kerato-derma blenorrhagica, progress to a chronic relapsing course with resultant joint damage, particularly of the knees and forefeet. Chronic heel pain carries a poor functional prognosis. Between 15 and 20 per cent of patients will develop ankylosing spondylitis, and nearly all in this group will have the tissue type B27.

Treatment with appropriate antibiotics may be used initially and at the onset of disease flare-ups, although its long-term benefit is unproven. Principles of treatment are otherwise identical to psoriatic arthritis. Both azathioprine and methotrexate have been advocated for severe persistent disease.

Arthritis associated with gut infection

Salmonellae are the most common organisms isolated from patients with arthritis following attacks of gastroenteritis. Approximately 2.4 per cent of patients develop an acute polyarthritis occurring 5 to 14 days after the initial gut infection. The arthritis can mimic rheumatoid disease but seldom lasts more than a few weeks and settles without any sequelae. In some patients, an acute monoarthritis is seen; occasionally these patients are found to have a true septic arthritis and the causative salmonella can be cultured from the joint fluid. Treatment with systemic antibiotics is usually curative.

Yersinia infections of the gastrointestinal tract can also lead to a reactive arthritis. The arthritis closely resembles that seen in sal-monella infections but the course may be more prolonged and the arthritis may be recurrent. Large, lower limb joints are most commonly affected, and sacro-iliitis with progressive signs of ankylosing spondylitis occasionally occurs. Occasionally the full clinical picture of Reiter's disease occurs following yersinia infection. The diagnosis is made by culturing yersinia from the faeces or demonstrating rising titres of antibodies to the organisms in the blood. Indium leucocyte scanning suggests that occult enteritis may persist during the arthritic phase.

More recently, campylobacter has been implicated as an additional infective cause (abdominal pain is often a prominent feature with this organism), and *Clostridium difficile* has also been isolated in a few patients.

Pathogenesis

The mechanism causing the synovitis is not understood, but impaired cell-mediated responses to the infecting organisms have been demonstrated, and a clear HLA B27 association exists. It has been suggested that a plasmid carried by these several enteric organisms may be the triggering factor common to dysenteric arthritides, but no evidence has yet been provided to support this hypothesis. Circulating immune complexes have not been implicated in pathogenesis.

Arthritis associated with acne

An arthritis clinically resembling seronegative spondarthritides with particular features of Reiter's disease, has been reported in association with acne fulminans and less commonly acne conglobata and hydradenitis suppurativa. No increase in HLA B27 carriage has been identified in these patients.

Enteropathic arthropathy

Definition

Any arthritis associated with primary bowel disease of whatever cause could be considered as an enteropathic arthritis. The two main members of this group are the arthritis associated with Crohn's disease (see page 12.121) and with ulcerative colitis (see page 12.126), but it is also seen in patients with Whipple's disease. Ankylosing spondylitis is also seen with increased frequency in these patients, both with and without peripheral arthritis. Arthritis following intestinal bypass operation for morbid obesity is discussed below.

Aetiology

The cause of enteropathic arthritis is unknown. The concept that bowel antigens escape across the damaged intestinal mucosa and form soluble antigen–antibody complexes in the circulation which then enter the joints and stimulate synovitis has yet to be proved conclusively. There is evidence that patients who develop arthritis after intestinal bypass operations for morbid obesity form circulating cryoprecipitable immune complexes containing bacterial antigens, and similar complexes have been isolated in patients with inflammatory bowel disease, but such complexes have not yet been demonstrated within the joints of patients with inflammatory bowel disease. Reconstruction of the normal bowel anatomy in intestinal bypass patients results in complete resolution of their chronic polyarthritis. Similarly, the arthritis associated with ulcerative colitis can be abolished by resection of the diseased bowel. Both these facts suggest that absorption of bacterial antigens into the circulation are a prerequisite for the development and chronicity of the arthritis. There is no particular tissue type associated with the peripheral arthritis, or with the associated bowel disease, but patients developing ankylosing spondylitis show an increased frequency of B27. In one series 13 out of 18 patients with spondylitis and ulcerative colitis were B27 positive. In Crohn's disease and associated ankylosing spondylitis the association with B27 is not as strong as it is in idiopathic ankylosing spondylitis.

Arthritis associated with ulcerative colitis

Clinical features

This commonly presents as a monoarthritis, usually of the knee, but a polyarticular presentation involving the ankles, elbows, small joints of the hands and feet, shoulders, and hips (in decreasing order of frequency) is occasionally seen. The sex ratio is equal. There is a close temporal relationship between the peripheral arthritis and exacerbations of the gut disease. When the gut disease goes into remission, the arthritis usually settles without any sequelae. Erythema nodosum sometimes occurs with the arthritis. There is a higher incidence of arthritis in those patients with more extensive gut involvement and a feature of the peripheral arthritis is that it settles when the diseased gut is resected. Peripheral arthritis can occasionally be a presenting feature of ulcerative colitis. Clubbing is a well-recognized complication and a periosteal reaction identical to that seen in hypertrophic pulmonary osteoarthropathy has been reported. An increased prevalence of ankylosing spondylitis has been found in several studies of patients with ulcerative colitis. In an unselected group of 234 patients with ulcerative

colitis, 6.4 per cent had ankylosing spondylitis, and a further 14 per cent had asymptomatic sacro-iliitis. Ankylosing spondylitis can antedate the colitis and is identical in its clinical presentation and spectrum of complications to the idiopathic variety. Unlike the peripheral arthritis, there is no relationship between exacerbations of the bowel disease and the ankylosing spondylitis.

Investigations
Radiology

The peripheral arthritis does not show any specific radiological features and usually leaves the articular surfaces undamaged. The spinal disease can often be detected on abdominal X-rays taken during barium studies for the gastrointestinal disease and the changes are identical to those seen in idiopathic ankylosing spondylitis. An erosive joint disease, particularly of the hips, is sometimes seen in these patients.

Laboratory tests

There are no specific laboratory tests that help in the diagnosis of the arthritis. The ESR is elevated and serological tests for rheumatoid factor are uniformly negative. Synovial fluid analysis and synovial histology show the changes of acute inflammation and are also non-specific.

Arthritis associated with Crohn's disease

Clinical features

The pattern and behaviour of the peripheral arthritis associated with Crohn's disease is similar to that seen in ulcerative colitis. However, it differs in one important feature in that resection of diseased gut often does not lead to a resolution of the arthritis and indeed the arthritis can have a postoperative onset. Erythema nodosum, as in ulcerative colitis, is occasionally associated with the arthritis. Arthritis is more common in those patients with large bowel disease and it would seem from two comparative studies that the arthritis is more common in Crohn's disease than it is in ulcerative colitis. About 16 per cent of Crohn's disease patients show radiological sacro-iliitis and approximately 6 per cent have ankylosing spondylitis. As in ulcerative colitis, the ankylosing spondylitis can antedate the Crohn's disease and is not associated with disease in any particular part of the gut, nor is there a temporal association between spondylitis and exacerbations of the bowel disease.

Clubbing is more common in Crohn's disease than in ulcerative colitis, and periosteal new bone formation, similar to that seen in hypertrophic pulmonary osteo-arthropathy, has been reported.

Investigations
Radiology

The peripheral arthritis is not associated with any specific radiological change, even after repeated attacks of synovitis. However, as in colitic arthritis, when the peripheral arthritis is seen in the presence of ankylosing spondylitis, erosive changes sometimes occur, mainly in the hips. The radiological changes of ankylosing spondylitis are identical to those seen in the idiopathic type.

Laboratory tests

Synovial fluid analysis and synovial biopsy usually reflect the acute inflammatory nature of the arthritis, though occasionally granulomata, similar to those seen in the gut, are found on synovial biopsy. Rheumatoid factors are not found in the blood.

Whipple's disease (intestinal lipodystrophy)

This is a rare disease with protean clinical manifestations including weight loss, pyrexia, skin pigmentation, abdominal pain, lymphadenopathy, and migratory polyarthritis. It shows a male predominance. The polyarthritis, often the first symptom of the disease, is a common association (68 per cent of patients in one series), but is usually self-limiting and residual deformity is rare. Ankylosing spondylitis has been reported in 18 of 64 patients with Whipple's disease but, as only two of them had sacro-iliitis, the diagnosis must be regarded as doubtful and the association still remains speculative. For this reason, the inclusion of Whipple's disease in the seronegative spondarthritides is somewhat tentative. The arthritis is probably best regarded simply as 'enteropathic'.

Aetiology

The aetiology of the arthritis is unknown. Studies of the synovial membrane are rare but those that have been performed have failed to show an excess of periodic acid–Schiff (PAS) positive granules within synovial macrophages such as seen so characteristically in the macrophages of the small intestinal mucosa on jejunal biopsy. However, rod-shaped organisms identical to those found in the small bowel mucosa have occasionally been identified in synovium and also in subcutaneous nodules, permitting definite diagnosis. The invariable response of the disease, including its joint manifestations, to prolonged antibiotic therapy would certainly argue in favour of an infective aetiology. As yet, there is insufficient evidence to implicate a specific tissue type predisposing to the disease.

Arthritis associated with jejuno-ileal bypass

This syndrome follows bypass of substantial amounts of the small bowel for control of obesity. Sacro-iliitis, associated with polyarthritis, has been reported. Additional features of dermatitis, episcleritis, and fever may occur. Reversal of the bypass is usually curative. Immune complex formation and circulation have been implicated in the pathogenesis of this arthropathy.

Behçet's syndrome

(See also Section 20.)

This is a rare symptom complex comprising recurrent oral and genital ulceration and relapsing iritis. It is more common in countries bordering the eastern Mediterranean, particularly Turkey, and also in Japan, and it has been suggested that the geographical distribution of the disease tends to follow the old silk routes from the East. Other clinical manifestations of the disease are superficial or deep venous thrombosis, and rarely arterial thrombosis; peripheral arthritis; central nervous system involvement such as meningo-encephalitis, cranial nerve palsies, and hemiparesis; and skin lesions including vasculitis with ulceration, erythema nodosum, and erythema multiforme. The peripheral arthritis can affect any synovial joint but the knees, ankles, and wrists are most commonly involved. Sixty-eight per cent of arthritic episodes in a recent study were monoarticular and 80 per cent oligoarticular (less than five joints). Joint involvement is usually a later manifestation of the disease, and permanent changes rarely develop. The

'pathergy' test (skin hypersensitivity to needle puncture) has been described as a useful adjunct to diagnosis, but it appears to be confined to the Turkish cases, and is not observed in English patients. It is not clear whether sacro-iliitis is more frequent in Behçet's patients than in the normal population.

Aetiology

HLA typing indicates a clear association with B5 in Behçet's patients, particularly those with ocular involvement. Weaker associations between B27 and joint involvement, and B12 and mucocutaneous involvement have been described. In addition to this evidence of genetic predisposition, an association with herpes simplex type I virus infection has been demonstrated using DNA hybridization, and abnormal responses between HSV-1 and Behçet's lymphocytes in culture provides some support for the hypothesis that an impaired immune response to HSV infection may be associated with persistent (intranuclear) virus survival and resultant disease. Evidence for endothelial dysfunction, and for a circulating 'lupus anticoagulant' may explain the thrombotic tendency.

Treatment

The arthritis can usually be controlled by simple anti-inflammatory drugs. Local (intraorbital) corticosteroid treatment is often beneficial for mild to moderate uveitis, but in severe uveitis, retinal vasculitis, and severe systemic disease systemic corticosteroids or immunosuppressive agents may be required.

References

Berens, D. L. (1971). Roentgen features of ankylosing spondylitis. *Clin. Orthopaed.* **74**, 20–33.
Bitter, T., Calin, A. and Hughes, G. R. V. (1979). Symposium on Reiter's syndrome. *Ann. rheum. Dis.* **38** (Suppl. 1), 84–91.
Brewerton, D. A., Caffrey, M. F. P., Nicholls, A. and James, D.C.O. (1974). The histocompatability antigen (HLA B27) and its relation to disease. *J. Rheum.* **1**, 249.
Caughey, D. E. and Bywaters, E. G. L. (1963). The arthritis of Whipple's syndrome. *Ann. rheum. Dis.* **22**, 327–335.
Ebringer, R. (1979). Symposium on the spondarthritides, spondarthritis and the postinfectious syndromes. *Rheum. Rehab.* **18**, 218–226.
Eglin, R. P., Lehner T. and Subak-Sharpe, J. H. (1982). Detection of RNA complementary to herpes-simplex virus in mononuclear cells from patients with Behçet's syndrome and recurrent oral ulcers. *Lancet* ii, 1356–1360.
Emery, A. E. H. and Lawrence, J. S. (1967). Genetics of ankylosing spondylitis. *J. Med. Genet.* **4**, 239–244.
Moll, J. M. H. (ed.) (1980). *Ankylosing spondylitis.* Churchill Livingstone, Edinburgh.
Wright, V. (1979). A unifying concept for the spondyloarthropathies. *Clin. Orthopaed.* **143**, 8–14.
—— and Moll, J. M. H. (1976). *Seronegative polyarthritis.* North Holland, Amsterdam.

SYSTEMIC LUPUS ERYTHEMATOSUS

M. A. BYRON AND G. R. V. HUGHES

Introduction

Systemic lupus erythematosus (SLE) is a multisystem disease, characterized by circulating autoantibodies, and a variety of immunological abnormalities which participate in the mediation of tissue damage. It is not a rare disease, prevalence rates of 1 per 2000 population being reported in the United States. There is evidence of racial differences in prevalence and severity. In the United States the disease may be found in 1 in 250 Black women, but only 1 in 700 for all women. It is commoner and more resistant to treatment in parts of Southeast Asia. SLE

occurs in children and the elderly, but the peak age at onset is in the third decade. The disease is nine times more common in females than males, and during childbearing years this ratio rises to 15:1.

Aetiology and pathogenesis

The aetiology of SLE remains a mystery, not least because the syndromes comprising it may not be a single disease, but a constellation of symptoms and signs produced by a variety of aetiological factors.

Table 1 Autoantibodies in SLE

Non-organ-specific: Common
Anti-DNA (dsDNA; ssDNA)
Antihistone
Antiextractable nuclear antigen (ENA) (Ro, La, Ribonucleoprotein Sm)
Antiphospholipid (cardiolipin, lupus anticoagulant, VDRL)
Rheumatoid factors
Cytotoxic antibodies (lymphocytes, neutrophils, platelets)
Coombs antibodies

Organ–specific: Uncommon
Thyroid
Gastric parietal cell
Mitochondrial
Smooth muscle

Pattern	Appearance	Disease association	Antigen
Homogeneous (diffuse)		Common pattern	Deoxyribonucleoprotien
Rim of nucleus (peripheral; annular)		SLE	Double-stranded DNA (ds DNA)
Flame	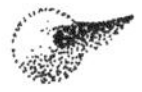	SLE	?dsDNA
Nuceolar		Scleroderma SLE	Nucleoli
Speckled		SLE Sjögren's syndrome Mixed connective tissue disease	Extractable nuclear antigens (ENA)

Fig. 1 Patterns of immunofluorescence showing antinuclear antibody on rat liver substrate. (Reproduced from Chapel, 1984, *Essentials of clinical immunology*. Blackwell Scientific Publications, Oxford by permission.)

Immunopathology

Mechanisms of autoimmunity are discussed in Section 4. In SLE, the presence of autoantibodies, hypergammaglobulinaemia and elevated viral antibody titres are indications of B cell hyperactivity, and abnormalities of T cell function (helper or suppressor) may facilitate this defect. Subsequent antigen–antibody complex formation results in deposition of immune complexes, activation of the complement cascade, both classical and alternate pathways, and cell injury. Activated complement components also affect vascular permeability and promote the inflammatory response. Circulating immune complexes are detectable in SLE serum, and immune complex deposits can be seen by electron microscopy and immunofluorescence antibody techniques, e.g. in the glomerulus, and at the dermoepidermal junction.

Range of autoantibody production

The enormous array of non-organ-specific autoantibodies found in SLE (Table 1) has been termed an 'autoimmune thunderstorm'. These antibodies, however, are directed at relatively few macromolecules which are components of the cell, and it is becoming recognized that the diversity of antibody reaction detectable in SLE serum, may be due to a quite limited number of antibodies which react with an antigenic determinant shared by many molecules, e.g. the phosphodiester backbone of DNA, RNA, and phospholipids.

The presence of antinuclear antibody (ANA) and antibody to double-stranded DNA (dsDNA) remain the mainstay of the diagnosis of SLE, although about 5 per cent of patients do remain persistently ANA-negative. Several patterns of nuclear fluorescence are seen when rat or mouse liver is used as the substrate for the ANA (Fig. 1) but when rapidly dividing cells of a human epithelioid line are used, different patterns can be identified and ANA-negative sera will show positivity. Antibodies against cytoplasmic or extractable nuclear antigens are usually characterized by methods such as counter-immunoelectrophoresis. Besides having diagnostic value some of these antibodies are believed to be pathogenetic, though antibody titres do not correlate with disease activity (see later). Clinical interest has centred around defining subsets of SLE by antibody typing. However, the conversion of a 'serological subset' into a clinical 'subset' may rely more heavily on statistics than clinical observations. Despite these reservations, certain antibodies do appear to be associated with certain clinical features; anti-Ro antibodies are associated with the development of congenital heart block in the offspring of SLE patients; antiphospholipid antibodies (cardiolipin antibodies), responsible for the false-positive VDRL and the circulating lupus anticoagulant are associated paradoxically with an increased thrombotic tendency and a high incidence of recurrent abortion; and anti-RNP antibodies may be associated with Raynaud's phenomenon.

Immunoregulation

Although autoantibody production may be initiated by antigen (probably not DNA), disturbed immunoregulation may allow chronic production. Hyperreactivity of B cells, depressed T-suppressor and enhanced T-helper functions have been variously reported, and in murine models of SLE the abnormalities described are species related. These functional disturbances augment each other, and in addition autoantibodies to lymphocytes are cytotoxic for T cells. Similar abnormalities are, however, described in disorders not associated with autoantibody production, suggesting that other factors, genetic or environmental are also important. Also, autoantibody production *per se*, need not be pathogenetic, and it appears that only antibodies with certain immunochemical properties form immune complexes which deposit in tissues. Factors such as avidity, ability to bind complement, and isoelectric point may be important in this respect. It is now being appreciated that the study of deposited, rather than circulating immune complexes is likely to be more informative.

Equally important are factors affecting the handling of immune complexes, such as reduced erythrocyte complement–receptor numbers and diminished Fc-receptor function of splenic macrophages. Recent research has also centred on the role played by immune mediators, particularly interleukin-1 (IL-1), interleukin-2 (IL-2), and immune interferon (IFN). IL-1 is a polypeptide produced by macrophages, which stimulates IL-2 production by activated T cells, as well as having other effects (Table 2). The T cells in turn produce IL-2 which promotes T cell proliferation and B cell production of immunoglobulin. Both IL-1 and IL-2 production, as well as the expression of IL-2 receptors on T cells, have been found to be deficient in SLE. Immune interferon levels, however, are high, and this glycoprotein also has widespread functions. As well as influencing lymphocyte function these mediators may well play a direct role in the pathogenesis of joint and other tissue injury. Patients differ from one another with regard to type and degree of cellular and humoral abnormality, and recognition of this heterogeneity will be of great importance for future investigations.

Genetic factors

Genetic susceptibility to SLE is suggested by several observations. SLE occurs in the relatives of patients in a frequency several hundred-fold that of the general population. Immunological abnormalities are also more common in SLE family members, though also in non-consanguineous household contacts, suggesting an environmental factor. Twin studies show a greater than 60 per cent concordance of SLE in monozygotic twins, whereas the frequency in dizygotic twins is no different from that of first degree relatives. Racial differences in prevalence also point to a genetic factor.

The genes that control immune responsiveness are found at the

Table 2 Immune mediators in SLE

Mediator	Source	Target cells	Action
Interleukin 1 (1L-1)	Monocytes Macrophages	T and B cells synovium	Proliferation and differentiation of all target cells
		Fibroblasts Chondrocytes	Collagenase and prostaglandins
		Hepatocytes	Acute phase proteins
Interleukin 2 (1L-2)	T cells helper/ suppressor	T and B cells	Promotes cell growth and differentiation, e.g. release of lymphokines, antibody, etc.
Immune interferon (IFN)	T cells, natural killer cells	All cells	Antiviral Antiproliferative Induces HLA surface markers B cell differentiation Macrophage activation

Table 3 Major clinical manifestations of SLE

Manifestation	Percentage
Musculo-articular	95
Cutaneous	81
Fever	77
Neuropsychiatric	59
Renal	53
Pulmonary	48
Cardiac	38

Estes and Christian (1971).

major histocompatibility complex (MHC) of the sixth chromosome. These genes give rise to the human leucocyte antigens (HLA-antigens) which are expressed on various cells. SLE is not associated with a particular HLA antigen, but associations have been described most consistently with HLA-A1, B5, B7, B8 DR2, and DR3. The relevant gene need not belong to one of these products, but may be sited near to them, so that they are inherited in linkage disequilibrium. The haplotype B8 DR3 is frequently associated with a variety of autoimmune diseases (e.g. diabetes mellitus, coeliac disease, and chronic active hepatitis) and it may be that this haplotype is inherited with a gene allowing polyclonal B cell activation, and SLE is just one of a number of possible consequences of this.

Genes controlling production of several complement components also map in the MHC, and homozygous deficiency of the early components especially C2 are frequently associated with SLE. Acquired deficiencies of C2 and C4 also predispose to SLE. In a family study of idiopathic SLE there was an increased prevalence of null (silent) alleles for C4 in patients, a finding in strong linkage disequilibrium with the presence of DR3, and suggesting a directly inherited subtle complement defect in this disease. A homozygous or heterozygous deficiency of complement may result in abnormal handling of immune complexes with greater tissue deposition.

Acetylator status is genetically determined, and slow acetylators are at greater risk of developing drug-induced SLE. In idiopathic SLE, however, no consistent results for acetylator status have been found. In mouse models of SLE breeding experiments with normal mice have failed to show the segregation of a particular phenotype with disease.

Sex hormones
That sex hormones influence SLE is illustrated by the high female preponderance, the fact that hormonal preparations and menses can adversely influence symptoms, and that pregnancy and the puerperium are times when disease flare is likely to occur. Reports of SLE in Klinefelter's syndrome (men with XXY chromosomes) would bear this out and some studies have shown that males with SLE are hormonally indistinguishable from women. In one mouse model of SLE (the NZB/W mouse) the females develop the disease earlier and more severely than the males. Treating the females with androgens delays the onset of the disease and castrating the males results in disease activity as in the females, suggesting a protective effect of male hormones. There is also evidence of direct effects of hormones on macrophages, other reticuloendothelial cells, and thymic epithelium. Thus in SLE the effects of sex hormones may represent physiological effects on a disordered immune system. However, the effect of anti-oestrogen or synthetic androgen treatment on human SLE is either disappointing or inconclusive.

Viral infection
The finding of 'virus-inclusions' in glomerular endothelial cells in 1973 rekindled interest in a viral aetiology for SLE. These tubulo-reticular structures are now considered to be a non-specific manifestation of cell injury. Attempts to isolate a virus from human SLE tissue has as yet been unsuccessful, although type C RNA oncornavirus has been isolated from mice with a lupus-like disease, and transfer of virus to uninfected animals may lead to immune complex nephritis depending on the genetic susceptibility of the strain. The finding of type C RNA antigens on SLE peripheral blood leucocytes and in various tissues, by immunofluorescence, remains a subject of controversy.

Clinical features
SLE is a multisystem disorder characterized by exacerbations and remissions. The incidence of major features is listed in Table 3 and the common physical findings in Fig. 2. In addition, there is often malaise, tiredness, and tendency to drug allergy.

Musculoskeletal
Tenosynovitis is the prominent feature in SLE. It may be mild and recurrent or may progress relentlessly to cause joint deformity which mimics chronic rheumatoid arthritis and is seen in about 15 per cent of patients. Arthralgia or arthritis occurs in 90–100 per cent of lupus patients, and may frequently predate the diagnosis. The pain often appears out of proportion to the degree of synovitis, and erosions are usually absent even in patients who develop a deforming arthritis. Severe tense synovitis of joints is unusual. The joints most commonly involved are the proximal interphalangeal (PIP), the metacarpophalangeal (MCP), the wrist, and the knee, with other joints less frequently involved. Septic arthritis may occur and an infective aetiology should be sought especially when one joint flares.

Aseptic bone necrosis may occur in SLE, usually related to corticosteroid therapy. The distinctive X-ray appearance of an area of 'ground-glass' necrotic bone may be seen, though scanning with ^{99}technetium compounds (^{99}Tc) may show abnormalities at an earlier stage. With a more conservative approach to management, the incidence of this complication has fallen. Myalgia is very common and a true myositis with raised muscle enzymes occurs in 5 per cent of SLE patients. A myopathy has also been described, not always associated with therapy, but occasionally produced or exacerbated by corticosteroids.

Cutaneous
Skin manifestations are protean in SLE.

Discoid lesions Chronic discoid lupus may be the only manifestation of SLE, less than 10 per cent of patients with lesions sub-

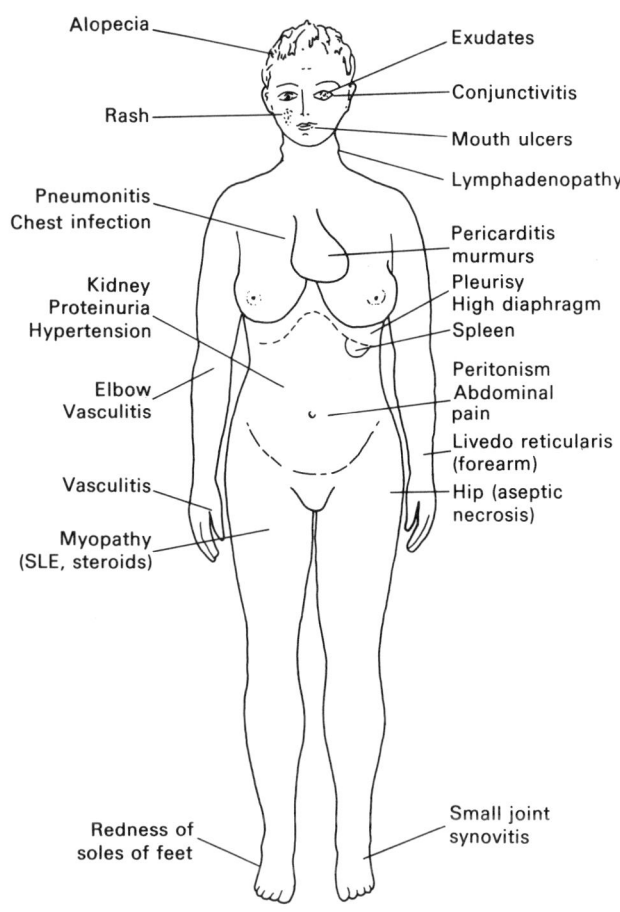

Fig. 2 Frequent findings in SLE.

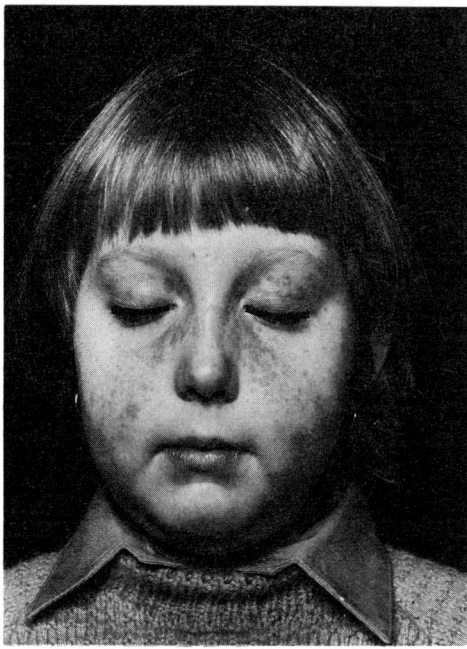

Fig. 3 Butterfly rash in SLE.

sequently developing overt extracutaneous disease. Conversely, 15–20 per cent of patients with well-documented SLE will have typical discoid skin lesions at some time during the course of their disease. The typical lesions show three stages of development: erythema, hyperkeratosis, and finally atrophy. Lesions usually start with one or more sharply defined papules in the butterfly area of the face, other common sites being scalp, ears, forehead, chest, back, and upper arms. The mature lesions show erythema, oedema, and elevation of the central area with follicular plugging. Eventually the central area becomes depressed and atrophic, and finally a scar is left with hyperpigmentation at the edges. Scalp lesions result in scarring alopecia.

Subacute cutaneous LE   The subacute variety of cutaneous LE (SCLE) has a widespread distribution: face, neck, upper trunk, extensor surfaces of arms and hands. It is similar to discoid lupus but is non-scarring, less persistent, and has less prominent scaling and follicular plugging. The lesions have a tendency to coalesce, usually follow a course of exacerbation and remission and are particularly photosensitive. Patients with this type of skin involvement frequently manifest multisystem disease, but as a group have a lower frequency of nephritis and neuropsychiatric disease. Serologically they may be negative for the standard ANA test. They usually possess precipitating antibodies to the cytoplasmic antigen, Ro.

Acute cutaneous LE   The classic malar butterfly rash (Fig. 3) or the more extensive morbiliform eruption of acute cutaneous LE occurs in 30–40 per cent of SLE patients. The lesions are abrupt in onset, last for hours or days, and frequently coincide with exacerbations of systemic disease. This acute erythematous eruption is sometimes the presenting symptom of SLE and it occurs fre-

quently after exposure to sunlight. The widespread morbiliform rash may resemble a drug reaction, erythema multiforme or toxic epidermal necrolysis.

Immunoglobulin and complement deposition may be found at the dermal epidermal junction on immunofluorescence of these lesions, and form the basis of the 'lupus-band' test. Although positive in most forms of cutaneous LE, fluorescence is found least often in subacute cutaneous LE, and most often in acute LE where it may be found in clinically uninvolved skin (75 per cent). False-positive tests are infrequent.

Vascular lesions   Raynaud's phenomenon is common but generally milder than that seen in scleroderma. Vasculitic lesions may occur in 20 per cent of patients. These tender indurated nodules commonly occur on finger-tips, and on the elbows. Livedo reticularis is not uncommon and may fluctuate with disease activity.

Other lesions   Alopecia may occur at some time in 60 per cent of patients but is often seen at the onset of disease. Mild hair fall may be associated with corticosteroid therapy. Mouth ulcers occur in 30–40 per cent of patients. They are frequently painless and may herald an impending exacerbation. Epiglottitis and laryngeal involvement, although rare, may be life-threatening.

Central nervous system
CNS involvement occurs in up to 60 per cent of patients, and is a major cause of morbidity. There is no universally acceptable classification of CNS lupus but a practical one is to differentiate between primary nervous system disease and complications arising from other organ involvement or therapy. The primary disease can be further divided into neurological, psychiatric or mixed neuropsychiatric disease, the latter being the most common.

Primary CNS involvement
Neurological
The neurological features are summarized in Table 4. Each may occur as an isolated event, but is usually accompanied by other clinical features of disease activity. Seizures and EEG abnormalities are common and may precede the diagnosis by many years. Movement disorder such as chorea may also be an early manifestation. Thrombotic vascular episodes are occasional presenting features, and may be associated with the presence of the circulating lupus anticoagulant (see later). Spinal involvement with mono- or para-

Table 4 Neurological manifestations of CNS disease in SLE

Seizures (grand mal, petit mal, Jacksonian, temporal lobe)
Chorea
Aseptic meningitis
Vascular episodes (migraine, strokes)
Cortical atrophy
Transverse myelitis
Neuritis (cranial and peripheral sensory and motor neuropathies, mononeuritis multiplex, Guillain-Barré syndrome)
Apparent demyelination
Neuromuscular junction disorder (myasthenia gravis)
Cerebellar disorders (ataxia)
Extrapyramidal disorders (rigidity, tremor)
Pseudotumour cerebri
Hypothalamic–pituitary disorders (inappropriate ADH secretion)

Table 5 Secondary CNS involvement in SLE

Primary disorder	Neurological and psychiatric features
Uraemia	Headache, confusion, drowsiness, restlessness, insomnia, seizures, coma, polyneuropathy
Hypertension	Headache, confusion, seizures, visual impairment, focal lesions, coma
Infection	Meningitis, intracerebral abscess
Coagulopathy	Intracerebral haemorrhage/infarction
Corticosteroids	Depression, sleep disturbance, psychosis, euphoria

paresis, is rare but may occur as the only feature of neurological disease, and clinical pictures similar to multiple sclerosis but with lupus serology have been described. Peripheral neuropathy occurs in 10 per cent of cases. The other features in Table 4 are uncommon but well described. A major feature of SLE is headache, and both typical and atypical migraine are often troublesome and sometimes incapacitating.

Psychiatric
Between 20 and 40 per cent of SLE patients develop organic psychiatric disease, although this is probably a gross underestimate. Clinical presentations vary from mild depressive attacks and phobias to behaviour disorders and even severe schizophrenia-like syndromes. Fortunately, psychiatric disease in SLE rarely leaves permanent sequelae.

Secondary CNS involvement
Neuropsychiatric features secondary to other organ involvement are summarized in Table 5. Corticosteroids are an uncommon cause of psychiatric problems, especially with the lower doses now recommended. Intracranial infection is a serious and sometimes fatal complication, particularly in patients receiving corticosteroids or immunosuppressive drugs. Meningism may not always be due to infection, but SLE patients are prone to a form of aseptic meningitis associated with the ingestion of certain anti-inflammatory drugs, e.g. ibuprofen and indomethacin.

Pathology
There is no single characteristic feature. Gross lesions may not be obvious, but microscopic abnormalities are common, especially multiple microinfarcts. Significantly, vasculitis is a relatively uncommon feature. Immune complex deposits have been found in the choroid plexus of a few patients with CNS disease, and it is speculated that disturbances of the blood–brain barrier integrity may also be of pathogenetic importance.

Renal
Clinical nephritis (see page 18.48) occurs in up to 75 per cent of SLE patients, occurring usually within 5 years of onset, and more rarely as a presenting feature. However, almost all patients show

Table 6 Histopathological features of lupus nephritis

Description	Histological features	Electron microscopic features
Minimal change	Normal or mesangial hyperplasia	Immune deposits in mesangium
Focal glomerulonephritis	Glomerular hypercellularity focal and segmental proliferative changes in minority of glomeruli	Subendothelial deposits
Membranous glomerulonephritis	Evenly thickened glomerular capillary basement membrane	Subepithelial and mesangial deposits
Diffuse proliferative glomerulonephritis	Diffuse endothelial and mesangial thickening Most glomeruli involved 'Wire-loop' lesions and crescent formation	Widespread large subepithelial and subendothelial deposits giving rise to wire-loop appearance

glomerular abnormalities on biopsy even when urine and renal function are normal. In over 90 per cent of patients the clinical presentation of lupus nephritis is proteinuria with full nephrotic syndrome in 50 per cent. Most patients have microscopic haematuria, but the macroscopic haematuria of acute nephrotic syndrome is rare. Mild hypertension accompanies renal presentation in about 25 per cent. Rapidly progressive glomerulonephritis or acute renal failure are occasional modes of presentation, or they may develop as a feature of already diagnosed disease. Reduction in glomerular filtration rate and presence of casts, hyaline, granular, and red cell casts, accompany these complications.

Clinical features at the onset of nephritis, including nephrotic syndrome, do not discriminate between patients with a good or bad prognosis. However, age of onset less than 20 years does carry a slightly better prognosis. Overall 10-year survival rates from the onset of nephritis are 65 per cent, and are no different for patients with mild or severe forms at first biopsy, presumably because treatment of severe disease has improved survival. Renal failure is usually a late event. Whilst high titres of anti-DNA antibodies and low serum complement are usually found in patients with active renal involvement, changes in them do not necessarily parallel activity of the nephritis. The timing of renal biopsy in SLE is still controversial, but is generally indicated in patients with marked proteinuria or abnormal urinary sediment. Histologically there are four main patterns (Table 6). Proliferative glomerulonephritis (focal or diffuse) is the most commonly seen and membranous the least common. Immunofluorescence may show deposition of IgG, IgM, and C3 mainly, but also IgA, C1q, and C4. Only 25 per cent of specimens demonstrate all these reactions. Properdin and factor B may also be deposited, suggesting involvement of both direct and alternate pathways of complement activation. Fibrin may be deposited especially in the crescents of severe disease and in association with thrombi. These features are associated with progression to glomerulosclerosis, i.e. irreversible nephron loss and renal failure. Histological transformation from one pattern to another is probably quite common. Treatment may also result in regression of histological features, usually with clinical improvement.

A degree of interstitial nephritis often co-exists with the glomerular changes of SLE, and may be associated with immune deposits in the basement membranes of the renal tubules. If interstitial changes are the only pathological feature, urinary findings may be minimal or absent, although renal tubular acidosis may be found.

Pulmonary
Respiratory symptoms occur very commonly in SLE and dyspnoea may be due to lung or extrapulmonary disease. Pleurisy with

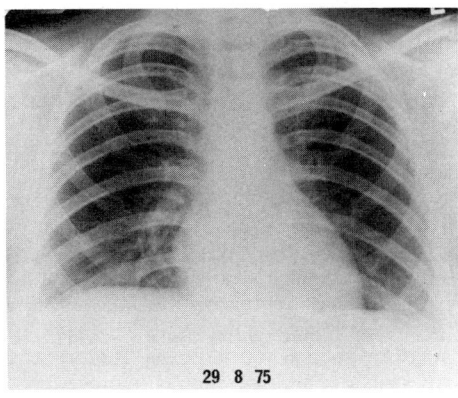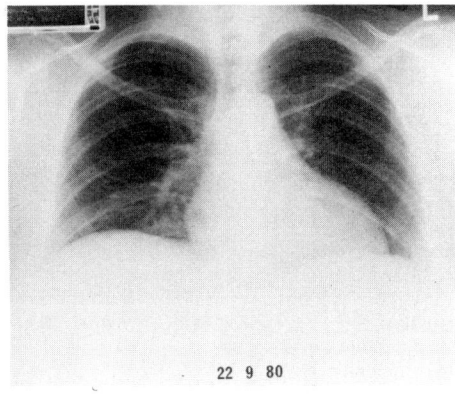

Fig. 4 Progressive elevation of the diaphragms in SLE ('shrinking lung').

pleural effusion is the commonest manifestation. The fluid is an exudate with an excess of neutrophils or lymphocytes, but unlike rheumatoid arthritis, the glucose concentration is normal. The pleurisy may be dry, and cause recurrent or persistent pain often without radiographic changes. Gradual elevation of the diaphragms, with obliteration of costophrenic angles is a well-recognized X-ray finding resulting in 'shrinking lungs' (Fig. 4). The restrictive defect on lung function tests in this situation is due to diaphragmatic abnormality rather than interstitial lung disease. Acute or chronic lung disease is less common, but acute pneumonitis, recurrent atelectasis, pulmonary infiltrates or fibrosis are occasionally encountered. Infections are a frequent problem especially in immunosuppressed patients where unusual infective agents should be sought, e.g. nocardia, legionnaire's, pneumocystis etc. Pulmonary hypertension, once thought uncommon, is now being recognized more frequently and may be associated with anticardiolipin antibodies and thrombosis.

Cardiovascular

The commonest cardiac lesion is pericarditis reported in 20–30 per cent of SLE patients. Asymptomatic pericardial effusions may be detected by echocardiography in up to 60 per cent of patients with active disease. Substernal pain aggravated by leaning forward or coughing is the usual complaint, and pleuritis is a frequent accompanying feature. A friction rub may be heard and electrocardiography may confirm the diagnosis. Constrictive pericarditis and tamponade are rare complications.

Mild myocarditis with focal fibrinoid change in the walls of small arteries and septa is a fairly common post-mortem finding. Clinically the diagnosis is based on tachycardia out of proportion to fever, gallop rhythm, and cardiomegaly. There is often concomitant pericarditis and an ECG may show a prolonged PR interval or other conduction abnormalities. The condition rarely results in cardiac failure. A distinctive non-infective endocarditis (Libman–Sacks endocarditis) may occur in SLE but again this is largely a post-mortem finding, with rarely any clinical significance. Systolic murmurs which may occur in up to 70 per cent of lupus patients can often be attributed to fever, anaemia, and tachycardia. Infective endocarditis is rare.

'Early' coronary artery disease may occur. While the pathogenesis of this accelerated arterial disease has been associated with corticosteroid therapy in some cases, it may be a manifestation of the thrombotic tendency associated with anticardiolpin antibodies.

Haematological

Haematological features are very common, especially in patients with active disease. Mild to moderate normochromic, normocytic anaemia is most frequently encountered, with haemolysis, either Coombs positive or negative, being seen less often. Leucopenia occurs in up to 65 per cent of patients and lymphopenia is common even when total white cell count is normal. This contrasts with other vasculitides where the white cell count is usually elevated.

Mild thrombocytopenia is a frequent occurrence but levels below 50 000/mm are uncommon. Apparent 'idiopathic' thrombocytopenia may antedate the development of SLE by years. Direct and/or indirect antiplatelet antibodies occur in over 80 per cent of patients, but their presence does not correlate with platelet numbers. Bone marrow examination may help to differentiate between immune and drug-induced thrombocytopenia. More rarely a dyserythropoeitic marrow may follow the prolonged use of cytotoxic drugs such as chlorambucil.

The lupus anticoagulant is detected by its prolongation of coagulation tests, particularly those of the intrinsic pathway. Prolongation is not corrected by addition of an equal volume of normal plasma, excluding a factor deficiency. It is an antibody interfering with prothrombin activator complex, and is found in 30–40 per cent of patients, if more sensitive tests are used. Its presence is associated with a false-positive test for syphilis, and high titres of antibodies against cardiolipin, this cross-reactivity being explained by its antiphospholipid activity. Presence of the anticoagulant is not associated with a bleeding tendency, unless there is concomitant severe thrombocytopenia or prothrombin deficiency, and biopsies and surgery can be carried out without problem. Paradoxically it is associated with a high risk of either arterial or venous thrombosis and recurrent abortion (see page 11.10). The exact mechanism is unknown, but a block of the metabolism of arachidonic acid to prostacyclin (PG_{12}), a potent inhibitor of platelet aggregation has been suggested. Antibodies against clotting factors are rare but those against factor VIII may cause severe haemorrhagic problems. These anticoagulants are usually corticosteroid sensitive.

The ESR and other acute phase reactants are usually elevated in periods of disease activity, including complement levels especially C3. C-reactive protein (CRP) levels, however, are usually normal or near normal except in the presence of infection. A frequent and striking finding in the SLE patient is an ESR in excess of 100 and a CRP of zero.

Other systems

Gastrointestinal symptoms such as anorexia and nausea may accompany other manifestations of SLE. Crampy intermittent non-specific abdominal pain occasionally occurs with active disease, but localizing signs must be treated as an emergency, as mesenteric arteritis may lead to bowel infarction. Clinical ascites is rarely found but serositis is a frequent post-mortem finding, with or without pancreatitis.

Hepatomegaly or splenomegaly occur in 20–30 per cent of patients. Jaundice is rare. Mild elevations or transaminases may parallel disease activity, though higher enzyme levels may result

Table 7 Features suggesting a diagnosis of SLE

Female > male
Negro > white
< 40 years old
No joint erosions after two years
Lymphopenia
Drug allergy
Alopecia
Neuropsychiatric disturbance
Livedo reticularis
Vascular thrombosis (venous or arterial)
Photosensitivity
False-positive tests for syphilis
Low serum complement

---

from salicylate ingestion or from CMV infection. Non-tender lymphadenopathy occurs in up to 50 per cent of patients, whereas parotid enlargement is much less common.

Differential diagnosis

Mild forms of SLE may masquerade as other diseases for many years, especially the joint complaints or neuropsychiatric problems. The American Rheumatism Association 1982 revised criteria for the diagnosis of SLE provides a useful check list of features to look for when SLE is suspected. However, they were designed for classification for use in clinical and therapeutic studies, rather than clinical diagnosis, and using these criteria mild cases will be missed. Table 7 shows useful pointers to the diagnosis of SLE, and screening for autoantibodies should be a standard investigation, where these features are encountered. The immunofluorescence test for ANA is a valuable screening test and has replaced the LE cell test. It is not specific for SLE, however, being found frequently in other connective tissue diseases, in other autoimmune diseases and in approximately 5 per cent of the normal population. Antibodies to native DNA are found in over 60 per cent of SLE patients and rarely in other conditions such as chronic active hepatitis and Sjögren's syndrome. Antibodies to certain ribonucleoproteins and cytoplasmic antigens (see Table 1) may support the diagnosis of SLE when antibodies to DNA are absent. The main conditions in the differential diagnosis of SLE are rheumatoid arthritis, other connective tissue diseases, subacute bacterial endocarditis, lymphoma, idiopathic thrombocytopenia, thrombotic thrombocytopenia, gonococcal septicaemia, and sarcoidosis.

Management

General measures

Monitoring disease activity SLE is a chronic disease of exacerbation and remission and patients do require long-term support. It is not known whether treatment during remission alters prognosis. An important step forward in the treatment of SLE has been the realization that it is not a uniformly fatal disease requiring large doses of toxic drugs. Assessing disease activity can be difficult as serological abnormalities do not necessarily reflect clinical features. However, rising titres of antinuclear activity or DNA-binding and falling complement levels suggest an exacerbation. An infective episode can mimic a flare of SLE, and in this situation a raised CRP is an indicator of infection. Infection is still one of the major causes of death and atypical pathogens should be specifically sought. In practice, however, a flare frequently accompanies or follows infection. Exacerbation is also more common during the puerperium. The foundation of good management of SLE is careful monitoring, of all the systems which could be involved, and the treatment of new problems along conventional lines. Steroids need not be prescribed simply because the diagnosis is SLE, when other therapies exist for the particular problem encountered.

Specific problems Ultraviolet light barrier creams provide protection from photosensitivity and other skin lesions can sometimes be treated with topical preparations. Antigenic stimuli such as immunization should be avoided in patients with active disease or in those receiving immunosuppressive therapy. Drug sensitivity is common, but certain drugs should be used with care as they may provoke exacerbation in some individuals, e.g. sulphonamides, penicillin, and oral contraceptives. However, the majority of SLE patients can use the low oestrogen contraceptive pill without problems. Drugs known to induce lupus syndromes, e.g. hydralazine and anticonvulsants, are not specifically contraindicated in idiopathic SLE. Patients with Raynaud's syndrome should be advised to stop smoking and symptoms may be controlled by simple measures such as warm gloves. If more severe, conventional therapy such as nifedipine should be prescribed.

End-stage renal disease requires management along the usual lines. Often at this stage SLE activity is quiescent, and this may explain why the recurrence of lupus nephritis in transplanted kidneys is rare, survival of grafts into lupus recipients being similar to that in other individuals.

Drugs

Spontaneous remission is common in SLE, and many patients can be managed without drugs, or only require simple medication such as non-steroidal anti-inflammatory drugs for musculoskeletal manifestations. A proportion of patients develop hepatotoxicity on aspirin, but other anti-inflammatory agents are generally well tolerated.

Antimalarials Chloroquine salts are still considered first-line agents for SLE, especially where cutaneous and joint manifestations predominate. With the prolonged medication required for SLE side-effects such as headache, gastrointestinal disturbance, skin eruptions, and hair fall may be encountered, but the major concern with those drugs is ocular toxicity. Transient impairment of accommodation is a common early side-effect, and rarely requires discontinuation of the drug, though patients should be warned regarding driving or operating machinery. Subepithelial corneal deposits of unchanged material compound may occur, but these are not a marker of incipient retinal toxicity and disappear completely when the drug is stopped.

As retinal damage may be asymptomatic until toxicity is advanced and irreversible, baseline and annual ophthalmological examination is recommended. With daily maintenance doses not exceeding 200 mg for hydroxychloroquine and 250 mg for chloroquine, the risk of ocular toxicity is low. Chloroquine salts are probably underutilized in SLE.

Corticosteroids Many patients can be managed without corticosteroids, or on a low-dose or even alternate-day regime. There are two major reasons for prescribing corticosteroids. They may occasionally be required when non-life-threatening features fail to respond to other measures and are causing severe morbidity. In this situation, features such as arthritis, rash, fever, pleurisy, pericarditis, and haemolytic anaemia may respond dramatically, and doses of prednisolone greater than 0.5 mg/kg/day are rarely required. This dose, however, may need to be doubled (1 mg/kg/day) when major life-threatening manifestations develop such as severe nephritis, seizures, coma, widespread organic brain disease, severe thrombocytopenia or vasculitis involving major organs or peripheral nerves. Response to therapy is very variable, but high doses should not be continued for long periods. Above all else, steroid dosage exceeding 40 mg prednisolone daily is associated with an increased incidence of infection as well as aseptic bone necrosis. The side-effects of long-term therapy are well known, and whatever the indication for steroid therapy, once clinical response is achieved the dose should be tapered to the lowest required to control symptoms. Side-effects can be further minimized by once daily morning doses, or alternate day therapy.

Pulsed methyl prednisolone The use of intermittent high-dose intravenous methyl prednisolone was developed to avoid the side-effects of prolonged oral steroids. The 'pulse' usually consists of 1 g of methyl prednisolone by slow i.v. infusion, administered on three consecutive days. Favourable results have been reported in patients with rapidly deteriorating renal function and diffuse proliferative nephritis but there is no evidence yet for its effectiveness in non-renal disease. Furthermore, side-effects are still encountered. Some are those associated with oral therapy, e.g. hyperglycaemia, sodium retention, and acute psychosis, but others are unique to this form of therapy, such as flushing, a metallic taste in the mouth, and painful joints a few days later, with non-inflammatory effusions. There is some evidence that there are fewer infections associated with pulse therapy.

Immunosuppressives The most frequently used cytotoxic agents are azathioprine, cyclophosphamide, and chlorambucil. They are rarely used alone, as they are too slow acting, and various studies have suggested that combinations of these drugs with prednisolone are more effective than either alone. The major indications are severe active lupus nephritis, and for a 'steroid-sparing' effect in patients requiring large doses of corticosteroids and developing side-effects.

Azathioprine with its lower ratio of toxicity is used most often, though controlled clinical trials of its effectiveness are inconclusive. At a daily dose of 1–2 mg/kg/day, bone marrow toxicity may occur, and occasionally allergic hepatitis is seen, necessitating withdrawal of the drug. The risk of developing malignancies following administration of azathioprine is not known but appears small.

Cyclophosphamide and chlorambucil, both alkylating agents, have a higher ratio of toxicity and are usually reserved for the minority of severely ill patients unresponsive to other drugs. Oral cyclophosphamide is associated with a high level of toxicity, and intermittent i.v. regimes of 0.5–1.0 g/m² are advocated to minimize this, with particular success in renal disease. Chlorambucil is usually prescribed at a dose of 0.05–0.2 mg/kg/day, but with both of these agents, the benefit of treatment, even if demonstrable must be balanced against the potential toxicity which include malignancies (particularly lymphomas and acute leukaemias), fatal infections, infertility, and with cyclophosphamide, bladder dysfunction.

Plasma exchange (plasmapheresis) Plasma exchange is successful in removing damaging circulating antibody in patients with Goodpasture's syndrome and myasthenia gravis. A controlled trial in SLE showed plasmapheresis to be effective in reducing circulating immune complexes and reducing DNA binding and other serological features, but rapid rebound to pretreatment levels occurred, and the frequency and degree of clinical improvement was the same in both plasma exchange and control groups. There is some anecdotal evidence that plasma exchange accompanied by other forms of immunosuppression might be beneficial. Several deaths have been reported due to cardiac dysrhythmia or occlusion of the pulmonary vascular bed. This form of therapy is limited to severe and potentially fatal disease states.

Prognosis

This has improved with recognition of milder forms of disease, and a more conservative approach to treatment. Recent data showed an estimated mean five-year survival of 98 per cent, and even in nephritis survival has been calculated at 76 per cent for five years and 65 per cent at ten years from the onset of clinical nephritis. Renal disease still carries the gravest prognosis, with CNS disease coming a close second, and assuming an increasing role in morbidity and mortality after five years of disease. Until recently, SLE was regarded with dread, but it is now recognized that the disease may be milder than rheumatoid arthritis, and is certainly milder than many other connective tissue diseases.

Table 8 Drugs implicated in drug-induced lupus

Frequent	Rare
Hydralazine	Aminosalicylic acid
Procainamide	D-penicillamine
Anticonvulsants (phenytoin, hydantoins, primidone)	L-dopa
	Methyldopa
Isoniazid	Methylthiouracil
Chlorpromazine	Propylthiouracil
Oral contraceptives (may exacerbate pre-existing SLE)	Phenylbutazone
	Practolol
	Quinidine
	Reserpine
	Sulphonamides
	Allopurinol
	Gold salts

Table 9 Differentiation between drug-induced and idiopathic SLE

Feature	Drug-induced	Idiopathic
Clinical		
Peak age at onset (years)	50–60	20–30
Race	White > black	Black > white
Female:male	5:4	9:1
Joint symptoms	Very common	Very common
Cutaneous	Uncommon	Very common
Pulmonary	Very common	Common
Renal ⎫		
CNS ⎭	Rare	Common
Laboratory		
ANF	+ve	+ve
DNA antibody	−ve	+ve
Antihistone antibody	+ve	+ve
Serum complement	Normal	Usually low

Drug-induced lupus

Drug-induced lupus is rare, and the drugs most frequently implicated are listed in Table 8. Although more than 25 drugs have been reported to induce this syndrome, there are some doubts about their true association, e.g. anticonvulsants may be used in treatment of early manifestations of idiopathic SLE, and sulphonamides may exacerbate SLE or unmask a subclinical state. Hydralazine and procainamide are the most frequently encountered offenders in drug-induced lupus. Prolonged therapy with either agent results in the appearance of a positive ANF in a high proportion of patients, but the full blown picture of lupus-like syndrome is much less common, occurring in approximately 10 per cent of patients on hydralazine and 20 per cent on procainamide. Factors increasing the incidence of the syndrome include large daily and total doses administered, slow drug-acetylator status, and in hydralazine-induced disease, presence of the HLA–DR4 phenotype. One suggested mechanism for the induction of autoantibody was a molecular similarity between the drug and nuclear antigens, resulting in cross-reacting antibodies, but it is now thought more likely that the drugs may react with nuclear antigens, such that the drug–antigen complex is immunogenic. Some of the drugs are known to inhibit T lymphocyte function *in vitro*, and *in vivo* may indirectly alter lymphocyte function by the induction of antilymphocyte antibodies. As in idiopathic SLE, immune complex deposition is a pathological feature of the drug-induced syndrome. Certain drugs, e.g. hydralazine and isoniazid (hydrazine derivatives) inhibit the binding of C4 to antigen–antibody complexes, and in this way may affect the solubilization of complexes and their removal from the circulation. Acetylated metabolites of these drugs show no such inhibition of complement function. Several of these mechanisms may be operating. The main features distinguishing drug-induced from idiopathic SLE are shown in Table 9. Discontinuation of the drug usually results in prompt resolution of the syndrome, though occasionally symptoms may persist for months and steroid therapy may be necessary. It is not necessary to discontinue the drug in asymptomatic patients with ANA, as the majority will never develop clinical symptoms. Some of the drugs thought to induce lupus, may also exacerbate idiopathic SLE, e.g. sulphonamides and oral contraceptives, but hydralazine may be used in idiopathic SLE without adverse effect.

References

Barnett, E. V., Dornfield, L., Lee, D. and Leibling, M. R. (1978). Long term survival of lupus nephritis patients treated with azathioprine and prednisone. *J. Rheumatol.* (5) 3, 275–287.

Batchelor, J. R., Welsh, K I., Tinoco, R. M., Dollery, C. T., Hughes, G. R. V., Bernstein, R., Ryan, P., Naish, P. F., Aber, G. M., Bing, R. F. and Russell G. I. (1980). Hydralazine-induced systemic lupus erythematosus: influence of HLA-DR and sex on susceptibility. *Lancet* i, 1107–1110.

Cameron, J. S., Turner, D. R., Ogg, C. S., Williams, D. G., Lessof, M. H., Chantler, C. and Leibowitz, S. (1979). Systemic lupus with nephritis: a long term study. *Q. J. Med.* 48, 1–24.

Fessel, W. J. (1974). SLE in the community. *Arch. Intern. Med.* 134, 1027–1035.

Fielder, A. H. L., Walport, M. J., Batchelor, J. R., Rynes, R. I., Black, C. M., Dodi, I. A. and Hughes G. R. V. (1983). Family study of the major histocompatibility complex in patients with systemic lupus erythematosus: importance of null alleles of C4A and C4B in determining disease susceptibility. *Br. Med. J.* 286, 425–428.

Ginzler, E. M., Diamond, H. S., Weiner, M., Schlesinger, M., Fries, J. F., Wasner, C., Medsger, T. A., Zeigler, G., Klippel, J. H., Hadler, N. M., Albert, D. A., Hess, E. V., Spencer–Green, G., Grayzel A., Worth, D., Hahn, B. H. and Barnett, E. V. (1982). A multicentre study of outcome in systemic lupus erythematosus. I Entry variables as predictors of prognosis. *Arth. Rheum.* 25, 601–611, 612–617.

Hochberg, M. C., Boyd, R. E., Ahearn, J. M., Arnett, F. C. and Stevens, M. B. (1985). Systemic lupus erythematosus: A review of clinico-laboratory features and immunogenetic markers in 150 patients with emphasis on demographic subsets. *Medicine* 64, 285–295.

Hughes, G. R. V. (cd.) (1982). Systemic lupus erythematosus. *Clinics in rheumatic diseases* Vol. 8, p. 1. W. B. Saunders, Philadephia.

Kant, K. S., Pollak, V. E., Weiss, M. A., Glueck, H. I., Miller, M. A. and Hess, E. V. (1981). Glomerular thrombosis in systemic lupus erythematosus prevalence and significance. *Medicine* 60, 71–86.

Leibling, M. R., McLaughlin, K., Boonsne, S., Kasdin, J. and Barnett, E. V. (1982). Monthly pulses of methyl prednisolone in SLE nephritis. *J. Rheum.* 9, 543–548.

Maddison, P. J., Provost, T. T. and Reichlin, M. (1984). Serological findings in patients with ANA-negative systemic lupus erythematosus. *Medicine* 60, 87–94.

Perry, H. M., Tan, E. M., Carmody, S. and Nakamoto, A. (1970). Relationship of acetyl transferase activity to anti-nuclear antibodies and toxic symptoms in hypertensive patients treated with hydralazine. *J. Lab. clin. Med.* 76, 114–125.

Shoenfeld, Y. and Schwarz, R. S. (1984). Immunologic and genetic factors in autoimmune disease. *N. Engl. J. Med.* 311, 1019–1029.

Sim, E., Gill, E. W. and Sim, R. B. (1984). Drugs that induce systemic lupus erythematosus inhibit complement component C4. *Lancet* ii, 422–423.

Tan, E. M., Cohen, A. S., Fries, J. F., Masi, A. T., McShane, D. J., Rothfield, N. F., Schaller, J. G., Talal, N. and Winchester, R. J. (1982). The 1982 revised criteria for the classification of systemic lupus erythematosus. *Arth. Rheum.* 25, 1271–1277.

Urowitz, M. B., Bookman, A. A. M., Koehler, B. E., Gordon, D. A., Smythe, H. A. and Ogryzlo, M. A. (1976). The biomodal mortality pattern of systemic lupus erythematosus. *Am. J. Med.* 60, 221–225.

Wei, N., Klippel, J. H., Huston, D. P. *et al.* (1983). Randomised trial of plasma exchange in mild SLE. *Lancet* i, 17–21.

Weinstein, A. (1980). Drug-induced systemic lupus erythematosus. *Prog. Clin. Immunol.* 4, 1–21.

POLYARTERITIS AND RELATED SYNDROMES

G. H. NEILD AND D. G. WILLIAMS

Introduction

There are several diseases in which the underlying lesion is inflammation of the vessel wall, i.e. vasculitis or, since it is usually the arteries or arterioles which are affected, polyarteritis. Vasculitis may occur as part of a systemic disease such as systemic lupus erythematosus (SLE), rheumatoid arthritis, and angio-immunoblastic lymphadenopathy, or the vasculitis itself may be the primary disorder. This section will be devoted mainly to describing the latter systemic variety; those forms of vasculitis confined to the skin alone will not be considered.

Virtually nothing is known about the aetiology or pathogenesis of polyarteritis. Traditionally, attempts to classify this condition have related to clinical syndromes, histological definitions of the size of the vessels involved, or the clinicopathological correlations between these two schemes. In practice patients often do not fit easily into one category or the other. Since it is clear that prompt treatment with steroids and immunosuppressive drugs can halt or, in some cases, induce remission of polyarteritis, it is of the utmost importance that the disorder is diagnosed without delay so that appropriate treatment can begin. Therefore, in this description of the clinical features of polyarteritis, priority has been given to an account of the many features which may be seen without at first considering the subgroups into which they may be divided; brief descriptions of these are given later.

Pathology

The term polyarteritis (periarteritis) describes an inflammation of the full thickness of the arterial wall, i.e. adventitia, media, and intima. The term vasculitis extends this definition to include all types of blood vessel. The predominant cells in the inflammatory reaction are mononuclear. In some forms of arteritis, giant cells may be seen ('*giant cell arteritis*') or the mononuclear cells may form granulomata adjacent to the damaged vessel wall ('*granulomatous arteritis*'). An important practical point is that the inflammatory changes are not continuously present along the length of a vessel (Fig. 1), so that histological preparations may miss the affected portion of the vessel and fail to demonstrate the vasculitis.

Inflammation associated with fibrinoid necrosis of the media is described as a necrotizing vasculitis. Fibrinoid, a term deprecated by many pathologists but too widely used to change, indicates that the staining characteristics of fibrin are demonstrable. A polymorph neutrophil reaction accompanies fibrinoid necrosis and the presence of fragmented neutrophils, nuclear debris or karyorrhexis is termed 'leucocytoclasis' by dermatologists. Fibrinoid necrosis is associated with dissolution of the elastic lamina and loss of this structure is an essential finding in making the diagnosis of necrotizing arteritis. Necrosis will heal with fibrosis and scarring but the elastic lamina remains interrupted. Aneurysms may form at points where the elastic lamina has been breached.

Rarely, inflammation of the vessel wall may be confined to the intima. This intimal thickening may lead to luminal stenosis or obstruction and this process is often referred to as an 'endarteritis obliterans'. This process is not an arteritis, in the true sense.

Pathogenesis

The pathogenesis of polyarteritis is poorly understood. The histological changes indicate two main components: cellular infiltration and necrosis of the vessel wall. The mononuclear cell infiltration, especially prominent in the granulomatous forms of polyarteritis, may indicate that a cell-mediated reaction has caused the damage and there is some experimental evidence to support this. In some forms of arteritis, necrosis of the vessel wall is very prominent. In such cases, polymorphs are the predominant cell, and there may be few mononuclear cells. In other forms, for example, drug-related, necrosis is very rare and polymorphs are not seen. Thus, there may be at least two major and distinct components to the injury, one which is cell mediated and the other humorally mediated.

Since a lesion similar to polyarteritis in humans may be seen in animals with immune complex disease, e.g. experimental acute serum sickness and murine SLE with arteritis, and in humans with acute serum sickness the proposal has been made that polyarteritis too is an immune complex disease. Immune complexes can be found in the circulation of some patients but by no means all. Complement and immunoglobulins may be found in the wall of affected vessels, but there is no consistent pattern and deposition may be due to non-specific trapping. Better evidence of immune complex injury come from studies of a small number of patients with polyarteritis associated with hepatitis B in whom the antigen was found in the affected vessel wall and in circulating immune complexes.

Although the general clinical setting of polyarteritis leads one to assume that immunopathogenetic mechanisms cause the tissue damage, other possible mechanisms, e.g. cytotoxins produced by infectious organisms with a secondary inflammatory response, cannot be excluded.

Aetiology

The cause of most cases of polyarteritis is unknown, but there are some associations which suggest possible mechanisms.

1. Occasionally, the illness follows administration of drugs which may act as an antigen or hapten and initiate an immune response. Those most commonly implicated include sulphonamides, penicillins, gold salts, amphetamines, and, more rarely, drugs used by addicts. The evidence that drugs play an aetiological role is, however, circumstantial, and it must be remembered that many patients have a prodromal period with symptoms which may

be interpreted as an infection, for which the incriminating drug(s) is given.

2. More obvious examples of foreign antigens are those due to infections, such as hepatitis B virus, which is assumed to cause an immune complex disease. Evidence of hepatitis B infection is found in less than 10 per cent of cases, contrary to early reports suggesting infection in 30 per cent. Polyarteritis has also been described following streptococcal infections.

3. Very rarely today, a true serum sickness may follow the administration of a foreign protein, such as horse antilymphocyte globulin.

4. Finally, polyarteritis may be associated with lymphoproliferative disorders such as myeloma, lymphoma, hairy cell leukaemia, and angio-immunoblastic lymphadenopathy. It is not known why this should be. It has been suggested that hairy cell leukaemia is associated with reticuloendothelial cell blockade and hence the persistence of immune complexes, but there is no experimental evidence to support this sequence of events.

Clinical features

Polyarteritis most commonly occurs in Caucasians (80–90 per cent of cases). It is slightly more common in males. The overt presentation is usually preceded by a prodromal illness lasting weeks or months consisting of malaise, anorexia, intermittent fever up to 40 °C (40–80 per cent of cases), night sweats, and considerable weight loss (30–70 per cent of cases). Myalgia and arthralgia often accompany this phase. Hypertension is not a major feature at presentation, but becomes more prominent as a sequel to renal injury. The diagnosis may be very difficult before focal signs develop. The different forms of polyarteritis involve the various parts of the body in similar ways although some organs are involved more commonly in specific forms of arteritis. The ways in which different organs are involved is now described.

Ear, nose, and throat

Upper respiratory tract involvement is common, occurring in 30–60 per cent of cases, and may be the sole presenting feature.

Ear There may be a secretory otitis media with earache and conductive deafness. Sensorineural deafness and tinnitus can also occur. The mechanism of the otitis media is unknown, although rarely it is associated with obstruction of the Eustachian tube by granuloma. The pinna may be painful and inflamed due to chondritis.

Nose Epistaxis, nasal obstruction, rhinorrhoea or pain from sinuses may occur. These are all very much more common with the granulomatous vasculitides. Thickening of the sinus mucosa is common; polyps are found particularly with the Churg–Strauss syndrome. Granulomata may cause ulceration of any part of the nasal cavity. If chondritis occurs, the nasal cartilage may be painful and inflamed, and later there may be complete collapse of the cartilaginous nose.

Throat Ulceration of the hard or soft palate, often very painful, but occasionally painless, may be seen. Granulomatous involvement of the cord or inflammation of the crico-arytenoid joints can cause hoarseness and rarely, stridor.

Lung

Lower respiratory tract involvement occurs in 40–65 per cent of patients. Dyspnoea, cough, haemoptysis, and pleuritic pain are the more common symptoms. Radiological opacities may be due to granulomata, alveolar haemorrhage or infarction. Small vessel disease may lead to pneumonitis and pulmonary fibrosis. Large granulomata may cavitate and can become colonized by fungi. Haemoptysis varies from slight streaking of sputum to massive haemorrhage. Lung haemorrhage, without haemoptysis resembles pulmonary oedema radiologically and may be difficult to diagnose; one may be alerted by an unaccountably low haemoglobin. When fresh alveolar haemorrhage is present, the K_{CO} (rate con-

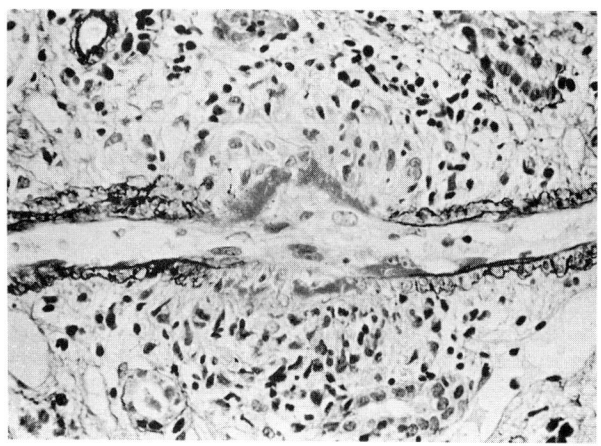

Fig. 1 Longtitudinal section through a medium-sized artery from a patient with polyarteritis showing the segmental nature of the inflammation (× 125).

stant for CO transfer corrected for haemoglobin) is usually raised. The K_{CO} is normal or reduced in pulmonary oedema and low in pulmonary fibrosis. Lung haemorrhage may also be demonstrated by the detection of haemosiderin in alveolar lavage.

Joints
Joint symptoms occur in about 60 per cent. A migratory polyarthralgia is a common symptom in the prodrome. Arthritis (synovitis) is uncommon (10–15 per cent). A periostitis with typical radiological features may also occur.

Muscle
Muscle involvement may present as myalgia or weakness, and is found in 30–80 per cent of patients. Diffuse myositis with elevated levels of CPK is very uncommon. A muscle biopsy, frequently performed for diagnostic purposes, is pointless unless the muscle is painful or inflamed. Electromyography may be useful to localize injured muscle.

Eye
Eye involvement is common (40–80 per cent of cases), but may be subtle and overlooked. The eye may be red and painful. Redness is usually due to episcleritis, not conjunctivitis. Scleritis is less common but potentially more serious as it may lead to perforation of the sclera. Anterior uveitis is uncommon and is suggested by pain and loss of visual acuity in addition to redness. Retinal vasculitis is common. Small haemorrhages and exudates may be seen in 10–20 per cent of cases and rarely there may be small infarcts, but these fundal changes are non-specific. Fluorescein angiography will show diffuse vessel leakage and infarcts.

In the absence of severe hypertension and uveitis, loss of visual acuity may be due to retinal vasculitis at the macula, optic nerve involvement due to posterior ciliary arteritis, involvement of the central retinal artery which supplies the retina, or vasculitis of the choroidal circulation. The latter may be very difficult to diagnose. The patient presents with loss of visual acuity and oedema of the macula (serous maculopathy). Subtle changes on the fluorescein angiogram may demonstrate the changes in the choroidal circulation.

Rarely, the orbit may be involved by a granuloma which can lead to proptosis, diplopia, and loss of visual acuity.

Nervous system
Peripheral nervous system Peripheral nerves are involved in 50–70 per cent of patients. There are two forms of peripheral nerve disease. Vasculitis of the vessels supplying the peripheral nerves causes an ischaemic injury and leads to mononeuritis multiplex. The nerves to the extremities are most commonly involved and the lower limbs more frequently than the upper. The second form is a symmetrical lower limb polyneuropathy with a cutaneous sensory loss in a stocking distribution. Nerve involvement is typically slow to improve and any recovery may be incomplete.

Central nervous system Cerebral and vertebral artery involvement occurs in about 25 per cent of cases. The higher mental functions may be affected with loss of short-term memory, loss of intellect, and change in personality. Focal lesions may occur in the cerebrum, cerebellum, and brain stem with accompanying fits. Isolated cranial nerve lesions and focal involvement of the spinal cord may occur rarely.

Genitourinary tract
Involvement of the kidneys is common, occurring in 65–80 per cent of cases and is associated with a poor prognosis. Patients may present with extrarenal symptoms but be found to have asymptomatic renal disease manifest as microscopic haematuria and proteinuria with or without a raised plasma creatinine concentration. A rapidly progressive renal failure, developing from normal renal function to anuria over a matter of days or weeks is usually due to a severe necrotizing glomerulonephritis, often accompanied by crescent formation. Very rarely, patients present with a nephrotic

syndrome. A less common cause of renal failure is infarction of the kidneys. Hypertension, which particularly accompanies classical polyarteritis nodosa, can probably contribute to the renal damage.

Vasculitis of the ureter, bladder, epididymis, and testis are rare, but may lead to pain, haematuria, haemospermia, and even infarction of these organs.

Skin
A wide range of skin lesions is found in 20–50 per cent of patients, but the majority are non-specific. Specific lesions include skin necrosis, subcutaneous nodules with or without ulceration and necrosis, and livedo reticularis. Cutaneous nodules are more common with the granulomatous vasculitides. They are found most commonly on extensor aspects of the elbows, then on the fingers and thumbs. On the digits, they are often multiple and symmetrical over the distal phalanx. They are also found on the scalp as immobile indurated lesions. Nodules may ulcerate and become infected. Indolent, chronic ulceration of the skin is common with rheumatoid vasculitis.

The non-specific lesions include macular erythema, erythema multiforme, erythema nodosum, petechial haemorrhage, subungual or splinter haemorrhages, purpura which may be macular or papular, urticaria in the form of vesicles, bullae or pustules, and alopecia. All these lesions may show morphological evidence of vasculitis.

Cardiovascular system
All parts of the heart may be involved, and involvement is seen in 10–50 per cent of patients. Coronary arteritis and thrombosis may lead to massive myocardial infarction and sudden death. Smaller vessel disease will cause a more diffuse muscle injury with ischaemia, multiple foci of necrosis, and fibrosis which lead to ventricular failure. Myocardial involvement is very common when an eosinophilia is present and there may be eosinophilic myocarditis. Pericarditis is also common.

Raynaud's phenomenon is a common accompaniment of vasculitis. Arteritis of limb vessels is not common, but may occur leading to peripheral ischaemia. Rarely, arteritis of the vasa vasorum can lead to rupture or a dissecting aneurysm of the major vessels.

Gastrointestinal tract
This system is involved in 25–30 per cent of patients. In the mouth, ulceration is common and may be extensive. Haemorrhages and infarcts of the mucosa may be seen. Very rarely, infarction of the pulp of the teeth may occur. Gastrointestinal symptoms are usually vague and non-specific and include abdominal pain, diarrhoea, and haemorrhage. Mesenteric arteritis may lead to abdominal catastrophy in the form of gut or pancreatic infarction. In Henoch–Schönlein purpura, protein-losing enteropathy may be severe and the protein loss may lead to hypovolaemia.

Hepatic involvement is usually an incidental finding although arteritis can involve the liver or the gall bladder causing perforation and biliary peritonitis. Hepatomegaly occurs in 40 per cent of cases. Liver function tests may be mildly abnormal in 50 per cent but there are no diagnostic features.

Clinical subgroups of polyarteritis
Polyarteritis nodosa
In classic polyarteritis nodosa the larger sized vessels are affected and the inflammation produces the characteristic 'nodules'. The onset may be acute and devastating with arteritis leading to ischaemia and infarction of the involved organ. Mortality is usually related to coronary involvement and myocardial infarction, pancreatic involvement and pancreatitis, mesenteric involvement and bowel ischaemia or infarction, or renal involvement and uraemia.

Microscopic polyarteritis
This condition, also known as hypersensitivity angiitis, refers to polyarteritis affecting the smaller arteries. It is the most common

form of arteritis. The whole range of clinical features may be seen and it is this form in particular which may present with renal involvement.

Wegener's granulomatosis

Wegener described this condition as 'a variant of polyarteritis in which nasal or paranasal granulomata were prominent features'. The brunt of the disease falls upon the upper and lower respiratory tract and the kidneys. An association with chronic suppurative disease of the respiratory tract has been described. Morphologically the vasculitis is associated with granulomata which may also occur in extravascular sites.

Patients usually present with upper respiratory tract symptoms, particularly rhinorrhoea or sinusitis, and at presentation 70 per cent have radiological evidence of pulmonary infiltration. Their other manifestations of systemic vasculitis are no different, nor less serious, than other patients with microscopic polyarteritis. However, demographically, patients with this syndrome are a well-characterized and homogenous group. There is a male-to-female ratio of approximately 1.6:1 and the condition appears to be very uncommon in non-whites.

The strict diagnosis of this clinico-pathological syndrome depends on the histological demonstration of granulomata in the respiraory tract. In clinical practice, this may not be possible and, when performed, biopsy of nasal lesions often reveals merely necrotic debris and chronic inflammatory tissue. This means that many physicians accept 'polyarteritis plus lung involvement' as an *a priori* diagnosis of 'Wegener's granulomatosis', which in turn means that in some published series, 'polyarteritis' does not appear to involve the lungs. Since both conditions respond to steroids and immunosuppressive drugs, this diagnostic dilemma is not of major importance, although some authors have claimed that Wegener's granulomatosis responds to cyclophosphamide better than azathioprine.

Churg–Strauss syndrome

Churg and Strauss described another variant of polyarteritis in which patients had asthma and eosinophilia (more than $1.5 \times 10^9/l$). Histologically, they found both a granulomatous vasculitis and extravascular granulomata with giant cells and necrotic collagen at the centre of the granuloma, a syndrome they called 'allergic granulomatosis'.

Patients with this syndrome characteristically have a long prodrome of allergic disease; the sexes are equally affected. Most patients have had allergic rhinitis, with a mean age of onset of 28 years, and this associated with nasal polyposis, nasal obstruction, and recurrent sinusitis. Asthma commences at a mean age of 35 years, and vasculitis three years later. During the prodromal period, episodes of asthma, and eosinophilia may be associated with transient pulmonary infiltrates (Loeffler's eosinophilic pneumonia). The vasculitis has a predilection for the heart and may be associated with myocarditis; 48 per cent of deaths have a cardiac cause. Like Wegener's granulomatosis, the systemic manifestations of the vasculitis are no different from those of polyarteritis (see above).

Henoch–Schönlein purpura (page 18.36 and Section 20)

This syndrome is typically a disease of prepubertal boys; with the majority aged six months to six years. It is characterized by the tetrad of a purpuric rash, colicky abdominal pain with or without bloody diarrhoea, arthralgia, and glomerulonephritis. The organ involvement may develop in any chronological order. The symptoms are due to a necrotizing vasculitis affecting arterioles, capillaries, and venules. The distribution of the rash is characteristic and involves feet, extensor surfaces of the legs, and the buttocks. Histological examination of the skin shows that the postcapillary venule is most frequently affected. Joint pains occur in two-thirds, with ankles and knees, then hips, wrists, and fingers, being involved most commonly. Gastrointestinal symptoms occur in 60–70 per cent of cases, although they are less common in those

under two years. The jejunum and ileum are most commonly involved. A protein-losing enteropathy may occur. The glomerulonephritis presents as a nephritic illness, usually with just proteinuria and haematuria but some may develop a nephrotic syndrome or even crescentic nephritis with rapidly progressive renal failure. The glomerular lesion is characterized by deposits of IgA in the mesangium, and IgA may be found in vessel walls in fresh areas of vasculitis.

The condition is rare in adults in whom the diagnosis of Henoch–Schönlein purpura should not be used unless glomerular or vascular IgA is demonstrated. Often, adults given a clinical diagnosis of Henoch–Schönlein purpura are found to have polyarteritis.

Essential cryoglobulinaemia (Section 19)

This condition may be associated with a typical necrotizing polyarteritis and is characterized by palpable purpura, weakness, arthralgia, and hepatosplenomegaly. Renal involvement is common and characterized by a diffuse proliferative glomerulonephritis with glomerular deposits of immunoglobulins and complement, in contrast to the segmental necrotizing glomerulonephritis that is most commonly seen with polyarteritis.

Cryoglobulins, serum proteins which precipitate at temperatures below 37 °C, are usually found in conjunction with a systemic illness; the term *essential* implies that no underlying condition has been identified. The commonest underlying conditions fall into three groups: connective tissue diseases, lympho-proliferative neoplasms including angio-immunoblastic lymphadenopathy, and chronic infections, which are usually bacterial (prosthetic infections, visceral abscesses), lepromatous leprosy or secondary syphilis. Cryoglobulins are divided into three types depending on their immunochemical characteristics: Type I, in which the cryoglobulin is a monoclonal Ig of Bence-Jones protein; type II, a mixed form with a monoclonal component acting as an antibody (rheumatoid factor) against polyclonal IgG; type III, a mixed form with one or more classes of polyclonal Ig.

In one series of patients from New York with essential cryoglobulinaemia and hepatic dysfunction 75 per cent had evidence of hepatitis B infection with HBs antigen or antibody in their serum or cryoglobulin. This had not been found in series from other parts of the United States or elsewhere.

Kawasaki's syndrome (mucocutaneous lymph-node syndrome)

This syndrome (page 24.1) is very rare in the west, but is common in Japan where it was first described by Kawasaki. Its frequency in the Japanese is partly explained by its association with an HLA haplotype peculiar to this race. It is an acute, febrile illness of young children, characterized by hyperaemia of the oropharynx and ocular conjunctivae, a strawberry tongue, and cervical lymphadenopathy. There is also peripheral oedema and erythema of the soles and palms which later desquamate. In these respects, this illness is very similar to scarlet fever or the more recently described 'toxic shock' syndrome. The disease, the cause of which is unknown, is usually self-limiting but may be followed by an arteritis with a predilection for the coronary arteries. There is a 1–2 per cent mortality due to cardiac causes. The coronary arteritis is associated with aneurysm formation. Deaths occur 3–5 weeks after the onset of the illness and may be due to myocarditis, myocardial infarction or rupture of an aneurysm. This condition is probably the same as so-called 'infantile polyarteritis nodosa'.

Giant cell ('temporal' or 'cranial') arteritis

In this form of necrotizing arteritis, giant cells are found adjacent to the ruptured internal elastic lamina. The disease is usually confined to branches of the carotid artery, although rarely it may behave as a systemic arteritis. It affects persons over 55 years and occurs equally in men and women. It is characterized by fever, weakness, headaches with tender scalp arteries, and loss of visual acuity due to involvement of the opthalmic artery. It frequently occurs in conjunction with polymyalgia rheumatica. The diagnosis must be made early since visual loss may be sudden and the condition responds well and rapidly to high-dose oral steroids. Although the prodromal symptoms may be vague, the clinician can be alerted to the diagnosis by the finding of a normochromic normocytic anaemia and a high ESR in excess of what may seem appropriate to the symptoms.

Involvement of the arch of the aorta (aortitis) may occur in 10–15 per cent and can rarely be associated with aneurysmal dilation of the ascending aorta and aortic valve incompetence.

Takayasu's ('pulseless') disease (page 13.193)
This is an aortitis that involves the aortic arch and its branches, and the abdominal aorta. Inflammation of the vessel wall leads to thrombosis and either stenosis of the lumen or complete occlusion. This is in contrast to other forms of aortitis, such as those due to giant cell arteritis, syphilis or associated with chronic seronegative arthritis, in which aortic dilation occurs.

The disease is very rare in the west and characteristically affects young, southeast Asian women. When the vasculitis is active, the patient is unwell, with weight loss, arthralgia, and localized chest tenderness corresponding to areas of diseased vessel. The ESR is raised. Patients may present when the vasculitis is inactive and they have already lost pulses. Constitutional symptoms may be conspicuous by their absence and the ESR normal. At this point in the disease, steroids will not be efficacious.

Familial granulomatous arteritis
A familial form of arteritis has been described recently, manifest by fever, hypertension, polyarthritis of juvenile onset together with non-caseating granulomata in both vascular and extravascular sites. It appears to be dominantly inherited with variable penetration.

Hypocomplementaemic vasculitis
In this condition, recurrent skin vasculitis, usually manifested as urticaria, is associated with hypocomplementaemia which is not a feature of the other subgroups. It usually affects females. Systemic involvement is not severe, consisting of arthralgia in some cases and rarely a mild proliferative glomerulonephritis. The ESR is elevated in distinction to more common forms of recurrent urticaria.

Relapsing polychondritis
This condition is rare and the tissues affected are those with a high glycosaminoglycan content, such as cartilage, aorta, sclera, cornea, and parts of the ear. The clinical features are recurrent chondritis of the auricles, nasal cartilage, and laryngeal and tracheal cartilage; a non-erosive polyarthritis; inflammation of the eye including conjunctivitis, keratitis, scleritis, episcleritis, and uveitis, and aural injury involving the cochlea and vestibule.

In 30 per cent of cases, there is an associated autoimmune disease. Sixty per cent have evidence of involvement which may be either a polyarteritis or aortitis. There is a 25 per cent mortality at five years due predominantly to tracheal collapse or vascular disease.

Immunoblastic lymphadenopathy
A hypocomplementaemic vasculitis may be associated with this lymphoproliferative disorder. The condition is characterized by fever, generalized lymphadenopathy, hepatosplenomegaly, polyclonal gammopathy, and a Coombe's positive haemolytic anaemia. Thrombocytopenia may also occur. Histologically, there is diffuse obliteration of the lymph-node architecture due to proliferation of small vessels and immunoblasts. Progression to a malignant lymphoma may occur.

Polymorphic reticulosis
This is a lymphoproliferative disorder, probably a malignant lymphoma, which has some clinical features in common with Wegener's granuloma. This disorder is sometimes localized to the upper respiratory tract ('lethal midline granuloma'). It may be disseminated, involving skin, lung, kidney, and gastrointestinal tract and tends to invade blood vessels ('lymphomatoid granulomatosis'). The localized form may respond to radiotherapy. The disseminated form has been successfully treated with prednisolone and cyclophosphamide.

Rheumatoid vasculitis
Systemic necrotizing vasculitis may occur in patients with rheumatoid arthritis, especially those with long-standing seropositive nodular disease. Skin involvement is common (85 per cent) with deep cutaneous ulcers and digital and nailfold infarcts. Activity of the vasculitis is associated with raised levels of serum IgG, rheumatoid factor, and low levels of complement. Eighty eight per cent of patients are reported to have the tissue type HLA DR4.

SLE and systemic sclerosis
Both these conditions may be accompanied by a polyarteritis.

Behçet's syndrome
This syndrome is a triad of relapsing uveitis with recurrent oral and genital ulceration. In this condition a phlebitis occurs, which may lead to superficial thrombophlebitis or occlusion of major, central veins. However, an arteritis may occur and a retinal or choroidal vasculitis is common (see pages 16.20 and 24.13).

Differential diagnosis of polyarteritis
There are other disorders, mostly rare, which can mimic polyarteritis but which are not accompanied by histological evidence of vasculitis. Nonetheless, they enter the differential diagnosis and are described briefly as follows.

Weber–Christian disease (nodular, non-suppurative panniculitis)
This condition is characterized by recurrent bouts of fever, with crops of subcutaneous nodules on thighs, arms, abdomen, back, and legs. These are usually painful and red, become indurated and lead to lipoatrophy. Histology shows necrosis of subcutaneous fat with neutrophils and later lipid-filled macrophages. This skin condition may be associated with a systemic illness, which is usually a polyserositis.

Degos' disease (malignant atrophic papulosis)
This is a rare and lethal condition that involves skin, gut, and the nervous system. The skin lesion is pathognomonic with a circular, porcelain-white depressed centre of 4–8 mm diameter, with a slightly elevated, erythematous margin. The arterial lesion consists of luminal stenosis or occlusion due to endothelial swelling, intimal proliferation, and thrombosis. There may be fibrinoid necrosis of the wall. Death is frequently related to intestinal perforation.

Hypereosinophilia syndrome (page 24.8)
Idiopathic hypereosinophilia (eosinophil count greater than $1.5 \times 10^9/l$) is a rare condition. It is associated with a cardiac lesion characterized by endomyocardial fibrosis (Loeffler's endocarditis), which leads to thrombosis and a restrictive cardiomyopathy. It typically affects young men (M:F = 9:1) at a mean age of 33 years (range 20–50). It is associated with a systemic disease which may mimic polyarteritis. Involvement of skin, central nervous system, kidneys, and gut occurs in addition to the cardiac pathology. Eosinophil counts range from 1.5 to $150 \times 10^9/l$. Disease activity may be associated with thrombocytopenia. Histologically, vessels show intimal proliferation and thrombosis leading to luminal stenosis. These lesions have, erroneously, been considered to be due to the sequelae of emboli from the heart, although embolization of ventricular thrombus can occur.

Infective endocarditis (page 13.314)
The involvement of extracardiac organs, including vasculitic lesions in the skin, may mimic polyarteritis, particularly in those cases in which the presence of a cardiac lesion is difficult to diagnose.

Septicaemia

When the source of sepsis is occult and there is dysfunction of one or more major organs, polyarteritis may appear to be the diagnosis, especially when a vasculitis of hands and feet accompanies septicaemia.

Diagnosis

The most crucial step is to be aware of the possibility of polyarteritis. Very often the diagnosis rests on clinical grounds alone, based on the features described above. Biopsy of an affected organ can provide histological proof but the inflammation affecting the vessel wall is usually not continuously present along its length. A section from a biopsy specimen, even if it does include an appropriately sized vessel, may therefore not demonstrate the inflammatory lesion. The histological findings are then normal or 'consistent with the diagnosis of polyarteritis', this depending on the interpretation of secondary or associated changes, e.g. a crescentic glomerulonephritis with segmental infarction of glomeruli.

Arteriography, particularly of the splanchnic vessels, can demonstrate small aneurysms and vessels blocked by thrombi even when there may not be clinical or laboratory evidence of damage to organs supplied by the vessels. The value of this investigation depends on familiarity with the diagnostic features and on the size of arteries affected being appropriate. This investigation has low sensitivity and a negative coeliac or renal angiogram does not exclude the diagnosis.

There are no diagnostic laboratory tests. Haematological investigations may provide diagnostic clues. The ESR may be raised, but is not invariably so. The haemoglobin is usually reduced to 9–11 g/dl and the cells are normochromic and normocytic. A lower value should raise the possibility of gut or lung haemorrhage. A neutrophil leucocytosis is the rule and counts of up to 40 $\times 10^9/1$ may occur. Eosinophilia occurs in 10–20 per cent of all cases of polyarteritis; patients with counts above $1.5 \times 10^9/1$ are likely to have a Churg–Strauss syndrome. Hypocomplementaemia is not a feature of microscopic polyarteritis and the presence of rheumatoid factor and immune complexes is neither common nor specific enough to be helpful.

Treatment

It is now accepted that the mainstay of treatment of severe cases of polyarteritis is the combination of steroids and immunosuppressive drugs. There are no properly conducted trials to prove that either of these agents is efficacious, let alone to determine the correct dose of steroid treatment, its optimum route of administration, or the immunosuppressive drug of choice. A retrospective survey of the mortality of polyarteritis during the phases of treatment with no immunosuppressive drugs, steroids alone, and steroids with immunosuppressive drugs showed a progressive increase of five-year survival rate, namely, 13, 50, and 80 per cent, respectively. It is for these reasons and the clinical observation that the disease can be halted, reversed, and even undergo remission when steroids and immunosuppressive drugs are used together that these drugs are now the best available treatment for severely affected patients.

Steroids may be given orally, or in severe cases, intravenously in high-dose boluses, so-called 'pulse therapy'. The choice of immunosuppressive drug lies between cyclophosphamide and azathioprine. There are no clinical studies pointing to any one of these as the correct choice, although some authors have the impression that cyclophosphamide is more effective than azathioprine and have noted a small number of cases who did not respond to azathioprine, but did so when this drug was replaced by cyclophosphamide. On the other hand, cyclophosphamide is in general more toxic than azathioprine, causing greater bone marrow suppression, gonadal failure, alopecia, and haemorrhagic cystitis. Two particular traps for the unwary using cyclophosphamide are its diminished excretion in renal failure and its pulmonary toxicity, which could be misinterpreted as continuation or relapse of pulmonary vasculitis.

A recent addition to the therapy of severe polyarteritis is plasma exchange, which may be viewed as an immunosuppressive process as well as a means of removing antigens, antibodies, antigen–antibody complexes, and humoral mediators of inflammation. There have been no studies which have defined its role. Anticoagulants and drugs altering platelet function have been used, particularly in the treatment of nephritis, but there is no evidence to support their use, and they are now much less frequently employed.

Schemes of treatment

In order to give some guidance to the treatment of particular manifestations of polyarteritis, a variety of schemes of treatment according to the severity of the disease are described here. Two general comments need emphasis. First, the speed at which treatment is begun, particularly in severe cases, is as important as the components of the treatment; delays of hours, let alone days, can have disastrous consequences. Second, the schemes which follow are not to be interpreted as rigid. Individual clinicians will have experience of regimens which differ in detail but which are just as effective. Familiarity with and constant use of a particular combination of drugs are important ingredients for success.

Treatment at presentation Dosages of drugs are for an average-sized person.

1. *Severe polyarteritis* e.g. rapid deterioration in function of the brain, kidneys, heart, or a marked but static degree of impairment of function of vital organs: high-dose steroids either orally, 60–80 mg prednisolone daily, or intravenous methylprednisolone 1 g daily for three days, repeated if necessary on days 8, 9, and 10 with a background oral steroid dose of 20–40 mg/day; oral immunosuppressive drugs: either cyclophosphamide (2–2.5 mg/kg/day) or azathioprine (2–3 mg/kg/day). Cyclophosphamide can be given intravenously in the first few days of treatment, and has obvious advantages if the patient is too ill to take drugs orally. It is in this group of patients that plasma exchange could be considered, either as initiating treatment, or as a 'reserve' treatment should the initial steroids and immunosuppressive drugs fail to induce a response (3–4 litres of plasma exchanged daily for 7–10 days).

2. *Moderate polyarteritis* e.g. stable and less severe dysfunction of vital organs: oral prednisolone 40–60 mg/day with increase of dose if there is no response; immunosuppression with either azathioprine 2–3 mg/kg/day (preferred) or cyclophosphamide 2–2.5 mg/kg/day (reserved if there is no response to azathioprine).

3. *Mild polyarteritis* e.g. no or slight dysfunction of vital organs: steroids alone may be tried as prednisolone 20–40 mg/day; immunosuppressive drugs may be held in reserve (doses as above) if there is no improvement or may be used alone as first choice, especially in the elderly because of their susceptibility to the side effects of steroids.

Continuation of treatment Once treatment has begun a consequent problem is the correct dosage of drugs to maintain the patient in as complete a remission as possible. To discuss this comprehensively it is necessary to describe how activity of disease can be estimated, and the possible outcomes for individual patients other than death. These may be summarized as:

(*a*) *Complete remission*: this is not common, and is recognized by a continuing remission on no treatment.

(*b*) *Relapsing*: patients have apparent remission on very little or no treatment but the disease reappears from time to time (and not always with the same presenting symptoms) requiring treatment *de novo*.

(*c*) *Suppressed or smouldering*: the disease requires continuous treatment to suppress its activity which reappears as soon as steroids and/or immunosuppression are reduced below a threshold level. These subdivisions are obviously not clearcut, but they provide a useful framework within which the physician can manoeuvre.

The assessment of activity of the disease is easy when continuation or relapses are florid, but becomes more difficult as the patient responds to treatment. There are no specific guides to activity, and reliance has to be placed on assessment by a combination of methods:

1. *Clinical*: Continuation or fresh appearance of any of the clinical features described above obviously imply active disease.

2. Measurement of function of affected organs when appropriate, e.g. liver or kidney involvement, is a convenient monitor of activity. A disadvantage of both of these methods is that in acute stages of the disease it is not necessarily apparent how much dysfunction is due to permanent damage and how much to reversible changes.

3. *Laboratory assessment*: The ESR is raised in 90–95 per cent of patients with active disease, but is often less than 100 mm/hour and may be normal. The serum concentration of C-reactive protein, an acute-phase protein, is raised during active disease and is a more accurate sensitive index of disease activity than the ESR, (page 9.157). The haematological abnormalities described in the section on diagnosis indicate activity if they develop or recur. The presence or amount of rheumatoid factor and circulating immune complexes are poor guides to activity.

Reduction of treatment As the disease is controlled, the dose of steroids can be reduced, obviously as quickly as possible in the early stages if high doses have been used, aiming approximately at 20 mg prednisolone daily at 2–3 months. Plasma exchange should generally not be considered for more than two weeks as by then it can be seen to be effective or not, and continuation at the rate of exchange described above may be dangerous. If cyclophosphamide has been used as the first choice for immunosuppression then its conversion to azathioprine can be considered at 1–3 months, particularly in younger patients.

Once the acute phase is over and the patient's condition is stable on, for example, prednisolone 20 mg/day plus azathioprine 150 mg/day the prednisolone can be gradually reduced in steps of 2.5 mg every four to six weeks. After 1–2 years of disease inactivity an attempt can be made to wean the patient off steroids and then the immunosuppression.

It must be emphasized that the schemes of treatment described above must be tailored to the individual patient's needs. They form only a general guide to management and many variations on the details of treatment can be found.

Hypertension must be adequately controlled. Regular dialysis and/or renal transplantation are successful treatments for those patients who develop end-stage renal failure.

Outcome

It is difficult to give an exact overall prognosis for polyarteritis because of the wide variation in the disease and the bias inevitable in published figures because of selection of patients according to the special interest of the unit to which they were referred. The survival at five years is approximately 80 per cent; a feature with a bad prognosis is the serious involvement of vital organs. Nonetheless, the prognosis for this group has improved with the wider use of steroids and immunosuppressive drugs, recognition of the urgency with which treatment should be begun, and better management of the complications of therapy, particularly infections.

References

Churg, J. and Strauss, L. (1951). Allergic granulomatosis, allergic angiitis and periarteritis nodosa. *Am. J. Pathol.* **27**, 277–294.

Cohen, R. D., Conn, D. L. and Illstrup, D. M. (1980). Clinical features, prognosis and response to treatment in polyarteritis. *Mayo Clin. Proc.* **55**, 146–155.

Fauci, A. S., Haynes, B. F. and Katz, P. (1978). The spectrum of vasculitis. Clinical, pathologic, immunologic and therapeutic considerations. *Ann. Int. Med.* **89**, 660–676.

—— and Wolff, S. M. (1983). Wegener's granulomatosis: prospective clinical and therapeutic experience with 85 patients for 21 years. *Ann. int. Med.* **98**, 76–85.

Frohnert, P. P. and Sheps, S. G. (1967). Long term follow up study of periarteritis nodosa. *Am. J. Med.* **43**, 8–14.

Gorevic, P. D., Kassab, H. J., Levo, Y., Kohn, R., Meltzer, M., Prose, P. and Franklin, E. C. (1980). Mixed cryoglobulinaemia: clinical aspects and long term follow up of 40 patients. *Am. J. Med.* **69**, 287–308.

Lanham, J. G., Elkon, K. B., Pusey, C. D. and Hughes, G. R. (1984). Systemic vasculitis with asthma and eosinophilia: a clinical approach to Churg–Strauss syndrome. *Medicine* **63**, 65–81.

Lieb, E. S., Restivo, C. and Paulus, H. E. (1979). Immunosuppressive and corticosteroid therapy of polyarteritis nodosa. *Am. J. Med.* **67**, 941–947.

Lupi-Herrera, E., Sanchez-Torres, G., Marcushamer, J. *et al.* (1977). Takayasu's arteritis: clinical study of 107 cases. *Am. Heart J.* **93**, 94–103.

McAdam, L. P., O'Hanlan, M. A., Bluestone, R. and Pearson, C. M. (1976). Relapsing polychondritis. *Medicine* **55**, 193–215.

Moore, P. M. and Cupps, T. R. (1983). Neurological complications of vasculitis. *Ann. Neurol.* **14**, 155–167.

Rose, G. A. and Spencer, H. (1957). Polyarteritis nodosa. *Q. J. Med.* **26**, 43–81.

Rotenstein, D., Gibbas, D. L., Majmudar, B. and Chastain, E. A. (1982). Familial granulomatous arteritis with polyarthritis of juvenile onset. *N. Engl. J. Med.* **306**. 86–90.

Scott, D. G. I., Bacon, P. A. and Tribe, C. R. (1981). Systemic rheumatoid vasculitis: a clinical and laboratory study of 50 cases. *Medicine* **60**, 288–297.

——, —— and Elliott, P. J. (1982). Systemic vasculitis in a district general hospital 1972-1980: clinical and laboratory features, classification and prognosis of 80 cases. *Q. J. Med.* **51**, 292–311.

Serra, A., Cameron, J. S., Turner, D. R., Hartley, B., Ogg, C. S., Neild, G. H., Williams, D. G., Taube, D., Brown, C. B. and Hicks, J. A. (1984). Vasculitis affecting the kidney: presentation, histopathology and long-term outcome. *Q. J. Med.* **53**, 181–207.

Spry, C. J. F. (1982). The hypereosinophilic syndrome: clinical features, laboratory findings and treatment. *Allergy* **37**, 539–551.

Tanaka, N., Sekimoto, K. and Naoe, S. (1976). Kawasaki disease. Relationship with infantile periarteritis nodosa. *Arch. Pathol. Lab. Med.* **100**, 81–86.

Weisenberger, D., Armitage, J and Dick, F. (1977). Immunoblastic lymphadenopathy with pulmonary infiltrates, hypocomplementaemia and vasculitis. *Am. J. Med.* **63**, 849–854.

SYSTEMIC SCLEROSIS

M. I. V. JAYSON

Introduction

Systemic sclerosis, also known as progressive systemic sclerosis and scleroderma, is a multisystem disease in which the characteristic features are collagen proliferation, mild inflammatory cell infiltration, obstruction of small blood vessels, and ischaemic atrophy. The term 'systemic sclerosis' is preferred as 'progressive systemic sclerosis' implies continued activity of the disease which is not always the case and 'scleroderma' suggests the disease involves the skin alone. Indeed in some cases systemic sclerosis may not affect the skin. The term scleroderma should be reserved for the purely cutaneous features. 'Morphoea' is a form of scleroderma in which there are well-demarcated plaques of fibrosis restricted to the skin. Morphoea is a separate disease from systemic sclerosis and visceral involvement hardly ever occurs. Some patients may have extensive confluent areas of skin involvement giving rise to generalized morphoea.

The various causes of scleroderma may be classified as shown in Table 1. Although there may be considerable overlap between the various types of systemic sclerosis on the whole the disease pattern is usually distinct within each subgroup. This classification is helpful for assessing the likely prognosis.

Diagnostic criteria for the presence of definite systemic sclerosis have now been established (Table 2).

Prevalence and incidence

Systemic sclerosis is relatively uncommon with estimates of the annual incidence varying between 2.3 and 12 cases per million population. It may develop at any age with a peak incidence in the fourth or fifth decade. It is rare in children. In young people there is relatively a much higher incidence in females than males being 15:1 whereas in adults over 45 years the female to male ratio is only 2:1. It affects all races but the prognosis is somewhat worse for Negroes than Caucasians. Associations have been described with being married, excessive alcohol intake, and performing manual and less skilled work.

Exposure to various environmental factors may be associated with systemic sclerosis. An increased incidence has been reported in stone masons, coal miners, and gold miners. Systemic sclerosis-like conditions have developed following exposure to vinyl chloride, other chlorinated hydrocarbons, epoxy resins, and as part of the connective tissue problems in Spain thought to be due to adulterated cooking oil. Some drugs may produce scleroderma-like conditions. In particular bleomycin, and tryptophan and carbidopa have been identified. This may be analogous to the peritoneal fibrosis and retroperitoneal fibrosis associated with practolol and methysergide, respectively. Features of scleroderma have been reported after paraffin wax implantations for cosmetic surgery.

There have been a number of familial cases. There is an increased incidence of tissue types HLA A1, B8, DR3, and of DR5. DR5 may be associated with the CREST syndrome and B8 may be a marker for rapidly progressive disease with widespread visceral involvement.

Acrosclerotic features may occur in association with diabetes mellitus and in particular with insulin-dependent childhood diabetes. There is an uncertain association with malignancy except possibly for carcinoma of the lung which may occur as an end-stage event in advanced pulmonary fibrosis.

Pathological and clinical features

The pathological changes and clinical features of systemic sclerosis are due to a variable combination in the different organ systems of mild chronic inflammatory cell infiltration, connective tissue proliferation, vascular obstruction, and ischaemic atrophy.

Presentation

The first features of the disorder usually appear between 30 and 50 years of age but it can develop in any age group. Raynaud's phenomenon is by far the most common mode of onset and may be the only feature for many years. Raynaud's patients who develop signs of ischaemic damage with necrotic skin ulceration are likely to have systemic sclerosis or some other connective tissue disorder as the underlying diagnosis. Thereafter there may be progressive induration and stiffening of the skin with loss of movements of the fingers. Much less frequently the presenting features may be polyarthritis, dysphagia, small bowel or other problems.

Although visceral involvement may not be obvious at presen-

Table 1 Classification of causes of scleroderma

1 Localized cutaneous
    Morphea – single or multiple plaques
    Generalized
    Linear scleroderma
2 Systemic sclerosis
    CREST syndrome
    Diffuse
    Overlap syndromes
3 Eosinophilic fasciitis
4 Drug and chemical induced

Table 2 Preliminary criteria for the diagnosis of systemic sclerosis

Major criterion
    Proximal scleroderma (to MCPs and MTPs)

Minor criteria
    Sclerodactyly
    Digital tip pitting or loss of substance of distal fingerpad
    Bibasilar pulmonary fibrosis

At least the major or two or more minor criteria required for the diagnosis of systematic sclerosis

Masi *et al.* 1980

Table 3 Prevalence of organ involvement (per cent)

	Pathological (D'Angelo et al., 1969)	Clinical (LeRoy, 1976)
Skin	98	90
Oesophagus	74	52
Small intestine	48	
Large intestine	39	15
Lungs	81	
Pleura	81	43
Heart	81	40
Pericardium	53	11
Muscle	41	20
Kidney	58	35

tation, pathological changes are frequently widespread. Table 3 compares the prevalence of clinical and pathological evidence of organ system involvement in patients with systemic sclerosis.

Raynaud's phenomenon and peripheral vascular disease

Raynaud's phenomenon is a syndrome of reversible peripheral ischaemia occurring predominantly in the hands but also in the feet and sometimes elsewhere. It is usually precipitated by cold and only a slight temperature change may be required. Attacks can be caused by emotion or other poorly recognized events. The fingers turn white, icy cold, and then may become deeply cyanosed. During the rewarming stage they may turn bright red due to profound vasodilation. Pain with numbness and paraesthesiae is common and often most marked during the rewarming phase.

When Raynaud's phenomenon has been present for several years without evidence of any other underlying disorder it is called primary Raynaud's disease. Frequently Raynaud's phenomenon is the presenting feature of connective tissue disease and in particular systemic sclerosis but the other features making the diagnosis only become apparent on long-term follow up. Other conditions associated with Raynaud's phenomenon include cervical rib and thoracic outlet syndromes, atherosclerosis, administration of certain drugs such as β-blockers, and the prolonged use of vibrating hand tools.

With more severe peripheral ischaemia, the systemic sclerosis patient develops small areas of infarction at the finger tips. Small areas of ulceration develop which heal giving the appearance of pitting and atrophy of the pulps of the fingertips (Fig. 1). Radiographs may show lysis of the tips of the terminal phalanges (Fig. 2). Larger areas of ulceration may develop at the finger tips (Fig. 3) and also elsewhere and particularly over the extensor surfaces of the finger joints. There is a risk of secondary infection due to poor peripheral vascular supply and some patients may develop gangrene of the digits. Infections of the fingers may require surgical drainage or eventually amputation. Some patients may lose several digits.

Dilated capillaries are prominent as telangiectasia on the face (Fig. 4), palms of the hands, and elsewhere. The nailbeds may appear swollen and it is possible to see dilated capillaries which on capillary microscopy show a characteristic pattern of enlarged and deformed capillary loops surrounded by avascular areas. There is

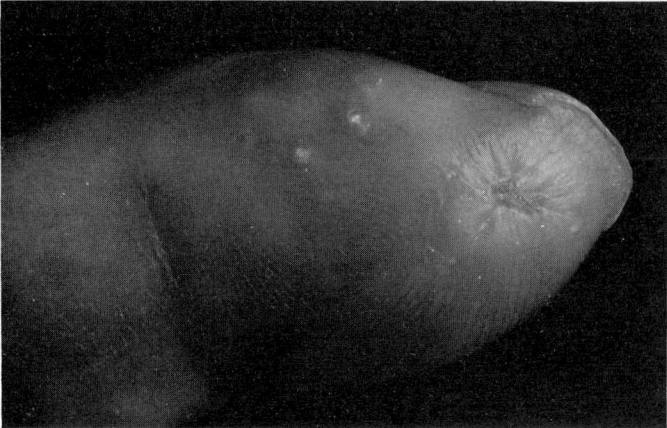

Fig. 1 Fingertip showing atrophy, pitting and scarring of the finger pulp.

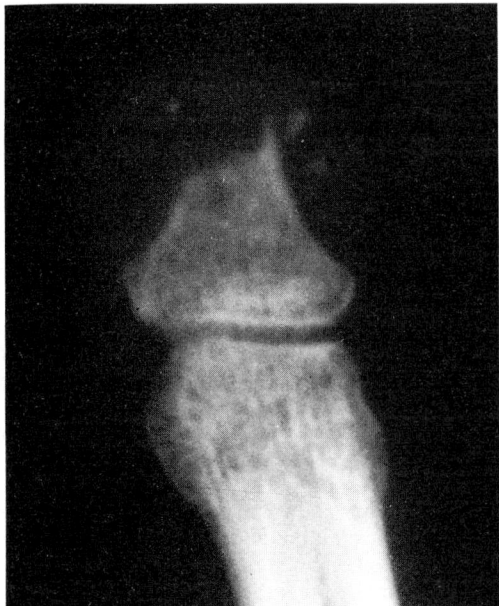

Fig. 2 Osteolysis of the tip of the terminal phalanx.

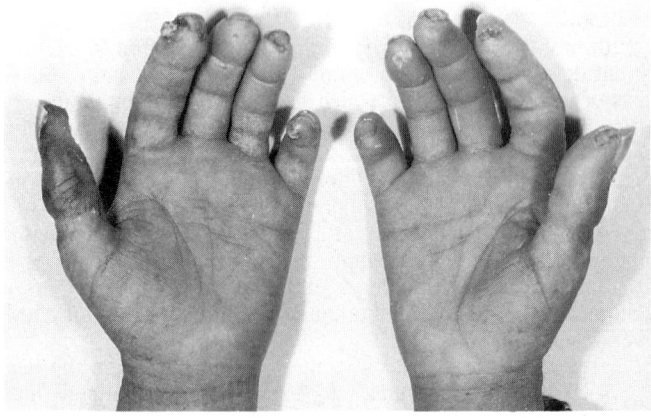

Fig. 3 Multiple areas of digital tip ischaemia with ulceration, atrophy, and scarring.

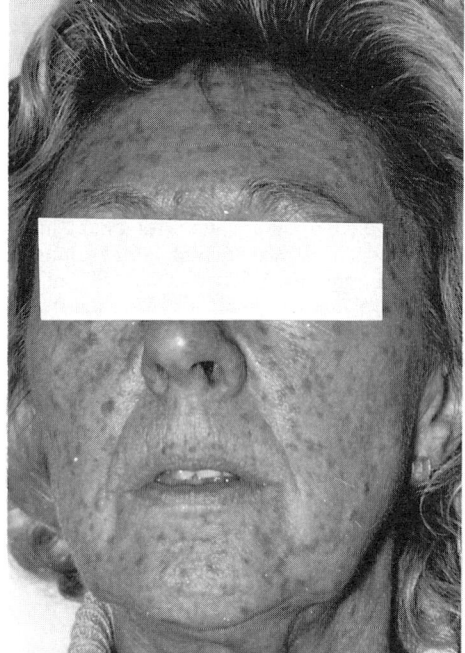

Fig. 4 Telangiectasia of the face.

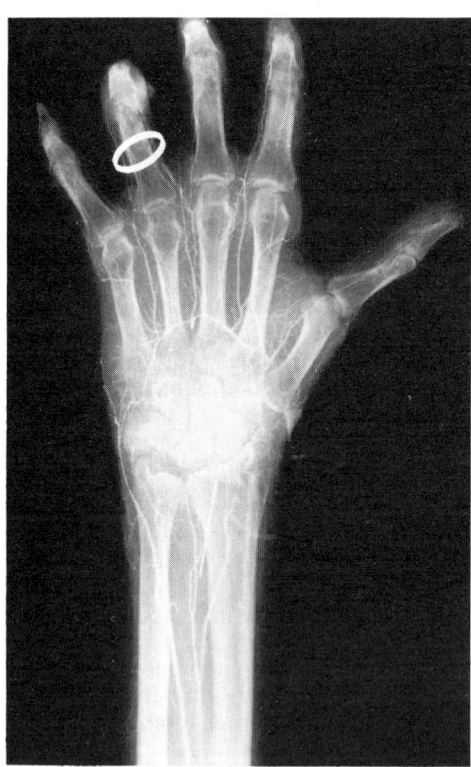

Fig. 5 Arteriogram showing attenuation and segmental obstruction of the digital vessels.

some correlation between these nailbed capillary changes and visceral involvement by systemic sclerosis. On arteriography, in advanced cases, the lumina of the digital vessels are attenuated with segmental blocks producing loss of the more distal circulation (Fig. 5).

Skin changes

These vary from minimal changes in the fingers with minor tethering of the skin to extensive involvement of the whole body which

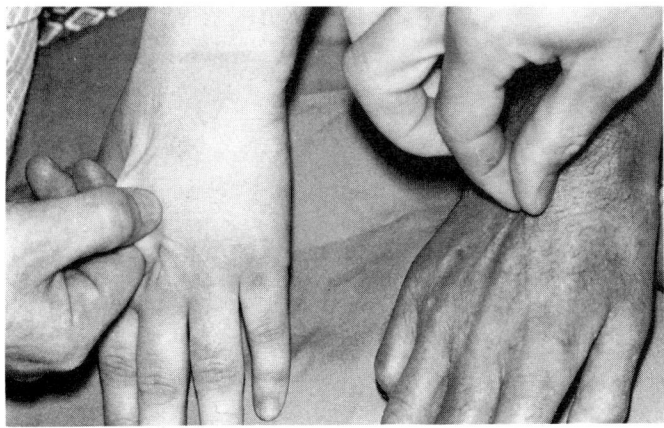

Fig. 6 The difficulty in pinching up the indurated skin of a patient with systemic sclerosis (right) compared with normal skin (left).

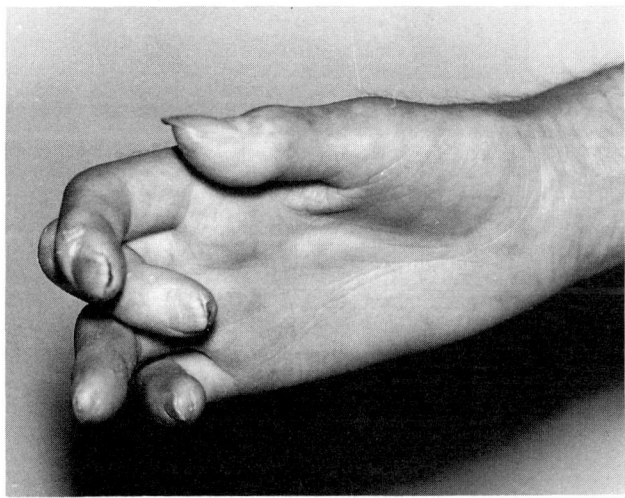

Fig. 7 Advanced sclerodermatous changes in the hands with tight indurated skin and inability to straighten the fingers properly.

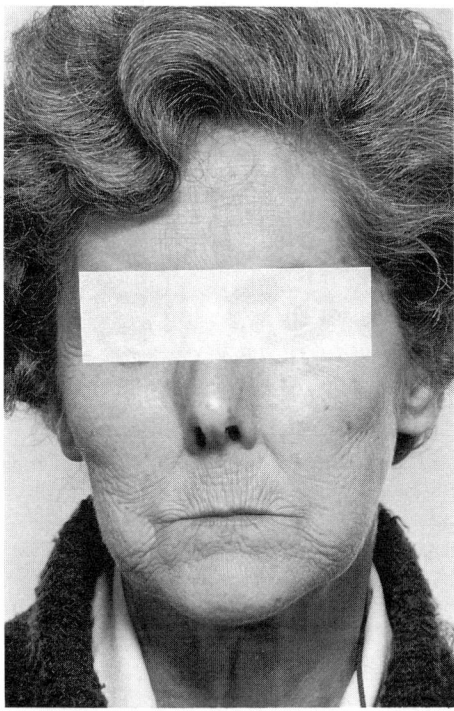

Fig. 8 Radial furrowing around the mouth with thin pursed lips. There are also telangiectasia of the face.

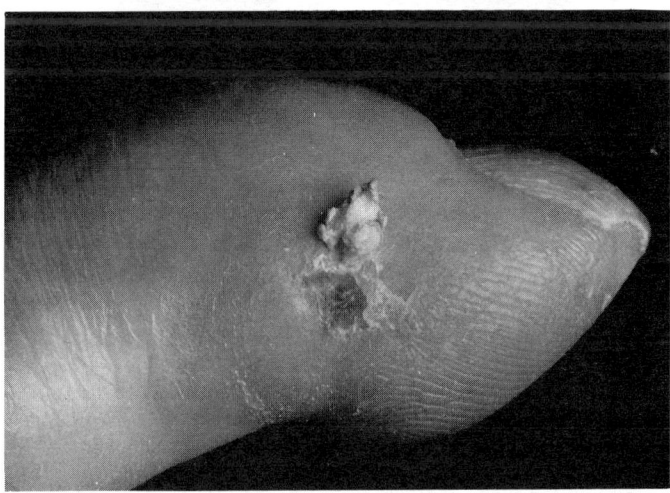

Fig. 9 Calcinotic material discharged from a small ulcer on the finger. There is also atrophy of the pulp of the finger tip.

may appear as if encased in a suit of armour. The term 'sclerodactyly' refers to changes limited to the fingers and not spreading proximal to the metacarpophalangeal joints. 'Acrosclerosis' describes the skin changes occurring predominantly in a peripheral distribution particularly the hands, feet, distal forearms, and legs but also may include the face around the mouth. The term 'proximal scleroderma' indicates that the disease has involved skin proximal to the metacarpophalangeal joints and 'diffuse scleroderma' implies involvement of the trunk.

There may be a transient oedematous phase in the skin which may not be obvious before being replaced by the typical tethered and indurated skin of scleroderma. The skin appears swollen and pressure with the thumb may leave a finger print on the skin surface.

The skin becomes tight and indurated and difficult to pinch up (Fig. 6). This may lead to limitation of joint movements and commonly patients are unable to straighten their fingers properly and so they lie curled with slight flexion deformities (Fig. 7). In involved areas there may be loss of hair and patches of depigmentation and hyperpigmentation.

The patient may have difficulty in opening the mouth because of tightness around the lips which appear narrowed and radial furrows in the surrounding skin produce a pursed lip appearance (Fig. 8). The tightness of the skin may make the nose look beak-

like and these changes, together with telangiectasia, make the facial appearances of scleroderma easily recognizable.

These skin changes are not necessarily permanent or progressive. In some patients sclerodermatous changes can improve and on occasions return almost to normal.

Calcinosis may develop in involved areas in the skin and subcutaneous tissues. In particular calcinotic lesions develop in the fingers but also elsewhere and the skin may ulcerate and discharge this material (Fig. 9). This process may be painful and some patients describe picking out this chalky material from the lesions. Calcinotic deposits are easily recognized on radiographs (Fig. 10).

In early skin involvement a biopsy may appear relatively normal except for a sparse infiltration of chronic inflammatory cells deep in the dermis which may be concentrated around small blood vessels. This is a very non-specific pattern in contrast with the later indurated phase in which there are diagnostic changes of atrophy

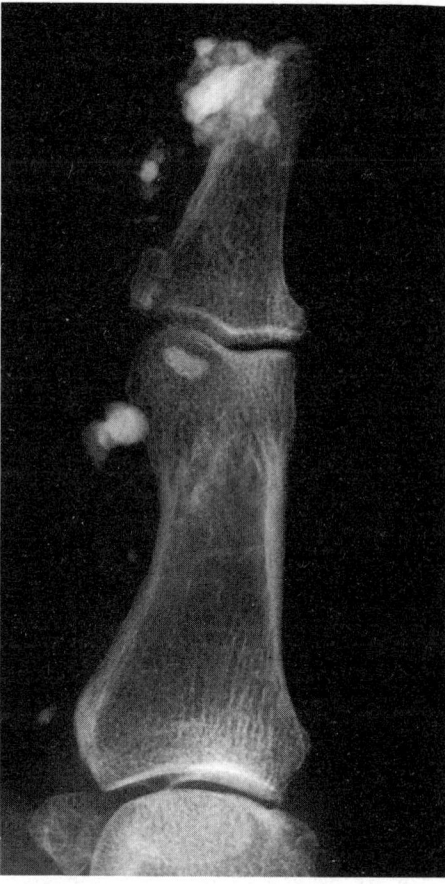

Fig. 10 Radiograph of a finger showing multiple areas of calcinosis.

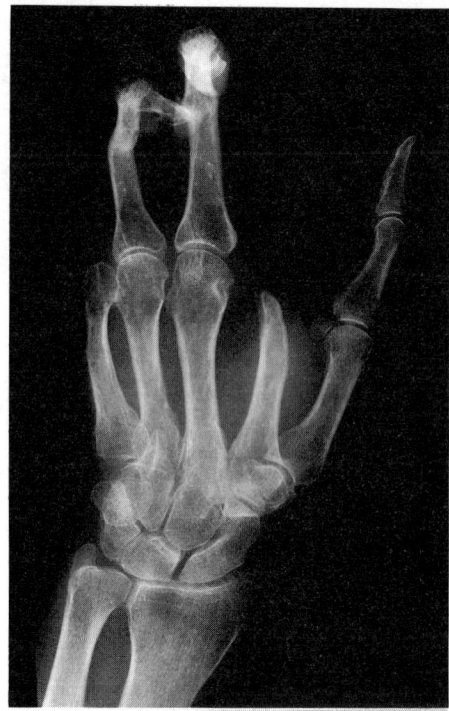

Fig. 11 Radiograph of hand in advanced systemic sclerosis showing multiple amputations, fusion of proximal interphalangeal joints, and fixed flexion deformities of the fingers.

and disappearance of the hair follicles and sweat glands, thinning of the epidermis, and thickening of the dermis due to gross collagen proliferation.

Joints and tendons
Although involvement of the joints and tendons is common it may be difficult to distinguish from stiffness and joint contractures produced by changes in the skin. Mild synovitis and fibrosis of the capsules of the joints and tendon sheaths can produce pain, tenderness, and loss of function. It may be possible to palpate and hear a coarse leathery crepitus during movements. This is most obvious in the patello-femoral joint and the tendons of the distal forearms and legs. Radiographs show deformity, loss of joint space, subluxation, and occasionally fusion of damaged joints (Fig. 11). Histological examination usually shows relatively mild inflammatory changes in the synovium with dense capsular fibrosis and a thick layer of fibrin on the synovial surface.

Muscle and nerve changes
Mild myositis is common. Pathological examination reveals a mild chronic inflammatory cell infiltration usually in a perivascular distribution with muscle fibre atrophy and fibrous replacement. This principally occurs in the limb girdle muscles with weakness but little pain and seems more common in those patients with overlap connective tissue disease syndromes. There may be appropriate electromyographic abnormalities with elevation of the serum creatine phosphokinase and aldolase. Neurological involvement is rare but there is an association with trigeminal neuralgia.

Gastrointestinal involvement
Oesophageal changes occur in up to 90 per cent of patients. There is atrophy of the muscle coats and dilation of the lumen with loss of neuromuscular co-ordination and loss of tone in the lower oesophageal sphincter. The principal symptoms are of lower oesopha-

geal dysphagia with difficulty in swallowing particularly if lying flat. Reflux and severe heart burn may develop and in severe cases a secondary stricture may develop exacerbating the dysphagia. Barium swallow examination and oesophageal manometry may show disordered peristalsis, oesophageal reflux, stricture formation, and a dilated oesophagus (Fig. 12). Involvement of the upper oesophagus fortunately is rare but can lead to incompetence of the cricopharyngeal apparatus and inhalation of food into the trachea.

In the small intestine, disordered mobility may lead to secondary bacterial overgrowth and a malabsorption syndrome. Many patients are symptom free but those with more severe disease may develop steatorrhoea and weight loss. On barium examination, the passage of food is delayed with flocculation, dilated intestinal loops, thickened folds, and a wire spring appearance of the small bowel when not distended. Rarely there is complete loss of peristalsis and the small bowel becomes grossly distended. In some cases there is also a volvulus. This is known as intestinal pseudo-obstruction and may be fatal complication. In the large intestine the walls may balloon out to give the appearance of pseudo-diverticulosis (Fig. 13). Perforation can occur. Large bowel disease may also present with obstruction or infarction of the colon. In pneumatosis cystoides intestinalis, cysts or streaks of gas occur in the bowel wall or mesentery.

Sjögren's syndrome
The lacrimal, parotid, and submandibular glands may be affected by inflammatory cell infiltration, collagen deposition, and glandular atrophy. Although frank Sjogren's syndrome (see page 16.41) only occurs in a small proportion, careful testing will show some evidence in most patients.

Respiratory involvement
On testing lung function it is common to find a mixture of restrictive, obstructive, and small airway changes frequently with the ventilation/perfusion mismatching. The diffusing capacity decreases in the cold seasons and also on cold challenge suggesting a form of Raynaud's phenomenon affecting the lungs.

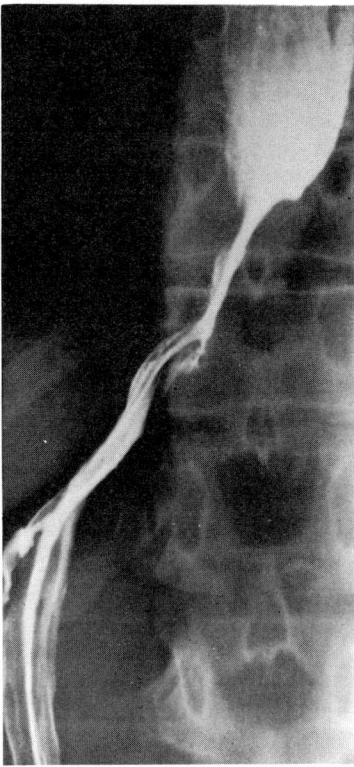

Fig. 12 Barium swallow examination showing an oesophageal stricture and dilation of the oesophagus above.

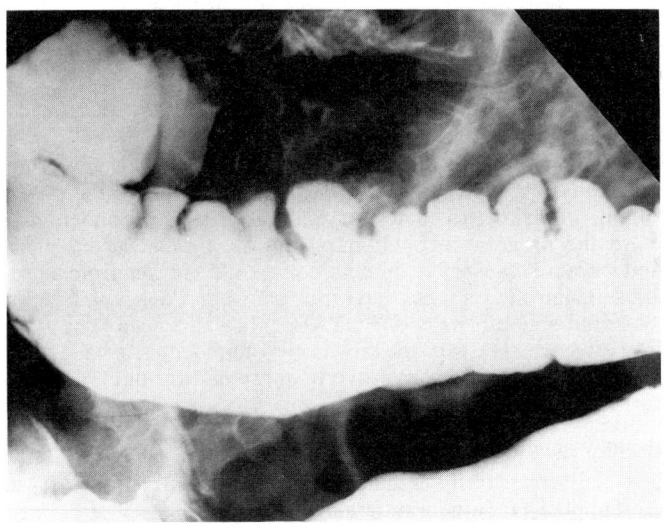

Fig. 13 Transverse colon showing multiple wide necked pseudo-diverticulae.

Fibrosing alveolitis (diffuse interstitial pulmonary fibrosis) usually starts in the lower lung fields and spreads gradually upwards. There is progressive development of dyspnoea with fine basal rales and radiographs show fine reticular changes with a honeycomb appearance in more severe cases. Alveolar cell carcinoma has been reported but is believed to be the result of hyperplastic changes in advanced pulmonary fibrosis rather than to have a specific relationship with systemic sclerosis.

Intimal proliferation in the smaller pulmonary arteries and arterioles can lead to the development of pulmonary hypertension. This complication seems particularly associated with the CREST variant of systemic sclerosis and is the principal fatal complication of this form of the disease.

Cardiac involvement

Pathological evidence of pericarditis is common but is only recognized in about 7 per cent of patients in life. Myocardial fibrosis can lead to a cardiomyopathy with intractable congestive cardiac failure, rhythm changes, angina pectoris despite normal major coronary arteries, and sudden death.

Kidney involvement

Renal disease is the principal fatal complication of systemic sclerosis. The majority of these deaths occur in the cold seasons. In contrast with a normal increase there is a decrease in renal perfusion on cold challenge of the skin suggesting that a form of renal Raynaud's phenomenon plays a part in the pathogenesis of permanent renal damage.

The patients with proximal and diffuse scleroderma are particularly at risk and renal failure occurs rarely in the CREST syndrome. Malignant hypertension and acute renal failure can develop suddenly and histological examination of the kidneys shows changes similar to those of malignant hypertension with mucoid intimal proliferation and thickening of the small arteries producing vascular obstruction and fibrinoid necrosis of arterioles and glomeruli. An elevation in the blood renin levels provides the basis for treatment with an angiotensin-converting enzyme inhibitor.

Systemic sclerosis variants

There are a number of subtypes of the disease. Classification of patients is helpful for indicating prognosis although in any individual the disease pattern can include the full range of features.

The CREST syndrome refers to a combination of Calcinosis, Raynaud's phenomenon, oEsophageal involvement, Sclerodactyly, and Telangiectasia. Most patients have a long history of Raynaud's phenomenon and subsequently may develop ulceration, pitting, and occasionally gangrene in the fingers. The disease progresses extremely slowly and the long-term prognosis for life is relatively good. However, these patients may develop severe pulmonary hypertension and there is an association with primary biliary cirrhosis. The CREST syndrome is associated with the presence of anticentromere antibody in the serum which provides a helpful diagnostic and prognostic test.

In contrast in diffuse scleroderma the skin of the trunk and limbs is involved at an early stage. These patients are at much greater risk of visceral involvement and in particular of acute renal failure and have a considerably worse prognosis.

Mixed connective tissue and undifferentiated connective tissue disease are terms used for an overlap syndrome with a variable combination of features of systemic sclerosis, systemic lupus erythematosus, dermatomyositis, and other autoimmune problems. On the whole the prognosis is better than for the individual diseases separately. The presence of an antibody to an extractable nuclear antigen is helpful for identifying this condition.

Eosinophilic fasciitis is a syndrome of sclerodermatous change occurring in the skin of the limbs and trunk but usually sparing the hands and feet. Raynaud's phenomenon does not occur and there are no visceral complications. The erythrocyte sedimentation rate is increased and there may be eosinophilia and hypergammaglobulinaemia. On skin biopsy there is marked thickening of the deep fascia with hypertrophy of collagen and a mild chronic cell inflammatory infiltration. The cause of this syndrome is unknown although anecdotal accounts suggest that in some cases excessive physical exertion may precipitate its onset. The skin changes will usually respond to steroid therapy.

Pathogenesis

The most striking feature of the disease is gross overproduction of collagen by fibroblasts in the deeper layers of the dermis. Lymphokines from chronic inflammatory cells, mitogens for fibroblasts in the serum, and the selective suppression of low collagen-producing fibroblasts have been suggested as mechanisms underlying this collagen overproduction. There is also evidence of increased formation of glycosaminoglycan particularly in the earliest stages of the disease. This suggests that there is a generalized propensity to overproduction of connective tissue components.

Microcirculatory damage occurs in virtually all cases of systemic sclerosis. The numbers of capillaries are grossly reduced and those remaining become dilated and distorted. In the arterioles there is intimal proliferation with fibrin deposition and platelet adhesion leading to obstruction of the lumen. The vascular damage may be mediated by a circulating endothelial cell cytotoxic factor or by abnormalities of serotonin metabolism. There is evidence of defective fibrinolytic activity in the blood leading towards hyperfibrinogenaemia and hyperviscosity as well as failure to clear fibrin deposits from the vessel walls. These factors will exacerbate the poor peripheral vascular flow.

An immunological basis for the disorder is suggested by the combination in overlap syndromes of features of systemic sclerosis with those of systemic lupus erythematosus, dermatomyositis, and rheumatoid arthritis. A scleroderma-like syndrome can develop as a consequence of graft versus host disease – a clear example of an immunological disorder. Circulating antinuclear antibodies are found in virtually all patients. Antinuclear factor is usually of the speckled or nucleolar patterns but bears little or no correlation with disease severity or outcome. An antibody against a nuclear protein Scl 70 is found in about 20 per cent of systemic sclerosis patients but seems restricted to this disorder. The anticentromere antibody is helpful for identifying the CREST syndrome. Alterations in cell-mediated immunity may also be found with reductions in numbers of circulating T-lymphocytes and an excess of T-lymphocytes in the chronic inflammatory infiltration in the skin. These factors suggest that altered immunity plays a role in the pathogenesis of this disease.

There are clear examples of systemic sclerosis-like syndromes produced after exposure to certain drugs or chemicals. It remains possible that many other cases, at present of unknown cause, are due to exposure to some environmental agent perhaps in genetically predisposed individuals.

Prognosis

The overall survival rate is about 70 to 80 per cent at 5 years. The patients with the CREST pattern have a much better prognosis than those with diffuse scleroderma. Factors indicating a markedly adverse prognosis include early involvement of the skin of the trunk, rapid progress of the skin lesions, and the development of cardiac, pulmonary, and renal disease. Other identified adverse factors include Negroid rather than Caucasian race, older age at presentation, excess alcohol intake, cigarette smoking, elevated ESR, and anaemia. The principal cause of death as a consequence of systemic sclerosis is acute renal failure and malignant hypertension. Other potentially fatal complications include pulmonary hypertension, respiratory failure, intestinal pseudo-obstruction, and occasionally other problems.

Treatment

This includes general management and symptomatic relief, measures to improve the peripheral blood flow, forms of treatment aimed at reducing inflammation and fibrosis, and treatment of specific organ system problems.

General and symptomatic treatments

The patient must protect the hands and feet against cold exposure. Warm clothes and gloves with thermal linings are important and, for some patients, electrically heated gloves and socks powered by a rechargeable battery carried on a waist band are very helpful. The first signs of infection or ulceration must be treated promptly and trauma to the fingers and toes should be avoided. Patients must stop smoking and drugs known to precipitate Raynaud's phenomenon such as β-blockers and ergotamine should be stopped. Some patients find lanolin and other creams helpful for softening the skin and if telangiectasia are unsightly and distress the patient, cosmetic skin preparations are helpful. Physiotherapy, exercises, and splinting to try to prevent and control deformities and improve mobility are often prescribed but seem of doubtful value.

Improvement of peripheral microcirculation

Peripheral vasodilators are used with the object of increasing the nutritional microcirculation. Although in acute studies they appear effective their long-term value is somewhat uncertain and in particular it remains to be determined whether they will prevent the development of fibrotic features of the disease. For acute peripheral ischaemia and in particular to avert infections and incipient gangrene of the digits, intravenous infusions of prostaglandin E_1 or I_2, or low molecular weight dextran may be used. Intra-arterial reserpine can produce local vasodilation in an ischaemic limb.

For long-term treatment agents available include reserpine, guanethidine, methyldopa, and nifedipine. One per cent topical glyceryl trinitrate may also improve the circulation locally. Sympathectomy may provide symptomatic relief but does not seem to alter the long-term course of the disease. The fibrinolytic abnormalities, with failure to clear fibrin deposits in the vessel walls and hyperfibrinaemia and hyperviscosity of the blood, can be corrected using the non-virilizing anabolic steroid stanozolol. This agent does show some promise for the long-term management of this disorder. Low molecular weight dextran probably works in the same way. Plasmapheresis has also been used to reduce fibrinogen levels but also improves red cell deformability.

Anti-inflammatory and immunosuppressive therapy

Non-steroidal anti-inflammatory drugs do not offer any benefit other than relieving the mild joint synovitis. In general steroids seem disappointing although there may be benefit for those patients with marked inflammatory cell infiltration of skin if treated early and for those with overlap syndromes. There is no evidence that immunosuppressive therapy is of any help.

Antifibrotic drugs

Penicillamine interferes with the cross-linking of collagen producing a lathyritic effect. It does appear to be useful for the purely dermal problems provided it is administered early and it may retard the progress of pulmonary fibrosis. Colchicine has been used because *in vitro* it inhibits collagen excretion from fibroblasts. Controlled studies have not shown it to be of benefit. Potassium amino-benzoate (POTABA) has also been shown not to be effective. The weak oestrogen cyclofenil seems to have some influence by reducing connective tissue synthesis but is of uncertain value.

Specific organ involvement

Careful assessment of the individual organ systems is necessary in order to plan a treatment programme.

Metoclopramide improves oesophageal motility and may relieve dysphagia. Reflux leads to heartburn and to stricture formation. H2 antagonists may be effective. In the presence of a stricture oesophageal dilation may be required and there are reconstructive procedures for reflux at the oesophageal–gastric junction. Malabsorption may be due to secondary bacterial overgrowth and should be treated with oral antibiotics. Intestinal pseudo obstruction may respond to conservative treatment. Surgery may be indicated for a volvulus, resection of an isolated loop of non-peristaltic bowel or to exclude some other organic obstruction. Occasionally the ileum is totally resected and the patient managed on a parenteral nutrition regime. For large bowel disease dietary regulation is essential to avoid diarrhoea and constipation.

Cardiac failure is usually resistant to treatment but pericarditis may respond to steroid therapy and rhythm and conduction defects should be treated in the appropriate ways. Fibrosing alveo-litis and pulmonary hypertension are managed as such and lung infections are treated vigorously. However, the prognosis is often poor.

Acute renal failure and malignant hypertension is the most feared complication. Vigorous antihypertensive treatment, in particular with oral angiotensin-converting enzyme inhibitors such as captopril or enalapril can be dramatically effective in reversing these systemic sclerosis renal crises. It is important to treat patients promptly at the onset of acute renal failure and hypertension before permanent renal damage has developed. Some patients are treated by dialysis, or by nephrectomy and renal transplantation. However, the extensive skin changes commonly present in these subjects produce formidable practical problems. There may be some improvement in other features of the disease following successful control of the renal problem. This remains uncertain.

References

D'Angelo, W. A., Fries, J. F., Masi, A. T. and Schulman, L. E. (1969). Pathologic observations in systemic sclerosis (scleroderma). *Am. J. Med.* **46**, 428–440.

Jayson, M. I. V. (1985). Systemic sclerosis. *Copeman's textbook of rheumatology* (ed. J. T. Scott) (in press).

LeRoy, E. C. (1976). Scleroderma (systemic sclerosis). *Modern topics in rheumatology*, Heinemann, London.

Masi, A. T. *et al.* (1980). Preliminary criteria for the classification of systemic sclerosis (scleroderma). *Arth. Rheum.* **23**, 581–590.

Rodnan, G. P. (Ed.) (1979). Progressive systemic sclerosis. *Clinics in rheumatic diseases*. W. B. Saunders, London.

SJÖGREN'S SYNDROME

M. L. SNAITH

History and definition of terms

The eponym acknowledges the contribution of Henrik Sjögren, a Swedish ophthalmologist. Previous authors had recognized the entity underlying pathological dryness of mouth and eyes and its association with inflammatory arthritis. Sjögren, however, emphasized the importance of that association and the simultaneous occurrence of other clinical manifestations which could be related directly or indirectly to it. There is now, however, a problem of definition as newer clinical and immunopathological data have indicated the pivotal but essentially non-specific nature of Sjögren's syndrome in relation to the other autoimmune connective tissue diseases. This chapter assumes the following definitions.

Kerato-conjunctivitis sicca (KCS): pathological deficiency of the aqueous tear film, leading to an increased concentration of mucin, adherent epithelial strands, and patchy loss of integrity of the conjunctiva.

Xerostomia: pathological reduction in salivary flow with or without salivary gland enlargement.

Primary glandular sicca syndrome: consists of the above, not necessarily to an equal degree.

Primary extraglandular sicca syndrome: consists of patients with sicca syndrome who also manifest such features as hyperglobulinaemic purpura, vasculitis, Raynaud's syndrome or pseudolymphoma (see below).

Secondary Sjögren's syndrome: this term describes patients who have a recognizable disease entity such as rheumatoid arthritis (RA) or systemic lupus erythematosus (SLE) concurrently with the sicca syndrome. Abbreviations such as SS-RA or SS-SLE denote these.

It will be apparent that there are some discrepancies with these definitions. For example, KCS is pathognomonic of Sjögren's syndrome yet is frequently allied with xerostomia which is merely a descriptive term for the symptoms due to loss of saliva. Hence it will probably be preferable to insist upon the appropriate histopathological appearance on salivary gland biopsy. The situation can therefore rapidly become too academic. There are other problems, particularly with regard to secondary Sjögren's syndrome. This depends upon the criteria used to diagnose the accompanying disease. Thus a patient with sicca syndrome, arthralgia, one or two swollen joints, high titre rheumatoid factor, lymphadenopathy but no erosions might easily be classified variably as primary extra-glandular sicca syndrome or as secondary Sjögren's syndrome with rheumatoid arthritis. This is perhaps pedantic but recent data indicate that there may be immunogenetic differences between these groups (see below).

Clinical manifestations

Patients may present in many different ways; for example, with dental problems, joint pain, rashes or Raynaud's syndrome. The fact that the patient has Sjögren's syndrome may be only discerned as an incidental finding to a major disease association such as rheumatoid arthritis. The respective components and appropriate investigations may be conveniently discussed together.

Kerato-conjunctivitis sicca (KCS)

A patient presenting with xerophthalmia due to KCS has an eye that looks so irritable that it should be, but is not, watering. Grittiness, discomfort, fatigue, and stickiness of the eye are common complaints. A dry dusty atmosphere makes matters worse and superimposed infection such as with staphylococci may occur. 'Dry eyes' is a not uncommon complaint especially in post-menopausal women and positive diagnosis must be sought.

Methods of substantiating a diagnosis of KCS include Schirmer's test; Bengal Rose staining of the conjunctiva and cornea; slit lamp examination; tear film break-up time; tear protein profiles, (e.g. lysosyme concentration); tear film osmolality; fluorescein dilution; and lacrimal gland biopsy.

Of these the first three are the most widely used and the others will not be discussed here. The Schirmer's and Bengal Rose tests are easily applied by the non-ophthalmologist and, provided their limitations are observed, provide clinically useful information. For the Schirmer's test, the folded end of a 5 × 22 mm strip of No. 41 filter paper (available in packs) is inserted into the conjunctival sac and the patient closes the eyelids. If after 5 min (or before) the whole of the paper is well soaked, abnormal tear secretion is most unlikely. If less than 10 mm of paper is wet it is worth while waving smelling salts or ammonia beneath the patient's nose and moving the paper slightly to another site in the sac. If after 5 min there is still no more than 10 mm of wetting, further investigation is warranted (6 mm is more often used for the purpose of research surveys). Bengal Rose stains the pathological mucin an unmistakable pink (Fig. 1). However, many ophthalmologists maintain that the abnormal epithelial strands (filamentary keratitis) and debris seen with the slit lamp are the most characteristic features.

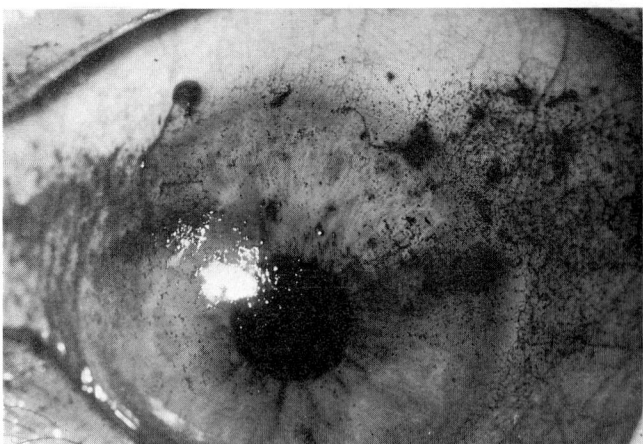

Fig. 1 Bengal Rose staining of conjunctiva.

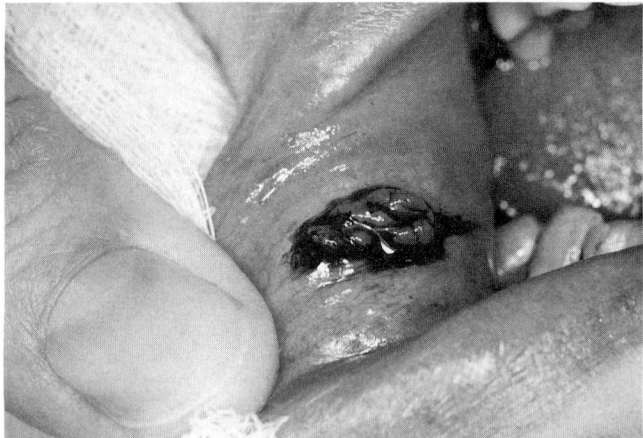

Fig. 2 Minor salivary glands of lower lip revealed for excision.

Xerostomia

Patients may not complain of a dry mouth despite subnormal salivary function or pathological change revealed by biopsy (see below). There are also diverse causes for real or perceived dryness of the mouth, e.g. advancing age, habitual mouth breathing, anxiety, antidepressants or heavy smoking. It is seldom that such as these lead to the extreme dryness which may be seen in Sjögren's syndrome, the patient being unable to eat dry food without recourse to water (the 'cracker' biscuit test). Dental problems with dental pain, gingivitis, mouth odour, and severe caries may be paramount. Distorted canaliculi and inspissated secretions may cause duct blockage and retrograde infection. Angular stomatitis and tongue fissuring occur. Swellings of the parotid or submandibular gland may be quite transient and painless but there is an increased risk of lymphoma in Sjögren's syndrome (see below) and rapid or painful swelling, particularly if unilateral, may be an indication for direct biopsy of the affected gland. The dryness may be so apparent as to obviate investigation. Where doubt exists, or a measure of change is sought, several investigations are available. These include measurements of salivary flow rate (function); sialography (anatomy); scintigraphy (function) and biopsy (pathology).

Salivary flow rate Salivary flow is measured by stimulating the glands and collecting saliva over a fixed time. Methods vary from chewing rubber bands and spitting out the saliva to cannulating the ducts. One method involves intravenous pilocarpine as a maximal stimulus; a special double suction cup is placed over each parotid duct as being representative of the whole secretory apparatus.

Sialography Sialography involves the injection of 0.5 to 2.0 ml of water-soluble contrast via a cannulated duct into each parotid gland in turn. Duct dilation and other abnormalities occur in up to 15 per cent of the general population and can be confused with the sclerosis and dilation of acini and ductuli which result from the lymphoid infiltration of Sjögren's syndrome. Sarcoid is the main differential diagnosis. Sialography is of special relevance when parotid lymphoma is suspected. The opportunity of cannulation can be taken to analyse the saliva obtained (if it is not too viscid and meagre as it is in severe Sjögren's syndrome). To date the disease specificity of changes in composition is not established.

Sequential salivary scintigraphy Sodium pertechnetate, 5–10 mCi (technetium-99) is injected intravenously, with sequential gamma imaging of head and neck. Salivary uptake may be compared with that of the normal thyroid gland. The test may be made sensitive and semiquantitive in experienced hands but it is time consuming and involves a dose of irradiation however modest.

Salivary gland biopsy Scintigraphy, sialography, and flow rates assess major salivary gland function. Clearly the site of suspected

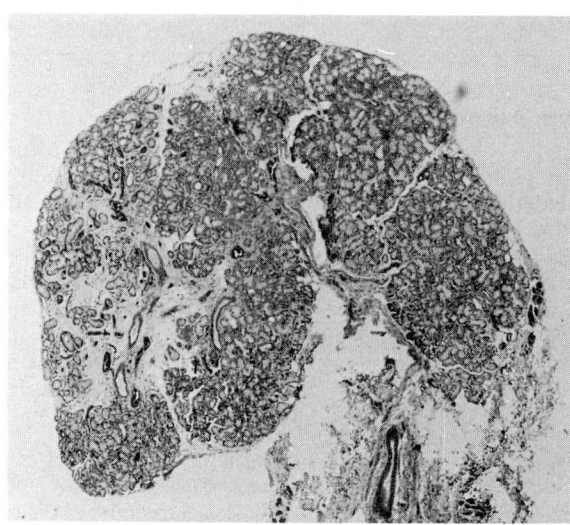

Fig. 3 Normal salivary gland (haematoxylin and eosin).

malignancy must be biopsied directly, but minor salivary gland morphology reflects that of the major gland (at least as far as the pathology of Sjögren's syndrome is concerned). The technique of minor salivary gland biopsy is simple but must be adhered to for safe reliable results (Fig. 2). The incision is closed with absorbable sutures and soreness rarely lasts for more than a few days. Chisholm and Mason's scheme for grading histological changes is widely used: normally (Fig. 3) no foci (an aggregate of more than 50 lymphocytes) of lymphocytes are seen. Four or more foci per 4 mm^2 of tissue (Fig. 4) implies unequivocal pathology. Plasma cell infiltrate may be important. A recent review emphasizes the value of this procedure as a crucial index of Sjögren's syndrome.

Other aspects of sicca disease

The term autoimmune exocrinopathy has been suggested to indicate the potential involvement of the glands of the skin and gastrointestinal or genital tracts. The patient may not think to complain of vaginal dryness as well as discomfort in the eye and it is probable that the more assiduous the clinical examination and investigation of patients with Sjögren's syndrome the more widespread such involvement will be found.

The clinical spectrum of patients with Sjögren's syndrome
Arthritis

Rheumatoid arthritis (RA) affects about half of all patients with Sjögren's syndrome and a further 15 per cent will have arthralgia

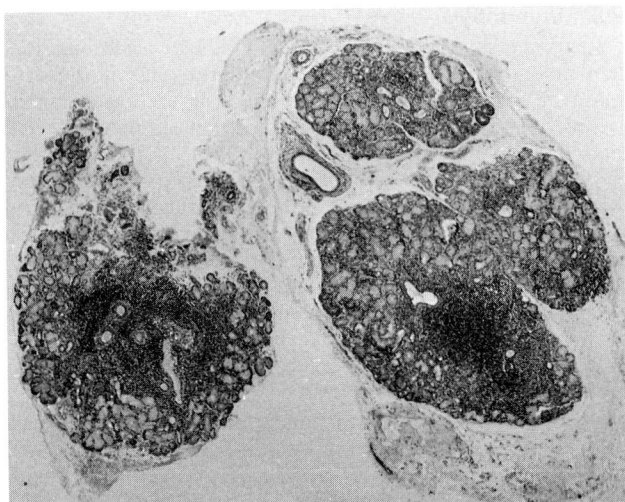

Fig. 4 Grade 4 salivary gland biopsy (see text).

or mild inflammatory arthritis, not fulfilling criteria for RA. Most patients with SLE or scleroderma are likely in addition to have relevant rheumatic symptoms. Conversely, taking patients with RA as the denominator, Sjögren's syndrome has been found in between 20 and 30 per cent. A large post-mortem study of patients with RA indicated that lymphocytic infiltration may be ubiquitous. Sjögren's syndrome usually presents symptomatically in patients with well-established RA but may occasionally precede it for several years. There seems to be no clinical difference between the arthritis of those patients with RA who do have and those who do not have Sjögren's syndrome but the sicca symptoms tend to be much milder than in patients with SLE or scleroderma.

Iatrogenic Sjögren's syndrome
In any chronic immunologically mediated disease such as RA the influence of medication must be considered (recalling such disorders as penicillamine-induced myasthenia gravis and the salivary gland enlargement occasionally caused by phenylbutazone); but, to date, no such conclusive evidence has been found of induced sicca syndrome.

Raynaud's phenomenon and disease
Raynaud's phenomenon is associated with connective tissue diseases in general and particularly scleroderma. It is also quite common in the general population. The association with Sjögren's syndrome is therefore difficult to assess but there does seem to be a genuine increase especially in primary sicca syndrome, compared to rheumatoid arthritis.

Muscle disease
Muscle biopsies in patients with Sjögren's syndrome may reveal asymptomatic abnormalities and a frank clinical polymyositis has been reported. Polymyositis is not a common disease and no comprehensive search for Sjögren's syndrome in such patients has been described. This would be of interest in view of the clinical differences between childhood dermatomyositis, adult 'autoimmune' polymyositis, and adult neoplasm-associated dermatomyositis.

Gastrointestinal disease
Gastrointestinal symptoms might be expected to arise from salivary pathology. It is, however, rare for this to be a major problem. Indeed it is important to ensure that symptoms such as dysphagia are not due to associated but undetected scleroderma. Hypochlorhydria, atrophic gastritis, and parietal cell antibodies have been found frequently, serum pepsinogen levels are reduced and pernicious anaemia may be rather more common.

Liver involvement seems to be infrequent in primary Sjögren's syndrome. Antimitochondrial antibodies were found in only 6 per cent of one series and against smooth muscle, mitochondrial or liver cell in one-third of another. Conversely when SS is sought in autoimmune liver disease (i.e. secondary Sjögren's syndrome) it is commonly found: e.g. 52 per cent of a combined series of chronic active hepatitis and primary biliary cirrhosis, and all 14 in a series of patients with primary biliary cirrhosis.

Renal disease
The distinction must be made between renal pathology due to an associated disease (e.g. lupus nephritis, amyloid due to RA, analgesic nephropathy) and any more specific nephropathy. However, these having been accounted for, there remains a group of patients with nephropathy. There is no unique Sjögren's lesion, but tubular disorders are common if sought. Hyperglobulinaemia is probably not primarily responsible. Azotaemia or nephrotic syndrome are rare. Renal biopsy, when it has been performed, usually reveals mild interstitial nephritis, although extramembranous deposits indicating immune complex involvement have been occasionally noted.

Skin manifestations
The skin is often dry, but not ichthyotic. Patients with SS may develop cutaneous vasculitis, as may other patients with connective tissue diseases. Again, there is no vasculitic pathology unique to Sjögren's syndrome although hyperglobulinaemic purpura is rather characteristic: benign in itself but uncomfortable and unsightly. Visceral vasculitis is rare. The frequency of Sjögren's syndrome in scleroderma is, for reasons which may reflect patient selection or pathological criteria, variably reported from 0 to 90 per cent. Salivary gland fibrosis, without leucocyte infiltration has been reported to indicate a poor prognosis in scleroderma.

Nervous system
A series of 16 patients with primary SS complicated by CNS involvement was reported in 1982. Four patients had spinal cord disorders, including subarachnoid haemorrhage. Cerebral involvement was focal and intermittent and did not resemble the diffuse, often protracted cerebral disease of SLE. Peripheral sensory neuropathy is uncommon, usually mild, and may have a vasculitic basis (as may the cerebral lesion). Twelve of the 16 patients of the above series had an accompanying vasculitis.

Pulmonary involvement
An array of clinical problems has been described: chronic bronchitis, bronchiectasis, asthma, irreversible airways obstruction, diffuse interstitial pneumonia, and fibrosing alveolitis. As ever, if secondary to another disease, one may ascribed the complication to one or other component with equal logic. Restrictive defects predominate.

The 'sicca' component, with viscid mucus and secondary infection may lead to crusting in the pharynx, sore throats, and a hoarse voice. 'Bronchitis sicca' denotes patients with a chronic dry cough due to inspissated secretions and intermittent, secondary infection. Diminished aerosol penetrance of radiolabelled polystyrene particles to the whole lung, but normal central airways clearance, has been reported, implying peripheral plugging analogous to that which may occur in asthma. On the other hand, obstruction could be due to the lymphoproliferative pneumonitis. Lymphoma or pseudo lymphoma may involve the lung. Cardiac disease is rare but pericarditis as part of associated connective tissue disease is not.

Differential diagnosis of Sjögren's syndrome
Amyloid, hyperlipoproteinaemia and haemochromatosis can occasionally produce a sicca syndrome, but the true picture may be established quickly by biopsy.

Laboratory investigations in Sjögren's syndrome
A mild normocytic hypochromic or normochromic anaemia is common, leucopenia, thrombocytopenia, and haemolytic anaemia less so. One can expect a raised sedimentation rate. Perhaps the most typical pathological finding is hyperglobulinaemia, usually

IgG. Otherwise laboratory variables will reflect target organ involvement.

Immunopathology of Sjögren's syndrome

There is evidence of considerable immune hyperreactivity in all people with SS with hyperglobulinaemia (which may be symptomatic with hyperviscosity syndromes or purpura), elevated levels of immune complexes, and autoantibodies and disturbed cellular immunity.

Humoral immunity

Eighty eight per cent of an early series of patients with primary SS had antinuclear antibodies (ANA) compared to the SS-RA patients with a frequency of 56 per cent. Other authors have since reported similar findings, with perhaps a rather lower prevalence. The fluorescent staining patterns are variably diffuse, speckled or occasionally nucleolar. The titre seems to bear no clear relationship to disease activity.

The Ouchterlony method of antibody detection defined a number of different systems often identified by the initials of an index patient. It is now apparent that those termed Ro, SjD, and SSA are the same or very similar, as are La, SjT, SSB, and Ha. The macromolecular antigens concerned, whilst sharing common determinants, are not necessarily physicochemically identical, especially if derived from a different tissue or a cultured cell line. The antigens can now be purified and used in specific assay systems, such as an enzyme-linked immunosorbent assay (ELISA). They are soluble complexes of protein with small RNA nucleotides. Ro has a molecular weight of about 150 kD, and La one of 100. Ro is probably cytoplasmic and La cytoplasmic and nuclear. Their intracellular functions are unclear, but monoclonal antibodies raised against these purified antigens are of interest to the cell biologist. The naturally occurring autoantibodies may be of any immunoglobulin class.

Anti-Ro antibodies occur in about one-third of all patients with SS, the frequency of anti-La being more variably reported. The prevalence seems greatest in primary SS and in SS-SLE. Anti-Ro has been associated with vasculitis in SS and also in SS-SLE. Anti-La in patients with undiagnosed arthralgia may predict for SS rather than RA.

Antibodies to DNA or DNA protein are found in about a quarter of patients with primary SS or SS-RA. High titres of antibodies to double-stranded DNA will probably indicate associated SLE with concurrent or impending nephritis. Some rheumatoid factors have antinuclear binding specificity. Interestingly, a positive Rose-Waaler is found in close to 100 per cent of SS patients, whether or not there is an associated erosive synovitis. IgG and IgA antiglobulins are also found in excess, in the blood and saliva of patients with RA, systemic SS or SS-RA.

Circulating immune complexes are elevated in most patients with SS, irrespective of type. Levels are said not to correlate with disease activity. Such complexes may be handled abnormally by the reticuloendothelial system in SS as judged by the clearance of radiolabelled antibody-coated erythrocytes. Ro/anti-Ro complexes may be pathogenic.

Organ-specific autoantibodies are frequent (about 30 per cent) in patients with SS: specificities include thyroid, ovary, pancreas, parietal cell, liver cell, membrane, skeletal muscle, and smooth muscle. This frequency does not seem to be matched by organ-specific disease and may in part reflect polyclonal activation. Thyroid may be the exception – pathological similarities between autoimmune thyroiditis and the salivary gland in SS have been pointed out although there may be no increased prevalence of thyroid disease amongst patients with KCS.

Antibodies to salivary duct are commoner in SS-RA (50–70 per cent) than in primary SS (10–20 per cent) or RA alone (20–30 per cent). This, if anything, reverse ratio between target organ disease severity and antibody level permits of varying interpretation as to its role in pathogenesis.

Cellular immunity

The humoral evidence might be taken to indicate a combination of general clonal expansion and reduced suppression, but there is no increase in circulating B cells spontaneously secreting immunoglobulin. Lymphopenia is relatively uncommon and there is no overall T cell lymphopenia. These are all in relative contrast to SLE. Suppressor T cells with an IgG Fc receptor are depleted in blood and lip biopsy specimens. Mitogen-induced plaque formation is reduced in some patients, as is the autologous mixed lymphocyte reaction (by inference, affecting the generation of suppressor T lymphocytes). Humoral and cellular factors interact: for example, sera from SS patients with extraglandular SS blocked the expression of the Fc receptor on normal lymphocytes.

Genetics of Sjögren's syndrome

In view of the evidence, both human and animal, that genetic influences bear upon the expression of disease such as rheumatoid arthritis and SLE, it would not be surprising if such were found to be the case in Sjögren's syndrome. An association with DR4 is found in SS-RA: DR3 tends to be increased in patients with primary SS, as are certain B cell alloantigens. DR2 and DR3 may also be associated with higher titres of antibody to the autoantigen La.

Malignancy in Sjögren's syndrome

It has been suggested that SS encompasses a continuous spectrum of lymphoproliferation, from hyperglobulinaemia, with autoantibodies and immune complexes, to malignant lymphoproliferation. Indeed of 136 patients with SS traced retrospectively, 7 cases of non-Hodgkins lymphoma were found, giving a relative risk of 44 compared to the normal. An intermediate stage, of 'pseudolymphoma' has been identified involving enlarging lymphadenopathy, hyperglobulinaemia, and extraglandular, benign, but sometimes massive lymphoreticular hyperplasia. Considerable parotid enlargement was occasionally treated with irradiation and this seems to have been associated with a yet greater risk of subsequent malignancy. There may already be an increased risk of lymphoreticular malignancy among patients with rheumatoid arthritis, although the contribution from drug-induced oncogenesis is uncertain.

Whether the so-called Benign Lymphoreticular Lesion of Sjögren's glands is really so benign or not, a policy of early biopsy should be maintained if a patient has enlarging lymph-nodes or salivary glands. Malignant lymphoma of Sjögren's has been shown to be of B cell phenotype, but pseudolymphoma may be predominantly of T cell phenotype.

Treatment of Sjögren's syndrome
Symptomatic

A problem-orientated approach to the management of patients with Sjögren's syndrome is appropriate in most. Symptomatic treatment is safe and reasonably successful. The dry eye is managed with some form of tear substitute, methylcellulose being the most commonly used. The drops are applied as required for ease, usually two to four times a day. A 20 per cent solution of the mucolytic acetylcysteine is useful in more severe cases, as are the slow-release rods for night times. Oral bromhexine has been advocated for xerophthalmia. Surgical obliteration of the naso-lacrimal duct in order to reduce drainage is occasionally required. Supervening infection, often staphylococcal, should be treated appropriately. Mouth infections should be treated promptly. Teeth must be preserved if at all possible, as dentures become ill-fitting.

Other secretions are less of a problem: a bland lubricant may be used for the vagina, or one of the many proprietary preparations for the skin.

Systemic treatment

In secondary SS the nature of the treatment will be dictated largely by the accompanying disease. Even in primary SS, where the sicca features predominate, it is relatively unusual for them to be so severe and unresponsive to symptomatic management that systemic treatment is needed on the grounds of reduced glandular secretions alone. The extraglandular complications may also be treated individually: non-steroidal anti-inflammatory drugs for arthralgia, alkalis for renal tubular acidosis, various vasodilating drugs for Raynaud's, and so on. More serious features such as myositis or lung infiltrates may warrant corticosteroids: usually 30–60 mg, daily of prednisolone, tapering according to response. Pseudolymphoma is reported to respond well to steroids, but unacceptable steroid toxicity may be an indication for the addition of a cytotoxic drug such as azathioprine. Controlled trials are lacking. The rare long-term malignant complications of SS will of course require the opinion of an oncologist.

Aetiology

It seems inherently unlikely that so protean a condition is a homogenous pathological entity. Perhaps it represents variable modes of expression of lymphoid hyperplasia resulting from autoimmune stimulation, with secondary clinical features due to local manifestations such as immune complex vasculitis.

An indication of the central position of Sjögren's syndrome in relation to autoimmune disease is given by the comparison with other forms of chronic inflammatory arthritis: Sjögren's syndrome does NOT complicate psoriatic arthritis, ankylosing spondylitis or Reiter's syndrome. Why there is such an inextricable link with the exocrine glands remains unclear.

References

Alarcon–Segovia, D., Diaz-Jonenen, E. and Fishbein, E. (1973). Features of Sjögren's syndrome in primary biliary cirrhosis. *Ann. int. Med.* **779**, 31–36.
Alspaugh, M. A. and Tan, E. M. (1975). Antibodies to cellular antigens in Sjögren's syndrome. *J. Clin. Invest.* **55**, 1067–1073.
Anderson, J. R., Cray, K. G., Beck, J. S. and Kinnear, W. F. (1961). Precipitating auto-antibodies in Sjögren's disease. *Lancet* **2**, 456–460.
Anderson, L. G. and Talal, N. (1982). The spectrum of benign to malignant lympho-proliferation in Sjögren's syndrome. *Clin. Exp. Immun.* **10**, 199–224.
Bloch, K. J., Buchanan, W. W., Wohl, M. J. and Bunim, J. J. (1965). Sjögren's syndrome: A clinical, pathological and serological study of 62 cases. *Medicine* **44**, 187–231.
Cipoletti, J. F., Buckingham, R. B., Barnes, E. L., Peel, R. L., Mahmood, K., Cignettis, F. E., Pierce, J. M., Rabin, B. S. and Rodnan, G. P. (1977). Sjögren's syndrome in progressive systemic sclerosis. *Ann. Int. Med.* **87**, 535–541.
Denko, C. W. and Old, J. W. (1969). Myopathy in the sicca syndrome. (Sjögren's syndrome). A study of sixteen cases. *Arch. Int. Med.* **105**, 849–858.
Dijkstra, P. F. (1980). Classification and differential diagnosis of sialographic characteristics in Sjögren's syndrome. *Sem. Arthr. Rheum.* **10**, 10–17.
Fairfax, A. J., Haslam, P. L., Pavia, D., Sheahan, N. F., Bateman, J. R. M., Agnew, J. E., Clarke, S. W. and Turner-Warwick, M. (1981). Pulmonary disorders associated with Sjögren's syndrome. *Q. J. Med.* **50**, 279–295.
Fox, R. I., Adamson, T. C., Fong, S., Robinson, C. A., Morgan, E. L., Robb, J. A. and Howell, F. V. (1983). Lymphocyte phenotype and function in pseudolymphoma associated with Sjögren's syndrome. *J. Clin. Invest.* **72**, 52–62.
Golding, P. L., Brown, R., Mason, A. M. S. and Taylor E. (1970). Sicca complex in liver disease. *Br. Med. J.* **4**, 340–342.
Isenberg, D. A., Hammond, L., Fisher, C., Griffiths, M., Stewart, J. and Bottazzo, G. F. (1982). Predictive value of SS-B precipitating antibodies in Sjögren's syndrome. *Br. Med. J.* **284**, 1738–1740.
Kassan, S. S. and Gardy, M. (1978). Sjögren's syndrome: an update and overview. *Am. J. Med.* **64**, 1037–1046.
MacSween, R. N. M., Goudie, R. B. and Amderson, J. R. (1967). Occurrence of antibody to salivary duct epithelium in Sjögren's disease, rheumatoid arthritis and other arthritides. *Ann. Rheum. Dis.* **26**, 402–411.
Maddison, P. J. (1985). Dry eyes: autoimmunity and relationship to other systemic disease. *Trans. Ophthalmol. Soc. UK* **104**, 458–461.
Malinow, K. L., Molina, R., Gordon, B., Selnes, O. A., Provost, T. T. and Alexander, E. L. (1985). Neuropsychiatric dysfunction in primary Sjögren's syndrome. *Ann. Intern. Med.* **103**, 344–350.
Manthorpe, R., Frost-Larsen, K., Isager, H. and Prause, J. U. (1981). Sjögren's syndrome: a review with emphasis on immunological features. *Allergy* **36**, 139–153.
Molina, R., Provost, T. T. and Alexander, E. L. (1985). Two types of inflammatory vascular disease in Sjögren's syndrome. *Arthr. Rheum.* **28**, 1251–1258.
Moutsopoulos, H. M., Chused, T. M., Mann, L., Klippel, J. H., Fauci, A. S., Frank, M. M., Lawley, T. J. and Hamburger, M. I. (1980). Sjögren's syndrome (sicca syndrome): current Issues. *Ann. Int. Med.* **92**, 212–226.
Oxholm, P., Bundgaard, A., Madsen, E. B., Manthorpe, R. and Rasmussen, F. V. (1982). Pulmonary function in patients with primary Sjögren's syndrome. *Rheum. Int.* **2**, 179–181.
Penner, E. and Reichlin, M. (1982). Primary biliary cirrhosis associated with Sjögren's syndrome: evidence for circulating and tissue-deposited Ro/anti-Ro immune complexes. *Arthr. Rheum.* **25**, 1250–1253.
Shearn, M. A. (1971). Sjögren's syndrome. In *Major problems in internal medicine* Vol. 2 (ed. L. H. Smith Jr), pp. 617–671. W. B. Saunders Co, Philadelphia.
Strand, V. and Talal, N. (1980). Advances in the diagnosis and concept of Sjögren's syndrome (auto-immune exocrinopathy). *Bull. Rheum. Dis.* **30**, 1046–1052.
Yoshinoya, S., McDuffy, S., Alarcon-Segovia, D. and Pope, R. M. (1982). Detection and partial characterization of immune complexes in patients with rheumatoid arthritis plus Sjögren's syndrome and with Sjögren's syndrome alone. *Clin. Exp. Immun.* **48**, 339–347.

MIXED CONNECTIVE TISSUE DISEASE (MCTD)

M. L. SNAITH

Patients are said to have MCTD when there are overlapping features of systemic lupus erythematosus (SLE), polymyositis, scleroderma or rheumatoid arthritis, to differing extents; a necessary criterion is the presence of antibodies in high titre to ribonucleoprotein (RNP), giving rise to a speckled pattern antinuclear antibody (ANA). There is however no necessary pathological end point. Whether it is clinically or conceptually useful to so define a group of patients remains a debated subject. In order to set this in perspective, it is worthwhile recalling the process by which the concept evolved.

In the late 1960s Sharp and co-workers observed that there was a group of patients whose serum sustained a high titre of antinuclear antibodies throughout periods of remission and relapse, by contrast with patients with SLE, whose titres often became negative during remission. Upon reviewing the clinical data, it became apparent that these patients had features of several conditions conventionally regarded as rather separate: SLE, polymyositis etc. as above. The antinuclear antibodies were at the time detected using complement fixation and a crude extract of calf thymus nuclei. It further became apparent, using a haemagglutination method, that high titres of a particular antibody were characteristic of this group of patients. The antigen was present in a saline extract of calf thymus (hence ENA–extractable nuclear antigen). Patients with definite SLE often also had antibodies against this ENA, in a titre which was barely affected when the ENA-coated erythrocytes were treated with ribonuclease, and moderately reduced by trypsin digestion. This antigen became known as Sm, after Smith, the index patient.

The group of patients with the 'mixed' clinical features seemed to share an antibody specificity which was also moderately affected by trypsin, but completely abolished by digestion of the antigen with ribonuclease (hence RNP, for ribonucleoprotein). The name MCTD was applied to this group of patients. Their clinical characteristics were as follows:

Characteristic	Per cent
Arthritis/arthralgia	96
Swollen hands	88
Raynaud's phenomenon	84
Abnormal oesophageal motility	77
Myositic	72
Lymphadenopathy	68
Fever	32
Hepatomegaly	28
Serositis	24
Splenomegaly	21
Renal disease	0
Anaemia	48
Leucopenia	52
Hypergammaglobulinaemia	80

(after Sharp et al., 1972)

The most distinctive clinical feature of this early group of patients appeared to be their tendency to have swollen, puffy hands, similar to those with which physicians were familiar in patients with early scleroderma. The MCTD patients, at least initially, failed to proceed to the more fibrotic and severe form of that disease. The other prominent feature was the rarity of severe renal disease and a concomitant absence of high titre anti-DNA antibodies.

At first it seemed that the anti-RNP antibody would prove to be an early marker for this disorder and that the patients could be assured of a reasonably complete and rapid improvement in their symptoms in response to quite moderate doses of steroids, with little likelihood of renal disease. However, it became apparent that patients with undoubted SLE could have anti-RNP. Thus this antibody as a necessary criterion had to be matched by the absence of, or at most low titres of, antibodies to DNA. There are therefore no absolute criteria for MCTD. This might not have been too unsatisfactory a state of affairs if the patients had remained as a group, with a rather characteristic cluster of features: but this is not the case despite the puffy 'sausage' fingers of a patient with MCTD which are indeed quite striking.

The problem has been that an increasing number of patients have been described with all the features of MCTD but with additional features such as severe glomerulonephritis and DNA antibodies. One then had to say that this was just an unusual manifestation of MCTD, or that the patient also had SLE: clearly, to many, an unsatisfactory state of affairs. An additional complication has been that with the passage of time patients with MCTD have evolved into more definite entities such as scleroderma. Several useful surveys have been published, approaching the problem of definition from different standpoints: some patients may present with rheumatoid arthritis (RA) but evolve later to typical MCTD. Another report showed that, of 20 patients diagnosed as having MCTD, half could initially be said to have RA and on retrospective review or follow up over up to 30 years, 11 could be reclassified as having scleroderma. On the other hand, by applying the 1974 American Rheumatism Criteria for SLE, all 20 could be said to have that disease. By the 1982 criteria, with Raynaud's phenomenon removed, the situation changes once again. Rheumatological nosology is indeed lacking in pathological specificity. Twenty two of the original 1972 series of 25 patients with MCTD were traced in 1982 and only five could still be so classified. Five had evolved into definite scleroderma.

Clinical aspects of MCTD

Arthritis is a very common component; indeed, a diagnosis of RA is commonly made, but there is an impression that it does not follow the normal course of RA. The synovitis tends to be milder, the erosions smaller, and the degree of functional impairment less. It is uncommon for drugs such as gold to be required to control symptoms, as either non-steroidal, anti-inflammatory drugs or steroids given for other manifestations suffice to control the joint disease.

Over 90 per cent of patients suffer from Raynaud's disease, which may be very troublesome, with digital gangrene. Rashes tend to be erythematous, although perhaps with fewer atrophic or discoid lesions than in SLE. Deposition of IgG in epidermal nuclei in a speckled pattern has been claimed to be characteristic, but this may be a laboratory artefact.

Pleuropericardial involvement seems to occur in much the same way as in SLE. Attention has been drawn to the development of lung disease and pulmonary hypertension.

Myositis is a prominent feature; it does not seem to have any unique aspects compared with those in 'primary' or SLE-associated myositis. Immunoglobulin deposition has been observed around normal vessels as well as in association with sarcolemma and perimysium.

Although the absence of nephropathy was a *sine qua non* for the diagnosis of MCTD, some patients with apparent MCTD develop renal disease and azotaemia, with no DNA antibodies. The number of patients who fall into this category is too small to permit more than a passing comment, but immune complex nephropathy has been described.

Oesophageal involvement was common in the earlier series and the progression to classical systemic sclerosis has already been emphasized. Hepatitis seems to be rather unusual.

Cerebral involvement seems to be less common and less severe than in SLE. No characteristic features have been defined, although trigeminal nerve palsies appear to be unusually frequent and apparent precipitation by anti-inflammatory drugs has been noted.

As in SLE, females are more commonly affected than males (between 6 and 9 to 1). Children appear to have a notable tendency to develop proliferative vascular lesions. Nephritis seems to be relatively more common in children than in adults.

Pathological aspects of MCTD

Antinuclear antibodies

A positive fluorescent and antinuclear antibody test, often to remarkably high titre (i.e. 1 : 10 000 or more) is virtually necessary for the diagnosis of MCTD. The pattern is speckled but this is common to SLE and Sjögren's syndrome. Its abolition by treatment of the substrate with ribonuclease is confirmation of the nature of the binding antigen, but is not as sensitive a technique as immunoprecipitation (*vide infra*).

Antibodies to RNP

The clinical records of 44 patients found to have high titres (>1 : 10 000) of anti-RNP antibodies have been examined. In those studied, within 5 years of onset there were fewer 'overlap' features; eventually over half the patients developed a more traditionally definable connective tissue disease, principally fibrotic scleroderma. Eleven patients developed nephritis, with negative tests for anti-DNA antibodies. Thus, not only is there some doubt about there being necessary and sufficient clinical criteria for MCTD, the same may be said to apply to antibodies to RNP. Nevertheless, high titres are striking and the phenomenon is worth examining in a little greater detail.

Throughout the early years of the history of MCTD, identification of the antibody/antigen system was achieved using standard sera in gel precipitation (Ouchterlony) and relying upon lines of identity to show that sera had the same specificity. A modification of this technique, immunoelectrophoresis, is speedier and more sparing of sera. The haemagglutination method, using calf or rabbit thymus extract, is more taxing technically but allows great sensitivity. The antigen has always been found to be complexed to some extent with the Sm antigen, but recent work has shown that there are at least two species of nuclear RNP involved.

Since these antibodies are the most consistent laboratory characteristic of MCTD, what could be their role in pathogenesis?

This is uncertain, but they are normally of IgG subclass, speckled intranuclear fluorescence has been noted in the skin of such patients, and anti-RNP antibodies may penetrate living cells through Fc receptors. Nuclear matrix proteins have been shown to be the targets of the autoimmune reaction in some patients.

Other laboratory findings in MCTD

In active disease, a normocytic anaemia of 'chronic disease' is usual, together with other non-specific findings such as hyperglobulinaemia, elevated acute phase proteins, and mild leucopenia. Thrombocytopenia of the immune consumptive type is occasionally found, as is haemolytic anaemia. Lymphopenia does not seem common. As emphasized above, antibodies to single or double-stranded DNA are found less usually than in SLE; where they are noted, it is usually in low titre or, if in high titre, then one tends to find a more 'SLE-like' clinical syndrome, with nephritis becoming more apparent. Serum complement levels are usually normal, in the absence of advancing glomerulonephritis. Increased concentrations of circulating immune complexes may be detected.

The presence of immunoglobulin and complement, demonstrable at the dermo-epidermal junction by immunofluorescence and termed the lupus 'band' test, is considered rather specific for SLE. A 'speckled' pattern of epidermal staining has been described as being characteristic of MCTD, but positive 'bands' have also been noted.

Since a large minority, or majority, of patients have features of rheumatoid arthritis at one or other stage of their clinical course, one might expect to find rheumatoid factors: 37 per cent in one series. There have been no other published data on the nature of these antiglobulins.

The inference from the presence of high titre auto-antibodies in MCTD and associated disease is that immunoregulation is disordered: T suppressor cell circuitry has been shown to be abnormal in SLE although whether this is a primary T cell defect or secondary to null cell control is as yet unclear. Similar but not identical T subset abnormalities have been shown in patients with MCTD; which is a pointer in favour of there being some genuine immunopathological identity for MCTD.

Treatment and prognosis of patients with MCTD

Clinical features such as arthritis may be treated with nonsteroidal anti-inflammatory drugs (or such measures as intralesional corticosteroids and physical treatment for contractures). Pleuritis, arthralgia, rashes, and malaise may respond to antimalarials as in SLE. Oral corticosteroids remain the mainstay of the management of patients with more severe disease, much as those with SLE. There is no published evidence that D-penicillamine or colchicine prevent the progression to fibrotic scleroderma, although that would be an appealing strategy. The use of the more toxic regimens of steroids or immunosuppressives is dictated by the severity of end-organ involvement. Thus, if myositis is either not responding to prednisolone in adequate dosage (i.e. 1–1.5 mg/kg body weight/day), or steroid myopathy is developing, then one would consider adding azathioprine, 2.5 mg/kg/day (or another cytotoxic drug), endeavouring progressively to reduce the steroid dosage thereafter.

There is no evidence that patients with MCTD who develop features, for example, of SLE or scleroderma, should be treated any differently from patients not passing through a MCTD 'stage'.

It remains possible that high titre anti-RNP antibody, as the main serological abnormality, is associated with a cluster of myositis, swollen hands, Raynaud's phenomenon, arthritis, a negative association with renal disease and a relatively good prognosis. However, until techniques are available for more specific immunomodulation, the identification of such clusters of clinical manifestations is more of theoretical than therapeutic value.

The prognosis of patients with MCTD remains a vexed question. Undoubtedly some patients go into clinical and serological remission, particularly if they remain in the classical mould: but then the potential functional recovery of muscle or joints is very different from fibrotic scleroderma or diffuse glomerulonephritis. It is nice to be able to reassure a patient that she does have a potentially reversible illness. Female patients may want to know what their chances are of having children normally. It seems that the outlook is much the same as for patients with SLE (page 16.20); there is an abnormally high fetal wastage for a variety of reasons. Children with MCTD are reported as having a worse prognosis than adults perhaps because of the greater frequency of nephritis and vascular pathology.

References

Alarcon-Segovia, D. (1983). Mixed connective tissue disease: A disorder of immune regulation. *Sem. Arthr. Rheum.* **13** (Suppl. 1), 114–120.

——, Lorente, L. and Ruiz-Argelles, A. (1979). Antibody penetration into living cells II; Antiribonucleoprotein IgG penetrates into T lymphocytes causing their deletion and the abrogation of their suppressor function. *J. Immun.* **122**, 1855–1862.

Bennett, R. M. and O'Connell, D. J. (1980). Mixed connective tissue disease; A clinicopathologic study of 20 cases. *Sem. Arthr. Rheum.* **10**, 25–51.

—— and Spargo, B. H. (1977). Immune complex nephropathy in mixed connective tissue disease. *Am. J. Med.* **63**, 535–541.

Bernstein, R. F. (1980). Ibuprofen-related meningitis in mixed connective tissue disease. *Ann. Intern. Med.* **92**, 206–207.

Cohen, A S., Reynolds, W. E., Franklin, E. C., Kulka, J. P., Ropes, M. W., Shulman, L. E. and Wallace, S. L. (1971). Preliminary criteria for the classification of SLE. *Bull. Rheum. Dis.* **21**, 643–648.

Fritzler, M. J., Ali, R. and Tan, E. M. (1984). Antibodies from patients with mixed connective tissue disease react with heterogenous nuclear ribonucleoprotein or ribonucleic acid (hn RNP/RNA) of the nuclear matrix. *J. Immun.* **132**, 1216–1221.

Gilliam, J. N. and Prystowsky, S. D. (1977). Mixed connective tissue disease syndrome. *Arch. Derm.* **113**, 583–587.

Glassock, R. J. and Goldstein, D. A. (1982). Recurrent acute renal failure in a patient with mixed connective tissue disease. *Am. J. Nephrol.* **2**, 282–290.

Hench, P. K., Edgington, T. S. and Tan, E. M. (1975). The evolving clinical spectrum of mixed connective tissue disease. *Arthr. Rheum.* **18**, 404.

Iwatsuki, K., Tagami, H., Imaizumi, S., Ginoza, M. and Yamada, M. (1982). The speckled epidermal nuclear immunofluorescence of mixed connective tissue disease seems to develop as an *in vitro* phenomenon. *Br. J. Derm.* **107**, 653–657.

Lemmer, J. P., Curry, N. H., Mallory, J. H. and Waller, M. V. (1982). Clinical characteristics and course in patients with high titre RNP antibodies. *J. Rheum.* **9**, 536–542.

Leroy, E. C., Maricq, H. R. and Kahaleh, M. B. (1980). Undifferentiated connective tissue syndromes. *Arthr. Rheum.* **23**, 341–343.

Levitan, P. M., Weary, P. E. and Guiliano, V. J. (1975). The immunofluorescent 'band' test in mixed connective tissue disease. *Ann. intern. Med.* **83**, 53–55.

Nimelstein, S. H., Brody, S., McShane, D. and Holman, H. R. (1980). Mixed connective tissue disease; a subsequent evaluation of the original 25 patients. *Medicine* **59**, 239–248.

Oxenhandler, R., Hart, M., Corman, L., Sharp, G. C. and Adelstein, E. (1977). Pathology of skeletal muscle in mixed connective tissue disease *Arthr. Rheum.* **20**, 985–988.

Reichlin, M. and Mattioli, M. (1972). Correlation of a precipitin reaction to an RNA protein antigen and a low prevalence of nephritis in patients with systemic lupus erythematosus. *N. Engl. T. Med.* 908–911.

Sakane, T., Steinberg, A. D., Reeves, J. P. and Green, I. (1979). Studies of immune function of patients with systemic lupus erythematosus. *J. Clin. Invest.* **64**, 1260–1269.

Sharp, G. C., Irvin, W. S., Tan, E. M., Gould, G. R. and Holman, H. R. (1972). Mixed tissue disease - an apparently distinct rheumatic disease syndrome associated with a specific antibody to an extractable nuclear antigen (ENA). *Am. J. Med.* **52**, 148–158.

Singsen, B. H., Swanson, V. L., Bernstein, B. H., Henser, E. T., Hanson, B. and Landing, B. (1980). A histologic evaluation of mixed connective tissue disease in childhood. *Am. J. Med.* **68**, 710–717.

Sullivan, W. D., Hurst, D. J., Harmon, C. E., Esther, J. H., Agia, G. A., Maltby, J. D., Lillard, S. B., Held, C. H., Wolfe, J. F., Sunderrajan, E. V., Maricq, H. R. and Sharp, G. C. (1984). A prospective evaluation emphasizing pulmonary involvement in patients with mixed connective tissue disease. *Medicine* **63**, 92–107.

Tan, E. M., Cohen, A. S., Fries, J. F., Masi, A. T., McShane, D. J., Rothfield, N. F., Schaller, J. G., Talal, N. and Winchester, R. J. (1982). The 1982 revised criteria for the classification of systemic lupus erythematosus. *Arthr. Rheum.* **25**, 1271–1277.

POLYMYOSITIS AND DERMATOMYOSITIS

M. A. BYRON

Introduction

Polymyositis (PM) and dermatomyositis (DM) form part of a heterogeneous group of inflammatory muscle disorders of unknown aetiology. The conditions are characterized by muscular weakness, with or without wasting, associated with pain and tenderness in the muscles in the acute phase, and atrophy and contraction in the more chronic phase. The incidence has been estimated in the USA as 0.5 cases per 100 000 population, with the highest rate in negro females. In northeast England a prevalence of 8 per 100 000 has been reported. There is a female preponderance under the age of 55 years, with little or no skin involvement. These features are reversed in older patients with associated neoplasms. Several clinical types of polymyositis are recognized and are shown in Table 1.

Aetiology

Viral

The descriptions of syndromes resembling polymyositis, in association with acute viral infections suggests that such infections could provoke chronic immunopathological disorders in susceptible individuals. Although electron microscopic (EM) studies have shown virus-like inclusion particles in muscles of patients, these have rarely been confirmed by isolating the suspected virus. One exception is the isolation of echovirus from the cerebrospinal fluid of hypogammaglobulinaemic patients with chronic echovirus infection and an atypical myositis (see later). Coxsackie B virus has been implicated indirectly, as high levels of IgM antibody against coxsackie B have been found in 37 per cent of patients with acute myocarditis or pericarditis (important features of polymyositis). Also a murine model of polymyositis is induced by coxsackie B1. In this model inflammation persists long after the infecting virus can be isolated. New progress is being made now that it is appreciated that subtle differences exist in the properties and virulence of different virus strains which may appear identical by conventional antisera.

Immunological

One of the prominent histological features of PM is a chronic inflammatory infiltrate, characterized by monoclonal antibodies as predominantly inducer T cells; and circulating lymphocytes from patients are cytotoxic to human fetal muscle cells. Humoral antibodies have now been identified by immunoprecipitation (Table 2), and antinuclear antibodies can be detected. Analysis of the chemical nature of the antigens may reveal the possible stimuli for

Table 1 Classification of polymyositis and dermatomyositis

Primary idiopathic polymyositis

Primary idiopathic dermatomyositis

Dermatomyositis (or polymyositis) with neoplasm

Childhood dermatomyositis with vasculitis

Dermatomyositis (or polymyositis) with collagen vascular disease (overlap syndrome)

Table 2 Autoantibodies in polymyositis and dermatomyositis

Antibody	Specificity	Antigen
Jo-1	30% PM patients	Histidyl-t-RNA synthetase
Mi-2	25% DM patients	Nuclear protein 50–58 Kd
n-RNP	10–15% PM patients with features of SLE or PSS	
PM-1 or PM-Sc1	8% PM patients and overlap syndromes	Nucleolar antigen

autoimmune reactions. Sera with anti-Jo-1 activity bind histidyl-t-RNA and block its aminoacylation. This suggests that certain RNA viruses which become specifically aminoacylated, could act as the inciting antigen.

Genetic

A number of cases of familial polymyositis have been reported, and there is a weak association with HLA B8 and DR3. The latter association is much stronger in patients possessing anti-Jo-1 antibody, which may identify a subgroup of patients particularly at risk of interstitial lung disease.

Pathology

The characteristic histological picture is one of muscle fibre degeneration and necrosis, with infiltration by inflammatory cells. The mainly perivascular cellular infiltrate consists predominantly of lymphocytes and macrophages, with a few plasma cells and occasional polymorphs. Degeneration of muscle fibres affects both type I (red) and type II (white) and the proportion of damaged fibres is reflected in the number showing centrally placed nuclei. In the chronic phase necrotic fibres are replaced by scar and adipose tissue and regeneration of less damaged fibres occurs, either from surviving parts or from satellite cells. A striking feature is the variability in size of individual fibres in cross section, as degeneration and regeneration occur side by side. These findings are not specific for polymyositis, and up to 15 per cent of biopsies from patients with the disease appear normal.

Vascular changes may be important features, especially in children in whom vasculitis is common. The vessels affected are the arteries and arterioles of the endomysium and perimysium. An uncommon feature, again more frequently seen in children, is calcification in fibrous tissue between affected muscle bundles and occasionally in the skin. The histology of affected skin in DM has no specific features. There is oedema and basal cell vacuolation, but no immunoglobulin deposition.

Clinical features

There is a bimodal distribution in age of onset of myositis, with a peak at 5–14 years, and again at 45–64 years. The childhood illness has characteristic features and will be dealt with separately.

In adults the most frequently encountered mode of presentation is that of progressive or fluctuating proximal weakness over a period of months, often commencing in the shoulder girdle and cervical muscles. Weakness is usually disproportionately severe in comparison with muscle atrophy in the early stages, and is often accompanied by mild pain and muscular tenderness. Dermatomyositis is diagnosed if certain skin manifestations are also present. The most characteristic is the heliotrope discoloration and oedema of the eyelids, which occurs in 25 per cent of patients, and tends to wax and wane, not always with disease activity. A similar purplish dusky appearance may be seen on the cheeks and other light exposed areas, although true photosensitivity is rare. Violaceous and scaly rashes may occur on knees, elbows, and knuckles in 30–50 per cent of patients. These become atrophic leaving pale plaques particularly over the knuckles (collodian patches or Gottron's papules). Similar skin lesions may be seen in systemic lupus erythematosus (SLE), but detection of immune globulins by immunofluorescence on skin biopsy in the latter should help in differentiation.

Nailfold changes (cuticular hypertrophy), periungual erythema, and telangiectasia are non-specific indicators of myositis, and occur in other connective tissue diseases. Microscopy of nailfold capillaries may show a bushy branching appearance in dermatomyositis, but prominent vascular dilation and small nailfold infarcts are not specific for DM.

Less often patients present with a short history (average of 4 weeks) of intense and unremitting pain with exquisite tenderness in proximal and trunk musculature, and rapidly evolving proximal weakness which often involves bulbar and ventilatory functions. Subcutaneous oedema is present and may be gross. The clinical features reflect massive muscle fibre necrosis which may be severe enough to produce myoglobulinuria and impairment of renal function. Skin is not usually involved.

A chronic form is also recognized, which encompasses cases previously described as 'late progressive muscular dystrophy' or 'menopausal muscular dystrophy'. Patients present with a slowly progressive proximal myopathy without skin involvement or stigmata of autoimmunity. These patients usually respond to immunosuppressive therapy and may remit spontaneously.

Systemic features such as weight loss and fever account for 5 per cent of presentations. Dysphagia and oesophageal dysfunction may be prominent as in scleroderma. Cardiac involvement, as assessed by echocardiography, thallium-scanning, and 24-hour cardiac monitoring is very common, though the majority of patients are asymptomatic. Reported abnormalities include various types of heart block, cardiac arrhythmias, myocardial infarction, prolapsed mitral valve, and pericarditis. Routine electrocardiography may indicate definite abnormalities, but subtle changes, such as non-specific ST abnormalities and infrequent premature contractions should be further investigated. Raynaud's phenomenon (often antedating the diagnosis) occurs in about 30 per cent of patients, and a similar proportion develop mild or transient arthritis. The incidence of lung involvement is unknown, but is of two types; an acute infiltrative lesion, associated with a good response to steroids, and a chronic fibrosing alveolitis. Aspiration pneumonia carries a high mortality especially when accompanied by ventilatory failure. Renal involvement is rare, but renal failure due to myoglobinuria may occur.

Juvenile dermatomyositis

In childhood, dermatomyositis is seen much more frequently than polymyositis and is more common in girls. The two specific features which separate this type from adult disease are the presence of vasculitis and the late development of calcinosis. Other features more common in childhood disease are severity of rash, high incidence of pain and oedema, rapid development of contractures and tendon nodules. Approximately 50 per cent of children present with rapid onset proximal muscle weakness with severe constitutional symptoms, oedematous skin, and violaceous rash affecting eyelids, knuckles, and proximal interphalangeal joints. Progressive weakness may lead to difficulty with swallowing, pho-

Table 3 Criteria for the diagnosis of polymyositis/dermatomyositis

1 A characteristic clinical presentation
2 Muscle biopsy evidence of fibre necrosis and inflammation
3 Elevated serum muscle enzymes, particularly creatine kinase
4 A mixed electromyographic picture in which myopathic and denervating features can be seen

Modified from Bohan and Peter (1975).

nation, and respiration. Vasculitis probably accounts for the frequency of serious skin ulceration, and when affecting the gastrointestinal tract can lead to haematemesis, melaena, and perforation. Retinitis, characterized by extensive exudative deposition mimicking the cytoid bodies of SLE have been recorded. Cardiac involvement is quite common.

Those children who do not present in this acute way may suffer an insidious onset of weakness or the development of contractures. Calcinosis, rash or vasculitis may occasionally be presenting features. Calcinosis usually appears after 2–3 years, but is on occasion a very late complication. It is usually subcutaneous, and may extrude through the skin giving rise to necrosis. Occasionally calcium is deposited in the fascial planes where it further interferes with function.

IgG, IgM and C3 are deposited in the vessel walls of skeletal muscle in children with dermatomyositis, much more commonly than in adults. Prognosis is generally better in children, and it is rare for the myositis to be still active after 2–3 years, though the morbidity from calcinosis may be great.

Investigations and differential diagnosis

All patients suspected of having polymyositis should have a full blood count, sedimentation rate, chest X-ray, autoantibody screen, muscle enzyme estimation, electromyography, and muscle biopsy. The value of detecting specific antibodies (see Table 2) has yet to be clarified.

Criteria for the diagnosis of polymyositis or dermatomyositis are shown in Table 3. According to Bohan and Peter all four criteria should be satisfied before the diagnosis is established, but in practice some features may be absent.

The muscle enzymes creatine kinase (CK), SGOT, and aldolase are usually raised, although any one of these may be normal even in acute disease. Biopsies should be taken from clinically involved but not severely weakened muscle, and open biopsy is preferable to needle biopsy in view of the patchy nature of involvement. Electron microscopy is only useful to exclude rarer myopathies and metabolic dystrophies.

Electromyography is important in differentiating myositis from non-inflammatory myopathy, although at presentation 10 per cent of those with myositis may show no abnormality. The triad of findings almost pathognomonic of PM includes (*a*) short polyphasic small motor units, (*b*) spontaneous fibrillation, and (*c*) bizarre high-frequency repetitive discharges, but the patterns found differ with the stage of the disease.

In a prospective study of electromyography, muscle strength testing, and serum enzyme estimation before treatment and every 2 months during the first year of therapy, the three methods were found to be complementary, but muscle strength testing was of the greatest practical value. Table 4 lists the main disorders in the differential diagnosis of inflammatory muscle disease. Dermatomyositis is usually sufficiently characteristic in its clinical manifestations to present little problem. Only a small minority of patients with polymyositis present genuine difficulty in diagnosis.

Management

General measures

In the acute phase the patient will require bed rest and splinting of affected limbs in a good position to prevent contractions. Muscle

Table 4 Differential diagnosis of inflammatory muscle disease

Polymyositis (PM)
Dermatomyositis (DM)
Mixed connective tissue disease (MCTD)
Systemic lupus erythematosus (SLE)
Progressive systemic sclerosis (PSS)
Rheumatoid arthritis (RA)
Polyarteritis nodosa (PAN)
Polymyalgia rheumatica (PMR)
Myasthenia gravis (MG) and myasthenic myopathy
Muscular dystrophy
Endocrine myopathy – thyrotoxicosis
Metabolic myopathy – osteomalacia
Drug and toxic myopathies – penicillamine, chloroquine, corticosteroids
                tamoxifen, alcohol, isoniazid, sulfa drugs

Neurogenic atrophy
Granulomatous myopathy
Carcinomatous myopathy
Infective and parasitic myositis
Glycogenoses – rare

strength should be assessed regularly using MRC assessments. As muscle strength begins to improve and muscle enzyme levels fall active physiotherapy can begin.

Regular palatal and respiratory muscle assessment is important, and serial peak flow measurements are useful. Respiratory failure is usually preceded by tachypnoea and associated with dysphonia and nasal regurgitation. Assisted ventilation may be required for weeks and pulmonary infections require prompt treatment. Dysphagia can contribute to aspiration pneumonia, and may be severe enough to require tube feeding.

Drug therapy

Corticosteroids remain the drugs of first choice, in initial doses of 40–80 mg prednisolone daily (maximum: 1 mg/kg/day), until the patient demonstrates unequivocal clinical and laboratory evidence of remission. As strength returns and plasma levels of creatine kinase fall prednisolone dosage is slowly reduced. A good response usually occurs within 6 weeks, but a 2 month trial is justifiable before adding in other immunosuppressive agents. An alternate day regimen is not suitable for establishing a remission but is valuable thereafter.

In those patients who do not respond to steroids or who develop unacceptable side-effects, cytotoxic therapy may be necessary. Azathioprine is used most frequently in doses up to 2.5 mg/kg/day, with careful monitoring of the white cell count. The drug is administered orally, but nausea and dyspepsia may be troublesome, and liver dysfunction may occur with elevated plasma enzyme administration. Methotrexate has also been given intermittently by line intravenous route at doses of 0.5–0.8 mg/kg with a good response in 75 per cent of patients. There is, however, a high rate of side-effects, including stomatitis, rash, purpura, fever, and gastrointestinal upset. Other therapies recommended for unresponsive patients include intensive immunosuppression (anti-lymphocyte globulin, azathioprine, and steroids), plasmapheresis, and total body irradiation. The results of such therapy are variable and favourable observations have been uncontrolled or anecdotal.

Special problems

There is no specific treatment for the skin although pruritis may be helped by simple creams. Vasculitis is usually an indication for cytotoxic therapy. Calcinosis, although usually a sequela of juvenile DM, can occur as late as 30 years after the onset of the disease. Drug therapy does not prevent its development, but surgical removal is possible in some cases. Fibrosing alveolitis is a late complication for which it may be worth trying treatment with cyclophosphamide. Digoxin may cause or aggravate atrioventricular conducting defects in patients with myocardial involvement, for which pacemakers are occasionally required.

Prognosis

The highest mortality is within the first year (5–20 per cent). Poor prognostic features are symptomatic cardiac involvement and pneumonitis, especially if associated with aspiration. The majority of patients become asymptomatic within 3–4 years of starting steroids, but persistence of disease is variable. Children suffer long-term morbidity largely as a result of calcinosis.

Myositis and malignancy

Some controversy still exists over the exact association between polymyositis/dermatomyositis and malignancy. The reported incidence of malignancy varies from 6 to 50 per cent, some studies finding a higher incidence in dermatomyositis than polymyositis. If a true association exists between a dermatosis and malignancy, one might expect (Curth's criteria) (a) a statistically significant relationship between the malignancy and the skin complaint, (b) a concurrent onset of the tumour and dermatosis, (c) that the two conditions follow a parallel course, and (d) that a specific tumour type should be involved. These criteria are rarely met for dermatomyositis: the majority of patients with dermatomyositis do not have or develop a malignancy; in only a few patients is the malignancy and skin problem concurrent. The courses of the two conditions do not always run parallel to each other, and finally a wide variety of tumours (both carcinoma and lymphoma) have been described in association with myositis.

In practical terms a malignancy should be sought if there are any unexplained symptoms, physical findings or laboratory tests. Exhaustive searches are not justified in view of the fact that the most frequently encountered tumours are in breast, lung, ovary, colon, stomach, and uterus. An increased suspicion and careful evaluation are warranted in patients with unrelenting course, lack of response to therapy, and in the older age group (over 50 years of age). Similarly all exacerbations of disease should be thoroughly evaluated. One skin manifestation, more specifically linked with malignancy is 'malignant erythema', which is a fiery red suffusion overlying the more chronic lesions of dermatomyositis.

Echovirus dermatomyositis

Echovirus usually produces a mild disease in immunocompetent individuals, i.e. self-limiting diarrhoea, mild hepatitis or rarely meningitis. In patients with hypogammaglobulinaemia, however, especially males with the X-linked variety who are incapable of producing antibodies, a very characteristic illness is produced. The main features are of a myositis, though not typical of classical dermatomyositis, and central nervous system disease.

The onset is insidious and signs of muscle involvement may be missed for years. Non-pitting oedema of the lower legs and rarely thighs and forearms may be the presenting feature.

A transient non-pruritic rash may appear on the limbs, but it is only occasionally violaceous. The degree of muscle involvement is very variable. Muscles are not painful and it is rare for patients to complain of muscle weakness. Stiffness of knees and elbows may be a complaint and flexion deformities of these joints gives rise to a characteristic stooped posture which may be associated with cachexia due to loss of muscle mass. Histological examination of of muscle usually shows some abnormality, ranging from a mild infiltrate of mononuclear cells around vessels between muscle bundles to obvious muscle fibre atrophy, and extensive fibrosis. Electromyography may show the changes of mild patchy myositis, with progression to a myopathic pattern in more chronic cases.

Eventually nearly all patients develop central nervous system features, the commonest being headaches, convulsions, and VIIIth nerve deafness. Spastic paraplegia and other cranial nerve palsies may occur, and death is often due to brain stem involvement. Post-mortem study reveals a vasculitis of the spinal vessels with gross fibrotic thickening of the meninges.

Diagnosis is made by isolating echovirus from the cerebrospinal fluid, and treatment is with antiserum specific for the serotype. Mortality is high.

References

Ansell, B. M. (ed.) (1984). Inflammatory disorders of muscle. *Clin. Rheum. Dis.* **10**(1), 1–216.

Bohan, A. and Peter, J. B. (1975). Polymyositis and dermatomyositis. *N. Engl. J. Med.* **292**, 344–348.

Bohan, A., Peter, J. B., Bowman, R. L. and Pearson, C. M. (1977). A computer-assisted analysis of 153 patients with polymyositis and dermatomyositis. *Medicine (Balt.)* **56**, 255–286.

Callen, J. P. (1982). The value of malignancy evaluation in patients with dermatomyositis. *J. Am. Acad. Dermatol.* **6**, 253–259.

——, Hyle, J. F., Bole, G. G., Jr and Kay, D. R. (1980). The relationship of dermatomyositis and polymyositis to internal malignancy. *Arch. Dermatol.* **116**, 295–298, 403–407.

Curth, H. O. (1976). Skin lesions and internal carcinoma. In *Cancer of the skin* (eds R. Andrade, S. L. Grimpart, G. L. Popkin and T. D. Rees), pp. 1308–1341. W. B. Saunders, Philadelphia.

Reichlin, M. (1984). Seroreactivity in myositis patients. *J. Rheumatol.* **11**, 591–592.

Whitaker, J. N. (1982). Inflammatory myopathy; a review of aetiologic and pathogenetic factors. *Muscle Nerve* **5**, 573–592.

POLYMYALGIA RHEUMATICA AND GIANT CELL ARTERITIS

A. G. MOWAT

Polymyalgia rheumatica (PMR) and giant cell arteritis (GCA) may represent opposite ends of a disease spectrum, a possibility that is examined in this chapter, but since they appear to present with different clinical symptoms and signs and demand rather different treatment, it is convenient to describe the conditions separately.

Polymyalgia rheumatica

PMR is a clinical condition occurring predominantly in patients over the age of 60 years in which there is prominent pain and stiffness in the shoulder and pelvic girdles associated with variable systemic symptoms and an elevated eythrocyte sedimentation rate (ESR). The incidence has been difficult to establish, partly because firm diagnostic criteria do not exist and partly because, with wide-ranging symptoms, patients present to several hospital departments. While an incidence of some 50/100 000 of the population has been accepted for hospital referrals on both sides of the Atlantic, careful study of defined elderly populations has shown an incidence of 1.5 per cent which exceeds that of any other inflammatory rheumatic disease in the elderly.

Disease characteristics

Although the commonest age group involved is that between 60 and 70 years, a third of patients are under 60 years and the disease is recognized in those under 30 years. The male:female ratio is 1:2. Although recorded in most races and populations it has a peculiar predilection to those of Scandinavian descent.

The onset is often dramatic, some patients giving the date of their first symptom and in most it is fully developed within a month. The source of pain and stiffness is usually localized to the muscles although tenderness is not as severe as in myositis. There may be additional tenderness involving periarticular structures such as bursae, tendons, and joint capsules. The onset is commonest in the shoulder girdle spreading to involve both shoulders, pelvic girdle, and proximal muscles with striking symmetry. Although a range of variants is possible, involvement of distal muscles is unusual. Immobility is most severe on waking, a characteristic complaint being a need to roll out of bed often with the aid of a spouse. Such morning stiffness may persist for hours making the patient totally dependent.

The extent of joint involvement is disputed. Osteoarthritis is common in the affected age group but an incidence of mild inflammatory polyarthritis varying from 0 to 100 per cent has been recorded. Almost any joint may be affected, but particularly the knee and small finger joints. However, because the arthritis is mild and non-deforming some argue that proximal and central joint involvement, which may be the basis for the referred pain patterns, is underdiagnosed. Recent arthroscopic, radiographic, and scintigraphic studies of the shoulder and sternoclavicular joints would seem to support this contention originally claimed by Bruk in 1967. Carpal tunnel syndrome is an occasional accompaniment. Despite the prominent muscle symptoms electromyographic (EMG) studies and serum muscle enzyme values are normal while changes on sequential muscle biopsy are non-specific and largely due to disuse.

Most patients look unwell and complain of general malaise, fatigue, and depression. Anorexia and weight loss (mean 6 kg) can be striking, often suggesting neoplasia, while night sweats and fever are frequent, occasionally being the presenting feature. Serum values of liver enzymes, alkaline phosphatase, and gammaglutamyl transferase, are elevated in most patients and can be correlated with the ESR and disease severity. Liver biopsy shows only a mild cellular infiltrate and minor changes in the bile caniculi, perhaps surprising when an association with primary biliary cirrhosis is claimed. All these general and abnormal liver features clear rapidly with corticosteroid therapy.

Laboratory findings

The most consistent abnormality is a raised ESR, often to over 100 mm/hour, but this should not be overinterpreted since PMR accounts for only 2 per cent of such high values. Although untreated patients with a normal ESR do exist in whom C-reactive protein values may be helpful, an ESR of 40 mm/hour has good diagnostic value. A mild hypochromic, normocytic anaemia (mean 12.2 g/dl; range 8.0–14.5 g/dl) is common with a normal marrow and low plasma iron values. Iron therapy is ineffective, the haemoglobin rising with disease control. Other cell counts are normal, there are no consistent changes in protein electrophoresis, immunoglobulins or complement values, and rheumatoid factor shows a low incidence of positivity consistent with the patients age. Claims of increases in circulating immune complexes and decreases in the number of OKT8 T cells, although they might explain an underlying arteritis need confirmation, particularly since earlier, apparently specific lymphocyte transformation to arterial antigen could not be confirmed.

Differential diagnosis

In the absence of a unique feature or confirmatory laboratory test PMR remains a clinical diagnosis; thus it is axiomatic that a careful history is taken and a full examination carried out. Diagnostic criteria have been validated and the seven best discriminatory features are shown in Table 1. A patient should be considered to have PMR if three or more criteria are fulfilled. Until recently there was a mean delay in diagnosis of six months, the striking features being ascribed to osteoarthritis or psychological illness, but greater awareness has led to earlier and overdiagnosis. This has been compounded by an overreliance on the specificity of the corticosteroid response. Many elderly patients feel better with corticosteroids and most rheumatic diseases including osteoarthritis respond dramatically to these drugs.

Differential diagnosis will include a wide range of conditions (Table 2). Infection may be viral or bacterial with miliary tuberculosis and infective endocarditis causing confusion. Bone diseases may be difficult to separate as they are common incidental findings in this elderly group and the alkaline phosphatase is raised in PMR. Similarly with neoplastic disease, which may be associated with myalgia even in the absence of secondary spread to bone and related tissues. Primary muscle disease can be distinguished by EMG, biopsy, and enzyme values, but inflammatory joint disease, particularly osteoarthritis, rheumatoid arthritis, and other connective tissue diseases, e.g. polyarteritis, scleroderma (all of which may start with a polymyalgic pattern lasting some months in older patients) cause confusion though appropriate serological tests should help. Lastly, the fibromyalgic syndrome (fibrositis), parkinsonian akinesia, perhaps drug induced, and hypothyroidism should be considered.

Aetiology and pathogenesis

While the arteritis in GCA ensures a homogeneous group it is possible that PMR includes several different conditions, one of which is due to arteritis. A distinct prodromal malaise noted by many patients and a possible summer/winter peak incidence has prompted an unrewarding search for infective causes although psittacosis and hepatitis B have had support. The disease's infrequency in spouses argues against environmental factors. There is increasing evidence from follow-up studies, arthroscopy, and scintigraphy that a central arthritis affecting chiefly clavicular, shoulder, and sacro-iliac joints explains PMR and in one elegant study the typical pain distribution was produced by hypertonic saline injection into these joints and surrounding ligaments. In those with proven arteritis, an arteritis which need not be confined to the temporal and other central vessels, but rather one found in larger arteries all over the body associated with bruits and tenderness, a similar pattern of referred pain can be implicated. An immune destruction of the internal elastic lamina is proposed and supported by finding circulating immune complexes, together with immunoglobulins, complement deposition, and a mononuclear cell infiltrate adjacent to the lamina (Fig. 1).

Although found worldwide, PMR is commoner in populations of Scandinavian extraction while familial aggregation has also suggested the possibility of genetic factors, however, despite many reports of tissue typing, not always with appropriate age and race matched controls, no consistent pattern has emerged.

Treatment

Once the diagnosis is secure there is no justification for treating PMR with non-steroidal anti-inflammatory drugs; all should receive prednisolone. The dose should be just sufficient to abolish symptoms, e.g. 10–20 mg/day in two divided doses, and it is rarely necessary to use an arteritic suppressing dose (60–100 mg) since those patients at risk of visual and neurological complication can be separated by symptoms and signs (see below). The initial ESR value is no guide to disease type or steroid dose but can be a useful measure in deciding upon dose reduction. It is usually possible to reduce the dose to 10 mg/day within 2–3 months but thereafter the rate must be slow, some requiring a small dose for years. Alternate day therapy is ineffective while withdrawal at any time may be followed by a relapse perhaps months later. Such low dose

Table 1 Validation of diagnostic criteria for polymyalgia

Discriminatory features	Sensitivity* (%)	Relative value†
Shoulder pain and/or stiffness bilaterally	86	155
Onset duration 2 weeks or less	88	151
Initial ESR > 40 mm/h	74	149
Stiffness duration > 1h	80	141
Age 65+ years	70	139
Depression and/or weight loss	58	130
Upper arm tenderness bilaterally	36	132

* Sensitivity (%) = $\dfrac{\text{Individuals with disease with positive test}}{\text{All individuals with disease}}$

Specificity (%) = $\dfrac{\text{Individuals with disease with positive test}}{\text{All individuals without disease}}$

† Relative value = Sensitivity + Specificity (range 0–200)
After Bird *et al* (1979).

Table 2 Differential diagnosis of polymyalgia rheumatica

Infection	Viral
	Brucellosis
	Tuberculosis
	Endocarditis
Bone disease	Osteoporosis
	Osteomalacia
	Paget's disease
	Senile hyperostotic spinal ankylosis
Joint disease	Osteoarthritis
	Rheumatoid arthritis
	Connective tissue diseases
Others	Neoplasia
	Muscle disease
	Fibromyalgia syndrome
	Parkinsonism
	Hypothyroidism

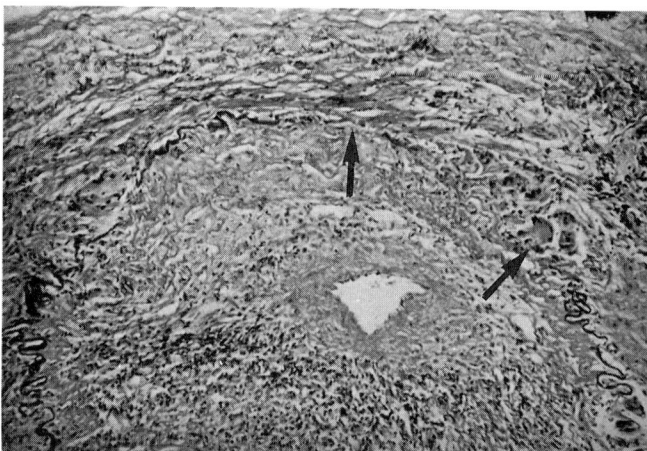

Fig. 1 Photomicrograph of a temporal artery biopsy showing giant cells, a monocellular infiltrate, and disruption of the internal elastic lamina.

therapy, although associated with occasional osteoporosis and vertebral collapse for which some recommend prophylactic calcium supplements, appears safe with no excess incidence of fluid retention, diabetes or avascular hip disease.

Relationship of polymyalgia rheumatica to giant cell arteritis

William Bruce, a physician practising in Strathpeffer Spa, Scotland, described PMR in 1888 using the term senile rheumatic gout, while Jonathan Hutchison described GCA in 1890, the current names being applied much later. For more than 20 years a common cause has been suggested, emphasized by the term polymyalgia arteritica based upon the following:

1. The age and sex distribution is the same. Caucasians (Scandinavians) are mostly affected.

2. The similarity of the myalgia and associated systemic features.

3. The similarity of the laboratory features even though many represent non-specific inflammatory features.

4. The positive biopsy findings show an identical pattern of giant cell arteritis with disintegration of the internal elastic lamina affecting the aorta and larger arteries (Fig. 1).

5. The similarity in the corticosteroid response.

6. The failure to demonstrate differences in disease cause between biopsy positive and negative patients with PMR (Table 3).

Table 3 Biopsy findings in 148 patients with polymyalgia/giant cell arteritis

Symptoms	Biopsy findings		No biopsy	Total
	Positive	Negative		
Local syptoms of TA* without myalgia	27	1	0	28
Local symptoms of TA with myalgia	42	4	1	47
Myalgia without local symptoms of TA	29	39	5	73

* TA, temporal arteritis.

Table 4 Clinical presentation and features of giant cell arteritis (percentage of cases affected)

Chief presentation	%	Clinical features	%
Symptoms of temporal arteritis	30	Symptoms of temporal arteritis	90
PMR	27	PMR	55
Weight loss, malaise	14	Weight loss, malaise	50
Fever	13	Visual disturbance	40
Visual disturbance	6	Fever	32
Headache	4	Cranial features	24
Anaemia	4	Peripheral neuropathy	12
Claudication (leg)	2	Claudication (leg)	7

The last finding may be explained by the patchy involvement that can be missed even in long specimens from temporal or occipital arteries. Angiography at the time of biopsy has not increased the sensitivity. The importance of a positive biopsy to a clinician is less of a guide to initial steroid dosage which reflects clinical and not laboratory features but rather as reassurance about later questioning over the diagnosis and true need for steroid treatment.

Giant cell arteritis

Giant cell (cranial, senile or temporal) arteritis (GCA), rare before the age of 50 years, chiefly affects those between 65 and 75 years with a male:female ratio of 1:2. An annual incidence of biopsy proven disease of 17/100 000 and prevalence of 133/100 000 has been recorded for a Minnesota community, similar values being noted elsewhere, and the condition has a predeliction for Caucasians especially those of Scandinavian extraction.

Disease characteristics

The features of GCA are protean, variable in presentation and on examination, but typical series are shown (Table 4). The diagnosis depends upon a high degree of clinical suspicion in less typical cases. As with PMR the onset may be dramatic and always becomes fully developed over a few weeks although the delay in diagnosis may be months. The malaise, fever, and anaemia are similar to those in PMR, the differences being in the vascular symptoms. The majority have temporal features with headache, scalp sensitivity, and tender, thickened arteries; the classical nodular red streaks being unusual. Overwhelming generalized headache and the feared complication of irreversible loss of vision are more readily recognized. The listed clinical features emphasize the developing arteritis (Table 4). A wide range of cranial manifestations reflects the involvement of larger arteries with an internal elastic lamina in the face, neck, and brain base but not cerebral vessels. These include headaches, scalp tenderness, and skin necrosis, jaw claudication while talking or chewing, tongue pain and claudication, and face and neck pain with nerve damage. The visual manifestations which include blurred vision, amaurosis fujax, transient and permanent blindness, diplopia, and visual hallucinations are due to ischaemic changes in the ciliary arteries causing optic neuritis or infarction with a smaller number of cases being due to central retinal artery thrombosis. A few patients may have evidence of arteritis elsewhere with intermittent claudication, peripheral neuropathy, widespread vessel tenderness with bruits, myocardial ischaemia and damage, and occasionally an aortic arch syndrome with valve disease.

Laboratory features

These are exactly the same as in PMR. Biopsy confirmation of the diagnosis is important but should not be a reason for withholding steroids since characteristic pathological features persist for about one week after treatment has begun. In contradistinction to other vasculitides renal involvement is rare. Angiography perhaps with computerized tomographic (CT) scanning may add to the diagnosis and explain apparently bizarre features.

Differential diagnosis

Since the diagnosis of GCA depends upon a positive biopsy, the differential diagnosis does not include other causes of headache, neck pain, anaemia, and weight loss. The vasculitis of rheumatoid arthritis or systemic lupus erythematosus affects arterioles, and is associated with other disease features especially arthritis and characteristic immunological tests. Polyarteritis, although not always nodular, affects small arteries with cutaneous, abdominal, and renal rather than cranial features and the histology is distinctive. Although cranial and central nervous system features occur in Wegener's granulomatosis, involvement of many systems includes characteristic lesions of the respiratory tract with diagnostic histologic features. Takayasu's arteritis, in which the pathological lesions mimic those of GCA, is confined to the aortic arch and its major branches chiefly in young oriental women.

Treatment

The only treatment is corticosteroid; immunosuppressive therapy having no direct effect and the modest steroid sparing rarely warrants the additional hazard. With clear arteritic features 60–100 mg of prednisolone in two to four divided doses per day is required, reductions being gradual depending upon clinical features and a falling or normal ESR. The initial ESR is no guide to disease severity or corticosteroid dose and no clear prognostic feature or laboratory test has emerged to identify those who are likely to have the feared visual complications. All patients need to be monitored carefully anticipating that low doses (<20 mg/day) may be required for several years with all the potential hazards of such long-term therapy in the elderly. GCA does not reduce life expectancy.

References

Allison, M. C. and Gallagher, P. J. (1984). Temporal artery biopsy and corticosteroid treatment. *Ann. Rheum. Dis.* **43**, 416–417.

Behn, A. R., Perara, T. and Myles, A. B. (1983). Polymyalgia rheumatica and corticosteroids: how much for how long? *Ann. Rhuem. Dis.* **42**, 374–378.

Bird, H. A., Esselinckx, W., Dixon, A. ST. J., Mowat, A. G. and Wood, P. H. N. (1979). An evaluation of criteria for polymyalgia rheumatica. *Ann. Rheum. Dis.* **38**, 434–439.

Bruk, M. I. (1967). Articular and vascular manifestations of polymyalgia rheumatica. *Ann. Rheum. Dis.* **26**, 103–113.

Coombes, E. N. and Sharp, J. (1961). Polymyalgia rheumatica. A misnomer? *Lancet* **ii**, 1328–1331

Healey, L. A. and Wilske, K. R. (1978). *The systemic manifestations of temporal arteritis.* Grune and Stratton, New York.

Hussaini, A. S. AL. and Swannell, A. J. (1985). Peripheral joint involvement in polymyalgia rheumatica: a clinical study of 56 cases. *Br. J. Rheum.* **24**, 27–30.

Jones, J. G. and Hazleman, B. L. (1981). Prognosis and management of polymyalgia rheumatica. *Ann. Rheum. Dis.* **40**, 1–5.

Mowat, A. G. (1979). Generalized rheumatism: polymyalgia rheumatica and its differential diagnosis. *Clin. Rheum. Dis.* **5**, 775–795.

Smith, C. A., Fidler W. J. and Pinals, R. S. (1983). The epidemiology of giant cell arteritis. *Arthr. Rheum.* **26**, 1214–1219.

OTHER INFLAMMATORY ARTHRITIDES

B. L. HAZLEMAN

Joint symptoms may be either the presenting feature or major component of many conditions. These include infections, metabolic disorders, blood dyscrasias, sarcoidosis, neoplasia, and amyloidosis. Certain types of arthritis tend to be more common in particular age and sex groups. Because of differences in prognosis and management, it is important to distinguish between them. The patterns of joint involvement and the accompanying systemic features help in this differentiation and require a careful assessment of the history and physical signs and an accurate interpretation of laboratory tests. Since no systematic review of these conditions is possible, they are outlined in alphabetical order for ease of reference.

Acne arthralgia

Severe acne may be associated with myalgias, arthralgia, and nonseptic joint effusions. Large joints are usually involved. Most reported cases have been in young males. There is a tendency for improvement with resolution of the acne.

Amyloid arthropathy

Articular involvement has been described most frequently in cases of myeloma associated amyloidosis, and is also present in primary generalized amyloidosis (see page 9.145). In most instances, the associated monoclonal protein is either a kappa Bence Jones protein or an intact immunoglobulin with a kappa light chain. Arthropathy is not a significant feature of secondary amyloidosis nor familial amyloidosis.

Amyloid arthritis can mimic a number of rheumatic diseases due to the fact that it can present as a symmetrical peripheral arthritis associated with nodules, morning stiffness, and fatigue. This may lead to an erroneous diagnosis of rheumatoid arthritis. Amyloid should be considered in patients with nodules and non-erosive disease. Small and large joint involvement can occur. The initial symptoms are usually pain and stiffness, associated with soft tissue flexion contractures of the hands. The joints are often swollen, firm, and occasionally tender but redness and severe tenderness are not noted. The shoulder may be prominently involved giving the appearance of a 'padded shoulder'. Subcutaneous nodules are present in 70 per cent of patients. An associated carpal tunnel syndrome is often present and amyloidosis should be excluded in cases of idiopathic carpal tunnel syndrome occurring in middle-aged and elderly men, by examining tissue removed at operation.

Synovial fluid analysis usually reveals a non-inflammatory fluid and examination of Congo red-stained sediments under polarized microscopy may reveal amyloid deposits in fragments of synovial villi. X-rays show osteoporosis or lytic lesions, but erosions are rare. Large deposits in bone stimulate neoplasms and can lead to pathological features.

Anaphylactoid (Henoch–Schönlein) purpura

The syndrome is due to a widespread vasculitis involving arterioles and small capillaries. It can occur at any age but primarily in children, especially boys. The disease occurs most often in the spring and usually follows an upper respiratory tract infection. The onset is acute with fever, headache, and rash. Initially, macules or urticarial papules occur on the buttocks and the extensor aspects of the limbs. These become flat, purpuric, and may coalesce or even ulcerate. Localized oedema of the face, scalp, hands, and feet occurs; in young children it can mimic arthritis. Haemorrhage into the gut wall can cause colic, melaena or haematemesis.

In general the joint involvement is mild, consisting of transient, non-migratory synovitis with synovial swelling, pain, and stiffness, usually affecting more than one joint. The ankles, knees, hips, wrists, and elbows are usually affected, with a tendency to lower limb involvement. The synovial fluid is inflammatory in character. Joint destruction does not occur.

A mild focal glomerulonephritis producing proteinuria and microscopic haematuria occurs in 50 per cent of cases. Occasionally it progresses to the nephrotic syndrome and rarely to renal failure. The disease usually settles in 4–6 weeks without sequelae, but may recur.

Carcinoma polyarthritis

A polyarthritis resembling rheumatoid arthritis may be the presenting manifestation of malignancy. This is a distinct entity separate from hypertrophic osteoarthropathy and from symmetrical metastases. Although most often confused with rheumatoid disease, it has been mistaken for adult Still's disease when associated with unexplained fever. There is a close temporal relationship between the onset of a low-grade, seronegative polyarthritis and discovery of the malignancy; improvement of the joint symptoms parallels the successful treatment of the underlying tumour and recurrence of the joint symptoms is associated with reappearance of the tumour. Arthritis is most common in patients with carcinoma of the bronchus, prostate or breast. It is more common in elderly men.

Other rheumatic disorders which may be complications of malignancy include polymyositis, secondary gout, necrotizing vasculitis, systemic sclerosis, and a syndrome resembling polymyalgia rheumatica.

Coagulation defects (see Section 19)

Acute haemarthrosis is the most constant feature of severe haemophilia and in the majority, preceding trauma does not occur. Up to 90 per cent of patients suffer numerous episodes of joint bleeding. Patients with moderate and mild forms of haemophilia (plasma factor VIII levels more than 1 per cent) rarely present with 'spontaneous' intra-articular bleeding, although they may bleed following injury. The incidence and severity of joint disease are directly related to the severity of the coagulation defect. Nearly all patients with less than 5 per cent activity of deficient factor experience haemarthrosis, while less than half the patients with greater than 5 per cent activity bleed into their joints. Patients with Christmas disease behave in a similar manner. Joint bleeding usually begins before the age of 5 years but is rare before the child begins to walk and tends to recur repeatedly during childhood, after which it becomes less frequent. The preponderance of knee, elbow, and ankle bleeds over those into other joints is pronounced, and is presumably because these are hinge articulations, subject to angulatory and rotatory strain. Patients often comment that haemarthroses occur in cycles; this is probably due to chronic hypertrophy and vascularity of the synovial membrane. If a haemarthrosis is not treated early enough or adequately with factor VIII replacement the haemarthrosis progresses due to synovial proliferation and vascularity and also because of atrophy of surrounding muscles.

In acute haemarthrosis the joint becomes hot, painful, swollen, and very tender. Most severe haemophiliacs will volunteer that often before the onset of pain they are aware of an abnormal sensation of prickling, increased warmth, and stiffness in the joint. Prompt treatment is so important that the haemophiliac will act on these premonitory symptoms and obtain treatment. Pain is the most disabling complaint in acute joint haemorrhage and is due to a local irritant effect of blood and also to joint distension. The joint is usually held in flexion and the degree assumed is that in which the volume of the joints is maximal and the intrascapular pressure minimal.

Within a few hours of haemorrhage into a joint a cellular reaction with exudation of polymorphonuclear leucocytes and increase in the synovial lining cells takes place. Within a few days hyperplasia of the synovial cells is seen. Haemosiderin pigment is soon present both in the synovial lining and in the deeper tissues.

Immediate treatment is indicated at the earliest symptoms suggestive of joint haemorrhage, long before the development of any physical findings. There are four aims of treatment: to stop bleeding, to relieve pain, to maintain and restore joint function, and to prevent chronic joint changes. These aims are achieved by some or all of the following measures: clotting factor replacement, immobilization, local measures such as ice packs and elevation of the limb, aspiration, and rehabilitation. Many of these procedures can be avoided by prompt replacement therapy and in the majority factor replacement is sufficient. Pain is relieved by replacement therapy, splinting, and analgesics. Joint aspiration may be required if the haemarthrosis is under tension.

Permanent joint damage depends upon the frequency of bleeding into a joint and the length of time that blood remains in a joint. The end stages of haemophilic arthropathy have features in common with both degenerative joint disease and long-standing rheumatoid arthritis. Joint function is lost and motion is severely restricted. There is often an associated flexion deformity, and subluxation, joint laxity, and alignment abnormalities are not uncommon. Hyperaemia of epiphyseal plates with resultant irregular overgrowth and periarticular fibrosis, both contribute to the deformity and loss of function. Once established joint changes are present, treatment falls into four categories: physiotherapy, orthotic appliances, corrective plasters/traction, and reconstructive surgery.

Erythema nodosum

Joint manifestations occur in about 75 per cent of patients with erythema nodosum. Arthralgia is more common than a synovitis and can precede the appearance of skin lesions. A symmetrical synovitis occurs in one-third of patients usually involving the knees and ankles but can involve wrists, elbows, small joints of the hands, and shoulders. The affected joints are painful, tender, and stiff with synovial thickening and effusion. The presence of erythema nodosum around the ankles may be confused with involvement of these joints, because of the redness and swelling with pain and stiffness on movement which arise from the skin and subcutaneous lesions.

Erythema nodosum is considered to be an allergic cutaneous vasculitis or a hypersensitivity response to a number of agents, including streptococcal infection, sarcoidosis, tuberculosis, meningococcal and fungal infections, Crohn's disease, and ulcerative colitis and drug therapy, particularly sulphonamides.

The synovitis is self-limiting and non-erosive. Anti-inflammatory drugs usually provide effective relief but corticosteroid therapy may be necessary.

Familial mediterranean fever (see page 24.4)

This disease, inherited as an autosomal recessive trait affects mainly Sephardic Jews and Armenians. The onset is commonly in childhood or early adult life. It is characterized by fever and attacks of abdominal pain due to peritonitis lasting 1–3 days. Secondary amyloidosis is a well-recognized complication.

The joint symptoms consist of episodic, recurrent attacks of synovitis marked by pain and swelling of the joint. Although less frequent than the peritoneal attacks they are experienced by 75 per cent of patients and in one-third they are the presenting feature. In some patients they may be the only feature for years, in others they dominate the clinical picture because of their severity and the resulting incapacity. Protracted attacks persisting for months sometimes occur. The joints most commonly affected are the knees, ankles, and hips; occasionally more than one joint is involved and recurrent attacks usually involve the site affected originally. Fluid from the peritoneum or joint shows a high polymorphonuclear cell count and is sterile.

One of the typical features of the disease is the propensity for recovery of the joints after what appears to have been a poten-

tially damaging arthritis. There is no treatment available to abort an attack once it has started and complete bedrest and anti-inflammatory drugs, including corticosteroids, provide no demonstrable effect. Colchicine therapy prevents attacks and secondary amyloidosis is a rare disease in Israel now that prophylactic colchicine is used routinely.

Haemangioma of synovium

True haemangiomas of the synovium or joint capsule are rare and most are associated with soft tissue vascular abnormalities, particularly arteriovenous malformations or skin vascular lesions. The most common symptoms include unilateral intermittent joint pain and enlargement with subsequent limitation of movement.

Therapy for a localized haemangioma of the joint is excision of the tumour. However, those lesions associated with soft tissue vascular malformations may have recurrences due to the extensive vascular abnormalities. Radiation therapy has been advocated in such cases with mixed results.

Haemochromatosis (see Section 19)

The patient who develops arthritis is nearly always a man over the age of 50 years, and, although other clinical features of haemochromatosis usually antedate the onset of arthritis, it can occasionally be the presenting complaint. The first symptoms of arthritis usually occur in the 2nd and 3rd metacarpophalangeal joints and they become more severe on the dominant hand. The patient notices minor pain on flexion of the fingers with bony swelling of the involved joints as in degenerative arthritis. Later other small joints in both hands may be involved with resulting bony swelling and deformity, but ulnar deviation does not occur. The arthritis causes little in the way of symptoms. In a few patients more severe progressive changes take place, especially in the hip joints. Superimposed on this slowly progressive degenerative joint disease there may be attacks of acute synovitis due to pyrophosphate arthropathy; this usually involves the knees, but can involve several joints at the same time leading to a mistaken diagnosis of rheumatoid arthritis.

The earliest radiological change is the appearance of small cysts in the metacarpal heads; prominent cystic changes can be seen in the carpal bones. In the shoulder subchondral sclerosis occurs and in the hips cystic changes with loss of cartilage. The most striking change is that of chondrocalcinosis affecting the knee most commonly; extra-articular sites of calcification include the tendo achilles, the ligamentum flavum, and intervertebral discs.

The development of arthritis is not related to the length of time the patient has had symptoms of haemochromatosis, but the age of the patient when the first symptom of haemochromatosis appears is an important determining factor, those with a later onset developing arthritis. Venesection therapy is not thought to influence the arthritis.

The calcification that occurs in articular cartilage in the intervertebral disc is calcium pyrophosphate dihydrate. Iron and haemosiderin can be found in the chondrocytes and synovium of untreated cases. The mechanism by which the arthritis occurs is unknown. A direct relationship with iron overload is supported by reports of identical joint lesions in secondary haemochromatosis. Pyrophosphatase inhibition by metal ions has been cited as a possible mechanism but does not explain the distribution of the joint changes in haemochromatosis with the predilection for the metacarpophalangeal joints which differs from that seen in other types of idiopathic chondrocalcinosis.

Haemoglobinopathies

Sickle cell disease is by far the most common haemoglobinopathy to produce rheumatic symptoms, but most problems can be seen not only in homozygous sickle cell disease but also in patients with sickle-C haemoglobin, sickle-thalassaemia and sickle-F haemoglobin (see Section 19).

Expansion of the bone marrow occurs in all haemoglobinopathies associated with haemolysis but except where secondary mechanical problems develop these changes seem to be asymptomatic. *Gout and hyperuricaemia* occurs in about 40 per cent of adults with sickle cell disease. *Sickle cell dactylitis* may be seen in children from six months to two years. This consists of diffuse, symmetrical, tender, warm swelling of hands and/or feet. Infarction of marrow, cortical bone, periosteum, and periarticular tissues appear most likely to be the underlying mechanism. Patients with sickle cell disease are susceptible to *bacterial infections* or osteomyelitis or less frequently septic arthritis.

Bone infarction and *avascular necrosis* is a prominent feature of sickle cell disease. The bone pains in sickle cell crises are felt to be largely due to infarction. Aseptic necrosis of the head of the femur is the most disabling complication. Similar aseptic necrosis occurs at the humeral head, tibial condyles, and occasionally other sites.

Joint effusions involving the knee usually occur during crises and are far more common than gout or septic arthritis. Synovial effusions are usually non-inflammatory and result from infarction of the synovium. Haemarthrosis is not uncommon.

Hepatic disorders and arthritis

The association of hepatic disorders and arthritis is well described. Polyarthritis or arthralgia occurs in 25 per cent of patients with chronic active hepatitis. An acute self-limiting arthritis affecting large joints is described with viral hepatitis and about 4 per cent of patients with alcoholic cirrhosis suffer from arthropathy during their illness. An erosive inflammatory arthritis commonly accompanies primary biliary cirrhosis. The arthritis is non-deforming and usually asymptomatic. The erosions are symmetrical and involve the distal small joints of the hands. An association with progressive systemic sclerosis has been described. Bone lesions similar to those seen in hyperlipoproteinaemia have been described and tend to be periarticular rather than true joint lesions.

Hyperlipoproteinaemia and joint symptoms (see page 9.114)

Articular symptoms may occur with type II and type IV hyperlipoproteinaemia. Type II hyperlipoproteinaemia may cause a migratory polyarthritis affecting small and large peripheral joints which resembles rheumatic fever. Xanthomata may produce tendon nodules and involve bone with the formation of para-articular bone cysts. Features include a corneal arcus and premature atherosclerosis. The condition is inherited as an autosomal dominant, and plasma low-density lipoprotein and cholesterol concentrations are raised.

Type IV hyperlipoproteinaemia is characterized by an increase in plasma triglyceride and very low-density lipoprotein levels and is probably inherited as an autosomal dominant. This disorder predisposes to premature vascular disease. The onset of musculoskeletal symptoms occur later than those in type II, most usually in the early forties. The most frequent joint complaints are of morning stiffness, pain on movement or joint tenderness. There is little evidence of joint inflammation, despite the intensity of joint pain.

Hypogammaglobulinaemias

These immune deficiency syndromes arise from either failure of synthesis (primary) or increased breakdown (secondary) of the gammaglobulins. Primary hypogammaglobulinaemia is associated with a non-erosive inflammatory synovitis in 10 to 30 per cent of patients. The arthritis resembles rheumatoid arthritis with symmetrical pain, stiffness, tenderness, and synovial swelling occurring in the small and medium-sized peripheral joints.

The natural history is variable in that the synovitis can be transient or persist for many years with continuing tenderness and effusion. Little evidence of permanent joint damage is seen. Subcutaneous nodules are occasionally found. The histology of synovium and subcutaneous nodules differs from that of rheumatoid arthritis in that plasma cells are absent. Tests for rheumatoid factor are negative. Patients with hypogammaglobulinaemia are also prone to develop septic arthritis.

Infective arthritis

Arthritis may arise from direct infection of joints by micro-organisms, or less commonly as a reaction to a preceding infection (Table 1).

In bacterial arthritis it is usually possible to find the organism in the joint, although this is not the case with the meningococcus. Infections with salmonella can be type I or occur after the infection in the bowel has cleared when the arthritis is termed reactive and belongs to type III. Arthropathy due to syphilis belongs in type II, and viral infections probably also fall in this group. In this section only type I and type II infections will be discussed.

Bacterial arthritis

Most cases of bacterial arthritis result from haematogenous spread from infection; much less frequently infection results from joint aspiration or injection or spread from osteomyelitis. Certain organisms predominate and *Staphylococcus aureus, Streptococcus pyogenes, Diplococcus pneumoniae*, and *Neisseria gonorrhoeae* are found most frequently. In children *Haemophilus influenzae* is often found. 'Main Line' drug addicts may develop septicaemia and septic arthritis with less common Gram-negative organisms. Certain organisms appear to exhibit a tropism for joints: for instance, septic arthritis complicates about 1 per cent of pneumococcal and salmonella septicaemia when treatment is delayed, whereas 80 per cent of patients with gonococcal septicaemia develop arthritis. Factors that influence the susceptibility of the host include debilitating disease, hypogammaglobulinaemia, corticosteroids, and immunosuppressive therapy. In rheumatoid arthritis both local factors as well as a reduced resistance to infection may be important. Other local factors, including non-penetrating joint trauma, may predispose to infection in healthy individuals.

The identification of a septic joint in rheumatoid arthritis can prove difficult but the possibility should be kept in mind whenever there is an increase in pain, swelling or other evidence of local inflammation in one or a limited number of joints. A problem of increasing frequency is the development of low-grade infection complicating prosthetic joint replacement, and the recognition of this may be delayed many months. Organisms of low virulence, especially *Staphylococcus albus*, predominate.

Infection must be considered in all cases of acute arthritis particularly when only one joint is affected. Delay in treatment may lead to death, or at best, permanent joint damage. Septic arthritis may occur at any age, but is particularly common under the age of 15 years and in the elderly. Severe monoarticular inflammation, characterized by marked pain, tenderness, erythema, and swelling strongly suggests septic arthritis, but it is important to remember that there may be minimal signs of inflammation and in patients on corticosteroids or in debilitating illness or in an infant, there may be almost no systemic illness. A child may present with sudden refusal to move a limb. An infected joint is commonly associated with a fever often accompanied by rigors and the patient looks ill. When the organism is the gonococcus a migratory polyarthritis may precede localization in a single joint. In children under five years of age more than one joint may be involved but at any age between 10 and 20 per cent of staphylococcal infections and 75 to 85 per cent of gonococcal infections involve two or more joints.

A definite diagnosis can only be made by demonstrating the organism in the joint fluid or tissue. Synovial fluid glucose is often

Table 1 Association between microbial infection and arthritis

Type	Infection known	Microbes in joints	Antigens in joints	Syndrome
I	+	+	+	Infective
II	+	−	+	Postinfective
III	+	−	−	Reactive
IV	−	−	−	Inflammatory

reduced but can be normal, particularly in the case of gonococcal infections. An elevated joint fluid lactic acid can be helpful in diagnosis. Smears of joint fluid may reveal organisms and is most likely to be positive in staphylococcal, streptococcal, and coliform infections but is only occasionally positive in gonococcal and meningococcal arthritis. Synovial fluid and blood should be sent immediately for culture. In addition to routine aerobic and anaerobic cultures, special media are needed for the isolation of *N. gonorrhoeae* and culture of sputum, urine, and cervical mucus may prove helpful in special circumstances.

High dose, parenteral antibiotic therapy should be commenced as soon as cultures have been taken. The Gram-stained film may offer some guidance to initial therapy. Any alteration can be made once the sensitivities are known. Drugs reach adequate levels within the joint when given systemically and intra-articular therapy is not required. However, the joint should be splinted in a suitable position to relieve pain until the inflammation has subsided.

Although osteomyelitis usually results in sterile joint effusions it can lead to a septic arthritis. Osteomyelitis should be considered if the site of maximal tenderness extends beyond the joint. If there is any doubt about the bone adjacent to an infected joint, bone scanning will isolate an osteomyelitis lesion. The management is the same as in septic arthritis.

Synovial fluid should be aspirated when it reaccumulates, since the presence of purulent material may inhibit the action of antibiotics. Gross joint destruction and the presence of contiguous osteomyelitis are indications for surgical drainage, as is failure of response to therapy within 72 hours of treatment. Surgical drainage is often necessary for joints which are difficult to aspirate and drain, such as the hips and sacro-iliac joints. Once the acute inflammation has subsided, passive exercises graded into active exercises can be tailored for each patient. Weight bearing can be resumed when all signs of inflammation have subsided.

The duration of antibiotic therapy should be continued for four to six weeks after clinical response; if infection has complicated pre-existing disease or caused joint destruction prior to diagnosis, 12 or more weeks therapy is required. The prognosis for full recovery is good when effective therapy commences quickly.

Transient synovitis of the hip can prove a difficult differential diagnosis. No definite cause has been established and it may represent a number of conditions. Children of both sexes between the ages of 2 and 12 years develop acute pain, often in the knee, and inability to stand. A low-grade fever and slight elevation of the ESR may be present but the child is fit. If in doubt it is better to treat as an infection until the results of investigations are known.

Gonococcal arthritis

This usually affects females and homosexual males, as the primary infection if often asymptomatic. In North America gonococcal arthritis is the most frequent cause of septic arthritis in young adults. The symptoms vary but the most common pattern is a migratory polyarthritis associated with tenosynovitis; the infection localizes in one or two joints; there may be fever and rigors. The upper limbs are more often involved as are smaller rather than larger joints, although the knee is frequently swollen. The gonococcus may be identified in the joint fluid in only 25 per cent of infected patients. Erythematous skin lesions which may be macular, vesicular or pustular occur in one-third of cases and are found adjacent to involved joints; these appear before or within a few days of the arthritis and may be painful at the outset. Signs of venereal infection in pharyngeal and anal as well as genital areas should be looked for, but their absence does not exclude the diagnosis. Table 2 illustrates the difference between gonococcal and non-gonococcal arthritis.

There should be little difficulty in distinguishing between Reiter's disease and gonococcal arthritis. There is an 80 per cent female preponderance of gonococcal arthritis, compared with the high incidence of males with Reiter's disease. In gonococcal arth-

Table 2 Differences between gonococcal and non-gonococcal arthritis

	Gonococcal arthritis	Non-gonococcal arthritis
Age group affected	Teens and Young Adults	All ages
Sex most frequently affected	Females	Males
Medical predisposition	No	Yes
Pattern	Polyarthritis	Usually monoarthritis
Joints most frequently involved	Small joints of hands and wrists	Lower limbs and large joints
Tenosynovitis	Yes	No

ritis, pyrexia is more common, the upper limb joints being involved more frequently and there is less symmetry in the arthritis compared with Reiter's disease. Penicillin is still the drug of choice and during the acute stage the joint should be rested in a splint. Penicillinase-producing strains are common in Asia and North America, but less common in Britain.

Meningococcal arthritis

A purulent arthritis involving a single joint, often the knee, can occur in the septicaemic phase and also during treatment. An acute transient polyarthritis associated with marked pain and tenderness can develop at the time of the petechial rash. Chronic meningococcaemia can cause difficulty in diagnosis; it usually affects young adults and is characterized by rigors, fevers, rash, headaches, and joint pains, the latter often flitting.

Syphilitic arthritis

Direct invasion of the synovium by *Treponema pallidum* is relatively uncommon. Congenital syphilis may cause (*a*) acute epiphysitis or osteochondritis which usually occurs in the first few weeks of life and most commonly affects the upper portion of the humerus, resulting in a painful para-articular swelling; (*b*) Clutton's joints, a painless bilateral hydrarthrosis of the knees which develops between the ages of eight and sixteen years, the onset is insidious and pursues a benign self-limiting course; and (*c*) rarely neuropathic arthropathy secondary to tabes dorsalis occurs.

Migratory polyarthralgia occurs infrequently during the secondary stage of acquired syphilis and may resemble rheumatic fever.

Lyme arthritis

This was first described in Connecticut in 1972. Clinical features include a recurrent asymmetrical arthritis involving a few large joints. The arthritis follows 1–24 weeks after an erythematous rash called erythema chronicum migrans. This epidemic form of arthritis was originally thought to be caused by an arbovirus transmitted by a tick of the genus *Ixodes*. There is now good evidence that the tick-borne causative agent is a spirochaete. Penicillin or tetracycline therapy given at the time of the rash may shorten the early illness and prevent arthritis.

Tuberculous arthritis

Despite the decline of bone and joint tuberculosis, this disease must still be considered in the differential diagnosis of chronic joint disease and over 300 new cases are seen each year in England and Wales. It is most common among immigrants under the age of 30 years and in the middle aged or elderly, and its presentation may be somewhat atypical. Knees and hips are most commonly involved and also sometimes tendon sheaths and carpal bones. Biopsy of the synovial membrane is the most reliable method of diagnosis because the bacilli are rarely cultured from synovial fluid.

About 1 per cent of patients with tuberculosis have skeletal involvement; of these approximately 50 per cent have spinal disease, 30 per cent inflammation of hips or knees, and 20 per cent arthritis of other joints, particularly the sacroiliac joints. Around half do not have active pulmonary disease. It is assumed that haematogenous dissemination infects subchondral bone adjacent to the joint or to a spinal intervertebral disc. The resulting osteomyelitis may remain dormant for years before there is activation. Alcoholism, diabetes mellitus, local trauma, and chronic debilitating states may predispose to activation.

In peripheral joint involvement a caseating granulomatous synovitis is produced. Destruction of cartilage occurs relatively late in contrast to pyogenic arthritis; involvement is usually monarticular. When the vertebral column is involved dissection along fascial planes may cause a psoas abscess; involvement of two adjacent vertebrae, if untreated, may lead to a kyphosis. The anterior portions of the vertebrae between the VIth thoracic and Vth lumbar level are usually involved. Severe anterior wedging may lead to compression of the spinal cord. Tuberculous involvement of the knee is more frequent in adults, while spine and hips are more often affected in children. Knee involvement begins insidiously and is much less painful than hip involvement.

Extra-articular tuberculosis can induce an allergic polyarthritis involving the knees, elbows, and small joints of the hands and feet. Patients are usually febrile but the joints involved do not develop radiological changes. Indian and Pakistani immigrants are most frequently affected in United Kingdom populations. The illness runs an acute course although in 25 per cent of cases the sedimentation rate is less than 20 mm/hour . Although *Mycobacterium tuberculosis* is the usual organism isolated in Britain, the atypical *Myobacterium kansasii* has been isolated from infected joints and the bovine strain has been implicated in carpal tunnel infection.

Synovial fluid should be stained by Z–N stain for acid fast bacilli and cultured. Negative cultures of synovial fluid do not exclude the diagnosis, and if infection is suspected a biopsy is necessary. Usually an open synovial biopsy is required as a closed biopsy does not usually provide sufficient material for analysis.

Drug therapy should include at least two agents given for at least 18 months. Surgical decompression may be required if there is impending cord involvement from spinal disease.

Fungal infections

Fungal infections of joints rarely occur. There is variable joint pain and muscle spasm; skin tests with the appropriate fungal antigens are usually strongly positive. Culture of pus, synovial fluid or biopsy material permits definitive diagnosis. Surgical drainage and excision of necrotic tissue may facilitate recovery.

Actinomycosis commonly affects the mandible but involvement of vertebrae occasionally occurs from local spread; bone abscesses develop. Blastomycosis may cause punched out lesions in the neighbourhood of joints or produce vertebral collapse. The organisms can be identified in the joint fluid. Coccidioidomycosis may cause a benign polyarthritis occasionally associated with erythema nodosum, a chronic arthritis occasionally develops. Histoplasmosis may also be associated with erythema nodosum and a monarticular destructive arthritis has been described. Sporotrichosis may also affect joints causing disruptive local lesions.

Viral infections

Several viral infections may be accompanied or followed by an arthropathy. These include rubella and rubella vaccination, infectious hepatitis, mumps, infectious mononucleosis, vaccinia, varicella, and adenovirus and arbovirus injections. A viral arthritis should be suspected if the patient has a low white cell count with a relative lymphocytosis. Joint symptoms may coincide with, follow or even precede the onset of other signs and symptoms, are usually mild, and tend to resolve spontaneously in a few weeks. In contrast to bacterial infections viral arthropathies are usually polyarticular. It is thought that the synovitis results from immune complex deposition. Only in rubella arthritis has the virus been isolated from an affected joint, but in arthritis caused by infection with type B viral hepatitis and adenovirus, low levels of C_3, C_4, and CH_{50} have been observed, which return to normal during con-

valescence, and immune complexes have been detected in both serum and synovial fluid.

Rubella

The highest incidence of rubella arthritis is in adolescent girls, the disease being less frequent in childhood. Joint symptoms may accompany, precede or follow the rash which may be so faint or transient that it is easily missed. The occurrence of a rubella epidemic or contact in the family, the rash, and occipital lymphadenopathy all aid diagnosis.

The arthritis involves the metacarpophalangeal or proximal interphalangeal joints (85 per cent), elbows, wrists, and knees in a symmetrical fashion. Morning stiffness, painful tenosynovitis, the occasional occurrence of carpal tunnel syndrome, and a positive latex test for rheumatoid factor may make the resemblance to rheumatoid arthritis even more striking, and differentiation between the two conditions in the early stages may not be possible on clinical grounds alone. The erythrocyte sedimentation rate may be normal or slightly elevated. Rubella antibodies may be demonstrable in high titre.

Complete resolution of the arthritis occurs within a few weeks to a few months. Only in rare cases are symptoms so severe that a short course of corticosteroids is required. Arthralgia may persist for several months.

Rubella vaccination This produces musculoskeletal symptoms in up to 20 per cent of cases. An arthritis similar to that associated with the natural infection occurs two to four weeks afterwards and usually lasts for a few days but may occasionally persist for several weeks. Occasionally synovitis persists for months. Joint pain affecting the arms or legs two to ten weeks after rubella vaccination is caused by radiculoneuritis and may be associated with paraesthesiae.

Infectious hepatitis

During the early incubation period of viral hepatitis, some patients may experience joint symptoms which may be mild and transient (usually type A infections) or acute and prolonged (usually type B infections).

Symptoms include symmetrical synovitis associated with fever, anorexia, malaise, and occasional urticarial rash. The arthritis usually resolves with the appearance of jaundice. Joint disturbance can also be prominent in anicteric cases. This type of arthritis is rare before adolescence.

Mumps

Arthritis caused by mumps is commoner in male teenagers. Less than 1 per cent of those affected by mumps developed arthritis, usually two weeks (range: four days to four weeks) after the start of the illness. It is usually migratory and asymmetrical, involving large joints. When pericarditis is also present it can resemble rheumatic fever. During an epidemic children may have an arthritis but no parotitis. The presence of rising antibody titres to mumps virus may help to confirm the diagnosis.

Chickenpox (varicella)

This may be complicated by bacterial arthritis with spread from infected scabs. A transcient, acute arthritis may occur at the time of the rash.

Adenoviral arthritis

The arthritis usually occurs in infected children. It begins with fever, coryza, and pharyngitis, followed by a macular erythematous rash and symmetrical arthritis.

Infectious mononucleosis

Widespread lymphadenopathy, splenomegaly, rash, fever, and transient arthritis or arthralgia may mimic both rheumatic fever and systemic juvenile chronic arthritis. However, the rash tends to be larger and raised and does not recur as often as juvenile arthritis. This is a disorder of adolescents. In children, cytomegalovirus can cause a similar picture.

Arboviruses

Arboviruses (arthropod borne) are associated with arthritis in certain parts of the world; the Ross River virus in Australia and the O'nyong-nyong virus in Africa. Symptoms include fever, rash, and arthritis or arthralgia.

Kawasaki's disease (mucocutaneous lymph-node syndrome) (see page 24.1)

This is an uncommon acute inflammatory disease which occurs under the age of 5 years. Clinical features include (a) fever lasting more than 5 days, (b) bilateral conjunctivitis, (c) diffuse redness of mouth and pharynx, (d) erythema of palms and soles with oedema, and (e) lymphadenopathy.

Usually the disease is self-limiting but sudden death can occur from acute myocardial ischaemia. It has been suggested that the vasculitis of Kawasaki's disease may be a response to an antigen carried by house dust mite.

Leukaemia

Joint symptoms include symmetrical or occasionally migratory polyarthritis, arthralgias, and bone pain and tenderness. Sixty per cent of patients with lymphocytic leukaemia have joint symptoms, usually involving large peripheral joints.

Acute lymphoblastic leukaemia occurs mainly in young children where it can mimic Still's disease with fever, lymphadenopathy, and splenomegaly. An acute suppurative arthritis or haemarthrosis can occur; but aching in the limbs is more commonly due to subperiosteal infiltration. A leukaemoid reaction, with or without immature cells in the peripheral blood, may lead to diagnostic confusion. This occurs particularly in young children with infections, lymphoma or neuroblastoma, all of which can be associated with joint symptoms.

Lymphoma

Bone pain is the most common symptom. Synovial reaction is rarely caused by direct invasion; it is most often attributed to adjacent bone disease. Articular symptoms are less frequent than one might expect in view of the frequency of skeletal invasion.

Multicentric reticulohistiocytosis

This is a rare systemic disease of unknown aetiology, with a large number of synonyms. There are fewer than 50 reported cases. It is characterized by an infiltration of lipid laden histiocytes and multinucleated giant cells into various tissues. Skin nodules and a destructive polyarthritis are the most common findings.

The onset of the disease is usually insidious with almost two-thirds presenting with a polyarthritis. Skin nodules may precede the arthritis or appear concurrently. Middle-aged females are most commonly affected.

One of the most characteristic features is the rapid development of a severe incapacitating, deforming arthritis. The interphalangeal joints are most frequently involved but other joints, including the spine, may be affected. The distal interphalangeal joints, in contrast with rheumatoid arthritis are commonly involved. Radiographs show in the early stages 'punched out' bone lesions, followed later by severe destructive changes.

Nodules appear most frequently on the face and hands, but can occur in any part of the body. They can range in number from a few to hundreds and are light copper to reddish-brown in colour. Mucosal surfaces are also frequently involved. Associated malignant disease has been reported in 20–30 per cent of patients. There is no satisfactory treatment for the condition.

Neuropathic joints (synonym Charcot's joints)

Any loss of joint sensation renders that joint liable to develop a gross osteo-arthrosis with prolific new bone formation and marked

instability. In practice Charcot's joints are seen in association with tabes dorsalis, syringomyelia, and diabetes mellitus. They may also occur in association with paraplegia, Charcot–Marie–Tooth disease, myelomeningocele, and leprosy. An associated pyrophosphate arthropathy leads to inflammation. The joints are usually painless, although the diabetic tarsal neuropathic joint may be painful and present a clinical and radiological appearance suggestive of sepsis.

Ochronosis

In ochronosis or alkaptonuria, homogentisic acid accumulates in cartilage causing it to become leathery and rigid, and thus prone to rapid degeneration. This affects the spinal joints in particular, the disc spaces becoming thin and ragged. Any peripheral joint may also be affected and severe disability may result.

The diagnosis is usually obvious, homogentisic acid appearing in the urine causing it to go black on exposure to the light or on alkalinization. The deposits in the cartilage of the ear or in the sclera also become blackened when exposed to light.

The treatment is that of osteoarthrosis but in the absence of the capacity to correct the underlying metabolic abnormality it is largely ineffective.

Osteitis pubis

This is an uncommon, self-limiting condition of adults, characterized by pain and tenderness in the pubic rami adjacent to the symphysis. The pain is aggravated by walking or standing and is relieved by rest. The condition can follow retropubic prostatectomy or gynaecological procedures and is seen in athletes. Radiographs may show patchy increased density of both pubic rami associated with mottled areas or rarefaction.

Palindromic rheumatism

Described in 1941 and derived from the Greek word meaning to recur this episodic synovitis consists of attacks of joint pain, swelling, redness, tenderness, and stiffness developing spontaneously and lasting from three to seven days. Joints most commonly involved are the wrists and hands, knees, ankles and elbows, with only one or two joints being involved at any one time. During the interval between attacks the joints appear normal. Up to one-third progress to develop a more typical pattern of rheumatoid arthritis. Treatment consists of anti-inflammatory drugs and in those with frequent attacks, treatment with gold salts or penicillamine is often effective.

Pyoderma gangrenosum

This painful non-infective ulcerating skin lesion of unknown aetiology may be associated with ulcerative colitis, rheumatoid arthritis, a paraproteinaemia or occur without an identifiable underlying disorder. A seronegative, progressive, symmetrical erosive polyarthritis has been described and about 30 per cent of patients have arthralgia or arthritis. The arthritis may develop before and is unrelated to the activity of the skin lesion. It is unlike rheumatoid arthritis in that the joints involved include the first carpometacarpal and terminal interphalangeal joints in addition to the elbows, temporomandibular joints, and cervical spine. Synovial fluid shows a depressed complement level suggesting immune complex deposition, but skin histology does not reveal arteritis nor immune complex deposition.

Renal transplantation and haemodialysis

Joint complaints during haemodialysis include septic arthritis, acute synovitis, and acute calcific periarthritis. In those undergoing renal transplantation a transient synovitis may develop in the early postoperative period. Avascular necrosis affecting the head of the femur or lower femoral condyle may be a later complication.

Rheumatic fever and Jaccoud's syndrome

Polyarthritis is the commonest clinical feature of rheumatic fever, and is usually the presenting symptom. It occurs in some 75 per cent of initial attacks and involves large and medium-sized joints. The skin over the affected joints is hot and red, and the joints themselves are swollen and extremely painful and tender. The arthritis almost always affects more than one joint and is migratory; it affects each joint for a few days. The older the child the smaller the joints involved. There is some round cell infiltration of the synovium and no erosions are seen on X-ray.

Rarely the synovitis becomes chronic and may last several years, before subsiding completely. In others the process may lead to a chronic deformity superficially resembling rheumatoid arthritis which was described originally by Jaccoud in 1869. The following are the characteristics of Jaccoud's syndrome: (a) multiple attacks of rheumatic fever, (b) delayed recovery with stiffness and subsequent deformity of the metacarpophalangeal joints, (c) deformity due to soft tissue fibrosis rather than synovitis, (d) flexion at metacarpophalangeal joints with correctable ulnar deviation of fingers. There may be hyperextension at the PIP joints; tendon crepitus may be present, (e) inactive joint disease with few symptoms and good function, and (f) radiological 'hook-like' erosion of the metacarpal head. The ESR and tests for rheumatoid factor are normal.

Sarcoidosis

Arthritis is the most frequent rheumatological manifestation of sarcoidosis, occurring in up to 37 per cent of patients. It is three times more common in females. Two distinct clinical patterns, acute and chronic, have been recognized in adults. An acute onset is most common. Frequently associated with erythema nodosum and hilar lymphadenopathy (Löfgren's syndrome), the synovitis is symmetrical, migratory, and most frequently affects the knees and ankles, proximal interphalangeal joints, and wrists and elbows. Monoarthritis is unusual. The arthritis reaches maximal intensity within three days and may last from two weeks to four months. Joint deformity and destruction does not occur.

Chronic sarcoid arthritis may occur at any time in the course of the disease and may occur with acute exacerbations over a period of years. This is more common in Blacks and is usually accompanied by other signs of sarcoidosis. Synovial membrane biopsy may reveal granuloma. Radiological changes appear late and therefore are of limited diagnostic value. The joint space is narrowed and mottled rarefactions and multiple 'punched out' cystic lesions may be seen in the metacarpals and phalanges.

Acute synovitis responds to salicylates or, if necessary, corticosteroids. The response to corticosteroid therapy in the chronic group is poor.

Serum sickness

A generalized polyarthritis may be associated with serum sickness usually following the therapeutic injection of foreign serum. After some 2 to 16 days an acute reaction develops consisting of fever, rash, and headache. Arthritis and arthralgia, usually of the larger joints occurs in 50 per cent of cases. There may be transient proteinuria. These patients should be treated with antihistamines or corticosteroids.

Sweet's syndrome

The characteristic tender, red or purple, discrete skin plaques are associated with myalgias, arthralgias, or non-inflammatory joint effusions. All manifestations usually resolve over 2–3 months. Sjögren's syndrome and a facial rash have been reported causing confusion with systemic lupus erythematosus.

Tietze's syndrome and costochondritis

Both disorders are characterized by inflammation of one or more costal cartilages at the costochondral junction but the less common Tietze's syndrome is associated with local swelling whilst costochondritis is not. The cause is unknown; violent coughing and direct trauma are suspected of playing a role, although there is often no history of trauma. All ages can be affected, including children.

One or more tender lumps of the upper costal cartilages gradually develop. A single costal cartilage is involved in 80 per cent of patients, the second and third being most affected. Deep breathing and coughing may produce local pain. On examination the lumps are firm and somewhat tender, but not warm. The onset of pain is either acute or insidious. Special investigations show no evidence of a generalized disorder. Biopsy shows minor inflammatory changes. The course is variable; there may be spontaneous remission, or painless lumps may persist for years. If the pain is troublesome, local injections of lignocaine and/or corticosteroid preparations may give relief.

The diffuse nature of costochondritis and its occurrence in an older age group make it more likely that it will be confused with visceral pain. Costochondritis is too diffuse to inject but anti-inflammatory drugs are often effective. These syndromes must not be confused with sepsis or rheumatoid arthritis involving the manubriosternal joint.

Wilson's disease (see page 9.47)

The disease not infrequently presents in childhood and this may be a reason why joint damage is less obvious than in haemochromatosis where the mean age of onset is much later, and where age changes in cartilage may be contributory factors. Chondrocalcinosis occurs as does bone fragmentation at the joint margins with irregularity and sclerosis of the underlying bone. Osteochondritis and chondromalacia patellae have also been described.

The pathogenesis of the arthropathy is not understood although copper inhibits pyrophosphatase. Joint manifestations do not correlate with other features of the disease. A lupus-like syndrome with an inflammatory polyarthritis is a known but rare accompaniment of penicillamine therapy, which is the mainstay of treatment in Wilson's disease.

References

Barrow, M. V. and Holubar, K. (1969). Multicentre reticulohistiocytosis. *Medicine* **48**, 287.

Burgdorfer, W., Barbour, A. G., Hayes, S. F., Benach, J. L., Grunwald, E. and Davis, J. P. (1982). Lyme disease – a tick borne spirochetosis? *Science* **216**, 1317.

Bywaters, E. G. L. (1950). The relation between heart and joint disease including 'rheumatoid heart disease' and chronic post-rheumatic arthritis (type Jaccoud). *Br. Heart J.* **12**, 101.

Cohen, A. S. and Canoso, J. J. (1975). Rheumatological aspects of amyloid disease. *Clin. Rheum. Dis.* **1**, 149.

Cream, J. J., Gumpel, J. M. and Peachey, R. D. G. (1970). Schönlein–Henoch purpura in the adult: a study of 77 adults with anaphylactoid or Schonlein–Henoch purpura. *Q. J. Med.* **39**, 461.

Dumonde, D. C. and Steward, M. W. (1979). Role of microbial infection in rheumatic disease. In *Textbook of the rheumatic diseases* (ed. W. S. C. Copeman), pp. 244, Churchill Livingstone, Edinburgh.

Duthie, R. B., Matthews, J. M., Rizza, C. R. and Steel, W. M. (1972). *The management of musculoskeletal problems in the haemophilias.* Blackwell Scientific Publications, Oxford.

Golding, D. N. and Walshe, J. M. (1977). Arthropathy of Wilson's disease. *Ann. Rheum. Dis.* **36**, 99.

Halsey, J. P., Reeback, J. S. and Barnes, C. G. (1982). A decade of skeletal tuberculosis. *Ann. Rheum. Dis.* **41**, 7–10.

Hamilton, E., Williams, R., Barlow, K. A. and Smith, P. M. (1968). The arthropathy of idiopathic haemochromatosis. *Q. J. Med.* **37**, 171.

Hench, P. S. and Rosenberg, E. F. (1941). Palindromic rheumatism. *Proc. Mayo Clin.* **16**, 808.

Holt, P., Davies, M. G. and Nuki, G. (1977). Polyarthritis in association with pyoderma gangrenosum. *Ann. Rheum. Dis.* **36**, 285.

Khachadurion, A. K. (1968). Migratory polyarthritis in familial hypercholesterolemia (type II hyperlipoproteinemia). *Arth. Rheum.* **11**, 385.

Lansbury, J. C. (1953). Collagen disease complicating malignancy. *Ann. Rheum. Dis.* **12**, 301.

Loewi, G., Webster, A. D. B. and Asherson, G. L. (1975). Arthritis in immune deficiency. *Scand. J. Rheum.* **4** (suppl. 8) 11.

Manshady, B. M., Thompson, G. R. and Weiss, J. J. (1980). Septic arthritis in a general hospital. *J. Rheum.* **7**, 523.

Marx, W. and O'Connell, D. (1979). Arthritis of primary biliary cirrhosis. *Arch. intern. Med.* **139**, 213.

Newman, J. H. (1976). Review of septic arthritis throughout the antibiotic era. *Ann. Rheum. Dis.* **35**, 198.

O'Brien, W. M., LaDu, B. N. and Bunn, J. J. (1963). Biochemical, pathological and clinical aspects of alcaptonuria, ochronosis and ochronotic arthropathy: Review of the world literature (1584–1962). *Am. J. Med.* **34**, 813.

Rooney, P., Ballantyne, D. and Watson Buchanan, W. (1975). Disorders of the locomotor system associated with abnormalities of lipid metabolism and the lipoidoses. *Clin. Rheum. Dis.* **1**, 163.

Schumacher, H. R. (1975). Rheumatological manifestations of sickle-cell disease and other hereditary haemoglobinopathies. *Clin. Rheum. Dis.* **1**, 37.

Seifert, M. H., Warin, A. P. and Miller, A. (1974). Articular and cutaneous manifestations of gonorrhoea. *Ann. Rheum. Dis.* **33**, 140.

Spilberg, I., Silzbach, L. E. and McEwen, C. E. (1969). The arthritis of sarcoidosis. *Arth. Rheum.* **12**, 126.

Sohar, E., Pras, M. and Gafric, J. (1975). Familial Mediterranean fever and its articular manifestations. *Clin. Rheum. Dis.* **1**, 195.

Truelove, C. H. (1960). Articular manifestations of erythema nodosum. *Ann. Rheum. Dis.* **19**, 174.

THE MANAGEMENT OF INFLAMMATORY JOINT DISEASE

A. G. MOWAT

Introduction

The same general principles of management apply to all forms of inflammatory joint disease in which the cause is unknown. However, the extent to which these principles are applied will depend upon the natural history, severity, and chronicity of the disease. It is convenient to describe the general management of rheumatoid arthritis and such treatment can be modified to suit each individual patient and disease. It is important that the nature of the disease and the aims of a careful management plan be fully understood by the patient, the family, and the medical advisers from the outset.

There are considerable advantages in treating patients with inflammatory joint disease in a separate ward or unit as they can often help and advise each other and are not subjected to the pressures of bed turnover which inevitably prevail in general medical or surgical wards. These patients progress slowly and indeed may not improve if their treatment programmes are hurried. Further, since the diseases produce complex disabilities and are usually associated with domestic, economic, employment, and social factors, team work is essential in their management. The team is composed of general practitioner, physician, orthopaedic surgeon, physiotherapist, occupational therapist, nursing staff, and medical social worker. A psychiatrist may often be added. A close liaison must be continued with the various domiciliary services.

The aim of management of chronic joint disease is simply to allow the patient to achieve and maintain the maximum functional capacity. This will entail not only an accurate assessment of the initial status of the patient but a continuing assessment of the changing status of the disease and of the patient's reaction to it. It is important to appreciate that the patient's problem is not so much the arthritis but rather the disability that it produces. Many patients, especially the elderly, are subjected to unnecessary hospital visits for examination and treatment when all they require is a simple, commonsense approach to their domestic difficulties.

Whilst each patient must be treated as an individual, with a quite different approach being adopted for children, it is convenient to consider rheumatoid arthritis as a three-stage disease:

1. Potentially reversible soft tissue proliferation.
2. Controllable (but irreversible) soft tissue destruction and early cartilage erosion.
3. Skeletal collapse with mechanical changes when mechanical and not drug solutions must be sought.

This simple concept, with the appropriate plan of treatment (Table 1), must be interpreted with caution since the disease affects and advances in different joints and in different patients at different rates.

Analgesics

Analgesics have always had limited value in inflammatory conditions. Recently the recognition of inflammatory processes in osteoarthritis (page 16.76) and the satisfactory side-effect profiles of the new non-steroidal anti-inflammatory drugs, which are also peripherally acting analgesics, has further reduced their usage.

For acute gout, injury or joint haemorrhage including haemophilia short-term usage of adequate doses of potent narcotics is justified (dipipanone 10 mg, morphine 10 mg, pethidine 100 mg). For longer term use paracetamol (1–1.5 g), codeine (60–90 mg), dextropropoxyphene (65–130 mg), nefopam (30–60 mg), and pentazocine (50–100 mg), together with variants and combinations are safe and have the advantage of not exacerbating a haemorrhagic problem by altering platelet aggregation. New, safer narcotics (buprenorphine, nalbuphine), although useful in sublingual form

Table 1 Staged therapy in rheumatoid arthritis

	Medical	Surgical	Therapist
Stage 1	SAARD	Synovectomy	Advice
	NSAID		Simple aids
	Local steroid injections		Simple exercises
	Radioactive synovectomy		
Stage 2	NSAID	Tendon repair	Simple aids
	SAARD	Limited bone excision	Splints
Stage 3	NSAID	Arthroplasty	Splints
		Joint replacement	Domestic/walking aids
		Arthrodesis	House conversions

NSAID : Non-steroidal anti-inflammatory drugs.
SAARD : Slow acting antirheumatic drugs.

for postoperative pain in orthopaedic surgery are less useful for sustained prescription in rheumatological practice.

Non-steroidal anti-inflammatory drugs (NSAIDs)

The worldwide use of these drugs, the logical first step in the treatment of inflammatory arthritis, gout, osteoarthritis with its increasingly recognized inflammatory component, and a wide range of soft tissue lesions including those in sportsmen, has increased enormously in the past decade. There is little evidence that a peak has been reached, the introduction of a new drug being accompanied by a growth in the market with minimal change in the prescription of established agents. However, in recent years important changes have taken place. Although development of NSAIDs continues unabated, the introduction of new drugs has been delayed while several have been withdrawn worldwide after limited adverse experience in one country. Some of these decisions by the Drug Regulatory Authorities reflect genuine problems and concerns (e.g. phenylbutazone and related fluid retaining and marrow toxic pyrazolones) but in other cases bad prescribing practices fuelled by inaccurate advertising have highlighted the expected side-effects of these agents and led to the loss of useful drugs (e.g. benoxaprofen, zomepirac). It has become easy to expect that a freely available NSAID is effective and safe and that its use requires no special consideration by patient or physician.

These unreal expectations are largely confounded by the complexity of the inflammatory process, much of which is still being elucidated. Thus any discussion of the action of NSAID tends to concentrate upon the inhibition of the cyclo-oxygenate breakdown pathway of arachidonic acid and hence changes in the production of prostaglandins and related compounds, and details of *in vitro* activity of a drug are paraded as evidence of its potential in human disease. In reality the inflammatory process has many facets. Thus the cyclo-oxygenase pathway is mirrored by the alternative lipoxygenase breakdown pathway for arachidonic acid leading to the production of equally damaging products, superoxide radicals, and the leukotrienes; a pathway unaffected by the majority of NSAIDs. Further, arachidonic acid and its products are not the only chemicals released by the interaction of a variety of cells, neutrophils, macrophages, and synovial cells, with immune complexes, crystals, and tissue breakdown products. Such released chemicals include histamine, kinins, proteases, and superoxide radicals for some of which natural inhibitors have been identified. Finally, while in some conditions the response may be largely chemical, in others, for instance, rheumatoid arthritis, there are complex cellular and immunological events leading to chronic inflammation. Clearly with so many potential sites of action for NSAIDs it would be unwise to assume that firstly a single action, prostaglandin synthetase inhibition, was paramount particularly when antihistamines have been shown to be ineffective in arthritis and that secondly all NSAIDs have the same spectrum of activity.

It can be postulated that the complexity of an inflammatory process is reflected in the variability of the drug response and the incidence of side-effects (Table 2). Thus gout and soft tissue lesions represent a fairly simple inflammatory process, responsive to most NSAIDs with only modest differences in efficacy and a low incidence of side-effects. Indeed the failure of a new drug to work in acute gout might occasion more interest than its success. Ankylosing spondylitis is associated with some differences in drug effect but with a moderate incidence of side-effects; incidentally there is no evidence that phenylbutazone has a specific or diagnostic action in this disease. Osteoarthritis exhibits increasing complexity with clear interpatient differences, while the intricate inflammation of rheumatoid arthritis and related connective tissue diseases is amply matched by differing patient responses and a high incidence of side-effects.

Testing in animal models of inflammation and pain, although indicating the basic activity and safety of a drug, does not define its level of activity in humans. This level, while it can be measured

Table 2 Implications for NSAIDs in different diseases

Disease	Inflammatory process	Patient preference	Side-effects
Soft tissue lesions	Simple	Little	Few
Gout	Simple	Little	Few
Ankylosing spondylitis	Confused	Modest	Occasional
Osteoarthritis	Complicated	Moderate	Frequent
Rheumatoid arthritis	Complex	Great	Multiple

Table 3 Assessment of analgesic anti-inflammatory drugs in humans

Pain : Visual analogue scale (10 cm line)
        Four point grading
Morning stiffness duration
Ring size of proximal interphalangeal joints
Articular index (standard score for inflamed joints)
Range of large joint movement
Grip strength
Walking time (standard distance)
Functional tests

Side-effect profile
Laboratory toxicity data

Global scores
Patient preferences

using standardized techniques (Table 3) shows marked inter-patient variation and in many cases the results of clinical trials are dependent upon some global score: a score that balances clinical benefit and side-effects and expresses the result as patient preference.

The chemical grouping of the NSAID is shown in Fig. 1. Despite chemical similarity individual responses to different group members can show marked variation, indicating that failure to respond to one does not invalidate all (e.g. propionic acids). Further, while a variable incidence of dyspepsia and other gastrointestinal side-effects occurs with all these drugs, there is some consistency in the type of other side-effects associated with each group although patients do not necessarily develop it with all drugs of the group (e.g. skin rash with phenylacetic acids and central nervous system effects of headache, dizziness, and depression with cyclic acetic acids). It is, therefore, impossible to indicate a 'best buy' or to exclude the remainder of a group on the basis of the inefficacy or toxicity of one member. However, remembering the essential contribution of patient compliance, it is possible to provide some advice:

1. *Make a small selection* from a range of chemical groupings *for regular prescription* as familiarity improves usage (Table 4 and Fig. 1).

2. *Defer usage of older aspirin preparations and indomethacin.* They are regarded as being stronger than most of the newer drugs. This is reflected in a higher incidence of responding patients but also a higher incidence of side-effects; problems which tend to outweigh their cost advantages.

3. *Prescribe only one drug at a time* since there is little evidence of synergism or reduced toxicity with two or more. However, one drug by day and a different drug by night is acceptable. With a greater understanding of the inflammatory process and individual drug actions, such purity of prescription may be challenged.

4. *Prescribe an adequate dose.* Some drugs (e.g. aspirin and naproxen) show some relationship between blood levels and efficacy, with the opportunity for laboratory monitoring of blood levels in the case of aspirin, but higher doses of many other NSAID tend to produce more responders with little increase in toxicity.

5. *Prescribe for a limited time.* Drugs given twice or more fre-

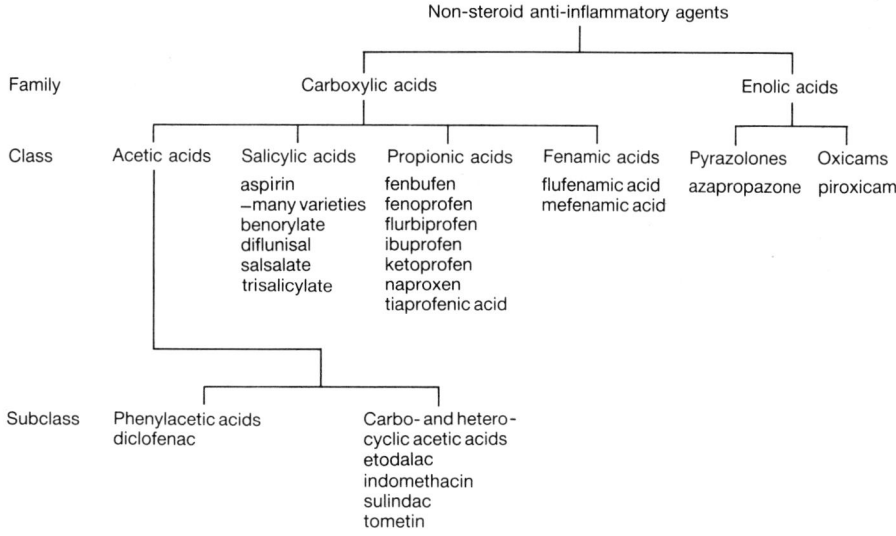

Fig. 1 Non-steroidal anti-inflammatory drugs.

Table 4 Non-steroidal anti-inflammatory drugs

Drugs	Dose	Frequency (times daily)
Diclofenac	50 mg	3–4
Etodolac	200 mg	2
Indomethacin	75 mg (slow release)	2
Sulindac	200 mg	2
Tolmetin	400 mg	4
Aspirin	600–900 mg	6
Aloxiprin	1200 mg	4
Benorylate	10 ml	2
Diflunisal	500 mg	2
Salsalate	1–1.5 g	2
Trilisate	1–1.5 g	2
Fenbufen	600 mg	1–2
Fenoprofen	600 mg	4
Flurbiprofen	100 mg	3
Ibuprofen	400–800 mg	4
Ketoprofen	100 mg (slow release)	1–2
Naproxen	500 mg	2
Tiaprofenic acid	200 mg	2–3
Flufenamic acid	200 mg	4
Mefenamic acid	500 mg	4
Azapropazone	600 mg	2
Piroxicam	20 mg	1

quently per day will produce stable blood and tissue levels and hence a clinical effect, within one week, while those with a longer half-life given once a day require 2–3 weeks. The timing of drug changes should reflect these facts.

Problems with NSAIDs
As with any drug the findings from initial clinical trials of NSAIDs can lead to mistakes perpetuated in subsequent prescribing.

The wrong dose may be selected   The history of these drugs abounds with examples of dramatic increases in initially recommended dosages and the subsequent introduction of double-strength tablets. Indeed physicians have come to expect that the dose can be and probably should be doubled. However, since not all NSAIDs enjoy a wide therapeutic safety range such behaviour has contributed to unexpected side-effects and the withdrawal of useful drugs.

The wrong regime may be selected   Blood levels may not mimic synovial tissue levels or indicate the true effect of the drug. There

may be delays in transfer into synovial tissue, local concentration of drug or diurnal variations in drug effect. Thus twice daily treatment often works well with good patient compliance when plasma half-life studies suggest more frequent administration. Conversely the claimed convenience of once daily medication for drugs with a long half-life may have less relevance in a painful condition when most patients like access to a drug with a discernible speed of action more than once in 24 hours.

The wrong patient may be selected   The elderly and the very young may handle tahese drugs quite differently from normal controls. It is important that appropriate pharmokinetic studies are undertaken in diseased patients of all ages since the findings may be quite different. While clinical studies are usually required in the young it has only recently been appreciated that the marked differences in drug handling in the elderly combined with changes in body weight, fat, and water can significantly alter plasma levels. Certainly unless specific information is available, NSAIDs should be given with caution to underweight and elderly patients.

Gastrointestinal side-effects
While a wide range of side-effects can be expected with NSAIDs, some being more frequent with one chemical group than another, gastrointestinal intolerance remains a major problem. Although the relationship between NSAIDs and dyspepsia, often accompanied by florid superficial mucosal changes demonstrated by sequential gastroscopic examination, is accepted, the relationship between NSAIDs and peptic ulceration is still debated due to the difficulties of finding an adequate control group. Some evidence suggests that patients with inflammatory joint disease have an inherently higher incidence of peptic ulceration independent of drug therapy. Further, even if occasional patients show an important idiosyncratic blood loss with a NSAID which means they should never receive that drug again, the majority of studies of gastrointestinal blood loss with these drugs show only modest daily increases over baseline values, losses that will not contribute to clinical anaemia.

Acidic NSAIDs tend to be concentrated in sites where the pH is lower. This is beneficial in joints but also means concentration in gastric parietal cells. Since this concentration occurs by both local and systemic mechanisms slow-release preparations designed to deliver the drug in a controlled way beyond the stomach, pro-drugs with an inactive and non-irritant compound being absorbed and converted to active drug in the liver and suppositories are not necessarily the answer to dyspepsia in the arthritic.

In diseases that demand more than analgesia it is unacceptable to withdraw all anti-inflammatory drugs because of gastrointestinal side-effects and for the patients to be severely cautioned against their future use. There is an increasing range of drugs available for the neutralization or reduction in gastric acid. These will reduce the pH gradient between gastric contents and the lining cells limiting drug uptake. In addition a series of widely differing mucoprotective agents are becoming available which should control the damage induced by the local prostaglandin inhibitory effect of NSAIDs. There is little evidence of interaction between these drugs and NSAIDs and although questions about the safety of long-term combined usage are unanswered, in the short term such combination therapy is very effective.

Finally a contribution from the patient is important so that standard dyspeptic advice in respect of smoking, alcohol, proper meals, and drug taking with food is followed.

Patient education

Patients must understand the likely benefits and possible side-effects of NSAID treatment. These drugs largely control the symptoms of pain and stiffness associated with musculoskeletal inflammation while having a modest effect upon the underlying process so that tenderness and joint swelling are slower to settle. In chronic inflammatory disorders like rheumatoid arthritis NSAIDs will produce little alteration in the erythrocyte sedimentation rate and other acute phase proteins and will not alter the values of immunoglobulins or rheumatoid factor. Thus it is unrealistic to expect the removal of all pain and stiffness, a perfect night's sleep and striking improvement in function. Patients need to understand their disease, measuring gain rather than expecting cure.

Suggested prescribing pattern

In the early management of the patient with arthritis or soft-tissue rheumatism these sequential changes might be initiated in the event of lack of response or the development of side-effects.

(a) Propionic acid derivative alone
(b) Try another propionic acid ± 75–100 mg indomethacin at night
(c) Try another NSAID ± indomethacin at night
(d) Salicylic acid preparation with 12-hour action or indomethacin by day and night
(e) Consider other NSAIDs ± combinations of earlier therapy
(f) Review diagnosis and need for more 'specific' therapy.

Existing NSAIDs should be used thoughtfully recognizing the problems and limitations described above. New NSAIDs should be used cautiously. They are unlikely to have fewer side-effects or a unique action and will certainly be more expensive. While it is tempting, it is also unwise to overprescribe new drugs to patients with a long history of intolerance or lack of efficacy with NSAIDs. 'Difficult to treat' patients are likely to remain so.

Slow acting antirheumatic drugs (SAARDs)

These drugs are most commonly used in patients with rheumatoid arthritis, partly because this condition outnumbers all other forms of inflammatory arthritis put together, but more importantly because many of these drugs or therapies, due to lack of specific effect, have limited application in other conditions e.g. penicillamine. Gold therapy seems the most effective agent in psoriatic arthropathy with no propensity to exaggerate the skin features, and methotrexate may have occasional application in cases of resistant reactive arthritis. Immunosuppressive drugs and various forms of cell separation may be utilized in systemic lupus erythematosus. Slow acting antirheumatic drugs have the capacity to control the disease and occasionally induce remission. They are best used in patients whose disease is unlikely to go into natural remission and when there is the maximum potential benefit. Thus

Table 5 Slow-acting antirheumatic drugs

Group I	Drugs of proven value and widely used
	Azathioprine
	Chloroquine
	D-Penicillamine
	Gold salts
Group II	Clinically active drugs under continuing investigation
	Auranofin
	Chlorambucil
	Dapsone
	Levamisole
	Methylprednisolone pulsing
	Methotrexate
	Sulphasalazine
	Thiols
	Thymopoietin
Group III	Less practical or unproven treatments
	Plasmapheresis
	Selective cellular centrifugation
	Thoracic duct drainage
	Antilymphocytic globulin
	Interferon

patients with seropositive, stage 1 rheumatoid arthritis (Table 1) in whom there is synovial proliferation of 6–12 months' duration (and perhaps early radiographic change), should, even if symptoms are controlled by NSAIDs, be considered for SAARDs. The severity and rate of progression will determine decisions in seronegative and stage 2 disease, while the use of SAARDs in stage 3 disease, except perhaps to influence lesions based upon overt vasculitis, is rarely indicated.

The range of SAARDs is considerable (Table 5) and despite much experimental work, their mode(s) of action is largely unknown and beyond the scope of this chapter. Thus the physical removal of a cell or protein does not imply that its pathogenic role is understood. In general, although there may be no direct action, a fall in rheumatoid factor titres almost invariably accompanies a clinical response.

Clinical decisions and drug choice are best made after consultation with a specialist rheumatologist. There is no 'best buy', treatments being mentioned alphabetically, and the final choice depends upon clinical experience, patient characteristics, their likely sensitivities, and their previous drug experience. A failure to respond after six months shown as improvement in the clinical indices in Table 3 together with a fall in erythrocyte sedimentation rate and other acute phase proteins, and a rise in haemoglobin values, demands the use of another drug. A clinical response may also be associated with a fall in the platelet count and serum immunoglobulin values to normal. All treatments must be closely monitored with appropriate blood and urine tests at 2–4 weekly intervals (perhaps less frequently in the third year of a treatment) and the patient should have direct access to the clinician at all times lest typical early features of toxicity are ignored. Eventually tissue typing (e.g. the presence of DR3) may identify both likely responders and those with special sensitivities.

While, in general, it is sensible to move from less to more toxic drugs, there is no evidence that the order of use of SAARDs influences the eventual chance of successful disease control. Once achieved there is a natural reluctance on the part of both patient and physician to discontinue therapy lest the disease, which is almost always merely suppressed rather than pushed into true remission, flares and proves difficult to control. This reluctance is encouraged by the knowledge that the risk of side-effects diminishes with time. However, it is sensible to attempt gradual dose reduction or the use of interval therapy such as 1–3 days per week. Although radiographic evidence of disease control with the healing of erosions is the ideal, this has proved to be a disputed phenomenon for most drugs partly because it is difficult to set up a satisfactory long-term clinical trial with adequate control groups.

Table 6 D-Penicillamine therapy

Problem (frequency)		Time (months)	Action and outcome
Ineffective	(25–30%)	6	Another drug
Early 'drug' rash	(10%)	1–2	Stop; desensitize
Loss of taste	(20%)	1–2	Continue. Clears 1–2 months
Nausea	(20%)	1–2	Hold dose. Clears
Thrombocytopenia	(10%)	Anytime	Repeat count if falling
			Stop if below 50 x 10^9/l
			Desensitize when recovered
Pancytopenia	(Rare)	Anytime	Stop. Never re-use
Proteinuria	(10%)	4–24	<5 g/day – continue – clears over 12 months
	(Rare)		5 g/day ± oedema – stop
			Close renal monitoring in both
Late 'pemphigus' rash	(5%)	6–18	Continue if mild

Table 7 Gold therapy

Problem (frequency)		Time (months)	Action and outcome
Ineffective	(25–30%)	6	Another drug
Rash–various	(20%)	2–6	Stop. If mild, desensitize
Mouth ulcers	(20%)	2–6	Stop. If mild, desensitize
Thrombocytopenia	(1%)	Anytime	Stop. Deaths even with
Pancytopenia	(Rare)	Anytime	prompt withdrawal. Never re-use
Proteinuria	(5%)	4–12	> 1g/day–stop
			Do not reuse

Group I

Azathioprine

This is the safest 'immunosuppressive' which is as effective, but less toxic, in a daily dose of 1 mg/kg compared with the traditional 2.5 mg/kg. Some 70 per cent of patients will show clinical benefit with neutropenia and gastrointestinal complaints being the commonest side-effects. There is an increased incidence of herpes zoster, unusual with other popular SAARDs. It does not cause infertility but should be avoided in those of child-bearing age. There is an approximately 50 per cent increase in the frequency of all tumours, non-Hodgkin's lymphoma, and squamous carcinoma of the skin being the most common, perhaps due to altered immune surveillance. These risks should be considered before starting azathioprine. It has a traditional role as a corticosteroid sparer although other SAARDs are equally effective.

Chloroquine

Available in several forms (phosphate, sulphate 250 mg/day: hydroxysulphate 200–400 mg/day) chloroquine is probably the least effective but the least toxic SAARD and is a useful first drug for many patients since routine blood and urine tests are not mandatory. About half the patients will show benefit varying as with all SAARDs from modest to disease remission. The bitter taste and dyspepsia can be overcome by taking the tablets with food, while eye side-effects are rare with current low doses. Corneal deposition leading to blurred vision is reversed by drug withdrawal and is no contraindication to future use. Largely irreversible retinopathy, which produces a characteristic 'bulls eye' macula in its later stages, is detected by specialist visual field examination particularly with a red light. There is no agreement over the required frequency of examination although initial and six monthly ones are suggested. Similarly concern over continuous, long-term usage, since side-effects are partly dose related, may also reflect older reports. Chloroquine is being re-evaluated in clinical trials and is frequently being used as a second drug in combination with other SAARDs, particularly gold and D-penicillamine, as this approach to intractable cases develops.

D-Penicillamine

D-Penicillamine (Table 6) enjoys equal popularity with gold with 70 per cent of patients showing improvement. Since the first controlled trial in 1973 its rate of introduction and final dosage have decreased. With the password 'Go slow – go low' side-effects have been fewer although some are only delayed. With patients safely able to take the drug over many years, it is sensible to alter the dose either up or down approximately in time with expected clinical responses e.g. 125–250 mg increments at 2–3 monthly intervals with a maximum dose of 750 mg/day. If gastric tolerance allows, the drug should be given remote from meals and iron supplements since it binds to metals and other thiols.

The side-effects have occasioned as much interest as its clinical benefit since many, including the nephropathy, are immunologically generated and yet they may regress and clear despite continued treatment. Of the rarer side-effects, drug-induced lupus and myasthenia should be remembered as they may be confused with a flare in the rheumatoid arthritis.

Gold salts

A variety of salts both water and oil based are available for intramuscular injection with no clear differences in beneficial or toxic effects (Table 7). Despite 50 years of use the ideal way to use gold has probably not been determined. Most advocate 50 mg i. m. weekly without preceding test doses and a decrease in frequency to 2-, 3-, and finally 4-weekly intervals when the patient shows a clear clinical response (2–4 months) and at similar times thereafter. A response is unlikely beyond 20 weeks (1 g). Some employ lower doses (10 mg) since efficacy and toxicity are not clearly related to serum levels, although presumably they may be related to tissue levels which are immeasurable *in vivo*. Many rheumatologists consider that responding patients should be maintained indefinitely on gold since there is the impression (disputed) that a second course is less successful. However, breakthrough disease can be controlled by increasing the frequency of the injections.

The wide range of side-effects, many serious but rare, which are similar to those of penicillamine suggests a common action. However, failure to respond to one does not exclude benefit from the other although occasionally the same side-effect may occur.

Gold is unique among SAARDs in having no upper gastrointestinal side-effects although rarely it causes a colitis. It is also particularly useful for those patients who forget to take or do not like oral medication, the doctor or nurse being in complete control.

Group II

Auranofin

Auranofin is an oral form of gold in which the less prominent thiol component may explain its different action. A daily dose of 6 mg will produce clinical benefit in approximately 50 per cent of patients with a lower incidence of haematological and renal side-effects than with injectable gold salts. Diarrhoea in some 35 per cent of patients remains the most inconvenient side-effect. The cellular and humoral interactions of the drug have been extensively investigated and there is adequate experimental evidence to expect the drug to work. It may find a place alongside chloroquine as a useful initial drug.

Chlorambucil

This 'immunosuppressive' drug has been widely used in Europe, particularly France, for the treatment of rheumatoid arthritis and other connective tissue disorders but for no clear reason has not gained acceptance in Britain or North America. The laboratory studies indicate a similar effectiveness to azathioprine with a similar incidence of side-effects in patients, although a low incidence of gastrointestinal irritation, a high incidence of intercurrent infections especially herpes zoster and the risk of future malignancy merit special consideration. A daily dose of 0.2 mg/kg (approximately 12 mg) is required.

Cyclophosphamide

This is an alkylating agent with cytotoxic, immunosuppressive, and anti-inflammatory properties that improves some 70–75 per cent of patients and which has been shown to heal radiological lesions. The high incidence of often distressing side-effects on 150 mg/day has led to several trials of lower doses with conflicting results. A dose of 75 mg/day appears effective with few cases of alopecia and leucopenia but many patients suffer nausea, vomiting, stomatitis, haematuria, and intercurrent respiratory infections. However, the withdrawal rate may be lower than with some apparently safer agents perhaps suggesting patient satisfaction. There are serious concerns over long-term usage which may cause haemorrhagic cystitis, neoplasia and sterility. Cyclophosphamide is best reserved for those patients with rheumatoid arthritis and other connective disorders with life-threatening complications based upon vasculitis.

Dapsone

The considerable similarities in the immune response in leprosy and rheumatoid arthritis encouraged the first trials of dapsone in 1976. The results supported by formal placebo and drug comparison studies suggest clinical benefit in up to 50 per cent with the main side-effects being nausea, rash, and a significant but transient, haemolytic anaemia which peaks after 6 weeks of treatment. Dapsone has been given at the rate of 100–50 mg/day for the first week.

Levamisole

Levamisole is a widely available anthelmintic with interesting and well-investigated immunomodulatory activities, although these may prove irrelevant in rheumatoid arthritis. Effective as 150 mg on one day each week, it has been shown to be superior to placebo and equal to gold and penicillamine. The side-effects, dominated by rashes and neutropenia, have discouraged its use even though they are no worse than with other agents. Severe neutropenia which occurs in 3–5 per cent of cases is especially common in seropositive women who carry the HLA B27 antigen.

Methylprednisolone

Short intravenous infusions of large doses (1 g) of this potent steroid are widely and often uncritically used. With initial studies in transplant patients confirming the safety of the technique which is remarkably free of traditional steroid side-effects, it was first used in patients with life-threatening complications and then increasingly as an adjunct to other therapies. It may be used as a method of sparing oral steroids or overcoming the lag period while other SAARDs become effective. Infusions may be given on two or three consecutive days in severe cases and at 4–6 weekly intervals for longer term disease control.

Methotrexate

As a folic acid antagonist the inhibitory effect of this drug on a number of amino acid pathways is well established. While this forms the basis of an immunosuppressive action there are independent anti-inflammatory activities. The drug has an established if limited place in the treatment of polymyositis and psoriatic arthropathy although the effect upon the joints is less dramatic than upon the skin. A variety of regimes are under study in these diseases and rheumatoid arthritis with no clear indication that oral therapy is accompanied by fewer side-effects than intravenous dosing. Side-effects are numerous with bone marrow and liver damage being the most serious but in general are milder than those encountered in the treatment of malignancy due to the lower doses employed.

Sulphasalazine

Originally introduced in the early 1940s for both rheumatoid arthritis and ulcerative colitis because of its theoretical antibacterial and anti-inflammatory activity, sulphasalazine succeeded in the latter but failed in the former chiefly due to errors in trial design and modest toxicity. It was reconsidered following the success of dapsone which it chemically resembles and with which it shares a number of side-effects including nausea, rash, and haemolytic anaemia. The clinical trialist as well as the historian can learn from this episode. Recent clinical trials have shown significant clinical improvement in 60 per cent of patients and side-effects have been reduced by increments in doses of 0.5 g/day during the early weeks to a maximum of 2 g/day.

Others

Thymopoietin is under study since it may represent the basis of action of levamisole and hence have clinical benefit but few side-effects, while a number of thiols have been tried in the hope that not only will the side-effects of penicillamine be avoided but also the mechanism of action of these agents be elucidated.

Group III

Antilymphocytic globulin and transfer factor have not yet proved to be practical or reliable methods of treatment while the use of interferon, an agent from which the popular press has told patients to expect much, must await wider availability of supplies.

A return to mediaeval blood letting forms the basis of three expensive and demanding physical treatments under evaluation. The oldest, the removal of lymphocytes by thoracic duct drainage, has a dramatic effect upon clinical and vasculitic features of the disease that cannot be explained simply on immunosuppressive grounds. A variation on the technique is the removal of lymphocytes by centrifugation (lymphapheresis). Plasmapheresis with the concept of removal of inflammatory immune complexes is perhaps less effective in rheumatoid arthritis than other related diseases.

In conclusion, SAARDs are an advancing and exciting field in rheumatological practice, a field that offers considerable advantages to the patient if he can co-operate with a knowledgeable and conscientious physician. In most cases the knowledge that he is treating a chronic inflammatory rather than a malignant disease means that the physician must temper his enthusiasm to employ combinations of toxic drugs whose actions are largely unexplained. Nevertheless combinations of established SAARDs are now being studied with some exciting results and without any evidence of side-effect excess. For the future there are exciting treatments on the horizon. Monoclonal antibodies directed at T lymphocytes or DR antigens, cyclosporin, and total body irradiation are at an early stage of evaluation. Androgenic steroids may have application in predominantly female diseases such as rheumatoid arthritis and systemic lupus. Finally more sophisticated and highly targeted drug delivery systems will have a ready application in the field of rheumatic diseases.

Corticosteroids

Amid all the adverse publicity for corticosteroids their dramatic effect in inflammatory joint disease has been almost forgotten. They possess potent anti-inflammatory activity and have a SAARD-like action since they influence extra-articular features and slow the radiographic progression of rheumatoid arthritis. There are few advantages and no greater safety with the use of depot injections or newer oral preparations over ACTH or prednisolone.

In rheumatoid arthritis the side-effects outweigh the anti-inflammatory benefit and the drug should be avoided. Whilst the side-effects of corticosteroids are well known, in patients with rheumatoid arthritis the exaggeration of the normal skin thinning and osteoporosis is undesirable as is the increased risk of gastrointestinal problems due to the combined effects of NSAIDs and of superadded infection particularly in joints. With the wide range of NSAIDs available night time corticosteroid therapy for the control of morning stiffness is unnecessary while alternate day therapy has not proved very effective. A few patients with life-threatening disease will require these drugs but the dose should be minimized by concurrent administration of a SAARD. Interestingly corticosteroids appear less effective in the seronegative spondarthritides and their use is consequently contraindicated. Further, it is always unwise to prescribe corticosteroids for an undetermined arthritis or myalgia; but it is often done out of a misplaced wish to give the patient some relief.

Local corticosteroid therapy

Local injections of a corticosteroid preparation into joints or surrounding soft tissues can be helpful in controlling inflammation. Such injections carry the risk of superinfection, a crystal reaction and bone necrosis, but these risks are minimized if a simple, clean, non-touch technique is employed and clear indications for their use are recognized. These include:

1. Intra-articular injections for the patient with one or two inflamed joints
2. Tendonitis or tendon nodules, although the benefit with nodules may be transitory and surgical clearance eventually be required
3. Capsular and ligamentous involvement
4. As a temporary measure in the treatment of median or other nerve compression syndromes.

Contraindications to the use of local corticosteroids include:

1. Uncertain diagnosis
2. Proven or possible infection in the joint
3. Severe joint damage, since they will be ineffective and may increase joint damage
4. A neurological deficit: because there is a risk of producing Charcot-type arthropathy.

Other drugs

Depression is a common accompaniment of chronic disease. In general patients do better if they can, with the help of the treatment team, come to terms with their disability rather than waste physical and emotional energy in fighting it. Most respond to sympathetic, informed advice; a few require drug therapy to assist them over difficult periods.

Muscle spasm around a joint is a normal reaction to pain and inflammation. The treatment must be directed at the cause, the inflammation, rather than the result and hence additional muscle relaxants should rarely be required. The same applies to night sedation. A small dose of a benzodiazepine will allow the patient to get to sleep while an adequate, slow-acting NSAID should ensure that pain, which often comes from the shoulder as they roll over, does not wake them.

Anaemia is a common feature of chronic inflammatory joint disease and has a complex aetiology. Although a small number of patients have genuine iron deficiency either due to drug-induced gastrointestinal blood loss or to a poor diet brought about by their inability to or lack of interest in preparing proper meals, the majority will show no response to oral iron therapy which merely adds to their drug burden and often increases their tendency to constipation. A careful assessment of iron status or a brief clinical trial is therefore required. Control of disease is accompanied by an improvement in haemoglobin values.

Osteoporosis, largely due to disuse, but partly exacerbated by corticosteroid therapy, is a frequent finding and in some areas, e.g. the hands, may be used as a measure of disease severity since it will improve as joint symptoms are controlled and function returns. Since arthritis is common in middle-aged women who are already subjected to osteoporosis secondary to hormonal imbalance the problem may become severe with early vertebral fracture and collapse and hence increased pain and dysfunction. Such patients will require appropriate drug therapy (page 17.9).

Medical synovectomy

A variety of chemicals and isotopes have been injected into one or two joints to control synovitis and recurrent effusion when systemic drugs and local corticosteroid injections have failed. The technique which is as successful as surgical synovectomy (page 16.68) avoids the need for such surgery, can often be done on outpatients, and is associated with few side-effects. In the United Kingdom isotopes are preferred, each being chosen to have suitable beta-emission characteristics for a given joint, e.g. 5 mCu of yttrium-90 for a knee. A small proportion of the isotope leaves the joint concentrating chiefly in the regional lymph-nodes and chromosomal abnormalities can subsequently be found in circulating lymphocytes. The long-term effects of this are unknown but the potential dangers can be minimized by splinting the injected joint for 2–3 days and confining the treatment to those over the age of 45 years.

The contribution of the therapist

The physiotherapists and occupational therapists are important members of the treatment team. Their contribution includes:

(*a*) Advice and encouragement about the disease and its treatment
(*b*) Advice about rest
(*c*) Exercises and other physical methods including walking aids
(*d*) The provision of various appliances designed to overcome disability and dependence upon others
(*e*) Advice about changes in employment and in the pattern of daily living.

Rest

A period of rest each day may allow increased and more economical function during the remainder of the day. Such a rest may be combined with the use of a suitable splint and periods of prone and supine lying to prevent and/or correct deformity in the spine, hips, and knees. For the patient with active disease rest in hospital is required. Use of joints during the phase of active disease increases pain, muscle spasm, and wasting, exaggerates systemic symptoms, and causes flexion deformities in weight-bearing joints. Bed rest relieves these symptoms and improves general well being. There are dangers, however, in uncontrolled bed rest in the form of general physical deterioration, muscle weakness, and joint contractures. To ensure adequate support, proper posture, and comfort a firm mattress and back rest are used, and splints for arms and legs provided. A bed cage or continental quilt removes the weight of bedclothes from inflamed joints.

Exercise, physical therapy, splints, and walking aids

Due to pain inhibition, exercises will not improve muscle bulk or strength around an inflamed joint. Once inflammation has settled, a programme of simple graduated exercises is essential as considerable muscle wasting occurs with joint disease. Certainly all patients with ankylosing spondylitis should be taught (and periodically retaught) a series of exercises to maintain spinal and chest mobility and posture. Passive movements cause protective muscle spasm and are discouraged, while in general, active, isotonic, exercises against increasing resistance are the most satisfactory. Such exercises can be performed in a heated pool when the absence of gravity and reduced muscle spasm hastens recovery.

The application of ice, various forms of heat, and ultrasound relieves pain so allowing exercises to be performed and probably speeds the healing of soft tissue lesions partly by altering vascularity. Different patients respond better to one modality than another.

Splints, made out of plaster of paris, or an increasing range of easy to use, light, durable, and inexpensive materials, can be used:

(*a*) In combination with rest in the acute phases of a polyarthritis when it is often beneficial to immobilize the patient in the splint by the use of cuffs. Such immobilization is maintained until inflammation has settled (1–2 weeks) during which time they are not removed for exercises or toilet purposes.

(*b*) In serial fashion to correct flexion deformities, usually at the knee. Such deformities soon become fixed and accelerate joint destruction so every effort should be made to achieve correction early in the disease course when continued use of a resting splint at night at home and a rigorous exercise programme will allow the corrected position to be maintained.

(*c*) As aids to everyday function. A painful wrist inhibits function in the uninvolved hand beyond, an inflamed knee prevents the use of other lower limb joints. Splintage in a good position allows both the inflammation to settle and increased function from other joints to be realized.

Many patients require a walking aid – stick, crutch or frame – although pride may lead to early resistance. Careful selection and instruction in the use of an aid is essential. Grandfather's old stick, with its worn ferrule, which is too short and is used in the wrong hand will not do. The therapist can advise on a wide range of other splints and appliances and alterations to footwear.

Domestic and occupational factors

Domestic and occupational problems caused by joint disease are chiefly the responsibility of the occupational therapist and social worker, but satisfactory adaptation to disease depends upon the efforts of the whole team with full co-operation from the patient and family. Any patient who has functional difficulties should be considered for assessment, ideally in their own home although access to facilities for the practice of routine activities such as dressing, bathing, cooking, ironing, etc. is useful. A wide range of simple aids to assist patients with such tasks can be readily provided. Patients with hip or knee disease have difficulty in using chairs, beds, and toilets or normal height and suitable raises will be required. Furniture should be moved to provide a clear floor area for walking while an extra banister may be needed. More major alterations may be necessary to allow a patient to remain independent at home and close liaison with the local authority is essential.

Transport and travel may become an increasing problem for the arthritic and those with very limited walking ability may be eligible

for mobility allowance. For some the careful selection of a wheelchair for indoor or outdoor use may be invaluable. The therapist and/or the nearest Department of Health and Social Security Appliance Centre can give the necessary advice.

Many patients will require advice in planning an economical pattern of daily living so that heavier and more difficult tasks are spread over the week. Patients are reluctant to accept that routine tasks such as washing need not be done on fixed days, and that there are different ways of ironing, cooking, etc. They must learn to adjust constantly to their disease. Finally, advice about a change of employment should not be given hurriedly as lighter jobs are usually less well paid. The prognosis in many forms of joint disease is often better than is imagined and patients should be encouraged to return to their original employment. When the patient is determined on a change of job every help should be given him. A personal approach to an employer is always worthwhile. The Disablement Resettlement Officer can help with re-employment, assessment of employment potential, and retraining.

Orthopaedic surgical treatment

It is impossible to provide adequate care for patients with rheumatic disease without ready access to the services of an orthopaedic surgical department. Some 10 per cent of patients with rheumatoid arthritis attending a clinic would benefit from an orthopaedic procedure although for a variety of reasons it may not be possible to carry out all the operations deemed beneficial. In osteoarthritis the patient load is even greater. Although exact numbers are hard to determine, more than 100 000 total joint arthroplasties are performed annually in the United States with the numbers continuing to grow. In much of the developed world the success of surgical treatment for arthritis has not been paralleled by an expansion in the surgical service. The true demand may be even higher based upon surveys of the disabled in the community but with long waiting lists many patients are simply not referred. Problems will be compounded if the revision rate for such surgery, currently contributing one-quarter of the patient load in some specialized American centres is reflected in other national practices. It is therefore important that careful selection of the patients who are likely to gain the most benefit is undertaken. Orthopaedic surgery is part of the management programme (Table 1) and others in the medical team need to be aware of the range of procedures available, the likely results, and the optimum time for their consideration. Combined clinics can be used to provide such information while discussing patients with a wide range of functional and mechanical problems. It is impossible to answer the question 'when should a patient be referred for surgical treatment?' since the moment varies greatly depending upon the stage and severity of the disease and the arthritis team's interpretation of that patient's need.

Surgical aims

1. An improvement in function related to the domestic, social, economic, employment or sexual implications of the patient's deformity and disability.

2. Relief of pain. Many will argue that this is the prime reason for operation, but this merely reflects greater difficulty in demonstrating improved postoperative function than pain relief. In most cases pain relief leads to a functional improvement, although occasionally, particularly when a joint is arthrodesed, surgery may simply allow the patient to sit or sleep without pain.

3. Improvement in appearance. Since deterioration occurs slowly, it is uncommon, except in young women and some patients with juvenile chronic polyarthritis, to operate for cosmetic reasons alone.

Preoperative assessment

The surgical decision whether to operate, and if so upon which joint, is often difficult to make. This is partly due to the complex disabilities arising from multiple joint disease and partly because almost all orthopaedic surgery, in contrast to other surgery, is both elective and demanding upon the patient. Thus, except in the case of stabilization of the upper cervical spine, it has no effect upon the patient's general health or life expectancy.

The patient's needs must be clearly defined and often a home visit will demonstrate that nothing can improve function sufficiently to enable her to climb the stair or visit the shop. The extent of the arthritis may require that upper limb surgery is first performed so that walking aids can be used for mobilizing after subsequent lower limb surgery or that a hip should be replaced before a knee since this allows the easier recovery. The patient's and her family's reaction must also be evaluated since patients may have unrealistic dreams accompanied by poor resolve while the family may have become so adapted to a patient's disability that they will not allow her to utilize improvement.

As with any elective operation the patient must have adequate cardiorespiratory reserve. While improving anaesthetic techniques allow major surgery to be performed on less fit patients, it should be appreciated that the improved mechanics of walking after total hip replacement may be associated with a 50 per cent reduction in oxygen consumption and hence considerably less cardiac strain. Anaemia may need correction. In patients with severe long-standing rheumatoid, amyloidosis with a low serum albumin, and marked osteoporosis are factors which may affect postoperative recovery. The reduced life expectancy in rheumatoid arthritis may also influence surgical decisions. Although analgesics can be withdrawn from patients with osteoarthritis, those with inflammatory arthritis should have all therapy continued lest there be an increase in general disease symptoms; it is usual to perhaps double the dose of any corticosteroid for 48 hours using intramuscular hydrocortisone.

Thromboembolic disease

Major hip and knee surgery is associated with an increased incidence of deep venous thrombosis and pulmonary embolism and many orthopaedic surgeons employ some form of anticoagulation. Although there is no general agreement over the best method it appears that subcutaneous heparin, probably the best method in general surgical practice, is less successful in orthopaedic surgery and that warfarin is the easiest to administer and control provided that the theoretical interaction between the drug and NSAID is remembered. In practice, although all NSAIDs alter platelet adhesiveness with possible bleeding consequences, competition for protein binding with warfarin only occurs with aspirin preparations and most other NSAIDs, particularly naproxen and diclofenac, can be given with safety. In general, patients with osteoarthritis undergoing these procedures should be anticoagulated while for reasons that are ill understood such anticoagulation is unnecessary in patients with rheumatoid arthritis and other inflammatory disorders unless there is a past history of thromboembolic disease. In patients with systemic lupus erythematosus who may require major joint replacement, particularly of the hip for avascular necrosis, the possibility that there is a disease-related circulating anticoagulant should be remembered (page 16.25).

Anaesthetic difficulties

The anaesthetist and all who handle the cervical spine of the unconscious rheumatoid patient must remember that many have an unstable neck. Since the majority of patients are symptomless and radiographs are unhelpful in predicting those that are likely to have trouble, all must be handled carefully.

Occasionally involvement of the temporomandibular joint will limit mouth opening, while in a few patients, usually those with ankylosing spondylitis and juvenile chronic polyarthritis which has extended into adult life, the cervical spine may have ankylosed presenting even greater difficulties with intubation.

Perversely the early loss of teeth and their replacement by dentures in many patients with inflammatory joint diseases reduces the problems with intubation. Teeth are lost partly because dental hygiene is inadequate with poor upper limb function and partly due to accelerated dental caries with Sjögren's syndrome.

Technical considerations

When surgery has been decided upon the surgeon must consider a number of technical factors. The range of movement available with some operations may be greater than with others but may be achieved with some reduction in stability. In general, excision arthroplasty leads to less stability than prosthetic arthoplasty and this is particularly the case in the hip and elbow. Such considerations may also be important if it becomes necessary to remove an infected prothesis leaving a joint with a good range of movement but considerable instability. A tourniquet normally employed for operations distal to the shoulder and hip joints, restricts the operative time to approximately 1.5 hours with a further reduction if the patient has significant peripheral arteriosclerosis or vasculitis. Generalized osteoporosis is common in inflammatory arthritis. Its relationship to age, disease, disease activity, disuse, and corticosteroid therapy is disputed. It may be a factor in the progression of joint disease and can provide technical difficulties with prosthetic fixation.

Skin problems

Patients with inflammatory arthritis, particularly rheumatoid arthritis and systemic lupus erythematosus, have thinning of the skin with some loss of subcutaneous fat and connective tissues supporting blood vessels, changes which are exaggerated by corticosteroid therapy and which lead to easy bruising of the limbs with careless handling. Vulnerable areas must be protected during surgery. Despite these skin changes and the slight tendency for such patients to have an increased incidence of bacterial infection, there is no evidence that wound healing is delayed and they can have their sutures removed and be allowed to mobilize at the same time as those with osteoarthritis.

Infection

Patients with rheumatoid arthritis and systemic lupus erythematosus have a higher incidence of prosthetic infection than do patients with osteoarthritis; although the incidence is greater in both groups if the joint has been the site of a previous operation, whether or not a prosthesis was employed. While there is still debate over the need for special operating theatres for prosthetic surgery, the recognition that clean orthopaedic cases must be separated from all other surgical cases together with more careful techniques has led to a lowering of infection rates in conventional theatres. An important recent survey covering over 8000 total hip and knee operations carried out in conventional or ultraclean theatres has shown joint sepsis, confirmed at re-operation a mean of 2.5 years later, in 63 of 4133 operations (1.5 per cent) in the conventional group and in 23 of 3922 operations (0.6 per cent) in the ultraclean group. The study supported the use of an antibiotic regimen over the operative period with 3.4 per cent of cases becoming infected in conventional theatres without antibiotics compared with 0.3 per cent of cases in ultraclean theatres with antibiotics. The possibility of infection of a prosthesis from a septic focus elsewhere in the body must always be considered, as it constitutes a major surgical disaster. Certainly infection more than five years after the operation is likely to be due to haematogenous spread rather than being a manifestation of infection at the time of surgery. It follows that septic foci in nails and rheumatoid nodules should be eradicated and infection of the urinary tract or chest treated energetically, not only preoperatively but whenever they occur in a patient with a metal implant. Dental sepsis, more likely in the younger rheumatoid patients than the older osteoarthritic patient with dentures, also needs to be considered. As many as 10 per cent of patients with arthritis of the feet have infected lesions in whom overenthusiastic chiropody can lead to bleeding and systemic infection.

The painful prosthetic joint

Despite the success of prosthetic surgery in arthritis, with sustained follow-up an increasing number of patients begin to complain of pain in their arthoplasty. It has been suggested that 10 per cent of patients will require revision surgery within 10 years of their initial surgery while a further 10 per cent of patients with minor symptoms ignored by themselves and their surgeons might also benefit from such revision. Pain in a prosthetic joint may be due to infection, loosening, ligamentous instability, prosthetic fracture, stress fracture in bone or the presence of cement loose bodies. While in some careful clinical examinations and sequential radiographs will provide the diagnosis, in many it will require the measurement of plasma acute phase proteins, the determination of possible metal hypersensitivity, joint aspiration, arthography and bone scanning using both technetium-99m labelled diphosphonates and gallium-67 citrate. Prosthesis loosening for whatever cause is commonest in patients with osteoarthritis who have had a single damaged joint replaced which they have subjected to considerable stress as they attempt to maintain their social and sporting lifestyle. In contrast the in-built restraints provided by polyarticular rheumatoid and related disease accompanied by a measure of general ill health are sure to restrict the patient's activity and the strain imposed upon the prosthesis. Ways of combating these problems using different materials and methods of fixation to bone, antibiotic impregnated cement and sensitive immunological tests and new radiographic techniques are under continuing study.

Types of operation

There are four major types of operation currently used in the joints of patients with arthritis: synovectomy/debridement, arthroplasty, osteotomy, and arthrodesis.

Synovectomy/debridement

In osteorarthritis loose bodies, osteophytes or menisci which are causing joint locking or impeding motion usually of the knee or elbow may be removed. Synovectomy is undertaken in inflammatory arthritis for pain and swelling unresponsive to medical therapy. The operation is of value in finger, wrist, elbow, and knee joints, with the best results, and possibly a prophylactic effect, after 6–12 months of persistent disease, before significant cartilage damage has occurred. Thus 80 per cent of patients will have relief of pain and swelling one year after surgery falling to 50 per cent at five years. The alternative of radioisotope synovectomy has been mentioned earlier. Synovectomy of tendon sheaths, particularly those of the fingers, provides long-term pain relief and improved function and may be required urgently to prevent stretching or rupture.

Arthroplasty

This described any operation which reconstitutes a joint. In a few cases the operation consists simply of excision of the damaged joint surfaces and synovial tissue, e.g. metacarpophalangeal and metatarsophalangeal joints. However, with the success of total hip replacement prostheses are being increasingly used to replace part or the whole of a joint. Such prostheses should fulfil the following criteria:

(a) Clinical criteria
Relieve pain
Restore movement and stability
Correct deformity
(b) Technical criteria
Be chemically and physically inert
Be long wearing
Produce minimal wear particles
Have low friction characteristics
Be firmly fixed to bone
Have inherent stability
Should mimic normal joint function

While there is a wide range of replacements, more than 300 for the knee alone, most have two non-linked metal and high-density polyethylene components, both of which are bonded to bone using methylmethacrylate cement.

Osteotomy

Division of a bone near to a joint, but outside joint capsule, is useful in osteoarthritis, e.g. knee. The operation allows weight to be carried through a different, largely undamaged portion of the articular cartilage and also relieves pain, particularly night pain, by reducing intra-osseous venous pressure. Since in patients with inflammatory arthritis the whole joint is affected by the disease process, changes in load bearing have little application.

Arthrodesis

The pathological process in inflammatory arthritis may lead to fibrous and occasionally bony ankylosis, particularly at the wrist. Since such ankylosis leads to improved function, it may be produced surgically, there being good clinical indications at the wrist, elbow, knee, ankle, and subtalar joints, provided the correct position for arthrodesis and the possible difficulties for the patient have been adequately assessed and explained beforehand. Arthodesis of these joints should not be dismissed as outdated in an age of prosthetic surgery.

Details of the very wide range of surgical procedures available is beyond the scope of this chapter. A few common types will be mentioned while those interested should consult specialist texts.

Forefeet

Hallux valgus occurs almost exclusively in shoe wearers, 90 per cent being female, although genetic, anatomical, and dynamic factors with muscle and bone imbalance are also involved. While it may occur in the young, the increasing presentation with age is accompanied by an increasing incidence of osteoarthritis and the development of bursitis (bunion).

Osteoarthritis of the first metatarsophalangeal joint occurs independently of hallux valgus with an equal sex incidence. There is pain, accentuated by non-supportive footwear, and loss of movement leading to hallux rigidus.

Prevention and treatment of these disorders by the use of sensible footwear is an unattainable goal. A rigid hallux may be arthrodesed but the excision arthroplasties of Keller (proximal phalanx) and Mayo (metatarsal) relieve pain while maintaining some function. In rheumatoid arthritis a combination of initial changes and secondary mechanical factors at the metatarsophalangeal joints produces the characteristic broadening and rigidity of the forefoot with hallux valgus, deviation of the other toes in a lateral direction, subluxation of the toes on to the dorsum of the foot, and the development of callosities over the prominent metatarsal heads in the sole. If alteration of footwear fails to relieve symptoms, excision arthroplasty at the metatarsophalangeal joints should be considered. The 90 per cent good results by a variety of techniques have largely removed the need for joint replacement (Fig. 2a, b).

Midtarsal, subtalar, and ankle joints

Involvement of these joints is best treated by provision of suitable shoes with valgus insoles while various forms of anklet, custom-made orthosis or a leg iron may adequately support these joints. Occasionally, manipulation under anaesthesia following by ice treatment and exercises reduces pain and restores movement.

Arthrodesis is the surgical treatment of choice for severe arthritis of any cause. Whatever combination of arthrodesis for the three joints is chosen patient satisfaction is high even though delays in skin healing and bony union may mean the use of a walking plaster for three months. The joints should be fused in neutral, or perhaps a few degrees of plantar flexion at the female ankle.

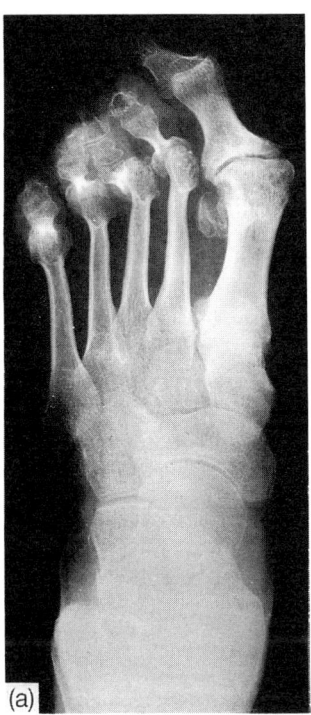 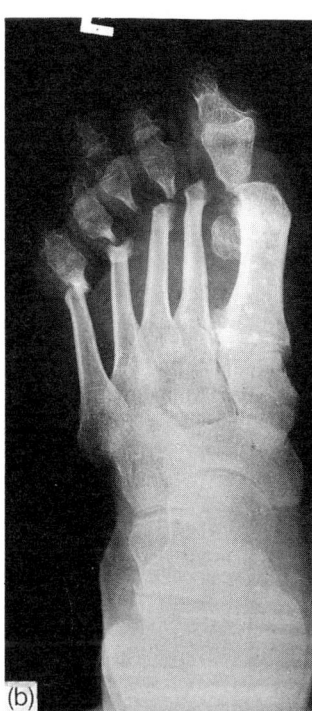

Fig. 2 (a) Preoperative radiograph of the left foot of a rheumatoid patient showing extensive erosion of the metatarsal phalangeal joints with subluxation at the lateral forejoints. (b) Radiograph of the same foot postoperatively showing the bone excision. Despite the failure to restore normal bone alignment, which is usual, the relief of pain and return of function is excellent.

Although prostheses for the ankle joint exist, experience is still limited.

Knee joint

Apart from flexion and extension, anteroposterior glide, abduction, adduction, and rotation are all possible at the knee, the last being particularly important. Owing to the shape of the femoral condyles flexion and extension occur around a continuously changing axis. Movement of the knee is further complicated by the presence of the menisci which are important in joint lubrication, have a shock absorbing role and carry 70 per cent of the load across the joint. Finally, the patella contributes to the function of the quadriceps mechanism. These observations mean that

1. Menisci are not removed unless they are severely damaged, and then usually just the damaged portion;
2. Surgeons are reluctant to undertake patellectomy;
3. There has been a marked swing away from linked rigidly bone-fixed hinge prostheses towards non-linked, carefully designed prostheses which maintain the changing centre of axis of movement and which allow the rotation of the femur medially on the tibia as the knee approaches full extension.

The arthroscope, which has greatest application at the knee, has extended the range of 'day-case' surgery, has reduced the morbidity and difficulties of postoperative mobilization associated with operations such as partial meniscectomy, now done entirely via the arthroscope, and has allowed a greater understanding of normal and abnormal joint function. The instrument, used in theatre under general anaesthesia, offers the chance of diagnosis, selective biopsy, and joint lavage as well as a range of procedures such as removal of cartilage and bone fragments, limited synovectomy and division of adhesions. In early inflammatory arthritis synovectomy relieves pain and swelling often for several years and may have a prophylactic effect upon joint damage. Although less used since the advent of isotopic therapy surgical synovectomy is still useful in those with an enlarged posterior cyst. Such cysts, which

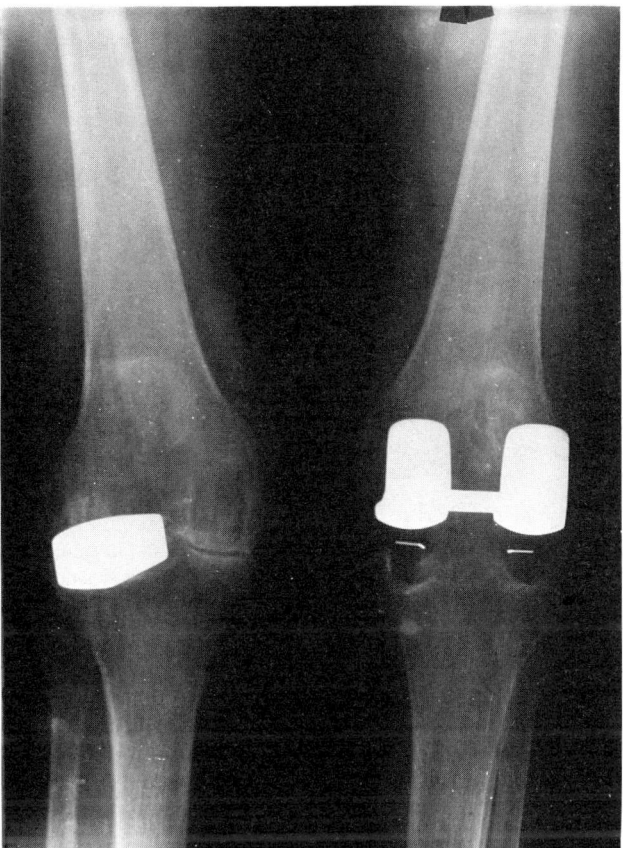

Fig. 3 Standing antero-posterior radiographs of the knees of a rheumatoid patient. On the left a MacIntosh arthroplasty, the introduction of a variable height, non-cemented spacer, has been undertaken on the lateral compartment. On the right a Geomedic total knee replacement has been performed; the metal femoral capping and the markers in the non-linked high-density polyethylene can be seen.

are usually extensions of the normal semimembranosus-gastrocnemius bursae may become grossly enlarged, prevent full knee extension, and cause venous obstruction. In addition, since they are connected to the knee joint by a one-way valvular mechanism, they are subjected to markedly increased fluid pressures. This may result in the enlargement of the cyst into the calf or the sudden rupture of the cyst with the release of irritant synovial fluid. Symptoms and signs of joint rupture, which have also been recorded at the wrists and elbow, mimic those of a deep venous thrombosis. Arthrography or ultrasonography rather than venography in conjunction with a full history and examination should establish the diagnosis. Rupture of the cyst should be treated by rest and local steroid injections. A large cyst may be excised but synovectomy of the joint treats the cause of both a small cyst and rupture.

Although not quite emulating the success of hip arthroplasty, the rapid progress in total knee surgery over recent years, which has left many mechanically unsound prostheses discarded in its wake, means that experienced surgeons who carefully select their patients can achieve pain relief, joint stability, correction of deformity, and more than 90° of flexion (adequate for normal seating and getting on public transport) in some 85 per cent of cases (Fig. 3). A wide range of devices, all of which can produce the above results, are available so that each can be matched to the correct clinical situation. When failure is due to loosening or infection, the aim is to achieve sound fixation with the minimum of bone excision. Treatment of such failures by the insertion of another prosthesis or arthrodesis is technically difficult and unreliable. Such factors tend to favour the use of total knee arthroplasty in those who are less likely to overload the joint, the older underweight patient, and those with polyarticular disease. High tibial

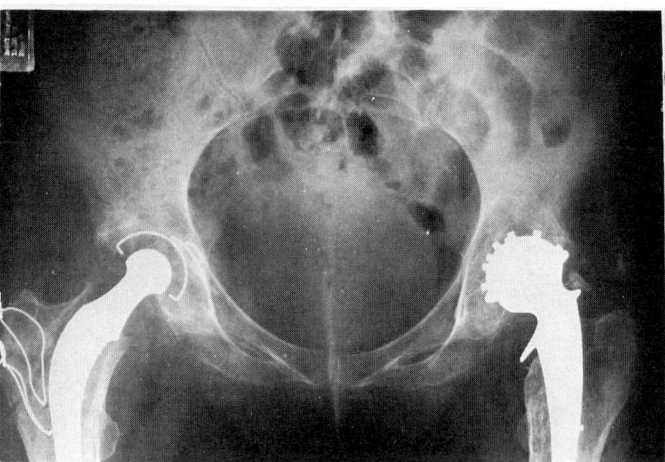

Fig. 4 Bilateral total hip replacement. On the right a McKee-Farrar, a metal upon metal device which has proved to have high friction wear characteristics, leading to loosening of one or both components and hence its discontinued usage. On the left a Charnley device with a metal femoral stem and a high-density polyethylene acetabular cup with in-built marker wire to estimate position and wear. Wires have been used to refix the greater trochanter, removed to facilitate correct prosthesis insertion. A small wire mesh cap retains cement at the base of the acetabulum.

osteotomy will relieve pain in three-quarters of those with osteoarthritis, particularly those with a varus deformity, and does not preclude future arthroplasty. The operation is not suitable for inflammatory arthritis when the whole joint is affected. While the osteotomy will require 6–8 weeks support, modern cast bracing avoids the vascular complications of plaster and allows early movement. Arthrodesis which may require up to three months' immobilization in plaster of Paris, should be used with caution particularly in younger patients and those with rheumatoid arthritis in whom the operation may accentuate the rate of damage in the other major lower limb joints and eventually become a functional handicap. The great advantage of the operation is the production of a pain-free, stable limb and it may be combined with arthroplasty of the other knee.

Hip

Operative treatment of hip disease in almost any type of arthritis should be by total hip replacement. There is little justification, except in the face of sepsis or loosening of a prosthesis, or occasionally in the very young for undertaking earlier operations such as synovectomy, osteotomy, excision or cup arthroplasty. Excision arthroplasty (Girdlestone pseudarthrosis), is valuable as a salvage procedure, although the result is rather unstable with up to 2.5 in (6 cm) of leg shortening. It is also useful when quick pain relief and increased range of motion is required for patients confined to a wheelchair.

Total hip replacement offers patients a 95 per cent chance of complete or almost complete pain relief. The range of movement will be increased in most patients, probably more predictably in rheumatoid than osteoarthritis (Fig. 4). A disappointing patient group are those with ankylosing spondylitis, even though hip involvement still merits surgical treatment. The disappointment (only 80 per cent sustained good results) is partly due to heterotopic ossification and partly because the preoperative stiffness results in only 90° of total movement compared with 150° for other diseases. Low friction prostheses with a metal femoral and a plastic acetabular component (Charnley and variants) are used. Patients can expect to bear weight after five days and leave hospital using one stick after stitch removal at 12–14 days. Normal activities can be resumed within six weeks. Short-term complications include wound infection (4 per cent), wound haematoma (3 per cent), thromboembolic disease with pulmonary embolism (2

per cent), and cardiovascular complications; both the latter may be fatal. These problems are almost inevitable in elderly patients with osteoarthritis, however well they are assessed and managed because this is a major operation requiring a four unit blood transfusion. Later complications include heterotopic ossification which significantly limits movement in 2 per cent of cases, prosthesis dislocation (1–2 per cent), deep infection (5 per cent), and prosthesis loosening. The relationship between infection and other causes of loosening and the difficulties of diagnosis have been discussed above. With time the risks of prosthesis failure increases and is related to the transmitted stresses but it is calculated that 75 per cent of prostheses will survive intact for 20 years.

Despite these problems the success of the operation remains outstanding since it dramatically alters the level of patient dependence and for many restores function almost to normal. Since it may be impossible to undertake such surgery on all suitable cases, careful selection of those likely to show the greatest gain may be necessary.

Shoulder

Any operative procedure on the shoulder joint is liable to induce capsulitis (frozen shoulder) with persisting postoperative pain and limited movement. Excision of the acromion and the underlying bursa relieves pain and improves movement, but often at the expense of stability. Arthrodesis may improve upper limb function if the optimum position for fusion is carefully chosen. There are an increasing number of total shoulder prostheses of widely differing design. The operations are technically difficult and may only relieve pain having no effect upon an already limited range of movement. The results of longer term follow-up, particularly the incidence of complications including loosening are keenly awaited.

Elbow

In inflammatory arthritis, synovectomy, particularly when combined with excision of the radial head, relieves pain and increases movement, especially hinge motion. In osteoarthritis removal of loose bodies often dramatically improves movement by removing the mechanical block. In a few patients with both rheumatoid and osteoarthritis, there is severe damage of the humeral-ulnar compartment for which surgical treatment is less certain.

As at the knee, a clearer understanding of joint mechanics and the forces involved has led to the abandonment of rigid hinges which inevitably loosened and the gradual introduction of a range of metal/plastic unconstrained surface replacements (Fig. 5a–c). Complications, including loosening, remain more frequent than with hip and knee surgery so that such surgery is not widely available. Salvage arthrodesis may be difficult due to bone loss while an external splint to support the unstable joint can be cumbersome and unsightly since it needs to be worn over most clothes. Primary arthrodesis with the elbow in 90° of flexion and neutral rotation can provide excellent pain-free function provided other upper limb joints are not seriously damaged. Surgical treatment is occasionally required for persistent common extensor tendonitis (tennis elbow).

Wrist and tendon sheaths

Median nerve compression at the wrist from whatever cause will require surgical relief if rest, splintage, diuretics, and local corticosteroid injections fail. While the conditions is common in the early phases of inflammatory arthritis this only accounts for 5 per cent of cases. Even with early surgical decompression one-third of cases will take three years to recover fully. Poor results reflect delay in diagnosis and once motor signs are present recovery is unlikely.

Synovectomy of the dorsum of the wrist should always include synovectomy of the related extensor tendons and usually excision of the lower end of ulna. This operation, which is indicated when there is reduced hand and wrist function due to persistent pain in the distal radio-ulnar joint or evidence of extensor tendon rupture, stretching or weakness, relieves pain and improves hand

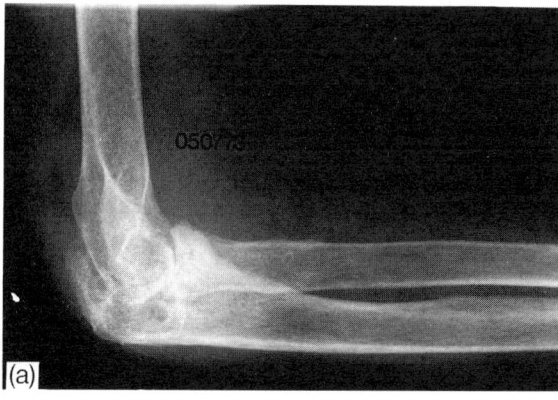

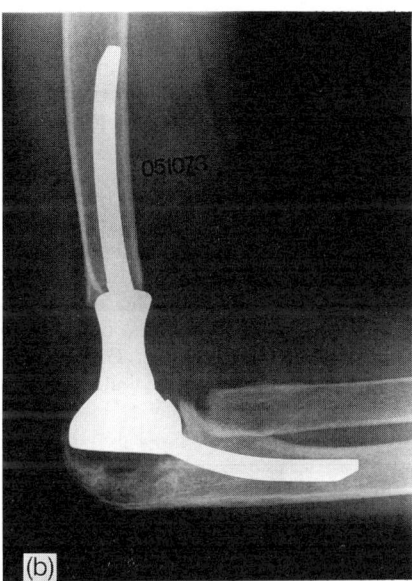

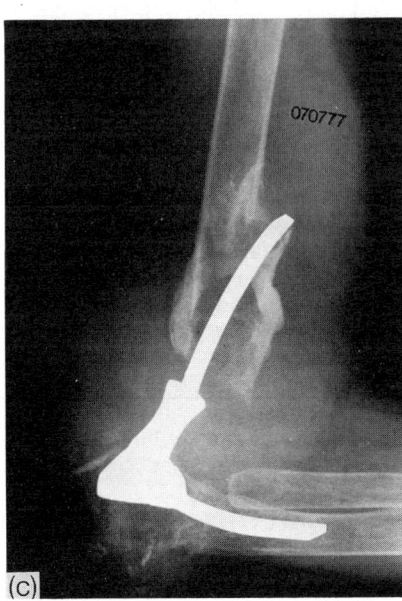

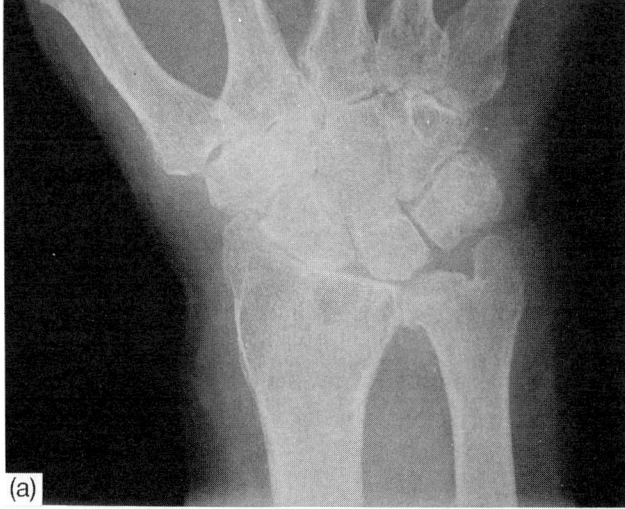

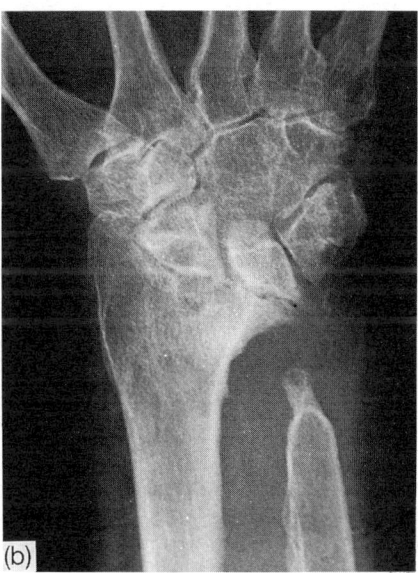

Fig. 5 (a–c) Sequential lateral radiographs of the right elbow in a rheumatoid patient over a period of four years. The extensive humeral-ulnar disease was treated with a hinge replacement. This type of rigid, linked, cemented device has proved to be biomechanically unsound and in this, as in all patients, it became loose producing gross bone destruction and loss of function. This is beyond salvage and the patient needs to wear an external support.

Fig. 6 (a) Preoperative radiograph of the right wrist in rheumatoid arthritis showing erosive change and synovial proliferation at the distal radio-ulnar joint which led to symptomatically and functionally successful excision of the lower end of ulna. (b) The same wrist several years later showing the bone excision. The erosive disease has been uncontrolled and led to a loss of cartilage in the radiocarpal joint while the common broadening of the radius to support the lunate bone has occurred.

function in over 90 per cent of patients (Fig. 6, a b). A variety of techniques exists for arthrodesis of the severely damaged wrist which produce satisfactory results particularly when patients have only a limited range of painful movements. Most patients find that arthrodesis in a neutral position or in a few degrees of flexion is best, particularly for toilet purposes. These good results mean that replacement arthroplasty, as yet in an early phase of development, will probably never have wide usage.

Tendon repairs

Flexor tendons rarely rupture although the sheaths may require clearance because of diffuse pain and impaired movement at the wrist, in the palm where nodules are particularly apt to develop, and in the fingers (Fig. 7). Although drug therapy or prophylactic surgery should prevent extensor tendon rupture, surgical treatment is often required. The tendon defects cannot be repaired and tendons must be joined to each other or tendon transfers undertaken. Full recovery is often delayed.

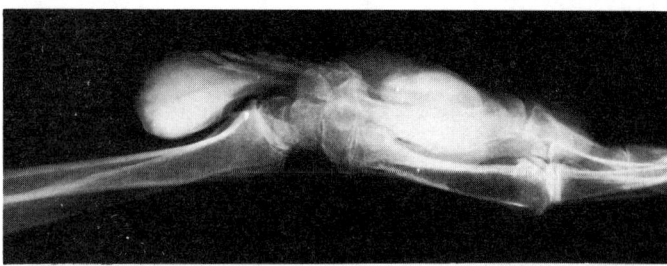

Fig. 7 Radiograph of opaque dye in a grossly enlarged flexor tendon sheath, the dye passing beneath the retinaculum at the wrist. Such gross synovial proliferation and effusion required surgical clearance to restore tendon function and prevent rupture.

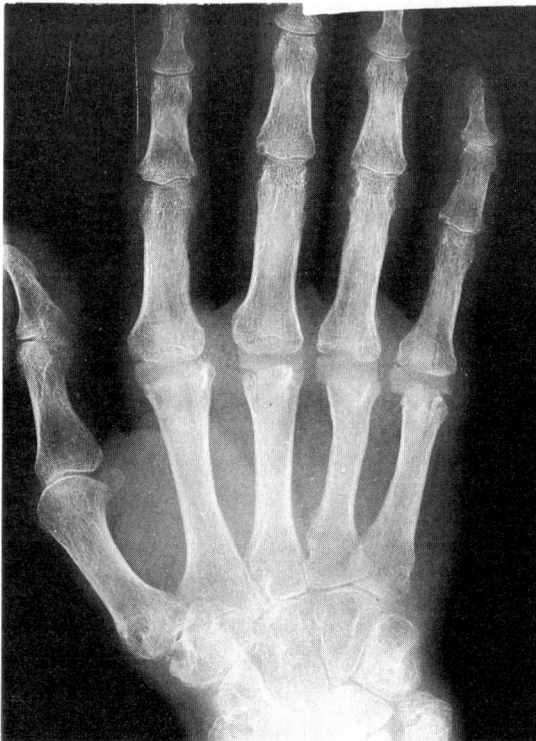

Fig. 8 Radiograph of a rheumatoid hand showing silastic Swanson prostheses in the finger metacarpal phalangeal joints associated with correction of ulnar deviation. Moderate movement was maintained but accompanied by full movement at the undamaged proximal interphalangeal joints good function was restored.

Fingers

In the fingers of rheumatoid patients peri-articular, tendon, and muscle involvement as well as joint disease, contribute to the symptoms and to the characteristic ulnar deviation, swan neck, and boutonniere deformities. In addition to synovectomy of the metacarpal and proximal interphalangeal joints, soft tissue release, repair of the extensor apparatus, and realignment of the tendons may be required. Although such procedures produce cosmetically satisfactory results, there is usually some loss of movement and finger function is not always improved (Fig. 8). Many surgeons prefer to delay operating until more extensive changes have taken place, often with subluxation of the metacarpophalangeal joints, since an improvement in function is then achieved.

In all hand surgery it is vital to undertake a practical assessment of hand function to determine the patient's real wishes and needs. Subsequent surgery must be planned on a very individual basis because, for example, it is often difficult to combine both a good grip and good pinch movement and some surgeons will elect to provide one function in each hand. It is essential that the potential gains in pain relief, function, and appearance are balanced against the risk of a bad result. In no other branch of orthopaedic surgery is it so vital to have available skilled therapists to assist with preoperative assessment, to make splints, and undertake slow and time-consuming postoperative mobilization and retraining.

There are various types of prosthesis available particularly for the metacarpophalangeal joints (Swanson, Calnan-Nichol, etc.) but none of them is entirely satisfactory, since they result in some loss of movement, may not achieve long-term correction of deformity or may fracture and require removal or replacement. Arthrodesis of a painful, deformed or unstable proximal interphalangeal joint of the fingers and any of the three thumb joints will correct deformity and may substantially improve pinch movements and relieve pain.

Surgical treatment for osteoarthritis of the hand, whether due to overuse, trauma or as part of Heberden node-associated generalized disease may involve similar small joint surgery. However, disease at the carpometacarpal joint of the thumb is much commoner than in inflammatory arthritis. Excision of the trapezium and the use of a silastic replacement combined with adequate soft tissue release provides a mobile joint with inherent stability that satisfies the requirements of more patients although a few men engaged in heavy work may be better served by an arthrodesis.

Spine

Although pain and instability at various levels may suggest surgical treatment, usually some form of fusion, in patients with arthritis it is usually the combination of pain and clearcut neurological complications that leads to surgery, pain alone being treated with drugs and suitable support, e.g. cervical collar, lumbar corset.

In the cervical spine instability of the atlanto-axial joint is common in rheumatoid arthritis and occasionally found in other inflammatory diseases including ankylosing spondylitis. A variety of different mechanisms are responsible for the instability with the potential for differing neurological features. Thus anterior subluxation of the atlas on the axis may be accompanied by upper cervical root pain and irritation and long tract signs in arms and legs while destruction of the lateral masses of the atlas with downward movement of the skull is associated with medullary damage as the odontoid peg goes through the foramen magnum. In some patients the complaints may be bizarre not necessarily suggesting neurological involvement: a bursting sensation in the upper limbs, painful lower limb spasm or more usually a sudden deterioration in walking ability and balance. Further, the presence of widespread joint disease with attendant muscle wasting and perhaps some peripheral neuropathy due to vasculitis can make formal neurological assessment very difficult. When cervical involvement is suspected the patient must be handled with great care and should be put in a protective collar until radiographic studies are available. Standard lateral radiographs of the neck in flexion and extension and a through-mouth view of the odontoid peg may need to be supplemented by myelography and CT scanning. If satisfactory improvement in neurological features can be achieved by carefully controlled traction and fixation, fusion either anteriorly or posteriorly using wires and/or bone graft should be undertaken and this will usually require continued postoperative immobilization for several weeks.

Subluxation at lower levels, e.g cervical 3 and 4, is common but often ignored; in inflammatory arthritis and in the presence of radiographic lesions at more than one level, most careful neurological examination and myelography is needed. In osteoarthritis surgical fusion or removal of osteophytes may be required, the commonest levels being C5–6–7.

In the lumbar spine degenerative change in both intervertebral discs and posterior interfacetal joints may lead to nerve root or cauda equina compression. Once again surgery is undertaken for neurological features rather than pain and these must be clearly demonstrated and persistently present. Spinal stenosis, an increas-

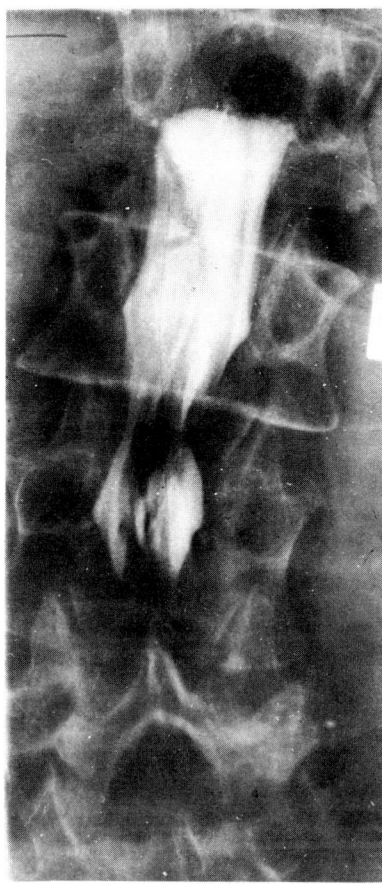

Fig. 9 Myelogram showing a complete block to the passage of the dye at the middle of the fourth lumbar vertebra and a partial block at the lumbar 3–4 junction. The patient presented with spinal stenosis due to florid osteophyte formation partly induced by the long-standing scoliosis.

14 days. Full neurological recovery may take much longer and in some may never occur.

Osteotomy of the spine in ankylosing spondylitis both at the cervical and lumbar levels was once popular but is now rarely undertaken, partly because it is technically difficult and fraught with complications and partly because increasingly early diagnosis and good treatment largely prevents serious deformity. In any event if the patient has good hip and knee flexion the problems of such deformity can be largely overcome. Since severe spinal disease is often accompanied by hip disease with loss of movement there is a tendency to consider total hip replacement in these patients.

ingly commonly recognized condition, does not always present with the typical story of exercise-induced pain and neurological features in the legs often accompanied by paraesthesiae and altered sensation in the perineum; the symptoms clearing quickly with rest and often avoided by exercise in flexion, e.g. bicycle riding. Spinal stenosis is usually due to narrowing of the canal by ingrowth of osteophytes or a central protrusion of a degenerate disc (Fig. 9). Myelography and CT should be used as a preliminary to surgery when it will delineate the lesion and its site more clearly rather than as an uncritical test in patients with vague backache even though modern materials cause little irritation or morbidity. Various grades of compression will be needed from simple removal of an osteophyte or part of a disc to more extensive laminectomy often at several levels. In all the postoperative recovery is rapid, the patient being fully ambulant with stitches removed by

References

Ahern, M. J., Hall, N. D., Case, K. and Maddison, P. J. (1984). D-Penicillamine withdrawal in rheumatoid arthritis. *Ann. Rheum. Dis.* **43**, 213–217.

Arden, G. P. and Ansell, B. M. (1978). *Surgical management of juvenile chronic polyarthritis*. Academic Press, London.

Benjamin, A. and Helal, B. (1980). *Surgical repair and reconstruction in rheumatoid disease*. Macmillan, London.

Field, E. H., Strober, S., Hoppe, R. T., Calin, A., Engleman, E. G., Kotzin, B. L., Tanay, A. S., Calin, H. J., Terrell, C. P. and Kaplan, H. S. (1983). Sustained improvement of intractable rheumatoid arthritis after total lymphoid irradiation. *Arth. Rheum.* **26**, 937–946.

Fowler, P. D., Shadforth, M. F., Crook, P. R. and Lawton, A. (1984). Report on chloroquine and dapsone in the treatment of rheumatoid arthritis. *Ann. Rheum. Dis.* **43**, 200–204.

Gumpel, J.M. (1978). Radiosynoviorthesis. *Clin. Rheum. Dis.* **4**, 311–326.

Huskisson, E.C. (1980). Anti-rheumatic drugs. *Clin. Rheum. Dis.* **5**, 351–733.

—— (1980). Anti-rheumatic drugs II. *Clin.Rheum.Dis.* **6**, 463–695.

—— (1984). Anti-rheumatic drugs III. *Clin. Rheum. Dis.* **10**, 217–432.

Lancet (1980). Editorial. Inducing remission in rheumatoid arthritis. *Lancet* **i**, 193–194.

Lidwell, O. M., Lowbury, E. J. L., Whyte, W., Blowers, R., Stanley, S. J. and Lowe, D. (1982). Effect of ultraclean air in operating theatres on deep sepsis in the joint after total hip or knee replacement: a randomised study. *Br. Med. J.* **2**, 10–15.

Marks, J. S. (1982). Chloroquine retinopathy: is there a safe daily dose? *Ann. Rheum. Dis.* **41**, 52–58.

Mowat, A. G. (1986). Surgical treatment of arthritis. In *Copeman's textbook of rheumatic diseases* (ed. J. T. Scott). Churchill Livingstone, Edinburgh.

Nicolle, F. V. and Dickson, R. A. (1979). *Surgery of the rheumatoid hand: a practical manual*. Heinemann, London.

Pullar, T. and Capell, H. A. (1984). Sulphasalazine: a 'new' anti-rheumatic drug. *Br. J. Rheumatol.* **23**, 26–34.

Verdickt, W., Dequeker, J., Ceuppens, J. L., Stevens, E., Gautama, K. and Vermylen, C. (1983). Effect of lymphoplasmapheresis on clinical indices and T cell subsets in rheumatoid arthritis: A double-blind controlled study. *Arth. Rheum.* **26**, 1419–1426.

Williams, H. J., Reading, J. C., Ward, J. R. and O'Brien, W. M. (1980). Comparison of high and low dose cyclophosphamide therapy in rheumatoid arthritis. *Arth. Rheum.* **23**, 521–527.

Wilkins, R. F., Watson, M. A. and Paxson, C. S. (1980). Low dose pulse methotrexate therapy in rheumatoid arthritis. *J. Rheumatol.* **7**, 501–505.

OSTEOARTHRITIS AND RELATED DISORDERS

P. DIEPPE

This chapter describes the pathological and clinical features of osteoarthritis (OA) and some important related diseases. It covers an immensely common, painful and disabling group of rheumatic conditions that remain ill understood. Until recently OA was thought to be an inevitable consequence of ageing and of 'wear and tear'. However, modern research has started to uncover a fascinating set of complex biophysical and biochemical processes. Further work could lead to more fundamental understanding of cartilage and connective tissues in general, as well as of OA in particular.

OA affects both axial (spinal) and peripheral joints, but the clinical features and associations are quite different at the two sites. The chapter is therefore divided so that the spinal diseases can be treated separately. Calcification of articular cartilage (chondrocalcinosis) is a frequent phenomenon associated with increasing age and with osteoarthritis of both peripheral and axial joints. It sometimes results in a distinctive type of joint disease, and is described at the end of the chapter.

Osteoarthritis of peripheral joints

Definition and terminology

The term osteoarthritis (OA) is used to describe a group of conditions affecting the synovial joints and characterized by loss of articular cartilage with overgrowth and remodelling of the underlying bone.

A number of synonyms are in use (e.g. osteoarthritis, arthrosis, hypertrophic arthritis); some, such as 'degenerative joint disease' are frankly misleading, implying a manifest, passive process associated with old age. In fact, OA is a multifactorial, metabolically active condition which usually starts in middle-age. The key to future understanding of OA is the recognition that it includes several distinct but as yet ill-defined diseases, and that it can result from many different mechanical, inflammatory or metabolic processes. The term 'joint failure' (cf. heart failure), which emphasizes the pathophysiology of the condition and the concept of OA as a final common pathway of many diseases, is preferable.

Epidemiology

OA is extremely common. It is difficult to estimate its true incidence, but radiological surveys suggest that about 10 per cent of all adults have moderate or severe joint disease. This is especially frequent in women (F:M ratio about 2:1) and the elderly. However, X-rays and symptoms correlate poorly: only about 30 per cent of those with significant pathological changes are symptomatic and even fewer become significantly handicapped. Nevertheless, three-quarters of those disabled by arthritis are said to have OA and about 30 per cent of sickness incapacity from rheumatic diseases is attributed to this condition. Because symptomatic OA is more prevalent in the elderly and the natural history is often one of slow progression, the lives of many middle-aged and elderly people are made miserable by OA. The challenge to a medical profession caring for an ageing population is clear.

Osteoarthritis (joint failure) occurs throughout the animal kingdom and there is skeletal evidence that it has been common throughout man's history (unlike rheumatoid arthritis and some other joint diseases which may be of more recent origin and are only found in *homo sapiens*). However, there are racial and geographical differences in frequency and in disease expression; for example OA of the hand is common in Caucasian women, and

OA of the hip is rare in the Chinese. Genetic factors are particularly obvious in some subsets of OA, especially the generalized 'nodal' form, in which a polygenic inheritance is postulated. Employment also affects OA; it is particularly frequent in the hips and backs of miners and in the hands and necks of cotton workers. Similarly, trauma or certain special activities can result in premature OA of a particular joint (e.g. wicket-keeper's hand, ticket-collector's thumb or Zulu dancer's hip!).

Many other factors influence the development of symptoms in a damaged joint, including the demands made on, and the mechanics of, a limb, as well as intercurrent disease and socio-economic considerations (e.g. the 'threshold' at which patients complain about joint pain). Symptomatic OA must therefore be distinguished from pathological joint failure.

Aetiology

OA is a multifactorial condition of unknown aetiology and pathogenesis.

Five major aetiological factors are implicated (Table 1). The prevalence of OA rises with increasing *age*, but age alone is an insufficient explanation. It has been estimated that we would have to live for at least 200 years before the natural age changes in connective tissue (which differ biochemically from those seen in OA) would lead to joint failure on their own. The importance of an *inherited predisposition* has already been mentioned and genetic factors stand out as the single most critical factor in some patients (e.g. those with nodal, generalized OA). *Mechanical stresses* can cause OA, but only if abnormal and repetitive. Normal joint use, even if in excess as in some sportsmen, does not on its own cause OA, but severe trauma, surgery or a mechanical anomaly of a joint will predispose to failure. *Biochemical changes* in the cartilage, leading to a weakened collagen matrix, altered proteoglycans and excess release of degradative enzymes are also implicated and are of primary importance in some patients, (e.g. ochronosis). *Previous inflammatory joint disease* can damage the cartilage so that joint failure results from normal joint loading. Thus the later result of rheumatoid arthritis can produce a pathological picture which is similar to that seen in OA of other causes.

OA can be viewed as the failure of articular cartilage to cope wih normal stress, or as cartilage destruction resulting from abnormal joint stress. The interaction of the five aetiological factors mentioned is well illustrated by postmeniscectomy OA of the knee. About 40 per cent of patients who have had a meniscectomy (which produces an inflammatory response as well as altered joint mechanisms) will develop OA after 15 years. This is most likely to

Table 1 Osteoarthritis: Definition and aetiopathogenesis

Definition	A condition of synovial joints characterized by degradation of articular cartilage and increased activity of subchondral bone
Pathophysiology	A disturbance of the balance between the stresses applied to a joint and its capacity to withstand them. Joint failure can result from abnormal mechanical loading, or decreased resistance of the cartilage and subchondral bone
Aetiological factors include	Ageing of connective tissue An inherited predisposition Abnormal joint loading Biochemical anomalies of cartilage Previous inflammatory joint disease

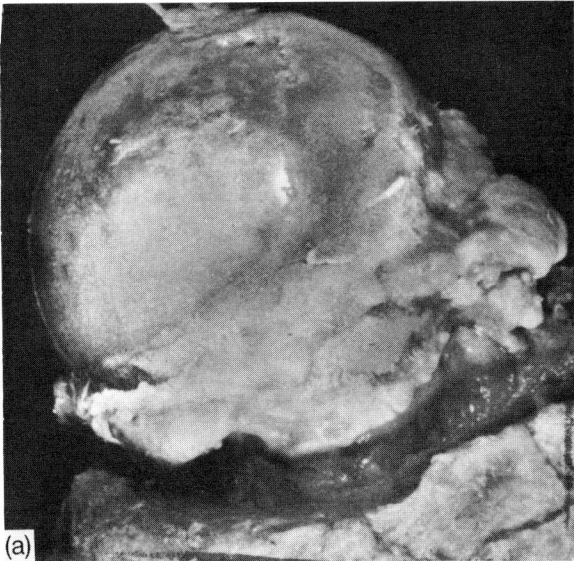
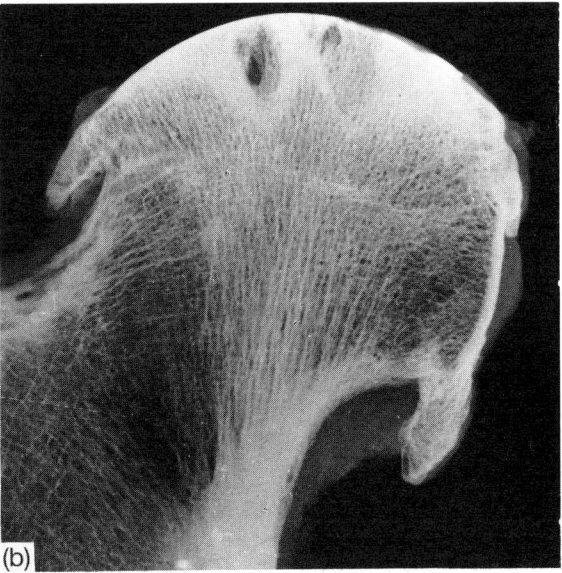
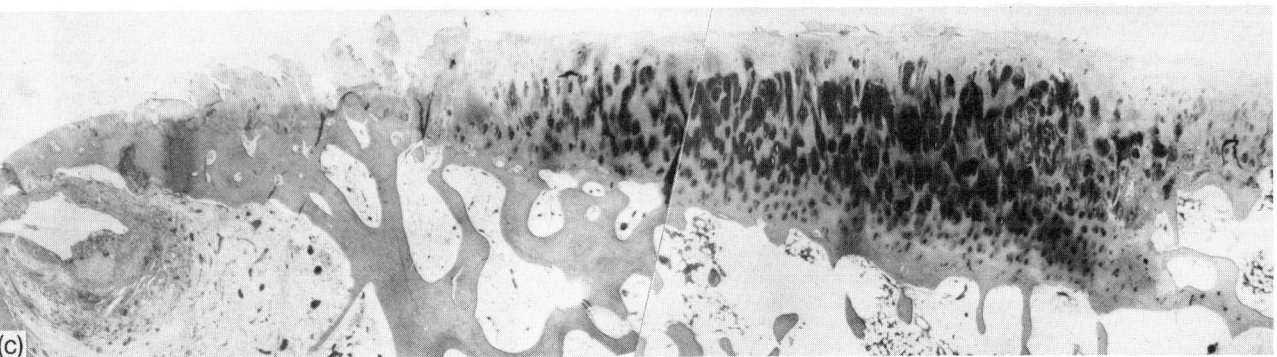

Fig. 1 An osteoarthritic femoral head obtained at post mortem. The left-hand picture shows an ovoid area of exposed eburnated bone surrounded by a broad zone of thinned fibrillated cartilage; marginal osteophytes are prominent. The right-hand picture is an X-ray of a slab cut from the centre of the specimen in the plane of the photograph; the loss of cartilage and osteophytosis are clearly shown. The bone below the exposed region has reacted with increased density, but two osteolytic 'bone cysts' have also developed.

The photomicrograph shows some of the range of changes in advanced OA. On the far right there is ossification of the cartilage (subsequent to vascular penetration); from there, moving left, the cartilage progressively thins and disappears. There is coarse fibrillation on parts of the surface. The volume of bone under the thinned areas is increased, but fibrous proliferation has led to bone resorption and degeneration to produce a bone cyst seen on the X-ray. (Illustrations and caption by Dr P. D. Byers, Institute of Orthopaedics, London.)

occur in the older subjects and those with a family history or evidence of generalized OA at other sites, suggesting interactions of abnormal mechanics and inflammation with an inherited predisposition or a metabolic abnormality.

Pathology

All tissues of the joint are affected by osteoarthritis, but the most striking and distinctive features are: (1) destruction of the cartilage in the absence of severe synovial inflammation, and (2) sclerosis and remodelling of the subchondral bone.

Articular cartilage

Normal articular cartilage is 2–4 mm thick and the main constituents are water (70 per cent), collagen fibres (15 per cent) and proteoglycan ground substance (10 per cent). Its integrity is maintained by the hydrophilic proteoglycans which keep the ordered collagen network under constant tension. There is a slow turnover of components, due to the activity of small numbers of cells (chondrocytes) found mainly in the middle and lower zones. The weight-bearing surface is smooth and undulating, and only the transitional, calcified zone that binds cartilage to bone is vascularized.

Early *biochemical* changes in OA include an increase in the water content of cartilage and a change in chemistry of the proteoglycans. Later the collagen network fails and cartilage integrity is lost. The chondrocytes increase in activity, and probably in number, and minute deposits of mineral are often found in the perichondrocytic region. It remains to be seen which, if any, of these changes initiate cartilage destruction.

At a *morphological* level, early cartilage damage is reflected by superficial flaking and splitting (fibrillation), and a reduction in uptake of stain. If the condition progresses, large fissures and cracks appear, a reduction in volume of cartilage follows; and finally the underlying bone may be uncovered (Fig. 1). Clusters of active chondrocytes ('brood nests') or cellular degeneration may also be seen. At a macroscopic level Indian-ink staining may help to pick out areas of early superficial damage, and late changes are obvious; the softening and disintegrating cartilage crumbling to expose the eburnated bone beneath (Fig. 1).

Fibrillation of cartilage only occurs in some areas of the joint and does not develop over its whole surface. It is also clear that only some areas which become fibrillated progress to florid OA, some early cartilage changes being non-progressive. Furthermore, advanced OA is accompanied by regeneration of new fibrocartilage in and around the areas of hyaline cartilage destruction. The final pathological picture is that of a battleground, in which active regenerative processes are combating the disintegration of some areas of the damaged surface.

Bone

The subchondral bone is more active, sclerotic and vascular than normal. As the disease progresses remodelling occurs, with a consequent change in joint contour and congruity. Bony osteophytes appear at the joint margins, and form lips, tending to splint movement. Small trabecular microfractures are sometimes seen and may help stimulate the patchy subchondral sclerosis, which can result in immensely hard, smooth bone in some areas and relatively porotic regions elsewhere (bone cysts). The striking feature of OA bone is its active, regenerative nature, changing the contour of the joint (Fig. 1). Both animal experiments and scintigraphic studies in humans suggest that changes in the activity of subchondral bone are a very early feature of OA.

The soft tissues

In early OA the only soft tissue changes seen are mild, non-specific, patchy inflammatory infiltrates in the synovium. In late joint failure more florid changes may occur. The capsule becomes thickened with increased fibrosis, and the synovium may contain aggregates of lymphocytes, giant cells and plasma cells as well as engulfed particles of cartilage and mineral. It may be difficult to distinguish advanced OA from rheumatoid disease, although the marked capsular fibrosis, amount of joint debris, and relative paucity of immunological features are helpful distinguishing points. Most authorities regard the soft tissue changes of OA as being secondary to cartilage damage, although experimental studies emphasize the early nature of synovial disease.

The synovial fluid is usually increased in quantity, but has a relatively low count in which mononuclear cells predominate $(0.2-3.0 \times 10^9$ cells/l). In about 30 per cent of aspirated fluids microcrystalline hydroxyapatite or calcium pyrophosphate can be detected, and numerous cartilage fragments are present in the joint space of the majority.

Radiology

The pathological features described are reflected in the typical radiological changes of osteoarthritis (Table 2). Loss of joint space is characteristic, but also occurs in many other diseases. The bony changes are more specific for OA and include subchondral sclerosis, cyst formation, and osteophytosis (Fig. 2). Osteophytes tend to be of two types: (1) small, dense areas around the joint margin, and (2) larger more porotic protrusions ('molten wax' osteophytes). The excess mineralization of OA may result in linear deposits of calcific density in the cartilage ('chondrocalcinosis', usually due to pyrophosphate deposition), or rounded, sometimes trabeculated deposits in the soft tissues (usually hydroxyapatite). The latter are commonest in the hands ('ossicles') or knees (usually called 'loose bodies'). The soft tissue component of OA may be reflected by minimal soft tissue swelling around the joint. In advanced OA destruction of bone, subluxation and avascular necrosis may complicate the radiological picture, and specific changes in the pattern and distribution of OA are seen at different joint sites.

The plane radiograph remains the 'gold-standard' in diagnosing and assessing severity and progression of osteoarthritis. However, other imaging techniques are now being used to investigate and assess the disease. Computerized tomography and ultrasound can be used to assess joint spaces and the spinal canal. Scintigraphy (bone scans) illustrates the activity of subchondral bone and may indicate prognosis.

Clinical features

The most frequent presenting feature of OA is *pain*. There are no nerve fibres in cartilage, and few pain receptors in subchondral bone, so it is not surprising that most people with radiological evidence of the condition are asymptomatic. Pain probably arises

Table 2 The pathology and radiology of osteoarthritis (Figs. 1, 2, 3)

Pathological features include	Radiological features include
Destruction of articular cartilage	Loss of joint space
Increased activity and remodelling of subchondral bone	Sclerosis Cysts Osteophytes
Mild synovial reaction and excess fluid	Mild soft tissue swelling
Mineralization	Linear cartilage deposits ('chondrocalcinosis') Spotty soft tissue deposits ('ossicles' or 'loose bodies')

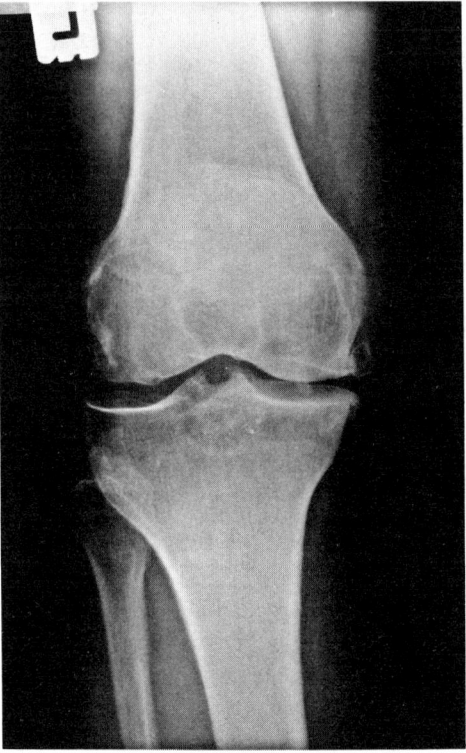

Fig. 2 X-ray of a knee joint showing mild osteoarthritis associated with severe chondrocalcinosis. The linear calcification of the menisci and hyaline cartilage within the joint space are clearly shown, and represent deposits of calcium pyrophosphate dihydrate in the cartilage.

from the development of some secondary change: possibilities include raised intraosseous pressure, synovitis, and mechanical strain on capsular and ligamentous insertions. After pain, the most important clinical feature of OA is *loss of function*, usually caused either by the pain itself or loss of joint movement.

Clinical assessment of a patient with OA involves history taking, physical examination and investigations (Table 3). Particular points to note in the history include a strong family history (especially of 'nodal' or premature OA), any previous disease or trauma that might predispose to joint failure, the symptoms, and the effect of the disease on the patient's life. The examination must include a careful assessment of joint movement and function as well as a general examination for intercurrent disease and other possible causes of the symptoms. Investigations are often unnecessary and are only done to exclude other conditions and confirm the radiological presence of OA.

Patients diagnosed as suffering from OA are usually in their sixth or seventh decade, and women outnumber men by three to one (a rather higher female preponderance than that found in radiological surveys). The mean age of onset of symptoms is about

Table 3 Clinical features of osteoarthritis

Mean age of onset	About 55 (wide range)
Ratio, women:men	About 3:1 (higher for hand disease, lower for hip OA)
Main joint sites	Hands (distal interphalangeal joints and thumb base)
	Knees
	Hips
	Feet (first metatarsophalangeal joint)
Symptoms	Pain on joint use
	Inactivity stiffness
	Loss of movement
	Cracking of joints
Signs	Bony swelling
	Tenderness (joint line or periarticular spots)
	Small, cool effusions
	Painful limitation of movement
	Joint crepitus
Investigations	Radiology: confirms presence of OA, helps exclude other bone or joint disease
	Others: all haematology, biochemical and serological assays are normal. Invasive tests are generally unhelpful and unwarranted

55 years, but the condition can start in the twenties or thirties, or may first present in later life. Although some cases resolve spontaneously, many are slowly progressive, with intermittent exacerbations and remissions of pain lasting days, weeks or months. Exacerbations can sometimes be related to overuse or trauma, but are just as often spontaneous and inexplicable. Because of the relationship of OA to increasing age and the effect of other disorders on pain and function, symptoms, signs and disability become most apparent in the elderly.

Symptoms

The cardinal symptoms of OA are pain, stiffness, immobility and 'cracking' of the joints. As already mentioned, the *pain* is variable, but is usually the dominant symptom. It tends to occur on use of the joint, and is worst at the end of the day. It is often described as a deep 'aching' sensation. Rest pain sometimes occurs in severe OA, perhaps as a result of raised intraosseous pressure. Mild early morning *stiffness*, lasting from 5 to 30 minutes usually occurs but inactivity stiffness is more severe and more diagnostic. The patient typically 'gells' or 'seizes-up' after periods of inactivity, and may take several painful, embarrassing minutes to loosen up. Loss of the *full range of movement* of the affected joints occurs and progressive deterioration leads to complaints and disability dependent upon the site and severity of involvement. Patients often also notice that joints *creak* and crack; a sensation that can be appreciated by palpation of joint crepitus, which is sometimes frankly audible as patients enter the consulting room!

Signs

The physical signs of an osteoarthritic joint include tenderness, bony swelling around the joint line, pain and crepitus on movement, loss of range of movement, and mild signs of inflammation. Careful *palpation* of an OA joint is an important and rewarding examination. Osteophytosis and remodelling lead to bony swelling, and a certain amount of soft tissue swelling and small effusions may also be palpable. More important is definition of the areas of tenderness, which may be over the joint line, but may be restricted to small, circumscribed, periarticular regions near to bursae or ligament and capsular insertions. These tender areas may respond to local injections, completely relieving symptoms of an OA 'joint', and are therefore very significant. *Moving* an affected joint, with one hand over the joint line itself, will help to detect crepitus (which is not specific to OA), pain on motion, and the range of movement, which are important functional considerations.

Investigations

There is no laboratory test for osteoarthritis. All haematological, biochemical and serological tests are normal. The disorder affects joints alone, so that only imaging techniques, arthroscopy, or joint biopsy will reveal pathology. A plane radiograph is always helpful in assessing joint damage and excluding other pathology. Other imaging or invasive investigations are neither necessary nor likely to provide information that is helpful or specific. Other tests should only be performed if there is doubt about the diagnosis.

Osteoarthritis of particular joint sites

The knee

OA of the knee usually presents with pain. A good history and examination should ascertain three things: (1) the source of the pain, (2) the degree and cause of any disability, and (3) the presence or absence of any inflammation or associated joint conditions.

Knee pain can arise from the hip or spine (see below), from the numerous bursae and ligaments around the joint, or from the joint itself. The different compartments of the joint give rise to different symptoms: the patellofemoral joint causes pain on flexion – typically on walking downstairs – and on compression of the patella against the femur (patella compression test); tibiofemoral OA causes pain on weight-bearing and tenderness over the medial (more commonly) or lateral joint line.

Disability can arise from a variety of problems. Flexion deformities are common and result in a bad gait; loss of flexion can cause difficulty with steps, stairs and buses. Wasting and weakness of the quadriceps apparatus usually accompanies knee OA and can lead to instability. Ligamentous laxity, or varus (common) and valgus (rare) deformities due to tibial plateau collapse also occur and can result in crippling disabilities.

A low-grade inflammatory reaction resulting in effusions, warmth, and 'Baker's' cysts (synovial cysts in the popliteal fossa originating from the knee) are often present. Exacerbations of a more obvious inflammatory nature are not uncommon, but should alert one to the possible presence of an associated condition such as chondrocalcinosis (see below).

The radiograph is helpful in ascertaining compartmental involvement, the degree of joint damage and presence or absence of chondrocalcinosis. The film should be taken with the patient standing.

The hands

The distribution of hand involvement in OA is characteristic: the trapezometacarpal joint (carpometacarpal joint of the thumb) and distal interphalangeal (DIP) joints (especially the index finger) are most often affected, with proximal interphalangeal, metacarpophalangeal and wrist involvement being respectively less common. Swelling of the finger ends and base of thumb result in the typical 'square hand' shown in Fig. 3. Involvement of the DIPs results in hard swellings on the dorsum of the joint; these 'Heberden's nodes' are thought of as a specific feature of OA, although in fact other conditions affecting this joint result in a similar deformity (Table 4). Inflammation, with redness of the overlying skin is common in the early stage of development of a Heberden's node; later, cystic swellings containing jelly-like material (hyaluronate) may arise, and angulation deformities and loss of movement develop. Symptoms and disability vary, but are usually mild. OA at the base of the thumb, however, can be both very painful and quite a handicap, preventing a proper pinch-grip. It is sometimes relieved by intra-articular steroid injections.

The hip

Pain is the dominant symptom, although stiffness and difficulty in walking can be the presenting complaints. Hip pain is usually felt

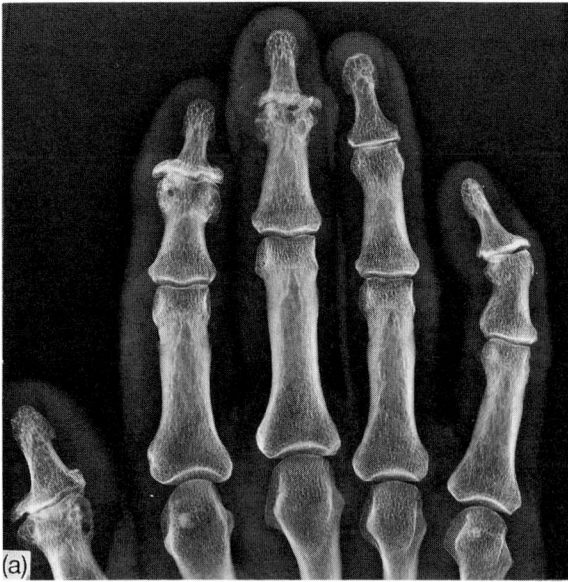

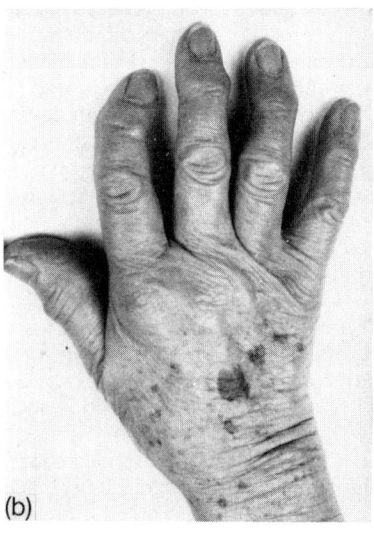

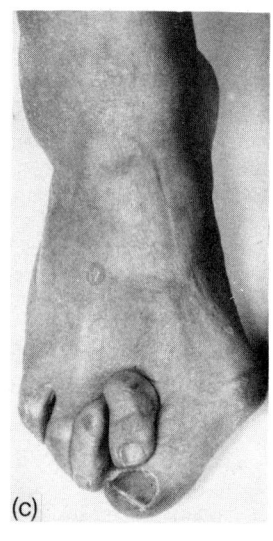

Fig. 3 Peripheral osteoarthritis. The swelling of the distal interphalangeal joints of the hand (Heberden's nodes), and hallux valgus in the foot are shown. The X-ray shows advanced OA of the interphalangeal joint of the thumb, and distal joints of the index and middle finger. Joint space narrowing, osteophytes, bone sclerosis, and cysts are all present. There is also a little soft tissue swelling.

Table 4 Diseases affecting the terminal interphalangeal joints

Common	Osteoarthritis (look for disease at base of thumbs and knees)
	Psoriatic arthropathy (usually associated with nail pits, nail dystrophy and typical rash)
	Gout (asymmetrical, associated with acute attacks; look for tophi)
Uncommon	Juvenile chronic polyarthritis
	Sarcoidosis
	Septic arthritis
	Calcific periarthritis
	Rheumatoid arthritis

in the groin and front of the thigh, although referral to the knee can cause diagnostic confusion. Reproduction of the pain on hip rotation, rather than knee flexion, is an important sign. Range of

Table 5 Conditions that may complicate OA, or mimic it clinically

1 Bone and joint diseases
    Inflammatory arthropathies
    Periarticular soft tissue lesions
    Osteopaenia
    Paget's disease of bone
    Neoplasia of bone (primary or secondary)
    Hypertrophic pulmonary osteopathy
2 Miscellaneous conditions
    Polymyalgia rheumatica
    Depression
    Thyroid disease
    Peripheral vascular disease
    Carcinomatosis

movement becomes restricted, and internal rotation is usually lost first, and affected most; loss of extension and full flexion are often very disabling. As the disease progresses, collapse of the femoral head may result in shortening of the leg. The characteristic gait involves a downward tilt of the pelvis when weight is taken on the affected side (the 'Trendelenburg' sign).

Careful radiological assessment is very important in hip OA. The X-ray may reveal the cause (such as hip dysplasia – see below); the distribution of disease – usually upper-pole only, or concentric; complications such as avascular necrosis or protrusio acetabulae, and any other associated bone or joint disease.

The foot

OA of the ankle and hindfoot are surprisingly rare. The usual joint to be affected is the first metatarsophalangeal joint. This may be asymptomatic. It can result in loss of movement ('hallux rigidus'), and pressure on the prominent metatarsal of hallux valgus can result in soft tissue swelling, inflammation, and even ulceration, if shoes are too tight ('bunions' or 'poor man's gout', Fig. 3).

Differential diagnosis

OA is frequently present in elderly people who may be suffering from more than one disease. It is therefore important to look for other causes of local or generalized pain and stiffness (Table 5). A good history and clinical examination will usually provide clues to the presence of such diseases, particularly as OA is never responsible for any systemic or extra-articular features.

Investigations are often misleading, especially in the older patient. Because radiological changes are almost universal in the elderly it is all too easy to 'confirm' a lazy diagnosis of OA as the cause of musculoskeletal symptoms, perhaps missing the more important intercurrent depression, Parkinsonism, thyroid disease or polymyalgia rheumatica. Conversely, older subjects may have a mildly elevated ESR or uric acid, or weakly positive rheumatoid and antinuclear factor, leading to the erroneous diagnosis of a separate arthropathy.

The history and clinical examination are critical, both to make the correct diagnosis and to help delineate the cause of symptoms related to an osteoarthritic joint.

Classification and clinical subsets

Traditional classifications of OA have separated a 'primary' group (in whom no cause is apparent) from a 'secondary' group where a single aetiological agent is implicated (such as a previous fracture or operation). As our understanding of the condition increases, the primary group may get smaller and the list of secondary types increase. However, it is likely that in most cases OA is multifactorial. In many patients, one fairly obvious, dominant mechanical, metabolic or inflammatory component can be recognized, and a revised provisional classification, based on this approach, is shown in Table 6. Two particular, distinctive clinical subsets are frequently seen in Caucasian patients.

Table 6 Subsets of OA based on the dominant clinical or aetiological features

A	Primary	No apparent predisposing factor (often polyarticular)
B	Secondary	(Sometimes monoarticular)
1	Associated with mechanical factors	
	Any joint	Post-traumatic (e.g. fracture or unstable joint)
		Joint hypermobility
		Occupational arthropathies (e.g. wicket-keepers thumb)
	Knee joint	Postmeniscectomy (40% 15 yrs after operation)
		Long-leg arthropathy (OA knee of the longer leg)
		Chondromalacia patellae
	Hip joint	Epiphyseal dysplasia
		Slipped epiphysis
		Perthes' disease
		Congenital dislocation
		Hip OA in manual workers
		Leg-length inequality
2	Associated with a metabolic abnormality	
		Chondrocalcinosis (pyrophosphate arthropathy)
		Acromegaly
		Ochronosis
		Kashin-Beck disease
		Gout
		Lathyrism
3	Associated with an inflammatory or familial component	
		Secondary to another inflammatory arthropathy
		Primary generalized osteoarthritis
		Familial OA of the hip or other joint site

'Secondary' OA of the hip

Epidemiological evidence suggests that hip osteoarthritis behaves as a separate disease entity. It often occurs in younger people, is more common in men, and shows less correlation with changes in other peripheral joints and more correlation with spinal disease than OA at other joint sites.

Radiological surveys suggest that a large proportion of OA isolated to one or both hip joints is due to pre-existing anatomical or mechanical abnormalities. Minor degrees of dysplasia of the femoral head or acetabulum, previous slipped epiphyses, Perthes disease, or congenital dislocation can all be responsible. Pain and stiffness may develop slowly during early adulthood, and symptoms are often variable, relative asymptomatic periods being interrupted by days or weeks of unusually intense discomfort. As the damage progresses, the loss of articular cartilage with remodelling and flattening of the femoral head may cause, or accentuate, any pre-existing inequality in leg length. Secondary pain in the back often develops. Symptoms may respond to non-steroidal anti-inflammatory drugs and physiotherapy (especially hydrotherapy), and a stick held in the opposite hand to reduce weight bearing. However, many cases come to surgery, and total hip replacements have revolutionized the treatment of this disease.

The radiograph usually shows damage at the superior pole of the hip joint and the femoral head tends to move upwards and laterally as the condition progresses.

Primary generalized osteoarthritis

(Synonyms: 'nodal osteoarthritis', 'inflammatory osteoarthritis', 'interphalangeal osteoarthritis', 'erosive osteoarthritis'.)

Various synonyms have been applied to this entity, which appears to be a distinct subset of OA especially common in Caucasian women.

The onset of the disease is usually gradual, beginning around the age of 50 years. The hands become stiff and ache and the joints then develop swelling and tenderness. The overlying skin is often red, and cysts may form. The distal interphalangeal joints are most often involved, but the proximal interphalangeal (PIP) joints and carpometacarpal joints of the thumb, as well as the knees and other large joints, are often affected as well. The initial inflammatory element is sometimes severe and dramatic enough to cause

confusion with rheumatoid disease or other arthropathies. As the disease progresses, however, the inflammation tends to subside, but the swelling of the joints and the fingers becomes more pronounced and firmer, forming the characteristic Heberden's (DIPs) or Bouchard's (PIPs) nodes (Fig. 3). Early on, X-rays show soft tissue swelling and joint-space narrowing, and a little sclerosis underlying bone; but later ossicles and then osteophytes form around the interphalangeal joints, cysts may appear, and occasionally erosions are found. The late stage of the disease consists of relatively painless, bony swelling of the interphalangeal joints, which may be markedly restricted in movement, and someties angulated, causing difficulty with simple household tasks. Bone scans pick out the active joints in the hand and correlate with progressive clinical and radiographic changes. Progressive osteoarthritis in other joints may occur concurrently, particularly medial-compartment disease of the knee. If the hips are involved the radiographs usually show bilateral concentric joint-space narrowing, distinguishing it from the superior-pole disease described above.

There is a strong genetic element to this subset, family studies suggesting either polygenic inheritance, or possibly a dominant trait with variable penetrance. Mechanical factors also play a part, dictating the distribution and severity of joint involvement in some cases. Men are occasionally affected (M:F ratio approximately 10:1). The age of onset varies, it often seems to coincide with the female menopause ('menopausal arthritis'), but shows no clear correlation with hormone levels and oestrogens do not appear to have any beneficial therapeutic effect.

Prognosis and management

The natural history of OA is unknown. Symptoms sometimes resolve spontaneously and radiological evidence of repair is occasionally seen. More often symptoms persist and joint function slowly deteriorates. In a few cases the disease takes a rapid course, especially if associated with chondrocalcinosis or complicated by avascular necrosis of bone. A rare atrophic form with rapid progression is also described.

There is no specific or disease-modifying therapy. The aims of management include education (especially to reduce anxiety about crippling disease and its inevitable progression to a wheelchair), alleviation of symptoms, and the maintenance of joint function (Table 7). It is important to identify and treat any obvious factor which may exacerbate pain, such as obesity or a secondary periarticular disorder. Patients should be encouraged to keep as active as they can, without abusing their joints. Functional aids such as a walking stick can help considerably and the physiotherapist may be able to improve muscles and movement as well as providing temporary symptomatic relief. Drugs (analgesics or non-steroidal anti-inflammatory agents) should only be used sparingly to relieve symptoms, and surgery (e.g. hip replacement) may be necessary in severe cases. Specific therapeutic measures are considered in more detail on page 16.61.

Spinal osteoarthritis

Back pain is so common that few escape it. Unfortunately the cause is often mysterious, and OA may be blamed in the absence of corroborative evidence. Radiological studies show that spinal OA becomes almost universal as age advances, but the disparity between X-rays and symptoms is even more marked than in peripheral OA. However, some distinct pathological and clinical entities do exist, and these will be described.

There are two principal joints in the spine: the intervertebral (disc) joints which are secondary cartilaginous articulations, and the apophyseal (posterior, interfacetal) joints which are of synovial type. OA of each can be defined in the same way as before – as a condition characterized by loss of cartilage and increased activity of bone. Intervertebral joint OA is known as spondylosis,

Table 7 Management of patients with osteoarthritis

1 Patient education
E.g. reassure that it is not crippling RA, may not progress, and that symptoms may improve. Advise to keep active
2 Physical therapy
Consider physiotherapy to maintain optimum muscle power, movement and function. A walking stick (opposite hand) often helps in hip or knee disease
3 Identify and treat specific causes of pain
E.g. identify specific periarticular tender spots and consider local injection, reduce obesity, look out for 'flares' caused by synovitis, examine for instability of joints
4 Drugs
Judicious use of simple, safer analgesics and non-steroidal anti-inflammatory drugs during symptomatic exacerbations of disease
5 Occupational therapy
Aids and appliances to improve function in severe cases
6 Surgery
Consider osteotomy or arthroplasty in severe cases

and is pathologically distinct from apophyseal joint OA, although the two usually coexist.

Pathology

Disc disease and spondylosis

The intervertebral discs consist of a ring of strong fibrocartilage (annulus) and a central area of hydrophilic, pressured ground substance (nucleus). They sustain immense pressures, particularly on bending and lifting. The central nucleus pulposis often herniates, and the disc prolapses ('slipped disc'), moves vertically into bone, or posteriorly into the neural canal. Vertical herniation, forming bone cysts (Schmorl's nodes) is very common, and relatively unimportant. Posterior herniation often occurs in young people in the cervical (especially C5/6) and lumbar (L4/5 and L5/S1) regions if a tear exists in the annulus. The gelatinous nuclear material is then squeezed out like toothpaste, and may in some cases move in and out of the disc space with different movements. More commonly it is pushed out laterally, to be slowly absorbed over a period of weeks or months. Disc herniation or prolapse is followed by a loss of height (narrowing of the disc space), and a secondary osteophytic reaction at the margins of the bone (spondylosis).

Spondylosis (i.e. loss of disc material and bone sclerosis and osteophytes) is important in an older age group, and can occur in the absence of herniation of the nucleus pulposis. Loss of hydration of the nucleus, and splits and damage to the annulus may occur, resulting in loss of total cartilage volume, and altered mechanical properties. Sclerosis and osteophytosis of bone accompanies these changes, and bone may encroach on the neural canal, causing narrowing (spinal stenosis).

Apophyseal joint OA

Pathological changes in these joints are identical to those of OA in any other synovial articulation, and have already been described.

The apophyseal joints work in conjunction with the intervertebral joints, one cannot move without the other. OA tends to coexist in the two areas and mechanical factors probably play an important role in their aetiology. Thus 'slipped discs', back pain and spondylosis are commoner in people doing manual labour than in sedentary workers. Some jobs involving heavy lifting have a very high turnover of employees simply because of the frequent occurrence of back injuries and slipped discs.

Clinical syndromes

Prolapsed intervertebral disc

'Slipped discs' are common in the lower lumbar spine, may occur in the neck, and occasionally occur elsewhere in the spine. Young working men are particularly susceptible, and minor trauma, such as lifting a heavy weight, often precipitates the incident. Symp-

toms arise from the stretched or torn posterior longitudinal ligament (back pain or 'lumbago'), and from damage to nerve roots caused by direct pressure or vascular occlusion (root pain, e.g. 'sciatica'). The onset is often sudden, and back pain may precede the development of root pain by hours or days. Pain is severe, and exacerbated by coughing or sneezing ('impulse pain' produced by raised intrathecal pressure). Parasthesiae, numbness and weakenss of the affected dermatome may appear, producing, for example, pain and numbness in the back of the calf and sole of the foot, reduced dorsiflexion of the foot, and a reduced ankle jerk in the typical L5/S1 lesion. Back movements are painful and limited by paraspinal muscle spasm, and a scoliosis (concave to the side of the lesion) may appear. Pain can be reproduced by stretching the affected nerve root, as in the straight leg-raising test for L5/S1 compression.

The vast majority of prolapsed discs slowly resolve over a period of weeks or months, and most treatment has little or no effect on the outcome. A minority come to surgery, which should always be considered if weakness or other significant neurological problems arise. Central protrusions, high lumbar or thoracic lesions, and some cervical discs can cause diagnostic difficulty and serious spinal cord compression.

Although spontaneous resolution is the rule, recurrences are common, and may lead to chronic back pain. Spondylosis and osteoarthritis often occur in later years.

Spinal stenosis

The width of the spinal canal varies. If it is relatively narrow, encroachment by a central disc protrusion, by osteophytes or by a spondylolisthesis (anteroposterior slip of one vertebra on another) may result in significant stenosis.

The typical syndrome resembles vascular claudication, the patient acquiring leg pain with or without neurological signs and symptoms, on walking. Symptoms are relieved by rest, and frequently by bending forward, and probably arise from occlusion of the spinal arteries (classically bicycle riding is not limited). 'Intermittent claudication of the cauda equina' may be difficult to differentiate from peripheral vascular disease.

Cervical spondylosis

This term strictly refers to symptomatic OA of the intervertebral joints in the neck. In practice it is used to label middle-aged or elderly patients with neck pain, radiological evidence of OA, and no other obvious cause of symptoms.

The pain and stiffness in the neck tend to wax and wane, and to radiate into the back of the head or shoulders. Neck movements are restricted and painful, and tender areas over apophyseal joints may be palpable. A background of mild discomfort may be interrupted by episodes of severe pain lasting days, weeks or months before resolving. Maintenance of neck mobility is a good rule unless root compression or other neurological problems arise. Symptoms bear little or no relationship to the severity of the universal X-ray changes.

Lumbar spondylosis

Chronic, variable low back pain with radiological OA is often diagnosed as lumbar spondylosis; the syndrome is similar to that of the neck, and the same problems and reservations apply to the diagnosis.

Pain may radiate into the buttocks or legs, and tends to be aggravated by prolonged sitting or standing. The spine gets stiff after immobility, and movements are limited and painful. As in the neck, the symptoms are very variable, and not predictable from radiographic appearances.

Vertebral hyperostosis

This is an interesting condition that may be related to OA. It is a radiological diagnosis, defined as the presence of large anterior osteophytes in four or more disc spaces in the absence of signifi-

Table 8 A clinical classification of some of the causes of back pain

Clinical description	Some causes
1 Mechanical – pain affected by movement, and worse on prolonged sitting or standing. Often chronic and relatively mild	Spondylosis Apophyseal OA Vertebral hyperostosis Spondylolisthesis Congenital and other structural anomalies Idiopathic
2 Inflammatory – associated with morning stiffness, often relieved by exercise	Ankylosing spondylitis Other 'Spondarthropathies' (Spondylosis and OA)
3 Neurological – impulse pain, root radiation and/or neurological signs	Disc prolapse Spinal stenosis
4 Sinister – clues may include ill-health, systemic signs and symptoms, isolated areas of severe tenderness, weight loss, fever etc.	Infection – tuberculous, Staphylococcal, Brucella and others Neoplasia – primary or secondary deposits Metabolic bone disease
5 Referred – pain radiating to the back from another source	Numerous thoracic and abdominal causes, e.g. posterior erosion of peptic ulcer
6 Unclassified – all too common	Numerous structural and psychogenic causes

cant disc-space narrowing. The bony overgrowths are commonest in the thoracolumbar junction, and may coalesce to result in segments of spinal fusion. The sacroiliac joints are normal (contrasting with ankylosing spondylitis and related disorders), but osteophytosis and bony overgrowth, with or without OA, are common elsewhere. (Synonyms: 'diffuse idiopathic skeletal hyperostosis', 'Forrestier's disease'.)

Symptoms are usually absent or minimal, but fusion can result in severe immobility, and rarely areas of severe pain or spinal stenosis occur.

Sorting out back pain

Although most people get back pain, and although there are many possible causes, a precise diagnosis can only be made in a minority. Important principles include observing the discipline of a good history and examination, avoidance of over-investigation, and being aware of the occasional 'sinister' cause of back pain, such as myelomatosis.

A working classification of some of the common causes of back pain is shown in Table 8.

The history is of utmost importance, differentiating mechanical, neurological and inflammatory elements, as well as defining the duration and degree of disability endured by the patient. A careful examination should include spinal movements, palpation for tender areas, measurement of leg length, a neurological examination, and a general examination for signs of a causative condition (e.g. carcinoma with spinal deposits). Investigations are usually unhelpful and must depend on duration and severity of pain and the index of suspicion. An ESR, plasma calcium, and alkaline phosphatase (for metabolic bone disease), acid phosphatase in men (prostatic Ca) or protein electrophoresis (myeloma) are generally more than enough. A plain radiograph is usually taken, and special oblique, flexion–extension, or other views may occasionally help. Disc disease can be further investigated and visualized by CT scanning, radiculography, and occasionally discography or spinal venography. Malignant or septic foci may be revealed by scintigraphy. Other investigative techniques such as magnetic resonance imaging and spectroscopy are being used in much needed research into the causes of back pain.

Back pain, like osteoarthritis, presents an enormous challenge to the medical profession.

Chondrocalcinosis

Crystal deposition diseases of joints

The formation of mineral outside the skeleton is sometimes the result of a disease (e.g. calcification of old tuberculous foci), and sometimes its cause (e.g. renal calculi). Joints are particularly susceptible to mineral deposition. Age, metabolic disturbances and connective tissue damage predispose to crystal formation in articular cartilage. The crystals may cause no damage, but can trigger attacks of acute inflammation or contribute to chronic joint disease. Gout (page 9.123) is the best known crystal deposition disease of joints, but several others have been described (Table 9).

Calcification of articular cartilage (Chondrocalcinosis – CCA)

Two main calcium salts can be deposited in articular cartilage. (1) Calcium pyrophosphate dihydrate ($Ca_2P_2O_7$. $2H_2O$) is deposited in the mid-zone as aggregates of monoclinic or triclinic crystals. Inorganic pyrophosphate ($P_2O_7^{4-}$, PP_1) is a product of all cellular metabolism, and is a natural inhibitor of basic calcium phosphate deposition, but the formation of calcium crystals is a very singular event – occurring only in articular cartilage. (2) Hydroxyapatite ($Ca_{10}(PO_4)_6$.OH: HA or 'bone mineral') is the main constituent of a range of apatites and other basic calcium phosphates found in the skeleton, but sometimes deposited elsewhere, especially in damaged or avascular tissues. Periarticular deposits are common, but aggregates of the tiny crystals can also form in the perichondrocyte of articular cartilage.

Calcium pyrophosphate deposition (CPPD)

Incidence

CPPD is a common, age-related phenomenon. Radiological surveys show that it is rare in people under 50 (< 1 per cent prevalence), but the incidence rises steadily with increasing age so that about 40 per cent of 90-year-olds have extensive deposits. The salt has a predilection for fibrocartilage and is found mainly in knee menisci, the triangular ligament of the wrist, pubic symphysis, and spinal discs; in severe cases deposition is more widespread and also affects hyaline cartilage.

Classification and causes

Age alone is the main predisposing factor (Table 10). Occasional cases are familial, and a few are due to a metabolic disease such as hyperparathyroidism, which alters calcium or PP_1 metabolism. In both familial and metabolic disease widespread deposits form in young adults. Previous joints damage also predisposes to early CPPD, found at the site of damage only.

Identification

The susceptibility of the mid-zone of fibrocartilage to CPPD results in its characteristic radiological sign – linear chondrocalcinosis (Fig. 2). Crystals are often shed into the synovial fluid and can be identified by polarized light microscopy. The small rod-shaped particles, about 1–5 μm long, are positively birefringent, aiding distinction from the negatively birefringent urate needles found in gout.

Disease associations

Most deposits are *asymptomatic*. Because of its high prevalence in the elderly, radiological chondrocalcinosis is a frequent chance finding which is sometimes misinterpreted as the cause of an unrelated disorder.

Acute pseudogout

This is a self-limiting inflammatory synovitis caused by crystal shedding from the CPPD deposits. It is one of the commonest causes of acute arthritis in the elderly, affects the sexes equally,

Table 9 Crystal deposition diseases of joints

Crystal deposited	Distribution	Disease associations
Monosodium urate monohydrate	Peripheral; hands and feet especially	1 Acute gout 2 Chronic tophaceous gout
Calcium pyrophosphate dihydrate	Intermediate; knees, wrists, ankles etc.	1 Acute pseudogout 2 Chronic pyrophosphate arthropathy
Hydroxyapatite and other basic calcium phosphates	Central; shoulders, hips, spine	1 Acute calcific periarthritis (acute synovitis) 2 Osteoarthritis – especially advanced progressive disease

Other crystals occasionally found in joints include cholesterol, other lipids, and calcium oxalate.

Table 10 Causes and classification of calcium pyrophosphate deposition

1 Age-associated, sporadic form (very common in the elderly)
2 Related to previous joint damage (common)
3 Metabolic (uncommon) – including:
    Hyperparathyroidism
    Hypothyroidism
    Haemochromatosis
    Hypomagnesaemia
    Hypophosphatasia
4 Familial (rare)

and is rare in the under 60s. Like gout, attacks can be precipitated by trauma or intercurrent disease, and occur spontaneously. The knee (70 per cent) is the commonest site of attacks, but wrists, ankles and elbows may be affected, and most joints are occasionally involved. The synovitis is usually monoarticular and lasts for about two weeks before slowly subsiding; it may be associated with a mild fever. Aspiration of joint fluid allows the crystals to be identified, confirming the diagnosis, and also relieves symptoms. Non-steroidal anti-inflammatory drugs or intra-articular steroids (if sepsis has been excluded) are also effective.

Chronic pyrophosphate arthropathy

This is a distinct variant of OA associated with CPPD. It is common in elderly patients (70+) and affects more women than men. The commonest joints to be affected are the knees (90 per cent), wrists, ankles, elbows, hips, and shoulders. Radiographs show exuberant new bone formation in addition to chondrocalcinosis, and extensive patellofemoral joint disease is characteristic. Some patients develop rapidly progressive joint destruction, but in many the condition appears to stabilize. Therapy is the same as for OA.

Apatite deposition

Incidence and causes

Most extraskeletal soft tissue calcific deposits contain apatite, are caused by previous tissue damage, and are of little significance. *Periarticular* deposition is common around the shoulder, but also occurs at the hips, knees, and other joints. Most of these deposits are idiopathic, but occasional familial cases are seen; the incidence is increased in diabetes, and hypercalcaemic or hyperphosphataemic states can result in widespread deposition. The incidence of

intra-articular deposition is unknown but it is probably common in the elderly and in OA.

Identification

Large periarticular deposits are seen on radiographs. Small deposits and most intra-articular aggregates, cannot be visualized. The individual crystals are small (around 500 Å long) and can only be identified by electron microscopy, but a variety of less specific staining and labelling techniques have been used to try and identify articular crystals.

Disease associations

As with CPPD, most deposits probably remain asymptomatic.

Acute calcific periarthritis

This is a rare condition occurring in both sexes and at any age. The shoulder is the commonest site. Rapid onset of severe pain is associated with the shedding of crystals from a periarticular deposit – usually in the supraspinatus tendon. The pain slowly subsides and is helped by anti-inflammatory therapy.

Occasional cases of synovitis are also due to apatite-crystal shedding. Apatite crystals are frequently found in OA joints, but their contribution to the condition remains unclear. Unlike CPPD, no distinct OA subset has been identified, although there are recent reports of a rapidly progressive, atrophic form of the disease which may be related to excess apatite deposition.

References

Ali, S. Y. (1978). New knowledge of osteoarthrosis. *J. clin. Path.* **31**, suppl. (Roy. Coll. Path.) **12**, 191.

Dieppe, P. A. (1978). New knowledge of chondrocalcinosis. *J. clin. Path.* **31**, suppl. (Roy. Coll. Path.) **12**, 214.

Jayson, M. I. V. (1981). *The lumbar spine and back pain*, 2nd edn. Pitman Medical, London.

Moskowitz, R., Howell, D., Goldberg, V. and Mankin, H. (eds) (1984). *Osteoarthritis: diagnosis and management.* W. B. Saunders, Philadelphia.

Muir H. (1977). Molecular approach to the understanding of osteoarthrosis. *Ann. rheum. Dis.* **36**, 199.

Nuki, G. (1980). *The aetiopathogenesis of osteoarthrosis.* Pitman Medical, London.

Sokoloff, L. (ed.) (1985). Osteoarthritis. *Clin. rheum. Dis.*

Wright, V. (ed.) (1976). Osteoarthrosis. *Clin. rheum. Dis.* **2**, 3.

NON-INFLAMMATORY ARTHROPATHIES AND SOFT TISSUE RHEUMATISM

I. HASLOCK

Non-inflammatory arthropathies

Aches and pains in the locomotor systems are suffered by everyone at some time. When they are precipitated by a day in the garden or the first training session of the rugby season, they are generally accepted as 'normal'. Similarly their association with a bout of influenza is such an expected phenomenon that the aches and pains of febrile illnesses usually attract little attention – they are just part of the disease. However, when similar non-specific symptoms occur without any obvious precipitating cause, they are perceived by the sufferer as abnormal and hence in need of medical explanation. Unfortunately many are never explained adequately, but careful history taking and examination, with attention paid to other systems as well as the musculo-skeletal system, may reveal a specific cause for symptoms which at first seem ill-defined and nebulous.

Locomotor symptoms associated with malignancy

Polyarthritis

Almost any malignancy, especially carcinomas of the breast and lung, may present as a non-specific polyarthralgia, with symptoms similar to those of early rheumatoid arthritis. Other signs of malignancy may be absent for up to two years from development of joint symptoms, though many patients in whom a malignancy is said to have been inapparent have not, in fact, had a comprehensive physical examination and appropriate haematological, biochemical, and radiological screening tests undertaken.

Leukaemia especially in children, is associated with arthritis in about 15 per cent of cases. This may be the presenting feature, although physical and haematological abnormalities are almost invariably found along with the joint symptoms. Chemotherapy used in the treatment of leukaemia lowers resistance to infection, and septic arthritis may occur. This should be differentiated from the non-specific type of monoarthritis or polyarthritis described above by aspiration of any joint showing florid inflammatory signs and culture of the synovial fluid.

Myeloma is associated with a similar polyarthritis which may also be the presenting feature of the disease. In some patients the clinical presentation closely mimics rheumatoid arthritis, and it is essential that globulin abnormalities are not assumed to be part of the rheumatoid process, especially in seronegative cases, but are sufficiently investigated to exclude a paraproteinaemia. Back pain is also a feature of myelomatosis even in the absence of radiological bony lesions.

Secondary deposits near joints may mimic arthritis. Pain, local heat, and swelling may all be present although careful clinical examination will often reveal the site of the lesion to be distant from the joint. Radiology or scintigraphy may show the presence of other secondaries and general examination may reveal the site of the primary tumour or other signs of disseminated malignancy. Secondaries in the synovium are very rare considering its rich blood supply.

Spinal secondaries are the commonest locomotor malignancies, and are particularly found in association with carcinomas of the breast, prostate, kidney, bronchus, and thyroid. Patients with secondaries will only be distinguished from the morass of patients with back pain by careful general history taking and observation and examination of the whole patient, not just the back, supplemented by haematological, radiological, and scintigraphic investigation when suspicion is aroused.

Pigmented villonodular synovitis

This is a condition of uncertain aetiology which produces brown-pigmented thickening in the synovial membrane of joints and, more rarely, tendon sheaths and bursae. Low-grade malignancy, benign haemangioma formation, viral infection, and chronic inflammation have all been suggested as causes. The disease predominantly affects young adults and usually presents as a painless monoarticular swelling affecting a large joint, usually the knee. The swelling becomes more persistent with the passage of time, and aspiration reveals heavily blood-stained synovial fluid. Less commonly, the disease is diffuse with prominent involvement of tendon sheaths as well as one or more joints. Treatment is by surgical removal although incomplete excision is often followed by a florid recurrence. Patients with diffuse disease or in whom synovectomy has failed should be treated by radiotherapy.

Benign synovial tumours

These are rare causes of monoarticular swelling. They are usually haemangiomas or lipomas and very rarely fibromas. Treatment is by local excision.

Primary malignant tumours

Primary malignancies in joints are fortunately rare, and although generally called synoviomas are more properly synovial carcinomas. They present as swelling in or adjacent to a large joint and, although most common in adolescents and young adults, they have been reported in all age groups. The primary site of the tumour is rarely within the joint but is closely associated with it and tends to invade the joint rapidly. Diagnosis is by biopsy; if the joint is aspirated the fluid is often blood-stained, and these malignancies must be considered in the differential diagnosis of a blood-stained effusion. Synoviomas are highly malignant and not only invade the joint and local bone but metastasize early and widely to lymph-nodes, bone, and lungs. Treatment is by radical excision coupled with radiotherapy. The prognosis is poor.

Clubbing

Clubbing of the fingers and, more rarely, the toes may accompany intrathoracic malignancy as well as chronic lung sepsis, cyanotic congenital heart disease, liver disease, and inflammatory bowel disease. In about five per cent of cases of carcinoma of the lung, hypertrophic osteoarthropathy occurs. This is an inflammatory polyarthritis, particularly affecting the wrists. Examination reveals tenderness of the associated long bones and X-ray shows periosteal elevation along the shaft of the affected bones, starting at the distal end. Treatment is by control of the underlying malignancy, successful excision being accompanied by remission of the hypertrophic osteoarthropathy and regression of the clubbing. Despite the frequency of clubbing associated with inflammatory bowel disease, hypertrophic osteoarthropathy is exceptionally rare in these conditions.

Referred pain

Referred pain from malignancy most frequently affects the shoulder joint. Carcinoma of the lung or malignancy involving the diaphragm may present as shoulder pain, and direct invasion of the joint or brachial plexus by an apical tumour produces similar symptoms (Pancoast's syndrome).

Rheumatic complaints associated with endocrine disorders

The thyroid

Untreated hyperthyroidism does not cause rheumatic symptoms, but rarely after treatment the condition of thyroid acropachy develops. Fluffy periosteal new bone formation is accompanied by soft tissue swelling in the fingers and toes and by pretibial myxoedema. No treatment alters the condition, which is rarely more than a mild nuisance.

In contrast, hypothyroidism is frequently accompanied by locomotor symptoms. These most frequently consist of vague aches and pains related to muscles and joints, and the diagnosis of hypothyroidism must be considered in all patients with such symptoms. Diagnosis is confirmed by finding other clinical features of the endocrine disorder and a low plasma T_4 concentration. Carpal tunnel syndrome is also found in myxoedematous patients and is frequently bilateral. All the locomotor symptoms of hypothyroidism are relieved by appropriate replacement therapy, and require no other specific treatment.

The parathyroid

Hyperparathyroidism of any type may be associated with, and sometimes presents as, rheumatic symptoms. These are often vague aches and pains but may be a well-defined polyarthritis affecting the wrists, hands, feet, and knees particularly. X-ray shows erosive changes in the joints and also subperiosteal resorption, giving the involved bones a rat-bitten appearance, and some fluffy new bone formation. Pain may also arise from the thin bones found in hyperparathyroid patients and fractures in the feet may follow minimal trauma. Chondrocalcinosis may be a complication of hyperparathyroidism. Definitive treatment of the endocrine disorder produces remission of the rheumatic symptoms which may be slow, as bony healing is involved.

Metabolic bone disease

Other forms of metabolic bone disease also give rise to locomotor symptoms. Osteoporosis may be the only finding on investigation of a patient with back pain, and often produces symptoms before radiological evidence of vertebral collapse appears. There is controversy regarding the efficacy of treatment of osteoporosis, but some patients certainly appear to derive symptomatic relief from such empirical therapies as supplementary calcium, with or without anabolic steroids or vitamin D, even though their use is not associated with demonstrable remineralization of the spine. Exercise may help both to decrease the occurrence of osteoporosis and to relieve its symptoms. Osteomalacia produces less well-defined rheumatic symptoms with poorly localized bone pain and muscle weakness. Radiology may reveal pseudofractures, but the diagnosis in each form of metabolic bone disease rests primarily on clinical suspicion leading to appropriate biochemical studies and bone biopsy.

Paget's disease

Paget's disease of bone is often an incidental radiological finding. However, the bone pain it produces may cause ill-defined 'rheumatic' pains, and involvement of bone ends may produce accelerated osteoarthritis in associated joints. Treatment with etidronate disodium (Didronel®) or calcitonin is often successful in reducing bone pain but is rarely accompanied by sufficient remodelling to affect the progress of superimposed joint disease.

The pituitary

Hypersecretion of growth hormone in adults, usually as a result of a pituitary adenoma, leads to acromegaly which is characterized not only by visible enlargement of bones, especially of the head, hands, and feet, but also by a characteristic arthropathy. Almost any joint may be affected, with overgrowth of the bone ends and synovium leading to swelling, pain and stiffness usually of symme-

trical distribution. Symptoms are episodic, but if the underlying disease is not treated a severe disabling arthritis, similar to advanced osteoarthritis, may occur. Treatment with non-steroidal anti-inflammatory drugs may be needed in addition to treatment of the underlying disease.

The adrenal

Cushing's syndrome produces osteoporosis, which may cause backache and muscular weakness which is occasionally mistaken for 'rheumatism'. More prominent rheumatological problems are produced by pharmacological corticosteroid administration. As well as generalized osteoporosis, aseptic bone necrosis especially of the femoral heads occurs, particularly where high doses of corticosteroids are employed, e.g. after renal transplantation. Intra-articular corticosteroid injections may lead to local necrosis of cartilage and bone (steroid arthropathy) especially when the dramatic pain relief which this form of treatment affords leads the patient to undertake an extravagant amount of exercise.

Diabetes

Several rheumatic diseases are more prevalent in diabetes than the general population, including ankylosing vertebral hypertosis, neuroarthropathy, especially affecting the feet and leading to distal osteolysis, and periarthritis of the shoulder. This shoulder stiffness may be accompanied by changes in the hand to produce the shoulder–hand syndrome. The hand becomes shiny, oedematous, warm, and moist as a result of autonomic dysfunction. X-rays show spotty osteoporosis. The same condition can be produced by other causes of secondary shoulder disease, especially myocardial infarction, epilepsy, and treatment with barbiturates. Similar changes in the hand or foot following trauma are known as Sudeck's atrophy (page 16.89) and these, along with other rarer syndromes such as hip–foot syndrome and transient painful osteoporosis are grouped under the general term algodystrophy.

Treatment is with analgesic/anti-inflammatory drugs and vigorous physiotherapy. Prednisolone, 10–15 mg daily, controls symptoms in many patients.

The syndrome of diabetic cheiroarthropathy is now recognized as being much more common than previously thought. Alterations in collagen produce waxy thickening in the skin and tendon sheaths which pulls the fingers into flexion. The inability to extend the fingers fully is best demonstrated by the 'prayer sign', in which opposition of the hands in a praying position reveals an inability to oppose the flexor surfaces of the fingers. Cheiroarthropathy is associated with other signs of poor diabetic control such as neuropathy and retinopathy. Although the fingers feel stiff and clumsy they rarely curl sufficiently to produce severe handicap. In contrast, Dupuytren's contracture, which may also be associated with diabetes as well as liver disease and epilepsy, may be very disabling and require surgical treatment. The major structure involved is the palmar fascia, which binds the flexor tendons and produces severe flexion of the fingers into the palm. Interference with the digital vessels by the thickened fascia may lead to gangrene.

Rheumatic complaints associated with neurological disorders

Pain or weakness in muscles, whatever the cause, may be called 'rheumatism' by the patient, and should be clinically distinguished from joint disease. Muscle weakness leading to instability of joints may cause both pain and premature osteoarthritis.

Hemiplegia

Hemiplegia produes a diminution in the severity of both rheumatoid arthritis and osteoarthritis in the affected limbs, which may be completely spared if the rheumatic disease comes on after the stroke. Hemiplegic patients suffer from capsulitis, and occasional dislocation, of the shoulder because of stretching or tearing of the capsule by poor lifting techniques when the limb is incapable of producing protective muscle spasm. This condition can only be prevented by constant awareness of the problem by all staff dealing with hemiplegic patients and immaculate lifting techniques.

Paraplegic patients develop sacro-iliac joint changes and also soft tissue calcification, usually around the femora and pelvis, but these findings are of little clinical significance.

Neuroarthropathy (neuropathic joints; Charcot joints)

This is a severe disorganization of one or more joints secondary to neurological disease. It was originally described in patients with tabes dorsalis and was attributed to lack of pain sensation leading to repeated trauma and consequent joint damage. It is now appreciated that neuroarthropathy may be intensely painful. Other causes include diabetes mellitus, syringomyelia, and, more rarely, leprosy, Charcot–Marie–Tooth disease, myelomeningocoele, subacute combined degeneration of the cord, and congenital indifference to pain. Affected joints undergo a combination of destructive changes and profuse new bone formation. X-rays show loss of joint space, irregularity of the subchondral bone with some areas of bone loss, and others of marked sclerosis, and extensive new bone formation leading to deformity and loose body formation. Charcot joints are often unstable and require splintage both for stability and to relieve pain when it is present.

Soft tissue rheumatism

Some people seem prone to non-specific aches and pains of unknown aetiology which tend to be termed 'muscular rheumatism', 'non-articular rheumatism' or 'myofascial pain'. Such labels simply reflect ignorance of the underlying pathophysiology of these conditions. The term 'fibrositis', which has previously been used as a non-specific name for muscular rheumatic pain, especially in the back, has recently been defined as a syndrome of diffuse musculo-skeletal pain associated with tenderness over a series of well-defined 'trigger spots'. Patients with fibrositis are also prone to tension headaches and irritable bowel syndrome and some have evidence of psychological disturbance. This definition encompasses a wide spectrum of patients some of whom appear to have a distinct physical syndrome and others whose locomotor symptoms appear to be entirely produced by psychological stress. Better delineation of specific syndromes within this continuum is obviously necessary, but some other non-articular rheumatological problems are well characterized clinically even though their pathology is often poorly defined. It should be remembered in examining patients presenting with localized soft tissue problems that the various syndromes often either overlap or coincide. Thus in the upper limb conditions such as carpal tunnel syndrome, tennis elbow, and capsulitis of the shoulder occur not only in isolation but in combination with each other. This may reflect their association with narrow cervical canal diameter either congenital or acquired as a result of cervical spondylosis. Several of these conditions are commonly associated with overuse, so that restriction of shoulder movement occurring as the initial soft tissue lesion may lead to compensatory overuse of the elbow leading to tennis elbow as a secondary phenomenon.

The upper limb

The shoulder

The complex interrelationships of the muscles, tendons, and bursae related to the shoulder joint together with its wide range of movement appear to make it particularly vulnerable to the development of pain and restriction. Unfortunately, there is considerable confusion in the nomenclature of shoulder disease, with different authorities referring to the painful restricted shoulder syndrome as capsulitis of the shoulder, periarthritis, adhesive capsulitis, frozen shoulder, rotator cuff lesion, and subacromial or subdeltoid bursitis. Subtle differences among these 'different' entities are often described but appear to be of little practical importance.

Examination of the painful shoulder usually reveals diminished adduction and rotation, both active and passive, with reversal of the normal scapulo-humeral rhythm of movement. Tenderness may be related to the anterior part of the shoulder joint, the subacromial region or the posterior aspect of the shoulder. There is often muscle spasm, particularly of the upper fibres of trapezius, leading to pain in the neck, and pain may also be referred to the deltoid muscle or the medial condyle of the elbow as well as being felt diffusely around the whole of the shoulder girdle.

Pathologically the primary lesion appears to be tearing of fibres at the insertion of the rotator cuff with secondary inflammation both in relation to the healing fibres and in the subacromial bursa. As movement may exacerbate the pain, the limb tends to be held to the patient's side with consequent adhesion formation both within the joint and between the surrounding soft tissue structures.

Treatment is by reduction of pain, muscle spasm, and inflammation using non-steroidal anti-inflammatory agents and physical methods such as infrared radiation or ice. Thereafter the shoulder is remobilized, the accent being on teaching the patient an active home exercise regime which gradually but progressively increases the range of pain-free movement. Full relief of symptoms takes up to two years to accomplish and the range of movement is rarely normal after an episode of capsulitis although an adequate functional range is usually achieved. Resolution of symptoms may be accelerated by local corticosteroid injection into the rotator cuff, the joint itself or into the subacromial bursa. Occasionally manipulation, either under the influence of intravenous diazepam or general anaesthesia, is used to regain movement in a recalcitrant joint.

More localized lesions occasionally form part or all of the painful stiff shoulder syndrome. A painful arc of adduction between about 45° and 90° is associated with calcification in the supraspinatus tendon, the pain being related to the position in which the calcified portion is squeezed between the humeral head and the acromion. Patients with this condition can hold their arm fully elevated if it is passively moved to that position, but are inhibited from achieving elevation by the painful arc, and tend to drop the arm suddenly as the pain strikes rather than achieving smooth depression from an elevated position. Treatment is by local corticosteroid injection, ultrasound application to disrupt the calcium deposit or, occasionally, surgical removal of the deposit.

Bicipital tendinitis is differentiated by the finding of local tenderness over the insertion of the long head of the biceps and pain on resisted flexion of the pronated forearm. Local corticosteroid infiltration into the paratenon is usually effective but care must be exercised not to inject into the body of the tendon as this may lead to tendon rupture.

The elbow

Pain related to the common extensor origin on the lateral epicondyle is called tennis elbow and the less common syndrome of pain related to the common flexor origin on the medial epicondyle is called golfers' elbow. Both these are overuse phenomena usually relating to easily identifiable, often sporting, activities as their names imply. Tearing of muscle fibres near the bony insertions, or pulling up of the periosteum in that area, sets off a low-grade inflammatory reaction. There is local tenderness, and pain occurs when the muscles are brought into action. Ideally the precipitating movement should be avoided and the elbow rested, but this is usually advice the patient will not, or cannot, follow. It is very important in relation to all overuse injuries in sportsmen to examine the player's technique in conjunction with an experienced coach. Many such overuse injuries are the result of bad technique, and coaching to correct the technique is as important as medical treatment, for if faulty style is not eliminated recurrence is inevitable. Local corticosteroid injection is often helpful in reducing the pain although several injections may be necessary. Both manual frictions, applied by a physiotherapist, and ultrasound have also been used effectively in these conditions. Rarely surgery is required to achieve full symptom relief, especially where lifting of the periosteum has led to formation of a spicule of new bone which is often both palpable and visible on X-ray.

The wrist and hand

Tenosynovitis of the wrist and hand occurs as part of inflammatory disease such as rheumatoid arthritis, but may occur as a discrete entity as the result of overuse. The extreme example of this is cane-cutters' disease, a severe form of tenosynovitis of the wrist extensors suffered by sugar-cane cutters in the harvesting season. Lesser degrees of the same condition are associated with racquet sports or unaccustomed house-painting. As the thumb is, functionally, half the hand, the extensors of the thumb are particularly prone to develop overuse inflammation. Clinically the affected tendon sheath becomes painful, especially on use, tender, and swollen, and exhibits soft crepitus on movement. The overlying skin is often red and warm. The thickening induced by swelling of the tendon sheath may become sufficient, especially as it becomes more chronic, to prevent smooth running of the tendon. This condition is known as stenosing tenovaginitis or, in relation to the thumb extensors and abductors, de Quervain's disease. Treatment of simple tenosynovitis is by rest either in a splint or a plaster cast. Resolution may be aided by injection of corticosteroid into the tendon sheath, but significant obstruction requires surgical release of the stenotic sheath.

Nerve entrapment syndromes in the upper limb

Tenosynovitis in the wrist flexors may cause carpal tunnel syndrome. The carpal tunnel is formed in the concavity of the carpus by the anterior annular ligament on its volar aspect. The tunnel contains the flexor tendons and the median nerve, the latter being the structure prejudiced by any condition leading to diminution in the amount of space available in the tunnel. In addition to tenosynovitis, this condition may be caused by inflammatory or degenerative arthritis in the wrist, myxoedema, acromegaly, pregnancy, and oral contraceptive use. However, the commonest form is idiopathic carpal tunnel syndrome found predominantly in middle-aged women. The symptoms comprise burning pain related to the sensory supply of the median nerve, that is, the palmar surface of the thumb, index and middle fingers, with occasional involvement of part or all of the ring finger. The symptoms are characteristically worse at night, waking the patient from sleep and being relieved by shaking the hand and arm. The pain of carpal tunnel syndrome often extends proximally into the forearm. The thumb abductors in the thenar eminence may become wasted and weak, although such obvious muscle involvement usually occurs only later in the disease. Other aids to diagnosis include percussion over the carpal tunnel, which produces pain in the median nerve distribution in some patients (Tinel's sign), and flexing the patient's wrist, which may also reproduce the pain (Phalen's sign). The best diagnostic test is direct measurement of median nerve conduction, which is slowed by nerve compression. Treatment is of the underlying cause where possible. Symptomatic relief is often obtained by wearing splints with the wrist in slight extension at night and is the only treatment required in, for example, pregnancy. Other measures include local corticosteroid injection into the carpal tunnel and surgical decompression.

Compression of the ulnar nerve is less common. It usually occurs at the elbow where the nerve crosses the medial epicondyle and is associated either with arthritis in the joint producing local pressure, or stretching of the nerve by prolonged flexion. Tingling and numbness are experienced in the little, and sometimes ring, finger but motor dysfunction is a late feature. Treatment is by avoidance of damaging prolonged flexion or surgical removal of the compressive lesion, with transfer of the nerve where significant deformity is stretching it. More rarely ulnar compression takes place in the wrist; the site of the lesion is identified by nerve conduction studies.

Radial palsy is rare, involving mainly the posterior interosseous branch at the elbow. The muscles supplied become weak, reduced power of wrist extension being the best clinical sign. Treatment is by surgical release of the nerve.

The lower limb

The thigh and knee

Subtrochanteric bursitis produces symptoms which are often diagnosed as hip pain. The pain is felt in the lateral side of the thigh and is exacerbated by hip movement. Examination reveals local tenderness just distal to the greater trochanter, and the symptoms are relieved by local corticosteroid injection which may need to be repeated two or three times to achieve complete resolution. The prepatellar bursa becomes inflamed when subjected to repeated trauma – bent knee of miners, housemaids' knee or clergyman's knee – producing painful swelling distal to the lower pole of the patella. This area becomes red and oedematous and secondary infection may occur. Local injection is less effective in this site and excision is frequently required.

Ligamentous injuries to the knee are common accompaniments of sport and recreation. Pain may be accurately located at the medial or lateral side, but more diffuse pain and swelling may make differentiation from an internal derangement difficult. Local tenderness and swelling occurs, usually related to the tibial attachments of the medial or lateral ligaments, and pain may be produced on stressing the appropriate ligament by flexing the knee to about 20° and then forcibly abducting or adducting the leg with the thigh fixed. Local corticosteroid injection, frictions, ultrasound, and muscle strengthening may all be effective, but severe strains require a period of immobilization in a Robert–Jones bandage, or plaster of Paris. Muscle wasting, in the quadriceps especially, takes place with extreme rapidity when the knee is immobilized. To some extent this can be prevented by isometric exercises in the plaster, but it is of great importance not to allow vigorous use of the leg either in sport or at work until muscle strength and bulk have been progressively restored by graded exercise, or further sprains around the knee will almost inevitably occur.

The leg and ankle

In contrast to the partial tears seen elsewhere, the calf is the site of sudden rupture of tendons, usually the plantaris, or of parts of the gastrocnemius muscle belly. The patients feels sudden pain in the calf, with local tenderness and swelling. Plantaris rupture is of no significance and requires only an antalgesic heel-raise until the pain subsides. Achilles tendon or gastrocnemius rupture requires surgical repair. The ankle is prone to sporting ligamentous injuries and also those arising from accidents such as stepping awkwardly off kerbs. The stability of the ankle joint is almost entirely dependent on the integrity of the surrounding ligaments, and minor tears in them may produce serious problems resulting in a chronically 'weak' or unstable ankle. The ankle is also particularly prone to swelling after injury, as the hydrostatic pressure here is very high, and ligaments may be stretched or disrupted as a result of this. Strains or partial tears of the ankle ligaments should, therefore, be treated by immobilization in a tight bandage or plaster of Paris for a short period (two to three days) followed by an assessment of the severity of the damage and subsequent therapy aimed to reduce oedema and improve muscle tone. Posttraumatic rehabilitation with especial attention to fine balancing movements, most easily stimulated by use of a wobble-board, is essential if recurrent strains are to be avoided.

The foot

Bursal lesions in the foot are common. The great toe is subject to valgus deviation, especially when ill-fitting shoes are worn which force the great toe into valgus and cause rubbing on the lateral surface of the metatarso-phalangeal joint. Inflammation of the bursa at this position produces a bunion. Treatment is by prophylaxis – avoiding ill-fitting shoes – local pressure relief by padding, or surgical correction of the hallux valgus. The calcaneal bursa, between the achilles tendon and the calcaneum, may become inflamed, often in conjunction with achilles tendinitis. This latter condition produces heel pain and the swollen achilles tendon sheath is easily visible and palpable and is often red. This condition usually arises as a result of overuse, and may be exacerbated or caused by local pressure. Unfortunately the heel-tabs on running shoes which are often claimed to protect against this problem appear to be a prime cause of it. Rest and infiltration of corticosteroid into the paratenon are effective forms of treatment but, especially in sportsmen, it is important to modify the footwear to prevent recurrence. A rarer overuse condition is central core degeneration of the achilles tendon. Here the tendon itself is swollen and at operation is found to contain a degenerate central core which requires excision.

The longitudinal arch of the foot is maintained by the long plantar (spring) ligament. Laxity of this ligament produces a flat foot. Pain felt at the insertion of the ligament into the calcaneum occurs as part of the enthesopathy of seronegative spondarthritis but also as an isolated, idiopathic condition. Plantar spurs may be seen on X-ray in these patients, but well-defined spurs are of no pathological significance occurring as often in normal subjects as in patients with heel pain; in contrast, fluffy spurs are indicative of the presence of an inflammatory process. Initially treatment is by removing impact trauma by use of sorbo heel pads. If this fails local corticosteroid injection may be effective, although this procedure is painful. Surgery may be necessary.

Metatarsalgia or pain felt under the metatarsal heads is a common accompaniment of rheumatoid arthritis but also occurs as an isolated, idiopathic complaint. Overuse and inappropriate footwear are the usual precipitating causes. Treatment is by use of a metatarsal bar attached to the sole of the shoe or appropriately padded insoles. Morton's metatarsalgia is a variant of this condition caused by neuroma formation in the digital nerves at the level of the metatarsal heads. Careful examination reveals the tenderness to be located in the web space between the toes rather than under the metatarsal heads. Treatment is by surgical excision.

Nerve entrapment syndromes in the lower limb
Meralgia paraesthetica
Meralgia paraesthetica is a patch of numbness and tingling over the antero-lateral aspect of the thigh. It is caused by pressure on the lateral cutaneous nerve of the thigh and often resolves spontaneously.

The commonest nerve entrapment syndrome in the lower limb is interference with the common peroneal nerve as it winds around the neck of the fibula. Cysts, tumours or fractures in this region may cause this syndrome, as may prolonged cross-legged sitting, but the commonest cause is external pressure from plaster of Paris. There is pain and tingling on the outer border of the lower leg and the dorsum of the foot with weakness of dorsiflexion and eversion. The only confirmatory clinical sign of this condition available to the examiner when the patient is in a plaster is loss of sensation in the first web-space. Treatment is by removal of pressure.

Hypermobility syndrome
Hypermobility in joints has until recently only attracted attention as a part of the heritable disorders of connective disease such as Ehlers–Danlos syndrome. It is now apparent that some people have greater than normal flexibility of their joints, and that this produces symptoms. Chronic backache (the loose back syndrome) accompanies spinal hypermobility, and most other symptoms are of pain, aching, and, paradoxically, a feeling of stiffness usually in the fingers and knees. Diagnosis is by examination for the signs of hypermobility which are ability to (1) appose the thumb to the ipsilateral forearm, (2) passively extend the little finger to 90° from the dorsum of the wrist, (3) hyperextend the elbows (4) hyperextend the knees, (5) bend forward and place the hands flat on the floor with the knees straight. The presence of the appropriate feature in each affected joint is scored one, giving a possible total of nine, a score of six indicating generalized hypermobility. Treatment is by explanation, avoiding excessive movements, especially in children who are prone to demonstrate their 'double-joints' to their friends, and isometric exercises, especially where the back is involved, to splint and limit the affected joints with bulky muscles. The chronic discomfort is often such that long-term non-steroidal anti-inflammatory medication is required. Hypermobility is a precipitating cause of osteoarthritis.

References
Beighton, P. Grahame, R. and Bird, H. (1983). *Hypermobility of joints.* Springer-Verlag, Berlin.
Cyriax, J. H. and Cyriax, P. J. (1983). *Illustrated manual of orthopaedic medicine.* Butterworth, London.
Dixon, A. St. J. (ed.) (1979). Soft tissue rheumatism. *Clinics in rheumatic diseases* Vol. 5. W. B. Saunders, London.
Holt, P. J. L. (ed.) (1981). Endocrine aspects of rheumatic diseases. *Clinics in rheumatic diseases* Vol. 7. W. B. Saunders, London.
Williams, J. G. P. (1979). *A colour atlas of injuries in sport.* Wolfe, London.

ALGODYSTROPHY
(reflex sympathetic dystrophy or Sudeck's atrophy)
R. M. ATKINS AND R. B. DUTHIE

Introduction
Algodystrophy is a syndrome consisting of pain, vasomotor and sudomotor instability, early subcutaneous swelling followed by late atrophy, and loss of joint movement (Fig. 1). It is associated with focal juxta-articular osteoporosis and its uncertain aetiology is reflected by its many synonyms (Table 1).

The condition typically follows minor trauma, although some patients remember no precipitating event. It may follow painful medical conditions such as myocardial infarction or herpes zoster. It has recently been shown that a transient form of the syndrome occurs very commonly following Colles' fracture.

Aetiology
The aetiology is obscure, and there is no suitable model for the condition. The most widely accepted hypothesis suggests the existence of an abnormal reflex arc mediated by the sympathetic nervous system. Following trauma there are alterations in the vasomotor status of the affected region due to a self-limiting sympathetic reflex. It is suggested that in algodystrophy this reflex is abnormally sustained and intense leading to a prolonged disturbance of the microcirculation. At capillary level there is inadequate tissue nutrition which causes local acidosis and dystrophy. The acid metabolites may then contribute to the increased osteoclastic

activity which may also be a direct effect of the sympathetic response. The mechanism by which the abnormal sympathetic state is maintained is controversial. One suggestion is that an abnormal synapse is set up peripherally between injured efferent and afferent nerve fibres in an area where destruction of the myelin sheath allows 'short-circuiting' of the impulses. Alternatively, potentiation of the normal feedback mechanism may occur in the internuncial pool in the spinal cord due to prolonged and continuous pain impulses which are carried by afferents in the sympathetic nervous system. Finally, the abnormal personality of many patients with the severe syndrome may give rise to unusual efferent impulses from the cerebral cortex, which potentiate the sympathetic reflex by modulation of the pain pathway in the substantia gelatinosa of the dorsal horn.

Clinical features

The most common sites of involvement are the distal parts of the limbs, although it is well recognized in the knee and it has been reported in both the hip and the spine. The elbow is the least commonly involved limb joint. When the shoulder only is involved, the condition is commonly termed a 'frozen shoulder', whereas involvement of both the shoulder and the hand, especially following myocardial infarction, is called the shoulder–hand syndrome. Vasomotor instability and swelling are most marked when the algodystrophic process affects the distal portion of a limb and when a hip or shoulder alone is involved, these signs may be absent.

There are several characteristics of the natural history of the dis-

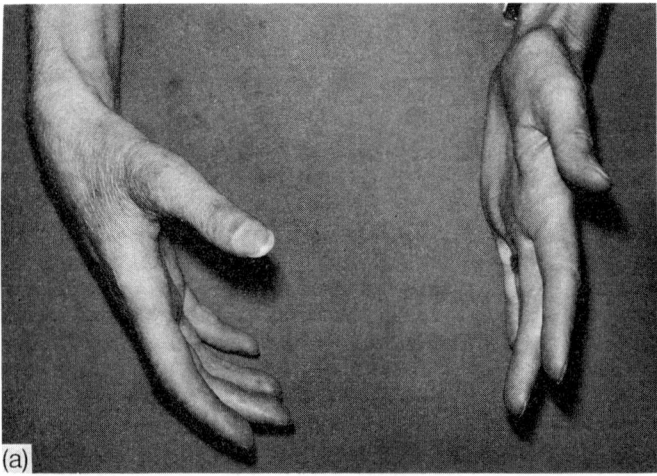

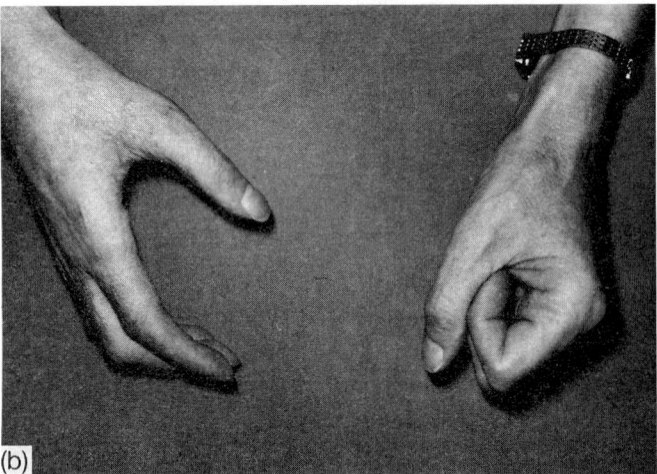

Fig. 1 Algodystrophy of the right hand with the normal left hand for comparison. The limitation of movement is shown in full finger (a) extension and (b) flexion. Note also the atrophic spindle-like appearance of the fingers with loss of the joint crease.

Table 1 Synonyms for algodystrophy

Algodystrophy
Sudeck's atrophy
Sudeck's post-traumatic osteodystrophy
Reflex sympathetic dystrophy syndrome
Post-traumatic sympathetic atrophy
Post-traumatic painful osteoporosis
Shoulder–hand syndrome
Minor causalgia

order, irrespective of the aetiology or the affected site. Its onset is usually gradual with increasing pain in the region of a joint or joints which is more severe and long-lasting than would be expected from the nature of the precipitating event. In the case of a fracture, the joints affected are not those involved in the fracture, and, for example, in a Colles' fracture the pain is commonly most marked in the fingers and shoulder and begins some weeks after the fracture.

The type of pain is variable, occurring initially only at the extremes of movement, but as the condition progresses it becomes more constant and in the case of the hand particularly, proximal radiation occurs. The intensity and nature of the pain also vary from a dull ache to causalgic pain or to a severe lancinating pain which may be completely incapacitating. In severe cases the patient will avoid contact of the affected part with any form of covering. Occasionally a small trigger zone is found, which when touched induces severe pain in the whole limb. The patient may be so frightened of the limb being knocked that in the case of the upper limb the affected part is held in a characteristic position protected by the other hand. In this case the shoulder is internally rotated, the elbow flexed with the wrist palmar flexed in half pronation. The limb may be held in this position for so long that contractures occur giving rise to a characteristic appearance.

The vasomotor instability may take several forms. Classically early in the condition, there is a 'hot phase' which lasts for a few days to a few weeks. At this time the skin is warm, red, and swollen, and there may be local sweating. Later on a 'cold phase' supervenes, with a cool, clammy, cyanotic appearance. Finally, the vasomotor instability disappears completely. Other patients may complain of abnormal temperature sensitivity of the affected part, the limb being warm and red in hot surroundings and cool and cyanotic in a cold environment. Excess sweating of the affected area may occur at any stage but tends to return to normal late in the condition.

In the beginning there is a variable degree of subcutaneous oedema which may pit but as this subsides the skin and subcutaneous tissues become atrophic. It is the combination of oedema, atrophy, and vasomotor instability which gives rise to the classical shiny, discoloured appearance of the affected part.

From an early stage joint movements are limited. Initially, full passive movement is possible, and the finding of a patient with a limited range of movement while awake which becomes full under anaesthetic, may erroneously lead to suspicion of malingering. As the condition progresses, the joint limitation becomes more fixed due to collateral ligament contracture and tendinous adhesions, and a degree of muscle wasting occurs.

Systemic signs of inflammation are almost universally lacking. The patient is not toxic, has a normal pulse rate, and is apyrexial. There is no regional lymphadenopathy. The peripheral pulses are normal and neurological examination is unremarkable, apart from occasional hyperreflexia. White cell count and ESR are invariably normal.

Patients suffering severely from the syndrome often show a particular personality type, being very dependent, anxious, and depressed, and appearing to overreact to the pain and disability of the syndrome. It is not clear whether these personality traits predate the onset of the syndrome but it may be that a refusal to mobilize the painful involved joints leads to a poorer late result.

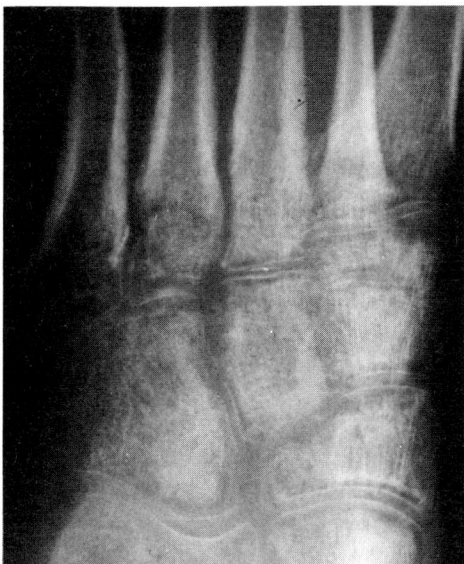

Fig. 2 Patchy osteoporosis with subchondral lysis and maintenance of the joint space in a case of algodystrophy of the foot.

Radiographic changes are late, lagging behind the symptoms by up to two months and, in the case of the mild and transient form of the disorder, changes may not be seen. The classical appearance, seen in severe cases, is of patchy osteoporosis with a subchondral lucent line (Fig. 2) changing after a time to severe local osteoporosis, giving a 'washed out' appearance. At no stage of the disorder is there any narrowing of the joint space or thinning of the articular cartilage. This is an important negative sign for the diagnosis of algodystrophy. None of these radiographic features is diagnostic of the disorder.

In contrast to the late and variable appearances on X-ray, bone scintigraphy with technetium-99-labelled diphosphonate gives a characteristic appearance on delayed films early in the disorder. Uniformly increased uptake of tracer is seen throughout the bones of the region involved in the algodystrophic process, but the increased uptake is most marked in the periarticular regions (Fig. 3).

Algodystrophy is nearly always a transient condition, resolving after a few months to two years. Long-term sequelae occur more frequently in the upper limb. These include joint contractures, most commonly flexion contracture of the proximal interphalangeal joints of the hand, and diminished abduction and external rotation of the shoulder. Permanent thinning of the skin and loss of subcutaneous tissue may occur. After the acute osteoporotic phase has passed, bone density may be visibly increased on serial X-rays but in more severe or chronic cases, permanent changes in trabecular bone structure are seen. Bone scintigraphy ceases to be abnormal after a variable period.

Treatment

The treatment of algodystrophy is controversial, because of its transient nature, uncertain aetiology, and protean manifestations. The mainstay is physiotherapy, the aim of which is to maintain passive joint movement and to encourage active use of the affected part until the underlying condition resolves. Paraffin wax baths may be particularly helpful in mobilization. In this way late contractures are minimized, but there is no evidence to suggest that giving physiotherapy either before or after the condition has started has any effect on the underlying natural history. Non-steroidal anti-inflammatory agents seem to provide better relief from pain than narcotic drugs.

Manipulation of the sympathetic nervous system has been used in various forms for many years. Leriche was the first to note relief of pain by local femoral sympathectomy. This radical technique

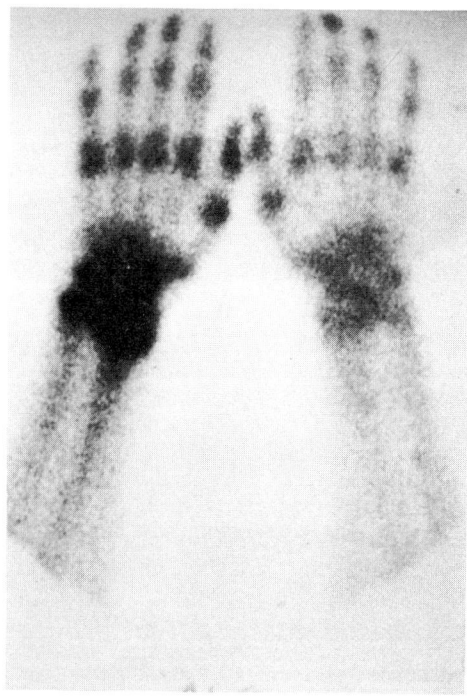

Fig. 3 Characteristic bone scan appearance in algodystrophy. Note the uniform increase in uptake in the periarticular regions of the finger joints compared with the normal side. The increased uptake at the wrist is due to trauma.

has given way to the use of ganglion blockade using local anaesthetic. Steinbrocker studied a series of 69 patients and noted complete recovery in 32 per cent, appreciable benefit in 49 per cent, and failure in 19 per cent of patients following ganglion blockade. The most important determinant of success is treatment of the patient in the early stage of the disease before the appearance of trophic changes. For the upper limb, stellate ganglion blockade is used, whereas the lumbar sympathetic chain is infiltrated for the leg. Injections are repeated as necessary depending on the patient's response.

Postganglionic, sympathetic blockade using guanethidine infusion intravenously with a tourniquet inflated proximally on the limb has been shown by some to give good relief. Local anaesthetic may be added to the infusion.

Systemic therapy using β-blockade, e.g. propanolol, has been shown to work in some cases. It is not known whether the action of the drug is due to a local effect on the algodystrophic process or due to a central anxiolytic effect permitting the patient to be more co-operative with physical therapy.

Subcutaneous injection of calcitonin daily for 4–8 weeks has been shown to be effective, particularly in lower limb algodystrophy. Calcitonin is a naturally occurring polypeptide which inhibits bone resorption by osteoclasts, but which also has vasomotor and analgesic effects. It is not clear to which of these properties calcitonin owes its efficacy in the condition. Systemic corticosteroids have been used by some with variable results. However, local corticosteroid injection has been shown to be particularly useful in adhesive capsulitis of the shoulder.

References

Doury, P., Dirheimer, Y. and Pattin, S. (1981). *Algodystrophy*. Springer-Verlag, Berlin.

Lee Lankford, L. and Thompson, J. E. (1977). Sympathetic dystrophy, upper and lower extremity: diagnosis and management. *American Academy of Orthopaedic Surgeons Instructional Course Lectures 1977* **26**, 163–178.

—— (1982). Reflex sympathetic dystrophy. In *Operative hand surgery* (ed. D. P. Green), pp. 539–563. Churchill Livingstone, Edinburgh.

SECTION 17
DISORDERS OF THE SKELETON

DISORDERS OF THE SKELETON

R. SMITH

Introduction

Teeth excluded, bone is the only tissue which is normally mineralized, and this enables it to perform an obvious and important structural function. The presence of mineral should not encourage one to believe that bone is inert, or to neglect the considerable cellular and metabolic activity which occurs within it. Many disorders affect the skeleton and only some can be dealt with here. Therefore a number of localized or acquired conditions such as fractures, deformities, infections, and tumours often dealt with by orthopaedic surgeons are excluded. The descriptions which follow consider first, conditions such as osteoporosis, osteomalacia, parathyroid bone disease, and Paget's disease, generally thought of as metabolic; second, those which appear to arise from disorders of collagen synthesis and mucopolysaccharide breakdown; and third, some rare inherited and familial disorders of bone where the cause is often obscure. Mineralization and ossification occurring in non-skeletal sites will also be discussed.

To understand these diseases a brief account of bone physiology and a summary of some clinical features are given. Parathyroid hormone and calcitonin are dealt with in detail elsewhere (see page 10.51 *et seq.*).

Physiology of bone

In the last few years, our understanding of bone physiology has widened. There is much interest in the cells of bone and how they communicate; and in non-collagen as well as collagen components of bone matrix. Advances of knowledge in bone disease such as osteoporosis, osteopetrosis, osteogenesis imperfecta, and Paget's disease reflect this.

The mammalian skeleton serves two main functions. The first is structural; the second is to act as an accessible mineral store. Bone is a metabolically active tissue apparently enclosed in a cellular envelope thought to separate the extracellular fluid space from a specialized fluid particular to bone. The formation, resorption, and composition of the skeleton is controlled by bone cells whose activity is modified by many factors. These include circulating hormones such as calcitonin, parathyroid hormone, and vitamin D metabolites, local factors such as prostaglandins, and mechanical forces.

There are still many unanswered questions in bone physiology. They include the control of mineralization and the factors determining the size, shape, and internal structure of the skeleton.

Bone cells

These are osteoblasts, osteoclasts, and osteocytes. Osteoblasts are bone-forming cells derived from precursor stromal cells which have several functions. Probably the most important of these are the formation and secretion of collagen and non-collagen proteins to form bone matrix, and its subsequent mineralization. The way in which mineralization occurs is not fully understood but the osteoblast contains enzymes such as alkaline phosphatase, which is also a pyrophosphatase, which are important in this process. An additional role of osteoblasts now appears to be the control of osteoclastic activity. Osteoclasts are multinucleated bone-resorbing cells derived from haemopoietic monocyte/macrophage pre-

cursors which resorb intact bone by mechanisms which are disputed.

Osteocytes are derived from osteoblasts and can be found either on the surface of bone or within the mineralized bone in lacunae. The lacunae of separate osteocytes are connected by canaliculi, through which run the osteocyte processes. In neither of these positions is the osteocyte inert, although the extent of its effect on perilacunar bone is controversial.

The anatomical relationship between these cells is shown in Fig. 1. Recent studies on isolated bone cells and cultured osteoblast-like populations show that cells contain receptors for many hormones, and that the hormonal relationships between bone cells are very complex. Bone fluid has not been directly analysed, so that although its composition is thought to be different from that of the general extracellular fluid, actual figures are not known.

Bone matrix

The organic matrix of bone is 90 per cent collagen. Collagen is the main extracellular protein in the body; more than 50 per cent of it is in the skeleton and the strength of bone depends on it. The remaining 10 per cent of bone matrix contains a variety of non-collagen substances. These include osteocalcin (or gla protein), sialoprotein, bone-specific proteoglycans, and several phosphoproteins of which osteonectin may be particularly important. Bone also contains non-collagen substances apparently concentrated from plasma, such as α2HS glycoprotein.

Collagen

The collagens are a family of molecules characterized by protease-resistant triple-helical Gly X Y repetitive sequences. Collagen is synthesized (Fig. 2) within fibroblasts (or osteoblasts) from long polypeptides or α-chains. Each collagen molecule consists of a helix of three α-chains. There are at least 10 genetically different collagens. The important fibrillar collagens and their α-chain composition are shown in Table 1. Each type of α-chain has its own genetic control and its own specific mRNA. During its formation

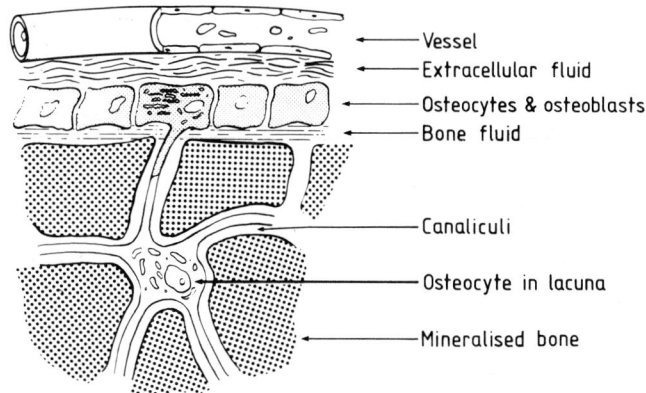

Fig. 1 To demonstrate the normal relationship between bone, bone cells, extracellular fluid, and blood vessels. Transfer of ions may occur through or between the cells covering the bone. The bone fluid is continuous with that in the canaliculi and separated from the general extracellular fluid. The osteoid layer covering the newly formed bone is omitted.

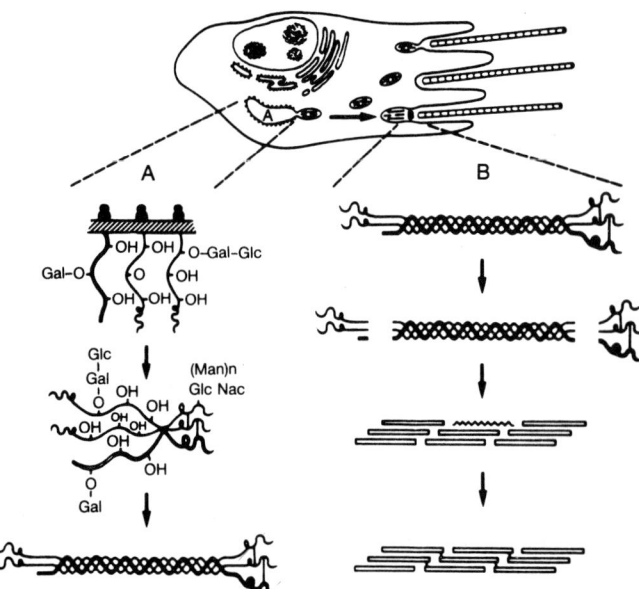

Fig. 2 To show synthesis and assembly of collagen molecules from the individual pro α-chains. Within the fibroblast (A) these chains are modified, assembled, and folded into the triple helix. In (B) the pro collagen chains are exported and shortened and self assemble into fibrils which cross link. Gal, galactose; Glc, glucose; GlcNac, N-acetylglucosamine; and (Man)$_n$ mannose residues. (Reprinted by permission of The *New England Journal of Medicine* and the authors, Prockop and Kivirikko, **311**, 376–386.)

within the cell the large precursor molecule undergoes important posttranslational modifications; it is then secreted from the cell and molecular self assembly and fibre formation is completed.

The structure of the precursor or pro α-chain contains enough information and equipment to ensure that these chains form molecules and that the molecules self assemble into microfibrils or fibrils. The result of this complex series of metabolic steps is a cross-linked fibre formed from an array of genetically specific rope-like triple-helical collagen molecules. These different genetic collagens have specific tissue distributions, and different properties apparently suited to their function. A striking example is the difference between the loosely organized collagen of basement membrane and the strong oriented fibres in bone. The synthesis of the α-chains of collagen is controlled by specific genes whose chromosomal location is different for each chain (thus the gene for α1(I) is on chromosome 17, and for α2(I) on chromosome 7). These genes are large and have a striking and highly conserved structure. In the three fibrillar collagens the 4.5 kb of coding sequence is dispersed in 51 exons separated by non-coding sequences (introns) of varying length, and the longest gene is 38 kb. Repetitive 54 bp exons, sometimes replaced by 108, 45 or 99 bp, code for 6 Gly X Y triplets in the helical region.

The clinical effect of inherited disorders of collagen is dealt with later (page 17.25). In bone, collagen is broken down predominantly by a specific collagenase which splits the native triple-helical molecule three-quarters of the way along its length into two unequal fragments; subsequently these large polypeptide fragments can be attacked by a variety of additional enzymes. When collagen is degraded some of its peptide fragments are excreted in the urine; these contain amino acids such as hydroxyproline and hydroxylysine previously formed by posttranslational modification of proline and lysine already incorporated into the protein chain. These modified amino acids cannot be used for further protein synthesis and their excretion rate indicates the rate of collagen turnover, particularly that of bone. This is so because the skeleton contains relatively so much of the body's collagen, and bone colla-

gen is metabolically more active than many other collagens. Since bone resorption and formation are closely linked, the excretion of hydroxyproline is closely related to the plasma alkaline phosphatase concentration, a measure of osteoblastic activity.

In bone the arrangement of collagen is such that there are spaces or 'hole' zones within the three-dimensional staggered array of the collagen molecules, in which the first crystals of bone mineral appear to be laid down. The collagen fibres are normally arranged in concentric lamellae on bone surfaces and because of their regular arrangement they are birefringent. When present in excess they produce the characteristic histological appearance of osteomalacia (see page 17.15). Where the turnover of bone is considerably increased, as in Paget's disease and osteitis fibrosa cystica, or where the collagen is abnormal as in severe osteogenesis imperfecta, the arrangement of some of the collagen is random (fibre or woven bone).

Proteoglycans
These complex macromolecules occupy a considerable amount of space in many tissues, and because of their size control hydration and structure. They consist of a protein core with carbohydrate side chains attached to it by linkage regions, but the structure and composition varies considerably from one proteoglycan to another. In the skeleton, bone proteoglycans are smaller than those in cartilage; in both they may modify collagen synthesis and fibre formation. A series of inherited enzyme defects leads to the accumulation of partially degraded proteoglycans, and causes the group of disorders called the mucopolysaccharidoses (see page 17.30, in which there are important skeletal abnormalities.

Non-collagen proteins
Analysis of the non-collagen proteins of bone matrix depends on the source and type of bone and the methods used. In adult cortical bone, sialoprotein (which contains a large amount of sialic acid) is abundant; in fetal bone a number of phosphoproteins may be identified. It has been considered that one of these, osteonectin, specifically links calcium to collagen but this now seems unlikely. Bone gla protein (osteocalcin) is of interest because of the vitamin K dependent carboxylation of its peptide-bound glutamic acid. The synthesis of this abundant product of the osteoblast appears to depend on $1,25(OH)_2D_3$, and its plasma levels are apparently related to bone formation rate, but its function is unknown.

Bone mineral and mineralization
The specific feature which distinguishes bone from all other tissues except dentine is the presence of mineral. This is a calcium phosphate complex with the overall composition of hydroxyapatite, initially present in an amorphous form which soon becomes crystalline (the importance of the amorphous phase in early mineralization may have been overemphasized). Mineral is deposited on the collagenous matrix of bone to which it adds structural rigidity and it constitutes about 99 per cent of the body's calcium. For these reasons it is of considerable importance; where mineralization of the bone matrix is defective, as in osteomalacia, the bone is soft and easily deformed; and in any disturbance of calcium metabolism the skeletal mineral must play an important part (Fig. 3).

The factors which control mineralization are not fully understood but must be both chemical and cellular. Until the precise composition of bone fluid is known the physicochemical processes will remain obscure. However, the concentrations of calcium and phosphorus in the general extra-cellular fluid appear to be sufficient to maintain crystallization, if not to initiate it, and this mineralization may normally be prevented by the action of inhibitors. One such potential inhibitor is pyrophosphate, which can *in vitro* prevent the formation and subsequent development of hydroxyapatite crystals. The body contains considerable amounts of pyrophosphate which appear to be continually and rapidly removed by the action of naturally occurring pyrophosphatases.

Table 1 Characteristics of the major human fibrillar collagens

Collagen type	Subunits	Chromosomal assignment	Known molecular configurations	Major tissue distribution (human)
I	$\alpha1(I)$	17q2l-qter	$[\alpha1(I)]_2\alpha2(I)$	All tissues except cartilage and vitreous. Very high concentrations in major stress-bearing structures such as tendons, bone and dentine, ligaments, skin, blood vessels
	$\alpha2(I)$	7q22	and $[\alpha1(I)]_3$	
II	$\alpha1(II)$	12q	$[\alpha1(II)]_3$	Cartilage, vitreous of the eye
III	$\alpha1(III)$	2q23	$[\alpha1(III)]_3$	Most tissues except bone and dentine. Highest concentrations in pliable tissues such as skin, gut and blood vessel walls, lung

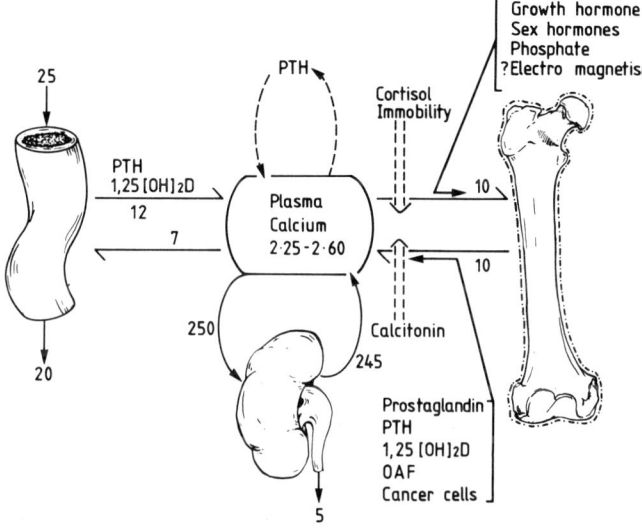

Fig. 3 An outline of calcium balance. The figures represent the daily exchange in adults in mmol, and the concentration in the plasma in mmol/l. To convert to mg multiply by 40. The considerable (but unknown) exchange between bone fluid and general extracellular fluid is not shown.

Therefore one mechanism by which mineralization might occur is by the local enzymatic removal of pyrophosphate. Since osteoblasts (and matrix vesicles) produce alkaline phosphatase, and also a pyrophosphatase, they could control mineralization of bone in this way. A central role for the osteoblast in mineralization would also explain why the collagen of bone mineralizes whilst that of other tissues without osteoblasts normally does not. Another difference between these tissues is the presence in bone of the specific non-collagen proteins.

Recent work has further emphasized the importance of cells in mineralization. In mineralizing cartilage and bone, and probably in all mineralizing tissues, so-called calcifying vesicles have been found which also contain alkaline phosphatase and pyrophosphatase, and in which the early crystals of bone appear to be laid down. The role of matrix vesicles (apparently derived from chondrocytes and osteoblasts) remains controversial. It seems that they are important in the mineralization of cartilage, woven bone, and various non-skeletal tissues, but it is difficult to see where they could contribute to the mineralization of lamellar bone.

Bone growth, modelling, and remodelling

The shape of the bone alters rapidly during growth and slowly in adult life, and the factors which control it are little understood. In childhood and adolescence the most dramatic changes occur in linear growth by a series of alterations at the growth plate; but bone is also subject to continual processes of remodelling, with osteo-clastic bone resorption and osteoblastic new bone formation, which give the adult bone its shape. In later life these processes are very slow; and in long bones the rate of endosteal bone resorption exceeds the rate of periosteal new bone formation, so that the width of the cortex is progressively narrowed whilst the external diameter slowly increases.

The events which occur at the growth plates are complex; in effect regular rows of cartilage cells arranged parallel to the long axis of the bone undergo a series of specific changes to produce a tissue in which columns of chondrocytes are separated by columns of calcified cartilage matrix. In the formation of bone this area of preliminary calcification is removed (together with the chondrocytes) by the action of chondroclasts, and bone tissue is laid down and mineralized in its place. This regular but complex succession of events may be altered by many factors of which rickets produced by vitamin D deficiency is a classic example.

Following the formation of the new bone in the metaphyseal areas, osteoclastic modelling continues; where the osteoclasts are ineffective, as in osteopetrosis, a club-shaped appearance results. Bone formation and bone resorption continue to be closely linked throughout life. Most disorders which affect one will also affect another; for example, in Paget's disease of bone where bone turnover may be increased by some 50 times above normal the rates of resorption and formation remain balanced. In contrast sudden immobilization, which rapidly reduces the rate of bone formation without a similar fall in resorption, causes considerable net loss of bone. During life overall bone formation must exceed resorption in childhood and adolescence; and in early adult life the processes are equal. However from about the age of 30 years bone formation rate progressively falls behind that of bone resorption so that increasing age is one of the most important factors leading to structural collapse of the skeleton.

The way in which formation and resorption of bone are linked remains unknown, but the mechanisms presumably involve the bone cells; likewise it is not known how stress on bone stimulates osteoblastic activity, although small electric signals (piezoelectricity) may be important. Recent work identifies so-called coupling factors thought to link bone resorption and formation. Cultured osteoblastic bone cells subjected to deformation produce prostaglandins as do similar cells exposed to electromagnetic fields.

It is important to recognize the continual cellular activity within bone and the effect of physical forces upon it. This is not only a feature of the growing skeleton and of young bone. The anatomical basis for this activity has been defined as the BMU (bone multicellular unit) which goes through a well-defined cycle of cellular events, beginning with activation of bone resorbing cells, followed by a phase of reversal and the formation of new bone by osteoblasts. What causes recruitment of the osteoclasts and why resorption is followed by formation is only dimly perceived, and the cellular events are complex. Clearly the amount of bone eventually produced will depend on many factors, for example, the number of cells involved, the extent and duration of their activity, and the length of the reversal phase.

Control of bone composition

More is known about the factors which control the mineral content of bone and are related to changes in calcium and phosphate metabolism than those which control its matrix. Changes in mineral will necessarily be associated with changes in matrix; examples of this are bone resorption and bone growth. The main hormones known to affect mineral homeostasis are vitamin D, parathyroid hormone (PTH), and calcitonin, but there are many others of considerable importance, such as the somatomedins (derived from growth hormone), the sex hormones, and locally acting agents such as prostaglandins and osteoclast-stimulating factors. Since the parathyroids and calcitonin are dealt with elsewhere (see page 10.51 *et seq.*), they will only be considered briefly here.

Calcium and phosphorus

The movements of calcium within the body and the factors which control them in the adult human are shown in Fig. 3. These will be different during times of growth and physiological stress such as pregnancy and lactation. Normally only a fraction of the calcium in the diet is retained, and the greatest daily movements are through the kidneys and the cellular envelope which supposedly surrounds the skeleton. The skeleton contains approximately 1 kg (25 000 mmol) of calcium. The relative importance of these renal and skeletal contributions to overall calcium homeostasis may differ in different disorders. Within this system of control the total plasma calcium is closely regulated between about 2.25 and 2.60 mmol/l (9.0 and 10.2 mg/100 ml). Calcium in the plasma is either ionized (47 per cent of total calcium), protein-bound (46 per cent), or complexed. It is the ionized fraction which is important in the control of parathyroid hormone and calcitonin secretion. Precise control of the plasma concentration is essential. Recent work continues to emphasize the importance of calcium in many functions of the body. These include muscle contraction, endocytosis, and exocytosis, cell mobility, the movement of chromosomes, and the release of neurotransmitters. Calcium is the most abundant and versatile intracellular messenger. A major receptor which appears to mediate and modulate most of its activities is the protein calmodulin which is almost universally present in cells above the level of bacteria.

The mechanisms which control phosphate metabolism are less well understood; in the past its absorption across the intestine has been thought to follow passively that of calcium. Three factors determine the plasma phosphate; the flow into the extracellular space from gut, bone, and soft tissue; the renal tubular reabsorption of phosphate; and the glomerular filtration rate (GFR). In steady-state conditions with a normal GFR the main determinant of plasma phosphate is the rate of reabsorption by the kidney which is particularly influenced by parathyroid hormone. There are inherited disorders with low and high tubular reabsorption of phosphate (hypophosphataemic rickets and tumoral calcinosis, respectively). Phosphate should be considered as an ion of importance in its own right, and not as a poor relation to calcium as has been the case.

Vitamin D

Knowledge of vitamin D has increased very rapidly within the last decade. It was initially identified as a necessary constituent of food and called a vitamin, but it is now more often considered as a prohormone manufactured from precursors in the skin when exposed to ultraviolet light and converted to metabolically active steroid-like metabolites according to the needs of the target tissues. There are two forms of vitamin D. One, vitamin D_3, cholecalciferol, is synthesized in the skin by the action of ultraviolet light on the precursor 7-dehydrocholesterol (pro vitamin D). The other, vitamin D_2, ergocalciferol, is made artificially by the irradiation of ergosterol, a plant sterol, and is used to fortify foods with vitamin D. The main dietary sources of vitamin D_3 are the oily fishes and dairy products. Vitamin D_2 is added in particular to margarine.

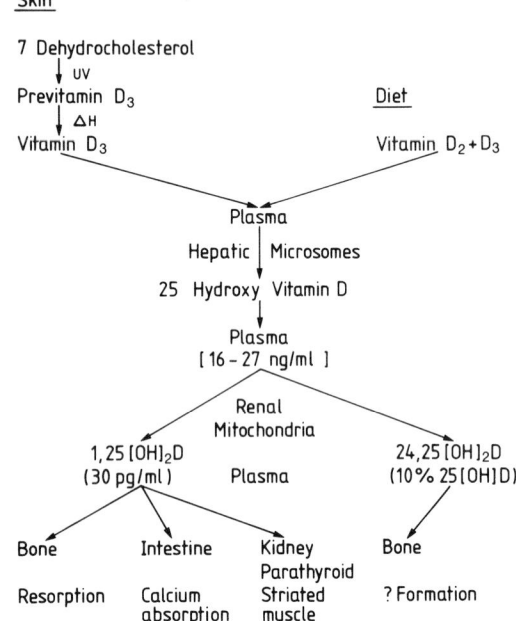

Fig. 4 An outline of the metabolism of vitamin D. The figures in brackets indicate the normal range of mean concentration in the plasma; that of 24,25 (OH) $_2$D is given as a percentage of circulating 25(OH)D concentration which itself shows seasonal differences.

The biosynthesis of vitamin D_3 in the skin is complex and it is not exactly known where it occurs. The effect of ultraviolet light on its precursors is to form a previtamin D_3 which slowly isomerizes to vitamin D_3 at body temperature (Fig. 4). Only vitamin D_3, and not previtamin D_3, is bound to a specific protein which transports it to the liver for the first of its metabolic modifications. Both vitamins D_3 and D_2 undergo a 25-hydroxylation in the hepatic microsomes. This 25-hydroxylated derivative circulates in the plasma, can be readily measured, and is a good index of vitamin D status; thus it is increased by sunlight and by oral vitamin D, and tends to be low in the elderly and those with osteomalacia.

The next important step in vitamin D metabolism is the renal formation of the dihydroxylated derivatives 1,25(OH)$_2$D and 24,25(OH)$_2$D. Whether 1 or 24 hydroxylation occurs appears to depend particularly on the prevailing level of plasma calcium. 1,25(OH)$_2$D, considered to be the most active metabolite of vitamin D, is synthesized particularly when there is hypocalcaemia. The activity of the renal-1-α-hydroxylase, which is located in the mitochondria of the cells of the renal tubules, is stimulated by low plasma calcium, low plasma phosphate, and parathyroid hormone. It also appears to be affected by the oestrogens, prolactin, and somatomedins which could provide a way of increasing calcium absorption during physiological need. The production of 1,25(OH)$_2$D is closely controlled by a negative feedback mechanism, and is integrated with the action of parathyroid hormone. 1,25(OH)$_2$D itself increases plasma calcium by stimulating bone resorption and increasing calcium absorption across the small intestine, in part by controlling the synthesis of a calcium-binding protein within the small intestinal cell. Thus when PTH secretion is increased by hypocalcaemia the subsequent stimulation of 1-α-hydroxylation produces an increase in 1,25(OH)$_2$D and an increase in plasma calcium which effectively removes the stimulus to further 1-α-hydroxylation.

Since one of the most striking effects of 1,25(OH)$_2$D on bone is to produce osteoclastic bone resorption it is difficult to understand how giving its precursor (vitamin D) cures rickets; however, the administration of vitamin D or the exposure of skin to ultraviolet light in effect increases the concentration of a number of vitamin

D metabolites, and there is some evidence that $24,25(OH)_2D$ has effects on bone which are different from those of $1,25(OH)_2D$. Although the main target tissues of vitamin D and its metabolites are bone and the small intestine, they are probably not the only ones. Thus when highly radioactive $1,25(OH)_2D$ is given it may be demonstrated in tissues such as the parathyroid, the renal tubular cells, the glomeruli of the kidney, and the basal cells of the skin.

Recent work on vitamin D metabolism has been concerned with its formation in the skin, its effect on myeloid cell lines, and the formation of $1,25(OH)_2D$ in granulomatous tissue. Comparison of the effects of simulated equatorial solar radiation and appropriate monochromatic ultraviolet sources on the human epidermis shows that the maximum formation of vitamin D is less with the first source. Interestingly pigmentation by the skin reduces the amount of vitamin D (not 25OHD) produced by a single standard dose of ultraviolet light. Thus the effect of sunlight is not predictable from the ultraviolet radiation in its spectrum; additionally after exposure to sunlight, circulating levels of vitamin D tend to plateau whereas those of biologically inactive derivatives increase.

One of the most interesting extraskeletal effects of $1,25(OH)_2D_3$ is to induce the differentiation of myeloid cell lines which suggests the possibility of treating leukaemia derived from such cells. Another interesting observation is the extra renal 1-α-hydroxylation of $25(OH)D$ by a variety of granulomatous tissues, especially sarcoid. The reason why this occurs is unknown. In the case of sarcoid, treatment with corticosteroids rapidly reduces the high concentration of $1,25(OH)_2D_3$ and the associated hypercalcaemia.

Parathyroid hormone (see also page 10.51 *et seq.*)
Synthesis of this 84 amino acid hormone within the parathyroid gland begins with a precursor molecule containing two additions which are subsequently removed. Study of the nucleotide sequence of cloned DNAs has provided information on the amino acid sequence of the parathyroid precursor molecule. The formation of PTH from this precursor molecule begins with the removal of the pre and pro sequences. Secretion of the 1–84 PTH molecule occurs via secretory granules. Some PTH may be degraded within the parathyroid gland itself, but the specific cleavage of PTH between residues 33 and 34 occurs mainly in the liver and may be regarded as an activation step. This provides the major circulating fragments which are –C terminal which are biologically inactive and have a long half-life, and –N terminal which are the reverse. This situation initially led to considerable disagreement in the interpretation of PTH assays. In diagnosis it is always important to know which assays are being used, –C or–N terminal or middle molecule.

Secretion of parathyroid hormone is stimulated by hypocalcaemia, and its effects tend to restore the plasma calcium to normal. PTH secretion is also sensitive to changes in circulating magnesium concentration; and other factors such as prostaglandins, catecholamines, and hydroxylated vitamin D metabolites may have a modulating effect under certain circumstances. PTH causes an increase in the intestinal absorption and renal reabsorption of calcium and an increase in bone resorption. It also has an independent effect in decreasing renal tubular reabsorption of phosphate. The effect on the small intestinal cell may be partly due to stimulation of the renal-1-α-hydroxylase, increasing the production of $1,25(OH)_2D$. Such an effect would also increase bone resorption, but parathyroid hormone also itself stimulates osteoclastic bone resorption, probably via receptors on the osteoblasts.

Defects in the synthesis, metabolism, and effects of parathyroid hormone may produce various forms of hypoparathyroidism (see page 10.51 *et seq.*). Since the parathyroids are stimulated by hypocalcaemia, secondary hyperparathyroidism is a common feature of osteomalacia. In at least some of the forms of hypoparathyroidism there is a reduction of the G unit which is a guanine nucleotide-binding protein which normally couples hormone receptors to the catalytic unit of the adenylate cyclase complex.

Calcitonin (see also page 10.51 *et seq.*)
The short polypeptide calcitonin, or thyrocalcitonin, is secreted by the C cells of the thyroid gland. Its main effect on bone is to reduce osteoclastic bone resorption, but it has other non-skeletal effects including those on sodium metabolism. The cells which synthesize calcitonin are neuroectodermal which accounts for the secretion on occasion by carcinoid tumours and by phaeochromocytomas. The occurrence of a medullary cell carcinoma of the thyroid with hypercalcitoninaemia may be a clue to the dominantly inherited multiple endocrine adenoma syndrome type II (Sipple's syndrome, see page 13.382 *et seq.*).

The most striking effect of exogenous calcitonin on the skeleton is to suppress osteoclastic bone resorption, especially in those patients where bone turnover is rapid, as in Paget's disease (see page 17.19). Although the role of calcitonin is still obscure it is now possible to measure physiological changes in its concentrations; according to some these appear to increase in growth and pregnancy and to fall in postmenopausal women. The parafollicular C cells of the thyroid also produce substances related to calcitonin, namely, katacalcin and calcitonin gene-related peptide (CGRP) whose functions are obscure.

Other hormones and local factors
The growth and composition of the skeleton is affected by many other hormones. Growth hormone, through its active derivative somatomedin, stimulates the proliferation of cartilage and the growth of bone and soft tissue; deficiency leads to dwarfism and osteoporosis; excess during childhood leads to gigantism, and in the adult to acromegaly. Since the epiphyses are fused in adult life, growth in length is no longer possible, but new bone is added to periosteal surfaces.

The thyroid hormones stimulate bone turnover and prolonged thyrotoxicosis is associated with osteoporosis, with bone resorption in excess of bone formation. The sex hormones also have an effect on the skeleton: in the male hypogonadism is associated with osteoporosis; and in the female it is thought that oestrogens prevent parathyroid-mediated bone resorption, so that bone resorption increases after the menopause. Since oestrogens also stimulate the renal-1α-hydroxylase, and calcitonin levels are low after the menopause, the causes of postmenopausal osteoporosis (see page 17.12) are complex.

Bone is also subject to a large number of local factors; some of these, such as mechanical strain may contribute to bone formation; others may lead to the excessive resorption of bone especially around secondary tumour deposits. These include a group of osteoclast-stimulating factors (together known as OAF) which are produced particularly by myeloma cells, and prostaglandins. The prostaglandins are a large family of compounds with a 20-carbon fatty acid structure, of which the E series has been particularly associated with bone resorption. Resorption of bone around metastatic deposits such as those of cancer of the breast may occur for a number of reasons: these include production of prostaglandins and their metabolites, and of the OAFs and the direct effect of the tumour itself. There is also evidence that human breast cancer cells have receptors for $1,25(OH)_2D$, and this might contribute to bone resorption.

Whilst cancers of haematological origin may cause bone resorption and hypercalcaemia by the release of OAF, the hypercalcaemia of solid tumours without bone metastases ('humoral hypercalcaemia of cancer') may be due to tumour-derived transforming growth factors (especially TG Fα) which stimulate osteoclastic bone resorption.

References
Avioli, L. V. and Krane, S. M. (1977/8). *Metabolic bone disease* 2 volumes. Academic Press, London.
—— and Haddad, J. G. (1984). The vitamin D family revisited. *N. Engl. J. Med.* **331**, 47–49.

Table 2 Some examples of short stature

Cause	Example	Condition	Genetics	Clinical features
(a) Proportionate		*(b) Disproportionate (short-limbed)*		
Genetic	Familial	Achondroplasia	Dominant	Very short limbs
	Late puberty	Diastrophic dwarfism	Recessive	Club feet, ossified ears, hitch-hiker's thumb, scoliosis
Endocrine	Growth hormone lack			
	Corticosteroid excess			
	Hypothyroidism	Thanatophoric dwarfism	Unknown	Short limbs, small chest, early death
Metabolic	Hepatic and renal disease			
	Mucopolysaccharidoses	Ellis–van Creveld syndrome	Recessive	Additional digits, congenital heart disease
Chronic disease	Cyanotic heart disease			
	Fibrocystic disease	Achondrogenesis	Recessive	Die in perinatal period; very little ossification of limbs, vertebrae or pelvis
Nutritional	Coeliac disease			
	Starvation			
Intrauterine	Low birth weight dwarfism (multiple)	Severe osteogenesis	Sporadic	Multiple fractures, abnormal
Chromosomal	Turner's syndrome	imperfecta	? Recessive	dentine
Social	Emotional deprivation	Cartilage-hair hypoplasia	Recessive	Very short; sparse hair
		Hypophosphatasia	Recessive	Neonatal forms most severe; phosphoethanolamine in urine
		Hypophosphataemic rickets	X-linked	Low phosphate
		Metaphyseal dysostosis	Dominant	May resemble severe rickets

Baron, R., Vignery, A. and Horowitz, M. (1983). Lymphocytes, macrophages and the regulation of bone remodelling. *Bone and mineral research* Annual 2 (ed. W. A. Peck), pp. 175–243. Excerpta Medica, Amsterdam.

Coccia, P. F. (1984). Cells that resorb bone. *N. Engl. J. Med.* **310**, 456–458.

Heath, D. and Marx, S. J. (1982). Calcium disorders. *Clinical endocrinology 2 Butterworths international medical reviews*. Butterworth Scientific, London.

Manolagas, S. C. and Deftos, L. J. (1984). The vitamin D endocrine system and haematolymphopoietic tissue. *Ann. inter. Med.* **100**, 145–146.

McKusick, V. A. (1972). *Heritable disorders of connective tissue* 4th edn C. V. Mosby, St. Louis.

Muir, H. (1983). Proteoglycans as organisers of the intercellular matrix. *Biochem. Soc. Trans.* **11**, 613–622.

Mundy, G. R., Ibbotson, K. J., D'Souza, S. M., Simpson, E. L., Jacobs, J. W. and Martin, T. J. (1984). The hypercalcaemia of cancer. *N. Engl. J. Med.* **310**, 1718–1727.

Nordin, B. E. C. (1984). *Metabolic bone and stone disease* 2nd edn. Churchill Livingstone, Edinburgh.

Prockop, D. J. and Kivirikko, K. I. (1984). Heritable diseases of collagen. *N. Engl. J. Med.* **311**, 376–386.

Raisz, L. G. and Kream, B. E. (1983). Regulation of bone formation. *N. Engl. J. Med.* **309**, 29–35, 83–89.

Smith, R. (1979). *Biochemical disorders of the skeleton*. Butterworth Scientific, London.

—— (1984). Recent advances in the metabolism and physiology of bone. In *Recent advances in physiology* Vol. 10 (ed. P. F. Baker), pp. 317–348. Churchill Livingstone, Edinburgh.

Sykes, B. and Smith, R. (1985). Collagen and collagen gene disorders. *Q. J. Med* **56**, 533–547.

The diagnosis of bone disease

In the diagnosis of a skeletal disorder the history and physical signs are of first importance, but radiology and biochemistry have particularly useful roles. Direct examination of bone, often obtained at biopsy, should not be neglected.

History

Deformity, pain, and fracture are common features. To these may be added proximal myopathy (in osteomalacia and rickets) and the symptoms of any underlying disease. The family history is important.

Deformity

Deformity in bone disease suggests previous skeletal disorders especially if there is a disturbance of growth. The main disturbances of growth are short stature and disproportion, but excessive height can also cause problems. In children a knowledge of growth is essential; in the normal adult the height and span are approximately equal and the crown to pubis measurement is also equal to the pubis to heel. Patients with short stature may be roughly divided into those in whom the short stature is proportionate and those in which it is disproportionate; in the latter group the commonest is short-limbed dwarfism. Proportionate short stature is often only one feature of a generalized disorder. In contrast the causes of short-limbed dwarfism primarily affect the skeleton. Further, proportionate short stature may occur in children who appear to be otherwise normal, whereas subjects with disproportionate short stature usually appear abnormal from birth. Some cases of proportionate and disproportionate short stature are given in Table 2. Achondroplasia and related syndromes are dealt with further on page 17.34.

Kyphosis, with loss of trunk height, as in osteoporosis and osteomalacia, is the commonest acquired deformity. It is often noticed because clothes no longer fit. Other deformities are characteristic of the underlying disease; for instance, active childhood rickets produces knock knees, bowed legs, enlarged epiphyses, and bossing of the skull; Paget's disease produces thick long bones and an enlarged skull vault; and severe osteogenesis imperfecta can produce very short limbs.

Bone pain and fracture

The cause of bone pain is usually not understood. In osteomalacia it may be generalized with tenderness to pressure; more often it is localized over the site of a fracture. It may be due to excessive vascularity, with stretching of the periosteum; certainly it can be rapidly relieved by appropriate treatment such as calcitonin for Paget's disease, or parathyroidectomy for parathyroid bone disease. Fractures commonly occur in generalized skeletal disorders of the skeleton: examples are the partial, multiple, and painful microfractures on the convexity of Pagetic bone; and the repetitive vertebral compression fractures of osteoporosis.

Myopathy

Proximal muscle weakness is a well-described feature of osteomalacia and rickets but its cause is unknown. The symptoms commonly result from weakness of the pelvic girdle muscles and include a waddling gait and inability to rise from a chair or to climb stairs. The legs may be described as stiff rather than weak. Weakness of the shoulder muscles may be noticed when attempting to lift objects off high shelves.

Underlying disease

In any patients with skeletal disorders it is necessary to be alert for the symptoms of the underlying disease such as renal failure, steatorrhoea or myeloma and to enquire particularly about previous operations such as partial gastrectomy or hysterectomy and oophorectomy.

Physical signs

Important physical signs of skeletal disorders are found in the appearance, particularly of the face and skull, the proportions of the skeleton, and the shape of the bones. These are best seen when the patient is out of bed, when an abnormal gait may also be noted. There may be vital clues for instance in the large vault of Paget's disease, the coarse features, large nose, big lower jaw, and the widely spaced teeth of acromegaly, and the round face, simplicity of expression, and cataracts of pseudohypoparathyroidism. Those endocrine disorders which affect the skeleton such as hypogonadism and hypopituitarism are also readily recognizable.

Specific features of the face should receive particular attention; these particularly include the eyes where such signs as corneal calcification or arcus juvenilis or dislocation of the lens are important. The shimmering of the unsupported iris, iridodinesis, is an important sign of lens dislocation. Corneal clouding occurs in some of the mucopolysaccharidoses and cystine crystals can be seen in cystinosis. Attention should also be paid to the teeth since the matrix of dentine and bone are chemically similar and an abnormal skeleton may be associated with abnormal teeth. This is not always so, but dentinogenesis imperfecta is found often in association with severe osteogenesis imperfecta; the teeth have an abnormal shape, tend to be transparent, and vary from yellow to grey. Enamel defects occur in hypoparathyroidism and teeth are lost early in hypophosphatasia.

The hands and feet require particular examination. The fingers may be abnormally long and thin, as in Marfan's syndrome, or excessively mobile; or alternatively they may be short, wide, and stiff in some of the mucopolysaccharidoses; or the hands may have short metacarpals as in pseudohypoparathyroidism or additional digits, as in the Ellis–Van Creveld syndrome. The monophalangic big toe is characteristic of myositis ossificans progressiva (see page 17.37). Abnormal body proportions may be found (Table 2); thus the limbs are relatively longer than the trunk in Marfan's syndrome and hypogonadism; or the trunk may be relatively short due to vertebral collapse with a thoracic kyphosis. Scoliosis is less common and often dates from adolescence; occasionally it may be a clue to an inherited connective tissue disorder. The thoraco-lumbar gibbus is a particular feature (although not an exclusive one) of the mucopolysaccharidoses. Deformity of the spine will be associated with changes in the rest of the trunk, so that the patient with severe osteoporosis, for instance, will develop a prominent sternum with ribs which touch the iliac crest and a transverse crease across the front of the abdomen.

Finally, one should look for clues of the underlying disorder and also for hypocalcaemia. Although spontaneous tetany is rare there are two recognized tests for latent tetany; of these, Chvostek's sign is more convenient but that of Trousseau more reliable. The first involves tapping the branches of the facial nerves as they spread out from within the parotid gland. If positive this will produce a twitching of the appropriate facial muscle. In the second the forearm is made ischaemic with a sphygmomanometer cuff for up to 3 min; if positive carpal spasm will occur.

Biochemical investigations

In some generalized disorders of the skeleton such as achondroplasia, osteogenesis imperfecta, and the epiphyseal dysplasias the biochemistry is normal; in others there are characteristic changes (Table 3).

In normal persons the fasting plasma calcium concentration remains virtually constant throughout life; the plasma phosphate declines with adolescence and the plasma alkaline phosphatase increases during the phase of rapid growth. Seasonal changes may also occur associated with the lack of vitamin D in the winter. Since the total plasma calcium includes a protein-bound fraction it is usual to relate it to the plasma albumin and if necessary correct it to a plasma albumin of 4 g/100 ml. Acceptable corrections include: corrected calcium (mg/100 ml) = measured calcium − albumin (g/100 ml) +4; or, in SI units, 0.02 mmol/l for every 1 g/l change of albumin from 40 g/l. The fasting plasma calcium is normal in osteoporosis and also in Paget's disease unless the patient is immobilized when it may be increased. It is also increased in primary hyperparathyroidism, various neoplasms, in sarcoidosis, in vitamin D overdosage, and in a number of other states, including acromegaly and thyrotoxicosis (see Table 10). It is often low in osteomalacia but may be restored towards normal by secondary hyperparathyroidism and is low in parathyroid insufficiency. Normal values are to be expected in vitamin D-resistant hypophosphataemic rickets and in other forms of renal tubular rickets.

Since the main determinant of the fasting plasma phosphate concentration is its renal tubular reabsorption, hypophosphataemia is a feature of primary hyperparathyroidism and vitamin D-resistant rickets; but it is also reduced by giving oral aluminium hydroxide and during prolonged intravenous nutrition. The plasma phosphate increases in hypoparathyroidism and in renal glomerular failure, and also in the rare recessively inherited form of tumoral calcinosis.

The plasma alkaline phosphatase normally increases in adolescence; and is usually elevated in osteomalacia particularly in young patients, but it may be near normal in renal tubular osteomalacia. Considerable increases can occur in primary hyperparathyroidism but only where there is co-existent bone disease. The greatest increases in plasma alkaline phosphatase are found in Paget's disease, and in idiopathic hyperphosphatasia. In hypophosphatasia it is characteristically low.

In the patient with bone disease examination of the urine is important but is often omitted. In a random specimen the presence of glucose may suggest multiple renal tubular defects in a patient with inherited rickets, and proteinuria is an important clue to myeloma. In a 24-hour urine important changes may be found in calcium and hydroxyproline excretion.

The amount of calcium excreted in the urine is related both to the plasma levels and to the percentage of the filtered load reabsorbed by the renal tubules, itself altered by parathyroid hormone. In the presence of hypocalcaemia urine calcium is therefore low, particularly in osteomalacia and rickets; and is increased by hypercalcaemia, especially where this is due to rapid bone loss as in neoplastic disease of the skeleton, leukaemia, myeloma, and immobilization. Because parathyroid hormone promotes renal tubular reabsorption of calcium the normal relationship between plasma and urine calcium is disturbed in parathyroid disease; however, most hypercalcaemic hyperparathyroid patients excrete more calcium than normal.

Total hydroxyproline in the urine (after acid hydrolysis of the peptides) is a good index of collagen turnover in bone, provided the patient is on a low gelatin diet. The physiological changes in hydroxyproline excretion are striking with a particularly sharp peak in adolescence coinciding with the maximum height velocity. The highest values are seen in active Paget's disease, where the excretion may be up to 50-fold the normal value. Hydroxyproline excretion correlates well with plasma alkaline phosphatase, and is therefore increased in some forms of osteomalacia and in hyperparathyroidism with bone disease. Since thyroxine increases collagen turnover urinary hydroxyproline is also abnormally high in thyrotoxicosis and abnormally low in myxoedema (either primary or secondary).

Radiology

The diagnosis of a bone disease often depends on the radiographic appearances, especially where there are no demonstrable biochemical changes. Conventional radiographs demonstrate well structural changes such as fractures, deformity, areas of resorption, and alteration in size, but are unreliable for the assessment of bone density. As radiographic techniques develop, increasing use is made of isotope bone scans and computerized tomography (CT) scans. Diphosphonate-labelled scanning agents are selectively taken up in areas of increased vascularity or turnover. They are very useful in demonstrating the extent of Paget's disease of bone, the presence of bony metastases, the pathological fractures of osteoporosis, and Looser's zones in osteomalacia. An isotope scan is preferable to multiple radiographs to assess the distribution (but not the structure) of abnormal bone.

CT scanning can also be very useful in bone disease. Examples include the delineation of ectopic ossification, of spinal cord compression, and of bone tumours.

Bone biopsy

Direct examination of bone is a valuable but underused investigation. The bone can be taken by a transiliac trephine (using a local anaesthetic) and sections should be examined with and without decalcification. In the metabolic bone diseases the appearances are characteristic with the excess osteoid of osteomalacia, the disorganized mosaic pattern, excessive cellular activity, and fibrosis of Paget's disease, and the changes of osteitis fibrosis cystica in hyperparathyroid bone disease. In mild osteogenesis imperfecta there is typically an increase in the number of osteocytes and in the more severe form a considerable increase in the amount of fibre bone. A normal biopsy will exclude these diseases except where they are patchy. Where possible, histological examination should now include transmission and scanning electron microscopy.

Further investigation

The measurement of external calcium and phosphorus balance is a classic way of investigating generalized bone disease and the effects of treatment upon it, but it is also tedious. The use of isotopes to measure calcium absorption and apparent bone formation and resorption rates is less direct and also depends on a number of assumptions. Methods for measuring bone mass are considered with osteoporosis (page 17.20).

Diagnosis

The diagnosis of a skeletal disorder is not difficult when there are

Table 3 Biochemical and other features in disorders of the skeleton

Disorder	Commonest symptom	Plasma			Urine		Other biochemical features	Comments
		Ca	P	Alkaline phosphatase	Ca	THP		
Osteoporosis	Fracture	N	N	N	N	N	None	Hypercalcuria if immobilized
Osteomalacia (and rickets)	Bone pain; proximal weakness	N or L	L	N or H	L	N or H	Depends on cause	Plasma P increased in renal glomerular failure
Paget's disease	Pain; deformity	N	N	H	N	H	None	Hypercalcaemia if immobilized
Hyperparathyroidism (with bone disease)	Bone pain; hypercalcaemic symptoms	H	L	H	H	H	Aminoaciduria	P'ase and THP normal if clinical bone disease absent
Osteogenesis imperfecta	Brittle bones	N	N	N	N	N	Many described, none confirmed (see page 17.11)	
Marfan's syndrome	Tall with scoliosis; dislocated lenses; aortic dissection	N	N	N	N	±H	None	Dominant inheritance; clinically heterogeneous
Homocystinuria	Mentally subnormal; look like Marfan's syndrome	N	N	N	N	N	Homocystine in urine	
Alkaptonuria	Back pain; early arthritis; dark urine	N	N	N	N	N	Homogentisic acid in the urine	Calcified intervertebral discs
Mucopolysaccharidoses	Short stature; thoracolumbar gibbus; mentally subnormal (depends on type)	N	N	N	N	N	Characteristic mucopolysaccharide in urine	See page 17.30 et seq.
Osteopetrosis (marble bones disease)	Anaemia; blindness, deafness, (severe form)	±H	N	N	Low	N	Increase in acid phosphatase	Mild form fractures only
Hypophosphatasia	Lethal short-limbed dwarfism; bone disease like rickets	N	N	Low	N	N	Phosphoethanolamine in urine	Fractures in adult
Hyperphosphatasia	Large head, bowing of long bones; occurs in childhood	N	N	Very high	N	Very high	None	Similar to Paget's disease
Fibrous dysplasia	Fracture; sexual precocity in girls; pigmentation	N	N	Slight increase	N	Slight increase	Biochemical changes in polyostotic form only	Occasional hypophosphataemic osteomalacia
Myositis ossificans progressiva	Pain and swelling in muscles; fixation of joints	N	N	? Increased during myositis	N	N	None	Monophalangic big toe

clear biochemical disturbances (Table 3) although, as in osteomalacia, its causes may be multiple. In cases in which the biochemical measurements are apparently normal it may sometimes be impossible to make an exact diagnosis; this is particularly so in some of the rare heritable disorders. Some guidance based on the age of the patient and frequency of the disorder is given in Table 4.

References

Byers, P. D. (1977). The diagnostic value of bone biopsies. In *Metabolic bone disease* Vol. 1 (eds L. V. Avioli and S. M. Krane), pp. 183–236. Academic Press, New York.

Nordin, B. E. C. (1984). *Metabolic bone and stone disease* 2nd edn. Churchill Livingstone, Edinburgh.

Paterson, C. R. (1974). *Metabolic disorders of bone.* Blackwell Scientific Publications, Oxford.

Smith, R. (1979). *Biochemical disorders of the skeleton.* Butterworth Scientific, London.

Osteoporosis

In osteoporosis the mass of bone is reduced but its composition is normal. This reduction results from an imbalance between the formation and resorption of bone. This imbalance most commonly occurs with increasing age, and osteoporotic bones are therefore a feature of old age. Osteoporosis (or osteopenia, see below) is only of clinical importance when it leads to fracture, most often of the vertebrae, femur or radius. However, fracture rate is not closely related to the incidence of osteoporosis since other factors, particularly the frequency of falls, are also important.

The development of osteoporosis with age is far more rapid in women than in men. This is associated with the decline in female hormones at the menopause; but is is also related to the original adult mass of the skeleton and to the variable immobility of increasing years.

Osteoporosis is by far the most common metabolic bone disease, and is also the most difficult to treat. The increasing incidence of femoral neck fractures, thought to be related to osteoporosis also make this disorder financially very important. Progress in our understanding of osteoporosis has been limited by the slowness at which this disorder progresses, by the many factors which cause it, and by the fact that various parts of the skeleton behave differently. For instance, trabecular and cortical bone, and the vertebrae and long bones, may develop osteoporosis at different rates. Significant advances have been made in methods for measurement of vertebral bone mass.

Table 4 Diagnosis of disorders of the skeleton

Age	Main presenting symptom	Most likely diagnosis	Frequency	Exclude
Over 50 years	Pain in the back loss of height fracture	Osteoporosis commonest in women	Common	Myeloma (especially in men) Secondary deposits Coexistent osteomalacia
	Deformity of long bones pain in hips and pelvis fracture	Paget's disease of bone commonest in men	Common	Osteomalacia Hyperparathyroid bone disease Skeletal metastases
	Bone pain and tenderness difficulty in walking unable to climb stairs pathological fracture	Osteomalacia	Uncommon, especially in the adult	Carcinoma Polymyalgia rheumatica
	Bone pain and deformity thirst, nocturia, depression vomiting, constipation	Osteitis fibrosa cystica commonest in women	Rare	Carcinoma with hypercalcaemia myeloma
20–50 years	Loss of height	Probably secondary deposits, or myeloma	Rare	Osteomalacia Idiopathic osteoporosis
	Muscle weakness loss of height bone pain	Osteomalacia	Rare	Late muscular dystrophy Neoplastic neuromyopathy
0–20 years	Bowing of bones deformity weakness	'Nutritional' rickets	Commonest in Asian immigrants in Northern cities	Other causes of rickets Hypophosphatasia
	Multiple fractures bruising	In infants, inflicted by parents, 'battered baby'	Not uncommon	Osteogenesis imperfecta
	Bone pain ill health	Leukaemia	Uncommon	Osteomyelitis Rickets
	Pain in back difficulty in walking pain in ankles less rapid growth	Juvenile osteoporosis	Rare	Leukaemia
	Failure to grow (dwarfism)	Many causes (Table 2)	Common	Particularly hypothyroidism, Turner's syndrome, and coeliac disease
	Excessive or disproportionate growth	Several causes, often familial	Less common than short stature	Particularly pituitary tumour Marfan's syndrome Homocystinuria Hypogonadism and chromosomal abnormalities
	Fracture and deformity at birth	Severe osteogenesis imperfecta	Uncommon	Hypophosphatasia Achondrogenesis Thanatophoric dwarfism

Definition

An accurate definition of osteoporosis is not easy. Some would regard it merely as a particular form of osteopenia, where osteopenia is defined as 'too little calcified bone'. Unfortunately in this sense osteomalacia is also a form of osteopenia, which is confusing. The term osteopenia has been widely applied to the normal reduction in bone mass with increasing age ('physiological osteopenia'). Osteoporosis is then identified as a loss of bone mass greater than that for normal individuals of comparable age, race, and sex. In practice it is much more simple to note that with increasing age loss of bone occurs to a variable extent in all individuals (physiological osteoporosis); that in some people rapid bone loss may occur irrespective of age (accelerated osteoporosis); and that in some this bone loss may lead to its only important clinical consequence, fracture. These definitions are quantitative. With increasing use of bone mass measurements, osteoporosis may be defined as a bone mass of less than the 5th centile (i.e. −2 S.D.) of the bone mass at maturity for that population. The actual incidence of fracture in subjects with osteoporosis defined in this way is not known, and opinions differ about the relationship between reduced bone mass and fracture rate.

Pathophysiology

The control of bone mass at tissue level depends on the bone remodelling cycle. Bone continues to turn over throughout life, although at a decreasing rate. New bone is formed periosteally and resorption is endosteal. These processes are normally balanced in early adult life but from about the age of 30 years the rate of bone formation is less than that of resorption. The eventual result for a long bone is that its external diameter is greater than in early adulthood, but its cortical thickness is diminished. The thickness and number of trabeculae are also diminished. Under appropriate circumstances these changes will lead to structural collapse.

There are variations in these processes with age and throughout the skeleton. Thus the most rapid increases in bone mass occur in infancy and later in adolescence, and at the end of this time the differences in bone mass between the sexes is well established, for instance, the ratio of the metacarpal cortical area to body weight is 20 per cent lower in girls than in boys. The mass of bone of the young adult is also influenced by racial characteristics, degrees of nutrition, and physical activity. These are important since a major factor influencing subsequent structural failure is the initial adult size of the skeleton. Furthermore, the rate of bone turnover varies from one part of the skeleton to another, being highest in the cancellous or trabecular bones of the vertebrae, the ribs, and the iliac bones.

Assuming that osteoporosis is an inevitable result of ageing, why is it more marked in some patients than others? There appear to be at least two reasons. The first is that bone loss is more rapid in females than in males, for a number of causes, and the second is that the degree of osteoporosis depends on the mature bone mass of the adult skeleton, itself the result of genetic and acquired factors (see below).

In population studies it seems that for each gender the decline of bone mass and the development of osteoporosis is normally distributed, and further that those who develop fractures have, on the whole, a bone mass significantly less (−2 S.D.) than the mean for early adult bone. This trend does not of course prevent fractures in elderly patients in whom bone mass is normal and the association between osteoporosis and femoral neck fracture rate is a poor one emphasizing the importance of other factors, particularly falls, in contributing to such fractures.

Bone mass

It is difficult to measure bone mass. It cannot be done directly in life except by bone biopsy; indirect methods assume that the osteoporotic bone is fully mineralized, and that therefore the mineral content of bone indicates its mass. Subjective assessment of bone density on radiographs is very inaccurate. If the definition of osteoporosis includes fracture it requires radiological evidence of this. Loss of trabeculae, as in the femoral neck, may be graded to give a reasonable index of bone mass and quantitative measurements may be made on fractured vertebrae. In the absence of structural collapse, loss of bone may be indicated by measurements of cortical bone thickness, by gamma ray absorption densitometry, by neutron activation analysis, and by CT scanning. Each of these have their protagonists. Measurement of the thickness of the metacarpal cortex from radiographs is a well-established way of measuring bone mass, which has been refined by taking the mean measurements of three metacarpals on each hand using accurate calipers and micrometers. The unmodified cortical thickness may be used as an index or it may be expressed in relation to the length of the bone. Photon absorptiometry measures the absorption by bone mineral of photons from gamma-emitting isotopes. Using a single photon source it can be applied to the lower end of the radius and to other accessible parts of the peripheral skeleton such as metacarpal and calcaneum.

Errors may arise from difficulties in positioning and from the presence of calcium in the soft tissues. In neutron activation analysis, ^{49}Ca with a half-life of 8.8 min, is one of the products of neutron bombardment. Measurement of this short-lived isotope will give an index of the amount of calcium present. The method may be applied to different bones in the body including the spine. These last three methods are all capable of giving useful sequential data and have approximately the same errors. In practice this means that the changes which normally occur in age-related osteoporosis and during its treatment cannot in general be detected in less than about two years. It will be appreciated that these methods measure changes either in trabecular or in cortical bone, which are not closely related. More recently the use of dual photon absorptiometry or of CT scanning makes it possible to measure vertebral bone density with a comparable degree of accuracy.

Causes of osteoporosis

The main recognized causes of osteoporosis are shown in Table 5. Many patients have more than one cause for osteoporosis which occurs most commonly in postmenopausal and elderly women, and is classified then as age-related bone loss. It could be argued that osteoporosis after the menopause is not idiopathic (and this would reflect current thought) but this would draw a possibly artificial distinction between postmenopausal and elderly osteoporosis. Osteoporosis not clearly related to age can be grouped under the heading of 'accelerated bone loss'. Rarely this occurs in childhood, in adolescence, and also in young adults, and it is sometimes associated with pregnancy. Accelerated bone loss not related to age may also occur as the result of immobility, endocrine disease, chromosomal disturbances, and a number of other conditions. It is possible to make a very long list of the causes of osteoporosis but this is often done more for the sake of completeness than for any practical reason. To include other bone diseases such as those due to secondary malignant deposits or to parathyroid overactivity, where loss of bone is merely one feature of the bone disorder, is confusing. However it is important to remember these disorders in the differential diagnosis of osteoporosis (Table 6).

Symptoms and signs

The symptoms of osteoporosis are deformity, localized pain, and fracture. They are typically seen in age-related bone loss. The commonest deformity is loss of height due to vertebral collapse. This may be noticed more by others than by the patient, who rarely knows her original height. However, this may be determined by measurement of the span (since in the young adult height and span are approximately equal). In the younger person the kyphosis is accompanied by deformity of the chest and protrusion of the manubrium sterni. In osteoporosis, most of the pain occurs in the back and is associated with collapse of the vertebrae.

Table 5 The main types of osteoporosis

Causes unknown (idiopathic)
  Age-related bone loss (common)
    Post-menopausal
    Elderly
  *Not related to age (rare)
    Osteoporosis of pregnancy
    Idiopathic juvenile osteoporosis
    Osteoporosis in young adults

Causes known or postulated*
  Immobility: general or local
  Endocrine
    Hypogonadism, including oophorectomy
    Cushing's syndrome—spontaneous or iatrogenic
    Thyrotoxicosis
    Hypopituitarism
  Chromosomal: Turner's syndrome (XO)
  Other
    Rheumatoid arthritis
    Heparin and cytotoxic agents
    Scurvy
    Inherited
      Osteogenesis imperfecta
      Homocystinuria

With osteomalacia
  Coeliac disease, partial gastrectomy, renal
  osteodystrophy, liver disease

* These are associated with accelerated net bone loss.

Table 6 The main differential diagnosis of osteoporosis

Osteomalacia: may co-exist with osteoporosis. Distinguish by bone biopsy and biochemistry
Hyperparathyroidism: can occasionally be associated with generalized 'osteoporosis'. Biochemistry (Table 3) is diagnostic
Multiple myeloma: distinguish by high ESR and light chains in the urine
Metastatic carcinoma: particularly from breast, bronchus, prostate, kidney, and thyroid
Osteogenesis imperfecta: in childhood distinguish from idiopathic juvenile osteoporosis, multiple fractures due to child abuse, and leukaemia

At first this is clearly related to a recognized stress, for instance, moving heavy furniture; it is severe and localized, and the vertebrae are tender to percussion. Some believe that vertebral collapse often occurs without symptoms. In established vertebral collapse, pain-free intervals become shorter. Examination of the patient will confirm loss of trunk height, thoracic kyphosis, proximity of the ribs to the iliac crest, and a transverse abdominal crease, and may give some clue about the cause of the structural collapse. For instance, bone tenderness, anaemia, and general ill health might suggest multiple myeloma or secondary carcinoma, while in children leukaemia may mimic juvenile osteoporosis. Clues to the various endocrine causes of osteoporosis should always be sought.

Radiology
Structural collapse provides the most convincing radiological sign of osteoporosis. In the vertebrae this appears as irregular anterior wedging affecting some vertebrae and not others (Fig. 5). The end plates may be biconcave but this change does not have the uniformity of distribution seen in osteomalacia, except where it occurs in juvenile osteoporosis or in osteogenesis imperfecta. Various changes are described in osteoporotic bones before fracture. These include loss of the less important (horizontal) trabeculae in the vertebrae with apparent accentuation of those in the vertical direction; reduction of cortical thickness in the long bones; and progressive loss of trabeculae also in these bones, par-

ticularly at the upper end of the femur. In the vertebrae herniation of the disc through the end plate causes a 'Schmorl's' node; it is said by some that this is unrelated to osteoporosis.

In the peripheral bones the cortex is thinned and especially in severe or acute osteoporosis (as with immobilization) the endosteal surface may appear scalloped, and the mineral loss has a 'spotty' or 'rain-drop' appearance. Osteoporosis is said not to affect the skull except where it is due to an excess of adrenal cortical steroids.

Biochemistry
Biochemical measurements in osteoporosis are usually normal; but recent immobility in a young person considerably increases the urinary calcium and after the menopause the ratios of calcium and hydroxyproline to creatinine measured in the urine after an overnight fast may both be increased, which implies increased bone resorption.

Recent long bone fracture may slightly increase plasma alkaline phosphatase. When the osteoporosis is due to some underlying disorder, the biochemical changes reflect this; for example, in thyrotoxic bone disease the plasma calcium, phosphate, and alkaline phosphatase, and the urinary hydroxyproline excretion, may all be increased. Patients with active osteoporosis may be in negative calcium balance with a high urine calcium and/or reduced intestinal absorption of calcium.

Other investigations
Bone biopsy is not a useful or necessary way of confirming osteoporosis, but it helps to identify underlying causes, to exclude co-existing metabolic bone disease such as osteomalacia, and other disorders with similar presentation. It should also probably be combined with bone marrow aspiration to exclude haematological disorders, especially in the young. In osteoporosis the reduction in trabecular volume may be associated with a reduction in mean wall thickness, a measure of bone formation rate.

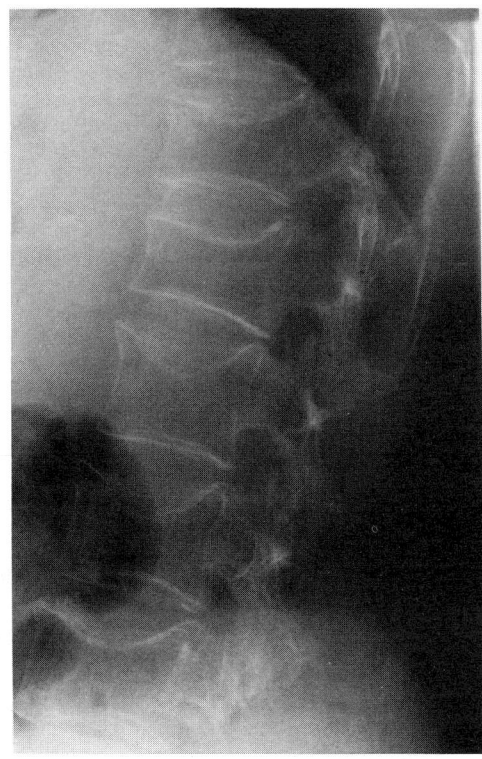

Fig. 5 The appearance of an osteoporotic spine. There is unequal collapse with variable wedging of the vertebrae. Some end-plates have also given way.

Isotope scanning may be useful to show the presence of fresh fractures, and to exclude such obvious features as multiple secondary deposits. For research sequential measurements of spinal density (dual photon absorptiometry or CT scanning) are widely used. Although further investigations are not usually necessary it may be useful for future treatment to know whether intestinal malabsorption of calcium or excessive urinary calcium loss predominate.

Diagnosis

There are two steps in the diagnosis of osteoporosis: first, to establish that osteoporosis is present and that other significant bone diseases are absent, and, second, to try to establish its cause since amongst these are some which can be improved by treatment. Osteoporosis itself will be readily excluded from other forms of metabolic bone disease because of its usually normal biochemistry, and from other causes of loss of trunk height and vertebral collapse by examination of the patient, the peripheral blood, the bone marrow, and the bone itself (Table 6). To establish the exact reason for osteoporosis can be difficult, since the causes are often multiple.

TYPES OF OSTEOPOROSIS

The commonest type of osteoporosis is that which occurs in women after the menopause. For clinical purposes it may be artificial to separate so-called 'postmenopausal' from 'senile' or 'elderly' osteoporosis, but the causes are probably different. In both there is age-related bone loss. In postmenopausal osteoporosis the main abnormality is excess bone resorption, in later years, defective new bone formation is the most important.

Age-related bone loss

The rapid loss of bone in women after the menopause is well documented, but its causes are still obscure. Osteoporosis is generally considered to be the main cause of fractures in postmenopausal women and as such is an enormous (and potentially preventable) health problem; thus of approximately one million fractures per year in women over 45 years of age in the United States, it is said that 700 000 occur in those with osteoporosis. It has also been estimated that the annual expenditure on acute medical care alone for elderly patients with fractured hips is more than 1 billion dollars a year.

The reasons why the bone mass in some postmenopausal women is so much less than in others are not known. Some women have a greater bone mass at the time of the menopause than others; if subsequent bone loss occurs at a constant rate, osteoporosis sufficient to contribute to fracture will occur later in such individuals. However, current work does not readily identify a separate group of postmenopausal women with a bone mass significantly lower than the rest of the population. Further, the relationship between fracture rate and osteoporosis is not close. However, careful studies have shown that, after the menopause, cortical bone loss is continuous whereas trabecular (iliac crest) bone loss which is initially rapid, later slows, and that the rates of femoral neck fracture and forearm fracture show similar respective trends. Observations such as these suggest that the type and frequency of postmenopausal fracture sustained is related to the loss of either trabecular or cortical bone.

It is difficult to distinguish a subpopulation of postmenopausal women whose greatly reduced bone mass is outside the normal distribution in the postmenopausal population as a whole, but there is evidence that the mass of bone at the time of the menopause and its subsequent loss may be highly variable. In an individual the maximum bone mass depends on genetic factors and previous use of the skeleton.

Excessively fast postmenopausal loss of bone has been attributed to malabsorption of calcium and to low levels of androstene-

dione, normally derived from the adrenal and converted peripherally into oestrogens. Other hormonal causes have been suggested, of which two are thought important: oestrogen deficiency and calcitonin deficiency. Young women who have oophorectomies at the time of hysterectomy lose bone far more readily than those who have a hysterectomy alone; and treatment of the first group with oestrogen restores bone mass so long as oestrogens are continued. Lack of oestrogen could contribute to loss of bone by allowing parathyroid-mediated bone resorption or by leading to a reduction in $1,25(OH)_2D$ because of its effect on renal l-α-hydroxylation. Further, the calcitonin levels in postmenopausal women are lower than normal, which could lead to excessive bone resorption; but the basal values (at least) are not significantly different in osteoporotic and non-osteoporotic females in this age group, and some of the data are controversial.

Apart from the obvious lack of oestrogen after the menopause, and the role of calcium deficiency or malabsorption, loss of bone from the mature skeleton may be increased by a high protein diet, excessive alcohol, caffeine intake, cigarette smoking, and lack of exercise. Amenorrhoea or oligomenorrhoea in young women before the menopause also contributes to bone loss from the mature skeleton, whereas pregnancy or the use of oral contraceptives are said to decrease it.

Treatment

The most important aspect of the treatment of age-related bone loss is its prevention.

Prevention

In theory osteoporosis may be prevented by building up a large skeleton in youth, by continuing physical activity and mobility in adult life, by an adequate (about 1500 mg) daily intake of calcium, and probably by the administration of oestrogens from the time of the menopause in females. This last point is controversial.

Sexual maturity and a well-defined growth spurt are important in determining adult bone mass, and the use of oral contraceptives or subsequent pregnancies appear to protect premenopausal women from bone loss. Further, women who lose bone rapidly in the early postmenopausal phase have the lowest endogenous sex hormone levels. Current evidence now clearly shows that young women whose ovaries have been removed at hysterectomy lose bone more rapidly than those who have had a hysterectomy alone, and that both peripheral and central (spinal) bone loss may be prevented or reversed by oestrogens. It is still doubtful how far this experience can be directly applied to the natural menopause; in oophorectomied patients loss of bone may resume if oestrogens are discontinued, so that replacement oestrogen once started needs to be continued.

There are dangers in giving oestrogens alone to postmenopausal women. These include an increased risk of thrombosis and uterine cancer. It is possible that their incidence has been overstressed and in any case such side effects have to be balanced against the considerable morbidity and mortality from fractures associated with untreated osteoporosis in a large number of women over the age of 45 years. Whether or not there is an increased risk of cardiovascular mortality or morbidity is controversial. At present it seems that oestrogens will be more widely used in future to prevent postmenopausal osteoporosis. Their use is more acceptable in women who have had hysterectomies, and in those who have not, the incidence of uterine cancer appears to be less if the oestrogens are combined with progesterones. Since it is impracticable to offer oestrogen therapy to all women around the menopause, their use should be considered primarily for certain groups. These include small, thin, white or oriental women; those with an early menopause or surgical oophorectomy; those with a strong family history of osteoporosis, and those with prolonged amenorrhoea or oligomenorrhoea during the normally fertile period of life.

Treatment of established osteoporosis

Some forms of treatment are obvious, others are controversial. The patient with pain due to vertebral collapse requires analgesics, and peripheral fractures require orthopaedic attention. Within the limitations of fracture it is important to maintain mobility to prevent further osteoporosis; this advice may conflict with the use of spinal supports to relieve pain.

Oral calcium, vitamin D, and oestrogens are variously used. Although calcium deficiency is not thought to be a cause of osteoporosis in humans there is some evidence that its administration may reduce bone loss, and it may be most effective when given in the evening to prevent nocturnal bone resorption. Westernized diets contain less calcium and more fibre than previously, and the intestinal absorption of calcium is reduced after the menopause. It is therefore often necessary to prescribe calcium to increase the oral intake to 1500–2000 mg daily.

Vitamin D or its metabolites alone are not effective treatment for osteoporosis, but they cure co-existent osteomalacia and appear to be effective when given with oestrogens to osteoporotic patients with malabsorption of calcium. One study showed that the three most effective of six forms of treatment in the prevention of further bone loss and reduction of vertebral crush fractures were oral calcium, oestrogens, or oestrogen plus vitamin D. Of agents which can stimulate new bone formation, oral sodium fluoride has been widely used; but calcium and vitamin D need to be given at the same time to mineralize the new bone, and there is also some doubt about its structural integrity.

The evidence that anabolic steroids, which increase muscle mass, can also prevent the loss of bone is not convincing; and detailed work has yet to establish the usefulness of the 1–34 fragments of parathyroid hormone. The recent demonstration that calcitonin levels are very low in postmenopausal women may renew attempts to use it in postmenopausal osteoporosis, but there is no good evidence of consistent improvement in bone mass. Other agents which are being examined include the newer diphosphonates and 24,25 dihydroxy vitamin D.

Two recent studies on the treatment of postmenopausal osteoporosis are relevant. One (from the United States) showed that the combination of sodium fluoride, oral calcium, and oestrogen was more effective than any other regimen in reducing the occurrence of vertebral fracture. Fluoride is known to increase new bone matrix formation, but additional calcium is necessary to mineralize the new bone, and fluoride produces significant gastrointestinal side effects. Another study (from Denmark) failed to show any increase in forearm bone mineral content in patients treated with fluoride, or with oral calcium, and concluded that oestrogen/progesterone was the only effective treatment.

Accelerated bone loss

This term covers the rapid bone loss of immobilization, osteoporosis associated with pregnancy, idiopathic osteoporosis in young people, and the osteoporosis of endocrine disease and of chromosomal abnormalities. Osteogenesis imperfecta, an inherited form of osteoporosis, is dealt with later (page 17.25).

Osteoporosis and immobilization

Immobility contributes to many forms of osteoporosis, particularly with increasing age. In such instances it is difficult to define exactly its importance relative to other factors. There are other situations, especially in the young, when the contribution of immobilization to bone loss is clearly very significant. This immobility may be local, around inflamed joints or fractured limbs, or it may be general. Thus rapidly progressive osteoporosis follows severe injury in the young associated with enforced immobilization. This is due to a sudden 'uncoupling' of bone resorption and formation. It may produce hypercalcaemia or hypercalcuria; radiographically there is a spotty 'rain-drop' form of rarefaction. Similar events probably occur in satellite travel. Much effort is being directed towards the prevention of this loss of bone in space travellers. Treatment is difficult but the osteoporosis will partially improve when mobility is resumed. Two localized forms of osteoporosis whose cause is unknown are a self-limiting transient osteoporosis which tends to affect the bones adjacent to larger joints, and that associated with Sudek's atrophy (page 16.89).

Osteoporosis and pregnancy

Women occasionally develop vertebral fractures during pregnancy. Pain in the back and kyphosis are noticed near term or shortly after delivery. The pain generally improves after two or three months and the loss of height may cease, but the bones remain osteoporotic. Further vertebral collapse in subsequent pregnancies does not necessarily occur.

It is possible that this very rare form of osteoporosis is associated with failure of the normal changes in calciotrophic hormones which appear to protect the maternal skeleton during pregnancy.

Osteoporosis in the young

Occasionally osteoporosis with structural collapse occurs during growth. The particular form which occurs around puberty (idiopathic juvenile osteoporosis) is usually self-limiting. Growth rate is reduced and shortness of the trunk with kyphosis due to vertebral fracture may develop. There is pain in the back which may follow injury. In this condition there may be metaphyseal fractures at the ends of the long bones which can be confused with Looser's zones (see page 17.16). Such fractures (Fig. 6) are associated with pain in the ankles and difficulty in walking. Excessive bone resorption has been reported but decreased bone formation also occurs. The cause of the condition is unknown. Although it is generally associated with the rapid growth of adolescence similar conditions occur in earlier childhood. Except in rare cases it is not progressive and the bones may return to a nearly normal structure within a few years, although spinal deformity persists. The real incidence of this condition may be underestimated; it could account for a number of cases of idiopathic kyphosis. The condition most difficult to distinguish it from is mild osteogenesis imperfecta, especially where the characteristic family history and blue sclerae are absent.

Osteoporosis and endocrine disease

The skeleton is affected by many hormones (page 17.5). In some conditions, for instance, thyrotoxicosis, the clinical effects are minor, but in others, such as Cushing's syndrome and hypogonadism, osteoporotic collapse of the skeleton is a significant feature.

Thyroid bone disease

In thyrotoxicosis bone turnover is excessive, bone resorption is more increased than bone formation and after many years of thyroid overactivity significant osteoporosis may occur. Biochemically there may be hypercalcaemia, hyperphosphataemia and an increase in plasma alkaline phosphatase; hypercalcuria and increased urinary hydroxyproline also occur. Since thyrotoxicosis is often recognized early, significant bone disease is uncommon; rarely it may be seen in patients who are thyroid addicts. It should be considered in all cases of obscure osteoporosis. Histologically there is an increase in the amount of bone surfaces covered by osteoid, and in fibrous tissue, osteoclasts, and osteoblasts; mineralization is normal.

Corticosteroids and osteoporosis

One of the commonest endocrine bone diseases is iatrogenic osteoporosis due to prolonged administration of corticosteroids. Osteoporosis may also occur in naturally occurring Cushing's syndrome. In patients treated with corticosteroids there is not a close association between corticosteroid dose and osteoporosis, although the duration of treatment and reduction in bone mass are significantly related. The effects of glucocorticoids are growth fail-

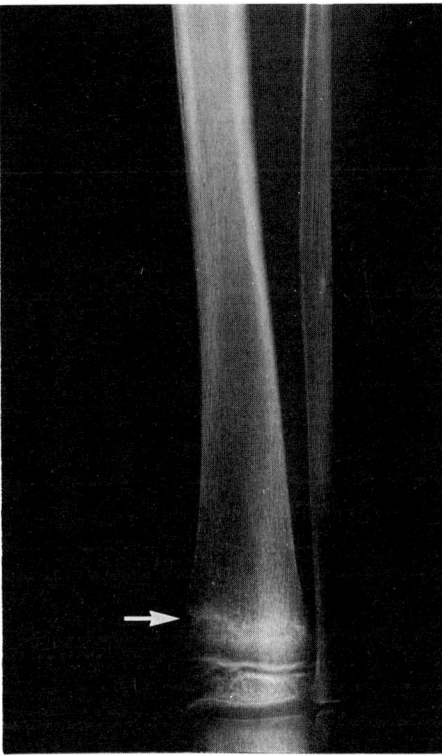

Fig. 6 Changes in the tibial metaphysis (arrowed) in an adolescent girl with idiopathic juvenile osteoporosis. Other metaphyses were affected and there was vertebral collapse.

ure in children, decreased intestinal calcium absorption, deficient synthesis of bone matrix, and delayed repair and remodelling of fractures. Osteoporosis particularly affects the vertebrae and, in contrast to other forms, the skull. There is also excessive callus formation around fractures. Such fractures may occur in the same regions as Looser's zones, i.e. pubic rami, ribs, and be relatively painless. Another skeletal feature is necrosis of the femoral heads.

The pituitary and osteoporosis

Osteoporosis is a feature of hypopituitarism. In childhood the lack of growth hormone and later of sex hormones produces infantilism. The epiphyses fuse very late and the rarefied bones tend to collapse in adult life. Acromegaly, due to excessive secretion of growth hormone after growth has ceased, is often said to be a cause of osteoporosis because of the radiographic appearance of the skeleton, but there is little other evidence of this. Reactivation of endochondral growth at certain cartilage bone junctions and stimulation of periosteal bone formation increases the size of the bones, particularly the vertebrae. An increase in plasma phosphate and urine calcium occurs; when the plasma calcium is increased this may be part of a multiple endocrine adenoma syndrome.

Hypogonadism

Hypogonadism in the female can be difficult to recognize although loss of sex hormones after the menopause is an important factor in postmenopausal osteoporosis. It has recently been recognized that the vertebral bone mass in young women athletes who have amenorrhoea is abnormally low, showing that the increase in stress through the skeleton does not counteract the effect of oestrogen deficiency. Similarly bone mass is reduced in women with anorexia nervosa.

In men hypogonadism is a potentially reversible cause of osteoporosis and should always be considered in a young patient. Clues are provided by the relatively long extremities, low hair line,

smooth skin, high-pitched voice, and absence of secondary sexual characteristics. There may also be a past history of surgical attempts to correct cryptorchidism. Treatment with testosterone derivatives is important.

Osteoporosis and chromosomal abnormalities

The commonest chromosomal cause of osteoporosis is probably Turner's syndrome, the XO anomaly. Classically such patients are girls with growth retardation, webbing of the neck, cubitus valgus, cardiac lesions, and lack of sexual development; but many patients with Turner's syndrome may be chromosomal mosaics with no symptoms apart from growth failure and apparently delayed puberty. In Down's syndrome osteopenia is described in childhood but does not persist after adolescence.

Other possible causes of osteoporosis

Osteoporosis may occur in association with alcoholism, liver disease, diabetes, heparin administration, and rheumatoid arthritis. It is said to occur more frequently in cigarette smokers and in thin people. The evidence for these statements varies. There are many reasons why alcoholics should have osteoporosis but little to suggest that alcohol has a direct effect on the skeleton. Recent studies demonstrate that diabetics do not have clinically significant osteoporosis. The relation to heparin administration is of interest since systemic mastocytosis is a rare cause of osteoporosis. The osteoporosis of rheumatoid arthritis may be mainly due to local immobilization. Osteoporosis in osteogenesis imperfecta, homocystinuria, and scurvy are dealt with separately.

References

Aitken, M. (1984). *Osteoporosis in clinical practice*. Wright, Bristol.
Boyce, W. J. and Vessey, M. P. (1985). Rising incidence of fracture of the proximal femur. *Lancet* **i**, 150–151.
Lindsay, R., Hart, D. M., Forrest, C., and Baird, C. (1980). Prevention of spinal osteoporosis in oophorectomised women. *Lancet* **ii**, 1151–1154.
Riggs, B. L., Seeman, E., Hodgson, S. F., Taves, D. R., and O'Fallon, W. M. (1982). Effect of the fluoride/calcium regimen on vertebral fracture occurrence in postmenopausal osteoporosis. *N. Engl. J. Med.* **306**, 446–450.
Smith, R., Stevenson, J. C., Winearls, C. G., Woods, C. G., and Wordsworth, B. P. (1985). Osteoporosis of pregnancy. *Lancet* **i**, 1178–1180.
—— (1985). Exercise and osteoporosis. *Br. Med. J.* **290**, 1163–1164.
Weinstein, M. C. (1980). Estrogen use in post-menopausal women – costs, risks and benefits. *N. Engl. J. Med.* **303**, 308–316.

Osteomalacia and rickets

Osteomalacia is the condition which results from a lack of vitamin D or a disturbance of its metabolism; in the growing skeleton it is referred to as rickets, and the terms are often used interchangeably. Inherited hypophosphataemia and a number of other renal tubular disorders may also cause rickets without clear evidence of abnormal vitamin D metabolism.

The main histological feature of osteomalacia is defecive mineralization of bone matrix. Our present understanding of osteomalacia relies largely on recent advances in knowledge of vitamin D metabolism (Fig. 4). For clinical purposes two aspects of the physiology of vitamin D require emphasis. The first is the quantitative importance of vitamin D synthesis in the skin in comparison with that in the diet, and the second concerns the relative role of different vitamin D metabolites. The measurement of circulating concentrations of 25(OH)D as an index of vitamin D status has identified those groups (Asian immigrants and the elderly) most at risk from vitamin D deficiency; importantly it has also shown the large amounts of vitamin D which can be synthesized in the human skin when exposed to ultraviolet light. The causes of osteomalacia can now be partly understood in terms of its metabolites, and the major importance of $1,25(OH)_2D$ is established. However, the effects of giving vitamin D cannot be ascribed to the actions of

1,25(OH)$_2$D alone, and probably include other biologically active derivatives, such as 25(OH)D and 24,25(OH)$_2$D.

Pathophysiology

The features of osteomalacia can be largely predicted from the known effects of vitamin D. Examination of undecalcified bone shows wide osteoid seams with many birefringent lamellae of collagen (Fig. 7) covering more of the bone surface than normal, and absence of the 'calcification front'. The absence of this front is important since excessive osteoid may also be found in conditions other than osteomalacia, such as hypophosphatasia, Paget's disease of bone, and thyrotoxicosis, where the calcification front is normal; in these disorders the increase tends to be in the amount of bone surface covered rather than in the thickness of osteoid. Excess osteoid also occurs when disphosphonate or aluminium accumulate in the skeleton (bone disease due to aluminium intoxication has occurred in some centres after chronic haemodialysis and parenteral nutrition). In rickets the main changes occur in the growth plate, which is disorganized.

Since there is intestinal malabsorption of calcium in vitamin D deficiency, both the plasma and urine calcium are lower than normal; absorption of phosphorus is also defective, with resultant hypophosphataemia. Since hypocalcaemia stimulates the secretion of parathyroid hormone this tends to correct the low plasma calcium and to exaggerate the hypophosphataemia. In osteomalacia osteoblastic activity is increased and the plasma alkaline phosphatase is therefore also increased. There appears to be no difficulty in laying down bone matrix collagen, but it cannot be properly mineralized. The effects of vitamin D deficiency are probably not confined to the skeleton, although they are clinically most obvious in this tissue.

Causes

There are many causes of osteomalacia (and rickets), some of which are very rare. They may conveniently be divided into three main groups: nutritional, malabsorptive, and renal (Table 7). The majority can be understood in terms of vitamin D metabolism (Fig. 8). In the elderly and immigrant the intake of vitamin D in the food is often deficient; its absorption is poor in coeliac disease, after partial gastrectomy, intestinal resection or bypass, and in biliary disease; and the absorption of calcium (but not vitamin D) may be reduced by phytate and chapattis. Endogenous synthesis of vitamin D in the skin is poor in northern cities, and is probably reduced by pigmentation of the skin. The 25-hydroxylation of cal-

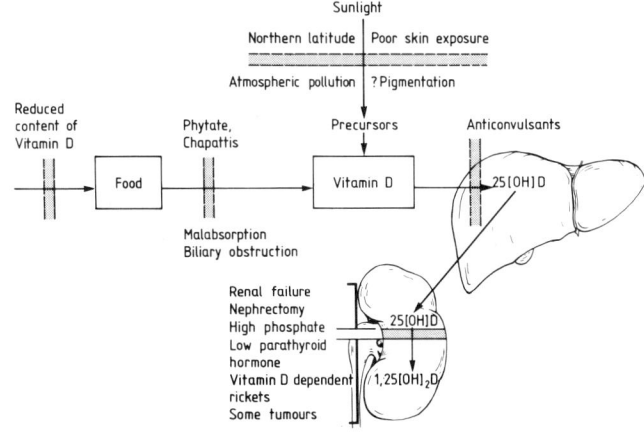

Fig. 8 The causes of osteomalacia in relation to the metabolism of vitamin D. Shaded bars indicate factors which may lead to a deficiency of vitamin D or to a disturbance of its metabolism.

Table 7 The main causes of rickets and osteomalacia

Lack of vitamin D
    Deficient synthesis in the skin
    Low dietary intake

Malabsorption
    Gluten-sensitive enteropathy (coeliac disease)
    Gastric surgery
    Bowel resection
    Intestinal bypass operations
    Biliary cirrhosis

Renal disease
    Renal-tubular disorders
        Familial hypophosphataemic rickets (Vitamin D-resistant rickets)
        Others*
    Renal glomerular failure
        Renal osteodystrophy
        Dialysis bone disease (aluminium intoxication)

Others
    Anticonvulsant osteomalacia
    Tumour rickets
    Vitamin D-dependent rickets
    Phosphate-deficiency rickets

* See Table 8.

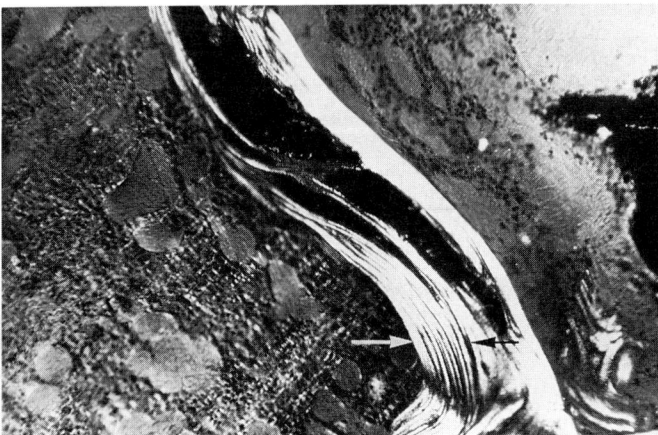

Fig. 7 Bone from a patient with osteomalacia. The birefringent osteoid seam is abnormally thick (up to 12 lamellae, arrows) and covers all bone surfaces. The bone preparation is undecalcified and viewed under polarized light (stain Von Kossa; magnification × 300). (Reproduced from Smith, 1979, *Biochemical disorders of the skeleton*, Butterworth, London, with permission.)

ciferol may be impaired in some liver diseases and probably also by anticonvulsants; and the 1-α-hydroxylation of 25(OH)D is reduced or absent in renal failure, after nephrectomy, in hyperphosphataemia, parathyroid insufficiency, in some forms of vitamin D-dependent rickets, and probably in some bone tumours. Many patients have more than one cause of osteomalacia; the elderly person may have a poor intake of vitamin D, reduced exposure to sunlight, and increasing renal failure. Reduced exposure to sunlight is a frequent consequence of physical disability. It may contribute to osteomalacia in rheumatoid arthritis, for instance.

The effects of renal glomerular failure on the skeleton are complex (page 18.156 *et seq.*). Two main events occur; one is an increase in plasma phosphate which leads to a fall in plasma calcium and to secondary hyperparathyroidism with excessive bone resorption, the other is reduced formation of 1,25(OH)$_2$D with defective intestinal absorption of calcium and defective mineralization of bone. The combination of these events rapidly produces severe deformity, especially in the growing skeleton. In some patients on dialysis a specific bone disease resembling osteomalacia has resulted from aluminium intoxication (page 18.156 *et seq.*).

Clinical features

The main symptoms of osteomalacia are bone pain and tenderness, skeletal deformity, and weakness of the proximal muscles. These may be accompanied by the features of the underlying disorder and by those of hypocalcaemia. In severe osteomalacia all the bones are painful and tender, often sufficiently so to disturb sleep. The tenderness can be particularly marked in the lower ribs and may also be accentuated over Looser's zones. Deformity is most often seen in rickets when the effects of vitamin D deficiency are superimposed on a growing skeleton. The linear growth rate is reduced, there is bowing of the long bones, enlargement of the costochondral junctions (rickety rosary), and bossing of the frontal and parietal bones. Later osteomalacia may produce a triradiate pelvis, a gross kyphosis, and corresponding deformities of the chest.

Proximal muscle weakness is an important symptom. Its cause is unknown and it is more marked in some forms of osteomalacia than in others. Most commonly there is a waddling gait, a difficulty in getting up and down stairs, out of low chairs, and in and out of small cars. In the elderly weakness may make walking impossible and suggest paraplegia. In younger subjects muscular dystrophy may be stimulated.

Features of the underlying disorder include anaemia, tiredness, and steatorrhoea in coeliac disease, pigmentation, thirst, and nocturia in renal failure. Occasionally hypocalcaemia may cause spontaneous tetany; in children the manifestations of carpopedal spasm, stridor, and fits are more dramatic than in the adult.

Examination of the patient with osteomalacia or rickets confirms the main symptoms. Measurement of the body proportions is useful. Thus patients with hypophosphataemic type I resistant rickets (see below) may have relatively short limbs whereas those with late-onset osteomalacia will have a relatively short trunk. It is important to look for clues of the cause of the osteomalacia, particularly the scars of previous gastric or intestinal surgery.

Biochemistry

Since there are many causes of osteomalacia the biochemical changes differ in detail from one another. The commonest changes which result from vitamin D deficiency or malabsorption are a low plasma calcium and phosphate, a low urine calcium, and an increase in the plasma alkaline phosphatase.

However, these vary with the stage of the disease. Initially hypocalcaemia may be the only abnormality. Later, when secondary hyperparathyroidism occurs the plasma calcium returns towards normal, but the plasma phosphate will fall and the alkaline phosphate increase. In vitamin D-resistant hypophosphataemic rickets the plasma phosphate is low, but the plasma calcium is normal and the alkaline phosphatase may also be normal. In renal glomerular failure the plasma phosphate, urea, and creatinine are all increased, and in the rare renal tubular syndromes there may be a marked systemic acidosis. In patients with osteomalacia the urine should always be examined for the presence of glucose and protein and (if these are present) amino acids.

Radiology

The radiological appearances differ according to whether growth has ceased or not. In rickets the main abnormalities are at the ends of the long bones where the width of the growth plate is increased, and the metaphysis is widened, cupped, and ragged (Fig. 9). Osteomalacia may show the deformities previously described but the radiological hallmark of active osteomalacia is the Looser zone (Fig. 10). This is a ribbon-like area of demineralization which may be found in almost any bone but is seen particularly in the long bones, the pelvis, and the ribs, and also around the scapulae. Looser's zones may be bilateral and symmetrical; in bones such as the femur they occur on the concavity of bone and are usually

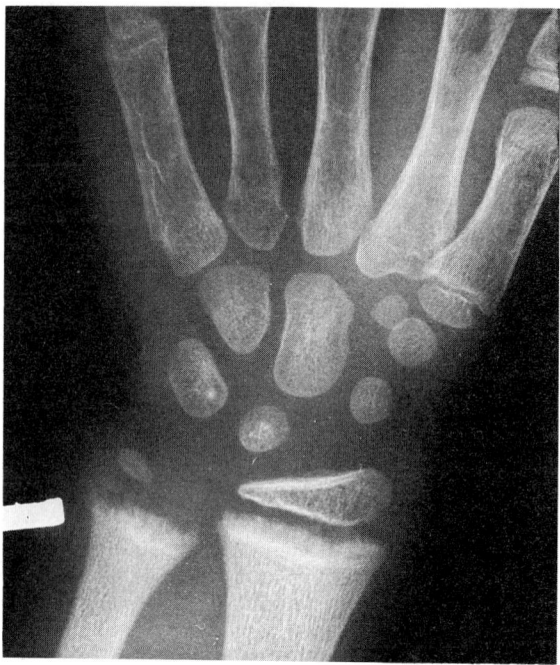

Fig. 9 Rickets in a child with cystinosis. The growth plate is widened and the metaphyses cupped and ragged. (Reproduced from Smith, 1979, *Biochemical disorders of the skeleton*, Butterworth, London, with permission.)

single, in contrast to the multiple fissure fractures on the convexity of the bone in Paget's disease. In osteomalacia the vertebral bodies often become uniformly biconcave to produce an appearance likened to a fish spine. In renal glomerular osteodystrophy, the end plates may become relatively more dense than the rest of the vertebral body to produce the so-called 'rugger jersey' spine. In hypophosphataemic vitamin D-resistant rickets the bones may also become very dense; in addition in this disorder calcification of the vertebral ligaments produces an appearance not unlike that of ankylosing spondylitis. The narrowing of the spinal canal this produces is well shown by CT scanning. In most patients with osteomalacia who have hypocalcaemia the radiological features of secondary hyperparathyroidism appear with subperiosteal bone resorption which affects the phalanges, the pubic symphysis, and the outer ends of the clavicles. In rickets, periostitis of the distal ends of the long bones such as the radius and ulna often occur. The most extreme effects of parathyroid overactivity are seen in the skeleton of the child with renal osteodystrophy where the region of the growth plate and metaphyses may fracture (an appearance likened to a 'rotting stump'). An isotope scan may be very useful in osteomalacia, demonstrating multiple pathological fractures often not seen on the plain films. The appearance needs to be distinguished from that of bony metastases.

Bone biopsy

Often the diagnosis of osteomalacia is clear without examining the bone, and in most patients this is done merely to confirm the diagnosis. Bone should be taken by transiliac biopsy and examined before and after decalcification to demonstrate the failure of mineralization and the wide osteoid seams. It is important to take all opportunities for the histological examination of bone; this particularly includes bone obtained at operation on fractured femurs in the elderly. In some situations bone biopsy may be useful as a guide to treatment.

Other investigations

Further investigation is not usually needed to diagnose osteomalacia, but may be necessary to identify its cause.

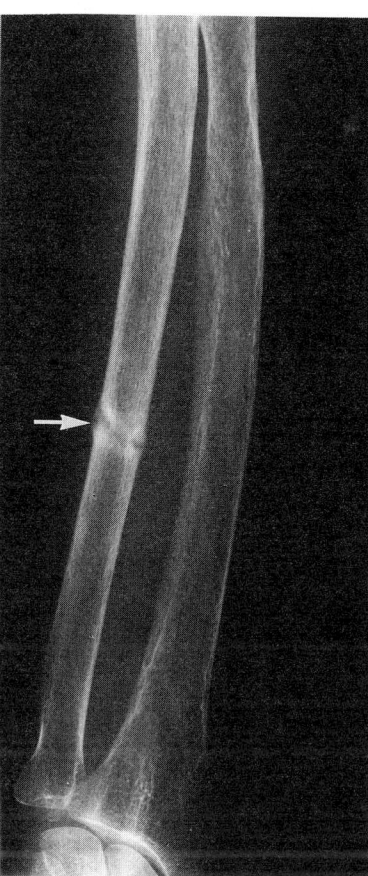

Fig. 10 The appearance of a Looser's zone (arrowed) in the ulna of a 74-year-old woman 13 years after a partial gastrectomy. The appearances in the other forearm were identical.

Diagnosis

The diagnosis of osteomalacia is not difficult once it is thought of. It should be distinguished from other forms of metabolic bone disease (Table 3), from other causes of proximal muscle weakness, and from other disorders causing bone pain. In patients with proximal muscle weakness, polymyalgia rheumatica, thyrotoxic myopathy, muscular dystrophy, neoplastic neuropathy, dermatomyositis, and polymyositis all need to be considered. Multiple myeloma and leukaemia may need to be excluded as causes of bone pain. Provided that the plasma calcium, phosphorus, and alkaline phosphatase are always measured in patients with these symptoms, those with osteomalacia should be easily identified. Patients with psychological illness may have an abnormal gait and complain of pain and weakness in their limbs; but in such patients the biochemistry will be normal. In practice the symptoms of pain and stiffness often first lead the patient with osteomalacia to a rheumatologist.

Treatment

The patient with rickets or osteomalacia will respond rapidly to vitamin D (or to its metabolites) in an appropriate dose, which is a useful way of confirming the diagnosis. Increased mobility with alleviation of the muscle weakness may be the first clinical response, despite a temporary increase in bone pain. Biochemically the plasma phosphate and urine hydroxyproline are the first to increase. The alkaline phosphatase may show a temporary rise and then fall slowly to normal levels. As the plasma calcium and 25(OH)D concentrations increase towards normal, the parathyroid hormone concentration falls.

The effective dose and preparation of vitamin D depends on the cause of the osteomalacia. That due to vitamin D deficiency will

respond to microgram doses but it is often useful to give considerably more than this, such as calciferol 1.25 mg daily for one to two weeks only. Where there is doubt about compliance, vitamin D may be injected intramuscularly in one large dose (up to 15 mg = 600 000 units). Lack of response to microgram doses suggests that the osteomalacia is not due to simple vitamin D deficiency but, for instance, to malabsorption or renal failure. It is particularly in the last group that the l-α-hydroxylated metabolites of vitamin D are effective. Clearly underlying disorders must be treated at the same time. For example, patients with coeliac disease will need a gluten-free diet.

Particular forms of osteomalacia and rickets

Nutritional osteomalacia

In the United Kingdom nutritional osteomalacia occurs particularly amongst the elderly and in Asian immigrants of all ages. In the elderly the high incidence of osteomalacia is mainly due to poor exposure to sunlight and to a low intake of vitamin D; and may be contributed to by the effects of drugs such as anticonvulsants and by increasing renal glomerular failure. Since the elderly are often housebound they may develop osteomalacia despite a sunny climate. Certainly the prevalence of osteomalacia in the elderly population is significant. The frequency of osteomalacia in patients with fractures of the femoral neck is also higher than previously suspected but figures up to 30 per cent which have been given (according to the histological definition used) are probably overestimates. Osteomalacia should always be excluded in elderly people with bone disease, and particularly in those with femoral neck fractures. Where possible this should be done by histological examination of bone taken at operation or by biopsy. Where this is not appropriate a therapeutic trial with vitamin D is often useful. Since it is often difficult to define osteomalacia accurately in elderly people such empirical treatment is important. In the geriatric population the mean concentration of 25(OH)D is much lower than in non-elderly patients; it shows the usual seasonal variation with lowest values in the winter and early spring and highest in late summer.

Asian immigrants to the United Kingdom develop osteomalacia and rickets more often than the indigenous population. They tend to live in northern cities away from sunlight and continue to take a diet low in vitamin D. Deficiency of vitamin D is more likely to occur in Asian women than in men because the women do not get out so much and eat a less varied diet. It has been suggested that chapattis contribute to the high incidence of osteomalacia and rickets but the evidence is not clear.

Pigmentation of the skin has only minor importance and osteomalacia due to lack of vitamin D will heal in both Blacks and Asians when they are exposed to sufficient ultraviolet light. As in the elderly, 25(OH)D levels are very low in Asian immigrants; they increase in the summer when there may be spontaneous healing of rickets. The rickets of Asiatic immigrants may be best prevented by fortifying food such as chapatti flour with vitamin D.

The causes of osteomalacia and rickets in Asian immigrants continue to be investigated, and are not fully explained by current knowledge of vitamin D metabolism. Measurements of 25(OH)D concentrations have shown that vitamin D status is normally determined by exposure to sunlight and the contribution of dietary vitamin D is largely irrelevant. However, follow-up studies on Asian communities living in northern cities in the United Kingdom now show a considerable decline in rickets in children although the incidence of adult osteomalacia continues to be high. This is attributed to the more ready adaptation of children to the Western way of life, and implies both an increase in dietary vitamin D and also an increase in sunlight exposure.

Osteomalacia and malabsorption

Coeliac disease (gluten-sensitive enteropathy) is a relatively common cause of osteomalacia. It should be suspected at any age and confirmed by a small intestinal biopsy showing an atrophic mucosa. Other causes of malabsorption vary in their frequency according to surgical practice. Thus it is well established that osteomalacia follows classic partial gastrectomy but the actual incidence is debated, its cause is probably multifactorial, and post-gastrectomy subjects tend to take little vitamin D in their diet. Available evidence suggests that clinical osteomalacia is rare after vagotomy and pyloroplasty. Osteomalacia can also follow removal of long segments of small intestine for conditions such as Crohn's disease, and complicates the currently used intestinal bypass operations for extreme obesity.

Osteomalacia and liver disease

In liver disease osteomalacia is uncommon; when it occurs it may be due to a number of factors such as malabsorption of vitamin D and its defective 25-hydroxylation. Most recent work is concerned with the osteomalacia of biliary cirrhosis, and osteomalacia in chronic liver disease appears to be a complication related to prolonged cholestasis.

Osteomalacia and renal disease

It is important to distinguish the osteomalacia and rickets of renal glomerular failure from that attributable to renal tubular disorders. Bone disease in renal glomerular failure (renal osteodystrophy) is dealt with elsewhere (see page 18.156 *et seq.*); this includes bone disease in the dialysed patient and the effects of aluminium. Renal glomerular osteodystrophy is a complex disease with excessive bone resorption, defective bone mineralization, and in some cases osteoporosis. Previously it was treated with large doses of native vitamin D; current therapy now includes 1-α-hydroxycholecalciferol or 1,25(OH)$_2$D.

Many renal tubular disorders lead to osteomalacia (Table 8). Of these the most common is the so-called hypophosphataemic vitamin D-resistant rickets (VDRR), which is normally inherited as an X-linked dominant characteristic, and in which the main abnormality is hypophosphataemia due to a reduction in the maximum renal tubular reabsorption rate of phosphate. Some patients in a family will have hypophosphataemia alone whilst others will have hypophosphataemia with accompanying bone disease. The cause of the renal abnormality has not been established. It does not seem to be due to overactivity of the parathyroids, and there is no convincing evidence of a deficiency or a disturbance of vitamin D metabolism. Children with hypophosphataemic rickets or osteomalacia are clinically and biochemically unlike patients with other forms of rickets. They present with deformity but are otherwise well, without muscle weakness; however, growth is defective and eventual height is usually less than 150 cm. Apart from hypophosphataemia there may also be no other detectable biochemical abnormality and the plasma alkaline phosphatase can be normal for age. Childhood radiographs show severe rickets and later the bones are often dense with buttressing and exostoses. In the adult a rare but well-recognized complication is calcification and ossification of the ligamenta flava, whose extent can be well shown by CT scanning which can lead to paraplegia. Ligamentous calcification may also contribute to deafness.

Treatment of inherited hypophosphataemia is controversial. For many years its mainstay has been large doses of vitamin D. This does not correct the eventual short stature and there is the continuing danger of vitamin D overdosage. Often oral phosphate is given in addition to vitamin D, and claims of improvement in growth rate have been made. The condition does not appear to respond to phosphate alone. More recently it has been shown that oral phosphate and 1,25(OH)$_2$D produces healing of both epiphyseal and trabecular bone.

It is important that parents should know the genetics of this condition. Because the defect in phosphate transport is inherited as a dominant on the X chromosome, an affected mother transmits the condition to 50 per cent of her children regardless of their sex. All the daughters of an affected father will have the disease, but none

Table 8   Rickets, osteomalacia, and renal-tubular disorders

Familial hypophosphataemic rickets
   (vitamin D-resistant rickets)

Adult-onset hypophosphataemic osteomalacia

Renal tubular acidosis
   Inherited
      Proximal (bicarbonate wastage)
      Distal   (H+ gradient defect)
   Acquired
      Ureterocolic anastomosis

Multiple renal-tubular defects (Fanconi syndrome)
   Inherited
      Cystinosis
      Oculocerebrorenal syndrome
      Wilson's disease
      Galactosaemia
   Acquired*
      Cadmium poisoning
      Multiple myeloma

* A common feature of these forms of Fanconi syndrome appears to be an increase in the excretion of lysosyme in the urine.

of his sons. In general affected sons have a more severe disease and some affected daughters may be asymptomatic. Diagnosis can be made from birth but demands accurate knowledge of the normal plasma phosphate at that age.

Other renal tubular osteomalacia syndromes include hypophosphataemic osteomalacia presenting in adult life which may be due to a tumour (see below), inherited, and acquired forms of renal tubular acidosis, and rickets associated with multiple renal tubular defects and generalized aminoaciduria (the Fanconi syndrome; see page 18.171 *et seq.* and Section 9). Renal tubular acidosis may be proximal or distal, with inability to reabsorb bicarbonate or to acidify the urine. The associated osteomalacia may be cured by giving bicarbonate alone or with vitamin D. A persistent acidosis with resultant osteomalacia may also result from uretero-sigmoid anastomosis. The commonest cause of the Fanconi syndrome in childhood is cystinosis or cystine-storage disease, where there is a widespread deposition of cystine crystals throughout the tissues and in which thirst, polyuria, dehydration, photophobia, and loss of weight begin at about the age of one year. The rickets will heal with the correction of the acidosis, and the administration of phosphate and 1-α-(OH)D; renal transplantation may also be effective.

Other rare causes of renal tubular osteomalacia include Wilson's disease, cadmium poisoning, and the X-linked oculocerebral renal syndrome.

Anticonvulsant osteomalacia

In patients treated with anticonvulsants the incidence of rickets and osteomalacia is higher than normal. This has been attributed to the induction by the anticonvulsants of hepatic enzymes which metabolize vitamin D to biologically inactive derivatives. However, epileptic patients in institutions are often deficient of vitamin D because they are deprived of sunlight, and osteomalacia in such patients probably has several causes.

Tumour rickets

An interesting but rare form of hypophosphataemic rickets or osteomalacia occurs in patients who have tumours often of a particular pathological type, namely, sclerosing haemangiomas or non-ossifying fibromas. In any adult who develops hypophosphataemic osteomalacia, particularly with prominent myopathy, a tumour should be considered. The disorder is improved by oral phosphate and cured by removal of the tumour. The way in which the tumour induces hypophosphataemia and subsequent osteomalacia is unknown but current evidence suggests that it interferes with renal l-α-hydroxylation of 25(OH)D, since the circulating levels of 1,25(OH)$_2$D are abnormally low. Oncogenic osteomalacia has also been described in prostatic and oat-cell carcinoma.

Vitamin D dependent rickets

Patients with this rare inherited form of rickets show the features of severe rickets without vitamin D deficiency. It is now recognized that there are at least two forms of vitamin D-dependent rickets (VDDR). In type I the l-α-hydroxylation of 25 OHD is defective so that the concentration of 1,25(OH)$_2$D is abnormally low. However, it can be increased by large doses of the native vitamin, which shows that the enzyme block is not complete; in type II there is an end-organ resistance to 1,25(OH)$_2$D which is present in high concentrations. In both forms there are severe rickets and myopathy from infancy; in type II lifelong total alopecia is a striking feature. VDDR type I responds to very large doses of vitamin D or physiological doses of 1,25(OH)$_2$D; type II may also respond to large doses of vitamin D or its metabolites, but some recorded cases suggest that recovery occurs spontaneously with age.

Phosphate-deficiency rickets

If patients take a large amount of phosphate-binding drugs such as aluminium hydroxide, a form of hypophosphataemic osteomalacia may develop. This differs clinically from inherited hypophosphataemic osteomalacia by the presence of severe muscle weakness. Other biochemical features include increased calcium absorption with hypercalcuria, associated with an increase above normal in the concentration of 1,25(OH)$_2$D.

References

Alfrey, A. C. (1984). Aluminium intoxication. *N. Engl. J. Med.* **310**, 1113–1115.

Dunningham, M. G., McIntosh, W. B., Ford, J. A. and Robertson, I. (1982). Acquired disorders of vitamin D metabolism. In *Calcium disorders*. Butterworths International Medical Reviews. *Clinical endocrinology* Vol. 2 (eds D. Heath and S. J. Marx), pp. 125–150. Butterworth Scientific, London.

Glorieux, F. H., Marie, P. J., Pettifer, J. M. and Delvin, E. E. (1980). Bone response to phosphate salts, ergocalciferol and calcitriol in hypophosphataemic vitamin D-resistant rickets. *N. Engl. J. Med.* **303**, 1023–1031.

Hosking, D. J., Campbell, G. A., Kemm, J. R., Cotton, R. E., Knight, M. E., Berryman, R. and Boyd, R. V. (1983). Screening for subclinical osteomalacia in the elderly: normal ranges or pragmatism? *Lancet* **ii**, 1290–1292.

Scriver, C. R., Fraser, D. and Kooh, S. W. (1982). Hereditary rickets. In *Calcium disorders*. Butterworth International Medical Reviews. *Clinical endocrinology* Vol. 2. (eds D. Heath and S. J. Marx), pp. 125–150. Butterworth Scientific, London.

Paget's disease of bone

Paget's disease of bone is also known as osteitis deformans. It was first described a century ago, but undoubtedly existed for many years before. Next to osteoporosis it is the commonest of the 'metabolic' bone diseases. Its hallmark is excessive and disorganized resorption and formation of bone. Its cause is unknown, but recent studies on its epidemiology and on the ultrastructure of Pagetic osteoclasts provide clues.

Incidence

Paget's disease occurs in about 3–4 per cent of subjects over 40 years of age, is commoner in men than in women, and its frequency increases with age. It is not unknown in younger people. In Britain about 650 000 people may have Paget's disease, but less than 5 per cent of them have symptoms. It seems to be an Anglo-Saxon affliction, being very rare in countries such as Scandinavia and Japan. Within England radiological surveys have shown that it

Table 9 The radiological prevalence of Paget's disease among hospital patients aged 55 years and over in some British towns

Town	Prevalence (%) of Paget's disease	
	Men	Women
Preston	8.6	6.3
Bolton	7.7	6.4
Blackburn	8.8	3.8
Bradford	7.9	3.6
Hull	7.6	3.1
Southampton	6.6	3.6
Bath	5.3	4.7
Stoke	4.7	4.2
York	5.8	2.5

These data are based on more than 500 patients in each town. The age-standardized incidence is always higher in men than in women. The high incidence in Lancashire towns is not explained. (Modified from Barker *et al.*, 1977.)

occurs most often in Lancashire towns and in northern industrial regions (Table 9). It is also more frequent in recent British immigrants to Western Australia than in the Western Australian population, but less frequent than in those relatives who remained in Britain. Such studies do not necessarily distinguish between the effect of environment and heredity. In a disorder as common as Paget's disease a high incidence in some families will occur by chance and many striking examples of 'familial' Paget's disease exist.

Cause

The high frequency of Paget's disease in the north of England led to the suggestion that it follows nutritional rickets, but there is no other evidence for this. Its behaviour is similar to that of a multicentric neoplasm or slow virus disease. Some evidence of the latter is provided by the discovery of virus-like inclusion bodies in the osteoclasts of patients with Paget's disease. The original contention that these represented the measles virus now seems unlikely; a respiratory syncitial virus seems a more likely candidate.

Pathophysiology

Histologically Pagetic bone shows abnormal-looking osteoclasts with many nuclei which appear to be actively resorbing bone, and busy osteoblasts which appear to be replacing it; these activities are closely linked. Fibrosis occurs in the marrow. The bone matrix is laid down in all directions and partially loses its birefringence. Mineralization of the matrix may be defective, probably because of the rate at which the matrix is laid down. The cement lines and the mosaic appearances of the bone result from the tidemarks of resorption followed by formation. Osteosarcoma may complicate Paget's disease and presumably results from the excessive and prolonged activity of the bone cells. Pagetic bone is larger and more vascular than normal and often deformed. Its physical characteristics depend on the stage of the disorder, and it may be hard or soft. In any case it fractures more readily than normal.

Signs and symptoms
Pain, deformity, fracture

In Paget's disease the bone itself may be painful, or pain may be due to arthritis of a nearby joint, to an associated fracture or to the development of sarcoma. It has been suggested that there is a specific type of hip joint disorder associated with Paget's disease. Bone pain could be due to distension of the periosteum since it is this part of the bone (and the vessels within bone) which contain nerves sensitive to pain. Clinically the affected bones are enlarged, deformed, and warm. The enlargement is well seen in bones such as the tibia and the skull; in the former the bone is typically bowed forwards; the latter shows a characteristic enlarge-

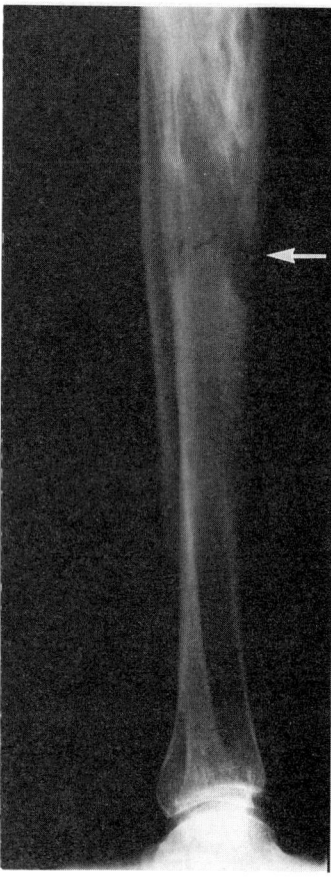

Fig. 11 A fracture in the region of a resorbing front in a Pagetic bone (arrowed). Proximal to the area of bone resorption the cortex is thickened and the bone widened by disorganized formation of new bone.

ment of the vault which is said to look like a soft beret, or 'tam-o-shanter', which appears to descend over the ears. Other long bones may become bent and a kyphosis may develop. Although any of the bones can be affected, including the maxilla and the phalanges, the most common sites for Paget's disease are the pelvis and the spine. Fracture may be the first symptom of undiagnosed Paget's disease, for instance, at the junction of a resorbing front with normal bone (Fig. 11), or across a microfracture (see Fig. 12).

Deafness and nerve compression
The deafness in Paget's disease is one of its most disabling symptoms and responds little to treatment. It has many causes of which nerve compression is only one.

Most nerves can be compressed by enlarging Pagetic bone. The spinal cord is particularly at risk, due to the combined effects of increased bone mass, vertebral collapse, and excessive vascularity. Paraplegia or cauda equina lesions may occur. Alterations in the shape of the skull may produce multiple cranial nerve palsies and brain stem lesions, with dysphagia, dysarthia, and ataxia. Basilar invagination with obstruction of cerebrospinal fluid drainage can lead to internal hydrocephalus, raised intracranial pressure, and confusion.

Heart failure
In severe Paget's disease cardiac output may be considerably increased, and with effective treatment this can be reduced towards normal. The increase is related to the excessive vascularity of the affected bones, but there is no convincing evidence of large arteriovenous shunts within the skeleton. The heart failure which results may be of the 'high output' variety but this is rare.

Both heart failure and Paget's disease of bone are common in the elderly, and their occurrence together is usually coincidental.

Sarcoma
The incidence of sarcoma in Paget's disease has probably been overestimated and appears to be 1 per cent or less of those with symptoms. Paget's sarcoma is said to occur often in the humerus, although Paget's disease itself is most common in the pelvis and spine; the diagnosis should be considered in a patient known to have Paget's disease if pain has developed for the first time, or worsened, or if deformity has altered. The radiographic appearance of the Pagetic bone alters, with evidence of bone destruction (Fig. 13); the tumours probably occur most often in the medulla of the bone. A recent review of 85 bone sarcomas associated with Paget's disease confirmed the humerus as a high-risk site. Rapidly worsening pain was the main symptom; lytic lesions were commoner than sclerotic; periosteal reaction was uncommon; and radionuclide diphosphonate scans often showed areas of decreased uptake (contrasting with the underlying Pagetic bone).

Associated disorders
It is often stated that Paget's disease is associated with an increase in many other disorders such as osteoarthritis, gout, vascular calcification, and articular chondrocalcinosis. All these occur more often in the elderly and the associations probably have little significance.

Biochemistry
The most striking biochemical change is a considerable increase in the plasma alkaline phosphatase. This enzyme is largely derived from the osteoblasts and reflects the intense overactivity of Pagetic bone. It is roughly related to the extent of clinical and radiological involvement; in contrast the acid phosphatase (derived partly

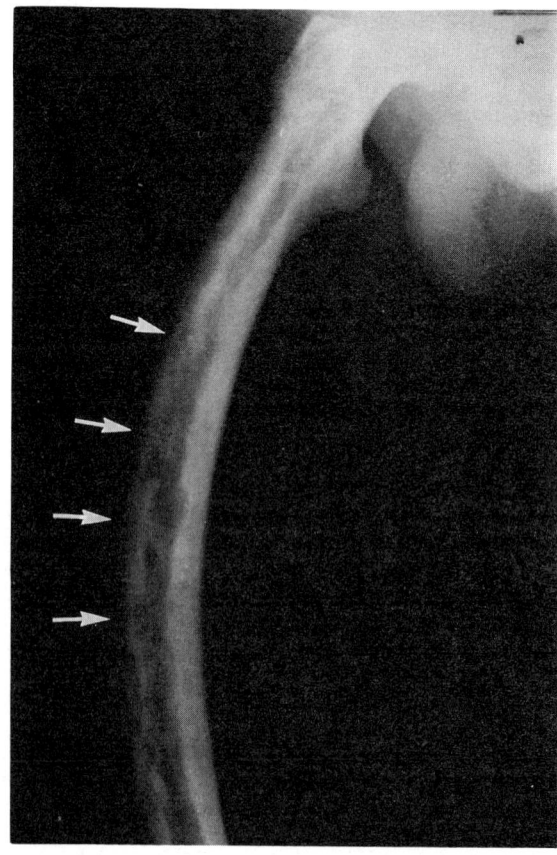

Fig. 12 Multiple microfractures ('fissure fractures' arrowed) on the convex surface of a Pagetic femur.

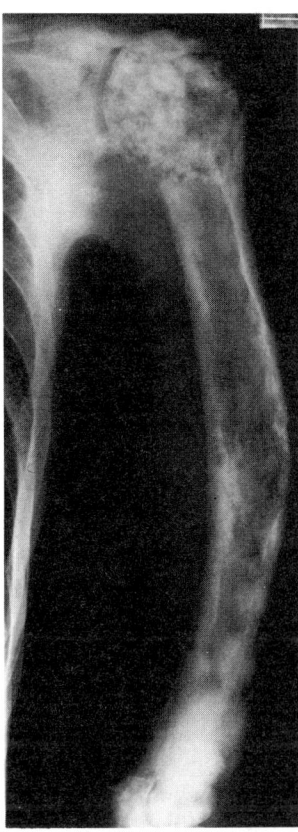

Fig. 13 A sarcoma in the upper end of the left humerus in a man of 70 with Paget's disease. The destructive lesion in the proximal humerus has been treated with radiotherapy; there are secondary deposits around the distal end of the bone. (Reproduced from Smith, 1979, *Biochemical disorders of the skeleton*, Butterworth, London, with permission.)

from osteoclasts) is only slightly increased. The rapid turnover of bone matrix collagen increases the urinary hydroxyproline (and hydroxylysine), in proportion to the increase in alkaline phosphatase. The plasma calcium and phosphate are usually normal; an increase in plasma calcium suggests co-existent hyperparathyroidism or may result from immobility.

Radiology
Plain films
The radiological appearances of Paget's disease are legion. The most characteristic is an increase in size of the affected bone. It is generally true that resorption predominates early in the disease and in the young patient. A resorbing front may be seen in a long bone (as a flame-shaped area) or in the skull (as 'osteoporosis circumscripta'). Excessive resorption is inevitably followed by disordered formation and at this stage that bone becomes thick and deformed. In elderly subjects the affected bone may be very osteoporotic and liable to fracture. Multiple partial fractures (microfractures, fissure fractures) are common on the deformed convex surface of long bones (Fig. 12), particularly the femur and tibia.

Radionuclide scans
The use of bone scanning agents (such as ^{99m}Tc EHDP) has been particularly informative in Paget's disease. Affected bones take up the scan avidly, which demonstrates both the extent of the bone lesions and the effects of treatment. In a recent study, scintigraphy was performed in 180 patients with Paget's disease and 826 lesions were identified. One-third of the patients had only one lesion, and only 10 had no symptoms. The increase in plasma alkaline phosphatase and urinary total hydroxyproline was proportional to scin-

tigraphic involvement, and those with skull involvement had the highest values. The distinction between monostotic and polyostotic disease appeared to be artificial.

Other investigations
The diagnosis of Paget's disease is usually obvious. If it is not, additional investigations may be helpful. These include iliac bone biopsy which is useful to exclude other generalized bone diseases such as osteomalacia, as well as to confirm Paget's disease. Patients with active Paget's disease are also normally in negative calcium balance and demonstrate a high skeletal turnover rate.

Diagnosis
Paget's disease should be differentiated from other forms of metabolic bone disease. It may be confused with osteomalacia because of the high plasma alkaline phosphatase; rarely an elevated plasma calcium may suggest additional hyperparathyroidism. Since Paget's disease is very common it may co-exist with many other conditions. It is important to differentiate it from prostatic carcinoma with osteoblastic bone secondaries. In this latter condition the dense bones are not enlarged (as they are in Paget's disease) and the acid phosphatase is considerably and disproportionately increased in relation to the alkaline phosphatase. Of the many other conditions with similar radiological appearance, fibrous dysplasia (see page 17.33), in which the alkaline phosphatase may also be slightly increased, may be difficult to distinguish; in the generalized form the unilateral bone lesions, pigmentation, and sexual precocity (in the female) are characteristic. Another rare disorder which is usually mistaken for Paget's disease is fibrogenesis imperfecta ossium (see page 17.36) in which there is generalized thickening of bone trabeculae without bony enlargement and multiple abnormal fractures.

Treatment
Most patients with Paget's disease require no treatment. Treatment is given for symptoms, to suppress the activity of the disease, and to prevent its further progression. Indications therefore include bone pain, nerve compression, and the suppression of vascularity before elective orthopaedic surgery.

Medical treatment
Patients with pain associated with Paget's disease should first be treated with a simple analgesic. If possible it should be determined whether the pain is directly due to the bone disease or to associated arthritis. In those patients who have pain due to bone disease which persists despite analgesia, or have the complications of deformity, nerve compression, deafness, or heart failure, specific treatment aimed at the Pagetic bone should be considered. This should also be considered to prevent further progress of the disease, especially in the young person with Paget's disease. There is no evidence that the rapid course of Pagetic sarcoma is altered by any treatment. Of the many agents previously tried in Paget's disease, such as aspirin, fluoride, and corticosteroids, only three are currently in use; mithramycin, phosphonates, and calcitonin. Mithramycin (like actinomycin) is an antimitotic given intravenously and is hepatotoxic in high doses. It is said to abolish pain rapidly in Paget's disease, and also to reduce the plasma alkaline phosphatase, but the effect is usually temporary. Mithramycin should probably only be used to treat painful Paget's disease in the elderly. It can be given on its own or in combination with diphosphonates or calcitonin. The usual daily dose is 15–25 μg/kg body weight either given as a 10-day course or once weekly.

The diphosphonates are a series of compounds with a P-C-P backbone resistant to the naturally occurring phosphatases and pyrophosphatases. They are effective orally and reduce excessive bone turnover in Paget's disease. The first diphosphonate to be used (and the only one commercially available), ethane-1-hydroxy-1,1-diphosphonate (disodium etidronate, EHDP) also interferes with mineralization if given in high doses (20 mg/kg body weight); subsequent derivatives, dichloromethylene diphosphonate (Cl$_2$ MDP) and 3-amino-1-hydroxypropylidine-1,1-*bis*-phosphonate (APD) do not appear to do this. According to their dose the phosphonates may take up to six months to produce their effect on symptoms, histology, and biochemistry. The recommended dose for EHDP is 5 mg/kg/day for up to six months. EHDP may also be given intravenously. It has also been used in combination with calcitonin and together these agents suppress Paget's disease more effectively than when given alone. The biochemical effects of EHDP appear to last for a long time (possibly several years) after the drug is stopped. Recent work shows that Cl$_2$MDP effectively suppresses resorption in Paget's disease without disturbing mineralization.

The calcitonins are the most widely used drugs for the treatment of Paget's disease and salmon calcitonin is the most effective commercially available form. Various dose regimens have been used, of which 100 MRC units three times a week is average. Calcitonin is injected intramuscularly or subcutaneously and may produce nausea and vomiting; if side effects are troublesome it is best given in the evening with an antiemetic. Its main effects, like those of the phosphonates, occur in the first 3 months of treatment, and continued injection is ineffective, especially when the alkaline phosphatase level has ceased to decline. Antibodies to calcitonin do develop but appear not to be related to calcitonin 'resistance'. It is becoming clear that the indications for the diphosphonates (now also known as bisphosphonates) and calcitonins are different. Calcitonin is preferred to treat bone pain, for osteolytic Paget's disease, and for preoperative treatment (below). The effect of these agents on deafness and nerve compression is not yet fully defined. Some evidence suggests that calcitonin may halt the progression of deafness. Since the main cause of the spinal cord compression is bony enlargement, it would be surprising if treatment of Paget's disease produced a significant improvement. However, several reports suggest that improvement does occur, particularly with Cl$_2$MDP. In one, treatment of eight patients with paraparesis due to Pagetic vertebrae with calcitonin or diphosphonates produced marked clinical improvement, which was at least comparable to the results of surgical decompression.

Finally calcitonin is increasingly given preoperatively to reduce excessive bleeding when operations such as total hip replacement have to be done on Pagetic bone.

Surgical treatment
Fractures through Pagetic bone require surgical treatment as if the bone was normal, although union may be delayed. In addition, osteotomy and intramedullary nailing may be considered for severe long bone deformity. Spinal cord compression not responding to medical treatment requires laminectomy. Rarely hydrocephalus may require a ventriculo-jugular shunt. Whatever form of surgery is undertaken, it is important that the period of immobility is as short as possible to avoid hypercalcuria and hypercalcaemia.

References
Barker, D. J. P., Clough, P. W. L., Guyer, P. B., and Gardner, M. J. (1977). Paget's disease of bone in 14 British towns. *Br. Med. J.* **1**, 1181–1183.

Douglas, D. L., Duckworth, T., Kanis, J. A., Jefferson, A. A., Martin, T. J. and Russell, R. G. G. (1981). Spinal cord dysfunction in Paget's disease of bone. *J. Bone Joint Surg.* **63B**, 495–503.

Hamdy, R. C. (1981). *Paget's disease of bone. Assessment and management.* Praeger Publishers, New York.

Harinck, H. I. J., Bijvoet, O. L. M., Vellanga, C. J. L. R., Blanksma, H. J., Frijlink, W. B. and Te Velde, J. (1986). The relation between signs and symptoms in Paget's disease of bone. *Q. J. Med.* **58**, 133–151.

Krane, S. M. (1982). Etidronate sodium in Paget's disease of bone. *Ann. inter. Med.* **96**, 619–625.

Smith, J., Botet, J. F. and Yeh, S. D. J. (1984). Bone sarcomas in Paget's disease: a study of 85 patients. *Radiology* **152**, 583–590.

Parathyroids and bone disease

Knowledge of the physiology of the parathyroid hormone (see page 10.51 *et seq.*) has expanded so rapidly that it now occupies a large part of any clinical description of parathyroid disorders. With increasing recognition of the many alternative ways in which parathyroid disorders may present the close relationship between these endocrine glands and the skeleton may be forgotten. However, primary hyperparathyroidism was first identified because of its effects on the skeleton and only later was it realized that parathyroid overactivity might more often present with renal stones, with pancreatitis, and with the signs and symptoms of hypercalcaemia, or be discovered by multichannel biochemical screening of plasma. It is important to emphasize the effect of hyperparathyroidism on the skeleton, and also to note that in its several forms hypoparathyroidism is also associated with skeletal abnormality.

Hyperparathyroidism
Pathophysiology
The clinical effects of hyperparathyroidism are due to an increase in secretion of parathyroid hormone and its fragments; these increase the intestinal absorption of calcium, the renal reabsorption of calcium, and the resorption of bone. The excessive production of parathyroid hormone may be primary (due to a parathyroid adenoma, to hyperplasia, and rarely to parathyroid carcinoma), secondary to prolonged hypocalcaemia with renal failure or steatorrhea, or rarely as part of an inherited endocrine adenoma syndrome. The effects of this increase in parathyroid hormone on bone and kidney are apparently mediated through cyclic AMP; and on the intestine partly by its effect on the renal 1-α-hydroxylase. Eighty per cent of patients with primary hyperparathyroidism have a parathyroid adenoma. In the remaining 20 per cent the parathyroids show primary chief or water clear hyperplasia or carcinoma. Variable hyperplasia also occurs in the dominantly inherited condition of benign familial hypercalcaemia (see below). Parathyroid carcinoma may be difficult to diagnose but it tends to have a different clinical picture from that of parathyroid adenoma; bone disease is frequent; occasionally there is a palpable mass in the neck; and often there is recurrence after operation.

The histological features of parathyroid bone disease (osteitis fibrosa cystica) include increased osteoclastic resorption, excess osteoid, fibrosis of the marrow, and where bone turnover is very rapid, an increase in woven bone. Whilst quantitative histological studies show that the bone in primary hyperparathyroidism is nearly always abnormal, clinical bone disease tends to occur only in those patients with the biggest parathyroid tumours and most marked hypercalcaemia.

Clinical features, symptoms, and signs
The annual incidence of primary hyperparathyroidism has been put at 25 per 100 000 of the population. Before multichannel biochemical screening a typical distribution of the clinical features was as follows: renal stones and nephrocalcinosis, 47 per cent; osteitis fibrosa 13 per cent; gastrointestinal manifestations, 12 per cent; hypercalcaemic symptoms, 7 per cent; hypertension, 4 per cent; psychiatric disorder, 2 per cent. Renal stones occur more often than bone disease, and psychological abnormalities are probably commoner than usually recorded. Recent reviews have suggested that more than half the patients with primary hyperparathyroidism are now diagnosed by biochemical screening; and that hypercalcaemia, dehydration, and confusion is a significant mode of presentation in the elderly. It is also clear that the likelihood of hypercalcaemia being due to hyperparathyroidism varies widely according to the sampled population (with or without symptoms; outpatients or inpatients) (Table 10). When osteitis fibrosa is the presenting symptom it produces bone pain and tenderness, deformity and pathological fractures. It may first be

Table 10 The causes of hypercalcaemia

Diagnosis	Features	Comments
Neoplastic disease* (usually hydrocortisone sensitive)	Common. With or without secondary deposits. Biochemistry like hyperparathyroidism. Multiple myeloma	Including tumours of lung, breast, and others High ESR, Bence–Jones (light chain) proteinuria
	Lymphoma, leukemia	
Hyperparathyroidism	Multiple (see text); does not respond to corticosteroids	
Vitamin D overdosage	May give acute hypercalcaemic symptoms; thirst, vomiting, sore eyes	Most often in patients treated with vitamin D
Sarcoidosis (and other granulomas)	Nephrocalcinosis, splenomegaly, hilar lymphadenopathy. Precipitated by sunlight or physiological amounts of vitamin D	May be due to inappropriate formation of $1,25(OH)_2D$
Immobility	Especially in young people or in Paget's disease	
Thyrotoxicosis	Increased bone turnover Plasma phosphate increased	Alkaline phosphatase and hydroxyproline increased
Milk alkali syndrome	Associated with milk and alkali ingestion for peptic ulceration; more commonly due to 'indigestion' tablets	Very uncommon in acute forms
Thiazide diuretics Hypoadrenalism Acute renal failure		

* The relative frequency of neoplastic disease and hyperparathyroidism as a cause for hypercalcaemia varies with the population. In screening of healthy outpatients more than 85 per cent of patients with hypercalcaemia have primary hyperparathyroidism; with symptomatic inpatients neoplastic disease is the most common cause.

discovered radiologically by the presence of subperiosteal bone resorption, resorption of the terminal phalanges, and occasionally 'cysts' or 'brown tumours' in the long bones or ribs. The patient with hyperparathyroidism may also have other musculoskeletal symptoms with difficulty in walking, stiffness in the joints, and proximal muscle weakness; the last of these could be related to an associated vitamin D deficiency.

Of the non-skeletal symptoms, those of renal stones, peptic ulceration, and pancreatitis are dealt with in more detail elsewhere (see page 10.51 *et seq.*). Symptoms of hypercalcaemia are nocturia, thirst, anorexia vomiting, constipation, and depression. Nocturia follows from inability to concentrate the urine, which is one of the reversible effects of hypercalcaemia. In a series of 61 patients with parathyroid carcinoma the presenting signs and symptoms were bone disease in 39, a palpable mass in the neck 19, and renal stones 18.

Biochemistry

The essential feature in primary hyperparathyroidism is a persistent and significant (2 S.D. above the mean) increase in the plasma calcium concentration. This estimation should be done at least twice on fasting blood and corrected for the level of plasma albumin. Its significance should be assessed against the range from the hospital laboratory. In most laboratories a value above 10.5 mg/100 ml or 2.6 mol/l would be considered abnormally high. In addition hypophosphataemia is common but not invariable. The alkaline phosphatase is raised in proportion to the extent of clinical bone disease and in the majority of patients is therefore normal. Other biochemical abnormalities may include a raised blood urea (in those patients with renal failure) and a hyperchloraemic acidosis. Analysis of multiple biochemical measurements to suggest the probability of hypercalcaemia being due to hyperparathyroidism has not generally proved to be useful, but a low serum albumin indicates malignancy. The urine calcium is often increased. The urinary hydroxyproline is increased in proportion to the alkaline phosphatase and there may be a generalized aminoaciduria. All these biochemical features are reversible.

Radiology

The commonest radiographic change in hyperparathyroidism, whether it is primary or secondary, is subperiosteal resorption of

the phalanges, said to occur more often in the fingers of the hand which is most used. Resorption of the tufts of the phalanges also occurs but this is a more difficult sign to interpret. Subperiosteal resorption can also occur in many other bones and may, for example, be seen at the ends of the clavicles, around the sacroiliac joints or the pubic symphysis, and around the medial aspects of the upper tibia. Localized areas of osteoclastic bone resorption with fibrosis (osteitis fibrosa cystica; brown tumours), may be seen in the long bones, ribs, and elsewhere (Fig. 14). The vault of the skull may show multiple small osteolytic lesions. It is also said that the lamina dura of the teeth are absent but this is not a useful sign. Cysts in the jaws may represent localized areas of osteitis fibrosa. Radiographs of the skeleton in hyperparathyroidism may also show generalized bone loss, suggesting osteoporosis.

In hyperparathyroidism secondary to prolonged hypocalcaemia, osteitis fibrosa is associated with osteomalacia and particularly contributes to the features of renal glomerular osteodystrophy.

Immunoassay and diagnosis

Recent work has made the diagnosis of hyperparathyroidism by immunoassay more reliable. However, the values in patients with hyperparathyroidism still overlap with the normal range, and are increased in patients with renal failure. This is particularly because of the reduced excretion of fragments of parathyroid hormone. The level of immunoreactive parathyroid hormone (iPTH) must be interpreted in relation to the plasma calcium concentration; this is because hypercalcaemia normally suppresses the secretion of parathyroid hormone. Thus when hypercalcaemia is due to primary hyperparathyroidism the iPTH level is normal or high; whereas if the hypercalcaemia is due to other causes such as malignant disease or vitamin D overdosage, it will be reduced.

The steps in the diagnosis of primary hyperparathyroidism are to establish that sustained hypercalcaemia exists, to distinguish it from other causes of hypercalcaemia, to demonstrate, if necessary by immunoassay, that there is overactivity of the parathyroids, and (again if necessary) to localize the tumour preoperatively. Immunoassay is being increasingly used in the diagnosis of primary hyperparathyroidism. However, it is usually possible to make the diagnosis without it and many patients were successfully treated before such assays were available. Similarly, the localization of a tumour is not necessary as a routine before neck explo-

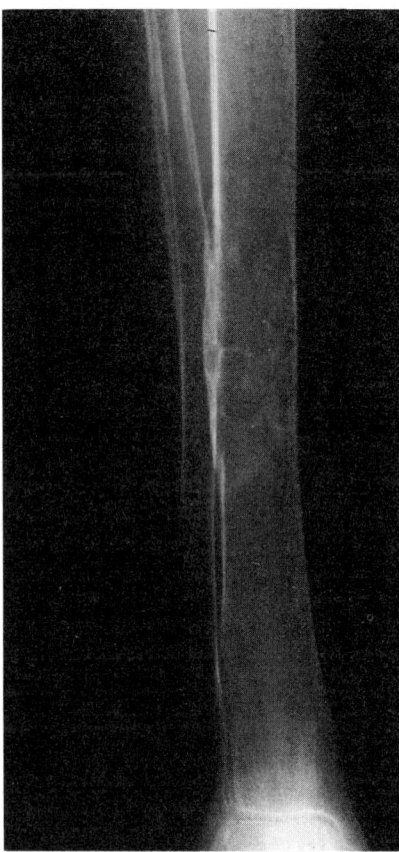

Fig. 14 Osteitis fibrosa cystica forming an expanding lesion in the tibia of a woman with a surgically proven parathyroid tumour. The plasma alkaline phosphatase was 555 IU/l.

ration, but is very useful where a second operation is necessary. This is done by measuring iPTH levels in blood obtained by selective catheterization of veins draining the tumour site. The reliability of the preoperative detection of parathyroid tumours by isotope scanning or by ultrasound still depends on the experience and enthusiasm of the investigator.

Of the known causes of hypercalcaemia in hospital inpatients, neoplasm is the most important (Table 10). It should always be considered and excluded clinically. It is important to note that the apparent cause of hypercalcaemia varies according to the population studied. Thus in healthy subjects primary hyperparathyroidism is its most frequent cause. In those patients with primary hyperparathyroidism, with hypercalcaemia, hypophosphataemia, hyperphosphatasia, and radiological evidence of osteitis fibrosa, and without clinical evidence of neoplasm, no further investigation is needed. Since only a few patients with hyperparathyroidism have clinical bone disease further differentiation from other causes of hypercalcaemia is usually necessary. In practice this means the exclusion of neoplasm, sarcoidosis, thyrotoxicosis, vitamin D overdosage, treatment with thiazide diuretics or the 'milk alkali' syndrome.

Hypercalcaemia in sarcoidosis provides the most frequent example of excessive formation of $1,25(OH)_2D$ apparently in the granulomatous tissues themselves (other examples are tuberculosis and disseminated candidiasis). Vitamin D overdosage usually occurs in patients being treated with this vitamin or its metabolites, but may also result from self-administration or industrial exposure. In its classic form the 'milk alkali' syndrome is rare, but hypercalcaemia due to the same combination of excess oral calcium and alkali still occurs, especially in the elderly, where there is an insidious onset of confusion and dehydration. Often the cause

of the hypercalcaemia cannot be readily diagnosed. Measurement of iPTH is important but may not available. In such circumstances the hydrocortisone suppression test is useful, although the way in which it works is not known. If the plasma calcium concentration remains high and unaltered after ten days of oral hydrocortisone (40 mg every 8 hours) this is in favour of hyperparathyroidism (prednisone is sometimes used instead of hydrocortisone).

Hypercalcaemia associated with neoplastic disease may occur with or without bone metastases. In most patients with malignant disease and hypercalcaemia there are secondary deposits in bone, with local destruction. Carcinoma of the breast and lung are the commonest tumours responsible for hypercalcaemia. Osteolytic activity of tumour tissue can be demonstrated *in vitro* and may sometimes be suppressed by aspirin or indomethacin. Similar findings have been reported with myeloma, where hypercalcaemia is approximately proportional to the degree of bone involvement and bone resorption is related to the production of osteoclast-activating factors by the malignant cells. Solid tumours may produce hypercalcaemia associated with multiple secondary deposits within the skeleton (shown by plain radiographs or isotope scanning).

Hypercalcaemia in the absence of metastases presents interesting problems. The biochemistry may be similar to that of primary hyperparathyroidism, particularly with a low plasma phosphate, and this condition has been called pseudohyperparathyroidism (which is confusing). The commonest tumour associated with this syndrome is a squamous-cell carcinoma of the lung. Differentiation of pseudohyperparathyroidism from primary hyperparathyroidism may be difficult because of the similarity of the biochemical findings and even of the bone histology. However, most of the patients with malignant disease and non-metastatic hypercalcaemia have low circulating levels of iPTH and of $1,25(OH)_2D$, despite often significant increases in nephrogenous cAMP. It has been suggested that such tumours produce a form of humoral hypercalcaemia by the synthesis of transforming growth factors which stimulate osteoclastic bone resorption.

Treatment
Exploration of the neck with removal of the adenoma and identification of the remaining parathyroid glands is the accepted treatment for symptomatic primary hyperparathyroidism. In patients with mild hypercalcaemia (for instance, less than 2.8 to 3.0 mmol/l) and no symptoms operation may be delayed, especially in the elderly, but follow up is necessary and operation may be preferable; but those with obvious clinical bone disease usually have large tumours and require urgent attention. Other significant symptoms such as renal stones, decreased renal function, and psychiatric disturbances attributable to hypercalcaemia are also indications for operation. Within the last decade the need for surgery in all patients with primary hyperparathyroidism has been questioned. Whilst operation may be economically preferable to prolonged medical follow up, and may prevent complications such as progressive bone loss, the outcome in patients who have not had surgery (for a variety of reasons) has been unexpectedly good.

It is important to control postoperative hypocalcaemia which may lead to tetany and fits with fracture of the softened bones. In the past this was done with large doses of vitamin D or DHT in the region of 4–8 mg daily, begun 48 hours before operation, but treatment with 1-α-hydroxycholecalciferol is far more effective and easy to control. Since it works rapidly it need not be given before operation; postoperatively daily doses of 2–4 μg are appropriate.

Familial benign hypercalcaemia

This rare condition is dominantly inherited. Mild hypercalcaemia occurs without hypercalcuria and is not improved by parathyroid surgery. Symptoms are few and include mild fatigue, sleepiness, and amnesia.

Multiple endocrine adenoma syndromes

Overactivity of the parathyroid may be familial, and may also be associated with overactivity of other endocrine organs. Two particular associations are recognized. Type I multiple endocrine adenoma (MEA) syndrome includes hyperparathyroidism, pituitary adenomata, insulin, and gastrin-secreting tumours of the pancreas and gastric hyperacidity (Zollinger–Ellison syndrome): type II MEA syndrome, also known as Sipple's syndrome, includes hyperparathyroidism, medullary carcinoma of the thyroid, and phaeochromocytoma. It has been proposed that these associations occur because the cells have a common origin from the neural crest, and form part of a general endocrine system.

Secondary (and tertiary) hyperparathyroidism

Where hypocalcaemia is prolonged, most often due to renal glomerular failure or gluten-sensitive enteropathy, the parathyroid glands increase both their size and activity in an attempt to restore the plasma calcium to normal. This increases bone resorption and is a particular feature of renal glomerular osteodystrophy. Occasionally in such patients hypercalcaemia develops and persists. It has been proposed that one of the hyperplastic parathyroid glands becomes autonomous, and the label 'tertiary hyperparathyroidism' has been given to this. Hypercalcaemia may also occur after renal transplantation.

Hypoparathyroidism

Parathyroid insufficiency may occur after surgical removal of the parathyroids, in idopathic hypoparathyroidism, and in a familial form of hypoparathyroidism which is often associated with manifestations of autoimmune disease, including moniliasis, malabsorption, thyroid, and adrenal failure, and pernicious anaemia. In such patients the levels of iPTH are undetectably low but the cAMP response to exogenous PTH is maintained. This distinguishes parathyroid insufficiency from pseudohypoparathyroidism (PHP), in which the biochemical features of hypoparathyroidism are associated with characteristic skeletal abnormalities. PHP is inherited and in the most common form the production of cAMP is defective. Hypocalcaemia leads to compensatory overactivity and enlargement of the parathyroids. Thus the cAMP response to exogenous PTH is absent or blunted while the circulating level of iPTH is high. Variations of PHP appear to exist, and disorders are described in which the cAMP response is present but there is still end-organ resistance (PHP type II), and also where the cAMP response is restored by giving vitamin D. Patients who have the skeletal manifestations of PHP but with normal biochemistry may be found in families with PHP, and to them the term pseudopseudohypoparathyroidism (PPHP) is applied.

So far as the skeleton is concerned the most striking changes are found in PHP. This condition is often familial, and the commonest form of inheritance appears to be as an X-linked dominant. Clinical features include mental simplicity, short stature, round face, short neck, and abnormal metacarpals (or metatarsals) of which the most common change is shortness of the fourth and fifth. The bones may be excessively dense, and widespread ectopic calcification may also occur, particularly in the basal ganglia and the subcutaneous tissues (Fig. 15). Treatment of the hypocalcaemia is the same as for idiopathic hypoparathyroidism, with $1-\alpha$-hydroxycholecalciferol.

References

Heath, D. and Marx, S. J. (1982). *Calcium disorders. Butterworths International Medical Reviews. Clinical Endocrinology* Vol. 2. Butterworth Scientific, London.
Kanis, J. A. and Yates, A. J. P. (1985). Measuring serum calcium. *Br. Med. J.* **290**, 728–729.

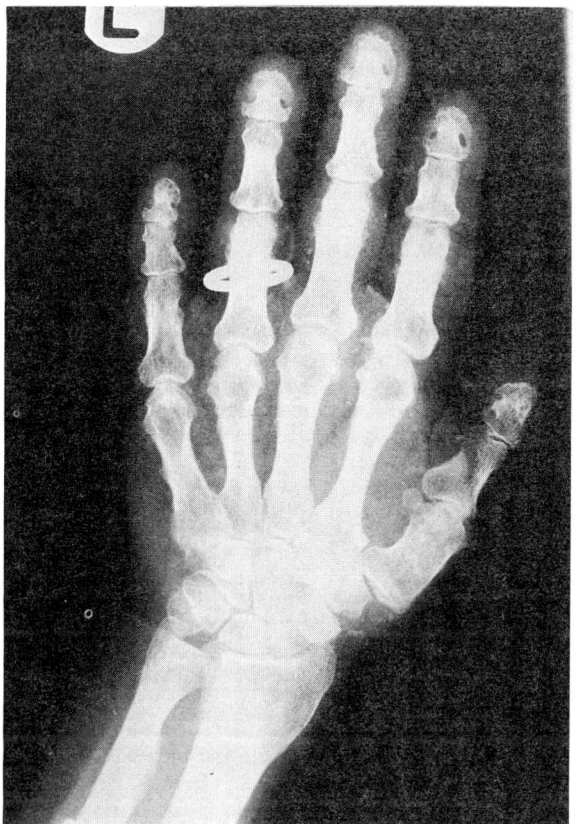

Fig. 15 Subcutaneous calcification in the hand of a woman with pseudo-hypoparathyroidism. The bones are also dense. (Reproduced from Smith, 1979, *Biochemical disorders of the skeleton*, Butterworths, London, with permission.)

Lancet (1984). Medical management of primary hyperparathyroidism (Editorial). *Lancet* **ii**, 727–728.
—— (1985). Determining the cause of hypercalcaemia (Editorial). *Lancet* **i**, 376–377.
Marx, S. J. (1980). Familial hypercalciuric hypercalcaemia. *N. Engl. J. Med.* **303**, 810–811.
Paterson, C. R., Burns, J. and Mowat, E. (1984). Long term follow up of untreated primary hyperparathyroidism. *Br. Med. J.* **289**, 1261–1263.

Osteogenesis imperfecta: the brittle bone syndrome

The term osteogenesis imperfecta (fragilitas ossium; the brittle bone syndrome) refers to a rare inherited group of disorders of connective tissue with the common feature of excessive fragility of bones. A number of extraskeletal collagen-containing tissues, particularly the sclerae, dentine, tendons, and skin are also involved. There is clinical and biochemical evidence of several defects of collagen synthesis (page 17.2).

Classification and genetics

The overall incidence of osteogenesis imperfecta is between 1:20 000 to 1:50 000 of the population. This is about the same as haemophilia, and is a significant cause of inherited crippling disease. Currently four main types are recognized (Table 11); this division is useful but many patients are difficult to classify. Types I and IV are dominantly inherited. Type II (lethal perinatal form) most often results from a new mutation. Some survivors from type II are included amongst the progressively deforming type of disorder with white sclerae (type III). In this very heterogenous group there is sometimes evidence of recessive inheritance. Subdi-

Table 11 Provisional classification of the brittle bone syndrome (osteogenesis imperfecta)

Type	Clinical features	Inheritance	Biochemistry* (see text)
I	Commonest form Mild with blue sclerae, insignificant bone deformity, stature often normal, fractures typically late, deafness common, dentinogenesis imperfecta in some	Dominant	Defective formation Type I collagen, half normal amounts of $\alpha1(I)$ chains
II	Lethal perinatal form, multiple fractures at birth, including ribs, one cause of lethal neonatal dwarfism, sclerae often deep blue	Most new mutations	Variable, probably many mutations causing delayed helix formation and overmodification
III	Fractures at birth, progressive deformity and kyphoscoliosis, bones often very narrow, sclerae often normal in adult life, dentinogenesis imperfecta common	Some recessive	Most unknown
IV	Fragile bones, short stature, normal sclerae, teeth often abnormal	Dominant	Some evidence of link to $\alpha2(I)$ gene

* In many patients no biochemical defect can be demonstrated.

visions have been described, according to the presence or absence of dentinogenesis imperfecta.

Pathophysiology

Current evidence suggests that osteogenesis imperfecta arises from abnormal synthesis of type I collagen, which is the only collagen of adult bone. In type I disorder there is a mild inherited osteoporosis with a reduction in bone mass. Bone formation is reduced; each osteoblast makes less collagen leading to an apparent increase in the number of osteocytes; in severe osteogenesis imperfecta there is disorganization of the bone matrix with large amounts of fibre bone. Outside the skeleton other collagen-containing tissues are affected. The sclerae and skin are thin and the dentine is abnormal with short branched dentinal tubules; there is also late-onset multifactorial deafness, hypermobility, and rarely cardiac valve lesions.

Biochemically the most consistently described defect is a reduced formation of type I collagen relative to type III, demonstrated in the fibroblasts and tissues. Rare abnormalities are the absence of the $\alpha2$-chain from type I collagen and excessive hydroxylation of lysine. Since bone contains type I collagen only, a relative lack of this genetic type would explain why the skeleton is predominantly affected.

Within the last few years mutations have been described in the collagen genes in lethally affected infants and also in survivors. These lead to the formation of abnormal (often short) α-chains, which are either incorporated into the triple helix making it unstable or rapidly degraded without incorporation. Harmless variations in collagen gene structure are being used to trace the inheritance of collagen genes in the brittle bone (and related) syndromes and to identify or exclude the mutant genes.

Clinical features

In type I osteogenesis imperfecta fractures may be few and of late onset and significant bone deformity does not occur. The sclerae are blue often with a prominent early arcus juvenilis. Dentinogenesis imperfecta may be present; the enamel breaks off the defective dentine and the teeth become transparent and discoloured, the roots are thin, and the pulp chambers are obliterated. Early onset nerve deafness resembling otosclerosis is common; it is due to a combination of causes including fractures of the ossicles. Hypermobility of the joints is common and tendon rupture rare. In the cardiovascular system aortic incompetence and redundant mitral valves are described. In perinatal lethal osteogenesis imperfecta (type II) there are multiple fractures at birth with gross deformity and shortening of the limbs (osteogenesis imperfecta

congenita; Fig. 16). The most typical form has structureless broad ribs and long bones ('broad-boned' lethal) but other variations do occur. The condition is usually sporadic without a family history. Although perinatal death is usual, some survive through infancy, and are then included in the progressively deforming disorder (type III). In this heterogeneous group, the limbs are short and bowed, there is kyphoscoliosis and a misshapen skull. Such individuals are unable to walk. Hyperplastic callus (Fig. 17) is an occasional feature; excessive amounts of callus are produced either following a small fracture or apparently spontaneously. Since this formation of callus is associated with pain and signs of inflammation and the mass of new tissue appears to be attached to the bone an initial diagnosis of sarcoma is often made.

Radiology

Radiographs of patients with osteogenesis imperfecta reflect the heterogeneity of this disease. In the mild type I form the cortex and the whole bone may appear thin but despite repeated fractures there is no significant deformity. In the most severe form the ribs and long bones are broad, deformed, and concertina-shaped (Fig. 16). Less severely affected patients show bowing of the long bones with some attempts at buttressing. The skull is often misshapen with a relatively large vault, with defective or almost completely absent mineralization at birth, and with multiple small bones (Wormian bones) particularly in the occipital region.

Biochemistry

There are no consistent biochemical changes in osteogenesis imperfecta, apart from those to do with collagen; many have been described but not subsequently confirmed. These include changes in urinary total hydroxyproline; plasma protein-bound hydroxyproline (hyprotein) and plasma pyrophosphate; in thyroid function; and in white cell metabolism.

Diagnosis

There is usually no difficulty in diagnosing osteogenesis imperfecta. In type I the presence of a positive family history, blue sclerae, and brittle bones are diagnostic; and in severely affected infants with intrauterine fractures there is no difficulty once the radiographs are seen. At birth severe osteogenesis imperfecta must be distinguished from other forms of lethal short-limbed dwarfism such as hypophosphatasia, achondrogenesis, and thanatophoric dwarfism; and from achondroplasia, which is rarely lethal. In childhood it is clinically and legally important to distinguish the battered-baby syndrome (non-accidental injury); and in adolescence, idiopathic juvenile osteoporosis may simulate late-

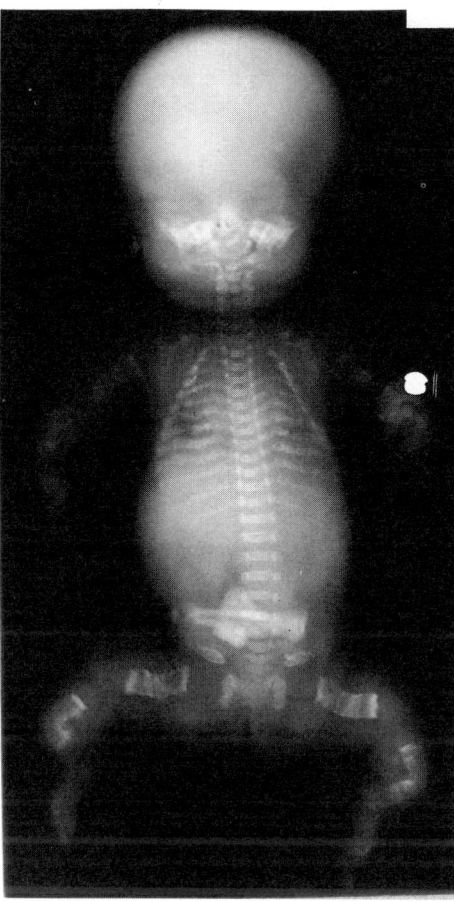

Fig. 16 Radiographic appearances of a baby who died at birth with osteogenesis imperfecta type II. The vault of the skull is not calcified and there are multiple fractures in the ribs and all the long bones. The femora are broad and the tibiae bowed. There was no family history.

onset osteogenesis imperfecta. Non-accidental injury is suggested by multiple fractures at varying stages and of particular sorts, together with signs of neglect. The diagnosis is rarely straightforward.

Treatment

Since the cause of osteogenesis imperfecta is unknown medical treatment is largely ineffective; and orthopaedic treatment is directed towards the healing of fractures and the prevention and correction of deformity. Medically, a large number of agents have been tried including various diets, sex hormones, magnesium, growth hormone, and calcitonin. Calcitonin is given because of the idea (held by some) that osteogenesis imperfecta is basically a disease of excessive bone resorption, but existing evidence suggests the opposite, namely, that the primary defect is in the osteoblast. Calcitonin can produce troublesome side effects especially after repeated injections in small children, and there seems little indication for its use. In mild osteogenesis imperfecta fractures heal well. When there is severe deformity attempts may be made to straighten the limbs by multiple operations using intramedullary rods. The skeleton may also be supported externally by the use of inflatable 'space suits'. In the severely affected case an alternative approach is to accept that the child will never walk and that he or she should be adapted to the environment by the provision of suitable electrically powered wheelchairs. Whatever line of treatment is adopted for the severely affected child it is important that mobility should be encouraged from the earliest age and that education is not neglected.

Prognosis

In any given child with osteogenesis imperfecta it may be difficult to assess the outcome, because of the heterogeneity of the disease. In general its severity tends to be constant in families. In type I osteogenesis imperfecta there is often little eventual deformity or disability although multiple fractures may occur in childhood. Short stature and some deformity occurs in type IV disease. The outcome in infants born with multiple fractures can be partly predicted from the appearance of the limb bones, ribs, and skull. Survival is most likely where there are few or no rib fractures, and at least some mineralization of the cranial vault. Some infants may survive for many years despite gross disability. However, death in infancy and childhood from respiratory infections is common.

Antenatal diagnosis and genetic advice

A severely affected fetus may be suspected by ultrasound and confirmed by appropriate radiographs at about 20 weeks of gestation. There is no accurate biochemical method at present for prenatal diagnosis. In types I and IV 50 per cent of the offspring of an affected parent are likely to be similarly affected. In lethal perinatal osteogenesis imperfecta the likelihood of a further affected child is very low; likewise the recurrence risk in type III disease is less than 25 per cent (the percentage risk of a recessively inherited disorder).

References

Prockop, D. J. and Kivirikko, K. I. (1984). Heritable disease of collagen. *N. Engl. J. Med.* **311**, 376–386.
Smith, R. (1984). Osteogenesis Imperfecta 1984. *Br. Med. J.* **289**, 394–396.
——, Francis, M. J. O. and Houghton, G. R. (1981). *The brittle bone syndrome*. Butterworth Scientific, London.
Sykes, B. and Smith, R. (1985). Collagen and collagen gene disorders. *Q. J. Med.* **56**, 533–547.

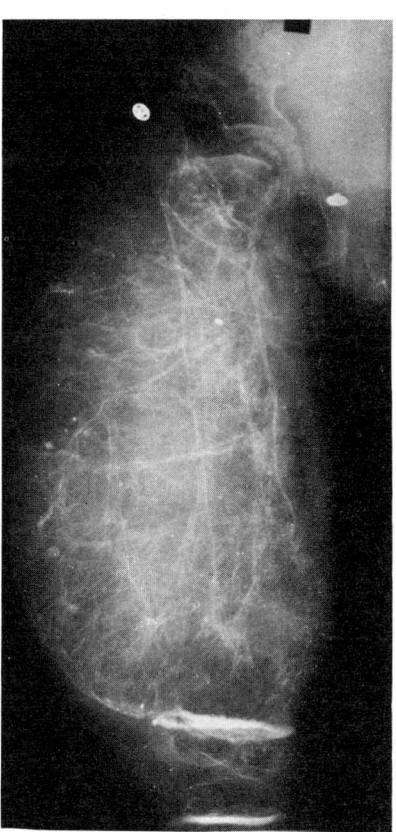

Fig. 17 Hyperplastic callus in a girl with severe osteogenesis imperfecta. The outline of the deformed and enlarged femur can be identified within the mass of new bone. (Reproduced from Smith, 1979, *Biochemical disorders of the skeleton*, Butterworths, London, with permission.)

Table 12 Primary and secondary inherited disorders of collagen which affect the skeleton

Disorder	Biochemical defect
Primary	
Osteogenesis imperfecta	See page 17.25
Ehlers–Danlos syndrome: Type VI	Lysyl hydroxylase deficiency
Type VII	Amino acid defect in procollagen extension
Marfan's syndrome	Unknown
Secondary	
Homocystinuria	Chelation of aldehydes with homocysteine
Alkaptonuria	Effect of homogentisic acid; mechanism disputed
Menkes' kinky hair syndrome	Copper deficiency reduces concentration of amino acid oxidase and subsequent cross linking

The Marfan and Ehlers–Danlos syndromes

Some inherited disorders of connective tissue affect the skeleton more than others. This is related to the type of collagen affected. Thus in osteogenesis imperfecta the biochemical defects affect that type of collagen (type I) contained in bone; in contrast Ehlers–Danlos syndrome type IV in which type III synthesis of collagen is often defective has no clinical effect on the skeleton. However, recent work has also shown that apparently similar mutations in the same collagen gene may be associated with markedly different phenotypes.

Disorders of collagen synthesis may be primary or may be secondary to other biochemical abnormalities, as in homocystinuria or alkaptonuria (Table 12). In many of the inherited disorders of connective tissue the biochemical lesion is not known, and the reason for the clinical features is therefore obscure.

The Marfan syndrome

This is a dominantly inherited disorder and is phenotypically heterogeneous. Despite intense investigation its cause is unknown (minor changes in $\alpha2(I)$ collagen have been described). The main clinical features are skeletal, vascular, and ocular. In the skeleton the extremities are long and thin (so that span exceeds height and the lower segment is longer than the upper), the fingers and toes are spidery (arachnodactyly), and overall height is often increased; the sternum is often depressed and twisted, and scoliosis is common; the palate is high arched. The main cardiovascular abnormalities are aortic incompetence and dissecting aneurysm, the latter arising from a necrosis of the aortic media. Mitral valve prolapse is also common. In the eyes upward or sideways dislocation of the lens is characteristic. The joint capsules, ligaments, tendons, and fascia may be weak, leading to dislocations and herniae. Some patients with the Marfan syndrome are excessively thin (asthenic form) whilst others are not. The combination of long thin extremities and loose-jointedness forms the basis of many of the physical 'tests' for Marfan's syndrome. For instance, the flexed thumb can extend across and beyond the ulnar margin of the hand, and the thumb and fourth finger of the hand overlap when the opposite wrist is grasped.

Diagnosis

Diagnosis of the Marfan syndrome is usually first suggested by excessive height and/or skeletal disproportion, and confirmed by the ocular and cardiac findings. Since it is inherited as a dominant disorder one parent should be clinically affected, but this need not be obvious because of the very variable expression of the gene. It is important to see the parents and any siblings in order to judge whether the height and proportions of an individual are abnormal or not. In doubtful cases there is no certain clinical way of excluding the Marfan syndrome. Marfan's syndrome should be distinguished from homocystinuria and congenital contractural arachnodactyly (Table 13). Disproportionately long limbs may also occur in hypogonadism, Kleinfelter's syndrome (XXY chromosomal abnormality), sickle cell anaemia and in some Black races. Scoliosis in the adolescent is often idiopathic and rarely due to the Marfan syndrome; dominantly inherited neurofibromatosis may cause a characteristic sharp kyphoscoliosis and disproportion. Arachnodactyly is not uncommon on its own, and the same applies to dislocation of the lens. Finally a Marfanoid appearance is described in some patients with Sipple's syndrome (see page 13.382 *et seq.*). There are no biochemical tests which help to diagnose the Marfan syndrome, but the urinary hydroxyproline may sometimes be slightly increased.

Treatment

The main problems which require attention in a patient with the Marfan syndrome are scoliosis, excessive height, and aortic valve disease and its complications. The scoliosis may be sufficiently severe and progressive to require surgical correction. Excessive height can be surgically corrected by suitably timed bilateral epiphysiodesis. In girls, where such height may be particularly troublesome a combined oestrogen–progesterone regimen has been used to start puberty early and close the epiphyses. Aortic dilation and its complications are the main cause of death in patients with the Marfan syndrome. It is said that the nature of the pulse wave in this disorder contributes to the extension and eventual rupture of the dissecting aneurysm; possibly the rate of aortic dilation may be reduced by giving β blocking agents such as propanolol. Surgical replacement of the aorta and its valves is increasingly successful.

The Ehlers–Danlos syndrome

This term is applied to a group of conditions with the common clinical features of abnormal velvety skin which heals poorly, hyperextensibility of the joints, and lax ligaments; different forms have additional features such as prolonged or spontaneous bleeding, rupture of the large blood vessels, ocular abnormalities and kyphoscoliosis. The distribution of these features can be partly explained on the basis of the tissue distribution of different collagens; thus in type IV Ehlers–Danlos syndrome, type III collagen, which is a component of blood vessels, may be reduced or absent and vascular catastrophes are a prominent feature. There has been

Table 13 The differential diagnosis of the Marfan syndrome (MS) from homocystinuria (H) and congenital contractural arachnodactyly (CCA)

	MS	H	CCA
Dislocated lens	+	+	−
Mental backwardness	−	+ (Variable)	−
Aortic dilation	+	−	−
'Floppy' mitral valve	+	−	−
Thrombosis	−	+	−
Arachnodactyly	+	+	+
Scoliosis	+	+	+
Osteoporosis	−	+	+
Contractures	Rarely	−	Always
Inheritance	D	R	D
Homocystine in urine	−	+	−
Excess hydroxproline in urine	Sometimes	−	−
Other	−	Fair hair, malar flush	Abnormal helix of ear

much recent work on the causes of the Ehlers–Danlos syndrome, and the number of described forms continues to increase (Table 14). However, in only a few are there significant skeletal features. Types IV and VII Ehlers–Danlos syndrome particularly affect the skeleton. Infants with type VI Ehlers–Danlos syndrome are 'floppy' at birth and may subsequently develop severe kyphoscoliosis; they also have ocular abnormalities, with microcornea and fragility of the eyeballs. The disorder is recessively inherited and due to lysyl hydroxylase deficiency producing defective cross-linking of collagen.

In type VII Ehlers–Danlos syndrome the main clinical feature is severe loose jointedness. Such patients have short stature and repeated dislocation of the hips.

Congenital contractural arachnodactyly

Patients with the Marfan syndrome may develop contractures of the extremities; there is a very rare condition which superficially resembles it in which contractures of many joints are present from birth and tend to improve with age. This is called congenital contractural arachnodactyly. It is dominantly inherited, there are no central nervous system abnormalities, the lenses do not dislocate and cardiac valve lesions are unusual. Scoliosis, osteoporosis, and abnormal external ears are described (Table 13).

Idiopathic scoliosis

Scoliosis commonly develops during the rapid growth of adolescence, particularly in girls, but its cause remains unknown. Abnormal collagen has been described in various tissues from such patients and scoliosis is a striking feature of some inherited disorders which affect collagen. Thus idiopathic adolescent scoliosis may in part be the result of an abnormality of collagen; alternatively the described changes in collagen may merely reflect the excessively rapid changes in growth rate during adolescence in these patients.

References

Pope, F. M. and Nicholls, A. C. (1984). Molecular abnormalities of collagen proteins and genes. In *Molecular medicine* Vol. 1 (ed. A. D. B. Malcolm). IRL Press, Oxford.
——, ——, Dorling, J. and Webb, J. (1983). Molecular abnormalities of collagen: a review. *J. R. Soc. Med.* **76**, 1050–1062.
Pyeritz, R. E. (1981). Maternal and fetal complications of pregnancy in the Marfan syndrome. *Am. J. Med.* **71**, 784–790.
—— and McKusick, V. A. (1979). The Marfan syndrome: diagnosis and management. *N. Engl. J. Med.* **300**, 772–777.

Homocystinuria and alkaptonuria

The correct formation of collagen fibres and the strength of the tissues which depend on them can be markedly disturbed by any agent which affects the cross-linking of collagen. An example of this is the effect of the lathyrogen aminoproprionitrile which prevents such cross-linking and produces scoliosis and aortic dissection in animals. In humans homocystinuria, alkaptonuria, and Menkes' steely hair syndrome are further examples. The latter condition is related to copper deficiency and is often classified with type IX Ehlers–Danlos syndrome (see above). Impaired growth, multiple Wormian bones, and cupping of the ends of the long bones are the skeletal features; central nervous system degeneration and arterial tortuosity and fragmentation are others.

Homocystinuria

In classic vitamin B_6-dependent homocystinuria (see page 9.11 *et seq.*) the skeletal features simulate those of Marfan's syndrome. The

Table 14 Clinical features in the Ehlers–Danlos syndrome

	Type	Inheritance	Skin extensibility and fragility	Bruising	Joint mobility	Other significant features	Biochemical defects
I	Gravis	Dominant (+? recessive)	Gross	Severe	Generalized gross	Prematurity Molluscoid pseudo-tumours Musculoskeletal deformity	?Abnormal collagen fibrils and fibre packing
II	Mitis	Dominant	Mild	Mild	Moderate, often limited to hands and feet	None	Not known
III	Benign hypermobile	Dominant	Variable, usually minimal	Mild	Generalized gross	Recurrent joint dislocations Osteoarthritis Skilled contortionists	Not known
IV	Ecchymotic (arterial or Sack-Barabas type; includes acrogeria)	Dominant or recessive	Thin pale skin with prominent veins	Gross	Minimal limited to digits	Rupture of great vessels and bowel Elastosis perforans serpiginosa	In synthesis of type III collagen
V	X-linked	X-linked	Moderate with variable fragility	Variable	Mild	Floppy valve syndrome	Lysyl oxidase deficiency (unconfirmed in other patients)
VI	Ocularscoliotic (hydroxylysine deficient disease)	Recessive	Moderate	Moderate	Generalized gross	Scoliosis Microcornea Ocular fragility	Procollagen lysyl hydroxylase deficiency
VII	Arthrochalasis multiplex congenita	Recessive	Moderate	Moderate	Severe	Short stature Congenital dislocations	N terminal cleavage site for pro collagen peptidase mutated
VIII	Periodontitis	Dominant	Minimal with marked fragility	Mild	Moderate limited to digits	Advanced generalized periodontitis	Not known
IX	X-linked skeletal	X-linked recessive	Moderate	Moderate	Moderate	Occipital exostoses Deformed clavicles Bowed long bones	Abnormal copper metabolism

recessively inherited defect in cystathionine synthase leads to the accumulation of homocysteine behind the metabolic block with the excretion of its disulphide form, homocystine, in the urine. Beyond the metabolic block, cystathionine and cysteine are deficient. Homocysteine itself appears to act as *in vivo* lathyrogen, and contributes to the progressive skeletal deformity with scoliosis, to the lens dislocation, and to the instability of the skin collagen. The thrombotic tendency, vascular damage, and platelet stickiness are probably also due to the excessive homocyst(e)ine, although the available evidence is controversial; and the variable damage to the central nervous system may be due to a number of factors. Characteristically the patient is mentally simple with light-coloured hair and has skeletal features of the Marfan syndrome; the lenses are often dislocated downwards and there is no evidence of aortic incompetence. Since the disorder is inherited as a recessive siblings, but not parents, are affected. Apart from the disproportion, the radiographic findings are not diagnostic but a form of 'osteoporosis' is described, with posterior biconcavity of the vertebrae; sometimes bones such as the femoral head appear disproportionately large.

It is important to establish the diagnosis, particularly where an operation such as for knock knees or scoliosis is contemplated, since extensive venous thrombosis may follow. The presence of homocystine (or cystine) in the urine is detected by the nitroprusside test, in which sodium cyanide is added to the urine to reduce homocystine to homocysteine, which then gives a purple-red reaction with freshly prepared sodium nitroprusside. It is important to note that homocystinuria is very variable in its clinical features, and the degree of mental backwardness may be mild or severe. Patients whose biochemical abnormality is corrected by pyridoxine (vitamin B_6) are less severely affected. Apart from pyridoxine dependency there are other causes of homocystinuria.

Alkaptonuria

This is one of the classic inborn errors of metabolism (see page 9.11 *et seq.*) which has significant effects on the skeleton. The inherited deficiency of homogentisic acid oxidase leads to the accumulation of homogentisic acid (and its polymers) in the tissues, and to its increased excretion in the urine. The way in which this biochemical abnormality produces the early arthritis in the larger joints is unknown; it has been suggested that the homogentisic acid acts as an *in vivo* tanning agent, increasing the cross-linking of collagen, but there is work which suggests the opposite.

Alkaptonuria is rare, but has an increased incidence in some inbred communities. Its main characteristics are dark urine, pigmentation of connective tissue, and an early progressive characteristic arthropathy.

The urine becomes dark on standing, more rapidly when alkaline, and because of the excessive homogentisic acid gives a positive reaction when tested for reducing substances, but not with glucose oxidase. The sclerae and the cartilages of the ears and nose take on a blue-black colouration, and pigmentation is found in cerumen and sweat. Tissues such as cartilage, tendons, and ligaments become darkly stained. The main troublesome effects of this disorder arise from early intervertebral disc degeneration with calcification and pain in the back and from an early degenerative arthritis of the larger joints, which may need surgical treatment (Fig. 18). At operation the articular cartilage over the femoral head is dark brown to black in colour and the bone beneath it is said to be very hard. Attempts to reduce the excessive homogentisic acid by dietary restriction of the precursor tyrosine or protein produce no clinical benefit.

References

La Du E. N. (1978). Alkaptonuria In *The metabolic basis of inherited disease* 4th edn (eds J. B. Stanbury, J. B. Wyngaarden, and D. S. Fredrickson), pp. 268–282. McGraw Hill, New York.

Mudd, S. H. and Levy, H. L. (1978). Disorders of transulfuration. In *The*

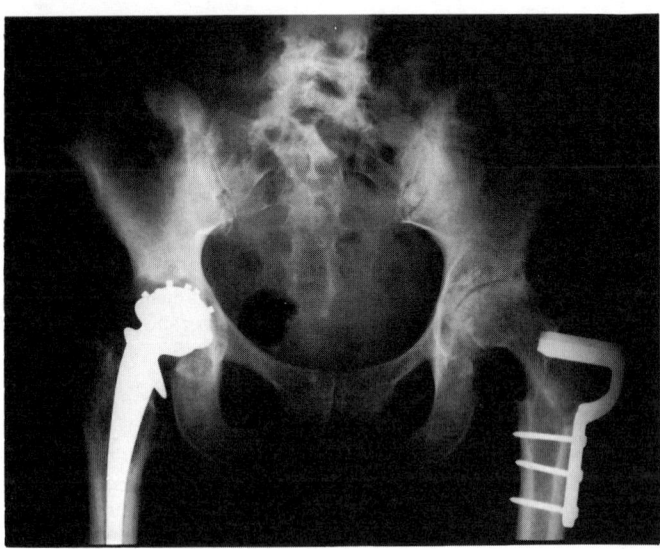

Fig. 18 The presence and results of extensive degenerative arthritis in a 54-year-old woman with alkaptonuria. The osteotomy was done at the age of 42 years and the total hip replacement two years later. Spinal radiographs (not shown) demonstrated calcified intervertebral discs.

metabolic basis of inherited disease 4th edn (eds. J. B. Stanbury, J. B. Wyngaarden and D. S. Fredrickson), pp. 458–503. McGraw Hill, New York.

——, Scovby, F., Levy, H. L., Pettigrew, K. D., Wilcken, B., Pyeritz, R. E., Andria, G., Boers, G. H. J., Bromberg, I. L., Cerone, R., Fowler, B., Grobe, H., Schmidt, H. and Schweitzer, L. (1985). The natural history of homocystinuria due to cystathionine β-synthase deficiency. *Am. J. Gen.* **37**, 1–31.

The mucopolysaccharidoses

Failure of the normal breakdown of complex carbohydrates leads to their accumulation in the tissues, and produces many clinical abnormalities. The disorders may be divided into two main groups, according to the chemistry of the accumulated substance, namely, the mucopolysaccharidoses and the mucolipidoses. The biochemical defects are described elsewhere in this book (see Section 9). Since some of these disorders have a prominent effect on the skeleton, they should also be briefly mentioned here; they are the Hurler syndrome (MPS IH), the Hunter syndrome (MP II), and the Morquio syndrome (MPS IV). With certain exceptions the bone changes themselves do not permit precise diagnosis of the type of dysplasia present, or distinction from the mucolipidoses.

The Hurler syndrome (MPS IH)

This is the most severe type of mucopolysaccharidosis and causes death at an early age. The enzyme defect is inherited as a recessive and all patients have the same appearance, to which the term gargoylism was previously applied.

Affected infants appear to develop normally in the first few months of life, but then deteriorate mentally and physically. Death often occurs in late childhood, commonly due to pneumonia or to coronary artery disease associated with mucopolysaccharide deposits.

The physical features include proportionate short stature (Table 2), a typical facial appearance, a short neck with a lumbar gibbus and chest deformity, and a protruberant abdomen. The facial features are coarse and ugly, with flattening of the nasal bridge, with large open mouth and tongue, and often with hypertrophied gums over enlarged alveolar ridges. The eyes are prominent with corneal clouding. There is noisy breathing and variable deafness.

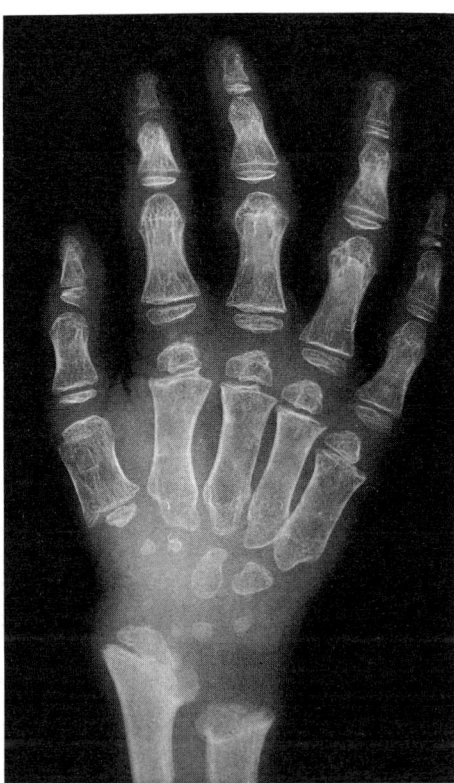

Fig. 19 The appearance of the hands in MPS type IV (Morquio syndrome). (Reproduced from Smith, 1979, *Biochemical disorders of the skeleton*, Butterworths, London, with permission.)

The vault of the skull may show scaphocephaly or acrocephaly. Other striking features include the stiff broad trident hands and the large abdomen with hepatosplenomegaly. Radiographs show the abnormal shape of the skull, the slipper-shaped sella turcica, the beaking of the vertebrae with the thoracolumbar kyphosis, and the bullet-shaped phalanges. Similar but less severe features are seen in the Hunter syndrome, inherited as an X-linked recessive.

The Morquio syndrome (MPS IV)

In this disorder the orthopaedic manifestations are striking, and intelligence is normal. Although the disorder is probably heterogeneous and only a proportion of the cases excrete an excess of keratan sulphate in the urine, the skeletal changes are uniform. In the first years of life the child becomes progressively more deformed and dwarfed. Characteristically the neck is short, the sternum is protruberant and there may be a flexed stance with knock knees. There is a striking loss of muscle tone in comparison to the stiffness of MPS IH; hypermobility and a loose skin are features. Radiographs in infancy show a spine similar to that of Hurler's syndrome, but later flattening of the vertebrae with anterior beaking leads to relative shortening of the trunk. The small bones of the hands are very different from those of MPS IH and the metacarpals show diaphyseal constriction (Fig. 19).

Importantly the odontoid may be hypoplastic, leading to atlantoaxial instability, compression of the long spinal tracts, and paraplegia.

The osteopetroses

There are a number of disorders characterized by an increase in the amount of bone in the skeleton associated with changes in modelling or with overgrowth of bone. These conditions are rare, often familial, and may be grouped together as the osteopetroses (Table 15). Probably the commonest is osteopetrosis itself, also known as marble bones or Albers–Schonberg disease. This has now been widely studied and in its most severe form appears to result from inherited defects in osteoclast functions.

Osteopetrosis (Marble bones disease)

There are two main genetically distinct types; one is recessively inherited and severe, the other is dominantly inherited and mild. However, as in the animal disease, intermediate forms appear to exist.

Severe osteopetrosis

In this condition (also referred to as infantile malignant osteopetrosis) there is severe bony overgrowth from early infancy, and rarely the diagnosis can be made *in utero*. The radiographic appearances are remarkable and diagnostic. Bone is increased throughout the skeleton, including the skull, and defects of modelling occur which particularly produce a club-shaped appearance in the metaphyses. Inexplicable variations occur in the density of the bones with striations seen across the metaphyses, concentrically on the iliac bones, and on the top and bottom of each vertebral body. In the vertebrae and phalanges these may produce an appearance of one bone within another ('endobone'). Involvement of the bone marrow leads to leucoerythroblastic anaemia, cranial nerve compression, and optic atrophy. In the severe infantile form the clinical appearance is characteristic; proptosis, overgrowth of the frontal bones, loss of hearing, poor growth, mental retardation, and hepatosplenomegaly all occur. The bones fracture easily and the frequency of osteomyelitis is increased. Death from haemorrhage or infection in early childhood is usual.

Biochemically there is a consistent increase in the plasma acid phosphatase whilst the plasma alkaline phosphatase remains within normal limits for age. The urine calcium may be very low whilst the calcium balance is excessively positive even for a growing child.

Table 15 Features of the osteopetroses

Osteoscleroses (sclerosis predominates, minor changes in bony shape)

Osteopetrosis	Severe recessive and mild dominant
Pycnodysostosis	Recessive, anterior fontanelle patent, short terminal phalanges

Craniotubular dysplasias (sclerosis of cranium; abnormal modelling of long bones)

Metaphyseal dysplasia (Pyle's disease)	Recessive, knock knee, muscle weakness, scoliosis, Erlenmeyer flask-shaped bones
Craniometaphyseal dysplasia	Progressive thickening of the skull, face and mandible, with disfigurement; most marked in the recessive form

Craniotubular hyperostoses (skeletal deformity due to overgrowth rather than to defective modelling)

Endosteal hyperostosis (Van Buchem's disease)	Large sclerosed mandible; bilateral facial paralysis and deafness; endosteal thickening of long bones
Diaphyseal dysplasia (Englemann's disease)	Dominantly inherited, severe hyperostosis, particularly in the diaphyses
Idiopathic hyperphosphatasia	Large head, fragility and bowing of the long bones

Miscellaneous
Osteopathia striata
Melorheostosis

Cause and treatment

The logical treatment of this condition will depend on increasing knowledge of its cause. The spontaneous variation in density of the bones suggests that this may be affected by environmental changes; and strict calcium restriction can decrease the density and improve the modelling of bone. It seems likely that at least some forms of osteopetrosis result from an inherited defect of osteoclasts, with defective resorption of bone. This has been increased by giving large doses of 1,25(OH)$_2$D to an infant on a low calcium diet, but without improvement.

Detailed studies of the animal models of the osteopetrotic grey lethal mouse, and the closely related microphthalmic mouse, have shown that bone resorption can be restored by the transfusion of splenic or bone marrow cells from a normal animal to a previously irradiated affected host, and in contrast that the disease can be transmitted to a normal animal. It has also been shown that under appropriate conditions the transplantation from a sibling of bone marrow containing normal osteoclasts and their precursors into an osteopetrotic infant can successfully restore normal bone resorption. A recipient, a 5-month-old girl with recessively inherited osteopetrosis who had been prepared with cyclophosphamide and modified total body irradiation, received a bone marrow transplant from her compatible 5-year old brother. The long-term results in other infants given bone marrow transplantation have not been uniform, but in some patients prolonged survival seems likely. Whilst such important measures aim at permanent correction of the underlying defect, supportive treatment such as blood transfusion and antibiotics may be necessary to maintain life. Corticosteroids have also been given.

Mild osteopetrosis

In this dominantly inherited disorder which varies in its expression the only detectable abnormality may be radiographic (Fig. 20), but fractures, osteomyelitis, nerve compression, and anaemia (at times of increased requirement such as growth and pregnancy) may occur. The diagnosis of the various forms of osteopetrosis is usually not difficult, since the radiographic appearances are so characteristic, as is the isolated increase in acid phosphatase. Apart from other hyperostoses (Table 15), in infancy the disorder may be confused with idiopathic infantile cortical hyperostosis and in later life with acquired myelofibrosis and fluorosis.

Other osteopetroses

These are all excessively rare. Some, such as craniometaphyseal dysplasia, are significant and disfiguring disorders; in others, such as osteopathia striata, the only significant abnormality is radiographic. The generalized form of diaphyseal dysplasia (Camurati–Engelmann disease) has received some attention because of its striking clinical features, which are not limited to the skeleton. To frontal bossing, proptosis, deafness, blindness, and bone pain associated with extensive hyperostosis can be added difficulty in walking, wasting and weakness of the muscles, skeletal disproportion, and delayed puberty.

References

Beighton, P., Horan, F. and Hamersma, H. (1977). A review of the osteopetroses. *Postgrad. Med. J.* **53**, 507–515.

Coccia, P. F. (1984). Cells that resorb bone. *N. Engl. J. Med.* **310**, 456–458.

——, Krivit, W., Cervenka, J., Clawson, C., Kersey, J. H., Kim, T. M., Nesbit, M. E., Ramsay, M. K. C., Warkentin, P. I., Teitelbaum, S. L., Khan, A. J. and Brown, D. M. (1980). Successful bone marrow transplantation for infantile malignant osteopetrosis. *N. Engl. J. Med.* **302**, 701–708.

Johnston, C. C., Lavy, N., Lord, T., Vellios, F., Merritt, A. D. and Deiss, W. P. (1968). Osteopetrosis. A clinical, genetic, metabolic and morphologic study of the dominantly inherited form. *Medicine* **47**, 149–167.

Smith, R., Walton, R. J., Corner, D. D. and Gordon, I. R. S. (1977). Clinical and biochemical studies in Engelmann's disease (progressive diaphyseal dysplasia). *Q. J. Med.* **46**, 273–294.

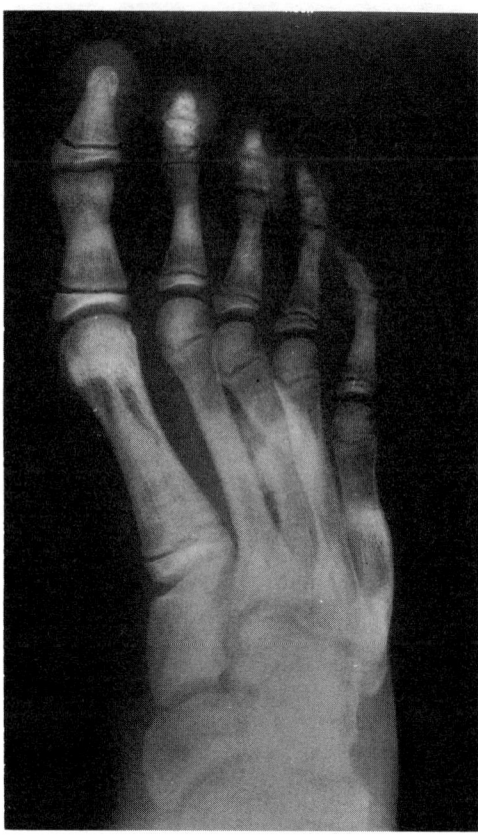

Fig. 20 The appearance of the bones in a boy with dominantly inherited osteopetrosis. There are considerable variations in density with evidence of recent and old pathological fractures, especially in the metatarsals.

Disorders of alkaline phosphatase

There are two very rare disorders named after changes in the circulating alkaline phosphatase concentration, hypophosphatasia and hyperphosphatasia. In neither of these conditions is the cause known and the changes in alkaline phosphatase are probably secondary rather than primary. In both there are well-defined changes in the skeleton.

Hypophosphatasia

This disorder has two biochemical abnormalities, a low plasma alkaline phosphatase and an increase in phosphoethanolamine in the urine. The connection between them is not understood. The severe disorder appears to be recessively inherited, but hypophosphatasia has very variable clinical features and time of presentation. Thus patients have been described with the skeletal features of hypophosphatasia but with a normal plasma alkaline phosphatase. Its incidence is therefore difficult to assess but it has been put at 1 in 100 000 births. The pathology, which closely resembles that of rickets, is explicable on the demonstrated increase in plasma pyrophosphate, a known inhibitor of mineralization. It is not known why the levels of alkaline phosphatase and pyrophosphatase are low, or if the primary defect is in the osteoblast.

The clinical severity of hypophosphatasia is greatest when the onset occurs early. The most severe form may be diagnosed *in utero* or soon after birth. Typically the ends of the long bones are not visible on radiographs and the skull shows wide unmineralized areas. Since the clinical appearances can include blue sclerae, severe osteogenesis imperfecta may be suggested at birth. Early death can occur and hypophosphatasia should be included in the differential diagnosis of lethal short-limbed dwarfism. In survivors, features include neuromuscular irritability, vomiting, dehydration, fever, occasional hypercalcaemia, and growth failure.

These less severely affected infants come to medical attention during or after the first six months of life with a widespread form of bone disease resembling rickets. Additionally there is premature loss of hypoplastic deciduous and permanent teeth, early synostosis of the cranial sutures, and exophthalmos. The dental changes, which may arise from abnormal cementogenesis, can be the only clinical feature. Radiographs of the skeleton show grossly defective mineralization with ragged metaphyses in the long bones.

Hypophosphatasia in adult life, which may be of dominant or recessive inheritance, produces a tendency to fracture particularly affecting the long bones. Partial fractures which resemble the Looser's zones of osteomalacia also occur but on the outer convex border of the affected bone (such as the femur) rather than on its medial aspect.

The diagnosis of hypophosphatasia depends on the characteristic changes in the bones, the low plasma alkaline phosphatase, the increase in phosphoethanolamine in the urine, and sometimes on family studies. In childhood, rickets is the main disorder to be distinguished. The irregular widened metaphyses are more grossly affected than in rickets and tooth structure is abnormal. Rarely phosphoethanolamine excretion may be increased in other conditions, such as coeliac disease and hypothyroidism. Affected heterozygote parents are usually clinically normal, but may have reduced plasma alkaline phosphatase levels and an excretion of phosphoethanolamine which is between that of normal and homozygote individuals.

Treatment is unsatisfactory and directed towards the complications of the disease. Although in the severe form there are wide areas of unmineralized osteoid in the skull early synostosis of the sutures occurs and craniectomy may be necessary. Prenatal diagnosis of the recessively inherited severe disorder is at present restricted to the attempted detection of the severe intrauterine skeletal defects by radiography and ultrasound, although measurement of the alkaline phosphatase produced by cultured amniotic fluid cells is feasible.

Hyperphosphatasia

This is a recessively inherited disorder with progressive bone deformity from infancy and a very high plasma alkaline phosphatase. The urinary total hydroxyproline is similarly very high; other reported biochemical abnormalities include an increase in the serum acid phosphatase and a low plasma urate. Characteristically the onset is in infancy, the patient becomes dwarfed, the head is large, and the long bones become progressively bowed. An associated bony fragility and sometimes blue sclerae may simulate osteogenesis imperfecta; but there are also features such as progressive irregular thickening of the skull and of the long bones which suggest the alternative name, juvenile Paget's disease. Radiographs of these bones show loss of the cortex with a cobweb trabecular pattern. Pathologically the bone shows considerable cellular activity, replacement of the cortex with trabecular bone, and extensive fibrosis. The condition may be heterogeneous and its treatment is not established; calcitonin has been used with considerable success in juvenile Paget's disease.

References

Eyring, E. J. and Eisenberg, E. (1968). Congenital hyperphosphatasia. A clinical, pathological and biochemical study of two cases. *J. Bone Joint Surg.* **50A**, 1099–1117.

Davies, M. and Stanbury, S. W. (1981). Rheumatic manifestations of metabolic bone disease. *Clin. Rheum. Dis.* **7**, 595–646.

Rasmussen, H. and Bartter, F. C. (1978). Hypophosphatasia. In *The metabolic basis of inherited disease* 4th edn (eds J. B. Stanbury, J. B. Wyngaarden, and D. S. Fredrickson), pp. 1340–1349. McGraw Hill Book Co. New York.

Whyte, M. P., Teitelbaum, S. L., Murphy, W. A., Bergfeld, M. A. and Avioli, L. V. (1979). Adult hypophosphatasia. *Medicine* **58**, 329–347.

Woodhouse, N. J. Y., Fisher, M. T., Sigurdsson, G., Joplin, G. F. and MacIntyre, I. (1972). Paget's disease in a 5-year old: acute response to human calcitonin. *Br. Med. J.* **4**, 267–269.

Fibrous dysplasia

Fibrous dysplasia of bone is a condition in which areas of fibrous tissue, either single or multiple, are found within the skeleton. The cause is unknown and the condition does not appear to be inherited; the polyostotic form is associated with characteristic endocrine abnormalities.

Monostotic fibrous dysplasia

This disorder is relatively common in orthopaedic practice. Although the lesions may occur in any bones, and particularly in the facial bones and ribs, the most frequent presenting symptom at any age is a fracture, often of the upper end of the femur (Fig. 21). The biochemistry is usually normal, and the diagnosis is made from the radiographic and pathological appearances. There is a smooth-walled translucent area within the bone, often with thinning of the cortex and sometimes with associated deformity. Pathologically, areas of fibrous tissue area are found, with the appearance of fibromata, associated with fibre bone and wide osteoid seams. The differential diagnosis is from other causes of bone cysts, from Paget's disease, and from hyperparathyroidism with osteitis fibrosa cystica. In the monostotic form treatment is largely orthopaedic. However, the large size of some of the defects in the shafts of the long bones may make conventional stabilization of fractures very difficult.

Polyostotic fibrous dysplasia

In this condition, which is often labelled as Albright's syndrome, multiple bony lesions occur together with pigmentation and with sexual precocity in females. It is commoner in girls than in boys and is usually manifest between the ages of 3 and 10 years. The bone lesions and the brown pigmentation are typically associated in position (but not in extent), and restricted to one side of the body. Sexual precocity is present in about 50 per cent of females with polyostotic disease, and is then the presenting complaint. It may occur at a very early age, with menstruation and appearance of secondary sexual characteristics from infancy. Where sexual precocity is not a feature (with rare exceptions it does not occur in boys) deformity and fracture are often the first symptoms. Gross deformity of the upper femur and femoral neck produce the 'shepherd's crook' deformity. Asymmetry of the long bones and of the skull is also seen; and in about half of the cases the base of the skull is thickened. The macular pigmentation tends to have smooth borders (in contrast to those of neurofibromatosis) and does not cross the mid-line. There are a number of other features which, like the sexual precocity, are inexplicable. These include thyrotoxicosis, acromegaly, and Cushing's syndrome. The skeletal lesions may cause complications such as spinal cord compression, and may be associated with hypophosphataemic osteomalacia. Sarcoma formation has been reported, but only after irradiation.

In the polyostotic disease both the plasma alkaline phosphatase and the urinary hydroxyproline may be slightly increased and the plasma phosphate slightly reduced. The pathology is similar to the monostotic form but it is said that cartilage and fluid-filled cysts are more common. Microscopically there is an abundance of woven bone and an increase in osteoblasts and osteoclasts. The cortex and marrow may be virtually replaced by fibrous tissue, so that the bones are fragile. Healing is rapid with abundant callus

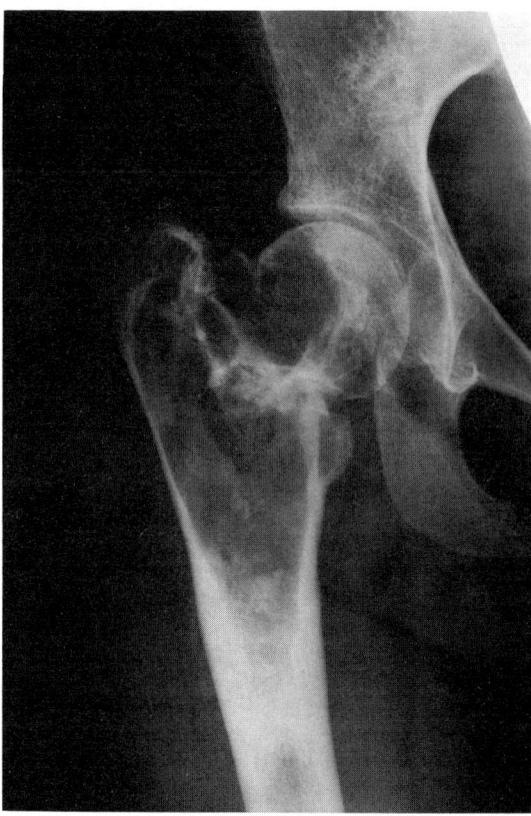

Fig. 21 Polyostotic fibrous dysplasia in a woman of 23 years. A large 'cyst' in the upper femora led to spontaneous fracture of the femoral neck which subsequently united with conservative treatment. Two ribs on the same side of the body show similar abnormalities. Puberty was precocious but pigmentation absent.

formation. Radiologically the bones are deformed, the cortex may be difficult to detect, and the medullary bone takes on a 'ground glass' or 'smoky' appearance. The main differential diagnosis is from osseous neurofibromatosis; in this condition there is also pigmentation, bone deformity, and sometimes hypophosphataemic osteomalacia. The borders of the pigmentation are less smooth than in fibrous dysplasia, and there are the other cutaneous features of neurofibromatosis; the bone deformity in neurofibromatosis can be quite bizarre, with overgrowth or undergrowth of isolated bones. In neurofibromatosis the characteristic spinal change is a very sharp upper thoracic kyphoscoliosis. Finally neurofibromatosis often shows clear evidence of dominant inheritance. The medical treatment of polyostotic fibrous dysplasia is particularly unsatisfactory, especially since its cause is unknown. Calcitonin has been used in an attempt to prevent progression of the bone lesions but without significant result.

References

De George, A. M. (1975). Albright syndrome: is it coming of age? *J. Ped.* **87**, 1018–1020.

Dent, C. E. and Gertner, J. M. (1976). Hypophosphataemic osteomalacia in fibrous dysplasia. *Q. J. Med.* **45**, 411–420.

Harris, W. H., Dudley, H. R. and Parry, R. J. (1962). The natural history of fibrous dysplasia. An orthopaedic, pathological and roentgenographic study. *J. Bone Joint Surg.* **44A**, 207–233.

Skeletal dysplasias

There is a considerable number of disorders which appear to affect only bone and cartilage, and whose cause and biochemistry are largely unknown. This may soon change with advances in our

Table 16 An outline classification of skeletal dysplasias

Dysplasias with short stature
Disproportionate short stature
  Short-limbed dwarfism
    Achondroplasia
    Hypochondroplasia
    Achondroplasia-like syndromes
      Achondroplastic forms of spondyloepiphyseal dysplasia
      Thanatophoric dwarfism
      Achondrogenesis
      Hypophosphatasia
      Severe osteogenesis imperfecta
      Other short-limbed dwarfs
  Short trunk dwarfism
    Spondyloepiphyseal dysplasia
Proportionate short stature
  Mucopolysaccharidoses
  Mucolipidoses
  Other proportionate dwarfs

Dysplasias without conspicuous dwarfism
  Multiple epiphyseal dysplasias
  Metaphyseal dysostosis (some forms only)
  Diaphyseal dysplasias

knowledge of bone matrix biochemistry. Meanwhile the classification of these dysplasias remains difficult and is made on clinical or radiological grounds. Clinically these disorders may be grouped into those with dwarfism or short stature and those without (Table 16). Short stature can affect predominantly the limbs or the trunk, or it may be proportionate. In the short-limbed group achondroplasia and achondroplasia-like dwarfs are the most typical. Those without conspicuous dwarfing include various inherited epiphyseal dysplasias, diaphyseal dysplasias (also included in the osteopetroses), and some of the metaphyseal dysplasias. An alternative classification, not based on height, groups the dysplasias according to whether the dysplasia is predominantly epiphyseal or metaphyseal, whether the spine is predominantly involved, and whether single limbs or segments are involved.

Achondroplasia

This is the prototype of short-limbed dwarfism. It is inherited as an autosomal dominant, with a high mutation rate. The incidence increases with paternal age. The cause is unknown, but apparent defects in type II (cartilage) collagen have been described. Until recently any patient with excessively short limbs in whom the cause was unknown tended to have the label of achondroplasia. This approach accounted for the apparently high frequency of achondroplasia and also for its apparently high mortality, since it included under this label many forms of lethal short-limbed dwarfism. It is now realized that there are several disorders which closely resemble achondroplasia but are clinically distinct from it.

Because the clinical definition of achondroplasia has not always been exact, its incidence and natural history is not well defined. In classic achondroplasia the pathological changes arise from a failure of the epiphyseal growth cartilage. Bulbous masses of cartilage appear at the end of the long bones. In contrast the formation of periosteal and membrane bone and the repair of bone is normal. It is this selective effect on growth cartilage which accounts for the skeletal deformity.

The diagnosis of achondroplasia can be made at birth or within the first year of life, when the disparity between the large skull and short limbs becomes obvious. The striking disproportion is between the trunk, which is of normal length, and the short arms and legs. Thus the finger tips may only come down to the iliac crest. The shortness of the limbs particularly affects the proximal segment. The limbs themselves look very broad, with abnormally deep creases, and the hands are trident-like. In contrast to the short limbs is the enlarged bulging vault of the skull, the small face, and flat nasal bridge or 'scooped out' glabella. The spine shows a lumbar lordosis and also sometimes some wedging of the upper lumbar vertebrae (which may later lead to a thoraco-lumbar kyphosis). Radiological appearances include metaphyseal irregularity and flaring in the long bones, irregular and late-appearing epiphyses, a pelvis which is narrow in its antero-posterior diameter, with short iliac wings and deep sacro-iliac notches, and a spine which shows progressive narrowing of the interpeduncular distance from above downwards, which is the reverse of normal.

Children with achondroplasia are of normal intelligence and the complications of this disease arise particularly from the skeletal disproportion. This may lead to early osteoarthritis, to obstetric difficulties, and the need for Caesarian section, to hydrocephalus and to paraplegia. Eventual height can vary from about 80 to 150 cm. Recent reviews emphasize how often narrowing of the spinal canal produces symptoms of spinal stenosis.

Homozygous achondroplasia (i.e. the offspring of two affected parents) is very rare and the bone disease is severe. In contrast the condition of hypochondroplasia is probably inherited independently from achondroplasia; the skeletal disproportion and the spinal abnormalities are less and the skull is unaffected.

Achondroplasia-like dwarfs

For the details of these and other short-limbed dwarfs the reader should consult more specialized texts (see also Table 16). Those which most closely resemble achondroplasia at birth are thanatophoric dwarfism, achondrogenesis, severe hypophosphatasia, and osteogenesis imperfecta congenita. All can be readily distinguished by their radiological features.

Spondyloepiphyseal dysplasias

This is a heterogeneous group of disorders in which the spine is predominantly affected and the short stature is due to shortness of the trunk. The most severe type is spondyloepiphyseal dysplasia (SED) congenita; milder forms are referred to as SED tarda. There are various forms of inheritance.

SED tarda is often inherited as an X-linked recessive, so that males only are affected. Small stature and pain in the back are noted from late childhood, and early osteoarthritis may occur. The vertebrae have a characteristic appearance due to failure of ossification in the anterior part of the so-called ring epiphysis, leading to central and posterior humps on the upper and lower parts of the flattened bodies (the appearance superficially resembles that of alkaptonuria). The condition needs to be distinguished from multiple epiphyseal dysplasia where the spine is generally less affected, and the inheritance is dominant.

SED congenita can be diagnosed at birth because of the short stature associated with a short trunk. There may be a close resemblance to Morquio's disease (MPS IV). The severe form may be distinguished from the age of about 4 years. There is considerable delay in the appearance of the capital femoral epiphysis (in some patients it may never be seen, except by arthrography). Marked lumbar lordosis, waddling gait, back pain, and progressive disproportion occur. The odontoid is hypoplastic, kyphoscoliosis may develop, and the interpeduncular distance of the vertebrae do not increase in the lumbar region. Because of all these changes paraplegia may occur.

There is a form of SED which resembles achondroplasia because of the short limbs (pseudoachondroplasia). Shortness of stature becomes obvious from about two years of age. Lumbar lordosis and scoliosis may develop. The tubular bones are short with irregular metaphyses and small deformed epiphyses. Hypermobility and early osteoarthritis occur.

Proportionate dwarfism

These include particularly the mucopolysaccharidoses (see page 17.30 and Section 9) and various other disorders discussed else-

where in this book (see Table 2). Although it is very useful to classify short stature into proportionate and disproportionate, there are many conditions in which this distinction is difficult to make. For instance, hypophosphataemic rickets, vitamin D-dependent rickets, and osteogenesis imperfecta may come into both categories.

Bone dysplasias without conspicuous short stature

Within this group of disorders are those which primarily affect the epiphyses, metaphyses or diaphyses. Patients with multiple epiphyseal dysplasia may be short but not severely so. Many epiphyses are affected but the spine is normal or nearly so. There are variable forms of inheritance. In patients with multiple hereditary exostoses (often also referred to as diaphyseal aclasis) there is a juxta-epiphyseal disorder of bone growth, limited to bones developed in cartilage, which gives rise to cartilage-capped exostoses which point away from the joint. Inheritance is autosomal dominant.

The metaphyseal disorders are rare; some, such as the Jansen type of metaphyseal dysostosis do cause severe dwarfing. In others with less severe growth disturbance rickets is simulated. In progressive diaphyseal dysplasia (Camurati–Engelmann's disease) which resembles in some ways marble bones disease, the dysplasia is only one of the clinical features.

Finally there is a disorder which affects membrane bone only. This is cleido-cranial dysostosis, in which the clavicles (and their associated muscles) are hypoplastic or absent, so that the shoulders can touch in front of the body. the skull is abnormal with frontal bulging; there are Wormian bones and open fontanelles in childhood.

References

McKusick, V. A. (1972). *Heritable disorders of connective tissue.* 4th edn. C. V. Mosby Co., St. Louis.
Rimoin, D. L., and Lachmann, R. S. (1983). The chondrodysplasias. In *Principles and practice of medical genetics* Vol. 2. (eds A. E. H. Emery and D. L. Rimoin), pp. 703–735. Churchill Livingstone, Edinburgh.
Spranger, J. W., Langer, L. O. and Wiedmann, H. R. (1974). *Bone dysplasias. An atlas of constitutional disorders of skeletal development.* W. B. Saunders Co, Philadelphia.
Wynne-Davies, R. (1973). *Heritable disorders in orthopaedic practice.* Blackwell Scientific Publications, Oxford.
—— and Hall, C. (1982). Two clinical variants of spondyloepiphyseal dysplasia congenita. *J. Bone Joint Surg.* **64B**, 435–441.
——, —— and Apley, A. G. (1985). *Atlas of skeletal dysplasias* 1st edn. Churchill Livingstone, Edinburgh.
——, Walsh, W. K. and Gormley, J. (1981). Achondroplasia and hypochondroplasia. *J. Bone Joint Surg.* **63B**, 508–515.

Assorted bone diseases

The skeleton is affected in many systemic diseases and also by the methods used to treat them. In some, the skeletal changes are clinically important; in others, they are a minor aspect of the general illness. Examples of the first are fluorosis and scurvy; and of the second the bone disease of thalassaemia and of prolonged parenteral nutrition.

Fluorosis

Fluorine is incorporated into bone and stimulates osteoblastic activity. For this reason sodium fluoride is used in the treatment of osteoporosis. However, continued exposure to high concentrations of fluorine during industrial processes or, more often, in the drinking water produces a pathological increase in the amount and density of bone with the important consequences of spinal cord compression. Where this chronic fluorosis is endemic, as in certain areas of India, the symptoms begin insidiously in adult life, with pain and stiffness in the back and progressive weakness of the extremities. Radiographs show sclerosis throughout the skeleton, with the most pronounced changes in the vertebrae and pelvis; the spinal canal and intervertebral foramina are narrowed. The cortex of the long bones is thickened and the metaphyses are wide. The intervertebral ligaments calcify as do muscle insertions around the hips, elbows, and ribs; and there is osteophyte formation. The appearance may superficially resemble that of ankylosing spondylitis; it is also to be distinguished from the osteopetroses. The histological appearances have some similarities to Paget's disease; there is disordered lamellar orientation and enlarged Haversian systems in the compact bone and spongy irregular peripheral bone, some of which extends into muscle attachments. The permanent teeth may show characteristic changes with white opaque patches and dark pigmentation of the enamel which may also be pitted.

Scurvy

Ascorbic acid is necessary for the intracellular hydroxylation of peptide-bound proline. In its absence formation of the collagen molecule is defective, structurally incompetent precursors accumulate within the cell, and collagen-containing tissues are weak. The clinical condition of scurvy which results is very rare, and occurs most often in neglected infants who do not receive fruit juice or ascorbic acid for several months. Extensive subperiosteal haemorrage leads to pain and immobility; the legs are held in a 'frog-like' position. Other features are perifollicular haemorrhage, purpura, swelling of the costochondral junctions, and bleeding gums. Radiographs show a widened zone of provisional calcification in the metaphyses with a proximal disordered area representing the destroyed primary spongiosa and failure of new bone formation. The edges of the metaphyses may show small spurs, and epiphyseolysis may occur. With healing the subperiosteal haematoma calcifies.

The clinical picture of scurvy resembles that of a 'battered baby' but scurvy is far less common. Similar radiographic appearances have been described in copper deficiency.

The haemoglobinopathies

In the inherited disorders of haemoglobin (see Section 19) the skeleton is often abnormal. This may result from a hyperplastic bone marrow, and overactivity of the osteoblasts so that the skull, facial bones, and long bones are thickened. Additional features include collapse of the weight-bearing bones and disorganization of the joints following bone infarction. In β-thalassaemia an increase in osteoid thickness has been described which resembles that of osteomalacia.

Parenteral nutrition

The increasing use of prolonged parenteral nutrition (see Section 8) has produced a number of unexpected deficiencies, such as those of phosphate and copper, and some inexplicable disorders. One of these is a form of bone disease with some similarities to osteomalacia. The main symptom has been periarticular bone pain, particularly in the ankles. Histology shows impaired mineralization of bone, and biochemistry shows an increase in plasma alkaline phosphatase, in urinary calcium, and sometimes in plasma calcium. The radiographic appearances suggest osteoporosis. There are normal levels of 25(OH)D and a negative calcium balance. Since patients on total parenteral nutrition are invariably ill to begin with and many have malabsorption there are several probable causes for this disorder. There is some evidence that it results from aluminium toxicity.

Fibrogenesis imperfecta ossium

This is a very rare apparently acquired disorder affecting particularly the bone matrix. Bone pain and pathological fractures begin in middle age or later. Radiographs characteristically show uniform coarse trabeculation with apparent thickening and widening of weight-bearing trabeculae as in the vertebrae and femoral necks. There is also ectopic mineralization around large joints and tendon insertions. Routine biochemical measurements show an increase in plasma alkaline phosphatase and often abnormal plasma proteins. The diagnosis is confirmed by bone biopsy which shows large areas of unmineralized bone matrix which is not (unlike osteomalacic osteoid) birefringent; electron microscopy shows that the normal lamellar collagen has apparently been replaced by an amorphous tissue containing very few fibres.

Fibrogenesis imperfecta ossium is usually initially mistaken for Paget's disease, fluorosis or myelofibrosis, but the bone biopsy is diagnostic. The disorder leads to progressive disability due to multiple fractures. The bone itself becomes excessively fragile and may be broken off at tendon insertions (at the tibial tubercules or olecranon processes).

The cause is unknown and most treatments have been ineffective. However, the presence of abnormal proteins has led to the use of melphalan with corticosteroids and also l-α-hydroxycholecalciferol, with reported improvement.

Vitamin A overdosage

Excessive ingestion of vitamin A can cause striking hyperostoses in the growing skeleton, and recently hyperostosis has been described in patients treated with retinoids for refractory ichthyosis. In four such patients long term 13-cis-retinoic acid therapy produced an ossification disorder resembling diffuse idiopathic skeletal hyperostosis (Forestier's disease). Stiffness and musculoskeletal pain particularly related to the spine is associated with ossification of the anterior longitudinal ligament, localized hyperostosis around the vertebral bodies, ossification of tendon insertions, and of the ilio-lumbar ligament. Initially the condition can be confused with ankylosing spondylitis. The long-term effects of synthetic retinoids on the skeleton are unknown.

Other disorders

The skeleton is also affected by lead and radiation; it is abnormal in shape and structure in a number of the storage disorders (in addition to the mucopolysaccharidoses), such as Gaucher's disease; and the metaphyses are dense in idiopathic hypercalcaemia, a disorder possibly related to excessive intake or abnormal metabolism of vitamin D.

References

British Medical Journal (1981). Chronic fluorosis. *Br. Med. J.* **i**, 253–254.

Burge, S. and Ryan, T. (1985). Diffuse hyperostosis associated with etretinate. *Lancet* **ii**, 397–398.

Fourman, P. and Royer, P. (1968). *Calcium metabolism and the bone.* 2nd edn. Blackwell Scientific Publications, Oxford.

Gratwick, G. M., Bullough, P. G., Bohne, W. O., Markenson, A. L. and Peterson, C. M. (1978). Thalassemic osteoarthropathy. *Ann. inter. Med.* **88**, 494–501.

Pittsley, R. A. and Yoder, F. W. (1983). Retinoid hyperostosis. *N. Engl. J. Med.* **308**, 1012–1014.

Shike, M., Harrison, J. E., Sturtridge, W. C., Tam, C. B., Bobechko, P. E., Jones, G., Murray, T. M. and Jeejeebhoy, K. M. (1980). Metabolic bone disease in patients receiving long-term parenteral nutrition. *Ann. inter. Med.* **92**, 343–350.

Singh, A. and Jolly, S. S. (1961). Endemic fluorosis. *Q. J. Med.* **30**, 357–372.

Stamp, T. C. B., Byers, P. D., Ali, S. Y., Jenkins, M. V., and Willoughby, J. M. T. (1985). Fibrogenesis imperfecta ossium: remission with melphalan. *Lancet* **i**, 582–583.

Swan, C. H. J., Shah, K., Brewer, D. B. and Cooke, W. T. (1976). Fibrogenesis imperfecta ossium. *Q. J. Med.* **45**, 233–253.

Table 17 The main causes of ectopic mineralization

Calcification without bone formation
  1 Secondary to biochemical abnormalities;
    Hyperparathyroidism, renal failure, idiopathic hyperphosphataemia, hypoparathyroidism and pseudohypoparathyroidism
  2 Secondary to tissue damage;
    Dermatomyositis, scleroderma or without known cause

Calcification with bone formation (ectopic ossification);
  1 Acquired
    Trauma, head injury, surgery, paraplegia
  2 Inherited
    Myositis (fibrodysplasia) ossificans progressiva

Ectopic mineralization

The deposition of calcium in the soft tissues (ectopic mineralization), sometimes associated with the formation of bone, is nearly always pathological, and often its cause is unknown. However, in the elderly calcification in tissues such as the arteries is so common that it may be regarded as one of the features of ageing, in the same way as age-related bone loss. There are recognized causes of ectopic mineralization, and it is important to divide them into those with ossification and those without. Since there are mysteries about normal mineralization it is rarely possible to explain satisfactorily why soft tissue calcification occurs. However, there are a group of disorders in which such calcification is associated with biochemical abnormalities.

Ectopic calcification without bone formation

Where the circulating level of calcium and/or phosphate is consistently high, with an increase in the calcium:phosphate product (Table 17) mineralization can occur in many soft tissues. The tissues affected include the blood vessels, the cornea, the conjunctivae, skin, brain, and kidneys. The distribution varies inexplicably with the cause; thus in parathyroid insufficiency calcification is particularly prominent in the basal ganglia and also in the skin; whereas in primary or secondary hyperparathyroidism calcification occurs in the blood vessels and periarticular tissues. One form of ectopic mineralization is characterized by the presence of large masses of calcium around the large joints. This may be referred to as 'tumoral calcinosis' and the term has been applied to this appearance from any cause. However, it is probably best restricted to the rare recessively inherited disease in which there is an isolated increase in the plasma phosphate due to an increase in its renal tubular reabsorption. In this condition masses of ectopic mineral which appear in childhood may require surgical removal; this should be combined with treatment with aluminium hydroxide, which binds phosphate in the gut and prevents its absorption, thus reducing the plasma phosphate towards normal and diminishing tumoral deposits.

Striking calcification can occur in tissues affected by acquired connective tissue disorders such as scleroderma and dermatomyositis (see Section 16), in which there is no detectable biochemical change, and these provide examples of dystrophic calcification. The form associated with scleroderma is more common, where the calcinosis may occur in association with Raynaud's phenomena, scleroderma, and telangiectases (CRST syndrome). Mineral is distributed subcutaneously around the phalanges and peripheral joints, but may also be found over pressure areas, such as knees and elbows. Large amounts may accumulate and discharge through the skin from time to time, producing a substance with the consistency of firm toothpaste and the chemistry of hydroxyapatite. More impressive is the generalized subcutaneous calcification which may follow shortly after an episode of dermatomyositis, and is seen in children. Typically there is a history of a generalized illness with painful weak proximal muscles, difficulty in walking, and often a rash; the diagnosis of dermatomyositis is confirmed by muscle biopsy and increased phosphocreatine kinase levels, and steroids or immunosuppresive drugs are started. Subsequently, often during a time of apparent slow improvement, extensive deposits of calcium may form in the subcutaneous tissues (Fig. 22), and sometimes apparently between the muscles, sufficient to provide a form of calcinosis universalis. The blood vessels are not involved. There are no consistently beneficial forms of treatment for these types of dystrophic calcification but treatment has been tried with diphosphonates, sodium ethylene diamine tetraacetate (EDTA) (to increase calcium excretion), aluminium hydroxide, or probenecid (to increase phosphate excretion and to lower plasma phosphate), with very occasional success. Fortunately calcinosis associated with dermatomyositis tends to improve spontaneously, often at puberty.

Ectopic calcification with bone formation: ectopic ossification

In this condition true bone forms outside the skeleton, often within the connective tissue of muscles. The formation of extra-skeletal bone matrix is followed by its mineralization. The main disability comes from progressive fixation of the joints.

Acquired ectopic ossification

Ectopic ossification may follow accidental injury, elective orthopaedic surgery (such as total hip replacement), neurological injury, and paraplegia. Whilst that after surgery may be the direct result of damage to the tissues, including the periosteum, the cause of ectopic ossification in paraplegia (where it is said to occur in up to 50 per cent of patients) is quite unknown.

The diphosphonate EHDP has been tried in these patients. There is some evidence that if EHDP is given immediately after a total hip replacement it may slow the onset of ectopic mineralization and improve the eventual mobility of the joint, compared with untreated controls. Likewise, if EHDP is given to patients such as those with neurological injury to cover the removal of ectopic bone, recurrence of mineralization may sometimes appear to be delayed. Unfortunately EHDP does not prevent the formation of new ectopic matrix in the operated site and this rapidly mineralizes when the phosphonate is discontinued (EHDP cannot be given for very long periods in therapeutic dose because of the deleterious effect on the normal skeleton). Treatment with corticosteroids or with radiotherapy, both of which have been tried, presumably reduce osteoblastic activity and new bone matrix formation.

Inherited ectopic ossification

There is one striking form of inherited ectopic ossification known as myositis (or fibrodysplasia) ossificans progressiva. This is a rare

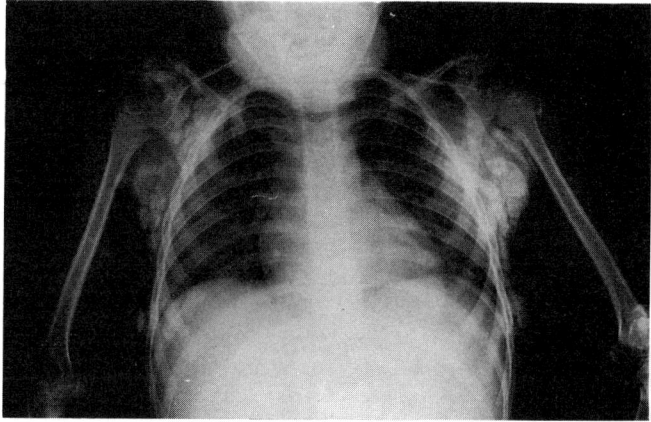

Fig. 22 Extensive subcutaneous calcification in a girl with dermatomyositis.

condition (approximate prevalence 1 per million) which is classified as an inherited disorder of connective tissue, with dominant inheritance but variable penetrance. Characteristic are progressive ossification within muscles and specific skeletal abnormalities, of which monophalangic big toes are the hallmark. The skeletal abnormality is present at birth but may not be recognized until later. The ossification centres are abnormal, and 'congenital hallux valgus' may be diagnosed. Later the main abnormality is shortness of the big toes but many variations exist. The thumbs are also said to be short but this is difficult to be certain of. Exostoses, abnormal shape of the long bones, and fusion of the cervical vertebrae are other features. Recent surveys have shown the extent of the radiological abnormalities. In the hands short first metacarpals and malformed phalanges of the fifth finger (leading to clinodactyly) occur; in the feet the changes are more variable and alter with age, and occasionally there are severe reduction defects in all digits; in the neck the cervical vertebrae are abnormal from birth, and there is progressive fusion, first of the laminae and later of the bodies.

The ossification within muscle is preceded by episodes of 'myositis' in which large muscles, often first of the back and neck, become painful, red, and hard; biopsy at this time will show considerable oedema with cellular infiltration and fragmentation of muscle fibres. A clinical diagnosis of infection or sarcoma may be made, and it is often thought that the lesions are associated with trauma and bruising. This is, however, difficult to establish. Likely precipitating causes are intramuscular injection, biopsy, removal of ectopic bone, accidental injury, dental treatment, and careless venepuncture. When a large area of muscle is involved the patient is ill and has a fever. Pain and swelling subside within a week or so, but with apparent improvement there is radiological evidence of progressive mineralization within the region of affected muscles. Blocks or bars of bone occur (Fig. 23) which eventually fix most joints. Ossification has a predilection for certain sites. Characteristically the neck and back are involved in early childhood; later the shoulders and arms; and in adolescence or earlier, ossification of muscles around the hip leads to progressive disability. Eventually the subject is unable to walk and is completely stiff. Fortunately the small muscles of the hands and feet are not involved; it is of interest that cardiac and smooth muscle are also unaffected.

The diagnosis of myositis ossificans progressiva in its typical form should not be difficult. However, it is very rare and its features are therefore often not known or remain unrecognized; occasionally, progressive stiffness rather than intermittent myositis may occur. The short big toes provide valuable clues and will prevent such erroneous diagnoses as Still's disease or the Klippel–Feil syndrome. Rare additional features in some patients include deafness and diffuse baldness of the scalp (often in women).

The cause of myositis ossificans progressiva is entirely unknown. Although the skeletal defects are present from birth, the episodes of 'myositis' come later. Some consider that these pri-

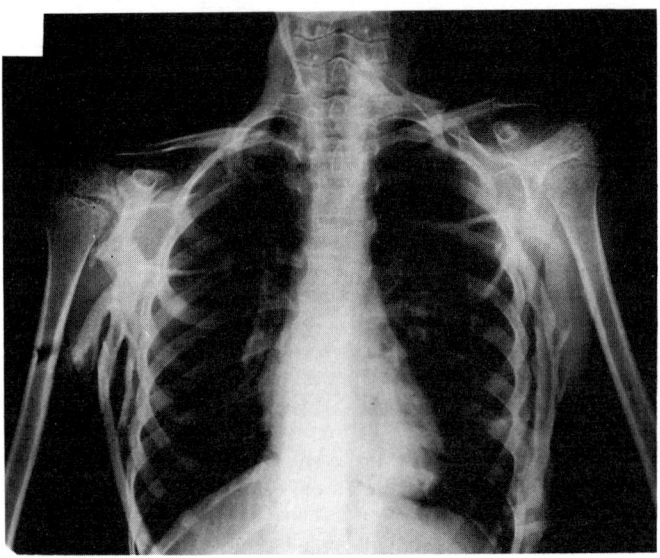

Fig. 23 Myositis ossificans progressiva in a girl. Extensive bars of ectopic bone have fixed the neck, chest, and shoulders.

marily involve the connective tissue within muscle (hence the term fibrodysplasia ossificans progressiva). No biochemical abnormalities have been described, except an increase in plasma alkaline phophatase during acute myositis. The chromosomes, when examined, have been normal.

Pathologically the ectopic bone contains all the components of skeletal bone, including cartilage; there is also evidence of active bone formation and resorption.

The treatment of myositis ossificans progressiva is not satisfactory. There is no known way of preventing the acute episodes of myositis and the subsequent formation of ectopic bone matrix. There is some evidence that if EHDP is given before, during, and for several months after removal of ectopic bone its recurrence is delayed. However, the effects of EHDP in this disease are not predictable and the improvement in mobility after operation is usually disappointing.

References

Connor, J. M. (1983). *Soft tissue ossification.* Springer–Verlag, Berlin.
—— and Evans, D. A. P. (1982). Fibrodysplasia ossificans progressiva: clinical features and natural history of 34 patients from the UK. *J. Bone Joint Surg.* **64B**, 76–83.
Smith, R. (1975). Myositis ossificans progressiva: A review of current problems. *Sem. Arthr. Rheum.* **4**, 369–380.
——, Russell, R. G. G. and Woods, C. G. (1976). Myositis ossificans progressiva. Clinical features of eight patients and their response to treatment. *J. Bone Joint Surg.* **58B**, 48–57.

SECTION 18
NEPHROLOGY

CLINICAL PHYSIOLOGY OF THE KIDNEY: TESTS OF RENAL FUNCTION AND STRUCTURE

R. B. I. MORRISON, J. M. DAVISON, AND D. N. S. KERR

Assessment of the function of the kidneys and the urinary tract

There are many more tests of renal function available than are necessary for the detection and management of most patients with renal disease and many of them are costly, troublesome, and available only in specialist hospitals and laboratories. In this contribution we deal with the tests that are available to general physicians, in the order that they are used in clinical practice, and give only enough information about the more specialized investigations to indicate what they involve for the patient and when they should be sought, by referral to a renal unit if necessary.

Urinalysis and urine microscopy

These simple procedures often give the first clue to the presence of renal disease and their value cannot be overemphasized.

Sample collection

A reliable mid-stream urine sample can be collected from males after retraction of the foreskin and from females with the labia separated by their fingers. This requires careful instruction of the woman and some agility; contamination is almost inevitable when samples are collected by the obese, the elderly, and those in late pregnancy. Ideally the genitalia should be swabbed with sterile saline but this is often impracticable. Antiseptics should be avoided if a sample is required for culture. The patient should have a full bladder and should move the container in and out of a free-flowing stream.

Bladder puncture, a well-accepted and safe procedure, is especially valuable in young children, but its usefulness must not be forgotten when investigating adults. The bladder should be sufficiently full to be easily palpable in the slim adult and dull to percussion well above the pubes in the obese. If there is any doubt, a potent diuretic should be given to fill the bladder before aspiration. No local anaesthetic is needed; the urine is aspirated through a thin, preferably all-metal, needle. The bladder sample is free of vulval contamination and therefore easier to interpret microscopically and less subject to overgrowth by contaminant bacteria than mid-stream urine, if there is a delay in transport to the laboratory.

In infants, urine samples may be collected in an adhesive perineal bag. A negative culture may be very helpful if infection is suspected and the sample is useful for urinalysis and microscopy but positive cultures often need to be confirmed by bladder puncture. Toddlers pose the biggest challenge; they do not accept bladder puncture readily. They will sometimes micturate in response to stimuli like stroking the abdomen or chilling the back, allowing the doctor with quick reflexes to catch a mid-stream urine, but it is usually necessary to instruct the mother in the technique.

Diagnostic catheterization should be reserved for the infirm. The risk of introducing infection is reduced by instilling 120 ml of 0.2 per cent neomycin before withdrawing the catheter.

The urine sample must be sent promptly to the laboratory to avoid growth of contaminant organisms and the dissolution of cellular elements and casts. It should be cooled in a 4 °C refrigerator if the transportation delay is greater than 2 hours. The introduction of the dip-slide or dip-spoon culture has increased the opportunity for bacteriological examination of the urine. It is a convenient technique for samples collected in doctors' surgeries and for the well-instructed patient at home, especially at night and at weekends. However, it has two limitations; some fastidious organisms do not grow on dip-slides and the laboratory receives no urine sample for microscopy. Consequently a dip-slide should always be accompanied by a form detailing the patient's symptoms and recent antibiotic therapy. Persistent discrepancies between symptoms and culture results should be checked by recalling the patient to the clinic or laboratory where a fresh urine sample can be collected and examined.

Urinalysis

The versatile dip-stick is the only method in common use today. We refer to one widely used variety (Ames' Labstix, Multistix etc.) to which there are several commercial alternatives available.

Protein

The detector square contains the indicators methyl red and bromophenol blue, with buffering salts. When the latter dissolve on contact with urine they stabilize the pH of the paper at a level which keeps the colour of the indicators a pale yellow-green. Protein in the urine lowers the pH at which the indicators change colour, so the detector becomes progressively green in response to increasing protein concentrations. The test is particularly sensitive to albumin, which is the main constituent of most pathological proteinurias, but is insensitive to Bence Jones protein. The concentration of protein in the urine of normal individuals can rise to about 150 mg/l which is sufficient to give a trace positive result with the dip-stick.

False-positive results can occur with very alkaline urine, e.g. during infection with urea-splitting organisms. There is considerable observer error when poorly trained hospital staff use the dip-stick as a semi-quantitative test of proteinuria but patients taught to test their own urine (for relapsing nephrotic syndrome) become adept at detecting the onset of proteinuria. Doubtful positive tests, and those in alkaline urine, should be checked with 25 per cent sulphosalicylic acid which is a little less sensitive.

Blood

The detector turns green in the presence of very low concentrations of haem pigments, either hemoglobin or myoglobin. Haematuria is usually accompanied by lysis of some red cells and therefore commonly produces a uniform positive test for haemoglobin. Scanty intact red cells produce small green spots by lysis on contact with the detector. However the chemical test should always be complemented by microscopy to detect minimal haematuria.

Dextrose

The test square contains glucose oxidase and is specific for dextrose. Although the colour depth is a semi-quantitative test it is not sufficiently accurate for the assessment of control of diabetes mellitus. In the absence of diabetes, dextrose may be found in the urine during pregnancy, in association with heavy proteinuria or in patients with tubular disorders such as Fanconi syndrome and renal glycosuria.

Urine pH

Random urine pH readings are of little diagnostic value. The pH detector square is useful in detecting infection with urea-splitting organisms, which raise urine pH to 8 or above, in alerting the observer to false-positive tests for proteinuria and in ensuring that the urine is being kept alkaline in patients with salicylate poisoning, uric acid calculi, cystinuria, and urinary infection during treatment with aminoglycosides.

Nitrate

An extended dip-stick (N-multistix, Ames) or a separate commercial stick can be used to detect nitrates. Most of the Gram-negative organisms reduce nitrates to nitrites and produce a red colour in the reagent square. False-negative tests are common (about 30 per cent), partly because some patients do not excrete sufficient nitrate and partly because of non-nitrate-reducing bacteria. However, the test has some use in giving immediate confirmation of urinary infection and in screening large populations. Its low cost compensates for a detection rate well below 100 per cent.

Leucocytes

Dipsticks which detect significant pyuria depend on the release of esterases. They give results in close accord with quantitative microscopy but have the disadvantage of a 15 min wait before the result can be read; all other detectors can be read within 1 min.

Urine microscopy

Together with detection of protein and blood in the urine, the careful examination of the urine sediment is of the greatest value in deciding whether the patient has renal disease, either primary or associated with a systemic illness. The urine sample should be fresh. If this is not possible, a trace of formalin will preserve cells and casts while boric acid 0.5 g per 30 ml of urine will also inhibit bacterial growth while maintaining viability, allowing both microscopy and culture after a delay of some hours.

The microscope must be of good quality, preferably binocular, and well maintained. Slides and cover slips must be free of dust and grease. Cleansing them inevitably leaves a few cellulose fibres which are often mistaken for casts by the untutored. They are easily distinguished by their sharper edges, greater length, and different refractive index.

The commonest indication for urine microscopy is the diagnosis of acute urinary infection. It should be performed by the doctor in his surgery or clinic when time is at a premium. A drop of urine under a cover slip can be examined under high power (×40 objective) within about one minute, since the answer is usually obvious (Fig. 1). The heavy pyuria, often accompanied by some haema-

turia and visible bacilluria, is readily distinguishable from normal urine without quantitative tests. When the answer is not so clear cut, the unspun urine may be examined in a counting chamber and the findings expressed quantitatively.

If renal disease is suspected a centrifuged urine is examined. The Kova system (Boehringer, Mannheim) facilitates recognition of formed elements and gives quantitative results if the urine is a timed specimen. Urine, 12 ml, is spun in a disposable tube. A bulbous pipette is pushed down the tube to isolate the last 1 ml and the supernatant is poured off. One drop of stain is mixed with the last 1 ml. A drop is placed in a disposable plastic slide with built-in coverslip and counting chamber. Experienced microscopists can obtain much the same information from a qualitative examination of an unstained sediment. A thick uncovered drop is scanned for casts then a cover slip is added and the high power used to distinguish cells, bacillia, yeasts, and trichomonads. Illumination is kept down by lowering the condenser and closing the diaphragm. Phase contrast is necessary for the study of red cell morphology. Polarized light for urinary lipids and crystals is rarely of diagnostic importance.

White cells

In the uncentrifuged urine, less than 3 leucocytes per cubic millilitre is normal, 3–10 of doubtful significance, and greater than 10 abnormal. However, these figures only apply to well-taken midstream urine, free of gross vulval contamination, which can be judged by the absence, or scanty presence, of squamous epithelial cells. When squames are numerous one can only make a guess, from experience, whether the leucocytes are out of proportion to the squames; there is little point in expressing this guess quantitatively; the best solution is to obtain a cleaner sample. It is abnormal to find any leucocytes in a bladder-puncture sample.

Not all pyuria is due to infection nor is bacteriuria always accompanied by pyuria; the causes of a dissociation between the two are summarized in Table 1.

Red cells

Although there are a few red cells in normal urine, if there are sufficient to produce any count in unspun urine they are almost certainly pathological. There is considerable observer error in detecting slight haematuria; scanty red cells are often confused with small oxalate crystals, yeasts, and small air bubbles. Their presence should always be confirmed under high power.

Red cells entering the urine through the glomerulus often show great variation in size and shape, whereas those arising from the collecting system appear more uniform. Several expert microscopists have demonstrated their ability to distinguish renal from bladder haematuria on this criterion in 'blind' studies using phase contrast microscopy.

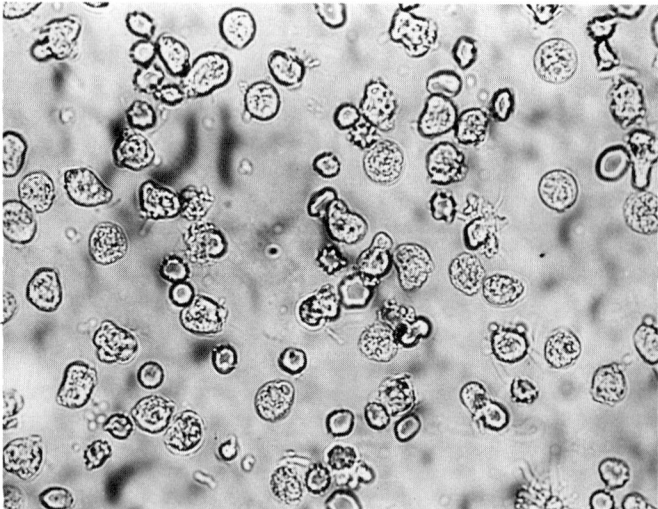

Fig. 1 Pus cells, red cells, and bacteria in an unspun urine sample from a patient with an acute urinary infection. High power.

Table 1 Dissociation between bacteriuria and pyuria

A. Bacteriuria without pyuria
  1 Asymptomatic bacteriuria
  2 Contamination
B. True heavy pyuria without bacteriuria
  1 Culture inhibited by:
    (a) Antibacterial agent
    (b) Specimen contaminated by antiseptic
    (c) Wrong growth conditions for fastidious organisms
  2 Urinary tuberculosis
  3 Renal or bladder calculi
  4 Analgesic nephropathy
  5 Chemical cystitis, e.g. cyclophosphamide
  6 Acute glomerulonephritis
  7 Non-bacterial (e.g. chlamydial) infections of the urethra
C. True light pyuria without bacteriuria
  1 Many chronic renal diseases (glomerulonephritis, polycystic disease, interstitial nephritis, etc.)
D. False pyuria (not confirmed on bladder puncture)
  1 Vaginal discharge

Casts

These are cylindrical bodies formed in the lumen of the distal tubule, particularly the collecting tubule, where flow and pH are low and osmolality high. Their matrix is formed from Tamm–Horsfall mucoprotein, a viscous glycoprotein with a molecular weight of about 23 000 000 daltons, which is secreted by the cells lining the distal convoluted tubule. Cells, cell debris, and other proteins in the tubular lumen may be agglomerated and caught up in the gel to form the different varieties of cast discussed below.

Hyaline casts

These consist entirely of Tamm–Horsfall protein. They are the clear, colourless cylinders, close to the refractive index of urine, which are occasionally seen in the urine of normal people, particularly when it is concentrated, or after exercise. Showers of hyaline casts appear in the urine during any febrile illness and after the administration of loop diuretics.

Granular casts

The granules in these casts are formed from disintegrated cells or from aggregated serum proteins; immunofluorescence studies have identified albumin, lipoproteins, and immunoglobulins in the granules. It is therefore surprising that they are not seen more often with the heavy proteinuria of nephrotic syndrome due to minimal change nephropathy.

Finely granular casts (Fig. 2) occur in much the same situations as hyaline casts and have similar significance. They are found with hyaline casts in the urine of normal subjects after exercise. Densely granular casts (Fig. 3) are always pathological. When the granules are very coarse they are often misidentified as red cell casts. They are found in many types of renal disease but are particularly characteristic of chronic proliferative or membranous glomerulonephritis, diabetic nephropathy and amyloidosis.

Fatty casts

These are composed of highly refractile fat globules of varying size, some of which may be mistaken for red cells. They are often accompanied by oval fat bodies which are epithelial cells stuffed full of fat granules, and by the presence of free fat globules in the urine; they are most commonly seen when there is moderate to heavy proteinuria. Such a sediment when viewed with polarized light reveals the classical Maltese crosses which are thought to be due to cholesterol esters.

Red cell casts

These are pathognomonic of glomerular bleeding. The cells may be densely packed (Fig. 4) and appear red but more commonly a

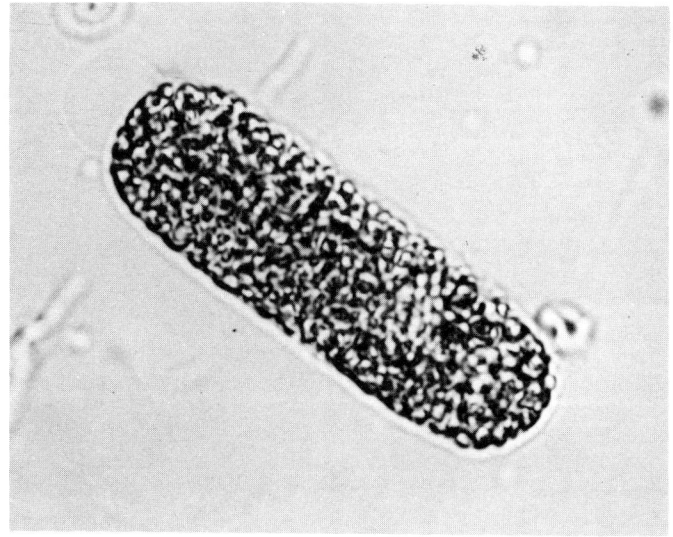

Fig. 3 A densely granular cast. High power.

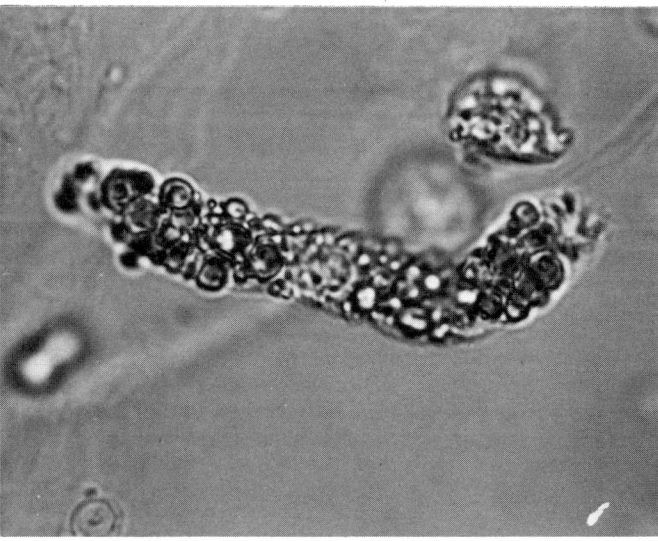

Fig. 4 A red cell cast from the urinary deposit of a patient with acute glomerulonephritis. High power.

few cells are trapped in a hyaline or granular cast (Fig. 5); when the cells degenerate, a rusty coloured granular cast is formed, called a haemoglobin cast. Commonly seen in large numbers at the height of an attack of acute nephritis, they may be found in any condition in which there is a continuing glomerulonephritis or vasculitis. They may be found in malignant hypertension, in company with red cells and granular casts.

Scanty red cell casts and granular casts are found in association with microscopic haematuria in several forms of focal proliferative glomerulonephritis. The discovery of even one red cell cast is of great diagnostic value, indicating a renal cause for the haematuria. A thorough search of the deposit from several concentrated urine samples is well worth undertaking and may be supplemented by the examination of a urine filtrate, which is stained and examined on the filter paper.

White cell casts

White cell casts are relatively rare but may appear in considerable numbers during an episode of acute pyelonephritis. A few may be found in the urine in chronic pyelonephritis and their numbers may increase if the patient develops a pyrexia for any cause.

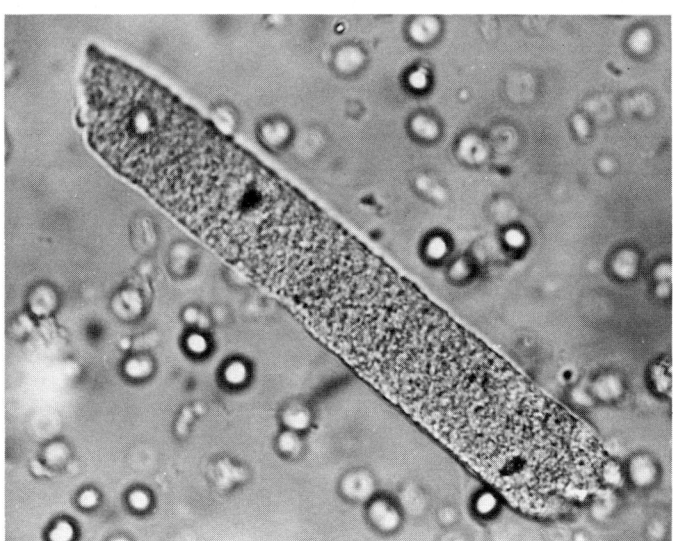

Fig. 2 A finely granular cast surrounded by red cells. High power.

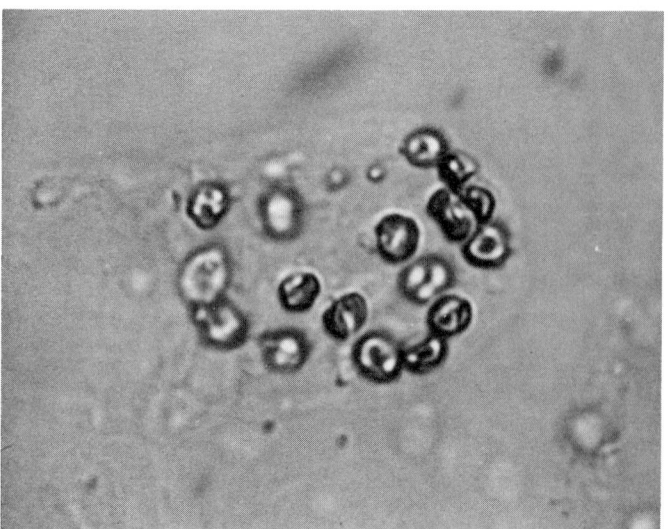

Fig. 5 One end of a cast predominantly hyaline but with a few red cells enmeshed in it. High power. Diagnostically this ranks as a red cell cast.

Sheets of leucocytes, or leucocytes clumped around other objects in urine, may be mistaken for white cell casts.

Epithelial cell casts

Casts with a regular arrangement of epithelial cells, suggesting that the epithelium has been shed in one piece, are found in the urine of patients with acute tubular necrosis or the more acute forms of glomerulonephritis. A commoner phenomenon is a hyaline or finely granular cast with one or two epithelial cells attached; these are seen in many forms of chronic renal disease.

Transitional epithelial cells

These are smaller than vulvar squames and of a more uniform, oval shape. They are seen in small numbers in normal urine and are sometimes plentiful in the presence of urinary infection. Clumps of transitional cells, often with bizarre nuclei, are found in the urine of patients with bladder cancer or papilloma; they give a clue to this diagnosis but their absence does not exclude it. When there is reason to suspect cancer of the urinary tract, formal cytology and other appropriate investigations are required.

Crystals

Cystine crystals (Fig. 6) may be found in freshly passed urine but more consistently if a concentrated sample is acidified and cooled in a refrigerator; their presence is diagnostic of cystinuria. Oxalate crystals (Fig. 7) are common in urine from normal individuals when it has stood for an hour or two. When present in freshly passed urine, in large numbers or in aggregates, they may indicate an increased liability to form oxalate stone, but firm conclusions can only be drawn if the urine is kept at 37 °C until examined on a warm-stage microscope.

It must be emphasized that although urinalysis and urine microscopy yield valuable information, it is possible for significant renal disease to be present without anything abnormal being detected in the urine.

Estimation of glomerular filtration rate (GFR)

Inulin clearance

GFR can be measured accurately with the aid of a substance which is completely filtered at the glomerulus, not secreted or reabsorbed in the renal tubule, stable in urine, and readily measured. The traditional choice has been inulin, a polymer of fructose with a molecular weight of about 5200. A wealth of investigation has confirmed its physiological suitability, but it has several disadvantages. It is poorly soluble and so must be dissolved by heating, which may partly hydrolyse it to fructose; it activates complement when injected, though no harm to patients has yet been reported; the chemical estimation is tedious and poorly reproducible in inexpert hands. Consequently it is the gold standard against which all other methods are measured but is seldom employed in clinical practice. A more soluble and homogeneous analogue, Polyfructosan-S (MW about 2700), and inulin labelled with ^{14}C are available and offer advantages over the parent compound but have never become popular.

GFR is measured by infusing inulin intravenously at a constant rate until it is evenly distributed in the extracellular space and the plasma concentration is almost steady, typically after 90–120 minutes. GFR is then equal to the renal clearance of inulin, defined as:

$$\text{Clearance} = \frac{\text{Urinary excretion rate}}{\text{Plasma concentration}} = \frac{UV}{P}$$

where U and P are the inulin concentrations in urine and plasma and V the *urinary flow rate*. To measure this flow rate it is necessary to induce a moderate diuresis by regular administration of fluid before and during the test. The patient is asked to void several timed urine samples and plasma samples are taken at the beginning and end of each. Catheterization is necessary if there is doubt about the patient's ability to empty the bladder completely, and is one of the unattractive features of the test.

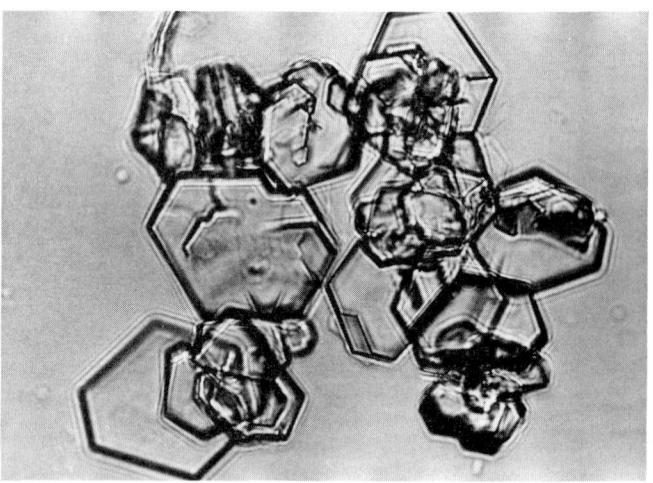

Fig. 6 Crystals of cystine in the urinary deposit of a patient with cystinuria and calculi. High power.

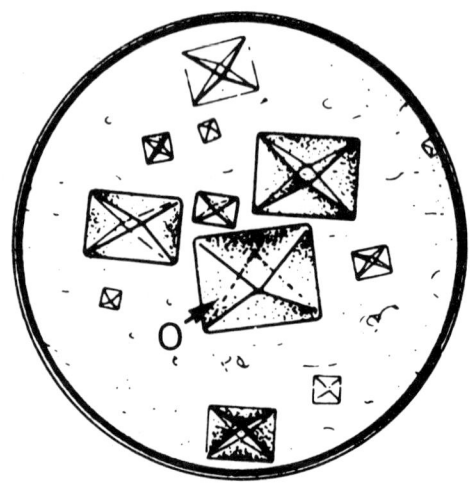

Fig. 7 Oxalate crystals, sketched from a urinary deposit.

Since the extrarenal clearance of inulin is very low (about 2 ml/min) urinary excretion is virtually equal to infusion rate once a steady state has been achieved. Consequently GFR can be calculated from the infusion rate and the plasma concentration. This method is preferred in children and others who have difficulty with complete bladder emptying. However, the infusion period must be prolonged to ensure complete stability of the plasma level; unlike the classical method it cannot be corrected for a slowly changing plasma level. A three-hour infusion is sufficient in most patients.

Clearance of EDTA and other radiopharmaceuticals

The problem of measuring inulin can be circumvented by substituting a radioactive substance with similar properties. The most extensively studied, and the most popular in Britain, is [51Cr]–EDTA. It is not protein bound, has an extrarenal clearance of about 4 ml/min in health and disease, and is handled by the kidney in a similar manner to inulin. Many comparisons have shown that estimates of GFR with inulin and EDTA are in close agreement over a wide range. Most authors have found that EDTA clearance slightly underestimates GFR and some have recommended that it should be multiplied by a correction factor such as 1.1 but in practice the clearance is usually reported uncorrected. The sodium and meglumide salts of iothalamic acid, labelled with 125I, have similar properties to EDTA and have remained popular in the USA. It is likely that both will be replaced by [99Tc]-Sn-DTPA which has a short physical half-life of 6 hours, reducing the radiation dose and permitting repeat observations daily when needed, yet is readily available in departments of nuclear medicine because it is used for brain and kidney imaging.

These radiopharmaceuticals can be substituted for inulin in the standard infusion test, with timed urine samples, with the added advantage that an external count over the bladder confirms complete voiding. They can also be used in the constant infusion technique without urine collection or for single injection followed by timed plasma and urine samples over the exponential phase of the plasma–activity curve. However, these techniques are seldom used outside research laboratories.

The usual method provided for routine hospital use is single intravenous injection followed by timed plasma samples. Plasma radioactivity falls steeply initially, reflecting diffusion into extracellular space. An exponential fall follows from about 2 hours post-injection. The slope of this part of the line is determined by GFR plus extrarenal clearance. The latter term is usually ignored since it is small and fairly constant. GFR is calculated by multiplying the slope of the exponential part of the curve by the volume of distribution, which is calculated by dividing the injected dose by the plasma activity at zero time.

Three blood samples are drawn at intervals determined by the expected result, judged from plasma creatinine. If renal function is close to normal, samples are drawn at 2, 3, and 4 hours; if it is thought to be between 30 and 60 per cent of normal, at 2, 4, and 6 hours; if renal function is below 30 per cent of normal, at 3, 6, 9, and 12 hours. If the patient is oedematous but has nearly normal renal function, samples are taken at 3, 4, and 5 hours to allow time for diffusion into the expanded extracellular volume, but the test becomes unreliable in the presence of gross oedema.

Clearance of EDTA and other radiopharmaceuticals is most reliably measured when renal function is normal or moderately reduced. It then has a reproducibility of about ± 5 per cent which is adequate for clinical purposes since GFR has a circadian rhythm, varying by about 10 per cent between its peak in midafternoon and its trough during the night, and is disturbed by emotion or exercise, EDTA clearance is therefore used to confirm the normality of renal function in patients with isolated proteinuria or haematuria, or other minor abnormalities which interfere in employment, superannuation and insurance, and in the selection of kidney donors. It is measured repeatedly to assess the results of procedures like surgery for obstruction or drug therapy for glo-

merulonephritis, and to plot the progress of renal diseases for which treatment, with undesirable side-effects is given only in the presence of declining function.

In late renal failure the test is inapplicable to outpatients and is decreasingly reliable as GFR declines; the extrarenal clearance assumes greater importance and the error in calculating the slope increases as it approaches the horizontal. At this stage in renal disease clinicians are forced to rely on plasma creatinine, despite the limitations discussed below.

Endogenous creatinine clearance

Creatinine is excreted largely by glomerular filtration. The endogenous production of creatinine from muscle maintains a nearly constant plasma concentration throughout the 24 hours. Consequently creatinine clearance can be measured from a timed collection of urine and a single plasma sample taken at any time during the collection period. One hour creatinine clearance permits supervised urine collection in outpatients and is popular in some countries but it involves a potentially large error from variable bladder emptying and wash-out effects. Twenty-four hour creatinine clearance reduces these errors and has been the standard method of estimating GFR in clinical practice for the last few decades. When performed punctiliously it gives an estimate of GFR very close to that provided by inulin clearance in health and many diseases. Thorough instruction of outpatients is essential to avoid errors from loss of part of the 24 hour collection. The importance of urination before defecation needs particular emphasis, to avoid accidental loss of urine. If diuretic therapy cannot be discontinued for the day before and during the collection, diuretics should be taken shortly after the start of the urine collection. Outpatients find it convenient to close their collection just before leaving for the hospital and provided renal function is stable it is permissible to draw the blood sample an hour or two later.

Endogenous creatinine clearance is useful as a single estimation of GFR when the radioactive methods are contra-indicated (pregnancy and young children) or inaccurate (oedema, renal failure) and when calculation of GFR from plasma creatinine is likely to be inaccurate (oedema, wasting, diseases causing muscle atrophy, obesity, pregnancy). It is best performed on two successive 24 hour collections; this reduces bladder emptying errors, if the results are averaged. It also gives some idea of the reproducibility of the test in the individual. When creatinine clearance is estimated in a metabolic ward, on patients with stable renal function, a reproducibility of ±10 per cent can be achieved but when it is collected under routine conditions on ordinary wards or in outpatients, typical reproducibility averages ±20–25 per cent. Patients can be divided into 'good collectors' (about two-thirds in our experience) whose paired collections typically agree within 15 per cent and 'bad collectors' whose paired collections differ widely.

The popularity of this test has declined in the last few years since it has been shown that it gives no better an estimate of GFR than calculation from the plasma creatinine, except in the special circumstances listed above. As a method of following changes in renal function with time it has few advantages over the much simpler measurement of plasma creatinine.

Creatinine clearance substantially overestimates GFR because of tubular secretion of creatinine in chronic renal failure, nephrotic syndrome and in renal transplant recipients. The overestimate varies from a few per cent to over 50 per cent in published reports. This variation is partly due to the methods used to measure creatinine, which should be known when interpreting creatinine clearance.

Calculation of creatinine clearance from plasma creatinine

If the production of creatinine remains constant, plasma creatinine is determined by the GFR (Fig. 8). As GFR declines plasma creatinine rises on a hyperbolic curve and its reciprocal falls along a straight line parallel to the GFR. This statement is not quite true because there is a small extrarenal clearance of creatinine, typically about 2.5 ml/min, due to bacterial degradation of creatinine in the gut. Consequently the plasma creatinine does not rise to infinity as the GFR falls to zero. The production of creatinine does remain fairly constant as renal disease advances, until the terminal stage when anorexia, nausea, and vomiting lead to loss of muscle mass. Consequently a plot of the plasma creatinine gives a good indication of changing GFR in most patients. The steep rise in plasma creatinine as the GFR approaches zero is disconcerting so some clinicians plot the reciprocal value as in Fig. 8. Over half of all patients with chronic renal failure lose their renal function at a roughly constant rate as shown diagrammatically in Fig. 8. Extrapolation of the reciprocal creatinine plot permits a rough forecast of when intervention like regular haemodialysis will be required.

Some caution is needed in interpreting plots of plasma creatinine. The laboratory error is proportionally higher when plasma creatinine is in the normal range. Even the best laboratories using automated equipment can only achieve a reproducibility of about ±10 per cent in the lower normal range, which imposes an equal error on any estimate of GFR. Although plasma creatinine is constant in the fasting subject and is little affected by the average British diet, a modest rise occurs after a meal of cooked red meat. This is typically about 20 μmol/1 but may be several times this figure after a large serving of goulash. Consequently if plasma creatinine rises abruptly in a situation where this alone calls for corrective action (e.g. following renal transplantation) the measurement should be repeated after 3 or 4 hours, during which cooked meat is withheld. The effect of diet on plasma creatinine is proportionally smaller when the level is raised in chronic renal failure. Consequently many nephrologists rely on a single accurate measurement of GFR when the patient first attends the clinic followed by serial measurements of plasma creatinine to assess progress. However, there are occasional pitfalls; a very small minority of patients do not display the expected rise in plasma creatinine as GFR falls and may become severely uraemic with a plasma creatinine as low as 400 μmol/1, a phenomenon attributed to unusually rapid secretion of creatinine by the tubules.

The production rate for creatinine varies widely between individuals in rough proportion to their muscle mass. The young have more muscle for a given weight than the old and men more than women; this is reflected in the plasma creatinine. In a fit young man a plasma creatinine of 120 μmol/1 probably indicates a normal GFR whereas in an elderly lady with rheumatoid arthritis a plasma creatinine of 80 μmol/1 may indicate a GFR of only half normal. However, the handling of creatinine by the kidney is unaffected by age, sex, or body build so one should be able to predict creatinine clearance from plasma creatinine with the aid of a formula or nomogram that estimates creatinine production from age, sex, and size. Several formulae have been devised and four of

these have recently been assessed in an independent comparison; the two which were most successful across the whole range of renal function are reproduced in Table 2. They are most reliable when GFR is moderately reduced and their main use is providing a quick approximate estimation of GFR to guide drug therapy in patients who have not recently had a more accurate measurement. However, it must be remembered that the calculation assumes constant renal function and the result can be misleading if the patient has suffered a recent depression of GFR from acute illness.

The formulae in Table 2 are least useful when plasma creatinine is in the normal range; a more accurate method is required to confirm normality of renal function for insurance and medico-legal purposes.

Table 2 Formulae for calculating creatinine clearance from serum or plasma creatinine

Males

Creatinine clearance in ml/min per 70 kg

$$= \left(\frac{145 - \text{age in years}}{\text{serum creatinine in mg/dl}}\right) - 3$$

$$= \left(\frac{88 \,(145 - \text{age in years})}{\text{serum creatinine in } \mu\text{mol/l}}\right) - 3$$

Females

Creatinine clearance in ml/min per 70 kg

$$= \left(\frac{0.85 \,(145 - \text{age in years})}{\text{serum creatinine in mg/dl}}\right) - 3$$

$$= \left(\frac{75 \,(145 - \text{age in years})}{\text{serum creatinine in } \mu\text{mol/l}}\right) - 3$$

Note: These formulae and all others studied by Hull *et al.* (1981) are inaccurate in the presence of liver disease.
Source: Hull, J.H. *et al.* (1981).

References
Hull, J. H., Hak, L. J., Koch, G. G., Wargin, W. A., Chi, S. L. and Mattocks, A. M. (1981). Influence of range of renal function and liver disease on predictability of creatinine clearance. *Clin. Pharmacol. Ther.* **29**, 516.

Cockcroft, D. W. and Gault, M. H. (1976). Prediction of creatinine clearance from serum creatinine. *Nephron* **16**, 31.

Estimation of GFR from plasma urea
There are still a few hospitals which do not provide plasma creatinine measurements. Doctors labouring under this disadvantage have to rely on plasma urea as the first indicator of depressed renal function, despite the disadvantages that it is rapidly affected by diet, rising in proportion to protein intake and fluctuating more widely during the day than plasma creatinine, and is dependent on

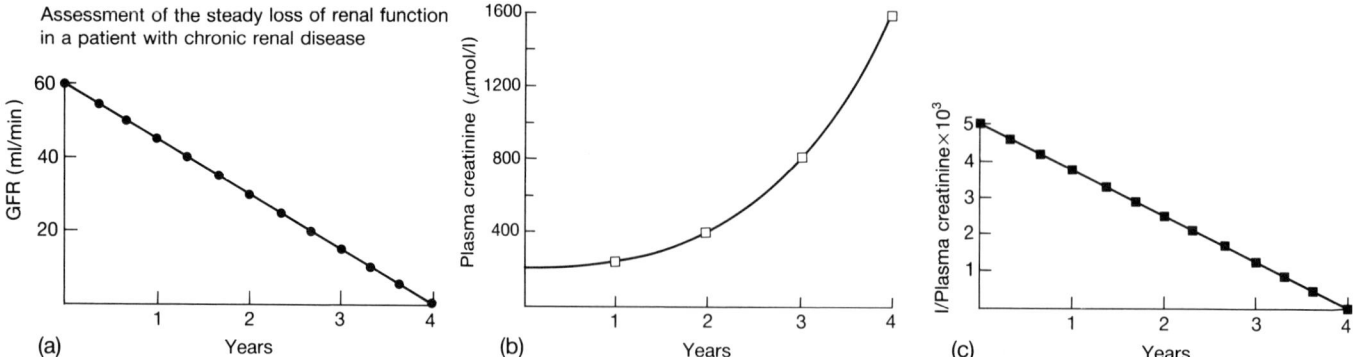

Fig. 8 The decline in glomerular filtration rate (GFR), rise in plasma creatinine and fall in the reciprocal of plasma creatinine in a patient with steady loss of renal function from chronic renal disease. The graphs of plasma creatinine and its reciprocal are calculated on the assumption that creatinine is not secreted by the tubules or degraded in the gut. The real life curves deviate slightly from this pattern. (Reproduced from *Medicine* Number 25, p. 1273, by permission of the publisher.)

urinary flow rate. Urea clearance rises from about 30 per cent of GFR at minimum urine flow rate to about 70 per cent of GFR at flow rates over 2 ml/min. The inferior diagnostic value of plasma urea has been confirmed; in one study, 65 per cent of patients with GFR 52–75 per cent of normal, 18 per cent of those with 28–52 per cent of normal, and 7 per cent of those with GFR less than 28 per cent of normal were misdiagnosed as having normal renal function on the basis of plasma urea.

The more fortunate physician who receives simultaneous reports of plasma urea and creatinine can derive some diagnostic clues from comparing the two (Table 3). A plot of plasma urea and creatinine is particularly helpful in distinguishing renal and pre-renal causes of uraemia.

Estimation of GFR from plasma β_2 microglobulin

Beta-2 microglobulin is a low molecular weight protein of about 11 800 daltons which is a surface constituent of most cells, thought to represent the constant zone of HLA antigens. It is filtered at the glomerulus, reabsorbed almost completely in the renal tubule but catabolized in the process. It is produced at a nearly constant rate, unaffected by diet, so its plasma concentration reflects the GFR; it rises with age as GFR declines since its production rate does not fall, like that of creatinine, with declining muscle mass. Plasma β_2 microglobulin is raised, probably as a result of overproduction, in some malignant, immunological, and hepatic diseases; in the absence of these it is probably a better guide to changes in GFR than is plasma creatinine, but is unlikely to replace the latter in clinical practice since its radioimmunoassay is far more tedious and expensive than the automated chemical test for creatinine.

There are three situations in which the extra expense of measuring plasma β_2 microglobulin is justified, where it is available. It is a more sensitive indicator of a slight fall in GFR than is plasma creatinine, e.g. in monitoring nephrotoxic drug therapy, or detecting the onset of transplant rejection or diabetic nephropathy. It remains a useful guide to GFR in terminal renal failure, when variable tubular secretion of creatinine makes the latter less reliable. It can be used as a measure of residual renal function in patients receiving regular haemodialysis since it is scarcely removed by haemodialysis with conventional cellulose membranes.

Estimation of renal plasma flow

Renal plasma flow is more subject to variation with physical or emotional stress than is GFR but it has a similar and parallel circadian rhythm. Its measurement is an important research investigation but it is seldom requested in clinical medicine.

Estimation of renal plasma flow from clearance of para-aminohippurate

Renal plasma flow can be measured with the aid of an agent which is completely removed from plasma in one passage through the kidney by a combination of glomerular filtration and tubular secretion. Para-aminohippurate (PAH) approaches this ideal since about 92 per cent of plasma PAH is removed by the time it reaches the renal vein, in healthy subjects. It diffuses rapidly through its volume of distribution and a steady plasma level can be achieved more quickly than with inulin. PAH clearance is therefore a convenient and reliable test of renal plasma flow for physiological studies. The result is corrected by assuming that the test subject has the usual 92 per cent extraction rate and is converted to renal blood flow on the assumption that the haematocrit in the kidney is the same as that in the peripheral blood (an approximation to the truth).

In renal disease the extraction of PAH during one passage through the kidney falls substantially and unpredictably so it is necessary to measure renal vein PAH concentration by cannulating the renal vein with a Seldinger catheter, rendering the test unsuitable for routine use.

Estimation of renal plasma flow by radiohippurate clearance

Hippurate (hippuran) has a slightly lower extraction rate on single passage through the kidney than PAH and has the same limitation that its extraction rate falls in the presence of renal disease. In other respects it is a suitable agent for measuring renal plasma flow and can be labelled with any of the radioisotopes of iodine. It can then be used by the single-shot technique on the same principles as measuring GFR by EDTA-clearance. Simultaneous administration of two agents, labelled with different isotopes, permits simultaneous measurement of GFR and renal blood flow and therefore the calculation of filtration fraction (the proportion of blood perfusing the kidney which passes into glomerular filtrate). The crude ratio 'clearance of EDTA or iothalamate/clearance to hippurate' is often referred to as filtration fraction, no account being taken of the unknown extraction rate for hippurate in the patient. This misnomer should be avoided but the crude ratio may have some diagnostic value, e.g. in the detection of transplant rejection, which causes a high ratio (high 'filtration fraction').

Correction for body size

Both GFR and renal plasma flow are determined by body size and in the adult they correlate better with surface area than with other measures of body size such as height or weight. Consequently they are often expressed per 1.73 m^2, calculated as: actual clearance $\times$ 1.73/surface area in m^2. Surface area is estimated from height and weight by the nomogram in Documenta Geigy. Since 1.73 m^2 is an out-of-date mean size in a population which is growing larger, it would be more logical to express the results per m^2 and this practice is gaining ground.

Investigation of proteinuria (see also page 18.56)

Healthy individuals excrete each day in their urine about 400 mg of non-dialysable solids, of which almost half are thought to be proteins. Identified proteins add up to about 150 mg per 24 hours which is taken conventionally as the upper limit of normal. The largest single constituent (40–70 mg) is Tamm-Horsfall mucoprotein (uromucoid). Albumin contributes about 10–20 mg and low molecular weight proteins, mainly unidentified, a further 30 mg. About 30 plasma proteins larger than albumin and over 30 enzymes have been identified but are present only in trace amounts. Other constituents are derived from prostatic and seminal secretions.

In concentrated urine these normal proteins attain a sufficient

Table 3 Diagnostic significance of differential changes in plasma urea and creatinine

---

Plasma urea raised out of proportion to plasma creatinine
  Sodium and water depletion
  Heart failure
  Gastrointestinal haemorrhage
  High protein intake (oral or i.v.) in presence of renal disease
  Protein catabolism
    Corticosteroid therapy
    Tetracycline in overdose or in presence of renal disease
  Following trauma
  Pure water depletion (modest effect)
Plasma creatinine raised out of proportion to plasma urea
  Some cases of rhabdomyolysis
  Drugs that block creatinine secretion (aspirin, cotrimoxazole) or increase creatinine production (penacemide): (modest effect)
Plasma urea depressed out of proportion to plasma creatinine
  Pregnancy
  Liver failure
  High fluid intake
  Low protein diet
Plasma urea and creatinine raised in parallel
  Chronic renal failure
  Established acute renal failure

concentration to give a trace-positive reaction to dipsticks; such reactions are ignored unless the urine is dilute. Early morning urine from young men often gives a positive reaction because of contamination with ejaculate easily recognized because there are numerous spermatozoa in the deposit. All other reactions of + or above call for further investigation.

Measurement of tubular functions

Measurement of urinary concentrating ability

In the course of any chronic renal disease, the tubules of surviving nephrons are exposed to an increased osmotic load, partly because the GFR per nephron is increased and partly because the plasma concentration of solutes such as urea, sulphate, and phosphate is elevated. Consequently the patient's ability to concentrate the urine declines, even if tubular function is preserved in the remaining nephrons. It is possible to relate urinary concentrating ability to the patient's GFR and deduce whether the concentrating ability is disproportionately reduced, indicating tubular disease. This test has been advocated for the differentiation of advanced chronic nephritis from chronic pyelonephritis or analgesic nephropathy (concentrating ability being best preserved in glomerulonephritis and worst affected in analgesic nephropathy). However the typical ranges for these groups of diseases at each level of renal function have not been well enough defined to make the test of much practical value at present. Special precautions are needed if fluid is withheld from patients in renal failure. Consequently concentrating ability is only tested in patients with normal or nearly normal GFR. The indications for its use are now restricted to a few specific circumstances where isolated distal tubular damage is suspected, e.g. in monitoring lithium therapy or detecting early analgesic nephropathy.

Maximum concentration is achieved only after all fluids have been withheld for more than 24 hours, an uncomfortable test which requires hospital admission to ensure compliance. Consequently it is usual to accept evidence of a sub-maximal concentrating ability above the lower limit of normal for the patient's age, tested for by three simpler manoeuvres. A few random early morning urine samples are collected and their osmolality tested. If none of these achieves the required level (e.g. 550 mosmol/kg) the patient is tested by fluid withdrawal or vasopressin.

Fluid withdrawal is imposed by asking the patient to avoid drinks after 4 p.m., taking a dry supper and no bed-time or morning drinks. The first two urine samples passed after rising are tested. This is a test of both the pituitary's ability to secrete ADH and the kidney's ability to respond.

The vasopressin tests investigate only the response of the kidney. The traditional stimulus is 5 units of pitressin tannate in oil intramuscularly at 8 a.m. The ampoule must be warmed and shaken before the contents are withdrawn. All urine samples passed over the next 8 hours are tested. In those countries where pitressin tannate is no longer available (including Britain) desmopressin is given intranasally; 20 μg are instilled into each nostril at 5 p.m. and the last evening and first morning samples are tested. Fluid intake should be kept low during these tests but total abstention from drinks is not necessary.

We tested 30 healthy adults and found that all achieved a urine osmolality of 750 mosmol/kg in one of the samples in these tests. The lower limit of normal falls with age to reach about 600 in the 60s. Subjects on a high-fluid intake (e.g. those with compulsive water drinking) require a more prolonged stimulus before reaching maximum urinary concentration.

Measurement of urinary acidification (see also pages 18.28, 18.171, and 9.164)

The kidney helps to maintain daily hydrogen ion balance by the reabsorption of bicarbonate (approximately 4000 mmol), the production and excretion of ammonium and the excretion of titra-

table acid. The latter two processes represent the regeneration of 60–100 mmol bicarbonate. Renal acidosis may be due to inefficient bicarbonate reabsorption, inability of the distal tubule to secrete hydrogen ion against a high concentration gradient (the gradient between blood at pH 7.4 and urine at pH 5.4 is 1:100), or reduced nephron mass.

Failure to reabsorb bicarbonate from the proximal tubule is a relatively common cause for mildly impaired urinary acidification but its detection requires the measurement of tubular reabsorptive capacity for bicarbonate, a test seldom performed in clinical practice and which is described in specialist textbooks of renal medicine.

In distal tubular acidosis, the classical form of renal tubular acidosis, the distal tubule is unable to maintain a high concentration gradient for hydrogen ion, so a very acid urine cannot be produced, no matter how acidaemic the patient becomes. If there is spontaneous acidosis, shown by a depressed plasma bicarbonate concentration, and urine pH is above 5.3, impaired urinary acidification is apparent and there is no need to proceed further.

To identify patients with incomplete renal tubular acidosis the short test of Wrong and Davies is employed. Ammonium chloride 100 mg per kg body weight is given either in capsules or as a flavoured mixture with breakfast and urine pH is measured in all urine samples collected over the next 8 hours. Blood samples are taken at the start and end of the test to confirm that sufficient ammonium chloride was given and absorbed to cause a significant fall in plasma bicarbonate. Provided that has happened, at least one urine sample should have a pH of 5.3 or below.

Measurement of phosphate clearance

About 13 per cent of plasma phosphate is protein bound but the concentrations of phosphate in plasma and glomerular filtrate are about the same because of the Donnan effect and because the volume occupied by plasma proteins is usually ignored when plasma concentrations are measured. Normally about 80 per cent of the filtered phosphate is reabsorbed by active transport in the proximal tubule and to a small extent in the distal tubule. Two processes, one parathormone dependent, appear to be responsible.

Phosphate excretion is described by the equation

Tubular reabsorption of phosphate = filtered phosphate − excreted phosphate.

As the filtered load rises during a phosphate infusion, the transport system becomes saturated and any further increase in filtered phosphate is promptly excreted. In practice, the moment of saturation is not a sharp end-point, possibly because nephrons vary in length and enzyme activity; the gradual slowing in the rate of increase as tubular absorption approaches its maximum is called splay (Fig. 9). By extrapolation back to zero excretion, a theoretical threshold is obtained; this is the level below which all phosphate would be reabsorbed, were it not for the presence of splay. At this plasma level, the phosphate reabsorption has reached the tubular maximum and

$$\text{Maximum tubular reabsorption of phosphate} = \text{Phosphate threshold} \times \text{GFR}$$

or

$$\text{Phosphate threshold} = \frac{\text{Maximum tubular reabsorption}}{\text{GFR}}$$

The plasma phosphate in normal individuals tends to remain close to the threshold value. However, it follows a circadian rhythm, rising during the morning, largely as a result of meals, and falling in the evening. It rises during acidosis and falls during alkalosis.

Phosphate threshold can be measured by giving a phosphate

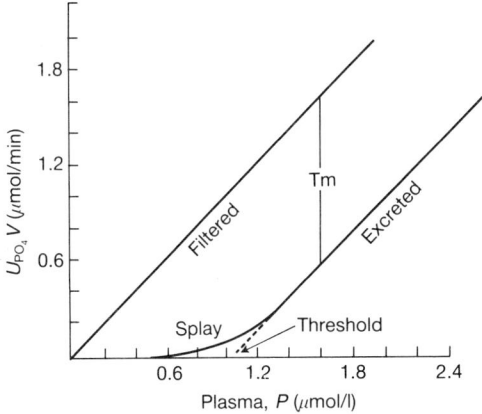

Fig. 9 The relationship between phosphate excretion and plasma phosphate when phosphate is infused into a normal subject. Filtered phosphate rises in a linear manner; it is calculated from creatinine (or inulin) clearance and plasma phosphate. Excreted phosphate starts almost at zero, rises gradually through the splay then runs parallel to filtered phosphate. The vertical distance between the two graphs is the maximum tubular reabsorption of phosphate.

infusion at a steadily increasing rate, measuring plasma and urinary phosphate and creatinine at set intervals and constructing a graph as in Fig. 9. This is too cumbersome for clinical practice and a simpler, less accurate, test is often employed. Because of the rhythm, the test is performed in the morning. After an overnight fast, the patient passes urine at 8 a.m., drinks 200 ml water and passes the test urine sample at 10 a.m.; a blood sample is drawn at the same time. The ratio of phosphate clearance to creatinine clearance is then calculated

$$\frac{\text{Phosphate clearance}}{\text{Creatinine clearance}} = \frac{\text{Urinary phosphate} \times \text{plasma creatinine}}{\text{Urinary creatinine} \times \text{plasma phosphate}}$$

$$\text{TRP} = 1 - \frac{\text{Phosphate clearance}}{\text{Creatinine clearance}}$$

Using either of these values, one can read the phosphate threshold off a nomogram constructed from the results on 200 normal subjects (Bijvoet, 1977).

If the original calculations show that tubular reabsorption is beyond the splay (TRP > 0.80) the threshold can be calculated by the equation

$$\text{Threshold} = \text{TRP} \times \text{plasma phosphate}$$

Ninety-five per cent of normal individuals have a phosphate threshold between 0.8 and 1.35 mmol/l (2.5–4.2 mg/dl).

Measurement of phosphate clearance and threshold is used to detect proximal tubular damage, to study the effect of other substances on phosphate transport or as an indirect test for hyperparathyroidism. Tubular damage increases phosphate excretion, lowering plasma phosphate until a new equilibrium is reached, with a low plasma phosphate, a normal daily excretion rate and a low phosphate threshold. A similar equilibrium state is found in primary hyperparathyroidism and in the rare condition of hypophosphataemic osteomalacia due to soft bone tumours. Clinical differentiation between these conditions is usually straightforward. If doubt exists, a raised serum ionized calcium and/or serum PTH favours hyperparathyroidism.

Measurement of phosphate threshold is not totally reliable in distinguishing primary hyperparathyroidism from idiopathic hypercalciuria, which is a major differential diagnosis, since some patients with the latter condition also have low phosphate thresholds. Additional confirmatory tests include the measurement

$$\frac{\text{Phosphate clearance}}{\text{Creatinine clearance}}$$

of before and after phosphate loading (in organic phosphate salts, 2 g per day for three days then 3 g per day for two days); the ratio rises further in patients with hyperparathyroidism than in normals or idiopathic stone formers.

The causes of some common abnormalities of phosphate excretion are summarized in Table 4.

Investigation of glycosuria

Glucose is freely filtered by the glomerulus and reabsorbed actively by the proximal tubule. Under normal circumstances, reabsorption is almost complete but, if the blood glucose rises sufficiently, a plasma level is reached at which the transport mechanism is saturated and glucose starts to spill into the urine—the glucose threshold. Glucose handling by the kidneys resembles that of phosphate in exhibiting threshold, splay, and maximum tubular reabsorption (see Fig. 9). The absorption of both substances parallels the absorption of sodium and water by the proximal tubule in response to expansion or contraction of the extracellular volume. In diabetes mellitus, the blood glucose rises above the threshold, either spontaneously or after a glucose load, causing glycosuria.

Glycosuria occurs at a blood glucose level below the threshold when the proximal tubule is damaged by cystinosis, Wilson's disease, heavy metals, and other tubular toxins and even when its function is disturbed by very heavy protein reabsorption in the nephrotic syndrome. It is a feature of genetic syndromes affecting proximal tubular function (Fanconi syndrome) and also occurs as an isolated inherited defect.

Isolated renal glycosuria may cause pruritus vulvae as in diabetes mellitus, but is usually asymptomatic. The diagnosis should only be made if the glycosuria is substantial. Suggested criteria are:

1. Glucosuria over 500 mg per 24 h/1.73 m² surface area while on a diet with 50 per cent of the calories from carbohydrate.
2. Normal blood glucose levels in a standard 50 g oral glucose tolerance test, accompanied by glycosuria.
3. No other evidence of tubular disease or of glomerular damage.

Measurement of urate clearance

Urate is freely filtered at the glomerulus and both reabsorbed and secreted by the tubules. Reabsorption occurs mainly in the proximal tubule by active organic acid transport and passive net movement along a concentration gradient. As the tubular fluid is acidified in the distal tubule most of the urate changes to undissociated uric acid and its solubility decreases. Uric acid excretion is rather insensitive to rapid changes in filtered load but it adapts efficiently to more chronic changes. The clearance of urate falls when urine flow rate drops below 1 ml/min and particularly when the reabsorption of sodium and water by the proximal tubule are enhanced as a result of ECF volume depletion. Many drugs affect the tubular handling of uric acid. Defective urate reabsorption is a feature of proximal tubular disorders such as Wilson's disease and cadmium poisoning.

The assessment of urate clearance is straightforward if the subject has a normal GFR and a normal or low plasma urate; these are the conditons that usually pertain when it is measured in a patient with suspected proximal tubular damage. Care should be taken to exclude sodium depletion, which decreases urate clearance, or sodium overload, which increases it, and to withdraw any drugs such as diuretics or analgesics which affect urate clearance. Urinary uric acid and creatinine are measured on a 24 hour collection and plasma urate and creatinine on a blood sample drawn during the 24 hours. In normal subjects urate clearance is less than 10 per cent of GFR, i.e. more than 90 per cent of filtered urate is reabsorbed. The use of a spot urine sample in place of a 24 hour collection has proved too unreliable to be of use in identifying tubular leaks.

Table 4 Some causes of abnormalities of phosphate excretion

Cause	Plasma phosphate	Phosphate threshold
Daily phosphate excretion low		
Low dietary intake	Low normal or low	Normal
Consumption of phosphate binders	Low normal or low	Normal
Malabsorption	Low normal or low	Normal, low if secondary hyperparathyroidism
Contracted ECF volume	Depends on cause	Normal, low if secondary hyperparathyroidism
Vitamin D deficiency	Low	
Daily phosphate excretion high		
High dietary intake	High normal or high	Normal
Muscle damage	High	Normal
Bone destruction	High	Normal
Vitamin D therapy	High	Normal
Daily phosphate excretion normal		
Proximal tubular damage	Low normal or low	Low
Primary hyperparathyroidism	Low normal or low	Low
Osteomalacia of bone tumours	Low	Low

Measurements of amino acid clearance

Amino acids are filtered at the glomerulus and reabsorbed actively in the proximal tubule. They display the same features of maximal tubular absorption, splay, and threshold as do phosphate and glucose but for some amino acids the splay is wide. At least five separate pathways of absorption exist. The best known affects the absorption of cystine, lysine, ornithine, and arginine; isolated genetic defects of this pathway cause classical cystinuria in which all four amino acids appear in the urine. The four other pathways are for alpha-amino neutral compounds (serine, leucine, etc.; defects cause Hartnup disease); beta-amino neutral compounds (taurine, alanine, etc.); dicarboxylic acids (glutamic, aspartic; defects cause dicarboxylic aminoaciduria); and glycine, proline, and hydroxyproline (defects cause familial iminoglycinuria). Acquired proximal tubular damage has a non-specific effect and causes generalized amino aciduria.

Formal measurement of amino acid clearance is too complicated for use in the clinic. It is usual to request a simple measurement of total amino aciduria and a qualitative assessment of the contribution of different amino acids by two-dimensional chromatography.

Urinary enzyme excretion

Enzymuria is usually measured as an early indication of tubular damage during clinical trials of new drugs; during treatment with drugs of known nephrotoxicity (e.g. aminoglycoside antibiotics, antitumour agents such as cis-platinum); as an early warning of overexposure to chromates, cadmium, and other industrial toxins. The enzyme chosen should be present in tubular cells and readily released by minor injury. The most popular is N-acetyl-β-glucosaminidase (NAG: EC 3.2.1.31). It is measured on a spot urine taken at a constant time of day, to allow for diurnal fluctuation, and expressed per gram (or millimole) of creatinine, to correct for urinary concentration. A dipstick for NAG has been devised and has proved useful in early detection of renal transplant rejection in pre-marketing trials.

Other causes of enzymuria include: increased glomerular permeability alone (Goodpasture's syndrome) or with raised blood level (pancreatitis); pyuria; urinary neoplasm. Diagnostic accuracy is increased if isoenzymes are identified by ion-exchange chromotography.

Excretion of small proteins and cellular antigens

An alternative to measuring urinary enzymes is the detection of low molecular weight proteins which are normally filtered by the glomerulus and reabsorbed almost completely by the tubules. There appearance in urine, if plasma level is not increased, indicates proximal tubular damage. The best studied is β_2-microglobulin which is more sensitive than plasma creatinine but less sensitive than urinary NAG in detecting early aminoglycoside toxicity.

A monoclonal antibody to brush border from tubular cells detects release of this antigen during proximal tubular damage. It appears to be the most sensitive test for such damage but is not yet commercially available.

Assessment of individual renal function, regional function, and renal structure

Straight radiography of the urinary tract

A straight radiograph of the kidneys, ureters, and bladder is referred to as a KUB and is an essential preliminary to urography. On this film it is often possible to trace the renal outlines and measure the renal size. The renal mass is roughly proportional to the cube of renal length and the latter is a more reliable guide than renal area on the film, since the kidneys are variably rotated on their vertical axes. If the outlines are obscured by bowel gas they are often clarified by tomography. The left kidney is normally about 1 cm longer than the right. The length should be recorded in cm for comparison with subsequent films but the normal range is wide (11–16 cm in the adult) so substantial reduction in renal mass must take place before it is possible to say with confidence that the kidneys are small. In children, the renal length is approximately equal to that of the first four lumbar vertebrae and their intervening discs. The other main function of a KUB is to detect calcification in the kidneys or radio-opaque calculi in the ureters or bladder, that may be obscured in the subsequent pyelogram. Oblique views and films taken in inspiration and expiration may be necessary to confirm that suspected calculi are in kidneys. The film may yield other diagnostic information; gallstones are often detected on a KUB and renal osteodystrophy or myelomatosis may be recognized in the skeleton.

Excretion urography

Synonyms Intravenous pyelography; IVP; IVU.

Modern contrast media are iodine-containing compounds such as diatrizoate, metrizoate, and iothalamate; the non-ionic compounds iopamidol and iohexol are less irritant to endothelia and are preferred by those who can afford the substantial extra cost. The agent is injected slowly over 2 min to avoid the unpleasant flush, nausea, and headache that accompany rapid injection. Occasional reactions include hypotension, asthma, urticaria or angioedema, convulsions, and cardiac arrythmia; the fatality rate of the procedure is about 1:40,000. The injection is therefore given through a butterfly needle which is left in place for 10 min for injection of hydrocortisone if a severe reaction occurs. A doctor and a resuscitation trolley should be available during the procedure.

The contrast medium is excreted almost entirely by glomerular filtration. A film taken at the end of the injection or 1 min later shows the kidneys opacified by contrast in the tubules, an appearance known as nephrogram. This film gives the best view of the renal outlines. The density of the nephrogram should give a measure of GFR and comparison of the two sides or of different parts of the kidney should be useful in assessing regional variations in GFR. In the conventional IVU this information is only qualitative since the density of radiographic film is difficult to quantify and bears a complex relationship to radiation dose. The new technique of digital imaging is expected to yield much more quantitative information. At present the crude impression of the relative contribution of the two kidneys to overall renal function, provided by the IVU, must be supplemented by isotopic studies if a therapeutic decision hinges on it.

Films are taken in rapid sequence over the next 5 min if the IVU is performed in the investigation of hypertension; they show the rate at which contrast reaches the calyces and pelves on the two sides; the nephrogram and pyelogram typically appear late on the side of a unilateral renal artery stenosis.

Films from 5 to 30 min show the collecting system if renal function is close to normal. If there is obstruction of the upper urinary tract it is essential to visualize the whole length of both ureters. This is sometimes facilitated by taking films with the patient prone, when a baggy pelvis will empty by gravity. If calyceal detail is inadequate, the pelvis and calyces may be distended by applying compression over the lower ureters with an abdominal belt. The contrast medium causes an osmotic diuresis, so the bladder is usually well filled by 30 to 45 min, allowing inspection of its outline and detection of diverticula or indentation by tumour, prostatic enlargement or extrinsic swelling. A post-micturition film is often taken to assess bladder emptying. Speed is essential since a 2 min delay in taking the post-micturition film during an osmotic diuresis gives a false impression of a substantial residual urine volume.

Late films are taken if there is evidence of obstruction or if the pyelograms are delayed because of impaired renal function. Films as late as 12 to 24 hours after injection are valuable if there is severe obstruction or advanced renal failure. Films taken over the next few days in patients with renal failure may show opacifiction of the gall-bladder or bowel due to excretion of the contrast by alternative routees.

One of the few defects of the IVU is its inability to indicate the site of complete obstruction. Some idea can be obtained by ultrasound but exact location often calls for retrograde or antegrade pyelography.

Retrograde pyelography
If the cystoscopy room is equipped for fluoroscopy and radiography, a bulb catheter is impacted in the ureteric orifice at cystoscopy and constrast is injected up the ureter under fluoroscopic control. If the patient must be moved to the X-ray department, a ureteric catheter is passed to the renal pelvis and securely taped; the contrast is then injected under screen control. If an obstruction is shown, the catheter may be left in as temporary drainage pending surgery.

Retrograde ureterography or pyelography give better detail than excretion urography and may be used to confirm suspected non-opaque calculi, epithelial tumours, or sloughed papillae. They provide additional information through cystoscopy and collection of urine direct from one kidney. However, complications are not infrequent; they include renal colic, temporary ureteric

obstruction from mucosal oedema, perforation of the pelvis, intrarenal or extrapelvic extravasation of contrast, and infection of the upper urinary tract, plus the complications of anaesthesia.

Antegrade pyelography
If a retrograde catheter cannot be passed, e.g. because the ureteric orifice is obstructed by carcinoma, a needle can be inserted percutaneously into the renal pelvis. It is a procedure calling for skill and best performed under the guidance of high-dose urography or ultrasound to locate the dilated pelvis. Urine is aspirated and contrast medium injected. A thin tube may be passed through or over the needle to be left *in situ* as a temporary nephrostomy, to allow infusion of fluid and measurement of pressure change (the Whittaker test for the severity of obstruction) or to infuse fluids such as Renacidin to dissolve calculi.

The complications include haematuria, extravasation of urine, and infection of the urinary tract.

Renal arteriography
Renal arteriography (Table 5) is a procedure which involves hospital admission, discomfort, and a substantially greater risk than excretion urography, ultrasound, or isotopic studies.

The aorta is catheterized by the Seldinger technique. A guide wire is threaded up the femoral artery and a radio-opaque catheter is passed over it to the level of the renal arteries. If the femoral arteries are blocked or very tortuous, a needle can be inserted percutaneously into the aorta but this carries a small risk of damaging the blood supply to the spinal cord. Contrast medium, as for urography, is injected rapidly into the aorta and serial films are taken to show the origins of the renal arteries and any accessory arteries. This injection also fills the other branches of the aorta, obscuring the view of the renal vasculature. If the renal circulation is not shown in sufficient detail, the catheter is advanced into each of the renal arteries in turn and further injection of contrast is given. This provides a better picture of the renal arteries, without confusion from other vascular trees, and a chance to observe the venous phase in greater detail. The price of this better definition is exposure of the kidneys to a higher concentration of contrast, with a greater risk of producing acute renal failure, and an enhanced risk of the more permanent insult of atheroembolism from dislodgement of arterial plaques. The femoral artery is carefully observed after aortography for haematoma, thrombosis, or later aneurysm.

Digital imaging is a new alternative to aortography; the faint arterial shadows that follow the intravenous injection of a large dose of contrast are enhanced electronically to give final pictures, as good as those on conventional films following intra-aortic injection. It will probably replace aortography for many of its present indications when the equipment becomes more widely available.

Renal venography
Renal vein thrombosis in infancy can often be diagnosed from the history, the presence of a loin mass, and a large, non-functioning kidney on excretion urography. In adult life renal vein thrombosis is usually a complication of nephrotic syndrome, beginning in the small vessels, and best shown on the venous phase of a renal arteriogram. Renal venography is used to detect thrombosis of the main renal veins or extension of renal tumours along the veins. A Seldinger catheter is passed from the femoral vein into the inferior vena cava and contrast is injected rapidly while the patient performs a Valsalva manoeuvre, which forces blood back into the renal veins. If necessary, the catheter is turned into the orifice of each renal vein in turn and further contrast injections are given.

Micturating cystourethrography (MCU)
The usual purpose of an MCU is the demonstration of vesico-ureteric reflux but it can also be used to display abnormalities of the bladder neck and urethra. Contrast is injected into the bladder via a urethral catheter; the alternative methods – suprapubic injection

Table 5 Major indications for aortography and renal arteriography

Indication	Usual place in sequence of imaging tests	Abnormalities sought
Hypertension:		
Suspected renal artery stenosis	Follows IVU, gamma scan	Stenosis Post-stenotic dilatation
Suspected renin-secreting tumour	Follows IVU	Tumour circulation
Space-occupying lesion of kidney	Follows IVU, ultrasound	Tumour circulation
Acute renal failure:		
Suspected renal artery thrombosis or embolism	First	Arterial occlusion
Suspected polyarteritis nodosa	Follows IVU	Arterial aneurysms
Loin pain, haematuria syndrome	Follows IVU	Small arterial occlusion*
Renal trauma / Bleeding after renal biopsy	Follows IVU ultrasound, and sometimes CT scan	Bleeding point To define renal circulation before surgery
Proposed partial nephrectomy or anatrophic nephrolithotomy	Follows IVU	To display renal circulation
Proposed live donation of kidney graft	Follows IVU	Renal circulation

*The specificity of this lesion is disputed.

or retrograde injection up the male urethra – are seldom employed in practice. The patient voids while sitting on a commode in front of the radiographic screen, and the reflux is recorded on spot films or cineradiography. The risk of subsequent urinary infection is substantial so it is common practice to administer an antibacterial for two or three days after the procedure.

Computer-assisted tomography (CT scanning)

CAT scanning of the trunk displays the kidneys particularly well in contrast to the surrounding perinephric fat and the enclosed peripelvic fat. A series of transverse sections of the trunk are displayed, cutting the kidneys at different vertical levels, one of them passing along the renal veins. Tumour extension into the renal veins is clearly shown. Other uses of the CT scan are the demonstration of renal cysts and tumours, perinephric haematomas, and other perinephric swellings, spread of renal and prostatic tumours into para-aortic lymph-nodes and abnormalities of renal shape such as horse-shoe kidney or polycystic disease. However, many of these objectives can be achieved, a little less elegantly, by cheaper and more widely available techniques such as ultrasound.

Ultrasonography

This is now the initial investigation for the majority of patients in renal failure and is likely to displace radiology as the leading structural investigation of the urinary tract. High-resolution real-time (moving picture) scans are becoming standard equipment.

Tissue density is the major determinant of acoustic impedence and when sound waves are passed into tissues of widely different acoustic impedences most of the waves are reflected, e.g. tissue/gas 99 per cent echo, tissue/bone 70 per cent echo. Fat is highly reflective and thick subcutaneous tissues lengthen the distance from the probe to the kidney, making ultrasonography difficult and occasionally impossible in obese patients.

Ultrasound findings are independent of renal function. They can therefore be used to study patients with renal failure, measuring with considerable accuracy the shape, depth from the surface, and internal architecture of the kidney and upper urinary tract

(Fig. 10). Ultrasound detects reliably the dilated calyces, pelvis, and ureter of the obstructed kidney and displays the normal or increased size and cortical thickness of other diseases causing acute renal failure. It can differentiate these from the small kidneys with decreased cortical thickness of most chronic renal diseases, telling the physician whether or not renal biopsy is indicated in the diagnosis of unexplained renal failure.

Ultrasound is frequently employed after renal transplantation. When there is delayed function the echo pattern of the kidney is of some help in distinguishing acute tubular necrosis from rejection, though more reliance is placed on serial gamma scans. If there is a later decline in renal function ultrasound may distinguish between the large kidney of acute rejection and that caused by hydronephrosis (Fig. 11). However, its most important role is in the detection of extrarenal collections of blood, pus, and lymph.

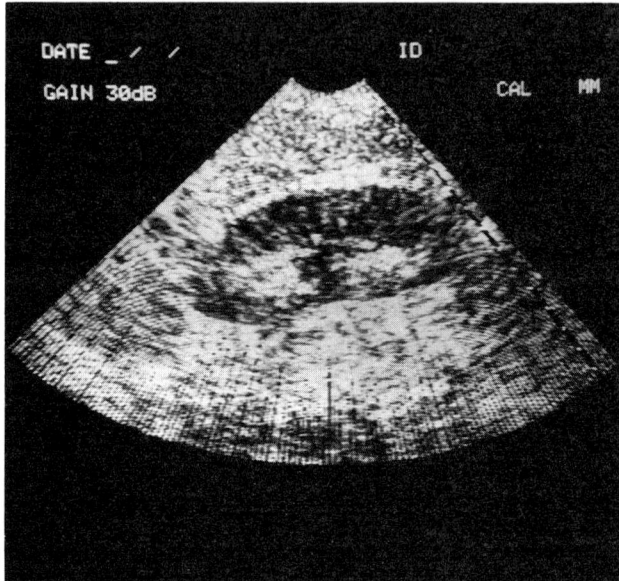

Fig. 10 Normal kidney displayed by ultrasonography, in longitudinal section. The small curved upper edge of the wedge represents the skin of the back, to which the probe is applied. The high-echo areas in the kidney are the calyces.

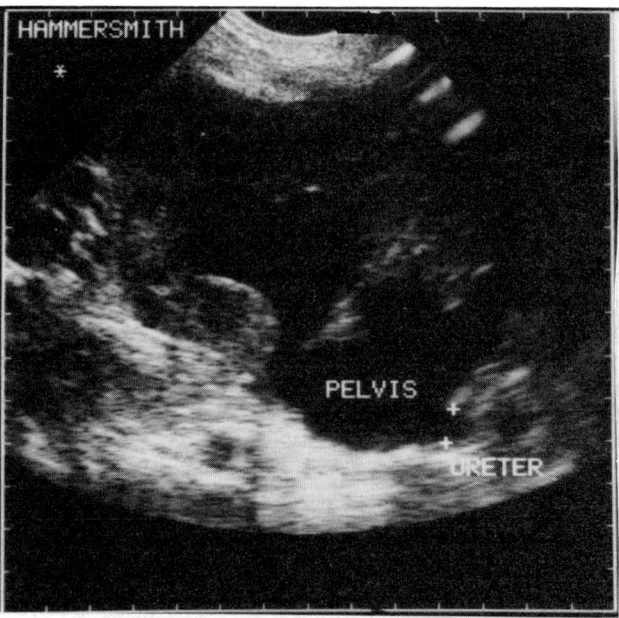

Fig. 11 Ultrasonogram of transplanted kidney showing dilation of renal pelvis and widening of ureter due to obstruction.

Ultrasound is often helpful in identifying the cause of abnormalities detected on the IVU. It may show whether an enlarged kidney is the site of hydronephrosis, an infiltrative process or a space-occupying lesion. It is particularly useful in deciding whether a localized swelling detected on IVU is cystic (and probably benign) or solid (and probably malignant). Very homogeneous solid tumours and those with necrotic centres may be misinterpreted as cysts while multilocular cysts and those which contain blood or are calcified may be mistaken for tumours. A suspected cyst is therefore often displayed by cyst puncture and injection of contrast to show its smooth interior wall. Suspected solid tumours are confirmed by aortography or selective renal arteriography.

Ultrasonography has replaced excretion urography as the screening test for polycystic disease; the two techniques are comparable in accuracy but ultrasonography is faster, cheaper, and devoid of the risks·of contrast injection and irradiation, but cysts and tumours below 1 cm diameter are not detected reliably by either ultrasound or excretion urography so polycystic disease cannot be excluded confidently below the age of about 20.

Perinephric lesions are readily displayed by ultrasound; it is used to detect extravasation of blood after trauma or renal biopsy. It is probably the best initial investigation for analgesic nephropathy if renal function is impaired; it shows a 'rosary' of calcified papillae, casting sound shadows. Ultrasonography is the first test for radiolucent calculi; it is also useful in detecting radio-opaque calculi but straight radiography remains the first investigation.

Radionuclide examination

Radionuclides

Three radionuclides are in common use. The best isotope of iodine is ^{123}I which has a short half-life of 13 hours and a suitable radiation energy of 159 keV but it is not universally available. ^{131}I with a half-life of eight days and a radiation energy of 364 keV is therefore still used. Two metals are in common clinical use: chromium as ^{51}Cr and technetium as ^{99m}Tc. The latter is an attractive agent for clinical purposes with a short half-life of six hours and a pure, moderate-energy (144 keV) gamma emission.

Radiopharmaceuticals

The radiopharmaceutical to which the radionuclide is attached may be excreted by glomerular filtration, by tubular excretion or by a combination of both; or it may be taken up by the tubule but excreted into the urine only in small amounts. A chelate of ethylene diamine tetra-acetic acid with chromium ($[^{51}$Cr]–EDTA) excreted by glomerular filtration and iodine-labelled o-iodohippurate (hippuran) have been described (on pages 18.6 and 18.9).

Several agents which are handled in different ways by the kidney have been chelated with ^{99m}Tc: gluconate as an alternative to hippuran; diethylene triamine penta-acetic acid (DTPA) as an alternative to $[^{51}$Cr]–EDTA and dimercaptosuccinic acid (DMSA), which is taken up by the tubules but not excreted to any significant degree, for estimating renal blood flow and static cortical imaging.

Measurement

For studies of individual or regional renal function, the gamma radiation is measured by external probes or a gamma camera. The probes are more sensitive but are difficult to place accurately over the kidneys and they give only an integrated measurement from the whole kidney and collecting system. The gamma camera is a large sodium iodide crystal (e.g. 50 cm diameter and 1.25 cm thick) surmounted by a battery of photomultiplier tubes. Gamma rays are directed to small areas of the lower surface of the crystal by a series of channels through a lead plate, called the collimator. When the electrons in the sodium iodide crystal have been excited by gamma rays they emit light photons and fall back into their original orbits. The photons are converted back into electrons at the photocathode and multiplied into an easily measurable

impulse which is proportional to the amount of light produced by the original encounter. The gamma camera produces both static and dynamic images quickly. It is combined with a digital computer which corrects the images for background activity (which is particularly important when renal function is impaired or when quantitative measurements are required) and stores and processes data. Areas of interest can be selected from the renal image displayed on a TV screen and activity curves drawn for individual areas such as renal cortex or renal pelvis. This modification of the renogram has largely replaced renography with external probes in centres possessing a gamma camera.

Renography

The patient must be well hydrated and is instructed to drink one litre of fluid in the hour before the procedure. He empties his bladder and is given a rapid intravenous injection of $[^{123}$I]–hippuran or $[^{99m}$Tc]–DTPA. Counts are taken continuously over both kidneys by probes or the gamma camera.

The typical curve is shown diagrammatically in Fig. 12. During phase 1, which lasts about 30 seconds, the count rate rises rapidly as the bolus of radionuclide enters the renal circulation. During phase 2, which lasts 2.5 to 5 min, the count rate rises more slowly as the tracer is taken up by tubular cells, secreted into the tubular lumen, and flushed into the renal pelvis. Phase 2 ends in a fairly sharp peak which coincides, in the normal, with the appearance of activity in the bladder. During phase 3 the count rate falls as loss of tracer from the kidney to the ureter and bladder outpaces the declining input from the bloodstream.

A normal renogram is shown in Fig. 13. The original graph is a series of dots each representing the total counts from the whole kidney in a fixed time interval. The smoothed lines are drawn through the points by computer. In this, as in many renograms, the division between phases 1 and 2 is poorly defined.

The main uses of the renogram are the detection of unilateral renal artery stenosis, which produces a delayed and sometimes

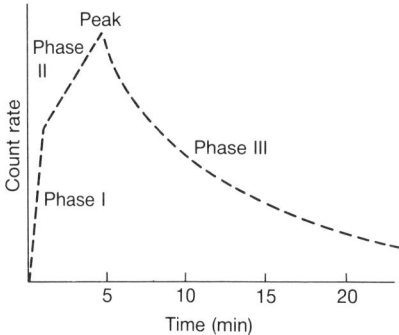

Fig. 12 Diagram of normal renogram, showing the phases which are explained in the text.

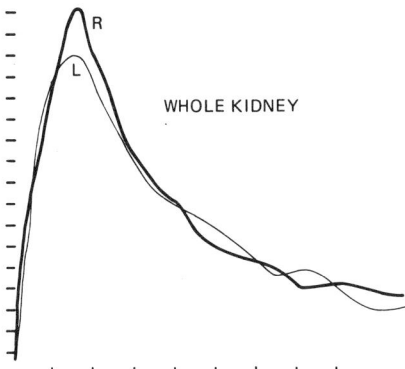

Fig. 13 Normal renogram. Vertical scale, count rate. Horizontal scale, time in 2 min intervals.

depressed peak and a prolonged phase 3 on the affected side, and the demonstration of obstruction. Figure 14 shows the whole kidney renogram of a patient with unilateral obstruction. A similar appearance may be found in patients with a large dilated pelvis which is no longer obsructed; the two can be distinguished by an injection of frusemide which rapidly clears tracer from a delated pelvis but not from one with fixed obstruction.

Imaging with the gamma camera: dynamic

The preparation is the same as for renography. Fluid loading is omitted if the patient is in renal failure. Hippuran is preferred to [^{99m}Tc]–DTPA if renal function is very poor, since it is concentrated by tubular secretion as well as glomerular filtration. After the bolus injection, counts are summated over intervals of 3–6 seconds over the first minute and every minute for the next 20 or more. The images at 30 seconds reflect arterial perfusion while those at 2 min largely reflect GFR. Late images show the excretion phase. The major clinical indications for use of the gamma camera are the following:

Assessment of the contribution of each kidney or of one region

The relative blood flow through the two kidneys is calculated from the 30 second images with hippuran. The total counts over each kidney are proportional to its blood flow, after background correction. If the total renal blood flow has been measured, the absolute blood flow through each kidney can be calculated. The clinician is more often concerned about the relative contributions to GFR, which are calculated on the same principle from the 2 min images. In a similar manner, the contribution of different parts of the kidney can be estimated to guide decisions on partial nephrectomy.

Detection or assessment of obstruction

The IVU is usually the best test to show the site of obstruction, if it is not complete, but the gamma camera is a better guide to the severity of obstruction. Serial images are recorded (Fig. 15a and b) from the same data as are used to constuct the renogram curves shown in Figs 13 and 14. The early images appear late on the obstructed side since the reduction in GFR and blood flow reduce initial uptake of the tracer. Later images show persistence of the renal and pelvic shadows and poor display of the ureters as tracer is cleared at a slower rate on the obstructed side. After an injection of frusemide (Fig. 15c) the unobstructed side rapidly clears while tracer persists on the obstructed side. The renogram curve gives an indication of the severity of obstruction. Initially there is flattening of the usually concave phase 3; as obstruction increases, there is a gradual rise in phase 3 (Fig. 14) until it becomes continuous with phase 2 so that the curve continues to rise throughout the 20 min observation period.

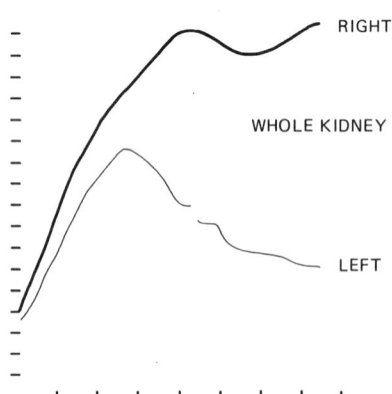

Fig. 14 Whole kidney renogram in unilateral obstruction. Axes as in Fig. 13.

In *chronic* obstruction the GFR contributed by each kidney should be calculated. If the obstructed kidney contributes less than 10 per cent of total GFR reparative surgery is unlikely to restore useful function and nephrectomy is usually indicated. However, in *recent* obstruction considerable recovery can be expected from conservative surgery even if the initial scan shows no renal function on the obstructed side. Following relief of obstruction phase 3 of the renogram may remain absent or elevated for several months.

Detection of vesicoureteric reflux

Reflux may be demonstrated at the end of a [^{99m}Tc]-DTPA scan but is more reliably detected by instilling [^{99m}Tc]-DTPA through a urethral catheter, as for micturating cystography. This technique only detects the more severe degrees of reflux but as it involves only 1 per cent of the radiation caused by X-ray cystography it may have a role in screening families or in following the progress of patients with severe reflux.

Differential diagnosis of acute renal failure

Pre-renal factors should be corrected before imaging. A [^{99m}Tc]-DTPA study shows mild to moderate reduction of perfusion, and no excretion, in patients with acute tubular necrosis. The lack of an excretion phase differentiates it from acute obstruction. Cortical necrosis, e.g. in the haemolytic uraemic syndrome is shown by the absence of perfusion, concentration, or excretion. Imaging is particularly useful in evaluating the reason for primary non-function of a kidney transplant. Infarction of the kidney, following renal artery thrombosis, is readily recognized because the kidney causes a negative shadow against the background radiation. In some transplant units, a gamma scan is performed on the first post-operative day if the transplant is not functioning normally, to confirm that it is well perfused and to provide a baseline from which to measure changes during the period of oliguria. During the perfusion scan, activity in the kidney can be compared with that in the neighbouring iliac artery to provide a 'perfusion index'. In uncomplicated acute tubular necrosis renal perfusion gradually improves through the oliguric period; if transplant rejection is superimposed, perfusion decreases. The gamma scan is complementary to ultrasound in detecting other causes of transplant malfunction such as obstruction and lymphocoele.

Investigation of hypertension

Dynamic imaging has its greatest use in detecting renal artery stenosis, a condition which may be missed on the IVU. The patient must be taken off diuretics for a week and well hydrated. Following a bolus injection of [^{123}I]-hippuran or [^{99m}Tc]-DTPA the arterial obstruction may be shown on the earliest perfusion scans. Later frames show reduced perfusion and smaller size of the affected kidney. A focal area of underperfusion may be shown if a branch artery is affected. If a unilateral renal artery stenosis is significant the kidney supplied by it will usually contribute less than 42 per cent of total GFR.

Imaging with the gamma camera: static

[^{99m}Tc]-DMSA is rapidly taken up by the tubular cells but little of it is excreted in the urine. At three hours about half of the dose is concentrated in the kidneys and no activity is seen in the ureters or bladder. Comparison of the activity over the two kidneys gives an estimate of their relative function, though not a true measure of GFR. In obstruction the 10 per cent of tracer which is normally excreted over three hours may be retained and falsely elevate the calculated renal function on that side.

The static scan gives a good view of renal anatomy. It has largely replaced rectilinear scanning but for the detection of space-occupying lesions, excretion urography and ultrasonography are usually chosen as the primary investigations.

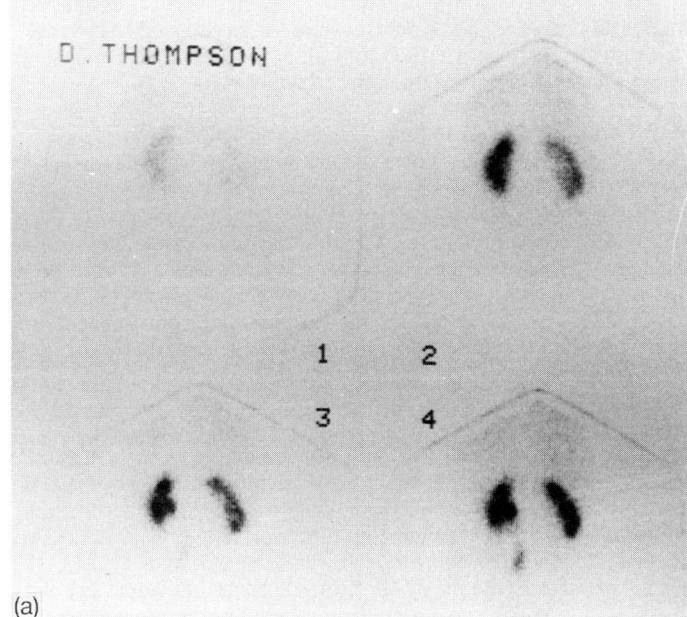

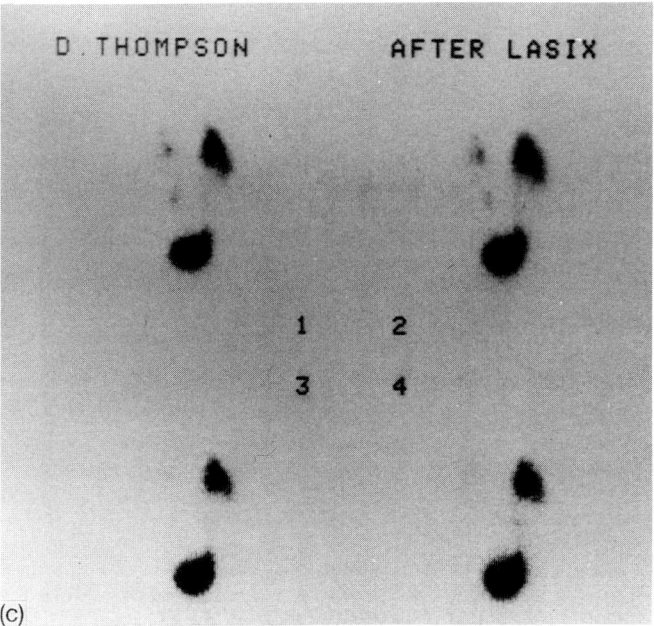

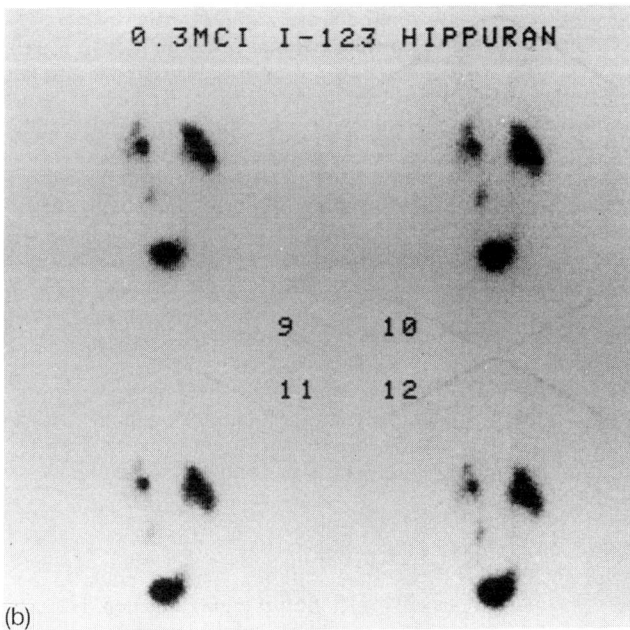

Fig. 15 (a) Gamma camera scan of a patient with right pelvi-ureteric obstruction. The right renal tract is on the right of the picture (mirror image of an IVU). Images at 1–4 min show slow appearance of radioactivity in parenchyma and pelvis of obstructed side. (b) Later images of scan shown in Fig. 15. Poor display of right ureter and persistence of radioactivity in right renal pelvis. (c) Frusemide test at the end of the scan shown in (a) and (b). Rapid clearing of radioactivity from the normal left side and persistence on the obstructed right side.

Changes in renal function with age

The infant's kidney is immature. GFR and renal plasma flow are about one-fifth of adult normal, when related to surface area in the neonate. This is partly an artefact since the infant's surface area is high in relationship to its lean body mass, but it is partly a true immaturity. The GFR doubles over the first two weeks of life and reaches adult levels by three months, as does the renal plasma flow. There is a rapid growth in glomerular surface area and an even more rapid growth in proximal tubular length over the first

year of life. Thereafter GFR and renal plasma flow, per unit surface area, remain constant until the third or fourth decades when a steady almost linear decline sets in (Fig. 16).

As renal function declines with age there are simultaneous changes in renal anatomy, even in subjects who are normal by the definition of 'no hypertension and no known renal or systemic disease that affects renal function'. The elastic layer of small arteries becomes thicker and reduplicated, encroaching on the lumen. The average size of nephrons shrinks and this change affects the juxtamedullary nephrons, which are responsible for maximum urinary concentration, disproportionately. The basement membranes of Bowman's capsule and the renal tubules are irregularly thickened,

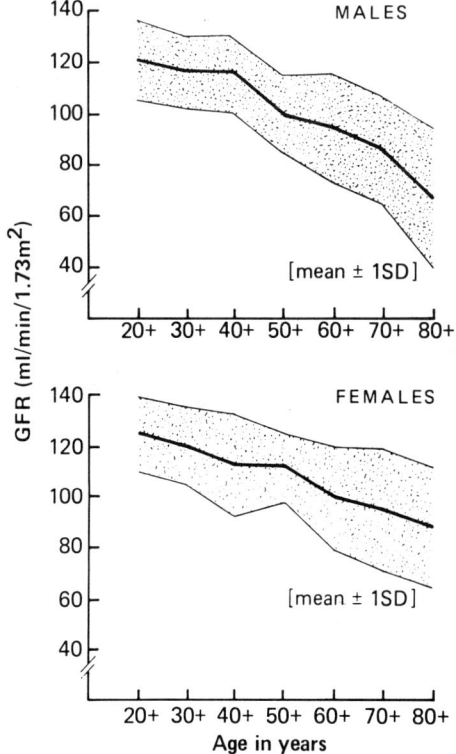

Fig. 16 Decline in GFR with age.

possibly as a respose to ischaemia. With increasing age, normality is enjoyed only by a minority. In one classic study of the aging kidney performed on the victims of sudden death, two-thirds had to be discarded because the subjects did not meet the definition of normality given above. The decline in GFR and renal plasma flow (which is less well documented but roughly parallel) is faster in patients with urinary infection and prostatic enlargement who make up a high proportion of the geriatric population.

Plasma biochemistry

Despite the decline in GFR, plasma creatinine remains in the normal range for young adults, because creatinine production falls as muscle mass shrinks with age (see page 18.5). Plasma urea also often remains in the normal range as protein intake falls in the elderly. When unstressed, elderly subjects also retain normal concentrations of plasma sodium, potassium, chloride, and bicarbonate and blood pH and $PaCO_2$. However, the old, like the very young, have a diminished abiltiy to maintain homeostasis under stress.

Urinary concentration

Infants have a lower maximum urinary concentration than adults. The mean normal is about 550 mosm/kg in the desmopressin test at two months but it rises steadily through the first year of life to reach about 1000 mosmol/kg at one year. This is partly due to the low urea production of the growing infant but non-urea solutes are also poorly concentrated in infancy. These changes are paralleled by growth of the renal tubules, lengthening of Henle's loop, and fall in medullary blood flow.

Maximum concentration remains constant until the third decade then falls by about 30 mosmol/kg per decade into old age. However, the scatter of results at all ages is high and published series contain rather few subjects in the later decades so the 95 per cent confidence limits are wide and the lower limit of normal in the elderly, quoted in the section on urinary concentrating ability, may be falsely low. Inability to handle a large water load is none the less characteristic of the very young and the very old.

Urinary acidification

Renal production of ammonia per unit time falls in old age, partly as a result of declining GFR but probably also as a reflection of diminished tubular mass. Consequently the elderly are less able than the young to correct an acidosis by renal excretion and they take longer to restore blood pH to normal after a metabolic insult.

Changes in renal structure and function during pregnancy (see also page 11.9)

Kidney length increases approximately 1 cm during pregnancy. The calyces, renal pelvis and ureter dilate, often giving the impression of obstructive uropathy. It has been assumed that this dilatation is accompanied by hypotonicity and hypomotility but modern urometry has shown that there is increased tone in the upper ureter and no decrease in the frequency and amplitude of ureteral contractions in pregnancy. Furthermore there is hypertrophy of the ureteral smooth muscle and hyperplasia of its connective tissue so the concept of toneless, floppy ureters with smooth muscle paralysed by the hormonal milieu of pregnancy is no longer tenable. Vesico-ureteric reflux probably occurs sporadically during pregnancy and may be present more frequently than the 3 per cent incidence documented by present techniques.

These anatomical changes have important clinical implications. Dilatation of the urinary tract may lead to collection errors in tests based on timed urine volume, e.g. 24-hour oestriol, creatinine, or protein excretion, and the error will be more important in shorter collection periods. Stasis within the ureters, and vesico-ureteric reflux, may contribute to the propensity of pregnant women with asymptomatic bacteriuria to develop acute pyelonephritis. Normal values for kidney length should be increased by 1 cm if the mea-

surement is made during pregnancy or immediately after delivery. Since dilatation of the ureters may persist until the 12th–16th post-partum week, elective radiological examination of the urinary tract should be deferred until after this period.

GFR and renal plasma flow

GFR and renal plasma flow (usually measured without correction for PAH or hippuran extraction) increase to levels 40–60 per cent above the non-pregnant norm (Fig. 17). The increments occur soon after conception and are evident throughout the first two trimesters. Similar changes, albeit on a smaller scale, occur in pregnant women with chronic renal disease, a single normal kidney or even a denervated ectopic kidney transplanted from a male donor showing that they can be superimposed on apparently maximal compensatory hypertrophy.

GFR falls significantly in the last three or four weeks of pregnancy even in normal women going about their usual activities. It is necessary to relate GFR to this normal falling rate when using it to assess high-risk pregnancy approaching term. There is no general agreement about the changes in GFR at term, some authors describing changes just before delivery while others believe they occur at the very start of the puerperium.

Serial measurements of GFR in the same individual are very helpful in pregnancy and ideally one should obtain a measurement before conception; this is our standard practice for planned pregnancy in women with renal disease and other high-risk pregnancies. Single estimations during pregnancy are harder to interpret because there is a wide range of normality. In non-pregnant women this range is narrowed by correcting GFR for surface area; the correction is invalid in pregnancy although it has been the basis for much interpretation of published data.

There are technical difficulties in performing clearance studies in pregnancy. A pregnant woman may have difficulty in emptying her bladder completely. This may be eased by giving her a water load and allowing her to rest on one side for an hour before the start and end of the collection. This standardizes the procedure and produces a modest water diuresis so that residual bladder urine is dilute. Pregnant women are particularly sensitive to salt intake which has a greater effect on renal function than in the non-pregnant woman. They are probably also more sensitive to changes in renal function from the volume-expanding effect of intravenous fluids. They are particularly sensitive to posture; in the supine position the gravid uterus compresses the great vessels and depresses GFR.

Plasma biochemistry

The plasma levels of creatinine and urea, which average 73 μmol/l and 4.4 mmol/l, respectively, in non-pregnant women decrease to

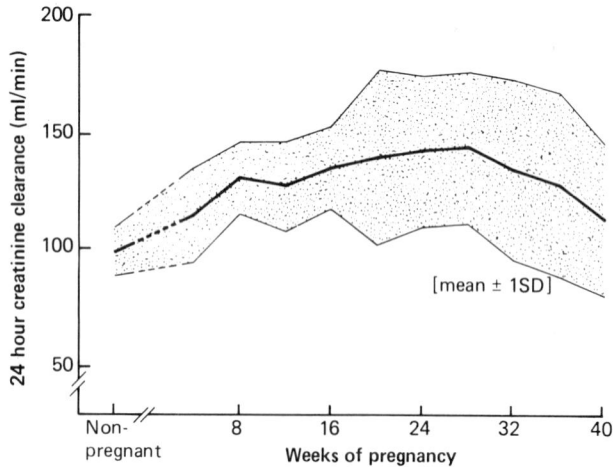

Fig. 17 Change in creatinine clearance during normal pregnancy.

mean values of 51 μmol/l and 3.2 mmol/l in pregnancy. Awareness of these changes is important because values considered normal in non-pregnant women may reflect decreased renal function in pregnancy. Plasma levels of creatinine and urea exceeding 75 μmol/l and 4.6 mmol/l, respectively, should alert the clinician to investigate renal function in more detail.

Renal regulation of acid-base is altered in pregnancy. The blood level of hydrogen ion decreases by 2–4 mmol/l early in pregnancy and this decrement is sustained until term. Thus arterial blood pH averages 7.44 in pregnant, compared to 7.40 in non-pregnant, women. Plasma bicarbonate concentration falls by about 4 mmol/l so that the normal range is 20–25 mmol/l in pregnancy. The mild alkalaemia is believed to be respiratory in origin; pregnant women normally hyperventilate and their arterial PCO_2 decreases from a mean of 5.2 kPa before pregnancy to 4.1 kPa during it. Consequently the pregnant woman is at a disadvantage when threatened by sudden metabolic acidosis.

An alkaline urine is formed at substantially lower plasma bicarbonate levels in pregnancy and there are high circulating levels of aldosterone and other potent mineralocorticoids. These phenomena might be expected to cause increased potassium loss in the urine. They do not; there is even a gradual retention of about 350 mmol of potassium, most of which enters the tissues of the enlarging fetus, placenta, and uterus. Moreover pregnant women lose less potassium in the urine than non-pregnant women when high-sodium diet and mineralocorticoids are administered. This tendency to conserve potassium despite high levels of circulating mineralocorticoids has been ascribed to the raised blood progesterone level. Plasma potassium remains in the normal range in pregnancy and the hypokalaemia of patients with Conn's syndrome and Bartter's syndrome may be ameliorated. Plasma sodium, on the other hand, falls by 3–6 mmol/l because of the changes in sodium and water handling discussed below.

Body fluid volume regulation; sodium and water excretion
The average primigravida gains about 12.5 kg body weight during pregnancy, the average multipara somewhat less. The gain is partly due to fluid since total body water increases by 6–8 litres, the majority entering the extracellular fluid. There are increases in plasma volume, which is greatest during the second trimester when the increment approaches 50 per cent, and in fluid within maternal and fetal interstitial spaces, which is greatest in late pregnancy. During normal pregnancy there is a gradual retention of 900 mmol of sodium, distributed between the products of conception and the maternal extracellular space. These alterations produce a physiological hypervolaemia but the mother's volume receptors sense these changes as normal; if the physiological expansion is limited by salt restriction or diuretic therapy, the maternal response resembles that of a salt-depleted non-pregnant subject.

Retention of salt and water occurs in spite of the 40–50 per cent increase in GFR which results in an extra load of 6000–10 000 mmol of sodium being filtered daily. Sodium depletion would quickly ensue if this were not accompanied by a parallel increase in the quantity absorbed. The increase in renal tubular reabsorption is the largest renal adaptation during pregnancy and is responsible for a considerable proportion of the increased basal energy expenditure during pregnancy. The mechanisms responsible are uncertain.

Soon after conception, plasma osmolality falls to a level about 10 mosmol/kg below that of the non-pregnant woman. This can be accounted for by a concomitant fall in plasma sodium and associated anions. Pregnant women might therefore be expected to stop secreting antidiuretic hormone and be in a state of continuous diuresis. This does not happen because there is a resetting of the osmoreceptor system to accept and preserve the new low level of plasma osmolality. Pregnant women can concentrate their urine as well as non-pregnant women except when they are lying on their sides when urinary concentrating ability falls. However, the ability to excrete a water load is altered. Pregnant women when sitting have an increased diuretic response to water loading, which declines during the third trimester so that at term they have a slower diuresis than non-pregnant women. The upright position is more antidiuretic in pregnancy and changing from lateral recumbency to the supine position also decreases urine flow.

Renal tubular functions
Excretion of glucose increases soon after conception and may exceed non-pregnant values by a factor of ten. The glycosuria varies widely from day to day and within the 24 hours; this intermittency is not related to blood dextrose concentrations or to the stage of pregnancy. Normal pre-pregnant levels are re-established within a week of delivery. The glycosuria is caused by a combination of the increased filtered load of glucose, caused by the rise in GFR, and a change in the reabsorptive capacity of the proximal tubule.

Plasma urate concentration has decreased by over 25 per cent by the eighth week of pregnancy, probably because of decreased renal tubular reabsorption. It rises again in the third trimester, to reach at least the non-pregnant mean, because of increasing tubular reabsorption of uric acid. Plasma urate and renal reabsorption are higher in pregnancies complicated by pre-eclampsia or intrauterine growth retardation. When plasma urate exceeds 350 μmol/l in hypertensive women there is a significant rise in perinatal mortality; serial measurements of plasma urate can be used to monitor progress.

The renal handling of nutrients is altered in pregnancy. There is an increased excretion of lactose, fructose, xylose, ribose, fucose, vitamin C, folic acid, nicotinic acid, and most of the amino acids. Total amino acid loss may reach 2 g per day. Some oligosaccharides of mammary origin appear in the urine. Lactose in the urine is also derived from the mammary gland. Lactosuria is a benign condition of pregnancy of no clinical importance except as a possible source of confusion with glycosuria if non-specific tests like Clinitest are employed. The two are readily distinguished by dipsticks such as Labstix which contain glucose oxidase and therefore give negative results with lactose.

References
Bijvoet, O. L. M. (1977). In *Metabolic bone disease* (ed. L. V. Avioli and S.M. Krane) Vol. 1, p. 60. Academic Press, New York.

Black, D. A. K. and Jones, N. F. (1979). *Renal disease*, 4th edn. Blackwell Scientific Publications, Oxford. Chapters 9 (Radiological investigation of renal disease), 10 (Radionuclides in the investigation of renal disease), and 11 (Urinalysis and assessment of renal function).

Brenner, B. M. and Rector. F. C. (1986). *The kidney*, 3rd edn. W. B. Saunders, Philadelphia. Chapters 4 (Glomerular filtration), 7 (Renal acidification), 16 (Renal handling of phosphates), and 18 (Clinical and laboratory assessment of the patient with renal disease).

Lindheimer, M. D. and Katz, A. I. (1978). *Kidney function and disease in pregnancy*. Lea and Febiger, Philadelphia.

O'Reilly, P. H., Shields, R. A. and Testa, H. J. (1986). *Nuclear medicine in urology and nephrology* 2nd edn. Butterworths, London.

Schumann, G. B. (1980). *Urine sediment examination*. Williams and Wilkins, Baltimore.

WATER AND ELECTROLYTE DISORDERS

Water and sodium homeostasis

J. G. G. LEDINGHAM

Body water

Water comprises some 50 to 60 per cent of body weight in adults, the proportion being less in individuals with more adipose tissue. About one-third of this large volume constitutes extracellular fluid, whilst two-thirds of it is intracellular. The two compartments are separated by a variety of cell membranes. The vast majority of these are freely permeable to water, so that fluid movements tend to maintain near isotonicity between intracellular and extracellular fluids.

Osmolality

Osmolality is a measure of the number of osmoles of solute *per kilogram* of solvent while osmolarity depends on the number of osmoles *per litre* of fluid. In clinical work substances are measured in molar rather than molal terms but osmometers measure osmolality rather than osmolarity. The two approximate each other so closely in body fluids at body temperature that no correction is necessary. One mmol of a non-polar solute provides 1 mosmol, but 1 mmol of a salt which dissociates completely into 2 ions yields 2 mosmol.

The major contributors to osmolality of the extracellular fluid are sodium and its corresponding anions, glucose and urea. A close approximation to measured plasma osmolality can be made by adding the molar concentrations of glucose and urea in plasma to twice the sodium concentration. Where glucose and urea concentrations are still reported in mg per 100 ml, the glucose concentration can be converted to mmol/l by dividing by 18, the urea nitrogen by 2.8, and the blood urea by 5.6. These calculations have been shown to provide a figure corresponding with measured osmolality in plasma or serum with an error of only some 5 or 10 mosmol/kg. This relationship only holds if other low molecular weight solutes are not present. The method is therefore inappropriate for urinary measurements. In practice, it is rare for calculated and measured plasma osmolality to differ much. Gross hyperlipidaemia or hyperproteinaemia can reduce the water content per unit volume of plasma, and in these circumstances measured sodium concentration is low (although not below 120 mmol/l), calculated osmolality therefore is also low, but measured osmolality is normal (around 285–290 mosmol/kg of water). Another reason for calculated osmolality falling short of measured osmolality is the presence in blood of large quantities of ethanol or more rarely other substances such as ethylene glycol, methyl alcohol, mannitol, isopropanol, ethyl ether, acetone, trichlorethane, and paraldehyde. In these rare situations calculated osmolality is likely to fall within the normal range, but measured concentration will normally exceed 300 mosmol/kg, the difference reflecting the concentration of foreign solute present.

Tonicity

This is a term used to express a measure of the force favouring a movement of water across a membrane which is permeable to water but impermeable to the solutes on either side which contribute to an osmotic gradient. In the clinical context extracellular fluid is hypertonic if an increase in osmolality is caused by an impermeable substance such as sodium chloride or mannitol while a rise in urea or alcohol increases osmolality equally within and without cells, resulting therefore in no fluid shifts from one compartment to the other.

Water homeostasis

Water intake in normal health is determined by a number of influences which come under the broad heading of 'thirst'. Output, variable from skin, lungs, and gastrointestinal tract, normally balances input precisely by way of haemodynamic and hormonal regulation of the excretion of water by the kidneys. When intake is less than excretion for whatever reason, the kidney can minimize the degree of resulting dehydration, but balance can then be restored only by further ingestion of water. Receptors which receive signals reflecting small changes in intracellular hydration, larger changes in extracellular fluid volume and perhaps in plasma angiotensin II concentrations, lie closely adjacent to one another in the anterior hypothalamus, some regulating antidiuretic hormone (ADH) release and others thirst. In general, stimuli which promote secretion of ADH also stimulate drinking and vice versa.

Water intake

Normal thirst: primary drinking in response to water deficit

Water deprivation stimulates thirst primarily by increasing intracellular osmolality. Any cause of intracellular water depletion results in drinking, whether caused by an absolute deficit or by a shift of water from intracellular fluid to the extracellular space, as occurs for instance after infusion of hypertonic saline or mannitol. Infusions of hypertonic urea or glucose do not cause thirst or significant release of ADH because these solutes readily enter cells, whereas mannitol and sodium do not. The osmotic threshold above which thirst occurs is variable between individuals, reproducible in an individual and higher by some 4 to 5 mosmol/kg than the osmotic threshold for ADH release.

Loss of intracellular fluid is probably sensed by osmotic changes and not by more specific changes in sodium concentration in the cerebrospinal fluid, as was once suggested. Osmoreceptors subserving thirst have been found in animals in the lateral hypothalamus close to those regulating ADH secretion. Additional peripheral receptors have been postulated in the portal venous system, the stomach, and the gut.

Loss of extracellular fluid and blood volume also stimulate thirst (which may be a prominent feature of acute major blood loss for instance) but the loss must be more than 10 per cent and the mechanism is much less sensitive than that of osmoregulation. Some 60–80 per cent of drinking after water deprivation in animals is stimulated by intracellular dehydration and 15–25 per cent by loss of extracellular volume. In humans there may be a greater contribution from change in extracellular fluid volume. The receptors which detect hypovolaemia and stimulate thirst have not been identifed precisely but probably lie in the walls of the capacitance vessels near the heart and in the pulmonary veins and left atrium.

Angiotensin II is known to stimulate thirst in animals, acting on vascular receptors in the pre-optic area, subfornical organ, and organum vasculosum of the lamina terminalis. Whether or not angiotensin II is dipsogenic in humans can be disputed. Circumstantial evidence suggests that it might be. Some patients in whom renin activity has been markedly elevated develop extreme thirst despite dilutional hyponatraemia. Rare examples have been reported among patients with renal failure undergoing regular haemodialysis, others with renin-secreting tumours, and in a few with the hyponatraemic hypertensive syndrome caused by reno-vascular disease. Removal of the source of renin by nephrectomy or relief of stenosis has relieved both thirst and hyponatraemia in these cases. However, infusion of angiotensin II into normal volume-replete subjects does not cause thirst or drinking in humans as it does in animals.

Age may affect thirst mechanisms adversely. Whereas the secretory response of ADH to water deprivation in the elderly is enhanced compared to that of younger subjects, thirst is markedly blunted. This, together with the reduced capacity of kidneys to conserve water with age must contribute to the common clinical experience that elderly patients readily become dehydrated.

Secondary drinking

When water is freely available, drinking is regulated by mechanisms less easy to research. Most people drink more than they need, regularly excreting a dilute urine to maintain homeostasis. Drinking in normal circumstances (secondary drinking) depends on habit, circadian rhythms, the need to drink with food, the palatability of the fluid available, and social occasions when coffee, tea, or alcohol become habit. Many of these stimuli depend on some pleasurable oropharyngeal sensation. Inhibitory signals from overhydration are relatively weak antagonists to pleasurable drinking. The mechanisms by which drinking is stopped – satiation – are not well understood. Signals from the oropharynx, oesophagus, stomach, and duodenum have been described.

Antidiuretic hormone (ADH): arginine vasopressin (AVP)

Antidiuretic hormone (page 10.23), by its effect on the collecting ducts of the kidney, is the hormone controlling the rate at which the kidney excretes or retains free water. It is a cyclic nonapeptide in which the first six amino acids form a ring structure by the junction of two cystine moieties in positions 1 and 6 by a disulphide bond (Fig. 1). In humans, because arginine occupies position 8 in the molecule (as opposed to lysine in other species) this hormone is often referred to as arginine vasopressin (AVP).

Synthesis

Vasopressin is synthesized with its carrying protein (neurophysin) in specialized cells in the anterior hypothalamus, clustered together mainly in the supraoptic and paraventricular nuclei. The axons of these neurosecretory cells extend from their origin by three separate pathways to deliver the granules of neurophysin and vasopressin to the neurohypophysis, to the median eminence, and to the third ventricle. Granules reaching the posterior pituitary (neurohypophysis) are stored there or released to the systemic circulation by exocytosis in response to appropriate stimuli. The functions of vasopressin reaching the third ventricle or anter-

ior pituitary from the median eminence via the portal venous system have not been settled.

Release

The factors promoting ADH release from the neurohypophysis include osmotic and neurogenic stimuli which, by inducing potentials in the neurosecretory cells, lead to exocytosis of stored granules linked to influx of calcium ions in the axons. Endorphins and perhaps angiotensin also appear to act directly, although there is some evidence that the effects of angiotensin are indirect, perhaps mediated by way of baroceptor function.

Osmoregulation of ADH release

There is an exquisitely sensitive relationship between plasma osmolality, plasma ADH, and the concentration of urine in health, such that very small changes in osmolality above a set point (near 280 mosmol/kg), characteristic for an individual but variable between individuals, results in changes in plasma ADH which produce major changes in the renal handling of water (Fig. 2). The osmoreceptors subserving this system lie in the anterior hypothalamus near to those regulating thirst but separate from the neurosecretory cells which synthesize ADH. The relationship between plasma osmolality and ADH release holds only if the major contribution to osmolality comes from a solute which does not readily enter the cell fluid of the osmoreceptor (e.g. sodium or mannitol). Hyperosmolality due to urea and/or glucose will not stimulate either ADH release or thirst significantly.

The relationship between osmolality and plasma concentrations of ADH is altered by changes in blood and extracellular fluid volume such that the osmolal set point for ADH secretion is lowered when volume is compromised and increased in volume expansion but there is no change in the sensitivity (slope) of the relationship. This change has been described as a 'resetting of the osmostat'.

The relationship is also sensitive to the rate of change of osmolality, precipitous change enhancing the response, with less marked effects when changes occur more gradually.

Volume receptors

Changes in haemodynamic forces without change in osmolal factors can also alter ADH release. The mechanisms involved are likely to be dependent on stretch receptors in the capacitance vessels near the heart in the pulmonary veins and left atrium, arterial baroceptors, and perhaps the renin–angiotensin system. The newly described atrial natriuretic factor is not part of this system which mediates ADH release and thirst in response to a reduced blood volume, and suppression when volume is expanded. Clinical and experimental observations indicate this to be a less sensitive mechanism for controlling plasma ADH concentrations than is the osmoreceptor system. Among patients with hypothalamic or

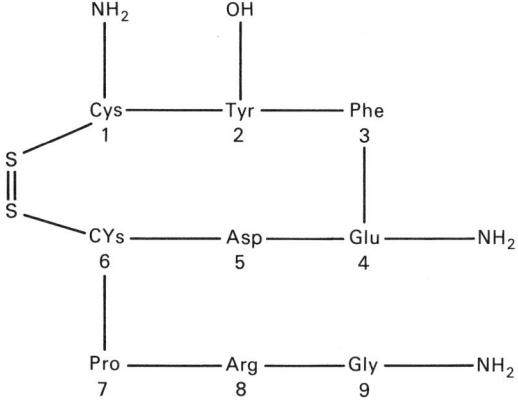

Fig. 1 Antidiuretic hormone, arginine vasopressin.

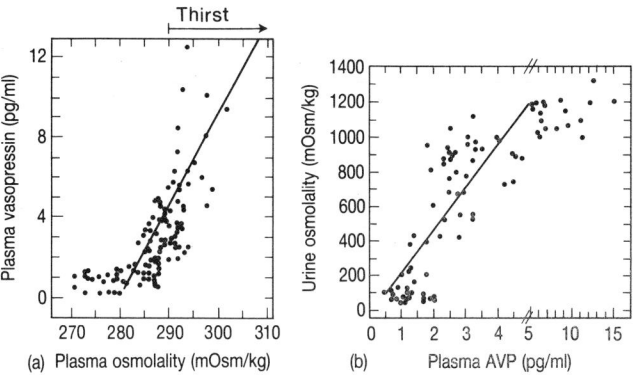

Fig. 2 Relationships between plasma osmolality, plasma AVP and urinary osmolality, in healthy adults in varying states of water balance. (Reproduced from Robertson, 1983, *J. Lab. Clin. Med.* **1**, 351–371, with permission.)

neurohypophyseal lesions, some have been shown to regulate ADH secretion by changes in extracellular fluid (ECF) volume without response to change in osmolality. Disease has distinguished the two mechanisms in such patients in whom there is a tendency to hypernatraemia with plasma osmolality in one reported case varying widely from day-to-day between 298 and 323 mosmol/kg, depending on the state of plasma and ECF volume.

Other non-osmolar factors
Other factors influencing ADH release and plasma concentrations include nausea (but not vomiting without nausea), hypoglycaemia, and hypotension. Pain and trauma are associated with very high levels of ADH, most probably not a direct consequence but mediated through hypotension and nausea. Mediators are likely to include angiotensin II, noradrenaline, acetyl choline, and endorphins.

Assay of ADH
Reliable assays for ADH in plasma and urine are now more widely available. They have elucidated the relationships between plasma osmolality and volume on the one hand and plasma ADH on the other. They are of value in distinguishing with certainty cranial diabetes insipidus from compulsive polydipsia and other thirst disorders and nephrogenic diabetes insipidus. Water deprivation or hypertonic saline studies interpreted by plasma and urinary osmolality alone can be misleading on occasion, unless ADH assays are included in the data. Measurements are of particular value in the diagnosis of syndromes of inappropriate secretion of ADH.

Normal ranges vary between laboratories. When blood volume and osmolality is normal, values of around 3 pg/ml (3.1 pmol/l) are reported. When osmolality is low, concentrations fall below 1 pg/ml and in hyperosmolar states levels exceed those required to produce a maximally concentrated urine and may reach 20 pg/ml (20.8 pmol/l). Much higher concentrations are seen in hypovolaemia or after hypoglycaemia or nausea. Values as high as 500 pg/ml (520 pmol/l) may accompany severe haemorrhage.

Effects of ADH on the kidney
The main effect of ADH is to allow permeability to water of the cells of the terminal distal tubules and collecting ducts of the kidney. Transport of water from tubular fluid is facilitated by ADH and is achieved by osmotic forces created by the countercurrent system and by other factors especially the medullary urea concentration which contribute to the maintenance of medullary interstitial hypertonicity. In the absence of ADH the cells of the distal nephron are poorly permeable to water; in the absence of medullary hypertonicity, the effects of ADH are blunted or absent. In both situations urinary concentration is prevented and dilute urine is excreted. Recent reports that hepatic urea synthesis is stimulated by ADH *in vitro* indicates another mechanism by which the hormone may facilitate water reabsorption by the renal medulla. ADH exerts its effects by the following sequence of events. The circulating hormone binds to specific receptors in the basal and lateral (serosal) aspects of the cells lining the late distal nephrons and collecting ducts. The receptors, activated by binding with ADH, stimulate the intracellular formation of cyclic AMP (cAMP) which, before degradation by phosphodiesterase, increases permeability of the luminal membrane of the tubular cells by phosphorylation of specific membrane proteins and by mechanisms in which the microtubules and microfilaments of these specialized cells participate.

Prostaglandins and ADH
ADH appears to stimulate the production of prostaglandins by the renal medulla, and there is considerable experimental evidence that renal medullary prostaglandins moderate the tubular effects of ADH by inhibiting the generation of cAMP. In humans, indomethacin and other prostaglandin synthetase inhibitors enhance the effects of exogenous vasopressin. Potassium depletion is associated with increased prostaglandin production by the kidney and with polyuria, both abnormalities being improved by treatment with inhibitors of prostaglandin synthetase.

Other effects of ADH
The terms 'antidiuretic hormone' and 'vasopressin' have been used as synonyms for years and this usage reflects long known observations on the pressor effects of larger doses of the peptide. Renal tubular receptors for ADH have been designated V_2 receptors. These differ from V_1 receptors which are found on vascular smooth muscle to promote contraction, and on hepatocytes to promote glycogenolysis. Activated V_1 receptors increase phosphatidylinositol turnover in membranes to increase cytosolic calcium concentration. There is an important, but unresolved controversy about the importance of ADH as a pressor hormone, particularly in malignant and mineralocorticoid hypertension, but it probably does play an important part in maintaining arterial pressure in hypovolaemic and hypotensive states. ADH at high concentrations may also facilitate haemostasis by increasing factor VIII activity in blood, as synthetic analogues of the hormone are known to do in the treatment of Von Willebrand's disease and uraemic bleeding.

Sodium homeostasis

Sodium is the major cation of the extracellular fluid which forms about one-third of total body water in adults. A reduction in body sodium content leads to contraction of extracellular fluid and plasma volumes, while an excess, not excreted by the kidney, results in volume expansion. Changes in sodium balance then affect volume rather than sodium concentration in most circumstances and this reflects the thirst–ADH–renal response to small changes in plasma sodium concentration in the extracellular fluid. A tendency toward hyponatraemia suppresses ADH secretion and the resulting renal loss of water restores the sodium concentration at the expense of volume. Hypernatraemia will promote thirst with increased water intake and ADH secretion with renal water retention. Again osmolar homeostasis is preserved at the expense of volume change. These mechanisms predominate unless volume changes are large (more than 10 per cent) when ADH and thirst are affected by volume as well as osmotic stimuli. There is therefore very little change in plasma sodium concentrations unless volume changes are very large, or thirst/antidiuretic hormone mechanisms are disturbed. It follows that changes in plasma sodium concentrations are more commonly reflections of abnormalities of water than of sodium metabolism (see below).

Sodium homeostasis in health depends very largely on renal regulation of urinary excretion which can balance intake over a range of 1–500 mmol or more daily. Losses of sodium from the bowel are small in health. Sweat contains sodium in a concentration around 50 mmol/l. Skin losses of salt and water may be very considerable in hot dry climates, but sweat sodium concentration is reduced after acclimatization.

Dietary salt
Dietary intake of salt (100–200 mmol/day in the United Kingdom) exceeds requirements enormously in many parts of the world, particularly in Japan, North America, and Europe. Hollenberg has argued persuasively against the common concept that a conventional low salt diet leaves healthy individuals 'sodium depleted'. The pattern of renal sodium conservation in the face of a low salt intake indicates conclusively that the 'set point' at which homeostatic mechanisms conserve sodium efficiently is to be found in normal humans when they are in balance on a 'low salt' intake. Balance studies indicate a loss of some 200–300 mmol of sodium between the steady state of balance on conventional 'normal' and 'low salt' intakes. It follows that most people live in a state of

sodium excess. Persuasive arguments have been put forward linking high salt intakes and essential hypertension, but the hypothesis remains unproven and continues to provoke controversy (see page 13.360).

Renal regulation of sodium homeostasis

The mechanisms by which changes in sodium balance and therefore in ECF and plasma volumes result in appropriate changes in urinary sodium excretion remain difficult to elucidate. In general efferent mechanisms are better understood than afferent ones but there are still areas of doubt despite so much work in this field.

Regulation by glomerular filtration rate

The potential for altering sodium excretion by change in glomerular filtration rate (GFR) is enormous if one considers that the normal adult kidneys filter fluid containing about 140 mmol sodium per litre at a rate of some 170 litres per 24 hours. The balance of evidence, however, suggests that it is by alteration in renal tubular handling of salt that homeostasis is achieved in health, although extreme reductions in filtration rate may promote sodium retention in renal failure. Alterations in the relationships between renal blood flow and glomerular filtration (filtration fraction) are important in determining tubular events by promoting changes in osmotic and hydrostatic forces and in viscosity in postglomerular peritubular fluid and in proximal glomerular filtrate. Acute changes in GFR are accompanied by appropriate changes in proximal tubular reabsorption (glomerulotubular balance) which may be mediated in part by these physical forces as well as perhaps by mechanisms involving feedback from macula densa cells and intrarenal hormonal systems involving angiotensin II, prostaglandins, and the kallikrein–kinin system (see pages 13.82 and 13.83).

Tubular reabsorption

Although, quantitatively, most of the reabsorption of filtered sodium takes place isosmotically in the proximal tubule, absorption in Henle's loop and in the distal tubule and collecting duct may ultimately determine the balance of sodium excretion. In the thick ascending limb of Henle's loop, reabsorption of sodium without water is active and mediated by the sodium/potassium co-transport mechanism. Decreased reabsorption at this site has been postulated as one of the mechanisms of Bartter's syndrome (see page 18.32) and increased reabsorption for some cases of hyporeninaemic hypoaldosteronism (see page 18.35).

Distal tubular reabsorption of sodium is probably of critical importance in regulating overall sodium balance. It is here that the putative atrial natriuretic factor (ANF, see below) is thought to work, and here also that increased sodium reabsorption may occur in such oedematous states as the nephrotic syndrome. The electrical changes resulting from active sodium reabsorption at this site contribute to the mechanisms whereby sodium ions exchange for potassium and hydrogen ions. Activity of sodium reabsorption in the distal nephron depends greatly on the rate of delivery of sodium, and on tubular fluid flow rates from more proximal sites as well as on local effects of aldosterone.

Control mechanisms

Evidence has been found for volume receptors in the capacitance vessels, pulmonary veins, and the walls of the atria of the heart (low pressure receptors) as well as in the arterial baroceptors. These are likely to sense changes in central blood volume, 'effective' blood volume, and cardiac performance, such that, by neurogenic and hormonal mechanisms, appropriate changes are brought about in the renal tubular handling of sodium.

The sympathetic nervous system, dopamine, the renin–angiotensin system, antidiuretic hormone, aldosterone, and renal haemodynamic events have long been implicated on the efferent side of the control mechanisms. But these taken together do not provide an adequate explanation particularly of the natriuresis which

follows volume expansion. Since the work of de Wardener and Mills 25 years ago there has been evidence of an existence of a natriuretic hormone or hormones. Until recently a discrete substance generally agreed to be the natriuretic hormone could not be identified, despite the detection by several laboratories of a variety of substances in plasma or urine of volume expanded and uraemic subjects capable of promoting natriuresis in rats and impairment of sodium transport in toad bladder and frog skin. In 1979 structures resembling secretory granules in heart atria were observed. Their number varied with sodium balance and extracts of rat atria given intravenously were shown to induce natriuresis. Since then events have moved apace. A low molecular weight peptide of 73 amino acids and a higher molecular weight one of 152 amino acids have been isolated from atrial extracts, and a 26 amino acid natriuretic substance has been synthesized. These atrial natriuretic factors (ANF) are both vasoactive and natriuretic. They oppose the vasoconstrictive effects of angiotensin II, noradrenaline, potassium, and histamine, and tend to reduce aldosterone secretion and lower arterial pressure. They increase renal blood flow, have little effect on glomerular filtration rate, and inhibit renal tubular sodium reabsorption in the collecting tubules and collecting ducts. They have no inhibitory effect on Na/K–ATPase. To date, data are scanty on changes in plasma concentrations in health and disease and these may not be the only natriuretic hormones, nor are they yet proven to provide the missing links in the chain of understanding of the control of sodium excretion.

Disorders of salt and water homeostasis

DIABETES INSIPIDUS

Neurogenic (cranial) (see page 10.24)

The close juxtaposition between the neuronal structures concerned with synthesis, storage, and release of ADH and centres concerned with thirst allows disorders of the hypothalamus to present a variety of clinical problems depending on the site, size, and nature of the lesion. There may be partial, moderate or total loss of neurosecretory function giving a wide range of 'severity'. Some patients unable to mount an osmotic-induced rise in ADH, can do so to non-osmotic stimuli such as an injection of apomorphine, or induced hypoglycaemia. There may be disturbances of the threshold of release of ADH with a 'reset osmostat'. There may be complete loss of osmoregulation but with responses to volume stimuli preserved. Uncommonly there may be primary abnormalities in thirst due to hypothalamic disease and closely resembling diabetes insipidus. Loss of both thirst and ADH secretion presents formidable problems. Loss of thirst with maintained ADH secretion has been described recently. Impaired ACTH secretion with cortisol deficiency may mask the polyuria of cranial diabetes insipidus.

Aetiology

Primary neurogenic diabetes insipidus

Idiopathic disease is one of the commonest diagnoses made in neurogenic diabetes insipidus. It can present at any age beyond infancy and in either sex. It is usually an isolated abnormality, but there is occasionally other evidence of hypothalamic disease such as hypopituitarism, narcolepsy, galactorrhoea, or growth failure in children.

Familial neurogenic diabetes insipidus is extremely rare, comprising perhaps 1 per cent of patients with primary disease. Inherited as a Mendelian autosomal dominant, it has been traced through seven generations in one family, presenting in infancy or early childhood.

Another primary form of neurogenic diabetes insipidus is the DIDMOAD syndrome (diabetes insipidus, diabetes mellitus, optic atrophy, and deafness). This syndrome which is also extremely rare is inherited as an autosomal recessive condition.

Histological evidence of diminished numbers of neurosecretory cells in the supraoptic nuclei can be found in each of these primary forms of cranial diabetes insipidus.

Secondary neurogenic diabetes insipidus

Trauma is now perhaps the commonest cause in this category, arising from head injury with rupture of the pituitary stalk, from pituitary surgery, or irradiation by yttrium-90 or heavy particles, or on occasion from birth injury. In these traumatic cases, diabetes insipidus may be temporary or permanent and varies considerably in severity. Lesions of the neurohypophysis itself, or of the stalk below the median eminence, allow recovery by virtue of surviving neurosecretory cells in the supraoptic and lateral hypothalamic nuclei. Lesions above the eminence cause more permanent and more severe disease. Water excretion after traumatic lesions often follows a three-phase course. Polyuria lasting hours or days begins 1–6 days after injury. The situation may then reverse with a short period in which urine is concentrated and its volume small. Diabetes insipidus then returns temporarily or permanently. The antidiuretic phase has been attributed to release of ADH previously stored in the neurohypophysis.

Primary or secondary tumours are the other main causes of secondary diabetes insipidus. Among carcinomas, those of lung and breast metastasize to the hypothalamus most commonly. Other causes listed in Table 1 are well recognized but rare.

Sheehan's syndrome may be a more common cause of partial pituitary diabetes insipidus than was once thought.

Clinical features

The onset of polyuria with polydipsia and thirst is usually sudden in contrast to the more insidious onset of symptoms in patients with psychogenic polydipsia. There may be other symptoms and signs reflecting the underlying cause of impaired ADH secretion such as evidence of a space-occupying lesion or disturbance in anterior pituitary function. Urine volumes are highest in those in whom ADH secretion in response to osmotic stimuli is totally absent, reaching 10–20 litres per 24 hours. Urinary osmolality is low (50–100 mosmol/kg) but if thirst mechanisms are intact and there is access to water, plasma sodium concentrations and osmolalities remain within the normal range. On occasion patients with the grossest polyuria may, if not treated, develop much increased bladder capacity and hydronephrosis, especially if there is a coincident undetected obstruction to bladder emptying (e.g. mild prostatic enlargement).

In milder forms of neurogenic diabetes insipidus the degree of polyuria and polydipsia is less, ranging from asymptomatic disease to the common presentation with urine volumes of 3–6 litres in 24

hours. These classical presentations may be modified by particular lesions in the hypothalamic–pituitary area.

Anterior pituitary disease

When diabetes insipidus is combined with hypopituitarism, polyuria and thirst may be mild or absent because of the antidiuretic effects of cortisol deficiency. In such cases cortisol treatment unmasks the underlying diabetes insipidus. The mechanism by which cortisol deficiency reduces the excretion of free water is not known.

Hypernatraemia in diabetes insipidus

When thirst mechanisms are intact, hypernatraemia does not occur unless the patient becomes confused or comatose, or is given insufficient postoperative fluid to replace urinary losses. Disturbances of thirst complicating diabetes insipidus produce marked hypernatraemia and a dangerous degree of dehydration unless patients are reminded constantly of the need to drink.

Avoidance of overhydration or dehydration with corresponding changes in plasma sodium concentration is remarkably difficult in this situation of combined hypodipsia and ADH deficiency. Perhaps the best approach is to provide regular treatment with synthetic ADH (DDAVP, see below) while closely regulating fluid intake according to needs demonstrated in hospital by monitoring of daily weight, fluid intake, urine output, and plasma sodium or osmolality. Robertson has suggested a daily schedule for treatment of such patients, illustrated in Table 2.

In some patients with hypothalamic disease, osmoregulation of ADH release and of thirst is lost while volume regulation remains intact. Volume regulatory mechanisms are relatively insensitive requiring a change of 10 per cent or more in either direction to stimulate or inhibit ADH release. The clinical picture is then one of fluctuating plasma sodium concentration and osmolality, ranging in one reported case from 298 to 323 mosmol/kg.

A number of patients have been described in whom the threshold plasma osmolality required to stimulate ADH release and cause thirst are both increased. In this disorder of regulation rather than deficiency of ADH the new steady state of chronic hypernatraemia and hyperosmolality has been described as 'resetting of the osmostat'.

Differential diagnosis

The conditions associated with thirst, polydipsia, and polyuria which more or less resemble cerebral diabetes insipidus are shown in Table 3.

Table 1 Causes of secondary neurogenic diabetes insipidus

Trauma	Head injury
	Birth trauma
Iatrogenic	Pituitary surgery
	Yttrium–90 implantation
	Heavy particle irradiation
Tumour	Primary pituitary
	Secondary carcinoma (esp. lung, breast)
	Lymphoma
	Leukaemia
	Teratoma
	Ectopic pinealoma
	Craniopharyngioma
Granuloma	Sarcoid, eosinophilic granuloma, tuberculosis, brucellosis, syphilis
Infection	Pyogenic abscess
	Meningitis
	Encephalitis
Vascular	Haemorrhage/thrombosis
	Sheehan's syndrome
	Sickle cell haemoglobinopathy

Table 2 Typical schedule for management of a patient with adipsic hypernatremia*

Target weight: 70 kg			
Average minimum daily output			2000 ml
Source:	Renal	1000 ml	
	Extrarenal	1000 ml	
Standard daily prescribed intake			2000 ml
Source:	Food	1000 ml	
	Drink	1000 ml	

Daily adjustments for changes in weight

Weight (kg)	Adjustment (ml)	Total intake (including food)
Below target		
1 kg	+1000 ml	3000 ml
2 kg	+2000 ml	4000 ml
3 kg	+3000 ml	5000 ml
4 kg	+4000 ml	6000 ml
5 kg or more:	Contact physician	
Above target		
1 kg	−1000 ml	1000 ml
2 kg	−2000 ml	Dry food only
3 kg or more:	Contact physician	

* Reproduced from Robertson (1984). *Kid. Int.* **25**, 460, with permission.

Table 3 Thirst–polyuria syndromes

Neurogenic diabetes insipidus	
Drinking abnormalities	Psychogenic polydipsia
	Hypothalamic polydipsia
	Drug-induced (phenothiazines)
Renal resistance to ADH	Inherited nephrogenic diabetes insipidus
	Potassium depletion
	Hypercalcaemia
	Drugs (see Table 4)
Kidney diseases	Fanconi syndrome
	Nephronophthisis
	Analgesic nephropathy
	Postobstructive
	Hyperglobulinaemia
	Myeloma
	Sarcoid
	Sjögren's syndrome
	Amyloidosis
	SLE
	Sickle haemoglobinopathy
Solute diuresis	Diabetes mellitus
	Uraemia
	High protein feeding
	Hypertonic enemas

Psychogenic polydipsia

A number of clinical features help to distinguish the more common psychogenic polydipsia from true diabetes insipidus. The patient is often female, of middle age, and with other features of psychological illness. The onset of symptoms is less abrupt than in diabetes insipidus; drinking bouts alternate with more normal periods to produce a stuttering pattern. Drinking in established psychogenic polydipsia is erratic compared with the very constant pattern in diabetes insipidus, and nocturnal polyuria is often absent. This fluctuating water intake results in a fluctuating plasma osmolality which also tends to be lower (265–280 mosmol/kg) than in diabetes insipidus (290–295 mosmol/kg). Primary polydipsia may be a feature of patients with emotional disorder or frank psychosis, and in some such patients water intake may exceed 40 litres a day, with hyponatraemia and plasma osmolality falling as low as 240 mosmol/kg despite suppression of ADH release. Maximal free water clearance is around 12–15 ml/min but can reach as much as 30 litres per day. In some polydipsic patients, hyponatraemia is related to a resetting of the osmostat, such that ADH release occurs at lower plasma osmolality than normal. A number of drugs have been associated with hyponatraemia and water intoxication in patients with compulsive polydipsia including chlorpromazine, fluphenazine, thioridazine, and amitriptyline. Despite these reports hyponatraemia is rare in compulsive polydipsia provided renal function is intact.

Hypothalamic polydipsia

Extreme thirst and polydipsia without abnormality in ADH metabolism has been reported in sarcoidosis, eosinophilic granuloma, internal hydrocephalus, or after encephalitis affecting the anterior hypothalamus. One recent report suggests that primary thirst disorders are more common than abnormal ADH release in hypothalamic sarcoid.

Drug-induced polydipsia

As described above, a number of psychoactive drugs have been thought to cause overdrinking in susceptible subjects, but the diseases for which the drugs are used (schizophrenia for instance) are themselves associated with polydipsia. As well as thiothixene, fluphenazine, thioridazine, amitriptyline, and chlorpromazine, lithium carbonate has been described as an occasionally dipsogenic substance.

Nephrogenic diabetes insipidus

Familial nephrogenic diabetes insipidus is an extremely rare disorder presenting soon after birth with polyuria, fever, vomiting, dehydration, constipation, and failure to thrive. Urine cannot be concentrated above 100 mosmol/l and osmolality is not increased by ADH treatment. Plasma concentrations of endogenous ADH are high. Untreated, the disease leads to impaired mental and physical development. The bladder enlarges and hydronephrosis may occur. The disease is an X-linked recessive disorder. Only males are affected clinically. Female carriers can be shown to have impaired urinary concentration on formal testing. The cause of the disease is probably a genetic defect of the mechanism whereby ADH stimulates adenyl cyclase in the distal nephron. Early diagnosis and prompt treatment by high fluid intake and benzothiadiazine diuretics (see below) allows a good prognosis (see page 18.98).

Hypercalcaemia

Hypercalcaemic nephropathy is discussed on page 18.95. Impaired conservation of water by the kidney, resistant to ADH, and its analogues is due to defective sodium–potassium co-transport in the thick ascending limb of Henle's loop. The result is reduced renal medullary hypertonicity and therefore reduced water transport along a concentration gradient across collecting ducts. In addition hypercalcaemia also interferes with activation of adenyl cyclase by ADH. Chronic scarring of the interstitial tissue of the medulla may also contribute.

Hypokalaemia

Hypokalaemia (see pages 18.31 and 18.96) also causes nephrogenic diabetes insipidus by more than one mechanism. Sodium-potassium co-transport in Henle's loop and adenyl cyclase activation by ADH are impaired as in hypercalcaemic nephropathy, but in addition hypokalaemia is associated with increased renal synthesis of prostaglandins which antagonize the effect of ADH on the distal nephron. Protein kinase stimulation by cAMP within cells of the collecting duct is also inhibited.

Drug-induced nephrogenic diabetes insipidus

Table 4 lists the drugs which may induce nephrogenic diabetes insipidus. The most important of these are lithium carbonate and demethylchlortetracycline.

Lithium

Polyuria from lithium treatment is well recognized and occurs despite plasma concentrations within the therapeutic range. Some 40 per cent of treated patients develop thirst but urine volumes exceeding 3 litres per day are less common (12 per cent in one series). It is clear that in most affected patients the mechanism is that of lithium-induced nephrogenic diabetes insipidus with plasma ADH levels markedly raised in relation to urinary osmolality. Animal studies suggest that lithium impairs the formation and utilization of cAMP induced by ADH in the distal nephron. There have also been some reports of disordered ADH release in individuals taking lithium (cranial diabetes insipidus). Others suggest

Table 4 Drug-induced states of nephrogenic diabetes insipidus

Lithium carbonate*
Demethylchlortetracycline* (demeclocycline)
Amphotericin B
Methoxyfluorane anaesthesia
Propoxyphene
Glibenclamide
Outdated parenteral tetracycline
Gentamicin

* Used to treat the syndrome of inappropriate ADH secretion (SIADH).

lithium may stimulate hypothalamic thirst centres on occasion, and in some polyuric patients taking lithium, compulsive polydipsia is a feature of the affective disorder for which the drug has been prescribed.

In most patients with lithium-induced nephrogenic diabetes insipidus, polyuria improves within three weeks of withdrawal of the drug but in some the response is more sluggish and there is evidence of a more permanent defect in a few patients. Incomplete renal tubular acidosis has also been described as a renal complication of lithium therapy.

Demethylchlortetracycline

This long acting tetracycline produces a dose-dependent nephrogenic diabetes insipidus resulting from interference with ADH activation of adenyl cyclase and with cAMP-induced production of protein kinase in distal tubular cells. In doses of 600–1200 mg daily, this drug induces diabetes insipidus in some 5–8 days. The effects of the drug last some three weeks after withdrawal, suggesting binding to intracellular proteins. It has been used successfully to treat the syndrome of inappropriate ADH secretion, but its use in hyponatraemia complicating heart failure and liver cirrhosis may lead to undesirable increases in blood urea.

Diagnostic tests of suspected diabetes insipidus

Water deprivation with serial measurements of weight, plasma osmolality, urine volume, and osmolality and, if possible, immunoassay of plasma ADH remain the best tests for most cases. Patients should be deprived of fluids for periods of 6–18 hours depending on clinical features. If severe diabetes insipidus is likely, water deprivation overnight may be dangerous. If psychogenic polydipsia is suspected, fluid restriction might have to be prolonged beyond 18 hours. In the standard test fluids are withheld overnight after baseline measurements of weight and plasma osmolality. The following morning hourly measurements are taken of weight, urine volume, and osmolality until 5 per cent of body weight has been lost or until a constant figure in sequential measurements of urine osmolality is achieved. Plasma osmolality should be seen to increase above 290 mosmol/kg to be sure of an adequate stimulus for ADH release. An analogue of ADH is then given to assess the real tubular response and observations continued for a further 2 hours. In the United Kingdom desmopressin (dDAVP) 2–4 µg is given intramuscularly. Elsewhere aqueous vasopressin is still available and is given in a dose of 5 units subcutaneously. Results from one series are shown in Table 5. Difficulties in interpretation may arise in patients with partial diabetes insipidus, in those with abnormal thirst secondary to hypothalamic disease, and in psychogenic polydipsia. In these cases more prolonged water deprivation may be helpful, but measurements of plasma ADH levels in relation to urine and plasma osmolality after hypertonic saline challenge is the investigation of choice (see below).

Hypertonic saline infusion

Infusions of 5 per cent saline with serial measurements of plasma osmolality and ADH concentration is of particular value in

Table 5 Water deprivation followed by ADH

Diagnosis	Urine osmolality mosmol/kg (mean ± S.D.)	
	Dehydration	Change post-ADH
Hospital inpatients	760 ± 220	−60 ± 110
Cerebral DI		
Complete	170 ± 60	+280 ± 220
Incomplete	450 ± 130	+220 ± 40
Nephrogenic DI	120 ± 40	+50 ± 10
Psychogenic polydipsia	740 ± 120	+40 ± 50

Reproduced from Miller *et al.* (1970). *Ann. Int. Med.* **73**, 721.

patients with partial diabetes insipidus, in psychogenic polydipsia which is not clearcut clinically, or after the water deprivation test. Five per cent saline should be infused at a constant rate of 0.06 ml/kg/min for 2 hours, using a pump. Blood samples are taken at 20 min intervals for measurement of ADH and osmolality for 2 hours, and the urine volume and osmolality is monitored hourly. Plasma osmolality rises smoothly to some 305 mosmol/kg and a plot of plasma osmolality against ADH concentration identifies the osmotic threshold for ADH release and the relationships between osmotic stimulus and ADH response. The normal range and subnormal responses are illustrated in Fig. 3.

Treatment of diabetes insipidus

A number of analogues are available for replacement therapy in cranial diabetes insipidus.

dDAVP

dDAVP (1-desamino-8-D[1]-arginine vasopressin) is a synthetic preparation with greater antidiuretic and less pressor activity than the natural substance. It is most conveniently administered as a nasal spray. dDAVP, 5–20 µg allows 8–20 hours of antidiuresis in patients with complete lack of ADH. Smaller doses successfully control less severe disease. This is the drug of choice for chronic neurogenic diabetes insipidus.

Aqueous vasopressin

Subcutaneous injections of aqueous vasopressin 5–10 units reduce urine flow in neurogenic diabetes insipidus for 3–6 hours. This is the drug of choice for transient states such as occur after head injury or pituitary surgery. The short duration of action is particularly valuable in reducing the risk of cerebral oedema in an unconscious patient in whom recovery of ADH secretion is expected.

Lysine vasopressin

This preparation, given by nasal spray (50 IU/ml) controls urine volumes for some 4–6 hours but rarely lasts overnight. It is absorbed poorly when the nasal mucosa is congested and resistance may develop. The newer synthetic analogue dDAVP has largely supplanted this drug.

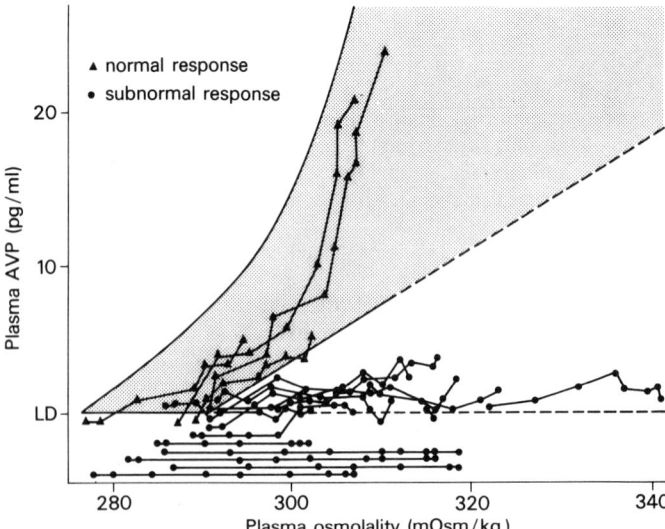

Fig. 3 Result of hypertonic saline infusion in 10 polyuric patients. The left panel shows normal response (shaded area represents normal range), and the right panel shows subnormal responses. (Reproduced from Baylis and Robertson, 1980, Plasma vasopressin response to hypertonic saline infusion to assess posterior pituitary function. *J. R. Soc. Med.* **73**, 255–260, by permission.)

Table 6 Miscellaneous drugs used in treatment of diabetes insipidus

Drug	ADH release	ADH action on tubules
Chlorpropamide	+	+
Biguanides	?	?
Clofibrate	+	–
Carbamazepine	+	–

Pitressin tannate in oil

This preparation is no longer available in the United Kingdom. It was the standard preparation for many years, and is still used in other parts of the world. It should be given in a dose of 2.5–5 units daily by intramuscular injection, or at longer intervals up to 72 hours. The ampoule should be warmed and thoroughly shaken before administration. Injection sites should be varied to prevent irregular absorption.

Benzothiadiazine diuretics

Thiazides probably reduce urine volume in *nephrogenic* diabetes insipidus by producing mild sodium depletion with resultant increased proximal tubular reabsorption and reduced delivery of sodium chloride to the ascending limb of Henle's loop where tubular fluid is diluted by reabsorption of salt without water. Thiazides are very effective treatment for nephrogenic diabetes insipidus, reducing urine volume from 6–10 litres per day to perhaps 2–4 litres. Efficacy is lost unless sodium intake is restricted.

Chlorpropamide

This can be a useful treatment for patients with partial cranial diabetes insipidus (Table 6). It appears to stimulate ADH release and to potentiate the actions of circulating ADH on the collecting ducts. Hypoglycaemia is an obvious risk, particularly dangerous in the elderly. Doses of 200–500 mg daily may be used. The effect of this drug is additive to that of thiazide diuretics or carbamazepine in cranial diabetes insipidus. It is of no value in nephrogenic disease. Tolbutamide is ineffective and glibenclamide enhances water excretion in patients with diabetes insipidus.

Phenformin and metformin

These have been shown to reduce urine volumes in hypokalaemic diabetes insipidus. The mechanism is uncertain.

Clofibrate

This appears to promote the release of ADH in patients with partial cranial diabetes insipidus. It is not useful in nephrogenic disease.

Carbamazepine

This also increases plasma ADH levels in patients with partial disease. It does not augment ADH at renal tubular level, nor is it effective in nephrogenic disease.

The effects of chlorpropamide, clofibrate, carbamazepine, and thiazide diuretics are additive. Only thiazides are effective in nephrogenic disease.

Indomethacin and other prostaglandin synthetase inhibitors

These also reduce urine volumes in diabetes insipidus, of both cranial and nephrogenic origin.

Hyponatraemia and hypernatraemia

HYPONATRAEMIA

A low concentration of sodium in plasma is not an uncommon finding in hospital practice. It is now most often associated with an excess of water without sodium deficit, although mild degrees of sodium depletion complicate the dilutional picture in some cases. More rarely, hyponatraemia results from primary salt deficiency with relative renal retention of water. Redistribution of water between cells and extracellular compartments is another cause. The condition of 'pseudohyponatraemia' may mislead clinicians in diagnosis and management.

Pseudohyponatraemia

Sodium concentration is measured in the laboratory in whole plasma, but sodium ions are present only in the aqueous phase. In conditions in which lipid components in plasma are greatly increased (e.g. diabetic ketosis or nephrotic syndrome) laboratory reports of hyponatraemia may simply reflect that increase, with the true plasma sodium concentration normal. Suspicion of pseudohyponatraemia can be confirmed by measurement of plasma osmolality (which is not affected) or by separate estimation of lipid concentrations. Paraproteinaemia with a massive increase of abnormal plasma protein concentration may occasionally cause pseudohyponatraemia, but is most unlikely to reduce the apparent sodium concentration below 130 mmol/l.

Hyponatraemia in sodium deficiency

Renal conservation of sodium is so efficient that the lowest of salt intakes alone is never enough to promote sodium depletion; there must be additional abnormal losses from gut or kidney or elsewhere.

Pathophysiology

Loss of sodium from the extracellular fluid leads initially to suppression of ADH secretion and an increase in free water clearance by the kidney. Osmolality is preserved at the expense of volume. More severe sodium deficits reduce renal perfusion and glomerular filtration; proximal tubular salt reabsorption is increased, with reduced delivery to the two diluting sites, impairing urinary dilution. Volume deficits of 10 per cent or more also stimulate ADH release and thirst by volume receptor pathways. Increased activity of the renin–angiotensin system may also stimulate thirst which, with the decreased renal excretion of free water, results in hyponatraemia, unless the sodium deficit is corrected. In this situation the diagnostic label sometimes used, 'syndrome of inappropriate ADH secretion (SIADH)' is clearly inaccurate, since the passage of a concentrated urine is entirely appropriate to the loss of volume, if not to the osmotic status of the patient. Hyponatraemia in this situation is the result of a very considerable deficit of sodium, in which the need for maintenance of volume overcomes the mechanisms normally controlling osmolar homeostasis.

Aetiology

The common sources of massive sodium losses are from the gut or the kidneys. Gastrointestinal losses from repeated vomiting, diarrhoea, or sequestration of fluid within the bowel are associated with major losses of potassium and alkalosis, or acidosis if there has been a bicarbonate loss. Renal salt loss is more occult, occurring particularly in the recovery phase of acute tubular necrosis, after relief of bilateral ureteric obstruction, and in conditions in which there are structural changes in medullary tissues, e.g. nephronophthisis, analgesic nephropathy, pyelonephritis or polycystic disease. Sodium depletion is a particular risk in patients with renal damage unable to conserve sodium normally, whose disease is accompanied by diarrhoea, vomiting or wrong advice to take a low salt diet. Abnormal losses of sodium may also be the result of overuse of potent diuretics and are to be expected in uncontrolled diabetes mellitus, and in the various syndromes of adrenocortical insufficiency (see page 10.76).

Clinical features

Sodium depletion should be diagnosed easily enough from the history in patients in whom the source of loss is the gastrointestinal tract, diabetes mellitus, or diuretic abuse. Sodium losses from intrinsic renal disease may be more difficult. Depletion sufficient to cause hyponatraemia, whatever the cause, is likely to produce the physical signs of reduced skin turgor and postural hypotension. There may be evidence of circulatory insufficiency with cold extremities, tachycardia, and venoconstriction. Simple investigations confirm the diagnosis; haematocrit, plasma proteins, blood urea, creatinine, and uric acid are raised. The urinary sodium concentration is less than 20 mmol/l and usually nearer 5 mmol/l provided renal function is normal.

Management

Increased dietary salt may suffice to correct the deficit in relatively healthy patients who can eat normally. More commonly, intravenous replacement by infusion of 0.9 per cent sodium chloride is required. In ill patients with threatened renal perfusion, replacement should be rapid with the insertion of a right atrial line to monitor central venous pressure in those with suspect cardiac function. Potassium supplements will be necessary in patients in whom there have been major gastrointestinal losses, but should be given with caution until the renal response to volume replacement is known to be satisfactory.

Hyponatraemia due to water excess

Pathophysiology

Dilutional hyponatraemia results from an intake of fluid which exceeds the maximal rate at which the kidneys can excrete it. Fluid can be ingested or administered so fast that the normal kidney cannot keep pace; more often the problem arises because of an impairment in renal water excretion. The capacity of the kidney to dilute urine depends on the glomerular filtration rate (GFR); an adequate delivery of sodium to the diluting sites in Henle's loop and distal tubules; normal function of the two diluting sites, and absence of circulating ADH. Dilutional hyponatraemia should still not arise despite abnormalities in each or all of these factors unless the intake of fluid is excessive for the maintenance of normal volume and osmolality of extracellular fluid. In some cases thirst is abnormal, in others the over-high intake of fluid is iatrogenic.

Dilutional hyponatraemia with normal renal function

The normal adult kidney excretes free water at a maximal rate of 10–20 ml/min, but massive amounts of water may be drunk by patients with acute psychoses, with psychogenic polydipsia, and in some with anterior hypothalamic disease. Acute hyponatraemia may also occur in some beer drinkers who manage to take in as much as 11–17 litres (20–30 pints) daily, much of that in a period of a few hours (beer drinkers' potomania).

Dilutional hyponatraemia with impaired water excretion

Aetiology

Overgenerous intravenous 5 per cent glucose given to patients after surgery is one of the commonest causes of a low plasma sodium in hospital practice. In acute renal failure with oliguria some degree of dilutional hyponatraemia is common and may become serious if fluid intake is not restricted.

The problem is less in chronic renal failure but bad advice to 'push fluids' is all too common a cause of hyponatraemia in patients in whom creatinine clearance is below 20 ml/min.

Dilutional hyponatraemia is also a common feature of severe heart failure and of cirrhosis of the liver and nephrotic syndrome. The mechanism is probably multifactoral. In each of these GFR is reduced and proximal tubular sodium reabsorption increased. There is, therefore, a much reduced delivery of sodium chloride to the ascending limb of Henle's loop and the distal tubules resulting in a marked reduction in the kidney's capacity to excrete free water. This is aggravated by high plasma levels of ADH, inappropriate to plasma osmolality and perhaps in response to volume stimuli. Thirst in these conditions may also be inappropriate. Suggestions that this may be secondary to high plasma angiotensin

II concentrations gain support from reports of restoration of more normal plasma sodium values in some (but not all) patients treated with the angiotensin-converting enzyme inhibitors captopril or enalapril.

The 'loop' diuretics frusemide, ethacrynic acid, and bumetanide inhibit sodium–potassium co-transport in the ascending limb of Henle's loop (diluting site 1). Thiazides inhibit sodium transport in the distal tubule (site 2). Both classes of diuretic therefore impair urinary dilution and both stimulate renin activity and increase in plasma angiotensin II which is likely to stimulate ADH release and perhaps thirst as well, so that fluid intake may exceed excretory capacity. Adrenal insufficiency and isolated hypoaldosteronism induce hyponatraemia by a variety of mechanisms, including reduced renal perfusion, defective tubular reabsorption of sodium in the distal nephron, reduced extracellular fluid volume, and continued secretion of ADH despite hypotonicity of plasma.

Dilutional hyponatraemia may also be seen in hypothyroidism. The inability of the kidneys to excrete free water normally in this condition may relate to reports of increased plasma ADH concentrations despite hyponatraemia.

Plasma sodium concentrations fall in pregnancy and there is evidence not only of volume expansion in this state, but also of a fall in the plasma osmotic threshold for ADH release (reset osmostat).

Syndrome of inappropriate ADH secretion (SIADH)

There are some patients for which this is a useful description of their disorder. ADH secretion despite hypotonicity and normal or expanded extracellular fluid volume *is* inappropriate (see page 18.25). The resulting hyponatraemia depends mainly on the high ADH levels, but also reflects continued water intake which is also inappropriate to osmolality. In some patients there is evidence of inappropriate thirst as well as ADH secretion, and in them water deprivation to increase plasma sodium is difficult to achieve and is accompanied by extreme thirst. In others hyponatraemia is the result of inappropriate ADH secretion and habitual social drinking. The causes of truly inappropriate ADH secretion are shown in Table 7. Most important among them are the malignant disorders, chest infections, and disturbances of central nervous function. Oat cell carcinoma of the bronchus is the commonest tumour to secrete ADH apparently identical in structure to endogenous ADH. Neurophysin has also been identified in tumour cells. Ectopic production of ADH is not the only mechanism by which tumours may be associated with dilutional hyponatraemia. In some cases the ADH excess is related to a marked fall in osmotic threshold for both thirst and ADH secretion from the neurohypophysis rather than the tumour itself. Hyponatraemia due to resetting of the osmostat has also been described in various nonmalignant conditions.

Of the drugs associated with inappropriate ADH secretion, the most common and important are chlorpropamide, carbamazepine, vincristine, and cyclophosphamide.

Clinical features of SIADH

The clinician is alerted to the possible diagnosis by hyponatraemia associated or not with neurological consequences. Confirmation of diagnosis requires that both renal and adrenal functions are normal and that there is evidence of hypervolaemia rather than hypovolaemia or hypotension which might reflect sodium depletion. The demonstration of hypotonicity of plasma and urinary osmolality exceeding that of plasma is not enough on its own. Evidence is needed of volume expansion, and this is best reflected by the urinary sodium excretion. In true SIADH urinary sodium concentration always exceeds 20 mmol/l and often 50 mmol/l, whereas in sodium depletion much lower values are to be expected unless renal function is abnormal. Haematocrit and plasma protein concentrations tend to be low in SIADH and blood urea, creatinine,

Table 7 True inappropriate ADH secretion (SIADH)

1	Malignant disease	
	Carcinoma	Lung (oat-cell), pancreas, duodenum thymus, prostate, adrenal, ureter, colon, nasopharynx
	Lymphoma/leukaemia	Hodgkin's, non-Hodgkin's, acute myeloid leukaemia
2	Nervous system	Meningitis, cerebral abscess, encephalitis, stroke, subarachnoid haemorrhage, vasculitis (SLE), head injury, subdural haematoma, Guillain-Barré, peripheral neuritis, central pontine myelinosis
3	Chest	Pneumonia, tuberculosis, lung abscess, aspergillosis, cystic fibrosis, intermittent positive pressure ventilation
4	Psychiatric	Schizophrenia, acute psychosis
5	Metabolic	Acute intermittent porphyria, trauma, 'ill' patients
6	Drugs	Chlorpropamide, carbamazepine, amitriptyline, desipramine, tranylcypromine, fluphenazine, indomethacin, cyclophosphamide, vincristine, opiates, barbiturates, oxytocin, bromocriptine
7	Surgery	After the second week of transsphenoidal pituitary surgery

and uric acid concentrations are also low, with increased fractional excretion of uric acid and phosphate.

Adrenal failure should always be carefully considered in the differential diagnosis but is usually obvious from clinical features, hyperkalaemia, and acidosis. The diagnosis is usually clinched by measurements of plasma cortisol before and after ACTH stimulation (see page 10.76), but isolated hypoaldosteronism is more difficult to exclude without measurements of plasma or urinary aldosterone. Hypothyroidism is not always clinically obvious but can be excluded by measurements of T_4 and TSH.

The hyponatraemia may be a symptomless laboratory finding, or may produce symptoms ranging from lassitude and anorexia to headache, confusion, muscle twitching, coma, and fits.

Treatment of SIADH

For many years water restriction has been imposed on patients with chronic hyponatraemia. The treatment is unpleasant. It should not be given to patients without symptoms, and is not always effective in those who do have symptoms. If the underlying cause cannot be removed (withdrawal of drugs inducing ADH release, treatment of infection in the chest or nervous system, removal of tumours or chemotherapy) and symptoms are persistent, lithium carbonate or demethylchlortetracycline have been used to antagonize the effects of ADH on the distal tubules. Demethylchlortetracycline is the better drug and should be given in a dose of 600–1200 mg daily. Its effects on the kidney are usually evident within a few days and reverse some three weeks after stopping treatment.

Frusemide and other loop agents interfere with tubular reabsorption of sodium and chloride in Henle's loop and thus impair urinary concentration. Chronic frusemide treatment, given with sodium supplements to maintain volume, may be effective in patients who cannot tolerate demethylchlortetracycline or water restriction. Oral urea 30–60 g daily has also been reported to increase free water clearance and raise plasma sodium concentrations by way of osmotic diuresis in patients with SIADH.

Water intoxication and oxytocin

Severe and dangerous water intoxication may follow oxytocin infusions given to women with a variety of obstetric problems, most commonly in a prolonged attempt to empty the uterus in missed abortion or mid-trimester termination of pregnancy. Hyponatraemia is the consequence of the antidiuretic effect of oxytocin itself, of an antidiuretic effect of pethidine and morphine which are often used for analgesia, and of the high volume of 5 per cent glucose in which the oxytocin is commonly given. More than 3.5 l of fluid have been given in each case reported in the literature.

Symptoms and treatment of water intoxication

Symptoms of water intoxication are unlikely until the plasma sodium concentration falls below 120 mmol/l. At and below that level the clinical picture depends on the rate at which water overload has developed with the most severe consequences following a rapid fall in osmolality. Confusion and headache are common early symptoms to be followed by coma and fits. These phenomena are likely to be caused by a combination of cerebral oedema and a fall in intracellular potassium concentration. Treatment is best undertaken with intravenous hypertonic saline (5 per cent) infused at a rate of 0.05 ml/kg/min with concurrent frusemide or other loop diuretic. Such an infusion has been shown to increase plasma osmolality by some 12–15 mosmol/kg and sodium by some 7 mmol/l over 2 hours. The aim should be to bring the plasma sodium up to 125 mmol/l. More rapid infusion than this carries risks which include heart failure, subdural haemorrhage, and central pontine myelinosis due to tortional stresses in response to variable water shifts in different parts of the brain. However, 50 ml of 29.2 per cent saline delivered through a central venous catheter over 10 min has been given successfully in patients with acute hyponatraemia sufficient to induce epileptiform seizures. The place of dexamethasone in the treatment of cerebral oedema caused by water intoxication is unclear.

Hyponatraemia due to fluid shifts

Hyperglycaemia, by producing an osmotic gradient between extracellular and intracellular fluid, will tend to draw water out of cells and thus induce hyponatraemia. Because glucose enters brain cells rapidly this fluid shift is not accompanied by significant change in ADH secretion or thirst. Hyperglycaemia is a common cause of hyponatraemia in hospital practice and was the cause of nearly 20 per cent of cases in a recent series. Intravenous mannitol also causes fluid shifts, but in this case associated with an increase in ADH and thirst since mannitol does not enter osmoreceptor cells in the brain.

The sick cell syndrome

Some terminally ill malnourished patients suffering from pulmonary tuberculosis, malignancy or profound cardiac, renal or hepatic failure may be found to have symptomless hyponatraemia (plasma sodium 120–130 mmol/l) without evidence of sodium depletion or water excess. Early reports emphasized a depletion of total body potassium and invoked the concept of 'sick' cell membranes with a resultant shift of sodium from extracellular to intracellular fluid. This is not a diagnosis to make with frequency or confidence but the syndrome may be a true entity. Infusions of hypertonic saline in such cases do not improve the patient's clinical state, and renal responses to increased or reduced sodium intake are appropriate around the new lower sodium concentration. Reports of improvement from potassium loading are difficult to substantiate.

HYPERNATRAEMIA

Pathophysiology

An increase in plasma sodium concentration is most commonly due to massive depletion of water, exceeding that of sodium. A true excess of sodium is rare and is always iatrogenic. There must be a component of deficient water intake in patients with hypernatraemia.

Loss of water from the extracellular fluid, by increasing osmolality, results in transfer of water from the relatively hypotonic intracellular compartment to the extracellular fluid. Water loss from plasma is 'buffered', therefore, and losses sufficient to cause hypernatraemia must be massive, since only some 10 per cent of the deficit is borne by the plasma volume. The morbid effects of intracellular dehydration are found largely in the brain, and of extracellular dehydration in a tendency towards venous or arterial thrombosis in young children.

Aetiology

Deficient water intake

The common reasons for grossly inadequate fluid intake are that the patient has no access to fluid, or is confused or comatose. Infants and unconscious patients are at particular risk as are the elderly sick. The recent demonstration that thirst (although not ADH secretion) is deficient in healthy old people is important, although hypernatraemia must be prevented in most of them by habitual social drinking. More rarely the problem lies in a lesion of the anterior hypothalamus interfering with normal thirst. In any of these situations an additional diabetes insipidus adds greatly to the risk.

Water loss

Gastrointestinal

Gastrointestinal fluids are hypotonic to plasma so that unreplaced losses from vomiting or diarrhoea result in hypernatraemia. Diarrhoea is a particular risk in neonates and infants.

Skin and lungs

Sweat sodium concentration varies between 50 and 100 mmol/l. Litres of hypotonic fluid can be lost rapidly from skin and lungs in hot, dry climates particularly if exercise is strenuous or underlying illness has caused high fever. Infants are particularly prone to develop hypernatraemia because of their large surface area in relation to body fluid volumes.

Weeping skin lesions are occasionally sources of significant losses of water, and in burns involving a large proportion of the body surface area, hypernatraemia is a common complication.

Kidney

Losses of water from the kidney in sufficient amounts to threaten hypernatraemia are likely in only two situations: in diabetes insipidus, cranial or nephrogenic, and in the presence of solute diuresis. Glucose in urine in uncontrolled diabetes mellitus inhibits proximal tubular sodium reabsorption. The increased delivery of chloride and sodium to the distal nephron enhances free water clearance even in the presence of ADH. Water losses exceed those of sodium by a considerable amount. Similar mechanisms underlie renal water losses in uraemia and in mannitol-induced diuresis. Hypernatraemia in unconscious patients used to be common when tube feeds contained a gross excess of protein and insufficient water. The products of protein catabolism induced solute diuresis and water losses causing hypernatraemia, particularly in the neurosurgical wards. The problem is still seen occasionally in hypercatabolic patients whose rate of urea production is much increased.

Excess of sodium

Plasma sodium concentrations are at or just above the upper limit of normal in some patients with primary aldosteronism, and less commonly in Cushing's syndrome. The precise cause is unknown in both disorders although there is some evidence that changes in volume of extracellular fluid may increase the osmotic threshold for ADH release and perhaps thirst too.

Greater rises in plasma sodium concentration due to true excess of sodium are always iatrogenic. The causes include overgenerous replacement of hypertonic salt solutions in hyponatraemic states, or of bicarbonate in the treatment of cardiac arrest or other causes

of lactic acidosis. Disasters have occurred when salt is added to milk for infant feeding in mistake for sugar. Infant feeding with high solute milk (National Dried Milk in the United Kingdom), which has a higher content of protein and salt than breast milk, may contribute to hypernatraemia both by excess salt intake and solute diuresis. Other ways in which excess salt can be introduced include the use of saline enemas, emetics, and inadvertent introduction of 5 per cent saline into the circulation during uterine administration to induce abortion. Hypernatraemia may complicate haemodialysis or peritoneal dialysis when concentrated dialysate solutions are incorrectly proportioned with water.

Essential hypernatraemia

Essential hypernatraemia has been used as a term to describe an altered relationship between osmolality or volume and ADH release. When the osmotic threshold is 'reset' as a result of hypothalamic disease, there may be a true reset of the threshold at a higher level of osmolality. A variant of this syndrome is the loss of osmolar control with intact control by volume receptors. In this situation ADH release is not stimulated until a 10 per cent or more contraction of volume has occurred, a state of affairs characteristically associated with a fluctuating hypernatraemia.

Pathophysiology of hypernatraemia and clinical signs

Hypernatraemia is particularly dangerous when the change is acute. In dehydrated infants it may cause venous or arterial thrombosis. The brunt of the damage otherwise falls on the brain. Despite protection against cerebral dehydration afforded by the build-up of unknown osmotically active solutes in the brain tissue during prolonged hyperosmolar states, particularly in hyperglycaemia, the physical contraction of brain cells results in shifts which may result in the rupture of vessels and petechial haemorrhage, subdural, subarachnoid, and intracerebral haemorrhage.

Thirst is less prominent than would be expected even in conscious subjects. Neurological changes include lethargy, drowsiness, muscle twitching, and coma.

Treatment

The aim of treatment should be the *gradual* correction of the hyperosmolar state. Fluid should be given by mouth whenever possible, but intravenous infusions are usually necessary. Hypotonic solutions are often advocated, but since the aim is *gradual* correction, normal saline at a concentration of 150 mmol/l may be more suitable when plasma sodium exceeds 170 mmol/l. The precise rate at which to infuse fluids is a matter of debate but full correction in a period of *not less than* 48 hours is a good rule. Not more than one-third of the excess of sodium concentration should be reduced in the first 8 hours. Overrapid infusion of hypotonic solutions may induce cerebral oedema in place of dehydration when the risk of aggravating any tendency whereby fluid shifts promote haemorrhage.

References

Arieff, A. I. and Guisado, R. (1976). Effects on the central nervous system of hypernatraemic and hyponatraemic states. *Kid. Int.* **10**, 104–116.

Ayus, J. C., Krothapalli, R. K. and Arieff, A. I. (1985). Changing concepts in treatment of severe symptomatic hyponatremia: rapid correction and possible relations to central pontine myelinosis. *Am. J. Med.* **78**, 897–902.

Baran, D. and Hutchinson, T. A. (1984). Outcome of hyponatraemia in a general hospital population. *Clin. Nephrol.* **22**, 72–76.

Beil, T. (1984). Water metabolism. *Sem. Nephrol.* **4**, 287–362.

De Rubertis, F. R., Michelis, M. F. and Davis, B. B. (1974). 'Essential' hypernatraemia. *Arch. Int. Med.* **134**, 889–895.

Dousa, T. P. and Valtin, H. (1976). Cellular actions of vasopressin in the mammalian kidney. *Kid. Int.* **10**, 46–63.

Forest, J. N., Cox, M., Hong, C., Morrison, G., Bia, M. and Singer, I. (1978). Superiority of demeclocycline over lithium in the treatment of the chronic syndrome of inappropriate secretion of antidiuretic hormone. *N. Engl. J. Med.* **298**, 173–177.

Hays, R. M. (1976). Antidiuretic hormone. *N. Engl. J. Med.* **295**, 659–665.

Herbert, S. C., Friedman, P. A., Culpepper, R. M. and Andreoli, T. E. (1982). Salt absorption in the thick ascending limb of Henle's loop: NaCl cotransport mechanisms. *Sem. Nephrol.* **2**, 316–327.

Kirkland, J. L., Pearson, D. J., Goddard, C. and Davies, J. (1983). Polyuria and inappropriate secretion of arginine vasopressin in hypothalamic sarcoidosis. *J. Clin. Endocrinol. Metab.* **56**, 269–272.

Lancet (1986). Atrial natriuretic peptide. *Lancet* ii, 371–372.

Leaf, A. (1984). Dehydration in the elderly. *N. Engl. J. Med.* **311**, 791–792.

Levine, S. D. and Schlordorff, D. (1984). Role of calcium in the action of vasopressin. *Sem. Nephrol.* **4**, 144–158.

Liard, J. F. (1984). Vasopressin in cardiovascular control: role of circulating vasopressin. *Clin. Sci.* **67**, 473–481.

Lifshitz, M. D. and Stein, J. H. (1983). Hormonal regulation of salt excretion. *Sem. Nephrol.* **3**, 196–204.

Maack, T., Camargo, M. J. F., Kleinert, H. D., Laragh, J. H. and Atlas, S. A. (1985). Atrial natriuretic factor: Structure and functional properties. *Kid. Int.* **27**, 607–615.

Morgan, D. B., Penney, M. D., Hullin, R. P., Thomas, T. H. and Srinivasan, D. P. (1982). The response to water deprivation in lithium treated patients with and without polydipsia. *Clin. Sci.* **63**, 549–554.

Robertson, G. L. (1983). Thirst and vasopressin function in normal and disordered states of water balance. *J. Lab. Clin. Med.* **101**, 351–371.

—— (1984). Abnormalities of thirst regulation. *Kid. Int.* **25**, 460–469.

Rolls, B. J., Wood, R. J. and Rolls, E. T. (1980). Thirst: the initiation maintenance and termination of drinking. In *Progress in psychology and physiological psychology* Vol. 9 (eds J. M. Sorague and A. N. Epstein), p. 263. Academic Press, New York.

Schrier, R. W. (1985).Treatment of hyponatraemia. *N. Engl. J. Med.* **312**, 1121–1122.

Singer, I. and Forrest, J. N. (1976). Drug-induced states of nephrogenic diabetes insipidus. *Kid. Int.* **10**, 82–95.

Wade, J. B. (1985). Membrane structural studies of the action of vasopressin. *Fed. Proc.* **44**, 2687–2692.

Zerbe, R. L. and Robertson, G. L. (1983). Osmoregulation of thirst and vasopressin secretion in human subjects: effects of various solutes. *Am. J. Physiol.* **244**, E. 607–614.

Idiopathic oedema of women

J. G. G. LEDINGHAM

Fluid retention unrelated to cardiac, hepatic, renal, allergic, hypoproteinaemic, obstructive venous, or lymphatic disease, and occurring in the absence of sodium-retaining drugs occurs not uncommonly in women and has been labelled idiopathic oedema, cyclical oedema, or periodic oedema. The first is the best name, since in only a proportion of cases is the condition truly cyclical. There is no clear relationship between this condition and premenstrual tension.

Clinical features

The cardinal features are of episodic or more constant fluid retention, aggravated by standing, with diurnal weight fluctuations exceeding 1.4 kg/day and day-to-day weight changes sometimes as much as 4–5 kg. During periods of weight gain, urine volumes may be as low as 300–500 ml/24 hours, containing minimal amounts (1–20 mmol/l) of sodium. The retained fluid accumulates in the face, hands, breasts, thighs, buttocks, and tissues of the abdominal wall. Rings do not fit over the swollen fingers and the expansion in waist and breast measurements results in some sufferers keeping two sizes of brassiere and girdle. Pitting ankle oedema is uncommon but may be observed after prolonged standing. Orthopnoea and pulmonary oedema are rare complications. Constipation is common. Episodes of fluid retention or of exacerbation of a more chronic state may occur unpredictably, but emotional stress, obesity, food high in carbohydrate, as well as prolonged standing, are recognized triggers.

The condition occurs only after menarche, is seen more often in the third and fourth decade but may persist with amennorrhoea, after oophorectomy, and may continue after the menopause. Sufferers are characteristically emotionally labile, prone to neurosis and depression. Extreme physical and mental lethargy are usual and the patient's misery during periods of retention is aggravated by the sense of bloated ugliness and distortion of appearance that she feels. Most, but not all, patients have found access to diuretics when first seen in hospital practice. Hypokalaemic hypochloraemic alkalosis with hyperuricaemia may reflect diuretic abuse, and rare patients abuse purgatives as well.

Pathophysiology

There is no strong consensus of opinion about pathophysiology. It may be that this is a heterogeneous condition. Certainly there is a subset of women in whom overconcern with weight and appearance leads to diuretic abuse and rebound oedema when diuretics are stopped, as described by de Wardener. Some of this group have features in common with anorexia nervosa. Whilst diuretic abuse may be an aggravating factor in some women and the primary factor in others, it cannot be the whole story since cases were described before potent diuretics became available and because withdrawal of diuretics in hospital over two to three weeks reverses the condition in only a few patients.

No good evidence exists of *primary* abnormalities in the renin–angiotensin–aldosterone system, nor in the metabolism of oestrogens or progestogens. Hyperprolactinaemia, dopamine deficiency and high plasma adenosine monophosphate have been described in a few cases, but it is unlikely that these changes are of aetiological significance in many patients. There is evidence of an orthostatic leak of plasma volume and plasma proteins into the tissue fluids in women subject to idiopathic oedema. The increase in venous blood haematocrit on standing is greater than normal, and reflects a fall in plasma volume which initiates renal salt and water retention, probably through enhanced proximal tubular reabsorption since there is a fall in fractional free water clearance and osmolar clearance. The renal response is then entirely *appropriate* to changes in plasma volume. Diurnal weight gains amounting to 4–5 kg must reflect an abnormally high fluid intake during periods of fluid retention, perhaps because of thirst stimulated by volume receptors. The mechanism of the presumed increase in capillary permeability is unknown, but could relate to abnormal arteriolar regulation of capillary hydrostatic pressures.

The distribution of oedema is an odd feature of this disorder, if it is indeed due to an abnormality of capillary permeability however caused. Such an abnormality would explain the aggravation of fluid retention on standing and its relief by lying flat, but does not explain why fluid is so predominantly distributed in face, breasts, fingers, abdomen, and thighs, while ankle oedema of the kind seen in nephrotic states, for instance, is remarkably rare.

Management

Sympathetic explanation of the nature of the problem helps management. Patients should be advised to avoid long periods of standing and to use supine rest to relieve oedema instead of diuretics whenever possible. Elastic stockings, put on before getting up, help to reduce the orthostatic loss of plasma volume. Clothes fitting tightly around the waist may aggravate the condition by increasing venous pressure in the legs and should be avoided. Obesity increases the tendency to fluid retention and some women associate exacerbation with an increase in dietary carbohydrate. Diuretics, by further decreasing an already reduced plasma volume, are an illogical treatment and should be used as sparingly as possible; but most patients' symptoms are unacceptable without some diuretic treatment. Resistance develops quickly and many patients are very difficult to wean from massive doses of loop agents, often combined with amiloride or spironolactone. Psychotherapy may help the neurotic and depressive traits but is of no proven benefit in reducing the frequency or severity of episodes of oedema.

Drugs have little to offer in this condition. Among those that have been tried occasional success has been reported with L-dopa, combined with carbidopa, bromocriptine, and most recently the tricyclic drug nomifensine but all must be considered of unproven value.

References
de Wardener, H. E. (1981). Idiopathic edema: role of diuretic abuse. *Kid. Int.* **19**, 881–892.

Edwards, O. M. and Bayliss, R. I. S. (1976). Idiopathic oedema of women. *Q. J. Med.* **45**, 125–144.

Gill, J. R. (1983). Idiopathic edema. *Sem. Nephol.* **3**, 205–210.

Disorders of potassium metabolism

J. G. G. LEDINGHAM

Hypokalaemia and hyperkalaemia

Physiological considerations

Potassium, the chief intracellular anion, is present in cells in a concentration near 160 mmol/l; 98 per cent of total body potassium is intracellular. The ratio of intracellular to extracellular potassium is a critical determinant of the membrane potential of excitable tissues. The passage of potassium into cells and its retention there against a concentration gradient requires the activity of the Na/K ATPase enzyme.

The plasma potassium concentration depends on intake, excretion and the distribution between extracellular and intracellular fluids. Dietary potassium intake commonly varies between 80 and 150 mmol daily. In normal circumstances the kidney is the only important route of excretion, with only some 5–15 mmol appearing daily in the stools. Plasma potassium concentration is regulated by homeostatic mechanisms controlling *internal* as well as *external* balance. External balance, which determines total body potassium, is largely controlled by the kidney with a small but sometimes important contribution by the gut. Internal balance determines the proportion of intracellular and extracellular potassium under the influence of pH, aldosterone, insulin, and the adrenergic nervous system.

Internal balance

pH and bicarbonate

The ratio of intracellular to extracellular potassium appears to be influenced by pH and plasma bicarbonate concentrations separately, with a rise in either increasing intracellular at the expense of extracellular potassium. The hyperkalaemia of acidosis has long been attributed to an exchange of hydrogen ions for potassium in cells. In most clinical states of acidosis, there is hyperkalaemia or a high plasma potassium concentration in relation to external balance; but hyperkalaemia is not a feature of postictal lactic acidosis, nor does infusion of organic acids (as opposed to mineral acids) in dogs induce hyperkalaemia. The reasons for these observations are not clear but it may be that potassium shifts are not induced in organic acidaemic states when the origin of the excess acid is intracellular.

Aldosterone

A rise in plasma potassium stimulates aldosterone secretion and a fall retards it. Although the major contribution of aldosterone in protecting against hyperkalaemia is to increase renal and to a much lesser extent colonic potassium excretion, it is possible that aldosterone also affects internal potassium balance. The adrenal gland is known to be essential for the phenomenon whereby acute

potassium loads are taken up by cells in animals accustomed to high potassium diet ('potassium adaptation') but more direct evidence for increased cellular uptake of potassium under the influence of aldosterone is lacking. One mechanism of potassium adaptation is by an increase in the activity of cell membrane Na/K ATPase in response to major increases in dietary intake.

Insulin

An increase in plasma potassium stimulates insulin release which might be expected to induce a net uptake of potassium into cells. High concentrations of insulin given intravenously certainly lower plasma potassium by promoting uptake into the liver and muscle. The much lower concentrations of endogenous insulin have not yet been proven to influence internal potassium balance significantly, but it may be that the larger amounts present in portal vein blood influence potassium uptake by the liver. Tolerance of potassium loads is impaired in insulin-deficient diabetes and in normal subjects infused with somatostatin, suggesting at least a permissive role for insulin in the regulation of cellular uptake of potassium.

The adrenergic nervous system

The rise in plasma potassium concentrations resulting from an infusion of potassium chloride is increased in the presence of the non-selective beta-adrenergic blocking drug propranolol or of the alpha agonist phenylephrine. Adrenaline infusions induce hypokalaemia by increasing potassium flux into skeletal muscle by beta-2 activation of membrane-bound adenylate cyclase and subsequent stimulation of Na/K ATPase. Sympathetic nervous discharge may also promote a shift in potassium from extra to intracellular fluid since tolerance of intravenous potassium is reduced in animals which have been chemically sympathectomized. Heavy muscular exercise results in loss of potassium from muscle to extracellular fluid and plasma concentrations can rise as much as 50 per cent after 10–15 min, falling precipitously in the postexercise period. Beta-blocking drugs exaggerate the hyperkalaemia of exercise while phentolamine reduces it. Adrenergic agonists are well recognized to promote hypokalaemia, particularly the beta-2 selective agents such as salbutamol and terbutamine. Theophylline derivations also induce the entry of potassium into cells and it has been suggested that one reason for sudden death in asthmatics may be a hypokalaemia-associated dysrhythmia induced by high endrogenous adrenaline and the use of salbutamol and theophylline derivatives together.

Plasma concentrations of adrenaline may rise to levels known to promote hypokalaemia after the pain and anxiety of myocardial infarction and it is not surprising that there are increasing reports of hypokalaemia in patients in coronary care units who have not yet been treated with potassium-losing diuretics. The hypokalaemia which may complicate delirium tremens after alcohol withdrawal is likely also to be beta-adrenergically mediated.

Non-selective beta-blockings drugs may increase plasma potassium significantly in some patients with chronic renal failure, or with insulin-deficient diabetes mellitus.

External balance

External potassium balance is regulated mainly by the kidney with a small contribution by the gastrointestinal tract in health. The colon can be an important route of potassium excretion in renal failure.

Renal control of external potassium balance

The classical concepts of renal tubular handling of potassium have changed in recent years and are in a complex state, but the ultimate control of urinary potassium excretion is still believed to lie in the mechanisms of potassium secretion in the distal nephron.

Proximal tubular reabsorption is at least in part an active process and appears complete by the end of the proximal segment. Potassium then re-enters tubular fluid in the pars recta and descending limb of Henle's loop to be reabsorbed in the ascending limb by Na/K co-transport. Potassium present in the descending limb may come from reabsorption in the collecting ducts via medullary tissue, thereby contributing to medullary hypertonicity by a recycling process.

In the early distal tubule there are mechanisms of active transport of potassium into cells on both the peritubular and luminal surfaces. Movement of potassium into tubular urine at this site is dependent on electrical and chemical gradients and is therefore passive. The luminal concentration of sodium and the nature of its accompanying anion are important factors in controlling these gradients.

Further down the nephron in the cortical collecting ducts potassium transport into tubular fluid is active, not strictly linked to sodium reabsorption but in some way dependant on intraluminal sodium concentration and the rate of flow of tubular fluid. Further secretion of potassium may occur in the medullary collecting ducts under conditions of metabolic alkalosis, solute diuresis, potassium loading, and facilitated by antidiuretic hormone (ADH).

A number of factors influence distal nephron potassium secretion and determine the rate of potassium excretion in urine.

Potassium adaptation
A chronic high potassium intake enhances potassium secretion probably by increasing intracellular uptake at the peritubular surface of the cells of the distal nephron. This strictly renal mechanism which increases the intracellular transport pool of potassium is enhanced by the hyperaldosteronism caused by potassium loading.

Sodium delivery to the distal nephron
Any condition which increases sodium delivery to the distal nephron (e.g. loop diuretics, osmotic diuretics, or salt loading) enhances urinary potassium excretion. The precise mechanisms by which this phenomenon occurs are not clear but relate to sodium concentration and tubular flow rate in the distal tubules.

Aldosterone
Mineralocorticoids enhance sodium reabsorption and potassium secretion in the distal tubules, probably by increasing the permeability of the luminal cell membranes and by increasing active transport of potassium across the peritubular membranes into the distal tubular cells.

pH changes
The effects of acidosis and alkalosis on *internal* potassium involve renal tubular cells so that there is an increase in intracellular potassium and therefore enhanced distal tubular potassium loss in alkalosis and the reverse in acidosis. In addition, the mechanism whereby potassium and hydrogen may exchange one for the other favours renal potassium wasting in alkalosis and retention in acidosis.

Flow rates of tubular fluid
There is good evidence from micropuncture studies that increased rates of flow in distal tubular fluid enhance potassium secretion in potassium replete but not deplete animals.

Antidiuretic hormone (ADH)
A significant stimulation of distal tubular potassium secretion by ADH suggests that this hormone may help to prevent potassium retention and hyperkalaemia in oliguria secondary to dehydration.

Hypokalaemia

Severe hypokalaemia (plasma potassium less than 2.4 mmol/l) occurred in 1 per cent of patients admitted to hospital in one recent series. Malignant disease, especially acute myeloid leukaemia, was a surprisingly frequent association attributed in some cases to the sodium load given with massive doses of carbenicillin or penicillin. These and other causes of hypokalaemia are listed in Table 1. Dietary deficiency alone is an uncommon cause but a high intake may prevent or a low one exacerbate changes in internal or external balance.

Pathophysiological effects of hypokalaemia
Marked potassium wasting impairs muscle function with weakness sometimes progressing to paralysis, absent reflexes, and on occasion acute rhabdomyolysis, particularly after exercise. The smooth muscle of the gut is also affected with reduced motility or frank ileus complicating hypokalaemia. The force of myocardial contraction is increased *in vitro* when the bath fluid potassium concentration is low, but in *in vivo* hypokalaemia may be associated with cardiac failure. Myocardial excitability is increased with hyperpolarization of membrane potentials and digitalis toxicity is enhanced. Arrhythmias associated with hypokalaemia include atrial tachycardia with block, atrioventricular dissociation, ventricular tachycardia or fibrillation.

The effects of hypokalaemia on the kidney include nephrogenic diabetes insipidus, a fall in glomerular filtration rate, and a tendency towards sodium retention. Failure to concentrate urine appears to be related to a reduction in medullary solute concentration as well as to resistance to ADH secondary to renal overproduction of prostaglandins. The mechanism whereby a low potassium diet results in renal sodium retention and sometimes oedema are not understood.

Chronic hypokalaemia is associated with morphological changes in the kidney, and the appearance of vacuoles in both proximal and distal tubular cells. Although it is often claimed that prolonged potassium deficiency causes irreversible and progressive renal damage, there is no good evidence that this is so.

Potassium deficiency *per se* is popularly supposed to result in metabolic alkalosis. The assumption is probably true but difficult to prove since in most clinical states of hypokalaemia there are usually other factors to consider. Deficits of up to 200 mmol of potassium alone do not induce alkalosis in normal subjects under experimental conditions.

Potassium deficiency with hypokalaemia also impairs renal tubular reabsorption of phosphate, with resultant hypophosphataemia being an occasional finding.

There are commonly no symptoms of hypokalaemia in otherwise healthy subjects. Muscle weakness or paralysis are features of

Table 1 Causes of hypokalaemia

1 Intracellular shifts	
Alkalosis	Theophylline overdose
High dose insulin	Periodic paralysis
Beta-2 adrenergic stimulation	? Aldosterone
2 Renal wasting	
Alkalosis (metabolic and	
respiratory)	Cushing's syndrome
Diuretics	Adrenogenital syndromes
Solute diuresis	Bartter's syndrome
Glucose	Liddle's disease
Urea	Magnesium depletion
Mannitol	Carbenoxolone sodium
Saline	Liquorice addiction
Carbenicillin	Renal tubular acidosis
Penicillin	Ureterosigmoidostomy
Aldosteronism	Gentamicin
Primary	Amikacin
Secondary	Acute leukaemia
Renin secreting tumours	
3 Gastrointestinal	
Pyloric stenosis	Chloride-diarrhoea
Bulimia nervosa	Villous adenoma of the rectum
Ileostomy	Purgative abuse

extreme depletion, but may affect respiratory muscles. In surgical wards the commonest manifestation is of paralytic ileus. The polyuria and polydipsia described as a result of poor renal water conservation due to potassium depletion are again relatively rare and late features. Paraesthesiae and in very rare cases tetany have also been described.

Specific syndromes of hypokalaemia

Gastrointestinal

Vomiting

The concentration of potassium in gastric and upper intestinal secretions varies between 5 and 10 mmol/l, so that direct losses in vomitus contribute only partially to potassium deficiency. Major losses of chloride and gastric acid result in hypochloraemic alkalosis, which induces a renal potassium leak. This, together with the shift of potassium from the extracellular to the intracellular fluid spaces, is largely responsible for the hypokalaemia. Patients with pyloric stenosis may present with deficits of sodium and potassium exceeding 500 mmol, of chloride rather more, and of water in excess of 5 l. In such extreme cases with massive chloride depletion the urine may be 'paradoxically' acid despite profound metabolic alkalosis. The excretion of an alkaline urine is not possible then until the chloride deficit is reduced by rapid intravenous infusion of sodium chloride with added supplements of potassium chloride.

Covert vomiting is a cardinal feature of bulimia nervosa which may in many respects resemble Bartter's syndrome (*vide infra*).

Diarrhoea

There is more potassium (50–100 mmol/l) in liquid stools than in vomitus so that potassium deficiency from diarrhoea does not require an additional renal leak. Any condition in which stool volumes are high may cause hypokalaemia (e.g. cholera or enteritis caused by *Escherichia coli*). A villous adenoma of the colon or rectum may result in profound hypokalaemia believed to be due to disturbance of ion transport in the colonic mucosa mediated by the tumour. Similar disturbances underlie the hypokalaemia of patients with non-insulin secreting islet cell tumours (Verner–Morrison syndrome, see Section 12). More common than these rarities is laxative abuse in which hypokalaemia is usual. Ureterosigmoidostomy may lead to profound hypokalaemia if urine is allowed to remain stagnant in the colon and is not evacuated regularly.

Renal

Diuretics

(See page 13.98.) All diuretics other than those acting directly on the distal tubules (amiloride, triamterene, and spironolactone) tend to increase urinary potassium excretion in an amount dependent on the dose, the natriuretic response, and the degree of prevailing secondary hyperaldosteronism. Hypokalaemia may or may not occur. It is most commonly observed early in treatment and potassium concentrations seldom fall below 3.0 mmol/l. In an analysis of published data, the average fall after treatment with benzothiadiazones or chlorthalidone was 0.69 mmol/l. In some 48 per cent of treated patients a level below 3.5 mmol/l was described. The tendency to hypokalaemia can be minimized by using the minimal effective dose, avoiding the longer acting agents (e.g. chlorthalidone) reducing sodium intake and using potassium-retaining diuretic–thiazide combinations. The need to prescribe potassium supplements routinely or not has been much debated. Risks of hypokalaemia are of cardiac arrhythmias and enhancement of digoxin toxicity. In the longer term, impairment of carbohydrate tolerance is a recognized problem related to an impaired insulin secretory response to hyperglycaemia rather than insulin resistance. An excellent correlation between total body potassium and impairment of insulin secretion has been described. On the other hand most patients with modest hypokalaemia come to no

particular harm and potassium supplements are variably absorbed, a nuisance to take, and can on very rare occasions cause jejunal ulceration and stricture formation. Most physicians would prescribe supplements of the chloride in patients who are prone to cardiac arrhythmias and in patients with severe liver disease in whom electrolyte imbalance may precipitate encephalopathy.

Bartter's syndrome

The first description of the syndrome which now bears his name was made by Bartter in 1962. Two Negro patients aged 5 and 25 years were reported, in whom there was profound hypokalaemic alkalosis, pitressin-resistant diabetes insipidus, secondary aldosteronism without hypertension, resistance to the pressor effects of angiotensin II, and hypertrophy and hyperplasia of the juxtaglomerular apparatus of the kidneys. Since then, many further cases have been described, more in children than in adults, but presenting at any age from the neonatal period to the opposite extreme of life. Reports of the disorder in siblings and in the first generation of children of consanguinious parents have been taken to suggest an occasional autosomal recessive inheritance, but most cases are not familial. Disorders of red cell cation transport have been described in Bartter's patients and in otherwise unaffected relatives (see below). The sexes are probably equally susceptible and evidence that the syndrome may be more common in Blacks than in other races is inconclusive.

Clinical findings

There is considerable heterogeneity in clinical and biochemical features which reflects the heterogeneity of causative mechanisms. In some patients the condition may be asymptomatic, with biochemical abnormalities detected by chance. At the other extreme there are marked features of hypokalaemia, including muscle weakness, polydipsia, polyuria, tetany, fits, vomiting, and in young children marked stunting of growth. While the cardinal features of the disorder are hypokalaemic alkalosis with urinary potassium wasting and a normal or marginally low arterial pressure, a proportion of cases show additional abnormalities including hyponatraemia, hypophosphataemia (with or without rickets), hypercalciuria, hypercalcaemia, nephrocalcinosis, hypomagnesaemia, and hyperuricaemia. Blood urea and plasma creatinine are usually normal. Urinary potassium wasting is a contrast feature and losses may exceed the filtered load, reaching amounts as high as 400–600 mmol/24 hours in rare patients. Plasma renin activity and angiotensin II levels are high, as is aldosterone secretion, unless retarded by profound hypokalaemia.

Renal histology

A variety of abnormalities of renal histology have been described, including, apart from juxtaglomerular cell hyperplasia, some examples of hypercellularity of glomeruli, periglomerular fibrosis, arteriolar sclerosis, and chronic interstitial nephritis. Primary renal damage may in some cases coincide with Bartter's syndrome if not be its underlying cause. Medullary interstitial cell hyperplasia, first observed by Verbeckmoes, is not now considered a feature confined to true Bartter's patients.

Theories of pathogenesis

Theories continue to abound, and none has yet found general acceptance. Bartter's original hypothesis was of a primary lack of response to angiotensin II by arteriolar smooth muscle, but pressor insensitivity to angiotensin II is now known to be a feature of any patient with persistent high renin activity because of a reduced number or avidity of vascular receptors for angiotensin II. Pressor insensitivity to noradrenaline is also a non-specific feature. Profound falls of arterial pressure in Bartter patients given saralasin (angiotensin II antagonist) or captopril (converting enzyme inhibitor) indicate the inaccuracy of the original idea and the important contribution made by angiotensin to the maintenance of blood pressure in these patients. Recently strong support has been given to the concept of disordered chloride transport in the ascending limb of Henle's loop, or of sodium in the distal nephron; but sodium can be conserved normally in most cases and indirect methods of assessing tubular function in Henle's loop or the distal nephron using free water clearance under conditions of water loading cannot be considered conclusive.

A variety of different abnormalities in cation transport have been described in the red cells of Bartter patients and their otherwise unaffected first degree relatives, resulting in increased sodium and decreased potassium concentration in their erythrocytes. But the inconsistencies in the abnormalities described and reports of similar phenomena in disorders as disparate as essential hypertension and thyrotoxicosis make these findings difficult to interpret. A report that changes in erythrocyte sodium transport can be reversed by correction of hypokalaemia adds to uncertainty in this area.

A number of different observations indicate overproduction of prostaglandins (PG) as one of the major if not primary features of the syndrome. Plasma PGA concentrations and urinary PGE_2, 6-keto $PFG_{1\alpha}$, kallekrein, and bradykinin are increased. Renal interstitial cells, a site of PG synthesis in the medulla are hyperplastic. Abnormalities of platelet aggregation appear to be caused by a circulating prostaglandin or a PG metabolite. Clinical and biochemical abnormalities are improved by treatment with prostaglandin-synthetase inhibitors and platelet function can be restored to normal. But overproduction of prostaglandins is now recognized to be a secondary phenomenon which occurs in any condition of profound and prolonged potassium depletion.

If the postulated defect in sodium chloride transport in the ascending limb of Henle's group is not proven it is the most widely quoted hypothesis, and its acceptance is implicit in recommended methods of differential diagnosis.

Differential diagnosis

Primary renal tubular disorders such as cystinosis can present as Bartter's syndrome. Laxative and diuretic abuse, together with vomiting produce all the features, including urinary potassium wasting if alkalosis or potassium depletion are extreme. Urinary chloride estimations will detect covert vomiting as occurs in bulimia nervosa. In that condition, in purgative abuse and in the 'rebound' chloride retaining state *after* diuretic abuse, urinary chloride on a high chloride intake is as low as 1–3 mmol/24 hours. Indexing of urinary chloride loss by GFR and free water clearance has been shown in the Bartter's syndrome to indicate an *increase* in fractional chloride excretion together with a reduction in maximal free water clearance.

Diuretic abuse mimics Bartter's syndrome precisely but can be detected by urinary assays for benzothiadiazines or loop agents. Villous adenoma of the rectum, renal tubular acidosis, chronic pyloric stenosis, and the effects of liquorice or carbenoxolone sodium are more easily detected but the diagnosis of a proximal tubulopathy of familial origin presents more difficulty. In this syndrome described in four siblings in 1983 all the classical features of Bartter's syndrome were present, but fractional delivery of solute and ascending limb reabsorption of chloride was normal. Paradoxically, although histological changes were prominent in proximal tubules (without change in juxtaglomerular cells) physiological changes were thought to be distal tubular.

Treatment

In some asymptomatic patients with mild biochemical disturbance, an increase in dietary potassium and supplements of potassium chloride (150–200 mmol/day) may suffice. Others can be improved by the addition of spironolactone, amiloride, or triamterene. Propranolol has been advocated to reduce the activity of the renin–angiotensin–aldosterone system, but in severe cases, particularly in children with stunted growth, prostaglandin synthetase inhibitors should be prescribed. There is most experience with indomethacin which should be given in a dose up to 2 mg/kg per day. Secondary aldosteronism is always improved, but some degree of hypokalaemia usually persists. Remarkable improvement in clinical features can be expected.

Other causes of renal potassium wasting

In primary aldosteronism hypokalaemia is more severe in adenoma than in hyperplasia (see page 13.390). Secondary hyperaldosteronism with hypokalaemia may complicate malignant hypertension, renal artery stenosis and the fluid retention of heart failure, cirrhosis of the liver, and nephrotic syndrome treated by diuretic agents. Cushing's syndrome may be associated with renal potassium wasting, especially if caused by carcinoma of the adrenal cortex or to by a non-endocrine tumour. Adrenogenital syndromes due to 11β-hydroxylase or 17α-hydroxylase deficiency result in hypokalaemia due to overproduction of deoxycorticosterone. Renin-secreting tumours increase urinary potassium loss by stimulating hyperaldosteronism. Liquorice consumed in large amounts or carbenoxolone sodium prescribed for peptic ulcer have aldosterone-like effects on renal tubules and may, as a result, induce hypokalaemia and hypertension. Renal tubular acidosis is discussed on page 18.171.

Liddle's syndrome

Hypokalaemia in this rare syndrome is accompanied by hypertension, but with a low aldosterone secretion. The condition may be caused by increased sodium–potassium exchange in the distal renal tubules, and both hypertension and hypokalaemia respond to triamterene treatment.

The effects of amiloride in this condition are unknown, but there is no response to spironolactone. It is possible that this syndrome and 11β-hydroxysteroid dehydrogenase deficiency are the same.

11β-hydroxysteroid dehydrogenase deficiency

A number of children with hypertension, hypokalaemia, and suppression of both renin and aldosterone have now been described. In them a defect of the peripheral metabolism of cortisol has been detected. The hypertension and hypokalaemia are worsened by hydrocortisone therapy. It is suggested that impaired metabolism of cortisol prolongs its half-life and allows it to act as a mineralocorticoid. Spironolactone improves both hypertension and hypokalaemia in these patients (see page 13.392).

Acute leukaemias

Renal potassium wasting and hypokalaemia may complicate acute myeloid, monocytic, and myelomonocytic leukaemias. Increased urinary lysozyme excretion either causing or reflecting renal tubular damage is found in many but not all cases.

In some cases gentamicin or amikacin renal tubular damage may be the cause (*vide infra*) and in others there is avid membrane activity in the leukaemic cells which take up potassium from plasma after venesection.

Antimicrobials

Amphotericin B, gentamicin, and amikacin may cause renal tubular damage leading on occasion to urinary potassium wasting and hypokalaemia.

Hypokalaemic periodic paralysis

In this rare condition, episodes of muscle weakness or paralysis lasting up to 24 or even 72 hours occur sporadically or at more regular intervals. In most cases there is a family history reflecting a Mendelian dominant inheritance. Symptoms first appear late in the first or in the second decade. Attacks appear to be caused by a shift in potassium from the extracellular to the intracellular fluid with profound hypokalaemia, although on occasion the plasma potassium can be normal. Precipitating factors may include rest after severe exercise, large carbohydrate meals, tension, and anxiety. Attacks may also occur during sleep with the patient awaking weak or paralysed. Histological changes in affected muscles include vacuolation and sometimes evidence of damage to myofibrils.

The mechanism of the disease is not known, but attacks can be provoked by administration of glucose and insulin, and prevented by diazoxide which blocks insulin release. Long-term treatment by diazoxide is considered to be too toxic for use in this condition.

A number of other treatments have been recommended including potassium supplements, spironolactone, amiloride, and propranolol or other non-selective beta-adrenergic blocking drugs. Acetazolamide or ammonium chloride may also prevent attacks by inducing extracellular fluid acidosis, but their long-term use may be associated with nephrocalcinosis.

A very similar hypokalaemia syndrome may complicate thyrotoxicosis particularly in oriental races (see page 10.48). This variant of the condition is always corrected by reversal of the hyperthyroidism.

Treatment of hypokalaemia

In most conditions in which oral potassium supplements are required there is an associated alkalosis making bicarbonate or citrate salts of little value. Potassium chloride can be given as an elixir but it is more acceptable embedded in a wax medium (Slow K). Enteric coated potassium chloride preparations cause occasional ulceration and stricture formation in the jejunum and should be avoided.

Indications for rapid elevation of plasma potassium by parenteral infusion are few, but include hypokalaemic cardiac arrhythmias, paralysis, and hypokalaemic diabetic keto-acidosis. In every case care should be taken to assess the adequacy of renal function. No rule is absolute, but it is rarely wise to infuse potassium in a concentration exceeding 40 mmol/l, at a rate exceeding 40 mmol/hour or 200 mmol/day. Care must be taken to monitor plasma levels closely, particularly in patients treated at these or faster rates.

Hyperkalaemia

Hyperkalaemia is less common than hypokalaemia but more dangerous. Very rarely, hyperkalaemic patients may complain of muscle weakness, but cardiac arrest is the only likely clinical manifestation. Diagnosis depends, therefore, on clinical suspicion, on measurement of potassium in plasma, and on the electrocardiogram.

The more important causes of hyperkalaemia are listed in Table 2. A recent report records hyperkalaemia in 406 of 29 000 patients

Table 2 Causes of hyperkalaemia

1 Excessive intake

2 Impaired renal excretion
Acute renal failure	Isolated hypoaldosteronism
Chronic renal failure	Renal tubular disorders
Potassium retaining diuretics	Treatment with angiotensin converting enzyme inhibitors
Adrenal insufficiency	

3 Changes in internal balance
Acidosis	Hyperkalaemic periodic paralysis
Crush injuries, burns, rhabdomyolysis	Succinyl choline
	Digoxin poisoning
Massive death of tumour cells	Familial hyperkalaemic acidosis

4 Pseudohyperkalaemia
    Haemolysed blood sample
    Leukaemia with very high
       white cell counts
    Familial pseudohyperkalaemia

admitted to a teaching hospital in one year. Renal dysfunction was present in 43 per cent of these and in 37 per cent hyperkalaemia was due to treatment (potassium supplement or potassium retaining diuretics).

Excessive intake

Examples of hyperkalaemia due to excessive intake of potassium by mouth in healthy people are rare but have been described after overdosage with slow-release potassium preparations (Navidrex K, Neonaclex K, and Slow K). Hyperkalaemia of dietary origin is a common enough problem in the presence of renal failure, and may complicate mineralocorticoid deficiency, or the inappropriate prescription of potassium-retaining diuretics. Parenteral infusion of potassium may cause dangerous hyperkalaemia if rates of infusion exceed 20 mmol/hour, or concentrations of potassium exceed 40 mmol/l, or less in the presence of renal insufficiency. There is a particular risk of hyperkalaemia if patients with impaired renal function are transfused with stored blood, or treated with large doses of potassium salts of penicillin.

Acute renal failure

Hyperkalaemia is to be expected in any case of acute renal failure (see page 18.129), especially when the condition is associated with muscle injury, tissue necrosis, gastrointestinal bleeding, or severe infection. The excess potassium is derived only partly from the diet, sometimes from unwise infusion of crystalloid or stored blood, from catabolism and necrosis of cells, and from intracellular stores in the presence of acidosis.

Chronic renal failure

Hyperkalaemia is rarely a problem in chronic renal failure (see page 18.136) until the glomerular filtration rate falls below 15–20ml/min. At lower levels of function, plasma potassium can usually be maintained at normal or near normal concentration by restriction in dietary intake, treatment of acidosis, and avoidance of potassium-retaining diuretics. The adaptive mechanism whereby potassium excretion per nephron is increased in chronic renal failure appears to involve increased activity of Na/K ATPase in the distal nephron. A similar change in colonic mucosa may contribute to increased faecal excretion of potassium in renal failure, and animal studies suggest an increased capacity of the intracellular space to take up potassium by a mechanism which requires the presence of the adrenal cortex, but does not depend on increased secretion rates of glucocorticoid or mineralocorticoid.

Pseudohyperkalaemia

Samples in which plasma or serum have not been promptly separated from red cells will contain excessive amounts of potassium derived from leakage out of red cells after venesection. This problem is well known and easily circumvented. Less common and less known is the pseudohyperkalaemia associated with leukaemias when the total white cell count is so high that leakage from white and red cells together induce pseudohyperkalaemia in a few minutes after venesection.

The usual cause of pseudohyperkalaemia is that blood samples have been taken some distance away from the laboratory. The red cells and plasma have then not been separated for many hours and the resulting leak of potassium from red cells does result in a falsely elevated plasma potassium. Haemolysed samples of course also show hyperkalaemia without long storage. In addtion to these well-recognized problems, occasional patients are seen with myeloproliferative disorders and very high white cell counts in whom the high plasma potassium derives from leakage in vitro from white cells in unseparated blood samples. Another cause of pseudohyperkalaemia is so-called 'familial pseudohyperkalaemia', a condition which may be familial with an autosomal dominant inheritance of abnormal cation transport across red cell membranes. The prime feature of this condition is that there is an abnormal net efflux of potassium from red cells stored over 2–6 hours at room temperature. The leak can be prevented by storing the cells at 37 °C rather than at room temperature. Radioisotope cation studies *in vitro* show a decreased temperature sensitivity by the 'passive leak' transport mechanism for potassium, accounting for the potassium leak at low temperatures. The blood film of these patients may show a few target cells and there is evidence of a mild compensated haemolytic state.

Potassium retaining diuretics
Large doses of amiloride or triamterene (and to a lesser degree of spironolactone) may cause severe hyperkalaemia, even in healthy people with normal renal function. These drugs are particularly to be avoided in renal failure.

Adrenal insufficiency
Addison's disease (see page 10.76) is commonly associated with modest hyperkalaemia (plasma potassium 5.0–6.5 mmol/l), hyponatraemia, and a rise in blood urea. Other clinical features are likely to suggest the diagnosis, which is commonly further investigated by measurements of cortisol and its response to stimulation of the cortex by synthetic ACTH (see page 10.78). This approach is satisfactory enough in most cases but will miss the diagnosis of isolated hypoaldosteronism, a condition which may occur more frequently than is currently recognized (see below).

Angiotensin-converting enzyme inhibitors
These agents (captopril and enalapril) are used in the treatment of hypertension and to reduce afterload in congestive heart failure. The fall in angiotensin II concentrations induced by these drugs results in a much reduced aldosterone secretion (at least in the short term) and low plasma and urinary aldosterone. Some elevation of plasma potassium occurs but severe hyperkalaemia (K>6.0 mmol/l) is only likely when ACE inhibitors are given to patients with creatinine clearance less than 20 ml/min.

Isolated hypoaldosteronism
The commonest cause of *chronic* hyperkalaemia without severe renal failure is probably hyporeninaemic hypoaldosteronism. The condition is caused by a relative or absolute deficiency of aldosterone. In many cases plasma renin activity is low and unresponsive to the erect posture and sodium depletion; in others there is evidence of an acquired enzymatic defect rate in the biosynthetic pathway of aldosterone, perhaps related to low plasma concentrations or antiotensin II. In this context, the response of aldosterone secretion to potassium infusion is reduced by captopril treatment. Aldosterone concentrations may be 'normal' or low but can be considered reduced in every case when indexed by the plasma potassium concentration (hyperkalaemia being normally a very potent stimulus to aldosterone secretion). Glucocorticoid metabolism in these patients is normal.

Clinical features
Patients are usually over the age of 60 years, although younger cases have been described. Vascular and ischaemic heart disease are common. Some 50 per cent of patients have been diabetic and 70 per cent have evidence of renal disease, most commonly some form of chronic interstitial nephritis, with modest impairment of glomerular filtration rate. Symptoms may include muscle weakness, but in most cases hyperkalaemia with hyperchloraemic acidosis is detected during laboratory investigation, or the disorder declares itself more dramatically with episodes of hyperkalaemia heart block, or cardiac arrest often precipitated by vomiting or diarrhoea which tends to reduce sodium delivery and flow in the distal tubules and thus reduce renal potassium excretion. A similar course of events may follow discontinuation of potent diuretics previously overgenerously prescribed. Blood pressure is normal or even high.

The associations of this disorder with old age, diabetes, and renal disease may reflect the decreasing activity of the renin–angiotensin system with age, reduced sensitivity of the renal stretch receptors with increasing rigidity of anteriolar walls, insulin deficiency, and autonomic neuropathy.

The condition should be suspected in any patient with hyperkalaemia without other obvious explanation. Investigation is complex and requires measurements of renin activity and plasma aldosterone in response to sodium deprivation, with assessment in addition of the aldosterone response to infusions of angiotensin and ACTH.

Cyclosporin treatment
In some patients treated by cyclosporin after renal transplantation hyperkalaemia (serum potassium 6.0–7.1 mmol/l) and acidosis may occur quite disproportionate to glomerular filtration rate and dietary intake. This condition is probably another variant of hyporeninaemic hypoaldosteronism and responds to treatment by fludrocortisone (*vide infra*).

Treatment
Most patients with hypoaldosteronism respond well to replacement therapy of 0.1–0.2 mg daily of fludrocortisone, but doses as high as 0.4 or even 1.0 mg may be needed to reduce potassium concentration to normal, often at the cost of inducing oedema, hypertension, or cardiac failure. The failure of normal replacement doses to correct hypokalaemia indicates a renal tubular component to the disease in some patients. In those in whom mineralocorticoids alone do not suffice, the combination of 9α-fluoro-hydrocortisone with a benzothiadiazine diuretic may be successful. Supplements of sodium bicarbonate may correct acidosis and facilitate renal potassium excretion.

Renal tubular disorders
Hyperkalaemia with impaired renal excretion of potassium may be a feature of any cause of renal tubular acidosis (see page 10.171). Much more rare are the conditions of type I and type II pseudohypoaldosteronism. In type I disease, hyperkalaemia of renal origin is associated with salt wasting and hypotension, features absent from type II cases. In neither condition is there evidence of aldosterone deficiency and in neither does mineralocorticoid in high dosage correct hyperkalaemia (in contrast to true hypoaldosteronism). Type I disease may be due to a specific defect in the renal tubular response to mineralocorticoid. In type II disease in which there is hyperkalaemia and hyperchloraemic acidosis, hypertension and suppression of plasma renin activity, there is evidence that the primary abnormality is increased chloride and thereby sodium reabsorption in Henle's loop. This, by limiting sodium delivery to the distal tubules, impairs secretion of both potassium and hydrogen ions. Potassium clearance in type II disease is not increased by mineralocorticoid nor by sodium loading, but can be corrected by the infusion of non-reabsorbable anions in the form of sodium sulphate.

Hyperkalaemic periodic paralysis
Even more rare than hypokalaemic periodic paralysis, this disease is familial with an autosomal dominant mode of inheritance. Attacks of paralysis begin in the first decade of life, usually precipitated by rest after exercise, when pronounced hyperkalaemia is associated with a flaccid paralysis lasting from a few minutes to several hours. Bulbar muscles may be involved. Myotonia may be a striking feature and can be demonstrated by McArdle's sign. Established attacks can be reversed by salbutamol inhalation but treatment is best given prophylactically by use of benzothiadiazine diuretics of fludrocortisone. Both are effective.

Succinyl choline
Agents that depolarize muscle membranes increase plasma potassium by some 0.5 mmol/l in healthy subjects. In patients already at risk of hyperkalaemia because of renal failure, complicating burns, crush injuries, or other hypercatabolic states, the rise after

muscle relaxants may be much greater and should be considered when such patients need general anaesthesia.

Digitalis

Severe hyperkalaemia may occur in patients who have taken an overdose of digitalis, presumably secondary to loss of intracellular potassium, following massive inhibition of Na/K ATPase.

Treatment of hyperkalaemia

Concentrations of potassium exceeding 7.0 mmol/l constitute a medical emergency. ECG abnormalities in order of severity include tenting of T waves, diminution or absence of P waves, widening of the QRS complex, slurring of the ST segment into the T waves, and a sine wave pattern immediately preceding cardiac arrest (see page 18.129).

If ECG changes are absent or involve only changes in P and T waves, intravenous glucose (50 g) and insulin (10–20 units soluble or actrapid) will lower plasma potassium by approximately 1.0 mmol/l within 30 min, the effect persisting some 1 to 2 hours; 50–100 ml 4.2 per cent sodium bicarbonate increases intracellular at the expense of extracellular potassium and is particularly effective when hyperkalaemia and acidosis are combined.

When the ECG changes are more advanced, with widening of the QRS complexes, intravenous 10 per cent calcium gluconate should be given over 2 to 5 min in whatever dose (usually 10–30 ml) is required to correct the ECG. The beneficial effects of calcium salts are evident within 2 min of infusion of infusion but are short-lived.

A combination of calcium gluconate, glucose and insulin, and hypertonic bicarbonate provides control of hyperkalaemia for 2 to 3 hours and can be supplemented when necessary by haemodialysis, peritoneal dialysis, or by cation exchange resins in the calcium or sodium phase. These agents in a dose of 15–20 g three or four times daily can be given by mouth or as a retention enema. Constipation, or worse, faecal impaction, may be avoided by adding 10–30 ml of a 70 per cent solution of sorbitol with each dose. Exchange resins begin to exert an effect on external potassium balance in some 1 or 2 hours.

References

Adu, D., Michael, J., Turney, J. and McMaster. P. (1983). Hyperkalaemia in cyclosporin-treated renal allograft recipients. *Lancet* ii, 370–372.

Carmine, Z., Ettore, B., Guiseppe, C. and Quirino, M. (1982). The renal tubular defect of Bartter's syndrome. *Nephron* 32, 140–148.

DeFronzo, R. A. (1980). Hyperkalaemia and hyporeninaemic hypoaldosteronism. *Kid. Int.* 17, 118–134.

Delaney, V. B., Oliver, J. F., Simms, M., Costello, J. and Bourke, E. (1981). Bartter's syndrome: physiological and pharmacological studies. *Q. J. Med.* 50, 213–232.

Epstein, F. H. and Rosa, R. M. (1983). Adrenergic control of serum potassium. *N. Engl. J. Med.* 309, 1450–1451.

Glassock, R. J., Goldstone, D. A., Goldstone, R. and Hsuch, W. A. (1983). Diabetes mellitus, moderate renal insufficiency and hyperkalaemia. *Am. J. Nephrol.* 3, 233–240.

Kaplan, N. M. (1984). Our appropriate concern about hypokalaemia. *Am. J. Med.* 77, 1–3.

Kokka, J. P. (1985). Primary acquired hypoaldsteronism. *Kidney Inter.* 27, 690–702.

Korff, J. M., Siebens, A. W. and Gill, J. R. (1984). Correction of hypokalaemia corrects the abnormalities in erythrocyte sodium transport in Bartter's syndrome. *J. clin. Invest.* 74, 1724–1729.

Kunau, R. T. and Stein, J. H. (1977). Disorders of hypo and hyperkalaemia. *Clin. Nephrol.* 7, 173–190.

Lancet (1981). Hypokalaemic periodic paralysis. *Lancet* i, 1140–1141.

Lancet (1983). Adrenaline and potassium: Everything in flux. *Lancet* ii, 1401–1403.

Layzer, R. B. I. (1982). Periodic paralysis and the sodium potassium pump. *Ann. Neurol.* II, 547–552.

Licht, J. H., Amundson, D., Hsuch, W. A. and Lombardo, J. V. (1985). Familial hyperkalaemic acidosis. *Q. J. Med.* 54, 161–176.

Medical Research Council Working Party on Mild to Moderate Hypertension (1983). Ventricular extrasystoles during thiazide treatment; substudy of MRC mild hypertension trial. *Br. Med. J.* 287, 1249–1253.

Morgan, D. B. and Davidson, C. (1980). Hypokalaemia and diuretics: an analysis of publications. *Br. Med. J.* 280, 905–908.

Oberfeld, S. E., Levine, L. S., Carey, R. M., Greig, F., Mick, S. and New, M. I. (1983). Metabolic and blood pressure responses to hydrocortisone in the syndrome or apparent mineralocorticoid excess. *J. clin. Endocrinol.* 56, 332–339.

Schamerlan, M., Sebastian, A. and Rector, F. C. (1981). Mineralocorticoid-resistant renal hyperkalaemia without salt wasting (type II pseudo-hypoaldosteronism). Role of increased renal chloride reabsorption. *Kid. Int.* 19, 716–727.

Stewart, G. W., Corrall, R. F. M., Fyffe, J. W., Stockdill, G. and Strong, J. A. (1979). Familial pseudohyperkalaemia. *Lancet* ii, 175–177.

Sufit, C. R. and Jamison, R. L. (1982). Potassium recycling in the renal medulla and newer aspects of potassium transport. *Sem. Nephrol.* 2, 328–335.

Veldhuis, J. D. (1983). The many faces of hypokalaemia. *Arch. int. Med.* 143, 1521–1522.

Whang, R., Flink, E. B., Dyckner, T., Wester, P. O. and Ryan, M. P. (1985). Magnesium depletion as a cause of refractory potassium repletion. *Arch. intern. Med* 145, 1686–1689.

Williams, F. A., Schambelan, M., Biglieu, E. G. and Care, R. M. (1983). Acquired primary hypoaldosteronism due to isolated zone glomerulosa defect. *N. Engl. J. Med.* 309, 1623–1627.

Ypersele de Strihou, C. van (1977). Potassium homeostasis in renal failure. *Kid. Int.* II, 491–504.

GLOMERULONEPHRITIS AND RENAL MANIFESTATIONS OF SYSTEMIC DISEASE

D. G. WILLIAMS AND D. K. PETERS

GLOMERULONEPHRITIS

Introduction

Glomerulonephritis is a major cause of morbidity and death from kidney disease, accounting for over one-third of patients with terminal renal failure requiring dialysis or transplantation. Effective treatment or prevention would contribute greatly to the health of the community and reduce the considerable and escalating costs associated with treatment of these patients. It is recognized that many forms of nephritis reflect disturbances in immune function and more precise delineation of these has played a general role in the understanding of immune-mediated disease.

Classification

The aetiology of nephritis is usually unknown. Although accumulation of immune complexes in renal tissues appear to be responsible in most conditions, insufficient is known about pathogenetic mechanisms for these to be the basis of classification. Morphological classification is limited because the glomerulus can respond to injury in only a relatively small number of ways: experimental studies in animals show that the same pathogenetic mechanism, for example, immune complex deposition involving one defined antigen, can produce glomerular disease with a wide range of functional and histological abnormalities, depending on a variety of such factors as the duration and rate of deposition of complexes in the kidney.

The widespread use of percutaneous renal biopsy in the 1960s led to a histological classification, which was modified to take account of pathogenetic mechanisms when immunofluorescent techniques were applied to renal biopsies. This approach has proved useful and workable, although it still leaves many phenomena to be explained. Histology and immunohistology were of particular help in advancing understanding of conditions such as crescentic nephritis, where a proportion of patients have the characteristic fixation of antibody to glomerular basement membrane (GBM), and in focal nephritis, where mesangial deposits of IgA identify an important subgroup. An aetiological description is rarely possible, e.g. acute exudative nephritis following streptococcal infection. The difficulties caused by a histologically based classification are readily exemplified: focal proliferative nephritis may be the first histological manifestation of fixation of antibody to GBM, but the same appearance can result from immune complex disease in SLE, or infective endocarditis.

As with other diseases, nephritis requires analysis which takes into account aetiology, pathogenic mechanisms, and prognosis, including responses to treatment. Examples of some typical abnormalities in glomerular histology are shown in Figs 1–8.

Clinical syndromes of glomerulonephritis

The many disorders involving the glomerulus have limited clinical expression and during its course a particular glomerular disease may cause more than one clinical syndrome. A strong clinicopathological correlation is therefore not found. Glomerular disease may produce the following:

1. *Reduction of glomerular filtration,* retention of salt and water, expansion of the intravascular volume and hypertension. The acute development of these features constitutes the *nephritic syndrome.* In severe instances acute oliguric renal failure may occur.

2. *Haematuria* Macroscopic haematuria is a feature of acute poststreptococcal nephritis and rapidly progressive glomerulonephritis; recurrent macroscopic haematuria is a symptom of idiopathic focal nephritis and membranoproliferative glomerulonephritis. Microscopic haematuria is common in glomerular disease.

3. *Proteinuria* This may vary from slight when it is asymptomatic, to heavy when it leads to the *nephrotic syndrome.*

4. *Loin pain* This is usually only a feature of acute diseases such as acute nephritis and crescentic nephritis.

5. *Chronic renal failure* This usually occurs with high blood pressure.

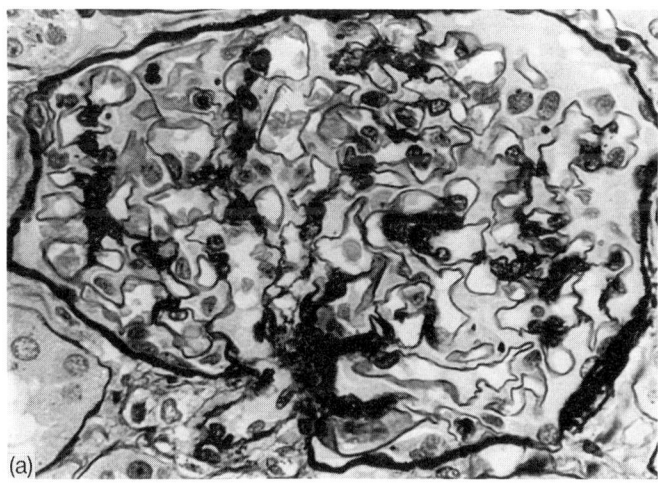

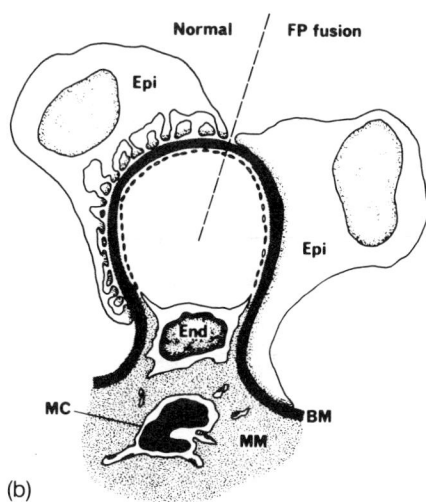

Fig. 1 (a) Normal glomerulus. Silver stain. × 400. (b) Diagram of a capillary loop illustrating normal foot process (on the left) and fusion (on the right). Epi = epithelial cell: End = endothelial cell; MC = mesangial cell; MM = mesangial matrix; BM = basement membrane.

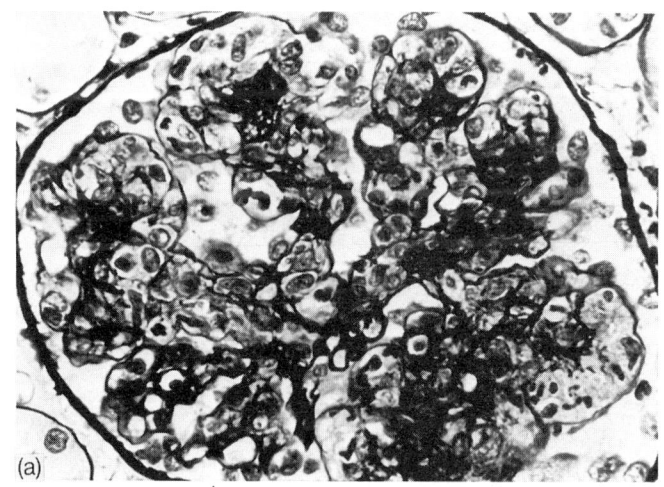

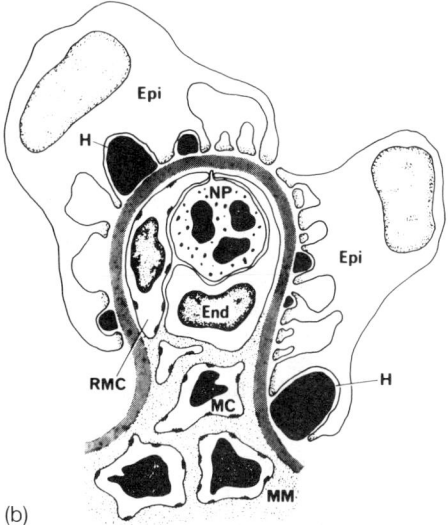

Fig. 2 (a) Postinfective glomerulonephritis with endocapillary hypercellularity and polymorphs in capillary lumina. Silver stain. × 400. (b) Diagram of loop with subendothelial deposit and lumen narrowed by swollen endothelial cell. H = hump; NP = neutrophil polymorph; RMC = reactive mesangial cell; Epi, End, MC, MM as in Fig.1b.

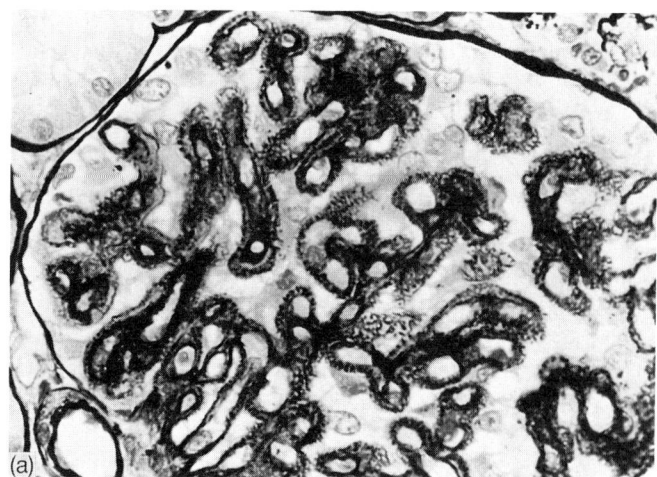

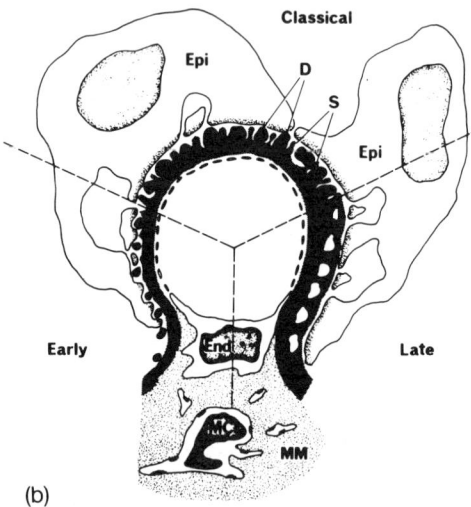

Fig. 3 (a) Membranous change showing 'spikes' or 'bristles' projecting from external capillary walls. Silver stain. × 400. (b) Diagram showing various stages of membranous change. The alteraion of spikes (S) of basement membrane with subepithelial deposits (D) is shown in the classical stage.

Immunopathogenetic mechanisms in glomerulonephritis

Two major mechanisms of glomerular injury have been identified by experimental studies and by examination of human renal material by immunofluorescence. The first and much the commonest in animals and humans is due to the glomerular accumulation of antigen–antibody complexes – *immune-complex disease*. This is recognized by a characteristic pattern of granular deposits containing immunoglobulins and complement in the glomerular capillary walls. The second mechanism of injury is glomerular fixation of antibody directed against the glomerular basement membrane (GBM); this gives rise to typically smooth linear deposition of antibody in a continuous distribution along the glomerular basement membrane.

Immune complex disease

The study of experimental models in which nephritis is brought about by single or repeated injections of foreign serum protein (serum sickness) has illustrated the potential for immune complexes to cause a wide variety of histological changes in the glomeruli. In acute *'one-shot' serum sickness* a single large dose of bovine serum albumin (BSA) injected into a rabbit results in acute disease characterized by nephritis, arthritis, and vasculitis, the

lesions developing at a time when soluble complexes of antigen and antibody, formed in antigen excess, are present in the circulation, and healing rapidly after antigen elimination, when antibody appears free in the circulation. Chronic progressive nephritis can be induced by repeated injections of smaller amounts of antigen so that immune complexes are present in the circulation over much longer periods. Various histological patterns of nephritis can be produced depending upon the proportions of antigen and antibody in the complexes (which determines the size of the immune complex) and the rate of deposition of complexes in the kidney. These patterns range from a *membranous nephropathy* which is brought about by the slow deposition of relatively small-molecular-weight complexes, to *rapidly progressive nephritis*, with glomerular proliferation, crescent formation and renal failure.

The development and pattern of glomerular disease depends particularly on the size of the immune complexes. Large complexes are rapidly taken up by the reticuloendothelial system, and very small complexes formed in great antigen excess cause little tissue damage; nephritogenic immune complexes are formed only over a relatively narrow range of complex size. Thus, the host's antibody response can be the major determinant in immune-complex disease, and in these simple experimental systems, the wide range of histological and clinical consequences are ultimately related to the host's immune response.

Understanding of factors determining variation in host response

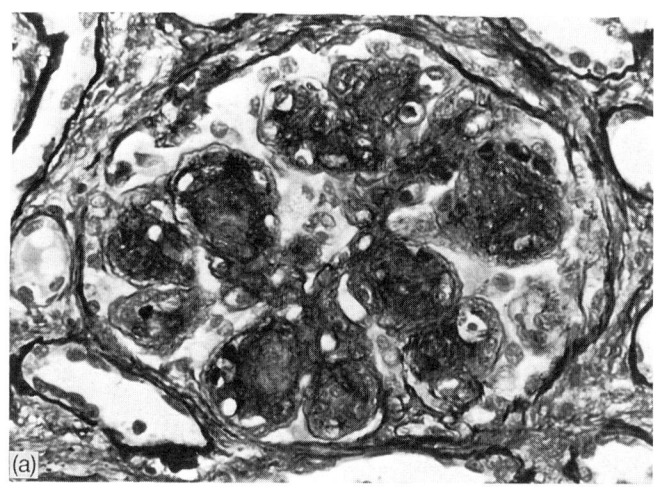

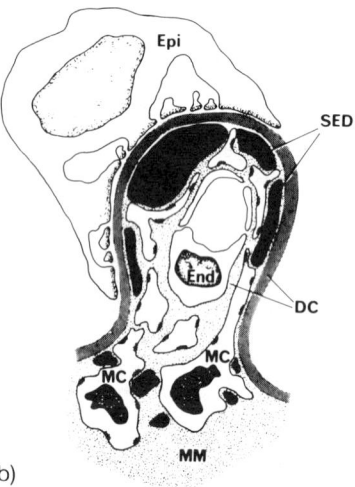

Fig. 4 (a) Mesangiocapillary glomerulonephritis showing a lobular appearance of the tuft and double contour appearance of peripheral capillary walls. Silver stain. × 400. (b) Diagram showing subendothelial deposits (SED) and mesangial cell (MC) cytoplasm in the subendothelial space, together producing the double contour (DC) seen in (a).

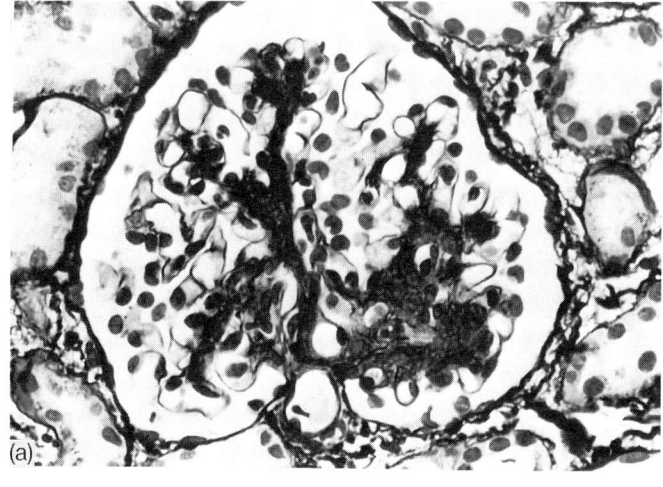

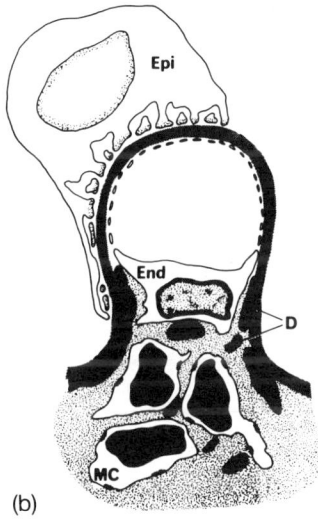

Fig. 5 (a) Mesangial proliferation showing thickening of the mesangial stalk. Silver stain. × 400. (b) Diagram of deposit (D) in the mesangial stalk. Larger paramesangial deposits extend towards the subendothelial region of the loop.

is therefore of central importance in nephritis. Recent evidence has emphasized the importance of genetic influence – the genes concerned being sited in the major histocompatibility complex (MHC) – and in this connection it is of interest that associations between certain immune-complex nephritides and HLA geno-types are being recognized. Another important host factor is the capacity to clear immune complexes from the circulation. This is illustrated by the very rare patients with congenital deficiencies of components of the complement system who have an increased tendency to develop immune-complex disease such as glomerulo-nephritis and systemic lupus erythematosus. Such complement deficiencies probably predispose to disease by impairing the capacity of the reticulophagocytic system to clear circulating immune complexes, since complement contributes to this process by opsonization. Deficiencies of complement associated with nephritis are listed in Table 1. The glomerular localization of anti-gen–antibody complexes is enhanced by factors which increase glomerular capillary permeability, such as haemodynamic factors, e.g. increased blood pressure, and release of vasoactive amines, e.g. histamine, which may be brought about by allergic mechan-isms. Recent studies have established that the charge of antigen may be a major determinant in the glomerular accumulation of immune complexes. Positively charged (cationic) agents bind to the (normal) anionic sites in the glomerulus, and serve to localize antigen, or complexes.

Immune complex nephritis in humans

Immunofluorescence microscopy shows that in the majority of human nephritides there are discrete deposits of immunoglobulins and complement in a pattern similar to that seen in experimental immune complex nephritis. In a small proportion of patients, cir-culating material with the characteristics of antigen–antibody com-plexes has been identified by a variety of tests. However, only in a minority of diseases in humans has the antigen responsible been identified in the deposits or in the circulating complexes. Indirect evidence of a role of particular antigen may be provided by resolu-tion of nephritis following its elimination, for example, in infective endocarditis following antibiotic treatment or replacement of an infected valve, or in patients with tumour-associated nephropathy by removal of tumour. The amount of immune complex producing severe glomerulonephritis can be very small and therefore may not be detected in the circulation, and recent work has established that in humans circulating antigen–antibody complexes may be bound to blood cells, such as erythrocytes. The complexes which accumulated in the kidney are of greatest importance, and their characteristics cannot be directly inferred from studies of circulat-ing complexes. However, the failure to demonstrate circulating antigen–antibody complexes in patients with putative immune complex nephritis has lent weight to the idea that a proportion of patients have granular deposits because of the reaction between circulating antibody and discrete glomerular antigens. In an exper-imental form of nephritis in rats (Heymann nephritis) this mech-anism has been shown to be responsible for the production of a membranous nephropathy.

Table 1 Complement deficiency and disease

Deficiency	Disease
C1q C1r C1s C4	High frequency of GN, vasculitis, and atypical SLE
C2	Approximately 50 per cent of affected subjects have GN, vasculitis, and related disorders
C1INH deficiency	Presents as hereditary angio-oedema. A few patients have immune-complex disease (probably due to secondary C4 and C2 deficiency)
C3	Recurrent infection Nephritis
I, H	Recurrent infection from C3 deficiency (due to C3 consumption from unrestrained activation of the alternative pathway)
C5–9	Recurrent infection, especially meningococcal and neisserial; a few patients with SLE

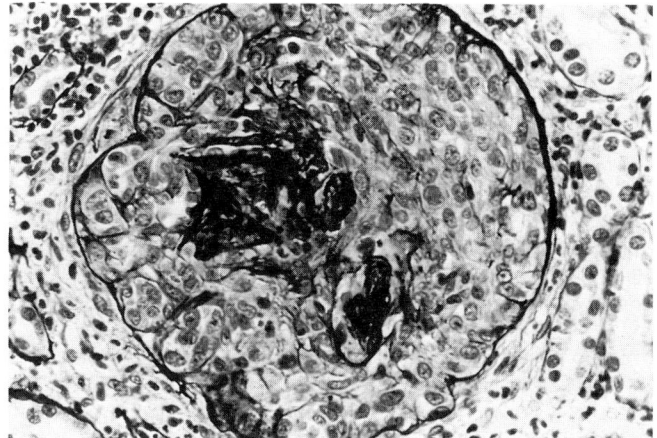

Fig. 6 Crescentic glomerulonephritis with concentric proliferation of cells lining Bowman's capsule and obliteration of the tuft. The darkly staining area is fibrinoid. Silver stain. × 400.

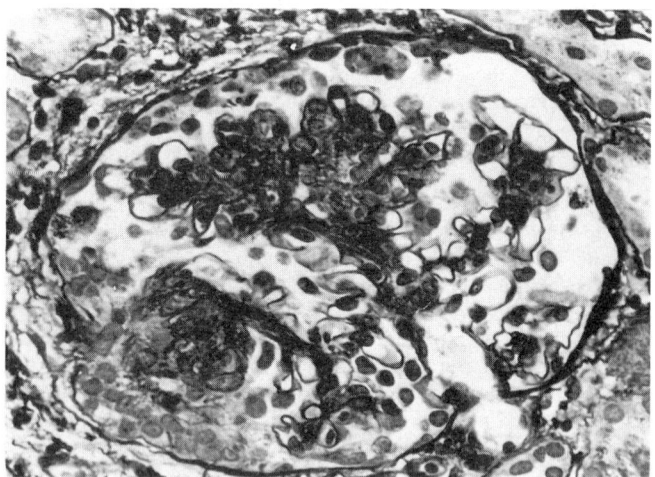

Fig. 7 Focal proliferation; increased mesangial cells and matrix affecting only part of the tuft. Capsular reaction and an adhesion at the bottom left. Silver stain. × 400.

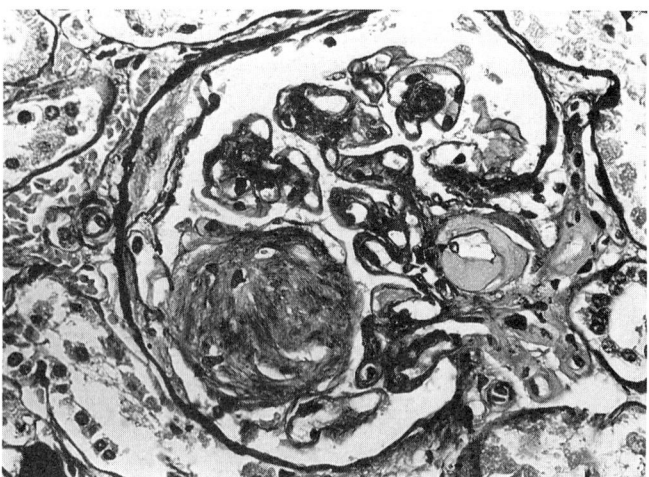

Fig. 8 Diabetic glomerulosclerosis with a sclerotic nodule, capsular drop (on the left) and hyaline in the afferent arteriole (right). Silver stain. × 400.

Antigens implicated in human immune complex disease

Great difficulty has been experienced in identifying antigens in most putative immune complex diseases in humans. In experimental animals various chronic infections, particularly persistent virus infections, can be complicated by immune complex nephritis, and the infection shown to be a source of antigen–antibody complexes. In man a large number of infections, viral, bacterial, fungal, and protozoal, can also be complicated by immune complex disease. In general however, it has proved difficult to establish concentration of antigen in renal tissue, and the evidence directly implicating infection as the cause of nephritis is largely based on the response to its eradication. Other evidence of circulating immune complexes, such as hypocomplementaemia, positive rheumatoid factor, and material reacting in the various assays from immune complexes may be present, although none of these findings is antigen specific; an exception is in chronic hepatitis B virus infection, where virus-derived material coated with antibody and complement can be seen by electron microscopic examination of plasma. There is, however, little doubt that infection is a major cause of immune-complex disease, especially in the Third World, where social and other conditions make infection common. Important examples of post-infectious nephritis are shown in Table 2.

Other antigens have also been implicated, mainly on indirect evidence: these include drugs (see below and Table 3), tumours (where immunofluorescence suggests immune-complex disease, and nephritis responds to successful eradication of tumour), and a variety of endogenous antigens of which the best-recognized are the nuclear antigen–antibody complex systems characterizing systemic lupus erythematosus and related disorders. Also worth mentioning are thyroglobulin in nephritis associated with Hashimoto's disease, and immunoglobulin itself in the mixed cryoglobulinaemia syndromes which will be considered in more detail later.

Table 2 Infectious organisms in human nephritis

Organism	
Bacteria	*Streptococcus*—GpA haemolytic
	Streptococcus viridans
	Staphycoloccus aureus and *albus*
	Diplococcus pneumoniae
	Meningococcus
	Salmonella typhi
	Klebsiella pneumoniae
	Mycobacterium tuberculosis
	Mycobacterium leprae
	Treponema pallidum
	Brucella
	Yersinia enterocolitica
	Leptospira
Viruses	EB
	HB$_s$ Ag
	Oncornavirus
	Mumps
	Measles
	Rubella
	CMV
	Coxsackie
	Variola
	Varicella
	Vaccinia
	? Guillain-Barré 'agent'
Rickettsiae	Coxiella
Mycoplasma	*Mycoplasma pneumoniae*
Fungi	*Candida albicans*
	Coccidioides immitis
Parasites	*Plasmodium malariae*
	Plasmodium falciparum
	Schistosoma mansoni
	Schistosoma haematobium
	Toxoplasma
	Filariae

Table 3 Common drugs and chemicals implicated in human nephritis

Drug	Histological type of nephritis
Gold	
Mercury	Membranous
Captopril	
Penicillamine	Membranous usually, crescentic rarely, anti-GBM very rarely
Penicillins	Interstitial; rarely acute proliferative
Non-steroidal anti-inflammatory drugs	
Sulphonamides	
Rifampicin	Interstitial
Cephalosporins	
Thiazides	
Frusemide	
Hydrocarbons	Anti-GBM
Heroin (or contaminants)	Focal sclerosis

Anti-GBM nephritis

Experimental nephritis is readily induced by injection of heterologous antibody to glomerular basement membrane (GBM) or by active immunization of the animal with heterologous GBM or the antigenically similar lung basement membrane. Fixation of antibody to the GBM leads to a local allergic reaction with fixation of complement and adherence of polymorphs. Immunofluorescence shows a characteristic intense linear fixation of antibody along the GBM. In humans such linear staining is the hallmark of anti-GBM disease, although similar appearances can be seen in diabetic nephropathy, probably due to absorption of circulating IgG onto diseased capillaries. The diagnosis of anti-GBM disease should therefore be confirmed by the demonstration of circulating antibody to GBM, which is now possible by radioimmunoassay techniques.

Anti-GBM nephritis accounts for only about 2–3 per cent of human nephritis. Most, though not all, patients develop a severe nephritis rapidly progressive in type, and many patients have concomitant intra-alveolar haemorrhage (Goodpasture's syndrome) probably due to fixation of antibodies on the alveolar basement membranes.

Cell-mediated immunity

The presence of monocytes in the glomeruli, interstitium, and crescents of nephritic kidneys has been interpreted as evidence that cell-mediated immunity (type IV reaction) is contributing to tissue damage, and this mechanism can be shown to be responsible for renal injury in experimental systems. It is uncertain whether or not a type IV reaction accounts for the failure to identify humoral immune reactants such as antibody or complement in a considerable proportion of patients with severe glomerular disease.

For the purpose of this chapter we shall consider the various forms of glomerulonephritis in two broad sections: the first concentrating on 'primary' glomerulonephritis in which the kidney is the principal subject of injury, the second where it is involved as part of a multisystem disease.

THE PRIMARY GLOMERULOPATHIES

Acute glomerulonephritis

The association between streptococcal infection (scarlet fever) and the development of acute nephritis was recognized by Blackwell in the early part of the 19th century and for many years poststreptococcal nephritis was regarded as the main cause of human acute nephritis.

This is now not the case, and indeed acute poststreptococcal nephritis of sufficient severity to cause admission to hospital is rare in northern Europe and North America. This presumably reflects better health and hygiene in the population, and possibly a change in the nature of the streptococcus itself. By contrast, poststreptococcal nephritis is still common in underdeveloped and tropical countries where it is often a sequel to skin infection.

Clinical features

Although characteristically a disease of children and young adults poststreptococcal nephritis may occur at any age. Males are more commonly affected than females in a ratio of 2:1. The characteristic clinical manifestation of poststreptococcal nephritis is the development of an acute nephritic syndrome: salt and water retention with mild generalized oedema; hypertension; usually slight to moderate proteinuria; variable impairment of glomerular filtration, and microscopic or macroscopic haematuria. The urine sediment shows red cells, red cell and granular casts, and occasionally leukocyte casts. Salt and water retention in poststreptococcal nephritis is associated with expansion in intravascular volume with elevation of jugular venous pressure and bradycardia. Elevation of blood pressure is variable and may not be evident in some patients especially children, until follow-up studies

reveal their true baseline blood pressures. In others, severe hypertension leading to hypertensive encephalopathy or pulmonary oedema may develop. Proteinuria is usually moderate, in the majority of patients being less that 5 g/24 hours. There is therefore only a moderate fall in the serum albumin, although haemodilution may also contribute to this. A small proportion may develop heavier proteinuria leading to nephrotic syndrome, although this is generally transient. Rarely, the acute nephritic syndrome may develop without any abnormality of the urine sediment.

Prognosis

In children the prognosis is excellent. The only risks are in the acute stage from hypertensive encephalopathy, pulmonary oedema or acute renal failure. In adults the prognosis is less certain, although clinical resolution is the usual short- to medium-term result. However, small amounts of proteinuria and abnormalities of the urine sediment may persist for long periods. Some workers have provided histological evidence suggesting that scarring continues to take place for many years after the initial episode of glomerular inflammation in up to half of their patients, but there is as yet no convincing data to indicate that such changes are clinically important in the vast majority of patients. Although regularly reported in earlier accounts of this disease, the development of an early progressive glomerulonephritis leading to renal failure in weeks or months (rapidly progressive or subacute glomerulonephritis) is rare. As mentioned, the transient nephrotic syndrome which develops in a minority of patients generally resolves.

Pathology (Figs 2a, b)

Renal biopsy shows proliferative glomerulonephritis with infiltration of polymorphonuclear leukocytes (PML) into the glomerulus (exudative proliferative nephritis). The proliferating cells are of mesangial and endothelial origin. In severe cases crescents may develop, probably as a result of proliferation of cells in Bowman's capsule or ingress of macrophages into the glomerulus. Immunofluorescence preparations show characteristic granular deposits of immunoglobulins and complement, although in mild cases and in biopsies take during resolution. C_3 only may be detected. The characteristic feature on electron microscopy is the so-called 'hump', a large subepithelial deposit containing immunoglobulins and complement. Humps disappear within a few months of the acute attack. However, mesangial increase in cellularity can persist for periods of six months or longer, leaving an appearance of mesangial ('stalk') thickening, which is highly suggestive, although not pathognomonic, of poststreptococcal nephritis. Of the various histological features, only crescent formation appears to have any prognostic significance but even extensive formation may resolve completely in this disease.

Circulating immune complexes are usually detectable, and hypocomplementaemia is frequent and profound. The cause of the latter has not been established. A low C_3 is found in most patients; other components of this classical pathway, C_1, C_4, C_2, may also be low. A serum factor which activates C_3 has been demonstrated in some patients.

Aetiology

Only certain strains of Group A haemolytic streptococci appear to be nephritogenic, particularly types 12, 4, and 1. Type 49 was the strain responsible for the much-studied outbreaks in the Red Lake Reservation. Type 12 may not necessarily produce beta-haemolysis or secrete streptolysin O or S. Therefore, poststreptococcal nephritis may occur following apparently non-haemolytic streptococcal infection, and the absence of an elevated titre of antistreptolysin O and S antibodies does not indicate that infection has not taken place. Long-lasting type-specific immunity appears to follow streptococcal infection: in the second outbreak of acute nephritis in the Red Lake Reservation, 12 years after the first, all original patients were spared.

Pathogenetic mechanisms

There is compelling evidence that this form of nephritis is mediated by the glomerular accumulation of antigen–antibody complexes. Nephritis characteristically develops after a latent interval of about 10 days (range 7–28) following streptococcal infection (in acute serum sickness immune complex nephritis occurs after a similar interval). The immunohistological patterns of acute serum sickness and acute poststreptococcal nephritis are strikingly similar. Serological features such as hypocomplementaemia, circulating mixed cryoglobulins, and hyperglobulinaemia suggest immune complex disease. Proof of immune complex pathogenesis, i.e. the identification of streptococcal antigen in glomeruli, has been difficult, although two groups have identified streptococcal plasma membrane in glomeruli. The reasons for the localization of this form of immune-complex disease to the kidney are uncertain, but increasing attention is being paid to the possibility that nephritogenic streptococci generate antigens with specific affinity for glomerular tissue.

Management

A short course of penicillin should be administered to eliminate residual streptococcal infection. Salt and water retention and high blood pressure should be controlled with diuretics and appropriate antihypertensive therapy; acute renal failure may require dialysis. Neither steroids nor cytotoxic drugs are indicated, nor is prophylactic penicillin following the attack. Bed rest seems a reasonable measure during the acute illness.

It is important that the patient and his relatives are encouraged to regard the outcome as good. Undue anxiety should not be created by persistent moderate proteinuria or abnormalities of the urine sediment.

Other infections leading to nephritis

That an immune-complex type nephritis follows infection is not surprising considering that infectious organisms constitute a major source of antigen. This complication, although well documented following a variety of infections – viral, bacterial, fungal, and protozoal – is surprisingly rare. Table 2 lists the principal organisms implicated. Although glomerular changes predominate, the interstitium and tubules of the kidney may be affected and in a minority of patients are the main lesion. Certain conditions will be described in more detail.

Infective endocarditis (subacute bacterial endocarditis, SBE) (see page 13.314)

Clinical features

In most patients, renal manifestations of endocarditis are of asymptomatic proteinuria and haematuria, with or without renal impairment. The latter can cause acute renal failure – an event which has received insufficient emphasis. A further point of clinical importance is that renal disease is often of greatest severity in those patients in whom endocarditis is occult or difficult to establish by routine bacteriological analysis. This may reflect the longstanding generation of antigen–antibody complexes brought about by chronic infection of the heart valves that does not lead to their destruction.

Pathology

The most frequent finding is a focal and segmental proliferative lesion of the glomeruli. A more severe picture of diffuse proliferative nephritis with or without crescents is seen less frequently. Intracapillary thrombi are a typical finding and their presence gave rise to the early concepts of focal emboli arising from the vegetations.

Immunofluorescent examination shows deposits of C_3, IgG, and IgM in the capillaries and mesangium, with subendothelial and subepithelial deposits revealed by electron microscopy.

Serum levels of C_4 and C_3 are frequently reduced and tests for circulating immune complexes are usually positive. Hypocomplementaemia should raise the possibility of infective endocarditis in patients with heart disease and nephritis, and is a useful method of monitoring therapy. Reduction in complement may also provide the earliest evidence of relapse.

Aetiology

The nephritis arises as a result of deposition of complexes of antigens from the infecting organism and antibody to those antigens. Almost any organism capable of causing SBE may be involved.

Treatment

The principle of treatment is to remove the source of antigen, i.e. cure the endocarditis by antimicrobials or surgery.

Shunt nephritis

This complicates infection of shunts used to drain hydrocephalus. The organism responsible is usually *Staphylococcus albus*; the nephritis is usually histologically similar to mesangiocapillary glomerulonephritis Type 1 (see page 18.46), although other forms such as diffuse and focal proliferative and focal segmental nephritis have been reported.

Shunt nephritis may cause proteinuria, haematuria, nephrotic syndrome, and renal failure. Its immune-complex nature has been demonstrated by the finding of staphylococcal antigens in the affected glomeruli and in circulating complexes. This condition responds to eradication of the infection which usually requires replacement of the infected shunt.

Visceral sepsis

A diffuse proliferative nephritis with or without crescents, or a focal proliferative nephritis occurs in association with deep-seated abscesses and sepsis. Resolution of the nephritis follows effective treatment.

Malaria and the nephrotic syndrome

There is strong epidemiological evidence of an association between *Plasmodium malariae* and nephritis. Data indicate historical and geographical associations between prevalence of *P. malariae* and admission to hospital with nephrotic syndrome. If this association is causative, *P. malariae* is an important cause of nephritis. More direct evidence is provided by the identification of *P. malariae* antigen in glomerular deposits in about 25 per cent of renal biopsies examined; but an important finding is that eradication of organisms by appropriate therapy appears to have no effect on the renal disease, which is usually progressive. This argues against a role of immune complex of malarial origin.

A variety of histological appearances have been reported. A major difficulty in interpreting these, and indeed other aspects of the disorder, is the lack of any firm definition of what constitutes malarial nephropathy, except its occurrence in an endemic area, and the absence of features of other well recognized types of nephritis.

Crescentic glomerulonephritis, rapidly progressive glomerulonephritis (RPGN) 'malignant' glomerulonephritis

These mixed pathological and clinical terms describe a heterologous group of conditions with the common feature of extensive proliferation of the cells in Bowman's capsule – crescent formation – usually affecting at least half the glomeruli (Fig. 6). Fibrinoid necrosis affecting the vessels in the glomerular tuft is a common finding. The term 'rapidly progressive' describes the tendency for acute and rapid deterioration to occur leading to renal failure in weeks or months; in exceptional patients, anuria can develop within days of onset.

Crescentic nephritis may develop against a background of different pathogenetic mechanisms: in experimental animals both anti-GBM disease and immune complex disease can cause crescentic nephritis; in humans crescentic nephritis is a frequent finding in both anti-GBM disease and immune complex-mediated diseases such as Henoch–Schönlein purpura or mixed cryoglobulinaemia. Crescent formation and focal necrotizing glomerulonephritis are also features of polyarteritis and Wegener's syndrome, in which the pathogenetic mechanism is less certain, as immunofluorescent studies frequently show paucity of the immune reactants Ig and C_3 in glomeruli. Only rarely does crescentic nephritis follow acute poststreptococcal nephritis, and most patients with RPGN have no antecedent streptococcal infection nor any of the other features of poststreptococcal nephritis.

Clinical features

Rapid loss of renal function, sometimes leading to renal failure in a few weeks dominates the presentation. The onset of disease may be associated with loin pain and macroscopic haematuria.

Clinical feature of associated systemic disease may be present and dominate the clinical picture. Constitutional symptoms such as fever, myalgia, and weight loss are common. In the majority of patients with crescentic nephritis the blood pressure is normal until glomerular scarring supervenes.

Pathology (Fig. 6)

Necrosis of the glomerular tuft, extensive crescent formation and breaks in basement membrane with the extravasation of red cells and fibrin into Bowman's space are common features. Some authors draw a distinction between forms of crescentic nephritis in which no involvement of the tuft can be detected – the glomerular tuft itself simply being compressed by the proliferating epithelial cells – and cases in which tuft proliferation can be detected, claiming a better prognosis in the latter group of patients. Vessels may occasionally show changes of hypertension or, rarely, evidence of microscopic polyarteritis.

Linear antibody can be detected by immunofluorescent techniques in the anti-GBM groups of diseases, and variable patterns of granular deposition are seen in the remainder. Fibrin deposition is found in areas of necrosis and crescent formation.

Measurement of serum complement is of value in differential diagnosis of RPGN, for hypocomplementaemia is a feature of poststreptococcal nephritis, diffuse lupus nephritis, mixed cryoglobulinaemia, and patients with chronic mesangiocapillary glomerulonephritis (who may have an exacerbation of disease resembling RPGN), but not of most other disorders associated with this syndrome, nor of the idiopathic form.

Management

Evaluation of treatment in this group of conditions is difficult because of their rarity and also their heterogeneity and variable rates of progression. Satisfactory controlled trials have not been undertaken.

There is evidence to indicate that patients with polyarteritis, Wegener's syndrome, and diffuse lupus nephritis benefit from steroids and cytotoxic drugs. Evaluation of treatment of other forms of RPGN is much more difficult. Some observers believe that a combination of cyclophosphamide with anticoagulant (dipyridamole and warfarin) is of value: the theoretical basis for using anticoagulants is that fibrin deposition in Bowman's space causes crescent formation in experimental forms of nephritis. Anticoagulants are particularly hazardous in uraemic patients because of the impairment of platelet function associated with uraemia. In anti-GBM nephritis success has been reported following intensive plasma exchange aimed at removing circulating antibody, combined with steroids and immunosuppressive drugs to control its synthesis (see later).

Nephritis associated with antibodies to glomerular basement membrane (GBM)

Anti-GBM antibody mediated nephritis is rare but has attracted interest because it is one of the few nephritic diseases in which the pathogenetic mechanism is defined and, with the development of radioimmunoassay for circulating antibody, it allows relationships between antibody and disease and the effects of various treatments to be explored.

Clinical features

The disease affects both sexes and all ages. It has so far been reported mainly in Caucasians and immunogenetic studies have established a close linkage with HLA DR2. There are suggestions that both infection and extensive exposure to hydrocarbon solvents may precipitate disease. About two-thirds of patients have pulmonary haemorrhage. The term Goodpasture's syndrome is widely used to describe the syndrome of lung haemorrhage and nephritis with anti-GBM antibody, of which anti-GBM disease is only one cause. Lung haemorrhage, which may be severe and life-threatening, is attributed to the pathogenetic effect of antibody on lung basement membrane, which is antigenically similar to GBM. A recent finding is that the majority of patients with pulmonary haemorrhage are cigarette smokers, and the majority of those with isolated nephritis due to antibasement-membrane antibodies are non-smokers. Nephritis is generally severe and rapidly progressive, although a minority of patients present with indolent disease and slowly progressive renal failure, and a few patients are reported with lung haemorrhage but histologically and functionally normal kidneys. In patients with rapidly progressive nephritis the features are those of rapid loss of renal function, sometimes with loin pain and macroscopic haematuria, and symptoms and signs of lung haemorrhage and anaemia. Lung haemorrhage can be missed, for extensive alveolar bleeding can occur without haemoptysis, and sometimes with little radiographic change or changes which may be misdiagnosed as pulmonary oedema. The blood pressure is generally normal and proteinuria moderate, although with the development of glomerular scarring hypertension and heavy proteinuria may develop. The feature which distinguishes anti-GBM disease from other causes of rapidly progressive nephritis is that except for evidence of lung disease and anaemia there is little in the way of generalized systemic disturbance: fever, myalgia, arthralgia, etc., are not prominent features. In a proportion of patients lung haemorrhage may long antedate the development of the nephritis.

Pathology

The usual finding is of crescentic nephritis but, depending on the stage at which biopsy is taken, the appearances range from focal nephritis with capsular adhesions and early crescent formation to 100 per cent circumferential crescents with collapse of the glomerular tuft. Linear deposition of IgG, sometimes with IgA (which in one case was the sole immunoglobulin), and C_3 in about 50 per cent of patients are seen on immunofluorescence studies, frequently with extensive fibrinogen deposition in crescents; in the few cases presenting with lung haemorrhage and normal renal function, biopsies have shown linear IgG deposition on the GBM. Patients presenting with more gradual loss of renal function show changes of chronic nephritis with glomerular sclerosis and sometimes evidence of sclerosed crescents. Similar changes may be seen after successful control of anti-GBM antibody production.

Serology

Anti-GBM antibody can be detected by indirect immunofluorescence, although measurement by radioimmunoassay is more reliable and quantitative. Otherwise serology is unremarkable: tests for non-organ-specific antibodies, immune complexes, cryoglobulins, and complement components are generally normal.

Treatment

The introduction of intensive plasma exchange, aimed at removing circulating antibody, and immunosuppression with cytotoxic drugs and steroids has radically improved the prognosis of this disease. It appears that the natural history of anti-GBM disease is the loss of circulating antibody over periods ranging from months to (more usually) several years, and that this process can be greatly accelerated by treatment. The clinical outcome depends largely on how much renal damage has taken place before antibody levels can be controlled; when because of glomerular injury, oliguria supervenes or the serum creatinine rises over 6–700 μmol/l, renal failure is nearly always irreversible. Lung haemorrhage can be controlled in the majority of patients, although patients presenting with massive lung haemorrhage may succumb before treatment can be effective. A feature which has emerged is that disease may become quiescent in the face of significantly elevated titres of antibody, and under such circumstances intercurrent infection has been shown to be the most important cause of relapse. Early diagnosis and treatment of intercurrent infection is therefore important in the management of these patients.

Bilateral nephrectomy had a vogue in the treatment of severe lung haemorrhage in anti-GBM disease, on the theoretical but unproven ground that removal of the source of the GBM antigen might hasten the decline in antibody production. Although some patients with fulminating lung haemorrhage appeared to have benefited from this procedure, there has been no supportive data from quantitative assays, i.e. no evidence of accelerated loss of anti-GBM antibody after operation. With the success of the regimen of plasma exchange and immunosuppressive drugs, which control lung haemorrhage in almost all patients, there is now no justification for this radical and dangerous approach.

Membranous nephropathy (epimembranous or extramembranous nephropathy)

This is a disease predominantly of adults in the United Kingdom and North America, although French nephrologists report it in approximately 10 per cent of biopsies in children. Males are more commonly affected than females. It is an insidious disorder, sometimes detected as asymptomatic proteinuria but more usually diagnosed when proteinuria has become heavy, causing the nephrotic syndrome.

Clinical features

Proteinuria, characteristically non-selective, is the main feature, usually causing a nephrotic syndrome. The blood pressure is normal in the early stages of disease. The urine sediment may show red cells and casts although these are often absent, and macroscopic haematuria is rare.

About 30 per cent of patients undergo spontaneous remission, and a similar proportion progress over several years. The remainder continue with proteinuria with or without impairment in renal function.

Pathology (Figs 3a, b)

Renal biopsy shows characteristic diffuse thickening of basement membranes. Its mechanism is shown by immunofluorescence and electron microscopic studies. The earliest event is accumulation of immunoglobulins and complement in a subepithelial position on the basement membrane. At this stage no thickening of the basement membrane may be evident on light microscopy, although the characteristic granular deposits are readily seen by immunofluorescence. The thickening of basement membrane is due to 'spiky' outgrowths which occur between the deposits. These spiky outgrowths give rise (on silver stains) to a characteristic comblike appearance. Especially in cases undergoing spontaneous remissions the complexes may be lost leaving 'holes' in the basement membrane.

Serological investigation is generally unhelpful: serum comple-

ment is normal, immunoglobulins may be reduced because of nonselective loss of IgG in the urine, cryoglobulins are usually absent and tests for circulating immune complexes are generally negative.

Aetiology

Membranous nephropathy is usually idiopathic, although a similar picture is sometimes seen in SLE (lupus membranous nephropathy), in heavy-metal intoxications, e.g. gold and mercury, and following use of drugs such as penicillamine. Persistent infection with hepatitis B virus has been identified in some patients, but a causal connection has not been firmly established.

There is a well-documented association between membranous nephropathy and solid tumour, especially carcinoma of the bronchus and gastrointestinal tract. Membranous nephropathy is also occasionally seen in lymphoma and leukaemia. The causal relationship between tumour and renal disease is indicated by the response to successful treatment of tumour, when proteinuria disappears.

Long regarded as having an immune-complex pathogenesis (the same histology was observed in some animals with chronic serum sickness) there is now much evidence suggesting an autoimmune pathogenesis involving a reaction between circulating antibody and a glomerular antigen: in Heymann nephritis, an experimental nephritis in rats, indistinguishable histologically from human membranous nephropathy, such a system has been demonstrated. Neither the equivalent glomerular antigen in humans nor the putative responsible antibody have as yet been identified. The human disease is strongly associated with HLA DR3.

Management

Nephrotic syndrome and hypertension should be treated appropriately. Steroids and immunosuppressive drugs were long considered to be without effect, but recent trials suggested that courses of high-dose, alternate-day steroids or steroids with cytotoxic drugs reduced progression to renal failure. However, at present there is no consensus on the value of these therapies, and further trials are being carried out. Pending the results of these trials it seems reasonable to reserve steroid therapy, with or without cytototoxic drugs, for those patients showing evidence of declining renal function.

Minimal change nephropathy (MCN)

The hallmark of this disorder is the complete loss of proteinuria following treatment with steroids. The histologically based terminology reflects the usual lack of change on light microscopy. It is the commonest cause of nephrotic syndrome in childhood. The disorder remains an enigma, for despite its response to steroid, MCN is devoid of features of inflammation, and any part played by immunological mechanisms in its pathogenesis is unclear (see page 18.59).

Clinical features

MCN is predominantly a disease of children, in whom it accounts for 80–90 per cent of cases of the nephrotic syndrome, and has its highest incidence at 2–4 years. It causes about 10 per cent of cases in adults. Most patients present with the nephrotic syndrome. In children ascites may dominate the picture, and rarely, acute renal failure occurs (see later).

The prognosis is excellent and mortality is low. Relapse is frequent. Patients who relapse frequently have been shown to benefit from treatment with cyclophosphamide or chlorambucil. A minority of patients who are resistant to steroids may also respond to these agents. Relapse frequently follows intercurrent infections, but measles infection may lead to remission – probably because of the well-established immunosuppressive effects of the virus.

Pathology

The disorder is characterized histologically by the paucity of abnormalities in the glomeruli and absence of immune reactants detected by immunofluorescence. However, the following changes may be seen: (*a*) a slight degree of mesangial proliferation, but not sufficient for the diagnosis of mesangial proliferative glomerulonephritis, and (*b*) mesangial deposits of IgM, which have been associated with the above proliferative changes. A further abnormality can be revealed by electron microscopy – fusion of the foot processes of the glomerular epithelial cells.

Proteinuria is characteristically highly selective – protein-clearance studies indicate the loss of predominantly lower molecular weight plasma proteins such as albumin into the urine, whereas large molecular weight proteins such as gamma-globulins are retained.

There are no characteristic serological changes. Circulating immune complexes are found in a proportion of patients, and serum complement is normal.

Pathogenesis

The pathogenesis of the condition is unknown. Various clinical observations and certain abnormalities of the immune system suggest an immunopathological basis. The clinical observations include: (*a*) that there is a good response to steroids and immunosuppressive drugs; (*b*) that occurrence of a nephrotic syndrome with histology identical to MCN in Hodgkin's disease may respond to successful treatment of lymphoma, but not to steroids alone, suggesting that lymphocytes or their products play a pathogenetic role; (*c*) that an MCN may coincide with atopy, and remit following desensitization or avoidance of antigen.

Immunological abnormalities in MCN comprise reduced transformation of lymphocytes to mitogens during relapse, sensitization of lymphocytes to renal antigens, the production of lymphokines altering capillary permeability, the presence of circulating immune complexes in relapse, and raised serum levels of IgM with low levels of IgG (not explicable by urinary loss) persisting into remission. Many of these abnormalities are not specific for MCN, occurring in other forms of nephrotic syndrome. At present the mechanisms involved are uncertain, but the likeliest seems to involve the production of a factor altering glomerular permeability by lymphocytes or similar steroid and cytotoxic drug-sensitive cells.

Management

Overall the prognosis is good, although a number of patients continue to relapse. The usual practice is to induce remission by relatively large doses of steroids such as prenisolone 60 mg/day. Most patients will lose proteinuria within 2–4 weeks, after which steroid doses can be gradually reduced, and eventually stopped. In patients who repeatedly relapse, a course of cyclophosphamide has been shown to be effective. Remission is induced with steroids and then cyclophosphamide is given in a dose 3 mg/kg body weight daily for 8 weeks. Generally, because of the dangers of this treatment, cyclophosphamide should not be considered unless the patient is suffering from serious complications of steroid therapy. In many relapsing patients, slow reduction in therapy leading to alternate-day therapy can be effective, while minimizing the harmful side-effects of steroids. Because of the frequency of MCN as a cause of nephrotic syndrome in childhood it is not necessary to perform a renal biopsy in children presenting with nephrotic syndrome until they have been shown to be steroid-resistant, or have features suggesting some other form of nephropathy (such as macroscopic haematuria or hypocomplementaemia.)

Complications

The most important are acute renal failure, infection, and thrombosis (see page 18.63). Insufficiently recognized is the syndrome of acute renal failure which is sometimes due to hypovolaemia, although in adults it occurs in patients without good evidence of volume depletion sufficient to cause renal failure. In such circumstances the association of glomerular disease and rapidly failing renal function may lead to the mistaken diagnosis of rapidly progressive nephritis. A further source of confusion is that in minimal-change nephrotic syndrome moderate hypertension is sometimes observed. Its mechanism is uncertain though it may be related to the renin response to hypovolaemia. Children appear to be particularly prone to develop pneumococcal peritonitis. This susceptibility may be due to hypoimmunoglobulinaemia, loss of complement factors in the urine, and disordered cellular immunity.

Focal glomerulosclerosis

Focal glomerulosclerosis (FGS) (focal hyalinosis) is a histologically based term initially applied to a nephropathy resembling that of minimal change, but characteristically steroid-resistant. However, its definition, by clinical or histological criteria is unsatisfactory (see later) and its aetiology and pathogenesis are unknown.

Clinical features

The typical patient presents with proteinuria or nephrotic syndrome, often accompanied by hypertension. The proteinuria is characteristically non-selective and fails to respond to steroids. All age groups are affected. Most progress to terminal renal failure, 50 per cent within 10 years. A small number of patients, particularly those who are not nephrotic and who are children, remit.

Pathology

The characteristic lesion is a focal sclerosing lesion with hyaline deposits (hyalinosis) which initially affects only a segment of the glomerulus before progressing to global sclerosis. In the early stages of the disease the glomeruli affected are those at the corticomedullary junction, and these may be missed on needle biopsy, leading to the mistaken diagnosis of minimal change nephropathy.

A further histological problem arises: it can be difficult in individual cases to distinguish this disorder from focal proliferative nephritis which has proceeded to scarring. That there is no proliferative phase in focal sclerosis is confirmed when the disorder recurs after transplantation, in which situation early biopsies show an identical sclerosing lesion.

Immunofluorescence microscopy usually shows deposits of C_3 and IgM in the affected segments, which may be due to non-specific fixation in damaged tissues. Circulating immune complexes are only occasionally found.

Pathogenesis

The cause of FGS is unknown. It may represent the final result of various processes. There is little information on what these might be.

Heroin abuse is the only condition associated with FGS. The nature of the link is unknown, and it is not clear whether the heroin itself, a vehicle, or infection due to intravenous injections is the responsible agent. Patients with acquired immune deficiency syndrome (AIDS) have lately been reported to have FGS without, apparently, any history of heroin abuse.

The relationships between minimal change nephropathy and focal sclerosis have been the subject of interest and controversy. Sometimes patients with steroid-responsive minimal change disease appear to develop steroid-resistant FGS; and some patients with FGS achieve a remission with steroids; yet others who are steroid-resistant respond to cyclophosphamide. There is therefore much merit in using a therapeutically based classification for this group of disorders, regarding them as having at either extreme a steroid-responsive nephrotic syndrome ('minimal change'), or a steroid-resistant, cyclophosphamide-resistant nephrotic syndrome ('focal sclerosis'); between these are steroid-resistant, but cyclophosphamide-responsive patients with histologies which may show minimal change or FGS. There is therefore no justification for using renal histology to determine therapy in this uncertain area.

Any explanation for the cause of FGS must also take account of the predeliction of the lesion, with proteinuria and the nephrotic syndrome, to recur in transplanted kidneys. A striking feature is the immediate proteinuria – within hours of grafting – which occurs in some patients.

Management

Care must be exercised before it is assumed that nephrotic patients with FGS will be steroid-resistant, for some will respond to steroids and others to a combination of steroids and cyclophosphamide. Unresponsiveness to steroids must therefore be established, and when this has been shown to be the case, a therapeutic trial of cyclophosphamide in a dose of 3 mg/kg for six to eight weeks is justified. In patients who fail to respond, management has to be symptomatic; very exceptionally a life-threatening nephrotic syndrome may require bilateral nephrectomy.

Mesangiocapillary glomerulonephritis (MCGN)

It is now clear that this form of nephritis should be considered to comprise at least two different types according to histological appearances; subendothelial MCGN (type I) and dense-deposit MCGN (type II). The differentiation is important since there are distinctive immunopathological differences.

Clinical features

MCGN affects mainly adolescents and young adults, type II having a higher incidence in younger patients. The presentation is usually with nephrotic syndrome or proteinuria, often with haematuria. Renal impairment may already be apparent, and some patients present with renal failure. Progression to renal failure occurs in about 50 per cent of patients in seven years.

A striking but rare feature is partial lipodystrophy – the loss of subcutaneous fat from various parts of the body, usually from any one or more of the face, upper limbs, and trunk. Although partial lipodystrophy occurs with other histological types of nephritis it is mainly associated with MCGN type II. The reasons for this close association are not known, but are probably linked with the abnormalities of the complement system common to MCGN type II, and to partial lipodystrophy, even when nephritis has not developed (see below).

Pathology (Figs 4a, b, page 18.38)

There is proliferation of mesangial cells in both forms, and in type I the capillary basement membranes are split by the extension of the proliferation into the capillary loops, giving a characteristic 'double contour' or 'tramline' effect. In type I MCGN, discrete deposits are seen by light and electron microscopy in the subendothelial position. In type II MCGN, an electron-dense ribbon-like deposit is seen between the layers of the glomerular basement membrane, and in the basement membrane of the tubules and Bowman's capsule.

Immunofluorescent microscopy reveals further differences between the two forms. In type I the deposits contain C_3 in all cases, and IgG in 80 per cent; IgM, C1q and C_4 are found in 30 per cent. In type II the deposits contain C_3 in all cases, and IgG in less than 50 per cent; other proteins have not been identified.

Complement

Both histological forms of MCGN are associated with profound abnormalities of the complement system. The original abnormality found was a persistent and marked reduction in C_3, which gave the condition its name of 'hypocomplementaemic nephritis'. The hypocomplementaemia can last months or years, but can also be intermittent, and may disappear eventually; adults with MCGN often have normal serum complement. Earlier studies showed striking reductions in C_3 but normal C1, C_4, C_2 – the early components of the classical pathway – suggesting a distinctive system of complement activation, now known to involve the alternative pathway. However, a proportion of patients with MCGN type I are recognized to have low serum levels of C1q and C_4, suggesting

activation of the classical pathway. Fresh plasma samples from hypocomplementaemic patients contain breakdown products of C_3, and radioisotope turnover studies show accelerated catabolism of C_3, but also suggest that reduction in C_3 synthesis contributes to hypocomplementaemia.

Nephritic factor

A striking feature of MCGN is the serum factor known as the C_3 nephritic factor (C_3NeF). This was initially detected by the ability of nephritic serum to break down the C_3 in normal human serum, and later shown to do this by activating the alternative pathway. It is known to be a unique IgG autoantibody directed against C_3bBb, the convertase of the alternative pathway, and acts by stabilizing and preventing its physiological breakdown – thereby causing protracted complement activation and hypocomplementaemia. It is found more frequently in MCGN type II than in type I, may be intermittent, and is usually detected in patients with profound hypocomplementaemia.

The presence of C_3NeF has no identifiable effect on the outcome of the disease. It persists after bilateral nephrectomy and in the transplanted patient, although it often disappears during the early phase of the post-transplant course. Since it occurs in partial lipodystrophy without nephritis and since partial lipodystrophy antedates nephritis in those cases in which the latter develops, it seems the C_3NeF is not a consequence of the nephritis, but precedes it. The consequent hypocomplementaemia could therefore predispose to the development of the nephritis by an associated defect in the clearing of antigens or the solubilization of immune complexes. Other possible explanations linking C_3NeF with MCGN are that the complement activation it causes is itself directly injurious to the kidney, or that it is an expression of a particular genetic make-up which itself predisposes in some way to the development of the nephritis. In this regard, an association of MCGN type II with DR7 HLA B12 has been reported.

Aetiology

In both types of MCGN the cause is unknown. Type I has histological similarities with immune-complex disease and the detection of immune complexes in the serum coupled with antecedent infections in certain cases suggests that MCGN type I is due to circulating immune complexes. The complexes may develop and/or persist on a background of immune deficiency in those patients with preceding hypocomplementaemia.

Type II MCGN does not present the accepted appearances of immune complex deposition, although immune complexes have been detected in the circulation. The nature of the dense deposit is unknown.

C_3NeF has been found in patients with partial lipodystrophy. Such patients, although prone to develop nephritis, do not normally do so – and the presence of C_3NeF in patients with partial lipodystrophy and normal kidneys provides strong evidence that complement activation is not directly nephrotoxic. While it seems clear that C_3NeF and associated hypocomplementaemia predispose to nephritis, other factors are clearly influential in its development and progression. These are unknown.

A histological appearance undistinguishable from type I MCGN is found in a variety of systemic disorders. These include shunt nephritis, in which the infecting organism is usually Staphylococcus albus and postinfectious nephritis (most cases having been poststreptococcal) neoplasia, sickle-cell disease, alpha-l-antitrypsin deficiency, and SLE.

Focal proliferative glomerulonephritis

In focal proliferative glomerulonephritis only a portion of glomeruli show abnormalities under the light microscope, and characteristically the affected glomeruli show segmental involvement of the tuft (Fig. 7, page 18.40).

It is clear that the focal proliferative change is a non-specific histological response. Both immune-complex deposition and anti-GBM antibody fixation can produce this pattern. It is, for example, found in conditions such as subacute infective endocarditis and systemic lupus erythematosus, and in the early stages of anti-GBM nephritis. It is also a feature of disorders where pathogenetic mechanisms are less well defined; for example, severe focal necrotizing glomerulonephritis is characteristic of microscopic polyarteritis nodosa and Wegener's granulomatosis. Focal nephritis is also a feature of disorders characterized by mesangial deposits of IgA. Henoch–Schönlein purpura, and idiopathic focal nephritis which, because they constitute major causes of GN in most parts of the world, will now be considered in more detail.

Idiopathic focal nephritis with mesangial deposits of IgA (IgA disease, Berger's disease)

Clinical features

Children and young adults are principally affected, and present with recurrent haematuria, usually macroscopic, frequently during upper respiratory tract infections, although the condition is not associated with any particular organism. Proteinuria is usually slight or absent. Older patients may present with hypertension or other indications of chronic glomerular disease. A small proportion of patients give a strong family history of renal disease and a number of reports identify IgA nephropathy in relatives.

Other forms of glomerular disease may also present with recurrent haematuria, for example, hereditary nephropathy associated with deafness (Alport's syndrome), membranoproliferative glomerulonephritis, and a histologically indistinguishable focal proliferative glomerulonephritis without mesangial deposits of IgA. Nevertheless, the combination of recurrent haematuria, focal nephritis, and mesangial deposits of IgA occurs sufficiently frequently for it to be considered a distinct clinical syndrome.

A form of IgA nephropathy is associated with chronic liver disease, particularly alcoholic cirrhosis, although this group does not generally present with recurrent haematuria.

A proportion of patients, amounting to 5–8 per cent, develop progressive disease leading to renal failure.

Pathology

The glomeruli show focal changes of mesangial proliferation, which are sometimes diffuse, rarely with crescents. The distinctive finding is the diffuse deposition of IgA in the mesangium, usually accompanied by IgG. All glomeruli, including those which are normal histologically, show the deposits. IgG, C_3, and properdin are found in a similar distribution to the IgA; IgA secretory piece is not present.

Raised levels of serum IgA are found in about 60 per cent of patients. Immunofluorescent study of skin which is clinically and histologically normal, shows IgA deposits associated with C_3. Serum levels of complement are normal. Circulating immune complexes have been detected, with a preponderance of IgA among them, and an excess of lymphocytes bearing IgA on their surface has been identified.

Henoch–Schönlein purpura

Clinical features

This well-recognized illness is characterized by involvement of skin, with non-thrombocytopenic purpura affecting the extremities and buttocks, joints with pain and swelling, gastrointestinal tract with pain and sometimes bleeding, and kidneys with haematuria, which may be gross or microscopic, and occasionally acute renal failure. Chilren and adolescents are mostly affected, males outnumbering females by 2 to 1. It is rare in adults. Infection, usually respiratory, frequently precedes the illness, although no particular organs are involved; drugs, e.g. sulphonamides and penicillins, have also been implicated as initiating agents. Attacks may be continuous or recurring, over weeks, months, or even

years, with complete recovery between. Follow-up studies have revealed that renal failure follows in 5–10 per cent of patients, even though the episode(s) of the syndrome may have become quiescent some years previously.

Pathology

Histological appearances range from mild mesangial hypercellularity to a crescentic nephritis. Mesangial IgA, C_3, and properdin are found by immunofluorescence.

Serum levels of IgA are often raised, complement components remain normal. IgA, with C_3 and properdin, can be found in the skin at both affected and unaffected sites.

Immune complexes have been detected in the sera by various methods and have been shown to contain IgA.

An association of HLA-BW35 with Henoch–Schönlein purpura has been reported. There is evidently a strong pathogenetic relationship between Henoch–Schönlein purpura and IgA nephropathy, and the two conditions cannot be distinguished by immunological or histological study of renal tissue.

Pathogenesis

The sequence of respiratory-tract infections and a disorder characterized by raised serum levels of IgA, IgA-containing complexes in the circulation, and IgA deposition in tissues suggests that the disease is caused by immune complexes formed in response to an antigen entering through the respiratory or gastrointestinal epithelium and so provoking an IgA response, but the true cause is unknown.

In the case of the IgA disease associated with cirrhosis of the liver, the antigen may have entered by default of the diseased liver and its deficient reticuloendothelial function.

No exogenous antigens have been defined in the circulating complexes, and it is not clear why such complexes have a predilection of deposition in the skin or kidneys. Any explanation for the pathogenesis of these conditions must also account for the recurrence of the disease in transplanted kidneys.

Other presentations of mesangial IgA nephropathy

IgA is found occasionally in the mesangial tissue of adults who present with asymptomatic proteinuria or hypertension without a history of antecedent recurrent haematuria. It is not yet clear if these patients represent the end stage of IgA disease in which clinical manifestations were less florid and therefore unnoticed, or have a different disease with mesangial deposition of IgA as a common pathogenetic mechanism.

Idiopathic focal glomerulonephritis without deposits of IgA

Some patients present with a typical syndrome of recurrent haematuria and a histologically identical focal proliferative nephritis, but show IgG, IgM, and C_3 deposits in the mesangium. The aetiology of this variant of focal nephritis is not known.

Management

No specific treatment has been shown to be of value in these diseases. A short course of high-dose steroids and cyclophosphamide is probably justifiable in treating those presenting with the severe crescentic form of the disease.

Alport's syndrome

Alport's syndrome, the commonest of the hereditary nephropathies, is a familial disorder characterized by nephritis and nerve deafness, a variable occurrence of ocular and other abnormalities, and a preponderance in males (see page 18.81).

Clinical features

The disease usually presents in childhood or young adults with haematuria; microscopic haematuria and proteinuria may also lead to diagnosis, but nephrotic syndrome is rare. Males may present with renal failure, but in women, in whom the disease is generally less severe, the diagnosis may be made following the development of pregnancy-associated hypertension. Sensory deafness is overt in about 40 per cent of patients, but detectable in others by audiometry. Other components of the syndrome include myopia, lenticonus, retinitis pigmentosa, and thrombocytopenia with giant forms of platelets.

The inheritance of Alport's syndrome is variable; there is a predominant autosomal dominant pattern with variable penetrance but X-linked inheritance has also been described.

Pathology

Diagnostic changes are found on electron microscopy of the kidney, which shows widespread thickening and splitting of the glomerular basement membrane. Neither light microscopic nor immunofluorescent appearances are specific, glomerular sclerosis being seen eventually in the former, and only occasional deposits of C_3 in a focal pattern in the latter. An antigenic abnormality in GBM has been identified: affected patients show greatly reduced binding to sera obtained from patients with Goodpasture's syndrome. Loss of the so-called Goodpasture's antigen is therefore a feature of the disorder, although it is not clear that this represents the primary genetic abnormality.

Diagnosis

This rests on the family history, clinical, and biopsy findings. The condition should always be considered in young patients presenting with recurrent haematuria.

Treatment

There is none for the disease process; chronic renal failure should be treated appropriately.

Other hereditary nephritides

A variety of genetically determined and inherited disorders may predispose to or cause nephritis. These range from the disorders associated with deficiencies of complement components to inborn errors of cholesterol metabolism. They are rare but of considerable interest as experiments of nature (see page 18.81).

Recurrence of nephritis in transplanted kidneys

Patients with anti-GBM antibody nephritis, mesangiocapillary glomerulonephritis type II (dense deposit disease), focal glomerulosclerosis, and mesangial IgA nephritis are those most likely to suffer a recurrence in grafted kidneys. Recurrence is reported but appears to be less common in patients with mesangiocapillary glomerulonephritis type I (subendothelial deposits), and membranous nephropathy.

In practice the risk of recurrence, which in itself does not usually lead to rapid destruction of the graft, does not contra-indicate transplantation, as graft survival in patients in whom the original disease was nephritis is not reduced compared to other groups. However, in the case of anti-GBM disease in which recurrent crescentic nephritis might develop, transplantation should be delayed until anti-GBM antibody is no longer detectable in the circulation.

Histological appearances of both mesangiocapillary nephritis (type I) and membranous nephropathy have been found in transplanted kidneys in patients whose original disease was neither of these conditions, nor indeed nephritis of any kind. This development of nephritis *de novo* may *presumably* represent *immune-complex disease* brought about by antibody formation against transplant antigens.

NEPHRITIS IN SYSTEMIC DISEASE

Systemic lupus erythematosus

Systemic lupus erythematosus (SLE) affords an excellent example in human disease of immune complexes causing nephritis. The apparent incidence of nephritis in SLE depends upon the vigour of the approach to diagnosis. If patients with SLE undergo renal biopsy in the absence of clinical evidence of renal disease, i.e. without even proteinuria and/or haematuria, nearly all exhibit immunohistological abnormalities consistent with SLE. On the other hand, only some 40 per cent of patients show clinical evidence of renal involvement at presentation (see page 16.20).

Clinical features

As with the disease in general, SLE with renal involvement is ten times more common in women than in men, and most patients affected are in their reproductive years. There is a higher frequency in Blacks than Whites in the same environments, in both the United States and the United Kingdom.

The presenting signs and symptoms comprise the gamut of clinical renal disease; haematuria and/or asymptomatic proteinuria; the nephrotic syndrome; rapidly progressive nephritis due to diffuse lupus nephritis; and, depending on the stage of diagnosis, varying degrees of renal failure. Any of the other clinical features of SLE may occur with renal disease, the commonest being arthritis and skin involvement. A frequent accompaniment of the more severe renal lesions is hypertension, which itself can contribute to renal damage.

There have been numerous reports that the prognosis of SLE nephritis has improved over the last two decades. This is not only due to the increased recognition of more mildly affected patients being diagnosed by the application of new tests such as DNA binding (DNAB), as mortality rates for patients with severe nephritis have improved. Although the reasons for this improvement cannot be identified with certainty, they probably reflect the better use of corticosteroids which, with cytotoxic agents, have brought about an increased survival in patients with severe disease. Diagnosis and treatment of infection – an important and common complication of SLE – is also probably much improved.

Pathology

All varieties of histological abnormality may be seen in SLE, ranging from normal appearance on light microscopy but with deposits of immunoglobulin and complement, to crescentic nephritis; there is no histological pattern specific to the disease. Most workers agree that histological appearances have prognostic value. Those patients in whom glomeruli look normal and those with focal proliferative or membranous nephritis, have a better prognosis than those with diffuse proliferation, with or without crescents. A recent report, however, indicated no difference in outcome between these groups (to death or terminal renal failure), which probably reflects the fact that the histological appearances in an individual may change during the illness. In a small but as yet uncertain proportion there may be such change, from focal to diffuse, for example, and the reverse is seen with successful treatment.

Immunofluorescent microscopy characteristically shows the presence of IgG, IgA, IgM, C_3, C_4, and Clq. Their distribution varies; it is generally diffuse, even though the histological changes are focal; it may be focal; it may follow the glomerular basement membrane in the membranous type, with or without mesangial deposits. The large number of proteins detected in SLE compared to other forms of nephritis can provide a diagnostic clue if SLE has not otherwise been considered.

Electron microscopy frequently reveals electron-dense deposits; their site varies according to the appearance on light microscopy. Thus, they are found in the mesangium in cases with normal, mild proliferative, or membranous appearances, but in the capillary loops in those with focal or diffuse proliferation, the deposits being subendothelial or subepithelial or both.

Serology

SLE is characterized by circulating antibody to nucleoproteins, anti-double-stranded (ds DNA) being that most commonly measured and used diagnostically, and hypocomplementaemia. Low serum levels of Clq, C_4, and C_3 are commonly detected, but low levels of C_2, C_5, and factor B as well as low haemolytic complement are also present. Other abnormalities of the complement system include circulating breakdown products of C_3, and increased catabolism of C_4, and C_3. The sera of some patients' can activate complement *in vitro*. These changes have been suggested as circumstantial evidence of complement-activating circulating immune complexes in SLE, and indeed many tests for circulating immune complexes are positive in a high proportion of SLE sera.

Two problems provide constant difficulty for the nephrologist caring for patients with SLE. These are the questions of how to predict acute exacerbations of the disease so that prophylactic treatment can be given, and how to give a long-term prognosis. Laboratory tests are frequently invoked in attempts to solve these problems.

Acute exacerbations

Much effort has been spent on the analysis of the relationship between serum complement levels (mainly C_4 and C_3), DNAB, and more recently, the level of circulating immune complexes on the one hand and the disease activity on the other. No consistent picture has emerged. While there is no doubt that exacerbations tend to be accompanied by hypocomplementaemia and a rise in DNAB, with a reversal in these trends during improvement, it is clear that disease can worsen without change in these variables; and, conversely, persistent hypocomplementaemia and high DNAB is consistent with remission. However, individual patients can be identified where changes in serum complement and DNAB correlate with disease activity. It is therefore important in any patient to establish the value of these tests so that unnecesary treatment is avoided.

Pathogenesis

Although the broad framework that SLE is an immune complex disease characterized by antibody formation against autoantigens, particularly nuclear antigens is established, many details in this process remain unclear.

Antigens

DNA DNA in its double-stranded form (dsDNA) and antibody formation to it have long been thought to play a central role in a pathogenic immune complex mechanism specific for SLE. This concept rests on the original observations that DNA and anti-DNA could be eluted from affected kidney, and the more recent observations that DNA and anti-DNA comprise circulating immune complexes in SLE. In addition, it has been shown that DNA fixes to basement membranes; circulating antibody may attach to it *in situ*, allowing complexes to deposit without necessarily being present as such in the circulation.

Viruses

Evidence that C type viruses are an important source of immune complexes in murine lupus has led to much work on the importance of similar virus infection in human SLE. However, only circumstantial evidence exists. This includes the finding of raised titres of lymphocytotoxic antibodies in household contacts, and reports of antisera to type C virus proteins giving positive reactions in diseased glomeruli from patients with SLE. These findings are controversial, and there are also reports of failure to demonstrate C virus antigens in tissues from SLE patients, or of finding such antigens in normals.

Antibody formation

Antibodies to DNA may be found in in the sera of normal people, and their higher concentration in those of SLE has been related to diminished T-cell suppressor function, which allows uncontrolled antibody production by B-cells. Although there is a tendency to accord the failure of suppressor T-cells a primary role in SLE, there is no good evidence for this, and the phenomenon may be secondary.

Another factor which may control antibody production to DNA is the oestrogen/testosterone secretion in the host. It has been shown in lupus-like disease of NZB/NZW mice that androgen increases survival and decreases antibody formation to DNA and the severity of the nephritis, whereas oestrogen has the opposite effect. This observation clearly has a bearing on the propensity for women to develop SLE, and for the higher female incidence to be more apparent between menarche and menopause.

Immune deficiency

There is a clear association between the development of SLE or SLE-like syndrome (the latter lacking the characteristic anti-DNA antibody), and complement deficiency affecting mainly the early components of the classical pathway. Deficiencies implicated have been Clr, Cls, C_4, C_2, C_5, and C_8. It is not known precisely how the complement deficiency is related to the development of SLE, but possibilities include effects of complement in generating immune complexes which are safely and efficiently cleared, impaired viral neutralization, and linkage of the gene loci controlling complement synthesis with the gene loci controlling the immune response. In support of the latter, C_2 and C_4 deficiency are in linkage disequilibrium with various HLA genes, and the latter are themselves presumed to be linked with immune-response genes.

The development of nephritis in SLE

Although histological evidence of renal disease may be found in the absence of any clinical evidence of renal damage, certain factors seem to influence the development of overt glomerular disease. Thus, nephritis is more prone to occur with high concentrations of antibody and higher avidity of the antibody to DNA, since nephritis is associated with smaller complexes than arteritis. Differences in the properties of the antibodies have been associated with different types of nephritis. Thus, a predominance of IgM over IgG has been found in diffuse proliferative forms of nephritis compared to focal proliferative forms. A low serum titre of non-precipitating antibody to DNA has been associated with the membranous form of SLE nephritis.

Treatment

This is a controversial and difficult matter. Much of the difficulty arises from the variation of the disease from patient to patient, and the changes which may occur during the course of the disease in any individual. In addition there are few data on controlled trials of the drugs used. From the practical standpoint the modes of treatment are best considered in relation to particular clinical problems; even so it must be emphasized that the following is a generalized guideline which must be tailored to each patient's vagaries.

(a) Acute SLE with severe renal involvement, i.e. diffuse proliferative nephritis± crescents/acute renal failure High doses of steroids, e.g. 60–100 mg prednisolone daily with either azathioprine or cyclophosphamide, are usually effective. There has been a recent tendency to treat such patients with high doses of intravenous methylprednisolone, e.g. 1 g daily for three days (the so-called 'pulse' therapy) and even more recently plasma exchange. Neither of these approaches has been validated, although institution of either has reversed a previous failure to respond to conventional therapy.

The use of anticoagulant drugs and agents to modify platelet function has not been critically studied; their use rests on the occurrence of intracapillary thrombi in the glomeruli and evidence of platelet activation, as well as the presence of crescents in some of these patients.

As the disease responds to treatment the aim should be to reduce the dosage of steroids to acceptable levels. If cyclophosphamide has been used in the acute stage, it should be withdrawn, and if an immunosuppressive drug is required, then azathioprine substituted because of the former's long-term effects.

(b) Mesangial, membranous or focal glomerulonephritis The treatment of these patients is usually governed by the severity of their extrarenal manifestations and the degree of proteinuria. If the former are severe or the patient nephrotic then steroids are required; immunosuppressive drugs are not indicated. If extrarenal manifestations and renal disease are mild, it is uncertain whether steroids, with or without immunosuppressive drugs, alter the natural history of the disease.

(c) Quiescent disease A major problem in the management of SLE nephritis is the long-term treatment of the patient who, having had moderate or severe renal involvement, now has evidence of stable renal disease without clinical or immunological evidence of activity. It is not clearly known whether prolonged treatment with steroids, with or without immunosuppressive drugs, alters the outcome. Controlled trials of azathioprine and cyclophosphamide have been performed with conclusions both in favour of and against their use. It has been suggested that use of azathioprine allows the reduction of steroids to lower levels; against this possible advantage must be placed the possible long-term ill-effects of azathioprine.

The use of laboratory tests in the management of these patients has been discussed above (see Pathology).

Mixed connective tissue disease

This rare condition has features in common with systemic lupus, systemic sclerosis and polymyositis (see page 16.45). Renal disease is not a frequent complication, but membranous or diffuse proliferative nephritis can occasionally be progressive or severe. The disorder is characterized by high titre of antibody to the so-called extractable nuclear antigen (ENA) but the relation of this to nephropathy is unclear.

Glomerular disease in polyarteritis nodosa (PAN) and Wegener's granulomatosis (page 16.28)

Polyarteritis is a multisystem disorder due to inflammation involving muscular arteries. Two broad types are recognized. The first (polyarteritis nodosa) involves medium-sized vessels, leading to aneurysmal dilatation which can be diagnosed in life by angiography. In the second type the vasculitic process involves small arteries, arterioles, and veins, and is often accompanied by severe necrotizing glomerulitis of the crescentic (rapidly progressive glomerulonephritis) type. This form is often termed 'microscopic polyarteritis'. Another variant, which will not be discussed in detail here because renal involvement is rare, is the Churg–Strauss syndrome (see page 16.31) characterized by asthma, hypereosinophilia, and nasal polyps.

Clinical features

Males predominate and the disease is commoner in the elderly. Constitutional symptoms such as fever, malaise, and weight loss are prominent, and the signs reflect the multisystem nature of the disorder. In the classic macroscopic kind (PAN) moderate or severe hypertension is common, and kidney involvement is due to the effects of high blood pressure or to infarction. Gut and liver involvement are common. In the microscopic varieties the blood pressure is more often normal, and glomerular disease is common, with a focal necrotizing glomerulonephritis, often leading to crescent formation and renal failure. The microscopic form is often

accompanied by other neurological disease, vasculitic purpuric rash, myalgia, and mononeuritis multiplex.

Pathology

The hallmarks of the condition are inflammation of the arterial wall and periarterial tissues with fibrinoid change in the wall. Infarction or ischaemic changes of tissue supplied by the diseased arteries may occur. In the microscopic form there is a crescentic glomerulonephritis with infarction and fibrinoid necrosis of the glomeruli.

Since the disease is frequently intermittent along the course of the artery, normal arterial tissue may be seen in biopsy material. Many features of the microscopic kind are also seen in Wegener's granulomatosis.

A higher ESR, anaemia and leucocytosis, with an eosinophilia in a third of patients, are characteristic.

Wegener's granulomatosis (page 16.31)

This is a closely related disorder. In addition to features of microscopic polyarteritis there are characteristic necrotizing granulomatous lesions affecting the upper respiratory tract, including the nasopharyngeal sinuses and lung. These lesions may cause presentation with epistaxis or haemoptysis. The histology of this granulomatous lesion shows an important vasculitic element with cellular infiltrates of small blood vessels, arterioles, and veins.

Management

The diagnosis ultimately rests upon the histological demonstration of arteritis, although in practice it may be clinically obvious without histology when the presentation is typical. A difficulty in confirmation is that arteries in biopsy specimens may all too often appear normal.

Although there are no good controlled trials, there is widespread support for the idea that cyclophosphamide is of particular benefit in the management of Wegener's granulomatosis and the microscopic form of polyarteritis. Generally, it is given in a dose of 3 mg/kg/day in association with steroids in moderate to high dose (40–60 mg/day). The position in polyarteritis nodosa is less certain, although retrospective data suggests that steroids have improved survival. Control of hypertension is important. Recent therapeutic developments include the usage of 'pulse' doses of methyl prednisolone and plasmapheresis, although the role of either of these approaches is uncertain.

Anticoagulants and drugs altering platelet function, e.g. dipyridamole, have been employed but there is no evidence to either support or discredit their use.

Where control is achieved it is often necessary to continue treating with steroids, although there is much to gain by substituting azathioprine for cyclophosphamide if long-term cytotoxic drugs appear to be required.

Pathogenesis

Vasculitis is a feature of experimental serum sickness and in man there is circumstantial evidence suggesting immune-complex pathogenesis. Although accounting for only a minority of patients, PAN has developed in association with persistent infection with hepatitis B virus (Australia antigen), and this antigen has been demonstrated in the vascular lesions themselves.

Many drugs, e.g. penicillins and sulphonamides, have been blamed for causing polyarteritis, In fact, exacting proof for drugs causing a 'hypersensitivity angiitis' has been provided in only a small number of instances, and it must be remembered that antibiotics will frequently be prescribed for the prodromal symptoms, thus making for the possibility that their association may be fortuitous rather than causative.

Systemic sclerosis

See page 16.34.

Clinical features

This is a disease which generally presents in the 4th or 5th decade, affecting women three times as often as men.

Renal involvement is uncommon at presentation but may develop during the course of the disease. It is usually manifested by high blood pressure and proteinuria, with or without uraemia; the urine sediment is often unremarkable. Accelerated hypertension, microangiopathic haemolytic anaemia and oliguric renal failure (renal scleroderma crisis) may occur.

High blood pressure is frequently severe, difficult to treat, and has a major influence on the progression of the disease. Hypertension and renal failure denote a poor prognosis, most patients developing end-stage renal failure or dying in one year from the onset of uraemia.

Renal involvement, which occasionally may predominate, usually develops against the background of the other features of systemic sclerosis affecting the skin, heart, gastrointestinal tract, and lungs.

Pathology

In the kidney, the characteristic changes are in the interlobular arteries. The intima is thickened by the deposition of a substance consisting of glycoproteins and micropolysaccharides and by proliferation of intimal cells. Fibrinoid changes are seen in afferent arterioles. These changes produce a marked narrowing or complete occlusion of the vessels. They resemble those of malignant hypertension but may occur in scleroderma with normal blood pressure.

Glomerular changes are non-specific. They include mesangial proliferation, localized thickening of the basement membranes, crescent formation, and glomerular necrosis due to ischaemia.

Diagnosis

The background evidence of systemic disease is all important, although the renal arterial changes, particularly in the presence of normal blood pressure, may be highly suggestive.

Pathogenesis

See page 16.38.

Treatment

Steroids and immunosuppressive drugs have no effect on the lesion or progress of systemic sclerosis. Control of the blood pressure is vital, and improvement of renal lesions has been reported when this is achieved. Angiotensin-converting enzyme inhibitors have been suggested as being specifically useful in this respect.

End-stage renal failure has been treated with dialysis and transplantation, with some, but not regular, success. Hypertension may continue to be a problem, and has led to early bilateral nephrectomy. The necessity for this extreme treatment has, however, been reduced and perhaps eradicated by improvements in antihypertensive drugs. Recent reports of return of some renal function in a few patients after periods of prolonged dialysis emphasize the need to avoid nephrectomy in this condition.

Sjögren's syndrome (page 16.41)

Renal involvement in this disorder more usually takes the form of a renal tubular disorder, with failure of acidification of the urine, and interstitial nephritis. Glomerular disease, of membranous or focal proliferative type, with immunofluorescent appearances of granular deposits of Ig and complement is also reported. Some patients have cryoimmunoglobulinaemia, with its associated histological features. In the severe forms of Sjögren's syndrome with renal involvement, there are anecdotal data suggesting that steroids and cytotoxic drugs may be of value.

Rheumatoid arthritis (page 16.3)

Despite the frequency of circulating immune complexes in rheumatoid arthritis, they would seem to be not nephritogenic, as glomerulonephritis is a rare accompaniment of this disease, apart from its occurrence as a complication of gold or penicillamine therapy. These cases and those of amyloidosis excepted, there have been descriptions of a small number of patients with glomerular changes of membranous nephropathy or mesangial proliferative nephritis.

Neoplasia and nephritis

Neoplasms of various kinds, but particularly adenocarcinomata lymphomata and leukaemias are occasionally associated with nephritis. Evidence for a causal relationship is provided by the remission of nephritis which follows successful treatment of the underlying neoplasm. Two principal histologies are found: membranous nephropathy is the usual form of nephritis to complicate carcinoma; minimal-change histology is that usually found in lymphoma. Occasional cases of membranous nephropathy associated with leukaemia have been reported. Carcinoma of bronchus, stomach, colon, pancreas, uterus, and the ovary are the commonest tumours reported with membranous nephropathy; its presentation from a renal point of view is indistinguishable from idiopathic membranous nephropathy. The response to surgical removal of tumour can be striking, with loss of proteinuria over several weeks; and reappearance of proteinuria may be the first indication of recurrence of tumour. It is widely believed – although not firmly established – that tumour-associated antigen is responsible for the generation of nepritis by an immune-complex mechanism.

The position in lymphoma-associated nephropathy is less clear; here the histology is of minimal change which, however, is steroid-resistant except in the circumstances where the underlying lymphoma is itself also susceptible to steroids. The pathogenetic mechanism although obscure, is of great theoretical interest in that the association hints that a lymphocyte product may be responsible for renal injury.

HAEMOLYTIC URAEMIC SYNDROMES: MICROANGIOPATHIC HAEMOLYTIC ANAEMIA

These two terms describe the essential clinical and pathogenetic features of a group of conditions characterized by severe intravascular haemolysis and the rapid development of renal failure. The sequence of events in these conditions is believed to be (1) damage to endothelium; (2) activation of coagulation with fibrin deposition and consumption of coagulation factors and platelets; and (3) damage to red cells caused by their contact with the abnormal vessel wall, giving rise to the characteristic 'helmet cells', 'burr cells', or 'fragmented red cells'. The initiating arteriolar damage may occur in malignant hypertension, pre-eclampsia, and eclampsia, i.e. disorders in which damage is probably primarily brought about by high blood pressure, but in other disorders the initial cause of the endothelial damage is unknown. These syndromes are (a) the haemolytic uraemic syndrome of childhood; (b) a closely similar syndrome (possibly a variant of (a)) developing in the puerperium – giving rise to the syndrome of postpartum renal failure; and (c) thrombotic thrombocytopenic purpura (TTP) – Moschcowitz' syndrome.

Haemolytic uraemic syndrome (HUS) and postpartum renal failure

Haemolytic uraemic syndrome classically occurs in infants, children, and young adults, presenting with severe anaemia, renal failure, and bleeding due to thrombocytopenia. The disorder is frequently preceded by diarrhoea or upper respiratory tract infection. The overlap between this syndrome and thrombotic thrombocytopenia (see below) is emphasized by the occasional occurrence in the former of involvement of other organs, e.g. brain and gastrointestinal tract.

Although originally described in infants, a similar syndrome occurs in older patients, particularly in women in the puerperium, up to 8 months or occasionally longer after delivery, following an apparently normal pregnancy. In addition, an identical syndrome can develop following the taking of the contraceptive pill.

The cause remains unknown, although various factors suggest an infective aetiology, such as the tendency for outbreaks of the infantile forms to occur in clusters and in certain geographical areas, especially South America, and sometimes in more than one member of the family. Recurrent attacks are described. Severe hypertension is a frequent late complication.

Pathology

The renal arterioles are occluded by fibrin-like material with fibrinoid necrosis of their walls. The glomeruli show ischaemic changes and thickening of capillary loops.

In addition to thrombocytopenia, laboratory tests may show other evidence of consumption of coagulation factors such as elevated levels of fibrin derivatives.

Thrombotic thrombocytopenic purpura (Moschcowitz' syndrome)

This rare disorder, which occurs principally in adults, has all the features of the haemolytic uraemic syndrome, together with more widespread evidence of vasculitic disease, particularly neurological manifestations. Characteristically it has a sudden onset associated with high fever, muscle pains, headache, and varied and often fluctuating neurological signs. Renal failure is present in most patients although varying degrees of renal involvement occur. The mortality rate is high, due to the neurological involvement (see Section 19).

Pathology

This is similar to that described in the haemolytic uraemic syndrome, except that vascular involvement is more widespread.

Treatment

Because of the consumptive coagulopathy, anticoagulants have been widely used. However, assessment of their value is difficult because the natural history of the disease varies widely – some children with haemolytic uraemic syndrome recover completely without therapy, others rapidly develop anuria and irreversible renal failure.

Steroids and immunosuppressive drugs have been used, particularly in thrombotic thrombocytopenic purpura with its graver prognosis, but their value is unproven.

More recently, there has been preliminary evidence of improvement in both conditions following plasma infusion or plasma exchange. It has been postulated that in such patients there is deficiency or depletion of an alpha-globulin specifically involved in the generation of prostacyclin (which prevents aggregation of platelets to the vascular endothelium) and that plasma infusion or plasma exchange corrects this deficiency.

Sarcoidosis

Proteinuria and the nephrotic syndrome with a variety of glomerular lesions – membranous nephropathy, focal segmental sclerosis, proliferative, and crescentic nephritis – have been described with granular immunoglobulin and complement deposits in sarcoidosis. Occasionally, sarcoid granulomata can be found in renal tissue, although they can easily be missed on a biopsy sample. The renal aspect of this syndrome responds well to steroids. Only exceptionally does progression to chronic renal failure occur.

Dysproteinaemias (page 18.132)

Abnormal production of plasma proteins may cause a number of different renal lesions by affecting tubules, glomeruli, or renal vasculature. The conditions falling under this heading are: myeloma, Waldenström's macroglobulinaemia, and mixed essential cryoglobulinaemia – characterized by clonal proliferation of immunoglobulin-producing cells; amyloidosis and light-chain disease, the latter due to specific deposition of light chains in glomerular and tubular basement membranes.

Clinical features

Most patients present with features of the underlying disorder, although renal involvement may dominate the illness or be the sole presenting feature.

Acute oliguric renal failure or chronic renal failure may develop in myeloma or Waldenström's macroglobulinaemia. Both of these conditions, as well as light-chain disease and idiopathic cryoglobulinaemia may present with proteinuria or nephrotic syndrome. Defects in tubular function may be found in a small number of patients but these rarely account for the presenting features.

Pathogenesis

The renal disease in dysproteinaemias may arise from a number of mechanisms:

(*a*) Light chains are probably toxic to tubular cells, causing them to undergo degeneration with subsequent interstitial inflammation and fibrosis. Heavy chains are not nephrotoxic.

(*b*) Intratubular cast formation of myeloma proteins may lead to obstruction, perhaps precipitated by dehydration, or by large doses of radiographic contrast media.

(*c*) Amyloidosis is a complication of myeloma; amyloid may be deposited in the glomeruli, vessels, and tubules.

(*d*) Intracapillary occlusion by deposits of IgM in Waldenström's macroglobulinaemia.

(*e*) Rarely, specific glomerular lesions arise in myeloma, where a nodular glomerular lesion can develop, and in light-chain disease where there is an intramembranous deposit with a proliferative glomerulonephritis. The latter resembles type II mesangiocapillary glomerulonephritis (dense-deposit disease).

(*f*) Hypercalcaemia in myeloma.

(*g*) Renal failure may also occur as a complication of therapy causing hyperuricaemia, extreme hyperphosphataemia, or may occasionally be due to nephrotoxic drugs.

Pathology

Histologically, a variety of appearances may be seen. Some are distinctive, e.g. capillary occlusion in macroglobulinaemia and cryoglobulinaemia, and ulcerative casts in myeloma; and the PAS-positive stained material in light-chain disease. The casts and eosinophilia are homogeneous, lie in dilated tubules, and may be surrounded by giant cells.

The various abnormalities in the blood and urine proteins, and in bone marrow are described elsewhere.

Diagnosis

This rests upon the demonstration of the abnormal serum protein, or Bence Jones proteinuria, and bone-marrow infiltration by plasma cells: these are not necessarily obvious investigations in a patient with renal failure or proteinuria.

Management

This is that of the underlying disease (see page 18.133 and Section 19). When cytotoxic treatment is used there is a risk that acute hyperuricaemia may occur and itself cause renal failure; allopurinol should be given prophylactically, but in reduced dose if renal failure is already present because of its depressive effect on the bone marrow.

The variable prognosis of the malignant dysproteinaemias has provided a problem in the treatment of those patients who have developed chronic renal failure and need dialysis or transplantation. Decisions are best taken in the light of the expected prognosis of the extrarenal manifestations of the disease.

Amyloidosis

The kidney is commonly affected in primary and secondary amyloidosis (see page 9.145).

Clinical features

Renal involvement manifests itself as proteinuria, which is usually poorly selective and may contain a paraprotein, and is severe enough to lead to the nephrotic syndrome in a third of cases. A minority of patients will have developed symptomatic renal failure at the time of presentation. The blood pressure is usually normal. Uncommon presenting features are diabetes insipidus due to involvement of the vasa recta and interference with the counter-current mechanism, and renal-vein thrombosis.

Systemic effects from involvement of other organs, and in secondary amyloid, evidence of the underlying disease, may also be present. Primary amyloid affects the middle-aged and elderly, males predominating, and may be accompanied by disease of the heart, liver, gastrointestinal tract, carpal tunnel syndrome, and splenomegaly. Secondary amyloid can occur at any age and in association with:

1. Chronic inflammation and infection. Rheumatoid arthritis, bronchiectasis, osteomyelitis, leprosy, ulcerative colitis, Crohn's disease, and paraplegia with its chronic infection of the bladder and skin ulcers.

2. Neoplasia: 10 per cent of patients with multiple myeloma develop amyloid. Other neoplasms such as lymphomas and carcinomas are also associated with amyloidosis.

3. Heredofamilial diseases. The commonest is familial Mediterranean fever, in which renal amyloidosis is the commonest cause of death. Other familial forms of amyloid renal involvement are those occurring with neurosensory deafness and recurrent urticaria, with neuropathy, found in Portugal, and the familial form of Ostertag.

The prognosis is poor, particularly when renal involvement is clinically evident. Progression of disease is usually inevitable, and in primary amyloid the survival rate is some 20 per cent at 5 years.

Pathology

By light microscopy deposits of amyloid may be seen in the mesangium, capillary and arteriolar walls, tubules, and collecting ducts. The amyloid substance characteristically stains pink-red with Congo red and exhibits a pale green birefringence under polarized light; thioflavin T stains cause fluorescence under ultraviolet light. Occasionally, even with marked proteinuria, there may be only a slight deposition of amyloid in the kidney, which may be missed, leading to an erroneous diagnosis of minimal-change nephropathy. Primary and secondary forms of amyloid are not distinguishable by light microscopy.

Electron microscopy reveals the characteristic fibrillar structure of amyloid.

Immunofluorescence is not helpful; the amyloid deposits may stain for immunogobulins and C_3, but there are no consistent or characteristic features.

Diagnosis

The kidneys are usually enlarged radiologically, but may be small in patients presenting with renal failure. Renal biopsy allows definitive diagnosis, but a presumptive diagnosis of renal amyloid can be made in a patient with the clinical features of renal amyloid and histological evidence of amyloid at a more accessible site. Such sites are the rectum, where it is necessary to obtain a specimen which includes the lamina propria; the gum; and involved skin.

Rectal and gum biopsies can, however, occasionally be negative in the presence of renal amyloid.

Pathogenesis

See page 9.154.

Treatment

In secondary amyloid successful treatment of the underlying cause can sometimes but not always result in renal improvement, but other forms of treatment are not helpful. Steroids and immunosuppressive drugs are without effect. Colchicine delays the development of amyloid in familial Mediterranean fever, but is without effect in other forms of the disease. More recently dimethyl sulphoxide has been used in treatment, but benefit is at best only marginal.

Terminal renal failure has been treated successfully by chronic dialysis and transplantation – the prognosis is governed by the involvement of other organs. Recurrence in transplanted kidneys is infrequent.

Cryoglobulinaemia

Cryoglobulins (see Section 19) are classified according to the proteins involved. Type I is a cryoprecipitable, monoclonal immunoglobulin; type II has a monoclonal component, usually IgM, directed against determinants on a polyclonal immunoglobulin such as IgG; and in type III both immunoglobulin components are polyclonal. Cryoglobulins with a monoclonal component are features of lymphoproliferative disease, whereas polyclonal cryoglobulins are found in diseases such as SLE, chronic infections, and poststreptococcal nephritis – disorders in which immune complexes feature. Renal disease, usually affecting the glomerulus, can occur in all types, and the appearances range from capillary occlusion with homogeneous protein, to a proliferative disorder suggesting immune-complex nephritis.

Mixed essential cryoglobulinaemia

This is a rare disorder of the middle-aged or elderly in which the cryoglobulin usually consists of a monoclonal IgM and IgG. The renal disease presents as asymptomatic proteinuria, with or without haematuria, nephrotic syndrome or occasionally as acute oliguric renal failure, renal changes developing against a background of purpura, particularly on the legs, Raynaud's phenomenon, arthralgia, hepatosplenomegaly, and fever. IgM (monoclonal) antigen is most common found, but other patterns including IgA and IgG, and anti-IgG are reported.

Pathology

The renal lesion is a diffuse proliferative lesion with frequent membranous deposits. Electron microscopy shows deposits with a characteristic crystalline structure, and immunofluorescence reveals deposits of IgG, IgM, and C_3.

Treatment

The condition is not responsive to steroids, and the role of immunosuppressive drugs is uncertain. Penicillamine has been used but with little evidence of benefit. Reports of plasmapheresis have indicated that this may produce an improvement, particularly in patients with severe peripheral vascular lesions.

Sickle-cell disease

Among the other renal complications of sickle-cell disease is a glomerulopathy, not seen in patients with sickle-cell trait (see Section 19).

Clinical features

The glomerulopathy causes proteinuria, which uncommonly may be sufficient to cause a nephrotic syndrome, and in some leads to end-stage renal failure. The renal disease may obviously occur against the background of the other manifestations of sickle-cell disease.

Pathology

Microscopic examination generally shows a mesangiocapillary glomerulonephritis, with mesangial-cell proliferation and splitting of the basement membrane. Immunofluorescent studies give variable results ranging from no abnormality to granular glomerular deposits of IgG, IgM, and C_3.

Pathogenesis

Claims that circulating complexes of renal-tubule epithelial antigen, released due to ischaemia, and antibody to it are responsible, have not been substantiated. Other suggestions include the deposition of complexes of iron and protein arising from the haemolysis, and that immune-complex disease is related to a deficiency of alternative pathway function found in this disease.

Treatment

Proteinuria is generally steroid-resistant although isolated instances of improvement have been reported. Despite the potential problems, chronic haemodialysis has met with moderate success.

Diabetes mellitus

Thirty to fifty per cent of juvenile- or maturity-onset diabetics develop nephropathy within 20 years, and about 60 per cent of those whose onset appears to be less than 15 years previously, develop renal failure. Diabetes is therefore an important cause of chronic renal failure, currently providing about 5 per cent of patients admitted to dialysis and transplant programmes and an even greater number who are presently not being so treated (at least in the the United Kingdom). The principal change is a diffuse, although heteromorphic sclerosing lesion of the glomeruli. Capillary necrosis is a rarer complication. Although it was long held to be the case it now seems unlikely that patients with diabetes are particularly prone to develop pyelonephritis (see page 9.81).

Pathology and pathogenesis (Fig. 8)

Thickening of the glomerular basement membrane, accompanied later in the disease by thickening of the tubular basement membrane and the basement membrane of Bowman's capsule, appears to be the fundamental pathological change. An accumulation of mesangial matrix ultimately results in diffuse and nodular (Kimmelstiel–Wilson) glomerular sclerosis. Hyaline nodular deposits and hyaline arteriolar degeneration are frequent. The pathogenetic mechanisms underlying these abnormalities are unclear, but increasing glomerular permeability to plasma proteins, (especially to IgG and albumin) is characteristic. Diffuse and nodular glomerular sclerosis can be produced, or occurs in various experimental or spontaneous forms of diabetes, in animals. The evidence strongly indicates that the renal lesion is a consequence of the diabetic state: in rats, transplantation of normal kidneys in animals with streptocytocin-induced diabetes is followed by the development in the transplanted kidney of changes characteristic of rat diabetic nephropathy; transplantation of diabetic kidneys into syngeneic, non-diabetic litter mates is followed by recovery; and successful islet-cell transplantation is followed by resolution of the lesions within two or three months.

The critical question of the nature and mechanism of the increased glomerular basement thickening in diabetes is unanswered. In juvenile-onset diabetes in humans and experimental diabetes in the rat, GBM thickness is normal at onset of disease but increases progressively with time. Studies on the chemical composition of GBM have been conflicting; in diabetic man a much-quoted report of increased hydroxylation of lysine has not been confirmed, and in rats the position is also unclear.

Haemodynamic factors, perhaps causing hyperfiltration damage, appear to play an important role in pathogenesis; unilateral nephrectomy in rats results in accelerated development of diabetic glomerular lesions; in man hypertension is often associated with accelerated deterioration of renal function, and interestingly in the case of renal-artery stenosis, the ischaemic kidney is apparently protected from the development of diabetic nephropathy.

Clinical features

Principal features of clinical diabetic nephropathy are slowly progressive deterioration of renal function, with proteinuria which may be heavy even when renal failure has developed. Patients will generally show other features of diabetic microangiopathy, particularly retinopathy which is present in almost every case. Blood pressure may be normal, but even mild degrees of hypertension are associated with accelerated loss of renal function. More severe hypertension is often a late or terminal development. Reversible proteinuria is a feature of diabetic ketoacidosis but is otherwise not a feature of early, well-controlled diabetes, although even moderate loss of control has been shown to be associated with increased albumin excretion when this is measured by sensitive, quantitative immunological techniques. Strenuous exercise is also shown to cause a marked increase in albumin excretion in diabetes early in the course of disease. The development of a nephrotic syndrome is prognostically important – the majority of those affected going on to end-stage renal failure in 3–4 years. Diabetes, amyloid disease, and focal sclerosis are the principal causes of nephrotic syndrome associated with end-stage renal failure. A point which may occasionally be important is that other causes of nephrotic syndrome may occur in diabetes and so may respond to other appropriate treatment.

Prophylaxis and treatment

There has been much discussion over the past several decades on the question of whether the microangiopathic complications of diabetes can be prevented by good diabetic control. The opinion of most workers, and the work on experimental diabetes cited already, indicates that the lesions are secondary to insulin deficiency, hyperglycaemia, or their consequences. However, it has yet to be demonstrated that good control does reduce the incidence of these complications, probably because of the difficulty in conducting clinical experimental work over the required period and indeed of effecting 'good control'. A central, unresolved question is what constitutes 'good control', and whether the departures from the physiological range of blood sugars which are inevitable with intermittent subcutaneous insulin are sufficient to lead to microangiopathy. The introduction of subcutaneous insulin by infusion or the use of the artificial pancreas does not, as yet, appear to have any identifiable benefit in respect of microangiopathy.

Treatment of established nephropathy

When disease is established it seems reasonable to make extra efforts to control blood sugar levels, preferably by giving several daily injections of soluble insulin. Arterial hypertension must be treated early and effectively. Good control can be shown to retard the rate of loss of renal function. Otherwise treatment is symptomatic. When sudden deterioration of renal function is observed, it is important to exclude obstructive uropathy due to papillary necrosis.

Treatment of end-stage renal failure

Patients are being treated by regular dialysis and transplantation with increasing success, although the results are still substantially worse than those of non-diabetic patients with end-stage renal failure: about one-third of patients survive three years of dialysis. The principal problems relate to the extent and severity of systemic complications, especially vascular and cardiovascular disease, which are the principal causes of death. Both peritoneal and haemodialysis are used and transplantation is at present mainly carried out in younger patients. However, it seems likely that newer immunosuppressive agents such as cyclosporin, which may reduce the need for steroids, will carry advantages and renal transplantation at an early stage before the problems of uraemia and hypertension supervene will lead to better results. Simultaneous pancreatic and renal transplantation has been tried at a few centres although at present with little success.

Drugs and chemicals

A large number of drugs and chemicals have been implicated in causing nephritis. Table 3 (page 18.127) shows those drugs for which there is acceptable evidence that this is so.

Interstitial nephritis

This form of nephritis mainly affects the interstitium, the glomeruli being spared or only slightly affected; but it has also lately been realized that clinically important interstitial disease may also accompany or complicate glomerulonephritis. There is a suspicion that the incidence of this disorder is growing, and there are increasing numbers of cases reported associated with drugs, such as non-steroid anti-inflammatory drugs (NSAID), diuretics, and antimicrobials (see pages 18.111 and 18.132).

Clinical features

Most patients present with renal impairment which may be acute or chronic. A small number are detected by asymptomatic proteinuria or haematuria. A nephrotic syndrome is reported in many cases of NSAID-associated nephritis, indicating an accompanying glomerular pathology. There may be associated systemic manifestations due to underlying disease, as in SLE or infection, or if the nephritis is a manifestation of hypersensitivity there may be a rash, and eosinophilia.

In many cases recovery of renal function follows elimination or suppression of an underlying cause and/or treatment with steroids. A minority of patients progress to chronic renal failure despite steroid treatment.

Pathology

The diagnosis is made by histological appearances. The interstitial tissue is infiltrated with leucocytes, usually lymphocytes, plasma cells, and macrophages. Eosinophils may be seen in some cases. Where interstitial nephritis is related to septicaemia, the infiltrate may consist of predominantly polymorphonuclear leucocytes. This should not be confused with pyelonephritis, where direct bacterial invasion of the renal parenchyma is responsible for the inflammation – indeed it is likely that many cases of interstitial nephritis were previously misdiagnosed as pyelonephritis.

Immunofluorescent microscopy is negative in most cases. In a minority there may be deposits of C_3, IgG, and IgM in the mesangium, and in others linear deposits of IgG and C_3 may be seen on the tubular basement membrane, suggesting the presence of antitubular basement membrane antibodies (anti-TBM antibodies).

Anti-TBM antibodies may accompany anti-GBM antibodies, but also occur in immune-complex nephritis and rejection. A few well-documented cases of drug-induced nephritis have been shown to be mediated by this mechanism, but it is responsible for only a minority, including those associated with drugs, rejection and primary glomerular disease.

Raised serum levels of IgE have been found in some patients with drug-associated interstitial nephritis, suggesting a type I reaction.

Diagnosis and management

The diagnosis is made histologically. Treatment of an associated infection or withdrawal of an offending drug may be curative, but

steroids should also be given. They often reduce the active inflammatory infiltrate, and stabilize or improve renal function. It is important to be aware of interstitial nephritis, for its development may explain sudden deterioration of renal function in patients with known glomerular disease, and also may account for renal failure in a variety of systemic disorders.

Cholesterol lecithin acyltransferase (LCAT) deficiency and nephritis (see page 9.118)

A rare inherited inborn error of lipid metabolism associated with deficiency of the enzyme LCAT (which is responsible for the conversion of cholesterol to its esterified form) is associated with widespread accumulation of lipid, particularly in the cornea and glomeruli. Typically, patients present in the second or third decade with corneal opacification and proteinuria, but renal failure may be delayed for many years. Not all metabolically affected subjects develop renal disease, and factors other than the genetic deficiency are indirectly involved. The disorder, although excessively rare, is of considerable interest.

The use of immunological tests in the management of nephritis

The development of the large number of laboratory immunological techniques originally applied to research in nephritis and other diseases has provided a tempting picture of easy solutions to the difficult clinical problems often arising in the management of nephritis. In fact the aid afforded by such tests is limited to a small number of diagnostic questions and even fewer therapeutic ones.

Specific antibodies

Detection of serum antibodies to DNA plays a crucial role in the diagnosis of SLE, but their measurement is of less definite help in the management of chronic SLE nephritis (see page 18.49). Raised serum concentrations of antibody to streptococcal antigens, and other organisms when suspected and applicable, provide circumstantial evidence for the organism as the cause of the nephritis. The most valuable antibody measurement is that of anti-GBM antibody, which has allowed accurate diagnosis of anti-GBM disease, the monitoring of the effects of treatment, the detection of recurrence, and the prediction of an opportune period for transplantation.

Serum complement

Hypocomplementaemia is a helpful diagnostic feature in poststreptococcal nephritis and other nephritides (such as infective endocarditis) associated with bacterial infection, SLE and mesangiocapillary nephritis type I and II – low serum concentrations of C_3, C_4, or haemolytic complement not being a feature of other forms of nephritis. Serial measurement of complement may be helpful in the management of SLE where low levels have some association with activity of disease, and in poststreptococcal nephritis in which persistent hypocomplementaemia has been associated with progressive disease.

Immune complexes

The value, if any, of determining serum levels of circulating immune complexes is not evident. Tests are of little diagnostic value and there is generally a poor correlation and disease activity.

References

Glassock, R. J. and Cohen, A. T. (1976). Secondary glomerular diseases. In *The kidney* 2nd edn (eds B. M. Brenner and F. C. Rector), Vol. II, p. 1493. W. B. Saunders, Philadelphia.
Williams, D. G. and Peters, D. K. (1982). The immunology of nephritis. In *Clinical aspects of immunology* 4th edn (eds P. J. Lachmann and D. K. Peters), Vol. II, p. 853. Blackwell Scientific Publications, Oxford.

PROTEINURIA AND THE NEPHROTIC SYNDROME

J. S. CAMERON

Proteinuria

Although proteinuria has been studied for almost 300 years, the structural and functional events which determine the appearance of excess protein in the urine are still poorly understood. Normal urine contains only a trace of protein; less than 200 mg per day in most individuals, of which only about 50 mg is albumin (75–150 mg/l and 10–20 mg/l respectively). This can be compared with the 70 g/l of protein found in normal plasma, of which 35–50 g/l is albumin. How does the kidney virtually exclude proteins from the glomerular filtrate whilst allowing 180 1/24 hours of plasma water and contained electrolytes to pass through the glomeruli? If there was a complete answer to this question, we could understand better how proteinuria in excess of the normal range appears in various diseases of the kidney. At the moment, there are only partial answers to this question, and much remains in the field of speculation.

However it is clear, principally from experimental work in laboratory animals that two factors are important in excluding proteins at the glomerular level. The first of these is *molecular size* (for most purposes shape can be ignored and all protein molecules treated as approximately spherical). The normal glomerular capillary wall structure filters molecules of a molecular size up to around 30 000 dalton (approximately) as water is filtered. Above this molecular weight, there is a rapid cut-off in the penetration of proteins into the filtrate, so that at the molecular weight of albumin (67 000 dalton) the penetration of protein is only about 0.01 per cent of water. What little albumin *is* filtered is then available for reabsorption and catabolism in the proximal renal tubules, so that the kidney is an important site of albumin catabolism in health; this catabolic role increases with increased delivery of protein to the renal tubules in disease.

The other factor which limits the penetration of proteins into the glomerular filtrate is molecular *charge*. Almost all physiological proteins are, at the pH of plasma, negatively charged: that is, they behave as anions. The glomerular capillary wall is rich in anionic glycoproteins, which are concentrated just underneath the endothelial cell, on the inside of the capillary wall; and also at the outer aspect of the basement membrane, just beneath the foot processes of the epithelial cell or podocyte. These charges repel the negative charges on the proteins so that the passage of negatively charged proteins is hindered compared with unchanged molecules. Conversely, the passage of positively charged, cationic molecules is facilitated.

The appearance of abnormal amounts of protein in the urine may be explained, therefore, by postulating either a change in the structure of the capillary wall such that it becomes more permeable to large molecules, that it has lost some or all of the anionic glycoprotein coat which is present in health, or both. However, our understanding of the function of the glomerular capillaries is incomplete, and other factors may be important which are not yet understood – for example, function of the epithelial celll, or podocyte.

Before considering the common problem, proteinuria of glomerular origin, the much less common proteinuria originating from *tubular* disease is considered.

'Tubular' proteinuria

It was mentioned above that normal glomeruli are almost as permeable to low molecular weight protein as they are to water. Thus, physiological proteins of low molecular weight together with pathological proteins, such as immunoglobulin light chains,

are normally filtered and thus are present in the plasma in only very low concentrations. These proteins are almost completely reabsorbed in the proximal tubule and catabolized there. In health, therefore, the tubular fluid is the only site where these proteins of a low molecular weight can be detected in any quantity. However, in renal failure they will accumulate in the plasma along with other substances normally cleared mainly by glomerular filtration, and in disease affecting the proximal tubule they will appear in the urine in relatively large amounts.

Tubular proteinuria consists principally of α- and β-globulins with a molecular weight from 5000 to 50 000 dalton, including some peptide hormones (insulin, growth hormone) enzymes such as lysozyme (molecular weight 11 500 dalton) and ribonuclease, and a number of microglobulins. These include β_2 microglobulin (molecular weight 13 500 dalton) which is a fragment of the HLA class 1 surface protein markers on cells, and β-thromboglobulin (molecular) weight 30 000 dalton) which is secreted by activated platelets. There is also a little albumin, but usually only 10–20 per cent of the total. Tubular proteinuria in the presence of normal renal function usually amounts from 0.5 to 1.0 g/24 hours and never exceeds 2.0 g/24 hours. The majority of the protein excreted reacts poorly or not at all with Albustix (see below) and some may not precipitate well on heating. The best methods of screening are either cellulose acetate electrophoresis of the urine, which will readily distinguish the tubular proteinuria from glomerular proteinuria (90–99 per cent albumin); or a test for one of the microglobulins which make up the bulk of 'tubular' proteinuria. Enzymes such as lysozyme can be assayed, and one test readily available in kit form is the Phadebas β_2 micro test (Pharmacia Ltd.) which measures the quantity of β_2 microglobulin in the urine. In urine from normal individuals < 0.1–0.4 μg/ml is found, whereas in individuals with tubular proteinuria 40–200 μg/ml may be detected.

The *causes* of 'tubular' proteinuria include all those conditions which lead to generalized disease of the proximal tubule – the Debré–de Toni–Fanconi syndrome (usually called the Fanconi syndrome for brevity). These include inherited metabolic disease leading to toxic effects on the proximal tubule – cystinosis, galactosaemia, tyrosinosis, idiopathic cases, etc. (Section 9) with heavy metals such as cadmium, lead, or uranium (see page 18.109) and some other acquired tubulopathies, such as analgesic abuse. Usually in the latter there is sufficient glomerular damage as a secondary event that the urinary protein is principally albumin. Finally, in the curious endemic Balkan nephropathy, interstitial renal disease is accompanied by the finding of a proteinuria of 'tubular' pattern early in the course of the condition. This may be used as a screening test for the early phases of the disease.

Proteinuria of glomerular origin

Proteinuria which results from damage or functional alterations within the glomeruli is predominantly albumin, in part because this is the major protein of the plasma, and also because the molecular weight of albumin is only a little above that at which protein is excluded from the urine in health. There is evidence from animal experiments that in glomeruli damaged by glomerulonephritis of soluble complex type, the loss of protein occurs focally in the capillary wall at the site of deposition (for formation) of the immune complexes. In so-called 'minimal change' disease (lipoid nephrosis) (see page 18.44) it appears more likely that a diffuse reversible functional alteration in the ability of the glomerulus to retain protein has occurred. This involves little structural change in the capillary wall, but the anionic charge on the basement membrane appears to be lost. Whether this is the cause of the proteinuria, or a result of it, like the fusion and loss of the delicate foot process structure of the podocytes, is not known.

Testing for proteinuria is usually done today by employing one or other 'stick' tests, of which Albustix is the best known. This exploits the shift in the titration curve of dyes in the presence of albumin. The stick also contains a buffer to keep the pH constant in the test environment (the stick's test pad) since otherwise variations in the pH of the urine might also cause change in colour. The dye usually employed is bromcresol green, which is yellow at the pH of the stick in the absence of albumin, but in its presence turns green with an intensity roughly proportionate to the amount of albumin present. The stick tests do not detect 'tubular' proteins, nor myeloma proteins with any sensitivity. More important is the fact that their level of sensitivity for albumin – about 30–40 mg/l – is only just above that found in many normal individuals, even at rest. Thus 'trace' readings with Albustix are common in healthy individuals and should be ignored. Even '+' readings may be found quite frequently (see below). However, it is now known that sensitive radioimmunoassays will detect *abnormal* albuminuria (microalbuminuria) but at a level below that detectable on Albustix®. This has been best studied in type I (juvenile insulin-dependent) diabetes (see page 9.80).

An alternative, slightly less convenient method is to mix equal volumes of 3 per cent sulphosalicylic acid (SSA) and urine. This test also may not detect proteins of 'tubular' origin, or myeloma proteins, and is slightly more sensitive than Albustix for albumin (10–20 mg albumin). A positive reads as a faint or definite haze in the mixture, indicative of precipitated protein.

It is usual to recommend (but rare to ensure) that positive tests with either of these methods should be confirmed using the classical heating of acidified urine (a few drops of urine plus 5–10 ml 5 per cent acetic acid). This step may be necessary because both the 'stick' tests and SSA test may give false positives, with radiographic contrast media and some drugs (such as tolbutamide and penicillins). Turbid urines are difficult to read in the SSA test.

Because of the great variation in concentration of protein in the urine throughout the 24 hours of the day, it is usual to quantitate proteinuria in 24-hour urines. This carries with it the inconvenience and inaccuracy of a 24-hour urine, and an alternative is to use the albumin/creatinine ratio on random 'spot' urines. The U_A/U_C ratio (each in mg/ml) is less than 0.2 in children and 0.1 in adults, if the albumin is measured accurately using an immunochemical method.

The finding of albuminuria in symptomless individuals

Albuminuria in the setting of dependent or generalized swelling is discussed below in the section on the nephrotic syndrome. What of the finding of proteinuria in an otherwise healthy individual examined for routine health check, insurance, or employment purposes, or in the course of investigation of other disease states?

Proteinuria in excess of 'normal' is a very common finding, especially in the young, and the principal problem is in whom, and how far, to investigate the finding. Depending upon the definition of what constitutes a positive urine test, between 1 and 5 per cent of school children will be found to be 'proteinuric' and almost as many young adults. The first step, in any individual found to have a positive test for protein, is to *repeat the test* for at least a further two specimens. More than half, especially those showing only '+' on their initial test, will be negative on subsequent testing. Several incidental medical conditions also must be noted. *Fever* is associated with proteinuria in 5 per cent of children – there are no data from adults. Much of this 'febrile' proteinuria probably results from innocuous renal deposition of immune complexes formed in the course of an infectious fever to various viral and bacterial agents (see page 18.38). This 'febrile' proteinuria is of no consequence and disappears as the fever resolves. *Congestive cardiac*

failure is accompanied by proteinuria of 0.5–1.5 g/24 hours in a considerable number of patients, and resolves as cardiac output improves; its origin is not understood. It is not necessary to assume coincident renal disease if this level of proteinuria is found. Coincident *hypertension* is more difficult to manage. Certainly a number of hypertensive individuals have a similar degree of proteinuria to that just discussed, which resolves when the blood pressure is treated adequately. However, the coincidence of proteinuria and high blood pressure should make one suspicious that more disease is present than essential hypertension (see below). *Exercise* is also discussed below.

If protein is present on repeated testing in three or more urines, then of course a physical examination is required, if not already performed. Particular attention should be paid to the level of blood pressure, bearing in mind the subject's age and sex, the presence of minor degrees of oedema, or the stigmata of uraemia (see page 18.139). Some basic chemical tests are needed, including plasma electrolytes, urea and creatinine, serum protein concentrations in children, an ASO titre (or equivalent investigation for streptococcal infection) repeated as necessary, and in girls especially, an antinuclear antibody test on serum.

At this point it is necessary to assess whether protein is present also in urine formed whilst recumbent.

A good proportion – 22 per cent of young college males in Levitt's classic study – will be found to have *postural (orthostatic) proteinuria*. In this state protein is regularly found in the daytime urine, sometimes even in concentrations of several grams per litre, whilst it is absent from the early morning urine formed during the night. The cause of this observation is unknown. Certainly it has nothing to do with recumbency or the erect posture, since quiet standing *reduces* the amount of physiological proteinuria in normal individuals; the effect of lordosis in causing kinking of the renal veins is often quoted but seems unlikely. Activity, on the other hand, especially *violent exercise*, leads to a fall in renal blood flow and reproducible proteinuria, even in healthy individuals normally without proteinuria. This old observation has recently received revived attention under the heading of 'jogger's nephritis', since haematuria is usually also present after exhausting effort. The proteinuria of 'postural' proteinuric individuals contains proteins of all sizes, not only albumin and other low-molecular weights. This observation is surprising, since it is usual in benign forms of profuse proteinuria for the proteinuria to be 'selective', i.e. only albumin and low molecular weight proteins. However, the proteinuria is usually slight, and this observation breaks down in minor proteinuric states.

The prognosis for a young individual with reproducible postural proteinuria is that of a normal individual up to 40 years following diagnosis. Interestingly many such individuals continue to show proteinuria, either postural or persistent proteinuria of minor degrees for several decades. They do not, however, develop high blood pressure or renal impairment, and we must conclude this is a variant of normal. A number of individuals with well documented postural proteinuria have haematuria also, but this does not influence the good prognosis.

Further investigation of the child/or young adult with postural proteinuria is not justified, but the remainder with recumbent proteinuria as well as proteinuria by day come under suspicion of having significant glomerular disease. Some more detailed assessment of renal function, such as a creatinine clearance, or a glomerular filtration rate measurement employing ^{125}I iothalamate or [51]Credetate, is useful as a baseline, and if abnormally low may suggest further investigations. The serum level of the third component of complement (C_3) should be measured also, and an intravenous urogram (IVU) performed. This is needed because structural disorders, such as reflux nephropathy, analgesic nephropathy, and polycystic kidneys may present through the finding of proteinuria, usually accompanied by leucocyturia and haematuria. The most useful prognostic procedure is to test the urine for blood repeatedly. If haematuria *and* proteinuria are found together, the chances of some significant renal abnormality being present is increased. On the other hand, *renal biopsy* studies of children or adults with isolated proteinuria – even when 1–3 g protein are excreted daily – usually show normal or nearly normal patterns. Membranous nephropathy may be found in a minority. The outlook in patients with isolated proteinuria without haematuria is excellent for renal function and survival. A biopsy may be needed, however, to establish with certainty that the kidneys are not damaged, for insurance or employment purposes.

If, on the other hand, the proteinuric individual has reduced renal function, persistent haematuria as well as proteinuria, is hypocomplementaemic, or has hypertension, then a renal biopsy will be considered by most physicians at this point. It is still possible that the urinary abnormalities will disappear, and it may be useful to wait some months before going ahead with a renal biopsy. This is particularly so in children who may be recovering from an undiagnosed acute post-infectious nephritis in whom haematuria and proteinuria persists for six months or two years before recovery (see page 18.41). On the other hand renal biopsy may show mesangiocapillary glomerulonephritis, local segmental glomerulosclerosis, or membranous nephropathy. The prognosis for patients with these histological appearances in their renal biopsies who are never nephrotic is much better than for their fellow patients with similar histological appearances who have an initial, and above all a persistent nephrotic syndrome (see Fig. 4, page 18.66).

The nephrotic syndrome

Definition

This rather meaningless term is part of the clumsy terminology of patients with glomerular disease. It is usually employed to describe patients whose proteinuria is of sufficient magnitude and duration to lower their serum albumin below the level at which normal renal perfusion and salt excretion can be maintained. The result is an expansion of body sodium and water, mostly distributed into the interstitial space, and visible as oedema. A common definition of the nephrotic syndrome is:

1. The presence of detectable oedema, usually dependent
2. Proteinuria > 3.0 g/24 h
   (or > 0.05 g/kg/24 h in children)
3. A serum albumin < 30 g/l

A few comments on this definition are necessary. First, some patients have such a low serum albumin that their urinary protein excretion in g/24 h is *less* than patients not so severely affected; this is revealed if the urine/plasma ratio of albumin is considered. Secondly, with increasing age, patients are progressively more vulnerable to proteinuria and develop hypoalbuminaemia more easily. Thus, a child or adult taking a good diet may maintain a normal serum albumin and remain oedema-free, even though excreting well above 3 g protein/24 h. Thirdly, when the serum albumin falls, older patients are much more likely to form oedema at *higher* serum albumin concentrations than younger patients or children. The latter rarely form oedema unless their serum albumin is less than 25 g/l, whereas in old age, oedema may form even at a serum albumin around 30–32 g/l. Finally, the presence of oedema is dependent upon salt intake, diuretic treatment, and posture.

All this implies that there is no clearcut, definitive boundary between a patient with persistent, profuse but symptomless proteinuria, and one with a nephrotic syndrome. A single patient may traverse this boundary in either direction, spontaneously or in response to treatment. Which patient should be labelled 'nephrotic' is finally a matter of taste in many cases, and it is perhaps better to draw this line fairly critically, including patients with a definite, unequivocal nephrotic syndrome only, who may require the management outlined below. Otherwise, patients who can manage without interference may be treated energetically but

unnecessarily. There is also no mention in the definition given above of plasma cholesterol levels, nor of oval fat bodies in the urine. Both seem to be secondary phenomena, and oval fat bodies maybe found in patients with progressive glomerular disease of several types but without oedema, in the presence of proteinuria insufficient to produce a nephrotic syndrome. Finally, the ugly term 'biochemical nephrotic syndrome' is sometimes encountered. This is used for a patient who has not developed oedema, either because of diuretic treatment, or because of ability to withstand a low serum albumin, but who otherwise satisfies the criteria of > 3g proteinuria/24 h and a serum albumin of less than 30 g/l.

Disordered physiology

Why does loss of protein in the urine lead to the accumulation of oedema? This is another question that cannot be answered with certainty because there is still no complete picture of the regulation of salt and water homeostasis in health. However, the conventional story is illustrated in Fig. 1. In essence, this description suggests that the nephrotic patient 'purchases' a relatively normal circulating plasma volume, tissue perfusion, and blood pressure at the expense of the accumulation of interstitial volume so that oedema becomes obvious. In extreme cases the patient may labour under 30–40 l of extra salt and water, almost all of it in the interstitial space.

Therre are many problems with this 'conventional' description of the nephrotic state, some of which have been discussed recently by Mees and colleagues. The most obvious of these are the lack of correlation, whether within or between patient comparisons are made of plasma albumin, circulating volume, and renal function. An extreme example of this discordance is the rare patient who is born analbuminaemic, but who can excrete sodium in a relatively normal fashion, and suffers only occasional mild ankle oedema if upright for prolonged periods. The loss of rather small amounts of albumin – 3 g/24 h for instance – is accompanied in the nephrotic syndrome by dramatic falls in the level of serum albumin and the presence of oedema which are not seen in other states of protein loss, for example, in the course of peritoneal dialysis, when much larger amounts of protein are lost each day in the peritoneal fluid.

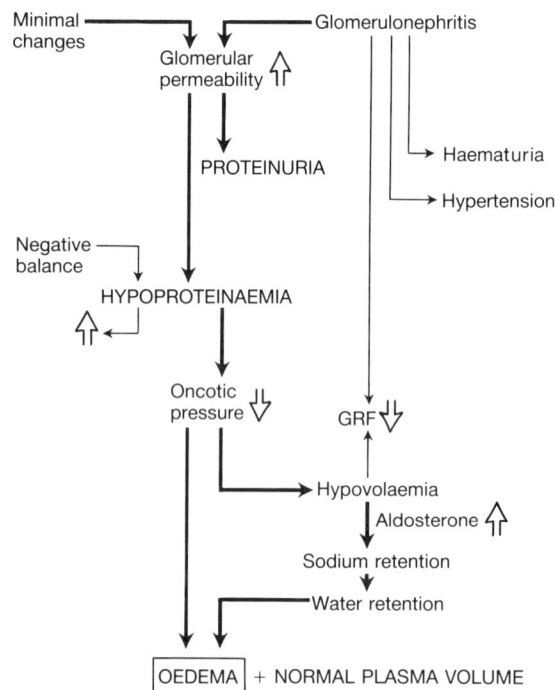

Fig. 1 A scheme to explain the relationship between loss of albumin in the urine and the accumulation of oedema in nephrotic patients (see text). GFR = glomerular filtration rate.

We must suppose that in the nephrotic syndrome much larger amounts of albumin are being catabolized than usual after reabsorption in the renal tubules but this has not been proved. A problem in the investigation of this area is the failure of nephrotic patients to satisfy the basic criteria for turnover studies of labelled proteins and doubts about the validity of albumin spaces as indicating plasma volume. After energetic treatment, it is often possible to maintain nephrotic patients free of oedema on the same dose of diuretic even though the serum albumin concentration and protein excretion are unchanged from their former state of extreme oedema and resistance to moderate doses of diuretics.

However, several points in practical management emerge from this tentative scheme which are borne out by clinical observation. The first is that, whilst oedema is forming and the patient is hypovolaemic, energetic treatment with diuretics may lead to further depletion of circulating volume and circulatory collapse. Secondly, once equilibrium has been established with a normal or even expanded plasma volume, then rapid intravenous infusion of albumin alone to achieve a diuresis may be followed by circulatory overload and pulmonary oedema. Thirdly, the ability of a nephrotic patient to excrete a water load will be very limited. There is little distal tubular delivery of sodium and hypovolaemia may stimulate ADH secretion even if osmotic considerations do not warrant its release.

Causes of the nephrotic syndrome

As in any clinical syndrome, there are a number of events which may damage the kidney so that proteinuria of dimensions sufficient to bring on a nephrotic syndrome is induced. These are listed in summary in Table 1, together with the relative proportions in an unselected series of nephrotics in adults and children. Figure 2 shows the different proportions at different ages. Most of these glomerular appearances are believed to result from the deposition or formation of immune (antibody–antigen) complexes in the glomeruli, and are discussed in the section on glomerulonephritis (see page 18.38). Although many articles and texts include very long lists of 'causes' of the nephrotic syndrome, most of these are single case reports, or only from a handful of patients, and more than 99 per cent of nephrotic patients fall into one of the groups listed. Under the heading 'miscellaneous' are included these many rare reports.

The question of *drug-induced nephrotic syndromes* is discussed in more detail in the section on toxic nephropathies (see page 18.108). In the majority (mercury and mercurial drugs, penicillamine, tridione, gold, captopril) the glomerular lesion is one of membranous nephropathy. A number of other drugs, including perchlorate, ethosuximade, propanolol, oral contraceptives, bismuth, phenindione, tolbutamide, phenylbutazone, and pyrithioxine, have been associated in single case reports with a nephrotic syndrome. These associations are much more doubtful.

Another group of patients show 'minimal changes' on their renal biopsies, and their condition apparently relates to specific allergies, most commonly pollens but also some drugs (e.g. penicillin), bee stings, foods, or poison oak and ivy. Finally, it is worth mentioning, in view of the common finding of minor proteinuria in heart failure, the rare association of the nephrotic syndrome with constrictive pericarditis, relieved by its surgical correction.

The difference in pattern of underlying histopathology in children and adults is immediately apparent from Table 1 and Fig. 2, and well known. The 'minimal change' lesion is predominant under the age of 15 years, overwhelmingly so in children between the ages of one and six years. An important part of the early management of any nephrotic patient is to establish, or guess, which of the appearances or disease listed in Table 1 may be present. This is not only because this information may influence immediate treatment, but because the likelihood of ultimate renal failure varies from negligible (minimal changes) to almost invariable (primary amyloidosis), whilst the chances of remission vary inversely with these observations (Table 1). In most forms of glomerulonephri-

Table 1 Underlying glomerular disease in the nephrotic syndrome[1]

	Children[2,3] (% of all nephrotics)	Adults[2] (% of all nephrotics)	Proportion of each group going into remission (%)
Apparently primary glomerular disease			
'Minimal change' lesion	80	25	65*
Focal segmental glomerulosclerosis	7	9	15–20
Membranous nephropathy	1	22	50
Proliferate g.n.			
Mesangiocapillary	5	14 } 26%	5
Other[4]	5	12 }	10–90 (see text)
Glomerular disease in systemic conditions			
Lupus[5]	–	8	25†
Amyloid[5]	–	7	0
Diabetes[5]	–	3	0
Henoch-Schönlein purpura	2	<1	75
Miscellaneous[6]	<<1	<<1	
Overall remission rate	(80%)	(36%)	

* Plus another 30% maintained in remission by treatment.
† Maintained in remission on treatment.
Notes:
1. These data refer only to Western communities such as Europe and North America. In tropical areas, the proportion of children and adults with 'minimal change' is much smaller – perhaps 10 per cent or less in children.
2. Children and adults refer to an onset of the nephrotic syndrome less than or greater than 15 years of age respectively.
3. Data for children are mainly those of the international study of the nephrotic syndrome in children (500 children): for adults, those seen at Guy's up to 1979 (400 adults).
4. 'Other' proliferative include: acute exudative glomerulonephritis: mesangial and focal proliferative glomerulonephritis, with and without IgA; proliferative g.n. with extensive crescent formation.
5. The absence of an entry for amyloid, diabetes, and lupus in the children's column indicates that, although rare patients with these conditions and a nephrotic syndrome may be seen, the number is insignificant.
6. 'Miscellaneous' includes the congenital nephrotic syndrome of the Finnish type in children, specific allergies, sickle cell disease, myeloma, drug intoxications, etc.

tis, those patients who develop a full nephrotic syndrome do worse in this respect than their luckier brethren who have proteinuria of lesser degree (Fig. 4, page 18.66). But even in conditions such as mesangiocapillary glomerulonephritis, a few patients appear to heal completely, even after prolonged nephrotic syndrome, although this event is rare (Table 1). Perhaps a quarter of patients with membranous nephropathy and a nephrotic syndrome become completely well after one to five years, and up to 50 per cent after 15 years. About 20 per cent of children – perhaps a lower proportion of adults – with focal segmental glomerulosclerosis also go into remission. The proportion of other types of proliferative glomerulonephritis remitting varies greatly: in acute post-infectious nephritis, the remission rate approaches 95 per cent, whilst in nephritis with extensive crescent formation (extracapillary proliferation) almost no patient remits completely, and few survive with renal function. Overall, 80 per cent of nephrotic children and 36 per cent of adults can be expected to be in remission after 5–15 years; the proportion dependent upon the presence of 'minimal change' patients is 70 per cent and 24 per cent respectively.

The nephrotic syndrome, aside from being inconvenient and unpleasant, is also dangerous in itself, quite apart from the risk of hypertension and renal failure complicating the underlying condition. The management of the major complications of the nephrotic state will be considered later, but one important point is that many of these can be made worse by treatment employed for the primary condition, so that a balance of profit and loss for intervention must be considered carefully for each patient.

The examination and investigation of the nephrotic patient

The differential diagnosis of generalized or dependent oedema must, of course, be gone through: it is a chastening thought for nephrologists that for every nephrotic patient, there must be several thousands with swollen ankles from varicose veins. Other causes of hypoalbuminaemia, such as nutritional problems, liver disease, and protein-losing enteropathy need to be excluded.

A number of preceding events have to be kept in mind when taking the history and completing the examination of a patient known, or suspected of having a nephrotic syndrome. These include the bacterial, parasitic, viral, and other infections known to be associated with immune complex disease. The possibility of tumours must be borne in mind, especially in patients over the age of 50 years, and association of lymphomas (both Hodgkin's and non-Hodgkin's) with a nephrotic syndrome and minimal change appearances in the glomeruli must not be forgotten. Other sources of autologous antigens such as thyroglobulin in thyroid disorders, IgG in essential mixed cryoglobulinaemia, and DNA in systemic lupus must be considered. Amyloidosis may be present, and if secondary there may be a history of osteomyelitis or tuberculosis. An occasional patient with diabetic nephropathy presents with renal disease rather than in a more conventional fashion. Others have disease related to heroin addiction, and in neonates the recessive inherited Finnish form of nephrotic syndrome may be present at birth. A few patients with massive obesity have been reported with a nephrotic syndrome, and proteinuria has been said to be present in 40 per cent of severely obese subjects. Finally, proteinuria and a full nephrotic syndrome may be found in congenital cyanotic heart disease.

Obviously, not all these apply equally to patients at different ages, and as indicated in Table 1, the renal biopsy appearances will differ greatly in adults and children. However, the following points are worth enquiring about directly in *all* patients:

1. Allergies: patients with 'minimal change' lesions have a much higher incidence of allergy, or histories of atopy in childhood than the general population.

2. Solvent exposure: there is growing evidence that a wide range of glomerulonephritis may be precipitated, perhaps in genetically susceptible individuals, by exposure to hydrocarbon fuels and solvents.

3. Drug exposure: a careful drug history is needed in view of the well-documented and more doubtful associations mentioned above.

4. Family history: a family history of nephritis, even in those patients without classical familial nephritides such as Alport's syndrome, is distinctly more common than was thought previously. This again may reflect a common genetic vulnerability.

In the *physical examination*, the key finding is oedema. This may be slight, and noticed only in the ankles in the evening, and around the eyes on rising. It may be asymmetric in the legs, perhaps in association with a secondary calf vein thrombosis. In children the oedema tends to be less dependent upon gravity, and frequently rather mild ankle oedema may be associated with a very puffy face, an abdomen distended with ascites, and 'Popeye' arms with swelling collected around the elbows; the appearance is enhanced by the muscle wasting, which can be extreme under cover of the oedema, and which is visible in the upper arm. Pleural effusions and ascites are present in many patients, if the oedema is severe. On occasion even the top of the head may be oedematous. In those kept in bed – which is not advisable in view of the risk of thromboses – the bulk of the oedema will be found in the upper thighs and over the sacrum. Genital oedema is often present, may be massive, and the source of a good deal of distress. Striae may appear from protein depletion and swelling even in nephrotic patients never treated with corticosteroids. Xanthomata may be present in patients with extreme hypercholesterolaemia. The liver may be enlarged, and in adult patients this may lead the unwary physician, seeing oedema and proteinuria (which occurs reversibly

in heart failure, as already noted) to diagnose and even treat with digitalis. The normal jugular venous pressure and the dimensions of the proteinuria should leave little room for doubt. The blood pressure measurement (taken standing and lying) is useful in several respects. Sustained diastolic hypertension suggests renal hypertension and structurally altered kidneys, but it is nice to remember that even 'minimal change' nephrotics may become hypertensive when critically hypovolaemic – perhaps a result of intense renin secretion and vasoconstriction. A fall of more than 15 mmHg on standing may also indicate critical hypovolaemia.

Investigations

Investigations in the nephrotic patient should be directed towards:

1. Assessing the severity of the nephrotic syndrome:
    (a) Haemoglobin and packed cell volume. Assuming a normal red cell production this will give some idea of hypovolaemia.
    (b) 24-hour urine protein, repeated several times.
    (c) Serum albumin concentration (remember that Auto Analyser automated dye binding methods *overestimate* albumin by about 5 g/l throughout the whole range).
    (d) Fasting plasma lipids, cholesterol, and electrophoretic strip.
    (e) Urine volume and Na^+ concentration – useless if patient has already received diuretics. Usually a low urine volume and a Na^+ concentration < 10 mmol/l will be found.
2. Assessing the degree of renal function impairment:
    (a) Estimation of plasma creatinine and urea.
    (b) Creatinine clearance; this may grossly overestimate the GFR in some nephrotic patients.
    (c) Glomerular filtration rate (^{51}Cr EDTA or ^{125}I iothalamate clearance). The results obtained may, of course, reflect more the reversible renal hypoperfusion of the nephrotic patient than the true degree of renal damage.
3. Estimating the nature of the underlying renal pathology:
    (a) Serum C_3 (and perhaps C_4 complement concentration).
    (b) Differential protein clearance measurement.
    (c) *Careful* examination of *fresh* urine for red cells and casts on more than one occasion (see page 18.2). The strategy here is to try to pick out patients with 'minimal change' lesions who will probably respond to corticosteroids: see below for discussion.
4. Specific tests for individual diseases:
    (a) HB_s and HB_e antigen.
    (b) Anti-nuclear factor; if +ve, measure double-stranded (d.s.) DNA binding or do *Crithidia* kinetoplast test.
    (c) ASO titre or other test for streptococcal infections.
    These will, of course, give information on possible specific aetiologies, and should be performed on all nephrotic patients.
5. Preparation for possible renal biopsy:
    (a) IVU.
    (b) Platelet count.
    (c) Prothrombin and cephalin–kaolin times.

Renal biopsy and other special tests in the nephrotic patient

Given the diversity of underlying disease, and the variable outcome of the several conditions, a tissue diagnosis is *desirable* in any nephrotic patient. But how *necessary* is it to perform a biopsy in nephrotic patients? Biopsy is not without risk. Although in skilled hands the risk of losing a kidney is negligible, bleeding profuse enough to require transfusion occurs about once in every hundred biopsies. The principal goals of biopsy are: (a) to establish whether a 'minimal change' lesion is present, with the implication that a rapid loss of proteinuria will occur if corticosteroids are given; and (b) if this is not the case, to determine the pattern of glomerular injury so that a prognosis can be given (Table 1) particularly with regard to the likelihood and possible timing of renal failure.

A glance at Table 1 and Fig. 2 suggests that an identical policy for patients of all ages is not likely to be the best strategy. In *adults*, the proportion of patients with 'minimal change' is low, so that giving corticosteroids without biopsy would result in three out of four patients being treated unnecessarily. Biopsy, therefore, is best done as early as possible in all nephrotic adults. In children, especially between the ages of one and six years, the majority of patients have 'minimal change' disease and will respond to corticosteroids. It is therefore reasonable to treat the majority of nephrotic children at this age with these agents *without* doing a renal biopsy, performing one if the child fails to respond with loss of proteinuria within four weeks of beginning treatment (see below). The exception to this rule will be the child aged one to six who shows features which suggest that disease other than minimal change may be present. First, he (the condition is commoner in males) may have Henoch–Schönlein purpura. There is no evidence that corticosteroids benefit the kidney in this condition. Secondly, some features although not definitive in themselves (except perhaps a low serum complement concentration) may suggest disease other than minimal change:

1. Persistent microscopic haematuria (i.e. in three or more urines)
2. Persistent diastolic hypertension, given a reasonable circulating volume
3. A low serum C_3 complement concentration
4. Poorly selective differential protein clearance

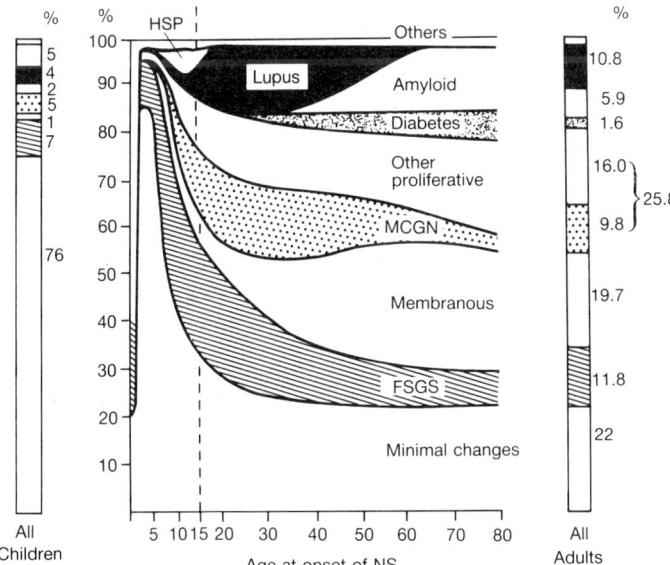

Fig. 2 The underlying histopathology of the glomerulus as revealed in biopsy studies of unselected nephrotic patients of different ages at onset. It can be seen that the proportion of patients with minimal change disease falls during childhood, from 85 per cent to about the adult proportion (20–25 per cent) by 20 years of age. In adults, other forms of glomerular disease underly the majority of nephrotic syndromes, amyloidosis taking the place of lupus in older patients, and membranous nephropathy becoming steadily more common. (HSP = Henoch Schonlein purpura nephritis; MCGN = mesangiocapillary glomerulonephritis; FSGS = focal segmental glomerulosclerosis. Others = other rarer causes of a nephrotic syndrome, e.g. paraproteinaemias, microscopic polyarteritis, Alport's syndrome etc.) The data are from over 500 adult and 200 childhood-onset nephrotic patients seen during 1963–84 at Guy's Hospital. Data from the children are from 1963–70 only, since after this time only selected patients were biopsied, as described in the text. (Taken from Cameron and Glassock, eds, 1986, The natural history and outcome of the nephrotic syndrome. In *The nephrotic syndrome*, Marcel Dekker, New York, in press.)

If more than two of these are present together, it suggests rather strongly that some structural abnormality of the glomerulus will be found on renal biopsy.

Some of these tests deserve a word of explanation. *The serum C_3 concentration* is depressed below its lower limit (55–60 per cent of reference normal pooled serum) in three common conditions: acute post-infectious glomerulonephritis, in which it returns to normal from a few days to no more than eight weeks later; mesangiocapillary (membranoproliferative) glomerulonephritis (MCGN, MPGN), in which it is low in about two-thirds of patients at some time, and remains so for months or years; and systemic lupus erythematosus (SLE) in which it is variably depressed, especially in patients with untreated active disease. The C_4 component is part of the main pathway leading to C_3 consumption, and is usually normal in both acute nephritis and MCGN, but almost always depressed equally or more than the C_3 in SLE. Two rarer forms of glomerulonephritis may show persistent or intermittently low C_3 concentrations, usually accompanied by a low C_4. These are the glomerulonephritis complicating subacute bacterial endocarditis (see pages 13.314 and 18.42) and essential cryoglobulinaemia (see Section 19) which are often mesangiocapillary in pattern. Thus, a low C_3 or C_4 is of value, a normal reading is useless.

The *differential protein clearance* test can be done on a spot urine and plasma sample, taken the same day. The idea behind the test is that patients with 'minimal change' lesions leak almost exclusively albumin into their urine, whilst proteins of higher molecular weight are virtually excluded. In contrast, in many forms of glomerulonephritis, these larger molecular weight proteins leak into the urine in significant amounts, although still forming less than 10 per cent of the proteinuria. One cannot simply measure the concentrations in the urine, however, because of the varying concentrations of the proteins in the plasma. What is done is to measure the concentrations in plasma (P) as well as urine (U) and measure the clearance ratio for at least two proteins, 1 and 2:

$$U_1V/P_1 \div U_2V/P_2$$

If we take albumin as the second (reference) protein (P_2) and IgG as the larger one (P_1), then we can get a clearance ratio which varies from 0.01 in the most 'selective' proteinuria in a patient with minimal changes, to 0.20 or even 1.00 in very 'non-selective' proteinuria in a patient with severe nephritis. The volume of urine (V) cancels out in the question above, so that a 'spot' urine sample and a serum sample from the same day can be used. In practice, a ratio of more than about 0.15 can be regarded as 'non-selective', and against the diagnosis of minimal change – although it by no means excludes it.

Microscopic haematuria is seen as an occasional finding in about one third of patients with 'minimal changes', but persistent haematuria in all specimens is very rare. It often indicates coincident urinary tract infection.

As mentioned earlier, measurement of glomerular filtration rate is a surprisingly poor discriminant between 'minimal change' disease in children or adults, and other causes of the nephrotic state.

Children over the age of ten, if nephrotic, should have a renal biopsy since, as Fig. 2 showed, the proportion benefited by 'blind' corticosteroid therapy falls below one half at this age. The children with onset below one year of age deserve a special mention. Although a 'minimal change' nephrotic syndrome may be seen in the first three months of life, it is distinctly rare in the first year, and very rare in the first six months. Some of the nephrotic children with a neonatal onset have inherited forms of nephrotic syndrome, particularly the usually fatal Finnish form, of which sporadic cases occur outside Finland, see page 18.81. Also, another inherited form of nephritis characterized by progressive mesangial sclerosis may present in the first year of life. Occasional infants have membranous nephropathy in association with congenital syphilis, and this must be looked for.

Investigation of specific complications

Thrombosis of the renal vein

This used to be considered a cause of the nephrotic syndrome, but is now recognized as a complication as a result of the hypercoagulable state present in the nephrotic syndrome. For unknown reasons, patients with amyloidosis, membranous nephropathy, and (to a lesser extent) mesangiocapillary glomerulonephritis are particularly susceptible to renal venous thrombosis and thus it is rare in childhood nephrotics. It may be unilateral, bilateral, or involve the inferior vena cava as well. How common renal venous thrombosis may be in adult nephrotic patients, particularly those with membranous nephropathy, is a source of controversy. Estimates vary from 1 or 2 per cent of all nephrotics diagnosed at a clinical level, to 50 per cent or more if careful renal venography is performed in all instances. Our own studies suggest the former low figure is correct. Whether symptomless, minor degrees of renal venous thrombosis influence prognosis is a further point for debate. At the moment, it seems reasonable to perform *renal venograms* only in nephrotic patients in whom there is some clinical suspicion of thrombosis, particularly membranous nephropathy and mesangiocapillary disease. Clinical suspicion usually arises if renal function falls off unexpectedly, especially with the appearance of haematuria (sometimes macroscopic) and loin pain. The IVU frequently shows asymmetry in size of the kidneys, the thrombosed organ being the larger. In other patients there may be few signs beyond asymmetry of leg oedema, or signs of caval thrombosis such as a collateral venous circulation. Ultrasonic examination, especially employing 'real time' techniques may enable the non-invasive diagnosis of renal vein thrombosis, but not that affecting minor renal veins. A negative result does not exclude thrombosis.

Search for underlying malignant disease

A variety of tumours have been reported to be associated with a nephrotic syndrome. Some of these patients have had amyloidosis, but the majority show patterns of presumed immune complex disease, usually membranous nephropathy. The exception to this is those associated with lymphomata, which usually show 'minimal changes' on renal biopsy. Carcinoma of the lung and colon were present in the majority of the adult patients, Wilms' tumour in the children. The question arises: in what circumstances is it useful to search for malignancy in nephrotic patients? The available evidence suggests that a search is rarely justified even in patients over the age of 50 years with membranous nephropathy; and that in other patients the return does not justify the inconvenience, expense, and possible morbidity. The screen should include a careful chest X-ray with hilar tomography, a barium enema, a barium meal and follow-through. A Wilms' tumour should be picked up on careful examination of the IVU.

General management of the nephrotic patient

Whatever the underlying causes, the nephrotic state itself can be treated. (Measures aimed at eliminating the proteinuria, and hence the syndrome altogether, are dealt with in the next section under the heading 'specific treatment'.) These general measures are, of course, of particular importance in patients whose underlying disease cannot be eliminated or repressed.

The *psychological* effects of the gross distortion of the body, both by the nephrotic syndrome itself, and the corticosteroids which may be used to treat it, must not be forgotten. Prolonged hospital admissions take their toll of morale. Fears of renal failure may be present, but not revealed. First, therefore, the individual patient's reaction (and his family's) must be assessed and dealt with, and employment, school, or other difficulties sorted out.

The main *physical* problem of the nephrotic syndrome is the excessive retention of salt and water within the interstitial space. Measures to limit intake and increase output of water are therefore obvious lines of attack. *Salt intake* should be limited to about 60 mmol/24 h in adult patients, i.e. about 1 mmol/kg/24 h. In patients with resistant oedema, reduction should be to 40 mmol/24 h (0.7 mmol/kg/24 h); more rigid restrictions are rarely (if ever) followed even in the hospital, and by and large are unnecessary. The former level (60 mmol/24 h) involves only adding no salt at table, using a moderate amount of cooking, and avoiding the obvious and not-so-obvious salt-rich foods. This is usually sufficient. *Water intake* need not be restricted in the stable outpatient, but in the early phases of oedema accumulation in severely ill patients, it will be noticed that the plasma sodium is often low. Some of this is 'false' hyponatraemia, because of replacement of plasma water by lipid in nephrotic plasma; but in many patients this represents a true retention of water in excess of sodium because of intense ADH secretion and inability to excrete a water load because of failure to deliver Na^+ to the distal nephron. Temporary limitation of water intake is therefore useful in the acute phase of some patients.

The main weapon in removing oedema is, however, *diuretics* (see page 13.98). How much of what diuretic should be given, and in what circumstances? In the stable outpatient with moderate oedema and no evidence of severe hypovolaemia, a moderate dose of frusemide (40–80 mg twice daily for an adult) alone or together with amiloride (5 mg daily) is usually sufficient to induce diuresis and maintain the patient oedema-free. Other loop-acting diuretics can also be used. The use of this combination prevents the potassium loss and depletion of total body potassium seen if thiazides or loop agents alone are used, and in the presence of a more proximal acting diuretic (frusemide or thiazide) the amiloride (which blocks distal tubular exchange of potassium for sodium) is able to act on the increased amounts of sodium reaching the distal nephron. Moduretic (a combination of thiazide and amiloride) can also be used, alone or better with a small dose of frusemide. The nephrotic patient is already wasting potassium from the severe secondary hyperaldosteronism which he often suffers, so that the use of a potassium-sparing diuretic in the regimen has advantages.

In more severely-ill patients with massive oedema, much larger doses of diuretic may be needed in the early phases. These can be given with safety only in hospital. Up to 500 mg of frusemide twice a day may be required in adult patients to remove the 20–40 l of oedema under which the patient may be labouring. Spironolactone can also be employed, but doses of as high as 400 mg daily may be needed to overcome the intense secondary hyperaldosteronism; it is better to start with 100 mg in adults, since this drug induces nausea quite frequently. Metolazone may also be used as an adjunct, in a dose of 10–40 mg daily. Again, dangers of too rapid removal of oedema by diuretics include hypovolaemic collapse and even acute renal failure. This danger is discussed in more detail below.

Alternatively, the oedema can be removed rapidly and safely by the use of intravenous frusemide *given into an intravenous infusion* of plasma or of albumin. The latter is preferable on theoretical grounds, since it contains little or no sodium, but in practice both are effective. Doses of 250–500 mg of frusemide intravenously may be needed in adults, but should *never* be given unless colloid is being run in at the same time. In this fashion, up to 5 l or more of oedema can be removed each day. The risk is, of course, critical hypovolaemia, since diuretics alone will reduce the circulating volume still further; hence the need for intravenous protein or albumin. It is worth mentioning again that in critical hypovolaemia the blood pressure may be *high* just before collapse occurs, presumably from intense vasoconstricton, perhaps due to increased angiotensin. We use intravenous albumin as a short cut in any severely oedematous patient requiring more than (say) 160 mg/day of frusemide to obtain a diuresis. The interesting observation is that, once having become free of oedema, many patients can maintain this oedema-free state taking only moderate doses of diuretics, which previously were ineffective. The dose of diuretic must be titrated for each patient, using daily weights as the end point. For children, smaller doses on a body weight basis (ideal weight for height, because of oedema) may be used.

It is traditional to feed nephrotic patients a *high-protein* diet, rich in animal protein (up to 100–120 g/day). Whether the addition of more protein to a diet already adequate in amino acids induces extra hepatic synthesis of albumin is unknown, but most clinicians have felt it more secure to err in this direction. Little attention also has been paid to the energy intake of nephrotic patients. It is our practice to try and supplement this also, on the basis of work in other fields, which suggests that utilization of protein is more efficient in the presence of higher energy intake. There are few data which suggest that the nephrotic patient resembles the uraemic patient in this respect, when a high protein intake is being fed. The possible effect of the energy supplement on plasma lipids needs to be considered (see below). If the patient is taking corticosteroids, the problem is usually to *limit* intake and prevent obesity.

Reduction of proteinuria with indomethacin

Indomethacin, by interfering with the production of prostaglandin E_2 and other prostaglandins in the renal medulla, produces a fall in outer cortical renal blood flow. This in turn leads to a reversible fall in the glomerular filtration rate, and in some patients, to a reversible decrease in proteinuria. Even though few now believe that this reduction in proteinuria is the result of a specific action on the glomerulonephritic process itself, the effect would seem to have therapeutic potential in reducing massive proteinuria in corticosteroid-resistant nephrotic patients. Despite several reports outlining success with this drug, we have failed, both in membranous nephropathy and in focal segmental sclerosis, to detect any consistent effect of the drug on protein excretion. In adults, doses of 150 mg/day must be given, which some patients cannot tolerate because of side-effects, and a few unlucky patients suffer gastrointestinal bleeds. However, in the occasional patient whose nephrotic syndrome is so severe that they cannot leave hospital, this drug is worth a try. It must also be remembered that indomethacin can induce acute renal failure.

Management of complications

Infections

The use of prophylactic antibiotics is contentious. Nephrotic patients are very susceptible to infections, both from 'classical' and opportunistic organisms. The reasons for this are not clear, apart from the low IgG levels that many suffer. There seems to be a particular susceptibility to encapsulated organisms such as pneumococci possibly because of the loss of components of the alternative pathway of complement into the urine. In view of the devastating effect of *pneumococcal peritonitis* and *septicaemia* – which still occur in children and adolescents, but can now be treated – it is our usual practice to put all active, severely oedematous childhood nephrotics on prophylactic penicillin. This can be stopped on remission or lessening of proteinuria. An unexplained feature of pneumococcal disease is that, although not by any means confined to 'minimal change' nephrotics, it does not occur in adults; the oldest patient we have seen with primary pneumococcal peritonitis was 17 years old. The diagnosis of pneumococcal peritonitis is not always easy; nephrotic patients, particularly children, may have severe abdominal pain in association with sterile ascites, perhaps associated with episodes of hypovolaemia. It is better to treat it if in doubt, and aspiration of ascitic fluid with a fine (e.g. lumbar puncture) needle for an immediate Gram stain may be of great help.

Established infections should, of course, be treated with appropriate antibiotics. These should be bactericidal wherever possible, because of the generally poor state of most nephrotic patients. This is particularly true of *cellulitis*, which is, in a nephrotic patient, a medical emergency. It can spread with terrifying rapidity, hour by hour; the blood culture is usually positive, and cardiovascular collapse frequently follows. Further, in addition to the more usual coccal organisms, cellulitis may be seen in nephrotic

patients from *Escherichia coli* or other Gram-negative rods. Antibiotic therapy should therefore be prompt, intravenous to start with, bactericidal and cover a broad spectrum of organisms. It is usually impossible to recover the organism from the cellulitis, but often it can be found in the blood; in any case, by the time the cultures are available the drama is usually over. In patients who are taking corticosteroids one should give hydrocortisone intravenously in the acute phase, since adrenal suppression is always present to some extent.

Hypercholesterolaemia is almost invariable in nephrotics, accompanied by hypertriglyceridaemia in almost half the cases; the lower the serum albumin the higher the cholesterol, which may given a clue to the pathogenesis. Two theories have been proposed. The first is that fatty acids are normally carried on albumin, which is reduced. The second is that lipoprotein (apoprotein) synthesis is increased as part of the protein hypersynthesis common to all nephrotics. Congenitally analbuminaemic subjects also show high plasma cholesterol concentrations. In nephrotics, although LDL (and in some instances VLDL) cholesterols are raised, HDL cholesterols are normal or raised despite some loss in the urine. Whether any treatment should be given for this hyperlipidaemia of the nephrotic syndrome is still being debated. It has been alleged that there is an excess of myocardial infarction (and possibly other vascular disease) in patients with a persistent nephrotic syndrome, but we have been unable to confirm this in an extensive long-term study, which is in accord with the normal HDL cholesterols found in almost all nephrotics. The agents that might be used – cholestyramine and clofibrate – are well known to have side effects. Clofibrate, in particular, is toxic in nephrotics, unless the dose is carefully titrated, because it is normally bound to albumin. Excessive levels of free clofibrate can lead to muscle necrosis, and this is a recognized complication in states of low albumin, or where other compounds displace clofibrate from its albumin-bound sites. At the moment, we do not give anti-hyperlipidaemic drugs to chronic nephrotic patients. Whether the lipid levels can be modified by a change to polyunsaturated fats, or a diminution of carbohydrate intakes has never been studied adequately. The latter might have the disadvantage of making the negative nitrogen balance worse, and we do not practise it.

Thromboses

Thromboses, both arterial and venous, are a frequent source of complications and mortality in nephrotic patients and may occur in almost any vessel, including the pulmonary artery. The sources of this hypercoagulability are complex: coagulation factors such as fibrinogen and factor VIII are increased in the plasma in the nephrotic syndrome, while anti-thrombin III is lost in the urine, and plasminogen activator release and tissue fibrinolysis are reduced. Haemoconcentration is often present, and the patients are often relatively immobilized. The platelets are more active in the presence of a low serum albumin, so that fatty acids are freely available to form thromboxane. Therefore, it seems reasonable to use prophylactic heparin in a dose of 5000 i.u. twice a day subcutaneously in patients with an active nephrotic syndrome in hospital, remembering that if anti-thrombin III levels are very low, heparin will be relatively ineffective. Long-term anticoagulation with warfarin may be confined to those with diagnosed thrombotic episodes.

Hypovolaemia, shock, and acute renal failure

Patients with a nephrotic syndrome, both children and adults, may experience severe enough hypotension – or enough renal hypoperfusion without hypotension – to become temporarily oliguric, with increasing uraemia. The urine passed by these patients is almost devoid of sodium, (< 10 mmol/l if diuretics have not just been given), and highly concentrated with respect to plasma (U_{osm}/P_{osm} 1.5–3.5:1, U/P creatinine and urea $> 10:1$). A prompt response can be expected in such a patient to volume replacement and diuretics, *in that order*. A frequent mistake is to give large doses of frusemide (or other loop-acting diuretic) *before* starting the intravenous protein infusion. Also, some of these patients are in this state because of coincident septicaemia, and a broad spectrum bactericidal antibiotic should be given intravenously after blood cultures have been taken.

In a few unfortunae nephrotics, however, events may have progressed further, and the urine may be dilute (U/P_{osm} <1:1, U/P urea < 3:1) with a sodium concentration of 20–50 mmol/l. This urine composition is similar to that found in acute intrinsic renal failure ('acute tubular necrosis') from any cause (see page 18.125) and a prolonged oliguria can be expected. Because of ascites and protein depletion, it is preferable to manage these patients by haemodialysis rather than peritoneal dialysis, so that intensive ultrafiltration and intravenous nutrition can be applied. The oliguric period in these patients may be as long as 8–12 weeks, for reasons which are not clear. Many patients who suffer this complication, both children and adults, have initially normal renal function and massive proteinuria, and so the majority have 'minimal change' disease. It seems reasonable to continue treating their primary complaint with corticosteroids even whilst the patient is oliguric, although the extra risks of infection in a uraemic individual must be remembered.

The treatment of associated hypertension
(See pages 13.374 and 13.388.)

This may form an important part in minimizing a decline in renal function caused by progressive disease. We have preferred a combination of vasodilator (hydrallazine, prazosin) with a beta-blocker (preferably one with renin antagonistic effects such as propanolol) as our treatment of first choice. It may be that ACE inhibitors such as captopril or enalapril, of Ca^{2+} blockers such as infedipine will be more effective in limiting glomerular drainage because of differential effects on afferent and efferent glomerular arteriolar tone, but this has not been shown in humans. The level of diastolic or mean blood pressure to be attained is also controversial.

Miscellaneous complications in nephrotic patients
Because patients with the nephrotic syndrome are pale and puffy and sometimes rather immobile, the question of *hypothyroidism* may be raised. There may be a reduction in thyroxine-binding globulin (TBG) which will depress both T_3 and T_4 levels. However, significant TBG reduction occurs only when proteinuria is severe or the patient is very ill. Depression of the monodeiodination of T_4 to T_3 in ill patients, or those severely lacking in appetite, would lead to a disproportionate lowering of serum T_3. T_3 uptake and TSH are normal in uncomplicated nephrotic syndromes. There is no reason for suspecting hypothyroidism in nephrotic patients, unless clinical tests other than T_3 or TBG levels are abnormal, such as slow-relaxing reflexes.

Although the majority of nephrotics are hypercoagulable, in some the pre-biopsy screen may reveal a *bleeding tendency*. Rarely is this accompanied by actual bleeding, but deficiencies of factors VII, IX, XI and XII resulting from massive urinary losses, have all been described in occasional patients. Patients with systemic lupus may show antibodies to clotting factors and platelet phospholipids which act as circulating anticoagulants. It is usually safe to do a renal biopsy on such patients under an infusion of fresh frozen plasma, maintained for four to six hours after biopsy.

Occasionally losses of iron and transferrin in the urine may be sufficient to induce an *iron deficiency anaemia*. This is very rare, and simply treated.

Finally, patients with the nephrotic syndrome have been known for some time to have very low urinary calcium excretion rates as well as low total and ionized plasma calcium concentrations and defective calcium absorption. It is now known that vitamin D-binding globulin is lost in the urine, and that *plasma vitamin D concentrations* are very low in nephrotics. Whether this matters in the long term in patients, especially children, with a prolonged

nephrotic syndrome is not clear. Both normal and osteroporotic bones have been reported in nephrotic patients, but most have no obvious problems of this kind.

Specific treatment of the nephrotic patient
Corticosteroids
The use of corticosteroids in the nephrotic syndrome has been shown to be of consistent value only in those patients proven or suspected to have the 'minimal change' lesion in their glomeruli. Why these patients respond to corticosteroids is as unknown as the nature of the condition itself. In addition, about one in five or fewer patients (usually children) with a nephrotic syndrome and focal segmental glomerulosclerosis (FSGS) will also respond, and may subsequently run a relapsing course like the minimal change patient may do. The response in these patients with FSGS has prognostic as well as therapeutic value (see below).

If a patient has had an established nephrotic syndrome for ten days or more, and has a minimal change lesion, then it is reasonable to treat with corticosteroids. The principal justification is that the nephrotic state is dangerous, as outlined above. However, the only controlled evidence is from two trials in adults, which showed no mortality in either corticosteroid-treated or control groups managed with diuretics alone during four years' follow-up. No controlled trials have ever been done in children but it is most workers' impression – including our own – that the nephrotic child is more frequently subject to a very severe nephrotic syndrome than are adults, and few paediatricians would be willing to withold treatment for too long in a very nephrotic child. However, there has been a general realization that there is no need always to rush in with corticosteroid treatment, if the patient's proteinuria is moderate, and oedema easily controlled with diuretics. One can wait, and keep corticosteroids in reserve.

The regimen in *children* which has been best studied is 60 mg/m^2/day (calculated on the ideal weight for height) of prednisone. By the end of the weeks on this dose, 88 per cent of those who will ultimately go into complete remission with loss of proteinuria have already done so. This is followed by four weeks on 60 mg/m^2 on alternate days. Longer term treatment has been alleged to decrease the relapse rate subsequent to withdrawal, but there is no good evidence that this is so. Given the mounting toxicity of corticosteroids with time, there seems no justification for a course of prednisone longer than about six weeks altogether. There are no data as to whether it is safe to withdraw treatment earlier in patients who respond quickly – the mode week for response in one trial was the second, and 11 days' treatment the mean response time; the trial protocol did not permit this question to be answered. On this dose, we may expect that some 94 per cent of children with a minimal change nephrotic syndrome will lose their proteinuria. The proportion of *adults* who achieve loss of proteinuria is a little lower, perhaps 85–90 per cent, but physicians have, in general, used lower doses in relation to body weight. A popular regimen in adults has been 60 mg of prednisone for a week, followed by gradually decreasing amounts for a further six to eight weeks, tapering the dose independent of whether an early response is obtained or not. By six to eight weeks, the percentage response is almost the same as in children, but the response rate is lower.

Relapses Of those patients (both children and adults) responding with complete loss of proteinuria, perhaps half will remain in remission, or at most have a single further relapse. Clearly, this presents no problems. The remainder, however, fall into the group of *persistently relapsing* 'minimal change' nephrotic syndrome. This may occur at any age, although the majority of patients are children. The first question is: when should one treat a relapse with corticosteroids? It is certainly worth waiting 7–10 days (unless severe hypovolaemia is already present), since a number of patients will go into spontaneous remission during this time. Then, the same course of prednisone as for the initial attack can be employed. Thereafter, the relapses may be absent or infrequent, so that diuretics alone can be used, with occasional recourse to corticosteroids. In contrast, the relapses may be so frequent that the patient is receiving large doses of corticosteroids most of the time, may even relapse against moderate or large doses of the drug, or immediately it is withdrawn, or the dose reduced ('corticosteroid-dependent' nephrotic syndrome).

These patients are at risk for all the well recognized side-effects of corticosteroid treatment. In children, the most serious of these in the long term is growth retardation, but the exaggeration of the osteoporosis, protein depletion, susceptibility to infection, and thrombosis already present in the nephrotic patient must not be forgotten. It is in these patients that treatment with cytotoxic drugs may be considered.

Immunosuppressive (cytotoxic) drugs
As well as responding to corticosteroids, most 'minimal change' nephrotic syndromes both in children and in adults will also respond to mustard-like drugs (nitrogen mustard, cyclophosphamide, chlorambucil) and also purine antagonists (6-mercaptopurine, 6-thioguanine, azathioprine). The few patients with 'minimal change' lesions who fail to lose proteinuria with conventional corticosteroid treatment also respond to these drugs. When the purine antagonists are used, remission is no more prolonged than with corticosteroids, so that (apart from a steroid-sparing effect), they have no great advantage over corticosteroids themselves. When mustard-like drugs are used, however, the remission obtained in frequently relapsing patients is prolonged, and may be permanent (Fig. 3) in about one third of children treated. Children who are corticosteroid-dependent do worse, however, than those who have proteinuria-free periods off treatment between relapses.

Cyclophosphamide has been the drug most extensively investigated. At the moment, chlorambucil does not seem to have an advantage, unless very prolonged (6 months) high dose (0.2 mg/kg day) courses are used, which have appreciable side-effects. With cyclophosphamide, a dose of 3 mg/kg/day may be used, which produced little or no obvious side-effects. Careful studies have shown that a course of six to eight weeks must be given to produce the effect shown in Fig. 3 but that longer treatments confer no advantage. That is important, because the side-effects of the drug (as of nitrogen mustard itself, and chlorambucil) include gonadal damage (Table 2). At the moment, it seems that a dose of cyclo-

phosphamide of 3 mg/kg/day (ideal weight for height) for up to eight weeks is devoid of gonadal effects, but that with longer courses males are much more susceptible than females (Table 2). A further consideration of mustard-like drugs is their oncogenic potential. A number of patients, usually treated for periods of many months or years, have developed solid tumours or leukaemias following treatment with either cyclophosphamide or chlorambucil. Immediate toxicity, seen with higher dosages (such as cystitis and hair loss) are rarely (if ever) found with the brief course discussed here. However, these risks suggest that cyclophosphamide should *never* be used as primary treatment of minimal change nephrotic syndrome. An exception may perhaps be the elderly patient with 'minimal change' disease, in whom the effect of the nephrotic syndrome may be devastating, with a significant mortality from infection and hypovolaemia, and in whom the gonadal risks are less important. In children the tendency is to use cyclophosphamide less and less as we learn how to best employ individualized corticosteroid regimens.

These data further suggest that only a single six or eight week course should be used in an individual nephrotic, and that if he or she should relapse following the course, as two-thirds do ultimately (Fig. 3), then a return should be made to corticosteroid treatment. It is often found that smaller doses of corticosteroids can be employed to control the disease after cyclophosphamide, compared to those required before. Alternate day corticosteroid regimens (which we use) have been suggested to allow better growth in children, but although this has never been proved in a controlled study in nephrotic patients, they may be used in either children or adults. However, three times a week regimens do not prevent relapses, at least in children.

Corticosteroid and cyclophosphamide treatment of patients with focal and segmental glomerulosclerosis
The finding of segmental sclerosing lesions, particularly in glomeruli deep in the cortex near medulla (juxtamedullary glomeruli) immediately alters the likely prognosis of patients with a nephrotic syndrome away from the excellent outlook enjoyed by those with 'minimal change' disease. Whether these sclerosing lesions are a complication of the 'minimal change' lesion, or a distinct lesion of differing pathogenesis (both attitudes have their strong advocates), the practical significance of the finding in an otherwise relatively normal biopsy is immediately clear. Some two-thirds of these patients with sclerosing lesions will end up in renal failure within 15 years, whilst about 20 per cent will go into remission during the same period; the remainder will persist with disease and their outcome is unknown. Can we distinguish these two very different outcomes at onset? The clinical features of the patients do not help us at all, neither does the histopathology. On the other

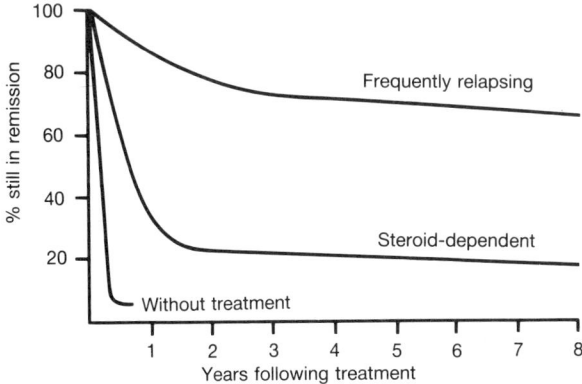

Fig. 3 The proportion of frequently-relapsing 'minimal change' childhood nephrotics remaining in remission following treatment with a brief course of cyclophosphamide or chlorambucil. Untreated, 100 per cent would be in relapse within a few months. About two-thirds of patients eventually experience a relapse of their condition, but thereafter, in our own data, no further relapse has occurred between 7 and 12 years of follow-up. The data summarizes six recently published series of patients, and the proportion of remission was calculated using the actuarial method. The difference in response between 'corticosteroid dependent' and 'multiple relapsing' patients is evident (see text for definitions).

Table 2 The effects of cyclophosphamide on the gonads

	Males	Females
Prepubertal	Azoöspermia, probably permanent, with 12 weeks' treatment or longer; this has not been observed with treatment of eight weeks or less, but sperm counts are permanently lowered after only eight weeks' treatment	Most children treated menstruate normally and are fertile; no sterility recorded
Postpubertal	Azoöspermia usually seen within 12 weeks' treatment or more; occasionally reversible	No sterility or interruption in menstruation with 12 weeks or less; over 12 weeks, menstruation stops; and if treatment continues ovarian fibrosis may be seen

hand, the result of a six week course of corticosteroids is highly predictive. If a patient loses proteinuria on this treatment, then it is very unlikely that he or she will suffer a decline in renal function and go into renal failure. On the other hand, if the patient falls within the 80 per cent who do *not* so respond, their chances of remission fall not to zero, but to about 5 per cent, whilst more than half of these 'non-responders' (40 per cent of the original 100 per cent) will be in renal failure within 5–10 years. Treatment of patients with focal segmental glomerulosclerosis using a brief course of corticosteroids is therefore worthwhile to establish likely prognosis. There is no evidence, as yet, that more patients will go into remission with cyclophosphamide than do with cortico-steroids; although those that respond to steroids will also respond to cyclophosphamide.

Corticosteroids and cytotoxic agents and membranous nephropathy

Until recently, it seemed clear that patients with nephrotic syndromes and membranous nephropathy did not respond to cortico-steroid treatment, and that initial enthusiasm had attributed an unrecognized 25 per cent spontaneous remission rate in adults within five years (50 per cent in children) to the treatment. About half the patients go into renal failure over 15 years from onset – almost all with a nephrotic syndrome. In addition, several small controlled trials demonstrated no short-term benefit.

However, a trial from the Interhospital study of nephrotic syndrome in adults from the USA has shown that patients treated with high dose alternate-day corticosteroids (120 mg/alt. day) for only eight weeks ran a significantly better course over the next four years than similar untreated controls, many fewer showing decline in renal function or entry into renal failure. These data are controversial at the moment, but it begins to look as though a sub-group of idiopathic membranous nephropathy patients, with a particularly rapid entry into renal failure (one to three years) compared with the usual rather indolent course of the disease, may be responsive to corticosteroids. Our present policy is to identify these patients by serial function tests, and to treat those who show a rapid fall off in glomerular filtration rate. Further trials may help to clarify this important question. More recently, impressive results have been obtained using a 6-month treatment alternating steroids and chlorambucil, month and month about. How necessary the chlorambucil may be in obtaining this result is not clear, and given the potential toxicity of even 3 months' chlorambucil, we are not, at the moment, using this regime.

Anticoagulants in mesangiocapillary glomerulonephritis (MCGN)

Neither corticosteroids nor cytotoxic agents, alone or in combination, seem to have any effect upon the long-term evolution of patients with this serious form of glomerulonephritis, which leads to renal failure in over three-quarters of those affected within 15 years, and in almost all of those with a nephrotic syndrome (Fig. 4). Several groups (including our own) have been encouraged to try the effect of combined anticoagulation and immunosuppression in carefully selected patients with severe forms of MCGN and rapid evolution towards renal failure, in an attempt to extend the apparent success of this treatment in some patients with very aggressive forms of crescentic nephritis. Results to date have been encouraging, with reversal of renal failure in the majority of over a dozen patients, but on withdrawal of treatment several patients have shown a rapid irreversible decline in function. The use of antiplatelet agents alone, which are of course safe, needs support from a controlled trial.

The management of patients with nephritis and *systemic lupus erythematosus* and *Henoch–Schönlein purpura* are dealt with in the section on glomerulonephritis (see page 18.36) and those with diabetes on page 9.80). However, it is worth discussing the indications for renal biopsy in nephrotic diabetes. In general, this is not necessary, but having diabetes is no bar to developing other forms of glomerulonephritis. If retinopathy is mild or absent, or haema-

turia or other unusual features present, then a renal biopsy is justified in view of the poor prognosis of diabetic nephropathy accompanied by a nephrotic syndrome: renal failure in an average of two to three years.

Other side-effects of treatment

Several of the many side-effects of corticosteroids have been mentioned above, but one practical problem not so far mentioned is the *leucocytosis* which they may induce, and which may confuse the diagnosis of infection in nephrotic patients. Total white counts of up to $25 \times 10^9/l$ may be observed in perfectly fit nephrotic patients on high-dose steroid treatment.

Again, the deleterious effects of diuretics on hypovolaemia have been mentioned, but another problem is a fall-off in renal function in a patient who has been taking diuretics. In a small but important minority this is the result, not of the primary disease or of hypovolaemia, but of an *allergic interstitial nephritis* induced by the drug. Both frusemide and thiazides seem capable of inducing this reaction, and since the condition responds dramatically to withdrawal of the drug and treatment with corticosteroids, it is important to think of it and identify the problem by further renal biopsy. Both bumetanide and ethacrynic acid can be used safely in such patients, if a diuretic is essential to continued management.

The long-term outlook for the nephrotic patient

In countries with good facilities for treating end-stage renal failure, no patient should die of uraemia and thus the mortality of the nephrotic syndrome should be zero. In practice, the lack of facilities for all patients in renal failure which disfigures the British medical scene ensures that some, mostly older patients do die of renal failure. However, the main unavoidable causes of death in nephrotic patients are the complications. Even a few patients with 'minimal change' disease may succumb to a major thrombosis, more rarely to sepsis or circulatory collapse. The nephrotic syndrome in the older patient is often devastating, and in the seventies and eighties, or even the sixties, patients may be lost from apparently avoidable complications, however vigilant their care may be.

In general, however, the outlook for the nephrotic patient is determined much more by the underlying nephritis than by the initial severity of his or her nephrotic syndrome. Despite this, for each form of progressive glomerular histopathology that has been

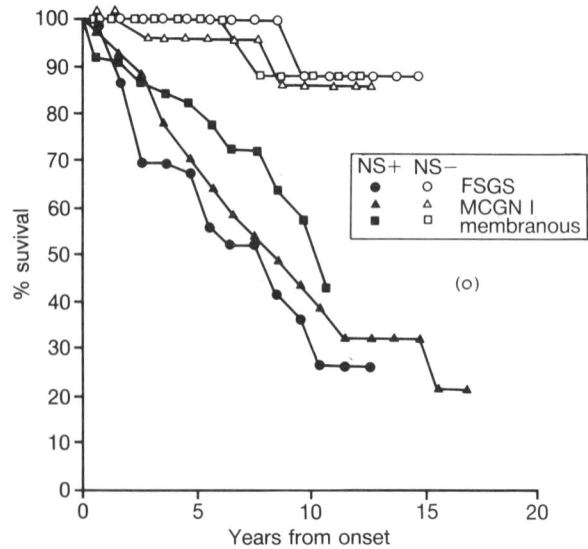

Fig. 4 Prognosis of patients showing membranous nephropathy, focal segmental sclerosis (FSGS) or mesangiocapillary glomerulonephritis (MCGN) with and without a nephrotic syndrome at onset. Data are presented as actuarially calculated estimates of survival of renal function.

studied, the outlook for the patient with a full nephrotic syndrome – even if it does not persist, as is often the case – is much poorer than the patient with similar histology who presents with haematuria or with proteinuria below the nephrotic range (Fig. 4). The broad prognosis for all the major groups of idiopathic glomerulonephritis with a nephrotic syndrome has been outlined above (Table 1). The gloomy news is that, with present management, and excepting these patients with a 'minimal change' lesion, more than half will have entered renal failure within a decade from onset. For children the outlook is better, but even for them more than one-third of those without 'minimal change' lesions will run a similar course. This confronts us with a therapeutic challenge we are still unable to meet. The only consolation for the patient is that, as he loses renal filtering surface, his proteinuria diminishes and so his nephrotic syndrome frequently – but not invariably – remits as uraemia supervenes. In fact, it is unusual for a full nephrotic syndrome to persist for more than five years: either remission occurs (or is induced) or proteinuria diminishes spontaneously, with or without reduction in renal function.

References

Albright, R., Brensilver, J. and Cortell, S. (1983). Proteinuria in congestive heart failure. *Am. J. Nephrol.* **3**, 272–275.
Barratt, T. M. (1983). Proteinuria (Editorial). *Br. Med. J.* **287**, 1489–1490.
Brenner, B. M., Hostetter, T. H. and Humes, K. D. (1978). Molecular basis of proteinuria of glomerular origin. *N. Engl. J. Med.* **298**, 826–833.
—— and Stein, J. H. (1982). *The nephrotic syndrome.* Churchill, New York.
Cameron, J. S. (1979). The natural history of glomerulonephritis. In *Renal disease* 4th edn (eds D. A. K. Black and N. F. Jones), p. 329. Blackwell Scientific Publications, Oxford.
—— and Glassock, R. J. (eds) (1986). *The nephrotic syndrome.* Marcel Dekker, New York (in press).
Collaborative study of the adult idiopathic nephrotic syndrome (1979).

Short-term prednisone treatment in adults with membranous nephropathy. *N. Engl. J. Med.* **301**, 1201–1211.
Dodge, W. F., West, E. F., Smith, E. H. and Bunce, H. (1976) Proteinuria and hematuria in schoolchildren: epidemiology and early natural history. *J. Pediat.* **88**, 327–347.
Dorhout Mees, E. G., Geers, A. B. and Koomans, H. A. (1984). Blood volume and sodium retention in the nephrotic syndrome: a controversial patho-physiological concept. *Nephron* **36**, 201–211.
Ginsburg, J. M., Chang, B. S., Matarese, R. A. and Garella, S. (1983). Use of single voided urine samples to estimate quantitative proteinuria. *N. Engl. J. Med.* **309**, 1543–1546.
Glassock, R. J., Cohen, A. H. and Martinez-Maldonado, M. (1985). Primary glomerular disease. In *The kidney* 3rd edn (eds B. M. Brenner and F. C. Rector) W. B. Saunders, Philadelphia (in press).
—— (1986). The pathophysiology of proteinuria. In *The nephrotic syndrome* (eds J. S. Cameron and R. J. Glassock). Marcel Dekker, New York (in press).
Kanwar, Y. S. (1984). Biology of disease. Biophysiology of glomerular filtration and proteinuria. *Lab. Invest.* **51**, 7–21.
Levitt, J. I. (1967). The prognostic significance of proteinuria in young college students. *Ann. intern. Med.* **66**, 685–696.
Lewis, E. J. (1985). The management of the nephrotic syndrome in adults. In *The nephrotic syndrome* (eds J. S. Cameron and R. J. Glassock). Marcel Dekker, New York (in press).
Llach, F. (1983). *Renal vein thrombosis.* Futura, New York.
Pesce, J. and First, M. F. (1979). *Proteinuria – an integrated review.* Marcel Dekker, New York.
Robinson, R. R. (1980). Isolated proteinuria in asymptomatic patients (Nephrology Forum). *Kidney Int.* **18**, 395–406.
Springberg, P. D., Garrett, L. E., Thompson, A. L. *et al.* (1982). Fixed and reproducible orthostatic proteinuria: results of a 20 year follow-up study. *Ann. intern. Med.* **97**, 516–519.
Strauss, J. (1979). Pediatric nephrology. *The nephrotic syndrome.* Vol. 5. Garland Press, New York.
Sumpio, B. E. and Hayslett, J. P. (1985). Renal handling of proteins in normal and diseased states. *Q. J. Med.* **57**, 611–635.
Trompeter, R. and Barratt, T. M. (1986). The management of the nephrotic syndrome in children. In *The nephrotic syndrome* (eds J. S. Cameron and R. J. Glassock). Marcel Dekker, New York (in press).

INTERSTITIAL NEPHRITIS AND URINARY TRACT INFECTIONS

A. W. ASSCHER

Interstitial nephritis

General considerations

Inflammatory disease which primarily involves the renal interstitium has many causes. Some of the most important of these are shown in Table 1. In many instances the aetiology of interstitial renal disease is still obscure. Until recently the view was held that bacterial infection of the urinary tract was the principal cause of interstitial nephritis. The results of long-term follow-up studies of patients with urinary tract infection have shown that renal infection in the absence of obstruction rarely produces progressive kidney damage. Renal infection only produces kidney damage in childhood, when infection and vesico ureteric reflux co-exist (see page 18.75). It is now apparent that the cause of the previous confusion was that chronic interstitial nephritis, whatever its cause, may present with superimposed bacterial infection. In these instances the urinary tract infection is the result rather than the cause of the underlying kidney damage.

Interstitial nephritis may present acutely, usually, with oliguric kidney failure (see below and page 18.132), or it may present with slowly progressive kidney failure, so called 'chronic interstitial nephritis'. In both its acute and chronic forms tubular dysfunction is a prominent feature. Thus low molecular weight proteinuria

(see page 18.56), β-microglobulinuria, urinary acidification and concentrating defects, and sodium and potassium losing nephropathies occur more commonly and earlier in the course of disease of the interstitium than in the case of glomerular inflammatory disease. In the individual patient, however, these features of primary interstitial disease are of little help in diagnosis and the most certain way of establishing the diagnosis of primary interstitial disease is by renal biopsy. In most kidney diseases, including the glomerular diseases, interstitial fibrosis contributes to progressive deterioration of kidney function, but in this section only those diseases which primarily affect the renal insterstitium will be considered.

Chronic interstitial diseases due to chemicals and drugs including analgesics are considered on page 18.108, and here only the acute forms of interstitial nephritis and two examples of chronic interstitial disease, namely Balkan (endemic) nephropathy and irradiation nephritis will be considered.

Acute interstitial nephritis

This condition (see also page 18.132) is most commonly due to drug sensitivity reactions. Examples of the more important causes of the disease are shown in Table 1. The pathogenetic mechanism(s) involved in these sensitivity reactions is not fully understood. In some instances (e.g. methicillin-induced interstitial

Table 1 Principal causes of interstitial nephritis

Congenital	Mechanical
Alport's disease	Reflux nephropathy
Medullary cystic disease	
(nephronopthisis)	Toxin-induced
	Balkan nephropathy
Immunological	
Sjögren's syndrome	Vascular
Methicillin nephritis*	Ageing kidney
Kidney graft rejection*	Diabetes
	Sickle cell disease
Metabolic	
Potassium depletion	Bacterial
	Chronic (childhood)
	pyelonephritis
Chemical	
Cadmium intoxication	
Lead nephropathy	Drugs
Lithium nephropathy	Analgesics
	Anticonvulsants*
Physical	Anticoagulants*
X-irradiation	Antibacterial agents*
Crystal nephropathies	Non-steroidal anti-inflammatory
	drugs*
	Radiomimetic drugs

* Denotes aetiological factors which is the main lead to acute interstitial nephritis.

disease) circulating antitubular basement membrane antibody can be demonstrated but it is not known whether these antibodies play a role in pathogenesis or whether their appearance is merely an epiphenomenon.

Clinically, acute interstitial nephritis usually presents with acute oliguric kidney failure, fever, sometimes arthralgia, eosinophiluria, and peripheral eosinophilia. Renal biopsy reveals a marked interstitial cellular infiltrate with acute inflammatory cells many of which may be eosinophils. In addition tubular necrosis is present. In the case of methicillin nephritis linear deposition of IgG can be shown along the tubular basement membranes; in other cases the immunofluorescent studies are negative. In some cases extra-tubular interstitial deposits of Tamm-Horsfall protein are found, and it is possible that the extrusion of this protein from the tubules elicits an acute inflammatory response which may either be the primary cause of the interstitial disease or may contribute to its progression.

The management of patients with kidney failure due to suspected acute interstitial nephritis includes early confirmation of the diagnosis by renal biopsy followed by high dose steroid treatment (either as oral prednisolone 60 mg/day or as a series of daily bolus injections of methyl prenisolone given intravenously in a dose of 1–2 g for 6–10 days). In addition the other routine measures for the treatment of acute kidney failure including dialysis should be instituted.

The outcome of the condition is usually favourable, although a number of cases have now been recorded in which progression to chronic interstitial nephritis has occurred.

Chronic interstitial nephritis

Chronic interstitial nephritis may well be a more important cause of end-stage kidney failure than has so far been realized. In most renal units the precise diagnosis of the cause of end-stage renal disease is seldom made. When the kidneys are smooth and small, it is assumed that kidney failure resulted from chronic glomerulonephritis whereas coarsely scarred kidneys are thought to be the end result of chronic pyelonephritis. This diagnostic approach leaves much to be desired because most types of chronic interstitial disease, other than those due to bacterial infection and analgesic nephropathy, lead to the development of small, smooth kidneys just as in the case of chronic glomerulonephritis. Some of the known causes of chronic interstitial nephritis are shown in

Table 1. It seems almost certain that others will be discovered because the main excretory pathway for many of the nephrotoxic substances in our environment is the kidney, which filters and concentrates them and so exposes the renal tubules to high concentrations of the unbound nephrotoxins. With the increase in use of nephrotoxic drugs, it is not surprising that interstitial nephropathy is becoming a more important cause of kidney failure. This subject is dealt with on page 18.108 *et seq.*

Balkan nephropathy (endemic nephropathy)

This form of chronic interstitial nephritis is endemic in certain restricted areas in Yugoslavia, Bulgaria, and Romania. All affected areas lie within the central Danube basin. The condition is almost entirely restricted to rural populations in these areas. It has been estimated that there are some 20 000 cases of this disease in the region. Despite many studies, the aetiology of the condition remains obscure although some evidence has pointed to the possibility that the disease may be due to a potent nephrotoxic mycotoxin derived from the fungus *Penicillium verrucosum var. cyclopium* which grows on stored foodstuffs, particularly maize when it is harvested during wet seasons and stored in moist conditions. The onset of the disease is insidious with mild proteinuria, β_2-microglobulinuria, features of progressive renal impairment and anaemia. The condition usually manifests in the third and fourth decades. Hypertension is not a prominent feature. The skin shows a coppery pigmentation. An unusually high incidence of uroepithelial tumours has been recorded in the endemic areas. The kidneys are small and smooth on X-ray of the abdomen. The prognosis is poor, with survival ranging from only a few months to as long as ten years (average three years) after initial diagnosis. The treatment is that of chronic kidney failure (q.v.).

Irradiation nephritis

Although the kidneys are relatively resistant to the harmful effects of ionizing radiations, kidney damage can occur following massive exposure of the renal areas, in the course of radiotherapy, or following administration of radio-mimetic drugs. A dose of the order of 20 Gy delivered over a period of six weeks is the minimum which has been recorded to produce kidney damage. The danger usually manifests after a prolonged latent interval which may range from six months to many years. The patient presents with an acute nephritic syndrome, with malignant phase hypertension, or with evidence of chronic progressive renal failure.

With the advent of newer radiotherapeutic techniques, it is now usually possible to shield the kidneys from excessive irradiation exposure and the condition is therefore much less commonly seen than previously. Once it is established there is little that can be done to alter its progression and the treatment is that of control of blood pressure together with the treatment of chronic kidney failure.

Infections of the urinary tract

General considerations

Urinary tract infections are a common source of morbidity. Twelve per 1000 consultations in general practice are on account of them and they are a common cause of absenteeism from work. The mortality associated with these infections is most difficult to estimate. Twenty per cent of adults and up to 30 per cent of children with end-stage kidney failure have been classified as suffering from chronic pyelonephritis which may be the end result of kidney infection. Infections of the urinary tract are also an important source of Gram-negative septicaemia. Approximately 20 per cent of all cases of Gram-negative septicaemia arise from the urinary tract and the condition is frequently fatal. This complication of urinary tract infection arises particularly after instrumentation of the urinary tract, or in patients in whom the defensive mechanisms are impaired, e.g. patients receiving immunosuppressive drugs or those suffering from lymphoproliferative disorders.

The introduction of antibacterial agents in the treatment of urinary tract infections has greatly reduced their morbidity. Surprisingly, the mortality of these infections has remained unchanged (Fig. 1). This may be because infection on its own in the absence of obstruction or back-pressure does not commonly lead to progressive kidney damage. Alternatively, it is possible that urinary tract infections frequently remain undetected and untreated because so often they produce few symptoms. Moreover, the symptoms of urinary tract infection are particularly vague in the childhood period, a time when the kidney is especially liable to damage from bacterial infection where infection and vesico-ureteric reflux co-exist.

The urinary tract is an anatomical unit. Infection of one part readily spreads to involve other parts. Although symptoms, particularly in childhood, are not a reliable guide either to the presence of infection or its localization, a number of clinical syndromes can be delineated. These are shown in Table 2.

Aetiology

Table 3 shows the prevalence of the various urinary pathogens in hospital and domestic environments. More recent studies using the technique of suprapubic aspiration of urine show that *Staphylococcus saprophyticus* infections particularly in young women account for up to 20 per cent of infections in domestic practice.

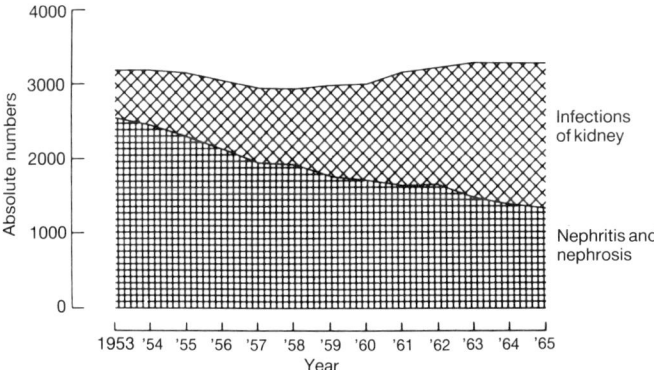

Fig. 1 Number of deaths from nephritis and nephrosis (ICD 590–94) and infections of the kidney (ICD 600) in females in England and Wales 1958–1965. (Reproduced by kind permission of Professor W. E. Waters and the Editor of *The Lancet*.)

Table 2 Clinical syndromes of urinary tract infection

Urethritis
Urethral syndrome ('abacterial' cystitis)
Prostatitis (acute and chronic)
Cystitis
Pyelonephritis (acute and chronic)
Necrotizing papillitis
Asymptomatic or covert infections

Table 3 Percentage prevalence of urinary pathogens in hospital and domiciliary practice

Organism	Inpatients ($n = 17411$)	Outpatients ($n = 220$)
Escherichia coli	47	64
'Coliforms'	17	9
Proteus mirabilis	21	15
Klebsiella aerogenes	7	4
Streptococcus faecalis	8	8

From McAllister, T. A. *et al.* (1971) *Postgrad. med. J.* **47**, suppl 7.

Infections due to the less common pathogens usually occur in the presence of gross structural abnormalities of the urinary tract or neurogenic defects, e.g. *Pseudomonas pyocyaneus* infection in patients with neurogenic disorders of the bladder. Tuberculous infections of the urinary tract are now uncommon but they still take their toll and will be considered separately (q.v.).

The source of the common *Escherichia coli* infection in women is the faecal flora. The organisms reach the urinary tract by the ascending route. Introital colonization precedes the development of urinary tract infection and in women and girls with recurrent infection, the periurethral cells have a greater number of bacterial receptor sites to which organisms may adhere by their fimbriae (Fig. 2) than in healthy controls. In boys, the organisms frequently originate from the sub-prepucial sac, whereas in the adult male the bacteria that produce infection commonly originate from the prostate gland. The higher prevalence of urinary tract infection in females compared with males is attributable to the shortness of the female urethra. Other factors facilitate the entry of organisms into the bladder of women such as the effects of sexual intercourse ('honeymoon cystitis'), the turbulence of the urinary stream, which leads to retrograde flow of its peripheral portions, and the absence of prostatic antibacterial factor which protects the male. In both sexes instrumentation of the urinary tract is an important factor in the pathogenesis of urinary tract infection; chief amongst these is the indwelling catheter.

In the bladder, urinary pathogens are able to multiply rapidly because human urine is a good culture medium. Whether or not infection is established depends on the balance between the multiplication rate of the bacteria and the effectiveness of the host defensive mechanisms. There are two kinds of defensive mechanism namely *hydrokinetic* and *mucosal*. The term hydrokinetic defence refers to the washout of bacteria by periodic voiding and dilution by the flow of urine from the kidneys. The number of bacteria in the bladder urine depends on the bacterial growth rate, the urine flow rate, the residual urine volume, and the frequency of micturition. The bacterial growth rate in turn is profoundly influenced by the urinary pH and to a lesser extent by its osmolality. The relationship between these variables has been studied in mechanical and computer models and it has been shown that clearance of bacteria from the bladder far exceeds that found in models. This finding suggests that in addition to the hydrokinetic defences, the bladder possesses an antibacterial effect which is usually referred to as the mucosal defensive mechanism. The nature of this mucosal mechanism remains to be elucidated but it seems likely that it involves the local production of secretory IgA which prevents the attachment of organisms to the uroepithelium. The phagocytic properties of urothelial cells may also play an important part in the mucosal defence.

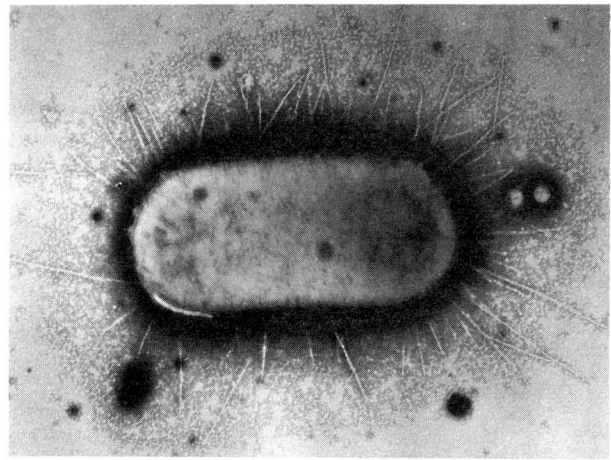

Fig. 2 Electron micrograph showing *Escherichia coli* fimbriae protruding from its surface.

Infection ascends to the kidney by several mechanisms. The most important pathway is intraluminal, organisms being carried to the kidney as a result of vesico-ureteric reflux. Such intraluminal ascent is further facilitated by the inhibitory effect of bacterial endotoxin on ureteric motility and possibly also by the motility of the invading bacterial strain. The ability of bacteria to persist in the kidney appears to depend on their capsular (K) antigen content since K-antigen prevents phagocytosis of the bacteria by leucocytes. Other bacterial virulence factors include the adhesiveness of the bacterial strain, its ability to produce haemolysin, its degree of fimbriation, and its ability to produce agglutination of blood group P positive human red cells which in turn is related to the possession of P or other mannose-resistant fimbriae. A possible alternative means of ascent of infection from bladder to kidney is via the periureteric lymphatics and this may be particularly involved in tuberculous infection.

Renal involvement may be diagnosed on clinical grounds but this is not reliable. Culture of ureteric urine is the most direct way to determine whether or not renal involvement exists. Since it is rarely possible to obtain ureteric urine, various indirect methods have been elaborated (Table 4). Of these the most promising non-invasive method is the detection of an antibody coating on bacteria which derive from the kidney in contrast to those of bladder origin which do not have such a coating. Unfortunately the method lacks both specificity and sensitivity. Precise location of urinary tract infection may be of clinical importance in relation both to the likelihood of recurrent infection and to the possible long-term sequelae of urinary tract infection. It has been suggested that the most practical method of locating UTI is to study the response to single dose treatment. If infection relapses upper tract infection must be suspected.

Non-specific urethritis in the male (NSU)

Non-specific urethritis is by far and away the commonest form of venereal disease in Britain today. As its name implies, there is still some dispute concerning its pathogenesis. Both ureaplasma urealyticium and chlamydial infections may cause the condition. More rarely the urethritis is due to infection with trichomonads.

Clinical

There is usually a history of sexual exposure followed by dysuria, difficulty in micturition, and a penile discharge. The discharge is most marked in the mornings. It may be clear, milky, or even yellow in the more acute form of the disease.

Diagnosis

The most important differential diagnosis is from gonococcal urethritis. It depends on examination of a Gram-stained film of the discharge and culture. In patients with Neisserial infection,

Table 4 Methods of localization or urinary tract infection

Direct	Indirect
Culture of renal biopsy	Serum antibody titres
Culture of ureteric urine	Antibody coating of pathogens
Bladder wash-out methods	Measurement of anti-Tamm–Horsfall antibody in serum
	Measurement of urinary β_2-microglobulin
	Measurement of renal concentrating power
	Urinary enzyme excretion, e.g. N-acetyl glucosaminidase
	White cell provocation test

Gram-negative diplococci are present in the pus cells whereas these are not found in patients with NSU. Culture further confirms the absence of gonococci. In a high proportion of these cases ureaplasma urealyticeum and Chlamydiae can be isolated both from the patients and their sexual partners.

Treatment

Patients with NSU frequently respond to treatment with tetracycline (500 mg four times daily for seven days) or erythromycin (500 mg four times daily for seven days). Complications may occur; these include the development of prostatitis in 20 per cent of cases and epididymitis in 3 per cent. Reiter's syndrome occurs in some 2 per cent of cases of NSU. Careful follow-up should be arranged so that concomitant syphilitic infection is not over-looked; serological testing for syphilis should therefore be undertaken six weeks after first presentation with urethritis.

Urethritis in the female

In about 50 per cent of women who present with symptoms of frequency and dysuria, urine culture is sterile. This puzzling condition is referred to by various names, e.g. urethral syndrome, abacterial cystitis, frequency and dysuria syndrome, or most clumsily symptomatic abacteriuria. When patients with this complaint are followed, approximately half of them develop bacteriuria and can thus be considered as showing intermittent bacteriuria. The remainder are permanently abacteriuric. It has been suggested that slow growing micro-aerophilic bacteria such as lactobacilli, corynebacteria, and *Streptococcus milleri* may be involved in the pathogenesis of the urethral syndrome. It is possible that these organisms are entrenched in the periurethral glands, the female equivalent of the prostate gland, but the role of these micro-aerophilic bacteria in the pathogenesis of the urethral syndrome remains in doubt.

Clinical features

The symptoms of the condition are indistinguishable from those of cystitis of bacterial origin except that nocturnal frequency is not so common. Urine culture is sterile. Some of the patients are found to have pyuria whereas others never have pyuria. In many cases the symptoms are precipitated by sexual intercourse. In these patients discomfort and anxiety may be considerable since the condition may lead to marital disharmony.

Diagnosis

The diagnosis depends on the finding of a negative routine culture in the presence of frequency and dysuria. In the differential diagnosis, tuberculosis of the urinary tract should be considered in particular in those women in whom sterile pyuria is found. Also gonococcal infection should be excluded and a search should be made for vaginal and cervical infections since these may present with symptoms of frequency and dysuria, possibly due to trauma of the external urethral orifice as a result of pruritis vulvae.

Treatment

The importance of recognizing the urethral syndrome is that most of these women would otherwise be considered to suffer from urinary tract infection and would then be studied extensively and often unnecessarily treated with costly and/or toxic antibacterial agents.

Therapy should consist of reassurance and attendance to vaginal and/or cervical infection. Attention to perineal hygiene and detection of sensitivity to rubber, vaginal sprays, or spermicidal jellies may lead to effective avoidance of these precipitating factors. In patients in whom symptoms are related to sexual intercourse a trial of post-intercourse antibacterial therapy is worthwhile. Cotrimoxazole (1 tablet), trimethoprim (50 mg), or nitrofurantoin (50 mg) may be used. Sometimes anxiolytic agents such as diazepam 5 mg three times daily bring relief.

Prostatitis

Urinary tract infections in males most commonly originate from an infection of the prostate gland. The commonest infecting organisms are *Escherichia coli*, enterobacter, klebsiella, *Proteus* spp., and enterococci, in that order of frequency. Occasionally a staphylococcal infection of the prostate occurs and may lead to the formation of a prostatic abscess. The infection may follow urethral instrumentation.

Clinical features

In the *acute* form of the disease the patient complains of severe perineal and low back pain which may be accompanied by fever due to an associated bacteraemia. In the *chronic* form the patient complains of a sensation of perineal fullness which may be associated with low back pain. Sometimes dysuria is also present and there may be a urethral discharge. There are usually no constitutional symptoms. The symptoms may be relieved by ejaculation, in other patients the symptoms are aggravated by sexual intercourse. Rectal massage can either relieve or exacerbate the symptoms. Clinically, the prostate feels enlarged and softened. In the acute form it is very tender to touch, in the chronic form lesser degrees of prostatic tenderness can be elicited.

Diagnosis and treatment

Confirmation of the diagnosis depends on culture of the causative organisms by obtaining a specimen of urine or urethral discharge after prostatic massage. Treatment of the condition is difficult because few antibacterial agents penetrate the prostatic fluid. Those that do penetrate the prostatic secretion, include trimethoprim, erythromycin, tetracyclines, and novobiocin. These are, therefore, the drugs of choice. Trimethoprim 200 mg twice daily or erythromycin 500 mg four times daily should be prescribed for at least 10 days, longer in the case of chronic infections. Recurrent infections may require long-term low dose suppressive treatment. In acute prostatitis due to staphylococcal infection surgical drainage of prostatic abscesses may be necessary.

Bacterial cystitis

Cystitis is usually due to bacterial infection but it may result from viral or fungal infection, toxic chemicals drugs (e.g. haemorrhagic cystitis due to cyclophosphamide) or X-irradiation. The commonest infecting organism is *Escherichia coli* but micrococcal infections may account for up to 10 or even 20 per cent of cases in sexually active women. More rarely the infection is due to *Klebsiella* spp., *Proteus* spp., *Streptococcus faecalis*, and pseudomonads. Infection reaches the bladder by the ascending route. The role of instrumentation (including catheterization) in the pathogenesis of cystitis must not be underestimated.

Clinical features

The main symptoms of cystitis are frequency, dysuria, and haematuria. Foul smelling urine may also have been noted by the patient or relatives and the patient may complain of suprapubic discomfort. In these patients in whom the symptoms are precipitated by sexual intercourse ('honeymoon cystitis'), marital disharmony, and anxiety may be a consequence of cystitis. In children the symptoms are less clearly defined and include crying attacks on micturition, vague abdominal pains, failure to thrive, and foul-smelling nappies.

Diagnosis

Diagnosis depends on the clinical findings and the results of urine microscopy and culture. Microscopy reveals pyuria and the causative organism can be identified both in the film and from stained preparation of the urine (Fig. 3). Culture confirms the presence of infection. Pyuria in the absence of bacteriuria should suggest tuberculous infection (q.v.) In adult women with cystitis, radiolo-

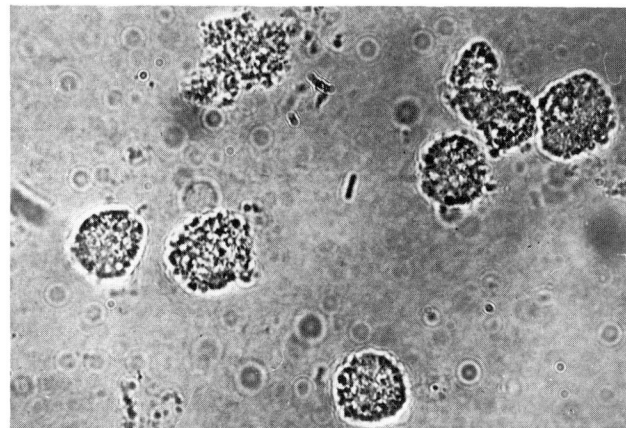

Fig. 3 Unstained film of urine obtained from patient with acute *Escherichia coli* bacterial cystitis. Note numerous pus cells and cocco-bacilli (magnification × 320).

gical examination rarely reveals abnormalities of the urinary tract which are amenable to treatment. In children of both sexes radiological abnormalities are more frequent, even in children examined on first presentation. It was generally accepted that excretion urography and micturating cystography should be performed in children, particularly under the age of four. As first-line investigation ultrasound and dimethylsuccinic acid (DMSA) scanning have now replaced these investigations as they are less invasive and involve less irradiation exposure. In women in whom infection relapses repeatedly an excretion urogram should also be carried out. Bacterial cystitis in males not precipitated by instrumentation, is nearly always associated with anatomical abnormalities of the urinary tract and excretion urography is therefore essential.

Treatment

The severity of symptoms frequently necessitates treatment before the bacteriological findings and sensitivity pattern of the urinary pathogens are known. In these circumstances the choice of antibacterial agent should be based on a knowledge of the prevailing sensitivity pattern of the common urinary pathogens in the environment in which the infection was acquired. Table 5 illustrates how the sensitivity pattern of urinary pathogens differs when hospital and general practice environments are compared; it shows that even within the hospital there is variation in the antibiogram of urinary pathogens from one department to another.

Amongst the drugs which might be used as first choice treatment the following may be mentioned: co-trimoxazole (2 tablets twice daily), trimethoprim (200 mg twice daily), ampicillin (250 mg four times daily), nitofurantoin (50 mg three times daily), and nalidixic acid (100 mg three times daily). Treatment need not exceed one week. It has recently been shown that even a single dose (amoxycillin 3 g) can cure lower tract infection. Symptoms should subside 24–48 hours after starting treatment. If there is no response within this time, the treatment should be changed to a

Table 5 Sensitivity patterns of urinary pathogens

Source of patient	Percentage of organisms resistant to				
	Sulphon-amides	Ampicillin	Co-tri-moxazole	Nitrofur-antoin	Nali-dixic
General practice	23	12	3	15	14
Antenatal clinic	29	25	1	6	2
Hospital inpatient	42	49	21	37	22
Urological dept.	57	56	20	46	52

After Williams, J. D. *et al.* (1973).

different antibacterial agent to which the infecting strain is sensitive. Since bacterial cystitis frequently recurs careful follow-up with repeat urine cultures must be arranged. Two types of recurrence may be distinguished, namely relapse and reinfection. Relapse of the infection occurs soon after cessation of treatment and the recurrent infection is due to the same organism as that which was isolated originally. Relapsing infection indicates a failure of treatment and is more common in patients in whom the infection involves the kidney. In contrast, reinfections occur usually not less than six weeks after cessation of treatment, and are due to different organisms from the original isolate. Reinfection, therefore, indicates a failure of host defensive mechanisms. The causes of relapsing infection together with suggested methods of management are shown in Table 6. If these remedies should fail, frequently relapsing symptomatic infections may need to be suppressed by long-term low-dose nightly antibacterial therapy (i.e. nitrofurantoin 50 mg, trimethoprim 100 mg, co-trimoxazole 1 tablet or cephalexin 125 nightly). This will prevent overnight multiplication of bacteria in the bladder and so allay symptoms. Again where infections are related to sexual intercourse, a single dose of one of the above antibacterial agents after intercourse may prove highly effective in controlling the symptoms. Long-term treatment of this kind is usually continued for one year. Thereafter, symptoms may not return. In all long-term treatment it is important that the drug which is used is so chosen as not to affect the resistance pattern of the bowel flora so that 'breakthrough' infections are reduced to a minimum. The success of trimethoprim in long-term treatment appears to be due to its ability to eliminate enterobacteraciae from the faeces and perineal floor. It is important also to advise a high fluid intake. This aids the hydrokinetic defences. The high urinary concentration of urinary antibacterial agents, which is far in excess of their minimal inhibitory concentration for most urinary pathogens, more than compensates for the dilution of drug due to the high fluid intake. Symptomatic reinfections which tend to be more widely spaced, can often be managed without the need for long-term suppressive treatment, by providing the patients with a one-week course of treatment to be taken at the first evidence of a recurrence. In women a surgically remediable cause for recurrent infection is rarely found but in older men prostatic enlargement is frequently the cause and in such cases appropriate surgical treatment will prevent recurrent infections.

Acute pyelonephritis

Acute pyelonephritis results from bacterial infection involving the pelvis (pyelon) of the kidney and spreading into the renal parenchyma. The commonest infecting organism is *Escherichia coli* although the less common urinary pathogens detailed in Table 3 may also be responsible. In the case of proteus infections renal involvement is almost invariable, whereas with *E. coli* infection only 30–50 per cent of infections involve the kidney. As in the case of bladder infection, infection of the renal parenchyma does not invariably produce symptoms. In fact asymptomatic infections are much more frequent than symptomatic pyelonephritis. Factors which predispose to the development of acute symptomatic pyelonephritis include pregnancy, diabetes mellitus, and obstructive uropathy, as well as the possession of 'p' fibriae by the infecting strains of *E. coli*.

The kidney shows swelling of pelvic epithelium together with acute inflammatory infiltration of the subepithelial tissue. Irregular streaks of pus extend outwards from the pelvis through the medulla to the cortex. The tubules in the affected areas are distended and filled with pus debris. In the presence of diabetes mellitus or obstructive uropathy, the inflammatory process may be so severe as to lead to necrosis of papillary tips (see necrotizing papillitis).

Clinical features

Loin pain and fever are the cardinal manifestations of acute pyelonephritis. The fever, usually sudden in onset and accompanied by rigors, is often a prominent feature. There are usually few complaints related to the lower urinary tract; the urine may be malodorous. On physical examination fever, tachycardia, and extreme tenderness in one or both renal angles are found. If, as rarely happens, a perirenal abscess has formed, the waist on that side may be lost and spasm of spinal musculature on the affected side may lead to a scoliosis with its concavity towards the affected side (Fig. 4). In severe bilateral cases, oliguria and acute renal failure may be present, due to occlusion of collecting ducts secondary to oedema of the pelvic epithelium and submucosa. In patients with diabetes mellitus, severe acute pyelonephritis with or without necrotizing papillitis may lead to diabetic precoma or coma and this may then be the presenting feature.

Diagnosis

Except in young children, the clinical diagnosis usually presents no difficulties. It is confirmed by examination of the urine deposit and urine culture. The deposit shows pus cell casts and organisms and culture allows identification of the pathogens. Blood culture may also be positive and a leucocytosis commonly accompanies the ill-

Table 6 Causes of relapsing infection and suggested management

Cause of relapse	Remedial action
Wrong choice of drug	When treatment is started before antibiotic sensitivity of pathogen is known choose drug on 'best guess' principle after consultation with local bacteriologist
Inadequate duration of treatment	A 7-day course of treatment should be used—if compliance is likely to be poor use long-acting drug
Emergence of minority resistant strain	Retreat
Inadequate concentration of drug at site of infection	Use high-dose treatment
Stones	Removal of stones

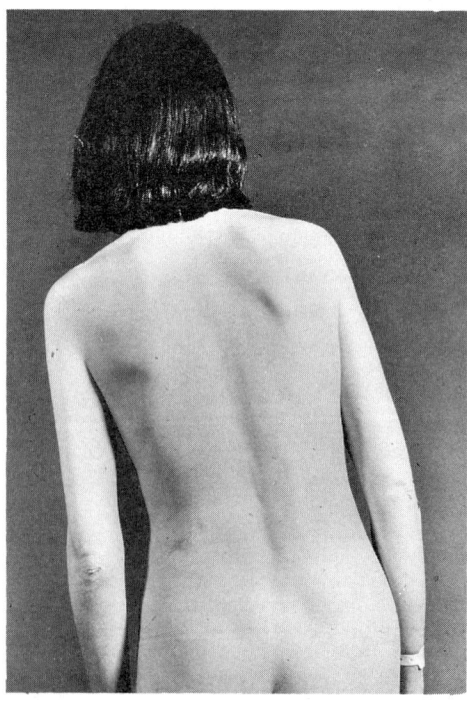

Fig. 4 Disappearance of concavity of left flank and scoliosis in patient with left-sided perirenal abscess.

ness. Excretion urography during the acute attack usually shows enlargement of the affected kidney and poor excretion of contrast medium. After the acute phase is over, the radiological findings are of greater value since underlying predisposing causes may be revealed, e.g. urolithiasis or congenital malformations. In the presence of perirenal abscess, the psoas shadow will be obscured and gas may accumulate around the kidney (Fig. 5). This complication is readily detected by ultrasound techniques. When papillary necrosis has occurred, papillary tips may be found in the urine deposit and the radiological findings will be characteristic of necrotizing papillitis (see below).

Treatment

In the pregnant woman, acute symptomatic pyelonephritis can be prevented by detection and treatment of asymptomatic bacteriuria in early pregnancy. The established case usually requires treatment before the results of urine culture and the sensitivity of pathogens to antibacterial agents are known. Treatment must therefore be based on a 'best guess' principle until such time that the bacteriological findings are available. Amoxycillin (500 mg four times daily) and trimethoprim (200 mg twice daily) are the best treatments available (at present). When resistance of the infecting strain is due to β-lactamase production Augmentin 375 mg three times daily may be used. This drug is a combination of amoxycillin (250 mg) and the β-lactamase inhibitor clavulanic acid (125 mg). Other treatments include ampicillin (500 mg four times daily). The duration of treatment need not exceed one week. A high (3 litre) fluid intake is advisable. If improvement has not taken place within 48 hours, the choice of drug may have been incorrect and will need to be reappraised according to the bacteriological findings. Alternatively, if the infection has led to formation of a perirenal abscess or there is an obstructive uropathy, appropriate drainage may be required. If severe oliguria accompanies the illness, adjustment of the dose of antibacterial agent may be required and peritoneal dialysis may be needed rarely. As in the case of bacterial cystitis (see above), infections frequently recur after treatment. Such recurrences may be either due to the same organism (relapse), or due to a different pathogen (reinfection). It is necessary, therefore, to arrange for careful follow-up of patients with acute pyelonephritis.

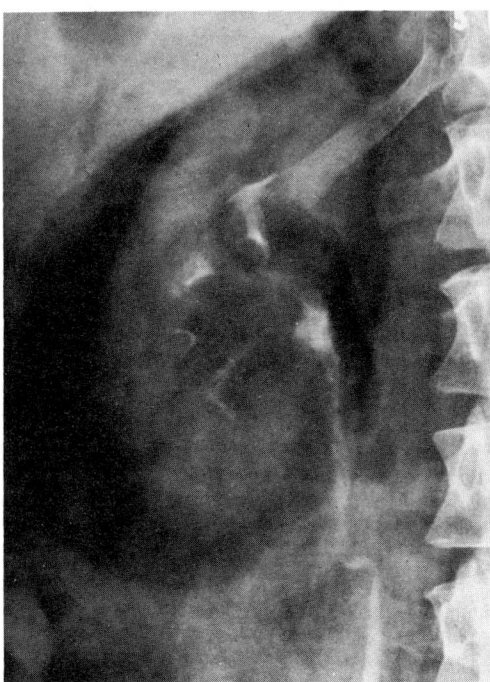

Fig. 5 Excretion urogram showing gas around right kidney in a patient with a perirenal abscess. (By courtesy of Dr L. A. Williams.)

Relapsing infections account for 20 per cent of the recurrences. They are due to a failure of treatment. The causes of such relapsing infections are shown in Table 6 and they should be identified and dealt with. Reinfections account for 80 per cent of the recurrent infections. They are due to a failure of host defensive mechanisms. Long-term low dose suppressive treatment may be necessary to strengthen the host defences and avoid symptomatic infections. The drugs which may be used are identical to those used for the treatment of bacterial cystitis (see above). Alternatively, if recurrent attacks are not very frequent, the patient may be provided with a seven day course of suitable antibacterial agent to be taken at the first evidence of a recurrent infection. The patient is also instructed to inoculate a 'dip-slide' before starting treatment and to send this to the laboratory. In this way morbidity is reduced to a minimum yet bacteriological control is retained.

Perirenal abscess

Perirenal abscesses are located between the renal capsule and the connective tissue which surrounds the kidney. They usually arise by direct extension of infection from the kidney and unlike renal carbuncles (see below) they are rarely the result of a septicaemia. Since a perinephric abscess is deeply situated, it is usually very large before it produces signs such as swelling, tenderness, and redness. Fever, loin pain, and malaise persisting after treatment of an attack of acute pyelonephritis are the early symptoms. Flattening of the concavity of the loin is a valuable clinical sign (Fig. 4).

The diagnosis is made when persistent loin pain, fever, and leucocytosis occur after apparently adequate treatment of acute pyelonephritis. The urine deposit usually shows pus cells and pus cell casts but culture may be sterile. Abdominal X-ray reveals a loss of psoas shadow on the affected side, the diaphragm on the affected side may be displaced upwards and fixed and perirenal gas may be seen (Fig. 5). Scanning with the use of ^{59}Ga can be very helpful in diagnosis since the gallium is taken up by the polymorphs in the abscess. A perinephric abscess usually requires surgical drainage together with antibacterial therapy.

Carbuncle of the kidney

A carbuncle of the kidney is a staphylococcal infection of the renal parenchyma. The condition commonly follows a staphylococcal skin infection. The organisms reach the kidney by the haematogenous route. The abscess cavities are usually confined to the renal cortex. They do not communicate with the renal pelvis but they may extend into the perirenal tissue leading to the formation of a coexisting perirenal abscess.

The patient presents with a high swinging fever some two weeks after a staphylococcal infection of the skin such as a boil or carbuncle or following infection of an intravenous cannula or cannulation site. On examination fever, loin pain, and tenderness are present. The waist may be filled in on the affected side and lumbar scoliosis with its concavity to the affected side may be present.

The urine deposit usually shows no abnormality unlike the findings in patients with a perinephric abscess. This is because the abscess does not communicate with the renal pelvis. Excretion urography may show a space occupying lesion. The psoas shadow is usually retained. The carbuncle can be detected by ultrasound techniques. The absence of vascularity on arteriography may help to distinguish a carbuncle from a malignant tumour of the kidney. Surgical drainage and antibacterial therapy are the mainstays of treatment.

Xanthogranulomatous pyelonephritis

This rare condition is usually the result of chronic recurrent infection due to *Proteus* spp. The kidney is enlarged and adherent to the surrounding tissues. The dilated pelvis often contains a 'matrix' or staghorn calculus and the renal parenchyma contains an abscess cavity or cavities which is (are) surrounded by a yellow zone(s) (Fig. 6). Histologically this yellow zone contains foam cells, multi-nucleate giant cells, and macrophages laden with periodic acid–Schiff positive staining granules.

Presenting féatures include fever, weight loss, loin pain, and a palpable mass in the loin. The main importance of this rare condition is in the differential diagnosis from adenocarcinoma of the kidney. Nephrotomograms may reveal lucent areas in the centre of the xanthogranulomatous lesion and arteriography shows absence of vascularity in the inflammatory mass. Nephrectomy is the treatment of choice.

Megalocytic interstitial nephritis

This condition is an interstitial nephritis in which the renal cortex contains greyish yellow foci of various sizes. Histologically these foci consist of large polygonal cells with coarsely granular eosinophilic cytoplasm which are intensely positive when stained with the periodic acid–Schiff stain. They are similar to the Michaelis–Gutmann bodies found in malakoplakia. The condition is almost certainly some form of chronic inflammatory process. Its main clinical importance is that the discrete cortical lesions may, as in the case of xanthogranulomatous pyelonephritis, be mistaken for a neoplasm of the kidney.

Renal papillary necrosis (see also page 18.112)

Aetiology

Papillary necrosis may arise as a result of severe infection as in the presence of obstructive uropathy or diabetes mellitus. It may also be a consequence of long-term medication with nephrotoxic agents such as phenacetin or it may be the consequence of sickle cell disease or sickle cell trait. The renal papilla is very susceptible to ischaemic damage because skimming of plasma into the blood cells which supply the medulla results in a low oxygen tension in the papillary region. The precise damaging agent(s) in analgesic mixtures are still unknown. Phenacetin or one of its breakdown products, possibly 1-phenetidine, appears to be the main culprit. It has been estimated that an intake in excess of 1 kg of phenacetin may lead to the condition.

Pathology

The necrosis usually involves several papillary tips and in cases due to excessive analgesic intake the condition is almost invariably bilateral. The necrotic papillae may remain *in situ*; where this is the case excretion urography may not show any abnormalities. They may calcify *in situ* or they may slough and calcify. Sloughed papillae may produce ureteric obstruction or they may be recovered from the urine. In patients with papillary necrosis due

to high analgesic intake there is an increased incidence of tumours of the uroepithelium as well as ureteric strictures.

Clinical features

When necrotizing papillitis is primarily infective in origin, the clinical features are those of severe acute pyelonephritis (see above). Infections of this degree of severity are particularly likely to occur in the presence of obstructive uropathy or in patients with diabetes mellitus, and if bilateral are often associated with oliguria. Diabetic patients with infective necrotizing papillitis not infrequently present in diabetic coma or precoma. In patients with high analgesic intake first presentation may be on account of urinary tract infection, renal colic, or the symptoms of chronic kidney failure. Analgesic consumption may have been high because of painful conditions such as migraine or arthropathy. Alternatively analgesics may have been taken in excess for less well-defined reasons, e.g. 'for nerves', insomnia, or even 'for kicks'. It is also common to meet secretive analgesic takers.

Diagnosis

This depends on recognition of the predisposing causes together with the finding of papillary material on urine microscopy and the appearance on the excretion urogram. The various findings are illustrated diagrammatically in Fig. 7. The urogram may be normal but usually it shows ulceration of the papilla at the tip or base, amputation and/or calcification of papillae, and undulation of the renal outline due to hypertrophy of the columns of Bertin (see Fig. 8). In patients in whom infection is the primary cause, the urine is infected and usually reveals a heavy bacterial growth.

Treatment

Prophylaxis is important. Unnecessary self-medication with analgesics must be discouraged and urinary tract infections in patients with diabetes mellitus and haemoglobinopathies require prompt attention and more careful follow-up than for patients who are not predisposed to necrotizing papillitis. In the established case, infection should be treated and the use of nephrotoxic analgesics must be stopped. The latter measure may lead to improvement of kidney function. Surgical treatment may be necessary to relieve obstructive uropathy.

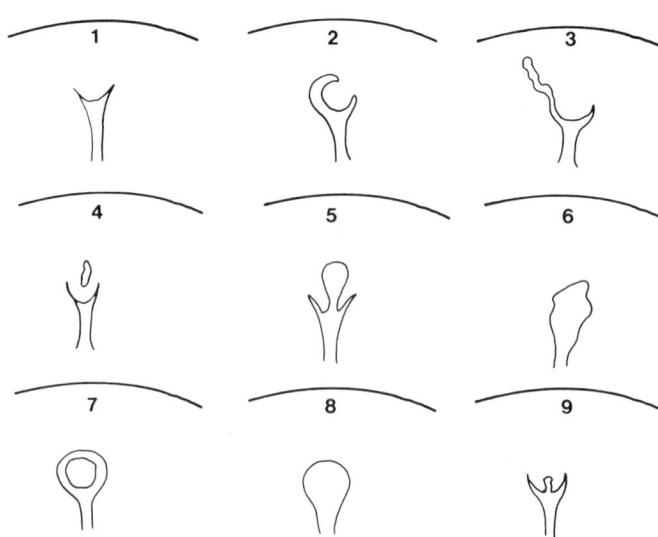

Fig. 7 Diagrammatic representation of renal damage to analgesics. 1. Normal papilla. 2–3. 'Sinus'-like cavitation. 4. Central papillary sloughing, mild. 5. Central papillary sloughing, moderate. 6. Sloughing involving both papilla and medulla. 7. Dissection of whole papillary tip with latter remaining *in situ*. 8. As in (7) only papilla has been passed down the ureter. 9. Papillary tip excavation. (By kind permission of the late Professor C. J. Hodson.)

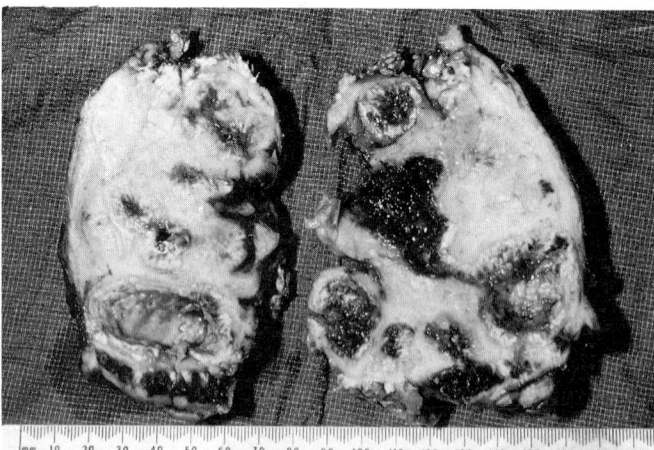

Fig. 6 Gross appearance of kidney showing xanthogranulomatous pyelonephritis. The whole kidney is replaced by abscess cavities which are surrounded by yellow lipid-containing zones.

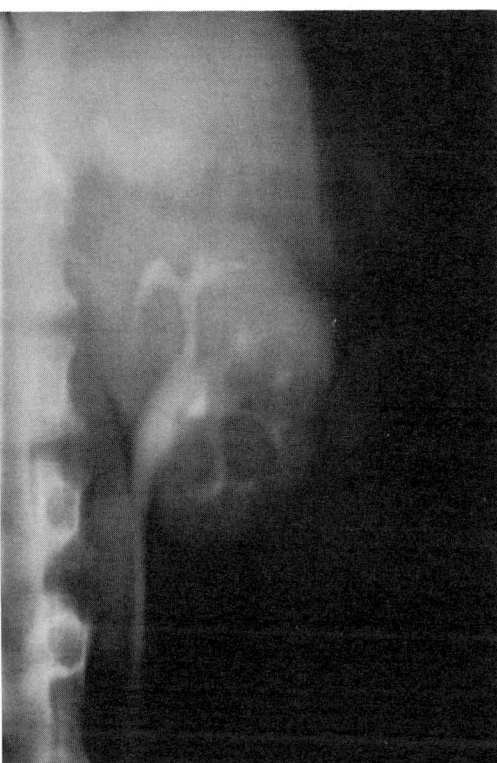

Fig. 8 Excretion urogram showing some of the features of analgesic nephropathy. Note undulation of renal outline due to hypertrophy of columns of Bertin. A detached papilla is seen in the renal pelvis and there is marked excavation of the calyceal fornices.

Chronic pyelonephritis

There is a divergence of opinion on the definition of chronic pyelonephritis. The most generally accepted definition is that chronic pyelonephritis is a form of chronic interstitial nephritis which results from long standing or recurrent bacterial infection of the kidney. It may occur in the presence of urinary tract obstruction (obstructive chronic pyelonephritis) or it may occur without obstruction.

Prevalence

It has been estimated that up to 20 per cent of adults and 30 per cent of children with end-stage kidney failure suffer from chronic pyelonephritis. Since approximately 70 per million of the population die from kidney failure each year, it is apparent that between 15 to 20 per million may die of chronic pyelonephritis. These figures must be viewed with caution since patients with end-stage kidney failure are rarely investigated in great detail with regard to the cause of their kidney failure. Figures of the prevalence of chronic pyelonephritis which are based on post-mortem findings must be interpreted with even greater caution. It has been suggested that the kidneys obtained from 3 to 5 per cent of all post-mortem examinations, show histological evidence of chronic pyelonephritis; the majority of these having been unrecognized in life. Whereas urinary tract infection is at least ten times more common in women than in men, the chronic pyelonephritis found post-mortem appears to be equally distributed between the sexes. This is but one of the many inconsistencies which casts doubt on the precise nature of the relationship between urinary tract infection and chronic pyelonephritis.

Pathogenesis

It is now becoming clear that in the absence of obstruction kidney damage due to ascending urinary tract infection mainly occurs in young children in whom infection and severe degrees of vesico-

ureteric reflux (VUR) coexist. In such cases, the intrarenal influx due to pyelo-tubular backflow which accompanies the most severe degrees of VUR, carries organisms into the renal parenchyma (Fig. 9). The importance of VUR and intrarenal reflux is such that it has even been suggested that VUR can produce kidney scarring in the absence of infection. To underline this the term *reflux nephropathy* has been coined. Since this term implies a prime role for VUR in the pathogenesis of kidney scarring and since its use might unleash a wave of unnecessary surgical repairs of VUR, it is not recommended. It is generally considered that both VUR and infection are necessary to produce kidney scars and that such scars develop only if the VUR is associated with intrarenal reflux (IRR). Since IRR only occurs in children below the age of four, the kidney scarring due to infection is nowadays aptly referred to as *chronic childhood pyelonephritis*. When organisms are carried into the kidney, two effects are produced, focal scarring and impairment of kidney growth. These effects are rarely sufficient to lead to kidney failure in themselves. They may, however, lead to a rise of blood pressure which in its turn may contribute to the deterioration of kidney function. It has also been postulated that severe VUR can lead to glomerular damage, so called alterative glomerulitis. Certainly glomerular proteinuria is invariably found in patients in whom chronic childhood pyelonephritis progresses to renal impairment. The cause of the glomeral lesions in reflux nephropathy is not known. It may be due to hyperfiltration by the glomeruli in the non-scarred portions of the kidney or it may be caused by reflux of kidney antigens into the circulation and subsequent deposition of kidney antigen-antibody immune complexes in the glomeruli. In some instances the back pressure resulting from severe VUR may lead to hydronephrosis and back pressure atrophy and this effect of VUR may also contribute to impairment of kidney function. Most commonly, however, the focal scars produced by infection and reflux persist into adult life and remain asymptomatic. The presence of kidney scars leads to a greater susceptibility to urinary tract infection and there is also a greater liab-

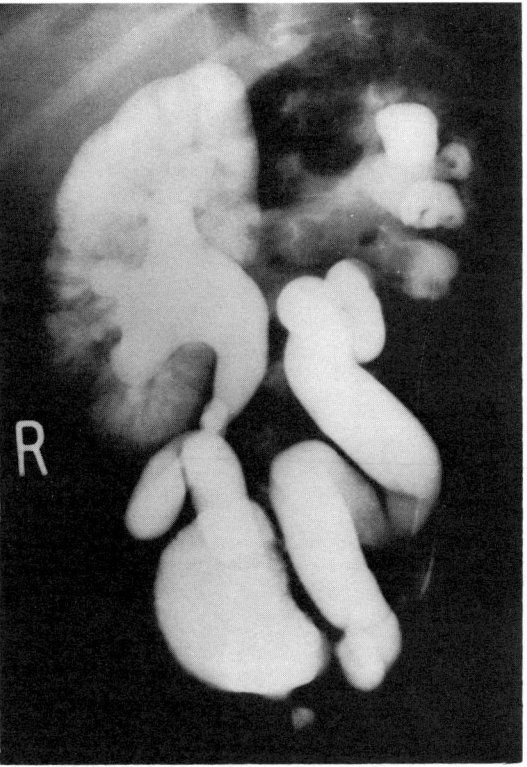

Fig. 9 Micturating cystogram in a girl aged three showing severe grade 3 vesico-ureteric reflux with intrarenal reflux on the right side and failure of kidney growth and hydronephrosis of the left kidney.

ility to a rise of blood pressure particularly during pregnancy. In adult women, scars acquired in childhood do not appear to progress and infection is a consequence of the scars rather than their cause.

Macroscopically, the pyelonephritic kidney is small and coarsely scarred (Fig. 10). Each of the scars is juxtaposed to a dilated calix (Fig. 11). Histological examination confirms the patchy scarring of the renal parenchyma which extends from the pelvis to the surface of the kidney. In the scarred areas there is a dense interstitial fibrosis and the tubules are dilated and filled with eosinophilic casts, to form so called thyroid-like areas which can be seen in Fig. 11. There may also be evidence of hypertensive vascular damage.

Clinical features

Most patients with chronic pyelonephritis are asymptomatic and can only be detected by screening for asymptomatic urinary tract infection in apparently healthy populations. The commonest presentation is with raised blood pressure; less commonly, recurrent symptomatic infections draw attention to the condition, and a few patients unfortunately present with the symptoms of end-stage kidney failure such as nocturia, lethargy, weakness, nausea, and vomiting.

Diagnosis

The diagnosis of chronic pyelonephritis is based on the radiological findings (Fig. 12). The juxtaposition of a cortical scar and a dilated calix is the hallmark of a pyelonephritic scar. The scars are usually most marked in the upper or lower poles of the kidney. In patients with pyelonephritic scars, micturating cystography frequently reveals vesico-ureteric reflux. This is particularly the case in children and in them pyelo-tubular back-flow of contrast medium may also be in evidence. Urine culture is usually sterile. In some instances bacteriuria is present and in others pyuria and pus cell casts are present. The condition must be distinguished from analgesic nephropathy. The findings on excretion urography are most helpful in drawing this distinction.

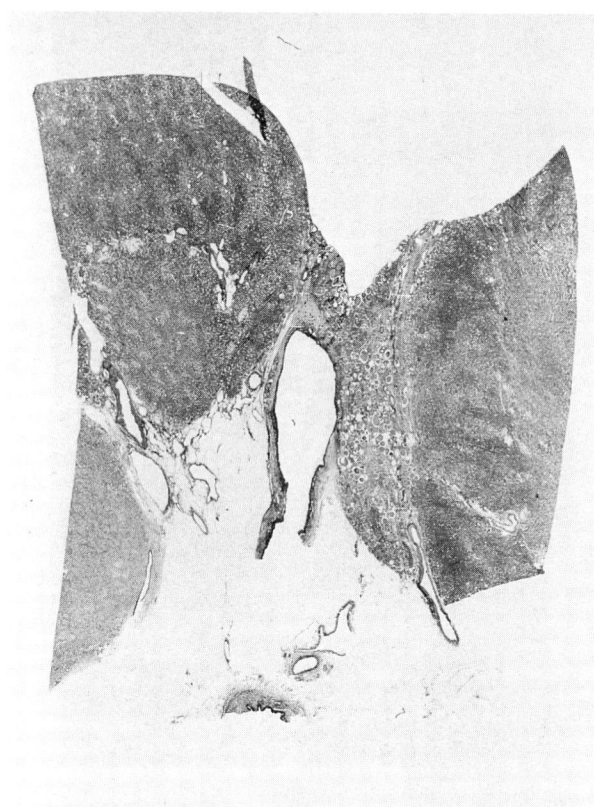

Fig. 11 Section through coarse kidney scar showing dilated calix with adjoining scar. The 'thyroid-like areas' in the scar are also visible (haematoxylin and eosin).

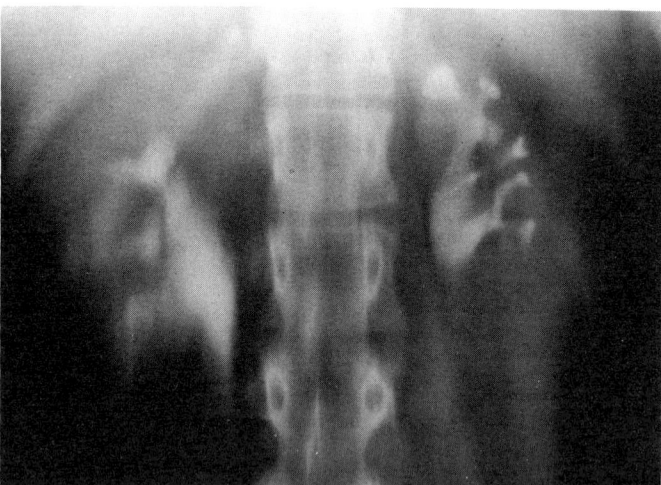

Fig. 12 Excretion urogram showing a coarsely scarred, contracted 'chronic pyelonephritic' left kidney and hypertrophy of the right kidney.

Treatment

In children in whom infection, VUR, and IRR coexist every effort should be made to eradicate the bacteriuria. This is best achieved by long-term low dose suppressive treatment. Instruction in the practice of double micturition may help to minimize residual urine and thus aid in the control of infection. The role of surgery in the correction of VUR is very doubtful particularly since VUR tends to clear spontaneously as the child grows older. In the adult, the management of chronic pyelonephritis should consist of careful observation of the blood pressure and prompt treatment of hypertension should it arise. Symptomatic episodes of infection should

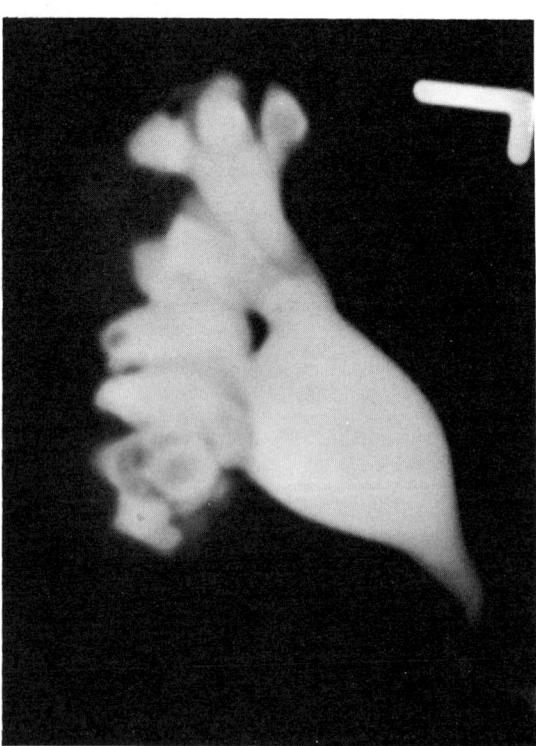

Fig. 10 Retrograde pyelogram on nephrectomy specimen of patient with chronic pyelonephritis. Note juxtaposition of scars and dilated calices.

be treated with appropriate antibacterial therapy as detailed in the treatment of acute pyelonephritis. Provided there is no obstructive uropathy the patient can be reassured that progressive kidney damage is highly unlikely to occur. Obstructive lesions should be dealt with surgically.

Asymptomatic bacteriuria

Asymptomatic bacteriuria or covert bacteriuria is a term which refers to the presence and multiplication of bacteria in the bladder urine in the absence of symptoms which are of a sufficient severity to require medical attention. It is, therefore, usually detected during screening of apparently healthy populations or it may be found in the course of follow-up of patients previously treated for symptomatic infections.

Prevalence

Asymptomatic bacteriuria is a common finding. Between 1–2 per cent of schoolgirls and 3–5 per cent of adult women are found to have asymptomatic bacteriuria. In males the condition is much less common; 0.05 per cent of schoolboys and 0.5 per cent of adult males show bacteriuria. The condition increases in prevalence with advancing age and in males the prevalence rises in the elderly in consequence of prostatic hypertrophy. In women the condition also increases in prevalence with increasing parity.

Pathogenesis

Escherichia coli is the causative organism in at least 90 per cent of cases of asymptomatic bacteriuria. They are derived from the bowel flora and reach the urinary tract by the ascending route. It is not known why in some subjects invasion of the bladder by strains of *E. coli* produces a bout of cystitis whereas in others asymptomatic infection is established. Differences in 'host–parasite' relationship may account for this. Patients with covert infections are more frequently infected with rough untypeable strains of *E. coli* than subjects with symptomatic infection. It may be that such rough strains are formed as a result of local antibody production and that they are less able to elicit an inflammatory response. The site of asymptomatic infections can be determined by ureteric catheterization, by the bladder washout technique or by the detection of antibody coating on the infection strain. Using these techniques it has been shown that asymptomatic bacteriuria originates from the kidneys in 30 to 50 per cent of the subjects.

Clinical features

By definition, asymptomatic bacteriuria produces no symptoms but close enquiry reveals that a recent past history of symptoms such as frequency and dysuria is common. The clinical significance of asymptomatic bacteriuria is not yet fully elucidated. In pregnant women the condition predisposes to the development of acute symptomatic pyelonephritis. Thirty per cent of women found to have ASB early in pregnancy develop symptomatic infection later on in pregnancy. Eradication of the asymptomatic infection prevents this. In non-pregnant women the value of detecting and treating ASB is not established since the condition is often transient and does not commonly lead to the development of symptomatic infection, rise of blood pressure, or progressive kidney damage. In children the value of detection and treatment of ASB has not been established either. It seems likely that in those children in whom bacteriuria and severe vesico-ureteric reflux coexist, treatment is indicated since this combination predisposes to the development of kidney scars.

Diagnosis

Bacteriuria literally means the presence of bacteria in the urine. This may result from contamination or infection and the distinction between these can be made by quantitative urine culture. Contaminants which are added to the urine during or after voiding are usually present in small numbers (less than 100 000 organisms per ml of urine) whereas organisms which are present in the bladder urine are present in high numbers (usually more than 100 000 organisms per ml) because they have multiplied in the urine between successive acts of micturition (Fig. 13). The distinction between bacteriuria due to contamination and that due to infection demands careful collection of mid-stream specimens and requires that multiplication of bacteria in the urine once voided is prevented by immediate culture or by cooling the urine to 4 °C during transport or by adding a preservative such as boric acid which prevents growth without killing the bacteria. The best method of quantitative urine culture is by the 'pour plate' technique. Since this is time consuming various semi-quantitative methods have been introduced of which the 'dip-slide' method is the best (Fig. 14). The slide which is coated with culture medium

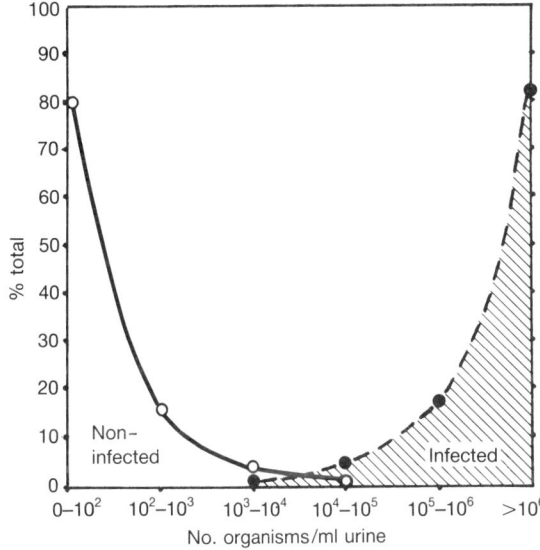

Fig. 13 Diagram showing the theoretical distribution of viable bacterial count (horizontal axis) in early morning specimens of urine obtained from large populations of subjects with asymptomatic bacteriuria (●– – –●) and uninfected controls (○——○).

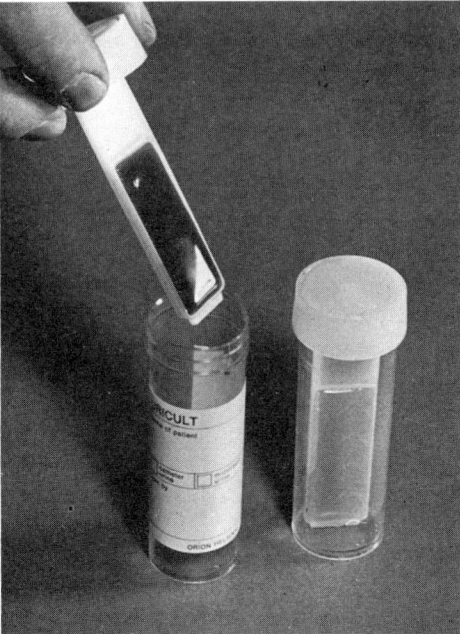

Fig. 14 The dip-slide. The slide can be inoculated wetting it on both sides whilst it is held in the urinary stream. Both sides are coated with culture media, one side being covered with a selective medium, e.g. MacConkey or CLED agar, and the other is covered with a non-selective medium, e.g. nutrient agar.

can be held directly in the urinary stream and may then be sent by post to the laboratory where it can be incubated and read off against a standard scale (Fig. 15). Several chemical methods for detection of significant bacteriuria have been introduced but these are less satisfactory.

Treatment

Significant bacteriuria only requires detection and treatment in pregnancy. There is some evidence that its detection and treatment can benefit the elderly and in those receiving immunosuppressive treatment. In all other instances, it has not so far been shown that screening for, and treatment of, symptomless infections is worthwhile. The treatment is identical with that which is used in symptomatic infection, but particular attention should be paid to embryopathic effects of the drugs used. Tetracyclines should be avoided because of their adverse effects on skeletal and tooth development. Sulphonamides should be avoided in late pregnancy since these may increase neonatal jaundice whereas nalidixic acid should not be used because it may produce neonatal hydrocephalus.

Tuberculosis of the urinary tract

Tuberculosis of the urinary tract (see also page 18.175) is less common in the United Kingdom than it used to be but its prompt detection remains a matter of utmost importance, since highly effective treatment is now available and kidney damage can therefore be avoided if treatment is given at an early stage of the disease.

Aetiology

Tuberculosis of the urinary tract is a consequence of haematogenous spread which occurs after primary infection. In most cases healing occurs and no progressive disease develops. Both kidneys may be seeded with tubercle bacilli but progressive disease is usually confined to one kidney and does not manifest clinically until 5–15 years after the primary infection. Hence clinical manifestation of tuberculous disease of the urinary tract are very rare in childhood. The initial focus of infection is the cortex. From there the disease spreads to the renal papilla and caseation of the papillary lesion leads to discharge of tubercle bacilli in the urine. In this manner tuberculous disease may spread to the ureter and bladder with the formation of ureteric strictures and the development of a contracted scarred bladder. Obstructive uropathy may follow and the kidney may be completely replaced by calcified caseous material, a condition which is referred to as a tuberculous autonephrectomy. In males, the epididymis, seminal vesicles, and vas deferens may also be infected but the testis is rarely involved. The

importance of stricture formation cannot be overemphasized since stricture formation causes kidney damage more often than spread of tuberculous infection within the kidney.

Clinical features

The disease usually presents with symptoms suggesting cystitis, particularly frequency of micturition; the constant interruption of sleep which this produces may lead to tiredness and irritability. Dysuria and haematuria are other presenting features. Rarely a single episode of gross haematuria is the presenting feature in similar fashion to the haemoptysis which may be the presenting feature of pulmonary tuberculosis. Renal colic may be due to the passage of blood clot or debris from ulceration of the kidney substance. Loin pain made worse by high fluid intake may also be a feature in patients in whom a tuberculous hydronephrosis has developed. Renal tuberculosis rarely presents with a cold abscess in the loin. In the male, involvement of the genital tract may call attention to co-existing renal tuberculosis which should always be looked for in cases of genital tuberculosis. Exceptionally patients with renal tuberculosis first present with end-stage kidney failure or with hypertension. Constitutional symptoms are rare in patients with renal tuberculosis.

Diagnosis

Urinalysis is the key to diagnosis. In the early stages of the disease the only abnormality may be sterile pyuria. As the disease progresses proteinuria may be observed and varying amounts of haematuria may be present. Tubercle bacilli may be seen on smears. Such a finding is not however diagnostic since acid-fast bacilli other than tubercle bacilli may be found in the urine of healthy subjects (e.g. *Mycobacterium hominis*). Repeated early morning urine sample culture of tubercle bacilli usually settles the issue. Guinea-pig inoculation is now only rarely necessary. In the urine, tubercle bacilli are often scanty; they may also be excreted intermittently. For these reasons numerous specimens should be cultured. A negative tuberculin test casts serious doubt on the diagnosis of renal tuberculosis. Excretion urography also plays an important part in the diagnosis. The earliest abnormalities consist of irregularities of the papillary tip. Later, calcification and ulceration may be noted and stricture of the neck of the calix (Figs 16 and 17) or of the ureter together with evidence of back pressure may be seen. Contraction of the bladder may also be present. Retrograde pyelography has a place in the detailed pre-operative analysis of obstructive lesions and is also necessary to delineate the extent of the disease when impairment of kidney function leads to poor excretion of contrast medium by the affected kidney. Renography has a place in follow-up of patients with obstructive disease. It is important to perform a chest X-ray since 50 per cent of patients with renal tuberculosis have concurrent active pulmonary tuberculosis. The genital tract should be carefully examined for concomitant infection.

Treatment

Accurate initial assessment of the extent of the disease, the presence of obstructive uropathy and the state of kidney function are essential and collaboration between physician, urologist, and radiologist is vital. Most patients can now be treated out of hospital. Chemotherapy has revolutionized the management and prognosis of renal tuberculosis. Until the drug sensitivity of the tubercle bacilli is known treatment should be with three of the following drugs: streptomycin, 0.75–1 g daily; sodium paraminosalicylate (PAS), 10–15 g daily; isoniazid (INAH), 200–300 mg daily; ethambutol, 15 mg per kg body weight daily; and rifampicin 450–600 mg daily. Such combined therapy prevents the emergence of bacterial resistance. After the sensitivity pattern is known, therapy with two of the drugs is continued, e.g. PAS and INAH, ethambutol and INAH, or rifampicin and INAH. In the presence of impaired kidney function or in the elderly, extreme care must be taken over the use of streptomycin and ethambutol since these

Density patterns of colonies corresponding to different concentrations of bacteria per ml of urine

MacConkey's Agar

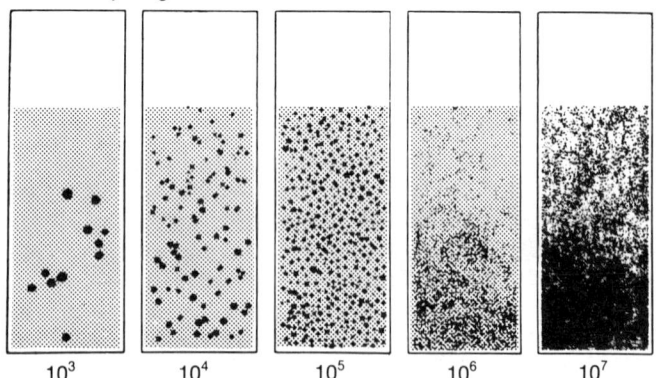

10^3 10^4 10^5 10^6 10^7

Fig. 15 Standard chart used to quantitate dip-slide cultures:

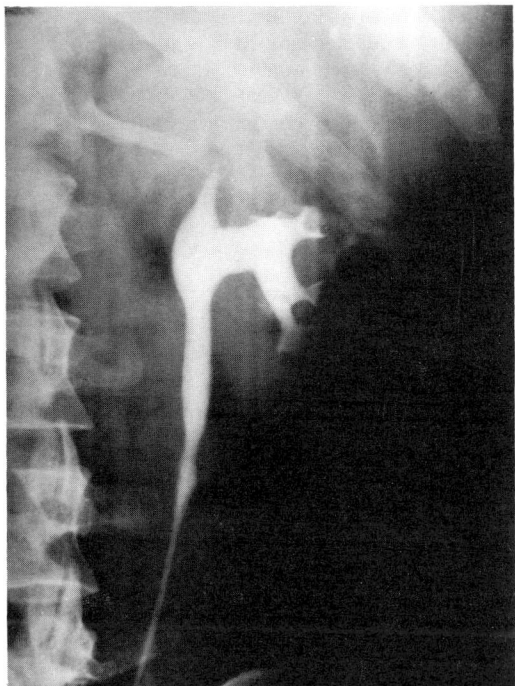

Fig. 16 Excretion urogram showing a tuberculous stricture of upper pole calix. (By courtesy of the late Mr R. A. Mogg.)

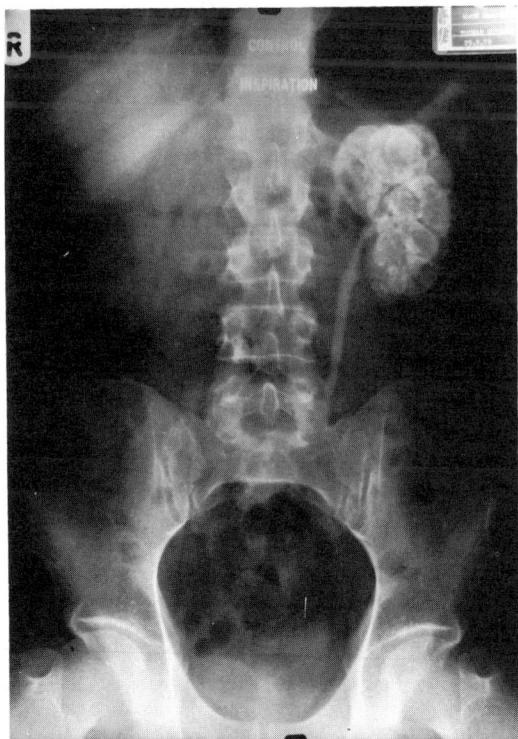

Fig. 17 Straight X-ray of abdomen showing calcification of tuberculous left kidney and ureter, the so-called 'plaster-cast' kidney.

drugs may be retained and produce severe toxicity. Regular monitoring of serum levels should be undertaken and the dosage of drugs should be adjusted accordingly. Rifampicin and INAH are the safest drugs in the presence of kidney failure. Treatment should be continued for six months to one year. In the presence of strictures simultaneous treatment with corticosteroids has been used to avoid more severe cicatrization. There is doubt about its value and surgical dilatation of ureteric strictures may be under-

taken or even a ureterostomy, cutaneous or via an ileal loop, may be required. Nephrectomy is only rarely necessary and where it is undertaken the whole length of the ureter should also be removed. It may be required when one kidney is already largely destroyed or when hypertension is due to unilateral renal tuberculosis.

Since the introduction of chemotherapy there has been a remarkable improvement in prognosis. The five-year survival is now of the order of 96 per cent.

Nosocomial urinary tract infections

The seeds and the soil
Unfortunately patients sometimes acquire UTI in the course of investigative, therapeutic or operative procedures. Such nosocomial (νοσοσ = illness; κομεω = to nurse) infections may be endogenous when the infection is derived from the patient's own bowel flora or they may be exogenous by infection from other persons or the hospital environment. There are several reasons why nosocomial infections are more serious and more difficult to treat than those acquired outside the hospital. The susceptibility of hospital patients, and in particular urological cases to urinary tract infection, is greater. Whereas the normal urinary tract can rid itself of small numbers of invading bacteria, interference with normal drainage or trauma caused by instrumentation may increase the liability to infection. Secondly, the infecting organisms are more often resistant to antimicrobials because the bowel flora in patients admitted to hospital changes to a more resistant pattern soon after admission as a result of entry of resistant organisms often derived from the hospital kitchens. Also when the infection is derived from the ward environment it tends to be due to more resistant strains because hospital bacteria are exposed to numerous antimicrobials and have therefore been subjected to a prolonged selection pressure leading to the emergence of bacterial strains which are resistant to most of the commonly used drugs. Nosocomial infections are caused by a wider range of organisms than those which occur in the community.

In addition to *E. coli*, *Proteus* spp, *Klebsiella*, *Pseudomonads*, *Alcaligenes*, *Serratia*, and *Providencia* are just some of the bacterial species that may be encountered singly or in combination. Gram-positive organisms are also met such as *Staph. aureus* and epidermidis as well as *Strep. faecalis*. Even anaerobic infections may occur though this is usually only in patients with fistulae between bowel and bladder resulting from neoplasia or diverticular disease.

Pathogenesis
The urinary catheter is the chief culprit in nosocomial infections and the most important source of infection is contaminated urine. Since urine is an excellent culture medium, drainage vessels may become heavily contaminated and act as the source of infection. Infection may be introduced during instrumentation or after catheter drainage has been established. The organisms may ascend to the bladder either in the lumen along with air bubbles or in the film of fluid which forms between the outside of the catheter and the urethral mucosa. In women with catheters, movements of the catheter can also carry organisms from the introitus into the bladder and in this case the catheter-induced infection will be due to organisms derived from the patient's own bowel flora.

Consequences of hospital infections
The consequences of nosocomial infections depend both on the nature of the patient's urological disorder and on the infecting organism. Provided that the urologist succeeds in correcting the drainage abnormality, the outlook for nosocomial infections is excellent. Most infections clear spontaneously or after simple antimicrobial treatment. However, in a minority, particularly in those patients in whom restoration of drainage has been unsuccessful,

more serious sequelae occur: these include the development of suppurative epididymitis, ascending acute pyelonephritis or most serious of all septicaemia. The latter may be rapidly fatal as a result of endotoxin shock or it may lead to widespread pyaemic abscesses including the development of bacterial endocarditis.

Preventive measures

Skilful surgery, avoidance of unnecessary catheterization, good ward hygiene, effective disinfection of vessels which contain or have contained infected urine, are important general measures. The incorporation of chlorhexidine in lubricating jellies used during instrumentation of the urinary tract is another worthwhile measure. This may be supplemented by installation of chlorhexidine solution into the bladder after insertion and before removal of the catheter. In this regard it is most important to remember that chlorhexidine solutions are not self-sterilizing and stock bottles may become contaminated. It is imperative that chlorhexidine solutions are supplied in sealed bottles.

Catheters and endoscopes must be sterile and handled with scrupulous aseptic technique. Catheter drainage should be of the 'closed' variety the tubing being fitted with non-return, flutter valves to prevent the ascent of air bubbles. The drainage bag should be emptied frequently through a tap at its lower end and the drainage once established should remain closed, and if clots cause obstruction they should be dislodged through the side arm of the catheter in which a Higginson's syringe is ready-fixed. Given these precautions, infection rates can be reduced from 90 per cent of post-prostatectomy cases to less than 15 per cent. Even if the urine is infected at the start, the same precautions should apply, because bacterial complications are almost invariably due to the most recent invaders of the urinary tract rather than the pre-existing infection to which an immune response has already been established. There is no place for prophylactic antibacterial therapy to lessen nosocomial infections with one exception, namely the practice of covering a single episode of catheterization, e.g. to avoid infection after voiding cystourography. When surgery has to be undertaken on an already infected urinary tract, it is wise to treat the infection in order to reduce the risk of bacteraemia.

Urinary tract infections in the transplanted kidney

UTI is common in kidney transplant recipients. Estimates vary between 28 and 80 per cent of the patients. It is most commonly encountered during the early weeks after transplantation. The pathogens are akin to those encountered in other nosocomial infections. Some 60 per cent are due to *Esch. coli* and the remainder due to the rarer pathogens such as *Strep. faecalis, Proteus* spp., *Pseudomonads* and in some instances *Candida albicans*. These early infections are worth detecting and treating since they are an important source of septicaemia and since it has also been claimed that they may trigger episodes of rejection, particularly in the case of *Strep. faecalis* infection. Early post-operative UTI is more common in patients with poor graft function but it seems unlikely that this is a cause and effect relationship and the probable explanation for the association is that poor graft function leads to defective wash-out of invading pathogens. When graft function is satisfactory, the early post-operative infections usually clear spontaneously once indwelling catheters are removed. In some patients, however, infection persists or recurs. Graft survival in such patients is no different from that in the non-infected subjects. These late infections are more common in patients in whom the urine had been infected before operation and there is therefore a marked female predominance. It follows that whereas eradication or suppression of early post-operative infection is essential, late infections appear harmless and are probably best left untreated provided they are symptomless.

References

Asscher, A. W. (1964). The delayed effects of renal irradiation. *Clin. Radiol.* **15**, 320.
—— (1980). *The challenge of urinary tract infections.* Academic Press, London.
Austwick, P. K. C. (1979). Endemic (Balkan) nephropathy. In *Renal Disease* 4th edn (eds D. A. K. Black and N. F. Jones), p. 879. Blackwell Scientific Publications, Oxford.
Brumfitt, W. (1972). Bacteriological aspects of renal disease. In *Renal Disease* 3rd edn (ed. D. A. K. Black). Blackwell Scientific Publications, Oxford.
—— and Asscher, A. W. (eds) (1973). *Urinary tract infection.* Oxford University Press, London.
Charlton, C. A. C., Cattell, W. R., Canti, G., Grottick, J., and O'Grady, F. W. (1973). The non-urethral syndrome. In *Urinary tract infection* (eds W. Brumfitt and A. W. Asscher). Oxford University Press, London.
Freedman, L. R. (1971). *Urinary tract infection and other forms of chronic interstitial nephritis.*
—— (1979). In *Diseases of the kidney* Vol. 2 (eds M. B. Strauss and L. G. Welt) p. 817. Little, Brown, Boston.
Galpin, J. E. (1973). Acute interstitial nephritis due to methicillin. *Am. J. Med.* **65**, 756.
Heptinstall, R. H. (1983). *Pathology of the kidney* 3rd edn, Vol. 3 pp. 1149–1397. Little, Brown, Boston.
Kass, E. H,. (1965). *Progress in pyelonephritis.* F. A. Davis, Philadelphia.
Kaufman, R. E. and Wiesner, P. J. (1974). Non-specific urethritis. *N. Engl. J. Med.* **291**, 1175.
Kilmartin, A. (1973). *Understanding cystitis.* Heinemann, London.
Kunin, C. M. (1979). *Detection, prevention, and management of urinary tract infections* 3rd edn. Lea and Febiger, Philadelphia.
Maskell, R. (1982). Urinary tract infections. Edward Arnold, London.
O'Grady, F. W. and Brumfitt, W. (1968). *Urinary tract infection.* Oxford University Press, London.
Quinn, E. L. and Kass, E. H. (1960). *Biology of pyelonephritis.* Little, Brown, Boston.
Relman, A. S. (1972). Pyelonephritis. In *Renal disease* 3rd edn. (ed. D. A. K. Black), p. 399. Blackwell Scientific Publications, Oxford.
Smellie, J. M. and Grüneberg, R. N. (1980). The treatment of childhood urinary tract infection with special reference to the use of trimethoprim and talampicillin for prophylaxis. In *Pyelonephritis*, Vol. 4 (eds H. Losse, A. W. Asscher and A. Lison), p. 162. Georg Thieme Verlag, Stuttgart.
Stamey, T. A. (1980). *Urinary infections* 2nd edn. Williams and Wilkins, Philadelphia.
—— (1980). A clinical classification of prostatitis with therapeutic implications. In *Management of urinary tract infections* (ed. A. W. Asscher). Medical Education (Services), Oxford.
Sussman, M. and Asscher, A. W. (1979). Urinary tract infection. In *Renal disease* 4th edn (eds D. A. K. Black and N. F. Jones), p. 400. Blackwell Scientific Publications, Oxford.
Wechslers, H. (1971). Renal tuberculosis. In *Diseases of the kidney* (eds M. B. Strauss and L. G. Welt), p. 1309. Little, Brown, Boston.
Williams, J. D., Kosmidis, J. and Geddes, A. M. (1973). Chemotherapy of urinary tract infections. In *Current antibiotic therapy* (eds A. M. Geddes and J. D. Williams), p. 99. Churchill Livingstone, London.

FAMILIAL RENAL DISEASE

C. CHANTLER

Introduction

Whilst familial renal disease is rare, there are a large number of familial conditions which involve the kidney primarily and an even larger number of essentially non-renal conditions which nevertheless have a renal component. The classification of familial renal disease used here is to some extent arbitrary but all important conditions with a renal component are either discussed in this chapter or referred to elsewhere in the book. Rare, essentially paediatric, syndromes are mentioned but not discussed but the references in the tables and those for further reading at the end of the chapter will enable most conditions to be traced.

Glomerular disorders

Hereditary nephritis (Alport's syndrome) (see page 18.47)

Hereditary nephritis with haematuria, progressive renal insufficiency, and deafness was first described by Guthrie in 1902 and the description of the same family was expanded by Alport in 1927. The condition accounts for about 5 per cent of all cases of terminal renal failure in children and adolescents. It is transmitted through generations with about 20 per cent of cases being apparently due to new mutations. Men are affected much more severely than women and usually develop terminal renal failure before the age of 20 years, whilst affected women may only show intermittent haematuria or develop renal insufficiency in later life; however, severe cases in young women have been recorded. Men with the disease appear to father affected daughters rather than affected sons but apparent transmission to sons has been recorded. More commonly the disease is transmitted by females perhaps because of the early deaths of the males. Some pedigrees suggest recessive autosomal inheritance while others are compatible with an autosomal dominant trait. In most instances, however, the transmission is compatible with an X-linked trait. Genetic theory and counselling has to take into account the greater severity of hereditary nephritis in males than in females, the fact that affected as well as unaffected sons and daughters can be born to healthy and to diseased mothers and that healthy fathers appear to produce only unaffected children. In one study diseased fathers produced only daughters two-thirds of whom were affected with the condition. Genetic counselling for individual families therefore is extremely complicated and must consider the pedigree of the family concerned. The primary defect is thought to be an abnormality in the structure of the glomerular basement membrane which has an abnormal protein composition. Electron microscopy shows typically split and lamellated glomerular capillary basement membranes with small granular densities within. In addition, marked attentuation of the basement membrane with discontinuity of the lamella densa is common though not specific to Alport's syndrome. In early cases the glomerulus may appear normal by light microscopy; later, mesangial proliferation, interstitial foam cells, and glomerular sclerosis appear; immunofluorescent studies are usually negative. The typical basement membrane splitting is relatively specific and usually present in early cases, and renal biopsy, therefore, is important for diagnosis.

The initial and the most important clinical feature is haematuria, sometimes intermittent early in the disease but later persistent. Exacerbations with upper respiratory infections or after exercise are common. Whilst microscopic haematuria with red cell casts in the urinary sediment is usually persistent, heavy haematuria with abdominal pain and renal colic can occur; proteinuria usually develops within the first 10 years in affected boys and

hypertension is almost invariable and severe as renal failure progresses. There is no specific treatment apart from the control of the hypertension and the management of chronic renal failure as it develops. Bilateral nephrectomy has sometimes been required for the control of hypertension after regular haemodialysis has been started or after renal transplantation.

The majority of affected persons do not have deafness but about a third may develop a high frequency loss. In any pedigree some individuals may be deaf without renal disease whereas others will have severe renal disease without hearing loss. About 15 per cent have ocular abnormalities such as cataracts, keratoconus or spherophakia, and myopia and nystagmus may be present.

Alport variants

Hyperprolinaemia with increased urinary excretion of proline, hydroxyproline, and glycine, which share a common tubular transport mechanism, is inherited as an autosomal recessive characteristic and associated in some cases with deafness and progressive renal damage. The histological changes are less well defined with some features of a chronic inflammatory interstitial nephritis and foam cells without the typical splitting of the basement membrane. It is important to note that hyperprolinaemia is not a feature of Alport's syndrome. Hereditary macrothrombocytopathia, nephritis, and deafness have been described and appear to be inherited as an autosomal dominant. A similar problem was apparent in another family with progressive nephritis but without nerve deafness where the megathrombocytes were associated with white blood cell cytoplasmic inclusions.

Familial benign haematuria

In some families suspected of having Alport's syndrome deafness and proteinuria do not occur and renal function is well maintained over many years. The haematuria is usually but not always microscopic and may be intermittent or persistent. Familial haematuria is usually transmitted as an autosomal dominant but a recessive pattern has been identified. A renal biopsy is usually necessary to exclude Alport's syndrome; the basement membrane may be attenuated but the typical splitting characteristic of Alport's is not seen.

Acute poststreptococcal nephritis

A high attack rate for familial contacts of individuals with acute poststreptococcal nephritis is partly due to exposure to the infecting organism but increased susceptibility to nephritis inherited as a family trait has also been suggested.

Congenital nephrotic syndrome

Congenital nephrotic syndrome (see page 18.61) may be familial, sporadic, or secondary to congenital infections such as syphilis, toxoplasmosis, cytomegalic inclusion disease etc. The sporadic variety is extremely rare and is probably simply an example of nephrotic syndrome as it occurs in infants and older children affecting very young babies. The familial varieties are the Finnish type, diffuse mesangial sclerosis, and focal glomerular sclerosis.

Finnish-type nephrotic syndrome is inherited in an autosomal recessive manner; the proteinuria is present before birth and affected infants can be diagnosed from the raised levels of alphafetoprotein in amniotic fluid obtained by amniocentesis in time to allow termination by the 20th week of gestation. The condition, as its name implies, is especially common in Finland with an incidence of 100 per million live babies but lack of Finnish ancestry does not preclude the diagnosis; we have seen it in two non-identical twins of Indian parentage. Most affected infants are born early and the placenta is large with a weight on average of 40 per cent of the baby's birth weight. Oedema is present either at birth or within the first week of life in 50 per cent of cases and in all by the end of the third month of life. The major feature on renal biopsy is cyst-like dilation of the tubules, so marked that in the past it has been given the unfortunate name of microcystic disease. The glomeruli are usually large due to the dilation of Bowman's space but otherwise normal on light microscopy though mesangial proliferation may be an early feature which progresses. The inherited abnormality appears to be a defect of the glomerular basement membrane. Later glomerular interstitial inflammation and sclerosis occur. Immunofluorescence is negative. The treatment is symptomatic and the prognosis poor with no response to steroids or immunosuppressive drugs. Most infants die of an intercurrent infection to which they are especially prone.

Diffuse mesangial sclerosis or focal glomerular sclerosis may be found on renal biopsy of children with congenital nephrotic syndrome. The onset of the nephrotic syndrome in these infants is often less severe than in the Finnish type and may not occur until the end of the first year of life. We have observed one family with two affected siblings with focal glomerular sclerosis where the proteinuria, whilst present soon after birth in one child did not occur in the other until 6 months of age. The progression of renal failure is also slower and survival to late childhood with the possibility of successful renal transplantation may occur. No specific therapy is effective in reducing the proteinuria. Whilst sporadic cases may occur, a high familial incidence compatible with an autosomal recessive inheritance has been recorded and the genetic prognosis must be guarded. The difficulties of providing accurate genetic and prognostic advice are complicated by the occasional case of steroid-sensitive nephrotic syndrome with minimal changes on biopsy that presents early in life and in addition we have observed two siblings with minimal change nephrotic syndrome who did not respond to steroids or immunosuppressive drugs. It seems reasonable if doubt exists over the nature of the renal biopsy appearance to undertake a trial of steroids. A syndrome of pulmonary stenosis and congenital nephrotic syndrome has been described in four of five children in a family.

Minimal change nephrotic syndrome

In about 4 per cent of cases of steroid-sensitive minimal change nephrotic syndrome (see pages 18.44 and 18.59), the condition is familial and about 3 per cent of affected children have a sibling with the disease. The contributions of genetic and environmental factors to this pattern are not known, an association with the inheritance of HLA-B12 has been postulated.

Hereditary onycho-osteodysplasia (Nail patella syndrome)

The nail of the thumb and great toe especially are hypoplastic with hemiatrophy and longitudinal ridging; the patellas are small or absent, the radial capitellum is malformed with impaired extension of the forearm and sometimes dislocation of the radius, and osseous spurs, extending medially from the ileum as iliac horns, are present. About a third of affected individuals have renal disease with proteinuria and intermittent nephrotic syndrome and 8 per cent die of renal failure. The condition is inherited as an autosomal dominant.

Hereditary osteolysis

Osseous lesions appear in early childhood with episodes of arthralgia in the wrists and ankles. Later the involved bones collapse and gradually disappear by a process histologically resembling avascular necrosis. In early adult life the progressive bone destruction appears to cease but deformities are severe. Hypertension with renal arteriosclerosis is common and chronic nephritis, nephrotic syndrome, and amyloid disease have been described. The inheritance is not clear; it may be as an autosomal dominant with variable expression but many cases are sporadic.

Complement abnormalities

(See page 18.46.)

Various autosomal recessive inherited deficiencies of complement components are associated with glomerulonephritis. It is believed that these deficiencies in complement predispose to glomerulonephritis by making the patient more susceptible to infections and to the formation of antibody–antigen complexes.

Sickle cell disease

(See Section 19.)

Both sickle cell disease and sickle cell trait are associated with renal disease. Haematuria especially during a sickle cell crisis, is common, so is hyposthenuria and an acidification defect. Nephrotic syndrome, in one case apparently due to immune complexes containing antigen released from the damaged tubules, or more modest proteinuria are occasional features of the disease. Haematuria is less frequent in association with the trait. Whether sickle cell disease or trait leads to early renal failure is not yet clear.

Balkan nephropathy

This curious nephropathy (see page 18.68) affects 10–75 per cent of households in agricultural communities in a small area on the borders of Bulgaria, Yugoslavia, and Rumania. The cause is unknown but some genetic predisposition to an environmental factor has been suggested. The early stages suggest tubular dysfunction with polydipsia, polyuria, and tubular proteinuria; later glomerular proteinuria and insufficiency develops.

Haemolytic uraemic syndrome

This rare condition (see page 18.51) is nonetheless a common cause of acute and chronic renal failure in childhood. It is characterized by the sudden onset of a microangiopathic haemolytic uraemia with disseminated or local intravascular coagulation in the kidney and acute renal failure which follows a gastrointestinal disturbance. Cases are usually sporadic but familial cases associated with an intermittent defect in prostacyclin metabolism have been described.

Goodpasture's syndrome

Familial incidence is rare but a strong association between HLA-DRW2 and Goodpasture's syndrome has been demonstrated (see page 18.43). Other more rare conditions which primarily involve the glomerulus are summerized in Table 1.

Tubular transport disorders

The following disorders which are, or occasionally may be, familial and which either primarily involve the renal tubule or may occasionally affect it are discussed elsewhere in the book: cystinuria, Hartnup disease, iminoglycinuria, blue diaper syndrome, cystinosis, adult Fanconi syndrome, Lowe's syndrome, galactosaemia, Wilson's disease, tyrosinaemia, glycogen storgage disease, oxalosis, hypophosphatasia, disorders of vitamin D metabolism, abnormalities of parathyroid function, and nephrogenic diabetes insipidus.

Renal glycosuria

The presence of persistent glycosuria with normal blood glucose levels in the absence of starvation and without evidence of abnormal renal loss of other sugars or other renal insufficiency suggests renal glycosuria. Both autosomal dominant and recessive inheritance has been postulated. Two types of defect have been identified involving either a reduction in the tubular maximum capacity for glucose reabsorption or an isolated reduction in tubular threshold alone. This primary glycosuria must be distinguished from the autosomal recessive syndrome of congenital malabsorption of glucose and galactose which presents with watery diarrhoea and an associated defect in the renal tubular reabsorption of glucose. Glycosuria as part of a Fanconi syndrome or secondary to tubular damage

Table 1 Selected other rare glomerular disorders (for full list see Berry *et al.*, 1986)

Title	Renal manifestation	Other features	Inheritance	Reference
Hypoparathyroidism with deafness	Proteinuria, nephrotic syndrome, renal failure	Congenital absence or hypofunction of parathyroids and nerve deafness	Aut rec	Barakat *et al.* (1977). *J. Paed.* **91**, 61
Charcot-Marie-Tooth disease	Progressive nephropathy with focal glomerular sclerosis	Progressive peripheral neuropathy	?Aut dom	Lemieux *et al.* (1967). *Can. Med. Assn. J.* **97**, 1193
Juvenile pernicious anaemia	Proteinuria	Defective ileal transport of vitamin B12	Aut rec	Spurling *et al.* (1964). *New. Engl. J. Med.* **271**, 995
Mitochondrial cytopathy (ragged red fibre disease)	Chronic renal failure with tubular atrophy, glomerular sclerosis	Abnormal mitochondria on muscle biopsy, vomiting, failure to thrive, anaemia cerebellar ataxia, retinitis pigmentosa, opthalmoplegia, convulsions	Aut rec	Egger *et al.* (1964). *Arch. Dis. Childhd.* **56**, 741
Alpha-1 anti-trypsin deficiency	Mesangiocapillary nephritis (rare)	Chronic emphysema, infantile hepatic cirrhosis	Aut rec	Moraz *et al.* (1976). *J. Pediat.* **57**, 232
Cockayne syndrome	Albuminuria, glomerulo-nephritis, renal insufficiency	Small stature, microcephaly, deafness, retinal dysplasia photosensitivity, mental retardation	Aut rec	Higginbottom *et al.* (1975), *Pediatrics* **64**, 929
Alstrom syndrome	Albuminuria, renal failure	Blindness, nerve deafness, obesity, diabetes mellitus	Aut rec	Goldstein *et al.* (1973). *Med.* **52**, 53
	Progressive deafness, cataracts, myopia, marfanoid habitus	Proteinuria, renal insufficiency	?Aut dom	Sohar (1956). *Arch. Int. Med.* **97**, 627
Kartagener syndrome	Mesangio-capillary glomerulonephritis	Bronchiectasis, sinusitis, situs viscerum inversus	Aut rec	Egbert *et al.* (1977). *Arch. Pathol. Lab. Med.* **101**, 95
	Proteinuria, membrano-proliferative glomerulonephritis	Small liver with hepatocellular damage, splenomegaly with hypersplenism dermatitis	Aut rec	Dobrin *et al.* (1977). *J. Pediat.* **90**, 901
Epidermolysis bullosa dystrophica	Amyloid	Subepidermal blisters, ulceration of mucosae	Aut dom Aut rec	Kretowski (1973). *Pediatrics* **51**, 938
	Proliferative glomerulonephritis	Thyrotoxicosis, absent frontal sinuses	?Aut rec	Wehner (1969). *Clin. Res.* **17**, 530
Lecthin cholesterol acyl transferase deficiency (LCAT)	Proteinuria, renal failure	Normochronic anaemia, corneal opacities	Aut rec	Flatmark (1977). *Transplant Proc.* **9**, 1665
Fabry disease angiokeratoma corpora diffusum	Glomerulonephritis, renal failure	Skin angioma, recurrent abdominal and limb pain	X-linked	Wise *et al.* (1962). *Q. J. Med.* **31**, 177
Primary amyloidosis	Renal amyloidosis, proteinuria, renal failure	Generalized amyloid, duodenal ulcer, neuropathy, urticarial rashes, deafness	Aut dom	Cohen (1972). *Metabolic basis of inherited disease.* McGraw Hill, New York
Familial mediterranean fever	Renal amyloid, proteinuria, renal failure	Recurrent fever and abdominal pain	Aut rec	Reuben *et al.* (1977). *Q.J. Med.* **46**, 243
	Steroid resistant nephrotic syndrome, renal failure	Hydrocephalus, peculiar facies, blue sclerae, thin skin, abnormal T cell function	?Aut rec ?X-linked	Daentl *et al.* (1978). *Birth defects* **14/6B**, 315
Meltzer	Proteinuria, haematuria, renal insufficiency	Cryoglobulinaemia, renal damage	Aut dom	Nightingale *et al.* (1977). *John Hopkins Med. J.* **140**, 267
Wiskott Aldrich	Thrombocytopenia, recurrent infections, elevated IgA levels	Nephrotic syndrome, glomerulonephritis	X-linked	Spitler *et al.* (1980). *Pediatrics* **66**, 391

associated with focal segmental glomerular sclerosis must be excluded. Glycosuria due to a lowered renal threshold for reabsorption associated with a raised GFR can also occur during pregnancy. Other rare tubular disorders are summarized in Table 2.

Metabolic diseases

Bartter's syndrome, Liddle's syndrome, pseudohyperaldosteronism, and various forms of familial disease causing amyloid and affecting the kidney are discussed elsewhere.

Magnesium wasting

Secondary hypermagnesuria can complicate gentamicin poisoning and occurs also with Bartter's syndrome, following diuretic therapy, and with hyperthyroidism, hypoaldosteronism, hyperparathyroidism, and renal tubular acidosis. Two familial forms of excessive renal loss of magnesium have been described, one with associated hypokalaemia and other occasional defects in tubular

reabsorption and in the other involving magnesium alone; both appear to be inherited in an autosomal recessive way. Nephrocalcinosis and renal acidosis may occur. In addition there is an X-linked recessive form of hypomagnesaemia due to impaired intestinal magnesium absorption but without excessive renal loss of magnesium. Clinical features are variable and have included convulsions in the newborn period, tetany, failure to thrive, and a non-specific dermatitis. Treatment consists of dietary supplements of magnesium gluconate, oxide or acetate to provide 1–2 mmol/kg/day. Extra potassium may be required and any co-existant acidosis should be corrected.

Diabetes mellitus

Familial aspects of diabetes mellitus are discussed on page 9.51 *et seq.* A rare autosomal recessive condition of pituitary diabetes insipidus, diabetes mellitus, optic atrophy, and deafness has been described (Wolfram's syndrome; DIDMOAD syndrome). The diabetes insipidus may lead to dilation of the urinary tract.

Table 2 Selected other rare tubular/interstitial disease (for full list see Berry *et al.*, 1986)

Title	Renal manifestation	Other features	Inheritance	Reference
Swachman's syndrome	Renal glycosuria (glactose fructose, lactose glucose), renal acidosis, aminoaciduria nephrocalcinosis	Pancreatic exocrine deficiency, neutropaenia, thrombocytopenia infections, growth retardation skeletal abnormalities, retinitis pigmentosa, developmental retardation	Aut rec	Aggett *et al.* (1980). *Arch. Dis. Childhd.* **55**, 331
Renal tubular acidosis with nerve deafness	Distal tubular acidosis	Congenital nerve deafness	Aut rec	Donckerwolke *et al.* (1976). *Acta paediat. Scand.* **65**, 100
Low molecular weight proteinuria	Tubular proteinuria	Mental retardation, hyper-beta-lipoproteinaemia	Aut rec	Eksmyr *et al.* (1976). *Acta paediat. Scand.* **65**, 251
Marble brain disease	Distal tubular acidosis	Osteopetrosis, cerebral calcifications, stunted growth	Aut rec	Ohlsson (1980). *Develop. Med. Child. Neurol.* **22**, 72
Oculocerebro renal syndrome	Tubular dysfunction, small glomeruli, renal failure	Corneal opacities, nystagmus brain abnormalities, mental retardation, absent testes	?Aut rec ?X-linked	McCance (1960). *Arch. Dis. Childhd.* **35**, 240
Senior-Loken	Nephrophthiasis	Tapeto retinal degeneration, metaphyseal dysplasia, chronic hepatitis etc.	Aut rec	Senior (1973). *Am. J. Dis. Child.* **125**, 442
Jeunne's syndrome	Juvenile nephrophthiasis, renal failure	Asphyxiating thoracic dystrophy	Aut rec	Donaldson *et al.* (1985) *Arch. Dis. Childhd.* **60**, 426
	Tubulo-interstitial nephritis	Chronic diarrhoea, villous atrophy of small intestine, chronic pancreatitis, elevated IgE and IgA levels, dermatitis	?Aut rec	Ellis *et al.* (1982). *Amr. J. Dis. Child.* **136**, 323
Congenital licthyosis	Aminoaciduria, glomerulosclerosis, renal failure, structural anomalies	Coarse hair, short stature, mental retardation, deafness etc	Aut rec	Rayner *et al.* (1978). *J. Pediat.* **92**, 776
Elliptocytosis	Renal tubular acidosis	Mild anaemia	Aut dom	Baehner *et al.* (1968). *Am. J. Dis. Child.* **115**, 414
Thyrocerebro renal	Interstitial nephritis	Goitre, cerebellar ataxia, seizures, deafness, muscle wasting, thrombocytopenia	?Aut rec	Cutler *et al.* (1978). *Birth Defects* **14/6B**, 265
Hypophosphatasia	Nephrocalcinosis	Low alkaline phosphatase, hypercalcaemia, rickets	Aut rec	Kozlowski *et al.* (1976). *Pediat. Radiol.* **5**, 103

The following disorders are discussed elsewhere: Fabry's disease, glycogen storage disease, mucopolysaccharide storage disease, LCAT deficiency, Refsum's disease, familial metachromatic leukodystrophy and Gaucher's disease, and Nieman–Pick disease. In most of these conditions the accumulation of abnormal material in the cells of the kidney whether vascular endothelial, glomerular, tubular or interstitial cells does not affect function. An exception is Fabry's disease in which the glomerular capillaries are progressively blocked by the accumulation of ceramide trihexoside leading to renal failure. Amino aciduria has been described in Hurler's syndrome. Renal insufficiency can occur in glycogen storage disease due to glucose-6-phosphatase deficiency. Glycogenolysis leads to high concentrations of lactic acid which interfere with the renal clearance of uric acid and can lead to the development of urate nephropathy. There is also evidence of increased uric acid biosynthesis in this condition. Most patients with glycogen storage disease do not develop Fanconi syndrome, and where it occurs the glycogen storage is usually of a special autosomal recessive type and not due to glucose-6-phosphatase deficiency or one of the other known varieties.

Renal and urinary tract calculus disease

The following disorders are discussed elsewhere: hypercalcuria, xanthinuria, glycosuria, uricosuria, adeninuria, and cystinuria. Uric acid urolithiasis due to hyperuricuria and not primarly due to hyperuricaemia has been described. It is inherited as an autosomal dominant and stone formation can be prevented with oral alkali and a high fluid intake. In contrast, hereditary nephropathy with hyperuricaemia, not apparently due to renal insufficiency, over-production of uric acid as in the Lesch–Nyhan syndrome (see page 9.123 *et seq.*) or primary gout has been described. It was thought to be due to decreased clearance of renal uric acid and inherited as an autosomal dominant. The importance of measuring plasma and urine uric acid in any patient with undiagnosed haematuria or chronic renal insufficiency is emphasized by these syndromes.

Structural anomalies

Dysplasia and hypoplasia

Abnormal renal development in the fetus can lead to either a deficiency in the number of nephrons in a small hypoplastic kidney or to altered structural differentiation of the metanephros with abnormal organization causing dysplasia. The collecting ductal epithelium may be columnar forming primitive ducts and the mesenchyme of the metanephric blastoma may differentiate into cartilage. The primitive ducts frequently undergo cystic dilation. The glomeruli may be incompletely differentiated and the glomeruli and tubules appear primitive. Most instances of renal dysplasia with or without gross cyst formation, and renal hypoplasia are sporadic and non-familial. In such cases the lesion is usually but not always isolated, the two kidneys are not symmetrically involved, and cystic dysplasia is frequently associated with obstructive uropathy. Familial examples of cystic dysplasia and less commonly hypoplasia are found in conjunction with other non-renal malformations. Familial isolated renal dysplasia, inherited as an autosomal recessive, has been described. The kidneys are usually symmetrically involved with or without polydactyly and it is sometimes confused with infantile polycystic disease though the typical liver pathology of infantile polycystic disease is absent. Histological confirmaton of the diagnosis is necessary, and the possibility of this heritable form of dysplasia should always be considered in a child with bilateral symmetrical dysplasia.

Autosomal recessive polycystic disease

This condition is generally termed infantile polycystic disease (IPCD) and distinguished from adult polycystic disease (APCD) which is inherited as an autosomal dominant. The terms are traditional but unsatisfactory because IPCD can present in the neonate, infant or older child, and whilst often leading to renal failure in early life, the progress is sometimes slow so that survival to adult life is possible. Likewise, APCD may be present in the neonate and we have the curious experience of making the diagnosis in an infant and then finding that the father who was previously undiagnosed had severe renal insufficiency from the same condition.

The cardinal pathological feature of IPCD is of dilated collecting ducts or medullary ductal ectasia. The dilated ducts appear as cysts radially arranged from the medulla to the subcapsular cortex. The kidneys are symmetrically enlarged and the calyces are stretched but not distorted by the cysts whose smaller size and symmetrical radial distribution distinguish the condition radiologically from APCD. The cysts opacify with contrast media on intravenous urography and a typical radiographic appearance enables a confident diagnosis (Fig. 1). The severity of the condition varies between affected families but generally breeds true within a family. The liver is always involved, even at birth where intrahepatic biliary malformation with bile duct hyperplasia and portal fibrosis progressing to cyst formation are seen throughout. Liver biopsy serves to distinguish IPCD from APCD in cases where doubt exists. The severity of the renal involvement determines the renal prognosis; in some families the babies die in the perinatal period with huge renal masses, in some presentation is in the neonatal period with progression to renal failure in the first year of life, whilst in others death occurs in infancy or in childhood (juvenile form) or not until well into adult life. The liver disease is progressive leading to portal hypertension and bleeding from oesophageal varices requiring operations to reduce portal press-

ure. In some families the liver disease predominates with congenital hepatic fibrosis and the renal involvement may be limited to medullary ductal ectasia and cyst formation only. The intravenous urogram in such cases shows only distortion of the calyces as in medullary sponge kidney or Laurence–Moon–Biedl syndrome (see page 18.166). Hypertension usually develops with IPCD as the renal failure progresses and can be severe. Treatment is limited to controlling hypertension and the metabolic consequences of renal insufficiency. A few of these children have undergone renal transplantation with or without prior surgery for portal hypertension, but in such cases the prognosis must be guarded because of the possibility of eventual hepatic failure.

Adult polycystic disease

Early onset of adult polycystic disease is an important differential diagnosis in any infant or child with bilateral renal enlargement and needs to be distinguished from infantile polycystic disease, tuberose sclerosis, bilateral Wilm's tumours, cystic dysplasia, and other cystic diseases, and any cause of diffuse parenchymal renal enlargement such as renal venous thrombosis or nephrotic syndrome which produces stretching and distortion of the calyces. It is discussed on page 18.164.

Cystic disease associated with chromosomal disorders

Renal cortical cysts which do not cause much functional disturbance are encountered in many chromosomal imbalance syndromes such as trisomy 13, 18, and 21; cystic dysplasia has been reported in trisomy 8. Renal agenesis, other renal anomalies, and anal atresia occur in over 60 per cent of the cat eye syndrome cases involving chromosome 22. Horse shoe kidney has been reported in trisomy 18 and in Turner's XO syndrome where renal cortical cysts also occur. It is reasonable to consider the possibility of renal anomalies in all chromosomal syndromes though most cases are sporadic unless they involve translocations.

Medullary sponge kidney

Medullary sponge kidney (see page 18.160) is usually a disease of adults and occurs sporadically. It has, however, been described in six members of a family and occasionally presents in childhood. Radiologically similar appearances of calyceal distortion with medullary cysts associated with dilation of the collecting ducts occur in infantile polycystic disease, congenital hepatic fibrosis, Laurence–Moon–Biedl syndrome, and Beckwith's syndrome discussed above. It is also occasionally found in association with congenital hemihypertrophy, and with Ehlers–Danlos syndrome (see Section 17) where renal cysts and renal tubular acidosis can also occur. Renal tuberculosis is an important differential diagnosis.

Neurofibromatosis

The renal involvement in neurofibromatosis which is inherited as an autosomal dominant condition comprises renal artery stenosis, due to intimal and medial hyperplasia or to extrinsic compression on the artery, or there may be an association phaeochromocytoma.

Vesico-ureteric reflux

Reflux nephropathy is the commonest single cause of end-stage renal failure in children, common in adults, and perhaps the only largely preventable cause of end-stage renal failure in both age groups. It is therefore extremely important to recognize that vesico-ureteric reflux is 10–20 times more frequent in first degree relatives of affected individuals with an incidence of 15 per cent.

Nephroblastoma

Wilm's tumour has an increased incidence in children with pseudohermaphroditism, congenital hemihypertrophy where adrenal tumours are also associated, and especially with congenital aniridia. The risk of Wilm's tumour with aniridia is associated with an abnormality of the short arm of chromosome 11 and all children

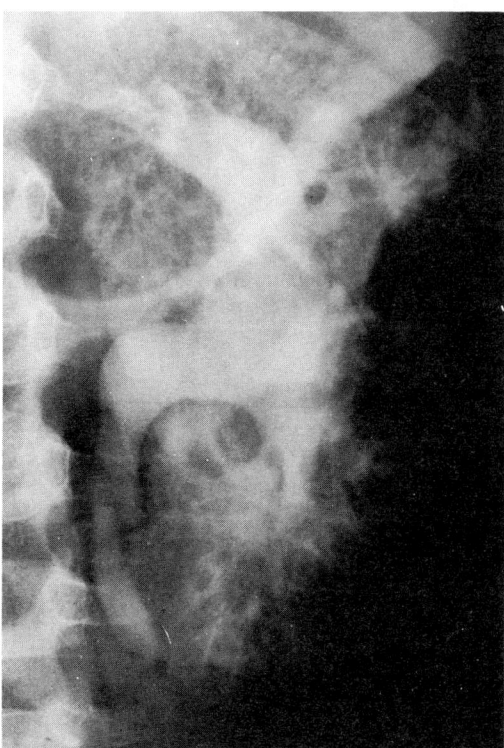

Fig. 1 Intravenous urogram of a child with infantile polycystic disease of the kidney.

Table 3 Selected other rare structural disorders (for full list see Berry *et al.*, 1986)

Title	Renal manifestation	Other features	Inheritance	Reference
Vater association	Renal dysplasia, persistent urachus	Vertebral defects, anal atresia, tracheoesophageal fistula, oesophageal atresia, renal dysplasia, hypospadius polydactyly	Sporadic ?Aut dom	Barry *et al.* (1974). *Am. J. Dis. Child.* **128**, 769
Brachio-oto-renal syndrome	Renal dysplasia, chronic renal failure	Congenital deafness with preauricular pits	Aut dom	Fraser *et al.* (1980). *Am. J. med. Genet.* **17**, 136
Beckwith's syndrome	Medullary dysplasia, distal tubular ductal ectasia, vesicoureteric reflux, nephroblastoma	Intra-uterine gigantism, hypoglycaemia, hyperinsulinaemia, exomphalos macroglossia	Aut rec Sporadic	Berry *et al.* (1980). *J. med. Genet.* **17**, 136
Zellweger's cerebro-hepato-renal syndrome	Cystic dysplasia	Abnormal skull and face development, hypotonia, intrahepatic bilary dysgenesis	Aut rec	Bowen *et al.* (1964). *John Hopkins med. J.* **114**, 402
Tuberose sclerosis	Benign hamartomas, angiomyolipomas, polycystic disease	Developmental retardation, fibroadenomas of sebaceous glands, cortical nodules etc	Aut dom	Anderson *et al.* (1969). *Am. J. Med.* **47**, 163
Meckel's syndrome	Cystic dysplasia	Posterior encephalocele, sloping forehead, polydactyly, hydrocephalus	Aut rec	Hsia *et al.* (1971). *Pediatrics* **48**, 237
Von Hippel-Lindau	Cysts	Haemangiomas of retina, cerebellum spinal cord, etc.	Aut dom	Christoferson *et al.* (1961). *J. Am. med. Assn.* **178**, 280 Kaplan *et al.* (1961). *J. Urol.* **83**, 36
Apert's syndrome	Polycystic kidneys	Craniosynostosis, syndactyly	Aut dom	Smith (1970). In *Recognizable pattern of human malformation.* W. B. Saunders, Philadelphia
	Polycystic kidneys, hydronephrosis	Unilateral ichthyosis, limb anomalies	Aut rec	Cullen *et al.* (1969). *Arch. Derm* **99**, 724
Dandy-Walker syndrome	Polycystic kidneys	Cystic dilatation of fourth ventricle	Aut rec	Goldston *et al.* (1963). *Am. J. Dis. Child.* **106**, 484
Leopard syndrome	Renal agenesis	Multiple lentigenes, ECG changes, pulmonary valvar disease, ocular, genital growth anomalies, deafness	Aut dom	Swanson *et al.* (1971). *J. Pediat.* **78**, 1037
Lacrimo, auricular dento-digital syndrome	Unilateral renal agenesis	Nasolacrimal duct obstruction, cup-shaped ears, enamel dysplasia, digital malformations	Aut dom	Hollister *et al.* (1973). *J. Pediat.* **83**, 438
Marfans syndrome	Ectopia, duplex kidneys	Arachnodactyly	Aut dom	Loughridge *et al.* (1959). *Q. J. Med.* **28**, 531
Klippel–Feil syndrome	Renal agenesis, ectopia	Short neck, vertebral fusion, winged scapula	Aut dom	Moore *et al.* (1975). *J. Bone Joint Surg.* **57A**, 335
Fanconi's anaemia	Duplication, unilateral agenesis, hydronephrosis, ectopia, horseshoe kidney	Congenital pancytopaenia, radial aplasia	Aut rec	McDonald *et al.* (1960). *Arch. Dis. Childhd.* **35**, 367
Ehlers–Danlos syndrome	Pelviureteric junction obstruction	Cutis hyperelastica	Aut dom	McKusick (1966). *Hereditable disorders of connective tissue*, 3rd edn. Mosby, St Louis
	Pelviureteric junction obstruction, vesicoureteric junction obstruction (both rare)		Aut dom	Aaron *et al.* (1948). *J. Urol.* **60**, 702 Simpson *et al.* (1970). *J. Am. Med. Assn.* **212**, 2264
	Horseshoe kidney (rare)		Aut rec	David (1974). *Br. Med. J.* **IV**, 571
	Duplex ureters		Aut rec	Atwell *et al.* (1974). *Arch. Dis. Childhd.* **49**, 390
Short rib polydactyly	Polycystic kidneys, hypoplasia	Short limbed dwarfism, short ribs, polydactyly, metaphyseal dysplasia, cleft palate, imperforate anus	Aut rec	Cherstrov *et al.* (1980). *Eur. J. Pediatr.* **133**, 57

with aniridia should be karyotyped. If the karotype is normal there is no increased risk of Wilm's tumour. An increased incidence of Wilm's tumour is also found in Beckwith's syndrome (see Table 3) and in the related autosomal recessive syndrome of congenital renal hamartoma, nephroblastomatosis, and fetal gigantism.

An increased risk of Wilm's tumour even without these other associated features has been suggested for families with one affected member, largely based on theoretical rather than empirical studies. These figures suggest a 5 per cent chance of a further sibling being affected when one child has a unilateral Wilm's tumour and a 10 per cent risk if the Wilm's tumour is bilateral. If a parent has had a bilateral tumour, the risk to the children is given as 30 per cent. Other rare structural anomalies are outlined in Table 3.

References

Berry, C., Gilli, G. and Chantler, C. (1986). Syndromes with a renal component in *Paediatric nephrology* 2nd edn (eds M. A. Holliday, T. M. Barratt and R. Vernier) Williams and Wilkins, Baltimore.

McKusick, V. A. (1978). *Mendelian inheritance in man*, 5th edn. Johns Hopkins Press, Baltimore.

Smith, D. W. (1970). *Recognisable patterns of human malformation*. W. B. Saunders, Philadelphia.

Stanbury, J. B., Wyngaardn, J. B. and Fredrickson, D. S. (1972). *The metabolic basis of inherited disease* 3rd edn. McGraw Hill, New York.

Further reading

Alport, A. C. (1927). Hereditary familial congenital haemorrhagic nephritis. *Br. Med. J.* **1**, 504–506.

Bennett, W. M., Musgrave, J. L., Campbell, R. A., Elliott, D., Cox, R., Brooks, R. E., Lovrien, E. W., Beals, R. K. and Porter,·G. A. (1973). The nephropathy of the nail patella syndrome: clinicopathological analysis of 11 kindreds. *Am. J. Med.* **54**. 304–319.

Bluett, N. H., Chantler, C., Singer, J. D. and Saxton, H. M. (1977). Congenital renal abnormalities in the Laurence–Moon–Biedl syndrome. *Arch. Dis. Childhd* **52**, 968–970.

Blythe, H. and Ockenden, B. G. (1971). Polycystic disease of kidneys and liver presenting in childhood. *J. Med. Genet.* **8**, 257–284.

Brivet, F., Girst, R., Barbanel, C., Gazengel, C., Maier, M. and Crosnier, J. (1981). Hereditary nephritis associated with May Hegglin anomaly. *Nephron* **29**, 59.

Brodehl, J. (1978). Renal glucosuria. In *Pediatric nephrology* (ed. C. S. M. Edelmann), p. 1036. Little Brown Co., Boston.

Cole, B. R., Kaufman, R. L., McAllister, W. H. and Kissane, J. M. (1976). Bilateral renal dysplasia in three siblings: report of a survivor. *Clin. Nephrol.* **5**, 83.

Counahan, R., Simmons, M. J. and Charlwood, G. J. (1976). Multifocal osteolysis with nephropathy. *Arch. Dis. Childhd* **51**, 717–719.

Egli, F. and Stalder, G. (1973). Malformations of kidney and urinary tract in common chromosomal aberrations. *Human Genet.* **18**, 1.

Eisenberg, R. L. and Pfister, R. C. (1972). Medullary sponge kidney associated with congenital hemihypertrophy (asymmetry). *Am. J. Roent. radium nucl. Med.* **116**, 773.

Epstein, C. J., Sahud, M. A., Piel, C. F. Goodman, J. R., Bernfield, M. R., Kushner, J. H. and Ablin, A. R. (1972). Hereditary macrothrombocytopathia, nephritis and deafness. *Am. J. Med.* **52**, 299–310.

Fournier, A., Paget, M., Pauli, A. and Devin, P. (1963). Syndromes nephrotiques familiaux. Syndrome nephrotique associee a une cardiopathie congenitale chez quatre soeurs. *Pediatrie* **18**, 677–685.

Grunfeld, J.-P. (1985). The clinical spectrum of hereditary nephritis. *Kid. Int.* **27**, 83–92.

Gubler, M. C., Levy, M., Broyer, M., Naizot, C., Gonzales, G., Perrin, D. and Habib, R. (1981). Alport's syndrome. A report of 58 cases and a review of the literature. *Am. J. Med.* **70**, 493–505.

Manz, F., Scharer, K., Janka, P. and Lombeck, J. (1978). Renal magnesium wasting, incomplete tubular acidosis, hypercalciuria and nephrocalcinosis in siblings. *Eur. J. Paediat.* **128**, 67–69.

Page, M., Asmal, A. C. and Edwards, C. R. (1976). Recessive inheritance of diabetes: the syndrome of diabetes insipidus, diabetes mellitus, optic atrophy and deafness. *Q. J. Med.* **45**, 505–520.

Perlman, M., Goldberg, G. M., Barziz, J. and Danovitch, G. (1973). Renal hamartomas and nephroblastomatosis with fetal gigantism. A familial syndrome. *J. Pediat.* **83**, 414–418.

Pyrah, L. N. (1966). Medullary sponge kidney. *J. Urol.* **95**, 274.

Rodriguez-Iturbe, B., Rubio, L. and Garcia, R. (1981). Attack rate of post-streptococcal nephritis in families *Lancet* **i**, 401–403.

Rogers, P. W., Kurtzman, N. A., Burn, S. M. and White, M. G. (1973). Familial benign essential hematuria. *Arch. Int. Med.* **131**, 257–262.

Scriver, C. R. and Efron, M. L. (1972). Disorders of proline and hydroxyproline metabolism. In *The metabolic basis of inherited disease* (eds J. B. Stanbury, J. B. Wyngaardon, and D. S. Fredrickson). McGraw Hill, New York.

Sibley, R. K., Mahan, J., Mauer, S. M. and Vernier, R. L. (1985). A clinicopatholgic study of 48 infants with nephrotic syndrome. *Kid. Int* **27**, 544–552.

Simmonds, H. A., Warren, D. J., Cameron, J. S., Potter, C. F. and Farebrother, D. A. (1980). Familial gout and renal failure in young women. *Clin. Nephrol.* **14**, 176.

Vargas, A., Evans, K., Ransley, P., Rosenberg, A. R., Rothwell, D., Sherwood, T., William, D. I., Barratt, T. M. and Carter, C. O. (1978). A family study of vesicoureteric reflux. *J. Med. Genet.* **15**, 85–96.

URINARY STONE DISEASE (UROLITHIASIS)

R. W. E. WATTS

Introduction

A urinary stone (calculus) consists of crystal aggregates with a small amount of associated protein and glycoprotein matrix material. Stones form in the urine outside the renal parenchyma and the smallest crystal aggregates probably begin within the collecting ducts. The term nephrocalcinosis refers to the deposition of calcium salts in the renal parenchyma and it may be associated with urolithiasis.

Incidence and geographic distribution

Urolithiasis is a common worldwide problem and Table 1 indicates its high incidence in the United Kingdom. There are many occasions when a clear aetiology or predisposing factors cannot be identified, and the recurrence rate after spontaneous passage or surgical removal is high, approaching 70 per cent by 10 years after the first stone episode. Idiopathic urolithiasis almost certainly includes several aetiologically separate entities.

Industrialization, the introduction of mixed as opposed to purely agrarian farming, economic improvement, and some degree of urbanization are associated with a decrease in childhood bladder stone disease and a progressive increase in renal stone disease in adults as living standards rise. The bladder stone disease in children which is hyperendemic in Third World countries is heterogeneous and resembles that seen in Europe in earlier times. X-ray crystallography has shown that calcium oxalate, ammonium urate, and uric acid were, and still are, the main components. Urate stones predominate in some parts of the Middle East, India, and North Africa. Calcium oxalate stones predominate in some parts of Southeast Asia, although both ammonium acid urate and calcium oxalate or calcium phospate stones occur in all areas. Calcium oxalate or mixed calcium oxalate and calcium phosphate renal stones in adults are the predominant stone type in Europe, North America, Australasia, and South Africa.

The epidemiological studies on which these generalizations are based suggest that urolithiasis may be regarded as a hazard of both affluence and deprivation. Dietary factors seem to be important in both groups, high protein, high carbohydrate diets are incriminated as risk factors for the upper urinary tract calcium oxalate stones in the relatively affluent industrial societies, and protein

Table 1 Incidence of urinary stones in the United Kingdom

Patients discharged from hospital with diagnosis of stones	1.8 per 10 000
Incidence of stones in general practice	7 per 10 000
General practice incidence of stones in males aged 45 to 60 years	21 per 10 000

deprivation, although not protein-calorie malnutrition (Kwashior-kor), in the underdeveloped regions. The 'stone waves' (epidemics of urinary stone) in Europe during times of extreme deprivation after major wars are also well documented. However, it should be emphasized that these associations do not imply established cause and effect relationships.

The cause of the extremely high incidence of pure calcium oxalate bladder stones in boys in Northern Thailand and adjacent areas is a special case. Here, the practice of partly replacing breast feeds with premasticated glutinous rice (Oryza glutinosa) from the early neonatal period increases urinary oxalate excretion partly because the rice contains a large amount of hydroxyproline which is metabolized to glyoxylate and hence to oxalate. It also decreases the fluid intake and urine volume, and lowers urinary phosphate. The Thai villagers eat leafy vegetables which are a direct source of additional dietary oxalate. It has been shown that lowered urinary phosphate excretion favours calcium oxalate crystallization and microlith formation, and supplementing the infants' diet with orthophosphate appears to be reducing the incidence of stone formation in the very young children in the region. The mechanisms by which orthophosphate may reduce stone formation are discussed on page 18.92. Inadequate milk feeding in infancy was recognized as being associated with urinary stones in childhood in England during the early nineteenth century. Except for occupations likely to cause underhydration and increased vitamin D due to prolonged exposure to sunlight, industrial exposure to beryllium and cadmium are the only well-recognized industrial hazards associated with an increased incidence of urinary stone.

Pathophysiology

Calcium-containing stones are the commonest type in the United Kingdom (Table 2). Even apparently pure calcium oxalate stones commonly contain a small central core of calcium phosphate or uric acid. This is due to the phenomenon of epitaxy whereby a crystal can grow on a chemically different crystal because, in one or more particular orientations of the two crystals, there is a nearly geometrically accurate fit between the parts that are in contact.

The proposition that stone formation begins intracellularly and leads first to localized areas of calcification on the renal papillae (Randall's plaques) has been generally abandoned. It has recently been proposed that Tamm-Horsfall glycoprotein aggregates and precipitates as the urine becomes concentrated during its passage along the renal tubule. Desialylation makes the precipitated glycoprotein (uromucoid) permanently insoluble and it enmeshes the microcrystals of calcium oxalate and calcium phosphate which migrate to the pelvicalyceal system and grow into stones.

Table 2 The composition of a series of approximately 1000 present day renal calculi studied at the Institute of Urology, London

Type of stone	Whole sample (%)	Adult	
		Males (%)	Females (%)
Pure calcium oxalate	39.4	47.9	22.2
Mixed calcium oxalate/phosphate	13.8	16.0	9.4
Magnesium ammonium phosphate	15.4	8.1	35.1
Stones which were virtually wholly composed of calcium and phosphate	13.2	11.3	17.8
Mixed stones containing:			
calcium, magnesium, ammonium, oxalate, phosphate and uric acid	6.4	6.0	8.4
All or predominantly uric acid	8.0	8.9	1.0
Cystine	2.8	1.5	5.9
Total	99.0	99.7	99.8

Data kindly supplied by Dr G. A. Rose, Institute of Urology, London, UK.

The urine of non-stone formers is in such a physicochemical state that although crystallization of stone-forming salts will not begin spontaneously it is likely to progress once it has been initiated. This arises because the concentrations of the ions, which contribute to calcium-containing stones, are such that the observed activity products for octacalcium phosphate $[(Ca^{2+})_3(H^+)(PO_4^{3-})_4]$, hydroxyapatite $[(Ca^{2+})_{10}(OH)_2(PO_4^{3-})_6]$ calcium oxalate $[(Ca^{2+}) (C_2O_4^{2-})]$, and magnesium ammonium phosphate $[(Mg^{2+}) (NH_4^+) (PO_4^{3-})]$ are between their solubility products and their formation products, or at the most only a little above their formation products. The solubility product is the product of the activities of the ions of a salt in a saturated solution at equilibrium, and the formation product is the product of the activities of the ions at which precipitation spontaneously occurs in a supersaturated solution of the salt. The calculation is complicated in order to allow for all the possible interacting ion species in urine, some of which are not stone constituents. Calcium oxalate is the salt which is most likely to precipitate from normal urine on the basis of the physicochemical criteria, and this agrees with the clinical observation that calcium oxalate is the commonest constituent to urinary stones. Brushite $(CaHPO_42H_2O)$ is the most likely salt to crystallize from persistently acidic urine.

Normal urine contains one or more physiological inhibitors of crystallization. These prevent the growth and aggregation of crystals. The propensity to stone formation in a particular urine depends on a balance between the degree of saturation with stone-forming salts and the protective effect of these physiological inhibitors of crystallization. There appear to be two such compounds in normal urine, the main one being a high molecular weight acidic glycosaminoglycan (mucopolysaccharide) and the other a low molecular weight polyphosphate which is probably pyrophosphate.

The simultaneous measurement of the degree of saturation and inhibitory potency of a urine specimen and their combination as a saturation-inhibitor index using a discriminant function analysis shows differences between normal subjects and idiopathic recurrent calcium stone formers (i.e. subjects who do not have an overt metabolic cause for the urolithiasis), and between stone-forming and non-stone-forming patients with hyperparathyroidism. The sizes of the crystal aggregates and the frequency of stone episodes can be correlated with the saturation-inhibitor index.

Small postprandial and diurnal variations in the urinary calcium and oxalate excretions, as well as longer term cyclic and seasonal variations occur. These can be quite small in absolute terms, but exert a marked effect on the degree of urine saturation which is quantifiable by measuring the activity products. The increased calcium and oxalate excretions in the summer months, with low values in the winter, are not associated with seasonal variations in urine pH, volume, creatinine, phosphate or magnesium excretion. There is a trend towards higher saturation levels of octacalcium phosphate as well as a significant increase in the saturation with calcium oxalate. These changes depend only on the seasonal variations in calcium and oxalate excretion, and not on urine volume. They are thought to reflect increased vitamin D synthesis in the skin during the summer months. This would promote increased absorption of calcium from the gut leaving more oxalate available for absorption and excretion. They correlate with the 50 per cent higher rate of stone formation by recurrent stone formers in the summer than in the winter. There is not a significant increase in the number of large stones requiring surgical removal in the summer, and this suggests that a short-term factor, such as a seasonal increase in urine saturation, promotes growth of normal small crystal aggregates into large agglomerations which form small stones. The diurnal variations in the degree of urine saturation due to changes in urine flow rate and pH as well as to changes in calcium and oxalate excretion, are superimposed on the seasonal variations. The diurnal and seasonal factors summate to increase the liability to crystallization at certain times in a 24-hour cycle and emphasize that calcium-containing stone-formers like other patients with urolithiasis must maintain a water diuresis. Decreasing the calcium intake only, may actually increase the degree of urine saturation with respect to calcium oxalate by allowing more oxalate to be absorbed and therefore excreted. This arises because the oxalate ion has a greater effect than the calcium ion on the activity product which measures the degree of urine saturation.

Most calcium-containing stones are of multifactorial origin. The risk factors are epidemiological and urinary and they summate in different degrees and combinations in the individual patients. The epidemiological risk factors are: age, sex, occupation, overall nutritional status, diet, fluid intake, climate, and the presence of specific metabolic disorders. The urinary risk factors are: high concentrations of calcium, oxalate, and uric acid, lack of the normal diurnal rhythm of urine pH, deficiency of crystallization-inhibiting glycosaminoglycans and a low urine volume. Of these, the urine volume and the urinary oxalate excretion are the most important.

The pathological findings in urolithiasis are those of urinary tract obstruction and complicating pyelonephritis. Renal fibrosis with ischaemia and renal hypertension only occurs if there is long-standing complicating pyelonephritis and/or nephrocalcinosis. The intrarenal deposits of calcium oxalate and hydroxyapatite in nephrocalcinosis excite relatively little inflammatory cell infiltration.

Many cases of urolithiasis are not associated with any overt biochemical changes although subtle physicochemical changes in the urine are ultimately responsible for their formation. The chemical findings which characterize the individual specific causes of urolithiasis are described with the diseases concerned. Cases of extensive bilateral stone disease with renal destruction also display the typical biochemical and other findings of uraemia.

Clinical aspects

Small stones which are voided spontaneously are generally composed of calcium oxalate. The larger calcium-containing stones which need surgical removal usually contain appreciable amounts of phosphate. Predominantly phosphatic stones indicate past or present urinary tract infection. Patients with primary hyperparathyroidism and renal tubular acidosis pass oxalate stones which generally contain some phosphate.

Urinary stones may be clinically silent or present as summarized in Table 3. Pain due to urinary stones is either a dull ache in the renal angle due to pelvicalyceal distension, or colicky (ureteric colic) in the lateral part of the abdomen, from the loin to the groin, perineum, scrotum, or penis. An attack of renal colic is often associated with retching and vomiting. Stones sometimes migrate down the ureter without pain and are occasionally passed *per urethram* with little or no discomfort. A history of recurrent urinary infections, which relapse after treatment, suggests the presence of a predisposing anatomical abnormality of the urinary tract, and this is commonly a stone. Occasional patients present with fever and rigors due to severe infection proximal to an obstructing calculus. Patients with impacted bilateral ureteric stones present with acute oliguric renal failure and uraemia. About 40 per cent of urinary stones are passed spontaneously, 20–25 per cent have to be removed from either the kidney or ureter, and 10–15 per cent lodge in the bladder.

Diagnosis

Urolithiasis presents four diagnostic problems: (*a*) the differentiation of the presenting symptoms from other types of renal disease and other causes of acute abdominal pain; (*b*) the differential diagnosis of patients with calculus anuria or oliguria; (*c*) the differentiation of the different types of urinary stone from one another; (*d*) aetiology.

Renal colic has to be differentiated from other causes of acute abdominal pain, notably intestinal colic, appendicitis, biliary colic, torsion of an ovarian cyst, and a ruptured ectopic pregnancy. Presentation with asymptomatic proteinuria may lead to initial confusion with chronic glomerulonephritis or chronic pyelonephritis. Painless haematuria as a presenting symptom suggests a renal tract neoplasm rather than a stone. A history beginning with increased frequency of micturition, accompanied by sterile pyuria and mild proteinuria (especially if the urine is acidic) will suggest renal tract tuberculosis as the provisional diagnosis, although such a picture can be produced by a stone particularly if it is impacted in the intramural part of the ureter causing bladder irritation. Anuria due to stone impaction (calculus anuria) may be preceded by remarkably little pain as the stones move down the ureter. The presence of a single functionless kidney can sometimes be traced retrospectively to such a painless obstructive episode. Calculus anuria and oliguria have to be distinguished from the prerenal, renal, and other postrenal causes of acute renal failure. Some of the important conditions to be considered in this context are: severe underhydration and sodium depletion, hypovolaemic shock, acute tubular necrosis, vasculitic and glomerular lesions, acute interstitial nephritis, obstructive uropathy due to other causes.

The patient should be investigated *immediately* if he presents with ureteric colic because spasm around a small stone greatly facilitates diagnosis. Ultrasonography is a sensitive technique for demonstrating dilated ureters and hydronephroses and its availability greatly reduces the need for emergency intravenous urography which is otherwise essential. Intravenous urography and other imaging investigations after the acute episode show the overall state of the urinary tract and a persistent obstructive lesion, but they do not demonstrate the small stones which pass easily because the local spasm relaxes. Plain abdominal films with tomography and computed tomography (CT) may give additional information about the nature of an obstructive lesion. However, collecting system dilation in the presence of either stag-horn calculi or multiple cysts, can only be excluded by intravenous urography. Percutaneous antegrade urography is a valuable way of locating the level of an obstructive lesion where this cannot be achieved by ultrasonography. It may be possible to dislodge or remove an obstructive lesion via this route and the renal pelvis can be drained immediately while definitive treatment is being planned.

The investigation of the patients who present with acute oliguric renal failure is simplified by the availability of imaging techniques additional to X-radiography. Under these circumstances the first-line investigation can be plain abdominal radiograph with tomography and ultrasonography. Computed tomography is used for cases where the ultrasound is not diagnostic or where the cause of an obstruction has not been defined. With this approach, less than 20 per cent of patients presenting with impaired renal function require either high-dose urography or retrograde ureterograms. The kidneys can be measured accurately by ultrasound, although the absolute measurements are less than those obtained by urography because of the absence of magnification. Although ultrasonography and computed tomography can simplify the immediate

Table 3 Urinary stones: clinical presentations

Pain
   Ureteric coli
   Lumbar ache
   On micturition
Haematuria
Sterile pyuria
Asymptomatic proteinuria
Dysuria and increased urinary frequency
Urinary tract infections
   Acute (single or recurrent attack)
   Chronic
   Pyonephrosis
Calculus anuria
Strangury and interruption of urine stream

diagnosis of urolithiasis and its complications they do not completely replace plain radiography and urography. The need for experienced interpretation as well as technical expertize and financial constraints are important considerations in relation to the introduction of the newer imaging methods.

Calcium oxalate stones are characteristically spiky and discoloured by altered blood, whereas phosphatic stones are generally larger, smoother, and more friable. Cystine stones are pale yellow and look crystalline. Xanthine stones are smooth, brownish yellow, and rather soft. The composition of urinary stones is markedly altered by complicating urinary infections. For example, a cystinuric patient may pass magnesium ammonium phosphate stones as well as cystine stones if there has been much infection. Similarly, the stone matrix which remains after a cystine stone has been dissolved medically may provide the basis on which a calcium oxalate stone develops subsequently.

Uric acid, xanthine, and 2,8-dihydroxyadenine and oxipurinol stones are radiotranslucent, as are pieces of stone matrix, aggregates of orotic acid and uric acid crystals, detached renal papillae, tumour tissue, and blood clots, all of which also occasionally cause ureteric obstruction and colic. The nature and cause of the radio-opaque stones, that is, the stones which contain calcium salts and the cystine stones, cannot be established by their radiographic appearance. The presence of multiple stones simultaneously, especially if they are bilateral, is generally held to indicate that they are likely to arise from a metabolic cause, but the presence of a single stone does not contraindicate investigation to identify a specific cause, and some patients repeatedly form stones for reasons which cannot be identified at present.

Ultrasonography, computed tomography, nuclear magnetic resonance (NMR) imaging, and static imaging with the gamma-camera after the injection of [^{99m}Tc]dimercaptosuccinic acid (DMSA) also give information about renal anatomy in the non-acute situation (page 18.1). Comparison of the two kidneys gives an estimate of their relative function although this should not be equated with GFR. About 10 per cent of the tracer is normally excreted over 3 hours. This proportion is increased in obstructive uropathy and therefore gives an erroneously high impression of the renal function in this situation. Static scanning with [^{99m}Tc] DMSA is particularly useful for the detection of renal cortical scars but is inferior to ultrasonography and urography for tumours, cysts, and other space-occupying lesions. Isotope renography with external probes, and dynamic imaging with the gamma-camera after the injection of [^{123}I]hippuran or [^{99m}Tc]diethylenetriamine pentaacetate (DTPA) are used in the investigation of urinary tract obstruction. The gamma-camera is the more versatile method and has largely replaced the use of external probes. Although the intravenous urogram is the most reliable guide to the level of an obstruction, the gamma-camera is a better guide to its severity. The different imaging techniques are complementary to one another. Intravenous urography retains a place even where the more recent developments are available and circumspectly used. It is particularly important as part of the preoperative assessment when definitive surgical treatment is to be undertaken.

Urinary stone patients should be investigated medically after the acute episode. Any stones which the patient may have passed must be analysed. Classical wet chemical methods are usually used, but thermogravimetric and infrared analytical methods are available and have advantages. Ideally, the analysis should be quantitative and include calcium, magnesium, ammonium, oxalate, urate, phosphate, and carbonate. Magnesium ammonium phosphate stones indicate past or present infections. The stones should be tested qualitatively for cystine and analysed quantitatively if the qualitive test is positive. The detection and determination of uric acid should be by an enzymatic differential spectrophotometric method using uricase in order to distinguish uric acid from 2,8-dihydroxyadenine. Specific enzymatic and ultraviolet spectroscopic methods are available for the identification of xanthine stones. The absolute identification of a 2,8-dihydroxyadenine stone requires either infrared spectroscopy of mass spectrometry.

Table 4 summarizes the radiographic and other imaging results in patients presenting with renal colic. As a generalization, finely stippled nephrocalcinosis suggests the presence of long-standing hypercalcaemia, whereas dense coarse nephrocalcinosis suggests primary hyperoxaluria or renal tubular acidosis. The causes of nephrocalcinosis are listed in Table 5. The minimum biochemical evaluation for a patient with urolithiasis is: (*a*) analysis of the stone; (*b*) microbiological and microscopic examination of the urine; (*c*) measurement of serum calcium, phosphorus, total protein and albumin, creatinine, sodium, and potassium; (*d*) a qualitative test for cystine and measurement of the pH of the first morning urine, this should be in the range pH 5.3–6.8; (*e*) measurement of the 24-hour excretion of calcium, creatinine, and uric acid with the patient ambulant and taking the usual diet. Attempts to assess the patient's 24-hour urinary volume as an outpatient are difficult and likely to be unreliable but the urinary creatinine value gives a rough indication of the completeness of the supposedly 24-hour collection. Ideally the urinary oxalate excretion should be measured as part of the initial evaluation. However, this may present difficulties because automated methods are not available. It should certainly be undertaken if there are multiple stones or nephrocalcinosis and the other parameters are normal (see page 9.41 for a discussion of the primary and secondary hyperoxaluria). The comprehensive biochemical investigation of stone-forming patients is summarized in Table 6. The serum calcium determinations should be made on blood which has been collected after an overnight fast, without venous occlusion, and with the patient lying recumbent. It is advisable to repeat the serum calcium, phosphorus, and protein determinations on more than one occasion. The protocol should include chest X-ray, a full blood count, and ESR.

Table 4 Diagnostic imaging findings in patients presenting with renal colic

Obstructive uropathy due to
   Radio-opaque stone*
   Radiotranslucent obstructive lesion (stone†, crystals, papilla, clot, carcinoma)
Generalized nephrocalcinosis
Medullary sponge kidney
Renal papillary necrosis (± sloughed papilla)
Cortical scars due to chronic pyelonephritis
Renal carcinoma (source of 'clot colic')
Coincidental calcific lesions (e.g. tuberculosis, Randall's plaques)

  * Sites of calcific lesions which may be confused with radio-opaque calculi: gallstones, costal cartilages, mesenteric lymph-nodes, adrenals, pancreas, renal and splenic arteries, pelvic veins.

  † The radiotranslucent stones are: uric acid, xanthine 2,8-dihydroxyadenine, orotic acid.

Table 5 Causes of generalized nephrocalcinosis

Mainly medullary (usual location)
   Primary hyperparathyroidism
   Idiopathic hypercalciuria
   Primary renal tubular acidosis
   Hypervitaminosis D
   Milk alkali syndrome
   Primary hyperoxaluria
   Sarcoidosis
   Chronic berylliosis
   Thyrotoxicosis
   Sulphonamide injury

Mainly cortical (very rare)
   Chronic glomeruloneophritis
   Renal cortical necrosis with recovery ('tram-line' calcification)

Table 6 Detailed biochemical investigation of patients presenting with urinary stones

Stone:	Inorganic constituents, uric acid, cystine, xanthine, 2,8-dihydroxyadenine*, orotic acid*
Blood:	(Collect fasting, recumbent, without venous occlusion.) Calcium, phosphorus, total protein, albumin, plasma protein electrophoresis, and quantitative immunoelectrophoresis, uric acid, alkaline phosphatase, urea, creatinine, Na, K, HCO$_3$, Cl
Urine:	Calcium†, phosphorus, oxalate, urate, creatinine (24-hour excretion) pH‡ after NH$_4$Cl load (0.1 g/kg body weight) Qualitative test for cystine Tests* for xanthine if serum uric acid < 1 mg/100 ml (59 μmol/l) Crystal* counts (freshly voided warm urine) Saturation* – inhibitor index Immunoelectrophoresis of any urinary protein

* Only rarely needed.

† These measurements should be made with the patient taking his usual diet. They should be repeated on more than one occasion. The urinary creatinine assesses the consistency of the 24-hour urine collections and allows the creatinine clearance to be calculated. Measuring the urine uric acid excretion after 5 days on a purine-free diet will identify uric acid overexcretors and therefore some of the patients with an excessive rate of uric acid synthesis.

‡ Measure urine pH hourly from 08.00 to 18.00 hours, give NH$_4$Cl at 10.00 hours.

The dietary history should be reviewed with particular reference to the intake of vitamins C (an oxalate precursor) and D, meat, milk, oxalate, and calcium. The volumes of fluid drunk and urine passed should be assessed. A history of exposure to the environmental factors, which predispose to urinary stones, should also be sought.

The principal systemic and metabolic causes of renal stones and nephrocalcinosis are summarized in Table 7. Urolithiasis and nephrocalcinosis can complicate any condition which causes prolonged hypercalciuria, the less common causes of which include Paget's disease of bone, tertiary hyperparathyroidism, thyrotoxicosis, and malignant disease. These conditions, and those listed in Table 7 except for idiopathic hypercalciuria and renal tubular acidosis, are associated with hypercalcaemia. Malignant disease mobilizes calcium by direct bone involvement with metastases, the production of a parathyroid hormone-like peptide, and possibly prostaglandins and steroidal compounds with vitamin D-like activity.

Sustained hypercalcaemia should lead to a review of the patient's clinical history for systemic symptoms of hypercalcaemia (Table 8), and circumcorneal calcification should be sought by careful visual inspection using a well-collimated beam of light shone tangentially across the cornea. Sustained hypercalcaemia raises the possibility that the patient may be suffering from primary hyperparathyroidism. The main differential diagnoses are sarcoidosis, multiple myelomatosis, malignant disease with hypercalcaemia, hypervitaminosis D, and milk alkali syndrome, and they have to be excluded by a careful re-evaluation of the *whole* clinical history, physical findings, and other data.

The prevalence of primary hyperparathyroidism (page 10.51 *et seq.*) approaches 1 per 1000 of the population, it occurs with greater frequency in women aged 30–60 years and is responsible for 5–10 per cent of cases of calcium-containing urinary stones. Conversely, about 50 per cent of patients with primary hyperparathyroidism have urolithiasis. The stones are most often calcium phosphate, the formation of which is favoured by the slightly alkaline urine as well as by the hypercalciuria. The estimation of systemic venous parathyroid hormone (PTH) levels and the results of the 12-day hydrocortisone suppression test (40 mg hydrocortisone 8 hourly) with measurement of the serum calcium, phosphorus, and urinary calcium levels 3 days before the test and on the 10th, 11th, and 12th day of hydrocortisone administration provide positive support for the diagnosis of primary hyperparathyroidism.

Table 7 The principle systemic and metabolic causes of renal stones and nephrocalcinosis

Primary hyperparathyroidism
Idiopathic hypercalciuria
Sarcoidosis
Milk-alkali syndrome
Hypervitaminosis D
Renal tubular acidosis
Prolonged immobilization
Multiple myelomatosis
Primary and secondary hyperoxaluria

Table 8 Systemic symptoms of hypercalcaemia

Neuropsychiatric
  Depression
  Irritability
  Malaise
  Muscle weakness
  Confusion and coma
Gastrointestinal
  Anorexia
  Nausea and vomiting
  Abdominal pain (acute pancreatitis)
Renal
  Polyuria
  Polydipsia

Classically, primary hyperparathyroidism produces hypercalcaemia with an elevated PTH. However, normocalcaemic primary hyperparathyroidism exists but a high PTH level establishes the diagnosis. Conversely, some patients with hypercalcaemic primary hyperparathyroidism have normal PTH concentrations. This combination is diagnostic because hypercalcaemia due to other causes suppresses the PTH to negligible levels. Primary hyperparathyroidism has been defined as a level of circulating PTH which is inappropriately high for the prevailing plasma calcium concentrations. It should also be noted that although the serum concentration of calcium ions controls PTH release from the gland it is the plasma total calcium concentration that is measured.

Caution is needed in interpreting the results of PTH assays in the presence of renal failure because this slows the rate of PTH inactivation and degradation (page 18.161). Also, the different radioimmunoassay methods give different results. The diagnosis of hyperparathyroidism often relies on several separate pieces of evidence which must all be given appropriate weight. Measurements of central venous parathyroid hormone levels are only recommended as preliminary to a second operation after a negative exploration when the anterior mediastinum will have to be explored.

Hypercalcaemia other than that due to primary hyperparathyroidism is suppressed by hydrocortisone. It may be necessary to adjust the serum calcium concentration for the effects of plasma albumin concentrations which deviate markedly from the mean normal value of 47 g/l (4.7 g/100 ml) by 0.02 mmol/1.0 g albumin observed concentration above or below the mean normal value (0.8 mg/100 ml for each 1.0 g albumin observed concentration above or below the mean normal value of 4.7 g/100 ml). A mild degree of hyperchloraemic acidosis commonly occurs in primary hyperparathyroidism. Measurement of cAMP excretion and the renal tubular reabsorption of phosphate give, at most, only collateral support to a diagnosis which is essentially based on the critical appraisal of calcium and PTH levels. When a diagnosis of primary hyperparathyroidism has been made, it should be reviewed from the viewpoint of its being either part of a multiple endocrine adenomatosis syndrome or one of the rare autosomal dominant inherited forms.

Idiopathic hypercalciuria is an important cause of urinary stones and is discussed separately on page 18.95.

Two groups of patients with intestinal disease are predisposed to urolithiasis because of their primary disease. Continuous loss of alkaline intestinal secretions from an ileostomy and in chronic diarrhoea makes the urine concentrated and persistently acid. This predisposes to uric acid stone formation. Malabsorption due to diffuse small intestine disease or resection leaves increased concentrations of long chain fatty acids in the bowel lumen. These bind calcium-liberating oxalate ions which are absorbed and excreted in the urine. This predisposes to calcium oxalate urolithiasis.

Treatment

The acute episode

A stone which is causing renal colic need only be removed immediately if infection is trapped above it. Otherwise, and provided it does not cause obstruction between attacks of colic, a ureteric stone can be treated conservatively. Stones less than 5 mm in diameter on a standard abdominal X-ray film usually either pass or migrate to the lowest part of the ureter from whence they can usually be removed endoscopically. Stones which are causing obstruction between attacks of colic should be removed surgically. The presence of obstruction and not the size and position of a stone is the major factor which decides the correct line of treatment. Cases of ureteric stone which are being treated conservatively need regular supervision with abdominal radiography every 6 to 8 weeks in order to assess the migration of the stone. In the absence of obstruction it is reasonable to wait 6–8 weeks after stone migration ceases before performing a lithotomy. Recurrence of renal colic indicates further ultrasound and/or intravenous urography after the attack to determine if obstruction has developed.

A single kidney, impaired, and especially deteriorating overall renal function, and bilateral ureteric stones indicate early surgical intervention. The spontaneous passage of stones is aided by maintaining a high fluid intake if necessary intravenously, and the effect of this may be augmented by a short burst of vigorous diuretic therapy by, for example, intravenous frusemide. Pelvicalyceal stones should not be treated surgically unless they are more than 5 mm in diameter or are causing obstruction to some part of the pelvicalyceal system. They should, however, be kept under surveillance. Urinary infection in the presence of partial ureteric obstruction requires vigorous continuous antibiotic therapy with bacteriological control, and vigilance lest a pyonephrosis develops behind the stone. Pethidine is satisfactory for the symptomatic treatment of renal colic. The overall philosophy in the management of patients with urinary stones is to relieve, or prevent, obstruction and infection without sacrificing functioning kidney tissue. The dissolution of pelvicalyceal stones by continous irrigation either from below or through a percutaneous nephrostomy has not gained wide acceptance. Calcium phosphate, magnesium ammonium phosphate urate, and cystine, but not calcium oxalate stones have been dissolved in this way.

The destruction and removal of stones under direct vision using a percutaneous nephroscope and an ultrasonic lithotrite probe is a major advance which reduces trauma to the kidney and shortens convalescence. The non-invasive dissolution of stones in the kidney and upper one-third of the ureter by focussed shock waves generated extracorporeally (lithotripsy) is another major therapeutic advance.

Stone prevention

Identifiable *biochemical causes* of the stone *and anatomical abnormalities* which obstruct the free flow of urine *should be treated*. The management of patients with urinary stones for which no cause has been found depends partly on the composition of the stone, which is usually calcium oxalate, mixed calcium oxalate/

phosphate, or more rarely uric acid. All patients who have had a stone should drink enough (about 3 litres in temperate climates) to maintain a urine volume of at least 3 litres per 24 hours. The patients should check this themselves. Some of the extra fluid should be taken late at night and larger volumes are needed in tropical climates and by those who work in hot environments. It is unnecessary to specify softened water, the final urine calcium concentrations achieved with hard tap water being only slightly higher than those with calcium-free water.

Uric acid stone formers should have the diurnal change in their urine pH assessed. If they excrete persistently acid urine and do not have hyperuric aciduria it is sufficient, in the first instance, to give enough alkali to keep the urine pH above 6. They should check the pH of their urine with a wide-range pH indicator paper. Allopurinol is recommended if there is proven hyperuric aciduria or if an alkalinizing regime fails or is inappropriate for other reasons. Lack of response to alkali indicates poor ability to inhibit crystal formation in the urine, undetected intermittently elevated uric acid excretion values or non-compliance. The degree of dietary restriction of animal protein and other purine-containing food necessary to lower uric acid excretion greatly is unacceptable to most European patients.

Patients who have had only one calcium-containing stone for which no cause was found need only be advised to maintain a high rate of urine flow, to avoid self medication with vitamins D and C, and calcium-containing antacids, and to avoid more than average intakes of dairy products and oxalate-rich beverages and fruits.

The responsiveness of urinary calcium excretion to dietary calcium restriction is variable and decreasing the concentration of calcium in the intestinal lumen increases the oxalate absorption and excretion. Dietary calcium restriction therefore needs to be accompanied by dietary oxalate restriction.

Patients with recurrent idiopathic calcium-containing stones require more vigorous treatment. Some have intermittent mild hypercalciuria and if this can be demonstrated, they should be treated as described under idiopathic hypercalciuria. Others have a mild degree of hyperoxaluria, which may be intermittent and result from hyperabsorption, and dietary restriction of oxalate to less than 100 mg/day is indicated (tea is the main source of dietary oxalate in England). The intake of lean meat should be reduced to less than 225 g/day (this reduces calcium and urate excretions), and that of milk to 300 ml/day or less. Allopurinol has been advocated for the treatment of idiopathic calcium oxalate stone-formers on the grounds that such stones may form on a nidus of uric acid. The value of this approach is as yet unproven.

Orthophosphates and magnesium oxide (or hydroxide) are used as non-specific inhibitors of crystallization when stones recur in spite of apparently adequate treatment or when no more specific treatment is available. Orthophosphates act by: (*a*) increasing the excretion of pyrophosphate; (*b*) binding some calcium in the gut; (*c*) increasing thirst; (*d*) competing with oxalate ions for excreted calcium ions in the urine. A dose equivalent to between about 1 and 2 g of elemental phosphorus per day is given in effervescent tablets (Phosphate Sandoz). Magnesium ions inhibit the growth of calcium oxalate crystals *in vitro*, and there are reports that stone development *in vivo* is inhibited by the prolonged administration of magnesium oxide. The dose used should be sufficient (for example, 200 mg daily) to increase materially the urinary magnesium excretion.

Course and prognosis

Urinary stones tend to recur even when a specific cause cannot be identified. Such recurrences may be separated by as much as ten years, the total recurrence rate after this period being about 70 per cent. The treatability of a systemic or metabolic cause (Table 7) determines the immediate prognosis with respect to non-renal morbidity and mortality, and influences that for further stone formation in the future. The amount of renal damage caused by the stones or nephrocalcinosis determine the prognosis with respect to renal function and hypertension. Urolithiasis does not cause hypertension unless it is complicated by pyelonephritis and renal fibrosis. Nephrocalcinosis worsens the prognosis even if the underlying cause can be treated as in primary hyperparathyroidism.

Idiopathic hypercalciuria

The term idiopathic hypercalciuria describes a situation in which no cause can be found for excessive urinary calcium excretion, and the serum calcium is consistently normal. The diagnosis depends on the exclusion of several major disorders and is therefore one which should be kept under review. It occurs more often in men than women and is the commonest identified cause of urolithiasis in Europe and North America. The plasma calcium is consistently normal, but the plasma phosphate levels may be a little low [about 0.8 mmol/l (0.5 mg/dl) less than normal] and there is often a mild hyperuricaemia [usually about 0.03 mmol/l (0.5 mg/dl) above the normal range].

Pathophysiology

The metabolic lesion in idiopathic hypercalciuria is unknown. Three pathophysiological subtypes have been proposed: (*a*) absorptive (excessive intestinal absorption of calcium); (*b*) renal (decreased renal tubular reabsorption of calcium); (*c*) resorptive (excessive mobilization of calcium from the skeleton). Further subdivisions of the absorptive group are: (*a*) hyperabsorption at all calcium intake levels; (*b*) hyperabsorption in the presence of high calcium intake only; (*c*) associated with a renal phosphate leak. The resorptive group may be only an extension of the renal group in whom parathyroid activity has increased in response to the chronic calcium loss in the urine. The increased parathyroid hormone secretion may be either suppressible by measures which raise the plasma calcium concentration ('secondary hyperparathyroidism') or nonsuppressible ('tertiary hyperparathyroidism'). These patients may also be classified initially as having normocalcaemic primary hyperparathyroidism. However, their renal calcium leak persists after removal of the parathyroid gland and suppressible hyperparathyroidism reappears after several years. It may be that patients diagnosed as having primary hyperparathyroidism due to symmetrical enlargement of all of the parathyroids or with more than one adenoma really have the renal type of idiopathic hypercalciuria.

The rate at which the urinary calcium excretion decreases in response to dietary restriction varies widely between different individuals. It has been suggested that the different responses to an arbitrarily fixed period of low calcium intake shown by individual patients with absorptive idiopathic hypercalciuria reflects this variability and not a fundamental difference between the patients. Some investigators maintain that the results of their pathophysiological studies indicate that all cases are of the renal type. A study of the kinetics of calcium ion transport across the small intestinal mucosa *in vitro* showed increased calcium uptake in both absorptive and renal idiopathic hypercalciurics suggesting that idiopathic hypercalciuria is a homogeneous disorder. This general conclusion agrees with the results of a recent study of the effects of low calcium diets on parathyroid function, and 1,25-dihydroxycholecalciferol levels which also suggested that idiopathic hypercalciuria may be an homogeneous disorder with a uniform elevation of calcium absorption and a variable defect of renal calcium reabsorption. The functionally reverse metabolic lesion occurs in familial benign hypercalcaemia, where the only abnormality is increased renal tubular calcium reabsorption, parathyroid function being normal. Familial benign hypercalcaemia is inherited as an autosomal dominant.

In spite of these pathophysiological and taxonomic problems the diagnosis of idiopathic hypercalciuria is the only one which fits a large proportion of calcium-containing stone-formers, at least in

Europe and North America. The normal urinary calcium excretion is 2.5 – 8.75 mmol (100 – 350 mg) per 24 hours and 2.0 – 7.5 mmol (80 – 300 mg) per 24 hours for men and women, respectively. Higher values are not always associated with stone formation and some intractable calcium-containing stone-formers excrete consistently normal amounts of calcium. Table 9 lists factors which modify the urinary calcium excretion. Prolonged studies have shown that some patients who would previously have been classified as normocalciuric idiopathic calcium-containing stone-formers excrete, *on average*, about 20 per cent more calcium and 20 per cent more oxalate than a corresponding group of non-stone-formers and the absolute amounts of calcium and oxalate which they excrete increase in the summer months. The oxalate is the more important risk factor for urolithiasis.

The morbid anatomical and histopathological findings in idiopathic hypercalciuria are those of urolithiasis and its complications.

Clinical aspects

Patients with idiopathic hypercalciuria usually present in the fourth and fifth decades with stones which usually recur. Idiopathic hypercalciuria is very common in women who have a higher incidence of primary hyperparathyroidism than men. Primary hyperparathyroidism is the most important differential diagnosis in both sexes. Idiopathic hypercalciuria is not an early stage in the evolution of primary hyperparathyroidism as has sometimes been suggested, although it can lead to secondary and tertiary hyperparathyroidism. Some cases of medullary sponge kidney have hypercalciuria and/or inability to acidify their urine normally. Hypercalciuria is also sometimes associated with primary renal tubular acidosis. These associations increase the likelihood of stone formation. The renal tubular dysfunction in chronic cadmium poisoning, berylliosis, and Wilson's disease also causes normocalcaemic hypercalciuria. Although it classically causes

Table 9 Factors affecting the average urinary calcium excretion. (In general these effects are variable from one individual to another. Individually they are usually small by comparison with the total daily calcium excretion but their results are additive and cogniscence of them may be helpful to patients with idiopathic hypercalciuria and to other patients with recurrent calcium containing calculi.)

Sex	Calcium excretion is lower in women than in men
Age	Calcium excretion is lower in children and the geriatric age group than in others
Environment	Exposure to sunlight increases calcium excretion in light-skinned subjects due to increased vitamin D synthesis. There are geographical differences which are independent of this effect, e.g. the higher urinary calcium excretion in the USA than in Europe
Associated diseases	Renal failure, nephrotic syndrome and intestinal malabsorption syndromes reduce the urinary calcium excretion
Diet	*Calcium*: high levels increase the urinary calcium excretion
	Vitamin D: high levels increase the urinary calcium excretion
	Inorganic phosphate: high levels reduce calcium absorption and excretion
	Fibre: high levels reduce calcium absorption and excretion
	Sodium content: high levels increase urinary sodium excretion. This is associated with an increase in urinary calcium
	Carbohydrate: high carbodydrate (glucose, sucrose, galactose) diets, increase urinary calcium (and magnesium) in parallel with an increased hydrogen ion excretion
	Protein: High protein diets increase urinary calcium (and urate) excretion

hypercalcaemia, sarcoidosis can be associated with normocalcae-mic hypercalciuria.

The associated hyperuricaemia, occasional aminoaciduria, and mild hypophosphataemia are attributed to renal tubule dysfunction caused by the hypercalciuria.

Idiopathic hypercalciuria in children appears to be a separate entity in which the hypercalciuria, nephrolithiasis, and nephrocalcinosis are associated with vasopressin-resistant diabetes insipidus, some impaired skeletal calcification, and hypercalciuria in the sibs and parents.

Treatment

Idiopathic hypercalciuria does not require treatment unless it is associated with urolithiasis. Hydration and dietary measures should be tried in the first instance (Table 10).

Even in hard water areas, the use of softened water has only a marginal effect. Special bread with a low calcium content is expensive, inconvenient, and inconsistent in its effect. Therefore, if the measures summarized in Table 2 do not control the hypercalciuria, it is more convenient to prescribe a pharmacological agent to reduce the urinary calcium excretion. A thiazide diuretic with a potassium supplement [for example, bendrofluazide 5 – 10 mg and potassium chloride 6.5 – 13 mmol (500 – 1000 mg) daily] is often effective. This does not change the faecal calcium but the plasma calcium may rise slightly. Long-term thiazide diuretics sometimes precipitate diabetes mellitus. Failure to maintain an initial good response to a thiazide is sometimes associated with a high excretion of sodium in the urine. This can be corrected by restricting the intake of sodium chloride. Cellulose phosphate (15 – 30 g daily), which acts by binding calcium in the gut, is an effective but more expensive agent, and is used if thiazide diuretics fail. Cellulose phosphate is a bulky powder taken with meals. It sometimes causes diarrhoea and bulky offensive stools. Idiopathic hypercalciuria must be treated continuously and the treatment controlled by measuring the 24-hour urine excretion of calcium. This should be kept within the normal range. A conscientiously applied dietary regime plus a thiazide and/or cellulose phosphate achieves this and reduces the frequency of stone forma-tion in most patients. If stone formation continues, orthophosphate or magnesium oxide (or hydroxide) may be added to the regime as non-specific inhibitors of crystal growth and aggregation (page 18.92). Allopurinol has been recommended for the treatment of recurrent hypercalciuric calcium oxalate stone-formers. This is unjustified in the vast majority of cases unless there is an associated hyperuricaciduria.

References

Boyd, J. C. and Ladenson, J. H. (1984). Value of laboratory tests in differential diagnosis of hypercalcaemia. *Am. J. Med.* **77**, 863–872.

Broadus, A. E. and Rasmussen, H. (1981). Clinical evaluation of parathyroid function. *Am. J. Med.* **70**, 475–478.

Brockis, J. G. and Finlayson, B. (eds) (1981). *Urinary calculus.* PSG Publishing Company, Littleton, Massachusetts.

Chaussy, C., Brendel, W. and Schmiedt, E. (1980). Extracorporeally induced destruction of kidney stones by shock waves. *Lancet* ii, 1265–1267.

Coe, F. L. (1981). Prevention of kidney stones. *Am. J. Med.* **71**, 514–516.

Dretler, S. P. and Pfister, R. C. (1983). Percutaneous dissolution of renal calculi. *Ann. Rev. Med.* **34**, 359–366.

Editorial (1982). Extracorporeal shock-wave lithotripsy. *Ann. inter. Med.* **101**, 387–389.

Finlayson, B. (1980). The treatment of urinary stone disease. *Austral. New Zealand J. Surg.* **50**, 13–17.

Fiskin, R. A., Heath, D. A. and Bold, A. M. (1980). Hypercalcaemia – a Hospital survey. *Q. J. Med. New Series* **71**, 405–419.

Pak, C. Y. C., Peters, P., Hurt, G., Kadesky, M., Fine, M., Reisman, D., Splann, F., Caramela, C., Freeman, A., Britton, F., Sakhaee, K. and Breslau, N. A. (1981). Is selective therapy of recurrent nephrolithiasis possible. *Am. J. Med.* **71**, 615–622.

Robertson, W. G. and Peacock, M. (1982). Risk factors in the formation of urinary stones. In *Scientific foundations of urology* 2nd edn (eds G. D. Chisholm and D. I. Williams), pp. 267–278. Heinemann Medical Books Ltd, London.

Rose, G. A. (1982). *Urinary stones: clinical and laboratory aspects.* MTP Press Limited, Lancaster, England.

Van Reen, R. (1980). Idiopathic urinary bladder stones of childhood. *Austral. New Zealand J. Sur.* **50**, 18–22.

Watts, R. W. E. (1980). The clinical approach to the aetiology of recurrent urinary calculi. *Austral. New Zealand J. Surg.* **50**, 8–12.

Webb, J. A. W., Reznek, R. H., White, F. E., Cattell, W. R., Fry, L. K. and Baker, L. R. I. (1984). Can ultrasound and computed tomography replace high-dose urography in patients with impaired renal runction? *Q. J. Med. New Series* **53**, 411–425.

Idiopathic hypercalciuria

Brockis, J. G. and Finlayson, B. (eds) (1981). *Urinary calculus.* PSG Publishing Co. Ltd., Littleton, Massachusetts.

Bordier, P., Ryckewart, A., Gueris, J. and Rasmussen, H. (1977) On the pathogenesis of so-called idiopathic hypercalciuria. *Am. J. Med.* **63**, 398–409.

Coe, F. L., Favus, M. J., Crockett, T., Strauss, A. L., Parks, J. H., Porat, A., Gantt, C. L. and Sherwood, L. M. (1982). Effects of a low-calcium diet on urine calcium excretion, parathyroid function and serum 1,25(OH)$_2$D$_3$ levels in patients with idiopathic hypercalciuria and in normal subjects. *Am. J. Med.* **72**, 25–32.

—— (1981). Prevention of kidney stones. *Am. J. Med.* **71**, 514–516.

Duncombe, V. M., Watts, R. W. E. and Peters, T. J. (1984). Studies on intestinal calcium absorption in patients with idiopathic hypercalciuria. *Q. J. Med. New Series* **53**, 69–79.

Finlayson, B. (1980). The treatment of stone disease. (1980) *Austral. New Zealand J. Surg.* **50**, 13–17.

Lemann, J., Adams, N. D. and Gray, R. W. (1979) Urinary calcium excretion in human beings. *N. Engl. J. Med.* **301**, 535–541.

Maschio, G., Tessitore, N., D'Angelo, A., Fabris, A., Pagano, F., Tasca, A., Grazani, G., Aroldi, A., Surian, M., Colussi, G., Mandressi, A., Trinchieri, A., Rocco, F., Ponticelli, C. and Mineti, L. (1981). Prevention of calcium nephrolithiasis with low dose thiazide, amiloride and allopurinol. *Am. J. Med.* **71**, 623–633.

Menko, F. H., Bijvoet, O. L. M., Fronen, J. L. H. H., Sandler, L. M., Adami, S., O'Riordan, J. L. H., Schopman, W. and Heynen, G. (1983). Familial benign hypercalcaemia. *Q. J. Med. New Series* **52**, 120–140.

Table 10 Dietary management of idiopathic hypercalciuria

1	Fluid intake	Sufficient to produce 3 litres of urine divided approximately uniformly over the 24-hour period. Tap water is satisfactory. Increase fluid intake in hot environments. Check 24-hour urine volume
2	Calcium	Minimize milk intake, this also reduces lactose intake. Omit cheese and yoghourt. Aim at an approximate 17.5 mmol (700 mg) per day calcium intake
3	Oxalate	Restrict intake because a low calcium diet increases oxalate absorption and excretion; urinary oxalate is a major risk factor for urolithiasis. Omit rhubarb, spinach, beetroot, strawberries, nuts, chocolate, cocoa, and tea (or limit to 2 cups per day)
4	Fruits and fruit juices	Omit those which are rich in vitamin C (an oxalate precursor). These are oranges, lemons, grapefruit, and Ribena syrup
5	Protein	Limit lean meat to 225 g/day
6	Carbohydrate	Sufficient for estimated calorie needs
7	Fibre	Include high fibre foods
8	Salt	Reduce dietary sodium chloride if urinary sodium >350 mmol/24 hours
9	Vitamin preparations	Omit vitamin D (promotes calcium absorption) Omit vitamin C (oxalate precursor)
10	Pharmaceuticals	Omit any which are calcium salts or which contain calcium salts unless they are needed for the treatment of another disease. Examples are: calcium aspirin, and many antacid preparations including aluminium hydroxide preparations

Muldowney, F. P., Freaney, R. and Ryan, J. G. (1980). The pathogenesis of idiopathic hypercalciuria: evidence for renal tubular calcium leak. Q. J. Med. New Series 49, 87–94.

Pak, C. Y. C., Britton, F., Peterson, R., Ward, D., Northcutt, C., Breslau, N. A., McGuire, J., Sakhaee, K., Bush, S., Nicar, M., Nor-

man, D. A. and Peters, P. (1980). Ambulatory evaluation of nephrolithiasis. Classification, clinical presentation and diagnostic criteria. Am. J. Med. 69, 19–30.

Rose, G. A. (1982). Urinary stones: clinical and laboratory aspects. MTP Press, Lancaster.

METABOLIC DISORDERS OF THE KIDNEY

R. W. E. WATTS

The renal transport defects, Fabry disease and primary renal tubular acidosis are dealt with on page 18.171 and Section 9.

Hypercalcaemic nephropathy

Pathophysiology

Acute hypercalcaemia causes epithelial cell degeneration, necrosis, and calcification, and the tubules become obstructed. There is marked impairment of urine concentrating ability, with resistance to vasopressin. This initial nephrogenic diabetes insipidus-like state causes underhydration which is aggravated by the nausea and vomiting associated with sodium and chloride depletion. Chronic hypercalcaemia leads to interstitial calcification and fibrosis which are most marked in the medulla. It is particularly associated with potassium depletion and acidosis. Chronic pyelonephritis and hypertension may be superadded.

Clinical aspects

Hypercalcaemic nephropathy is most often associated with malignancy. Other causes are primary hyperparathyroidism, multiple myelomatosis, sarcoidosis, and rarely vitamin D intoxication, milk alkali syndrome, immobilization (especially if the patient has Paget's disease), tertiary hyperparathyroidism, and hyperthyroidism.

The severity of the manifestations of hypercalcaemic nephropathy roughly parallel the degree of hypercalcaemia: serum total calcium concentrations greater than 3·5 mmol/l (14 mg/dl) indicate a grave risk of a hypercalcaemic crisis developing. If gross hypercalcaemia is found in a patient with renal failure it should be assumed that the hypercalcaemia is causing the impaired renal function. Tertiary hyperparathyroidism is very rare in chronic renal disease, although it occurs more often after a successful renal transplantation, and the hypercalcaemia may damage the grafted kidney. Transient hypercalcaemia occurs occasionally during recovery from acute renal failure (page 18.128).

The manifestations of calcium nephropathy may form only a small part of the overall clinical picture of the primary disease. An hypercalcaemic crisis may arise suddenly and be life-threatening in a patient, with, for example, primary hyperparathyroidism or malignant disease, who was previously in an otherwise relatively stable clinical state. Circumcorneal calcification indicates relatively long-standing antecedent hypercalcaemia.

Impaired urine concentrating ability with polyuria and polydipsia is usually the earliest manifestation. Dehydration, oliguria, and uraemia follow and the systemic manifestations of hypercalcaemia (anorexia, vomiting, lethargy, stupor, coma) appear. There may be proteinuria, haematuria, and pyuria even in the absence of pyelonephritis or nephrolithiasis. Medullary nephrocalcinosis and stones may be visible radiologically as complications of long-standing hypercalcaemia and hypercalciuria.

Treatment

The underlying disease should be treated urgently. Hypercalcae-

mia of 3.5 mmol/l (14 mg/dl) or greater must be treated in its own right by rapidly infusing sufficient isotonic sodium chloride solution to correct the dehydration and promote a vigorous diuresis. An intravenous dose of a loop diuretic (frusemide, bumetanide, ethacrynic acid) should be given. Thiazide diuretics should not be used. Prednisolone (20 mg, every 8 hours by mouth) or hydrocortisone (150 mg every 8 hours intravenously) is also commenced immediately unless the hypercalcaemia is due to hyperparathyroidism. In the rare cases where these measures are unsuccessful and the serum calcium has not begun to decrease within 12 hours of establishing a diuresis the regime can be supplemented by the infusion of orthophosphate [500 ml of Na_2HPO_4–KH_2PO_4 buffer solution (100 mmol/l with respect to phosphate, pH 7.4) over the course of 6 hours]. Oral effervescent phosphate preparations and oral fluids cannot usually be given because of nausea and vomiting, but they may be useful if significant hypercalcaemia persists after the symptoms subside. Intravenous sodium sulphate and sodium lactate have also been used in the emergency treatment of hypercalcaemia. The recommended doses of sodium sulphate is 2–3 litres of a solution containing 121 mmol/l administered over a period of 9 hours. The cytotoxic drug mithramycin inhibits bone resorption and lowers the serum calcium concentration within 1–2 days, the effect lasting for several days. It has been used for the treatment of acute hypercalcaemic crises in a dose of 25 μg/kg body weight given by intravenous infusion over a 4–24 hour period. The infusion can be repeated, but this increases the risk of myelotoxic, hepatotoxic, and nephrotoxic side-effects. Calcitonin which inhibits bone resorption, and increases the renal clearance of calcium is also of value as an adjunct to the main lines of treatment. Intravenous ethylene diamine tetra-acetic acid (EDTA) lowers the blood calcium rapidly, but the EDTA–calcium chelate is nephrotoxic and EDTA is not recommended for this purpose. Diphosphonate compounds (e.g. aminohydroxypropylidene diphosphonate) lower calcium concentrations by inhibiting osteoclastic bone resorption and may be more effective in the long run (if slower in onset) than these latter remedies. Close supervision and frequent biochemical monitoring of blood and urine is necessary during the management of hypercalcaemic crisis.

Most patients survive the acute episode provided an adequate rate of urine flow can be established and the hypercalcaemia corrected without overloading the circulation with salt and water. Calcium nephropathy of short duration may be completely reversible, although total recovery may take many months after removal of the cause. The extent of the structural renal damage cannot be assessed during the acute episode, and some cases continue to deteriorate in spite of biochemically effective treatment. Others remain oliguric and hypercalcaemic, and require treatment by peritoneal dialysis or haemodialysis. In general, the early diagnosed cases with a short total period of hypercalcaemia have the best prognosis. Apparently complete recovery may be followed by a gradual deterioration in renal function due to slowly progressive irreversible renal fibrosis initiated by nephrocalcinosis during the hypercalcaemic periods.

Hypokalaemic nephropathy

Pathophysiology

Hypokalaemic nephropathy (pages 18.23 and 18.31) usually follows several weeks or months of negative potassium balance. Table 1 lists the causes of chronic potassium depletion. The extracellular pool of potassium (about 50 mmol in the adult) is only a small part of the corresponding total body pool (2500–3000 mmol), and the plasma potassium concentration is a poor indicator of potassium homeostasis. A decrease of serum potassium by 1 mmol/l below the bottom of the normal range reflects a total body deficit of the order of 100–200 mmol.

Histologically, the renal tubule epithelium appears vacuolated and the mitochondria are damaged. These changes, which particularly affect the proximal convoluted tubules, are associated with impaired energy-dependent ion transport from the tubule lumen and a reduced osmotic pressure in the renal medulla. This decreases the kidney's sensitivity to vasopressin. Potassium repletion corrects the functional and structural abnormalities.

The normal dietary intake of 60–120 per 24 hours is small by comparison with the total body potassium pool and excessive potassium losses are usually the main cause of hypokalaemic nephropathy. Intractable vomiting causes a metabolic alkalosis which is partly compensated by the enhanced exchange of hydrogen ions in the lumen of the distal convoluted tubule for potassium ions in the renal tubule epithelium, and this causes a kaliuresis. As the state of potassium depletion develops there is a general exchange of intracellular potassium ions for extracellular hydrogen ions in order to maintain the concentration of potassium ions in the extracellular fluid. This produces an extracellular alkalosis with a generalized intracellular acidosis. The urine remains slightly acid, presumably because, at this stage, the supply of potassium ions for exchange with hydrogen ions in the tubule lumen is limited.

Clinical aspects

The main clinical manifestations of severe potassium depletion are muscular weakness, intestinal atony, and increased sensitivity to digitalis. These tend to overshadow the renal effects. There may be polyuria and polydipsia, and the picture occasionally resembles diabetes insipidus. Intermittent proteinuria and cylindruria sometimes occur and amino aciduria has been noted occasionally. The blood urea and serum creatinine are normal or only slightly increased in pure potassium depletion, and appreciable alterations

Table 1 Causes of potassium depletion

Gastrointestinal losses
Vomiting*
Continuous aspiration (for example, treatment or paralytic ileus)
Fistulae (biliary, pancreatic, gastrocolic)
Faecal [diarrhoea*, excessive purgation, use of potassium binding ion
    exchange resins, repeated enemata, uretero-sigmoid anastomosis, some
    villous tumours of the colon, APUDoma with raised vasoactive
    intestinal polypeptide secretion (Verner-Morrison syndrome)]
Urinary losses
Therapy with the thiazides and 'loop' diuretics (frusemide bumetanide,
    ethacrynic acid)
Primary renal disease (renal tubular acidosis, Fanconi syndrome, diuretic
    phase of recovery from acute tubular necrosis, chronic pyelonephritis)
Endocrine [primary hyperaldosteronism, secondary hyperaldosteronism
    (including Bartter's syndrome and juxtaglomerular cell tumour),
    Cushing's syndrome, corticosteroid therapy, islet-cell tumours of the
    pancreas]
Secondary to tissue breakdown (trauma, diabetic ketoacidosis)
Alkalosis (metabolic and respiratory)

---

*Gastric and upper intestinal secretors contain 5–10 mmol of potassium per litre and the kaliuresis due to hydrogen ion conservation in the distal renal tubule is a major factor in the production of potassium depletion by vomiting. Fluid faeces contain 50–100 mmol of potassium per litre and direct losses are the major determinant of potassium depletion due to diarrhoea.

in these parameters indicate the presence of other factors such as pyelonephritis, sodium depletion or hypotension. Although kaliuresis as a part of the physiological response to extrarenal losses of hydrogen ions can contribute to a negative potassium balance and therefore be a factor leading to hypokalaemic nephropathy, this type of renal lesion is not itself associated with excessive potassium losses in the urine. Except within the context of a metabolic alkalosis, such losses indicate that the negative potassium balance is due to either another type of renal disease or one of the endocrinopathies listed in Table 1.

It has been claimed that potassium depletion predisposes to pyelonephritis but this association is unproven.

Treatment

The cause of the negative potassium balance should be ascertained and corrected. Oral replacement should be used if possible except in emergency situations. Symptoms of potassium depletion occur only when the deficit is of the order of 300–1000 mmol. Therefore larger doses (150–200 mmol/day) than the conventional prophylactic 600 mg (8.1 mmol) of potassium chloride every 8 hours are needed for its correction. Potassium chloride is also used for intravenous therapy. It must be given slowly and in dilute solution (*maximum* rate: 40 mmol in 1 litre over 4–6 hours with careful biochemical control and, if the maximum rates of infusion are used, ECG monitoring). A concentrated solution of potassium chloride [the contents of a sterile ampoule containing 20 mmol (1.5 g) of potassium chloride] is added to 500 ml isotonic saline, dextrose-saline or dextrose solution as required, and *mixed thoroughly* before the infusion is begun.

Renal complications of excessive uric acid production

See also page 9.123 *et seq.*

Sodium urate nephropathy (gouty or chronic hyperuricaemic nephropathy)

Macroscopically, the kidneys are shrunken and feel firm. The histological lesions are interstitial deposits of monosodium urate (microtophi), particularly in the pyramid regions, segmental destruction of renal tissue (incorrectly referred to as urate infarcts), interstitial fibrosis, epithelial necrosis, glomerulosclerosis with uniform fibrillar thickening of the capillary basement membrane, atrophic dilation with pigmentary epithelial degeneration of the loops of Henle. Pyelonephritic and hypertensive lesions may also be present. Before the use of uricosuric drugs and allopurinol and before reliable serum uric acid measurements were readily available, the kidneys of virtually all cases of untreated gout showed either sodium urate crystals, pyelonephritis, and/or hypertensive vascular changes at post-mortem. There was usually a strong correlation between the clinical severity of the gout and the extent of the pathological changes in the kidneys. Because of early diagnosis on the basis of mild joint disease and the recognition of hyperuricaemia, the degree of functional renal impairment does not now correlate well with the degree of hyperuricaemia. Sodium urate nephropathy is rarely seen, but the associated renal vascular disease, uric acid calculi, and pyelonephritis are still important. The parenchymal and interstitial damage is not necessarily associated with either uric acid stones, or with microliths in the collecting tubules. Although they are interrelated, a high concentration of uric acid in the renal tubule appears to be a more important pathophysiological determinant of renal damage than the concentration of urate in the blood perfusing the kidney.

Clinical aspects

Except for the coexistence of gouty arthritis, uric acid calculi and early inability to alkalinize the urine the clinical features of patients with sodium urate nephropathy are the same as those of other patients with chronic renal failure. Before the introduction of uricosuric drugs, allopurinol, and reliable plasma uric acid measurements, the incidence of albuminuria and hypertension were between 20 and 40 per cent in patients whose hyperuricaemia was of sufficient degree and duration for them to have presented with gouty arthritis. About 25 per cent of these patients are said to have died from uraemia. These complications are now rarely seen.

Patients with sodium urate nephropathy present with asymptomatic proteinuria accompanied by hyperuricaemia, or with renal failure and hyperuricaemia which is disproportionate to the degree of renal failure. Occasionally, severe renal failure due to sodium urate nephropathy occurs in patients who have never suffered from gouty arthritis. A plasma uric acid concentration consistently greater than 0.55 mmol (9.24 mg/dl) in association with renal failure suggests either sodium urate nephropathy, or renal failure due to another cause in a patient who also has essential hyperuricaemia (i.e. without either primary gouty arthritis or another identifiable cause for the hyperuricaemia). This diagnostic uncertainty may be unresolvable because both the renal biopsy and the post-mortem histology show only non-specific chronic inflammatory and vascular changes; and imaging techniques show only small symmetrically shrunken kidneys. However, either increased uric acid excretion or the presence of monosodium urate crystals in a specimen of kidney tissue (fixed in alcohol) make the diagnosis much more probable.

The increasing practice of routine biochemical screening raises the question of the possible adverse affects of relatively minor degrees of hyperuricaemia on renal function in the future. A recent survey has shown that among asymptomatic individuals in whom azotaemia and hyperuricaemia were found on routine screening, the azotaemia was generally mild and probably of no clinical importance until serum acid values reached 0.821 mmol/l (13 mg/dl) in men and 0.595 mmol/l (9 mg/dl) in women. These findings and the results of other modern studies support the view that asymptomatic hyperuricaemia only very rarely requires treatment on the grounds that it materially increases the risk of renal failure in the future.

The commonest practical problem nowadays, is the asymptomatic patient in whom hyperuricaemia and proteinuria are detected on routine examination. In almost all of these there is a cause for the proteinuria other than the hyperuricaemia. These patients are commonly hypertensive and the high serum urate is thought to be in some way associated with the hypertension. The mechanism of this is uncertain but one suggestion is that minor vascular damage impairs the tubular re-excretion of urate.

Treatment

A patient with established renal failure, asymptomatic hyperuricaemia, and without present or past hyperuric aciduria only needs allopurinol if the plasma uric acid concentration consistently exceeds 0.8 mmol/l (12.7 mg/dl). The dose of allopurinol should be reduced in renal failure because it may have unusually severe toxic side-effects in this situation. Hyperuric aciduria, the presence of crystals in the kidney tissue or attacks of proven acute gouty arthritis, indicate allopurinol at lower plasma uric acid concentrations. Any loss of renal function attributable to renal deposits of sodium urate can be arrested, but not reversed, by allopurinol treatment. Patients with renal failure and marked hyperuricaemia usually die within a few years unless the uraemia is treated. In patients on chronic haemodialysis, the serum uric acid rises more rapidly than the blood urea between dialyses.

Urinary stones

Pathophysiology

Between 5 and 33 per cent of untreated primary gout patients in different series in Europe and North America have urinary stones, the incidence in the control population being about 0.1 per cent. This high incidence is now decreasing. Most of these stones (84 per cent) are pure uric acid, 4 per cent are a mixture of uric acid and calcium oxalate, and 12 per cent are mixed calcium oxalate–

phosphate stones. The incidence of stones is higher in secondary than in primary gout. The risk of asymptomatic hyperuricaemia patients developing a stone is about three times greater than in the non-hyperuricaemic subjects. Uric acid renal calculi begin as intratubular microliths and the impaired ability to alkalinize their urine displayed by some gout patients favours stone formation. The gross purine overproduction which occurs with hypoxanthine guanine phosphoribosyltransferase (HPRT) deficiency and in phosphoribosylpyrophosphate synthetase (PRPP-Sy) deficiency is associated with a high risk of urolithiasis (page 9.123 et seq.). Both of these inborn errors of metabolism are inherited as sex-linked recessives. Virtually complete HPRT deficiency causes the Lesch–Nyhan syndrome. Less severe degrees of HPRT deficiency and PRPP-Sy deficiency cause the X-linked recessive gout–nephrolithiasis–renal failure syndrome. The other familial hyperuricaemia syndrome (autosomal dominant hyperuricaemic nephropathy) comprises severe gout, hyperuricaemia, and renal failure which usually begins in the second decade, but no stones. The rate of purine de novo synthesis is not accelerated in this disease and it has recently been proposed that the metabolic lesion may be in the secretory component of the bidirectional transport of urate across the renal tubule epithelium.

Uric acid excretion should not exceed 3.66 mmol (600 mg) per 24 hours after 5 days on a purine-free diet. In the absence of dietary restriction, in the United Kingdom, a urinary uric acid excretion of 4.87 mmol (800 mg) per 24 hours indicates a significant degree of hyperuric aciduria.

Clinical aspects

The clinical features of uric acid stones are the same as those of other types of radiotranslucent urinary stone (see page 18.87 et seq.).

Hyperuric aciduria should not be treated unless it is associated with recurrent urolithiasis, except in HPRT and PRPP-Sy deficiencies where there is massive overproduction of uric acid.

Acute uric acid nephropathy

Pathophysiology

Acute uric acid nephropathy is an uncommon complication of cancer chemotherapy. It arises when extensive malignant disease is treated with cytotoxic drugs and/or irradiation. A large quantity of nucleic acid is rapidly degraded to urate and uric acid precipitates in the renal tubules, the pelvicalceal system and ureters, causing acute oliguric renal failure. The following may be contributory factors: (a) essential hyperuricaemia and hyperuricaciduria due to increased uric acid synthesis which is independent of, but increased by, the malignant process; (b) the excretion of a persistently acid urine due to the metabolic acidosis associated with a high level of anaerobic metabolism in the tumour and the catabolism of large amounts of tissue protein; this decreases the solubility of uric acid; (c) pre-existing inability to secrete an alkaline urine; (d) dehydration; and (e) the use of carcinostatic and other drugs which either stimulate the rate of purine de novo synthesis or are uricosuric.

Clinical aspects

The patient develops anuria or gross oliguria and azotaemia usually during the course of treatment of a reticulosis of myeloproliferative disorder. This arises in the latter case shortly after the leukocyte count has fallen most rapidly. The patient is febrile, dehydrated, and may have had flank pain or ureteric colic. Catheterization of the bladder yields only a small volume of blood-stained urine, which contains protein and sometimes uric acid crystals. The plasma urate and urine uric acid levels may be as high as 4.77 mmol/l (80 mg.dl) and 30 mmol (5000 mg) per 24 hours, respectively. Ultrasonography is the first investigation and will reliably detect the presence of hydroureters and hydronephroses due to bilateral impacted ureteric calculi, provided there has been a sufficient flow of urine and enough time has elapsed for dilation to occur. Ultrasonography can distinguish radiotranslucent pure uric acid stones from soft tissue shadows such as tumours and sloughed renal papillae. Intravenous urography is still necessary in this situation when ultrasonography gives negative or equivocal results as would be expected were the pelvicalyceal systems and ureters full of loose uric acid sludge. Intravenous urograms in acute uric acid nephropathy show an immediate dense and persistent nephelogram and the radiocontrast agent does not enter the renal pelves and ureters.

It is difficult to predict which patients will develop the acute obstructive urinary complications of cytotoxic drug therapy. The following may be pointers to their occurrence: (a) the presence of a large mass of malignant tissue; (b) a previous similar obstructive episode; (c) difficulty in maintaining an output of about 3 litres of alkaline urine per 24 hours; (d) pretreatment urinary uric acid concentrations approaching 11.9 mmol/l (200 mg/dl) (this is the solubility of sodium urate in urine at pH 7.0); (e) marked hyperuricaemia [serum uric acid greater than 0.714 mmol/1 (12 mg/dl)].

Acute uric acid nephropathy has also occurred after multiple epileptic seizures, the suggested source of the uric acid being the large amount of inosinic acid produced during violent protracted ischaemic muscle contraction, and nucleic acids liberated by muscle cell injury.

Treatment

Acute uric acid nephropathy can be prevented by giving allopurinol (for example, 200 mg 8 hourly) for 5 days before, as well as during the course of cytotoxic drug therapy or irradiation. A high rate of flow of alkaline urine should also be maintained. Allopurinol spreads the total urinary purine load between three compounds each with its own solubility [the solubilities of uric acid, hypoxanthine, and xanthine in urine at pH 7.0 are 11.9, 11.0, and 0.8 mmol/l (200, 150, and 13 mg/dl), respectively]. Obstructive uropathy due to either xanthine or oxipurinol (the metabolite of allopurinol) crystals and stones has been reported, but it is very rare and should not deter the use of allopurinol in this situation.

If an alkaline diuresis cannot be achieved with mannitol infusion [200 ml of a 20 per cent (w/v) solution over the course of 15–30 min] plus intravenous sodium bicarbonate, frusemide, and acetazolamide (a carbonic anhydrase inhibitor which stimulates the production of an alkaline urine) it may be necessary to catheterize the ureters and irrigate with a bicarbonate solution. An alternative may be to insert fine plastic catheters into the renal pelves percutaneously under imaging control and to irrigate the renal pelvis and ureters from above. The use of a intravenous urography to guide the placement of the pelvic catheters may be impossible because of failure of a radio-opaque agent to enter the pelvicalyceal system in sufficient concentrations. Allopurinol does not help the established case although it may be given after the urine flow has been re-established in order to prevent a recurrence. If the uraemia cannot be managed conservatively, haemodialysis will be required. A decision to adopt these additional measures will depend on the patient's general suitability with respect to the manifestations and prognosis of the primary disease. Provided a diuresis can be achieved, the outlook for the recovery of renal function is good.

Hereditary nephrogenic diabetes insipidus (page 18.23)

Pathophysiology

The nature of the metabolic defect which makes the cells of the distal convoluted and collecting tubules of the kidney resistant to the action of vasopressin is unknown. Hereditary nephrogenic diabetes insipidus is inherited as a sex-linked recessive. Minor degrees of impaired responsiveness to vasopressin (antidiuretic hormone) can also be demonstrated in the carrier females. There are no characteristic morbid anatomical or histopathological find-

ings related to the kidney in this disorder. Shortening of the proximal convoluted tubules has been reported on the basis of single nephron microdissection.

Antidiuretic hormone binds to the contraluminal plasma membranes of the collecting duct cells and activates adenylcyclase. This increases the production of cyclic adenosine-3′,5′monophosphate (cyclic AMP or cAMP) which increases the rate of water transport across the cells. The precise mechanism by which the solubility of water in the cell membrane is increased is not known. It is suggested that in hereditary nephrogenic diabetes insipidus, there is inability to accumulate cAMP.

Clinical aspects

Vasopressin-resistant diabetes insipidus presents in the affected males soon after birth with polyuria, dehydration, vomiting, fever, and convulsions. Failure to thrive and polydipsia are apparent in slightly older children. The patients may die in infancy if the episodes of severe dehydration are not recognized and treated promptly. They are unable to concentrate their urine beyond a specific gravity of about 1005 or between 50 and 100 mosmol/kg water although during solute diuresis the urine osmolality may approach isotonicity with the plasma (285–295 mosmol/kg water). If untreated the condition is associated with impaired mental and physical development, which is ascribed to polydipsia. This interferes with adequate food intake, rest, and play. Bladder distension and hydronephrosis occur in older children.

The characteristic syndrome of polydipsia, polyuria, and persistent hyposthenuria is only apparent when hydration is adequate. Nephrogenic diabetes insipidus is differentiated from the neurohypophyseal type by the inability of the well-hydrated individual to respond to vasopressin. The condition is particularly likely to be missed if there is no ascertainable family history of the condition. Repeated unexplained episodes of fever, dehydration, and constipation with failure to thrive in male infants should suggest the diagnosis. Persistent hypotonicity of the urine is the only specific laboratory finding; any other abnormalities in the plasma and urine composition are due to dehydration or associated disorders. The incompletely expressed form of the disease in the female carriers has to be differentiated from other types of renal disease in which there is a marked impairment of urine concentrating ability.

The affected boys are at risk in early life from the acute episodes described above. Intercurrent infection worsens the immediate prognosis. Life expectancy is normal and, if the episodes of dehydration can be avoided, it should also be possible to achieve normal physical and mental development. The female carriers do not usually require any special treatment.

Treatment

The acute episodes require vigorous fluid replacement. Although 5 per cent dextrose intravenously is usually appropriate in the treatment of pure water depletion it may aggravate the hypertonicity in this situation, and 2.5 or 3 per cent dextrose is recommended. Water should be administered by mouth as soon as possible. The plasma osmolality should be monitored during treatment.

The patient should always drink enough to avoid underhydration. A moderate degree of sodium depletion, produced by a low sodium diet, and a thiazide diuretic (with potassium supplements), reduces the chronic polyuria.

References

Bayliss, R., Clarke, C., Whitehead, T. P. and Whitfield, A. G. W. (1982). The management of hyperuricaemia. *J. R. Coll. Phys.* **18**, 144–146.

Culpepper, R. M., Herbert, S. C. and Andreoli, T. E. (1983). Nephrogenic diabetes insipidus. In *The metabolic basis of inherited disease* 5th edn (eds J. B. Stanbury, J. B. Wyngaarden, D. S. Fredrickson, J. L. Goldstein and M. S. Brown), pp. 1867–1888. McGraw-Hill, New York.

Emmerson, B. T. (1983). *Hyperuricaemia and gout in clinical practice.* ADIS Health Science Press, Sydney.

Fessel, W. J. (1979). Renal outcomes of gout and hyperuricaemia. *Am. J. Med.* **67**, 74–82.

Hande, K. R., Noone, R. M. and Stone, W. J. (1984). Severe allopurinol toxicity. Description and guidelines for prevention in patients' with renal insufficiency. *Am. J. Med.* **76**, 47–56.

Ralson, S. H., Gardner, M. D., Dryburgh, F. J., Jenkins, A. S., Cowan, R. A. and Boyle, I. T. (1985). A comparison of aminohydroxypropylidene diphosphonate, mithramycin and corticosteroid/calcitonin in the treatment of cancer-associated hypercalcaemia. *Lancet* **ii**, 907–910.

Wyngaarden, J. B. and Kelly, W. N. (1983). Gout. In *The metabolic basis of inherited disease* 5th edn (eds J. B. Stanbury, J. B. Wyngaarden, D. S. Frederickson, J. L. Goldstein and M. S. Brown), pp. 1043–1114. McGraw-Hill, New York.

Yü, T-F., Berger, L., Dorph, D. J. and Smith, H. (1979). Renal function in gout. V. Factors influencing renal haemodynamics. *Am. J. Med.* **67**, 766–771.

Yü, T-F. and Berger, L. (1982). *The kidney in gout and hyperuricaemia.* Futura Publishing Co., New York.

URINARY TRACT OBSTRUCTION

L. R. I. BAKER

Synonyms

Obstructive uropathy. The term 'hydronephrosis' is here taken to mean dilation of the renal pelvis. Here the term 'obstructive nephropathy' is taken to mean urinary tract obstruction causing prolongation of the transit time of glomerular filtrate down the nephron.

Definition

If the flow of urine is impeded at any point in its course from renal calyces to the exterior, urinary tract obstruction is present.

Obstruction may be partial or complete. Dilation of the outflow system proximal to the site of obstruction is a characteristic finding. The condition is remediable in most cases and is often a serious threat to life if undiagnosed and untreated. Bilateral obstruction or obstruction of a single kidney is a greater threat than unilateral obstruction. Complete obstruction is a greater threat than partial obstruction.

Aetiology

Obstructing lesions may lie within the lumen or the wall of the urinary tract, or may cause obstruction by pressure from outside. The major causes in each group are listed in Table 1.

Calculi and neuromuscular dysfunction at the junction of renal pelvis and ureter are common causes of unilateral obstruction. Prostatic obstruction, stone disease, and bladder tumours account for approximately 75 per cent of cases of bilateral obstruction in developed countries. Wide geographical variations occur in the relative incidence of some causes of obstruction, for example, schistosomiasis.

Urinary tract obstruction has been found in 3.8 per cent of a large series of routine autopsies and 25 per cent of autopsies carried out upon uraemic patients. Obstruction is a relatively common cause of renal failure in infants and children, owing to congenital anomalies, and in elderly men owing to prostatic obstruction. The overall frequency of urinary tract obstruction is the same in men and women. Between 20 and 60 years of age, obstruction is more frequent in women. Over the age of 60 years, the reverse is the case.

Pathophysiology

Obstruction with continuing urine formation results in a progressive rise in intraluminal pressure and dilation of the system proximal to the site of obstruction. The nearer intraluminal pressure approaches to glomerular filtration pressure, the lower becomes the glomerular filtration rate (GFR). Dilation of the urinary tract tends to protect nephrons from the damaging effects of backpressure but only to a limited extent.

In the early phase of obstruction, the kidney becomes oedematous and haemorrhagic. If obstruction persists, the kidney enlarges because of dilation of the renal pelvis. Such dilation causes compression and thinning of the renal parenchyma. Initially, the papillae and medulla bear the main brunt of compression but the renal cortex is also affected. With long-standing

Table 1 Causes of urinary tract obstruction

Within the lumen	Within the wall	Pressure from outside
Calculus	Pelvi-ureteric neuromuscular dysfunction (congenital, 10 per cent bilateral)	Pelvi-ureteric compression (bands, aberrant vessels)
Blood clot		
Sloughed papilla (diabetes, analgesic abuse, sickle cell disease)	Ureteral stricture (tuberculosis, especially after treatment; postoperative calculus)	Tumours, e.g. retroperitoneal growth or glands, carcinoma of colon, diverticulitis, aortic aneurysm
Tumour of renal pelvis or ureter	Uretero-vesical stricture (congenital, ureterocoele, calculus, schistosomiasis)	Retroperitoneal fibrosis
Bladder tumour		Accidental ligation of ureter
	Congenital megaureter	Retrocaval ureter (right-sided obstruction)
	Congenital bladder neck obstruction	Prostatic obstruction
	Neuropathic bladder	Tumours in pelvis, e.g. carcinoma of cervix
	Urethral stricture (calculus, gonococcal, after instrumentation)	Phimosis
	Congenital urethral valve	
	Pinhole meatus	

obstruction, the dilated calyces and pelvis are surrounded by only a thin rim of renal parenchyma. Reduction in size of the kidney, due to postobstructive atrophy, is a frequent occurrence in the long term. Slowly progressive partial obstruction tends to lead to gross dilation of the collecting system. In acute complete obstruction, dilation tends to be less.

An early histological change is tubular dilation involving first the collecting ducts and later the distal and proximal convoluted tubules. Flattening and eventual atrophy of tubular lining cells occurs. In advanced cases, patchy fibrosis involves collapsed tubules and glomeruli. The changes of pyelonephritis and of papillary necrosis may be superimposed.

The time-course of these events in humans is not known with certainty. Four factors influence the rate at which kidney damage occurs, its extent, and the degree and rapidity of recovery of renal function after relief of obstruction. These are: (a) whether obstruction is partial or complete; (b) the duration of obstruction; (c) whether or not infection occurs; and (d) the site of obstruction.

Complete obstruction for several weeks will lead to irreversible or only partially reversible kidney damage. Complete obstruction for several months spells total, irreversible destruction of the affected kidney. Partial obstruction carries a better prognosis, depending upon its severity. Bacterial infection commonly occurs, coincident with obstruction and stasis, rapidly hastening kidney damage. Obstruction at or below the bladder neck may induce hypertrophy and trabeculation of the bladder without a rise in pressure within the upper urinary tract, in which case the kidneys are protected from the effects of back-pressure. This is not the case with obstruction at more proximal sites.

Clinical features

Clinical features may be divided into those of upper tract obstruction and those of bladder outflow obstruction. Either may be complicated by urinary tract infection.

Upper tract obstruction may be symptomless or give rise to vague, mild symptoms such as backache and malaise. Loin pain may be dull or sharp, colicky or intermittent. It may be provoked by a high fluid intake, alcohol or diuretics, measures which increase urinary volume and hence distension of the collecting system, particularly in pelvi-ureteric junction obstruction. Loin tenderness may be present and an enlarged hydronephrotic kidney palpable. Upper urinary tract infection with malaise, fever, loin pain, and tenderness, and symptoms and signs of septicaemia may dominate the clinical picture.

Complete anuria is strongly suggestive of complete bilateral obstruction or complete obstruction of a single kidney. The differential diagnosis includes bilateral total renal cortical necrosis, acute anuric glomerulonephritis, and bilateral renal arterial occlusion. Conversely, polyuria may occur in partial obstruction due to impairment of renal tubular concentrating capacity. Intermittent anuria and polyuria indicate intermittent complete obstruction. Occasionally, hypertension and erythraemia occur in association with hydronephrosis. Improvement after relief of obstruction has been described in each case.

In bladder outflow obstruction, symptoms may be minimal or may be accepted by the patient as within normal limits. Hesitancy, narrowing, and diminished force of the urinary stream, terminal dribbling and a sense of incomplete bladder emptying are typical features. If a large volume of residual urine remains in the bladder after urination, the frequent passage of small volumes of urine may be a prominent symptom even in the absence of infection. Incontinence of such small volumes of urine is termed overflow incontinence or retention with overflow. Acute complete retention of urine, usually with severe suprapubic and perineal pain, may occur. In acute or chronic retention, the enlarged bladder can be felt or percussed after an attempt at voiding.

Lower urinary tract infection occurs commonly in association with bladder outflow obstruction. Frequency, urgency, urge incontinence, dysuria, strangury, suprapubic pain, haematuria,

and cloudy, smelly urine may be present. Asymptomatic bacteriuria is common.

Examination of genitalia, and rectal and vaginal examination are essential. It should be noted that the apparent size of the prostate is a poor guide to the presence of prostatic obstruction. Median lobe enlargement of a palpably normal prostate may give rise to severe obstruction, whereas an apparently grossly enlarged gland may cause little or no obstruction.

Diagnosis

It is essential that obstruction be excluded in all patients with unexplained renal failure. In patients with known renal disease, rapid deterioration in renal function unexplained by the primary renal problem likewise demands investigation. The occurrence of recurrent or relapsing urinary tract infections should raise the possibility of an associated obstructing lesion. The diagnosis of partial obstruction should not be discounted simply because urine volume is normal or increased.

The history should include enquiry as to analgesic abuse (associated with papillary necrosis, transitional cell tumours, and periureteric fibrosis), vitamin D consumption (associated with calculus formation), consumption of methysergide (associated with retroperitoneal fibrosis), and employment history and smoking habits (because of the increased incidence of bladder cancer in, for example, aniline dye workers and cigarette smokers). A history or family history of gout, diabetes or renal stone formation should be obtained.

The diagnosis of obstruction cannot be made by biochemical tests or examination of the urine. Particular attention should be

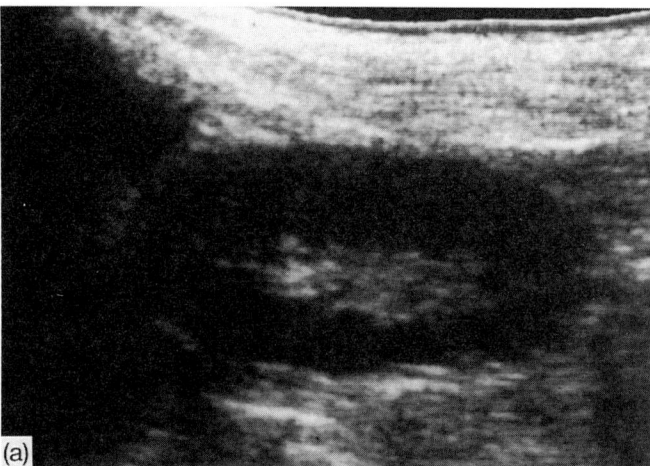

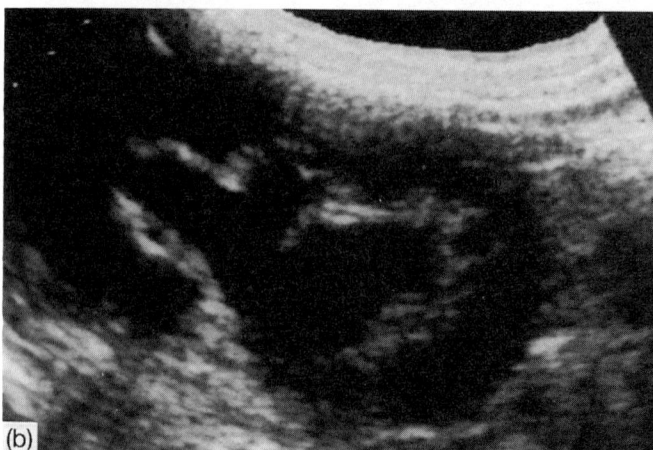

Fig. 1 (a) Longitudinal scan of normal kidney showing central sinus echoes. (b) Longitudinal scan of obstructed kidney showing dilated collecting system surrounded by sinus echoes.

paid in the physical examination to the possibility of a neurological lesion or a pelvic neoplasm (particularly prostate or cervix uteri) causing bladder or ureteric obstruction.

Diagnostic ultrasonography

Renal echograms obtained with commercially available grey scale equipment can detect upper urinary tract dilation. Not surprisingly in view of the great variability of normal collecting systems and renal pelvic anatomy, false-positive diagnoses are common. In one report 20 out of 71 examinations were false-positive but this is not a fatal drawback to the use of ultrasound as a *screening* test. It has now been demonstrated that ultrasonography can be relied upon in screening for upper urinary tract obstruction, provided appropriate facilities and expertise are available. It is possible therefore safely to dispense with urography in a substantial proportion of patients who would previously have required this investigation. Ultrasonography is non-invasive, painless, and without risk. It is especially helpful when intravenous urography is undesirable owing to allergy to radiographic contrast media or pregnancy.

Given appropriate facilities and expertise, initial investigation of the patient with unexplained impairment of renal function should comprise ultrasonography, together with plain abdominal X-ray and renal tomography to screen for urinary tract calculi. Tomography may be necessary to detect low-density calculi. In about 50 per cent of cases, unobstructed kidneys will be demonstrated (Fig. 1) and other means of detecting upper tract dilation, such as high-dose excretion urography and computer assisted tomography (CT) will be unnecessary. Judicious use of CT in addition to ultrasonography and plain X-rays will render urography unnecessary in more than 80 per cent of cases. Computer assisted tomography is of particular value in the assessment of ultrasound false-positive results, in the demonstration of calculi, including uric acid calculi (Fig. 2), and in demonstrating the cause of obstruction in patients with malignant disease and retroperitoneal fibrosis (Fig. 3).

Use of radionuclides

Radioactive iodine-labelled *o*-iodohippurate (hippuran) may be injected intravenously and the uptake of radioactivity by the kidney, its concentration therein, and its excretion assessed by scintillation detectors placed over the kidneys. The excretory phase is delayed in acute obstruction and the technique may be used as a screening test for this condition. Such delay is not diagnostic of obstruction, being seen, for example, in some cases of acute tubular necrosis and in the presence of a baggy, dilated but unobstructed collecting system. An 'obstructed' pattern may also be seen for some time *after* obstruction has been relieved and is difficult to interpret in long-standing obstruction. This, and the fact that the method does not provide anatomical information, limits its usefulness. Provided computer assisted subtraction of blood background radioactivity is performed, absence of uptake of radioactive hippuran indicates renal damage sufficiently severe to render correction of obstruction unprofitable. Relative renal blood-flow rates may similarly be deduced by background subtraction renography and this information can be helpful when a decision must be made as to whether or not to operate upon a kidney damaged by long-standing obstruction.

More detailed information, including anatomical information, is provided by dynamic renal scintigraphy. In this technique DTPA labelled with ^{99m}Tc (technetium-99m) is injected and gamma-camera imaging of the kidneys is carried out followed by computer analysis. Scintigraphy allows a distinction to be made between retention of isotope within the renal pelvis and prolongation of nephron transit time (obstructive nephropathy) hence permitting the distinction of a baggy unobstructed renal pelvis from an obstructive lesion which may require surgical treatment.

Whether ultrasonography or radionuclides are used to screen

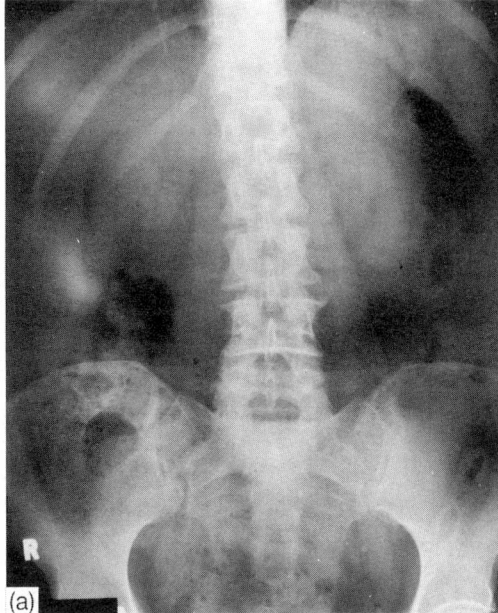

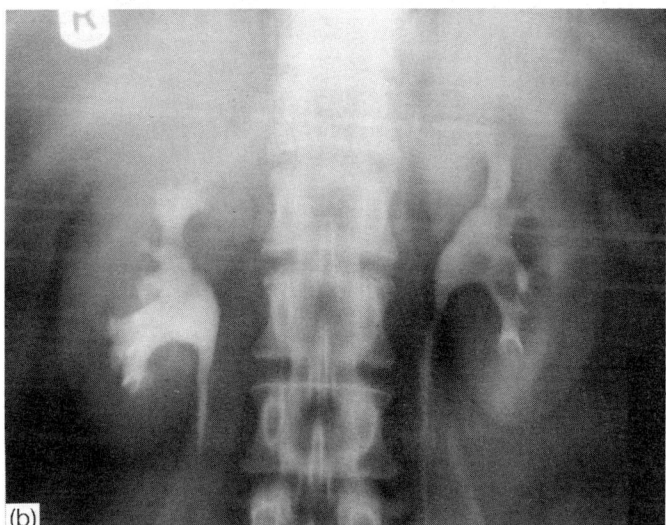

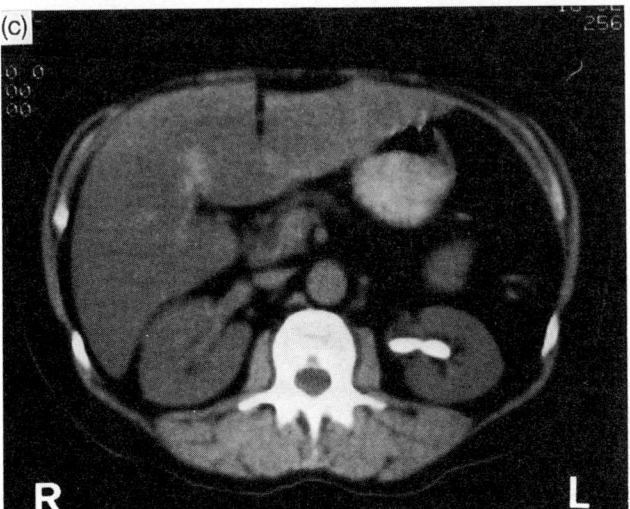

Fig. 2 (a) Plain abdominal X-ray in patient with left flank pain. (b) Same patient after injection of contrast. Note filling defects in collecting system on left side. (c) CT scan in same patient. Calculi in left collecting system are clearly seen. Subsequent chemical analysis showed calculi to be composed of uric acid.

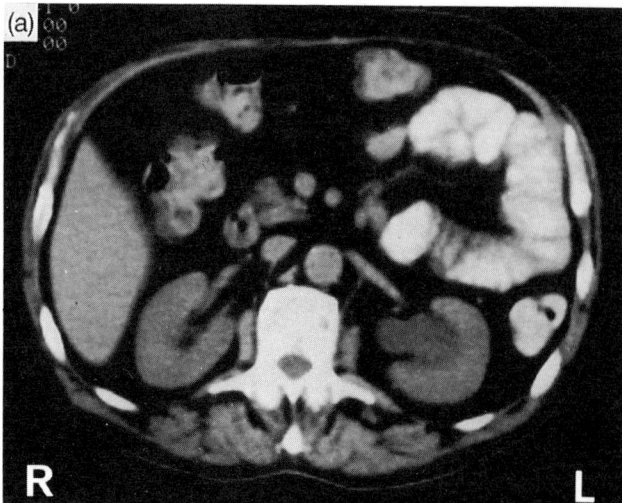

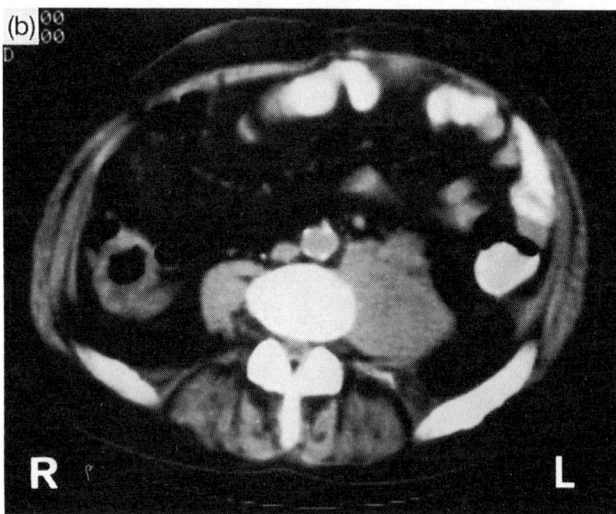

Fig. 3 (a) Abdominal CT scan in patient with ureteric obstruction due to malignancy. Note dilation of collecting system of left kidney. (b) Same CT scan as (a) at a different level showing malignant growth in left psoas region.

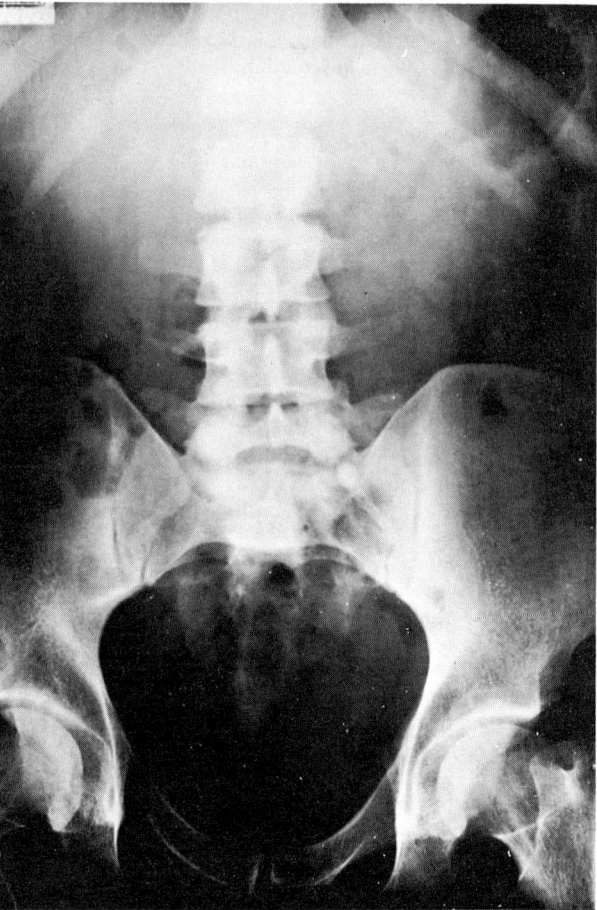

Fig. 4 Calculus overlying sacrum on left side is easily missed.

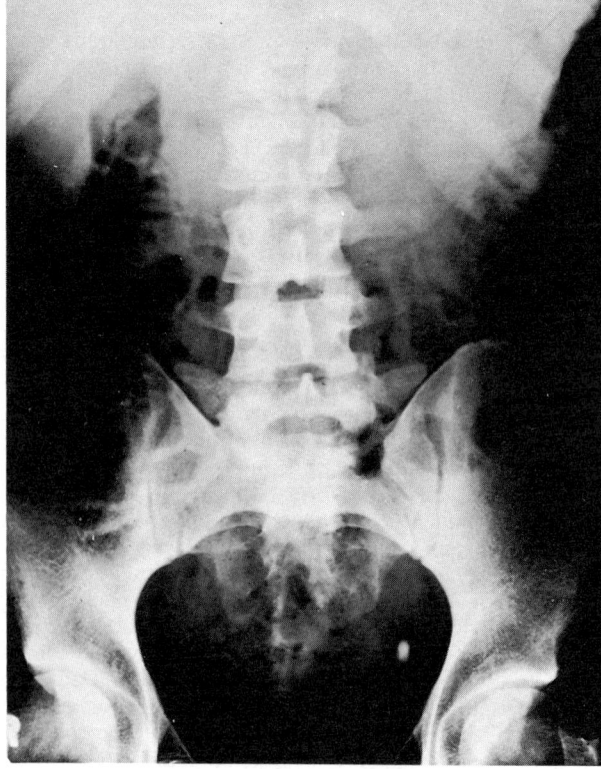

Fig. 5 Same patient as in Fig. 4 one week later. The calculus has descended and is now readily seen in the left side of the pelvis.

for urinary tract obstruction will depend in any given institution upon the availability of particular techniques and expertise.

Excretion urography (intravenous urography, IVU)

Excretion urography is still widely used in the diagnosis of urinary tract obstruction. Properly carried out, urography can usually exclude the diagnosis of obstruction even in the presence of severe renal failure (GFR less than 5 ml/min). Previous statements that a satisfactory examination cannot be carried out if the blood urea exceeds 16.5 mmol/1 (100 mg/dl) are untrue, provided that a high dose of a contrast medium such as sodium diatrizoate is given (usually as a single intravenous injection) and tomography of the renal areas is carried out if necessary. Late films over a period of 24 hours after injection of contrast may need to be taken. In patients with renal failure, prior dehydration must be avoided before excretion urography. Given this precaution and the use of modern contrast media, deterioration of kidney function attributable to the investigation rarely occurs. Patients with myelomatosis and diabetes mellitus are currently considered to be an exception to this rule. The films should be studied with the following questions in mind:

1. Are calculi or nephrocalcinosis visible on the plain film taken before injection of contrast?
2. Are two kidneys present?

3. What is their size?

4. What is the pattern of development of the nephrogram?

5. Is the collecting system shown sufficiently well, whether filled with contrast or as a negative shadow, to allow a conclusion as to the presence or absence of dilation?

6. Is there renal cortical thinning?

7. Is the ureter dilated and to what level? Is it displaced?

8. Does the bladder contain a filling defect?

9. Is bladder emptying complete on the after-voiding radiograph?

The plain film is an essential part of the examination. Calculi overlying bone are easily missed (Figs 4 and 5).

In recent unilateral obstruction, the affected kidney is enlarged and smooth in outline. The nephrogram is delayed owing to reduction in GFR and the calyces and pelvis fill with contrast later than occurs on the normal side. In time, an increasingly dense nephrogram develops on the affected side, eventually becoming denser than normal owing to the prolonged nephron transit time which allows greater than normal concentration of contrast medium within the tubules. In time, the site of obstruction may become obvious owing to dilation of the system to the level of the block (Figs 6–9).

Vesico-ureteric reflux results in dilation of the ureter and pelvicalyceal system in the absence of obstruction. Dilation of the *lower* ureter is a typical feature. Reflux can be demonstrated by micturating cystography. Observation of the free drainage of contrast medium from ureter to bladder on screening excludes the diagnosis of obstruction.

In women who have been pregnant, particularly those who have suffered pregnancy bacteriuria, one or both upper ureters (more often the right) may be dilated to the pelvic brim (Fig. 10). Obstruction is excluded by observing emptying of the system on a full-length postmicturition film (Fig. 11). Dilation of pelvis and calyces will not be present.

Typical radiographic appearances in obstruction at the pelviureteric junction due to neuromuscular dysfunction are shown in Fig. 12). The appearances may be accentuated by copious drinking of water or injection of frusemide during the examination.

The value of delayed renal tomography is illustrated in Fig. 13.

Excretion urography should include a full-length film taken after an attempt at bladder emptying by the patient. Complete emptying of the bladder indicates either that no obstruction to bladder outflow exists or that intravesical pressure can be raised sufficiently to overcome it. Apparent failure to empty may indi-

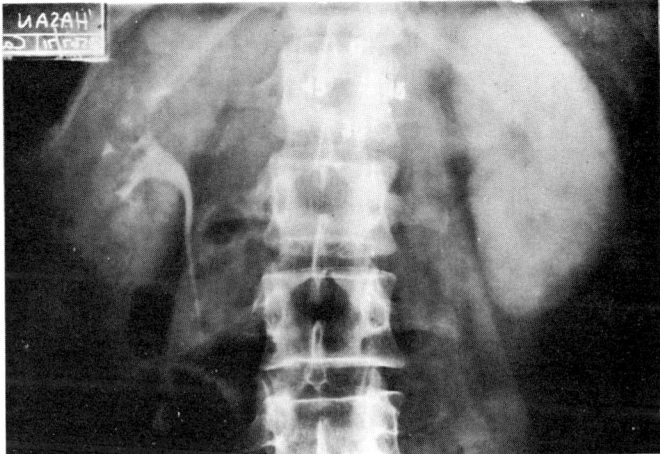

Fig. 6 Acute left ureteric obstruction. Note increased density of the nephrogram and absence of pyelogram on the left side 15 min after injection of contrast.

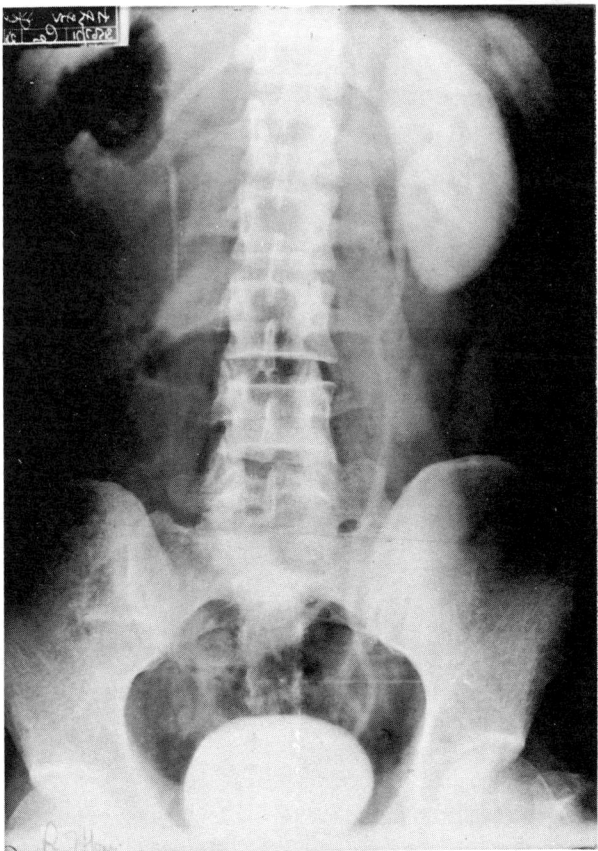

Fig. 7 Same patient as in Fig. 6. Later radiograph showing persistent dense nephrogram on the left. The pelvi-calyceal system and ureter which have now filled are only slightly dilated owing to very recent onset of obstruction. Obstructing calculus at the left ureteric orifice is not visible.

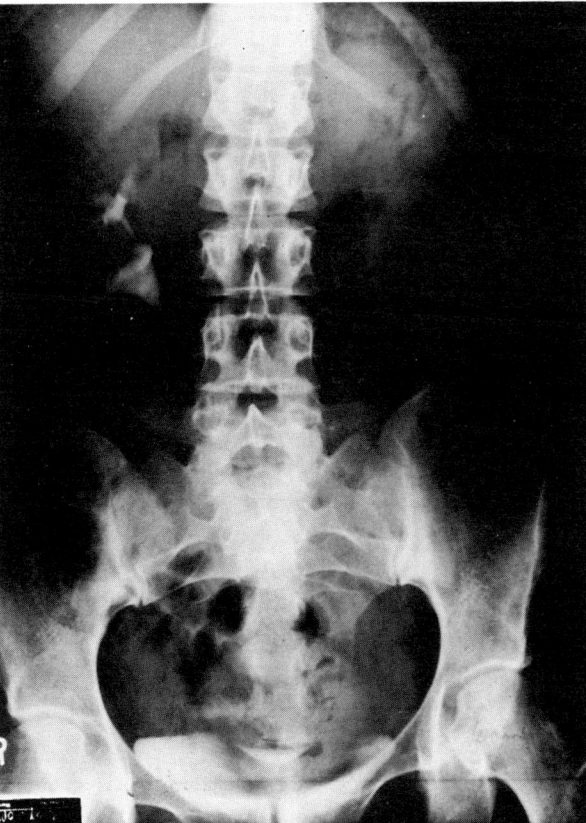

Fig. 8 More long-standing calculus obstruction on the left side. The nephrogram on the left has not appeared 10 min after injection of contrast.

cate a poor attempt at emptying by a nervous, embarrassed patient, failure to carry out the X-ray before the bladder has refilled with contrast from above, a hypotonic, non-obstructed bladder, vesico-ureteric reflux (in which condition contrast returns to the bladder from the collecting system), or outflow obstruction.

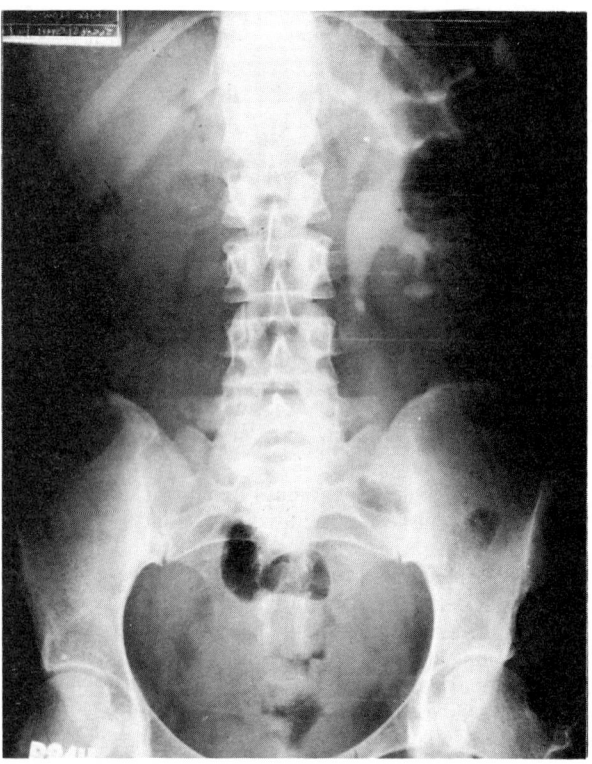

Fig. 9 Same patient as in Fig. 8. Radiograph taken 24 hours after injection shows delayed nephrogram and pyelogram on the left side. By this time, no contrast medium is visible on the normal right side.

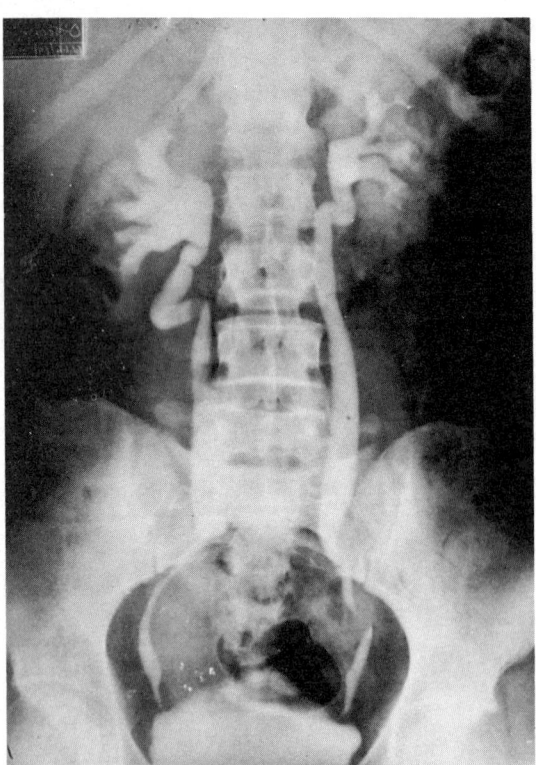

Fig. 10 Ureters dilated to level of pelvic brim following pregnancy bacteriuria.

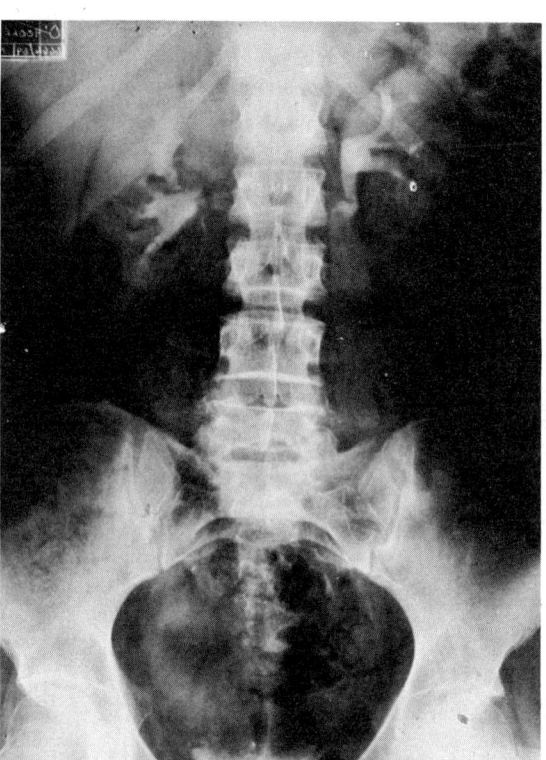

Fig. 11 Same patient as in Fig. 10. After-voiding radiograph. Note good emptying of ureters.

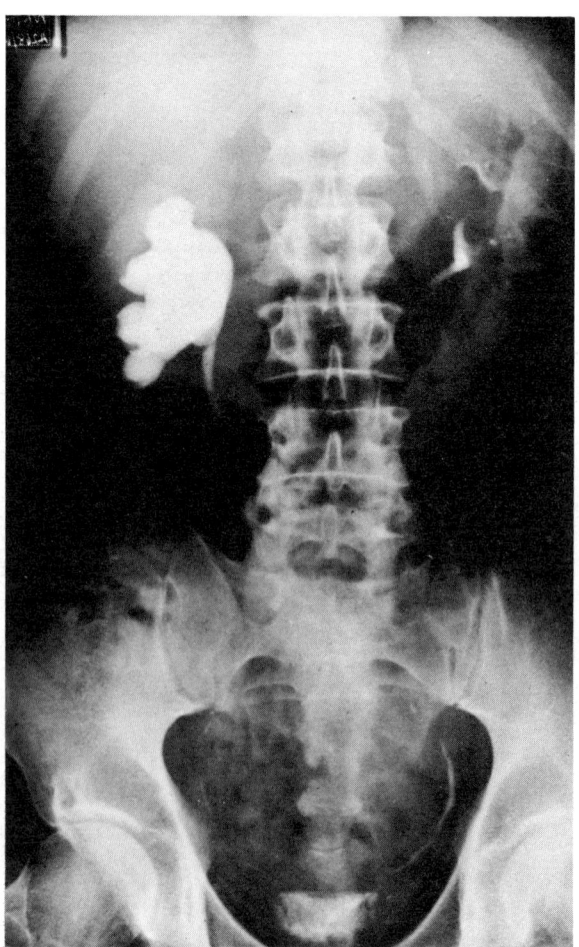

Fig. 12 Right pelvi-ureteric junctional obstruction. No mechanical obstructing lesion present.

A search for bladder tumours, tuberculosis, calculi, and trabeculation should be made. The size of the prostatic impression upon the base of the bladder is a very poor guide to the actual size of the gland.

Significant incomplete obstruction
There is no generally accepted definition of significant incomplete obstruction to outflow. Dilation of the collecting system is not diagnostic. Incomplete obstruction is only important clinically if it causes deterioration in kidney function which can be halted or corrected by surgery. Patients with one kidney or with bilateral obstruction may show a decline in serial measurements of GFR attributable to significant obstruction and there may be a similar change in uptake of radioactive hippuran or DTPA in unilateral obstruction. Other proposed methods of detecting significant incomplete obstruction are shown in Table 2. Further careful evaluation and comparison of these methods is necessary. The place of each of them in routine clinical practice is at present uncertain.

Antegrade pyelography and ureterography
Percutaneous introduction of contrast medium directly into the renal pelvis or a calyx via a needle with subsequent X-ray examination of the pelvi-calyceal system and ureter (antegrade pyelography and ureterography) is used increasingly to define the site and cause of obstruction (Fig. 14). Introduction of a needle into the system allows direct measurement of the pressure developing within it after infusion of fluid at a known flow rate. This may be of value in differentiating a baggy, low-pressure collecting system from an obstructed high-pressure one and allows a logical decision to be made as to whether operation is indicated. Diagnostic antegrade examination can be combined with the therapeutic

Table 2 Detection of significant incomplete obstruction

Introduction of a needle into the renal pelvis with direct measurement of the pressure developing after infusion of fluid at a known flow rate (antegrade pressure flow measurement)
Urographic observation of the degree of distension of the renal pelvis induced by intravenous frusemide (frusemide urography)
Observation of the effect of intravenous frusemide upon the isotope renogram (frusemide renography)
Comparison of activity/time curves after injection of ^{99m}Tc-DTPA in whole kidney versus renal pelvis (retention function analysis)
Measurement of the nephron transit time of a non-reabsorbable tracer (outflow obstruction may increase the transit time)

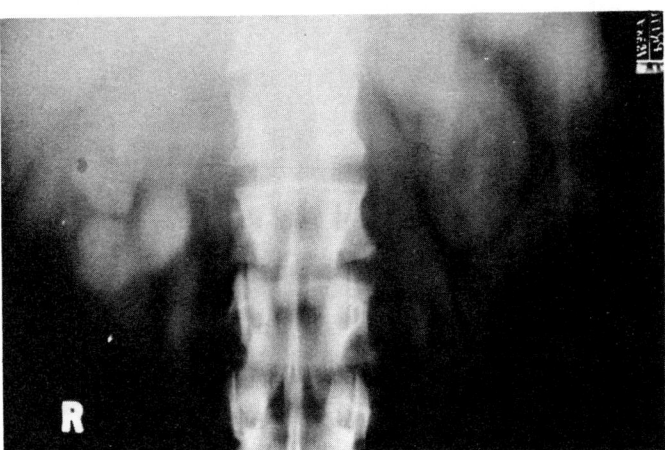

Fig. 13 Delayed renal tomogram carried out during high-dose excretion urography in a patient with unexplained renal failure showing obvious dilation of pelvi-calyceal system on the right side. Plain radiographs and early tomograms were uninformative. Diagnosis of obstruction due to retroperitoneal fibrosis was established subsequently.

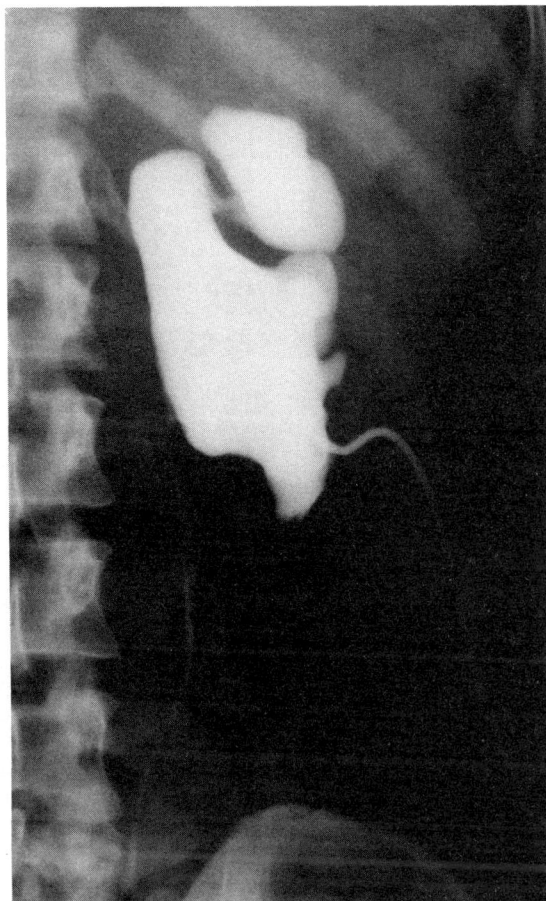

Fig. 14 Antegrade pyelogram in a patient with obstruction at the pelvi-ureteric junction. Antegrade examination was carried out to establish the site of obstruction and nephrostomy drainage was established at the same time, pending surgical correction of the problem.

manoeuvre of drainage of the collecting system by percutaneous needle nephrostomy.

Retrograde ureterography
Cystoscopy and catheterization of one or both of the ureters from below, followed by retrograde injection of contrast medium (retrograde ureterography) is indicated if antegrade examination cannot be carried out or there is a prospect of dealing with ureteric obstruction from below at the time of retrograde examination. The technique carries the risks of introducing infection into an obstructed urinary tract and of septicaemia and should be performed only when absolutely necessary. In obstruction due to neuromuscular dysfunction at the pelvi-ureteric junction and in retroperitoneal fibrosis, the collecting system may fill normally from below (Fig. 15).

Cystoscopy, urethroscopy, and urethrography
Obstructing lesions within the bladder and urethra can be seen directly by endoscopic examination. After introduction of contrast into the bladder by catheterization or by suprapubic bladder puncture, X-ray films taken during voiding will show obstructing lesions in the urethra. Urethrography is of particular value in the diagnosis of urethral valves and strictures (Fig. 16).

Pressure flow studies
Pressure changes within the bladder during filling and emptying may be recorded. A larger filling catheter and a smaller measuring catheter are employed and rectal pressure is measured concur-

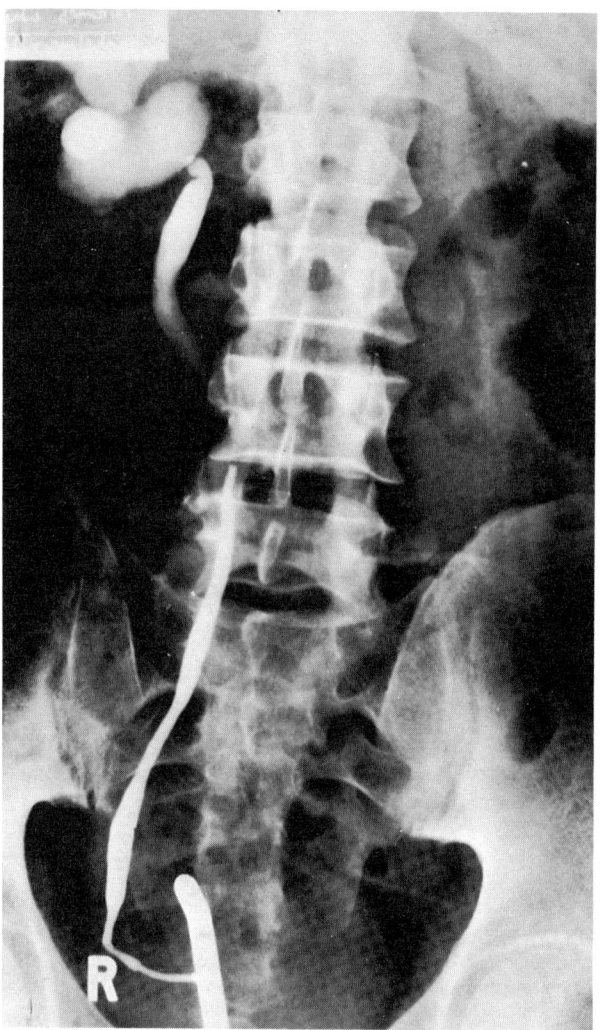

Fig. 15 Same patient as in Fig. 13. Retrograde ureterogram and pyelogram in retroperitoneal fibrosis. Characteristically for this condition, it has been possible to advance the ureteric catheter and to fill the system from below. Note dilation of calyces, pelvis and upper ureter.

rently as a gauge of intra-abdominal pressure. True bladder pressure is the pressure measured by the measuring catheter minus rectal pressure. Demonstration that a high voiding pressure is required to maintain flow is indicative of bladder outflow obstruction. Pressure flow studies may be combined with video cystography and urethrography which assist in defining the site of obstruction. For example, obstruction resulting from distal sphincter dysfunction may be distinguished from bladder neck obstruction in this way.

Normally, while the bladder is being filled, there is only a small pressure rise before the voluntary initiation of urination. Uninhibited contractions of the detrusor muscle during filling may be seen in upper motor neurone bladder neuropathy such as occurs in multiple sclerosis. Less commonly, a neuropathic bladder may be 'hypotonic', readily accepting large volumes of fluid before the initiation of weak contractions at low intravesical pressure. A common cause of such lower motor neurone bladder neuropathy is diabetes mellitus. Similar urodynamic findings are seen when long-standing bladder outflow obstruction has resulted in severe damage to bladder function.

Pressure flow and video studies may be indicated in patients with unexplained frequency and urgency of urination, in those with a poor symptomatic result after prostatectomy, after failed attempts to repair a cystocele or to cure urinary incontinence and when the presence of a neuropathic bladder is suspected. Such studies enable a logical decision to be taken as to whether surgery to relieve bladder outflow impairment should be carried out.

Treatment

Treatment is aimed at the relief of obstruction, treatment of the underlying cause, and prevention and treatment of infection. The ultimate aim is to relieve symptoms and preserve renal function.

Account must be taken of the degree of renal functional impairment present in deciding the type and dosage of antimicrobial to be used. It must be remembered that urine culture may be sterile when upper urinary tract infection is associated with complete obstruction. Severely ill patients with salt and water overload or uraemia will need dialysis before corrective surgery is carried out. When the site and nature of the obstructing lesion is uncertain, doubt exists as to the viability of the obstructed kidney or immediate definitive surgery would be hazardous, temporary external diversion of urine by, for example, nephrostomy may be valuable, allowing time for further investigation and treatment.

Nephrectomy or nephro-ureterectomy is justified: (a) when obstruction is due to malignant disease involving the urinary tract; and (b) when it is judged that no worthwhile amount of renal excretory function will be conserved by or will return after relief of obstruction. This is the case, for example, when extensive renal damage or complete destruction of the kidney follows prolonged obstruction or pyonephrosis.

Recent complete upper urinary tract obstruction demands urgent relief to preserve kidney function, the more so if infection is present. Provided that infection is absent, a more deliberate approach can be adopted in partial urinary tract obstruction, particularly if spontaneous relief is expected.

Typically, diuresis follows relief of obstruction at any site. Massive diuresis occurs in some patients due to previous sodium and water overload, the osmotic effect of retained solutes and defective renal tubular reabsorptive capacity (cf. diuretic phase of recovering acute tubular necrosis). This may be self-limiting. A minority of patients develop sodium and water depletion and require intravenous saline replacement. Hypokalaemia may occur. Renal tubular sodium, potassium, and water wasting may persist for weeks or months after relief of long-standing obstruction. Appropriate oral replacement is necessary.

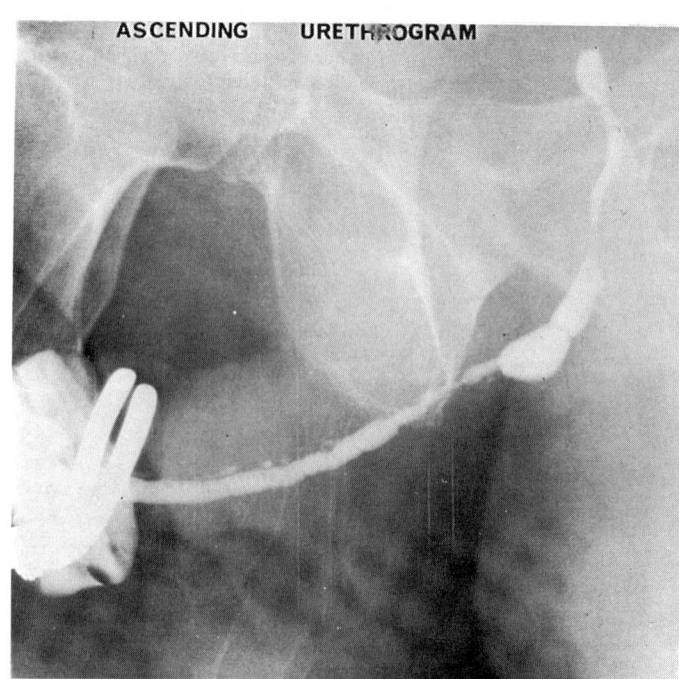

Fig. 16 Ascending urethrogram demonstrating long urethral stricture.

Calculi

Calculi causing complete obstruction should be dealt with if they have not moved spontaneously over a period of a few days. Provided infection is absent, intervention can be deferred in partial obstruction if it seems likely that the calculus will pass spontaneously. Calculi 5 mm or less in diameter usually do so. Plain abdominal X-rays should be taken every few days. The continuing presence and degree of obstruction is assessed periodically by renography, ultrasonography or excretion urography. If the latter method is used, the number of films taken should be limited to that needed to address this question. Failure of a calculus to pass or progress within at most four weeks in the presence of partial obstruction is an indication for intervention.

A revolution is in progress in the management of urinary tract calculi. With the exception of bladder calculi which could be gripped and crushed through a cystoscope by a lithotrite and calculi at the vesico-ureteric junction which could likewise be extracted endoscopically, the majority of urinary tract stones have, until recently, been removed by a cutting operation. Large bladder calculi, ureteric calculi, and calculi in the renal pelvis have been removed by cystotomy, ureterolithotomy, and pyelolithotomy, respectively. Open operation for renal stones can however now be avoided in many cases by creating a nephrostomy track to the calculus, dilating the track to a diameter of 9–10 mm and then either removing the calculus endoscopically via the track or causing it to disintegrate by direct application of an ultrasound probe. It is possible to extract ureteric stones endoscopically with the assistance of a ureteroscope and bladder calculi may be disintegrated by the endoscopic application of electrohydraulically produced shock waves. At the time of writing it appears certain that these promising techniques will be more widely used in future years.

A novel approach to the treatment of calculi employs externally delivered shock waves to shatter calculi into many fragments which are then passed spontaneously (Fig. 17). Extracorporeal shock wave lithotripsy (ESWL) offers a solution to the problem of the presence of a calculus or calculi within the kidney without the need for a surgical operation, with the promise of a reduction in morbidity and perhaps mortality, a much shorter hospital stay for the patient and a more rapid return to work. In addition, a number of patients who might have been unfit for conventional surgery may be suitable for shock wave lithotripsy. The technique is unsuitable for hard uric acid and cystine stones, for very large

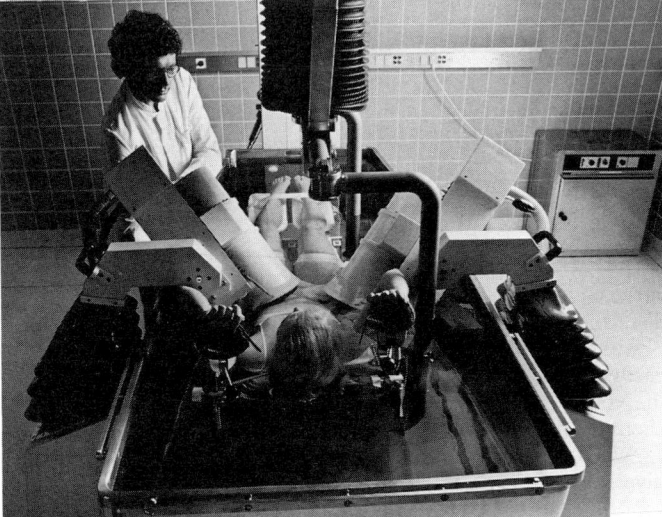

Fig. 17 Patient undergoing extracorporeal shock wave lithotripsy. Shock waves are generated by a spark discharge between two electrode tips sited within an ellipsoidal reflector at the base of a stainless steel bath containing de-gassed water. Paired X-ray image intensifiers guide the positioning of the patient through a computerized hydraulic system to bring the kidney stone within the focus of the shock waves.

stones (which must be 'de-bulked' percutaneously before lithotripsy), and for ureteric stones (although a proportion of these can be manoeuvred into the upper collecting system endoscopically and then dealt with by ESWL). Other disadvantages include the high capital cost of the necessary equipment, its size, the continued need for anaesthesia, and the need for further intervention in 10–15 per cent of patients in whom stone fragments do not pass. Such fragments can, in general, be removed endoscopically. Despite these problems, it seems likely that non-operative dissolution of calculi will be used increasingly in the developed world in future years provided stone recurrence rate in the long term proves to be no higher than after open surgery and no so-far unforeseen long-term complication emerges. Large staghorn calculi are still usually removed by a cutting procedure. Surface cooling of the kidney at the time of operation allows time for more complete clearance of stones with the renal artery clamped and protects against the development of ischaemic damage to the kidney. Infusion of inosine into the renal artery of the kidney to be operated upon may also protect against ischaemic damage.

Uric acid calculi are radiolucent. Their progress cannot be followed by a plain abdominal X-ray and repeated limited excretion urography is usually necessary. Repeated CT scanning is not, in general, appropriate. Small uric acid calculi or sludge may be rendered soluble by alkalinization of the urine by administration of sodium bicarbonate and/or acetazolamide. Occasionally, uric acid sludge can be removed from the ureter by retrograde catheterization followed by irrigation with sodium bicarbonate solution.

The underlying cause for calculus formation should be sought and appropriate preventive measures taken, e.g. long-term allopurinol prophylaxis in uric acid lithiasis.

Obstruction at the pelvi-ureteric junction

Commonly, this appears to result from a functional disturbance in peristalsis of the collecting system in the absence of mechanical obstruction. Surgical attempts at correction of obstruction by open or by percutaneous pyeloplasty are limited to patients with recurrent loin pain and those in whom serial excretion urography, background-subtraction isotope renography, or measurements of GFR indicate progressive kidney damage. Patients with unilateral obstruction should be followed up since the condition may become bilateral.

Retroperitoneal fibrosis

In this condition, the ureters become embedded in dense fibrous tissue, with resultant unilateral or bilateral obstruction, usually at the junction of middle and lower thirds of the ureter. The condition is progressive. Occasionally it is associated with mediastinal fibrosis and sclerosing cholangitis. The large majority of cases are of unknown aetiology and in these it has been suggested that the fundamental problem is an immunologically mediated periaortitis. Recognized associations are with retroperitoneal lymphoma, carcinoma of the bladder or colon, abdominal aortic aneurysm, and prolonged exposure to the drug methysergide. Dull backache, normochromic anaemia, and a raised erythrocyte sedimentation rate are typical features and may antedate obvious radiological evidence of obstruction. The earliest abnormality on excretion urography is medial deviation of one or both ureters, but this may be a normal finding. The diagnosis may be made on CT scanning if the typical periaortic mass is present.

Obstruction may be relieved surgically by ureterolysis. Biopsy of fibrous tissue should be performed at operation to determine whether or not there is an underlying lymphoma or carcinoma. Controlled trials are lacking but it appears that corticosteroids are of benefit in idiopathic retroperitoneal fibrosis. If bilateral obstruction is present and there is residual function in both kidneys, bilateral ureterolysis followed by steroid therapy is indicated except in high-risk patients in whom the less traumatic unilateral operation may be preferred. Operation alone or steroid therapy alone should be considered in those in whom steroids or surgery present particular hazards. Response to treatment and activity of disease may be assessed by serial measurements of erythrocyte sedimentation rate and GFR supplemented by isotopic and imaging techniques. Relapse after withdrawal of corticosteroid therapy may occur and such treatment may need to be continued for years. Long-term follow-up is mandatory.

Bladder outflow obstruction

Whatever the cause, upper tract dilation, declining kidney function, or severe symptoms are indications for surgical relief.

Benign prostatic hypertrophy

In acute retention or retention with overflow, the first priorities are to relieve pain and establish catheter drainage. A strict aseptic technique is essential. The bladder should be decompressed slowly to prevent bleeding from the mucosa. If urethral catheterization is impossible, suprapubic catheter drainage is established. Choice of management then lies between immediate prostatectomy, a period of catheter drainage followed by prostatectomy, or the acceptance of a permanent indwelling suprapubic or urethral catheter.

Patients complaining only of prostatism who do not have upper tract dilation require prostatectomy if symptoms are severe. Operation may be deferred if symptoms are mild. Eradication of lower urinary tract infection may relieve symptoms originally attributed to outflow obstruction. Periodic measurement of GFR and ultrasonography, isotope studies or excretion urography are carried out. Declining kidney function, upper tract dilation or increasing severity of symptoms demand surgery.

Unless the gland is very large, transurethral resection through a resectoscope is usually successful, carries a lower morbidity and mortality and demands a shorter stay in hospital than open prostatectomy.

Urinary diversion

This is required when obstruction cannot otherwise be relieved and when effective treatment is inconsistent with preservation of an intact urinary tract, e.g. after cystectomy for bladder cancer. High obstruction may render permanent nephrostomy unavoidable. Ureteric anastomosis to an ileal conduit opening on to the abdominal wall is a satisfactory method of diversion with no metabolic consequences. Ureteric anastomosis to colon or rectum should be abandoned owing to the consequent metabolic complications of hyperchloraemic acidosis, hypokalaemia, and osteomalacia. In some patients, obstruction is best relieved by the insertion of indwelling catheters or stents (double J stents) into the ureter and upper urinary tract, thus avoiding the need for external diversion of urine.

In obstruction due to untreatable malignant disease, it is wise to consider carefully whether urinary diversion is justified since this may exchange a pain-free death from renal failure for a painful one with malignant invasion of bones or nerves.

Prognosis

Prognosis depends upon the underlying cause, the duration, and degree of obstruction prior to relief, and whether or not infection has been present.

Animal experiments show that complete obstruction for one week results in irreversible reduction in GFR by 50 per cent. Clinical experience in humans indicates that return of useful kidney function is very unlikely if complete obstruction has been present for more than four to six months. Lesser degrees of obstruction carry a better prognosis.

References

Baker, L. R. I., Mallinson, W. J. W., Gregory, M. C., Menzies, E. A. D., Cattell, W. R., Whitfield, H. N., Hendry, W. F., Wickham, J. E. A. and Joekes, A. M. (1987). Iodiopathic retroperitoneal fibrosis: a retrospective analysis of sixty cases. *Br. J. Urol.* in press.

Chaussy, C. and Schmiedt, E. (1983). Shock wave treatment for stone in the upper urinary tract. In *Urologic clinics of North America* (ed. M. I. Resnick), pp. 743–750. W. B. Saunders, Philadelphia.

Federle, M. P., McAninch, J. W., Kaiser, J. A., Goodman, P. C., Roberts, J. and Mall, J. C. (1981). Computed tomography of urinary calculi. *Am. J. Roentgenol.* **136**, 255–258.

Keuhnelian, J. G., Bartone, F. and Marshall, V. F. (1964). Practical considerations from autopsies in uraemic patients. *J. Urol.* **91**, 467–473.

Talner, L. B., Scheible, W., Ellenbogen, P. H., Beck, C. H. and Gosink, B. B. (1981). How accurate is ultrasonography in detecting hydronephrosis in azotemic patients? *Urol. Radiol.* **3**, 1–6.

Webb, J. A. W., Reznek, R. H., White, F. E., Cattell, W. R., Kelsey Fry, I. and Baker, L. R. I. (1984). Can ultrasound and computed tomography replace high-dose urography in patients with impaired renal function? *Q. J. Med.* **211**, 411–425.

Whitaker, R. H. (1973). Methods of assessing obstruction in dilated ureters. *Br. J. Urol.* **45**, 15–22.

—— (1976). Equivocal pelvi-ureteric obstruction. *Br. J. Urol.* **47**, 771–779.

Wickham, J. E. A. and Miller, R. A. (1983). *Percutaneous renal surgery.* Churchill Livingstone, London.

TOXIC NEPHROPATHIES

F. P. MARSH

Alteration of renal structure and function caused by poisonous substances is common for a number of reasons. The kidneys are largely responsible for removing toxic substances and their metabolites from the body. Their exposure to blood-born toxins is favoured by a blood supply which is 60 times greater than might be expected from their weight; and also by the large endothelial surface area of their capillaries which, in relation to weight, is greater than that of any other organ. The glomerular mesangium can phagocytose macromolecules and the glomerulus is notoriously susceptible to immunologically mediated damage. Glomerular filtration and tubular absorption and secretion may produce concentrations of chemicals adjacent and within the tubular epithelium which are damaging to it; and the countercurrent mechanism of urinary concentration exposes the medullary interstitium to exceptional levels. Finally, metabolic and enzymatic processes are very active in the kidney, with, consequently, ample potential for disturbance.

Although the damage should be capable of recognition more easily than in many other organs because of the facility with which the volume and contents of the urine can be measured, and biochemical functions of the kidneys monitored, it often goes unrecognized or attributed to other causes. Numerous substances as diverse as heavy metals, organic chemicals, snake and insect venoms, and even plant matter have been shown to damage the kidneys, and there is increasing concern over the effects of long-continued exposure to occupational and other environmental hazards. The clinician, however, is most likely to encounter drug-induced nephropathy.

Toxic damage may be dose dependent, or may occur unexpectedly, perhaps reflecting constitutional or iatrogenic variations in metabolism or excretion of toxins, immunological responsiveness, or simultaneous exposure to other damaging agents, Clinically acute or chronic renal failure, haematuria, proteinuria, nephrotic syndrome, or disturbance of tubular function may result. The clinical manifestations generally reflect the severity and rate of progression of the morphological damage, but do not necessarily reflect its type. Thus acute glomerulonephritis, tubular necrosis, interstitial nephritis, and vascular damage may all present with oliguric renal failure and drug-induced nephrotic syndrome may be associated with minimal or gross alterations in the glomeruli, as seen by light microscopy. The nature of the clinical presentation is sometimes dose-related; for instance, a minor insult may cause minor tubular defects, heavier and more prolonged exposure may cause proteinuria and perhaps some reduction in glomerular filtration, whilst sudden serious insult may precipitate acute renal failure.

The kidneys may also suffer less directly from the effects of drugs or toxic agents; for instance, from hypotension, from hypovolaemia caused by diarrhoea and vomiting or excessive diuresis, from hypercalcaemia, or from obstruction of tubules by crystals, or of ureters by stones or fibrosis. Acute myoglobinuric renal failure secondary to rhabdomyolysis can be caused by drugs such as opiates, amphetamines, and alcohol.

Renal damage due to environmental and occupational toxins

Metals
Metals are not uncommon causes of toxic nephropathy. They may be encountered through occupational or general environmental exposure, or in drugs. Renal disturbances which individual metals can produce are shown in Table 1. The clinical manifestations depend on the chemical form of the metal, its dose, and the way in which it is presented. Gold, lithium, and platinum compounds which are medically useful will be discussed later (page 18.116). Mercury and bismuth are now rarely used in drugs but, like lead and cadmium, are potentially dangerous industrial toxins.

Mercury
Mercury is used extensively in industry. Mercurial compounds are still used by doctors, but to a diminishing extent, as diuretics, surface antiseptics, and, at operation, to kill seeded cancer cells. Dental fillings are usually made of silver–tin amalgams and mercury has been found in skin-lightening creams used by dark races. The injection of mercuric chloride is a well-known way of producing acute tubular necrosis experimentally; and acute exposure to metallic mercury or its compounds by ingestion, inhalation or injection, causes acute renal failure in humans. Recovery usually occurs spontaneously but heavy proteinuria may persist for months. Several cases, some fatal, have been recorded after peritoneal lavage with mercuric chloride during operations for abdominal cancer. Chronic exposure to mercurial compounds or metallic mercury can cause the nephrotic syndrome, sometimes with aminoaciduria and tubular glycosuria. In this event the histology is that of minimal change or membranous nephropathy.

Lead
The ingestion by children of lead in powdered paint from the blistering verandahs of Queensland in the late nineteenth and early twentieth centuries caused the development in them of uraemia and hypertension, due to chronic interstitial nephritis, many years later. The uses of lead in modern industry, and the opportunities for exposure to it, are enormous. Fortunately, lead poisoning is uncommon. Acute renal failure, tubular necrosis, and hypertension have followed acute exposure. Chronic renal failure, hypertension, and tubular dysfunction (tubular proteinuria, glycosuria, phosphaturia, and amino aciduria) can be caused by chronic exposure in adults. It has also been suggested that mild chronic occupational or environmental exposure to lead (for instance, in tap-water) may, even now, impair renal function or raise blood pressure. This suggestion remains controversial.

Cadmium
The industrial use of cadmium is widespread and inhalation of cadmium fume or dust has caused acute renal failure due to tubular or cortical necrosis, chronic renal failure with interstitial fibrosis, tubular proteinuria and abnormalities of the Fanconi type, and renal stones. The presentation depends on the severity and duration of exposure. Lead smelters and coppersmith braziers can be poisoned by fumes from cadmium contaminating the main metal. The addition of minute quantities of cadmium to the drinking water of dogs and certain strains of rats raises their blood pressure although the mechanism is unknown. These factors, and the knowledge that it is concentrated and tightly bound in the kidney as a metallothioneine, have led to the suggestion that cadmium ingested in vegetables or drinking water, or inhaled from cigarettes, may be involved in the causation of hypertension in humans. This is controversial and not yet supported by adequate epidemiological evidence. Likewise, although kidney tissue concentrations of cadmium similar to those found in humans cause chronic renal tubular and interstitial damage in birds and mice, long-term studies of populations exposed to small amounts for long periods have not shown any increase in deaths from kidney disease or hypertension.

Table 1 Varieties of renal disease caused by metals

Metal	Acute tubular necrosis	Nephrotic syndrome	Chronic renal failure ± hypertension	Isolated proteinuria	Tubular dysfunction
Arsenic	+		+	+	+
Bismuth	+		+	+	+
Cadmium	+		+	+	+
Copper	+		+*		+*
Gold	+	+		+	
Lead	+		+		+
Lithium	+		?		+
Mercury					
inorganic	+	+	+	+	+
organic	+	+			
Platinum	+				
Silver	+				
Thallium		+	+	+	
Uranium	+		+	+	+

* Deposited in the kidney in Wilson's disease.

Arsenic

Arsenic is another metal used extensively in the making of glass, alloys, colouring agents, insecticides, rodenticides, and fungicides. It is also used in sheep-dips, given to animals to promote their growth, and prescribed by veterinary surgeons for the treatment of haemobartonella and heartworm. Although hardly used by orthodox doctors, in India it is found in Ayurvedic, homeopathic, and Unani medicine, and arsenical tonics are still sold to improve libido and sexual performance and taken by pregnant women to ensure the birth of a male child. It has been found as an adulterant in opium and as a contaminant in beer, 'moonshine' whisky, drinking water from wells, and herbal preparations. According to their nature arsenical compounds can be absorbed through skin, mucosae, gut, and lung but excretion is mainly through the kidneys. Acute poisoning can cause prerenal uraemia (secondary to diarrhoea and vomiting), acute tubular necrosis, and cortical necrosis. Recovery may be incomplete and chronic renal failure may ensue due to glomerulosclerosis and interstitial fibrosis. Chronic arsenical poisoning can cause glycosuria, proteinuria, haematuria, and renal failure.

Bismuth

Bismuth is mainly used in emollient ointments or suppositories and to treat indigestion, although its oral use has been restricted in several countries because of the unpredictable development of encephalopathy and dementia in regular consumers. Proteinuria, Fanconi syndrome, and oliguric renal failure have been described after acute overdoses as well as in patients taking tablets regularly for months. Renal function improves within a few weeks of stopping the treatment, but recovery may be incomplete. Histologically, there is tubular necrosis and eosinophilic inclusion bodies have been found in the cytoplasm and nuclei of proximal convoluted tubules.

Dimercaprol, sodium calcium edetate, and penicillamine reduce the toxicity of some metals by forming complexes with them, and they may be valuable in the treatment of acute metal poisoning. The complexes can theoretically be removed from anuric patients by haemodialysis but the amount removed thereby may be paltry. Mild chronic nephropathy due to metals often improves when exposure to them is stopped, but unfortunately severe nephropathy may progress regardless.

Hydrocarbons and organic solvents

Carbon tetrachloride is a readily available household and industrial solvent and is also used as a fire extinguisher. It may cause poisoning by inhalation or ingestion and, being heavier than air, its vapour tends to persist in poorly ventilated rooms. Its toxicity is potentiated by alcohol. The commonest presenting symptoms are abdominal (pain, vomiting, and diarrhoea) and neurological (drowsiness, fits, and coma). Later, jaundice and a large tender liver may distract attention from oliguria, whose onset may be delayed for several days. The renal failure is potentially reversible, and death is most often due to hepatic failure. Intravenous acetylcysteine has been suggested to prevent the formation of toxic metabolites and improve the prognosis. *Tetrachloroethane* and *trichloroethylene* are also used as industrial solvents and cleaners; trichloroethylene is the anaesthetic trilene. Overexposure to them, and to many other halogenated hydrocarbons, causes symptoms like those of carbon tetrachloride poisoning.

Ethylene glycol, present in antifreeze, is another easily available nephrotoxic agent, although the lethal dose usually exceeds 100 ml. It is rapidly metabolized to oxalic acid. If the initial acute neurological symptoms, gastrointestinal haemorrhage, and cardiopulmonary failure are survived, the deposition of calcium oxalate crystals in the renal tubules may cause acute tubular necrosis (Fig. 1). *Diethylene glycol*, used over 30 years ago as an excipient for sulphanilamide, is more toxic and caused many deaths from acute cortical necrosis. It is uncertain how this was produced. *Propylene glycol* is not metabolized to oxalic acid and is less toxic than ethylene glycol, but may produce acute renal failure due to intravascular haemolysis.

Abuse of *petroleum products* can cause renal damage. Thus oliguria due to tubular necrosis has been described after washing the skin with diesel oil or inhaling its fumes. People addicted to sniffing glue, paint, or toluene can develop proteinuria, haematuria, pyuria, and distal tubular acidosis, as well as proximal tubular dysfunction like that of the Fanconi syndrome.

Recently there has been interest in an apparent relationship between exposure to hydrocarbons and glomerulonephritis. This rests on individual case reports and on epidemiological evidence of greater exposure to hydrocarbons in patients with Goodpasture's syndrome or idiopathic proliferative or membranous glomerulonephritis than in patients with hypertension or other renal diseases. Many of the clinical studies have methodological deficiencies and this important possible association is not yet proven. However, it is also possible to produce proliferative glomerulonephritis in rats by feeding them N,N'-diacetylbenzidine or exposing them to petrol vapour. The mechanism is unknown. It has been suggested that hydrocarbons may alter alveolar and glomerular basement membranes, rendering them antigenic and able to provoke the formation of antiglomerular basement membrane antibodies. Another possibility is the production of immune complexes containing antibodies to altered plasma protein or tubular antigen.

Paraquat

Paraquat is an easily obtained, highly effective but dangerous herbicide. Serious toxicity is rare after ingestion of paraquat granules, and unreported after exposure to the aerosol. However, the liquid concentrate (20–40 per cent) causes death in up to half of those who drink it; even a mouthful may be lethal. The minor effects are those of proximal tubular dysfunction, causing aminoaciduria, glycosuria, phosphaturia, and uricosuria. More serious is the frank renal failure developing in the first few days after ingestion; although this is reversible, pulmonary oedema and progressive pulmonary fibrosis are often fatal. Attempts to remove the paraquat by dialysis or charcoal haemoperfusion, or to antagonize its toxicity at cellular level, have been clinically unsuccessful.

Plant and animal toxins

Toxins of plant and animal origin are well established, if uncommon, causes of renal damage. Snake, spider, and hornet venoms may cause acute tubular or cortical necrosis due to a direct neph-

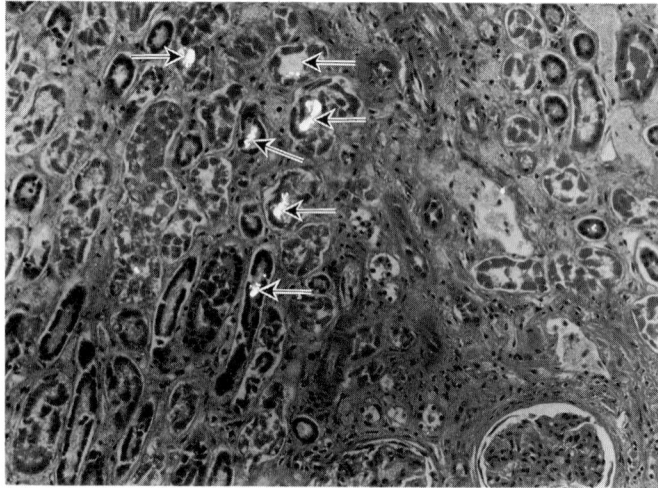

Fig. 1 Ethylene glycol poisoning. Deposition of birefringent calcium oxalate crystals, visible here under polarized light as densely white irregular deposits, in the renal tubular lumina of a man who had died after drinking ethylene glycol. H & E x 120. (Reproduced by courtesy of Dr S. M. Dodd.)

rotoxic effect in some cases, but secondary to shock, intravascular coagulation, and haemolysis, or muscle necrosis in others. Acute renal failure has also followed mushroom poisoning, and early dialysis to remove the toxin may be life-saving. Bee stings and idiosyncratic reactions to poison ivy and poison oak are often quoted, though rare, causes of the nephrotic syndrome.

Renal damage due to drugs

In modern medical practice drugs are by far the commonest causes of toxic nephropathy and if a patient's renal function alters unexpectedly the drug intake should be reviewed. Drugs which individually are only slightly nephrotoxic may be markedly so when taking in combination, and doses which are acceptable for patients with normal renal function may be excessive when given to those with pre-existing renal disease.

It is often difficult to prove how often and under what conditions a drug damages the kidney. Patients are often prescribed several drugs which individually or together may be nephrotoxic, but the conditions for which they are prescribed may themselves affect renal function. The results of animal experiments may not accord with the conclusions of subsequent clinical trials. Occasional, though serious, side-effects may not be encountered or recognized until a drug has been in clinical use for a considerable time. Recently introduced drugs are often claimed to be less toxic than their predecessors, but a wise doctor will treat such claims with a healthy scepticism.

Not all alterations in renal function caused by drugs are deleterious. Thus steroids greatly increase the glomerular filtration rate of the normal kidney, and this must be remembered when assessing their effects on renal disease. Even the damaging effects of certain drugs on renal cellular function may be put to therapeutic use, as with diuretics.

Effects on the kidney of some drugs which are often used, or are of particular importance, are discussed in the following paragraphs.

Antimicrobial agents
Aminoglycosides
Injections of neomycin, kanamycin, and streptomycin have long been known to be nephrotoxic. Reversible proteinuria, azotaemia, and occasionally acute tubular necrosis have also been ascribed to gentamicin. The risk is significant, but difficulty to quantify because this drug tends to be used especially in ill patients whose renal function may deteriorate for other reasons. The risk is dose related and greatest in the old and those with renal failure, who excrete aminoglycosides poorly; it is particularly important to avoid overdosage in these patients by serial measurements of serum gentamicin concentration. Clinical studies suggest that combinations of gentamicin with frusemide, a cephalosporin, or clindamyin are more nephrotoxic than gentamicin alone. The toxicity of recently introduced aminoglycosides is not established but some, such as tobramycin, netilmicin and amikacin, may damage the kidney less.

Amphotericin
Intravenous amphotericin, invaluable in the treatment of systemic mycoses, almost always causes some renal damage. Serial tests of renal function should be made during treatment. The drug reduces renal blood flow and glomerular filtration, often markedly; it also affects distal tubular function, diminishing urinary concentrating and acidifying capacity, and increasing urinary sodium and potassium losses. There is little proteinuria. It probably damages renal tubules and fungi in the same way, by creating pores, lined by amphotericin molecules, in their cell membranes which become excessively permeable to fluid and electrolytes. Histologically tubular atrophy, interstitial inflammation and calcification, arteriolar vacuolization, and calcified intratubular casts are found. Damage is related to the total dose, and is often reversible if the

drug is withdrawn or its daily dose is reduced. Most sensitive systemic mycoses are cured by total doses of 2–4 g, which is fortunate because plasma urea and creatinine concentrations remain elevated in over 40 per cent of patients treated with more than 4 g. Intravenous mannitol and bicarbonate have been advocated to reduce the nephrotoxic consequences, but their effectiveness is not proved in humans.

Cephalosporins
Cephaloridine in doses exceeding 5 g/day often causes proteinuria and cast excretion, less often diminishes glomerular filtration, and occasionally causes acute tubular necrosis. Probenecid and penicillin reduce its active transport into tubular cells and, presumably by this means, reduce its concentration in the renal cortex and its nephrotoxicity. Cephalothin causes acute renal failure only occasionally, and this is less clearly dose related. Other cephalosporins and cefoxitin (a cephamycin) do not seem to cause serious renal damage in humans, although some are nephrotoxic in animals. Pre-existing renal failure, or the simultaneous prescription of loop diuretics or of other nephrotoxic agents such as aminoglycosides or colistin, potentiate cephalosporin nephrotoxicity. In patients taking cefoxitin, glomerular filtration rate cannot be measured reliably using creatinine clearance. This is because urinary cefoxitin reacts in the same way as creatinine in the Jaffé reaction, causing a spuriously high apparent clearance. It is uncertain to what extent other cephalosporins do this.

Co-trimoxazole
Like other sulphonamides, the sulphamethoxazole component of co-trimoxazole may rarely cause acute renal failure (Fig. 2). It has been claimed that the combination of sulphamethoxazole and trimethoprim is a frequent cause of sudden deterioration in renal function, especially if the dose is not reduced in patients with renal failure. The extent of the risk is not generally agreed. Reversible reduction in creatinine clearance, without change in glomerular filtration rate as measured by other techniques, has been reported in normal subjects given co-trimoxazole. This may be due to trimethoprim-induced diminution in the tubular secretion of creatinine.

Penicillins
Occasionally methicillin, and even less often other penicillins, cause an acute illness a few days to six weeks after the start of treatment. It is characterized by fever, haematuria, and proteinuria, and sometimes renal failure, oliguria, maculopapular rash, and arthralgia. There is almost always an increase in blood and

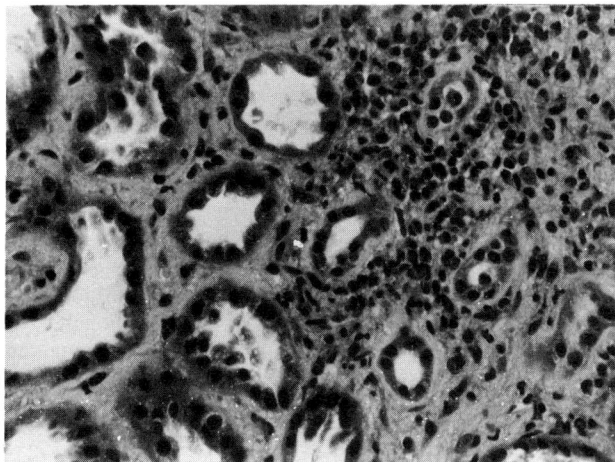

Fig. 2 Acute drug-induced interstitial nephritis. Renal biopsy showing lymphocytic interstitial infiltration in a woman who developed acute self reversing renal failure following administration of co-trimoxazole. H & E x 300. (Reproduced by courtesy of Dr S. M. Dodd.)

urine eosinophil counts. Recovery usually occurs rapidly when the drug is stopped but is sometimes incomplete. Pathologically there is an acute mononuclear and eosinophilic interstitial nephritis with marked peritubular filtration. Glomerulonephritis, arteritis, and polyarteritis nodosa-like syndromes may also occur. Immunoglobulins and complement components are sometimes found in glomeruli, tubules or interstitium, but electron microscopy does not reveal dense deposits suggestive of immune complexes. Although the presentation suggests a hypersensitivity reaction, the actual mechanism is unknown and the condition does not occur more often in those who are allergic to penicillin.

Rifampicin

Rifampicin rarely causes renal damage except when given on a twice or thrice weekly basis; or when the drug has been restarted after an interruption of a few days to several months. Oliguria occurs as part of a systemic reaction, with rigors, myalgia, diarrhoea, and vomiting, and sometimes hepatocellular jaundice. There is eosinophilia, and red and white cells are seen on urine microscopy. Recovery usually occurs within two weeks, provided no more rifampicin is taken. The renal pathology is that of an acute interstitial nephritis. The cause of the reaction is unknown, although an immunological mechanism is suggested by the presentation. However, immunoglobulins and complements are not typically found on immunofluorescent examination of the renal tissue and serum complements are usually normal.

Sulphonamides

Modern sulphonamides, correctly prescribed to adequately hydrated patients, are unlikely to crystallize out in renal tubules and obstruct them. Rarely they may cause an acute interstitial nephritis, precipitate a polyarteritis nodosa-like syndrome, or (like penicillin) activate systemic lupus erythematosus.

Tetracyclines

Tetracyclines, with the possible exception of doxycycline, should not be given to uraemic patients in whom they markedly increase plasma urea concentrations. Although this is mainly due to their anti-anabolic effect, glomerular filtration may be markedly reduced and the deterioration is not always reversible. An additional prerenal element may be superimposed due to tetracycline-induced anorexia and vomiting, natriuresis, and diminished urinary concentrating ability. This last has been utilized therapeutically in the treatment of inappropriate antidiuretic hormone secretion with demeclocycline. Unlike other tetracyclines, doxycycline does not usually accumulate in patients with mild or moderate renal failure. It can probably be given to them with safety, but their renal function should be monitored.

Anhydro-4-epitetracycline, a degradation product of tetracycline stored under excessively hot, humid conditions, has occasionally caused a Fanconi-like syndrome which is reversible on withdrawal of the drug.

In pregnancy, large intravenous doses of tetracycline can cause severe hepatic and renal failure.

Analgesics
Weak analgesics

Paracetamol overdose causes *acute renal failure* which, like the jaundice, is thought to be due to depletion of glutathione which conjugates cytotoxic metabolites of paracetamol and, therefore, to be treatable with acetylcysteine. Non-steroidal anti-inflammatory drugs sometimes cause acute renal failure which rapidly improves when the offending agent is stopped and is not associated with any specific glomerular or interstitial abnormality. The effect is probably due to suppression of renal vasodilator prostaglandin synthesis in patients with a stimulated renin–angiotensin system. Predisposing factors include old age, pre-existing renal disease (including nephrotic syndrome), atherosclerotic cardiovascular disease, hypertension, heart failure, diabetes mellitus, cir-

hosis with ascites, acute gout, and concomitant diuretic therapy. Several non-steroidal anti-inflammatory drugs have been shown to cause acute renal failure or nephrotic syndrome due to glomerulonephritis or interstitial nephritis, often with systemic manifestations such as fever, skin rashes, and eosinophilia. Such complications are uncommon, but important because they are potentially reversible after withdrawal of the drug and may recur if the drug is reintroduced.

Chronic interstitial nephritis

Chronic interstitial nephritis due to prolonged consumption of weak analgesics was first described in 1950. Since then the regular ingestion of analgesic mixtures has been recognized as an important cause of chronic renal failure. There is a rough correlation between the occurrence of the characteristic renal disease in a community and the consumption of analgesics in that community. The condition has been found most often in Australia, Switzerland, Scandinavian countries, and some parts of the United States, and least often in the United Kingdom and other European countries. Phenacetin is generally believed to be the most injurious agent, because until recently it was the common constituent of analgesic mixtures readily available to the public in the different countries. However, other analgesics have also been incriminated for several reasons. First, the same renal disease has been reported occasionally in patients taking other analgesics. Secondly, progression of renal failure in patients with nephropathy apparently due to phenacetin often ceases if they stop taking all analgesics, but is said to continue if other analgesics are substituted for phenacetin; this evidence is uncontrolled. Thirdly, numerous non-steroidal anti-inflammatory drugs can induce renal papillary necrosis in the rat and, in this animal, it is easier to produce papillary necrosis with aspirin, or mixtures of aspirin and phenacetin, than with phenacetin alone. Pigs, however, which metabolize aspirin like humans and also have multi-papillate kidneys, appear to be more resistant to the nephrotoxic effects of this drug.

The relevance of animal studies to human susceptibility to various analgesics is arguable, but epidemiological evidence concerning susceptibility has been difficult to obtain. Studies in New Zealand, the United States, and Wales, in which regular analgesic takers have been compared with non-consumers, have not shown a greater prevalence of renal impairment in those taking analgesic mixtures or aspirin. However, in an important prospective eleven-year study by Dubach in Switzerland, women with a large phenacetin intake at the start of the study were more likely than matched controls to develop impaired urinary concentrating ability or an increased serum creatinine concentration. Although these become abnormal in only a minority, the risk of death due to renal or urogenital causes was about six times greater than in the controls, after adjustment for age, cigarette smoking, and length of follow-up.

Two other diseases of the urinary tract have been attributed to analgesics, but they are much less common than the changes in the kidney parenchyma. The first is transitional cell carcinoma, usually of the renal pelvis but sometimes of ureter or bladder, which may develop at several sites, is often bilateral, and often recurs. It is a late complication with an average induction time of about 20 years. Its cause is uncertain, but some of the metabolites of phenacetin are carcinogenic, and cause urothelial hyperplasia in rats. The second disorder is a curious fibrotic infiltration of the ureters, which obstructs them.

Pathology

Early in the disease the external surface of the kidney appears normal, the cut surface showing yellow discolouration of the papillae. In advanced cases the kidneys are small, the papillae shrunken and black, and often separated from the rest of the pyramids. They sometimes contain calcium or bone, and act as a nidus for stone formation. The cortex over these papillae is thin, but it is unusual to find definite focal scars. Microscopically the papillae are partially or completely necrosed and may contain calcium or bone (Fig. 3a). The tubules are atrophic, the glomeruli sclerosed, and the interstitium shows changes of chronic inflammation and fibrosis. The walls of the arteries and capillaries show a characteristic hyaline thickening, although this is not specific (Fig. 3b). Although the cortical changes have been considered to be consequent on the papillary damage, experimental work suggests this may not be the case. In rats given aspirin the first electron microscopically detectable changes are in the medullary interstitial cells. These cells are thought to be concerned with prostaglandin synthesis, and their destruction might alter medullary blood flow. Toxic damage to tubular epithelium and papillary ischaemia from occlusive lesions in the vasa recta have also been postulated.

Clinical features

Analgesic nephropathy most often presents in middle age, twice as often in women as in men. It is especially likely to be found in three groups of people. First, depressed or neurotic women who appear to derive comfort from the sedative or stimulant properties of the analgesic mixtures rather than from their pain-relieving qualities. They often have social problems, a history of heavy cigarette or psychotropic drug consumption, and a family history of analgesic or alcohol abuse. They also deny their analgesic consumption. Secondly, people whose occupations involve precise,

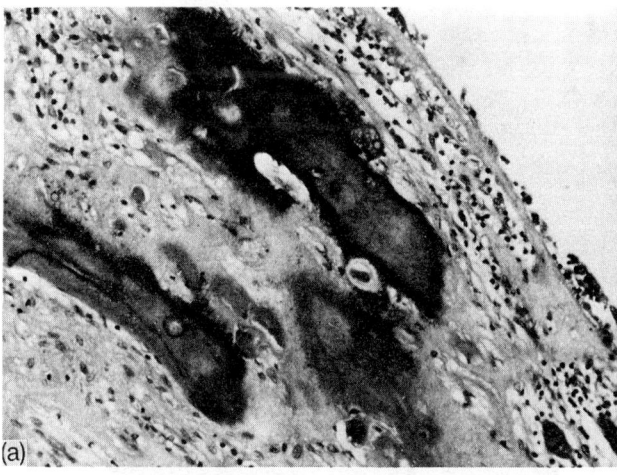

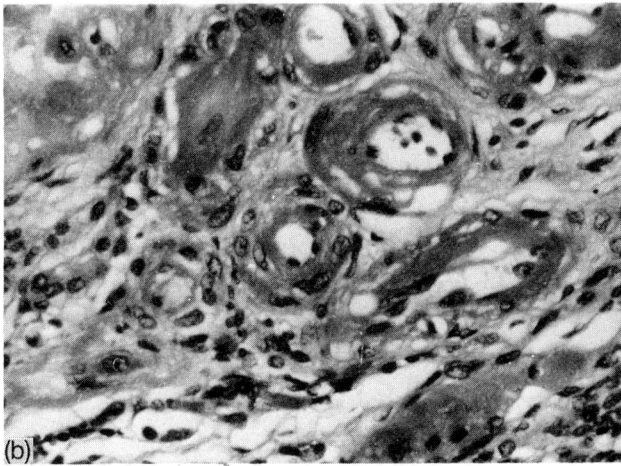

Fig. 3 Analgesic nephropathy. (a) Calcium and bone deposited in the renal medulla of a man with analgesic nephropathy; he later developed carcinoma of the bladder. Transitional epithelium of the renal pelvis is shown top right. H & E x 120. (b) Hyaline thickening of the walls of arterioles. H & E × 300.

concentrated work causing tension headaches. Thirdly, arthritic patients who require regular analgesics.

The commonest presentation is with symptoms and signs of chronic renal failure. Anaemia is often more than warranted by the degree of uraemia, probably because of aspirin-induced gastric bleeding; and it should be noted that phenacetin itself may cause methaemoglobinaemia or sulphaemoglobinaemia. Indigestion is frequent, gastric and duodenal ulcer less so, but occurring in perhaps a third; sometimes it is uncertain whether these cause, or result from, the analgesic intake. One-third of the patients is hypertensive, but there is a greater tendency to salt wastage than in glomerulonephritis; many are unable to conserve sodium and water in the face of dietary restriction or diarrhoea and vomiting, and are prone to develop prerenal uraemia. Occasionally regular sodium supplements are necessary to maintain sodium balance. Other patients present with urine infection, flank pain, renal colic or haematuria. Bacteriuria or sterile pyuria is often found. Proteinuria is usually slight and nearly always less than 3 g per 24 hours. Hypoalbuminaemia and the nephrotic syndrome are, therefore, not to be expected. Gross haematuria is usually due to the recent separation of a papilla but its appearance, or reappearance after several years' freedom, or the repeated finding of microscopic haematuria, should lead to a search for complicating carcinoma of the renal pelvis, ureter or bladder. Renal colic may be due to the impaction of a separated papilla or stone in ureter, or to carcinoma. Acute or chronic renal failure may be precipitated by renal obstruction, salt and water depletion, or intercurrent surgery; in the latter case hypovolaemia and an alteration in medullary blood flow are probably responsible.

Diagnosis

This depends on suspecting analgesic abuse in a patient with impaired renal function or relevant radiographic abnormalities. Unfortunately habitual analgesic consumers often deny their addiction. Suspicion of this may be strengthened by the finding of salicylate, or of phenacetin metabolites (the principal one being paracetamol), in the urine. Accumulative consumption of over 1 kg of phenacetin is potentially harmful to the kidneys; this sounds a lot but is reached within two years by the daily taking of six tablets, each containing 250 mg of phenacetin. It is uncertain whether the rate of consumption is important. The amount of aspirin or other analgesic needed to produce chronic renal damage is uncertain.

There is little characteristic about the renal failure: impairment of urinary concentrating and acidifying ability occur earlier in the course of the disease than in primary glomerular disorders, and there is a tendency to salt wastage.

Radiological investigation

Radiological investigation may show calcified papillae in both kidneys (Fig. 4) even before renal function has deteriorated or the kidneys have shrunk. They must be distinguished from the often finer nephrocalcinosis of renal tubular acidosis (Fig. 5), medullary sponge kidney, hyperparathyroidism, and irregular calcification associated with tuberculosis. Later the kidneys both shrink, and the papillae may separate. Detached calcified papillae may look like stones (Fig. 6) but they sometimes have radiolucent centres. However, the kidneys may look quite normal and classical evidence of renal papillary necrosis is seen in under half the cases. The calyceal changes may not be visible because a necrotic but unseparated and uncalcified papilla appears radiologically undistorted. When separation does occur, it allows contrast medium to track along the line of cleavage (Fig. 4b).

Eventually the papilla becomes surrounded by contrast medium, leaving behind a ragged cavity which becomes smooth and clubbed through re-epithelialization. Contrast medium may also track through necrotic medulla towards the cortico-medullary junction. Filling defects in the renal pelvis may be due to papilla, calculus, or complicating carcinoma, which may obstruct and cause a hydronephrosis. Bilateral hydronephrosis may be due to fibrosis of the ureteric wall.

These urographic changes must be distinguished from those of fetal lobulation, chronic pyelonephritis, and reflux nephropathy, other causes of papillary necrosis and chronic interstitial nephritis (such as irradiation and Balkan nephropathy) and from chronic obstructive atrophy, tuberculosis, cortical ischaemic scars, and bilateral renal artery stenosis. In fetal lobulation there is inden-

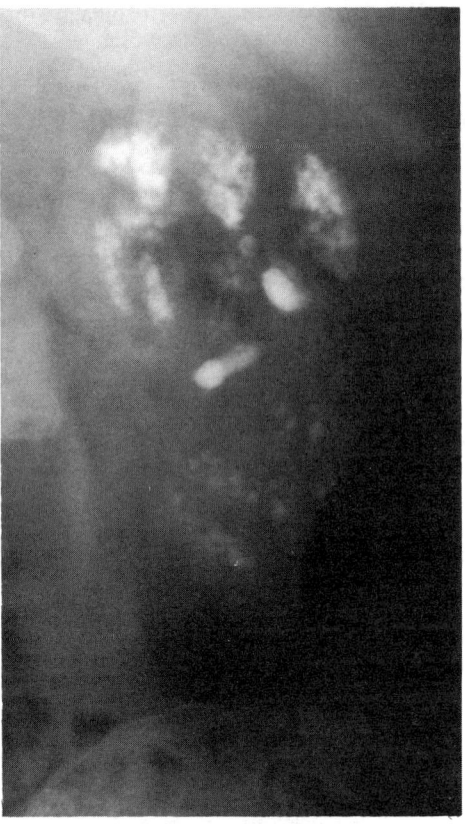

Fig. 5 Plain radiograph showing medullary calcification and stone formation in a woman with renal tubular acidosis.

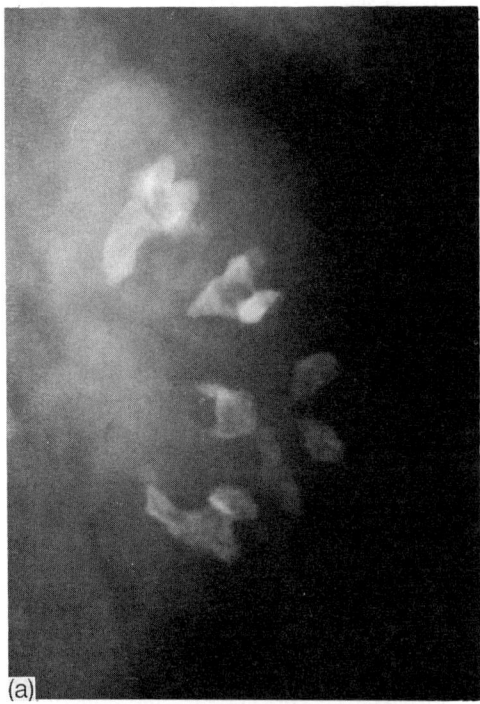

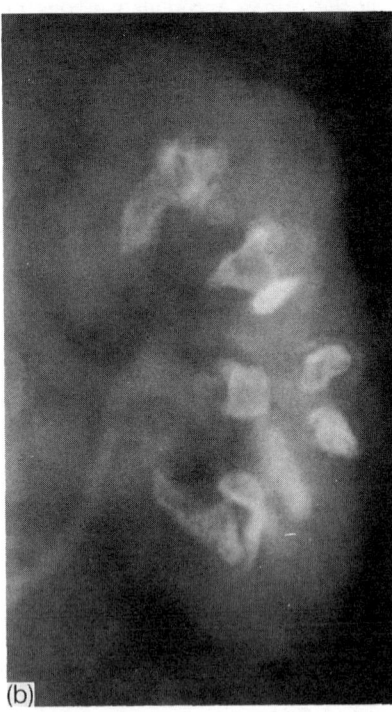

Fig. 4 (a) Plain radiograph showing calcified papillae in the left kidney of a 54-year-old man with a history of long-standing chronic analgesic consumption and previous right renal colic. The papillae in the right kidney were also calcified. (b) The IVU revealed that some of the papillae had separated, allowing contrast medium to pass behind them. The renal cortex is coarsely scarred.

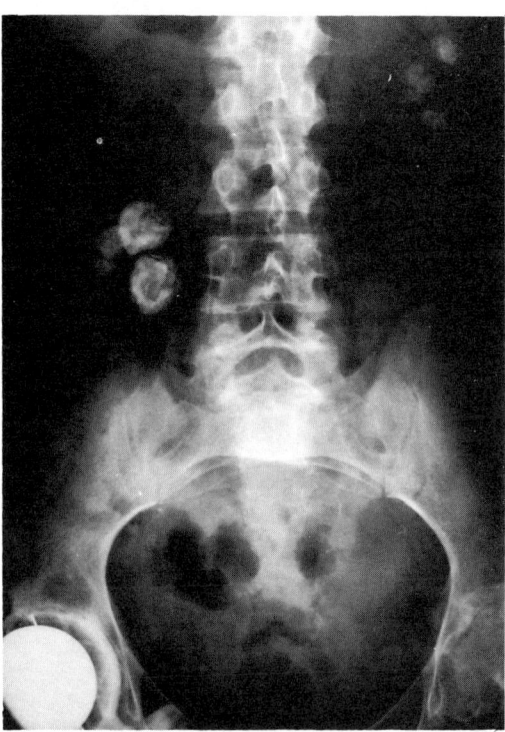

Fig. 6 Plain abdominal radiograph showing bilateral renal calculi in a 63-year-old woman with nephropathy due to long-standing analgesic consumption for painful hips. The right femoral head has been replaced by a prosthesis.

tation of the interpapillary cortex but the papillae are normal. Chronic pyelonephritis and reflux nephropathy cause asymmetrical renal contraction with focal cortical scarring; calyceal clubbing is rarely generalized (as is often the case in analgesic nephropathy), the papillae do not separate, and medullary cavitation is not found (Fig. 7). Chronic obstructive atrophy, particularly if the original obstruction has been relieved, may produce changes very similar to those of analgesic abuse. The ragged calyces caused by papillary separation in analgesic nephropathy may suggest tuberculosis, but this is unlikely to produce bilateral generalized calyceal changes. The finding of calyceal strictures should suggest tuberculosis, and in doubtful cases the urine should be cultured repeatedly for *Mycobacterium tuberculosis*. Ischaemic scars may affect any part of the cortical outline, but are unaccompanied by papillary abnormalities. In bilateral renal artery stenosis, a rare condition, the papillae are normal in shape and the kidneys may be normal in size, or small.

Renal papillae occasionally necrose in patients with urine infection complicating diabetes mellitus or obstructive uropathy. The presentation is usually acute with renal colic, haematuria, or renal failure. Papillae may necrose insidiously in patients with sickle cell disease or trait (Fig. 8); the radiological findings are then as described for analgesic nephropathy.

Renal biopsy
Biopsy is not usually helpful because inner medullary tissue is not often present in the biopsy specimen and changes in the more superficial tissue are not specific.

Cystoscopy
Cystoscopy and cytological examination of the urine for neoplastic cells should be carried out if urothelial carcinoma is suspected. Cytological abnormalities may precede other evidence of carcinoma by many months, and a case can be made for regular screening.

Prevention
Several countries have placed legal restrictions on the availability of phenacetin. However, the inessential use of all analgesics should be discouraged. No analgesic can be regarded as without danger, although only a very small proportion of treated persons suffer significant renal damage. If regular long-term analgesia is necessary, phenacetin-containing drugs should be avoided; the possible dangers of other analgesics should not be forgotten, although adequate relief from genuine pain must be the dominant consideration.

Treatment
Acute analgesic nephrotoxicity usually subsides rapidly when the drug is withdrawn, although it may recur if the same drug is given again. In patients with chronic nephropathy regular analgesic consumption must be stopped and only those quantities allowed which are necessary for the control of genuine pain. Hypertension and urinary infection should be treated for they may produce further impairment of renal function. The adequacy of dietary salt and fluid intake must be reconsidered periodically because of the tendency to sodium depletion, which may cause prerenal uraemia and further papillary necrosis; salt requirements may change with time. Surgery may be necessary to relieve obstruction from

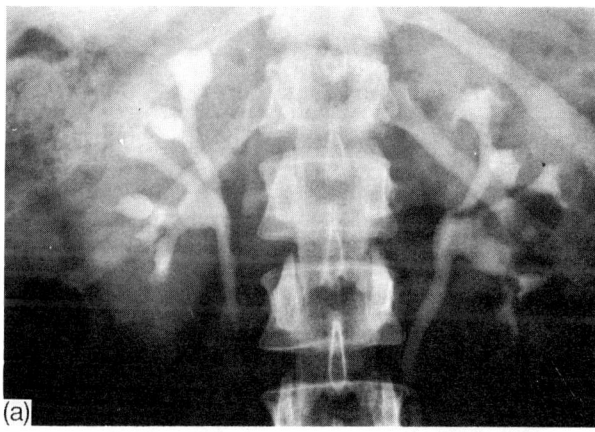

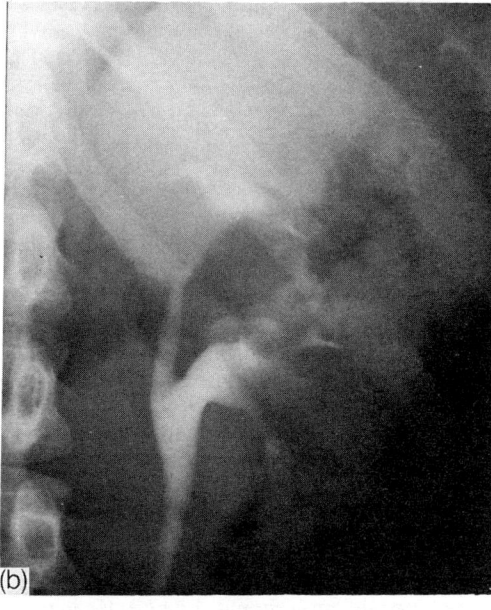

Fig. 8 IVUs in two patients with sickle cell trait. (a) The calyces of the left kidney are distorted and contrast medium can be seen tracking towards the cortex. Calyceal dilation in the right kidney, may, however, be accounted for by recent pregnancy. (b) The calyces are distorted, there is tracking of contrast medium towards the cortex and a pool of contrast medium in the lowest papilla suggests that this has separated. Reproduced from *Postgraduate Nephrology*; ed. F. P. Marsh, by permission of the publishers.)

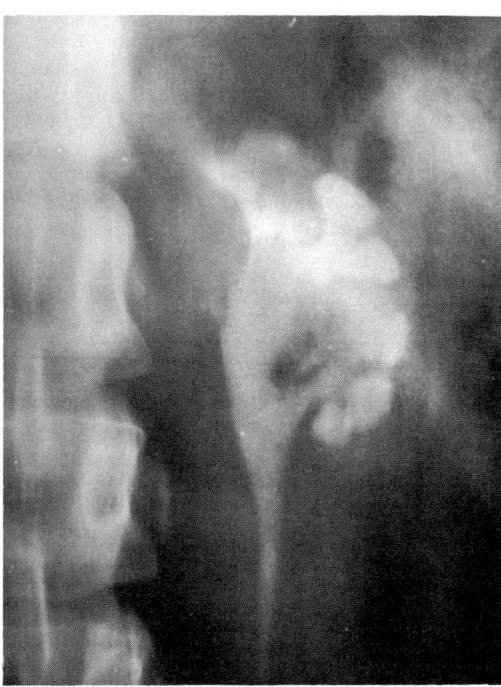

Fig. 7 Tomogram from an IVU showing severe cortical scarring and calyceal clubbing due to reflux nephropathy. In this condition the calyceal changes are not usually so generalized.

impacted renal papilla or stone, or due to peri-ureteric fibrosis. Particular care is necessary to minimize haemorrhage and avoid hypotension and saline depletion during and after surgery, for these may cause acute deterioration in renal function. Nephroureterectomy may be needed for complicating carcinoma. Unfortunately this has a poor prognosis, only a quarter of affected patients surviving five years. This is probably because renal failure often makes adequate removal of the tumour impossible, because the tumours tend to recur, and because metastases develop in almost half the patients.

Narcotic analgesics
Septicaemia, bacterial endocarditis, and chronic hepatitis B infection may cause immune complex glomerulonephritis in drug addicts.

An increased incidence of proteinuria, nephrotic syndrome, and chronic renal failure with a poor prognosis has been described in users of intravenous narcotics, especially heroin, who do not have such obvious bacterial or viral infections. Black addicts are said to be particularly susceptible. Focal glomerulosclerosis is most often found on biopsy but mesangiocapillary glomerulonephritis has also been observed. Focal deposits of IgM and C3 are usually found in the mesangium and along capillary loops using immunofluorescence microscopy. It is uncertain whether heroin itself, its diluents or contaminants, or the recurrent infection associated with its use by addicts, is responsible. Focal glomerulosclerosis causing nephrotic syndrome and rapidly deteriorating renal function has also been found in patients with the acquired immunodeficiency syndrome (AIDS). However, the association of this glomerular lesion with narcotics seems to be an independent one, for it was noted before AIDS became prevalent.

Acute renal failure due to necrotizing angiitis or to rhabdomyolysis and myoglobinuria has also been described in adults injecting narcotics intravenously.

Slowly acting agents used in rheumatoid arthritis
Gold
The urine of patients receiving gold therapy for rheumatoid arthritis should be tested regularly for protein. Proteinuria probably develops in 1 to 10 per cent, although in some cases a condition other than gold-induced damage, such as renal amyloid, is the cause. Nephrotic syndrome occurs much less often. The nephropathy is unrelated to other side-effects of gold, may present at any time and at any dose, and cannot be predicted from serum or urine gold concentrations. Histologically it is a membranous glomerulonephritis, although changes on light microscopy may be minimal. Electron and immunofluorescence microscopy of the glomeruli show subepithelial electron-dense deposits and granular deposition of IgG, C3, and sometimes IgM on the capillary basement membrane.

Although the deposits are presumed to be immune complexes, there is no proof of this. They contain neither gold nor sulphur, but gold has been found in other parts of the glomeruli, and in proximal tubules and the interstitium of the kidney.

Gold treatment should be stopped if the protein concentration in the urine exceeds 2 g/l; the proteinuria then usually subsides over a few months to a few years. It has been claimed that the treatment can later be cautiously reintroduced; and even that lesser amounts of proteinuria may subside even if chrysotherapy is continued.

Penicillamine
Regular tests for proteinuria should also be made in patients being treated with penicillamine because it develops in 7 to 30 per cent. Although found most often in the first year of treatment, it can present at any time and at any dose. Changes in the glomeruli are usually minimal as seen by light microscopy, but electron and immunofluorescence microscopy show evidence of a membranous glomerulonephritis of presumed immune complex nature, with small subepithelial electron-dense deposits, and granular deposits of IgG and C3 in the capillary loops. The prognosis is uncertain. The development of impaired renal function is uncommon, and it has been claimed that penicillamine need not be stopped if the proteinuria is only slight. However, mild proteinuria often precedes a nephrotic syndrome in these patients and despite cessation of treatment the urinary abnormality and the electron-dense deposits in the kidneys may persist for many months.

Much less often a crescentic proliferative glomerulonephritis has been described, associated with pulmonary haemorrhage in a very few patients; this has a much more serious prognosis.

Oral contraceptives
That oral contraceptives can produce hypertension, reversible on their withdrawal, is widely recognized. It is less well-appreciated that some increase in blood pressure occurs in almost all who take them, and that about 5 per cent of users will develop frank hypertension within five years, an incidence over twice that in nonusers. The mechanism is uncertain and attempts to predict those at special risk have been disappointing. Both oestrogen and progestogen components contribute to the abnormality, and it is not established that the low-dose oestrogen–progestogen contraceptives are less harmful.

Rarely malignant hypertension, or acute and irreversible renal failure occur. Attenuation of intrarenal vessels, intrarenal microthrombi, and microangiopathic haemolytic anaemia have been detected in patients with such complications. Multiple major arterial thromboses and renal infarction have also been described.

Metals
Lithium
Long-term lithium treatment is often used to prevent relapse in psychiatric patients with recurrent affective disorders. Close clinical supervision, with repeated estimation of serum lithium concentration, is necessary to avoid troublesome side-effects. There has been controversy over the importance of the drug's effects on the kidney, through which it is excreted.

Severe lithium intoxication can cause acute renal failure. Prolonged treatment, even when well controlled, often reduces the ability of the tubules to concentrate urine in response to vasopressin, but troublesome polyuria is uncommon. Concern has arisen over reports that renal interstitial fibrosis, glomerulosclerosis, and tubular atrophy were much more often found in people treated with lithium for several years than in matched non-psychiatric control patients; and that glomerular filtration rates sometimes fell in the former. Recent studies have suggested that the risk of renal failure developing during well-controlled lithium therapy is very small, and similar functional and pathological changes have been found in psychiatric patients treated with other psychotropic agents.

Platinum
Platinum is nephrotoxic, like other heavy metals. The effect is dose related and limits the use of inorganic cis-platinum complexes, such as cisplatin, in the management of refractory tumours. Proteinuria, cast excretion, and raised blood urea concentrations may develop within a few days of administration and magnesuria may cause hypomagnesaemia; subsequent recovery of renal function takes several weeks and may be incomplete. Histologically there is tubular damage and sometimes frank necrosis. Renal damage is favoured by the repeated administration of cisplatin over short periods and by co-administration of other potentially nephrotoxic agents such as aminoglycosides; it is reduced by giving saline infusions before and during treatment, and possibly by the simultaneous administration of mannitol or frusemide. Several less toxic analogues of cisplatin are being evaluated.

Radiographic contrast media
The safety of modern radiographic contrast media is often taken for granted. However, transient minor reduction in urine flow and

renal function is probably quite frequent after angiography, intravenous urography, and radiographic investigation of the biliary tract. It is uncertain how often this merely results from dehydration, and its incidence is said to be much reduced by preventing this. Serious nephrotoxicity is uncommon. Diabetics, patients with prerenal uraemia, existing hepatic or renal damage, or myeloma are claimed to be particularly susceptible as, to a less extent, are those with generalized vascular disease, proteinuria or hypoalbuminaemia. The repeated administration of contrast within a few days increases the risk and should be avoided as far as possible. Myelomatosis used to be considered an absolute contraindication to intravenous urography because of the danger of intratubular precipitation of myeloma protein by contrast medium. However, the low protein binding of modern media reduces the risk considerably provided dehydration is avoided.

Antihypertensive drugs

It is difficult to summarize the effects of antihypertensives on renal function because their acute effects often differ from those found during prolonged therapy, and patients with hypertension or renal failure may respond differently from those with normal renal function and blood pressure. The changes produced during long-term treatment with various classes of antihypertensives have been summarized by Bauer (1984). In general diuretics, direct acting vasodilators and converting enzyme inhibitors do not reduce glomerular filtration rate, whereas beta-blockers, central alpha II-adrenoceptor agonists, and adrenergic neurone blocking agents (central or peripheral) do so. In the long term, control of blood pressure is important in preventing unnecessarily rapid deterioration of renal function.

Several antihypertensives have specific nephrotoxic effects. Thiazides and loop diuretics occasionally cause acute interstitial nephritis or necrotizing vasculitis. Hydralazine can cause a lupus-like syndrome, usually considered to spare the kidney and to be uncommon if the dose is restricted to not more than 200 mg daily. However, its incidence is probably much greater than generally realized, even in patients taking only modest amounts of the drug. Renal involvement is also probably quite common. Rapidly progressive renal failure, reversible on withdrawal of hydralazine, has been described in a number of patients; the histology is that of a segmental proliferative glomerulonephritis.

Proteinuria has been reported in some 1 per cent of patients taking captopril, and about a fifth of these develop a nephrotic syndrome. The proteinuria occurs particularly amongst those with pre-existing renal disease or who are taking more than 150 mg of the drug each day. It resolves in most patients whether or not the drug is continued and renal function does not deteriorate. Renal biopsy has shown membranous nephropathy in some cases, but evidence that captopril was responsible for this is not conclusive. On present evidence enalapril is less likely to cause proteinuria. Converting enzyme inhibitors often produce a slight reduction in overall creatinine clearance in patients with a unilateral renal artery stenosis. Radioisotopic scanning, however, often shows a severe decrease in glomerular filtration rate on the affected side, due to a preferential reduction in postglomerular arteriolar resistance, with consequent diminution in filtration fraction. This is particularly important in those with bilateral stenoses or with stenosis of the arterial supply of a solitary kidney, such as a kidney graft, whose function may fail dramatically and permanently.

Miscellaneous agents

Clofibrate

Clofibrate should only be given in markedly reduced dosage, if at all, to uraemic patients, in whom it may cause severe and sometimes irreversible deterioration in renal function. They may also develop gross muscular weakness and pain due to an accumulation of unbound chlorphenoxyisobutyric acid, a metabolite. A reversible acute interstitial nephritis has also been attributed to the drug.

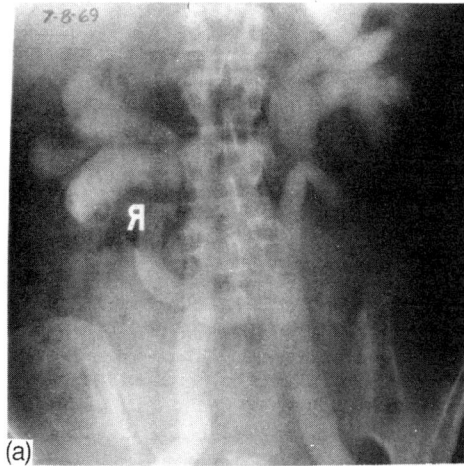

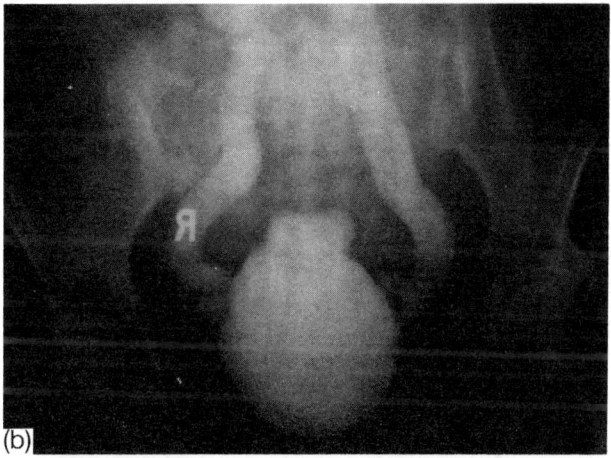

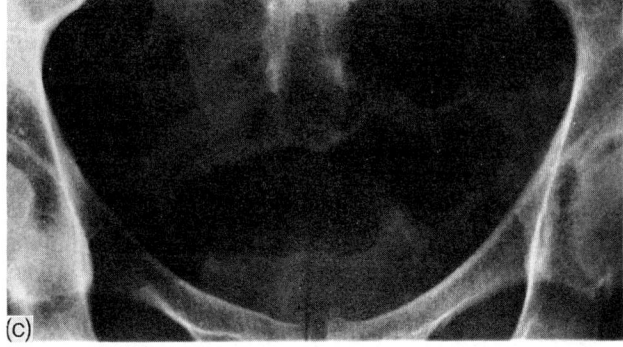

Fig. 9 IVU showing some late affects of cyclophosphamide cystitis in one patient. (a) Bilateral hydronephrosis due to vesico-ureteric reflux. (b) Dilated ureters and bladder diverticula. (c) Bladder wall calcification.

Cyclosporin

Cyclosporin A has become popular for preventing the rejection of transplanted organs, because graft survival during the first few years is greater than when classical immunosuppressants are used. Unfortunately, the drug is deposited in renal tubular cells and is nephrotoxic, causing glomerular damage, renal arteriolar changes, vacuolation, and atrophy of the proximal tubules and interstitial fibrosis. During cyclosporin therapy glomerular filtration is less than during treatment with prednisolone and azathioprine alone, although it improves when cyclosporin is stopped. The long-term effects of this new immunosuppressant are unknown.

Acute deterioration of renal function, the mechanism of which is uncertain, can occur at any time during the first year after transplantation and, in the case of kidney transplants, can be difficult to distinguish from rejection. Fortunately it improves within a day or so when the dose of cyclosporin is reduced. Acute nephrotoxicity is particularly common when high doses are used and in patients with high blood cyclosporin levels, but can occur when the concentration is relatively low. Ischaemic kidneys are particularly susceptible. Certain drugs, such as frusemide, aminoglycosides, and ketoconazole appear to increase the risk of acute nephrotoxicity, and steroids may reduce it.

Cyclophosphamide
Cyclophosphamide is unique among cytotoxic drugs in its ability to cause severe ulcerative haemorrhagic cystitis, which may result in bladder contraction and the development of gross vesico-ureteric reflux (Fig. 9). The development of carcinoma of the bladder several years later has been reported.

Mitomycin
Mitomycin can cause proteinuria, microscopic haematuria, and renal failure. The presentation is often indolent, several months after the end of treatment with the drug, but severe microangiopathic haemolytic anaemia, acute renal failure, hypertension, and dyspnoea may supervene, sometimes precipitated by blood transfusion. The pathological changes are those of a haemolytic uraemic syndrome, with focal glomerular proliferation and necrosis, capillary and arteriolar thrombi, and tubular necrosis. In the lungs alveolar haemorrhage and fibrin and intimal thickening of pulmonary arterioles are found. Glomerular sclerosis and renal interstitial fibrosis may become prominent. The cause is unknown. No treatment improves the renal lesions, although plasmapheresis has been reported to help the haematological manifestations.

Methoxyflurane
Inorganic fluoride and oxalic acid are produced by the metabolism of methoxyflurane. The fluoride is mainly responsible for the acute, often polyuric, renal failure which this anaesthetic may cause, although the deposition of calcium oxalate crystals in tubules and interstitium may contribute to this. Recovery usually occurs within a few days, but may be delayed for several months and occasionally does not occur. There appear to be differences in the susceptibility of individuals to the nephrotoxic effects, and patients with existing renal impairment or receiving methoxyflurane repeatedly may be particularly at risk. The likelihood of acute renal failure occurring is increased by high concentrations of the anaesthetic, prolonged anaesthesia, and by alcohol, phenobarbitone, and perhaps other enzyme inducers, as well as by other nephrotoxic agents such as gentamicin or tetracycline. Enflurane, a related anaesthetic, seems to be less nephrotoxic.

References
Barza, M. (1978). The nephrotoxicity of cephalosporins; an overview. *J. infect. Dis.* **137**, S 60–73.
Bauer, J. H. (1984). Role of angiotensin converting enzyme inhibitors in essential and renal hypertension. *Am. J. Med.* **77** (2A), 43–51.
Blackshear, J. L., Davidman, M. and Stillman, T. (1983). Identification of risk for renal insufficiency from non-steroidal anti-inflammatory drugs. *Arch. intern. Med.* **143**, 1130–1134.

British Medical Journal (1981). Penicillamine nephropathy. *Br. Med. J.* **282**, 761–762.
Butler, W. I., Bennett, J. E., Alling, D. W., Wertlake, P. T., Utz, J. P., and Hill, G. J. (1964). Nephrotoxicity of amphotericin B. Early and late effects in 81 patients. *Ann. intern. Med.* **61**, 175–187.
Churchill, D. N., Fine, A. and Gault, M. H. (1983). Association between hydrocarbon exposure and glomerulonephritis. An appraisal of the evidence. *Nephron.* **33**, 169–172.
Cunningham, E. E., Brentjens, J. R., Zielezny, M. A., Andres, G. A. and Venuto, R. C. (1980). Heroin nephropathy. A clinicopathologic and epidemiologic study. *Am. J. Med.* **68**, 47–53.
Dubach, U. C., Rosner, B. and Pfister, E. (1983). Epidemiological study of abuse of analgesics containing phenacetin. *N. Engl. J. Med.* **308**, 357–362.
Galpin, J. E., Shinaberger, J. H., Stanley, T. M., Blumenkrantz, M. J., Bayer, A. S., Friedman, G. S., Montgomerie, J. Z., Guze, L. B., Coburn, J. W. and Glassock, R. J. (1978). Acute interstitial nephritis due to methicillin. *Am. J. Med.* **65**, 756–765.
Hamner, R. W., Verami, R. and Weinman, E. J. (1983). Mitomycin-associated renal failure. Case report and review. *Arch. int. Med.* **143**, 803–807.
Ingles, J. A., Henderson, D. A. and Emmerson, B. T. (1978). The pathology and pathogenesis of chronic lead nephropathy occurring in Queensland. *J. Pathol.* **124**, 65–76.
Kannel, W. B. (1979). Oral contraceptive hypertension and thromboembolism. *Int. J. Gyn. Obs.* **16**, 466–472.
Kidney International (1978). Analgesic nephropathy. *Kidney Int.* **13**, 1–113.
Lancet (1976). Cadmium, lead and hypertension. *Lancet* ii, 1230–1231.
—— (1979). Lithium nephropathy. *Lancet* ii, 619–620.
—— (1979). Lithium and the kidney: grounds for cautious optimism. *Lancet* ii, 1056–1057.
—— (1983). Cadmium-continuing enigma. *Lancet* i, 1421.
Madias, N. E. and Harrington, J. T. (1978). Platinum nephrotoxicity. *Am. J. Med.* **65**, 307–314.
Marsh, F. P. (1985). Toxic nephropathies. In *Postgraduate nephrology* (ed. F. P. Marsh), pp. 425–447. Heinemann, London.
Mazze, R. I. (1976). Methoxyflurane nephropathy. *Environ. Hlth Perspect.* **15**, 111–119.
Nessi, R., Bonoldi, G. L., Redaelli, B. and di Filippo, G. (1976). Acute renal failure after rifampicin: a case report and survey of the literature. *Nephron.* **16**, 148–159.
Newton, P., Swinburn, W. R. and Swinson, D. R. (1983). Proteinuria with gold therapy: when should gold be permanently stopped? *Br. J. Rheumatol.* **22**, 11–17.
Pierides, A. M., Alvarez-Ude, F., Kerr, D. N. S. and Skillen, W. N. (1975). Clofibrate-induced muscle damage in patients with chronic renal failure. *Lancet* ii, 1279–1282.
Ruprah, M., Mant, T. G. L. and Flanagan, R. J. (1985). Acute carbon tetrachloride poisoning in 19 patients: implications for diagnosis and treatment. *Lancet* i, 1027–1029.
Shaper, A. G. and Pocock, S. J. (1985). Blood lead and blood pressure. *Br. Med. J.* **291**, 1147–1149.
Wenting, G. J., Tan–Tjiong, H. L., Derkx, F. H. M., de Bruyn, J. H. B. Man in'T Veld, A. J. and Schalekamp, M. A. D. H. (1984). Split renal function after captopril in unilateral renal artery stenosis. *Br. Med. J.* **288**, 886–890.
Winship, K. A. (1983). Toxicity of bismuth salts. *Adv. Drug. React. Ac. Pois. Rev.* **2**, 103–121.
—— (1984). Toxicity of inorganic arsenic salts. *Adv. Drug. React. Ac. Pois. Rev.* **3**, 129–160.
—— (1985). Toxicity of mercury and its inorganic salts. *Adv. Drug. React. Ac. Pois. Rev.* **4**, 129–160.

DRUGS AND THE KIDNEY

F. P. MARSH

General considerations

The kidneys eliminate most drugs or their metabolites from the body. When they fail, such substances may accumulate and cause unwanted effects. If repeated doses of a drug have to be given to a uraemic patient, the normal dose plan will probably have to be altered, unless the drug and its metabolites are unusually non-toxic. This is done by reference to the severity of renal failure as estimated by creatinine clearance or plasma creatinine concentration. However, creatinine clearance may overestimate the true glomerular filtration rate considerably in severe renal failure and in the nephrotic syndrome. Plasma creatinine by itself is a poor index of glomerular filtration in old or wasted patients, although several formulae and nomograms have been devised to allow for the effects of age, weight, and sex and, thereby, to relate creatinine concentration to clearance more closely in such people.

Factors other than reduced glomerular filtration may alter the effectiveness of drugs in renal failure. These include changes in tubular secretion or reabsorption, renal or hepatic metabolism, protein binding, receptor sensitivity, and gastrointestinal absorption. The combined effect of these is often uncertain in an individual patient and any prediction of an acceptable dose can only be approximate, even with the help of nomograms and computer-based calculations.

Serial estimations of drug concentration in relevant body fluids (usually plasma) may be of help in determining the proper dose, but are of less use than might be anticipated. Firstly, techniques are available for the routine assay of only a few drugs. Even less often is it feasible to measure that fraction of a drug which is unbound to plasma proteins and is, therefore, available for diffusion and attachment to receptor sites. Secondly, the measurements often do not take separate account of active or inactive drug metabolites which themselves may accumulate in uraemia. Finally, although the effects of many drugs are related to their concentrations in plasma, those of some, such as propranolol and hydralazine, are not.

It is important that recommendations about drug dosage in a patient with renal failure are recognized for what they are – approximations; and that the clinical response of each patient is carefully assessed.

The handling of drugs by renal tubules

All drugs (or their metabolites) which are excreted by the kidney are filtered to a greater or lesser extent by the glomeruli. Some are also actively secreted by the tubules or reabsorbed, usually passively, by them.

There are at least two separate pathways for the *active* proximal renal tubular secretion of drugs and their metabolites. The first handles organic acids such as penicillins, cephalosporins, nitrofurantoin, acyclovir, sulphonamides, chlorpropamide, frusemide and thiazide diuretics, phenobarbitone, salicylates, phenylbutazone, indomethacin, and probenecid. The second deals with organic bases, such as amiloride, mecamylamine, mepacrine, procainamide, triamterene, and quinidine. Drugs may compete for the same excretory pathway, which is how, for example, probenecid diminishes the excretion of penicillins, cephalosporins, nitrofurantoin, and acyclovir. *Passive* diffusion of lipid-soluble drugs can occur across tubular epithelial cells, theoretically in either direction. As urine containing a drug passes along the nephron, the concentration of that drug within the tubule increases as sodium and water are absorbed. A lipid-soluble drug can diffuse back to the plasma down the concentration gradient so created. A water-soluble drug is less able to cross the tubular epithelium in this way and is more readily excreted in the urine. Weakly acidic or basic drugs exist in the urine in ionized and unionized forms; the ratio between them depends on the pH of the urine and the ionization constant (Ka) of the drug. The latter is often expressed as pKa, which is the negative logarithm of the ionization constant. Because the unionized form is more lipid-soluble than the ionized, it more easily diffuses from tubule to blood. Any change in the urinary pH which favours ionization will therefore hinder such 'non-ionic diffusion' and enhance excretion of the drug. This is the basis for the treatment of salicylate and phenobarbitone overdosage by forced alkaline diuresis.

In chronic renal failure glomerular filtration and tubular function are both reduced. Sometimes the latter is disproportionately altered, as in the sodium wasting which may occur in polycystic renal disease, analgesic nephropathy, and chronic pyelonephritis. It is uncertain how much this affects the renal excretion of drugs.

Metabolism of drugs

The metabolism of most drugs takes place in the smooth endoplasmic reticulum of the liver, usually producing derivatives which are less active and more water soluble (and therefore more easily excreted in the urine). The effect of uraemia on the hepatic metabolism of individual drugs is difficult to determine; their metabolism may be unchanged, or reduced or (as with phenytoin) increased, and may be altered by the duration of treatment and the presence of other drugs.

Some drugs are metabolized by the kidney itself. Thus, effects on calcium metabolism previously attributed to cholecalciferol are now known to be due to hydroxylated derivatives, particularly 1,25-dihydroxycholecalciferol. This is produced in the kidney from the less active metabolite 25-hydroxycholecalciferol, itself formed in the liver from cholecalciferol. The diminished conversion of 25-hydroxy- to 1,25-dihydroxycholecalciferol in the failing kidney contributes to the development of osteomalacia and secondary hyperparathyroidism. The effects of these are resistant to calciferol given in anything less than huge amounts. Many of them, however, can be prevented or improved, at least temporarily, by minute doses of 1,25-dihydroxycholecalciferol (calcitriol), or 1-α-hydroxycholecalciferol (alfacalcidol) which is converted to the former compound in the liver. The long-term results and safety of such treatment are still being investigated.

Some opiates, notably morphine, codeine, and hydrocodeine (but not pethidine) were thought to be metabolized mainly by the renal tubules. Accumulation of the parent drug was believed to cause the prolonged respiratory failure and coma which sometimes occurs in patients with renal failure given normal doses. However, recent work suggests that the apparent sensitivity to morphine is due to accumulation of morphine 6-glucosamide, a metabolite which is normally excreted by the kidney and which cross-reacts with morphine in some assays.

Wherever metabolites are produced, they still have to be eliminated from the body. They are usually excreted by the kidneys, whose failure causes their concentrations to increase. Many cause or contribute significantly to the therapeutic or toxic effects superficially due to the parent drug, and their accumulation in uraemia may be dangerous. Examples of drugs whose active metabolites are retained in renal failure are given in Table 1. The retention of even inactive metabolites may have pharmacokinetic effects, although the clinical importance of this is uncertain. For example, an inactive metabolite may potentially modify the activity of its parent drug by competing for its binding sites, prolonging its half-life in plasma, or undergoing dissociation in the intestine after biliary excretion with subsequent reabsorption of the active moiety. Of more obvious therapeutic relevance is the cross-reaction of some metabolites with their parent compounds in diagnostic assays, causing false results. This is unimportant if the metabolite concentration is low, but may be misleading if it is high due to renal failure, as has been found in assays of digoxin, isoniazid, procainamide, and sulphadimidine. Similarly, the cross-reaction between bilirubin and metabolites of propranolol in spectrophotometric assays has led to the mistaken diagnosis of hyperbilirubinaemia in hypertensive dialysis patients.

Binding of drugs to plasma proteins

In plasma, only that part of a drug which is unbound to protein is diffusible and pharmacologically active. Acidic drugs, such as those shown in Table 2, bind mainly to the same receptor on the albumin molecule as binds bilirubin. Basic drugs (Table 3) bind mainly to other serum proteins such as α_1-acid glycoprotein (orosomucoid), gamma globulin, and lipoproteins; some receptors on albumin can accept neutral drugs (such as digitoxin) and basic ones. As might be expected, the number of free receptor sites is reduced by hypoalbuminaemia. In uraemia, acid radicals, including fatty acids, accumulate and compete for albumin receptor sites with acidic drugs, whose binding is, therefore, reduced. In contrast, the binding of basic or neutral drugs is normal or only slightly impaired in patients with renal failure.

Reduced binding of a drug to plasma proteins might be expected to potentiate its activity, enhance its toxicity, and promote its metabolism. However, the actual consequences for an individual drug are complex and poorly understood. They are likely to be of pharmacokinetic and clinical significance only for drugs which are highly protein bound (over 70 per cent), and have a low volume of distribution and a low therapeutic ratio. One important consequence is that measurement of such a drug's total plasma concentration (bound and unbound) may no longer be used satisfactorily to predict its activity.

Phenytoin, valproic acid, prednisone, and diazoxide are examples of drugs whose binding is significantly interfered with by uraemia and hypoproteinaemia. The serum concentration of phenytoin needed to produce an anti-epileptic effect is 10–20 mg/l in non-uraemic patients, whereas 3–6 mg/l has the same effect in those with end-stage renal failure. The effective serum concentration of valproic acid is also reduced in uraemia. Side effects of phenytoin and prednisone are more frequent in hypoalbuminaemic patients, and the antihypertensive action of intravenous diazoxide is said to be exaggerated in uraemic ones.

Drugs may bind to albumin in urine. The reduced natriuretic effect of frusemide in nephrotic patients has been attributed to this, less free frusemide being available to inhibit the absorption of chloride in the ascending limb of Henle's loop.

End-organ sensitivity

Little is known about the effect of renal failure on the sensitivity of cell receptors for drugs. It is difficult to separate such a direct effect from indirect ones, such as those caused by alterations in drug metabolism and protein binding. Changes in receptor sensitivity may contribute to the exaggerated toxicity in uraemic patients of colistin and certain narcotics, sedatives, and tranquillizers, and to the diminished effect of erythropoietin on marrow and parathyroid hormone on bone.

Absorption of drugs

Uraemia, short of that causing diarrhoea and vomiting, probably has no marked general effect on drug absorption. However, absorption of frusemide has been found impaired in end-stage renal failure, and the absorption of calcium is reduced because of failure to metabolize vitamin D. Inorganic iron absorption is normal.

Adverse drug reactions in renal failure

Patients with renal failure are far more likely to suffer from the side effects of drugs than those with normal kidney function. In one study of 900 patients in hospital, those with a plasma urea concentration exceeding 14 mmol/l (84 mg/dl) were two and a half times more likely to develop adverse drug reactions than those with a normal plasma urea. In another study one-third of 178 acute neuropsychiatric illnesses in patients with renal failure were attributed to drugs. The main reasons for such susceptibility are:

1. Most drugs and their metabolites are excreted in the urine and accumulate when the kidneys fail, unless dosage is altered appropriately.

2. Patients with renal failure often receive unmodified doses of drugs because practitioners are insufficiently aware of the dangers of prescribing them. Sometimes the existence of previously undiagnosed renal failure is brought to light by drug-induced toxicity.

3. The pharmacokinetics of many drugs, and the effects of uraemia on them, are poorly understood. This is, paradoxically, more likely to be so for long-established favourites than for recently developed preparations. It is particularly difficult to prescribe properly drugs which are eliminated partly by the kidneys and partly by the liver, and to allow for the results of combined hepatic and renal failure.

4. As in non-uraemic patients, it is often difficult to determine and monitor the end-point of therapy. In such a circumstance the effect of dosage alteration made because of uraemia is difficult to ascertain.

5. Symptoms of drug toxicity may be mistaken for those of uraemia or the underlying disease, and so pass unrecognized for what they are; they may even lead to the giving of other toxic medicines in an attempt to control them.

6. Patients with renal failure are often prescribed so many drugs in different amounts to be taken at different times that even those whose senses are not dulled by uraemia are likely to get confused and to take incorrect doses. Some drugs may antagonize or potentiate others.

Table 1 Examples of drugs whose active metabolites accumulate in uraemia

Acebutolol	Methyldopa	Pethidine
Allopurinol	Metoprolol	Propoxyphene
Clofibrate	Morphine	Sulphonamides
Digoxin		

Table 2 Examples of acidic drugs

Barbiturates	Indomethacin	Salicylates
Cephalosporins	Naproxen	Sulphonamides
Clofibrate	Penicillins	Theophylline
Diazoxide	Phenylbutazone	Thiazides
Diflunisal	Phenytoin	Thyroxine
Frusemide	Probenecid	Valproic acid
		Warfarin

Table 3 Examples of basic drugs

Alprenolol	Imipramine	Propranolol
Chlorpromazine	Morphine	Quinidine
Dapsone	Oxazepam	Triamterene
Diazepam	Pindolol	Trimethoprim
Dipyridamole	Prazosin	Verapamil
Disopyramide	Propoxyphene	

Prescribing for patients with renal failure

In theory

After a single dose of a drug, its plasma concentration changes in a manner which depends on the drug's absorption, distribution, metabolism, and excretion. At its simplest the fall from maximum concentration becomes exponential (Fig. 1), and the time taken for the plasma concentration of the drug to fall by half during this phase is called the plasma elimination half-life ($t_{\frac{1}{2}}$). If the same dose is repeated regularly, the maximum and minimum concentrations at first gradually increase, but after four half-lives they remain constant (Fig. 2). This stable state will continue unless the dose, frequency of administration, absorption, volume of distribution, or rate of elimination of the drug is changed.

In uraemia, the half-life of the drug will probably be prolonged. The results of making no alteration in dosage and frequency of administration are shown in Fig. 3. They are: (*a*) the time taken for drug concentrations in plasma to reach a stable state is increased, although still equal to four (new) half-lives; and (*b*) the maximum and minimum plasma concentrations are increased.

In order to prevent the development of excessive plasma levels, with consequent toxicity, the drug may be given less frequently or in smaller doses.

Reduction of dose frequency

The frequency of administration may be reduced, ideally in proportion to the increase in half-life of the drug (Fig. 4).

The time then taken to reach a stable state does not depend on the frequency of administration: it is still four half-lives. However, because the interval between doses is increased, plasma concentrations fluctuate more slowly, which may result in long periods when they are too high or low. Therefore, this method is unsuitable if the difference between therapeutically effective and toxic concentrations is small; or if continuously effective levels are required.

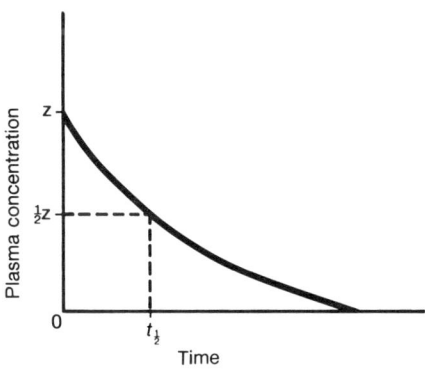

Fig. 1 Plasma elimination half-life of a drug. The half-life ($t_{\frac{1}{2}}$) of a drug is the time needed for its plasma concentration to fall by half.

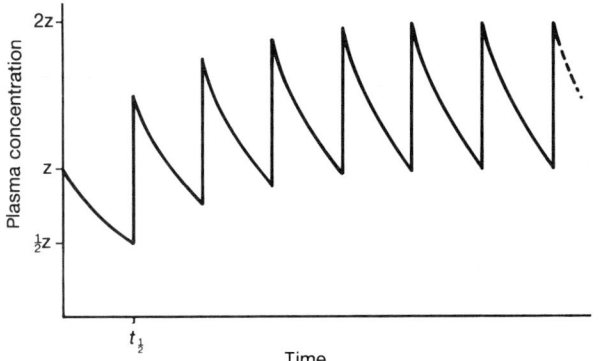

Fig. 2 Administration of a drug in constant dosage at intervals corresponding to its half-life. Diagram to show that after four half-lives the maximum and minimum concentrations achieved after each dose are constant. The curves obtained in life are usually more complex than shown.

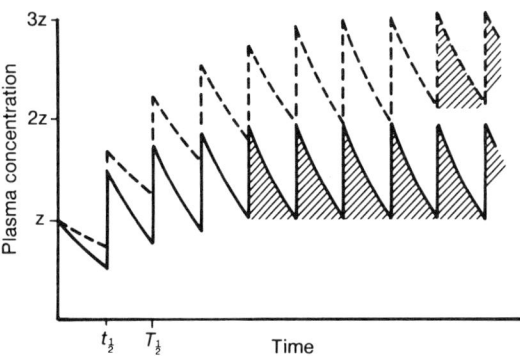

Fig. 3 Effect of increasing the half-life of a drug. Half-life doubled from $t_{\frac{1}{2}}$ to $T_{\frac{1}{2}}$; frequency of drug administration unchanged; dose unchanged; no loading dose. Solid line: plasma concentrations when half-life is $t_{\frac{1}{2}}$. Dashed line: plasma concentrations when half-life is $T_{\frac{1}{2}}$. The shaded areas under the diagrammatic curves indicate that the maximum and minimum concentrations occurring after each dose have become constant.

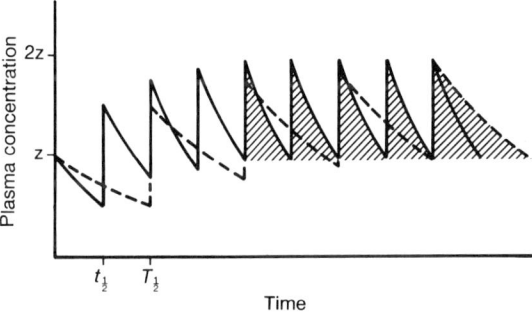

Fig. 4 Effect of increasing the half-life of a drug. Half-life doubled from $t_{\frac{1}{2}}$ to $T_{\frac{1}{2}}$; frequency of drug administration halved; dose unchanged; no loading dose. Solid line: plasma concentrations when half-life is $t_{\frac{1}{2}}$. Dashed line: plasma concentrations when half-life is $T_{\frac{1}{2}}$. The shaded areas under the diagrammatic curves indicate that the maximum and minimum concentrations occurring after each dose have become constant.

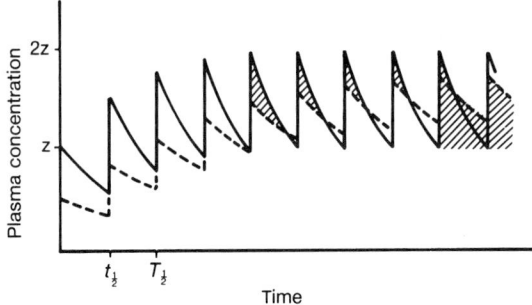

Fig. 5 Effect of increasing the half-life of a drug. Half-life doubled from $t_{\frac{1}{2}}$ to $T_{\frac{1}{2}}$; frequency of drug administration unchanged; dose halved; no loading dose. Solid line: plasma concentrations when half-life is $t_{\frac{1}{2}}$. Dashed line: plasma concentrations when half-life is $T_{\frac{1}{2}}$. The shaded areas under the diagrammatic curves indicate that the maximum and minimum concentrations occurring after each dose have become constant.

Reduction in dose size

The size of the dose, rather than the frequency with which it is given, may be reduced in proportion to the increase in half-life (Fig. 5). This is often more practicable, because dose intervals in uraemic and non-uraemic persons tend to be dictated by convenience as much as by pharmacokinetics. The fluctuations in plasma concentration being relatively little, the method is particularly suitable when the difference between therapeutically useful and toxic concentrations is small; and when continuously effective plasma levels are required.

More complex approaches, in which both dose frequency and size are altered, may be used for certain drugs such as aminoglycosides, in an attempt to maximize effectiveness and minimize toxicity. Their determination is often difficult, and there are often so many factors which affect the half-life that this is difficult to predict accurately, even with the help of nomograms or computer programs. Fortunately the half-life of a drug excreted entirely by glomerular filtration is related hyperbolically, not linearly, to glomerular filtration rate (Fig. 6), so that minor degrees of renal failure are unlikely to call for an alteration in drug administration.

Whichever of the modified dose regimes is used, the time taken to achieve stable (and hopefully therapeutic) plasma concentrations is likely to be increased in severe renal failure and will be four (new) half-lives. Therefore, if the half-life is long and an early action is important, a loading dose is necessary. Usually the normal one can be given, although digoxin is a possible exception. In the opinion of some, the loading dose of digoxin should be reduced by a third in patients with severe renal failure.

In practice

The simple concepts discussed above are useful as a basis for thinking, but do not do justice to an often complex situation. For instance, the half-life may be altered by factors other than glomerular filtration, as discussed earlier, and can usually only be estimated very approximately. The decline in plasma concentration is often not a single exponential function, and a drug may have two or more half-lives, depending on the part of the time–concentration curve under scrutiny. Metabolites of the prescribed drug may be biologically active, with beneficial and toxic effects, and their half-lives may be different from those of the parent substances. Elimination rates and volumes of distribution may vary with duration of treatment or the presence of other drugs. Finally, biological activity often, but by no means necessarily, parallels changes in chemical concentration of a drug in plasma.

Therapy should be based on pharmacological principles. However, some uncertainty as to the appropriate dose often remains, and mathematical calculations of doubtful applicability must not be allowed to replace careful clinical observation.

The most important rule is not to give a drug without good reason. If treatment is necessary, answers to the following questions should be sought:

1. Is it likely that dosage alteration will be necessary? Most drugs can be given in unchanged dose to patients whose creatinine clearance exceeds 50 ml/min. Even if this is less, dosage modification is usually unnecessary for a drug which is normally (*a*) given at intervals considerably exceeding its plasma elimination half-life (so that its plasma concentration is effectively zero before each dose), or (*b*) eliminated through other organs more rapidly than through the kidneys. This advice may not apply to a drug with a low therapeutic ratio, or if both hepatic and renal function are impaired.

2. Can the proposed drug reach the place where its action is desired? There is no point in prescribing a urinary antiseptic such as nitrofurantoin to a patient if impaired excretion prevents bacteristatic concentrations being attained in the urine.

3. Can the end-organ respond? Thiazide diuretics have little effect on sodium excretion in markedly uraemic patients, and to produce a diuresis even the powerful 'loop' diuretics (such as frusemide and bumetanide) may have to be given in massive doses.

4. Is the metabolism of the drug altered in uraemia? Normal doses of calciferol are ineffective in the treatment of renal osteodystrophy because the formation of its most active metabolite is reduced.

5. Does the drug interfere with measurements of renal function? Cefoxitin increases the apparent concentration of creatinine when measured by the Jaffé reaction. Because the interference lasts longer in urine than in blood it causes a spurious increase in the creatinine clearance. Conversely, co-trimoxazole, trimethoprim, and cimetidine can reduce creatinine clearance without affecting glomerular filtration rate as measured by other techniques, probably because they diminish the tubular secretion of creatinine. Such factors may cause incorrect deductions to be made about renal function, leading to incorrect drug dosage.

6. Is a rapid result required? In this case a loading dose may be necessary.

7. How long is the treatment likely to last? Compliance with dosage, and clinical observations, are more difficult during prolonged therapy, and extraneous factors are more likely to interfere.

8. Is the end-point of successful therapy easily recognizable? If not, a way of controlling therapy, and determining whether it is still required, should be sought.

9. Is the difference between an effective dose and a toxic dose small or large? If it is small, especial care is necessary.

10. Is it advisable and practicable to control treatment by serially measuring drug concentrations in the relevant body fluids? Proper interpretation requires knowledge of whether the results refer to free (unbound) or total drug, and whether active or inactive metabolites are included. It is also necessary to know some kinetics of the drug being measured, in order that samples may be taken at the proper times, and accurate deductions made from their analysis. For instance, gentamicin has a half-life of about two hours in normal people, and is usually given by injection three times daily for short periods only. Serum gentamicin concentration changes markedly in the interval between injections, and assessment of likely efficacy, toxicity, and dosage depends on measurements of the highest (postdose) and lowest (predose) concentrations. On the other hand digoxin has a prolonged distribution phase and a half-life of one and a half to two days when renal function is normal and is usually given twice daily for long periods; the timing of blood samples for its estimation is less critical, but they should be taken at least four hours after an oral dose, possibly longer in uraemic patients.

11. Are the toxic effects of the drug and its metabolites clinically recognizable? Can they be confused with symptoms of uraemia or the underlying disease, and they do subside rapidly when the drug is withdrawn? Particular care is necessary if the medicine is nephrotoxic or causes extrarenal uraemia.

12. Are side effects which are minor in patients with normal renal function likely to be hazardous in those with renal failure? For instance, spironolactone and amiloride can cause dangerous hyperkalaemia in patients with renal failure, whose ability to excrete potassium is reduced.

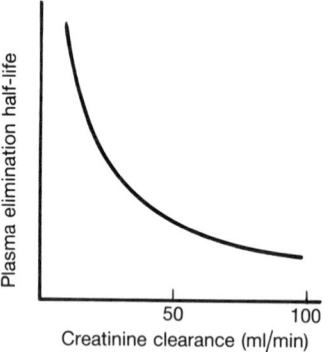

Fig. 6 Relationship between plasma elimination half-life and creatinine clearance. Diagram to show that small reductions in creatinine clearance have a marked effect on the half-life of a drug eliminated entirely by the kidneys in patients with considerable impairment of renal function, but little effect in patients whose renal function is only slight diminished.

Table 4 Adjustment of maintenance dose in renal failure

Drug	Factor by which normal dose amount should be divided, or by which normal dose interval should be multiplied[1]		Need for modification of dosage in dialysed patients[9]	Drug	Factor by which normal dose amount should be divided, or by which normal dose interval should be multiplied[1]		Need for modification of dosage in dialysed patients[9]
	Moderate renal failure[2]	Severe renal failure[3]			Moderate renal failure[2]	Severe renal failure[3]	
Acyclovir	1.5–3	3–6	Yes; H	Ibuprofen	1?	1?	No; H
Allopurinol	1	2	Yes; H	Imipramine	1	1	No; H and P
Amantadine	Avoid?	Avoid	No; H and P	Indomethacin	1	1?[5]	No; H
Amikacin	4	4	Yes; H and P	Insulin	1.3	2	? H no; P
Amiloride	3–7[10]	Avoid	–	Isoniazid	1	1–1.5	Yes; H and P
Amitriptyline	1	1	No; H and P	Isosorbide dinitrate	1	1	–
Amoxycillin	1	2	Yes; H no; P	Ketoconazole	1	1	No; H
Amphotericin B	1	1	No; H and P	Labetalol	1	1	–
Aspirin	1.5	Avoid[5]	Yes; H and P	Latamoxef	2	3	Yes; H
Atenolol	2	4	–	Lincomycin	2	4	No; H and P
Azapropazone	1?	3?	–	Lithium	2? Avoid[4]	Avoid	–
Azathioprine	1	1–1.5	Yes; H	Lorazepam	1	1	No; H?
Azlocillin	1–2	2	Yes; H no; P	Mecillinam	2	4	Yes; H
Benzhexol	1	1	–	Metformin	Avoid	Avoid	–
Captopril	1.5–6	Avoid?	Yes; H	Methenamine	Avoid	Avoid	–
Carbamazepine	1	1.5	No; H	Methyldopa	2	4	Yes; H and P
Carbenicillin	1.5	3	Yes; H and P	Metoclopramide	1.5	2	–
Carbidopa	1	1	–	Metolazone	1	1	No; H
Cefamandole	1–1.5	1.5	Yes; H	Metoprolol	1	1	Yes; H
Cefotaxime	1–1.5[6]	2[6]	Yes; H	Metronidazole	1	1.5–3	Yes; H no; P
Cefoxitin	1–3	3–6	Yes; H	Mezlocillin	1	1.5–2	Yes; H
Ceftazidime	1–2	4	Yes; H	Miconazole	1	1	No; H and P
Cefuroxime	3	6	Yes; H and P	Minocycline	1	1	No; H and P
Cephalexin	1	1–2	Yes; H no; P	Minoxidil	1	1	Yes; H
Cephalothin	1	1.5–2	Yes; H and P	Nadolol	1–2	2–3	Yes; H
Cephazolin	3	6	Yes; H no; P	Nalidixic acid	1	Avoid	–
Chlordiazepoxide	1	1	No; H	Naloxone	1	1	–
Chloroquine	1	2	No; H	Naproxen	1?	Reduce ?	No; H
Chlorpheniramine	1	1	–	Netilmicin	4	4	Yes; H and P
Chlorpromazine	1	1	No; H and P	Nifedipine	1	1	–
Chlorpropamide	Avoid	Avoid	No; P	Nitrofurantoin	Avoid	Avoid	–
Cholestyramine	1	1	–	Nortriptyline	1	1	No; H and P
Cimetidine	1.7	2	No; H and P	Opiates	7	7	Variable
Clindamycin	1	1–2	No; H and P	Pancuronium	1	Reduce	–
Clofibrate	2–3	Avoid	No; H	Paracetamol	1.5	2	Yes; H no; P
Cloxacillin	1	1	No; H	Penicillamine	Avoid	Avoid	–
Colestipol	1	1	–	Penicillin	1[8]	2[8]	Yes; H
Colistin	2	4	No; H and P	Phenelzine	1	1	–
Cyclophosphamide	1	1.5–2	Yes; H	Phenformin	Avoid	Avoid	–
Diazepam	1	1	No; H	Phenytoin	1	1	No; H
Diclofenac	1?	1?	–	Piroxicam	1?	1?	?
Diflunisal	1?	2?	–	Prazosin	Reduce	Reduce	No; H and P
Digitoxin	1	1–2	No; H and P	Prednisolone	1	1	Yes; H
Digoxin	2[4]	4–8[4]	No; H and P	Propranolol	1	1	No; H
Disopyramide	2	4	No; H	Ranitidine	1–2	2	–
Doxycycline	1	Avoid	No; H and P	Rifampicin	1	1	No; H
Enalapril	Reduce	Reduce	–	Sodium aurothiomalate	Avoid	Avoid	No; H
Erythromycin	1	1	No; H and P	Sodium valproate	1	1	No; H and P
Ethambutol	1–1.5	2	Yes; H and P	Spironolactone	2–4[10]	Avoid	–
Fenbufen	1?	?	–	Sulphamethoxazole	1.5	2	Yes; H no; P
Flucytosine	2–4	>4[4]	Yes; H and P	Tetracycline	Avoid	Avoid	–
Flurazepam	?	Avoid		Thiazides	1	Avoid	–
Fusidate sodium	1	1	No; P	Ticarcillin	1.5–2	3–4	Yes; H and P
Gentamicin	4	4	Yes; H and P	Tobramycin	4	4	Yes; H and P
Glibenclamide	1?	Avoid	–	Tolbutamide	1	Avoid	No; H
Glibornuride	1	Avoid	–	Trimethoprim	1.5	2	Yes; H no; P
Gliclazide	1	Avoid	–	Tubocurarine	1	Reduce	–
Glipizide	1	Avoid	–	Vancomycin (intravenous)	3	10	No; H and P
Heparin	1	1[5]	No; H and P	Verapamil	1	1	No; H
Hydralazine	1	1?	No; H and P	Warfarin	1	1[5]	No; H

[1] Factor of 1 indicates that the normal dose amount and interval are unchanged.
[2] Creatinine clearance 10–50 ml/min.
[3] Creatinine clearance <10 ml/min.
[4] Use regular estimations of serum drug concentration ± nomograms.
[5] Danger of gastrointestinal bleeding in uraemia.
[6] Further reduction needed if given with azlocillin, which diminishes its excretion.
[7] Pharmacodynamics poorly understood. Normal doses may cause prolonged respiratory failure and coma.
[8] Avoid very high doses.
[9] H = haemodialysis; P = peritoneal dialysis.
[10] May cause hyperkalaemia.

13. Is the patient's existing treatment likely to diminish the effectiveness or enhance the toxicity of a new drug? Will the new prescription likewise alter the actions of medicine already being taken? For example, lithium clearance is diminished and its toxicity enhanced by thiazides and indomethacin.

14. Does account have to be taken of restrictions on the patient's fluid and electrolyte intake?

15. Can the patient and relatives cope with all the tablets? It has been shown repeatedly that even in hospital, medicines are often given incorrectly.

Two groups of uraemic patients pose additional problems. The first consists of those whose renal function is changing rapidly, for instance, during recovery from acute tubular necrosis. In these, changes in plasma creatinine concentration lag behind those in glomerular filtration. Although recently described formulae have been claimed to enable creatinine clearance to be estimated from serial plasma creatinine determinations, even in patients with unstable renal function, changes in distribution volume and protein binding may add to the difficulty of predicting correct doses of drugs. In the second group are patients undergoing peritoneal dialysis, haemodialysis or haemofiltration. Some drugs, but not all, pass readily across peritoneal or haemodialysis membranes and this may necessitate an alteration in dosage. Peritoneal dialysis is performed for longer periods than haemodialysis, and drugs generally pass less readily across the peritoneum than across haemodialysis membranes. Therefore, quantities appropriate for patients receiving peritoneal dialysis may not be so for those on haemodialysis. Continuous ambulatory peritoneal dialysis is likely to differ from intermittent peritoneal dialysis in its effects on drug disposition, but the differences between them have not been fully explored. Drugs given in peritoneal dialysate may be absorbed and can accumulate and cause adverse reactions. There is little information about the effects of haemofiltration on drug dosage. The membranes used are highly permeable and would be expected to allow the free passage of drugs with a molecular weight up to 6000–12 000 daltons.

Dialysis patients usually have restricted sodium, potassium, and fluid allowances, which are particulary easily exceeded during intravenous therapy. The drug, as well as the vehicle in which it is administered, must be considered; thus 5.4 mmol of sodium are contained in every gram of carbenicillin or ticarcillin.

Table 4 gives a selection of drugs with recommendations concerning their use in patients with moderate and severe renal failure and those receiving dialysis. Most can be prescribed in normal doses to patients with mild impairment of kidney function. Clinical judgement must supplement the guidelines, as discussed above. It is particularly important to measure plasma concentrations when drugs whose toxic concentrations are only slightly greater than beneficial ones have to be used: these include digoxin, aminoglycosides, and lithium.

References

Bennett, W. M., Aronoff, G. R., Morrison, G., Golper, T. A., Pulliam, J., Wolfson, M. and Singer, I. (1983). Drug prescribing in renal failure: dosing guidelines for adults. *Am. J. Kid. Dis.* **3**, 155–193.

Bjornsson, T. D., Cocchetto, D. M., McGowan, F. X., Verghese, C. P. and Sedor, F. (1983). Nomogram for estimating creatinine clearance. *Clin. Pharmacokinet.* **8**, 365–369.

Chennavasin, P. and Craig Brater, D. (1981). Nomograms for drug use in renal disease. *Clin. Pharmacokinet.* **6**, 193–214.

Hallynck, T., Soep, H. H., Thomis, J., Boelaert, J., Daneels, R., Fillastre, J. P., Rosa, F. de., Rubinstein, E., Hatala, M., Spousta, J. and Dettli, L. (1981). Prediction of creatinine clearance from serum creatinine concentration based on lean body mass. *Clin. Pharmacol. Ther.* **30**, 414–421.

Marsh, F. P. (1985). Drugs and the kidney. In *Postgraduate nephrology* (ed. F. P. Marsh), pp. 448–458. Heinemann. London.

Reidenberg, M. M. and Drayer, D. E. (1984). Alteration of drug-protein binding in renal disease. *Clin. Pharmacokinet.* **9**, 18–26.

Rowland, M. (1984). Protein binding and drug clearance. *Clin. Pharmacokinet.* **9**, 10–17.

Verbeeck, R. K., Branch, R. A. and Wilkinson, G. R. (1981). Drug metabolites in renal failure: pharmacokinetic and clinical implications. *Clin. Pharmacokinet.* **6**, 329–345.

ACUTE RENAL FAILURE

J. G. G. LEDINGHAM

Introduction

The term 'acute renal failure' is an imprecise one, used to describe an abrupt loss of glomerular filtration rate (GFR) with a resultant rise in plasma urea and creatinine concentrations. Oliguria is common, but by no means invariable. This course of events may arise *de novo* but more commonly presents as a complication of serious illness or injury.

Causes

The causes of an abrupt loss of renal excretory function are legion (Table 1) but the true differential diagnosis can be quite narrow in the individual case when account is taken of the clinical setting in which acute renal failure has arisen. The commonest causes include extrarenal uraemia (poor renal perfusion), tubular necrosis, obstruction, glomerulonephritis, and acute interstitial nephritis. Renal failure caused by nephrotoxic drugs is increasingly recognized.

In one report based on observations over one year in a laboratory serving 750 000 people, raised blood urea concentrations were attributed to prerenal causes in 1500 cases, chronic renal failure in 200, obstruction in 150, and acute tubular necrosis in 60. In another series, also reported over a year but from a renal unit rather than from a biochemical laboratory, of 139 patients, 30 had prerenal uraemia, 10 obstruction, 7 acute parenchymal disease, and 92 acute tubular necrosis, mostly traumatic or surgical in origin. Both these reports came from the United Kingdom. In Boston, USA, some degree of renal dysfunction occurred in 5 per cent of 2216 medical and surgical patients admitted to one hospital over 5 months. The major causes were reported to be decreased renal perfusion (hypotension, volume depletion or cardiac failure), radiocontrast and aminoglycoside toxicity. In over half of these patients, impairment of renal function was thought to have been iatrogenic. Of those in whom the rise in plasma creatinine exceeded 3.0 mg/100 ml (265 μmol/l), 64 per cent died.

In general the traditional subdivision of patients into those with prerenal, renal, and postrenal causes is useful, if oversimple. The distinctions can be obvious, but commonly they are blurred. Abnormalities of fluid and electrolyte balance are to be expected in most cases and contribute to the degree of renal dysfunction whatever its cause.

Chronic renal disease with superimposed acute deterioration may mimic acute renal failure closely. The haemoglobin concentration is not always a good guide. It is nearly always low in chronic renal failure, but can be normal, for example, in polycystic

Table 1 Some causes of acute renal failure

Prerenal uraemia	Acute pyelonephritis
Acute tubular necrosis	Obstructive nephropathy
Acute cortical necrosis	Acute interstitial nephritis
Haemorrhage	(see Table 4)
Burns	Leptospirosis
GI losses	The acute glomerulonephritides
Crush injuries	Crystalluria (urate/phosphate/sulphonamide)
Rhabdomyolysis	Myeloma kidney
Heat stroke	Hypercalcaemia
Haemolysis	Renal artery occlusion
Septicaemia	Malignant hypertension
Pancreatitis	Systemic sclerosis
Hepatic failure	Haemolytic uraemic syndrome
Cardiac failure	Thrombotic thrombocytopenic purpura
Tetanus	Postpartum renal failure
Snake bite	Renal graft rejection
Amanita phalloides	Renal vein thrombosis
A. Verna cortinarius	
Drugs and chemicals	
(see Table 3)	

disease, and can fall with remarkable speed in acute renal disease. A history of troublesome pruritus, the presence of uraemic pigmentation or evidence in the optic fundi of long-standing hypertension all suggest a chronic process. Biochemical or radiological evidence of osteodystrophy is only likely when there has been uraemia over a period of years. Chronic renal disease can be diagnosed with confidence if the infusion urogram or ultrasound shows contracted kidneys, but in some patients with chronic disease the kidneys remain of normal size.

Prerenal uraemia

Any condition which threatens the perfusion of the kidneys may be associated with an acute deterioration of renal function which is reversible when perfusion is restored. The causes of prerenal uraemia overlap with those causing acute tubular necrosis and include trauma, burns, haemorrhage, major gastrointestinal or other unreplaced fluid losses, septicaemia, acute pancreatitis, and obstetric disaster; indeed any cause of circulatory failure. While the haemodynamic disturbance resulting in renal failure is usually obvious and major, measurements of brachial artery pressure and clinical estimates of the adequacy of the circulation do not always reflect the state of the *renal* circulation with accuracy.

The diagnosis of prerenal uraemia carries with it the implication that restoration of renal perfusion will reverse renal failure. The diagnosis is confirmed by observation of the effects of treatment and can, therefore, be made with certainty only retrospectively. Renal failure attributable to poor renal perfusion, but not reversed by restoring the circulation, implies acute tubular necrosis or more rarely acute cortical necrosis (see below).

Hypercalcaemia may result in acute prerenal uraemia by impairment of renal conservation of water, complicated by anor-

exia and vomiting (see page 18.95). A degree of direct damage to glomeruli and tubules is also likely if hypercalcaemia is prolonged.

Clinical features

The traditional signs of salt and water depletion are tachycardia, hypotension, postural hypotension, reduced skin turgor, reduced ocular tension, collapsed peripheral veins, and cold extremities (including nose and ears). But these are late signs and deficits of several litres may be present without any of them, especially in the young. In the old, signs are difficult to interpret. When the question of sodium and water depletion is raised and clinical evidence is dubious, fluid charts may be called in evidence. They are usually misleading; charts suggesting a patient to be 'in balance' are too often wildly incorrect. Records of daily weight are more reliable, but are rarely available before renal failure is diagnosed. Salt and water depletion is to be suspected in every patient with acute renal failure. Even when the central venous pressure appears normal by inspection or by direct measurement, fluid deficits may be present masked by constriction of the venous capacitance vessels.

The kidney is the first organ whose perfusion is reduced when the circulation is compromised. A healthy kidney when modestly underperfused increases its filtration fraction (i.e. preserves GFR when renal blood flow falls), but both urine volume and urinary sodium concentration are much reduced by increased tubular reabsorption of glomerular filtrate. This response is commonly used to distinguish prerenal uraemia from established renal damage.

Prerenal uraemia or established renal disease?

In uncomplicated prerenal uraemia, the urine is classically free of protein, low in volume and sodium concentration, and high in osmolality urea and creatinine concentrations. When renal damage has occurred urinary urea, creatinine, and osmolality tend to be lower and sodium concentration higher. These trends are useful clinically, but do not discriminate in every case. An index of fractional sodium excretion (urine to plasma sodium ratio divided by urine to plasma creatinine ratio multiplied by 100) is less than 1 per cent in most patients with poor perfusion of healthy kidneys, but may also be low in other conditions such as glomerulonephritis, cardiac and hepatic failure, myoglobinuric or haemoglobinuric renal failure, radiocontrast-induced renal failure, acute interstitial nephritis, and in a few cases of acute obstruction. Despite these limitations and recent suggestions in the literature that measurement of fractional sodium excretion may be of no prognostic value in acute renal failure, most physicians have found the approach reflected in Table 2 helpful. The data were derived from a prospective study in which simple measurement of urinary osmolality, sodium, and creatinine distinguished prerenal from renal uraemia in 80 per cent of cases but failed to do so in the remaining 20 per cent. Improved accuracy was achieved using the fractional sodium excretion index (see above) and the 'renal failure index'.

$$\text{Renal failure index} = \frac{\text{Urinary sodium (mmol/l)}}{\text{Urine/plasma creatinine ratio}}$$

Table 2 Acute renal failure. Indices ($\pm$ S.E.M. for the diagnosis of prerenal uraemia compared with acute tubular necrosis (ATN), acute glomerulonephritis and obstruction

Index	Prerenal uraemia	Oliguric ATN	Polyuric ATN	Acute obstruction	Acute glomerulonephritis
Urine osmolality (mosm/kg)	518.0 ± 35.0	369.0 ± 20.0	343 ± 17.0	393 ± 39.0	385.0 ± 61.0
Urine sodium (mmol/l)	18.0 ± 3.0	68.0 ± 5.0	50 ± 5.0	68 ± 10.0	22.0 ± 6.0
Urine/plasma urea ratio	18.0 ± 7.0	3.0 ± 0.5	7 ± 1.0	8 ± 4.0	11.0 ± 4.0
Urine/plasma creatinine ratio	45.0 ± 6.0	17.0 ± 2.0	17 ± 2.0	16 ± 4.0	43.0 ± 7.0
Renal failure index*	0.6 ± 0.1	10.0 ± 2.0	4 ± 0.6	8 ± 3.0	0.4 ± 0.1
Fractional excretion of sodium (%)*	0.4 ± 0.1	7.0 ± 1.4	3 ± 0.5	6 ± 2.0	0.6 ± 0.2

*See text.

From Miller, T.R. *et al.* (1978). *Ann. intern. Med.* **89**, 47–50, with permission.

The main deficiency of these urinary and plasma indices is the close resemblance between prerenal uraemia and acute glomerulonephritis, but microscopy of fresh urine distinguishes readily by the nature of the deposit in acute glomerulonephritis.

Management of prerenal uraemia and incipient acute tubular necrosis

The urgent requirement is to restore renal perfusion. When hypovolaemia is the cause, the need is to replace plasma volume by infusion of crystalloid or colloid. In the rarer cases of cardiogenic shock, the aim should be to increase cardiac output by pharmacological means.

Volume replacement

A central venous pressure (CVP) line is desirable but not essential. The CVP will be low in volume depletion and should be increased to some 5 to 8 cm of water. Normal (0.9 per cent) saline or colloid (e.g. plasma protein fraction) should be infused rapidly (initially 500 ml in the first half hour) watching the response in urine volume and venous pressure. If urine flow is reestablished, further volume replacement can be achieved without undue urgency. If the initial saline or colloid challenge does not restore urine flow, intravenous fluids should be continued as fast as clinical circumstances allow until the CVP reaches 6–8 cm water. Requirements may amount to as much as 2 or even 3 litres in the hour. If, at this stage, there is still oliguria most physicians will proceed to the use of loop diuretics (usually frusemide) and/or infusion of dopamine (*vide infra*).

In the uraemia of cardiogenic shock a Swann Ganz catheter is to be preferred to a central venous line since the critical measurement during treatment is then left rather than right atrial pressure.

The increased risk of sepsis in uraemic patients dictates that central venous lines should not be left *in situ* for longer than 12–24 hours unless inserted by the special surgical techniques which allow chronic implantation without infection.

Incipient acute tubular necrosis

When oliguria is not reversed by volume expansion, it is common clinical practice to try other measures to turn possible incipient acute tubular necrosis towards recovery and away from established acute tubular necrosis.

Mannitol may increase tubular flow rates with the potential for washing out tubular debris and casts, postulated to contribute to oliguria by mechanical obstruction. There is evidence too that mannitol may reduce renal vascular resistance. An intravenous infusion of 20–30 g is commonly advocated, but without sound evidence of efficacy. Dangers of mannitol treatment in the presence of oliguria include pulmonary oedema, cerebral dehydration, and haemolysis.

Large doses of mannitol have also been reported to cause renal damage. Alternative agents, probably now more widely used are the loop diuretics (of which there is most experience with frusemide) and dopamine, or both given together.

Frusemide There are a number of theoretical reasons why frusemide might improve renal function compromised by poor perfusion. First is the possibility that increased flow rates in distal fluid might wash out obstructive material. Second, loop agents can decrease renal vascular resistance, thus improving perfusion perhaps by stimulation of the release of local prostaglandins and/or by inhibition of tubuloglomerular feedback regulation of afferent arteriolar tone (see below). Thirdly, frusemide, by inhibiting active sodium transport, will reduce the oxygen requirements of a metabolically active area of the kidney which in health may operate on the verge of anoxia thereby reducing the risk of metabolic and structual damage while perfusion is critically reduced. The renal haemodynamic effects of frusemide are inhibited by indomethacin and by other drugs which reduce the activity of the cyclo-oxygenase system.

Doses of 100–500 mg of frusemide are given intravenously. Evidence that incipient acute tubular necrosis is ever truly reversed is difficult to find, but in a number of patients oliguric acute renal failure is converted to polyuric acute renal failure. The increased volumes of urine simplify management, reducing the risk of fluid overload and more importantly of hyperkalaemia. Deafness which is not always reversible has long been recognized as a risk of high-dose ethacrynic acid in renal failure and the same problem may arise on occasion with frusemide. The risk is minimal if these large doses are given over 10 to 15 min rather than in one large bolus.

Dopamine Doses of dopamine of 1 µg/kg/min dilate the renal and mesenteric circulation; cardiac output is increased by inotropic effects at slightly increased dosage, but vasoconstriction follows high dose treatment (page 13.111 *et seq.*). Low-dose dopamine infusion in patients in whom saline challenge or frusemide has not restored urine flow is increasingly practised in intensive care units, but without firm evidence that the procedure prevents established renal failure or improves prognosis. An increase in urine *volume* can be produced in most patients, as can occur after frusemide. This simplifies management, but there is no controlled evidence that requirements for dialysis or mortality have been reduced. There has been a recent trend towards combining low-dose dopamine with intravenous frusemide with apparent good effect, but again studies have been uncontrolled and this approach must still be regarded as unproven.

Alkali Infusion of sodium bicarbonate or citrate have been used since 1925 to alkalinize urine after incompatible blood transfusion or other conditions provoking massive intravascular haemolysis. Alkali is also recommended in the management of myoglobinuria and of myeloma kidney (light chain nephrotoxicity, see below).

It is difficult to be logical about treatment when the mechanism of oliguria is unknown. The rationale for alkali is to reduce precipitation of haemoglobin (or myoglobin) in renal tubules. The procedure is of unproven value. Beneficial effects may relate to the restoration of plasma volume and renal perfusion, but the risk of fluid overload must always be considered. Exchange transfusion, undertaken early after incompatible blood transfusion may be useful.

Prophylaxis against acute tubular necrosis

There is an increased risk of developing acute tubular necrosis in certain conditions, for instance in medical patients with hepatic failure or septicaemia and in surgical patients undergoing bile duct operations, resection of aortic aneurysm, cardiac bypass, or other comparably major procedures. The risk is greater in those in whom renal damage is already present. Salt and water intake in these patients must be more than usually closely observed and major fluid deficits avoided. Prophylactic infusions of mannitol, 20–25 g intravenously, probably reduces the risk of subsequent tubular necrosis, particularly in jaundiced patients, but cannot be expected to help unless deficits of plasma and extracellular fluid volume are prevented or rapidly corrected.

Established acute tubular necrosis

The term is imprecise, implying a pathology which is rarely confirmed by biopsy, is not often detected when biopsy has been done, but has become hallowed by usage. Kerr has described it as 'acute renal failure without obstruction and with no arterial, venous, glomerular or interstitial lesions sufficient to explain it'. The diagnosis is commonly made when renal function is acutely but not reversibly (in the short term) impaired by any cause of renal ischaemia, by intravascular haemolysis, and a variety of other nephrotoxic mechanisms. The term conveys the expectation that renal function will recover within any period from a few days to some three to six weeks. If it does not do so, possible diagnoses include acute cortical necrosis and acute interstitial nephritis. These and other conditions may be detected at renal biopsy performed in those whose renal function has not recovered as expected. Other conditions may be included in the too vague title of 'tubular necrosis'. A wide variety of poisons and drugs (Tables 3 and 4) can damage the kidneys acutely with reversible or irreversible acute renal failure.

Pathology

The kidneys are enlarged and oedematous. The glomeruli and vessels are usually normal and the major pathological processes occur in the tubules. These changes are patchy with damaged and normal areas adjacent to one another. In the proximal tubules of affected areas, changes range from flattening of the epithelial cells to frank necrosis. The distal tubules appear dilated and mitotic figures may be seen in both proximal and distal tubules. Interstitial oedema with infiltration by inflammatory cells is common.

Acute cortical necrosis

Acute cortical necrosis may follow any course of particularly intense or prolonged ischaemia, but is rare, amounting to 1–2 per cent of all patients with apparent acute tubular necrosis. Cortical necrosis is a recognized complication of acute renal failure occurring in pregnancy, particularly after *abruptio placentae*, eclampsia, or after septic abortion, and occasionally after acute pyelonephritis. The pathology is a patchy necrosis of glomeruli, tubules, interstitium, and small vessels of the renal cortex. The renal medulla and juxta-medullary glomeruli remain intact. Return of renal function, if it occurs, does so very slowly and is attributable to the survival of islands of intact cortical tissue. About 50 per cent of

patients recover enough function to sustain life without dialysis, but the GFR rarely exceeds 10–20 ml/min and hypertension, sometimes in the malignant phase, follows in many cases. Kidneys tend to contract with calcification of the necrotic cortex becoming evident at some six weeks. When confluent, the calcification outlines the kidney giving an egg shell or sometimes tramline appearance (Fig. 1). Because the lesions may be patchy and calcify in only about 50 per cent of patients, the diagnosis may not be proven by biopsy or tomography of the kidneys. Renal angiograms are more accurate, showing attenuation of interlobular arteries, an increase in the subcapsular vessels, and a negative nephrogram in the outer cortical zone.

Pathophysiology of acute tubular necrosis

The reasons for the prolonged oliguria of patients with acute tubular necrosis remain unsettled in spite of great attention focused on this problem over the last 40 years. Controversy persists about the possible mechanisms which include prolonged renal vasoconstriction, tubular obstruction by casts and cellular debris, changes in glomerular permeability, passive back flow of filtrate in the renal tubules, and the development of aglomerular shunts. Different animal models provide data to support each of these alternatives, and it is possible that any or all may contribute. But no animal model satisfactorily reflects the condition which occurs in humans. The balance of recent evidence suggests that intense

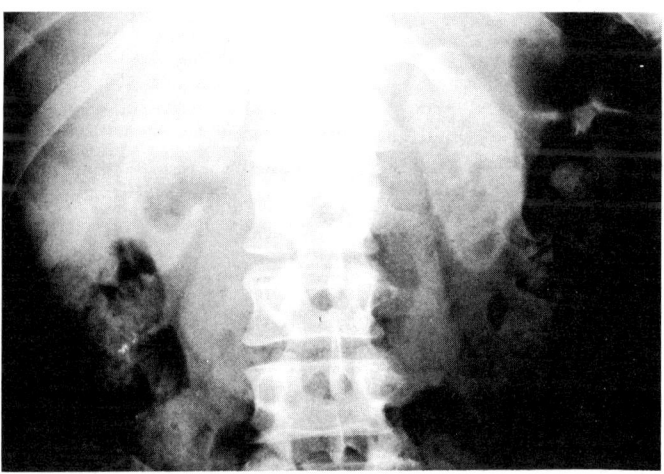

Fig. 1 Calcification of the renal cortex in acute cortical necrosis.

Table 3 Nephrotoxic chemicals and drugs (excluding drugs inducing acute interstitial nephritis)

Aniline	Adulterated heroin	Methoxyfluorane
Arsenic	Aminoglycosides	Methyl alcohol
Arsine	Amphotericin	Paraquat
Bismuth	Cantharides	Phenol
Cadmium	Carbon tetrachloride	Phosphorus
Copper	Colomycin	Polymyxin
Gold	Ethylene glycol	Radiocontrast media
Lead	Herbal remedies	Sodium chlorate
Lithium	Insecticides	Toluene
Mercury		Vancomycin
Platinum		
Silver		
Uranium		

Table 4 Drugs causing acute interstitial nephritis

Antimicrobials	Anti-inflammatory	Diuretics	Anticonvulsants
Penicillin	Fenoprofen*	Benzothiadiazines	Phenytoin
Methicillin	Ibuprofen*	Frusemide	Carbamazepine
Ampicillin*	Naproxen*	Triamterene	Phenobarbitone
Amoxycillin	Indomethacin*		
Carbenicillin	Phenylbutazone	*Metal salts*	*Miscellaneous*
Oxacillin	Mefanamic acid	Gold	Allopurinol
Nafcillin	Tolmetin*	Lithium	Aminocaproic acid
Cephalothin	Zomepirac*	Bismuth	Azathioprine
Cephalexin	Sulindac*		Cimetidine
Cephradrine	Glafenin		Clofibrate
Erythromycin	Aspirin		Cyclosporin
Sulphonamides	Diflunisal		Phenindione
Co-trimoxazole	Acetaminophen		Propranolol
Rifampicin	Paracetamol		Recombinant leucocyte A
Gentamicin			interferon
Minocycline			
Isoniazid			
Para-aminosalicylic acid			

*Associated with coincident minimal change nephrotic syndrome.

vasoconstriction is the trigger of the syndrome, and that persistent oliguria then results from diminished glomerular filtration, in spite of the return of apparently adequate perfusion. The paradox of continued renal blood flow without significant glomerular filtration might be explained by a combination of afferent arteriolar vasoconstriction and efferent vasodilation, but more favoured are changes in the glomerular ultrafiltration coefficient and/or an increase in intratubular hydrostatic pressure opposing the forces of glomerular filtration. Reduced glomerular ultrafiltration is unlikely to be due to structural damage to glomerular capillaries, although there are some reports of such damage in some animal models. More likely is a reduction in the surface area of glomerular membranes caused by mesangial cell contraction under the influences of a variety of local stimuli, perhaps angiotensin II in particular. One area of the kidney which may be most exquisitely sensitive to ischaemic damage is the thick ascending limb of Henle's loop. This site of sodium–potassium–chloride co-transport is situated in the outer medulla, an area in which blood flow is known to be much reduced after ischaemic injury in experimental animals, and which is thought to be in a state of precarious balance of supply and demand for oxygen even in health. Ischaemic damage here would be expected to reduce glomerular filtration by tubuloglomerular feedback at the macula densa. Such a state of affairs could pertain until repair of the cells of the loop could reduce the stimulus by restoring to normal the delivery of tubular fluid to the macula densa. This mechanism might explain the apparently favourable effects of high-dose frusemide in incipient renal failure, in that reduced oxygen supply could be balanced by a reduced demand as a result of inhibition of active transport by the drug.

Local intravascular coagulation and defective secretion of vasodilator substances such renal prostaglandins have also been suggested as important mediators of ischaemic renal damage, but no one mechanism is the proven aetiology of acute renal failure in humans. The answer to the problem remains elusive.

Clinical findings

In the immediate stages of acute renal failure, symptoms are few. The patient may notice oliguria, but the picture is likely to be dominated by the primary condition of which acute renal failure is a complication. Although urine volumes are usually less than 400 ml/24 hours, polyuric renal failure comprises as many as 50 per cent of all cases in some series. The later manifestations are largely those of uraemia in which gastrointestinal symptoms predominate, with anorexia, nausea, vomiting, but less often diarrhoea.

Muscle cramps can be troublesome, and when nitrogen retention is marked a characteristic 'flapping tremor' (asterixis) identical to that of carbon dioxide narcosis or of hepatic failure may be evident. Skin bruising and gastrointestinal bleeding occur. Uraemic haemorrhagic pericarditis with effusion is dangerous when it occurs but complicates acute renal failure much less frequently than chronic renal failure. Disorders of consciousness and coma are uncommon but epileptic fits may be observed. Measurement of arterial pressure may be useful in diagnosis. Hypertension suggests the presence of a renal glomerular or arterial lesion and is *not* a feature of acute tubular necrosis even when the patient is overloaded with salt and water. A low blood pressure or one that falls on standing indicates a major deficit of extracellular fluid volume, requiring urgent correction. Pulmonary oedema, although most commonly a manifestation of overhydration, can also be the result of increased pulmonary capillary permeability in uraemic patients.

Biochemical changes

A rise in blood urea and plasma creatinine concentration are the hallmarks of renal failure, acute or chronic. The plasma creatinine is a good guide to the GFR, but estimates of blood urea, dependent as they are on diet, and the rate of protein catabolism are less

precise. A logarithmic plot of creatinine or a direct plot of its reciprocal against time provides useful estimates of the rate of loss of GFR and any trend for the better or worse.

Hyperkalaemia is a particular problem in acute renal failure. The rate of rise of plasma potassium concentration, as of urea, is dependent not only on reduced urinary excretion, but also on the rate at which potassium is released from cells. Particularly rapid rises are to be expected when there is extensive tissue damage, as in crush injury, rhabdomyolysis, burns, sepsis, starvation, and other hypercatabolic states. Acidosis will aggravate the situation promoting leakage of potassium from healthy cells. Transfusion of stored blood in oliguric patients can cause dangerous rises in plasma potassium concentrations.

Hypocalcaemia with phosphate retention and hyperphosphataemia is usual. Calcium malabsorption, probably secondary to disordered vitamin D metabolism, occurs early in acute renal failure. It is usually asymptomatic, but tetany and fits may be provoked by over-rapid correction of acidosis with resultant depression of ionised calcium. The transient hypercalcaemia which may arise in the recovery phase of acute renal failure is related to a degree of secondary hyperparathyroidism, and may be more prolonged and accompanied by metastatic calcification in some patients in whom there has been extensive muscle injury (see below).

Hyponatraemia in renal failure usually reflects an intake of water inappropiately high for its excretion, a dilutional phenomenon which does not reflect sodium depletion (see page 18.25). Deficits of sodium are usually matched by those of water, with loss of extracellular fluid volume and the concentration of plasma sodium maintained normal.

The retention of uric acid, sulphate, and magnesium which occur in acute renal failure do not generally cause symptoms, but uric acid measurements may be helpful in assessing catabolic rates and muscle necrosis.

Criteria for the diagnosis of hypercatabolism in acute renal failure include a rate of rise of urea of 10 mmol/l or more, of creatinine of 100 μmol/l or more and of potassium 1 mmol/l or more daily, despite proper conservative management. Plasma bicarbonate falls exceed 2 mmol/l per day. Plasma phosphate reaches the unusually high concentrations of 2–3 mmol/l, and plasma calcium is unusually low at figures less than 1.5 mmol/l.

Non-traumatic rhabdomyolysis may not be clinically evident; it usually causes a pattern with particular elevation of phosphate and urate with depression of calcium. Aldolase, creatine phosphokinase, and lactic dehydrogenase concentrations in plasma are always clearly elevated in renal failure secondary to rhabdomyolysis. The combination of dark brown urine, positive for 'blood' on a reagent strip but without red cells on microscopy is suggestive of myoglobinuria.

Management

Diagnostic difficulties concerning the cause of acute renal failure usually involve the differentiation of prerenal uraemia and acute tubular necrosis, but on occasion there is doubt about the possibility of obstructive uropathy, acute interstitial nephritis or glomerulonephritis, or myeloma. A high-dose infusion pyelogram with tomography and, if necessary, films at 12 and 24 hours, is likely to confirm or refute the diagnosis of obstruction without the need for retrograde examination. Antegrade pyelography can then be used to provide more detailed information if obstruction is confirmed. Ultrasound techniques are now remarkably accurate in detecting dilation of the lower urinary tract and should be used in combination with high-dose urography. Renal biopsy should be undertaken early for diagnosis of glomerulonephritis or interstitial nephritis. Myeloma is most quickly diagnosed by bone marrow examination as well as by examination of concentrated urine for free light chains and of plasma for a monoclonal band.

Conservative management
Diet
The ideal diet for the undialysed patient with acute renal failure should provide all the essential aminoacids in a total protein intake of 0.3–0.5 g/kg body weight daily, with fat and carbohydrate to bring up the energy intake to at least 2000 calories (8.5 kJ) or 4000 calories (17 kJ) in hypercatabolic cases. When dialysis treatment is given, particularly peritoneal dialysis, protein intake must be increased to at least 1 g/kg body weight/day. In patients too unwell to take adequate food by mouth, tube feeding or parenteral nutrition should be given early; adequate nutrition is of particular importance in hypercatabolic cases, often the patients who are least inclined to eat. There is too often a tendency in general medical wards and in many renal units to pay lip service to the nutritional problems of acute renal failure, in spite of the evidence that good nutrition reduces mortality.

Water and electrolytes
In the absence of renal function the greatest care must be taken to regulate the intake of water and electrolytes in accordance with losses in the urine, from the gastrointestinal tract, from sweat, expired air, and other sources. Fluid intake is regulated to the volume of the previous day's output of urine plus 500 ml in temperate climates. This is a good working rule, but it must be used with flexibility and larger amounts are needed if the patient is febrile or is nursed in hot environments. Assessments of fluid requirements should be based not only on accurate fluid charts (they are rarely accurate) but more on records of daily weight and on clinical signs of over- or underhydration. In patients in whom nutrition is inadequate (most cases in practice) some allowance must be made for loss of tissue from catabolism in the assessment of daily weight. Losses of up to 0.5 kg/day are not uncommon.

Sodium
The intake of sodium must also be regulated by output, with due attention to the possibility of sequestration of sodium in the tissues, for instance, in crush or burn injury. Requirements are usually very small (17–30 mmol/day) but may be higher in polyuric cases. Daily measurements of 24-hour urinary losses give good guidance. Excess of sodium and water in most patients with tubular necrosis results in peripheral or pulmonary oedema. In those with glomerulonephritis, hypertension is likely to be the predominant ill effect of overload.

Potassium
The hyperkalaemia characteristic of acute oliguric renal failure constitutes one of the most important problems in management. It is essential to check plasma levels at least daily and in hypercatabolic cases more frequently than that. No potassium should be allowed parenterally or by mouth until potassium levels are known. Thereafter dietary consumption should be limited to the minimum compatible with an adequate intake of protein and essential aminoacids (20–30 mmol/day). Excretion of potassium can sometimes be increased by the use of frusemide in high doses (0.5–2.0 g daily by mouth or 100–400 mg parenterally). Distal tubular diuretics such as spironolactone, amiloride, and triamterene promote potassium retention and should never be used in renal failure. Blood for transfusion should be fresh and antimicrobials containing potassium avoided.

Ion exchange may be used to increase faecal excretion of potassium in exchange for sodium (Resonium A 15 g six-hourly orally or rectally) or for calcium (calcium Zeocarb in the same dose). They are best used prophylactically to prevent dangerous hyperkalaemia in patients at risk or to buy time when dialysis facilities are not immediately available.

Hyperkalaemia may produce muscle weakness or paralysis, but most commonly causes no symptoms. Cardiac arrest may occur when plasma concentrations exceed 7 mmol/l but there is no *precise* relationship between potassium levels and cardiac effects. The best guide to cardiac toxicity is the electrocardiogram (ECG). The characteristic findings are listed in Table 5 and are illustrated in Figs 2 and 3.

Treatment of hyperkalaemia
When ECG changes are evident, urgent action must be taken to reduce hyperkalaemia or its cardiac effects. Dialysis, whether peritoneal or haemodialysis, and ion exchange resins take some hours to work. The situation can be held in the short term by one or more of the following emergency treatments.

Glucose and insulin
An intravenous injection of 50 g of glucose covered by 10–20 units of soluble (regular) or Actrapid insulin will promote transport of extracellular potassium into cells. Plasma potassium may fall by 1 mmol/l or so and the effect may last some one or two hours.

Hypertonic sodium bicarbonate
Sodium bicarbonate, 50–100 ml 4.2 per cent, will also increase intracellular at the expense of extracellular potassium. It is an effective treatment, particularly in the presence of acidosis, but carries the risk of sodium overload and pulmonary oedema in patients already overhydrated or with suspect cardiac function.

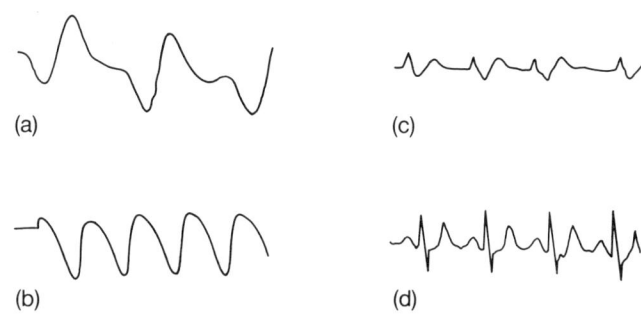

Fig. 2 (a) Plasma K^+ = 9.5 mmol/l. (b) Plasma K^+ = 9.5 mmol/l 2 min later. (c) After 40 ml 20 per cent CaCl i.v. (d) Plasma K^+ = 6.5 mmol/l after 90 min haemodialysis.

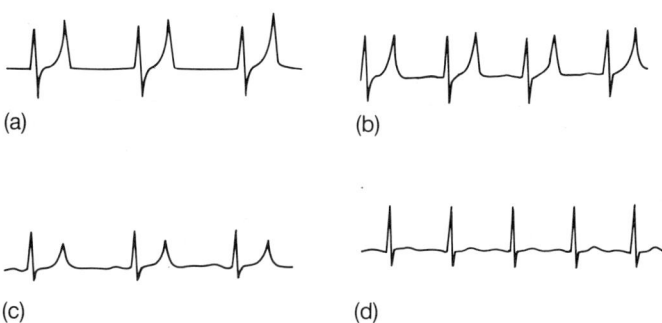

Fig. 3 Serial ECG changes in treated hyperkalaemia: lead V_4. (a) Note peaked T waves, broadened QRS complex, and absent p waves. Plasma $[K^+]$ = 9.2 mmol/l. (b) Effects of 20 ml 10 per cent calcium glutonate i.v. Note return of p waves. Plasma $[K^+]$ = 9.2 mmol/l. (c) Plasma $[K^+]$ lowered to 7.9 mmol/l. Note reduction in T waves. (d) Plasma $[K^+]$ restored to 4.4 mmol/l by dialysis.

Table 5 ECG signs of hyperkalaemia

1 Peaked T waves (tent-shaped)
2 Disappearance of P waves
3 Broadened QRS complex
4 Slurring of ST segments into T waves
5 Sine wave leading to cardiac arrest

Intravenous calcium

When the ECG changes include widening of the QRS complexes with slurring of ST segments, intravenous calcium must be given *immediately* and continued until the ECG has returned to normal. Although the standard dose of 10 ml of 10 per cent calcium gluconate is usually effective, more should be given without hesitation in resistant cases. On rare occasions up to 90 ml of 10 per cent gluconate salt has been required and a dose of 30 ml is not uncommon.

These short term measurements allow time for dialysis to be started. Peritoneal dialysis will control plasma potassium levels adequately in most cases of renal failure, but in some patients with hypercatabolic disease, especially when there is extensive tissue necrosis, control can only be achieved by intensive haemodialysis.

Acidosis

The metabolic acidosis of acute renal failure is not of itself a serious problem, but requires correction when obviously contributing to hyperkalaemia. If fluid and sodium balance preclude the use of sodium bicarbonate, extreme acidosis (plasma bicarbonate of less than 10 mmol/l) is best treated by dialysis.

Bleeding and infection

The commonest causes of death in acute renal failure are gastrointestinal bleeding and sepsis. The greatest care should therefore be taken with indwelling lines and catheters. Daily blood cultures are a sensible routine. Proven infection must be treated promptly with appropriate antimicrobials with due modification in dosage in those in whom renal failure increases the risks of toxicity. Cimetidine or ranitidine are often given for prophylaxis against upper gastrointestinal bleeding but there is no good evidence that this approach improves prognosis.

Dialysis in acute renal failure

There is no doubt that earlier and frequent dialysis improves the prognosis in patients with acute renal failure. At one time the indications for dialysis were accepted to be a blood urea concentration exceeding 60 mmol/l (BUN 180 mg/100 ml), a plasma potassium over 7 mmol/l, a plasma bicarbonate under 10 mmol/l, or the presence of fluid overload, symptomatic uraemia, bleeding, or pericarditis. These criteria are no longer acceptable and patients should be dialysed long before such gross uraemia has developed. Ideally, dialysis should be begun prophylactically, before the blood urea reaches 30 mmol/l (BUN 90 mg/100 ml) or creatinine 500 μmol/l (5 mg/100 ml) and should be repeated frequently enough to keep them below those figures. Such a prophylactic approach reduces complications and mortality.

Haemodialysis allows short periods of treatment, better biochemical control in hypercatabolic patients, and is more comfortable, but in some areas facilities are limited and the risk of haemorrhage is increased. Peritoneal dialysis is more generally available, less demanding of technical resources, cheaper, and is effective in most patients. It is, however, incapable of controlling hypercatabolic cases and abdominal pathology, respiratory complications, ascites, and extensive previous abdominal surgery may make it impossible.

Drugs in acute renal failure

Many drugs are excreted by glomerular filtration or tubular secretion and must be given in reduced dosage or at longer intervals than normal in renal failure patients (see page 18.123). Protein binding and extrarenal metabolism of drugs may be altered by the uraemic state. Drugs prescribed in renal failure should be reduced strictly to those that are essential and preferably to those whose pharmacokinetics in uraemia are known. The changes in doses recommended in renal failure should be regarded as a guide at best and whenever possible plasma levels should be monitored regularly to avoid toxicity. The particular agents to avoid include tetracyclines (increased protein catabolism) and a combination of frusemide and cephaloridine or of gentamicin with cephaloridine (nephrotoxicity). Despite its known nephrotoxicity, gentamicin is commonly used in patients with renal failure complicating Gram-negative sepsis; doses must be widely spaced according to the glomerular filtration rate; plasma levels must be checked before and 15–30 min after each dose.

Clinical course, complications, and prognosis

Renal failure with a low glomerular filtration rate and nitrogen retention lasts any time between a few days to three weeks or more after ischaemic or toxic insult. Recovery is occasionally even longer delayed and there have been reports of oliguria as long as 40 days before recovery of renal function. On the whole the duration of renal failure is shorter in those with polyuric renal failure in whom initial damage may have been less severe. Renal biopsy should be undertaken in those in whom recovery is not proceeding at four weeks to confirm diagnosis and to seek evidence of cortical necrosis.

Recovery of renal function is classically associated with stepwise increases in urine volume and improvement in creatinine clearance and blood urea following shortly afterwards. Most young patients who recover from tubular necrosis do so near enough completely, so that renal function is only distinguishable from normal by accurate clearance measurements. The GFR never returns completely, however. Some 10–20 per cent of nephrons fail to recover. In some, recovery is much less complete and in them a minor degree of cortical necrosis may have occurred. The elderly recover function more slowly and less completely.

Much attention is given to the polyuric phase of tubular necrosis, with emphasis on the possibility that large urine volumes and uncontrolled sodium loss may lead to significant volume depletion and the risk of re-establishment of renal failure. The condition is widely recognized but rarely seen these days. It is easily controlled by adjusting intakes of water, salt, and potassium to output.

Mortality

The mortality of acute renal failure varies according to its cause and to the extent of disease or injury outside the kidney. Deaths are much more common in patients whose age exceeds 60 years. The lowest rates (10–20 per cent mortality) are reported in renal failure complicating pregnancy or abortion. Results in surgical renal failure, including transfusion reactions, are appreciably worse (50–60 per cent mortality). Death when tubular necrosis is caused by burns or extensive trauma is to be expected in 70 per cent of patients. Medical conditions in which renal failure is secondary to nephrotoxins or septicaemia do better on the whole than surgical, with a mortality of some 30–50 per cent of patients at risk.

Death in acute tubular necrosis patients is now extremely uncommonly related to uraemia or hyperkalaemia. Sepsis and gastrointestinal haemorrhage are the major causes, particularly sepsis which is all too common a complication, introduced through burns, sites of trauma, the lungs, or by way of a catheter in the bladder, peritoneum, or central veins.

Some specific causes of acute renal failure

Hepatorenal failure

Renal failure may complicate advanced liver failure of any cause; the mechanism would appear to be that the renal cortex is underperfused (vasomotor nephropathy) in such cases. Septicaemia, endotoxaemia, fluid and electrolyte imbalance or hypovolaemia from gastrointestinal haemorrhage or overvigorous use of diuretics or paracentesis appear to be common precipitant causes. Hepatorenal failure rarely recovers unless liver function improves, but the reversibility of the renal failure is well illustrated by the good performance of kidneys taken from patients with hepatorenal failure and transplanted into recipients with normal hepatic function but end-stage renal disease.

Rhabdomyolysis

Myoglobinuria is a more common cause of acute renal failure than was once appreciated, but the mechanism of renal damage, as with intravascular haemolysis, is unclear. The association with crush injury or other trauma is obvious, but non-traumatic rhabdomyolysis escapes diagnosis more easily; muscle pain, swelling, and tenderness are not always present, even when necrosis is extensive. Recognized causes are increasing in number and include ischaemia, inflammatory disorders such as polymyositis and viral necrotizing myositis (glandular fever, influenza, coxsackie virus), carbon monoxide poisoning, heat stroke, prolonged convulsions, marathon running, and comparable severe exercise, barbiturate, alcohol, and heroin abuse, hypersensitivity to aminocaproic acid, hypokalaemia, acute hypophosphataemia, and metabolic disorders such as McArdle's syndrome (phosphorylase deficiency) and Tarius' syndrome (phosphofructokinase deficiency).

Malignant hyperpyrexia is also associated with rhabdomyolysis, disseminated intravascular coagulation, metabolic acidosis, hyperkalaemia, and renal failure. Episodes follow exposure to inhaled anaesthetic agents such as halothane, cyclopropane, ether or muscle relaxants. Rhabdomyolysis is dependent on the provocation of massive release of calcium from sarcoplasmic reticulum into cytosol in muscle, with resultant breakdown of ATP, inhibition of troponin, increased glycolysis, muscle contraction, pyrexia, and muscle necrosis. A similar course of events may rarely complicate the neuroleptic malignant syndrome.

Gram-negative septicaemia

Endotoxins of Gram-negative organisms damage the vascular endothelium of capillaries and of venules; lipid A component may be important in this respect. Complications of such damage include hypovolaemic shock, disseminated intravascular coagulation, gastrointestinal bleeding, acute renal failure, and adult respiratory distress syndrome (see page 15.161 and Section 14). The full blown picture is not difficult to detect, and treat with broad-spectrum antimicrobials and urgent volume replacement. Less obvious cases are quite common, and Gram-negative septicaemia must be considered to be a possible diagnosis in any patient in whom the cause of acute renal failure is obscure.

Radiocontrast-induced renal failure

The incidence of acute renal failure associated with iodinated contrast media has increased with the frequency of their use in radiology, reaching 0.5 per cent after angiography and 0.15 per cent after computerized tomography or urography. Impairment of glomerular filtration is more common than clinical renal failure, which, when it occurs, is usually transient with recovery after a few days. Prolonged renal failure is rare, but may be more likely to occur when uraemia follows the use of cholecystographic drugs. Patients with diabetes, myeloma, heart failure, dehydration, or with pre-existing renal disease are most at risk. An apparent association with increasing age probably only reflects increased exposure in the elderly. The mechanisms of renal impairment are uncertain; suggestions that damage relates to hyperosmolality (tri-iodinated compounds are four or five times isotonic) are unproven, as is the suggestion of tubular obstruction by the precipitation of casts containing Tamm–Horsfall protein.

Drug nephrotoxicity

Some drugs are known to damage the kidney by provoking an acute interstitial nephritis (see below), others by less well defined mechanisms. The list of potential nephrotoxic drugs is a long one (Table 3) but some are more frequently implicated than others. Amphotericin, colistin, bacitracin and polymyxins are predictably nephrotoxic. In other drugs the risk is much less (see page 18.108).

Aminoglycosides

Gentamicin, amikacin, kanamycin, and streptomycin are all potentially nephrotoxic, as are tobramycin and netilmicin to a lesser degree. These drugs are usually prescribed for seriously ill patients suspected to be suffering from dangerous Gram-negative infections. In clinical practice it is not easy to separate harmful effects of aminoglycosides from those of the underlying disease or of other drugs used to combat it. The risk of nephrotoxicity is increased with high dosage, prolonged treatment, and combined treatment with other nephrotoxic drugs. A combination of aminoglycoside and a loop diuretic increases toxicity, but evidence that cephalosporins also increase the risk is controversial. Impairment of renal function is usually mild, and unassociated with oliguria. It is most likely to be detected 10–14 days after starting treatment and it may be because of prolonged binding of the drug to renal cortical tissues that dysfunction may be demonstrable some days after the drug has been stopped. Apart from the risks of systemically administered drugs, irrigation of operation sites with neomycin, polymyxin, and bacitracin may be associated with acute renal failure. The risk of toxicity appears to be increased in older patients, when extracellular fluid volumes are low, and in the presence of pre-existing renal disease. Proteinuria and impaired concentration of water precede loss of glomerular filtration rate, which is rarely severe and usually slow in onset. Proximal tubular damage involves the brush border and its enzymes and is reflected by increased urinary excretion of lysosomal enzymes and of gamma-glutamyl transferase and alanine aminopeptidase.

The ill effects of tetracyclines (other than doxycycline) and of other drugs are more fully discussed elsewhere (see page 18.108).

Vascular causes – large vessels

Occlusion of the main renal arteries by trauma, thrombosis, or embolism may occasionally be the reason for acute renal failure. There may be few symptoms but loin pain resembling renal colic may occur, commonly with fever. Proteinuria and haematuria are not invariable. Early diagnosis is important because renovascular surgery can be surprisingly effective in restoring function, even when undertaken as late as 24 hours after onset. When arterial insufficiency is suspected, it can be confirmed by renography and arteriography should be undertaken as a matter of urgency.

Renal vein thrombosis is often clinically silent in the adult, but in infants may cause acute renal failure. Treatment by anticoagulation is the usual practice.

Small vessels, malignant hypertension

In accelerated hypertension, fibrinoid necrosis of renal arterioles secondary to the physical effects of the rate and degree of rise in arterial pressure commonly results in acute renal failure. Fibrinoid heals where arterial pressure is lowered but loss of autoregulation with such vascular damage results in reduced renal perfusion in the early days of antihypertensive treatment. Very often therefore there is a transient or more prolonged period of worse renal function after pressure is lowered. A small proportion of those coming to dialysis recover enough renal function over weeks or months to be ultimately free of the need for renal replacement treatment.

Systemic sclerosis

This disease (see page 16.34) does not normally involve the kidney enough to cause clinical concern, but in the malignant scleroderma syndrome fibrinoid necrosis, closely resembling that seen in malignant hypertension, affects interlobular arteries as well as small arterioles in the renal circulation. The result is severe cortical ischaemia with areas of glomerular sclerosis. The acute renal failure resulting usually runs a particularly severe and rapid course. It is not always accompanied by hypertension, but when arterial pressure is raised, it is often resistant to treatment with antihypertensive drugs. There have been a number of case reports of arrest or reversal of the syndrome after treatment with angiotensin converting enzyme inhibitors or nifedipine. These drugs should always be tried in patients with malignant scleroderma syndrome and renal failure, but results are often disappointing with relentless and rapid progression of renal failure to end-stage.

Idiopathic postpartum acute renal failure

This is one of a group of diseases with localized or more generalized intravascular coagulation with plugging of small arterioles or glomerular capillaries by fibrin and platelet microthrombi with resultant renal failure. This pattern of events is characteristic of the haemolytic-uraemic syndrome of children, eclampsia, and thrombotic thrombocytopenic purpura as well as of the rare condition of idiopathic postpartum acute renal failure. The condition begins within 24 hours or up to several weeks after normal pregnancy and delivery; a few cases have been described in which oliguria began before pregnancy was complete. The onset of renal failure is acute with oliguria or anuria. Microangiopathic haemolytic anaemia and hypertension are common but not invariable complications. Some two-thirds of affected women never recover renal function, but variable degrees of improvement may occur in the remainder. In some cases there are extrarenal manifestations resembling those of thrombotic thrombocytopenic purpura, and cardiac failure was a prominent feature in some reports. The pathology of the condition includes microthrombi in arterioles and capillaries of the kidneys with glomeruli ischaemic or occasionally necrotic. Treatment by heparin or fibrinolytic agents has been tried but does not appear to be effective. Hypertension should be controlled and renal failure treated by peritoneal or haemodialysis. There is no certainty of the value or otherwise of infusions of fresh frozen plasma or of treatment by plasma exchange.

On rare occasions a precisely similar syndrome complicates treatment by oral contraceptive drugs.

Acute glomerulonephritis

(See also page 18.41.)

Acute glomerular disease can on occasion result in complete or near complete loss of previously normal renal function in a matter of 10 days to 3 weeks. This rapidly progressive course of events can occur in idiopathic crescentic glomerulonephritis, in anti-glomerular basement membrane disease (anti-GBM disease; Goodpasture's syndrome) in polyarteritis nodosa, Wegener's granulomatosis, systemic lupus erythematosus, mixed cryoglobulinaemia, and very rarely after streptococcal infection. Urine microscopy makes the diagnosis of florid glomerular disease with detection of proteinuria, misshapen red cells, and red cell casts abundant in fresh urine samples. The precise diagnosis is made from assessment of the extrarenal manifestations and renal histology.

Hypocomplementaemia suggests poststreptococcal disease, lupus or mixed cryoglobulinaemia. Anti-GBM disease can be detected reliably by measurement of anti-GBM antibody in many centres now. The test takes only a few hours and allows early detection of this rare but very important cause of acute renal failure. Polyarteritis nodosa may be a much more difficult diagnosis to prove. If histology does not provide an answer, mesenteric and renal angiography are often disappointing and treatment has to be begun on clinical grounds (see page 16.28).

Precise diagnosis in rapidly progressive glomerulonephritis is a medical emergency. Anti-GBM disease responds well to immunosuppression with prednisolone and cyclophosphamide plus plasma exchange but only if treatment is begun before oliguria has occurred. Similar immunosuppressive treatment should be given as early as possible in the course of acute renal failure complicating polyarteritis nodosa, systemic lupus or Wegener's granuloma, and is often successful in halting or reversing renal failure.

Acute interstitial nephritis

This condition occurs much more commonly than was once recognized, and must be considered in any patient with acute or sub-acute renal failure in whom the cause is not already known. It is probable that many patients with this condition were in the past diagnosed as glomerulonephritis or acute tubular necrosis. Although most cases follow exposure to drugs, others arise without obvious cause and still others are complications of infective diseases. The number of drugs now known to be able to cause acute interstitial nephritis is already large, and increases year by year (Table 4). The drugs most commonly associated are the β-lactam antimicrobials, non-steroidal anti-inflammatory agents, and diuretics. Many infections can cause a very similar clinical and pathological picture and these include those due to streptococcus, salmonella, staphylococcus, brucella, meningococcus, legionella, diphtheria, mycoplasma, mycobacteria, leptospirosis, toxoplasmosis, and many viral disorders including mononucleosis and measles. Sarcoidosis has also been identified as a cause of acute interstitial nephritis.

Clinical features

Renal dysfunction after exposure to a causative drug may occur within a few hours in some cases, but only after weeks or months in others. Apart from acute loss of glomerular filtration rate (oliguric or polyuric) renal manifestations include macroscopic or microscopic haematuria, pyuria, and considerable proteinuria. Nephrotic rates of urinary protein loss have been reported in cases associated with some non-steroidal anti-inflammatory drugs, despite absence of detectable glomerular lesions on histological examinations. Minimal change nephrotic syndrome without interstitial nephritis has also been reported. There may be no extrarenal manifestations, but in some of the acute reactions to drugs there may be fever, arthralgia, skin rash, disturbed liver function and/or occasionally interstitial pneumonia. Flank pain probably relects acute oedema in kidneys which on ultrasound or radiological examination can often be shown to be enlarged. Plasma levels of IgE may be high in some 50 per cent of patients. Eosinophilia and eosinophiluria are well recognized but are often not present.

Pathology and pathophysiology

Histological examination of renal biopsy material shows tubulo-interstitial disease, with focal tubular atrophy, peritubular oedema, and infiltration with mononuclear cells, predominantly lymphocytes and plasma cells, but also with polymorphs and in some cases eosinophils, or basophils. Epithelioid macrophages have also been reported. Glomeruli are for the most part normal. Immunofluorescent examination most commonly shows nonspecific deposition of C_3 but in a small number of cases IgG antitubular basement membrane antibody has been detected; and may be a secondary rather than primary phenomenon.

Monoclonal techniques have shown that the predominant lymphocyte in the cellular infiltrate is the T_4 cytotoxic T cell, although T_8 T cells and B cells may also be found in some cases. It has been suggested, but not proven, that the heavy proteinuria seen in some patients with this syndrome is mediated by lymphokines of T cell origin acting to increase glomerular capillary permeability.

Treatment and prognosis

In many cases of drug-associated disease recovery of renal function over 1 to 12 months follows withdrawal of the offending agent. Prednisolone treatment is given by most physicians. It probably accelerates recovery and may induce it in some patients in whom it might not otherwise have occurred; proof of the efficacy of steroid treatment is hard to find, and occasional patients do not respond. Others relapse after withdrawal of prednisolone treatment. Permanent impairment of renal function, sufficient to require maintenance haemodialysis or transplantation can occur.

Myeloma

Acute or subacute renal failure is increasingly recognized as a presenting feature of myelomatosis otherwise occult. Some 2–8 per cent of patients with myeloma develop acute renal failure. Chronic renal insufficiency is associated with amyloidosis in relation to myeloma, but more acute deterioration in renal function is most likely to be due to hypercalcaemia (see page 18.95) and/or light chain nephropathy (myeloma kidney). Hyperuricaemia may contribute to renal dysfunction.

Pathology and pathophysiology of 'myeloma kidney'

The classical appearance of myeloma kidney is of a tubulo-interstitial nephritis. Atrophic tubules contain laminated casts of Tamm–Horsfall mucoprotein, immunoglobulin, and light chains. Interstitial tissue is oedematous and/or fibrotic with collections of inflammatory cells and characteristically multinuclear giant cells around tubules and sometimes extending into the tubular casts. On occasion casts and interstitial infiltration are not seen, and the appearances may be identical to those of acute tubular necrosis, an appearance which may confuse and which is seen more commonly when renal failure has apparently been precipitated by the use of radiocontrast media.

Myeloma kidney is associated with the excretion of free kappa or lambda light chains and it is likely that these damage the kidney either by cast formation or more likely by nephrotoxic effects on tubular cells and peritubular tissues consequent on reabsorption. A paradox is that many patients excrete large amounts of light chain without evidence of renal dysfunction. There is evidence that kappa light chains are more often nephrotoxic than are lambda. This may relate to the isoelectric point (Pi) which together with urine pH determines whether light chains in tubular fluid will be in cationic, anionic or neutral state. Cationic proteins are more easily filtered at the glomerulus and more avidly reabsorbed in the proximal tubules. The Pi of most light chains lies between pH 5.5 and 6.6. The true explanation as to why some light chains are nephrotoxic and others not, has yet to be discovered.

Management

The quickest and most accurate way to confirm a possible diagnosis of myeloma in a case of acute renal failure of obscure origin is by bone marrow biopsy for immunochemical analysis of plasma cell population and by examination of the urine for free kappa or lambda light chains.

In most cases, acute renal failure will have been precipitated by infection, by hypercalcaemia or other causes of loss of salt and water and, more rarely now than before, by the use of radiocontrast media. An urgent need therefore is for rapid and adequate replacement of sodium and water. The improved renal prognosis achieved in the latest Medical Research Council treatment trial in myeloma by the use of intravenous sodium bicarbonate is more likely to have been due to the improvement of circulating volume and renal perfusion than to the alkalinization of the urine for which the treatment was intended.

Fluid replacement may not restore renal function. The question of peritoneal or haemodialysis then arises. Recent results of such therapy plus or minus plasmapheresis in patients with acute renal failure in myeloma have been much more encouraging than previously. All such patients should be given *short-term* dialysis treatment whenever it is available; a few will do well and renal function may be restored to a remarkable degree. Prognosis is likely to be good when acute renal failure occurs in the course of already diagnosed and treated disease. The place for more chronic replacement treatment in those in whom renal failure becomes chronic is more debateable and must depend on the extrarenal manifestations of the disease. There is, sadly, no evidence that chemotherapy with melphelan or corticosteroids influences the renal prognosis favourably.

Acute pyelonephritis

Although acute pyelonephritis usually has little effect on renal excretory function, severe attacks, particularly in pregnant or diabetic subjects and particularly if treated late, may lead to oliguria and impaired filtration rates sufficient to require a period of dialysis. In diabetes, oliguria complicating pyelonephritis may be due to obstruction from detachment of a necrotic renal papilla which has impacted in one or both ureters.

Intratubular obstructive lesions

A rapid rise in plasma uric acid concentration complicating treatment of lymphoma, leukaemia, myeloma, or following starvation, may result in tubular urate deposition and oliguric renal failure. Hyperuricaemia and renal failure have also been observed after recurrent epileptic seizures. The rise in plasma urate, which occurs after traumatic or non-traumatic rhabdomyolysis, may also contribute to renal failure complicating that disorder. Prophylactic allopurinol ought to prevent the hyperuricaemia of tumour cell destruction, but the conventional dose of 300mg/day may be inadequate when the tumour mass is large. Dehydration in patients in pain and given sedating analgesics is another contributing factor to extreme hyperuricaemia in these cases. Established uric acid nephropathy is best treated by alkalinization of the urine by bicarbonate infusion, supplemented by diuretic treatment, perhaps most logically with acetazolamide or dichlorphenamide, both of which will alkalinize tubular fluid.

More uncommon even than intratubular obstruction by urate crystals is similar obstruction by *phosphate*, also delivered in massive amounts into extracellular fluid as a result of cell destruction in the course of treatment of malignant disease. Adequate hydration is again the safeguard against this complication. Phosphate is more soluble in acid than alkaline urine, and bicarbonate infusion may be unwise in those rare cases in which there is likely to be both urate and phosphate obstructing the renal tubules.

Sulphonamide crystalluria is now rare but can be associated with sulphadiazine treatment. Retrograde catheterization of the ureters with lavage is usually effective and should be combined with a high fluid intake and diuretics to increase urine flow.

Acute renal failure due to obstruction

Although occult obstruction is an uncommon cause of acute renal failure, it is an important one because reversible. Most obstructive lesions cause a chronic form of renal failure but acute cases do occur and are traditionally (but not always accurately) suspected when anuria is complete. Among important causes are renal calculi, retroperitoneal fibrosis, and malignant diseases especially of the cervix uteri, prostate, bladder and rectum. The subject is dealt with fully elsewhere (see page 18.99).

References

Anderson, R. J., Linas, S. L., Berns, A. S., Henrich, W. L., Miller, T. R., Gabow, P. A. and Schrier, R. W. (1977). Non-oliguric acute renal failure. *N. Engl. J. Med.* **296**, 1134–1138.

Bennett, W. M. (1983). Aminoglycoside nephrotoxicity. *Nephron* **35**, 73–77.

——, Aronoff, G. R., Morrison, G., Golper, T. A., Pullrain, J., Wolfson, M. and Singer, T. (1983). Drug prescribing in renal failure: Dosing guidelines for adults. *Am. J. Kid. Dis.* **3**, 155–157.

Brezis, M., Rosen, S., Silva, P. and Epstein, F. M. (1984). Renal ischaemia: A new perspective. *Kid. Int.* **26**, 375–383.

Clive, D. M. and Stoft, J. S. (1984). Renal syndromes associated with non-steroidal anti-inflammatory drugs. *N. Engl. J. Med.* **310**, 563–572.

Carmichael, J., Shankel, S. W. (1985). Effects of non-steroidal anti-inflammatory drugs on prostaglandins and renal function. *Am. J. Med.* **78**. 992–1000.

Cohen, D. J., Sherman, W. H., Osserman, E. F. and Appel, G. B. (1984). Acute renal failure in patients with multiple myeloma. *Am. J. Med.* **76**, 247–256.

de Fronzo, R. A., Cooke, C. R., Wright, J. R. and Humphrey, R. L. (1978). Renal function in patients with multiple myeloma. *Medicine (Balt.)* **57**, 151–166.

Gerber, J. G. and Nies, A. S. (1980). Furosemide-induced vasodilatation: importance of the state of hydration and filtration. *Kid. Int.* **18**, 454–459.

Goldstein, M. B. (1983). Acute renal failure. *Med. Clin. N. Am.* **67**, 1325–1341.

Graziani, G., Cantaluppi, A., Casati, S., Citterio, A., Scalamogna, A., Aroldi, A., Silenzio, R., Brancaccio, D. and Ponticelli, C. (1984). Dopamine and frusemide in oliguric renal failure. *Nephron* **37**, 39–42.

Grunfeld, J-P., Ganeval, D. and Bournerias, F. (1980). Acute renal failure in pregnancy. *Kid. Int.* **18**, 179–191.

Hayslett, J. P. (1985). Post-partum renal failure. *N. Engl. J. Med.* **312**, 1556–1559.

Harkonen, S. and Kjellstrand, C. (1981). Contrast nephropathy. *Am. J. Nephrol.* **1**, 69–77.

Honda, N. (1983). Acute renal failure and rhabdomyolysis. *Kid. Int.* **23** 888–898.

Henderson, I. S., Beattie, T. J. and Kennedy, A. C. (1980). Dopamine hydrochloride in oliguric states. *Lancet* **ii**, 827–828.

Isles, C. G., Mclay, A. and Boulton-Jones, J. M. (1984). Recovery in malignant hypertension presenting as renal failure. *Q. J. Med.* **53**, 439–452.

Kerr, D. N. S. (1979). Acute renal failure. In *Renal disease* 4th edn (eds D. A. K. Black and N. F. Jones), p. 437. Blackwell Scientific Publications, Oxford.

Kleinknecht, D., Grunfeld, J-P., Gomez, P. C., Moreau, J-F. and Garcia-Tores, R. (1973) Diagnostic procedure and long term prognosis in bilateral renal cortical necrosis. *Kid. Int.* **4**, 390–400.

Knapp, M. S. (1983). Renal failure after contrast radiography. *Br. Med. J.* **287**, 3–4.

Myers, B. D. and Moran, S. M. (1986). Hemodynamically mediated acute renal failure. *N. Engl. J. Med.* **314**, 97–105.

Pru, C. and Kjellstrand, C. M. (1984). The FE$_{Na}$ test is of no prognostic value in acute renal failure. *Nephron* **36**, 20–23.

Pusey, C. D., Saltissi, S., Bloodworth, L., Raniford, D. J. and Christie, J. L. (1983). Drug associated acute interstitial nephritis: Clinical and pathological features, and the response to high dose steroid therapy. *Q. J. Med.* **52**, 194–211.

Schrier, R. W. (1979). Acute renal failure. *Kid. Int.* **15**, 205–216.

Sitprija, V., Pipatanagul, V., Mertowidjojo, K., Boonpucknavig, V. and Boonpucknavig, S. (1980). Pathogenesis of renal disease in leptospirosis: clinical and experimental studies. *Kid. Int.* **17**, 827–836.

Tiller, D. J. and Mudge, G. H. (1980). Pharmacologic agents used in the management of acute renal failure. *Kid. Int.* **18**, 700–711.

CHRONIC RENAL FAILURE, DIALYSIS, AND TRANSPLANTATION

D. O. OLIVER AND A. J. WING

Chronic renal failure

Definition

In chronic renal failure progressive loss of nephrons causes permanently impaired renal function. *Diminished renal reserve* is the first stage of chronic renal failure; plasma biochemistry is normal and the abnormality in renal function is detected as a decrease in glomerular filtration rate (GFR). Diminished renal reserve becomes *early renal failure* at GFR about 30 ml/min, *late renal failure* at 10 ml/min, and *end-stage renal failure* (ESRF) at 5 ml/min.

The term *azotaemia* is used to indicate that the measured products of nitrogen metabolism, usually urea and creatinine, exceed normal blood levels. *Uraemia* is the illness which results from renal failure and it presents as a spectrum of symptoms resulting from the metabolic poisoning of each of the body's organs and systems. Many diseases causing progressive loss of renal function do so slowly and the symptoms of uraemia may therefore develop insidiously. Approximately one-third of patients presenting in ESRF do so as relative emergencies, their kidney failure being diagnosed only days or weeks before some form of renal replacement therapy (RRT) is necessary if death is to be prevented.

Presenting symptoms may be as non-specific as tiredness resulting from anaemia and the drowsiness of neurological depression, headaches due to the development of hypertension, nausea and dyspepsia suggesting peptic ulceration and pruritus. More dramatically, a heavy epistaxis or gastrointestinal haemorrhage, or an epileptic convulsion may lead to the biochemical tests which disclose renal failure. Occasionally, proteinuria or hypertension discovered at a routine medical examination is the first clue to serious renal disease.

Incidence and epidemiology

The incidence of chronic renal failure in patients selected for dialysis and transplantation is extensively documented in National and International Registries, but these sources do not include patients who fail the selection process or are not referred for treatment. Furthermore, mortality statistics may not differentiate between deaths among patients treated by dialysis and transplantation and others dying from chronic renal failure without treatment; defects which do not apply to mortality data compiled before dialysis and transplantation affected survival (Fig. 1).

Death from renal disease in the neonatal period and first year of life is often associated with other abnormalities incompatible with survival. From the first year to the end of the fourth decade there are about 30 deaths from chronic renal failure per million of population each year. In this age group other diseases which adversely affect survival are unusual, and excellent results are obtained by dialysis and transplantation. The incidence of chronic renal failure increases with age in such a manner that deaths from chronic renal failure among those aged 55–70 years almost equals those occurring between 1 and 55 years. Analysis of all deaths up to 70 years suggests about 150 new patients per million population each year who require conservative management, of which about half are suitable for dialysis and a lesser number for transplantation.

The incidence of chronic renal failure is probably at least twice as high in countries such as China, India, Southeast Asia, Africa, and South America where glomerulonephritis occurs more commonly than in Europe and North America. In the United Kingdom nephritis, which accounted for 7000 deaths in 1900, caused only 1000 in 1980. Diabetes is said to contribute about 25 per cent of patients treated by RRT in the United States, but in Europe it reaches this proportion in Scandinavian countries only. Hypertension is a frequent cause of renal failure in Blacks who make a disproportionate contribution to the end-stage renal disease programme in the United States.

In Australia, Belgium, and Switzerland analgesic nephropathy

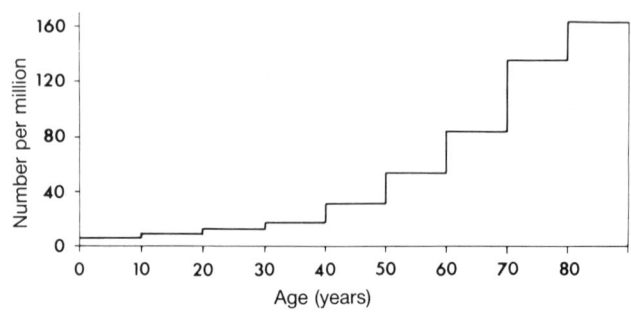

Fig. 1 Death rates from chronic renal failure according to age. Registrar General's report, England and Wales, 1967.

increases the incidence of ESRF in middle-aged women by about 40 per cent. Balkan nephropathy is another condition which is important in a limited geographical region.

Pathophysiology of chronic renal failure

In chronic renal failure, compensatory and adaptive mechanisms maintain acceptable health until GFR is about 10–15 ml/min and life-sustaining renal excretory and homeostatic functions continue until GFR is less than 5 ml/min. The relationship between the blood urea and GFR is shown in Fig. 2. The popular explanation for continuing function in remaining nephrons is the 'intact nephron hypothesis'; i.e. that most nephrons are non-functioning, while the remaining few function normally. These functioning nephrons produce an increased volume of filtrate and their tubules respond appropriately by excreting fluid and solutes in amounts which maintain external balance. For sodium and potassium some balance exists at GFR 5 ml/min and plasma values are commonly normal. For phosphate and urate, adaptation is less precise and plasma concentrations are increased in many patients at GFR 20 ml/min and in almost all at 5–10 ml/min.

The 'trade off' hypothesis is to be considered together with the intact nephron hypothesis, i.e. the concept that adaptations arising in chronic renal failure may control one abnormality, but only in such a way as to produce other changes characteristic of the uraemic syndrome. Although the mechanisms involved are largely unknown, examples are parathormone in phosphorus balance, vasopressin in free water clearance and natriuretic hormone and atrial natriuretic peptide in the control of sodium excretion. The established example of 'trade off' is excess parathormone essential for phosphate excretion; as GFR falls plasma phosphate rises, PTH secretion increases, and plasma phosphate is lowered by decreased tubular reabsorption. The cost of normal plasma phosphate is elevated PTH, secondary hyperparathyroidism, and metastatic calcification. Other abnormalities attributed to excess PTH include central and peripheral nervous disease, impotence, myopathy, carbohydrate intolerance, and lipid disorders. It is also suggested that there are 'trade offs' associated with the homeostasis of sodium, potassium, and other solutes.

Loss of nephrons from any cause initiates a process of progressive nephron destruction which continues independently of the original cause(s) of the renal disease. It appears that hyperperfusion of the remaining intact nephrons causes hyperfiltration and

damage which reveals itself first as mesangial thickening. This subsequently evolves into glomerulosclerosis. Hypertension and phosphate retention may also play a part in this process. This leads to consideration of a third hypothesis which is related to the pathogenesis of chronic renal failure. It states that hyperfiltration in residual nephrons is increased by a high load of protein metabolites, resulting in the more rapid exhaustion of nephrons. Work in experimental animals with diminished renal mass indicates that low protein diets permit increased survival with remnant kidneys. Evaluation of this hypothesis in clinical practice is difficult but early evidence suggests that the rate of progression of renal failure in some diseases can be slowed by the institution of low protein diets.

Water Inability to concentrate urine in the presence of dehydration is often the first symptom of chronic renal failure resulting in polyuria, nocturia, and thirst when GFR is about 30 ml/min. Diluting capacity is preserved until renal failure is advanced, the asymmetrical narrowing of the range of urinary osmolality eventually producing the fixed osmolality of chronic renal failure with its obligatory polyuria (Fig. 3). Diseases which affect predominantly the medulla such as pyelonephritis, interstitial nephritis, and medullary cystic disease may present with a concentration defect at an earlier stage of chronic renal failure. Defective urine concentration is due to increased solute load in surviving nephrons, with minor contributions from decreased tubular function and increased GFR per nephron. As a result urine osmolality is fixed at 300 mOsm/kg. Thirst accompanies polyuria and water balance is maintained provided there is free access to fluid. As obligatory water loss is increased there is need for careful attention to fluid balance in the presence of anorexia, fever, surgery, and other sources of extra-renal loss if dehydration, hypotension, and further impairment of renal function are to be avoided. Urinary dilution is maintained until late in chronic renal failure but large water loads are excreted more slowly than in normal subjects and excessive fluid results in hyponatraemia, mental disturbances, and convulsions.

Sodium As renal function decreases hormonal mechanisms increase the fraction of filtered sodium excreted so that sodium balance and extracellular fluid (ECF) volume are maintained until GFR is less than 10 ml/min. The extent of this adaptation is such that the 1 per cent or less of filtered sodium excreted by normal subjects increases to 30 per cent in late chronic renal failure.

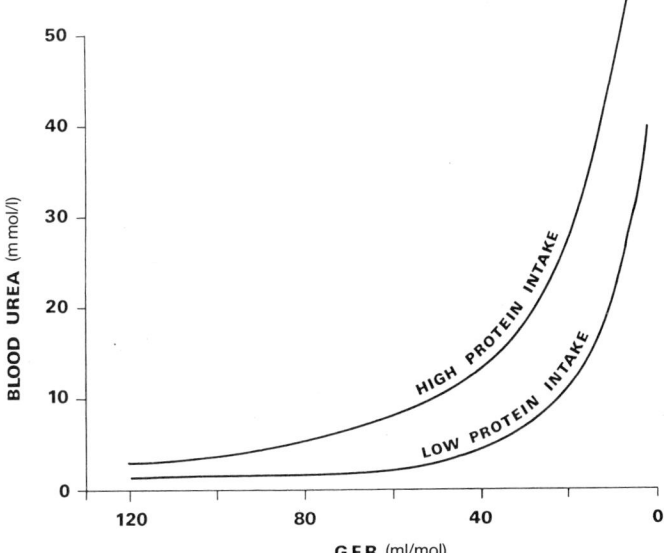

Fig. 2 Relationship between GFR (measured by creatinine clearance) and blood urea comparing the results in African subjects studied in Kampala (low protein intake) with British subjects studied in London (high protein intake).

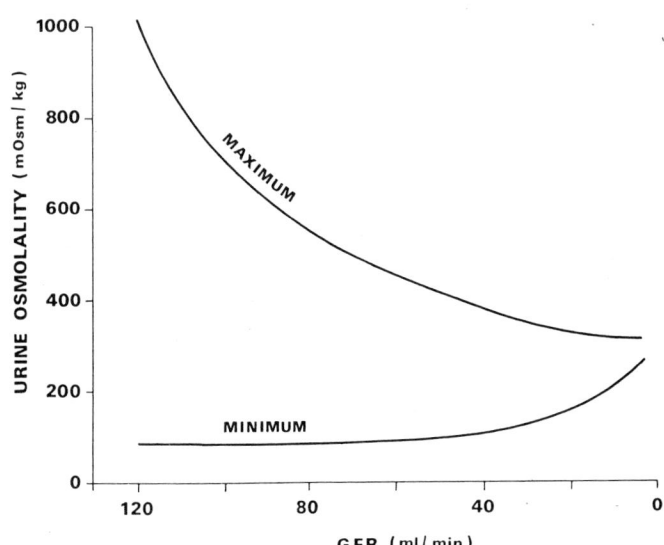

Fig. 3 Progressive loss of flexibility in water handling as renal failure worsens. Concentrating ability is impaired earlier than the ability to excrete a dilute urine.

Adaptive mechanisms are not unlimited; in late renal failure increased total body sodium, with water to maintain osmotic equilibrium presents as fluid overload and hypertension. Initially excess ECF does not cause oedema, but maintains normal body contours and may mask tissue wasting. In late renal failure there is often leg oedema, elevated jugular venous pressure, pulmonary congestion, and functional incompetence of mitral and aortic valves. The major consequence of sodium and fluid excess is hypertension, present in 80 per cent of patients in late chronic renal failure and often presenting in the malignant phase. Increased ECF volume is thought to increase blood pressure in renal disease initially by an increase in cardiac output, and later by an increase in peripheral resistance. In the presence of dietary sodium restriction or of loss of sodium by various routes functioning nephrons cannot restrict sodium excretion promptly so that ECF, plasma volume, and GFR all decrease. Although this sodium and fluid loss has been attributed to an osmotic diuresis, other mechanisms are involved and may dominate; thus, if sodium restriction is induced slowly over months patients reduce urinary sodium to less than 10 mmol/l without significant reduction in GFR. A small number of patients with early chronic renal failure usually with disease affecting the renal medulla present with a urinary sodium leak and sodium depletion on a normal sodium diet. In these patients blood pressure is normal or low, often with a postural drop and sodium supplements may be needed.

Potassium Most patients maintain normal external potassium balance until GFR is less than 5 ml/min but capacity to excrete potassium is limited and severe hyperkalaemia may follow a sudden reduction in residual GFR, excess dietary potassium (chocolate, nuts, instant coffee, some fruits and their juices, wine), potassium sparing diuretics (spironolactone, amiloride, triamterene), medication with high potassium content, surgery, and hypercatabolic states. Acidosis raises serum potassium by ion transfer out of cells and interference with renal excretion. Hypoxia causes hyperkalaemia by impaired uptake of potassium from ECF. In some patients, particularly those with diabetes mellitus and/or interstitial nephritis, and sometimes in early chronic renal failure hyperkalaemia may be due to selective aldosterone deficiency (hyporeninaemic hypoaldosteronism) (page 18.35) which responds to 9α-fluorohydrocortisone. Tubular resistance to aldosterone is another rare cause of hyperkalaemia. Complications occur at plasma potassium concentrations greater than 7.0 mmol/l; weakness in pelvic and shoulder girdle muscles may be the presenting symptom, but in most patients serious electrocardiographic abnormalities and fatal cardiac arrhythmias are the first signs of hyperkalaemia.

Acid–base The kidney is the principal organ to maintain acid–base balance by reabsorption of filtered bicarbonate, acidification of urinary buffers, and excretion of ammonia. As renal failure progresses, intact nephrons increase fractional reabsorption of filtered bicarbonate and excretion of hydrogen ion, which, with intracellular buffers and respiration, prevent acidosis, until GFR is less than 20 ml/min. Increasing acidosis, variable between patients, occurs at GFR less than 10 ml/min; normal net acid production exceeds the excretory capacity of remaining nephrons and diminished tubule function impairs ammonia synthesis and bicarbonate regeneration. Renal diseases which principally affect tubules and interstitial tissues are associated with acidosis quite early in chronic renal failure. Acidosis seldom requires treatment unless bicarbonate is less than 15 mmol/l and pH less than 7.30, except in children in whom prevention of severe acidosis with bicarbonate supplements may have a beneficial effect on renal osteodystrophy and growth retardation. Delayed excretion of excess base is also a feature of late chronic renal failure so that metabolic alkalosis may occur more easily and resolve more slowly after prolonged gastric aspiration, for instance.

Calcium and phosphate The role of the kidney regulating calcium and phosphate in body fluids and tissues is described in the chapter concerning renal osteodystrophy (page 18.156).

Endocrine Patients with chronic renal failure present a variety of endocrine disorders which include decreased erythropoietin as the principal cause of anaemia; abnormal cholecalciferol metabolism resulting in secondary hyperparathyroidism, osteomalacia, and ectopic calcification; hyperreninaemia and hyperaldosteronism as uncommon causes of hypertension; abnormal glucose tolerance from a disturbance of peripheral utilization; and hypothalamic–pituitary–gonadal dysfunction. Endocrine abnormalities found in uraemia which are not known to be associated with clinical disorders include increased serum concentration of growth hormone, luteinizing hormone, somatomedin, prolactin, gastrin, vasoactive hormone, glucagon, and melanophore-stimulating hormone. Follicle stimulating hormone and testosterone are generally decreased. Abnormal concentrations of hormones are explained by decreased production or degradation, overproduction in response to normal physiological stimuli, abnormal peripheral activity, deranged feedback control and end-organ failure.

Lipids Two-thirds of uraemic individuals have hypertriglyceridaemia and several lipoprotein abnormalities – increased very low-density lipoprotein (VLDL) with cholesterol enrichment and prevalence of VLDL subclass late pre-β lipoprotein, an increase in particle size and triglyceride content of low-density lipoprotein (LDL), and reduced concentration of high-density lipoprotein (HDL) cholesterol. Depressed lipoprotein lipase activity, found in uraemia suggests impaired peripheral metabolism as a likely cause for dyslipoproteinaemia. If an association between accelerated atherosclerosis and hyperlipidaemia is established, and at present this is not universally accepted, management of lipid abnormalities will become important in patients with chronic renal failure. Carnitine which plays a part in the oxidation of fatty acids, may be deficient in patients with chronic renal failure due to poor nutrition, diminished renal synthesis, and loss in the dialysate. Its administration as a dietary supplement may reduce cholesterol and triglyceride levels but is not yet routinely recommended because of unpredictable results and side-effects.

Uraemic toxins The retention of toxic waste products from impaired excretion was considered formerly to be important in the aetiology of the manifestations of chronic renal failure. In addition to urea, creatinine, phosphate, and sulphate, other compounds elevated in uraemic plasma are guanidines (methylguanidine, guanidinosuccinic acid), products of nucleic acid metabolism (uric acid, cyclic AMP, pyridine derivatives), amines from bacterial action in gut (aliphatic, aromatic, polyamines), phenol compounds, carbohydrate derivatives (myoinositol, mannitol, sorbitol, and glucuronic acid), hormones, and a large number of compounds of unknown composition varying from 500 to 5000 daltons termed 'middle molecules'. Retention of uraemic toxins, adaptations in intact nephrons, or trade offs do not explain all aspects of uraemia which presents as combined failure of renal excretory, metabolic, and endocrine functions. However, the known disturbances considered in the pathogenesis of uraemia provide a rational basis for therapy: (i) maintain optimal function in remaining nephrons; (ii) restrict dietary potassium, sodium, phosphate, water, and protein to amounts which can be balanced by excretion; (iii) restore abnormal calcium/phosphate metabolism by appropriate vitamin D medication, treatment for hyperphosphataemia and subtotal parathyroidectomy.

Diagnosis of chronic renal failure

Comprehensive diagnosis of the patient with renal failure has three components:

1. The doctor must establish that the renal failure is long-standing and not an episode of acute recoverable disease;
2. The possible cause or causes of the renal disease must be considered;
3. Any reversible factor(s) must be detected.

There is usually some urgency to reach conclusions on each of these aspects because correct immediate management may salvage critical orders of renal function and important decisions may have to be taken quickly concerning renal replacement therapy.

Chronic versus acute uraemia

At the first examination it is not always certain whether the patient has chronic irreversible or acute recoverable renal failure. Symptoms of poor health over the preceding 3–4 months, polyuria, nocturia, thirst, and normochromic anaemia indicate chronic kidney disease. Stunted growth, history of nephritic or nephrotic illness, longstanding hypertension, records of proteinuria from insurance or employment examinations, diabetes or other systemic diseases associated with renal disorders and hospital admissions for nephrological and urological disease suggest that renal failure is chronic. The presence of polycystic kidneys on clinical examination, renal calculi or shrunken kidneys in a standard intravenous pyelogram (IVU) indicate longstanding disease. Uraemic complications which appear late in the course of chronic renal failure such as secondary hyperparathyroidism, osteomalacia, and peripheral neuritis are features of established renal failure. Acute renal disorders may irreversibly damage both kidneys in rapidly progressive glomerulonephritis, cortical necrosis, haemolytic-uraemic syndrome, postpartum renal failure, and embolic disease.

Aetiology

The causes of ESRF given in Table 1 are those used to classify patients reported to the EDTA Registry since 1971. Selection of a diagnosis is based on clinical history, including family history in the case of inherited conditions, general examination for systemic diseases, investigation by ultrasound, radiology, and renal biopsy if indicated. The proportional contributions of these diseases to British and European programmes of RRT are shown for patients

Table 1 Causes of end-stage renal failure as recorded by the EDTA Registry showing percentages diagnosed in patients commencing treatment in 1984 aged under and over 65 years in the United Kingdom and other countries on the Register

Causes of end-stage renal failure	Per cent of new patients 1984			
	United Kingdom		Other countries	
	<65 years	>65 years	<65 years	>65 years
Chronic renal failure, aetiology uncertain	13.9	32.4	12.5	20.5
Glomerulonephritis: Histologically *not* examined	8.1	4.9	17.8	11.0
Histologically examined	13.0	9.0	11.1	3.8
Pyelonephritis/interstitial nephritis: Cause not specified	6.5	4.5	9.2	13.3
Associated with neurogenic bladder	1.4	0	0.5	<0.1
Due to congenital obstructive uropathy				
With or without vesico-ureteric reflux	2.1	0	1.5	0.4
Due to acquired obstructive uropathy	1.7	5.7	1.3	3.4
Due to vesico-ureteric reflux without obstruction	2.8		1.6	0.3
Due to urolithiasis	1.0	2.0	2.4	3.8
Due to another cause	0.7	0	1.0	1.2
Nephropathy: Caused by drugs or nephrotoxic agents, cause not specified	0.4	0	0.5	0.8
Due to analgesic drugs	0.9	1.6	2.9	3.4
Cystic kidney disease, type unspecified	0.2	0.4	1.2	0.9
Polycystic kidney: Adult type	10.2	3.4	7.5	4.7
Infantile and juvenile types	0.1	0	0.2	0.1
Medullary cystic disease, including nephronophthisis	0.1	0	0.4	0.1
Hereditary/familial nephropathy, type unspecified	1.5	0.4	1.9	0.4
Hereditary nephritis with nerve deafness (Alport's syndrome)	1.1	0	0.7	0.1
Cystinosis	0.1	0	0.1	0
Oxalosis	0.1	0	0.1	<0.1
Renal vascular disease: Type unspecified	1.7	2.5	1.7	4.5
Due to malignant hypertension (*no* primary renal disease)	2.8	1.2	1.9	0.9
Due to hypertension (*no* primary renal disease)	7.0	8.2	3.6	7.4
Due to polyarteritis	0.5	2.5	0.2	0.5
Wegener's granulomatosis	0.5	0.8	0.2	<0.1
Diabetes: Insulin dependent (type I)	9.2	2.9	7.4	5.6
Non-insulin dependent (type II)	2.7	3.3	2.3	4.8
Myelomatosis	1.1	4.1	0.5	1.5
Amyloid	1.6	2.0	1.7	1.7
Lupus erythematosus	1.3	0.8	1.0	0.1
Henoch–Schönlein purpura	1.1	0	0.3	<0.1
Goodpasture's syndrome	0.5	1.2	0.3	0.1
Scleroderma	0.5	0	0.1	0.2
Haemolytic uraemic syndrome (Moschcowitz syndrome)	0.2	0.4	0.3	<0.1
Multi-system disease, other	0.3	0	0.3	0.3
Cortical or tubular necrosis	0.4	0.4	0.3	0.5
Tuberculosis	0.5	0.4	0.8	1.0
Gout	0.3	0.8	0.6	0.9
Nephrocalcinosis and hypercalcaemic nephropathy	0.5	0.4	0.2	0.1
Balkan nephropathy	0	0	0.7	0.2
Kidney tumour	0.3	0	0.4	0.5
Traumatic or surgical loss of kidney	0.1	0	0.2	0.1
Other identified renal disorders	1.2	3.3	0.5	0.7
Total patients with diagnosis available	1500	244	14 332	3628

aged less than and more than 65 years in Table 1. There are some recognized geographical variations in the incidence of causes which were discussed above (page 18.134) but other apparent differences could be due to differences in patient selection or diagnostic practice. Thus diabetics are not invariably offered treatment because of inferior results and the clinical diagnosis of pyelonephritis/interstitial nephritis does not appear to be made on uniform criteria in all countries.

The history of patients in chronic renal failure should review all abnormalities from infancy with particular attention to enuresis, nephritic and nephrotic illness, disorders of micturition, urinary infections, loin pain, renal calculi or tissue in urine, haematuria, toxaemia of pregnancy, hypertension, drug ingestion, systemic disease, chronic sepsis, gout, and occupation. The history of familial kidney disease, of obvious importance in polycystic kidneys, is also essential in the less common hereditary disorders; deafness with glomerulonephritis in Alport's syndrome; glomerulonephritis with optic disc and retinal abnormalities; familial glomerulonephritis without associated diseases; concentration defect, anaemia, and acidosis early in the course of medullary cystic disease.

Physical signs of chronic uraemia are anaemia, pigmentation, brown arcs in nail beds, and skin excoriation. There may be evidence of malignant hypertension, polycystic disease, hydronephrosis, lower urinary tract obstruction, neurogenic bladder, or of systemic disease with renal involvement. Amyloidosis may be suggested by the finding of chronic sepsis or non-bacterial inflammation, oxalate calculi may be associated with longstanding bowel disease.

Urinalysis early in the course of chronic renal failure provides valuable information, but late in renal failure urinary abnormalities are less conspicuous. Proteinuria exceeding 3 g daily indicates a glomerular lesion – glomerulonephritis, diabetic nephropathy, malignant hypertension, collagen disease, or amyloidosis. Other chronic renal disorders are associated with less proteinuria which is seldom absent. Red cells are present in urinary sediment in proliferative glomerulonephritis, systemic diseases associated with glomerulonephritis, malignant hypertension, and intermittently in polycystic kidney disease. Red cell casts occur in rapidly progressive glomerulonephritis, glomerular involvement in systemic disease and malignant hypertension. Many granular and hyaline casts are found in renal diseases with predominant glomerular involvement, and a feature of amyloidosis is the large numbers and variety of casts. Large 'chronic renal failure casts' originate in the dilated nephrons present in chronic renal failure. Urinary infection is always sought but seldom found except in the presence of calculi, obstruction, and following instrumentation of the urinary tract. Glycosuria is persistent and heavy in diabetic nephropathy, and present in trace amounts in many other renal diseases due to reduced renal tubular threshold for glucose reabsorption.

Ultrasonography is progressively replacing intravenous urography for imaging the kidneys and urinary tract in the patient with advanced chronic renal failure. In the hands of a skilled operator, modern equipment usually, but not always, provides the information needed for management of the patient. Obstruction in the urinary tract can be excluded by measurement of ureteric, pelvic, and calyceal diameters. If obstruction is detected pelvic scanning may reveal the cause and drainage can be effected immediately by percutaneous nephrostomies performed under ultrasound control. Renal size and cortical thickness can be recorded using callipers on both longitudinal and transverse scanning. Bilaterally small kidneys with reduced renal parenchyma suggest the diagnosis of glomerulonephritis or hypertensive/vascular disease. Fat in the renal hila, cysts, abscesses, and renal masses is identified. Ultrasound is the preferred investigation to diagnose polycystic kidneys. Unfortunately, the permanent record of an ultrasound investigation is often unsatisfactory and it does not demonstrate the renal outline and show scars as well as radiology. Anatomical detail such as the appearance of papillary necrosis which the clinician sometimes requires for diagnosis of the cause of renal failure

is thus not so precise as that obtained with a good quality high dose IVU with nephrotomography. Technical problems arise from obesity, gas in the stomach and bowel, and a short gap between the 12th rib and iliac crest and may make ultrasonography of the kidneys unsatisfactory. However, radiographic contrast media may aggravate renal failure in any patient and particularly in those with arteriosclerotic vascular disease, diabetes, and myeloma, although the risk may be reduced by avoiding dehydration. Renal angiography has the same risk to function but is necessary to demonstrate reno-vascular disease particularly if surgery is contemplated. Digital subtraction angiography (DSA) is rapidly replacing conventional angiography. If contrast medium is given nephrotomography should be obtained.

Micturating cystourethrography (MCU) reveals vesico-ureteric reflux in more adult patients than have scarred kidneys. This is important when planning future transplantation but does not necessarily prove that the renal failure is due to reflux nephropathy which is characterized by scarred kidneys. Both the MCU and dynamic bladder studies are helpful in providing information on bladder emptying and the urethra.

A renal biopsy taken early in the course of chronic renal disease is more likely to make the diagnosis than one taken when failure is advanced. The biopsy must be examined by an experienced renal pathologist using light and immunofluoresent microscopy and who also has electron microscopy available if required. Renal histology of 'end-stage' kidneys is often not helpful in establishing primary renal disease, since many diseases result in a similar final appearance of glomerular obliteration and interstitial scarring. Therefore, it is not unusual for the cause of chronic renal failure to be uncertain and this is particularly likely to be the case in elderly patients (Table 1).

Assessment of renal function and biochemical disorders
Methods used are discussed on pages 18.4–18.17. In some disorders, particularly polycystic disease, loss of glomerular filtration may be predictable and illustrated by a plot of the reciprocal of the plasma creatinine against time (Fig. 4).

Reversible factors
Renal diseases and associated disorders which may be reversed by appropriate therapy are listed in Table 2. Group 1 lists the primary renal disorders which are sometimes amenable to treatment. Obstructive uropathy is the most important of the reversible lesions (see page 18.99). Surgical treatment of early obstructive uropathy frequently allows complete recovery; in obstructions of longer duration recovery is incomplete but worthwhile, but in late obstruction repair is seldom followed by useful return of renal function. Treatment of the other primary renal disorders listed in group 1 are

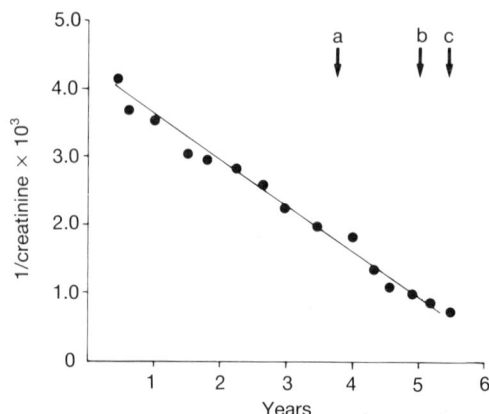

Fig. 4 Plot of reciprocal plasma creatinine (μmol/l) against time in adult polycystic disease patient: (a) work promotion, (b) arteriovenous fistula, (c) haemodialysis.

given in the chapters describing glomerulonephritis (page 18.36), nephropathy due to drugs and chemicals (page 18.108), hypertension, and collagen disorders (page 18.48). Steroids and other immunosuppressive agents have been used indiscriminatly for many renal diseases without good evidence of efficacy. Their use may be complicated by drug side-effects which impair subsequent restoration of health by dialysis and transplantation.

Aggravating factors listed in group 2 are sought at the initial examination and whenever there is an unexpected fall in renal function. Careful attention to salt and water balance and treatment of heart failure using loop diuretics are important. A single haemodialysis or peritoneal dialysis to relieve fluid overload may restore diuretic effectiveness. It is important to discontinue nephrotoxic drugs. These measures allow modest improvements in renal function less dramatic than in group 1, but some symptoms are relieved and time is gained to allow preparation for dialysis and transplantation; and life is prolonged for those patients for whom therapy is limited to conservative measures.

Diet and drugs in chronic renal failure

Reduction of protein content of the diet has two objectives: (1) to ameliorate the symptoms of uraemia and (2) to prolong survival. These objectives must be pursued in the context of plans for eventual dialysis and transplantation. If RRT is not available or is considered inappropriate dietary management can be followed to the ultimate even if the patient begins to become malnourished; whereas malnourishment would be a serious hazard at the time a patient is commencing dialysis and transplantation.

Low protein diets require accurate titration to the patient's level of renal function taking account of proteinuria and body size and are best prescribed and monitored by a specialist dietitian. A protein allowance of 0.6 g/kg body weight usually maintains a positive

Table 2 Reversible factors in chronic renal failure

1 Chronic renal diseases:
    Recent obstruction
    Analgesic nephropathy
    Hypertension
    Urinary infection
        Primary
        Secondary to obstruction
    Tuberculosis
    Glomerulonephritis with anti-GBM antibody
        (Goodpasture's syndrome)
    Glomerulonephritis secondary to infection
    Secondary amyloidosis
    Renal vein thrombosis

2 Disorders aggravating chronic renal failure
    Fluid and electrolyte imbalance
        Dehydration
        Sodium deficit
        Hypokalaemia
    Haemodynamic disturbance
        Congestive heart failure
        Hypotension
        Shock
    Malignant hypertension
    Urinary tract infection
    Nephrotoxins
        Tetracyclines
        Aminoglycosides
        Amphotericin B
        Non-steroidal analgesics
        Radiographic contrast material
    Metabolic disorders
        Hypercalcaemia
        Hyperphosphataemia
        Hyperuricaemia
        Hyperoxaluria

nitrogen balance and calorie intake of 35–40 kcal/kg body weight should be ensured so that the protein taken is not metabolized to provide energy. Protein contains potassium and phosphate and lowering the protein intake helps to control these also. The patient will require instruction in the avoidance of high potassium foods (e.g. instant coffee, chocolate, nuts, dried fruits and vegetables, salt substitute, wines, and beers) and may also need to take phosphate binders, either aluminium hydroxide or calcium carbonate to control plasma phosphate levels. There should usually be concurrent administration of vitamin supplements, possibly including 1,25 or 1-α-hydroxycholecalciferol if the bone disease requires this (see page 18.156). Surveillance includes regular weighing, blood chemistry, and sometimes measurement of urea excretion. Ideally this management is co-ordinated in a low clearance clinic operated in conjunction with renal replacement therapy, the availability of which reassures patients whose renal failure is rapidly progressive and encourages compliance from those for whom protein restriction may prove valuable conservative treatment.

Drugs in renal failure require particular care (see page 18.119) and it is not uncommon to find that symptoms attributed to uraemia were iatrogenic. An example of this is the drowsiness and depression sometimes caused by methyldopa which is so often prescribed for hypertension in patients with renal disease.

Complications and management

Early in chronic renal failure the clinical manifestations are those of the underlying renal disorder. Late and end-stage renal failure are dominated by uraemic complications which involve all body systems. Complications which affect morbidity and survival occur in cardiovascular, haemopoietic, musculo skeletal, and nervous systems. Uraemic complications which reduce the quality of life affect gastrointestinal, skin, endocrine, and immune systems.

Hypertension is present in most patients with chronic renal failure and its absence suggests dehydration or sodium depletion often related to a salt losing nephropathy. Raised arterial pressure contributes to nephrosclerosis and accelerated atherosclerosis with morbidity and death from cardiovascular disease. Renal function may improve after the treatment of malignant hypertension, but not so often after successful control of lesser degrees of raised pressure. Over-rapid reduction of pressure may result in impairment of renal perfusion and decline in renal function. Correction of excess body fluid and sodium, if necessary with loop diuretics, alone or together with beta-blockers and vasodilators controls hypertension in most patients. Angiotensin-converting enzyme inhibitors (captopril, enalapril) can be used successfully to lower arterial pressure even in patients resistant to other drugs, but since both agents are renally excreted, only low doses are permissible. These drugs may also cause worsening of function and even cessation of glomerular filtration in a kidney with renal artery stenosis (page 13.382 et seq.). Minoxodil is an effective hypotensive agent for initial treatment in severe hypertension, and sometimes as long-term therapy for males who are not troubled by hypertrichosis.

Pulmonary oedema and congestive heart failure are common in the late stages of chronic renal failure, and deterioration from early to life-threatening pulmonary oedema may occur over a few hours. Signs and symptoms of early pulmonary oedema are often sparse or absent but chest radiographs invariably show congestion sometimes with a peri-hilar 'bats wing' distribution. Many factors contribute; impaired excretion of sodium and water are paramount, but ischaemic heart disease, increased cardiac work from anaemia, hypoproteinaemia, increased pulmonary vascular permeability, and myocardial damage by deposits of calcium, phosphate, oxalate, and urate also contribute. A uraemic cardiomyopathy has been suggested but not proven. Treatment consists of loop diuretics in high doses by oral or intravenous routes, supplemented in severe pulmonary oedema by a single haemofiltration which removes 1–2 litres of fluid hourly, haemodialysis or more slowly by peritoneal dialysis.

Digoxin can be used for atrial fibrillation, but the dose should be greatly reduced in renal failure and plasma levels must be monitored because of the risk of dysrhythmias especially when hypocalcaemia is induced by diuretics or dialysis.

Pericarditis is rarely painless and usually manifests as central chest and shoulder-tip pain which varies with respiration and position. A pericardial friction rub is diagnostic. This is a late complication of chronic renal failure and indicates the need for maintenance dialysis. Electrocardiographic changes are transient or absent. Haemorrhagic pericardial effusion is a feature of uraemic pericarditis accompanied by a decrease in haematocrit, fever, and rapid increase in size of the heart shadow in chest radiographs. Cardiac tamponade occurs if an effusion accumulates rapidly. Ultrasonography detects small pericardial effusions and is the preferred investigation. Signs of tamponade regress as the parietal pericardium distends and pericardial aspiration or surgical drainage are seldom needed. In cardiac tamponade the maintenance of cardiac output depends on a high central venous pressure; dehydration and diuretic therapy should be avoided. Pain is relieved by non-steroidal analgesics which may also have an anti-inflammatory action. Constrictive pericarditis is a rare and late complication of uraemic pericarditis.

Anaemia is one of the earliest laboratory abnormalities in chronic renal failure and may overshadow other uraemic manifestations. Renal erythropoietin is deficient except in some patients with polycystic kidney disease who may have almost normal erythropoiesis. Haemolysis, depression of erythropoiesis by uraemia, and haemorrhage aggravate anaemia in late renal failure. Anaemia is characteristically normochromic and normocytic with marked anisocytosis (burr cells). The deleterious effects are partially compensated by a shift in the oxygen dissociation curve to the right related to increased concentrations of 2, 3-diphosphoglycerate and phosphates in red cells. Management is limited to the treatment of iron deficiency (low MCV, MCH, and ferritin), bleeding (menorrhagia, peptic ulceration), and the avoidance of excessive blood sampling for laboratory investigations. Androgenic steroids may improve anaemia, but acne, virilism, and the risk of hepatic damage are unacceptable side-effects for many patients.

Blood transfusions may be necessitated by severe symptoms such as angina but the benefit is temporary and they may further depress erythropoiesis. Further hazards of blood transfusion are iron overload and infections (hepatitis B, hepatitis non-A, non-B, and cytomegalovirus) which may have long-term implications for patients destined for RRT. Blood transfusions were thought to make subsequent transplantation difficult because of the provocation of antibodies, but there is less concern about this now that the benefit of pretransplant transfusion is appreciated.

A haemorrhagic disorder in end-stage chronic renal failure presents as bruising, excessive bleeding during surgery, epistaxis, increased gastrointestinal blood losses, menorrhagia, haemorrhagic pericardial effusion, and probably accounts for a low incidence of venous thrombosis and pulmonary embolism. Coagulation disorders are attributed to uraemia which decreases platelet factor 3, and depresses platelet aggregation and prothrombin consumption. Fibrin degradation products are increased moderately suggesting intravascular coagulation. Bleeding is managed by careful haemostasis during surgery, by fibrinolytic inhibitors, and in severe cases by dialysis which corrects abnormal platelet function. Uraemic bleeding can also be arrested by infusions of arginine vasopressin (AVP).

Gastrointestinal
Morning anorexia with nausea is one of the earliest symptoms of chronic renal failure. This develops into profound nausea, retching, and vomiting in ESRF. Reduction of the dietary protein may dramatically relieve these gastrointestinal symptoms. Hiccups used to be a classical hallmark of renal failure but are rare in the patient whose diet has been tailored to his or her level of renal function.

An increased incidence of hiatus hernia, oesophageal mucosal tears with haemorrhage induced by vomiting, and peptic ulceration are found during investigation for upper gastrointestinal disturbances in patients with chronic renal failure. Large bowel disturbances are uncommon in chronic uraemia; diarrhoea and constipation are likely to be side-effects from antibiotic, hypotensive, and hypophosphataemic therapy.

Musculo-skeletal problems
Retarded growth in children, renal osteodystrophy (osteitis fibrosa, osteomalacia, osteosclerosis, osteoporosis, and ectopic calcification), proximal myopathy, and their management are described on pages 18.156.

Skin
Pigmentation of skin and distal nail beds, due to melanin and lipochromes which darken on exposure to sunlight, are characteristic of chronic renal failure. Reduced sebum secretion contributes to dry skin and hair. Pruritus is a troublesome symptom which has been attributed to either secondary hyperparathyroidism or a saturated Ca × P product, but correction of these abnormalities is not always followed by resolution which suggests that other factors are involved. Therapy with antihistamines, oral cholestyramine or ultraviolet light sometimes relieves pruritus. Wound healing is delayed in uraemia. Tension sutures are used for large wounds and skin sutures are retained for 2–3 weeks to avoid wound rupture and incisional hernias.

Endocrine
Endocrine disturbances in uraemia principally affect erythropoietin and parathormone. Hyperreninaemia is a rare cause of hypertension. Other endocrine disturbances described in the pathophysiology of uraemia do not result in clinical disorders, and neither correction of deficiency nor excess of hormones relieves uraemic abnormalities. Facial appearances suggest hypothyroidism which is usually not confirmed by tests of thyroid function. Puberty is delayed. Ovulation is suppressed and amenorrhoea occurs in late chronic renal failure. Although conception may occur, the uraemic environment usually results in spontaneous abortion but rare reports of delivery of small but otherwise normal infants indicates the need for contraception in chronic renal failure. Males have decreased libido and sperm counts. Suppression of hyperprolactinaemia with bromocriptine or treatment with androgens does not have any beneficial effect on sexual function.

Immune system
Defects in uraemia involve cellular and humoral defence mechanisms. Leucocyte count is normal and increases with infection, but capacity to ingest and kill bacteria is decreased. A moderate lymphocytopenia is due to decrease in T and B lymphocytes. Tests of lymphocyte response to mitogens are impaired in the presence of uraemic serum with normal responses in control serum. Interferon production is also depressed. Immunoglobulins are normal unless there is profound hypoproteinaemia. The anamnestic reaction is normal, but response to new antigen is delayed and reduced. Impaired delayed hypersensitivity makes a negative Mantoux test difficult to interpret.

Although the immune system is depressed in uraemia to levels corresponding to the immunosuppressed transplant recipient who is susceptible to bacterial, viral, and protozoal infections, and to opportunistic organisms, these infections are not a particular feature of uraemia. There is, however, an altered response to some infections, such as the persistence of chronic hepatitis B infection (see complications of dialysis treatment) and perhaps slight increased frequency of herpes simplex–varicella infections and tuberculosis.

Dialysis and transplantation

Introduction

Probably a quarter of a million patients worldwide owed their lives to dialysis or renal transplantation at the close of 1984. Treatment programmes represent a large investment of resources and provide work for many specialized physicans, surgeons, nurses, and paramedical staff. An estimate of the personnel involved can be made from the number of specialized centres which are now active. Countries included in the European Dialysis and Transplant Association (EDTA) Registry have a total population of 579 million and an average of 3.3 centres per million. In the United States and Japan there are probably over 5 centres per million population.

Over 100 000 patients were alive on RRT on 31 December 1984 in the 33 countries covered by the annual survey of the EDTA Registry. Of these 62 per cent were treated by haemodialysis in hospital, 8 per cent by home haemodialysis, 2 per cent by intermittent peritoneal dialysis (IPD), 6 per cent by continuous ambulatory peritoneal dialysis (CAPD), and 22 per cent had functioning graphs. These treatments are used in an integrated sequence (Fig. 5), patients moving between different therapies as opportunities present, their personal choices often constrained by economic and medical factors. Facilities for dialysis and the availability of organs for transplantation vary between countries and this has resulted in different criteria for admitting patients to treatment, for instance, the exclusion of elderly patients in the United Kingdom and the German Democratic Republic when compared to other Western European countries (Fig. 6). International comparison also shows different proportional contributions from the various treatment modalities (Fig. 7). Hospital haemodialysis is the most costly method of treatment and successful transplantation the least costly and therefore programmes with a large component of hospital haemodialysis and a small contribution from transplantation are likely to be the more expensive per patient-year.

Haemodialysis and peritoneal dialysis relieve many uraemic

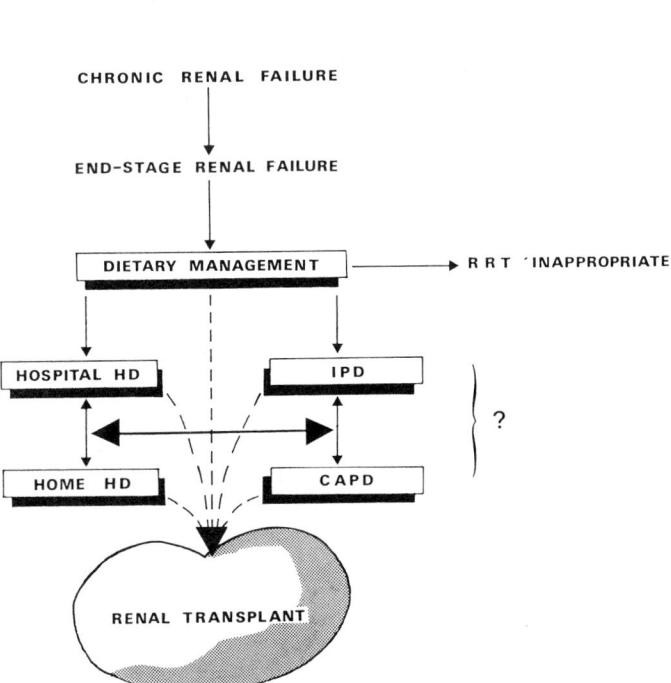

Fig. 5 Scheme to show choices of clinical strategies in the overall management of ESRF.

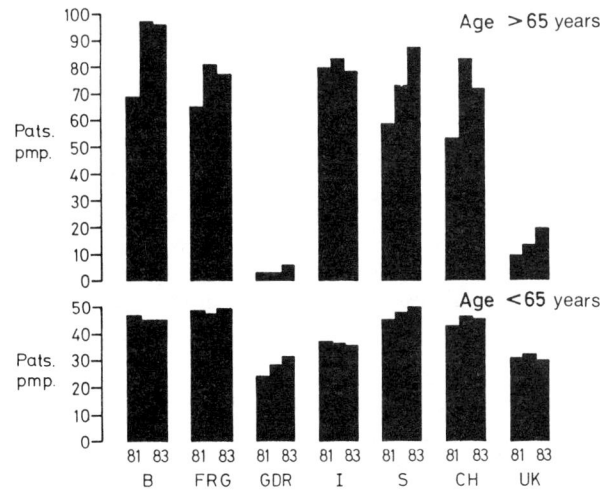

Fig. 6 Age-specific acceptance rates per million population (pmp) for RRT between 1981 and 1983 in Belgium (B), the Federal Republic of Germany (FRG), the German Democratic Republic (GDR), Italy (I), Sweden (S), Switzerland (CH), and the United Kingdom (UK). (Reproduced from Brunner et al., Proceedings EDTA, 1985, with permission of the Editor and the Publisher.)

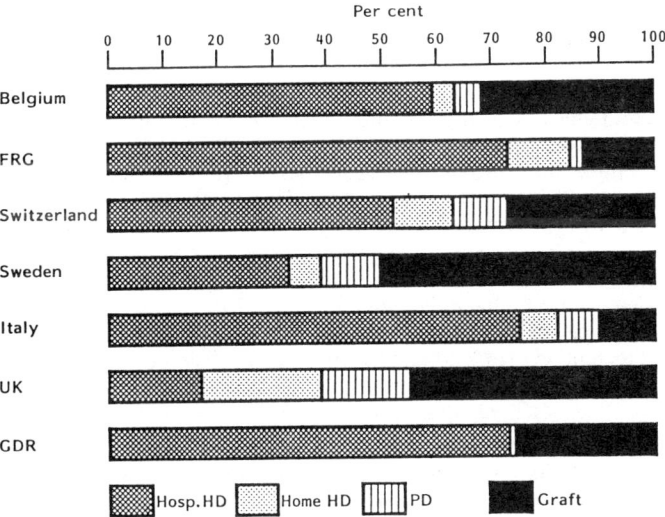

Fig. 7 Stock of patients alive on different forms of RRT on 31st December 1983 in seven countries. (Reproduced from Brunner et al., 1985, Proceedings EDTA, with permission.)

symptoms and restore electrolyte, acid–base, and fluid homeostasis but anaemia, metabolic, and endocrine changes are not reversed by current dialysis techniques and modified uraemia continues. Despite these limitations, dialysis patients achieve acceptable health for many years and 50–70 per cent return to work. A successful kidney transplant restores renal function and corrects uraemic abnormalities provided irreversible structural damage has been avoided. There are benefits if kidney transplantation is performed before the need for dialysis, but practical difficulties such as the waiting period to achieve an acceptable match between recipients and donors, shortage of kidneys, and inability to store donor kidneys for longer than 48 hours prevents such an approach at this time, except for patients who are able to receive a well-matched kidney from a healthy sibling or parent. Dialysis is needed as long-term treatment for patients who are unsuitable for kidney transplantation because of age or associated diseases which result in an unacceptable risk from immunosuppressive drugs used to prevent rejection. There are also individuals who recurrently reject grafts.

Dialysis

Starting dialysis

The decision to begin dialysis depends on clinical features, biochemical abnormalities and resources for treatment. Uraemic symptoms which do not respond to conservative measures e.g. nausea, vomiting, lethargy or difficulty at work or change in lifestyle indicate the need for treatment. Dialysis is rarely essential before creatinine clearance has fallen below 5 ml/min at plasma creatinine concentrations of 500–1500 μmol/l and blood urea greater than 30 mmol/l on a restricted protein diet. An earlier start is needed in the presence of refractory hypertension, heart failure, pericarditis, peripheral neuritis, and for most diabetic patients.

Principles of dialysis

The essential features of dialysis are similar for haemodialysis and peritoneal dialysis. In each technique solutes which have accumulated in uraemic plasma, extracellular and intracellular fluid diffuse across a semipermeable membrane towards the low concentrations present in dialysis fluid, and this gradient is maintained by replacing used dialysis fluid with fresh solution. For solutes for which neither gain nor loss is required, dialysis fluid concentrations are similar to those of normal plasma. Net gain of solute is achieved by preparing dialysis fluid with an increased concentration compared to plasma. Extracellular fluid is removed by ultrafiltration; in haemodialysis by a transmembrane pressure difference; and in peritoneal dialysis by a variable increase in dialysis fluid osmotic pressure depending on dextrose content.

Haemodialysis

Haemodialysis is the common replacement therapy in Europe with 70 per cent of patients receiving this treatment. The short duration of each treatment (e.g. four hours three times weekly) allows time for work and leisure. Disadvantages are the complexity of the extracorporeal dialysis system and the need for vascular access. Some older patients cannot tolerate the rapid changes in fluid and solute balance and major logistic problems arise if hospital haemodialysis is allowed to become the principal treatment for end-stage renal failure. Refinements in haemodialysis technique (Table 3) have been introduced largely to counteract the morbity of the procedure.

Dialysis fluid

Sodium content ranges from 120 to 145 mmol/l with 130–135 most commonly used, a concentration usually lower than that of plasma to allow correction of excess salt and water, hypertension and thirst. If fluid of inappropriately low sodium content is used osmotic equilibrium results in a shift of water into cells. Cerebral oedema from this response, aggravated by shifts of other solutes and pH changes, may cause headaches, vomiting, and seizures from 'dialysis disequilibrium'. These problems can be prevented by increasing the dialysate sodium content, or by using monitors which prepare dialysis fluid of variable sodium content.

Potassium concentrations in dialysis fluid of 1.0 mmol/l maintain plasma potassium in the normal range when dietary intake is 60–80 mmol/day. Potassium is lost into dialysate and moves into cells as metabolic acidosis is corrected. Hyperkalaemia remains an important cause of death in patients treated by dialysis and frequent measurements of plasma potassium are essential if dialysis schedules are disturbed because of problems with vascular access in hypercatabolic states, in young patients prone to dietary indiscretions, or if missed dialysis is suspected in home dialysis patients. When plasma potassium exceeds 7 mmol/l, intravenous calcium gluconate and sodium bicarbonate are given prior to emergency dialysis using dialysate of potassium content lower than normal (0.0–0.15 mmol/l). When hyperkalaemia persists despite adequate dialysis, there is need to review diet for foods of high potassium content, for reduction in dialysate potassium concentrations, and occasionally administration of potassium-binding cation-exchange resins.

Calcium Positive calcium balance during dialysis partly corrects the impaired intestinal calcium absorption and calcium losses in fluid removed by ultrafiltration. The concentration of calcium in dialysis fluid should therefore be set above plasma ultrafilterable calcium. A concentration of 1.6–1.75 mmol/l is recommended to correct and retard the progress of renal osteodystrophy (page 18.160).

Magnesium at 0.5 mmol/l equilibrates with plasma-ionized magnesium and there is net loss of magnesium during treatment. Paradoxically hypermagnesaemia occurs in many dialysis patients without recognized clinical results. Additional magnesium such as magnesium trisilicate antacids are best avoided.

Acetate and lactate The physiological anion bicarbonate cannot be added to bulk supplies of dialysis fluid because it forms insoluble carbonate salts with calcium and magnesium unless the pH of the solution is controlled by continuously bubbling CO_2 through it. Acetate is rapidly converted by the healthy liver into bicarbonate and has therefore become widely used in haemodialysis solutions as a source of anion to correct metabolic acidosis and to replace bicarbonate lost down the concentration gradient into the dialysis fluid. Lactate is used more often in peritoneal dialysis solutions.

Recently, attention has been drawn to the pharmacological actions of acetate which is a vasodilator and has a mild cardiodepressant action. It has therefore been blamed for dialysis hypotension particularly when large surface area (2.5 m^2) dialysers have been used or in patients who are slow metabolizers of acetate. Monitors which mix bicarbonate dialysis solutions provide an attractive alternative but add to the cost of therapy. Their use seems likely to be restricted to patients who have demonstrated a particular requirement.

Glucose was formerly important in dialysis fluid as an osmotic agent which removed fluid, prevented hypoglycaemia during long dialysis sessions, provided calories for patients on restricted diets, and was used in treatment for dialysis disequilibrium. Glucose may be omitted from dialysis fluid since weight is effectively removed by negative hydrostatic pressure, disequilibrium is managed by short dialysis sessions and the avoidance of large surface area dialysers and hyponatraemia. Glucose in dialysate is still needed by diabetic patients who may otherwise experience hypoglycaemia and for the same reason by many patients who cannot eat during dialysis.

Water from the domestic supply requires treatment by softeners, de-ionization or reverse osmosis before it is suitable for dialysis. The preferred preparation is reverse osmosis which removes almost all solutes, additives, contaminants, and particulate matter found in domestic water. Important dialysis-induced disorders due to calcium and aluminium in water are respectively,

Table 3 Techniques for blood purification used in the treatment of uraemia. All methods are dependent on the physical properties of the semipermeable membrane

Technique	Principles	
Haemodialysis	Diffusion down concentration gradients	(Usually simultaneous)
Ultrafiltration	Convective transport with water removal	
Sequential ultra-filtration-haemodialysis	Ultrafiltration performed with 'dry' dialyser (i.e. no dialysis fluid) either before or after haemodialysis	
Haemofiltration	Ultrafiltrated fluid replaced by substitution fluid infused either upstream or downstream of the filter (high permeability membranes)	
Haemodiafiltration	A combination of haemodialysis and haemofiltration	

the hard-water syndrome and dialysis dementia or encephalopathy, the latter also associated with osteomalacia and anaemia. Hard-water syndrome from malfunction of the water-treatment system causes acute hypercalcaemia, headaches, nausea, vomiting and hypertension during dialysis. Dialysis dementia, an osteomalacia-like disorder and anaemia are due to aluminium accumulation from prolonged treatment with water containing aluminium in a concentration usually greater than 50 μg/l from natural sources or when aluminium sulphate has been added to precipitate particular matter in domestic water. Encephalopathy is characterized by dysarthria, dyspraxia, myoclonus, dementia, spike and wave patterns on the electroencephalogram, and death 6–9 months after the onset of symptoms. Elimination of aluminium from dialysis fluid heals bone disease, improves anaemia, and may arrest encephalopathy early in the course of neurological disease. Other disorders associated with water for haemodialysis are haemolytic anaemia from chloramines and copper, methaemoglobinaemia from nitrates, fluoride accumulation in bone, and febrile reactions from pyrogens.

Vascular access
Problems associated with permanent access to the circulation to provide blood flows of 200–300 ml/min are the main reason for hospital admission, inadequate dialysis, incomplete rehabilitation and anxiety, and may reduce survival. A strategy for vascular access is essential for all patients with chronic renal disease. It includes the conservation of veins and arteries, the use of techniques for temporary access, for primary access in new patients with intact vessels, and secondary procedures for use in difficult circumstances.

Conservation of vessels
Important forearm and leg veins essential for haemodialysis are destroyed or damaged by infusions and repeated venepunctures which should be avoided in those at risk of renal failure. The prevention of premature atherosclerosis or the vascular calcification associated with renal osteodystrophy and hyperphosphataemia is an unimportant aspect of care of patients approaching end-stage uraemia.

Temporary access
Temporary access involves internal jugular, subclavian and femoral vein catheters introduced by the Seldinger technique. Subclavian catheters provide access for several weeks. Risks of infection are greater with femoral catheters which are used for short periods. Complications of temporary access are infection, thrombus in catheter and veins, and rarely perforation of large veins. Infections are avoided by meticulous techniques, occlusive dressings, and prohibition of the use of this catheter for blood samples and infusions. For clinical or suspected infections during prolonged subclavian catheterization, which are commonly due to *Staphylococcus aureus* and cause septicaemia, the catheter is removed and antibiotics are administered for 2–3 weeks. After 24–48 hours of antibiotic therapy a new catheter is inserted in the contralateral subclavian vein. Heparin left in the catheter after each dialysis prevents irreversible obstruction of the catheter lumen by thrombus; however, large mural thrombi around the catheter tip frequently impair flow, resulting in loss of this vein for access, and pulmonary embolism is a potential hazard. A poorly functioning catheter is replaced over a guide wire inserted through the original catheter.

Primary vascular access
Primary access for long-term haemodialysis is an *arteriovenous* (AV) *fistula* between the radial artery and cephalic vein near the wrist of the non-dominant arm. After a period of maturation which varies from a few days to several months, blood flow in forearm veins exceeds 300 ml/min. Blood is pumped to and from the dialyser using two 13–16 gauge needles, a needle with double lumina, or a single needle and blood-cycling device. The advantages of the AV fistula are free use of the arm, uninterrupted treatment for several years, and relative freedom from complications. Fistulae frequently remain patent after transplantation for use if the graft fails. Inadequate fistulae can be re-fashioned between the radial artery and cephalic vein at a proximal site, or between the ulnar artery and basilic vein, in the antecubital fossa, or upper-arm vessels. All potential sites should be exhausted in the original arm before changing to the other limb.

An access system which is now rarely used is an *arteriovenous* (AV) *cannula* ('shunt') of silastic tubing with teflon vessel tips inserted surgically between an adjacent limb artery and vein. The junction between arterial and venous cannulae is open during the interdialysis period and closed during dialysis, so that arterial blood is pumped to the dialyser and returns through the venous cannula. Disadvantages of the AV cannula are the need for surgical revision withing 6–12 months for repair of stenosis in the cannulated vein, thrombosis, infection, limited use of this limb, loss of limb veins and arteries, and thrombosis with loss of the AV cannula soon after transplantation. Although it was common to obtain 3–5 years of dialysis from each limb using cannulae, in some patients most sites were exhausted within one year. An advantage of the AV cannula is its availability for immediate use but improved temporary vascular access and peritoneal dialysis generally avoids the need on this ground. AV cannulas are now used only for small children and for some adults treated by home dialysis who are unable to insert needles into an AV fistula.

Secondary vascular access
The preferred secondary access is constructed from autologous vein grafts (saphenous, cephalic, external jugular) fashioned as a straight or looped AV fistula between large proximal arteries and veins in the forearm, antecubital fossa, upper arm, or thigh. If suitable veins for grafting are absent fistulae are made from expanded polytetrofluorethylene, bovine carotid arteries, or glutaraldehyde treated umbilical veins. Complications in fistulae made from foreign materials are more frequent than in autologous vein access systems.

Complications of vascular access
These include inadequate function, thrombosis, infection, circulatory disorders, and skin problems.

Reduced arterial flow, increased resistance to venous return or recirculation in the fistula may occur, the latter because of poor outflow from the fistula. An acceptable level of recirculation is about 10 per cent. Angiograms demonstrate the lesions responsible for inadequate vascular access and provide valuable information for surgical repair.

Occlusion by thrombus is usually preceded by a period of inadequate function. Thrombosed fistulae require immediate surgical repair. Occlusion of AV cannulae following excessive use of the cannulated limb, exposure to cold, hypotension, or during operations may be reversed by removal of thrombus by aspiration or embolectomy catheter followed by intravenous heparin (which may be given via an injection insert placed at the junction of cannulae) until the next haemodialysis. If flow is unsatisfactory after declotting a fibrinolytic agent (urokinase) is left in both limbs of a clamped shunt for 2–4 hours. AV cannula function is tested by dialysis as soon as possible after declotting; if poor function continues surgical repair is required.

Poor techniques allow skin organisms (*Staphylococcus aureus, Staphylococcus epidermidis*) to invade fistula needle wounds and shunt exit sites. Cellulitis responds to antimicrobials given for 10–14 days. Deep infections cause septicaemia, septic emboli, and local haemorrhage; response to antimicrobial therapy is poor and vascular access is usually lost.

Local circulatory complications of AV connections include ischaemia or excess flow. Tingling, numbness, and cold aggravated by exercise indicate ischaemia from either diseased or ligated arteries, or an arterial 'steal' through a large AV fistula.

On occasion there is ulceration and necrosis of finger tips. Pain, swelling, erythema, and dermatitis from venous hypertension is termed 'fistula thumb'.

Increased cardiac output occurs in all large AV fistulae; aggravates raised cardiac output from anaemia, and may contribute to congestive heart failure.

Ischaemia is avoided by careful evaluation of limb vessels before undertaking surgery. Steal syndromes and excessive flow are indications for reduction in size of the fistula. Carpal-tunnel syndrome has been attributed to congestion and ischaemia but is frequently bilateral which suggests that other factors are involved and the deposition of amyloid related to β_2-microglubulin has been described.

Skin may erode over the AV cannula in thin patients, after infections, and in those taking corticosteroids. Dermatitis frequently results from the use of skin antiseptics and tapes to secure needles during dialysis.

Membranes and dialysers

Dialysers consist of sterile blood compartments, prepared from membranes of Cuprophan, cellulose acetate or polyacrylonitrile fashioned as hollow fibres, sheets or coils, within a dialysis fluid chamber. Membrane thickness is between 7 and 70 μm with most dialysers employing membranes of 11–15 μm. Surface area of commonly used dialysers is 0.9–1.2 m^2 with smaller models available for children and bigger for unusual dialysis strategies. Design features variably reduce problems such as resistance to dialysis from stagnant fluid films on membrane surfaces, small blood volume, resistance to blood flow, thrombogenicity, and the volume of saline needed to return blood at the end of dialysis. Variations in membranes, surface areas, and construction provide a range of dialysers with different properties. Disposable dialysers are sterilized by ethylene oxide or gamma irradiation. Costs may be reduced by reuse of 'disposable' dialysers or, for instance, the Kiil dialyser. Hazards of reuse are pyrogenic reactions, septicaemia, administration of formaldehyde, formaldehyde allergy, and cold-reacting anti-N red-cell antibodies from this sterilizing agent.

The artificial kidney removes small molecules at rates related inversely to size and directly to blood and dialysate flow. Clearance of middle molecules is directly related to surface area, duration of dialysis, and membrane permeability. Dialysis clearance is measured by a formula similiar to that used in the estimation of GFR:

$$C = \frac{K_d \times t_d}{168} + K_r$$

where C is clearance ml/min; K_d is dialyser clearance ml/min (clearance by diffusion + clearance by ultrafiltration or convection); t_d is dialysis time (hours per week); K_r is residual renal clearance ml/min; and 168 is total hours in one week.

Adequate dialysis is provided by creatinine clearance 5 ml/min and middle molecule clearance of 3 ml/min each week. Clearance values for a 1.2 m^2 dialyser at blood flow 200 ml/min and dialysate flow 500 ml/min are: urea 160, creatinine 130, uric acid 120, phosphate 100, and vitamin B_{12} (middle molecule size) 40 ml/min. Fluid loss is at 300–500 ml/h, but 1000–2000 ml/h can be removed when necessary.

Biocompatibility of membranes has been cause for some concern. Cuprophan membranes promote coagulation and activate complement; they rupture and leak amino acids and water-soluble vitamins. Chemical leached from membranes may result in cardiac and skin disorders. Heparin administered during dialysis prevents massive thrombosis in the extracorporeal circuit, but despite an adequate anticoagulant effect as measured by clotting times, platelets, fibrin, leucocytes, and red cells are deposited on membranes and contribute to blood losses of 5–50 ml during each dialysis. Prostacyclin has been shown to prevent both platelet aggregation and coagulation. Large amounts of heparin are avoided during dialysis as cerebral haemorrhage and bleeding after surgery may occur during or soon after dialysis and heparin is the likely culprit; 1000–1500 units hourly is adequate for most patients, and if there is risk from haemorrhage, 500 units each hour provides sufficient anticoagulant for short dialysis provided blood flow is rapid. Aggregation of leucocytes in lungs by dialysis membranes activating the complement system causes leucopenia, hypoxia, and pulmonary hypertension in the first 30 min of dialysis, but there are no long-term pulmonary abnormalities associated with this phenomenon.

Haemodialysis monitors

The haemodialysis monitor in common use is a single-patient machine which prepares dialysis fluid at body temperature from a concentrate of electrolytes and treated water. It varies blood flows and dialysate pressures to achieve satisfactory solute clearance and fluid losses, tests for blood in dialysate from membrane rupture, and for air in blood. Abnormalities outside fixed or adjustable limits activate visual and audible alarms, and treatment stops until the fault is corrected. For hospital dialysis, a central source of dialysis fluid and individual patient monitors may replace single-patient systems. A portable dialysis system which does not need a constant source of water regenerates 4.5 litres of dialysate using a cartridge of resins, sorbents, and urease.

Haemodialysis treatment

Haemodialysis is performed three times each week for 4–6 hours with blood flow 200–300 ml/min and dialysate flow 500 ml/min. Twice weekly haemodialysis for eight or more hours provides adequate dialysis for some patients with residual renal function, and for short periods when thrice weekly treatment presents difficulties because of vascular access problems, work, or vacations. Dialysis schedules are tailored for the individual; short dialysis for small patients and those with residual renal function, longer for larger patients, and the choice of a dialyser which provides satisfactory clearance of solutes and fluid.

Hospital haemodialysis

Hospital haemodialysis is provided by centres with expert staff. It is essential at the start of dialysis, during complications, at the time of transplantation, and as long-term therapy for patients unable to transfer to home or limited-care dialysis. Hospital haemodialysis has inherent limitations as the principal treatment in end-stage renal failure: each hospital bed treats only 2–4 patients; treatment is seldom at times which suit patients; there is the expense of and time taken for travel, and difficulty in obtaining staff. Annual costs exceed those of the first year of home dialysis and are three times the cost of home dialysis in subsequent years.

Home haemodialysis

The lengthy training needed for self dialysis at home is worthwhile if the waiting period for a transplant is greater than six months or for patients unsuitable for transplantation. Home treatment allows improved patient survival and dialysis at times which suits patients at one-half the cost of hospital treatment. Factors which encourage home dialysis are: (i) simple vascular access; (ii) training periods adjusted to suit patients; (iii) patients responsible for their own treatment, except in the case of children; (iv)return to hospital dialysis for medical, technical, and social problems; (v) a room or cabin for dialysis; (vi) a dialysis nurse or technician resident in areas with more than 20 home-dialysis patients; (vii) high-quality monitors repaired and maintained by expert technicians, and (viii) funds to pay for home-dialysis assistants and to offset the cost of home dialysis for families with income reduced by chronic disease.

Limited-care haemodialysis

There are social and economic advantages if stable patients without need for the resources of the hospital unit receive treatment in a limited-care unit in which patients are responsible for dialysis with minimal supervision. Cost is less than hospital treatment but greater than home dialysis, travel is reduced, and the increase in dialysis places allows treatment at times suitable to most patients. The hospital unit supervises initial treatment and training, manages vascular access, and the patients return to the hospital centre when complications arise.

Peritoneal dialysis

There are a number of advantages in peritoneal dialysis. The peritoneal membrane is superior to those currently used in haemodialysis. Treatment is simple and requires less complex equipment. Access to the peritoneum is not difficult. Patients are less anaemic than in haemodialysis. Slow correction of fluid and solute abnormalities are better tolerated by children and the elderly and, treatment is easily undertaken at home. There are disadvantages, chiefly the long duration of treatment, peritonitis, the expense of recurrent hospital admissions, and the large volumes of commercially prepared fluid required.

Dialysis fluid

Peritoneal dialysis fluid is sterile, pyrogen-free, and presented in polyvinylchloride bags of 1–3 litres; older formulation in glass bottles and 10 litre containers being largely obsolete. A typical peritoneal dialysate contains sodium 132, potassium 0, glucose 75 (1.36 per cent) or 311 (3.86 per cent), calcium 1.75, magnesium 0.75, and lactate 35 mmol/l. Glucose increases oncotic pressure in dialysis fluid; 1.36 per cent for standard dialysis and 3.86 per cent to remove excess fluid. Problems associated with frequent use of 3.86 per cent glucose are hyperglycaemia, excessive calories which may amount to 600–800 daily, increased protein losses in dialysate, and hypertriglyceridaemia. Potassium is omitted from peritoneal dialysis fluid as potassium clearance is less than in haemodialysis.

Peritoneal access

Conservation of the peritoneal cavity is essential whether access is gained by temporary or by permanent procedures.

Conservation of the peritoneal cavity An intact peritoneal cavity is important for long-term management of end-stage renal failure in order that peritoneal dialysis may be used either as a long-term therapy or to complement haemodialysis for short periods. The peritoneal cavity is lost during intraabdominal sepsis, after abdominal surgery or peritonitis from peritoneal dialysis. After abdominal surgery 500 ml of peritoneal dialysis fluid left in the peritoneal cavity may prevent surgical adhesions. Antibiotic lavage may leave the peritoneal cavity available for dialysis despite infection. Sclerosing encapsulated peritonitis is a rare complication, thought to be related to repeated infection or chemical contamination, and is almost invariably fatal.

Temporary peritoneal access A rigid plastic or silastic catheter is inserted into the peritoneal cavity for temporary peritoneal access. Plastic catheters must be inserted for each treatment and are removed after each dialysis. Silastic catheters can remain *in situ* between dialyses and are preferred by patients and staff.

Permanent peritoneal access Permanent intraperitoneal access is provided by silastic catheters. Infections and leaks around the catheter are avoided by ingrowth of fibrous tissue into dacron cuffs external to peritoneum and 1–2 cm beneath the skin exit site. Infection introduced through the catheter lumen is partly prevented by special connectors, meticulous techniques taught and supervised by special staff. Catheters are inserted using either local or general anaesthetic in surgical theatres through a 3–5 cm incision over the lina alba or rectus muscle. They are placed in the pelvis by either a percutaneous trocar and cannula technique or by minilaparotomy. The latter is preferred, allowing a purse-string suture in peritoneum around the catheter for immediate dialysis without leaks of dialysis fluid.

Complications of peritoneal access

The risks are of leaks, malfunction, and infection.

Leaks of dialysis fluid around the catheter occur soon after implantation by the trocar method, in the presence of poor drainage with accumulation of fluid, after steroid therapy, and in obese or elderly patients. Most stop after draining the abdomen and discontinuing dialysis for three to five days.

Malfunction of the catheter presents as failure to drain dialysate or less frequently as impaired inflow. Malfunction occurs during the first week from incorrect placement, encasement by omentum, or from constipation. A catheter which lies transversely in the abdominal cavity indicates encasement with omentum, and an injection of contrast material shows adherent omentum or obstruction of the catheter pores. Laxatives may restore drainage when such obstruction cannot be demonstrated. Surgical revision is necessary for malpositioned catheters which do not drain satisfactorily, and sub-total omentectomy is needed for recurrent obstruction by omental adherence.

Infection Peritonitis is the most frequent and serious complication of peritoneal diaylsis. Protein losses in dialysis fluid increase, ultrafiltration decreases, and delayed treatment or recurrent infections may result in loss of the peritoneal cavity for dialysis. Clinical signs of peritonitis are cloudy dialysate, diffuse or localized abdominal pain, rebound tenderness, fever, and a count of neutrophil leucocytes greater than 50 per ml in peritoneal fluid. Organisms responsible are *Staphylococcus aureus, Staphylococcus epidermidis, Streptococcus viridans, Streptococcus faecalis, Pseudomonas, Enterococci,* and *Escherichia coli.* Fungal peritonitis is usually a complication of antimicrobial therapy. Peritonitis with negative cultures, 'sterile peritonitis', is uncommon if 250 ml of cloudy peritoneal fluid is collected and concentrated for bacteriological examination using enriched culture media before antimicrobial treatment is begun. A condition presenting as mild peritonitis soon after starting treatment, in which sterile fluid contains many eosinophils, is probably an allergic reaction to substances in fluid or from plastic containers.

Peritonitis should be treated at the first sign of infection before the results of Gram stain or culture are known. Two or three rapid exchanges are performed without antibiotics to reduce bacterial counts and then vancomycin 50 mg/l with a cephalosporin (e.g. ceftazidime 50 mg/l) are added to each exchange. A positive identification of the infecting organism may permit one of these drugs to be withdrawn, otherwise it is recommended that they are continued for 10 days. If there is a poor response a change of treatment is determined by results of culture and sensitivities. Concentrations (mg/l) of various antimicrobials recommended for dialysis fluid are: cloxacillin 50, amicillin 50, carbenicillin 100, cephaloridine 50, cephalothin 60, gentamicin 10, and kanamycin 20. The catheter should be removed if a fungal infection develops and will usually have to be taken out if a pseudomonas infection becomes established. It is also important to consider infection from an inflamed appendix, gall bladder, or diverticulitis. During peritonitis heparin 500 units/l are added to dialysate to inhibit fibrin deposition which may occlude the catheter. Cellulitis around the catheter exit responds to prompt treatment with antibiotics, but if a local abscess forms the catheter is removed to allow drainage of pus.

Peritoneal dialysis treatment

Peritoneal rather than haemodialysis is preferred in children, in those aged more than 60 years, in the presence of cardiovascular instability, during the waiting period for AV fistula maturation or transplantation, when vascular access for haemodialysis has been lost, when there is risk of haemorrhage from heparin, with diabetes mellitus, and in patients who live alone or are unable to manage haemodialysis.

Continuous ambulatory peritoneal dialysis (CAPD)

In CAPD 2 litres of peritoneal dialysis solution, supplied in collapsible containers, remains in the peritoneal cavity except during fluid exchanges. After filling the peritoneal cavity, the empty bag attached to the catheter is worn in the belt or waistband until the next exchange when it is used to drain peritoneal fluid. The minimum period between changes is four hours and one exchange remains in the peritoneal cavity overnight. Small molecules such as urea and electrolytes equilibrate between plasma and dialysis fluid in four hours, but creatinine equilibration is achieved only in the overnight exchange. Adequate dialysis for the majority of patients is provided by four exchanges of 2 litres daily. For larger patients, five exchanges are needed, and some also need a single haemodialysis each week. In small patients and if there is residual renal function three exchanges may be sufficient. Safe connections between the catheter and containers of dialysis fluid and the use of meticulous aseptic methods prevent infection at home, work, and during travel.

CAPD effectively controls uraemic symptoms, biochemical abnormalities, and there are theoretical advantages of improved middle-molecule clearance. Compared to haemodialysis, there is improved sense of well-being from increased haematocrit, more physiological steady-state biochchemistry and correction of fluid overload. Control of phosphate will almost always require continuous administration of phosphate binders. Hypertension is usually controlled by dialysis alone. Diet is normal and compensates for protein losses in dialysis effluent of about 8 g daily. The short training period does not interrupt work or family life, and there is independence for travel and vacations superior to other forms of dialysis at annual costs greater than for home haemodialysis, but less than for hospital treatment.

There are particular benefits from treating end-stage diabetic nephropathy for CAPD. Stable blood glucose concentrations result from addition of short-acting insulins to peritoneal dialysis fluid. Excellent control of uraemia and hypertension can be achieved without use of heparin, which may aggravate proliferative retinopathy. Vascular access for haemodialysis may be difficult in diabetic patients because of peripheral vascular disease or veins damaged by venesections and infusions. Diabetic patients do not have an increased frequency of peritonitis and inadequate peritoneal clearances from peritoneal vascular disease has not been encountered.

Continuous cyclic peritoneal dialysis (CCPD)

Continuous cyclic peritoneal dialysis is a variant of CAPD performed at night during sleep. Eight two-litre bags of peritoneal dialysis solution are dispensed through the night by an automatic cycler as three exchanges of 2 litres for 3 hours, and 2 litres remain in the peritoneal cavity for 14–15 hours during the day. The single connection and disconnection each day reduces the incidence of peritonitis by 50 per cent compared to CAPD but the need for equipment results in loss of independence and mobility. CCPD provides some of the advantages of CAPD for patients who are unable or unwilling to perform fluid exchanges during the day.

Intermittent peritoneal dialysis (IPD)

Treatment by intermittent peritoneal dialysis involves 2 litre exchanges each hour for 10–14 hours using an automatic cycler which dispenses and drains dialysis fluid. For patients with residual GFR greater than 3 ml/min, this treatment for three nights each week is adequate, but as residual renal function declines, IPD for 50 or more hours each week is needed. IPD patients are less well and require more dietary restriction than patients managed by continuous peritoneal dialysis or haemodialysis. This limits this treatment to short periods in patients waiting for a transplant, during maturation of an AV fistula for haemodialysis, for some small patients (less than 55 kg) who are unsuitable for haemodialysis, and in those who cannot cope with the ritual of CAPD or CCPD.

Complications of haemodialysis and peritoneal dialysis

The major complications associated with haemodialysis and peritoneal dialysis, and some minor ones, are listed in Table 4. Complications in Group 1, the result of haemodialysis, frequently occur during treatment or are a consequence of vascular access problems. Group 2 describes the complications associated with peritoneal dialysis and the catheter required for this treatment. Group 3 illustrates continuing uraemia during dialysis treatment; better dialysis and additional measures arrest or improve many of these complications.

Anaemia

In patients who have not been made anephric, haematrocrit increases from 15–20 per cent at the start of haemodialysis to 20–30 per cent over 6–12 months, while on CAPD haematocrits of 30–40 per cent are common by the fourth month of dialysis. Erythropoietin remains inappropriately low but inhibitors of erythropoiesis are probably more efficiently cleared by peritoneum. Haemolysis continues and may be aggravated by hypersplenism. Haemodialysis is associated with blood losses which are not replaced by suppressed marrow. Benefits of blood transfusion are brief due to haemolysis, and loss of the hypoxic stimulus to erythropoiesis. Regular transfusions (and excess parenteral iron) cause iron overload which is probably not amenable to chelating agents.

Bilateral nephrectomy should be avoided whenever possible, since haematocrit falls to about 15 per cent in anephric patients.

The objectives in management of anaemia are to promote erythropoiesis and to minimize blood losses. Optimal erythropoiesis depends on adequate dialysis and assessment of the need for iron. Iron deficiency is indicated by a hypochromic blood film, with MCH less than 27 pg and MCV less than 79 fl; serum ferritin is low. Iron absorption is normal in chronic renal failure but deficiency should be treated with oral preparations administered at times different from phosphate binding gels which may combine with iron and reduce absorption.

Folic acid 1 mg daily replaces folate removed by dialysis and prevents folate deficiency during periods of decreased dietary protein.

Androgen therapy is considered if symptomatic anaemia persists after six months of dialysis. Nandrolone decanoate 3 mg/kg per week or testosterone enanthate 4 mg/kg per week by intramuscular injection for men, and nandrolone decanoate only for women, increases haematocrit by about 5 per cent after six months of therapy in the 50 per cent of patients who tolerate treatment. Oral androgens are less effective than those given by the parenteral route, and anephric patients do not respond at all. Acne in both sexes and virilization in women result in 25 per cent discontinuing androgen treatment before a response can be expected, but serious toxicity such as jaundice and hepatoma have not been described. Treatment is stopped after six months if there is no response, and after 12 months in those with a satisfactory result among whom haemoglobin concentrations frequently remain at the new level.

In a very few patients, particularly in the anephric subjects severe symptoms of anaemia persist. In them regular transfusions of single units of blood are needed. It is hoped that erythropoietin may become available for therapeutic use during the next few years.

Bleeding disorders

Bleeding time and platelet function are restored to normal by peritoneal dialysis, less completely by haemodialysis. This response suggests that disturbed platelet function is due to retained substances of molecular weight of 10–15 000 Daltons, which are removed more effectively by peritoneal dialysis. The use of heparin in haemodialysis aggravates any bleeding state, and patients at risk should rather be treated by peritoneal dialysis. If this is not possible, short haemodialysis schedules with very low dose heparin, or regional heparinization is used, and at the end of

Table 4 Complications of haemodialysis and peritoneal dialysis

1 Disorders related to haemodialysis
   (*a*) Haemodialysis treatment
       Hypotension
       Haemorrhagic – membrane, blood line, vascular access, from
           heparin
       Air embolism
       Hypernatraemia
       Hyponatraemia
       Disequilibrium syndrome
       Muscle cramps
       Abnormal losses – vitamins, amino acids, carnitine
       Pyrogenic reactions
       Priapism
       Complement – leucocyte-induced pulmonary dysfunction
       Allergy and granulomas associated with synthetic materials
       Hard-water syndrome
       Dialysis dementia
       Fluorosis
       Haemolysis (hyponatraemia, overheated dialysate, chloramines,
           copper, formaldehyde)
   (*b*) Vascular access
       Inadequate flow
       Recirculation
       Infection – cellulitis, endarteritis, septicaemia
       Thrombosis
       Haemorrhage
       Aneurysm
       Raised cardiac output
       Fistula thumb
       Vascular steal syndromes
       Ischaemia
       Carpal tunnel syndrome
       Skin erosion
       Dermatitis

2 Disorders related to peritoneal dialysis
       Infection – peritonitis, tunnel abscess, cellulitis
       Catheter malfunction – obstruction, leaks, separation
       Loss of peritoneal ultrafiltration
       Sclerosing encapsulated peritonitis
       Obesity
       Pleural effusion
       Hernias – inguinal, umbilical, cystocoele, hiatus hernia
       Haemorrhoids
       Low back pain
3 Disorders related to unresolved uraemia during treatment with
   haemodialysis and peritoneal dialysis
       Anaemia
       Abnormal bleeding
       Hypertension
       Hypotension
       Pericarditis
       Heart failure
       Artherosclerosis
       Hyperlipidaemia
       Renal osteodystrophy
       Endocrine disorders
       Infections
       Malignancy

dialysis heparin effects are reversed with protamine sulphate. Uraemic bleeding which does not respond to dialysis commonly does so to infusions of vasopressin.

Hypertension

Hypertension persists in 25–30 per cent of patients treated by haemodialysis and to a lesser extent among patients treated by CAPD. Before resorting to long-term drug therapy, a further trial of sodium and water depletion is worthwhile. For patients on haemodialysis this is achieved without inducing acute transient hypotension by sequential haemofiltration-haemodialysis, in which extracellular fluid is filtered through the dialyser acting as an ultrafilter, followed by haemodialysis to correct solute and electrolyte disturbances. In peritoneal dialysis hypertonic dialysate is used to achieve negative balance. Water restriction is sometimes necessary.

The use of hypotensive therapy in resistant hypertension is the same as in essential hypertension. Beta-blockers and vasodilators are used alone or in combination with captopril or enalapril and minoxidil reserved for refractory cases.

Severe hypertension resistant to dialysis and most hypotensive drugs has been described in 5–10 per cent of haemodialysis patients. The clinical picture is of hypertension often in the malignant phase with marked dehydration; plasma renin is high. Bilateral nephrectomy always relieves hypertension but at the cost of severe anaemia and loss of any residual renal function. The need for this drastic treatment has been greatly reduced by the introduction of sequential ultrafiltration-haemodialysis (Table 3), minoxidil and angiotensin converting enzyme (ACE) inhibitors.

Pericarditis

Pericarditis is usually due to inadequate dialysis, rarely from cytomegalovirus infection. Heparin treatment and platelet defects associated with haemodialysis may result in haemorrhagic effusion which is not a feature of peritoneal dialysis.

In treatment pericardial pain is relieved by indomethacin. Haemodialysis is increased to short daily treatments of 2–3 hours with very low heparin dosage reversed by protamine sulphate, regional heparinization, or haemodialysis is replaced by peritoneal dialysis. In the early stage of pericardial effusion it is important to maintain cardiac output by an elevated central venous pressure; later, after a few days, parietal pericardium stretches with restoration of cardiac output and blood pressure. Excess body fluid and the effusion can then be removed by ultrafiltration during haemodialysis or by intensive two-hourly exchanges of 2 litres in peritoneal dialysis.

If pericardiocentesis is needed for cardiac tamponade, replacement of the effusion by three-quarters of its volume of air relieves pain and may prevent fluid re-accumulation.

Heart failure

Principal reasons for heart failure in dialysed patients are excessive fluid intake, inadequate ultrafiltration, increased cardiac output because of the AV fistula, anaemia, hypertension, and coronary artery disease. Early failure is often insidious with absent or few clincial signs but vascular congestion in chest radiographs is always present. Prevention is best achieved by an accurate assessment of 'dry' body weight and appropriate adjustment of fluid intake, and the amount of fluid to be removed by dialysis. Severe pulmonary oedema is treated with oxygen, diamorphine, and immediate haemofiltration-haemodialysis until symptoms and signs subside. It is usual to repeat dialysis within 24 hours, assess resolution of pulmonary congestion by chest radiographs, and reassess 'dry weight'. For chronic heart failure regular sequential haemofiltration-haemodialysis may correct fluid excess without hypotension. Reduction of excessive flow in an AV fistula is needed if this is an important factor contributing to heart failure.

Atherosclerosis and hyperlipidaemia

Half of the deaths of patients on RRT are due to cardiovascular complications (Table 5). Death rate due to myocardial ischaemia and infarction amongst patients aged 35–54 years is 20 times as high as in the general population of the same age and amongst those aged over 55 years it is 10 times as high. For cerebrovascular accident the rates are 50 times and 20 times for these age groups respectively.

The value of lipid lowering measures are not established; dietary management is suggested but drug therapy (e.g. clofibrate) is not usually prescribed. General dietary advice should consist of lowering fat to 35 per cent of energy intake with at least half provided as polyunsaturated fatty acids. Carbohydrates should pro-

vide 50 per cent of energy aiming for polysaccharides, high fibre foods, and avoiding sugars.

Nutrition

An important proportion of deaths are attributed to cachexia. Dialysis must be adequate to abolish nausea and anorexia so that the patient can eat a good diet. Energy intake should be 30–35 kcal/kg for haemodialysis patients who are not obese. If obese a lower energy intake should be given. Patients on CAPD obtain 400 kcal/day from the dialysis fluid and the energy content of food should be proportionately reduced. Haemodialysis patients should have 1.2 g protein/kg ideal body weight/day and peritoneal dialysis patients 1.5 g protein/day. Water-soluble vitamins are lost into

Table 5 Causes of death in patients on RRT as recorded by the EDTA Registry, showing percentages diagnosed in patients who died in 1984 in the United Kingdom and other countries according to age at start of treatment

Causes of death on renal replacement therapy		United Kingdom <65 years	United Kingdom >65 years	Other countries <65 years	Other countries >65 years
Cause of death uncertain/not determined/unknown		5.7	7.2	6.0	7.6
Cardiac:	Myocardial ischaemia and infarction	17.8	14.4	13.2	12.4
	Hyperkalaemia	1.4	0.9	2.7	1.3
	Haemorrhagic pericarditis	0.4	0	1.1	0.4
	Other causes of cardiac failure	5.5	5.4	7.6	9.7
	Cardiac arrest, cause unknown	9.2	1.8	10.3	10.0
	Hypertensive cardiac failure	1.6	1.8	3.5	2.1
	Hypokalaemia	0.2	0	0.3	0
	Fluid overload	1.2	0.9	2.3	1.1
Vascular:	Pulmonary embolus	1.2	0	1.2	1.0
	Cerebrovascular accident	6.5	7.2	10.7	12.2
	Haemorrhage from graft site	0.2	0	0.2	0.1
	Haemorrhage from vascular access or dialysis circuit	0	0	0.2	0.3
	Haemorrhage from ruptured vascular aneurysm	1.2	0.9	0.8	0.3
	Haemorrhage from surgery	0.4	0	0.2	0
	Other haemorrhage	0.7	0	0.7	0.2
Infection:	Pulmonary infection (bacterial)	4.6	9.9	2.8	3.3
	Pulmonary infection (viral)	1.2	0.9	0.4	0.5
	Pulmonary infection (fungal)	0.2	0	0.3	0.2
	Infections elsewhere	1.1	0.9	0.8	0.4
	Septicaemia	9.5	8.1	7.5	4.4
	Tuberculosis	0.2	0	0.6	0.4
	Generalized viral infection	0.7	0	0.4	0.1
	Peritonitis	4.1	3.6	1.4	1.9
Liver disease:	Viral hepatitis	0	0	1.3	0.3
	Drug toxicity	0	0	0.1	0.1
	Cirrhosis, not viral	0	0	1.0	0.5
	Cystic liver disease	0	0	0.1	0
	Liver failure, cause unknown	0	0	0.5	0.2
Gastrointestinal:	Gastrointestinal haemorrhage	1.1	3.6	2.1	1.7
	Mesenteric infarction	0.5	0	0.7	0.9
	Pancreatitis	1.2	0.9	0.9	0.1
	Sclerosing (or adhesive) peritoneal disease	1.1	0.9	0.4	0.2
	Perforation of peptic ulcer	0.4	2.7	0.2	0.2
	Perforation of colon	0.7	0	0.5	0.6
Social:	Patient refused further treatment	1.4	4.5	0.7	1.9
	Suicide	0.4	0	0.6	0.6
	Therapy ceased for any other reason	3.2	6.3	0.4	1.6
Miscellaneous:	Uraemia caused by graft failure	0.5	0	0.3	0
	Bone marrow depression	0	0	0.1	0.4
	Cachexia	1.9	4.5	3.6	9.9
	Malignant disease	5.7	8.1	5.5	5.8
	Dementia	0.7	0.9	1.1	1.9
Accident:	Accident related to treatment	0.4	0	0.3	0.3
	Accident unrelated to treatment	0.2	0	0.8	0.5
Other identified cause of death		6.0	3.6	3.7	3.0
Total patients with cause of death data available		566	111	5897	1986

dialysis fluid and must be replaced. These include folic acid and all other B group vitamins and vitamin C.

Renal osteodystrophy
Bone disorders associated with chronic renal failure and their treatment are described on page 18.156.

Neuropathy
The occurrence of severe peripheral neuritis during haemodialysis or peritoneal dialysis indicates either inadequate dialysis or a severely malnourished state. Adequate haemodialysis or peritoneal dialysis arrests or cures minor degrees of peripheral neuritis, but it is unusual for severe neuropathy to improve. Progressive neuropathy is an indication for renal transplantation, which reverses this disorder provided axonal degeneration has not occurred.

Endocrine
Of the numerous endocrine disturbances in uraemia only peripheral resistance to the action of insulin is reversed by dialysis. Impotence is present to some degree in 80 per cent of men and is complete in 55 per cent. Disturbed hypothalamic–pituitary–gonadal function with abnormalities of testosterone, FSH, LH, and prolactin, zinc deficiency, hyperparathyroidism, autonomic neuropathy, chronic ill-health, anxiety, and depression could each result in impotence but measures which correct these changes are not followed by improved potency. Amenorrhoea during end-stage renal failure is often followed by regular menstruation after several weeks dialysis, but it is unknown whether ovulation occurs regularly. The rare examples of pregnancy during dialysis which have progressed to term have resulted in small but otherwise normal infants.

Infection
Despite altered humoral, lymphocyte, and polymorphonuclear cell function in uraemia which continue during dialysis, the inflammatory reaction to bacterial infection and response to antimicrobial therapy are normal. In contrast, the incidence and nature of some viral infections are altered during dialysis treatment.

Hepatitis B (HBV) and hepatitis non-A, non-B (Section 5)
The principal infections affecting dialysis patients are hepatitis B (HVB) and hepatitis non-A, non-B. Hepatitis B infection and carrier state are recognized by the presence of hepatitis surface antigen (HBsAg), and previous HBV infections are detected by antibody to HBsAg (antiHBs). Hepatitis B infection runs a mild clinical course in some patients and in others HBsAg is present without symptoms. There is an increased incidence of persistent HBsAg antigenaemia; cross infection may arise in patients and staff, and death from acute hepatitis may result in both. HBsAg and liver function tests should be checked before entry into the dialysis programme and at regular intervals thereafter. Blood for transfusion must be negative for HBsAg. Cross infection precautions should be rigorous. Patients with hepatitis and carriers should be isolated and treated in a separate unit. Those at risk may be given passive and active immunization.

Hepatitis non-A, non-B is a mild clinical disorder to be considered in patients in whom a modest increase in AST is not explained by hepatitis B or A or by cardiac disease, toxic hepatitis, cytomegalovirus, or Epstein–Barr virus infection. Uncertainties in diagnosis and epidemiology will continue until a serological test detects this infection. Hepatitis non-A, non-B is transmitted by blood transfusion; cross infection occurs between haemodialysis patients, and chronic active hepatitis has been described. Patient to staff transmission has not been established with certainty. Precautions which control HBV infection are also important in the managament of this less infectious disease. Passive immunization with immune globulin has a protective effect. The incidence of hepatitis non-A, non-B will increase as a result of blood transfusions given to prevent transplant rejection.

Malignant diseases
The incidence of malignant diseases is about three times higher in uraemic patients on dialysis than in age–sex matched controls. Evidence from a study in six English renal units found that non-Hodgkin's lymphoma occurred more commonly in dialysed patients than in the general population. Some of the tumours are related to the cause of the renal disease, notably uroepithelial tumours in patients with analgesic nephropathy and renal carcinoma in patients with analgesic and Balkan nephropathy. Multiple renal adenocarcinoma also occur in the acquired cystic disease of end-stage kidneys. In this disorder, which presents as renal or perirenal haemorrhage, multiple renal cysts and tumours are found after several years of dialysis, and death from metastatic malignancy has occurred.

Renal transplantation

Selection
Present trends suggest that renal transplantation will be made available to almost all patients on dialysis programmes. Careful selection of recipients achieves the best results but at the cost of excluding high-risk patients from the potential improvement in quality of life which transplantation offers.

Long-term dialysis patients not infrequently confide that they are carrying on in the hope of a successful transplant and this is certainly a more pleasant choice for the physician than deliberate euthanasia (Fig. 5). Opportunities for transplantation are limited chiefly by the shortage of donor organs.

When a patient is placed on a waiting list for renal transplantation he joins a pool of patients from which the most suitable recipient can be selected when an organ becomes available. The chance of obtaining well-matched kidneys is better if the pool is large and the surgeons contributing to it are committed to a policy of organ sharing. The United Kingdom Transplant Service organizes the matching and distribution of grafts throughout the United Kingdom and Ireland. It has links with other major European transplant sharing organizations, Eurotransplant (serving the Netherlands, Belgium, Germany, and Austria), France transplant, and Scandia transplant. The EDTA Registry recorded 7724 grafts during 1984.

Patients on waiting lists are given priority if they are clinically urgent cases and in the absence of an exact match the graft is offered according to these clinical criteria. As an increasing proportion of cases have cytotoxic antibodies, plates of sera from these difficult cases are distributed to widely dispersed tissue typing laboratories so that cross-match tests may be performed as well as tissue typing.

High-risk patients include the elderly, diabetics, hypertensives, and those with multisystem diseases. Patients with bladder abnormalities, a history of peptic ulcer or malignancies have often been excluded from transplant programmes in the past but will probably come to be regarded along with other high-risk patients particularly if they express a strong personal risk to be transplanted despite the hazards. Primary renal disease and general health should be assessed carefully.

Renal disease
It is important that the primary renal disease is established before transplantation. In 80 per cent of patients the diagnosis is chronic glomerulonephritis, pyleonephritis, nephrosclerosis, or adult polycystic kidney disease, all associated with a straightforward transplant course. Rapid loss of function is unusual, and transplantation worthwhile in the less common disorders in which the original disease may recur in some 30–50 per cent of grafts (Table 6), but in this group it is exceptional to use a living related kidney for the first graft. After cadaver transplantation, loss of function or proteinuria may be due to rejection or recurrence of the original glomerulonephritis; biopsy and examination by light, immunofluorescence, and electron microscopy will determine. If

Table 6 Renal diseases which
recur in transplants

Glomerulonephritis:
    Mesangiocapillary:
        Dense deposits
        Subendothelial deposits
    Focal glomerulosclerosis
    IgA nephropathy
    Anti-GBM antibody
Oxalosis
Cystinosis
Amyloidosis
Diabetes

---

this graft is subsequently lost by rejection a second transplant from a related donor can be considered.

The diabetic patient presents difficult problems of vascular disease, blindness, and infection. In obstructive uropathy it is important to assess bladder and urethral function. Bladder neck resection or urethroplasty if needed are performed before transplantation. Bilateral nephrectomy is needed for frequent urinary infections despite relief of obstruction or associated with vesicoureteric reflux. Severe disorders of the lower urinary tract not amenable to surgical correction require an ileal conduit or caecal bladder. Collagen vascular diseases do not recur in grafts, and the results of transplantation are similar to those in other renal disease provided involvement of other systems does not prevent rehabilitation. Oxalosis frequently destroys grafts within a few months so that transplantation is seldom recommended in this disorder. For tumour in solitary kidneys or bilateral Wilm's tumour, patients remain on dialysis for one year following nephrectomy, irradiation or chemotherapy, with subsequent careful review for local recurrence or metastases before transplantation is considered.

Assessment of general health

A careful history and examination to seek potential sources of serious infection after immunosuppressive therapy is essential. Gall-bladder disease, localized diverticulitis, and other infective conditions amenable to surgery are treated before transplantation. A history of tuberculosis indicates the need for prophylactic antituberculous therapy for 6–9 months after transplantation. Generalized bronchiectasis is a contraindication to transplantation. Patients with heart failure, widespread vascular disease, or severe angina which cannot be corrected by coronary artery bypass surgery are more appropriately treated by dialysis. Renal osteodystrophy is treated before transplantation, but may be complicated by hypercalcaemia after surgery in some cases.

Peptic ulcer occurs frequently in uraemia. Haemorrhage or perforation following transplantation is associated with a mortality as high as 50 per cent, so that a barium examination or endoscopy should be performed before transplantation. Identified ulcers may be treated by vagotomy and pyloroplasty or by a course of cimetidine. Surgery is indicated for those ulcers which do not heal on medical treatment. Cimetidine or ranitidine may also be given as a prophylactic measure for three months following transplantation in patients with a history of recent peptic ulceration.

Hepatitis B

The hepatitis carrier state continues following transplantation and some patients with past infection become HBsAg positive after engraftment. There are two policies for HBsAg positive dialysis patients otherwise eligible for transplantation. In the first, all receive grafts with stringent precautions against the spread of infection to staff. In the second, all continue dialysis either at home or in an isolation hospital unit. For patients with non-A, non-B hepatitis precautions against cross infection prevents spread among patients and staff after transplantation.

Acquired immunodeficiency syndrome

The chief reason for transplanting patients with AIDS is to remove them from dialysis programmes. The natural history of AIDS limits the survival which can be achieved and does not appear to facilitate acceptance of the graft.

Psychological problems

Depression and anxiety are common during dialysis and generally resolve or improve following a successful graft. Before transplantation it is important to discuss with the patient and family the problems of immunosuppression, the possibility of losing the graft from rejection, the possible need to return to dialysis, and the good results which follow most second transplants.

Preparation for transplantation

Dialysis

If the graft is from a living relative there is ample time to prepare for surgery, but most cadaver transplants must take place at 24 hours notice or less. For those awaiting a cadaver graft, dialysis must maintain good health, normal levels of potassium and blood pressure, freedom from heart failure, and proper nutrition. Urea and creatinine concentrations are relatively unimportant. These conditions are more consistently achieved by CAPD, which can be continued in the early posttransplant period, without risk of haemorrhage from heparin if graft function is delayed. Preoperative dialysis must be necessary for those on haemodialysis who have not received treatment within the preceding 24 hours, in order to reduce potassium to about 4 mmol/l and adjust fluid balance to accommodate blood transfusion during surgery. It is important to avoid dehydration in case hypotension should occur during induction of anaesthesia, impair renal perfusion, and prevent diuresis in an otherwise well-functioning graft.

Patients treated by CAPD are generally better hydrated than those on haemodialysis who require several litres of saline at the time of surgery.

Blood transfusion

Blood transfusion before first cadaver transplants improves graft survival by about 20 per cent in the first year by a mechanism which is unknown. One hypothesis suggests induced 'tolerance' in the recipient's immune system, another invokes protective 'enhancing' antibodies, or there may be stimulation of recipient 'suppressor' lymphocytes which protect the graft. One unit of blood may give protection but 3–5 units are used commonly and more than 20 units are needed for maximum effect. It is likely that leucocytes rather than erythrocytes are responsible for the beneficial effect, but this is uncertain. Optimum timing of transfusion in relation to transplantation is also unknown; preoperative blood has been successful in some centres but not others, and in practice it is usual to give transfusions over 1–3 months after starting dialysis. Disadvantages of transfusion are the formation of cytotoxic antibodies against the HLA antigens which make subsequent transplantation difficult, and transmission of hepatitis B or hepatitis non-A, non-B. The incidence of cytotoxic antibodies is low after only 3–5 units and hepatitis B is not a problem when blood for transfusion comes from volunteers rather than commercial donors and precise methods are used for detection of HBsAg.

HLA antibody tests

Sera are examined regularly for cytotoxic antibodies against HLA antigens. Antibodies may appear briefly 2–4 weeks after blood transfusion and failed transplants as well as after pregnancy so that sera should be examined particularly at these times. Results are expressed in terms of per cent reactivity against a random panel of donor cells. Positive specimens should be stored but opinion is divided as to whether or not it is necessary to have a negative cross-match against the most strongly positive sera. Some centres are prepared to transplant if the reactivity percentage has fallen for 6 months and the most recent sample gives a negative cross-match. Exceptionally, plasmapheresis and cytotoxic therapy have been used to deplete the patient of antibodies so that grafting can be performed.

Nephrectomy, splenectomy, thymectomy
Bilateral nephrectomy, in preparation for transplantation, has decreased during the past decade from 40 per cent to about 5 per cent of patients, because a mortality as high as 10 per cent was reported in some series, and hypertension can be controlled without nephrectomy, by improved sodium and water homeostasis during dialysis and by potent hypotensive agents. In addition, bilateral nephrectomy always impairs health on dialysis; haematocrit falls to 15 per cent, and increased dialysis or dietary restriction is needed for fluid and sodium balance. Graft survival following nephrectomy is not improved but indications which remain are persistent urinary tract infection and renal calculi. Surgery should be performed through a loin or lumbar incision which leaves the peritoneal cavity intact for peritoneal dialysis, but on occasion an anterior approach through the peritoneal cavity is needed to remove a very large cystic kidney to make space for the transplant.

Splenectomy and thymectomy do not improve graft survival

Transplant histocompatibility
ABO compatibility is essential, but the main obstacle to successful kidney transplantation is an incompatibility between recipient and donor HLA antigens which elicits a response in the recipient's immune system resulting in graft rejection. This problem is overcome imperfectly by matching recipient and donor for histocompatibility antigens, and by non-specific immunosuppression using cyclosporin with or without prednisolone and azathioprine. Other factors are preformed antibodies against tissue antigens from previous transfusion, transplantation or pregnancy. A schema for the immune response involved in graft rejection is shown in Fig. 8.

Histocompatibility antigens
HLA (human leucocyte-locus A) antigens present on all nucleated cells are determined genetically by four alleles – HLA-A, B, C, and D – located on chromosome 6. HLA-A, B, C are detected on lymphocytes by serological methods. HLA-D, important as the antigen first recognized as foreign by the host's immune system,

can be determined by the mixed lymphocyte reaction but this requires several days and is not available for prospective cadaver kidney matching. A new group of antigens DR (D-related) can be detected by serological methods on B lymphocytes. They are believed to be either closely related to HLA-D, or identical, so that prospective matching for D locus antigens is now possible.

Each individual inherits one chromosome 6 from each parent providing two HLA antigens for each HLA locus. Among siblings 25 per cent inherit the same HLA haplotypes (HLA identical), 50 per cent share one haplotype, and 25 per cent have no common antigens unless parents share an antigen. One haplotype difference is to be expected between parents and children. Matching of individual antigens for unrelated cadaver grafting is made difficult by the presence of more than 40 HLA-A, B, and D antigens. To some extent the problem is simplified by a higher frequency of and linking together of some antigens, but the chances of finding a perfectly matched cadaver donor for any recipient vary from one in a hundred to one in several thousand depending on antigen frequency. The problem is less if the aim is matching of the nine antigens recognized by DR typing.

Effect of HLA matching
The importance of HLA matching for A and B antigens is demonstrated by graft survival at one year in sibling–sibling and parent–sibling donor–recipient pairs; for HLA identical siblings graft survival at one year is 95 per cent, for one haplotype disparity 90–95 per cent, and for complete HLA mismatches 75–85 per cent, which is similar to cadaver graft survival. It has been more difficult to establish a definite effect of HLA-A and B matching on cadaver graft survival, but latest data from large Registries all appear to point to the benefit of a 'full house' match (all 6 HLA-A, B, and D antigens) and of a single mismatch. The better results accruing from such good compatibility also appear to be demonstrable in transfused patients and when cyclosporin is used. To obtain a 60 per cent chance of such good matches requires a recipient pool of around 3000. Several factors other than histocompatibility and blood transfusion affect cadaver graft survival. One year first cadaver graft survival varies from 40 to 65 per cent in different centres. HLA-A and HLA-B matching improves results among men with non-O blood groups. Survival is better in children and adolescents than in adults, and may improve with length of time on dialysis.

Cross-match tests between donor lymphocytes and recipient sera detect cytotoxic antibodies to HLA antigens from previous blood transfusion, failed grafts or pregnancy which may result in immediate 'hyperacute' rejection. Potential graft recipients are examined for lymphocytoxins using the most recent and past serum containing cytoxic antibodies. For positive cross-matches it is important to determine whether recipient antibodies are directed against donor T and B lymphocytes; those against T cells result in hyperacute rejection, but antibodies restricted to B cells do not have harmful effects so that grafts can be successful despite a positive B cell cross-match.

Donor kidneys
Live related donors
Well-matched kidneys from siblings, parents, or children account for 30 per cent of transplants in centres with a policy of active recruitment of family donors. Advantages of live related grafts are superior matching, optimal preparation of the recipient, likely immediate graft function, and a planned operation under ideal conditions. Donor age varies from 18 to the sixth decade, but some units allow an identical twin below the age of consent to give a kidney.

All living donors undergo a meticulous examination which includes assessment of motivation, confirmation of normal general health and renal function determined preferably by a physician responsible for the donors interests, and not a member of the transplant team. Investigations include careful urinalysis, measure-

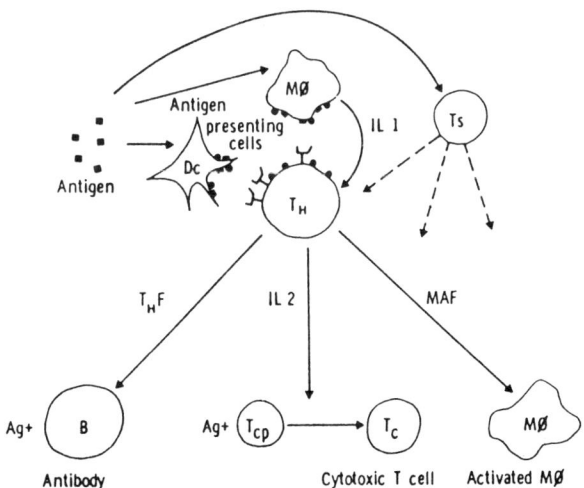

Fig. 8 A simplified version of the immune response to an antigen. Antigen is presented to the helper T cell (T_H) by the antigen presenting cells (APC) of the host, either macrophages (MØ) or dendritic cells (DG). The APC of the host must share the same Class II antigens with the T_H for the antigen to be recognized (MHC restriction). Once triggered the T_H produces a number of lymphokines, such as factors (T_HF) which makes B cells produce antibody, L-2, which is necessary for the maturation of the cytotoxic T cell precursor (T_{CP}) to the mature cytotoxic T cell (T_c) and the MAF which arms macrophages (MØ). Furthermore suppressor T cells (T_s) may be activated which can damp down this response at several levels. (Reproduced from Morris, 1985, *Kidney transplantation, principles and practice.* Grune and Stratton, London, with permission.)

ment of GFR, IVU, and renal anteriogram (or digital subtraction angiogram, DSA) as well as a search for hepatitis B antigen and antibody. Absolute contraindications to kidney donation are renal disease, multiple small renal arteries, coronary or cerebrovascular disease, hypertension, marked obesity, or any significant medical disorder. Complications from nephrectomy occur in 20–40 per cent of kidney donors depending on criteria used; deaths have occurred and a conclusion that nephrectomy has not been harmful cannot be made with certainty until the donor's death from causes unrelated to loss of one kidney has been confirmed. Following nephrectomy the remaining kidney hypertrophies, so that after several weeks glomerular filtration rate is more than 70 per cent of normal. For insurance and employment purposes kidney donors are accepted as normal risks. There is some evidence that donors have an increased chance of becoming hypertensive but no excess long-term mortality.

Cadaver donors and brain death

Cadaver kidneys come from donors supported by respirators, in whom brain death has occurred. Brain death has been defined in the United Kingdom by the Medical Royal Colleges and their Faculties (1976) as followsq:

1. *Conditions for considering brain deaths*
   (a) *Deep coma.* Exclude: (i) all depressant drugs and secondary hypothermia; (ii) primary hypothermia; (iii) metabolic or endocrine cause – establish near normal blood glucose, serum electrolytes, and acid–base status.
   (b) *Ventilatory support for absent respiration.* Exclude muscle relaxants and other drugs with neuromuscular blocking action.
   (c) *Establish, unequivocally, the primary disorder which has caused brain death.*
2. *Test of brain death*

All brain-stem reflexes are absent: (i) fixed dilated pupils; (ii) absent corneal reflexes; (iii) absent vestibulo-ocular reflexes; (iv) absent cranial nerve motor response to any painful stimulus; (v) no gag reflex; and (vi) no spontaneous respiratory movements after discontinuing ventilation with P_2CO_2 above the respiratory threshold of 6.7 kPa (50 mmHg).

3. *Other considerations*

It is usual for two senior doctors who are not members of the transplant team to test for brain death independently at 12–24 hour intervals, but there are conditions, such as massive cerebral haemorrhage or trauma, for which one examination is adequate. Kidneys for cadaver transplantation come largely from patients with cerebral trauma or haemorrhage, histologically proven primary brain tumour, or after cardiac or respiratory arrest in the age group 3–65 years. Kidneys are unacceptable in the presence of renal disease, systemic infection, severe hypertension, non-cerebral tumours, or if there is acute renal failure unresponsive to correction of hypovolaemia, hypotension, or treatment with diuretics. Measures which maintain blood pressure and organ perfusion in the unconscious patient – intravenous fluids, vasopressor agents, mannitol, and frusemide – are continued after brain death to maintain a urine volume of about 50 ml/h. Immediately before donor nephrectomy, renal tubular cell membranes are stabilized and coagulation and vasospasm reduced respectively by treatment with methylprednisolone 1 g, heparin 10 000 units, and phentolamine 50 mg. It has recently been suggested that calcium-blocking agents reduce the incidence of oliguria following grafting and administration of cyclosporin. All donors should be tested for hepatitis B antigen, cytomegalovirus status, and for HTLV-3/LAV.

Kidney preservation

The aims of kidney preservation are two-fold. First, to maintain viability of the kidney between removal and reimplantation. Second, to allow time for tissue typing, matching, transport of kidneys between national and international centres, preparation of

the recipient, and to permit the transplant operation to become a semi-elective procedure. Of paramount importance is the period of warm ischaemia timed from cardiac arrest or clamping of the renal artery until the kidney is uniformly cooled to 5 °C. The effect of warm ischaemia is such that 30 min is associated with brief, reversible loss of function, 30–60 min with severe loss of function which recovers over 1–2 weeks, and 60–120 min with severe, permanent functional impairment or death of the kidney. Preservation employs either short perfusion with cold, hypertonic electrolyte solutions and subsequent storage in sterile, saline ice slush, or complex and expensive apparatus which constantly perfuses the kidney with cooled albumin or plasma. Both methods allow cold storage (cold ischaemia time) for over 24 hours for kidneys which are usually removed with a zero warm ischaemia time (i.e. kidney removed while donor's heart is still beating or has just stopped) or at most 30 min of warm ischaemia. Machine preservation has now been abandoned, its extra complexity having been shown not to improve results over long-term storage on ice using special perfusing solutions (Marshall's or EuroCollins). Immediate graft function is expected in over 60 per cent of kidneys used within 36 hours, but this percentage drops if cold ischaemia is more prolonged. Kidneys have been used successfully up to 96 hours after removal. If acute tubular necrosis develops it is likely to be prolonged if cyclosporin has been used as the immunosuppresive.

Transplant operation

Meticulous attention to detail is essential for successful surgery in the uraemic, immune-incompetent state which reduces limits of safety. Features for special consideration are strict asepsis, careful haemostasis, ligation of lymphatics, and consideration of poor wound healing. Kidney grafts are placed in a retroperitoneal site in either iliac fossa adjacent to large peripheral vessels and the bladder. The graft is easily accessible for palpation and biopsy, and the peritoneal cavity remains intact should peritoneal dialysis be needed. A variety of techniques are employed in the anastomosis of normal, small, single, multiple or moderately atheromatous graft arteries to host common, external or internal iliac arteries. The graft vein is anastomosed to the common or external iliac vein (Fig. 9). The graft ureter is implanted in the bladder using a mucosal tunnel which prevents reflux, but if the graft ureter is short or has impaired blood supply the anastomosis is to host ureter or renal pelvis. Within both iliac fossae there are sites for four transplants, two on each side, a provision which is more than sufficient

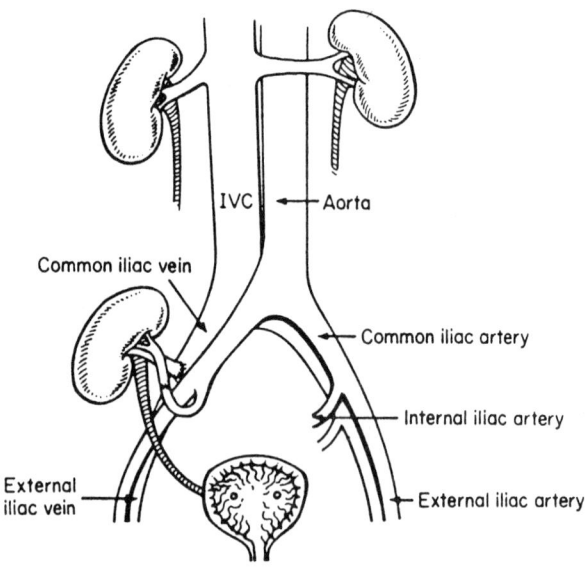

Fig. 9 Renal transplant in the right iliac fossa. (Reproduced from Wing and McGowan, 1975, *The renal unit*, MacMillan, with permission.)

for most chronic renal failure patients when well-matched, viable grafts are implanted by experienced surgeons. Immunosuppression with cyclosporin and prednisolone begins with intravenous administration at the time of transplantation or even prior to transplantation if time allows as in elective live donor grafting.

A perioperative wide-spectrum bactericidal antimicrobial reduces the incidence of wound and urinary tract infection, and treats organisms which may have gained access to the graft during the agonal period, graft harvesting, or preservation.

Management after transplantation

After nearly all living donor and 60 per cent of cadaver transplants there is immediate graft function. In the remainder, renal function is restored over 1–3 weeks as tubular necrosis recovers. GFR increases to 30–40 ml/min and may exceed 50 ml/min due to compensatory hypertrophy. Thus, most transplants rapidly reverse uraemia, the most gratifying change being an increase in haematocrit with resolution of anaemic symptoms. After kidney transplantation good management requires careful measurement of graft function to detect rejection or urological complications and surveillance for infections and other problems associated with immunosuppression. The uncomplicated patient is discharged to outpatient care after two weeks, initially to three outpatient visits each week, weekly after three months, and monthly after one year. All complaints, even 'minor illness', must receive careful attention so that rejection, potentially serious infections, and other conditions associated with kidney transplantation have appropriate investigation and treatment. For these reasons transplant recipients remain under the care of the transplant units for minor as well as major illness.

Evaluation of graft function

The superficial position of the graft in the iliac fossa permits clinical evaluation of size and turgor. Bruits from either normal intrarenal blood flow or graft artery stenosis are easily detected. A decline in urine volume may be the first sign of hypovolaemia, rejection, or a urological problem such as obstruction or urine leak. Examination of urine is essential for the detection of infection. An increase in proteinuria indicates rejection, venous obstruction or recurrent glomerulonephritis. Absence of proteinuria in a failing graft suggests obstruction. The electrolyte content of graft urine is determined by several factors and seldom provides information of diagnostic value. Measurement of plasma creatinine is the crucial test of graft function; a rise of 20–30 μmol/l or the absence of decline in creatinine at a time when graft function should improve indicates the need for further investigation. Noninvasive tests are preferred in the immunosuppressed patient because of the risk of infection. Ultrasonography demonstrates obstruction to the ureter, collections of lymph which may obstruct the ureter or iliac vein, urine leaks, or an abscess. Isotope renography assesses graft blood flow, tubular function, and obstruction. An IVU in a well-functioning graft gives more precise detail of obstruction or urine extravasation. Angiography is needed for evaluation of the vascular anastomosis. Percutaneous biopsy of the single functioning kidney graft is a safe procedure in experienced hands. Indications for biopsy are to distinguish tubular necrosis from rejection as the cause of poor graft function by the third post-transplant week, the investigation of loss of graft function not due to obstruction or urine leaks or the failure of antirejection therapy to improve graft function, or to distinguish chronic rejection from recurrent disease. Unfortunately, renal biopsy does not reliably distinguish rejection from cyclosporin nephrotoxicity in all cases. Some centres have used repeated fine needle aspiration biopsy to follow the cellular infiltrate in the graft.

Immunosuppression

Immunosuppression modifies or suppresses the immune response which would otherwise result in loss of grafts by rejection. Therapy is life-long and even brief discontinuation has been associated with prompt loss of the graft. The principal defect of current immunosuppression is its non-specific effects which also depress immune responses against bacteria, viruses, fungi, and even malignant cells.

Recent years have seen the almost universal adoption of cyclosporin as chief immunosuppressive agent. Improved graft survivals are widely reported following the acquisition of skills in handling the drug which occurred in most centres in 1982 (Fig. 10). The major disadvantage of cyclosporin is its nephrotoxicity and most centres use it in combination with prednisolone in low dosage. A major contribution to graft survival comes about from reducing the incidence of death with a functioning transplant frequently due to excessive immunosuppression. Because of this, lower doses of prednisolone were becoming popular before cyclosporin became available and this change in practice must share the credit for improved results during the last few years.

Cyclosporin inhibits the proliferative response of lymphocytes and there is growing evidence that this activity is directed predominantly against the T helper lymphocytes, preventing the production of lymphokines, especially IL–2, and so arresting the generation of cytotoxic T cells (Fig. 8). It appears to exert its effects at an early stage after exposure of the recipient to a tissue allograft. Most centres give between 15 and 11 mg/kg/day during the first week and by the one year point reduce this to 4 to 8 mg/kg/day. Many centres use blood levels to help determine dosage although there are technical problems in the measurement and the evidence that management is improved is weak. Side-effects are common, the most critical being nephrotoxicity, but abnormalities of liver function, gingival hyperplasia, hirsutism, and a variety of neurological complaints may all dictate a reduction in dosage. Nevertheless, despite its narrow therapeutic range, cyclosporin has proved a real advance in transplantation and it must be recommended over conventional immunosuppressives although it has a high cost. It is hoped that it may prove to be the forerunner of a new group of immunosuppressive drugs.

Azathioprine retards rejection by inhibiting recognition of foreign material and the primary antibody response by immunologically competent lymphoid cells. This agent does not have an effect on either established rejection or existing delayed hypersensitivity. The maintenance dose of azathioprine is 1–3 mg/kg/day which does not need modification in moderate renal impairment. An excess of azathioprine results in leucopenia, hepatitis, and alopecia. The dose should be reduced in the presence of leucopenia, severe infection, and in patients taking allopurinol. Splenectomy has been used when persistent leucopenia prevents the use of adequate doses of azathioprine. Cyclophosphamide replaces azathioprine if hepatocellular damage occurs with doses essential for immunosuppression or in those patients in whom idiosyncratic reactions to azathioprine develop.

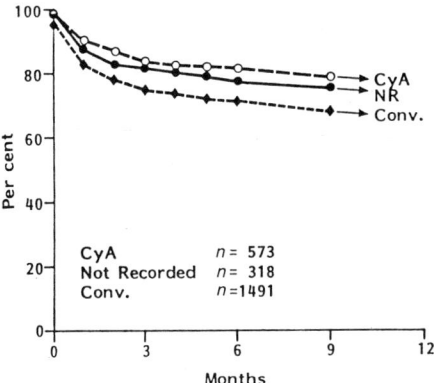

Fig. 10 Graft survival in first cadaver grafts in 1983, recipients aged 15 to 45 years, diabetics excluded. CyA, cyclosporin; NR, immunosuppression not recorded; Conv, conventional (azathioprine plus prednisolone). (Reproduced from Kramer *et al.*, 1984, *Proceedings EDTA*, with permission.)

Prednisolone reverses rejection by reducing the numbers of circulating T and B lymphocytes and by inhibition of cellular immunity. Thus, prednisolone and azathioprine together depress both cellular and humoral immunity and prednisolone has an additional anti-inflammatory effect on the rejection process. Prednisolone has been given regularly in doses of 0.5–1.5 mg/kg/day, but recent experience indicates that a maintenance dose of 20 mg/day for the first 60 days is associated with less infection, particularly overwhelming sepsis, prevents osteonecrosis, and a marked reduction in all side-effects. After 60 days the dose is gradually reduced to reach a maintenance level of 10 mg/day at six months and thereafter. Alternate day steroids are sometimes used, particularly in children in whom this method for giving steroids results in less growth retardation. For acute rejection intravenous methylprednisolone is given in 250–1000 mg doses over 15 min at intervals of 12–24 hours for 3–5 days. Alternatively, oral prednisolone 200 mg daily for three days is reduced to maintenance therapy over five days. Continuing or repeated episodes of acute rejection are usually resistant to steroids and treatment should not ordinarily exceed two or, at most three, courses during the six months following transplantation.

Other immunosuppressive agents under investigation as treatments for rejection include cyclosporin A, total lymphoid irradiation, and antilymphocyte and antithymocyte globulin. All these have potent immunosuppressive activity in the short term and there has recently been some interest in using them as therapy adjuvant to maintenance immunosuppression and even in the form of a protocol of triple or quadruple therapy. Early reports suggest that little advantage can be demonstrated and that the risks of infections and malignancy are increased.

Rejection

The histology of rejection has been extensively studied in graft biopsies. In *acute* rejection the changes are predominantly vascular with intravascular thrombosis, endothelial swelling and proliferation, fibrinoid necrosis, areas of tubular necrosis, and a focal interstitial infiltrate of mononuclear cells. In *chronic* rejection the vascular changes have progressed to extensive intimal fibrosis with obliteration of vessel lumen, glomerular fibrosis, and ischaemia, extensive interstitial fibrosis, and glomerular and mesangial changes which resemble mesangiocapillary glomerulonephritis ('transplant glomerulopathy'). *Hyperacute rejection* is defined as rejection occurring either during or within 48 hours of grafting. The graft is lost from intravascular thrombosis initiated by preformed cytoxic antibodies which were not detected by crossmatch test. *Acute rejection* is expected 1–12 weeks after all cadaver transplants. Early diagnosis and treatment of acute rejection is essential to arrest decline in graft function and prevent irreversible damage. In the absence of specific tests for rejection, diagnosis depends on swelling and pain in the graft, decreased urine volume, fever, and impaired graft function measured by an increase in plasma creatinine. Hypovolaemia, obstruction, urine leaks, graft infection, or a complication of the vascular anastomosis should be excluded. Acute rejection is confirmed by prompt resolution of symptoms and signs and improved graft function following either methylprednisolone or increased oral prednisolone therapy. Graft biopsy is performed if there is an incomplete or absent response; the presence of cellular infiltration suggests that further increased corticosteroid treatment may help, but extensive intimal proliferation indicates that steroids will be ineffective and that the graft should be abandoned.

Chronic rejection is considered when there is slow decline in graft function more than three months after the transplantation. It is important to confirm this diagnosis by biopsy which also excludes recurrence of the original kidney disease. Steroids do not have any beneficial effect on chronic rejection. Chronically rejecting patients are placed on the transplant waiting list and prepared for dialysis which is resumed before creatinine clearance is 5 ml/min.

Complications and management
Technical complications
Technical complications following transplantation may be vascular or urological. In experienced transplant centres such complications occur in less than 5 per cent of graft operations. These disorders must be differentiated from acute rejection. Many technical problems arise from difficulties and errors during donor nephrectomy such as severed multiple renal arteries, intimal tears from forceful traction, or interruption of the ureter's blood supply by close dissection of the renal pelvis and ureter. *Arterial complications*, thrombosis, and haemorrhage, are uncommon and result in loss of the graft. Graft artery stenosis is a late complication which results in hypertension, graft bruit, and loss of function if arterial narrowing is severe. The stenosis is demonstrated by angiography, which also indicates whether the lesion is amenable to surgical or transluminal angioplastic repair. *Venous* obstruction is a rare complication secondary to thrombosis from legs of iliac veins, diagnosed by arteriography or venography and treated with long-term anticoagulation. Severed *lymphatics* result in an accumulation of lymph (lymphocele) which may obstruct ureter and iliac veins, the former presenting as a cause of reduced urine volume and function, the latter in proteinuria and a swollen leg which simulates leg vein thrombosis. Lymphoceles are detected by rectal examination and demonstrated by ultrasonography. Conservative management is safest but if surgery is necessary, aspiration may be effective, and for recurrent lymphoceles it is necessary to create a wide surgical fistula which allows lymph to drain into the peritoneal cavity where it is absorbed. *Urological complications* include bladder *leaks* from cystotomy during implantation of the ureter, from a ureteric anastomosis created under tension, or from necrosis of an ischaemic ureter. Extravasated urine is easily differentiated from lymph or a serous discharge by finding elevated creatinine concentrations compared to plasma. Surgical repair is essential for all major leaks if infection and the loss of the graft are to be avoided. Small leaks may be treated conservatively but several weeks of bladder or wound drainage are needed. *Obstruction* of the ureter results from clots in the lumen, mechanical obstruction at the bladder anastomosis, or is a late consequence of ischaemia to the lower ureter. Treatment is surgical repair. For repairs of some leaks and obstructions the recipient's ureter is anastomosed to the graft ureter or renal pelvis. Repeated urological manoeuvres are associated with a very bad prognosis.

Infection
Minor infections are frequent in the early months following transplantation and serious infection is the principal cause of death (Table 5) in transplant recipients. Several factors contribute to susceptibility to infection; immunosuppression is the main one, but surgery involving the bladder, azotaemia, anaemia, coagulation defects, leucopenia, and hyperglycaemia may all play a part. Infections occur most frequently in the urinary tract, wound, lungs, blood, and skin. Corticosteroids may suppress clinical manifestations of infection so that peritonitis presents as slight abdominal pain with distension, and meningitis as headache with altered cerebration and minor or absent neck rigidity. Bacterial infections predominate with relatively more Gram-negative than Gram-positive organisms compared to the general population. Other infections to be considered are viruses (cytomegalovirus, herpes simplex, varicella-zoster, hepatitis B, influenza, adrenoviruses, and Epstein–Barr virus), fungi (*Aspergillus fumigatus, Candida albicans*) and protozoa (*Pneumocystis carinii*). Infections may arise from opportunistic organisms of the normal body flora and there may be mixed organisms. Infections are sometimes related to the treatment of rejection, but rejection can also be provoked by infection.

Careful measures have resulted in a significant reduction in mortality and morbidity from sepsis. Prevention has been described in sections concerned with patient selection, preparation, intraoperative antimicrobials, surgical techniques, low-dose maintenance steroids, and the limitation of courses of steroids for acute rejection. Principles for managing infection in graft recipients are similar to those for other individuals, but in diagnosis a particular vigilance should be kept for atypical organisms, tuberculosis, viruses, fungi, and protozoa. Investigations associated with some risk are justified in the transplant patient, such as tracheal aspiration, transbronchial drill lung biopsy, aspiration, or surgical exploration of inflamed tissues. Antimicrobial therapy should be bactericidal, determined when possible by sensitivity tests, and limited to the short effective courses which avoid emergence of resistant strains and infections due to opportunistic organisms. On occasion there may be doubt whether there is bacterial infection with negative cultures or virus disease in which diagnosis is delayed for lack of serological evidence. Differentiation is seldom difficult, but in suspected severe bacterial infection it is sometimes necessary to give wide-spectrum antibiotics by the parenteral route. An expectant policy is proper for most viral infections, among which cytomegalovirus is the most common.

Acyclovir is indicated intravenously (a reduced dose of 5 mg/kg/day is suitable if creatinine clearance is below 50 ml/min) for severe herpes simplex infections of the mouth and anus. Herpes zoster infections require a higher dose and response is equivocal. Cytomegalovirus infections can lead to agranulocytosis and further dire consequences and should be treated with hyperimmune globulin and, possibly, one of the new antiviral agents. In the face of severe viral infection it may be necsessary to stop immunosuppression and even to abandon the graft.

Other complications
The incidence of *hypertension* after transplantation varies from 20 to 80 per cent depending on the criteria for diagnosis and the interval after engraftment. Several mechanisms have been suggested including volume expansion, steroids and cyclosporin, acute and chronic rejection, graft artery stenosis, a hypertensive effect from the patient's own kidneys, or combinations of these factors. Renal artery stenosis is suggested by a rapid onset of severe hypertension and the presence of a loud bruit over the graft, the diagnosis being confirmed by angiography and restoration of normal blood pressure after surgical correction. Benefit from surgical repair is incomplete or absent if there is renal impairment from chronic rejection or recurrent renal disease, and drug therapy alone is used in these circumstances. Hypertension caused by the patient's diseased kidneys may be suggested by elevated renin activity in renal venous blood. Removal of the patient's own kidneys by surgery or therapeutic embolization gives the best results in patients with normal graft function, but if the graft fails the problems of dialysis in the anephric stage must be anticipated. Drug therapy is usually effective in hypertension associated with transplantation regardless of the aetiology of raised arterial pressure, but may be difficult in some with renal artery stenosis.

Administration of ACE inhibitors is potentially hazardous in the presence of graft arterial stenosis. They should be introduced cautiously under close observation. Abrupt cessation of urine flow proves that important arterial stenosis is present within the renal artery itself or at a microscopic level; fortunately, it appears to be reversible but a rapid rise in plasma potassium may occur.

Atherosclerosis affecting cerebral and coronary artery vessels has become a major cause of death in transplant recipients (Table 5). Factors responsible for atherosclerosis in chronic renal failure and during dialysis treatment may persist after transplantation; hypertension is the main factor with less well-defined roles for hyperlipidaemia and glucose intolerance. Ectopic calcification may also contribute to vascular injury. Pretransplant hypertriglyceridaemia and decreased high-density lipoprotein cholesterol persists in some patients after transplantation, and steroids may induce hypercholesterolaemia. In the majority of patients who achieve prolonged normal graft function plasma triglyceride and cholesterol become normal, but abnormalities may persist in older

patients, in the obese, and in those with glucose intolerance. Patients maintained on low dose or alternate day steroids who have well-tolerated grafts and normal renal function are least likely to show lipid abnormalities.

There is an increased incidence of *upper gastrointestinal ulceration and haemorrhage*, which is reduced by steroids in low dosage. Endoscopy provides exact diagnosis and assesses response to therapy. *Ischaemic necrosis* is a hazardous disorder affecting the large or small bowel, or there are multiple lesions throughout the gastrointestinal tract. Presenting symptoms are watery diarrhoea, mild abdominal pain, and distension. The diagnosis is confirmed by the finding of haemorrhagic ulcerated mucosa at sigmoidoscopy or colonoscopy. Resection of affected bowel is essential for survival but it is often difficult to determine the extent of the disease and repeat laparotomy may be needed if resection is not followed promptly by return of bowel activity. Pseudomembranous colitis must be differentiated from ischaemic colitis by the characteristic mucosal lesions and the presence of *Clostridium difficile* toxin in faeces. *Diverticular disease* is frequent among older transplant patients, particularly those with polycystic kidney disease; early treatment with antibiotics is needed to prevent septicaemia, abscess or perforation, and surgical treatment is occasionally necessary.

Acute pancreatitis is a particularly dread abdominal complication.

Renal osteodystrophy Successful renal transplantation reverses those abnormalities which cause secondary hyperparathyroidism and osteomalacia during chronic renal failure and dialysis treatment, but corticosteroid treatment tends to cause *osteoporosis* and *osteonecrosis* in a dose-related manner. Osteonecrosis is the most troublesome bone disorder following transplantation affecting weight-bearing joints, hips, knees, and shoulders. Although the exact cause is unknown, steroid-induced osteoporosis is an important factor; low-dose treatment is associated with a decrease in femoral head necrosis from 15 to 2 per cent. Hyperparathyroidism may result in hypercalcaemia for several months after transplantation until hyperplastic parathyroid glands involute during the first post-transplant year. Subtotal parathyroidectomy is required for prolonged severe hypercalcaemia which impairs graft function and for autonomous hyperparathyroidism. Hypophosphataemia from graft tubular phosphate leak may cause osteomalacia, and in this circumstance phosphate supplements are needed.

Malignancy is a late complication of transplantation, occurring approximately 100 times more frequently than expected in an age-matched population, probably the result of immunosuppression. Cancer discovered during the first transplant year suggests pre-existing malignancy or tumour transmitted with the graft. The most frequent malignancies are those of facial skin, lymphoma, reticulum cell sarcoma of the meninges, uterine cervix, uterus, bladder, kidney, breast, and colon. Localized tumours are treated by excision and irradiation. Growth of the primary tumour or of metastases may decline after stopping immunosuppression, although the graft is likely to be lost from rejection.

Combined treatment by dialysis and transplantation

Forecasts indicate that growth in the size of the patient population is not likely to level out until around 450 patients are on treatment per million population.

Patient survival on integrated programmes of dialysis and transplantation have shown some improvement in recent years, but are dependent on the age of the patients at the start of treatment (Fig. 11). The results represent a notable achievement of a generation of specialized nephrologists who have pioneered these treatments during the 25 years since the arteriovenous fistula was first described and during 20 years of clinical renal transplantation.

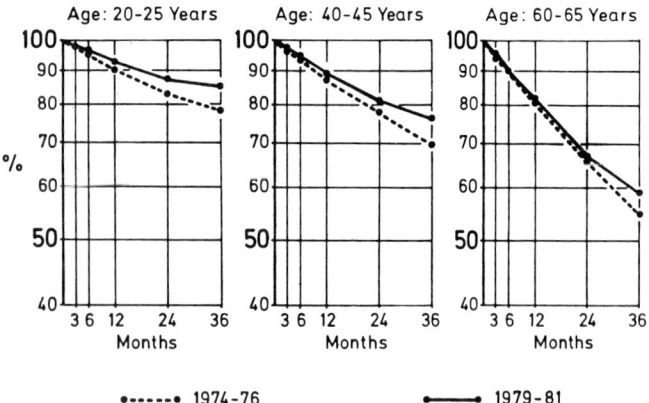

Fig. 11 Overall survival on RRT, 1974 to 1976 and 1979 to 1981. Numbers of patients for 1974 to 1976 and 1979 to 1981 were: aged 20 to 25 years, 1792 and 2217, respectively; aged 40 to 45 years, 3323 and 4316; aged 60 to 65 years, 2050 and 3799. (Reproduced from Kramer *et al.*, 1982, *Proceedings EDTA*, with permission.)

Preventive measures include the elimination of analgesic nephropathy and identification of other nephrotoxic agents and the removal of chronic antigenic stimulation by malaria and schistosomiasis in those parts of the world where these infections are endemic.

There are many alternative dialysis techniques from which to choose. Development has often been motivated by commercial opportunity. It is hoped that more attention may be given to developing less expensive methods of blood purification. The possibility of using the gut as a dialysing surface in conjunction with ingested sorbent granules remains a long-term hope.

Transplantation offers the best quality of life to the patient with ESRF. The supply of donor organs does not keep pace with the swelling waiting lists. Blood transfusion and cyclosporin have improved results and lower steroid requirements bring the ben-

efits of transplantation within the reach of many patients for whom its risks were previously thought too high. It seems likely that the care of chronic renal failure and ESRF will provide a continuing and large workload for hospital medicine for years to come.

References

Bell, P. R. F. and Calman, K. C. (1974). *Surgical aspects of haemodialysis*. Churchill Livingstone, Edinburgh.

Challah, S. and Wing, A. J. (1985). The epidemiology of genito-urinary disease. In *Oxford textbook of public health* (eds W. H. Holland, R. Detals and G. Knox), pp. 181–202. Oxford University Press, Oxford.

Conference of Medical Royal Colleges and their faculties in the UK (1979). *Br. med. J.* **1**, 322.

Drukker, W., Parsons, F. M, and Maher, J. F. (1983). *Replacement of renal function by dialysis* 2nd edn. Martinus Nijhoff, The Hague.

European Dialysis and Transplant Association (1971–85). *Combined report on dialysis and transplantation*, I–XV, Proceedings EDTA, 1971–1985, Vols 7–22.

Friedman, E. A. (1978) *Perspectives in nephrology and hypertension; strategy in renal failure*. John Wiley, New York.

Hamburger, J., Crosnier, J., Durmont, J. and Bach, J.-F. (1981). *Renal transplantation, theory and practice* 2nd edn. Williams and Wilkins, Baltimore.

Klahr, S. and Massry, S. G. (1981). *Contemporary nephrology*. Plenum Publishing, New York.

Legrain, M. (1980). *Continuous ambulatory peritoneal dialysis: Proceedings of an International Symposium*, Paris, 1979. Excerpta Medica, Amsterdam.

Marsh, F. P. (1985). *Postgraduate nephrology*. Heinemann, London.

Massry, S. G. and Sellers, A. L. (1976). *Clinical aspects of uraemia and dialysis*. Thomas, Springfield Ill.

Moncrief, J. W. and Popovitch, R. P. (1981). CAPD *update: continuous ambulatory peritoneal dialysis*. Masson, New York.

Morris, P. J. (1985). *Kidney transplantation, principles and practice* 2nd edn. Grune Straton, London.

Nolph, K. D. (1985) *Peritoneal dialysis* 2nd edn. Martinus Nijhoff, The Hague.

Terasaki, P. I. (1985). *Clinical kidney transplants*. ULCA Tissue typing Laboratory, California 90024.

RENAL BONE DISEASE

J. A. KANIS

Introduction

In the disorders affecting survivors with chronic renal disease, much attention has been directed to the disturbances in mineral metabolism which give rise to skeletal disease, since a high proportion of patients develop bone disease which is not favourably altered by dialysis treatment. Advances in the past few years have led to an understanding of some of the mechanisms by which renal bone disease arises, with the result that, despite their complexity, the objectives of treatment and the way in which these objectives might be realized have become more accurately defined.

Features of renal bone disease

The skeletal disorders found in chronic renal failure (Table 1) are collectively termed renal osteodystrophy, and may occur singly or in various combinations. None of these disorders is unique to renal failure nor to particular populations of patients, such as those managed conservatively, those on haemodialysis or indeed transplanted patients. But there are differences in the incidence of the various abnormalities, not only within these populations but also between various renal units. The variable prevalence of bone disease reflects in part the use of differing histological and radio-

graphic criteria for diagnosis, but other important factors include age, the nature, and duration of renal disease, and the treatment given.

By the time patients with progressive chronic renal failure are about to start dialysis treatment, the majority have histological abnormalities of bone but skeletal symptoms are found in a minority (less than 10 per cent). However, the biochemical disturbances which give rise to bone disease commonly give rise to extraskeletal manifestations in addition (Table 1).

Bone turnover

Bone is continually remodelled by synthesis of bone matrix (osteoid formation), mineralization of this osteoid matrix, and its subsequent resorption. These processes are governed by the activity of bone cells, which include osteoblasts (the bone forming cells), osteoclasts (the bone resorbing cells), and osteocytes, which are probably osteoblasts buried in bone matrix (see Section 17). Increased secretion of parathyroid hormone (PTH) is thought to be of major importance in renal bone disease by increasing the activity and the numbers of these bone cells and so increasing bone turnover. Rapid rates of bone turnover are associated with

Table 1 Features of renal bone disease and some clinical manifestations of disturbed calcium and phosphate metabolism in chronic renal failure

Feature	Clinical consequence
1 Hyperparathyroidism and osteitis fibrosa	Skeletal deformity, bone pain, pruritis ? Anaemia, impotence, neuropathy etc.
2 Osteomalacia and decreased availability of vitamin D, calcium and phosphate	Skeletal deformity, bone pain and tenderness pathological fracture*, proximal myopathy encephalopathy, microcytic anaemia*, haemolytic anaemia
3 Osteoporosis	Pathological fracture skeletal deformity
4 Osteonecrosis	Joint pain
5 Osteosclerosis and periosteal new bone formation	None known
6 Extraskeletal calcification	Depends on site – skin ulcers, pruritis, vascular disease, cardiac failure, pseudogout etc.

* Characteristic of aluminium toxicity.

deposition of fibrous tissue in the marrow spaces (osteitis fibrosa) and the formation of new bone matrix which is not lamellar but disorganized in structure (woven bone). This impairs its strength and occasionally gives rise to serious mechanical consequences (Fig. 1) particularly in the young. If hyperparathyroid bone disease is severe, an imbalance between bone formation and bone resorption occurs and skeletal mass diminishes, particularly that of cortical bone. In adolescents severe hyperparathyroid bone disease may resemble rickets on skeletal X-rays. Bone loss is not invariable and patchy osteosclerosis of trabecular bone (e.g. vertebral bodies) is also found. Biochemical indices of bone cell activity include serum measurements of parathyroid hormone (PTH), alkaline phosphatases (derived from bone-forming cells), and hydroxyproline (derived from the breakdown of collagen). Concentrations of all three are higher in patients with osteitis fibrosa than those without.

Osteomalacia is characterized by an increase in the amount of unmineralized bone matrix. It is important to distinguish increased amounts of osteoid due to augmented bone turnover from that due to a defect in its mineralization. Osteomalacia arises because of an abnormal delay between the onset of bone matrix formation and its subsequent mineralization. Increased osteoid mass due to increased bone turnover is found in many other disorders including Paget's disease, hyperparathyroidism, fracture repair, and hyperthyroidism. In chronic renal failure, osteomalacia and hyperparathyroidism commonly co-exist. They can be distinguished by histological measurements on bone biopsy which estimate the rate of mineralization. The most direct method is to administer two pulses of tetracycline before bone biopsy which are incorporated into bone at the site of mineralization. Since tetracyclines fluoresce under ultraviolet light, the rate and extent of bone mineralization can be measured. An accurate assessment is important for the diagnosis and the assessment of treatment.

Changes in bone mass are common in renal failure. There is commonly a redistribution of skeletal mass so that osteosclerosis and osteoporosis may co-exist in the same patient. Severe osteoporosis is rarely found in patients not yet requiring dialysis treatment but is common in the dialysis-treated population and after transplantation.

Clinical features

Disturbed mineral and skeletal metabolism has many consequences other than those affecting bone (see Table 1). The skeletal manifestations of renal bone disease include bone pain, bone

tenderness, fractures, retardation of growth, joint disease and soft tissue calcification.

Both osteomalacia and osteitis fibrosa may be associated with bone pain, tenderness, and muscle weakness. Pain in the lower limbs, pelvis, and back are particularly common and may be worse on exercise. Muscle weakness is frequently proximal. Symptoms are unusual in patients with developing renal failure unless the duration of renal failure is long. In patients receiving dialysis treatment there is, however, great variability in the prevalence of symptoms between dialysis units, ranging from 10 per cent to nearly 100 per cent of those treated.

In dialysis centres with a very high incidence of osteomalacia (reflecting a dialysis-induced cause, probably aluminium intoxication), indolent fractures occur, particularly of the ribs, spine, pelvis, and femoral neck. Multiple rib fractures may result in respiratory failure.

Osteosclerosis and periosteal new bone formation are not associated with symptoms and are therefore only incidental radiographic findings.

Extraskeletal calcification is characteristically found in the vascular tree and periarticular soft tissues (Fig. 2). A predisposing factor is an increase in the plasma calcium i.e. multiplication, phosphate product which induces precipitation when its solubility product is exceeded. Calcification occurs commonly in the eye, as band keratopathy or in the conjunctiva. Acute conjunctival precipitation may cause a chemical conjunctivitis, the 'red-eye' of renal failure. It has been suggested that deposition of calcium in the skin may contribute to pruritus, frequently an unpleasant condition in patients with chronic renal failure.

The abdominal aorta, femoral, and digital arteries are the most common sites of vascular calcification (usually medial) visible on X-rays. Ischaemic necrosis is unusual but disabling.

Avascular necrosis of bone occurs rarely in chronic renal failure but is a significant cause of morbidity in transplant recipients. The hip joint is the most commonly affected and presents with joint pain.

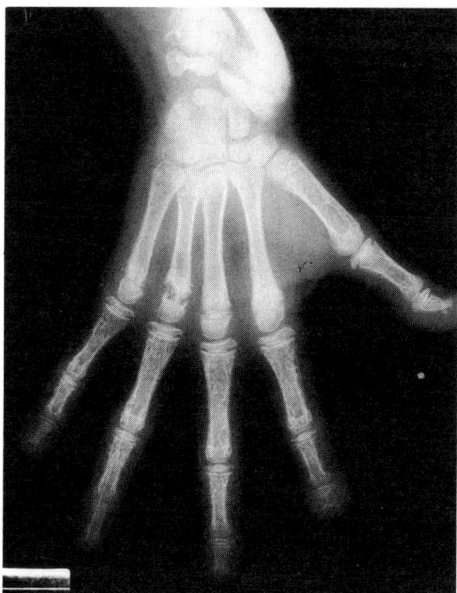

Fig. 1 Radiographic features of hyperparathyroid bone disease in an adolescent with chronic renal failure. Note the marked subperiosteal erosions of the phalanges. Erosion of the terminal phalange has resulted in the collapse of soft tissue giving a drumstick appearance of the fingers. Severe osteitis fibrosa at the wrist is indicated by the marked metaphyseal resorption giving rise to skeletal deformity. Less marked hyperparathyroid bone disease may give rise to radiographic features resembling rickets.

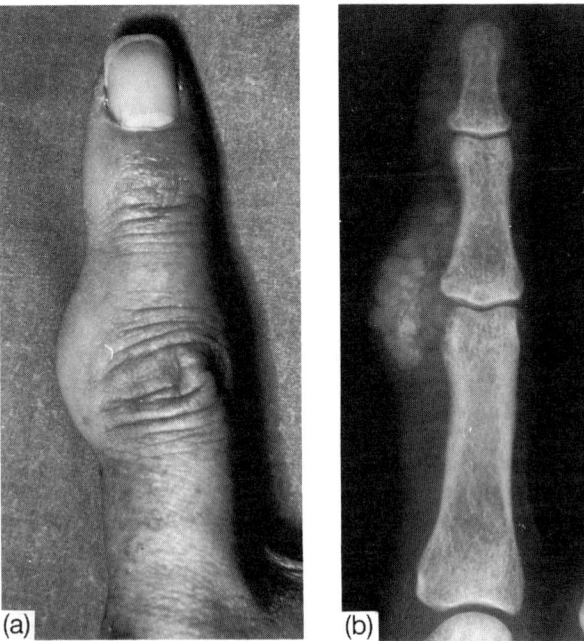

Fig. 2 Radiographic and clinical photograph of periarticular calcification due to hyperphosphataemia in a patient treated by intermittent haemodialysis.

Radiographic features

Radiography is much used in the assessment of renal bone disease but is relatively insensitive since many patients with significant skeletal abnormalities may have normal radiographic appearances.

The characteristic radiographic feature of hyperparathyroid bone disease is subperiosteal erosion of bone (Fig. 3). For reasons which are unclear, the sites of bone erosion most commonly affected include the radial aspect of the middle phalanges of the hand, the tufts of the terminal phalanges, and the distal ends of the clavicles. Gross erosion may result in collapse of soft tissue normally supported by bone. In the terminal phalanges this may give rise to the appearance of pseudoclubbing (see Fig. 1).

Radiographic features are uncommon in osteomalacia, and a negative radiographic survey is therefore not helpful in excluding it. There may be a generalized radiolucency of bone. Looser's zones (Fig. 3) are characteristic of osteomalacia and are most frequently seen in the pelvis. The presence of coarse trabecular markings, osteosclerosis, and periosteal new bone formation (Fig. 3) has been attributed to hyperparathyroidism, but their appearance appears to be more consistently associated with osteomalacia. The radiographic features of osteosclerosis bear only a superficial resemblance to those of avascular necrosis.

Children are particularly prone to renal bone disease and some may show radiographic features that resemble rickets. There are, however, important differences between uraemic 'rickets' and nutritional vitamin D deficiency which are more evident on histological than radiographic examination: in uraemia there is often no widening of the metaphyseal zone, and the width of the growth plate is not as thick as in vitamin D deficiency (though it may appear so radiographically because of metaphyseal fibrosis and resorption below the growth plate).

The radiographic features of extraskeletal calcification (see Fig. 2) depend on its site. Clinically significant extraskeletal calcification may occur in the absence of radiographic abnormalities and is occasionally detectable by radionuclide scanning.

Biochemical features

The classical biochemical findings related to skeletal metabolism in chronic renal failure include a low serum calcium, hyperphos-

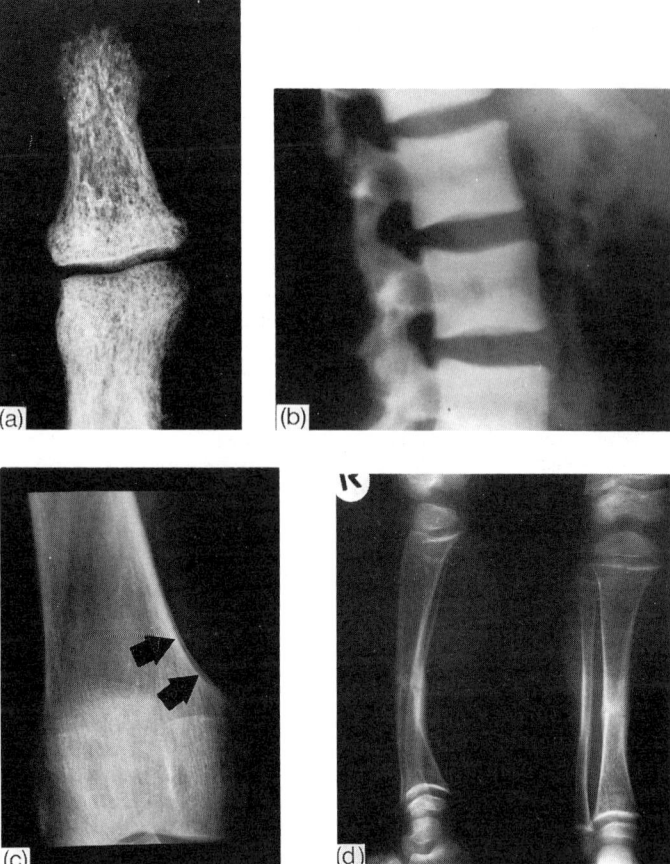

Fig. 3 Some of the radiographic features of renal bone disease: (a) subperiosteal bone resorption of the terminal phalanx due to secondary hyperparathyroidism; (b) changes in the lumbar spine manifest as alternate bands of increased and reduced radiodensity ('Rugger jersey spine'); (c) periosteal new bone formation. The periosteal separation from the mineralized cortex of the femur is shown by the arrows; (d) radiographic characteristics of osteomalacia. A Looser's zone is present in the midshaft of the tibia. There is widening of both of the epiphyseal plate and metaphysis.

phataemia, diminished intestinal absorption of calcium, raised plasma activity of alkaline phosphatase, and increased serum values of immunoassayable PTH. Serum concentrations of calcium are lower in chronic renal failure than in health, particularly in children, and may be lower in patients with osteomalacia than those without. These differences persist in patients on intermittent haemodialysis, though are less marked. Hypercalcaemia is less common but is found in dialysis-treated patients with severe hyperparathyroidism (so-called tertiary or autonomous hyperparathyroidism), in vitamin D toxicity, and in some patients with aluminium bone disease. The occurrence of mild or moderate renal failure and hypercalcaemia is sufficiently unusual that the diagnosis of primary hyperparathyroidism and secondary renal failure should always be considered. Transient hypercalcaemia also occurs rarely shortly after starting haemodialysis, and may be due to the resorption of pre-existing extraskeletal calcification.

Hyperphosphataemia occurs when the glomerular filtration rate falls below approximately 30 ml/min. The serum phosphate concentration is determined partly by the diet, the glomerular filtration rate, the tubular reabsorption of phosphate, the use of oral phosphate binding agents, and the dialysis regime. Patients with severe chronic renal failure also malabsorb phosphate, and hypophosphataemia may occasionally be noted despite the absence of renal function. As in the case of serum calcium, those patients with osteomalacia tend to have the lower values of serum phosphate (Fig. 4), but neither the serum calcium nor phosphate are sufficiently different from patients without osteomalacia to provide effective clinical discrimination.

Serum activity of alkaline phosphatase is commonly increased in chronic renal failure, but the increase is not always due to the bone-derived enzyme. Other sources in patients with renal failure are the gut and liver. The determination of hepatic enzymes such as 5'-nucleotidase activity may be helpful in excluding a hepatic source. In the absence of liver disease, hyperphosphatasia suggests increased bone cell activity as seen in secondary hyperparathyroidism. In osteomalacia associated with secondary hyperparathyroidism, alkaline phosphatase is also increased; but in osteomalacia in the absence of hyperparathyroidism, serum activity of alkaline phosphatase is commonly normal.

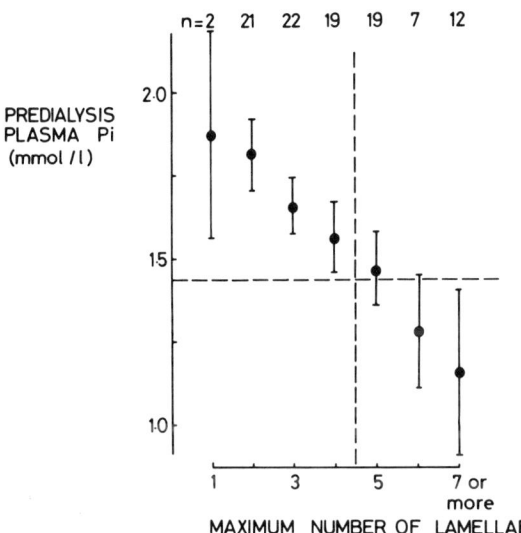

Fig. 4 Relationship between plasma phosphate (Pi) and a histological index of osteomalacia in patients with renal failure receiving dialysis treatment. Osteomalacia (five or more osteoid lamellae) was uncommon in patients with high plasma values of phosphate. Evidence of osteomalacia was commonly noted in patients whose plasma phosphate lay below the upper limit of the normal range (indicated by the dashed line).

Table 2 Factors of possible importance in the pathogenesis of renal bone disease

1 Disturbances in endocrine function
    Defective production of dihydroxy metabolites of vitamin D_3
    Impaired metabolism or urinary losses of 25-hydroxyvitamin D_3
      (nephrotic syndrome)
    Secondary hyperparathyroidism: PTH resistance
    Secretion, degradation or action of other hormones, e.g. calcitonin,
      thyroxine, gonadal steroids, prolactin and others
2 Accumulation of toxic products
    Aluminium, magnesium, and possibly other metals, e.g. iron,
      cadmium, beryllium, aluminium, manganese
    Products of metabolism such as hydrogen ions, middle molecules etc.
3 Drugs
    Phosphate binding agents
    Anticonvulsants and barbiturates
    Corticosteroids and cytotoxic agents
    Vitamins A, C, and D
    Heparin
4 Deficiency states
    Phosphate
    Availability of calcium (diet, dialysis, malabsorption)
    Dietary protein
    Vitamin C, pyridoxin, vitamin D
5 Other
    Age (adolescence), female sex
    Duration and nature of renal disease

Radioimmunoassays for parathyroid hormone (PTH) are becoming increasingly available, but there are several problems in interpreting immunoassayable PTH (iPTH) in chronic renal failure. The kidney is an important site of degradation of some of the biologically inactive fragments of PTH (see page 10.51 *et seq.*) and in some assay systems, values of iPTH in serum may be 20- or 40-fold higher than normal, even in the absence of significant secondary hyperparathyroidism as judged by other criteria. Nevertheless, serum values of iPTH are higher in patients with hyperparathyroid bone disease and renal failure than those without.

The absence of abnormal radiographic or biochemical findings does not exclude the presence of significant bone disease, particularly osteomalacia and osteoporosis. Methods of measuring bone mass include measurement of cortical width, photon absorption, and neutron activation analysis, which are becoming more widely available and provide a useful adjunct in the diagnosis and management of osteoporosis. Bone biopsy is the only certain way to exclude the presence of osteomalacia.

Pathophysiology

The biochemical and endocrinological disturbances giving rise to renal bone disease include abnormalities in the excretory function of the kidney, alterations of its endocrine function, and the effects of drugs, diet or differing dialysis regimens (Table 2).

Metabolism of vitamin D

It has been recognized for a long time that large doses of vitamin D (calciferol) may increase the intestinal absorption of calcium and heal osteomalacia and osteitis fibrosa in some patients with renal failure. The bone disease is 'vitamin D resistant' in the sense that the doses of vitamin D required are greater than physiological. There is now considerable evidence that this resistance in renal failure is due to defective metabolism of vitamin D. The kidney is involved critically in the metabolism of vitamin D since it is the major site of production of calcitriol [1,25-dihydroxy vitamin D_3 or $1,25(OH)_2D_3$] and $24,25(OH)_2D_3$. Defective production of calcitriol accounts for the vitamin D resistance but there are additional aspects of vitamin D metabolism important in renal bone disease.

The first step in the metabolism of vitamin D_3 is its conversion to calcidiol (25-hydroxyvitamin D or 25-OHD$_3$) which occurs mainly in the liver (see page 10.51 *et seq.*). In most patients with chronic renal failure, serum calcidiol is normal but low values, when present, are usually due to inadequate diet or reduced exposure to sunlight, particularly before the start of dialysis treatment. Serum values of calcidiol may also be low in patients with the nephrotic syndrome due to urinary losses, and give rise to bone disease. A number of patients take anticonvulsants including barbiturates, which induce hepatic microsomal enzymes, and might, therefore, increase the metabolism of calcidiol to inert products. There is little direct evidence for this and a more important effect of anticonvulsants may be to block the action of vitamin D metabolites on gut and bone. Low values of calcidiol may contribute to osteomalacia, particularly when the degree of renal failure is modest.

It is now commonly accepted that most of the actions of vitamin D_3 are mediated by metabolism of calcidiol to calcitrol. Since the kidney is probably the sole site of synthesis of calcitriol (apart from the placenta in pregnancy), the development of bone disease and its resistance to vitamin D and to calcidiol may result from impaired production of calcitriol due to loss of renal tissue and perhaps also to the inhibitory effects of hyperphosphataemia on the renal 1-α-hydroxylase enzyme. Serum values of calcitriol decrease when the GFR is less than 40 ml/min and are very low in end-stage renal failure.

Deficiency of calcitriol in humans retards skeletal growth and results in defective mineralization of matrix produced both by chondrocytes and osteoblasts. It also induces intestinal malabsorption of calcium and aggravates hypocalcaemia and secondary hyperparathyroidism. Reversal of many of these abnormalities by physiological doses of calcitriol provides convincing evidence for its importance in skeletal metabolism. However, it is not yet clear whether or not formation and mineralization of bone and cartilage are *direct* actions of the vitamin D metabolites (see page 10.51 *et seq.*).

The view that lack of calcitriol is the major cause of osteomalacia and secondary hyperparathyroidism in renal failure may be an oversimplification. Thus, not all patients with osteomalacia respond to treatment with 1-α-hydroxylated metabolites, and healing is commonly incomplete when histological indices of response are used. Moreover, the prevalence of osteomalacia is low in some renal units despite the ubiquity of defective calcitriol production (Fig. 5). These observations suggest that factors other than defective production of calcitriol must contribute significantly to the bone disease of chronic renal failure.

The production of $24,25(OH)_2D_3$ may also be deficient in renal failure since the kidney converts calcifidiol to this metabolite. In chronic renal failure, serum values of $24,25(OH)_2D_3$ are low but the administration of $24,25(OH)_2D_3$ alone does not heal bone disease. There is some evidence that both calcitriol and $24,25(OH)_2D_3$ are required for the actions of vitamin D on bone to be complete.

Phosphate metabolism

From animal experiments the hypothesis has been derived that the tendency for serum phosphate to rise as renal failure occurs, stimulates the secretion of PTH by decreasing the ionized fraction of serum calcium. The increase in PTH so induced decreases tubular reabsorption of phosphate and hence serum phosphate and increases serum calcium. Thus, during the course of progressive renal failure, serum values of calcium and phosphate may be kept relatively normal, but at the expense of an ever-increasing secretion rate of parathyroid hormone and its resultant skeletal effect – osteitis fibrosa. When the decrement in glomerular filtration rate is too great, the number of residual nephrons is not sufficient to lower serum phosphate, and hyperphosphataemia and hypocalcaemia ensue (Fig. 6). Hyperphosphataemia may be one of the reasons for reduced synthesis of calcitriol.

The importance of disturbed phosphate metabolism has not been fully evaluated in humans. However, the administration of phosphate in chronic renal failure does induce hypocalcaemia and hyperparathyroidism. In many disorders, including chronic renal failure, antacid abuse, and renal tubular disorders, the concen-

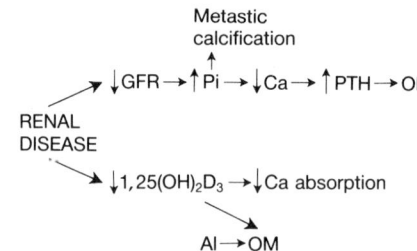

Fig. 6 The role of vitamin D, aluminium (A1), and parathyroid hormone (PTH) in the pathogenesis of renal bone disease. Progressive renal disease induces decrements in glomerular filtration rate (GFR) and synthetic capacity for calciferol [$1,25(OH)_2D_3$]. An increase in serum phosphate (Pi) due to the fall in GFR stimulates the secretion of PTH indirectly by decreasing serum calcium concentrations (Ca). During progressive renal failure serum calcium and phosphate tend to remain normal (because of the renal and skeletal effects of PTH) at the expense of an increasing secretion rate of PTH and its skeletal consequence, osteitis fibrosa (OF). When the compensatory abilities of the kidney are compromised by renal failure, hyperphosphataemia and hypocalcaemia prevail. Hyperphosphataemia may further inhibit synthesis of calcitriol and cause osteomalacia (OM). Malabsorption of calcium may contribute to secondary hyperparathyroidism.

tration of serum phosphate appears to be an important determinant of osteomalacia. Serum phosphate concentrations in dialysis-treated patients correlate inversely with the degree of osteomalacia, such that those patients with normal amounts of osteoid have the higher values of serum phosphate. It may be relevant that serum phosphate in such patients are considerably higher than the upper limit of normal in health, and a degree of hyperphosphataemia may therefore protect the patient from osteomalacia, despite defective vitamin D metabolism.

Calcium metabolism

It is probable that the skeletal effects of vitamin D are not solely dependent upon direct actions of the metabolites on bone itself but also due to consequent changes in extracellular concentrations of calcium, phosphate, and parathyroid hormone. One of the reasons why this question remains open is the difficulty in studying mineralization *in vitro*, whereas the effects of vitamin D metabolites *in vivo* are complex. Severe dietary deficiency of calcium appears to render patients with chronic renal failure unresponsive to calcitriol, whereas healing of osteomalacia occurs when the diet is adequately supplemented.

The dialysis membrane provides a site for the loss or the incorporation of calcium into the body. The net transfer is dependent on shifts in extracellular pH and serum protein concentrations, and on the respective calcium concentrations of serum and dialysis fluid. The use of a low dialysate calcium (e.g. 1.25 mmol/l) induces osteoporosis but calcium-rich dialysis fluids (e.g. 2.0 mmol/l) are not advised; extraskeletal calcification may be accentuated and, despite reports of decreased secretion of parathyroid hormone, the long-term skeletal response is disappointing. The ideal calcium concentration of dialysis fluid lies somewhere between 1.63 and 1.75 mmol/l. In view of the uncertain effects of vitamin D on bone, it is unknown whether the combination of a low-dialysate calcium and calcitriol would be advantageous.

Trace elements and water contaminants

A number of trace elements accumulate in chronic renal failure due either to impaired excretory function or to their entry from the dialysate fluid during dialysis. These include arsenic, strontium, molybdenum, magnesium, manganese, copper, aluminium, and fluoride, but, with the exception of aluminium, their role, if any, in the evolution of dialysis bone disease is not known. Patients with osteomalacia on haemodialysis treatment do not respond uniformly to treatment with vitamin D or related compounds, despite adequate control of serum phosphate and the

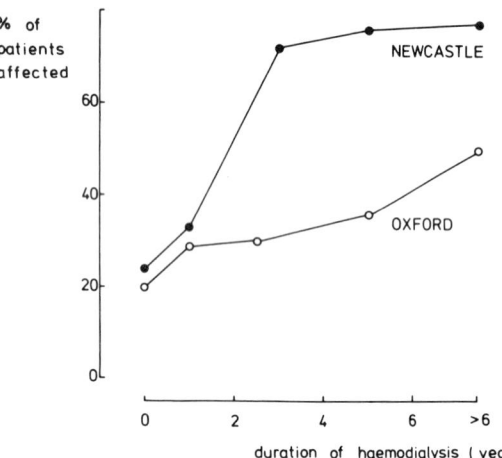

Fig. 5 The prevalence of osteomalacia in patients established on long-term intermittent haemodialysis as assessed by repeated bone biopsy. Note the large difference between Newcastle (a high aluminium area) and Oxford (low aluminium in the dialysate fluid) but a similar prevalence of osteomalacia at the time of starting dialysis. Patients from the Oxford Renal Unit do not invariably develop osteomalacia even after many years of haemodialysis.

administration of calcium supplements. Indeed the failure to respond to calcitriol may be one method of separating patients in whom osteomalacia is due to other causes.

Aluminium retention is an important factor in the pathogenesis of osteomalacia in some dialysis-treated patients. A form of osteomalacia associated with a high incidence of bone pain and fracture is common in certain geographical locations with a high aluminium content in the water (see Fig. 5), and its incidence appears to decrease with deionization of the water. There is also a good correlation (in the United Kingdom) between osteomalacia associated with fracture and the aluminium content of the water used for dialysis. Skeletal retention of aluminium and fracture are not always associated with osteomalacia and low rates of bone formation are the probable cause of pathological fracture.

The question arises whether the phosphate-binding agents containing aluminium salts may themselves give rise to aluminium toxicity. Waterborne, rather than oral aluminium, was the major source of skeletal aluminium in the past, but oral aluminium is now a significant cause of aluminium retention.

Aluminium toxicity should be suspected in patients with bone pain and muscle weakness who have little radiographic or biochemical evidence for hyperparathyroid bone disease. The presence of hypercalcaemia or pathological fracture are additional features. The diagnosis can be confirmed by bone biopsy which show focal aluminium accumulation by specific histochemical stains and low rates of bone formation. Osteomalacia when present is characterized by a paucity of active-looking osteoblasts – aplastic osteomalacia.

Acidosis
The role of acidosis in contributing to renal bone disease has been advocated for many years. It has been suggested that bone acts as a buffer by releasing alkaline bone salts and this is supported by the finding of a decrease in the bicarbonate content of bone from uraemic patients. The acute administration of acid loads to normal humans results in a negative calcium balance and it has been noted that the rate of mineralization increases acutely when alkalis are administered to acidotic patients with osteomalacia. The long-term effects of metabolic acidosis on bone are, however, less clear and it has not been regarded as a major factor, since the correction of acidosis appears to influence renal bone disease in only a minority of patients.

Parathyroid hormone metabolism
Not only is the kidney an important site of action for parathyroid hormone but the kidney is a major site for its degradation. Serum concentrations of iPTH are increased in early renal impairment, but it is difficult to know how much this reflects delayed degradation of inert fragments or increased secretion. Hypocalcaemia is a common finding in chronic renal failure, and it is generally accepted that this provides the major stimulus for the secretion of PTH. It is also possible that some vitamin D metabolites may exert direct effects on the parathyroid gland, and in chronic renal failure disturbed metabolism of vitamin D and possibly of magnesium may contribute to hypersecretion and hyperplasia of the parathyroids.

Although the major stimulus for parathyroid hormone secretion is hypocalcaemia, the mechanisms by which hypocalcaemia arise in chronic renal failure are ill-understood. Factors of possible importance include hyperphosphataemia (see phosphate metabolism), intestinal malabsorption of calcium, decreased renal tubular reabsorption of calcium, and 'skeletal resistance' to the action of PTH. Skeletal resistance to PTH is suggested by the finding of high concentrations of iPTH irrespective of the prevailing concentration of serum calcium. However, not all the fragments detected by immunoassay possess biological activity. Impairment of the calcaemic response to exogenous parathyroid extract in chronic renal failure has been cited as evidence for skeletal resistance to PTH possibly due to deficiency of calcitriol, but the relevance of such

observations made in acute studies to long-term effects on bone are not clear.

In contrast, there is abundant evidence that PTH is an important determinant of hyperparathyroid bone disease. The finding of hyperplastic glands and the effects of parathyroidectomy in affected patients are clinical indications of increased secretion and activity of PTH. Concentrations of iPTH in chronic renal failure also correlate with indirect and histological indices of bone resorption. These observations do not however exclude the possibility that a variety of factors may modify the response of skeletal tissue to PTH.

The influence of PTH on mineralization is less clear. Some patients develop osteomalacia after total parathyroidectomy when osteitis fibrosa has healed. The relative ease with which the woven osteoid (found in hyperparathyroidism) calcifies, compared to lamellar osteoid may explain the appearance of osteomalacia since lamellar bone is laid down after parathyroidectomy. A corollary is that osteitis fibrosa may protect against osteomalacia.

Other factors
It has been known for many years that uraemic plasma contained a factor which inhibits the calcification of rat cartilage. The nature of this uraemic factor has not been elucidated but there are many possibilities. One candidate might be pyrophosphate which is an inhibitor of calcium phosphate nucleation *in vitro*. Increased values are found in patients with hypophosphatasia and in patients with chronic renal failure, and it is conceivable but uncertain that these might cause failure of mineralization in both conditions.

Renal failure is associated with retention of many potential toxins such as guanidines, phenols, aliphatic amines, and other 'middle molecules' yet to be identified. Substances normally found in trace amounts such as fluoride, aluminium, vitamin A, and cadmium also accumulate and may contribute to disordered skeletal metabolism. Disturbances of acid–base balance and of the metabolism of hormones other than parathyroid hormone and vitamin D occur in chronic renal failure; affected hormones include calcitonin, growth hormone, insulin, sex hormones, prolactin, and thyroid hormone, all of which may variously influence skeletal tissue itself or the metabolism of its regulating hormones. In addition, protein-deficient diets tend to restrict the intake of vitamin C and pyridoxine, both of which may act as essential co-factors in the formation and maturation of collagen. The relative importance of these many factors is unknown.

Drugs and diet
The management of chronic renal failure, particularly before the advent of haemodialysis treatment, commonly included severe dietary restrictions. Vitamin C, pyridoxine, and vitamin D deficiency occur commonly in chronic renal failure and may cause bone disease in patients with moderate renal impairment. Severe phosphate restriction may induce osteomalacia and calcium-deficient diets will decrease the net intestinal absorption of calcium irrespective of the activity of the intestinal transport process.

Many drugs are known to affect skeletal metabolism, in addition to the effects of anticonvulsants and barbiturates on skeletal metabolism. Heparin, which is commonly used during dialysis treatment, causes increased bone resorption when very high doses are used. Avascular necrosis occurs most commonly when steroids are used in the treatment of the underlying renal disorder and after transplantation. It is likely that the combination of corticosteroids and chronic renal failure are additive risk factors, since avascular necrosis is relatively uncommon in patients with chronic renal impairment not exposed to steroids, and in steroid-treated patients with normal renal function. It seems probable that the presence of osteoporosis also predisposes to the development of the disorder but the pathogenesis of avascular necrosis is unknown and this is reflected by the large number of causative factors which have been proposed. The incidence of avascular necrosis appears lowest in those transplant units which avoid very high doses of intravenous corticosteroids for transplant rejection.

Treatment of renal bone disease

Treatment strategy should be based not only on the presence of bone disease or associated symptoms but also on a careful assessment of the other non-skeletal effects of disturbed mineral metabolism (see Table 1) and the mechanisms responsible for the disorder (see Table 2). The proposed management of the chronic renal disease itself should also be considered since, for example, therapeutic approaches may depend on the probability of subsequent transplantation.

There are a number of preventative measures which should be considered in all patients with advanced renal impairment. It is probable that the severe restriction of dietary protein, as sometimes practised, is a greater factor in inducing morbidity than it is in achieving beneficial effects. Though low protein diets restrict the amount of phosphate, this is better achieved with the use of phosphate-binding agents. Both vitamins C and B_6 should be given as dietary supplements, particularly in dialysis-treated patients. It is reasonable to ensure that the dietary intake of calcium and vitamin D are at least normal with the use of appropriate dietary supplements.

Plasma values of vitamin A are high in renal failure but may be due to increased binding by retinol-binding protein. Since vitamin A increases bone resorption and may augment PTH secretion, supplements containing vitamin A should be avoided.

Phosphate metabolism

Serum phosphate is nearly always markedly increased in patients with severe renal impairment. Control of serum phosphate concentrations probably contributes to the prevention of hyperparathyroid bone disease and is also important in the management and prevention of extraskeletal calcification. It is impractical to limit the dietary intake of phosphate, but decreased availability of phosphate for absorption can be achieved with the use of phosphate-binding agents. The most commonly used agent is aluminium hydroxide prescribed as a gel, in biscuits or in capsule form. Calcium carbonate also binds phosphate in the gut and has potential advantages in correcting acidosis when present, increasing the dietary calcium load, and avoiding the ingestion of aluminium; but in practice the amounts of calcium carbonate required are large. It is advisable to withdraw aluminium-containing drugs when aluminium toxicity is suspected.

Phosphate-binding agents should be given *before* meals and the dose regulated according to their effects on serum phosphate. Predialysis values of serum phosphate should be less than 2.2 mmol/l to avoid extraskeletal calcification. Factors which influence the dose required include the dietary intake of phosphate, concurrent treatment with vitamin D and its analogues or metabolites, and the haemodialysis treatment schedule prescribed. Profound hypophosphataemia should also be avoided since it is associated with osteomalacia (see Fig. 4). The concentrations of serum phosphate associated with osteomalacia (approximately 1.4 mmol/l) are considerably higher than those which cause impaired mineralization in patients with normal renal function. Thus the values of serum phosphate which best balance the risks of metastatic calcification and osteomalacia probably lie between 1.4 and 2.2 mmol/l in dialysis-treated patients.

Calcium metabolism

Unlike the net intestinal absorption of phosphate which is largely dependent on the dietary load, the net absorption of calcium is more critically dependent on the presence of the vitamin D metabolites, particularly calcitriol. Nevertheless, net intestinal transport of calcium can be augmented by large amounts of calcium carbonate (5–20 g daily) and this may improve osteomalacia. It is often more practicable to give vitamin D or one of its metabolites (discussed later) but net intestinal absorption of calcium cannot be greatly augmented if the diet is severely deficient in calcium. Moreover, calcium deficiency appears to impair the response to vitamin D. It is important, therefore, to ensure at least a normal dietary intake of calcium with the use of calcium supplements if necessary.

In patients receiving dialysis treatment, the dialysis membrane is an important site for the loss or incorporation of calcium into the body. The dialysate calcium which best balances the risks of osteoporosis and metastatic calcification lies between 1.6 and 1.75 mol/l.

Vitamin D and related compounds

A variety of vitamin D compounds are available for use in chronic renal failure. These include vitamin D_2 (calciferol), D_3 cholecalciferol, dihydrotachysterol, calcitriol, and alfacalcidol (1-α-hydroxy vitamin D_3). A great deal of clinical interest has focussed on calcitriol and its synthetic analogue alfacalcidol since they bypass the metabolic block caused by uraemia: but dihydrotachysterol (DHT) is also biologically active without the necessity for 1-α-hydroxylation by the kidney. DHT and alfacalcidol undergo hepatic hydroxylation and the 25-OHDHT or calcitriol so formed are the major circulating forms of these agents.

All the vitamin D-like compounds available for use are effective in augmenting calcium absorption, relieving symptoms of bone pain and muscle weakness, in increasing serum calcium, and in the majority of patients they suppress elevated serum values of alkaline phosphatase and correct radiographic abnormalities (Fig. 7). Skeletal deformity in the young can probably be prevented and growth partly restored. There is no evidence to suggest that patients who fail to respond to one agent respond favourably with the use of another.

The histological response to treatment is often less marked than the clinical, biochemical or radiographic responses, particularly in patients maintained on intermittent haemodialysis, where factors other than disturbed vitamin D metabolism presumably play a dominant role in the pathophysiology. Both osteitis fibrosa and osteomalacia appear to respond more readily when associated with each other. Once again this may be related to the different pathogenic mechanisms.

Although most patients with end-stage chronic renal failure have histological evidence of bone disease, they are often symptomless. In patients on dialysis treatment, considerable differences exist in the incidence and natural history of bone disease between renal units. Whether to treat asymptomatic patients with vitamin D metabolites will therefore depend on several factors,

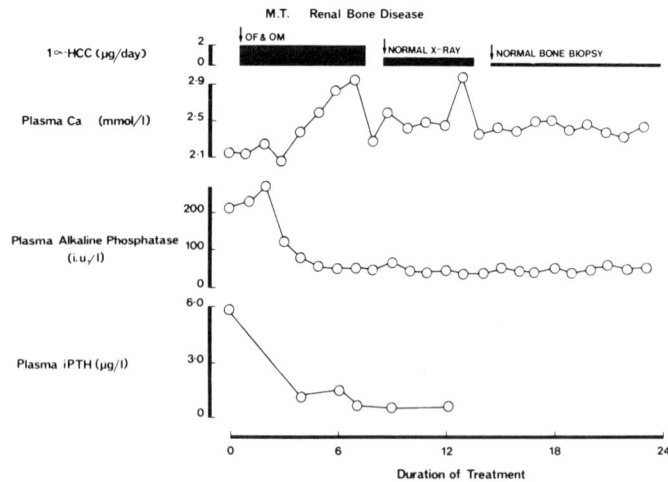

Fig. 7 Long-term treatment of renal bone disease with alfacalcidol (1-α-HCC) in a dialysis-treated patient. Healing of osteomalacia and osteitis fibrosa (OM and OF) occurred within 15 months. Episodes of hypercalcaemia occurred suddenly and the dose of alfacalcidol tolerated decreased progressively once plasma alkaline phosphatase had fallen to normal values. Remission from bone disease was maintained using a dose of 1-α-HCC of 1 μg thrice weekly.

but should be considered particularly in children in whom skeletal disease may progress rapidly.

Doses of the various agents required to maintain serum calcium within the normal range and to reverse bone disease are indicated in Table 3. In general, the dose tolerated in order to avoid hypercalcaemia decreases with time (Fig. 7). The greatest risks of hypercalcaemia occur at the start of treatment, particularly in patients who ultimately respond poorly to treatment, and in others, later when biochemical responses are nearing completion. Serum calcium should be monitored frequently during these risk periods. It is also important to note that these agents increase the absorption of phosphate and the requirements for phosphate-binding agents may be increased.

Despite claims to the contrary, there is no clinical evidence that calcitriol, alfacalcidol or DHT have any particular therapeutic actions not also possessed by other agents such as calcidiol or vitamin D. The advantages of the 1-α-hydroxylated derivatives of vitamin D and DHT lie in the ease with which doses are titrated according to requirements and the rapidity with which toxic effects are reversed on stopping treatment.

Treatment with vitamin D or its metabolites is not without risk. Prolonged increases in plasma calcium and phosphate give rise to extraskeletal calcification. Patients with pre-existing hypercalcaemia and osteomalacia should be treated cautiously, if at all, since such patients often respond poorly to treatment. Prolonged hypercalcaemia may also impair renal function, sometimes irreversibly, and there has been concern that vitamin D compounds may themselves be nephrotoxic. It is difficult, however, to be sure how much any deterioration of renal function reflects the natural history of the disorder or the effects of the hypercalcaemia or hyperphosphataemia. Close control of serum calcium and phosphate, and serial measurement of serum creatinine in patients not yet established on dialysis treatment are particularly important when any form of vitamin D is prescribed.

Aluminium toxicity

This severely disabling condition does not respond to treatment with vitamin D or its metabolites. It may respond slowly to transplantation or adequate removal of aluminium from the dialysis fluid. This probably reflects the prolonged skeletal retention of aluminium and the difficulty with which it is removed by haemodialysis, and indicates the importance of prophylaxis. Thus, where aluminium levels in the dialysate exceed 20 μg/l, the water should be treated by reverse osmosis or possibly by deionization.

Aluminium-containing antacids should not be prescribed except for the regulation of serum phosphate. They are most efficient

Table 3 Usual dose requirements of vitamin D, dihydrotachysterol (DHT), alfacalcidol, and calcitriol in dietary deficiency rickets and in vitamin D resistance due to chronic renal failure

	D$_3$	DHT	Alfacalcidol	Calcitriol
Approximate daily dose required to treat or prevent rickets (μg)	2.5–25	Up to 200	Up to 1.0	Up to 0.5
Potency relative to vitamin D$_3$	100	10	250	500
Approximate daily dose required to treat renal bone disease (μg)	750–10 000	200–1000	0.5–2.0	0.25–2.0
Potency relative to vitamin D$_3$	100	1000	500 000	500 000

Potencies are shown relative to that of vitamin D (=100 per cent). Note that, though larger amounts of DHT than vitamin D are required to treat simple rickets, only slightly higher doses are required to treat renal bone disease with DHT (or with alfacalcidol or calcitriol – up to four times) whereas much larger doses of vitamin D (up to 400 times) are required. Note 1 μg D$_3$ or calcitriol is equivalent to approximately 40 iu.

when given immediately before meals, and requirements may be minimized by use in combination with calcium salts such as calcium carbonate. The need for aluminium hydroxide can also be reduced by increasing the hours of dialysis treatment or the use of more efficient artificial kidneys.

The chelating agent desferrioxamine (DFO) is being increasingly used to decrease the body burden of aluminium. A typical regime is to give DFO (15 mg/kg/hour) by intravenous infusion during the first 2 hours of each haemodialysis treatment or to add a similar weekly dose (85 mg/kg) once weekly to the fluid used for peritoneal dialysis. In patients with significant aluminium retention, serum aluminium rises acutely due to its mobilization from tissues and chelation in the extracellular fluid. The rise in aluminium can be used as a diagnostic test and to judge the duration of treatment required. The amount of aluminium removed during each dialysis depends on the serum value and the type of dialyser used. Treatment is associated with clinical improvement (reduction in bone pain, muscle weakness) as well as improvements in the formation and mineralization of bone.

Parathyroidectomy

Surgical removal of parathyroid glands is an effective and rapid method of treating hyperparathyroid bone disease. It also improves extraskeletal calcification, but vascular calcification improves less readily than periarticular calcification. It should be considered in patients who fail to respond to medical treatment, particularly those with so-called tertiary or autonomous hyperparathyroidism – hyperparathyroid bone disease and a high serum calcium. Other indications include ischaemic necrosis of skin and intractable pruritis.

There are advocates both for subtotal and total parathyroidectomy. Recurrence of hyperparathyroidism is common following subtotal parathyroidectomy and it has been suggested that total parathyroidectomy should be considered in patients who are unlikely to receive renal transplants. The combination of vitamin D metabolites and subtotal parathyroidectomy does not avoid the risks of recurrence. The argument for total parathyroidectomy is that of avoiding recurrence but the occurrence (or unmasking) of osteomalacia resistant to vitamin D treatment is one of the reasons why partial parathyroidectomy may be preferable.

The main management problem is the immediate postoperative control of serum calcium when severe bone disease is present. Large intravenous doses of calcium (up to 6 g daily) may be required to avoid postoperative tetany. Prior treatment of patients with 1-α-hydroxylated derivatives of vitamin D appears to diminish the degree and duration of hypocalcaemia and in some may even avoid the need for surgery.

Renal transplantation

Theoretically, renal transplantation would be the treatment of choice for patients with bone disease. This rapidly restores the capacity to form calcitriol and of course reverses uraemia. Osteomalacia is often slow to heal, particularly when associated with aluminium retention. Bone disease, including osteomalacia and avascular necrosis may arise *de novo* in the transplanted population. There is a high incidence of hypercalcaemia and hypophosphataemia in the transplant population and this may be partly related to phosphate depletion by the use of antacids, the persistence of hyperparathyroidism which is slow to regress after transplantation, and the effects of corticosteroids to decrease renal tubular reabsorption of phosphate.

Experimental approaches

There are several agents which block or antagonize the effects of parathyroid hormone and bone, which include calcitonin and the diphosphonates. These might be of value in the management of renal osteodystrophy, either to prevent ectopic calcification in the case of diphosphonates or to reduce the hyperparathyroid or osteopenic component. Calcitonin appears to be effective in the management of patients with hypercalcaemia which occasionally occurs spontaneously in patients just starting dialysis treatment. Few data are available concerning the long-term use of these agents in controlling disturbed skeletal metabolism but the available information suggests that their place may be limited.

There has been recent interest in the possibility that high intravenous doses of calcitriol might suppress directly the secretion of PTH without raising serum calcium concentrations. It is also possible that some of the metabolites of vitamin D other than calcitriol may also have effects either directly on the parathyroid gland to suppress its secretion, or on bone to increase bone formation. One such candidate is 24,25-dihydroxy vitamin D_3 and it has been suggested that the combination of calcitriol and $24,25(OH)_2D_3$ may have more favourable effects on hyperparathyroid bone disease than the use of either agent alone.

Aluminium-containing antacids are the most efficient way of regulating phosphate metabolism but a small fraction of aluminium is absorbed. In some patients this contributes significantly to aluminium toxicity. Magnesium salts have been used to bind intestinal phosphate in combination with low dialysate magnesium concentrations, but may cause troublesome diarrhoea. Other aluminium-free phosphate-binding agents currently being evaluated are iron salts and synthetic polymers which deliver ionic calcium in the gastrointestinal tract.

References

David, D. S. (1977). *Calcium metabolism in renal failure and nephrolithiasis*. John Wiley and Sons, New York.

CYSTIC AND CONGENITAL ABNORMALITIES OF THE KIDNEYS

D. B. EVANS

Adult polycystic disease

The pathogenesis of this relatively common inherited condition is unknown. The mode of inheritance appears to be autosomally dominant. The condition can remain dormant for many years and normal kidney function is usually retained until middle life. Bilateral cyst formation occurs synchronously although the kidneys themselves are usually asymmetrical. Although the majority of patients with polycystic disease present with evidence of impaired renal function in the third or fourth decade, some may survive to old age. In rare cases the 'adult' disease may present in infancy (see page 18.85).

Pathology

At the time of diagnosis polycystic kidneys are almost invariably enlarged but retain their 'kidney' shape. Their surfaces are studded with cystic swellings, the cut surfaces revealing a collection of cysts of varying sizes throughout both cortex and medulla (Fig. 1). These cysts may be filled with clear uriniferous fluid, altered blood, or purulent material. Small areas of recognizable though disturbed renal tissue may survive between the cysts, and the pelves and calyces are stretched and distorted.

Histologically normal glomerular and tubular structures can be recognized in amongst the cysts, and micropuncture studies have

shown that the cysts participate both in solute absorption and active secretion.

Approximately one-third of patients with polycystic kidneys have hepatic cysts and rarely pancreatic, splenic, uterine, ovarian, and pulmonary cysts have been reported. Renal calculi occur in approximately 10 per cent of patients.

Berry aneurysms of the cerebral arteries are not infrequently associated, and in patients with polycystic disease intracranial haemorrhage will cause death in approximately 10 per cent. Neoplastic changes, though rare, are well recognized and should be suspected if recurrent haematuria, pain, fever, and weight loss occur in a patient with polycystic disease and no evidence of infection. Occasionally metastases may be prominent.

Clinical manifestations

Abdominal pain is a common presenting feature. In many cases this may be no more than a discomfort or an ache in the abdomen, but in some cases it may be more severe and situated in the abdomen or the loin. An increase in abdominal girth may draw the attention of some patients to their condition, particularly if they are aware of a family history of cystic renal disease. Haematuria, which may be painless or associated with clot colic, may also occur. Hypertension, urinary tract infections, haematuria, renal or ureteric colic, and acute or chronic renal insufficiency are all possible ways of presentation. If renal failure develops, urinary output often remains surprisingly high due presumably to the inability of the tubules to conserve salt and water in some patients with this disease. They are, therefore, particularly susceptible to dehydration and electrolyte imbalance as a result of gastrointestinal upsets and environmental changes. Rarely a fatal subarachnoid haemorrhage may be the first expression of this condition.

Diagnosis

In a slim patient with large, easily palpable polycystic kidneys, the diagnosis is rarely in doubt. However, in obese patients, even though the kidneys are considerably enlarged, they may be difficult to feel.

Intravenous urography (IVU) has been the main diagnostic tool.

The enlarged kidneys can usually be seen in the early nephrographic phase where the opacification tends to be patchy (Fig. 2). Later, the elongated compressed pelves and calyces become apparent (Fig. 3). However, urography and even ultrasound are too insensitive for the early identification of this condition for neither will recognize cysts measuring less than 1.5 cm in dia-

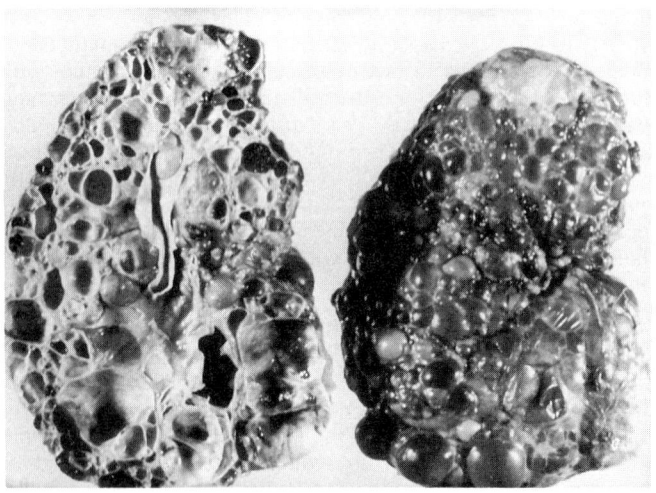

Fig. 1 Polycystic disease showing cut and uncut surfaces.

meter. Computed tomography can detect cysts down to 0.5 cm but even with this highly sophisticated development a clean bill of health cannot be given to relatives of affected persons much before the age of 30 years. This is a very important problem from the point of view of genetic counselling as well as in choosing suitable related living kidney donors. The possibility of histological examination has been suggested by certain American workers to be justifiable under certain circumstances.

The diagnosis is usually made earlier in females than in males for the disease will often be revealed during pregnancy or in the investigation of recurrent urinary infections. An important report by Reeders and others has shown by means of highly polymorphic DNA probes that the locus of the genetic defect in adult polycystic disease is closely linked to the α-globin locus on the short arm of chromosome 16. This advance will help presymptomatic and fetal diagnosis, and may ultimately allow a better understanding of the pathogenesis of the condition.

No specific abnormalities in blood or urine have been found in polycystic disease although, as renal tubular function declines, the failure to acidify and concentrate the urine may lead to profound acidosis and dehydration despite a relatively adequate GFR.

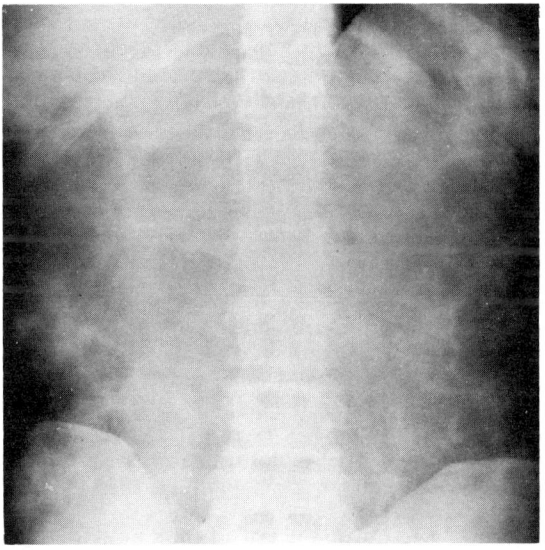

Fig. 2 Adult polycystic disease. Early nephrographic appearance.

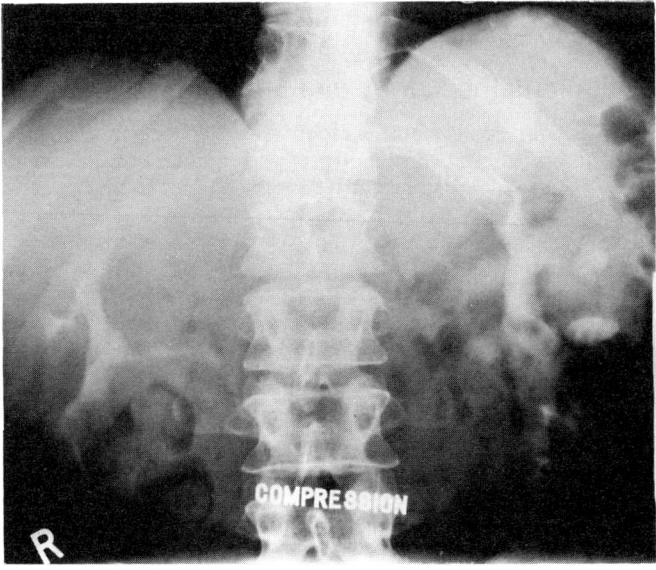

Fig. 3 Bilateral polycystic disease. Intravenous urogram showing elongation and compression of calyces and pelves.

Course and treatment

There is no specific treatment for this condition. Cyst puncture used to be practiced but with little benefit (Rovsing's operation).

Prompt treatment of urinary infections and hypertension may be beneficial in postponing the stage of renal failure. These patients usually maintain good urinary output despite failing renal function, but they are often vulnerable to conditions leading to fluid depletion, e.g. vomiting or diarrhoea.

Recurrent spontaneous haematuria may be particularly troublesome but usually responds to bed rest. Direct renal trauma, e.g. the wearing of seat belts in cars, can also result in haematuria. When chronic renal failure develops, dialysis and transplantation are indicated.

Prior to the advent of dialysis and transplantation, the majority of patients with polycystic disease died at approximately 40–50 years, either of chronic renal failure or of such associated conditions as hypertensive heart disease or cerebral haemorrhage.

Polycystic disease is one of the four commonest causes of chronic renal failure in the United Kingdom in the 30–50 year group, and consequently dialysis and transplantation are usually offered to these patients with very favourable results.

Bilateral polycystic disease of infancy

This is a rare condition with a reported incidence of between 1 in 6000 and 1 in 14 000 live births. A familial incidence has been shown and inheritance is autosomally recessive.

Many infants with this condition are stillborn, others may have such enlargement of the kidneys that labour may be obstructed. Those that are born alive tend to survive only for a short time. Clinically bilaterally enlarged lobulated kidneys can be felt on abdominal examination. Elevation of plasma urea and creatinine are common and hypertension may be present. The differential diagnosis lies between a renal tumour and hydronephrosis. The diagnosis can be confirmed radiologically.

Associated cysts of the liver, pancreas, spleen, and ovaries have been reported along with various bizarre neuroskeletal anomalies (see page 18.81).

Simple cysts

Simple retention cysts in the cortex of the kidneys are commonplace and in themselves are of little significance. However, occasionally they enlarge and cause symptoms such as pain and swelling. If large enough, they are susceptible to trauma and may rupture or bleed. Polycythaemia and hypertension have been ascribed to them. Radiologically a simple cyst may be confused with a hypernephroma. Nephrotomography, ultrasound, and cyst puncture may be necessary to differentiate the two conditions. Renal cysts are sometimes found secondary to such pathological entities as calculus disease, chronic infection, or haematomas.

Juvenile nephronophthisis (medullary cystic disease)

Juvenile nephronophthisis (JN), whilst rare, is a common cause of terminal renal failure in childhood accounting for 10–12 per cent of cases; 7 per cent of children starting dialysis in Europe in 1976 had JN. It is inherited as an autosomal recessive. Clinically and histologically it is similar to an autosomal dominant disease which presents in late childhood and adult life and which has been termed medullary cystic disease (MCD). The distinction between the two diseases is difficult because examples are recorded of apparently autosomal recessive JN occurring in families where some affected members have been children whilst in others the onset has been in late adolescence. Sporadic adult cases, presumably new dominant mutations, are recorded. The pathogenesis is unknown but the primary defect appears to be tubular with secondary glomerular and interstitial changes. The presenting clinical features in both JN and MCD are polyuria and polydypsia which usually are more severe than would be expected with the severity of the renal failure. Growth retardation is common but hypertension is variable at least until the terminal stages. The urinary concentrating defect is independent of the renal failure and there is usually an increased urinary sodium loss; hypokalaemia has been described and renal tubular acidosis is variable. Proteinuria is slight and haematuria uncommon. Glomerular filtration rate declines steadily and secondary consequences of renal failure such as renal osteodystrophy appear.

The kidneys are not usually enlarged and eventually may be small. Cysts are often not visualized on intravenous urography because cyst formation is variable and the concentration of contrast media may be poor. Segmental scarring and ureteral abnormalities are not a feature.

The main histological feature is interstitial inflammation with lymphocyte infiltration and tubular atrophy. Later medullary cysts located within distal tubules and collecting ducts appear and the renal cortex shrinks with widespread glomerular obsolescence. Cysts are not invariable even in late cases, and in the absence of a family history and the typical clinical features distinction from other forms of interstitial nephritis may be difficult. Treatment is restricted to correcting the electrolyte water and hydrogen ion excretion problems and controlling the metabolic consequences of renal insufficiency. Dialysis and transplantation are eventually required.

Many, sometimes confusing, variants of JN have been described. The commonest is the combination of JN with retinitis pigmentosa (Senior Loken syndrome). Visual acuity may be affected with tunnel vision but the eye lesion is not usually progressive or only slowly so. Presentation with severe tapetoretinal degeneration, optic atrophy, and blindness in early life (Leber's optic atrophy) is recorded. Congenital hepatic fibrosis and proliferation of bile ducts have been described in some families. Skeletal abnormalities with metaphysial chondoplasia of the femoral necks and cone-shaped epiphyses of the phalanges have been found. Mental retardation and cerebellar ataxia in association with JN and retinitis pigmentosa is also found but it is possible that some cases have been confused with the syndrome of mitochondrial cytopathy (see above). Another possibly autosomal recessive condition which

may be related is the combination of JN with chronic cholestatic liver disease.

Medullary sponge kidneys

This is a condition that rarely gives rise to significant symptoms. The diagnosis is made radiologically. Plain abdominal films may show characteristic clusters of small radio-opaque calculi on the tips of the renal papillae, and on intravenous urography the terminal collecting ducts and their cystic cavities show up as linear or cystic shadows radiating outwards from the calyceal cups (Fig. 4). The density of the contrast in these dilated tubules is higher than in the rest of the kidney. Any number of calyces may be affected and the condition may be unilateral. Grossly, the medulla of the kidney resembles a sponge, and histologically there is dilation of the terminal collecting ducts which are in connection with small cysts many of which contain small calculi. Inflammatory changes are usually seen in the surrounding tissues.

Clinical presentation depends upon complications. The vast majority are symptomless, but haematuria, renal colic due to the passage of stones, and infections of the urinary tract usually draw attention to the condition. Hemihypertrophy of limbs is sometimes associated. Overall renal function is usually normal though distal tubular function may be somewhat impaired. The prognosis is excellent and treatment of complications should be as conservative as possible. Rarely will partial or total nephrectomy be necessary for severe haemorrhage. The condition may on occasion be familial.

Multicystic renal dysplasia

Dysplastic changes in kidneys present in infancy and are due to abnormal parenchymal differentiation. Structural disorganization results in the presence of primitive tubular structures, dilated ducts lined by cuboidal epithelium, fat deposits, haemopoietic tissue, abnormal blood vessels, and hyaline cartilage. The cystic nature of the condition sometimes presents as a palpable abdominal mass in newborn infants. The condition is commonly unilateral, the affected kidney being non-functional. Rarely both kidneys may be involved.

Anomalies such as gastrointestinal atresias, interventricular septal defects, and lumbar meningomyelocoeles are sometimes associated.

Furthermore, many differing renal lesions have been described in association with genetic, hereditary, and other cerebral and skeletal malformation syndromes. By far the commonest renal abnormalities are cystic, often in association with dysplasia.

Tumours of the kidney and urinary tract

Although numerically renal tumours appear low down the cancer 'league table', their diverse modes of presentation and their sometimes unexpected response to therapy enhances their clinical importance.

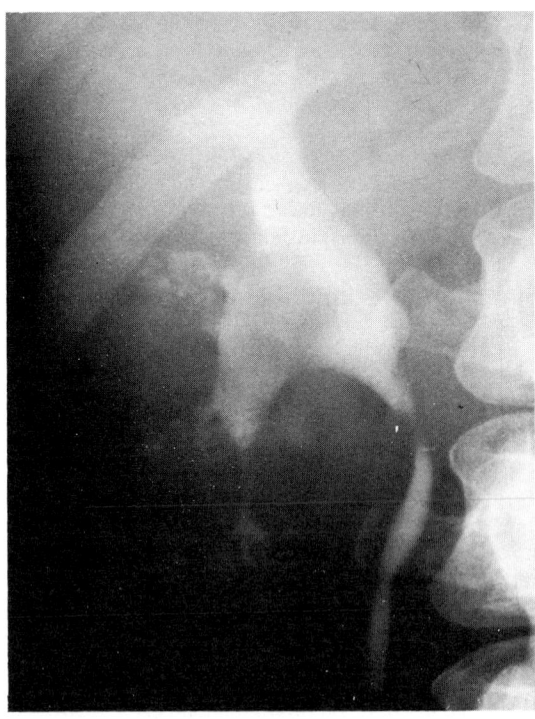

Fig. 4 IVU showing medullary sponge kidney.

Table 1 Renal tumours

Benign	Primary malignant	Metastatic
Adenoma	Hypernephroma	From lung, breast, or
Fibroma	(Renal cell carcinoma) (Grawitz)	stomach
Leiomyoma	Transitional or squamous cell tumours	
Angioma		
Hamartoma	Nephroblastoma (Wilms')	Lymphoma
Juxtaglomerular		Melanoma
cell tumour	Sarcoma	Sarcoma

Benign tumours such as adenomata are often only found at necropsy but others, such as haemangiomata, may cause significant haemorrhage during life.

The most important malignant tumours are the hypernephroma, the transitional cell tumour and Wilms' tumour although sarcomatous changes can develop in hamartomata and in cystic kidneys. Metastatic spread to the kidneys from the lung, breast, and stomach occur not infrequently, but they rarely produce any renal symptoms or signs.

Benign tumours

Adenomata

These are commonly found at post mortem and in surgical specimens. They rarely cause symptoms unless they grow to considerable size. Urographically, they may be difficult to distinguish from a renal cell carcinoma.

Hamartomata (angiomyolipomata)

These tumours are commonly found (and are usually multiple) in patients with tuberose sclerosis and consequently pose no great diagnostic difficulty. Occasionally, however, they occur as solitary tumours in otherwise healthy individuals. As they are very vascular, haemorrhage is not an uncommon feature.

Fibromata, leiomyomata, and neurogenic tumours

These sometimes grow to considerable size and may be highly vascular.

Juxtaglomerular cell tumour (haemangiopericytoma)

This is an exceedingly rare tumour in children and young adults, and its main interest lies in the fact that its cells secrete renin, resulting in hypertension (see page 13.382 *et seq.*) and hyperaldosteronism. Removal of the tumour leads to a resolution of the hypertension.

MALIGNANT TUMOURS

Renal cell carcinoma (hypernephroma).

These tumours probably originate from renal tubular epithelium and were first described by Grawitz in 1883. They are by far the commonest renal tumours in adults and males are affected more often than females.

Pathology

They vary in size and usually seem to be well demarcated from the rest of the renal tissue. They may be solitary or multiple and are sometimes present in both kidneys simultaneously. They appear whitish yellow and are covered with dilated veins. When bisected they are seen to be highly vascular and areas of haemorrhagic necrosis can occur within them. Invasion occurs into the renal veins and tumour emboli tend to get carried by the bloodstream into the lungs. Spread to lymph nodes, bone, liver, and the opposite kidney can also occur. Despite appearing well encapsulated, direct invasion into adjacent renal and perinephric tissues occurs. Microscopically they are composed of large clear cells sometimes mixed with smaller granular cells. These are arranged in sheets, or papillary or tubular patterns, and calcification is relatively common.

Histological classifications are notoriously difficult for the patterns of cell differentiation vary from one part of the tumour to the next. Staging of the tumour therefore must be gauged grossly on whether it is localized to the kidney or spread outside.

Clinical features

It is claimed that the triad of symptoms, haematuria, pain, and swelling are the classical symptoms of renal cell carcinoma. Haematuria certainly is the presenting symptom in approximately 50 per cent of cases, but pain and swelling tend to be less frequent and occur only when the mass is of considerable size and is invading surrounding structures. The commonest pain is a dull ache felt in the loin, but acute renal or ureteric pain may accompany bleeding and clot formation. The ability to palpate a mass depends on the size and site of the tumour as well as on the physique of the patient.

Non-specific symptoms such as anorexia, weight loss, weakness, and fatigue often antedate the above.

Of particular interest to physicians are the fascinatingly diverse modes of presentation of these tumours.

Fever Any patient with a fever for which no other cause can be found should merit an intravenous urogram. About 20 per cent of all hypernephromata are accompanied by a non-remitting fever caused probably by the secretion of a pyrogenic substance by the tumour.

High output cardiac failure may result from an arteriovenous anastomosis within the tumour itself.

Left varicocoele Due to its propensity to invade the renal veins occlusion of the left testicular vein may result, leading to a left-sided varicocoele.

Hormonal effects These tumours are sometimes capable of secreting polypeptides which have specific 'endocrine-like' effects. An erythropoietic factor is believed to be responsible for the polycythaemia syndrome which occurs in 2–3 per cent of cases and a parathyroid-like substance has been found which causes hypercalcaemia. Of course hypercalcaemia may occur when skeletal metastases are present. Prolactin, gonadotrophin, and corticosteroid secretion have also been ascribed to some renal carcinomas.

Hypertension occurs in about one-third of cases and some tumours have been shown to secrete renin. Immune complex glomerulonephritis may also occur in the non-malignant portion of the kidney.

Diagnosis

The investigation of any patient presenting with haematuria, loin pain or a swelling will undoubtedly include urine examination, cystoscopy and intravenous urography. Plain abdominal X-rays may show enlargement, irregularity or displacement of one or both renal outlines. Calcification within the tumours occurs in approximately 10 per cent of cases. After intravenously injected contrast, the mass will be better delineated, often causing distortion of the pelvicalyceal system. Occasionally it may be difficult to assess whether a space-occupying lesion in the kidney is cystic or solid, and ultrasound or CT scanning may be helpful in differentiating the two.

The most specific investigation is renal arteriography, for these tumours have characteristic appearances. It is important to perform bilateral renal arteriography so that small contralateral tumours are not missed and information derived thus may be helpful in planning surgery. Inferior vena cavography and renal venography are usually performed in addition to ascertain the extent, if any, of venous involvement by tumours.

Further pre-operative evaluation of the patient should include chest X-rays (and, if possible, whole lung tomography), bone, liver, and brain scans as well as lymphangiography.

Treatment

Where only one kidney is affected, its complete removal is advocated. Where bilateral tumours occur, or in the presence of a hypoplastic contralateral kidney, partial nephrectomy and conservation of as much normal renal tissue as possible can be achieved. If conservation of renal tissue is not possible, dialysis and transplantation have been shown to be successful.

A recent radiological innovation has shown that by introducing an embolus into the branches of the renal artery supplying the tumours and causing tumour infarction pre-operatively, surgery can be more easily accomplished in a bloodless field.

The presence of solitary metastases should not deter one from removing the primary tumour. Although regression of metastases have been reported, this is by no means universal. However, removal of solitary lung metastases after removal of the primary tumours has resulted in long term survival.

The value of radiotherapy and chemotherapy is not proven but they are often given. Relief of pain from bony metastases will often result from local irradiation.

Prognosis

The overall five-year survival rate is 30–50 per cent but with well differentiated tumour confined to the kidney, this figure will approach 60 per cent. Even at 10 years 25 per cent would be expected to survive.

Wilms' tumours (nephroblastomata)

These tumours of infancy and childhood are derived from embryonic renal tissues and contain a mixture of epithelial and connective tissue, and muscle elements. They grow rapidly to enormous dimensions, directly invade surrounding structures, and metastasize early via the bloodstream. Although usually unilateral, in approximately 5 per cent of cases tumours may be found in both kidneys. Morphologically they are solid but may undergo necrosis or haemorrhage and cystic degeneration. Histologically they consist mainly of spindle shaped epithelial cells, round cells, smooth and striated muscle cells, and sometimes cartilage or bone.

Clinical features

The majority of patients with Wilms' tumour are discovered before the age of three years. Abdominal distension usually causes a mother to seek medical advice and a palpable mass will be present in nearly all cases. Pain, fever, haematuria, and hypertension may also occur. Ascites and oedema may be detected if inferior venacaval thrombosis is present.

Diagnosis

Intravenous urography will show distortion or displacement of normal renal tissue but will not necessarily distinguish it from a cyst or large abscess. Ultrasound and CT scanning may be helpful, but arteriography and intravenous cavography will be necessary to confirm the diagnosis.

Treatment and prognosis

Nephrectomy is the treatment of choice followed by radiotherapy or chemotherapy. A recent study has shown that the combination of nephrectomy and actinomycin D gave the best results with a three-year survival rate for all stages of tumour of 83 per cent. Overall three-year survival rates were 65 per cent, and only 1 of 49 children who survived three years died subsequently from a Wilms' tumour.

Tumours of the urothelial tract

The majority of these tumours arise from transitional cells and may be papillary or solid. Squamous carcinoma is much rarer. Any part of the urothelial tract may be involved but the commonest tumours are benign or malignant papillomata of the bladder.

Transitional cell carcinoma usually is papillary in type and, if it arises in the renal pelvis, it will invade surrounding renal tissue, lymphatics, and the renal vein. Retroperitoneal, lung, liver, and bony metastases are common. If one urothelial tumour is discovered, the whole of the urothelial tract should be investigated for further tumours as they are often multiple.

It has been suggested that exogenous or endogenous carcinogens may play an important part in their aetiology, and certainly there is a high incidence of bladder carcinoma in workers in the dye industry who are exposed to aromatic amines. Patients with analgesic nephropathy and papillary necrosis occasionally develop pelvic tumours. Schistosomiasis, calculus disease, and chronic inflammation (sometimes related to indwelling bladder catheters) may predispose to urothelial cancer.

Symptoms and signs

Haematuria is a prominent feature and is usually intermittent and painless. Pain may be a feature if bleeding is brisk and clots are formed, or if the tumour obstructs the renal pelvis or ureter. These tumours are rarely large enough to be palpable. Bladder tumours on the other hand may give rise to frequency and urgency in addition to haematuria. Unilateral or bilateral ureteric obstruction can occur. Symptoms can therefore be very prominent even if the tumour is small. Large bladder tumours are usually palpable suprapubically or on rectal examination.

Diagnosis

Combination of urinary cytology, cystoscopy, and radiology will usually confirm the diagnosis, although clots or non-opaque stones in the pelvi-ureteric systems may cause considerable diagnostic difficulty. Angiography and venography may also be helpful in planning surgery.

Treatment and prognosis

Nephro-ureterectomy is the treatment of choice. In the case of bladder tumours the extent of surgery will depend on the stage of the tumour and in extreme cases, removal of bladder and urethral mucosa may be necessary. It is customary to combine surgery with radiotherapy but the value of the latter is not entirely clear.

Five-year survival figures for transitional tumours are less than 50 per cent overall, but the better differentiated they are the better the prognosis. Squamous tumours carry a far worse prognosis.

Congenital abnormalities of the kidneys and urinary tract

Approximately 10 per cent of the population possess some congenital malformation of the kidneys and urogenital tract. The spectrum varies from minor, insignificant anomalies to those that are so severe as to be incompatible with extra-uterine life. The importance of these abnormalities, however, lies in their predisposition to acquired conditions such as infection, stone formation, hypertension, and renal failure.

Congenital abnormalities occur as a result of defective embryological development resulting in: (a) inadequate renal tissue; (b) malpositioning; (c) malformation; and (d) abnormal differentiation of renal tissues.

Embryology

To understand more clearly these possible developmental anomalies it is essential to remind oneself of the embryology of the kidney. The basic elements derive from the mesoderm of the intermediate cell mass and the endoderm of the cloaca. When the embryo is 2.5 mm long, two longitudinal ducts develop lateral to the mesodermal somites on each side of the body and grow down to reach the cloaca. The pronephros and mesonephros develop in association with this duct (the Wolffian duct), the pronephros appears very early and regresses rapidly but the mesonephros develops into a primitive excretory organ. It later atrophies as the permanent kidney (the metanephros) develops, and in the male a portion of it is retained as the excretory apparatus of the testis. In the female it remains as a vestigial remnant in the broad ligament. The secretory portion of the permanent kidney eventually develops from the metanephros and the collecting ducts from the ureteric bud of the mesonephric duct. This bud grows in a cephalic direction towards the metanephros and then branches to produce calyces and collecting ducts which connect to the metanephrogenic tubules, the proximal ends of which are invaginated by capillary tufts to form glomeruli. These organs, which develop opposite the third lumbar vertebrum, appear to move in a cephalic direction eventually to lie opposite D12 L1/2. They also rotate medially through 90° so that the pelves face medially. Their blood supply, originally from the internal iliac arteries, is eventually derived from the abdominal aorta.

Renal abnormalities
Renal agenesis
Total renal agenesis is incompatible with extra-uterine survival. It is a very rare condition associated usually with other congenital abnormalities such as low set, poorly developed ears, 'parrot beak' nose, hypoplastic chin, spadelike hands and excessive skin over the nape of the neck, and pulmonary hypoplasia (Potter's syndrome).

Unilateral agenesis is of more importance and occurs in 1 in 1000 of the population. The contralateral kidney is comparatively hypertrophied and renal function is usually normal. The danger of trauma to such a solitary kidney is obvious. In approximately half these patients the ureter is absent, in which case half the bladder trigone may be missing.

Renal hypoplasia (miniature kidney)
This is a condition where the renal tissue is normal but the kidney is abnormally small. This abnormality occurs sporadically and is probably due either to a deficiency of metanephrogenic tissue or to defective branching of the ureteric bud.

It is difficult to differentiate radiologically between the small kidney of hypoplasia and a dysplastic or secondarily atrophied kidney. The only certain way is by histological examination. The contralateral kidney would be expected to be hypertrophied and renal function should be normal. Segmental hypoplasia causing malignant hypertension in children was described by Ask-Upmark in 1929. Radiologically the kidney resembles chronic pyelonephritis and micturating cystography usually reveals vesico-ureteric reflux. Arteriographically the renal arteries appear disproportionately small. Histologically the structures are hypoplastic and scarred, and intrarenal arterioles are thickened, fibrosed, and necrotic. Partial or total removal of the affected kidney may resolve the hypertension.

Bilateral hypoplasia is very uncommon but may present with multiple tubular defects, salt wastage, failure of growth, hypertension, and renal insufficiency.

Another rare form of hypoplasia known as oligomeganephronic renal hypoplasia results in progressive renal failure in children. Life expectancy is approximately 12 years.

Ectopic kidneys
During intra-uterine life the development of the kidneys from the metanephros takes place caudally and as the embryo develops, its hind portion elongates with the result that the developing kidney appears to 'ascend' and simultaneously rotates medially through 90°. Any interference with this ascent will lead to a caudally positioned or ectopic kidney with a ventrally placed pelvis. The normal kidney acquires its characteristic shape due to the moulding influences of its neighbouring structures – the ectopic organ consequently remains a flat amorphous mass, and if both kidneys fail to ascend, they fuse to form a flat 'cake'-like mass ventral to the sacral promontory (Fig. 5).

Crossed ectopia occurs when the renal mass drains via a collecting system that crosses the midline to enter the bladder normally or in an ectopic position. A crossed ectopic kidney lies below its orthotopic partner and sometimes becomes fused to it (Fig. 6).

The consequences of and problems relating to these anatomical anomalies are: (*a*) urinary infections, obstruction, and calculus formation which occur because of abnormal drainage and reflux; (*b*) a pelvic kidney may interfere with parturition; and (*c*) patients

may be operated upon unnecessarily because of the finding of a mass in the pelvis or loin, and inadvertent nephrectomy may be performed.

Acquired ectopy may occur in association with congenital diaphragmatic abnormalities, so that the kidneys may be situated in the thorax.

Horseshoe kidneys
The fusion of the lower poles of normally positioned kidneys gives a horseshoe appearance (Fig. 7). The isthmus between the kidneys may be composed of recognizable renal tissue or of a fibrous band. Occasionally the upper poles may be connected, and very rarely both lower and upper poles may be fused giving a doughnut appearance. Normally the fused portion of the kidneys lies anterior to the great vessels but occasionally it may lie behind or

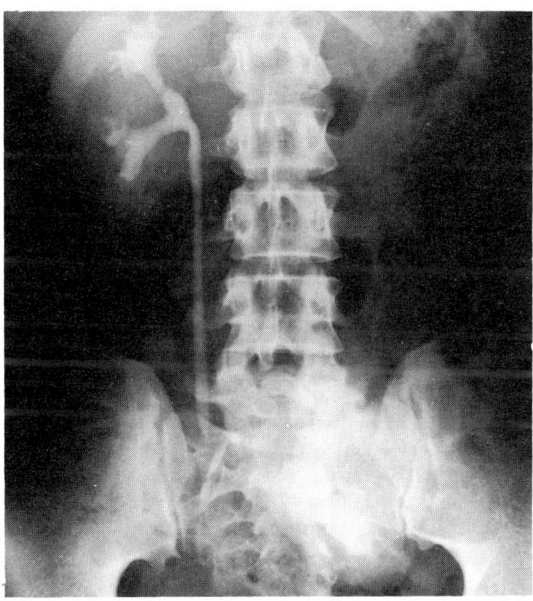

Fig. 5 IVU showing normal right kidney and ureter, and left pelvic kidney.

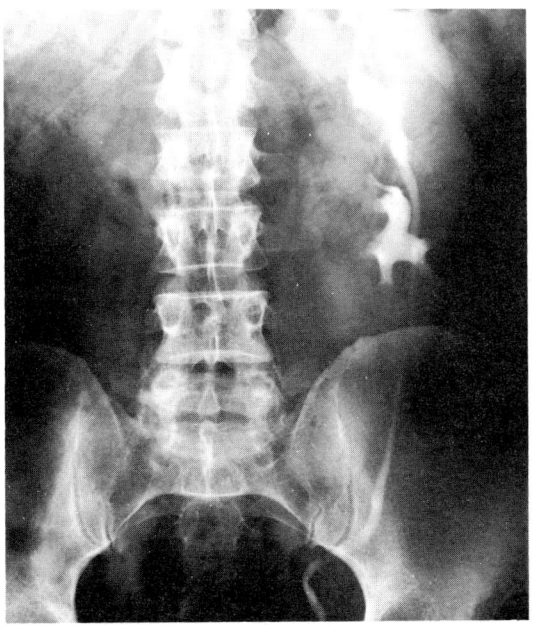

Fig. 6 IVU showing crossed ectopia.

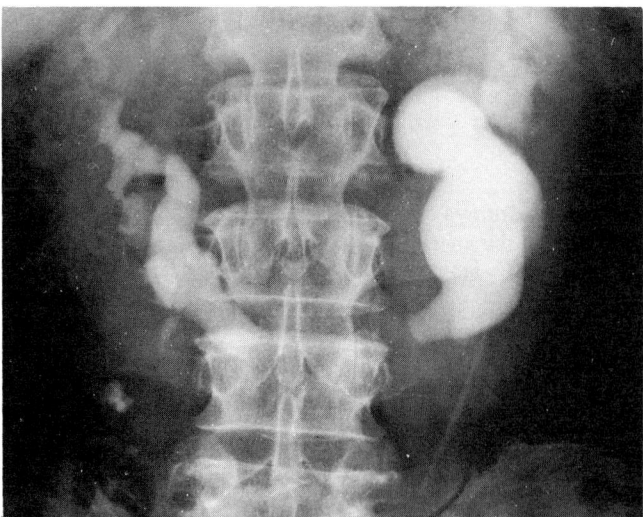

Fig. 7 IVU showing horseshoe kidney. Dilation of left calyces and pelvis.

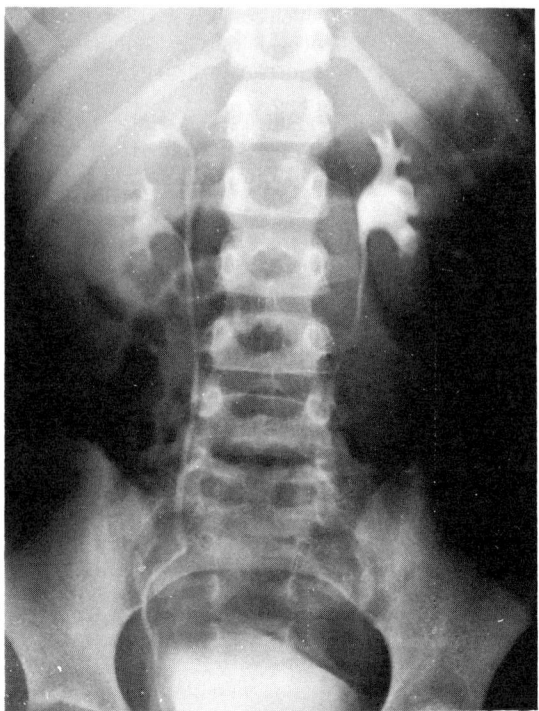

Fig. 8 IVU showing duplex right kidney and normal left kidney.

between the aorta and inferior vena cava. Some degree of malrotation of the kidneys is associated with fusion, and one or both ureters may lie behind the isthmus.

Complications of this condition are related to urinary drainage, so that infection, obstruction, and stones occur.

Renal dysplasia

Defective differentiation of the parenchyma during nephrogenesis results in morphological disorganization with the development of abnormal primitive tubular and mesenchymal structures, rudimentary glomeruli, and often cyst formation. Renal dysplasia may affect one or both kidneys partially or totally. Dysplastic tissues are non-functional and are often associated with ureteric ectopia. Developmental abnormalities of the gastrointestinal tract, heart, and the neural tube are sometimes associated.

Abnormalities of the pelvis and ureters

There are many developmental anomalies of these structures which are mainly of interest to urologists; many of them are amenable to surgical correction.

Pelvi-ureteric junction obstruction

This is due either to obstruction by an aberrant branch of the renal artery crossing the pelvi-ureteric junction or to disorganization of neuromuscular tissues at the pelvi-ureteric junction. The result may be massive dilation of the calyces and pelvis which, if long-standing, will destroy renal function on that side. Pain, swelling, infection, and haematuria may be the presenting symptoms.

Duplication of the pelvis and ureter

This is a common abnormality and occurs more frequently in females than in males. Ureteric duplication may be partial or complete (Fig. 8). Partial duplication rarely causes trouble, although reflux can occur from one segment to the other with resulting pain. In complete duplication the ureter from the upper renal moiety enters the bladder in an ectopic position low in the bladder, in the urethra, or vagina. Incontinence or reflux and infection are common complications. The diagnosis is made radiologically – the renal mass appearing larger than expected but with atrophy and scarring usually of the upper portion. In the presence of repeated infections, hypertension or pain, careful consideration should be given to the possibility of surgical removal of the affected moiety of the kidney with its accompanying ureter. In the totally asymptomatic person in whom this is found purely accidentally, there is no indication for immediate surgical intervention.

Ureterocoéle

An ectopic ureter is frequently associated with an ureterocoele – a cystic dilation of the intravesical portion of the ureter. This dilation may reach quite large proportions and is usually associated with vesico-ureteric reflux. In ureteric duplication the ectopic ureter is often associated with an ureterocoele which may result in obstruction to both ureters.

Chronic ureteric dilation

Obstruction due to defective function of the muscular coat of the lower end of the ureter can lead to gross dilation and tortuosity of the upper ureter. This condition can be distinguished radiologically from ureteric dilation associated with the 'prune belly' and 'megacystis megaureter' syndromes. If obstruction is proved by pressure-flow studies, excision of the lower ureter and reimplantation is indicated.

Congenital bladder and urethral abnormalities

Failure of development of the anterior abdominal wall and pubic bones is associated with malformation of the anterior bladder wall resulting in *ectopia vesicae* and *epispadias*. The bladder mucosa, ureteric orifices, and trigone are exposed. *Persistence* of the *urachus*, which is the embryonic tube connecting the bladder and allantois, leads to a urinary fistula from the umbilicus. If partial closure occurs, urachal cysts may develop.

Absence of abdominal musculature gives rise to the characteristic 'prune belly' syndrome which is invariably associated with dilation of the whole urinary tract and cryptorchidism.

Congenital urethral valves commonly cause urinary obstruction in male infants. If the condition is not recognized and treated, chronic renal failure will supervene. Diagnosis can usually be made by intravenous urography and the surgical correction is a very simple procedure.

References

Polycystic disease
Bricker, N. S. and Patton, J. F. (1955). Cystic disease of the kidneys: a study of dynamics and chemical composition of cyst fluid. *Am. J. Med.* **18**, 207–219.

British Medical Journal (1981). Adult polycystic disease of the kidneys. *Br. med J.* **282**, 1097–1098.

Dalgaard, O. Z. (1957). Bilateral polycystic disease of the kidneys. *Acta med. scand.* **158**, suppl. 328, 13–250.

De Bono, D. P. and Evans, D. B. (1977). The management of polycystic kidney disease with special reference to dialysis and transplantation. *Q. J. Med.* **46**, 353–363.

Kissane, J. M. (1979). Adult polycystic disease. In *Nephrology* (ed. Hamburger, Crosnier, and Grünfeld. Published by Wiley-Flammarion.

Kumar, S., Cederbaum, A. I., and Pletka, P. G. (1980). Renal cell carcinoma in polycystic kidneys: case report and review of literature. *J. Urol.* **124**, 708–709.

Ng, R. C. K. and Suki, W. N. (1980). Renal cell carcinoma occurring in a polycystic kidney of a transplant recipient. *J. Urol.* **124**, 710–712.

Reeders, S. T., Breuning, M. H., Davies, K. E., Nicholls, R. D., Jarman, A. P., Higgs, D. R., Pearson, P. L. and Weatherall, D. J. (1985). A highly polymorphic DNA marker linked to adult polycystic kidney disease on chromosome 16. *Nature* **317**, 542–544.

Tumours

Brown, J. J., Lever, A. F., Robertson, J. S., Fraser, R., Morton, J. J., Tree, M., Bell, P. R. F., Davidson, J. K., and Ruthven, I. S. (1973). Hypertension and secondary hyperaldosteronism associated with a renin secreting renal juxtaglomerular tumour. *Lancet* ii, 1228–1232.

Calne, R. Y. (1973). Treatment of bilateral hypernephromas by nephrectomy, excision of tumour and autotransplantation. *Lancet* ii, 1164–1167.

Cronin, R. E., Kaehny, W. D., Miller, P. D., Stables, D. P., Gablow, P. A., Ostroy, P. R., and Schrier, R. W. (1976). Renal cell carcinoma. Unusual systemic manifestations. *Medicine (Balt.)* **55**, 291–311.

Grawitz, P. (1883). Die sogenannten lipone der niere. *Virchows Archs.* **93**, 39.

Riches, E. W. (1963). Carcinoma of the kidney (lecture) *Ann. R. Coll. Surg. Eng.* **32**, 201–218.

Woodruff, M. F. A. (1969). Immunosuppression and cancer. *Lancet* i, 672.

Congenital abnormalities

Williams, D. I. (1974). Urology in childhood. In *Encyclopaedia of urology*. New York.

THE RENAL TUBULAR ACIDOSES

R. D. COHEN

Introduction

Renal tubular acidosis (RTA) is the term used to describe metabolic acidoses whose cause is a disorder of the renal tubules. The designation distinguishes this type of acidosis from that accompanying generalized glomerulotubular failure (uraemic acidosis). It is, however, of considerable importance that glomerular failure may supervene in chronic renal tubular acidosis – an outcome which may in some instances be prevented by treatment. The pathogenesis of uraemic acidosis has been described on pages 18.136 and 9.172.

Normal acid–base function of the kidney

In normal acid-base function of the kidney (Fig. 1a) both the proximal and distal nephron normally actively secrete hydrogen ions (H^+). A major function of H^+ secretion in the proximal tubule is the reabsorption of filtered bicarbonate. In the healthy adult about 4500 mmol of bicarbonate are filtered per day, and all but 10–15 per cent of this is titrated by secreted H^+ in the proximal tubule to form carbonic acid, which is rapidly dehydrated to carbon dioxide and water by brush border carbonic anhydrase. The CO_2 diffuses into the proximal tubular cells; here it combines with hydroxyl ions (generated when the original H^+ was pumped out into the lumen) to form bicarbonate, which then passes into the peritubular capillaries. Thus for each H^+ secreted, a single HCO_3^- ion is effectively reabsorbed.

That HCO_3^-, which escapes reabsorption by the above mechanism in the proximal nephron, passes to the distal nephron, where, in the common situation where final urine pH is less than 6.5, it is completely reabsorbed by further H^+ secretion. Events so far described have thus used H^+ secretion to reclaim filtered bicarbonate, and have done nothing to dispose of H^+ in response to any acid burden that requires correction. Nearly all authors describe how further H^+ secretion titrates phosphate buffer in the tubular lumen thus:

$$HPO_4^{2-} + H^+ \rightarrow H_2PO_4^-$$

and ammonia (NH_3), which has been formed in the tubular cells and has passed into the lumen by non-ionic diffusion, as follows:

$$NH_3 + H^+ \rightarrow NH_4^+$$

The amount of H^+ 'locked up' in $H_2PO_4^-$ can be approximately determined by titrating the urine back to pH 7.4, and is known as 'titratable acidity'. The total amount of net acid excreted by the kidney is therefore conventionally regarded as the excretion of

(titratable acid + ammonium − bicarbonate)

The bicarbonate term has been included to cover the situation where an alkaline urine is passed and bicarbonate has not been completely reclaimed. The total net acid excretion in the urine calculated in this way amounts to 50–100 mmol/day, the contribution of ammonium being typically 2–3 times greater than that of titratable acidity and that of bicarbonate very small. During any tendency to acidosis, H^+ secretion is enhanced; the phosphate buffer is more completely titrated, resulting in an increase in titratable acidity and lowering of urine pH. Furthermore, ammonia synthesis and diffusion into the urine is increased by a variety of mechanisms, so more H^+ is excreted as NH_4^+. Bicarbonate excretion is reduced to zero and, given sufficient stimulus, the urine reaches its minimum possible pH which varies between normal individuals in the range 4.4–5.3. The final acidification is achieved in the medullary collecting duct. The acidoses seen in different types of RTA are in conventional descriptions regarded as being ultimately due to various defects leading to inappropriately low excretion of H^+ buffered either as titratable acidity or NH_4^+ and/or to excessive excretion of bicarbonate.

However, in the past decade a major reinterpretation of the role of the kidney in acid–base homeostasis has been proposed by Oliver and Bourke and by Atkinson and Camien (see page 9.165 onwards). As explained there in more detail, they point out that, since ammonium is generated from glutamine virtually entirely as NH_4^+, there is no possibility of it acting as a significant buffer for H^+. This means that the ammonium term has to be deleted from the expression for net renal acid excretion, which now becomes:

(titratable acid − bicarbonate)

Nevertheless, renal excretion of NH_4^+ still remains of major importance for acid–base status, but *indirectly* in the following way. If one considers the total daily nitrogen load to be excreted, the majority of this excretion takes place by conversion to urea in

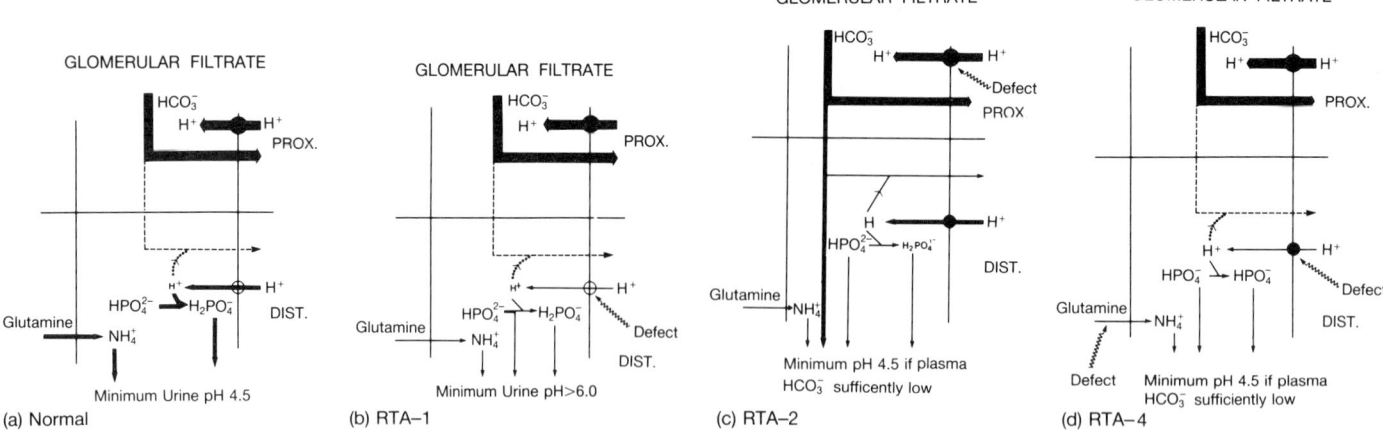

Fig. 1 Diagrams to indicate the site of the defects in different types of RTA. (a) Normal, (b) RTA-1—gradient defect in distal nephron, (c) RTA-2—proximal HCO_3^- reabsorption defect due to reduced H^+ secretion, (d) RTA-4—defects in NH_4^+ production and in capacity of H^+ pump in distal nephron due to hypoaldosteronism. The thickness of the arrows indicates the magnitude of the ionic fluxes (not to scale). See text for further explanation.

the liver and subsequent urinary excretion, most of the remaining nitrogen being excreted as NH_4^+ in the urine. Now, whenever a molecule of urea is synthesized, two H^+ ions are produced as byproducts. These H^+ are normally used to neutralize the large quantity of bicarbonate produced by metabolism of the non-amino portions of the amino acids constituting the proteins from which the urea was derived. If, however, there is a defect in the renal excretion of ammonium, the liver is forced to increase urea synthesis, with the consequent production of more H^+ than is needed to neutralize the amino acid-derived bicarbonate. Acidosis therefore results. Under this interpretation, therefore, that part of the acidosis in RTA which is due to underexcretion of NH_4^+ in the urine results from overproduction of urea, not from failure of excretion of H^+ buffered as NH_4^+. It is not known, however, how precisely the liver responds reciprocally by increasing urea synthesis when confronted with a decrease in urinary excretion of NH_4^+. The reader should bear this reinterpretation in mind when reading the extensive literature on RTA, which almost invariably regards the conventional calculation given above as a precise estimate of renal excretion of acid. The present author has yet to see a convincing argument against the above reinterpretation.

In the following description, RTA is broken down into three main categories, on the basis of clearly identifiable differences in pathogenesis.

Distal renal tubular acidosis ('classical' RTA, 'gradient RTA', RTA type 1)

This form of RTA (RTA-1) is characterized by an inability to generate a normal minimum urinary pH even in the presence of severe systemic acidosis. It may present in infancy, childhood or adult life, most typically with acute acidosis and hyperventilation, often accompanied by muscular weakness due to hypokalaemia. In most patients the attacks of acute acidosis represent a worsening of a mild chronic hyperchloraemic metabolic acidosis which may have been fully compensated until presentation. About 70 per cent of patients are found to have either nephrocalcinosis or calcium-containing renal calculi. Rickets and growth stunting in childhood are frequent features and osteomalacia may be seen in adults. Though glomerular filtration rate is characteristically normal or nearly so at the outset, progressive nephrocalcinosis, obstructive uropathy related to calculi, and recurrent urinary tract infections may eventually result in glomerular failure.

The *diagnosis* in the acute state is usually simple and depends on the observation of a urinary pH greater than 5.5 (and usually greater than 6) in the presence of a normal anion gap metabolic acidosis (see page 9.167), hyperchloraemia, and normal or nearly normal plasma urea and creatinine. Severe hypokalaemia, evidence of renal calcification, and the presence of clinical features related to one of the aetiologies discussed below may provide further evidence. The failure to acidify the urine maximally in the presence of severe acidosis (plasma bicarbonate < 12 mmol/l) serves to distinguish the condition from RTA types 2 and 4. Nephrocalcinosis is virtually confined to RTA-1. In the chronic non-acute state, which often presents with renal stones, incidental discovery of nephrocalcinosis, failure of growth, anorexia or lethargy, the diagnosis may be confirmed by the short acid load test (Wrong and Davies), the critical finding being the failure to achieve normal minimum urinary pH after ingestion of a standard body weight-related dose of ammonium chloride. Wrong and Davies also draw attention to a group of patients with nephrocalcinosis and failure to acidify the urine normally on ammonium chloride challenge, but did not have systemic acidosis ('incomplete syndrome of RTA'). It should be noted that it is neither necessary nor safe to administer the acid load test if the plasma bicarbonate is below 19 mmol/l. Under such conditions comparison of urinary pH with plasma bicarbonate, and arterial pH and PCO_2 should suffice.

Pathophysiology

RTA-1 is due to a failure of the distal nephron and collecting duct, to generate the 800–900:1 H^+ gradient between tubular lumen and blood that a normal subject can achieve under acidifying conditions. Except in rare patients with mixed syndromes, proximal tubular function is normal in terms of H^+ secretion and bicarbonate reabsorption. In RTA-1, the distal nephron defect is variable in severity, but if the urine pH cannot be lowered below 6–6.5 increasingly large quantities of bicarbonate may appear in the urine. This bicarbonate represents that proportion of the 10–15 per cent of filtered bicarbonate which has reached the distal nephron, but has not been reabsorbed because of failure of distal H^+ secretion. The H^+ secretion defect also results in the failure of titration of phosphate buffer. Because NH_4^+ excretion is lessened in alkaline urine, it may be lower than appropriate for systemic pH; under the reinterpretation discussed above, failure of NH_4^+ excretion would encourage increased urea synthesis and H^+ generation. All these factors, which are direct consequences of the distal tubular defect, lead to acidosis (see Fig. 1b). In children in particular, loss of bicarbonate may be a major contributor.

The precise nature of the defect which results in failure to establish the normal H^+ gradient is in most instances unknown. Theoretically, it could result from a failure of active H^+ secretion in the distal nephron, or, alternatively, an abnormal permeability of the distal nephron to H^+, resulting in leak-back of H^+ after secretion. The latter mechanism is clearly seen in RTA-1 occurring during amphotericin B therapy. This antifungal agent acts as a protonophore, i.e. it inserts itself into the luminal cell membrane in the distal nephron and provides a channel for back leakage of H^+ into the cell. Another possible mechanism is deficiency of distal cellular carbonic anhydrase; the isoenzyme present is carbonic anhydrase II and hereditary deficiency has been described in association with osteopetrosis and RTA-1. However, carbonic anhydrase is normal in the vast majority of cases.

A marked reduction in urinary citrate excretion is seen in RTA-1 and has been considered to be an indication of abnormal mitochondrial function in distal nephron cells, but there is no direct evidence to substantiate this view.

The hypokalaemia frequently present has two origins. Firstly, lack of H^+ flux out of the tubular cell into the lumen encourages K^+ exchange for luminal Na^+ in the distal nephron; even so, overall distal Na^+ reabsorption is impaired, leading to secondary aldosteronism, which provides the second reason for renal K^+ wasting. Correction of the acidosis, which raises distal luminal pH and therefore permits more H^+ secretion, results in amelioration of Na^+ and K^+ wasting (in contrast to RTA-2, see below).

Renal lithiasis is generally attributed to the hypercalcuria and hypocitraturia. Citrate complexes with calcium ions to form the $CaCit^-$ ion, which is partly responsible for maintaining calcium ions in solution in the urine and a situation in which there is both lack of citrate and increased calcium is likely to be lithogenic. The pathogenesis of the nephrocalcinosis is unclear. So is that of osteomalacia/rickets, which can be corrected by treatment of the chronic acidosis without vitamin D therapy. There is no evidence in humans for interference with vitamin D metabolism in acidosis, though transient depression of renal 1-hydroxylation of vitamin D by acidosis has been observed in animals.

Causes of RTA-1

RTA-1 may occur as a primary disorder, or secondary to a whole range of conditions which in one way or another affect distal nephron function.

The primary disorder may be clearly hereditary, or may be sporadic. The hereditary form behaves as an autosomal dominant and may present in childhood or in adult life. There is, however, an infantile form of the condition which is transient and may occur in siblings without other family history. It is not clear whether this is a recessive disorder, or due to environmental factors. The rare hereditary carbonic anhydrase deficiency has been referred to earlier.

In the acquired category, RTA-1 associated with presumptively autoimmune disorders account for a significant proportion of cases. Sjögren's syndrome is the most prominent association in this group, but other dysglobulinaemic or hypergammaglobulinaemic conditions also give rise to RTA-1. It does not appear, however, that the raised plasma globulin itself is the determining factor. RTA-1 is occasionally seen in primary biliary cirrhosis and, rarely, in fibrosing alveolitis. Although RTA-1 is a cause of nephrocalcinosis it seems fairly clear that nephrocalcinosis itself can, by causing medullary damage, give rise to RTA-1. Thus, for instance, hyperparathyroidism and chronic vitamin D poisoning may cause RTA-1 because of nephrocalcinosis. Conditions directly damaging the renal medulla, such as pyelonephritis, papillary necrosis, chronic obstructive uropathy, medullary sponge kidney, and sickle cell anaemia may also give rise to varying degrees of RTA-1. Amongst drug-related causes, analgesic nephropathy presumably acts through papillary damage; the RTA-1 associated with amphotericin B therapy has been explained above.

Treatment

The acutely acidotic patient will usually have moderate to very marked hypokalaemia. It is essential that the hypokalaemia be corrected *before* the acidosis. If, mistakenly, the acidosis is dealt with before the hypokalaemia, movement of K^+ into cells will further lower plasma K^+ and cardiac arrest may occur. Potassium, and then isotonic sodium bicarbonate are administered intravenously, aiming to restore the abnormalities over a few hours. If hypokalaemia has caused muscular weakness leading to respiratory insufficiency, artificial ventilation is imperative.

In the chronic condition, therapy with oral sodium bicarbonate has markedly beneficial effects. Not only will it prevent recurrent exacerbations of acidosis, but renal potassium loss will be curtailed, hypercalcuria will be diminished and hypocitraturia improved, osteomalacia or rickets healed and growth restored in children.

In addition, progression of nephrocalcinosis and nephrolithiasis and consequent renal damage may be halted. The daily bicarbonate requirement is usually in the range 1–3 mmol/kg body weight. Not infrequently, potassium supplements are required in addition to sodium bicarbonate.

Proximal renal tubular acidosis (RTA Type 2; bicarbonate wasting RTA.)

This form of RTA (Fig. 1c) is superficially clinically similar to RTA-1, but there are notable distinguishing features. It is rare as an isolated defect and in the great majority of patients is associated with multiple abnormalities of proximal tubular function, e.g. glycosuria, aminoaciduria, hyperphosphaturia, and uricosuria. Provided the patient is sufficiently acidotic, the urine pH falls to the normal minimum. Nephrocalcinosis and renal calculi are virtually never present. Bicarbonate leakage into the urine is much greater than in RTA-1 and, in consequence, very large quantities of sodium bicarbonate may be required for therapy. There may be marked polyuria and polydipsia, especially in those patients in whom the acidosis has been fully controlled by bicarbonate therapy. Proximal myopathy, osteomalacia or rickets are common associations of RTA-2, probably largely because of the frequent aetiological involvement of disorders of vitamin D supply or metabolism. RTA-2 resembles RTA-1 in that it presents with a chronic (or acute exacerbation of) normal anion gap hyperchloraemic acidosis with a marked tendency to potassium deficiency due to renal potassium loss.

Pathophysiology

The basic lesion in RTA-2 is a depression of the capacity of the proximal tubule to secrete H^+ and thus to reabsorb bicarbonate. In a normal individual or in a patient with RTA-1, bicarbonate does not appear in the urine until the plasma bicarbonate is above 25–28 mmol/l. In RTA-2 this bicarbonate 'threshold' is lowered, often markedly so, due to the proximal tubular defect. The result is that the distal nephron is flooded with bicarbonate which has escaped proximal reabsorption, and the low capacity (but high gradient) distal H^+ secreting mechanism cannot produce enough H^+ to reabsorb this bicarbonate, which therefore spills over into the urine. However, when, in consequence of the bicarbonate leak, plasma bicarbonate falls to a level which reduces the filtered bicarbonate load to one with which the defective proximal tubule can cope, then the distal nephron is fully capable of producing a normally minimal urinary pH of 4.5–5.3 (Fig. 1c). The acidosis in RTA-2 is predominantly due to the bicarbonate leak, but it is to a lesser extent related to failure of titration of phosphate and failure of appropriate NH_4^+ excretion due to the inappropriately high urine pH—at least while plasma bicarbonate remains above the renal threshold. The high distal load of sodium bicarbonate is also responsible for sodium wastage. This leads to secondary aldosteronism, which, together with the high demand created for Na^+/K^+ exchange in the distal nephron, results in potassium wastage and hypokalaemia. The polyuria is due both to the distal sodium bicarbonate load and to the effects of potassium deficiency on the renal concentrating mechanism. When osteomalacia/rickets is seen in RTA-2 it may be related both to the basic cause of the syndrome (see below) and possibly to the acidosis itself.

Causes of RTA-2

Nearly always some factor which damages proximal tubular function can be identified. However, familial autosomal dominant RTA-2 has been reported as an isolated lesion. Isolated damage to the proximal tubular H^+ secretion mechanism occurs during treatment with the carbonic anhydrase inhibitor acetazolamide and in carbonic anhydrase II deficiency, in which there is also an element of RTA-1.

More usually RTA-2 occurs as a part of more generalized proximal tubular damage with reabsorption defects for glucose, amino acids, and phosphate, i.e. the Fanconi syndrome. There are many causes of the Fanconi syndrome—in the genetic category are included cystinosis, Wilson's disease, hereditary fructose intolerance as well as the idiopathic variety. Amongst acquired causes of RTA-2/Fanconi syndrome may be listed vitamin D deficiency, lead poisoning, multiple myeloma, thereapy with outdated tetracycline, hyperparathyroidism, and the nephrotic syndrome. A more comprehensive list has been compiled by Sebastian and Morris. The precise mechanisms of damage in patients with RTA-2/Fanconi syndrome are not usually clear. However, in hereditary fructose intolerance the absence of fructose-1-phosphate aldolase in the proximal tubular cells results in the accumulation of fructose-1-phosphate during fructose ingestion. Fructose phosphorylation depletes ATP stores markedly and the generalized tubular malfunction may be due to this perturbation of energy metabolism. In vitamin D deficiency, the lesion is probably contributed to both by the deficiency itself and by the accompanying secondary hyperparathyroidism.

Therapy

The bicarbonate leak is much more severe in RTA-2 than in RTA-1, and the daily dose of sodium bicarbonate needed to prevent acidosis may be very large (3–20 mmol/kg body weight). In contrast to RTA-1, effective treatment of the acidosis in RTA-2 does not help, and may worsen the potassium deficiency and polyuria, by providing an even greater sodium bicarbonate load to the distal tubule. If glomerular failure ensues, as for example in cystinosis, then the bicarbonate requirement may lessen. Potassium supplements in the form of oral bicarbonate will be required. If the amount of oral bicarbonate needed is intolerable, hydrochlorthiazide may be added. This agent appears to increase proximal bicarbonate reabsorption and diminish the bicarbonate requirement but may necessitate an increase in potassium supplementation.

Hyperkalaemic renal tubular acidosis (RTA type 4)

During the past decade attention has been increasingly drawn to a form of renal tubular acidosis characterized by hyperkalaemia rather than hypokalaemia. As in RTA-1 and RTA-2, patients present with metabolic acidosis in which the anion gap is normal or nearly so and there is a similar tendency to hyperchloraemia. As in RTA-2, if the plasma bicarbonate falls sufficiently, then the distal tubule is able to amount to a normal blood/urine pH gradient. These patients frequently have slight or moderate glomerular impairment, but the degree of hyperkalaemia is quite out of proportion to this (see page 18.35).

Pathophysiology

It is clear that the basic abnormality behind the many aetiologies of RTA-4 is either hypoaldosteronism or failure of aldosterone action. Mineralocorticoid deficiency diminishes the capacity of the

H^+ secreting mechanism in the distal nephron, but not its power to sustain a pH gradient if bicarbonate delivery from the proximal tubule is small. There is no evidence of a proximal tubular defect in H^+ secretion and bicarbonate reabsorption. The hyperkalaemia is a direct consequence of the mineralocorticoid deficiency and has the additional effect of suppressing renal production of NH_4^+, the excretion of which is diminished in RTA-4. The nitrogen not thus excreted is converted to urea and H^+ in the liver. In this way the failure of NH_4^+ excretion in RTA-4 is largely responsible for the acidosis (Fig. 1d).

Causes

Aldosterone deficiency leading to RTA-4 may be due to primary adrenal disease, as in Addison's disease and certain inborn errors of steroid synthesis. However, much more commonly it is related to deficient renin production, which may be seen in many chronic renal disorders, most notably in diabetes and chronic tubulo-interstitial disease, including pyelonephritis. Renin production is to some extent dependent on prostaglandin synthesis, and increasingly commonly RTA-4 is being seen in patients receiving prostaglandin synthetase inhibitors in the form of non-steroidal anti-inflammatory agents. Finally, RTA-4 is seen in patients receiving aldosterone antagonists and in infants with pseudo-hypoaldosteronism; in both these circumstances there is a renal insensitivity to aldosterone action.

Treatment

Patients with RTA-4 in which acidosis is significant or hyperkalaemia is potentially dangerous should be treated with a mineralocorticoid. Typically 0.05–0.15 mg fludrocortisone daily improves NH_4^+ excretion, and restores hyperkalaemia and acidosis towards normal.

Differential diagnosis of the different types of renal tubular acidosis

For convenience, the points of distinction between the different types of RTA have been summarized in Table 1, the contents of which have been restricted to the simpler clinical considerations.

Table 1

	RTA-1	RTA-2	RTA-4
Urine pH when plasma HCO_3^- <13 mmol/l	>6	<5.4	<5.4
Plasma potassium	Low	Low	Raised
Nephrocalcinosis or renal lithiasis	+	−	−
Therapeutic requirement For bicarbonate For mineralocorticoid	Modest −	Large −	Modest +

References

Morris, R. C. and Sebastian, A. (1983). Renal tubular acidosis and the Fanconi syndrome. In *The metabolic basis of inherited disease* 5th edn (eds J. B. Stanbury, J. B. Wyngaarden, D. S. Frederickson, J. L. Goldstein and M. S. Brown). McGraw-Hill, New York.

Sebastian, A. and Morris, R. C. (1977). Renal tubular acidosis. *Clin. Nephrol.* **7**, 216–230.

Seldin, D. W. and Wilson, J. D. (1978). Renal tubular acidosis. In *The metabolic basis of inherited disease* 4th edn (eds J. B. Stanbury, J. B. Wyngaarden and D. S. Frederickson). McGraw-Hill, New York.

Wrong, O. M. and Davies, H. E. F. (1959). The excretion of acid in renal disease. *Q. J. Med.* **28**, 259–313.

GENITOURINARY TUBERCULOSIS

J. C. SMITH

Tuberculosis of the genitourinary tract (GUTB), although declining in incidence, still remains an important clinical problem in both the indigent and immigrant populations in the United Kingdom. As it becomes rare, clinicians become less alert diagnostically and the disease may be missed, especially in its early stages. It remains more common in Eastern Europe and in developing countries. It probably develops in some 3–4 per cent of cases of pulmonary tuberculosis (see also page 18.78).

Presentation

Most cases present with frequency of micturition and dysuria and are usually treated as 'difficult cases of cystitis'. Haematuria is not uncommon. Other manifestations include a renal mass, pain or swelling of the epididymis, or, more rarely, hypertension. However, the condition may be symptomless and a calcified tuberculosis pyonephrosis may be found on routine X-rays of patients who deny any previous urinary symptoms. Tuberculous prostatitis and urethritis are rare.

Investigation

Urine examination

GUTB should be suspected in any case of pyuria where an organism cannot readily be cultured. 'Sterile pyuria', once the hallmark of GUTB, is now much more common as the result of antimicrobial therapy of other types of bacterial infections or of analgesic nephropathy.

The organisms of *Mycobacterium tuberculosis* are excreted in the urine in scanty numbers and are best found by repeated microscopy and culture of early morning specimens of urine (at least three and possibly up to six specimens). The diagnosis should never be made solely on the finding of acid-fast bacilli in the urine as smegma bacilli may give a similar appearance. Cultures may take several weeks to grow but the diagnosis is rarely of urgent importance and treatment should be withheld until the positive confirmation by culture is obtained.

Radiology

An intravenous urogram is essential in all cases of suspected GUTB. The plain X-ray may show areas of calcification and excretion pictures will reveal the two main causes of renal damage, destruction of the parenchyma and obstruction of the drainage system (Figs 1–3). Both of these are manifestations of late disease but tuberculosis should be suspected in all cases of renal scarring where there is also ureteric obstruction. Arteriography is rarely indicated.

All cases of renal tuberculosis are initially bilateral as spread of the organism occurs via the blood stream. Many of the resulting small areas of infection heal spontaneously, but others progress to form closed abscess cavities. Still others nearer the calyces will ulcerate and discharge their contents into the collecting systems forming communicating cavities.

Obstruction of the collecting system may result in calyceal stenosis with 'silent' areas in the kidney, pelvi-ureteric junction obstruction with hydronephrosis, or obstruction further down in the ureter particularly at the uretero-vesical junction.

Tuberculous cystitis is always secondary to renal tuberculosis and results in a small capacity bladder possibly associated with vesicoureteric reflux. *Cystoscopy* is rarely necessary to make the diagnosis but should be performed in all cases of haematuria. Tubercles may be seen around an affected ureter but all unusual lesions should be biopsied. Not only may this give a rapid histolo-

gical diagnosis of tuberculosis but it may also exclude (or confirm) the presence of a bladder neoplasm which may occasionally mimic tuberculosis.

Indication for therapy

Treatment should usually be withheld until a positive culture and sensitivities of the organism have been obtained. However, when classical radiological appearances are accompanied by acid-fast bacilli in the urine or there has been a positive bladder biopsy treatment may be begun immediately, particularly if the disease is advanced. Therapy should never be started on weak diagnostic grounds since once it has been started, it may be impossible to obtain confirmation and the diagnosis will forever be in doubt.

Medical treatment

Antimicrobial therapy

Medical treatment is by the use of standard antituberculous therapy (see Section 5 and page 18.78) with particular care if there is any evidence of renal impairment. Traditionally long courses of treatment (one to two years) were advised but with increasing experience and new drugs, shorter courses (six months) have been advocated.

The addition of corticosteroid drugs has been suggested to prevent the complication of healing fibrosis with either obstruction of the upper tracts or reduction in the capacity of the bladder. If the initial intravenous urogram shows obstruction, a further urogram should be obtained four or six weeks later. This may show no change, improvement, or deterioration, and if the last, a course of corticosteroids with repeated urograms may lessen the need for later surgery to correct obstruction.

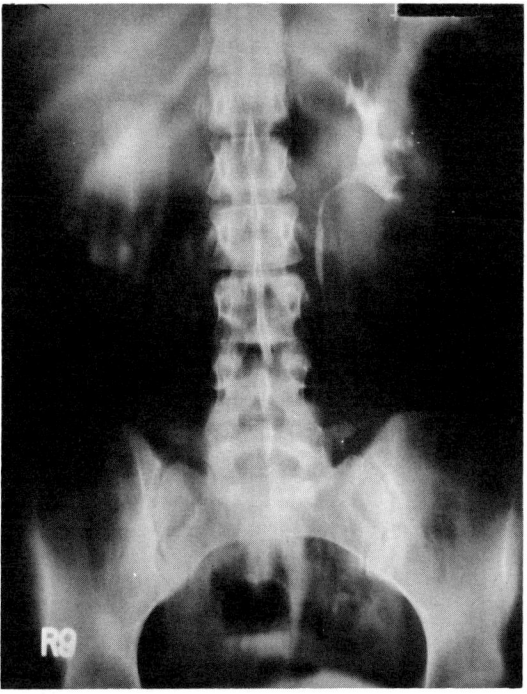

Fig. 1 Bilateral renal tuberculosis showing right hydronephrosis secondary to obstruction of the lower ureter and a closed cavity. Note the absence of normal calyces in the lower pole of the left kidney.

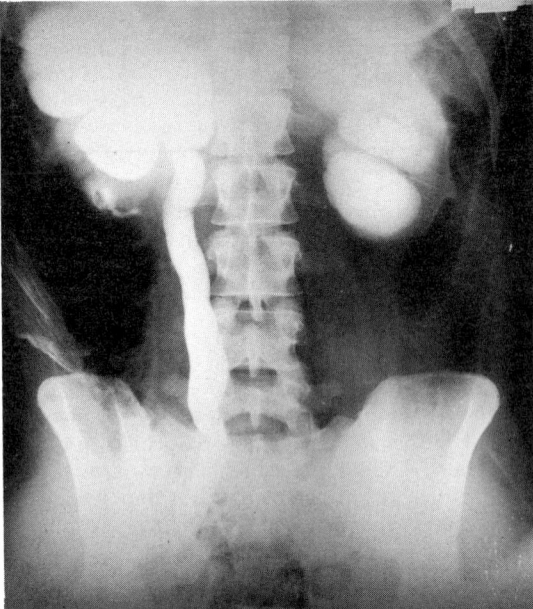

Fig. 2 Shows clearer detail outlined by right antegrade (percutaneous) pyelogram and left cyst puncture. Surgical treatment consisted of reimplantation of the right ureter and excision of the lower pole of the left kidney (cavernostomy).

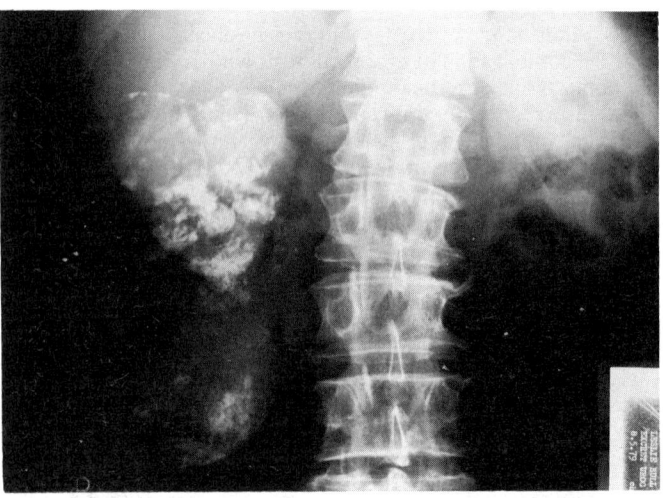

Fig. 3 Calcified tuberculous pyonephrosis. Nephrectomy is usually advisable in this condition as miliary spread otherwise remains a threat for the future. The operation should be covered by a short course (six weeks) of appropriate antimicrobial therapy.

Surgical treatment

Surgery has three main roles in the treatment of GUTB.

1. Excision of destroyed tissue which has failed to respond to antimicrobial therapy. This includes nephrectomy for functionless tuberculous pyonephrosis and, much less commonly, polar nephrectomy for more localized disease. Tuberculous renal abscesses may now be treated with aspiration and instillation of antimicrobials.

Excision of epididymal masses which fail to resolve on antibiotic treatment may be necessary.

These surgical procedures may be performed after a few weeks of antimicrobial therapy given in adequate dosage.

2. Correction of obstruction in the upper urinary tract. As mentioned above, tuberculosis produces obstruction of the calyces or ureters by inflammation and fibrosis. On many occasions the obstruction will resolve with antimicrobial treatment with or without the addition of corticosteroids. If the obstruction persists or increases, surgical treatment may be necessary to correct pelviureteric junction obstruction (pyeloplasty) or uretero-vesical junction obstruction (reimplantation of the ureter). These operations should be done during the course of medical therapy, timing depending on the radiological progress of the obstruction, and overall renal function.

3. Enlargement of the contracted bladder by enterocystoplasty (ileo, colo, or caecocystoplasty) is necessary in severe bladder tuberculosis where the healing process results in a contracted bladder with resultant great frequency and nocturia. It should rarely be performed early in the period of treatment for sometimes surprising improvement follows the use of antituberculous drugs. In most instances, the trigone can be preserved and the bowel simply used to increase the bladder capacity leaving the uretero-vesical valve in situ.

Follow up

After all treatment, but especially after short courses of therapy, careful follow up is desirable with urine cultures and further radiology when indicated.

Most authors record at least five years of follow up but others report relapses after many years, particularly among patients treated with inadequate drug combinations given in the early days of antituberculous therapy.

References

Butler, M. R. and O'Flynn, J. D. (1975). Reactivation of genito-urinary tuberculosis. *Eur. Urol.* **1**, 14–17.
Gow, J. G. (1976). Genito-urinary tuberculosis. In *Urology* (ed. J. P. Blandy), pp. 226–260. Blackwell Scientific Publications, Oxford.
—— (1979). Genito-urinary tuberculosis. *Br. J. Hosp. Med.* **22**, 556.
Skutil, V. and Gow, J. G. (1977). Urogenital tuberculosis. *Eur. Urol.* **3**, 257–272.

GEOGRAPHICAL VARIATION IN RENAL DISEASE

SOUTHEAST ASIA

V. SITPRIJA

The spectrum of renal diseases in southeast Asia, in general, does not differ from that in other geographical areas. However, because of the tropical environment, difference in socio-economy, culture, and genetic variation, certain diseases are prevalent, and some are unique, e.g. tropical nephropathy. Attention will therefore be focused on these renal diseases.

Glomerulonephritis

The pattern of glomerular diseases in southeast Asia differs somewhat from that of the western world. Mesangial IgM proliferative glomerulonephritis, IgA nephropathy, and focal glomerulosclerosis are common while minimal change lesion is less frequent. Lupus nephritis has a high incidence. A mild form of glomerulonephritis following infection is often observed.

Mesangial IgM proliferative glomerulonephritis

This glomerular disease constitutes 35 to 40 per cent of all idiopathic glomerulonephritis in Thailand. It is the common cause of nephrotic syndrome and asymptomatic proteinuria. The disease is male preponderant and usually occurs in young adults. Glomerular filtration rate is normal and the patient is normotensive. Occasionally, haematuria is the presenting symptom. The lesions resemble those observed in infectious diseases, and this raises the question of the role of tropical infections in the pathogenesis. A number of cases are associated with parasitic infection, but no relevant antigen can be identified in the glomeruli. Yet, the primary role of infection in the pathogenesis of the lesion cannot be totally excluded; for instance autoimmune mechanisms could play a secondary role in the development of the lesion, and evidence of impaired cell-mediated immune response has been shown; T helper cells are decreased while T suppressor cells are increased. The response to steroids is favourable in 80 per cent of cases. Those who do not respond to steroids may improve on antiplatelet agents or cyclophosphamide. Platelet survival is reduced in some 50 per cent. Some cases may progress slowly to chronic renal failure; hypertension is a bad prognostic sign. The relationship between this disease and focal glomerulosclerosis remains uncertain.

IgA nephropathy

The disease has a high incidence in Singapore and the Far East especially among those with asymptomatic glomerular disease. In Thailand it is less common than mesangial IgM nephropathy. How much race plays a role has not been established. Early surveys show no particular HLA association. The disease usually presents as asymptomatic haematuria often associated with respiratory infection. Occasionally, it may present with nephrotic syndrome, hypertension or even impaired renal function. The clinical course is often benign unless the patient is hypertensive. Platelet survival is usually normal. Treatment does not alter outcome but corticosteroids are often used when there is nephrotic syndrome. Of interest are the transient forms of IgA nephropathy in patients with typhoid fever, intestinal tuberculosis or ingestion of cantharidine in which the lesions readily resolve when the basic disease is under control.

Focal and segmental glomerulosclerosis

This histological lesion which includes glomerular hyalinosis accounts for 15 to 20 per cent of glomerulonephritis in Thailand. Nephrotic syndrome and sometimes asymptomatic proteinuria are common. There is a male preponderance. Hypertension may occur when the disease progresses. Hyperchloraemic acidosis is usually associated with interstitial changes. Although the evolution of the disease is far from clear, in some patients it seems to have evolved from a steroid-responsive or steroid-dependent nephrotic syndrome. The results of treatment have been disappointing. Some believe that a hypercoagulability state exists in these patients, and platelet survival and fibrinogen half-life are shortened. Because of this the combined use of steroids, cyclophosphamide, antiplatelet agents, and anticoagulants has been instituted by some clinicians. The results, however, vary among different series. The disease generally progresses to renal failure.

Lupus nephritis

Lupus nephritis is a common secondary glomerular disease. As in Western countries there is a preponderance of affected females. The clinical pictures in general do not differ from those observed in the West. Although in Singapore the disease affects mainly Chinese, in Thailand it is commoner in Thai people of poor socio-economy, suggesting an environmental factor in aetiology. There is a diversity of presentation and clinical course of the disease. Nephrotic syndrome occurs in over 50 per cent of cases. Diffuse proliferative glomerulonephritis is the most common renal pathological change.

The response to steroids is usually good in mild cases but in the severe form a combination of corticosteroid and immunosuppressive agents is required. Not all kidney diseases in lupus patients are the result of lupus erythematosus. Since drugs can be easily obtained in the market without prescription, the use of potentially nephrotoxic drugs such as non-steroidal anti-inflammatory agents must be considered in clinical assessment of any lupus patient who has impaired renal function.

The mortality of lupus nephritis has greatly fallen over the past decade, and the pattern of deaths appears to be changing. Death from cerebral involvement and renal involvement has declined with increasing mortality due to infection and complications resulting from treatment. Glomerular sclerosis, tubular atrophy, and interstitial mononuclear cell infiltration are usually associated with a bad outcome.

Postinfectious glomerulonephritis

A number of cases occur following infection. Besides poststreptococcal glomerulonephritis which is seen mostly in children, mild glomerular disease characterized by mild proteinuria with benign urinary sediment change is commonly observed following tropical infection. Histologically, there is either thickening of the mesangial area or hyperplasia of mesangial cells with deposition of IgM and C3 mainly in the mesangial region. These changes disappear when the basic disease is under control, usually within 4 to 6 weeks. Transient mesangial IgM glomerulonephritis has been observed in trichinosis, malaria, salmonellosis, and a number of infectious diseases. Transient IgA mesangial proliferative glomerulonephritis may follow intestinal infections such as typhoid fever and tuberculosis. In chronic infections glomerular lesions may persist, for instance, in leprosy with a varying spectrum of glomerular disease. Glomerulonephritis due to hepatitis B is occasionally observed.

Renal stone disease

Renal stones cause an important health problem. Calculi are calcium salts in 90 per cent of cases. The cause is not apparent. In children bladder stones are related to low phosphate intake, but the mechanism in adults seems to be different. Hypercalciuria is observed in the minority of renal stone patients. Distal renal tubular acidosis is not uncommon. Of interest is djenkolic acid stone development following ingestion of djenkol bean (*Pithecolobium lobatum*) in the southern part of Thailand, Indonesia, and Burma.

Thiazides remain the drugs of choice in the prevention of recurrent stone formation. The use of young coconut water (buko water) in the treatment of urinary tract stone in Philippines deserves further scientific investigation.

Tubulo-interstitial diseases

Besides drug-induced interstitial nephritis, tropical infection can be responsible for the renal lesions. Leptospirosis is a common cause of interstitial nephritis in the tropics. The renal lesion is observed even in patients without renal failure with interstitial changes preceding tubular damage. The infiltrate consists mainly of mononuclear cells, plasma cells and few eosinophils.

Scrub typhus is another tropical infectious cause of interstitial nephritis. Interstitial changes are focal. In the majority of cases there are only mild urinary sediment changes without impaired renal function.

The other less common infectious causes of interstitial nephritis include measles, leprosy, and infectious mononucleosis. Renal tuberculosis is not uncommon, but the disease is often overlooked. Although diphtheria and scarlet fever have long been quoted in the literature as the causes of interstitial nephritis, they are perhaps rare.

Animal toxins may occasionally cause interstitial nephritis. This has been shown in Russell's viper bite. Renal failure is severe with prolonged oliguria. The condition is fortunately not common, and could represent a severe form of envenomation.

Acute renal failure

Acute renal failure is common in the tropics, and tubular necrosis is the usual cause. Several predisposing factors are incriminated in its development. The hot climate causes volume contraction and salt depletion; low socio-economy leads to poor nutritional status and infection; the use of some traditional medicines can sometimes cause renal damage; and, finally, the high incidence of glucose-6-phosphate dehydrogenase deficiency predisposes to intravascular haemolysis. Two mechanisms are involved in the pathogenesis of renal failure. The first is ischaemia from non-specific effects including hypotension, hypovolaemia, blood hyperviscosity, catecholamine release, intravascular coagulation, intravascular haemolysis, myoglobinuria, jaundice, and fever. Second, certain bacteria and their toxins can directly damage the renal tissue. This is seen in leptospirosis, snake bite, and some plant toxins. Renal failure due to infection is usually hypercatabolic in type with a rapid rise in blood urea nitrogen and serum creatinine. Hyperuricaemia, hyperphosphataemia, and hyperkalaemia may be present. Jaundice may be observed when infection is severe. Renal failure may be associated with a haemoglobinuria and myoglobinuria. Treatment is concentrated on the basic disease. Renal failure usually resolves when the underlying disease is under control. Dialysis, when indicated, should be performed frequently because of hypercatabolism. Exchange blood transfusion is useful in patients with gross hyperbilirubinaemia.

Leptospirosis

Renal failure complicates 40 to 67 per cent of leptospirosis cases during the period of leptospiraemia and immunologic phase. Renal failure is often hypercatabolic. Hyperphosphataemia and hyperuricaemia may be noted. Jaundice may or may not be present. Icteric renal failure, known as Weil's syndrome, represents a severe form of infection, and need not be associated with icterohaemorrhagiae infection. Haemolytic uraemic syndrome may occasionally occur. In most cases renal failure is non-oliguric, but oliguria can occur in severe infection or in hyperbilirubinaemia. In mild cases prerenal azotaemia may be seen. Serotype bataviae is common in this geographical region. Renal pathological changes include interstitial nephritis and tubular necrosis. Renal failure is attributed to leptospire migration and non-specific effects of the infection.

Falciparum malaria

Renal failure in falciparum malaria is usually associated with heavy parasitaemia or intravascular haemolysis. Blackwater fever is uncommon. Rather, intravascular haemolysis is due to drugs and glucose-6-phosphate dehydrogenase deficiency. Unlike leptospirosis in which jaundice is variable, jaundice is usually present in malarial renal failure. Hyperkalaemia can be alarming when associated with intravascular haemolysis. Acute tubular necrosis is the main pathological finding. In severe cases with heavy parasitaemia exchange blood transfusion has been fruitful in reducing the degree of parasitaemia, removal of chemical mediators, and lowering the degree of jaundice which may further compromise the already impaired renal function. Renal failure appears to be the consequence of ischaemia secondary to non-specific effects and a compromised microcirculation by parasitized red blood cells.

Other tropical infections

Renal failure is occasionally observed in typhoid fever. The patient is usually jaundiced and has intravascular haemolysis due to glucose-6-phosphate dehydrogenase deficiency. The same is true for scrub typhus. Renal failure may be noted in trichinosis when the disease remains undiagnosed and untreated, but is usually mild secondary to hypovolaemia. Diphtheria may occasionally cause acute renal failure, attributed to renal ischaemia secondary to cardiotoxicity. In cholera, in addition to tubular necrosis, hypokalaemic nephropathy may be a striking pathological finding, but it is not common nowadays. In shigellosis haemolytic uraemic syndrome has been documented. Cortical necrosis may be observed, and renal failure may be severe.

Snake bite

Renal failure occurs following envenomation of Russell's viper (*Vipera russellii*), sea snake (*Enhydrina schistosa*), and occasionally green pit viper. Russell's viper bite is the most common cause. In fact, any kind of snake bite with severe systemic symptoms is capable of causing acute renal failure by non-specific effects. Although tubular necrosis is a common pathological change, a broad spectrum of renal changes can be seen. Arteritis, thrombophlebitis, interstitial nephritis, extracapillary proliferative glomerulonephritis, and even cortical necrosis have been described in Russell's viper bite. In green pit viper bite diffuse proliferative glomerulonephritis without immune complex deposition has been reported. It is believed that viper venom is vasculotoxic. Myoglobinuria is common in sea snake bite. In general, mild mesangial proliferative glomerulonephritis is commonly seen. Mesangiolysis described in animal experiments has not been observed in renal biopsy material from humans. Management is focused on antivenom therapy. Haemodialysis in sea snake bite has been reported to improve muscular symptoms.

Other animal toxins

Hornet and wasp stings can cause acute renal failure. Multiple stings, rather than a single sting, are responsible. Clinically, myonecrosis and myoglobinuria are common and intravascular haemolysis may occur with haemoglobinuria. Plasma levels of muscle enzymes are elevated. Hyperkalaemia, hyperuricaemia, and hyperphosphataemia are frequently observed. The urine is dark, and in most cases there is oligo-anuria. The renal pathology is of acute tubular necrosis. The causes of renal failure are multiple, but myoglobinuria is probably the main cause. Although nephrotic syndrome has been reported following bee sting, a cause–effect relationship has not been proven.

Finally, raw bile of grass carp is another cause of renal failure. A traditional Chinese way of improving visual acuity is by ingestion of raw gall bladder of grass carp (*Ctenopharyngodon idellus*) which is believed to be tubulotoxic.

Plant toxins

Little is known about nephrotoxic plants. Although several kinds of plants have been described as being nephrotoxic, very few have been proven by scientific study. Djenkol bean from the southern part of Thailand, Malay Peninsula, Indonesia, and Burma is known for its nephrotoxicity. The principle ingredient is djenkolic acid which is capable of causing tubular injury, crystalluria, and stone formation. The patient may present with oliguria or anuria. It is a common experience that a number of patients with already compromised renal function develop renal failure following the ingestion of Chinese herbal medicine, but the responsible ingredient is unknown.

Other toxins

The other causes of renal failure such as nephrotoxic antibiotics and non-steroidal anti-inflammatory agents do not differ from those observed in Western countries. Paraquat is however an important fatal cause of acute renal failure. Mortality is over 70 per cent depending upon the amount ingested with respiratory failure as the usual mode of death.

Chronic renal failure

Chronic glomerulonephritis is the major cause of chronic renal failure. Analgesic nephropathy is not common. Chronic renal failure poses a problem in management. Although haemodialysis and renal transplantation are available, because of the high cost and limited man power they can only be performed in a small selected group of patients. Continuous ambulatory peritoneal dialysis has recently been used in the hope of reducing costs but this also requires support from a strong haemodialysis unit and is complicated by infection.

Conservative treatment thus remains the cornerstone in the management of chronic renal failure. The present aim is rather to prevent renal disease and to recognize it earlier. If a low protein intake is truly a protective mechanism against the progress of chronic renal disease, the diet of people with low socio-economy in certain geographic areas may convey an advantage. Whether or not the clinical course of renal failure in this group of patients is longer than that of higher socio-economic groups warrants further observation.

References

Areekul, S. (1979). Djenkol bean, djenkolic acid and djenkolism *J. Med. Assoc. Thai.* **62**, 529–531.

Boonpucknavig, V. and Boonpucknavig, S. (1982). Glomerulonephritis: pathogenesis, pathology and incidence in Thailand. *Ramathibodi Med. J.* **5**, 16–35.

Futrakul, P., Poshyachinda, M. and Mitrakul, C. (1978). Focal sclerosing glomerulonephritis: a kinetic evaluation of hemostasis and the effect of anticoagulant therapy: a control study. *Clin. Nephrol.* **10**, 180–186.

Sidabutar R. P., Lumenta, N. A. and Suling, R. C. (1978). Chlorthalidone in prevention of urinary calcium stone. *J. Med. Assoc. Thai.* **61** (Suppl. 1), 195–198.

Sinniah, R. and Feng, P. H. (1976). Lupus nephritis: correlation between light, electron microscopic and immunofluorescent findings and renal function. *Clin. Nephrol.* **6**, 340–351.

Sitprija, V. (1979). Mechanisms of renal involvement in tropical diseases. *Proceedings of the Third Colloquium in Nephrology*, Tokyo, 1979, (eds K. Oshima and T. Takeuchi), pp. 104–107. Sasaki Printing and Publishing Co. Ltd., Sendai.

Sitprija, V. and Boonpucknavig, V. (1977). The kidney in tropical snake-bite. *Clin. Nephrol.* **8**, 377–383.

RANGOON, BURMA

HLA MON

Table 1 shows the causes of acute renal failure admitted to Rangoon General Hospital, Burma, from 1 June 1973 to 30 September 1984.

Patterns of acute renal failure in Burma

Burma is still a developing agricultural country and the occupational hazard her farmers are exposed to most commonly (70 per cent, 391 out of 553) is acute renal failure due to bites by Russell's viper (*Vipera russelli*) (Table 1). The overall mortality is still about 39 per cent (152 out of 391). The pattern of acute renal failure in Burma is different from other parts of Southeast Asia. Of the infective causes, most are due to public health problems related to vector-borne diseases and their sequelae. Some of them are related to rodents which are prevalent.

Almost all the cases due to drugs and chemicals relate to self-medication or prescription by doctors for desperate clinical conditions (e.g. nephrotoxic antibiotics for septicaemia). The easy availability of medicines on the open market and the moderately high cost of private consultation lead to self-medication which gives rise to this problem. Legislative control with its enforcement should reduce these problems significantly.

Proper measures should be taken to eradicate the Russell's viper (with due consideration given to its ecological disturbance) and to upgrade public health systems.

Table 1

Primary disease	Number of cases
Russell's viper bite	391
Glucose-6-phosphate dehydrogenase deficiency	39
Post gastroenteritis	19
Nephrotic syndrome	18
Viral hepatitis and massive liver necrosis	17
Acute pyelonephritis	13
Leptospirosis	9
Unknown septicaemia	8
Non-cerebral malaria	7
Nephrotoxic antibiotics	5
Djenkol bean (pithecolobium) poisoning	4
Cirrhosis liver and hepatoma	3
Viral infections	3
Cerebral malaria	2
Overdose of	
Dapsone	2
Methyl bromide	1
Salicylate	1
Sodium nitrite	1
Indigenous medicine	1
Throat infection (*Pseudomonas pyocyaneae*)	1
Paroxysmal nocturnal haemoglobinuria	1
Steven–Johnson syndrome	1
Renal tuberculosis	1
Histiocytic lymphoma	1
Primary hyperuricaemia	1
Polycystic kidneys	1
Unknown cause	2
Total	553

Africa

F. J. MILNE AND J. L. SEGGIE

Introduction

Although there is reasonable documentation of the current patterns of renal disease in Africa, the size and heterogeneity of the populations of this continent make it difficult in a short chapter to present more than major trends. The trends discussed should be considered against the background of population explosion with rapid urbanization and thus some of the patterns of disease described may change rapidly.

Urinary tract infections
Bacterial cystitis and acute pyelonephritis

Urinary tract infection in African populations does not differ significantly from that in Western European populations. Women are more frequently affected than men and asymptomatic bacteriuria is found in 10 per cent of pregnant women. The true prevalence of infection in children is unknown, although such community surveys as have been carried out indicate that asymptomatic bacteriuria may be found in 6 to 10 per cent. It is uncertain whether primary vesico-ureteric reflux occurs in Black children to the same extent as in White children. Potential predisposing causes of urinary tract infection include: kwashiorkor in young children; bladder and renal calculus disease which, although rare in most African populations, is common in boys and adult males in the Sudan and Nigeria; urethral stricture as a sequel of gonococcal urethritis in males; chronic vesical schistosomiasis and sickle cell disease in which papillary necrosis predisposes to pyelonephritis.

Tuberculosis of the renal tract

Considering that pulmonary tuberculosis is rife throughout Africa, it is astonishing that renal tuberculosis is seldom diagnosed. In spite of autopsy evidence that miliary tubercles frequently involve the renal parenchyma, overt clinical renal and lower urinary tract tuberculosis is rare.

Schistosomiasis haematobium
Vesical schistosomiasis may lead to severe fibrosis and calcification of the bladder with stenosis of the intramural portions of the ureters. Radiological studies have disclosed the presence of hydroureter and hydronephrosis in approximately 15 per cent and of a non-functioning kidney in up to 20 per cent of unselected patients with *Schistosoma haemotobium* infection. Vesicoureteric reflux is a further complication which may predispose to pyelonephritis.

Glomerulonephritis
Whereas in Europe or America glomerulonephritis is commonly idiopathic or a manifestation of systemic disease, in Africa it is frequently causally linked to infections prevalent within the African environment. The extremely high incidence of glomerulonephritis in African populations is partly attributable to this fact.

Acute poststreptococcal glomerulonephritis
In contrast to developed countries where it is a vanishing disease, poststreptococcal glomerulonephritis is extremely common. It is usually associated with impetigo, often itself a complication of scabies, rather than with pharyngitis or tonsillitis. In the considerable experience of the paediatric renal service of the University of Natal, South Africa, most young patients recover rapidly but 15 per cent develop serious complications (severe pulmonary oedema, renal failure, and hypertensive encephalopathy) and 2 per cent die. Occasionally, in older children and adults nephritis evolves into a true nephrotic syndrome, followed by a rapidly progressive course to end-stage renal failure.

As a confirmatory test of streptococcal infection the antistreptolysin test (ASOT) is frequently negative in cases of nephritis following on skin sepsis. The antideoxyribonuclease B (anti-DNAse B) and antihyaluronidase tests are then much more reliable.

Quartan malarial nephropathy
(See page 18.42.)

The role of *Plasmodium malariae* in the genesis of glomerular disease may have been overemphasized, especially as the histopathological lesion, thought originally to be pathognomonic of quartan malarial nephropathy, has since been identified in the absence of malarial parasitaemia. This lesion, beginning with focal glomerular sclerosis with a curious splitting or flaking of the glomerular basement membrane and progressing with obliteration of capillary lumina by basement membrane-like material to global sclerosis, is probably best viewed as a variety of 'tropical nephropathy' for which there are likely to be several causes.

As may be inferred from the above description of the progress of the glomerular lesion, the clinical course is one of advancing renal failure uninfluenced by therapy with either antimalarial or immunosuppressive agents.

Glomerulonephritis and hepatitis B
A striking feature of the nephrotic syndrome in Black children is the rarity with which minimal change glomerulonephritis is seen. Instead membranous glomerulonephritis assumes major importance.

Recently surveys of glomerulonephritis in Zimbabwean and South African Blacks have highlighted the aetiologic role of hepatitis B virus infection in the genesis of membranous disease in both children and young adults. Nephropathy is associated with carriage of the hepatitis B surface antigen rather than with active hepatitis and usually resolves spontaneously over a period of 6 to 12 months.

Other infections prevalent in Africa and deserving of mention since they too are linked to development of glomerular disease are detailed in Table 1.

Two additional non-infective glomerulopathies need to be considered in Black subjects:

Table 1 Para-infectious glomerulonephritides

Infective organism	Nature of renal lesion	Clinical manifestations
Viral		
Hepatitis B	Membranous GN	Proteinuria; haematuria → nephrotic syndrome → spontaneous remission
Bacterial		
Group B haemolytic streptococci	Diffuse proliferative (exudative) GN	Acute nephritic syndrome, occasionally nephrotic syndrome; occasionally acute renal failure; rarely evolution to end-stage renal failure
Treponema pallidum	Membranous and proliferative GN	Proteinuria → nephrotic syndrome; mild to moderate renal dysfunction. Consider: young adult (complication of secondary syphilis) infant (complication of congenital syphilis) child (complication of endemic syphilis still common in West Africa)
Mycobacterium leprae	Diffuse proliferative GN	Haematuria, proteinuria, mild to moderate renal dysfunction (in setting of erythema nodosum leprosum) [ENL] (reaction)
	Amyloidosis	Nephrotic syndrome → chronic renal failure in lepromatous leprosy (clinical course punctuated by ENL reactions) and tuberculoid leprosy (complicated by chronic, suppurating trophic ulceration)
Salmonella typhi	Diffuse proliferative GN	Transient proteinuria and haematuria (especially in G6PD-deficient individuals)
Streptococcus viridans (and others in infective endocarditis)	Focal proliferative GN (often with crescents)	Haematuria and proteinuria; variable renal dysfunction; occasionally acute renal failure
Parasitic		
Plasmodium falciparum	Diffuse proliferative GN	Transient haematuria and proteinuria
Plasmodium malariae	Sclerosing GN = 'tropical nephropathy' (see text)	Nephrotic syndrome → end-stage renal failure
Schistosoma mansoni	Proliferative and sclerosing GN*	Nephrotic syndrome
Schistosoma haematobium	Proliferative GN	
	Amyloidosis	Nephrotic syndrome in young adults

*Egyptian studies documenting this glomerulopathy link pathogenesis of the lesion to concomitant chronic *Salmonella typhi* infection.

Mercurial nephropathy The nephrotic syndrome, reflecting an underlying membranous lesion, may rarely develop after prolonged use of skin 'whitening' cosmetics which contain mercury. The disease is confined to women and usually remits spontaneously, although over several months, provided that patients can be persuaded that such cosmetics are both unnecessary and harmful.

Sickle cell glomerulopathy (see Section 19) This entity is not often encountered in practice, despite the high incidence of sickle cell anaemia in tropical Africa. In fact, most reported cases of sickle cell glomerular disease (encompassing mesangial expansion and manifesting as heavy proteinuria with progressive renal dysfunction) have been in North American and West Indian Blacks.

Acute renal failure

Shock, secondary to fluid depletion, blood loss, burns, and/or septicaemia underlies the majority of cases of acute renal failure in Africa as in the developed world. The spectrum of causes of acute renal failure is, however, wider and again infections play a major pathogenetic role. Glucose-6-phosphate dehydrogenase (G6PD) deficiency, which predisposes to intravascular haemolysis and haemoglobinuria and ingestion of nephrotoxic agents contained in traditional herbal medicaments must also be considered.

Malaria (page 5.474)

In falciparum malaria intravascular haemolysis and haemoglobinuria and heavy parasitaemia operate in the genesis of acute renal failure which may be oliguric or non-oliguric. Since chloroquine and quinine are cleared by the kidneys it is recommended that dosage of both these drugs in the presence of renal failure be reduced to 10 mg/kg/day administered as an intravenous infusion in 5 per cent dextrose water over 4 hours.

Typhoid (page 5.218)

Typhoid regularly produces most of its victims during the rainy season when water contamination is most likely to occur and it is a common cause of acute renal failure. Pathogenetic factors include septicaemic shock, disseminated intravascular coagulation, massive intestinal haemorrhage, and haemoglobinuria resulting from haemolysis in G6PD-deficient individuals. Acute proliferative glomerulonephritis and interstitial nephritis have been documented, but neither is likely to be important since these histological changes do not correlate with the degree of renal impairment.

Leptospirosis (page 5.327)

This is an important cause of hepatitis accompanied by renal dysfunction. Wild and domestic animals serve as reservoirs of infection and water sources such as dams and wells, as well as stagnant pools and puddles, are frequently contaminated.

Renal failure occurs on the basis of an interstitial nephritis induced as leptospires migrate from peritubular capillaries through the renal interstitium and are excreted in the urine. Disseminated intravascular coagulation, myoglobinuria, jaundice, and hypovolaemia are probably contributing factors in severely affected patients.

Viral haemorrhagic fevers

Major causes of death due to disease associated with the Congo fever arbovirus, and the Lassa, Marburg, and Ebola viruses include haemorrhage, shock, acute renal failure, and hepatorenal failure.

Nephrotoxins

Several surveys of acute renal failure, notably those from Central and Southern Africa, testify to the frequency of nephrotoxin-induced acute renal failure. Medicaments are either administered by the traditional herbalist or are purchased as patent remedies without prescription. These may be taken orally or administered

per rectum or per vaginam and for a variety of indications which include 'impotence', infertility, menstrual disorders, procurement of abortion, and constipation. Vomiting, cramping abdominal pains, and diarrhoea are followed by diffuse bleeding (haematemesis, bloody diarrhoea, haemoptysis, and epistaxis). Jaundice is a common additional finding.

Pregnancy-related acute renal failure

Self-induced abortion with supervening sepsis, eclampsia, and post-partum and ante-partum haemorrhage account for approximately 25 per cent of all cases of acute renal failure and for the majority of cases in women. In abortion-related cases ingestion or vaginal administration of abortifacient substances is frequently contributory. As might be anticipated renal failure complicating septic abortion carries a mortality rate of about 50 per cent whilst that following vaginal haemorrhage and uncomplicated by sepsis has a good prognosis provided bilateral cortical necrosis does not occur.

Hypertension

Hypertension is a problem of major importance in Africa. The rural prevalence of this disease is low, but it is increasingly encountered in the cities and with current demographic trends hypertension may assume alarming proportions in the future.

In those countries of North Africa where bilharzia and chronic pyelonephritis are common, 30 per cent of hypertensives have underlying renal disease. However, in Southern Africa, East Africa, and Nigeria no underlying cause can be found in the great majority. Takayashu's disease is common in North Africa, but renal artery stenosis is rarely found in the Blacks of Southern Africa.

Morbidity and mortality in Blacks is mainly related to pressure effects and atheromatous complications are rare. Thus, death occurs from cerebrovascular haemorrhage, congestive cardiac failure, and uraemia, rather than thrombotic stroke, ischaemic heart disease or peripheral vascular disease.

Malignant hypertension

The development of the malignant phase of hypertension is common in urban South Africa amongst Blacks. While the disease is declining in developed countries, it accounts for about 40 per cent of Blacks who develop end-stage renal failure requiring dialysis in urban South Africa and is the commonest cause of end-stage renal failure in Nigeria. In most of these patients essential hypertension and not underlying chronic renal disease seems to be the cause. As with the American Black essential malignant hypertension probably accounts for an excess of chronic renal failure compared to Whites.

Patients may present as a medical emergency with severe pulmonary oedema, encephalopathy, stroke or uraemia, or they may be largely asymptomatic despite the very high blood pressure and malignant retinopathy. Typically, haematuria is microscopic and proteinuria mild, while the renal size is normal to slightly reduced. The renal outcome depends on the initial serum creatinine and control of hypertension. There is usually a deterioration of renal function with initiation of therapy but this frequently improves with time and blood pressure control. In our experience patients presenting with a serum creatinine greater than 500 μmol/l invariably deteriorate and most require dialysis, whilst the renal function of those with an initial serum creatinine less than 500 μmol/l improves or remains stable.

Many reports have appeared in recent years on the adverse effects, particularly upon the nervous system, of lowering the blood pressure too rapidly in patients with malignant hypertension. The rapidity with which blood pressure should be lowered depends on whether life-threatening complications exist at presentation: any encephalopathy or severe pulmonary oedema requires aggressive therapy which aims to reduce the blood pressure within

10 to 30 min, but not below a diastolic pressure of 110 mm Hg in the first 24 hours. The asymptomatic patients or those with mild pulmonary oedema should have their blood pressure lowered gradually to ±150/110 mm Hg over 24 to 48 hours and then maintained at or below 140/90 mm Hg.

Renal failure must be managed as it presents. Some patients may require immediate dialysis whilst others develop deteriorating renal function. Whilst some patients will continue on permanent dialysis, a small number may regain sufficient renal function over time and dialysis can be discontinued.

End-stage renal failure

In a review of the conditions causing death in seven African hospitals the two commonest groups of chronic diseases were cardiac disease and chronic renal failure. The commonest cause of end-stage renal failure remains chronic glomerulonephritis. However, in areas where bilharzia is endemic, chronic pyelonephritis and obstructive uropathy assume importance. As mentioned, essential malignant hypertension is a major cause in certain areas. Diabetes mellitus is prevalent throughout Africa, but there is some evidence that the development of diabetic nephropathy is less common amongst Blacks.

Patients with chronic renal failure tend to present late. They remain remarkably well, probably because of their staple low-protein high-carbohydrate diets, despite serum creatinines over 1000 μmol/l, until advanced uraemia supervenes. In the investigation of chronic renal failure it is important to exclude potentially treatable conditions such as hypertension, urinary tract obstruction, either due to urethral strictures or bilharzia, and urinary tract infections. Because patients often present with uraemia, initial peritoneal dialysis is warranted in order to allow time for investigation and treatment of potentially reversible causes.

Intermittent peritoneal dialysis is simple, relatively inexpensive, and available in many parts of Africa. However, haemodialysis is restricted to major centres in a limited number of countries. Rightly, maintenance haemodialysis does not enjoy a high priority in most African health budgets. Even continuous ambulatory peritoneal dialysis (CAPD), although less expensive than haemodialysis, requires back-up haemodialysis facilities and cannot be viewed in the same light as the prevention and treatment of malaria or bilharzia. However, in time and with progressive urbanization, such facilities will become available. If end-stage renal failure management is undertaken, the goal must be successful transplantation. Provided the donor kidneys come from a homogeneous population pool, transplantation is as successful as in developed countries.

References

Adu, D., Anim-Addo, Y., Foli, A. K., Yeboah, E. D., Quartey, J. K. M. and Ribeiro, B. F. (1976). Acute renal failure in tropical Africa. *Br. Med. J.* **1**, 890–892.
Barsoum, R. S., Bassily, S., Baligh, O. K., Eissa, M., El-Sheemy, N., Affify, N. and Hassaballa, A. M. (1977). Renal disease in hepatosplenic schistosomiasis: a clinicopathological study. *Trans. R. Soc. hyg. trop. Med.* **71**, 387–391.
Gold, C. H. (1980). Acute renal failure from herbal and patient remedies in blacks. *Clin. Nephrol.* **14**, 128–134.
——, Isaacson, C. and Levin, J. (1982). The pathological basis of end-stage renal disease in blacks. *S. Afr. Med. J.* **61**, 263–265.
Hallett, A. F., Adhikari, M., Cooper, R. and Coovadia, H. M. (1977). Post-streptococcal glomerulonephritis in African children. *Trans. R. Soc. hyg. trop. Med.* **71**, 241–246.
Hendrickse, R. G., Adeniyi, A., Edington, G. U., Glasgow, E. F., White, R. H. R. and Houba, V. (1972). Quartan malarial nephrotic syndrome. Collaborative clinico-pathological study in Nigerian children. *Lancet* i, 1143–1149.
Jhetam, D., Dansey, R., Morar, C. and Milne, F. J. (1982). The malignant phase of essential hypertension in Johannesburg blacks. *S. Afr. Med. J.* **61**, 899–902.
Morel-Maroger, L., Saimot, A. G., Sloper, J. C., Woodrow, D. F., Adam, C., Niang, I. and Payet, M. (1975). 'Tropical nephropathy' and 'tropical extramembranous glomerulonephritis' of unknown aetiology in Senegal. *Br. Med. J.* **1**, 541–546.
Poonpucknavig, V. and Sitiprija, V. (1979). Renal disease in acute *Plasmodium falciparum* infection in man. *Kid. Int.* **16**, 44–52.
Seedat, Y. K., Naicker, S., Rawat, R. and Parsoo, I. (1984). Racial differences in the causes of end-stage renal failure in Natal. *S. Afr. Med. J.* **65**, 956–958.
Seggie, J., Nathoo, K. and Davies, P. G. (1984). Association of hepatitis B antigenaemia and membranous glomerulonephritis in Zimbabwean children. *Nephron* **38**, 115–119.
Smith, J. H., Kamel, I. A., Elwi, A. and von Lichtenberg, F. (1974). A quantitative post mortem analysis of urinary schistosomiasis in Egypt. I. Pathology and pathogenesis. *Am. J. trop. med. Hyg.* **23**, 1054–1071.

SECTION 19
DISORDERS OF THE BLOOD

INTRODUCTION

D. J. WEATHERALL

The study of blood is one of the most fascinating branches of clinical medicine. There are very few diseases which do not produce changes in the blood at some time during the course of the illness. Furthermore, the primary disorders of the blood and blood-forming tissues can give rise to extremely diverse clinical manifestations which may involve any of the organ systems. Textbooks often give their readers an unbalanced picture of haematology in the real world. Even in specialist haematological practice primary disorders of the blood and blood-forming organs make up only a small fraction of the workload; most patients that are referred with haematological abnormalities have diseases in other systems. Anaemia is a good example. The bulk of anaemias seen in medical wards are due to blood loss, infection, renal failure, malignant disease, and, in many parts of the world, malnutrition and parasitic infestation. Anaemia may be the first indication of a chronic urinary tract infection, hypothyroidism, pituitary failure, bacterial endocarditis, polymyalgia rheumatica, or even that endemic disease of 'medical grand rounds', atrial myxoma.

Thus, although this section concentrates heavily on the primary diseases of the blood and blood-forming organs, the reader should be aware that many of these conditions are relatively uncommon. Hopefully, the summary of the haematological manifestations of non-haematological diseases which appears later in the section will leave the reader with a more balanced view of the scope of this absorbing subject.

An approach to patients with haematological disorders

The diagnosis of blood diseases follows the same process as any other condition; expertise in the laboratory will never make up for an inadequate history and clinical examination. It should be remembered that many patients who are referred to hospital for a specialist opinion on their blood are worried about the possibility of leukaemia, although they will rarely say so. It is important to reassure them as soon as possible if this is not the diagnosis. Where leukaemia is suspected no time should be lost in arriving at an accurate diagnosis and in developing a well-worked out plan of management. The situation can then be discussed frankly with the patient and their family; knowledge of what they are up against and precisely what form of treatment is to be instituted often engenders a great sense of relief after weeks or months of fearing the worst.

History

In taking a history from a patient who is suspected of having a haematological disorder certain factors are of particular importance. The symptoms of anaemia are described in detail later in this section. However, it should be remembered that a slowly developing anaemia may be completely asymptomatic, even when the haemoglobin level is extremely low. Individuals who are otherwise healthy should be able to compensate for a relatively mild anaemia; a young woman with a haemoglobin level of 10.5 g/dl who complains of tiredness and inability to cope with life is more likely to be suffering from the effects of chronic anxiety due to marital problems than from mild anaemia. Other general symptoms are of great importance, particularly weight loss, night sweats, bone pain, and pruritis. While moderate nocturnal sweating is common in anxiety states, drenching sweats requiring several changes of nightclothes and sheets is a more ominous symptom, often associated with infection or lymphoproliferative disease. Pruritis occurs with many disorders of the blood. When associated with lymphoma it is non-specific, but when it accompanies the myeloproliferative disorders it is often precipitated by warmth such as getting into bed or a hot bath. A detailed drug history is also essential; there are very few drugs that do not produce haematological side-effects.

Although a complete systematic history must be taken, gastrointestinal and haemostatic functions are particularly relevant to diseases of the blood. When investigating anaemia a detailed dietetic history is essential and it is important to ask specifically about symptoms such as a sore tongue, bleeding gums, dysphagia, dyspepsia, disturbance of bowel habit suggestive of malabsorption, and rectal bleeding. Patients are often referred to haematological departments for investigation of easy bruising. Many people, particularly women, bruise easily and the key question is whether the bruising is *unusual* for them. Is it spontaneous or related to only mild trauma? It is also extremely helpful to enquire into certain key episodes in a patient's life which may provide a clue as to whether there is an inborn bleeding tendency. These include circumcision, dental extraction (was a return to the dentist for stitching or packing ever required?), menstruation, surgical procedures, and so on.

Assessment of menstrual blood loss is an important part of the history in women with iron deficiency, as well as for assessing haemostatic function. It is not enough to ask a woman whether she considers that her periods are normal. If she uses only internal tampons, she probably does not have menorrhagia. However, the use of one or more packets of the more absorbent brands of external pads, or having to get up at night to change pads or to stay at home during the menstrual period, suggests a heavy loss.

Family histories are particularly important for the diagnosis of blood diseases. It is not only essential to ask for a family history of anaemia or bleeding disorders; the racial origin of the patient's ancestors may also give valuable clues for the cause of anaemia. The long forgotten Italian great-grandparent may have been the source of the thalassaemia gene which is responsible for a refractory hypochromic anaemia or the red cell enzyme deficiency which leads to a haemolytic drug reaction. A detailed personal history is also essential. Cigarette or cigar smoking is probably the commonest cause of mild polycythaemia and alcohol can produce remarkably diverse haematological changes. A detailed occupational history may reveal exposure to industrial solvents or other agents responsible for bone marrow depression; unusual hobbies may also result in contact with toxic agents.

Physical examination

The examination of a patient with a haematological disorder follows the same pattern as any physical examination but there are certain aspects of particular importance. On general inspection it is essential to examine the skin carefully for evidence of bruising, purpura, infiltration or ulceration. The distribution and pattern of bruising or petechiae may be diagnostic, particularly in disorders such as Henoch–Schönlein purpura, senile purpura, scurvy, purpura due to venous obstruction, and the painful bruising syndrome. Thrombocytopenic purpura is often seen most easily over pressure areas; a few lesions in these regions are easily overlooked. Cutaneous lymphoma may mimic a variety of skin diseases. Chronic leg ulceration is a common finding in sickle cell anaemia; it occurs occasionally with other genetic haemolytic anaemias. The perianal region and perineum should be carefully inspected. There may be perianal infiltration, particularly in the monocytic leukaemias, and it is very important to recognize perianal infection early in neutropenic patients. Rectal examination should be avoided in the latter for fear of disseminating infection. Potential sites of infection is compromised patients must be examined daily. They include the skin, intravenous infusion sites, the mouth and throat, and the perineum. The mucous membranes, nail beds, and palmar creases should be examined carefully for pallor, always remembering that the clinical assessment of anaemia is very inaccurate. Pigmentation of the face is sometimes a feature of folic acid deficiency. Mild jaundice may be a useful indicator of haemolysis, while a greyish pigmentation of the skin is common in patients with iron overload, both primary and secondary to repeated transfusion. There is an association between vitiligo and pernicious anaemia. In patients with polycythaemia there may be suffusion of the conjunctivae, a high colour, and prominence of the vessels over the face, neck and upper part of the chest. The nails should be examined for unusual fragility; flattened spoon-shaped nails, koilonychia, which are supposed to be diagnostic of chronic iron deficiency, are now rarely seen.

An assessment of the size of the lymph-nodes and an inspection of other lymphatic tissue is a major part of the examination of patients with haematological disorders. It is most important to develop a systematic approach to lymph-node examination. Each group of nodes in the head and neck, axillae and groins together with the epitrochlear nodes must be examined in detail. In the head and neck it is useful to start with the occipital nodes, then move to the preauricular and postauricular nodes, and, finally, to examine systematically the anterior and posterior triangles and supraclavicular regions. The scalp should be inspected for signs of infestation and secondary infection due to scratching in children with enlarged occipital or posterior cervical nodes. A simple way of describing enlarged lymph-nodes should be used, without the use of too many adjectives. Nodes should be labelled as hard, firm or soft, and tender or non-tender. Ambiguous terms such as 'rubbery' should be avoided. Soft, tender nodes usually indicate infection. Large, firm nodes are characteristic of lymphoma. Hard nodes occur in secondary carcinoma, although calcified nodes, matted together and attached to skin, are still encountered in patients with tuberculous adenitis. The approximate size of the nodes should be recorded together with whether they are mobile, attached deep or superficially, and discrete or matted together. It is also very important to examine the tonsils and adenoids, particularly in a patient suspected of having a lymphoproliferative disease.

A detailed examination of the mouth should include the state of the tongue, mucous membranes, gums, teeth, and fauces. Glossitis, as evidenced by a smooth, depapillated tongue occurs in iron deficiency and megaloblastic anaemia. Small black bullae (blood blisters) on the tongue or mucous membranes, which burst and leave superficial ulcers, are characteristic of thrombocytopenic purpura. Gum hypertrophy is sometimes found in patients with acute leukaemia, particularly the monocytic type, and in some individuals with megaloblastic anaemia due to phenytoin therapy. Ulcers of the mouth and fauces occur in all forms of acute leukaemia. Oral infection, often associated with ulceration, is very common in neutropenic patients. Monilia may be seen on the fauces, tongue or mucous membranes. Monilial infection of the throat, associated with dysphagia, should raise the suspicion of oesophageal moniliasis. The teeth may be badly formed and the bite may be abnormal in patients with severe forms of thalassaemia. Dental abscesses are common in patients with neutropenia; suspect teeth should be gently percussed for evidence of apical infection. Telangiectases may be found on the lips and oral mucous membranes of patients with hereditary telangiectasia.

On abdominal examination the most important questions are the size of the liver, whether there is splenomegaly, and if there are any palpable para-aortic lymph-nodes. It is not possible to learn how to examine the spleen from a textbook, but a few hints may be helpful. Large spleens can often be seen to move up and down on respiration if the abdomen is well illuminated and the observer stands at the end of the bed. Very large spleens tend to move downwards and medially towards the right iliac fossa and can be missed if the examiner does not start palpating from this region, moving upwards and medially towards the left subcostal region. A sure way to miss a moderately enlarged spleen is to go digging in with the fingers without eliciting the patient's help. With the left-hand hooked round the region above the left costal margin, and the right hand resting lightly on the abdomen, the patient should be asked to gently breathe in and out through their mouth. The secret of success is to persuade the patient to breathe just deeply enough to move the spleen down without contracting the abdominal muscles. The examiner should wait for the spleen tip to meet their fingers rather than to try to find it by deep palpation. Once defined, the position of the lower border of the spleen should be recorded in centimetres, vertically below the costal margin. Manoeuvres designed to facilitate the palpation of a slightly enlarged spleen such as turning the patient on their right side, while useful for impressing clinical examiners, are rarely of much help in practice. Be gentle! The author has seen two malignant spleens ruptured by overenthusiastic medical students. If there is pain over the spleen or referred to the left shoulder, don't forget to listen for a rub. Finally, remember that spleens come in all sizes and shapes, and often lie more laterally than expected. Do not be disappointed not to feel the much publicized notch; it happens once or twice in a clinical lifetime! The differential diagnosis of palpable masses in the region of the spleen is considered later in this section.

The eyes are a mine of information in patients with haematological disorders. Periorbital oedema is sometimes seen in infectious mononucleosis. The conjunctivae may show mild icterus which is not obvious in the skin, and there may be haemorrhages in bleeding disorders. Pingueculae of the conjunctivae are seen in Gaucher's disease. Retinal haemorrhages are common in patients who have had a sudden fall in haemoglobin level. They are less frequent in severely thrombocytopenic patients with normal haemoglobin levels; the combination of anaemia and thrombocytopenia is particularly likely to lead to severe retinal bleeding. Papilloedema occurs commonly in patients with leukaemia involving the central nervous system. Proliferative abnormalities of the retinal vessels are often seen in patients with sickling disorders, particularly haemoglobin SC disease. The hyperviscosity syndrome associated with macroglobulinaemia and some forms of myeloma is characterized by fullness of the retinal veins which are sometimes broken up into segments like a string of sausages. These changes are often associated with widespread retinal haemorrhages. Optic atrophy may occur in patients with severe vitamin B_{12} deficiency. Unilateral exophthalmos occurs occasionally in patients with myeloma deposits or lymphoma involving the orbit.

Examination of the musculoskeletal system may be particularly rewarding in patients suspected of having genetic disorders of blood. In patients with coagulation defects such as haemophilia or Christmas disease recurrent bleeding into joints may produce a chronic deforming arthritis. Muscle haematomata are also common and are easily missed. For example, bleeding into the psoas sheath may produce a discrete swelling above the inguinal ligament which may later be associated with nerve compression leading to weakness of the quadriceps and anaesthesia over the anterior aspect of the thigh. If muscle pain is the presenting symptom it is very important to palpate the muscle groups carefully for cystic swellings which may occur in haemophiliacs after bleeding into muscles. The joints have other important associations with blood disorders. A mild refractory anaemia is a very common accompaniment of rheumatoid arthritis. Painful arthritis of the large joints may be the presenting symptom of primary haemochromatosis. Gout is a common complication of all the myeloproliferative diseases; the ears should be examined carefully for tophi in addition to a full assessment of the joints. The value of bone tenderness in the diagnosis of acute leukaemia has been overemphasized. It is often absent. When present it is best elicited by carefully palpating the sternum or tibiae, or by rib compression. Be gentle, because sometimes the tenderness is quite exquisite. Bone tenderness or local swelling is also found in patients with myeloma or sickle cell anaemia. In children with thalassaemia or other hereditary haemolytic anaemias there may be reduced growth, bossing of the skull, and facial deformities. A wide variety of skeletal changes may occur with congenital hypoplastic anaemia.

The use of the laboratory

Finally, the diagnosis and management of blood disease requires an examination of the blood and, if appropriate, the bone marrow. Clinicians will obtain the maximum information from their colleagues in the laboratory if they ask the right questions. Scribbling down 'full blood count' on a laboratory request form is useless. It is essential to ask for an examination of the blood film in any patient who is suspected of having a haematological disorder. More can be learnt from the help of an experienced morphologist than any other investigation in clinical haematology. Some haematological investigations are underused; others are requested far too often. For example, the often forgotten reticulocyte count is an invaluable guide to the response of the bone marrow to anaemia and for the recognition of bleeding or mild haemolysis. On the other hand, bone marrow examination, while invaluable in many cases, is an unpleasant investigation and should only be requested with very clear indications. For example, clinicians should stop and think why they are ordering a bone marrow examination in an elderly patient with a peripheral blood lymphocyte count of $80\,000 \times 10^9/1$. This can only be chronic lymphatic leukaemia; the bone marrow will be infiltrated with lymphocytes. Why put the patient through this traumatic investigation? The result is predictable and will not help in their management.

In the section which follows we shall describe briefly the normal blood count and what can be learnt from a peripheral blood film and bone marrow examination. It cannot be emphasized too strongly that the most useful information is obtained by very close liaison between the laboratory and the ward. Clinicians should visit the haematology laboratory regularly, review films and haematological data with their laboratory colleagues, and be very precise in setting out the reasons for the investigations which they order. Much valuable information is lost because of lack of good liaison between the bedside and the laboratory.

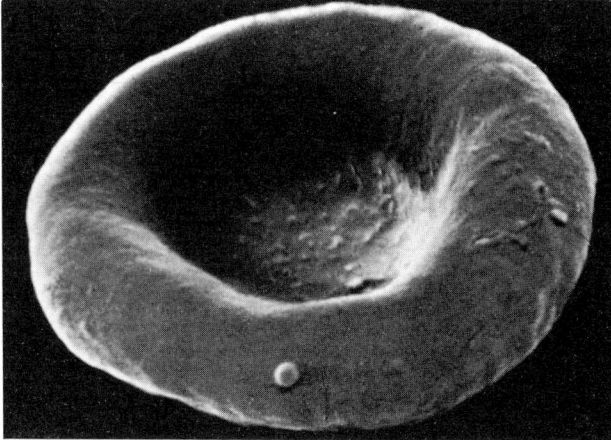

Fig. 1 A human erythrocyte as viewed through the scanning electron microscope. (By kind permission of Dr S. M. Lewis.)

Table 1 Significance of morphological and staining variations of the red cells

Change	Clinical significance
Hypochromia	Defective haemoglobinization; usually iron deficiency or defective haemoglobin synthesis
Microcytosis	As above
Macrocytosis	Dyserythropoiesis or premature release; may indicate megaloblastic erythropoiesis or haemolysis
Anisochromia	Variability of haemoglobinization or presence of young red cell populations, e.g. in haemolysis
Spherocytosis	Usually indicates damage to membrane; may result from a genetic disorder of the membrane or an acquired defect often due to antibody or other damage to the cell
Target cells	Large 'floppy' cells which occur with deficient haemoglobinization or in liver disease; also occur in hyposplenism
Elliptocytes	May result from a genetic defect in the red cell membrane but also occur in a variety of acquired conditions including iron deficiency
Poikilocytes: include burr cells, helmet cells, schistocytes, fragmented forms, etc.	Usually indicates trauma to red cells in microcirculation or severe oxidant damage
Sickle cells	Occur in the sickling disorders
Acanthocytes	Occur in genetic disorders of lipid metabolism
Inclusions: iron granules (siderocytes). Howell-Jolly bodies and Cabot's rings (nuclear remnants), basophilic stippling, and Heinz bodies	Iron granules and nuclear remnants are often seen after splenectomy. Basophilic stippling indicates accelerated erythropoiesis or defective haemoglobin synthesis. Heinz bodies are precipitated haemoglobin or globin subunits

Examination of the blood

Constituents of normal blood

Blood consists of several different types of cells suspended in plasma. The classification and morphological analysis of blood cells was made possible by the studies of Ehrlich who, in 1877, described the use of aniline dyes for staining dried blood films. This approach has been refined over the years with the gradual improvement of the microscope, and the fine structure of the blood cells has been analysed in greater detail with the electron microscope and, more recently, with the scanning electron microscope (Fig. 1).

The formed elements of the blood, or blood cells, consist of the red cells, white cells, and platelets. The red cells are biconcave discs which measure approximately 7–8 μm in diameter (Fig. 1). They consist of a membrane which contains a concentrated solution of haemoglobin and a variety of other proteins, salts, and vitamins. Normally they are of a uniform shape and size and contain similar amounts of haemoglobin. On supravital staining, approximately 1 per cent of the red cells show a reticular appearance. These are newly released cells and because of their staining characteristics are called reticulocytes.

The white cells are classified according to their morphological appearances into granulocytes (polymorphonuclear leucocytes), monocytes, and lymphocytes. The granulocytes and monocytes are phagocytic cells while the lymphocytes are involved in a variety of immune mechanisms. The granulocytes can be further classified according to their maturity. In the newly produced forms, band cells or juvenile polymorphonuclear leucocytes, the

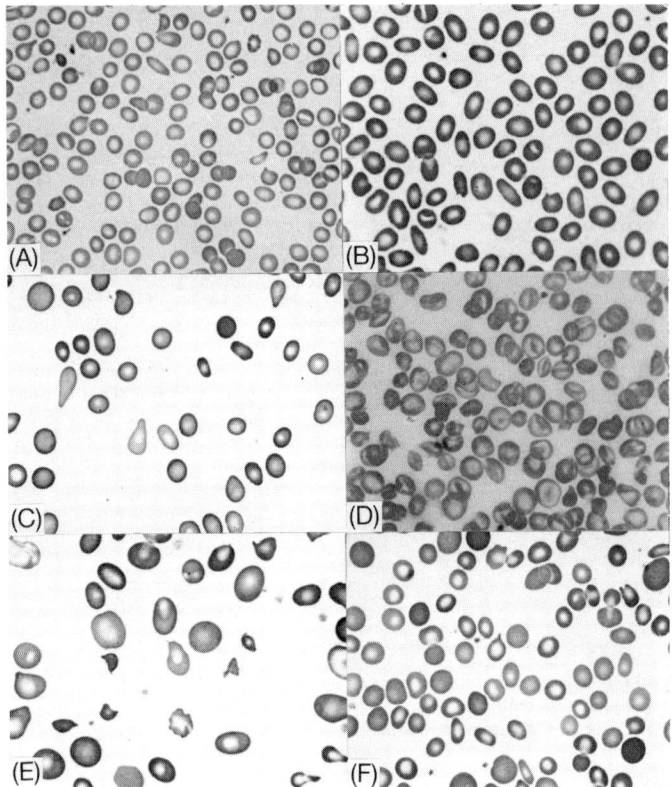

Fig. 2 Morphological changes of the red cells (× 600–800). (A) Hypochromia and microcytosis. (B) Elliptocytosis. (C) Poikilocytosis (myelosclerosis). (D) Target cells and intracellular crystals (haemoglobin C disease). (E) Macrocytosis and anisocytosis (pernicious anaemia). (F) Dimorphic picture – normochromic and hypochromic (sideroblastic anaemia).

nucleus is horseshoe-shaped but single. In a normal blood film the majority of the granulocytes have matured beyond this stage and their nuclei consist of two or more lobes separated by thin, filamentous chromatin strands. These cells are about 12–15 μm in diameter. The granulocyte series is further classified according to the staining characteristics of the granules into neutrophils, eosinophils, and basophils. The monocytes are of similar size to the granulocytes but have oval nuclei with a slate coloured cytoplasm which may contain some fine granules.

There are two morphologically distinct forms of lymphocyte; a large cell with a diameter of 8–16 μm and a smaller one measuring 7–9 μm. Both forms are round and have a light blue cytoplasm. In the large lymphocytes the nucleus fills about half of the cell whereas in the small lymphocytes it almost completely fills the cell.

The platelets are disc-shaped cells measuring approximately 2–3 μm in diameter. In normal blood they are relatively homogeneous in structure; their fine structure cannot be distinguished by conventional light microscopy.

A more detailed description of the structure and function of these different blood cells and their precursors appears later in this chapter.

Investigation of the blood – the normal blood count

A full blood count can be carried out on a 5 ml anticoagulated blood sample. A stained blood film is prepared for examination of the morphology of the different cells. Using either chemical and physical methods, or the more accurate electronic cell counters, the relative volume of packed red cells and white cells, the haemoglobin level, and the red cell, white cell, and platelet counts can be determined. From a series of calculations relating the volume of packed cells, haemoglobin level, and red cell count, it is poss-

Table 2 Normal haematological data

Measurement	Male	Female
White cell count (x10⁹/l)	7.25 (3.9–10.6)	7.28 (3.5–11.0)
Red cell count (x10¹²/l)	5.11 (4.4–5.9)	4.51 (3.8–5.2)
Haemoglobin (g/dl)	15.5 (13.3–17.7)	13.7 (11.7–15.7)
Packed cell volume (%)	46.0 (39.8–52.2)	40.9 (34.9–46.9)
Mean cell volume (fl)	90.1 (80.5–99.7)	90.4 (80.8–100.0)
Mean cell haemoglobin (pg)	30.2 (26.6–33.8)	30.2 (26.4–34.1)
Mean cell haemoglobin concentration (g/dl)	33.9 (31.5–36.3)	33.6 (32.4–35.8)
Platelets (10⁹/l)	295 (150–440)	295 (150–440)

From Lewis (1982) and Williams (1983).

Table 3 Calculation of the absolute indices

Mean cell volume (MCV) = PCV ÷ RBC (per 1) × 10^{15}
    expressed as femtolitres (fl)
Mean cell haemoglobin (MCH) = Hb (g/dl) ÷ RBC (per 1) × 10^{12}
    expressed as picograms (pg)
Mean cell haemoglobin concentration (MCHC) = Hb (g/dl) ÷ PCV
    expressed as g/dl

Table 4 Mean haemoglobin values and range of red cell indices during development

	Birth	3 months	12 months	10 years	Adults
Haemoglobin (g/dl)	19.5	13.0	11.0	12.0	♂ 15.5 ♀ 13.7
MCV (fl)	109–128	83–110	77–101	77–95	80.99
MCH (pg)	26–33	24–34	23–31	24–30	27–33
MCHC (g/dl)	30–34	27–34	28–33	30–30	31–36

From Lewis (1982) and Wood (1982).

ible to derive a series of absolute indices which provide useful information about the size and degree of haemoglobinization of the red cells. Finally, the relative numbers of reticulocytes and the erythrocyte sedimentation rate can be determined.

The stained blood film

An examination of the stained blood film is the most important investigation in haematology. Each of the cell types are studied separately.

The red cells are examined to assess their degree of haemoglobinization and their shape; if both are normal, they are described as normochromic and normocytic. Disorders of the red cell are frequently associated with changes in their morphology or staining properties. These include variation in size or anisocytosis; an increase in size or macrocytosis; a reduction in size or microcytosis; variability in shape or poikilocytosis; pale-staining or hypochromia which suggests under-haemoglobinization; and variation in the degree of staining from cell to cell which is called anisochromia. In addition to these changes there may be more specific alterations in the morphology of the red cells. Some of these, together with the different clinical disorders with which they are associated, are summarized in Table 1 and illustrated in Fig. 2.

Table 5 The normal white cell count and differential white cell count at different ages

Age (years)	Leucocytes (total)	Neutrophils			Eosinophils	Basophils	Monocytes	Lymphocytes
		Total	Juvenile	Segmented				
1	11.4 (6.0–17.5)	3.5 (1.5–8.5)	0.35	3.2	0.3 (0.05–0.70)	0.05 (0–0.20)	0.55 (0.05–1.1)	7.0 (4.0–10.5)
4	9.1 (5.5–15.5)	3.8 (1.5–8.5)	0.27 (0–1.0)	3.5 (1.5–7.5)	0.25 (0.02–0.65)	0.05 (0–0.20)	0.45 (0–0.8)	4.5 (2.0–8.0)
6	8.5 (5.0–14.5)	4.3 (1.5–8.0)	6.25 (0–1.0)	4.0 (1.5–7.0)	0.23 (0–0.65)	0.05 (0–0.20)	0.40 (0–0.8)	3.5 (1.5–7.0)
10	8.1 (4.5–13.5)	4.4 (1.8–8.0)	0.24 (0–1.0)	4.2 (1.8–7.0)	0.20 (0–0.60)	0.04 (0–0.20)	0.35 (0–0.8)	3.1 (1.5–6.5)
21	7.4 (4.5–11.0)	4.4 (1.8–7.7)	0.22 (0–0.7)	4.2 (1.8–7.0)	0.20 (0–0.45)	0.04 (0–0.20)	0.30 (0–0.8)	2.5 (1.0–4.8)

Modified from Williams (1983).

The white cells may be abnormal in number or morphology. An increased white cell count is called a leucocytosis. If this involves the polymorphonuclear series, it is called a polymorphonuclear leucocytosis or granulocytosis. An elevated eosinophil, basophil, monocyte, or lymphocyte count is called an eosinophilia, basophilia, monocytosis, or lymphocytosis respectively. A reduced white count is called a neutropenia or lymphopenia, depending on the cell type involved. An absence of granulocytes in the blood is called agranulocytosis. As is the case for the red cell series, much can be learned by morphological examination of the white cells. A blood film is said to show a 'shift to the left' if there are relatively more 'young' polymorphonuclear leucocytes present than normal. This is reflected by an increased proportion of band forms and, in more extreme cases, by a variable number of myelocytes or metamyelocytes. In acute bacterial infections vacuoles may appear in the cytoplasm of polymorphonuclear leucocytes. In addition, the granules may become morphologically abnormal; heavy granulation of this type is called toxic granulation. This change is sometimes associated with the presence of small (1–2 μm) oval bodies called Döhle bodies. A variety of genetic changes of nuclear configuration or of the granules of the polymorphonuclear leucocytes have been described; these are discussed later in this section.

The packed cell volume, haemoglobin level, and red cell indices

A great deal can be learnt about the character of an anaemia from a few simple haematological tests. The volume of packed red cells (PCV or haematocrit) can be estimated either by centrifugation of a blood sample or by a conductivity method in which it is derived from measurement of the red cell volume and the number of red cells using an electronic counting system. The haemoglobin concentration is usually determined spectrophotometrically by comparing a test sample with a stable standard, usually of the cyanmethaemoglobin derivative. Although for many years red cell counting fell into disrepute, it has now become part of a standard blood count because of the accuracy of electronic cell counters.

Normal values for the PCV, haemoglobin level, and red cell count are shown in Table 2. It is important to become familiar with the variability of these figures at different stages of development and between the sexes (Tables 2, 4, and 5). Furthermore, it should be emphasized that the accuracy of these measurements relies very much on the method which is used for their determination. For example, using an electronic cell counter, extremely reproducible results for all three measurements can be obtained, whereas a red cell count carried out using a counting chamber is of little value. By combining information obtained from these measurements the red cell indices can be estimated (Table 3). The mean cell haemoglobin (MCH), which is derived from the haemoglobin value and the red cell count and is expressed in picograms (pg), gives a reliable indication of the mount of haemoglobin per cell. The mean cell haemoglobin concentration (MCHC) represents the concentration of haemoglobin in g/dl (100 ml) of erythrocytes. The mean cell volume (MCV), calculated in femtolitres (fl), gives an indication of the size of the erythrocytes. Hence it is elevated in patients with macrocytic disorders and

Table 6 Normal values for red cell, plasma and blood volumes

	Value (ml/kg)
Red cell volume	
Men	30 ± 5
Women	25 ± 5
Plasma volume	45 ± 5
Total blood volume	70 ± 10

Lewis (1982).

reduced in the presence of microcytic red cells. The normal values at different stages of development are summarized in Table 4.

It should be emphasized that the red cell indices give an indication of the *average* size and degree of haemoglobinization of the red cells. Thus they are only of value if combined with an examination of a blood film to provide information about the relative uniformity of any changes in size or haemoglobin concentration.

The total and differential leucocyte count

The leucocyte count can be determined either using a counting chamber or electronically. The differential count is obtained from analysing the different types of white cells in a total of 200–300 cells, or more if the total white cell count is unusually low. It should be remembered that the total white cell count shows remarkable variability even in the same individual at different times. There are variations during the menstrual cycle and a marked diurnal rhythm with minimum counts in the morning with subjects at rest. Activity may increase the white cell count slightly as may emotional stress and eating. Furthermore, the differential white cell count varies considerably during normal human development. There is a preponderance of lymphocytes during the first few years of life and of polymorphonuclear leucocytes during later development and in adult life. These normal variations are shown in Table 5.

The platelet count

This is most accurately determined using an electronic cell counter although a rough approximation can be obtained using a counting chamber. There is marked variation in the normal platelet count and the range in health is approximately 150–400 × 10^9/l. A slight drop in the count occurs before menstruation but on the whole it varies less within an individual than the white cell count.

Blood volume, red cell mass, and plasma volume

Because the haemoglobin level or PCV may vary due to expansion or contraction of the plasma volume, it is sometimes necessary to measure the red cell mass and plasma volume directly. This is usually done by radio-isotope dilution. The red cell volume (RCV) is measured by labelling the red cells with ^{51}Cr and the plasma volume (PV) by the use of isotope-labelled albumin. These measurements are fraught with difficulties because of the variation of vascularity and PCV between different organs, and because fat is a relatively avascular tissue. There is still considerable contro-

Table 7 Clinical significance of variable relationship between red cell and plasma volumes

Red cell volume	Plasma volume	Cause	Effect
Normal	High	Pregnancy (2nd–3rd trimesters) cirrhosis nephritis congestive cardiac failure	Relative anaemia
Normal	Low	'Stress' peripheral circulatory failure dehydration high altitude (1st 2 weeks) prolonged bed rest	Relative polycythaemia
Low	Normal	Anaemia	Accurate reflection of degree of anaemia
Low	High	Anaemia	Clinical anaemia less severe than indicated by blood count
Low	Low	Haemorrhage severe anaemia	Clinical anaemia more severe than indicated by blood count
High	Normal to low	Polycythaemia vera secondary polycythaemia ('erythrocytosis')	Accurate reflection of clinical state or polycythaemia less severe than apparent
High	High	Polycythaemia	Polycythaemia more severe than apparent
Normal or high	High	Marked splenomegaly	Pseudo-anaemia

Modified from Lewis (1982).

Table 8 Normal range for differential count on aspirated bone marrow

	Percentage
Reticulum cells	0.1–2
Haemocytoblasts	0.1–1
Myeloblasts	0.1–3.5
Promyelocytes	0.5–5
Myelocytes	
Neutrophil	5–20
Eosinophil	0.1–3
Basophil	0.5–0
Metamyelocytes	10–30
Polymorphonuclears	
Neutrophil	7–25
Eosinophil	0.2–3
Basophil	0–0.5
Lymphocytes	5–20
Monocytes	0–0.2
Megakaryocytes	0.1–0.5
Plasma cells	0.1–3.5
Pronormoblasts	0.5–5
Basophilic and polychromatic normoblasts	2–20
Pyknotic normoblasts	2–10

From Lewis (1982).

versy about how best to express the results. A variety of correction factors have been derived which attempt to relate the measured RCV or PV to an ideal body weight. In practice it is usual to simply calculate the RCV or PCV in ml/kg. The wide range of normal values are summarized in Table 6 and the changes in various disease states in Table 7.

The erythrocyte sedimentation rate (ESR)
The ESR is a measure of the suspension stability of red cells in blood. It is usually expressed in mm and is obtained by measuring the distance from the surface meniscus to the upper limit of the red cell layer in a column of blood after 60 min. The ESR depends on the difference in specific gravity between the red cells and plasma but is influenced by many other factors, particularly the rate at which the red cells clump or form rouleaux. The increased sedimentation rate of clusters of cells reflects reduced fluid friction resulting from a decreased surface : volume ratio. Rouleaux form-

ation is related to the concentration of fibrinogen and, to a lesser extent, of α_2 and γ globulins in the plasma. Unfortunately, the ESR is also subject to many technical difficulties including the dimensions of the tube, the nature of the anticoagulant used, and any degree of tilt of the tube from the horizontal.

The ESR is still widely used as a non-specific index of organic disease. It is elevated in many acute or chronic infections, neoplastic diseases, collagen diseases, renal insufficiency, and any disorder associated with a significant change in the plasma proteins. Anaemia may cause an increased rate of sedimentation, and although many attempts have been made to develop correction factors to allow for this variable, none is satisfactory. Like all haematological measurements, the ESR changes in certain physiological states, particularly in pregnancy and with increasing age. In men and women over the age of 60 a slightly elevated ESR is often found without an obvious cause.

Other haematological investigations
The simple tests that have been outlined in this section form the general screening investigations for all haematological disorders. In later sections we will describe the more specialized investigations which are often required to diagnose specific disorders of the red cells, white cells, and platelets, or of haemostasis and coagulation.

Examination of the marrow
Bone marrow can be examined by needle aspiration, closed needle biopsy, or open surgical biopsy. In adults the sites most easily available are the sternum and the anterior or posterior iliac crests, although the marrow at the latter sites tends to become rather fatty in elderly subjects. In children of less than a year old the anterior surface of the tibia is the site of choice, but in older children the iliac crest or the lumbar vertebral spines are suitable. After aspiration of the marrow, films are made and stained with a Romanowsky stain. Needle or surgical biopsy samples are fixed and sectioned by standard methods.

The marrow films are examined initially under low power to assess the overall cellularity and for the presence of abnormal cells. It is sometimes useful to obtain a differential count (Table 8) and from this the myeloid/erythroid (M/E) ratio can be determined. This is approximately 3:1 in health although, if there is increased erythroid activity, it may fall to unity or less. It should be remembered that differential counts may be quite inaccurate because the precursors may not be distributed homogeneously. This is a particular problem in disorders in which there are abnormal cells in the marrow. Having determined the overall cellularity, the morphology of the individual cells is examined. The degree of maturation of the red cells, white cells, and megakaryocyte series is assessed and the marrow is examined carefully for the presence of any abnormal cells.

A biopsy specimen is particularly useful for looking at overall cellularity and relating the amount of haemopoiesis to the amount of fatty tissue. It is of particular value if an aspiration yields a 'dry tap' when it may show replacement by fibrous or tumour tissue which may not aspirate readily. Using appropriate stains it is possible to estimate the amount of iron and reticulin in the marrow.

Assessment of bone marrow activity and distribution

Some indication of marrow function is obtained from its morphological appearances and from the M/E ratio. It is also possible to measure the rates of production and turnover of the red cell series using radioactive iron (see page 19.82). It is sometimes necessary to attempt to estimate the distribution of the haemopoietic marrow, and this is usually done by using isotopes to produce scintograms that show the distribution of erythropoietic or reticuloendothelial marrow throughout the body. Erythropoietic marrow can be visualized using the short-lived positron emitting isotope ^{52}Fe with a scintillation camera. In health this shows erythropoietic marrow in the ribs, spine, pelvis, scapula, and clavicle with a variable amount in the skull. The reticuloendothelial portion of the marrow can be labelled with a radiocolloid with an appropriate particle size; the most effective and commonly used is ^{99}Tc^{m}-sulphurcolloid.

References

General haematology texts

Dacie, J. V. and Lewis, S. M. (1984). *Practical haematology*, 6th edn. Churchill Livingstone, Edinburgh.

Hardisty, R. M. and Weatherall, D. J. (1982). *Blood and its disorders*, 2nd edn. Blackwell Scientific Publications, Oxford.

Nathan, D. G. and Oski, F. A. (1981). *Haematology in infancy and childhood*, 2nd edn. W. B. Saunders, Philadelphia, London, Toronto.

Penington, D. G., Rush, B. and Castaldi, P. (1978). *Clinical haematology in medical practice*. Blackwell Scientific Publications, Oxford.

Williams, W. J., Beutler, E., Erslev, A. J. and Lichtman, M. A. (1983). *Hematology*, 3rd edn. McGraw-Hill Book Co., New York.

Normal haematological data

Lewis, S. M. (1982). The constituents of normal blood and marrow. In *Blood and its disorders* 2nd edn (eds R. M. Hardisty and D. J. Weatherall), pp. 3–56. Blackwell Scientific Publications, Oxford.

Williams, W. J. (1983). Examination of the blood. In *Hematology*, 3rd edn (eds W. J. Williams, E. Beutler, A. J. Erslev and M. A. Lichtman), pp. 9–24. McGraw-Hill Book Co., New York.

Wood, W. G. (1982). Developmental haemopoiesis. In *Blood and its disorders*, 2nd edn (eds R. M. Hardisty and D. J. Weatherall), pp. 75–100. Blackwell Scientific Publications, Oxford.

HAEMATOPOIETIC STEM CELLS

Stem cells and haematopoiesis

D. G. NATHAN

Introduction

Normal haematopoiesis in the adult is regulated by the production of blood cells from their recognizable precursors in the bone marrow, their survival in the vasculature and their demise in the reticuloendothelial system, predominantly in the spleen, the liver, the lung, and the marrow itself. Though the concentration of cells in the blood oscillates, it is notable that the values observed in normal individuals are, in fact, remarkably consistent, particularly considering the vast differences in the life-spans of these cells. For example, the mean life-span of granulocytes in the peripheral blood may be measured in hours. In contrast, platelets survive for 7–10 days. Though platelets are removed from the blood in part by random forces, most of their life-span is dictated by metabolic changes within them that lead to predetermined death in about 7–10 days. Normally, red cells are almost entirely lost by a process of metabolic decay that begins after the erythrocyte has attained an age of approximately 100 days. Lymphocytes have very dramatic differences in life-span. Some are removed from the circulation in two or three weeks by a process that is not at all understood. Others, particularly certain T-lymphocytes, are thought to survive for the entire life-span of the individual, carrying within them the programmes embossed upon them by the thymus prior to its atrophy.

Though steady-state concentrations of the blood cells vary from each other by three logs or more, the actual marrow production rates that maintain them are very similar. Approximately 5×10^4 red cells, 2×10^4 platelets and 2×10^4 granulocytes must be produced per μl of blood per day to maintain a normal blood count. Lymphocyte production must be considerably lower because of the bulk of lymphocytes in the peripheral blood are the long-lived T-lymphocytes described above.

These relatively constant production rates of blood cells are regulated by a highly complex marrow tissue characterized morphologically by recognizable differentiating precursor cells that are themselves partially renewed by a widely variable population of invisible progenitor cells, some of which have the characteristics of stem cells. These differentiating precursor cells and their progenitors are packed together into fronds surrounded by endothelial cells that separate the marrow cells from the venous sinuses. The completed blood cells find apertures through the endothelial cells and migrate between them to fall into the sinuses, the currents of which carry them into the peripheral blood.

In this chapter, we shall describe some of the important aspects of the physiology of haematopoiesis in the marrow. To understand this process, we must first review its ontogeny and comparative development.

Phylogeny and ontogeny

John Hunter was a remarkable surgeon, but in this writer's opinion he was wrong when he decided that the red cell is the least important element in the blood. Adaptation to terrestrial existence, accompanied by the development of a cardiorespiratory system, demanded that haemoglobin be encapsulated within erythrocytes rather than float free in the vasculature. This permits high oxygen delivery and acceptable blood viscosity. The renewal rate of red cells is a function of metabolic rate. Thus, turtles and crocodiles have remarkably low red cell production rates whereas pygmy shrews renew their red cells very rapidly. Marmots exhibit a marked reduction in red cell renewal when they hibernate at cold temperatures. In the juvenile state, European eels lack erythrocytes but when they swim against the current of the rivers in northern Europe, nucleated erythrocytes appear. This is one of the most primitive demonstrations of the role of oxygen demand on erythropoiesis and is also observed in non-red-cell-producing organisms such as Daphnia, the English water flea that produces high molecular haemoglobin in its ovaries when exposed to low oxygen tension in stagnant ponds.

In the developing human, haematopoiesis moves through several overlapping anatomical and functional stages, beginning in the yolk sac, entering the hepatic phase at 6 weeks, and the marrow phase at 20 weeks gestation. Transfer to the bone marrow phase is generally complete at birth. These anatomical shifts in sites of haematopoiesis are associated with marked alterations in functional properties, particularly with respect to the red cell. These changes, which are described in detail on page 19.108, are referred to as the 'fetal switch'. Clearly this transition is not a single event involving the gamma chains of fetal haemoglobin alone, but is instead polygenic involving a series of enzymes that are regulated in a programmed fashion. The mechanism of this co-ordinated series of changes of gene expression is as yet undetermined, but it appears to be mediated at the level of the progenitors of haematopoietic cells and is strongly influenced by site-specific regulatory factors.

Marrow anatomy

The relative red (active) marrow space of a child is much greater than that of an adult, presumably because the high requirements for red cell production during neonatal life demand the resources of the entire production potential of the marrow. During postnatal life the demands for red cell production ebb, and much of the marrow space is slowly and progressively filled with fat (Fig. 1). In certain diseases that are usually associated with anaemia, such as myeloid metaplasia, haematopoiesis may return to its former sites in the liver, spleen, and lymph nodes and may also be found in the adrenals, cartilage, adipose tissue, thoracic paravertebral gutters, and even in the kidneys.

The micro-environment of the marrow cavity is a vast network of vascular channels or sinusoids that separate clumps of haematopoietic cells, including fat cells. The cells are found in the intrasinusoidal spaces. The vascular and haematopoietic compartments are separated by reticular cells (presumably fibroblasts) that form the adventitial surfaces of the vascular sinuses and extend cytoplasmic processes to create a fibronectin-rich lattice on which blood cells are found. The latter is demonstrated by reticulin stains of marrow sections (Fig. 2) as well as by flourescent antibody stains. The conformation of the meshwork of fibroblast cytoplasmic extension and fibronectin, and the location of haematopoietic cells in the network of vascular sinuses are best illustrated by scanning electron microscopy (Fig. 3).

A schema of the marrow circulation is shown in Fig. 4. The central and radial arteries ramify in the cortical capillaries, which in turn join the marrow sinusoids and drain into the central sinus. Cells that egress from the marrow sinusoids then join the venous circulation through concomitant veins. The inner, or luminal, surface of the vascular sinusoids is lined with endothelial cells, the cytoplasmic extensions of which overlap, or interdigitate, with one another. The escape of developing haematopoietic cells into the sinus for transport to the circulation occurs through gaps that develop in this endothelial lining and even through endothelial cell cytoplasmic pores.

The location of the different haematopoietic cells is not random. Clumps of megakaryocytes are found adjacent to marrow sinuses. They shed platelets, the fragments of their cytoplasm, directly into the lumen. This reduces the requirement for movement of bulky mature megakaryocytes, a mobility characteristic of the granuloid- and erythroid-differentiated precursors as they approach the point at which they egress from the marrow. A schema that illustrates the transfer of haematopoietic cells into the sinuses is shown in Fig. 5.

The micro-environment just described must have cells that

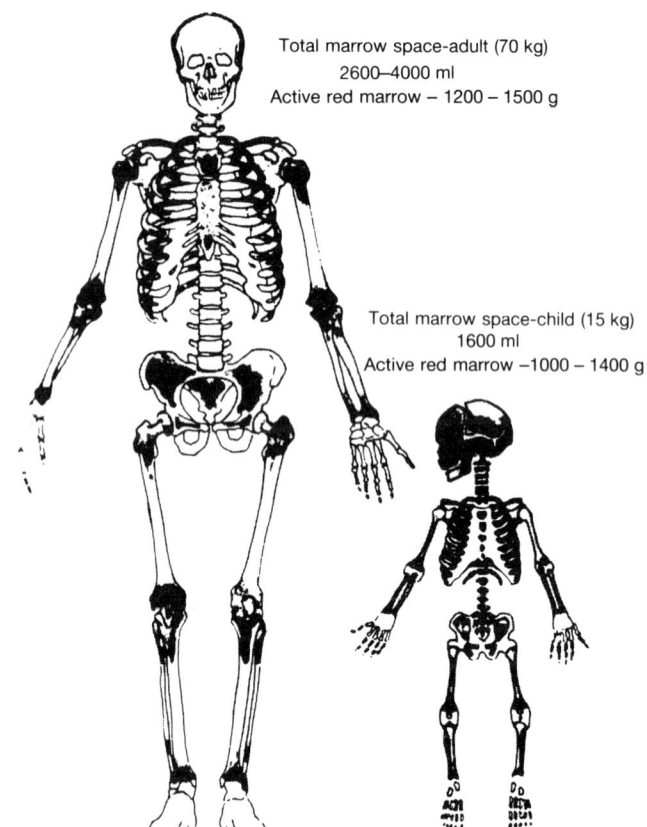

Total marrow space-adult (70 kg)
2600–4000 ml
Active red marrow – 1200 – 1500 g

Total marrow space-child (15 kg)
1600 ml
Active red marrow –1000 – 1400 g

Fig. 1 A comparison of active red marrow-bearing areas in a child and adult. Note the almost identical amount of active red marrow in the child and adult despite a fivefold discrepancy in body weight. (Reproduced from MacFarlane and Robb-Smith (eds), 1961, *Functions of the blood*, p. 357. Blackwell Scientific Publications, Oxford.)

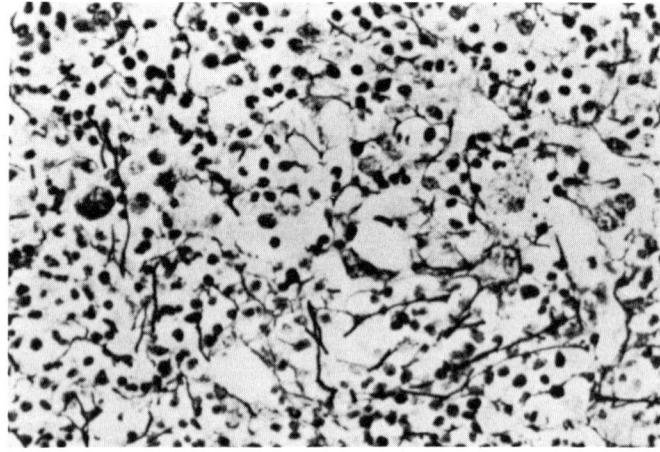

Fig. 2 Bone marrow biopsy of a patient with mild myelofibrosis. A slight increase in the number of reticulin fibres in a delicate discontinuous fibre network is present. (Gomori stain × 350.) (Reproduced from Lennert, Nagai, *et al.*, 1975, *Clin. Haematol.* **4**, 335.)

transfer information-containing replicative signals to the marrow progenitor and precursor cells. The nature of these signals and the cells that produce them are described briefly below. The loss of this information transfer system may be responsible for some types of aplastic anaemia.

As mentioned above, the formed elements of blood in verte-

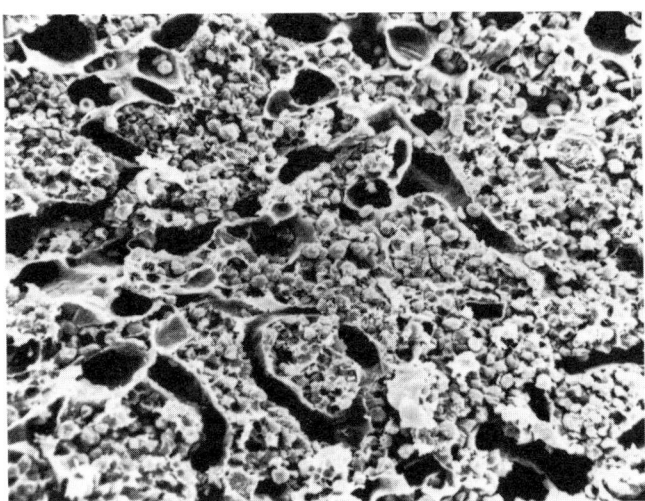

Fig. 3 Scanning electronmicrograph of rat femoral marrow. The haemato-poietic cells are grouped between the interlacing network of vascular sinuses. Many cells are dislodged when the marrow is transected, and separate spaces are present where cells had been. (Reproduced from Lichtman, Chamberlain *et al.*, 1978, Factors thought to contribute to the regulation of egress of cells from marrow. In *The year in hematology*, (eds) K. Silber, J. LoBue *et al.*, pp. 243–279. Plenum Medical Book Company, New York.)

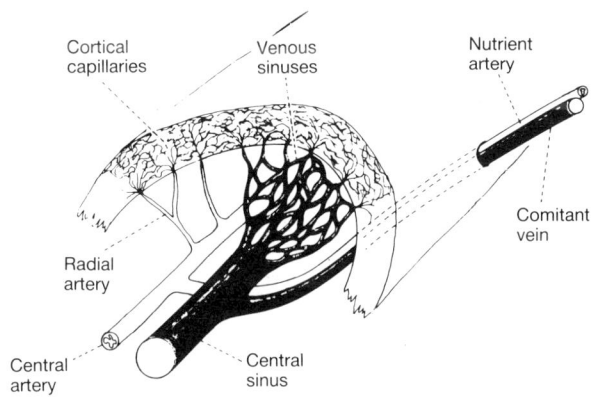

Fig. 4 A schematic representation of the circulation of the marrow. The nutrient artery, central arteries, and radial arteries feed the cortical capillaries. The cortical capillaries anastomose with the marrow sinuses, which drain into the large central sinus. The central sinus enters the comitant vein by which the marrow effluent enters the systemic venous circulation. An interesting feature of the circulation of marrow is the transit of nearly all arterial blood through cortical capillaries before entering the marrow sinuses. Not shown are the arterial communications from muscular arteries that feed the periosteum and penetrate the cortex to anastomose with intracortical vessels. (Reproduced from Lichtman, Chamberlain *et al.*, 1978, Factors thought to contribute to the regulation of egress of cells from marrow. In *The year in hematology*, (eds) K. Silber, J. LoBue *et al.*, pp. 243–279. Plenum Medical Book Company, New York.)

brates, including humans, continuously undergo replacement to maintain a constant number of red cells, white cells and platelets. The number of cells of each type is maintained in a very narrow range in normal adults – approximately 5000 granulocytes, 5×10^6 red blood cells, and 150 000 – 300 000 platelets per μl of whole blood. In the following section we shall examine the normal regulatory mechanisms that maintain a balanced production of new blood cells. They are still not completely understood, but present evidence strongly supports the following basic principles.

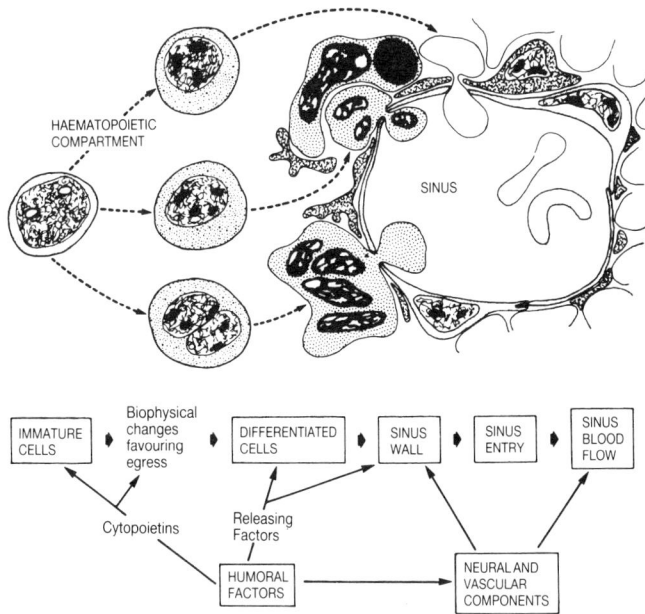

Fig. 5 A schematic diagram of the factors that may be involved in controlling the release of marrow cells. The central relationship between the haematopoietic compartment and the marrow sinus is depicted. The drawing highlights the similarity of the egress process for the three major haematopoietic cells: reticulocytes in the top pathway, granulocytes and monocytes in the centre pathway, and platelets in the lower pathway. Immature cells undergo physical changes under the influence of cytopoietins that favour egress. In the case of the reticulocyte, enucleation precedes egress. This is shown by the solid black inclusion in the perisinal macrophage representing nucleophagocytosis antecedent to digestion of the erythroblast nucleus. The cytoplasmic protrusion of the megakaryocyte presumably detaches itself from the cell and will further fragment into platelets in the circulation. (Reproduced from Lichtman, Chamberlain *et al.*, 1978, Factors thought to contribute to the regulation of egress of cells from marrow. In *The year in hematology*, (eds) K. Silber, J. LoBue *et al.*, pp. 243–279. Plenum Medical Book Company, New York.)

Function of progenitors

The progenitors of the recognizable precursor cells are non descript primitive cells present at extremely low frequencies, approximately 1 in 1000 marrow cells. A single pluripotent stem cell is capable of giving rise, in a stochastic fashion, to increasingly committed progenitor cells according to the schema outlined in Fig. 6. These committed progenitors are destined to form differentiated recognizable precursors of the specific types of blood cells. There is no clear evidence that environmental stimuli influence the inherent programme of maturation of primitive progenitors to more committed progenitors.

Pluripotent stem cell progenitors are so defined because they are capable of self-renewal and under appropriate conditions can differentiate *in vitro* into a broad array of marrow precursors. The committed progenitor cells are limited in proliferative potential and are not capable of indefinite self-renewal. Their proliferative as well as their differentiative potentials are influenced by growth factors that are products of monocytes, thymocytes or certain stromal cells, probably fibroblasts. When pluripotent progenitors mature to committed progenitors they 'die by differentiation'. The maintainence of their numbers depends on influx from the pluripotent stem cell pool.

Committed progenitor cells are capable of response to humoral regulators produced in response to the circulating levels of particular differentiated cell types. Therefore, amplification of production occurs at the committed progenitor cell level.

Haematopoietic differentiation requires an appropriate microenvironment. In normal adult humans, this is confined to the bone

THE PROGENITOR BASIS OF HAEMATOPOIESIS

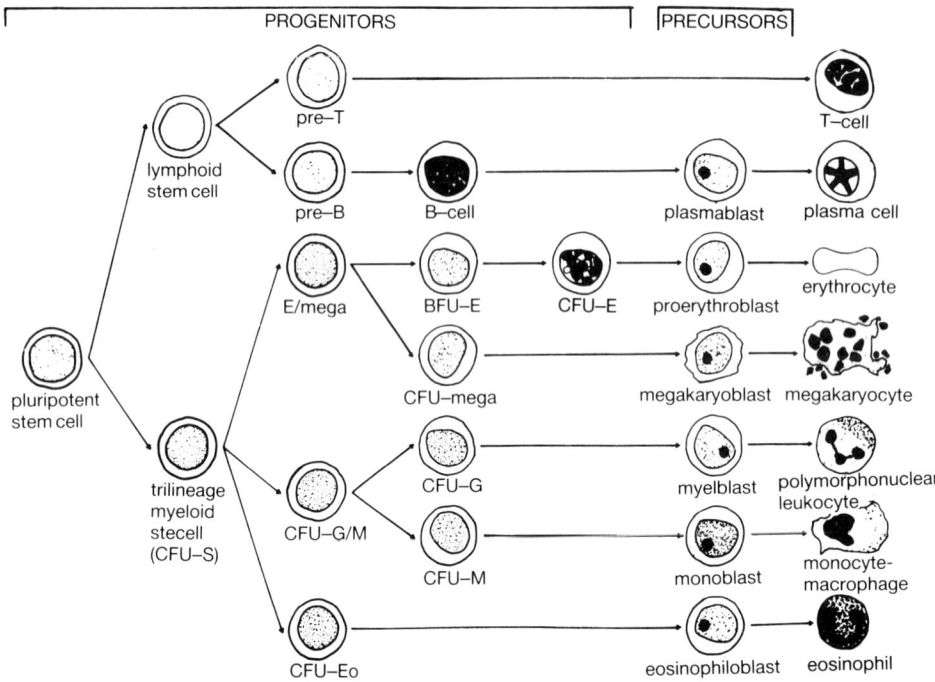

Fig. 6 The maturation sequence of progenitor cells. Progression advances from left to right. The sequence is characterized by a progressive approach to single lineage commitment. The term stem cell connotes high capacity for self-renewal, but all progenitors have some self-renewal capacity.

marrow, whereas in the mouse it includes both the spleen and bone marrow. The existence of certain strains of mice that exhibit a deficiency in the haematopoietic micro-environment suggests that the interactions between haematopoietic cells and the bone marrow micro-environment involve very specific molecular mechanisms. However, progenitors can exist outside the marrow. A number of early haematopoietic cells, including the pluripotent stem cells and certain committed progenitor cells, have been demonstrated in the peripheral circulation of normal individuals and experimental animals. The capacity of haematopoietic stem cells to negotiate the peripheral circulation is especially significant in relation to bone marrow transplantation which is carried out by infusion of bone marrow cells from the donor into the peripheral circulation of the recipient.

The relatively limited production of lymphocyte progenitors has made it difficult to demonstrate that the lymphocyte is derived from the same population of stem cells as the other cellular elements of blood. Present evidence indicates, however, that both T- and B-lymphocytes are in fact derived from a pluripotent stem cell that has the capacity to give rise to a tripotent stem cell that in turn matures to form the committed progenitors of red blood cells, phagocytes, and megakaryocytes.

The pluripotent stem cell

Till and McCulloch demonstrated that colonies of haematopoietic cells could be observed in the spleen in bone-marrow transplanted, irradiated recipient mice within 10 days after the transplant. These spleen colony-forming units (CFU-S) produce colonies that contain precursors to erythrocytes, granulocytes, macrophages, and megakaryocytes. Subsequent experiments using karyotypically matched donor cells confirmed the clonal origin of the differentiated cells and recent experiments in which foreign genes have been inserted into spleen colony-forming cells have further substantiated this finding. It was also shown that each

colony contains a number of stem cells that could form secondary colonies of differentiated progeny in a second irradiated recipient. The demonstration of a stem cell that can differentiate to form progenitor cells for erythropoiesis, granulopoiesis, and megakaryopoiesis is completely consistent with subsequent observations in diseases such as chronic myeloid leukaemia (CML) and polycythaemia vera in which a clonal origin of abnormal erythroid, granulocytic, and megakaryocytic precursor cells can be demonstrated (see page 19.13). In addition, these studies of CML have demonstrated a pluripotent stem cell that gives rise to B-cells as well as to the aforementioned blood cells. More recent studies provide a model of the CFU-S compartment in which CFU-S is viewed as a continuum of cells with a decreasing capacity for self-renewal, increasing likelihood for differentiation, and increasing proliferative activity. The cells progress in a unidirectional fashion in this continuum. The growth of a particular CFU-S in the marrow requires a 'niche'; thus isogeneic marrow infusions are not successful unless the recipient is irradiated or treated with sufficient doses of cytotoxic drugs to create an adequate number of niches. Therefore, reports of failure of engraftment in aplastic anaemia using identical twin donors do not necessarily suggest an immunologic basis for the disease but, equally as likely, imply persistence of non-functional pluripotent progenitors in the aplastic marrow niches. These abnormal cells must be destroyed in order to allow implantation of transfused normal progenitors.

Erythropoiesis

The least mature committed erythroid progenitor is known as an erythroid burst-forming unit or BFU-E because when it differentiates *in vitro* it forms large colonies of erythroblasts and reticulocytes that may contain as many as 50 000 cells. The colonies, derived from single cells, have a burst-like appearance because they may be composed of multiple subcolonies. Thus one BFU-E may initially divide in culture to form subcolony-forming cells which then differentiate into colonies of erythroblasts and reticulocytes. Much work has been devoted toward an understanding of the conditions which induce the formation of BFU-E-derived colonies *in vitro*. Two ingredients in addition to certain factors in serum are required. There must be continuously available a source of glycoprotein with a molecular weight of approximately 25 000, currently referred to as burst-promoting activity (BPA). This activity can be derived from T-cells, monocytes, and macrophages. More recently the activity has also been shown to reside in a tiny subfraction of non-adherent, non-T, FC receptor-positive cells and in certain fibroblastoid cells derived from the sites of haematopoiesis. Burst-promoting activity appears to induce the division and migration of BFU-E *in vitro* as well as to increase their sensitivity to the differentiating hormone, erythropoietin. The latter, largely derived from the kidney in man, interacts with the cell membrane of BFU-E exposed to BPA and induces the process of terminal differentiation to proerythroblasts and on to reticulocytes. The mechanisms by which erythropoietin induces this process of differentiation is not known, but it presumably triggers a cascade of erythroid cell-specific gene expression via its interaction with a receptor on the progenitor cell surface or within it. Conceivably, BPA renders the receptor more accessible to erythropoietin, perhaps by interacting with a neighbouring receptor. Though BPA has been characterized by its role in erythropoiesis, it is possible that its erythroid activity is only one such function. Recent studies of murine T-cells have shown that these cells are capable of producing a molecule called interleukin 3, the gene for which has been cloned, sequenced, and expressed *in vitro*. The resulting material can induce the differentiation of committed erythroid, phagocyte, and megakaryocyte progenitors *in vitro*. The search is now on for such a master haematopoietin in humans. A strong candidate is granulocyte macrophage colony stimulating factor (GMCSF). This material, the gene for which has been cloned and expressed, has BPA and trilineage colony stimulating activity as well.

Erythroid burst-forming units progressively mature during their sojourn in the marrow and in doing so, lose their capacity to divide and migrate *in vitro* but gain in apparent sensitivity to erythropoietin until they reach the stage at which they are known as erythroid colony units (CFU-E) which, in culture in the presence of erythropoietin, form small, single erythroid colonies within 7 d. Erythroid colony units also require BPA to respond to erythropoietin, but their sensitivity to both hormones make this difficult to demonstrate in the laboratory. Erythroid colony units and mature BFU-E are also highly responsive to the mitogenic effect of erythropoietin as well as to its differentiating role. Therefore, in haemorrhagic or haemolytic anaemias with elevated levels of erythropoietin, the numbers of CFU-E and mature BFU-E may rise remarkably in the marrow. Immature BFU-E are less responsive to the mitogenic effect of erythropoietin, and therefore, the frequency of this subset of BFU-E changes little in anaemia. Proerythroblasts represent the ultimate stage of differentiation of committed erythroid progenitors. In contrast to the progenitors, which comprise less than one 10th of a per cent of the marrow cell population, proerythroblasts are present at 3 – 5 per cent, and their daughters, the recognizable erythroid precursors, comprise 30 per cent of the population.

Estimates of reticulocyte production and erythroblast content of marrows, together with measurements of the rate at which the proerythroblast compartment is renewed from the progenitor pool suggest that approximately 10 per cent of the daily reticulocyte production is derived from the terminal differentiation of proerythroblasts newly developed from the progenitor department. During anaemic stress the rate at which progenitors differentiate to proerythroblasts may increase ten-fold or more. This increase in the rate of proerythroblast formation from progenitors is associated with an increase in the production of fetal haemoglobin in a large fraction of the erythroid cells derived from them. The basis of this reactivation of fetal haemoglobin synthesis in proerythroblasts newly derived from progenitors is not understood and the extent to which fetal haemoglobin may be increased in such settings could be genetically controlled. In any case, it is an important phenomenon since those with the capacity to develop large increases in fetal haemoglobin and are also homozygous for major beta-chain haemoglobinopathies may have a remarkably mild course (see page 19.110). Fetal haemoglobin elevation occurs in many forms of accelerated erythropoiesis and is indeed a marker of such a condition.

The downward regulation of erythropoiesis is influenced by levels of erythropoietin but also by direct suppression of erythroid progenitors by certain classes of T-lymphocytes. Overactivity or proliferation of the latter may lead to erythroid aplasia.

Phagocytopoiesis

The development of a clonal assay for granulocyte and macrophage progenitors preceded the development of erythroid progenitor assays by nearly a decade, yet a clear understanding of the regulation of myeloid differentiation remains elusive. Figure 6 describes the development and regulation of granulocyte, monocyte, and macrophage production from the pluripotent stem cell. The colony-forming-unit-granulocyte-macrophage (CFU-GM) derived from the pluripotent progenitor gives rise to separate granulocyte and monocyte progenitors which, under the influence of unique colony stimulating factors, differentiate to mature granulocytes and/or monocytes respectively. Monocytes leave the circulation and differentiate further to fixed tissue macrophages. These tissue macrophages include alveolar macrophages and hepatic Kupffer cells, dermal Langerhans cells, osteoclasts, peritoneal macrophages, pleural macrophages, and possibly brain microglial cells, though the origin of the latter is still uncertain. Thus, the wide variety of cells with diverse functions which must be supplied from the granulocyte–macrophage progenitor requires that this system be highly regulated at many levels of differentiation.

The granulocyte compartment itself is more complex than either the erythroid or megakaryocyte compartments. The circulating half-life of the newly rapidly deployed granulocyte is only 6.5 h. In order to meet sudden demands, an additional non-circulating granulocyte pool exists in the spleen, marginated around blood vessels, and in a readily releasable bone marrow pool.

The myriad of chemotactic and other factors that are responsible for the rapid release of granulocytes from the marrow and tissue pools are distinct from colony-stimulating activity (CSA). The latter is the generic term for a series of glycoproteins of molecular weight, approximately 20 000, that are produced mainly by both T-cells and macrophages or by an interaction between them. There are several colony-stimulating activities, the most important ones being those responsible for the production of granulocytes and macrophages by the relatively immature CFU-GM progenitor, by granulocytes and macrophages from the more mature CFU-G and CFU-M progenitors, and by eosinophils from the CFU-EO progenitor. The rate at which new myeloblasts or monoblasts are produced by progenitors *in vivo* is not known, but exhaustion of progenitors in infection, particularly in the newborn period, is associated with a fatal outcome due to a failure of granulocyte production.

As mentioned in the discussion of erythropoiesis, a single master colony-stimulating activity capable of inducing the differentiation of erythroid, phagocyte, and megakaryocyte progenitors exists in mice, and is known as interleukin 3; it is largely the product of T-cells. Such a master haematopoietin might exist in man and initiate the differentiation of all the committed progenitors. It is as likely, however, that two haematopoietins are required to induce the differentiation of phagocyte progenitors, one a compound such as GMCSF that prepares the surface of the progenitor to interact with a second and more specific molecule directed toward the differentiation of a more completely committed cell. In the next five years, as purified progenitors and inducing hormones become available the physiology will surely be clarified.

Suppression of phagocyte production An elaborate system of suppression of granulocyte and macrophage production involving T-lymphocytes and their products, particularly interferon, monocytes, and perhaps acidic isoferritins can be demonstrated *in vitro* and in some circumstances, clones of T-cells that suppress granulocyte production *in vitro* and *in vivo* have caused profound granulocytopenia. Clearly, a twin regulatory system exists that contributes to the fine control of phagocyte production by close control between progenitors and adventitial cells that secrete inducer and suppressor molecules. It is well established that T-lymphocytes capable of the suppression of phagocyte colony formation may be present in human marrow and induce neutropenia.

Megakaryocytopoiesis

Details concerning megakaryocyte progenitors are still being accumulated in man. Recent studies suggest that the regulation of thrombopoiesis parallels that of erythropoiesis to a certain extent. Megakaryocyte colony-stimulating activity (Meg CSA) appears to regulate early events in differentiation, while a hormone called thrombopoietin is responsible for the amplification of platelet production by directly stimulating the megakaryocyte to produce greater numbers of platelets. Thus Meg CSA and thrombopoietin appear to be analogous to BPA and erythropoietin in their roles as inducer and amplifier, respectively. Megakaryocyte precursors differ, however, from erythroid or myeloid cells in that, as their maturation proceeds, an increase in DNA content, i.e. mitosis without cell division, occurs. In the mouse, megakaryocyte differentiation can be stimulated by pokeweed mitogen-stimulated spleen-cell-conditioned medium, but the cell of origin of Meg CSA remains unknown.

Summary

Haematopoiesis is the process of terminal differentiation of recognizable immature precursors of the formed elements of the blood. Renewal of the precursor pool is accomplished by the differentiation of committed progenitor cells that are themselves renewed by a process of stochastic maturation of stem cells. A group of haematopoietins derived from T-cells, monocytes, and fibroblasts govern the differentiation of committed progenitor cells by mechanisms yet to be defined. A master haematopoietin is known to be produced in mice. It lacks erythropoietin actively but induces the capacity of committed erythroid progenitors to respond to erythropoietin.

The melange of marrow cells described above exists in delicate fronds thrust into the venous sinuses. Cells are packed in close proximity within the fronds, held together by extensions of fibroblast-like cytoplasm and fibronectin. Such a delicate anatomy is subject to a myriad of abnormalities that can disturb the orderly progress of cell–cell interactions that govern the system. The multiple symptoms of bone marrow failure are the results of these disturbances.

References

Dexter, T. M. (1984). The message in the medium. *Nature* **309**, 746–747.

Golde, D. W. and Takaku, F. (eds) (1985) *Hematopoietic stem cells.* Marcel Dekker, New York.

Graber, S. E. and Krantz, S. B. (1978). Erythropoietin and the control of red cell production. *Ann. Rev. Med.* **29**, 51–66.

Lajtha, L. G. (1982). Cellular kinetics of erythropoiesis. In *Blood and its disorders*, 2nd edn, (eds. R. M. Hardisty, and D. J. Weatherall), pp. 57–74. Blackwell Scientific Publications, Oxford.

McCulloch, E. A. (ed.) (1984). Culture techniques. *Clinics in haematology*, Vol. 13, pp. 307–519. W. B. Saunders, London.

Metcalf, D. and Moore, M. A. S. (1971). Hematopoietic cells. In *Frontiers of biology, Vol. 24*, (eds A. Neuberger, and E. G. Tatum). North Holland Publishing Company, Amsterdam.

Mladenovic, J. and Adamson, J. W. (1982). Erythroid colony growth in culture: analysis of erythroid differentiation and studies in human disease states. *Rec. Adv. Haematol.* **3**, 95–108.

Moore, M. A. S. (1982). Bone marrow culture: leucopoiesis and stem cells. *Rec. Adv. Haematol.* **3**, 109–142.

Quesenberry, P. (1979). Hematopoietic stem cells. *New Eng. J. Med.* **301**, 755–761.

Weiss, R. E. and Reddi, A. H. (1981). Appearance of fibronectin during the differentiation of cartilage, bone and bone marrow. *J. cell. Biol.* **88**, 630–636.

Classification of stem cell disorders

D. J. WEATHERALL

Since we know so little about the mechanisms of haematopoiesis, some readers may be surprised that we have devoted a section of a textbook of medicine to diseases of stem cells. However, provided it is remembered that when we talk about 'stem cells' we are never quite sure about the stage of commitment and differentiation of the cell population that we are trying to define, it is helpful to consider diseases which affect more than one type of blood cell under this heading. At least this approach provides us with a framework on which to try to understand what has long been an extremely puzzling and diverse group of disorders.

In order to introduce the idea of stem cell disorders we must consider how it arose and briefly examine the evidence that these conditions are due to abnormal proliferation of early haematopoietic progenitors.

The concept of stem cell disorders

In the previous chapter we discussed the properties of the pluripotent stem cell population which gives rise to the early progenitors of the haematopoietic and lymphopoietic systems. Very little is known about the regulation of these pluripotent cells or about the way in which their further differentiation down particular cell lines is controlled. What is clear, however, is that there is a hierarchy of haematopoietic progenitors at different levels of commitment and differentiation, together with several potential regulatory proteins, each with different, but possibly overlapping, specificities.

The idea that certain haematological disorders might result from defects of cells with the capacity for differentiation into more than one type of blood cell arose from studies of patients with either hypoplastic of hyperplastic conditions of the bone marrow. For example, in the aplastic anaemias white cells and platelets are affected as well as the red cells. Similarly, there are several hyperplastic disorders of the marrow in which more than one type of blood cell is involved. Thus it has always seemed likely that these diseases reflect lesions of early progenitor cells at a stage before they have been programmed to differentiate down a maturation pathway for one type of blood cell. Recent studies using cell culture, cytogenetics, and isoenzymes, have provided a more solid basis for these speculations.

It is not known whether all disorders of stem cells occur at the level of the pluripotential stem cell. This may not be the case. Many of them seem to involve progenitors at a later stage which, although they still have the capacity to produce more than one type of blood cell, are already restricted to the haematopoietic or lymphopoietic differentiation pathways.

The results of abnormal proliferation of progenitors at different levels of commitment can be anticipated from Fig. 1. A lesion of the pluripotent stem cell (level 1) should produce an abnormal clone capable of giving rise to all the formed elements of the blood, both haematopoietic and lymphopoietic. On the other hand, a disorder involving level 2 of commitment will produce cell lines of mixed progeny, but limited to haematopoietic or lymphopoietic lineages. Disorders of the later stages of commitment (stage 3) would involve only single cell types such as red cells, granulocytes or B lymphocytes. In fact, most of the diseases which are phenotypically myeloid appear to involve a stem cell which is common to both haematopoiesis and lymphopoiesis. On the other

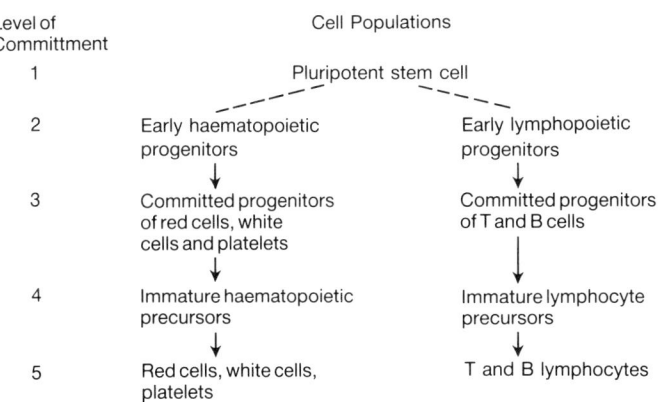

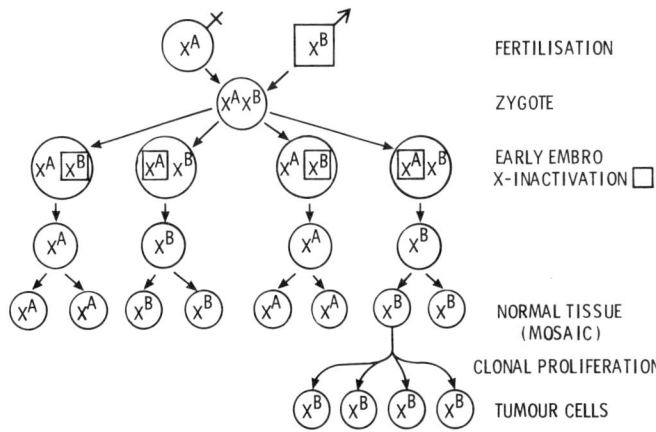

Fig. 1 A schematic representation of the levels of commitment of the haematopoietic and lymphopoietic progenitor cells. (Modified from Lichtman, 1983.)

Fig. 2 Diagramatic representation of the results of X inactivation in females heterozygous for glucose-6-phosphate dehydrogenase types A and B. The normal tissues of such individuals contain either the A or B form of the enzyme. Neoplastic cell lines derived from a mutation in a single cell will contain either A or B types, but not both.

hand, with a few exceptions, lymphoid neoplasms seem to arise from progenitors with a more limited differentiation potential.

If these ideas are correct, and the evidence cited below suggests that they might be, at least in outline, it is clear that the hierarchy of levels of progenitor-cell commitment that characterizes normal haematopoiesis provides the basis for an extraordinarily diverse series of blood diseases. When looked at in this way it is possible to make sense of many haematological disorders, the nature of which has hitherto been completely obscure.

A word of caution is necessary, however. The hyperplastic stem cell disorders are, in effect, neoplasms of the haematopoietic system. Thus it may be naive to relate the products of a *neoplastic* cell line to a particular stage in the *normal* haematopoietic maturation cycle. The neoplastic change could *per se* cause the activation of genes which might not be expressed in normal haematopoietic progenitors; we should not always assume that the presence of a particular marker on a cancer cell is a reliable guide to its lineage in terms of normal haematopoiesis. Another problem is why these haematological disorders appear to involve progenitors with different capacities for differentiation, and why the mutations that cause them provide their target cells with a proliferative advantage over their normal fellows. In part, these uncertainties reflect our lack of knowledge about the properties of cell populations at different levels of commitment, and doubts about the validity of models like those shown in Fig. 1.

Evidence for defects of the pluripotent stem cells or their immediate progeny

The most useful approach to analysing the origin of haematopoietic cells in patients with haematological diseases is to study markers which can be used to 'tag' the progeny of single cells. So far, most of the information which has been derived about the level of commitment of abnormal haematopoietic cells has come from the use of chromosome and enzyme markers.

The most useful marker chromosome in this field is the Philadelphia or Ph[1] chromosome. This is a chromosome 22 which has lost part of its long arm which is translocated onto the long arm of another chromosome, usually No. 9; in addition, part of chromosome 9 is translocated onto chromosome 22. In other words, the Ph[1] chromosome is the result of a reciprocal translocation between chromosomes 9 and 22 (9:22)(q34:q11). The nomenclature for chromosome abnormalities is described in Section 4.

Originally it was thought that the Ph[1] chromosome was specific for chronic myeloid leukaemia (CML), a condition which is described later in this section (page 19.27). The abnormal chromosome is found in the white cell and red cell precursors and in megakaryocytes but not in phytohaemagglutinin-stimulated lymphocytes, which are mainly T lymphocytes. This suggests that

CML is derived from a progenitor which has the capability of differentiating into red cells, white cells, and platelets but not into the lymphocyte series. However, in some cases a much earlier progenitor cell, possibly a pluripotent stem cell, may be involved. For example, some patients with CML develop a much more aggressive illness with a lymphoblastic type of metamorphosis. In such cases the Ph[1] chromosome can be found in the lymphoblastic cells which can also be shown to be of B cell origin. Furthermore, the Ph[1] chromosome has been found in a number of patients with *de novo* acute lymphoblastic leukaemia. More recently it has been found that peripheral blood or bone marrow cells of patients with CML which have been induced to proliferate *in vitro* by Epstein–Barr (EB) virus, and hence which are thought to be B lymphocytes, contain the Ph[1] chromosome, as do B lymphocytes isolated from the blood of some patients with this disorder. These observations suggest that at least some forms of CML arise from very early progenitors with the capacity for differentiating down both haematopoietic and lymphopoietic lines. Thus, although the reason for the remarkable clinical diversity of the Ph[1] chromosome disorders is not known it is apparent that at least some of them result from the production of a clone of abnormal cells derived from an early progenitor population at stage 1 of commitment (Fig. 1), that is, before the diversion of the haematopoietic and lymphopoietic progenitor compartments.

Another very useful tool for studying the origins of peripheral blood cells in patients with haematopoietic disorders is a polymorphism of the enzyme glucose-6-phosphate dehydrogenase (G6PD). There are many structural variants of this enzyme (see page 19.140). The wild type (normal enzyme) is designated B. There is a particularly common variant which differs from normal by a single amino acid substitution, and which is found mainly in African Negro populations, called the A type. Because the gene which controls the structure of G6PD is on the X chromosome, males show either the A or B types but never both. On the other hand, females may be homozygous for the A type (AA), heterozygous for A and B (AB), or homozygous for B (BB). However, in females one X chromosome in each cell is inactivated at an early stage of embryonic development, a mechanism for modifying dosage of genes on the X chromosome described first by Mary Lyon, and hence called Lyonization. Since this process is random, females who are heterozygous for G6PD types A and B have two cell populations, one expressing the A enzyme, the other the B. In other words they are mosaics (Fig. 2).

It follows, therefore, that a G6PD AB female heterozygote will, on average, have 50 per cent of red cells which express the A enzyme, and 50 per cent which express the B enzyme. Of course,

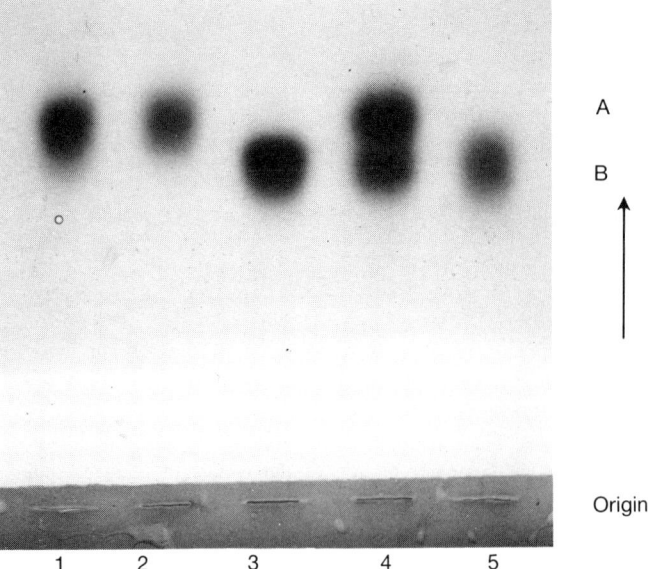

Table 1 Disorders of pluripotential progenitor cells.

Aplastic anaemia
Myeloproliferative disorders
    Acute
        Acute myeloid leukaemia (AML)
        Other variants of AML
        Promyelocytic leukaemia
        Acute myelomonocytic leukaemia
        Acute erythroleukaemia
        Some forms of acute undifferentiated leukaemia
        *Some lymphoblastic leukaemias

    Chronic
        Polycythaemia vera
        Chronic myeloid leukaemia
        Primary thrombocythaemia
        Primary myelosclerosis

Myelodysplastic syndrome
Paroxysmal nocturnal haemoglobinuria
Unclassified disorders

* The problems of the relationship of the acute undifferentiated and lymphoblastic leukaemias to the haematopoietic system is discussed in the text.

Fig. 3 Glucose-6-phosphate dehydrogenase patterns (starch gel electrophoresis) of the blood cells of patients with haematological malignancies. (1) Blood cells from a woman with chronic myeloid leukaemia, heterozygous for G6PD types A and B; her blood cells show only the A-type; skin cells showed both A and B types. (2) Blood cells from an AB female with chronic myeloid leukaemia; again only the A-enzyme appears in the blood cells. (3) Blood cells from an AB female with chronic myeloid leukaemia; in this case only the B-enzyme appears in the blood cells. (4) Blood cells from an AB female with acute lymphoblastic leukaemia in remission; both A and B-enzymes are present in the blood cells. (5) Blood cells from a BB female with acute lymphoblastic leukaemia in remission; only the B enzyme is detected. (Kindly prepared by Dr Philip Fialkow of the Department of Medicine, University of Washington.)

this will vary considerably because of the statistical chance that the random inactivation process may affect more A chromosomes than B chromosomes, or vice versa. But on average their cells will contain about 50 per cent of each form of the enzyme. If such a heterozygous woman has a haematological disorder which is due to the abnormal proliferation of a clone of cells derived from a single stem cell, the progeny of which populate the marrow and peripheral blood at the expense of their normal counterparts, most of her peripheral blood red cells will be of either the A or B variety (Fig. 2). On the other hand, it will be clear from analysis of the enzymes in other tissues that she is a genetic heterozygote, despite the presence of only one form of G6PD in her red cells (Fig. 3). Furthermore, if the single G6PD enzyme is also found in her peripheral blood white cells and platelets it must be inferred that the neoplastic transformation has occurred in a progenitor with the capacity for differentiating into all the haematopoietic elements. If both T and B lymphocytes also show a single G6PD type, the transformation must have occurred at the pluripotent stem cell level, before the haematopoietic/lymphopoietic progenitor diversion.

The G6PD polymorphism has been an extremely valuable tool for analysing disorders of haematopoietic stem cells. As we shall see later it has provided good evidence that polycythaemia vera, chronic myeloid leukaemia, and some forms of preleukaemia are derived from early pluripotent progenitors. It is possible to analyse the G6PD variants both in marrow and peripheral blood cells and in the *in vitro* colony systems which were described in the previous chapter. Its major disadvantage is that its use is restricted to females who are heterozygous for the G6PD variant. Of course, any common X-linked enzyme variants could be used for this purpose but unfortunately none has been found which is equally polymorphic or as amenable to electrophoretic analysis as G6PD.

As well as these cytogenetic and enzyme markers for studying the cellular origin of peripheral blood cells there are many antigenic markers which are specific for different classes of granulocytes and lymphocytes. These are considered in the appropriate chapters later in this section. When used in combination with cytogenetic and enzyme studies it is possible to begin to build up a picture of the levels of commitment of the progenitor cells in a number of haematological disorders.

The classification of stem cell disorders

A tentative classification of the disorders of haematopoietic stem cells is shown in Table 1; they fall into three main groups: aplastic anaemias; myeloproliferative disorders; and the myelodysplastic syndrome. The major characteristic which all these conditions have in common is that there are quantitative and qualitative abnormalities of more than one type of blood cell; this is the *sine qua non* of a stem cell disorder.

Aplastic anaemia

Aplastic anaemia is an unfortunate term because this condition is nearly always characterized by pancytopenia, i.e. defective production of red cells, white cells, and platelets. There are examples of selective cytopenias, but the term 'aplastic anaemia' is used to describe a pancytopenia which may occur *de novo* or following exposure to a variety of toxic agents. Since lymphocytes may also be involved it appears that, at least in some cases, the target cells are progenitors which are early in the maturation pathway, before the division into haematopoietic and lymphopoietic precursors.

Myeloproliferative disorders

The concept of myeloproliferative disorders is not new. It was a term invented by Dameshek and others in the 1950s in an attempt to explain some of the variability of the haematological findings in patients with polycythaemia vera, chronic myeloid leukaemia, and myelosclerosis. Because there is so much overlap between these conditions with regard to the cell lines which are involved, and because disorders like polycythaemia vera and chronic myeloid leukaemia often terminate in myelosclerosis, it was suggested that they all result from abnormal proliferation of cells derived from a common precursor. The concept of myeloproliferation has been very useful. Although some revision has been necessary with increasing knowledge about the properties of haematopoietic stem cells and with the availability of cell markers, Dameshek's original concept still holds true, at least in outline. He did not suggest that because these conditions have haematological features in common they must have the same aetiology. But the idea of abnormal proliferation of pluripotent progenitors as the basis for these diverse conditions has allowed their further classification and has formed a firm basis for their exploration by the more sophisticated techniques outlined earlier.

The term 'myeloproliferative disorder' is still in regular use and covers any neoplastic conditions of the bone marrow in which there is abnormal proliferation of pluripotent haematopoietic progenitors. A classification of these conditions is included in Table 1. Based on clinical observation they fall into two major groups: acute and chronic. The chronic myeloproliferative disorders are those which have been grouped together under this general heading since Dameshek's early papers. They include polycythaemia vera, chronic myeloid leukaemia, primary thromocythaemia, and myelosclerosis. Originally it was thought that myelosclerosis results from abnormal proliferation of the connective tissue elements of the marrow. It is now believed that the fibrosis of the marrow which characterizes this condition is a reaction to the products of an abnormal line of haematopoietic cells, probably platelets. These conditions have in common the fact that at any time during the illness there may be abnormally high numbers of red cells, white cells or platelets, myeloid metaplasia of the spleen, liver, and lymph-nodes, and a terminal phase of myelosclerosis or acute leukaemia.

There are several acute forms of myeloproliferative disorder. The acute leukaemias fall into three main groups, myeloblastic, lymphoblastic, and acute undifferentiated forms. There is evidence from the patterns of cellular proliferation and enzyme analyses that acute myeloid leukaemia is heterogeneous with regards to the level of commitment of the target cell; in some cases the abnormal cell line seems to involve only the white cells; in others all the formed elements. More work is required on this subject. The relationship of the lymphoblastic and undifferentiated leukaemias to bone marrow progenitors is unclear. Recent evidence suggests that the forms associated with the Philadelphia chromosome are related to definable haematopoietic progenitors but the cellular origins of the common forms of acute lymphoblastic leukaemia and their relationship to the cells of the haematopoietic hierarchy has not been defined.

Finally, there are some other rare acute myeloproliferative syndromes including acute erythroleukaemia and megakaryocytic leukaemia.

In grouping all these neoplastic blood disorders together under the heading of myeloproliferative disorders we are doing no more than making the assumption that many of them are derived from haematopoietic progenitors at different levels of commitment and differentiation. It should be emphasized that we are not suggesting that they have a common aetiology, only that they have enough features in common to make the general concept of myeloproliferation a useful approach to classifying these conditions in day-to-day clinical practice.

Myelodysplastic syndrome

The myelodysplastic syndrome is a subgroup of haematopoietic stem cell diseases in which dyshaemopoiesis is the predominant finding. Dyshaemopoiesis is a term used to describe abnormalities of differentiation or maturation of haematopoietic cells that lead to striking morphological changes of the bone marrow, and usually to anaemia, thrombocytopenia, and neutropenia, or various combinations of cytopenias. In many of these conditions there is ineffective erythropoiesis or granulopoiesis, i.e. intramedullary destruction of developing red cells or white cells. The bone marrow may be hypoplastic or hyperplastic. Very little is known about the pathogenesis of these disorders and we are still at the stage of attempting to classify them on cytological and cytogenetic grounds. At least some of them are preleukaemic.

Paroxysmal nocturnal haemoglobinuria

The strange syndrome of paroxysmal nocturnal haemoglobinuria is also thought to be a disorder of early haematopoietic progeni-

tors. Although this condition is characterized by an acquired defect of the red cell membrane there is good evidence that the white cells and platelets are also affected, probably by the same basic membrane abnormality. Enzyme marker studies have suggested that this condition results from the acquisition of an abnormal clone of haematopoietic progenitors, the progeny of which, in this case, are characterized by primary abnormalities of their cell membranes.

Unclassifiable disorders assumed to be of stem cell origin

It is quite common to encounter haematological disorders which are not classifiable into any particular myeloproliferative or myelodysplastic syndrome. Patients may be encountered who have unusually high white cell or platelet counts together with myelodysplasia. Clearly they have a primary abnormality of haemopoiesis with features of both myeloproliferation and myelodysplasia. Because more than one type of haematopoietic cell progenitor must be involved in the pathogenesis it is current practice simply to designate them as an unclassifiable myeloproliferative or myelodysplastic disorder and to treat them symptomatically. No doubt as these conditions are studied with the various cell markers outlined earlier in this chapter it will be possible to classify them more rationally.

In the sections that follow we shall examine each of these groups of stem cell disorders in more detail. It must be emphasized again that the concepts outlined in this introduction are relatively new and it is very likely that many of them will require revision as more sophisticated techniques for analysing the origins of different cell populations are developed.

References

Adamson, J. W. (1984). Analysis of haemopoiesis: the use of cell markers and *in vitro* culture techniques in studies of clonal haemopathies in man. *Clin. Haemat.* **13**, 489–502.

Adamson, J. W. and Fialkow, P. J. (1978). Pathogenesis of the myeloproliferative syndromes. *Br. J. Haemat.* **38**, 299–304.

Fialkow, P. J. (1979). Clonal origin of human tumours. *Ann. Rev. Med.* **30**, 135–143.

—— (1983). Hierarchal hematologic stem cell relationships studied with glucose-6-phosphate dehydrogenase enzymes. In *Hemopoietic stem cells* (eds Sv.-Aa. Killmann, E. P. Cronkite and C. N. Muller-Berat), pp. 174–186. Munksgaard, Copenhagen.

—— (1984). Clonal evolution of human myeloid leukaemias. In *Genes and cancer*, pp. 215–226. Alan R. Liss, Inc., New York.

Jacobson, R. J., Temple, M. J., Singer, J. W., Raskind, W., Powell, J. and Fialkow, P. J. (1984). A clonal complete remission in a patient with acute nonlymphocytic leukemia originating in a multipotent stem cell. *N. Engl. J. Med.* **310**, 1513–1517.

Lichtman, M. A. (1983). Classification of the hemopoietic stem cell disorders. In *Hematology*, 3rd edn (eds W. J. Williams, E. Beutler, A. J. Erslev and M. A. Lichtman), pp. 144–150. McGraw-Hill, New York.

Mladenovic, J. and Adamson, J. W. (1982). Erythroid colonies in culture: Analysis of erythroid differentiation and studies in human disease states. *Rec. Adv. Haemat.* **3**, 95–108.

Moore, M. A. S. (1982). Bone marrow culture: leucopoiesis and stem cells. *Rec. Adv. Haemat.* **3**, 109–142.

Raskind, W. H., Tirumali, N., Jacobson, R., Singer, J. and Fialkow, P. J. (1984). Evidence for a multistep pathogenesus of a myelodysplastic syndrome. *Blood* **63**, 1318–1323.

Rowley, J. D. (1980). Ph[1]-positive leukaemia, including chronic myelogenous leukaemia. *Clin. Haemat.* **9**, 55–86.

The leukaemias

S. T. CALLENDER AND C. BUNCH

The leukaemias are neoplastic disorders characterized by an uncontrolled clonal proliferation of haemopoietic cells derived from a malignantly transformed progenitor, resulting in replacement of the normal bone marrow and often infiltration of other

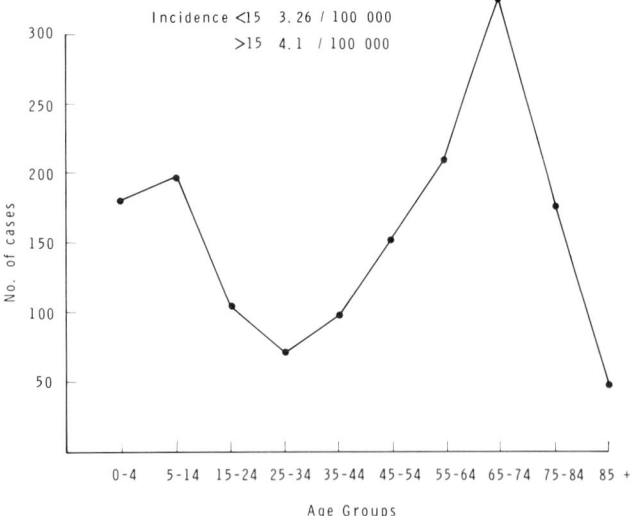

Fig. 1 Incidence of acute leukaemias in different age groups expressed as new cases registered in England and Wales in 1973.

organs. The leukaemias are conventionally classified by their kinetic behaviour as acute or chronic, and by their pattern of differentiation as myeloid or lymphatic. Although we shall describe these conditions together in this chapter, it should be remembered that in many cases their precise cellular origins and relationships to the developmental hierarchy of haematopoietic stem cells, as described in earlier chapters, is still uncertain. Indeed, the chronic lymphatic leukaemias have many features in common with the lymphomas which are described in later chapters (pages 19.169 *et seq.*).

History

Bennett in Scotland and Virchow in Germany are credited with the first descriptions of leukaemia in 1845. The former described a case in which death was attributed to 'the presence of purulent matter in the blood'. The latter entitled his paper 'Weisses blut' (white blood) but later described the condition as 'leukaemia'.

After Ehrlich developed his tri-acid stain for blood films, the diversity of the blood picture was recognized. The more precise diagnosis and classification of the different forms of leukaemia was made possible by the examination of fresh bone marrow smears obtained by the technique of marrow puncture. It has been further refined by cytochemical, electron microscopic, immunological, cytogenetic and, most recently, by molecular biological techniques.

Age incidence

The acute leukaemias show two peaks of incidence, in children in the 5–14 year age group and in adults between 55 and 75 years (Fig. 1). When, however, the distinction is made between acute lymphoblastic leukaemias (ALL) and the acute myeloid and monocytic leukaemias, it can be seen that the lymphoblastic leukaemias occur primarily in children and have a male predominance whereas the non-lymphoblastic leukaemias have their highest incidence in adult life and the sex incidence is equal (Figs. 2 and 3). The chronic leukaemias occur most commonly in the over-40 age group, chronic lymphatic leukaemia (CLL) being more than twice as common as chronic granulocytic leukaemia (CGL) (Fig. 4).

Aetiology

In the majority of cases of leukaemia there is no clue as to the aetiology of the condition. An increased incidence has, however, been found in relation to certain factors.

Radiation injury

In the early years of this century before stringent safety precautions were introduced, it was recognized that radiologists had an increased mortality from leukaemia. The risk from radiation

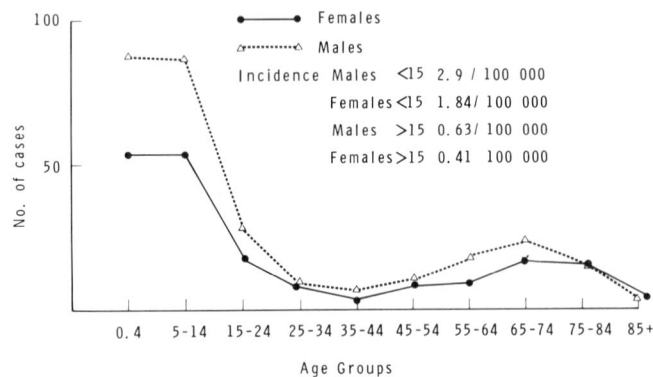

Fig. 2 Incidence of ALL in different age groups expressed as new cases registered in England and Wales in 1973.

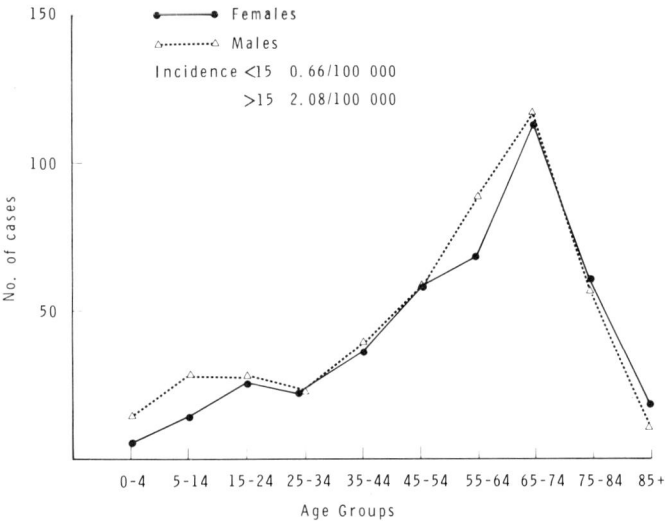

Fig. 3 Incidence of AML in different age groups expressed as new cases registered in England and Wales in 1973.

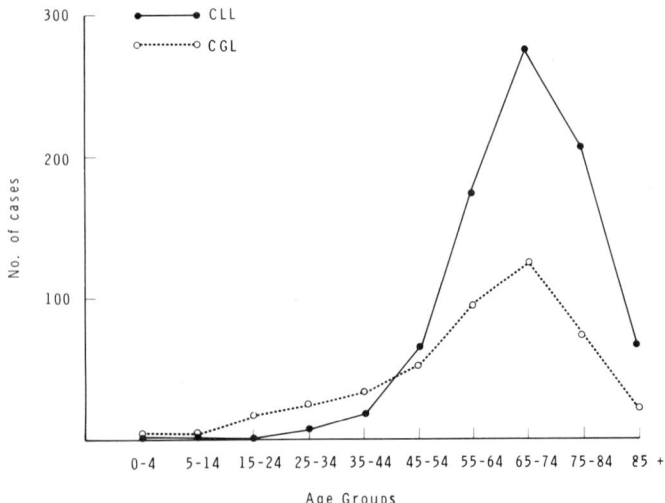

Fig. 4 Incidence of CGL and CLL in different age groups expressed as new cases registered in England and Wales in 1973.

injury was further highlighted by the observed increase in leukae-mia following the atomic bomb explosions at Hiroshima and Nagasaki. The incidence was greatest in Hiroshima where the exposure was primarily due to high energy neutron irradiation. The number of cases was directly related to the distance from the explosion, indicating that the risk was related to the dose received. The peak incidence of leukaemia occurred about 6 years after exposure.

Further evidence for the effect of radiation injury was found in a study of patients who had received X-ray therapy for ankylosing spondylitis. Such patients showed an increased incidence of both aplastic anaemia and leukaemia, whereas patients treated by other means showed no such increase. The peak incidence was 4–5 years after irradiation and it showed a direct relationship with the age at exposure.

The question of whether there is a safe threshold for irradiation has been debated ever since an increased risk of developing leuk-aemia was found in children born to mothers who had been X-rayed in pregnancy. However, in the survivors of the atomic bomb explosions there was apparently no increased incidence of leukae-mia below an exposure of 100 cGy at Nagasaki or 20 cGy at Hiro-shima, the latter being largely high energy neutron irradiation. Furthermore, children who were exposed *in utero* at the time of the explosions did not show an increase in leukaemia.

The leukaemias associated with radiation injury have been acute leukaemias or chronic granulocytic leukaemias. The inci-dence of chronic lymphocytic leukaemia is not increased. The occurrence of leukaemia may be preceded by a myelodysplastic or frankly aplastic phase.

Chemical injury

A number of chemicals may contribute to the development of leukaemia. Occupational exposure to benzene is a well-recognized hazard – for example, leukaemia has been described in shoe-makers using adhesives containing benzene and in workers exposed to benzene in the rubber film industry. Again, the leukae-mia is often preceded by a dysplastic phase.

Leukaemogenic factors in medical treatment

The use of chemotherapeutic agents, particularly the alkylating drugs, in treatment of other conditions, for example Hodgkin's disease and myeloma, has resulted in an increased incidence of secondary malignancies including leukaemia. The risk appears to be greater in those who have received radiotherapy as well as che-motherapy. In Hodgkin's disease it has been estimated that the risk of developing leukaemia within 10 years of the primary diag-nosis is almost 30 times that in the general population.

Genetic factors and syndromes of immune deficiency

Sibship studies have shown that if one child in the family has leuk-aemia there is about twice the risk of another child developing the disease as in the general population. This, of course, does not necessarily indicate genetic predisposition as environmental fac-tors in common might also be responsible.

Conditions associated with chromosomal damage such as Down's syndrome and Fanconi's anaemia have an increased inci-dence of leukaemia. Earlier studies suggested that the incidence in Down's syndrome might be increased 10–20 times but later obser-vations have shown that in many instances where leukaemia has been diagnosed it has proved to be a leukaemoid reaction which subsequently disappeared.

A greatly increased incidence of leukaemia is found in a number of the rare inherited disorders in which immune deficiency is a prominent feature. For example, in ataxia telangiectasia between a half to two-thirds of the children develop malignancies, the majority of which are leukaemias or lymphomas, whilst in the Wisckott–Aldrich and Bloom's syndromes some 8–9 per cent only develop leukaemia. Furthermore, in ataxia telangiectasia and Bloom's syndrome chromosomal abnormalities may also occur, and it seems likely that in these conditions the immune deficiency

and/or the chromosomal abnormalities may render the individual susceptible to some other induction factor.

Infection

Although it is well-recognized that many animal leukaemias are caused by retroviruses, there is no evidence of transmission of such leukaemias to man, and the search for similar viruses in human leukaemias has largely been unsuccessful. Recently, how-ever, an RNA C type virus has been isolated from a particular form of human T cell leukaemia/lymphoma first recognized in clusters of Japanese and latterly Caribbean and other populations (see page 19.260). This virus is biologically distinct from all known animal retroviruses, and has been designated the human T cell lymphotrophic virus 1, HTLV-1. A similar though distinct virus (HTLV-2) has even more recently been shown to be associated with the rare 'hairy-cell' leukaemia (page 19.35).

Cytogenetic abnormalities and oncogenes

Chromosomal abnormalities are commonly found in all forms of leukaemia and there is an increasing suspicion that in many instances these may be intimately involved in the pathogenesis of the malignant transformation. This seems particularly likely in the case of two well-defined abnormalities, the 8 ; 14 translocation seen in certain B cell lymphomas (page 19.168) and the 9 ; 22 translocation pathognomonic of CGL (page 19.28). In both instances, cellular oncogenes are located on one of the translo-cated segments and may be activated or otherwise modified by the rearrangement process. In the 8 ; 14 translocation, the c-*myc* gene is juxtaposed to one of the three immunoglobulin genes which are, of course, actively transcribed in B cells. The properties of the cel-lular oncogenes and their possible role in malignant transforma-tion is considered in Section 4.

In other leukaemias such clear-cut relationships between chro-mosomal rearrangements and oncogene activation have not yet been found. In acute myeloid leukaemia, for example, evidence for activation of the N-*ras* oncogene has recently been produced, and in four out of five cases studied this was associated with a specific mutation within the gene itself. However, this is likely to be but one step in the process of malignant transformation, as other patients with AML may have chromosomal rearrangements which do not involve the N-*ras* gene.

Pathophysiology

The functional defect in acute leukaemia appears to be a failure of normal differentiation and maturation of a population of leuco-cyte precursors which proliferate uncontrollably at the expense of the normal marrow population. A limited capacity for differentia-tion is retained, at least in the acute myelogenous leukaemias. Unexpectedly, the leukaemic cells proliferate at a slower rate than normal precursors, leading to a progressive accumulation of immature cells. At the same time there is a failure of marrow func-tion, which results in anaemia, thrombocytopenia, and neutrope-nia. This is probably not due to simple 'crowding out' by leukaemic cells, but may result from a more subtle disturbance of normal regulatory mechanisms, possibly by the production of inhi-bitors of cell proliferation by the leukaemic cells themselves.

It appears that a critical mass of leukaemic precursors, about 10^{12}, must be present in children with acute leukaemia before symptoms appear. Most of the clinical manifestations of acute leukaemia can in fact be related to bone marrow failure leading to infection, anaemia, and bleeding, together with the metabolic consequences of a large tumour mass and the effects of infiltration of various organs by the malignant cell population.

The chronic leukaemias differ from the acute leukaemias in that during the early part of the illness at least the capacity for differen-tiation in the neoplastic cell remains more or less intact. The basic defect seems to be an inappropriate input of cells into the amplify-ing and differentiating compartments so that there is a huge expansion of the cell line involved. In chronic granulocytic leukaemia (CGL) this is reflected by the presence in the marrow, blood, liver, and spleen of large numbers of myeloid cells at all stages of development, a variable proportion of which are mature neutrophils. The leukaemic cells all have a specific chromosome abnormality, the Philadelphia chromosome, indicating that they are the progeny of a single stem cell. Similarly, in chronic lymphatic leukaemia (CLL) the marrow, lymph nodes, liver, and spleen are infiltrated with large numbers of small and large lymphocytes; again these appear to arise from a particular class of lymphocytes, although no single specific chromosomal marker is associated with this condition.

Marrow failure is not a feature of the early phases of the chronic leukaemias. Rather, the clinical manifestations mainly reflect the metabolic consequences of a high cell turnover, the effects of the enlargement of the spleen and liver on the circulating red cell mass (see page 19.188), and the results of abnormal neutrophil or platelet function in CGL and humoral immunity in CLL. On the other hand, marrow failure commonly occurs in the later stages of CGL, either as a result of progressive fibrosis of the marrow or due to transformation into acute leukaemia. Similarly, marrow failure is also a late feature of CLL, but although this is often ascribed to 'crowding out' of the marrow with lymphocytes, this is probably too simplistic an explanation, and the mechanism is not really understood.

ACUTE LEUKAEMIA

Clinical features
Most of the clinical features of acute leukaemia are common to all types of the disease as they are related to the replacement of normal bone marrow by leukaemic cells. The onset may be insidious, with gradually increasing lethargy and malaise over a period of weeks. Sometimes, an initial diagnosis of infectious mononucleosis or a non-specific viral illness is made, particularly when the first symptoms are those of a sore throat, fever, and lymphadenopathy. Apart from anaemia the principle features are infection and haemorrhage, due to neutropenia and thrombocytopenia respectively.

Infective lesions
Focal infection occurs most commonly in the lungs, mucous membranes and skin. Pulmonary infections are the most serious, and are particularly troublesome in patients with pre-existing lung disease. Oropharyngeal ulceration is extremely common, varying from shallow ulcers to deep necrotic areas, and may be complicated by candida or herpes simplex infection. Perianal ulceration may occur, and rectal examination should be avoided for fear of producing a fissure or spreading infection.

Some patients have skin lesions which they have attributed to boils or insect bites but which have failed to heal, or they may have trivial cuts which have developed into spreading infection. Infected lesions are often atypical since there is no pus formation in the absence of granulocytes (Fig. 5).

The most serious infectious problem is septicaemia, which may occur in the absence of focal sepsis and prove rapidly fatal if not recognized immediately. It is commonly due to Gram-negative organisms, e.g. *Escherichia coli*, *Pseudomonas* spp., *Proteus*, and *Klebsiella*.

Haemorrhagic lesions
Purpura, bruising, mucous membrane bleeding, and menorrhagia may all be presenting features. Occasionally, prolonged haemorrhage following dental extraction leads to the diagnosis. Fundal haemorrhages occur most frequently when there is profound anaemia. Widespread ecchymosis and excessive bleeding from venepuncture sites should suggest the possibility of disseminated intravascular coagulation (DIC). This may complicate septicaemia, but is particularly a feature of the promyelocytic variety of AML (Fig. 6). It may result in fatal cerebral haemorrhage early in the course of the disease.

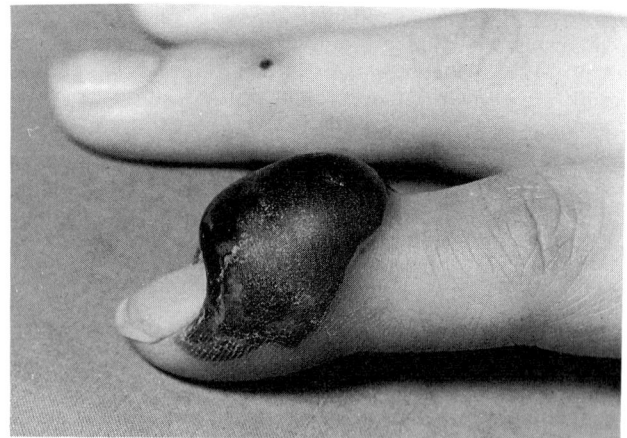

Fig. 5 Haemorrhagic infected lesion on the finger of a patient with acute myeloid leukaemia.

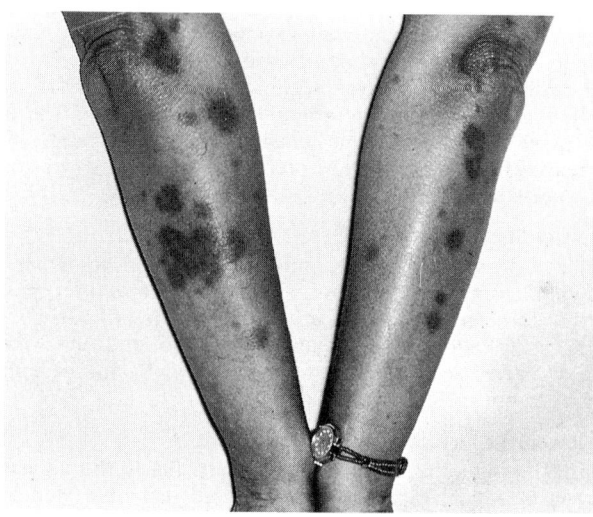

Fig. 6 Symmetrical haemorrhagic lesions in a patient with disseminated intravascular coagulation complicating acute promyelocytic leukaemia.

Other presenting features
Marked generalized lymphadenopathy and hepatosplenomegaly may all occur in ALL, but massive mediastinal lymphadenopathy is a particular feature of T cell ALL, and may lead to dyspnoea or other obstructive symptoms (Fig. 7).

Extramedullary infiltration occurs early in some cases, particularly in AML. Hypertrophy of the gums due to a combination of infection and infiltration with malignant cells is a feature of the monocytic variety of AML and may be so gross as almost to obscure the teeth (Fig. 8). Skin infiltration in the form of widespread pinkish plaques is also a feature of monocytic leukaemia (Figs. 9 and 10).

Localized bony deposits, particularly in the orbit, may occur early in AML, sometimes producing proptosis.

Involvement of the CNS is usually a later manifestation but occasionally is seen at the onset and may produce cranial nerve lesions, spinal nerve root involvement or meningeal disease.

Infiltration of the testes, ovaries, or breasts can occur early but, again, these sites are more likely to be affected as a late feature.

Severe bone pain, due in some cases to expanding tumour and in others to infarction of the bone marrow, may in a febrile, acutely ill patient, simulate acute osteomyelitis, and a presentation with painful, swollen joints may suggest the diagnosis of acute rheumatic fever.

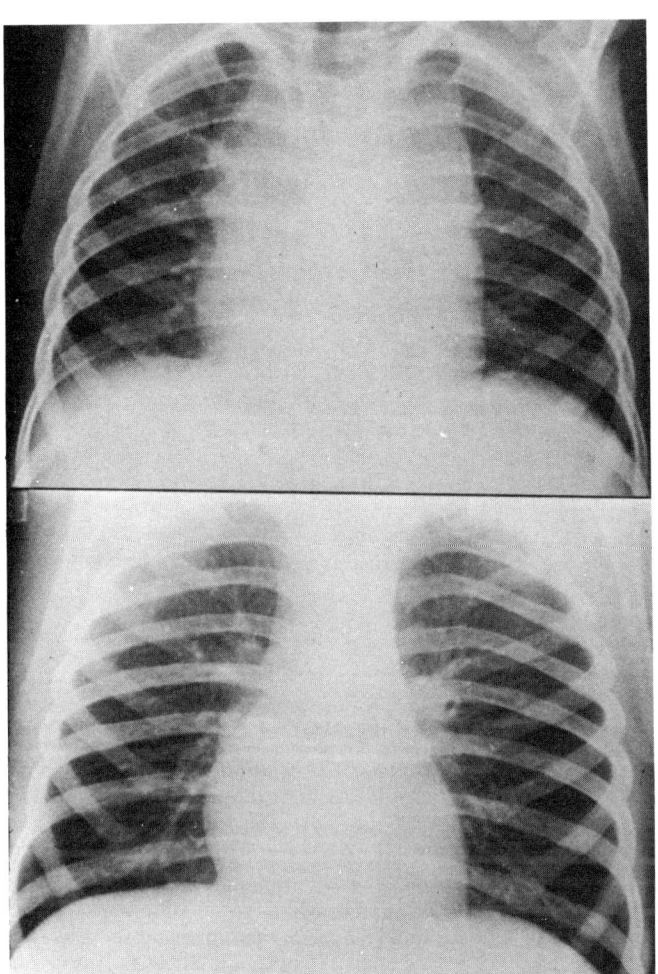

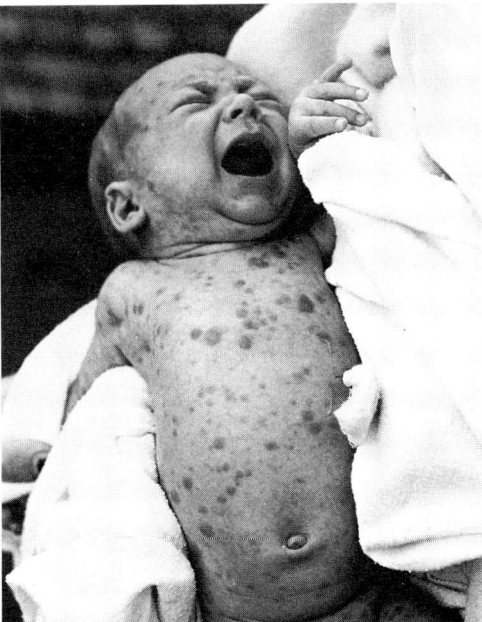

Fig. 9 Skin infiltration in a neonatal acute monocytic leukaemia; in contrast to acute leukaemia in older children, the disease in neonates is usually of the AML type, and is frequently accompanied by skin infiltration.

Fig. 7 Massive mediastinal lymphadenopathy in a 5-year-old boy with T cell ALL before (above) and after (below) treatment with steroids; the leucocyte count was $608 \times 10^9/l$ at presentation.

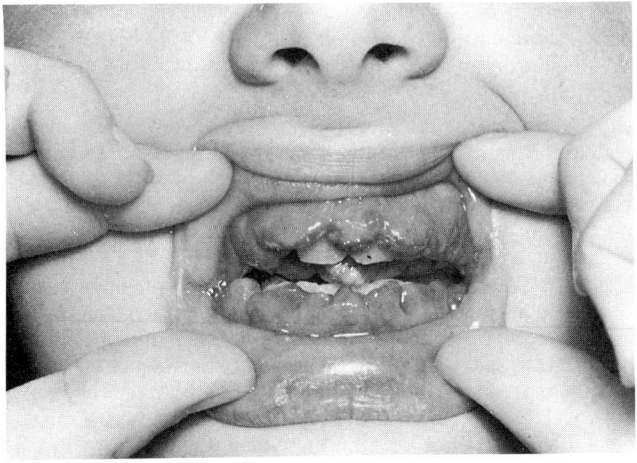

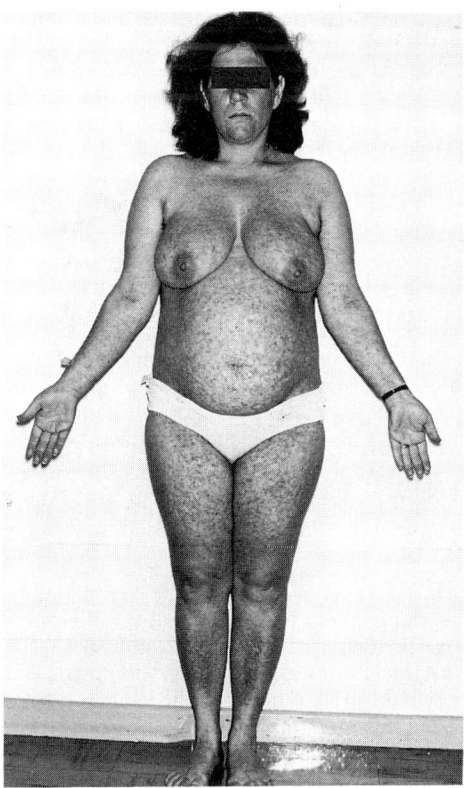

Fig. 8 Gum hypertrophy in a patient with acute monocytic leukaemia.

Fig. 10 Widespread skin infiltration in an adult patient with acute monocytic leukaemia.

Diagnosis

Although the initial clinical picture may suggest a viral illness or other disorder, once a blood count has been done there can be little doubt about the diagnosis. Anaemia is usually severe and the platelets reduced. The total leucocyte count is very variable but normal granulocytes are greatly reduced or absent. A careful examination of the blood film usually reveals the presence of blast cells, although these may be few in number, and the diagnosis should be confirmed by examination of the bone marrow. In addition to making marrow smears it is important to take samples for immunological markers and chromosome studies. The marrow is usually hypercellular and easy to aspirate but it may occasionally

Table 1 Classification of acute leukaemias by surface markers, histochemistry, and enzymes

	Morphologically identifiable as lymphoid or myeloid				Sudan black, Peroxidase	Frequency (per cent)†
	Reaction with anti-ALL serum	Surface IgG	E rosettes	TdT*		
Lymphoblastic (ALL)						
common ALL	+	−	−	+	−	75
T Cell	−	−	+	+	−	10
B Cell	−	+	−	−	−	<5
null Cell	−	−	−	±	−	10
Myelogenous (AML)‡						
M1: Myeloblastic (undifferentiated)	−	−	−	−	±	} 62
M2: Myeloblastic (differentiated)	−	−	−	−	±	
M3: Promyelocytic	−	−	−	−	+	5
M4: Myelomonocytic	−	−	−	−	+	20
M5: Monocytic	−	−	−	−	+	<5
M6: Erythroleukemia	−	−	−	−	±	<5
Morphologically unclassifiable (<5% of all acute leukaemias):	Some patients may show evidence of lymphoid origin with antiALL or positive TdT.					
Acute transformation of chronic granulocytic leukaemia:	Patients have positive Ph¹ chromosome but may be classified as either lymphoblastic or myeloblastic by the morphologic and functional criteria given above.					

* Elevated levels of terminal deoxynucleotidyl transferase.
† Data from Chessels *et al.* (1977). ALL. *Lancet* **ii**, 1307; and Crowther *et al.* (1973). AML. *Br. Med. J.* **1**, 131.
‡ M1 to M6 correspond to the FAB classification.

be difficult to obtain a sample at first. The predominant cells are blast cells and there is usually little or no evidence of normal erythropoiesis or myelopoiesis, and megakaryocytes are scant.

Differentiation between ALL and AML
The distinction between the lymphoblastic and myeloblastic leukaemias is often clear from the examination of blood and bone marrow films stained by one of the Romanowsky methods. Features to note are the presence of specific granules in a proportion of the cells which will indicate myeloid origin and, in particular, the presence of *Auer rods* which are virtually diagnostic of AML. These are azurophil rod-shaped bodies found in the cytoplasm which probably result from the fusion of several azurophil granules.

Cytochemical techniques may also be helpful. Specific granules in AML cells may be more apparent after staining with Sudan black or myeloperoxidase methods, whilst coarse, block positivity in the PAS (periodic acid-Schiff) reaction is typical of ALL.

The FAB classification of the acute leukaemias A French/American/British cooperative group has made proposals for the more detailed morphological classification of the acute leukaemias (the FAB classification) based on standard Romanowsky stains. This defines three groups of lymphoblastic leukaemia, six of myeloid (non-lymphoblastic) leukaemia.

L1, the common type in children The cells have a high nuclear-cytoplasmic ratio; nuclei are usually regular with inconspicuous nucleoli.

L2, commoner in adults More than half the cells are of large size (at least twice the diameter of a small lymphocyte), there is a low nuclear-cytoplasmic ratio, the cytoplasm occupying 20 per cent or more of the surface area of the cell. The nucleus is often cleft with an irregular nuclear membrane, and the nucleoli are often prominent.

L3, occurring in both children and adults Lymphoblasts are large, more homogeneous in size, with oval or round nuclei and prominent nucleoli. Cytoplasmic vacuolation is a marked feature. Cells of this type are of B cell origin and have chromosomal translocation (t:[18 ; 14]) similar to that of Burkitt's lymphoma (page 19.183). L3 represents only about 5 per cent of all cases, but it is important to recognize because it has a particularly bad prognosis.

The six AML subgroups are designated M1–M6:

M1, myeloblastic leukaemia without maturation In this group,

3 per cent or more of the blasts are peroxidase positive. A few have azurophil granules and/or Auer rods.

M2, myeloblastic leukaemia with maturation More than 50 per cent of the cells are myeloblasts or promyelocytes. Single Auer rods are common.

M3, hypergranular promyelocytic leukaemia In this group the majority of cells show heavy granulation and multiple Auer rods, so-called 'faggots'. A variation of M3 has been described in which the nucleus is bilobed, multilobed, or reniform and there may be only a small proportion of typical hypergranular cells. This variant is often erroneously diagnosed as 'monocytic'. The bone marrow is likely to be more typical than the peripheral blood.

M4, myelomonocytic leukaemia This is similar to M2 but monocytes and promonocytes exceed 20 per cent of the cells. Occasional Auer rods may be seen.

M5, monocytic leukaemia In this group monocytoid cells predominate. There may be occasional Auer rods. Both M4 and M5 are characterized by the presence of a high serum lysozyme concentration.

M6, erythroleukaemia Here, bizarre dyserythropoietic red cell precursors constitute more than 50 per cent of the cells. There is also usually an increased proportion of myeloblasts and promyelocytes and Auer rods may be seen. The abnormal erythroblasts show heavy PAS positivity which can be either granular or diffuse.

Immunological and biochemical analysis The phenotype of the leukaemic cell can be further defined by immunological, enzymatic, and molecular techniques (Table 1). In the majority of cases of ALL the cells lack the surface characteristics of mature B or T cells but express an antigen known as CALLA (common ALL antigen). This was originally detected in heteroantisera raised in rabbits to ALL blast cells, but monoclonal reagents are now available. The antigen is not leukaemia-specific, and is expressed on a small population of normal bone marrow cells. More recently, it has been demonstrated that CALLA-positive leukaemic cells have rearranged immunoglobulin genes, indicating their early differentiation into B cell lineage.

In about 5 per cent of cases the ALL blasts have a more mature B cell phenotype in that they express surface immunoglobulin. These cases correspond to the L3 FAB classification and have characteristics in common with the malignant cells of Burkitt's lymphoma (page 19.183).

Table 2 Consistent chromosome defects in patients with leukaemia

Chromosome defect	Disease
	Unique chromosomal defects
t(4;11)(q21;q23)	Acute 'lymphocytic' leukaemia, L2*
t(8;21)(q22.1;q22.3)	Acute myelogenous leukaemia, M2
t(15;17)(q22;q11.2)	Acute promyelocytic leukaemia, M3
inv(16)(p13.2q22)	Acute myelomonocytic leukaemia, M4
	Shared chromosomal defects
del(5)(q22q23)	Acute myeloid leukaemia, subtypes M1, M2, M4, M5, M6
del(7)(q33q36)	Acute myeloid leukaemia, subtypes M1, M2, M4, M5, M6
+8	Acute myeloid leukaemia, subtypes M1, M2, M4, M5, M6
t(8;14)(q24.1;q32.3)	Burkitt's lymphoma Acute lymphoblastic leukaemia—L3
t(9;11)(p22;q23)	Acute monocytic leukaemia Acute myelomonocytic leukaemia
t(9;22)(q34.1;q11.2)	Chronic myelogenous leukaemia Acute myelogenous leukaemia—M1 Acute lymphoblastic leukaemia—L1, L2
t(11;14)(q13;q32)†	Chronic lymphocytic leukaemia

* Recently suspected to represent an undifferentiated M4 acute nonlymphocytic leukemia.

Adapted from Yunis (1983).

A T cell phenotype can be demonstrated in about 10 per cent of cases of ALL. This presentation is more common in older children and young adults and is associated with a high leucocyte count, gross mediastinal involvement and hepatosplenomegaly—features it shares with T cell lymphoblastic lymphoma (page 19.178).

With the exception of B cell ALL mentioned above there is little correlation between the immunological phenotype and the FAB classification: CALL and T cell types occur in both the L1 and L2 FAB groups. Despite rigorous attempts, a small proportion of all cases of ALL remain difficult to classify.

The subclassification of the leukaemias is important in that it has some bearing on response to treatment and prognosis. As already mentioned, B cell ALL has a bad prognosis with a poor response to current treatment. T cell ALL may show an initial good response but the ultimate prognosis is poor unless aggressive therapy is maintained. The common type of ALL has the most favourable prognosis, and the unclassified group is intermediate between T cell and common ALL.

Chromosomal abnormalities in acute leukaemia

Chromosomal abnormalities are common in the acute leukaemias, and with more refined banding techniques it is becoming apparent that, at least in AML, most if not all patients will have some abnormality or another. Although a consistent abnormality such as the Ph^I chromosome in CGL is not found, two-thirds of patients show one of several distinctive abnormalities (Table 2).

As discussed earlier in this chapter the presence of major chromosomal alterations sheds some light on the pathogenesis of the leukaemias, and there is considerable interest in the possibility that cellular proto-oncogenes might be activated or enhanced as a result of such abnormalities. Certain chromosomal abnormalities may also have a degree of prognostic significance. For example, in ALL the presence of the same Ph^1 chromosome found in CGL is associated with a poor response to treatment.

Treatment of acute leukaemia

In 1948 Dr Sidney Farber and his colleagues published the results of some remarkable observations on the effect of a folic acid antagonist, aminopterin, on 16 children with acute leukaemia. The claims were cautious but ten of the patients 'showed clinical, haematological, and pathological evidence of improvement of important nature'. This work was the stimulus for the development of a series of agents which interfere in one way or another

with the proliferation of the malignant cell, with the result that 20 years later the schedule of treatment used by Pinkel's group in Tennessee was resulting in a 50 per cent survival of children with ALL in first remission 4 years from diagnosis.

The remarkable advances which have been achieved in the treatment of leukaemia have been made possible by the formation of collaborative study groups, particularly in the United States and Europe, and by the treatment of patients in special centres.

There are two elements to the achievement of improved prognosis; first the carefully controlled trials of various treatment schedules, and secondly and equally important the steady improvement in supportive treatment and awareness throughout of the complications of both the disease and therapy. Both chemotherapy and supportive therapy require special experience and suitable facilities, particularly good bacteriological and transfusion services.

The aims of treatment are to eliminate the abnormal clone of leukaemic cells from both blood and bone marrow and from all possible extramedullary sites, and to allow repopulation of the marrow with normal haemopoietic cells. Remission is defined as absence of leukaemic cells from the peripheral blood, a normal or recovering blood count, and less than 5 per cent of blast cells in a normal regenerating bone marrow. This, strictly speaking, should be termed 'haematological remission' since it does not exclude the possibility of residual disease in extramedullary sites such as CNS and testes.

Over the years it has become apparent first that combinations of drugs are generally more effective than the same drugs used separately, and secondly that some drugs are more useful in the early stages of induction of remission and others for maintenance treatment.

Various principles have been evolved for the management of different types of leukaemia; progress has been relatively fast in the treatment of the common type of childhood ALL, so that a considerable proportion of such children may be 'cured' of the disease, although long-term survival is still relatively rare in the poor-prognosis childhood ALL, in adult ALL, and in all forms of AML.

General approach to management

Management of patients with leukaemia is made much easier by free and open discussion of the diagnosis and the problems which may be involved in treatment. It is obviously wise to be certain of the diagnosis before arranging for such a discussion. Although prognosis differs in the different forms of these diseases, it is justifiable, especially in the childhood ALL, to take a reasonably optimistic view but to emphasize that treatment requires the close co-operation of the patient and the family for a prolonged period of time.

Although leukaemia is a rare condition, it now ranks as one of the principal causes of death in childhood, and publicity in press and television and in books and films has made leukaemia a dreaded disease. The time spent in explaining that control of the condition or even cure is often possible, particularly in children, and in trying to allay anxiety is an extremely important part of management.

Both parents of a child should be seen together so that there is no confusion between them as to what they have been told, and they should be given every opportunity to ask questions, not only at the initial interview but at any other time during treatment. The parents may want their child to be kept in total ignorance of the seriousness of the condition, but many quite young children may want to know the reasons for their different treatments; no child should be made to feel excluded from discussion, and simple practical explanations should be given to their questions.

Relatives also sometimes request that the diagnosis should be kept from teenage or adult patients. The doctor should always respect the wishes of the family, but attempts should be made to persuade them that the patient may benefit by being able to discuss the problem openly. In some cases this enables a much closer relationship to develop, for example, between a husband and wife, enabling them to give each other mutual support.

At the outset of treatment it is important to make it clear to both patient and family doctor that there will be free access to the hospital for advice or admission at any time. The increased susceptibility to infection associated first with neutropenia and later with immunosuppression should be explained and, particularly with children, any contact with viral illnesses, especially measles or chickenpox, should be reported immediately. Open access to the hospital centre will allow the patient to remain at home for most of the time; this has both a beneficial psychological effect and reduces exposure to antibiotic-resistant organisms in the hospital environment.

Drugs used in the treatment of acute leukaemias

Prednisolone Prednisolone is one of the most effective drugs in the induction of remission in ALL. Used alone it will achieve a remission in some 60 per cent of cases, but in combination with vincristine the remission rate is about 95 per cent. It is not myelotoxic but has a lytic reaction on lymphoblasts.

Vinca-alkaloids The vinca-alkaloids are microtubular poisons which inhibit mitotic spindle formation and thus arrest cells in metaphase. Vincristine is used in ALL in preference to vinblastine as it is less myelotoxic. It is however neurotoxic and may produce paraesthesiae, loss of reflexes, weakness and constipation. Severe jaw pain and pains in the legs occur sometimes. Rare cases of convulsions and coma have been reported.

Methotrexate Methotrexate is a folic acid antagonist. It is myelotoxic and produces mucosal damage and mouth ulceration. Longer-term effects are fibrosis of the liver and osteoporosis. Methotrexate is used by oral, intravenous, intrathecal, and intraventricular route. It is the principal drug used in prophylaxis and treatment of CNS leukaemia, and it is also included in maintenance regimens for ALL and some maintenance regimens for AML. Chemical meningitis is an occasional complication of intrathecal administration.

6-Mercaptopurine (6MP) This is a purine analogue which interferes with DNA synthesis. It is myelosuppressive and hepatotoxic. Its effect is enhanced by allopurinol and the dose should be halved when the latter is given at the same time. It is given by mouth and is used in maintenance chemotherapy of ALL.

6-Thioguanine (6TG) This purine has largely replaced 6MP in treatment of AML and is used both in induction and maintenance treatment. It is also myelosuppressive and hepatotoxic and may produce nausea and vomiting. The dose is not affected by allopurinol.

Anthracyclines Daunorubicin (rubidomycin) and doxorubicin (Adriamycin) are both inhibitors of DNA replication and synthesis. They are myelotoxic and may produce severe marrow hypoplasia. They are also cardiotoxic; the toxic effect on the myocardium is cumulative and is uncommon below a total dose of 500 mg/m^2 of daunorubicin. Nausea and vomiting are common during and following intravenous doses of these drugs. Anthracyclines are primarily used to induce remission in AML but are also used in induction regimes for poor prognosis ALL.

Cytosine arabinoside (ara-C) This is a pyrimidine analogue which has proved especially valuable in the induction of remission in AML. It is myelosuppressive and also produces nausea and vomiting. The drug crosses the blood–brain barrier to some extent, and has been used in high doses for prophylaxis against CNS leukaemia, although acute cerebellar toxicity may be a complication. It can be given subcutaneously, intravenously or intrathecally, and is used in this manner for prophylaxis or treatment of CNS leukaemia.

L-Asparaginase This is an enzyme derived either from *Escherichia coli* or *Erwinia*. Blasts cells in ALL are dependent on asparagine and they undergo lysis when deprived of asparagine by L-asparaginase. Toxicity is partly related to the degree of purity of the enzyme and includes anaphylaxis, fever, and pancreatic damage. L-asparaginase also produces deficiencies of antithrombin, plasminogen, fibrinogen, and factors IX and XI, which has been thought possibly to account for the rare occurrence of cerebral thrombosis and bleeding leading to stroke early in treatment. The main use of L-asparaginase is in remission induction in ALL.

Cyclophosphamide This alkylating agent has been included in some combinations of chemotherapy, particularly COAP (cyclophosphamide, Oncovin [vincristine], ara-C, and prednisolone). It is myelosuppressive, produces alopecia, and occasionally heamorrhagic cystitis. COAP may be useful in patients who have failed other standard treatment, as a more intensive induction treatment for poor-risk ALL, or in maintenance treatment in AML. High-dose cyclophosphamide is also commonly used in conditioning regimens for marrow transplantation.

General conduct of therapy

Although in the last few years certain principles of treatment have been evolved for the different forms of leukaemia, treatment protocols are constantly under review and are modified according to the knowledge gained in carefully controlled clinical trials. Treatment may involve some or all of the following phases:

1. Remission induction.
2. Consolidation.
3. Prophylaxis against CNS leukaemia, especially in ALL.
4. Remission maintenance.
5. Intensification.

Throughout treatment a balance has to be kept between the desirable effect of reducing the abnormal tissue and unacceptable toxicity or side-effects of the drugs used.

Before commencing treatment the patient should be carefully examined for signs of bleeding or infection or for the presence of other conditions, such as cardiac failure, which might influence their treatment. A full blood count and bone marrow examination will have been done to establish the diagnosis, but in addition renal and hepatic biochemical profiles should be obtained including calcium and uric acid estimation. A chest X-ray and ECG should also be performed. The patient should be well-hydrated, with intravenous fluids if necessary. If significant tumour lysis is anticipated or the uric acid is raised, allopurinol 10 mg/kg per day should be started 24–48 hours before specific treatment.

Supportive care Adequate supportive care is critical to the success of antileukaemia therapy. The patient is not only at risk from bleeding and infection as a consequence of his disease but also from the myelotoxic effects of therapy. These are generally less severe in ALL then in AML, in which the production of severe marrow hypoplasia is an essential part of the treatment approach. The problems encountered in patients undergoing treatment for acute leukaemia are varied and are best dealt with by physicians with special experience in this field.

Management of neutropenia and infection The successful management of infection in patients with acute leukaemia depends upon a thorough acquaintance with the types of infecting organism most frequently encountered, combined with prompt investigation and institution of appropriate therapy. This topic is fully covered in Section 5.

Blood and platelet transfusions Red cell transfusion may be necessary for a severe anaemia at the outset of treatment, particularly if the platelet count is low, since it is in these circumstances that bleeding into the optic fundi is most likely to occur. Patients with very high leucocyte counts are at particular risk from cerebral catastrophe due to hyperviscosity, and should be transfused with extreme caution only if absolutely necessary (see below, page 19.27).

Platelet transfusion is essential if thrombocytopenia is accompanied by purpura or bleeding. The question of prophylactic platelet transfusion when there is no evidence of haemorrhage is more debatable since there is some danger of producing platelet antibodies which may make use of platelets less effective in subsequent haemorrhagic episodes. Nevertheless, the widespread availability of platelet concentrates has greatly reduced the risk of early death from haemorrhage.

Psychological support Some 20–30 per cent of children with leukaemia develop depressive illness or anxiety states, and marital problems even leading to divorce are common. If one parent becomes too involved with the leukaemic child, others in the family may feel neglected and develop behaviour problems. Similarly, in adult patients difficulties already present in a marriage may be exacerbated, leading sometimes to separation, although others are drawn closer together by a shared problem. Every attempt should be made from the time of diagnosis to assess the relationships between family members and to anticipate problems. Continuity of management is important in building up confidence and supplying the necessary support. There should be emphasis on allowing the patient to lead as normal a life as possible between hospital visits, and the collaboration of schools or places of work may play an important part in management.

During remission in the leukaemia the tension is often relieved, but relapse may be an even greater emotional strain than the original illness.

Treatment of ALL

Risk factors

In the past few years factors have emerged as indicators of bad prognosis in ALL, and treatment may be modified according to whether patients conform to a standard risk or high-risk category.

A relatively poor prognosis is indicated by:

1. Age: less than 2 years or more than 10 years of age
2. Male sex
3. White cell count of over 20×10^9
4. The presence of a mediastinal mass
5. CNS disease at presentation
6. T cell ALL
7. B cell ALL

Factors 2, 3, and 4 are all features associated with T cell leukaemia.

Induction of remission

There is a fairly general agreement that in patients classified as having a standard risk, vincristine and corticosteroids should be used for induction of remission. Weekly injections of vincristine, 1–1.5 mg/m² (maximum 2 mg) plus prednisolone, 40 mg/m²/day by mouth will produce a haematological remission in over 90 per cent of children with common ALL. These two drugs have little myelotoxicity and regeneration of the normal marrow usually occurs rapidly as the leukaemic cells are destroyed. If there is no evidence of infection or bleeding, children can usually be allowed home within a few days of starting treatment, which can be continued on an outpatient basis.

The use of a third drug such as L-asparaginase or one of the anthracyclines may not increase the remission rate significantly but does have some effect on duration of remission. The latter are myelosuppressive, and are best used towards the end of the induction phase following normal bone marrow regeneration. So far attempts to improve results in the poor prognosis groups by the addition of further drugs during the induction phase have not been impressive.

Over 90 per cent of patients will be in haematological remission within about 4 weeks of starting treatment. Those who respond more slowly do not necessarily have a worse prognosis but the introduction of other drugs, such as L-asparaginase or an anthracycline if these have not already been used, should be considered.

Table 3 Infection in acute lymphoblastic leukaemia in childhood

Incidence of infection	Number	Per cent
Pyrexial during induction	73	40
Confirmed or probable infection	34	18
Doubtful infection	39	22
Serious infections	16	9
Death during first 8 weeks of treatment	3	1.6
Death primarily due to infection	1	
Microbiologically confirmed infections		
Bacteraemia		
Pseudomonas aeruginosa	6	
Escherichia coli	4	
Staphylococcus aureus	1	
Streptococcus pneumoniae	1	
β-Haemolytic streptococcus	–	
Klebsiella pneumoniae	–	
No bacteraemia		
Pseudomonas aeruginosa	1 (1)*	
Staphylococcus aureus	8 (4)	
β-Haemolytic streptococcus	2	
Escherichia coli	1	
Mycoplasma pneumoniae	–	
Candida albicans	1	

* Figures in brackets correspond to serious non-bacteraemic infections. Some children had multiple infections.
Data from Chessells and Leiper (1980). *Arch. Dis. Child.* **55**, 118–123.

Dangers during remission induction treatment Hyperkalaemia and hyperuricaemia resulting from massive destruction of leukaemic cells are particular hazards in patients with initial high leucocyte counts and organomegaly and may result in cardiac arrest or renal failure respectively. Such patients should be well hydrated intravenously before starting therapy and the use of a cardiac monitor is advisable. The effects of hyperuricaemia may be prevented by allopurinol (which takes several days to act) or mitigated by alkalinization of the urine with intravenous bicarbonate.

Infection during remission induction Studies at The Hospital for Sick Children, London showed that 40 per cent of children with ALL had an episode of pyrexia during remission induction but in only half of these was infection confirmed or probable. In children with high-risk factors who were treated with more intensive initial treatment such as COAP, infection was commoner and more serious but in only one of 184 patients was death within the first 8 weeks of treatment attributable to infection. The incidence of infection and microbiological findings are shown in Table 3.

CNS prophylaxis

In the earlier clinical trials a high proportion of children achieved a haematological remission, but it soon became obvious that in more than half the patients the site of first relapse was in the central nervous system and that the meninges constituted a sanctuary site from which leukaemic cells could not be eliminated by the available induction therapy.

Autopsy studies suggest that leukaemic cells reach the brain by penetrating the walls of the veins to invade the meninges. Thrombocytopenia resulting in microhaemorrhages may increase this risk. The arachnoid trabeculae are destroyed, and leukaemic cells can be found in the CSF. As the cells proliferate they penetrate into the deep arachnoid tissues, destroy the pia-glial membrane, and finally invade the brain parenchyma. In designing prophylactic treatment it was argued that intrathecal chemotherapy was unlikely to reach the areas deep in the cortex and white matter, and that radiation therapy would therefore provide more effective prophylaxis for CNS leukaemia.

Earlier studies showed that doses of 5 or 12 Gy (500 or 1200 rad) of craniospinal irradiation were insufficient to prevent CNS leukaemia, but 24 Gy (2400 rad) of craniospinal irradiation or 24 Gy (2400 rad) of cranial irradiation plus intrathecal methotrexate reduced the incidence of CNS relapse to about 5 per cent.

Unfortunately long-term follow up has revealed that there may be serious sequelae to the use of CNS irradiation, especially when combined with high doses of methotrexate, although the incidence is very variable in different series. The findings are sufficiently worrying for a number of other protocols for the prevention of CNS leukaemia to have been suggested, particularly using intrathecal methotrexate combined with high dose methotrexate followed by folinic acid rescue, starting during the induction phase. The results from some centres suggest that effective prophylaxis may be possible using chemotherapy only.

Although CNS prophylaxis has dramatically improved the survival of children with ALL, such treatment has its own hazards. Some of the complications are relatively minor, others are serious, particularly the long-term sequelae.

Early complications Alopecia CNS irradiation is invariably followed by total alopecia and it is important to warn both parents and the patient that this will occur. They should be reassured that the effect will not be permanent.

The somnolence syndrome About 60 per cent of children develop this syndrome following cranial irradiation some 20–50 days after the treatment. The onset is often abrupt and is characterized by drowsiness, anorexia, irritability, and lethargy, lasting 1–2 weeks and accompanied by changes in the electroencephalogram. The occurrence of the syndrome does not appear to affect the prognosis and the aetiology is uncertain.

Late complications Intellectual development There is very little hard evidence to suggest that there is any gross disturbance of intellectual development in children treated for leukaemia, although there is some suggestion that younger patients may fall behind particularly in relation to numerical skills.

Leucoencephalopathy This is the most serious complication, and is heralded by a variety of neurological symptoms, including lethargy, dysarthria, ataxia, fits, confusion, dysphagia, spasticity, decerebrate posture, and coma. It is commoner in patients who have had one or more episodes of CNS leukaemia, and it appears to be particularly associated with the use of higher doses of methotrexate (50 mg/m^2 or more) following 20–24 Gy of cranial irradiation.

It is suggested that the cranial irradiation alters the blood–brain barrier and allows the diffusion of methotrexate into the brain, causing necrosis of the white matter. Changes are most marked in the frontoparietal area but may also be found in the occipital and temporal regions. The pathological appearances are those of degeneration and necrosis, with reactive astrocytosis (Fig. 11).

Mineralizing microangiography This is a less serious complication and probably results from radiation damage to the microvasculature although it has been observed in the absence of cranial irradiation or intrathecal methotrexate. Degenerative changes in the endothelium and vessel walls lead to necrosis and calcification in surrounding tissue in the grey matter, particularly in the lenticular nuclei and areas of anastomosis between the anterior, middle, and posterior cerebral arteries. The clinical manifestations are those of fits, behaviour disorders, and lack of muscular co-ordination. Calcification may be demonstrated on skull X-ray. Young children appear to be particularly susceptible. The two conditions of leucoencephalopathy and mineralizing microangiography may occur together. The incidence is extremely variable in different centres, presumably due to variations in treatment protocols.

Maintenance treatment

Following CNS prophylaxis, treatment is required for some 2–3 years in order to maintain patients in remission. The principal agents used are 6-mercaptopurine (6MP) and methotrexate. 6MP is commonly given in a continuous dosage of 50–70 mg/m^2 daily, with weekly doses of 15–20 mg/m^2 of methotrexate. Tolerance to the treatment is variable but it is generally supposed that the dosage of the drugs used in maintenance should be sufficient to

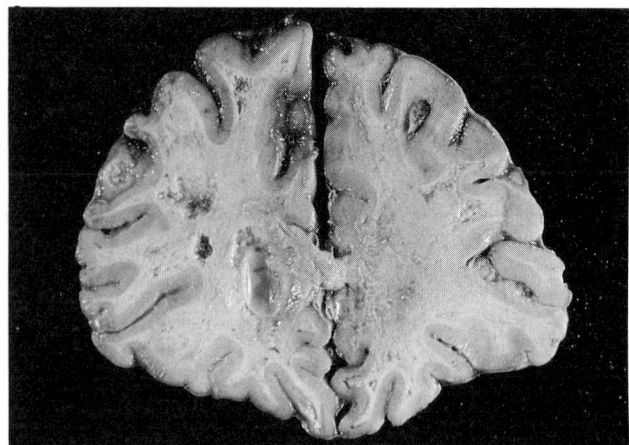

Fig. 11 Section of brain from a child with leucoencephalopathy. Common ALL was diagnosed at the age of 6 and remission induced with vincristine, prednisolone and asparaginase. CNS relapse occurred a year later despite prophylaxis with cranial irradiation and intrathecal methotrexate (IT MTX), and was treated with further intrathecal methotrexate via an Ommaya reservoir. She improved clinically, but a year later had an acute reaction to intrathecal methotrexate and subsequently developed encephalopathy and spastic paraparesis. She died 6 months later following haematological relapse. The white matter shows degenerative and cavitating changes and the cut surface has a granular appearance. (Photograph by courtesy of Drs T. Hughes and J. Durrant.)

produce mild toxicity, for example, a sore mouth or just short of that. In many protocols pulses of vincristine and prednisolone are introduced for 2 weeks every 10–12 weeks.

In some regimens, 6MP has been started during cranial irradiation and full maintenance treatment begun immediately after the end of the radiotherapy. Both irradiation and 6MP suppress lymphopoiesis and render the patient liable to infection. Thus one Medical Research Council UKALL Trial had to be modified when it was found that this type of regimen produced an unacceptable amount of infection in the post-induction period and during haematological remission. There was a notable improvement in results when the dose of 6MP during irradiation was reduced and a gap in treatment introduced after CNS treatment.

It has been suggested that it may be more logical to give intermittent maintenance treatment to allow better recovery of immunologically competent cells between courses and thus reduce the incidence of infection.

Hazards during maintenance treatment Intercurrent infection, which may be serious and lead to death, is the principal hazard for patients who are in remission during maintenance treatment.

Viral complications Viral infections are particularly hazardous in these children. It is useful to know which of the common viral infections the patient has previously encountered and it is thus wise to screen for antibodies to common viruses including herpes simplex, zoster, measles, CMV, and EB virus, at presentation.

Measles Children who have not been immunized for measles are at risk of developing the disease. The infection itself may be quite mild or even overlooked but it can be complicated by fatal pneumonia or be followed after an interval of 2–9 months by measles inclusion body encephalitis, which is almost invariably fatal. The child develops a variety of neurological symptoms such as fits, hemiplegia, athetosis, and lethargy proceeding to coma and death. Characteristic measles inclusion bodies can be detected in the brain at autopsy. Since there is no effective treatment, parents should be warned to bring children who have been in contact with measles to hospital *immediately* to be given high-dose immunoglobulin for prophylaxis.

Varicella and herpes zoster Primary chickenpox (varicella) is especially dangerous in the immunosuppressed, and patients who have not previously had the infection should be warned to avoid contact with other infected children. If contact does occur the patient should be given prophylactic hyperimmune globulin. If varicella or herpes zoster is diagnosed, acyclovir should be given as soon as possible and chemotherapy suspended temporarily.

Cytomegalovirus (CMV) infection If the patient has been shown to be CMV negative at the beginning of the illness all transfusion should, if possible, be from CMV negative donors. This is especially important if a later bone marrow transplant is contemplated. An acquired infection or reactivation of infection is not necessarily serious but it may give rise to anxiety if it produces hepatitis or prolonged fever. Occasionally death occurs from cytomegalovirus pneumonitis.

Pneumocystis carinii This is a notable complication and should be suspected in any immunosuppressed patient who develops chest signs, particularly extreme dyspnoea and cyanosis with little or no evidence of crepitations. The chest radiograph shows diffuse infiltration, usually of both lungs. Lung biopsy may be required to prove the diagnosis but since the condition responds well to high doses of co-trimoxazole, when the condition is suspected, treatment may be given blind.

Cessation of treatment Although some patients, particularly girls, may remain in remission after relatively short periods of treatment, most studies have indicated that the optimal length of maintenance treatment is probably of the order of 30–36 months. If treatment is then stopped, about 80 per cent of patients will thereafter continue in remission and the chances of relapse after about 4 years of continuous remission are quite small. The disadvantages of longer maintenance treatment are the toxicity of the drugs, resulting in liver and lung damage, and the hazard of intercurrent infections associated with the immunosuppression.

Relapse

Haematological relapse For those patients who have a haematological relapse during maintenance treatment the outlook is poor. Although a second remission may be reinduced it is likely to be shortlived, so that these are subjects in whom, if a second remission is obtained, the only likelihood of cure is by means of a bone marrow transplant if a suitable matched donor is available.

Relapse after stopping treatment is more readily brought under control a second time but, again, the ultimate prognosis is poor and consideration should be given to bone marrow transplant.

Extramedullary relapse in a 'sanctuary' site may occur without haematological relapse although it is frequently followed shortly after by evidence of bone marrow disease.

CNS relapse In spite of prophylactic treatment for CNS disease, some 5 per cent of patients with ALL develop CNS leukaemia. A lumbar puncture is essential in any patient who complains of headache or any other symptom referable to the central nervous system and the fluid should be examined for blast cells in a cytocentrifuge preparation. Temporary control of meningeal disease may be achieved by twice-weekly intrathecal injections of methotrexate (10 mg/m^2, maximum single dose 15 mg); longer-term remissions may be obtained following cranial irradiation. The risk of bone marrow relapse is high, and systemic 'reinduction' chemotherapy should probably be reinstituted concomitantly.

Testicular disease The difference in prognosis in ALL of children between boys and girls is, at least in part, due to the prevalence of testicular disease, which tends to occur predominantly within a short time of completing maintenance treatment. The incidence is some 10–30 per cent in different series.

Boys may be sensitive about complaining of testicular discomfort or swelling and care should be taken to examine the testes regularly as part of the overall supervision of the patient. Testicular infiltration can be treated by radiotherapy but bone marrow relapse is likely to occur concurrently or shortly afterwards.

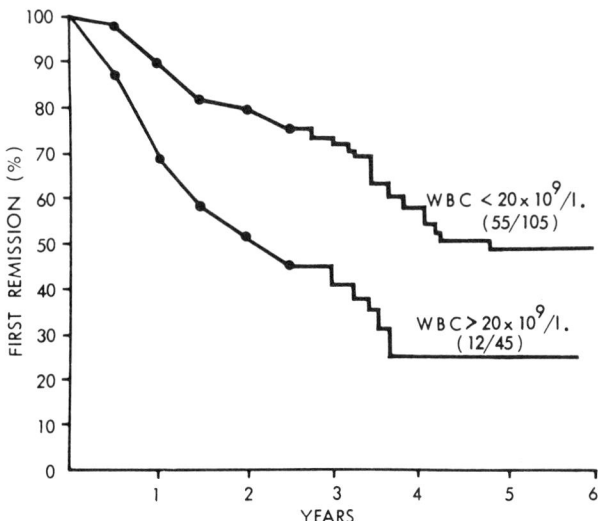

Fig. 12 Analysis of first complete remission in children with ALL in relation to presenting leucocyte count. Reproduced with permission from Chessels (1979).

Many centres now, as a routine, carry out testicular biopsy when maintenance treatment is to be discontinued. The biopsy is positive in about 10 per cent of clinically normal testes but a negative biopsy does not exclude the possibility of a few patients subsequently developing testicular disease. Fibrotic changes and reduction in spermatogenesis due to chemotherapy is evident in about 30 per cent of subjects. Because of the grave prognosis in those boys developing overt testicular disease, prophylactic testicular irradiation has been suggested, and in one trial appeared to have a beneficial effect.

A different approach to prophylaxis has been to give intravenous, intermediate dose methotrexate followed by folinic acid rescue combined with intrathecal methotrexate early in initial remission induction, with a view of getting a high concentration of methotrexate into all sanctuary sites, including the CNS and testes, early in the disease with the hope of preventing later relapse occurring in these sites.

Other sites of relapse The ovaries and breasts are other possible sites of relapse, and a few cases have been reported in which iritis with leukaemic hypopyon was the first indication of relapse.

Prognosis in ALL

Unfortunately since the spectacular improvement in prognosis following the introduction of prophylaxis for CNS disease, when it became evident that some 50 per cent of children entering remission might be expected to be 'cured' of the disease, there has been little improvement in outlook, particularly in those patients who are now recognized as being in the poor risk group.

Of the high-risk factors, age is only operative in the early stages of the disease. For those who are still alive and in remission at 2 months, the prognosis is the same at all ages. The outstanding feature which determines prognosis is the blood leucocyte count at presentation: the higher the count the worse the prognosis in all types of ALL (Fig. 12). The association of high leucocyte counts with T cell ALL is largely responsible for the worse prognosis in this group. The median duration of first remission in common ALL is more than 3½ years whereas that for T cell ALL is less than a year (Fig. 13).

The long-term prognosis is worse for boys than for girls, which is in part explained by the frequency of testicular relapse in boys. The sex difference is still clear even when the good-risk patients only are considered (Fig. 14).

The need now is to try and identify factors responsible for some

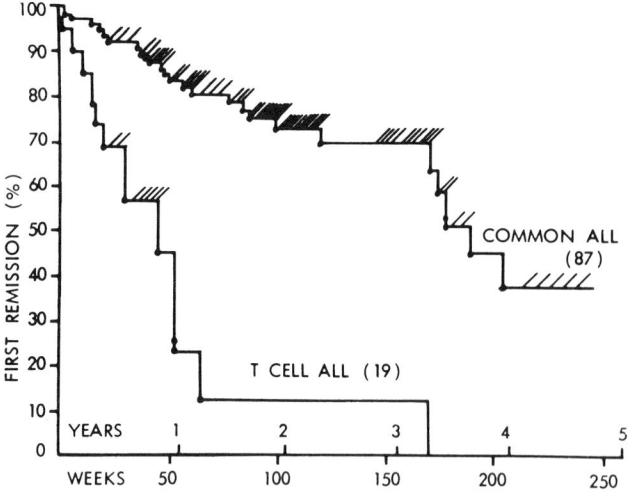

Fig. 13 Life-table analysis to show relative remission duration in common ALL and T cell ALL. Oblique lines indicate patients still in remission, black dots children who have relapsed. Reproduced with permission from Chessels (1979).

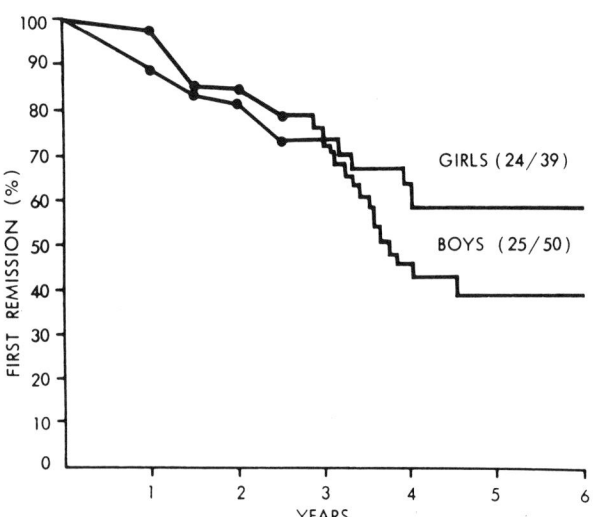

Fig. 14 Comparison of first remission in 'good risk' boys and girls (initial leucocyte count less than $20 \times 10^9/l$ and aged 2–10). Reproduced with permission from Chessels (1979).

patients in the good-risk group doing badly and to improve the response to treatment in the high-risk groups.

Growth and development

Most children, in spite of the necessary chemotherapy, grow and develop normally. Girls go through puberty and menstruate normally, and there are now several reports of normal children being born to girls 'cured' of ALL (Fig. 15). In view of the evidence of testicular damage shown on testicular biopsy (see below), it seems likely that male fertility may be reduced.

Treatment of AML

Remission induction

The induction of remission of AML is far more difficult and hazardous than in ALL as the aim is to produce severe marrow hypoplasia, in the hope that this will be followed by active regeneration of normal marrow. Throughout the induction phase the patient is at great risk of developing infection, which is increas-

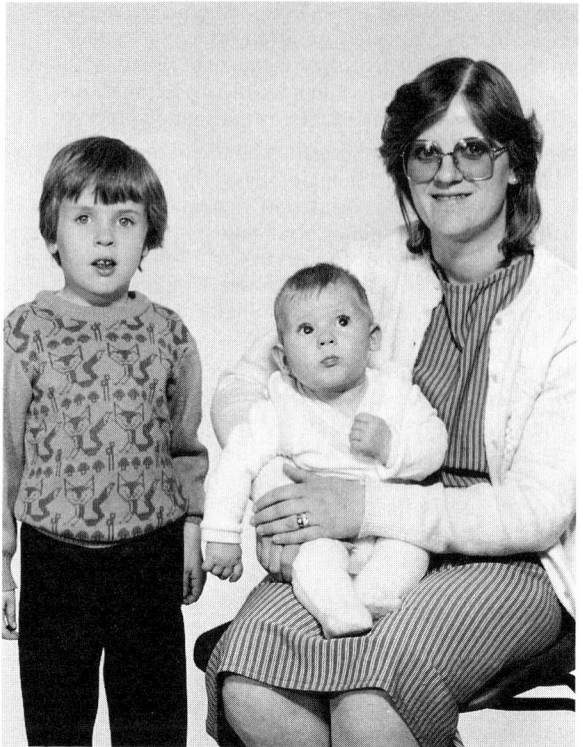

Fig. 15 GC and her two children, the first born 7 years after the diagnosis of ALL. She was treated for 3 years and has remained in continuous remission. Six years after diagnosis she had a stillbirth at 8 month's gestation: no congenital abnormality was found. A year later, in 1979, she had a normal delivery of a healthy boy. Her second child was born in 1984.

Table 4 DAT induction and consolidation treatment in AML*

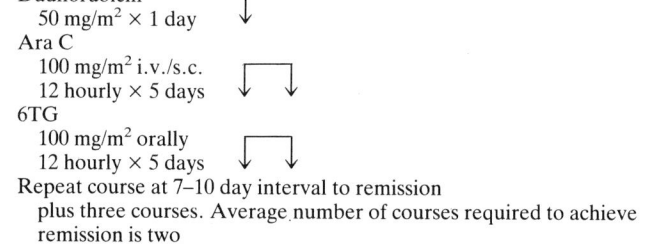

Daunorubicin
   50 mg/m^2 × 1 day
Ara C
   100 mg/m^2 i.v./s.c.
   12 hourly × 5 days
6TG
   100 mg/m^2 orally
   12 hourly × 5 days
Repeat course at 7–10 day interval to remission
   plus three courses. Average number of courses required to achieve remission is two

* The regime outlined is termed '1 + 5 DAT', indicating the number of days each drug is given. Other, more intensive variations (2 + 7, 3 + 10 DAT) are currently under evaluation.

ingly likely as the neutrophil count drops below $0.5 \times 10^9/l$, and bleeding which occurs particularly with platelet counts of less than $20 \times 10^9/l$.

Combinations of daunorubicin, cytosine arabinoside (ara-C) and 6-thioguanine (DAT) appear to be the most successful regimes to date for inducing remission in AML. An example of a protocol using these drugs is shown in Table 4. The interval between courses has to be adjusted according to the blood count and bone marrow. Since as many as 10^9 blast cells may remain in the bone marrow at a time when none can be recognized in the bone marrow smear, further consolidation courses should be given after the marrow is considered to be in remission before going on to maintenance treatment.

Remission can be achieved in some 60–80 per cent of patients with AML, particularly in the younger age groups. The remission rate, however, is highly dependent upon the standard of supportive treatment available.

Hazards during induction treatment Leucostasis If the leucocyte count is particularly high (over $10 \times 10^9/l$), there is a danger of the development of leucocyte thrombi in the brain, lungs, and heart. The blast cells have been shown to have a high viscosity and to be more rigid and less able to pass through small capillaries. At presentation the haemoglobin level is likely to be reduced and the whole blood viscosity therefore not increased. If, however, the patient is transfused to above a haemoglobin level of about 10.0 g/dl before the leucocyte count is reduced by chemotherapy, there may be a sharp increase in viscosity and consequent leucostasis. Special care should therefore be taken not to transfuse patients with very high blast counts at presentation unless they are dangerously anaemic, and even then the haemoglobin should not be raised above 10.0 g/dl.

Electrolyte disturbances This may be a hazard in the early stages of treatment. Hyperkalaemia and hyperuricaemia may result from massive destruction of cells, and a high fluid intake should be ensured and the renal function monitored. On the other hand, hypokalaemia occurs in some patients, particularly with the monocytic varieties of AML, in which there are high levels of serum and urinary lysozyme which are presumed to interfere with renal tubular function and increase potassium excretion. High-dose intravenous antibiotic therapy may contribute to hypokalaemia.

Disseminated intravascular coagulation (DIC) DIC is a common feature of the promyelocytic type of leukaemia – when it may be precipitated by cell breakdown at the start of treatment – or it may be a complication of septicaemia. Its management remains controversial: one view is that all patients with the diagnosis of promyelocytic (M3) leukaemia should be given heparin prophylactically, but the efficacy of heparin for established DIC is unproven. Large and frequent platelet transfusions and infusions of fresh-frozen plasma are though to be of some benefit. If there is evidence of septicaemia, appropriate antibiotic treatment should be started immediately.

Infection Even if infection has not been present initially it is extremely likely to occur during remission induction and is a major cause of death within the first 6 weeks of diagnosis. The management of fever and infection is discussed in Section 5.

Nutrition During the induction of remission, both because of infections and the nausea and vomiting produced by the cytotoxic drugs, patients may lose weight rapidly and there may be significant problems in maintaining nutrition; in some cases parenteral nutrition may be needed temporarily. Unfortunately hospital food is a potent source of antibiotic-resistant organisms which may colonize the bowel and give rise to troublesome infections. It is wise therefore to avoid fresh salads which may be heavily contaminated with such organisms, but there is no proof that actual sterilization of all food is beneficial.

Maintenance treatment

In ALL there is good evidence that maintenance treatment prolongs remission and survival but the situation in AML is much less clear. Traditionally patients have been offered maintenance treatment with, for example, monthly 5-day courses of cytosine arabinoside and 6-thioguanine, but with such regimes the median duration of remission has been only a few months and many patients have thus relapsed whilst still receiving treatment.

Currently, trends are towards much more aggressive remission induction followed by intensive consolidation for several months, alternating cycles which combine a number of different drugs known individually to have some effect in AML. 'Intensification' of treatment at intervals during or on completion of maintenance may confer additional benefit.

Bone marrow transplantation

One of the most disappointing aspects of the treatment of AML is the high relapse rate following even aggressive induction maintenance therapy. Even more intensive treatment can be employed

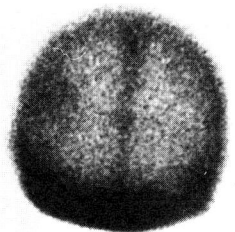
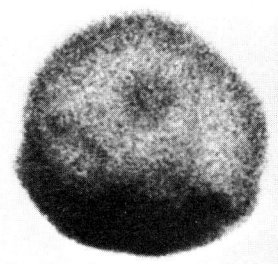

Fig. 16 Technetium-99 scans showing localized leukaemic deposit in the brain of a 56-year-old man presenting with headache and facial weakness 2 years after a diagnosis of AML (M3 type). The CNS relapse was treated with 33 Gy of cranial irradiation plus intrathecal cytosine arabinoside. Response was complete and a CT brain scan 5 years later was normal.

including whole body irradiation provided a suitable source of haemopoietic cells can be found to 'rescue' the patient from the effects of treatment. In conventional bone marrow transplantation (see page 19.256) the donor is an HLA identical sibling, or much less commonly an identical twin or a relation who is less well-matched. If a suitable donor is not available it may be reasonable to attempt an *autograft* using the patient's own bone marrow harvested before the period of intensive treatment.

Results of bone marrow transplantation have been very encouraging with up to half the patients in some series becoming long-term disease-free survivors. The role of autografting is less clear – there is the theoretical possibility that residual leukaemic cells in the harvested marrow might cause relapse. The procedure is, however, straightforward and initial results are at least comparable with conventional therapy.

CNS disease

Involvement of the CNS may occur early in AML with the patient presenting with cord compression, nerve root involvement, or a cranial nerve palsy. Lesions tend to be more focal than in ALL. In the majority of cases where CNS disease becomes evident it is accompanied by active marrow disease, and prophylaxis against CNS involvement is not generally included in treatment although the possible benefit is being investigated. Localized deposits may be radiosensitive and, if they do occur without haematological relapse, should certainly be treated with radiotherapy with or without the addition of intrathecal chemotherapy (Fig. 16).

Prognosis in AML

Although there has certainly been some improvement in the prognosis of AML the median survival is still only of the order of a year in most series. Recently the Medical Research Council completed a large multicentre treatment trial in AML: 1127 patients were entered; the overall median survival was just over 12 months and the 5-year survival is projected to be about 18 per cent, although the results vary considerably with age. A large proportion of patients in this study were treated at district general hospitals where the success rate was initially low. There was, however, significant trend towards longer survival as the trial progressed presumably reflecting improved efficiency of supportive care. The most significant prognostic factor in this study was age: remission was obtained in 85 per cent of those under the age of 14, 73 per cent of those aged 14–59, and 48 per cent in those aged 60 and over, with an overall remission rate of 67 per cent. The duration of remission was, however, less obviously influenced by age.

CHRONIC GRANULOCYTIC LEUKAEMIA

Chronic granulocytic leukaemia (CGL) is a rare disease with an incidence of about 1 : 100 000 of the population over the age of 15. It occurs most commonly between the ages of 30 and 50 years and is rare below the age of 10. There is an atypical juvenile form of granulocytic leukaemia seen in children below the age of 5.

Aetiology

Some cases of leukaemia occurring after exposure to ionizing radiation or chemicals such as benzene have the features of chronic granulocytic leukaemia but no other aetiological factors have been identified.

Pathogenesis

Chronic granulocytic leukaemia (CGL) is characterized by the uncontrolled proliferation of myeloid cells. In 1960 a specific chromosomal abnormality was identified, which has become known as the Philadelphia (Ph^1) chromosome. This results in fact from a reciprocal exchange (translocation) between chromosomes 9 and 22; the exchange always occurs at the same bands, q34 on chromosome 9 and q11 on chromosome 22, and produces an abnormally long chromosome 9 (9q+), and a shortened chromosome 22, the Philadelphia chromosome.

Perhaps the most exciting development in our understanding of the pathogenesis of this condition has been the discovery that the cellular proto-oncogenes *abl* and *sis* are located at or near the breakpoints on chromosomes 9 and 22 respectively, and are in fact included in the translocated segments. No evidence for transcription of *sis* has been found, but recently it has been shown that the translocation places the c-*abl* gene very close to what has become known as the *breakpoint cluster region* or *bcr* on chromosome 22. As a result a new gene is produced which is in effect a fusion of the *bcr* and *abl* genes. This 'gene' is actively transcribed in CGL patients; its product is a protein kinase similar to but different from the normal product of the c-*abl* gene, and the intriguing possibility is that this is in some way involved in the malignant transformation.

The Ph^1 chromosome is found in over 95 per cent of cases of CGL and is present in granulocyte, erythrocyte, and platelet precursors. In almost every case all cells are Ph^1-positive by the time of diagnosis and they usually remain so even during periods of clinical remission. These findings indicate that the mutant (clonogenic) cell in CGL is in fact a primitive progenitor common to erythroid, myeloid and megakaryocytic lines. Further confirmation for the clonal origin of CGL comes from studies in individuals heterozygous for glucose-6-phosphate dehydrogenase (G6PD) isoenzymes A and B (see page 19.13), in which haemopoietic cells are uniformly of either one G6PD type or the other, indicating their origin from a common progenitor. Although circulating lymphocytes are Ph^1-negative, these cells may derive from precursors which predate the malignant transformation, and the observation that about half the cases of acute transformation show a lymphoid phenotype (see below) suggests that the neoplastic mutation has occurred in a pluripotent haemopoietic stem cell or a very closely related progenitor.

In about one-third of cases additional chromosomal abnormalities are found, such as an absent Y, extra C group chromosome, duplication of the Ph^1, or additional translocations. A few clinically typical cases of CGL are Ph^1-negative but, interestingly, molecular analysis in such cases has shown rearrangements in the *bcr* region on chromosome 22.

In the course of CGL, the disease progresses from a chronic phase to a transformed phase. The stage at which this takes place is unpredictable. Whilst in about 20 per cent of cases no change in karyotype occurs, in the remainder additional chromosome abnormalities may presage the onset of metamorphosis, for example, an additional Ph^1 or other hyperdiploidy, or structural abnormalities. One pathognomonic abnormality is the appearance of an isochrome for the long arm of chromosome 17.

Particular interest has centred around those Ph^1-positive cases in which the acute transformation sees the emergence of clones of primitive cells with the phenotype of lymphoblasts rather than myeloblasts as might be intuitively expected. The lymphoid nature of these cells has been confirmed by the finding of immunoglobulin gene rearrangements as well as positivity for the common-ALL antigen (CALLA) and the enzyme TdT (see page 19.20).

Clinical features of classical CGL

Symptoms

About half the patients with CGL present with symptoms referable to the disease but these are often insidious in onset and may date back for a year or more. In just less than one-fifth of cases the diagnosis is found by chance during treatment for an unrelated condition, or during screening as a potential blood donor.

The more chronic symptoms are those of tiredness, abdominal discomfort or weight loss, and are related to the anaemia, splenomegaly, and hypermetabolism. More acute symptoms which lead to diagnosis are severe and acute abdominal pain from splenic infarction, haemorrhagic symptoms including the occurrence of large haematomata, and gout from hyperuricaemia. Fever and sweating may also be presenting symptoms. Priapism is a rare but dramatic feature.

Clinical signs

The dominant physical sign is splenomegaly, which is almost invariably present even in cases where the diagnosis is made by chance. The spleen may be only just palpable but in over 70 per cent of cases it is 10 cm or more below the costal margin at diagnosis, and occasionally extends down into the right iliac fossa and may be readily visible on inspection of the abdomen. Enlargement of the liver is more variable, but some hepatomegaly is usually present and is occasionally out of proportion to the splenomegaly. There may be evidence of anaemia, bruising, and/or purpura. Fundal haemorrhages may occur, particularly if the haemoglobin level is very low. If the white cell count is extremely high, a creamy appearance of the blood can be recognized in the fundal vessels.

Laboratory findings

Although in some cases there may be little or no anaemia and the leucocyte count may be only moderately raised, by the time of presentation the haematological changes in the majority are florid (Fig. 17). There is usually only a moderate anaemia, but in about 15 per cent of cases the haemoglobin level is less than 7.5 g/dl and the symptoms of anaemia may be prominent. The leucocyte count ranges from a modest increase in the region of 25×10^9/l to over 750×10^9/l, and is more than 100×10^9/l in the majority of cases. Thrombocytopenia is rare at presentation; on the other hand, thrombocytosis occurs in nearly half of the patients and values of over 1000×10^9/l are not uncommon. The blood film shows an increase in neutrophils and myelocytes with occasional earlier forms, and often some increase in basophils and eosinophils; if there is a thrombocytosis, large clumps of platelets may be prominent.

If there is any doubt about the diagnosis, a blood film should be stained for leucocyte alkaline phosphatase as the enzyme is almost always reduced in the granulocytes of CGL. Chromosomal analysis of the blood and/or bone marrow should finally confirm the diagnosis. The bone marrow shows extreme cellularity with a predominance of cells of the granulocytic series and often an increase in megakaryocytes. Red cell precursors are proportionately reduced.

Other features which may be found on investigation are a high uric acid and a raised serum alkaline phosphatase. The serum vitamin B_{12} binding protein transcobalamin 1 is produced by granulocytes, and is therefore greatly increased in association with the granulocytic proliferation. This results in an increased vitamin B_{12} binding capacity and high levels of serum vitamin B_{12}.

Differential diagnosis

There is little difficulty in making the diagnosis in a florid case of CGL when the classical features of a leucocyte count of more than

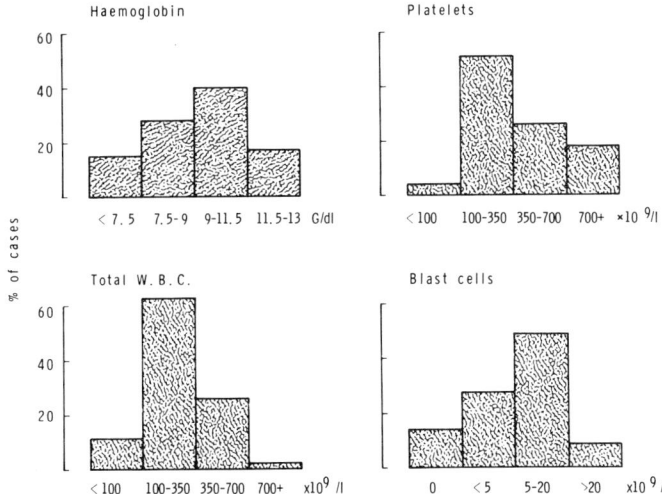

Fig. 17 Blood findings at presentation in 102 patients with CGL entered into a Medical Research Council trial (*Br. Med. J.* **1**, 201,1968).

100 × 10⁹/l with a preponderance of granulocytes and a few granulocyte precursors are seen in the blood film, and clinical examination reveals the presence of splenomegaly. In other patients in whom a leucocytosis is found by chance, and especially in those with counts in the region of $25-30 \times 10^9$/l, there may be some initial difficulty in distinguishing between CGL and a reactive leucocytosis, for example, from occult infection or infarction, or a *leukaemoid reaction* such as may occur in disseminated tuberculosis or widespread malignancy. The presence of splenomegaly which, although uncommon, may occur in either of the latter two conditions, may add to the confusion. A careful history is all-important in guiding the direction of further investigation.

Patients with myelofibrosis or polycythaemia vera provide more serious problems with differential diagnosis. Very occasional cases of polycythaemia vera have been observed to progress to CGL, and myelofibrosis is often a sequel to the chronic phase of CGL (see page 19.40). The principal features which distinguish the three conditions are shown in Table 5.

Course of the disease

Chronic granulocytic leukaemia has a very varied course but is ultimately fatal. There are usually two phases: first the *chronic phase*, during which the patient may become totally asymptomatic and able to lead a normal life. This phase is, however, usually followed by an *accelerated phase* during which the disease becomes more aggressive and difficult to control, or by frank transformation into an acute leukaemia – the so-called *blast crisis*.

The chronic phase

The duration of the chronic phase is variable – from a few weeks to 10–15 years or more. The median survival is, however, only about 3 years and although the quality of life during the chronic phase has been improved with treatment, the overall median survival has increased very little.

Because of the insidious onset of the disease, patients tend to present at different stages of its evolution, and as one might expect, this tends to be reflected in the duration of the chronic phase.

With conventional treatment there is no question of a cure of the disease or elimination of the abnormal clone. Even though the clinical signs may regress and the blood count return to normal, the Ph¹ chromosome almost always persists. Very rare cases have been described in which aggressive chemotherapy or inappropriately prolonged busulphan therapy has lead to a period of aplasia, followed by regeneration of normal marrow and loss of the Ph¹-positive clone. This can be more consistently (and reliably)

Table 5 Differential diagnosis of chronic myeloproliferative diseases

	CGL	Myelofibrosis	Polycythaemia vera
Haemoglobin	Normal or decreased	Normal or decreased	Increased (unless previous blood loss)
WBC	Increased frequently > 100 000/dl	Normal to moderate increase	Normal to moderate increase
Platelets	Decreased, normal or increased	Decreased, normal or increased	Normal or increased
Film	Neutrophil leucocytosis; some early forms; basophilia	'Teardrop' erythrocytes; leuco-erythroblastic picture	Normal or hypochromic; moderate neutrophilia
Marrow	Hypercellular; increased M/E ratio	Dry tap	Normal or hypercellular; M/E ratio normal
LAP score	Decreased	Normal or increased	Normal or increased
Commonest chromosome abnormality	95% Ph¹+	C Group aneuploidy	C Group aneuploidy
Spleen	+ to ++	Usually ++	Normal or +
Haemorrhagic symptoms	+	+	+
Thrombotic symptoms	(+)	(+)	+

achieved with bone marrow transplantation following high-dose chemotherapy and total body irradiation (see below and page 19.256).

During the chronic phase the function of the granulocytes is not impaired and susceptibility to infection is not increased unless neutropenia is induced by overtreatment. Haemorrhagic or thrombotic complications are rare once treatment has begun even in the continued presence of a high platelet count.

The accelerated phase

The onset of the accelerated phase is unpredictable. As already mentioned additional chromosome abnormalities may presage the onset of metamorphosis. In about 10 per cent of cases there is rapid onset of a blast cell crisis with all the clinical features of an acute leukaemia. Death from infection, haemorrhage or uncontrolled leukaemia may occur within a few weeks.

In the majority, however, the deterioration is more gradual. It may be indicated first by a lack of response to treatment which has formerly been effective or by the development of pancytopenia not attributable to the chemotherapy, or by a gradual increase in the proportion of blast cells. The blood findings may remain fairly stable for some months but the patient becomes ill, loses weight, and develops progressive splenomegaly and hepatomegaly. There is often fever, sweating, bone pain, and splenic pain, and there may be complications from infection or haemorrhage. Extramedullary masses may be a feature, with infiltration of the skin, lymphadenopathy, and local destructive bone lesions which may give rise to hypercalcaemia. CNS signs may occur, either as a result of invasion from local deposits in bone, or from meningeal leukaemia or intracranial haemorrhage.

The bone marrow during the transformation phase may be cellular with obvious increase in blast cells or, more usually, there is a dry tap with difficulty in obtaining marrow. The blood film will often show a leucoerythroblastic picture similar to that found in myelofibrosis, but may change terminally to a frankly blastic picture.

The duration of the accelerated phase may last sometimes for 1 or 2 years. The cachexia, gross splenomegaly, and constitutional symptoms are very distressing to the patient. Death usually results from a complicating infection or intracranial haemorrhage.

Occasionally patients present with a blast cell leukaemia with no preceding history of chronic disease but with the Ph[1] chromosome marker. Such patients differ clinically from ordinary acute leukaemia in having more organ involvement with lymphadenopathy and splenomegaly. Some of these have the haematological features of ALL and are positive with anti-ALL sera and for the enzyme TdT.

Treatment of CGL

Treatment of the chronic phase: busulphan

Splenic irradiation remained the treatment of choice for CGL until the 1940s when radioactive phosphorus was introduced as a means of controlling the condition. The treatment was, however, largely abandoned when the alkylating agent busulphan was found to be useful in CGL.

Various dosage regimens have been used with busulphan but the most generally acceptable is a daily dose of 4 mg/day. The haemoglobin level should begin to rise and the white cell count to fall within a few weeks of starting treatment, with accompanying clinical improvement (Fig. 18). It is rare for larger doses to be necessary, and certainly no change in dose should be contemplated unless there is a complete failure of response in the first 4 weeks. It is very important to monitor the progress of the haematological changes. Blood counts should be taken at 1–2 week intervals and the results obtained without delay so that the decision can be made whether or not to continue treatment. It is helpful in making these decisions if the blood counts are charted on a semilogarithmic scale since the continued fall in white count can usually be predicted. It is wise not to allow the leucocyte count to drop below about 15×10^9/l or platelets below 100×10^9/l in the first instance, since on stopping the drug a further fall may be expected over 2–3 weeks. The possible danger of inducing pancytopenia should always be kept in mind and, in particular, a reduction in the platelet count should be taken as a warning sign that treatment should be suspended immediately.

With a favourable response the spleen reduces in size and may become impalpable; hepatomegaly is also reduced. The dosage of busulphan may be adjusted to maintain a near normal count – for example, by giving 1–2 mg on alternate days or on 2 or 3 days per week – but it is probably preferable to give intermittent treatment and to reintroduce busulphan only when there has been a progressive tendency for the leucocyte count to rise again.

In the early stages of treatment, and particularly if the leucocyte count is very high, allopurinol, 300–600 mg/day, should be given, and the patient should be urged to take a high fluid intake in order to avoid the adverse effects of hyperuricaemia.

Complications of busulphan treatment

Pancytopenia Busulphan is the only cytotoxic drug with the capacity to damage the pluripotent haemopoietic stem cells permanently and, if treatment is not monitored carefully and at frequent intervals, the bone marrow may be irreversibly damaged. In most cases in which this has happened the warning signs have been ignored.

Amenorrhea This is usual in women of menstrual age and may lead to an early menopause. Testicular atrophy and gynaecomastia have also both been observed.

Pigmentation This is a fairly frequent finding in patients on busulphan treatment and is noticeable in about one-third of patients who have had the drug for more than 2 years.

Pseudo-Addison's disease An interesting but rare complication is the development of anorexia, weight loss, weakness, and fever which, together with the pigmentation, simulates Addison's disease. No evidence of adrenocortical failure can, however, be

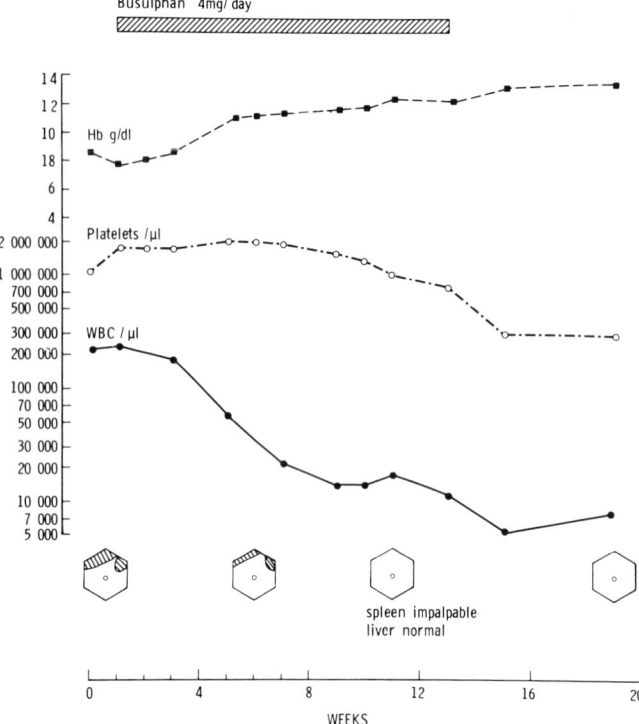

Fig. 18 Response to treatment with busulphan, 4 mg/day, in a patient with chronic granulocytic leukaemia.

demonstrated and the condition tends to recover spontaneously on stopping busulphan treatment.

Interstitial pulmonary fibrosis This is a serious complication. The symptoms are those of weight loss, dyspnoea, and dry cough. Again, the condition may be reversible if recognized early, and steroids have been found to relieve the symptoms in some cases.

Cytological dysplasia This has been described in some patients on busulphan treatment, and the increased incidence of cancer of the lung in patients receiving the drug may be related to the cytological changes.

Alternative chemotherapy

In patients who are poorly controlled by busulphan or who develop unacceptable toxicity, hydroxyurea is the most useful drug to use. It should be given in doses of 0.5–2 g/day with careful control of the blood count. It is not so toxic to the bone marrow as busulphan and its effects are quickly reversible.

Bone marrow transplantation

The recognition that busulphan therapy has had little impact on the duration of the chronic phase, and that evolution into a more rapidly progressive phase is inevitable, coupled with observations that on rare occasions excessive treatment has resulted in loss of the Ph[1]-positive clone, has led to the suggestion that high-dose chemoradiotherapy followed by bone marrow transplantation during the *chronic* phase might be a useful alternative approach. Recent studies have amply confirmed this. The procedure is well-tolerated and can result in prolonged disease-free survival with apparent elimination of the Ph[1] clone in many instances. Bone marrow transplantation is less well-tolerated by the elderly, but should be seriously considered in patients under 50 who have a suitable HLA identical sibling donor (page 19.256).

Splenectomy

A number of studies have been made in recent years in which splenectomy has been performed after the use of busulphan to reduce the size of the spleen and return the leucocyte count to normal. It has been suggested that early splenectomy might be beneficial, in that it would avoid the distress of gross splenomegaly in the terminal stages of the disease and that it might remove a major site of blast-cell transformation. No convincing evidence has ever been produced that the spleen is indeed the major site of such transformations, nor that splenectomy alters significantly the course of the disease or the quality of life.

Leucapheresis

Some centres have investigated the effect of repeated leucapheresis on patients with CGL. This not only directly reduces the circulating leucocyte count, but also has an indirect effect in reducing the high level of circulating myeloid progenitor cells. However, whilst producing general symptomatic improvement and reduction in splenomegaly, this treatment has not been shown to have any effect on long-term survival.

Treatment of transformed CGL

As has already been noted, one of the first signs of transformation in CGL is a diminishing response to therapy. In general, the response of patients in the transformed phase is poor, and in only a minority can a good remission be achieved. However, it has now become clear that two types of blast cell transformation occur, one myeloid and the other in which the blast cells have the features of lymphoblasts. Patients with lymphoblastic characteristics may respond well to treatment with vincristine and prednisolone, treatments effective in ordinary ALL, and some patients may return temporarily to a chronic phase. Treatment of myeloblastic transformation is much less satisfactory, but a few patients may respond to aggressive multidrug chemotherapy similar to that employed in AML.

In those patients who have accelerated disease without a frank blast cell crisis, relief may sometimes be given by the careful use of hydroxyurea in a dose of 0.5–1.5 g/day, combined with symptomatic support.

'JUVENILE' CGL

In children, Ph^1-positive CGL occurs very occasionally; the clinical features are similar to those found in the adult disease and response to treatment is much the same. There is, however, a particular 'juvenile' form of CGL seen in children under the age of 5 years. It is Ph^1-negative and has a number of distinct clinical and haematological features.

It represents about 2–3 per cent of all cases of childhood leukaemia, and differs clinically from the adult type of CGL in presenting with more lymphadenopathy, the lymph nodes showing a tendency to break down and suppurate. Skin rashes are a common presenting feature, particularly on the face, but also extending to other areas. There may be purpura and a tendency to bruise.

Thrombocytopenia is usually present and the leucocyte count is notably less than that found in the adult type CGL (usually less than $100 \times 10^9/l$) and the proportion of blasts, monocytes, and lymphocytes is higher than in the adult type where there are more mature granulocytes. This may be due in part to the younger age of the juvenile CGL patients. There may also be many nucleated red cells in the blood of the juvenile patient.

The most striking abnormality is a high level of haemoglobin F (up to 40–50 per cent). This contrasts with other forms of childhood leukaemia in which the haemoglobin F level is seldom more than 10 per cent. There are also other features of fetal red cells such as a reduced haemoglobin A_2 level, and a reduction in the isoenzymes B and C of carbonic anhydrase and an increase in G6PD.

It has been suggested that this type of CGL is essentially a congenital abnormality, perhaps arising from a structural or functional chromosomal change.

It is important to distinguish between the two types of childhood CGL as their prognosis is very different. Chromosome studies should therefore always be performed if possible on such children.

Treatment

The adult type of CGL shows much the same type of response in children to treatment with busulphan as do older patients. The juvenile type appears to be far more resistant to therapy: partial remissions have been reported with 6-mercaptopurine, but the overall median survival is less than 1 year. Marrow transplantation should be seriously considered if there is a suitable donor available.

PRE-LEUKAEMIA

These are various conditions in which there is an increased risk for the subsequent development of acute leukaemia. These include the myeloproliferative disorders (polycythaemia rubra vera, myelofibrosis, chronic granulocytic leukaemia and essential thrombocythaemia) described elsewhere in this section, and also a group of rare childhood disorders associated with chromosomal fragility including ataxia telangiectasia, Bloom's syndrome, and Fanconi's anaemia. Finally, there is an equally heterogeneous group of disorders encountered mainly in later life and characterized by varying degrees of refractory anaemia and pancytopenia. These latter conditions are known variously as pre-leukaemia, smouldering leukaemia, or myelodysplasia; a brief description is given here, and the topic is discussed more fully on page 19.58.

Pathogenesis

It is generally accepted that the majority are clonal disorders of haemopoiesis in which the abnormal clone shows abnormal differentiation and maturation characteristics but does not – at least initially – have much proliferative advantage over any remaining normal clones. In the majority of instances there are no predisposing factors, but it is noteworthy that many patients who develop acute leukaemia after radiation exposure or treatment for another malignancy do so after an initial myelodysplastic stage.

Clinical features

The condition usually presents with symptoms of anaemia/and or bleeding, but is not infrequently discovered as a result of a investigation of some other problem. There are no specific clinical findings, although the spleen may be palpable but is never grossly enlarged.

Haematological features

The anaemia may be normochromic and normocytic or macrocytic. There may be considerable variation in size and shape of the red cells with some macrocytes and oval cells, which initially may suggest a diagnosis of vitamin B_{12} or folate deficiency. There is sometimes a dimorphic picture, and occasional nucleated red cells may be seen. The leucocyte count is usually normal or low with a neutropenia and sometimes a monocytosis. There may be hypersegmentation of the neutrophils (pseudo-Pelger-Huet phenomenon) and defective granulation. Thrombocytopenia is a feature in about half the cases and there may be atypical giant platelets present.

The marrow is usually hyperplastic with dyserythropoiesis. Many of the nucleated red cells have multiple nuclei or resemble megaloblasts so that again an erroneous diagnosis of vitamin B_{12} or folate deficiency may be made. Ring sideroblasts are found in about 20 per cent of cases. The myeloid precursors often show poor granulation and there may be some increase in blast cells but not sufficient to make the diagnosis of overt leukaemia.

Other abnormal features

A moderate rise in haemoglobin F, up to about 10 per cent, may be found in pre-leukaemia and a few cases have been shown to have acquired haemoglobin H disease (see page 19.129). Some have been found to show the same defect in red cells as in paroxysmal nocturnal haemoglobinuria (PNH) with sensitivity to lysis by complement in acidified serum (Ham's test) or a positive sugar water test.

Cytogenetic abnormalities
Chromosomal abnormalities have been reported in 25–50 per cent, and are particularly common in patients with a history of previous radiation exposure or cytotoxic drug treatment. The abnormalities found have been similar to those reported in AML, with particular patterns tending to recur. These include partial or complete deletions of chromosomes 5 and 7, and trisomy 8. Evolution into a florid acute leukaemia may or may not be associated with further detectable abnormalities.

Differential diagnosis
The condition of pre-leukaemia has to be distinguished from any other cause of anaemia in the elderly, such as the anaemia of chronic disorders – including that due to renal failure and malignancy, vitamin B_{12} or folate deficiency, and other primary haematological disorders such as chronic lymphocytic leukaemia or one of the myeloproliferative disorders.

As already suggested, the most likely confusion is between pre-leukaemia and vitamin B_{12} or folate deficiency although the marrow appearances are not really those of a true megaloblastic anaemia. If there is any doubt, B_{12} and folate levels can be measured. The marrow appearances are the key to the diagnosis and it should not be necessary to subject these patients to further investigation.

Treatment and prognosis
Treatment is primarily supportive, that is, with blood transfusion and platelet transfusion when indicated, and antibiotics for intercurrent infection. Chemotherapy is generally not indicated, particularly as most of these patients are elderly and frail. The condition tends to evolve gradually into a frank AML, this occurring in about one-third of the cases within 6 months, in half within a year, and three-quarters within 2 years. However, a few cases may have a much slower evolution, over 5 years or more, whilst others may die of intercurrent infection or haemorrhage before the development of overt leukaemia.

CHRONIC LYMPHOCYTIC LEUKAEMIA

Chronic lymphocytic leukaemia (CLL) differs in many respects from the other forms of leukaemia and has more in common with the diffuse lymphocytic varieties of non-Hodgkin's lymphoma. The definition of CLL as a leukaemia depends upon the predominant infiltration of the bone marrow and invasion of the blood by small lymphocytes which have failed to mature normally and which are immunologically incompetent.

In most cases the lymphocytes in CLL show evidence of B cell differentiation. This, and their clonal origin is confirmed by the presence of monoclonal cell surface IgM and/or IgD and of a unique arrangement of the heavy and light chain immunoglobulin genes. In about 5 per cent of cases there is evidence of further maturation in that a monoclonal Ig is found in the serum, usually IgM and light chains may be excreted in the urine.

In a minority of cases no surface Ig can be demonstrated, and the lymphocytes have the surface characteristics of T cells and in addition show rearrangement of the T cell antigen-receptor genes.

Two other malignant lymphoproliferative conditions, hairy cell leukaemia and prolymphocytic leukaemia, are generally considered to be variants of CLL (Table 1), although the malignant cells have a distinct phenotype. A further condition, which is sometimes grouped with CLL, is the recently recognized *adult leukaemia-lymphoma syndrome* (ATL). This is probably a distinct entity, and runs a much more aggressive course than even T cell

CLL. ATL has the distinction of being the only form of human leukaemia in which a causative viral agent has been demonstrated.

Classical CLL
CLL is a disease of older age groups and has a male preponderance. It represents about 25 per cent of cases of leukaemia in the Western world but in some races, notably the Japanese and Chinese, it is rare. No specific aetiological factors have been identified and, in particular, it has not been related to previous radiation exposure.

Clinical findings
In about 25 per cent of cases, CLL is discovered by chance and is entirely symptomless although examination may reveal some enlarged nodes which have gone unnoticed by the patient and/or there may be splenomegaly. In other cases the patient may seek advice having noticed abnormalities such as lymphadenopathy, skin infiltration, or purpura.

About half the patients have some constitutional symptom such as weight loss, fatigue, general malaise, fever, or sweating, and there may be a history of frequent infection, especially chest infection. Occasionally there is a more acute onset associated with bone marrow failure when symptoms of anaemia and thrombocytopenia may be prominent.

There may be no abnormal physical signs or there may be lymphadenopathy of varying degree. The enlarged glands are discrete and non-tender and are usually symmetrical in distribution; large localized masses are more suggestive of lymphoma. The spleen may be palpable with or without lymph node enlargement and it is sometimes massive in size. Skin infiltration may occur either at presentation or later in the disease process, the lesions varying from macules to purplish-brown raised plaques (Fig. 1), which occasionally ulcerate.

Petechiae, bruising, bleeding from mucous membranes, and fundal haemorrhages are usually late features of the disease and are associated with thrombocytopenia. Herpes zoster is a frequent complication of CLL, especially in patients receiving chemotherapy, and the lesions may become haemorrhagic and/or generalized.

Chest symptoms are usually the result of complicating infection although pulmonary infiltration, hilar lymphadenopathy, and pleural effusions are features of advanced cases. Massive lymphadenopathy sometimes produces obstructive symptoms such as oedema of the legs.

Occasional patients have evidence of leukaemic infiltration of the gut, particularly of the stomach and small bowel, which may produce symptoms of ulceration and bleeding or malabsorption.

CNS involvement in CLL is rare and abnormalities in the central nervous system are more likely to be due to cerebral haemorrhage or infection – particularly bacterial, viral, or cryptococcal.

Leukaemic infiltration of the kidneys, although commonly found at autopsy, is seldom clinically evident. An obstructive nephropathy sometimes occurs with massive lymph node enlargement involving the ureters.

Haematological findings
The haemoglobin level is frequently normal, especially in those cases where the diagnosis is made by chance (Fig. 2). Anaemia,

Table 1 Classification of chronic lymphatic leukaemia

	B cell (per cent)	T cell (per cent)
Classical CLL	99	1
Hairy cell leukaemia	100	0
Prolymphocytic leukaemia	80	20

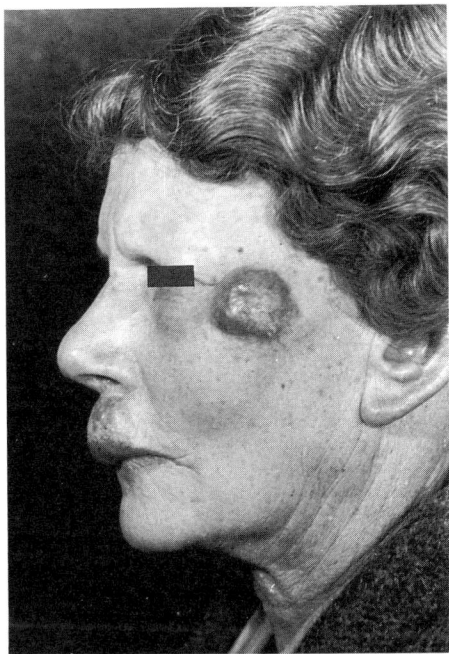

Fig. 1 Skin infiltration on the cheek and upper lip of a patient with CLL.

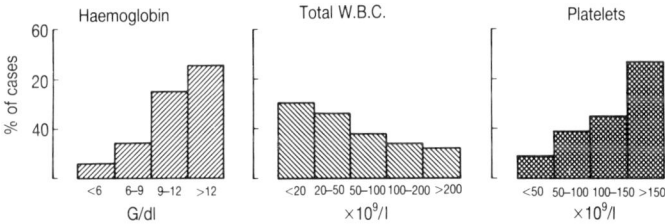

Fig. 2 Haematological findings at presentation in CLL.

when present, may be the result of marrow failure, hypersplenism (page 19.189), or due to a complicating autoimmune haemolytic anaemia (page 19.144). Where the latter complication arises there is usually a positive Coombs' test, the serological reactions being similar to those found in idiopathic autoimmune haemolytic anaemias. In several well-documented cases the haemolytic anaemia has antedated the onset of CLL but it may occur months or years after the onset of the lymphocytic leukaemia.

The leucocyte count is extremely variable but there is always a persistent lymphocytosis. Counts in the range of $200–600×10^9$ per litre are not uncommon even in asymptomatic patients. The majority of the cells are well differentiated small lymphocytes, but there may be a varying number of larger cells with a higher proportion of cytoplasm and poorly condensed chromatin. When the diagnosis is in doubt, particularly in patients with relatively low counts, immunofluorescent or immunoperoxidase techniques may be used to demonstrate the monoclonal nature of the cells from the cell surface immunoglobulin.

Thrombocytopenia is usually a late finding associated with marrow failure. Occasionally, however, it has an autoimmune basis.

It is seldom necessary to examine the bone marrow except in doubtful cases. It will, however, be found to be diffusely infiltrated with cells similar to those found in the peripheral blood. An arbitrary figure of 40 per cent or more lymphocytes in the total cell population is taken as confirmatory evidence of CLL.

Other laboratory findings

An important feature in CLL is that in 50–75 per cent of cases there is pronounced hypogammaglobulinaemia, the IgM being most affected. The depression in immunoglobulin tends to become more severe with advance of the disease. The consequent reduction in humoral immunity is responsible for the high incidence of chest infection, viral infections, particularly herpes zoster, and fungal infections.

In about 5 per cent of patients a paraprotein is found, usually of the IgM type but occasionally IgG or IgA. Monoclonal light chains may also be found in the urine. The presence of an IgM paraprotein may make the distinction from Waldenström's macroglobulinaemia difficult; in the latter condition the lymphocytosis is seldom marked and the morphology of the lymphocytes, particularly in the bone marrow, may be more plasmacytoid in type. Occasionally, the paraprotein is a cryoglobulin, or has cold agglutinin activity, in which case a cold haemolytic anaemia may occur.

Hyperuricaemia is sometimes seen in CLL and it may give rise to renal failure, particularly if treatment results in rapid destruction of cells.

Clinical course

It has long been recognized that CLL has an extremely variable course, many patients living for years in a stable condition with little trouble from their disease (Fig. 3) while others have a much more aggressive disease with a very limited prognosis.

Rai and his colleagues have suggested a scheme for staging patients with CLL on clinical and haematological grounds (Table 2). This staging was based on the concept that in CLL the neoplastic lymphocytes have a very long lifespan and the clinical picture is the result of a progressive accumulation of non-functioning cells.

Analysis of a large series of patients supported the validity of the classification. The median survival for the various stages diminished progressively from more than 150 months in stage 0 (bone marrow and blood lymphocytosis only) to 19 months in stages III and IV (complicated by anaemia and thrombocytopenia respectively). When the patient progressed from an earlier stage to a later one, the prognosis changed accordingly.

An International Workshop subsequently analysed data on over 900 patients with CLL, and as a result proposed a revised prognostic staging system suggesting that it could be integrated with the Rai system by using Roman numerals in parenthesis to indicate the Rai classification (Table 3).

The use of such a system makes it possible to compare the results of controlled clinical trials and it provides a basis for the investigation of such problems as the relationship of stage and clinical response to the lymphocyte characteristics, the pathogenesis of anaemia, and thrombocytopenia in CLL, and recognition of patients with stable as opposed to aggressive disease.

Treatment

The problem of when to treat a patient with CLL is a very real one. Most physicians would agree that treatment is indicated in

Table 2 Rai classification of chronic lymphatic leukaemia

Stage	Clinical features	Median survival from diagnosis (months)
0	$\geq 15 \times 10^9/1$ lymphocytes in blood $\geq 40\%$ lymphocytes in marrow	> 150
I	Lymphocytosis + enlarged lymph nodes	101
II	Lymphocytosis + enlarged spleen and/or liver $\pm$ enlarged lymph nodes	72
III	Lymphocytosis + Hb < 11g/d1 or PCV < 33% $\pm$ enlarged nodes, spleen, or liver	19
IV	Lymphocytosis + platelets $< 100 \times 10^9/1 \pm$ enlarged nodes, spleen, liver, or anaemia	19

Data from Rai *et al.* (1975). *Blood* **46**, 219.

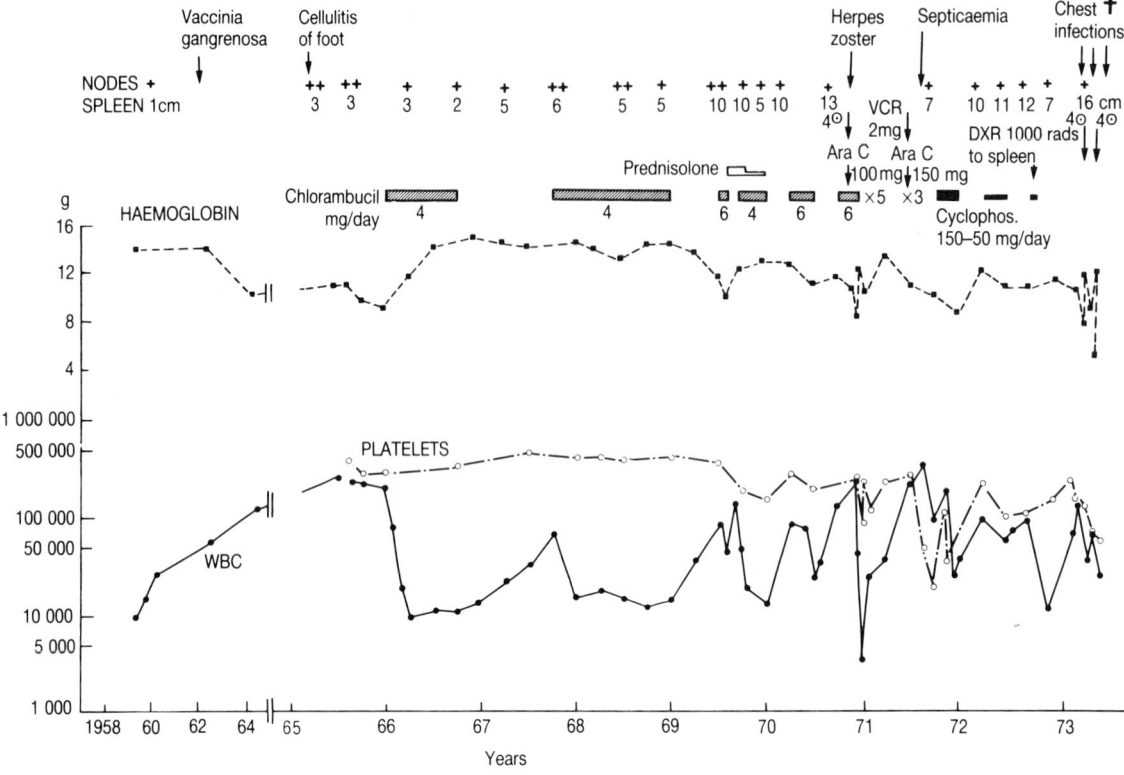

Fig. 3 Example of a patient with CLL who required no treatment and remained relatively well for six years, after which her disease became more aggressive. She subsequently had several complications associated with severe immunosuppression.

obvious advancing disease with the presence of complications such as haemolytic anaemia, but the diagnosis of CLL in an asymptomatic patient certainly does not from our present knowledge warrant therapeutic interference even in the presence of significant lymphocytosis. There is no convincing data to show that patients treated early in the disease fare better than those in whom treatment is delayed until clinical problems develop.

Only very rare instances of complete remission have been reported in CLL and the aim therefore is to control symptoms and improve the quality of life rather than cure the disease.

The accepted indications for treatment of CLL are:

1. Increasing or troublesome lymphadenopathy
2. Systemic symptoms
3. Marrow failure
4. Autoimmune complications, i.e. haemolytic anaemia and immune thrombocytopenia

Since the lymphocytes of CLL are effectively non-dividing and long-lived, radiotherapy or chemotherapy with agents which are non-cycle specific are used in treatment. Chlorambucil is usually the first choice. It is conventionally given in continuous daily doses of 0.1–0.15 mg/kg/day. The treatment must be controlled by regular blood counts at 2–3 week intervals, and the drug may need to

be suspended temporarily if there is evidence of marrow toxicity, e.g. a low platelet count; after an interval it may be re-introduced at a lower dose.

In about 20 per cent of cases there is an excellent response; lymphnodes and the spleen become inpalpable and the blood count returns to near normal. A further 40 per cent of patients respond less well, with a reduction in lymphadenopathy and splenomegaly but persistence of lymphocytosis. The remaining 40 per cent respond poorly if at all. There is no clear view as to whether treatment should be continued to get a maximum effect or whether it can be suspended when the patient has improved symptomatically.

Cyclophosphamide can be used as an alternative alkylating agent but it is usually less well tolerated and is unlikely to be effective if chlorambucil has failed. It has been suggested that intermittent treatment with higher doses of chlorambucil might produce less immunosuppression and less marrow toxicity than continuous therapy. In one such regimen chlorambucil in a dose of 0.2 mg/kg/day is given in cycles of 10–14 days, followed by a two-week interval. Other regimes use high doses of chlorambucil one every four weeks starting with an initial single dose of 0.4 mg/kg and increasing the dose every course by 0.1 mg/kg until there are signs of marrow toxicity or the lymphocytosis is brought under control. Such regimens appear to be effective but whether they produce better results than the more conventional regimens has yet to be proved.

In patients presenting with marrow failure, chlorambucil should be withheld initially, and prednisolone given in a dose of 40–60 mg/day. This causes rapid lysis of lymphocytes and, if there is bulky disease, allopurinol should be started 24 hours before the prednisolone and a high fluid intake ensured. A temporary increase in the lymphocyte count may be seen in the peripheral blood, possibly due to redistribution of lymphocytes. This, however, is usually followed by a fall in the leucocyte count and a rise in haemoglobin and platelets. Prednisolone should be used in the knowledge that prolonged administration is particularly hazardous

Table 3 Revised classification of CLL integrated with the Rai system

Clinical Stage A	No anaemia or thrombocytopenia and less than three areas of lymphoid enlargement A(0), A(I), A(II)
Clinical Stage B	No anaemia or thrombocytopenia, with three or more involved areas B(I) or B(II)
Clinical Stage C	Anaemia and/or thrombocytopenia regardless of the number of areas of lymphoid enlargement C(III) or C(IV)

in the elderly immunosuppressed patient, and should be tailed off and discontinued if possible within six to eight weeks. If the steroids have produced a good response, chlorambucil may be added to the treatment at a stage when normal marrow is regenerating.

The complications of autoimmune haemolytic anaemia and immune thrombocytopenia may respond to steroid treatment. If, however, they can be controlled only by continuing the steroid treatment for an unduly long time, splenectomy should be considered if the patient's general condition permits. It may be completely effective in controlling the symptoms and may avoid the need for alternative hazardous treatment. Splenectomy may also be useful in the treatment of patients in whom gross splenomegaly is a dominant feature.

Radiotherapy has an important place in the treatment of CLL, and may help to control localized lymphadenopathy which has not responded to chemotherapy. Local splenic irradiation may also be effective in controlling the disease, especially when splenomegaly is significant. Fractionated low-dose total body irradiation (TBI) has also been used in active CLL, sometimes with good effect, but this has not been widely adopted.

As in the management of all malignant blood conditions, supportive treatment makes a considerable contribution to the care of the patient. Anaemia and thrombocytopenia may need to be treated by red cell and platelet transfusion respectively, particularly in the stage of marrow failure.

One of the most important aspects, however, is the management of intercurrent infections to which these patients are particularly prone. Recurrent chest infections are often a feature and should be treated seriously. The possibility of infection with pneumococci, legionella or opportunistic organisms such as *Pneumocystis carinii* should always be borne in mind.

Viral and fungal infections are particularly dangerous. Herpes zoster is common and unfortunately is not always taken seriously. It may rapidly become generalized and secondarily infected, and should be treated promptly with intravenous acyclovir.

The use of intramuscular immunoglobulin for prophylaxis has unfortunately proved disappointing. Newer, concentrated immunoglobulin preparations suitable for intravenous use are currently under trial, but it remains to be seen whether they will effectively prevent infection in severely hypogammaglobulinaemic patients.

Causes of death

Infection is a major cause of death. Other causes are haemorrhage, progressive resistance to treatment, marrow failure, and other malignancy.

An association between CLL and other tumours has been repeatedly noted; particularly skin tumours and carcinomas of the lung and colon. Figures differ in different series but possibly up to 20 per cent of patients with CLL have another malignancy. The diagnosis of carcinoma often precedes that of the CLL and chemotherapy for the leukaemia cannot be implicated in the aetiology of the cancer. Possibly the increased lack of immune surveillance in the CLL patients renders them particularly susceptible to develop carcinoma.

'Hairy cell' leukaemia (HCL)

This condition was formerly called *leukaemic reticuloendotheliosis* and was thought to be due to a malignant proliferation of histiocytic cells. More recent studies have shown that the abnormal cells are usually of B cell origin, and the conditions should therefore be regarded as more closely allied to CLL.

Clinical features

The condition is commoner in males (M:F, 4:1) and most of the patients are aged between 40 and 50 years. Symptoms are those of general debility, a tendency to recurrent infections, and abdomi-

nal discomfort associated with splenomegaly, which is present in the majority and which is often gross. Hepatomegaly may be present, but there is usually little or no lymph node enlargement. Osteolytic bone lesions occur in some patients.

Haematological features

There is usually pancytopenia with a haemoglobin of less than 10.0 g/dl, a low total leukocyte count and moderate thrombocytopenia although the platelets are seldom low enough to produce haemorrhagic symptoms.

The pancytopenia is due to a combination of hypersplenism and bone marrow infiltration or fibrosis. Isotope studies show that the splenic red cell pool is much higher than in other conditions with a similar degree of splenomegaly. This relates to the particular splenic histology in HCL, with dilated cords of red pulp and the formation of pseudosinuses.

Examination of the blood film shows a preponderance of lymphoid cells with the typical 'hairy' appearance, i.e. cells 10–20 μm in diameter with oval or slightly folded nuclei and a mottled cytoplasm showing irregular spiky protrusions. The majority of the hairy cells are PAS positive and stain for acid phosphatase which is typically tartrate resistant.

The bone marrow is often hypocellular and difficult to aspirate so that a trephine biopsy may be necessary. The difficulty in aspiration is due to an increase in reticulin. The marrow is generally infiltrated with cells of similar appearance to those in the blood. In some patients pancytopenia occurs with little or no splenomegaly suggesting that their disease is principally confined to the marrow.

Immunology

In contrast to ordinary CLL, immunoglobulin deficiency is not usually a feature. A paraprotein has been noted in some cases, sometimes in association with osteolytic lesions.

Clinical course and treatment

The results of chemotherapy in this type of lymphoproliferation are disappointing and the treatment of choice for patients with marked enlargement of the spleen is splenectomy. Many patients treated by splenectomy survive for years with no further treatment whereas the prognosis in those not operated upon may be only one or two years.

Recently, significant responses have been reported following administration of alpha-interferon, either leukocyte derived or the recombinant DNA variety. This has been administered intramuscularly or subcutaneously in doses of around 3 million units a day for several weeks. Regression of splenomegaly and improvement of peripheral blood picture has been achieved, and in some instances the response has been sustained after withdrawal of therapy. The exact role of interferon has yet to be defined, but it appears to be particularly useful in patients with little or no splenomegaly (who may respond poorly to splenectomy) or in those in whom splenectomy may be contraindicated.

Prolymphocytic leukaemia (PLL)

This rare condition is generally considered as a variant of CLL although the immunological characteristics of the malignant cell are somewhat different.

Clinical features

PLL affects patients predominantly in the seventh decade of life and is twice as common in males as females. The dominant clinical feature is gross splenomegaly (and to a lesser extent, hepatomegaly) and patients may present with symptoms relating to the spleen or with marked constitutional symptoms such as malaise, weight loss, sweats and fever. There is usually little or no lymphadenopathy although this and skin nodules are sometimes present in patients with the T cell variety (see below).

Haematological findings

Anaemia is usually quite marked and the total white cell count is very high (usually $100-1000 \times 10^9/l$) with a high percentage of abnormal lymphoid cells. The platelets may be moderately reduced but severe thrombocytopenia is unusual. The blood film shows a preponderance of large lymphoid cells with rather more cytoplasm than is usual in the cells of classical CLL. There are often well-marked vesicular nucleoli, and the cytoplasm tends to be somewhat basophilic. The bone marrow shows infiltration with similar cells.

Immunology

Immunological studies suggest than in most of these patients the cells have B cell characteristics. Despite the term 'prolymphocytic', these cells have a higher density of membrane immunoglobulin, and are immunologically more mature than the lymphocytes of classical CLL. Normal immunoglobulin production may be depressed and in some patients a paraprotein may be found.

In about 20 per cent of cases the cells have a T cell phenotype; two-thirds of these have a helper phenotype (OKT4+) and one-third a suppressor phenotype (OKT8+).

Clinical course and treatment

In general patients with PLL fare far less well than those with CLL at every stage of the disease. PLL tends always to be progressive and an indolent phase is not seen. The disease is especially rapidly progressive in the T cell variety.

Treatment of PLL is difficult. Response to chemotherapy is usually poor, but useful responses may sometimes be obtained with an aggressive protocol such as CHOP. One must remember, however, that these patients are often frail and elderly, and may not tolerate such a regime. Splenectomy may be useful, especially when local symptoms or hypersplenism are prominent but is not without its risks at this age. Splenic irradiation is worth considering and may be a useful alternative.

References

Chronic granulocytic leukaemia

Champling, R. E. and Golde, D. W. (1985). Chronic myelogenous leukaemia: recent advances. *Blood* **65**, 1039–1047.

Gale, R. P. and Cannani, E. (1985). The molecular biology of chronic myelogenous leukaemia. *Br. J. Haematol.* **60**, 395–408.

Galton, D. A. G. (1982). The chronic leukaemias. In *Blood and its disorders* 2nd edn (eds R. M. Hardisty and D. J. Weatherall), pp. 877–917. Blackwell Scientific Publications, Oxford.

Hardisty, R. M., Speed, D. E. and Till, M. (1964). Granulocytic leukaemia in childhood. *Br. J. Haematol.* **10**, 551–566.

Marcus, R. E. and Goldman, J. M. (1986). Autografting in chronic granulocytic anaemia. *Sem. Hematol.* **15**, 235–248.

Chronic lymphocytic leukaemia

Brouet, J-L., Flandrin, G., Sasportes, M., Preud'Homme, J-L. and Seligman, M. (1975). Chronic lymphocytic leukaemia of T-cell origin. Immunological and clinical evaluation in eleven patients. *Lancet* **ii**, 890–893.

Catovsky, D. (1983). Prolymphocytic and hairy cell leukemias. In *Leukemia* 4th edn (eds F. W. Gunz and E. S. Henderson), pp. 759–781. Grune and Stratton, New York.

——, Linch, D. C. and Beverley, P. C. L. (1982). T cell disorders in haematological diseases. *Clin. Haematol.* **11**, 661–695.

——, Pettit, J. E., Galton, D. A. G., Spiers, A. S. D. and Harrison, C. V. (1974). Leukaemic reticuloendotheliosis ('hairy' cell leukaemia): a distinct clinico-pathological entity. *Br. J. Haematol.* **26**, 9–27.

Galton, D. A. G. (1982). The chronic leukaemias. In *Blood and its disorders* 2nd edn (eds R. M. Hardisty and D. J. Weatherall), pp. 877–917. Blackwell Scientific Publications, Oxford.

——, Goldman, J. M., Wiltshaw, E., Catovsky, D., Henry, K. and Goldenberg, G. J. (1974). Prolymphocytic leukaemia. *Br. J. Haematol.* **27**, 7–23.

Han, T., Ozer, H., Sadamori, N., Emrich, L., Gomez, G. A., Henderson, E. S., Bloom, M. L. and Sandberg, A. A. (1984). Prognostic importance of cytogenetic abnormalities in patients with chronic lymphocytic leukemia. *N. Engl. J. Med.* **310**, 288–292.

Janssen, J. T. P., De Pauw, B. E. and Holdrinet, R. S. G. (1984). Treatment of hairy-cell leukaemia with recombinant α_2-interferon. *Lancet* **i**, 1025–1026.

Quesada, J. R., Reuben, J., Manning, J. T., Hersh, E. M. and Gutterman, J. U. (1984). Alpha interferon for induction of remission in hairy-cell leukemia. *N. Engl. J. Med.* **310**, 15–18.

Rai, K. R., Sawitsky, A., Cronkite, E. P., Chanana, A. D., Levy, R. N. and Pasternack, B. S. (1975). Clinical staging of chronic lymphocytic leukemia. *Blood* **46**, 219–234.

Sonnier, J. A., Buchanan, G. R., Howard-Peebles, P. N., Rutledge, J. and Graham Smith, R. (1983). Chromosomal translocation involving the immunoglobulin kappa-chain and heavy-chain loci in a child with chronic lymphocytic leukemia. *N. Engl. J. Med.* **309**, 590–594.

General

Brodeur, G. M. (1986). Molecular correlates of cytogenetic abnormalities in human cancer cells: implications for oncogene activation. *Prog. Hematol.* **14**, 229–256.

Franchini, G. and Gallo, R. C. (1985). Viruses, *onc* genes and leukaemia. In *Recent advances in haematology* 4th edn (ed. A. V. Hoffbrand), pp. 221–238. Churchill Livingstone, Edinburgh.

Franks, L. M. and Teich, N. (eds) (1986). *Introduction to the cellular and molecular biology of cancer.* Oxford University Press, Oxford.

Gunz, F. W. and Henderson, E. S. (eds) (1983). *Leukemia* 4th edn. Grune and Stratton, New York.

Rowley, J. D. and Ultmann, J. E. (eds) (1983). *Chromosomes and cancer. From molecules to man.* Academic Press, New York.

Acute leukaemia

Chessels, J. M. (1982). The acute leukaemias. In *Blood and its disorders* 2nd edn (eds R. M. Hardisty and D. J. Weatherall), pp. 829–875. Blackwell Scientific Publications, Oxford.

—— (1985). Risks and benefits of intensive treatment of acute leukaemia. *Arch. Dis. Child.* **60**, 193–195.

Jacobs, A. D. and Gale, R. P. (1984). Recent advances in the biology and treatment of acute lymphoblastic leukemia in adults. *New. Engl. J. Med.* **311**, 1219–1232.

Johnson, F. L. and Thomas, E. D. (1984). Treatment of relapsed acute lymphoblastic leukemia in childhood. *New Engl. J. Med.* **310**, 263.

Kay, H. E. M. (1982). The leukaemias: pathogenesis and classification. In *Blood and its disorders*, 2nd edn (eds R. M. Hardisty and D. J. Weatherall), pp. 799–828. Blackwell Scientific Publications, Oxford.

Leukens, J. N. and Miles, M. R. (1970). Childhood leukemia: meeting the needs of patient and family. *Missouri Med.* **67**, 236–241.

Mauer, A. M. (1986). New directions in the treatment of acute lymphoblastic anemia of childhood. *New Engl. J. Med.* **315**, 316–317.

Priest, J. R., Robinson, L. L., McKenna, R. W., Lindquist, L. L., Warkentin, P. I., LeBien, T. W., Woods, W. G., Kersey, J. H., Coccia, P. F. and Nesbitt, M. E. Jr (1980). Philadelphia chromosome positive childhood acute lymphoblastic leukemia. *Blood* **56**, 15–22.

Report on behalf of the Medical Research Council's Working Party on Leukaemia in Childhood (1978). Testicular disease in acute lymphoblastic leukaemia in childhood. *Br. Med. J.* **i**, 334–338.

Rifkind, R. A. (1986). Acute leukemia and cell differentiation. *New Engl. J. Med.* **315**, 56–57.

Secker-Walker, L. M. (1984). The prognostic implications of chromosomal findings in acute lymphoblastic leukemia. *Can. Genet. Cytogenet.* **11**, 233–248.

Shalet, S. M. Hann, I. M., Lendon, M., Morris Jones, P. H. and Beardwell, C. G. (1981). Testicular function after combination chemotherapy in childhood for acute lymphoblastic leukaemia. *Arch. Dis. Child.* **56**, 275–278.

Sieff, C. A., Chessels, J. M., Harvey, B. A. M., Pickthall, V. J. and Lawler, S. D. (1981). Monosomy 7 in childhood: a myeloproliferative disorder. *Br. J. Haematol.* **49**, 235–249.

Whitehouse, J. M. A. and Kay, H. E. M. (eds) (1979). *CNS complications of malignant disease.* Macmillan, London.

Whittaker, J. A., Reizenstein, P., Callender, S. T., Cornwell, G. G., Delamore, I. W., Cale, R. P., Gobbi, M., Jacobs, P., Lantz, B., Maiolo, A. T., Rees, J. K. H., Van Slyck, E. J. and Vu Van, H. (1981). Long survival in acute myelogenous leukaemia: an international collaborative study. *Br. Med. J.* **282**, 692–695.

Polycythaemia vera

D. J. WEATHERALL

The term 'polycythaemia' is used to describe an increased red cell count, packed cell volume or haemoglobin level. In his early descriptions of the disease William Osler realized that there are two main types of what he called 'polyglobulism': (a) relative, in which there is a reduction in plasma volume with a normal red cell mass; and (b) true, in which there is a genuine increase in the red cell mass. It is now more usual to call these conditions relative and absolute polycythaemia. The absolute polycythaemias are divided into primary polycythaemia or polycythaemia rubra vera, usually shortened to polycythaemia vera (PV), which is a myeloproliferative disorder of unknown aetiology, and the secondary polycythaemias, which result from a variety of different pathological mechanisms.

Here we shall consider polycythaemia vera since there is good evidence that this condition results from the neoplastic proliferation of a multipotent haematopoietic progenitor cell. The relative and secondary polycythaemias, and the differential diagnosis of an increased haemoglobin level, are considered in a later chapter (page 19.152).

Aetiology

PV results from abnormal proliferation of red cell precursors derived from a single haemopoietic progenitor cell with the capacity for differentiation down red cell, white cell, and platelet lines. Evidence for this comes from studies of the red cell enzymes of African females with the disorder who are also heterozygous for the A and B glucose-6-phosphate dehydrogenase (G6PD) variants (see page 19.13). In excess of 90 per cent of their red blood cells carry only one G6PD-type, either A or B, whereas in other tissues a more or less equal number of cells containing A or B type enzymes are found. The lymphocytes do not appear to be involved in this abnormal proliferative process. Thus the basic mechanism of PV is a change in the genetic constitution of a single multipotent haemopoietic progenitor so that its progeny proliferate independent of the normal control mechanisms involved in haemopoiesis. It has been suggested that some of the abnormalities of the bone marrow in this condition, particularly the tendency to mysclerosis in the later stages of the illness, are the result of the production of growth factors, such as platelet-derived growth factor, by the abnormal megakaryocyte line

Erythropoietin levels are normal or low in the blood and urine of patients with PV and there is an appropriate rise after venesection. On in vitro culture, the red cell precursors from patients with this disorder show increased and prolonged unstimulated erythropoiesis and an unusual dose response curve to erythropoietin. These studies suggest that PV is not due to a primary abnormality of erythropoietin metabolism, because as the red cell mass increases the normal feedback reduction of erythropoietin output occurs. Thus it appears that the basic defect in PV is a proliferation of precursors which behave quite independently of the normal erythropoietin regulation system. Whether this is because they have an altered receptor state for the hormone remains to be determined. What is clear is that the abnormal clone of erythroid progenitors has the capacity to proliferate preferentially as compared with its normal counterparts.

There is a considerable incidence of acute leukaemic transformation in patients with PV. Many of them develop chromosomal abnormalities during the course of their illness, suggesting that the primary mutational event in the stem cell makes it more likely that unstable cell lines will develop with a tendency to leukaemic transformation. In this sense PV can be looked upon as a preleukaemic condition (see page 19.58). Indeed, the natural history of the disorder bears a strong resemblance to that of chronic myeloid leukaemia (see page 19.29).

Haemodynamics and oxygen transport

When measured in vitro, the viscosity of blood increases exponentially with an increasing packed cell volume. When the rate of flow is measured as a reciprocal of the viscosity at varying packed cell volume levels, it decreases in a linear function with an increasing packed cell volume. If the flow rate is multiplied by the oxygen content of the blood, the product provides a measure of the rate of oxygen transport at different packed cell volumes. Optimum oxygen transport occurs at packed cell volumes of between 40 and 50 per cent. If no compensatory mechanisms occurred, there would be a reduced rate of oxygen transport even with a moderate increase in the packed cell volume. In fact, even at relatively high packed cell volumes, oxygen transport is adequate because there is an increase in the total blood volume, particularly in the plasma volume, and an increased cardiac output together with an enlargement of the peripheral vascular bed leading to a fall in peripheral resistance. Indeed, at a packed cell volume of 60 per cent there may be some increase in oxygen delivery. As pointed out many years ago by William Castle, hyervolaemia per se increases oxygen transport because the increased blood oxygen content and cardiac output more than compensate for the increased viscosity of the blood. Unfortunately, however, PV is a disease of middle and old age and is frequently associated with cardiovascular disorders such as hypertension and coronary artery and cerebrovascular disease. Hence, these compensatory mechanisms tend to break down, and this is particularly likely to occur at packed cell volumes in excess of 60–65 per cent, at which level there may be a marked increase in the workload on both left and right sides of the heart because of the high viscosity in the systemic and pulmonary circulations. In addition there may be a marked reduction in the cerebral blood flow at high PCV levels, and this, together with associated cerebro-vascular disease and a high platelet count, makes the cerebral circulation particularly vunerable to occlusive episodes (see page 19.154).

While many of the complications of PV are related to the haemodynamic changes secondary to increased blood viscosity, there is the added factor of the abnormal function of the aberrant cell line. Thrombotic episodes probably result from reduced flow of thick, viscous blood together with the high platelet count that commonly accompanies the discorder. Damage to the intestinal mucosa following thrombotic episodes may account for the high incidence of mucosal ulceration. The abnormal platelets of PV and primary thrombocythaemia (see page 19.44) are able to produce microvascular changes which are distinct from the large-vessel thromboses characteristic of PV. There is also defective haemostasis, probably due to abnormal platelet function. The platelets do not aggregate in response to adrenaline or collagen, and show a reduced response to the aggregation inhibitor, PGD_2. Hence, PV is characterized by the bizarre association of both thrombotic and bleeding tendencies in the same individual, associated with cardiovascular complications consequent on increased cardiac work resulting from an increased blood viscosity. The effects of the latter depend on a complicated series of factors which include variability of shear rates in different vessels, the state of the vessel wall, the level of the PCV, and cardiovascular function.

Symptoms

The disorder sometimes starts insidiously. On the other hand, patients may first present with an acute, dramatic complication such as a cerebrovascular accident or major thrombotic episode.

Presenting symptoms may involve almost any organ system. Non-specific complaints, probably related to circulatory disturbances in the nervous system, are most common and include headache, dizziness, vertigo, tinnitus, and visual disturbances including blurring and diplopia. There may be a cardiovascular presentation with angina, intermittent claudication, or recurrent venous thrombosis or embolic disease. Other symptoms include an increased bruising tendency or more severe bleeding in the form of epistaxis or gastrointestinal haemorrhage, and abdominal pain due to a peptic ulceration or splenomegaly. The condition may be first recognized during the course of investigation for gout.

A particularly common symptom is severe and intractable pruritus. This has a very characterisitc relationship to warmth and frequently occurs after getting into bed at night or bathing. Some patients present with a burning sensation in the feet or toes. This may be associated with vascular lesions which cause small areas of gangrene on the tips of the toes, similar to those which occur in primary thrombocythaemia (see page 19.44).

Physical findings

Many patients with PV are plethoric and show a cyanotic tinge to the nose, ears, and lips. Typically there is injection of the conjuctivae and a flush over the neck and upper half of the trunk. At least 75 per cent of patients with PV have splenomegaly sometime during their illness. The size of the spleen varies greatly and in some cases a straight abdominal X-ray or an isotope scan may be necessary to demonstrate that it is enlarged. A moderate degree of hepatomegaly is present in about one-third to one-half of patients. Although arterial hypertension has been thought to be a common accompaniment of PV, it is difficult to be sure about this because PV occurs at an age when hypertension is extremely common in the population and it is far from clear whether the association is real.

Neurological examination is normal unless there has been a cerebrovascular accident, although some patients have engorged retinal veins at presentation.

Haematological changes

Typically there is an increase in the haemoglobin and packed cell volume levels; the latter may range from 50 to more than 70 per cent. These findings are associated with an absolute increase in the red cell mass. In the majority of patients there is an elevation of either the white cell or platelet count, or both. Bone marrow examination shows an active marrow, but erythropoiesis is normoblastic and there are no diagnostic features. A variety of abnormalities of platelet function have been demonstrated (see pages 19.37 and 19.44). The changes in splenic function in PV are considered on page 19.193).

There are several other laboratory findings which help in making the diagnosis of PV. Many patients are hyperuricaemic, and secondary gout is quite common. The arterial oxygen saturation is usually normal although, interestingly, mild degrees of unsaturation may occur occasionally in patients with otherwise well-documented PV. The leucocyte alkaline phosphatase (LAP) is usually increased, which helps to distinguish cases with very high white cell counts from chronic myeloid leukaemia in which it is reduced. The serum vitamin B_{12} content and the capacity of the serum to bind vitamin B_{12} is often markedly increased. There has been considerable interest in the last few years in the cytogenetic changes in PV. It is still not absolutely certain whether they are related to therapy, but there is increasing evidence that even patients who have not received radioactive phosphorus or cytotoxic drugs have an increased incidence of chromosomal abnormalities. These include aneuploidy and the presence of an extra C group chromosome. The chromosomal changes are more marked in those patients who develop marrow failure or leukaemia; occasionally the Philadelphia chromosome may appear during an acute leukaemic transformation.

Differential diagnosis

Usually there is little difficulty in diagnosing PV. The finding of an increased haemoglobin level and packed cell volume, an increased red cell mass, splenomegaly and an associated elevation in the

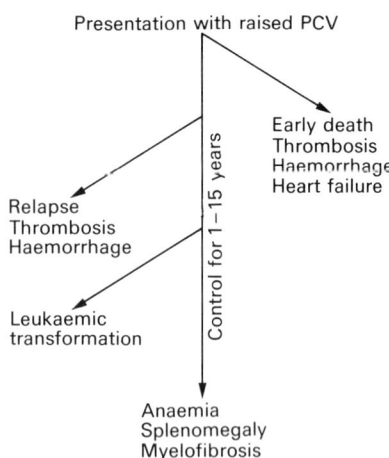

Fig. 1 Schematic representation of the natural history of polycythaemia vera.

white cell and/or platelet count is diagnostic. Provided that an absolute polycythaemia has been demonstrated by red cell mass estimation, the only difficulty is ruling out the various causes of secondary polycythaemia; this problem is considered in a later section (page 19.153).

Occasionally, difficulty is encountered in patients with what is apparently PV but in whom the spleen is not enlarged and the white cell and platelet counts are not elevated. Certainly, there is a small group of patients with persistently elevated red cell masses in whom there is no other abnormality consistent with the diagnosis of PV and in whom no cause for secondary polycythaemia can be found. These individuals should be followed carefully and their polycythaemia managed by venesection. In the author's experience some of them have developed the typical features of PV after several months or years, while in others a cause of secondary polycythaemia such as a tumour has shown itself after an equally long period. This problem is discussed further on page 19.152.

Course and prognosis

It is extremely difficult to give an accurate prognosis in this disorder. It appears that younger patients survive longer and that the prognosis for those who present with a major complication at the onset is considerably worse than those who present with minimal symptoms. There is still controversy about the relationship between different forms of therapy and prognosis (see below). Survival times range from months up to 15 or 20 years, and several series of patients treated with radioactive phosphorus have given median survival times of approximately 8 to 12 years. Unless there are major complications at the onset it is possible to give a reasonably good prognosis for this disorder.

During the course of the illness (Fig. 1) there may be vascular or thrombotic complications, particularly if the packed cell volume is allowed to remain in excess of 55 per cent or more; a very high platelet count is also associated with an increased incidence of thrombotic and haemorrhagic complications. Any blood vessel may be involved; the portal veins, fundal veins, cerebral circulation, and digital vessels of the hands and feet are often involved. In many of those patients who do not die of vascular complications, the polycythaemia gradually 'burns out' and is replaced by anaemia, massive splenomegaly, and progressive fibrosis of the bone marrow. At this stage the illness is indistinguishable from primary myelosclerosis (see page 19.40).

The other form of termination of PV is acute leukaemia. It is very difficult to obtain accurate figures for this complication, and in several large series collected from the literature the incidence ranges from 0 to 30 per cent of cases. It is possible, although not certain, that leukaemic transformation is more likely to occur in patients who have received some form of radiation therapy. Recent evidence suggests that chlorambucil therapy is associated with a significant increase in the number of cases of acute leukaemia. Leukaemic transformation is characterized by a sudden decline in general health, anaemia, thrombocytopenia, and the presence of variable numbers of primitive white cell precursors in the peripheral blood and bone marrow.

Management

The correct approach to the management of PV has been, and indeed still is, very controversial. There are several large-scale international and national trials under way to attempt to define the best way to control this condition; but because of its long course it will be many years before the answers are available. However, certain principles are clear.

Currently, PV is not curable and hence the objectives of management are to maintain well-being and to diminish the likelihood of complications for as long as possible. This is achieved by reducing dangerously high packed cell volumes into a safer range by venesection and then by maintaining this level, either by regular venesection or the use of myelosuppressive agents, or both. At the same time an attempt is made to maintain the platelet count at a safe level and to control other complications such as hyperuricaemia and secondary folate deficiency with appropriate drugs.

Since patients with high packed cell volumes are at great risk of thrombotic episodes it is important to initiate a venesection regime as soon as the diagnosis is clear. It is usually possible to remove 350–500 ml of blood every other day until the PCV is reduced to the normal range. In older patients who find venesection distressing, smaller quantities of blood, in the 200–300 ml range, may be removed. In emergencies, pre-operatively for example, more blood may be removed and replaced by an equal volume of plasma.

Once a normal PCV has been attained maintenance therapy should be started. In young patients in whom the platelet count is not dangerously high, it is better to try to maintain the PCV at a normal level by regular venesection. As mentioned earlier, it is important to keep the PCV below 50 per cent, and ideally below 45 per cent. After a while changes of iron deficiency will be observed. This does not matter, although some patients complain of glossitis, asthenia, and other symptoms which have been ascribed to iron deficiency. Thus it is customary to treat these patients with iron although this probably increases the frequency with which venesection is required.

In older patients who cannot tolerate regular venesection, or in younger patients in whom there is a very high platelet count, myelosuppressive therapy is indicated. The type of myelosuppressive treatment has been a major controversy for many years, mainly because of the fear that use of these agents might provoke leukaemic transformation. This is the basis for several clinical trials to assess the best way of treating PV. So far, the most important information has come from the Polycythaemia Vera Study Group. Their prospective randomized trial set out to compare treatment with venesection alone with the use of an alkylating agent (chlorambucil) supplemented by venesection, or ^{32}P supplemented by venesection. After 14 years there was no significant difference in survival between the various groups. However, the causes of death were stongly influenced by therapy (Fig. 2). The risk of acute leukaemia among patients treated with chlorambucil was 13.5 times greater than that among patients treated with ^{32}P. As mentioned elsewhere in this section, the leukaemogenic potential of alkylating agents is now well established from information about patients treated with these conditions for other disorders. However, another trial has suggested that busulphan given intermittently is less leukaemogenic, suggesting that leukaemic transformation may be dependent on both the alkylating agent employed and its mode of administration.

So which form of myelosuppressive therapy should be used in PV, given our current state of ignorance? In older patients it

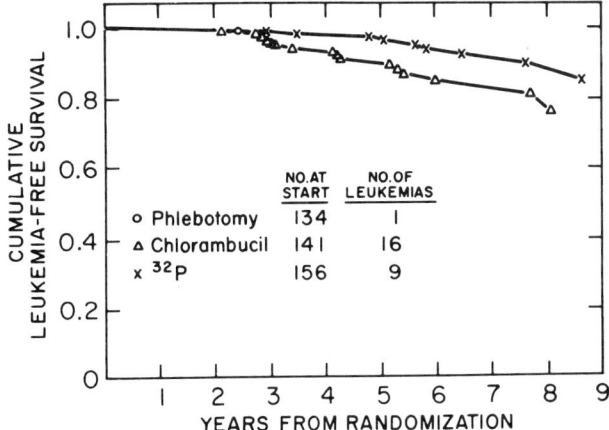

Fig. 2 Cumulative leukaemia-free survival of patients with polycythaemia vera following randomization to chlorambucil, phlebotomy or ^{32}P therapy. The difference in the risk of developing leukaemia between the chlorambucil group and the other two is significant. (Reproduced from Berk et al., 1981, with permission.)

seems reasonable to use ^{32}P. Following venesection to a normal PCV, a dose of ^{32}P, 3–5 mCi (2.3 mCi/m^2), should be given intravenously. Sometimes a second, smaller dose, 2–3 mCi ^{32}P, is required three to four months after the initial injection in order to bring the disease under complete control. The condition then often remains quiescent for months or even years. It is most unusual to produce severe marrow hypoplasia with this regime. In younger patients intermittent busulphan or hydroxyurea can be used. Busulphan should be given at a dose of 4–6 mg daily until the platelet count is approaching normal, at which time the dose should be reduced to 2 mg daily until a normal platelet count has been achieved. The drug should then be stopped and the patient carefully followed with regular blood counts. The count may remain under control for months or even years after a single course of busulphan although usually intermittent courses with gaps of several months in between are required. Hydroxyurea is also useful as a myelosuppressive agent. It should be started at a dose of 500 mg to 1 g daily and the dose tapered down as control is achieved. It is a very valuable drug for achieving rapid control of the platelet count. A recent report of the Polycythemia Vera Study Group suggests that hydroxyurea is probably now the drug of choice for myelosuppression in this condition.

A variety of agents have been reported to improve the pruritus of PV, none of which has been uniformly successful. This distressing symptom seems to respond best to myelosuppressive treatment. Additional relief may be obtained from the use of H$_1$ or H$_2$ histamine blockers. Suitable regimes are cyproheptadine 4 mg orally three times a day or cimetidine 300 mg orally three times a day, either alone or in combination. Hyperuricaemia should be managed with a xanthineoxidase inhibitor; allopurinol starting with 100 mg daily and gradually increasing until the uric acid level is controlled is an appropriate regime.

In the later, 'burnt out' stages of the illness, when there is massive splenomegaly and myelofibrosis, the management is similar to that for primary myelosclerosis (page 19.42). It consists of blood transfusion, iron and folate replacement, and, occasionally, splenectomy if there is gross hypersplenism. In patients who develop an acute leukaemic transformation the management is as described for acute leukaemia (page 19.26); acute leukaemia superimposed on PV is usually very refractory to treatment.

References

Adamson. J. W., Fialkow, P. J., Murphy, S., Prchal, J. F. and Steinmanm, L. (1976). Polycythemia vera: stem-cell and probable clonal origin of the disease. *N. Engl. J. Med.* **295**, 913–916.

Berk, P. D., Goldberg, J. D., Silverstein, M. N., Weinfeld, A., Donovan,

P. B., Ellis, J. T. Laszlo, J., Najean, Y., Pisciotta, A. V. and Wasserman, L. R. (1981). Increased incidence of acute leukemia in polycythemia vera associated with chlorambucil therapy. *N. Engl. J. Med.* **304**, 441–444.

Brodsky, I. (1982). Busulphan treatment of polycythaemia vera. *Br. J. Haematol.* **52**, 1–3.

Castle, W. B. and Jandl, J. H. (1966). Blood viscosity and blood volume: Opposing influences upon oxygen transport in polycythaemia. *Sem. Hematol.* **3**, 193–198.

Ellis, J. T. and Peterson, P. (1979). The bone marrow in polycythemia vera. *Pathol. Ann.* **14**, 383.

Goldberg, J. D., Donovan, P. B., Fructman, S. M., Berlin, N. I. and Wasserman, L. R. (1986). Therapeutic recommendations in polycythemia vera based on Polycythemia Vera Study Group protocols. *Sem. Hematol.* **23**, 132–143.

Murphy, S. (1983). Polycythaemia vera. In *Hematology*, 3rd edn (ed. W. J. Williams, E. Beutler, A. J. Erslev and M. A. Lichtman), pp. 185–195. McGraw-Hill, New York.

Loeb, V. (1975). Treatment of polycythaemia vera. *Clin. Haematol.* **4**, 441–448.

Modan, B. (1965). An epidemiological study of polycythemia vera. *Blood* **26**, 657–667.

Modan, B. (1975). Interrelationship between polycythaemia vera, leukaemia and myeloid metaplasia. *Clin. Haematol.* **4**, 427–440.

Pearson, T. C., and Guthrie, D. L. (1984). The interpretation of measured red cell mass and plasma volume in patients with elevated PC values. *Clin. Lab. Haematol.* **6**, 207–217.

Wetherley-Mein, G. and Pearson, T. C. (1982). Myeloproliferative disorders. In *Blood and its disorders*, 2nd edn (eds R. M. Hardisty and D. J. Weatherall), pp. 263–272. Blackwell Scientific Publications, Oxford.

Myelosclerosis

D. J. WEATHERALL

The term 'myelosclerosis' is used to describe progressive fibrous replacement of the bone marrow; it is used synonymously with *myelofibrosis*. The condition may be part of the myeloproliferative syndrome or may be secondary to the effects of other neoplastic disorders of the bone marrow, metabolic changes involving vitamin D or its metabolites, and a variety of other conditions which provoke a fibrous reaction by an unknown mechanism.

Primary myelosclerosis

Primary myelosclerosis is a myeloproliferative disorder characterized by anaemia and abnormal proliferation of haemopoietic precursors associated with a variable degree of fibrosis of the bone marrow and myeloid metaplasia in the spleen, liver, and other organs. This last characteristic is the reason why the condition has many alterative names, including *myeloid metaplasia, agnogenic myeloid metaplasia*, and *megakaryocytic splenomegaly*. Furthermore, the curious pathological association of myeloid metaplasia and progressive fibrosis of the marrow explains the extremely bizarre and variable clinical and haematological pictures which are associated with this interesting disorder.

Aetiology

The cause of myelosclerosis and myeloid metaplasia is unknown. It seems likely that the abnormal haemopoietic elements which constitute the myeloid metaplasia of the spleen, liver, and other organs result from the neoplastic proliferation of an abnormal stem cell population. Recent evidence in support of this notion has come from enzyme studies similar to those used to demonstrate the clonal origin of polycythaemia. Fibroblasts grown from bone marrows of females with primary myelosclerosis who are heterozygous for glucose-6-phosphate dehydrogenase types A and B show both forms of the enzyme, while platelets and other blood cells contain only one form. These findings suggest that the fibroblast proliferation occurs secondarily to the effects of abnormal proliferation of a clone of haemopoietic progenitor cells. Similar results have been obtained from cytogenetic analyses. It is currently believed that the fibrotic reaction results from the release of platelet-derived growth factor for fibroblasts, or related factors from the abnormal line of megakaryocytes.

The fibrous tissue in the bone marrow of patients with myelosclerosis is demonstrated with the silver stain for reticulin. This staining reaction highlights many proteins, but in the bone marrow identifies mainly collagen and fibronectin. Platelet-derived growth factor, as well as stimulating fibroblasts to proliferate, induces collagen synthesis. Myelofibrosis is a dynamic process and there are several collagenases released from monocytes and macrophages which may degrade the fibrous tissue.

During the evolution of myelosclerosis the two major pathological processes, progressive fibrosis of the bone marrow and myeloid metaplasia of the liver, spleen, and lymph-nodes, seem to occur simultaneously, although there is remarkable variability between patients in the rate and extent of these changes. The fibrosis of the marrow is extremely patchy and there may be areas of hyperplasia that can cause diagnostic difficulties. The hyperplasia involves all the precursor cells, particularly megakaryocytes. Indeed, megakaryocytic proliferation is a major feature of this disorder. Despite the existence of hyperplastic areas of the marrow, red cell production is diminished, and, while in the early stages of the illness there may be a raised white cell and platelet count, these tend to fall as fibrosis of the marrow progresses. Hence, a major factor in producing the clinical picture of myelosclerosis is progressive bone marrow failure. The second is hypersplenism due to increasing enlargement of the spleen. This process, and the associated hepatomcgaly, seems to be largely due to myeloid metaplasia. It is now considered that this extramedullary haematopoiesis is part of a neoplastic proliferation which characterizes myelosclerosis, but that it may also play a role in compensating for bone marrow failure; while possible, there is no definite evidence that this is the case. The mechanism by which the massively enlarged spleen causes worsening of the anaemia, hypervolaemia, thrombocytopenia, and neutropenia is described elsewhere in this section (see page 19.189).

Clinical features

The presenting symptoms in myelosclerosis are extremely variable. The disorder may first be recognized because an enlarged spleen is discovered accidentally by the patient or physician. Sometimes it is large enough to cause abdominal distension or a dragging sensation in the left upper quadrant. On the other hand, the first symptoms may be progressive anaemia, weight loss or general ill health, bone pain, or acute abdominal pain due to a splenic infarct. Some patients are first referred to dermatologists with pruritis which has the same distinctive relationship to warmth as occurs in polycythaemia vera. Occasionally, the early clinical picture reflects abnormal platelet function and there may be increased bruising, unexplained gastrointestinal blood loss, or bleeding after minor trauma (Fig. 1).

The only physical finding which is almost invariably present is splenomegaly. The spleen ranges in size from just palpable to massive, and this is one of the few disorders in which the patient may present for the first time with a spleen in the pelvis. There is usually some degree of hepatomegaly.

Finally, since about a third of patients with myelosclerosis have a patchy osteosclerosis, the condition may first be recognized by the finding of an unusual bone X-ray in a patient who is having a radiological examination for another cause.

Haematological changes

Anaemia is present in over two-thirds of all patients when they are first seen. In the early stage of the illness it may be quite mild but usually becomes more severe as the disorder progresses. The red cells are characteristically misshapen, with many tear-drop shaped forms, bizarre poikilocytes, and ovalocytes (Fig. 2). These changes are the real hallmark of myelosclerosis. Quite often there are nucleated red cells in the peripheral blood.

The white cell count is often elevated. The white cells consist mainly of mature neutrophils but there are usually some immature forms, metamyelocytes, myelocytes, or even a few myeloblasts

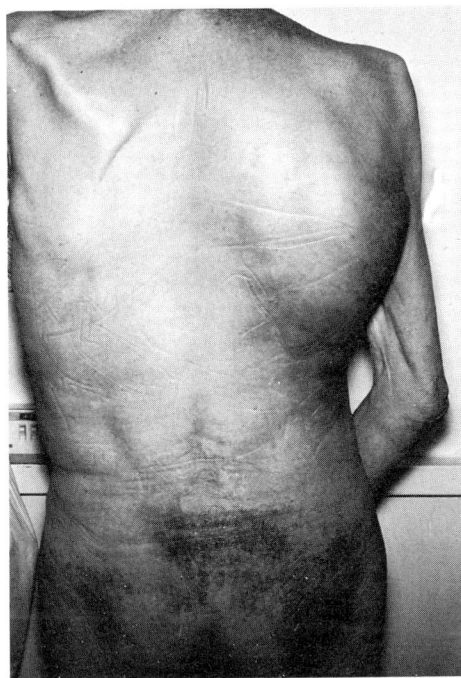

Fig. 1 A massive haematoma over the scapula region with tracking down in the tissue planes of the back in an 81-year-old patient with myelosclerosis and abnormal platelet function.

(Fig. 2). These changes, together with the presence of nucleated red cells, constitute a leucoerythroblastic reaction. The platelet count is variable. In the earlier stages of the illness there is quite often a moderate thrombocytosis. As the disease progresses and the spleen enlarges, the platelet count tends to fall and severe thrombocytopenia may be a troublesome feature in advanced myelosclerosis. The platelet morphology is abnormal; the changes are characterized by giant forms and occasional shreds of megakaryocyte cytoplasm in the peripheral blood (Fig. 2).

Bone marrow examination usually yields a 'dry' tap. However, it is always worthwhile looking carefully in the tail of such hypocellular preparations because there may be large platelet aggregates or scattered clumps of megakaryocytes which will give a clue to the diagnosis. A needle or open biopsy shows extensive fibrosis with islands of haemopoietic cells, and megakaryocytic hyperplasia. Because of the patchiness of the myelofibrotic process, it is possible to aspirate fragments of hypercellular marrow. Even in these cases, however, silver staining for reticulin will show a marked increase in fibre formation (Fig. 3). Although many cytogenetic abnormalities have been reported in this disorder, there are no specific chromosomal changes which are of diagnostic help.

Other laboratory findings

There is usually an elevated uric acid level. The neutrophil alkaline phosphatase is variable, and normal, high, or low levels may be found.

Abnormalities of haemostasis and coagulation are common. In addition to thrombocytopenia many patients show abnormal platelet aggregation in response to collagen and adrenalin. The prothrombin time may be prolonged, often as the result of a deficiency of factor V. In some patients there may be features of disseminated intravascular coagulation although, curiously, they do not have the marked bleeding tendency usually associated with these findings.

Splenic or lymph-node aspiration almost invariably shows myeloid metaplasia. However, any form of biopsy except of the bone marrow should be avoided in myelosclerotic patients because of their bleeding tendency.

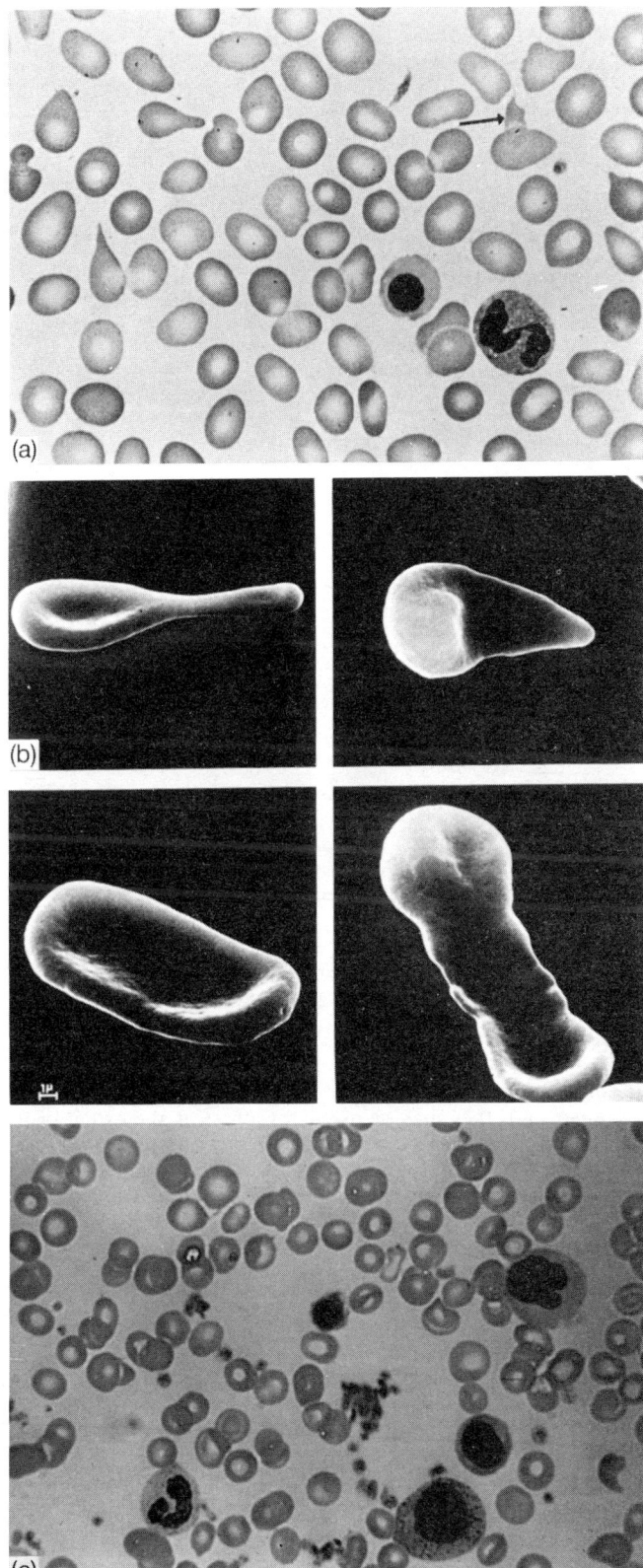

Fig. 2 Haematological changes in myelosclerosis. (a) A peripheral blood film showing tear drop cells, a nucleated red cell, and a grossly distorted cell marked by the arrow. (From Liebold, P. F. and Weed, R. I. (1975) *Clin. Haemat.* **4**, 353, with permission.) (b) A scanning electron microscope study showing characteristic poikilocytes. (From Liebold, P. F. and Weed, R. I. (1975). *Clin. Haemat.* **4**, 353, with permission.) (c) A leukoerythroblastic reaction in myelosclerosis showing young red cell precursors. Note, in addition, the abnormal platelet morphology and platelet clumps.

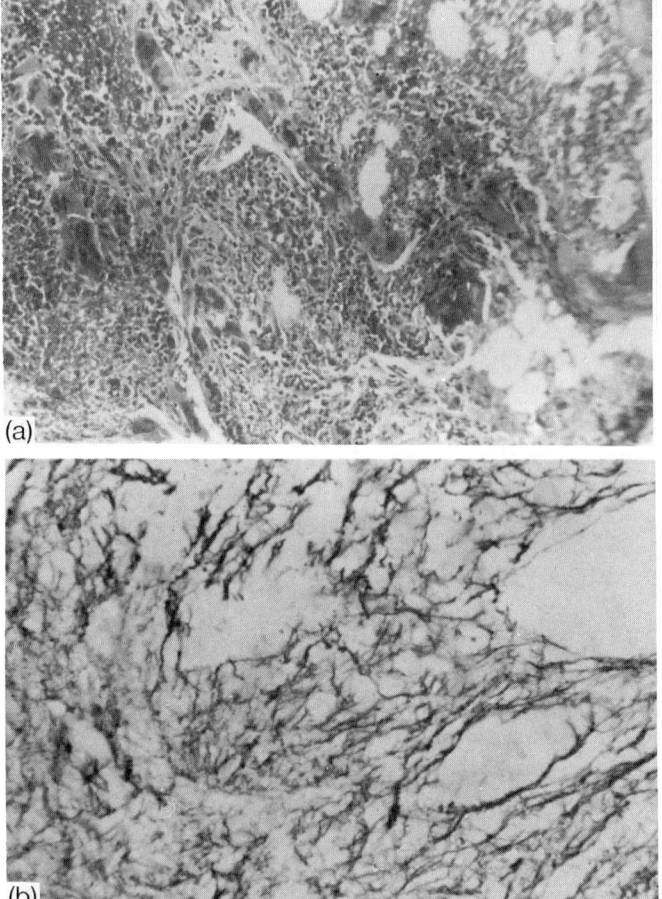

Fig. 3 Bone marrow appearances in myelosclerosis. (a) A biopsy showing a hyperplastic fragment with marked megakaryocytic hyperplasia. (b) A silver stain showing the marked increase in reticulin.

Ferrokinetic studies

Although it is rarely necessary to use iron kinetic studies for diagnostic purposes they may be useful for assessing the extent of the disease and the degree of effective splenic erythropoiesis, in cases in which splenectomy is being considered. This subject is considered in detail on page 19.191.

Differential diagnosis

The typical picture of myelosclerosis with a massive spleen and fibrosed bone marrow usually produces no diagnostic difficulty. However, in the earlier phases of the illness when myeloid metaplasia predominates and the peripheral blood shows a leucocytosis and thrombocytosis, it is easy to confuse the condition with chronic myeloid leukaemia. However, the bone marrow in the latter disorder shows a predominance of myelocytes and promyelocytes, the leucocyte alkaline phosphatase is low, and a Philadelphia chromosome is present. In addition, the disorder must be distinguished from the causes of secondary marrow fibrosis mentioned later in this section and from other causes of a leucoerythroblastic anaemia, especially secondary carcinoma, other myeloproliferative disorders, and disseminated tuberculosis.

Complications

The major complications of myelosclerosis relate to the massive splenomegaly. The development of progressive hypersplenism (see page 19.40) has already been mentioned. Splenic infarction (Fig. 4) with associated pain over the spleen or in the left shoulder tip is relatively common. Trauma to the large spleen may cause it to rupture, either into the abdominal cavity or with the production

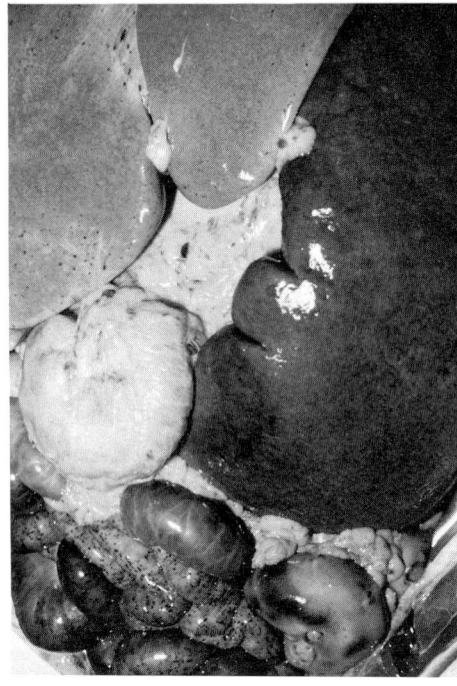

Fig. 4 Autopsy showing massive splenomegaly together with a splenic infarct on the medial surface of the spleen in a patient with advanced myelosclerosis.

of a perisplenic haematoma. Secondary gout is common. Because of the rapid turnover of the abnormal red cell precursors, secondary folate deficiency is also common and may cause a sudden worsening of the anaemia with a marked macrocytosis and the appearance of megaloblasts in the blood. Presumably because of abnormal platelet function or peptic ulceration, chronic gastrointestinal blood loss occurs and the anaemia of myelosclerosis may be made worse by co-existent iron deficiency. Serious bruising and haematoma formation may result from mild trauma (see Fig. 1).

There appears to be a genuine association between myelosclerosis and portal hypertension which may be accompanied by bleeding from oesophageal varices. The pathogenesis is not understood; presinusoidal obstruction due to infiltration of the hepatic sinusoids, portal or splenic vein thrombosis, and increased flow in the portal system have all been suggested.

Course and prognosis

The course of myelosclerosis is variable. Some patients retain a relatively normal haemoglobin level and have a minimal splenomegaly for many years. More commonly there is a gradual decline in the patient's general condition with a progressive worsening of the anaemia, and increasing splenomegaly which may reach enormous proportions. Although the median survival is usually given as approximately 5 years there is a very broad scatter and it is not at all uncommon for patients to live 10–20 years after myelosclerosis has been diagnosed. The usual cause of death is progressive anaemia which becomes refractory to blood transfusion, due at least in part to haemodilution caused by the massive spleen. Approximately 20 per cent of cases terminate in acute myeloblastic leukaemia. There is a sudden worsening of the anaemia and a marked increase in the number of blast cells in the peripheral blood.

Treatment

There is no definitive treatment for patients with myelosclerosis. They should be followed carefully and complications such as iron or folate deficiency corrected. If they become symptomatic due to progressive anaemia, they should be started on a blood transfusion programme, although particular care is required when transfusing patients with this disorder. Because of the high blood volume associated with hypersplenism, it is very easy to overload them and to precipitate acute pulmonary oedema. Although splenic irradiation and chemotherapy have been used in an attempt to reduce the size of the spleen, the results are equivocal. Local irradiation is usually ineffective in reducing its size but some benefit may be obtained from a judicious use of busulphan or hydroxyurea. The author favours the latter drug because of its fewer side-effects and the fact that it is easier to titrate the white cell and platelet counts than is the case with busulphan. It is wise to start with a low dose of hydroxyurea, 500 mg daily for example, and gradually to increase it keeping a careful watch on spleen size and white cell and platelet counts. Androgen therapy has been used to improve marrow function but the results are disappointing.

The place of splenectomy is controversial. It is argued that if the spleen is removed early on in the course of the illness, it may prevent the development of the problems of hypersplenism which occur as the disease progresses. Against this, however, is the fact that many patients with this disorder have many years of symptom-free life before the disease enters its terminal stage of massive splenomegaly. It is impossible to anticipate how long patients will take to develop symptoms referable to splenomegaly. Certainly when the spleen is large, surgery can be extremely hazardous. There are often multiple adhesions which make the operation technically difficult, and post-operatively there may be a massive rise in the platelet count with subsequent thrombotic and bleeding complications. Although it is possible to control the platelet rise by the administration of busulphan or hydroxyurea, post-operative thrombocytosis can still be extremely difficult to manage. Furthermore, some patients develop progressive hepatomegaly after splenectomy. For these reasons I prefer to manage myelosclerosis conservatively with careful iron and folate replacement therapy and the use of transfusion when required, and to reserve splenectomy for those rare cases in which splenic pain and severe hypersplenism becomes a major feature of the illness. The management of portal hypertension with bleeding oesophageal varices in patients with myelosclerosis is extremely difficult. Although there have been reports of successful shunt procedures, with or without splenectomy, surgery is so hazardous in these patients that it is better to try to manage the bleeding conservatively by sclerosing the varices (see Section 12).

Acute myelosclerosis and acute megakaryoblastic leukaemia

Although a very acute form of myelosclerosis has been recognized for a long time, it is only recently that evidence about its cellular origin has started to accumulate. Cytogenetic studies suggest that, as in chronic forms of myelosclerosis, the fibrotic reaction in the bone marrow is secondary to another pathological mechanism rather than the primary cause of the disease. Combined morphological and cytochemical analyses suggest that acute myelosclerosis is probably a myeloproliferative disorder which involves primarily the megakaryocyte or its precursor. For this reason it is preferable to call the condition *acute megakaryoblastic leukaemia*. It is currently believed that the myelofibrosis is mediated by growth factors released from the abnormal megakaryocytes, possibly platelet-derived growth factor. If this hypothesis is correct, acute myelofibrosis has the same basic pathophysiology as the more chronic form of the illness.

The condition has been seen in patients of all ages and is characterized by the rapid onset of symptoms of anaemia, low-grade fever, bleeding, proneness to infection, and, sometimes, generalized bone pain. On examination there is pallor and there may be a purpuric rash. The spleen is either impalpable or only slightly enlarged. There may be marked bone tenderness.

The blood picture is characterized by anaemia, neutropenia, and thrombocytopenia with a leucoerythroblastic reaction. Bone marrow aspiration almost invariably yields a dry tap and a tre-

Table 1 Disorders associated with myelofibrosis (full references are given by McCarthy, 1985)

Malignant
   Idiopathic myelosclerosis
   Acute myelosclerosis (acute megakaryoblastic leukaemia)
   Chronic myeloid leukaemia
   Acute lymphoblastic leukaemia
   Hairy cell leukaemia
   Polycythaemia vera
   Systemic mastocytosis
   Hodgkin's disease
   Myeloma
   Secondary carcinoma

Non-malignant
   Renal osteodystrophy
   Vitamin D deficiency
   Hypoparathyroidism
   Hyperparathyroidism
   Grey platelet syndrome
   Systemic lupus erythematosus
   Systemic sclerosis
   Thorium dioxide administration

phine biopsy shows increased reticulin, often accompanied by proliferation of bizarre cells which have the cytochemical characteristics of megakaryocytes.

The disease has an extremely poor prognosis and does not respond well to conventional leukaemia chemotherapy or radiotherapy. There has been one report of successful remissions following low-dose cytosine arabinoside (10 mg/m^2/day in twice daily subcutaneous injections). It is not clear whether this drug is working as a cytotoxic agent or has a more subtle action in stimulating the resolution of myelofibrosis. Recently, several patients have been treated successfully by bone marrow transplantation following intensive chemotherapy and radiotherapy. Without transplantation, the prognosis is extremely poor with survival of greater than a year being uncommon. Apart from the use of cytosine arabinoside, treatment is largely supportive with blood transfusion, platelet infusions, and appropriate management of infection.

Secondary myelosclerosis

There is a wide variety of disorders which may be associated with increased reticulin formation in the bone marrow. Secondary myelosclerosis is frequently associated with a *leucoerythroblastic anaemia*. This is characterized by a variable degree of anaemia, changes in shape and size of the red cells, and the presence of nucleated red cells or myelocytes, or even an occasional myeloblast, in the peripheral blood. As in primary myelosclerosis, bone marrow aspiration results in a 'dry tap', and a trephine biopsy is required to establish the cause of the fibrotic reaction. Some of these conditions are summarized in Table 1.

Neoplastic disorders

All forms of leukaemia and chronic myeloproliferative disorders may give rise to some degree of myelofibrosis. It is quite common for polycythaemia vera or chronic myeloid leukaemia to enter a terminal myelosclerotic phase. Occasionally Hodgkin's disease or non-Hodgkin's lymphoma may also result in marrow fibrosis. Disseminated carcinoma invading the marrow can also give rise to a variable degree of fibrosis.

Systemic mast cell disease

The mast cell disorders are rare conditions which range from solitary benign mast cell tumours to the bizarre syndrome of the malignant form of *systemic mastocytosis*. The syndrome of *cutaneous mastocytosis with urticaria pigmentosa* is described in Section 20.

The malignant form of systemic mastocytosis may develop *de novo* or superimposed on urticaria pigmentosa. It is a disease of the sixth and seventh decades and is more common in males. The symptoms are very varied and include general malaise, recurrent diarrhoea, pruritis, the skin manifestations of urticaria pigmentosa, hepatosplenomegaly, dense sclerotic bone changes, and an increased number of mast cells in the skin, liver, lymph nodes, and bone marrow. Rarely, mast cells spill into the peripheral blood in large numbers giving rise to the picture of *mast cell leukaemia*. The condition is diagnosed by demonstrating mast cell infiltration of a lymph node or bone marrow using special staining techniques. The disorder has a poor prognosis although symptoms can sometimes be controlled by the use of H1 or H2 receptor antagonists. In some cases there appears to be overproduction of prostaglandin D_2 and symptoms may be reduced with aspirin. There have also been reports of successful control by blocking the uptake of calcium ions necessary for degranulation of mast cells with cromoglycate. Standard antileukaemia agents are not effective. The prognosis from the time of diagnosis is usually less than 2 years, although the author has observed two patients with typical pathological features of the conditions who remained in reasonable health for over 5 years.

Myelofibrosis and vitamin D deficiency

There have now been a number of reports of children with rickets, myelofibrosis, and myeloid metaplasia. There was associated splenomegaly and leucoerythroblastic blood changes. These changes reverted to normal after treatment with vitamin D or 1,25-dihydroxy vitamin D_3. Interestingly, it has been shown that the active metabolite of vitamin D_3 inhibits the proliferation of human megakaryocytes *in vitro* and also induces myeloid cells from normal individuals or patients with chronic myeloid leukaemia to mature into monocytes and macrophages.

Renal failure

Myelofibrosis occasionally occurs in patients with renal failure with or without other features of renal osteodystrophy. It has been suggested that complication may also be caused by a deficiency of vitamin D although it has also been found that increased concentrations of parathyroid hormone, which occur in patients with renal failure, may also enhance the accumulation of collagen in the bone marrow.

Infection

It has been suggested that disseminated tuberculosis can produce a clinical picture very similar to myelosclerosis. However, it seems more likely that these are examples of tuberculous infection in patients with an underlying myeloproliferative disorder. There have been no really convincing cases of complete reversion to a normal blood picture after antituberculous therapy. This is a very confusing subject which requires further study. However, a sudden deterioration in a patient with a myeloproliferative disorder, with no evidence of an acute leukaemic transformation, should raise the possibility of disseminated tuberculosis.

Other rare causes of marrow fibrosis are summarized in Table 1.

References

Bain, B. J., Catovsky, D., O'Brien, M., Prentice, G., Lawlor, E., Kumaran, T. O., McCann, S. R., Matutes, E. and Galton, D. A. G. (1981). Megakaryoblastic leukaemia presenting as acute myelofibrosis – a study of four cases with platelet peroxidase reaction. *Blood* **58**, 206–213.

McCarthy, D. M. (1985). Fibrosis of the bone marrow: content and causes. *Br. J. Haematol.* **59**, 1–7.

Silverstein, M. N. (1983). Agnogenic myeloid metaplasia. In *Hematology*, 3rd edn (eds W. J. Williams, E. Beutler, A. J. Erslev and M. A. Lichtman), pp. 218–220. McGraw-Hill Book Company, New York.

Sultan, C., Sigaux, F., Imbert, M. and Reyes, F. (1981). Acute myelodysplasia with myelofibrosis: a report of eight cases. *Br. J. Haematol.* **49**, 11–16.

Takácsi-Magy, L. and Graf, F. (1975). Definition, clinical features and diagnosis of myelofibrosis. *Clin. Haematol.* **4**, 291–308.

Wetherley-Mein, G. and Pearson, T. C. (1982). The myeloproliferative disorders. In *Blood and its disorders*, 2nd edn (eds R. M. Hardisty and D. J. Weatherall), pp. 1239–1316. Blackwell Scientific Publications, Oxford.

Primary thrombocythaemia

D. J. WEATHERALL

Primary thrombocythaemia is a myeloproliferative disorder characterized by hyperplasia of the megakaryocytes and a marked increase in the platelet count. There may be an associated increase in the white cell count or even in the red cell count, and the dividing line between this disorder and polycythaemia vera may be indistinct. Based on its varied clinical features this condition has collected a variety of names over the years including *haemorrhagic thrombocythaemia*, *essential thrombocythaemia*, and *megakaryocytic leukaemia*.

Aetiology and pathogenesis

Recent evidence suggests that primary thrombocythaemia has a similar pathogenesis to the other myeloproliferative disorders and that it results from the abnormal proliferation of a stem cell line which, in this case, differentiates mainly towards the megakaryocyte/platelet compartments. It has been found that women with this disorder who are heterozygous for G6PD types A and B (see page 19.13) have platelets which show predominantly the A or B types, indicating that they are all derived from a single abnormal progenitor.

The platelets are morphologically abnormal and the platelet count is usually higher than that observed in *thrombocytosis*, i.e. an increased production of normal platelets. The clinical features of this disorder are the result of the high platelet count and the functional abnormalities of the platelets which are produced by the abnormal cell line. As expected, the very high platelet count is associated with a thrombotic tendency but, because of abnormal platelet function, bleeding is often a major feature of the disease. The platelets do not aggregate normally in response to adrenaline or collagen. On the other hand, they may aggregate spontaneously and they show a defective response to the inhibitory prostaglandin, PGD_2.

A few patients with primary thrombocythaemia have chromosome abnormalities, particularly a deletion of the long arm of chromosome 21.

Clinical features

The commonest symptom is abnormal bleeding, usually spontaneous. The most usual site is the gastrointestinal tract but haematuria and spontaneous bruising occur commonly. Interestingly, the disorder is not associated with genuine purpuric lesions. Thrombo-embolic phenomena are less frequent than bleeding. Thrombosis of the splenic vein and the superficial or deep veins of the legs have been reported and may be followed by pulmonary emboli and infarction. Not infrequently the disorder presents to the vascular surgeon with curious thrombotic lesions of the vessels of fingers and toes which cause small areas of gangrene not unlike those seen in the vasculitis of rheumatoid arthritis and collagen-vascular diseases (Fig. 1).

The spleen is often enlarged, at least in the early stages of the illness. Splenic atrophy has also been reported and is thought to follow thrombosis of the splenic vessels. When this occurs, or when the spleen is mistakenly removed before the diagnosis is recognized, the platelet count may rise to a value almost approaching that of the red cell count. Such patients are at particular risk of bleeding or thrombosis, or both.

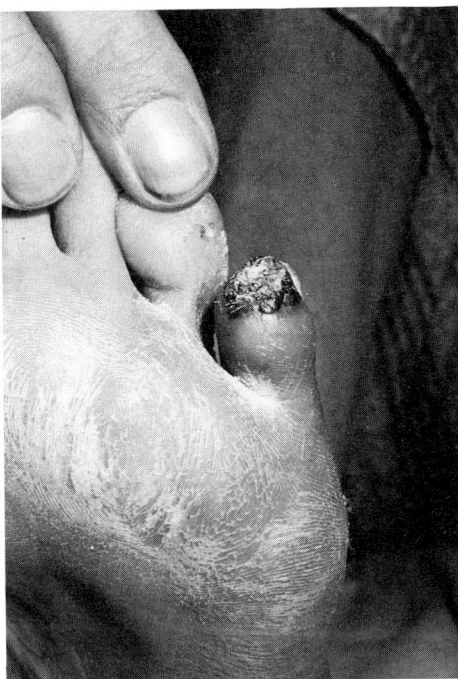

Fig. 1 A thrombotic lesion with infarction of the end of the toe in a patient with primary thrombocythaemia.

Laboratory findings

The main finding is a greatly elevated platelet count which is often in excess of $800-1000 \times 10^9/1$. The platelet morphology is abnormal, with many large and bizarre forms and aggregates in the peripheral blood. The bone marrow shows marked megakaryocytic hyperplasia. There is usually a mild polymorphonuclear leucocytosis and occasionally a slight elevation in the packed cell volume. Episodes of anaemia are quite common, almost certainly resulting from either acute or chronic blood loss. In patients whose spleens have atrophied typical changes of hyposplenism are found in the peripheral blood (see page 19.191).

Specialized tests of platelet function have shown a variety of abnormalities including reduced adhesiveness, reduced serotonin content and uptake, and reduced aggregation in response to ADP and adrenalin but not to collagen (see page 19.44).

Diagnosis

Thrombocythaemia must be distinguished from other causes of an elevated platelet count (Table 1). These include bleeding, malignant disease, rheumatoid arthritis, and infection. In the latter disorders it is very unusual to find platelet counts in excess of $800 \times 10^9/1$ and this, together with the remarkable morphological changes of the platelets usually serves to distinguish primary thrombocythaemia from thrombocytosis.

Course and prognosis

Because it is a relatively rare disease, very little is known about the natural history and prognosis of primary thrombocythaemia. Although many patients run a course punctuated by episodes of bleeding, thrombosis, embolism, and other complications, and the disease may be difficult to manage if the spleen has been mistakenly removed or if there is a thrombosis of the splenic vessels leading to splenic atrophy, the condition can also be surprisingly mild. Indeed, it is becoming apparent that young patients who present without symptoms may live for many years without suffering any ill effects. Furthermore, after a short course of alkylating agents or ^{32}P, many patients remain well for months or years before requiring another course of therapy when the platelet count finally rises again, as it always does.

For these reasons it is possible to give a reasonably good pro-gnosis for patients with this condition. If it is found by chance there may be a long period of freedom from symptoms. Even if the disease presents with a complication it is usually possible to control the platelet count for many years. There have been occasional reports of acute leukaemic transformation.

Table 1 Causes of a raised platelet count

Myeloproliferative disorders
  Primary thrombocythaemia
  Polycythaemias vera
  Myelosclerosis
  Chronic myeloid leukaemia

Secondary thrombocytosis
  Bleeding
  Inflammatory disorders
  Rheumatoid arthritis
  Malignant disease
  Post-splenectomy
  Splenic atrophy; sickle cell disease, coeliac disease
  Drugs: vincoids, epinephrine
  Post-thrombocytopenia
  Haemolytic anaemia

Treatment

Because this condition is rare there have been few opportunities to study large numbers of patients to assess the best form of treatment. However, certain facts seem to be emerging. First, because young patients with this disorder, even with very high platelet counts, often remain asymptomatic for many years it seems reasonable to leave them untreated under regular surveillance, and to initiate therapy only if symptoms occur or if the platelet count is progressively rising. In older patients there seems to be a genuine risk of vascular accidents and the platelet count should probably be reduced to below $500 \times 10^9/1$. Excellent control can usually be achieved using either ^{32}P or busulphan. In the author's experience younger patients respond well to a starting dose of busulphan 4 mg daily which is reduced to 2 mg daily as the platelet count approaches normal. Once the count is normal the drug must be stopped; the count will often remain at a normal level for months or even years. It is very important to stop the drug when the platelet count has reached a normal level and not to persist with treatment since a dangerous pancytopenia may result. In older patients, or in those who cannot be maintained under regular surveillance, ^{32}P therapy is the best approach. The dose regime is similar to that described for the management of polycythaemia vera (see page 19.39). Equally good results have been described by the use of phenylalanine mustard. If the platelet count needs reducing rapidly hydroxyurea at a dose of 15–30 mg/kg per day is extremely effective. In emergencies the platelet count can be lowered rapidly by plateletpheresis. In older patients who have had vascular occlusive episodes the use of platelet antiaggregating agents such as aspirin or dipyrimadole has been suggested, although their place in the management of this disease remains to be established. It should be remembered that thrombocythaemic platelets function abnormally and it is possible that the use of these agents may increase the risk of bleeding.

In young patients who are being kept under surveillance without treatment it is important to monitor the platelet count carefully throughout pregnancy. It may rise, and if elective surgery is needed, or prior to childbirth, the platelet count can be reduced by plateletpheresis.

References

Fialkow, P. J., Faguet, G. B., Jacobson, R. J., Vnrdya, K. and Murphy, S. (1981). Evidence that essential thrombocythemia is a clonal disorder with origin in a multipotent stem cell. *Blood* **58**, 916–919.

Hoagland, H. C. and Silverstein, M. N. (1978). Primary thrombocythemia in the young patient. *Mayo Clin. Proc.* **53**, 578–580.

Hussain, S., Schwartz, J. M., Friedman, S. A. and Chua, S. N. (1978). Arterial thrombosis in essential thrombocythemia. *Am. Heart J.* **96**, 31–36.

Pamlilio, A. L. and Reiss, R. F. (1979). Therapeutic plateletpheresis in thrombocythemia. *Transfusion* **19**, 147–149.

Singh, A. K. and Wetherley-Mein, G. (1977). Microvascular occlusive lesions in primary thrombocythaemia. *Br. J. Haemat.* **36**, 553–564.

Silverstein, M. N. (1968). Primary or hemorrhagic thrombocythemia. *Arch. Int. Med.* **122**, 18–22.

Weingeld, A., Branehog, I. and Kutti, J. (1975). Platelets in the myelo-proliferative syndrome. *Clin. Haemat.* **4**, 373–392.

Wetherley-Mein, G. and Pearson, T. C. (1982). The myeloproliferative disorders. In *Blood and its disorders*, 2nd edn (eds R. M. Hardisty and D. J. Weatherall), pp. 1269–1316. Blackwell Scientific Publications, Oxford.

Aplastic anaemia and other causes of bone marrow failure

E. C. GORDON-SMITH

Introduction

The concept of bone marrow failure as a cause of peripheral blood cytopenias is imprecise but convenient. Broadly, it indicates that the cause of the peripheral blood disturbance lies within the dividing pool of cells in the marrow itself. Fundamental to the classification of disorders within this group of bone marrow failures is the idea that normal development of cells within the bone marrow and release of normal cells into the peripheral blood depend upon an interaction between haematopoietic cells and the environment in which they proliferate and differentiate. The pathogenesis of most of these disorders is unknown and their separation depends mainly upon morphological criteria. In most instances the conditions are metastable, that is, other changes may occur on the background of the damaged marrow usually, though not always, in the direction of malignant change. The advent of powerful but toxic treatment such as bone marrow transplantation and massive chemotherapy for a variety of malignant and non-malignant conditions of the bone marrow has emphasized the need for definition and classification in this group of disorders so that suitable patients may be selected for these treatments and, equally important, those to whom such treatments offer no benefit are spared the unnecessary side-effects. Such a classification is shown in Table 1.

Aplastic anaemia

Definition

Aplastic anaemia is a syndrome characterized by peripheral blood pancytopenia associated with hypoplasia of the bone marrow in which there is neither fibrosis nor infiltration by malignant cells. Vitamin B_{12} and folate levels are normal, and the disorder is not associated with other dietary deficiencies.

Classification

As defined above, the syndrome of aplastic anaemia may occur in a number of ways. There is no universally acceptable classification but a number of more or less well-defined entities may be identified. These are summarized in Table 2. Inevitably, aplastic anaemia occurs following exposure to cytotoxic drugs or irradiation at a high enough dosage. The severity and duration of aplasia is dose-related and recovery usually occurs 1–6 weeks after the cytotoxic agent is discontinued. With very high dose radiation, stem cell killing is complete and recovery does not occur. When high dose radiation is used for a local lesion which includes an area of bone marrow, that area of bone marrow may later on become fibrosed and, again, recovery does not occur. Idiosyncratic

Table 1 Classification of bone marrow failure

Pathogenesis	Diseases
Haematopoietic cell failure	Aplastic anaemias Pure red cell aplasia Chronic neutropenia Amegakaryocytic thrombo-cytopenia
Proliferative dysplasias with abnormal differentiation	Refractory anaemia with excess of blasts Idiopathic acquired sideroblastic anaemia Myelodysplastic syndromes
Abnormal environment	Proliferative dysplasias with fibrosis Myelofibrosis
Infiltrations	Leukaemias Lymphomas Carcinoma Lipid storage diseases (for example, Gaucher's disease) Amyloid
Bone marrow necrosis	

Table 2 Classification of aplastic anaemias

Disease	Cause	Characteristics
Inevitable aplastic anaemia	Cytotoxic drugs Radiation	Dose-dependent: recovery in 2–6 weeks
Idiosyncratic aplastic anaemia	Drugs Viruses Idiopathic	Not dose-dependent; prolonged course
Immune aplastic anaemia	Drugs	Antibodies may be detected
	Viruses	Recovery 2–3 weeks after offending agent is removed
Inherited (congenital) aplastic anaemia	Autosomal recessive	Fanconi anaemia; other forms
'Malignant' aplastic anaemia		Pre-ALL* of childhood 'microleukaemia'

*ALL = acute lymphoblastic leukaemia.

acquired aplastic anaemia is the disease to which the term 'aplastic anaemia' is usually applied without further qualification. The disease arises spontaneously or may follow exposure to normal doses of a variety of drugs which do not usually cause haematological disturbances. The nature of these agents is discussed in greater detail below (page 19.47).

Aplastic anaemia may also follow a virus infection, particularly hepatitis. The disease is usually prolonged and recovery is unpredictable. Immune aplastic anaemia is an uncommon disorder which, again, may follow exposure to certain drugs or after some virus infections, particularly infectious mononucleosis. It may also be associated with other autoimmune disorders. Unlike the idiosyncratic aplastic anaemias, recovery usually occurs 2–3 weeks after withdrawal of the offending agent. In some instances it is possible to demonstrate inhibitors of granulopoiesis or erythropoiesis *in vitro*. Congenital aplastic anaemia (Fanconi anaemia) is an inherited disorder in which hypocellularity of the bone marrow and pancytopenia develop, usually during childhood. It is associated with skeletal and skin abnormalities, described in greater detail below (page 19.51). 'Leukaemic' aplastic anaemia occurs mainly in childhood. Acute lymphoblastic leukaemia of childhood may present in a form indistinguishable from aplastic anaemia.

Table 3 Drugs which are associated with aplastic anaemia

Class of drug	Association	
	Definite	Probable
Antibiotics	Chloramphenicol Sulphonamides	
Anti-inflammatory agents	Phenylbutazone Oxyphenbutazone Penicillamine Gold salts Amidopyrine	Indomethacin Propionic acid derivatives
Thyrostatic agents	Potassium perchlorate	Carbimazole Thiouracils
Anticonvulsants	Phenytoin	Trimethadione
Psychotropics	Chlorpromazine	Dothiepin Phenothiazines
Antiparasitics	Mepacrine Organic arsenicals	Chloroquine
Diuretics		Chlorthiazide Other thiazides Acetazolamide
Antidiabetic drugs	Chlorpropamide	
Antihistamines		Many different types

Idiosyncratic acquired aplastic anaemia

Aetiology
In about half of cases of aplastic anaemia it is not possible to define an aetiological agent. Amongst the rest, drugs, viruses and environmental toxins may be identified as probable causes. As yet there is no test which can pinpoint with certainty the cause of the aplastic anaemia. Drugs have been implicated in the aetiology of aplastic anaemia for 50 years or more. The list of drugs to which patients with aplastic anaemia have been exposed before the aplasia developed is long. In many cases multiple drugs have been given. The agents most commonly implicated are certain antibiotics, of which chloramphenicol is the best known, and anti-inflammatory drugs, where phenylbutazone and its derivatives are most commonly involved. Table 3 includes a list of the more frequently reported drugs. Aplastic anaemia is more likely to occur following a second or subsequent exposure to the drug than after the first exposure. Viruses are also implicated in the aetiology of aplastic anaemia, particularly hepatitis viruses.

About 10–20 per cent of patients with aplastic anaemia, particularly in the younger age group, give a history of jaundice and hepatitic symptoms some 6 weeks before the pancytopenia develops. In many instances disturbances of hepatocellular function have been demonstrated. The hepatitis is usually hepatitis B surface antigen negative, but the precise aetiology of the hepatitis is often unidentified. Various domestic and recreational drugs and chemicals have been implicated and may cause aplasia, although more commonly they produce a proliferative dysplasia of the marrow. Glues used in model-making may affect some susceptible individuals and there is a higher incidence of glue sniffers in patients with aplastic anaemia than in the general population. DDT and other insecticides have been associated with aplastic anaemia, although the solvent in which the DDT is dissolved before spraying may be equally to blame. Hair dyes have been incriminated in the past, but seem to be less commonly associated since aniline was discontinued as a constituent. The lack of suitable tests for possible aetiological agent together with the delay between exposure to that agent and the development of pancytopenia means that the list of substances thought to cause aplastic anaemia is long and may be inaccurate.

Incidence and epidemiology
Aplastic anaemia is a rare disease; figures for the incidence in different populations are not available. In Europe it is probably between 10 and 20 per million of the population per year. All age groups may be affected and there is a slight preponderance of males, possibly reflecting the greater risk of exposure to toxic substances at work amongst men. In the Far East the incidence of aplastic anaemia is much higher and the male preponderance much more obvious (see page 19.266). This may be related to the greater use of chloramphenicol and the increased risk of hepatitis. The risk of developing aplastic anaemia following exposure to one of the drugs known to cause this disorder is equally uncertain. With chloramphenicol the incidence is probably somewhere in the region of one in 20 000 patients at risk. A realization that chloramphenicol could cause aplastic anaemia and the wide publicity given to this risk means that chloramphenicol is much less commonly prescribed in the West than previously and it is no longer the single commonest cause of aplastic anaemia. Phenylbutazone and its derivatives became the more common cause but recently the danger has been recognized and the group has been withdrawn. Whatever the true risk of developing aplastic anaemia, it is clear that drugs should only be prescribed for specific purposes.

Pathogenesis
Even the way in which the various haematological agents bring about aplastic anaemia is unknown. There appears to be a failure of the pluripotent, haematopoietic stem cells in the bone marrow to proliferate and differentiate into mature blood cells. What is not clear is whether there is a defect in the environment which prevents their normal function. The abnormality might be in the marrow microenvironment or there might be inhibitors circulating in the blood. In about 50 per cent of cases where bone marrow cells from identical twins are transfused into patients with aplastic anaemia, recovery takes place without prior immunosuppression. This suggests that the environment is not grossly disordered otherwise the transfused stem cells would not be able to grow. It also suggests that an autoantibody is not the major cause of aplastic anaemia. Such engraftment does not always occur, however, and in some patients it is necessary to give immunosuppressive treatment before engraftment from an identical twin is successful. This suggests that disordered immunity may be a factor in the pathogenesis of a proportion of cases of aplastic anaemia. Cell culture techniques in humans are not sufficiently advanced to allow identification of stem cells, and tests for inhibitors of granulocyte colonies or red cell colonies in vitro have produced conflicting results. This is partly because many of these patients have received multiple transfusions and have been sensitized to a variety of cells, and in such circumstances it is difficult to identify specific inhibitors of haematopoiesis.

Diagnosis and pathology
The diagnosis of aplastic anaemia is made on the basis of the peripheral blood and bone marrow findings. In the peripheral blood there is pancytopenia with no abnormal cells present. The anaemia is usually normocytic at presentation but may be macrocytic, even strikingly so, particularly in chronic cases. The reticulocyte count is low. Neutrophils are invariably reduced and the count may be very low. Circulating neutrophils may have rather heavy granulation, so-called 'toxic' granulation, and have a high alkaline phosphatase content. The eosinophils and basophils are usually also grossly depleted and monocytopenia is usual. The reduction in the lymphocyte count is more variable; in children particularly it may be relatively high so that the total white cell count may be normal. It is only when the differential white cell count is carried out that the severe neutropenia is recognized. The platelet count is reduced and the relatively uniform small size of the platelet is an indication that production has failed.

Bone marrow aspiration is usually easy, fragments are obtained which are fatty, and there is a reduction of haemopoietic cells in the trials. The cellularity of the marrow may be judged to some extent from the marrow aspirate, but a so-called 'dry tap' (no material obtained from an aspirate) or a 'blood tap' (no fragments obtained) does not allow an assessment of bone marrow activity.

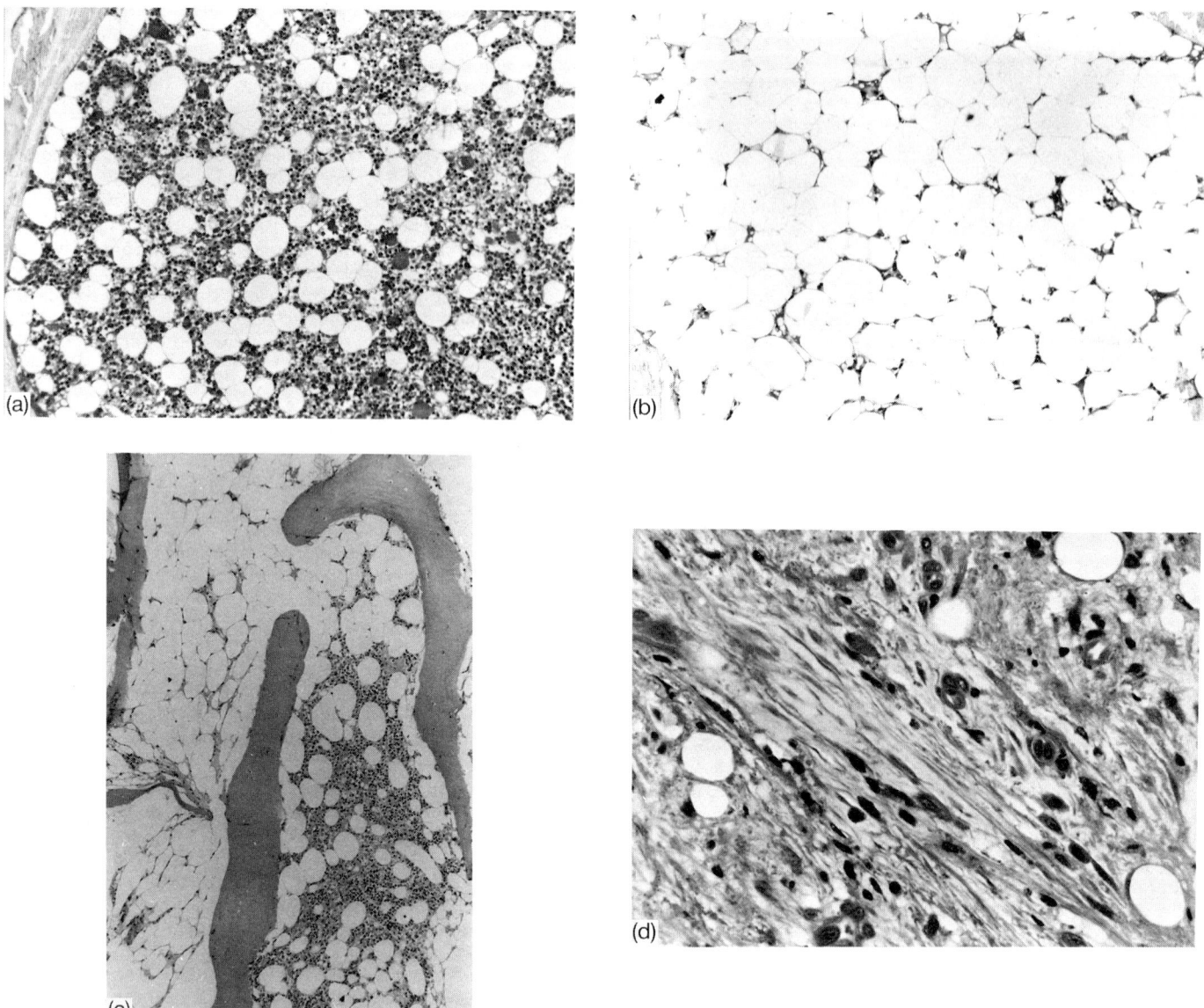

Fig. 1 Trephine biopsies of adult posterior iliac crest. (a) Normal marrow. (b) Severe aplastic anaemia. (c) Cellular focus in severe aplastic anaemia. (d) Proliferative dysplasia with fibrosis.

In aplastic anaemia there may be a patchy loss of cellularity throughout the marrow so that one aspirate may yield relatively normal-looking marrow. The diagnosis of aplastic anaemia should therefore not be made on a bone marrow aspirate alone, and assessment of cellularity should properly be made on a trephine biopsy; the latter shows replacement of the normal cellular marrow by fatty marrow. The reticulin network of the marrow is reduced commensurate with the reduction in the general overall cellularity. Focal areas of preserved cellularity may be seen in the bone marrow trephine, and it is one of the mysteries of aplastic anaemia that these focal areas of cellularity do not repopulate the remainder of the marrow (Fig. 1).

Dyserythropoiesis

In severe aplastic anaemia where normal haematopoiesis is almost completely abolished, there remains a cellular infiltrate within the marrow which in some cases may be quite prominent. This consists of normal lymphocytes, plasma cells, and reticulum cells, with the occasional blast cell. The appearances are similar to those seen in chronic inflammation. The infiltrates may be relatively uniform throughout the marrow or may occur in focal areas.

Malignant cells are not seen. Where haematopoiesis has not been completely abolished, the remaining areas may demonstrate abnormalities of differentiation, particularly in the red cell series. This abnormal differentiation is known as dyserythropoiesis.

Clinical features

The clinical features of aplastic anaemia arise from the results of the deficiencies of the cellular elements of the blood. Bleeding manifestations are often the first which take the patient to seek help from the doctor. The development of severe thrombocytopenia usually takes place over a matter of days or weeks so that catastrophic haemorrhage as a presenting feature is unusual; minor signs of the bleeding tendency present first. Excessive bruising or a petechial rash may be noticed. More commonly there is bleeding from the gums or from the nose. Haemorrhages in the buccal mucosa may occur, and haemorrhages in the retinae may be a portent of serious bleeding. The anaemia also develops slowly and the patient may complain only of mild fatigue or shortness of breath on marked exertion. Infections, particularly of the oropharynx or upper respiratory pathways may be a presenting feature. Infections anywhere aggravate the effect of thrombocyto-

Table 4 Criteria of severe aplastic anaemia*

Neutrophils	$<0.4 \times 10^9/l$
Platelets	$<10 \times 10^9/l$
Reticulocytes	$<10 \times 10^9/l$
Bone marrow	>80 per cent of remaining cells are non-myeloid

*Any three of the above four present for at least 2 weeks.

penia, particularly in the mouth. Good oral hygiene may reduce the amount of bleeding as well as clearing up local sepsis. There are no specific physical findings in aplastic anaemia, since any abnormalities resulting from the pancytopenia would be the same whatever the cause of the loss of cells. There is no lymphadeno-pathy except that associated with local infection. The liver and spleen are not enlarged. If the aplastic anaemia has followed an episode of apparent hepatitis, there may be some residual jaundice with enzyme abnormalities consistent with cholestasis.

The progression of the disease is variable and depends upon the severity and completeness of the marrow damage. In most large series of patients with aplastic anaemia where only support in the form of transfusions has been given, half the patients die within 3–6 months as a result of infection or haemorrhage. Patients alive at a year, however, have a very much better chance of surviving, at least for the next 2 or 3 years. This suggests that there is a group of patients with severe disease with a very poor chance of recovery and another group with a milder disorder. Various attempts have been made to determine which features indicate a poor prognosis (Table 4).

The identification of the group with severe aplastic anaemia is important since for these patients early bone marrow transplantation is the treatment of choice if a suitable donor is available. The subsequent course for patients who survive is variable. Spontaneous recovery, apparently to complete normality, may occur even after several years of pancytopenia. Other patients may remain stable for many years, and then gradually haematopoietic activity decreases further and they become anaemic and eventually die of infection or bleeding. Abnormal clones of cells may develop in these patients with a much greater frequency than in the normal population. An example of the development of an abnormal clone of cells developing in aplastic anaemia is paroxysmal nocturnal haemoglobinuria (PNH) (see page 19.54). Paroxysmal nocturnal haemoglobinuria red cells are especially sensitive to lysis by activated complement and are identified by the acidified serum lysis test (Ham's test). They may appear at any time during the course of aplastic anaemia. Acute myeloid leukaemia is also recognized as a complication of aplastic anaemia and may occur even after a period of apparent complete remission from the aplasia. This association between leukaemia and aplasia is discussed further below (page 19.51).

Until platelet transfusions became readily available, the usual cause of death in these patients was haemorrhage. Most patients now succumb to infection or a mixture of infection and haemorrhage, often after many months of treatment with antibiotics. It is virtually impossible to eradicate infection in the severely neutropenic patient until such time as neutrophil production returns.

Treatment

The treatment of aplastic anaemia has two main components. The first is to protect and support the patient from the consequences of pancytopenia and to keep him alive so that there may be a chance of spontaneous recovery. The second is to try to accelerate the recovery of the bone marrow by whatever means without eradicating the chance of spontaneous recovery.

Support and protection

For the aplastic patient this depends upon reducing potential sources of infection to a minimum and replacing deficient cells by transfusion (see Section 5 and page 19.248 *et seq.*). Infections may

arise from the environment or from sources of bacteria and other agents with the patient. As with all immunosuppressive patients, significant and lethal infections may arise from contamination with organisms which are not normally pathogenic. Exogenous infections are more likely in a hospital environment than at home, so any patient with aplastic anaemia admitted to hospital must be nursed in a clean and, preferably, sterile area. The precautions required to prevent spread of infection from one patient to another in hospital are not as rigorous as may be imagined, but must always be followed because once infection has been established in the severely neutropenic patient it cannot be eradicated until the neutropenia recovers. The two most important effective measures are for all medical and nursing staff to remove or cover outer garments which are likely to have been in contact with other infected patients, and for hands to be washed before entering the patient's room and, again, before touching the patient. Other more stringent measures probably add little more in the way of protection. Virus infections are not in themselves especially likely in the neutropenic host, but if they occur they produce an environment in which secondary bacterial infections may flourish. When the neutropenic patient is also immunosuppressed in other ways, virus infections assume a very important role in causing morbidity.

Endogenous infection arises from organisms carried within the patient, particularly the upper respiratory passages and the gastro-intestinal tract. Scrupulous skin and oral hygiene is essential. Repeated mouth washes with an antiseptic lotion such as chlorhexidine or hydrogen peroxide should be carried out regularly and after eating. The skin should be cleaned regularly with antiseptic. The extent to which potential pathogens should be removed from the gastrointestinal tract is debatable. Mostly these are aerobic organisms which are easily eliminated by antibiotics. Some would argue that removal of the anaerobic bacteria may actually be harmful. So-called complete decontamination of the gut is achieved by giving a variety of non-absorbable antibiotics together with antifungal agents such as nystatin or amphotericin. Co-tri-moxazole together with an antifungal agent may be equally effective in eliminating most aerobic pathogens although this has yet to be demonstrated conclusively. Recolonization of the bowel by potential pathogens can be avoided by using freshly cooked food and avoiding sources of hospital pathogens such as salads and fresh fruit. It must be remembered that patients with aplastic anaemia may require months of protective isolation and therefore measures must be practical as well as effective. Bowel decontamination is restricted to patients in hospital. In the outpatient department it is not possible to maintain a sterile gut, and patients are probably better protected by their own natural bowel flora than by non-absorbable antibiotics. They should, however, be advised to avoid both food with high bacterial content, and crowded places where they are liable to pick up infections.

Once an infection is established it is essential to treat it as soon as possible. Systemic antibiotics must be given as soon as fever or signs of infection occur and appropriate samples have been sent to the laboratory. If an organism is isolated the antibiotics should be changed, according to the sensitivities of the organism. Since the most common exogenous infections arise from *Pseudomonas* or *Klebsiella*, and the endogenous ones from aerobic organisms of the gastrointestinal tract, the antibiotics used in the first instance must be appropriate to those organisms. Most centres use a combination of aminoglycoside with a second antibiotic likely to have activity against *Pseudomonas* or a third-generation cephalosporin (suitable regimens are described in Section 5). Localized skin infections carry a particularly grave prognosis since it is difficult to achieve adequate antibiotic levels in the oedematous lesion. A major problem in aplastic anaemia is to decide when to discontinue the antibiotics. The patient may become afebrile and apparently well, but when the antibiotics are stopped, infection by the original organism is all too likely to return unless the neutropenia recovers. Transfusions of granulocytes may be helpful if the fever or infection does not resolve with antibiotics alone, but there is no place for prophylactic granulocyte transfusions in the management of aplastic anaemia (see Section 5 and page 19.254).

Transfusion of red cells and platelets is the other main standby in the management of aplasia. Red cell transfusions usually present few problems, but it must be remembered that the platelet count will fall and catastrophic haemorrhage may occur. Platelets should always be given before starting red cell transfusion and preferably also at the end in order to avoid this complication. Repeated platelet transfusions usually lead to the development of antibodies and resistance to platelet concentrates. The antibodies may be anti-HLA or antiplatelet specific antigens. Resistance is indicated by an inability to raise the platelet count by platelet transfusion. It may become impossible to control bleeding manifestations. It is also possible that, with the development of antibodies, immune complexes form which lead to a fall in the granulocyte count as well as the platelet count as resistance increases. Conventionally, platelets are only given when there is a clinical indication for their use. These indications include the rapid development of purpura, extensive bleeding from the gums and in the buccal mucosa, retinal haemorrhages, and headache. Major haemorrhage from any site is also an indication for platelets. In aplastic anaemia, particularly when the patient is being managed on an outpatient basis, catastrophic and fatal haemorrhage may be the first indication of severe bleeding, particularly so if the patient develops an infection. For this reason some centres manage their outpatients with regular platelet transfusions even though resistance may develop. This gives an opportunity for at least a weekly review of the patient and control of severe purpura. Sensitization to platelets may be avoided by using HLA-matched platelets or those that have been rendered free of white cells.

Further details of the management of patients with marrow failure are given in Section 5.

Specific measures

Androgens were the first drugs used in the treatment of aplastic anaemia which had any degree of success. High dose anabolic (androgenic) steroids are given by mouth. Only those which are alkylated in the 17α position are absorbed from the gastrointestinal tract, and their usefulness is limited by hepatotoxicity. This includes the development of hepatocellular carcinoma and the formation of multiple venous lakes called *peliosis hepatitis*. Other side-effects are associated with the virilizing action of androgenic steroids. Androgens may raise the responsiveness of the red cell precursors to erythropoietin and also have a direct effect on stem cell proliferation. In severe aplastic anaemia there has been no definite evidence that anabolic steroids improve survival, but when some marrow function remains, they may produce a significant rise in all cell lines. In patients who respond it takes about 3 months before effects are seen and recovery of the blood count is thereafter slow. Occasionally patients become androgen-dependent and stopping therapy leads to a relapse. For this reason androgens should be tailed off slowly and the dose adjusted to response.

Bone marrow transplantation

Replacement of the aplastic bone marrow by normal marrow from a suitable donor has long been considered the most rational treatment for aplastic anaemia (see also page 19.256). Early attempts to establish allogenic grafts were universally unsuccessful but transient engraftment could be demonstrated in some immunosuppressed recipients. In others, mild immunosuppression together with unmatched bone marrow was followed by recovery of the patient's own marrow. These observations have led to two major forms of therapy for aplastic anaemia. In young patients (under 40 years or so) with severe aplastic anaemia who have a suitable HLA-matched donor, early transplantation is the recommended treatment. The transplant should be carried out as soon as poss-

ible after the diagnosis of severe aplastic anaemia has been established, and before the patient has received multiple transfusions, which increase the chances of rejection, or becomes infected, which decreases the chances of surviving the transplant period. In bone marrow transplantation for severe aplastic anaemia relatively mild immunosuppression is sufficient to permit engraftment without using whole body irradiation. The incidence of graft failure or rejection was, however, in the order of 30 per cent, and additional measures have been tried to reduce this problem. These have included a modest amount of total body irradiation, the use of total nodal irradiation, the use of additional chemotherapy for immunosuppression and the administration of cyclosporin in the post-transplant period. Each of these measures reduces the incidence of graft failure or rejection but does not decrease the amount of graft-versus-host (GVH) disease. In addition, each of these measures carries its own side-effects and it is not yet clear which is the method of choice. The prospects for improvement in the success rate of transplantation for aplastic anaemia are, however, good; provided that a graft can be established and the problems of graft-versus-host disease overcome, the patients will be cured.

These problems are considered further on page 19.256.

Immunosuppression and androgens with or without mismatched marrow

The observation that some patients given modest immunosuppression and apparently mismatched marrow recovered from their own marrow function led to the use of antilymphocyte globulin (ALG), given for 5 days together with bone marrow from family members which was only partly matched with the recipient. The initial results of this form of therapy appeared to be promising. Later it was found that the marrow is unnecessary since, when antilymphocyte globulin and androgens alone are used, the survival rate is similar. The rate of recovery is usually slow with few patients showing a response before about 3 months, and in some instances much later. It is thus difficult to demonstrate with certainty that the immunosuppression had any effect. Many patients treated in this way who survive for a year or more may still require some form of transfusion support, and may indeed continue with neutropenia and or thrombocytopenia. It is worth achieving even modest improvement in aplastic anaemia since with neutrophil counts above 0.5×10^9/l and platelets about 30×10^9/l an independent and relatively safe existence is possible. If the patient fails to respond to the first course of antilymphocyte globulin (usually prepared in a horse) a second course using rabbit antihuman lymphocyte globulin may be given. Some 40–50 per cent of patients respond to the first course. About 40 per cent of non-responders to the horse protein will achieve some improvement. The best way of giving antilymphocyte globulin and the timing of a second course still has to be determined. There seems to be no advantage in giving more than a 5-day course in any event. Reactions during infusion of antilymphocyte globulin are common and serum sickness occurs in some 75 per cent of patients requiring treatment with corticosteroids.

Other forms of immunosuppression including high dose methylprednisone and cyclosporin have been used, with about equal success to antilymphocyte globulin in the first instance, and anecdotal success with cyclosporin. Other forms of therapy which have been used include drugs which are thought to stimulate granulopoiesis or granulocyte release, such as lithium or aetiocholanolone, and attempts to prolong the survival of such cells as do emerge, in particular by splenectomy. Reports on the use of these approaches are sporadic and it is difficult to assess their validity. The use of high dose corticosteroids other than in the circumstances outlined above is dangerous, but low dose corticosteroids, equivalent to 10 mg prednisolone, may reduce minor haemorrhage due to thrombocytopenia, although there is no definite evidence that this is the case.

Table 5 Abnormalities associated with Fanconi anaemia

Condition	Patients affected (%)*
Hyperpigmentation of the skin	75
Malformation of the skeleton	
all patients	66
aplasia or hypoplasia of the thumb	50
aplasia or hypoplasia of the radii	17
syndactyly	15
reduced number of carpal bones	30
Microsomy	60
Microcephaly	40
Malformation of kidneys	28
Strabismus (in males)	30
Hypogenitalism (in males)	20
Cryptorchidism	20
Mental retardation	17
Deafness	7
Short stature	80
Growth hormone deficiency†	Rare

* Percentages are approximate. Data derived mainly from Fanconi (1967).
† Most patients have normal levels despite short stature.

Congenital aplastic anaemia – Fanconi anaemia

The commonest of the inherited disorders which produce aplastic anaemia is that described by Fanconi in 1927. The disorder is inherited as an autosomal recessive and is associated with multiple developmental abnormalities, particularly of the skin and skeleton (Table 5).

Haematological features

Patients with Fanconi anaemia usually have a normal or nearly normal blood count at birth and during infancy. The disease presents with the effects of pancytopenia usually about the age of 5 years or later. Bleeding due to thrombocytopenia is the most common presentation, with anaemia second. The neutrophil count is often relatively well-preserved for some years after severe thrombocytopenia and anaemia develop. The bone marrow becomes progressively hypocellular over the years. In the initial stages macrophages showing active phagocytosis and an infiltrate of lymphocytes are prominent. Granulopoiesis may be relatively well-preserved. Dyserythropoiesis is common.

Chromosomal features

A characteristic finding in Fanconi anaemia is multiple non-specific abnormalities in the chromosomes. These consist mainly of chromatid breaks and aberrations. It is suggested that these lesions arise as a result of failure of one of the DNA repair systems (see Table 6). Although much work has been devoted to identifying such an enzyme defect, it has so far eluded definitive proof. Such a defect would explain the delay in the development of aplasia since this would be the result of cumulative damage to DNA which would not be repaired. However, it explains neither the inevitable nature of the aplasia nor the associated abnormalities of Fanconi anaemia.

Clinical features

The features of the full-blown Fanconi anaemia are characteristic. In some cases diagnosis may be difficult because of absence of the characteristic skeletal and skin features and formes frustes probably exist. The main features are listed in Table 5. Infants are of low birth weight and fail to grow normally. The skin is often mildly pigmented with areas of deeper pigmentation producing café-au-lait spots, often together with areas of depigmentation. Skeletal abnormalities involve particularly the bones of the forearm and thumbs. Abnormalities of the kidneys are also common. Mental development is only occasionally abnormal.

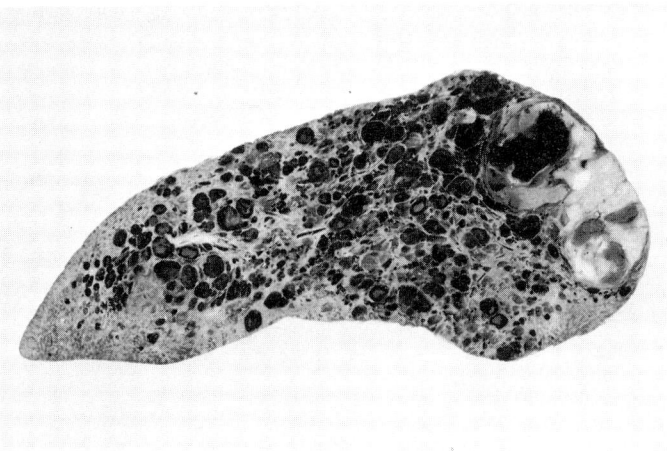

Fig. 2 Hepatocellular carcinoma in the liver of a patient with Fanconi anaemia treated for 4 years with anabolic steroids; the liver also shows multiple venous lakes (*peliosis hepatis*), another side-effect of anabolic steroids.

Prognosis and treatment

The outlook in Fanconi anaemia is poor. Untreated, the disease is usually relentless. Despite support with transfusions over many years most patients die of haemorrhage or infection. Treatment with anabolic steroids may bring about a remission of variable duration. Several years free from transfusion requirements may be obtained, but at the price of virilization and abnormalities of the liver. Hepatocellular carcinoma seems to be particularly common in children treated for years with 17α alkylated anabolic agents (Fig. 2). The development of acute leukaemia is also common and may be the presenting feature. Fanconi anaemia should be suspected in all children presenting with acute myeloid leukaemia under the age of 10 years. Its detection would be important at least for identifying the familial nature of the disease for the purpose of genetic counselling.

There are well-documented reports of patients with Fanconi anaemia going into spontaneous remission at the time of puberty, and complete recovery of normal bone marrow function has been described. Unfortunately this does not happen often and there is no way of predicting who will recover. In general, the severity of the disease and the rapidity with which pancytopenia develops is predictable within one particular family but there is marked variation between different families. Leukaemia and other malignant disease is more common in the relatives of patients with Fanconi anaemia than in the population at large.

Bone marrow transplantation is the only curative form of treatment for these patients but unfortunately it carries special risks. Severe skin reactions with epidermal necrolysis seem to be particularly common in patients with this disorder, and the success of transplantation is much lower than in acquired aplastic anaemia.

Aplastic anaemia and acute leukaemia

Aplastic anaemia is one response to bone marrow damage and acute leukaemia is another. As such the distinction between the two may not always be clear, at least on the histological and anatomical basis. There are a number of syndromes in which aplasia and acute leukaemia seem to be linked.

Acute lymphoblastic leukaemia of childhood

This may present in a form indistinguishable from aplastic anaemia. Blasts are not seen in the peripheral blood, and the bone marrow aspirate and trephine are hypocellular without any obvious infiltration by malignant cells. The aplasia in these children responds to treatment with prednisone and a swift remission may be obtained. Some 6–8 weeks later there is the emergence of leukaemic cells in the peripheral blood. It is suggested that the

Table 6 Disorders with possible defective DNA repair mechanisms associated with increased risk of leukaemic and other malignancies (see also Section 4)

Disease	Clinical features	Evidence for DNA repair defect	Malignancy
Fanconi anaemia	Aplastic anaemia Skeletal disorders Skin disorders	Chromatid breaks	Acute leukaemia ?Hepatocellular carcinoma
Xeroderma pigmentosa	Keratosis of skin Neurological disease Mental deficiency Bone marrow failure	Excessive chromatid fragility to ultraviolet light Excision repair defect	Skin cancers
Bloom's syndrome	Growth disorder Sun-sensitive eruptions Disturbed immune function	Chromatid breaks Sister chromatid exchanges	Acute leukaemia
Ataxia telangiectasia	Cerebellar ataxis Oculocutaneous telangiectasia Combined immune deficiency	Defective excision repair	Acute leukaemia and other lympho- reticular malignancies

aplasia is an early result of the leukaemia or possibly part of the body's reaction against leukaemia. It has also been suggested that corticosteroids should be given to all young children with aplastic anaemia as a diagnostic test for acute leukaemia. The acute leukaemia is of the lymphoblastic type and is not more severe than that seen in children who do not have the aplastic phase.

Microleukaemia

This is a term which has been applied to a disease characterized by a hypoplastic marrow in which a small proportion of blasts may be seen, usually with occasional blasts in the peripheral blood. The condition differs in a number of ways from aplastic anaemia, but the differences may be subtle. There is usually more reticulin present in the marrow and aspiration of the marrow may be difficult. The neutrophil alkaline phosphatase score may have low rather than high values as seen in aplastic anaemia. The condition may remain stable for months or years during which the patient requires transfusions but is otherwise well. Slowly the proportion of blasts in the bone marrow and peripheral blood increase and eventually this condition becomes frankly leukaemic. Mostly, these patients do not respond to antileukaemic therapy, but remissions may occasionally be obtained so that it is probably worth trying chemotherapy when the frankly leukaemic phase emerges. If a suitable bone marrow donor is available, transplantation is indicated, but under these circumstances additional chemotherapy and total body irradiation must be given to eradicate the leukaemic clone.

Acute leukaemia following aplastic anaemia

Some patients who survive for several years with aplastic anaemia may eventually develop acute leukaemia. Even in retrospect, no evidence of the leukaemic change may be found in the early stage of the illness. There may indeed be a period of apparent remission before the acute leukaemia develops. Sometimes other clones of abnormal cells such as paroxysmal nocturnal haemoglobinuria (PNH) cells are detected before the leukaemia is manifest. These patients are treated as for other cases of acute leukaemia though the prognosis is poor.

Drug-induced leukaemia

A number of drugs which more commonly produce aplastic anaemia may produce acute leukaemia directly. Acute leukaemia has been described following exposure to chloramphenicol and phenylbutazone. Benzene more commonly produces a myeloproliferative disorder or frank leukaemia rather than aplasia, but any of these responses are seen in different individuals.

Fanconi anaemia and acute leukaemia have already been mentioned (pages 19.51–19.52). A number of other disorders listed in Table 6, in which there is evidence of DNA repair deficit, are also associated with an increased risk of acute leukaemia (see also Section 4).

The proliferative bone marrow failures

There are a number of disorders characterized by peripheral blood pancytopenia in which the bone marrow is cellular but is ineffective in its production of normal peripheral blood cells (see also pages 19.58 and 19.130). Primitive cells are not usually present in the peripheral blood but there may be morphological, biochemical, or cytogenetic changes in the peripheral blood cells which are indicators of the disturbed haematopoiesis. These conditions have been given a number of names such as 'pre-leukaemia', 'smouldering leukaemia' and 'proliferative dysplasia'. It is particularly unsatisfactory to refer to this group as 'pre-leukaemia' since it suggests that these patients will inevitably develop leukaemia, whereas in certain circumstances the condition may be stable for many years and the problems which arise are not those of malignant change but of support for the patient. It is becoming apparent that there are various reasonably well-circumscribed syndromes within this major group of proliferative bone marrow failure. These are described in the section on the myelodysplastic syndromes (page 19.58).

Proliferative dysplasia with fibrosis

Occasionally fibrosis of the bone marrow appears without evident underlying cause and in the absence of hepatosplenomegaly or extramedullary haemopoiesis. The condition is characterized by increased pancytopenia sometimes with the presence of red cell and white cell precursors in the peripheral blood – the so-called leucoerythroblastic picture. Bone marrow aspirate is usually unsuccessful, and a trephine biopsy shows a variable degree of reduction in haemopoietic cells with the marrow replaced by reticulin and fibroblasts. Primitive cells are not seen at this stage of the illness. Ferrokinetic studies may indicate some remaining but ineffective erythropoiesis (see page 19.43).

Bone marrow failure affecting single cell lines

There are a number of conditions in which anaemia, neutropenia or thrombocytopenia develop in isolation as a result of the failure to produce these cells by the bone marrow. The conditions may be inherited or acquired and the main disorders are listed in Table 7.

Pure red cell aplasia

Pure red cell aplasia is characterized by an anaemia with a marked reduction or absence of reticulocytes in which the neutrophils and

Table 7 Bone marrow failure affecting single cell lines

Disease	Cause	Example
Red cell aplasia	Inherited	Diamond–Blackfan syndrome
	Idiopathic, acquired (?autoimmune)	With or without thymoma
		With other autoimmune disorders
	Drug induced	Penicillamine
		Diphenylhydantoin
		Chlorpropamide
		Chloramphenicol
	Virus induced	Aplastic crisis in haemolytic anaemia (Parvovirus)
		Transient erythroblastopenia in childhood
	Riboflavin deficiency	Experimental
Neutropenia	Inherited	Infantile genetic agranulocytosis (Kostmann syndrome)
		With pancreatic insufficiency (Schwachman–Diamond syndrome)
		Others
	Idiopathic, acquired (?autoimmune)	?Cyclical
	Drug induced	Thiazides
		Semi-synthetic penicillins
	Virus induced	Rubella
Amegakaryocytosis	Congenital	With total absence of radii
		Isolated
	Acquired	Variant of aplastic anaemia

platelet count are normal. The bone marrow is cellular with normal granulopoiesis and megakaryocytes, but in which one of two abnormalities of the red cell precursors exists. There may be a complete absence of red cell precursors or there may be red cell precursors present up to a certain stage of development but not beyond, the so-called 'maturation arrest'. Ferrokinetic studies show a grossly prolonged clearance time of radioactive iron from the peripheral blood and failure to incorporate this iron into the peripheral blood cells. Apart from the changes in the red cell series, there are no other abnormalities in the peripheral blood and there is no evidence of peripheral destruction of red cells. The patients are in other respects normal. Both congenital and acquired forms exist.

Congenital pure red cell aplasia

This has also been called rather confusingly, 'congenital hypoplastic anaemia', but is better known by its eponym, the *Diamond–Blackfan syndrome*. In most instances anaemia is present at birth or is detected shortly afterwards. There is a profound reticulocytopenia often with no reticulocytes present in the peripheral blood. There is no hepatosplenomegaly. The white count and platelet counts are normal. Skeletal abnormalities may be present of which triphalangeal thumb is the most common. There are no disturbances of growth, of the skin, or other organs as are seen in Fanconi anaemia. The disorder has an autosomal recessive inheritance.

Treatment presents many problems. Most of these children, if treated early enough with corticosteroids, will respond and the haemoglobin can be brought back to normal or maintained at normal levels after transfusion. However, the condition is steroid-dependent, and major problems result from the continued use of

corticosteroids in the doses necessary to maintain remission. Some of the side-effects may be reduced by using an intermittent regimen of corticosteroids on alternate days or even alternate weeks. Transfusion of the patients will permit normal growth but will, of course, produce all the other problems of iron overload (see page 19.87) and chelation therapy would be required from an early stage. Some patients fail to respond to corticosteroids, and this seems to be particularly true if the corticosteroids are instituted late in the illness. These patients rely on blood transfusions for survival.

During the course of the disease the spleen may enlarge and transfusion requirements increase. In these patients splenectomy may reduce transfusion requirements and occasionally is associated with a marked increase in steroid responsiveness or even complete remission. This only seems to apply to those patients whose spleen is enlarged.

Acquired pure red cell aplasia

This may occur *de novo* or following administration of various drugs. Between about one-third and one-half of the idiopathic cases are associated with a thymoma. The red cell aplasia may precede, accompany, or follow the development of the thymoma and excision of the tumour has variable effect with no guarantee of recovery of the anaemia. The haematological features of the disorder are similar to that seen in the congenital red cell aplasia with anaemia and reticulocytopenia associated with absence of red cell precursors or maturation arrest of the red cell series in the bone marrow. There is an unpredictable responsiveness to corticosteroids and there are reports of patients who are unresponsive to corticosteroids responding to immunosuppressive therapy with drugs such as cyclophosphamide. Autoantibodies have been thought to play a role in the genesis of this disease and occasionally immunoglobulins have been identified which inhibit haem synthesis or prevent the development of red cell colonies *in vitro*. Very rarely antierythropoietin antibodies have been found.

Apart from the association with thymoma, pure red cell aplasia may be seen in other conditions where there is a high incidence of autoimmune disease. It may occur in association with acquired idiopathic hypogammaglobulinaemia and in association with other autoimmune diseases. Occasionally the direct antiglobulin test (Coombs' test) may be weakly positive, usually with complement on the surface of the red cell. There may be severe thrombocytopenia in some cases. The presence of such autoimmune phenomena suggests that the patient has a better chance of responding to corticosteroids than in their absence. There is an increased incidence of malignant disease in association with acquired pure red cell aplasia. Apart from the expected incidence of lymphoma seen in patients with disorders of immune regulation, there also appears to be an increased incidence of acute myeloid leukaemia. In patients who fail to respond to corticosteroids, blood transfusion with chelation therapy is the main form of management. Occasionally, splenectomy may increase responsiveness to corticosteroids or immunosuppression. An enlarging spleen which increases transfusion requirements is an indication for splenectomy.

Erythroblastopenic anaemia in childhood

'Aplastic crises' may occur in patients with haemolytic anaemia. The term is confusing because only the red cell series is affected. Rapid anaemia develops as a consequence of failure of red cell production in the presence of increased destruction. In many of these cases infection with *parvovirus* seems to be the cause. Antibodies to the virus are absent at the time of crisis and the patient recovers as IgM antibodies appear followed by the IgG response. Urgent transfusion may be required during the crisis. Transient erythroblastopenia of childhood may also have a viral aetiology though this is not so clearly demonstrated. The anaemia with reticulocytopenia usually occurs in children from 18–26 months old (range 1–72 months). There is usually a history of preceding viral or bacterial illness. Recovery occurs within a few weeks of diagnosis though the patient may need transfusion in the meantime.

Isolated defects in white cell or platelet production

These conditions are described elsewhere and are summarized in Table 7.

References

Brooks, B. J. Jr, Broxmeyer, H. E., Bryan, C. F. and Leech, S. H. (1984). Serum inhibitor in systemic lupus erythematosus associated with aplastic anemia. *Arch. intern. Med.* **144**, 1474.

Camitta, B. M., Nathan, D. G., Forman, E. N., Parkman, R., Rappeport, J. M. and Orellana, T. D. (1974). Post-hepatitis aplastic anaemia – an indication for early bone marrow transplantation. *Blood* **43**, 473–483.

——, Thomas, E. D., Nathan, D. G., Santos, G., Gordon-Smith, E. C., Gale, R. P., Rappeport, J. M. and Storb, R. (1976). Severe aplastic anaemia: a prospective study of the effect of early bone marrow transplantation in acute mortality. *Blood* **48**, 63–70.

Champlin, R. E., Feig, S. A., Sparkes, R. S. and Gale R. P. (1984). Bone marrow transplantation from identical twins in the treatment of aplastic anaemia: implication for the pathogenesis of the disease. *Br. J. Haematol.* **56**, 455–463.

Davis, L. R. (1983). Aplastic crises in haemolytic anaemia: the role of parvovirus-like agent. *Br. J. Haematol.* **55**, 391–393.

Fanconi, G. (1967). Familial constitutional panmyelocytopathy: Fanconi's anaemia (FA). I. Clinical aspects. *Semin. Hematol.* **4**, 233–240.

Geary, C. J. (ed.) (1979). *Aplastic anaemia.* Baillière Tindall, London.

Heimpel, H., Gordon-Smith, E. C., Heit, W. and Kubanek, B. (eds) (1979). *Aplastic anemia. Pathophysiology and approaches to therapy.* Springer-Verlag, Berlin.

Kidson, C. (1980). Diseases of DNA repair. *Clin. Haematol.* **9**, 141–157.

Schroeder, R. M. and Kurth, R. (1971). Spontaneous chromosomal breakage and high incidence of leukemia in inherited disease. *Blood* **37**, 96–112.

Storb, R., Prentice, R. L., Thomas, E. D. *et al.* (1983). Factors associated with graft rejection after HLVA-identical marrow transplantation for aplastic anaemia. *Br. J. Haematol.* **55**, 573–585.

Thomas, E. D. (ed.) (1978). Aplastic anaemia. *Clin. Haematol.* **7**.

—— (1984). Acquired severe aplastic anemia: progress and perplexity. *Blood* **64**, 325–328.

Williams, D. M., Lynch, R. E. and Cartwright, G. E. (1973). Drug-induced aplastic anemia. *Semin. Hematol.* **10**, 195–223.

Paroxysmal nocturnal haemoglobinuria

J. V. DACIE

Paroxysmal nocturnal haemoglobinuria (PNH) is an uncommon acquired disorder characterized by the production of an abnormal line of red cells which are unusually prone to lysis by complement. It is of particular interest with respect to its clinical presentation and its relationship to aplastic anaemia. It affects both sexes and probably individuals of all racial groups. It is essentially a disease of adults, the majority of patients being between 20 and 40 years of age; it is rare but not unknown in childhood.

Aetiology and pathophysiology

PNH is an acquired disease of haemopoietic stem cells and it is possible to demonstrate that the patients' leucocytes and platelets are abnormal as well as their red cells. There is evidence, derived from red cell enzymes studies (page 19.13), that PNH is a clonal disease, arising apparently as the result of somatic mutation, and this being so it is particularly remarkable that a proportion of patients recover completely. Although at one time in the evolution of the disease, the PNH red cell progenitors appear to have some advantage over normal red cell progenitors and largely replace them – as happens in leukaemia – in PNH the abnormal clone gradually disappears in some patients, and if the patient has sufficient surviving normal stem cells he or she will eventually recover. The cause of the gradual elimination of the abnormal clone is uncertain; possibly it is the result of gradual ageing of the abnormal stem cell population.

The relationship between PNH and aplastic anaemia is intrigu-ing and likewise uncertain. There appears to be no connection with the cause of the aplasia. PNH has thus developed subsequent to marrow aplasia of idiopathic (unknown) origin, after marrow aplasia thought to be drug or chemically induced and in a least one instance after aplasia of genetic origin (as in Fanconi's anaemia). Possibly the marrow aplasia facilitates the growth of the not very vigorous PNH clone by reducing competition by normal stem cells.

The abnormal red cell line can be demonstrated by lysis in acidified serum, which reflects its increased sensitivity to complement. An interesting phenomenon is that not all the patient's red cells undergo lysis under these conditions or in any of the other tests which have been used to recognize PNH. The red cells thus vary considerably in their complement sensitivity. At least two populations of abnormal red cells can be demonstrated in most patients: Type II cells, 3–5 times as complement sensitive as normal cells, and Type III cells, 10–15 times as sensitive, as well as normal (Type I) red cells. The significance of more than one population is uncertain. The severity of a patient's illness can, however, be correlated with the proportion of highly complement sensitive Type III red cells that are formed.

The nature of the lesion(s) in the red cells (and in granulocytes and platelets) leading to this increased complement sensitivity has been the subject of much research. Type II cells have been shown to bind more C3b than normal cells and Type III cells to be abnormally sensitive to the terminal complement components C5b–C9 in addition. Recent work has shown that in PNH there is a deficiency in the decay accelerating factor of red cell stroma (DAF) which normally protects red cells from damage by C3b deposition.

Biochemical studies of PNH red cells

PNH red cells differ from normal red cells in several ways in addition to their remarkable increased sensitivity to lysis by complement: e.g. acetylcholinesterase activity is diminished or absent; exposure to H_2O_2 or ultraviolet light causes an increased formation of lipid peroxides; p-chloromercuribenzoate brings about increased lysis; the i antigen is prominent. No clear link between these abnormalities and the cells' increased sensitivity to complement lysis has, however, yet been established.

Creation of PNH-like red cells *in vitro*

Exposure to certain chemicals has been shown to affect normal cells in such a way that they undergo lysis *in vitro* under the same conditions as do PNH cells. The sulphhydryl compounds cysteine and AET (2-aminoethylisothiouronium bromide) in appropriate concentrations are particularly effective and can be employed as useful laboratory reagents; they act by increasing the complement sensitivity of the cells. But how exactly they bring this about and what relation there is (if any) between the lesion(s) produced by the chemicals and those of naturally occurring PNH cells are uncertain.

Mechanism of haemolysis

The increased haemolysis in PNH is primarily intravascular, hence the haemoglobinaemia, methaemalbuminaemia, ahaptoglobinaemia, haemoglobinuria, and the long-continuing haemosiderinuria. Lysis *in vivo* is thought to be determined by the continuous activation of the alternative complement pathway which occurs normally. PNH red cells pick up small amounts of activated C3 (C3b) (normal red cells probably do this also to some extent) and these small amounts are sufficient to bring about the lysis of the sensitive PNH cells although not causing lysis of normal red cells.

The increase in haemoglobinaemia which occurs during sleep, and which explains the nocturnal haemoglobinuria seen in seriously affected patients, is probably due to the activation of the alternative pathway during sleep resulting in an increased uptake of C3b by the red cells or the delivery from the marrow during sleep of cohorts of very sensitive cells. How the postulated activation is brought about is uncertain; increased acidaemia during sleep is probably not the cause. The acute haemolysis which may complicate infections or follow inoculations, transfusions or surgical interventions (e.g. splenectomy) also probably depends upon activation of the alternative pathway. Endotoxin derived from the gut seems likely to be an activating factor and to play a part in bringing about local haemolysis (and thrombosis) within the portal and hepatic venous systems.

As mentioned below, venous thrombosis poses a serious threat to life in PNH, particularly cerebral thrombosis and intrahepatic thrombosis resulting in the Budd–Chiari syndrome. It seems probable that the abnormal complement-sensitive platelets of PNH play a part in the genesis of the thrombosis. The increased proneness to bacterial infections that some PNH patients suffer from seems likely to be a consequence of the deficiency and abnormal function of neutrophils.

Clinical findings
Onset of the disease
This is usually insidious, with gradually increasing weakness and dyspnoea on exertion, accompanied by pallor and perhaps slight jaundice. In the typical case these symptoms are associated with the intermittent passage of dark urine (haemoglobinuria). This is, however, not a constant feature and the disease may run its course without it ever being noticed. Haemoglobinuria may, however, be a striking sign, and as the title paroxysmal *nocturnal* haemoglobinuria signifies it is in the urine formed at night and passed first thing in the morning that haemoglobin tends to be found. In a minority of patients rhythmic nocturnal haemoglobinuria persists for many days or weeks; occasionally, the haemoglobinuria is not obviously nocturnal. (Actually, as has been discussed, the haemoglobinuria is associated with sleep, not night-time.)

Physical signs
These are not distinctive. There is usually slight to moderate jaundice. The spleen is often palpable a few centimetres below the costal margin and the liver may be slightly enlarged also; it becomes markedly so if intrahepatic venous thrombosis develops. Skin purpura or other evidence of a haemorrhagic tendency may be noticeable in the presence of marked thrombocytopenia.

Urine
The urine is red-brown to almost black in colour if it contains haemoglobin and/or methaemoglobin. A constant finding, even in the absence of free haemoglobin, is haemosiderinuria, i.e. the presence in the urine deposit of numerous small granules giving a positive Prussian-blue reaction for free iron. The granules are derived from renal tubular cells which have taken in iron from the glomerular filtrate and, after the haemoglobin molecule has been broken down, retain the iron derived from haem in the form of haemosiderin. Despite the retention of iron, renal function is usually, although not invariably, well preserved.

Associated symptoms and signs
Abdominal pain
Many patients suffer from attacks of abdominal pain. This varies from a feeling of vague discomfort to severe colic or cramp and may be accompanied by vomiting which may persist for hours. Sometimes the symptoms are experienced when haemolysis is particularly active but this is not always the case. In a few patients the severity of the pain and doubt as to the diagnosis have led to laparotomy being undertaken. The pain is probably the result of thrombosis occurring within small veins in the portal system. Rarely thrombosis has led to infarction of part of the small intestine. In some patients abdominal pain has been the presenting feature of their illness and failure to recognize the possibility that PNH is responsible for their symptoms has led to delay in diagnosis.

Headaches
Some patients have suffered from distressing headaches, but this symptom seems to less common than that of abdominal pain. In a few instances headache has presaged a cerebral vascular accident.

Thombophlebitis and thrombo-embolism
Venous thrombosis (in addition to causing abdominal pain when small vessels are affected) can lead to serious consequences. Thrombosis and thrombo-embolism are in fact the most frequent immediate cause of death in PNH. Veins almost anywhere in the body may be involved; particularly serious is major thrombosis within the portal system and intrahepatic venous thombosis leading to the Budd–Chiari syndrome.

Factors which precipitate attacks of haemolysis
While haemolysis generally occurs for no apparent cause a number of factors can increase its severity and lead to intense and prolonged haemoglobinuria. Amongst such exacerbating factors are an infection, even a minor one such as the common cold, a blood transfusion, a surgical procedure, menstruation, the administration of medicinal iron (either orally or parenterally), exposure to cold, and inoculations.

Other clinical associations
Proneness to infections
Some patients seem to be unusually susceptible to bacterial infections. This is probably a consequence of granulocytopenia and/or defective neutrophil function.

Gallstones
As in other types of haemolytic anaemia, pigment gallstones frequently form in PNH patients and may lead to cholecystitis or obstructive jaundice.

Iron deficiency
As already mentioned, haemosiderinuria is a constant and persistent finding in PNH, even when the rate of haemolysis is insufficient to result in overt haemoglobinuria. As much as 10 mg of iron may be lost daily in this way. Patients have presented as cases of iron deficiency anaemia and the fact that there is, too, chronically increased haemolysis may be overlooked. At necropsy, it is characteristic of PNH that although the kidney is heavily loaded with iron, all other organs of the body are conspicuously free of iron.

Association of PNH with hypoplasia of the bone marrow
Many patients suffering from PNH give a history of pancytopenia and of having been diagnosed originally as suffering from aplastic anaemia. Thus of 80 personally observed patients, aplastic anaemia was the first diagnosis in 23 of them compared with haemolytic anaemia in 29. In 25 there was insufficient information to be certain as to the mode of onset and in three patients PNH had been preceded by myelosclerosis. The cause of the association between PNH and aplastic anaemia is not known for certain (see page 19.49).

This relationship takes several forms:

1. (Most common): marrow hypoplasia is present at the onset and then a variable but significant degree of recovery of marrow function occurs after which 'classical' haemolytic PNH develops.

2. (Less common): marrow hypoplasia is present at the onset, there is no recovery of marrow function, tests for PNH become weakly positive, and the patient remains pancytopenic without increased haemolysis being obvious.

3. (Least common): haemolytic PNH is present at the onset, marrow hypoplasia subsequently develops, and pancytopenia continues with or without signs of increased haemolysis.

In a small number of patients PNH has been complicated by the development of leukaemia and in a few patients, too, PNH has

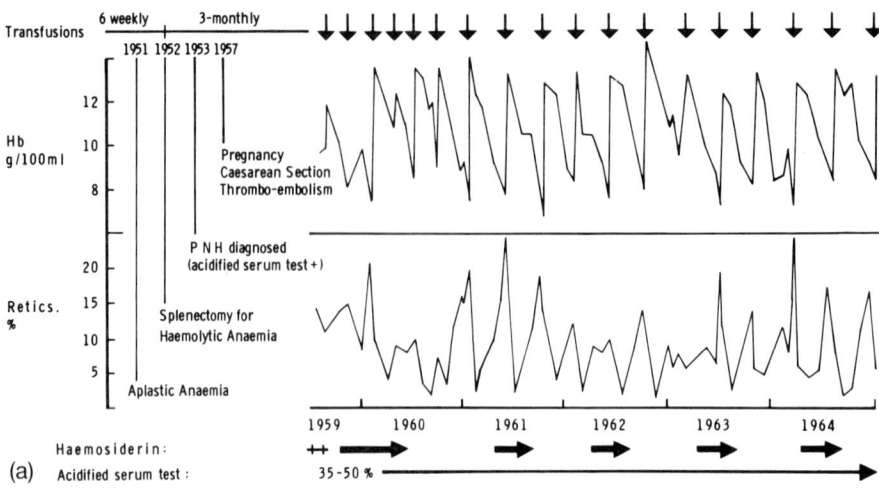

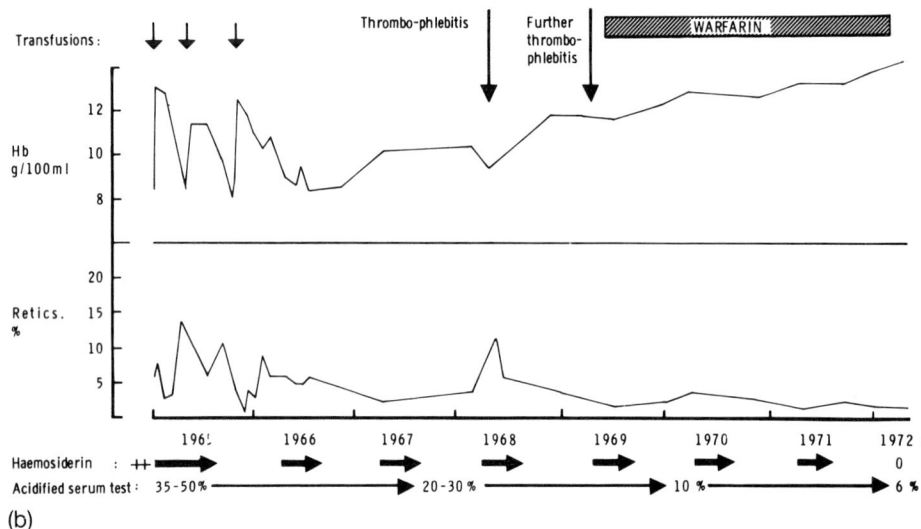

Fig. 1 (a, b) Clinical and haematological course of a female patient with PNH, illustrating recovery after an illness lasting 20 years. Aplastic anaemia had been diagnosed when she was aged 20 years, PNH two years later. The acidified serum test eventually became completely negative and when last heard of (in 1984) she was still well. (Reproduced from Dacie and Lewis, 1972, *Ser. Haemat.* **5**, 3–23, with permission.)

been preceded by myelosclerosis. The nature of these associations is uncertain; they are far less frequent than the association with aplastic anaemia. PNH appears to be far less common than leukaemia as an apparent sequel to excessive irradiation.

Course of the disease and chances of recovery

PNH is a very chronic disorder and some patients have survived for 20 years or even longer after diagnosis; many have survived more than 10 years. The median survival of 80 patients personally observed in London between 1946 and 1971 was 10 years. Of 85 patients studied by the author between 1939 and 1971, 47 are known to have died; six, however, recovered and became clinically well despite continuing weakly positive laboratory tests for PNH, while a further six patients also recovered completely both clinically and haematologically and eventually gave completely negative laboratory tests for PNH (Fig. 1). Thus an appreciable proportion of PNH patients (perhaps 10–15 per cent) recover

completely, a remarkable and encouraging fact taking into account that PNH is a clonal disease of marrow stem cells.

Blood picture

The characteristic finding is neutropenia, anaemia, and thrombocytopenia, accompanied by reticulocytosis. The severity of the changes depends upon the proportion of 'sensitive' PNH red cells the patient is forming and the degree to which the bone marrow is hypoplastic. In some patients anaemia is so severe that repeated blood transfusion is necessary; in others it is much less severe and transfusions are seldom if ever required. Reticulocyte counts vary widely from patient to patient and in individual patients from time to time. Thus counts range from less than 1 per cent to about 40 per cent depending upon the severity of haemolysis and the degree to which the marrow is able to respond to the consequent anaemia.

The neutrophil and platelet counts vary widely. Approximately

50 per cent of the patients may be expected to have $< 1.5 \times 10^9/1$ neutrophils and/or $< 50 \times 10^9/1$ platelets at one time or another. The neutrophils are unusual in that they lack alkaline phosphatase.

The appearance of the blood film is usually not remarkable. The red cells vary slightly to moderately in size and shape; polychromasia reflects the reticulocyte count. The MCV is normal or above normal (if the reticulocyte count is raised), the MCH is normal or less than normal where there is iron deficiency. The plasma contains free haemoglobin and is brownish in colour in cases in which haemolysis is active and methaemalbumin is present. Haptoglobins are typically absent. The haemoglobin pattern is typically normal on electrophoresis. However, raised haemoglobin F levels have been recorded in a few patients.

Diagnosis

A positive diagnosis of PNH depends on demonstrating that the patient's red cells are unusually sensitive to lysis by human complement. The 'classic' test is the acidified serum test, often referred to as the Ham test. In this test the red cells to be tested for the PNH abnormality are suspended in fresh normal ABO-compatible serum acidified to a pH of about 6.5. PNH red cells undergo lysis if the suspension is incubated at 37 °C for up to 30–60 min, while normal red cells do not. It is characteristic of PNH that not all the patient's red cells undergo lysis under these circumstances and little or no lysis occurs in unacidified fresh serum at about pH 7.8. PNH red cells are not more sensitive than normal red cells to lysis by acid in the absence of fresh serum. The role of acidification is to activate the alternative (Pillemer) complement pathway and this takes place in the absence of red cell–red cell antibody interaction.

The acidified serum test, if carried out with proper controls, is a sensitive and reliable test for PNH. Subsequent to its introduction, a series of other tests, e.g. the thrombin, sucrose low ionic strength (sugar water), inulin, cobra venom, and cold antibody lysis tests, have been introduced, all similarly depending upon demonstrating the increased sensitivity of PNH red cells to lysis by complement via the alternative or classical pathway. None of these tests, however, seems to have a clear advantage over the simple acidified serum test although they can provide useful confirmation of the diagnosis, and in the writer's view PNH should not be diagnosed unless a properly controlled acidified serum test is clearly positive.

From the clinical point of view it is important not to forget that PNH is a possible diagnosis in any patient presenting with anaemia of obscure origin, particularly if accompanied by a slight to moderate reticulocytosis, neutropenia, and thrombocytopenia, even if the patient's chief (or only) complaint is of abdominal pain. It is wise to carry out the acidified serum test (or the sucrose test) and to look for haemosiderinuria at an early stage in such a patient's investigation.

Treatment

At the time of writing there appears to be no way in which the fundamental defect in the PNH cells can be rectified or neutralized. Patients can, however, be helped in a number of ways. The aim should be to sustain the patient (without doing harm) until recovery takes place. The patient should be told that this is possible.

Blood transfusions

These are the mainstay of treatment for the seriously affected patient. The red cells should preferably be washed to remove as far as possible plasma, leucocytes, and platelets so as to avoid normally harmless antigen–antibody reactions leading to activation of complement by the alternative pathway and consequent exacerbation of haemolysis. This is particularly important in patients receiving a series of transfusions. Because of the haemosiderinuria there is no risk of generalized haemosiderosis.

Corticosteroids

In some acutely ill patients haemolysis has been reduced by their use, but their side-effects should be carefully considered before administering them to a patient with a long-continuing disease.

Androgens

These have been particularly recommended by Hartmann and coworkers. They act as marrow stimulants (useful if the marrow is hypoplastic) and they may also apparently depress haemolysis. However, their potential side-effects are a disadvantage.

Iron

Most, if not all, PNH patients, if seriously affected, eventually become iron deficient as the result of the constant haemosiderinuria. Replacement of the iron is thus necessary. This should be proceed with tentatively, as in some patients the oral or parenteral administration of iron leads to episodes of haemoglobinuria. This is probably the result of stimulation of erythropoiesis by the therapeutic iron and the relatively sudden delivery of complement-sensitive cells into the peripheral blood.

Anticoagulants

Oral anticoagulants or heparin have usually been given to patients suffering from thrombosis. They may be of value: they do not, however, seem to affect the haemolysis as was at one time thought.

Drugs

A variety of drugs has been tried, e.g. vitamin E, 6-mercaptopurine, and pencillamine, but none has been proved to be of value.

Splenectomy

This used to be undertaken quite frequently. It is of dubious value with respect to diminishing the rate of haemolysis and raising the platelet count, and as the procedure may be followed by thrombosis developing within the portal system, it is probably best avoided.

Bone marrow transplantation

Several patients have been treated successfully by allogeneic transplantation of normal bone marrow, and this procedure should certainly be considered if the patient is seriously affected and a suitable donor is available. In two instances where normal marrow from a healthy identical twin was transplanted the marrow was administered without prior chemotherapy aimed at destroying the PNH clone. In both cases, however, the patient's marrow was hypoplastic. Whether normal marrow from a healthy identical twin would gradually replace a PNH clone (in the absence of chemotherapy) if the affected patient's marrow at the time of the transplant was hyperplastic or normoplastic is uncertain. If some PNH clones are less vigorous than normal haemopoietic cells this could happen.

References

Dacie, J. V. and Lewis, S. M. (1972). Paroxysmal nocturnal haemoglobinuria: clinical manifestations, haematology and nature of the disease. *Ser. Haemat.* **5**, 3–23.

Fefer, A., Freeman, H., Storb, R., Hill, J., Singer, J., Edwards, A. and Thomas, E. (1976). Paroxysmal nocturnal hemoglobinuria and marrow failure treated by infusion of marrow from an identical twin. *Ann. intern. Med.* **84**, 692–695.

Hartmann, R. C. and Kolhouse, J. F. (1972). Viewpoints on the management of paroxysmal nocturnal haemoglobinuria (PNH). *Ser. Haemat.* **5**, 42–60.

——, Luther, A. B., Jenkins, D. E. Jnr, Tenorio, L. E. and Saba, H. I. (1980). Fulminent hepatic venous thrombosis (Budd–Chiari syndrome) in paroxysmal nocturnal hemoglobinuria: definition of a medical emergency. *Johns Hopk. med. J.* **146**, 247–254.

Hershko, C., Gale, R. P., Ho, W. G. and Cline, M. J. (1979). Cure of aplastic anaemia in paroxysmal nocturnal haemoglobinuria by marrow transfusion from identical twin: failure of peripheral-leucocyte transfusion to correct marrow aplasia. *Lancet* **i**, 945–947.

Nicholson-Weller, A., March, J. P., Rosenfield, S. I. and Austen, K. F. (1983). Affected erythrocytes of patients with paroxysmal nocturnal hemoglobinuria are deficient in the complement regulatory protein, decay accelerating factor. *Proc. natl. Acad. Sci.* USA **80**, 5066–5070.

Oni, S. B., Osunkoya, B. O. and Luzzatto, L. (1970). Paroxysmal nocturnal hemoglobinuria: evidence for monoclonal origin of abnormal red cells. *Blood* **36**, 145–152.

Pangburn, M. K., Schreiber, R. D. and Müller-Eberhard, H. (1983). Deficiency of an erythrocyte membrane protein with complement regulatory activity in paroxysmal nocturnal hemoglobinuria. *Proc. natl. Acad. Sci. USA* **80**, 5430–5434.

Rosse, W. F. (1973). Variations in the red cells in paroxysmal nocturnal haemoglobinuria. *Br. J. Haemat.* **24**, 327–342.

Storb, R., Evans, R. S., Thomas, E. D., Buckner, C. D., Clift, R. A., Fefer, A., Neiman, P. and Wright, S. E. (1973). Paroxysmal nocturnal haemoglobinuria and refractory marrow failure treated by marrow transplantation. *Br. J. Haemat.* **24**, 743–750.

Myelodysplastic syndromes

D. CATOVSKY

Myelodysplastic syndromes (MDS) are acquired, usually progressive, cytopenias associated with a cellular bone marrow and ineffective haemopoiesis. This pathogenesis should distinguish these disorders from cytopenias caused by peripheral destruction or resulting from aplastic bone marrows. As a rule two or three of the bone marrow cell lineages are involved in MDS but, rarely, only one may be affected. Because anaemia is the most common manifestation these disorders have been designated as refractory anaemias of various types, although the term refractory cytopenia may be more accurate.

Two major types of MDS can be recognized, both carrying an increased risk of transformation to acute myeloid leukaemia (AML): (1) *primary MDS*, the most common, has no known cause, and (2) *secondary MDS*, which results from the use of alkylating agents with or without radiotherapy for the treatment of lymphomas, multiple myeloma or solid tumours. Secondary MDS often precedes the development of overt AML and occurs with a frequency which is in direct relationship to the duration of the cytotoxic therapy often after 3–10 years from diagnosis of the original malignancy.

MDS have been described in the past under many names. Two, preleukaemic syndrome and smouldering acute leukaemia, have been widely used in the United States. The term *preleukaemia* was used to define refractory cytopenias involving two cell lineages but without showing an increase in blast cells in the bone marrow. *Smouldering leukaemia* was used to describe cases with an increase in blast cells but short of the values frequently found in established AML. Recently, a French, American and British (FAB) co-operative group has attempted to subclassify these heterogeneous conditions in order to learn more about their pathogenesis, and management. The new terms used by the FAB classification take into account the blood and bone marrow findings to define the various types of MDS and do not assume the development of AML as inevitable, recognizing that a high proportion of patients die as a consequence of the cytopenias without features of overt leukaemia. MDS are, on the other hand, clonal disorders affecting haemopoietic precursor cells and, as such, they bear a close relationship to AML. In contrast to the latter, myelodysplasia is characterized by functional and morphological abnormalities resulting from a defective haemopoiesis and is not, in its early stages, associated by the monomorphic cell proliferation characteristic of leukaemic processes.

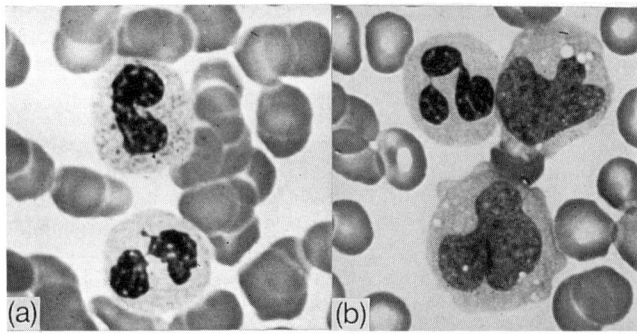

Fig. 1 Peripheral blood cells of MDS. (a) Neutrophils with the Pelger anomaly; (b) Monocytes and a neutrophil from a case of CMML (× 900).

Clinical and laboratory features

MDS affect almost always adults over the age of 50 years. The median age of patients with primary MDS is between 60 and 70 years. Secondary MDS affects, as a rule, younger patients. The disease is rare in children but some well-documented cases have been described.

Anaemia, fever or bleeding manifestations are the most common presenting symptoms. There are usually few, if any, significant physical signs. Splenomegaly is found in 20 per cent of cases, more often associated with one of the forms of MDS, chronic myelomonocytic leukaemia (CMML).

The key elements for diagnosis, in the presence of persistent and otherwise unexplained cytopenia, are the examination of peripheral blood and bone marrow.

Haematological findings

Anaemia (haemoglobin less than 12 g/dl) is the most constant feature; it is usually normocytic and normochromic, or moderately macrocytic (MCV greater than 104 fl). The red cells may show anisopoikylocytosis, polychromasia, punctate basophilia and, commonly, nucleated forms with dyserythropoietic features. Reticulocyte counts are, as a rule, low (< 0.5 per cent) (Fig. 1).

The white cell count is variable, often low (< 4×10^9/l) and, less commonly, normal. Leucocytosis with a monocytosis is only a feature of CMML. Neutropenia (< 1×10^9/l) is seen in one-third of cases depending on the type of MDS: it is almost always severe in cases in transformation to AML and it is rare in sideroblastic anaemia. A common finding in the blood films of MDS patients is the presence of abnormal neutrophils: (*a*) hypogranular or agranular forms, with absence or marked reduction of azurophil granules and/or specific secondary granules, (*b*) cells with a round or bilobed nucleus (acquired Pelger anomaly), and (*c*) hypersegmented neutrophils. A proportion of myelocytes and blasts may be present depending on the type of MDS. Cytochemical reactions for myeloperoxidase or Sudan Black B can highlight the neutrophil abnormalities by demonstrating two populations of neutrophils, positive, as normal cells, and negative, due to the absence of primary granules.

Thrombocytopenia (platelets less than 100×10^9/l) is less frequent than anaemia and neutropenia, again depending on the type of MDS. It is seen with higher frequency in CMML (two-thirds of cases) and in cases with increased bone marrow blasts or in transformation to AML. The blood film may show large or even giant platelets and, rarely, megakaryocyte fragments.

Bone marrow

The marrow is always normocellular or hypercellular displaying characteristic quantitative and qualitative changes with maturation defects in two or three of the cell lineages. These features are summarized in Table 1. The presence of ringed sideroblasts (detected by the Prussian blue stain) is a feature of acquired idiopathic sideroblastic anaemia (AISA) in which over 20 per cent of

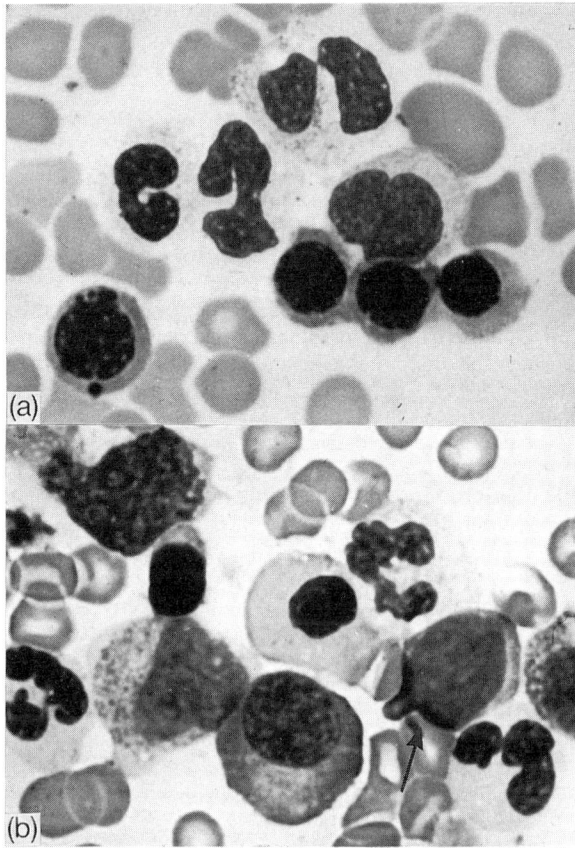

Fig. 2 Bone marrow appearances in MDS. (a) Erythroblasts from a case of refractory anaemia; one of them shows nuclear fragments. (b) Cells from a case of refractory anaemia with excess of blasts. Note a blast cell (arrow), hypogranular neutrophils and a late erythroblast with megaloblastic features (× 900).

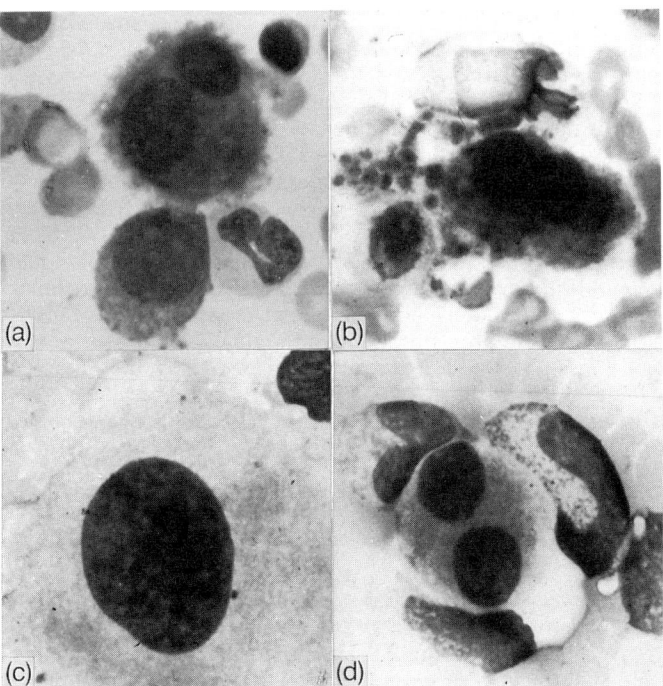

Fig. 3 Qualitative abnormalities of megakaryocytes. (a, b, d) Binucleated or trinucleated micromegakaryocytes. (c) Large mononuclear form (× 900).

Table 1 Features of myelodysplasia in the bone marrow cell lineages

Dyserythropoiesis: ringed sideroblasts; nuclear fragments; multinuclearity; abnormal nuclear shape; karyorrhexis; cytoplasmic vacuolation; megaloblastic changes (Fig. 2)

Dysgranulopoiesis: agranular or hypogranular neutrophils and myelocytes; hyposegmented nucleus (Pelger anomaly); hypersegmented forms with bizarre shapes; blasts with few or no granules; irregular distribution of the cytoplasmic basophilia

Dysmegakaryopoiesis: micromegakaryocytes; large mononuclear forms; megakaryocytes with multiple small round nuclei; small cells with bilobed nuclei (Fig. 3)

the erythroblasts display the typical ring perinuclear arrangement of siderotic granules (see page 19.130). Ringed sideroblasts are also seen in 20–30 per cent of cases of the other types of MDS. Ultrastructural studies have shown that these granules result from the deposition of iron in the mitochondria and from aggregates of ferritin particles in the cytoplasm (see page 19.131). Nuclear abnormalities in the erythroblasts, including cells with single, double, or more, indentations, and abnormal cytoplasmic features of various types are characteristic of dyserythropoiesis and are seen in the majority of patients with MDS (Fig. 2). Dysgranulopoiesis is more marked in cases with excess marrow blasts. In addition to the abnormalities seen in the neutrophils, promyelocytes, and myelocytes may show sparse granularity or coarse azurophil granules.

The presence of blast cells in the marrow is one of the main features considered for the classification of MDS. Two types of blasts have been recognized as significant: type I, with absent cytoplasmic granules, and type II with few azurophil granules. Promyelocytes are distinguished from blasts by their eccentric nucleus with a clear zone in its vicinity (corresponding to the Golgi zone at ultrastructural level), the presence of numerous azurophil granules, a low nuclear/cytoplasmic ratio and a more condensed nuclear chromatin pattern compared with that seen in both types of blast cells.

Megakaryocytes may be decreased in number or show the qualitative abnormalities listed in Table 1 (Fig. 3). The degree of dysmyelopoiesis, in particular dysgranulopoiesis and dysmegakaryopoiesis, has been shown to correlate with progression to AML.

Bone marrow trephine biopsy
With a cytopenia and a leucoerythroblastic blood picture a marrow biopsy is essential to exclude hypoplastic anaemia, chronic idiopathic myelofibrosis and infiltration by neoplastic cells (see page 19.43). The features of dysmyelopoiesis are best analysed in plastic-embedded marrow biopsy specimens and semithin sections (3 µm) which should include stains for reticulin fibres. Marrow fibrosis is not a feature of primary MDS but it is not rare in secondary MDS. The megakaryocytic abnormalities are better appreciated in these preparations than in films obtained from aspirates. The trephine biopsy is as a rule hypercellular in MDS, with little remaining fat spaces. The abnormal localization of immature precursors (ALIP), e.g. clusters of blasts in the central spaces of the marrow and not along the endosteal spaces where they are normally found, has been considered a distinct feature of MDS. The presence of ALIP correlates well with the presence of blasts as seen in aspirates in cases with more than 5 per cent blasts in the marrow. In addition, cases in which the aspirates do not show an excess of blasts may show ALIP clusters recognized only by trephine biopsies. This is important because the presence of ALIP seems to be associated with worse prognosis and with a higher probability of developing AML.

Classification of MDS

The FAB classification (Table 2) has been found to be reproducible and a basis for comparisons between different series. The

Table 2 FAB classification of MDS

Disease (abbreviation)	Percentage of blasts	
	BM	PB
Refractory anaemia (RA) RA with ringed sideroblasts (RAS)	< 5	< 5
RA with excess of blasts (RAEB) Chronic myelomonocytic leukaemia (CMML)*	5–20	< 5
RAEB in transformation (RAEB-t)	> 20–30	≥5[†]

Bennett *et al.* (1982).
* Absolute monocytosis (> 1×10^9/l).
[†] Or Auer rods in granulocyte precursors.
BM, bone marrow; PB, peripheral blood.

main features considered for the classification, in the presence of dysmyelopoiesis, are (*a*) the proportion of marrow blasts (< 5 per cent, 5–20 per cent and between 20 and 30 per cent), (*b*) the presence of ringed sideroblasts, (*c*) blood monocytosis, and (*d*) the presence of blasts in the blood and/or Auer rods (see Table 2).

The five categories of MDS should not be considered as rigid entities. Progression from one to another, usually from RA to RAEB and from RAEB to RAEB-t (see Table 2 for further explanation) is frequently seen. In addition, all of them have been shown to progress to AML although with different frequency.

Refractory anaemia (RA)
Patients with refractory anaemia (RA) often have a macrocytic anaemia with erythroid hyperplasia in the marrow but with ineffective erythropoiesis, as shown by ferrokinetic studies. Neutropenia and/or thrombocytopenia are frequently associated features although very rarely they can be seen without anaemia. Blast cells are rarely found in the blood and are not prominent in the marrow either. Ringed sideroblasts are absent or seen in less than 15 per cent of the nucleated red cells. Infections and bleeding are the main clinical problems and these depend on the severity of the cytopenia. Evolution to AML is not uncommon. The relative incidence of RA within MDS cases is between 20 and 30 per cent.

Refractory anaemia with ringed sideroblasts (RAS)
This condition is characterized by anaemia with erythroid hyperplasia and the presence of ringed sideroblasts in the marrow (see page 19.130). Deficient haemoglobinization of some of the red cell precursors results in a dimorphic blood picture; platelet and white cell counts are often normal. It has a chronic course with a lower risk of evolution to AML than other types of MDS. The risk may be greater in cases with abnormalities of platelets and/or granulocytes; it is low in cases involving only the erythroid series. The frequency of this disease within the MDS group has varied in different series according to whether pure erythroid cases or those with involvement of other cell lineages were included; the incidence in two recent studies was 14–15 per cent.

Refractory anaemia with excess of blasts (RAEB)
The characteristic of this group is the presence of 5 per cent or of more type I or II blasts in the marrow, up to 20 per cent. Cytopenias involving the three cell lineages are common and are associated with marked dysplastic changes in the marrow, particularly dysgranulopoiesis and dysmegakaryopoiesis (see Table 1). Ringed sideroblasts are present in one-third of cases. The frequency of RAEB has varied from 18 per cent to 34 per cent in different series. This condition has a higher incidence of bleeding complications, infections due to neutropenia and evolution to AML than RA and RAS. Patients with RAEB have an equal chance of dying as a result of marrow failure or leukaemic transformation. In a proportion of patients without severe cytopenia the condition may remain stable for many months or even years. It

is this group which has influenced the need to distinguish RAEB from *de novo* AML (> 30 per cent blasts in the marrow) and RAEB-t (> 20 per cent and up to 30 per cent blasts) because of their very different prognoses.

RAEB in transformation (RAEB-t)
This group differs from RAEB in that there are over 20 per cent (up to 30 per cent) of blasts in the marrow and/or 5 per cent or more blasts in the blood, and/or presence of Auer rods in the granulocyte precursors. RAEB-t has been described in order to define a group with intermediate features between MDS and AML. The incidence is of the order of 10 per cent and the poor prognosis of these patients, median survival of 3–5 months in three series, suggests that the clinical behaviour of RAEB-t, if untreated, is not very different from that of *de novo* AML. More information is still required to establish whether any of the specific features of RAEB-t carry the same ominous prognosis.

Chronic myelomonocytic leukaemia (CMML)
It is not generally agreed whether CMML should be considered a MDS or a myeloproliferative disorder. The appearances of the marrow are similar to RAEB, but with prominence of promonocytes which morphologically may resemble promyelocytes. The blood, on the other hand, is characterized by neutrophilia and monocytosis (> 1×10^9/l) and the only consistent cytopenia is thrombocytopenia which is often responsible for bleeding manifestations. In contrast to other MDS, 20 per cent of CMML patients have moderate splenomegaly. Gum hypertrophy and lymphadenopathy, a feature of acute myelomonocytic leukaemia (page 19.20) is not seen in CMML. The incidence of CMML within the various MDS series is between 5 and 20 per cent. Some patients of CMML are diagnosed as atypical (Ph negative) chronic myeloid leukaemia (see page 19.28), although in the latter condition a higher proportion of immature granulocytes are present in the blood and the clinical course is shorter than in CMML. CMML patients are often elderly and the disease runs a chronic course; but evolution to AML is always a possibility.

Differential diagnosis
MDS should be distinguished from other types of anaemias and from overt leukaemias. Other causes of aregenerative chronic anaemia, e.g. caused by renal or liver disease should always be excluded by appropriate investigations (page 19.91). In cases of RA it is important to exclude nutritional anaemias by measuring iron, vitamin B_{12} and folic acid levels. Even if this has been done it is customary to initiate a trial of treatment with vitamin B_{12}, folic acid, and/or pyridoxine. As a rule patients with MDS will not respond. The guidelines of the percentages of blasts in RAEB and RAEB-t are useful to distinguish these two conditions from established AML. One type of AML, erythroleukaemia, characterized by bizarre erythroid hyperplasia and increased numbers of blasts, may still present problems in the differential diagnosis with these two forms of MDS. This difficulty often arises from the variability in the overall percentage of erythroblasts in erythroleukaemia. To overcome this problem the FAB group has recently proposed that if more than 50 per cent of erythroblasts are present in the marrow, the diagnosis of erythroleukaemia may still be possible if 30 per cent or more of the non-erythroid cells (excluding erythroblasts) are blasts, even if the *total* percentage of blasts is less than 30 per cent.

Chromosome abnormalities
Clonal karyotypic abnormalities can be demonstrated in the marrows of 50–70 per cent of MDS patients. The incidence of chromosome abnormalities in secondary MDS is between 90 and 100 per cent. The most frequent abnormalities in MDS are listed in Table 3. These involve numerical or structural changes of chromosomes 5, 7 and 8 which are affected with equal frequency. All these chromosome changes are seen also in AML. On the other hand, none

Table 3 Chromosome abnormalities in MDS*

Monosomy or deletion of chromosome 5 (-5 or 5q$-$)
Monosomy or deletion of chromosome 7 (-7 or 7q$-$)
Trisomy 8 ($+8$)
Trisomy 19 or 21 ($+19$ or $+21$)
Deletion 20q$-$

 * *Second International Workshop* (1980); Nowell (1982).

Table 4 Prognostic factors in MDS

Age > 60 years
Severity of the cytopenias*
Degree of myelodysplasia[†]
Bone marrow and peripheral blood blasts > 5 per cent
FAB classification
ALIP[‡] in bone marrow biopsies
Karyotypic abnormalities
Pattern of growth in culture

 * Hb $\leq$ 10 g/dl, platelets $\leq$ 100 $\times$ 10^9/l and neutrophils $\leq$ 2.5 $\times$ 10^9/l in the Bournemouth score (Mufti *et al.*, 1985); varying levels of neutrophils and platelets in the FAB score (Varela *et al.*, 1985).
 [†] Dysgranulopoiesis and dysmegakaryopoiesis (Varela *et al.*, 1985).
 [‡] Abnormal localization of immature precursors, i.e. clusters of blast cells in the centre of the bone marrow spaces as opposed to their normal localization along the endosteal surface (Tricot *et al.*, 1984).

of the changes associated with specific types of AML, such as t(8; 21) in myeloblastic or t(15; 17) in promyelocytic leukaemia are found in MDS (see page 19.20). The Philadelphia chromosome, t(9; 22), is not found either in MDS patients. Some of the abnormalities have been described in association with particular types of MDS. For example 5q$-$ has been found mainly in RA or RAEB patients with macrocytic anaemia, normal white cell counts, normal or increased platelet counts, and dyserythropoiesis and distinct micromegakaryocytes in the marrow. Monosomy 7 has been associated with abnormal neutrophil function.

The frequency of abnormalities is greater in cases with more than 5 per cent blasts in the marrow, i.e. RAEB and RAEB-t. Similarly, the evolution to AML is high (75 per cent) in cases with complex karyotype abnormalities, and twice as high in MDS cases with abnormalities than in those without them. In addition to its prognostic significance, the presence of an abnormal karyotype is important in the differential diagnosis between MDS and non-preleukaemic anaemias.

Bone marrow culture studies

In vitro cultures in semisolid media that support the growth of haemopoietic precursor cells (see page 19.7), e.g. cells forming granulocyte/macrophage colonies or CFU-GM, have been used to predict the progression of MDS to AML. This is often associated with an increase in cluster formation and/or a decrease in the number of colonies formed. The abnormalities in *in vitro* growth observed in MDS are similar to those observed in acute leukaemia.

Prognosis

Despite the chronic course of some cases, most series have shown that the median survival of patients with MDS ranges between 15 and 27 months. The main causes of death are complications resulting from the cytopenias, i.e. bleeding and infections, and evolution to acute leukaemia.

A number of prognostic factors have been identified by several studies (Table 4). Most of them are closely interrelated so that it is difficult to identify which is the more important. The severity of the cytopenia, chiefly neutropenia and thrombocytopenia, will have a direct bearing in some of the complications. An increase in blast cells, which is one of the determinants of the FAB classification (see Table 2), is one of the bad prognostic features. Patients with < 5 per cent of marrow blasts, e.g. RA and RAS, have median survivals from 2 to 5 years in some series. The longest survivals are found in RAS when features of dyshaemopoiesis, other than the presence of ringed sideroblasts, are absent. The presence of ALIP (page 19.59) identified in marrow trephine biopsies is a poor prognostic finding in patients with RA and RAS even if the marrow aspirates show less than 5 per cent blasts; it is associated particularly with transformation to AML.

A simple scoring system has been proposed which takes into account the degree of cytopenia (Table 4) and the percentage of marrow blasts (above or below 5 per cent). In a series of 141 MDS patients, those with high scores had a statistically significant shorter survival than those with low scores. This system appears to recognize good and bad prognostic subgroups within patients with RA, RAS and RAEB. Another scoring system is based on the levels of neutrophils and platelets (quantitative components) and of dysgranulopoiesis and dysmegakaryopoiesis. The latter was found to be best for predicting the evolution to AML, whilst the overall score was important in predicting survival.

Complications

Infections due to neutropenia and bleeding due to thrombocytopenia are the main problems encountered in the management of MDS. Interestingly, these two factors are the most common causes of death in patients with RA and RAS. Patients with RAEB have an equal chance of dying of these complications or of a leukaemic evolution.

Progression to AML

An evolution towards AML is the inevitable outcome in 25–50 per cent of RAEB and CMML patients, and in greater than 50 per cent of those with RAEB-t. This course is less common in RA and RAS (5–15 per cent of cases); both in RA and RAS the findings of ALIP in marrow biopsy specimens may help predict the leukaemic evolution. Similarly, complex cytogenetic abnormalities and a high cluster to colony ratio in CFU-GM cultures, particularly if they progress, may precede the leukaemia changes.

Secondary MDS

This condition is seen now with increasing frequency in younger patients who have been treated for prolonged periods with alkylating agents for neoplastic or non-neoplastic conditions. Many cases of secondary AML evolve through a phase of MDS. Several factors may help to distinguish secondary from primary MDS. Secondary MDS show early macrocytosis, a hypocellular marrow or an increase in reticulin fibres leading, sometimes, to myelofibrosis. The risk of secondary MDS and AML increases with the duration of exposure and may vary according to the type of cytotoxic agent used. In myelomatosis the use of melphalan for more than 3 years is associated with a 10 per cent risk of MDS and AML in those surviving 5 years.

Treatment

Because of the life-threatening nature of MDS, the choice of active treatment to induce a remission or simple supportive care to protect the patient from the effects of the cytopenia must be made with extreme care. Anaemia without other evidence of marrow failure could always be supported by blood transfusions. As stated earlier, a therapeutic trial of folic acid, pyridoxine, and/or vitamin B$_{12}$ should always be considered to identify responsive anaemias. For moderate neutropenias, oral antibiotics or antifungal agents should be given at the first sign of infection. For patients with more than 5 per cent blasts, or with marked cytopenia, supportive measures may not be enough to prolong survival. Anabolic steroids and glucocorticosteroids, although widely used in the past, are not indicated for the treatment of MDS.

In the last few years a number of agents which induce differentiation and maturation of leukaemic cells have been used to treat patients with MDS. Some of these, like cytosine arabinoside (Ara-C), are already known to be effective in AML by their cytotoxic effect. Ara-C has been used in MDS at low doses (5–10 mg/m^2 twice a day), initially for 2 or 3 weeks, in order to induce haematological remissions. Although the exact mechanism of action of low-dose Ara-C is still not clear, i.e. inhibition of DNA synthesis and/or differentiation induction in myeloid cells, this agent has been shown to induce complete remissions in 20–30 per cent of cases. Despite its differentiating effect patients treated with low-dose Ara-C often undergo a transient deterioration of their cytopenia during the early stages of treatment, and should therefore receive effective supportive care with blood products and antibiotics until a full response is obtained.

Other agents that induce differentiation have also been used in MDS, e.g. cis-retinoic acid and 1,25-dihydroxyvitamin D3, but with only short-lived responses. Intensive combination chemotherapy, as used in AML, should be considered for younger patients, including those with MDS. The documentation of complete remissions with normal haematopoietic regeneration in patients treated by these regimens demonstrates that normal stem cells are still present in myelodysplastic bone marrows. Supralethal therapy with drugs and total body irradiation followed by a bone marrow transplant from an HLA-identical sibling has been tried with some success in younger patients with primary and secondary MDS.

The choice of treatment in MDS depends on a number of factors of which patients' age and prognostic features are the most important. Even if a decision for active treatment is considered it is not clear at the present time which are the best agents or drug combinations. Randomized control trials of conservative supportive care versus low-dose Ara-C or low-dose Ara-C in combination with cis-retinoic acid are being pursued at the present time.

References

Bennett, J. M., Catovsky, D., Daniel, M. T., Flandrin, G., Galton, D. A. G., Gralnick, H. R. and Sultan, C. (1982). Proposals for the classification of the myelodysplastic syndromes. Br. J. Haematol. 51, 189–199.

Coiffier, B., Adeleine, P., Viala, J. J., Bryon, P. A., Fiere, D., Gentilhomme, O. and Vuvan, H. (1983). Dysmyelopoietic syndromes. A search for prognostic factors in 193 patients. Cancer 52, 83–90.

Galton, D. A. G. (1984). The myelodysplastic syndromes. Clin. Lab. Haematol. 6, 99–112.

Juneja, S. K., Imbert, M., Jouault, H., Scoazec, J-Y, Sigaux, F. and Sultan, C. (1983). Haematological features of primary myelodysplastic syndromes (PMDS) at initial presentation: a study of 118 cases. J. Clin. Pathol. 36, 1129–1135.

Mufti, G. J., Stevens, J. R., Oscier, D. G., Hamblin, T. J. and Machin, D. (1985). Myelodysplastic syndromes: a scoring system with prognostic significance. Br. J. Haematol. 59, 425–433.

Nowell, P. C. (1982). Cytogenetics of preleukemia. Cancer Genet. Cytogenet. 5, 265–278.

Second International Workshop on Chromosomes in Leukemia, 1979 (1980). Chromosomes in preleukemia. Cancer Genet. Cytogenet. 2, 108–113.

Sokal, G., Michaux, J. L., Van den Berghe, H., Cordier, A., Rodhain, J., Ferrant, A., Moriau, M., De Bruyere, M. and Sonnet, J. (1975). A new haematologic syndrome with a distinct karyotype: The 5q– chromosome. Blood 46, 519–533.

Tricot, G., De Wolf-Peeters, C., Hendrickx, B. and Verwilghen, R. L. (1984). Bone marrow histology in myelodysplastic syndromes. I. Histological findings in myelodysplastic syndromes and comparison with bone marrow smears. Br. J. Haematol. 57, 423–430.

——, Vlietinck, R., Boogaerts, M. A., Hendrickx, B., De Wolf-Peeters, C., Van den Berghe, H. and Verwilghen, R. L. (1985). Prognostic factors in the myelodysplastic syndromes: importance of initial data on peripheral blood counts, bone marrow cytology, trephine biopsy and chromosomal analysis. Br. J. Haematol. 60, 19–32.

Varela, B. L., Chuang, C., Woll, J. E. and Bennett, J. M. (1985). Modifications in the classification of primary myelodysplastic syndromes: the addition of a scoring system. J. Hematol. Oncol. 3, 55–63.

THE RED CELL

Erythropoiesis and the normal red cell

D. J. WEATHERALL

The circulating red cells and their nucleated precursors in the bone marrow comprise a functional unit called the erythron. As an introduction to the disorders of the red cells we shall consider the morphological and biochemical characteristics of erythropoiesis, i.e. the formation of red cells, and what is known about the regulation of the erythron.

Erythropoiesis

In order to appreciate the pathophysiology of anaemia and the complex compensatory mechanisms which are brought into play to maintain oxygenation of the tissues in patients with anaemia it is necessary to have a broad understanding of the way in which red cells are produced and how this is regulated.

The early stages of erythropoiesis

As described in the previous section, the red cell precursors are derived fom pluripotential stem cells by a differentiation step, the regulation and nature of which is still not understood. Recently, different populations of erythroid precursors have been defined which are probably part of the early committed erythroid population but which cannot be recognized as such under the microscope. Using either plasma clots or methyl cellulose as supporting

media it has been possible to grow colonies of these erythroid precursors from mononuclear cells derived from human fetal or adult bone marrow or peripheral blood (see also page 19.10). The first colonies to appear are small and consist of about 8–16 cells; they are usually fully developed after a few days of incubation. After a longer period in culture larger colonies or 'bursts' appear that are made up of several thousand cells. The growth of these colonies depends on the presence of erythropoietin in the media. The cells which give rise to the small colonies are called CFU-E (colony-forming units, erythroid), and those which produce the 'bursts' are called erythropoietin-dependent burst forming units, or BFU-E. It seems very likely that the CFU-E are the more differentiated of the two and are probably close to proerythroblasts in the differentiation pathway. On the other hand, the BFU-E are probably a much earlier population and are less sensitive to erythropoietin.

Nothing is known about the stimulus for the differentiation of early BFU-E from pluripotential stem cells. They require a factor (or factors) termed 'burst promoting activity' for in vitro growth. Furthermore, under certain experimental conditions they require the presence of T lymphocytes for their growth in culture.

Current ideas about the function and regulation of BFU-E and CFU-E are shown in Fig. 1. It is believed that the BFU-E form an amplification compartment which can respond to the requirements for erythropoiesis by rapid contraction or expansion. During maturation of the BFU-E their sensitivity to erythropoietin increases; by the time they reach the CFU-E stage they are highly

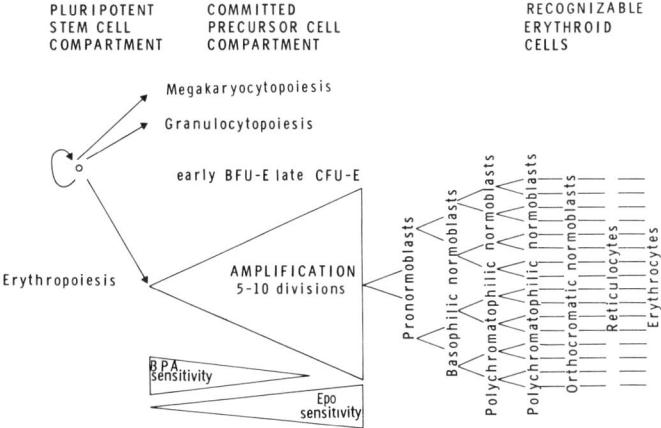

Fig. 1 Schematic representation of the various levels of erythropoiesis. (BPA = burst promoting activity; Epo = erythropoietin). The details of the different compartments are described in the text.

responsive to this hormone. The CFU-E mature directly into pronormoblasts which are the first cells in the erythroid maturation pathway that can be recognized morphologically.

Morphological and biochemical development of the red cell

The total maturation time of the identifiable red cell precursors in the bone marrow is approximately seven days. The first four days are spent in cell division; approximately 16 daughter cells are produced from each primitive red cell precursor (Fig. 2). The remaining three days are devoted to maturation and haemoglobin synthesis, and during this period the nucleus is extruded. The red cell precursor, which is now called a reticulocyte, remains in the marrow for a further 24 hours and then moves into the peripheral circulation where it matures into a red cell in approximately one day. Since about 1 per cent of the total red cell mass is destroyed every 24 hours, in normal individuals there is a comparable number of reticulocytes delivered daily into the circulation.

The earliest recognizable red cell precursor is the basophilic pronormoblast. This is a large cell with a diameter of about 24 μm. It has a deep-blue staining cytoplasm indicating that there is, as yet, no haemoglobin present. After several cell divisions there are well-marked maturation changes both in the nucleus and in the cytoplasm. The next maturation stage is the polychromatophilic normoblast, which has a pink cytoplasm indicating that haemoglobin synthesis has commenced. The nucleus is smaller than that of the pronormoblast and the chromatin is starting to clump. By the fourth maturation division the cells reach the orthochromatic normoblast stage, in which the cytoplasm is uniformly pink and the nuclear chromatin is highly condensed. The nucleus is then lost from the cell which becomes a reticulocyte, i.e. a cell containing some residual RNA and other organelles which, on supravital staining, clump and produce a characteristic appearance on light microscopy. It is estimated that between 5 and 10 per cent of the red cell precursors are lost during their passage through the marrow. As we shall see later, in certain disorders of red cell maturation this level of 'ineffective erythropoiesis' is considerably elevated above the normal baseline.

These morphological changes of red cell maturation are accompanied by important alterations in the chemistry of the red cell precursors. The early forms have a well-formed Golgi apparatus and mitochondria. They are capable of DNA, RNA, and protein synthesis, and oxidative metabolism. At the polychromatophilic normoblast phase of development, DNA and RNA synthesis cease. After further maturation the mitochondria and RNA are lost and the cell is then able to metabolize glucose only through

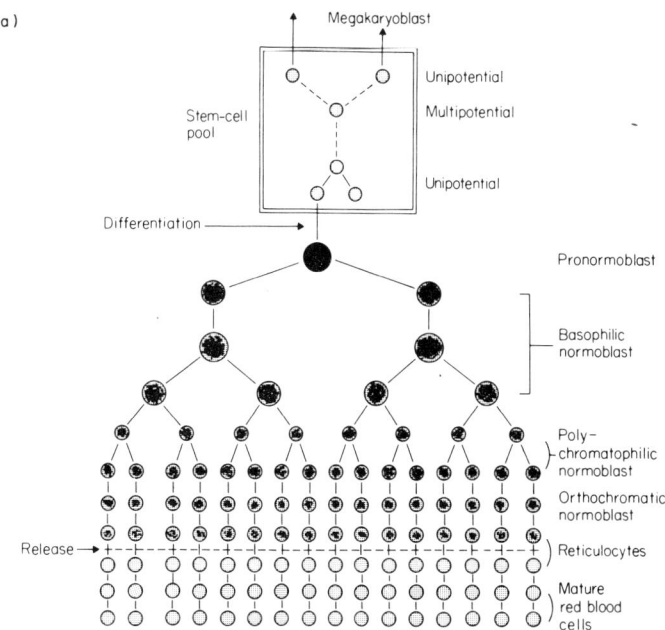

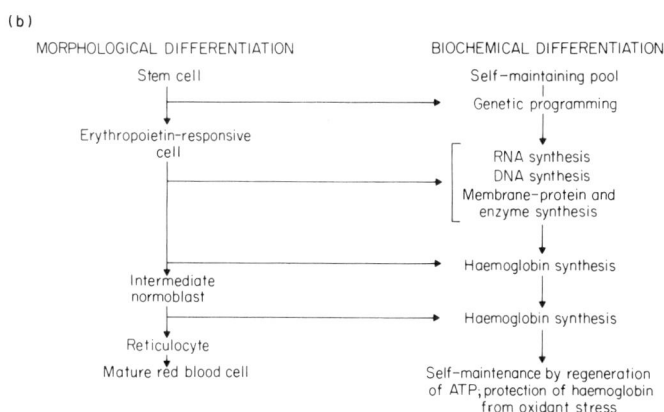

Fig. 2 Erythropoiesis. (a) A schematic representation of the main steps involved in the maturation of red cells. (Reproduced by permission of Dr A. Erslev.) (b) The relationship between morphological differentiation and biochemical differentiation.

the anaerobic Embden–Meyerhof pathway. In addition, the mature cell has a hexose monophosphate shunt which normally provides little energy but which is of great importance in protecting the cell against oxidative damage. At first sight this seems to be a very simple and unsophisticated biochemical factory with which to go out into the turbulent world of the peripheral circulation. But as we shall see later it is beautifully suited to the needs of a cell which has to traverse a microcirculation and deal with the metabolically unfavourable environment of the circulation and, particularly, the spleen.

Regulation of erythropoiesis

It has been known for many years that the main stimulus to erythropoiesis is the degree of oxygenation of the tissues. It is now clear that information on the level of tissue oxygenation is transferred to the blood-forming organs by the action of a hormone called erythropoietin which is capable of stimulating erythropoiesis.

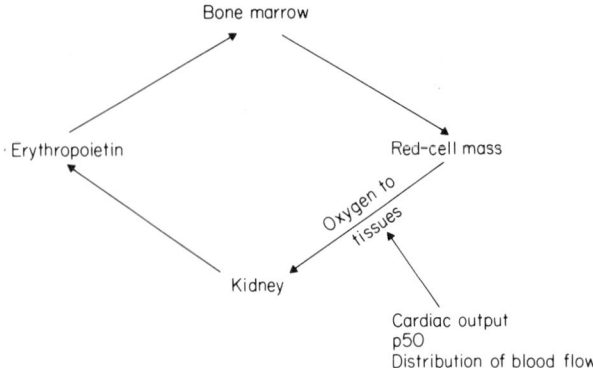

Fig. 3 The regulation of red cell production.

Thus, if the haemoglobin level falls or if the oxygen supply to the tissues is reduced in other ways, there is an increased production of erythropoietin which stimulates the bone marrow to increase the output of red cells until oxygen delivery is restored to normal. This is an elegant example of a biological feedback loop (Fig. 3).

Erythropoietin is a sialoglycoprotein with a molecular weight of approximately 33 000. Recently, it has been purified to homogeneity and the gene which regulates its structure has been cloned, introduced into micro-organisms, and persuaded to produce active erythropoietin. These remarkable advances should allow the development of an accurate radioimmune assay and the production of erythropoietin for therapeutic purposes. The normal concentration of erythropoitin in plasma has been estimated to be about 0.02 units/ml. Approximately 4.0 units are excreted in the urine daily. The half-life of erythropoietin in the plasma appears to be less than 5 hours; less than 10 per cent is excreted in the urine and the bulk is metabolized in the liver.

It is now believed that the kidney is the major site of erythropoietin production, although doubts remain as to whether the hormone is secreted in an active form or must first interact with a substrate in the plasma. During fetal life the liver is the major site of production. Anephric humans produce some erythropoietin although at a low rate. Extrarenal erythropoietin is immunologically identical to renal erythropoietin.

Erythropoietin does not act on stem cells but only on progenitors in the committed erythroid compartment. There is increasing sensitivity to the hormone during the transition from BFU-E to CFU-E. Its mode of action is not yet understood. It stimulates RNA synthesis and there is some evidence that its action requires the participation of a small protein messenger analagous to cytoplasmic steroid receptor molecules. It causes an increased rate of protein synthesis in red cell precursors, an increased rate of cell division, and a more rapid transit time of red cell precursors through the bone marrow. It appears to be the physiological regulator of erythropoiesis. However, there is evidence that other hormones and related agents affect red cell production. These include corticosteroids, androgens, growth hormone, thyroxine, β adrenergic agonists, cyclic AMP, and certain prostaglandins, all of which have a stimulatory effect on erythroid colony production. The existence of receptors for these agents on red cell progenitors provides a mechanism whereby modulation of response of the erythroid cells to erythropoietin may be mediated.

The fact that erythropoiesis is regulated by a hormone which is produced by the kidney has important clinical implications. For example, the anaemia of renal disease is at least in part due to defective production of erythropoietin. Some renal tumours synthesize erythropoietin and cause polycythaemia. Severe hypoxia, as occurs in chronic lung disease or congenital heart disease, is associated with a marked drive to erythropoietin production and hence a variable increase in red cell output. Further examples of the clinical importance of erythropoietin will be considered in later sections.

The factors required for normal erythropoiesis

There are several factors which are essential for the normal function of the bone marrow. Iron is required for haemoglobin synthesis and also seems to have a direct effect on the regulation of erythroid proliferation. Vitamin B_{12} and folate are required for normal DNA synthesis and hence for nuclear maturation. A detailed account of the metabolism of iron, vitamin B_{12}, and folate is given later in this section. It has been suggested that certain other vitamins including pyridoxine, ascorbic acid, riboflavin, and vitamin E are essential for erythropoiesis in humans, but it has been difficult to provide good evidence that this is the case. Similarly, certain trace elements such as copper, manganese, cobalt, and zinc may also be required; animals deprived of these metals show abnormalities of erythropoiesis. However, the relevance of these observations to human disease is not clear.

The red cell

The mature red cell is a biconcave disc, 7.5 μm in diameter, 2.5 μm thick at the periphery, and 1 μm thick at the centre. This shape provides an optimal surface area for respiratory exchange. The cell is composed of about 70 per cent water, the remainder consisting of haemoglobin and small amounts of lipid, sugar, and enzyme proteins.

The red cell has two main functions. First, it must maintain itself in the circulation for about 120 days. Second, it must maintain its haemoglobin in a state which is suitable for oxygen transport during this time. In describing the functions of the red cell we have to consider separately its three major components, membrane, haemoglobin, and metabolic pathways. However, it is important to appreciate that each of these are dependent on one another and can interact to modulate oxygen transport, protect haemoglobin from oxidant damage, and maintain the constancy of the osmotic environment of the cell.

Membrane

A diagram of the structure of the red cell membrane is shown in Fig. 4. It is composed of lipids, carbohydrates, and protein. Essentially, it consists of a lipid bilayer with intercollated proteins and glycoproteins. The carbohydrates are mainly glycolipids and glycoproteins. The mature red cell does not synthesize lipids *de novo*, and several lipid components, particularly cholesterol, exchange with lipids in the plasma. There are two main classes of membrane proteins, the peripheral proteins and the integral membrane proteins. The former make up an extensive submembranous reticulum called the red cell cytoskeleton which is responsible for the shape, integrity, and flexibility of the red cell membrane. The basic building block of the cytoskeleton is the spectrin tetramer. The integral membrane proteins consist of an anion transport protein, a glucose transport protein and the sialoglycoproteins, glycophorins A, B, and C. The anion transport protein is the predominant integral protein and makes up 25 per cent of the membrane protein which is equivalent to 1.2×10^6 copies per red cell. It is involved in the transport of HCO_3^- and Cl^-. The membrane also has a variety of transport systems, including Na^+, K^+–ATPase which is involved in the transport of Na^+ out of and K^+ into the cell, Ca^{2+}, Mg^{2+}–ATPase, and acetyl cholinesterase. These membrane pumps are of critical importance for maintaining electrolyte homeostasis in the red cell. Sodium is actively pumped from the cell against a concentration gradient of 10 mEq/1 inside the cell to 145 mEq/1 in the plasma. Potassium, on the other hand, is pumped into the cell against a concentration gradient of about 4.5 mEq/1 in the plasma to 100 mEq/1 in the cell. The calcium/magnesium pump mediates calcium efflux against a 50 to 100-fold concentration gradient, converting one molecule of ATP to ADP for each two molecules of Ca^{2+} extruded. The membrane also has several protein kinases.

The critical functions of the red cell of maintaining its shape and deformability are mediated by these different components of its

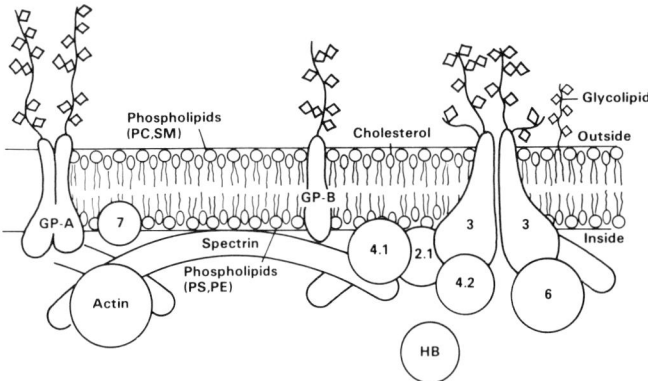

Fig. 4 A diagram of the red cell membrane showing the relationship of integral and internal membrane proteins to the lipid bilayer. The numbers refer to individual membrane proteins. GPA and GPB are glycophorins A and B; PC phosphatidylcholine; SM sphingomyelin; PS phosphatidylserine; PE phosphatidylethanolamine. (Reproduced with permission from Brain, M. C., 1982, *Blood and its disorders*, 2nd edn (eds R. M. Hardisty and D. J. Weatherall), p. 455. Blackwell Scientific Publications, Oxford.)

membrane. Considerable amounts of energy are required for the pumping activities needed to maintain the constancy of the electrolyte environment of the red cell. These functions can be modulated by hormones, cyclic nucleotides, calcium, and calmodulin. In later sections we shall see how primary or secondary abnormalities of the membrane lead to changes in function and hence to premature destruction of red cells.

Haemoglobin

The major haemoglobin of adult red cells, haemoglobin A, is a tetramer of two α and two β chains consisting of 141 and 146 amino acids, respectively. The heterogeneity and genetic control of haemoglobin is considered in a later section (page 19.108). Each globin chain is attached to a haem molecule, a protoporphyrin ring which contains an iron atom and which can reversibly bind oxygen. The oxygen binding of whole blood (Fig. 5) is ideally suited for oxygen transport. The sigmoid shape of the curve, which reflects the allosteric properties of haemoglobin, is beautifully adapted to oxygen transport. At relatively high oxygen tensions in the lungs oxygen is rapidly taken up and it can be released readily at tensions encountered in the tissues. The curve is quite different to that of myoglobin, a molecule which consists of a single globin chain with haem attached to it, and which has a hyperbolic oxygen dissociation curve. It has been realized for many years that the transition from a hyperbolic to a sigmoid curve must reflect co-operativity between the haem molecules. The molecular basis for this haem/haem interaction is now understood. When one haem molecule takes on oxygen the affinity for oxygen of the remaining haems of the tetramer increases markedly. This is because haemoglobin can exist in two configurations, deoxy (T) and oxy (R) (T and R stand for tight and relaxed states, respectively). The T form has a lower affinity than the R form for ligands such as oxygen. At some point during the sequential addition of oxygen to the four haems transition from the T to R configuration occurs; at this point the oxygen affinity of the partially liganded molecule increases dramatically. These allosteric changes involve a series of interactions between the iron of the haem groups and various bonds within the molecule that lead to subtle spatial alterations as oxygen is taken on and given up. We shall consider the clinical implications of haem/haem interaction later in this section.

The position of the oxygen dissociation curve can be modified in several ways. First, oxygen affinity is decreased with increasing CO_2 tensions. This phenomenon, which is largely pH dependent is called the Bohr effect. It facilitates oxygen unloading at tissue levels, where a drop in pH due to CO_2 influx lowers oxygen affi-

nity. In contrast, in the lungs efflux of CO_2 and increase in intracellular pH increases oxygen affinity, and hence uptake. Carbon dioxide influences haemoglobin in two ways. First, diffusion of CO_2 into the red cells, where carbonic anhydrase produces carbonic acid, decreases the pH, hence lowering the oxygen affinity by the Bohr effect. Second, by combining with the terminal amino acid groups to form carbamino compounds, CO_2 further lowers oxygen affinity.

The position of the oxygen dissociation curve is modified by factors other than pH and CO_2. For example, another important constituent of the red cell that can modify oxygen transport is 2,3-diphosphoglycerate (2,3-DPG). Increasing concentrations of 2,3-DPG shift the oxygen dissociation curve to the right, that is, cause a state of reduced oxygen affinity, while diminishing concentrations have the opposite effect. 2,3-DPG fits into the gap between the two β chains of haemoglobin when this becomes widened during deoxygenation, and interacts with several specific binding sites in the central cavity of the molecule. However, in the oxy configuration the gap between the two β chains narrows and the molecule cannot be accommodated. It follows that, with increasing concentrations of 2,3-DPG, more haemoglobin molecules tend to be held in the deoxy configuration and the oxygen dissociation curve is therefore shifted to the right.

Thus it is apparent that the red cell has a remarkable facility for adaptation to different requirements for oxygen transport. In the next chapter we shall consider how these various adaptive mechanisms are utilized to facilitate oxygen transport in various disease states.

Red cell metabolism

The mature red cell has no nucleus or mitochondria and no tricarboxylic acid cycle. Hence the major source of energy is the glycolytic Embden-Meyerhof pathway. Glucose is metabolized via this pathway with the production of lactate, with a net gain of 2 mol of ATP and the reduction of 2 mol of NAD to NADH per mol of glucose. The other energy pathway is the hexose monophosphate (HMP) shunt in which there is a reduction of 2 mol of NADP to NADPH per mol of glucose. In addition there is a 'metabolic siding' in the Embden-Meyerhof pathway which is regulated by diphosphoglycerate mutase and which generates 2,3-diphosphoglycerate. These different pathways are illustrated and described in detail on page 19.140.

The metabolic functions of the red cell can be summarized as follows. First, it must maintain its osmotic stability through the activity of its membrane pumps. This critical transport function is driven by ATP. Second, it must maintain the iron of haemoglobin in the reduced state, by reducing Fe^{3+} to Fe^{2+}. The enzyme system involved, methaemoglobin reductase, is driven by NADH. Third, 2,3-diphosphoglycerate must be generated to act as a modulator of haemoglobin function (see below). Fourth, the sulphydryl groups of haemoglobin and membrane proteins must be protected by maintaining adequate amounts of reduced glutathione. This system is dependent on NADPH generated from NADP via the pentose pathway. Finally, NAD must be synthesized from nicotinic acid, glutamine, glucose, and inorganic phosphate, and NADP formed by the reaction of NAD and ADP. As we shall see in a later section, a breakdown of any of these critical metabolic functions causes shortening of the red cell survival and/or abnormal oxygen transport.

The life span of red cells

The life span of red cells, normally about 120 days, can be assessed by several methods. These include the use of antigenically recognizable cells by the Ashby technique, cohort labelling of newly produced red cells, or labelling of a sample of circulating cells with ^{51}Cr or $DF^{32}P$. In clinical practice, ^{51}Cr labelling of blood samples is the most convenient technique. Elution of label from red cells in the circulation causes an exponential decay of radioactivity. Correction for elution may be made, but the more usual method is to

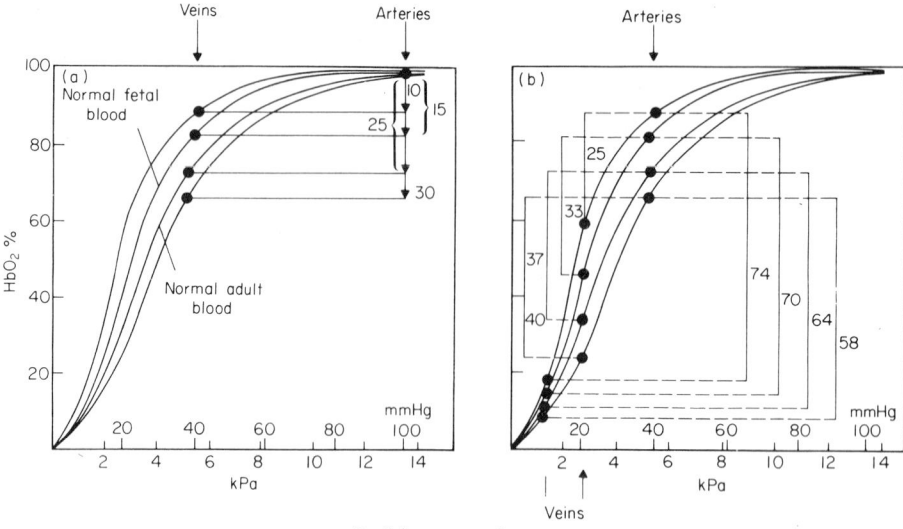

Fig. 5 Oxygen dissociation curves of human blood. (a) The curves for normal adult and fetal blood and the effect of changing the oxygen affinity with normal partial pressures of oxygen in the arteries and veins, PaO$_2$ and PvO$_2$. It is clear that lowering the oxygen affinity releases more oxygen to the tissues. (b) Effect of changing the oxygen affinity when there is a very low arterial PO$_2$ (40 mmHg). It is clear that if mean venous PO$_2$ is about 20 mmHg, lowering the oxygen affinity increases release. In contrast, with a low mean venous PO$_2$ less oxygen is released to the tissue as the curve shifts to the right. (Reproduced with permission from Huehns, E. R., 1982, *Blood and its disorders*. 2nd edn (eds R. M. Hardisty and D. J. Weatherall), p. 333. Blackwell Scientific Publications, Oxford.)

express the results in terms of half-life ($t_{\frac{1}{2}}$) of the label in circulation. The normal $t_{\frac{1}{2}}$ of ^{51}Cr labelled cells is 25–36 days. By the use of suitable external counters it is possible to determine the sites of red cell destruction.

Red cell destruction and the fate of haemoglobin

In health, erythrocytes are phagocytosed by the reticulo-endothelial cells of the spleen, liver, and elsewhere. The changes of the ageing red cell which allow them to be identified and removed from the circulation are still not fully understood.

Once in reticulo-endothelial cells, the haemoglobin liberated from the phagocytosed red cells is degraded. The first stage is the splitting up of haem and globin. The iron is split off from the haem molecule and reutilized for haemoglobin synthesis. Similarly, the globin fraction is broken down and the amino acids reutilized. Haem is converted to biliverdin by the enzyme haem oxygenase. One molecule of carbon monoxide is produced with each biliverdin molecule. The subsequent degradation of biliverdin via the action of biliverdin reductase, and the chemistry of the production and excretion of bilirubin is considered in detail in Section 12.

References

Beutler, E. (1983). Energy metabolism and maintenance of erythrocytes. In *Hematology*, 3rd edn (eds W. J. Williams, E. Beutler, A. J. Erslev and M. A. Lichtman), pp. 331–334, McGraw Hill, New York.

Bunn, H. F. and Forget, B. G. (1977). *Human hemoglobins* 2nd edn. W. B. Saunders, Philadelphia.

Clarkson, B., Marks, P. A. and Till, J. E. (1978). *Differentiation of normal and neoplastic hematopoietic cells, Books A and B*. Cold Spring Harbor Conferences on Cell Proliferation.

Dickerson, R. E. and Geis, I. (1983). *Hemoglobin*. The Benjamin/Cummings Publishing Company, Inc., Menlo Park, California.

Eaves, A. C. and Eaves, C. J. (1984). Erythropoiesis in culture. *Clin. Haemat.* **13**, 371–391.

Emerson, P. M. and Grimes, A. J. (1982). Red cell metabolism: hereditary enzymopathies. In *Blood and its disorders*, 2nd edn, (eds R. M. Hardisty and D. J. Weatherall), pp. 265–321. Blackwell Scientific Publications, Oxford.

Erslev, A. J., Caro, J., Miller, O. and Silver, R. (1980). Plasma erythropoietin in health and disease. *Ann. Clin. Lab. Sci.* **10**, 250–257.

Huehns, E. R. (1982). The structure and function of haemoglobin: clinical disorders due to abnormal haemoglobin structure. In *Blood and its disorders*, 2nd edn (eds R. M. Hardisty and D. J. Weatherall), pp. 323–400. Blackwell Scientific Publications, Oxford.

Izak, G. (1977). Erythroid cell differentiation and maturation. *Prog. Hemat.* **10**, 1–41.

Lajtha, L. G. (1979). Stem cell concepts. *Differentiation*, **14**, 23–34.

Lajtha, L. G. (1979). Haemopoietic stem cells; concepts and definitions. *Blood Cells* **5**, 477–491.

Lajtha, L. G. (1982). The cellular kinetics of haemopoiesis. In *Blood and its disorders*, 2nd edn (eds R.M. Hardisty and D.J. Weatherall), pp. 57–74. Blackwell Scientific Publications, Oxford.

Lewis, S. M. (1982). The constituents of normal blood and bone marrow. In *Blood and its disorders*, 2nd edn, (eds R. M. Hardisty and D. J. Weatherall), pp. 3–56. Blackwell Scientific Publications, Oxford.

Mladenovic, J. and Adamson, J. W. (1982). Erythroid colony growth in culture: analysis of erythroid differentiation and studies in human disease states. In *Recent advances in haematology, 3* (ed. A.V. Hoffbrand), pp. 94–107. Churchill Livingstone, Edinburgh.

Quensenbery, P. and Levitt, L. (1979). Hemopoietic stem cells, I, II and III. *N. Eng. J. Med.* **301**, 755–761, 819–823, 868–872.

Schrier, S. L. (1982). The red cell membrane and its abnormalites. In *Recent advances in haematology, 3* (ed. A. V. Hoffbrand), pp. 69–93. Churchill Livingstone, Edinburgh.

Anaemia: pathophysiology, classification, and clinical features

D. J. WEATHERALL

The main function of the red blood cells is oxygen transport. Hence a functional definition of anaemia is a state in which the circulating red cell mass is insufficient to meet the oxygen requirements of the tissues. However, there are many compensatory mechanisms that can be brought into play to restore the oxygen supply to the vital centres, and therefore in clinical practice this definition is of limited value. For this reason anaemia is usually defined as a reduction of the haemoglobin concentration, red cell count or packed cell volume to below normal levels.

The definition of anaemia

It has been extremely difficult to establish a normal range of haematological values, and hence the definition of anaemia usually involves the adoption of rather arbitrary criteria. For example, the World Health Organization recommends that anaemia should be considered to exist in adults whose haemoglobin levels are lower than 13 g/dl (males) or 12 g/dl (females). Children aged six months to six years are considered anaemic at haemoglobin levels below 11 g/dl and those aged six to 14 years below 12 g/dl. The disadvantage of such arbitrary criteria for defining anaemia is that there may be many apparently normal individuals whose haemoglobin concentration is below their optimal level. Furthermore, the published 'normal values' for adults (see page 19.4) indicate that there is such a large standard deviation that many adult females must be considered 'normal' even though they have haemoglobin levels below 12 g/dl.

It must not be assumed that haemoglobin values within the normal range denote 'normality' for the individual and they certainly do not exclude occult deficiencies such as latent iron or vitamin B_{12} deficiency, which are revealed only by specific assays. For example, in a random sample of the adult population in Wales investigated during 1967 there was clear evidence of iron deficiency in subjects with haemoglobin concentrations well within the conventional normal range.

Prevalence of anaemia

Anaemia is a major world health problem and its distribution and prevalence in the developing world is considered in detail in the next chapter.

The prevalence of anaemia has been studied in many populations but it is difficult to compare data from different sources because of variations in methodology and criteria adopted. Certain patterns emerge, however. An early survey carried out in Great Britain established that haemoglobin levels were low in a significant proportion of the population, particularly susceptible groups being children under the age of five years, pregnant women, and those in social classes IV and V. A later random population study in the United Kingdom reported a prevalence of anaemia of 14 per cent for women aged 55–64 years and 3 per cent for men aged 35–64 years. These and similar studies have shown that anaemia is commonest in women between the ages of 15 and 44 years and that it then becomes relatively less frequent, although the prevalence increases again in the 75-year-and-over age group. Interestingly, it is only in the latter group that the prevalence in males and females is almost the same. Where the cause of the anaemia has been analysed in these surveys, the majority of cases have been due to iron deficiency. No doubt this prevalence data varies considerably between the developed countries, but it is clear that nutritional anaemia is relatively common in most populations at certain periods during development and late in life.

Adaptation to anaemia

The function of the red cell is to carry oxygen between the lungs and the tissues. However, tissue oxygenation is the result of a complex series of interactions of different organ systems of which the red cell is only one (Table 1). Obviously the cardiac output, ventilatory function, and state of the capillaries are of great importance as well. Each of these oxygen supply systems are regulated differently. Ventilation responds to changes in pH, CO_2, and hypoxia. Cardiac output responds to the amount of blood entering the heart and this is regulated mainly by the effects of tissue metabolism as it modifies the resistance to blood flow in the microvasculature. The erythron itself responds to changes in haemoglobin concentration, arterial oxygen saturation, and to the oxygen affinity of the circulating haemoglobin. Thus a decreased capacity of any of these components may be compensated for by increased activity of the others in an attempt to maintain tissue oxygenation.

Table 1 The steps involved in the transport of oxygen to the tissues

Steps	Factors involved
Ambient O_2 tension	Altitude
Ventilation	Alveolar ventilation Gas to blood diffusion Ventilation/perfusion ratio Anatomical shunt
Circulation	Cardiac output Blood: haemoglobin concentration oxygen dissociation curve
Tissue diffusion	Inter-capillary distance

Oxygen diffuses across the alveolar membrane and into the blood which equilibrates with the alveolar gas; the approximate oxygen tension is 100 mmHg, at which the blood is fully saturated with an oxygen content of 20 vols per cent. As blood is pumped through the tissue capillaries oxygen diffuses out. Although the venous oxygen tension varies between organs, the oxygen tension of the pooled venous blood in the pulmonary artery, the 'mixed venous oxygen tension', is remarkably constant at 40 mmHg. At this oxygen tension the oxygen content is 15 vols per cent. Hence, oxygen delivery as measured by the arteriovenous oxygen difference is normally 5 vols per cent. By reducing the oxygen carrying capacity of blood, anaemia tends to reduce the arterial–venous oxygen difference and this may be compensated for by the following mechanisms: (a) modulation of oxygen affinity; (b) redistribution of flow between different organs; (c) increase in cardiac output; and (d) reduction of mixed venous oxygen tension to increase the arteriovenous oxygen difference.

Intrinsic red cell adaptation

The consequences of anaemia on the normal oxygen binding curve of blood are shown in Fig. 1. Anaemia, by lowering the haemoglobin concentration, reduces proportionately the oxygen carrying capacity of the blood. As a response to this there is an increase in 2,3-DPG concentration in the red cell, shifting the dissociation curve to the right, so significantly enhancing tissue oxygen delivery (Fig. 1).

With increasing severity of anaemia there is a progressive increase in 2,3-DPG which may increase oxygen delivery by as much as 40 per cent for the same haemoglobin concentration. It should be noted, however, that a consequence of this adaptation is a lower venous oxygen content and hence a lower reserve of oxygen available for further increase in oxygen demand, as might occur on exercise for example. Hence the increase in 2,3-DPG in anaemia tends to ameliorate the effects of diminished oxygen carrying capacity of the blood so reducing the adaptation required by other steps involved in tissue oxygen delivery (Fig. 2). 2,3-DPG levels vary in a variety of other clinical conditions; some of these are summarized in Table 2.

Local changes in tissue perfusion

The total blood volume does not change greatly in anaemia and therefore increased tissue perfusion has to be achieved by shunting of blood from less to more vital organs. There is vasoconstriction of the vessels of the skin and kidney; this mechanism has little effect on renal function. The organs which gain from the redistribution seem to be mainly the myocardium, brain, and muscle.

Cardiovascular changes

It seems likely that mild anaemia is compenstaed by shifts in the oxygen dissociation curve. Overall, oxygen consumption is

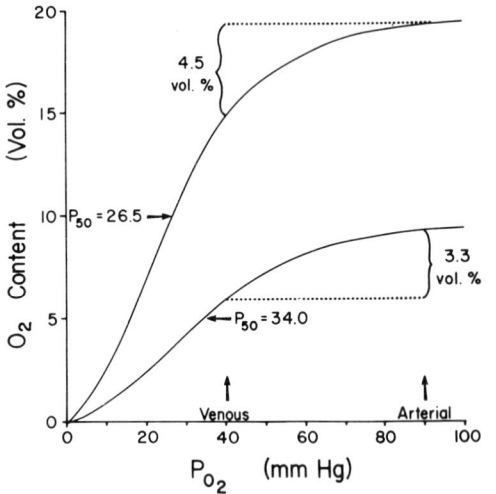

Fig. 1 Enhancement of oxygen loading by decreased red cell oxygen affinity in a patient with anaemia. An anaemic patient with 50 per cent reduction in haemoglobin concentration has only a 27 per cent reduction in oxygen unloading. (Based on Klocke, R. A., 1972, *Chest* **69**, 795.)

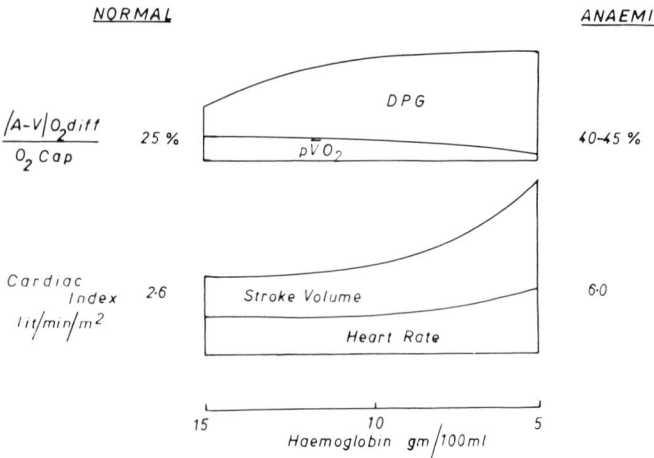

Fig. 2 The changes in factors involved in oxygen delivery with progressive anaemia. As anaemia becomes more severe cardiac compensation becomes more significant (pVO_2 = mixed venous oxygen tension). (From Bellingham, 1974.)

unchanged in anaemia. However, when the haemoglobin level falls below 7–8 g/dl, there is an increase in cardiac output, both at rest and after exercise (Fig. 2). There is an increase in the stroke rate, and a hyperkinetic circulation develops characterized by tachycardia, arterial and capillary pulsation, a wide pulse pressure, and haemic murmurs. The circulation time is shortened, left ventricular stroke work is increased, and coronary flow increases in proportion to the increased cardiac output. It has been found that there is an acute reversal of the high output state of chronic anaemia in response to orthostatic stress or pressor amines. This suggests that redistribution blood volume and vasodilatation with reduced afterload play a dominant role in the hyperkinetic circulatory responses to chronic anaemia. The mechanism of the vasodilatation is not known; it may be a direct result of tissue hypoxia. An additional factor which may be of some importance in increasing cardiac output is the reduction in blood viscosity produced by a relatively low red cell mass.

While the normal myocardium may tolerate sustained hyperactivity of this type indefinitely, patients with coronary artery disease or those with extreme anaemia may have impaired oxygenation of the myocardium. In such cases cardiomegaly, pul-

Table 2 Some conditions in which there is a change in red cell 2,3-diphosphoglycerate (DPG) levels leading to modification of oxygen transport

Increased 2,3-DPG; increased $p50$, reduced whole-blood oxygen affinity
　Anaemia
　Alkalosis
　Hyperphosphataemia
　Renal failure
　Hypoxia
　Pregnancy
　Cyanotic congenital heart disease
　Thyrotoxicosis
　Some red cell enzyme deficiencies
Decreased 2,3-DPG; decreased $p50$, increased whole-blood oxygen affinity
　Acidosis
　Cardiogenic or septicaemic shock
　Hypophosphataemia
　Hypothyroidism
　Hypopituitarism
　Following replacement with stored blood

monary oedema, ascites, and peripheral oedema may occur and a state of high output cardiac failure is established. At this stage the plasma volume is almost always increased.

Pulmonary function
Since blood, regardless of its oxygen carrying capacity, is almost completely oxygenated in the lungs, the oxygen pressure of arterial blood in an anaemic patient should be the same as that in a normal individual, and hence an increase in respiratory rate should not improve the oxygenation of the tissues. Curiously, however, severe anaemia is associated with dyspnoea. Although in some patients this may be related to incipient cardiac failure, in most cases it appears to be an inappropriate response to hypoxia which is centrally mediated.

Clinical manifestations and classification of anaemia

Clinical effects of anaemia
Since anaemia reduces tissue oxygenation, it is not surprising that it is associated with widespread organ dysfunction and hence an extremely varied clinical picture. The latter depends, of course, on whether the anaemia is of rapid or more insidious onset.

After acute blood loss the red cell mass and plasma volume are reduced proportionately and the symptoms are mainly of volume depletion. Depending on the amount of fluid replacement there may be a small fall in the PCV during the first 10 hours; volume replacement by the influx of albumin from the extravascular compartment takes between 60 and 90 hours. Hence the picture of rapid blood loss is characterized by the typical syndrome of shock, with collapse, dyspnoea, tachycardia, a poor volume pulse, reduced blood pressure, and marked peripheral vasoconstriction.

With anaemia of more insidious onset, the compensatory mechanisms outlined above have time to come into play. In mild anaemia there may be no symptoms or simply increased fatigue and slight pallor. As the anaemia becomes more marked the symptoms and signs gradually appear. Pallor is best discerned in the mucous membranes; the nail beds and palmar creases, although often said to be useful sites for detecting anaemia, are relatively insensitve for this purpose. Cardiorespiratory symptoms and signs include exertional dyspnoea, tachycardia, palpitations, angina or claudication, night cramps, increased arterial pulsation, capillary pulsation, a variety of cardiac bruits, reversible cardiac enlargement, and, if cardiac failure occurs, basal crepitations, peripheral oedema, and ascites. Neuromuscular involvement is reflected by headache, vertigo, lightheadedness, faintness, tinnitus, roaring in the ears, cramps, increased cold sensitivity, and haemorrhages in the retina. Acute anaemia may occasionally give rise to papilloe-

Table 3 The main groups of anaemias classified according to the underlying cause

Reduced red cell production
    Defective precursor proliferation
    Defective precursor maturation
    Defective proliferation and maturation
Increased rate of red cell destruction
    Haemolysis
Loss of red cells from the circulation
    Bleeding

Table 4 Main causes of anaemia due to defective production of red cells

Reduced proliferation of precursors
  Iron deficiency anaemia
  Anaemia of chronic disorders
    Infections, malignancy, collagen disease, etc.
  Reduced erythropoietin production
    Renal disease
    Reduced oxygen requirements
      Hypothyroidism
      Hypopituitarism
    Reduced O_2 affinity of haemoglobin
    Erythropoietin antibody production
  Primary disease of the bone marrow
    Aplastic anaemia
      Primary
      Secondary to drugs, irradiation, chemicals, toxins, etc.
    Pure red cell hypoplasia
    Infiltrative disorders
      Leukaemia
      Lymphoma
      Secondary carcinoma
      Myelofibrosis
Defective maturation of precursors
  Nuclear maturation
    Vitamin B_{12} deficiency
    Folate deficiency
    Erythroleukaemia
  Cytoplasmic maturation
    Iron deficiency
    Disorders of globin synthesis
    Disorders of haem and/or iron metabolism
    Disorders of porphyrin metabolism
  Unknown mechanism
    Congenital dyserythropoietic anaemias
    Myelodysplastic syndrome
    Infection
    Toxins and chemicals

dema. Gastrointestinal symptoms include loss of appetite, nausea, constipation and diarrhoea. Genitourinary involvement causes menstrual irregularities, urinary frequency, and loss of libido. There may be a low-grade fever.

In the elderly, in whom associated degenerative arterial disease is common, anaemia may present with the onset of cardiac failure. Alternatively, previously undiagnosed coronary narrowing may be unmasked by the onset of angina. Other symptoms of arterial degenerative disease may be also exacerbated or unmasked, e.g. intermittent claudication and a variety of neurological pictures associated with cerebral arteriosclerosis. It is important that anaemia is recognized as a contributing factor to the symptoms of these degenerative diseases as its correction may frequently bring about considerable symptomatic improvement.

Causes and classication of anaemia
A reduction in the red cell mass can result from either defective production of red cells or an increased rate of loss of cells, either by premature destruction or bleeding. Decreased production of red cells may result from a reduced rate of proliferation of red cell precursors in the bone marrow or from failure of maturation leading to their intramedullary destruciton, i.e. ineffective erythropoiesis. Based on this approach we can derive a very simple pathophysiological classification of anaemia as shown in Table 3 in which the causes are divided into failure of red cell proliferation, defective maturation, haemolysis, and blood loss.

Anaemia due to defective proliferation of red cell precursors
The major causes of this group of anaemias are an inadequate supply of iron, primary diseases of the bone marrow which involve stem cells or later erythroid precursors, or a reduction in the amount of erythropoietin reaching the red cell precursors (Table 4).

Iron deficiency results in defective erythroid proliferation and also in abnormal maturation of the red cell precursors due to defective haemoglobin synthesis. Red cell precursors require adequate iron supplies for normal proliferation, and the anaemia of iron deficiency tends to be hypoproliferative as well as dyserythropoietic. Chronic inflammatory disorders and related conditions also interfere with the iron supply to red cell precursors, probably by blocking the release of catabolized red cell iron from reticuloendothelial cells. The basic defect in iron deficiency anaemia and that due to inflammation is similar, therefore, in that the supply of iron is inadequate to meet the requirements for erythropoiesis.

Defective proliferation of red cell precursors can result from any of the causes of bone marrow failure including infiltration with leukaemic or other neoplastic cells, damage due to ionizing radiation, drugs, or infection, and various intrinsic lesions of the stem cells or red cell precursors. The latter disorders include the congenital hypoplastic anaemias, involving either all the formed elements or the red cell precursors alone.

Finally, decreased proliferation of the red cell precursors may result from erythropoietin deficiency. The commonest cause is chronic renal failure. A similar mechanism may be involved in conditions in which the tissue requirement for oxygen is reduced. These include various endocrine disorders such as hypothyroidism

and hypopituitarism. It may also explain the mild anaemia associated with haemoglobin variants with decreased oxygen affinity.

As a group, the hypoproliferative anaemias are associated with a low reticulocyte count and defective proliferation of the bone marrow precursors. The red cells are usually normochromic and normocytic although there may be a mild macrocytosis. If the anaemia is due to iron deficiency, the cells are hypochromic. If granulopoiesis is normal, the defect in red cell proliferation is reflected by an increase in the M/E ratio.

Defective red cell maturation
Defects of red cell maturation may involve primarily nuclear or cytoplasmic maturation (Table 4). Those involving nuclear maturation include vitamin B_{12} and folic acid deficiency and other causes of megaloblastic anaemia, and some of the primary marrow disorders including erythroleukaemia. The important causes of defective cytoplasmic maturation include the inherited disorders of globin synthesis, the thalassaemia syndromes, and the genetic and acquired defects of iron metabolism which characterize the sideroblastic anaemias. There are other genetic defects of red cell maturation, the congenital dyserythropoietic anaemias, in which the aetiology is unknown. Furthermore, agents such as drugs, chemicals, and infections may interfere with erythroid maturation.

The main pathological mechanism common to all the anaemias which result from maturation abnormalities is ineffective erythropoiesis. In other words, there is marked erythroid proliferation but many of the precursors are destroyed in the bone marrow before they enter the circulation. Hence, the characteristic finding is marked erythroid hyperplasia with a reduction in the M/E ratio associated with a low reticulocyte count. Because of the significant intramedullary destruction of precursors there is usually an elevated bilirubin and LDH level. Furthermore, there are nearly always morphological abnormalities of the red cell precursors. The anaemias which are associated with abnormal nuclear maturation such as those due to vitamin B_{12} and folic acid deficiency are characterized by megaloblastic erythropoiesis and macrocytic red cells, while those caused by abnormal cytoplasmic maturation are characterized by normoblastic hyperplasia and hypochromic and microcytic red cells. However, even in the latter conditions, there is marked anisocytosis and there may be a proportion of macrocytes in the peripheral circulation.

Blood loss

As mentioned earlier, the clinical picture associated with an acute loss of a large volume of blood is that of hypovolaemic shock.

Anaemias due to chronic blood loss may develop very insidiously and cause considerable diagnostic problems. Chronic blood loss from the gastrointestinal tract or uterus of more than 15–20 ml per day produces a state of negative iron balance. Assuming that the patient starts with a normal body store of iron, which is usually in the region of 1 g, the bone marrow will be able to maintain a normal haemoglobin level until the iron stores are totally depleted. At this stage there is no demonstrable iron in the bone marrow and the plasma iron level starts to fall but the patient is not anaemic. With a further fall in the plasma iron level, the haemoglobin level starts to fall although at this stage the erythrocyte morphology may be relatively normal, as are the red cell indices. It is only when iron deficiency anaemia is well established that the typical morphological appearances of the red cells develop, and only after extreme periods of iron depletion that the tissue changes of iron deficiency become manifest.

From these considerations it is apparent that there may be prolonged blood loss before a patient presents with the symptoms and signs of anaemia. During the earlier stages the peripheral blood film may not be helpful in diagnosis even though the serum iron level may be extremely low. Indeed, sometimes a dimorphic blood picture with normochromic and hypochromic cell populations may be seen. With chronic blood loss there is quite often a persistent thrombocytosis, and a hypochromic blood picture with thrombocytosis should always raise the possibility of chronic bleeding. In practice the commonest sites of such bleeding are a hiatus hernia, peptic ulcer, tumour of the large bowel, or the uterus.

Haemolytic anaemia (Table 5)

When the lifespan of red cells is shortened there is a reduction in the circulating red cell mass which leads to relative tissue hypoxia. This causes an increased output of erythropoietin with stimulation of the bone marrow and an increased rate of red cell production. This is reflected by a raised reticulocyte count and a macrocytosis due to the presence of young cells in the peripheral circulation. Because of the increased rate of red cell destruction, there is an increased production of bilirubin which leads to mild icterus and the presence of increased amounts of urobilinogen in the urine and stool. Thus the haemolytic anaemias are characterized by a variable degree of anaemia, a reticulocytosis, and hyperbilirubinaemia. Their pathophysiology is considered in detail on page 19.134.

Red cells are prematurely destroyed either because of an intrinsic lesion or as a result of the action of an extrinsic agent. The intrinsic abnormalities of the red cells which lead to their premature removal are nearly all genetic defects of either the membrane, haemoglobin, or metabolic pathways. The extrinsic agents which may cause premature destruction of the cells include a variety of antibodies, chemicals, drugs, and toxins, or bacteria and parasites. In addition, red cells may be damaged by direct trauma in the microcirculation or on body surfaces.

Premature destruction of red cells may take place either intravascularly or extravascularly, or, as occurs more commonly, in both sites. The site of destructon depends on the type and degree of damage to the red cell. For example, complement-damaged cells develop large holes in the membrane and are destroyed in the

Table 5 General classification of haemolytic anaemia. A more detailed classification is shown in Table 4, page 19.136.

Genetically determined
  Defects involving the structure and/or metabolism of the membrane
  Haemoglobin disorders
  Enzyme deficiencies involving the main metabolic pathways
Acquired
  Immune (iso- or auto)
  Non-immune
    Trauma
    Membrane defects
    Drugs, chemicals, toxins
    Bacteria, parasites
    Hypersplenism

circulation, whereas IgG coated cells are removed mainly in the reticulo-endothelial system.

Clearly, there are numerous causes of premature destruction of red cells. These will be considered in detail later in this section. Usually it is easy to recognize that a particular anaemia has a haemolytic basis by virtue of the reticulocytosis and macrocytosis associated with erythroid hyperplasia of the bone marrow, hyperbilirubinaemia, and increased urinary urobilinogen. However, it should be remembered that many anaemias associated with abnormal proliferation or maturation of red cells have a haemolytic component. For example, there may be a slightly shortened red cell survival in patients with pernicious anaemia or thalassaemia and yet there may be a very poor reticulocyte response. Similary, there is a haemolytic component in the anaemia due to inflammation or malignancy but again the marrow response is poor. In such cases it may be necessary to measure the lifespan of the red cells directly in order to determine the magnitude of the haemolytic component as compared with defective proliferation or maturation.

General approach to the anaemic patient

Clinical assessment

The clinical assessment of patients with anaemia has two main objectives. First, it is essential to determine the degree of disability caused by the anaemia and hence how quickly treatment must be started. Second, as much information as possible about the likely cause of the anaemia must be obtained from a detailed clinical history and physical examination. There is no place for the 'blind' treatment of anaemia without first establishing the cause.

In assessing the severity of the anaemia and how urgently treatment should be instituted a detailed history of the patient's exercise tolerance must be obtained. This should include a specific enquiry of symptoms suggestive of cardiac complications including angina, dysrhythmias, positional dyspnoea, cough, or ankle swelling. The clinical examination should include a careful assessment of the degree of pallor, the position of the neck veins, whether there are warm extremities and a bounding pulse with a large pulse pressure, the presence of ankle or sacral oedema, and whether there are basal crepitations. The finding of profound anaemia with signs of cardiac failure indicates that urgent treatment is required. If the anaemia is associated with marked splenomegaly there will almost certainly be an increased blood volume and, particularly if there are already signs of cardiac failure, the patient may well go into acute left ventricular failure if transfused. Severely ill patients with profound anaemia require immediate treatment in an environment where they can be under constant observation, have regular measurements of the central venous pressure, and where they can be managed by experienced clinical and nursing staff.

An account of history taking and clinical examination in patients with haematological disorders was given earlier in this section (page 19.1). It cannot be emphasized too strongly that in

Table 6 The main causes of anaemia classified according to the associated red cell changes

Hypochromic–microcytic (reduced MCV, MCH and MCHC)
  Genetic
    Thalassaemia
    Sideroblastic anaemia
  Acquired
    Iron deficiency
    Sideroblastic anaemia
    Chronic disorders (mildly hypochromic, occasionally)
Normochromic–macrocytic (increased MCV)
  With megaloblastic marrow
    Vitamin B_{12} or folate deficiency
  With normoblastic marrow
    Alcohol, myelodysplasia
Polychromatophilic–macrocytic (increased MCV)
  Haemolysis
Normochromic–normocytic (normal indices)
  Chronic disorders
    Infection, malignancy, collagen disease, rheumatoid arthritis
  Renal failure
  Hypothyroidism, hypopituitarism
  Aplastic anaemia or primary red cell hypoplasia
  Primary disease of bone marrow, leukaemia, myelosclerosis, infiltration
    with other tumours
Leukoerythroblastic (indices usually normal)
  Myelosclerosis
  Leukaemia
  Metastatic carcinoma

many cases the anaemia is a symptom of a non-haematological disorder. A detailed history and clinical examination will often provide a clue as to the likely cause of the anaemia and which laboratory investigations are likely to be most productive for confirming the diagnosis (see page 19.1).

Haematological investigation

A preliminary blood count and blood film examination should classify anaemia into hypochromic–microcytic, and macrocytic or normochromic, normocytic varieties (Table 6). In middle-aged females with a history of several pregnancies or heavy menstrual loss it is reasonable to assume that a hypochromic anaemia is due to iron deficiency and treat them with iron without further invesigation. However, hypochromic anaemia in males or young or postmenopausal females always suggests blood loss and should be investigated accordingly. If there is any doubt about a hypochromic anaemia being due to iron deficiency, the serum iron level and total iron binding capacity should be established. Hypochromic anaemia with a normal serum iron suggests a genetic or acquired defect in haemoglobin synthesis, common causes being thalassaemia and sideroblastic anaemia. The diagnosis of a macrocytic anaemia always requires further investigation and should be followed up with a bone marrow examination. A macrocytosis with a normoblastic bone marrow may result from alcohol abuse, haemolysis, or, occasionally, one of the refractory anaemias with hyperplastic bone marrow (see page 19.130). Macrocytic anaemias with megaloblastic bone marrows are usually due to vitamin B_{12} or folate deficiency and should be investigated accordingly. If there is macrocytosis with a reticulocytosis, hyperbilirubinaemia, and a normoblastic marrow, a haemolytic anaemia is likely; an approach to the further investigation of haemolysis is described on page 19.136.

The normochromic, normocytic anaemias often cause more diagnostic difficulty. Some help can be gained from a determination of whether the white cell and platelet counts are normal. If there is associated neutropenia and thrombocytopenia, a primary disease of the bone marrow is likely and bone marrow examination should be carried out to determine whether there is hypoplasia of the various precursor forms, hypoplastic or aplastic

anaemia, or whether the pancyptopenia results from infiltration of the bone marrow as occurs in the various forms of leukaemia. If there are nucleated red cells or young white cells on the peripheral film, i.e. a leucoerythroblastic picture, a bone marrow examination is essential as this type of reaction usually indicates infiltration of the bone marrow with abnormal cells, either as part of a primary marrow disease such as leukaemia, or metastatic carcinoma. In the normochromic–normocytic anaemias in which the white cell count and platelet count are normal, it is also helpful to carry out a bone marrow analysis. The commonest cause is anaemia of chronic disorders, the diagnosis of which is described in detail below. Another particularly common cause is chronic renal failure. After these conditions have been excluded, there remain the chronic anaemias associated with endocrine deficiencies (see page 19.91) or the primary red cell hypoplasias (see page 19.52).

The management of anaemia

The management of specific forms of anaemia is described in detail in subsequent sections. However, a few principles can be outlined here. In general, a cause should always be sought before treatment is instituted. There is no place whatever for treating anaemia 'blind' with multi-haematinic preparations. As mentioned above, most cases of iron deficiency anaemia require further investigation for a source of blood loss. If there is a clear-cut history of poor diet, multiple pregnancies, or obvious uterine bleeding, it is reasonable to start iron therapy and observe the haemoglobin level both during the period of treatment and for some months after iron therapy has been stopped. A rise in the haemoglobin level of approximately 1 g/dl per week indicates a full haematological response. In the megaloblastic anaemias it is quite reasonable to start treatment with vitamin B_{12} and folic acid once a diagnosis of a megaloblastic anaemia has been established and blood samples have been obtained for serum folate and B_{12} levels. The cause of the megaloblastic anaemia can be established at leisure once these samples have been obtained. A brisk reticulocyte response five to seven days after initiating therapy suggests that there will be a full restoration of the haemoglobin level to normal. Failure of response of a hypochromic anaemia to adequate iron therapy should be managed by first finding out whether the iron is being taken and, if so, by determining the serum iron level. If it is normal, causes of hypochromic anaemia which are not associated with iron deficiency, thalassaemia and sideroblastic anaemia for example, should be sought. Similary, refractory macrocytic anaemias require detailed analysis of the bone marrow morphology as there may be an underlying preleukaemic state.

Blood transfusion should always be avoided unless the haemoglobin level is dangerously low, when it is reasonable to transfuse the patient up to a safe level and then allow the haemoglobin to return to normal following appropriate treatment of the underlying cause. The decision whether to transfuse an anaemic patient depends mainly on the severity of the anaemia and its cause. For example, a young patient with a haemoglobin value of 5 g/dl who is shown to have an active duodenal ulcer should probably be transfused because they would be at severe risk from a further brisk bleed from the ulcer. On the other hand, a patient of similar age with a similar haemoglobin level due to chronic nutritional iron deficiency might well be allowed to restore their haemoglobin level on oral iron therapy.

Occasionally, patients present in gross congestive cardiac failure with profound anaemia. This picture is usually seen in elderly patients with long-standing pernicious anaemia or iron deficiency. This type of condition still carries a high mortality and requires urgent treatment. Such profoundly anaemic patients require transfusing up to a safe level, i.e. a haemoglobin value of 6–8 g/dl. This can usually be achieved by the slow transfusion of two or three units of red cells with the intravenous administration of a potent diuretic such as frusemide with each unit; the diuretic should never be mixed directly with the blood. A very careful check on the neck veins and lung bases should be carried out throughout the period of transfusion. Ideally, a central venous pressure line should be inserted before the transfusion is started. Occasionally, patients are encountered in such gross heart failure that the administration of packed cells and diuretics worsens the failure. In this situation it is possible to raise the circulating red cell mass by infusing packed cells or whole blood through one arm while removing an equal volume of blood from the other. By carrying out a two-to-three unit exchange transfusion of this type it may be possible to tide the patient over while treating the heart failure by conventional means.

References

Adamson, J. W. and Finch C. A. (1975). Haemoglobin function, oxygen affinity and erythropoietin. *Ann. Rev. Physiol.* **37**, 351–369.

Bellingham, A. J. (1974). The red cell in adaptation to anaemic hypoxia. *Clinics Haemat.* **3**, 577–594.

Grimes, A. J. and Emerson, P. M. (1982). Red cell metabolism: the hereditary enzymopathies. In *Blood and its disorders*, 2nd edn. (eds R. M. Hardisty and D. J. Weatherall), pp. 265–322. Blackwell Scientific Publications, Oxford.

Hjelm, M. and Wadman, B. (1974). Clinical symptoms, haemoglobin concentration and erythroctye biochemistry. *Clinics Haemat.* **3**, 689–704.

Heuhns, E. R. (1982). The structure and function of haemoglobin: clinical disorders due to abnormal haemoglobin. In *Blood and its disorders*, 2nd edn. (eds R. M. Hardisty and D. J. Weatherall), pp. 323–400. Blackwell Scientific Publications, Oxford.

Rorth, M. (1974). Hypoxia, red cell oxygen affinity and erythropoietin production. *Clinics Haemat.* **3**, 595–608.

Varat, M. A., Adolph, R. J. and Fowler, N. O. (1972). Cardiovascular effects of anemia. *Am. Heart J.* **83**, 415–426.

Viteri, F. E. and Torun, B. (1974). Anaemia and physical work capacity. *Clinics Haemat.* **3**, 609–626.

Wickramasinghe, S. M. and Weatherall, D. J. (1982). The pathophysiology of erythropoiesis. In *Blood and its disorders*, 2nd edn. (eds R. M. Hardisty and D. J. Weatherall), pp. 101–148. Blackwell Scientific Publications, Oxford.

Woodson, R. D. (1974). Red cell adaptation in cardiorespiratory disease. *Clinics Haemat.* **3**, 627–648.

Anaemia as a world health problem

A. F. FLEMING

Introduction

Homo sapiens evolved over millions of years as a relatively rare species of hunter-gatherers. Their lack of specialization allowed them to adapt to large variations of environment and diet, including the profound alterations introduced by the invention of agriculture and animal husbandry. Agriculture increased vastly the available energy-rich foods and permitted quantum leaps in the size of populations. Humans have adapted only partially to these self-imposed changes, which occurred recently in evolutionary terms, between about 300 generations ago in western Asia and 80 generations ago in the forests of Africa. The costs of agriculture, which include the commonest anaemias worldwide (Table 1), follow from (*a*) increased density of population, (*b*) alterations of the natural distribution of water, soil, and flora, and (*c*) changes in the food available.

Effects of density of population

Large populations carry the risk of famine, especially following natural disasters such as drought, or war. Secondly, density of population and inadequate disposal of waste intensifies the transmission of infections. In terms of evolution it is probable that sub-human primates, such as chimpanzees with population densities of about 4 per km^2, were the principal hosts for malaria, and that humans were infected as zoonoses only when their populations

Table 1 Causes of anaemia related to agriculture

Infection	Genetic	Nutritional
Malaria	α° thalassaemia hydrops fetalis	Iron deficiency
Hookworm	Hb-H disease	Folate deficiency
Schistosomiasis	β-thalassaemias	(Vitamin B$_{12}$ deficiency)
	Sickle cell disease Hb-E, Hb-D G6PD deficiency Elliptocytosis	(Protein-energy malnutrition)

were less than 1 per 10 km^2. As humans became numerous and replaced other primates, malarial species evolved and transferred to humans as their main host: it is postulated that *Plasmodium falciparum*, *P. ovale*, and *P. vivax* are related, respectively, to *P. knowlesi*, *P. gonderi*, and *P. cynomolgi* of Old World monkeys. *P. malariae* remains a parasite common to chimpanzees and humans.

Changes in the environment caused by agriculture

Clearing of the forest and bush by slashing and burning creates open sunlit pools of water preferred for breeding sites by *Anopheles gambiae*. Irrigation dams and channels produce the swampy ground and vegetated shady water-edges favoured by *A. funestus*. The numbers of these vectors of malaria can reach astonishing numbers; averages of over 250 bites per night and up to 145 sporozoite-positive bites per year per person have been recorded. Over 500 million people are exposed to malaria, and 100 million cases per year is certainly an underestimation. In the sudan savanna of Nigeria, the infant mortality rate was 245/1000 per year, and the death rate in the one-to four-year age group was 154/1000 per year: these figures were reduced by about two-thirds through anti-malarial intervention. Anaemia due to malaria is often profound (see page 19.241), and haemoglobin values of less than 2 g/dl are often seen in non-immune children and during first pregnancies. Recurrent malaria in the immune population causes more-or-less constant haemolysis and compensatory erythroid hyperplasia: control of malaria in areas of Africa and New Guinea have been followed by an increase of mean haemoglobin values in both sexes and at all ages of about 2 g/dl.

Hookworm and schistosomiasis are only two among the many other diseases, the transmission of which is favoured by agriculture, and both are major causes of anaemia. Hookworm is found throughout the tropical world and it is estimated that there are over 450 million infected people (see Section 5). There are about 40 million people infected by *Schistosoma haematobium* in Africa and western Asia, about 30 million with *S. mansoni* in Africa, tropical America and the Caribbean, and 46 million with *S. japonica* in eastern Asia.

Evolutionary adaptations to malaria

The immensely heavy biological burden of malaria has led to the selection for inherited variants of red cell haemoglobin, enzymes, and membrane, which confer partial protection against the worst effects of *P. falciparum* malaria. The advantage enjoyed by heterozygotes is balanced, however, by hereditary anaemias, often severe, in homozygotes or compound heterozygotes (Tables 1 and 2).

Haemoglobinopathies

(See page 19.108.)

The genes for α^0 thalassaemia, α$^+$ thalassaemia, the β thalassaemias, and haemoglobins S, C, D-Punjab (or Los Angeles), and E, all achieve polymorphic frequencies in areas where *P. falciparum* malaria is or was endemic (Figs 1–4). Migration and the slave-trade have carried the haemoglobinopathies, especially haemoglobin S and β thalassaemia, to the Americas, northern Europe, and Australasia. There are at least 240 million heterozygotes for the haemoglobinopathies in the world. More than 200 000 lethally affected homozygotes are born each year, equally divided between thalassaemias and sickle cell disease (Table 2). These diseases are most common in countries of low socio-economic development, where around half the population are below 15 years of age: the numbers born with severe haemoglobinopathies will double by AD 2000. Unlike the anaemias from infectious diseases and malnutrition, the burden on the health services from haemoglobinopathies will increase with improved standards of living, as the life-expectancies of the patients are prolonged.

α Thalassaemia
(See page 19.116.)

The total number of α^0 thalassaemia heterozygotes in Southeast Asia and southern China is about 30 million, with the highest frequencies in northern Thailand (Fig. 1). Homozygous inheritance occurs in at least 10 000 infants per annum; it is lethal, resulting in a hydropic fetus who is stillborn or dies soon after birth (page 19.118). Mothers bearing these infants suffer from toxaemia of pregnancy. The double heterozygous inheritance of α^0 thalassaemia with either α^+ thalassaemia or haemoglobin Constant Spring causes haemoglobin H disease (page 19.118), a thalassaemic condition of intermediate severity, most often presenting as acute haemolysis following infection. Haemoglobin H disease is seen commonly in Southeast Asia: for example, about 56 000 infants are affected annually in Thailand.

β Thalassaemia
(See page 19.110.)

Thalassaemia major arises from the homozygous or compound heterozygous inheritance of various genes for β^0 thalassaemia or β^+ thalassaemia (see page 19.111). Between 22 000 and 42 000 affected infants are born each year, the greatest number being in Asia (Table 2). The haemoglobin value is consistently less than 7 g/dl: without treatment, death is usual before six years of age, usually from infection or heart failure. Treatment with repeated blood transfusions and deferoxamine to reduce iron overload controls the disease, and prolongs near-normal life, at least into the third decade of life and probably much longer (page 19.121). However, about 25 units of blood are needed per patient per year, and the total cost per patient of US $5000–8000 per year presents an impossible burden on the health resources of developing countries.

Milder forms of β thalassaemia, or combinations of β thalassaemia and structural haemoglobin variants, are also extremely common (page 19.119). For example, haemoglobin E thalassaemia (Table 2; Figs 2 and 4) affects thousands of children throughout Southeast Asia, Burma, and the eastern half of the Indian subcontinent.

There are approximately 67.6 million heterozygotes for β thalassaemia in the world, including over 60 million in Asia (Fig. 2). The condition is essentially symptomless, but the haemoglobin level is about 2 g/dl lower than normal. Anaemia is more pronounced in pregnancy, and is associated with placental hypertrophy, intrauterine growth retardation, and about 15 per cent of infants being born with Apgar scores of three or less.

Sickle cell disease
(See page 19.122.)

Sickle cell trait is carried by about 60 million people in the world, of whom 50 million are in Africa (Fig. 3). The trait is harmless but over 100 000 infants are born each year with sickle cell disease, the great majority in Africa (Table 2). Sickle cell anaemia is by far the commonest and most severe form of the disease, but haemoglobin SC disease is important locally in West Africa, especially Ghana and Upper Volta, where the frequency of the haemoglobin C gene is up to 0.15 (Fig. 4), and sickle cell thalassaemia is not uncommon in Liberia, the Mediterranean basin, and in racially mixed populations of the Americas (Table 2).

Haemolysis, infarction, and infection result in death before the age of four years of the great majority of children with sickle cell anaemia in rural tropical Africa. Those with the milder sickling disorders, SC disease and S thalassaemia are likely to survive childhood, and females present with complications during pregnancy. With improved social conditions and the establishment of sickle cell clinics, more children will lead near-normal lives, and sickle cell disease will grow to be one of the greatest loads on the health services of tropical Africa.

Enzymopathies: glucose 6-phosphate dehydrogenase deficiency
(See page 19.140.)

There are numerous variants of the enzyme glucose 6-phosphate dehydrogenase (G6PD), but discussion is confined only to those which cause intermittent haemolysis and reach polymorphic frequency.

There are three zones of the Old World where G6PD deficiency occurs commonly, (a) the Mediterranean, western Asia, and the Indian subcontinent, (b) southern China, Southeast Asia, Indonesia, and Papua New Guinea, and (c) subsaharan Africa. Gd^{Mediterranean} is the common variant in the first zone: it occurs in up to 20 per cent of males in much of the Mediterranean basin, and can reach 50 per cent in certain communities in Sardinia. The frequency in Iran is around 10 per cent; in India, frequencies show wide variation, but are the highest in west Bengal

Table 2 Annual number of births of homozygotes or compound heterozygotes for the major haemoglobinopathies (conservative estimates)

Area	$\alpha^0\alpha^0$ thalassaemia (hydrops fetalis)	β-thalassaemia major	Hb-E/β-thalassaemia	Hb-S/β-thalassaemia	Hb SS and Hb SC	Total
Africa (subSaharan)	–	?	–	?	100 000	100 000
North Africa	–	850	–	300	100	1 250
Eastern Mediterranean	–	1 650	–	530	3 100	5 280
Asia	10 000	16 950	16 100	200	4 000	47 250
North America and Caribbean	–	100	?	200	2 300	2 600
South America	–	90	–	500	4 100	4 690
Oceania	?	?	?	–	–	?
Total minimum	10 000	21 990	16 100	1 830	113 700	163 620
Possible total	20 000	42 000	32 200	3 600	120 000	217 800

From WHO Working Group (1983). The conditions are described in detail on pages 19.108–19.130.

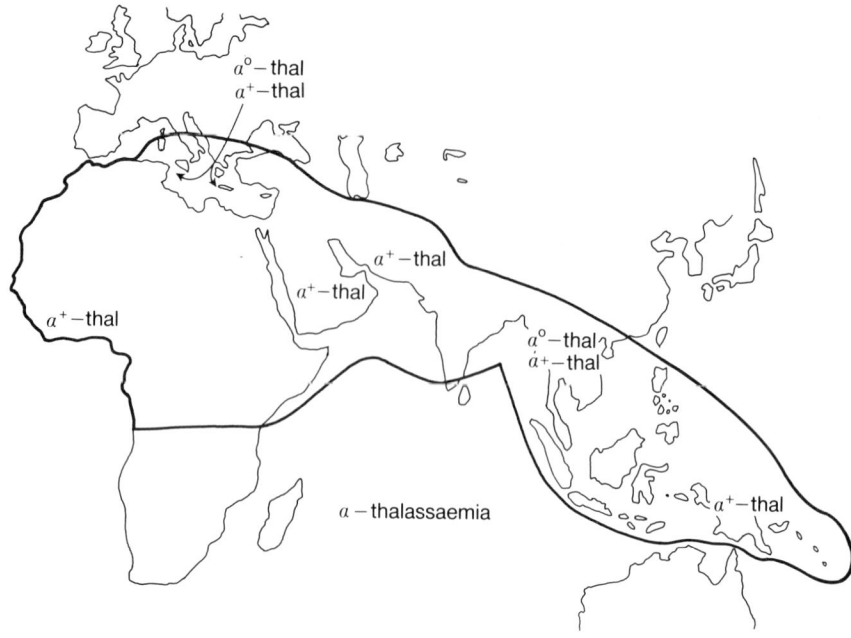

Fig. 1 Areas of the old world where the α thalassaemias occur commonly. The different types of α thalassaemia are described on page 19.116.

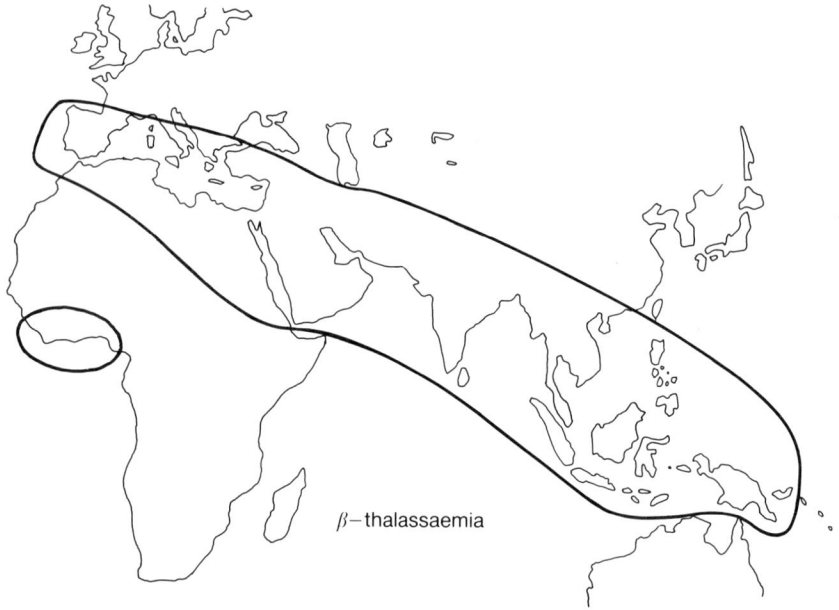

Fig. 2 Areas of the old world where the β thalassaemias occur commonly.

(14 per cent). There is a great heterogeneity of enzyme variants in the second zone: Gd^{Mediterranean} is common, but Gd^{Canton}, Gd^{Union}, and Gd^{Mahidol} also reach polymorphic frequencies. Deficiencies of all types occur in 12–15 per cent of males in Laos, Thailand, and Cambodia. GdA$^-$ is observed in up to 30 per cent of males in subsaharan Africa, including south of the Zambesi: GdA has even greater frequency, but it is not associated with haemolysis: Gd^{Mali} and Gd^{Gambia} are found locally at polymorphic frequency, the latter not causing disease.

The clinical and haematological manifestations of different G6PD deficiencies are discussed on page 19.140. They present major health problems primarily through their contribution to neonatal jaundice, secondly by causing haemolysis and jaundice during acute infections, and finally, with the severe deficiencies only, through haemolysis triggered by certain oxidant drugs.

Hereditary elliptocytosis

(See page 19.138.)

Elliptocytosis is widespread and common in Peninsular Malaysia, Borneo, Philippines, Indonesia, and Papua New Guinea. It is present in more than 20 per cent of Melanesians in some areas of lowland Papua New Guinea, and their red cells have been shown to be highly resistant to invasion by *P. falciparum*, *in vitro*. A similar variant is seen in about 3 per cent of northern and southern Nigerians.

About 80 per cent of subjects with elliptocytosis have otherwise

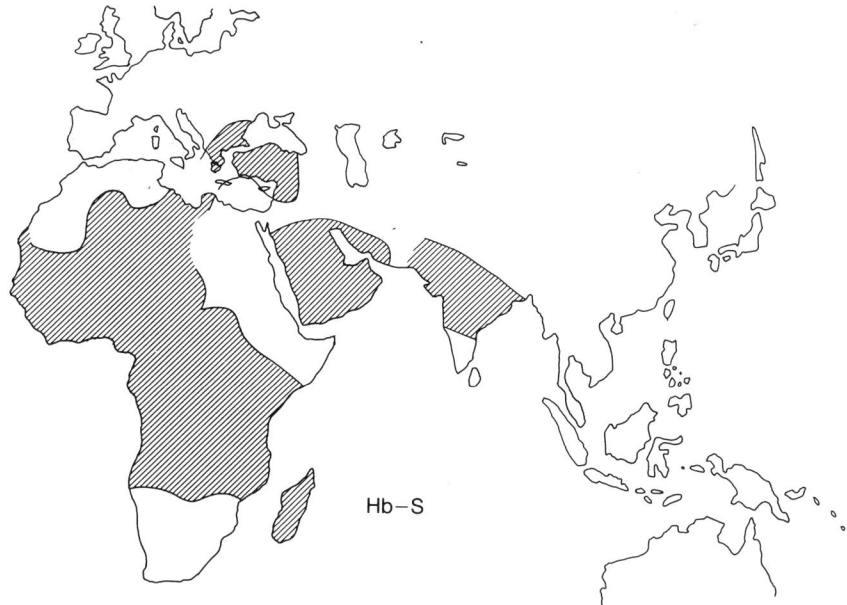

Fig. 3 Areas of the Old World where haemoglobin S gene occurs at frequency greater than 0.02.

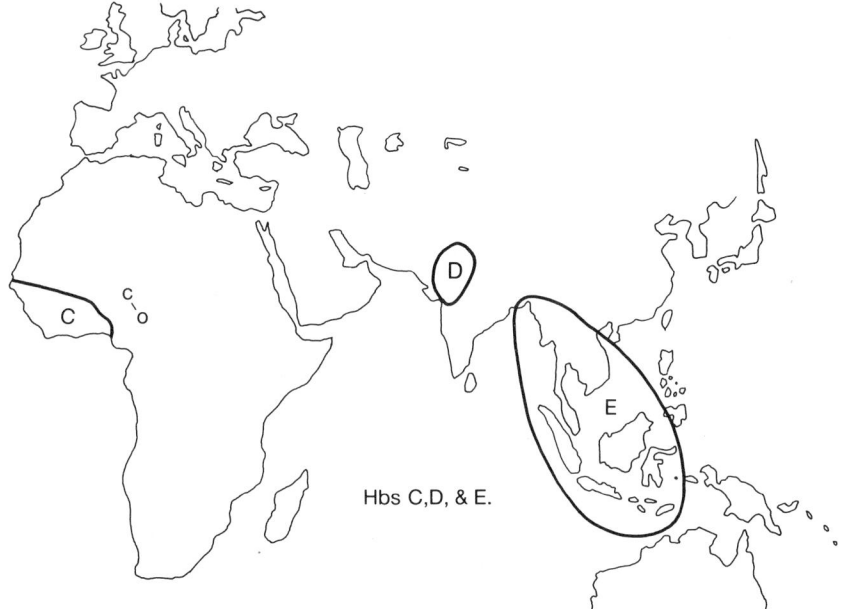

Fig. 4 Areas of the Old World where haemoglobins C, D-Punjab (or Los Angeles), and E occur commonly. (From Fleming, 1982, with permission.)

normal red cell indices. Others have a partially compensated haemolytic anaemia, with an average haemoglobin about 2 g/dl lower than normal. The occasional child has extremely severe life-threatening haemolytic anaemia, apparently triggered by the successful invasion by *P. falciparum*.

Changes in the diet following agriculture

The domestication of plants by agriculture resulted in a reduction of the contribution of animal food in the diet from about 70 to 5 per cent or less. This affected profoundly the intake of bioavailable iron, folate, and protein.

Iron deficiency

Humans are adapted to absorb haem efficiently as an intact metalloporphyrin, and to utilize the iron. As a consequence, iron deficiency and anaemia are uncommon amongst those groups who have persisted as hunter-gatherers, for example, the Hadza in Tanzania and the !Kung Bushmen in the Kalahari Desert, and amongst pastoralists who eat blood and meat, like the Masai in Kenya. In contrast, the absorption of non-haem iron (except from breast milk) is comparatively restricted, and iron deficiency and anaemia are common in communities whose food is predominantly of vegetable origin. The three great staples of humans are rice, wheat, and maize. Sorghum and millet are important in some

Table 3 Absorption of non-haem iron from meals

	Iron intake (mg)	Mean iron absorption (%)
Rice meals	14.6	6.9
Wheat meals	0.6	28
Maize meals	4.6	3.5
Sorghum porridge		2.8
Soya beans	0.5–4.0	2.6–11.0
Black beans		1.5–2.6

Modified from Bothwell *et al.* (1982).

Table 4 Prevalence of anaemia (per cent) in preschool children (Hb <11.0 g/dl), non-pregnant women (Hb <12.0 g/dl), pregnant women (Hb <11.0 g/dl) and men (Hb <13.0 g/dl)

Geographical area	Preschool children	Non-pregnant women	Pregnant women	Men
Latin America (7 countries)		17	24	4
Chile	35			
Nigeria	63	46	52	36
Northern India	90	84	80	48
Southern India	76	81	88	56
Burma	3–27	5–15	82	1–5
Philippines	42	37	72	7

From various sources including Baker and DeMaeyer (1979) and Fleming (1982).

Table 5 Prevalence (per cent) of anaemia (Hb <11.0 g/dl) and iron deficiency (saturation of transferrin <15 per cent) during pregnancy

Geographical area	Anaemia	Iron deficiency
Latin America	27	49
Nigeria	47	31
Northern India	80	52
Southern India	57	99
Philippines	63	35

From various sources including Baker and DeMaeyer (1979) and Fleming (1982).

drier areas of Africa and Asia. Soy and other legumes are essential sources of protein in many countries. Iron content is generally low, but more importantly, iron absorption is inhibited by fibre, phytates, phosphates, and polyphenols of these vegetable staples (Table 3). Ascorbic acid and amino acids (especially cysteine) from animal protein are the major enhancers of absorption of non-haem iron, but natural sources are expensive, and animal protein may be excluded from the food by religious beliefs, including Hinduism. Much of the world's population is restricted to a diet from which sufficient iron cannot be absorbed to meet physiological requirements, especially during infancy, early childhood, adolescence, menstruation, and pregnancy (Tables 4 and 5). Loss of iron from chronic haemorrhage due to hookworm or schistosomiasis contributes further to the high frequencies of iron deficiency and anaemia. Perhaps 20 per cent of the world's population are iron deficient.

Megaloblastic anaemias
(See page 19.93.)

Deficiency of active folate coenzymes is common, resulting from low intake, malabsorption, high requirements or metabolic blocks. Deficiency of vitamin B_{12}, which figures prominently in medical textbooks, is comparatively unimportant from a global view.

Table 6 Prevalence of megaloblastic erythropoiesis in samples of all pregnant women and anaemic pregnant women

	Country	Population sample	Percentage megaloblastic
All pregnant women	Nigeria	Primigravidae, Zaria	56
		Primigravidae protected against malaria	25
	Southern India	Rural and urban	66
	Indonesia	Rural	25
	Western Australia	Urban	18
Anaemic pregnant women	Nigeria	Rural and urban, Ibadan	75
	Pakistan	Urban	25
	Malaysia	Urban	25
	Singapore	Urban Indian	45
		Urban Malay	30
		Urban Chinese	7

From various sources, including Luzzatto (1981) and Fleming *et al.* (1985).

Folate deficiency

There is scanty information about the folate content of foods eaten commonly in the tropics. Yams, sweet potatoes, other tubers, plantain, fresh peppers, locust beans (*Parkia fillicoidea*), and green vegetables are all rich sources, but rice, maize, cassava, sorghum, and millet are poor. Folates are heat-labile so that prolonged cooking and repeated reheating are major factors contributing to the high prevalence of megaloblastic anaemia amongst Africans and Indians, as illustrated by the frequency in Indians in Singapore, compared to the Chinese, who cook vegetables lightly (Table 6). Low intake is not necessarily the result of a lack of folate in the food; the more-or-less continuous anorexia of recurrent infections such as malaria, or chronic infections like tuberculosis, is a most important cause of deficiency in children in the tropics.

Acute enteric infections, and also infections of other systems, for example, pneumonia, are important causes of malabsorption in childhood. In southern India, over 70 per cent of patients with sprue for three months or more, have megaloblastic marrows due to folate deficiency.

Children and pregnant women are particularly liable to depletion of folate because of high physiological requirements. Pathologically high demands result from erythroid hyperplasia secondary to haemolysis. The effects of recurrent malaria are seen most clearly during pregnancy: antenatal antimalarial prophylaxis alone in Nigeria was followed by higher serum folate levels, a reduction of the prevalence of megaloblastosis and the abolition of life-threatening anaemias (Table 6). Patients with sickle cell anaemia and thalassaemia major are almost invariably folate depleted on first presentation in rural areas.

Dihydrofolate reductase activity, and hence the conversion of folate to its active forms, is inhibited at 39 °C; pyrexia may lead to acute megaloblastic arrest of erythropoiesis, and may play a role in the megaloblastosis seen so often complicating infectious diseases.

Megaloblastic erythropoiesis is commonly a preanaemic state: 18 per cent of pregnant women in Western Australia showed frank megaloblastosis, but folate deficiency was associated only occasionally with anaemia (Table 6). However, once the haemoglobin starts to fall, profound anaemia, often with neutropenia and thrombocytopenia is liable to develop rapidly.

Thirty-nine per cent of Indian and 34 per cent of Nigerian children with kwashiorkor have megaloblastic erythopoiesis. In northern Nigeria 40 per cent, and in Cameroon 79 per cent of anaemic preschool children have megaloblastosis. The highest prevalence recorded during pregnancy is in West Africa (Table 6).

Vitamin B₁₂ deficiency

The requirements for vitamin B_{12} are so low (rising to only 3 μg per day during pregnancy), that they are met by the smallest intake of animal products. Serum levels and liver stores are lowest in Hindu vegetarians, but even amongst the poorest in southern India, purely dietary deficiency is uncommon, probably because bacterial contamination of water and food provides sufficient vitamin. (Dietary deficiency can occur when Indians migrate to the United Kingdom, where clean food and piped water removes this source of vitamin B_{12}.) Significant deficiency in the vegetarian adult is liable to develop if there is interference with absorption by the ileum following infection. Deficiency becomes progressively common with time of duration of tropical sprue (see Section 12). Infants of deficient Indian mothers are born with low stores and fed on breast milk containing insufficient vitamin B_{12}; after a few months they develop megaloblastic anaemia with locomotor complications, which may progress to coma and death.

Pernicious anaemia is rare in Asia and practically unknown in Africa.

Agriculture-related anaemias

There are three periods of life when anaemia is most prevalent and has the most serious consequences: (*a*) the neonatal period, (*b*) childhood, and (*c*) pregnancy. Maternal anaemia will be discussed first, as the frequency and severity of neonatal jaundice and anaemia in childhood are largely governed by intrauterine events. Although anaemia is less common in adult men and non-pregnant women, it reduces work capacity and hence has important economic consequences.

Anaemia in pregnancy

(See also Section 11.)

Women are liable to anaemia during pregnancy because they have higher requirements for iron and folate, and there is an increased susceptibility to infection, of which *P. falciparum* is by far the most important in endemic areas. Both frequency and density of parasitaemia increase progressively to reach a peak around mid-pregnancy especially in first pregnancies. The major causes of anaemia in pregnancy in the world are iron deficiency and folate deficiency, malaria, and the haemoglobinopathies. The relative importance of these factors will vary around the world: for example, iron deficiency predominates in India (Table 5), whereas malaria complicated by folate deficiency is the major cause of profound anaemia in West Africa (Table 6).

The impact of anaemia, dietary deficiency and malaria on the mother and the infant are shown schematically in Fig. 5. Deficiencies of iron and folate, and malaria lower further the immune responses, and the pregnant woman enters a vicious cycle of infection, nutritional deficiency, and depressed immunity. She is less able to withstand haemorrhage, and is breathless on exertion, or at rest when anaemia is severe. The full impact is seen if the haemoglobin level is less than about 3 g/dl, when congestive cardiac failure may develop and, without treatment, mortality is around 50 per cent: appropriate transfusion of concentrated red cells with a rapidly acting diuretic and medication reduces mortality to about two per cent.

The consequences to the infant are more often disastrous. If anaemia persists throughout pregnancy, as with the haemoglobinopathies or in the absence of treatment, fetal hypoxia results in compensatory placental hypertrophy and retarded intrauterine growth. Fetal distress is common and Apgar scores of three or less are observed in about 15 per cent if the mothers' haemoglobin level is below 10 g/dl. The prevalence of low birth weight is related directly to the severity of maternal anaemia; when Nigerian mothers' PCV values were 0.23 or less at the time of delivery, 50 per cent of infants weighed less than 2.0 kg and perinatal mortality

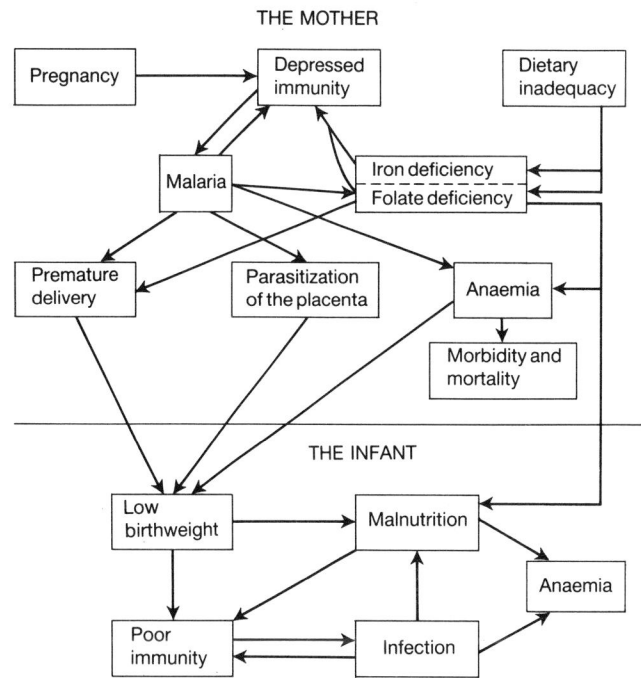

Fig. 5 The pathophysiology of malaria, iron deficiency, folate deficiency, and anaemia during pregnancy. (From Fleming *et al.*, 1985, with permission.)

was more than 30 per cent. Successful treatment of maternal anaemia for about six weeks before delivery results in a dramatic improvement of birth weight and other measures of infant health.

The causes of anaemia may themselves have directly adverse effects on the fetus. Malaria infects the placenta and causes low birth weight; pyrexia precipitates premature labour. Folate deficiency is itself a cause of premature delivery.

Infants of iron deficient mothers have low iron stores; their folate status at birth reflects that of the mother, and the folate content of breast milk is diminished by maternal deficiency and maternal malaria. Low birth weight is strongly associated with poor immunity: neonatal infections lead to further depression of immunity and the infant has completed the same cycle of poor immunity, infection, and malnutrition as the mother, but in the infant the cycle is much more vicious as the immune system is undeveloped and nutrition is critical.

Neonatal jaundice

Jaundice (serum bilirubin above 250 μmol1/1) during the first week of life is a common problem in hospitals in Asia and Africa, but estimates of its frequency are unreliable. Aetiology is nearly always multiple; four causes are most prevalent, sepsis, prematurity, G6PD deficiency, and ABO incompatibility. Less frequent causes include haematomas and elliptocytosis. Rhesus incompatibility is unusual except among Caucasians, and intrauterine infections by toxoplasmosis, cytomegalovirus, herpes, and malaria present no problem where the mothers have high levels of acquired immunity.

Awareness by mothers and doctors, and early treatment by exchange transfusion and phototherapy, reduces mortality dramatically, but despite treatment 26 per cent of affected Ghanaian infants showed subsequent psychomotor retardation.

Anaemia in childhood

Preschool children in the underdeveloped countries are liable to be anaemic from six months of age onwards for several reasons. They have lost protection from maternally derived antibodies and have not yet acquired active immunity, breast feeding may be replaced by inappropriate or inadequate solid foods, they may be exposed to hookworm infection once they start crawling, and the β-globin haemoglobinopathies become manifest. The common causes of anaemia are malaria, viral and bacterial infections, iron and folate deficiency, protein-energy malnutrition (PEM) (see Section 8), and haemoglobinopathies. Aetiology is almost always multiple; the children have been caught in a vicious cycle of infection, depressed immunity, and malnutrition, of which anaemia is only one major complication (as illustrated in the lower half of Fig. 5).

Infections suppress immunity
Many infections impair cell-mediated immunity especially, but also humoral immunity and phagocytic function. Measles and malaria in particular are commonly complicated by upper and lower respiratory tract and gastrointestinal infections frequently associated with anaemia in childhood.

Infections lead to anaemia and malnutrition
The anaemia of malaria has many mechanisms (page 19.241). Viral and bacterial infections depress erythropoiesis, immobilize iron in the reticulo-endothelial system, and cause toxic, microangiopathic or immune haemolysis, but the strongest link from infection to anaemia in childhood is through malnutrition. Anorexia causes rapid depletion of folate stores and a negative iron balance, and jeopardizes energy and protein balance. Gastrointestinal and other infections cause malabsorption of folate and other nutrients. Measles is further complicated by protein-loosing enteropathy. Demands for folate are increased by erythroid hyperplasia following haemolysis of malaria or other infections. Dihydrofolate reductase is inactivated by pyrexia.

Malnutrition causes anaemia and suppresses immunity
PEM is associated with a mild normochromic, normocytic anaemia unless complicated by iron or folate deficiency and infection. The most important feature of PEM in the aetiology of anaemia is impairment of resistance to infection. There are defects of the non-specific defences (skin, epithelial surfaces, secretions, complement, and function of the phagocytes), depletion of T lymphocytes, and some depression of humoral immunity. Iron deficiency results in depression of cell-mediated immunity and the bactericidal activity of neutrophils: this is offset partially by the bacteriostatic properties of unsaturated transferrin. Folate deficiency causes neutropenia and defective lymphocyte division, affecting cell-mediated more than humoral immunity.

Consequences of anaemia in childhood
The syndrome of infection, malnutrition, and anaemia in early life is commonly fatal, or leads to permanent defects of growth, development and intellectual function. Iron deficiency alone is associated with reduced weight gain and poor scholastic performance, both improving following the administration of iron supplements.

Anaemia and work capacity
Compensatory mechanisms (page 19.67) ensure that oxygenation of the tissues is adequate at rest while haemoglobin levels are above about 7 g/dl, but subjects will quickly become breathless on exertion. The performance of near-maximal work, as measured by the Havard step-test, shows a direct correlation to haemoglobin concentration, and the earning capacity of anaemic rural workers is reduced seriously. When the haemoglobin falls below about 7 g/dl, the compensatory mechanisms fail, lactic acid accumulates, and subjects are breathless even at rest. Self-employed farmers often do not present for treatment until they have reached this stage, when any heavy manual work is impossible. Iron deficiency *per se* limits physical exertion as depletion of the iron-containing enzyme α-glycerophosphate dehydrogenase impairs glycolysis and results in excessive production of lactic acid.

Anaemia effects the whole family through inability to care for children, loss of earnings or reduction of food production. The economy of the village suffers from a diminution of the area of ground under cultivation, and the national economy is effected by overall low productivity. The socio-economic consequences of the high prevalence of anaemia in rural tropical communities are enormous.

Prevention of anaemia
The global control of anaemia is an immense and complex problem. The first step is research into the prevalence of anaemia in infants, children, pregnant women, non-pregnant women, and adult men, and into the relative importance of the common causes of anaemia. Recommendations can then be made as to the initial treatment required. Maternal child health centres should be established. These will ensure the prevention of anaemia in pregnancy. Most of the causes of neonatal jaundice can be avoided by antenatal care, which reduces the frequency of low birth weight, birth trauma, and sepsis: oxidant drugs should not be prescribed without good reason, and ABO incompatibility can be anticipated. Antenatal care will go far to prevent anaemia in childhood by reducing prematurity, increasing average birthweight, and improving the nutritional status of the newborn. Anaemia will be controlled further by the encouragement of breast feeding, iron and folic acid supplementation for premature and other infants at risk, early detection and treatment of malnutrition and its prevention by education of mothers, prompt diagnosis and treatment of malaria, prevention by immunization and the early treatment of other infections, and the early diagnosis of haemoglobinopathies. The health of mothers and children will be enhanced by advice aimed at extending the intervals between births. Genetic counselling and prenatal diagnosis (see page 19.120) will reduce the frequency of haemoglobinopathies.

On a national or international level, the eradication of malaria now seems to be beyond our present capabilities, but the impact of malaria can be minimized by mosquito avoidance and control near to homes. Transmission of many diseases associated with anaemia will be broken by clean water and adequate disposal of sewage. Hookworm may be eliminated by the use of pit-latrines, abandoning the use of human faeces as fertilizer, and the wearing of cheap plastic sandals when in the fields; hookworm has been virtually eradicated from South Korea during the last 20 years by these simple methods.

Many countries are conducting trials of fortification with iron of commonly eaten foods: these include an acidified milk-formula for infants and biscuits (with bovine-haemoglobin) for children in Chile, sugar in Guatemala, salt in India, fish-sauce in Thailand, and soy-sauce in China. Results are promising and the global control of nutritional iron deficiency could be achieved in the foreseeable future.

Finally, there are many schemes, large and small, around the world aimed at boosting the production of food. Irrigation and agriculture will, however, increase the sum of human misery unless these plans include measures to avoid the transmission of the diseases which in turn cause malnutrition and anaemia.

References
Baker, S. J. and DeMaeyer, E. M. (1979). Nutritional anemia: its understanding and control with special reference to the work of the World Health Organization. *Am. J. clin. Nutrit.* **32**, 368–417.
Basta, S. S., Soekirman, M. S., Karyadi, D. and Scrimshaw, N. S. (1979). Iron deficiency anemia and the productivity of adult males in Indonesia. *Am. J. clin. Nutrit.* **32**, 916–925.
Bothwell, T. H., Charlton, R.W., Cook, J. D. and Finch, C. A. (1979). *Iron metabolism in Man.* Blackwell Scientific Publications, Oxford.
——, Clydesdale, F. M., Cook, J. D., Dallman, P. R., Hallberg, L., Van-Campen, D. and Wolf, W. J. (1982). *The effects of cereals and legumes on iron availability.* International Nutritional Anemia Consultative Group (INACG), Washington DC.

Brabin, B. J. (1983). An analysis of malaria in pregnancy in Africa. *Bull. Wld Hlth Org.* **61**, 1005–1016.

Burman, D. (1982). Iron deficiency in infancy and childhood. *Clinics Haemat.* **11**, 339–351.

Castelino, D., Saul, A., Myler, P., Kidson, C., Thomas, H. and Cooke, R. (1981). Ovalocytosis in Papua New Guinea – dominantly inherited resistance to malaria. *Southeast Asian J. trop. Med. Pub. Hlth.* **12**, 549–555.

Dallman, P. R., Siimes, M. A. and Stekel, A. (1980). Iron deficiency in infancy and childhood. *Am. J. clin. Nutrit.* **33**, 86–118.

Farid, Z., Patwardhan, V. N. and Darby, W. J. (1969). Parasitism and anemia. *Am. J. clin. Nutrit.* **22**, 498–503.

Finch, C. A. (1972). Iron nutrition. *Ann. N. Y. Acad. Sci.* **300**, 221–227.

Fleming, A. F. (ed.) (1982). *Sickle-cell disease: a handbook for the general clinician.* Churchill Livingstone, Edinburgh.

—— (1982). Iron deficiency in the tropics. *Clinics Haemat.* **11**, 365–388.

—— and Werblińksa, B. (1982). Anaemia in childhood in the guinea savanna of Nigeria. *Ann. trop. Paediat.* **2**, 161–173.

——, Ghatoura, G. B. S., Harrison, K. A., Briggs, N. D. and Dunn, D. T. (1985). The prevention of anaemia in pregnancy in primigravidae in the guinea savanna of Nigeria. *Ann. trop. Med. Parasitol.* **80**, 211–233.

Florencio, C. A. (1981). Effects of iron and ascorbic acid supplementation on hemoglobin level and work efficiency of anemic women. *J. occupat. Med.* **23**, 669–704.

Hågå, P. (l980). Plasma ferritin concentrations in preterm infants in cord blood and during the early anaemia of prematurity. *Acta paediatr. scand.* **69**, 637–641.

Huq, R. S., Abalaka, J. A. and Stafford, W. L. (1983). Folate content of various Nigerian foods. *J. Sci. Food Agric.* **34**, 404–406.

Jacobs, A. (1982). Non-haematological effects of iron deficiency. *Clinics Haemat.* **11**, 353–364.

Kidson, C., Lamont, G., Saul, A. and Nurse, G. T. (1981). Ovalocytic erythrocytes from Melanesians are resistant to invasion by malaria parasites in culture. *Proc. natl. Acad. Sci. USA* **78**, 5829–5832.

Livingstone, F. B. (1971). Malaria and human polymorphisms. *Ann. Rev. Genet.* **5**, 33–64.

Luzzatto, L. (ed.) (1981). *Haematology in tropical areas. Clinics Haemat.* **10**, 697–1073.

Macdougall, L. G., Moodley, G., Eyberg, C. and Quirk. M. (1982). Mechanisms of anemia in protein-energy malnutrition in Johannesburg. *Am. J. clin. Nutrit.* **35**, 229–235.

Molineaux, L. and Gramiccia, G. (1980). *The Garki project: research on the epidemiology and control of malaria in the sudan savanna of West Africa.* World Health Organization, Geneva.

Oppenheimer, S. J., Higgs, D. R., Weatherall, D.J., Barker, J. and Spark, R. A. (1984). α thalassaemia in Papua New Guinea. *Lancet* **i**, 424–426.

Weatherall, D. J. and Clegg, J. B. (1981). *The thalassaemia syndromes*, 3rd. edn. Blackwell Scientific Publications, Oxford.

Werblińska, B., Stankiewicz, H., Oduloju, M. O., Atuchukwu, C. M. and Fleming, A. F. (1981). Neonatal jaundice in Zaria, northern Nigeria. *Nigerian J. Paediat.* **8**, 3–10.

Wong, H. B. (1980). Singapore kernicterus. *Singapore Med. J.* **21**, 556–567.

Working Group on Fortification of Common Salt with Iron (1982). Use of common salt fortified with iron in the control and prevention of anemia- a collaborative study. *Am. J. clin. Nutrit*, **35**, 1442–1451.

World Health Organization Working Group (1983). Community control of hereditary anaemias: memorandum from a WHO meeting. *Bull. Wld. Hlth Org.* **61**, 63–80.

Iron metabolism

A. JACOBS

Biochemistry

Iron is an important element in human metabolism. It has a central role in erythropoiesis and is involved in intracellular processes in all the tissues of the body. Many of the known iron compounds in the body are haemoproteins, some of which are directly involved with oxygen transport. The haemoglobin molecule has a molecular weight of 64 500 and consists of four haem groups linked to four polypeptide chains. It can bind four molecules of oxygen (see page 19.65). Myoglobin has a molecular weight of 17 000 and consists of a single polypeptide chain with one haem group. It has a higher affinity for oxygen than haemoglobin and behaves as an oxygen store in muscle cells. When oxygen supply is limited, it is released to cytochrome oxidase which has a higher affinity for oxygen than myoglobin. Mitochondria contain a system for the transport of electrons from intracellular substrates to molecular oxygen with the simultaneous generation of ATP. This pathway contains a number of iron compounds, including the cytochromes, which transmit electrons by means of reversible valency changes of their iron atoms. Failure in this system due to lack of oxygen supply to the tissues, enzyme depletion, or blocking with metabolic inhibitors such as cyanide leads to failure of energy production and an accumulation of intermediate metabolites with eventual cell death. Iron enzymes are also involved in a diverse range of other metabolic processes such as the hydroxylation reactions associated with drug detoxication and sterol synthesis, DNA synthesis, catecholamine metabolism, and collagen formation.

When any cell takes up more iron than is needed for its specific metabolic requirements, the excess stimulates ferritin synthesis and a small intracellular store is formed. The storage iron compounds, ferritin and haemosiderin, are found mainly in the reticulo-endothelial cells of the liver, spleen, and bone marrow where iron has been released following haemoglobin breakdown, but they are also found in many parenchymal cells. Liver parenchymal cells contain visible amounts of iron and muscle contains storage iron both in muscle cells and in the reticulo-endothelial cells between the fibres. The storage compounds represent a reserve of iron that can be mobilized when requirements elsewhere in the body are increased.

Ferritin is a soluble protein with a unique configuration. It has an outer protein shell, consisting of 24 subunits of molecular weight 18 500, and an inner core consisting of a variable amount of iron deposited as a ferric hydroxyphosphate complex. Apoferritin has a molecular weight of about 48 000 and the complete molecule about 900 000 with an iron content of over 20 per cent. Synthesis of the protein is stimulated by the presence of iron and degradation occurs when no iron is incorporated. The formation of apoferritin is gradually followed by the accumulation of iron inside the shell, possibly by the passage of small iron complexes through channels formed between the subunits. There are two types of ferritin subunit, H and L, and different cells may contain different isoferritins whose biochemical and physiological properties are based on the proportion of the two subunits. The expressed gene for the H subunit is located on chromosome 11 and that for the L subunit on chromosome 19. Haemosiderin is an amorphous insoluble storage compound with a higher iron content than ferritin. It is probably formed by the partial digestion of ferritin protein shells with a consequent condensation of molecules. Its precise composition depends on the degree of protein denaturation and its iron content may be as high as 37 per cent. Both substances produce a Prussian Blue reaction which allows their identification in histological preparations.

Iron is transported through the plasma bound to transferrin. This is a beta-globulin with a molecular weight of about 80 000; it binds 1.3 μg of iron per mg protein. The plasma concentration of transferrin is about 2.3 g/l and normally a total of about 4 mg of iron circulates bound in this form. The molecule has two separate binding sites each capable of binding one atom of ferric iron, and one bicarbonate ion is normally bound with each iron atom. The equilibrium constants for the two sites at physiological pH are approximately equal and of the order of 10^{30}. Transferrin synthesis occurs primarily in the liver and appears to be related to the level of storage iron, being increased in iron deficiency and decreased when normal or increased stores are present.

Iron balance

The iron content of the body is normally kept constant by a delicate balance between the amount absorbed and the amount lost. Iron losses from the body are limited and there is no physiological mechanism for regulating the excretion of excess amounts. Small amounts are lost from epithelial surfaces through the exfoliation of cells and as insensible blood loss from the gastrointestinal tract. Relatively little is lost from the urinary tract or from the skin.

Attempts have been made to measure total iron losses by administering radioactive tracer and observing its rate of disappearance either from the peripheral blood or by whole-body counting. The data suggest an average daily iron loss of about 1 mg in men and non-menstruating women and about 2 mg in menstruating women. Data from different parts of the world show a remarkable consistency in those with a normal body load despite differences of race and climatic conditions. In South African Bantu a mean iron loss of about twice normal is probably related to increased iron load and a consequent increase in the iron content of exfoliating cells, particularly from the gut.

In young women there is a mean menstral loss of about 40 ml, equivalent to about 0.7 mg iron daily but more than 10 per cent of women have losses in excess of 80 ml, equivalent to over 1.4 mg daily and therefore a mean daily total iron loss in excess of 2.3 mg. Menstrual loss in excess of 80 ml is commonly associated with iron deficiency and amounts higher than this should be defined as menorrhagia.

Iron requirements should be a simple matter of replacement for iron lost. However, the availability of iron in different foods varies and this, together with differences in intraluminal reactions and the absorptive capacity of the intestinal mucosa, makes it difficult to determine the amount of food iron required. It is generally assumed that under normal conditions about 5–10 per cent of dietary iron is absorbed, and, as the average iron content of the British diet is about 14 mg daily, it should not be difficult for a man with normal iron losses to maintain himself in positive balance. When iron losses are minimal, a dietary iron absorption of less than 10 per cent may be adequate. If the iron requirements of a menstruating woman are in excess of 2 mg daily then the amount and availability of food iron must be enough to allow iron balance to be maintained by a compensatory increase in the level of intestinal absorption. Individual dietary iron intake is lower in families with children and decreases with the number of children, suggesting a more remote effect of pregnancy on iron balance. The iron absorption mechanism is extremely sensitive to changes in iron status and it seems likely that the majority of people in the population can adapt to different iron intakes. Iron deficiency anaemia is commonly found in menstruating women but it is usually possible to compensate for normal menstrual iron losses when dietary intake is about 11 mg daily. In normal women haemoglobin levels are only significantly reduced in those with a menstrual loss in excess of 80 ml.

Interaction between foods is an important source of variation in iron absorption. For instance, absorption is impaired by egg and potentiated by orange juice. Many countries have adopted enrichment of flour as a national policy in an attempt to maintain the level of intake. Prophylactic administration of iron is indeed widely adopted despite criticism of its effectiveness and lack of agreement regarding the harmful effects of minor degrees of iron overload.

There are a number of physiological situations such as pregnancy and lactation where iron requirements are greater than normal and negative iron balance can give rise to latent or clinical iron deficiency. When adequate iron is available the red cell mass may increase by about 30 per cent in pregnancy taking up an additional 500 mg iron as haemoglobin. In addition about 250–300 mg of iron is transferred across the placenta to the fetus. Both these processes occur largely during the second half of pregnancy. During delivery and the puerperium blood loss of 500 ml or more together

with placental iron may account for an additional deficit of about 300 mg iron. The net iron requirements are somewhat reduced as the expanded red cell mass returns to normal after delivery but the total cost may be about 500 mg. Iron requirements during pregnancy cannot be calculated easily as many non-pregnant women have little or no reserve iron and may already be overtly iron deficient. Supplementation with medicinal iron is necessary to ensure adequate iron status, and 30 mg of elemental iron given daily by mouth in the form of ferrous sulphate or fumarate is effective in maintaining haemoglobin levels throughout pregnancy.

Prematurity results in a shortening of the period when iron is transferred to the fetus. The total amount of iron in the newborn infant is closely related to birth weight. Most of this iron is in the form of circulating haemoglobin and late clamping of the cord after delivery can result in an increase of over 50 per cent in this fraction. In a well-nourished population the administration of either oral or parenteral iron to the mother during pregnancy has little effect on the haematological status or iron stores of the infant in the first 18 months of life. The most important factor in the infant's iron economy that can be influenced by medical treatment is its postnatal iron intake.

During growth from infancy to adult life the total body iron content increases approximately from 300 to 4000 mg and if there were a uniform rate of growth, this would mean a daily iron increment of 0.5 mg in addition to the normal replacement of physiological losses. In fact, there are considerable differences in iron metabolism and growth rate during this period which affect requirements. During the first six weeks of life there is a decrease in haemoglobin mass. Some of the iron from this source is probably utilized for myoglobin synthesis but most enters the storage pool and is reflected by the increase in liver iron content and serum ferritin concentration found at this time. Injected iron is poorly utilized for haemoglobin synthesis during the first eight weeks of life but after this time erythropoiesis becomes more active.

The redistribution of iron in the first three months of life with little increase in body content is in accord with the data on serum ferritin concentration which rises to a maximum at one month and then falls, reaching its lowest level at the age of 6–12 months. An intake of about 0.5 mg iron daily is needed in the first six months of life and 0.75 mg daily between six and twelve months. Requirements then drop until the onset of puberty when 1 mg daily may be necessary. Iron deficiency is sometimes found at this age. Dietary requirements in the second year of life are probably about 5–7 mg daily provided that there is a good state of nutrition at the end of the first year.

The previous considerations of iron balance apply largely to Western populations in which prevailing socio-economic conditions result in a moderately satisfactory nutritional status. In many tropical areas there may be an element of dietary iron deficiency, and the quantity of meat eaten and the level of iron absorption are often low. Hookworm infestation is often the prime cause of excess iron loss, the amount of blood lost from the intestine and the degree of anaemia being proportional to the worm load. Many other factors such as protein and riboflavin deficiency and infection are important in the aetiology of tropical anaemia but these do not interfere with iron balance. The major problem in these circumstances is one of socio-economic status rather than iron metabolism (see page 19.75).

Iron absorption

Physiological control over iron balance is normally maintained by the regulation of iron absorption. The intestinal epithelium is extremely sensitive to the iron requirements of the body and can reject unwanted dietary iron or absorb increased amounts when stores are low. The absorption of inorganic iron is highest when given alone in the fasting state and is reduced by food in proportion to the size of the meal. Food iron is released into the gastric juice either as Fe^{2+} and Fe^{3+} ions, or as a haem complex and the intraluminal behaviour of these is different. The amount of food iron available for absorption depends on its release during the digestive process and its interaction in the gastrointestinal lumen. Less than half the total amount of iron in food is released by peptic digestion and this is considerably reduced in subjects with gastric atrophy. Unpolymerized ferrous and ferric ions found in the stomach at pH 1–2 are chemically reactive and, when the gastric contents pass into the jejunum these form complexes which may be available for mucosal uptake. Both phytate and phosphate limit iron absorption through the formation of insoluble complexes. The stimulating effect of ascorbic acid on iron absorption is partly related to the reduction of iron to the more soluble ferrous form and partly to the formation of soluble iron–ascorbate chelates. Fructose and a number of other compounds also form iron chelates which remain soluble at an alkaline pH and may pass across the epithelial cell membrane. Food iron absorption may be reduced by orally administered desferrioxamine or by the tannin in tea. Abnormal components of the diet in patients with pica may sometimes remove iron from solution and make it unavailable. The simultaneous administration of iron salts and tetracycline results in a gross impairment of absorption of both substances probably due to the formation of unavailable iron chelates in the gut lumen.

Under normal circumstances most of the ionizable iron released from the food in the stomach either binds to the mucoprotein in the gastric secretions or becomes unavailable on neutralization. Only in exceptional circumstances when large amounts of a potential chelating agent such as ascorbic acid or citric acid are ingested do low molecular weight complexes form. The iron–mucoprotein complex behaves as an intraluminal carrier system enabling non-haem to reach the absorbing epithelium in a soluble state, though it is not absorbed in this form. There is no evidence that gastric secretions play any part in the physiological regulation of iron absorption or that pancreatic secretions have any specific effect on iron absorption.

Most of the haem iron liberated from food enters the absorbing cells as the intact haem complex. It takes rather longer to appear in the plasma than iron derived from non-haem sources and this lag is probably due to the metabolic splitting of haem within the cell. Iron released from haem within the epithelial cells is subsequently assumed to follow the same metabolic pathway as other forms of absorbed iron. Haem iron behaves as a stable chelate until it has entered the mucosa and its absorption is unaffected by the intraluminal factors which influence ionizable iron.

Most of the iron absorbed from the gut crosses the epithelial cells rapidly and the major phase is completed within two to three hours. Unwanted iron which enters the mucosal cells is sequestered there in the form of ferritin. Most of the mucosal ferritin is ultimately lost from the gut wall with the exfoliation of villous cells at the end of their normal life-span. The main factor influencing iron absorption is the iron status of the body. Absorption is increased in iron deficiency states, even in the absence of anaemia, and is reduced when iron stores are excessive.

The nature of the control mechanism for iron absorption is not understood. All the cells of the body require iron for the synthesis of iron-containing proteins and this is normally obtained from circulating transferrin. In the case of the small intestinal epithelial cell iron is taken up both from the serosal and luminal surface and enters a 'labile' cytoplasmic pool probably bound to a specific protein carrier from which most of it is utilized for iron–protein synthesis in mitochrondria. If the supply of iron is greater than necessary for mitrochondrial needs, then the excess in the 'labile' pool will be great enough to stimulate apoferritin synthesis with the secondary incorporation of iron into the protein. Iron uptake both at the serosal and mucosal pole of the cell appears to be related to the cell's metabolic requirements so that an excess is not usually present. However, when the intraluminal concentration of iron in the gut rises to a high level after food, while uptake by the

absorbing cell will still be influenced by local metabolic requirements, the total uptake may exceed needs and the surplus is sequestered in non-absorbed ferritin iron.

When the body's iron requirements and the iron status of intestinal cells are normal, iron uptake is low. In iron deficiency little iron is available within the body for epithelial cells and they are therefore depleted. The mitochondrial requirements for iron–enzyme synthesis are increased for as long as this depletion remains unsatisfied and this results in increased iron uptake from the gut lumen into the 'labile' intracellular pool. The increased requirements of the body result in a rapid transfer of iron from the labile pool to the plasma, only a small fraction being deviated to mitochondria, and the intracellular iron concentration never becomes high enough to stimulate apoferritin synthesis. The body's need for iron is reflected by the epithelial cells' need for iron and this is the major force controlling passage of iron from the lumen into the cell.

The control of iron transfer from the intestinal cell to the plasma may be explained as follows. Iron absorption is known to be sensitive to changes in iron storage levels within the body even when haemoglobin and serum iron concentrations remain normal, and presumably when the iron metabolism of the intestinal cells remains normal. Iron circulating in the plasma bound to transferrin exchanges with iron in all cells of the body. The intracellular iron in all tissues which is available for binding to transferrin may be called 'exchangeable' iron. In a stable metabolic state the number of iron atoms picked up by transferrin from 'exchangeable' iron in tissues must equal the number cleared from the plasma and this is reflected by the plasma iron turnover which can be measured clinically. A small part of the exchangeable iron is derived from the 'labile' pool in the intestinal cells. In general the total exchangeable iron in the body reflects the level of storage iron and if the plasma iron turnover remains constant then a decrease in storage iron must be accompanied by an increase in transfer from the intestinal epithelium to maintain the equilibrium. This type of equilibrium explains the observed inverse relationship between iron stores and absorption. It also explains why an increased plasma iron turnover, as in haemolytic disease, may result in increased absorption.

There is evidence that anaemia itself, possibly through the effect of anoxia, may act as a stimulus to iron absorption. Both in experimental animals and in patients with aplastic anaemia iron absorption is increased at low haemoglobin levels and this has been shown to be a direct effect of anoxia rather than an effect of erythropoietin. It does not depend on any change in plasma iron turnover and the mechanism is unknown.

Iron transport

Iron is transported round the body by the plasma and extravascular fluids. Plasma iron is bound to transferrin. Ferritin is normally present in plasma in small amounts but this form of the protein has a low iron content and does not provide a significant route for iron transport. Although only about 4 mg of iron is present in the plasma at any one time the daily turnover is about 30 mg. Most of the iron entering plasma is released from reticulo-endothelial cells following the breakdown of effete red cells. Smaller amounts enter the plasma pool from intestinal absorption, from the mobilization of storage compounds, and from parenchymal iron pools. Most of the iron leaving the plasma pool passes to developing red cell precursors in the bone marrow where it is incorporated into haemoglobin and finally appears in mature red cells in the peripheral blood. This process can be followed by a combination of plasma, whole blood, and surface counting after the intravenous injection of [^{59}Fe] transferrin [Fig. 1]. In normal subjects about 34 per cent of the iron leaving the plasma pool refluxes from extravascular sites and is incorporated in mature red cells only after recycling. Plasma iron concentrations are normally extremely labile and may fluctuate over a three- or four-fold range during the

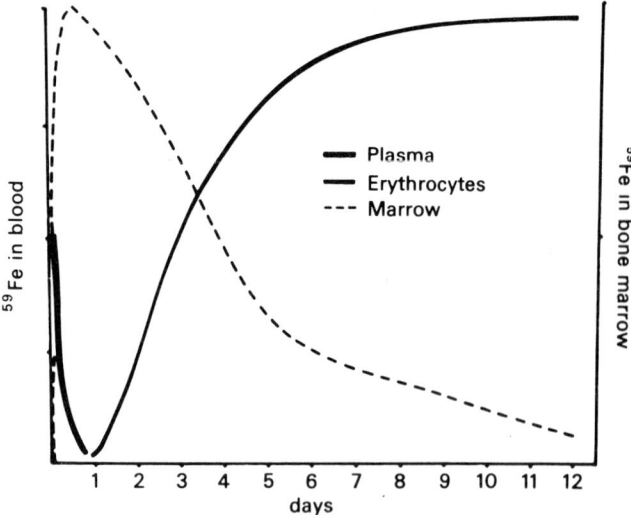

Fig. 1 The fate of [^{59}Fe] transferrin injected intravenously at zero time.

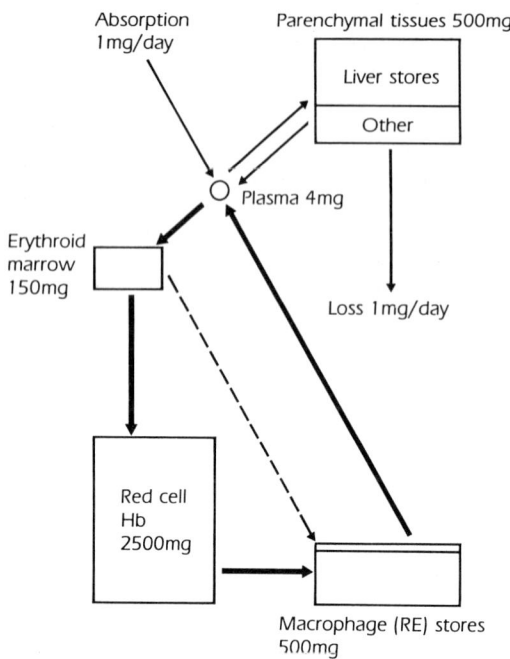

Fig. 2 The major metabolic pathways of iron. These are dominated by iron supply for erythropoiesis and turnover of iron from senescent red cells (heavy arrows). The normal minor component of ineffective marrow erythropoiesis is shown by the broken line.

day. Fluctuation is much less in severe iron deficiency or overload. The mean plasma iron in men is about 18 μmol/l and in women about 16 μmol/l. The difference between sexes appears at puberty and is not related to iron status. The values for total iron binding capacity (TIBC) found in normal adults varies from 50 to 70 μmol/l and this is usually about one-third saturated with iron. Levels are often slightly higher in women than in men and this may be related to the higher incidence of iron deficiency.

Changes in serum iron and iron-binding capacity may be found in a wide variety of disease states though their use for diagnostic purposes has limitations. Serum iron is generally decreased either because of iron deficiency when it follows depletion of storage iron, in chronic inflammatory conditions and malignancy, or more transiently following acute infections or surgery. Serum iron concentration may be increased in a number of conditions associated with decreased erythropoiesis, haemolytic anaemia, and ineffective erythropoiesis, or increase in the amount of iron in the body. The serum TIBC is invariably low in acute and chronic infection and this may be due either to an increase in catabolism or a decrease in transferrin synthesis, but the rapid fall in transferrin level following the injection of endotoxin indicates that some other mechanism may also be involved.

Systemic conditions associated with impaired protein synthesis or increased loss, such as kwashiorkor or the nephrotic syndrome, are also associated with low transferrin levels. The serum iron-binding capacity is frequently reduced in patients with iron overload. An abnormally high TIBC is seen as a characteristic feature of iron deficiency, in many cases in the absence of anaemia, and in patients taking oral contraceptives. Normally there appears to be approximately equal amounts of transferrin in the plasma and the extracellular fluid. Transferrin-bound iron is not taken up by mature red cells but becomes attached to receptors on the surface of nucleated red cells and reticulocytes. Similar receptors, though fewer in number, are present on all other cells, and represent the route for iron transfer to the intracellular space. Reticulocytes have a greater avidity for iron-saturated transferrin, possibly because of a structural modification resulting from the metal attachment to protein leading to changes in its reticulocyte-binding capacity. There is *in vitro* evidence that the two iron-binding sites of transferrin are functionally different and that this may play a part in the regulation of iron transport and absorption. In vivo evidence for functional differences between the two binding sites gives no clear indication that such differences are significant in humans.

Iron transport across the placenta is rapid and unidirectional.

During pregnancy the maternal serum iron level either remains constant or falls, but the transferrin concentration usually rises. This coincides with increased iron absorption and an increase in the mobilization of storage iron. If the placental receptor sites are more efficient in removing iron from transferrin than the receptor sites on red cells precursors when the transferrin saturation is low, then the diversion of iron to the fetus at the expense of the mother can be explained. Serum iron concentrations in the fetus are usually high and the transferrin level is low compared with those of the mother but this does not appear to be due to differences in the binding capacity of fetal and maternal transferrin. Transferrin does not cross the placenta in significant amounts and the placental transfer of iron is associated with the formation of haemosiderin and ferritin. Maximum transfer occurs in later pregnancy and is probably related to the growth of the fetus.

Ferrokinetics

Much of the existing information about the movement of iron in the body has been obtained by the use of radioactive tracers. The major pathways of iron metabolism are shown in Fig. 2. Iron–59, an easily counted gamma-emitting nuclide with a half-life of 45 days, is the most commonly used isotope. Particularly detailed studies have been made of the redistribution in radioactive transferrin-bound iron injected into the peripheral circulation. Information obtained in this way is useful in studying the plasma iron pool, marrow utilization of iron for erythropoiesis, and the distribution of iron in the tissues.

Most of the iron leaving the plasma is utilized for erythropoiesis in the bone marrow. In normal subjects there is a rapid exponential decrease in plasma radioactivity with removal of half the ^{59}Fe in about 60–90 min. If plasma radioactivity is followed over several days, a slower rate of clearance is found and analysis shows that the clearance curve can be broken down into two or more additional exponential components. It is possible to derive quantitative data on effective and ineffective erythropoiesis, red cell lifespan, and non-erythroid iron turnover.

Radioactive iron used for these studies should be firmly bound to transferrin before injection. The labelled preparation is injected intravenously and venous samples are taken for the measurement of plasma radioactivity. When accurate data are required, it is necessary to correct the plasma activity to the level corresponding to the initial plasma iron concentration. The fractional clearance rate of ^{59}Fe is the fraction of the plasma iron which leaves the plasma per unit time. This can be estimated by plotting activity against time on log-linear paper or by direct calculation of the regression line. The plasma iron turnover (PIT) may be calculated from the ^{59}Fe fractional clearance rate and the total plasma iron. In normal adults about 30 mg iron leaves the plasma each day, but this is largely dependent on the size and plasma volume of the subject. PIT is more usefully expressed as the turnover per litre whole blood as this allows meaningful comparisons between different individuals.

Over 80 per cent of the iron passing through the plasma is destined for the erythroid bone marrow. When the bone marrow is hyperplastic and particularly avid for iron, the fractional clearance rate of ^{59}Fe from the plasma is increased and plasma activity is often reduced to half its initial level in less than 30 min, but when erythropoiesis is depressed this may take several hours. Most [^{59}Fe] transferrin is removed from the plasma within 24 hours and shortly after this time ^{59}Fe begins to appear in circulating red cells. Red cell incorporation is usually complete within 14 days and in normal subjects about 80 per cent of injected iron is found in red cells at that time.

The main clinical use of ferrokinetics has been as an index of erythropoietic activity. The amount of iron destined for erythropoiesis can be calculated if the total reflux iron is subtracted from the total PIT. This is somewhat greater than the erythrocyte iron turnover which reflects only effective erythropoiesis, and the difference between the two values gives a measure of ineffective erythropoiesis. When erythropoietin production is unimpaired, the delivery of iron to the bone marrow is the limiting factor in erythropoiesis.

In anaemic patients the abnormalities that develop depend on the particular factor limiting erythropoiesis. In simple iron-deficiency anaemia the supply of iron is the limiting factor. Plasma ^{59}Fe clearance is rapid but, although a normal PIT may be maintained, this may not be adequate to allow the erythroid hyperplasia needed to compensate for the anaemia. In patients with inflammation or malignancy there is also a low PIT but there appear to be other factors limiting the bone marrow response in cases where anaemia is a feature. In patients with chronic renal disease the impaired production of erythropoietin and consequent marrow hypoplasia leads to a normal or low ^{59}Fe utilization but the PIT may not be reduced to the same extent and a considerable proportion of the injected iron may be taken up rapidly by the liver. Similar ferrokinetic abnormalities occur in primary marrow hypoplasia. In myelodysplasia a high degree of ineffective erythropoiesis is a predominating feature.

Intracellular iron metabolism

Most of the iron leaving the plasma pool is utilized by developing red cells for haemoglobin synthesis. There is some uncertainty regarding the way in which iron enters these cells and the possible intermediate steps that exist before its incorporation into haem. The transferrin receptor has been characterized as a transmembrane protein of molecular weight 176 000. The gene coding for the receptor is located on chromosome 3. There is some controversy regarding the mechanism of iron–transferrin–receptor dissociation. Good evidence points to endocytosis of the entire complex followed by externalization of the receptor with release of the iron-free transferrin to the extracellular space. However, conflicting data show that release of iron and its transfer to the cell interior occurs entirely at the cell membrane. The problem remains unresolved.

Ferritin has been demonstrated within nucleated red cells and

reticulocytes but as the cell reaches its full haemoglobin content the ferritin disappears. Electron microscopic examination of bone marrow has suggested that immature red cells cluster around macrophages and obtain their iron from them by a process analogous to pinocytosis which in this instance is called rhopheocytosis. In normal subjects an alternative mechanism probably operates. All stages of the developing red cell from the earliest differentiated precursors to the reticulocyte have the ability to take up transferrin-bound ^{59}Fe *in vitro* and this can occur long before haemoglobin synthesis commences. Apoferritin synthesis can be demonstrated *de novo* in normoblasts and reticulocytes and it is probable that ferritin observed in micropinocytotic vesicles on the surface of the erythroblast is synthesized at that site from iron released by transferrin rather than ingested from iron-loaded reticulo-endothelial cells.

The function of ferritin within red cell precursors is not clear. It may serve as an intermediate between iron uptake and haem synthesis but other experiments suggest that ferritin is not an active intermediate in haemoglobin synthesis but functions as an intracellular storage form of iron which is removed from the maturing cells before they are released in the circulation. The final stage in the biosynthesis of haem involves the incorporation of ferrous iron into protoporphyrin IX catalysed by the mitochondrial enzyme ferrochelatase which is part of the inner mitochondrial membrane. If haem synethesis is blocked, as in lead poisoning, iron accumulates and stimulates ferritin production. As the cell achieves its full haemoglobin content, ferritin disappears either through incorporation of ferritin into haem or through the expulsion of ferritin from the cell surface.

The major factors governing iron metabolism in reticulo-endothelial cells are the rates of red cell breakdown and erythropoiesis and the amount of storage iron. Most of the iron in reticulo-endothelial cells is derived from senescent red blood cells. The haem ring is split by a microsomal enzyme system producing bilirubin and releasing the iron for reutilization. The terminal oxidase is cytochrome P–450, and NADPH and oxygen are required. When haemoglobin is released in the circulation, it binds to haptoglobin and is taken up primarily by liver parenchymal cells.

Iron deficiency and overload

M. J. PIPPARD

Disturbances in iron balance result either in iron deficiency (which is manifest when the synthesis of physiologically active iron-containing compounds is limited) or, much less commonly, in iron overload (where there is excess accumulation of the iron reserve compounds, ferritin and haemosiderin). Iron status is assessed by considering the content of the main iron compartments shown in Fig. 2 (page 19.82). These consist of *storage iron*, in macrophages and hepatocytes, *transport iron*, supplying the tissues, and the main functional iron compounds which are dominated by *red cell iron* in the form of haemoglobin.

Measurement of iron status

There is no one test, or combination of tests, that is optimal for all clinical circumstances. This is because abnormalities may affect only one iron compartment or may develop sequentially. In addition, factors other than iron status affect many of the measurements (Table 1). Investigations useful at different stages of the development of iron deficiency and in iron overload, together with normal values, are shown in Tables 2 and 6, respectively.

Storage iron
Measurement of the serum ferritin concentration is reproducible and well correlated with iron stores in normal people. Values

Table 1 Factors influencing serum iron, total iron binding capacity (TIBC) and ferritin measurements

Measurement	Increase	Decrease
Serum iron (Normal 10–30 μmol/1)	Iron overload Liver disease Decreased erythropoiesis (e.g. aplastic anaemia) Haemolysis/dyserythropoiesis (e.g. pernicious anaemia)	Iron deficiency Infection/inflammation
Serum TIBC (Normal 45–70 μmol/l)	Iron deficiency Pregnancy Oral contraceptive	Iron overload Infection/inflammation Protein loss/ mulnutrition
Serum ferritin (Normal 20–300 μg/l, but age and sex dependent)	Iron overload Liver disease* Infection/inflammation Malignancy Haemolytic anaemia Hyperthyroidism Spleen or bone marrow infarction	Iron deficiency

*May be massive increase with severe hepatocellular damage.

slowly increase through adult life except in premenopausal women, who have lower mean concentrations (approximately 30 μg/l) than men (approximately 100 μg/l). These values correspond to iron stores of around 300 and 1000 mg, respectively. Concentrations below 20 μg/l are specific for storage iron depletion but values above 300 μg/l do not necessarily indicate iron overload. This is because ferritin synthesis is increased by factors other than iron, and because damage to ferritin-rich tissues can release large amounts into the circulation. Where doubt remains, it may be necessary to look for Prussian Blue stainable iron in bone marrow macrophages (in the differential diagnosis of iron deficiency) or in a liver biopsy (in the diagnosis of parenchymal iron overload). Iron stores have also been assessed by measuring urinary iron excretion in the 6 hours after a test dose of an iron chelating agent (e.g. desferrioxamine 500 mg i.m.). This is useful in assessing parenchymal iron overload, but, like the serum ferritin, may give falsely high values in haemolytic and dyserythropoietic anaemias. Non-invasive computerized tomography and magnetic studies to assess liver iron load may eventually prove valuable, particularly in monitoring response to treatment in iron overload.

Transport iron
The factors influencing serum iron and total iron binding capacity are discussed on page 19.82. The percentage saturation of the TIBC is the best measure of iron supply to the tissues. In iron deficiency similar information is given by the less labile measurement of free erythrocyte protoporphyrin concentration (see page 19.131). However, an increase in transferrin saturation is the first change in the development of parenchymal iron loading, and its measurement remains an essential part of screening for iron overload.

Red cell iron
A reduction in the amount of haemoglobin iron may be part of an overall reduction of body iron in iron-deficiency anaemia or acute blood loss. Other anaemias result in the movement of iron from red cells into macrophage stores: a corresponding increase in serum ferritin and bone marrow stainable iron should therefore be expected.

Iron deficiency

Physiological and pathological demands on iron reserves, combined with limited bioavailability of iron in the diet of much of the world's population, mean that iron balance is precarious for many hundreds of millions of people.

Prevalence
Population studies have defined iron deficiency using an arbitrary cut-off point for haemoglobin concentration, by a more quantitative approach that includes serum ferritin assay, or by assessing the haemopoietic response to a therapeutic trial of oral iron. Studies in the United States showed 5 per cent of children to have iron-deficiency anaemia, while 20 per cent of women of childbearing age had no storage iron (compared with only 3.3 per cent of men). In Sweden 17 per cent of premenopausal women had a significant rise in haemoglobin concentration after iron administration, while even after the menopause 14 per cent of women in South Wales remained anaemic (haemoglobin less than 12.0 g/dl).

Although iron deficiency is common in Western countries particularly in women and preschool children, in the tropics the majority of some populations are anaemic and many will respond to oral iron. Diet and blood loss from hookworm infestation are likely causes of this high prevalence of iron deficiency (see page 19.76 and Section 5).

Pathophysiology
Reduction in total body iron content can range in severity from diminished iron stores to severe anaemia and deficiency of tissue iron containing enzymes (Table 2). Only when iron stores have been utilized does a continuing negative iron balance lead to a reduction in iron supply to erythroid and non-erythroid tissues.

Haematological effects
In the early stages of iron-deficient erythropoiesis (latent iron deficiency) the haemoglobin concentration and red cell indices (MCV, mean corpuscular volume; and MCH, mean corpuscular haemoglobin) may still be in the normal range. However, a transferrin saturation below 16 per cent is insufficient to maintain normal erythropoiesis. In the bone marrow the number of Prussian Blue-staining, cytoplasmic ferritin granules in the erythroblasts (sideroblasts) is reduced. In addition, iron incorporation into haem is restricted leading to accumulation of the immediate precursor, protoporphyrin: since free erythrocyte protoporphyrin is lost only slowly from circulating red cells its measurement allows a retrospective view of iron supply over the preceding weeks.

Further iron depletion leads to increasingly severe dyserythropoiesis and anaemia. The bone marrow shows moderately increased numbers of red cell precursors with 'ragged' cytoplasm but there is no increase in circulating reticulocytes. Small, poorly haemoglobinized red cells are produced, some of which are distorted (Fig. 1) and have a shortened life-span. The platelet count is commonly increased.

Effects on other tissues

These are less well defined than the haematological effects though iron absorption is a sensitive measure of iron requirements and is increased even with minimal iron depletion. Anaemia and depletion of tissue iron-containing enzymes usually develop in parallel but either may be present without the other. Haem-containing cytochromes in epithelial cells, as well as muscle, liver, and kidney, are depleted and mitochondrial protein synthesis and integrity may also be dependent on iron. However, epithelial abnormalities, including atrophy of buccal and gastric mucosal surfaces, oesophageal postcricoid mucosal web formation, and koilonychia, are poorly correlated with tissue enzyme levels. In addition, atrophic gastritis and oesophageal webs may respond slowly or not at all to iron therapy. Whether gastric atrophy may sometimes be the cause rather than the effect of iron deficiency remains unclear. As with oesophageal webs, there is an association with circulating parietal cell antibodies, thyroid antibodies, achlorhydria, and an increased risk of pernicious anaemia, sug-

gesting that additional environmental or genetic factors may be involved besides iron deficiency. Lymphocyte function and immune response may also be impaired in iron deficiency, though conflicting roles for iron in protecting against or exacerbating the risk of infection have been proposed. Muscle dysfunction and impaired mental performance are even more controversial as possible non-haematological effects of iron deficiency.

Clinical features

There is no convincing evidence that depletion of storage iron has any deleterious effects apart from an inability to respond rapidly to increased physiological demands for iron (e.g. in pregnancy).

Features of iron deficiency anaemia are non-specific, and include pallor, breathlessness, and tachycardia. In severe cases angina or heart failure may develop. Up to 50 per cent of patients show glossitis, which may proceed to almost complete loss of lingual papillae. This is more common in older patients on a poor diet. Angular stomatitis is less specific for iron deficiency. Nails may be brittle and flattened though the almost diagnostic spoon-shaped deformity (koilonychia) is increasingly rare in United Kingdom practice. Dysphagia may be due to an oesophageal web (*Patterson-Kelly syndrome*). This is a premalignant condition which may occur in the absence of anaemia, usually in middle-aged women. Pica may occur in both children and adults with ingestion of ice, clay, soap or other unusual materials.

Diagnosis

In a microcytic anaemia with a clear cause for negative iron balance, measurement of either serum ferritin or transferrin saturation and subsequent haematological response to iron therapy will confirm the diagnosis. These measures of iron status will also help to distinguish iron deficiency from other causes of impaired haemoglobin synthesis and microcytic anaemia (e.g. thalassaemia trait, sideroblastic anaemia). This is particularly important in α-thalassaemia, where there are no diagnostic abnormalities of haemoglobin electrophoresis (see page 19.119). In hospital patients the major differential diagnosis is the anaemia of chronic disorders (page 19.91) in which inhibition of macrophage iron release may also give rise to mild, or occasionally severe, impairment of iron supply. This is typically a normocytic or mildly microcytic anaemia which has to be distinguished from the early stages of iron deficiency, before there are marked red cell changes. However, in severe chronic inflammatory disease the anaemia may be more markedly microcytic and here the question of possible co-existent iron-deficiency anaemia frequently arises. In both cases distinction depends upon demonstrating normal or increased iron stores, associated with reduced serum iron and TIBC, if the anaemia is due solely to inflammatory disease. Unfortunately, the serum fer-

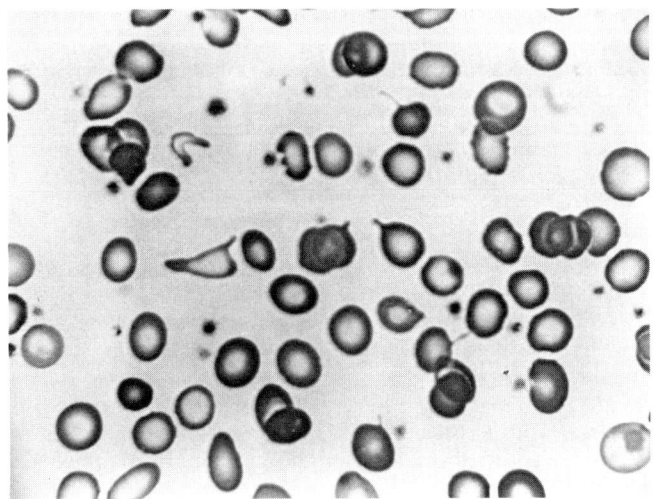

Fig. 1 The peripheral blood film in iron deficiency anaemia showing pale and distorted red cells (× 970, Leishman stain).

Table 2 Development of iron deficiency with gradual depletion of body iron content

	Normal	Storage iron depletion	Iron deficient erythropoiesis	Iron deficiency anaemia
Iron stores				
RE marrow iron	Present	Trace/absent	Absent	Absent
Serum ferritin (μg/l)	20–300	20	10	<10
Serum TIBC (μmol/l)	45–70	70	75	>75
Iron supply to tissues				
General: serum iron (μmol/l)	20 ± 9	20	<10	< 7
saturation of TIBC (%)	35 ± 15	30	<16	<10
Erythron: marrow sideroblasts (%)	30–50	30–50	<10	<10
red cell protoporphyrin (μg/dl red cells)	30	30	100	200
Red cell production				
Haemoglobin (g/dl)	>12	>12	>12	<12
Mean red cell volume, MCV (fl)	80–92	80–92	80	<80
Morphology	Normal	Normal	Normal	Microcytic/hypochromic

ritin is an acute phase reactant and in inflammatory disease values may be in the normal range despite co-existent iron deficiency: in practice a bone marrow stained for iron is often the quickest way to be certain of iron status. Nevertheless, in rheumatoid arthritis, chronic renal disease, and inflammatory bowel disease serum ferritin values below 50 μg/l are usually associated with iron deficiency. The serum ferritin may thus still be used to monitor iron status in these disorders, in which chronic blood loss due to therapy or disease is common, and where a fall in serum ferritin below this concentration may warrant oral iron treatment.

Other diagnostic problems may be seen in acute blood loss anaemia where there may be a reticulocytosis if iron stores are not completely exhausted, and the demand for iron may outstrip the rate at which stores can be mobilized. Previous parenteral iron therapy may also leave a residue of relatively unavailable iron in macrophages despite current evidence of inadequate iron supply to the tissues. Where patients have started oral iron therapy prior to investigation, the serum ferritin remains a good guide to iron stores (provided the dose of iron is less than 180 mg daily), and it does not increase until the haemoglobin compartment is replete.

Aetiology

It is vital that the underlying cause of negative iron balance should be identified, and where possible treated. The most likely cause depends on the age and sex of the patient. Dietary insufficiency is likely to play a part only at times of increased physiological demands for iron. These occur during rapid growth in infants between the age of 6 and 24 months (particularly if birthweight was low), adolescents (particularly girls), and in premenopausal women (particularly with heavy menstrual blood loss or multiple pregnancies). In the United Kingdom there is a high incidence of iron deficiency among Asian women of child-bearing age who eat a vegetarian diet containing poorly available iron. The increased demands for iron, and need for iron supplements in pregnancy, have been discussed on page 19.77 and in Section 11. In older children, men, and postmenopausal women there is likely to be a pathological cause, usually increased blood loss from the gut. Malabsorption of iron may occasionally be responsible.

Increased blood loss

In a review of 371 patients in the United Kingdom in 1965 gastrointestinal haemorrhage accounted for iron deficiency in 60 per cent of cases. There was a preponderance of women in this series among whom menorrhagia accounted for iron deficiency in 37 per cent of cases. An important additional finding was that a considerable number of patients had more than one source for blood loss. The most common alimentary causes were haemorrhoids (10 per cent), salicylate ingestion (8 per cent), peptic ulceration (7 per cent), hiatus hernia (7 per cent), and diverticulosis (4 per cent). A neoplasm was found in 2 per cent and in 16 per cent no cause for occult blood loss could be found. Other causes of gastrointestinal bleeding include oesophageal varices, gastritis, inflammatory bowel disease, familial telangiectasia, and haemorrhagic states. In children there may be bleeding from a Meckel's diverticulum and in the elderly angiodysplasia of the gut is increasingly recognized. Many non-steroidal anti-inflammatory drugs cause acute or chronic bleeding from the upper gastrointestinal tract. In the tropics the major cause of gastrointestinal blood loss is hookworm infestation where the blood loss is proportional to the number of parasites.

Gastrointestinal bleeding is usually clinically inapparent and its detection may be difficult. This is because it may be intermittent, and tests for faecal occult blood are relatively insensitive below a loss of 20 ml of blood daily. Several stool samples should therefore be tested. However, even if they are negative, and clinical examination does not suggest gut pathology, endoscopic and barium studies should be carried out in males and postmenopausal women. In premenopausal women, menstrual blood losses should first be assessed. These are notoriously difficult to estimate though some idea can be obtained from the number of towels used and

duration of each period. In difficult cases quantitative radioisotope studies of blood loss may be helpful, if time consuming. Stools and/or menstrual pads may be counted after injection of ^{51}Cr-labelled red cells though this test is insensitive below a faecal loss of 3 ml daily. Where doubt remains as to whether there is blood loss or some other cause for iron deficiency, whole body counting following oral administration of ^{59}Fe can determine both whether iron absorption is increased appropriately for iron deficiency and whether radioiron is lost from the body over the subsequent weeks. In patients in whom these investigations show no cause for gastrointestinal bleeding it is reasonable to follow-up carefully after iron therapy; it is not uncommon for anaemia to recur, but the development of serious underlying disease is rare. If there is recurrent severe bleeding additional investigation including angiography may be necessary, looking for vascular malformations, particularly in the colon, or rare small bowel tumours. Very occasionally only at laparotomy may the source of bleeding be identified.

Bleeding into the urinary tract is uncommon and is usually clinically obvious as in schistosomal infestation. Occult loss as haemosiderin may occur in chronic haemolysis due to a prosthetic heart valve or paroxysmal nocturnal haemoglobinuria. Regular blood donation should also be recognized as a drain on iron reserves.

Malabsorption

Both blood loss and impaired iron absorption may give rise to progressive iron deficiency following partial gastrectomy. These may be due to chronic gastritis, reduction in hydrochloric acid secretion, and loss of the normal 'hopper' function of the stomach. Iron deficiency is occasionally the sole manifestation of coeliac disease and though this may be diagnosed in childhood, it may present for the first time at any age. Evidence of hyposplenism may be detected by red cell changes on a blood film and should lead to consideration of jejunal biopsy.

Treatment

The essential search for the underlying cause of iron deficiency should not delay the start of iron treatment. Where iron deficiency has been attributed to increased physiological demands for iron, without extensive investigation, patients should be followed regularly to avoid missing a source of blood loss.

Oral iron should be used except in special circumstances since parenteral iron can have serious adverse effects and does not increase the speed of resolution of the anaemia. In adults 120–180 mg of elemental iron per day in divided doses should be given as one of the simple salts shown in Table 3. Absorption is best on an empty stomach, but side-effects are less if the tablets are taken with meals. Children can tolerate up to 5 mg/kg/day. Adverse effects include nausea, abdominal pain, diarrhoea, and constipation. They are related to the amount of available iron in the gut lumen. More expensive slow release preparations (which reduce availability by carrying the iron beyond the site of maximum absorption in the duodenum) and additives to enhance iron absorption (e.g. ascorbic and succinic acids) should not be used: the same effect in moderating adverse effects or increasing the amount of available iron can be obtained by reducing or increasing the dose of a simple iron salt.

The maximum response to treatment is a daily increase of 0.1– 0.2 g/dl in haemoglobin concentration. It will be slower where the dose of oral iron is less than 100 mg/day (though this is seldom clinically important) and where there is additional infection, or inflammatory disease. Treatment is arbitrarily continued for about 3 months after resolution of anaemia to provide a small reserve iron store.

Parenteral iron should be used only in those completely unable or unwilling to take oral iron, or where this cannot keep pace with continuing blood loss. It may also be useful where follow-up is likely to be inadequate, since iron repletion is assured. The deficit

Table 3 Iron content of therapeutic iron salts

Iron preparation	Amount	Iron content
Tablets		
Ferrous sulphate (dried), BP	200 mg	60 mg
Ferrous fumarate, BP	200 mg	65 mg
Ferrous gluconate, BP	300 mg	35 mg
Ferrous succinate, BP	100 mg	35 mg
Paediatric mixtures		
Ferrous sulphate mixture, BP	5 ml	12 mg
Ferrous fumarate mixture, BP	5 ml	45 mg

Table 4 Causes of iron overload

1	Blood transfusion	Congenital anaemias (e.g. β-thalassaemia major, sideroblastic anaemia, red cell aplasia)
		Acquired refractory anaemias (e.g. myelodysplasia, hypoplastic anaemia)
2	Excess iron absorption	Idiopathic haemochromatosis
		Ineffective erythropoiesis (e.g. β-thalassaemia intermedia, sideroblastic anaemia, congenital dyserythropoietic anaemia)
3	Excess iron intake	
	(a) from prolonged oral iron therapy	Patients in (2) are at particular risk
	(b) from high iron alcoholic drinks	Bantu siderosis
	(c) Excess parenteral iron therapy	
4	Secondary to liver disease	Alcoholic cirrhosis
		Portacaval anastamosis
5	Focal*	Idiopathic pulmonary haemosiderosis
		Renal tubular haemosiderosis

*In these rare circumstances bleeding into a single organ may give rise to local iron sequestration in the presence of a generalized iron deficiency.

of body iron should be calculated from the degree of anaemia. *Iron dextran* (Imferon®) may then be given as a course of intramuscular injections (50–100 mg iron/day) or as a single total dose intravenous infusion (1–2 g) over 6 hours. Anaphylaxis may occur and an infusion should not be used if there is a history of allergy: in any event a small test dose must be followed by administration under close medical supervision. Flushing and nausea may occur, as well as a syndrome of arthralgia, fever, and lymphadenopathy which may persist for several days. *Iron sorbitol* (Jectofer®) can be given only by intramuscular injection. Low molecular weight iron is released into circulation, causes a metallic taste in the mouth, and partial excretion in the urine may exacerbate urinary tract infection. Local skin staining can occur with both preparations. With iron dextran utilization may be incomplete because of sequestration at the injection site or in macrophages after clearance by the reticulo-endothelial system.

Refractory hypochromic anaemia

Failure of treatment is commonly due to the patient not taking oral iron. Continuing severe blood loss, associated inflammatory disease, or malabsorption may also limit the response. It is essential to reassess the diagnosis of iron deficiency since other causes of hypochromic anaemias include many of the iron-loading anaemias (see below).

Iron overload

The absence of a physiological pathway for the excretion of excess iron means that patients with an increased iron intake (Table 4) are at risk of progressive accumulation of iron and potentially lethal tissue damage. A primary inherited disorder of iron metabolism (idiopathic haemochromatosis) may be responsible, or iron overload may be secondary, usually to disordered erythropoiesis. Where excess iron is derived from regular blood transfusions it is easy to recognize and to quantify (each unit of 450 ml of whole blood contains approximately 200 mg of iron). Where the iron derives from inappropriate absorption from a normal diet, the risk may be concealed until the patient presents with established tissue damage.

Iron and tissue damage

The term 'haemochromatosis' is usually employed to describe the association of iron loading in parenchymal cells (especially in liver, heart, and endocrine glands) with tissue damage and fibrosis. Sequestration of iron in macrophages appears to be relatively harmless. Iron derived from blood transfusions is taken up as senescent red cells by macrophages and only subsequently redistributed to parenchymal cells. This redistribution to potentially more damaging sites occurs more slowly in patients with hypoplastic bone marrows (e.g. red cell aplasia) than in patients with active, dyserythropoietic marrows (e.g. thalassaemia disorders). In contrast, iron absorbed through the gut may be cleared preferentially by hepatic parenchymal cells as is any haemoglobin–haptoglobin complex in the circulation of patients with dyserythropoietic or

haemolytic anaemias. Such factors are likely to be important in determining the rate of development of tissue damage.

Pathogenesis of iron damage

Mechanisms by which iron produces cellular damage remain uncertain. The ability of iron to adopt either a ferrous or ferric state underlies its importance for cellular electron and oxygen transport systems. However, this very feature which makes iron essential may in excess generate oxygen free radicals leading to denaturation of cellular proteins and membrane damage through lipid peroxidation. Hepatocyte lysosomal fragility is increased in iron-loaded patients: their plasma may also contain a fraction of non-transferrin bound iron which could be particularly liable to cause damage through hydroxyl radical formation.

Idiopathic haemochromatosis

Aetiology and pathology

Idiopathic haemochromatosis results from an inborn error of iron metabolism, but the nature of the fault producing a chronic positive iron balance remains unknown. A defect of regulation of intestinal iron absorption, a more generalized defect resulting in an inability of macrophages as well as enterocytes to retain iron, and an increased affinity of liver cells for transferrin iron, have all been considered. Iron absorption is usually normal in established cases, but as iron stores are reduced by phlebotomy treatment absorption increases to above the normal range. Thus, as in normal subjects, iron absorption is inversely proportional to iron stores, but the point of equilibrium is 'set' at a much greater iron load. At post-mortem the destructive effect of the gradual accumulation of parenchymal iron over many years becomes clear. Concentrations of iron in the liver and pancreas may be 50–100 times normal and in the heart 10–15 times normal. Both liver and heart are usually enlarged with cirrhosis and myocardial fibrosis. When cirrhosis is marked, less iron is found in regenerating liver nodules, and hepatoma develops in some cases. The anterior pituitary, thyroid, parathyroid, and adrenal glands also show heavy iron deposition, but curiously the pancreatic islets, though scarred and reduced in number, may contain relatively little iron. There is much less iron in the macrophages of liver and bone marrow until the later stages of the disease, in contrast to most cases of secondary haemochromatosis. Synovial tissues may be heavily laden with haemosiderin, but the amount bears little relation to the severity of any arthopathy.

Table 5 Clinical features of idiopathic haemochromatosis (data from Milder *et al.*, 1980, based on 34 patients)

Symptoms	%	Signs	%
Weakness, lethargy	74	Skin pigmentation	82
Loss of libido	56	Hepatomegaly	76
Impotence	56	Testicular atrophy	50
Weight loss	53	Splenomegaly	38
Abdominal pain	50	Cardiac disease	35
Arthritis	47	Loss of body hair	32
Confusion, stupor	12	Ascites	15
Peripheral neuritis	9	Gynaecomastia	12
Vertigo	6		
Vomiting	6		

Inheritance

Detailed family studies have shown that at least one determinant of the disorder is closely linked with the HLA system on chromosome 6, particularly HLA-A3. Only homozygotes show full expression of the disease, though clinically insignificant increases in liver iron may occur in a minority of heterozygotes. Consistent with this autosomal recessive inheritance is the observation that the disease occurs much more frequently in siblings than in offspring. Those cases in which vertical transmission does occur may be attributed to the high frequency of the haemochromatosis allele (1 in 20 in some populations) and consequent chance homozygous–heterozygous matings.

Idiopathic haemochromatosis is rare before adult life, but in juvenile cases males and females have been equally affected. Differences in the rate of development of disease which run true in families suggest that there may be a number of different genetic defects causing varying severity of disease.

Clinical features

Around 70 per cent of patients first develop symptoms between the ages of 40 and 60 years, with a male to female incidence of 9:1. Excessive dietary iron intake or blood loss (including menstruation and regular donation of blood) will accelerate or delay manifestation of the disease: the latter presumably accounts for the lower incidence in women. The clinical features (Table 5) extend far beyond the classical triad of diabetes, hepatomegaly, and slate grey skin pigmentation (associated with increased deposits of melanin). Symptoms of diabetes, gonadal failure, and arthritis may be present for several years before the diagnosis becomes otherwise obvious. Nearly all patients develop some degree of glucose intolerance and many require insulin therapy. Hypogonadism is commonly hypogonadotrophic in origin. Arthritis is more frequent in older patients and is characterized by chondrocalcinosis of the articular cartilage, loss of joint space and periarticular subperiosteal bone resorption. The second and third metacarpal–phalangeal joints and the wrists are most consistently affected, and swelling, deformity, and limitation of movement may be mistaken for rheumatoid arthritis. The pathogenesis is poorly understood, though calcium pyrophosphate crystals may give attacks of acute 'pseudogout'. The hip and knee joints undergo destructive arthritis in up to 10 per cent of patients and surgical hip replacement may become necessary. Cardiac failure and arrhythmias may occur at any age but are a more common presenting feature in younger patients: rapid clinical deterioration and death may result. Abdominal pain may be related to hepatic enlargement but the possibility of hepatoma should be considered particularly in older patients. The function of the enlarged liver is usually only mildly disturbed, but severe hepatic failure carries a poor prognosis.

Diagnosis

A high degree of clinical suspicion is needed given the variety of clinical manifestations. Laboratory tests are centred on the dem-

onstration of parenchymal iron loading and assessment of the function of the main 'target' organs (Table 6). Liver biopsy is important both to confirm iron overload and to assess tissue damage. Where biopsy is not possible a desferrioxamine excretion test can provide further evidence of hepatocyte iron loading. Since the basic metabolic defect is unknown, diagnosis depends upon exclusion of causes of secondary iron overload. Liver disease, particularly when due to alcohol, may cause problems in differential diagnosis. It shares a number of clinical features with idiopathic haemochromatosis as well as having a serum transferrin saturation and ferritin concentration which may be increased out of proportion to iron stores. Further confusion can arise from the high prevalence of alcoholism (as much as one-third of patients in some series) in idiopathic haemochromatosis: the high iron content of some alcoholic drinks and enhancement of iron absorption by alcohol probably increase the likelihood of homozygous disease reaching full clinical expression. Liver biopsy usually distinguishes these conditions in that iron deposits in alcoholic liver disease are only moderate and tend to be in macrophages (Kupffer cells) rather than hepatocytes. Occasionally doubt remains, and family studies may then help with diagnosis. It is also important to exclude disorders of erythropoiesis in which iron loading may occur despite totally asymptomatic mild anaemia (see below). There are no specific haematological changes in idiopathic haemochromatosis though liver disease and hypersplenism may give rise to macrocytosis and low white cell or platelet counts.

Treatment and prognosis

Insulin treatment and later the removal of excess iron by regular phlebotomy, dramatically altered the causes of death in idiopathic haemochromatosis (Table 7). In a retrospective study of severely affected patients phlebotomy greatly reduced mortality from cardiac and hepatic failure, with a striking increase in five-year survival (66 per cent, $n=45$) compared with untreated patients (18 per cent, $n = 18$). However, neoplasia, which in some series has not been confined to hepatoma, now accounts for a large proportion of deaths. Earlier diagnosis may reduce this risk of neoplasia since there are no reports of hepatoma in patients identified and treated before the onset of cirrhosis of the liver. Iron removal improves the control of diabetes in a minority of patients, but in general, endocrine function, unlike cardiac and hepatic function, shows little benefit from phlebotomy. The arthritis is also unaffected by treatment and indeed may appear for the first time after the iron has been completely removed.

Most patients tolerate weekly phlebotomy of 450 ml (200 mg iron), maintaining a haemoglobin concentration above 12.0 g/dl. Where hepatic failure is present reinfusion of the patient's plasma, after separation of the red cells, may be necessary. Life-threatening cardiac failure may occasionally preclude phlebotomy and it would then appear reasonable to give desferrioxamine as a continuous intravenous infusion (100 mg/kg/24 hours) in an attempt to tide the patient over until cardiac function improves. Serum ferritin concentrations decline during treatment which may need to be continued for 2 to 3 years since total iron load is usually around 20 g, and may be as much as 40 g. As iron depletion approaches serum iron and haemoglobin concentration fall. The frequency of phlebotomy should then be decreased, with maintenance treatment at around 2–6 units removed each year for the rest of the patient's life. The aim should be to maintain a normal transferrin saturation and a serum ferritin below 200 $\mu g/l$.

Screening and early diagnosis

First degree relatives of patients with idiopathic haemochromatosis are at risk for the disease. All those over the age of 10 years should be tested for any increase in serum transferrin saturation and ferritin concentration at two-year intervals. Liver biopsy is needed if either becomes persistently abnormal. Siblings with the same HLA haplotypes as the propositus are also likely to be homozygous for the disease. This may help in identifying those too

Table 6 Diagnosis of symptomatic idiopathic haemochromatosis

		(Normal)
Parenchymal iron overload		
1 Serum transferrin saturation	>80%	(<60)
2 Serum ferritin concentration	>1000 μg/l	(<300)
3 Desferrioxamine test (500 mg i.m.)		
– urine iron excretion	>8 mg	(<1.5)
4 Liver biopsy: stainable iron	Hepatocytes	
iron concentration	>1% of dry weight	(<0.13)
5 Quantitative phlebotomy: iron removed	>10g	(0.2–1)
Tissue damage		
1 Liver: biochemical tests	Micronodular	
liver biopsy	cirrhosis	
2 Pancreas: blood glucose		
glucose tolerance test	Diabetes	
3 Pituitary: gonadotrophins	Hypogonadism	
4 Heart: echocardiogram	Cardiomyopathy	
radionucleotide scan		

young for iron loading to be manifest. Relatives thought to be heterozygous are probably not at risk of serious iron loading. However, with present uncertainty about possible genetic variants of idiopathic haemochromatosis, they also should be seen regularly and warned that alcohol and oral iron could increase their tendency to load iron. It seems likely that careful monitoring and institution of phlebotomy before there is tissue damage will avoid morbidity and give the prospect of a normal life expectancy.

Iron-loading anaemias

In chronic refractory anaemias iron overload may result from the need for regular blood transfusions or from excessive absorption of dietary iron (Table 4). In the wide spectrum of thalassaemia disorders (see page 19.110) both mechanisms are found. In severe homozygous β-thalassaemia blood transfusion is essential and tissue iron damage becomes evident by the second decade of life. In more mildly anaemic patients who do not require regular transfusions (β-thalassaemia intermedia) persistent erythroid marrow expansion is associated with a variable increase in iron absorption from the gut. In these cases pathological effects of iron overload may be delayed until middle life. The problems of assessment of iron overload are somewhat different in these two groups of patients.

Transfusion iron loading

Cardiac iron loading occurs in patients who have received more than 100 units of blood (20 g iron) and other parenchymal tissues are damaged in a pattern similar to that seen in idiopathic haemochromatosis. The rate of iron loading is predictable and blood transfusion records provide the best guide to total iron load. The serum ferritin may be much higher than is usually seen in idiopathic haemochromatosis and is a poor guide to precise amounts

of iron overload. Levels in excess of 4000 μg/l may reflect additional factors such as haemolysis, liver damage from iron, or transfusion-associated hepatitis. Liver biopsy is not justified as a routine, since the presence of iron overload is not in doubt. Other investigations to assess tissue damage may be needed as in Table 6.

Gastrointestinal iron loading

It is important to realize that the degree of anaemia is not helpful in predicting the risk of iron loading in patients with dyserythropoiesis who do not require blood transfusions. Indeed a virtually normal haemoglobin concentration may co-exist with severe iron overload and tissue damage (see Fig. 3). A much better guide is the degree of erythroid marrow expansion, which can be measured by morphological or ferrokinetic techniques in presymptomatic patients. Such patients should be followed-up regularly as described for the screening and early diagnosis of idiopathic haemochromatosis.

Patients with erythroid expansion due to chronic haemolytic anaemias are not normally at risk of iron overload from increased dietary iron absorption. However, occasional cases of iron excess in hereditary spherocytosis and pyruvate kinase deficiency have been described. There are unproven suggestions that coincidental inheritance of the heterozygous state for idiopathic haemochromatosis and a defect of erythropoiesis (e.g. hereditary spherocytosis, β-thalassaemia trait) might account for cases of severe iron overload in haematological disorders where this complication is otherwise rare.

Treatment

Where possible the rate of iron loading should be reduced. In β-thalassaemia major, splenectomy may reduce transfusion requirements if there is hypersplenism. The availability of dietary iron

Table 7 Effect of treatment on causes of death in idiopathic haemochromatosis

Causes of death	Sheldon (1935) (%)	Finch and Finch (1955) (%)	Bomford and Williams (1976) (%)
Diabetes	50	4	2
Bacterial infection (especially pneumonia)	20	13	5
Cardiac failure	—	31	9
Liver disease (cirrhosis, hepatic failure, haematemesis)	11	29	15
Hepatoma	7	14	29
Other neoplasms	—	—	22
Miscellaneous	12	9	18
Introduction of treatment*		Insulin	Venesection

*The effect of the introduction of insulin treatment was seen between 1935 and 1955, and of phlebotomy therapy to remove the excess iron between 1955 and 1976.

might be reduced by exclusion of meat and increased intake of foods containing phytate, phosphate, or tea. However, this source of iron loading is insignificant in transfused patients in whom the erythroid marrow is suppressed, and in patients with increased gastrointestinal iron absorption the occasional use of iron chelation therapy is likely to be less disruptive to lifestyle.

Iron chelation therapy

The only iron chelating agent in current clinical use is desferrioxamine (Desferal®). While highly specific for iron this drug has to be given by injection, with slow infusions (intravenous or subcutaneous) being much more effective in removing iron than intramuscular bolus injections. Infusions may have the additional advantage of continually chelating the most available, metabolically active iron, which is likely to be most toxic. On treatment the urine becomes discoloured due to excretion of the red iron chelate, ferrioxamine, but a major portion of the iron chelated from the liver is also excreted via the bile into the faeces. Urine iron excretion is highly variable, being increased with iron load and with the degree of anaemia in dyserythropoietic (but not hypoplastic) anaemias. In addition, repletion of any ascorbic acid deficiency associated with iron overload increases urine iron excretion, perhaps by mobilizing storage iron to a form or site where it is available to desferrioxamine. When used to enhance desferrioxamine treatment the dose of ascorbate should not exceed 100 mg/day because of concern that such iron mobilization may increase iron toxicity, particularly to the heart. Because treatment is burdensome and must be lifelong in transfusion-dependent patients, and desferrioxamine is very expensive, the indications and precise drug regimen should be carefully considered for each patient.

Planning chelation therapy

In elderly patients with acquired refractory anaemias, or where the underlying haematological disorder has a poor prognosis, chelation therapy which is designed to prevent the complications of iron overload several years later is likely to be inappropriate. Where iron overload is the main threat to life, as in the thalassaemia disorders, standard treatment now consists of subcutaneous infusions of desferrioxamine given over 10–12 hours usually on six nights each week, using a small infusion pump (Fig. 2). Initially, 24-hour urine collections for iron measurements should be made after increasing doses (0.5 to 3.0 g as 12-hour s.c. infusions) on successive days. In all but the most heavily iron loaded the urine iron excretion tends to level off at higher doses, and the optimal dose may be selected as that giving maximal iron chelation before the plateau is reached. In most cases this will be in the range 50–75 mg/kg body weight by 12-hour s.c. infusion each night. By contrast, stool iron excretion shows no tendency to plateau at higher doses, at which it forms a progressively larger proportion of total iron chelated. To take advantage of this it is worthwhile giving a single larger intravenous infusion (e.g. 150 mg/kg) at the time of each regular blood transfusion. Continuous intravenous high doses have been used to obtain more rapid iron removal in severely iron-loaded patients, but in some cases such therapy has led to visual impairment due to retinopathy. Auditory impairment has also been reported with continous therapy: despite the remarkable overall lack of toxicity with s.c. desferrioxamine, sight and hearing should therefore be monitored at least annually.

Response to treatment

There is frequently a rapid fall in serum ferritin concentration after starting regular chelation therapy and this probably reflects improved liver function as well as declining iron stores. Thalassaemic patients complying with therapy (and compliance can be a major problem, particularly in teenagers) have improved cardiac function. Prevention of pubertal growth failure due to iron loading in thalassaemia may be dependent on starting chelation early in life, and treatment should ideally begin before there is an appreci-

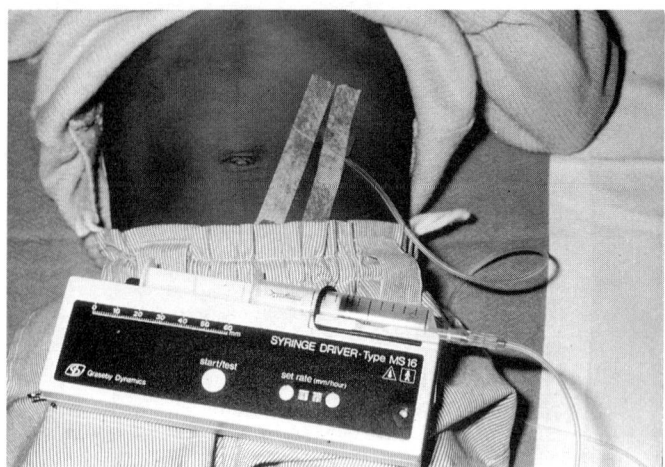

Fig. 2 Subcutaneous infusion of desferrioxamine in a thalassaemic child using a portable battery driven pump. The syringe is connected via narrow-bore tubing to a fine gauge butterfly needle inserted deeply into the subcutaneous fat of the anterior abdominal wall.

able iron burden, and certainly by the age of 4 years. The dose should be reassessed at annual intervals as patients grow. Urine iron excretion decreases after prolonged treatment and faecal iron loss assumes greater importance as iron load declines. Desferrioxamine therapy has obvious drawbacks, but offers the best hope of limiting iron damage until an effective oral iron chelating agent is developed: unfortunately this prospect remains remote.

Non-transfused patients

Iron overload due to excess iron absorption may be treated with subcutaneous desferrioxamine as described above. Occasional patients who are less anaemic may tolerate additional cautious phlebotomy, and reduction in iron stores is reflected in declining serum ferritin and eventually serum iron concentrations (Fig. 3). Normal iron stores should subsequently be maintained by occasional use of phlebotomy (where possible) or by intermittent desferrioxamine infusions. The latter approach is made feasible by the slower rate of iron loading from the gut than from blood transfusions and by the observation that fecal iron excretion after deferrioxamine remains considerable even when iron stores have been reduced to a low level.

Excess iron intake

Oral iron

Prolonged oral iron ingestion in normal people does not usually produce significant iron loading. However, in patients with idiopathic haemochromatosis or dyserythropoietic anaemias the rate of iron loading may be considerably increased. The fortification of foods with iron to deal with widespread iron deficiency carries an increased risk to patients with these iron loading states: the balance of risks and benefits will depend on the relative frequency of the conditions in particular populations.

Bantu siderosis

Over 20 years ago a majority of adults, particularly males, in the Johannesburg area were found to have increased iron stores, sometimes comparable to those of idiopathic haemochromatosis. This iron loading resulted from a high intake of iron in beer prepared in iron pots, with the low pH of the beer ensuring that the iron was in an ionized and readily absorbable form. In contrast to idiopathic haemochromatosis the excess iron is present in intestinal cells and both macrophages and parenchymal cells in the liver. Portal fibrosis and cirrhosis of the liver may be accompanied by pancreatic and cardiac iron loading. Ascorbic acid deficiency due to accelerated ascorbate metabolism is often present, together with osteoporosis. The serum transferrin may not be fully satur-

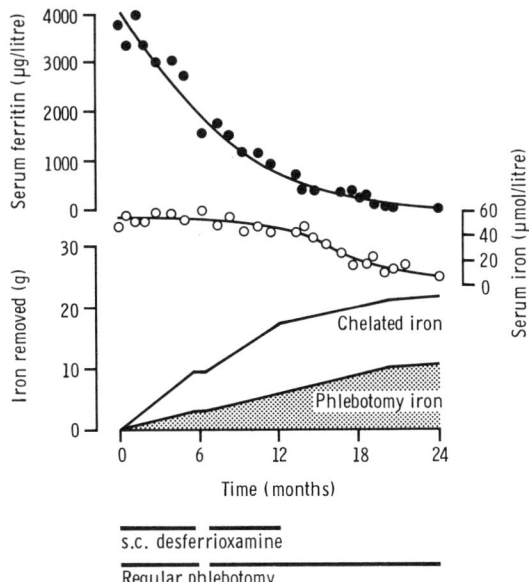

Fig. 3 Management of iron-loading anaemia. A 56-year-old man with asymptomatic congenital dyserythropoietic anaemia (Hb 11.0 g/dl; erythroid expansion 10 times normal) had never been transfused but had severe liver iron loading with cirrhosis. He tolerated intermittent phlebotomy (Hb maintained above 10 g/dl) combined with subcutaneous desferrioxamine infusions (6 g/24 hours twice per week) to remove approximately 20 g of iron over 18 months.

ated despite severe iron loading since ascorbate deficiency limits mobilization of macrophage iron (and may thus offer some protection against the toxicity of excess iron).

Parenteral iron therapy

This may occasionally give rise to iron overload, for example in patients on chronic haemodialysis where, without careful monitoring, intravenous iron may overcompensate for the regular blood losses. The demonstration that iron absorption is appropriately increased in patients with renal failure and iron deficiency suggests that if iron supplements are given by mouth this complication will be avoided. Serum ferritin measurements correlate well with bone marrow iron in such patients and may be used to monitor iron stores: a concentration of less than 50 μg/l is a realistic indicator of the need for oral iron supplements.

Iron overload and liver disease

The relationships between alcohol, liver disease, and iron overload are discussed in the sections dealing with idiopathic haemochromatosis and excess iron intake. However, iron stores can be mildly increased in other forms of chronic liver disease, this tendency being exacerbated by portacaval shunt. It remains controversial whether liver damage itself may potentiate iron absorption.

References

Bainton, D. F. and Finch, C. A. (1964). The diagnosis of iron deficiency anemia. *Am. J. Med.* **37**, 62–70.

Beveridge, B. R., Bannerman, R. M., Evanson, J. M. and Witts, L. J. (1965). Hypochromic anaemia. A retrospective study and follow-up of 378 in-patients. *Q. J. Med.* **34**, 145–161.

Bomford, A. and Williams, R. (1976). Long term results of venesection therapy in idiopathic haemochromatosis. *Q. J. Med.* **45**, 611–23.

Bothwell, T. H., Charlton, R. W., Cook, J. D. and Finch, C. A. (1979). *Iron metabolism in man*. Blackwell Scientific Publications, Oxford.

Callender, S. T. (1982). Treatment of iron deficiency. *Clin. Haemat.* **11**, 327–338.

Cartwright, G. E., Edwards, C. Q., Kravitz, K., Skolnick, M., Amos, D. B., Johnson, A. and Buskjaer, L. (1979). Hereditary hemochromatosis. Phenotypic expression of the disease. *N. Engl. J. Med.* **301**, 175–179.

Cook, J. D. (1982). Clinical evaluation of iron deficiency. *Sem. Hemat.* **19**, 6–18.

Finch, S. C. and Finch, C. A. (1955). Idiopathic hemochromatosis, an iron storage disease. *Medicine* **34**, 381–430.

Gutteridge, J. M. C., Rowley, D. A., Griffiths, E. and Halliwell, B. (1985). Low-molecular-weight iron complexes and oxygen radical reactions in idiopathic haemochromatosis. *Clin. Sci.* **68**, 463–467.

Jacobs, A. and Worwood, M. (eds) (1980). *Iron in biochemistry and medicine II*. Academic Press, London and New York.

Jacobs, A. (1982). Non-haematological effects of iron deficiency. *Clin. Haemat.* **11**, 353–364.

Ley, T. J., Griffith, P. and Neinhuis, A. W. (1982). Transfusion haemosiderosis and chelation therapy. *Clin. Haemat.* **11**, 437–464.

Milder, M. S., Cook, J. D., Stray, S. and Finch, C. A. (1980). Idiopathic hemochromatosis, an interim report. *Medicine* **59**, 34–49.

Niederau, C., Fischer, R., Sonnenberg, A., Stremmel, W., Trampisch, H. J. and Strohmeyer, G. (1985). Survival and causes of death in cirrhotic and noncirrhotic patients with primary hemochromatosis. *N. Engl. J. Med.* **313**, 1256–1262.

Pippard, M. J. and Callender, S. T. (1983). The management of iron chelation therapy. *Br. J. Haemat.* **54**, 503–507.

Sheldon, J. H. (1935). *Haemochromatosis*. Clarendon Press, Oxford.

Simon, M. (1985). Secondary iron overload and the haemochromatosis allele. *Br. J. Haemat.* **60**, 1–5.

Wolfe, L., Olivieri, N., Sallan, D., Colan, S., Rose, V., Propper, R., Freedman, M. H. and Nathan, D. G. (1985). Prevention of cardiac disease by subcutaneous deferoxamine in patients with thalassemia major. *N. Engl. J. Med.* **312**, 1600–1603.

Normochromic, normocytic anaemias

S. T. CALLENDER

With the increase in automation in laboratories, one of the principal investigations for any kind of complaint is a blood count and one of the commonest findings is that of a normochromic normocytic anaemia. The problem is then whether the anaemia is significant and how far it should be investigated.

In the first instance it is important to establish that the blood findings do in fact represent anaemia in the particular individual. In relation to this the variations with age must be taken into account as well as the wide range of 'normal' values. A knowledge of any previous blood count is clearly useful since a haemoglobin in the lower range of normal may represent anaemia in a patient known to have a higher haemoglobin when in good health.

Most of the normochromic, normocytic anaemias are secondary to another disease; a minority will prove to have a primary blood disorder. The possible causes are summarized in Table 1.

Anaemia of chronic disorders (ACD)

This is a rather unsatisfactory phrase used to cover the most common of the normochromic normocytic anaemias, namely, that found in chronic infections, in inflammatory conditions including the collagen vascular disorders, and in malignant disease.

Table 1 Causes of normochromic, normocytic anaemia

Chronic disorders	Infections, malignancy, collagen vascular disorders
Renal failure	
Endocrine failure	Hypopituitary and hypothyroid
Marrow failure	Aplastic anaemia, red cell aplasia, marrow infiltration
Acute blood loss and early iron deficiency	Gastrointestinal or genitourinary bleeding

Any infection may result in a temporary disturbance of erythropoiesis but in acute infections with rapid recovery this may be barely noticeable. In chronic disease processes, however, the anaemia develops gradually over a period of weeks and then becomes constant, fluctuating only with the severity of the disease or with complicating factors such as blood loss.

Pathogenesis

The precise mechanism of the anaemia of chronic disorders is still not clearly defined. Four elements have to be considered.

1. Reticuloendothelial sequestration of iron.
2. A reduction in red cell life span.
3. A defect in production of erythropoietin.
4. Factors inhibitory to erythropoiesis.

Reticuloendothelial sequestration of iron It has been widely accepted that there is sequestration of iron in the reticuloendothelial (RE) cells in ACD and that there is a block in the release of iron. This was first demonstrated experimentally in dogs in whom sterile abscesses had been produced by injection of turpentine. Iron given to the dogs in the form of labelled transferrin was incorporated normally into new red cells but when given in the form of non-viable red cells the iron utilization was about half that expected. Since the iron from non-viable red cells has to be processed by RE cells the findings indicated a hold up of iron delivery from these cells. This has been referred to as 'RE block'.

The cause of the diversion of iron to the RE system in ACD remains speculative. One hypothesis is that infection stimulates the production of 'leucocyte endogenous mediator' from macrophages. This substance, which is probably identical to interleukin-1, sets in train the acute phase reaction and release of leucocyte granules. These granules contain lactoferrin, and this iron-binding protein is found at high concentrations at sites of inflammation. It has been postulated that the lactoferrin competes with transferrin for iron and that the bound iron is then sequestered by the macrophages. This theory, though attractive in some respects and fitting some of the known facts, is as yet unproven.

A second hypothesis suggests that the diversion of iron from plasma to the RE system is the result of stimulation of apoferritin production in response to the inflammatory process. Although there is some experimental evidence which can be interpreted in this way it is not compatible with the generally accepted view that apoferritin synthesis is stimulated only by the presence of iron. The theory therefore awaits more definite proof.

Although the cause of the diversion of iron to RE cells and the consequent hypoferraemia is not clear it may be an adaptation which aids defence against infection. Most bacteria require iron for growth; hence limitation of available iron might limit bacterial proliferation.

Although limitation of supply of iron to the marrow caused by RE block can explain many of the haematological abnormalities in ACD ferrokinetic data obtained by different groups of workers have given conflicting results. Most, however, indicate that limitation of iron supply alone cannot explain the defect in erythropoiesis and other factors have to be considered.

Shortened red cell lifespan A number of investigators have shown that there is usually some shortening of the red cell lifespan in ACD. This is due to an extracorpuscular factor and not to an intrinsic abnormality of the red cells. The defect is not gross and the marrow response could normally readily compensate for the reduced red cell survival. A shortened red cell lifespan can therefore only be regarded as a contributory factor in the anaemia.

Failure of erythropoietin production Erythropoietin levels have been assayed in rheumatoid arthritis and a variety of other diseases including chronic infections and malignancy and in experimental models. In iron deficiency there is a highly significant inverse correlation between erythropoietin production and the degree of anaemia. This is not seen in the anaemia of chronic dis-

Table 2 Characteristics of the anaemia of chronic disorders compared with normal and iron deficiency anaemia

	Normal	Iron deficiency anaemia	Anaemia of chronic disorders
Morphology of blood	Normochromic normocytic	Hypochromic microcytic	Normo- or hypochromic normocytic: rarely microcytic
Plasma Fe (µmol/l)	20.6 ± 9	Low <7.2	Low <12.0
TIBC (µmol/l)	58.0 ± 4.5	High 71.6 ± 9	Low 44.8 ± 9
% transferrin saturation	35.0 ± 15	Low <15	Low 10–25
% sideroblasts	40–60	Low <10	Low 5–20
Serum ferritin (µg/l)	100 ± 60	Low <10	Often high >200
RE iron	Present	Absent	Increased
Erythrocyte protoporphyrin (nmol/l)	<700	Increased	Increased
Plasma copper (µmol/l)	16–31	Increased	Increased

orders although the marrow appears to be capable of responding to an adequate stimulus in that hypoxia and cobalt, and the injection of purified erythropoietin will produce a response. According to such studies the defect would therefore appear to be in erythropoietin production.

Factors inhibitory to erythropoiesis Developments in tissue culture techniques have stimulated interest in possible inhibitory factors in the anaemia of chronic disorders, and there is good evidence that such inhibitors do have a role in at least some types of ACD. Serum from anaemic patients with rheumatoid arthritis has been shown *in vitro* either to lack a normal stimulant effect or to inhibit erythropoiesis. In some types of malignancy, in both humans and rats, experiments suggest the presence of similar inhibitory factors.

From the above brief discussion it will be evident that there are many unsolved problems in the pathogenesis of ACD and it is probable that the factors concerned may not be the same in all cases.

Characteristics of the anaemia of chronic disorders

The anaemia is usually mild and the PCV is rarely less than 30 per cent. In some cases hypochromia may develop. Microcytosis is rarely seen but when it does occur it follows the development of hypochromia rather than preceding it as in iron deficiency. ACD is accompanied by characteristic changes in iron metabolism which have to be distinguished from those of iron deficiency (Table 2). A reduction in plasma iron is an early finding in all inflammatory conditions. It returns rapidly to normal with recovery from acute infections but more gradually with recovery from chronic disorders. The total iron-binding capacity is reduced, not increased as in iron deficiency, and the percentage saturation is also reduced although not usually to the degree seen in iron deficiency anaemia. In both conditions the percentage of sideroblasts in the bone marrow is diminished but in chronic disorders the RE iron is adequate or increased whereas in iron deficiency, unless parenteral iron has recently been given, the RE iron is reduced or absent. The serum ferritin is low in iron deficiency but frequently raised in chronic disorders. The free erythrocyte protoporphyrin is increased in both conditions but in ACD the increase is correlated with the duration of the underlying disorder and may take some weeks to become evident.

A number of other changes in the plasma of patients with ACD are characteristic of the 'acute phase response', e.g. an increase in ceruloplasmin and fibrinogen.

Conditions often associated with normochromic anaemia (Table 1)

Renal failure

Normochromic normocytic anaemia is a frequent presenting feature in renal disease which should always be considered as a possible cause. The anaemia of renal disease is discussed further in the section on blood changes in systemic disease (page 19.243).

Endocrine disease

Hypometabolism as seen in hypopituitary and hypothyroid states leads to reduced demand for oxygen in the tissues and a consequent reduction of output of erythropoietin. This is probably the major factor in the development of a mild normochromic normocytic anaemia in some patients with these conditions. This and other factors are discussed in a later section (page 19.247).

Bone marrow failure

While normochromic normocytic anaemia is a common feature of bone marrow failure, except in the pure red cell aplasias, there are usually other obvious changes in the blood. The white cells and platelets are reduced in aplastic anaemia and abnormal white cells are found in leukaemia. Where the marrow is infiltrated with malignant cells there may be a leucoerythroblastic reaction with resulting nucleated red cells and occasional immature white cells in the peripheral blood.

Acute blood loss and early iron deficiency

It is often overlooked that blood loss from the gastrointestinal or genitourinary tract may well be sufficient to cause anaemia but as long as iron stores are sufficient to maintain an output of normal red cells the anaemia will be normochromic and normocytic. An increase in reticulocytes may suggest blood loss as a cause of the anaemia since the other conditions considered here are all hypoproliferative anaemias and have a low reticulocyte count.

Polymyalgia rheumatica and giant-cell arteritis

The condition originally described as 'a rheumatoid syndrome occurring in the elderly' was later named polymyalgia rheumatica (see Section 16) and it included the feature of a refractory anaemia, usually of moderate degree, with a haemoglobin level of about 11.0 g/dl but which may be more severe and even as low as 6.0 g/dl. Giant-cell arteritis, which has some features in common with polymyalgia rheumatica, can sometimes present with anaemia and the pain in both conditions may be insignificant. Some elderly patients present with anaemia and high ESR. No cause can be found, and, like polymyalgia, the condition responds dramatically to corticosteroid treatment. This is probably a variant of the polymyalgic syndrome. It has also been called refractory anaemia with dysproteinaemia; there is, however, no evidence that these patients produce monoclonal or structurally abnormal polyclonal immune globulins. In all these conditions the anaemia has the features of the anaemia of chronic disorders. The awareness of these syndromes as a cause of chronic anaemia in the elderly is important since, when they are accompanied by symptoms such as anorexia, weight loss, and pain the condition may be erroneously attributed to malignancy.

Diagnosis in normochromic normocytic anaemia

In the majority of cases a careful history and physical examination will reveal evidence of an underlying disease. Special attention should be given to eliciting any possible history of fever, its nature, severity or periodicity which may point to an infection or perhaps lymphoma or other malignancy. In relation to fever the ethnic origin or recent residence in a tropical country may be significant. Enquiry into possible sources of recent blood loss is also important. In the physical examination such features as purpura, bruising, finger clubbing, mouth ulceration, minor joint changes, lymph-node enlargement, splenomegaly, palpable masses, and bony tenderness should be sought.

Where there are no obvious leads to diagnosis, in younger age groups occult infections, renal disease, blood loss, leukaemia, and marrow aplasia should be the first to consider. Not so long ago tuberculosis was among the most important causes to be eliminated, and in recent immigrants from countries where tuberculosis is common, this still applies.

In the elderly, malignancy and the polymyalgia-arteritis syndromes are the most important differential diagnoses since in addition to the anaemia they may show very similar features of anorexia and weight loss and the characteristic pains or stiffness of the vasculitic disorders may erroneously be attributed to malignant infiltration.

Investigation

Most of the causes of normochromic normocytic anaemia are readily identified by the history and physical examination. In patients in whom the diagnosis is more obscure chemical and microscopic examination of the urine and a careful review of the blood film may direct the lines of further investigation. If a primary blood disorder or neoplastic infiltration of the bone marrow is suspected it will need to be confirmed or excluded by examination of the bone marrow, including a trephine biopsy.

The most difficult problems arise in those patients in whom initial routine tests are unhelpful and yet the normochromic normocytic anaemia has the characteristics of ACD. Here the investigations will be along lines similar to those for a fever of unknown origin (see Section 5), taking into account, as already indicated, the age and ethnic origin of the patient and previous occupation or exposure to tropical illnesses.

Treatment

Treatment of normochromic normocytic anaemias is essentially that of the underlying disease. No haematinic will produce a response except in those cases where iron deficiency is also present, e.g. in rheumatoid arthritis where a blood loss anaemia may complicate the ACD. In such cases a partial improvement may be expected with iron therapy.

In many elderly patients presenting with the features of ACD it may be justifiable to give a therapeutic trial of steroids and to proceed to further investigations only if there is no immediate and dramatic response characteristic of the polymyalgia giant-cell arteritis syndromes. Early recognition of the true diagnosis may save weeks of fruitless investigation for a non-existent neoplasm.

References

Bunch, C. and Weatherall, D. J. (1982). The haematological manifestations of systemic disease. In *Blood and its disorders* 2nd edn (eds R. M. Hardisty and D. J. Weatherall). Blackwell Scientific Publications, Oxford.

Lee, G. R. (1983). The anemia of chronic disease. *Sem. Hematol.* **20**, 61–80.

Hume, R., Dagg, J. H. and Goldberg, A. (1973). Refractory anemia with dysproteinemia: long-term therapy with low-dose corticosteroids. *Blood* **41**, 27–35.

Megaloblastic anaemia and miscellaneous deficiency anaemias

A. V. HOFFBRAND

Introduction

The megaloblastic anaemias are a group of disorders characterized by a macrocytic anaemia and distinctive morphological abnormalities of the developing haemopoietic cells in the bone marrow. In severe cases, the anaemia may be associated with leucopenia and thrombocytopenia. Megaloblastic anaemia arises because of inhibition of DNA synthesis in the bone marrow and this is usually due to deficiency of one or other of two water-soluble B vitamins, vitamin B_{12} (B_{12}) or folate; B_{12} deficiency may also cause a severe neuropathy. In a minority of cases, megaloblastic anaemia arises because of a disturbance of DNA synthesis brought about by a drug or a congenital or acquired biochemical defect which causes a disturbance of B_{12} or folate metabolism or affects DNA synthesis independent of B_{12} or folate. B_{12} and folate are discussed first and the other rare megaloblastic anaemias are mentioned at the end of this chapter.

Biochemical and nutritional aspects of vitamin B_{12} and folate

Vitamin B_{12}

Biochemistry

Four major forms of the vitamin exist in humans, all with the same cobalamin nucleus which consists of a planar corrin ring (hence the term 'corrinoids' for B_{12} compounds) attached at right-angles to a nucleotide portion, 5, 6-dimethylbenzimidazole joined to ribose-phosphate (Table 1). *5'-Deoxyadenosylcobalamin* (ado-B_{12}) accounts for about 80 per cent of the vitamin inside human and other mammalian cells and is mainly in mitochondria; *methyl-cobalamin* (methyl-B_{12}) is a minor component in cells but the main form in plasma. Both these forms are extremely light-sensitive and are photolysed to *hydroxocobalamin* (hydroxo-B_{12}) within 10 seconds of exposure to daylight; *hydroxo-B_{12}* is present in small amounts in tissues and plasma and is available commercially for therapeutic use. The fourth form, *cyanocobalamin* (cyano-B_{12}), is present only in traces in nature, but is stable and is used radioactively labelled with cobalt-57 or cobalt-58 for *in vitro* and *in vivo* studies of B_{12} metabolism. Hydroxo- and cyano-B_{12} are converted after two reduction steps in cells of the body to the two biochemically active forms. The fully reduced compounds are termed Cob(I)alamins, and the oxidized compounds Cob(III)alamins. Analogues of B_{12} (pseudo-B_{12}s) exist in nature and differ by having a different sugar (cobamides) or no nucleotide portion (cobinamides), or alterations in the corrin ring. The source and identity of B_{12} analogues in human serum is unclear. Endogenous production is suggested by their presence in all sera (including fetal serum) and their fall in parallel with physiologically active B_{12} in B_{12} deficiency.

B_{12} is known to be involved in only three reactions in human tissues: as ado-B_{12} in the isomerization of methylmalonyl CoA to succinyl CoA and of α-leucine to β-leucine, and as methyl-B_{12} in the methylation of homocysteine to methionine, a reaction which also requires methyltetrahydrofolate (Fig. 1). In bacteria, B_{12} takes part in other reactions involving single carbon unit metabolism: isomerization reactions, or oxidation-reduction reactions. In some bacteria, but not in man, B_{12} has a direct role in DNA synthesis by virtue of its involvement in ribonucleotide reductase.

Nutrition

B_{12} is synthesized by micro-organisms; animals obtain it by eating parts of other animals or animal produce (milk, cheese, eggs, etc.), or vegetable foods contaminated by bacteria. Clean vegetables, fruit, nuts, and cereals do not contain B_{12} and cooking has little effect on it; a normal mixed diet contains between 5 and 30 μg daily, the amount increasing with the quality. In some species, but not in humans, B_{12} is absorbed after synthesis by bacteria in the large intestine. Total body B_{12} in man is about 3–5 mg, which is mainly stored in the liver (about 0.7–1.1 μg/g). There is no particular concentration in rapidly proliferating tissues. Adult daily losses are related to body stores; to maintain normal body stores, daily requirements are of the order of 2 μg. It takes 3–4 years on average for deficiency to develop if supplies are totally cut off by malabsorption. There is an enterohepatic circulation for B_{12}, variously estimated at 3–9 μg daily which is intact in vegans which may partly account for their tendency to maintain low body stores without progressing to severe deficiency,. The body is unable to degrade B_{12} and deficiency has not been shown to be due to excess utilization or loss.

Absorption

The vitamin is released from protein binding in food by proteolytic enzymes, heat, and acid, and combines one molecule to one molecule with *intrinsic factor* (IF), a glycoprotein with a molecular weight estimated at 44 000–63 000 daltons, produced by the parietal cells of the stomach (Table 2). The normal stomach produces a vast excess of IF, measured in units (1 unit binds 1 ng B_{12}). B_{12} in bile is also attached to IF and reabsorbed through the ileum. At neutral pH, in the presence of calcium ions, B_{12}-IF complex attaches passively to specific IF receptors on the brush border of the mucosal cells of the terminal ileum. The receptor consists of an outer α-unit and an inner β-unit. A second B_{12} binding protein in gastric juice, an 'R' binder (see below), also binds food B_{12} but does not facilitate its absorption. *Pancreatic trypsin* is needed to degrade this protein and so release B_{12} for attachment to IF and subsequent absorption. After a delay of 3–5 hours during which the vitamin may be in lysosomes, suggesting that uptake into the ileum occurs by pinocytosis, B_{12} appears in the portal blood, reaching a peak 8 hours after ingestion, mainly attached to one of its transport proteins, *transcobalamin II*. IF itself is digested by the cell, possibly in the brush border or lysosomes, and is not absorbed. Absorption of B_{12} by this process is limited by the

Table 1 Vitamin B_{12} and folate

	Vitamin B_{12}	Folate
Parent form	Cyanocobalamin (cyano-B_{12}) mol. wt. 1355	Folic acid (pteroylglutamic acid) mol. wt. 441.4
Crystals	Dark red needles	Yellow, spear-shaped

Natural forms	Deoxyadenosyl-cobalamin
	Methyl-cobalamin
	Hydroxo-cobalamin
		Reduced (di- or tetrahydro-), methylated, formylated,
		  other single carbon additions; mono- and
		  polyglutamates

Foods	Animal produce (especially liver) only	All, especially liver, kidney, yeast, greens, nuts
Adult daily requirements	2 μg	100 (50–200) μg
Adult body stores	3–5 mg	6–20 mg
Length of time to deficiency	3–4 years	4 months
Daily diet content	5–30 μg	About 400 μg
Cooking	Little effect	Easily destroyed
Absorption	IF (+ neutral pH + Ca^{2+}) via ileum	Deconjugation, reduction, and methylation via duodenum and jejunum
Plasma transport	Tightly and specifically bound to transcobalamins	One-third loosely bound albumin, other proteins; ? specific protein
Enterohepatic circulation	3–9 μg/day	60–90 μg/day

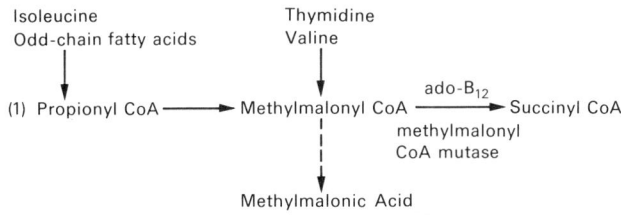

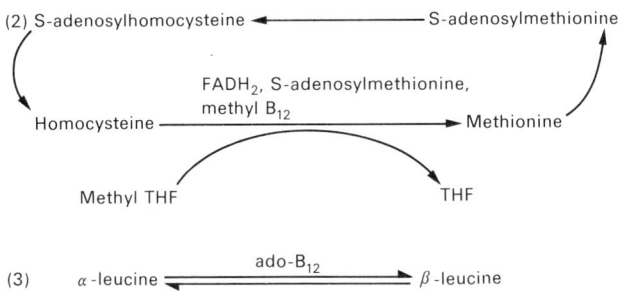

Fig. 1 Biochemical reactions of vitamin B_{12} in human tissues.

Table 2 Vitamin B_{12} binding proteins

	Intrinsic factor	Transcobalamin (TC) I and III*	Transcobalamin (TC) II
Present in source	Gastric juice Gastric parietal cell	Plasma Granulocytes ? other organs	Plasma, CSF Macrophages ? liver parenchyma, ileum
Molecular weight	44 000–63 000	60 000	38 000
Structure	Glycoprotein	Glycoprotein	Simple polypeptide
Normal total B_{12} binding capacity	30–110 μg/l	700–800 ng/l	900–1000 ng/l
B_{12} content	No B_{12}	300–400 ng/l B_{12}	30–60 ng/l B_{12}
Function	B_{12} absorption (not itself absorbed)	? Storage of B_{12} ? Protection of B_{12} ? Binding of B_{12} analogues	B_{12} delivery to marrow, placenta, brain, and other tissues

* Related 'R' in binders in other tissues and secretions, e.g. milk, gastric juice, saliva, tears.

number of ileal receptors to a few micrograms a day and although 80 per cent of a single dose of 1–2 μg may be absorbed, the proportion diminishes steeply at higher doses. A small (less than 1 per cent) trace of a large (1 mg or more) dose of B_{12} can be absorbed passively and rapidly through the buccal, gastric, and jejunal mucosae without IF participating.

Transport

B_{12} in plasma is 70–90 per cent attached to a glycoprotein, transcobalamin I (TC I). TC I does not enhance cell uptake of the vitamin, however, and accounts for only 0.4 per cent of total body cell B_{12} uptake (see Table 2). It is one of a group of glycoproteins, called 'R' binders, which are present in many tissues and fluids (e.g. gastric juice, saliva, tears, milk, and colostrum) and have the same amino acid composition but differ in the composition of the carbohydrate moiety of the molecule. The 'R' binders may have the role of binding analogues of B_{12}, derived from food or intestinal organisms and transporting them to the liver for excretion in the bile. A closely related 'R' protein, TC III, also occurs in human plasma and is probably derived from the specific granules of granulocytes; it normally carries only 0–10 per cent of plasma B_{12}. TC III may have a significant role in B_{12} transport but this is not established. The third plasma B_{12} binding protein, transcobalamin II (TC II), is synthesized in macrophages, liver, and possibly the ileum. It gains B_{12} from the ileum and by release of free B_{12} from the liver and other organs. It is normally almost completely unsaturated, however, since it actively enhances uptake of B_{12} by bone marrow, placenta, and other tissues of the body which contain receptors for TC II. TC II accounts for most of cell B_{12} uptake. At least five genetic variants of TC II exist, distinguished by their electrophoretic mobility, probably reflecting autosomal polymorphism with many co-dominant alleles at one locus. Serum TC II is normally higher in women than men and in blacks compared to whites.

The concentration of B_{12} in cerebrospinal fluid is low, with a mean of 19 ng/l in normal subjects. Most of this is attached to TC II. There is virtually no B_{12} in normal urine.

Folate

Biochemistry

This vitamin exists in nature in over 100 forms which are all derivatives of folic acid (pteroylglutamic acid) which consists of a pteridine, a para-amino benzoic acid moiety and L-glutamic acid (see Table 1). Naturate folates may differ from folic acid by: (*a*) being reduced in the pteridine ring to di- or tetrahydro-forms; (*b*) having

a single carbon moiety attached at positions N_5 or N_{10} (e.g. methyl, formyl, etc.); and (*c*) having a chain of glutamate moieties attached by γ-peptide bonds to the L-glutamate moiety. In human and other mammalian cells, the number of glutamates is mainly four, five, or six. In body fluids (plasma, cerebrospinal fluid, bile, milk, etc.), however, folates are invariably monoglutamate derivatives in plasma, 5-methyltetrahydrofolate (methyl-THF) predominates possibly with small amounts of 10-formyl-THF also present.

The biochemical reactions of folate are shown in Table 3. In each there is a transfer of a single carbon group (e.g. methyl (–CH_3), formyl (–CHOH), methenyl (=CH–), methylene (=CH_2) or formimino (–CHNH) from one compound to another. The folate compounds cycle in these reactions from one derivative to another. Three of the reactions are concerned in synthesis of DNA precursors (two in purine and one in pyrimidine synthesis). It is likely that it is the polyglutamate derivatives of folate inside cells that are the active folate co-enzymes involved in each of the reactions. During thymidylate synthesis, oxidation of folate to the dihydro-state occurs; the enzyme dihydrofolate reductase returns folate to the active tetrahydro-state (Fig. 2). During its reactions, folate is not completely re-utilized, some degradation at the C_9–N_{10} bond occurs to non-folate compounds. Thus, folate utilization is increased and folate deficiency likely when cell turnover and DNA synthesis is increased.

Nutrition

Folate occurs in most foods, the highest concentrations (more than 30 μg/100g wet weight) being found in liver (where, like B_{12}, it is stored), kidney, green vegetables, yeast, nuts, and fruit. It is easily destroyed by cooking, particularly if large volumes of water and high temperatures are used; vitamin C protects it from oxidative destruction so re-heating of food is particularly likely to reduce the folate content. Recent studies of a western diet suggest an average normal daily intake of 400 μg with 50 per cent or more in the polyglutamate form. Body stores are about 10–12 mg with a mean liver concentration of about 7 μg per g. Primitive or rapidly growing tissues have higher folate concentrations than corresponding mature tissues. Normal adult requirements are about 100 μg daily, although estimates as low as 50 μg and as high as 200 μg have been made.

Absorption

Folates are absorbed rapidly, mainly through the duodenum and jejunum. Polyglutamates are deconjugated to the monogluta-

Table 3 Main biochemical reactions of folates in human tissues

Reaction	Enzyme
1 Conjugation or deconjugation	
Hydrolysis of poly- to monoglutamates	Folate 'conjugase' (γ-glutamylcarboxypeptidase, pteroylpolyglutamate hydrolase)
Conjugation of monoglutamates to polyglutamates	Folate-polyglutamate synthetase
2 Oxidation-reduction	
Oxidized or dihydrofolates converted to tetrahydrofolates	Dihydrofolate reductase
3 Amino acid interconversions	
(a) homocysteine → methionine* + + methyl THF → THF	5-Methyl THF methyltransferase
(b) 5-formiminoglutamic acid → (Figlu) glutamic acid + + THF → formimino THF	Figlu transferase
(c) serine → glycine + + THF → 5,10-methylene THF	Serine-hydroxymethyltransferase
4 DNA synthesis	
Purine synthesis	
(a) GAR ⟶ formyl GAR 5,10-methenyl THF ⟶ THF	GAR transformylase
(b) AICAR ⟶ inosinic acid 10-formyl THF ⟶ THF	AICAR transformylase
Pyrimidine synthesis	
deoxyuridine monophosphate (dUMP) → thymidine monophosphate (TMP) 5,10-methylene THF → THF	Thymidylate synthetase
5 Formate fixation	
formic acid + ATP + THF → 10-formyl-THF + ADP	THF formylase
6 ? Methylation of biogenic amines	
e.g. dopamine → epinine methyl THF → THF	? Dopamine methyltransferase

* See Figs 1 and 2.
THF = tetrahydrofolate, DHF = dihydrofolate, GAR = glycinamide ribotide, AICAR = 5-amino-4-imidazolecarboxamide ribotide.
Reaction (6) has been demonstrated only *in vitro* and may not take place *in vivo*.

mate, possibly in the intestinal lumen, at the brush border, and possibly in lysosomes of intestinal cells by a deconjugating enzyme, 'folate conjugase' (γ-glutamylcarboxypeptidase, pteroyl-polyglutamate hydrolase), completely reduced to the tetrahydro-state and methylated at the N_5 position so that methyl-THF enters portal plasma whatever food folate is ingested (see Table 1). Folic acid itself, which is not present in food, but is used therapeutically, enters the portal blood largely unchanged since it is a poor substrate for reduction by dihydrofolate reductase. It does, however, share a specific folate uptake process through the intestine since in the rare disorder, specific malabsorption of folate, there is failure of absorption of all folates including folic acid. The small intestine has a large capacity to absorb folate; between 50 and 100 per cent of natural folate is absorbed whatever the dose. If excessive amounts are fed, the excess is largely excreted in urine as folates or their breakdown products after cleavage of the C_9–N_{10} bond. There is a substantial enterohepatic circulation for folate, estimated to contain up to 90 μg folate daily. If this is broken, plasma folate falls to about a third within 24 hours.

Transport

Folate is transported in plasma, two-thirds unbound and about one-third loosely bound to albumin and possibly other proteins.

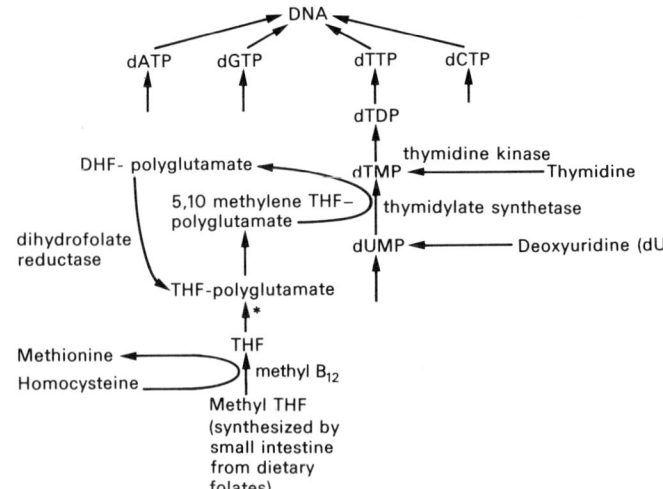

Fig. 2 Suggested mechanisms by which B_{12} deficiency affects folate metabolism and interferes with DNA synthesis. Indirect involvement of B_{12}, as methyl B_{12}, in DNA synthesis is suggested by the 'methylfolate' trap hypothesis. Methyl B_{12} is involved in formation of intracellular THF from plasma methyl THF*. THF and/or it formyl derivative are the 'ground substances' from which all folate coenzymes are made by glutamate addition and single carbon unit transfer (see text). 5,10 Methylene THF polyglutamate, is involved in thymidylate synthesis. D = deoxyribose, A = adenine, G = guanine, T = thymine, C = cytosine, TP = triphosphate, DP = diphosphate, U = uridine.

There is no specific plasma transport protein for folate which enhances cell uptake. An active transport mechanism exists, however, for getting folates into cells. In most cells the folates then remain until the cells die but the liver can probably release folate from intact cells. Specific binding proteins for folate have been described in milk, plasma, leucocytes, liver, and other tissues but the role these play, if any, in normal folate metabolism is unclear. Milk protein, however, may enhance intestinal folate uptake. In plasma the binding protein may take oxidized folates and breakdown products of folates to the liver for excretion or reconversion back to functional folates. Plasma folate is filtered by the glomerulus and mostly reabsorbed unless the renal tubular maximum is exceeded. Normal urine folate is 0–13 μg in 24 hours. Folate is secreted into cerebrospinal fluid (which has a mean concentration of 24 μg/l) and is present in bile. Human milk has a concentration of 50 μg/l.

Biochemical basis of megaloblastic anaemia

All known causes of megaloblastic anaemia, whether drugs, deficiencies, or inborn errors of metabolism, inhibit DNA synthesis by reducing the activity of one of the many enzymes concerned in purine or pyrimidine synthesis or by inhibiting DNA polymerization from its precursors. Folate deficiency, by reducing supply of the co-enzyme 5,10-methylene THF as its polyglutamate derivative, inhibits thymidylate synthesis, a rate-limiting reaction in DNA synthesis, but B_{12} does not have a direct role in this or any other reaction in mammalian DNA synthesis. B_{12} deficiency probably inhibits DNA synthesis indirectly by its effect on folate metabolism.

Clinical, laboratory, and biochemical observations have all shown that B_{12} deficiency disturbs folate metabolism. Patients with severe B_{12} deficiency may show a haematological response to folic acid in large doses, and in both folate and B_{12} deficiency the patient may show a haematological response to intravenously infused thymidine. Cell folate tends to be low, forminoglutamic acid (Figlu), and 5-amino-4-imidazole carboxamide (AICAR) excretion is raised, and serine–glycine interconversion reduced in B_{12} deficiency, as in folate deficiency. The deoxyuridine (dU) blocking test (see page 19.102) suggests a defect in thymidylate synthesis in B_{12} deficiency which can be corrected *in vitro* by folic acid as well as by B_{12}. On the other hand, cell uptake of methyl-THF is reduced, cell folate is reduced, and serum folate raised in B_{12} deficiency. The most anaemic patients with B_{12} deficiency, as in folate deficiency, show the lowest levels of serum and red cell folate and the greatest disturbance of folate biochemical reactions.

One explanation for these effects of B_{12} deficiency on folate metabolism is provided by the 'methylfolate trap' hypothesis (Fig. 2). This suggests that in B_{12} deficiency, folate is 'trapped' as methyl-THF, the form made by the intestine from food folate and circulating in plasma, because of the need for B_{12} (as methylcobalamin) in conversion of methyl-THF to THF, the reaction in which homocysteine is methylated to methionine. The 'trap' is supposed to lower the intracellular supply of the THF, the most reactive of the folate compounds from which the other folate co-enzymes are made. The natural folate co-enzymes are probably the reduced derivatives of the folate polyglutamates rather than monoglutamates. It is clear that methyl-THF cannot act as a substrate for folate polyglutamate synthesis in human cells. The preferred folate monoglutamate to which glutamate moieties are added is probably formyl-THF but *in vitro* studies suggest that THF may also act as substrate. It seems most probable that the main role of B_{12} in folate metabolism is in the 'demethylation' of methyl-THF so that THF and thus formyl-THF are formed and folate polyglutamate formation can occur (Fig. 2). Chanarin and coworkers propose that it is in the provision of the formyl moiety of formyl-THF, rather than THF or the THF moiety of formyl-THF that B_{12} has a crucial rate-limiting role. They suggest that the formyl group of formyl-THF is provided by methionine via S-adenosylmethionine and methylthioadenosine and it is the lack of synthesis of methionine from homocysteine which is the crucial defect in B_{12} deficiency. The methionine, they suggest, may also be needed directly for provision of the 5,10-methylene group of 5,10-methylene-THF. It seems unlikely that B_{12} is needed in haemopoiesis solely to provide 'activated' formate, but this may indeed be an additional role to the provision of THF. In any event the result is that B_{12} deficiency or inactivation puts a block between methyl-THF entering cells from plasma and the formation of intracellular folate polyglutamate coenzymes. This causes the rise in plasma folate, low level of intracellular folates and reduced activity of all reactions requiring folate coenzymes, including those involved in DNA synthesis, seen in patients with B_{12} deficiency.

Clinical features and causes of megaloblastic anaemia

Although pernicious anaemia is only one of many causes of megaloblastic anaemia (see Tables 4, 5, and 6), it is convenient to describe the general clinical features of the anaemia under this heading since pernicious anaemia is the most frequent cause of megaloblastic anaemia in western countries. The laboratory findings and treatment of pernicious anaemia and other megaloblastic anaemias are discussed later.

Acquired pernicious anaemia

(Addisonian pernicious anaemia, Biermer's anaemia.)

Definition

A disease of unknown origin in which there is atrophy of the stomach leading to severely reduced or absent intrinsic factor secretion with consequent severe malabsorption of B_{12}, and B_{12} deficiency.

Table 4 Causes of vitamin B_{12} deficiency and malabsorption of vitamin B_{12}

1 Causes of severe B_{12} deficiency
  (*a*) Nutritional
      Vegans
      Long-continued extremely poor diet (rarely)
  (*b*) Malabsorption
      Gastric causes
      Acquired (Addisonian) pernicious anaemia
      Congenital intrinsic factor deficiency or abnormality
      Total and partial gastrectomy
      Destructive lesions of stomach
      Intestinal causes
        Stagnant-loop syndrome (jejunal diverticulosis, ileocolic
          fistula, anatomical blind loop, stricture, etc.)
        Ileal resection and Crohn's disease
        Chronic tropical sprue
        Selective malabsorption with proteinuria
        Fish tapeworm
        TC II deficiency
2 Causes of malabsorption of B_{12} without severe B_{12} deficiency
    Simple atrophic gastritis, severe chronic pancreatitis
    Zollinger–Ellison syndrome, adult coeliac disease
    Drugs
      PAS, colchicine, neomycin, slow K, ethanol, metformin,
        phenformin, anticonvulsants
    Deficiencies of folate, B_{12}, protein

Table 5 Causes of folate deficiency

1 Poor diet
    Especially poverty, psychiatric disturbance, alcoholism, dietary
      fads, scurvy, kwashiorkor, goat's milk anaemia, partial
      gastrectomy, other gastrointestinal disease, intensive care units
2 Malabsorption
    Gluten-sensitive enteropathy (child or adult or associated with
      dermatitis herpetiformis)
    Tropical sprue
    Congenital specific malabsorption
    Minor factor: partial gastrectomy, jejunal resection, Crohn's
      disease, lymphoma, systemic infections
    Drugs: cholestyramine, sulphasalazine, ? others (see 5 below)
3 Excess requirements
    Physiological
      Pregnancy
      Prematurity and infancy
    Pathological
    (*a*) Malignancies—leukaemia, carcinoma, lymphoma, myeloma,
        sarcoma, etc.
    (*b*) Blood disorders—haemolytic anaemia (especially sickle cell
        anaemia, thalassaemia major)
        —chronic myelosclerosis, sideroblastic anaemia
    (*c*) Inflammatory—tuberculosis, malaria, Crohn's disease,
        psoriasis, exfoliative dermatitis, rheumatoid arthritis, etc.
    (*d*) Metabolic—homocystinuria (some cases)
  4 Excess urinary excretion
    Congestive heart failure, acute liver damage, chronic dialysis, ? B_{12}
      deficiency
5 Drugs
    Mechanism uncertain
      Anticonvulsants (diphenylhydantoin, primidone, barbiturates)
      ? Oral contraceptives
      ? Nitrofurantoin
      ? Alcohol
      Also drugs causing malabsorption of folate (see 2 above)
6 Liver diseases
    Mixed causes above, and poor storage

Aetiology and associated diseases

Although a disease of the stomach, pernicious anaemia (PA) is considered with blood diseases since it usually presents with anaemia; it is indeed the most common cause of megaloblastic anaemia

Table 6 Megaloblastic anaemia not due to vitamin B_{12} or folate deficiency

1 Abnormalities of B_{12} or folate metabolism
  Congenital
    Transcobalamin II deficiency
    Inborn errors of folate metabolism, e.g. methylfolate transferase,
      ? dihydrofolate reductase deficiency
    Homocystinuria and methylmalonic aciduria (some cases)
    Responding to large doses of B_{12} and folate
  Acquired
    Nitrous oxide
    Dihydrofolate reductase inhibitors: methotrexate,
      pyrimethamine, trimethoprim, ? pentamidine, triamterene
2 Independent of vitamin B_{12} or folate
  Congenital
    Orotic aciduria, responds to uridine
    Lesch–Nyhan syndrome, ? responds to adenine
    Thiamine-responsive
    Some cases of congenital dyserythropoietic anaemia
  Acquired
    Erythroleukaemia, other myeloid leukaemias (some cases)
    Primary acquired sideroblastic anaemia (50 per cent of cases) and
      other myelodysplastic syndromes
    Drugs
      Antimetabolites: 6-mercaptopurine, cytosine, arabinoside,
        hydroxyurea, 5-fluorouracil, azauridine, azaserine, etc.
      Alcohol
    ? Vitamin E deficiency

in many countries. It is a disease of older persons with a peak incidence of about 1:205 in the United Kingdom at 60 years and less than 10 per cent of cases are under 40 years; there is a female:male ratio in most (but not all) series of about 1.6:1. There is a higher incidence (about 44 per cent compared to 40 per cent) of blood group A compared with controls in Britain. No overall association between PA and HLA type has been found, but those with an endocrine disease also have a greater incidence of HLA-B8, B12, and BW15. There are regional differences in incidence in the United Kingdom, with over 200 cases per 100 000 in Scotland, less than 60 per 100 000 in Southeast England. It occurs in all races including Negro, Indian, Red Indian, Chinese, as well as Caucasians, but is most frequent in northern Europeans and persons with early greying and blue eyes. There is a higher incidence in close relatives of either sex (with a positive family history of about 30 per cent of cases) but the type of inheritance is not clear.

Carcinoma of the stomach occurs in about 4 per cent of patients with pernicious anaemia, an incidence of about three times the control rate. The disease may also be associated with other 'autoimmune' diseases, particularly *primary myxoedema, thyrotoxicosis, Hashimoto's disease, Addison's disease*, and *vitiligo*. About 55 per cent of patients show thyroid antibodies and 33 per cent of patients with primary myxoedema have parietal cell antibody. Close relatives also may show these diseases or their associated antibodies. There is probably no significant association with diabetes mellitus. Other evidence for an immune aetiology of the gastritis of pernicious anaemia is the improvement in mucosal appearance and function with corticosteroid therapy, the presence of antibodies in serum and gastric juice directed against parietal cells and IF, and of cell-mediated immunity to IF (see Section 12). Parietal cell antibody is present in the serum of 85–90 per cent of patients. Two antibodies to IF exist in serum. Type I ('blocking') occurs in about 50 per cent of the sera and is directed against the B_{12}-binding site. Type II (to the ileal binding site) occurs in 30–35 per cent of sera, but only if Type I antibody is also present. IF antibodies exist in gastric juice, and here they may neutralize the action of remaining IF. The IF antibodies are virtually specific for pernicious anaemia, but parietal cell antibody occurs in many subjects with atrophic gastritis without pernicious anaemia. Lymphocyte populations in IF-antibody positive patients show a T_4 to T_8 ratio higher than in controls or those negative for IF antibody. IF antibody may cross the placenta and cause temporary IF

deficiency in the newborn infant. Pernicious anaemia may also be associated with *hypogammaglobulinaemia* or with selective IgA deficiency when it tends to present at an early age and antibodies to parietal cell and IF may be absent.

The relation of pernicious anaemia to simple gastric atrophy which occurs in about 15 per cent of people between 40 and 60, and between 20–30 per cent of the older population is not clear. In many cases, simple gastric atrophy does not progress to pernicious anaemia after 10 or more years of follow-up. In a minority, however, IF deficiency severe enough to cause malabsorption of vitamin B_{12} and megaloblastic anaemia, glossitis, or vitamin B_{12} neuropathy occurs. In them, the development of IF antibody in the gastric juice may be important.

Pathology

(See also Section 12.)

There is a gastritis in which all layers of the body and fundus of the stomach are atrophied with loss of normal gastric glands, mucosal architecture, and absence of parietal and chief cells, but mucous cells lining the gastric pits are well preserved. An infiltrate of plasma cells and lymphocytes with an excess of T_8 (suppressor) cells occurs and intestinal metaplasia may be present. The antral mucosa is remarkably well-preserved and, like the fundus, shows an increased number of gastrin-secreting cells.

Clinical features

The general features of megaloblastic anaemia are similar, whatever the underlying cause, although the onset of megaloblastic anaemia due to folate deficiency is often more rapid than with B_{12} deficiency. Particular clinical features in the individual patient may point to the underlying disease, whether pernicious anaemia or some other cause. In pernicious anaemia, the anaemia usually develops gradually, perhaps over several years, and symptoms may not occur until it is severe. There is little relation between duration of symptoms and severity of anaemia. The most common complaints are those due to the anaemia (e.g. weakness, tiredness, dyspnoea on exertion), loss of mental and physical drive, or those due to a sore tongue. Paraesthesiae in the feet or hands, numbness, or difficulty in walking suggest B_{12} neuropathy. Psychiatric disturbances are common and range from mild neurosis to severe organic dementia. Mild jaundice is frequent, but is usually not noticed by the patient. Loss of appetite and weight, indigestion, and episodic diarrhoea are frequent. An intercurrent infection may precipitate severe anaemia and thus symptoms in patients with pre-existing asymptomatic B_{12} (or folate) deficiency. Older patients may present with congestive heart failure. In a few patients bruising due to thrombocytopenia is marked. On the other hand, many patients are diagnosed because a blood test is performed for an incidental purpose. This is particularly so now that electronic blood counting accurately shows the mean corpuscular volume.

The typical patient with pernicious anaemia has fair hair (prematurely grey), with blue eyes and wide cheekbones. Physical signs, if present, are those of anaemia, perhaps with mild jaundice, giving the patient a so-called 'lemon-yellow tint'. A few patients with either vitamin B_{12} or folate deficiency develop a widespread brown pigmentation, affecting nail-beds and skin creases particularly, but not mucous membranes, which is reversible with the appropriate therapy. The biochemical basis for this is not clear. It is not established, however, that B_{12} or folate deficiency is a cause of recurring aphthous ulcers. The tongue may be red, smooth, and shiny, occasionally with ulcers. A mild pyrexia up to 38 °C is common in patients with moderate to severe anaemia. The liver and spleen may be palpable in severe cases, while the cardiovascular system shows changes due to anaemia. Patients with pernicious anaemia may also have features of an associated disorder on presentation, most commonly myxoedema, but other thyroid disorders, vitiligo, carcinoma of the stomach, Addison's disease, and hypoparathyroidism, may also precede, occur simultaneously with, or follow the onset of the anaemia.

Vitamin B_{12} neuropathy

(This disorder is considered in detail in Section 21.)

B_{12} deficiency may cause a symmetrical neuropathy affecting the lower limbs more than upper (Section 21) which usually presents with paraesthesiae, difficulty in walking, or unsteadiness, particularly in the dark. In some cases an optic neuritis or psychiatric disturbance dominates. The neuropathy is due to severe B_{12} deficiency judged by serum B_{12} levels or methylmalonic acid excretion but may occur with mild or no anaemia. It may be due to any cause of severe B_{12} deficiency, most commonly pernicious anaemia. The biochemical explanation for the neuropathy is not clear. A defect in fatty acid metabolism in myelin tissue due to lack of ado-B_{12} has been suggested. More recent studies in nitrous oxide treated monkeys have suggested that the neuropathy results from deficiency of S-adenosyl methionine (SAM) in the brain caused by the block in conversion of homocysteine to methionine. Cycloleucine which inhibits SAM formation and produces a neuropathy in some animals resembling human B_{12} neuropathy, causes defective methylation of arginine in myelin basic protein but such a lesion has yet to be shown in vitamin B_{12} neuropathy occurring clinically in humans or induced experimentally by dietary deficiency in fruit bats or by N_2O exposure to monkeys or rats. The theory that inactivation of B_{12} as cyano-B_{12} by, e.g. smoking or diet, plays a part is no longer tenable.

General tissue effects of vitamin B_{12} (and folate) deficiencies

Both deficiencies cause macrocytosis and other abnormal features of proliferating epithelial cells throughout the body (e.g. bronchial, bladder, buccal, and uterine cervix), with glossitis and angular cheilosis, a mild malabsorption syndrome, and reduced regeneration of damaged liver cells. In both sexes sterility (reversible with B_{12} or folate therapy) may result from effects on the gonads. It is unlikely, however, that the deficiencies in children affect overall body growth. Whether abnormalities of pregnancy such as congenital malformations, pre- or post-partum haemorrhage, or abruptio placentae are precipitated by clinical folate deficiency is also uncertain, although there does seem to be a real association with prematurity. Generalized reversible melanin pigmentation occurs in a few patients with B_{12} or folate deficiency, the cause for which is uncertain. Defective bactericidal activity of phagocytes due to impaired intracellular killing has been described in B_{12} deficiency but not in folate deficiency.

Other causes of vitamin B_{12} deficiency

Juvenile pernicious anaemia

A few cases of pernicious anaemia with gastric atrophy and achlorhydria and IF antibodies have occurred in children. They may show associated ('autoimmune') conditions, e.g. myxoedema, hypoparathyroidism, Addison's disease, or chronic mucocutaneous candidiasis.

Congenital IF deficiency (congenital pernicious anaemia)

About 40 cases have been reported of a child being born with absent IF but an otherwise normal stomach on biopsy and secretion studies, e.g. of acid. Inheritance is autosomal recessive. In one case, IF was present in the gastric juice which could bind B_{12} but could not attach it to ileal receptors. These children tend to present with irritability, vomiting, diarrhoea, and loss of weight, and are found to have megaloblastic anaemia. The usual age of diagnosis is about two, although a few have been diagnosed as early as four months and others only in their teens.

Total gastrectomy

All patients who have this operation will develop B_{12} deficiency which usually presents between two and six years post-operatively, and they should be treated with prophylactic B_{12} injections from the time of the operation.

Partial gastrectomy

Iron deficiency usually accounts for the anaemia which occurs in up to 50 per cent of subjects following this operation. Subnormal serum B_{12} levels develop in about 18 per cent of patients from about two years postoperatively and about 6 per cent develop megaloblastic anaemia due to the deficiency. In most of these patients, the malabsorption of B_{12} is due to an abnormal jejunal flora. The exact incidence of B_{12} deficiency depends mainly on the size of the remnant, which tends to be smaller if the operation is subtotal, and the peptic ulcer gastric rather than duodenal. Nutritional folate deficiency may account for about a fifth of all cases of megaloblastic anaemia following partial gastrectomy. Vagotomy and pyloroplasty is not a cause of B_{12} deficiency.

Small intestinal lesions

Colonization of the upper small intestine with colonic bacteria, if sufficiently heavy as in the stagnant-loop syndrome, leads to malabsorption of B_{12}. The most common causes are listed in Table 4. It appears that the bacteria destroy IF. Infestation with the fish tapeworm (*Diphyllobothrium latum*) has a similar effect but is now almost completely eradicated and infestation is only sufficiently marked in Finland and around the lakes of Russia to cause megaloblastic anaemia frequently.

Resection of a metre or more of terminal ileum

This causes severe malabsorption of B_{12}. Other diseases which may affect ileal structure and function include tropical sprue, in which severe B_{12} deficiency with anaemia or rarely neuropathy is a manifestation only in the chronic phase, gluten-sensitive enteropathy in which megaloblastic anaemia, if it occurs, is always due to folate deficiency (and B_{12} deficiency, if it occurs, is mild), and Crohn's disease in which malabsorption of B_{12} is frequent, but severe B_{12} deficiency is unusual unless an ileal resection, or fistula or stagnant-loop occurs.

Selective malabsorption of vitamin B_{12} with proteinuria (Imerslund's disease, Imerslund–Gräsbeck syndrome)

This is a congenital disorder, with autosomal recessive inheritance. It has been reported in many countries of Europe and in the United States. The child secretes IF normally but is unable to transport B_{12} across the ileum to portal blood. In some but not all cases tested an abnormality in ileal receptors for IF-bound B_{12} has been found. The proteinuria, present in over 90 per cent of cases but not in all, is benign, non-specific, and persists after B_{12} therapy. The clinical presentation of the disease is identical to that of congenital IF deficiency.

Other causes of malabsorption of vitamin B_{12}

A number of other conditions and drugs may cause malabsorption of B_{12} but rarely cause B_{12} deficiency of clinical severity. PAS, colchicine, neomycin, 'slow' potassium tablets, metformin, and phenformin have all been reported to cause malabsorption of B_{12}. In chronic pancreatitis and the Zollinger–Ellison syndrome there is failure to release B_{12} from R protein due to absence of or inactivation of pancreatic trypsin. Malabsorption of B_{12} also occurs in inherited TC II deficiency.

Dietary B_{12} deficiency

This occurs most commonly in Hindus, who omit all animal produce from their diet. The incidence of overt megaloblastic anaemia is much lower than the incidence of subclinical deficiency assessed by the serum B_{12} assay, low figures often being accompanied by entirely normal health. These subjects have low B_{12} stores. In India, babies have been born B_{12}-deficient with megaloblastic anaemia caused by severe B_{12} deficiency (due to poor diet or sprue) in the mother. Dietary deficiency of B_{12} also occurs in non-Hindu vegans, and rarely in people living for some years on a totally inadequate diet because of poverty.

Folate deficiency

Clinical features

The main clinical features of megaloblastic anaemia due to folate deficiency are similar to those when the anaemia is due to B_{12} deficiency except a severe neuropathy does not occur and the underlying disease causing the deficiency tends to be different. Folate deficiency may develop rapidly, and although many mildly deficient patients do not progress for months or years, in some patients the deficiency may lead to a severe pancytopenia ('arrest of haemopoiesis') over a short period, particularly if an infection supervenes.

Folate deficiency has not been proved to cause an organic neuropathy, but a mild peripheral neuropathy has been found in about 20 per cent of patients with folate deficiency. The suggestion that folate therapy may precipitate fits in epileptics has not been confirmed by double-blind trials. Some studies suggest folate, as methyl-THF, may be involved in methylation of biogenic amines, e.g. dopamine, in the brain. If so, this may explain some of the psychiatric disturbances which seem to be more common in folate than B_{12} deficiency.

Nutritional folate deficiency

Minor degrees of nutritional folate deficiency are frequent in most countries, but severe megaloblastic anaemia is much less common. In England, nutritional folate deficiency may account for about 17 per cent of all cases of megaloblastic anaemia. In western communities, it occurs mainly in the old and poor living alone on an inadequate diet from which liver, fruit, and fresh vegetables are omitted; in many, barbiturate or alcohol consumption or a physical abnormality, e.g. partial gastrectomy, rheumatoid arthritis, or tuberculosis, may aggravate the effects of a poor diet. A few cases have developed because a special diet is taken, e.g. for phenylketonuria or for slimming. Scurvy is usually accompanied by severe folate deficiency while goat's milk anaemia is nutritional folate deficiency due to the low (6 μg/l) folate content of goat's milk. In less well-developed countries, where pernicious anaemia is rare, nutritional folate deficiency may be the main cause of megaloblastic anaemia, often presenting in pregnancy, e.g. in Burma, Malaysia, Africa, or India. Among Hindus, nutritional B_{12} deficiency is also common, however, and in many countries, e.g. Caribbean islands, Sri Lanka, and Southeast Asia, tropical sprue (see Section 12) is an important cause of both deficiencies and is difficult to distinguish from 'pure' nutritional deficiency.

Rapidly developing folate deficiency has recently been described in patients in intensive care units with infections, multiple organ failure and receiving drugs. Poor nutrition combined with excess demands and possibly alcohol infusion are the main factors.

Malabsorption

(See Section 12.)

Gluten-induced enteropathy (adult coeliac disease, idiopathic steatorrhoea)

Folate deficiency occurs in virtually all untreated patients, the serum folate being subnormal whether or not megaloblastic anaemia is present; red cell folate is subnormal in 80 per cent or more, normal results being found in very mild cases. Anaemia occurs in about 90 per cent of adult cases, due to folate deficiency alone in 30–50 per cent and due to mixed iron and folate deficiency in the remainder. Mild B_{12} deficiency may also occur but is not a cause of anaemia in uncomplicated cases. Spontaneous atrophy of the spleen occurs in most of the patients; in about 10–15 per cent of cases, the blood film shows the presence of Howell–Jolly bodies, siderotic granules, and target and crenated cells which do not disappear with either folic acid or a gluten-free diet. Malabsorption of folic acid and of folate polyglutamates has been demonstrated in almost all untreated patients. A gluten-free diet produces a spontaneous rise in serum and red cell folate and improved folate absorption in those patients who respond to this treatment.

Malabsorption of folate also occurs in children with gluten-induced enteropathy and virtually all show subnormal serum and red cell folate levels; anaemia is most often due to combined iron and folate deficiency but 'pure' megaloblastic anaemia also occurs.

Patients with *dermatitis herpetiformis* almost all show some degree of jejunal abnormality and the severity of folate malabsorption and deficiency correlates with the severity of the intestinal lesion (see Section 12).

Tropical sprue

(See Section 12.)

Malabsorption of folate occurs in all severe untreated patients in the acute phase and megaloblastic anaemia due to folate deficiency may develop within a few months. Not only does the anaemia respond to folate therapy but in many patients all the clinical features, and malabsorption of xylose, fat, B_{12}, and other substances, improve on folate therapy alone. Favourable responses to folic acid are most frequent in the first year of the disease when about 60 per cent of patients appear to be cured by folic acid alone. Long-standing cases are more likely to be B_{12} deficient and thus to require B_{12} as well as folate and antibiotic therapy.

Congenital specific malabsorption of folate

This is an abnormality reported in five children, including two sisters and the child of a consanguineous marriage. The children all showed features of damage to the central nervous system (mental retardation, fits, athetotic movements) and presented with megaloblastic anaemia responding to physiological doses of folic acid given parenterally but not orally. All forms of folate are poorly absorbed. Low levels of folate in cerebrospinal fluid also suggest a defect of folate transport through the choroid plexus.

Other causes

One study has reported that absorption of folate is impaired by systemic infections. Mild degrees of folate malabsorption have also been reported in patients following jejunal resection or partial gastrectomy, with Crohn's disease, and with lymphomas. In the intestinal stagnant-loop syndrome, folate levels tend to be high due to absorption of bacterially produced folate from the upper small intestine. A number of drugs including alcohol, anticonvulsants, oral contraceptives, antituberculous drugs, nitrofurantoin, sulphasalazine, bile salt metabolites, and sodium bromosulphopthalein have been suggested, on variable evidence, to cause malabsorption of folate in some subjects but none are definitely established except sulphasalazine.

Increased folate utilization

Pregnancy (see also Section 11)

This, associated with poor nutrition, is probably the commonest cause of megaloblastic anaemia in the world. The frequency of the anaemia was about 0.5 per cent in most western cities with incidences up to 5 per cent in some series and up to 50 per cent in some areas of Asia and Africa until the introduction of prophylactic folic acid. The incidence increases with parity, is higher in twin pregnancies, and in some but not all series the incidence has been highest at the end of the winter. Folate requirements in a normal pregnancy are thought to be increased to about 300–400 μg daily, some 200–300 μg above normal. Serum and red cell folate tends to fall as pregnancy progresses with about 30 per cent subnormal red cell folate levels in Britain in late pregnancy and to rise spontaneously about 6 weeks after delivery. Lactation may prove an additional cause of folate deficiency, however, which may precipitate megaloblastic anaemia in the post-partum period.

The cause of the deficiency in pregnancy is increased demand due to folate transfer to the fetus that cannot be met from body reserves or dietary intake. Malabsorption of folate and increased urine folate excretion may be minor factors in some patients and, in a few, megaloblastic anaemia of pregnancy is the first sign of adult coeliac disease. The statistical association of iron and folate deficiencies in pregnancy, as in partial gastrectomy patients, is probably due to the poor quality of the diet some of these subjects take, rather than to either deficiency predisposing to the other.

Prophylactic folic acid should now be given routinely in pregnancy. Most use a dose of about 350 μg daily. Conventional doses of 5 mg daily are equally satisfactory but have the theoretical drawback of being more likely to mask anaemia in the rare pregnant subject with untreated pernicious anaemia and thus allow B_{12} neuropathy to develop.

Prematurity

Newborn infants have higher serum and red cell folate levels than adults. These fall to a lowest value at about six weeks of age due to utilization (and possibly excessive urinary loss) exceeding intake. In normal infants, folate levels reach normal adult values when mixed feeding commences. In premature infants, the fall in folate levels after birth is particularly steep and a number of such infants have developed megaloblastic anaemia, particularly if infections, feeding difficulties, or haemolytic disease with exchange transfusion have occurred. Prophylactic folic acid, e.g. 1 mg weekly for the first 3–4 weeks of life, may be given, particularly to those babies weighing less than 1.5–1.8 kg at birth.

Malignant diseases

Mild folate deficiency is frequent in patients with all these conditions (Table 5). In general, the severity correlates with the extent and degree of dissemination of the underlying disease. Patients with megaloblastic anaemia due to folate deficiency are unusual and folic acid therapy often does not produce a satisfactory haematological response because of other factors depressing haemopoiesis. As folic acid might 'feed the tumour', it should be withheld unless there is a real indication for its use, e.g. gross megaloblastosis causing severe anaemia, leucopenia, or thrombocytopenia.

Blood disorders

Chronic haemolytic anaemia

Requirements for folate are increased in patients with increased erythropoiesis, particularly when there is ineffective erythropoiesis with a high turnover of primitive cells. Occasional patients, presumably those with a poor folate intake, develop megaloblastic anaemia particularly in sickle cell anaemia, thalassaemia major, hereditary spherocytosis, and warm-type autoimmune haemolytic anaemia, and prophylactic folic acid is usually used in these disorders.

Chronic myelosclerosis

Megaloblastic haemopoiesis was reported in as many as one-third of patients in a series in London with this disease but a lower incidence occurred in a large series in the United States. Circulating megaloblasts, increased transfusion requirements, severe thrombocytopenia, or pancytopenia may be the first indication that folate deficiency has developed. Polycythaemia vera is not a potent cause of folate deficiency, presumably because there is considerably less ineffective haemopoiesis.

Sideroblastic anaemia

Folate deficiency, usually mild, occurs in about 50 per cent of these patients, particularly those with the secondary acquired form. Megaloblastosis, refractory to folate or B_{12}, also occurs in the acquired forms as in other myelodysplastic diseases.

Inflammatory diseases

Folate deficiency has been described in patients with tuberculosis, malaria, Crohn's disease, psoriasis, widespread eczema, and rheumatoid arthritis. In each, the degree of deficiency is related to the extent and severity of the underlying disorder. Increased demand

for folate probably is a factor but reduced appetite is also important in those who develop megaloblastic anaemia.

Metabolic

Homocystinuria
(See Section 9.)

Patients with the most common form of this disorder due to cystathionase deficiency may show folate deficiency possibly due to excess conversion of homocysteine to methionine and thus excess utilization of the folate coenzyme concerned.

Excess urinary loss of folate

Urine folate excretion of 100 μg a day or more occurs in some patients with *congestive cardiac failure* or active *liver disease* causing necrosis of liver cells. It is presumed that losses are due to release of folate from damaged liver cells. *Haemodialysis* and *peritoneal dialysis* remove folate from plasma. The amounts of folate that can be lost in this way are small but folate deficiency has occurred in such patients, when such losses are combined with poor intake. Folic acid (e.g. 5 mg weekly) is now usually given prophylactically to patients with renal failure who require long-term dialysis.

Drugs

Dihydrofolate reductase (DHFR) inhibitors

Methotrexate, aminopterin, pyrimethamine, and trimethoprim all inhibit DHFR but have different relative activities against the human, malarial, and bacterial enzymes. They cause varying degrees of impairment of folate metabolism in humans. Trimethoprim, used as an antibacterial agent, may aggravate pre-existing folate or B_{12} deficiency but does not of itself cause megaloblastic anaemia.

Alcohol

Folate deficiency occurs in spirit-drinking alcoholics. The main factor is poor nutrition and it is likely that alcohol interrupts the enterohepatic circulation for folate. It also has a direct effect on haemopoiesis, causing vacuolation of normoblasts, impaired iron utilization, sideroblastic changes, macrocytosis, megaloblastosis, and thrombocytopenia, even in the absence of folate deficiency. Beer drinkers seem relatively immune from folate deficiency because of the high folate content of beer.

Anticonvulsants, barbiturates

Diphenylhydantoin, primidone, and barbiturate therapy are associated with some degree of folate deficiency varying from low serum folate without recognizable haematological abnormality to mild macrocytosis or to severe megaloblastic anaemia. The more severe degrees of deficiency are associated with poor dietary intake of folate and usually prolonged drug therapy at high doses.

The mechanism for the deficiency is undetermined. Malabsorption of folate, excess utilization due to induction of folate-requiring enzymes, displacement of folate from its binding protein, or competition for folate-requiring enzymes have all been suggested but not proven. Increased degradation of folate has been shown in mice exposed to diphenylhydantoin.

Oral contraceptives

It seems unlikely that the use of these drugs is associated with an increased incidence of subnormal serum and red cell folate levels. Individual women have been described who developed megaloblastic anaemia due to folate deficiency for no other apparent cause but where detailed studies were undertaken unsuspected adult coeliac disease or malnutrition was present.

Other drugs

Nitrofurantoin, triamterene, proguanil and pentamidine have been suggested to cause folate deficiency. Homofolates and carboxypeptidase G are two folate antagonists which have not been used in man.

Table 7 Laboratory diagnosis of megaloblastic anaemia

1 General tests
    Peripheral blood film and count
    Bone marrow
    Serum bilirubin, iron, LDH
    Urea, electrolytes, uric acid
2 Tests for B_{12} or folate deficiency
    Therapeutic trial
    Serum B_{12} and folate; red cell folate
    Urine excretion of methylmalonic acid after valine
    Deoxyuridine suppression test
3 Tests for cause of B_{12} or folate deficiency
    B_{12} deficiency
        Serum antibodies to parietal cell, IF; immunoglobulins
        Gastric secretion; IF, acid
        Gastric biopsy, endoscopy
        Barium meal + follow-through
        Radioactive B_{12} absorption tests (alone, with IF)
        Proteinuria, fish tapeworm ova, intestinal flora, etc.
    Folate deficiency
    Small intestinal function
        Xylose, glucose, vitamin A, fat, B_{12} absorption
        Jejunal biopsy
        Barium follow-through
    Tests for many underlying conditions

Liver disease

Folate deficiency occurs most commonly in alcoholic cirrhosis where alcohol, poor nutrition, poor storage, and excess urine losses may all be important. The deficiency is less frequent in other types of liver disease.

Laboratory investigation of megaloblastic anaemia

This consists of three stages: (a) recognition that megaloblastic anaemia is present; (b) distinction between B_{12} or folate deficiency (or rarely some other factor) as the cause of the anaemia; (c) diagnosis of the underlying disease causing the deficiency (Table 7).

Recognition of megaloblastic anaemia

The peripheral blood

The anaemia is usually suspected because of the presence of macrocytic red cells in the peripheral blood. There is a raised mean cell volume to between 100 fl and 140 fl and oval macrocytes are seen in the blood film. In mild cases, macrocytosis is present before anaemia has developed. Poikilocytosis and anisocytosis are also marked in severe cases, and Cabot rings (composed of arginine-rich histone and non-haemoglobin iron) and occasional Howell–Jolly bodies (DNA fragments) may be present in the red cells. A leucoerythroblastic blood picture may occur due to extramedullary haemopoiesis in the liver and spleen. The mean corpuscular volume may be normal if there is associated iron deficiency, when the blood film appears dimorphic or if the anaemia (usually due to folate deficiency or antimetabolite drug therapy) develops acutely over the course of a few weeks. The mean cell volume is also normal in some severely anaemic cases due to excess red cell fragmentation. The reticulocyte count is low for the degree of anaemia, usually of the order of 1–3 per cent.

The peripheral blood also shows hypersegmented neutrophils (which have nuclei with more than five lobes) and the leucocyte count is often moderately reduced in both neutrophils and lymphocytes, although the total leucocyte count rarely falls to less than $1.5 \times 10^9/l$. The T4/T8 lymphocyte ratio is reduced. The platelet count may be moderately reduced but rarely falls below $40 \times 10^9/l$.

Biochemical changes

These are confined to the anaemic patient and include a slight rise in serum bilirubin (up to 50 μmol/l), mainly unconjugated, a rise in serum lactic dehydrogenase of up to 10 000 i.u./l with less marked rises in serum lysozyme and serum transaminases. The serum iron is also raised and falls within 12–24 hours of effective treatment and the serum ferritin is mildly raised and falls over the first few days of therapy. The serum cholesterol is low and alkaline phosphatase mildly reduced. Absence of haptoglobins is usual. In severe cases, free haemoglobin may be present in plasma, Schumm's test for methaemalbumin in serum is positive, and haemosiderin and fibrin degradation products are present in urine. The direct Coombs' test is weakly positive in some patients, due to complement only on the surface of the cells.

Bone marrow

The bone marrow is hypercellular in moderate or severely anaemic cases and expanded along the lengths of the long bones. The myeloid–erythroid ratio is often reduced or reversed. The developing red cells are larger than normal and show a number of morphological abnormalities; there is asynchronous maturation of nucleus and cytoplasm, nuclear chromatin remaining primitive with an open, lacy, fine granular pattern despite normal maturation and haemoglobinization of the cytoplasm. Fully haemoglobinized cells with incompletely condensed nuclei may be seen. Excessive numbers of dying cells, and nuclear remnants including Howell–Jolly bodies, mitoses, and multinucleate cells may be present. Because of death of later cells, there is a disproportionate accumulation of early cells, especially pro- and basophilic megaloblasts. Giant and abnormally shaped metamyelocytes, and megakaryocytes with hypersegmented nuclear lobes are also usually present. Studies with labelled thymidine have shown an increase of cells in G_2 and mitosis and of cells with intermediate amounts of DNA between 2C and 4C but not synthesizing DNA, and presumably destined to die.

The severity of these changes tend to parallel the degree of anaemia. In milder cases, changes, described as 'intermediate', 'transitional', or 'moderate' are principally in the size and nuclear chromatin pattern of the individual developing erythroid cells, with giant metamyelocytes present; hypercellularity and gross dyserythropoiesis may be absent. In very mild cases, megaloblastic changes are difficult to recognize, so that the correlation between one observer and another is poor. In patients with severe anaemia but only mild megaloblastic changes, some additional cause for the anaemia should be sought.

Deoxyuridine suppression test

This is an *in vitro* biochemical test for B_{12} or folate deficiency based on the presence of a block in thymidylate synthesis (Fig. 2). Deoxyuridine added to normoblastic cells reduces the incorporation of radioactive thymidine into DNA. The deoxyuridine is converted into deoxyuridine monophosphate (dUMP) and hence to mono-, di-, and tri-thymidine phosphates which inhibit thymidine kinase and so uptake of the labelled thymidine. Uptake of labelled thymidine into DNA is not blocked as much by deoxyuridine in cells from patients with B_{12} or folate deficiency as in normoblastic cells because of the block in conversion of dUMP to TMP (thymidylate synthetase) in megaloblasts. Correction of the test *in vitro* with B_{12} or methyl-THF can be used to differentiate the two deficiencies since B_{12} will correct in B_{12} deficiency whereas methyl-THF does not; the reverse occurs in folate deficiency. The test is normal in cells from patients with megaloblastosis due to a block in DNA synthesis other than at thymidylate synthetase.

Chromosomes

Changes found in marrow and other proliferating cells include: (a) random chromatin breaks; (b) exaggeration of centromere constriction; and (c) thin, elongated, uncoiled chromosomes.

Ineffective haemopoiesis

The increased cellularity of the marrow with degenerate forms, and the low reticulocyte count for the degree of anaemia, suggest that many developing cells are dying in the marrow. Red cell survival is moderately shortened, and radio-iron studies show rapid clearance, with increased plasma iron turnover but poor red cell iron utilization. Further evidence for ineffective erythropoiesis are the increased stercobilin excretion in relation to the circulating haemoglobin mass, the marked increase in the early labelled peak of bilirubin excretion after (^{15}N) glycine administration, and high serum LDH levels. The ineffectiveness of leucopoiesis is suggested by raised serum lysosyme despite leucopenia.

Differential diagnosis

Other causes of macrocytosis include a high reticulocytosis (e.g. haemolytic anaemia or regeneration of blood after haemorrhage), aplastic anaemia, red cell aplasia, liver disease, alcoholism, myxoedema, acquired sideroblastic anaemia and the myelodysplastic syndromes, myeloid leukaemias, cytotoxic drug therapy, chronic respiratory failure, myelomatosis, and other causes of a leuco-erythroblastic anaemia. In these cases, the macrocytes tend to be circular not oval, the typical changes in neutrophils are not seen and megaloblastic marrow changes are not present (except in some alcoholics with anaemia solely due to alcohol, and in some cases of myelodysplastic syndromes) unless B_{12} or folate deficiency is also present. Once a bone marrow biopsy has been performed, the principal differentiation is from *other causes of megaloblastosis*, particularly: (*a*) *erythroleukaemia* in which megaloblastic changes, if present, are usually bizarre with many dyserythropoietic and multinucleate cells, an increase in myeloblasts without giant metamyelocyte formation, and the periodic acid-Schiff reaction may be positive, whereas it is negative in B_{12} or folate deficiency; and (*b*) *acquired sideroblastic anaemia* and other myelodysplastic syndromes. Other causes of megaloblastic anaemia not due to B_{12} or folate deficiency are listed in Table 6.

Some patients with rapidly developing megaloblastic anaemia, particularly due to folate deficiency, may develop almost complete aplasia of the red cell series and the peripheral blood and bone marrow may resemble that of acute myeloid or promyelocytic leukaemia. The presence of a few typical megaloblasts and giant metamyelocytes should point to the correct diagnosis; a trial of B_{12} and folic acid therapy should be given if there is real doubt.

Diagnosis of vitamin B_{12} or folate deficiency

The peripheral blood and bone marrow appearances are identical in folate or B_{12} deficiency. Special tests are, therefore, needed to distinguish between the two deficiencies. The deoxyuridine suppression test has been described already (see above) and is used for reliable and rapid diagnosis in some laboratories.

B_{12} deficiency

This may be established as the cause of megaloblastic anaemia by carrying out a therapeutic trial. A good response to a physiological dose (1–2 µg) of B_{12} administered daily while maintaining a diet low in B_{12} and folate indicates B_{12} deficiency while a response to 100–200 µg folate indicates folate deficiency (Fig. 3). If the B_{12} is given orally, a response indicates dietary B_{12} deficiency. This trial can be carried out successfully only in patients with moderately severe megaloblastic anaemia uncomplicated by other causes for anaemia.

A more widely applicable test is the assay of the B_{12} content of serum, which can be done microbiologically (using *Euglena gracilis* or *Lactobacillus leichmannii*) or by one or other radioisotopic assay. The normal ranges have been reported to be different, being higher with the radioassays (e.g. 200–1200 ng/l) than microbiological assays (e.g. 160–900 ng/l). Subnormal levels are found with microbiological assays in all cases of megaloblastic anaemia due to B_{12} deficiency, being extremely low in B_{12} neuropathy. Using the radioassays, false normal serum B_{12} levels have been reported in some cases of B_{12} deficiency. These have been ascribed to the presence in serum of analogues of B_{12} which are not active for the microbiological assay organisms but compete with B_{12} for the binding proteins other than pure IF used in the assay. Results with radioassays with B_{12} analogues added to block

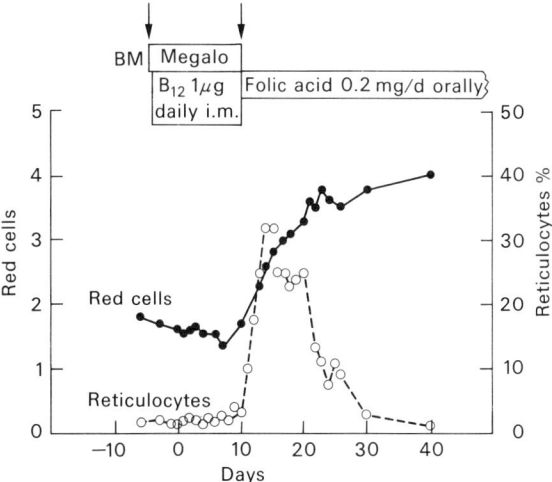

Fig. 3 Response to physiological doses of vitamin B_{12} and folic acid in a patient with megaloblastic anaemia due to folate deficiency. Red cell concentration units are $\times 10^{12}$/l. (Patient studied jointly with Professor D. L. Mollin.)

binding sites on the protein other than those for true B_{12} give results comparable to those of the microbiological assays. Subnormal serum B_{12} levels in the absence of tissue B_{12} deficiency have been reported in pregnancy, in patients with severe nutritional folate deficiency, in subjects taking large doses of vitamin C, and occasionally in iron deficiency. A false low result may also be found with the microbiological assays if the serum to be tested contains a drug, e.g. antibiotic or antimetabolite, which inhibits the growth of the assay organism.

Raised serum B_{12} levels, if not due to therapy or a contaminated serum, are most commonly caused by a raised B_{12} binding capacity due to a rise in TC I as in a leucocytosis due to a myeloproliferative disease, particularly chronic granulocytic leukaemia, myelosclerosis, polycythaemia rubra vera, and the hypereosinophilic syndrome. Raised levels of 'R' binder also occur in association with some tumours, especially hepatoma and fibrolamellar tumour of the liver. In benign leucocytosis, the rise is mainly in TC III and this is often not accompanied by a high serum B_{12} level. Raised levels of TC II occur in conditions where macrophages are stimulated, e.g. autoimmune diseases such as SLE, rheumatoid arthritis, in Gaûcher's disease and in some monocytic or monoblastic leukaemias, in histiocytic lymphomas and inflammatory bowel disease. In active liver diseases, serum B_{12} may be raised due to release of B_{12} from the liver with saturation of the serum B_{12} binders.

A third and less widely used test for B_{12} deficiency is the measurement of 24-hour urine excretion of methylmalonic acid after a loading dose of 10 g valine (normal 0–9 mg/24 hours). Excretion is raised in B_{12} deficiency but not in folate deficiency or any other acquired disorder so far tested. Rare cases of congenital methylmalonic aciduria have been described due to a variety of enzyme defects. The test is less sensitive than the serum B_{12} assay.

Folate deficiency

A therapeutic trial giving 50–200 µg folic acid daily can be carried out. Large doses of folic acid may produce a response in a B_{12}-deficient patient. Direct tests include the serum and red cell folate assay. In many laboratories, microbiological assay using *Lactobacillus casei* is still used but radioassays are also available. The serum folate is always low (less than 3.0 µg/l) in folate deficiency (and is normal or raised in B_{12} deficiency unless folate deficiency is also present). The serum folate assay does not accurately measure the severity of folate deficiency. Falsely low results are most frequently due to drug inhibition of the growth of *L. casei*. Raised levels occur after folate therapy and also in B_{12} deficiency and in the stagnant-loop syndrome. Red cell folate is a better guide than the serum folate to tissue folate stores but is also low (less than 160 μg/l) in a proportion of patients with megaloblastic anaemia solely due to B_{12} deficiency. The measurement of urinary Figlu excretion after an oral loading dose of L-histidine was used as a test for folate deficiency but is now obsolete.

Diagnosis of the cause of B_{12} deficiency

Although the clinical and family history and the clinical findings may point to pernicious anaemia or some other cause of B_{12} deficiency, it is important to establish this for certain. A brief dietary history will rapidly establish whether or not the patient is a vegan.

Radioactive B_{12} absorption tests are valuable to demonstrate malabsorption of B_{12} and to differentiate gastric from small intestinal lesions as the cause. The patient, after an overnight fast, is fed an oral radioactively labelled dose of cyanocobalamin, usually 1 μg, labelled with the cobalt-58 or cobalt-57 isotope. Absorption can be measured by whole body counting, liver uptake, faecal excretion, by 24-hour urinary excretion with a non-radioactive, parenteral flushing dose of 1 mg B_{12} (Schilling test), or by plasma radioactivity. Normal subjects absorb more than 30 per cent of the 1 μg dose. In patients with a gastric cause (e.g. pernicious anaemia or partial gastrectomy), malabsorption is corrected when the labelled B_{12} is given with a commercial preparation of IF, whereas if the lesion is small intestinal, the absorption does not improve with IF. Treatment with broad spectrum antibiotics may improve the absorption in the stagnant-loop syndrome. In some patients with pernicious anaemia, the absorption with IF only improves substantially after weeks of B_{12} therapy, possibly due to slow recovery of ileal function from the effects of B_{12} deficiency. A combined test 'Dicopac' has been devised in which B_{12} labelled with cobalt-57 is given simultaneously with (^{58}Co)-B_{12} attached to IF. This is particularly convenient for the urinary excretion test if urine collection is likely to be incomplete but because of isotope exchange it is not as accurate as two separately performed tests. A double isotope test has also been developed in which ^{58}Co-B_{12} is incorporated *in vitro* in egg yolk; ^{57}Co-B_{12} is given in crystalline form. It is aimed to give a more accurate guide to food B_{12} absorption. Some patients with atrophic gastritis or following partial gastrectomy and low serum B_{12} levels may show normal absorption of crystalline B_{12} but reduced absorption of food B_{12}. Patients with pernicious anaemia show malabsorption of both forms.

Gastric secretion studies, after pentagastrin stimulation reveal achlorhydria (resting pH 7.0 and not falling by more than 1.0 unit on stimulation) and grossly reduced or absent IF in gastric juice in pernicious anaemia.

A barium meal X-ray will show features of gastric atrophy (reduction of folds, long tubular shape) in between 70 and 100 per cent of cases and help to exclude gastric carcinoma. Follow-through examination of the small intestine will help to exclude a small intestinal lesion, e.g. duodenal or jejunal diverticulosis, which is particularly likely to become colonized with faecal bacteria in patients with achlorhydria. Endoscopy and gastric biopsy may be preferred.

The serum gastrin level is raised in most patients with gastric atrophy and the serum is tested for *antibodies to IF, parietal cells, and thyroid*, and *serum immunoglobulins* are measured in view of the association with hypogammaglobulinaemia.

Diagnosis of the cause of folate deficiency

An inadequate diet is usually at least partly implicated but an exact estimate of dietary intake from the clinical history is impossible because of variation in folate content of foods, losses in cooking, and size of portions. Often it is the general social circumstances that suggest a poor intake. Drug intake, particularly of barbiturates, is important. Many underlying inflammatory or malignant diseases may exaggerate the tendency to folate

deficiency in patients with inadequate diets. The main cause of malabsorption of folate in western communities is gluten-induced enteropathy and although tests of absorption of xylose, glucose, vitamins A and B_{12}, barium meal studies, and tests for reticulin antibody in serum may be done as screening procedures, in patients with severe folate deficiency, a jejunal biopsy is usually necessary. In certain tropical countries sprue may cause a generalized malabsorption syndrome in which folate deficiency commonly occurs. Tests of folate absorption have been devised, either by measuring the rise in serum folate after an oral dose of folic acid or of more natural folate derivatives, e.g. folate polyglutamates, or by measuring urinary or faecal excretion of radioactivity after feeding one or other labelled folate compound. None of these tests has achieved routine use.

Retrospective diagnosis of vitamin B_{12} or folate deficiency

It is not uncommon for haematology departments to be asked to make a retrospective diagnosis of the cause of vitamin B_{12} or folate deficiency in patients who have been treated 'blind' for megaloblastic anaemia or in whom low serum levels of folate or B_{12} have been found but the underlying cause of the deficiency has not been determined before treatment. If vitamin B_{12} deficiency is suspected an absorption test should be carried out without, and if appropriate, with intrinsic factor. If the results suggest true pernicious anaemia the patient should be given vitamin B_{12} for life. If not, efforts should be made to find other causes for vitamin B_{12} deficiency (see page 19.97 and the chapter on malabsorption in Section 12). Similarly, if folate deficiency is suspected or if it was not known which vitamin was deficient when treatment was started, it is important to exclude malabsorption provided that there are no other obvious causes of decreased folate intake or increased requirements.

Treatment of megaloblastic anaemia

Therapy is aimed at correcting the anaemia, completely replenishing the body of whichever vitamin is deficient, treatment of the underlying disorder, and prevention of relapse. In most cases, it is possible to diagnose which deficiency is present before starting therapy.

Vitamin B_{12} deficiency

Hydroxocobalamin 1000 μg intramuscularly given six times at several days' interval over the first few weeks will restore normal B_{12} stores. There is no evidence that patients with B_{12} neuropathy derive greater benefit from more frequent doses although many physicians use these for six months or so.

Response to therapy The patient feels better with increased appetite and well-being within 24–48 hours, and the mild fever, if not due to infection, falls to normal. A painful tongue and uncooperative disorientated state may also be improved in 48 hours. The reticulocyte count begins to rise on the second day and shows a peak after five to seven days of therapy, the height depending on the initial red cell count, being about 40–50 per cent at red cell counts of 1.0×10^{12}/l, 30–40 per cent at counts between 1.0 and 2.0×10^{12}/l, 10–20 per cent at counts between 2.0 and 3.0×10^{12}/l and up to 10 per cent at red cell counts of $3.0–4.0 \times 10^{12}$/l (Fig. 3). The red cell count rises to above 3.0×10^{12}/l by the third week while the white cell count becomes normal by the third to seventh day and the platelet count rises with the reticulocyte count and may reach levels of $500–1000 \times 10^9$/l before falling to normal at about 10–14 days. The bone marrow reverts to normoblastic by 36–48 hours, although giant metamyelocytes persist for 10–12 days. The serum iron falls within 24 hours, usually to subnormal levels, while the serum LDH falls more gradually during the first 14 days of therapy.

Maintenance Hydroxocobalamin 1000 μg intramuscularly are given once every three months for life in pernicious anaemia and most other causes of B_{12} deficiency, to prevent relapse. The life expectancy in pernicious anaemia, once treated, is as good as that in the general population in women, and slightly lower in men, probably due to the increased incidence of carcinoma of the stomach. In a few patients with B_{12} deficiency, the underlying cause can be reversed, e.g. expulsion of the fish tapeworm, improvement of a vegan diet, surgical correction of an intestinal stagnant-loop. A few micrograms of B_{12} can be absorbed each day in pernicious anaemia from oral doses of 1000 μg or more by passive diffusion, but this maintenance therapy is reserved for those who cannot have injections, e.g. with a bleeding disorder, or who refuse them, and for the extremely rare individual who is allergic to all injectable forms of B_{12}. Vegans may be maintained on much smaller oral doses of B_{12} each day, e.g. 50 μg as a tablet or syrup.

Prophylactic maintenance B_{12} therapy should be given from the time of operation after total gastrectomy, or after ileal resection if a B_{12} absorption test postoperatively reveals malabsorption of the vitamin. Patients with pernicious anaemia tend to develop iron deficiency anaemia and they may also develop thyroid disorders or carcinoma of the stomach. It is advisable that a regular blood count be performed once a year. Routine regular barium meal examination is not warranted but these diseases must be particularly borne in mind if relevant symptoms or signs develop.

Folate deficiency

This is corrected by giving 5 mg folic acid by mouth daily. It is usual to continue for at least four months, until there is a completely new set of red cells, although body stores will theoretically be normal within a few days of therapy. In patients with severe malabsorption of folate, larger oral doses of folic acid, e.g. 5 mg three times daily, may be used but it is not necessary to give parenteral folate except for those patients unable to swallow tablets. The response to therapy is as described after B_{12} therapy. The decision whether or not to continue folic acid beyond 4 months depends on whether or not the cause can be corrected. In practice, long-term folic acid is usually needed only in patients with severe haemolytic anaemias (e.g. sickle cell anaemia and thalassaemia major), myelosclerosis, and in gluten-induced enteropathy when a gluten-free diet is either unsuccessful or not feasible. In patients on a gluten-free diet, assessment of folate status is one simple way of following the improvement in absorption.

Prophylactic folic acid This should be given to all pregnant women (doses of 300–400 μg daily are used often combined with an iron preparation), to patients undergoing regular haemodialysis or peritoneal dialysis, and to premature infants weighing less than 1.5 kg at birth, and to selected patients in intensive care units or receiving parenteral nutrition.

Folinic acid (5-formyl THF) This, a reduced folate, is used to prevent or treat toxicity due to methotrexate or other dihydrofolate reductase inhibitors.

Folate therapy has been shown to improve chromosomal stability in the fragile X syndrome even though these patients do not have folate deficiency or a demonstrable defect of folate metabolism.

Severely ill patients

Some patients, usually elderly, are admitted to hospital severely ill with megaloblastic anaemia, perhaps in congestive heart failure, or with pneumonia. In this case, it is necessary to commence therapy immediately after obtaining blood for B_{12} and folate assay and performing bone marrow aspiration, before it is known which deficiency is present. Both vitamins should be given simultaneously in large doses. Heart failure and infection should be treated in conventional fashion but blood transfusion should be avoided except in cases of extreme anaemia when 1–2 units of packed cells may be given slowly, accompanied by removal of a similar volume of blood from the other arm, and diuretic therapy.

Other therapy

Hypokalaemia may occur during the response to therapy and oral potassium supplements should be given to those with initial heart failure or if severe hypokalaemia is demonstrated, but are not needed routinely. An attack of gout has been reported on the sixth to seventh day of therapy. Most patients develop hyperuricaemia at this stage but the clinical disease probably only occurs in those with a strong gouty tendency. Iron deficiency commonly develops in the first few weeks of therapy and this should be treated initially with oral ferrous sulphate in the usual way.

Megaloblastic anaemia due to inborn errors of folate or vitamin B_{12} metabolism

Folate

A number of babies have been described, mainly in Japan, with congenital deficiency of one or other enzyme concerned in folate metabolism, 5-methyltetrahydrofolate methyltransferase, methylene THF-reductase, Figlu transferase, methenyl-THF cyclohydrolase. Some of the babies had multiple congenital defects including the heart and cerebral ventricles and nearly all showed impaired mental development. In the methylfolate transferase deficiency, megaloblastic anaemia was present. Congenital dihydrofolate reductase deficiency has also been described but not definitely proven. Congenital specific malabsorption of folate is described on page 19.100.

Vitamin B_{12}

Congenital deficiency of transcobalamin II was first reported in 1971 in two siblings who developed megaloblastic anaemia requiring therapy with large daily doses of B_{12} at three and five weeks of age respectively. Similarly affected families have been described in which neuropathy developed in the absence of adequate therapy. One case has shown functionally inactive TC II in plasma. The serum B_{12} level is normal, B_{12} being bound to transcobalamin I. Absorption of B_{12} is impaired. Treatment is with massive doses of B_{12} (e.g. 1000 μg intramuscularly three times each week). In contrast, in subjects with low TC I levels, low serum vitamin B_{12} levels occur, but with normal haemopoiesis.

Children with one form of *congenital methylmalonic aciduria*, which responds to B_{12} therapy in large doses, have been shown to have a defect in conversion of hydroxocobalamin to ado-B_{12}. They do not show megaloblastic anaemia. In a few, this defect has been associated with a defect of formation of methyl-B_{12} and with homocystinuria but some of the children have also surprisingly not shown megaloblastic anaemia.

Megaloblastic anaemia due to acquired disturbances of folate or vitamin B_{12} metabolism

Folate

Therapy with dihydrofolate reductase inhibitors may cause megaloblastic anaemia. This is usual with methotrexate and less likely with pyrimethamine unless high doses are used or the patient is already folate deficient. Trimethoprim and triamterene are very weak folate antagonists in man, but may precipitate megaloblastic anaemia in patients already B_{12} or folate deficient (see page 19.101).

Vitamin B_{12}

Nitrous oxide (N_2O)

This anaesthetic gas oxidizes B_{12} from the active fully reduced cob (I) alamin form to the inactive cob (II) alamin and cob (III) alamin forms, inactivating methyl B_{12} and hence methionine synthetase. Megaloblastosis develops within several hours in humans and a fault in thymidylate synthetase can be demonstrated by the deoxyuridine suppression test in both human marrow and in the marrow cells of experimental animals exposed to N_2O. This recovers over several days when exposure to N_2O is discontinued. After many weeks exposure, monkeys develop a neuropathy resembling B_{12} neuropathy in humans, and peripheral neuropathies have also been described in humans (e.g. dentists and anaesthetists) repeatedly exposed to the gas. Methylmalonic aciduria has not been found in animals or humans exposed for short periods to N_2O.

Inactivation as cyano-B_{12}

The suggestion that B_{12} may be inactivated as cyano-B_{12} by smoking or ingestion of certain foods, and that this may be relevant to tobacco amblyopia or neuropathies in tropical areas, has not been substantiated.

Megaloblastic anaemia not due to folate or vitamin B_{12} deficiency or metabolic defect

Congenital

Disorders of DNA synthesis

Orotic aciduria This is a rare recessive disorder involving two consecutive enzymes (orotidylic pyrophosphorylase and orotidylic decarboxylase) in pyrimidine synthesis and presents with megaloblastic anaemia in the first few months of life. The diagnosis is made if needle-shaped, colourless crystals or orotic acid are found in the urine, daily excretion ranging from 0.5 to 1.5 g. Heterozygotes excrete slightly raised levels of orotic acid but show no haematological disorder. Treatment with uridine (1–1.5 g daily) leads to a haematological response, restoration of normal haemopoiesis and growth, and reduction in orotic acid excretion.

Lesch–Nyhan syndrome A few patients with this rare disorder of purine synthesis have shown megaloblastic change but whether this was due to associated folate deficiency or a direct result of reduced purine synthesis is not certain (see Section 9).

Vitamin E deficiency This has been reported to cause megaloblastosis in a group of children with kwashiorkor. However, many were also folate deficient.

Vitamin C deficiency Megaloblastosis appears to be due to associated folate deficiency.

Thiamine response Three cases have been well-documented but the biochemical explanation is not apparent.

Responding to large doses of vitamin B_{12} and folate A single case has been reported which needed both vitamins in large doses but the site of the defect was not elucidated.

Congenital dyserythropoietic anaemia Some cases of congenital dyserythropoietic anaemia show megaloblastic changes not due to B_{12} or folate deficiency (see page 19.133).

Acquired

Megaloblastic changes are often marked in erythroleukaemia and less commonly in other forms of acute myeloid leukaemia. They also occur in about 50 per cent of patients with primary acquired sideroblastic anaemia and in other myelodysplastic syndromes. The exact site of block in DNA synthesis in these syndromes is unknown but it is not at thymidylate synthetase.

Drugs which directly inhibit purine or pyrimidine synthesis (e.g. cytosine arabinoside, 5-fluorouracil, hydroxyurea, azauridine, or azaserine) may cause megaloblastic anaemia. Alcohol has also been found to have a direct effect on the bone marrow causing megaloblastosis in some cases even in the absence of B_{12} or folate deficiency. On the other hand, drugs which inhibit mitosis (e.g. colchicine or daunorubicin) or alkylate preformed DNA (e.g. cyclophosphamide, chlorambucil, or busulphan) do not cause megaloblastosis.

Other deficiency anaemias

Vitamin C

Anaemia is usual in scurvy but the pathogenesis is complicated. It is likely that vitamin C has a direct effect on erythropoiesis but folate and iron deficiencies, haemorrhage or haemolysis often complicate the picture.

Biochemical and nutritional aspects

Vitamin C is needed for collagen synthesis by its involvement in the hydroxylation of protein and for maintenance of intercellular substance of skin, cartilage, periosteum, and bone. It may also have a general role in oxidative–reduction systems, e.g. glutathione, cytochromes, pyridine, and flavin nucleotides. Although vitamin C is also thought to be needed for maintaining body folates in the reduced active state, the exact reactions involved are unclear. Vitamin C has a particular role in iron metabolism, iron excess causing increased utilization of vitamin C and in extreme cases clinical scurvy, whereas iron deficiency is associated with a raised leucocyte ascorbate concentration. Vitamin C is needed for incorporation of iron from transferrin into ferritin and for iron mobilization from ferritin. Vitamin C therapy increases iron excretion in patients receiving subcutaneous desferrioxamine infusions and also, at least in experimental animals, affects iron distribution by increasing parenchymal relative to reticuloendothelial iron. Minimum adult daily requirements for vitamin C are about 10 mg, but 30–70 mg is recommended; utilization and therefore requirement is relatively higher in infants, children, and pregnant and lactating women. Vitamin C may be excreted as such but is also broken down to oxalate.

Vitamin C is present in food as its reduced (ascorbic acid) and oxidized (dehydroascorbic acid) forms, the highest concentrations occurring in greens, fruits, tomatoes, liver and kidney. Potatoes are not a rich source but provide a substantial proportion of normal dietary intake. Cooking, particularly in alkaline conditions with large volumes of water, destroys the vitamin which is also lost on storage with exposure to the air. Absorption occurs through the length of the small intestine and deficiency is never solely due to malabsorption.

The anaemia of scurvy is typically normochromic, normocytic with a slightly raised reticulocyte count to 5–10 per cent and a normoblastic marrow with erythroid hyperplasia. This suggests a direct role for vitamin C in erythropoiesis but not all patients with clinical scurvy are anaemic. Extravascular haemolysis with mild jaundice and increased urinobilinogen excretion occurs in many of the patients. Moreover, in many the anaemia is complicated by folate deficiency (due to inadequate folate intake) with a megaloblastic marrow, or in a few by iron deficiency due to external haemorrhage, reduced diet intake, and possibly reduced iron absorption. In a few patients placed on a low folate diet, response of megaloblastic haemopoiesis to vitamin C alone has been described. In others, response of the megaloblastic anaemia to folic acid alone on a low vitamin C diet has occurred but in most such cases, both vitamin C and folic acid have been found necessary.

Vitamin B_6

This is involved as its coenzyme forms pyridoxal-5-phosphate in many reactions of the body especially for transaminases and decarboxylases. It is also a cofactor in the important rate-limiting reaction in haem synthesis, delta-aminolaevulinic acid (ALA)-synthetase (see page 19.120). It occurs in natural tissues in three major forms, pyridoxine, pyridoxamine, and pyridoxal phosphate. Red cells are capable of interconverting them. Anaemia due purely to vitamin B_6 deficiency has been produced in animals. It is hypochromic and microcytic with a raised serum iron and increased iron in erythroblasts with some partial or complete ring sideroblasts. A similar anaemia has occurred in humans with malabsorption, pregnancy or haemolysis but has not been fully documented to respond to physiological doses of vitamin B_6

alone. Vitamin B_6-responsive anaemia is, however, well documented among patients with sideroblastic anaemia of all types (see page 19.130). Pyridoxine responses occur particularly in the inherited form (when it is assumed that a fault in one or other enzyme of haem synthesis, e.g. ALA-synthetase, increases the need for pyridoxal-phosphate as cofactor) and when sideroblastic anaemia occurs in patients receiving pyridoxine antagonists, e.g. antituberculous drugs (see page 19.132).

Riboflavin

On the basis of studies in experimental animals and humans fed a deficient diet together with a riboflavin antagonist, deficiency of this vitamin is known to cause a normochromic, normocytic anaemia associated with a low reticulocyte count and red cell aplasia in the marrow, sometimes with vacuolated normoblasts. The exact biochemical basis is undecided. Clinically, a similar anaemia may occur in pure form but is usually associated with the anaemia due to protein deficiency as in kwaskiorkor or marasmus. Other clinical features of riboflavin deficiency, e.g. dermatitis, angular cheilosis, and glossitis may be present.

Thiamine

Thiamine-responsive anaemia has been reported in three infants with megaloblastic anaemia, in two with associated ring sideroblasts. There was no evidence of thiamine deficiency and the biochemical basis remains unclear.

Nicotinic acid, pantothenic acid, and niacin

Deficiencies of these vitamins cause anaemia in experimental animals but anaemia purely due to one or other of these deficiencies has not been established to occur in humans.

Vitamin E

This vitamin is needed for preventing peroxidation of cell membranes. A haemolytic anaemia responding to vitamin E has been reported in premature infants. Less well documented is a macrocytic anaemia due to vitamin E deficiency in protein-calorie deficient infants and aggravation of anaemia in patients with thalassaemia major because of vitamin E deficiency.

Protein deficiency

Anaemia is usual in both 'pure' protein deficiency, kwashiorkor, and in protein-calorie malnutrition (marasmus). It has been reported in many parts of the world where malnutrition, especially in children and pregnant women, is common. The anaemia also occurs in patients with gastrointestinal disease and severe malabsorption. The anaemia is typically normochromic, normocytic, and of the order of 8.0–9.0 g/dl. The reticulocyte count is usually reduced and the marrow may show a selective reduction in erythropoiesis. Experimental studies in animals suggest that the anaemia is largely due to reduced serum erythropoietin levels consequent on a lack of stimulus for erythropoietin secretion. Lack of amino acids for synthesis of erythropoietin or globin is not the cause. In many patients, the anaemia is complicated by infection, folate or iron deficiency and possibly other vitamin deficiencies, e.g. riboflavin, vitamin E, and then it may be more severe and show additional morphological abnormalities in the blood and marrow.

References

Carmel, R. (1983). Clinical laboratory features of the diagnosis of megaloblastic anemia. In *Nutrition in hematology* (ed. J. Lindenbaum), pp. 1–31. Churchill Livingstone, New York.

Chanarin, I. (1979). *The megaloblastic anaemias*, 2nd edn. Blackwell Scientific Publications, Oxford.

——, Deacon, R., Lumb, M., Muir, M. and Perry, J. (1985). Cobalamin–folate interrelations: a critical review. *Blood* **66**, 479–488.

Cooper, B. A. (1976). Megaloblastic anaemia and disorders affecting utilisation of vitamin B_{12} and folate in childhood. *Clin. Haematol.* **5**, 631–659.

Das, K. C. and Herbert, V. (1976). Vitamin B_{12}-folate interrelations. *Clin. Haematol.* **5**, 697–725.

Hoffbrand, A. V. (ed.) (1976). Megaloblastic anaemia. *Clin. Haematol.* **5**, no. 3.

—— and Wickremasinghe, R. G. (1982). Megaloblastic anaemia. In *Recent advances in haematology*, Vol 3 (ed. A. V. Hoffbrand). pp. 25–44. Churchill Livingstone, Edinburgh.

Lavoie, A., Tripp, E. and Hoffbrand, A. V. (1974). The effect of vitamin B_{12} deficiency in methylfolate metabolism and pteroylpolyglutamate synthesis in human cells. *Clin. Sci. Molec. Med.* **47**, 617–630.

Metz, J. (1983). The deoxyuridine suppression test. *CRC Crit. Rev. Clin. Lab. Sci.* **20**, 205–241.

Perry, J., Chanarin, I., Deacon, R. and Lumb, M. (1983). Chronic cobalamin inactivation impairs folate polyglutamate synthesis in the rat. *J. Clin. Invest.* **71**, 1183–1190.

Reynolds, E. H. (1976). Neurological and psychiatric aspects of vitamin B_{12} and folate deficiency. *Clin. Haematol.* **5**, 661–696.

Scott, J. M. and Weir, D. G. (1980). Drug-induced megaloblastic change. *Clin. Haematol.* **9**, 587–606.

Shorvon, S. D., Carney, M. W. P., Chanarin, I., and Reynolds, E. H. (1980). The neuropsychiatry of megaloblastic anaemia. *Br. Med. J.* **281**, 1036.

Vitamin B_{12}

Amess, J. A. L., Burman, J. F., Nancekievill, D. G., and Mollin, D. L. (1978). Megaloblastic haemopoiesis in patients receiving nitrous oxide. *Lancet* **ii**, 339–342.

Babior, B. M. (ed.) (1975). *Cobalamin: biochemistry and pathophysiology*. Wiley, New York.

Chanarin, I. (1982). The effects of nitrous oxide on cobalamins, folates and on related events. *CRC Crit. Rev. Toxicol.* **10**, 179–213.

Crang, A. J. and Jacobson, W. (1980). The methylation *in vitro* of myelin basic protein by arginine methylase from mouse spinal cord. *Biochem. Soc. Trans.* **8**, 619–620.

Dinn, J. J., Weir, D. G., McCann, S., Reed, B. B., and Scott, J. S. (1980). Methyl group deficiency in nerve tissue: a hypothesis to explain the lesion of subacute combined degeneration. *Irish J. Med. Sci.* **149**, 1–4.

Doscherholmen, A., Silvis, S. and McHahon, J. (1983). Dual isotope Schilling test for measuring absorption of food bound and free vitamin B_{12} simultaneously. *Am. J. Clin. Pathol.* **80**, 490–495.

Fish, D. T. and Dawson, D. W. (1983). Comparison of methods used in commercial kits for the assay of serum vitamin B_{12}. *Clin. Lab. Haematol.* **5**, 271–277.

Hall, C. A. (ed.) (1983). The Cobalamins, *Methods in hematology*, Churchill Livingstone, Edinburgh.

——, Begley, J. A. and Green-Colign, P. D. (1984). The availability of therapeutic hydroxocobalamin to cls. *Blood* **63**, 335–341.

Hoffbrand, A. V. (1983). Pernicious aemia. *Scot. Med. J.* **28**, 218–227.

Kapadia, C. R. and Donaldson, R. (1985). Disorders of cobalamin (vitamin B_{12}) absorption and transp Ann. Rev. Med. 93–110.

Kondo, H., Kolhouse, J. F., and Allen, R. H. (1980). Presence of cobalamin analogues in animal tissues Proc. Nat. Acad. Sci. **77**, 817–821.

Kuovonen, I, and Gräsbeck, R. (1981 opology of the hog intrinsic factor receptor in the intestine. *J. Biol. em.* **256**, (1), 154–158.

Marcoullis, G. and Nicholas, J. P. (1 . Interactions of cobalamins in the gastrointestinal tract. In *Progres gastroenterology*, vol 4 (eds G. B. J. Glass and P. Sherlock), pp. 172. Grune and Stratton, New York.

Matthews, D. M. and Linnell, J. C. 2). Cobalamin deficiency and related disorders in infancy and child. *Eur. J. Paediatr.* **138**, 6–16.

Mollin, D. L. Anderson, B. B., and En, S. F. (1976). The serum vitamin B_{12} level: its assay and signific Clin. Haematol. **5**, 521–546.

Scott, J. M. and Weir, D. G. (1981 methyl folate trap. *Lancet* **ii**, 337–340.

Smith, E. L. (1975). *Vitamin B_{12}*, 3rd ethuen, London.

Stenman, U.-H. (1976). Intrinsic fact the vitamin B_{12}-binding proteins. *Clin. Haematol.* **5**, 473–495.

Sweeney, B., Bingham, R. M., Amos Petty, A. C. and Cole P. V. (1985). Toxicity of bone marrow lts exposed to nitrous oxide. *Br. Med. J.* **291**, 567–569.

Taylor, K. B. (1976). Immune aspect icious anaemia and atrophic gastritis. *Clin. Haematol.* **5**, 497–51

Van der Westhuyzen, J., Fernandez-(and Metz, J. (1982). Cobalamin inactivation by nitrous ox duces severe physiological impairment in fruit bats: protection by methionine and aggravation by folates. *Life Sci.* **31**, 2001–2010.

Zagalak, B. and Friedrich, W. (eds) (1979). *Vitamin B₁₂*. Walter de Gruyter, Berlin and New York.

Zittoun, J., Farcet, J. P., Marquet, J., Sultan, C. and Zittoun, R. (1984). Cobalamin (vitamin B₁₂) and B₁₂ binding proteins in hypereosinophilic syndromes and secondary eosinophilia. *Blood* **63**, 779–783.

Folate

Botez, M. I. and Reynolds, E. H. (eds) (1979). Folic acid. In *Neurology, psychiatry, and internal medicine*. Raven Press, New York.

Colman, N. and Herbert, V. (1980). Folate binding proteins. *Ann. Rev. Med.* **31**, 433–439.

Cooper, B. A. (1984). Folate: its metabolism and utilization. *Clin. Biochem.* **17**, 95–98.

Halsted, C. H. (1980). Intestinal absorption and malabsorption of folates. *Ann. Rev. Med.* **31**, 79–87.

Hoffbrand, A. V. (1974). Anaemia in adult coeliac disease. *Clin. Gastroenterol.* **3**, 71–89.

Steinberg, S., Campbell, C. and Hillman, R. S. (1979). Kinetics of the normal folate enterohepatic cycle. *J. Clin. Invest.* **64**, 83–88.

Miscellaneous

Adams, E. B. (1970). Anemia associated with protein deficiency. *Semin. Hematol.* **7**, 55–66.

Cox, E. V. (1968). The anaemia of scurvy. *Vit. Horm.* **26**, 635–652.

Herbert, V. (ed.) (1980). Hematologic complications of alcoholism. *Semin. Hematol* **17**, 83–84.

Hillman, R. S. and Steinberg, S. E. (1982). The effects of alcohol on folate metabolism *Ann. Rev. Med.* **33**, 345–354.

O'Sullivan, W. J. (1973). Review: orotic acid. *Aust. NZ J. Med.* **3**, 417–422.

Disorders of the synthesis or function of haemoglobin

D. J. WEATHERALL

Disorders of the synthesis or structure of haemoglobin may be either inherited or acquired. The inherited disorders of haemoglobin are the commonest single gene disorders in the world population. Recent figures compiled by the World Health Organization suggest that there are hundreds of millions of carriers, and that each year 200 000–300 000 severely affected homozygotes or compound heterozygotes are born (see page 19.72). In many of the developing countries, where there is still a very high mortality from infection and malnutrition the first year of life, these conditions are not yet recognized an important public health problem. However, once economic conditions improve and infant death rates fall, the genetic disorders of haemoglobin start to place a major burden on the health services. This phenomenon has already been observed in parts of the Mediterranean region and Southeast Asia.

As a result of mass migrations of populations from high incidence areas of the haemoglobin disorders these conditions are being seen with increasing frequency in parts of the world where they have not been recognized previously. Because some of them, particularly sickle cell and and the more severe forms of thalassaemia, can produce threatening medical emergencies it is important for clinicians have at least a working knowledge of their clinical features, management, and prevention.

The other reason why haemoglobin disorders have become of particular interest in recent years is that they were the first group of diseases to be studied by the new methods of recombinant DNA technology. Is known about their molecular pathology than any other disorders and it is likely that their study has already given good idea of the overall repertoire of mutations that underlie inherited diseases.

Before describing haemoglobin disorders it is necessary to discuss briefly the structure and synthesis of haemoglobin and the way that it is genetically determined. Readers who are not familiar

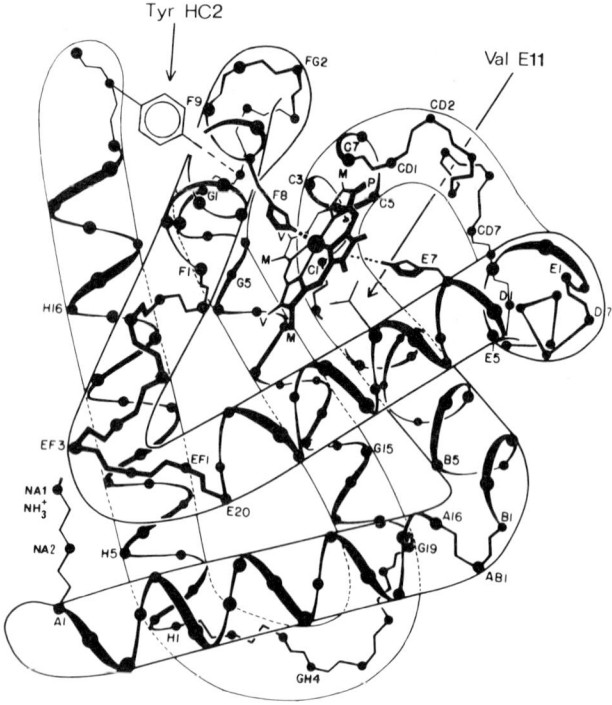

Fig. 1 The α chain subunit of human haemoglobin showing the position of the haem molecule in a cleft formed by the globin chain. The helical parts of the chain are given letters of the alphabet and each amino acid residue in each helical region has a specific number, e.g. val E11 is the eleventh amino acid in the E helical region. The non-helical regions of the amino and carboxyl terminal ends of the chains are labelled NA and HC respectively. (Reproduced by permission of Dr. M. F. Perutz and the Editors of the Cold Spring Harbor Symposia for Quantitative Biology.).

with the basics of DNA structure and the mechanisms of inheritance should consult Section 4 before tackling this brief account of haemoglobin genetics.

The structure, genetic control, and synthesis of haemoglobin

Structure

Human haemoglobin is heterogeneous at all stages of development; different haemoglobins are synthesized in the embryo, fetus, and adult, each adapted to the particular oxygen requirements of these changing environments.

The human haemoglobins all have a tetrameric structure made up of two different pairs of globin chains, each attached to one haem molecule (Fig 1). The reasons for this complex structure were considered earlier in this section (page 19.65). Adult and fetal haemoglobins have α chains combined with β chains (Hb A, $\alpha_2\beta_2$), δ chains (Hb A₂, $\alpha_2\delta_2$) or γ chains (Hb F, $\alpha_2\gamma_2$). In embryos, α-like chains called ζ chains combine with γ chains to produce Hb Portland ($\zeta_2\gamma_2$), or with ε chains to make Hb Gower 1 ($\zeta_2\varepsilon_2$), and α and ε chains combine to form Hb Gower 2 ($\alpha_2\varepsilon_2$). Fetal haemoglobin is itself heterogeneous; there are two kinds of γ chains which differ in their amino acid composition at position 136 where they have either a glycine or an alanine residue; those with glycine are called $^G\gamma$ chains, those with alanine $^A\gamma$. The $^G\gamma$ and $^A\gamma$ chains are the product of separate ($^G\gamma$ and $^A\gamma$) loci.

Genetic control

We now have a detailed picture of the arrangement and structure of the human globin genes. Initially this information came from studies of families with haemoglobin variants but more recently the individual genes have been cloned and their nucleotide

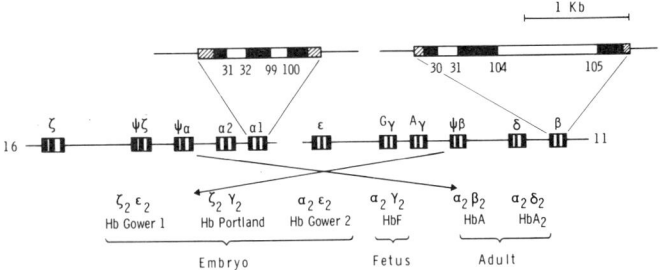

Fig. 2 The genetic control of human haemoglobin. Two of the genes are enlarged to show the introns (unshaded) and exons (dark staining). Kb = 1000 nucleotide bases.

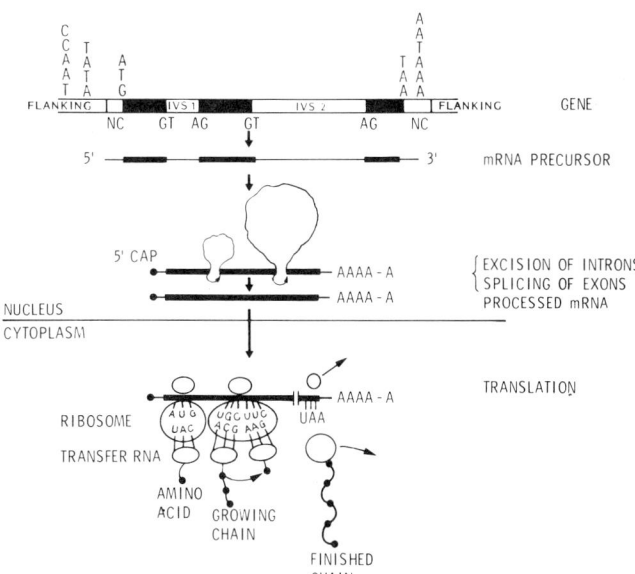

Fig. 3 Gene structure, messenger RNA processing, and protein synthesis. Each of the structures and steps illustrated are described in detail in the text.

sequence and that of their flanking regions has been determined. The arrangement of the two main families of globin genes is illustrated in Fig. 2. The β-like globin genes form a linked cluster on chromosome 11, which is spread over approximately 60 kb (kb = kilobase or one thousand nucleotide bases); they are arranged in the order $5'-\varepsilon-^{G}\gamma-^{A}\gamma-\psi\beta-\delta-\beta-3'$. The α-like globin genes also form a linked cluster, in this case on chromosome 16, in the order $5'-\zeta-\psi\zeta-\psi\alpha-\alpha2-\alpha1-3'$. The ψβ, ψζ, and ψα genes are pseudogenes, that is, they have sequences which resemble the β, ζ or α genes but contain mutations which prevent them from functioning as structural genes. They may be 'burnt out' remnants of genes which were functional at an earlier stage of evolution.

Some of the important structural aspects of the globin genes and their flanking sequences are illustrated in Figs 2 and 3. Like most mammalian genes they have one or more non-coding inserts called intervening sequences (IVS) or introns at the same position along their length. The non-α globin genes contain two introns of 122 to 130 and 850 to 900 base pairs between codons 30 and 31 and 104 and 105, respectively. Similar though smaller introns are found in the α and ζ globin genes. At the 5' non-coding (flanking) regions of the globin genes there are two blocks of nucleotide homology which are found in analogous positions in many species. The first is AG-rich and is called the Hogness box. The second, called the CCAAT box, is found about 70 base pairs upstream (to the left) from the 5' end of the genes. These sequences are involved in the initiation of transcription and hence play an important role in the regulation of the structural genes. As we shall see later, mutations in these regions can reduce the output of the related genes. At the 3' non-coding regions of all the globin genes there is a sequence AATAAA (Fig. 3) which is believed to be the signal for polyA addition to RNA transcripts; we shall discuss the significance of this when we consider the disorders of globin chain synthesis.

Synthesis

The synthesis of a globin chain follows the same pattern as any protein (Fig. 3). There is a flow of information from the DNA of the structural gene through an intermediary, a form of RNA called messenger RNA, to the cell cytoplasm where protein chains are assembled on a messenger RNA template which is a mirror image of the gene from which it was transcribed. When a globin gene is to be transcribed a messenger RNA molecule is synthesized from one of its strands by the action of an enzyme called RNA polymerase. The primary transcript of the globin genes is a large messenger RNA precursor molecule which contains both introns and coding regions (exons). While in the nucleus this molecule undergoes a number of modifications (Fig. 3). First, the introns are removed and the exons are spliced together. It should be noted that the exon/intron junctions always have the sequence GT at their 5' end, and AG at their 3' end. This appears to be essential for accurate splicing and, as we shall see later, if there is a mutation in these sites normal splicing cannot occur. The messenger RNAs are modified at their 5' end by the addition of a CAP structure, and at their 3' end by the addition of a string of adenylic

acid residues (polyA). The processed messenger RNA now moves into the cytoplasm to act as a template for globin chain production.

Since amino acids cannot interact directly with messenger RNA they are transported to the template on specific carrier molecules called transfer RNAs; there are specific transfer RNAs for each amino acid. The order of amino acids in a globin chain is determined by a triplet code, i.e. three bases (codons) code for a particular amino acid. The transfer RNAs also contain three bases, called anti-codons, which are complementary to messenger RNA codons for particular amino acids. The transfer RNAs carry the amino acids to the messenger RNA template where they find the right position by codon/anticodon base pairing. When the first transfer RNA is in position a second transfer RNA moves in alongside and the two amino acids which they carry form a peptide bond between them; the globin chain is now two amino acid residues long. Further transfer RNAs move in to appropriate positions and the growing globin chain is transferred to each in turn, gradually increasing in length as the messenger RNA is translated from the 5' to the 3' end (left to right). The transfer RNAs are held in appropriate steric conformation with the messenger RNA by the two subunits which make up the ribosomes. There are specific initiation (AUG) and termination (UAA, UAG, UGA) codons. When the ribosomes reach the termination codon translation ceases, the completed globin chain is released, and the ribosomal subunits fall apart and are recycled. Individual globin chains combine with haem, which is synthesized through a separate pathway (see page 19.131), and with themselves to form definitive haemoglobin molecules. Very little is known about the way in which the globin genes are regulated or switched on and off during development. Control seems to be mediated mainly at the transcriptional level with some fine tuning during translation.

Classification of the disorders of haemoglobin

The main groups of disorders of haemoglobin are shown in Table 1. The genetic disorders are divided into those in which there is a reduced rate of production of one or more of the globin chain, the thalassaemias, and those in which there is a structural change in a globin chain leading to instability or abnormal oxygen transport. In addition, there is a harmless group of mutations which interfere with the normal switching of fetal to adult haemoglobin production; these conditions are known collectively as hereditary persist-

Table 1 Disorders ot haemoglobin

Genetic
  Thalassaemia
  Structural variants
  Hereditary persistence of fetal haemoglobin
Acquired
  Methaemoglobin
  Carbonmonoxyhaemoglobin
  Sulphhaemoglobin
  Defective synthesis
    Haemoglobin H/leukaemia
    Haemoglobin H/mental retardation
    Reactivation of fetal haemoglobin production

Table 2 The thalassaemias

α thalassaemia
  α^o
  α^+
β thalassaemia
  β^o
  β^+
$\delta\beta$ thalassaemia
  $(\delta\beta)^o$
Haemoglobin Lepore
$(\gamma\delta\beta)^o$ thalassaemia
δ thalassaemia

ence of fetal haemoglobin. Although of no clinical significance, they are important models for studying the regulation of gene switching during development. The acquired disorders of haemoglobin can also be subdivided into those characterized by defective synthesis of the globin chain and those in which the structure of the haem molecules is altered, leading to inefficient oxygen transport.

Like all biological classifications this way of splitting up the haemoglobin disorders is not entirely satisfactory. For example, some structural variants are synthesized in reduced amounts and hence produce the clinical picture of thalassaemia.

The thalassaemias

Historical introduction

The thalassaemias are the commonest of the inherited haematological disorders and, indeed, are probably the commonest single gene disorders in the world population. The condition was first recognized in 1925 by a Detroit paediatrician called Thomas B. Cooley who described a series of infants who became profoundly anaemic and developed splenomegaly over the first year of life. Subsequently, further cases were identified and the disorder was variously called von Jaksch's anaemia, splenic anaemia, erythroblastosis, Mediterranean anaemia, or Cooley's anaemia. However, in 1936 George Whipple and Lesley Bradford, in describing the pathological changes of the condition for the first time, recognized that many of their patients came from the Mediterranean region and hence they invented the word 'thalassaemia' from the Greek $\theta\alpha\lambda\alpha\sigma\sigma\alpha$, meaning 'the sea'. Although more recently it has been realized that the disorder occurs throughout the world and is not localized to the Mediterranean region, the name has stuck.

During the last ten years it has become clear that thalassaemia is extremely heterogeneous and that its clinical picture can result from the interaction of many different genetic defects. The short account which follows concentrates mainly on the clinical and haematological aspects; readers who wish to learn more about the molecular pathology and population genetics of thalassaemia are referred to several reviews and monographs which cover the field more extensively and which are cited at the end of this section.

Definition and classification

The thalassaemias are a heterogeneous group of genetic disorders of haemoglobin synthesis, all of which result from a reduced rate of production of one or more of the globin chain(s) of haemoglobin. They are divided into the α, β, $\delta\beta$ or $\gamma\delta\beta$ thalassaemias according to which globin chain(s) is produced in reduced amounts (Table 2). In some thalassaemias no globin chain is synthesized at all, and hence they are called α^o or β^o thalassaemias, whereas in others some globin chain is produced but at a reduced rate; the latter conditions are called α^+ or β^+ thalassaemias. The $\delta\beta$ and $\gamma\delta\beta$ thalassaemias are always characterized by an absence

of chain synthesis; thus they are $(\delta\beta)^o$ and $(\gamma\delta\beta)^o$ thalassaemias. Because thalassaemia occurs in populations in which structural haemoglobin variants are common, it is not at all unusual for an individual to receive a thalassaemia gene from one parent and a gene for a structural haemoglobin variant from the other. Furthermore, both α and β thalassaemia occur commonly in some countries and hence individuals may receive genes for both types. These different interactions produce an extremely complex and clinically diverse series of genetic disorders which range in severity from death in utero to extremely mild, symptomless hypochromic anaemias.

The thalassaemias are inherited in a simple Mendelian codominant fashion. Heterozygotes are usually symptomless, although they can be easily recognized by simple haematological analysis. More severely affected patients are either homozygotes for α or β thalassaemia, compound heterozygotes for different molecular forms of α or β thalassaemia, or compound heterozygotes for one or other form of thalassaemia and a gene for a structural haemoglobin variant. Clinically, the thalassaemias are classified according to their severity into major, intermediate, and minor forms. *Thalassaemia major* is a severe transfusion dependent disorder. *Thalassaemia intermedia* is characterized by anaemia and splenomegaly though not of such severity as to require regular transfusion. *Thalassaemia minor* is the symptomless carrier state. While these descriptive terms do not have a precise genetic meaning, they remain useful in clinical practice.

THE β THALASSAEMIAS

The β thalassaemias are the most important types of thalassaemia because they are so common and produce severe anaemia in their homozygous and compound heterozygous states (Table 3).

Distribution

The β thalassaemias occur widely in a broad belt ranging from the Mediterranean and parts of north and west Africa through the Middle East and Indian subcontinent to Southeast Asia (see Fig. 2, page 19.74). The high incidence zone stretches north through Yugoslavia and Romania and the southern parts of the USSR and includes the southern regions of the People's Republic of China. The disease is particularly common in Southeast Asia where it occurs in a line starting in southern China and stretching down through Thailand and the Malay peninsula through Indonesia to some of the Pacific island populations. In these populations, and in some of the Mediterranean island and mainland countries, carrier frequencies for the various forms of β thalassaemia range between 2 and 30 per cent. In many of these regions the β thalassaemias cause a major public health problem and a drain on medical resources; this will become even greater as the incidence of infant or early childhood death due to infection and malnutrition declines. It should be remembered that β thalassaemia is not entirely confined to these high incidence regions; it occurs sporadically in every racial group.

Table 3 The β, δβ and γδβ thalassaemias

Type of thalassaemia	Findings in homozygote	Findings in heterozygote
β°	Thalassaemia major*† Hbs F and A$_2$	Thalassaemia minor Raised Hb A$_2$
β$^+$	Thalassaemia major*† Hbs F, A and A$_2$	Thalassaemia minor Raised Hb A$_2$
δβ	Thalassaemia intermedia Hb F only	Thalassaemia minor Hb F 5–15 per cent. Hb A$_2$ normal
δβ (Lepore)	Thalassaemia major or intermedia. Hbs F and Lepore	Thalassaemia minor Hb Lepore 5–15 per cent. Hb A$_2$ normal
γδβ	Not viable	Neonatal haemolysis. Thalassaemia minor in adults, with normal Hbs F and A$_2$

* Occasionally have thalassemia intermedia phenotype.
† Many patients with thalassaemia are compound heterozygotes for different molecular forms of β° or β$^+$, or for β° and β$^+$ thalassaemia.

Molecular pathology

During the last few years β globin genes from many patients with β thalassaemia have been cloned, grown in bacteria, and sequenced, and the molecular lesions responsible for the defective synthesis of the β globin chains have been determined. It turns out that the disease is extremely heterogeneous and that about 40 different mutations can produce the clinical phenotype of β thalassaemia. Some of these lesions completely inactivate the β globin genes leading to the phenotype of β° thalassaemia; others cause a reduced output from the genes and hence the picture of β$^+$ thalassaemia.

The main classes of mutations that cause β thalassaemia are summarized in Table 4 and in Fig. 4. One variety, which is common in certain Indian populations, results from a deletion of about 600 bases at the 3′ end of the β globin gene. The remainder of the β thalassaemia mutations are single base changes or small deletions or insertions of one or two bases at various points in the genes. As shown in Fig. 4 they occur in both introns and exons, and also in the flanking regions. Some of the exon substitutions are *nonsense mutations*, i.e. a single base change in a codon produces a stop codon in the middle of the coding part of the messenger RNA (Fig. 5a). This causes premature termination of globin chain synthesis and hence leads to the production of a shortened and non-viable β globin chain. Other exon mutations result in *frame-shifts*; that is, one or more bases are lost or inserted and the 'reading frame' of the genetic code beyond the lesion is thrown out of phase (Fig. 5b). Several mutations have been described, either within introns or at intron/exon junctions, which interfere with the mechanism of *splicing* the exons together after the introns have been removed during the processing of the messenger RNA precursor. Single base substitutions at the intron/exon junctions prevent splicing altogether and result in the phenotype of β° thalassaemia. Some intron mutations produce alterative splicing sites so that both normal and abnormal messenger RNA species are produced (Fig. 6). An incorrectly spliced messenger RNA is non-functional because it contains intron sequences; in some cases a nonsense mutation or frame-shift is generated. Thus, the messenger RNA cannot act as a template for the synthesis of a normal globin chain.

Single base substitutions have also been found in the flanking regions of the β globin genes of patients with β thalassaemia. Two are in the ATA box and others are further upstream, about 80–90 bases from the initiation codon. It seems likely that these mutations are in the regulatory regions which are involved in the initiation of transcription of the β globin genes. To put it into a more familiar context, if we think of these regulatory regions as signal

Table 4 Main classes of β thalassaemia mutations

1 Deletions
2 Premature chain termination ('nonsense')
3 Frameshift
4 Defective RNA processing
    Splice junction or consensus regions
    Alternative splice sites in introns
    Cryptic splice sites in exons
    Poly A addition
5 Transcription

boxes controlling the rate of traffic down the β globin gene 'track' these mutations act like an inefficient signalman who moves trains (RNA polymerases) onto the track at a reduced rate. These mutations are all associated with the clinical phenotype of β$^+$ thalassaemia; some β chains are made but at a reduced rate. Because there are so many different β thalassaemia mutations it follows that many patients who are apparently homozygous for β thalassaemia are, in fact, compound heterozygotes for two different molecular lesions.

Pathophysiology

The basic molecular defect in the β thalassaemia results in absent or reduced β chain production. Alpha chain synthesis proceeds at a normal rate and hence there is imbalanced globin chain synthesis with the production of an excess of α chains (Fig. 7). In the absence of their partner chains the latter are unstable and precipitate in the red cell precursors, giving rise to large intracellular inclusions. These interfere with red cell maturation, and hence there is a variable degree of intramedullary destruction of red cell precursors, i.e. ineffective erythropoiesis. Those red cells which do mature and enter the circulation contain α chain inclusions which interfere with their passage through the microcirculation, particularly in the spleen. These cells are prematurely destroyed and thus the anaemia of β thalassaemia results from both ineffective erythropoiesis *and* a shortened red cell survival. The anaemia is a stimulus to increased erythropoietin production from the kidneys and this causes massive expansion of the bone marrow which may lead to serious deformities of the skull and long bones. Because the spleen is being constantly bombarded with abnormal red cells, it hypertrophies and the resulting splenomegaly and bone marrow expansion gives rise to a massive increase of the plasma volume which causes an exacerbation of an already severe degree of anaemia.

As mentioned previously, fetal haemoglobin production largely ceases after birth. However, some adult red cell precursors (F cells) retain the ability to produce a small number of γ chains. Because the latter can combine with excess α chains to form haemoglobin F, cells which make relatively more γ chains in the bone marrow of β thalassaemics are partly protected against the deleterious effect of α chain precipitation. Hence, red cell precursors which produce haemoglobin F are selected in the marrow and peripheral blood of these patients, and thus they have relatively large amounts of haemoglobin F in their red cells. Furthermore, because δ chain synthesis is unaffected, the disorder is characterized by a relative or absolute increase in haemoglobin A$_2$ ($\alpha_2\delta_2$) production. These interactions are summarized in Fig. 7.

It follows that if the anaemia is corrected with blood transfusion the erythropoietic drive is shut off, growth and development are normal, and bone deformities do not occur. On the other hand, each unit of blood contains 200 mg of iron; with regular transfusion there is a steady accumulation of iron in the liver, endocrine glands and myocardium. Thus, although well-transfused thalassaemic children grow and develop normally, they die of iron overload unless steps are taken to remove iron.

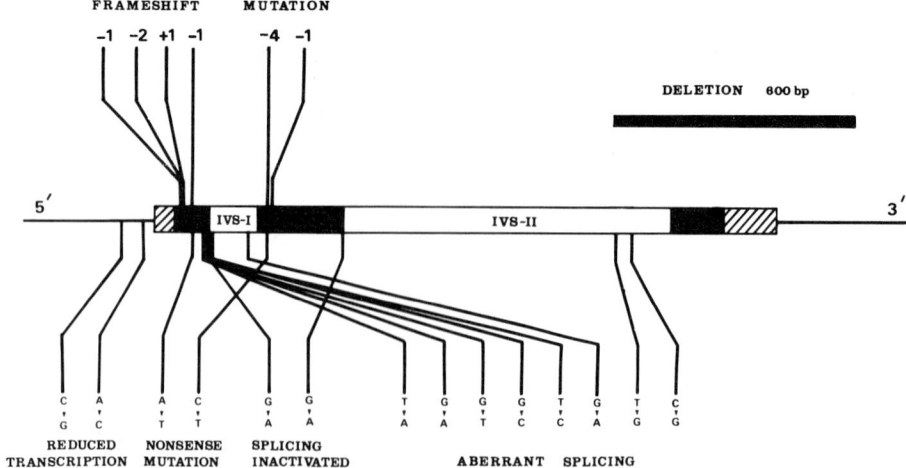

Fig. 4 A summary of some of the mutations which produce β thalassaemia. Each mutation is described in detail in the text.

NONSENSE MUTATION

HIS   LYS   TYR   HIS

- - - CAC AAG UAU CAC - - - - NORMAL

- - - HIS   LYS

      CAC AAG UAA - - - - - - MUTATION

                    STOP

(a)

FRAMESHIFT MUTATION

LYS   SER ILE THR LYS

- - - - AAG AGU AUC ACU AAG - - - - NORMAL

                    - 2 BASE DELETION

- - - - AAG AGU AUC --U AAG - - - - MUTATION

(b)   STOP

Fig. 5 Point mutations which cause β° thalassaemia. (a) Premature stop codon (nonsense mutation). (b) Frameshift mutation. See text for further details.

THE SEVERE HOMOZYGOUS OR COMPOUND HETEROZYGOUS FORMS OF β THALASSAEMIA

These are the commonest and most important forms of thalassaemia and give rise to a major public health problem in many parts of the world.

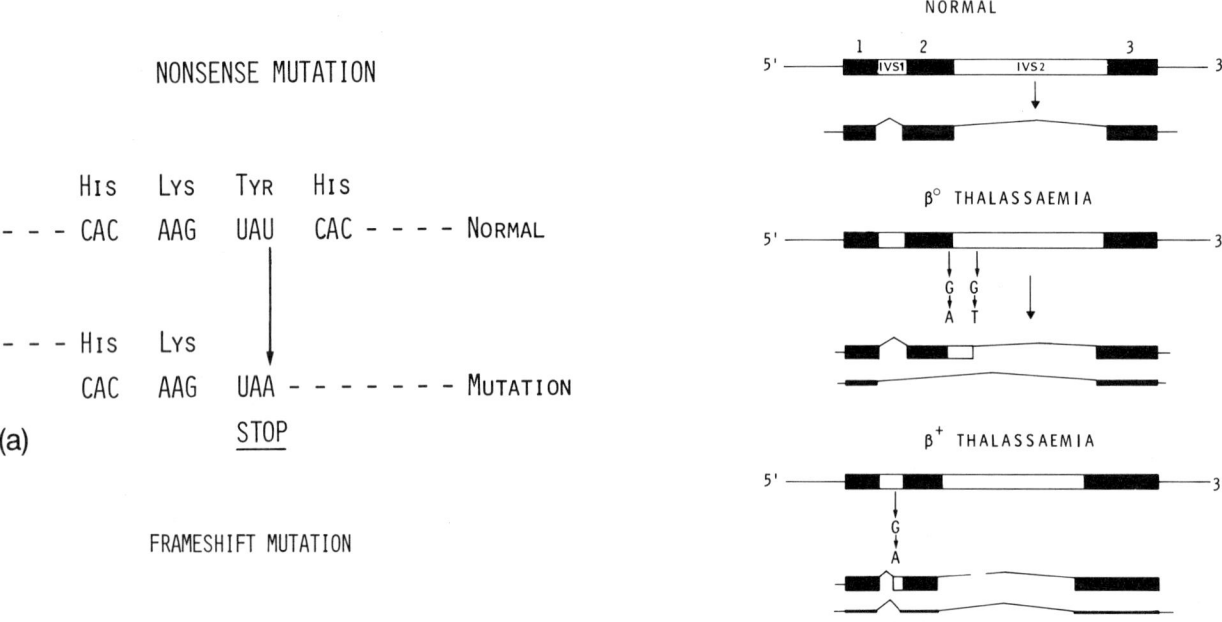

Fig. 6 A representation of the consequences of different splice site mutations. In the β° thalassaemia case there are two mutations, one which inactivates the normal splice site, and another which produces a new splice site. Two abnormal messenger RNA molecules are produced. In the β+ thalassaemia case a new splice site is produced in the first intron. Both normal and abnormal messenger RNAs are produced; the latter in greater amounts.

Clinical features

Most severe forms of β thalassaemia present within the first year of life with failure to thrive, poor feeding, intermittent bouts of fever, or failure to improve after an intercurrent infection. At this stage the affected infant looks pale, and in many cases splenomegaly is already present. There are no other specific clinical signs and the diagnosis depends on the haematological changes outlined below. If the infant is put on a regular blood transfusion regimen at this stage, early development is normal and further symptoms do not occur until puberty, when the effects of iron loading due to repeated blood transfusion start to appear. If, on the other hand, the affected infant is not adequately transfused, the typical clinical picture of homozygous β thalassaemia develops. Thus the clinical manifestations of the severe forms of β thalassaemia have to be described in two contexts, i.e. the well-transfused child, and the child with chronic anaemia throughout early life.

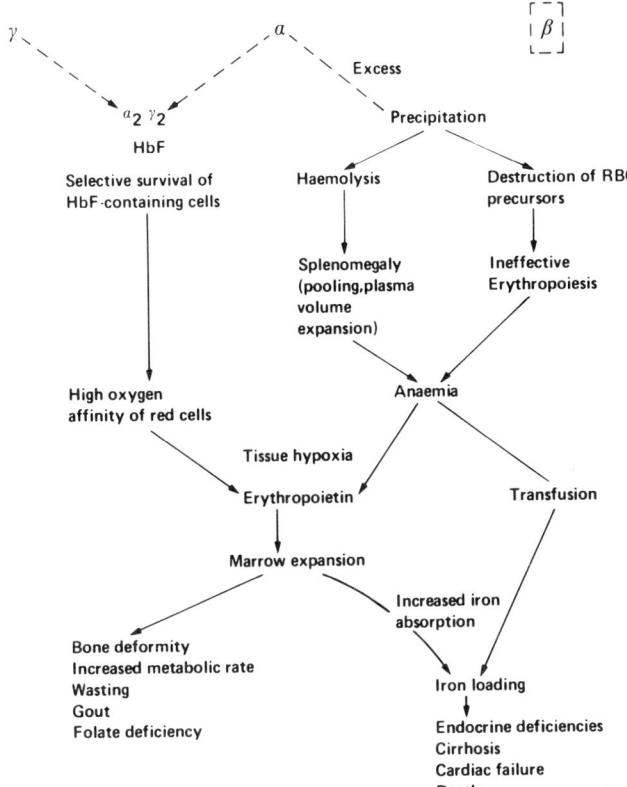

Fig. 7 The pathophysiology of β thalassaemia.

In the well-transfused thalassaemic child early growth and development is normal and splenomegaly is minimal. However, there is a gradual accumulation of iron and the effects of tissue siderosis start to appear by the end of the first decade. The normal adolescent growth spurt fails to occur and hepatic, endocrine, and cardiac complications of iron overloading produce a variety of problems including diabetes, hypoparathyroidism, adrenal insufficiency, and progressive liver failure. Secondary sexual development is delayed, or does not occur at all. The short stature and lack of sexual development may lead to serious psychological problems. By far the commonest cause of death, which usually occurs toward the end of the second or early in the third decade, is progressive cardiac damage. Ultimately these patients die either with protracted cardiac failure or suddenly due to an acute arrhythmia. The use of intensive chelation therapy may prevent or delay this distressing termination.

The clinical picture in children who are inadequately transfused is quite different. Early childhood is interspersed with a series of distressing complications and the overall rates of growth and development are markedly retarded. There is progressive splenomegaly, and hypersplenism may cause a worsening of the anaemia, sometimes associated with thrombocytopenia and a bleeding tendency. Because of the bone marrow expansion there may be hideous deformities of the skull with marked bossing and overgrowth of the zygomata giving rise to the classical mongoloid facies of β thalassaemia (Fig. 8a). These changes are reflected by striking radiological changes which include a lacy, trabecular pattern of the long bones and phalanges and a typical 'hair on end' appearance of the skull (Fig. 9). These bone changes may be associated with recurrent fractures. There is an increased proneness to infection which may cause a catastrophic drop in the haemoglobin level. Because of the massive marrow expansion resulting from the chronic anaemia, these chidren are hypermetabolic, run intermittent fevers, lose weight (Fig. 8b), have increased requirements for folic acid, and may become acutely folate depleted with worsening of their anaemia. Because of the

increased turnover of red cell precursors, hyperuricaemia and secondary gout occur occasionally. There is a bleeding tendency which, although partly due to thrombocytopenia secondary to hypersplenism, may also be exacerbated by liver damage associated with iron loading and extramedullary haemopoiesis. Because of the bone deformities of the skull, there may be distressing dental complications with poorly formed teeth and malocclusion, and inadequate drainage of the sinuses and middle ear may lead to chronic sinus infection and deafness. If these unfortunate children survive to puberty, they develop the same complications of iron loading as the well-transfused patients. In this case some of the iron accumulation results from an increased rate of gastrointestinal absorption as well as that derived from the inadequate transfusion regimen.

The prognosis for poorly transfused thalassaemic children is bad. If they receive no transfusions at all they die within the first two years, and if kept at a low haemoglobin level throughout early childhood, they usually succumb to an overwhelming infection. As already mentioned, if they reach puberty, they die of the effects of iron accumulation with acute or chronic cardiac failure of the same type as occurs in the well-transfused child.

Haematological changes

There is always a severe anaemia and the haemoglobin values on presentation range from 2 to 8 g/dl. Although the red cells are hypochromic and microcytic, the red cell indices, as derived from an electronic cell counter, may give surprisingly normal results, although usually the MCH and MCV are reduced. The appearance of the stained peripheral blood film is grossly abnormal (Fig. 10). The red cells show marked hypochromia and variation in shape and size. There are many hypochromic macrocytes and misshapen microcytes, some of which are mere fragments of cells. There is a moderate degree of anisochromia and basophilic stippling. There are always some nucleated red cells in the peripheral blood and, after splenectomy, these are found in large numbers. In the post-splenectomy film many of the nucleated cells and mature erythrocytes show ragged inclusions after incubation of the blood with methyl violet. There is usually a slight elevation in the reticulocyte count. The white cell and platelet counts are normal unless there is hypersplenism when they are reduced. The bone marrow shows marked erythroid hyperplasia with a myeloid/erythroid (M/E) ratio of unity or less. Many of the red cell precursors show ragged inclusions after incubation of the marrow with methyl violet.

There are biochemical changes of increased haemolysis and progressive iron loading. The bilirubin level is usually elevated and haptoglobins are absent. The ^{51}Cr red cell survival is shortened. The serum iron rises progressively and most transfusion-dependent children have a totally saturated iron binding capacity. This change is mirrored by a high plasma ferritin level, and liver biopsies show a marked increase in iron both in the reticulo-endothelial and parenchymal cells (Fig. 11).

Other biochemical changes

Many thalassaemic children are vitamin E and ascorbate depleted. Folic acid deficiency has already been mentioned. Frank diabetes may develop and endocrine function tests may reveal parathyroid or adrenal insufficiency, or inappropriate response by the pituitary to various release hormones; growth hormone levels are usually normal.

Haemoglobin changes (Table 3)

The haemoglobin F level is always elevated. In β° thalassaemia there is no haemoglobin A and the haemoglobin consists of F and A_2 only. In β^+ thalassaemia the level of haemoglobin F ranges from 30 to 90 per cent of the total haemoglobin. The haemoglobin A_2 level is usually normal and is of no diagnostic value.

Heterozygous β thalassaemia

Carriers for β thalassaemia are usually symptom free except in periods of stress such as pregnancy when they may become significantly anaemic. Splenomegaly is rarely present.

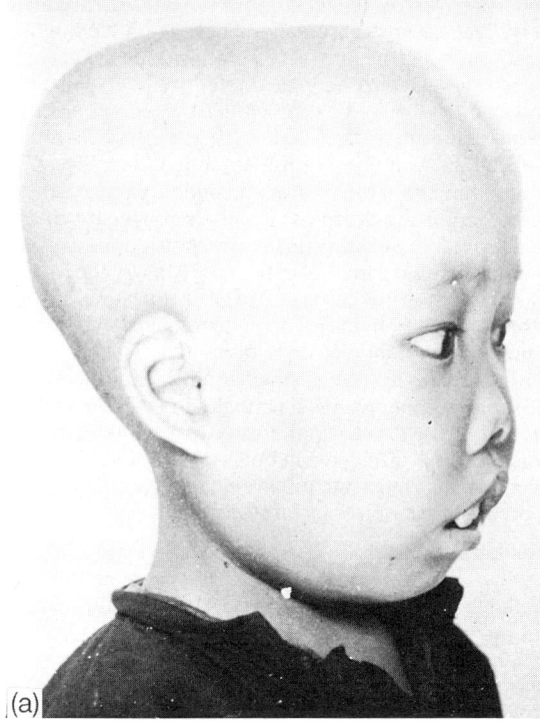

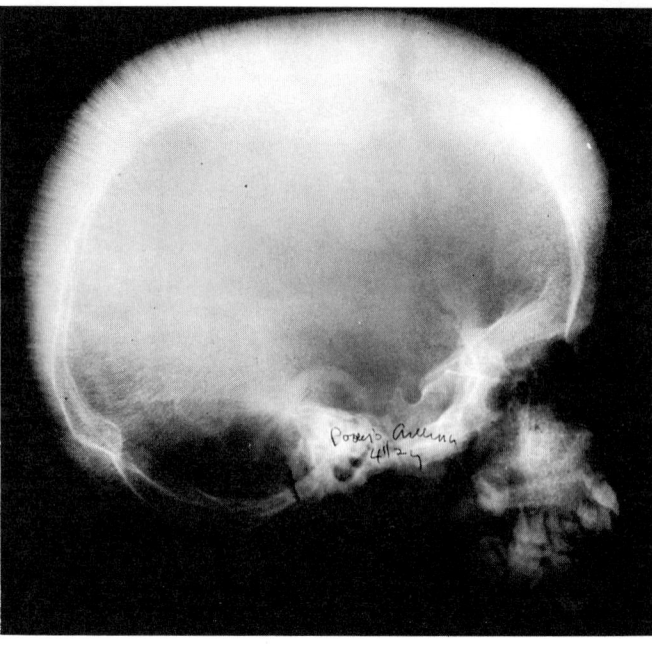

Fig. 9 Radiological changes of the skull in homozygous β thalassaemia.

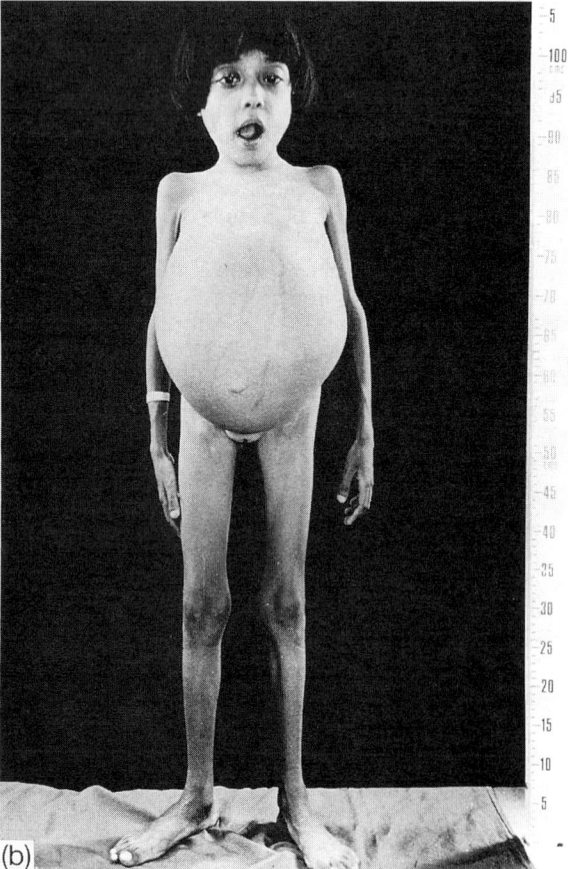

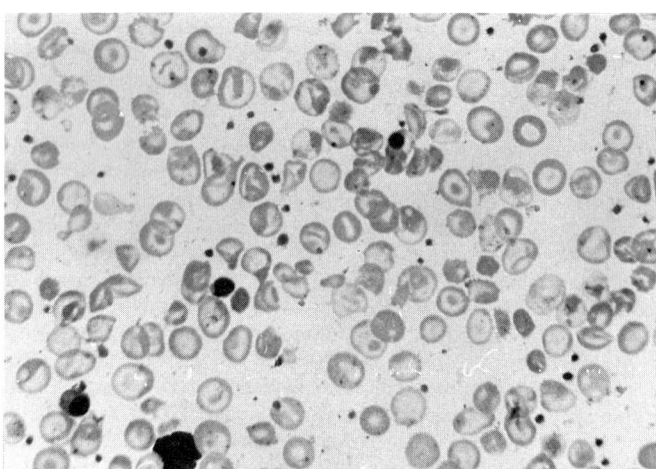

Fig. 10 Peripheral blood film in homozygous β ($\times$ 630, Leishman stain).

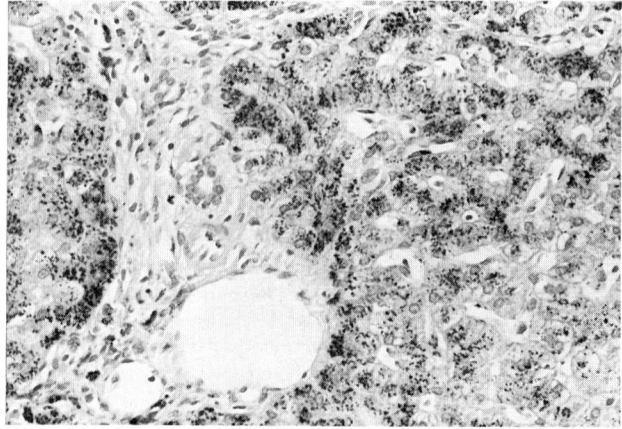

Fig. 8 Homozygous β thalassaemia. (a) Skull and facial deformity due to bone marrow expansion. (b) Gross wasting of the limbs and hepatomegaly in an undertransfused child.

Fig. 11 Histological appearances of the liver in homozygous β thalassaemia showing gross iron deposition ($\times$ 270, iron stain).

Haematological changes

There is a mild degree of anaemia with haemoglobin values in the 9–11 g/dl range. The red cells show hypochromia and microcytosis with characteristically low MCH and MCV values. The reticulocyte count is usually normal. The bone marrow shows moderate erythroid hyperplasia.

Haemoglobin changes

The characteristic finding is an elevated haemoglobin A_2 level in the 4–6 per cent range. There is a slight elevation of haemoglobin F in the 1–3 per cent range in about 50 per cent of cases. A less common form occurs in which the haemoglobin A_2 is not elevated.

β thalassaemia in association with haemoglobin variants

In many populations, because there is a high incidence of β thalassaemia and various haemoglobin variants, it is quite common for an individual to inherit a β thalassaemia gene from one parent and a gene for a structural haemoglobin variant from the other. Although numerous interactions of this type have been described, in clinical practice only three are of real importance, i.e. sickle cell β thalassaemia, haemoglobin C β thalassaemia, and haemoglobin E β thalassaemia.

Sickle cell β thalassaemia

The clinical manifestations which result from the interaction of the β thalassaemia and sickle cell genes vary considerably from race to race. In Negro populations there is an extremely mild form of β^+ thalassaemia which, when it interacts with the sickle cell gene, produces a condition characterized by mild anaemia and few sickling crises. This condition is compatible with normal survival and is often ascertained by chance haematological examination. On the other hand, in Mediterranean populations it is quite common for an individual to inherit a β° thalassaemia determinant from one parent and a sickle cell gene from the other. Sickle cell β° thalassaemia is often associated with a clinical picture which is indistinguishable from sickle cell anaemia (see page 19.122).

The diagnosis of sickle cell thalassaemia rests on the clinical features of a sickling disorder (see page 19.122) found in association with a peripheral blood picture with typical thalassaemic red cell changes, i.e. a low MCH and MCV. In the more severe forms of sickle cell β° thalassaemia there may be an elevated reticulocyte count, and sickled red cells are found on the peripheral blood film. The diagnosis can be confirmed by haemoglobin electrophoresis, which in sickle cell β^+ thalassaemia shows haemoglobin S together with 10–30 per cent haemoglobin A and an elevated haemoglobin A_2 value. In sickle cell β° thalassaemia the haemoglobin consists mainly of haemoglobin S with an elevated level of haemoglobins F and A_2. To be absolutely certain about the diagnosis it is necessary to examine the parents; one should have the sickle cell trait and the other the β thalassaemia trait.

Haemoglobin C thalassaemia

This disorder is restricted to West Africans and some North African and southern Mediterranean populations. It is characterized by a mild haemolytic anaemia associated with splenomegaly. The peripheral blood film shows numerous target cells and thalassaemic red cell changes with a moderately elevated reticulocyte count. Haemoglobin electrophoresis shows a preponderance of haemoglobin C. The diagnosis is confirmed by finding the haemoglobin C trait in one parent and the β thalassaemia trait in the other.

Haemoglobin E β thalassaemia

This is the commonest severe form of thalassaemia in Southeast Asia and throughout the Indian subcontinent. Recent work has shown that haemoglobin E is inefficiently synthesized, and hence, when a haemoglobin E gene is inherited together with a β° thalassaemia determinant, which is the commonest type of β thalassaemia in Southeast Asia, there is a marked deficiency of β chain

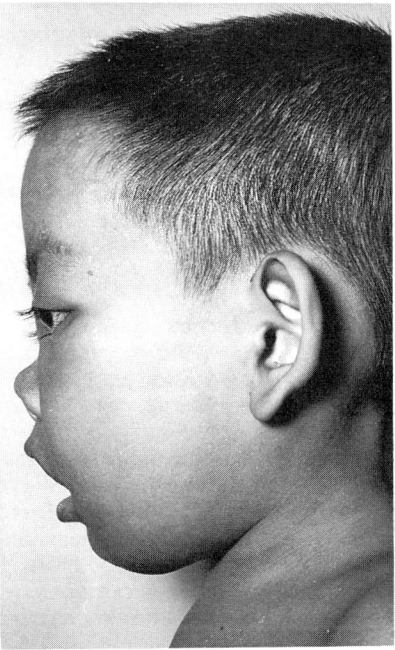

Fig. 12 Bossing of the skull in haemoglobin E thalassaemia.

production, and the resulting clinical picture can closely resemble homozygous β° thalassaemia.

The clinical and haematological changes in haemoglobin E thalassaemia are variable. There is usually a marked degree of anaemia and splenomegaly with typical thalassaemic bone changes (Fig. 12). Although not always transfusion dependent, patients with this disorder usually run low haemoglobin values in the 4–9 g/dl range with an average of 6–7 g/dl. The blood film shows typical thalassaemic red cell changes and the bone marrow shows marked erythroid hyperplasia with α chain inclusions in many of the red cell precursors.

Although very little is known about the natural history of this disorder, it seems likely that in many parts of Southeast Asia and India it causes a very high mortality in the early years of life. Complications include a marked proneness to infection, secondary hypersplenism, progressive iron loading leading to liver rather than cardiac damage, a variety of neurological lesions due to tumours caused by extramedullary erythropoiesis extending in from the inner tables of the skull or vertebrae, folate deficiency, and recurrent pathological fractures. On the other hand, some patients with haemoglobin E thalassaemia grow and develop normally with few complications and there are many recorded cases of pregnancy in women with this disorder.

The diagnosis of haemoglobin E thalassaemia is confirmed by finding only haemoglobins E and F on haemoglobin electrophoresis and by demonstrating the haemoglobin E trait in one parent and the β thalassaemia trait in the other.

THE $\delta\beta$ THALASSAEMIAS

(See Table 3.)

Molecular genetics and classification

Disorders due to reduced β and δ chain synthesis are much less common than those due to defective β chain production alone. Work carried out over the last few years has shown that these conditions are remarkably heterogeneous at the molecular level. In some cases they result from deletions of the β and δ globin genes, while in others there appears to have been mis-paired synapsis and unequal crossing over between the δ and β globin gene loci with the production of $\delta\beta$ fusion genes. The latter produce $\delta\beta$ fusion chains which combine with α chains to form haemoglobin variants called the *Lepore haemoglobins* (Lepore was the family name of the first patient to be recognized with this disorder). Hence it is usual to classify this group of conditions into the $\delta\beta$ *thalassaemias* and the *haemoglobin Lepore thalassaemias*.

Clinical and haematological changes

The $\delta\beta$ thalassaemias have been reported in many populations although there are no high frequency areas. In the homozygous state there is a mild degree of anaemia with haemoglobin values of 8–10 g/dl. There is often a moderate degree of splenomegaly but these patients are usually symptomless except during periods of stress such as infection or pregnancy. Haemoglobin analysis shows 100 per cent haemoglobin F. Heterozygous carriers for this condition have thalassaemic blood pictures, elevated levels of haemoglobin F of 5–20 per cent, and normal levels of haemoglobin A_2.

The homozygous state for haemoglobin Lepore is characterized by a clinical picture which is usually similar to that of homozygous β thalassaemia although in some cases it may be milder and non-transfusion dependent. The clinical and haematological findings are similar to those of β thalassaemia. The haemoglobin consists of F and Lepore only. Heterozygous carriers have thalassaemic blood pictures associated with about 5–15 per cent haemoglobin Lepore.

There is a group of genetic disorders of haemoglobin production encountered most commonly in Negro populations which are called collectively '*hereditary persistence of fetal haemoglobin*' (HPFH). Homozygotes have a mild thalassaemia-like blood picture but are not anaemic. They have 100 per cent haemoglobin F. Heterozygotes show no haematological abnormalities and carry 20–30 per cent haemoglobin F. These disorders are due to gene deletions involving the δ and β globin genes and therefore appear to be extremely mild forms of $\delta\beta$ thalassaemia in which the lack of δ and β chain production is almost entirely compensated by the synthesis of the γ chains of haemoglobin F.

THE $\gamma\delta\beta$ THALASSAEMIAS

There are several rare forms of thalassaemia which result from long deletions of the β globin gene cluster which, as well as removing the β genes, remove the δ, γ and, in some cases, embryonic ε genes. This means that there is no output of globin chains from this gene cluster at all. Clearly, the homozygous state for these disorders would not be compatible with survival. Heterozygotes have severe haemolytic disease of the newborn with anaemia and hyperbilirubinaemia. If they survive the neonatal period they grow and develop normally; in adult life they have the haematological picture of heterozygous β thalassaemia with mild anaemia, hypochromic microcytic red cells, and a haemoglobin pattern consisting of haemoglobin A, no elevation of haemoglobin F, and a normal level of haemoglobin A_2.

OTHER β THALASSAEMIA VARIANTS

It is not uncommon to encounter patients with the clinical features of heterozygous β thalassaemia who do not have an elevated haemoglobin A_2 level and yet who do not appear to have α thalassaemia. This condition occurs in some Mediterranean populations. It is important to recognize it because if it is inherited together with a typical β thalassaemia gene it can produce a severe transfusion dependent disorder. Hence this variant is important in antenatal screening programmes (see page 19.120). It can only be identified for certain by globin chain synthesis analysis in a specialized laboratory.

Families are encountered occasionally in which there is a more severe form of heterozygous β thalassaemia associated with anaemia, jaundice, and splenomegaly. In some of these families it is apparent that the affected individuals are in fact compound heterozygotes for β thalassaemia and the so-called 'silent' β thalassaemia gene, i.e. a determinant which cannot be identified haematologically in heterozygotes. In other families the severe form of β thalassaemia behaves as a single gene disorder with full expression in heterozygotes. In at least some of these families the disorder results from the synthesis of a highly unstable β globin chain variant.

THE α THALASSAEMIAS

Although the α thalassaemias are commoner than the β thalassaemias they pose less of a public health problem. This is because the severe homozygous forms cause death in utero or in the neonatal period and the milder forms do not produce major disability.

Distribution

(See Fig. 1, page 19.74.)

The α thalassaemias occur widely through the Mediterranean region, parts of West Africa, the Middle East, isolated parts of the Indian subcontinent, and throughout Southeast Asia in a line stretching from southern China through Thailand, the Malay peninsula, and Indonesia to the Pacific island populations. For reasons that will become apparent when we consider the molecular pathology of these disorders the serious forms of α thalassaemia are restricted to some of the Mediterranean island populations and Southeast Asia.

Definition and inheritance

The genetics of α thalassaemia is complicated, not least because the condition has collected such a confusing nomenclature over the years.

Because both haemoglobins A and F have α chains, genetic disorders of α chain synthesis result in defective fetal and adult haemoglobin production. In the fetus, deficiency of α chains leads to the production of excess γ chains which form γ_4 tetramers, or haemoglobin Bart's (Fig. 13). In adults, a deficiency of α chains leads to an excess of β chains which form β_4 tetramers, or haemoglobin H, which is the adult counterpart of haemoglobin Bart's. Thus, the presence of haemoglobins Bart's or H in red cells is the hallmark of α thalassaemia. If this was the whole story α thalassaemia would pose no problems. However, for reasons which are not yet clear a critical level of globin chain imbalance is required before detectable amounts of haemoglobin Bart's or H appear in the red cells. Unfortunately for clinicians, in persons heterozygous for different forms of α thalassaemia this level is not reached; significant amounts of these variants only occur in the red cells of patients who have inherited two or more α thalassaemia determinants and hence who have a severe degree of α chain deficiency. This means that the carrier states for different forms of α thalassaemia are difficult to diagnose.

The clinically important forms of α thalassaemia (Table 5) result from the interaction of two main classes of α thalassaemia determinants. It is still customary to define these conditions by the haematological changes in heterozygotes. First, there is a more severe form which produces a mild but recognizable hypochromic anaemia in heterozygotes. Because we now know that this condition results from a genetic lesion which causes a complete absence of α chain production from the affected chromosome, we call it α° *thalassaemia*. The second type is almost completely silent in carriers; their red cells are normal or only slightly hypochromic. We call this α^{+} *thalassaemia* because we know from molecular studies that the output of α chains from the affected chromosome is only partially reduced. To put it another way, the terms α° and α^{+} thalassaemia describe haplotypes – the products of *two* linked α chains on one of a pair of homologous chromosomes 16. Before we had all this information it was usual to call α° and α^{+} thalassaemia α *thalassaemia 1 and 2*, respectively.

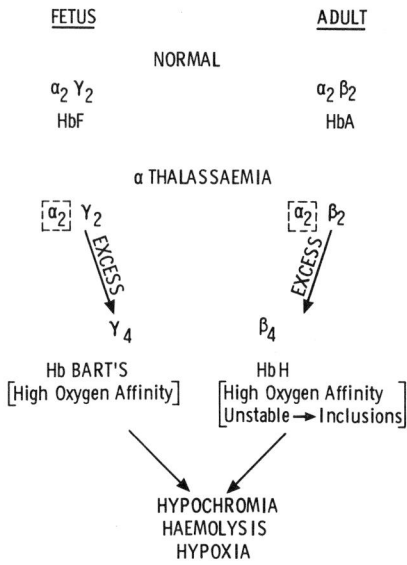

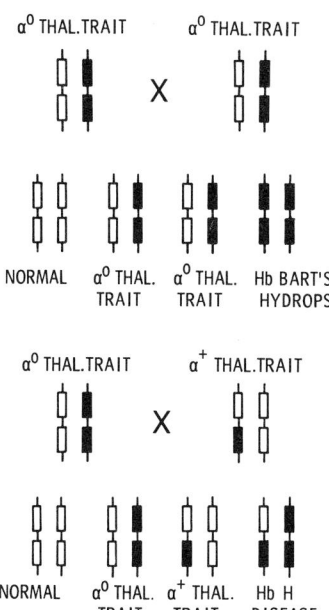

Fig. 13 The pathophysiology of α thalassaemia.

Fig. 14 The genetics of α thalassaemia. The black α genes represent gene deletions or otherwise inactivated genes. The open α genes represent normal genes. α° thalassaemia and α⁺ thalassaemia are defined in the text.

Table 5 The α thalassaemias

Type	Findings in Homozygotes	Findings in Heterozygotes
α°*	Hb Bart's hydrops Hbs Bart's and Portland	Thalassaemia minor Normal Hb A_2
α⁺*	Thalassaemia minor† Normal Hb A_2	'Silent' or mildly hypochromic red cells
α⁺ Constant Spring*	Moderate anaemia Splenomegaly. 5 per cent Hb Constant Spring	Silent ∾ 1 per cent Hb Constant Spring

* Haemoglobin H disease results from compound inheritance of α° thalassaemia and α⁺ thalassaemia of either variety.

† In Saudi Arabian populations haemoglobin H disease may result from homozygous inheritance of a severe α⁺ haplotype. This chromosome contains one inactivated α gene and another with a polyA addition mutation.

In clinical practice we encounter two symptomatic types of α thalassaemia, the haemoglobin Bart's hydrops syndrome and haemoglobin H disease. The former results from the homozygous inheritance of α° thalassaemia. On the other hand, haemoglobin H disease usually results from the co-inheritance of both α° and α⁺ thalassaemia. We now know that there are many different molecular types of both α° and α⁺ thalassaemia. These genetic interactions are summarized in Fig. 14.

Molecular pathology

The α° thalassaemias result from the deletion (loss) of both linked α globin genes. There are at least six different-sized deletions, one which is particularly common in Southeast Asia and another which occurs mainly in Mediterranean populations (Fig. 15). The molecular basis of the α⁺ thalassaemias is more complicated. In some cases they result from deletions which remove one of the linked pairs of α globin genes, leaving the other one intact. In others, both α globin genes are intact but one (or both) of them has a mutation which either partially or completely inactivates it. These mutations are rather like those which cause β thalassaemia. They may cause abnormal splicing or the production of a highly unstable α chain which is not capable of producing a viable haemoglobin. One particularly common form of non-deletion α⁺ thalassaemia occurs in Southeast Asia and results from a single

base change in the chain termination codon UAA, which changes to CAA. The latter is the codeword for the amino acid glutamine. Hence, when the ribosomes reach this point, instead of the chain terminating, messenger RNA which is not normally translated is 'read through' until another stop codon is reached. Thus an elongated α globin chain is produced which is synthesized at a reduced rate. The resulting variant with an unusually long α chain is called *haemoglobin Constant Spring* after the name of the town in Jamaica in which it was first discovered. It occurs in 2–5 per cent of the population of Thailand.

Another form of non-deletion α thalassaemia is very common in Saudi Arabia. It results from a single base change in the highly conserved sequence at the 3′ coding region of the α globin gene, AATAAA, which is changed to AATAAG. As mentioned earlier, this sequence is the polyA signal site; the mutation probably interferes with polyadenylation of α globin messenger RNA.

Genotype/phenotype relationships

These molecular studies explain much of the clinical variability of α thalassaemia in different populations. Since the haemoglobin Bart's hydrops syndrome requires the homozygous inheritance of α° thalassaemia, this condition will only occur in populations where α° thalassaemia is common. Because it is largely confined to Southeast Asia and the Mediterranean islands it is in these populations that the haemoglobin Bart's hydrops syndrome causes a public health problem. Similarly, because most forms of haemoglobin H disease are due to the inheritance of both α° and α⁺ thalassaemia, haemoglobin H disease is also restricted mainly to Mediterranean and Oriental populations. On the other hand, α⁺ thalassaemia occurs very commonly throughout parts of west Africa, the Indian subcontinent and the Pacific island populations. However, because α° thalassaemia does not occur in these regions the haemoglobin Bart's hydrops syndrome and haemoglobin H disease are not seen. The homozygous state for α⁺ thalassaemia is characterized by a mild hypochromic anaemia, very similar to the heterozygous state for α° thalassaemia; the results of having only two out of the normal four α genes seem to be the same whether the two genes are missing from the *same* chromosome or *opposite pairs* of homologous chromosomes.

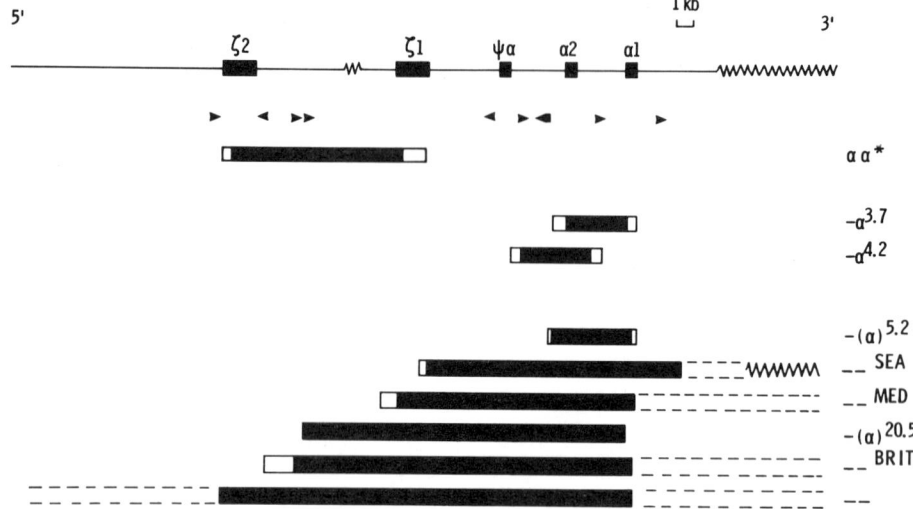

Fig. 15 The deletions which produce α thalassaemia. The missing DNA is indicated by dark areas. The approximate size of the deletions is given in kb (1000 nucleotide bases). SEA = Southeast Asian, Med = Mediterranean, Brit = British.

Pathophysiology

The pathophysiology of α thalassaemia is different to that of β thalassaemia. A deficiency of α chains leads to the production of excess γ chains or β chains which form haemoglobins Bart's and H, respectively (Fig. 13). These soluble tetramers do not precipitate in the bone marrow and hence erythropoiesis is more effective than in β thalassaemia, i.e. there is less intramedullary destruction of red cell precursors. However, haemoglobin H is unstable and precipitates in red cells as they age. The resulting inclusion bodies are trapped in the spleen and other parts of the microcirculation leading to a shortened red cell survival. Furthermore, both haemoglobins Bart's and H have a very high oxygen affinity; because they have no α chains there is no haem/haem interaction and their oxygen dissociation curves resemble myoglobin. Thus the pathophysiology of severe forms of α thalassaemia is based on defective haemoglobin production, the synthesis of homotetramers which are physiologically useless, and a haemolytic component due to their precipitation in older red cells.

The haemoglobin Bart's hydrops syndrome

This condition, which results from the homozygous state for α° thalassaemia is a common cause of fetal loss throughout Southeast Asia and in Greece and Cyprus. Affected infants produce no α chains at all and hence can make neither fetal nor adult haemoglobin.

The clinical picture is very characteristic (Fig. 16). These infants are usually stillborn between 28 and 40 weeks, or if they are live-born take a few gasping respirations and then expire within the first hour after birth. They show the typical picture of hydrops fetalis with gross pallor, generalized oedema, and massive hepatosplenomegaly. There is a very large friable placenta. All these findings are due to severe intrauterine anaemia. The haemoglobin values are in the 6–8 g/dl range and there are gross thalassaemic changes of the peripheral blood film with many nucleated red cells. The haemoglobin consists of approximately 80 per cent haemoglobin Bart's and 20 per cent of the embryonic haemoglobin, Portland ($\zeta_2\gamma_2$). It is believed that these infants survive to term because they continue to produce embryonic haemoglobin at this level; haemoglobin Bart's has an oxygen dissociation curve like myoglobin and is therefore useless as an oxygen carrier.

Apart from fetal death this syndrome is characterized by a high incidence of toxaemia of pregnancy and considerable obstetric difficulties due to the presence of the large, friable placenta. Both parents have thalassaemic red cell changes with normal haemoglobin A_2 values, i.e. the characteristic finding of the heterozygous state for α° thalassaemia.

Haemoglobin H disease

Molecular genetics and pathogenesis

As mentioned earlier, haemoglobin H is a tetramer of normal β chains with the formula β_4. It is produced when there is a marked reduction of α chain synthesis. Haemoglobin H disease usually results from the inheritance of α° thalassaemia from one parent and α^{+} from the other. It may also result from the inheritance of α° thalassaemia and haemoglobin Constant Spring or from the homozygous state for a severe non-deletion form of α thalassaemia. The latter form of inheritance is particularly common in Saudi Arabia.

Clinical features

There is a variable degree of anaemia and splenomegaly but it is most unusual to see severe thalassaemic bone changes or the growth retardation characteristic of homozygous β thalassaemia. Affected patients usually survive into adult life although the course may be interspersed with severe episodes of haemolysis associated with infection, or worsening of the anaemia due to progressive hypersplenism. In addition, oxidant drugs such as sulphonamides may increase the rate of precipitation of haemoglobin H and therefore exacerbate the anaemia.

Haematological changes

Haemoglobin values range from 7–10 g/dl and the blood film shows typical thalassaemic changes. There is a moderate reticulocytosis, and on incubation of the red cells with brilliant cresyl blue, numerous inclusion bodies are generated by precipitation of the haemoglobin H under the redox action of the dye. After splenectomy large, preformed inclusions can be demonstrated on incubation of blood with methyl violet. Haemoglobin analysis reveals from 5 to 40 per cent haemoglobin H together with haemoglobin A and a normal or reduced level of haemoglobin A_2.

Family findings

One parent is heterozygous for α° thalassaemia and the other is either heterozygous for α^{+} thalassaemia or haemoglobin Constant Spring. The latter is recognized by the finding of two or three faint bands following haemoglobin A_2 on haemoglobin electrophoresis

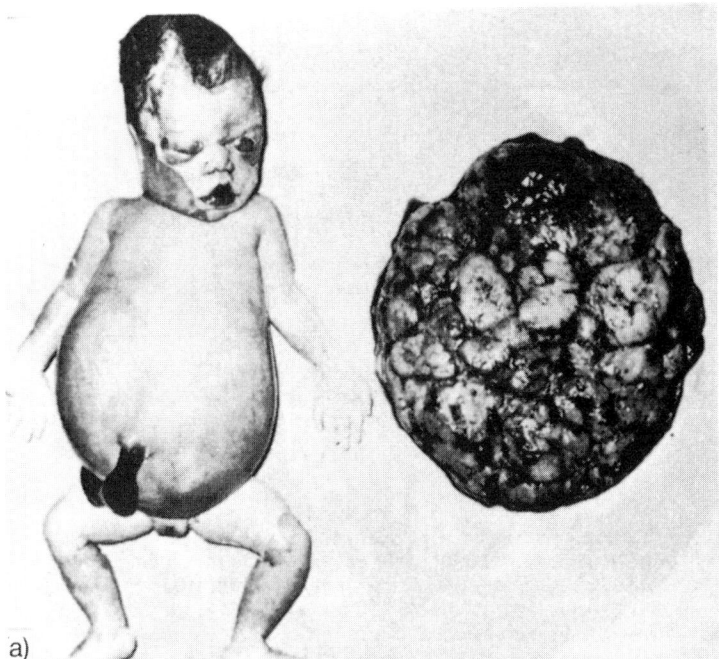

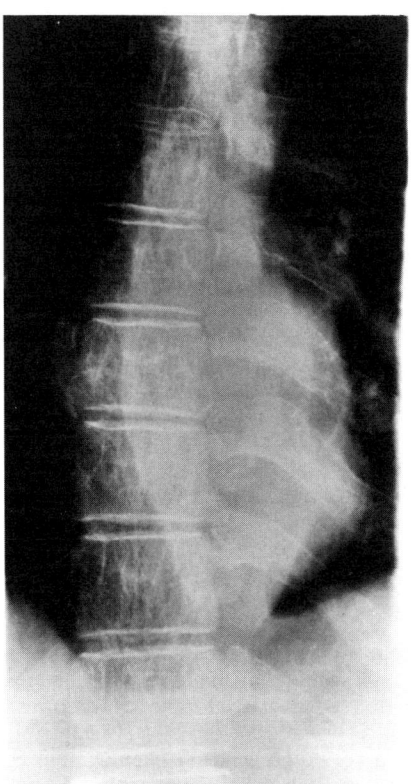

Fig. 17 An extramedullary haemopoietic mass in a patient with β thalassaemia intermedia.

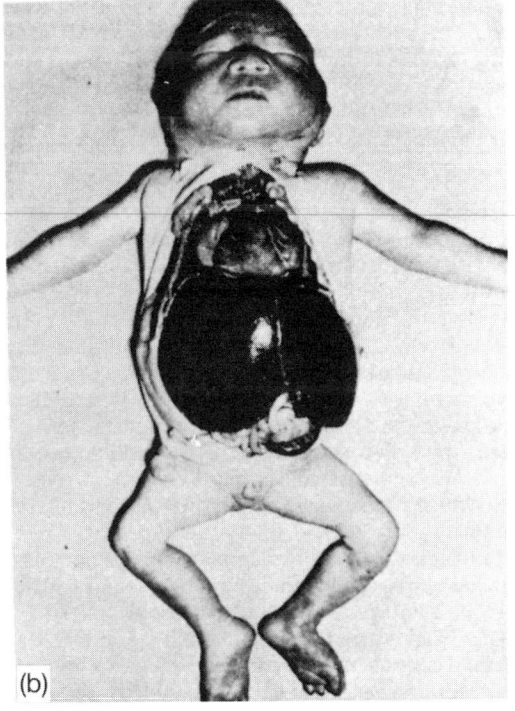

Fig. 16 The haemoglobin Bart's hydrops syndrome. (a) A hydropic infant with massively enlarged placenta; (b) Autopsy findings with an enlarged liver. (Reproduced by permission of Professor P. Wasi.)

using an alkaline buffer system. The haematological findings in the α^o and α^+ *thalassaemia traits* are summarized in Table 5.

THALASSAEMIA INTERMEDIA

Definition and pathogenesis

The term thalassaemia intermedia is used to describe patients with the clinical picture of thalassaemia which, although not transfusion dependent, is associated with a much more severe degree of anaemia than that found in heterozygous carriers for α or β thalassaemia. Many of the conditions which have been described previously in this section follow this clinical course, e.g. haemoglobin

C or E thalassaemia, the various $\delta\beta$ thalassaemias and haemoglobin Lepore disorders, and the wide variety of conditions which can result from the interactions of the different β and $\delta\beta$ thalassaemia determinants. However, some children with this condition have parents with typical heterozygous β thalassaemic blood pictures and elevated haemoglobin A_2 levels. These individuals appear to be homozygous for β thalassaemia yet run a much milder course than is usually the case with this condition (see page 19.112). There is increasing evidence that many of them have inherited an α thalassaemia determinant as well as being homozygous for β thalassaemia. This reduces the overall degree of globin chain imbalance and consequently the severity of the dyserythropoieses which usually accompanies homozygous β thalassaemia; hence these children run a milder clinical course. In other cases, particularly in the Negro races, relatively mild forms of homozygous β thalassaemia seem to reflect the action of less severe β thalassaemia mutations (see Table 4).

Clinical and haematological changes

The clinical features of the intermediate forms of thalassaemia are extremely variable. At one end of the spectrum are individuals who are virtually symptom-free, and except for moderate anaemia, are completely normal. At the other end there are patients who have haemoglobin values in the 5–7 g/dl range and who develop marked splenomegaly, severe skeletal deformities due to expansion of bone marrow, and, as they get older, become heavily iron-loaded because of increased intestinal absorption of iron. Recurrent leg ulceration, folate deficiency, symptoms due to extramedullary haemopoietic tumour masses in the chest and skull (Fig. 17), gallstones, and a marked proneness to infection are particularly characteristic of this group of thalassaemias.

Because of the heterogeneity of these disorders, it is only possible to determine the course that is likely to evolve in any individual patient by following the disorder very carefully from early childhood.

Differential diagnosis of the thalassaemias

There are few conditions which are likely to be confused with the more severe forms of homozygous β thalassaemia or haemoglobin H disease. The racial backgroud of the patient, the presence of anaemia from early in life, and the characteristic haematological changes make the diagnosis relatively easy. Once thalassaemia is suspected, the parents and near relatives should be examined for the carrier states for α or β thalassaemia. Both disorders can be distinguished from simple iron deficiency by the finding of a normal serum iron or ferritin level and by the associated changes in the haemoglobin pattern. It should be remembered, however, that in some races iron deficiency and heterozygous thalassaemia frequently occur together in the same person, particularly during pregnancy. Heterozygous β thalassaemics who are also iron deficient may drop their haemoglobin A_2 values which are restored after iron therapy. The sideroblastic anaemias can be easily distinguished from thalassaemia by the morphological appearances of the red cells and the presence of ring sideroblasts in the bone marrow. It should be remembered that there are some rare forms of *acquired haemoglobin H disease* in elderly patients with leukaemia or in mentally retarded children (see page 19.129).

The laboratory diagnosis of thalassaemia

The thalassaemias should be suspected when a typical thalassaemic blood picture is found in an individual of an appropriate racial group. The homozygous states for the severe forms of β thalassaemia are easily recognized by the typical haematological changes associated with very high levels of haemoglobin F; haemoglobin A_2 values vary so much that they are of no diagnostic value. The heterozygous states are recognized by microcytic hypochromic red cells and an elevated level of haemoglobin A_2. The $\delta\beta$ thalassaemias are characterized by the finding of 100 per cent haemoglobin F in homozygotes, and 5–15 per cent haemoglobin F together with a normal level of haemoglobin A_2 in heterozygotes (see Table 3).

When β thalassaemia is diagnosed, a quantitative haemoglobin electrophoresis should be carried out to exclude the presence of an abnormal haemoglobin variant such as haemoglobin E or Lepore.

The haemoglobin Bart's hydrops syndrome is recognized by the finding of a hydropic infant with a severe anaemia, a thalassaemic blood picture, and the presence of 80 per cent or more haemoglobin Bart's on haemoglobin electrophoresis. Haemoglobin H disease is identified by the finding of a typical thalassaemic blood picture with an elevated reticulocyte count, generation of multiple inclusion bodies in the red cells after incubation with brilliant cresyl blue, and the finding of variable amounts of haemoglobin H on haemoglobin electrophoresis. There are no really useful diagnostic tests for the different α thalassaemic carrier states although α^0 thalassaemia heterozygotes usually have typical thalassaemic red cell changes with a normal haemoglobin A_2 value.

A simple flow diagram showing the laboratory approach to the diagnosis of the thalassaemias is shown in Fig. 18.

Prevention and treatment

Thalassaemia produces a severe public health problem and a serious drain on medical resources in many populations. Since there is no definitive treatment, most countries in which the disease is common are putting a major effort into its prevention.

Prevention

There are two major approaches to the prevention of the thalassaemias. Since the carrier states for the β thalassaemias can be easily recognized, it is at least theoretically possible to screen populations and give genetic counselling about the choice of marriage partners. If β thalassaemia heterozygotes marry other carriers, one in four of their children will have the severe transfusion-dependent homozygous disorder. While large-scale programmes of this type have been set up in Italy, the results are not yet available,

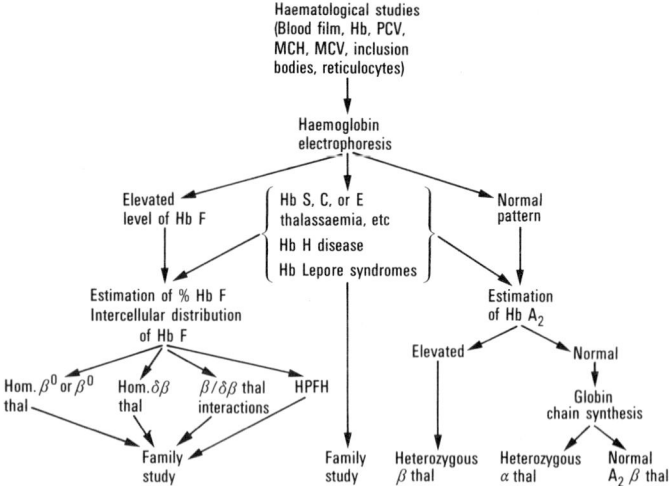

Fig. 18 A flow diagram showing an approach to the differential diagnosis of the thalassaemia syndromes. (Reproduced from Weatherall and Clegg, 1981.)

and in smaller pilot studies in Greece the outcome has not been encouraging. Until more is known about the usefulness of this form of prospective genetic counselling, most countries are developing screening programmes at antenatal clinics. When heterozygous carrier mothers are found, their husbands are tested and if they are also carriers the couple are offered the possiblity of prenatal diagnosis and termination of pregnancies carrying fetuses with severe forms of thalassaemia.

Prenatal diagnosis

Prenatal diagnosis should be offered to couples at risk for having children with severe forms of β thalassaemia. Because of the serious obstetric complications and the trauma of carrying a hydropic fetus to term there is also a good indication for prenatal diagnosis for the haemoglobin Bart's hydrops syndrome. Termination of pregnancies at risk for milder forms of thalassaemia is undertaken, but should only be considered after very careful counselling of the parents. Some children with intermediate forms of thalassaemia are symptom free and develop normally; others have more severe anaemia and bone deformity. We are currently trying to determine which particular molecular defects and interactions are associated with these different clinical courses.

Prenatal diagnosis of thalassaemia can be carried out in several ways. The diagnosis can be made by globin chain synthesis studies of fetal blood samples obtained by fetoscopy at 18–20 weeks gestation. The diagnosis can also be made by fetal DNA analysis on amniotic fluid cells obtained by amniocentesis earlier in the second trimester. More recently it has been possible to carry out prenatal diagnosis of thalassaemia and sickle cell anaemia by direct analysis of fetal DNA obtained by chorion biopsy at about the tenth week of gestation. If it turns out that this approach is not associated with an unacceptably high rate of fetal loss it will replace fetal blood sampling or amniocentesis for the prenatal diagnosis of the thalassaemias. Because it reduces the long period of uncertainty, during which the fetus is growing and the mother and her relatives and friends are coming to accept she is to have a child, and because late second trimester terminations are often difficult, first trimester diagnosis is much more acceptable to many women. Prenatal diagnosis of thalassaemia is now well established in many countries, and in Sardinia, Greece, and Cyprus has already significantly reduced the number of new cases of thalassaemia in the community.

Because prenatal diagnosis of thalassaemia is now well established it is very important to discuss the genetic implications of the condition when carriers are detected by chance, regardless of the individual's racial background. They should also be given a letter explaining, in simple terms, the pattern of inheritance and the dangers for their children. This approach should always be followed, even for sporadic cases in low-incidence regions, such as northern Europe. Because of the increasing movements of populations they might marry another carrier and have severely affected children. I have seen an English woman with two homozygous children; she was a known carrier but was not counselled and married a man of Italian extraction. Apart from the personal tragedy for such a family, in the future carelessness of this kind may have unfortunate medico-legal consequences.

Symptomatic treatment

The symptomatic management of severe β thalassaemia hangs on regular blood transfusion, the judicious use of splenectomy if hypersplenism develops, and the administration of chelating agents to attempt to deal with the problem of iron overload from regular blood transfusion. When the diagnosis of severe β thalassaemia is suspected during the first year of life, the infant should be followed for several weeks to make sure that the haemoglobin level is falling to a level at which regular transfusion will be necessary. It is difficult to be dogmatic about exactly when transfusions should be started, but if the infant is severely anaemic and it is feeding poorly or otherwise failing to thrive, it will almost certainly need to be transfused. The object should be to maintain the haemoglobin level between 9 and 14 g/dl and this usually requires transfusion every six to eight weeks. Either washed or frozen red cells should be used and whole blood should be avoided because of the danger of sensitization to serum or white cell components. A careful check on the pre- and post-transfusion haemoglobin level should be kept and the transfusion requirements carefully plotted. If there is a marked increase in blood requirement, hypersplenism should be suspected. It is becoming clear that any thalassaemic child with an easily palpable spleen probably has some degree of hypersplenism. Spenectomy should be carried out as late as is feasible and, if possible, not in the first five years because the incidence of post-splenectomy infection seems to be particularly high in early childhood. Apart from increased transfusion requirements, the presence of neutropenia or thrombocytopenia is a useful guide to the presence of hypersplenism. After the operation children should be maintained on prophylactic penicillin indefinitely and the parents warned about the dangers of overwhelming infection (see page 19.194).

The only useful chelating agent for the prevention or treatment of iron overload in thalassaemia is desferrioxamine (Desferal). The drug has to be administered systemically and there is convincing evidence that much better results are obtained by a slow subcutaneous infusion using some form of mechanical pump than by single bolus injections. Desferal therapy should be started as early as possible, but for practical purposes this usually means somewhere between the second or third year or later. The child should be admitted to hospital and a 12 hour, overnight Desferal infusion set up using a 'butterfly' needle placed subcutaneously in the anterior abdominal wall. The urinary iron excretion in the 24-hour period after the infusion is measured, after which, using the same technique, a dose-response curve is obtained starting with 0.5 g of Desferal and increasing the dose until a plateau of iron excretion is reached. This determines the dose which the child should receive on five nights a week with a rest at weekends. Much better iron excretion is obtained if the child is ascorbate replete which is achieved by giving 100–200 mg of ascorbic acid daily. Apart from some redness at the injection site there are no side effects of Desferal therapy except for the very rare occurrence of cataracts which seem to be reversible after stopping the drug. A careful ophthalmological surveillance should be maintained while on this regimen. For those children or parents who cannot cope with this complicated treatment, it is still worth giving daily bolus injections of Desferal with a dose schedule as outlined in Table 6. Whatever the route that is chosen for Desferal therapy, the urinary iron

Table 6 Approximate dose range (about 25 mg/kg) and method of administration of intramuscular desferrioxamine at different stages of development

Weight range (kg)	Age (years)	Dose (mg)	Distilled water (ml)
15–25	3–6	500	1.5–2
25–35	7–12	750	2
35–45	13–puberty	1000	2–3
45–65	Postpubertal	1500	4

From Modell (1977).

should be monitored from time to time to make sure that the drug is still effective. It should be remembered that a considerable amount of iron is also excreted through the faeces in this form of therapy. It is still too early to say for certain whether chelation therapy will prolong the life of transfusion-dependent thalassaemic children although this seems likely (see page 19.90).

The intermediate forms of β thalassaemia and haemoglobin H disease require careful surveillance and splenectomy if hypersplenism develops. Haemoglobin H disease is usually fairly innocuous although patients should be warned against the use of oxidant drugs which tend to precipitate haemoglobin H and worsen the anaemia. Children with β thalassaemia intermedia should be watched carefully in early childhood, and, if there are signs of growth retardation or increasing bone deformity, they should be placed on a transfusion regimen as outlined above.

Finally, it is most important that all thalassaemic children are under regular surveillance by an experienced paediatrician. Apart from the specific complications of the disorder, their proneness to infection and bony deformities lead to a series of general paediatric complications, particularly recurrent ear infection, deafness, sinus infection, emotional disturbances, and a variety of orthodontal problems. The families require constant encouragement and they should be told that the current form of chelation therapy is, in a sense, buying time until more active oral chelating agents become available or until a more definitive form of treatment is developed. If well looked after, these children can have a relatively normal childhood, and the recent advances in the use of chelating drugs may mean that some of the distressing side-effects of iron loading which occur at puberty may at least be delayed, and possibly prevented indefinitely.

Structural haemoglobin variants

Over 300 structural haemoglobin variants have been described, most of which result from single amino acid substitutions. Many of them are harmless and have been discovered during surveys of the electrophoretic patterns of human haemoglobin. Of course, this approach underestimates the number of variants because it only identifies those in which the amino acid substitution alters the charge of the haemoglobin molecule.

Single amino acid substitutions cause clinical disorders only if they alter the stability or functional properties of haemoglobin. A classification of the diseases which result from structural abnormalities of haemoglobin is shown in Table 7. They include the sickling disorders, the unstable haemoglobins associated with congenital non-spherocytic haemolytic anaemia, the high oxygen affinity variants which lead to hereditary polycythaemia, and a group which produce methaemoglobinaemia. We shall consider the different varieties of genetic methaemoglobinaemias at the end of this chapter.

Nomenclature

Originally, the structural haemoglobin variants were named by letters of the alphabet. By the late 1950s there were no letters of the alphabet left and it was decided to designate new haemoglobin

Table 7 Clinical disorders due to structural haemoglobin variants

Disorder	Variants
Haemolysis and tissue damage	Haemoglobin S
Drug-induced haemolysis	Haemoglobin Zürich and other unstable haemoglobins
Chronic haemolysis	Unstable haemoglobin variants Haemoglobin C
Congenital polycythaemia	High affinity variants
Congenital cyanosis	Haemoglobin(s) M Low affinity variants
Hypochromia. Thalassaemic phenotype	Haemoglobin E Haemoglobin Constant Spring

Table 8 The major sickling disorders

Disorder	Genotype (normal = $\alpha\alpha/\alpha\alpha$. β/β)	
SS disease (sickle cell anaemia)	$\alpha\alpha/\alpha\alpha$	β^S/β^S
SC disease	$\alpha\alpha/\alpha\alpha$	β^S/β^C
SD disease	$\alpha\alpha/\alpha\alpha$	β^S/β^D
S–β thalassaemia	$\alpha\alpha/\alpha\alpha$	$\beta^S\beta^o$ or β^S/β^+
S-hereditary persistence of fetal Hb	$\alpha\alpha/\alpha\alpha$	$\beta^S/-$ *
S–α thalassaemia	$\alpha-/\alpha\alpha$ or $\alpha-/\alpha-$	β^S/β^S

     * Indicates β gene deletion.

variants by the place of origin of the first patient in whom they were characterized. It is customary to call the heterozygous (carrier) state the 'trait' and the homozygous condition the 'disease'. For example, haemoglobin S heterozygotes (genotype AS) are said to have the sickle cell trait, while individuals homozygous for the sickle cell mutation (genotype SS) are said to have sickle cell disease. In practice it is very important to distinguish between the carrier state and the homozygous or compound heterozygous state for a sickle haemoglobin variant; carriers are always asymptomatic.

The sickling disorders

Sickling disorders (Table 8) consist of the heterozygous state for haemoglobin S or the sickle cell trait (AS), the homozygous state or sickle cell disease (SS), and the compound heterozygous state for haemoglobin S together with haemoglobins C, D, E, or other structural variants. In addition, there are several disorders which result from the inheritance of the sickle cell gene together with different forms of thalassaemia (see page 19.115).

Pathogenesis

Haemoglobin S differs from haemoglobin A by the substitution of valine for glutamic acid at position 6 in the β chain. Although this has been known since Vernon Ingram's work over a quarter of a century ago, it is still not absolutely clear how it gives rise to the sickling phenomenon. The latter appears to be due to the unusual solubility characteristics of haemoglobin S which undergoes liquid crystal (tactoid) formation as it becomes deoxygenated. In the latter state aggregates of sickled haemoglobin molecules arrange themselves in parallel, rod-like structures with a diameter of about 11.6 nm. The molecules of these strands are in a helical configuration. It seems likely that there is a tendency for normal haemoglobin molecules to become lined up in a similar way when haemoglobin is in the deoxy configuration, and in sickle cells the $\beta6$ valine substitution somehow stabilizes these molecular stacks. There is considerable variation with which different haemoglobins are able to participate with haemoglobin S in the sickling process. This accounts for some of the clinical variability of the different sickling conditions. For example, haemoglobin F is almost com-

pletely excluded from the sickling process and therefore increasing concentrations in the red cell tends to reduce the rate of sickling.

During their passage through the circulation, red cells containing haemoglobin S at a high concentration go through a series of cycles of sickling and desickling and finally, owing to loss of membrane and changes in membrane permeability, the cells become irreversibly sickled (Fig. 19). Sickling has two main effects. First, sickled erythrocytes have an increased mechanical fragility and hence a significantly shortened survival. This leads to a chronic haemolytic anaemia. Secondly, because of the formation of aggregates of sickled erythrocytes, particularly in the microvasculature, the viscosity of the blood increases, which leads to vascular stasis, local hypoxia, further sickling and, in extreme cases, to complete blockage of small vessels and tissue infarction.

Distribution

The sickling disorders occur very frequently in African Negro populations and, sporadically, throughout the Mediterranean region and the Middle East. There are extensive pockets in India but the disease has not been seen in Southeast Asia. It is thought that the high frequency of the sickle cell gene occurs because carriers are more resistant than normal individuals to *P. falciparum* malaria. This notion is supported by both epidemiological and *in vitro* culture studies (see Fig. 3, page 19.75).

Clinical features

Except in conditions of extreme anoxia such as flying in unpressurized aircraft, the *sickle cell trait* causes no clinical disability. However, it is possible for individuals to suffer vaso-occlusive episodes if they become unusually hypoxic under anaesthesia and therefore all individuals of the appropriate racial background should have a sickling test (see below) before receiving an anaesthetic. If the test is positive, the anaesthetic should be given with adequate oxygenation and special care should be taken to avoid post-operative dehydration.

Sickle cell anaemia

This is a condition which runs an extremely variable clinical course. At one end of the spectrum it is characterized by a crippling haemolytic anaemia interspersed with severe exacerbations or crises, while on the other hand it may be an extremely mild disorder which is only found by chance on routine haematological examination. The reason for these remarkable differences in phenotypic expression of what appears to be the same genetic defect, which are only partly understood, include the level of haemoglobin F, climate, and, probably most important, socio-economic factors such as availability of early treatment of infection.

Typically, sickle cell anaemia presents in infancy with a variable degree of anaemia and jaundice and most patients go through the rest of their life with a chronic haemolytic anaemia. A common presenting symptom is the so-called *hand and foot syndrome* which occurs early in infancy and is characterized by a painful dactylitis with swelling of the fingers or feet. Epiphyseal damage during one of these episodes may lead to chronic shortening of a digit. Infants are anaemic from about the third month of life and during early development often have significant splenomegaly. In most cases this gradually resolves due to repeated infarction of the spleen, a condition called autosplenectomy. Indeed, it is most unusual to feel the spleen after the end of the first decade. Typically, these children have haemoglobin levels in the 6–8 g/dl range with a reticulocyte count of 10–20 per cent. There is chronic, mild icterus with an elevated bilirubin level. Examination of the peripheral blood film shows anisochromia and poikilocytosis with a variable number of sickled erythrocytes (Fig. 19). As the children grow older the haematological changes of hyposplenism develop with the appearance of pits on the surface of the red cells, Howell–Jolly bodies, and distorted red cells. The while cell and platelet counts are usually normal or slightly elevated.

Apart from the signs mentioned above, growth and develop-

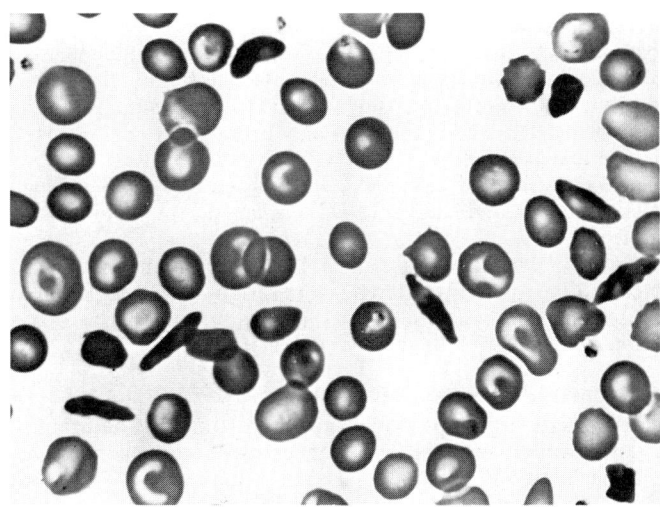

Fig. 19 Irreversibly sickled cells in the peripheral blood (× 1000, Leishman stain).

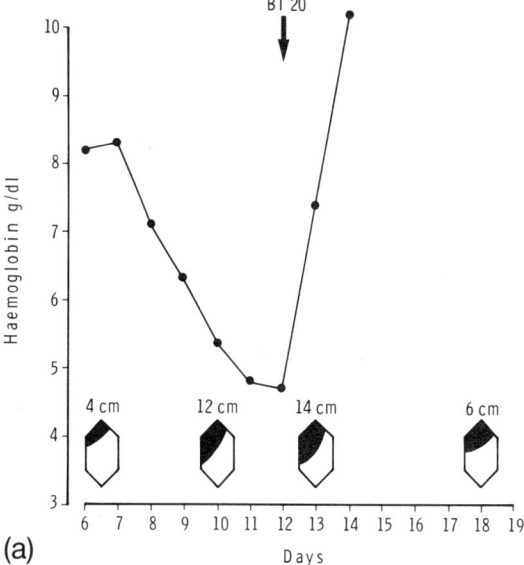

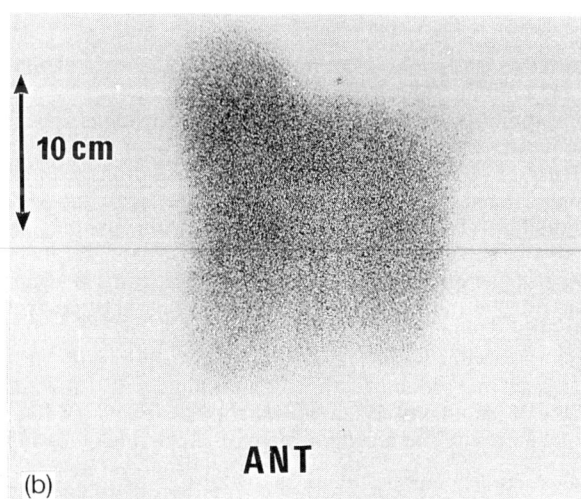

Fig. 20 Hepatic sequestration crisis in sickle cell anaemia. (a) Clinical course. (b) Liver scintigram. BT = Blood Transfusion.

ment are usually normal although there may be some skeletal deformities including frontal bossing of the skull due to expansion of the bone marrow. In some studies children have tended to be short for their age, while postadolescents were usually tall. Inequalities between upper and lower segments, stresses in the early literature, are unusual. The only other physical sign which is frequently present is chronic leg ulceration; this is discussed in a later section.

Complications

The chronic haemolysis of sickle cell disease is interspersed with acute exacerbations of the illness called sickling crises. Furthermore, there are a series of serious and life-threatening long-term complications which develop in many patients with symptomatic cell anaemia.

The different forms of sickle cell crises are summarized in Table 9. The commonest is the painful crisis. This is sometimes precipitated by infection and dehydration or exposure to cold, although quite often no underlying cause can be found. The episode starts with vague pain, often in the back or bones of the limbs. The pain gradually worsens and its bizarre distribution may cause a major diagnostic puzzle. The pain is almost certainly due to blockage of small vessels with sickled erythrocytes, and marrow aspiration over areas of bone tenderness reveals infarction of the marrow tissue. Occasionally, abdominal pain is the major symptom and this may be associated with distension and rigidity, a picture very similar to an acute abdominal emergency. The diagnostic difficulties in distinguishing between an *abdominal crisis* and a surgical abdomen are compounded by the fact that the bowel sounds are often very quiet during abdominal crises. Two other serious forms of thrombotic crises occur which are known as the 'lung' and 'brain' syndromes. The 'lung' syndrome is characterized by acute dyspnoea and pleuritic pain and is due to infarction of major pulmonary vessels. It is often preceded by a rapid fall in the PCV which may reflect sequestration of sickled cells in the pulmonary vessels. Neurological involvement may present in a variety of ways including fits with or without focal neurological signs.

During painful crises there may be a marked increase in the rate of haemolysis with a fall in the haemoglobin level. Such *haemolytic episodes* are relatively uncommon. Much more serious are periods of transient bone marrow aplasia called *aplastic crises*. These seem to result from intercurrent infection, particularly due to parvoviruses, and frequently affect more than one sibling in the same family.

Finally, and most serious, are the *sequestration crises*. These occur mainly in babies and young children and are characterized

Table 9 Acute exacerbations ('crises') in sickle cell (SS) disease

1 Thrombotic
   Generalized or localized bone pain
   Abdominal
   Pulmonary
   Neurological
2 Aplastic
3 Haemolytic
4 Sequestration
   Spleen
   Liver
   ?Lung
5 Various combinations of above

by a rapid enlargement of the spleen or liver which become engorged with sickled erythrocytes. As the crisis progresses a large proportion of the total red cell mass may be trapped in the spleen or liver, and death may occur due to gross anaemia. These episodes show a tendency to recur in the same individual. Hepatic

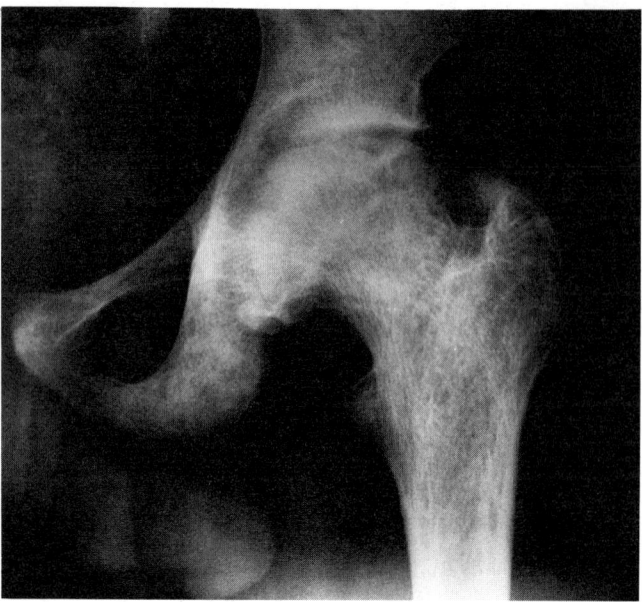

Fig. 21 Aseptic necrosis of the left femoral head in sickle cell thalassae-mia. (Reproduced by courtesy of Dr Graham Serjeant.)

sequestration which may occur in adults, is easily overlooked if the liver size is not monitored carefully (Fig. 20).

The commonest cause of death in sickle cell anaemia appears to be a sequestration crisis or acute infection, or both. It is not absolutely clear why patients with this disorder are so prone to infection although splenic malfunction may play a role (see page 19.194). Abnormalities of the alternate pathway of complement activation have also been described. A variety of organisms are involved, particularly the pneumococcus, and in some tropical countries typhoid infection of bone infarcts leads to typhoid osteomyelitis. Despite the relative resistance of heterozygotes to *P. falciparum* malaria, deaths due to malaria are extremely common in Africa.

Pregnancy may be uneventful, or associated with an increased incidence of painful crises. There is slightly increased incidence of maternal mortality and a definite increase in the rate of fetal loss.

Chronic complications

The chronic complications of sickle cell anaemia result largely from infarcts following repeated episodes of vascular occlusion. Almost any organ can be involved. Those of particular risk are areas which rely largely on small vessels for their blood supply. The bones are particularly prone to infarction. Aseptic necrosis of the humeral or femoral heads may lead to their destruction and to gross deformity of the shoulder and hip joints (Fig. 21). Bone infarcts may result in chronic sequestra formation which may become secondarily infected with the production of osteomyelitis. Infarction of the bone marrow does not seem to have any long-term sequelae, although occasionally pieces may break off and embolize to the lungs.

Another organ at particular risk is the kidney. During early childhood renal function may be impaired but this can be corrected by blood transfusion, suggesting that it is due to reversible changes in the renal vasculature. These alterations in renal function are not reversible in later life and chronic progressive renal failure due to damage of the renal vessels is one of the commonest causes of death in adults with sickle cell anaemia. A typical nephrotic syndrome may develop at some stage during the illness. Despite the fact that pulmonary infarction occurs quite frequently, repeated episodes leading to severe pulmonary hypertension and right heart failure are unusual, although this complication has been well documented.

The phenomenon of autosplenectomy and splenic hypofunction has already been mentioned. There is usually some degree of

cardiomegaly and a variety of flow murmurs may be heard but most of these signs seem to be the result of chronic anaemia, and myocardial infarction or fibrosis does not occur frequently. Recurrent attacks of painful priapism may lead to permanent deformity of the penis. Repeated infarction may lead to chronic fibrosis of the liver and liver failure.

Finally, there is increasing evidence that, unless the neurological crises are treated energetically, permanent brain damage may result.

Occular manifestations are also relatively common in sickle cell anaemia although they tend to be more serious in haemoglobin SC disease; they will be considered with the latter disorder in a later section (see page 19.126) and in detail on page 23.6.

Course and prognosis

There are still large gaps in our knowledge about the natural history of sickle cell anaemia. The prognosis seems to depend on the racial background of the patient, socio-economic and ill-defined genetic factors and, above all, the availability of good paediatric care in the early years.

Recent studies in rural East Africa indicate that this disease still has a high mortality in the first year or two of life. In Jamaica there appears to be a 10 per cent mortality in the early years although survival into adult life and old age is common. This is also the case in some urban parts of Africa and in the United States and Europe. In Saudi Arabia and India a particularly mild form of the condition occurs in which the mortality is extremely low in childhood, and a normal survival seems to be the rule. It is becoming increasingly apparent that the commonest cause of death in the first year or two of life is infection, often associated with splenic sequestration. In later life infection is still a frequent cause of death, although studies in Jamaica indicate that chronic, progressive renal failure may be responsible for a significant number of deaths in middle life.

Laboratory diagnosis

The sickle cell trait causes no haematological changes and is diagnosed by the finding of a positive sickling test together with haemoglobins A and S on electrophoresis (Fig. 22). Sickle cell anaemia is diagnosed by the finding of a variable degree of anaemia, an elevated reticulocyte count, sickled erythrocytes on the peripheral blood film, a positive sickling test, and a haemoglobin electrophoretic pattern characterized by the absence of haemoglobin A and a preponderance of haemoglobin S with a variable amount of haemoglobin F (Fig. 22). The diagnosis is confirmed by finding the sickle cell trait in both parents.

There are a variety of simple sickling tests available, but for ward laboratories the simplest is to take a drop of blood and mix it with a drop of freshly prepared 2 per cent sodium metabisulphite, place a coverslip over the mixture, seal the edges with vaseline, and examine the slide for sickling after one hour.

Management

Like all genetic diseases the first priority should be prevention. In the few places it has been tried, prospective genetic counselling and education of communities has not had much effect on the incidence of new cases. However, there are very effective methods for prenatal diagnosis of the condition and it is likely that programmes will be set up whereby women are screened at the antenatal clinic and at-risk couples advised about the possibility of therapeutic abortion of affected fetuses. However, before these programmes are fully developed, we need to know more about the natural history of sickle cell anaemia and the burden that is placed on families and individual patients in high incidence populations.

Apart from advice about anaesthesia and avoidance of unpressurized aircraft or deep-sea diving, individuals with the sickle trait require no treatment.

Most patients with sickle cell anaemia manage well with relatively low haemoglobin levels, and regular blood transfusion is not

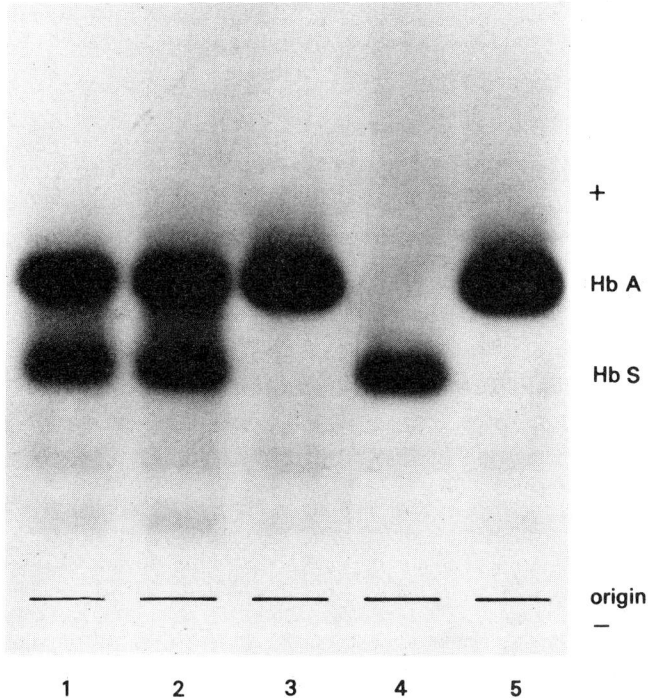

Hb A

Hb S

origin

1   2   3   4   5

Fig. 22 The haemoglobin pattern in the sickling disorders (starch gel electrophoresis, protein stain, pH 8.5). The following are shown (left to right): (1 and 2) the sickle cell trait; (3) normal; (4) sickle cell anaemia; (5) normal.

Table 10 General principles in managing sickle cell crises

1 Full clinical examination to find a source of infection
2 Rest, fluid replacement, oxygen, and analgesia
3 Once or twice daily PCV and reticulocyte estimations
4 Once or twice daily estimation of spleen and liver size
5 Transfusion* only if: (*a*) dangerous fall in PCV or reticulocytes
 (*b*) complications such as lung or brain syndrome
 (*c*) crises recur frequently, particularly in pregnancy
 (*d*) surgery is required

* After transfusion the percentage of sickle cells (using a sickling test or the level of haemoglobin S) should be below 30 per cent. This is achieved by either transfusion (if the initial PCV is very low) or by partial exchange transfusion.

ordinarily required. Adaptation to anaemia is particularly successful because of the low oxygen affinity of haemoglobin S. Episodes of infection should be treated early, and in populations in which the diet is low in folate, regular folate supplements should be added. Patients should be given access to a unit that is used to managing the disorder and advised to come early at the first sign of a painful crisis.

All but the mildest painful crises should be managed in hospital (Table 10). The patient should be fully examined for evidence of underlying infection and then given adequate intravenous fluids, oxygen, antibiotics, and analgesia. It should be remembered that the pain may be excruciating and strong analgesics should not be withheld because of fear of addiction; the episodes are usually short-lived. The packed cell volume or haemoglobin level, and reticulocyte count should be estimated at least daily, and perhaps twice daily, but unless there is a fall in the haemoglobin level or evidence of an impending aplastic crisis as evidenced by a drop in the reticulocyte count, transfusion is not required. If the haemoglobin level falls due to increased haemolysis or bone marrow failure, a blood transfusion should be given to restore the haemoglobin level to normal or slightly higher. A sequestration crisis is an indication for urgent transfusion and very close surveillance because profound anaemia may develop over a period of hours. Hence, patients with a sickling crisis should have regular examination of the abdomen to assess spleen and liver size to try and anticipate impending episodes of sequestration. Complications such as the brain or lung syndrome should be treated by partial exchange transfusion. The level of sickle cells should be reduced to below 30 per cent. If the initial haemoglobin level is lower than 5 – 6 g/dl, this can be achieved by transfusion up to 13/14 g/dl followed by regular 'top-up' transfusions to reduce endogenous erythropoiesis. If the initial haemoglobin value is unusually high, e.g. in excess of 9 g/dl, it is better to carry out a partial exchange transfusion.

Hypertransfusion or exchange transfusion can be used to cover major surgical procedures or in patients who are having recurrent crises. Occasionally, the spleen may enlarge to such a degree that secondary hypersplenism occurs. This complication usually occurs in young children with sickle cell disease, particularly in malarious areas. Splenectomy may be indicated in such cases. Similarly, because sequestration crises seem to recur in the same infant, this may also be an indication for splenectomy.

There is no special treatment required during pregnancy except for regular surveillance and folate supplementation. If the haemoglobin level drops significantly, or if there are recurrent crises, a regular transfusion regime should be started to cover pregnancy and delivery. This should maintain a normal haemoglobin level and less than 30 per cent sickle cells (or haemoglobin S).

Occular complications, particularly proliferative retinopathy, require expert opthalmological advice; early results of treatment of proliferative retinopathy with either zenon arc or argon laser indicate that the risk of vitreous haemorrhage is significantly reduced. Chronic hip pain and difficulty with walking due to *aseptic necrosis of the femoral heads* may require total hip replacement. It is frequently asked whether *oral contraceptives* are contraindicated in sickle cell anaemia. There is no evidence that they increase the number of veno-occlusive episodes and should certainly not be withheld; it is probably wiser to use a low oestrogen preparation. Any surgical procedure should be undertaken with great caution. It is critical to maintain high levels of oxygen and adequate hydration throughout the pre-operative and postoperative period. Limb tourniquets should be avoided and any major procedures are probably best carried out after exchange transfusion. *Haematuria* is a worrying symptom and although drugs such as ε-aminocaproic acid have been advocated there is no evidence that they shorten the period of bleeding. Terminal renal failure should be managed as for any other form of renal insufficiency.

Priapism occurs quite frequently in patients with sickle cell anaemia. It should be remembered that it occurs in other conditions such as chronic leukaemia, polycythaemia vera, renal failure treated by haemodialysis, and in association with disorders characterized by an increased tendency to thrombosis, particularly disseminated cancer. It may also occur for no apparent cause. In sickle cell anaemia it has been found that nearly two-thirds of major episodes of priapism are preceded by 'stuttering' attacks and therefore it has been suggested that effective therapy at this stage may reduce the risk of sustaining a major attack. Preliminary data suggest that stilboestrol 5 mg daily may be effective in preventing a major episode of priapism in patients who have had these spells of minor episodes. Fully developed priapism is a serious complication because if not relieved it frequently leads to permanent impotence. It has been suggested by the group in Jamaica, who have wide experience of this problem, that conservative treatment is restricted to 24 hours at the most. During this time the patient should be hydrated, given adequate analgesia, and transfused up to a level at which the number of sickleable cells is below about 30–40 per cent. If there is no improvement by these simple measures surgery should not be delayed. The most efficient procedure is a cavernosus-spongiosum shunt which is a relatively minor procedure and produces a very good cosmetic result. Anticoagulants have no role in the treatment of priapism associated with sickle cell anaemia; they have been advocated in cases of priapism associated with high platelet counts or hypercoagulable disorders; again, their role is uncertain. Whatever the cause of priapism the critical part of management seems to be to proceed to early surgery, rather than waiting in the hope of resolution, after 24 hours. In patients who have become impotent after a severe episode of priapism it may be necessary to insert a penile prosthesis.

Although numerous anti-sickling agents have been promoted over the years, none of them has stood the test of a properly designed clinical trial. Current research is directed to trying to prevent sickling by developing agents which inhibit polymerization of haemoglobin S by disrupting intermolecular bonds, decrease the intracellular concentration of deoxy haemoglobin S, or stabilize the red cell membrane. Several promising peptides have been produced which seem to reduce the rate of polymer formation. Cyanate, by reacting with free amino groups (carbamylation) maintains haemoglobin S in the oxy-configuration and this inhibits sickling. It is too toxic to give systemically, although there is still some interest in extra-corporeal carbamylation as a form of treatment for severely affected patients. Several drugs, including thioridezine and zinc compounds, are potent inhibitors of calmodulin, a membrane component involved in the formation of the irreversibly sickled cell in response to increased calcium concentration in the red cell membrane. Quite recently a completely different approach to the management of sickle cell anaemia has been investigated. As mentioned earlier high levels of fetal haemoglobin protect against sickling. For this reason patients have been treated with the agent 5-azacytidine in an attempt to stimulate fetal haemoglobin production. The rationale for this approach is that this drug is known to hypomethylate DNA. Active genes tend to be hypomethylated and therefore it was hoped that it might be possible to activate the γ globin genes in patients with sickle cell anaemia. Early reports indicate that this does occur. However, this agent has carcinogenic properties and could not be used for the long-term treatment of this disorder. However, this work will undoubtedly stimulate a search for safer agents which are capable of stimulating fetal haemoglobin synthesis.

Other sickling disorders

The other sickling disorders include the interaction of haemoglobin S with haemoglobins C, D, and some of the rarer haemoglobin variants. The interactions with the different forms of β thalassaemia were described earlier (see page 19.115). In many of these conditions the clinical manifestations are little different from the sickle cell trait, but haemoglobin SC disease and SD disease more closely resemble sickle cell anaemia.

Haemoglobin SC disease

This disease is relatively common in West Africans. It is characterized by a milder anaemia than sickle cell disease and many cases go unrecognized into adult life when they may present with one of the complications of the disorder. These are the result of damage to the microvasculature, probably because of the relatively high haemoglobin level and the combined effects of sickling and red cell rigidity caused by haemoglobin C (see below). Aseptic necrosis of the femoral or humeral heads or unexplained haematuria are two of the commonest complications. Widespread thrombotic episodes, particularly involving the lungs, may occur during intercurrent infection or in pregnancy or the puerperium. The other serious complication is the damage which may follow repeated blockage of the retinal vessels which leads to retinitis proliferans, retinal detachment, and permanent blindness. There is some evidence that patients with SC disease with an unusually high haemoglobin level are particularly at risk.

Haemoglobin SC disease is diagnosed by finding a mild anaemia with splenomegaly and characteristic morphological changes of the red cells including many target forms, intracellular crystals, and sickle cells. The sickling test is positive and haemoglobin electrophoresis shows haemoglobins S and C in about equal proportions. One parent shows the sickle cell trait and the other the haemoglobin C trait.

In severe thrombotic episodes patients with haemoglobin SC disease should be well hydrated and treated with anticoagulants. There is some evidence that regular venesection may help to delay the retinal changes in patients with unusually high haemoglobin levels, although this requires confirmation. Severe retinal disease is treated by coagulation therapy. In the life-threatening thrombotic episodes of pregnancy a partial exchange transfusion should be carried out.

Haemolysis due to other common haemoglobin variants

After haemoglobin S the second commonest variant in West Africa is haemoglobin C. Haemoglobin C, because of its relatively low solubility, appears to exist in a pre-crystalline state in red cells and hence causes their rigidity and premature destruction in the micro-circulation. The homozygous state for haemoglobin C, *haemoglobin C disease*, is characterized by a mild haemolytic anaemia with splenomegaly. The blood film shows 100 per cent target cells, and haemoglobin analysis shows haemoglobin C with small amounts of haemoglobin F. This is a mild disorder and no specific treatment is required.

The commonest haemoglobin variant throughout Southeast Asia and the Indian subcontinent is haemoglobin E. The homozygous state for this variant, *haemoglobin E disease*, is characterized by a very mild degree of anaemia with a slight reticulocytosis. The blood film shows mild morphological changes of the red cells which are hypochromic and microcytic, rather resembling the changes seen in some forms of thalassaemia. Again, no treatment is required for this mild anaemia.

Haemoglobin variants which migrate in the position of haemoglobin S but which do not sickle have been given the general title of *haemoglobin D*. There are several different molecular varieties of this variant. The homozygous state for some forms of haemoglobin D is associated with a moderately severe anaemia, splenomegaly, and a mild degree of haemolysis. The compound heterozygous state for haemoglobins S and D produces a disorder very similar to sickle cell anaemia. It is diagnosed by finding one parent with the haemoglobin D trait and the other with the sickle cell trait.

The unstable haemoglobin disorders

The unstable haemoglobin disorders are a rare group of inherited haemolytic anaemias which result from structural changes in the haemoglobin molecule which cause its intracellular precipitation with the formation of Heinz bodies. Their true incidence is not known and there have been several well-documented families in which patients with one of these haemoglobin variants have had no affected relatives, suggesting that the condition has arisen by a new mutation.

Aetiology and pathogenesis

Most of the unstable haemoglobin variants result from single amino acid substitutions at critical areas of the molecule. For example, substitutions in or around the haem pocket can disrupt the normal anatomy and allow in water with subsequent oxidative damage to haem which leads to precipitation of the haemoglobin. Some substitutions, such as those involving proline residues, cause marked disturbance of the secondary structure of a globin chains. A few of these variants result from deletions of either single amino acid residues or several residues. For example, in haemoglobin Gun Hill five amino acids are missing including the haem binding site. As the unstable haemoglobins precipitate in the red cells or their precursors, they produce intracellular inclusions or Heinz

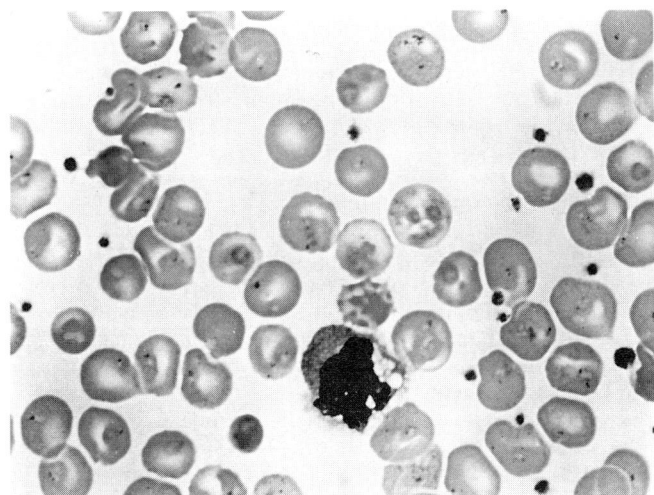

Fig. 23 The peripheral blood film of a patient with an unstable haemoglobin disorder, haemoglobin Hammersmith. This is a postsplenectomy film which shows small inclusions in many of the red cells ($\times$ 1000, Leishman stain.)

bodies which make the cells more rigid and hence cause their premature destruction in the microcirculation (Fig. 23).

Clinical features

All these conditions are characterized by a haemolytic anaemia of varying severity and splenomegaly. There may be a history of the passage of dark urine, particularly during episodes of infection. Like all chronic haemolytic anaemias, there is an increased incidence of pigment gallstones with their associated complications. The condition may become worse during periods of intercurrent infection and, in the more severe forms, such episodes are associated with life-threatening anaemia. Patients with unstable haemoglobins are at particular risk of haemolytic episodes following the administration of oxidant drugs such as sulphonamides.

Apart from intermittent icterus and splenomegaly there are no characteristic physical findings.

Laboratory diagnosis

This condition should be thought of in any familial haemolytic anaemia, particularly if a red cell enzyme deficiency cannot be demonstrated. The peripheral blood film shows the typical features of haemolysis but the red cell morphology may be relatively normal. Occasionally there is a mild degree of hypochromia and microcytosis. Unless splenectomy has been carried out, Heinz bodies are not seen in the peripheral blood (Fig. 23).

The most characteristic feature of the unstable haemoglobins is their heat instability. If a dilute haemoglobin solution is heated at 50 °C for 15 minutes, most of the unstable haemoglobins precipitate as a dense cloud. A similar phenomenon can be induced by such agents as isopropanol. Some of these variants can be characterized by haemoglobin electrophoresis but others, because they result from the substitution of a neutral amino acid, produce no electrophoretic changes and can only be demonstrated by the heat precipitation test.

Treatment

Because these conditions are so rare there has been very little experience of the effects of splenectomy. From the little information that is available from the literature, and from the author's personal experience, it appears that if a child has had several life-threatening episodes of anaemia or is running a steady-state haemoglobin level which is impairing development or well-being, splenectomy should be undertaken. It is interesting to note that some of these haemoglobin variants produce a 'right shift' in the oxygen dissociation curve, and a measurement of the $p50$ as part of the pre-splenectomy assessment may help to decide whether to proceed to surgery; a marked right shift, i.e. an increased $p50$, indicates that the anaemia should be more easily tolerated than if the oxygen dissociation curve is moved in the opposite direction with a low $p50$. An accurate history from the child or its parents is probably more helpful, however.

Haemoglobin variants which cause abnormal oxygen binding

In 1966 an 81-year-old man presented at Johns Hopkins Hospital, Baltimore, with mild angina and a haemoglobin value of 19.9 g/dl. No cause could be found for his polycythaemia but it was noted that he had an abnormal haemoglobin. The oxygen dissociation curve of his blood was found to be displaced to the left. This suggested that the abnormal haemoglobin might have a high oxygen affinity and that the patient's increased red cell count might be compensating for a primary defect in oxygen unloading. Further studies showed that this was the case and hence established a new cause for secondary polycythaemia. Since then over 20 haemoglobin variants of this type have been defined, all associated with familial polycythaemia.

Aetiology

The high oxygen affinity haemoglobin variants result from single amino acid substitutions at critical parts of the haemoglobin molecule which are involved in the configurational changes which underlie haem/haem interaction and the production of a sigmoid oxygen dissociation curve (see page 19.65). Many of them occur at the junctions between the α and β subunits. Others involve the amino acids which are involved with the binding of 2, 3-diphosphoglycerate (2, 3-DPG) to haemoglobin. As mentioned in an earlier chapter (page 19.65), increasing concentrations of 2, 3-DPG tend to push the oxygen dissociation curve to the right; fetal haemoglobin has a high oxygen affinity (left-shifted curve) because it cannot interact with 2, 3-DPG; mutations of the DPG binding sites have a similar effect.

Pathophysiology

All the high oxygen affinity variants have a left-shifted oxygen dissociation curve with a reduced $p50$. Thus the variant haemoglobin holds on to oxygen more avidly than normal haemoglobin and this leads to tissue hypoxia. This in turn causes an increased output of erythropoietin and an elevated red cell mass.

Clinical features

Many patients with high oxygen affinity variants are completely healthy and are only found to carry the variant when a routine haematological examination shows an unusually high haemoglobin level or packed cell volume. There have been one or two reports of arterial or venous thrombosis in these patients. However, this is uncommon and in most cases the patients are asymptomatic, there is no splenomegaly, and apart from a raised red cell mass there are no associated haematological findings. Although it might be expected that a high oxygen affinity haemoglobin would cause defective oxygenation of the fetus none of the reported families has had a history of frequent stillbirths.

Diagnosis

The condition should be suspected in any patient with a pure red cell polycythaemia associated with a left-shifted oxygen dissociation curve. The diagnosis can be confirmed by haemoglobin analysis.

Treatment

In asymptomatic patients with high oxygen affinity haemoglobin variants no treatment is necessary. The difficulty arises if the patient has associated vascular disease with symptoms of coronary or cerebral artery insufficiency. There is insufficient published information to make any dogmatic statements about how this complication should be managed. The author has seen two patients of this type who seem to have responded to venesection; more experience is required before this form of treatment can be recommended, however. These patients require a high haemoglobin level for oxygen transport; half their haemoglobin is physiologically useless.

Low oxygen affinity variants

At least six haemoglobin variants with reduced oxygen affinity have been reported. The first to be described, haemoglobin Kansas, was found in a mother and son with unexplained cyanosis. The subjects were asymptomatic and had normal haemoglobin levels without any evidence of haemolysis. Like many of the high affinity variants the amino acid substitution in this variant was at the interface between the α and β globin chains. For reasons which are not clear some substitutions in this region give rise to variants with a relatively low oxygen affinity. This condition should be thought of in any patient with an unexplained congenital cyanosis; the differential diagnosis is considered below.

METHAEMOGLOBINAEMIA, CARBOXYHAEMOGLOBINAEMIA, AND SULPHAEMOGLOBINAEMIA

Methaemoglobinaemia is a condition characterized by increased quantities of haemoglobin in which the iron of haem is oxidized to the ferric (Fe^{3+}) form.

Carboxyhaemoglobinaemia (carbonmonoxyhaemoglobinaemia) results from the binding of carbon monoxide to the haem molecules.

Sulphaemoglobinaemia is a rare condtion in which there is a mixture of haemoglobin derivatives whose structure is poorly characterized but which can be defined by their specific spectral characteristics.

Pathogenesis

As mentioned earlier in this Section, each haemoglobin molecule has four haem molecules. At first sight it is not clear why the oxidation of a proportion of the iron atoms, or the fact that they are liganded to carbon monoxide, should cause such profound changes in oxygen transport. However, oxidation of 30 per cent of the haem molecules has a much more serious effect on tissue oxygenation than a reduction of the haemoglobin level by the same amount. This is because, if a single haem is oxidized, it so alters the conformation of the haemoglobin molecule that the oxygen affinity of the other three haems is increased. Thus methaemoglobin, carboxyhaemoglobin, and cyanmethaemoglobin all have very high oxygen affinities with 'left shifted' oxygen dissociation curves, and hence are associated with impaired unloading of oxygen to the tissues.

Methaemoglobinaemia

Methaemoglobinaemia causes a variable degree of cyanosis and should be thought of in any patient with significant central cyanosis in whom there is no evidence of cardiorespiratory disease. The degree of cyanosis produced by 5 g/dl of deoxygenated haemoglobin can be produced by 1.5 g/dl methaemoglobin and 0.5 g/dl of sulphaemoglobin. Methaemoglobin concentrations of 10–20 per cent are tolerated quite well but, because it is useless as an oxygen carrier, levels above this are often associated with dyspnoea and headache. Much depends on the rapidity at which it is formed; many patients with lifelong methaemoglobinaemia are asymptommatic while individuals who have accumulated a similar level of methaemoglobin acutely after exposure to drugs or toxins may be acutely dyspnoeic. For reasons which are not clear it is unusual for patients with chronic methaemoglobinaemia to have an increased haemoglobin level or red cell count.

Methaemoglobinaemia may arise as a result of a genetic defect in red cell metabolism or haemoglobin structure, or may be acquired following the ingestion of various oxidant drugs and toxic agents.

Genetic methaemoglobinaemia

There are two forms of inherited methaemoglobinaemia. The first results from a deficiency of red cell NADH-diaphorase, the second from a structural alteration in either the α or β globin chains of haemoglobin.

NADH-diaphorase catalyses a step in the major pathway for methaemoglobin reduction. The enzyme reduces cytochrome b^5 using NADH as a hydrogen donor. The reduced cytochrome b^5 reduces, in turn, methaemoglobin to haemoglobin. There are several different molecular forms of *NADH-diaphorase deficiency* which have been identified by electrophoretic analysis of NADH-diaphorase in the red cells of affected patients. The condition is inherited as an autosomal recessive. Homozygotes have elevated levels of methaemoglobin and are cyanosed from birth. Heterozygotes do not have elevated levels of methaemoglobin but seem to be unusually susceptible to the oxidant action of drugs. For example, severe cyanosis has been precipitated in heterozygotes for NADH-diaphorase deficiency by the use of antimalarial drugs.

There are several abnormal haemoglobin variants which are associated with genetic methaemoglobinaemia, all of which are designated *haemoglobin M*, and further identified by their place of discovery, e.g. haemoglobin M Boston, M Milwaukee, etc. These varients usually result from amino acid substitutions near the haem pocket. Normally, haem lies between two histidine residues, one called the proximal histidine to which it is attached and the other called the distal histidine. Oxygen is bound to haem at a site opposite to the distal histidine. If the latter is substituted by tyrosine, as occurs in the α chain variant haemoglobin M Boston and in the β chain variant M Saskatoon, for example, a stable bond is formed between the haem iron and the phenolic ring of the tyrosine, and the iron atom is 'fixed' in the Fe^3 state. These haemoglobin variants are associated with cyanosis which is present from early life. In the case of the α chain variants it is present from birth, while the β chain haemoglobin variants only produce cyanosis after the first few months of life as adult haemoglobin synthesis becomes established. Unlike NADH-diaphorase deficiency, which is inherited as a recessive, the haemoglobin Ms have a dominant form of inheritance. Thus it is very simple to make the diagnosis of genetic methaemoglobinaemia and to determine the likely molecular basis by taking a good history; even the affected globin chain can be ascertained!

The diagnosis is confirmed by spectroscopic examination of the blood and by determination of methaemoglobin levels. The precise cause can be established by an assay of NADH-diaphorase or by haemoglobin analysis under appropriate conditions.

Genetic methaemoglobinaemia due to NADH-diaphorase deficiency is readily treated by the administration of ascorbic acid 300–600 mg daily by mouth in divided doses, or by the administation of methylene blue, either intravenously (1 mg/kg body weight) or by mouth, 60 mg three to four times daily. On the other hand, the genetic methaemoglobinaemias due to structural haemoglobin variants do not respond to ascorbic acid, methylene blue or any other treatment. In fact most affected individuals go through life asymptomatic and require no treatment.

Acquired methaemoglobinaemia

Acquired methaemoglobinaemia usually results from the administration of drugs or exposure to chemicals which cause oxidation of haemoglobin. There are many agents which are capable of exceeding the red cells' ability to reduce methaemoglobin. They include ferricyanide, bivalent copper, chromate, chlorate, quinones, and certain dyes with a high oxidation–reduction potential. Nitrite, often used as a preservative, is one of the most common methaemoglobin-forming agents and nitrates, after conversion to nitrites in the gut, may cause serious methaemoglobinaemia in infants. Other agents which commonly cause methaemoglobinaemia include phenacetin, primiquin, sulphonamides, and various aniline dye derivatives.

If any of the agents listed above is given in a low dose over a long period of time it may lead to chronic methaemoglobinaemia with or without a haemolytic anaemia. However, after exposure to a large amount of these agents, and the development of in excess of 50–60 per cent methaemoglobin, the symptoms of acute anaemia develop because methaemoglobin lacks the capacity to transport oxygen. Thus the clinical picture may be characterized by vascular collapse, coma, and death.

Methaemoglobinaemia with haemolytic anaemia

The haemolytic action of oxidant drugs is described later (page 19.147). Chronic methaemoglobinaemia with haemolytic anaemia characterized by Heinz body formation and fragmented red cells occurs commonly in patients receiving dapsone, salazopyrine, or phenacetin. This condition is usually innocuous and can be modified by adjusting the dose of the drug.

Occasionally, acute intravascular haemolysis associated with methaemoglobinaemia and intravascular coagulation occurs and may lead to renal failure. It usually follows the ingestion or infusion of a strong oxidizing agent such as chlorate or arsine. There is gross intravascular haemolysis and methaemoglobinaemia together with evidence of disseminated intravasular coagulation. The haemoglobin level may fall very rapidly and the condition may be complicated by renal failure.

Treatment

In cases of chronic acquired methaemoglobinaemia, the drug or chemical agent should be removed where possible. If continued therapy is required, it should be administered at a lower dose.

Acute toxic methaemoglobinaemia may present a serious medical emergency. Methylene blue should be administered in a dose of 1–2 mg per kg intravenously over a five-minute period. Repeated doses may be needed. Toxicity is uncommon although doses of over 15 mg per kg may cause haemolysis in young infants. The drug should not be used if the methaemoglobinaemia is due to chlorate poisoning as it may convert the chlorate to hypochlorite which is an even more toxic compound.

In those cases in which there is acute methaemoglobinaemia with intravascular haemolysis, haemodialysis with exchange transfusion is the treatment of choice.

Carboxyhaemoglobinaemia

Carbon monoxide (CO) has an affinity for haemoglobin approximately 210 times that of oxygen. Following acute exposure it is so tightly bound that it takes about four hours for an individual with normal ventilation to expel half of it. At levels of 5–10 per cent there may be no symptoms, but above 20 per cent there is usually headache and weakness. Levels of 40–60 per cent or more lead to unconsciousness and death.

Carbon monoxide poisoning is discussed in Section 6 and secondary polycythaemia due to chronic exposure is considered later in this Section (page 19.155).

Sulphaemoglobinaemia

This poorly-defined condition derives its name from the fact that it can be produced *in vitro* by the action of hydrogen sulphide on haemoglobin. It has not been reported as a genetic disorder and is usually associated with the administration of drugs, particularly sulphonamides or phenacetin. It has also been reported in patients with chronic constipation or malabsorption syndromes (*enterogenous cyanosis*) although its relationship to these disorders is far from clear.

Other acquired abnormalities of the structure or synthesis of haemoglobin

Glycosylated haemoglobin, haemoglobin Alc

Haemoglobin may undergo post translational modification in patients with diabetes. The abnormal haemoglobin, haemoglobin Alc, is formed by the non-enzymic combination of glucose with the N-terminus of the β chain, forming first a Schiff base which then undergoes a rearrangement to form a stable ketoamine. The level of haemoglobin Alc is raised in diabetics and is related to the blood sugar level over the previous weeks. The value of the estimation of haemoglobin Alc as an index of the control of diabetes is considered in Section 9.

Haemoglobin Pb

Some children with lead poisoning develop a modified haemoglobin which migrates rapidly on alkaline electrophoresis. The precise structural alteration is not known but, if present, this variant is a useful indicator of severe lead poisoning.

Haemoglobin H and mental retardation

A syndrome has been described which is comprised of mental retardation and the presence of the haematological changes of haemoglobin H disease or $\alpha°$ thalassaemia. Recent work suggests that this is an acquired disorder and that at least in some cases, defective α chain production is due to a large deletion of the α globin gene complex which is probably acquired in the parental germ cells and which may be associated with the retarded development seen in affected children. The condition is characterized by the haematological changes of $\alpha°$ thalassaemia or haemoglobin H disease, a variable degree of impaired intellectual development, and mild skeletal deformities of the feet with retardation of the descent of the testes.

Haemoglobin H and leukaemia

It is becoming apparent that a number of elderly patients may develop a cell line containing haemoglobin H during the course of the evolution of a myeloproliferative disorder or acute leukaemia. The mechanism is unknown. The presence of haemoglobin H or haemoglobin H inclusions in an elderly patient should raise the suspicion of a preleukaemic disorder.

Fetal haemoglobin production in adult life

A number of haematological disorders are associated with a reversion to fetal haemoglobin production after the neonatal period. These include juvenile myeloid leukaemia, other forms of leukaemia, and congenital hypoplastic anaemias. Haemoglobin F may also appear transitorily during rapid regeneration of the bone marrow after drug-induced hypoplasia, virus infection, or bone marrow transplantation.

References

Alter, B. P. (1984). Review: Advances in the prenatal diagnosis of hematologic disease. *Blood* **64**, 329–340.

Bellingham, A. J. (1976). Haemoglobins with altered oxygen affinity. *Br. Med. Bull.* **32**, 234–238.

Bookchin, R. M. and Lew, V. L. (1983). Red cell membrane abnormalities in sickle cell anemia. In *Progress in hematology* XIII (ed. E. B. Brown), pp. 1–24. Grune and Stratton, New York.

Bunn, H. F. and Forget, B. G. (1985). *Human hemoglobins* 2nd edn. W. B. Saunders, Philadelphia.

Dickerson, R. E. and Geis, I. (1983). *Hemoglobin*. The Benjamin/Cummings Publishing Company, Inc., Menlo Park, California.

Emerson, P. M. and Grimes, A. J. (1982). Red cell metabolism: hereditary enzymopathies. In *Blood and its disorders* 2nd edn (eds R. M. Hardisty and D. J. Weatherall), pp. 265–321. Blackwell Scientific Publications, Oxford.

Huehns, E. R. (1982). The structure and function of haemoglobin: clinical disorders due to abnormal haemoglobin structure. In *Blood and its disorders* 2nd edn (eds R. M. Hardisty and D. J. Weatherall), pp. 323–400. Blackwell Scientific Publications, Oxford.

Jaffe, R. (1981). Methaemoglobinaemia. *Clin. Haemat.* **10**, 99–122.

Milner, P. F. (1981) The clinical effects of Hb S: An overview. In *Progress in clinical and biological research*, Vol. 51, *The functions of red blood cells: Erythrocyte Pathobiology* (ed. D. F. H. Wallach), pp. 297–320. Alan R. Liss, Inc., New York.

Modell, C. B. (1977). Total management of thalassaemic major. *Arch. Dis. Child.* **52**, 489–497.

Nienhuis, A. W., Anagnou, N. P. and Ley, T. J. (1984). Review: advances in thalassemia research. *Blood* **63**, 738–758.

Orkin, S. H., Antonarakis, S. E. and Kazazian, H. H. (1983). Polymorphism and molecular pathology of the human beta-gene. In *Progress in hematology* XIII (ed. E. B. Brown), pp. 49–74. Grune and Stratton, New York.

Serjeant, G. R. (1985). *Sickle cell disease.* Oxford University Press, Oxford.

Taramelli, R., Grosveld, F. and Wright, S. (1985). The human β-globin genes. *Oxford Surveys on Eukaryotic Genes* **2**, 1–24.

Urbanetti, J. S. (1981). Carbon monoxide poisoning. In *Progress in clinical and biological research*, Vol. 51, *The functions of red blood cells: erythrocyte pathobiology*. (ed. D. F. H. Wallach), pp. 355–386. Alan R. Liss, Inc., New York.

Warth, J. A. and Rucknagel, D. L. (1983). The increasing complexity of sickle cell anemia. In *Progress in hematology*, XIII (ed. E. B. Brown), pp. 25–48. Grune and Stratton, New York.

Weatherall, D. J. (1985). Prenatal diagnosis of inherited blood diseases. *Clin. Haematol.* **14**, 747–774.

—— (1986). The regulation of the differential expression of the human globin genes during development. *J. Cell Sci.* Suppl. 4, 319–336.

—— and Clegg, J. B. (1981). *The thalassaemia syndromes* 3rd edn. Blackwell Scientific Publications, Oxford.

——, Higgs, D. R., Clegg, J. B. and Wood, W. G. (1982). Annotation. The significance of haemoglobin H disease in patients with mental retardation or myeloproliferative disease. *Br. J. Haemat.* **52**, 351–355.

—— and Wainscoat, J. S. (1985). The molecular pathology of thalassaemia. In *Recent advances in haematology*, Vol. 4 (ed. A. V. Hoffbrand), pp. 63–88. Churchill Livingstone, Edinburgh.

White, J. M. (1976). The unstable haemoglobins. *Br. Med. Bull.* **32**, 219–222.

World Health Organization (1983). Community control of hereditary anaemias. *Bull WHO* **61**, 63–80.

Other anaemias resulting from defective red cell maturation

D. J. WEATHERALL

In the previous sections we have considered anaemias which result from a reduced output of red cells due either to a lack of specific factors which are required for the nuclear or cytoplasmic maturation of their precursors, or from well-defined genetic defects of haemoglobin synthesis. However, in addition to these conditions there are other dyserythropoietic anaemias which are caused by either genetic or acquired disorders of red cell maturation but in which the precise defect is, as yet, unknown (Table 1).

Although the anaemias which are described in the following sections form a very diverse group, they have one major feature in common. In each case the marrow is able to respond to an increased output of erythropoietin by proliferation of its red cell precursors. However, because maturation is defective many of these cells are destroyed before they reach the circulation. This process results in a haematological picture characterized by erythroid hyperplasia of the bone marrow associated with a low and inappropriate reticulocyte response in the blood, a combination of findings which is the hallmark of *ineffective erythropoiesis*.

Table 1 Anaemias in which defective red cell maturation and increased ineffective erythropoiesis is a major factor

---

Abnormality of DNA synthesis
    Vitamin B$_{12}$ deficiency
    Folate deficiency
    Drugs (antipurines, antipyrimidines)

Defective cytoplasmic maturation
    Disorders of globin synthesis
        Thalassaemia
    Disorders of haem and/or iron metabolism
        Sideroblastic anaemia

Unknown mechanism
    Congenital dyserythropoietic anaemias
    Myelodysplastic syndrome (see page 19.58)
    Infection
    Chemicals and toxins (see page 19.46 on aplastic anaemia)

Table 2 The sideroblastic anaemias

Congenital
    X-linked
    ? others
Acquired
    Primary or idiopathic
    Secondary
        Drugs—INAH, chloramphenicol, etc.
        Alcohol
        Lead
        Malabsorption
        Myeloproliferative disorders
        Leukaemia
        Secondary carcinoma
        Other systemic disorders

The sideroblastic anaemias

The sideroblastic anaemias are a group of genetic or acquired disorders characterized by severe dyserythropoieses and marked iron loading of the red cell precursors and, in some cases, widespread haemosiderosis (Table 2).

Definition

The term sideroblastic anaemia is an unfortunate one. Normal red cell precursors are sideroblasts in that they contain small aggregations of ferritin iron scattered throughout the cytoplasm. These remain in the cells until they reach the peripheral blood after which they are removed in the spleen. Red cells which contain iron-staining granules, siderocytes, are only seen in the blood after splenectomy. In the sideroblastic anaemias there is an *abnormal* accumulation of iron in the erythroblasts. Much of the excess iron is situated in the mitochondria which lie in a circle round the nucleus of the red cell precursors, and hence on staining with Prussian blue or other iron stains, a ring or collar of heavy iron granules is seen in the perinuclear region (Fig. 1). Such red cell precursors are called abnormal or 'ring' sideroblasts and are the characteristic feature of all the sideroblastic anaemias. The iron loading of the mitochondria can be easily seen on electron microscopy (Fig. 2).

Aetiology and pathogenesis

The underlying aetiology of the sideroblastic anaemias has not been completely worked out. It is clear that there is a variable defect in erythroid maturation with intramedullary destruction of red cell precursors and a considerable degree of ineffective erythropoiesis. It is believed that the marked accumulation of iron, and the mitochondrial damage which results from this process, plays an important role in this maturation defect. Whether this is the

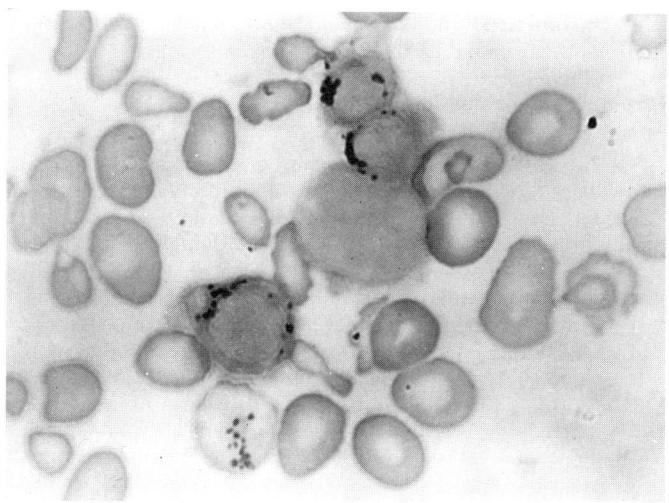

Fig. 1 Bone marrow treated with a stain specific for iron showing typical ring sideroblasts (× 800).

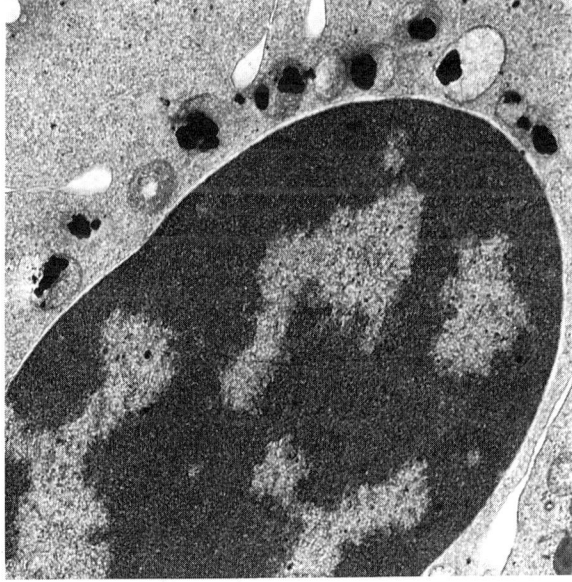

Fig. 2 Iron loading of the mitochondria in the perinuclear region in sideroblastic anaemia (electron microscopy × 20 000). (Reproduced by permission of Professor S. Wickramasinghe.)

primary abnormality in sideroblastic anaemia is uncertain, however.

The sideroblastic anaemias are all characterized by the curious anomaly of hypochromic red cells together with iron loading of their precursors. This suggests that there is underlying abnormality of haemoglobin synthesis and it is currently believed that at least some forms of sideroblastic anaemia may result from defective haem production. There is some evidence that the rate of iron movement into red cell precursors is regulated, at least to some degree, by the level of haem in the cells and, therefore, if there is a defect in haem synthesis, there may be increased movement of iron into the developing red cells. The synthetic pathway for the production of haem is summarized in Fig. 3. Two of the enzymes in the pathway, δ-amino laevulinic acid synthetase (ALA synthetase) and haem synthetase, are mitochondrial enzymes while the others are found in the cytoplasmic compartment of the red cell precursors. Pyridoxyl phosphate is an important co-factor for the early step in haem synthesis in which succinate and glycine con-

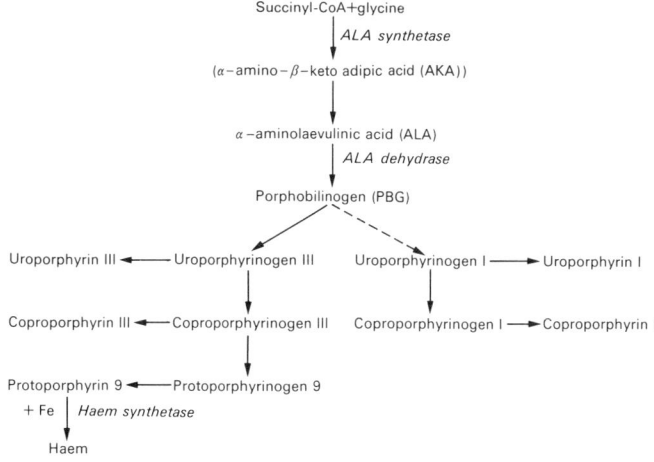

Fig. 3 The metabolic pathway for the synthesis of haem.

dense with the production of δ-amino laevulinic acid. In some of the genetic forms of sideroblastic anaemia a deficiency of ALA synthetase or haem synthetase has been demonstrated, although because these are mitochondrial enzymes, and because the mitochondria are probably damaged by excess iron, it is not clear whether the enzyme deficiency is the primary defect or whether abnormal iron loading and mitochondrial damage causes a secondary reduction in the activity of these enzymes.

In some forms of sideroblastic anaemia specific mitochondrial toxins can be implicated. These include chloramphenicol, phenacetin, and paracetamol. The sideroblastic anaemia of lead poisoning probably results from inhibition of ALA synthetase and haem synthetase by the action of lead. Agents such as alcohol and some of the antituberculous drugs may interfere with pyridoxine metabolism and hence with the early steps of haem synthesis.

In some of the primary idiopathic sideroblastic anaemias there is evidence that the disorder results from the proliferation of a clone of abnormal stem cells. They are thus considered to be part of the myelodysplastic syndrome (page 19.58).

Clearly, the sideroblastic anaemias have a heterogeneous basis and in no case has the underlying defect been defined precisely. The interesting possibility remains that at least some of these disorders result from a primary abnormality in iron transport and that the reported enzyme defects and haem deficiency are secondary to mitochondrial damage consequent upon iron loading.

The sideroblastic anaemias are a good example of what have been called 'iron loading anaemias'. In most anaemias in which there is marked erythroid hyperplasia *and* ineffective erythropoiesis, there is an increased rate of gastrointestinal iron absorption. This occurs in the thalassaemias (see page 19.113), sideroblastic anaemias, and in other dyserythropoietic disorders. The reason why patients with these conditions, who often have increased iron stores, continue to iron load is not clear. Ultimately they may develop generalized haemosiderosis with endocrine, liver, and cardiac damage (see page 19.89).

The genetic sideroblastic anaemias

These are extremely rare conditions. In most cases they follow a sex-linked pattern of inheritance with males showing anaemia and female carriers only mild morphological changes of their red cells. More severely affected females have been encountered, however. This may reflect variability of X-chromosome inactivation or genetic heterogeneity of the disorder. The anaemia usually appears in early childhood, although presentation later in life has been well documented.

The condition is characterized by a mild to moderate anaemia with haemoglobin values in the 6–9 g/dl range, and there is usually some degree of splenomegaly (Table 3). The peripheral blood film

Table 3 Clinical and haematological features of sideroblastic anaemia

Congenital	Acquired
Mainly males	Both sexes
Mild splenomegaly	Splenomegaly unusual unless part of a myeloproliferate disorder
Dimorphic blood picture with an extremely hypochromic population	Dimorphic blood picture; usually a population of moderately hypochromic cells
Reduced MCH and MCV	MCV often normal or increased and MCH normal or slightly reduced
Marrow hyperplasia with large percentage of ring sideroblasts	Marrow hyperplasia, normal cellularity, or hypoplasia; variable numbers of ring sideroblasts
Platelets and white cells normal	White cells usually normal; platelets reduced in 30% of cases; occasionally increased
Red cell protoporphyrin reduced	Red cell protoporphyrin elevated
Hb A_2 reduced, Hb F normal	Hb A_2 reduced or normal. Hb F normal

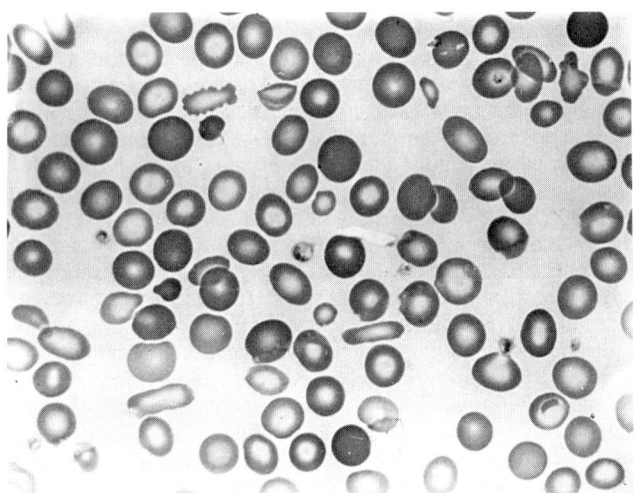

Fig. 4 Genetically determined sideroblastic anaemia. The peripheral blood film shows a dimorphic population with both normochromic and misshapen hypochromic microcytic red cells ($\times$ 800, Leishman stain).

shows hypochromic cells interspersed with a normochromic population (Fig. 4). The bone marrow shows erythroid hyperplasia with abnormal nuclear and cytoplasmic maturation and the presence of a large proportion of ring sideroblasts. The red cell protoporphyrin level is usually reduced.

In the typically X-linked form the mother of affected sons shows small numbers of hypochromic cells mixed in a predominantly normochromic population and a few ring sideroblasts in the bone marrow. Some, but not all patients with this disorder, show progressive iron loading as they grow older with a steady increase in serum iron and ferritin values. Ultimately, they may develop generalized haemosiderosis which may lead to diabetes, liver disease, and progressive cardiac failure.

There may be two other subgroups of hereditary sideroblastic anaemia, one characterized by a full haematological response to pyridoxine, and another in which there are increased levels of coproporphyrin and decreased levels of protoporphyrin in the red

cells. The latter condition has been called '*anaemia hypochromica sideroblastica hereditaria*' by European haematologists.

Acquired sideroblastic anaemia
Primary
By far the commonest form of acquired sideroblastic anaemia is the primary idiopathic type for which no underlying cause can be identified. This condition occurs equally in males and females and usually presents after the age of 50 years although the author has seen several cases presenting in early childhood. There is usually a mild degree of anaemia, and splenomegaly occurs in only a small proportion of cases. The haematological changes are characterized by haemoglobin values in the 7–10 g/dl range and a 'dimorphic' blood film with both normochromic and hypochromic populations of red cells. The red cell indices are often abnormal with an increased MCV in the 100–120 fl range. The platelet count is usually normal, but both thrombocytosis and thrombocytopenia have been observed. The bone marrow shows marked erythroid hyperplasia and the presence of increased numbers of ring sideroblasts.

Many patients with this condition run a long course with chronic anaemia as the only abnormal finding. In some cases there is a steady increase in the serum iron and ferritin values, and occasionally generalized haemosiderosis may occur with the development of diabetes, liver damage, and cardiac failure. A small proportion of patients develop leukaemia after many years of what appears to be a primary sideroblastic anaemia (see page 19.58 *et seq.*).

Secondary
In some individuals with acquired sideroblastic anaemia it is possible to demonstrate exposure to toxins or drugs. One of the commonest causes of the condition, certainly in the United States although less frequently in the United Kingdom, is acute alcoholic intoxication. These patients are usually seen following a very high intake of alcohol and their blood films are dimorphic with marked macrocytosis; the bone marrow shows both dyserythropoietic and megaloblastic changes and variable numbers of ring sideroblasts. There is a high incidence of associated folic acid deficiency (see page 19.97).

The antituberculous drugs, isoniazid, cycloserine, and pyrazinamide, given either alone or in combination, occasionally cause a secondary sideroblastic anaemia. The actual incidence of anaemia in patients receiving these drugs is low although several studies have shown that a high proportion of them have ring sideroblasts in their bone marrows. Isoniazid therapy is frequently associated with sideroblastic changes in the marrow but severe anaemia is rare. In contrast, cycloserine and pyrazinamide quite often produce anaemia with sideroblastic changes. Choloramphenicol also causes sideroblastic anaemia in a small proportion of patients. A sideroblastic reaction is seen commonly in patients with lead poisoning who are anaemic and who also have basophilic stippling of their red cells. There have been occasional reports of the association of sideroblastic anaemia with other drugs, phenacetin and paracetamol for example, but there has usually been evidence of associated haemolytic anaemia and folate deficiency.

Finally, sideroblastic changes are occasionally seen in a diverse series of systemic diseases. Among the non-haematological disorders in which a few ring sideroblasts occur are infections, hypothyroidism, rheumatoid arthritis, and collagen-vascular diseases. Among the haematological disorders in which ring sideroblasts are found are listed various haemolytic anaemias, pernicious anaemia, folic acid deficiency, different forms of leukaemia, myeloma, lymphoma, and the myeloproliferative diseases. In all these conditions the presence of ring sideroblasts is unexplained and the associated anaemia is clearly related to the underlying disorder rather than to the sideroblastic reaction.

There appears to be a distinct group of patients with sideroblastic anaemia who respond well to pyridoxine. Although, as mentioned earlier, many patients with acquired sideroblastic anaemia show some biochemical evidence of abnormal pyridoxine metabolism, the majority of them do not respond well to pyridoxyl phosphate. There are scattered reports of individuals who did have a full haematological response however, and whose haemoglobin values fell after withdrawal of pyridoxine. Whether this represents a separate and aetiologically distinct group of sideroblastic anaemias remains to be determined. True pyridoxine-deficiency has been reported in a few patients with an underlying malabsorption syndrome. Both the sideroblastic changes and the steatorrhoea remitted on a gluten-free diet.

The diagnosis of sideroblastic anaemia

The sideroblastic anaemias are often missed because the morphological appearances of the red cells are not adequately examined. Most of these conditions are associated with a moderate degree of anaemia but the red cell indices may be confusing. In the genetic group they usually show an overall hypochromic and microcytic picture with low MCH and MCV values, but in the acquired sideroblastic anaemias there may be a macrocytosis. The striking feature of all these conditions is the dimorphic blood picture with normochromic *and* hypochromic cells which, except in patients who are recovering from iron deficiency anaemia after iron therapy, is not seen in any other disorder. This haematological picture should always be followed by a bone marrow examinaton and a search for ring sideroblasts by appropriate staining techniques. The diagnosis of primary or secondary sideroblastic anaemia rests on the determination of exposure to drugs, lead, or other toxins, and the presence or absence of another general systemic or haematological disorder.

Treatment

The genetic sideroblastic anaemias usually require no treatment. It is worth giving a trial of pyridoxine (see below) although in most cases there is no response. Secondary folate deficiency should be excluded and the patient should be followed up carefully with regular serum iron and ferritin estimations. If there is evidence of iron accumulation, it is worth starting on a programme of regular venesections or, if the patient cannot tolerate this approach, using a chelating agent such as desferrioxamine (see page 19.90).

In the acquired sideroblastic anaemias a careful search for an underlying cause should be carried out. Particular care should be taken to obtain a good drug history and any evidence of exposure to toxins. Once an underlying disease has been excluded, these patients simply require regular surveillance. The haemoglobin level may remain constant for many years and no treatment is required. It is worth trying a course of pyridoxine and high doses in the order of 25–100 mg or even larger thrice daily may be required to obtain a haematological response. In the majority of cases this type of therapy produces either no response or a short-lived reticulocytosis with no increase in the haemoglobin level. Trials of pyridoxal phosphate have been found to be equally unsuccessful. It is important to rule out secondary folate deficiency by measuring the serum folate level, and, if this is low, folic acid should be administered. Splenectomy seems to have little place in the treatment of either genetic or acquired sideroblastic anaemia. Finally, if patients become symptomatic they should receive regular blood transfusions. In all cases of sideroblastic anaemia, whether under regular surveillance on no treatment or on regular transfusion therapy, it is important to monitor the serum iron and ferritin levels. If evidence of iron overload is obtained, these patients should be treated with desferrioxamine along the lines outlined on page 19.90. It is doubtful if adults require subcutaneous administration of the drug with a portable pump, but regular bolus injections should be given and the response monitored by measuring the urinary iron excretion. Suitable dose regimens are shown in Table 6 on page 19.121.

In the secondary sideroblastic anaemias due to drug therapy the drug should be stopped where possible. The management of lead poisoning is described in Section 6.

Other rare dyserythropoietic anaemias

To complete this review of anaemias due to defective erythropoiesis we must briefly describe some uncommon forms of congenital and acquired dyserythropoietic anaemia.

Congenital dyserythropoietic anaemias

In recent years a group of disorders called congenital dyserythropoietic anaemias (CDA) have been defined by their bizarre red cell precursor morphology and associated serological findings. These conditions usually although not always present early in life with anaemia and unusual red cell changes characterized by anisopoikilocytosis and, sometimes, macrocytosis. Bone marrow examination shows marked erythroid hyperplasia, the most striking feature being multinuclearity of the red cell precursors. The fact there is a very poor reticulocyte response indicates that these are primarily dyserythropoietic anaemias.

Several types of CDA are recognized. In Type 1 there are megaloblastoid erythroblasts with internuclear chromatin-bridge formation, i.e. the cell nuclei are incompletely separated from each other. Type 2 is characterized by erythroblastic multinuclearity and a positive acid-serum lysis test using the sera of some but not all individuals, and not (in contrast to paroxysmal nocturnal haemoglobinurea, see page 19.57) when using the patient's serum. This disorder has been called HEMPAS – Hereditary Erythroblastic Multinuclearity with Positive Acid Serum lysis. Type 3 CDA is characterized by erythroblast multinuclearity with large, abnormal erythroblasts which have been called gigantoblasts. At the time of writing the form of genetic transmission and underlying cellular defects in this group of disorders have not been determined and they can only be defined on morphological or serological grounds associated, in some cases, with a family history.

Acquired refractory anaemia with hyperplastic bone marrow

Occasionally, patients are encountered with mild to moderate anaemia whose marrows show a marked erythroid hyperplasia and dyserythropoiesis. When presented with such a problem the first step is to rule out easily identifiable causes as vitamin B_{12} or folate deficiency and the various genetic and acquired dyserythropoietic states defined earlier in this section. However, in some cases no obvious cause can be found and the condition falls into no clear-cut category. It should be remembered that severe dyserythropoiesis can occur in aplastic anaemia, myelosclerosis, or in association with certain infections such as chronic malaria. However, when these conditions have been ruled out there is a group of patients whose marrows show marked erythroid hyperplasia with dyserythropoiesis as evidenced by asynchrony of nuclear and cytoplasmic maturation of the red cell precursors, mild megaloblastic changes, mitotic abnormalities including nuclear fragmentation, karyorrhexis (abnormal lobulation of the nuclei), and binuclearity. Sometimes these changes are associated with a reduced white cell and platelet count and morphological abnormalities of the white cell and platelet precursors. In some cases the red cells show an increase in i-reactivity and there is an elevated level of haemoglobin F. (The i-antigen is normally expressed only on fetal erythrocytes.) In some patients with this variety of anaemia, acute leukaemia develops months or years after the onset.

Recently, it has become the custom to classify these disorders as part of the myelodysplastic syndrome, and to try to subclassify them further according to associated abnormalities of the white cells and platelets together with cytogenetic analysis. This syndrome is considered under the section on stem cell disorders (page 19.58). Whether all these conditions result from primary abnormalities of pluripotential haemopoietic stem cells, or whether at least some of them reflect defects in the marrow microenvironment, remains to be determined. In clinical practice it is important to identify these conditions as forming part of this syndrome, and, in particular, to rule out any of the treatable causes of dyserythropoiesis.

Dyserythropoiesis and infection

The haematological manifestations of infection are considered later in this chapter. The bone marrow response to infection has been a neglected area of haematology for many years. However, there is increasing evidence that dyserythropoiesis may occur in association with a variety of infections, particularly viral and parasitic. There have been sporadic reports of acute dyserythropoietic changes in the bone marrows of patients with severe bacterial infections although the incidence of this complication is uncertain. Similar changes may be found in patients with viral infections. The most extreme example of the association of viral infection and bone marrow damage is the recently described *virus haemophagocytic syndrome*. This disorder is usually seen in immune suppressed patients and is characterized by a rapidly progressive anaemia together with marked erythroid hyperplasia, dyserythropoiesis, and erythrophagocytosis of red cell precursors by bone marrow macrophages. Although little is known about the natural history of this disorder it seems to carry an extremely poor prognosis.

Dyserythropoiesis is also a feature of *Plasmodium falciparum* malaria infection. It is seen frequently in acute *P. falciparum* malaria infections in non-immune individuals and is also well documented in children with chronic malaria in West Africa. The bone marrows of these patients are often hyperplastic with marked abnormalities of red cell precursor maturation.

While, in general, very little is known about the bone marrow responses to infection it is becoming clear that in any severely ill patient with progressive anaemia in whom the marrow shows dyserythropoietic changes, an underlying infection should be suspected.

References

Galton, D. A. G. (1984). The myelodysplastic syndromes. *Clin. lab. Haemat.* **6**, 99–112.

Heimpel, H. (1976). Congenital dyserythropoietic anaemia type I: clinical and experimental aspects. In *Congenital disorders of erythropoiesis*, (eds R. Porter and D. W. Fitzsimons), Ciba Foundation Symposium 37, pp. 135–150. North-Holland, Amsterdam.

Hines, J. D. and Grasso, J. A. (1970). The sideroblastic anemias. *Sem. Hemat.* **7**, 86–106.

McKenna, R. W., Risdall, R. J. and Brunning, R. D. (1981). Virus associated hemophagocytic syndrome. *Hum. Path.* **12**, 395–398.

Mollin, D. L. (1965). A symposium on sideroblastic anaemia. Introduction: sideroblasts and sideroblastic anaemia. *Br. J. Haemat.* **11**, 41–48.

Peto, T. E. A., Pippard, M. J. and Weatherall, D. J. (1983). Iron overload in mild sideroblastic anaemia. *Lancet* **i**, 375–378.

Schafer, A. I., Cheron, R. G., Dluhy, R., Cooper, B., Gleason, R. E., Soeldner, J. S. and Bunn, H. F. (1981). Clinical consequences of acquired transfusional iron overload in adults. *N. Engl. J. Med.* **304**, 319–324.

Sokal, G., Michaux, J. L. and ven den Berghe, H. (1980). The karyotype in refractory anaemia and preleukaemia. *Clin. Haemat.* **9**, 129–140.

Verwilghen, R. L. (1976) Congenital dyserythropoietic anaemia type II (HEMPAS) In *Congenital disorders of erythropoiesis*, (eds R. Porter and D. W. Fitzsimons), Ciba Foundation Symposium 37, pp. 150–170. North-Holland, Amsterdam.

Valentine, W. N. (1983). Sideroblastic anemias. In *Hematology*, 3rd edn (eds W. J. Williams, E. Beutler, A. J. Erslev and M. A. Lichtman), pp. 537–546. McGraw-Hill, New York.

Weatherall, D. J. and Abdalla, S. (1982). The anaemia of *P. falciparum* malaria. *Br. Med. Bull.* **38**, 147–151.

White, J. M. and Nicholson, D. C. (1982). Haem and pyridoxine metabolism. In *Blood and its disorders*, 2nd edn (eds R. M. Hardisty and D. J. Weatherall), pp. 546–576. Blackwell Scientific Publications, Oxford.

Haemolytic anaemia

D. J. WEATHERALL AND E. C. GORDON-SMITH

Introduction

The normal red cell survives for approximately 120 days in the circulation. If its lifespan is significantly shortened, the red cell mass falls, relatively less oxygen is transported to the kidneys, and hence there is an increased output of erythropoietin which results in an increased rate of erythropoiesis. If the bone marrow is healthy, the red cell mass may be restored to normal in this way. This condition is called a *compensated haemolytic state*. If the marrow is healthy, the red cell survival can be reduced by as much as eight times without the development of significant anaemia. However, if the red cell survival time is less than 15 days even a healthy marrow cannot compensate and a *haemolytic anaemia* results. If the bone marrow is abnormal or if there is inadequate supply of iron or other agents required for red cell production, anaemia may result even if the red cell survival is considerably greater than 15 days.

The mechanisms and consequences of a shortened red cell survival

Before describing the different forms of haemolytic anaemia it is necessary to review briefly the mechanisms which cause a shortened red cell survival, the consequences of haemolysis, and the various compensatory mechanisms which are brought into action in order to attempt to restore the red cell mass to normal. The diagnosis of haemolytic anaemia depends on an understanding of these basic principles.

Haemolytic mechanisms

Premature destruction of red cells occurs either because the red cell membrane is abnormal in structure or function, the cells are subjected to excessive physical trauma in the circulation, or because they have become unusually rigid due to the precipitation or abnormal molecular configuration of haemoglobin (Table 1).

For a red cell to survive it must be capable of altering its shape to quite a remarkable degree as it passes through the microcirculation. This characteristic depends mainly on the surface-to-volume ratio of the red cell which is in turn related to the integrity of its

Table 1 Mechanisms of haemolysis

Mechanisms	Examples
Abnormalities or red cell membrane	
Genetic abnormality of membrane structure	Hereditary spherocytosis, elliptocytosis
Alteration in lipid constitution	Liver disease
Altered sulphydryl reactivity	Oxidant drugs
Altered properties resulting from interaction with complement or immunoglobulins	Immune haemolytic anaemia
Increased permeability, reduced plasticity	Glycolytic enzyme defects
Increased rigidity causing abnormal flow	
Aggregation of haemoglobin molecules	Sickle cell anaemia
Decreased solubility of haemoglobin	Haemoglobin C disease
Inclusion (Heinz) body formation	Thalassaemia, unstable haemoglobins, oxidant drugs
Direct physical trauma	
Direct external trauma	March and karate haemoglobinuria
Turbulent flow	Cardiac haemolytic anaemia
Cleavage by fibrin strands	Microangiopathic haemolytic anaemia

membrane. Normal red cell membrane function requires the production of energy for active transport of Na^+ and K^+ in and out of the cells and for maintenance of the membrane protein SH groups in a reduced state. It also depends on the constant renewal of membrane lipids for the preservation of a normal lipid composition. If these functions fail, the red cell tends to become spherical, i.e. it develops a small surface area relative to volume, and hence is not so easily deformed. This in turn leads to its selective sequestration in the spleen and other parts of the reticuloendothelial system. This is the type of haemolytic mechanism which occurs in genetic disorders of the red cell membrane such as hereditary spherocytosis, or in which there is a defect in its energy pathways. The membrane may also be damaged by interaction of antibodies on its surface with macrophages of the reticuloendothelial system or by the direct action of trauma, chemicals, bacteria, or parasites.

Direct trauma to the red cells may occur in several ways including turbulence created by cardiac valve prostheses, rigid fibrin strands in the microcirculation, or excessive pressure on body surfaces.

Red cells which contain abnormally aggregated or precipitated haemoglobin molecules become less deformable and may be damaged in the spleen or other parts of the microcirculation. This is the basis for the shortened red cell survival in the sickling and thalassaemia disorders. Precipitation of haemoglobin with the production of intracellular inclusions or Heinz bodies may result from the action of a variety of oxidant agents. Oxidative damage to the red cell may occur in several ways and the mechanisms are only partly understood. They include reduction in red cell glutathione levels, haemoglobin instability, generation of superoxides and other intermediates capable of causing peroxidation of the membrane lipids, deficiency of antioxidants such as vitamin E, and the accumulation of iron.

The site of red cell destruction depends on the type and degree of damage to the cells. For example, complement damaged cells develop large holes in their membrane and are destroyed in the circulation whereas IgG-coated cells are removed by interaction with macrophages in the reticuloendothelial elements of the spleen and liver. It should be remembered that the constant bombardment of the spleen by abnormal red cells results in splenomegaly, a phenomenon which is called 'work hypertrophy'. Thus many haemolytic anaemias are associated with progressive splenomegaly and secondary hypersplenism (see page 19.189).

The consequences of haemolysis

The haematological and biochemical changes which result from haemolysis reflect both compensatory mechanisms aimed at restoring the circulating red cell mass to normal, and the results of an increased rate of haemoglobin breakdown from the prematurely destroyed red cell population (Table 2).

Compensatory mechanisms

If there is a significant reduction in the circulating red cell mass, there is a compensatory increase in erythropoietin production from the kidney. Within a few days of the onset of haemolysis the reticulocyte count increases and erythroid hyperplasia of the bone marrow becomes measurable by a decrease in the myeloid/erythroid (M/E) ratio. If the haemolysis is sustained there is expansion of the erythroid marrow and within two to three months the rate of erythropoiesis may rise to 10–15 times normal. The increased rate of red cell production is reflected in the peripheral blood by a reticulocytosis and the presence of deep-blue staining macrocytes on the blood film. The reticulocytes are larger than normal and hence are called 'shift' or 'stress' reticulocytes; they may have skipped a terminal maturation division.

The increased rate of red cell turnover has some important consequences. There is a greater-than-normal demand for iron and folate. The spread of erythroid marrow down the long bones may lead to bone deformities similar to those observed in the severe dyserythropoietic anaemias (see page 19.113). If the haemolysis

Table 2 The main features of haemolytic anaemia

1 Increased red cell production
    Polychromasia
    Macrocytosis
    Reticulocytosis
    Erythroid hyperplasia; M/E ↓
    Increased folate requirements

2 Increased red cell destruction
    Bilirubin level raised
    Increased faecal and urinary urobilinogen
    Haptoglobin and haemopexin levels reduced
    Evidence of intravascular destruction:
        Methaemoglobinaemia
        Raised plasma haemoglobin
        Haemoglobinuria
        Haemosiderinuria

3 Short red cell survival
    Reduced $^{51}Cr\ t_{\frac{1}{2}}$

4 Secondary effects
    Splenomegaly
    Bone changes

has been present from early life, there is often extramedullary haemopoiesis in the spleen, liver, and lymph nodes.

Haemoglobin catabolism

After haemoglobin is liberated into the circulation, it is bound to haptoglobin, and haptoglobin/haemoglobin complex is rapidly removed into the reticuloendothelial system (Fig. 1). Since this process may occur more rapidly than the liver's capacity to produce haptoglobin, a reduction in the serum haptoglobin level provides an extremely sensitive index of intravascular haemolysis. Even when the haemolysis is primarily extravascular, the haptoglobin level tends to fall, possibly because there is a small leak of free haemoglobin into the circulation. If the binding capacity of haptoglobin is exceeded, haemoglobin appears in the plasma where it is degraded and the haem which is liberated binds to a β-glycoprotein called haemopexin. Normally, sufficient haptoglobin is present to bind 100–140 mg of haemoglobin per 100 ml of plasma. The normal concentration of haemopexin is approximately 80 mg/100 ml of plasma.

When the haemoglobin binding capacity of haptoglobin and the haem binding capacity of haemopexin is saturated, free haemoglobin appears in the plasma where it is rapidly oxidized to methaemoglobin, dissociated, and the haem bound to albumin to form methaemalbumin. The latter produces a dirty brown discoloration of the plasma. If there is severe intravascular haemolysis, haemoglobin may be liberated into the plasma in sufficient amounts to saturate its haptoglobin, haemopexin, and albumin binding capacities and hence may appear in the urine. This happens because tetrameric haemoglobin dissociates into $\alpha\beta$ dimers with a molecular weight of about 32 000. At a plasma haemoglobin level of 30 mg/dl or less no haemoglobin appears in the urine because it is reabsorbed in the proximal renal tubules. At levels in excess of this, free haemoglobin is found in the urine. Porphyrin and globin are rapidly catabolized in the renal tubular cells and much of the iron liberated is converted into haemosiderin. Cells containing the latter are cast off and appear in the urine; haemosiderinuria is the most reliable indication of chronic intravascular haemolysis.

There is increased production of bilirubin whenever the red cell survival is shortened. This is insoluble and is carried in the plasma bound to albumin. After conjugation in the liver cells it is excreted into the gut where it is converted by bacterial action to a group of compounds known collectively as faecal urobilinogen. Some is reabsorbed into the circulation and re-excreted via the enterohepatic circulation. However, being soluble these compounds pass through the glomeruli and appear in the urine as urinary urobilinogen where they can be demonstrated using Erlich's aldehyde

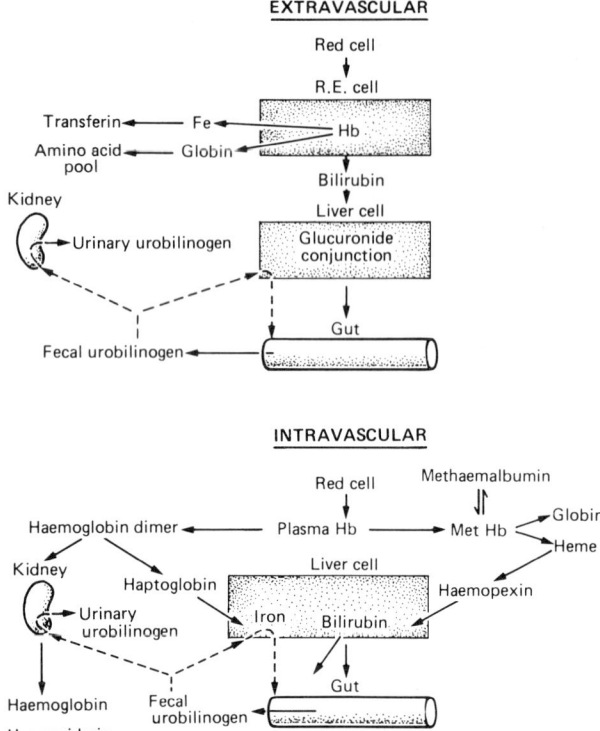

Fig. 1 Pathways of haemoglobin catabolism in haemolytic anaemia.

reagent. Thus in all haemolytic anaemias there is an increased production of faecal and urinary urobilinogen. Because the formation of the former is dependent on the bacterial state of the gut, its level is not a reliable indicator of the degree of haemolysis. Furthermore, faecal urobilinogen may be derived from ineffective erythropoiesis, i.e. direct breakdown of developing erythroid precursors in the marrow, rather than from the peripheral destruction of mature erythrocytes. Thus its level may be elevated in dyserythropoietic anaemias *as well* as in haemolytic anaemias.

Recognition of haemolysis

The clinical, haematological, and biochemical changes of haemolysis are easily understood if the principles outlined above have been followed. The degree of anaemia depends on the ability of the bone marrow to compensate by producing red cells at an increased rate, and the latter is recognized by the presence of deep-staining macrocytes on the blood film and by a variable reticulocytosis. The bone marrow shows variable erythroid hyperplasia with a decreased M/E ratio. There is an increased serum bilirubin level and serum haptoglobins are either reduced or absent. In the presence of severe intravascular haemolysis there may be free haemoglobin in the plasma and urine, and in all states of chronic intravascular haemolysis there is a variable degree of haemosiderinuria which can be identified by staining a spun-down urinary deposit with the Prussian blue reagent. In addition to these findings, which are present in all forms of severe haemolysis, there are specific morphological, serological, and biochemical changes of the red cells which accompany the different types of haemolytic anaemia and which are described in detail in later sections.

In the majority of haemolytic anaemias there is some enlargement of the spleen. In some cases it is useful to measure the red cell survival directly and to try to determine the site of red cell destruction. This is usually done by labelling a peripheral blood sample with ^{51}Cr, reinjecting the cells, and measuring the rate of disappearance of the labelled population. In clinical practice it is unnecessary to correct for elution of label from the cells and it is

Table 3   General approach to the diagnosis of haemolytic anaemia

1 Is there evidence of an increased rate of red cell production?
     Blood film—polychromasia; macrocytosis
     Reticulocyte count—elevated
     Marrow—erythroid hyperplasia

2 Is there evidence of an increased rate of red cell destruction?
     Bilirubin level—elevated
     Faecal and urinary urobilinogen—elevated
     Plasma haptoglobin and haemopexin—reduced
     ^{51}Cr $t_{\frac{1}{2}}$—reduced

3 Is the haemolysis mainly intravascular?
     Plasma haemoglobin—elevated
     Methaemalbumin—present
     Haemoglobinuria—present
     Haemosiderin in urine—present (if chronic)

4 Where are the red cells being destroyed?
     ^{51}Cr labelling and external counting

5 Why are the red cells being destroyed?
     Genetically determined
         Morphology spherocytes, ovalocytes, etc.
         Haemoglobin analysis
         Enzyme assay
     Acquired
         Immune — Coombs' test
         Non-immune — red cell morphology
         Associated disease
         Ham's test, etc.

usual to measure the time that it takes for 50 per cent of the label to disappear from the blood ($t_{\frac{1}{2}}$). The normal ^{51}Cr $t_{\frac{1}{2}}$ is 20–25 days. By using external counting and taking measurements over the heart as a background, it is possible to compare the rate of accumulation of radioactivity over the spleen and liver and to determine which site is most active in destruction of red cells. These data are usually converted to a simple spleen/liver radioactivity ratio. These procedures are usually carried out when splenectomy is contemplated, but otherwise are not often required for the recognition of haemolysis, which is based on the simple haematological and biochemical analyses outlined above.

An approach to the clinical and laboratory diagnosis of haemolysis is summarized in Table 3.

Classification of the haemolytic anaemias

The haemolytic anaemias are usually classified into two main groups: (*a*) genetically determined, and (*b*) acquired (Table 4). Like all biological classifications this is imperfect. For example, although certain genetically determined red cell enzyme defects lead to haemolysis, they may require the action of an external agent such as a drug or toxin before a haemolytic episode occurs. Despite this difficulty it is convenient to describe the different clinical forms of haemolytic anaemia under these two main headings.

The inherited haemolytic anaemias

The main groups of inherited haemolytic anaemias are summarized in Table 4. These disorders result from inherited defects in either the red cell membrane, the red cell enzyme systems, or the structure or synthethis of haemoglobin.

DISORDERS OF THE RED CELL MEMBRANE

The structure and function of the red cell membrane is described on page 19.64. There are a number of inherited haemolytic anaemias which are thought to be due to structural changes of the red cell membrane. As knowledge about the structure and organiz-

Table 4 Main groups of haemolytic anaemias

Genetic disorders of the red cell
  Membrane
    Hereditary spherocytosis
    Hereditary ovalocytosis
    Stomatocytosis
    Pyropoikilocytosis
    Other 'leaky' membrane disorders
    ?March haemoglobinuria
    Acanthocytosis
  Haemoglobin
    Sickling disorders
    Haemoglobins C, D, and E
    Unstable haemoglobins
    Thalassaemia syndromes
  Energy pathways
    Hexose-monophosphate shunt
    Embden–Meyerhof pathway
    Others
Acquired disorders of the red cell
  Immune
    Isoimmune; Rh or ABO incompatibility
    Autoimmune; warm or cold antibodies
  Non-immune
    Trauma
      Microangiopathy
      Valve prosthesis
      Body surface
    Membrane defects; PNH, liver disease
    Parasitic disorders
    Bacterial infection
    Physical agents, drugs, and chemicals
    Hypersplenism
    Defective red cell maturation

ation of the membrane has increased over the last few years it has been possible to make a start in determining the molecular basis for at least some of these conditions.

Hereditary spherocytosis

Hereditary spherocytosis (HS) is a form of familial haemolytic anaemia characterized by the presence of small spherocytic red cells in the peripheral blood. It occurs with a frequency of approximately 200–300 per million of the population of the United States and United Kingdom. It is inherited as an autosomal dominant. Several studies have attempted to define the chromosomal location of its genetic determinant. Although the short arm of chromosome 12, and in one family chromosome 14, have been possible candidates, its precise assignation remains to be clarified.

Aetiology

Despite many years of work the precise defect of the HS cell remains elusive. The membranes of HS cells have a diminished phospholipid and cholesterol content. This is presumably due to the loss of membrane from the cells which leads to a decrease in their surface-to-volume ratio and hence in the transformation from a disc to a sphere. Spherocytosis causes a decrease in red cell deformability and results in entrapment of the cells in the microcirculation, particularly the spleen. Spherocytes have increased osmotic fragility which can be accentuated by sterile incubation in the absence of glucose; this effect can be reduced by the addition of glucose to the incubation media. During incubation there is a rapid fall in intracellular ATP levels which is probably due to a marked increase in the activity of the membrane pumps in an attempt to overcome the increased movement of sodium into the cells. This permeability change is thought to be due to a primary defect in membrane protein structure. Human HS cells have many features in common with spectrin-deficient mouse cells. At least one form of HS has been found to be associated with a defect at

the distal end of spectrin leading to defective association of spectrin with membrane band 4.1 (see page 19.64), and hence with actin. Spectrin deficiency has been found in the membranes of one patient with atypical HS, but in many cases no defects in the membrane proteins have yet been demonstrated. It seems likely that HS will turn out to be heterogeneous at the molecular level.

The anaemia and shortened red cell survival characteristic of HS can be corrected by splenectomy. It seems likely that the mechanism whereby the spleen destroys HS cells is analogous to the changes which take place on prolonged sterile incubation of these cells *in vitro* where there is both metabolic depletion and a rise in pH from lactic acid formation. HS cells from the spleen have higher levels of Na$^+$ and lower levels of ATP, and the level of glucose in the spleen is lower than that in the peripheral blood. Thus, it appears that the leaky HS red cell is able to survive in the circulation, but when it is packed together with its fellows in the spleen, its inherent metabolic deficiencies are magnified and there is increased movement of sodium into the cell, further depletion of ATP, and loss of various membrane components. All these mechanisms interreact to cause an increasing degree of spherocytosis and hence sequestration and death of the cell.

Clinical features

The disorder commonly presents in childhood and may sometimes become apparent for the first time as an episode of neonatal jaundice. However, some patients go through the early years of life with the condition unrecognized and may present in middle or old age with a complication such as obstructive jaundice due to gallstones or a sudden worsening of their anaemia associated with an intercurrent infection. The main clinical features are mild and intermittent jaundice without bile in the urine (acholuric jaundice), mild anaemia, and splenomegaly. The continuous increase in bile pigment frequently leads to the formation of biliary calculi with biliary colic, recurrent cholecystitis, and, occasionally, obstructive jaundice. During episodes of intercurrent infection there may be a worsening of the anaemia with an increased rate of haemolysis. Rarely, an aplastic crisis occurs at which time the reticulocyte count falls and there is a temporary hypoplasia of what is usually hyperplastic bone marrow. Aplastic crises, which have recently been related to human parvovirus infection, are associated with extremely severe anaemia of rapid onset.

Other rare complications of HS include recurrent, intractable ulceration of the ankles and progressive iron loading with generalized haemosiderosis similar to that which occurs in some of the dyserythropoietic anaemias (page 19.113).

Finally, some patients with this condition go through life entirely asymptomatic and are only found during family studies.

Haematological changes

There is usually a mild anaemia with haemoglobin values in the 8–12 g/dl range. The reticulocyte count is elevated and examination of a stained blood film shows polychromasia and a variable number of spherocytes (Fig. 2). The bone marrow shows normoblastic hyperplasia. The red cell osmotic fragility is usually increased. The fragility curve may assume a variety of forms in which either the whole curve is 'shifted to the right' or the majority of it is normal but there is a small 'tail' of cells with increased osmotic fragility. The changes in osmotic fragility are more marked after blood is incubated for 24 hours and this effect can be corrected by the addition of glucose at the beginning of the incubation (Fig. 3). Similarly, there is an increased rate of haemolysis when the cells are incubated for 24 hours *in vitro*; this is partly corrected by glucose (Type I autohaemolysis; see page 19.139).

The serum bilirubin level is usually elevated, serum haptoglobins are reduced or absent, and there is an increased production of faecal and urinary urobilinogen. Occasionally, when HS is complicated by obstructive jaundice, the spherocytic changes of the red cells may become less marked and the condition may be missed if this interesting phenomenon is not thought about. It probably

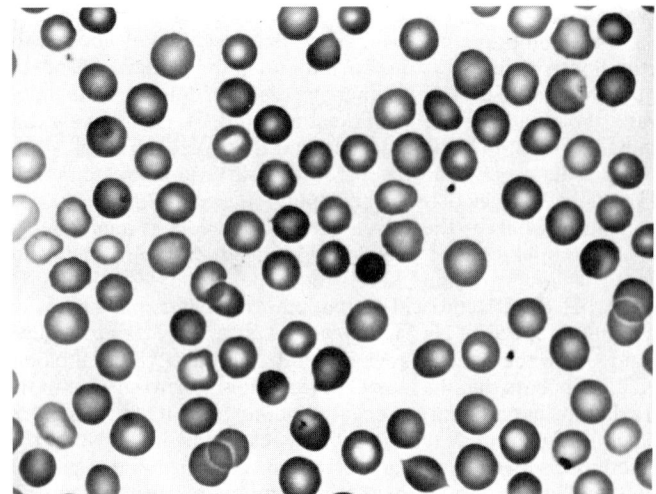

Fig. 2 The peripheral blood film in hereditary spherocytosis. Many dense spherocytes are present (× 1000, Leishman stain).

results from the increased movement of lipid into the red cell membrane due to the inhibition of acyl transferases by bile products.

Differential diagnosis

There are few disorders that can be confused with HS once the presence of spherocytes on the blood film is recognized and an osmotic fragility test confirms that the red cells show increased osmotic lysis. The only other inherited haemolytic anaemias which are associated with spherocytic red cells are the haemoglobin C disorders but the peripheral blood changes are quite different (see page 19.126). Acquired spherocytosis occurs in some of the autoimmune haemolytic anaemias (see page 19.143) and in other conditions associated with damage to the red cell membrane. The autoimmune haemolytic anaemias are easily recognized by the presence of a positive Coombs' test and the absence of other affected family members. If there is any doubt about the diagnosis of a mild form of HS, a full family study should be carried out.

Treatment

Except in the very mildest cases splenectomy should always be carried out once the diagnosis of HS is established. It is advisable to delay the operation until after the age of 5 years because of the risk of infection (see page 19.194). After splenectomy there is almost always a rise in the haemoglobin level to normal and the reticulocyte count declines to normal at the same time. The red cells retain their abnormal morphological and biochemical properties, but in the absence of the spleen have an almost normal survival time. Apart from occasional relapses due to hypertrophy of accessory spleens, the results of surgery are uniformly excellent.

Hereditary elliptocytosis (HE)

This condition is characterized by the presence of oval or elliptical red cells (Fig. 4). It has been realized for some time that it is genetically heterogeneous. For example, the determinant for one variety is linked to the loci which determine the rhesus blood group system whereas another is clearly not linked to this gene cluster. More recently three varieties have been defined. The first two, the common form of HE and so-called spherocytic HE (which has features of both HE and HS), are both autosomal dominant disorders with mild haemolysis. Homozygotes have severe haemolysis with fragmented cells. The third type is called stomatocytic HE and is inherited as an autosomal recessive. The latter condition is found almost exclusively in Polynesia where its high prevalence is thought to be due to resistance of the elliptical cells to *P. falciparum* malaria.

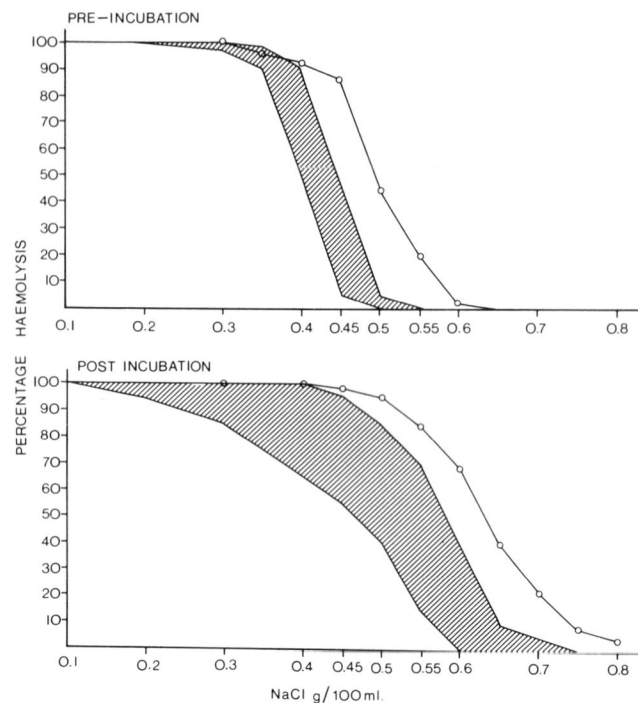

Fig. 3 Osmotic fragility changes in hereditary spherocytosis. The upper curve shows increased fragility in the cells of a patient with hereditary spherocytosis (open circles) as compared with the normal control range (hatched). The bottom figure shows the same result after sterile incubation of the blood for 24 hours.

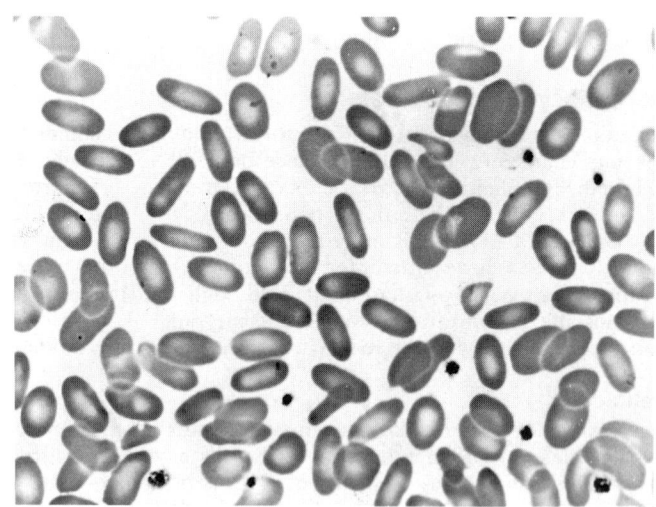

Fig. 4 The peripheral blood film in hereditary elliptocytosis (× 1000, Leishman stain).

Aetiology

Although it is now believed that HE results from a genetic defect of the red cell membrane, the molecular lesion has yet to be clearly defined. A complete deficiency of membrane protein 4.1 which links spectrin to actin has been found in one family with severe elliptocytosis, and a partial deficiency has been found in association with mild forms of the condition. However, the molecular basis of these deficiencies is not yet understood. It seems very likely that HE will turn out to be very heterogeneous at the molecular level.

Clinical and haematological features

In symptomatic HE there is a variable degree of anaemia and splenomegaly and the peripheral blood film shows a variety of morphological changes including oval cells, long 'pencil' cells, and other bizarre poikilocytes (Fig. 4). There is an elevated reticulocyte count and all the associated changes of haemolysis.

Differential diagnosis

It is difficult to confuse HE with any of the other genetically determined haemolytic anaemias, although it should be remembered that oval cells may be observed occasionally in the different forms of thalassaemia and in iron deficiency anaemias.

Treatment

Most heterozygous carriers of HE require no treatment although, if the anaemia is symptomatic, the condition seems to be at least partially corrected by splenectomy; the morphological changes of the red cells persist.

Stomatocytosis

The word 'stomatocyte' is used to describe red cells with longitudinal depression across their centres in contrast to the usual central circular depression seen in a normal discoid cell. This alteration is supposed to resemble a mouth! Stomatocytes have been described in association with a variety of disorders including alcoholism, red cell enzyme defects, lead poisoning, and thalassaemia. Not infrequently they are simply smear artefacts!

However, there is increasing interest in hereditary haemolytic anaemias characterized by the presence of many stomatocytes on the peripheral blood film. Well-documented families have had one or more affected members with a moderate degree of anaemia and reticulocytosis, and metabolic studies of the red cells have shown remarkable alterations in both cation content and transport. However, the nature of the membrane defect which gives rise to these changes remains to be determined. In several of these families the condition was inherited in a dominant fashion and homozygous individuals were identified who had a moderately severe haemolytic anaemia and approximately twice the normal red cell sodium content, with a marked increase in the rate of sodium efflux from their cells.

Hereditary pyropoikilocytosis

This genetically determined haemolytic anaemia is characterized by the presence of many microspherocytic red cells which have blunted projections or are triangular in shape. The disorder derives its name from the fact that these cells undergo marked fragmentation when the temperature is raised to approximately 45 °C, whereas normal red cells do not undergo such changes until the temperature reaches 49–50 °C. Recent work suggests that it results from a structural alteration in the alpha subunit of spectrin.

The condition, which seems to be extremely rare, is characterized by mild haemolytic anaemia with the very characteristic red cell changes.

March haemoglobinuria

This condition is described in detail later in this section (see page 19.151). However, because recent studies suggest that it may be associated with a structural defect in the red cell membrane, it may well be added to the list of genetically determined disorders of the membrane should these findings be confirmed and observed in relatives of affected individuals.

Acanthocytosis

Irregularly arranged, multiple spiny projections on the red cells are characteristic of the rare recessive disorder, *abetalipoproteinaemia*. The syndrome presents early in life with diarrhoea and steatorrhoea and is associated with progressive neurological involvement including ataxia, tremor, hyporeflexia, and nystagmus. Retinal degeneration with atypical retinitis pigmentosa leads to blindness; β lipoprotein is absent from the serum. There is a mild haemolytic anaemia and the peripheral blood film shows variable numbers of acanthocytes.

Several variants of this condition have been reported; notably, the association of the acanthocytes and mental retardation with normal β lipoprotein levels.

HAEMOLYSIS DUE TO RED CELL ENZYME DEFICIENCIES

Until a few years ago it was customary to use the term '*congenital non-spherocytic haemolytic anaemia*' to describe any haemolytic disorder which was present from early life, and which was not an example of such easily identified conditions as hereditary spherocytosis or sickle cell anaemia. As these anaemias were studied further, it became apparent that they could be divided into two subgroups according to the haemolytic effects of sterile incubation of the red cells in the presence or absence of glucose, i.e. those in which glucose partly corrects autohaemolysis (Type 1), and those in which it has no effect (Type 2). This finding suggested that at least some of these conditions might result from a metabolic disorder of the red cells. More recently it has been possible to analyse the chemical basis for these conditions in more detail and to demonstrate that some of them result from enzyme deficiencies or inherited haemoglobin variants.

Several different inherited haemolytic anaemias have been described which appear to be the result of a deficiency of specific red cell enzymes. However, it is interesting to note that, although the metabolic pathways of the red cell are understood, at least in outline, most centres which are able to screen for all the red cell enzymes are only able to demonstrate a deficiency of a specific enzyme in a very small proportion of cases of congenital non-spherocytic haemolytic anaemia. Clearly, there is a long way to go in this field before it is possible to characterize the underlying defect in the majority of the inherited haemolytic anaemias for which no abnormality of the membrane or haemoglobin structure can be defined.

Normal cell metabolism

During normal red cell development the mitochondria are lost at about the time as the nucleus is extruded, and, therefore, mature red cells have no capacity for oxidative energy production. They are delivered into the circulation with a relatively simple 'pay-as-you-go' energy-producing system which burns glucose as its main source of fuel (see page 19.65).

Glucose is metabolized mainly through the anaerobic Embden–Meyerhof (EM) pathway with the production of lactate as the end product (Fig. 5). There is a net production of 2 mol of ATP and the reduction of 2 mol of NAD^+ to NADH per mol of glucose. About half of the ATP produced in this way is used for the red cell to maintain its volume and the integrity of its membrane by pumping sodium and water out of the cell and potassium into the cell. The role of the remainder of the ATP which is produced is unknown. The reduction of NAD^+ plays an important role in preventing the oxidation of the iron of haem. The other major energy pathway is the hexose monophosphate (HMP) shunt (Fig. 6) in which there is reduction of $NADP^+$ to NADPH. This pathway is stimulated by certain redox compounds and oxidants. One of the major functions of the HMP is the maintenance of adequate levels of reduced glutathione in the red cell which is essential for protection against oxidant damage.

There is a 'metabolic siding' in the EM pathway called the Rapoport–Leubering shunt which is controlled by diphosphoglycerate mutase and which generates 2,3-diphosphoglycerate (2,3 DPG). The latter is the most abundant intracellular phosphate in human erythrocytes and plays an important role in controlling

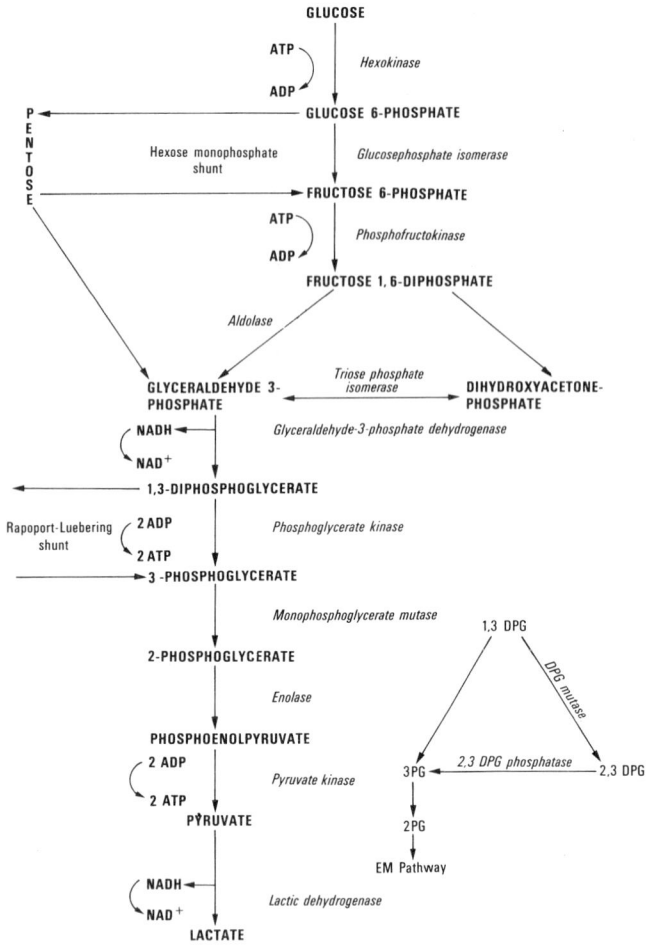

Fig. 5 The relationship between the main red cell glycolytic pathway (Embden–Meyerhof) and the other metabolic pathways. The insert shows the production of 2,3-DPG in the Rapoport–Luebering shunt.

oxygen transport (see page 19.65). Clearly, the rate of 2,3 DPG production is closely related to the rate of glycolysis. Blocks early in the EM pathway cause reduced DPG production, while blocks late in the pathway, pyruvate kinase deficiency for example, cause it to accumulate. Thus enzyme defects vary considerably in their effects on DPG production, and hence on oxygen transport and the degree of compensation for anaemia.

The red cell contains enzyme systems for the utilization of substrates other than glucose under unusual conditions; these include adenosine, inosine, fructose, manose, galactose, and lactate. Numerous other enzymes have been reported to be active in reticulocytes and mature red cells.

Inherited enzyme deficiencies

Many red cell enzyme deficiencies have been reported but usually as individual cases or in a few members of single families. The only two which have been well documented and which are relatively common are glucose-6-phosphate dehydrogenase deficiency and pyruvate kinase (PK) deficiency. We shall describe these disorders in detail, together with some other less common enzyme deficiencies of the HMP and EM pathways. Other enzyme deficiencies are listed in Table 5.

Glucose 6-phosphate dehydrogenase (G6PD) deficiency

G6PD deficiency is an inherited condition in which the activity of red cell G6PD is markedly diminished. The gene determining the structure of G6PD is carried on the X chromosome and, there-

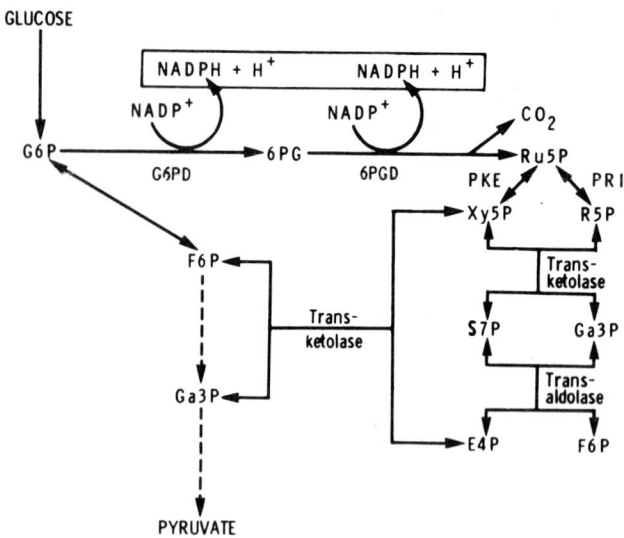

Fig. 6 The hexose-monophosphate pathway. Intermediates: G6P, glucose 6-phosphate; F6P, fructose 6-phosphate; Ga3P, glyceraldehyde 3-phosphate; 6PG, 6-phosphogluconate; Ru5P, ribulose 5-phosphate; R5P, ribose 5-phosphate; Xy5P, xylulose 5-phosphate; S7P, sedoheptulose 7-phosphate; E4P, erythrose 4-phosphate. Enzymes: G6PD, glucose 6-phosphate dehydrogenase; 6PGD, 6-phosphogluconate dehydrogenase; PKE, epimerase, PRI, phosphoribose isomerase. Cosubstrates: $NADP^+$ and $NADPH + H^+$, oxidized and reduced forms of nicotinamide-adenine dinucleotide phosphate.

fore, the defect is inherited in a sex-linked fashion. Hence, it is fully expressed in affected males. Because one X chromosome is inactivated during early development (lyonization), female heterozygotes have two populations of red cells, deficient and normal. Because the inactivation process is random, the total level of enzyme in the blood of female carriers varies markedly, ranging from normal to almost as low as that found in hemizygous males.

G6PD deficiency is widespread in the populations of Africa, the Mediterranean, the Middle East, and Southeast Asia. It has been estimated that there are more than 100 million affected individuals in the world population.

Pathogenesis

G6PD deficiency results from the inheritance of any one of a large number of G6PD variants which have been defined either by their electrophoretic mobility, thermal stability, pH optima, substrate affinity, or by other techniques of enzyme chemistry. Normal G6PD is called type B. In Africa there is a common variant called A. G6PD deficiency in this population results from the production of another mutant form of the enzyme called the A⁻ type. Although this is synthesized in normal quantities, it is unstable and its level rapidly declines as red cells age. The Mediterranean variant, which is also extremely common, appears to be a structural mutant with reduced enzyme activity. Some variants, e.g. G6PD Oklahoma, have a marked decrease in substrate affinity. In the Mediterranean form of the disease there are extremely low red cell enzyme values, whereas in the A⁻ variety of G6PD deficiency there may be easily detectable enzyme levels in affected males. Over 100 G6PD variants have now been discovered and are named after their place of origin. Although many are harmless, some of them are associated with drug-induced haemolysis or chronic haemolytic anaemia.

Mechanism of haemolysis

The haemolysis of G6PD deficiency is characterized by the formation of intracellular inclusions, called Heinz bodies, which consist of denatured haemoglobin and stromal protein. The precise mechanism whereby haemoglobin damage and precipitation occurs in

Table 5 Red cell enzyme deficiencies

Associated with significant haemolytic anaemia
  Enzymes of Embden–Meyerhof pathway
    Hexokinase (HK)
    Glucose phosphate isomerase (GPI)
    Phosphofructokinase (PFK)
    Aldolase (ALD)
    Triosephosphate isomerase (TPI)
    Diphosphoglycerate mutase (DPMG)
    Phosphoglycerate kinase (PGK)
    Pyruvate kinase (PK)

  Enzymes of the hexose monophosphate (HMP) shunt and
  glutathione metabolism
    Glucose 6-phosphate dehydrogenase (G6PD)
    Glutathione peroxidase (GSH-Px)
    GSH deficiency secondary to deficiency of:
      γ-Glutamyl cysteine synthetase
      GSH synthetase
    Glutathione reductase (GSSG-R)

  Enzymes of nucleotide metabolism
    Adenylate kinase
    Pyrimidine 5′-nucleotidase

Haemolytic anaemia absent or association with deficiency uncertain
  Enzymes related to HMP shunt, nucleotide metabolism, or glycolysis
    6-Phosphogluconate dehydrogenase (6-PGD)
    Adenosinetriphosphatase (ATPase)
    Glutathione reductase (GSSG-R)
    The 'high ATP' syndromes
    'High ITP'
    Lactate dehydrogenase (LDH)

  Other enzyme deficiencies detectable by red cell assay
    Catalase
    Galactose 1-phosphate uridyl transferase
    NADH-methaemoglobin reductase
    NADPH-methaemoglobin reductase
    Glyoxalase
    Adenosine deaminase
    Amylo-1, 6-glucosidase
    Hypoxanthine-guanine phosphoribosyl transferase

Associated with megaloblastic anaemia
  Orotidine 5′-phosphate pyrophosphorylase
  Orotidine 5′-phosphate decarboxylase
  5′-Phosphoribosyl 1-pyrophosphate (PRPP) synthetase

Modified from Valentine (1978).

G6PD-deficient cells is still uncertain. Some drugs and chemicals have a direct oxidant action on haemoglobin and also form free radicals which may oxidize reduced glutathione to the disulphide form (GSSG), or complex glutathione with haemoglobin to form mixed disulphides. When oxidation damage of this kind occurs, haemoglobin is irreversibly denatured and precipitates in the form of Heinz bodies. Normal red cells can defend themselves against this process by reducing GSSG to GSH via the HMP shunt (Fig. 6); this is not possible in G6PD deficient cells. It is emphasized that this description of oxidative damage to haemoglobin may be a gross oversimplification of what actually happens. For example, oxidative damage to red cells results in the production of irreversible and unstable intermediates of haemoglobin metabolism called haemichromes, and the generation of superoxides and other 'excited' intermediates capable of damaging red cell lipids, all of which are treated to methaemoglobin production which can be caused by many oxidant drugs. Furthermore, none of these mechanisms explain why neonatal haemolysis or sensitivity to fava beans occurs in G6PD-deficient individuals.

Clinical features

The clinical consequences of G6PD deficiency are summarized in Table 6. Haemolysis can occur after exposure to a variety of drugs

and other oxidants, in the neonatal period without the action of any apparent toxic agent, and after exposure to the bean *Vicia faba*. It has also been reported to occur during intercurrent illnesses.

A list of some of the more important drugs which can produce haemolysis in G6DP-deficient individuals is shown in Table 7. Sensitivity to individual agents varies depending on the type of enzyme deficiency and the size of the dose. For example, drugs such as chloramphenicol may induce haemolysis in individuals with the severe Mediterranean G6PD deficiency but not in Negroes with the milder A⁻ variant. Furthermore, haemolytic episodes tend to be self limiting in individuals with the A⁻ variant, whereas if the drug is continued in those with the Mediterranean form, there may be gross and sometimes fatal intravascular haemolysis.

Typically, an episode of drug-induced haemolysis begins one to three days after receiving the drug. There is a rapid onset of anaemia and jaundice and the peripheral blood picture shows all the characteristics of haemolysis with Heinz bodies in the red cells. In severe cases there may be shivering, backache, abdominal pain, and the passage of dark urine. As mentioned above, in the A⁻ type of G6PD deficiency the haemolytic reaction is self limiting. This is because the reticulocytes have relatively normal enzyme activity.

Severe haemolytic reactions due to the action of the bean *Vicia faba*, favism, are seen commonly in the Mediterranean region, the Middle East and indeed anywhere where G6PD-deficient patients are exposed to the bean. The pathogenesis of favism is not fully worked out. It has a seasonal incidence, a peak occurring in childhood although some individuals are exposed to the bean for years before the first attack, and seems to spare some G6PD families completely. The toxic factor in the bean has not been defined. Other genetic factors may be involved in addition to G6PD deficiency.

Jaundice and evidence of mild haemolysis may occur during the first week of life of G6PD-deficient infants and may occasionally lead to kernicterus. Despite much work it is not clear why newborn infants who are G6PD deficient develop hyperbilirubinaemia. The haemolytic component is relatively mild, and studies in Greece have suggested that this reaction may require the interaction of a second genetic factor, so far unidentified.

There have been numerous reports of the occurrence of severe haemolytic reaction in G6PD-deficient individuals during the course of intercurrent illness such as bacterial and virus infections, hepatitis, and diabetic ketoacidosis. Again, the mechanism is not clear.

Although a single structural gene codes G6PD in all tissues, including leucocytes, clinical manifestations of deficiency are nearly always limited to the red cells. A few families have been reported with complete or almost complete deficiency of leucocyte G6PD. The clinical manifestations are very similar to chronic granulomatous disease (see page 19.160), although less severe.

Finally, some of the rare types of G6PD deficiency are associated with a continuous haemolytic process and this forms one group of the hereditary non-spherocytic haemolytic anaemias. These patients usually present early in life, sometimes with neonatal jaundice, and haemolysis is exacerbated by infection or the administration of drugs. They commonly have splenomegaly and the clinical and haematological picture is like that observed in some of the other red cell enzyme defects mentioned later in this section.

Laboratory diagnosis

In the absence of haemolysis most G6PD deficient individuals have a normal haematological picture and the condition can only be identified by a specific enzyme assay. During haemolytic episodes the haematological changes are as described above with the presence of Heinz bodies in the red cells. It should be remembered that it may be difficult to make the diagnosis during an acute

Table 6 Clinical disorders associated with G6PD deficiency

1 Drug-induced haemolysis
2 Favism
3 Neonatal jaundice
4 Chronic haemolytic anaemia
5 Haemolysis associated with intercurrent illness

Table 7 Some drugs which may cause haemolysis in G6PD-deficient subjects

Aminoquinolines	Analgesics
Primaquine	Acetylsalicylic acid
Pamaquin (Plasmoquine)	Acetophenetidin (Phenacetin)
Chloroquine	Acetanilide
Sulphones	Miscellaneous
Dapsone (Avlosulphon)	Vitamin K (water-soluble
Sulphoxone (Diasone)	analogues)
Thiazosulphone (Promizole)	Naphthalene (moth balls)
	Probenecid (Benemid)
Sulphonamides	
Sulphanilamide	Dimercaprol (BAL)
Sulphacetamide (Albucid, Sulamyd)	Methylene blue
Sulphafurazole (Gantrisin)	Acetylphenylhydrazine
Sulphamethoxypyridazine	Phenylhydrazine
(Lederkyn, Midicel, Kynex)	P-aminosalicylic acid
Nitrofurans	
Nitrofurantoin (Furadantin)	Quinine*
Furazolidone (Furoxone)	Quinidine*
Nitrofurazone (Furacin)	Chloramphenicol*

* Not shown to be haemolytic in Negroes.
From Emerson and Grimes (1982).

haemolytic crisis in an individual with G6PD deficiency of the A⁻ variety. The high reticulocyte count may produce a normal enzyme assay and hence the test has to be repeated when the haemolytic episode is over. Although this is less of a problem with other varieties of G6PD deficiency, the Mediterranean type for example, red cell enzyme activity may still increase significantly during a haemolytic crisis.

The further classification of G6PD deficiency by subtype (e.g. A⁻, Mediterranean, Canton, etc.) requires a variety of sophisticated approaches including electrophoretic analysis, estimation of the Km for NADP and glucose 6-phosphate, pH optima, and utilization of substrate analogues.

Therapy

G6PD-deficient individuals should avoid any drugs which may provoke haemolysis and should be given a list of these agents (Table 7). In very severe episodes blood transfusion may be necessary. Splenectomy has been reported to be of some value in the rare subgroup with persistent haemolysis.

Pyruvate kinase deficiency

Pyruvate kinase (PK) deficiency is the commonest of the inherited red cell enzyme defects after G6PD deficiency. It has been reported in many different races, and the sexes are affected equally. The most commonly described form is inherited as an autosomal recessive. Homozygotes have haemolytic anaemia, splenomegaly, and a gross deficiency of red cell PK activity, while heterozygotes are clinically and haematologically normal and have about half the usual amount of PK activity in their red cells.

Aetiology and pathogenesis

As might be expected from its place in the EM pathway (see Fig. 5), deficiency of PK results in the accumulation of glycolytic inter-mediates, particularly 2,3-DPG and phosphoenol pyruvate. In the absence of efficient glycolysis the red cell must obtain its energy requirements by other means. In the severe PK deficient patient there is a marked reticulocytosis, and probably most of the red cells' energy is derived by oxidative pathways related to the residual mitochondria in the younger cell population. One of the most fascinating features of this disease is that after splenectomy the reticulocyte count rises; it appears that PK deficient patients are reliant on the presence of a young red cell population for survival. Perhaps mitochondrial phosphorylation is inhibited in the spleen and hence cells which depend on it survive longer after splenectomy.

PK deficiency shows a remarkable degree of molecular heterogeneity. In some cases there is simply a quantitative defect in the enzyme but in others mutant enzymes with abnormal kinetic properties have been described. It appears that many apparent homozygotes are in fact compound heterozygotes with different genetic lesions at each of their PK loci. *Acquired PK deficiency* has been observed in patients with acute leukaemia or refractory anaemia.

Clinical features

Severe PK deficiency often presents at birth with neonatal jaundice and haemolysis. There is a variable degree of chronic haemolysis throughout life with jaundice, anaemia, splenomegaly, and even bone changes similar to those seen in thalassaemia in the most severe cases. There is often a marked exacerbation of the anaemia during periods of stress such as infection. Interestingly, however, the anaemia is very well tolerated. This is probably because the high levels of red cell 2,3-DPG cause a right shift in the oxygen dissociation curve and hence a more efficient oxygenation of the tissues. Aplastic crises due to human parvovirus infection have been reported.

Laboratory diagnosis

The blood picture shows all the hallmarks of chronic haemolysis and the stained blood film shows polychromasia and macrocytosis with a varying number of irregularly contracted red cells. There is an increased rate of autohaemolysis which is not corrected by glucose (Type 2 autohaemolysis). The diagnosis is confirmed by a PK assay.

Therapy

There is no specific therapy but there have been many reports of improvement after splenectomy. As mentioned above, the reticulocyte count often remains elevated after the operation and indeed may even become set at a higher level than before splenectomy. Transfusion is required during periods of exacerbation of the haemolysis.

Pyrimidine 5′ nucleotidase deficiency

This condition, which is transmitted as an autosomal recessive trait, causes a variable haemolytic anaemia which is characterized by marked basophilic stippling of the red cells. It is of interest because it appears to be relatively common and by 1980 33 individuals from 24 separate kindreds had been reported. There appears to be a predisposition in Mediterranean, Jewish, and African populations. An acquired form of this enzyme deficiency occurs in severe lead poisoning and may be at least in part responsible for the haemolytic component of lead intoxication. Splenectomy does not appear to be effective in the genetic form of the condition.

Red cell enzyme deficiencies associated with multisystem disease

The other red cell enzyme deficiencies which cause haemolytic anaemia are summarized in Table 5. Most of these conditions are rare and have only been encountered in a few families. Usually there is chronic haemolysis without involvement of other systems but there is an increasing number of examples of red cell enzyme deficiencies which are associated with multisystem disease.

Triosephosphate isomerase (TPI) deficiency is characterized by a moderately severe haemolytic anaemia associated with a bizarre neurological disorder characterized by either progressive spasticity or flaccidity, diffuse muscle weakness, dysphasia, facial paresis, absent reflexes, fixed deformities of the hands, and tremor. Curiously, different neurological symptom complexes seem to occur in individuals with this disorder. Enzyme activity is greatly reduced in muscle, plasma, spinal fluid, skin fibroblasts, and white cells, suggesting that TPI deficiency involves most body tissues. Sudden unexplained death due to cardiac arrythmias has been described, and in some patients there is an unusual susceptibility to infection.

The syndrome of myopathy and congenital non-spherocytic haemolytic anaemia associated with *phosphofructokinase (PFK) deficiency* was first described by Tarui and his colleagues and is now sometimes known as *Tarui's disease.* The condition is also called *glycogenesis, type VII.* PFK is an allosteric enzyme which catalyses a major rate-limiting and regulatory reaction of anaerobic glycolysis. It exists as tetrameric isozymes composed of different combinations of three distinct subunits which are each under separate genetic control. These are called type M (muscle), L (liver), and P (platelet or fibroblast); the genetic determinants are on chromosomes 1, 21, and 10, respectively. Subunits are variably expressed in different tissues. For example, muscle PFK consists of M4 tetramers while erythrocytes contain five isozymes: M4, M3L, M2L2, ML3, and L4. Tarui's disease appears to be the homozygous state for deficiency of the M subunit. The disorder shows marked clinical variability and is characterized by muscle weakness, exercise intolerance, intermittent myoglobinuria, and a variable degree of haemolysis. Hyperuricaemia and gout is a common complication.

Phosphoglycerate kinase (PGK) deficiency is an X-linked disorder in which hemizygous males have a neurological syndrome characterized by seizures, variable mental retardation, emotional ability, speech impairment, and progressive extrapyramidal disease. There is severe chronic haemolytic anaemia which sometimes becomes transfusion dependent. There have been several reports of response to splenectomy. The haemolytic disorder is punctuated by severe exacerbations, often caused by infection, and characterized by worsening of the anaemia, jaundice, and a marked reticulocyte response.

Several patients with *gamma-glutamyl cysteine synthetase deficiency* have been reported in whom there were progressive neurological abnormalities including spinocerebellar ataxia, muscle weakness, absence of deep tendon reflexes, and impaired vibratory and position sense in all extremities. As the neurological disorder progressed speech became impaired and myoclonic spasms occurred.

Glutathione synthetase deficiency occurs in two forms, one with haemolytic anaemia as the sole manifestation, and one with haemolysis, metabolic acidosis, and, usually, though not always, neurological disease.

Several families have been reported in which there are patients with *pyrimidine-5-nucleotidase deficiency* associated with haemolytic anaemia and mild mental retardation. Red cell *aldolase deficiency* is also associated with dysmorphic features, and mental and growth retardation.

It seems likely that more of these rare syndromes will turn up. Presumably, whether or not a red cell enzyme deficiency is associated with multisystem disease, or whether it only causes haemolytic anaemia, depends on whether the particular enzyme that is defective is shared with other tissues. The recent studies on PFK deficiency outlined above underline the complexity of these relationships.

A general approach to congenital non-spherocytic haemolytic anaemia

When young children present with haemolysis, the first step is to look for one of the acquired causes of haemolytic anaemia mentioned later in this chapter. Once these have been excluded, and abnormalities of the red cell membrane and haemoglobin have been ruled out, the level of red cell G6PD and PK should be determined. This will leave a number of patients in whom no diagnosis can be made, and they should then be referred to centres capable of analysing all the red cell enzymes and glycolytic intermediates. In practice only a small proportion of cases of this type can be ascribed to a particular enzyme deficiency and in the majority no specific abnormality can be found.

GENETIC HAEMOLYTIC ANAEMIAS DUE TO ABNORMALITIES OF HAEMOGLOBIN

Some of the structural haemoglobin variants, and the thalassaemias, are associated with a variable degree of haemolysis. These conditions are described on pages 19.108–19.130.

Acquired haemolytic anaemia

The acquired haemolytic anaemias are caused by many different agents but the pathogenesis may be divided into three major groups: immune; physical and chemical changes in the environment; and damage to the membrane or contents of the cell by chemical agents (usually oxidant) or organisms (see Table 4, page 19.137).

THE IMMUNE HAEMOLYTIC ANAEMIAS

Pathogenesis

Immune haemolysis may occur when antibody or complement are attached to the red cell surface. Antibodies bound to the red cell membrane cause binding of the red cells to macrophages by the Fc receptors on the latter with subsequent phagocytosis. The antibodies may be IgG, IgA, or IgM, depending upon the aetiology. When IgG is bound, there is competition between free IgG in plasma and the bound IgG for the Fc receptor sites. In the spleen, the plasma skimming effect of the arteriolar network reduces the amount of free IgG so that destruction of IgG-coated red cells tends to be particularly active. IgM antibodies are bound most avidly at low temperatures and give rise to the cold autoimmune disorders (see below). IgM antibodies also fix complement to receptors on the red cell so that haemolysis occurs because of complement activation (see Section 4). Macrophages have receptors for the activated component of C3, C3b, which does not exist in significant amounts in plasma, so that destruction of cells takes place throughout the macrophage system, not just in the spleen. If sufficient complement is bound and activated on the membrane, intravascular lysis occurs as a direct result of the action of the late complement components. In the acquired disorder paroxysmal nocturnal haemoglobinuria (PNH), the red cell membrane is peculiarly susceptible to the action of activated complement, even in the absence of bound antibody (see page 19.54).

Antibody directed against red cell membrane may be provoked in a number of ways which will be discussed in more detail under the particular disorders. Briefly, antibodies may be directed against membrane components themselves, against components altered by binding of drugs, or against drug–plasma components, the antigen–antibody complex being passively bound to the membrane.

The presence of antibody or complement on the surface of the red cell is detected by the direct antiglobulin test (DAGT) or Coombs' test. Antibody which reacts against normal red cells of similar blood group may be detected in the serum by the indirect antiglobulin test and eluates may be prepared from the antibody-coated cells to test the specificity of the antibody. The temperature at which the antibody is most active and the class of immunoglobulin involved are also required for reaching a diagnosis.

Drug-induced immune haemolytic anaemia

Drugs may produce a haemolytic anaemia either as a result of antibodies directed against the red cell but provoked by the drug, or directly by an oxidant effect (see later). There are three major ways in which drugs cause the development of antibodies which bind to the red cell surface (Table 8).

Hapten-membrane association

Some drugs, of which penicillin is the best-understood example, are bound to red cell membrane proteins by covalent bonds. The drug complex then acts as an antigenic determinant which binds specific antibody which is mainly IgG in type. This type of haemolytic anaemia is produced by penicillin in high daily dosage (10-20 mega units per day) as used in the management of bacterial endocarditis but only occurs after prolonged exposure or following a second course of treatment. Cephalosporins have a similar property and will cross-react with penicillin-induced antibodies.

The haemolysis is gradual in onset but may be profound in its effect, particularly if there is a marrow depression due to chronic infection. The DAGT is strongly positive but antibodies in the serum will not react with normal red cells of the same type unless penicillin is also present. When the drug is withdrawn haemolysis ceases fairly promptly though the DAGT may remain positive for 60–80 days. The antibody reacts partially against breakdown products of penicillin but these patients rarely have the usual manifestations of penicillin sensitivity. There is no specificity of the antibody for normal blood group substances.

Immune complex formation

Many drugs have been incriminated in acute haemolytic anaemia (Table 8) but the number of case reports for most individual drugs is very small. An exception is rifampicin which regularly causes immune cytopenias if given in intermittent doses. The antibodies produced in most cases are IgM which activates complement components. Intravascular haemolysis may be profound with haemoglobinaemia and haemoglobinuria. Occasionally, acute renal failure ensues, though this is unlikely to be due to haemoglobinaemia by itself. The haemolysis follows a second or subsequent administration of a very small dose of the drug and is not seen after first exposure. The DAGT is positive due to complement on the surface of the red cells, but antibody is rarely detected. Antibodies which are lytic for normal red cells only in the presence of the drug are found in the serum. Once the drug is withdrawn the haemolysis stops and the haemoglobin rapidly returns to normal.

'Autoimmune' drug-induced haemolytic anaemia

Three drugs, α-methyldopa, mefenamic acid, and levodopa have been found to provoke the development of autoantibodies directed against red cell membrane constituents, occasionally producing haemolytic anaemia. The drugs have to be taken on a regular basis for 3–6 months before the DAGT becomes positive. If the drug is then discontinued the DAGT becomes negative after a variable period, usually between 7 and 24 months. If the drug is then restarted, a further 3–6 months elapse before the test becomes positive again. The antibody is IgG in type; complement is not bound.

Haemolysis is extravascular and usually moderate. Spherocytes may be seen in the blood film but in general there are no specific features. Haemolysis stops fairly rapidly after withdrawal of the drug and steroid therapy is rarely indicated.

Autoimmune haemolytic anaemia

Haemolytic anaemia due to antibodies directed against normal red cell membrane constituents may arise as a 'primary' event in otherwise healthy individuals or may be associated with a number of other diseases (Table 9). Why such antibodies arise is unknown though it is likely that several factors, including a genetic predisposition, are involved. Table 9 shows that most secondary cases are associated with either malignancy of the lymphoid system or with more generalized autoimmune disorders. Autoimmune haemolytic anaemia (AHA) may be further classified according to the temperature at which the antibodies are most active against normal red cells in vitro. In warm AHA the antibodies are most active at 37 °C while in cold AHA they are most active at low temperatures, e.g. 4 °C.

Warm autoimmune haemolytic anaemia

Warm AHA is an uncommon disorder which may arise at any age and which affects females slightly more than males (about 3:2). It is more common in older age groups because of its association with lymphoid neoplasms.

Table 8 Drug-induced immune haemolytic anaemia

Mechanism	Drugs	Dosage of drug which produces haemolysis	Coombs' test	Reaction of eluate	Haemolysis
Hapten–membrane association	Penicillin, cephalosporins, insulin	High; exposure for some weeks	Mainly IgG	Reacts against drug-coated cells only	Extravascular
Immune complex	Stibophen, quinidine and quinine, p-aminosalicylic acid, isoniazid, phenacetin, antazoline, sulphonamides, sulphonylureas, amidopyrine, dipyrone, rifampicin, insecticides	Low; second or subsequent exposure produces immediate haemolysis	Usually complement only	Reacts against drug-coated cells and sometimes against free drug	Intravascular acute
Autoimmune	α-Methyldopa, mefenamic acid, levodopa	Prolonged normal dosage	IgG	Reacts against normal red cells in the absence of the drug	Extravascular (usually slight)

Table 9 Autoimmune haemolytic anaemias (AHAs)

	Warm	Cold
Primary	Idiopathic AHA Evans' syndrome (AHA and thrombocytopenia)	Idiopathic, chronic cold haemagglutinin disease (CHAD)
Secondary	Systemic lupus erythematosus, other autoimmune disorders, lymphomes (pariculary chronic lymphocytic leukaemia and Hodgkin's disease), drugs, ovarian teratoma, other cancers	Lymphomas (particularly histiocytic), globinuria (PCH), paroxysmal cold haemoglobinuria infectious mononucleosis Mycoplasma pneumonia Other virus infections (rare)

Clinical features

The onset and severity of the disorder are variable. Most patients present with a progressive anaemia or mild jaundice but sometimes there is a fulminant illness with intravascular haemolysis, though this is rare in warm AHA. At the other extreme, the DAGT may be positive but insufficient antibody is present to produce a shortening of the red cell lifespan. Sometimes the symptoms and signs of the associated disorder dominate the clinical picture but the AHA equally commonly precedes the discovery of the primary disease, sometimes by months or years. The spleen is usually palpable in AHA but rarely attains a great size, except in association with a lymphoma.

Haematological features

Anaemia and reticulocytosis are the most marked features of the blood count. There may be neutrophilia, often with a left shift, accompanying the massive erythropoietic drive which follows the onset of anaemia. Nucleated red cells may be seen in the peripheral blood. In uncomplicated AHA the platelet count is normal or high, again a reflection of general marrow drive, but in some patients the platelets are also destroyed by antibody and the haemolysis is accompanied by thrombocytopenia (*Evans' syndrome*). AHA and immune thrombocytopenia may also occur at different times in the same person.

The peripheral blood film may suggest the diagnosis (Fig. 7). Spherocytosis occurs in many but not all cases of AHA and the cells may show autoagglutination. This is not always easy to identify in warm AHA, in contrast to the massive autoagglutination which occurs on slides made at room temperature from the blood of people with cold haemagglutinin disease (see below).

Red cell antibodies in warm AHA

The direct antiglobulin test is positive in virtually all cases of warm AHA. Table 10 shows the various types of DAGT which may be detected in warm AHA using specific antisera and the frequency

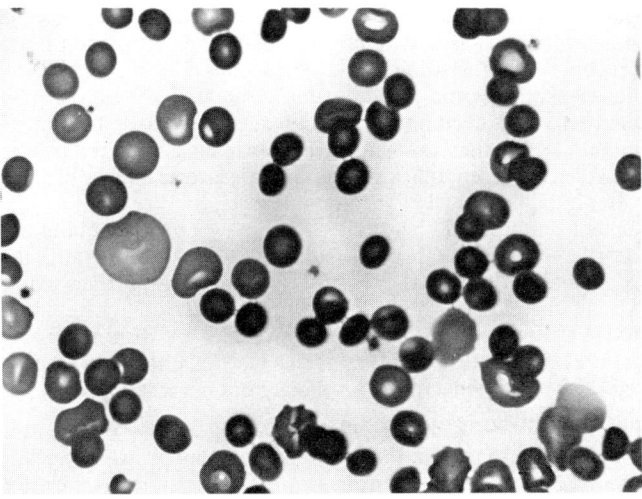

Fig. 7 The peripheral blood changes in autoimmune haemolytic anaemia. There is marked anisocytosis and anisochromia with many macrocytes and microspherocytes. The macrocytes reflect the reticulocytosis ($\times$ 1000, Leishman stain).

of each type in primary and secondary AHA. Except in systemic lupus erythematosus (SLE) there is no difference in the distribution or frequency of membrane-bound antibody. In SLE, IgG and complement are both present during the phase of haemolysis but the IgG component may become very weak and finally disappear as the patient recovers.

Pathogenesis

The site of destruction of red cells in AHA depends upon whether sufficient complement is fixed to cause intravascular haemolysis or whether the antibody coating promotes phagocytosis by macrophages. When IgG only is bound to the red cell, destruction takes place mainly in the spleen. If complement only is detected, intravascular haemolysis or generalized destruction throughout the macrophage system is likely. When both IgG and complement are present the situation is unpredictable and radioisotope studies with ^{51}Cr may be helpful in detecting the main site of red cell destruction.

Treatment

The aim of treatment in AHA is to keep the patient in the best possible health until the autoantibody disappears and haemolysis stops. In many patients with idiopathic AHA the antibodies disappear or diminish to insignificant levels after a period varying from a few months to more than 10 years. Transfusion may be life-saving in the acute phase of the disorder and should not be delayed because of apparent incompatibility of cross-match. ABO matched blood which appears least incompatible should be used.

Table 10 The types of Coombs' test in patients with warm autoimmune haemolytic anaemia

Reactions with antisera to	Idiopathic		Lymphoma		SLE		Other autoimmune disease	
	Number	%	Number	%	Number	%	Number	%
IgG only	28		7		0		6	
IgG + IgA	3	45	0	45	0	0	6	44
IgA only	2		1		0		0	
IgG + complement	29		9		6		7	
IgG + IgM + complement	2	42	1	50	2	100	1	50
Complement only	10	13	1	5	0	0	1	6

Figures from Worlledge, S.M. (1974). In *Blood and its disorders* (eds R. M. Hardisty and D. J. Weatherall). Blackwell Scientific Publications, Oxford.

Corticosteroids are the first measure used to control haemolysis. Prednisolone, 80 mg daily, is effective in most patients and there is rarely any benefit in using higher doses. This dose may usually be reduced over a period of two to three weeks to 20 mg daily but thereafter a more cautious reduction should be used to find the minimum controlling dose. A maintenance dose of 10 mg prednisolone daily is acceptable in adults and side effects may be reduced further if the drug is given on alternate days.

Splenectomy should be carried out only when an adequate trial of corticosteroids has proved ineffective. The type of antibody present and the results of ^{51}Cr survival studies with surface counting may sometimes provide some help in deciding whether to remove the spleen. Immunosuppressive therapy with drugs such as azathioprine is reserved for patients who have failed to respond to steroids and splenectomy, or who are not fit for surgery.

Cold autoantibody syndromes

Disorders due to autoantibodies which react most strongly at low temperatures may arise as primary (idiopathic) disorders or may be secondary to a variety of diseases (Table 9). The symptoms and signs of the diseases may result from agglutination of red cells or from haemolysis. Which of these occurs depends upon the titre of the antibody and the thermal range at which it is active.

Chronic cold haemagglutinin disease

Cold haemagglutinin disease (CHAD) in a chronic form is a disease of elderly patients, usually of unknown cause but occasionally associated with lymphoma. The patients have a chronic intravascular haemolytic anaemia which is made worse by a cold environment and which is often associated with Raynaud's phenomenon. Examination of a blood film made at room temperature shows gross autoagglutination which is absent if the blood is taken at 37 °C and the films prepared at this temperature. The DAGT is positive to complement bound to the red cell surface. IgM antibodies which are usually monoclonal, having $\varkappa$ light chains only and anti-I specificity, are found in the serum. CHAD from antibodies with other characteristics does occur but is rare. The disease progresses slowly with a gradual rise in titre of the cold antibody and may terminate with a malignant lymphoma after 10 years or more. The main treatment is to keep the patient warm, but intermittent treatment with chlorambucil may reduce the antibody level and lead to temporary improvement. Steroids and splenectomy are not of benefit. Blood transfusion should be avoided if possible; if absolutely necessary, it should be given slowly and via a warming coil.

Acute cold haemagglutinin disease

An acute intravascular haemolysis due to a rise in titre of anti-I antibodies may occur following *Mycoplasma pneumoniae* infection. The haemolysis appears about 10–14 days after the onset of respiratory symptoms and is usually transient but occasionally patients require transfusion which must be given through a warming coil.

A rise in anti-I IgM antibodies is found in infectious mononucleosis and rarely this may cause an acute haemolytic anaemia when the antibody reaches sufficient titre and thermal range. Serious consequences are rare.

Paroxysmal cold haemoglobinuria (PCH)

Paroxysmal cold haemoglobinuria is a rare disorder caused by a complement-fixing antibody, the Donath–Landsteiner antibody. The condition used to arise most commonly in congenital syphilis but most cases are now associated with virus infections such as mumps, measles, or chickenpox. The condition may also arise without apparent antecedent infection and in this case, as well as in congenital syphilis, attacks may occur over many years. Acute intravascular haemolysis accompanied by abdominal pain, peripheral cyanosis, and vascular symptoms of Raynaud type occurs a few minutes after exposure to cold. In addition to the haemoglobinaemia and haemoglobinuria there may be a transient leucopenia. The diagnosis is confirmed by identification of the Donath–Land-

steiner antibody which fixes itself to the red cell in the cold and binds on complement; this causes lysis as the cells are warmed.

Haemolytic disease of the newborn (HDN)

Haemolytic disease of the newborn occurs when IgG antibodies produced by the mother cross the placenta and react with fetal red cell antigens in sufficient quantities to cause destruction by the fixed macrophage system. Usually these antibodies belong to the Rh or ABO blood group systems but antibodies directed against many other antigens have caused HDN.

The most severe form of HDN is found in Rh haemolytic disease, but apart from differences in the blood film the clinical features are generally similar whatever the cause. In the most severe disorder, *hydrops fetalis*, the infant is usually born prematurely and both placenta and infant are grossly oedematous. The infant is very pale and usually dies. In less severe cases the child may appear normal at birth but develops progressive anaemia and jaundice over the first 24–48 hours. The bilirubin may quickly reach levels at which kernicterus threatens and exchange transfusions are urgently required. In milder cases still, anaemia develops during the second to eighth week of life. The anaemia may be marked but jaundice is not usually a problem. The old name for this disorder, *erythroblastosis fetalis*, emphasizes the most striking appearance of the blood film in these infants, namely, the presence of many nucleated red cells in the peripheral blood.

Rh haemolytic disease (see also page 19.249)

HDN may occur when an Rh-(D)-negative mother who has previously been exposed to the D antigen, either in an earlier pregnancy or by blood transfusion, has a Rh-(D)-positive child. Rh incompatibility is the commonest cause of HDN with an incidence, prior to preventive measures, of 5–7.5 per 1000 births and a mortality of about 20 per cent amongst affected infants. It is essential to identify families who are at risk and to prevent sensitization of the mother by the D antigen.

Identification of 'at-risk' families

All pregnant women should have their ABO and Rh blood groups identified as soon as they are known to be pregnant and should be screened for alloantibodies. Mothers who are Rh-(D)-negative should have their serum retested for anti-D antibodies at regular intervals (20 weeks and monthly in the third trimester). They are unlikely to form anti-D antibodies during their first pregnancy unless they have been previously transfused. A rising titre of anti-D antibody may be an indication for amniocentesis, a procedure which gives direct information about the amount of jaundice present in the fetus.

Management of the 'at-risk' fetus

If it is established that the fetus has a high risk of being severely affected by HDN, every effort should be made to prevent further damage. After about 36 weeks' gestation the risks of premature delivery are less than those of HDN so labour should be induced. Before 34 weeks the risks of prematurity are much greater than the risks of HDN. In this case intrauterine transfusions of blood which lacks the offending antigen are given in an attempt to decrease the effects of haemolysis. This procedure is particularly hazardous in the early part of pregnancy and is never free from risk. Once started, transfusions have to be given every 10–14 days.

Management of the affected infant

The DAGT is a useful indicator of affected infants and should be carried out on cord blood from all those 'at risk'. The indications for exchange transfusion are severe anaemia (haemoglobin less than 12 g/dl) or danger of kernicterus. The actual criteria for determining when to carry out an exchange transfusion vary between centres but a bilirubin level of 250 mmol/l (14.5 mg/dl) may be considered an absolute indication. The need for further exchange transfusions may be reduced by phototherapy which makes use of the property of light in the blue-green spectrum to convert bilirubin to water-soluble and harmless biliverdin.

Prevention of Rh sensitization

The discovery that IgG anti-D given intramuscularly to the mother in the postpartum period will protect against Rh immunization has revolutionized the management of Rh haemolytic disease. Immunization is caused by transplacental haemorrhage from fetus to mother which usually occurs during delivery. IgG anti-D (25 μg) will neutralize about 1 ml of fetal cells and 100 μg given within 72 hours of delivery will protect 99 per cent of mothers at risk. Increasing the dose improves the protection and at some centres IgG anti-D is given during pregnancy to guard against the rare situation where transplacental haemorrhage occurs early. Examination of the mother's blood for fetal red cells by the acid-elution technique for staining fetal haemoglobin will help to identify the size of the transplacental haemorrhage. If more than nine fetal cells are seen in five high-power fields then 200 μg of anti-D should be given.

ABO haemolysis of the newborn

HDN due to ABO incompatibility occurs when IgG antibodies against the child's blood group cross the placenta in high concentration and this may arise when a group O mother has a group A or B infant. Although 15 per cent of pregnancies are ABO incompatible, haemolysis is rare, hyperbilirubinaemia occurring in only about 1.5 per 1000 pregnancies and exchange transfusion being necessary in only about 1 in 1500 infants. In contrast to Rh HDN, ABO incompatibility occurs as commonly in the first pregnancy as in subsequent pregnancies and once it has occurred, further children are not necessarily affected. Hydrops fetalis probably never occurs from this cause. The DAGT is only weakly positive or is negative in the infant's blood but the infant's blood film may show spherocytosis. Treatment, when necessary is by transfusion of O cells from donors who do not have high titres of immune anti-A or anti-B.

NON-IMMUNE ACQUIRED HAEMOLYTIC ANAEMIAS

Damage to the red cell membrane leading to haemolysis may occur in certain infections, through oxidative damage brought about by various drugs and chemicals or through physical damage to the red cell. Except in infection where immune mechanisms probably play some part in the destruction of red cells, intravascular haemolysis is the usual result.

Infections causing haemolytic anaemia

Malaria
(See Section 5 and page 19.241.)

Toxoplasmosis
(See Section 5.)

Most infections with *Toxoplasma gondii* are symptomless or very mild. Infection of the fetus in utero, however, may give rise to a very severe disease resembling haemolytic disease of the newborn. Stillbirth and premature delivery are common and the infant may be hydropic and severely anaemic with erythroblasts in the peripheral blood. There are usually neurological symptoms due to the presence of cysts in the brain. Rarely, acquired toxoplasmosis produces a haemolytic anaemia in adults.

Bacterial infection
Depression of erythropoiesis is the common cause of the anaemia associated with bacterial infections (see page 19.240) but in some circumstances acute haemolysis is the dominant feature. Severe infections, particularly with Gram-negative organisms which produce endotoxin may lead to disseminated intravascular coagulation (DIC) and a mechanical haemolytic anaemia (see below). *Clostridium welchii septicaemia* is associated with an intense intravascular haemolysis, microspherocytosis, and fragmentation of the red cells. Renal failure usually occurs. Two mechanisms operate to produce the haemolysis, DIC and direct destruction of red cells by lecithinase and proteolytic toxins produced by the organism. *Bartonella bacilliformis* causes *Oroya fever* which is characterized by fever, chills, bone and muscle pain, and acute intravascular haemolysis. The organism occurs only in western South America and may be recognized on Romanowsky stained blood films as red micrococci on or just inside the red cell membrane (see Section 5).

Chemically induced haemolysis

Haemolysis may be caused by a number of drugs and chemicals because of their oxidant effect or that of their metabolites (Table 11).

Pathogenesis
The major pathways by which reducing power is generated in red cells were described earlier (page 19.140). Many drugs and chemicals are strong oxidants and may overcome these reduction mechanisms. There are several inherited conditions which make red cells more susceptible to oxidant damage. G6PD deficiency has already been described (see page 19.140). There is individual variability in the way in which some drugs are metabolized. For example, the oxidant metabolite of phenacetin, 2-OH phenetidine, is formed in small amounts in most individuals, but in subjects who develop chronic intravascular haemolysis or renal damage due to phenacetin a much higher proportion of the drug is metabolized into phenetidine. There is a relatively inefficient reduction system in the red cells of newborn infants and hence they are much more prone to develop haemolysis due to the administration of oxidants.

Variability in absorption of drugs seems to play a role in the development of drug-induced haemolytic anaemia. For example, partial gastrectomy may encourage overgrowth of bowel flora which may in turn increase the level of oxidant metabolites. The use of dapsone and salazopyrine in inflammatory disorders of the bowel may change the pattern of their absorption and hence increase their toxicity at varying times during the course of an illness.

Intravascular haemolysis with renal failure

Some strongly oxidizing chemicals such as arsine or chlorate, which may be encountered in industry or used for self-poisoning, produce an intense haemolysis together with DIC and acute renal failure. Constitutional symptoms occur and there may be cyanosis due to associated methaemoglobinaemia. The blood film is bizarre with red cell ghosts, fragments, and microspherocytes. The platelet count may fall. Treatment is urgent, the prime requirements being blood transfusion and the preservation of renal function. Haemodialysis and exchange transfusion have been used with success though mortality is high. The management of acute methaemoglobinaemia is discussed on pages 19.128 and 19.129.

Acute intravascular haemolysis

Haemoglobinaemia by itself is not a cause of renal failure and acute intravascular haemolysis may follow drug ingestion without renal impairment. This may occur in apparently normal patients who have ingested drugs such as phenylhydrazine which have an oxidant action. In patients with G6PD deficiency or in infants this is the common result of exposure to oxidant drugs (see page 19.140).

Chronic intravascular haemolysis

The usual result of normal individuals taking oxidant drugs such as dapsone or sulphasalazine for long periods, and an idiosyncratic effect in patients susceptible to phenacetin, is a chronic intravascular haemolysis. Cyanosis, due to the presence of methaemoglobin and sulphaemoglobin may be prominent. Renal impairment always occurs with phenacetin as a direct effect of the drug on the kidney but is not seen with the other drugs.

Laboratory findings
There are features of intravascular haemolysis and the peripheral blood film shows red cells which are irregular and contracted, often with only a segment of the membrane apparently normal. *Heinz bodies* (precipitated haemoglobin) may be seen but are uncommon unless the spleen has been removed.

Treatment
Withdrawal of the drug will terminate the haemolysis but it is not always possible to stop treatment, particularly with dapsone or sulphasalazine. Provided the haemolysis is well compensated it is reasonable to continue the treatment together with iron and folate supplements. If anaemia is a problem, reduction of the dose of the drug may be necessary.

MECHANICAL HAEMOLYTIC ANAEMIAS

Fragmentation of red cells by mechanical trauma occurs when foreign material has been introduced into major vessels at cardiac surgery and where small blood vessels have been partially blocked by fibrin strands. The former has been called cardiac haemolysis and the latter microangiopathic haemolytic anaemia.

Cardiac haemolysis

The insertion of prosthetic valves or patches into the heart or aorta usually leads to some destruction of circulating red cells. Under certain circumstances this process can be sufficient to produce severe haemolytic anaemia. The first detailed description of such a case by Sayed *et al.* (1961) contains most of the important clinical and laboratory findings.

Pathogenesis
Cardiac haemolysis is likely to develop where foreign material is present in a turbulent stream of blood. Homografts rarely produce marked haemolysis. Mitral valve prostheses produce severe haemolysis less commonly than aortic but when they do the anaemia is often profound. The usual cause is a failure of the anchorage points of the graft ring so that blood leaks in a small jet around the side between the high pressure left ventricle and low pressure left atrium.

Cardiac haemolysis is aggravated by an increase in cardiac output so that exercise and anaemia itself may increase the rate of cell destruction.

Cardiac surgery in patients with haemoglobinopathies or other congenital haemolytic anaemias presents special problems. The difficulties of surgery in patients with sickling disorders are dealt with elsewhere (see page 19.125) but, postoperatively, cardiac haemolysis may be greater in patients with mechanically fragile cells.

Clinical features
The onset of significant haemolysis depends upon the development of suitable circumstances for mechanical destruction. This may occur at any time but there are certain periods where these conditions are most likely to be met and the acuteness of the haemolysis may give some indication as to its cause. Severe haemolysis occurring immediately postoperatively suggests a surgical cause such as a defective stitch in the mitral valve ring or incomplete occlusion of a foramen with a patch. Gradually increasing haemolysis after the patient has left hospital suggests that exercise is promoting turbulence or possibly that iron deficiency is aggravating the anaemia and increasing the turbulence. Delayed onset of haemolysis, particularly after some years in patients with ball valve prosthesis, suggests distortion of the ball or other abnormalities of the prosthesis and reoperation may be necessary.

Laboratory findings
The peripheral blood film shows distorted and fragmented red cells with microspherocytes in most cases but in very acute lesions fragmentation may be hard to find and does not correlate well with the severity of the mechanical haemolysis. The platelet count is usually normal or high as is the white cell count. Other features of intravascular haemolysis are present.

Table 11 Chemically induced haemolysis

Drug or chemical	Probably haemolytic substance	Remarks
Phenacetin	2-Hydroxyphenetidin	Cyanosis and HB* haemolysis, renal papillary necrosis
Sulphonamides	Hydroxyamino derivatives	Acute haemolysis: hypersensitiity or G6PD deficiency: chronic haemolysis rare
Sulphones	4, Hydroxylamino derivatives	HB haemolysis, dose related
Salicylazosulphapyridine	Sulphapyridine	HB haemolysis, dose related
Phenothiazine	?	Overdose produces HR haemolysis
Phenazopyridine	?	Methaemoglobinaemia common, haemolytic HB anaemia may occur
Para amino-salicylic acid	*m*-Aminophenol	Solutions of PAS stored in warm become brown: *m*-NH$_2$ phenol
Phenylhydrazine and acetyl phenylhydrazine	Phenylhydrazine	No longer used in treatment of polycythaemia vera; self administration may occur; used as experimental oxidizing agent
Water soluble vitamin K analogues	2-Methyl-14-naphthoquinone	Premature infants at risk
Sodium or potassium chlorate	C10$_4$	Weed killer: DIC† as well as HB haemolysis and methaemoglobinaemia
Lead	—	The haemolytic component of lead poisoning is mild
Copper	—	Self poisoning or contaminated tubing
Naphthalene, naphthol	Naphthol	Moth balls, nappy sterilizer; may be absorbed through by infants
Wax crayons (red and orange)	*p*-Nitroaniline	Not permitted now in most countries: children and infants at risk
Well-water nitrates	Nitrite	Methaemoglobinaemia in infants; haemolysis may occur occasionally
Nitrobenzene derivatives	Aromatic nitro groups	Industrial workers, especially in munitions, at risk
Nitrotoluene TNT arsine	Arsine	Metal smelters at risk
Insect and snake bites	?	Haemolysis occurs occasionally after bites by spiders and some snakes

* HB: Heinz body. † DIC: Disseminated intravascular coagulation.

Table 12 Causes of microangiopathic haemolytic anaemia

Disease	Microangiopathy
Haemolytic-uraemic syndrome	Microthrombi in renal arteries and capillaries
Thrombotic thrombocytopenic purpura	Disseminated intravascular coagulation (DIC)
Renal cortical necrosis	Necrotizing arteritis
Acute glomerular nephritis	Necrotizing arteritis
Pre-eclampsia	Fibrinoid necrosis. DIC (?)
Malignant hypertension	Fibrinoid necrosis. Intimal proliferation in renal vessels
Disseminated carcinomatosis (especially mucinous types)	DIC tumour emoli (?)
Polyarteritis nodosa	Arteritis
Wegener's granulomatosis	Arteritis
Systemic lupus erythematosus	Arteritis
Homograft rejection	Microthrombi in transplanted organ
Meningococcaemia and other septicaemias	DIC
Cavernous haemangioma	?Local vascular anomalies or thrombosis
Purpura fulminans	?Microthrombi in skin vessels
Polycarboxylate interferon induction	DIC

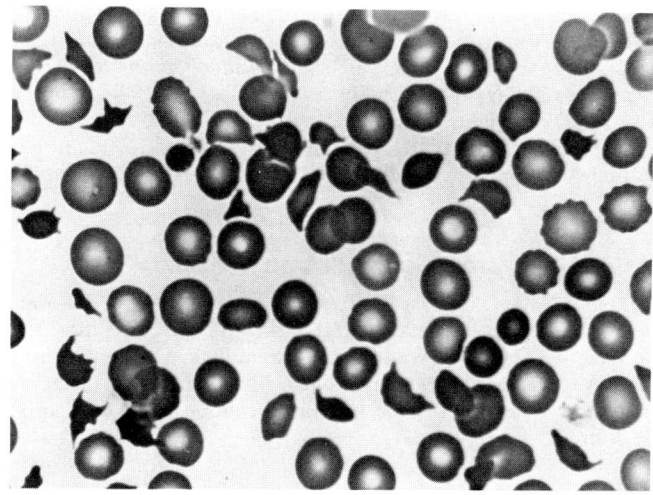

Fig. 8 The peripheral blood changes in microangiopathic haemolytic anaemia. This patient had recurrent thrombotic thrombocytopenic purpura and the marked fragmentation of the red cells together with microspherocytosis is evident on the blood film (× 1000, Leishman stain).

Management

Oral iron should be given so that iron deficiency does not develop as a result of haemosiderinuria. Intractable haemolysis may be an indication of surgical re-exploration.

Cardiac haemolysis and bacterial endocarditis

Bacterial endocarditis may cause a severe and rapid anaemia which is difficult to distinguish from mechanical haemolysis due simply to foreign material. The anaemia is caused by marrow depression usually associated with an increase in mechanical destruction of red cells. The mild hypochromia of infection may suggest iron deficiency but a low serum iron *and* a low iron-binding capacity, and the presence of iron in marrow macrophages indicate secondary anaemia (see page 19.92). There is usually a rise in α_2-macroglobulin in endocarditis in contradistinction to the reduced α_2 level in haemolysis. Serum complement components are normal in cardiac haemolysis but may be reduced in endocarditis. An enlarging spleen and the presence of red cells as well as haemoglobin in the urine points to bacterial endocarditis.

Microangiopathic haemolytic anaemia (MAHA)

Microangiopathic haemolytic anaemia is a term used to describe intravascular haemolysis due to mechanical destruction of red cells as a result of a variety of pathological changes in small blood vessels. The term was first used by Brain and his colleagues when they noted that fragmented red cells were associated with a wide range of conditions, all of which had in common damage to small blood vessels. The condition has been described in association with a variety of systemic disorders, some of which are summarized in Table 12.

Pathogenesis

MAHA develops in many different disorders associated with pathological changes in small vessels of which microthrombi in capillaries and arterioles, fibrinoid necrosis, necrotizing arteritis, and invasion of capillary walls by malignant cells are probably the most common.

Some of the disorders which produce MAHA are associated with disseminated intravascular coagulation (DIC) and it has been suggested that microthrombi cause haemolysis because the red cells are fragmented during their passage through the fibrin clots in the small vessels. While this is certainly true in some cases, the relationship between DIC and MAHA is far from clear cut. Some patients show evidence of a severe form of DIC and yet have virtually no fragmented red cells in their peripheral blood while others may have a severe MAHA and yet show no laboratory evidence of DIC. It is possible that these discrepancies reflect differences in the rate of fibrin deposition and the size of the vessels involved in the pathological process. However, there are still many gaps in our knowledge about the pathogenesis of this condition and its relationship to fibrin deposition is still uncertain.

Clinical features

MAHA is characterized by a haemolytic anaemia of varying severity. It is usually seen in a clinical setting of one of the disorders which are summarized in Table 12.

The haemolytic uraemic syndrome and thrombotic thrombocytopenic purpura are considered separately later in this section. The presence of renal disease, pre-eclampsia, or septicaemia usually presents no diagnostic difficulty. If a patient presents with MAHA with no obvious associated disease, it is important to rule out an underlying carcinoma or collagen vascular disease. The commonest tumours which are associated with this condition are mucus-secreting carcinomata of the stomach, lung, breast, and large bowel. These are nearly always widely disseminated and it is often possible to demonstrate tumour cells in the bone marrow. If disseminated carcinomatosis can be excluded, it is necessary to proceed to investigations for the various collagen vascular disorders summarized in Table 12.

Laboratory features

There is a variable degree of anaemia with a reticulocytosis and all the features characteristic of haemolytic anaemia. The diagnosis is made largely on the morphological appearances of the red cells which show marked fragmentation and many microspherocytes (Fig. 8); the Coombs' test is negative. A reduced platelet count suggests that there may be an associated DIC (see page 19.231).

Treatment

The only really successful approach to the treatment of MAHA is to find and eradicate the underlying cause. Severe anaemia requires blood transfusion. The use of heparin in the haemolytic uraemic syndrome and in thrombotic thrombocytopenic purpura is considered later. In other forms of MAHA its value is uncertain and it is the authors' experience that, unless the underlying cause can be dealt with, it is best to treat the condition symptomatically with blood transfusion. Certainly, heparin does not seem to be of value in the form of MAHA associated with disseminated carcinomatosis or collagen vascular disease. The subject of heparin therapy for DIC is considered further on page 19.231. The place of agents which reduce platelet aggregation is under investigation but at present there is no evidence that they are of value in this condition.

Haemolytic-uraemic syndrome (HUS)

In 1955 Gasser and his colleagues described five previously healthy children who developed acute renal failure and intravascular haemolysis. They gave the name haemolytic uraemic syndrome (HUS) to the association and since then many cases have been described. The renal aspects of the condition are considered in Section 18.

Pathogenesis

HUS is a disease of infancy although the peak incidence varies in different parts of the world, being about 13 months in Argentina and about 4 years in California, for example. There is also a seasonal variation and it is commoner in the northern hemisphere in the late spring and early summer. There are several reports of more than one family member being affected. These observations, together with the acute febrile nature of the illness, suggest an infectious basis, and viruses, rickettsiae, and bacteria have been variously indicated.

The delay between the febrile illness and the onset of haemolysis and renal failure has cast doubt on whether there is a direct cause-and-effect relationship between the infection and the onset of haemolysis and suggests that an immune response to the infecting organism triggers off intravascular coagulation. On the other hand it has been consistently impossible to detect any evidence for immune complex deposition in the microangiopathic lesions in this disorder. The latter consist of widespread damage to the vascular endothelium with secondary fibrin deposition involving particularly renal arterioles and glomerular capillaries. These changes are also found widely throughout all the organ systems. It is presumed that the red cell changes are secondary to damage during their passage through these small vessels. Laboratory evidence of a consumptive coagulopathy has been obtained although the results are inconsistent.

Clinical and haematological features

The syndrome usually develops following a febrile illness accompanied by diarrhoea and vomiting in a previously healthy child. There may be marked gastrointestinal symptoms including bloody diarrhoea and abdominal pain.

Evidence of acute intravascular haemolysis with rapidly developing anaemia develops during or shortly after the prodromal illness and may precede the onset of oliguria. Purpura and bleeding may also occur during the acute phase. Drowsiness, convulsions, and coma may develop and death may occur during the acute phase from uncontrollable anaemia, haemorrhage, or hypertension.

About a third of patients do not develop oliguria, and about a third have up to 10 days, and the remainder up to 4 weeks, of oliguria. The majority of patients without oliguria recover completely without treatment. The longer the perod of oliguria, the more likely it is that the condition will go on to a chronic renal failure.

The overall death rate from HUS syndrome varies from about 2 to 10 per cent. Widespread differences in prognosis between southern and northern hemispheres may reflect differences in aetiology and supportive care in these areas.

The peripheral blood film shows fragmentation and distortion of the red cells with occasional spherocytes. In contrast to cardiac haemolytic anaemia, thrombocytopenia is common although not invariable. There is often a moderate leucocytosis. Usually there is laboratory evidence of intravascular haemolysis with a raised plasma haemoglobin level, methaemalbumin, low or absent serum haptoglobins, and, sometimes haemoglobinuria. Coagulation studies (see page 19.231) give equivocal and often conflicting results although in some cases there is evidence for a consumptive coagulopathy.

Management

The mainstay of treatment is supportive care, transfusion, hydration, control of hypertension, and, if necessary, dialysis. These measures are considered in greater detail in Section 18.

There have been many reports of the use of heparin therapy in this disorder. The results are, at the best, equivocal. More recently there have been anecdotal reports of the use of inhibitors of platelet aggregation and synthetic prostacyclins. The numbers treated so far are so small that no conclusions can be drawn about the value of this treatment. Corticosteroid therapy is ineffective.

Thrombotic thrombocytopenic purpura (TTP)

Thrombotic thrombocytopenic purpura is a disorder which has many similarities to HUS but occurs mainly in adults and the central nervous system is involved more commonly than in HUS. The renal aspects are considered in Section 18.

Aetiology and pathogenesis

The aetiology of TTP is completely unknown although, because of the many similarities to HUS, an infective basis has been suggested.

The pathological changes in TTP include the presence of hyaline material within the lumen of small vessels, endothelial proliferation and aneurysmal dilation of the vessels. The first two changes may be the result of intravascular coagulation whereas the anatomical changes in the vessels have features in common with those seen in polyarteritis nodosa and systemic lupus erythematosus. Some patients with TTP have other pathological changes more commonly associated with systemic lupus erythematosus including periarticular fibrosis of the spleen, thickening of the glomerular basement membranes with the appearance of wire loops, atypical verrucous endocarditis, and occasionally positive LE preparations. It is clear that at least at the tissue level there is a marked overlap between HUS, TTP, and the collagen vascular disorders.

Recently it has been found that there is an increase in platelet adhesiveness in TTP which seems to be caused by a failure of prostacyclin production by the vascular endothelium. Some patients appear to lack a serum factor which allows the renewal of prostacyclin production as assayed by the rabbit aorta model. Furthermore, some patients with TTP show decreased excretion of the metabolite of prostacyclin, 6-keto-PGF$_{Ia}$. These observations require further evaluation.

Clinical features

The disorder affects females more commonly than males and may occur at any age with a peak incidence in young adults. The onset is often sudden with the development of fever and signs of neurological damage. The latter include convulsions, coma, transient or permanent paralyses, and bizarre psychiatric disturbances, sometimes with hallucinations. Purpura may accompany or follow the neurological signs and there may be severe bleeding, particularly from the gastrointestinal tract. Anaemia is not usually severe although occasionally there may be dramatic intravascular haemolysis with haemoglobinuria.

The illness may run a fluctuating course of days or weeks and some patients may have a series of acute episodes with apparent recovery in-between. The commonest causes of death are bleeding, a cerebrovascular accident or renal failure.

Haematological and biochemical changes
There is a mild to severe haemolytic anaemia with fragmentation and contraction of the red cells. This is associated with a variable degree of thrombocytopenia; in some cases the platelets may almost disappear from the peripheral blood. The bone marrow is cellular and megakaryocytes are present in increased numbers and have normal morphology. There is usually a neutrophil leucocytosis. In some cases coagulation studies show evidence of a consumption coagulopathy.

There is nearly always some proteinuria and often evidence of renal damage in the form of casts and red cells together with a raised blood urea and reduced creatinine clearance. In some cases there may be serological findings suggestive of systemic lupus erythematosus.

Chronic relapsing forms and TTP in pregnancy
There appears to be a subgroup of patients with a TTP-like illness who give a long history of relapses going back to childhood and often initiated by a disorder resembling the haemolytic uraemic syndrome.

TTP seems to be particularly prone to occur during pregnancy or in the post-partum period and this may account for the slight excess of young women affected by this disease. It is often associated with miscarriage. Removal of the fetus does not always lead to remission.

Treatment
Because TTP is a rare disease, there have been few extensive studies of its management and the literature is full of anecdotal case reports. It is extremely difficult to give a balanced view as to how this condition should be managed and, indeed, whether any form of therapy other than careful symptomatic treatment has any real effect on its outcome.

Symptomatic treatment includes transfusion for anaemia and the management of renal failure by dialysis. Many other approaches have been tried including the administration of heparin, drugs which reduce platelet aggregation such as aspirin and dipyridamole, dextran 70 infusion, splenectomy and, more recently, exchange transfusion and the administration of fresh frozen plasma. The rationale of the last approach is that plasma exchange might replace a missing prostacyclin-stimulating factor which also might be replaced by the blood products used in plasmapheresis. At least one patient who responded showed a rise in 6-keto-PGF_{Ia} levels after plasmapheresis.

With this rather anecdotal evidence as a basis it seems reasonable to start treatment with antiplatelet drugs and to maintain an adequate haemoglobin level and manage the renal failure appropriately. If there is no response plasma exchange should be initiated and, if the patient responds with a rise in platelet count and/or reduction in haemolysis, treatment should be continued with plasma infusion alone with the reintroduction of plasma exchange if the condition deteriorates. If there is no response to any of these measures within a few days, prostacyclin analogue infusion may be tried or splenectomy considered. As judged by the current literature on TTP it seems likely that the mortality will be of the order of 30 per cent or more whatever measures are adopted.

March haemoglobinuria
Haemoglobinuria following vigorous exercise in young men has been recognized for many years as a benign disorder but it was the studies of Davidson (1964) which showed that mechanical haemolysis was the cause. Haemoglobinuria follows walking or running on a hard surface and lasts for a few hours. There may be some systemic symptoms such as nausea and abdominal pain but usually the haemoglobinuria is symptomless. The haemolysis is produced by the interaction of a hard surface and red cells in the superficial vessels of the feet, but the blood film is normal in appearance and fragments are not seen. Treatment is not usually necessary but the insertion of a springy sole into running shoes will usually prevent haemolysis. As mentioned above (see page 19.139), recent studies on the red cell membrane suggest that a structural change may underlie the increased susceptibility to mechanisms of red cell destruction in this condition; these observations await confirmation.

Haemolytic anaemia of burns
Extensive burns produce intravascular haemolysis with microspherocytosis and fragmentation in the peripheral blood. The direct action of heat is probably important in the pathogenesis but intravascular coagulation in the postinjury period may play some part.

Acquired disorders of the cell membrane
Paroxysmal nocturnal haemoglobinuria is the commonest acquired disorder of the red cell membrane. Changes in the environment of the red cell, particularly the lipid environment, may induce membrane changes which lead to some shortening of red cell lifespan though haemolytic anaemia is uncommon.

Lipid disorders
The cholesterol and part of the phospholipid content of the red cell membrane are in equilibrium with plasma lipids. Changes in the latter influence the lipid content of the membrane and the shape and deformability of the red cell. Abnormalities of membrane lipid metabolism may contribute to the haemolysis of liver disease and disorders associated with hyperlipidaemia.

Liver disease
(See page 19.245.)

There is a shortening of the red cell lifespan in most patients with acute hepatitis, cirrhosis, and Gilbert's disease (see Section 12). In Gilbert's disease the decreased red cell survival and slight reticulocytosis suggests that haemolysis may contribute to the increased unconjugated bilirubin, but it seems probable that it is only a minor factor and that deficiency of the enzyme UDP-glucuronyl transferase is mainly responsible. In biliary obstruction and mild liver disease target cells are seen in the peripheral blood. In more severe disorders acanthocytosis is prominent.

Zieve's syndrome
This is the association of haemolytic anaemia with abdominal pain, cirrhosis, hyperlipidaemia, and jaundice in chronic alcoholics. The peripheral blood contains spherocytes and the osmotic fragility is increased unlike most liver disorders in which it is reduced.

Wilson's disease
(See Section 9.)

Acute haemolysis may be a presenting feature in Wilson's disease. It may be caused by the presence of free copper in the plasma.

Vitamin E deficiency
Vitamin E is necessary to prevent auto-oxidation of the unsaturated fatty acids in the red cell membrane. Deficiency may occur in premature infants fed polyunsaturated fatty acids in artificial foods. A haemolytic anaemia with acanthocytosis occurs together with thrombocytosis. There is a prompt response to vitamin E administration.

Congenital pyknocytosis
This is a rare condition seen in infants characterized by haemolytic anaemia and the presence of bizarre contracted red cells. The hae-

molysis may be marked but the disease is usually transient and the child recovers completely. The cause is unknown.

Hypersplenism

A significant enlargement of the spleen is frequently associated with a slightly shortened red cell survival even though the red cells are intrinsically normal. The mechanism and methods for identifying this form of haemolysis are considered on pages 19.189 and 19.191.

Anaemia of chronic disorders and renal disease

The haemolytic component of the anaemia of chronic disorders is described on page 19.92.

Physical agents

Haemolytic anaemia has been observed in astronauts exposed to 100 per cent oxygen. There have been occasional reports of acute haemolysis occurring in patients undergoing hyperbaric oxygen therapy. The mechanism for these changes is unknown. The shortened red cell survival which occurs after total body irradiation has a complex basis which is ill understood; red cells are remarkably resistant to the direct effects of ionizing radiation.

References

Adelman, R. D., Halsted, C. C. and Shiekolishlam, B. M. (1980). Hemolytic uremic syndrome: associated conditions. *J. Pediat.* **97**, 161–162.

Bateman, S. M., Hilgard, P. and Gordon-Smith, E. C. (1979). Thrombotic thrombocytopenic purpura: a possible plasma factor. *Br. J. Haematol.* **43**, 498.

Becker, P. S. and Lux, S. E. (1985). Hereditary spherocytosis and related disorders. *Clin. Haematol.* **14**, 15–44.

Beutler, E. (1983). Glucose 6-phosphate dehydrogenase deficiency. In *Hematology*, 3rd edn (eds W. J. Williams, E. Beutler, A. J. Erslev and M. A. Lichtman), pp. 561–573. McGraw-Hill, New York.

Brain, M. C. (1982). The red cell membrane; disorders of membrane structure and function. In *Blood and its disorders*, 2nd edn. (eds R. M. Hardisty and D. J. Weatherall), pp. 453–478. Blackwell Scientific Publications, Oxford.

——, Dacie, J. V. and Hourhane, D. O'B. (1962). Microangiopathic haemolytic anaemia: the possible role of vascular lesions in pathogenesis. *Br. J. Haematol.* **8**, 358.

Chevion, M., Navok, T. and Glaser, G. (1982). Favism inducing agents: biochemical and mechanistic considerations. In *Advances in red blood cell biology* (eds D. J. Weatherall, G. Fiorelli and S. Gorini), pp. 381–390. Raven Press, New York.

Clarke, C. A. and Whitfield, A. G. W. (1979). Deaths from rhesus haemolytic disease in England and Wales in 1977; accuracy of records and assessment of anti-D prophylaxis. *Br. Med. J.* **i**, 1665–1669.

Davidson, R. J. L. (1969). March or exertional hemoglobinuria. *Semin. Hematol.* **6**, 150.

Editorial *The Lancet* (1979). Plasma exchange in thrombotic thrombocytopenic purpura. *Lancet* **i**, 1065–1066.

Emerson, P. M. and Grimes, A. J. (1982). Red cell metabolism: the hereditary enzymopathies. In *Blood and its disorders*, 2nd edn (eds R. M. Hardisty and D. J. Weatherall), pp. 265–322. Blackwell Scientific Publications, Oxford.

Gordon-Smith, E. C. (1980). Drug induced oxidative haemolysis. *Clin. Haematol.* **9**, 557–586.

—— (1982). The non-immune acquired haemolytic anaemias. In *Blood and its disorders*, 2nd edn (eds R. M. Hardisty and D. J. Weatherall), pp. 515–544. Blackwell Scientific Publications, Oxford.

Gross, S. (1976). Hemolytic anemia in premature infants; relationship to vitamin E, selenium, glutathione peroxidase and erythrocyte lipids, *Semin. Hematol.* **13**, 187.

Hensby, C. N., Lewis, P. J. Hilgard, P., Nufti, G. J., Hows, J. and Webster, J. (1979). Prostacyclin deficiency in thrombotic thrombocytopenic purpura. *Lancet* **ii**, 748.

Hughes-Jones, N. and Bain, B. (1982). Immune haemolytic anaemia. In *Blood and its disorders*, 2nd edn (eds R. M. Hardisty and D. J. Weatherall), pp. 479–514. Blackwell Scientific Publications, Oxford.

Kaplan, B. S. and Drummon, K. V. (1978). The hemolytic-uremic syndrome as a syndrome. *New Engl. J. Med.* **298**, 964–966.

Kattamis, C. A., Kyriazakou, M., and Chiadis, S. (1969). Favism. Clinical and biochemical data. *J. Med. Genet.* **6**, 34–41.

Keitt, A. S. (1981). Diagnostic strategy in a suspected red cell enzymopathy. *Clin. Haematol.* **10**, 3–30.

Mackin, S. J. (1984). Thrombotic thrombocytopenic purpura. *Br. J. Haematol.* **56**, 191–198.

Magilligan, D. J., Fisher, E. and Alam, M. (1980). Hemolytic anemia with porcine xenograft aortic and mitral valves, *J. Thorac. Cardiovasc. Surg.* **79**, 628–631.

Marsh, G. W. and Lewis, S. M. (1969). Cardiac hemolytic anemia. *Semin. Hematol.* **6**, 133–145.

Miwa, S. (1981). Pyruvate kinase deficiency and other enzymopathies of the Embden Meyerhof pathway. *Clin. Haematol.* **10**, 57–80.

Mohandas, N., Phillips, W. M., and Bessis, M. (1979). Red blood cell deformability and hemolytic anemias. *Semin. Hematol.* **16**, 95.

Palek, J. (1985). Hereditary elliptocytosis and related disorders. *Clin. Haemat.* **14**, 45–88.

Rutkow, I. M. (1978). Thrombotic thrombocytopenic purpura (TTP) and splenectomy: A current appraisal. *Ann. Surg.* **188**, 701–705.

Sayed, H. M., Dacie, J. V., Handley, D. A., Lewis, S. M. and Cleland, W. P. (1961). Haemolytic anaemia of mechanical origin after open heart surgery. *Thorax*, **16**, 356–360.

Valentine, W. N. and Paglia, D. E. (1984). Erythrocyte enzymopathies, hemolytic anaemia and multisystem disease: an annotated review. *Blood* **64**, 583–591.

Walker, B. K., Ballas, S. K. and Martinez, J. (1980). Plasma infusion for thrombotic thrombocytopenic purpura during pregnancy. *Arch. Intern. Med.* **140**, 981–983.

The relative and secondary polycythaemias

D. J. WEATHERALL

The word 'polycythaemia' means an increased red cell count, packed cell volume, or haemoglobin level. In an earlier section we described the form of polycythaemia which is thought to be due to the neoplastic proliferation of a clone of haemopoietic red cell progenitors, polycythaemia vera (page 19.37). However, while it is quite common in clinical practice to encounter patients with a haemoglobin level which is above normal, this type of polycythaemia is quite rare. In this chapter we shall consider the more common causes of polycythaemia and how these are identified and managed.

Classification and pathogenesis

The mechanisms for the production of polycythaemia are summarized in Table 1. A high haemoglobin level can occur for two main reasons. First, there may be a reduction in the plasma volume with a normal red cell mass. Second, there may be a genuine increase in the red cell mass. Thus it is usual to divide the polycythaemias into relative and absolute. The causes of a contracted plasma volume which leads to a relative polycythaemia are considered later.

The mechanisms for the production of an increased red cell mass are best understood in terms of a breakdown of the normal regulation of erythropoiesis (see page 19.63). The rate of red cell production is controlled by the level of erythropoietin, the production of which is governed by the oxygen supply to the tissues. As well as the neoplastic proliferation of haemopoietic progenitors which occurs in polycythaemia vera there are several other ways in which the red cell mass can increase. First, there may be an appropriate response to an increased output of erythropoietin secondary to hypoxia. This is the mechanism of the polycythaemia of chronic obstructive airways disease, cyanotic congenital heart disease, altitude, hypoventilation, or defective release of oxygen by the red cells. The latter may result from chronic carboxyhaemoglobinaemia due to cigarette smoking or, much less commonly, from intrinsic abnormalities of haemoglobin or red cell enzymes.

Table 1 Mechanisms for the production of polycythaemia

Relative
  Reduced plasma volume

Absolute
  Normal or low erythropoietin levels; abnormal proliferation
    polycythaemia vera
  Increased erythropoietin levels
    Appropriate
      lung disease, cyanotic heart disease, altitude, abnormal
      haemoglobin, hypoventilation, decreased 2,3-DPG production
    Inappropriate
      renal tumour; other erythropoietin-secreting tumours, after renal
      transplant; genetic defect in erythropoietin regulation
    Mechanism unknown
      endocrine disease; Cushing's disease, phaeochromocytoma

Second, there may be inappropriate secretion of high levels of erythropoietin. This usually results from an erythropoietin-secreting renal tumour or from ectopic production of erythropoietin from extrarenal lesions. It may also occur as a transient phenomenon after renal transplantation, or in families with a genetic defect in erythropoietin regulation. Finally, there are some endocrine disorders such as Cushing's disease in which there may be a genuine increase in the red cell mass, the mechanism of which is not understood.

In clinical practice it is not uncommon to encounter patients with a genuine increase in the red cell mass who do not appear to fit into any of these categories. They do not have splenomegaly or an elevated white cell or platelet count characteristic of polycythaemia vera, and yet no other cause for polycythaemia can be found. They may have an elevated red cell mass of approximately the same magnitude for many years. This condition has been called *idiopathic* or *benign erythrocytosis*. However, it is becoming clear that some of these patients, if observed for long enough, develop splenomegaly or an elevated platelet or white cell count and other features which indicate that they have polycythaemia vera. However, this does not always happen and there appears to be a form of true polycythaemia which is not a myeloproliferative disorder and for which no cause can be found. It seems reasonable to retain the term *benign erythrocytosis* for this ill-defined condition.

An approach to the patient with polycythaemia

An unusually high haemoglobin level or packed cell volume (PCV) is one of the commonest reasons for the referral of patients to haematology departments. If a great deal of unnecessary worry for the patient and expensive investigation is to be avoided it is very important to develop a logical aproach to this problem (Fig. 1).

The first rule is that, unless the haemoglobin level is extremely high, it is wise never to diagnose polycythaemia on a single blood count. Care must be taken to ensure that a count is obtained when the patient is well hydrated, is not receiving large doses of diuretics, and has not had a heavy night's alcohol intake the day before the blood sample is taken. Heavy smokers who have a mild polycythaemia should be asked to stop smoking and their blood counts repeated several weeks later. Finally, it should be remembered that the haemoglobin level and PCV have a large standard deviation; many referrals for the investigation of polycythaemia stem from an ignorance of normal haematological values.

Having determined that the haemoglobin value or PCV is genuinely elevated the next step is to decide whether it is a true or relative polycythaemia. This requires a plasma volume and red cell mass determination. We shall return to the problem of interpreting these data when we consider the diagnosis of relative polycythaemia.

If the red cell mass determination shows that there is an absolute polycythaemia the next step is to decide whether this is a prim-

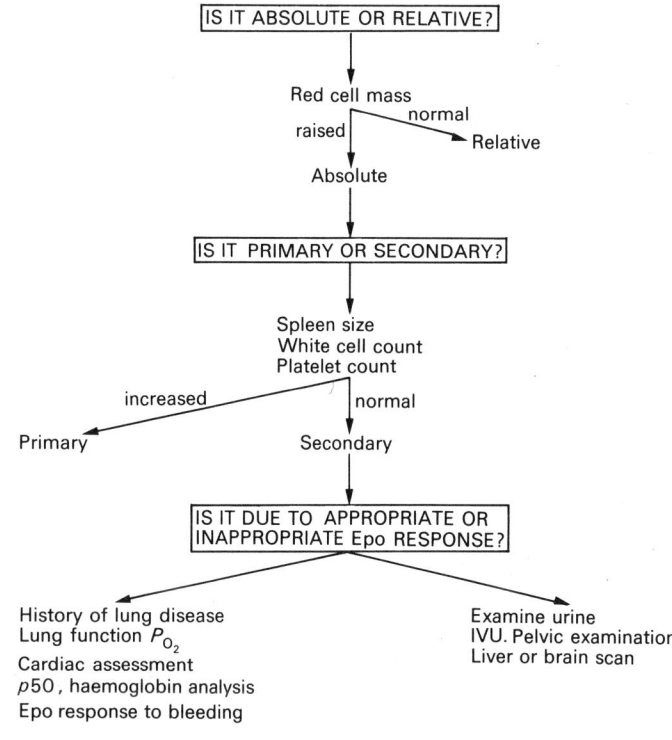

Fig. 1 Flow chart of investigations for polycythaemia.

ary myeloproliferative disorder or a pure red cell polycythaemia. The criteria for the diagnosis of polycythaemia vera are considered on page 19.38. In the absence of a raised platelet and/or white cell count, or splenomegaly, another case for the elevated red cell mass must be sought.

The causes of secondary polycythaemia are summarized in Table 2. Hypoxia due to chronic obstructive airways disease is by far the commonest. While this diagnosis can usually be made on clinical grounds this is not always the case and it may sometimes be necessary to resort to blood gas analysis, either at rest or after exercise, to rule out this diagnosis. Cyanotic heart disease usually presents no diagnostic problems but occasionally patients are encountered who have arteriovenous malformations which may not be obvious clinically. Again, analysis of the arterial oxygen saturation will provide a clue to the diagnosis. Before proceeding further it is very useful to carry out a P_{50} estimation. If the P_{50} is reduced, indicating a left shift in the oxygen dissociation curve, the carboxyhaemoglobin level should be estimated; patients are often unreliable about their smoking habits! If this is normal and the P_{50} is low there must be an intrinsic abnormality of the red cells, either of the haemoglobin or of the red cell enzymes. If the P_{50} is normal a source of inappropriate erythropoietin production should be looked for. The most likely site is the kidney, either a hypernephroma or a renal cyst. Thus a careful microscopic examination of the urine should be carried out followed by an ultrasound examination of the kidney, an IVU and, if indicated, a renal arteriogram. It may be necessary to carry out a CT scan of the liver and posterior fossa to exclude a hepatoma or haemangioblastoma of the cerebellum. In women, careful pelvic examination should be performed to search for uterine fibroids which are occasionally associated with polycythaemia. However, it should be emphasized that erythropoietin-secreting tumours are a *very rare* cause of polycythaemia and it is only necessary to go to these lengths in the minority of cases.

If the pathophysiology of secondary polycythaemia has been

Table 2   Clinical classification of polycythaemia

Relative or pseudopolycythaemia ('stress' polycythaemia)

True polycythaemia
  Primary
    polycythaemia rubra vera
  Secondary
    altitude
    chronic lung disease
    cyanotic congenital heart disease
    renal disease
      tumours, cysts, hydronephrosis, post-transplant
    non-renal tumours
      hepatoma, cerebellar haemangioma, uterine fibromata
    endocrine
      Cushing's disease, phaeochromocytoma
    genetic
      abnormal haemoglobin
      abnormal erythropoietin response
      abnormal 2,3-DPG metabolism
    obesity
      Pickwickian syndrome
    other causes of hypoventilation

---

appreciated it will be self-evident that this tedious series of investigations could be considerably simplified if we had a simple and reliable method for the estimation of the erythropoietin level. While an erythropoietin assay is not usually available, except in research laboratories, this should not be the case for long. The recent cloning of the gene for erythropoietin and its expression in micro-organisms should lead to the production of pure erythropoietin and the development of a reliable radioimmune assay within the near future.

Finally, when all these investigations have been carried out there remain a number of patients who have an increased red cell mass for which no cause can be found. It is worth assessing their close relatives to see if the condition falls into the rare group of hereditary polycythaemias due to abnormal erythropoietin control. Having excluded this diagnosis these patients should be kept under regular surveillance because, as mentioned earlier, at least some of them develop features of polycythaemia vera, sometimes after many years.

Relative polycythaemia

Relative polycythaemia has collected several names over the years, including apparent, spurious, pseudo, stress, or benign polycythaemia, and Gaisböck's syndrome. The term describes an elevated haemoglobin level or packed cell volume which results from a contraction of the plasma volume, and is not associated with an absolute increase in red cell mass. As will become apparent, the situation is not as simple as this definition might suggest.

Classification

There are two main groups of relative polycythaemias. The first is made up of patients who have a disturbance of fluid balance leading to a diminished plasma volume such as may occur in severe dehydration, following diuretic therapy, and in various endocrine disorders such as Addison's or Cushing's diseases. The second group is made up of patients who seem to have red cell masses at the upper limit of normal and a slightly contracted plasma volume. We shall confine this discussion to the second group.

Aetiology and pathogenesis

The relative polycythaemias in which there are no obvious fluid or electrolyte disturbances, although probably quite common, have been extremely difficult to define and virtually nothing is known about their pathogenesis. The real problem in this field is that it is extremely difficult to obtain accurate measurements of the red cell mass, or for that matter the plasma volume. Where these have

been done in a series of individuals labelled as having relative polycythaemia, the results have been inconsistent. In some cases the red cell mass is at the upper limit of what is accepted as 'normal' and the plasma volume is at the lower limit of normal, while in others the red cell mass may be normal and there may be a clear-cut reduction in the plasma volume. For technical reasons it is not possible to repeat these measurements very often in the same individual and hence to determine how constant the results are in the same person at different times. As a group these individuals tend to be obese, middle-aged males who are anxious and/or aggressive, overweight, and mildly hypertensive.

Against these rather spurious diagnostic criteria it has been difficult to demonstrate any clear-cut abnormalities of salt or water metabolism and the occasional reports of abnormal aldosterone or ADH patterns have been inconsistent. There is clearly a genetic component to this condition but at the moment it is ill-defined.

Relationship to thrombotic disease

There is increasing interest in the relationship of mildly elevated haemoglobin or PCV levels to cerebrovascular and coronary artery disease. There is some epidemiological data suggesting a relationship between the haemoglobin level and the incidence of arterial thrombotic disease. Cerebral blood flow studies suggest that there is a significant decrease in flow at PCV values ranging from 48–55 per cent, presumably due to increased blood viscosity. All these data indicate that a moderate elevation of the PCV may be an important risk factor in the pathogenesis of arterial disease, but more work is required before this is firmly established.

Clinical features

The typical clinical picture of relative polycythaemia is the overweight middle-aged male who is slightly hypertensive and has a haemoglobin value in the 18–20 g/dl range and a PCV of 49–55 per cent. There are no specific symptoms or signs which can be attributed to this 'disorder' and usually the presenting feature is an associated medical condition, most often cardiovascular disease or hypertension. An elevated haemoglobin level is found occasionally on routine investigation for a completely unassociated condition.

Laboratory findings

With the exception of an elevated haemoglobin and packed cell volume the rest of the haematological findings are completely normal. The red cell mass is usually normal, and as mentioned above the plasma volume may be moderately contracted. Sometimes the red cell mass is at the upper limit of normal and the plasma volume at the lower limit.

Differential diagnosis

This type of relative polycythaemia should be diagnosed with caution. It should be remembered that a high haemoglobin level may be encountered in patients who are receiving diuretic therapy, who are dehydrated for any cause (including a heavy night's drinking), or who have one of the causes of a genuine increase in the red cell mass. As emphasized earlier, tobacco smoking is one of the commonest of the latter conditions. Hence extensive investigation should not be carried out until it has been demonstrated that the haemoglobin value or packed cell volume are consistently elevated on two or three separate occasions. If this is the case, a red cell mass should be estimated and the diagnosis confirmed by finding a normal value. The clinician should always bear in mind that normal male packed cell volume is 47 per cent ± 6.2 per cent and therefore many normal men have packed cell volumes of 50–52 per cent and should not, therefore, be classified as abnormal and subjected to extensive investigation.

Management

In the past it was thought sufficient, once the diagnosis of relative polycythaemia was made, to reassure the patient strongly and to stop examining his or her blood. Suitable advice was given about weight reduction the control of hypertension, and stopping smoking. Although this is still the case, there is some recent evidence that the mild elevation of blood viscosity which occurs in patients with packed cell volumes in the 50–55 per cent range may predispose towards coronary artery and cerebrovascular disease. At the time of writing this is a controversial subject and more data are required before the place of regular venesection of these patients is firmly established. At the present time it seems reasonable to venesect patients who have had episodes of coronary artery or cerebrovascular disease and who have persistently elevated packed cell volumes, or those who have a particularly bad family history of cardiovascular disease. It is much more difficult to make a case for venesection in an asymptomatic middle-aged male with a slightly elevated PCV; if future studies show that these individuals are at considerable risk of developing vascular disease, a more aggressive approach will be required.

Secondary polycythaemia
Some of the causes of secondary polycythaemia are listed in Table 2.

Acute mountain sickness, Monge's disease
These conditions, and a description of the secondary polycythaemia that results as part of adaptation to altitude, are discussed in Section 6.

Respiratory disease
This is probably the commonest cause of secondary polycythaemia. The increased production of erythropoietin results from arterial hypoxia. There may be a right shift in the oxygen dissociation curve resulting from increased 2,3-DPG production secondary to hypoxia but this is probably of little functional significance. A curious feature of chronic pulmonary disease is that some patients do not show a compensatory polycythaemia, even if they are severely hypoxic. Although it has been suggested that this may be the result of bone marrow depression due to associated infection, this is not always the case and the lack of correlation between the PCV and degree of hypoxia in chronic chest disease remains unexplained. It should always be remembered that smoking may contribute to the polycythaemia of chronic lung disease.

The therapeutic value of venesection in patients with polycythaemia secondary to chronic obstructive airways disease remains controversial. There is some evidence for improvement in cardiac function and cerebral blood flow after venesection. Thus there may be a place for venesection in patients with PCV values of greater than 55–60 per cent, although this question requires further study.

Alveolar hypoventilation
Central alveolar hypoventilation due to an impaired response of the respiratory centre has been reported in patients with cerebrovascular accidents or in association with Parkinson's disease, encephalitis, and barbiturate overdosage. Alveolar hypoventilation may also result from mechanical impairment of the chest in patients with muscular dystrophies, poliomyelitis, or ankylosing spondylitis (see Sections 16 and 21). The *Pickwickian syndrome* is characterized by gross obesity and somnolence; the associated polycythaemia seems to be caused by a combination of both central and peripheral hypoventilation. The precise aetiology is unknown but the mechanism appears to involve a vicious circle of somnolence, hypercapnia, and hypoventilation which leads to lack of respiratory response, which is further aggravated by mechanical impairment of ventilation due to extreme obesity.

There has been considerable recent interest in the problem of *sleep apnoea*. Intermittent alveolar hypoventilation is frequently observed in normal males, and in patients who are already hypoxic due to lung disease it may cause severe arterial hypoxaemia, hypercapnia, cyanosis, and marked secondary polycythaemia. This subject is considered in detail in Section 15.

Cardiovascular disease
In any congenital heart disease with a right-to-left shunt there may be arterial oxygen unsaturation, severe cyanosis, finger clubbing, and extreme secondary polycythaemia. Some children with severe congenital heart disease of this type may have packed cell volumes in excess of 80 per cent. There is a genuine risk of thrombotic episodes, particularly if these children become dehydrated due to an intercurrent illness. There may be an indication for venesection, particularly before surgery, although the precise value of reduction of the haematocrit is not clear.

Hypoxaemia and secondary polycythaemia occurs in association with other types of right-to-left vascular shunts. For example, it is well recognized as a complication of pulmonary arteriovenous aneurysms, and hereditary telangiectasia. Shunting of this kind may also be the mechanism for the mild secondary polycythaemia which is sometimes observed in patients with cirrhosis of the liver. For this reason it is important to carry out a blood gas analysis in any patient with unexplained polycythaemia.

Defective oxygen transport
Carboxyhaemoglobin due to smoking is one of the commonest causes of secondary polycythaemia. Heavy smokers may have as much as 15 per cent of carboxyhaemoglobin, and because of the resulting increase in oxygen affinity there may be sufficient hypoxic drive to produce a moderate degree of polycythaemia. A mild degree of secondary polycythaemia is also seen in patients with genetic or acquired forms of methaemoglobinaemia (see page 19.128).

A variable degree of polycythaemia is found in patients and their affected family members with high oxygen affinity haemoglobin variants. These are described in detail on page 19.127. They can be identified by haemoglobin analysis and are all associated with a left-shifted oxygen dissociation curve and a reduced P_{50}. Polycythaemia P_{50} also occurs with red cell enzyme deficiencies associated with low levels of 2,3-DPG.

Tissue hypoxia
The only chemical that regularly produces secondary polycythaemia is cobalt. In the past this agent has been used to treat patients with refractory anaemias although it is no longer in vogue because of its side-effects. It is thought to act by inhibiting oxidative metabolism.

Inappropriate erythropoietin production
There is a variety of disorders which cause inappropriate erythropoietin production and hence a variable degree of polycythaemia. The hormone is produced by *renal tumours*, or occasionally by *tumours of the cerebellum or liver*. It has been estimated that about 2 per cent of all patients with hypernephromas have erythrocytosis. It is possible to demonstrate an increased level of erythropoietin in the serum and urine in such patients. The precise mechanism for increased erythropoietin production in patients with renal tumours remains to be determined. Although it has been suggested that the tumour secretes the hormone the finding of increased erythropoietin production in some patients with *Wilms' tumour*, or even *benign adenomas* of the kidney, suggests that mechanically induced hypoxia due to the pressure of the tumour may stimulate normal renal parenchyma to increase erythropoietin production. Once these tumours are removed the red cell mass returns to normal, although polycythaemia may recur in patients who develop metastatic tumours in the contralateral kidney.

There is a well-documented association between secondary polycythaemia and *cerebellar haemangiomata*. Cyst fluid has been shown to contain material with the properties of erythropoietin. Workers in Hong Kong, where *hepatocellular carcinoma* is common, have reported that up to 10 per cent of patients with these tumours have secondary polycythaemia. The mechanism is uncertain, since increased blood levels of erythropoietin have not been demonstrated.

There is also a well-documented association between mild polycythaemia and the presence of large *uterine myomas*. In some cases the polycythaemia regresses after removal of the tumour. The mechanism is not clear. It is possible that the large abdominal mass interferes with the vascular supply to the kidneys and so causes renal hypoxia. However, inappropriate erythropoietin secretion by the muscle cells of the tumour has been demonstrated in several patients and, interestingly, in a patient with cutaneous leiomyoma.

Mild polycythaemia has also been reported in patients with other forms of renal pathology including *hydronephrosis, polycystic disease, renal artery stenosis,* and *Bartter's syndrome.* Interestingly, it does not seem to be a common finding in patients with renal artery stenosis.

A transient polycythaemia occurs sometimes after *renal transplantation*. Although it was originally suggested that this might reflect a temporary overproduction of erythropoietin by the transplanted kidney there is recent evidence that the source of the erythropoietin is the patient's own kidney. The mechanism of this curious response to transplantation remains to be determined.

Endocrine disorders

Mild polycythaemia has been recorded in patients with phaeochromocytomas or aldosterone-producing adenomas. High levels of erythropoietin have been found in the serum of these patients and the polycythaemia regresses after removal of the tumour. The mechanism of increased erythropoietin production is unknown. A mild polycythaemia may occur in patients with Cushing's syndrome and is probably the result of non-specific stimulations of the marrow by steroid hormones; the platelets and white cells are often involved.

Genetic disorders of erythropoietin regulation

These rare conditions have been observed in a few families. In one variety the erythropoietin level is inappropriately high for the increased red cell mass and does not increase in response to venesection. Thus it appears that the renal sensor mechanism which

regulates erythropoietin production in response to hypoxia is defective. Another variety has been described in which erythropoietin production responds normally to venesection. In this case the condition is thought to result from an abnormal end-organ response to the hormone rather than a primary defect in the regulation of erythropoietin synthesis. These conditions seem to be harmless and the patients require no treatment once the true nature of the polycythaemia has been determined.

References

Adamson, J. W., Stamatoyannopoulos, G., Kontras, S., Lascari, A. and Detter, J. (1973). Recessive familial erythrocytosis: aspects of marrow regulation in two families. *Blood* **41**, 641–652.
Burge, P. S., Johnson, W. S. and Prankerd, T. A. J. (1975). Morbidity and mortality in pseudopolycythaemia. *Lancet* i, 1266–1269.
Erslev, A. J. (1983). Secondary polycythemia (erythrocytosis). In *Hematology* 3rd edn (eds W. J. Williams, E. Beutler, A. J. Erslev and M. A. Lichtman), pp. 673–686. McGraw-Hill Book Company, New York.
Kazal, L. A. and Erslev, A. J. (1975). Erythropoietin production in renal tumors. *Ann. Clin. Lab. Sci.* **5**, 98–109.
Murphy, G. P., and Kenny, G. M. and Mirand, E. A. (1970). Erythropoietin levels in patients with renal tumors or cysts. *Cancer* **26**, 191–194.
Nallan, R., Otis, P. and Martin, D. C. (1975). Polycythemia following renal transplantation. *Urology* **6**, 158–164.
Pearson, T. C. and Guthrie, D. L. (1984). The interpretation of measured red cell mass and plasma volume in patients with elevated PCV values. *Clin. Lab. Haematol.* **6**, 207–217.
Russell, R. P. and Conley, C. L. (1964). Benign polycythemia: Gaisbock's syndrome. *Arch. Intern. Med.* **114**, 734–740.
Smith, J. R. and Landaw, S. A. (1978). Smokers' polycythemia. *N. Engl. J. Med.* **298**, 6–10.
Weinreb, N. J. and Shih, C-F, 81975). Spurious polycythemia. *Sem. Hematol.* **12**, 397–407.
Wetherley-Mein, G. and Pearson, T. C. (1982). The myeloproliferative disorders. In *Blood and its disorders* 2nd edn (eds R. M. Hardisty and D. J. Weatherall), pp. 1269–1316. Blackwell Scientific Publications, Oxford.
Whitcomb, W. H., Peschle, C., Moore, M., Nitschke, R. and Adamson, J. W. (1980). Congenital erythrocytosis: a new form associated with an erythropoietin-dependent mechanism. *Br. J. Haematol.* **44**, 17–24.
Zwillich, C. W., Sutton, F. D., Pierson, D. J., Creagh, E. M. and Weil, J. V. (1975). Decreased hypoxic ventilatory drive in the obesity-hypoventilation syndrome. *Am. J. Med.* **59**, 343–348.

THE WHITE CELL AND THE LYMPHOPROLIFERATIVE DISORDERS

Leucocytes in health and disease

C. BUNCH

Although there are five different types of leucocyte in the peripheral blood, it is convenient to consider them in two main groups: *phagocytes*, which have the capacity to engulf microorganisms and other foreign material, and *lymphocytes* or *immunocytes* which are concerned with the immune response (see Section 4) (Fig. 1). The phagocytes can be further subdivided into the *polymorphonuclear* leucocytes, which are cells that have lost the capacity to replicate and whose nucleus has condensed into two or more separate lobes, and the *monocytes*, which are precursors of the much longer lived tissue macrophages. A characteristic feature of all phagocytes is the presence of a number of cytoplasmic granules; these are most prominent in the polymorphonuclear series, which are classified into three major types – neutrophil, eosinophil and basophil – on the basis of the staining characteristics of their cytoplasmic granules. The term *granulocyte* is often

used to refer to these cells or, more specifically, to the neutrophils which are by far the most numerous. The total and differential leucocyte counts at various ages from birth to adulthood are given in Table 5 on page 19.5.

Unlike erythrocytes and platelets, the leucocytes are merely passengers in the blood stream and carry out their major functions within the tissues. All leucocytes originate from the marrow where a common pluripotent stem cell gives rise not only to the phagocytes but also to erythrocytes, platelets, and most probably to lymphocytes as well. The phagocytes spend only a few hours in the bloodstream in transit from the marrow to the tissues, where the neutrophils survive for only a few days, whilst the monocytes proliferate and differentiate into various kinds of macrophages with lifespans ranging from months to years. Lymphocytes on the other hand are generally much longer lived and may recirculate many times between the lymphatic system and the bloodstream. The functions of the lymphocytes are discussed in detail in Section 4; here only the alterations in lymphocytes that are reflected in the peripheral blood will be reviewed.

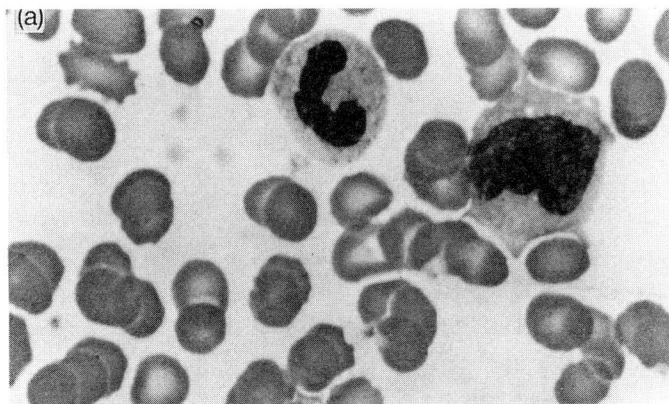

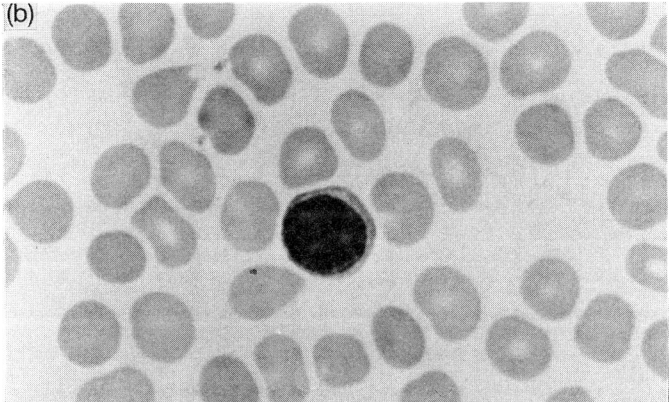

Fig. 1 Normal peripheral blood leucocytes. (a) A neutrophil (top) and a monocyte. (b) A lymphocyte.

Neutrophils

Physiology

Morphology and production

The mature neutrophil is 10–20 μm in diameter with a segmented nucleus of 2–5 lobes. In females, a drumstick-like nuclear appendage which contains the inactivated X chromosome is seen in about 6 per cent of neutrophils. There are several hundred cytoplasmic granules which are indistinct by light microscopy. The specific neutrophil granules stain faintly pink with Romanowsky dyes, and contain principally lysozyme (muramidase) and lactoferrin. There are a number of larger, azurophilic granules which stain more prominently at the promyelocyte and myelocyte stage of development. These are typical lysosomes and contain myeloperoxidase, lysozyme, acid hydrolases, and a variety of other bacteriocidal proteins.

The earliest recognizable myeloid cell is the myeloblast, and earlier stages of myeloid differentiation cannot be distinguished morphologically. Once a progenitor cell has been committed to myeloid differentiation, several amplifying divisions occur before the myeloblast stage is reached. Committed progenitor cells may be assayed by incubation of marrow or peripheral blood mononuclear cells in semi-solid media; under appropriate conditions groups of cells containing granulocytes and macrophages appear after a few days. Groups containing 50 or more cells are defined as colonies, each of which arises from a single progenitor known as a colony forming unit – CFU_{GM} (for granulocyte–macrophage). CFU_{GM} are thought to be early committed granulocyte progenitors one or more divisions before the myeloblast stage. Their growth in culture depends upon the presence of one or more of a variety of substances which are collectively known as colony-stimulating activity (CSA). Several of these substances have now been purified and cloned, and their role in the control of granulopoiesis *in vivo* is currently under evaluation (see below).

In 3–4 subsequent divisions, differentiation proceeds from the myeloblast, through the promyelocyte stage, at which the non-specific lysozomal granules appear, to the myelocyte, at which stage specific neutrophil granules appear. The capacity to divide is lost after the myelocyte stage, and with further development there is a progressive condensation and lobulation of the nucleus, through the metamyelocyte (band) stage to the mature neutrophil. In general, cells spend 5–10 days in the proliferating (mitotic) compartment and 3–7 days in the maturation (postmitotic) compartment within the marrow. The latter can be imagined as a storage pool which can be readily mobilized into the bloodstream in response to infection. In these circumstances, a larger proportion of band neutrophils and even some metamyelocytes may be released, producing the characteristic 'left-shifted' blood picture.

Only about one-half of the neutrophils in the blood are freely circulating; the remainder are to be found marginating, or rolling along the endothelial surface of the blood vessels, particularly in the lungs. Cells are thought to enter and leave the bloodstream via the marginating compartment, but can exchange freely between the circulating and marginating pools during their brief stay in the blood. The relative sizes of these two pools can be altered by a number of factors, and this may affect the peripheral blood neutrophil count which samples only the circulating compartment. A striking example is the leucocytosis that follows corticosteroid administration, which is mainly due to a shift in cells from the marginating to the circulating pool.

Neutrophils migrate from the bloodstream by squeezing between endothelial cells and penetrating the basement membrane. They do not return to the blood. Under normal conditions migration into and within the tissues is probably random, and only scanty neutrophils are found in normal histological tissue sections. On the other hand, phagocytic cells are actively attracted to and accumulate at sites of tissue injury, inflammation or infection.

During an acute inflammatory response there are alterations in local blood flow and vascular permeability which facilitate the migration of neutrophils into the area. Neutrophils show increased adherence to endothelial cells in postcapillary venules at or close to sites of injury, and at the same time a tendency to aggregate or clump together. It is not clear whether adherence is mediated principally by neutrophil factors, or due to changes within the endothelium. Some neutrophil degranulation occurs (which may facilitate penetration into the tissues), and there is evidence that lactoferrin is a potent stimulator of granulocyte adherence. In certain circumstances, however, release of neutrophil substances such as elastase and toxic oxygen radicals may actually produce endothelial or more extensive vascular damage (see below). Glycoprotein molecules on the neutrophil and endothelial surfaces are also thought to be important in the process of neutrophil adherence.

Interactions between bacteria, antibodies, neutrophils, and substances released by the phagocytes themselves, augment the inflammatory response and activate the complement, kinin, coagulation, and fibrinolytic cascades. As a result, specific chemotactic substances are generated which actively attract more neutrophils to the site. The most notable of these are C5a, prekallikrein, plasminogen activator, and prostaglandins.

Control of granulocyte production The rapid neutrophil response to tissue injury and infection, and its subsequent return to a remarkably constant steady-state level, indicate the involvement of some fairly close-coupled feedback mechanisms in the control of granulocyte production and release. Rapid mobilization of large numbers of phagocytic cells to sites of injury involves a number of mechanisms which together form part of the acute inflammatory response. These include alterations in regional blood flow, the attraction of phagocytes to injured sites along a 'diffusion gradient' of inflammatory mediators and tissue breakdown products, and increased margination of neutrophils (and possibly also release from the marrow) stimulated by endotoxin and other humoral mediators.

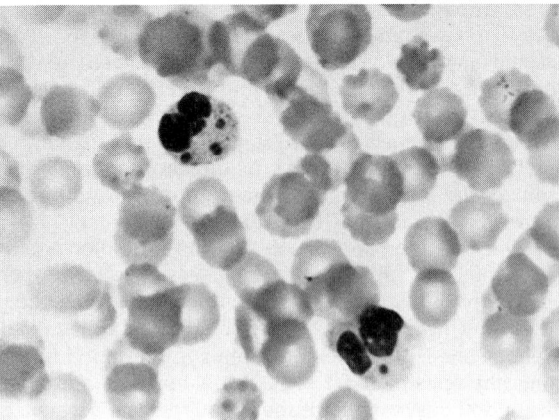

Fig. 2 Phagocytosis. Two neutrophils which have ingested pneumococci in the presence of immune serum. (Photograph by courtesy of Dr R. I. Vanhegan.)

These events are closely followed by a marked increase in marrow neutrophil production, and some of the mechanisms controlling the level of production have become apparent with the isolation and purification of a number of distinct growth factors. The requirement for such factors is apparent from *in vitro* colony-forming assays, hence the general term *colony-stimulating factor (CSF)*. CSF can be extracted from a variety of tissues, and is also elaborated by T cells and monocyte/macrophages, especially during interactions between the two.

More recently, at least four distinct colony-stimulating factors (CSFs) have been purified and subjected to molecular cloning. They are termed according to their principal stimulatory activity *in vitro* as G-CSF, M-CSF, GM-CSF, and interleukin (IL)-3, which stimulates production and differentiation of all classes of granulocyte. Although defined *in vitro*, the various CSFs are almost certainly relevant to the control of granulopoiesis *in vivo*, and the fact that CSF is elaborated by activated macrophages and T cells, which are abundant at sites of infection, is of particular interest. CSF may also have wider importance: a fascinating recent observation has been that the receptor for murine M-CSF closely resembles and may be identical to the product of the feline proto-oncogene c-*fms*. leading to the speculation that abnormal activation of these genes, perhaps as the result of chromosomal aberration, might play a part in the pathogenesis of certain leukaemias. The location of the human c-*fms* gene is on the long arm of chromosome 5; deletion of this arm (5q-) is a feature of a form of myelodysplasia (page 19.61) characterized by refractory anaemia, mild myeloid hyperplasia, abnormal thrombopoiesis, and a tendency to progress to acute leukaemia.

Functions of the neutrophils

The principal function of the neutrophil is to ingest and kill bacteria. *Phagocytosis* involves contact between organism and the neutrophil followed by membrane changes which engulf the bacterium together with some of its surrounding milieu, containing it within a plasma membrane-lined vesicle or phagosome (Fig. 2). Phagocytosis is greatly enhanced when bacteria are coated by immunoglobulin or the C3b component of complement. This process is known as *opsonization* and facilitates attachment of the organisms to specific IgG or complement receptors on the neutrophil surface. High levels of circulating IgG specific for the infecting agent are produced later in the course of active infection, but during the early stages opsonization can occur through activation of the alternate complement pathway with the production of C3b which 'fixes' on the microbial surface.

Phagocytosis stimulates several metabolic events within the neutrophil which together result in the death and digestion of any ingested microbes. Bacterial killing involves a number of mechan-

isms, and organisms differ in their susceptibility to each of them. Immediately after phagocytosis, cytoplasmic granules fuse with the phagocytic vacuole into which they discharge their contents, exposing bacteria to a wide variety of enzymes and cationic proteins. There is a sharp fall in intravacuolar pH which favours the action of acid hydrolases. These events are not sufficient to kill bacteria, and the most potent bacteriocidal mechanisms involve the generation of hydrogen peroxide and reactive oxygen radicals such as superoxide, singlet oxygen, and hydroxyl ions, all of which are highly toxic. These are generated as a result of a burst of oxidative metabolism (the so-called respiratory burst) which is stimulated by perturbations of the neutrophil membrane such as occur during phagocytosis. An electron transport chain comprising a flavoprotein dehydrogenase and cytochrome b_{-245} located in the membrane (and thus the wall of the phagocytic vacuole) takes electrons from NADPH and transfers them onto oxygen to generate superoxide within the vacuole.

The activity of hydrogen peroxide is further enhanced by the enzyme myeloperoxidase in the presence of halide ions. The digestive process is completed by the many enzymes discharged into the vacuole and is generally followed by the degeneration of the neutrophil itself with extracellular release of granular contents and other substances. The accumulation of neutrophils and their degeneration gives rise to the pus which characterizes acute inflammation.

Neutrophil disorders

Neutrophil may be abnormal in number, structure or function. Alterations in the numbers of circulating neutrophils generally reflect changes in the rate of production, although alterations in consumption or in the distribution between marginating and circulating pools may also be reflected in the neutrophil count. A simple classification of the quantitative neutrophil disorders is given in Table 1.

Neutrophilia

An increase in circulating neutrophils is termed a *neutrophil leucocytosis* or *neutrophilia*. It is most commonly due to a physiological increase in production in response to tissue infection or injury. The total leucocyte count is typically elevated into the $10–30 \times 10^9$ per litre range but may occasionally be higher. The differential count shows a predominance of neutrophils, and some less mature forms may be present reflecting premature marrow release. In very severe infections the neutrophil count may occasionally rise to 50×10^9 per litre or even higher, and differentiation from chronic granulocytic leukaemia (CGL) becomes important. This type of reaction, which has perhaps unfortunately been called *leukaemoid*, may occur with any severe infection. It is well recognized in disseminated tuberculosis, but is seen now more commonly in the presence of metastatic or necrotic tumours. In some instances, elaboration of CSF by such tumours has been demonstrated.

Table 1 Quantitative neutrophil disorders

Increased production
  Appropriate: infection, tissue damage etc.
  Inappropriate
    Benign: leukaemoid reactions
    Malignant: leukaemia, myeloproliferative disorders, disseminated carcinoma
Decreased production
  Reduced proliferation
    Primary: marrow failure (congenital or acquired)
    Secondary: drugs, toxins, irradiation, infiltration
  Ineffective myelopoiesis: megaloblastic anaemia, drugs, alcohol
Increased destruction or utilization
  Infection, hypersplenism, antibodies, drugs/antibody
Disturbance of circulating/marginating pool equilibrium
  Reduced margination: corticosteroids, exercise, adrenaline
  Increased margination: endotoxin, dialysis

Estimation of the amount of neutrophil cytoplasmic alkaline phosphatase is a useful way of distinguishing leukaemoid reactions from CGL as it is elevated in the former and decreased in the latter. Neutrophilia may occur in other disorders associated with tissue damage or necrosis, such as malignancy, myocardial infarction, and in some collagen vascular disorders.

There are a number of mechanisms by which drugs may produce a neutrophilia. For example, neutrophil production is enhanced by lithium therapy, and corticosteroids produce a shift from the marginating to the circulating blood pools and in very high doses may also increase mobilization from the marrow.

Neutropenia

Neutropenia is defined as a circulating neutrophil count below 1.5 $\times 10^9$ per litre and results most commonly from reduced proliferation of myeloid precursors, but may also be caused by ineffective myelopoiesis, or by increased utilization, destruction, or vascular margination. A complete absence of circulating neutrophils is termed *agranulocytosis*. Neutropenia is associated with an increased susceptibility to bacterial infection; the risk becomes progressively greater as the neutrophil count falls, and infection is commonly serious and may be rapidly fatal. The management of this problem is discussed in Section 5.

Acquired neutropenia The important causes of neutropenia are shown in Table 1. Neutropenia is most commonly a manifestation of marrow failure, which is most often due to infiltration with leukaemic or other malignant cells, or to cytotoxic drug administration. Isolated neutropenia has been described in association with virtually any *drug*, and the important offenders are shown in Table 2. In many instances the effect is not related to the dose of the drug but appears to be idiosyncratic. On the other hand some drugs, for example those used to treat malignant disease, are inherently cytotoxic and marrow depression is dose-related and generally involves other haemopoietic cell lines as well. Patients may complain of a sore throat or mouth ulceration, or may have symptoms and signs of infection elsewhere. The drug responsible should be withdrawn immediately. Haemopoietic recovery normally occurs within 1–2 weeks although the prognosis depends on whether or not the patient develops infection during this period. The outlook is particularly poor if serious infection is present when agranulocytosis is first discovered.

Paradoxically some *infections* may be accompanied by a mild leucopenia. This is commonly seen in the early stages of viral infections, but may also occur in the enteric fevers, bacillary dysentery and brucellosis. The mechanism is not understood. Normally the marrow contains a large reserve pool which is sufficient under normal circumstances for the majority of infections, although leucopenia may result from exhaustion of this reserve in the presence of overwhelming sepsis. A persistent leucopenia in the course of obvious bacterial infection indicates marrow failure.

Immune destruction of neutrophils within the circulation or the marrow is uncommon. By analogy with Rhesus haemolytic disease of the newborn, a transient *neonatal iso-immune* destruction has been described due to placental transfer of maternal cytotoxic antibodies. Autoantibodies, and/or damage by immune complexes have been implicated in the neutropenia of collagen vascular disorders including rheumatoid arthritis, SLE, and Felty's syndrome. In some instances, neutropenia may result from immune destruction of marrow granulocyte progenitors. Immune mechanisms have also been implicated in the neutropenia caused by certain drugs such as phenylbutazone, aminopyrine and methylthiouracil. It is likely that these drugs act as haptens in association with an unknown leucocyte antigen.

A striking but transient neutropenia has been observed during *haemodialysis* and when leucocytes have been harvested for transfusion by the circulation of blood through nylon–wool filters. These procedures are associated with complement activation, and the neutropenia is probably due to a massive margination and sequestration of neutrophils within the pulmonary circulation.

Genetic neutropenias There are a number of very rare genetic neutropenias. In *Kostmann's infantile agranulocytosis* severe neutropenia is present from birth and is associated with severe infections, which are often fatal in infancy. This is probably a heterogeneous condition: in some there are normal numbers of progenitors and the disorder may be one of defective maturation, possibly associated with a lack of a serum factor. In others, progenitor cell assays have been abnormal.

Reticular dysgenesis with congenital aleucocytosis is characterized by severe agranulocytosis and lymphopenia from birth together with hypogammaglobulinaemia, and may be associated with thymic aplasia or thymoma.

Neutropenia is also found in a rare association with *congenital pancreatic insufficiency* or in an autosomal dominant form.

Cyclical neutropenia is an interesting form of genetic neutropenia in which the neutrophil count undulates in 14–21 day cycles. Recurrent infections occur but the diagnosis may be difficult unless serial blood counts are performed. The defect appears to be in the pluripotent stem cell, and similar fluctuations in reticulocytes, erythroid progenitors and platelets can be detected. A similar disorder is seen in grey collie dogs which can be transferred by marrow transplantation into normal dogs or cured by transplantation of normal marrow.

Miscellaneous causes of neutropenia Neutropenia is also a feature of *megaloblastic anaemias*, in which myelopoiesis is ineffective and there is intramedullary destruction of myeloid as well as erythroid cells, excessive *alcohol* consumption, which may also produce ineffective myelopoiesis and may also damage neutrophils directly, and *splenomegaly*, in which neutropenia may co-exist with thrombocytopenia and anaemia due to excessive pooling or sequestration of cells within the enlarged spleen. The association of splenomegaly, rheumatoid arthritis and neutropenia is known as *Felty's syndrome* (Section 16). The mechanism for neutropenia in this condition is complex and autoimmune mechanisms have been suggested.

Functional neutrophil disorders (Table 3, see also Section 4)

An increased susceptibility to infection is well recognized in many systemic conditions including diabetes mellitus, uraemia, malnourishment, alcohol ingestion, corticosteroid therapy and the immune-complex-associated disorders such as rheumatoid arthritis and systemic lupus erythematosus. The exact mechanism is not fully understood, and although a number of minor defects in phagocytic function and in other aspects of the immune response have been demonstrated, it is doubtful if any of these are of particular

Table 2 Mechanisms of drug-induced neutropenia

Defective production
  Predictable
    Cytotoxic drugs
    Chloramphenicol
  Idiosyncratic
    Phenothiazines
    Antithyroid drugs
    Phenylbutazone
    Sulphonamides
    Many others
  Ineffective myelopoiesis
    Phenytoin
    Pyrimethamine
    Primidone
    Chloramphenicol
    Others
Immune destruction (drug-hapten-antibody interaction)
  Aminopyrine
  Many examples of single reports
Combinations of the above
  Suspected for many drugs but not proved

Table 3 Functional neutrophil disorders

Defect	Examples	Clinical features
Chemotaxis opsonization	Various antibody and complement deficiency states	Recurrent pyogenic infections
Migration, phagocytosis	Actin dysfunction (rare); a variety of systemic illnesses, including immune complex diseases, burns, diabetes mellitus, drugs e.g. alcohol, corticosteroids	Recurrent infection, failure of pus formation, or may be subclinical
Bacterial killing	Various enzyme deficiencies (e.g. of NADH oxidase G6PD) leading to failure of postphagocytic burst of oxidative metabolism	Chronic granulomatous disease (see text)
	Myeloperoxidase deficiency	Asymptomatic

clinical relevance. On the other hand there exists a group of well recognized but exceedingly rare inherited defects of phagocytic function in which the clinical picture is dominated by recurrent, often serious infection.

The most strikingly inherited defect of phagocyte function is *chronic granulomatous disease* (CGD) in which phagocytosis is normal but granulocytes are unable to kill ingested bacteria, which survive intracellularly resulting in chronic local granulomatous inflammation with damage to surrounding tissue. The disorder has a recessive inheritance which is usually sex-linked although an autosomal pattern is sometimes encountered. Curiously, a number of families have been reported in which the mothers of affected boys with the sex-linked variety have developed a disorder resembling lupus erythematosus. The defect in CGD is a deficiency of a component of the membrane-associated electron transport chain involved in the 'respiratory' burst of oxidative metabolism that accompanies phagocytosis. The affected cells are thus unable to kill catalase-positive micro-organisms such as staphylococci, serratia, candida and aspergillus. Catalase-negative organisms such as streptococci and most Gram-negative bacteria are killed normally; these organisms cannot inactivate endogenous peroxide which is lethal in the presence of myeloperoxidase released into the phagocytic vacuole.

The disorder typically presents in the first few weeks of life with superficial skin sepsis. Spread to regional lymph nodes follows, and this leads to painful swelling with eventual suppuration.

Biopsy of affected sites reveals non-caseating granulomas with giant cells so that tuberculosis may be suspected. Even with appropriate antibiotic therapy healing is slow, and a chronically discharging sinus often results. Infective episodes are usually accompanied by high swinging fever and the patient may look toxic although bacteraemia is uncommon. More deeply-situated infections are common, particularly in the lungs, liver and urinary tract, and lead to progressive damage and organ failure. Death is usual within the first few years of life and few children survive to young adulthood. Even then, the quality of life is poor, and there is no evidence for a milder course with increasing age. Repeated infections take a progressive toll and survival of more than 20 years is extremely uncommon.

Unless the disease has previously been recognized in the family the diagnosis is usually made when the clinical picture of recurrent infection prompts investigation of neutrophil and immune function. The simple nitroblue tetrazolium (NBT) test, in which affected neutrophils are unable to reduce NBT to a blue formazan dye, is adequate for screening purposes, although the exact metabolic lesion is usually more difficult to define. There is no specific treatment for this disorder and management rests on prophylactic therapy with anti-staphylococcal agents such as flucloxacillin. Long-term co-trimoxazole may also be of benefit. When infection occurs it should be treated vigorously with early surgical drainage of abscesses together with appropriate antibiotic therapy, which may have to be given intravenously for several weeks. Granulocyte transfusions have been used on occasions but there is only anecdotal evidence of their benefit in this disorder. Not surprisingly the disease is psychologically as well as organically disrupting, and pastoral problems with the affected child and the family are often severe.

Other inherited functional defects Rare patients have been described with inherited defects of neutrophil migration, chemotaxis, or phagocytosis, and with other enzyme deficiencies leading to defective bacterial killing. All are characterized by recurrent bacterial infection.

Structural abnormalities of the neutrophils

The commonest structural abnormality of the neutrophils is *toxic granulation* which is frequently seen in the course of severe infections. There is undue prominence of the azurophilic granules which are larger and stain more deeply than normal. The mechanism is unknown. Also seen quite commonly in severe infections are small bright blue elliptical bodies representing persistent rough endoplasmic reticulum. These are called *Döhle* bodies and occur in pregnancy, cancer, trauma and following cytotoxic drug administration. In the rare inherited *May–Heggelin anomaly*, Döhle bodies are found in all neutrophils in association with giant platelets. There is often a neutropenia and thrombocytopenia, and whilst there may be a mild bleeding diathesis, the disorder is otherwise benign.

The *Chediak–Steinbrink–Higashi anomaly* is an exceptionally rare autosomal recessive disorder in which there are massive abnormal cytoplasmic inclusions in the neutrophils and their precursors. The basic abnormality is in fact a much more widespread defect in lysosomal granule formation with systemic features that include progressive lymphadenopathy and hepatosplenomegaly, neurological abnormalities, and oculocutaneous albinism associated with abnormal giant melanosome formation. There is also neutropenia and thrombocytopenia and death from bleeding or infection occur in early childhood.

Auer rods are acquired cytoplasmic inclusions seen in the myeloblasts and promyelocytes of some patients with acute myeloid leukaemia. They are deep-red rod-like structures and are often associated with bizarre granulation. They stain positively with Sudan black and are particularly useful in the differentiation of acute myeloid leukaemia from the lymphoblastic form.

Failure of nuclear segmentation, the *Pelger–Huet anomaly*, is occasionally seen in leukaemias and lymphoreticular disorders although it is more commonly found as an autosomal dominant trait or during severe infections. The nucleus is round or dumbell-shaped but neutrophil function is unimpaired.

Hypersegmentation of the nucleus is common in megaloblastic anaemias and can occur as an autosomal dominant trait. The neutrophils may be larger than normal, up to twice the normal size.

Toxic damage by neutrophils

Neutrophils are potent cells and form part of a complex defence mechanism that is able to do a great deal of harm to invading micro-organisms. It should thus not be surprising if, on occasions, activation of neutrophils resulted in damage to the tissues they were designed to protect, and there is increasing evidence that in certain circumstances interactions between neutrophils and endothelial cells may have adverse effects and lead to significant tissue damage.

One example of this – complement-mediated neutrophil sequestration in the pulmonary circulation leading to dyspnoea and hypoxia – has been described above. There is also considerable evidence that neutrophils are an essential component of certain types of immune- or toxin-mediated vascular injury, such as the Schwartzman and local Arthus reactions, and serum sickness, and that they may play a part in the increased vascular permeability and lung damage associated with the adult respiratory distress syndrome (Section 15). Precisely how such adverse effects are mediated is not clear. Neutrophil degranulation releases many proteases including elastase, together with highly reactive radicals such as the hydroxyl ion, superoxide and hydrogen peroxide which could lead to endothelial cell damage by membrane lipid peroxidation.

Lymphocytes (see also Section 4)

The peripheral blood lymphocytes (Fig. 1) are small round cells measuring 8–12 μm. They represent 20–50 per cent of the total leucocytes and have a scanty pale blue-staining cytoplasm with some occasional vacuoles and azurophilic granules. The nucleus is round and slightly indented and occupies most of the cell volume. It contains densely packed chromatin and a nucleolus may be visible.

For many years these rather homogeneous appearing cells were largely ignored and their function was unknown. However, in the past 30 years or so it has become abundantly clear that they have a fundamental role in the immune response. Furthermore, it is now known that there are many subclasses of lymphocyte which interact in a highly orchestrated fashion in response to a variety of immunological challenges. This topic is fully explored in Section 4.

Lymphocytes are descended from cells originating in the bone marrow and are functionally divided into two classes, the thymus-dependent or *T cells*, which are principally concerned with cell-mediated immune processes, and *B cells*, which are concerned with humoral immunity and are the precursors of antibody-producing plasma cells. B cells are thought to have a relatively short lifespan and are found mainly in the lymph nodes, spleen and bone marrow. T cells, on the other hand, are an extremely heterogeneous group of cells with a variety of functions. They are thought to be much longer-lived and some may have a lifespan of several years. They recirculate extensively throughout the lymphatic system and blood stream and represent about 70 per cent of the peripheral blood lymphocytes.

Lymphocytosis

A mild peripheral blood lymphocytosis is an extremely common finding in the course of most viral illnesses. Some of the lymphocytes in these conditions may be large with an open nuclear chromatin structure and one or more nucleoli. These appearances are typical of lymphocytes transforming or, more correctly, proliferating in response to antigen stimulation, and this may give the erroneous impression of a less mature cell. This phenomenon is seen particularly in conditions such as infectious mononucleosis and cytomegalovirus infections, which are principally infections of the lymphocytes themselves. These disorders are described in detail in Section 5. Other infections in which lymphocytosis may be seen include tuberculosis, brucellosis, syphilis and pertussis.

Acute infectious lymphocytosis is a sporadic disorder of children and young adults which may be asymptomatic or associated with fever, upper respiratory symptoms, a morbilliform rash and some superficial lymphadenopathy. There is a marked leucocytosis which may reach 100×10^9 per litre, due to an increase in the number of small lymphocytes. The disorder is benign and resolves over a 3–5 week course. Although presumed to be infective, the responsible agent has not been identified.

An absolute lymphocytosis occurring in older patients is most commonly due to chronic lymphatic leukaemia (page 19.32).

Lymphopenia

Lymphocyte counts of less than 1.0×10^9 per litre are seen in about 5 per cent of normal adults. Lymphopenia may also be due

to stress, increased adrenocortical activity, the administration of corticosteroids, or to a malignant disorder of the lymphoid system.

Monocytes

It is widely accepted that peripheral blood monocytes are precursors of tissue macrophages in transit from the marrow, where they originate from committed myeloid stem cells. Like neutrophils, monocytes spend only a few hours in the blood and have circulating and marginating pools. In contrast, however, they continue to proliferate in the tissues where as macrophages their lifespan is measured in months or years. Macrophages are widely distributed with a predilection for lymph nodes, spleen, liver and marrow, where some are fixed to endothelial structures lining the sinusoids of these organs. This fixed phagocytic capacity is called the *reticulo-endothelial system*, although the phagocytic cells are not endothelial in origin and do not produce reticulin fibres. Other macrophages roam freely through the tissues and respond readily to chemotactic stimuli, arriving at inflammatory sites rather later than neutrophils.

Macrophages are large cells, measuring between 20 and 80 μm, and have a prodigious phagocytic capacity. They have membrane receptors for IgG and C'3 and can consume a wide variety of particulate matter. Under appropriate circumstances several macrophages may fuse together to form the multinucleate giant cells characteristic of chronic inflammation. An important role of the fixed macrophages of the reticuloendothelial system and in particular the spleen, is to clear unwanted particulate matter such as bacteria and effete blood cells from the circulation.

Macrophages are intimately involved in the immune response (Section 4) and are able to process ingested antigen and present it, in association with surface class II histocompatibility determinants, to antigen-reactive T cells. In addition, they produce a number of humoral mediators or *monokines*. Some of these are now well-characterized, and include the interleukins IL-1 and IL-3, and alpha-interferon. IL-1 enhances the activation of T cells responding to antigen presented by macrophages and other cells, such as the dendritic cells within the lymph node and the Langerhans cells in skin. These activated T cells produce another mediator, IL-2, which stimulates the expansion of a clone of antigen-specific T cells.

IL-1 is also able to activate antibody production by B cells, and has widespread effects on other cells and tissues. It has been identified as the 'endogenous pyrogen' of acute inflammation, producing fever by a direct hypothalamic effect, and one of the mediators inducing hepatic synthesis of acute-phase proteins. It activates neutrophils, and also their release from the marrow. Neutrophil activation results in the release of lactoferrin, and the sequestration of iron – lactoferrin complexes has been postulated as one of the factors contributing to the anaemia of chronic disorders (page 19.91).

Some other factors produced by macrophages, including IL-3, have important regulatory functions within the haemopoietic system (see above and page 19.11), whilst some can activate other macrophages to a state of enhanced phagocytic capacity. This may be important in the elimination of certain intracellular parasites such as protozoa, mycobacteria and listeria which are able to survive ingestion by unactivated macrophages.

Monocyte abnormalities

The circulating monocyte count is normally less than 0.8×10^9 per litre or up to 10 per cent of the total leucocytes. A lower limit is more difficult to define but decreased production of monocytes is most commonly associated with the administration of cytotoxic drugs or ionizing radiation. Neutropenia is also produced by these agents but macrophages are relatively insensitive, and a significant defect in the phagocytic capacity of the monocyte macrophage system is thus only seen after a prolonged and intensive cytotoxic therapy when it may be associated with deep seated fungal and protozoal as well as bacterial infections.

A *monocytosis* is usually due to increased monocyte production and occurs to a slight degree in the recovery phase of most infections and during the course of chronic infections such as tuberculosis and subacute bacterial endocarditis. In the latter condition, monocytosis is more pronounced in capillary blood obtained from the ear lobe. Increased numbers of monocytes are also seen in association with malignant disease and chronic non-infective inflammatory disorders such as ulcerative colitis and collagen–vascular diseases.

Eosinophils (see also Section 24)

The eosinophil granulocytes are characterized by the presence of 20 or so large refractile cytoplasmic granules which stain bright red with eosin. These granules contain typical lysosomal enzymes but about one half of their total protein is a strongly basic substance known as *major basic protein* (MBP). Its function is unknown although its basic properties enable it to neutralize heparin, which is a major constituent of the cytoplasmic granules of the basophil. Eosinophils constitute less than 6 per cent of the total circulating leucocytes with a diurnal variation that correlates inversely with adrenocortical activity. Despite intensive research the exact role of the eosinophil and the MBP in health and disease remains a mystery, although it has long been recognized that eosinophil production is increased in association with allergy and parasitic infestation.

Eosinophils share certain properties with neutrophils: both respond equally well to chemotactic stimuli, but eosinophils migrate selectively to sites of allergic reaction or parasitic infestation. Certain substances preferentially attract eosinophils, notably antigen–antibody complexes, lymphokines and a substance present in the cytoplasmic granules of the basophil which has been called the *eosinophil chemotactic factor of anaphylaxis*.

Eosinophils are phagocytic cells but are less efficient in this respect than neutrophils. Of particular interest is the fact that whilst the latter may secrete some of their granular contents to the exterior in the course of phagocytosis, eosinophils do this readily in the presence of helminths, which are too large for them to engulf. The parasites can be killed in this way and this may be one of the more important of the eosinophil's functions. The presence of eosinophils at sites of allergic reaction is less easily understood, although they may there act to contain or modulate the effects of basophil degranulation.

Eosinophilia

The principal causes of an increased eosinophil count are shown in Table 4. A blood and tissue eosinophilia is seen in virtually every invasive metazoan infection but is less predictable when infestation is confined to the gastrointestinal tract. With tissue invasion, eosinophilia may be extreme with persistent levels of in excess of 10×10^9 per litre.

Allergic disorders such as bronchial asthma, rhinitis, drug allergies, eczema, contact dermatitis and urticaria may also be accompanied by an eosinophilia though values seldom reach 10×10^9 per litre. Various pulmonary disorders are associated with eosinophilia, notably bronchial asthma and during the migration of metazoan larvae through the lungs, and it may also occur as a manifestation of allergy to inhaled organic dusts or with pulmonary involvement in polyarteritis nodosa.

Whilst eosinophils are usually absent from the blood during the course of acute bacterial infection, a slight eosinophilia has been described in scarlet fever, and may occur during recovery from bacterial infection or in the course of certain viral illnesses. Less common causes of eosinophilia include malignancy, particularly Hodgkin's disease and other lymphomas and it may occasionally be a manifestation of cancer, particularly in the presence of widespread necrotic metastases.

Table 4 Causes of eosinophilia

1 Parasitic infestations
2 Allergic disorders, e.g.
    Bronchial asthma
    Hay fever (allergic rhinitis)
    Other hypersensitivity reactions including drug reactions
3 Skin disorders, e.g.
    Urticaria
    Pemphigus
    Eczema
    Psoriasis
    Dermatitis herpetiformis
4 Pulmonary disorders
    Bronchial asthma
    Polyarteritis nodosa
    Parasitic infestations
5 Malignant disorders
    Lymphoma
    Carcinoma
    Melanoma
    Eosinophilic leukaemia
6 Miscellaneous, e.g.
    Hypereosinophilic syndrome
    Ulcerative colitis
    Sarcoidosis
    Hypoadrenalism

Massive eosinophilia is most commonly a manifestation of widespread parasitic invasion, but whilst the picture may suggest a leukaemic process, true eosinophilic leukaemia is extremely rare. Occasional patients have been reported in which massive eosinophilia is associated with progressive hepatosplenomegaly and congestive cardiac failure due to a restrictive cardiomyopathy. This condition has earned the title hypereosinophilic syndrome, although the associated 'fibroplastic endomyocarditis' was first described by Löffler (Sections 13 and 24). The aetiology is unknown and it is not clear if the eosinophilia is the cause of, or an exaggerated response to tissue injury. The outcome is ultimately fatal although treatment with cytotoxic drugs or steroids to reduce the eosinophilia, together with energetic treatment of heart failure, may produce a beneficial clinical response.

Eosinopenia

The circulating eosinophil level has a diurnal variation that inversely correlates with adrenocortical activity. Patients with excess circulating corticosteroids, whether exogenously administered or endogenously increased by stress or endocrine disease, have very low eosinophil counts. This is not normally of any practical value, except that it is perhaps unwise to diagnose Cushing's disease when eosinophils are clearly visible in the peripheral blood smear.

Basophils

The basophils are the least numerous of the peripheral blood leucocytes and are indeed often hard to find in a normal peripheral blood smear. They number between 0 and 0.08×10^9 per litre, i.e. less than 1 per cent of the total leucocyte count, and are similar in size to the neutrophil but with a number of strikingly basophilic granules. The granules contain principally heparin, histamine, the eosinophil chemotactic factor of anaphylaxis (see above) and a platelet-aggregating substance. In many ways the basophils resemble the tissue mast cells and may well be precursors of these cells, although the exact relationship is not clear. They are produced in the marrow where the earliest recognizable precursor is the basophil myelocyte.

Basophils and tissue mast cells play a crucial role in immediate hypersensitivity reactions. They have membrane receptors for the Fc proportion of IgE and the interaction of basophil-bound IgE with specific antigen produces basophil degranulation with release of granule contents into the surrounding tissues. The clinical effects are dramatic and immediate, with urticaria, bronchial asthma, rhinitis or in severe instances anaphylactic shock. Such reactions are fortunately uncommon but some individuals have an allergic or atopic tendency which may have a genetic component. These patients typically have increased amounts of basophil-bound IgE.

The importance of the basophil in health is unclear and a complete, isolated absence of basophils has not been described. An increase in blood basophils is characteristic of myeloproliferative disorders, particularly chronic myeloid leukaemia and myelosclerosis, and on some occasions may be striking. Less impressive increases have been described in myxoedema, ulcerative colitis, tuberculosis, haemolytic anaemias, carcinoma and after splenectomy, although these changes are not really of any clinical significance.

Systemic mastocytosis (page 19.43 and Section 20) is an exceptionally rare disorder of adult life in which there is widespread tissue infiltration with mast cells. The earliest manifestations are in the skin with the development of patchy or widespread pigmented nodules which are infiltrated with mast cells. There is often marked dermatographism and local urticaria can be provoked by minor trauma. At this stage the disorder is indistinguishable from urticaria pigmentosa (Section 20), but later in the course of this disease mast cells infiltrate the marrow, liver, spleen and other tissues. Symptoms may generally be attributed to infiltration of specific organs or be related to the release of histamine or heparin from mast cells. Thus patients may occasionally describe episodes of flushing, headache, urticaria, tachycardia or gastrointestinal symptoms. In its later stages the disorder resembles a leukaemia with generalized lymphadenopathy, splenomegaly, and hepatomegaly, and infiltration of the bone marrow leading to anaemia, leucopenia, and thrombocytopenia. Occasionally mast cells are found in large numbers in the peripheral blood giving rise to the description *mast cell leukaemia*.

References

Beeson, P. B. (1983). Cancer and eosinophilia. *N. Engl. J. Med.* **309**, 792–793.

Beeson, P. B. and Bass, D. A. (1977). *The eosinophil.* W. B. Saunders, Philadelphia.

Boggs, D. R. (1983). The haematopoietic effects of lithium. *Sem. Hemat.* **20**, 129–138.

—— and Winkelstein, D. R. (1983). *White cell manual* 4th edn. F. A. Davis, Philadelphia.

Boxer, L. A., Coates, T. D., Haak, R. A., Wolach, J. B., Hoffstein, S. and Baehner, R. L. (1982). Lactoferrin deficiency associated with altered granulocyte function. *N. Engl. J. Med.* **307**, 404–410.

——, Greenberg, M. S., Boxer, G. J. and Stossel, T. P. (1975). Autoimmune neutropenia. *N. Engl. J. Med.* **293**, 748–753.

——, Hedley-White, T. and Stossel, T. P. (1974). Neutrophil actin dysfunction and abnormal neutrophil behaviour. *N. Engl. J. Med.* **291**, 1093–1100.

Butterworth, A. E. and David, J. R. (1981). Eosinophil function. *N. Engl. J. Med.* **304**, 154–156.

Cawley, J. C. and Hayhoe, F. G. H. (1973). *Ultrastructure of haemic cells. A cytological atlas of normal and leukaemic blood and bone marrow.* W. B. Saunders, London.

Dale, D. C., Guerry, D., Wewerka, J. R., Bull, J. M. and Chusid, M. J. (1979). Chronic neutropenia. *Medicine (Balt.)* **58**, 128–144.

Fauci, A. S., Harley, J. B., Roberts, W. C., Ferrans, V. J., Gralnick, H. R. and Bjornson, B. H. (1982). The idiopathic hypereosinophilic syndrome: clinical, pathophysiologic, and therapeutic considerations. *Ann. intern. Med.* **97**, 78–92.

Harlan, J. M. (1985). Leukocyte–endothelial interactions. *Blood* **65**, 513–525.

Jacob, H. S. (1983). Complement-mediated leucoembolization: a mechanism of tissue damage during extracorporeal perfusions, myocardial infarction and in shock – a review. *Q. J. Med.* **52**, 289–296.

——, Craddock, P. R., Hammerschmidt, D. E. and Moldow, C. F. (1980). Complement-induced granulocyte aggregation. An unsuspected mechanism of disease. *N. Engl. J. Med.* **302**, 789–794.

Johnston, R. B. (1982). Defects of neutrophil function. *N. Engl. J. Med.* **307**, 434–436.

Kay, A. B. (1976). Functions of the eosinophil leucocyte. *Br. J. Haemat.* **33**, 313–318.

Logue, G. L. and Shimm, D. S. (1980). Autoimmune granulocytopenia. *Ann. Rev. Med.* **31**, 191–200.

Murphy, P. (1976). *The neutrophil.* Plenum Medical, New York.

Nathan, C. F., Murray, H. W. and Cohn, Z. A. (1980). The macrophage as an effector cell. *N. Engl. J. Med.* **303**, 622–626.

Segal, A. W. (1985). Variations on the theme of chronic granulomatous disease. *Lancet* **i**, 1378–1382.

Segal, A. W. and Peters, T. J. (1976). Characterisation of the enzyme defect in chronic granulomatous disease. *Lancet* **i**, 1363–1365.

Vincent, P. C. (1977). The measurement of granulocyte kinetics. *Br. J. Haemat.* **36**, 1–4.

Vincent, P. C., Levi, J. A. and MacQueen, A. (1974). The mechanism of neutropenia in Felty's syndrome. *Br. J. Haemat.* **27**, 463.

Introduction to the lymphoproliferative disorders

C. BUNCH AND K. C. GATTER

Proliferation of lymphocytes in response to antigenic stimuli is a central part of the immune response (see Section 4), and commonly leads to enlargement of lymph glands and other lymphoid tissue participating in the reaction. In most instances the antigenic stimulus is an infecting organism, the lymphadenopathy is short lived, and the glands return to their normal size after successful control of the infection responsible. Occasionally, however, the proliferative response is more prolonged and may itself give rise to clinical problems.

Persistent lymphadenopathy may simply reflect repeated antigenic challenge – as commonly occurs, for example, in young children suffering repeated upper respiratory infections during the winter months. Alternatively, it may be due to persistence of antigen, possibly because the immune response is inadequate for one reason or another, or because an infecting organism (such as the tubercle bacillus) is relatively inaccessible and difficult to eliminate. In other instances, for example, in rheumatoid arthritis and other collagen-vascular disorders, lymphadenopathy is associated with an abnormal immune response directed against 'self' antigens. Finally, and much less commonly, autonomous proliferation of a neoplastic clone of lymphoid cells may occur, giving rise to one of the malignant lymphoproliferative disorders considered later in this section.

Organization of the immune system

Many of the clinical features of lymphoproliferative disorders can be explained by the fact that lymphoid tissue is strategically placed throughout the body. In addition to a network of 500–600 or so discrete lymph nodes, lymphatic tissue is found extensively in the oropharynx (Waldeyer's ring), bronchial tree, and gastrointestinal tract. Lymphocytes are also found in the bone marrow, where they tend to form small follicles, and of course in the spleen.

Lymph-node structure (Fig. 1)

The lymph-nodes are loosely arranged into outer cortical and inner medullary areas within a connective tissue capsule. Lymph enters the node via afferent lymphatics and percolates through radial sinusoids to the hilum, where it leaves the node via efferent lymphatics. Blood enters and leaves the node through hilar vessels: an extensive vascular network extends throughout the node, and specialized post capillary venules allow extensive traffic of lymphocytes between the blood and lymphatic vessels.

Cells in the cortical areas are arranged into a number of spherical nodules or *follicles* with a pale centre known as the *germinal centre*. These comprise mainly B cells with a smaller number of T

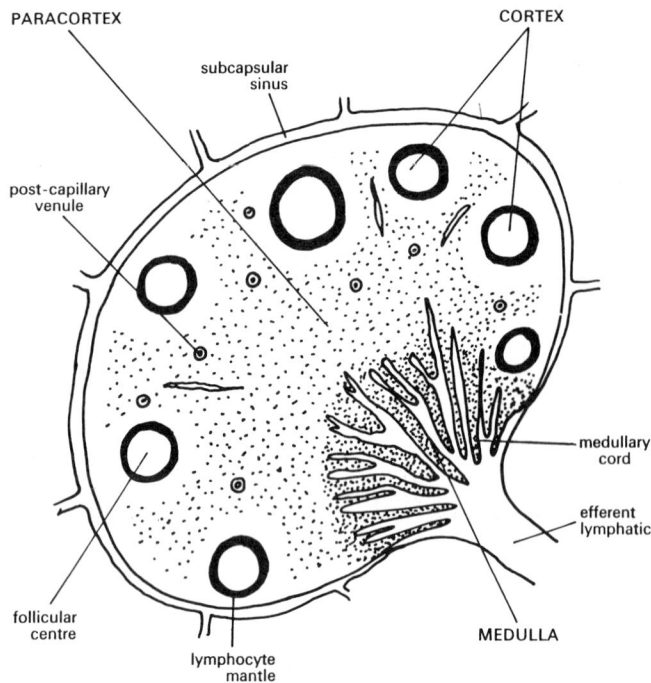

Fig. 1 Functional architecture of a normal lymph node. (Reproduced with permission from Arno, 1980, with permission of the author and MTP Press.)

Table 1 Principal causes of lymphadenopathy

Inflammatory	*Granulomatous*
Suppurating	Infective
Pyogenic infection	Tuberculosis
Non-suppurating	Syphilis
Infection – local or systemic	Toxoplasmosis
Immunologically-based	Histoplasmosis etc.
Collagen disease	Non-infective
Rheumatoid arthritis	Sarcoidosis
Serum sickness	
Dermatopathic	*Malignant*
Drugs e.g. phenytoin	Primary
Addison's disease	Lymphoma
Thyrotoxicosis	Leukaemia
	Secondary
	Carcinoma
	Melanoma
	Sarcoma
	Congenital
	Lymphangiomas
	Cystic hygroma

cells and non-lymphoid cells. The cuff surrounding the germinal centre consists of mature small lymphocytes. Within the centre itself, the most characteristic cell is a slightly larger small follicular lymphocyte known as a *centrocyte* or, because of its irregular nucleus, as a *small cleaved cell*. A number of larger cells can also be found, including macrophages (histiocytes), transformed lymphocytes or *immunoblasts*, and cells with a regular, centrally placed nucleus variously called *centroblasts* or *non-cleaved follicle-centre cells*. Also within the germinal centre are *follicular dendritic cells*, so called because of their network of interdigitating cytoplasmic processes that extend throughout the follicle. The origin of these dendritic cells is not clear, but they are thought to be involved in antigen processing and presentation.

Following antigenic challenge intense proliferative activity takes place in the germinal centre as B cells recognizing foreign antigens undergo clonal expansion and differentiation. The associated morphological changes give rise to the appearance of different types of cell within the germinal centre, and the various stages of B cell differentiation are also reflected in the expression of different antigens. This explains in part the diversity of lymphomas that can arise in the follicle centre, as the malignant cells retain a limited but variable capacity for differentiation reflected in their morphology and immunochemical phenotype.

The interfollicular and paracortical areas consist mainly of T cells. The medulla is comprised of cords of cells lining the sinusoids – the so-called *medullary cords*. These cells include fixed macrophages, plasma cells, lymphocytes, and connective tissue cells.

Lymphoid tissue in other sites is arranged in a broadly similar fashion. Gut-associated lymphoid tissue consists of a diffuse collection of lymphocytes throughout the submucosa which coalesces patchily to form more discrete nodules (e.g. Peyer's patches). Bronchial lymphoid tissue is similarly arranged. The structure of the spleen is described on page 19.186.

Lymphocyte recirculation

Lymphocytes are not static, and there is extensive movement or *recirculation* of cells throughout the lymphatic system. This occurs because only a small number of lymphocytes are capable of responding to a given antigen, and it explains to some extent the clinical patterns of involvement and spread of malignant lymphomas. Cells pass from the bloodstream to the lymphatic system through postcapillary venules within the lymph-nodes, and return to the blood stream by the thoracic duct. Part of the enlargement of lymph-nodes that occurs following immune stimulation can be accounted for by a marked increase in lymphocyte traffic through the node.

Lymphadenopathy

Normal lymph nodes are impalpable, except in some very thin subjects. Palpable enlargement is commonly referred to as lymphadenopathy, even though the nodes may be simply reacting in a normal fashion.

Causes

The main causes of lymphadenopathy are shown in Table 1. As indicated above, lymphadenopathy is most commonly due to infection, but other inflammatory disorders may be responsible. Lymphomas are relatively rare, and malignant involvement of a lymph-node is more commonly due to metastatic carcinoma.

Clinical management

In many instances the cause of lymphadenopathy will be apparent after taking a careful history and performing a thorough clinical examination. The history should encompass the patient's general health and past illnesses, possible exposure to infection including contact with animals or birds and travel abroad, and constitutional upsets such as fever, weight loss, sweats or pruritis. Alcohol-induced pain at sites of affected nodes is characteristic if not pathognomonic of Hodgkin's disease.

Physical examination should take note of the location and extent of the lymphadenopathy, and the characteristics of the nodes themselves (see page 19.171). Localized, tender lymphadenopathy should prompt a search for an infected lesion or portal of entry in the area drained by the node. Tender nodes are usually inflammatory or reactive, but rapid enlargement due to malignancy can stretch the capsule and produce pain. Hard nodes, especially if fixed and matted together, suggest malignancy. When there is cervical lymphadenopathy, the throat and pharynx should be carefully examined. A full general examination should be performed, with particular attention to the size of the liver and spleen.

Investigations should include a full blood count, ESR, and examination of the blood film. These may be diagnostic in cases of leukaemia, or may point to a viral cause such as glandular fever. Additional investigations might include a chest radiograph, biochemical profile, and antibody screens for an infective cause, together with specific cultures as appropriate.

Lymph-node biopsy

The cause of lymphadenopathy can be determined in the majority of instances by history, clinical examination, and the simple investigations outlined above. If this fails to yield a diagnosis, a lymph-node biopsy may be necessary, but knowing just when to do a lymph-node biopsy is often difficult and the usefulness of this investigation is reduced if it is performed indiscriminately. If the clinical suspicion of lymphoma is strong and there are good reasons why treatment should not be delayed, perhaps because the patient's condition is deteriorating, a biopsy should be taken as soon as possible. If the suspicion is less strong, then one should wait at least until the results of all the investigations are to hand: in this time a number of conditions will resolve spontaneously.

The diagnostic yield is improved by careful selection of the node to be biopsied. Supraclavicular nodes are preferred as axillary or inguinal nodes may be involved in reaction to local trauma or infection. Similarly, nodes peripheral to a malignant node, although enlarged themselves, may show only a reactive pattern and it is better to remove the largest node, even if this is technically more difficult. The biopsied specimen should not be put automatically into formalin: many of the techniques described below require fresh, unfixed tissue, and close liaison with the histopathologist is essential.

Methods for the study of lymphoproliferative disorders

Traditionally, the diagnosis of abnormal lymphoproliferative conditions, and especially the malignant lymphomas, has depended upon conventional histological evaluation of the tissues involved, the interpretation of which has been limited by the prevalent understanding of the structure and function of the lymphoid system. Less than 40 years ago, however, the function of lymphocytes was largely unknown, and many of the techniques devised by basic scientists to unravel the complexities of the immune system have now been successfully applied to clinical problems and as a result have greatly refined our diagnostic ability and our understanding of these conditions.

Histopathology

Conventional histological examination remains the cornerstone of diagnosis in a lymphoid biopsy. It is said that more errors are made in the diagnosis of lymph-nodes than in any other organ and that the commonest reason for this is poor preparation of the biopsied tissue. The clinician, by alerting the pathologist to an impending biopsy and providing fresh unfixed tissue, will ensure that material is received in an optimal state. Needle core biopsy, and more recently, fine needle aspiration have been advocated as a more convenient and rapid replacement to formal biopsy. They are often useful in the diagnosis of metastatic carcinomas, and may assume an increasingly important role as experience of them is gathered. At present, however, whenever there is clinical suspicion of lymphoma one must recommend removal of an entire node, in one piece, as the best means of obtaining an accurate diagnosis.

The histological evaluation of a lymph node depends on a systematic microscopic examination, taking into account the different compartments (capsule, follicles, paracortex, and sinuses) and cell types (lymphocytes, macrophages, plasma cells etc.) of which it is comprised. Although a few conditions can be diagnosed on the basis of a single abnormal feature, the major distinction between a benign and a malignant process can usually only be made after careful consideration of all the features mentioned above. Further details can be found in the discussion below on patterns of lymph-node reactivity and in the chapter on lymphomas (page 19.169).

The major limitation of a purely morphological approach to lymph-node diagnosis is that the cellular composition and structure of a node is largely related to its immunological function which can, at best, only be perceived indirectly in conventional histological preparations.

Immunocytochemistry

The introduction of reliable immunoenzymatic staining techniques coupled with the development of monoclonal antibodies has considerably refined the conventional histological examination of lymphoid tissue. The value of using an immunocytochemical technique such as the immunoperoxidase or immunoalkaline phosphatase method is that these provide permanent histological preparations which are similar to, and can be easily compared with, routine histological specimens. Monoclonal antibodies are invaluable because of the wide range of antigens that can be detected, the purity of the preparations, the homogeneity of the antibodies, and their wide availability. Using these techniques and reagents the histologist can now readily identify the different cell types (B cells, T cells, dendritic reticulum cells, macrophages etc.) within lymphoid tissue and can accurately classify the immunological origin of most lymphoproliferative disorders (Fig. 2).

The major application of these techniques has been in the study of lymphomas, in the hope of improving their classification and ultimately their treatment, but although this has generated a great deal of information it has as yet had little direct influence on patient management. This fact has unfortunately tended to obscure several genuine advances, one of which is the ability of a well-chosen panel of monoclonal antibodies to differentiate anaplastic tumours such as carcinoma, lymphoma, melanoma, and various sarcomas (see Fig. 3 and legend). The final diagnosis in such conditions has considerable bearing on management, and it is of particular interest that using these methods most pathologists have found cases of lymphoma which have been misdiagnosed as carcinoma or melanoma, with whose appearances they are more familiar.

Molecular approaches

One problem that puzzled immunologists for many years was how the body is able to respond to so many different antigens and yet produce a specific antibody for each new antigen encountered. It was clear that the total genome was not large enough to code for each possible antibody separately, and that there must be some mechanism to generate the necessary degree of antibody diversity. It is now known that this is achieved not by posttranslational modification of a primitive antibody molecule, but by the assembly of a 'supergene' from smaller coding segments in a process of gene 'rearrangement' that occurs at a very early stage of a lymphocyte's differentiation into the B cell lineage.

The process of rearrangement affects the immunoglobulin heavy and light chain genes sequentially and precedes their expression and thus the synthesis of immunoglobulin. It is shown schematically for the kappa light chain gene in Fig. 4. A similar mechanism for generating diversity in the T cell antigen receptor has recently been demonstrated. The state of the immunoglobulin genes within a given tissue can be analysed by hybridization of radioactive complimentary DNA (cDNA) probes for segments of the rearranged genes to digests of DNA extracted from the tissue in question (Fig. 5). In non-lymphoid tissues, whether normal or neoplastic, the immunoglobulin genes remain in their germ-line configuration in all the cells and the cDNA probe hybridizes only with DNA fragments of a single size. If cells from a single clone (for example, from a malignant B cell neoplasm) are analysed, the probe also hybridizes with large numbers of fragments containing the rearranged gene, but because the rearrangement effectively compresses the gene these fragments are of a different size and can readily be separated from those containing the germ-line genes. On the other hand normal and reactive lymph-nodes contain many clones of cells each capable of producing a different antibody; in these circumstances the probe hybridizes with small

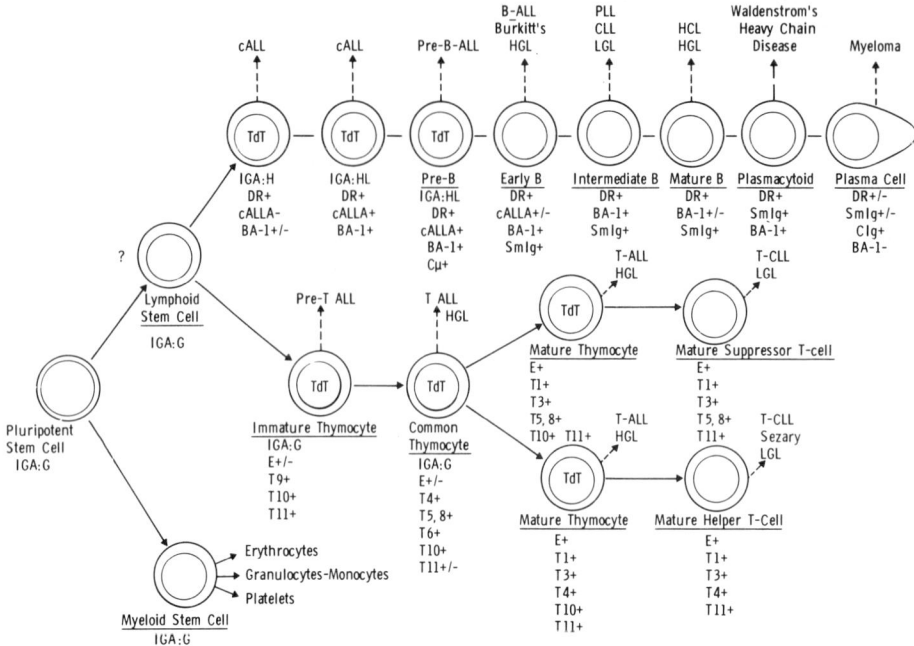

Fig. 2 A scheme of lymphocyte differentiation based on surface markers, enzyme, and molecular studies. Each 'cell' illustrated represents a phenotypically discrete stage in a continuum of differentiation. The pathways of differentiation are indicated by a solid arrow → and the relationship of various developmental stages with lymphomas and leukemias is indicated by a broken arrow (− − − →). The phenotypic characteristics are indicated beneath each cell. IGA indicates the arrangement of immunoglobulin genes as follows: G = germ line arrangement, H = heavy chain genes rearranged, L = light chain genes rearranged; T1, 3, 6, 8–11, and BA-1 represent reaction with monoclonal antibodies detecting various stages of T and B lymphocyte development, respectively; cALL = common acute lymphoblastic leukemia antigen; TdT = terminal transferase; DR = HLA DR expression; E = sheep erythrocyte, rosetting; Cμ = cytoplasmic μ heavy chain; SmIg = surface membrane Ig; CIg = cytoplasmic Ig (heavy and light chain); CLL = chronic lymphatic leukemia; PLL = prolymphocytic leukemia; HCL = hairy cell leukemia; HGL = non-Hodgkin's lymphoma (high grade); LGL = non-Hodgkin's lymphoma (low grade). (Modified from Foon, 1982).

numbers of many different-sized fragments, which cannot be readily distinguished from each other.

In addition to revealing how the immune system is able to respond to many different antigens, analyses of the immunoglobulin and T cell antigen receptor genes are proving to be a powerful tool in the investigation of lymphoproliferative disorders. For example, analysis of immunoglobulin genes has shown that the common variety of acute lymphoblastic leukaemia, previously thought to lack markers of B or T cell lineage, is in fact of early B cell origin. Similarly, hairy cell leukaemia, the cellular origin of which was argued for years, is now known to be a B cell neoplasm. These techniques can also help in diagnosis. Whilst the majority of lymphoproliferative disorders can be confidently diagnosed with conventional light microscopy, establishing a malignant as opposed to the reactive nature of a lymph node is difficult in a small proportion, even with the immunocytochemical techniques outlined above. This is particularly true in T cell malignancies, which lack any readily identifiable markers of monoclonality and in which analysis of the T cell receptor gene can provide objective evidence of monoclonal expansion.

Patterns of lymph-node reactivity

Lymph nodes can be divided into three functional areas; the follicles, the paracortex, and the medullary sinuses. When lymph-nodes respond to antigenic stimuli or invasion by infectious or neoplastic agents changes often predominate in one of these areas, leading to one of three basic reactive patterns (Fig. 6).

Follicular hyperplasia occurs when either increases in the size or number of lymphoid follicles contributes to significant lymph-node enlargement. This is a common histological finding in enlarged lymph nodes during childhood and adolescence. The condition is self-limiting and an underlying cause is rarely discovered. Specific causes of marked follicular hyperplasia include rheumatoid arthritis, measles, and toxoplasmosis.

Paracortical expansion is characteristically seen in many viral infections presumably due to a greatly increased stimulation of T lymphocytes. Florid persistent lymphadenopathy due to paracortical expansion is seen after vaccination for diseases such as smallpox, herpes zoster, whooping cough or influenza. It also commonly occurs in adolescents with infectious mononucleosis. Another cause of exaggerated paracortical expansion occurs in granulomatous responses to tuberculosis, yersinia infections or sarcoidosis. In these conditions the paracortex is filled with epithelioid histiocytes (cells of macrophage origin) rather than T lymphocytes.

Finally, *sinus hyperplasia*, which may overflow into the paracortex (leading to so-called 'passive' paracortical expansion), is commonly seen in nodes draining inflammatory or neoplastic conditions. Here the expansion and subsequent lymphadenopathy is caused by a greatly increased drainage of macrophages into the sinuses from the periphery as well as their proliferation in the sinuses themselves. Specific conditions giving rise to sinus hyperplasia include the lipidoses and Whipple's disease, and the condition may also be seen following lymphangiography.

In conclusion, it should be emphasized that many conditions cause changes in each of the three areas of a lymph-node so that distinction between the three basic reactive patterns described above is not always clear.

Non-malignant lymphoproliferative disorders

Generalized lymphoproliferation is a feature of several infections, which may occasionally present in an unusual fashion raising the possibility of something more sinister. The most obvious example

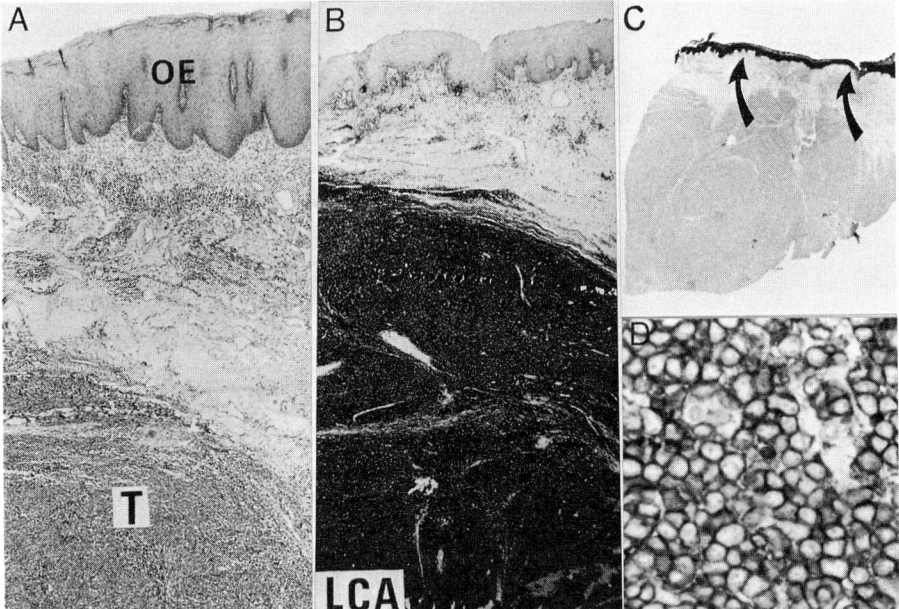

Fig. 3 This figure illustrates a typical problematical tumour biopsy. The patient, a middle-aged male, presented with a tumour in the oral cavity. A small biopsy was taken and, after considerable debate, reported as poorly differentiated squamous cell carcinoma. This led to an extensive resection involving hemimandibulectomy and deep neck dissection. However, it can be seen in (A) that the oral tumour (T) in the operation specimen lies deep to the epithelium (OE) and is not connected with it. A monoclonal antibody against the leucocyte common antigen (LCA) which stains leucocytes in conventionally-fixed paraffin sections shows (B) that the tumour is strongly positive. In contrast staining with anti-epithelial antibodies (C) gave no reaction with this tumour. Note that the oral epithelium (arrowed in C) gives a strong reaction with this anti-epithelial antibody providing a built-in control. The strong surface membrane labelling for LCA (shown in detail in D) in the absence of epithelial positivity is characteristic of lymphoma. On clinical reassessment this patient was found to have extensive mediastinal and abdominal lymphadenopathy. He was treated with systemic chemotherapy to which he made a good initial response although he died of his disease two years later. Undoubtedly the radical and mutilating operation was unnecessary. Subsequently other diagnostic errors of this type have been averted by similar immunocytochemical staining procedures performed in conjunction with routine histological examination of the biopsy specimen.

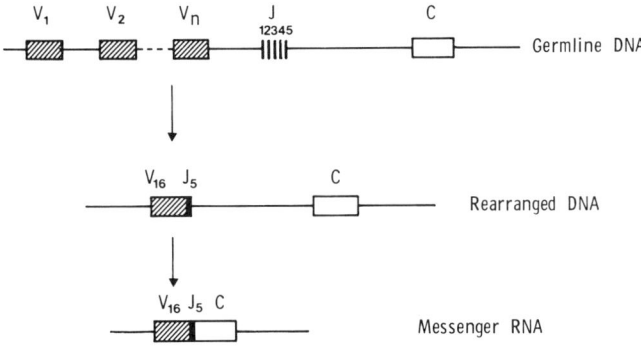

Fig. 4 The variable region of the kappa light chain gene is assembled from separately encoded V and J segments that are brought together by genomic rearrangement during B-cell differentiation. The germ-line kappa gene cluster contains in excess of 100 different V (variable region) segments and 5 J (joining) segments. In this example the rearranged DNA contains one V gene segment (V_{16}) and one J gene segment (J_5). The final messenger RNA containing the VJC sequence is produced by processing of the primary transcript from the rearranged gene segments. (Photograph by courtesy of Dr N. T. J. O'Connor.)

is infectious mononucleosis (glandular fever), but cytomegalovirus infections and toxoplasmosis are other conditions in this category (See Section 5).

Several other conditions which may be clinically confused with lymphoma are described on page 19.184. Some of these, such as angioimmunoblastic lymphadenopathy and lymphomatoid granulomatosis, whilst not necessarily neoplastic (at least in their early stages) may nevertheless progress to a true malignant lymphoma.

Infectious mononucleosis (see also Section 5)

Infectious mononucleosis (IM) is worthy of special mention as the virus responsible, the Epstein–Barr virus (EBV) preferentially infects B lymphocytes, and most of the clinical features of the disease can be ascribed to an intense proliferation of T cells attempting to eliminate the infected B cells. This is never fully achieved, and in common with other herpes viruses, the EBV lies dormant and may be reactivated at a later date in susceptible individuals. Whilst resolution of the clinical features of IM normally occurs within a few weeks, in some patients the T cell response is suboptimal and the condition may wax and wane, resolving eventually after several months.

One effect of EBV infection on B cells is to 'immortalize' the cell, that is, to confer the potential for unlimited proliferation. This is most readily apparent *in vitro*: cells from individuals who have had IM will proliferate quite easily in culture whilst it is generally impossible to encourage B cell proliferation *in vitro* from previously uninfected individuals. Normally this tendency is kept in check by suppressor T cells *in vivo*, but in some highly immunodeficient individuals such as transplant patients, uncontrolled B cell proliferation may occur. At first this is polyclonal, but in some instances (and sometimes more than once in a given individual), a particular clone 'takes-off' producing a condition indistinguishable from an immunoblastic lymphoma.

Pathogenesis of malignant transformation

It is now widely accepted that the majority of malignant neoplastic disorders result from the transformation of a single progenitor cell to a cell with abnormal potential for growth and differentiation, rather than from a general breakdown of homeostatic mechanisms, although the latter could conceivably contribute to the survival of an abnormal clone in some instances. What is less certain is

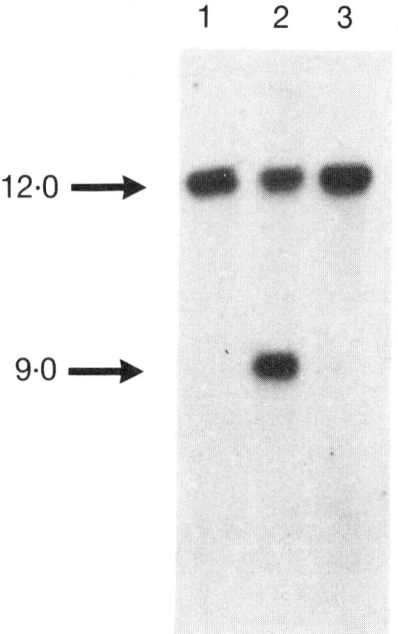

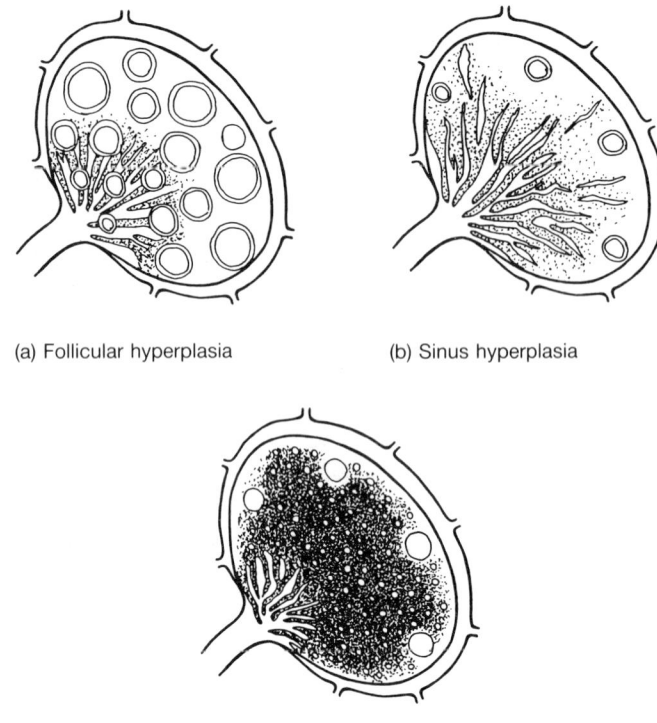

(a) Follicular hyperplasia   (b) Sinus hyperplasia

(c) 'Active' paracortical response

Fig. 5 Autoradiographs of DNA digested with *Bam*H1, a restriction endonuclease which reproducibly cuts DNA at sites of specific sequences giving rise to DNA fragments which can be separated according to size. The fragment containing the constant (C) region of the kappa gene is identified by hybridization with a probe consisting of a radioactively labelled complementary DNA sequence. Track 1 shows the pattern in normal DNA, in which the kappa genes remain in the germ-line configuration. The probe has hybridized with a single 12 kilobase fragment. Track 2 shows DNA extracted from a B cell lymphoma expressing kappa-chain synthesis. The single additional 9.0 Kb band indicates not only that the kappa genes have undergone rearrangement in this particular tumour, but also that a single rearrangement has occurred and that the tumour is monoclonal. Track 3 shows DNA extracted from a metastatic carcinoma: the kappa genes have not rearranged. (Photograph by courtesy of Dr N. T. J. O'Connor.)

the nature of the transforming event, and how it arises in the first place.

Evidence for clonality

The malignant nature of a wide range of neoplastic disorders has been inferred either from the observation that any associated cytogenic abnormalities (see below) consistently affect the majority or all of the neoplastic cells – suggesting that they arise from a common ancestor – or from the fact that when the condition develops in a female patient heterozygous for the A and B variants of the X-linked enzyme glucose-6-phosphate dehydrogenase, the affected cells express only one of the two variants (A *or* B), not both as would be expected if the neoplasm had not originated in a single cell (see also page 19.13).

In the case of lymphoid neoplasms, additional evidence for clonality comes from the clonal nature of the immune response itself, although some care is required in its interpretation. The most easily demonstrated examples are the paraproteinaemias (page 19.196), in which a single clone of B cells produces a single type of immunoglobulin with either kappa or lambda light chains, but not both. Similar observations can be extended to the majority of B cell neoplasms, and are carried to a greater degree of sophistication by the demonstration that each clone of B cells has a unique arrangement of its immunoglobulin genes as described above. Similarly, although the clonal nature of T cell neoplasms has been harder to demonstrate by other means, the recent discovery of analogous genetic rearrangements affecting the antigen–receptor genes has confirmed the clonal (and by inference the neoplastic) nature of many T cell disorders.

Fig. 6 Patterns of lymph-node reactivity. See text for description. (Reproduced with permission from Arno, 1980, with permission of the author and MTP Press.)

Cytogenetics

It has been known for some time that some human malignancies are consistently associated with chromosomal abnormalities. With the advent of high-resolution banding techniques it has become apparent that cytogenetic abnormalities occur in the vast majority of tumours, and that these are not necessarily random.

The most common defects are deletions of certain bands or in some circumstances of an entire chromosome, reciprocal translocations, or duplication of a chromosome (trisomy). Several examples are given in the chapters on leukaemias (page 19.17) and lymphomas (page 19.183). Of particular interest is the observation that many of these defects involve the sites of cellular proto-oncogenes. For example, in Burkitt's lymphomas (page 19.183) a consistent finding is a translocation between the long arms of chromosomes 8 and 14. One effect of this translocation is to move the c-*myc* gene from chromosome 8 and to juxtapose it to one of the immunoglobulin heavy chain genes (which are actively transcribed in B cells) on chromosome 14.

Aetiology (see also Section 4)

Although the precise nature of the alterations that occur within a cell to confer malignant properties remains unknown, a framework is beginning to emerge that helps us to understand in part the pathogenesis of malignant disorders. In many instances malignant transformation is associated with abnormal expression of one or more cellular proto-oncogenes. These are genes which show a great deal of homology with genes present in retroviruses associated with a number of animal and avian neoplasms. At first it was thought that the presence of these genes signified previous retroviral infection, but the converse is now thought to be true, that the genes have at some stage in evolution been 'captured' by the viruses from eukaryotic cells. The genes are in fact highly conserved, and in the majority of instances code for a protein (usually tyrosine) kinase that is thought to be intimately involved with the control of cell growth and proliferation.

It is thus not difficult to imagine how abnormal expression of such genes might play a part in the proliferation of malignant neoplasms. Evidence that oncogenes are directly related to malignant transformation has come from *in vitro* transfection experiments, in which certain (already abnormal) cell lines can be induced to proliferate uncontrollably by the introduction of genomic material from malignant tumours. As mentioned above, and elsewhere in this Section, abnormal expression of an oncogene may result from its translocation to a site of high transcriptional activity and/or by mutation – resulting in an abnormal gene product. Alternatively, increased expression could result from gene duplication, as could occur in trisomy states.

Such events are unlikely to account entirely for the process of malignant transformation, and it is believed that several discreet steps are required, with oncogene activation perhaps representing the last straw. The first step could involve an alteration in the kinetics or growth potential of a cell population that simply allows cells to go on growing indefinitely without altering their response to regulatory influences. An example is EBV infection of B cells which, as we have seen, enables these cells to proliferate indefinitely *in vitro*. This behaviour is suppressed by T cells *in vivo*, but uncontrolled proliferation may result if T cell activity is seriously impaired, as after tissue transplantation.

In areas of Africa where Burkitt's lymphoma is endemic, EBV infections are extremely common in infancy or early childhood, when they are often subclinical. It is of interest that the EBV was first isolated from cultures of Burkitt's lymphoma cells some years before its causative role in infectious mononucleosis was established. Although a direct aetiological association between the virus and this lymphoma has been postulated, it is most unlikely to be the sole factor. It has been suggested that persistent malarial infection, which has a similar geographical distribution to Burkitt's lymphoma chronically stimulates the immune system, increasing its susceptibility to somatic mutation or to some other transforming event.

References

Adams, J. M. (1985). Oncogene activation by fusion of chromosomes in leukaemia. *Nature* **315**, 542–543.

Arno, J. (1980). *Atlas of lymph node pathology*. MTP Press, Lancaster.

Desforges, J. F. (1985). T-cell receptors. *N. Engl. J. Med.* **313**, 476–577.

Foon, K. A., Schroff, R. W. and Gale, R. P. (1982). Surface markers on leukemia and lymphoma cells: recent advances. *Blood* **60**, 1–19.

Gatter, K. C., Alcock, C., Heryet, A. and Mason, D. Y. (1985). Clinical importance of analysing malignant tumours of uncertain origin with immunohistological techniques. *Lancet* i, 1302–1305.

Greaves, M. F., Myers, C. D., Katz, F. E., Schneider, C. and Sutherland, D. R. (1984). Cell-surface structures involved in haemopoietic cell differentiation and proliferation. *Br. Med. Bull.* **40**, 224–228.

Klein, G. (1975). The Epstein-Barr virus and neoplasia. *N. Engl. J. Med.* **293**, 1353–1357.

Klein, G. (1981). The role of gene dosage and genetic and genetic transpositions in carcinogenesis. *Nature* **294**, 313–318.

Korsmeyer, S. J., Arnold, A., Bakhshi, A., Ravetch, J. V., Siebenlist, U., Hieter, P. A., Sharrow, S. O., LeBien, T. W., Kersey, J. H., Poplack, D. G., Leder, P. and Waldmann, T. A. (1983). Immunoglobulin gene rearrangement and cell surface antigen expression in acute lymphocytic leukemias of T cell and B cell precursor origins. *J. clin. Invest.* **71**, 301–313.

Korsmeyer, S. J., Hieter, P. A., Ravetch, J. V., Poplack, D. G., Waldmann, T. A. and Leder, P. (1981). Developmental hierarchy of immunoglobulin gene rearrangements in human leukemic pre-B-cells. *Proc. Natl. Acad. Sci. USA* **78**, 7096–7100.

Louie, S., Daoust, P. R. and Schwartz, R. S. (1980). Immunodeficiency and the pathogenesis of Non-Hodgkin's lymphoma. *Sem. Oncol.* **7**, 267–284.

O'Connor, N. T. J., Wainscoat, J. S., Weatherall, D. J., Gatter, K. C., Feller, A. C., Isaacson, P., Jones, D., Lennert, K., Pallesen, G., Ramsey, A., Wright, D. H. and Mason, D. Y. (1985). Rearrangement of the T-cell-receptor β-chain gene in the diagnosis of lymphoproliferative disorders. *Lancet* i, 1295–1297.

Purtilo, D. T. (1980). Epstein-Barr-virus-induced oncogenesis in immune-deficient individuals. *Lancet* i, 300–302.

Warnke, R. A., Gatter, K. C., Falini, B., Hildreth, P., Woolston, R. E., Pulford, K., Cordell, J. L., Cohen, B., De Wolf-Peeters, C. and Mason, D. Y. (1983). Diagnosis of human lymphoma with monoclonal antileukocyte antibodies. *N. Engl. J. Med.* **309**, 1275–1281.

Yunis, J. J. (1983). The chromosomal basis of human neoplasia. *Science* **221**, 227–236.

The lymphomas

S. T. CALLENDER, C. BUNCH, AND R. I. VANHEGAN

Lymphoma is a term that has been applied rather loosely to cover the causes of swelling of lymph nodes and spleen, excluding those known to be infective and those due to spread of epithelial malignancy. As a result of careful classification of the biopsy appearances and follow-up of patients, it is apparent that there are 'malignant lymphomas' which, at presentation, are progressive, invasive and destructive conditions: these have been divided into two main groups, Hodgkin's disease and the non-Hodgkin's lymphomas (the latter being further subdivided into low and high grade malignancy). 'Benign lymphoma' has probably come to the end of its usefulness as a term describing a number of progressive hyperplasias, such as angio-immunoblastic lymphadenopathy (page 19.184) which may have a viral aetiology and which may run a self-limiting course or progress to a fatal outcome. Finally, there are a number of conditions which can have a clinical presentation simulating malignancy, associated with enlargement of a local group of nodes, where an infective aetiology is beyond dispute, e.g. toxoplasmosis, leishmania or cat scratch disease, while just occasionally tuberculosis is unexpectedly diagnosed in a lymph node biopsy.

The diagnosis of lymphoma rests on biopsy but, to put the incidence in perspective, lymphoma accounts for only a minor proportion of lymph-nodes biopsied in a district general hospital (Fig. 1). Lymphoma accounts for about 5 per cent of malignant disease in adult females (that is, one-fifth the incidence of breast cancer) and 6 per cent in males (that is, one-seventh the incidence of lung cancer). Overall, 60 per cent of the lymphomas can be expected to be of B lymphocyte origin; 10 per cent of T cell origin; 5 per cent of monocyte–macrophage lineage; and 14 per cent Hodgkin's disease origin. It should be borne in mind that about a quarter of all lymphomas present in an extranodal site such as the gut or skin. Because of its relative rarity, a lymphoma may be overlooked on a general medical unit as a treatable cause of a 'pyrexia of unknown origin' (PUO), ill-defined malaise, or unexplained weight loss. Conversely, lymphoma is not an uncommon incidental finding at an autopsy on an elderly patient dying of something else.

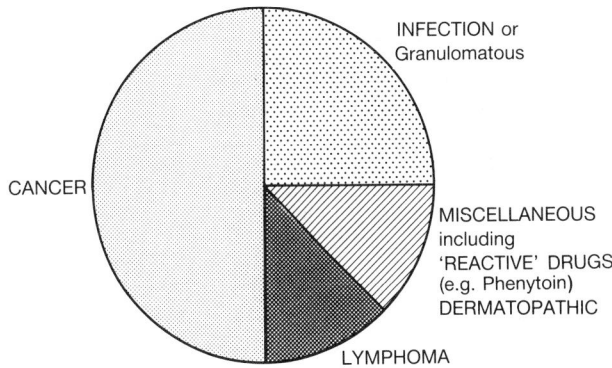

Fig. 1 Relative frequency of different histological diagnoses in surgical biopsies of suspect nodes in a district general hospital.

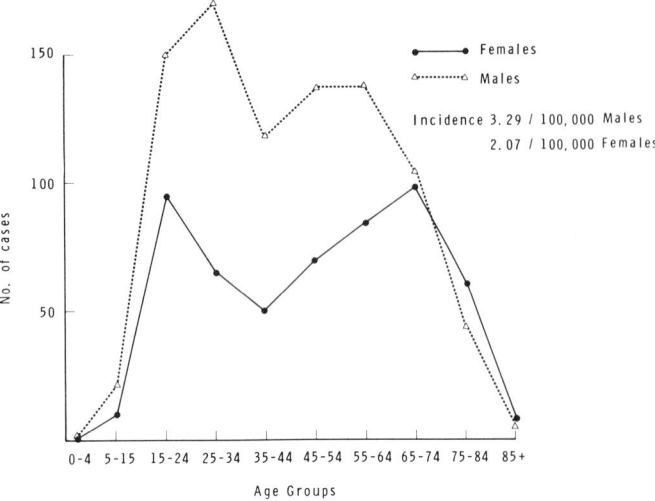

Fig. 2 Age distribution of Hodgkin's disease expressed as new cases registered in England and Wales in 1973.

HODGKIN'S DISEASE

In 1832 Thomas Hodgkin of Guy's Hospital, London, described the autopsy findings in seven patients who had died with a disorder characterized by generalized lymph node enlargement and splenomegaly. The earliest histopathological descriptions of what became known as Hodgkin's disease were published in 1878 by Greenfield. In 1892, Sternberg described characteristic giant cells and areas of necrosis in this condition, although he believed at the time that these changes represented an unusual reaction to tuberculosis. The recognition that the giant cells of Hodgkin's disease are an integral and diagnostic part of the pathological process was not made until the classic paper of Dorothy Reed of Johns Hopkins Hospital in 1902. Although surprisingly little has been learnt about the aetiology of Hodgkin's disease over the years, much progress has been made in its histological classification and management.

Incidence

Hodgkin's disease is about twice as common in males than females, and shows two peaks of incidence – one in young adults, the other in the elderly (Fig. 2). Interestingly, the nodular sclerosing form of the disease departs from this generalization in being more common in the younger age group, and in girls.

Aetiology and pathogenesis

Although in early descriptions Hodgkin's disease was considered to be an unusual reaction to tuberculosis, its malignant neoplastic nature is no longer in doubt. Chromosomal abnormalities have been detected in about two-thirds of cases studied: the most characteristic feature is aneuploidy with near triploidy or hypotetraploidy occurring in the most instances. No single characteristic abnormality has been detected but marker chromosomes have been found in nearly half, confirming the clonal origin of the neoplastic cells.

There remains considerable controversy surrounding the nature of the neoplastic mononuclear and multinuclear cells in Hodgkin's disease. Ultrastructurally the nuclei of the mononuclear cells resemble those of transformed lymphocytes, whilst the presence of cytoplasmic processes, small lysosomes and cytoplasmic microfibrils suggests a monocytic origin, although cytochemical staining for non-specific esterase (a characteristic of monocyte-derived cells) is consistently negative. The cells have receptors for immunoglobulin, which can be detected on their surface and occasionally within the cytoplasm. Studies with monoclonal antibodies, however, have shown that this immunoglobulin is polyclo-

nal, suggesting that it has been adsorbed and then ingested rather than synthesized by the cell itself.

More recently, cell marker studies with monoclonal antibodies have again shown conflicting results. It seems fairly clear, however, that the Hodgkin's cells do not carry markers of B-cell, T-cell or 'null-cell' differentiation, and many of the markers associated with monocytic origin are also absent. Studies with a monoclonal antibody (Ki–1), which detects an antigen on the neoplastic cells of Hodgkin's disease, have shown a population of small Ki–1 positive cells around and within the cortical follicles of normal lymph nodes. At present the origin and function of these cells is unknown.

The aetiology of Hodgkin's disease also remains unknown. As with other forms of malignancy, it is likely that no single event is responsible for the malignant transformation underlying the disease, and a series of possibly unrelated steps seems probable. Several lines of evidence suggest that at least one of these steps might involve an infectious agent, but although there have been several claims to have demonstrated such an agent, either directly by tissue culture or by inoculation of cell-free extracts into animals, no really convincing or reproducible evidence for a major infectious component has yet emerged.

An interesting association is the presence of significantly raised antibody titres to the Epstein–Barr (EB) virus in some patients, although the numbers involved suggest that the EB virus cannot have an important aetiological role. One possibility is that impairment of the immune response by EB virus infection could render the individual more susceptible to other, more significant agents.

There have been many reports of a familial incidence of Hodgkin's disease, but it is not certain whether these indicate a true increased genetic risk for the relatives of patients with the disease, or whether they reflect that family members are likely to be exposed to similar environmental hazards. Similarly, descriptions of clustering of cases, when looked at critically, do not necessarily indicate transmission from one case to another but could have occurred by chance alone.

Pathological features

Histological diagnosis

In Hodgkin's disease the lymph-node biopsy shows destruction of nodal architecture, best seen in reticulin preparations, with a proliferation of Hodgkin's mononuclear cells and the diagnostic Reed–Sternberg binucleate or multinucleate cells in a characteristic histological setting. In contrast to non-Hodgkin's lymphomas, early Hodgkin's disease may affect just part of a node, starting usually in the perifollicular areas.

The overall histological picture of Hodgkin's disease is somewhat heterogeneous, but four basic types are recognized.

Lymphocyte predominant The infiltrate consists mainly of small lymphocytes with a variable admixture of histiocytes but very few granulocytes or plasma cells and infrequent Reed–Sternberg cells. Approximately 10–15 per cent of cases are lymphocyte predominant at presentation.

Nodular sclerosing The nodular appearance is due to bands of collagenous connective tissue. The Hodgkin's mononuclear cells appear particularly well-hydrated and the cytoplasm shrinks away from the peripheral attachments during processing to leave 'lacunae'. Reed-Sternberg cells are usually easily found and there are variable proportions of lymphocytes, histiocytes, granulocytes (including eosinophils) and plasma cells within the tumour nodules. Approximately 20–50 per cent of patients present with this type of disease and the proportion of younger patients, often female and with mediastinal disease, is high.

Mixed cellularity The architecture of the lymph node is diffusely effaced by a mixed infiltrate with conspicuous granulocytes, especially eosinophils, plasma cells, lymphocytes and histiocytes,

Table 1 Percentage involvement of lymph node sites at presentation in Hodgkin's disease

Sites	Per cent
Cervical	51
Mediastinal	24
Axillary	18
Inguinal	16
Abdominal	9
Other nodes	2
Multiple sites	26

Adapted from Smithers (1967).

and plentiful Reed–Sternberg cells. This type accounts for 20–40 per cent of cases at presentation.

Lymphocyte depleted This is characterized by large numbers of atypical mononuclear cells, often pleomorphic with bizarre mitoses and many Reed–Sternberg cells, but a paucity of other cells. Often there is accompanying diffuse fibrosis. This form is rare at presentation accounting for 10 per cent or less.

In relapsed cases of nodular sclerosing disease the histological type tends to remain the same, whilst the pattern of the other three types may progress from lymphocyte-predominant through mixed cellularity to lymphocyte-depleted.

Clinical features

In the majority of patients the first complaint is of the discovery of an enlarged lymph node. Other patients may be referred because of the chance finding of mediastinal lymph node enlargement on a routine chest X-ray. Sometimes the patient has had a sore throat or a fever which has been attributed to a viral infection, but a gland first noted at the time has failed to disappear as the infection resolved. Patients are sometimes unaware of how long an enlarged node has been present. Some give a history dating back for several months; others may have noted fluctuation in the size of the nodes.

The commonest nodes to be enlarged are in the neck and axillae, less frequently in the groin (Table 1). The nodes are characteristically painless. Alcohol-induced pain in affected sites is a dramatic but rare feature.

About a quarter of the patients will have some constitutional symptoms, of which fever is the most important, indicating more extensive disease. The fever may be mild and indicated only by the occurrence of drenching night sweats, or it may have a swinging and hectic character. The Pel–Ebstein cyclical fever recurring at intervals of a few weeks, although considered characteristic of Hodgkin's disease, is in fact rarely encountered.

Other constitutional symptoms such as malaise, loss of energy, and weight loss are less specific but an inexplicable loss of weight of more than 10 per cent usually indicates extensive disease.

Severe skin itching is a feature of some cases of Hodgkin's disease and, indeed, of other malignant lymphomas and myeloproliferative disorders. It may precede the onset of other features so that the patient may be referred initially to a dermatologist, and may be so generalized and intolerable that it leads to a widespread excoriation. It may or may not be relieved by treatment of the underlying condition.

Massive lymph node enlargement may give rise to local problems, such as superior vena caval obstruction from mediastinal lymphadenopathy. Inferior vena-caval obstruction is much rarer.

Clinical evaluation

Because of its effect on prognosis and the selection of treatment, special care must be taken to determine whether or not the patient has any constitutional symptoms. In particular, if there is no clearly documented history of fever, it may be useful to get the

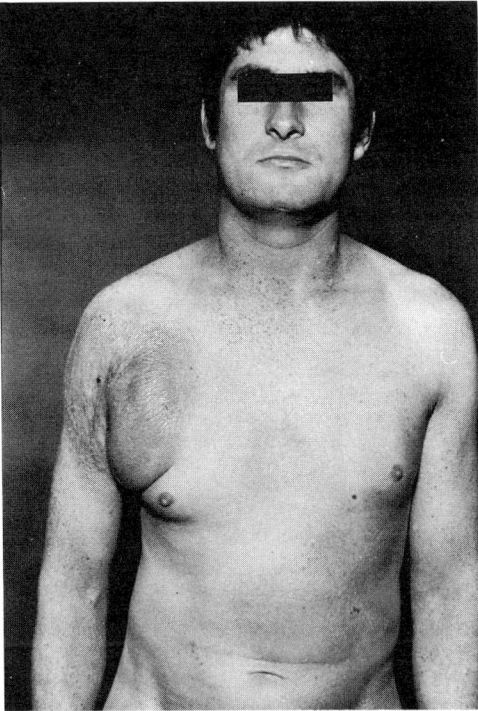

Fig. 3 Skin infiltration overlying large lymph nodes in a patient with Hodgkin's disease.

patient to record his temperature during the period of investigation.

Every patient should have a complete physical examination, particular note being made of the presence or absence of anaemia, weight loss, or evidence of signs of mediastinal obstruction. Examination for pathological lymph nodes must be done systematically. With the patient in a supine position the preauricular, submandibular, cervical, supraclavicular, and infraclavicular areas should be palpated, followed by the axillary, epitrochlear, inguinal, and femoral groups of nodes. In a thin patient the iliac nodes may also be palpable. The patient should then be asked to sit up and the physician should feel the occipital glands from behind and should re-examine the cervical, supraclavicular and axillary areas.

The area of Waldeyer's ring (tonsils, adenoids, and nasopharyngeal glands) is more likely to be involved with non-Hodgkin's disease but it should not be forgotten, particularly where there is upper cervical lymphadenopathy.

A note should be made of all enlarged nodes and their size measured for future reference. Other features, such as texture and mobility and attachment to other tissues, which may help to distinguish the lymphadenopathy from other causes of lymph node infiltration should also be noted.

The significance of lymphadenopathy in areas away from the original enlarged nodes is in some cases difficult to assess. This is particularly so in the case of small nodes palpable in the groins and axillae which may be enlarged secondary to infection or trauma of the feet or hands.

Splenomegaly should always be sought, although splenic enlargement does not always indicate involvement with Hodgkin's disease and conversely normal spleen size does not exclude involvement. Hepatomegaly is a feature of advanced disease.

Bone involvement is rare early in the disease, but may be suggested by local areas of pain and tenderness.

Local skin infiltration sometimes occurs, particularly in the thoracic wall as an extension from mediastinal or hilar node involvement, or in the region of massive lymph node enlargement (Fig. 3).

Extradural tumours occasionally produce cord compression and

Table 2 Ann Arbor classification of Hodgkin's disease*

Stage I	Involvement of a single lymph node region (I) or of a single extralymphatic organ or site (I_E)
Stage II	Involvement of two or more lymph node regions on the same side of the diaphragm (II) or localized involvement of extralymphatic organ or site and of one or more lymph node regions on the same side of the diaphragm (II_E)
Stage III	Involvement of nodes on both sides of the diaphragm (III). There may also be splenic involvement (III_S) or localized involvement of extralymphatic organ or site (III_E) or both (III_{ES})
Stage IV	Diffuse or disseminated involvement of one or more extralymphatic organs or tissues with or without associated lymph node enlargement

* Each stage is qualified according to whether or not the patient has systemic symptoms. **A** indicates no systemic symptoms, **B** indicates the presence of any of the following: unexplained weight loss of >10 per cent in the previous 6 months, unexplained fever over 38 °C, or night sweats. **E** is used to designate a *single* extralymphatic organ or site.
From Carbone *et al.* (1971).

very rarely there may be involvement of the meninges with Hodgkin's tissue, but these are usually late features.

Involvement of the kidneys is uncommon but an obstructive uropathy may occur secondary to pressure from enlarged glands which may also sometimes occlude the renal vein and produce a nephrotic syndrome. Other rare features are involvement of the pericardium and the gastrointestinal tract.

Staging of Hodgkin's disease

Involvement of the glands in Hodgkin's disease has been shown to spread from one group to the next directly connected by lymphatics. Recognition of this anatomical spread has made it possible to predict certain patterns of disease. Thus, for example, left lower cervical and supraclavicular lymphadenopathy is far more likely to be associated with upper para-aortic lymph node involvement and splenic or splenic hilar node involvement than is right supraclavicular lymph node disease, the spread being via the thoracic duct.

Since the disease does not spread in a random fashion it has become important in planning treatment to define accurately the extent of the disease at presentation. By agreement at a meeting at Ann Arbor a classification was devised which has been widely accepted (Table 2).

'B' symptoms are rare in stage I disease and if present a special effort should be made to exclude any other involvement, particularly of the mediastinal of para-aortic nodes. There does, however, appear to be a small proportion of patients with genuine stage I disease who have constitutional symptoms.

When the extent of disease has been determined by clinical examination and non-invasive investigations, the patient is said to have been *clinically staged*. However, this may not accurately reflect the true extent of the disease, particularly within the abdomen. This has led to the widespread use of laparotomy, including splenectomy, lymph node and liver biopsy to define the extent of involvement more accurately. Patients staged in this way are said to have been *pathologically staged*. The proportion of patients with different pathological stages in a consecutive series of over 1000 cases of newly diagnosed Hodgkin's disease at Stanford University is shown in Fig. 4.

Investigations

The history and clinical examination will already have aroused suspicion of a lymphoma, but lymph node biopsy will be required to establish diagnosis and to distinguish between Hodgkin's disease and non-Hodgkin's lymphoma. A drill biopsy or needle aspiration is seldom useful in distinguishing between lymph node pathologies and an adequate node biopsy is essential. This may be particularly difficult if the lymph nodes are not readily accessible, for example, in the case of mediastinal disease, and occasionally

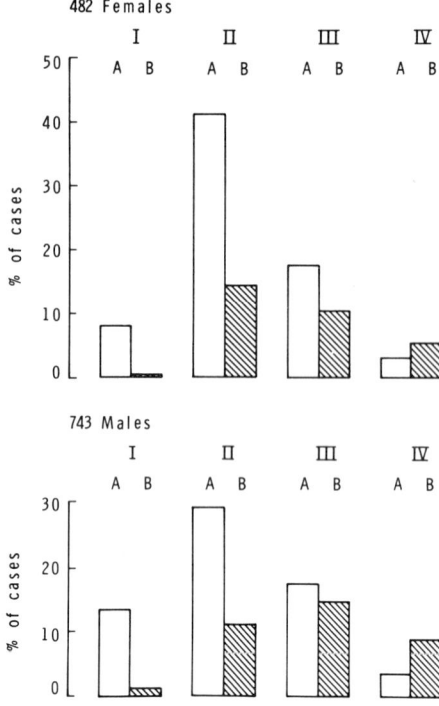

Fig. 4 Ann Arbor staging in relation to A and B symptoms in patients with Hodgkin's disease derived from data on 1225 consecutive untreated patients at Stanford University Medical Center, 1961–77. Reproduced by courtesy of Dr H. S. Kaplan.

more than one attempt may be necessary to obtain satisfactory tissue. In cases where there is a good deal of tissue necrosis sometimes a second or even a third biopsy may be necessary.

Once the diagnosis has been confirmed certain investigations are essential for the adequate staging of Hodgkin's disease. The importance of the history in relation to fever and weight loss has already been emphasized, as has the need for thorough examination of all the lymph node groups, spleen, liver, and areas of bony tenderness. Other investigations should proceed as follows.

Haematology

The blood count in patients with no constitutional symptoms is likely to be normal. Anaemia is uncommon and usually indicates widespread disease. An autoimmune haemolytic anaemia is a rare occurrence in Hodgkin's disease when it is usually a late feature and often associated with splenomegaly. The leucocyte count is variable, whilst a leucocytosis may indicate very active disease or tissue necrosis. Lymphopenia, when present, is a poor prognostic sign. Moderate eosinophilia is occasionally found but it is of no special significance. The platelet count is usually normal at presentation. The ESR is non-specific but may give some indication of the activity of the disease. It usually returns to normal during remission and serial estimates may be useful in that any rise in an otherwise asymptomatic patient may indicate relapse.

Biochemistry

This is useful for detecting disturbances of liver function which might be associated with liver involvement, or to look for isolated increases in serum alkaline phosphatase or a raised serum calcium level which may point to bone involvement. The uric acid level should also be measured as hyperuricaemia may occasionally be a hazard in the early stages of treatment, and rare cases of hypouricaemia associated with abnormal renal tubular secretion have been reported.

Chest radiograph

Assessment of the amount of mediastinal disease, hilar node involvement, and parenchymal lung involvement is particularly important in that involvement in these areas is recognized as a bad prognostic feature. A penetrated posteroanterior film may reveal retrocardiac glands not visible on an underpenetrated film, which may have been reported as normal. Any doubt about mediastinal or parenchymal lung involvement will usually be resolved by computed tomography.

Bone marrow examination

Ordinary bone marrow smears are less likely to reveal infiltration with Hodgkin's disease than a trephine biopsy, which should be taken from one, or preferably two, sites. If there is clear-cut evidence of marrow involvement the treatment of choice is chemotherapy. It may therefore be unnecessary to proceed with further investigation except from the point of view of having baseline data with which to compare future progress.

Computed tomography (CT)

In recent years CT has largely replaced lymphangiography as the major investigation in the lymphomas. It is non-invasive and has the advantage of simplicity. CT is particularly effective in revealing enlargement of retroperitoneal, iliac and mesenteric lymph-node groups, and can also detect enlarged nodes in the mediastinum which may not have been apparent on the plain radiograph. It may also detect large deposits in the liver and spleen, but cannot detect micronodular disease or distinguish this from reactive hyperplasia.

The main disadvantage of CT is that lymph-node enlargement is not the only criterion of abnormality, and the technique cannot detect disease in normal-sized nodes.

Lymphangiography

Bilateral lower-limb lymphangiography has in the past proved an excellent method for defining abnormalities in nodes in the femoral, inguinal, iliac, and para-aortic areas, and is reportedly accurate in detecting abnormalities in these areas in about 80 per cent of cases. However, the technique does not help with defining abdominal nodes above the level of the kidneys or mesenteric nodes which may, in part, account for the 10–25 per cent of equivocal or false-negative results. False-positives occur occasionally but are quite rare. One minor advantage is that the dye remaining can be used to follow the progress of the disease during therapy.

Excretion urography

This usually complements the lymphangiogram since the position of the kidneys or distortion of the line of the ureters may indicate the presence of large nodes which have not filled with the lymphangiogram contrast.

Radioisotopic scintigraphy

Technetium sulphur colloid scans of the liver and spleen are of limited value. They define the size of these organs and may show localized lesions although a negative scan does not exclude involvement. Bone scintigraphy may be useful if there is any indication of bony involvement such as local bone pain or tenderness, a raised alkaline phosphatase or hypercalcaemia.

Gallium-67 citrate has been described as a 'tumour-seeking' isotope and is occasionally useful in Hodgkin's disease. It is taken up by the majority of lesions greater than 2 cm in diameter and is most useful in the mediastinum where it can help distinguish between fibrosis and tumour. Unfortunately there is a significant false-positive rate as the isotope can be taken up by inflammatory lesions. Furthermore, excretion of the isotope into the bowel makes gallium scanning much less useful in the abdomen.

Ultrasonography

This may also be used to detect abdominal involvement, but its resolution is not as good as that obtained with CT. It is mainly useful as a quick guide to treatment response.

Staging laparotomy

Even careful clinical examination combined with the investigations outlined above will fail to reveal intra-abdominal disease in some patients, and it has been traditional to proceed to a staging laparotomy, unless the overt disease is so extensive that chemotherapy rather than radiotherapy is indicated. Before this operation, the nature of Hodgkin's disease should be clearly discussed with the patient and the reasons for laparotomy explained in detail.

An adequate staging laparotomy requires careful exploration with splenectomy, a systematic examination of all groups of glands, that is, para-aortic, coeliac, iliac, splenic hilar glands, and glands at the porta-hepatitis, with biopsy of representative glands from all areas and particularly of any that are suspect. A wedge biopsy of the liver is also taken. In young women, if total nodal irradiation is contemplated as treatment, the ovaries should if possible be moved to lie outside the planned radiotherapy field.

In experienced hands, staging laparotomy has a low morbidity. Prior to the widespread availability of CT scanning, laparotomy altered the stage in some 30–40 per cent of patients. In the majority staging was increased, whilst in a minority it was reduced. After CT scanning, the proportion of patients with clinical stages I or II who have a positive laparotomy is reduced (15–20 per cent). One of the major drawbacks of laparotomy is a small but worrying incidence of overwhelming post-splenectomy infection occurring sometimes many years after the operation.

An alternative approach is to forego laparotomy in patients who are clinically stage IA or IIA. Such patients can be treated with conventional radiotherapy provided that the small but significant risk of relapse outside the treatment field is accepted. This risk appears particularly slight with lymphocyte predominant disease, and a significant proportion of patients who relapse can in the event be salvaged with suitable chemotherapy, and possibly cured.

Treatment of Hodgkin's disease

The introduction of megavoltage radiotherapy and combination chemotherapy has revolutionized the outlook for patients with Hodgkin's disease, and cure is now a realistic goal for the majority. Whilst radiotherapy is appropriate for localized disease, in which it is highly effective and relatively free of troublesome side-effects, widespread disease is best treated with chemotherapy. Accurate staging of the extent of disease is therefore an essential preliminary to successful treatment.

Stages IA and IIA

Radiotherapy is usually considered to be the treatment of choice in patients staged pathologically as I or II. The usual treatment is by extended field, external beam megavoltage irradiation designed to treat *all* the major lymph node groups of the half of the body in which the disease is localized. Individually cast shielding blocks are used to protect the lungs from excessive radiation.

The rare patient with infradiaphragmatic stage I or II disease is treated in an analogous manner with an inverted Y-shaped field encompassing the para-aortic and iliac lymph node groups.

A dose of 35 Gy is given to the designated field, with a boost to a total of 40 Gy to the areas known to be affected. Treatment is given in daily fractions, treating on 5 days per week over 4 weeks.

Patients who present with a large mediastinal mass pose a special problem, as it may not be possible to treat their disease adequately with radiotherapy without damaging the lungs. They frequently have a nodular sclerosing histology and a poor prognosis. In these instances combined modality treatment is preferable, with chemotherapy given initially to produce regression or remission of disease, followed by mediastinal radiotherapy. This approach obviates the need for a staging laparotomy.

Stages IB and IIB

Patients with clinically localized disease but clear-cut B symptoms probably have more widespread involvement than is apparent and are best treated with chemotherapy from the outset.

Table 3 Chemotherapy of Hodgkin's disease

	Days		
	1	8	14
MOPP			
Nitrogen mustard (HN$_2$) 6 mg/m^2 i.v.	↓	↓	28 day cycle × 6
Vincristine 1.4 mg/m^2 i.v.	↓	↓	No treatment on days 15–28
Procarbazine 100 mg/m^2 oral	→————————→		
Prednisolone 40 mg/m^2 oral	→————————→		In cycles 1 and 4 only
De Vita *et al.* (1970)			

	Days		
	1	8	14
MVPP			
HN$_2$ 6 mg/m^2 i.v.	↓	↓	42 day cycle × 6
Vinblastine 6 mg/m^2 i.v. (maximum 10 mg)	↓	↓	No treatment on days 15–42
Procarbazine 100 mg/m^2 oral	→————————→		
Prednisolone 40 mg oral	→————————→		
Sutcliffe *et al.* (1978)			

	Days		
	1	8	14
ChlVPP			
Chlorambucil 6 mg/m^2 oral (maximum 10 mg)	→————————→		28 day cycle to remission + 5 cycles
Vinblastine 6 mg/m^2 i.v. (maximum 10 mg)	↓	↓	No treatment on days 15–28
Procarbazine 100 mg/m^2 oral (maximum 150 mg)	→————————→		
Prednisolone 40 mg oral	→————————→		
Dady *et al.* (1982)			

Stage IIIA

There has been considerable debate as to whether patients with stage IIIA disease are best treated with radiotherapy (either with a mantle field for supradiaphragmatic nodes together with an inverted Y for infradiaphragmatic nodes, or an extended mantle which includes any involved para-aortic nodes), or chemotherapy. If used, radiotherapy should be confined to patients with pathologically staged IIIA disease – that is, those who have undergone laparotomy and splendectomy – but most centres now favour chemotherapy for all patients with clinical stage III disease, obviating the need for a staging laparotomy.

Stages IIIB, IVA, and IVB

There is general agreement that patients with clinical stages IIIB and IV do not require staging laparotomy as the treatment of choice is combination chemotherapy in the first instance. The most useful cytotoxic combinations (Table 3) are the original MOPP regime (mustine, vincristine [Oncovin], procarbazine and prednisolone), first introduced in 1970; MVPP, in which vincristine is replaced by the less neurotoxic vinblastine, and ChlVPP or LOPP, in which nitrogen mustard is replaced by chlorambucil (Leukeran), which can be taken by mouth and which causes far less nausea and vomiting. There are many other combinations in current use including such drugs as doxorubicin, dacarbazine, and CCNU, but so far no protocol has produced convincingly better results than the original MOPP regime.

Management of chemotherapy

Treatment with chemotherapy can be carried out on an outpatient basis. Patients should be given an outline of the treatment, the possible side-effects should be mentioned but not over-emphasized, and they should be urged to return to work or to normal activity as soon as they feel able to do so.

Because of the nausea and vomiting which almost invariably accompany the administration of mustine, an antiemetic such as chlorpromazine, nabilone or domperidone should be given beforehand. Even then, vomiting may be severe. In these circumstances it is not surprising that many patients begin to question the need for chemotherapy, especially once the symptoms of the original disease have been controlled, and for this reason many centres now use chlorambucil in preference to mustine. This undoubtedly leads to better compliance, and in one multicentre study no difference in efficacy was found between a chlorambucil regime (LOPP) and MOPP, although long-term follow-up has not yet been reported.

If mustine is used, great care should be taken with its administration: it should be injected directly into the tubing of a fast-running intravenous infusion to prevent problems with leakage of the drug, as this may cause necrosis of the surrounding tissues. Similar care should be taken to avoid extravasation of vincristine or vinblastine, although these can usually be safely injected directly into a vein.

The importance of compliance and regular attendance needs to be emphasized, and many patients need constant encouragement, particularly those receiving mustine. Administration at a weekend often enables patients to continue at work without significant interruption.

It is essential to have a full blood count before starting each new course of treatment, and to modify the doses of drugs or the interval between courses accordingly. Patients should be told to contact the treatment centre immediately about any problems or should they need any advice. Details of treatment regimes and suitable dose modifications are shown in Table 3 and in the original publications.

Children Children with Hodgkin's disease pose special problems mainly because extensive treatment can impair their growth and development. Fortunately, Hodgkin's disease in childhood has a comparatively good prognosis, with the exception of girls with stage IV disease or bulky mediastinal disease of the nodular sclerosing pattern. Stage IA in high cervical or inguinal areas rarely relapses after radiotherapy alone, and local involved field radiation is appropriate. Laparotomy and splenectomy is best avoided because of the increased risk of postsplenectomy infection in children.

Duration of chemotherapy The optimal duration of treatment is still uncertain, though one should probably aim to give at least three courses after complete clinical resolution of the disease. Most physicians give at least six courses altogether, after which the majority of patients will be in clinical remission. At this point a limited restaging should be undertaken – this should include a CT scan but laparotomy is not necessary. In many instances restaging reveals significant residual lymph node enlargement, and the difficulty can be in distinguishing scarring from active disease. This is particularly a problem in patients whose original presentation was with bulky mediastinal disease. If there are no other signs of disease activity (such as symptoms or raised ESR) and the histology was favourable, an expectant policy is justified, but the CT scan should be repeated once or twice at 1–2 month intervals. If there is any doubt about disease activity then supplementary radiotherapy to residual sites of lymph node enlargement is warranted.

For patients in full remission there is no good evidence that any maintenance treatment is necessary, and indeed this may be harmful in view of the increased hazard of second malignancies in patients with Hodgkin's disease.

Treatment of relapse Patients who have achieved complete remission, either with radiotherapy or chemotherapy, but who subsequently relapse may well respond to further treatment. The extent of recurrence should be fully defined. Chemotherapy is indicated if it occurs within a previously irradiated area, otherwise there is a choice between further radiotherapy and chemotherapy although the latter is increasingly preferred.

Complications of treatment

With the majority of patients expecting to survive for many years after treatment, unwanted effects of therapy assume greater importance, especially if the quality of survival is permanently impaired in some way. In view of the appalling prognosis recorded in the days before effective treatment was available, these might arguably be a reasonable price to pay. Nevertheless, the potential hazards of treatment are now well understood, and with care can be reduced to a minimum.

Complications of radiotherapy

Radiation-induced cardiopulmonary disease The chest X-ray of patients who have received mantle irradiation generally shows some paramediastinal fibrosis which is, however, asymptomatic. A more widespread radiation pneumonitis may occasionally follow irradiation therapy, when it may be associated with dyspnoea and a dry cough. Serious pulmonary fibrosis may be a later development, although it is very uncommon with properly planned irradiation and prompt treatment of chest infections during radiotherapy. The lung changes have to be distinguished from intercurrent infection, such as with *Pneumocystis carinii*, although opportunistic infections are more likely to be seen late in the disease, especially in those who have received chemotherapy in addition to radiotherapy.

Cases of cardiomyopathy occurring several years after mediastinal irradiation have been reported. This complication is dose-related and is particularly associated with older age and concomitant administration of anthracycline drugs such as doxorubicin.

Radiation-produced myelosuppression Treatment by irradiation may be limited by leucopenia and thrombocytopenia, particularly in those who have received previous chemotherapy.

Hypothyroidism A proportion of patients develop overt hypothyroidism following upper mantle irradiation. In some series the incidence has been as much as 20 per cent. The thyroid gland is especially sensitive to radiation, and the incidence of thyroid carcinoma is also increased.

Complications of chemotherapy

Nausea and vomiting Several of the drugs used in the treatment of Hodgkin's disease cause nausea and vomiting. This is mainly a problem with mustine and doxorubicin, and most patients receiving combinations including one of these will have some degree of gastrointestinal upset. If severe, a change to a different regimen may make the treatment more tolerable and stop the patient from defaulting.

Alopecia Alopecia of some degree is common particularly when vincristine, cyclophosphamide or doxorubicin are used. Patients should be warned of this possibility but may be reassured that the effect is largely temporary.

Neurotoxicity The use of the vinca-alkaloids, but particularly vincristine, may produce troublesome neurotoxicity. Most patients get some paraesthesiae and lose their ankle jerks, and occasional patients get severe pains, particularly in the legs and in the jaw, which may be quite intolerable. A change to vinblastine is indicated if this occurs. Ileus of the bowel may sometimes also be produced, and constipation should be avoided in patients receiving the vinca-alkaloids.

Myelosuppression This is the most troublesome complication of chemotherapy and it may restrict its use. Particular care is required in giving chemotherapy after radiotherapy when the marrow reserves may already have been reduced. In these circumstances chemotherapy should be introduced at half the normal dose, and only stepped up when it is established that the treatment will not produce significant myelosuppression. Excessive myelosuppression can be largely avoided by the use of suitable dose modifications as indicated in Table 3.

Infertility This is a problem in male patients with chemotherapy, and the possibility of storing sperm for future artificial insemination should be considered. Unfortunately, viable sperm collections cannot always be obtained, but recent studies suggest that a complete return of normal spermatogenesis may occur in about a quarter of the patients who have remained in remission for more than 2 years. Chemotherapy is commonly associated with amenorrhoea, but in females ultimate fertility does not seem to be as frequently affected as is male fertility. Early menopausal symptoms may be encountered, and may indicate the need for hormone replacement.

Aseptic bone necrosis This has been noted particularly in the femoral head and has usually been attributed to corticosteroid treatment used during combination chemotherapy, but it may also be associated with local bony lesions for which radiotherapy has been required.

General complications

Second malignancies It is now well-recognized that patients successfully treated for Hodgkin's disease are at risk from second malignancies. A variety of malignancies has been encountered, but the most common is acute myeloid leukaemia (AML). The risk is relatively small but appears to be proportional to the duration and intensity of treatment, being highest in those receiving both radiotherapy and chemotherapy. Figures from the National Cancer Institute in the United States, suggest a 29-fold increase in risk overall.

Infections Because of the defects in cellular immunity associated with Hodgkin's disease, and the myelosuppressive and immunosuppressive effects of treatment, patients are particularly susceptible to infection (see Section 5). Bacterial infections are particularly common during chemotherapy, whilst herpes zoster is a frequent late complication. Opportunistic infections such as *Pneumocystis carinii* and fungal infections are seen occasionally in patients with resistant disease who have been extensively treated. There used to be a particular association with tuberculosis, but this is now rather rare.

Of particular note is an increased susceptibility to sudden, overwhelming infection following splenectomy. The causative organism is usually *Strep. pneumoniae*, but *Haemophilus influenzae* or *Neisseria meningitidis* are occasionally encountered. The danger of such infections is that they may be fatal within a few hours of onset: it is thus most important that patients undergoing staging laparotomy should be appraised of the risk, and advised to seek medical advice early in the course of any febrile illness. If this is likely to be difficult, they should be given a supply of a suitable antibiotic (such as ampicillin) to take themselves. The role of pneumococcal vaccines is currently being evaluated but the antibody response may be less effective after splenectomy, and this would not, of course, protect against other organisms. Overwhelming infections have been reported to occur in up to 10 per cent of patients, although in other series this has not been a feature.

Progressive multifocal leucoencephalopathy (Section 21) This is a serious demyelinating disorder caused by infection with the JC virus. It occurs in severely immunocompromised patients and occasionally complicates Hodgkin's and other lymphomas.

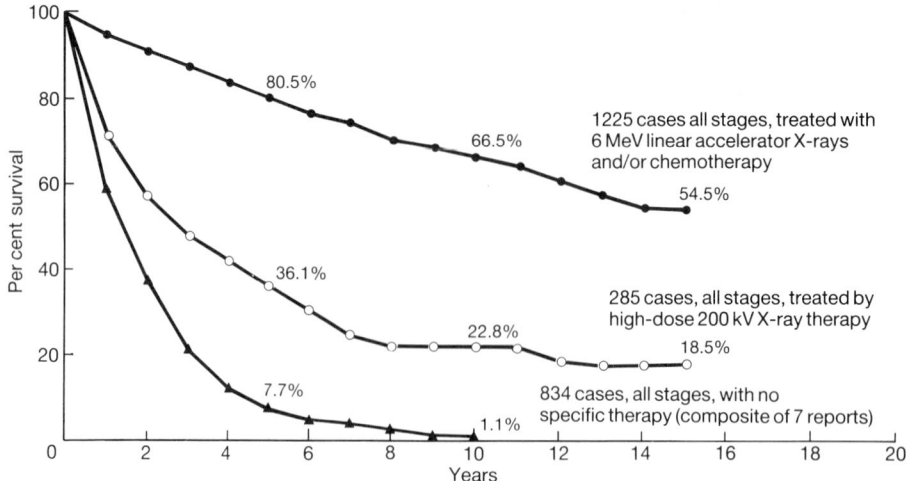

Fig. 5 Comparison of representative 5-year survival data from three different eras for patients with Hodgkin's disease of all stages: with no specific treatment, with the introduction of high dose kV radiotherapy, and with intensive MV radiotherapy and/or chemotherapy. (Reproduced with permission from Kaplan, 1980.)

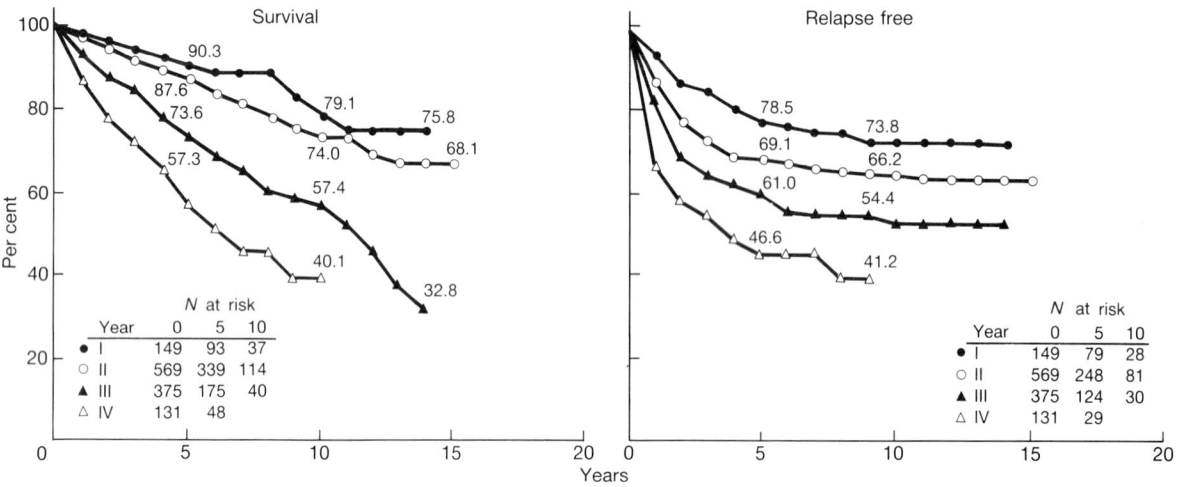

Fig. 6 Actuarial analysis of survival and freedom from relapse in the Stanford series of 1225 patients with Hodgkin's disease in relation to Ann Arbor clinical stage. (Reproduced with permission from Kaplan, 1980.)

Prognosis in Hodgkin's disease

Data derived from early series of patients with Hodgkin's disease who received no specific therapy show that the mean survival was less than 2 years and less than 10 per cent of the patients were alive at 5 years after diagnosis. The prognosis improved first with the introduction of low-dose and subsequently extended-field radiotherapy. Further improvements followed with the use of single chemotherapeutic agents and, later, combination chemotherapy, to the extent that some 70–80 per cent of patients will survive to 5 years, most of whom can probably be considered cured (Fig. 5). Prognosis depends on a number of factors:

1. The extent of the disease, stages IA and IIA having the best prognosis and IV the worst (Fig. 6).

2. The presence of systemic (B) symptoms, which at all stages indicate a worse prognosis.

3. The histology: lymphocyte predominant and nodular sclerotic histology have a better prognosis than mixed cellularity and lymphocyte depleted types. This may be influenced by the fact that the former group tends to be more frequent in the stage I and II diseases, whereas mixed cellularity and lymphocyte depletion tends to be found in more advanced cases. An exception to this

rule is bulky mediastinal nodular sclerosing disease occurring in young women, which has a much less favourable prognosis than other presentations with this histology.

4. Age has some influence on prognosis, particularly in the more advanced stages of the disease when older patients have a worse prognosis than young adults. This is at least in part due to older patients tolerating treatment less well than younger patients.

5. Sex: there is no sex difference with stage I and II disease, but male patients with stage III and IV disease have a worse prognosis than females with similar staging.

6. Relapse: although patients who relapse may respond to further therapy, their prognosis is not so good as in previously untreated cases. Salvage with chemotherapy is most successful in patients previously treated with radiotherapy.

NON-HODGKIN'S LYMPHOMA

The non-Hodgkin's lymphomas (NHL) comprise a group of malignant disorders which by definition include all lymphomas which lack the characteristic histopathological features of Hodgkin's disease – in other words, Reed–Sternberg cells are absent and desstruction of the normal architecture need not be present. There is now clear evidence that the majority if not all of these disorders have a clonal origin from a single mutant cell, and in most cases the malignant cells show characteristics of B cell differentiation with most of the remainder being of T cell origin. A rather loose definition of lymphoid tissue enables cells of the monocyte macrophage lineage to be included: these cells are frequently described as 'histiocytes' by pathologists, although in the context of lymphomas this term has not always been so precisely used.

The results of treatment for NHL have been much less satisfactory than in Hodgkin's disease. Considerable effort has been made in recent years to characterize these disorders, particularly with respect to their aetiology, cellular and molecular biology, natural history and response to treatment. Current concepts of aetiology and pathogenesis were described on page 19.168.

Classification and pathology

Both the clinical and histopathological features of NHL are diverse, and this has lead to a plethora of classifications. Until recently the most widely used classification was that of Rappaport in 1966; this scheme is clinically useful as it correlates well with prognosis, but it was produced at a time when our knowledge of the origin and functions of different cell types within normal and reactive lymph nodes was scanty, and its terminology is now frankly misleading.

In recent years our understanding of lymphoid differentiation has increased markedly, helped by immunological techniques which can pinpoint surface antigens on individual cells within suitable histological sections. This has led to a much clearer idea of the structure of normal lymph nodes, the traffic of cells through them and the changes that occur following antigenic stimulation. More recent classifications of NHL have attempted to relate the nature of the malignant cell to its normal counterpart. Several such schemes have evolved which vary mostly in their technical requirements and suitability for use with routine histopathological methods. All have prognostic significance, but it is unfortunately not possible to make direct translations between the various classifications, and this makes comparisons of therapeutic trials difficult to interpret.

In an attempt to circumvent this problem, an expert international panel reviewed in 1981 clinical and histological material from 1175 patients. All cases were classified by six systems: Rappaport, Kiel, British National Lymphoma Group, Lukes-Collins, WHO, and Dorfman. The result was a 'working formulation of non-Hodgkin lymphoma for clinical use' which can be readily translated into any one of the standard classifications. This scheme (Table 4) was not meant to supplant any of those in use already but is a common language through which, for example, comparison of results of clinical trials may be made.

It should be noted that in spite of all the efforts put into the classification of NHL, in all series up to 10 per cent of cases cannot be accurately classified with the material or techniques available.

The classification most widely used in European centres is that devised by Lennert's group in Kiel. This scheme uses information gained from cell-marker studies combined with a cytological/haematological approach, and enables a considerable consensus to be reached by non-specialist histopathologists working with routine biopsies. It has good prognostic correlations and, like other classifications, separates NHL into those with a relatively good prognosis (low-grade) and others with high-grade or poor prognostic features.

The relative frequency of the different subtypes of NHL in the Kiel classification are shown in Table 5. The commonest varieties are those of follicle centre-cell origin, referred to in the Kiel classification as centrocytic or centroblastic/centrocytic lymphomas.

Low-grade lymphomas

Lymphocytic lymphoma The common B cell type of lymphocytic lymphoma is often arbitrarily separated from chronic lymphatic leukaemia (CLL) on the basis of the degree of involvement of the circulating blood. As with CLL the pace of progression is variable, and in some patients proliferation may reach a plateau and remain stable for many years. In general the features are similar to those of CLL, described in detail on page 19.32, including impaired humoral immunity with paraprotein production in about 10 per cent of cases.

A particular feature of the T cell lymphocytic lymphomas is their predilection for the skin, which may be related to the known immunological functions of the skin and the fact that normal T cells interact dynamically with epidermal structures as part of the local immune response to invading antigen. The cutaneous T cell lymphomas are described on page 19.182.

Immunocytic lymphomas In this group there is an accumulation of cells, intermediate in morphology between lymphocytes and plasma cells, which contain monoclonal intracellular immunoglobulin. Lymph nodes, gut, or spleen may be involved singly or in combination, or plasmacytomas may develop, often in association with the respiratory tract. There may be a paraprotein in the serum. Both Waldenström's macroglobulinaemia and myeloma are included in this group (see page 19.196).

Follicle centre-cell lymphomas The normal reactive germinal follicle is comprised mainly of B lymphocytes (as judged by monoclonal immunoglobulin expression) in a high state of mitotic activity. Because the appearance of lymphocytes alters as they proliferate, this gives rise to the illusion of fairly distinct cell 'populations' within the follicle. Broadly, two main types of cell are recognized, *centrocytes*, which are of varying size and which have an irregular, cleaved nucleus, and *centroblasts*, which are larger cells with round, vesicular nuclei containing several nucleoli. Lymphomas are recognized in which the predominant cell has characteristics of centrocytes, centroblasts or, most commonly, both. Furthermore, these tumours may involve the lymph gland as a whole in a diffuse, monotonous fashion, or may retain some semblance of follicle-formation or nodularity.

Nodularity is most commonly seen in *centroblastic/centrocytic* lymphoma, and in extreme cases the follicles may be enormous (*giant follicular lymphoma* or *Brill-Symmers' disease*). Centroblastic/centrocytic lymphoma is probably the commonest type of NHL in the western world, but despite its relatively high mitotic index, the prognosis of this lymphoma is relatively good. This contrasts with the less common, purely *centrocytic lymphoma*, which although comprised of cytologically rather 'low-grade', inactive looking cells with few mitoses, has a rather poor prognosis, intermediate between the other low-grade and the high-grade lymphomas. Normal centrocytes recirculate between the blood and lymphoid tissues; the neoplastic cells may therefore be widely distributed at diagnosis, and their very low mitotic rate may render them less responsive to chemotherapy and radiotherapy.

High-grade lymphomas

Centroblastic lymphomas Low-grade follicle centre cell tumours may evolve into higher grade malignancies composed of monomorphic large cells (centroblasts) with non-cleaved nuclei and prominent nucleoli. Alternatively, centroblastic lymphomas may arise *de novo*. It is, however, often difficult to differentiate centroblasts histologically from immunoblasts, which may sometimes look very similar in routine preparations. The true centroblastic type of lymphoma has a rather better prognosis – only slightly worse than the mixed follicle centre-cell tumours and better than immunoblastic lymphomas.

Immunoblastic lymphomas These are aggressive tumours which may be comprised of either B or T immunoblasts. They have a poor prognosis although good responses and a small proportion of cures have been obtained following aggressive chemotherapy.

An interesting group of immunoblastic tumours has been des-

Table 4 A working formulation of non-Hodgkin's lymphomas for clinical usage (equivalent or related terms in the Kiel classification are shown)

Working formulation	Kiel equivalent or related terms
Low grade	
A. Malignant lymphoma	
Small lymphocytic	
consistent with CLL	ML lymphocytic, CLL
plasmacytoid	ML lymphoplasmacytic/lymphoplasmacytoid
B. Malignant lymphoma, follicular	
Predominantly small cleaved cell	
diffuse areas	
sclerosis	ML centroblastic-centrocytic (small), follicular ± diffuse
C. Malignant lymphoma, follicular	
Mixed, small cleaved and large cell	
diffuse areas	
sclerosis	
Intermediate grade	
D. Malignant lymphoma, follicular	
Predominantly large cell	
diffuse areas	
sclerosis	ML centroblastic-centrocytic (large), follicular ± diffuse
E. Malignant lymphoma, diffuse	
Small cleaved cell	
sclerosis	ML centrocytic (small)
F. Malignant lymphoma, diffuse	
Mixed, small and large cell	ML centroblastic-centrocytic (small), diffuse
sclerosis	ML lymphoplasmacytic/lymphoplasmacytoid, polymorphic
epithelioid cell component	
G. Malignant lymphoma, diffuse	
Large cell	ML centroblastic-centrocytic (large), diffuse
cleaved cell	ML centrocytic (large)
non-cleaved cell	ML centroblastic
sclerosis	
High grade	
H. Malignant lymphoma	
Large cell, immunoblastic	ML immunoblastic
plasmacytoid	
clear cell	
polymorphous	T zone lymphoma
epithelioid cell component	Lymphoepithelioid cell lymphoma
I. Malignant lymphoma	
Lymphoblastic	
convoluted cell	ML lymphoblastic, convoluted cell type
nonconvoluted cell	ML lymphoblastic, unclassified
J. Malignant lymphoma	
Small noncleaved cell	
Burkitt's	
follicular areas	ML lymphoblastic, Burkitt type and other B lymphoblastic
Miscellaneous	
Composite	—
Mycosis fungoides	Mycosis fungoides
Histiocytic	—
Extramedullary plasmacytoma	ML plasmacytic
Unclassifiable	—
Other	—

Reproduced with permission from the Non-Hodgkin's Lymphoma Pathologic Classification Project (1982).

cribed recently in patients with severe combined immunodeficiency, either inherited or due to intense immunosuppression following transplantation. In most instances the neoplastic cells have contained the EB virus, and molecular studies have shown that in some cases the proliferations are polyclonal, whilst in others they have been monoclonal. Occasionally both polyclonal and monoclonal proliferations have been seen in the same patient. Regression of tumours has sometimes followed withdrawal or reduction of immunosuppressive therapy. It seems most likely that these patients have gross impairment of normal T cell-mediated regulation of EB virus infected B cells, and that this may well predispose to malignant transformation.

Lymphoblastic lymphomas Unlike the other varieties of NHL, lymphoblastic lymphomas occur predominantly in a younger age group. The most characteristic presentation is with a mediastinal mass which may be large enough to produce superior vena caval obstruction. These mediastinal tumours are usually of T cell type and the disease has many features in common with T cell acute lymphoblastic leukaemia. Indeed, if not treated there is sooner or later invasion of blood and bone marrow with malignant lymphoblasts.

Adult T cell leukaemia/lymphoma syndrome (ATL) This is a more recently recognized condition of particular interest as it is the first

Table 5 Distribution of subtypes of non-Hodgkin's lymphoma using the Kiel classification

Histological subtype	Per cent of patients
Low grade non-Hodgkin's lymphoma	69.4
Lymphocytic (including CLL)	24.9
Lymphoplasmacytoid (immunocytoma)	18.9
Centrocytic	7.7
Centroblastic-centrocytic	13.9
Borderline/unclassifiable	4.0
High grade non-Hodgkin's lymphoma	30.2
Centroblastic	13.9
Immunoblastic	7.4
Lymphoblastic	5.3
Borderline/unclassifiable	3.6
Unclassifiable non-Hodgkin's lymphoma	0.4

Data on 1127 patients entered into a multi-centre study. From Brittinger *et al.* (1984).

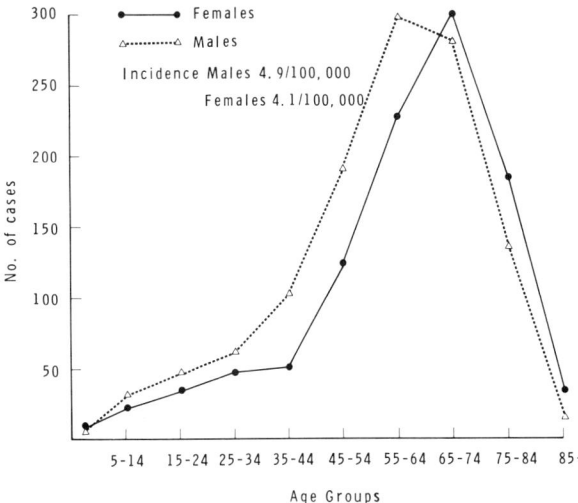

Fig. 7 Age distribution of non-Hodgkin's lymphomas expressed as new cases registered in England and Wales in 1973.

human malignancy to be shown to have a strong association with a type C retrovirus, in this instance designated HTLV1. As might be expected from this association, the condition tends to occur in clusters. It was first described in patients from Japan and subsequently in the Caribbean although it has now been detected in other populations. ATL is an aggressive systemic disorder characterized by widespread lymphadenopathy, bone lesions, refractory hypercalcaemia, bone marrow, peripheral blood, CNS and skin involvement.

Burkitt's lymphoma B cell lymphoblastic lymphomas are rare in the western world, but have cytological and cytogenetic similarities to a common type of lymphoma endemic in certain parts of Africa known as Burkitt's lymphoma. Both types commonly exhibit an 8:14 chromosomal translocation, but the association of the 'western' type with EB virus infection is less strong. These tumours are particularly aggressive and are amongst the fastest-growing human neoplasms. They are described more fully on page 19.183.

True histiocytic neoplasms
There has been considerable confusion over the term 'histiocytic lymphoma'. True histiocytic neoplasms are derived from cells of monocyte/macrophage lineage, but unfortunately markers for the clonal origin of macrophages are not yet available and it can be difficult to distinguish 'well-differentiated' neoplastic cells from reactive macrophages. Furthermore, the large eosinophilic cells which looked histiocytic to earlier workers and which were classified as such by Rappaport, have in most instances been shown by cell-marking techniques to be transformed B cells. It is therefore advisable to avoid the term 'histiocytic lymphoma' altogether but to use the term *malignant histiocytosis* for neoplastic malignant disorders of monocyte/macrophage (i.e. true histiocytic) origin.

Histiocytic medullary reticulosis The most striking example of malignant histiocytosis is the very rare condition sometimes called histiocytic medullary reticulosis. This is a disease of middle age characterized by a fever, a rash, hepatosplenomegaly and pancytopenia. Histiocytes in the splenic red pulp and hepatic sinusoidal cells show some erythrophagocytosis. As the disease progresses the architecture may be destroyed and tumour masses develop especially in the skin and bones.

Virus-induced haemophagocytic syndrome This condition must be carefully distinguished from a purely reactive disorder which is seen occasionally in immunosuppressed patients. This has been termed the virus-induced haemophagocytic syndrome (see also page 19.134). There is often a history of a viral-like illness during the previous few weeks and laboratory investigation may reveal evidence of EB virus or CMV infection. Despite its reactive nature this is a serious multisystem illness with a high mortality rate.

There is frequently an associated disseminated intravascular coagulation, and pancytopenia is invariable. The bone marrow shows increased numbers of histiocytes with prominent phagocytosis or red cells, platelets and nucleated cells. The histiocytes and cells are mature and morphologically normal. This contrasts with malignant histiocytosis in which the histiocytes are less mature in appearance and haemophagocytosis is less striking.

Malignant histiocytosis may present with local tumours in lymph nodes, extranodal sites and the gut. In the first two they are often fast-growing but a high cure rate may follow surgical excision. In the gut malignant histiocytic lesions may arise *de novo* presenting as one or more ulcers or with obstruction, or they may develop in association with long-standing coeliac disease.

Proliferation of cells with histiocytic features are evidence in the *histiocytosis X* group of tumours although some of these have a malignant clinical course there is no good evidence that they are neoplastic. They are described more fully on page 19.206.

Clinical features of non-Hodgkin's lymphomas
The non-Hodgkin's lymphomas, with the exception of the lymphoblastic lymphomas are all relatively uncommon under the age of 40 and have a peak incidence in the 60–70 year old age group (Fig. 7). In the commoner types the presenting features may be very similar to those of Hodgkin's disease with local or general lymph node enlargement, with or without systemic symptoms. The spread of the disease is, however, unlike that of Hodgkin's disease in that there is no clear anatomical spread from one area to the contiguous one.

Many cases cannot be distinguished clinically from Hodgkin's disease, for example, those presenting with a single group of enlarged glands, particularly in the neck or axilla. Others, however, may show involvement of nodes rarely enlarged in Hodgkin's disease, such as the epitrochlear or popliteal nodes, and involvement of pharyngeal lymphoid tissue (Waldeyer's ring) is relatively common. With the exception of T cell lymphoblastic tumours, mediastinal involvement is much less common than in Hodgkin's disease.

In contrast to Hodgkin's disease, non-Hodgkin's lymphomas frequently involve extranodal lymphoid tissue, either as the presenting feature or at a later stage of the disease. Extranodal disease is the primary site of presentation in some 20–30 per cent of patients. The organs most frequently involved are the skin, soft tissue, bone and bone marrow, and the gastrointestinal tract, particularly the stomach and small intestine. When the symptoms are those of a gastrointestinal haemorrhage or obstruction, the diagnosis may be made first at laparotomy. A possible background of coeliac disease should always be suspected in the intestinal lymphomas and the presence of clubbing of the fingers makes such an association particularly likely. In patients of Middle Eastern origin a primary gut lymphoma may be associated with alpha-chain disease (see pages 19.182 and 19.205).

Pleural effusions or ascites, not necessarily related to obstructive lesions, are sometimes a feature, particularly of the follicle centre cell tumours. In rare cases such effusions may be frankly chylous.

Occasionally patients present with CNS disease, for example with spinal cord compression or cranial nerve lesions, although this is usually found to be secondary to disease elsewhere. Other patients may develop CNS disease during the course of their illness; this is particularly common in the poor prognosis types of tumour and is seen most frequently in the lymphoblastic group. Very occasionally primary CNS lymphomas are encountered. These are usually cerebral but cerebellar or spinal cord lesions may be seen rarely. The testis is a primary site in a small proportion of cases and about 5 per cent all testicular tumours prove to be lymphomatous.

Anaemia, neutropenia, and thrombocytopenia are unusual in patients with follicle centre cell tumours but occur in a substantial proportion of patients in all other major groups. Blood changes are mainly associated with marrow involvement, but anaemia also occurs and tends to correlate with the degree of splenomegaly. Autoimmune haemolytic anaemia and thrombocytopenia may occur in some cases. Apart from the patients with lymphocytic lymphoma, leucopenia is rarely a feature. Paraproteins are found in a proportion of the B cell tumours. On the other hand, suppression of normal immunoglobulin production is common in B cell NHL, IgG being less frequently depressed than IgA or IgM. Because of these disturbances in immune function, a proportion of patients will present for the first time with infection.

Whilst skin involvement is occasionally seen in most types of NHL, primary skin lymphomas are almost always of T cell origin. The cutaneous lymphomas are described on page 19.182.

Diagnosis and investigation of non-Hodgkin's lymphomas

The diagnosis of non-Hodgkin's lymphoma depends primarily on obtaining an adequate biopsy. Histology of the lymphomas is frequently difficult to interpret and every effort should be made to obtain the maximum information from the biopsy. Much additional knowledge may be obtained about the origin of the lymphoma from immunocytochemistry which requires a specimen of fresh or frozen tissue. Biopsy samples should not, therefore, be placed in formalin or other fixative; it is usually helpful to alert the histopathologist *before* performing the biopsy to ensure prompt and correct handling. These immunohistological techniques are not yet widely available, but it should nevertheless be possible to preserve tissue by freezing and to send it to a reference centre if the diagnosis from routine histology remains in doubt. The appearances may be grossly altered by the administration of steroids, chemotherapy or radiotherapy, and all treatment should therefore be deferred if possible until after the biopsy has been taken.

Investigations should proceed along the same lines as those already described for Hodgkin's disease. A detailed history is essential, particularly in relation to the presence or absence of symptoms. A full physical examination is required including the nasopharyngeal area. The size and position of all involved nodes should be noted. A full blood count, ESR, tests of renal and liver function, uric acid, LDH (which in some cases is a useful marker of disease activity) and immunoglobulins should be estimated. Bone marrow aspirates and trephine specimens should be examined for evidence of marrow involvement.

The most useful radiological investigations are a chest radiograph and a CT scan of the chest and abdomen (Fig. 8). Other investigations will be determined by the type of presentation of the illness. As NHL is frequently widespread at presentation, staging laparotomy is less helpful than in Hodgkin's disease, and has now been largely abandoned.

Treatment of non-Hodgkin's lymphomas

Over the years there has been relatively little agreement about the optimal treatment for patients with NHL, but recent improvements in its classification, the introduction of less invasive investigations, and experience with different approaches to treatment are enabling a more rational approach to treatment to emerge, based on realistic goals. One must remember that many patients with NHL are elderly, and their expectation of life even without lymphoma may be limited. In many instances attention to the *quality* of life is at least as important as the duration of survival.

Low-grade tumours

It is now apparent that, despite their more indolent course, few patients with low-grade NHL can be cured, even with aggressive cytotoxic therapy. Exceptions are a minority with disease localized to one or two nodes who may be cured by surgical removal and/or radiotherapy. The aim of treatment in most patients with a low-grade NHL is therefore the control of symptoms and prolongation of survival rather than cure.

Some patients may not require treatment at first and can be safely watched and treated only if symptoms occur, or can be anticipated from progression of the disease. Patients with stage I or II disease may be treated with radiotherapy to involved areas, particularly if node enlargement is producing local symptoms. Radiotherapy will generally produce good local control but the majority of patients will relapse in other sites sooner or later.

A variety of chemotherapeutic schedules for low-grade NHL have been suggested. Whilst the time required to achieve a remission is usually shorter with combination chemotherapy such as COP (Table 6), randomized trials have shown that single agent therapy using cyclophosphamide or chlorambucil may achieve just as good results although taking longer to do so.

Splenectomy may sometimes be helpful, either in patients whose disease is largely confined to the spleen or where hypersplenism is a feature. It may also be useful in the occasional patient with an autoimmune haemolytic anaemia where steroids or immunosuppressive treatment has failed or produced undesirable side-effects.

High-grade tumours

In high-grade NHL (centroblastic, lymphoblastic and immunoblastic) the prognosis without treatment is extremely poor and aggressive combination chemotherapy is generally used. In contrast to low-grade NHL the early mortality of high-grade disease is high but paradoxically patients who do go into remission may have prolonged disease-free survival and may possibly be cured (Fig. 9). Lymphoblastic lymphomas are best treated in the same way as acute lymphoblastic leukaemia including CNS prophylaxis (see page 19.23). Centroblastic and immunoblastic tumours appear to do better with combination chemotherapy containing doxorubicin, for example CHOP (cyclophosphamide, hydroxydaunorubicin [Adriamycin], vincristine, [Oncovin] and prednisolone) (see Table 6).

As in other malignant haematological disorders supportive treatment in the form of blood and platelet transfusions when indicated, and prompt treatment of infections, is an important part of management. Even apparently minor infections should be treated seriously. The dangers of herpes zoster infection which may become generalized, or of infections with *Pneumocystis carinii* or *Pneumophilia legionella* should always be kept in mind.

Prognosis of non-Hodgkin's lymphomas

The prognosis of NHL is generally less good than that of Hodgkin's disease, and until recently very few patients could expect to

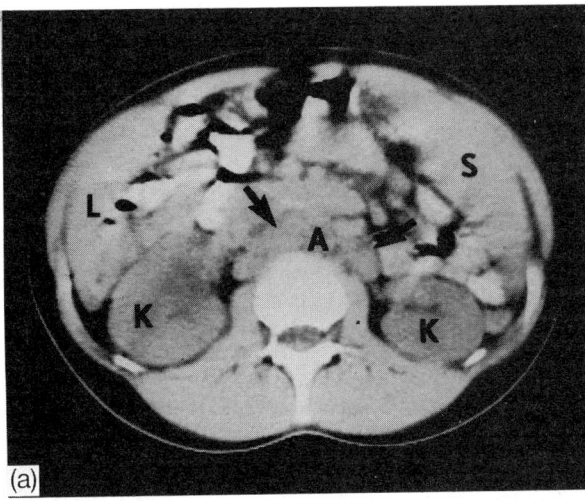

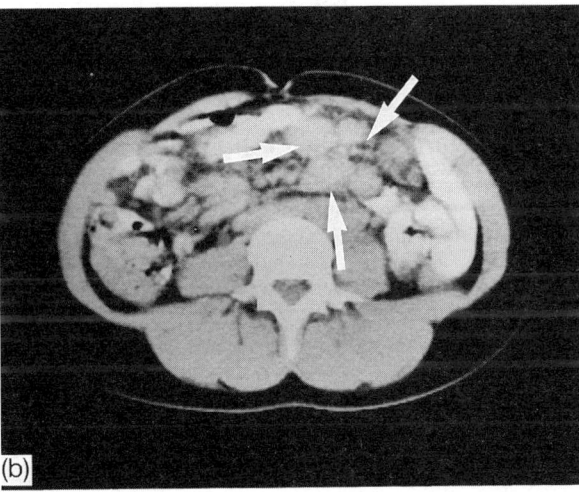

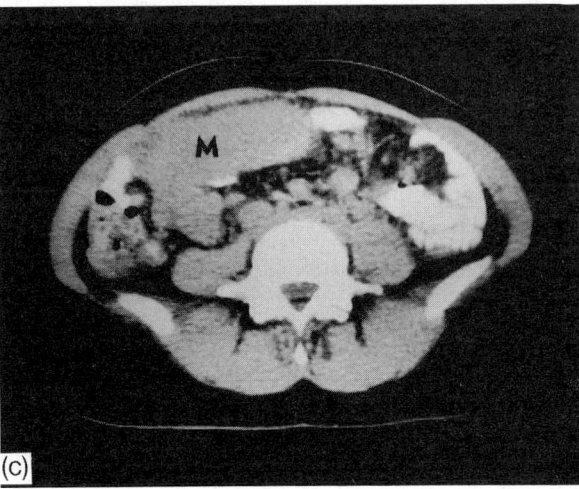

Fig. 8 The value of computed tomography in abdominal lymphoma. (a) A group of enlarged lymph nodes (arrowed) is seen surrounding the aorta (A); note the tip of an enlarged spleen (S), lying anteriorly. (L = liver; K = kidneys). (b) A few centimetres lower, a group of enlarged mesenteric nodes is seen (arrowed). (c) More inferiorly, there is a large soft-tissue mass (M) arising from the distal small bowel. Lymphangiography in this patient would have demonstrated the para-aortic lymphadenopathy, but not the disease in other areas. Reproduced by courtesy of Dr. S. Golding.

Table 6 Some chemotherapy schedules commonly used in the treatment of non-Hodgkin's lymphomas*

COP	
Cyclophosphamide	400 mg/m^2 oral for 5 days
Vincristine (Oncovin)	1.4 mg/m^2 day 1 i.v. (maximum 2 mg)
Prednisolone	100 mg/m^2 oral for 5 days

Course repeated every 3 weeks to remission or no further improvement

CHOP		
Cyclophosphamide	750 mg/m^2 i.v.	
Doxorubicin (hydroxydaunorubicin)	50 mg/m^2 i.v.	day 1
Vincristine (Oncovin)	1.4 mg/m^2 i.v.	
Prednisolone	100 mg/m^2 oral for 5 days	

Course repeated every 3–4 weeks until remission +3 courses

*With all schedules the dosage of drugs and/or frequency of treatment may need to be modified according to the blood counts. Elderly patients should generally be treated at half-dosage, at least for the first course. COP is sometimes referred to by the acronym CVP.

be cured. It must be remembered, however, that NHL represents a much more heterogeneous group of neoplasms, and this is reflected in the differing prognosis according to histological subtype, which is largely independent of the actual histological classification used (Fig. 10).

Intuitively, one might expect patients with low-grade lymphomas to have a better prognosis than those with histologically more malignant forms. This generally holds true for patients followed up for up to 5 years after diagnosis (Fig. 11), but it is now becoming clear that as in Hodgkin's disease a proportion of patients with high-grade histology may be cured with more aggressive approaches to treatment.

On the other hand, with low-grade tumours, a cure is possible for only a very small minority of patients with very localized forms of disease, even with aggressive treatment. Indeed the failure of a variety of aggressive approaches to alter the ultimate outcome in low-grade disease suggests that a much more gentle approach is appropriate for these patients especially as many are elderly.

Other factors are important in determining prognosis. Age is clearly significant: the incidence of most forms of NHL increases with age and the elderly tolerate aggressive treatment much less well. In a study of unselected patients in Oxford the most powerful prognostic factors that emerged were the histological grade and the presence or absence of systemic symptoms. These two factors were largely independent. Clinical stage I disease (all groups) carried a good prognosis but stages beyond this were of no further prognostic value. The level of haemoglobin at presentation may be of some prognostic use although the mechanism of anaemia is obscure and does not always appear to be related to marrow infiltration with tumour. Neutrophilia and changes in acute phase proteins were of weaker prognostic significance.

The major causes of death are advancing tumour which is refractory to all forms of treatment, and infection.

PRIMARY EXTRANODAL LYMPHOMAS

As discussed earlier in this chapter non-Hodgkin's lymphomas have a tendency to involve structures other than lymph nodes either by direct invasion (for example, from mediastinal node into pleura, lung or pericardium) or more remotely. Extranodal spread occurs in Hodgkin's disease, but is much less common. *Primary* extranodal presentations (without evidence of disease elsewhere) are much less common and are almost exclusively confined to the non-Hodgkin's group. A wide variety of tissues may be involved but those especially worthy of mention are the skin and gastrointestinal tract. For completeness, Burkitt's lymphoma is also described in this section.

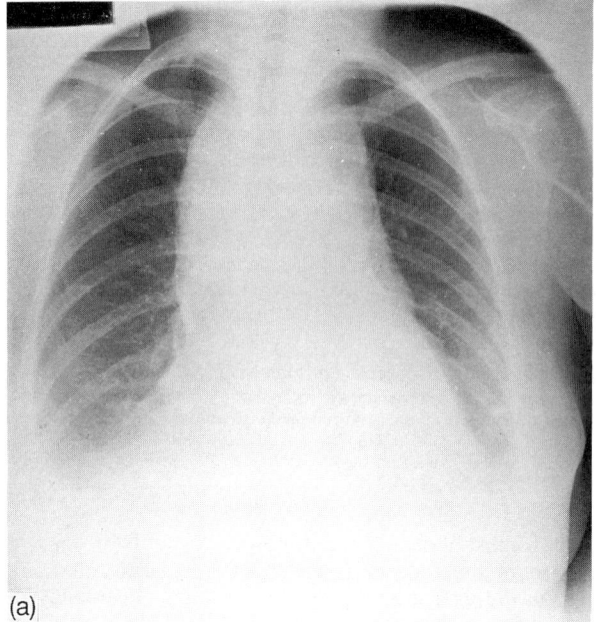

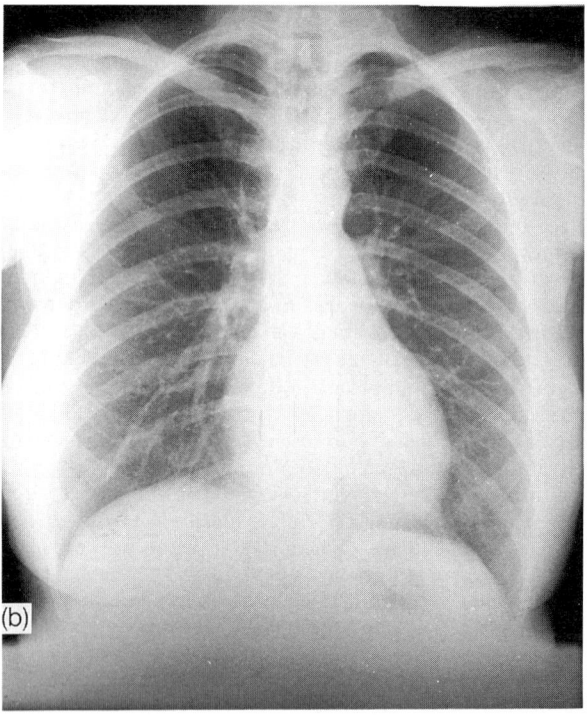

Fig. 9 JT, aged 31 at diagnosis, with malignant T-cell lymphoma associated with mediastinal obstruction, bilateral pleural effusions (which contained malignant T-cells) and involvement of the bone marrow but not of peripheral blood. Treated with aggressive chemotherapy on the lines of ALL, plus CNS prophylaxis with intrathecal methotrexate and 2 years maintenance chemotherapy. (a) chest X-ray at presentation; (b) 6 years later, when the patient remains well and in complete remission.

Primary cutaneous lymphomas

Primary lymphomas (see also Section 20) arising in the skin are almost always of T cell origin and generally show a helper T cell phenotype. High-grade (large-cell) lymphomas are rare; although of innocent and localized presentation they are difficult to treat and the relapse rate is high.

Mycosis fungoides (MF)

This is a progressive disorder which presents initially with a non-specific scaly eruption, progressing eventually to the formation of multiple skin tumours, some of which may ulcerate. The disease tends to affect middle-aged men, and may be present for 20 years or more before systemic spread follows with lymphadenopathy and visceral involvement. Death is often from unrelated causes, although internal organs may be found to be involved at autopsy.

The Sèzary syndrome (SS)

The Sèzary syndrome (which may be considered as a generalized though insidious leukaemic variant of MF) starts initially with a non-specific, eczematous or licheniform skin eruption which progresses to an intensely pruritic, generalized exfoliating erythroderma, with a particular predilection for the face, palms and soles. At this stage the condition bears a striking resemblance to acute graft-versus-host (GVH) disease. Patchy hyperpigmentation and also some degree of lymphadenopathy are common. Plaque formation resembling that of MF is often found, and the histology of the two conditions at this stage is similar. Spontaneous remissions and exacerbations do occur, but the disease is ultimately fatal with an average life expectancy of 5 years. In both mycosis fungoides and the Sèzary syndrome the malignant cell usually has a helper T cell phenotype. When chromosomal studies have been performed these have generally been abnormal, with marked aneuploidy. Occasionally marker chromosomes have been detected, confirming a clonal origin.

Primary gastrointestinal lymphomas

The gastrointestinal tract is the commonest primary 'extranodal' site for non-Hodgkin's lymphomas. These are not strictly extranodal as these tumours almost certainly arise within the abundant lymphatic tissues within the intestinal wall.

Gastric lymphoma

About 75 per cent of primary gastrointestinal lymphomas arise within the stomach, where lymphoma is responsible for about 5 per cent of all malignancies. Presenting features include pain, in 80 per cent of patients, weight loss in 40 per cent, and vomiting in 20 per cent. Overt haemorrhage occurs in about 20 per cent, but about half the patients may have occult bleeding which may lead to iron deficiency. A palpable epigastric mass is present in about one-third. The diagnosis is best made by endoscopy and biopsy. Treatment is conventionally by surgical resection followed by local radiotherapy, but the rate of occurrence outside the involved field is high and there is a strong case for considering systemic chemotherapy in these patients.

Primary small intestinal lymphoma (PSIL)

Lymphoma is the commonest neoplasm affecting the small intestine. In western countries the usual presentation is either with a solitary tumour which may cause obstruction or haemorrhage, or with more diffuse involvement associated with abdominal pain, weight loss, malabsorption, obstruction, bleeding or perforation. Such patients frequently show the histological appearances of *malignant histiocytosis of the intestine* (see page 19.179) with villous atrophy, crypt hypoplasia and a 'histiocytic' infiltrate. Indeed, this presentation occasionally complicates an existing gluten enteropathy.

A much stronger association with malabsorption is seen in the so-called *Mediterranean-type lymphoma* (see also Section 12). This was originally described in patients of Oriental, Jewish or Arabic extraction but has now been recognized in populations of low socioeconomic standards further afield. The histological pattern is one of lymphoma developing in a setting of dense plasma cell infiltration involving predominantly the lamina propria. Free alpha-chain protein can be demonstrated in the serum of a proportion of these patients (see page 19.205). It seems likely that these lymphomas arise in a setting of chronic immune stimulation within the gastrointestinal tract from repeated infections related to poor standards of hygiene.

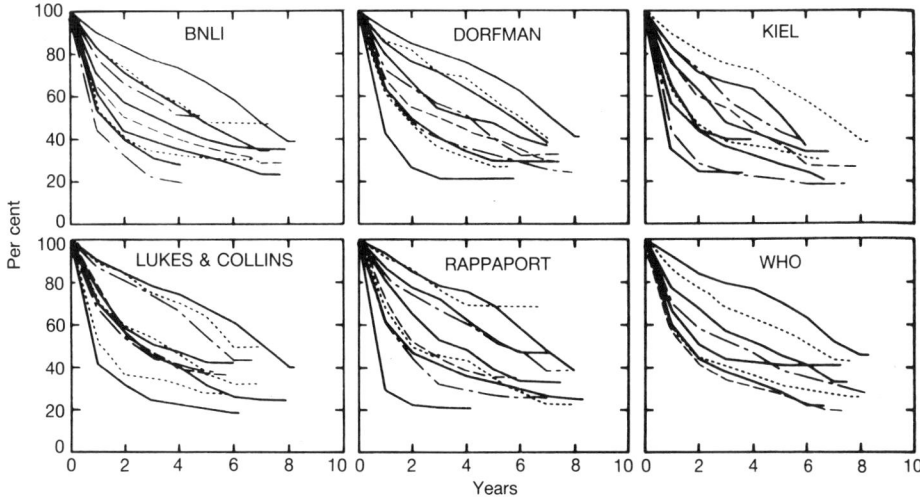

Fig. 10 Actuarial survival curves for six classifications of non-Hodgkin's lymphomas. (Reproduced with permission from The Non-Hodgkin's Lymphoma Pathologic Classification Project, 1982, *Cancer*.) Each curve represents a subtype within that particular classification (see original article for details).

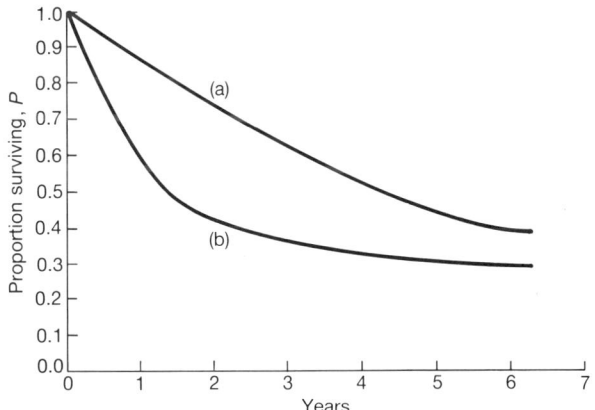

Fig. 11 Overall survival of (a) 782 patients with low-grade non-Hodgkin's lymphoma, and (b) 341 patients with high-grade non-Hodgkin's lymphoma, according to the Kiel classification adapted from Brittinger *et al.* (1984).

Burkitt's lymphoma

This very interesting lymphoma is the commonest neoplasm in children in a wide equatorial belt of Africa. It has also been recognized in New Guinea and sporadic cases have been described both in Europe and North America. The peak incidence is in the 4–7 year age group and over 80 per cent of cases occur between the ages of 3 and 12 years. The clinical picture varies somewhat with the age of the subject, the typical jaw tumours (Fig. 12) being commonest in the younger patients. These tumours arise in relation to molar or premolar teeth, leading to loosening of the teeth. They may involve the mandible or maxilla and in the latter case may extend up to involve the orbit.

Abdominal involvement is also present in the majority of cases; retroperitoneal masses, ovarian tumours, hepatic involvement, or gastrointestinal tumours being common. Involvement of the testes and breast may also occur. The masses may extend into the cranium or involve the spinal cord to give paraplegia. There may also be involvement of bones with tumour.

One of the reasons that Burkitt's lymphoma has aroused such

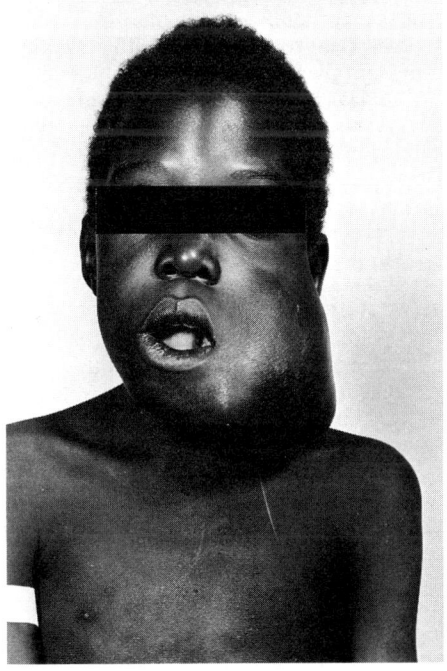

Fig. 12 Jaw tumour in a child with Burkitt's lymphoma. (Reproduced by courtesy of Professor D. H. Wright.)

interest is the close association between the tumour and high titres of antibodies against EB virus and the cellular antigens determined by it. Burkitt has drawn attention to the geographical distribution of the tumour and the importance of tumour-free gaps in tropical Africa, and has deduced that malarial infection may increase the tendency to neoplasia resulting from infection with a virus (the EB virus) which usually produces a non-malignant lymphoid proliferation. A translocation between chromosomes 8 and 14 (t[8;14][q24.13;q32.33]) is characteristic of Burkitt's lymphoma. The relationship to the presence of EB virus is not clear. It has, however, not been found in other conditions associated with the EB virus such as nasopharyngeal carcinoma. The abnormalities involving chromosome 14 have been found in relation to a variety of other lymphoma, particularly of B cell origin. Recent work describing the relationship between the chromosomal changes in this condition and the changes in cellular oncogenes is described on page 19.168 and in Section 4.

Burkitt's lymphoma is traditionally classified separately or as an undifferentiated lymphoblastic lymphoma. Some have argued that it could be regarded as a variant of follicle centre cell lymphoma. There are, however, strong arguments for separating Burkitt's lymphoma from the common follicle centre cell tumours. Burkitt's lymphomas show no evidence of cytoplasmic immunoglobulin and no follicular pattern, and lymph node and spleen involvement, which is common in follicle centre cell tumours, is relatively rare. Furthermore, the behaviour and response to therapy is quite different from that of centroblastic lymphoma in adults.

Treatment

The Burkitt tumours are extremely sensitive to chemotherapy and long-term remissions sometimes result from a single dose of cytotoxic treatment.

The prognosis is largely influenced by the extent of the disease at presentation. Tumours at a single site have an excellent prognosis, for example, early jaw tumours with no involvement elsewhere almost always regress completely. The regression is often evident even within 48 hours of starting treatment and if there is total or almost total disappearance of the mass long-term remission is likely. Partial remission, however, is usually followed by evidence of further tumour growth.

A variety of chemotherapeutic agents has been used but the alkylating agents appear to be the most effective. Cyclophosphamide, 30–40 mg/kg, given intravenously as a single injection or repeated in 10–14 days has produced a total remission of about 40 per cent and partial remission in a further 40 per cent of patients. Long-term remissions are obtained in about 21 per cent of cases including all stages. The survival curve for a series of 74 cases treated in Uganda suggested that the majority of patients remaining in complete remission for over a year could be considered as 'cured'.

Non-African (western) Burkitt's lymphoma

The rare, sporadic, non-African Burkitt's lymphoma has a broader age range extending over the first three decades, with a median age at diagnosis of about 11 years. Abdominal tumours predominate, two-thirds of the patients presenting with retroperitoneal, ileocaecal, or ovarian tumours. The jaw tumours so characteristic of the African type of Burkitt's lymphoma are seen in only about one-sixth of the cases as presenting or coexisting features. Some abnormal cells can be detected in the bone marrow or cerebrospinal fluid in a significant number of patients but diffuse infiltration is usually only seen as a preterminal event with massive extramedullary disease. The EB virus is not so clearly implicated in the genesis of the non-African cases but the characteristic chromosomal translocation is usually present.

The non-African patients may respond just as dramatically to intravenous cyclophosphamide as do the African patients, and attention has been drawn to the fact that the rapid lysis of tumour cells may give rise to biochemical complications and possible early death, for example, from hyperkalaemia. Despite an initial good response, the ultimate prognosis is extremely poor, and virtually all patients relapse within a few months. Bone marrow transplantation (allogeneic or autologous) should be considered.

Miscellaneous conditions related to lymphoma

There are several uncommon conditions in which there is progressive although often non-fatal enlargement of lymph nodes. These conditions are not necessarily malignant, but some may subsequently progress to lymphoma, and may in time produce clues as to its aetiology. A common denominator appears to be an alteration of the vascular structure of nodes through which lymphoid cells have to pass.

Angioimmunoblastic lymphadenopathy

This is a disease of older patients principally in the sixth or seventh decade, only some 10 per cent being under 40 years of age. They present with constitutional symptoms of fever, malaise, pruritis, polyarthralgia, anorexia, and weight loss. About half the patients have skin rashes which may be maculopapular, purpuric, or urticarial.

Lymphadenopathy is an almost invariable feature and it may involve both peripheral and internal lymph nodes. Hepatosplenomegaly is common, and lung involvement, arthritis, polyneuropathy, skin plaques and nodules, vasculitis, glomerulonephritis, oedema, and ascites have all been described in this condition.

An autoimmune haemolytic anaemia is often found and a leucocytosis with eosinophilia is common. The erythrocyte sedimentation rate (ESR) is usually raised, with a polyclonal hypergammaglobulinaemia.

The histological appearance of the glands is characterized by a proliferation of arborizing postcapillary venules (the epithelioid venules) in the paracortex. Initially, elements of reactive lymphoid tissue and germinal centres remain. In between the new vessels the interstitium is packed with transforming B cells (immunoblasts) which are polyclonal.

In some instances the process is related to the presence of a recognizable antigen and regresses when the stimulus is removed. In other circumstances the stimulus may be autoimmune or appear to follow infection by a variety of viruses.

In 30–50 per cent of cases the condition progresses to a malignant phase: a clone of immunoblasts, or cells so undifferentiated that they do not appear to synthesize or carry immunoglobulin, emerges and the condition changes into a high-grade, immunoblastic lymphoma with local invasion and destruction of the node.

Response to treatment is variable. Exposure to a known stimulus, for example, one which has produced an allergic drug reaction, should be avoided in future, and if the condition shows no tendency to regress spontaneously, treatment with prednisolone and possibly an immunosuppressive drug such as cyclophosphamide is indicated. Once the condition has entered the malignant phase treatment appropriate for a high-grade lymphoma may be tried, but the prognosis is poor.

Kaposi sarcoma

This condition shares a strikingly similar distribution in Africa to that of Burkitt's lymphoma and it accounts for approximately 16 per cent of all malignancies in some areas. It presents in children as a widespread lymphadenopathy. The lymph nodes are generally replaced by a sarcomatous proliferation of spindle cells which may be related to pericapillary fibroblasts although the histogenesis is not known. They form slit-like clefts containing red cells. When the process involves an organ such as the gut death may occur from massive haemorrhage.

In Europe Kaposi sarcoma is diagnosed when a much more indolent vascular spindle cell proliferation involves the skin, particularly of the extremities. Nodal and visceral involvement may supervene. It is uncertain to what extent the African childhood lymph node disease and the adult western skin tumour are identical.

Recently, a striking association between Kaposi sarcoma and the acquired immune deficiency syndrome (AIDS) has been recognized. This is described in Section 5.

Angiofollicular lymph node hyperplasia

This condition, which is also known as *giant lymph node hyperplasia* or *Castleman disease*, is held to be almost always benign. The majority present as mediastinal masses to be distinguished from thymoma, Hodgkin's disease, or a Sternberg sarcoma, but similar changes are described in cervical, retroperitoneal or mesenteric lymph nodes and much less commonly elsewhere. Approximately one in ten patients will have constitutional symptoms and signs such as sweating, fatigue, fever, a raised sedimentation rate, and possibly thrombocytopenia or anaemia.

The affected node shows 'follicles' of small lymphocytes surrounding a capillary, the wall of which shows a conspicuous concentric lamella arrangement of plump eosinophilic endothelial cells often resembling a Hassall's corpuscle in a normal thymus. Elements of normal node usually remain. Whether the process is a true benign neoplasm, possibly related to T cells, or represents a 'lymph node hamartoma' remains unsettled. It is important to recognize the condition since in the face of quite severe constitutional symptoms the clinical picture may suggest lymphoma. However, with the removal of the tumour all systemic symptoms disappear and the prognosis is universally good.

Lymphomatoid granulomatosis

This condition is characterized by a pleomorphic cellular infiltrate with atypical lymphocytoid and plasmacytoid cells, together with a granulomatous reaction. It affects adults between the third and sixth decades. The lungs are most commonly involved. Presenting features include cough, dyspnoea, pleuritic pain, fever, skin infiltrates, or neurological symptoms. A chest X-ray may show a nodular infiltrate. The diagnosis and distinction from Wegener's granulomatosis depends on biopsy.

The condition may progress towards a more florid lymphoma, usually of a high-grade variety. The disorder is responsive to combined chemotherapy with cyclophosphamide and prednisone; long remissions can be obtained.

References

Armitage, J. O., Fyfe, M. A. E. and Lewis, J. (1984). Long-term remission durability and functional status of patients treated for diffuse histiocytic lymphoma with the CHOP regimen. J. Clin. Oncol. 2, 898–902.
Berard, C. W., Greene, M. H., Jaffe, E. S., Magrath, I. and Zeigler, J. (1981). A multidisciplinary approach to non-Hodgkin's lymphomas. Ann. intern. Med. 94, 218–235.
Bergsagel, D. E., Alison, R. E., Bean, H. A., Brown, T. C., Bush, R. S., Clark, R. M., Chua, T., Dalley, D., DeBoer, G., Gospodarowicz, M., Hasselback, R., Perrault, D. and Rideout, D. F. (1982). Results of treating Hodgkin's disease without a policy of laparotomy staging. Cancer Treat. Rep. 66, 717–731.
Blattner, W. A., Kalyanaraman, V. S., Robert-Guroff, M., Lister, T. A., Galton, D. A. G., Sarin, P. S., Crawford, M. H., Catovsky, D., Greaves, M. and Gallo, R. C. (1982). The human type-C retrovirus HTLV, in blacks from the Caribbean region, and relationship to adult T-cell leukemia/lymphoma. Int. J. Cancer 30, 257–264.
Blayney, D. W., Jaffe, E. S., Blattner, W. A., Cossman, J., Robert-Guroff, M., Longo, D. L., Bunn, P. A. Jnr. and Gallo, R. C. (1983). The human T-cell leukemia/lymphoma virus associated with American adult T-cell leukemia/lymphoma. Blood 62, 401–405.
Brittinger, G., Bartels, H., Common, H., Duhmke, E., Fulle, H. H., Gunzer, U., Gyenes, T., Heinz, R., Konig, E., Meusers, P. et al. (1984). Clinical and prognostic relevance of the Kiel classification of non-Hodgkin's lymphomas results of prospective multicenter study by the Kiel lymphoma study group. Hemat. Oncol. 2, 269–306.
Burns, B. F. and Evans, W. K. (1982). Tumours of the mononuclear phagocyte system: a review of clinical and pathological features. Am. J. Hematol. 13, 171–184.
Canellos, G. P., Come, S. E. and Skarin, A. T. (1983). Chemotherapy in the treatment of Hodgkin's disease. Sem. Hemat. 20, 1–24.
Carbone, P. B., Kaplan, H. S., Musshof, K., Smithers, D. W. and Tubiana, M. (1971). Report on the committee on Hodgkin's disease staging classification. Cancer Res. 31, 1860–1861.
Catovsky, D., Linch, D. C. and Beverley, P. C. L. (1982). T cell disorders in haematological diseases. Clin. Haemat. 11, 661–695.
Chabner, B. A., Fisher, R. I., Young, R. C. and DeVita, V. T. (1980). Staging of non-Hodgkin's lymphoma. Sem. Oncol. 7, 285–291.
Coltman, C. A. (1980). Chemotherapy of advanced Hodgkin's disease. Sem. Oncol. 7, 155–173.
Dady, P. J., McElwain, T. J., Austin, D. E., Barrett, A. and Peckham, M. J. (1982). Five years' experience with ChlVPP: effective low-toxicity combination chemotherapy for Hodgkin's disease. Br. J. Cancer. 45, 851–859.
DeVita, V. T. (1981). The consequences of the chemotherapy of Hodgkin's disease: the 10th David A. Karnofsky Memorial Lecture. Cancer 47, 1–13.
——, Serpick, A. A. and Carbone, P. P. (1970). Combination chemotherapy in the treatment of advanced Hodgkin's disease. Ann. intern. Med. 73, 881–895.
Dorreen, M. S., Habeshaw, J. A., Stansfeld, A. G., Wrigley, P. F. M. and Lister, T. A. (1984). Characteristics of Sternberg-Reed, and related cells in Hodgkin's disease: an immunohistological study. Br. J. Cancer 49, 465–476.
Foon, K. A., Zighelboim, J. and Gale, R. P. (1981). Treatment of acute myelogenous leukemia in older patients. N. Engl. J. Med. 305, 1470.
Gray, G. M., Rosenberg, S. A., Cooper, A. D., Gregory, P. B., Stein, D. T. and Herzenberg, H. (1982). Lymphomas involving the gastrointestinal tract. Gastroenterology 82, 143–152.
Haghighi, P. (1983). Primary small intestinal lymphoma and immunoproliferative small intestinal disease: an update. In Malignant lymphomas (eds S. C. Sommers and P. P. Rosen), pp. 269–295. Appleton-Century-Crofts, Norvalk, Conn.
Isaacson, P. and Wright, D. H. (1978). Malignant histiocytosis of the intestine. Hum. Pathol. 9, 661–677.
Kaplan, H. S. (1980). Hodgkin's disease, 2nd edn. Harvard University Press, Cambridge, Massachusetts.
—— (1981). Hodgkin's disease: biology, treatment, prognosis. Blood 57, 813–822.
Kinzie, J. J., Hanks, G. E., Maclean, C. J. and Kramer, S. (1983). Patterns of care study: Hodgkin's disease relapse rates and adequacy of portals. Cancer 52, 2223–2226.
Lewin, K. J., Kahn, L. B. and Novis, B. H. (1976). Primary intestinal lymphoma of 'Western' and 'Mediterranean' type, alpha-chain disease and massive plasma cell infiltration: a comparative study of 37 cases. Cancer 38, 2511–2528.
Lukes, R. J. and Tindle, B. H. (1975). Immunoblastic lymphadenopathy: a hyperimmune entity resembling Hodgkin's disease. N. Engl. J. Med. 292, 1–8.
Lutzner, M., Edelson, R., Schein, P., Green, I., Kirkpatrick, C. and Ahmed. A. (1975). Cutaneous T-cell lymphomas: the Sèzary syndrome, mycosis fungoides, and related disorders. Ann. intern. Med. 83, 543–552.
McElwain, T. J. and Sloane, J. P. (1982). Malignant disorders of the lymph nodes. In Blood and its disorders 2nd edn (eds R. M. Hardisty and D. J. Weatherall), pp. 919–967. Blackwell Scientific Publications, Oxford.
McKenna, R. W., Risdall, R. J. and Brunning, R. D. (1981). Virus associated hemophagocytic syndrome. Human Pathol. 12, 395–398.
Mead, G. M., Macbeth, F. R., Williams, C. J., Ryall, R. D. H., Wright, D. H. and Whitehouse, J. M. A. (1984). Poor prognosis non-Hodgkin's lymphoma in the elderly: clinical presentation and management. Q. J. Med. 211, 381–390.
The Non-Hodgkin's Lymphoma Pathologic Classification Project (1982). National Cancer Institute sponsored study of classifications of non-Hodgkin's lymphomas. Summary and description of a working formulation for clinical usage. Cancer 49, 2112–2135.
Portlock, C. S., Rosenberg, S. A., Glatstein, E. and Kaplan, H. S. (1978). Impact of salvage treatment on initial relapses in patients with Hodgkin disease, stages I–III. Blood 51, 825–833.
Porzig, K. J., Portlock, C. S., Robertson, A. and Rosenberg, S. A. (1978). Treatment of advanced Hodgkin's disease with B-CAVe following MOPP failure. Cancer 41, 1670–1675.
Prchal, J. T., Crago, S. S., Mestecky, J., Okos, A. J. and Flint, A. (1981). Immunoblastic lymphoma: an immunologic study. Cancer 47, 2312–2318.
Robinson, B., Kingston, J., Costa, R. N., Malpas, J. S., Barrett, A. and McElwain, T. J. (1984). Chemotherapy and irradiation in childhood Hodgkin's disease. Arch. Dis. Child. 59, 1162–1167.
Rowley, J. D. and Fukuhara, S. (1980). Chromosome studies in non-Hodgkin's lymphomas. Sem. Oncol. 7, 255–266.

Safai, B. and Good, R. A. (1980). Lymphoproliferative disorders of the T-cell series. *Medicine (Balt.)* **59**, 335–351.

Santoro, A., Bonfante, V. and Bonadonna, G. (1982). Salvage chemotherapy with ABVD in MOPP-resistant Hodgkin's disease. *Ann. intern. Med.* **96**, 139–143.

Scott, G. L., Myles, A. B. and Bacon, P. A. (1968). Autoimmune haemolytic anaemia and mefenamic acid therapy. *Br. Med. J.* **3**, 534–536.

Shearer, W. T., Ritz, J., Finegold, M. J., Guerra, I. C., Rosenblatt, H. M., Lewis, D. E., Pollack, M. S., Taber, L. H., Sumaya, C. V., Grumet, F. C., Cleary, M. L., Warnke, R. and Sklar, J. (1985). Epstein-Barr virus-associated B-cell proliferations of diverse clonal origins after bone marrow transplantation in a 12-year-old patient with severe combined immunodeficiency. *N. Engl. J. Med.* **312**, 1151–1159.

Smithers, D. W. (1967) *Br. Med. J.* **2**, 263.

Stein, H., Gerdes, J., Schwab, U., Lemke, H., Mason, D. Y., Ziegler, A., Schienle, W. and Diehl, V. (1982). Identification of Hodgkin and Sternberg-Reed cells as a unique cell type derived from a newly detected small-cell population. *Int. J. Cancer* **30**, 445–459.

Stuart, A. E., Stansfeld, A. G. and Lauder, I. (eds.) (1981). *Lymphomas other than Hodgkin's disease.* Oxford University Press, Oxford.

Sutcliffe, S. B. *et al.* (1978). MVPP chemotherapy regimen for advanced Hodgkin's disease. *Br. Med. J.* **1**, 679–683.

Tester, W. J., Kinsella, T. J., Waller, B., Makuch, R. W., Kelley, P. A., Glatstein, E. and DeVita, V. T. (1984). Second malignant neoplasms complicating Hodgkin's disease: the National Cancer Institute Experience. *J. Clin. Oncol.* **2**, 762–768.

Watanabe, S., Shimosato, Y. and Nakajima, T. (1983). Proliferative disorders of histiocytes. In *Malignant lymphomas* (eds S. C. Sommers and P. P. Rosen), pp. 65–108. Appleton-Century-Crofts, Norwalk, Conn.

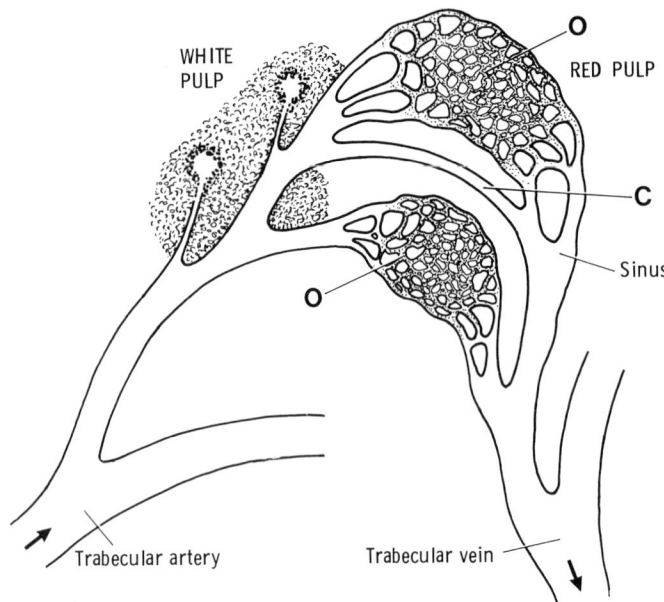

Fig. 1 Diagramatic illustration of the circulation of the spleen. The blood passes either directly into a sinus (C, closed system) or first into the cord spaces in the red pulp (O, open system).

Disorders of the spleen

S.M. LEWIS

Since Hippocratic times the role of the spleen has been controversial. Galen called it an organ of mystery; the elucidation of the mystery has been a long slow process! Its structure was described during the seventeenth and early eighteenth centuries by Harvey, Glisson, Wharton, Malpighi, and van Leeuwenhoek. In 1777, William Hewson recognized an association with the lymphatic system, and in 1846 Virchow demonstrated that the Malpighian follicles are concerned with the formation of white blood cells. In 1885, Ponfick showed that the spleen can remove particles from the blood and might be involved in its destruction. Two years later Spencer Wells performed a laparotomy on a 27-year-old woman with a lifelong history of the passage of dark urine with attacks of jaundice and who had an abdominal tumour which was thought to be a fibroid. This turned out to be a large spleen and its removal was followed by a complete remission. The retrospective diagnosis of hereditary spherocytosis was made by Lord Dawson of Penn some 40 years later, by which time splenectomy was being performed quite frequently for leukaemia, Hodgkin's disease, Banti's haemolytic jaundice, Gaucher's disease, polycythaemia, and thrombocytopenic purpura. The frequent success of the operation led Doan and Dameshek and their respective supporters to engage in a lively argument on the mechanisms whereby the spleen can destroy blood cells or suppress their formation, a process which Chauffard had earlier called 'hypersplenism'.

The past two decades have seen the resolution of many of these problems and there is now a much greater understanding of the functions of the spleen in health and its involvement in disease. Methods have been developed by which the various functions of the spleen can be defined and measured. Some of them have important clinical applications.

Structure of the spleen

At birth the spleen is about 4.5 cm in length, 2.5 cm wide, and 1.5 cm thick, and the mean weight is 11 g. By the age of one year the weight is 15–25 g; by five years it is 40–70 g, and by 10 years it

is 80–100 g. It reaches its maximum weight of about 200–300 g soon after puberty, and is slightly lighter throughout adult life until the age of 65 years when it decreases to 100–150 g or less. It is slightly heavier in the adult male than in the female. These figures have been derived from autopsy studies; they are probably underestimates. This is mainly due to the splenic red cell pool which will be described later. Ultrasound, computerized tomography, and scintigraphic radionuclide scans have shown that, *in vivo*, the normal adult spleen has a length of 8–13 cm, a width of 4.5–7 cm, a surface area of the order of 45–80 cm^2, and a volume less than 275 cm^3. A spleen greater than 14 cm long is usually palpable. It should be noted, however, that the spleen is mobile and palpation does not always provide a reliable guide to its size. Plain X-rays, too, are often unreliable for delineating the spleen.

The spleen has a complicated structure (Fig. 1). It consists of a connective tissue framework, vascular channels, lymphatic tissue, lymph drainage channels, and cellular components of the haemopoietic and reticulo-endothelial (RE) systems. Histologically, there are two main components: (*a*) the red pulp; and (*b*) the white pulp. The red pulp consists of sinuses and pulp cords. The sinuses, 20–40 μm in diameter, are lined by endothelial macrophages. The white pulp consists of peri-arteriolar lymphoid sheath and the adjoining follicles (Malpighian bodies) which contain a germinal centre and are structurally similar to lymphoid follicles. The outer capsule of the connective tissue framework consists of collagen tissue with elastic fibres covered by serous endothelium. From this come off a large number of lace-like trabeculae which extend into the pulp, carrying blood vessels, and autonomic nerve fibres. Within the spleen the trabeculae are in direct continuity with a mesh of reticular fibres which supports the pulp vessels, and which forms the basement membranes of arterial capillaries and the splenic sinuses. Along the reticular fibres lie adventitial reticular cells. These cells have an important role in regulating blood flow through the interendothelial slits of the vascular sinuses.

Blood is brought to the spleen via the splenic artery and thence, through the trabecular arteries, into the central arteries which are sited in the white pulp. The latter vessels run into the central axis of the peri-arteriolar lymphatic sheaths; they give off many arterioles and capillaries, some of which terminate in the white pulp whilst others go on to the red pulp. There they either connect directly with the sinuses and thence, via the collecting vein, to the trabecular vein (closed system), or they first pass into the cord spaces before joining up with the sinuses (open system).

Thus, as the blood flows through the spleen it will come into contact with the reticular fibres, and also with endothelial macrophages which lie in the interstices of the reticular mesh.

Blood flow in the spleen

Because the spleen has two vascular systems (closed and open) as described above, there are both rapid and slow transit components in the splenic circulation. The rapid transit (closed system) is of the order of 1–2 min and slow transit (open system) about 30–60 min. In normal subjects the open system has a minor role and the blood flows through the spleen as rapidly as through organs possessing a conventional vasculature, at a rate of 5–10 per cent of the blood volume per minute, so that each day the circulating blood has repeated passages through the spleen. In splenomegaly, the blood flow through the spleen increases up to 20 per cent or more of the blood volume per minute. At the same time, a certain proportion of the blood may be pooled in the cord spaces (see below). During the flow of the blood, the plasma and the leucocytes pass preferentially to the white pulp by a process of plasma skimming, and the plasma rapidly reaches the venous system, whilst blood with a relatively high-packed cell volume remains in the axial stream of the central artery. Some of the latter flows directly through the sinusoids to the venous system, while the remainder passes into the cords of the red pulp; the normally flexible red cells squeeze through endothelial slits into the sinuses whilst cells with fixed membranes or with inclusions which render them relatively inflexible remain in the cords where they either become conditioned for later transit or are destroyed.

Functions of the spleen

In this section the physiological functions of the spleen will be described together with the way in which these are changed in various pathological conditions.

Haematopoiesis

In the fetus the spleen plays a relatively minor role in haematopoiesis in comparison with the liver. There is, however, some erythropoiesis and granulopoiesis in the spleen from the 12th week; this continues until birth, after which there is normally no demonstrable haemopoiesis. However, the potential remains, and under severe haematological stress, e.g. in thalassaemia and in chronic haemolytic anaemias, extramedullary erythropoiesis may occur together with intensive erythroid hyperplasia of the bone marrow, presumably as a compensatory mechanism. This must be distinguished from myeloid metaplasia occurring in myelofibrosis (page 19.40) and occasionally in patients with leukaemia or secondary carcinoma. In these conditions foci of haemopoietic tissue become established in the spleen and elsewhere outside the bone marrow. They represent an abnormal proliferation which is distinct from compensatory erythropoiesis.

The spleen contains a large bulk of lymphoid tissue. It is not a major site of lymphopoiesis; most of the lymphocytes in the white pulp of the spleen migrate there from other sites of origin such as the bone marrow and thymus. However, the germinal centres of the spleen may respond to antigenic stimulus by proliferation of lymphocytes.

Experimental studies have demonstrated that there are as many multipotential haemopoietic stem cells (CFU-S) and erythroid progenitors (BFU-E) in the spleen as in the marrow. It is not clear whether the stem cells in the spleen and the marrow are identical and whether there is a direct line of development from splenic CFU-S to erythroid cells in the spleen; undoubtedly, normal haemopoietic development requires the cellular environment of the marrow. Splenic irradiation is known to cause leucopenia far more readily than a similar dose to other organs; it has been suggested that this is due to destruction of colony forming cells, precursors of myelopoiesis, which are present in the spleen. This provides a rationale for splenic irradiation in treating myeloproliferative diseases.

Humoral control of haemopoiesis

It has been suggested that the spleen elaborates humoral factors which control haemopoiesis, either by suppression or stimulation, as appropriate. The evidence is not convincing, although in some experimental studies the spleen has been shown to be a site of limited production or storage of erythropoietin.

Cell sequestration, phagocytosis, and pooling

The spleen has a remarkable ability to 'cleanse' or 'recondition' red cells for recirculation and also to remove from the circulation effete or damaged cells as well as foreign matter. Unfortunately, as the case is with so many physiological phenomena, these useful functions may become harmful under certain circumstances. It is important to distinguish between the three mechanisms which are involved: *sequestration* is a temporary (reversible) process whereby cells are held in the spleen before returning to the circulation; *phagocytosis* represents the irreversible uptake of nonviable cells by macrophages or destruction of viable cells which have been damaged in some way, perhaps by prolonged sequestration or by deposition of antibody on the cell surface; *pooling* is the presence in the spleen of an increased amount of blood (or some of its component parts). In contrast to sequestration, pooled cells are in continuous exchange with the circulation.

As blood flows through the sinuses and cords, effete and damaged cells, and particulate foreign matter are promptly phagocytosed by the endothelial macrophages. Intact cells are held up temporarily, during which time siderotic granules, Howell-Jolly bodies, and Heinz bodies are removed by 'pitting'. In this process the particles are taken out with a small amount of cell membrane but without destroying the cell. After the inclusions have been removed the red cells return to the circulation. Sequestration of reticulocytes also occurs, and they are retained in the splenic cords for part of their last two or three days of maturation while they lose their intracellular inclusions, alter their surface membrane composition, and become smaller. The spleen normally sequesters 30–45 per cent of the total circulating platelet content of the blood. This platelet pool is rapidly mobilizable under conditions of stress, and normally there is a constant transit between spleen and vascular pools.

As the blood becomes more viscous in the spleen, red cells are subjected to a further hazard. Because they are packed together in the presence of metabolically active macrophages, they are deprived of oxygen and glucose. This increases their membrane rigidity and reduces their deformability. Cells may become inflexible if: (*a*) they are metabolically abnormal (as in certain congenital haemolytic anaemias) and thus unduly sensitive to the unfavourable environment of the spleen; (*b*) if they are held up in the spleen for a prolonged period and are thus rendered metabolically abnormal; and (*c*) if they are already spherical (as in hereditary spherocytosis), fragmented (as in microangiopathic haemolytic anaemia), or misshapen in some other way (see page 19.134). This results in their being trapped in the cord spaces where they subsequently undergo phagocytosis. This is the process by which heat-damaged or chemically altered cells are taken up in the spleen. Cells which have been sequestered and damaged may also end their lives in this way. Identifying the role of the spleen in cell destruction is an important aspect of the management of patients with haemolytic anaemia.

Immunological function

The spleen contains the largest single accumulation of lymphoid tissue in the body; about 25 per cent of the total T lymphocyte pool and 10–15 per cent of the B lymphocyte pool. Micro-organisms or other antigens that find their way to the spleen are taken up by the cord macrophages and are delivered to immunocompetent cells in the lymphoid tissue. This stimulates antibody production and an increase in the size of lymphoid germinal centres of the spleen. Secondary stimulation with the antigen enhances antibody production, usually IgG. Red cells sensitized by IgG antibody do not, as a rule, agglutinate in the peripheral blood, but the environment in the spleen promotes local agglutination with consequent sequestration and destruction. At the same time the antibody-coated cells lose pieces of their membrane as they come in contact with Fc receptors on macrophages, and become spherical and less flexible each time they pass through the sinus vasculature, until finally they become too rigid to traverse the endothelial pores and thus are trapped, as described above. The rate of cell destruction in the spleen is influenced in opposite ways by two factors. On the one hand, increased cell destruction results in an expanding number of mononuclear macrophages in the splenic cords and hence in increased lysis. On the other hand, the damaged red cell load tends to blockade the reticulo-endothelial (RE) cells and thus reduce their phagocytic potential, at least temporarily.

Blood pool

The normal red cell content of the spleen is less than about 100 ml or 8 per cent of the total red cell mass and there is no significant red cell pool. However, enlarged spleens are capable of developing remarkably large pools with a relatively slow exchange of red cells with the general circulation. In the myeloproliferative disorders, as much as 40 per cent of the blood volume, representing a litre of blood, may be present in the spleen. Increased pools also occur in lymphoproliferative disorders, especially hairy cell leukaemia and prolymphocytic leukaemia.

In health there is a good correlation between the amount of blood in the spleen and its size. In myeloproliferative disorders the pool is disproportionately large and is a major cause of splenomegaly. In lymphomas, however, the splenomegaly is sometimes greater than can be accounted for by the pool alone, possibly because in such cases the increase in spleen size is due primarily to an expansion of the lymphoid components with replacement of splenic sinuses by tumour. In myelofibrosis, on the other hand, there is an increase of the reticular element with expansion of the closed system in the red pulp. A similar effect occurs in hairy cell leukaemia (see page 19.35).

Not unexpectedly, the red cell content of the spleen increases with increasing body haematocrit. There is a disproportionately increased pool in polycythaemia vera compared with secondary polycythaemia, where the pool remains small irrespective of the haematocrit level. This suggests that in polycythaemia vera there is a fundamental structural alteration in the spleen with an expansion of the closed system. Increased pools are also found in patients with hepatic cirrhosis. Here it is the increased portal pressure which leads to an increased splenic blood flow: the splenic arteries are dilated and the splenic pulp becomes expanded with prominent dilated sinuses. Conversely, it has been observed that portal hypertension is not uncommon as a secondary event in myeloproliferative disorders with splenomegaly (see page 19.43).

In myeloproliferative disorders and some other conditions an enlarged splenic blood pool may contribute significantly to the anaemia, so that direct measurement of splenic red cell volume makes it possible to predict the extent to which splenectomy will result in improvement in the anaemia and in reducing transfusion requirements.

Platelets also have a significant reservoir in the spleen, which is rapidly interchangeable with the circulation. In some cases of thrombocytopenia destruction occurs mainly in the spleen and it is essential to distinguish this from pooling. As far as granulocytes are concerned, no pool is demonstrable in the normal spleen but an abnormally large marginal pool has been found in cases of splenomegaly associated with neutropenia.

Table 1 Some characteristics of an enlarged spleen

Moves downward and medially on inspiration
Dull to percussion
A notch may be palpable on medial margin
Does not push through from left loin (cf. left kidney)
Is difficult to insert fingers above mass under left costal margin (cf. left kidney)

Plasma volume control

The mechanism by which plasma volume is controlled is not clear. There is a complex neurohumoral mechanism which controls the fluid equilibrium between interstitial and intracellular compartments, ensuring that the water volume and electrolyte concentration in the circulating blood are both kept within normal limits. Under normal conditions, the red cell volume is fairly constant while the plasma volume undergoes continual transient variations which trigger off the necessary adjustments which ensure that the total blood volume remains constant. There is no evidence that the spleen is involved in this mechanism. However, when the spleen is enlarged, it does play a role, and splenomegaly is frequently associated with an increased plasma volume which may lead to an apparent anaemia (so-called pseudo-anaemia or dilutional anaemia). Several possible mechanisms have been suggested to explain the expanded plasma volume in splenomegaly: (a) the enlarged organ requires an expansion of blood volume to fill the additional intravascular space; in conditions where marrow erythropoietic activity is reduced, as in myelosclerosis, it may not be possible to maintain the normal red-cell/plasma volume ratio and the additional volume is provided by plasma alone; (b) increased pressure in the portal vein and an increase in splanchnic blood volume resulting from obstructive or hyperkinetic portal hypertension; and (c) protein alterations, especially increased globulin levels with reduced albumin, resulting in an alteration in colloid oncotic pressure.

The last mechanism has been suggested as a factor in tropical splenomegalies and in cirrhosis. In blood dyscrasias, the increase in plasma volume is directly proportional to the size of the spleen; this is not so in cirrhosis.

Splenomegaly

A palpable spleen is usually enlarged. Occasionally a normal spleen is palpable if it is displaced downwards, by a pleural effusion for example. Useful information may be obtained from assessing the size of the spleen together with any related clinical and haematological findings, but a firm diagnosis often requires special investigations of splenic function and, occasionally, diagnostic laparotomy and splenectomy.

Clinical detection of splenomegaly (see also page 19.2)

As the spleen enlarges it moves forwards, downwards, and medially towards the right iliac fossa. The features which suggest that a left-sided mass is a spleen are summarized in Table 1.

The spleen has to be 1.5–2 times its normal size to be palpable; Imaging procedures provide more reliable methods for measuring the actual spleen size. These include radionuclide scans, ultrasonic scans, X-ray computerized tomography, and nuclear magnetic resonance. In clinical practice the usual method for expressing the extent of splenomegaly is in centimetres below the left costal margin. The differential diagnosis of a mass in the left hypochondrium is summarized in Table 2.

Causes of splenomegaly

So many conditions are associated with splenomegaly that it is impossible to give a comprehensive list. It is even more difficult to list the 'common' causes as these depend on geographical pathology; thus, in western Europe and the United States viral infection and portal hypertension are the commonest causes of spleno-

Table 2 Differential diagnosis of swellings in left upper quadrant of the abdomen

---

Spleen
Left kidney
Tumours of splenic flexure of colon
Masses arising from the stomach
Retroperitoneal masses

---

megaly and these together with leukaemias, malignant lymphomas, myeloproliferative disorders, haemolytic anaemias, and other infections account for most cases. Globally, however, the incidence of these haematological causes of splenomegaly is swamped by the great preponderance of splenic enlargement caused by the parasitic infections, particularly malaria, leishmaniasis, and schistosomiasis. In some countries haemoglobinopathies head the list. Portal hypertension is an important cause of splenomegaly in most tropical countries but it is especially prevalent in north-eastern India and southern China. The 'tropical splenomegaly syndrome' is seen commonly in New Guinea and central Africa.

Some of the causes of splenomegaly are listed in Table 3 which also gives some indication of the relative size of the spleen in various conditions. The spleen sizes indicated are only a rough guide; clearly, where the spleen is markedly enlarged, it may have been only just palpable at an earlier stage of the disease. Most of the conditions listed are described in other sections of the book. Those in which splenomegaly is the primary or an especially important feature are described below.

Hypersplenism

Hypersplenism is a clinical syndrome of varied aetiology. It is characterized by:

1. Splenomegaly, although this may be only moderate.
2. Pancytopenia or a reduction in the number of one or more types of the blood cells: neutropenia is less common than anaemia and thrombocytopenia.
3. Normal production or hyperplasia of the precursor cells in the marrow or a so-called maturation arrest with paucity of the more mature cells but orderly maturation in the earlier stages. Some of the megakaryocytes show unusual features of sharply demarcated cytoplasmic borders and no granularity or signs of platelet formation.
4. Premature release of cells into peripheral blood, resulting in a mild reticulocytosis with nucleated red cells and occasional immature granulocytes.

Other features are:

5. Decreased red cell survival.
6. Decreased platelet survival.
7. Hypervolaemia (i.e. increased plasma volume) if splenomegaly is marked.

The mechanisms which produce the various parts of the syndrome were considered earlier.

The haematological features may be obscured or dominated by the primary disease, especially if it involves the marrow. The diagnosis of hypersplenism is ultimately confirmed by response to splenectomy, although an immediate remission may be followed in the longer term by relapse with return of cytopenia.

Tropical splenomegaly syndrome (big spleen disease)

In areas where malaria is endemic, adults may present with moderate to massive splenomegaly, no obvious signs of active malaria, but all the features of hypersplenism including pancytopenia, expanded plasma volume, and haemolysis. It is apparently secondary to malaria, the evidence being its geographical incidence, the presence of raised titres of malaria antibody and the fact that, on continuous long-term antimalaria therapy, there is a marked and sustained reduction in spleen size, the pancytopenia remits, and the patient improves. The serum IgM level is usually high, and this decreases to normal concomitantly with response to antimalarial therapy. The spleen shows diffuse reticulo-endothelial hyperplasia. These features suggest that the pathogenesis is an intense immunological response to circulating antigens with immune complex formation and phagocytosis as a result of repeated exposure to the malarial parasite. It is not clear why this effect is only seen in a proportion of individuals in areas of the world where malaria is endemic (see above).

A similar degree of splenomegaly occurs in schistosomiasis (see Section 5) but in this condition there is the further complication that the eggs (especially *Schistosoma mansoni*) have a direct effect on the liver, resulting in hepatic fibrosis, and leading to portal hypertension.

Non-tropical idiopathic splenomegaly

A number of patients present with marked splenomegaly and the haematological features of hypersplenism, but without exposure to malaria or other parasitic disorders. There may be a positive antiglobulin test and other evidence of autoantibody production. Some of these patients have a malignant lymphoma at the time of presentation but in others the essential feature is non-neoplastic lymphoid hyperplasia which probably represents an immunological reaction to as yet unidentified stimuli. The chances of long-term cure after splenectomy appear to be good. However, a lymphoma may appear at periods ranging from months to years after splenectomy in this condition. The disorder is diagnosed by the finding of massive splenomegaly in the absence of any other cause and by the non-specific histological appearances of the spleen.

Storage diseases

Storage diseases (see Section 9) comprise a group of conditions in which the lysosomes of the reticulo-endothelial (RE) cells become grossly overloaded with undegraded metabolites because of a genetically determined deficiency of one or other of the lysosomal enzymes. There are some 30 enzymes active against protein, carbohydrates, and lipids, respectively. The spleen, together with bone marrow and liver, has a high content of RE cells which are involved in this process. Depending on the composition of the accumulated material, the storage diseases have been classified as lipidoses, mucopolysaccharides, etc. The main clinical features are described elsewhere (see Section 9); here the haematological aspects are summarized briefly.

Gaucher's disease

Irrespective of age, common presenting features of Gaucher's disease are splenomegaly, hepatosplenomegaly, and bone destruction. In the infantile form neurological signs may predominate. In the juvenile form the nervous system is involved only occasionally and the dominant features are gross splenomegaly and hepatomegaly. In the adult form splenomegaly may not be detected until the second decade or later. The first symptom is often bleeding due to thrombocytopenia, or infection from neutropenia.

Anaemia, thrombocytopenia, and neutropenia are frequent and the serum acid phosphatase level is markedly elevated. The bone marrow (and the spleen) contain numerous Gaucher cells. These are large (20–80 μm) cells with a small eccentric nucleus and a coarsely clumped cytoplasm filled with pale staining foamy lipid. They are refractile under polarized light, PAS, and acid phosphatase positive; Sudan black and oil red O negative. On electron microscopy they have a characteristic appearance of twisted bilayered rods. It should be remembered that Gaucher-like cells are also found, albeit in small numbers, if normally functioning lysosomes are faced with excessive cell destruction, e.g. in chronic

Table 3 Some causes of enlargement of the spleen

Acute bacterial, viral, and other infections	Chronic lymphatic leukaemia
Chronic bacterial infections: TB and brucellosis	Leukaemic reticulo-endotheliosis*
Chronic parasitic infections: malaria, kala azar, schistosomiasis*	Polycythaemia vera
Idiopathic non-tropical splenomegaly*	Myelosclerosis*
Tropical splenomegaly*	Megaloblastic anaemia
'Congestive'; portal and biliary cirrhosis; portal vein obstruction; splenic vein obstruction; Budd-Chiari syndrome; cardiac failure	
	Reticulosis
	Hodgkin's disease
Congenital haemolytic anaemia	Other reticuloses
Hereditary spherocytosis (HS)	
Symptomatic elliptocytosis	Miscellaneous
Structural haemoglobinopathy	Amyloid, sarcoidosis, tumour of the spleen
Thalassaemia	
Red cell enzyme defects	Connective tissue disorders
	Systemic lupus erythematosus
Acquired haemolytic anaemia	Felty's syndrome
Warm antibody haemolytic anaemia	
Cryopathic haemolytic syndrome	Storage diseases
	Gaucher's disease*
Primary blood dyscrasia	Niemann-Pick disease
Acute leukaemia	Histiocytosis X*
Chronic myeloid leukaemia*	

*May be associated with massive splenomegaly.

granulocytic leukaemia, congenital dyserythropoietic anaemias, and thalassaemia.

Niemann–Pick disease

The clinical picture of Niemann–Pick disease (see Section 9) is dominated by hepatosplenomegaly and mental retardation. The disorder presents in infancy, and death often occurs between the second and third years of age, but, as with Gaucher's disease, it may present later in life. In the older age groups hypersplenism becomes a feature, but in the childhood cases, anaemia and thrombocytopenia are uncommon and, if present, are mild. In contrast to Gaucher's disease, the serum acid phosphatase level is normal. The diagnosis depends on finding the characteristic Niemann-Pick cells in the bone marrow. These are 20–80 μm in size. The cytoplasm is engorged with globular droplets of sphingomyelin. The cells stain blue-green by Romanowsky stain and greenish yellow with haematoxylin and eosin. The PAS stain is variably positive, oil red O and Sudan black B are, as a rule, positive, and acid phosphatase is negative.

Other lipid storage diseases

Several other rare lipid storage diseases may cause hypersplenism. They include *Tangier's disease* in which cholesterol esters fill the histiocytes, and *Wolman's disease* which is associated with an accumulation of triglycerides and cholesterol esters. *Sea-blue histiocytosis* is characterized by splenomegaly, hepatomegaly, thrombocytopenia, and, occasionally, neurological damage. The bone marrow and spleen contain cells which have an accumulation of glycosphingolipids, phospholipids, and mucopolysaccharides. The cells stain blue-green by Romanowsky stain, but in contrast to those in Niemann-Pick's disease they stain brownish yellow with haematoxylin and eosin. It is not clear whether this is a specific disorder. Similar cells occur in a wide variety of conditions in which there is excessive breakdown of leucocytes, platelets, and red cells. However, in these disorders there are usually only a few of the abnormal cells in the marrow.

Inborn errors of lipid mechanism give rise to a variety of disorders in which there may be secondary proliferation of histiocytic cells. These include *Hand–Schüller–Christian disease, eosinophilic granuloma,* and *Letterer-Siewe disease* now usually referred to as *histiocytosis x.* The proliferaton of histiocytes is especially active in the spleen, lymph-nodes, and bone marrow. Splenomegaly is usually moderate, but occasionally it is more marked and may be associated with hypersplenism (see page 19.206).

Space-occupying lesions and injury of the spleen

The commonest cause of splenic masses are: trauma leading to haematoma or rupture, abscesses, tumours, and cysts.

Splenic injury

The spleen is relatively unprotected and easily injured. Spontaneous rupture has been reported in a number of conditions in which the spleen is enlarged: these include typhoid, malaria, leukaemia, Gaucher's disease, and polycythaemia. This may be restricted to a subcapsular haematoma or there may be rupture into the peritoneal cavity.

The diagnosis is suggested by the symptoms of shock, left upper quadrant guarding and tenderness, pain referred to the left shoulder, and clinical and laboratory evidence of bleeding. Straight abdominal X-ray is not, as a rule, helpful in diagnosis but X-ray computerized tomographic (CT) scanning, splenic arteriography, ultrasound examination, or isotope scanning may be more useful.

Abscess

Although the spleen is frequently enlarged in association with systemic infection, splenic abscesses are rare. They result from direct or haematogenous spread, or when a haematoma becomes infected. Conditions associated with splenic infarction such as sickle cell disease, are particularly likely to give rise to splenic abscesses. Almost any organism can be involved.

Metastatic tumour

Metastases in the spleen are uncommon by comparison to other organs; they occur late in the course of primary carcinoma and are not found in the absence of metastases elsewhere. Metastases in the spleen are most frequently derived from malignant lymphomas, especially Hodgkin's disease, and reticulum cell sarcoma. Lung, breast, prostate, colon, and stomach are the organs from which carcinoma is most likely to disseminate to the spleen. Melanoma is also a relatively frequent primary source.

Cysts

Splenic cysts are rare. The most frequent is due to *Taenia echinococcus* (hydatid); other causes include haemangiomas, lymphangiomas, and dermoids. Cysts may also develop in area of haemorrhage or infarction. A splenic scan is a particularly useful method for identifying a cyst and recognizing it as the cause of apparent splenomegaly (Fig. 2).

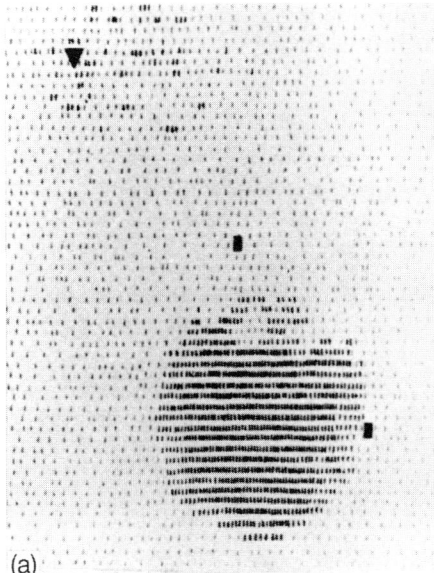

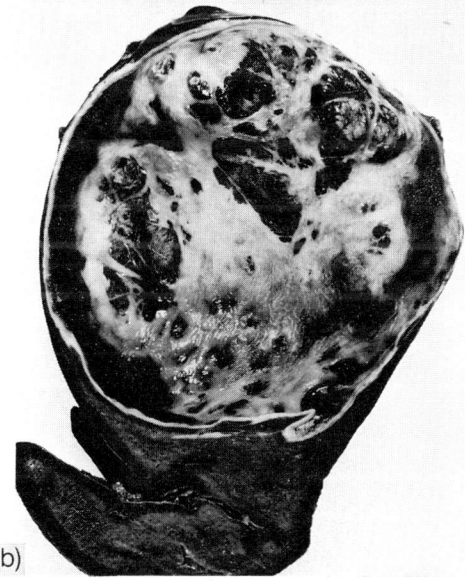

Fig. 2 Spleen scan (with radionuclide-labelled heat damaged cells) from a boy who presented with splenomegaly. (*a*) The scan showed uptake of the label predominantly in the area below the costal margin. (*b*) At laparotomy the upper two-thirds of the spleen was found to be occupied by a large splenic cyst. (Illustration by courtesy of Dr. J. Pettit: reproduced by permission of *Clinics Haemat.* **6**, 640, 1977).

Loss of spleen function and splenic infarction

Splenic hypoplasia or atrophy

Congenital hypoplasia is rare; in some cases it is associated with extensive developmental abnormalities of the heart and gut. *Splenic atrophy* may occur in a number of acquired conditions – sickle cell disease, coeliac disease, dermatitis herpetiformis, ulcerative colitis, Crohn's disease, essential thrombocythaemia, and Fanconi's anaemia. Steroid therapy and cytotoxic drugs cause atrophy of the white pulp, especially the germinal centres. The spleen shrinks in size in old age. Vascular blockade and infarction is the basis for splenic atrophy in sickle cell disease (see page 19.122) and this may also be the case in thrombocythaemia (see page 19.44). The mechanism of splenic atrophy in coeliac disease is not known. On histological examination, the spleen is seen to be encapsulated by thick fibrous tissue. The atrophy does not reverse even if the patient responds satisfactorily to a gluten-free diet. It is not related to the abnormality of jejunal mucosa.

Splenic atrophy is characterized by changes in the blood film appearances; the main features are the presence of Howell-Jolly bodies and siderotic granules in some of the red cells. This is due to loss of the spleen's pitting function. Depression of sequestering activity, which usually occurs at the same time, can be identified by a scan after administration of isotope-labelled damaged red cells, combined with the measurement of the rate of clearance of the cells from circulation (see below). Pitting and phagocytosis are, however, separate functions and there may be dissociation of these activities in an individual patient.

Splenic infarction

Splenic infarction occurs quite frequently in patients who have very large spleens. It is particularly common in association with myelosclerosis and chronic myeloid leukaemia. It also occurs in the majority of patients with sickle cell anaemia. In this disorder splenic infarction occurs early in life and repeated episodes result in an autosplenectomy (see page 19.122). Occasionally, when there is the rapid growth of the spleen in association with an aggressive form of non-Hodgkin's lymphoma, particularly histiocytic medullary reticulosis, there may be multiple infarctions and spontaneous rupture of the spleen with the signs mentioned in an earlier section.

Splenic infarction causes pain in the left upper quadrant. If the diaphragmatic surface of the spleen is involved, the pain may be referred to the left shoulder tip. The physical signs include tenderness over the spleen, and sometimes a loud splenic rub is heard. Treatment is by rest and analgesia. The occurrence of repeated splenic infarction may be an indication for splenectomy although it should be remembered that the history of episodes of this type usually indicates that there will be multiple adhesions between the spleen and the overlying peritoneum.

Investigation of splenic function

Assessment of splenic function is often required in investigating a haematological disorder, particularly if splenectomy is contemplated. In many conditions it is sufficient to assess the spleen size, examine the peripheral blood for evidence of pancytopenia or a reduction in the number of neutrophils and platelets, and to examine the bone marrow to determine whether haemopoiesis is normal. Often this simple approach combined with a knowledge of the likely effects of splenectomy for a particular haematological disorder will be all that is necessary to make a decision about whether to proceed to surgery. Sometimes, however, it is helpful to carry out more sophisticated studies to define more thoroughly the functions of the spleen. This approach is also useful occasionally for establishing an accurate haematological diagnosis.

Studies with radionuclides provide information about the extent of splenic involvement in a disease process, the role of the spleen in producing anaemia, and the likely benefits of splenectomy.

The following list summarizes the various *in vivo* tests which have been developed for investigating splenic function:

1. Delineation of functional splenic tissue
2. Estimation of spleen size
3. Measurement of splenic blood flow
4. Measurement of splenic red cell pool
5. Measurement of phagocytic function (irreversible extraction)
6. Identification of sites of red cell destruction ('surface counting')
7. Quantification of splenic red cell destruction
8. Plasma volume changes of splenomegaly
9. Identification and quantification of splenic extramedullary erythropoiesis
10. Role of spleen in platelet kinetics, especially in thrombocytopenia

Details of the methods used and analysis of results obtained in various conditions are to be found in specialized textbooks (e.g.

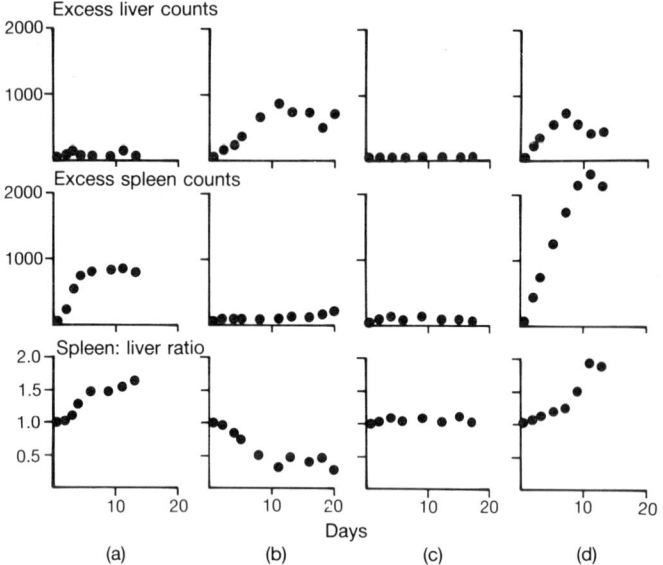

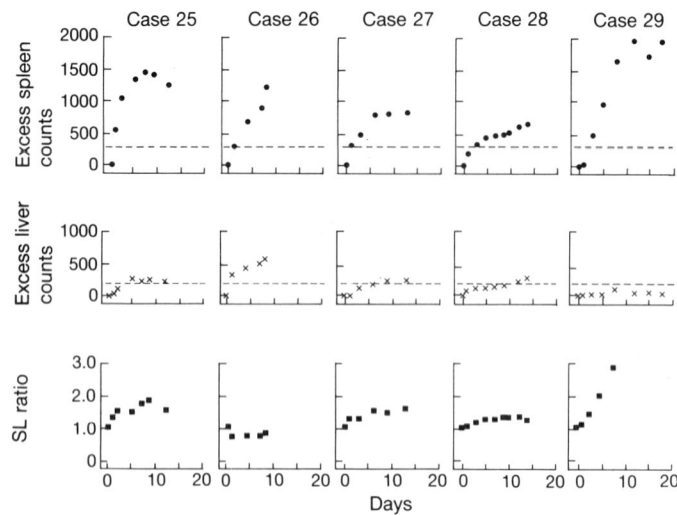

Fig. 3 Examples of surface counting patterns which have been found in: (*a*) hereditary spherocytosis, hereditary elliptocytosis, and some cases of autoimmune haemolytic anaemia; (*b*) sickle cell disease; (*c*) pyruvate kinase deficiency and intravascular haemolysis: (*d*) autoimmune haemolytic anaemia. The vertical axis shows arbitrary units of radioactivity, normalized to counts on the first day. Excess spleen counts increased to about 1000 or more without parallel liver activity indicate that splenectomy is likely to be beneficial in controlling haemolysis.

Fig. 4 Patterns of surface counting found in different patients with autoimmune haemolytic anaemia: red cell destruction was confined to the spleen in case 29; in the other cases the liver was also involved to a greater or lesser extent.

Dacie and Lewis, 1984). The combination of investigations used depends on the particular clinical problem. For example, spleen pool size measurement may help to distinguish secondary polycythaemia from polycythaemia vera. In many conditions associated with splenomegaly, it is important to distinguish increased reticulo-endothelial macrophage activity causing cell destruction from increased red cell accumulation in a large pool, and to what extent enlargement of the spleen is due to tumour infiltration. Surface counting following injection of ^{51}Cr-labelled erythrocytes provides a qualitative indication of splenic red cell destruction in various haemolytic anaemias (Figs 3 and 4); quantitative scanning provides a more accurate measurement of the actual proportion of the cells which are destroyed in the spleen and elsewhere. In myelofibrosis and hypersplenism, it may be helpful to determine the relative importance of the splenic red cell pool, red cell destruction, and extramedullary erythropoiesis (see below).

The most useful test is *delineation of functional splenic tissue*. The spleen can be visualized and its size estimated by scintillation scanning following injection of labelled red cells after they have been damaged artificially in a way which ensures that they will be removed from the circulation by the spleen, e.g. by heating to 50 °C. The picture obtained by a gamma camera or rectilinear scanner (Fig. 5) demonstrates whether a mass in the left upper abdomen is a spleen and whether there is accessory spleen tissue; it will help to diagnose space-occupying lesions of the spleen such as cysts (Fig. 2), haemangiomas, and haematomas. Infarcts and tumour deposits in the spleen are less easily demonstrated unless they are larger than 2–3 cm in diameter. Conversely, functional asplenia, previous splenectomy, or splenic atrophy is readily detected. Hypofunction may occur when a tumour or cyst obliterates a large part of the splenic tissue.

Recording the spleen size is useful for monitoring response to therapy and for staging in myeloproliferative disorders. In polycythaemia vera, splenomegaly is an important diagnostic feature; in some cases in which the spleen is not palpable it is possible to show that it is nonetheless enlarged using this approach.

A similar procedure with undamaged labelled red cells provides

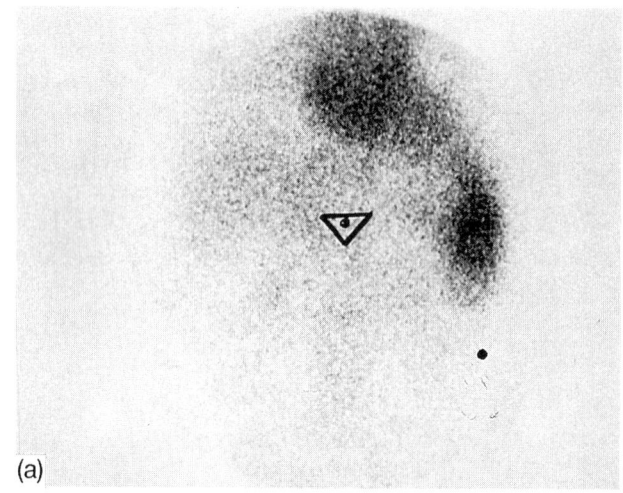

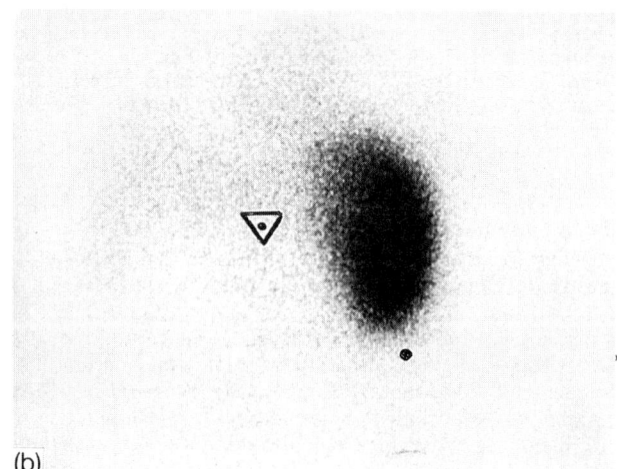

Fig. 5 Images obtained by scintillation camera following administration of (*a*) ^{99}Tc-labelled red cells and (*b*) ^{111}In-labelled heat-damaged red cells.

a measurement of the *splenic red cell pool*. It is a relatively simple procedure which can be carried out with standard scanning equipment. (Figs 5 and 6).

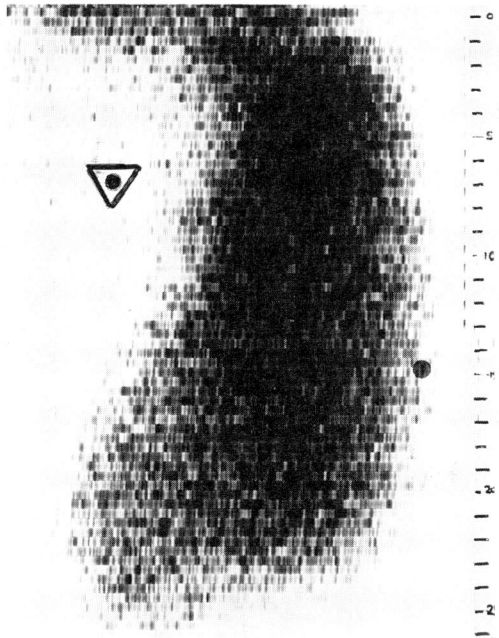

Fig. 6 Splenic enlargement and increased red cell pool in a patient with myelofibrosis. Demonstrated by scan after administration of ^{113m}In-labelled red cells. The markings indicate the costal margin. The upper pole of the spleen merges with the image produced by labelled blood in the heart.

The increased pool which occurs in the myeloproliferative and lymphoproliferative disorders has been described on page 19.188. The extent of splenic red cell pool should be taken into account when assessing the significance of associated anaemia. Measuring the pool is particularly useful for distinguishing polycythaemia vera from secondary polycythaemia (see page 19.153).

The rate at which heat-damaged red cells are cleared from circulation provides a rough guide to the *competence of splenic function*. A slow clearance ($t\frac{1}{2}$ greater than 15 min) is due to a combination of slow splenic blood flow and decreased phagocytic function. A slow clearance may identify splenic hypofunction before the blood film shows Howell-Jolly bodies and other morphological changes. Occasionally, there is the paradox of slow clearance and splenomegaly. This has been seen in children with sickle-cell disease, in malignant histiocytosis, and in amyloidosis.

Extramedullary erythropoiesis
Normally, transferrin-bound iron passes to the bone marrow where the iron is released and enters erythroblasts for incorporation into the haemoglobin of developing erythrocytes. In the normal spleen iron does not dissociate from transferrin. Hence uptake of iron, demonstrable by surface counts shortly after administration of ^{59}Fe, indicates that there is erythropoiesis in the spleen. The effectiveness of splenic erythropoiesis can be assessed by the fall in surface counts on subsequent days coupled with the increase in blood radioactivity as a measure of red cell production. Extramedullary erythropoiesis in the spleen occurs in the majority of patients with myelosclerosis. A different pattern of iron accumulation in the spleen is seen in patients with haemolytic anaemia with splenic destruction of red cells or in those with splenomegaly and red cell pooling: initially, surface counting shows no evidence of uptake, but radioactivity increases during the first and second week of the study as the newly formed cells are destroyed or sequestered in the spleen (Fig. 7).

A major limitation of surface counting as a means for measuring the extent of erythropoiesis at different sites is that, as only small segments of bone marrow and other organs are examined by a col-limated counter, the results may be unrepresentative. Also, radioactivity in the ribs may be confused with splenic activity. Moreover, even if surface counting demonstrates the occurrence of extramedullary erythropoiesis in the spleen, it will fail to measure its extent and is thus of little value in deciding whether splenectomy may be disadvantageous. These limitations can be overcome by quantitative scanning, using cyclotron-produced ^{52}Fe which has a half-life of only eight hours, and thus can be administered in relatively high doses and on repeated occasions for serial studies at conveniently short intervals. Thus, it is possible to assess the changes in erythropoiesis during the course of the disease, to define more accurately the fraction of an administered dose of labelled iron which is utilized in splenic erythropoiesis, and hence to distinguish splenomegaly due to myeloid metaplasia from that caused by red cell pooling (Fig. 8). For example, in patients with polycythaemia vera and myelosclerosis serial studies may be performed at conveniently short intervals to assess changes in erythropoiesis, and the effect of various forms of therapy on the clinical course in general and on the spleen in particular. ^{52}Fe studies are useful for detecting early stages of transition from polycythaemia vera to myelosclerosis and for diagnosing the syndrome of transitional myeloproliferative disorder (see page 19.38).

Platelet kinetics
About one-third of an injection of ^{51}Cr-labelled platelets disappear from circulation during their lifespan, mainly in the spleen pool. Splenomegaly is associated with a marked increase in pooling: by contrast, in asplenia, nearly 100 per cent of the labelled platelets are recovered in the circulating blood. Surface counting has been used to identify the role of the spleen in thrombocytopenia. In some cases the spleen and in others the liver has appeared to be the main site of destruction. However, the clinical usefulness of such counting data in predicting the results of splenectomy is debatable. More reliable information can be derived from quantitative scanning following injection of platelets labelled with ^{111}In oxine. The spleen appears to deal with platelets by pooling and destruction in a manner similar to the way it handles red cells; normally platelets at the end of their lifespan are destroyed to an equal extent by the macrophages of the spleen and bone marrow. In thrombocytopenia there are three patterns of platelet distribution and destruction: (*a*) platelets have a normal lifespan but there is increased splenic pooling; (*b*) there is accelerated destruction but this occurs to an equal degree in the spleen and marrow; (*c*) platelet survival is markedly reduced and there is abnormal destruction in the bone marrow. Thus, quantitative platelet kinetic studies with ^{111}In can provide useful information in deciding whether to advise splenectomy for a patient with thrombocytopenia.

Indications for splenectomy
The main indications for splenectomy are summarized in Table 4. The decision is usually based on knowledge of the likely result for a particular disease and on a simple assessment of abnormal splenic function which includes the degree of anaemia, the presence or absence of neutropenia or thrombocytopenia, and, in some cases, measurement of red cell survival combined with external counting, and blood volume estimation. Obviously it is impractical to carry out all the sophisticated tests of splenic function described in the previous section on every patient and they should be reserved for difficult cases when the information thus obtained, taken in conjunction with clinical factors, may influence the decision for or against splenectomy.

Clinical and haematological effects of splenectomy
Removal of the spleen is associated with certain immediate and delayed clinical complications and by the presence of permanent changes in the peripheral blood picture.

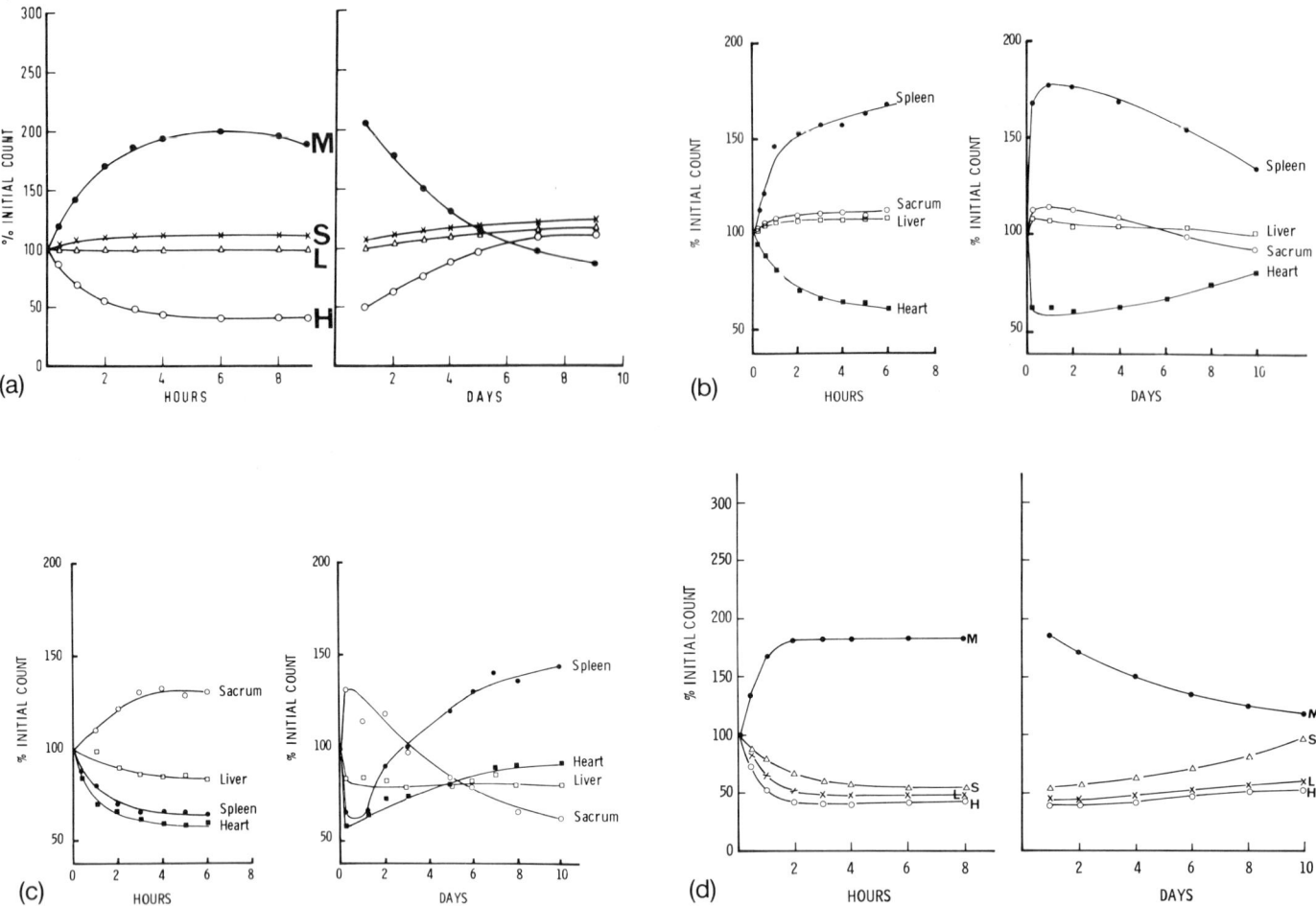

Fig. 7 ^{59}Fe ferrokinetic counting studies showing the patterns obtained in (a) a normal subject, (b) myelofibrosis with splenic extramedullary erythropoiesis, (c) hypersplenism with pronounced splenic red cell pooling, (d) dyserythropoiesis with splenic phagocytosis M = marrow, S = spleen, L = liver, H = heart (or blood) radioactivity, normalized to the count rate immediately after administration of the isotope.

Clinical complications

Immediate

In some splenectomies particularly when the spleen is bound down by adhesions following previous splenic infarction, there may be difficulty in achieving haemostasis. This is particularly so if the patient goes into surgery with a platelet count below 50 x 10^9/1. It is sometimes useful to administer platelets as soon as the spleen has been removed to try to achieve a dry splenic bed. Post-operative collections of blood often become secondarily infected with the production of a subphrenic abscess. Since the platelet count tends to rise immediately after the operation, there is an increased risk of thrombo-embolic disease in the first two or three weeks after splenectomy: this is increased by post-operative infection, and therefore the main lines of prevention are scrupulous attention to haemostasis at surgery and early mobilization and breathing exercises after the operation.

Long-term

Patients who have undergone splenectomy have an increased risk of serious, overwhelming infection. This is certainly the case when the operation is carried out within the first five years of life although even in adults the risk is still slightly increased.

The incidence of postsplenectomy infection seems to vary depending on the indications for the original operation. For example, it is much less common in patients who are splenectomized for trauma or hereditary spherocytosis and commoner in

those with chronic diseases such as thalassaemia, which do not respond fully to the operation.

Overwhelming septicaemia in a splenectomized patient may present with frightening rapidity; the interval between the onset of symptoms and death may be only a few hours. For this reason it is very important to warn parents of splenectomized children to seek medical attention immediately there are any unusual symptoms. Young children should all receive oral penicillin (250 mg twice daily) and this should be continued until the age of 18 years. This approach is probably not necessary in adults although they should be given appropriate warning about seeking medical attention if they have any unusual symptoms. Clinical trials are testing pneumococcal vaccine to reduce the incidence of postsplenectomy infection; its value is uncertain, especially as it does not contain a number of the pneumococcal subtypes which cause serious infection in children. Another approach to preventing infection is to repair the damaged spleen rather than remove it and, if this is impractical, to implant some of the excised spleen tissue.

Apart from bacterial infection splenectomized patients are at risk from parasitic disorders, particularly *falciparum* malaria. It is most important that they take malarial prophylactics when visiting endemic areas. A rare cause of relapse of a haematological disorder after initial response to splenectomy is the growth of *accessory spleens*. This has been well documented in patients with hereditary spherocytosis or thrombocytopenic purpura. With the easy availability of techniques for scanning the spleen (see page

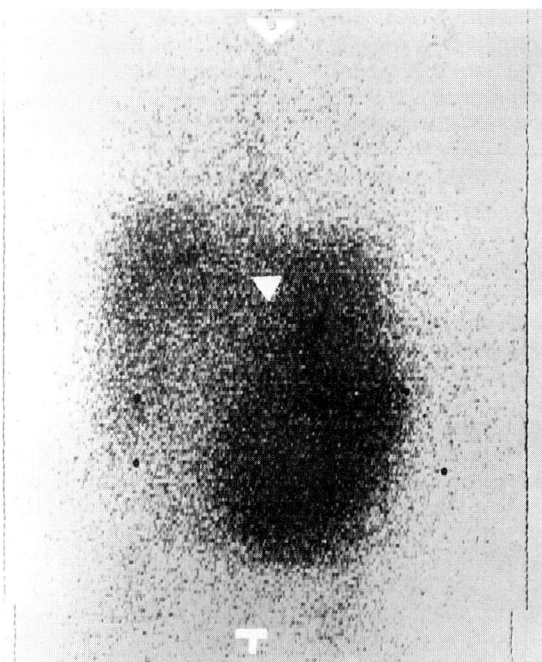

Fig. 8 ^{52}Fe scan in a patient with myelofibrosis showing the extent of splenic erythropoiesis. A small amount of erythropoiesis is demonstrable in the vertebral column.

Table 4 Indications for splenectomy

Definite
1 Trauma
2 Hereditary spherocytosis
3 Chronic idiopathic thrombocytopenia purpura
4 As part of staging laparotomy for Hodgkin's disease and non-Hodgkin's lymphoma

Occasional
1 Disorders in which hypersplenism becomes a major feature of the clinical picture, e.g. hereditary or acquired haemolytic anaemia, myeloproliferative disease, some lymphomas, portal hypertension, Felty's syndrome, parasitic disease, etc.
2 Carcinoma of colon, pancreas, etc. involving spleen
3 In cases in which the cause of the splenomegaly cannot be determined by other methods

19.192), it is worthwhile looking for accessory spleen in any patient with one of these disorders who relapses after splenectomy.

Platelets

In the immediate postoperative period the platelet count rises steeply usually to about 600–1000 x 10^9/1 with a peak at 7–12 days. The thrombocytosis is usually transitory and falls to near normal values over the following one or two months. However, during this period thrombo-embolism may occur. It is advisable to administer antiplatelet therapy (e.g. aspirin 100 mg daily) as long as the thrombocytosis persists. Occasionally, the thrombocytosis persists indefinitely after splenectomy; this is usually associated with continuing anaemia.

Other approaches to reducing the size of the spleen

Reduction of splenic size and function can also be achieved by splenic artery ligation or arterial embolization, and by irradiation. In the procedure for embolization, gel foam, silastic microspheres, or metallic coils are introduced by catheter into the splenic artery. It is an effective means of reducing the size and functions of the spleen. However, it carries the risk of infection of disseminated coagulopathy, while inaccurate delivery of the emboli may result in hepatic infarction. Because of the high risk of abscess formation and other complications, this procedure should be limited to patients needing splenectomy but unable to tolerate surgery, e.g. because of severe thrombocytopenia. Furthermore it should be followed by surgical removal of the spleen as soon as the patient's clinical condition allows.

References

Bateman, S., Lewis, S. M., Nicholas, A. and Zaafran, A. (1978). Splenic red cell pooling: a diagnostic feature in polycythaemia. *Br. J. Haemat.* **40**, 389–396.

Bowdler, A. J. (1982). The spleen in disorders of the blood. In *Blood and its disorders*, 2nd edn (eds R. M. Hardisty and D. J. Weatherall), pp.751–798. Blackwell Scientific Publications, Oxford.

Bowring, C. S. (1977). Quantitative radioisotope scanning and its use in haematology. *Clinics Haemat.* **6**, 625–637.

——, Ferrant, A. E., Glass, H. I., Lewis, S. M., and Szur, L. (1975). Quantitative measurement of splenic and hepatic red-cell destruction. *Br. J. Hamat.* **31**, 467–477.

Brubaker, L. H. and Johnson, C. A. (1978). Correlation of splenomegaly and abnormal neutrophil pooling (margination). *J. Lab. Clin. Med.* **92**, 508–515.

Castanada-Zuniga, W. R., Hammerschmidt, D. E., Sanchez, R. and Amplatz, K. (1977). Nonsurgical splenectomy. *Am. J. Roentgen.* **129**, 805–811.

Christensen, B. E. (1973). Erythrocyte pooling and sequestration in enlarged spleens. Estimations of splenic erythrocyte and plasma volume in splenomegalic patients. *Scand. J. Haemat.* **10**, 106–119.

Crane, C. G. (1981). Tropical splenomegaly. Part 2: Oceania. *Clinics Haemat.* **10**, 976–982.

Crosby, W. H. (1980). The spleen. In *Blood, pure and eloquent* (ed. M. M. Wintrobe), Ch. 5. McGraw Hill, New York.

Dacie, J. V. and Lewis, S. M. (1984). *Practical haematology, 6th edn*, Ch. 18–19. Churchill Livingstone, Edinburgh.

Davis, H. H., Varki, A., Heaton, W. A. and Siegel, B. A. (1980). Detection of accessory spleens with indium-111 labelled autologous platelets. *Am. J. Haemat.* **8**, 81–86.

Fakunle, Y. M. (1981). Tropical splenomegaly. Part 1: Tropical Africa. *Clinics Haemat.* **10**, 963–975.

Ferrant, A., Cauwe, F., Michaux, J. L., Beckers, C., Verwilghen, R. L. and Sokal, G. (1982). Assessment of the sites of red cell destruction using quantitative measurements of splenic and hepatic destruction. *Br. J. Haemat.* **50**, 591–598.

Heier, H. E. (1980). Splenectomy and serious infection. *Scand. J. Haemat.* **24**, 5–12.

Hocking, W. G., Machlede, H. I. and Golde, D. W. (1980). Splenic artery embolization prior to splenectomy in end stage polycythemia vera. *Am. J. Haemat.* **8**, 123–127.

Klonizakis, I., Peters, A. M., Fitzpatrick, M. L., Kensett, M. J., Lewis S. M. and Lavender, J. P. (1981). Spleen function and platelet kinetics. *J. clin. Path.* **34**, 377–380.

Koeffler, H. P., Cline, M. J. and Golde, D. W. (1979). Splenic irradiation in myelofibrosis: effect on circulating myeloid progenitor cells. *Br. J. Haemat.* **43**, 69–77.

Lewis, S. M. (1978). Newer method of assessment for splenectomy. In *Advanced medicine* vol. 14 (ed. D. J. Weatherall), pp. 200–209. Pitman, London.

Mitchell, A. and Morris, P. J. (1983). Surgery of the spleen. *Clinic Haemat.* **12**, 565–590.

Pettit, J. E. (1977). Spleen function. *Clinics Haemat.* **6**, 639–656.

——, Lewis, S. M., Williams, E. D., Grafton, C. A., Bowring, C. S. and Glass, H. I. (1976). Quantitative studies of splenic erythropoiesis in polycythaemia vera and myelofibrosis. *Br. J. Haemat.* **34**, 465–475.

Spencer, R. P. and Pearson, H. A. (1975). *Radionuclide studies of the spleen*. CRC Press, Cleveland.

Szur, L. (1970). Surface counting in assessment of sites of red cell destruction (annotation). *Br. J. Haemat.* **118**, 591–596.

——, Pettit, J. E., Lewis, S. M., Bruce-Tagoe, A. A. and Short, M. D. (1973). The effect of radiation on splenic function in myelosclerosis: studies with ^{52}Fe and ^{99}Tc^m. *Br. J. Radiol.* **46**, 295–301.

Videbaek, A., Christensen, B. E. and Jønsson, V. (1982). *The spleen in health and disease*. FADL's Forlag, Copenhagen.

Weiss, L. (1965). The structure of the normal spleen. *Sem. Hemat.* **2**, 205–228.

Weiss, L. (1974). A scanning electron microscope study of the spleen. *Blood* **43**, 665–691.

Weiss, L. (1983). The red pulp of the spleen: structural basis of blood flow. *Clinics Haemat.* **12**, 375–393.

——, and Tavassoli, M. (1970). Anatomic hazards to the passage of erythrocytes through the spleen. *Sem. Hemat.* **7**, 372–379.

Wennberg, E. and Weiss, L. (1969). The structure of the spleen and hemolysis. *Ann. Rev. Med.* **20**, 29–40.

Paraproteinaemia

D. Y. MASON, C. BUNCH, AND S. CALLENDER

Introduction

The term paraproteinaemia is used to describe the presence in the blood of increased amounts of a single immunoglobulin (antibody) which is derived from the monoclonal proliferation of B cells capable of terminal differentiation into antibody producing cells.

In some instances such proliferations are clinically benign in that they may be asymptomatic, progress slowly, if at all, and are not associated with impairment of normal antibody responses or of bone marrow function. In other instances, however, proliferation is progressive and autonomous, and gives rise to serious clinical problems. Two main clinical conditions are recognized and are discussed in this section – *myeloma*, in which the B cell clone differentiates to plasma cells and the monoclonal immunoglobulin may be of any class, and *Waldenström's macroglobulinaemia*, in which the clone differentiates to a lympho-plasmacytoid stage intermediate between lymphocyte and plasma cell, and the paraprotein is IgM.

The categories of human paraproteinaemia described in this section, together with their cardinal clinical, pathological, and immunochemical features are summarized in Table 1. Before describing the different types of human paraproteinaemia, it is helpful to review briefly relevant aspects of immunoglobulin structure and of B-cell maturation in man. These topics are considered further in Section 4.

The nature of immunoglobulin

The basic structure of the immunoglobulin molecule is illustrated in Fig. 1. The most important feature from the point of view of human paraproteinaemias is that the region of the molecule formed by the aposition of the N-terminal regions of its constituent heavy and light chains is highly variable in structure. The functional importance of this variability is that this region of the molecule is concerned with antigen binding. The ability of the immune system to recognize a very large number of different antigens (in excess of 10^6) is directly attributable to the wide range of configurations found in the variable region of the Ig molecule.

Classification of immunoglobulins

Immunoglobulin molecules are categorized on the basis of the type of heavy chain they contain into five major groups (Table 1). The five classes of heavy chains (γ, μ, α δ, ε) differ one from another in the structure of their constant regions. This accounts for the distinct functional properties associated with different classes of immunoglobulin (e.g. the ability of IgG to cross the placenta, the ability of IgE to bind to mast cells, etc.)

Light chains are of two types – kappa and lambda. Any individual immunoglobulin molecule contains two light chains of a single class, i.e. two kappa chains or two lambda chains but never one of each. Each of the five heavy chain classes may be associated with either kappa or lambda chains. There is an overall 2:1 predominance of kappa chains, except in the case of IgD, in which lambda chains are present in a 9:1 excess (Table 2).

Table 1 Human paraproteinaemia

Disease	Predominant cell type	Paraprotein type	Growth pattern	Clinical features	Treatment
Benign paraproteinaemia	Presumably plasma cells, but numbers too few to be identified	Usually IgG or IgM; light chains only very rarely found in urine	Neoplastic clone not clinically manifest	No symptoms (with the rare exception of antigen-binding paraprotein, e.g. anti-red cell antibodies)	nil
Multiple myeloma	Plasma cell	55% IgG ($\pm$ light chains) 25% IgA ($\pm$ light chains) 20% light chain only	Bone marrow infiltration; bone erosion	Bone pain, fractures, renal failure, anaemia, hypercalcaemia	Melphalan (L-phenylalanine mustard) cyclophosphamide multiple chemotherapy, radiotherapy
Waldenström's macroglobulinaemia	Lymphoplasmacytoid	IgM ($\pm$ small amounts of light chain)	Lymph nodes and spleen	Hyperviscosity, splenomegaly, lymphadenopathy	Chlorambucil
Paraproteinaemia in association with lymphoma and lymphoid leukaemia*	Immature B cells	Most frequently IgM ($\pm$ free light chains); occasionally light chains are produced alone	Predominantly in lymph nodes and spleen	Signs and symptoms of underlying lymphoma/leukaemia	Cytotoxic drugs, radiotherapy
Heavy chain diseases	Plasma cells, lymphoplasmacytoid cells or more primitive B cells	γ, μ, or α chains (usually incomplete), accompanied by free light chains in some cases of μ chain disease	Variable (see text)	Variable (see text)	Cytotoxic drugs; α chain disease may respond to antibiotic therapy

* Note that in these diseases (in contrast to those listed above) paraproteinaemia is only rarely encountered (incidence approximately 10 per cent).

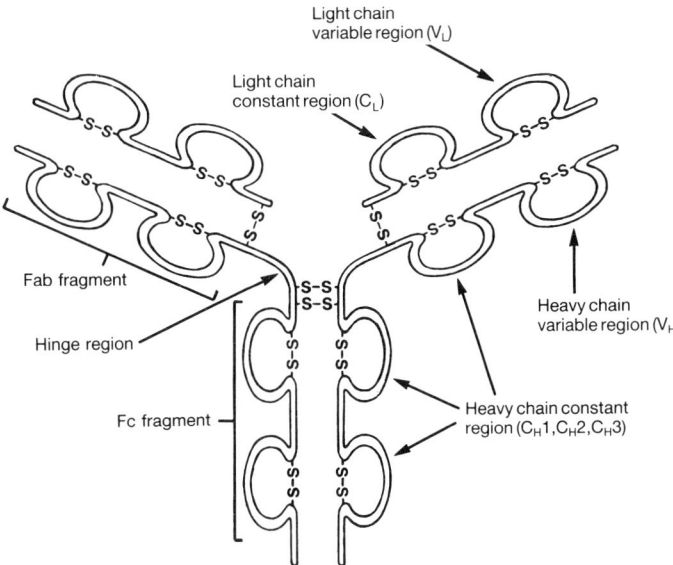

Fig. 1 The immunoglobulin molecule (illustrated schematically) has a molecular weight of approximately 160 000. IgG, IgD and IgE all show this basic structure (although minor variations occur). IgA is found both in this form and also as dimers (the form in which IgA appears in secretions) or higher molecular weight polymers (see Table 1). IgM is almost all in the form of a 19S pentamer (Table 1).

Table 2 Categories of human immunoglobulin

Class	Heavy chain	Light chain	Number of units	Molecular formula	Serum concentration (mg/ml)
IgG	γ	K or λ	Monomer	$\gamma_2 K_2$ or $\gamma_2 \lambda_2$	8–16
IgA	α	K or λ	Monomer, dimer, or polymers	$(\alpha_2 K_2)$ l-n or $(\alpha_2 \lambda_2)$ l-n	1.4–4.0
IgM	μ	K or λ	Pentamer	$(\mu_2 K_2)$ 5 or $(\mu_2 \lambda_2)$ 5	0.5–2.0
IgD	δ	K or λ	Monomer	$\delta_2 K_2$ or $\delta_2 \lambda_2$	<0.4
IgE	ε	K or λ	Monomer	$\varepsilon_2 K_2$ or $\varepsilon_2 \lambda_2$	0.02–0.45

Immunoglobulin production

Figure 2 illustrates the maturation pathways of human B cells and also indicates the capacity of B cells at each stage of their maturation to express cytoplasmic and/or surface immunoglobulin. In the early stages of this sequence, i.e. at the small B lymphocyte stage, the only detectable immunoglobulin is found on the cell surface, where it acts as receptor for antigen. Once the cell has been triggered to differentiate (by exposure to antigen), surface immunoglobulin begins to disappear and the synthesis of cytoplasmic immunoglobulin destined for secretion begins. Most of the immunoglobulin found in serum or secretions is released from B cells which have reached their terminal differentiation stage (the plasma cell, Fig. 2). However, it is important to realize that earlier stages in this maturation sequence (e.g. lymphoplasmacytoid cells and germinal centre cells) may also be capable of immunoglobulin secretion. This is of relevance in the context of paraproteinaemia associated with non-Hodgkin's lymphoma (see below).

The concept of lymphoid clones

As noted above, immunoglobulins show a remarkable degree of molecular heterogeneity. The basis of this phenomenon lies in the fact that the lymphoid system contains large numbers of different cell lines or 'clones', each of which is programmed to produce its own unique immunoglobulin molecule. This molecule retains the same variable region structure (although different constant regions may be expressed) throughout the maturation of the clone. In consequence, the antigen binding specificity of the molecules found on the surface of an immature cell is identical to that of the immunoglobulin released from the cell when it has reached its terminal maturation stage.

The existence of a large number of lymphoid clones, each with unique antigen binding specificity, and the constancy of this specificity during clonal maturation, are the two fundamental facts which explain the way in which the lymphoid system produces antibody in response to antigen. Exposure to antigen triggers only those clones on which the surface immunoglobulin is capable of binding determinants on the antigen. These clones then mature to secrete large amounts of antibodies specific for the triggering antigen.

Polyclonal and monoclonal Ig production

In the scheme described above a single antigen may be capable of stimulating a number of different clones. Furthermore, infecting organisms are likely to stimulate a response to a number of different antigens. Since each clone produces a unique immunoglobulin molecule, the 'polyclonal' antibody produced in response to antigenic stimulation will be heterogeneous when analysed by a technique such as electrophoresis, in which the mobility of molecules reflects their molecular structure. This accounts for the fact that normal human immunoglobulin shows a diffuse distribution pattern on serum electrophoresis (Figs. 3 and 4) reflecting the large number of different clones which contribute to its production.

In contrast, if a single clone is triggered to differentiate, the immunoglobulin which it secretes will be seen as a homogeneous protein band on electrophoresis (Figs. 3 and 4). This 'paraprotein' is the hallmark by which monoclonal proliferations of plasma cells, and of their precursors, are recognized. As will be apparent subsequently, a homogenous band is also seen when the monoclonal cell product is an incomplete molecule (e.g. free light chains).

The terms 'monoclonal gammopathy' or 'plasma cell dyscrasia' are sometimes used as synonyms for the term 'paraproteinaemia'.

Abnormalities of immunoglobulin production in paraproteinaemia

Paraproteins differ from normal polyclonal immunoglobulin in that they are of restricted electrophoretic mobility and of a single heavy and light chain class, e.g. IgG kappa, IgM lambda, etc. It should be emphasized that paraproteins are usually completely normal in terms of molecular structure and amino acid sequence, a fact which enabled protein chemists to gain their initial insight into immunoglobulin structure by studying monoclonal paraproteins. However, although neoplastic immunoglobulin-secreting clones usually produce paraproteins of normal molecular structure, there is frequently an imbalance between the rate of heavy and light chain production. In most cases this leads to the secretion of an excess of free light chains. This is of practical clinical relevance for two reasons. Firstly the detection of monoclonal urinary light chains is of diagnostic importance in many cases of paraproteinaemia. Secondly, light chain excretion is responsible for severe renal damage in a substantial proportion of myeloma patients.

In a minority of cases the neoplastic B cell clone loses the ability to produce heavy chains ('the light chain diseases' – see below). Further abnormalities which may occur much less frequently in paraproteinaemia include the production of two or more paraproteins (biclonal paraproteinaemia – see Fig. 4) and the non-secretion of immunoglobulin, despite the fact that the cells are morphologically mature plasma cells. This latter pattern ('non-secretory myeloma') is usually accounted for by a block in secretion of intracellular immunoglobulin rather than by a failure of immunoglobulin synthesis. An even rarer pattern of disordered immunoglobulin production is represented by cases in which free heavy chains are produced by the neoplastic B cells (see below under Heavy Chain Disease).

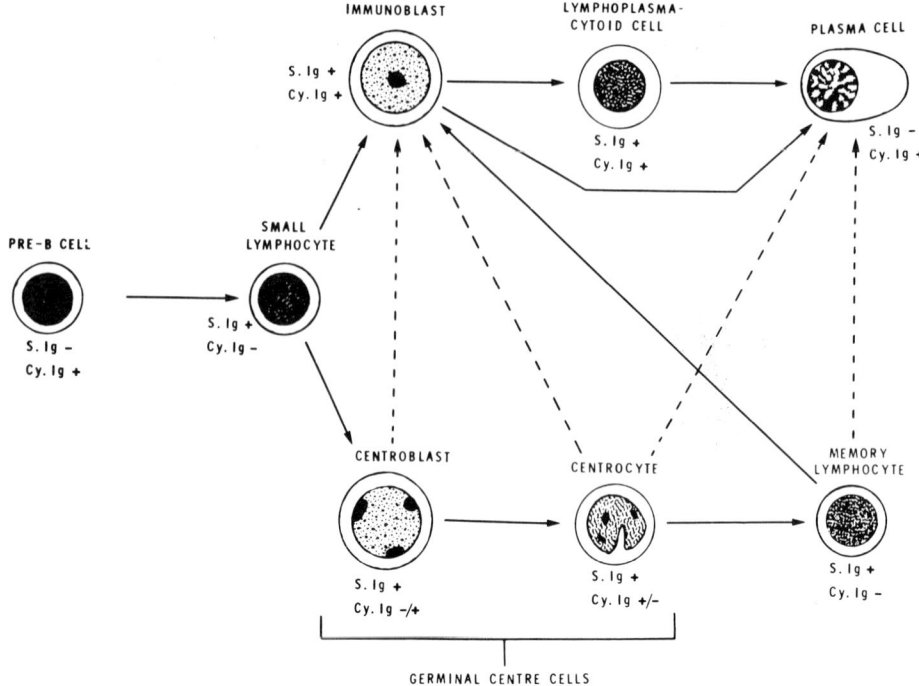

Fig. 2 Schematic illustration of B cell maturation (after Lennert *et al.*). The presence or absence of surface immunoglobulin (S Ig) and of cytoplasmic immunoglobulin (Cy Ig) at each maturation stage is indicated. Note that the capacity to secrete immunoglobulin (as indicated by the presence of cytoplasmic Ig) is not restricted to the plasma cell stage and in consequence neoplasms of cells such as immunoblasts or germinal centre cells may be associated with the presence of a paraprotein.

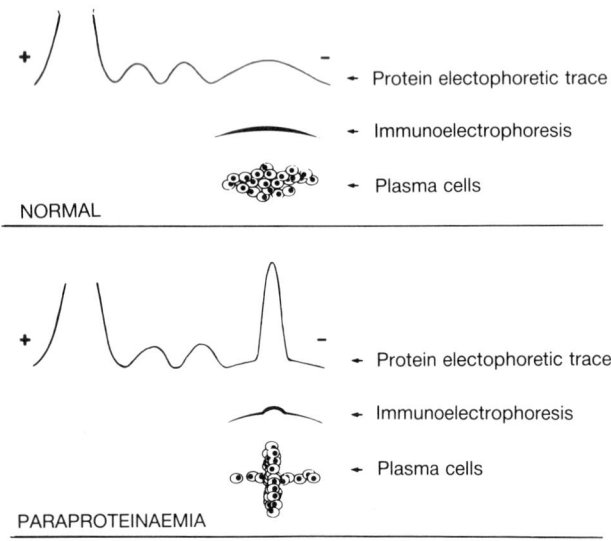

Fig. 3 Illustration of the difference between polyclonal and monoclonal plasma cell proliferation. In normal subjects immunoglobulin is secreted by a number of plasma cell clones and consequently shows a diffuse distribution on electrophoresis. In contrast a single plasma cell clone predominates in paraproteinaemia patients and its secreted Ig product appears as a homogeneous 'spike' of restricted mobility on electrophoresis. Immuno-electrophoresis against anti-serum specific for the heavy or light chain of the paraprotein shows deformation or kinking in the region of the paraprotein.

Benign paraproteinaemia

This type of paraproteinaemia (also referred to as 'essential' or 'asymptomatic' paraproteinaemia) may be found both in healthy subjects (sometimes referred to as 'primary' benign paraprotein-

aemia) and in hospital patients suffering from non-lymphoproliferative disorders ('secondary' benign paraproteinaemia).

Benign paraproteinaemia in normal subjects

Serum paraproteins may be found by routine screening in 0.1–1.0 per cent of the normal adult population. A few of these represent early cases of lymphoproliferative disease. However, in most instances the paraprotein shows no change over a period of time and these individuals remain asymptomatic. The frequency of benign paraproteinaemia in healthy subjects rises steeply with advancing age, being of the order of 3 per cent in subjects over the age of 70.

Benign paraproteinaemia in hospital patients

Paraproteins have been detected in patients suffering from a wide variety of clinical disorders, and in at least some cases the association is fortuitous, reflecting both the frequency with which the serum from hospital patients is analysed electrophoretically and also the fact that older individuals (who predominate among hospital patients) have the highest incidence of benign paraproteinaemia (see above).

However, a number of disorders, including chronic inflammatory states (particularly affecting the biliary tract), liver disease, connective tissue disorders, and neoplasms (especially of the colon, biliary system and lung) appear to be associated with an increased incidence of benign paraproteinaemia. This has led to suggestions that repeated antigenic stimulation of the lymphoreticular system (e.g. by bacterial, viral, neoplasia-associated, or autologous antigens) accounts for the emergence of the paraprotein-producing clone.

Diagnosis of benign paraproteinaemia

Whatever the explanation of benign paraproteinaemia, its chief clinical importance lies in the fact that it may lead to the patient being erroneously categorized as suffering from myeloma or other B cell neoplasm.

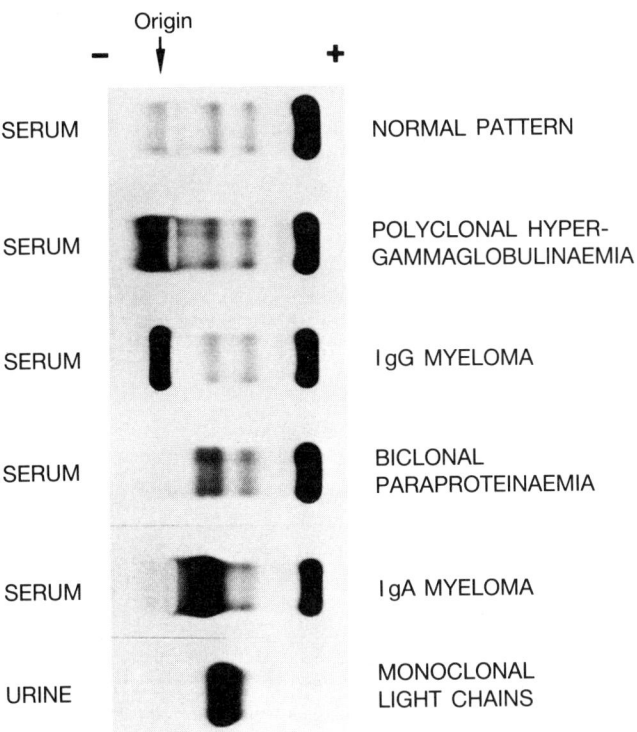

Origin

− +

SERUM — NORMAL PATTERN

SERUM — POLYCLONAL HYPER-GAMMAGLOBULINAEMIA

SERUM — IgG MYELOMA

SERUM — BICLONAL PARAPROTEINAEMIA

SERUM — IgA MYELOMA

URINE — MONOCLONAL LIGHT CHAINS

Fig. 4 Agarose electrophoresis of serum from a normal subject compared with polyclonal hypergammaglobulinaemia and different types of paraproteinaemia. Note the contrast between the diffuse Ig increase characteristic of polyclonal hypergammaglobulinaemia, and the restricted mobility of the serum paraprotein in IgG myeloma (see also Fig. 3) Marked depression of background immunoglobulin ('immune paresis') is also seen in this latter sample. The migration of the IgA paraprotein in the β-globulin region (and its relatively broad electrophoretic disribution) is frequently seen in this class of paraproteinaemia. Note that the monoclonal urinary light chains (sometimes referred to as Bence–Jones protein) migrate as a single protein band in the same way as serum paraproteins.

The following criteria usually allow cases of benign paraproteinaemia to be unequivocally distinguished from lymphoid neoplasia:

1. Absence of skeletal radiological evidence of bone marrow disease. Marrow aspiration may show a slight increase in the number of plasma cells but they do not show the morphological abnormalities seen in myeloma.

2. Maintenance of a constant concentration of paraprotein when the patient is observed over a period of time.

3. Absence of 'immune paresis' (suppression of normal serum immunoglobulin levels).

4. A relatively low concentration of serum paraprotein (less than 20 g/l).

5. Absence of urinary light chain excretion.

Occasionally diagnostic difficulty may arise over a case of myeloma or Waldenström's macroglobulinaemia which is detected early in the course of the disease (before the classical diagnostic features have emerged). In these circumstances it is justifiable to observe the patient for a period until the first symptoms appear. There is no evidence that delay in the initiation of therapy worsens the ultimate prognosis in these patients.

Myeloma

The cellular basis of myeloma

Myeloma may be defined as a plasma cell neoplasm although original mutation and much of the subsequent cell multiplication prob-

Table 3 Immunochemical classes of myeloma

Class of myeloma	Relative frequency (%)	Proportion of cases excreting light chains (%)*	K/λ ratio
IgG	55–60	50–70	2:1
IgA	20–25	50–70	2:1
Light chain disease	20	100	1.2:1
IgD	1	90	1:9
Other (IgM, biclonal, non-secretory)	1		

* The frequency with which light chains are detected is partly dependent upon technical factors, (e.g. the degree to which the urine is concentrated before testing, the sensitivity of the electrophoresis procedure, etc.) and this figure consequently shows considerable variation between different published reports.

ably occurs at an earlier stage in the B cell maturation sequence; the plasma cells found in the marrow aspirate represent a terminally differentiated non-dividing state. An analogy may be drawn with chronic granulocytic leukaemia in which the predominant cell type, the polymorph, is not capable of division.

Immunochemical classes of myeloma

Myeloma may be classified on the basis of the secreted paraprotein into a number of different immunochemical categories (Table 3). There is little clinical difference between these different groups, although those cases in which free light chains are excreted carry a risk of renal damage and, less frequently, of amyloid deposition. Furthermore, the presence of a serum paraprotein may, because of its high concentration and/or high molecular weight, lead to the development of hyperviscosity symptoms. For some reason the rare cases of IgD myeloma have a more aggressive clinical course than most cases of myeloma, with a higher risk of extra-osseous spread, plasma cell leukaemia, and renal failure.

Clinical features of myeloma (Fig. 5)

Myeloma resembles other malignancies in having its peak incidence in the seventh decade of life. Its frequency is of the order of 5 new cases per 100 000 and it is slightly more common in males. There appears to have been an increase in the incidence of myeloma over the past 35 years, which is only partly explained by improvements in diagnosis. In about 10 per cent of cases the diagnosis is made by chance, often during investigation of an unexplained high ESR. The patient may be asymptomatic or may have been suffering from mild and rather vague ill-health. The ease with which the diagnosis can be made in the laboratory means that many more relatively asymptomatic patients are now being diagnosed. Some estimates of the rate of growth of the abnormal clone of plasma cells indicate that the tumour may have been present for as long as 15–20 years before it becomes clinically evident. When symptoms do develop they are predominantly due to bone involvement by the neoplastic plasma cells, and to renal disease, classically associated with the excretion of monoclonal light chains – so-called *Bence–Jones proteinuria*.

Bone involvement

Some 60 per cent of patients present with skeletal pain as their major symptom. This particularly affects the back and ribs and is made worse by movement. The sudden onset of severe pain, either with or without an apparent precipitating cause such as a fall, may indicate collapse of a vertebra or spontaneous fracture of a rib. These pains are usually accompanied by some deterioration of general health with fatigue, weakness, and malaise.

Hypercalcaemia

Anorexia, depression, and vomiting leading to dehydration should suggest hypercalcaemia associated with widespread bone disease; it is present in about 30 per cent of patients, and if not recognized and treated, may lead to rapid deterioration and early death.

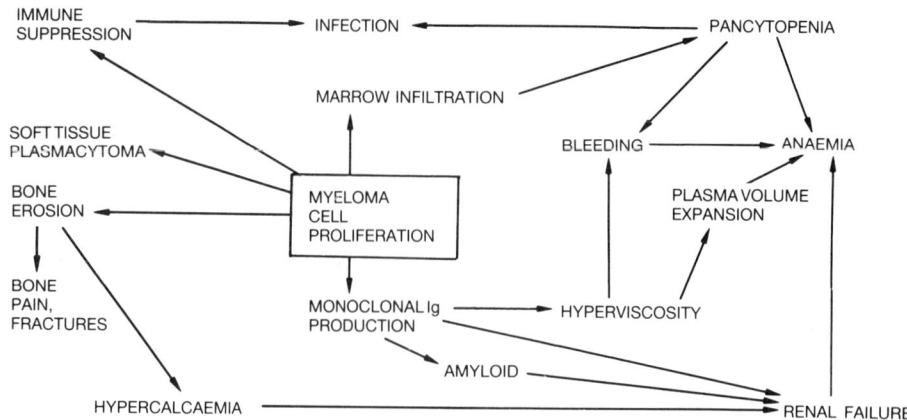

Fig. 5 Summary of the clinical features of myelomatosis.

Renal involvement

Almost 50 per cent of myeloma patients show some evidence of renal impairment at presentation. The classical histological lesion consists of eosinophilic hyaline casts within the lumen of proximal and distal tubules. These casts, which consist primarily of monoclonal light chains filtered by the glomeruli, excite a foreign body giant cell reaction around their periphery and lead to progressive tubular atrophy and destruction of renal tissue. The glomeruli are normally unaffected in myeloma although in a minority of patients amyloid deposition may be observed. Other histological features encountered in myeloma include nephrocalcinosis and infiltration of the kidney interstitium by myeloma cells and/or by chronic inflammatory cells.

Renal failure in myeloma usually progresses slowly over a long period. However, often at the time of presentation a combination of dehydration and hypercalcaemia may lead to marked exacerbation of the degree of renal impairment. In consequence the patient's renal function should be reassessed after adequate hydration and correction of hypercalcaemia.

Haemorrhagic symptoms

Bleeding may be a feature, e.g. bruising, purpura, and epistaxes. These may accompany renal failure or be due to thrombocytopenia, interference with platelet function or with clotting factors by the paraprotein, or to hyperviscosity. The latter is, however, less common in myeloma than in Waldenström's macroglobulinaemia.

Neurological symptoms

When *hyperviscosity* is present there may be some mental impairment and disturbed vision resulting from haemorrhages and exudates in the retina. Peripheral neuropathy may occur, particularly when there is associated amyloidosis and it may be an indication either of direct involvement of the peripheral nerves or, when confined to the median nerve distribution, of amyloid deposits producing a carpal tunnel syndrome. The polyneuropathy of the type found in other neoplasias may also sometimes occur and may precede the development of obvious myeloma. In such cases the CSF protein may be raised in the absence of an increased cell count.

Occasionally, a paraprotein is discovered during investigation of patients with peripheral neuropathy. This most often turns out to be a benign paraprotein and amyloidosis is unusual. Cases have been described in association with a solitary plasmacytoma, with clinical improvement after resection or local radiotherapy. In other instances treatment with cytotoxic drugs usually has little impact on the neuropathy. Rarely, specificity of the paraprotein for antigens in peripheral nerve tissues has been demonstrated.

About 10 per cent of patients present with paraplegia, the result of pressure from an epidural mass of plasmacytoma. In such cases the diagnosis is often made only at laminectomy. Spinal nerve root compression may be either the result of pressure from paravertebral masses of tumour or, more usually, from collapsed vertebrae.

Local masses

Soft tissue plasmacytomas Soft tissue deposits of myeloma may be encountered in cases of myelomatosis. In some cases these represent a direct extension from an underlying bony lesion, e.g. from cranial bones or ribs. In other patients the soft tissue tumour is not in continuity with bone.

When these tumours are encountered at presentation, they are of little prognostic significance. However, if they develop in a patient who is in clinical remission, they frequently herald relapse of the disease. It should be noted in the context of soft tissue plasmacytomas that tumours in this histological category can occur which are not associated with myelomatosis. The commonest site for these tumours is in association with the air passages and respiratory tract, although they may occur at almost any site in the body. Their pattern of clinical behaviour is quite distinct from that of myeloma and they show no tendency to spread to bone.

Solitary myeloma of bone Occasionally patients present with a solitary erosive bony deposit of myeloma. When investigated further, some of these patients show classical evidence of diffuse involvement by myeloma elsewhere in the skeleton. In other patients there is no evidence of disseminated disease, although a paraprotein may be detectable at a low level in the serum. Some of these patients, however, will develop multiple myelomatosis after a period of time, which may occasionally be as long as 20 years.

Infection

In myeloma there is an increased susceptibility to infection, associated with depression of normal serum immunoglobulin levels and a defective antibody response. In some patients the underlying diagnosis of myeloma may first be made at the time of an infection. Serious infection at presentation is most likely to be due to pneumococcus, but Gram-negative infections are more common later in the disease, especially if neutropenia complicates the picture.

Amyloid

The symptoms of amyloidosis, e.g. cardiac failure, nephrotic syndrome, macroglossia, are encountered in approximately 5–10 per cent of myeloma patients. Further details of this complication are given in Section 9.

Diagnosis

The diagnostic triad in myeloma consists of the presence of osteolytic lesions in the bones, atypical plasma cells in the bone marrow, and the demonstration of a paraprotein ('M'-band) on

Table 4 Common laboratory and radiological abnormalities in myeloma

1 Haematological abnormalities
      Blood count
         Anaemia
         Raised ESR
         Rouleaux on film
      Bone marrow
         Infiltration with plasma cells
2 Immunochemical abnormalities
      Serum electrophoresis
         Serum M band of a single heavy and light chain class
         Reduction of normal immunoglobulin
      Urine electrophoresis
         Light chain band of a single light chain class
      Serum immunoglobulins
         Elevation of IgG or IgA due to paraprotein
         Suppression of other Ig classes
3 Biochemical abnormalities
      Hypercalcaemia
      Uraemia, raised creatinine, hyperuricaemia, and hypoalbuminaemia
4 Radiological abnormalities
      Lytic lesions
      Pathological fractures
      Soft tissue masses

In the great majority of cases of suspected myeloma the diagnosis may be confirmed (or confidently excluded) on the basis of bone marrow aspiration, serum and protein electrophoresis, and X-rays of skull, chest, vertebral column, and pelvis.

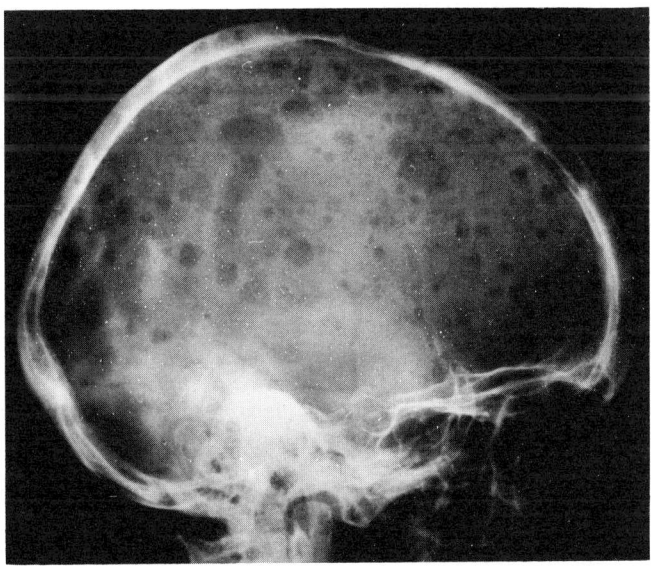

Fig. 6 Skull X-ray in a classical case of multiple myelomatosis. Note the numerous 'punched out' lytic lesions.

(immuno) electrophoresis of the serum and/or of light chains in the urine (see Table 4).

Radiological abnormalities

The myeloma cells produce an osteoclast activating factor (OAF) with the result that multiple skeletal erosions occur. In contrast to the lesions produced in metastatic carcinoma there is seldom any osteoblastic reaction. The radiological appearances are those of numerous punched-out lytic lesions, in the skull, the vertebral column, ribs, pelvis, and proximal long bones (Fig. 6). A chest X-ray often reveals pathological fractures associated with rib erosion. There is usually a background of diffuse osteoporosis, frequently with vertebral collapse. Soft tissue masses may be found, particularly in the chest where they probably arise by direct extension from the ribs.

Haematological investigations

The peripheral blood usually shows an anaemia which stems from one or more of the following causes: marrow infiltration, increased plasma volume associated with hyperviscosity, renal failure, and bleeding. The haemoglobin is less than 12 g/dl in some 60 per cent of patients and less than 8 g/dl in about 8 per cent.

Leucopenia is uncommon at presentation and in a series of over 700 cases the count was less than 4×10^9/l in only 16 per cent. Thrombocytopenia is even less frequent and counts of less than 100×10^9/l were recorded in only 13 per cent of patients. During chemotherapy both neutropenia and thrombocytopenia are more common and this is also the case in the rare aggressive type of myeloma characterized by peripheral blood invasion (plasma-cell leukaemia). Neutropenia and thrombocytopenia, if not attributable to chemotherapy, may herald the development of acute leukaemia which is being seen with increasing frequency in patients being treated for myeloma.

The presence of a circulating paraprotein is often indicated by the bluish staining protein background of the blood film, together with marked rouleaux formation. The tendency to develop rouleaux may cause difficulties in cross-matching blood for transfusion.

A high ESR is often the first pointer to the diagnosis of myeloma but it is not invariably raised and is less than 20 mm/hour in some 10 per cent of patients (most of whom suffer from light chain disease). If raised, the actual level of the ESR is of no additional significance.

The bone marrow usually shows a diffuse infiltration with plasma cells, although sometimes these tend to occur in clumps. To make a definite diagnosis it is generally accepted that there should be more than 10–15 per cent of plasma cells present. The mean number in some series is about 30 per cent but in many cases the myeloma cells dominate the picture. These cells are typically slightly larger than normal plasma cells and differ from them in that their nuclear chromatin is relatively poorly condensed and the cytoplasm is paler. Bi- and trinucleate forms may be seen although this is not diagnostic of myeloma. Other abnormalities which may be encountered in a minority of cases include areas of cytoplasmic eosinophilia ('flaming' cells) and a variety of cytoplasmic and nuclear inclusions.

The diagnosis of myeloma is usually readily made on the basis of the marrow aspirate which is positive in over 90 per cent of cases. False negative or equivocal samples are usually accounted for by the fact that the patient is at an early stage of the disease or because the aspirate is hypoplastic. A polyclonal reactive plasmacytosis, e.g. in cases of rheumatoid arthritis, may occasionally suggest the diagnosis of myeloma. However, the cytological features of reactive plasma cells should enable them to be recognized. If necessary the monoclonal nature of a plasma cell infiltrate may be demonstrated by immunocytochemical staining with heavy and light chain specific antisera. The lack of other clinical and laboratory features of myeloma, e.g. bone erosions, serum or urine paraproteins, and suppression of other immunoglobulin levels will enable most cases of reactive plasmacytosis to be distinguished from true myeloma.

Measurement of serum immunoglobulin levels

A variety of different patterns may be obtained in myelomatosis when serum immunoglobulin levels are measured (Table 5). These patterns are accounted for both by the presence of a paraprotein which causes a high reading for the relevant immunoglobulin class and by immune paresis which depresses Ig values.

Serum electrophoresis on cellulose acetate or agarose reveals a homogeneous band migrating in the γ- or β-globulin regions (Fig. 4). Suppression of normal immunoglobulins (immune paresis) is often visible on electrophoresis and may provide an important clue in distinguishing myeloma from benign paraproteinaemia, in which immune paresis is usually absent.

Light chains are not usually visible as a paraprotein in the serum

Table 5 Patterns of serum immunoglobulin levels in different immuno-chemical classes of myeloma

Table 5 Patterns of serum immunoglobulin levels in different immuno-chemical classes of myeloma

Myeloma class	Serum immunoglobulin levels		
	IgG	IgA	IgM
IgG	Raised	Low	Low
IgA	Low	Raised	Low
IgD	Low	Low	Low
Light chain disease	Low	Low	Low

Table 6 Common therapeutic regimes used in treating myeloma

	Continuous treatment	Intermittent treatment
Cyclophosphamide	150 mg/day or 2–3 mg/kg daily	600–1000 mg/m² i.v. or 250 mg/m² for 4 days orally every 3–4 weeks
Melphalan	1–4 mg/day orally	5–10 mg/day orally for 4–7 days every 4–6 weeks
Melphalan + prednisolone		As above, plus 40 mg/day prednisolone during each course
Chlorambucil	1–3 mg/day orally	
BCNU		150 mg/m² i.v. every 4–6 weeks

Note: Blood counts should be monitored at weekly intervals and the dosage reduced or interval between courses prolonged if the granulocyte count is $<1 \times 10^9$/l and/or the platelet count is $<100 \times 10^9$/l when the next course is due. As with all chemotherapy, a haematological chart should be kept to monitor progress.

Where renal impairment is present after hydration, the initial dosage of drugs (with the exception of prednisolone) should be halved and increased with care in subsequent courses.

on electrophoresis unless renal function is severely impaired. Urine electrophoresis is essential for their detection. It may be necessary to concentrate the urine sample 200-fold in order to detect low levels of light chain excretion.

Immuno-electrophoresis of serum and urine samples against specific anti-Ig antisera allows the heavy and light chain class of the paraproteins to be ascertained. However, care is necessary in interpreting the results of this investigation since there are a number of artefactual causes for a negative or weak precipitin reaction. A particularly common cause of confusion is the presence of small amounts of polyclonal serum Ig in the urine. This material may react more weakly with one anti-light chain antiserum than with the other (usually because these antisera are raised against free rather than bound light chains). This may be erroneously interpreted as representing the presence of free monoclonal light chains in the urine. Since urinary monoclonal light chain excretion is virtually diagnostic of a B cell neoplasm, a report of light chain excretion in the absence of other clinical and laboratory abnormalities should be interpreted with caution.

Biochemical investigations

Hypercalcaemia is found in 25–50 per cent of myeloma patients at presentation and is related to the extent of skeletal destruction. Symptoms may be absent, however, and in at least a proportion of patients this may be accounted for by binding of calcium to the serum paraprotein. Alkaline phosphatase levels are usually normal; high levels are usually accounted for either by healing of a pathological fracture or occasionally by amyloid liver damage.

Blood urea and creatinine levels are elevated in approximately 50 per cent of myeloma patients, reflecting renal impairment. Some automatic analysers give erroneously high urea readings in the presence of a paraprotein and the laboratory should be warned and if necessary use a manual technique. Serum uric acid levels are often also elevated probably because of renal damage rather than myeloma cell breakdown, although the latter may be a major factor at the initiation of chemotherapy.

A low serum sodium and/or a reduced anion gap is encountered in the minority of myeloma patients. These abnormalities are probably related to a decrease in plasma water secondary to a high serum protein level and also to retention of chloride and/or bicarbonate in compensation for a paraprotein.

There is often a reduction in serum albumin, and increased levels of β_2 microglobulin which may reflect rapid cell turnover and worse prognosis. The plasma viscosity may be elevated, usually in cases of IgA or IgM myeloma.

Investigation for amyloid

If amyloid is suspected as a complication of myeloma, rectal biopsy may provide confirmatory evidence.

Treatment

There is still some doubt as to whether the patient in whom the diagnosis has been made by chance requires active treatment. In some cases it may be difficult to decide initially whether the patient has a benign paraproteinaemia or myeloma, and it is therefore justified to wait and see whether the paraprotein level rises progressively.

Solitary plasmacytomas may be treated by radiotherapy and in a

proportion an apparent cure is achieved. However, the majority will subsequently develop disseminated disease and they should therefore be followed-up carefully.

In the symptomatic patient for whom chemotherapy is indicated the most important factor to establish at the time of diagnosis is the degree of renal failure. If renal failure is present, and particularly if it is associated with hypercalcaemia, energetic hydration is essential. In many patients raising the fluid intake up to 3 litres per day may improve renal function dramatically.

Dehydration is a potent factor in producing an exacerbation of the renal disease and special care should be taken not to dehydrate the patient for any investigative procedures, e.g. intravenous pyelography. Allopurinol should be started before any chemotherapy in patients with elevated uric acid levels.

Chemotherapy

Two alkylating agents, melphalan and cyclophosphamide, are the principal drugs used. The aim is to reduce the total tumour mass, with resultant reduction in the paraprotein and relief of symptoms. Treatment is certainly beneficial in many cases but it is rare for all evidence of disease, e.g. marrow infiltration, to be eradicated.

Cyclophosphamide and melphalan have been given both in intermittent dose regimens and continuously at lower dosages. Controlled trials have failed to establish clearly the superiority of any particular schedule, although intermittent dosage appears to lead to more rapid response than continuous therapy. A number of multiple drug regimens have been introduced, e.g. a combination of vincristine, adriamycin, cyclophosphamide, and prednisolone. The aim of this more aggressive form of therapy has been both to increase the proportion of responding patients and also to reduce the tumour cell mass to a greater degree and thereby to prolong the period of subsequent remission.

The value of multiple chemotherapeutic regimens is not clearly established, however. On the basis of existing evidence the most appropriate therapy for a newly diagnosed symptomatic case of myeloma is treatment with intermittent melphalan (see Table 6). Patients who show no evidence of clinical response after at least three courses of treatment may be switched to a multiple drug schedule.

All chemotherapy should be carefully monitored by regular blood counts, and the dosage reduced or intervals between courses lengthened if there is evidence of bone marrow suppression. The blood counts should be charted and the level of paraprotein regularly monitored, both in the serum and urine.

A favourable response should result in gradual reduction in the paraprotein. About one sixth of the patients fail to respond but the remainder show a reduction in the paraprotein level of variable degree. As the paraprotein falls, the haemoglobin may rise and clinical symptoms improve, but the radiological appearances show much less amelioration. Recently, encouraging results have been reported using very high doses of melphalan (100–140 mg/m^2). This is followed by a prolonged period of marrow hyperplasia after which a high proportion of patients show clinical and biochemical remission. This treatment should be considered for younger patients, but requires close supervision by a specialist team.

Radiotherapy

The use of radiotherapy in solitary plasmacytomas has already been referred to but local radiotherapy plays an additional important role in the relief of bone pain in case of multiple myeloma. Localized bone lesions are often highly radiosensitive and pain may be relieved dramatically by doses of the order of 12–15 Gy (1200–1500 rad). Laminectomy for removal of an extradural mass causing spinal cord compression should be followed up by radiotherapy to the area, and later by chemotherapy.

Spontaneous fractures of the limbs at the site of a lytic lesion may heal satisfactorily with a combination of plating and radiotherapy, although some remain ununited. As an alternative to chemotherapy, some centres have advocated the use of widefield, hemi- or total body irradiation, based on the known radiosensitivity of most bone lesions. This approach appears to be well tolerated and may be especially valuable in end-stage paliation with widespread bone disease. Its possible role as initial treatment requires evaluation.

General supportive measures

The general management of the patients is extremely important. Much can be done to relieve discomfort and pain with appropriate analgesic treatment. The patient should be encouraged to remain ambulant since inactivity may exacerbate the bone disease.

Infection is always a hazard and prompt treatment is needed for any intercurrent infection. The patients should be warned about their increased susceptibility to infection so that they may seek medical attention immediately.

Anaemia may require treatment with blood transfusion, and the occasional patient who has thrombocytopenia may need platelet transfusion. Symptoms of *hyperviscosity* (page 19.204) should be treated with plasmapheresis, repeated as required.

Hypercalcaemia is usually precipitated by bed rest, infection, or dehydration. It requires urgent treatment with forced saline diuresis using frusemide, as calcium excretion closely parallels sodium excretion by the kidney. The aim should be to give 4–6 litres of saline daily, with due attention to the problems of circulatory overload. It is usual also to give corticosteroids such as prednisolone 30 mg daily, or equivalent, and consideration should be given to cytotoxic treatment for the underlying myeloma. It may take several days for the calcium level to come under control, and even longer for the patient's mental state to improve, especially if elderly. Long-term control is facilitated by early mobilization. Occasional refractory cases may respond to calcitonin or to diphosphonates, although the latter are not widely available.

Maintenance treatment

There is no general agreement as to whether treatment should be maintained indefinitely or suspended when the paraprotein has reached a plateau level and re-introduced when there is evidence of deterioration. Studies by the South West Oncology Group in America showed that the median survival for patients who had responded to treatment was unaffected by maintenance treatment given after twelve months of initial chemotherapy but a recent MRC trial suggested that there might be marginal benefit from continuing treatment.

Table 7 Prognostic factors at diagnosis in myeloma

1 Good prognosis group	Blood urea ≤ 8 mmol/l	22% of patients
	Hb > 10 g/dl Asymptomatic	
2 Intermediate group	All not in (1) or (3)	56% of patients
3 Poor prognosis group	Hb ≤ 7.5 g/dl plus restricted activity or blood urea > 10 mmol/l plus restricted activity	22% of patients

Data from *Br. J. Cancer* (1980) **42**, 831–40.

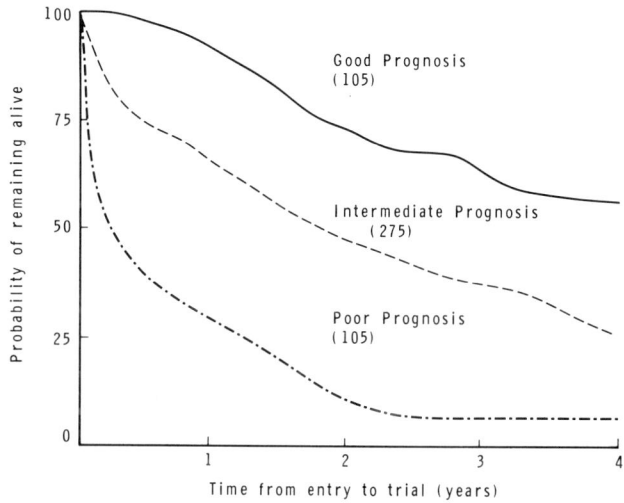

Fig. 7 Survival for patients in the prognostic groups I, II, and III. (Data from MRC trials, 1980, *Br. J. Cancer* **42**, 831–40.)

Prognosis

By the time the diagnosis of myeloma is made the abnormal clone may well have been growing for as long as 15–20 years. The rate of paraprotein production by myeloma cells in culture, together with the serum concentrations of paraprotein, has been used to estimate the size of the tumour mass in individual patients. When patients are divided into three groups with a low, high, and intermediate cell burden, the groups show a good correlation with prognosis. Thus the probability of survival for two years in the low tumour mass group has been reported in two series of patients as 76 and 85 per cent respectively, and in the high tumour mass 33 and 18 per cent.

A simpler approach has been used in the analysis of the patients included in the MRC myeloma trials. Factors present at the time of diagnosis have been analysed and three major prognostic factors have emerged, all of which are based on easily available data. The three major variables are the level of the blood urea, the haemoglobin, and the assessment of clinical disability (Table 7). The difference in prognosis in these three groups is shown in Fig. 7. The probability of surviving for two years is 76, 50, and 9 per cent in groups 1, 2, and 3 respectively.

It is clear that in assessing therapeutic trials, knowledge of the proportion of patients in the different sub-groups is essential before any proper comparisons can be made.

Sooner or later the patient's condition escapes from control. In some cases this is heralded by a sharp increase in the level of serum paraprotein. In a few patients light chain excretion unaccompanied by an increase in serum paraproteins may re-appear, or be observed for the first time in the disease, a phenomenon

Disorders of the blood

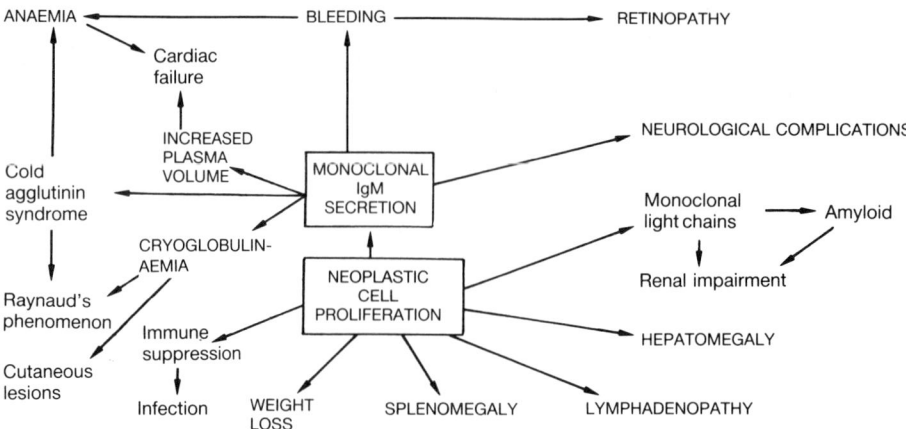

Fig. 8 Summary of the clinico-pathological features of Waldenström's macroglobulinaemia. The more important clinical features are printed in capitals.

which is thought to represent the emergence of a biochemically more primitive neoplastic clone ('Bence–Jones escape').

In a minority of patients there is a rapid terminal deterioration associated with the development of a acute myeloid leukaemia or an anaplastic lymphoid neoplasm, sometimes referred to as plasma cell reticulosarcoma. It is not clear how far the use of alkylating agents can be implicated in this terminal malignant phase. Supportive therapy in the form of blood and platelet transfusions is indicated, but aggressive chemotherapy is unjustified as the condition is resistant to treatment.

Death is ultimately due to one or other of the complications of the myeloma, particularly renal disease, infection, hyperviscosity or haemorrhage, all of which become increasingly frequent when the myeloma has escaped from control.

Waldenström's macroglobulinaemia

This disorder is named after the Swedish physician who first described it as a possible new syndrome in 1944. It is also referred to as 'primary macroglobulinaemia'. The condition affects mainly elderly subjects, and about two-thirds of the patients are male.

Clinical features (Fig. 8)

While many patients are asymptomatic, others complain of general tiredness and weakness. Evidence of bleeding particularly epistaxis and purpura, is common. Visual disturbance and neurological symptoms, particularly confusion which may progress to coma, may result from increased plasma viscosity. The latter may also cause great expansion of the plasma volume and consequent cardiac failure. Raynaud's phenomenon may also be a feature, particularly when the macroglobulin precipitates at low temperatures (cryoglobulinaemia). In these circumstances, the actual level of paraprotein may be underestimated unless care is taken to maintain the specimen at 37 °C from the time it is taken until the sample is analysed.

There may be no abnormal physical signs, particularly in the asymptomatic patients, but spleen and liver enlargement are found in about one-third of the subjects and there is often some lymphadenopathy. Examination of the fundi may show dilated tortuous vessels, clumping of erythrocytes and consequent appearance of segregation in the dilated vessels. Retinal haemorrhage may be a sequel to these changes. These signs and associated neurological symptoms constitute the hyperviscosity syndrome (see page 23.3).

Haematological abnormalities

Anaemia is often a feature and is, at least in part, due to haemodilution. Leucocytosis is uncommon but a relative lymphocytosis is usual. Thrombocytopenia is rare. Examination of a blood film may show marked rouleaux formation and protein staining in the background. The paraprotein may possess anti-red cell activity leading to auto-agglutination.

The bone marrow may be somewhat hypoplastic and difficult to obtain but it often shows an infiltration with pleomorphic cells which vary in morphology from small lymphocytes to plasma cells. These cells can be shown by immunological typing to belong to the same neoplastic clone as the peripheral lymphocytes.

Lymph node biopsy

In patients in whom the dominant symptom is lymphadenopathy the provisional diagnosis of lymphoma may have been made and the first tissue to be biopsied is a lymph node. The histological appearances are characteristic, showing diffuse infiltration with lymphoid cells which infiltrate through the capsule of the node. These cells show a limited degree of plasmacytic differentiation and frequently contain PAS positive cytoplasmic and intranuclear inclusions. Mast cells may be prominent. However, it should be noted that these histological appearances may occasionally be found in the absence of a serum paraprotein. In at least a proportion of such cases, IgM of a single light chain class is detectable in the neoplastic cells by immunocytochemical techniques. This picture may represent 'non-secretory' Waldenström's macroglobulinaemia.

Paraprotein production

The paraprotein is classically IgM in type although very occasionally the typical clinical and histological features of Waldenström's macroglobulinaemia may be associated with the presence of a serum IgG or IgA paraprotein. Excess free light chains may be produced by the neoplastic cells but renal damage is much less common than in myeloma. The plasma viscosity may be elevated.

Abnormalities of haemostasis

The haemorrhagic symptoms are associated with a number of abnormalities. Although the platelet count may be normal, platelet function is deranged. Some of the defects appear to be related to coating of the platelets with the macroglobulin. The IgM protein may also interact with some of the labile coagulation factors to inhibit coagulation, and a severe haemorrhagic picture is sometimes produced.

Treatment

Asymptomatic patients require no treatment and the condition may remain stable for many years. However, patients should be kept under supervision with regular blood counts and serum IgM estimation. If the latter value starts to rise, and particularly if the patient becomes symptomatic, chemotherapy will have to be considered.

There are a few reported series of small numbers of patients treated with chlorambucil, melphalan, or cyclophosphamide with apparent benefit and reduction of serum viscosity and IgM. Because of the great variability in the course of the disease, however, such treatment should probably not be given in the asymptomatic phase.

If hyperviscosity is a problem, plasmapheresis is indicated and may be of great if temporary benefit.

A terminal phase of rapidly accelerating disease may occur or death may result from intercurrent infection, haemorrhage, or thrombosis.

Paraproteinaemia in association with lymphoma and lymphoid leukaemia

In most (if not all) categories of B cell lymphoproliferative disease a paraprotein may occasionally be found. The frequency is highest in cases of chronic lymphatic leukaemia and in diffuse non-Hodgkin's lymphoma. In nodular lymphoma and hairy cell leukaemia paraproteins are considerably rarer.

The explanation of the association between lymphoproliferative disease and paraproteinaemia probably lies in the fact that the neoplastic cells in many of these diseases have a limited ability to undergo terminal differentiation towards the Ig-secreting plasma cell stage. However, whilst the predominant cell type in a case of non-Hodgkin's lymphoma is clearly not plasmacytoid, there may nevertheless be a 'tail-forward' of maturation by the neoplastic clone producing a minor population of cells capable of Ig synthesis. In this context it should be appreciated that serum or urinary electrophoresis is a relatively crude procedure for the detection of the production of Ig by neoplastic B cells. If more sensitive techniques are used (e.g. biosynthetic labelling or immunocytochemical analysis of intracellular immunoglobulin), evidence of monoclonal Ig production by neoplastic B cells may be found more frequently.

Heavy chain diseases

These rare conditions are characterized by the production of free Ig heavy chains. Three types of heavy chain disease (γ, μ, and α heavy chain disease) have been described corresponding to the three major classes of immunoglobulin. Cases of δ and ε heavy chain disease have yet to be described, presumably reflecting the rarity of the corresponding classes of Ig.

The clinical features of these three disorders are relatively distinct. However, it is important to realize that there is no absolute association between the production of a particular heavy chain by neoplastic cells and a specific pattern of clinical behaviour. This is illustrated by the fact that μ chains are produced by neoplastic cells in acute lymphoblastic leukaemia of the pre-B cell type as well as in 'classical' μ chain disease. Furthermore, the typical clinical pattern of α chain disease (see below) can occasionally be associated with the production of γ chains. This lack of congruence between immunochemical and clinicopathological categories is also found in other types of paraproteinaemia (e.g. free light chain production may be found in both myeloma and non-Hodgkin's lymphoma, IgG paraproteins may be found in otherwise typical examples of Waldenström's macroglobulinaemia) and should caution us against too rigid a biochemical categorization of these disorders.

γ Chain disease

This disorder was first described in 1964: since that time less than 100 further cases have been reported.

Paraprotein

Neoplastic cells usually produce dimers of γ heavy chains, each of which is of lower molecular weight than the normal γ chain. This reflects the presence of an internal deletion in the chain, involving predominantly the variable region.

Clinical features

The typical clinical picture is that of a non-Hodgkin's lymphoma presenting with lymphadenopathy, hepatosplenomegaly, malaise, anaemia, and fever. The disease usually progresses relatively rapidly causing death from infection or disseminated malignancy within a few months of diagnosis.

Diagnosis

Marrow aspiration usually reveals an increase in plasma cells and/or lymphoplasmacytoid cells, often associated with eosinophilia. A peripheral blood count frequently shows anaemia and eosinophilia. Circulating atypical lymphocytes and plasma cells may be found.

Serum electrophoresis reveals a band in the γ or β region, which is characteristically relatively broad in distribution. On immunoelectrophoresis the band reacts with anti-gamma-antisera but not with anti-light chain reagents.

α Chain disease

This disease (see also Section 12) is the commonest of the heavy chain diseases. It predominantly affects patients of near-Eastern or Mediterranean origin (principally from Tunisia, Algeria, Iran, Spain, Israel, southern Italy, and Turkey) and is especially associated with conditions of poor hygiene.

Paraprotein

As in γ heavy chain disease the neoplastic cells in α chain disease produce an incomplete heavy chain, probably because of an internal deletion involving between a quarter and a half of the chain.

Clinical features

α Chain disease usually occurs in a setting of immunoproliferative small intestine disease, features of which include a severe malabsorption syndrome with steatorrhoea, abdominal pain, marked weight loss, and finger clubbing. Barium studies show a malabsorption pattern in the small bowel.

Diagnosis

Small bowel biopsy shows diffuse infiltration of the lamina propria with plasma and/or plasmacytoid cells, usually throughout the duodenum and jejunum, with extensive involvement of the more distal small bowel. These cells may synthesize α chain but not light chain.

Serum electrophoresis reveals a broad band in the α_2 or β region in about 50 per cent of patients, and the same protein may be seen at low concentration in the urine. Immune-electrophoresis reveals a reaction with antisera to α chain but not with anti-light chain antisera. However, the failure of some IgA paraproteins to react with anti-light chain antisera constitutes a potential cause of false diagnosis of α chain disease, and suspected samples should be referred to a specialist laboratory.

Progress and clinical management

The disease may initially run an intermittent course in which there are spontaneous periods of partial or complete symptomatic remission. In most cases, however, if untreated, the patient's clinical state will deteriorate, often terminating in the development of one or more poorly differentiated lymphomas which may cause obstruction, intussusception, or perforation. These tumours are usually classified as immunoblastic and there is evidence that they arise as mutant clones within the original proliferating cell population.

In a number of patients treatment with broad spectrum antibiotics has been followed by remission sometimes lasting for several years, prompting speculation that the proliferating plasmacytoid cells are 'driven' by micro-organisms in the small bowel. Cytotoxic therapy (chlorambucil and cyclophosphamide) have also been used in some cases. The prognosis once a lymphoma has developed, however, is poor.

μ Chain disease

This is the rarest of the heavy chain diseases, less than 20 cases having been reported. The disease resembles γ and α chain disease in that μ chain may contain a deletion, but differs in that the neoplastic cells frequently produce free light chains in addition to μ chains. The light and heavy chains do not assemble, however, to form complete IgM molecules.

Most patients have been over the age of 40 and have either resided in parasite-infected areas (e.g. the Ivory Coast) or have had a clinical picture of chronic leukaemia or anaplastic lymphoma. Characteristically plasma cells containing one to three cytoplasmic vacuoles are seen in marrow aspirate.

References

Bergsagel, D. E., Bailey, A. J., Langley, G. R., MacDonald, R. N., White, D. F. and Miller, A. B. (1979). The chemotherapy of plasma-cell myeloma and the incidence of acute leukemia. *N. Engl. J. Med.* **301**, 743–748.

Callihan, T. R., Holbert, J. M. and Berard, C. W. (1983). Neoplasms of terminal B-cell differentiation: the morphologic basis of functional diversity. In *Malignant lymphomas* (eds S. C. Sommers and P. P. Rosen), pp. 169–268. Appleton-Century-Crofts, Norwalk, Conn.

Carter, P., Koval, J. J. and Hobbs, J. R. (1977). The relation of clinical and laboratory findings to the survival of patients with macroglobulinaemia. *Clin. Exp. Immunol.* **28**, 241–249.

Cuzick, J. (1981). Radiation-induced myelomatosis. *N. Engl. J. Med.* **304**, 204–210.

Delamore, I. W. (1982). Hypercalcaemia and myeloma. *Br. J. Haemat.* **51**, 507–509.

Durie, B. G. M., Russell, D. H. and Salmon, S. E. (1980). Reappraisal of plateau phase in myeloma. *Lancet* ii, 65–68.

—— and Salmon, S. E. (1975). A clinical staging system for multiple myeloma. Correlation of measured myeloma cell mass with presenting clinical features, response to treatment, and survival. *Cancer* **36**, 842–854.

Fine, J. M., Lambin, P. and Muller, J. Y. (1979). The evolution of asymptomatic monoclonal gammopathies. A follow-up of 20 cases over a period of 3–14 years. *Acta med. Scand.* **205**, 339–341.

Hewell, G. M. and Alexanian, R. (1976). Multiple myeloma in young persons. *Ann. Intern. Med.* **84**, 441–443.

Kyle, R. A. (1975). Multiple myeloma: review of 869 cases. *Mayo Clin. Proc.* **50**, 29–40.

—— (1983). Long-term survival in multiple myeloma. *N. Engl. J. Med.* **308**, 314–316.

—— and Greipp, P. R. (1980). Smouldering multiple myeloma. *N. Engl. J. Med.* **302**, 1347–1349.

Lewin, K. J., Kahn, L. B. and Novis, B. H. (1976). Primary intestinal lymphoma of 'Western' and 'Mediterranean' type, alpha chain disease and massive plasma cell infiltration: a comparative study of 37 cases. *Cancer* **38**, 2511–2528.

MacKenzie, M. R. and Fudenberg, H. H. (1972). Macroglobulinemia: an analysis for forty patients. *Blood* **39**, 874–889.

McIntyre, O. R. (1979). Current concepts in cancer: multiple myeloma. *N. Engl. J. Med.* **301**, 193–196.

Medical Research Council Working Party on Leukaemia in Adults (1980). Prognostic features in the third MRC myelomatosis trial. *Br. J. Cancer* **42**, 831–840.

Medical Research Council Working Party on Leukaemia in Adults (1984). Analysis and management of renal failure in the fourth MRC myelomatosis trial. *Br. Med. J.* **288**, 1411–1416.

Preston, F. E., Cooke, K. B., Foster, M. E., Winfield, D. A. and Lee, D. (1978). Myelomatosis and the hyperviscosity syndrome. *Br. J. Haemat.* **38**, 517–530.

Siris, E. S., Sherman, W. H., Bacquiran, D. C., Schlatterer, J. P., Osserman, E. F. and Canfield, R. E. (1980). Effects of dichloromethylene diphosphonate on skeletal mobilization of calcium in multiple myeloma. *N. Engl. J. Med.* **302**, 310–315.

Wiltshaw, E. (1976). The natural history of extramedullary plasmacytoma and its relation to solitary myeloma of bone and myelomatosis. *Medicine (Balt.)* **55**, 217–238.

Woodruff, R. K., Wadsworth, J., Malpas, J. S. and Tobias, J. S. (1979). Clinical staging in multiple myeloma. *Br. J. Haemat.* **42**, 199–205.

Zawadzki, Z. A., Kapadia, S. and Barnes, A. E. (1978). Leukemic myelomatosis (plasma cell leukemia). *Am. J. Clin. Path.* **70**, 605–611.

Histiocytosis X

J. PRITCHARD AND V. A. BROADBENT

Introduction

The term 'histiocytosis X' (H-X) was coined in 1953 by Lichtenstein to describe a disease process with numerous clinical manifestations but a fairly uniform histopathological appearance. Until that time three separate clinical entities were recognized: *eosinophilic granuloma* was used to describe single or multiple bone lesions, *Hand–Schüller–Christian disease* to indicate the triad of exophthalmos, diabetes insipidus, and multiple bone lesions, and *Letterer–Siwe disease* to denote multiple soft-tissue involvement. In practice, there is considerable overlap between these entities and, until there is evidence to the contrary, it seems reasonable to regard them as components of a clinical spectrum. Although other names, such as '*Langerhans cell granulomatosis*', have been proposed the familiar term 'histiocytosis X' is still in common use because it aptly indicates our continuing state of ignorance concerning the pathogenesis of the disorder. Recently it has been proposed that *Langerhans cell histiocytosis* might be a more precise designation.

Incidence

Various children's 'tumour' registers suggest an incidence of 30–50 cases per year in the United Kingdom, but that is almost certainly an underestimate for the following reasons: (*a*) the disease is almost certainly underdiagnosed, mild skin involvement being mistaken, for instance, for seborrhoeic eczema (see below), (*b*) patients present to many 'organ specialists' (ENT surgeons, ophthalmologists, orthopaedic surgeons, for instance) and notification is not, of course, obligatory, and (*c*) adult cases are not taken into account. The true incidence is probably well over 100 cases per annum.

Histopathology

Whatever organ is involved, the light microscopic appearance of H-X infiltrates is characterized by the presence of histiocytes and 'small round cells' in various proportions together with differing numbers of eosinophils (Fig. 1). The appearance of the histiocytes varies but they have no unequivocal features of malignancy and, more importantly, there appears to be no correlation between the histological grading of a biopsy and the clinical course of the disease. Electron microscopy, by revealing characteristic inclusion 'granules' (Birkbeck granules, Fig. 2) in the histiocytes, can be extremely helpful in identifying the cells as Langerhans cells; less 'differentiated' cells may, however, contain few or no granules. Immunohistochemical studies reveal that Langerhans cells stain positively with anti-Ia, peanut agglutinin, S-100, OKT4, and OKT6 antibodies. The enzymes α-mannosidase, ATPase, and acid phosphatase are positive in Langerhans cells and can be helpful in diagnosis.

Pathogenesis

The cause of H-X is unknown, but clinical and histopathological features virtually rule out a malignant process. No infective agent has ever been identified. Though standard immunological tests (serum immunoglobulin levels, PHA response) are invariably normal, a relative deficiency of suppressor (OKT8 positive) lymphocytes has been demonstrated in the blood of patients with

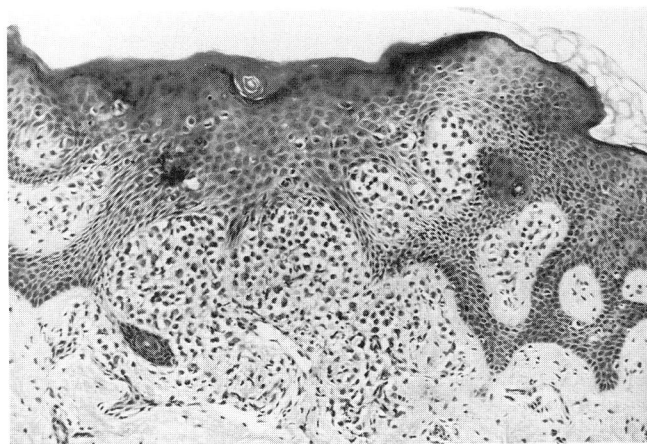

Fig. 1 Biopsy from skin involved by H-X. The infiltrate of histiocytes, eosinophils, and lymphocytes traverses the dermo-epidermal junction. In this case, the rash resolved spontaneously (H and E stain, × 125).

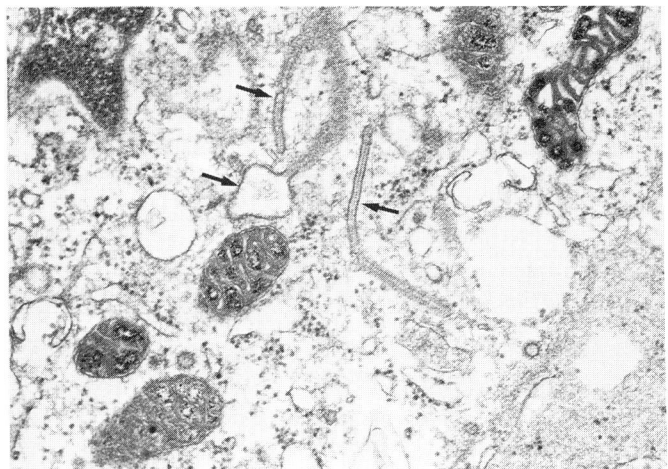

Fig. 2 Electron microphotograph showing Birbeck 'granules' (arrows) in Langerhans cells from an H-X skin infiltrate. The 'tennis racket' head and trilaminar structure of the racket 'handles' is clearly seen.

multisystem H-X. Some of these patients also had evidence of partial thymic atrophy and a primary immunodeficiency state was postulated. Despite evidence that suppressor cell numbers increased after *in vitro* incubation of blood with a crude thymic hormone preparation ('thymosin'), neither 'thymosin' nor synthetic thymic hormone preparations have been effective in clinical trials. Currently, research attention is turning to the histiocytes themselves, especially Langerhans cells. It seems likely that the underlying abnormality is one of faulty intercellular communication, perhaps because of abnormalities in production of lymphokines or other growth factors.

Clinical manifestations

General features

Sites of disease presentation vary enormously and, as a result, symptoms can vary. Table 1 lists the presenting symptoms of 30 children presenting to one large children's hospital over a three year period. Clinical features in adults are similar. The disease can present in the newborn period and in the elderly, but the peak age is around 2–4 years. Boys seem to be affected rather more frequently than girls (M:F 1.5–2:1) but with the same degree of severity. In 75 per cent of patients, many organs are obviously affected at presentation (multisystem disease); in the remainder only one organ or organ system is involved (single-system disease)

Table 1 Presenting symptoms of 30 children with histiocytosis X*

Symptom	Number
Skin rash	15
Recurrent aural discharge	8
Bone pain	5
Scalp lump(s)	5
Proptosis	4
Failure to thrive	3
Breathlessness	3
Lymphadenopathy	2
Hepatosplenomegaly	1
Spinal cord compression	1

* Numbers add up to more than 30 as some children had multiple symptoms.

though detailed investigation may reveal occult multisystem disease. Some 20–30 per cent of affected children grow poorly, falling below the tenth centile for height and weight. The cause is often multifactorial, the result of (*a*) a chronic disease process, (*b*) loss of height of involved vertebrae, (*c*) corticosteroid therapy, and (*d*) rarely, growth hormone deficiency.

Specific organs

Symptom frequency is given in Table 1: in this section, organ systems are listed alphabetically.

Bone marrow and blood The degree of bone marrow infiltration varies from zero to near-total replacement by H-X cells. Marrow trephines are a more sensitive test than aspirates, though α-D-mannosidase staining may help to reveal occasional invading cells in bone marrow smears. Evidence of bone marrow failure occurs where involvement is extensive and is manifest by anaemia, leucopenia (neutrophils are usually more profoundly affected than lymphocytes), and low platelet counts. Perhaps because bone marrow failure is often a preterminal event, resultant infections are unusual; bleeding is more common, especially into involved tissues, e.g. skin as purpura.

Although some authors have claimed that monocytosis, seen in some patients, represents dissemination into the bloodstream there has not, as yet, been an unequivocal demonstration of H-X cells circulating in the blood.

Bones Any bone may be affected (see Fig. 3) but, whereas involvement of the small bones of the hand and foot is rare, there seems to be an especial predilection for the bones of the skull. Lesions are typically lytic and it can be assumed that factors with bone-resorbing activity are released by H-X cells. Especially in young children, florid periosteal reaction to a lesion may mimic a malignant tumour. H-X deposits heal with a margin of sclerosis. In some patients, lesions of various 'ages' can be seen simultaneously.

Less than half of bone lesions are painful; invasion into adjacent tissues leads to the appearance of a soft-tissue swelling, a more common mode of presentation. Pathological fractures occur, but are unusual, and may provoke healing.

Ears Aural discharge can be the result either of otitis externa, when adjacent skin involvement extends into the external auditory canal, or of disease extension from the mastoid into the middle ear. The process is usually painless but troublesome aural discharge is common, with accompanying partial deafness. Secondary bacterial infection occurs frequently.

Eyes The reason why the H-X process favours the retro-orbital regions is unknown but proptosis is a relatively common manifestation of the disease. Usually a lytic lesion is present in the orbital wall, and the proptosis is due to soft tissue extension. Occasionally optic nerve function may be so compromised that emergency radiation therapy is needed but in most cases, because the orbital

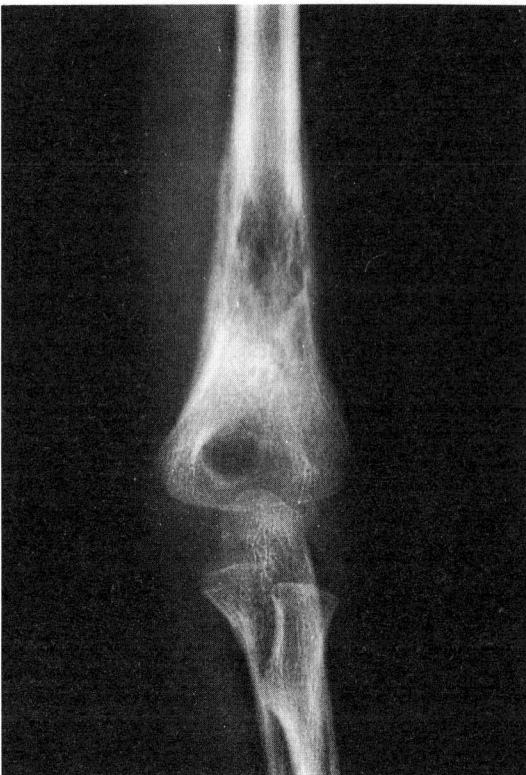

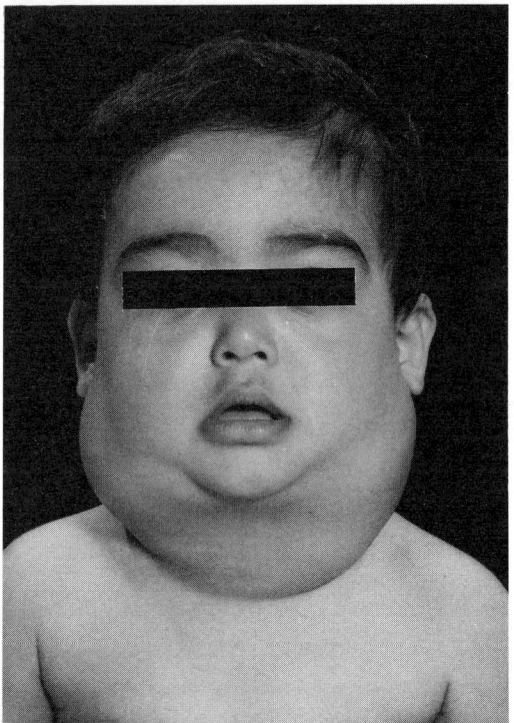

Fig. 4 Massive cervical lymphadenopathy due to H-X. Note the child's good general condition.

Fig. 3 Osteolytic lesion of the humerus in a five-year-old boy presenting with a painful arm. When the periosteal reaction is as florid as this, the differential diagnosis includes osteomyelitis and malignancy, especially Ewings sarcoma.

mass is usually extraconal, vision is unaffected. Other neuro-ophthalmic complications, such as optic or oculomotor neuropathies and papilloedema, and direct infiltration of intra-ocular structures such as the uveal tract and retina do occur but are very rare.

Liver and spleen The liver can be directly involved by the H-X process, resulting in hepatomegaly and, in more severe instances, jaundice and other evidence of liver failure such as hypoalbuminaemia and decreased synthesis of clotting factors. A distinct second entity must, however, be considered in H-X patients whose liver disease seems disproportionately severe: a histopathologically distinct form of hepatic fibrosis, which occurs almost exclusively in association with H-X, has been described. There is little follow-up information on this condition, nor is its aetiology understood, but fibrosis is usually severe and the prognosis, therefore, very guarded. Distortion of bile ducts can occur and lead to biliary stasis and obstructive jaundice.

Splenic enlargement is almost invariably due to infiltration by H-X but can also be a manifestation of portal hypertension in patients with severe liver disease. The incidence of 'hypersplenism' is uncertain because in most patients with pancytopenia heavy bone marrow infiltration and splenomegaly coincide, making it difficult to determine the relative contribution of the two organs.

Lungs and airways If lung function tests are used as criteria, involvement of lung parenchyma is relatively frequent, but pulmonary symptoms and signs occur in less than 10 per cent of patients. Functional abnormalities, indicating small 'stiff' lungs with reduced thoracic gas volume, decreased compliance and increased pulmonary resistance, may precede radiological changes. Spontaneous pneumothorax results when a lung cyst, represented by the honeycomb X-ray changes so characteristic of H-X, ruptures into the pleural cavity. Exercise intolerance, cough, and chest pain are unusual. In the sick febrile patient care must be

taken to distinguish X-ray changes that are the result of the primary disease process from those of a complicating infection, such as *Pneumocystis carinii*, cytomegalovirus or measles, especially in patients receiving immunosuppressive therapy. Upper airway obstruction due to tracheal infiltration has been reported.

Lymph-nodes The exact incidence of node involvement is difficult to establish but its severity can certainly vary. Regional lymphadenopathy is more common than generalized enlargement. Occasionally massive adenopathy (Fig. 4) can cause obstructive symptoms. Nodes are usually painless. Occasionally suppuration, mimicking infection, occurs; cultures are negative and the discharging necrotic material presumably consists of the degenerate contents of indolent lesions.

Mouth and gastrointestinal tract Early oral infiltration may be manifest by a 'granular' appearance of the buccal mucosa, or by thickening of the gingivae. Sometimes, by contrast, involvement may be so severe that ulceration occurs; exceptionally a palatal fistula may develop. Severe dental involvement may occur in the absence of lytic lesions in the mandible and maxilla and is presumably the consequence of direct invasion from involved oral mucosa. In infants teeth may erupt prematurely. Loss of the dental lamina dura is a typical radiological feature (Fig. 5); in severe cases, gum retraction and erosion of dental alveoli may cause loosening of teeth. Involvement of the lower gastrointestinal tract is probably underestimated. Malabsorption has occasionally been described but clinically significant involvement of the oesophagus, stomach, and colon has not.

Pituitary and brain: diabetes insipidus Around one-third of patients develop diabetes insipidus, one half as a presenting feature and the other half subsequently. A pituitary origin is evident from the prompt and complete responsiveness to exogenous antidiuretic hormone (ADH). X-ray abnormalities in the region of the pituitary fossa and adjacent skull base are present in only a minority of cases, making it unlikely that direct invasion from an adjacent bony lesion is responsible. If a local deposit is responsible, some very specific 'homing' signal must be involved. Recent

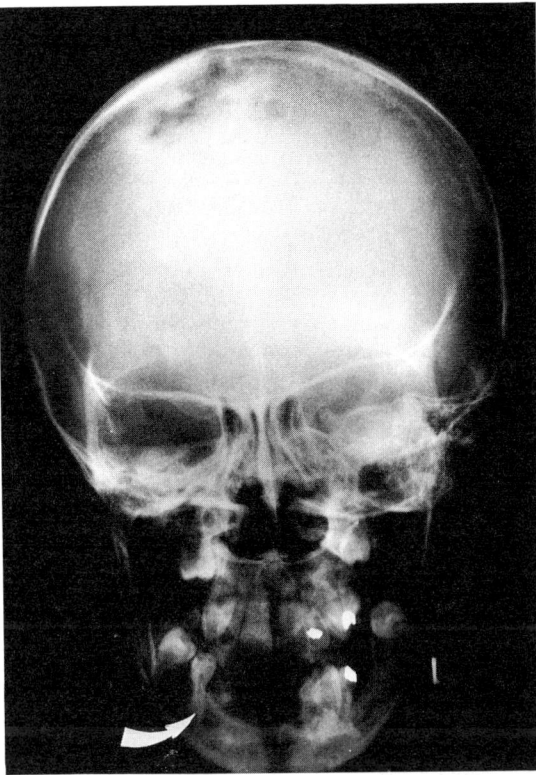

Fig. 5 Loss of dental lamina dura (arrow) resulting from bone destruction in the mandible: as a result, teeth may be lost prematurely. Lytic lesions are also seen in the skull vault.

CAT scanning and autopsy studies suggest that histiocyte infiltration of the pituitary stalk and/or gland is relatively common and presumably the cause of diabetes insipidus. Although diabetes insipidus remits in some patients, in most it appears to be a long-term, perhaps permanent, complication even when disease at other sites responds to therapy. Involvement of the posterior lobe of the pituitary gland is relatively specific; growth hormone (GH) deficiency has been recorded occasionally but only in association with diabetes insipidus. Deficiencies of other anterior pituitary hormones are extremely rare.

Meningeal infiltration has been reported in patients with widely disseminated disease but involvement of the brain itself is exceptional. Sometimes there may be direct intracranial extension of a lesion in the skull. Spinal cord compression, when it occurs, is invariably due to a soft tissue extension from an intact or collapsed vertebral body.

Skin Infiltration by H-X has a characteristic distribution (Fig. 6) with a predisposition for the mid-line trunk, especially the back, as well as the groin, napkin area, scalp, and postauricular areas. Frequently, there is a history of cradle-cap since birth. These features may have previously led to a mistaken diagnosis of seborrhoeic eczema.

Individual lesions are 1–5 mm brownish-pink maculopapules. In patients with apparently normal skin, these lesions should be diligently searched for, especially over the back. In severe cases, the rash can be confluent in some areas with ulceration. When the platelet count is <20 x 10^9/1 because of bone marrow involvement or hypersplenism, the rash may become haemorrhagic.

Rarely, skin ulceration from an underlying localized lesion in bone or lymph-node can occur (Fig. 7). Xanthelasmata are occasionally present.

Other organs Muscles including the heart, endocrine glands, excepting the pituitary, kidneys, and gonads are the only organs that regularly seem to escape involvement.

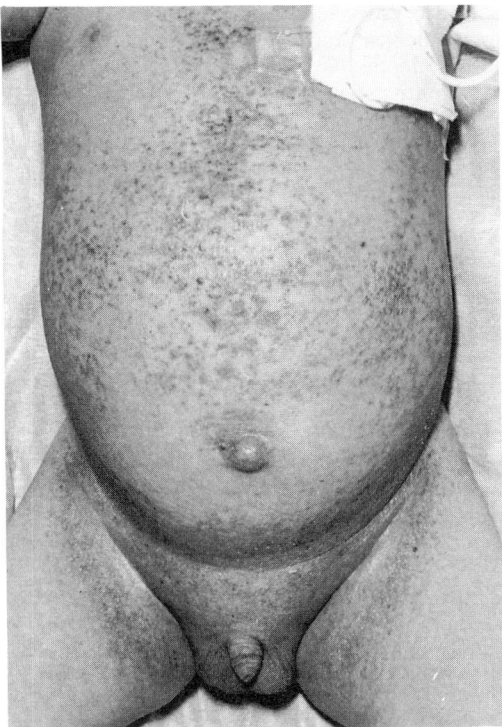

Fig. 6 Skin infiltration of characteristic distribution. Individual lesions are raised brownish-pink maculopapules. The rash is confluent in the groins and there are haemorrhagic areas on the anterior abdominal wall.

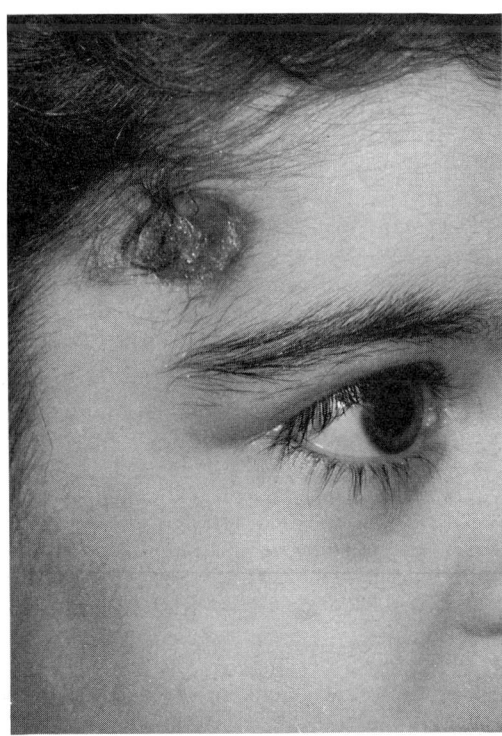

Fig. 7 Skin ulceration from an underlying bony lesion of the skull. This three-year-old girl also had diabetes insipidus but no other evidence of H-X.

Differential diagnosis

Especially when clinical presentation is unusual, delay in diagnosis is more commonly the result of failure to consider H-X as a possibility than of difficulty in distinguishing it from other conditions.

In the majority of cases an exact diagnosis can be made from standard histopathological studies with electron microscopy and histochemical and immunohistological techniques as adjuncts. In infants with multisystem involvement, differentiation from familial erythrophagocytic reticulosis (lymphohistiocytosis) may be difficult. Malignant histiocytosis (histiocyte medullary reticulosis), which occurs more commonly in adults than in children, has some clinical features – skin rash, node enlargement, hepatosplenomegaly, and pancytopenia – in common with H-X. Its relentlessly progressive nature is usually apparent, however, and histopathological appearances differ from those of H-X. In patients with massive cervical lymph-node enlargement, massive *sinus histiocytosis (the Rosai–Dorfman syndrome)* should be considered. In children with skin disease, the various forms of *juvenile (naevoid) xanthogranuloma* should be excluded.

Investigation and staging

Initial investigation should include full blood count, liver function tests with serum albumen, prothrombin time and partial thromboplastin time, chest radiographs, skeletal survey, bone marrow aspirate and trephine, lung function tests, and early morning urine osmolality.

A number of elaborate staging systems have been devised. Although such objective criteria may facilitate comparison of treatment results between centres, it is not clear that assignation of a stage is helpful in determining management of a particular patient, or in assessing prognosis. In practice, organ failure seems to be a more important prognostic factor than organ involvement; bone marrow failure, manifested by pancytopenia, and liver failure are particularly ominous.

Management

General principles

Ignorance of the pathogenesis of H-X preludes a scientifically rational approach to treatment but clinical observation and clinical trials have led to development of moderately effective measures.

Now that the disease is no longer regarded as a malignancy, the therapeutic strategy is a good deal more conservative than in the past; 'aggressive' chemotherapy, because of its immediate and delayed toxicity, is contraindicated.

Single-system disease

When H-X is apparently limited to one system it is the skeleton that is most often involved. Spontaneous resolution (Fig. 1) often occurs and a period of observation is appropriate unless the function of a vital structure (e.g. optic nerve or spinal cord) is threatened or if there is pain that cannot be controlled by simple analgesics. Intralesional corticosteroid injections [50–100 mg hydrocortisone (Solucortef[R]], repeated 2–3 times at 2–3 weekly intervals if necesary, are often effective when active intervention is needed. Rare soft tissue lesions are managed in a similar way, though intralesional injections are sometimes impractical. Because of the risk of induction of 'second tumours', radiation therapy should be used only when a site of disease is inaccessible to the needle or when vital organs (e.g. optic nerve or spinal cord) are threatened, and the dose should not exceed 10 Gy.

Multisystem disease

Spontaneous resolution can occur and an initial period of observation may be appropriate. Indications for systemic therapy are listed in Table 2. Agents active against cancer are generally used and responses are often impressive but published data suggest that steroids alone are as effective as 'cytotoxic' drugs, even when these are used in combination. By contrast there is strong evidence that 'aggressive' combination drug regimes are associated with a higher complication rate. Thus a relatively conservative approach is indicated. In most patients, there is response to daily prednisolone 2 mg/kg; after an arbitrary four weeks' induction therapy, and depending on the quality of the response, the regime can be modified with the intent of controlling disease by the smal-

Table 2 Indications for systemic therapy in multisystem histiocytosis X

Systemic symptoms – failure to thrive, fever, misery
Discomfort – especially if from multiple sources
Organ 'failure' – especially liver, bone marrow, lungs, reticulo-endothelial system

lest possible dose of steroids, and preferably none at all. If maintenance treatment is needed, alternate day administration is preferable so that there is less-than-complete suppression of adrenal function. In children, growth failure and immunosuppression are the most worrying features of chronic steroid therapy and diabetes mellitus, osteoporosis, and hypertension are uncommon.

When response to corticosteroids is unsatisfactory, a vinca alkaloid can be added. Vincristine (1.5 mg/M^2 (0.05 mg/kg for infants < 6 months), weekly for 4–6 weeks, then 2–3 weekly for a variable period) is preferred to vinblastine because vincristine is the less myelotoxic. There is some evidence that epipodophyllotoxin VP 16 (etoposide) is effective in some instances where disease is steroid resistant; the suggested dosage is 150 mg/M^2 (5 mg/kg for infants < 6 months) daily × three intravenously or 300 mg/M^2 (10 mg/kg for infants < 6 months) daily × three orally, every 3–4 weeks. Claims that methotrexate, cyclophosphamide, and 6-mercaptopurine are active agents in steroid-resistant H-X have not yet been substantiated.

Other measures may be helpful where specific organ systems are involved. The symptoms of diabetes insipidus are completely reversed by administration of DDAVP (a synthetic form of antidiuretic hormone) intranasally (5 μg b.d. or t.d.s.). Potassium permanganate soaks are helpful topically in the management of an ulcerated skin rash. Ung coco oil, followed by washing with a keratolytic shampoo, can be helpful in the removal of crusted lesions from the scalp; topical steroid lotion is then applied to inflamed areas. Topical nitrogen mustard can be very effective where other methods have failed to control skin rash, but expert dermatologic advice is needed. Steroid eardrops (Predsol[R]) can reduce the volume of discharge from otitis externa and antibiotics are indicated when secondary infection of the middle or external ear is suspected or proven. If gingival involvement is severe, surgical curettage can be helpful and may also reduce the incidence of later dental complications. Where the lungs are involved, and the patient is immunosuppressed, regular septrin (co-trimoxazole) should be considered as prophyllaxis against *P. carinii*. Pleurodesis may be needed for recurrent pneumothorax.

Response and outcome

The prognosis for patients with single-system disease is uniformly good. Progression to multisystem involvement is rare and mortality is close to zero. Some 10–20 per cent of patients develop chronic problems but there is a tendency for disease to 'burn itself out' over 1–5 years.

Patients with multisystem H-X fare less well, but the prognosis is better than some publications suggest. In a few patients spontaneous regression occurs. Almost all those receiving systemic therapy show some response. In most patients symptomatic and objective improvement is marked, sometimes with reversal of organ failure. Infections, including those with opportunistic organisms, are common treatment-related complications, especially with the more aggressive chemotherapy regimens.

Overall, 20–30 per cent of patients enter sustained complete remission and about 10 per cent, especially those who present with or develop organ failure, die. The remaining 60–70 per cent enter a chronic disease phase, with involvement of new organ systems in some cases. During this phase, problems include chronic discharging ears, deafness, lymph-node 'suppuration', recurrent pneumothorax, and dental and orthopaedic problems. Diabetes insipidus is usually permanent and growth hormone deficiency can occur.

The effects of chronic disease on the child and the family should not be underestimated. When proptosis and a skin rash are severe, the appearance of the child may be so grotesque as to lead to a degree of social rejection, compounding the child's sense of inadequacy that is an inevitable result of the physical abnormalities. During follow-up, consideration should be given to these problems as well as to specific medical complications.

References

Broadbent, V. and Pritchard, J. (1985). Histiocytosis-X – current controversies. *Arch. Dis. Childh.* **60**, 605–607.

Broadbent, V., Pritchard, J., Davies, E. G., Levinsky, R. J., Heaf, D., Atherton, D. J., Pincott, J. R. and Tucker, S. (1984). Spontaneous remission of multi-system histiocytosis X. *Lancet* 253–254.

Greenberger, J. S., Crocker, A. C., Vawter, G., Jaffe, N. and Cassady, J. R. (1981). Results of treatment of 127 patients with systemic histiocytosis (Letterer–Siwe syndrome, Schüller–Christian syndrome and multifocal eosinophilic granuloma). *Medicine* **60**, 311–338.

Groopman, J. E. and Golde, D. W. (1981). The histiocytic disorders – a pathophysiologic analysis. *Ann. intern. Med.* **94**, 95–107.

Komp, D. M. (1981). Long-term sequelae of histiocytosis X. *Am. J. Ped. Hemat./Onc.* **3**, 165–168.

Le Blanc, A., Hadchoel, M., Jehan, P., Odiévre, M. and Alagille, A. (1984). Obstructive jaundice in children with histiocytosis X. *Gastroenterology* **80**, 134–139.

Lichtenstein, L. (1953). Integration of eosinophilic granuloma of bone, Letterer-Siwe disease and Schüller-Christian disease as related in manifestations of a single nosologic entity. *Arch. Path.* **56**, 84–102.

Moore, A. T., Pritchard, J. and Taylor, D. S. I. (1985) Histiocytosis X, an ophthalmological review. *Br. J. Ophthalmol.* **69**, 7–14.

Nezelof, C. (1979). Histiocytosis X: a histological and histogenetic study. *Perspect. Paed. Pathol.* **5**, 153–178.

Smith, D. G., Nesbit, Jr, M. E., D'Angio, G. J. and Levitt, S. H. (1973). Histiocytosis X: role of radiation therapy in management with special reference to dose levels employed. *Radiology* **106**, 419–422.

HAEMOSTASIS AND THROMBOSIS

J. A. DAVIES AND E. G. D. TUDDENHAM

Introduction

Haemostasis may be defined as the sum of processes which lead to the arrest of haemorrhage. These processes are surface activated and are initiated by the contact of blood platelets and of plasma coagulation factors with subendothelial tissue. The endothelium of blood vessels is uniquely adapted to present to blood a non-reactive surface that also actively opposes haemostatic reactions. The smallest breach in the continuous lining of vascular endothelial cells, however, presents a surface on which coagulation and platelet aggregation will commence.

A highly responsive mechanism is clearly needed in order that a breach through which blood may be flowing out of a vessel under high pressure can be rapidly sealed. The mechanisms that have evolved to ensure rapid sealing are characterized by molecular and cellular amplification of small initial signals. The factors involved circulate in a precursor, non-reactive form which, upon surface contact, sequentially activate each other, with dramatic multiplicative enhancement. Such a system is inherently unstable and requires containment by inhibitors, negative feedback loops, and enzymic dissolution of coagulum to prevent the disastrous consequences of blocking patent vascular channels. It has been calculated that potentially there is enough thrombin in 10 ml of blood to clot the entire vascular tree in a few seconds if its action were unopposed.

Pathological haemostasis comprises those disorders in which inadequate response to injury leads to excessive haemorrhage and those disorders in which inappropriate or uncontrolled haemostatic responses lead to thrombosis. Though the processes of haemostasis and thrombosis are clearly interlinked, it is an oversimplification to regard one as merely an aberration of the other. Thrombi develop using the pathways of haemostasis, but the stimuli which initiate thrombosis are poorly understood. In most cases vascular insults are probably responsible, rather than faults in the haemostatic mechanism.

The coagulation mechanism

Two biochemical amplification pathways initiated by contact of blood with damaged tissue converge to generate thrombin. Thrombin is the enzyme which modifies fibrinogen so that it polymerizes to form a physically solid, fibrin clot. These two pathways, the intrinsic and extrinsic, are traditionally presented as separate and are tested *in vitro* in ways which preserve their apparent distinctiveness. However, there is good evidence that physiologically, interactions occur at several levels between the two pathways. Both are necessary for normal haemostasis, and deficiency in one cannot be compensated by normal function of the other. The enzymes and co-factors involved in coagulation and some of their properties are listed in Table 1.

The intrinsic pathway is an enzyme cascade triggered by contact of blood with any negatively charged surface. Following vascular injury blood comes in contact with elements of the subendothelial connective tissues such as collagen fibrils (Fig. 1) to which the contact factors adhere, with consequent activation. Factor XII in the presence of high molecular weight kininogen (HMWK) is adsorbed first, and can activate prekallikrein to kallikrein, which in turn activates factor XII to factor XIIa. This reciprocal activation generates significant quantities of factor XIIa after a lag of several minutes, which then activates factor XI to factor XIa by limited proteolysis (Fig. 1). Factors XII, XI and prekallikrein circulate as inactive zymogens that are converted to active protease enzymes by limited proteolysis, in a manner analogous to the activation of trypsinogen to trypsin. The analogy goes further since all the protease enzymes of the haemostatic and fibrinolytic systems are of the 'serine' type with strong sequence homology to trypsin and elastase and an identical catalytic mechanism. Specificity is conferred by the presence of specialized binding sites so that factor XIa, for example, will act only on factor IX, the next zymogen in the intrinsic pathway. This step requires ionized calcium to proceed efficiently. Calcium chelating agents such as trisodium citrate, therefore, stall the intrinsic pathway at this point. They are used to anticoagulate blood for processing, storage, and laboratory testing. Calcium ions are replaced to allow coagulation to proceed in assays of coagulation function.

Factor IXa next activates factor X. Three co-factors are needed for this to proceed at all rapidly: calcium ions, platelet membrane phospholipid, and factor VIII. Activation occurs on the surface of adherent activated platelets. In the presence of the co-factors the rate of factor Xa generation is 30 000-fold more rapid than in their absence. The next two steps, activation of prothrombin and fibrin monomer formation, are common to instrinsic and extrinsic pathways (Fig. 2). Factor Xa activates prothrombin to thrombin and requires three co-factors: calcium, platelet phospholipid, and factor V; the reaction again taking place on the platelet surface. Factor V and factor VIII subserve similar co-factor functions and are homologous in overall structure, amino acid sequence, and activation by thrombin. Although they are not protease enzymes they circulate in a precursor form that requires limited cleavage by thrombin for expression of co-factor activity. Hence thrombin, once generated even in minute amounts, provides a positive feedback loop to activate factors V and VIII.

Thrombin removes two pairs of small peptides from fibrinogen, fibrinopeptide A from the α-chains and fibrinopeptide B from the β-chains. This changes the charge structure sufficiently to allow the fibrin monomers immediately to polymerize (Fig. 3). Finally, polymerized fibrin held together only by hydrophobic and electrostatic bonds is stabilized by covalent cross-linking induced by the transamidating enzyme, factor XIII, which has to be first activated by thrombin to factor XIIIa.

The extrinsic pathway is initiated by tissue factor (sometimes designated factor III). Tissue factor is an apoprotein-lipid complex present in varying amounts in the cell walls of tissues, brain being a particularly good source. It has only recently been purified to homogeneity and is incompletely characterized biochemically. Tissue factor forms a complex with factor VII that directly activates factor X. There is reciprocal activation between the two factors generating factors VIIa and Xa. The earlier stages of the intrinsic pathway are by-passed, accounting for the apparently more rapid action *in vitro* of the extrinsic pathway. Nevertheless, both pathways are essential for normal haemostasis, probably due to the need for reciprocal activation of factor VII by factor Xa, and of factor IX by factor VIIa (Fig. 1).

The proteolytic activations which occur in the coagulation pathways are summarized in Fig. 4. Small changes in molecular structure, the cleavage of a single peptide bond or removal of an activation peptide converts inactive zymogens and co-factors to their fully active form. Occurring sequentially this produces dramatic molecular amplification. From one molecule of factor XIa, 2×10^8 molecules of fibrin can be generated in 1 min if all the factors are present at physiological concentrations. Conversely deficiency of a single factor will slow or halt the process.

Tests of coagulation function

Clot formation for technical reasons is tested *in vitro* independently of platelet function and by methods which fully separate the intrinsic and extrinsic pathways. Tests are carried out on citrated, platelet-poor plasma, separated without delay from blood collected by careful non-traumatic venepuncture into non-wettable plastic tubes. These precautions minimize preactivation of the clotting systems and decay of labile factors. The results will be invalid if these precautions are not observed. The reagents used need to be carefully standardized and a continuous check on results maintained by comparison with normal plasma in each test procedure.

The *prothrombin time* (PT) is measured by mixing saline extract of brain containing tissue factor/phospholipid complex with plasma. Calcium is added and the interval to appearance of a clot timed. This tests the extrinsic pathway and prolongation reflects deficiency or inhibition of the relevant factors (Table 2, Fig. 2). Using British comparative thromboplastin the normal range is 11–15 s. The *activated partial thromboplastin time* (APTT) is measured by first activating the contact factors with kaolin or similar dispersed, negatively charged particles. The interval to clot formation is recorded after phospholipid (to substitute for platelets) and calcium have been added. Two to eight minutes are allowed for activation in different procedures and this influences the normal range quoted by individual laboratories. The APTT is sensitive to deficiency or inhibition of factors in the pathway from prekallikrein to fibrinogen (Table 2, Fig. 2).

Comparison of results from PT and APTT allows partial localization of a particular defect. For example, factor VIII deficiency would cause a long APTT but the PT would remain normal.

The *thrombin clotting time* is performed by adding exogenous (usually bovine) thrombin to citrated plasma and recording the interval to clot formation. It is sensitive only to deficiency of fibrinogen, or inhibition of thrombin.

A modified thrombin time can be used to quantify fibrinogen or the resultant clot can be washed and weighed directly. Tests using mixtures of normal and abnormal plasmas are performed to detect an inhibitor. A test plasma found to have prolonged APTT or PT is mixed with an equal volume of normal plasma and the test repeated. If prolongation is due to simple deficiency then normal plasma will supply the lack and correct the clotting time. Conversely if the abnormal plasma contains an inhibitor it will inactivate the factor(s) in the normal plasma so that no shortening of the clotting time occurs.

Table 1 Some properties of plasma coagulation factors

Factor		Molecular weight	Concentration	$t_{\frac{1}{2}}$	Function
XII	Hageman factor	80 000	40 mg/l	40 h	Activates factor XI; also plasminogen
XI	Plasma thromboplastin antecedent	160 000	5 mg/l	80 h	Activates factor IX
IX*	Christmas factor	54 000	5–10 mg/l	18 h	Activates factor X
VIII	Antihaemophilic factor	360 000	200 μg/l	10 h	Co-factor for the activation of factor X by factor IXa
X*	Stuart Prower factor	55 000	10 mg/l	30 h	Activates factor II
V	Labile factor	330 000	10 mg/l	12 h	Co-factor for the activation of factor II by factor Xa
II*	Prothrombin	35 000	100 mg/l	3 days	Converts fibrinogen to fibrin; activates factors VIII, V, XIII, and protein C
III	Tissue factor	43 000 (apoprotein)	Zero (tissue derived)		Co-factor for the activation of factor X by factor VIIa
VII*	Proconvertin	53 000	500 μg/l	3 h	Activates factor X
I	Fibrinogen	340 000	2–4 g/l	4 days	Polymerizes to form the physical clot
XIII	Fibrin stabilizing factor	320 000	10 mg/l	13 days	Cross-links fibrin to stabilize it
Protein C	Autoprothrombin	56 000	5 mg/l	8 h	Inactivates factor VIII and factor V; may activate plasminogen
Protein S*	II A*	68 000	20 mg/l	?	Co-factor for protein C

* Vitamin K dependent proteins.

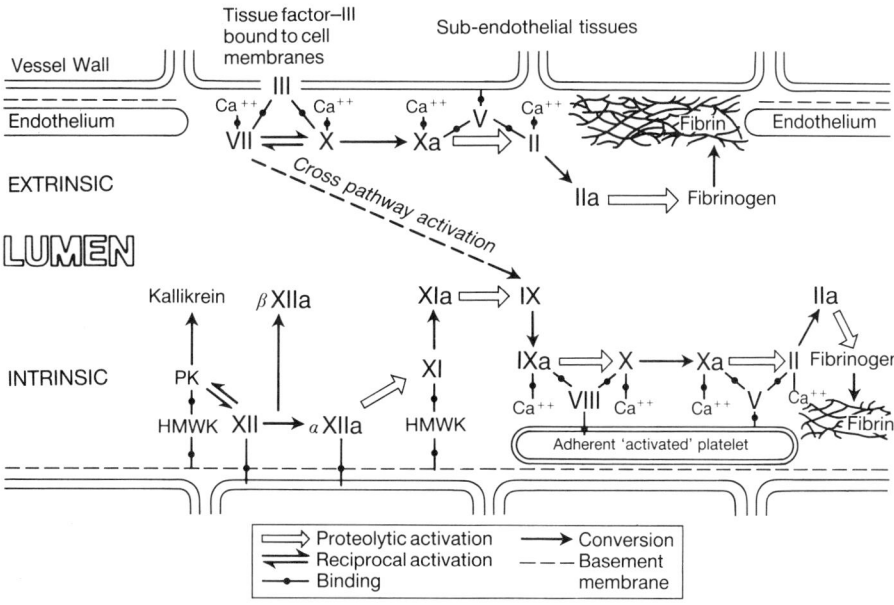

Fig. 1   Coagulation is activated by exposure to non-endothelial surfaces (intrinsic pathway) and tissue factor (extrinsic pathway). There is reciprocal activation between the pathways, which function as an integrated system. Coagulation is a surface-mediated phenomenon, the reactants binding to vascular components during contact activation and key steps in the activation sequence taking place on the platelet surface.

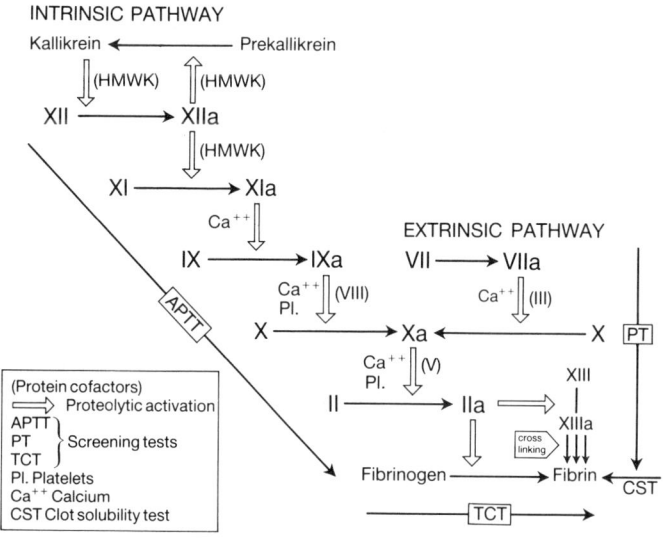

Fig. 2   The intrinsic and extrinsic pathways of blood coagulation. The activated partial thromboplastin time (APTT) utilizes the intrinsic route to fibrin. Prothrombin time (PT) utilizes the extrinsic route. The thrombin clotting time (TCT) tests fibrinogen–fibrin conversion.

Specific *factor assays* are carried out to pinpoint a defect. Most inherited coagulopathies are due to single factor deficiency. The assays commonly used rely on plasma that is completely devoid of one or the other factor (e.g. severe haemophilia A plasma, lacking factor VIII). The ability of the test plasma is compared with that of a control, normal plasma in its capacity to correct the defect, and this allows quantification of the specific factor.

Inherited disorders of blood coagulation

Haemophilia A (classical haemophilia, factor VIII deficiency)

This is the commonest of the hereditary bleeding disorders (Table 3) with an incidence of between 30 and 120 per million of the

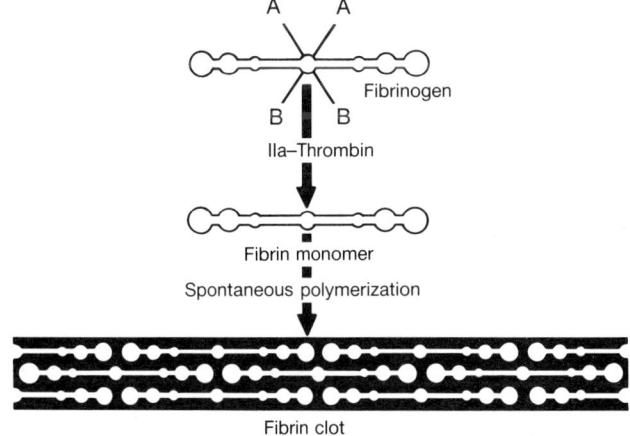

Fig. 3   Thrombin removes two pairs of short peptides from fibrinogen, yielding a fibrin monomer which then spontaneously polymerizes in long strands.

population. It occurs in all races and geographical areas. The United Kingdom had 4321 cases of haemophilia A registered by Haemophilia Centres in 1980. The condition is due to deficiency of factor VIII whose gene is located on chromosome Xq 2.8 and is therefore transmitted as a sex-linked recessive defect. Haemophilia is the classic example of this mode of inheritance (Fig. 5). There seems to be a high mutation rate since about a third of cases are apparently sporadic with no traceable affected relative. It is not known whether new mutations occur chiefly during spermatogenesis or oogenesis but this may soon be resolved by direct analysis using factor VIII gene probes. Several mutations causing haemophilia A have been identified including deletions and single base transitions. The disorder is heterogeneous at the molecular level. Therefore practical gene tracking for carrier detection and antenatal diagnosis depends on common restriction fragment length polymorphisms within or close to the factor VIII locus (Fig. 5).

Until recently the only method for detecting carriers of haemophilia A was to measure their level of coagulation factor VIII com-

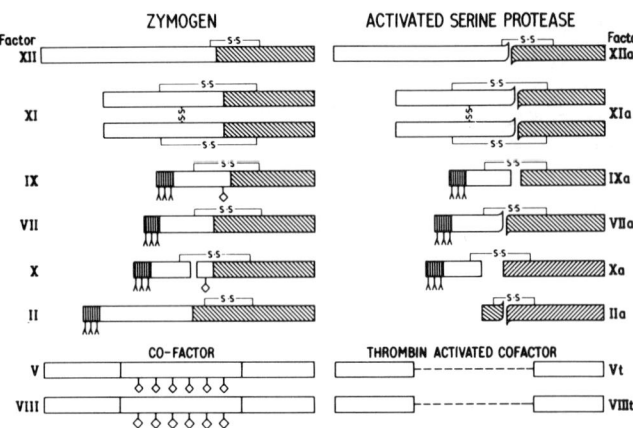

—S·S— Cystine disulphide linkage

▨▨▨▨ Chain containing active site of serine esterase

☐ Glycosylated activation peptide
   ◊◊◊

▥ Region of Vitamin K dependent factors containing ◊ Carboxy Glutamates
   ⋀⋀⋀

----- Non covalent linkage

Fig. 4 Proteolytic activation of zymogens in the coagulation pathway.

Table 2 Screening tests of haemostasis

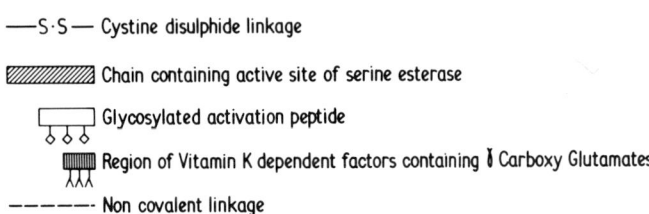

Name	System tested	Abnormalities indicated by prolongation
Activated partial thromboplastin time (APTT)	Intrinsic pathway	Deficiency or inhibition of one or more of the following factors: XII, XI, IX, VIII, X, V, II, I, pre Kallikrein, HMWK
Prothrombin time (PT)	Extrinsic pathway	Deficiency or inhibition of one or more of the following factors: VII, X, V, II, I
Thrombin clotting time (TCT)	Fibrinogen to fibrin conversion	Deficiency or abnormality of fibrin; inhibition of thrombin by heparin or fibrin degradation products
Fibrinogen	Total quantity of clottable fibrinogen	Hypofibrinogenaemia
Mixture tests (only if PT or PTT prolonged)	Correction of prolonged PT or APTT by normal plasma	Failure to correct indicates the presence of an inhibitor of coagulation, e.g. failure to correct APTT may indicate a factor VIII antibody

pared with that of von Willebrand factor which is autosomally coded. Due to random inactivation of the X chromosome (see page 19.13) this method could never totally exclude the carrier state. Recently, restriction fragment length polymorphisms (see Section 4) have been discovered within the factor VIII gene and in linked anonymous X gene probes. Direct fetal blood sampling for antenatal diagnosis by coagulation factor assay is also highly successful but cannot be performed until 18–20 weeks gestation.

All the problems and complications of haemophilia A are due to deficiency of factor VIII with consequent drastic slowing of throm-

Table 3 Relative frequency of congenital blood coagulation defects

Disorder	Number of cases registered*	Per cent
Haemophilia A	221	46.4
Von Willebrand's disease	148	31.1
Haemophilia B	53	11.1
Factor XI deficiency	46†	9.7
Factor V deficiency	3	0.6
Factor XII deficiency	3	0.6
Factor VII deficiency	2	0.4
Total	476	100

* Royal Free Hospital Haemophilia Centre 1984.
† Reflects presence of a large Jewish community in North London.

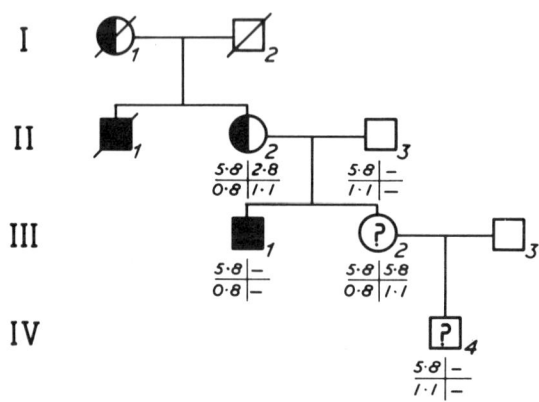

Fig. 5 Inheritance of haemophilia through four generations. □ ○ normal male and female, ∅ deceased, ■ severe haemophilia A, ◐ obligate carrier, ⑦ status unknown. II₁ (deceased) and III₁ had severe haemophilia A. Therefore it is clear that I₁ and II₂ are obligate carriers of haemophilia A. III₂ is a potential carrier who requested diagnosis when 8 weeks pregnant with IV₄. Diagnosis by means of gene tracking using two restriction fragment length polymorphisms (RFLPs) was undertaken. 5·8/2·8 are alleles detected by a linked probe (DX 13) and 0·8/1·1 are alleles within the factor VIII gene itself. Peripheral blood DNA from adults and a chorion biopsy from the fetus were tested with the results shown. III₂ is a carrier since she has X chromosome markers 5·8/0·8 present in her haemophilic brother. Her male fetus is normal since it received the X chromosome with 5·8/1·1 alleles that derive from II₃ who is normal. This prediction was confirmed later by direct blood sampling of the fetus at 18 weeks.

bin generation via the intrinsic pathway. The severity of bleeding is related to residual factor level (Table 4). Clots are slow to form, and once formed, break up easily. Bleeding continues for days or weeks after surgery such as dental extraction or after major trauma. Apparently spontaneous bleeding occurs into major joints with distressing frequency. This causes intense pain due to pressure within the joint capsule (Fig. 6). If untreated, each episode of haemarthrosis takes many days to resolve. The longer term consequence of repeatedly exposing joint surfaces to blood is accelerated destruction of cartilage and hypertrophic osteoarthropathy. This usually resembles severe osteoarthritis radiologically, with marked bony deformity and ultimate ankylosis particularly of the knees, elbows, and ankles. A florid proliferative synovial overgrowth is a feature of some cases and the joint damage may somewhat resemble that seen in rheumatoid arthritis.

Other frequent sites of bleeding are the large muscles, especially the psoas, and the renal and intestinal tracts. Intestinal bleeding can be intramural with signs mimicking appendicitis or obstruction. Central nervous system haemorrhage also occurs especially after trauma and used to be the commonest cause of death in haemophiliacs. Laboratory diagnosis is based on the finding of a prolonged partial thromboplastin time, normal bleeding

Table 4 Relationship between residual factor level and severity of haemophilia

Factor level* (per cent)	Clinical grade	Manifestations
< 2	Severe	Frequent spontaneous bleeds
2–5	Moderately severe	Occasional spontaneous bleeds. Bleeding after minor trauma
5–15	Mild	Bleeding only after trauma or surgery
15–35	Very mild (many carriers of haemophilia A or B in this group)	Excessive bleeding only after severe trauma or major surgery
35–45	'Grey area'	May or may not bleed abnormally
> 45	Normal	No abnormal bleeding

* Applicable to factors VIII, IX, VII, X, II. Not applicable to factors XI, XII, XIII, V (see text).

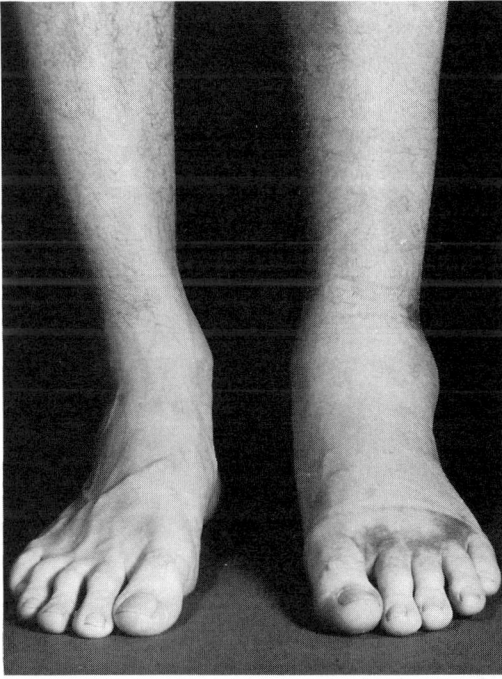

Fig. 6 Joint bleed into the ankle in a patient with haemophilia A.

time and specific factor assays demonstrating a deficiency of factor VIII coagulant activity with normal levels of von Willebrand factor, factor IX and factor XI.

Treatment of bleeding episodes is by means of intravenous factor VIII replacement (Tables 5–7) given as soon as possible after the onset of bleeding. Particularly dangerous sites of bleeding are intracranial, sublingual, pharyngeal, and iliopsoas. The latter presents as pain in the inguinal region with flexion at the hip on the affected side, and paraesthesia in the cutaneous distribution of the femoral nerve.

Any haemophiliac who has suffered significant trauma to the head should be admitted for observation and placed on full-dosage factor VIII to maintain plasma levels over 50 per cent for 24 hours. Bleeding in the oropharyngeal region likewise requires close observation and sufficiently intensive factor VIII therapy to arrest haemorrhage and avert the risk of asphyxia. Intramuscular haematomas, whether iliopsoas or elsewhere, require strict rest initially and prolonged therapy with factor VIII to arrest haemorrhage and permit reabsorption of haematoma, followed by graded physiotherapy to restore function. Failure to control muscle bleeding can lead to permanent ischaemic damage to nerves by entrapment and muscle necrosis (Volkmann's ischaemic contracture).

Often, inexperienced physicians and surgeons undertreat haemophilic bleeding, lulled into a false sense of security by the fact that bleeding may be delayed for many hours after trauma or temporarily arrested by local measures or inadequate doses of factor VIII.

Dental extraction in haemophiliacs without factor VIII cover is invariably followed by days or weeks of exsanguinating haemorrhage. A simple regime has now been shown highly effective in preventing bleeding after dental surgery. Immediately prior to dental extraction a single dose of factor VIII sufficient to raise the plasma level to 50 per cent is given together with tranexamic acid (1 g in adults, proportionately less in children). The antifibrinolytic is then continued by mouth three times daily for 5 days and usually no further factor VIII will be required.

The best analgesic for the pain of haemophilic bleeding is prompt therapy with adequate amounts of factor VIII. Formerly when no effective haemostatic agent was available many patients became addicted to morphine or its analogues, given as a palliative by despairing physicians who lacked alternative remedies. Chronic pain due to haemophilic arthropathy can be alleviated by ibuprofen or indomethacin in standard dosage. Aspirin is contraindicated because it definitely compounds the bleeding tendency and is especially prone to cause gastrointestinal bleeding. Paracetamol is a safe alternative mild analgesic. Any haemophiliac who requests regular supplies of stronger analgesics (pentazocine, pethidine, morphine etc.) for 'bleeding' is probably addicted to narcotics or very likely to become so and should be counselled and managed accordingly.

The practical problem of providing intravenous infusions of factor VIII at short notice for unpredictable bleeding episodes has been largely solved by training patients (or their relatives) in self therapy. 'Home treatment' has revolutionized the social, educational, and employment potential of haemophiliacs, giving them freedom undreamt of 20 years ago. However, continuing supervision by a Haemophilia Centre is mandatory. It is now widely accepted that management of haemophilia should be undertaken by specialized centres who will care for a sufficient number of patients to gain experience in all aspects of this uncommon disorder. The concept of 'comprehensive care' for haemophilia is based on such centres where the skills of the physician, the orthopaedic surgeon, the nurse, the social worker, the physiotherapist, and the laboratory scientist can be focused (whole or part time) on the special needs of haemophiliacs. Although comprehensive care at specialized centres remains the ideal, there will always be occasions when the general practitioner or casualty officer will be confronted with a haemophiliac requiring immediate attention. The following guidelines may be of assistance. Ask to see the patient's haemophilia card. This will record factor deficiency and level, presence or absence of inhibitors, allergic reactions, and blood group, together with the address and telephone number of the centre where he is registered, who should be contacted in any case for specific advice. Ask the patient whether he thinks he has bleeding at the time and what his usual treatment would be for the type of bleed in question. For example, a spontaneous bleed into the knee joint in a 70 kg adult haemophiliac if treated early will usually respond to a single infusion of 750 units of factor VIII. This dose is sufficient to raise the factor level to 15 per cent of normal and would be contained in about 10 bags of cryoprecipitate or about three bottles of National Health Service (UK) factor VIII concentrate (usual contents – 250 units per bottle). If the joint continues to be painful with limited movement then further doses may be necessary at 12- to 24-hour intervals. It would be quite unusual for an early spontaneous joint bleed to fail to respond to three treatments and this failure would suggest the presence of inhibitors. In the event of major trauma or surgical complications requiring operative intervention it is essential to transfer the

Table 5 Therapeutic materials for treatment of haemophilia A, B and von Willebrand's disease

Material	Purity units of factor/ml	Advantages	Applications	Limitations/disadvantages
Fresh frozen plasma	1	All factors present Single donor per pack Very simple to prepare	Haemophilia A or B	High volume, maximum dose in adult 1000 ml/12 h
Cryoprecipitate	5–15	Contains VIII, vWF, fibrinogen, and XIII Single donor per pack	Haemophilia A, von Willebrand's disease, afibrinogenaemia, XIII deficiency	Must be stored frozen Units vary in potency Inconvenient to draw up
Factor VIII* concentrate	15–30	Stored at 4 °C Assayed potency Relatively higher purity	Haemophilia A, severe von Willebrand's disease	1000–5000 donors per batch Hepatitis risk
Factor IX* concentrate	15–30	Stored at 4 °C Assayed potency Higher purity	Haemophilia B	1000–5000 donors per batch Hepatitis risk Thrombogenic potential
DDAVP	—	Not blood derived	Mild haemophilia A or von Willebrand's disease	Only effective for two doses Water retention

* All concentrates in use in 1986 are heat treated to diminish risk of transmitting hepatitis and AIDS viruses.

Table 6 Dosage calculation for factor replacement therapy

Factor	Formula		Example
VIII	Dose in units =	$\dfrac{\text{Percentage rise} \times \text{Patient's weight in kg}}{1.5}$	To obtain 30 per cent rise in a patient weighing 50 kg Dose = $\dfrac{30 \times 50}{1.5}$ = 1000 units
IX	Dose in units =	$\dfrac{\text{Percentage rise} \times \text{Patient's weight in kg}}{0.9}$	To obtain 45 per cent rise in a patient weighing 70 kg Dose = $\dfrac{45 \times 70}{0.9}$ = 3500 units

Table 7 Replacement level aimed to control or prevent bleeding in factor VIII or IX deficiency

Clinical problem	Percentage required	Treatment
Minor haemarthrosis	15	Single infusion usually adequate
Major haemarthrosis, muscle bleeding	25	May require repeated infusions over several days to a week
Head injury, surgery, major trauma	50	Minimum, maintained by repeated infusions

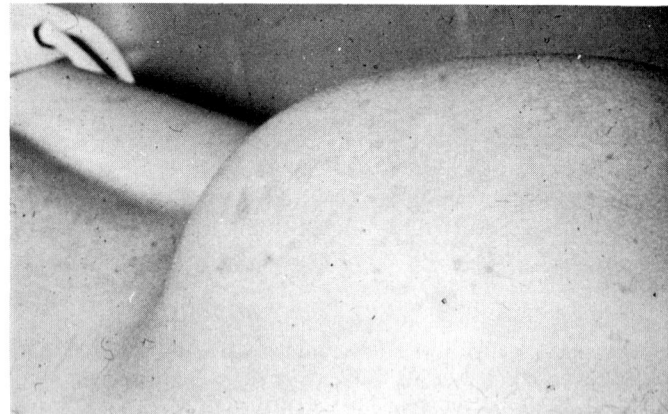

Fig. 7 Gluteal haemorrhage in a haemophiliac following an intramuscular injection given without adequate coverage with factor VIII replacement.

patient to a specialized centre where factor VIII can be monitored and maintained at the appropriate level (Table 6).

Younger patients who have received optimum therapy from infancy are now growing up without significant joint damage. Generally the older the patient the more severe and crippling his arthropathy will be. As the joint destruction progresses towards ankylosis, intra-articular bleeding becomes less frequent and pain due to osteoarthrosis predominates. Orthopaedic management of this situation includes joint replacement and arthrodesis.

Surgery must be covered by fully adequate replacement therapy (Tables 5, 6 and 7), closely monitored by specific factor VIII assays. The factor VIII level will need to be raised to the normal range (50–200 per cent) and maintained there for a week after major surgery and at somewhat lower levels until healing is completed. Since the half-life of factor VIII is 8 to 12 hours, twice-daily infusions are mandatory in the immediate postoperative period. Only Haemophilia Centres are experienced and equipped to give this type of cover for major surgery. However, provided that adequately monitored factor VIII replacement is given, normal haemostasis will be secured and no other special precautions should be needed.

Intramuscular injections are normally absolutely prohibited in the haemophiliac since they can cause dramatic and even life-threatening intramuscular haematomas (Fig. 7) though they are safe during the period for which full replacement therapy has been given.

Three complications of factor VIII replacement therapy have

Table 8 Complications of haemophilia treatment

Complication	Frequency (per cent)	Cause	Treatment
Antibodies to factor VIII	5–15	Unknown	High-dose human or porcine factor VIII. Activated factor IX complex 'Activated factor IX'
Antibodies to factor IX	1	Gene deletion in 50% of cases	
Acute hepatitis	50–100	Hepatitis B. Two types of non-A, non-B	Supportive
Chronic active hepatitis	5–50	Persistence of virus?	Interferon?
AIDS	1–2	Retrovirus HTLVIII	Supportive
Allergic reactions	5–20	Impurities	Antihistamine, steroids, higher purity concentrates

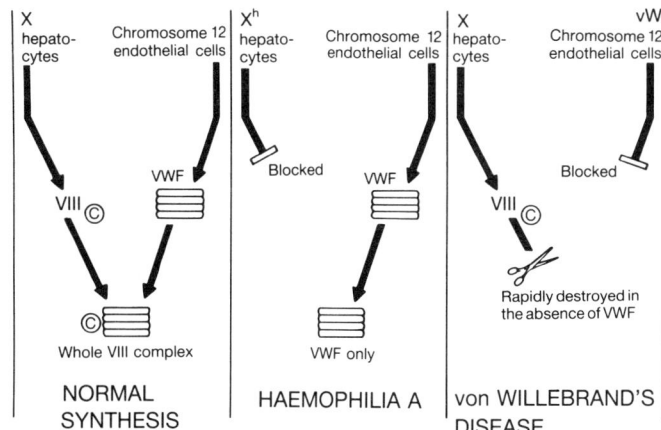

Fig. 8 Normal synthesis of factor VIII and von Willebrand factor to form the factor VIII complex, compared with defective synthesis of factor VIII in haemophilia A, and of vWF in von Willebrand's disease.

become prominent in recent years (Table 8). Some patients develop antibodies to factor VIII which their immune system treats as a foreign protein. Management of these patients is extraordinarily difficult and expensive, and involves a variety of treatments: very high doses of human factor VIII concentrate; porcine factor VIII (Hyate: C); factor IX concentrate; 'activated prothrombin complex'; and plasmapheresis. Elective surgery can be contemplated only if the antibody titre is low. A second problem arises because all coagulation factor concentrates derived from pooled plasma from multiple donors have the potential to transmit at least three hepatitis viruses. Hepatitis B, and two types of non-A, non-B virus could not, until recently, be inactivated by pasteurization without destroying the coagulation factors, which are trace proteins with a low stability when exposed to heat, or ultraviolet radiation. New heat-treated concentrates may be safer but this has not been firmly established by clinical trials. The attack rate for hepatitis non-A, non-B in a previously unexposed patient after a single factor concentrate infusion is 100 per cent. Therefore, concentrates should be given only where there is no alternative. The third complication arises from infection with human T-cell lymphotropic virus type III (HTLVIII, LAV), a retrovirus which causes acquired immune deficiency syndrome (AIDS) and is transmitted by factor concentrates (see Section 5). The majority of haemophiliacs treated with factor VIII concentrate obtained from the United States now have antibodies to HTLV III and have therefore been exposed to the virus. Although the attack rate is low (about 1 in 100 exposures) patients do not recover. It is accordingly essential that haemophiliacs are not *heedlessly* given factor concentrates. An alternative therapy which raises factor VIII levels in mild haemophilia is administration of the synthetic vasopressin, 1-deamino-8-D-arginine-vasopressin (DDAVP). Given intravenously at 0.4 μg/kg DDAVP causes a two- to four-fold short-term increase in plasma concentrations of factor VIII and von Willebrand factor. A patient with mild haemophilia A and a plasma factor VIII level of 15 per cent could therefore achieve a level of 45 per cent after DDAVP infusion, sufficient to cover minor surgery. DDAVP treatment needs to be monitored closely by factor VIII assay and since the synthetic hormone, although lacking pressor activity, retains weak antidiuretic activity fluid intake may need to be restricted. It also stimulates release of plasminogen activator and is therefore always given together with an inhibitor of fibrinolysis such as tranexamic acid.

Haemophilia B (factor IX deficiency, Christmas disease)
The genetic and clinical features of haemophilia B are identical to those of haemophilia A, so that the two disorders can only be distinguished on the basis of specific factor assays. The distinction is

crucial nevertheless as treatment is specific. The incidence of haemophilia B is about one-sixth that of haemophilia A, with 777 known cases in the United Kingdom in 1980.

Management with factor IX concentrates follows similar principles to those outlined for factor VIII, except that the longer half-life of factor IX (18 hours) allows therapy to be given less frequently. The incidence of antibodies to factor IX in haemophilia B is about 1 per cent, compared with that of antibodies to factor VIII in haemophilia A of between 5 and 10 per cent. The factor IX gene is located on chromosome Xq 2.7. Recently restriction fragment length polymorphisms have been identified within the gene so that carrier determination and antenatal diagnosis by chorion biopsy are now feasible.

Von Willebrand's disease
This usually mild bleeding disorder differs clinically and genetically from haemophilia A and B in that most kindreds exhibit autosomal dominant transmission. Rarer examples of autosomal recessive inheritance are encountered and the affected homozygous individuals then have a bleeding disorder resembling severe haemophilia A. Considerable confusion has arisen over the observation that factor VIII levels are low in both von Willebrand's disease and haemophilia A, but the distinct features of the two conditions can be clarified (Fig. 8, Table 9).

The fundamental lesion in von Willebrand's disease is insufficient or defective von Willebrand factor, a protein which promotes platelet adhesion (Fig. 1). Consequently, patients have prolonged skin bleeding times, a tendency to bruise, and are at risk of haemorrhage from mucous membranes (nose, mouth, gut, uterus). Von Willebrand factor also serves as a carrier molecule for factor VIII, protecting it from premature destruction. Hence, in von Willebrand's disease, levels of both von Willebrand factor and factor VIII are reduced. Standard concentrates of factor VIII (e.g. cryoprecipitate, freeze-dried concentrate) contain both von Willebrand factor and factor VIII in a bimolecular complex. Replacement therapy accordingly is similar to that used in haemophilia A, though cryoprecipitate is preferred since the labile element which enhances platelet adhesiveness is better preserved. Infusion of von Willebrand factor not only corrects the bleeding time but prolongs survival of the patient's own factor VIII, accounting for the 'overresponse' or *de novo synthesis* of factor VIII after such infusions. This cuts down the frequency with which infusions need to be given to cover surgery.

DDAVP (see above) is effective in most patients with mild von Willebrand's disease as in haemophilia A. There is marked variability in levels of factor VIII and von Willebrand factor in different cases, both from time to time and in different affected

Table 9 Comparison of haemophilia A and von Willebrand's disease

Haemophilia A	von Willebrand's disease
Sex-linked recessive	Autosomal dominant or recessive
Deficient or defective factor VIII synthesis	Deficient or defective von Willebrand factor synthesis
Delayed thrombin production via intrinsic pathway	Reduced platelet adhesion, reduced plasma levels of factor VIII
Bleeding in joints and muscles. Most cases severe	Bleeding from mucous membranes. Homozygous cases also have haemarthroses. Most cases mild
Incidence 30–100 per 10^6 population	Incidence 30–100 per 10^6 population
Treatment with cryoprecipitate, factor VIII concentrates, DDAVP for mild cases	Treatment with cryoprecipitate, DDAVP except severe cases

members of the same kindred, which can make diagnosis difficult. Five subtypes of von Willebrand's disease are now recognized, one of which is associated with thrombocytopenia (type IIB), and one of which is in fact due to a platelet defect (pseudo- or platelet-type von Willebrand's disease). It is important not to expose infrequently treated patients to large donor pool concentrates, if bleeding can be controlled or prevented by single donor cryoprecipitate or DDAVP, to minimize the risk of virus infection.

Bleeding from the uterus, nose, or mouth, can often be controlled using the fibrinolytic inhibitors tranexamic or aminocaproic acids (1 g six-hourly in adults). After dental surgery both in the haemophilias and von Willebrand's disease, fibrinolytic inhibitors given for five days greatly reduce or abolish the need for further factor replacement after an initial dose at the time of extraction or other operation. This is because saliva contains potent fibrinolytic activators, which otherwise cause rapid clot dissolution. Arthropathy occurs only in the rare homozygous cases who suffer from joint bleeds comparable to those of haemophilia A.

Factor XI deficiency
This disorder is inherited as an autosomal dominant and is quite common (about 4 per cent incidence) in Jews of Eastern European ancestry. In the heterozygous form, factor XI levels range from 4 to 40 per cent and bleeding only occurs after trauma or surgery. Homozygous cases have less than 1 per cent factor XI but even these individuals rarely bleed spontaneously. Since there is no factor XI concentrate available, treatment is with fresh frozen plasma. This factor has a long half-life and the level required for haemostasis is about 30 per cent, so in practice it is feasible to maintain adequate haemostasis with plasma infusions alone.

Deficiency of factor VII, factor X, factor V, and factor II
These are all rare autosomal recessive bleeding disorders which produce bleeding resembling haemophilia A, the severity depending on the residual level of the factor. Concentrates are available of factor VII, factor X, and factor II.

Afibrinogenaemia
This is a rare autosomal recessive bleeding disorder that is surprisingly mild clinically. Patients have prolonged bleeding times in addition to virtually incoagulable blood.

Cryoprecipitate contains a large amount of fibrinogen and so can be used to control bleeding when it occurs. Some cases develop antibodies to fibrinogen and become refractory to treatment.

Abnormal fibrinogens (dysfibrinogenaemia)
More than 20 variant fibrinogens have now been described. These are usually detected when a mild bleeding disorder is investigated

and a very prolonged thrombin clotting time is found despite normal quantities of fibrinogen determined by clot weight or immunological methods. More sophisticated investigation shows a reduced rate of release of fibrinopeptide A in some cases, usually due to the substitution of arginine by histidine at α-chain residue 14, the site of cleavage by thrombin. These defects are transmitted in an autosomal dominant manner, and perhaps because affected individuals produce normal as well as abnormal fibrinogen, bleeding is never a serious problem clinically.

Several abnormal fibrinogens have been associated with a thrombotic tendency. A likely aetiology for this apparent paradox is reduced susceptibility of the abnormal fibrin molecules to fibrinolysis.

Factor XIII deficiency
This rare autosomal recessive bleeding disorder has some intriguing additional features. Excessive umbilical cord bleeding is invariably reported. Affected women have repeated early spontaneous abortions. Wound healing is poor, leading to tissue-paper scars at sites of old injury. These problems, which are due to lack of stabilizing cross-links in the fibrin forming the wound coagulum, can be corrected by means of cryoprecipitate infusion, which is rich in factor XIII. As the half-life is long and only 2 per cent of the normal level is necessary for haemostasis, weekly infusions can be given prophylactically.

Combined factor V and factor VIII deficiency
This is a rare autosomal recessive bleeding disorder, of great theoretical interest, since it appears to be due to a single gene defect despite the undoubtedly separate loci for factors V and VIII. It has been suggested that it might be due to deficiency of an inhibitor to protein C, a plasma protein which normally inactivates factors V and VIII. At present clinical studies have not substantiated the hypothesis. Cryoprecipitate or fresh frozen plasma can be used to treat the usually mild bleeding problems in these patients.

Platelet function in haemostasis
Platelets reduce red cell leakage from the circulation, form haemostatic plugs to seal ruptured arterioles and capillaries, and interact with coagulant proteins to promote coagulation.

Platelet morphology
Inactive platelets circulate as biconvex discs which are about one-tenth the volume of red cells and 20 times less numerous. The outer, peripheral zone of the platelet consists of the unit membrane of the cell, the region lying immediately within it, and an outer halo, the glycocalyx, containing glycoproteins which modify platelet function. The unit membrane is a bilamellar structure composed of phospholipids and some 30 or more glycoproteins. It provides a surface for reactions in the coagulation sequence and a source of fatty acids (principally arachidonic acid) for certain metabolic processes. Membrane proteins can be analysed by gel electrophoresis of solubilized membrane fractions and major identifiable glycoproteins have been assigned Roman numerals. Amongst other possible functions, membrane glycoproteins act as surface receptors and the absence of specific glycoproteins in certain rare hereditary disorders has enabled their role to be partly defined. *Glycoprotein Ib* binds von Willebrand factor and is involved in platelet adhesion. *Glycoprotein IIb and IIIa* functionally form a complex, bind fibrinogen, and thereby support the bridging mechanism required for platelet aggregation. *Glycoprotein V* is probably the thrombin receptor on the platelet surface.

Stimulated platelets change shape from smooth, lentiform discs to spheres with spiky projections, produced by gelling and cross-linking of internal contractile proteins. The pseudopodia consist of insolubilized proteins extruded in parallel filaments and covered by the plasma membrane. Vigorous platelet activation results in centripetal movement and dissolution of organelles followed by cell contraction and extrusion of stored constituents. Platelets contain large amounts of the muscle protein actomyosin, which is probably the main effector of cell contraction, though the process is not well understood.

Platelets do not have a nucleus, but contain dense bodies which store adenosine diphosphate (ADP), serotonin, and calcium; and alpha granules containing fibrinogen, platelet factor 4, beta thromboglobulin, and a cell mitogen – the platelet-derived growth factor. There are also peroxisomes with catalase activity; lysosomes containing beta glucuronidase, acid phosphatase and n-acetyl glucosaminidase; glycogen granules; mitochrondria; and a few Golgi vesicles.

Adhesion of platelets to surfaces

Platelets adhere to surfaces which are not covered with endothelial cells. Flow in blood vessels is not a smooth orderly process and the cells jostle and collide with each other in the axial stream. These and other forces disperse platelets which intermittently strike the vessel wall. Where there is incomplete coverage with endothelial cells, platelets rapidly attach to the surface (Fig. 9a). Contact is followed by change from a disc-shape to a sphere, followed by extension of pseudopodia and flattening of the platelet on the surface. In this way, spreading platelets can cover a small break in the endothelium like a plaster. Platelets react much more vigorously when exposed to some foreign materials and to collagen fibrils in the media. Spreading is followed by extrusion of ADP, serotonin, and calcium, and arachidonate mobilized from the cell membrane is metabolized to endoperoxides and thromboxanes which are potent agonists of platelet aggregation (Fig. 9b). The released products activate neighbouring platelets which stick together and form a microthrombus.

Platelet interaction with collagen is partly mediated by von Willebrand factor. Experiments have shown that von Willebrand factor binds to exposed subendothelium, particularly collagen, and then interacts with glycoprotein Ib on the platelet surface. This reaction is important at high shear rates found in the microcirculation. At lower shear rates the molecular forces which bind platelets to surfaces are not known.

Platelet aggregation

Platelets adhere to each other (aggregation) following exposure to certain agonists. Physiologically, aggregation follows adhesion and activation of platelets exposed to damaged vessel surfaces. Aggregation is essential for the formation of the haemostatic plug, a mass of adherent and coalescent platelets which seals ruptured arterioles and capillaries.

The process has been extensively studied *in vitro*. If thrombin, for example, is added to a suspension of stirred platelets it binds to a surface receptor and induces transmission of a signal across the platelet membrane. This liberates arachidonate from membrane phospholipids, leading to synthesis of prostaglandins and mobilization of intracellular calcium. Internal calcium flux triggers contraction of proteins within the cell, which profoundly alters cell morphology and extrudes the contents of the storage organelles. Secretion, particularly of ADP, but also of other cell constituents in the platelet release reaction, activates nearby platelets which will adhere to one another if they come in contact. Fibrinogen forms a molecular bridge between adjacent cells, binding to a complex of glycoproteins IIb and IIIa which is exposed on the membrane during platelet activation. Agonists of platelet aggregation vary in potency, weak inducers failing to stimulate the release reaction or metabolism of arachidonate, forming loose, unstable aggregates. Exposure to strong inducers like thrombin results in irreversible aggregation and formation of a

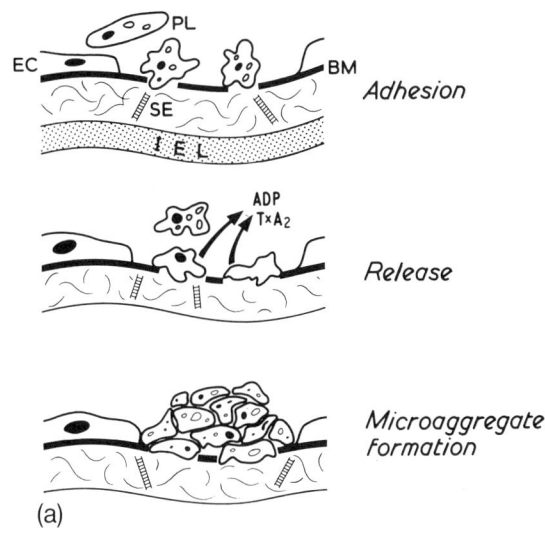

Adhesion

Release

Microaggregate formation

(a)

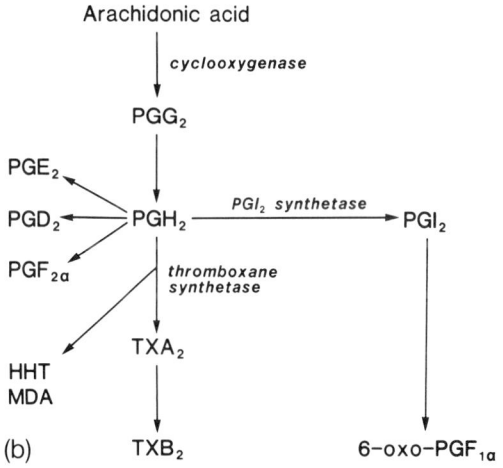

Arachidonic acid

cyclooxygenase

PGG₂

PGE₂

PGD₂ ← PGH₂ → PGI₂   *PGI₂ synthetase*

PGF₂ₐ

thromboxane synthetase

TXA₂

HHT
MDA

(b)   TXB₂   6-oxo-PGF₁ₐ

Fig. 9 Platelet interactions and synthetic activities. (a) At sites of endothelial cell (EC) loss, platelets (PL) adhere to components in the subendothelium (SE). The characteristic banded fibrils of collagen are scattered throughout the subendothelium and collagen is also an element of the basement membrane (BM). Deeper injury may breach the internal elastic lamina (IEL). Following adhesion, platelets release adenosine diphosphate (ADP) and thromboxane A₂ (TXA₂). Release of these and possibly other constituents attract surrounding platelets to form a microaggregate. (b) The substrate for prostaglandin synthesis is arachidonic acid released from phospholipids in the cell membrane. Thromboxane A₂ is the principal pro-aggregatory product of platelets. In contrast, vascular cells synthesize the platelet inhibitor prostacyclin (PGI₂).

mass of firmly adherent platelets. Most inhibitors of aggregation stimulate adenylate cyclase within platelets leading to increase in intraplatelet cAMP, which inhibits calcium mobilization and prostaglandin synthesis.

Platelets aggregate in response to thrombin, ADP, serotonin, arachidonate, and platelet-activating factor (produced by white blood cells and platelets) which are involved in physiological haemostasis. Bacterial lipids, immune complexes, some fatty acids and viruses are more likely to initiate pathological platelet activation.

Interactions with the coagulation mechanism

Platelets interact with the coagulation mechanism to accelerate thrombin generation. Platelets exposed to foreign surfaces generate factor XIa activity, by-passing factor XII. Activated factor X binds to the surface of platelets, factor V acting as a receptor. Generation of thrombin by the prothrombinase complex occurs many 1000-fold more rapidly on platelet surfaces than in a platelet-free artificial medium. The cell membrane of stimulated platelets is reorientated, and phosphatidylserine, which is negatively charged and on the inner aspect of the membrane in quiescent platelets, moves to the outer surface in what has been called the 'flip-flop' mechanism. Negatively charged phospholipids act as templates for organization of the factor X-activating and prothrombinase complexes. Several coagulant proteins bind to phospholipids by calcium bridges, activation of platelets, and exposure of phosphotidylserine acting as powerful catalysts of fibrin formation. This ensures that the loosely adherent platelet plug is stabilized by deposition of fibrin. Fibrin itself binds to platelets which contract, locking platelets and fibrin together in a firm, resilient coagulum at the site of vessel injury. Coagulation reactions on the platelet surface are physically protected from flow dispersion of reactants in the blood stream and inactivation by plasma inhibitors.

Platelet function tests

Measurement of the bleeding time is probably the best single test of platelet function. Reproducible results can be achieved using a standard cut like the one inflicted by the Simplate device. Bleeding time is prolonged when the platelet count falls below $100 \times 10^9/l$ and there is a rough inverse correlation with lower platelet counts. Bleeding time is also markedly prolonged in most functional platelet disorders, and to a variable extent by drugs which inhibit platelet function.

Methods for measuring *platelet adhesion* are time consuming and unsuitable for clinical application. *Platelet aggregation* is assessed by determining the density of platelet suspensions in plasma using modified photometry. Platelet-rich plasma is placed in a cuvette and the test agonist added while the platelets are stirred automatically. The change in platelet shape, and the increase in light transmission as platelets aggregate are recorded on chart paper. Aggregation is difficult to standardize and there is wide intersubject variation. As a result quantitative determination of aggregation is usually not helpful in diagnosis unless a gross defect is present. Characteristic aggregation patterns occur in the rare congenital disorders of platelet function (Fig. 10) and platelet-inhibitory drugs affect aggregation responses. Platelets in a normal plasma agglutinate in the presence of ristocetin (an antibiotic withdrawn from use because it caused platelet aggregation), von Willebrand factor serving as a molecular bridge, so that agglutination to ristocetin is defective in von Willebrand's disease. Agglutination of formaldehyde-treated platelets by ristocetin provides a semiquantitative measurement of von Willebrand factor in plasma. Assessment of platelet function in the routine hospital laboratory therefore depends on the appearance of the blood film, platelet count, bleeding time, and aggregation to some standard agonists. Diagnosis of suspected functional platelet defects should be carried out in specialized centres.

Bleeding due to platelet defects

Genetically determined platelet disorders

The hereditary disorders of platelet function (Table 10) can be broadly classified into membrane glycoprotein disorders and defects of platelet secretion. Von Willebrand's disease is not strictly a platelet disorder since the deficiency is in plasma von Willebrand factor. Figure 10 summarizes the *in vitro* aggregation response of platelet-rich plasma in various platelet disorders.

Bernard–Soulier syndrome

This is a rare autosomal recessive trait characterized by a moderate bleeding tendency with nose bleeds, menorrhagia, and bleed-

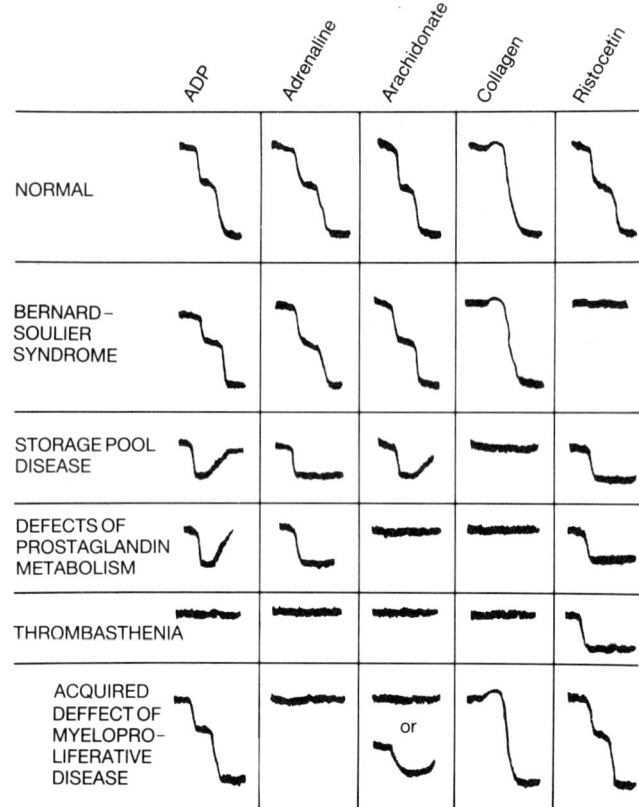

Fig. 10   Pattern of aggregation characteristic of some platelet disorders.

ing from the gastrointestinal tract. Purpura is not very common, probably because of some residual platelet function. Laboratory investigation shows marked prolongation of the bleeding time, giant platelets, and variable thrombocytopenia. Bernard–Soulier platelets lack a major membrane glycoprotein, glycoprotein Ib, which is the receptor for von Willebrand factor. This defect can be readily demonstrated by the failure of Bernard–Soulier platelets to agglutinate when exposed to ristocetin (Fig. 10). Ristocetin causes normal platelets in plasma containing von Willebrand factor to clump together by a mechanism which involves binding of von Willebrand factor to glycoprotein Ib. The defect can be reproduced by treating normal platelets with an antibody to glycoprotein Ib or resuspending them in plasma lacking von Willebrand factor. Aggregation to ADP and collagen is normal, but thrombin-induced aggregation is impaired for reasons which are not clear. Bernard–Soulier platelets exhibit reduced adhesion to subendothelium. The diagnosis is made if the investigation of a patient with life-long bleeding from mucosal surfaces and skin bruising reveals giant platelets on the blood film, thrombocytopenia, prolongation of the bleeding time, and platelets which fail to aggregate to ristocetin but aggregate normally to other agents. Detailed biochemical investigations are required to show absence of glycoprotein Ib on platelets. In serious bleeding episodes platelet transfusion is effective but its use should be restricted because antibodies develop to glycoprotein Ib.

Thrombasthenia (Glanzmann's disease)

This is a rare disorder with autosomal recessive inheritance. Patients have a life-long, moderate to severe bleeding tendency. Platelet count and morphology on light and electron microscopy are normal. There is prolongation of the bleeding time, defective clot retraction, and absent aggregation to ADP, collagen, and thrombin (Fig. 10). However, the platelets agglutinate normally to ristocetin and can bind ADP and collagen, change shape, and undergo the release reaction. Some of the patients lack platelet fibrinogen. Thrombasthenic platelets are defective in glycoproteins IIb and IIIa. These glycoproteins form a complex in the presence of calcium, which is activated during aggregation. The glycoprotein IIb–IIIa complex binds fibrinogen, which probably acts as a molecular bridge linking aggregating platelets together. Thrombasthenic platelets adhere normally to subendothelial structures, but fail to spread and do not excite platelet micro-aggregate formation. Diagnosis is usually straightforward in a patient with the appropriate history because of the striking absence of aggregation to standard agonists. Treatment is by use of platelet transfusion during serious bleeding episodes, although antifibrinolytic drugs can also be useful, particularly for menorrhagia.

Storage pool disease

This is the commonest of the congenital disorders of the release reaction and is due to lack of a releasable platelet storage pool of ADP. Some cases are familial, with either autosomal dominant or recessive inheritance; others are congenital with no clear-cut history to suggest a hereditary basis; and a few seem to be acquired. The severity of bleeding is variable, some cases coming to notice by excessive bleeding after surgery, others suffering mucosal bleeding, extensive bruising, and haemorrhage following minor trauma. Investigation shows prolongation of the bleeding time, a normal platelet count, and impaired aggregation to ADP and collegen (Fig. 10) because of failure to release the storage pool of ADP. Electron microscopy of the platelets shows absence of the dense granules which contain ADP and serotonin. Such platelets cannot release adenine nucleotides and are unable to store or release serotonin. As a result they agglutinate normally to ristocetin and adhere normally to subendothelium, but fail to promote subsequent aggregation and platelet plug formation. Treatment is limited to reassurance that serious spontaneous haemorrhage is unlikely and to advice on avoidance of non-steroidal anti-inflammatory drugs, which exaggerate the defect. Platelet transfusion restores haemostasis in severe bleeding or as prophylaxis for surgery.

Other defects of the release reaction

There are several rarer genetic disorders in which storage capacity is impaired in association with other abnormalities. The bleeding tendency in *Wiskott–Aldrich* and *Chediak–Higashi syndromes* is mild and due to a combination of thrombocytopenia and a reduced platelet content of adenine nucleotides. *Hermansky–Pudlak syndrome* is an autosomal recessive condition in which the storage pool defect is one element in a clinical triad also consisting of oculocutaneous albinism and abnormal pigmentation of bone-marrow macrophages. There is a group of defects in which storage organelles are normal but release fails to occur due to failure of normal prostaglandin synthesis (Fig. 10). In the 'aspirin-like defect' platelets behave as though exposed to aspirin and fail to undergo release after aggregation *in vitro* with ADP and collagen, due to deficiency of an enzyme, cyclo-oxygenase. *Thromboxane synthetase* deficiency similarly leads to defective release. The true frequency of these conditions is unknown due to the difficulty of reliably excluding exposure to non-steroidal anti-inflammatory drugs. Bleeding is usually mild.

A few families have been described in whom the alpha granules of platelets are absent, leading to the *grey platelet syndrome* (the platelets look grey on microscopy). Patients have a moderate bleeding tendency to which loss of platelet coagulant activity probably contributes. There is prolongation of bleeding time, thrombocytopenia, and enlarged, greyish-hued platelets on the blood film. Absent release of one of the α granule constituents, such as platelet factor 4, confirms the diagnosis.

Acquired platelet defects

Thrombocytopenia

Reduction of the platelet count may be due to decreased production, increased destruction (Table 11), or abnormal splenic sequestration.

Platelet production Platelets are released into the circulation from megakaryocytes in the bone marrow. Platelet production is partly controlled by a circulating agent, thrombopoietin, whose site of synthesis is unknown. Thrombocytopenia stimulates platelet production and release. Platelets form within megakaryocytes by invagination of a membrane which envelops small packages of the cytosol and organelles. The megakaryocyte cytoplasm then fragments, forming about 1000 platelets per cell which enter the circulation where they survive for 8 to 10 days before being removed by the reticuloendothelial system.

Failure of platelet production occurs in two ways. Infiltrative disease of the bone marrow or marrow hypoplasia reduce megakaryocyte numbers and hence platelet production. Leukaemias, aplastic anaemia, and malignant disease involving the marrow produce thrombocytopenia by this mechanism. Less commonly, megakaryocytes are present in normal numbers but do not produce platelets (ineffective thrombopoiesis). This occurs in chronic alcohol toxicity, megaloblastic anaemia, and some other dyshaemopoietic disorders (see page 19.58). Drugs, particularly the thiazide diuretics, can depress thrombopoiesis by direct interference with megakaryocyte maturation.

Platelet destruction Pathological shortening of platelet life-span involves one or more mechanisms: platelet consumption in mas-

Table 10 Hereditary disorders of platelet function

Membrane glycoprotein disorders		
Bernard–Soulier syndrome	Giant platelets; thrombocytopenia, reduced platelet adhesion, absent agglutination to ristocetin	Absence of glycoprotein Ib
Glanzmann's thrombasthenia	Absent aggregation, agglutinate with ristocetin, normal platelet count and morphology	Absent membrane glycoproteins IIb–IIIa; defective fibrinogen binding
(Von Willebrand's disease)*	Impaired platelet adhesion, reduced agglutination to ristocetin	Deficiency of vWF in plasma
Defects of platelet secretion		
Storage pool disease (SPD)	Defective release, impaired aggregation to ADP, collagen	Absent dense granules; defective release of ADP, calcium, serotonin
Aspirin-like defect	As SPD	Normal dense granules; defective release of ADP; absence of cyclo-oxygenase (PG synthesis)
Grey-platelet syndrome	Thrombocytopenia; agranular, large platelets; abnormal aggregation to collagen, thrombin	Absent α granules; defective release; possible defect of coagulation interaction

* No intrinsic platelet defect.

Table 11 Main causes of thrombocytopenia

Reduced platelet production

Marrow infiltration – leukaemia, myelofibrosis, etc.
Marrow hypoplasia – drugs, toxins, radiation, etc.
Infection – congenital rubella and other viral illnesses*
Congenital amegakaryocytic thrombocytopenia
Defective megakaryocytic maturation – megaloblastic anaemia, alcohol

Decreased platelet survival

Destruction
    Idiopathic thrombocytopenic purpura
    Drug-induced
    Infection*
    Post-transfusion
    Neonatal thrombocytopenia
    Secondary immune thrombocytopenia – SLE, lymphoma, etc.
Consumption
    DIC, TTP
    Infection*
    Haemangioma (Kasabach–Merritt syndrome)
Sequestration of platelets
    Splenomegaly

    * The thrombocytopenia of infections is probably the result of several different mechanisms.

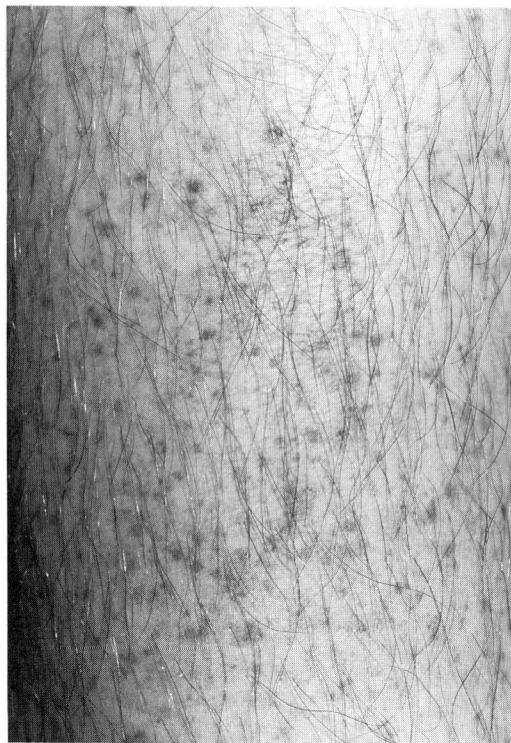

Fig. 11 The shin of a 16-year-old boy with idiopathic thrombocytopenic purpura, showing the discrete flat purpuric spots which fade from red through purple to brown in colour.

sive thrombosis; accelerated phagocytosis by cells of the reticuloendothelial system of platelets coated with immunoglobulin, platelets with adsorbed immune complexes on their surface, or platelets damaged by multiple impacts with non-endothelialized surfaces in the circulation; and, rarely, platelet destruction by complement-dependent lysis.

Acute thrombocytopenic purpura

In children, acute thrombocytopenia can develop 7–10 days after an infection, most often following infectious mononucleosis, mumps, rubella or rubeola and occasionally after immunization. Thrombocytopenia is rarely severe and usually disappears spontaneously over a few weeks, though it may persist longer after infectious mononucleosis. It probably results from adsorption of immune complexes on the platelet surface. The onset is sudden with widespread petechiae on the skin and mucosal surfaces, which occasionally form bullae in the mouth. Death from intracranial bleeding very occasionally occurs.

Acute idiopathic thrombocytopenic purpura is also seen, almost always in children and young adults. In three-quarters of cases there is an antecedent upper respiratory tract infection 2–3 weeks previously. The onset is sudden and thrombocytopenia often profound with extensive purpura. Mortality is from 1 to 2 per cent, resulting largely from intracranial haemorrhage. The mechanism of thrombocytopenia is thought to be similar to that which follows exanthematous virus infections due to adsorption of immune complexes by platelets. Diagnosis is rarely difficult: purpura develops in a child in the absence of serious underlying disease, the blood film simply shows thrombocytopenia and the bone marrow large numbers of immature megakaryocytes. Most cases will recover spontaneously within a few weeks. There is no evidence that steroids influence the course of the disease and they should not be used routinely. The guidelines given on the next page should be followed if it is thought that steroids must be given a trial because of a high risk of bleeding.

Chronic idiopathic thrombocytopenic purpura (ITP) (Werlhof's disease; purpura haemorrhagica; essential thrombocytopenia; autoimmune thrombocytopenic purpura)

In this condition, thrombocytopenia develops insidiously, usually without any obvious cause, though a few cases seem to develop from the acute form of the disease. Most patients are young or middle-aged women.

Typically the disorder presents with bruising or scattered purpura, particularly over areas of trauma or pressure (Fig. 11). Some patients present with menorrhagia, recurrent nose bleeds, or occasionally with unexplained gastrointestinal blood loss. There are variable numbers of petechial lesions in the skin and in more severe cases there may be haemorrhagic bullae in the mouth. More extensive ecchymoses can follow mild trauma. It is most unusual to be able to palpate the spleen in this condition, and splenomegaly suggests that there is underlying leukaemia, lymphoma or portal hypertension. Chronic ITP runs a waxing and waning course with recurrent crops of petechial haemorrhages, mucous membrane bleeding or, uncommonly, severe bleeding from the gastrointestinal tract. It is most unusual to see fundal haemorrhages unless the patient is also anaemic. Thrombocytopenia is variable but the rest of the blood count is normal unless there has been significant blood loss. Occasionally there is associated autoimmune haemolytic anaemia (Evans' syndrome). Bone marrow examination usually shows increased numbers of megakaryocytes, consistent with increased platelet turnover, which appear less granular than normal.

The immunological basis of ITP was first suspected from the observation that affected women frequently gave birth to children with transient neonatal thrombocytopenia. In Harrington's classical experiment plasma from affected patients caused thrombocytopenia when transfused into normal recipients. Further confirmation of the hypothesis was delayed by lack of reliable methods for detecting antibody on affected platelets but platelet associated IgG (PAIgG) can be demonstrated in more than 80 per cent of cases. Normal human platelets have plasma IgG non-specifically adsorbed to the surface, so that there is sometimes doubt whether the amount of PAIgG is pathological. Concentration of PAIgG tends to correlate inversely with platelet count. Since ITP platelets may have only twice the normal amount of PAIgG it is not clear why the antibody leads to accelerated platelet destruction. Some immunoglobulins might be directed at specific membrane components but current methodology cannot resolve this.

It is important to distinguish the idiopathic form of chronic immune thrombocytopenia from thrombocytopenia secondary to systemic lupus erythematosus (SLE), lymphoma, drug-induced immune thrombocytopenia, hypersplenism, and bone marrow suppression. Diagnostic difficulty is most likely in SLE and drug-induced thrombocytopenia, in both of which PAIgG is increased.

Treatment

Many patients do not require specific treatment. Although the platelet count is reduced, bleeding is often disproportionately slight, probably because the proportion of young, biochemically more efficient cells is increased. Patients with platelet counts above $50 \times 10^9/l$ do not require therapy in the absence of bleeding or significant purpura. Patients with counts in the range $20-50 \times 10^9/l$ should be given a trial of corticosteroid therapy as a few will achieve lasting remission. Whether splenectomy is justifiable in this group is debatable and is probably best decided on the basis of clinical evidence of a bleeding tendency and fitness for surgery, both of which would favour splenectomy. Patients with platelet counts below $20 \times 10^9/l$ are at considerable risk of bleeding. They should be treated as soon as the diagnosis is established with 80 mg prednisolone daily, gradually reducing so that a maintenance dose of less than 15 mg daily is attained within 3-4 weeks. Failure to maintain a platelet count above $50 \times 10^9/l$ or continued severe bleeding is an indication for splenectomy.

The decision on when to opt for splenectomy is sometimes difficult: many patients survive without serious bleeding for years with periodic remissions and relapses; there is an immediate 1-2 per cent mortality for the operation in fully fit patients and an increased risk of infection thereafter (which is greater in children); and although splenectomy results in a satisfactory degree of remission in about 80 per cent of patients, the operation is a high price to pay for failure in the remainder. However, the worst outcome is late splenectomy in the patient rendered Cushingoid and at high operative risk following an overextended and unsuccessful course of steroids. All patients should receive polyvalent pneumococcal vaccine before operation, prophylactic penicillin for a year thereafter or until they reach the age of 21 years, and be given prompt antibiotic treatment for bacterial infections. A few individuals with very low platelet counts before surgery may respond rapidly to a course of high-dose gammaglobulin intravenously, which enables splenectomy to be carried out more safely. Gammaglobulin is very expensive and as the treatment has not been properly evaluated, should be given only after careful thought to patients at high risk of bleeding. It probably works by saturating Fc receptors and blocking the reticuloendothelial system.

Many treatments have been tried in patients who do not respond to corticosteroids or splenectomy, and in whom either a very low platelet count or symptomatic bleeding remains a problem. Until recently immunosuppressive treatment using azathioprine in a dose of 100-300 mg daily was indicated. Response to immunosuppressive therapy sometimes occurs only after a few weeks or months and treatment should be continued for six weeks before abandoning it as ineffective. The response is rarely dramatic and the potential benefit from immunosuppressive therapy should be weighed against the well-known adverse effects. There does not seem to be an advantage for any particular immunosuppressive agent and enthusiasm for the use of vincristine in patients refractory to other forms of treatment has not been borne out by experience.

Administration of the steroid danazol can apparently induce remission in some cases refractory to corticosteroids and splenectomy. Danazol treatment has not been properly assessed and its value relative to other treatments is not yet certain. However, it should probably be tried first because of the most encouraging results so far obtained, and its low toxicity.

Other treatments which have been tried include plasmapheresis, colchicine, and high-dose gammaglobulin intravenously. The effect of gammaglobulin usually seems to be transient and it is likely to be more useful in preoperative management of a few

high-risk patients. Platelet infusions are rarely indicated though may be necessary in the emergency management of massive and life-threatening bleeding, or if there is uncontrollable oozing from the splenic bed during splenectomy. Oral tranexamic acid can be helpful in symptomatic management of menorrhagia though hysterectomy is occasionally necessary.

Drug-induced immune thrombocytopenia

Immune thrombocytopenia was first described in response to quinine, but the mechanism was worked out using the obsolete sedative carbromal (Sedormid). Susceptible individuals produced an antibody which in the presence of the drug, caused platelet agglutination. In nearly all instances the mechanism involves antibody production in response to the drug and adsorption onto the platelet surface of the drug – IgG immune complex. Although the antibody is not directed against a platelet component, the reaction is relatively specific: exposure to quinine can evoke an IgG immune complex which binds only to platelets and an IgM complex which binds to red cells. Drug-induced immune thrombocytopenia requires a minimum of about seven days to develop on first exposure, as antibody levels must attain a certain concentration for immune complexes to develop. Thereafter thrombocytopenia can occur unpredictably, sometimes following years of continuous exposure. Repeat administration of a drug to which the patient is sensitized induces an acute fall in platelet count. Drugs most frequently associated with this reaction include quinidine and quinine (often contained in proprietary medicines or soft drinks), heparin, PAS, methyldopa, and digitoxin. Repeat challenge to establish the diagnosis is potentially dangerous. Treatment is simply to stop the drug and advise the patient against taking it again.

Post-transfusion thrombocytopenia

This is a rare phenomenon in which thrombocytopenia develops about a week following blood transfusion. The mechanism involves production of antibodies directed against the Pl^{A1} antigen. About 3 per cent of the population who lack the Pl^{A1} antigen are theoretically at risk, but prior sensitization is required, occasionally from earlier transfusion and more commonly during pregnancy. In consequence, most patients are older women. There is widespread purpura and mucosal bleeding, with an approximate 10 per cent mortality. Exchange transfusion supplemented by platelet transfusion is indicated in severe cases. Subsequent blood transfusions in these patients should employ Pl^{A1} antigen negative blood.

Isoimmune neonatal thrombocytopenia

This rare condition (1 in 5000 births) is similar in its genesis to post-transfusion purpura. Fetal platelet antigens evoke antibody production in the mother and these return across the placenta. Unlike rhesus incompatibility and haemolytic disease of the newborn the syndrome frequently occurs in first pregnancies. The platelet Pl^{A1} antigen is the immunogen in most cases. Thrombocytopenia develops a few hours after birth, leading to fatal intracranial haemorrhage in 10-15 per cent of infants. Prompt platelet transfusion (preferably of cells lacking the offending antigen) is required to cover the period while the antibody is cleared.

Hypersplenism

Hypersplenism from any cause may result in thrombocytopenia, probably due to increased destruction in the enlarged spleen (see page 19.189). In addition sequestration of platelets in the splenic pool proportionately lowers the platelet count in the general circulation.

Disseminated intravascular coagulation (DIC)

Thrombocytopenia due to increased platelet destruction in a thrombotic process is usually seen only in fulminant cases of disseminated intravascular coagulation. Thrombocytopenia is only one factor in the bleeding tendency, recovery of the platelet count proving an early sign of improvement (see page 19.231).

Disorders of the blood

Acquired thrombocytopathy

Platelet function is frequently qualitatively abnormal in the myeloproliferative disorders (see page 19.44). Defects include loss of coagulation-promoting functions, failure of aggregation to standard aggregating agents (Fig. 10), and release defects due both to an acquired storage pool syndrome and to failure of the release mechanism. These abnormalities occur against a background of decreased, normal, or increased platelet count. Thrombocytopathy has been most clearly shown in patients with essential thrombocythaemia or polycythaemia vera in whom there is often a bleeding tendency, a prolonged bleeding time, and a variety of laboratory defects of platelet function (see page 19.38).

Platelets often function poorly in blood from patients with renal disease. Several defects have been described, including defective aggregation, reduced availability of phospholipid for acceleration of coagulation, and impaired clot retraction. The bleeding time is prolonged. Dialysable plasma factors, which are probably acid products of metabolism, are responsible and a functional defect of von Willebrand factor has also been claimed, which can be transiently corrected by infusion of DDAVP or cryoprecipitate.

A platelet function defect can be produced by the presence of certain pathological plasma proteins. Degradation products of fibrin and fibrinogen inhibit aggregation, possibly by blocking fibrinogen binding sites, and can enhance the bleeding tendency in states of excessive fibrinolysis. Macroglobulins affect platelet function non-specifically by coating the platelet surface and preventing agonist binding to the cell membrane, so contributing to the bleeding tendency associated with macroglobulinaemias.

Liver disease has been associated with thrombocytopathy but the aetiology is obscure. Acute alcohol intoxication causes depression of platelet function by blocking release. Chronic intoxication is associated with gross morphological abnormalities such as disorientation of the peripheral microtubules. These defects may contribute to the incidence of gastrointestinal haemorrhage in alcoholics. Cessation of alcohol is followed by a rebound to hyper-reactivity of platelet response.

Contribution of the vessel wall to haemostasis

The vessel wall contributes to haemostasis in three ways: vasomotor constriction of vessels limits blood loss; removal of endothelium exposes procoagulant and platelet-stimulating materials; and loss of the normal non-haemostatic properties of endothelium promotes haemostasis when vessels are damaged. Diseases of the vessel wall are discussed in Section 13.

Vasoconstriction

Injury to arteries and arterioles leads to prompt contraction mediated by local reflexes which are probably dependent upon stretch receptors in smooth muscle fibres. The stump of an avulsed limb often bleeds very little, although clean transection of the same artery would lead to catastrophic haemorrhage. Experimental injury to the muscle layer in the vessel wall provokes vigorous and persistent ring-like contractions which virtually obliterate the lumen. The contractile stimulus is transmitted between muscle cells in a narrow circumferential band which does not pass along the axial plane of the vessel. Violent forces expended in surrounding tissues may trigger the response, and can be observed in bullet wounds, for example, following which long sections of uninjured artery in the wounded area may go into intense spasm. Blood augments the effect and evokes powerful and sustained contractions as it tracks along an arterial wall, an action illustrated by the spasm of cerebral vessels in the region of a leaking aneurysm seen at angiography.

Chemical messengers which convey vasoconstrictor signals are poorly characterized. The artery wall releases vasoconstrictor substances (angiotensin II and metabolites of arachidonic acid) but serotonin and thromboxane A_2 liberated from activated platelets are probably more important. They are released close to the smooth muscle coat of the arterial wall as platelets coalesce into microthrombi.

Exposure of substances which promote haemostasis

Loss of endothelium, particularly if injury extends through the full thickness of the vessel wall, unmasks an array of materials which promote haemostatic plug formation. Tissue thromboplastin is a lipoprotein which interacts with factor VII leading to explosive generation of factor Xa and rapid formation of thrombin. A reciprocal activation mechanism occurs by which factor Xa cleaves factor VII to a more active form, factor VIIa. Factor VIIa also activates factor IX in the intrinsic pathway *in vitro*, and this has been proposed as a mechanism whereby tissue thromboplastin release could be a powerful and persistent stimulus to fibrin formation. Tissue thromboplastin is widely distributed in tissues and is even present on damaged endothelial cells. Experimental infusion of tissue thromboplastin in animals results in hypercoagulability, and massive release of tissue thromboplastin is probably a major causative factor in the development of disseminated intravascular coagulation following crush injuries.

Collagen and other connective tissue components, in addition to cell debris, initiate coagulation by contact activation. However, alternative pathways by which factor XI is activated must exist since deficiency of the other 'contact factors' (factor XII, high molecular weight kininogen and prekallikrein) does not cause a serious bleeding tendency. Exposure of collagen (particularly types I and III) causes platelets to adhere and release with secondary aggregation building up a platelet thrombus. Basement membrane and microfibrils associated with elastin are less reactive than collagen fibrils.

Endothelial cells synthesize von Willebrand factor, which promotes haemostasis by mediating platelet adhesion. Von Willebrand factor binds to vascular collagen and glycoprotein Ib on the platelet surface and thus physically cross-links platelets to exposed collagen. Release of von Willebrand factor from damaged endothelial cells probably augments plasma and platelet-released von Willebrand factor in haemostatic plug formation.

Loss of inhibitor systems

Endothelial cells have a surface coating of glycosaminoglycans, complex mucopolysaccharides carrying a strong negative charge. Human endothelium synthesizes mainly heparan sulphate, which has some properties similar to heparin, another glycosaminoglycan. Heparan sulphate could suppress contact activation of coagulation while the endothelial layer is intact. Heparans potentiate the action of antithrombin III (AT III), which binds irreversibly to the active site of thrombin and every other serine protease clotting factor, thus inactivating them. This mechanism is called into play as soon as activated factors are generated, whether at sites of injury or spontaneously within the blood column. A reduction of AT III below about 60 per cent of normal levels leads to a thrombotic tendency.

Endothelial cells synthesize at least two activators of the fibrinolytic system. Fibrinolysis has little effect on the early stage of haemostasis but acts to confine the coagulum to the site of injury by lysing fibrin spreading beyond the damaged zone. Endothelial cells have a surface receptor for thrombin called thrombomodulin. Thrombin bound to thrombomodulin does not cleave fibrinogen, but is preferentially directed towards activation of protein C, a plasma protein which inactivates factors V and VIII. Protein C is also involved in initiation of the fibrinolytic response. Deficiency of protein C (and of its regulatory protein, protein S) leads to a thrombotic tendency, underlining the importance of this controlling system in the haemostatic mechanism. Intact endothelium at the margin of a zone of vascular injury through these mechanisms can retard formation of the coagulum and stimulate the fibrinolytic response.

Blood platelets do not adhere to intact endothelial cells *in vivo*. Endothelial cells elaborate enzymes which degrade ADP (i.e.

Table 12 Aetiological classification of purpuras

Trauma	Mechanical purpura (cough purpura)
	Factitious purpura
	Painful bruising syndrome?
Coagulation defects	Severe haemophilia A or B
	von Willebrand's disease
Platelet defects	Thrombocytopenia
	Thrombocytopathy
	von Willebrand's disease
Direct endothelial damage	Anoxia
	Chemical injury
	Immunological reactions
	Henoch-Schönlein syndrome
	Drugs
	Infections
Decreased mechanical strength of the microcirculation	Hereditary haemorrhagic telangiectasia
	Hereditary connective tissue disorder
	Senile purpura
	Dysproteinaemias
	Scurvy
	Cushing's syndrome
	Amyloidosis
Micro-embolic damage	DIC, fat embolism, micro-organism emboli (e.g. SBE)
Psychosomatic	Psychogenic purpura
	Painful bruising syndrome?
Malignancy	Kaposi's sarcoma

ADPase activity) and this could limit interplatelet reactions evoked by vascular damage. Prostaglandin I_2, prostacyclin, is a more potent inhibitor of platelet reactions and a powerful vasodilator. Prostacyclin is synthesized in the vessel wall, principally by endothelial and smooth-muscle cells, and inhibits platelet adhesion and aggregation. PGI_2 release from endothelium is stimulated by thrombin and this might constitute a significant negative feedback mechanisim *in vivo*.

Vascular purpuras

Vascular defects account for some of the more unusual forms of purpura (Table 12). Bleeding is usually due to loss of normal mechanical stability of the vessel wall and haemostatic function is normal.

Hereditary haemorrhagic telangiectasia (Osler–Rendu–Weber syndrome)

This dominantly inherited condition usually becomes clinically manifest at puberty or later. The characteristic telangiectasis is a thin-walled, sack-like lesion formed of vascular cells and full of blood, resembling a small haemangioma. Multiple telangiectases are present in the skin and mucous surfaces. They appear as 2–3 mm diameter raised lesions, red in colour, which blanch on pressure. Patients often present with nose bleeds or iron-deficiency anaemia resulting from bleeding from one or more of the lesions in the stomach or elsewhere in the gastrointestinal tract. The diagnosis can usually be made from the appearance of typical telangiectases on the face, within the mouth, or proximal to the nail folds. It is important to examine family members for similar lesions. Very rarely death results from uncontrolled gastrointestinal haemorrhage.

Treatment is limited to blood or iron replacement, and application of pressure when possible to the bleeding site, for example by packing the nose. In serious cases, systemic inhibition of fibrinolysis or surgical attack on the bleeding point may be required. There is anecdotal evidence that oestrogen therapy reduces the frequency of attacks by an unknown mechanism. In about 15 per

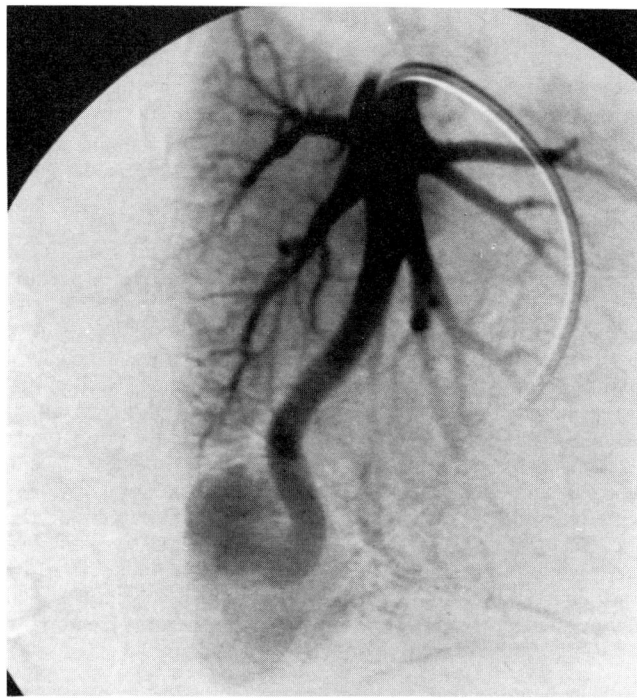

Fig. 12 Digital subtraction vascular angiogram of the left lung in a woman with hereditary haemorrhagic telangiectasia. There is a large arteriovenous malformation (AVM) in the posterobasal segment, with a feeding artery approximately 1 cm in diameter. The AVM was successfully embolized with multiple steel coils leading to significant reduction in right-to-left shunt and improved exercise tolerance. (Reproduced by courtesy of Dr D. J. Lintott.)

cent of patients arteriovenous malformations develop in the lungs, and can be sufficiently large to cause a right-to-left shunt (Fig. 12).

Connective tissue disorders

Bleeding is a significant feature of certain inherited disorders of connective tissue, for example, in some of the eight subgroups of the Ehlers–Danlos syndrome. Death from uncontrolled gastrointestinal haemorrhage or rupture of a major vessel occasionally occurs. Hyperextensibility of joints and easy deformability of skin, which are hallmarks of the syndrome, are a consequence of various defects in collagen synthesis (see Section 17). Bleeding probably results from rupture of small vessels inadequately supported in abnormally mobile tissues and structurally weakened by defective collagen. Laboratory tests of haemostatic function, including the bleeding time, are usually normal. Pseudoxanthoma elasticum can also present with bleeding into the skin and, occasionally, fatal gastrointestinal haemorrhage caused by similar mechanisms.

Easy bruising

Some individuals, usually women, present with a history of easy bruising. Inevitably some individuals will bruise more easily than others following minor trauma and further investigations should only be instigated if there has been significant bruising, in particular the occurrence of spontaneous bruises of an unusually large size.

Mechanical factors

Unusual pressure to skin occasionally produces purpuric lesions such as 'string vest purpura'. Acute venous obstruction can produce purpura, for example, *cough purpura* which occurs over the face of children with whooping cough and similar disorders. The striking confluent purpura which accompanies asphyxia, and the patches of purpura which can appear on the neck and behind the ears following breath-holding attacks are also due to acutely elevated venous pressure. Crops of purpura occur round the ankles of patients with venous insufficiency in the legs, particularly during warm weather.

The painful bruising syndrome (psychogenic purpura, autoerythrocyte sensitization)

This uncommon disorder of unknown aetiology is confined almost entirely to women between the ages of 20 and 50 years, with a predilection for those with some medical connection. It is characterized by bruises on the limbs or trunk, the patient giving a characteristic story of tingling or slight pain, followed by the appearance of a bruise which may grow in size over a period of hours. In severe cases the limbs are covered in bruises and there may be large confluent lesions on the trunk although rarely on the back. These attacks persist for months or years, though usually the condition remits spontaneously. Many of these women have strange personalities, and physical or emotional trauma frequently precede the onset of symptoms, though there are no distinctive psychiatric abnormalities. In some cases the lesions can be reproduced by injecting red cells or red-cell stroma subcutaneously, hence one of the alternative names for the condition, autoerythrocyte sensitization. There is probably an organic basis for some cases, while in others it is clearly artefactual and associated with self-inflicted skin wounds. Psychotherapy is not helpful and the disorder is best treated by reassurrance that serious bleeding will not occur and that spontaneous recovery is likely.

Senile purpura

Bruising on the forearms and back of the hands is extremely common in the elderly. The lesions are large, flat, purplish bruises with a sharp outline, due to weakening of vascular structures and loss of supporting subcutaneous tissue with advancing age. Almost identical bruises occur in some patients on corticosteroid therapy and in association with Cushing's syndrome.

Henoch–Schönlein purpura

The Henoch–Schönlein syndrome and the vascular purpuras which are precipitated by a number of infective agents and by certain drugs are likely to share common pathogenic features, although there are obvious differences. The purpuric and erythematous lesions of the skin are probably due to inflammation in the wall of small blood vessels from which red cells leak. Vascular damage is thought to be mediated by the immune system, involving immune complex deposition, or some form of hypersensitivity reaction. Low-grade intravascular coagulation may contribute particularly to purpura caused by infective agents.

Henoch–Schönlein syndrome is a relatively uncommon disorder which classically presents in male children, and occasionally in adults. There is seasonal variation in incidence and a preceding upper respiratory tract infection in about a third of cases. It is thought to result from an anaphylactic response to an infective agent, because of the sudden onset following an infection and the typical histology of a leukocytoclastic vasculitis with inflammation of the vessel wall and deposits of IgA-containing immune complexes. However, no specific allergen nor transferable factor has been identified. The fully developed syndrome consists of malaise, fever, myalgia, joint pains, abdominal pain, glomerulonephritis, and the characteristic rash. This is distributed on the extensor surfaces of the limbs and buttocks and appears as a purpuric eruption against a background of erythema. Abdominal pain follows involvement of small mesenteric vessels in the arteritic process and focal glomerulonephritis can occur (see Section 18). Periarticular swelling and angioedema of the hands and feet are occasionally seen. In about half the cases, and particularly in adults, the illness is limited to malaise and the typical rash. Diagnosis is based on the clinical features, and often on the characteristic appearance of the skin rash (see Section 20). Laboratory investigation is rarely helpful. Mild polymorphonuclear leucocytosis can occur and tests of urine and faeces may be positive for blood. In cases complicated by nephritis the urine contains protein, red cells, and casts.

Treatment does not alter the course of the disorder. Corticosteroids are sometimes used for symptomatic relief of joint pain and swelling, and are usually prescribed if renal involvement is suspected though their value is uncertain. Fatalities due to intussusception of the bowel, major gastrointestinal bleeding, or progressive glomerulonephritis with renal failure are rare. Relapses, usully consisting of the rash alone, are common, particularly in adults, and the disorder occasionally recurs at intervals over several years.

Vascular purpura due to infection or drugs

Purpura due to vasculitis occurring during acute infections is probably produced by a combination of vessel wall damage promoted by immune complex deposition and initiation of intravascular coagulation. Certain infective organisms seem particularly likely to initiate vascular purpura, for example, meningococci and rickettsiae.

Drugs, particularly aspirin, sulphonamides, and the benzothiadiazines, occasionally cause vascular purpura. Cross-reactivity between membrane components of vascular cells and antibodies induced by the drug, or damage by immune complexes resulting from sensitivity to the drug, are possible but unproven pathogenic factors.

Dysproteinaemias

Oozing from capillaries, and occasionally episodes of major bleeding, are recognized features of the dysproteinaemias. Abnormal immunoglobulins (characteristically IgM or IgA types) interfere with fibrin formation and platelet function, probably by forming a surface film which interferes with molecular interaction. In addition, there may be accelerated clearance of coagulation proteins following complex formation with the abnormal immunoglobulin. Damage to vascular cells, especially in the microcirculation, may result from heavy coating with abnormal protein and from hypoxia due to cell sludging in small vessels.

Scurvy

(See also Section 8.)

Customarily considered a colourful aspect of maritime history, mild scurvy is not infrequent amongst the old and undernourished sectors of the British population. Punctate haemorrhage and hyperkeratosis around hair follicles with a variable degree of bruising, particularly on the shins, is typical. Bleeding from mucosal surfaces and subperiosteal haemorrhage occurs only with more severe disease, now rarely seen in developed countries. Lack of vitamin C impairs synthesis of connective tissues and leads to abnormal fragility of blood vessels and supporting structures. Laboratory tests of haemostatic function are usually normal thought inconsistent abnormalities of platelet function have been described. The diagnosis of this disorder is considered in detail in Section 8.

Cushing's syndrome

Purpura due to increased vascular fragility is a feature of Cushing's syndrome (see also Section 10). Chronic exposure to abnormally high levels of glucocorticoid hormones inhibits normal protein synthesis and progressively weakens connective tissues. Loss of supporting subcutaneous fat in some areas and the poor tensile strength of the skin leads to abnormal tearing and stretching of small vessels with resulting purpura and bruising. Abnormal bleeding following trauma also occurs because of instability of thrombus related to poor wound healing. Similar changes occur in some patients who are treated with corticosteroid drugs.

Amyloidosis (see also Section 9)

Purpura occurs in cutaneous amyloidosis. It is found particularly in the periorbital region. Some patients with systemic amyloidosis exhibit selective factor X deficiency which is due to binding of factor X by amyloid fibrils (see also Section 9).

The fibrinolytic system

Blood contains a mechanism for fibrin dissolution and removal which is activated during haemostasis. The process is essential for remodelling of blood vessels following haemostatic plug formation and for removal of extravascular fibrin after wound healing.

Plasminogen activation

Plasmin is the end product of fibrinolytic activation. Plasmin, a two-chain molecule, is a potent proteolytic enzyme with a spectrum of activity similar to trypsin. It is formed from the proenzyme, plasminogen, a single-chain globulin, by the cleavage of a single arginine–valine bond. Two forms are found in plasma: native or glu-plasminogen which has a terminal glutamic acid, and a partly degraded form, lys-plasminogen, with a terminal lysine, produced by plasmin autocleavage of the parent molecule. Lys-plasminogen has greater affinity for binding to fibrin and is more susceptible to proteolytic activation than glu-plasminogen.

Plasmin is formed by proteolytic cleavage of plasminogen by activators. The intrinsic activation pathway generated entirely within the blood is probably of little physiological importance. Contact activation of blood generates fibrinolytic activity through a mechanism which involves factor XII, factor XI, high molecular weight kininogen and kallikrein. It has been proposed that factor XII deficiency might predispose to thrombosis because of defective intrinsic fibrinolytic activity but this is not certain. Defects of contact activation are uncommon so that it is difficult to establish definitely whether this pathway of fibrinolysis is more than a laboratory curiosity. Proteases released from activated leucocytes cause plasminogen activation directly and could contribute to the intense fibrinolysis observed in some cases of disseminated intravascular coagulation (DIC) and following trauma to blood in extracorporeal circulations.

Physiological fibrinolysis is almost entirely due to release of tissue-plasminogen activators from endothelial cells (Fig. 13). Immunological studies have revealed two types: tissue-type plasminogen activator (tPA) and urokinase-type activator. Tissue-type activator has been purified from material produced by a human melanoma cell-line and is now being synthesized using recombinant DNA technology. It is a serine protease with sequence homology to other coagulation proteases, though unlike coagulation zymogens it is active when released. Tissue plasminogen activator has a very strong affinity for fibrin, and bound to fibrin has an enchanced capacity to convert fibrin-bound plasminogen to plasmin. Urokinase-type activator does not bind to fibrin. However, streptokinase–activator complex (formed during therapeutic administration of streptokinase) binds to fibrin, though its activity is not enhanced. Since both tPA and plasminogen bind to fibrin there is a highly efficient generation of plasmin localized within the fibrin coagulum and virtually none outside the clot (Fig. 13). Plasma normally has a low level of activator activity which is markedly increased by exercise, stress, and venous occlusion. There is some circumstantial evidence that individuals who produce little activator activity under such circumstances have an increased risk of thrombosis.

Inhibitors of fibrinolysis

Fibrinolysis is checked by protease inhibitors which inhibit both activators of plasminogen and plasmin itself. A specific inhibitor of tPA has recently been identified in endothelial cells. A number of inhibitors in plasma can retard the intrinsic, contact-mediated fibrinolytic activation including C1 inactivator, antithrombin III, and α_2-macroglobulin, but are unlikely to be of clinical importance. Inhibition of free plasmin is vital for protection of several plasma proteins against uncontrolled proteolytic activity in plasma; plasmin can digest prothrombin, factors V and VIII, and

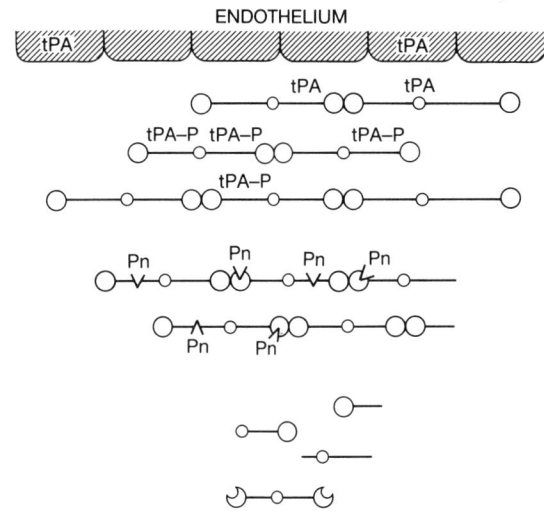

Fig. 13 Fibrin formation initiates release of tissue plasminogen activator (tPA) from endothelial cells. Plasminogen (P) and tPA bind to polymerizing fibrin. Plasmin (Pn) generated *in situ* cleaves fibrin at multiple sites, releasing soluble fibrin degradation products.

fibrinogen, in addition to fibrin. Antithrombin III and α_1-antitrypsin have weak antiplasmin activity but are of little importance in the control of fibrinolysis. Alpha$_2$-macroglobulin forms a slow-acting reservoir of antiplasmin activity which is particularly effective if the fast-acting antiplasmin is saturated.

It is now clear that α_2-antiplasmin is the most important antiplasmin in blood. It binds to plasmin in one of the fastest protein–protein interactions so far measured, initially in a reversible reaction, and more slowly forming a stable complex with a one-to-one molar ratio which is inactive. Lack of α_2-antiplasmin permits uncontrolled plasmin action and causes a rare but severe bleeding disorder. Formation of the plasmin–antiplasmin complex has two consequences: the inhibitor blocks the active site, preventing proteolysis; in addition, complex formation masks lysine-binding sites on plasmin which are necessary for binding to fibrin. Partitioning of formed plasmin between α_2-antiplasmin and fibrin constitutes part of the molecular control of fibrinolysis (Fig. 13).

Plasmin–fibrin interaction

Tissue plasminogen–activator and plasminogen bind avidly to fibrin as it forms. Plasminogen binds to fibrin through the lysine-binding site (so called because it binds lysine, one of a number of amino acids with antifibrinolytic activity). Hence physiological fibrinolysis is generated once tissue plasminogen activator, plasminogen, and the terminal reaction substrate, fibrin are found in close proximity. Plasmin remains bound to fibrin through its lysine binding sites and cannot bind to antiplasmin. The close molecular association which bars inactivation by antiplasmin accelerates proteolysis of fibrin. Hence self-destructive fibrinolytic potential is incorporated into thrombi during their formation (Fig. 13). Plasmin thus formed is committed to fibrin proteolysis; plasmin formed elsewhere is almost instantaneously inactivated by complex formation with α_2-antiplasmin.

Plasmin attacks fibrin at a number of different points. Fibrin is degraded and eventually the large dimeric molecule is reduced to an amino-terminal core, fragment E, about one-tenth the size of the parent molecule and to a major fragment designated D. Numerous intermediates are produced, two of the major forms being fragments X and Y. Early fibrin degradation products are clottable by thrombin and compete with fibrinogen for thrombin. Certain fragments retain the capacity to polymerize and may compete for fibrin polymerization sites. Excess fibrin degradation products thus inhibit clot formation. This does not affect normal haemostasis but leads to inhibition of coagulation during therapeutic or pathological fibrinolysis.

Tests of fibrinolytic activity

Plasma contains little or no free plasmin, and fibrinolytic activity is usually assessed by estimation of plasma activator activity and assay for breakdown products of fibrin. There are a number of different methods for assessing plasma activator, which depend on measuring the time taken for clot lysis after antiplasmins have been removed. In the most commonly used method, activators, plasminogen, and fibrinogen are precipitated with other proteins from plasma by acidification and dilution. The so-called euglobulin precipitate is redissolved, clotted with thrombin, and the time to clot lysis observed. The *euglobulin clot lysis time* (ECLT or ELT) is largely a measure of activator activity in plasma. Similarly, there are a number of different techniques available for measurement of *fibrin degradation products* (FDPs). Most depend on estimation of the concentration of fibrinogen and fibrin-related antigens in serum, (from which the clotting process will have removed thrombin-clottable fibrinogen). Most laboratories use commercial kits which utilize latex spheres coated with antisera to fibrinogen which agglutinate in the presence of the antigen.

Several different types of assay for tPA, tPA-inhibitor, plasminogen, plasmin, and α_2-antiplasmin are available but their use is currently largely restricted to specialized laboratories.

Anticoagulant, fibrinolytic and antiplatelet drugs

Iatrogenic bleeding caused by anticoagulants is one of the commoner causes of haemorrhagic disease. Heparin, oral anticoagulants, and fibrinolytic agents profoundly depress haemostatic activity and in overdose create a potentially lethal bleeding tendency. Serious bleeding resulting from antiplatelet treatment is uncommon.

Heparin

Heparin is a glycosaminoglycan consisting of repeated sequences of sulphated glucosamine and glucuronic or iduronic acid, linked to form a strongly negatively charged organic acid. Glycosaminoglycans are widely distributed in connective tissues. Heparan sulphate synthesized by endothelial cells and located on their surface probably contributes to their non-reactivity in the coagulation system. Heparin and heparin-like compounds are heterogeneous in molecular size, composition, and anticoagulant properties. Heparin is located mainly in mast cells but can be found in extracellular sites in aorta and lung. The physiological function of tissue heparin is not known.

Therapeutic heparin is prepared from bovine lung and pig intestinal mucosa and has proved difficult to standardize because of chemical heterogeneity. Potency is expressed in units which relate to anticoagulant activity but this is not a precise measurement because of differences between assay systems and batches of material.

The anticoagulant action of heparin depends on the presence in plasma of the natural coagulation inhibitors heparin co-factor II and antithrombin III. Activated factors II (i.e. thrombin), IX, X, and XI form 1:1 molar complexes with antithrombin III and are permanently inactivated. The reactions are accelerated a 1000-fold or more in the presence of heparin. Heparin also has some direct antithrombin activity. The kinetics of the reactions vary and accelerated inhibition of factor Xa, for example, proceeds at lower concentrations of heparin than others. This has been proposed to account for the efficacy of low-dose heparin in prophylaxis of deep venous thrombosis. There is minimal systemic anticoagulant effect measured by APTT (see page 19.214) during low-dose heparin therapy. Low molecular weight heparins and semisynthetic derivates of heparin-like molecules which have greater anti-Xa activity and little anticoagulant action measured by APTT are now being intro-

duced. Heparin also interferes with platelet function and this could contribute to unwanted episodes of bleeding.

Anticoagulant therapy is usually started with heparin because its action is rapid in onset. There is an impression, which is not well substantiated, that it is more potent than oral anticoagulants in suppressing thrombosis. In the United Kingdom, unlike the practice in North America where longer periods of infusion are used, heparin is commonly given for two to three days. This is almost certainly adequate in most cases. Heparin should be given as a loading dose of 5000 units, followed by continuous infusion of 1000 to 1500 units hourly, adjusted to keep the APTT at about twice the control value. Warfarin can be started at the same time, since heparin given at the dosage indicated prolongs the prothrombin time by only a second or two. This enables oral anticoagulation to be established before heparin is stopped.

Full intravenous heparinization produces a significant bleeding tendency but serious haemorrhage is uncommon. Bleeding is most likely to occur from the site of a previously unsuspected lesion such as a duodenal ulcer, from accidental overdose or a casual approach to control of therapy. Adjusting dosage by monitoring the APTT reduces the risk of serious overdose but in one large series there was no difference in mean APTT between patients who bled compared with those who did not. Stopping treatment is usually sufficient to allow arrest of haemorrhage because the average plasma half-life of heparin is only about 90 min (the half-life varies with concentration). In severe bleeding the action of heparin should be reversed by infusion of protamine sulphate. This is theoretically straightforward, as 1 mg protamine sulphate neutralizes the action of 1 mg heparin. In practice, it is impossible to calculate the level of heparin in the blood accurately during continuous infusion or several hours after a bolus injection, and a starting dose of protamine has to be chosen arbitrarily. It is better to start with a low dose and titrate the need for additional doses according to the effect on the APTT, since overdose of protamine can itself induce bleeding.

Oral anticoagulants

Drugs of the coumarin group were developed following observations that spoiled sweet clover caused a bleeding disorder in cattle. This was shown to be due to the presence of a coumarin compound from which synthetic derivatives were subsequently produced. Sodium warfarin has been the most widely used, but there are alternatives. Warfarin is a competitive inhibitor of vitamin K, which is required for the final stages of synthesis of factors II, VII, IX, X, and protein C in the liver. Vitamin K is required for the carboxylation of glutamic acid residues in the coagulant proteins. Gamma carboxyglutamic acid so formed binds calcium and is essential for protein binding to phospholipids necessary for normal coagulation. Inhibition of vitamin K results in a failure of carboxylation and production of functionally inert proteins. These were detected immunologically in the plasma of patients treated with warfarin before the biochemical basis of drug activity was understood and were designated by the acronym PIVKA, standing for Protein-Induced-by-Vitamin-K-Absence. The defect in coagulation function produced by coumarins is reflected in marked prolongation of the prothrombin time, which is used to monitor treatment.

Warfarin and congeners are well absorbed from the gastrointestinal tract. Anticoagulant effects are delayed in onset and persist for several days after cessation of treatment, both because of the nature of drug action on protein synthesis and because coumarins are strongly bound to plasma proteins. Many drugs interact with warfarin and increase the anticoagulant effect (Table 13). Warfarin is metabolized by the liver and consequently has a much more pronounced effect in patients with liver disease. Drugs which induce liver enzymes, for example, barbiturates, tend, conversely, to reduce its effect. Patients treated with warfarin should be prescribed a minimum of other drugs because of the frequency of drug interactions, and alterations in concurrent treatment

Table 13 Some drug interactions with warfarin

Increased response to warfarin	
Inhibition of coumarin metabolism	Chloramphenicol, cimetidine, amiodarone, metronidazole, dextropropoxyphene
Displacement from protein binding	Phenylbutazone, chloral hydrate, nalidixic acid
Receptor interactions	Clofibrate, anabolic steroids
Others	Thyroxine, co-trimoxazole
Reduced response to warfarin	
Increased coumarin metabolism	Barbiturates, primidone, griseofulvin, rifampicin, carbamazepine, phenytoin
Interference with absorption	Cholestyramine
Stimulation of protein synthesis	Oral contraceptives

Non-steroidal anti-inflammatory drugs increase the risk of bleeding because of co-incident effect on platelets and likelihood of gastric erosion.

should be made with careful monitoring of PT if interaction is possible. Warfarin therapy should be started with a single dose of 10 mg followed by 5 mg daily until adjusted in response to the prothrombin time. Larger loading doses achieve therapeutic levels quicker in patients with a daily requirement greater than 6 mg (median dose) but cause an overshoot in PT in the remainder which makes subsequent control time consuming. Several schemes have been devised for calculating dosage, but none is sufficiently reliable and convenient to have been adopted generally. Warfarin should be started while the patient is still receiving heparin, which prolongs the PT time only slightly at therapeutic levels. Prothrombin time should be measured before the first dose of warfarin is given and carried out daily until control is established. Results are usually expressed as the ratio of the time using patients' plasma relative to control. Most physicians accepted a ratio of 2.0–4.5 as optimal for PT, determined using the Manchester Comparative Reagent supplied to most British hospitals. This reagent has now been discontinued due to fears of contamination by viruses during processing of human brain. Rabbit brain thromboplastin will be used in future and the results adjusted to allow for a different sensitivity. The International Normalized Ratio (INR) should be maintained between 2.0 and 4.5. Higher ratios might have greater antithrombotic activity but demand more effective anticoagulant control services than are generally available.

Bleeding due to accidental overdosage with warfarin or its congeners is more difficult to control than bleeding during heparin administration. Patients remain anticoagulated for several days after treatment is stopped. The effect of warfarin should be reversed by intravenous injection of vitamin K_1 if bleeding is severe. Since warfarin and vitamin K are competitive antagonists the use of vitamin K_1 will make it difficult to reanticoagulate the patient for several days. For an average size adult with minor bleeding 5 mg vitamin K_1 given intravenously should restore the PT level to normal within 2–6 hours and will permit reinstitution of warfarin therapy within 48–72 hours. Major bleeding in a patient with markedly prolonged PT should be treated with 10–20 mg vitamin K_1 administered slowly intravenously, and infusion of fresh frozen plasma. In the very rare life-threatening case factor IX concentrate, which also contains factors II, VII, and X, should be given. There is inevitably a risk of transmitting hepatitis and of causing thrombosis.

Ancrod

Ancrod has been relatively little used, but has interesting properties. It was isolated from the venom of the Malayan pit viper following clinical observations that patients bitten by the snake had incoagulable blood but rarely suffered from severe bleeding.

Ancrod has a thrombin-like action reacting directly with fibrinogen to release fibrinopeptide A although it does not release the B peptide. Fibrin formed by ancrod is not cross-linked and is rapidly cleared from the circulation by a combination of secondary fibrinolysis and the reticuloendothelial system. The anticoagulant effect probably largely depends on fibrinogen depletion which secondarily lowers blood viscosity.

Drugs which activate fibrinolysis

Two drugs, urokinase and streptokinase, have been used to promote the rapid lysis of major thrombi. Urokinase is produced naturally by renal parenchymal cells and is present in human urine. It acts by direct proteolytic cleavage of plasminogen to form plasmin and there is a linear dose–response relationship which makes urokinase relatively safe and predictable. Unfortunately, it is very expensive, and in nearly all circumstances it is hard to justify its use in place of streptokinase.

Streptokinase is a purified exotoxin from type C streptococci. It forms a complex in plasma with plasminogen which develops activator activity. The activator complex then forms plasmin largely from unbound plasminogen. At the start of streptokinase infusion free plasminogen concentration is high and there is rapid plasmin formation which can saturate the inhibitor system, leading to a degree of uncontrolled proteolytic activity. However, plasminogen is rapidly used to form the complex, and thereafter small amounts of plasmin are released as fresh plasminogen is synthesized.

Urokinase is probably more efficient than streptokinase and infusions need be given only for 12 to 24 hours. Streptokinase requires three or four days to achieve a similar degree of thrombolysis. Both drugs need to be given by infusion, to which hydrocortisone should be added in the case of streptokinase because it is antigenic. Maintenance doses of streptokinase vary from 50 000 to 100 000 units/hour. Calculation of the loading dose varies, depending on the schedule followed. Dosage of urokinase is assessed on the basis of body weight and varies according to the preparation used. In both instances it is advisable to consult the detailed instructions supplied by the manufacturer. Fibrinolysis is induced systemically and in most cases there is probably little advantage to be gained by local infusion at the site of thrombosis. An exception to this is the use of streptokinase to lyse thrombi in coronary arteries by direct infusion through a coronary artery catheter. The high local concentration of activator and the small mass of thrombus enables lysis to be achieved in 30–60 min, although fibrinolytic action is detectable in the systemic circulation.

Bleeding following use of urokinase or streptokinase can be extremely severe. Neither drug should be given within 10 days of surgery; strokes within the previous 3 months or lesions such as peptic ulcer are absolute contraindications; and invasive procedures on the circulation or intramuscular injections should be avoided. Serious bleeding should be managed with infusion of the antifibrinolytic agent tranexamic acid and restoration of fibrinogen concentration with cryoprecipitate or human fibrinogen.

The most exciting development in therapeutic fibrinolysis since its inception has been the recent synthesis of human tissue-type plasminogen activator (tPA) by recombinant DNA technology. Activity of tPA is greatly enhanced by the presence of fibrin, unlike streptokinase and urokinase, and therefore it produces much less systemic fibrinogenolysis. Early evidence from animal experiments and studies in patients indicates that tPA is relatively selective for fibrin and thrombi can be lysed with minimal proteolysis in blood.

Orally active drugs which enhance fibrinolysis have weak activity. They were thought to act by increasing production or release of vascular activator but alternatively could lower levels of inhibitors of plasminogen activation. The diguanide phenformin and the anabolic steroid ethyloestrenol are active individually and synergistically; the anabolic steroid, stanozolol, has been used more recently. There is no evidence from clinical trials that these drugs have significant antithrombotic activity.

Non-steroidal, anti-inflammatory drugs with antiplatelet activity

Many non-steroidal, anti-inflammatory drugs inhibit platelet function measured *in vitro*, though only aspirin and sulphinpyrazone have been assessed in clinical trials. Sulphinpyrazone, although used originally as a uricosuric agent, was found to inhibit platelet function. Non-steroidal, anti-inflammatory drugs inhibit the enzyme cyclo-oxygenase, which catalyses the formation of endoperoxides (precursors of prostaglandins) from arachidonic acid. Inhibition of cyclo-oxygenase prevents the production of endoperoxides and thromboxane A_2, which induce the platelet release reaction. In the presence of inhibitors of cyclo-oxygenase, platelets aggregate poorly *in vitro* and experimental microthrombus formation is inhibited. Aspirin irreversibly acetylates the enzyme and single exposure results in inhibition of cyclo-oxygenase for the lifespan of the platelet. In contrast, sulphinpyrazone is a reversible, competitive inhibitor. Inhibition of prostaglandin synthesis in addition suppresses vascular prostacyclin synthesis and this might have deleterious consequences by reducing platelet-inhibitory activity of the vessel wall. There is debate whether the enzyme in platelets is more susceptible to inhibition than the enzyme in endothelial cells. However, the optimum dose of aspirin required to achieve an ideal balance between these effects is not known. Sulphinpyrazone, unlike aspirin, prolongs platelet survival in humans and since platelet survival has some predictive power for thromboembolic risk, this could indicate that other, unrecognized actions might be important.

Other drugs which inhibit platelet function

Dipyridamole was observed to inhibit white body formation in experimental animals after being used as a vasodilator. It impairs cell uptake of adenosine and raises intraplatelet concentrations of cyclic AMP thereby inhibiting the platelet release reaction, and reducing platelet adhesion in experimental systems.

The synthetic polysaccharide dextran prolongs the bleeding time and interferes with platelet function. It is a sticky molecule and probably coats the surface of both platelets and endothelial cells.

A range of drugs which inhibit platelet function is under development. Of these, ticlopidine, an agent which acts both on the megakaryocyte and the platelet, inhibits platelet aggregation and markedly prolongs the bleeding time. Unfortunately it can cause neutropenia and is currently unavailable in the United Kingdom though widely used elsewhere. Compounds which inhibit production of thromboxane A_2 or block its activity and analogues of prostacyclin are being evaluated.

Platelet inhibitory drugs rarely cause significant bleeding though they can probably provoke haemorrhage from peptic ulcers. In published clinical trials about twice as many episodes of bleeding occur during aspirin treatment as during placebo administration. Ticlopidine is the only platelet inhibitor which markedly prolongs the bleeding time and if combined with oral anticoagulant treatment can produce a serious haemorrhagic tendency.

Acquired bleeding disorders

Haemostatic failure due to inadequate levels of coagulation factors can arise from deficient or defective synthesis, increased destruction or pathologic inhibition. Sometimes several mechanisms operate simultaneously. Abnormal bleeding in the absence of a previously diagnosed coagulation disorder needs to be evaluated urgently in the light of the possible causes and clinical associations (Table 14).

Vitamin K deficiency

Vitamin K is essential for synthesis of functional factors II, VII, IX, X, and proteins C and S. In the absence of vitamin K these proteins are released from the liver lacking carboxyl groups and fail to bind to phospholipid, which is essential for their haemostatic reactions. The dominant clinical effect is a bleeding disorder resembling haemophilia B, with haematuria, haematomas, and haemarthroses. Vitamin K is a fat-soluble vitamin found in green vegetables but also synthesized by colonic flora. Pure dietary deficiency is rare, most cases encountered in clinical practice being due to malabsorption secondary to small-bowel disease or biliary obstruction. Gut sterilization by antibiotics might contribute but cannot alone cause a deficiency if dietary intake is normal. Premature infants have a critical vitamin K status since most placental transfer occurs late in pregnancy, their livers are immature with reduced capacity to synthesize coagulation factors, breast milk is low in vitamin K, and the infant colon contains no bacterial flora. Formerly this commonly led to a severe haemorrhagic state (*haemorrhagic disease of the newborn*, HDN) but universal use in developed countries of prophylactic intramuscular vitamin K injections to premature infants at birth has made the condition rare.

Diagnosis is based on the finding of prolonged PT and APTT which can be corrected by mixing with normal plasma and with very rapid return to normal of these tests after intravenous administration of soluble vitamin K 10 mg (less to infants and children). Patients with liver disease often respond only partially to vitamin K, since this treatment has no effect on the consequences of hepatocellular damage which have a complex effect on haemostasis.

Vitamin K antagonism

Inadvertent overdosage with warfarin regularly produces haemorrhagic problems and is often provoked by concurrent administration of drugs which displace warfarin from albumin binding or interfere with clearance (Table 13). It is important to monitor anticoagulant control carefully when new drugs are added to therapy in anticoagulated patients. Occasionally anticoagulants are taken surreptitiously by psychiatrically disturbed patients to induce a factitious bleeding state. This may be suspected when laboratory findings strongly suggest vitamin K deficiency but no cause can be identified. Plasma warfarin measurements can confirm this possibility.

Liver disease

Bleeding in liver disease is multifactorial. Impaired synthesis leads to reduced levels of all factors with the notable exception of factor VIII. Activated clotting factors that are not neutralized by interaction with endothelial cells are removed by the reticuloendothelial system (RES) in the liver, which probably recognizes desialated molecules that have lost their glycosylated activation peptides. Complexes of factors and antifactors are also removed by the RES. Laboratory tests frequently suggest the presence of DIC, with low fibrinogen, increased fibrin degradation products (FDP) and short clot lysis times (Table 15). Contributing to these findings are lowered levels of antiplasmin and reduced clearance of FDP. Abnormal fibrinogen (dysfibrinogenaemia) is sometimes demonstrable by a very prolonged thrombin and reptilase clotting times in the face of normal levels of fibrinogen antigen. This has been associated with hepatocellular carcinoma. In general, the severity of the bleeding tendency correlates best with the overall severity of hepatocellular disease. Because of the very short half-life and high turnover of factor VII, the prothrombin time is a sensitive index of hepatic synthetic function. It is unwise or dangerous to attempt liver biopsy when the prothrombin time is prolonged by more than 4 s compared with controls. Temporary correction can be achieved by plasma infusion in some cases. Thrombocytopenia due both to depressed marrow production and to hypersplenism is common in liver disease. Platelet function may also be disturbed

Table 14 Acquired bleeding syndromes

Condition	Mechanism	Clinical associations
Vitamin K deficiency	Failure to carboxylate factors II, VII, IX, X	Malabsorption, biliary obstruction, prematurity (HDN)
Vitamin K antagonism	Oral anticoagulants interfere with vitamin K metabolism	Warfarin overdose, surreptitious ingestion, potentiating drugs
Vitamin C deficiency	Defective collagen synthesis	Poor diet, alcoholism
Liver disease	Defective synthesis of clotting factors and inhibitors. Defective clearance of active factors	All forms of chronic and acute hepatocellular disease
Alcohol	Inhibits platelet function	Liver disease
Disseminated intravascular coagulation	Excess stimulus to coagulation overwhelms control, free thrombin produced and platelets and clotting factors consumed. Secondary fibrinolysis occurs	See Table 15
Haemolytic uraemic syndrome	Vascular injury to renal endothelium with renal failure and microangiopathic haemolysis	Infections?
Thrombotic thrombocytopenic purpura	Widespread vascular damage with hyalin microthrombi, platelet depletion and microangiopathic haemolysis	Infections?
Acquired haemophilia	Autoantibody to factor VIII or more rarely other factors	Pregnancy, rheumatoid arthritis, penicillamine

and adhesion impaired due to a functional von Willebrand factor defect. The resulting prolonged bleeding time can sometimes be corrected in the short term by administration of DDAVP (0.3 μg/kg). Investigation of patients with liver disease prior to surgery should include a full screen of haemostasis and a bleeding time. In practice, the most troublesome form of bleeding in liver disease is that from oesophageal varices, a local mechanical problem secondary to portal hypertension, exacerbated by coagulation defects and platelet deficiency. The haemostatic and coagulation problems associated with liver transplantation are discussed in Section 12.

Alcohol ingestion

Alcohol is a direct toxin on the marrow, inhibiting platelet production, and on platelets themselves, inhibiting their function. In the longer term, of course, alcoholism is associated with hepatic cirrhosis and all the complications of liver disease. Its action is synergistic with warfarin to produce a dangerous bleeding tendency if taken to excess.

Disseminated intravascular coagulation

Release of soluble thromboplastins, if sufficiently intense and prolonged, activates coagulation and can overwhelm the controlling systems leading to generalized coagulation in the circulation. Direct endothelial damage produces a similar effect which, through thrombin generation, leads to deposition of fibrin,

secondary fibrinolysis (a protective phenomenon), platelet aggregate formation, and finally, haemostatic failure with depletion of clotting factors. The rate and localization of the thrombotic stimulus will determine the clinical outcome. Tissues particularly susceptible to microvascular blockage and necrosis are the heart, kidney, brain, and liver.

DIC has been associated with a large and diverse group of clinical aetiologies (Table 16). Cases in which DIC is chronic with little depletion of coagulation factors, no obvious clinical signs of a bleeding tendency, and indicators of continuing consumption confined to laboratory tests (increased FDP, PT, and APTT slightly) can be treated with heparin pending definitive therapy (for example, evacuation of a dead fetus). Acute DIC presents with a severe bleeding tendency, usually in patients who are dangerously ill with one or more of the aetiologies in Table 16. The first sign is often continued bleeding from or massive bruising around intravenous access sites. Exsanguinating haemorrhage may occur during or after surgery and alarming extravasation may result from minor procedures such as bone marrow aspiration. Heparin is dangerous in this situation as it will exacerbate the bleeding. Correction of the haemostatic defect is essentially a holding operation until the underlying cause of DIC can be identified and treated. Fresh frozen plasma should be infused as a source of coagulation factors, all of which it contains. Response should be monitored by repeated assay of prothrombin time and partial thromboplastin time. If the fibrinogen level is markedly depressed cryoprecipitate can be given. Multiple donor concentrates are contraindicated at present because of the high risk of transmitting viral diseases and (in the case of prothrombin complex concentrates) of triggering further intravascular coagulation. Platelet concentrates should be infused if the count falls below 80×10^9/l.

Microangiopathic haemolysis is thought to occur as a result of red cells being forced through fibrin meshwork in the microcirculation. It remits as DIC is brought under control. Fibrinolysis is protective in DIC and so fibrinolytic inhibitors are dangerous and contraindicated.

Haemolytic uraemic syndrome

This may be regarded as a special case of DIC localized to the renal vasculature. The exact cause of the damage is most likely to be immunological, with deposition of immune complexes of a critical size between the glomerular endothelial cells and basement membrane and activation of complement. It presents most often in childhood with uraemia and haemolysis after a trivial infection (see page 19.150 and Section 18).

Thrombotic thrombocytopenia purpura

This syndrome, first described by Moschkowitz, consists of thrombocytopenia with widespread microvascular thrombi causing tissue damage and histologically containing hyalin thrombus. Clinical features of the syndrome include fever, leucocytosis, and progressive, multifocal neuropsychiatric disturbances. Usually laboratory investigation does not reveal the picture of DIC, though rarely this can occur as a late phenomenon. Most patients are young and female. Formerly the prognosis was very poor, but latterly has improved with the introduction of plasma therapy (either by simple infusion or by plasmapheresis) though the reason why this should be successful is as obscure as the aetiology (see page 19.150).

Acquired anticoagulants

Autoantibodies to coagulation factors are produced rarely but most often with specificity for factor VIII. The resulting clinical condition may be described as acquired haemophilia A. Patients sometimes have associated conditions such as rheumatoid arthritis or may be pregnant, but most often are elderly with no intercurrent illness. Treatment is by means of high-dose factor VIII to control bleeding episodes. Considerable success has been reported using porcine factor VIII concentrate, with which the acquired autoantibodies usually do not cross-react. Antibodies to von Willebrand factor have also been reported to produce acquired von Willebrand's syndrome.

An antibody to phospholipoprotein which interferes with several lipoprotein-dependent stages in coagulation has been termed the *lupus anticoagulant* because it was first detected in patients with systemic lupus. It usually prolongs the APTT by 5 to 30 s while the prothrombin time is often normal unless the antilipoprotein nature of the antibody is emphasized by diluting the thromboplastin reagent. Its inhibitory action is confirmed by using mixtures of patients' and normal plasmas in the APTT assay. The inhibitor can be detected in about 10 per cent of patients with SLE who frequently have antibodies to other lipid-containing antigens such as cardiolipin. In spite of the anticoagulant effect *in vitro* a bleeding tendency is most unusual and the antibody is associated with recurrent abortion and a (paradoxical) tendency to thrombosis (see page 19.243).

Approach to the bleeding patient

Clinicians and pathologists are asked to evaluate supposedly excessive bleeding in two different circumstances. Firstly, there is the outpatient consultation for a history of bleeding often because elective surgery is under consideration and the patient has warned the surgeon of undue bleeding in the past. A detailed history should be taken, paying attention to the site and character of bleeding episodes, their length and relationship to trauma or surgery, and age at onset. The effect of common surgical operations such as tonsillectomy and dental extraction should be noted. For example, bleeding for an hour after dental extraction is normal whereas bleeding for two days is highly abnormal. Easy bruising, frequent nosebleeds, menorrhagia, and prolonged bleeding from superficial cuts all suggest a platelet-mediated defect. Conversely haemarthroses and muscle bleeds strongly suggest haemophilia A or B. The family history should be taken, noting racial group, consanguinity, and evidence for sex-linked or autosomal transmission. A detailed drug history is essential.

Physical examination is often relatively unhelpful except in severe haemophilia where haemophilic arthropathy is obvious. The clinical features of vascular and connective tissue disorders should be sought, since laboratory investigation cannot diagnose these conditions. Likewise, features of endocrine disturbance should be looked for. A definite diagnosis will probably require laboratory assays of coagulation factors and platelet function.

The second type of consultation arises with the patient who is currently bleeding excessively often during or immediately after surgery, or who is under intensive care. These cases are much harder to diagnose accurately since the bleeding is often multifactorial in origin and the results of laboratory tests are changing rapidly as well as being influenced by intercurrent therapy with plasma, platelets, and anticoagulants. It is important to establish the time of onset of bleeding and how it related to therapeutic or surgical intervention. It may not be possible to elicit any history from the patient, but relatives should be questioned about bleeding in the past since mild haemophilia or von Willebrand's disease can present in adult life. Bleeding localized to a site of surgery may simply be due to local factors, a diagnosis which can be made more confidently when the laboratory screening tests are normal. Bleeding from drip sites as well as from the surgical wound indicates generalized haemostatic failure. Urgent investigations will include platelet count, examination of the blood film for evidence of microangiopathy, and measurement of PT, APTT, fibrinogen, and fibrin degradation products (see page 19.228). Disseminated intravascular coagulation (DIC) is the commonest finding in seriously ill patients developing a bleeding tendency for the first time but, occasionally, previously unsuspected coagulation inhibitors or specific factor deficiencies are encountered.

Venous thromboembolism

Between 2 and 5 per cent of the population suffer venous thrombosis at some time. Often morbidity will be minimal and risk of pulmonary embolism low. However, 3096 deaths from pulmonary embolism were certified in England and Wales in 1980; pulmonary embolism is now the commonest cause of maternal death; and the postphlebitic syndrome remains an intractable problem. The cost and effort devoted to prophylaxis against venous thromboembolism indicates the continuing potential seriousness of the condition.

Aetiology and pathogenesis

Deep vein thrombosis (DVT) probably develops through a combination of sluggish blood flow and hypercoagulability (an imprecise term denoting a reduced threshold for activation of haemostasis leading to accelerated fibrin formation). Recognized clinical risk factors (Table 17) largely fit this aetiological concept and it is supported by experimental studies.

Studies using the jugular vein thrombosis model have shown that infusion of a procoagulant, such as the contact activator ellagic acid, or trace amounts of activated clotting proteins, in rabbits and dogs, followed by venous occlusion, results in formation of homogeneous dark red thrombi. Neither stasis nor hypercoagulability alone results in thrombosis, but shorter periods of occlusion are required the stronger the procoagulant. Tissue trauma or sur-

Table 15 Laboratory tests in acquired bleeding disorders

	PT	APTT	TCT	Fbg	FDP	Platelets	Other tests
DIC	Long or N*	Long or N	Long	Low or N	Raised	Low	Red cell fragments; short ECLT
Vitamin K deficiency or antagonist	Long	Long	N	N	N	N	Factors II, VII, IX, X low
Liver disease	Long or N	Long or N	Long or N	Low or N	Raised or N	Low† or N	Factor VIII raised
Heparin	Long	Long	Long	N	N	N occasionally low	Reptilase time normal
Factor VIII antibody	N	Long	N	N	N	N	Mixing tests confirm inhibitor; low F VIII
Lupus‡ anticoagulant	Long or N	Long	N	N	N	N	Mixing tests confirm inhibitor; effect not increased by incubation; prolonged PT accentuated using dilute thromboplastin

* N, normal.
† FDP may cause erroneous low value.
‡ Associated with thrombosis and spontaneous abortion.

Table 16 Some clinical conditions associated with DIC*

Infective	Gram negative septicaemia
	Viruses
	Malaria
Malignant	Adenocarcinomas† (gut, ovary, prostate, pancreas etc.)
	Promyelocytic leukaemia
Circulatory	Mismatched transfusion
	Giant haemangioma†
	Aortic aneurysm
	Shock
	Allergic vasculitis†
Obstetric	Retained dead fetus†
	Pre-eclampsia†
	Amniotic fluid embolism
	Abruptio placentae
Toxic	Snake bites
	Heat stroke
Miscellaneous	Major trauma
	Head injury†

* Many other associations have been described in occasional cases.
† Conditions indicated tend to have a chronic course.

Table 17 Factors which predispose to venous thrombosis

Related to hypercoagulability	*Related to stasis*
Oestrogen administration	Cardiac failure
Puerperium	Stroke
Surgery	Pelvic obstruction
Malignancy	Prolonged
Myocardial infarction	immobility
Hereditary disorders of haemostasis	Nephrotic syndrome
Antithrombin III deficiency	Dehydration
Heparin co-factor II deficiency	
Protein C deficiency	*Unknown*
Protein S deficiency	
Abnormal plasminogen	Age
Abnormal fibrinogen	Behçet's syndrome
Coagulation factor concentrates	Lupus anticoagulant
Paroxysmal nocturnal haemoglobinuria	Sepsis
	Homocystinuria

gical procedures can substitute for direct activation of coagulation. Vascular injury is not required, consistent with observations from post-mortem examinations which rarely show primary vessel wall injury in deep vein thrombosis.

Oestrogens and venous thrombosis
Administration of oestrogen increases the risk of venous thrombosis and the effect is apparently dose related: low-oestrogen oral contraceptives carry a very low relative risk; large doses of oestrogen used in early clinical trials in prevention of myocardial infarction and metastatic prostatic carcinoma caused a marked increase in deaths from embolism. Pregnancy probably does not increase the incidence, but it rises about twenty-fold during the puerperium. Oestrogen increases plasma concentrations of fibrinogen and factors II, VII, VIII, IX, and X; depresses antithrombin III concentration; and reduces fibrinolytic activator in the vessel wall, changes which can be broadly interpreted as prothrombotic. Whether hypercoagulability alone is sufficient to account for the thrombotic risk from oestrogen is not known. Oestrogen also has profound metabolic effects, slows venous blood flow, and probably damages the vessel wall, each of which could contribute to a thrombotic tendency.

Surgery
Small calf-vein thrombi are common after surgical operations. Some procedures, for example, open prostatectomy and fixation of fractured neck of femur carry a pronounced risk (35 and 75 per cent incidence, respectively). The potential hazard of venous thrombi is indicated by the 6–10 per cent mortality from pulmonary embolism shown in autopsy studies on patients dying following surgery for fractured femoral neck. Unfortunately it is not possible to predict which patients will develop life-threatening ileo-femoral thrombi and which relatively harmless thrombi in small calf veins.

Tissue trauma at operation is likely to be an important aetiological factor; operations near the hip joint could also involve damage and obstruction to the femoral vein. Shortened APTT and reduced fibrinolytic activator activity measured preoperatively increase the risk of postoperative thrombosis. Small thrombi probably develop in calf veins or around valve cusps during operation and in some patients (perhaps those with intercurrent disease, poor mobility or inadequate defence mechanisms) the thrombi grow and become symptomatic 5–7 days postoperatively. Increasing age is the most important independent risk factor for postoperative DVT, but the reason is not known.

Malignancy
Patients with cancer have a three- to five-fold excess risk of venous thrombosis overall, although malignancy is not a strong independent risk factor for postoperative DVT. Cancers of the lung, pancreas, breast, prostate, and gut are particularly likely to be associated with thromboembolism (and DIC). Mucin from adenocarcinomas and proteases isolated from colonic and breast cancers can activate factor X; in addition patients with malignancy frequently have minor abnormalities of haemostatic function which could promote thrombogenesis. Transient superficial thrombophlebitis is a rare complication of malignancy: lesions are typically painful, discoloured, and tender, lasting for a few days and occurring in superficial veins usually in the limbs. As DVT often occurs in these patients, hypercoagulability is presumed to be a significant factor.

Myocardial infarction
At the time anticoagulants were introduced into treatment of acute myocardial infarction, 20 per cent of hospital deaths were due to venous and arterial thromboembolism. The incidence of DVT assessed by leg scanning is still about 30 per cent, but due to routine prophylaxis and early mobilization, massive thrombosis or significant pulmonary embolism is now rare.

Hereditary disorders of haemostasis
Recurrent DVT, spontaneous thrombosis in patients below 30 years of age, episodes of thrombosis in unusual sites, or a strong family history, should lead to screening for hereditary defects in plasma coagulation proteins associated with a high risk of thromboembolism.

Protein C deficiency This is probably the commonest form of familial thrombophilia. The defect shows autosomal dominant transmission in most kindreds although a few homozygous cases have been detected, presenting with severe DIC and purpura fulminans in neonates. A characteristic clinical sign is the development of skin necrosis on first being treated with warfarin. Blood tests in heterozygotes show protein C antigen concentrations ranging from 30 to 60 per cent of normal. Many cases when first studied are already on treatment with warfarin which depresses levels of protein C antigen, and this can make diagnosis difficult. The concentration of another vitamin K-dependent protein such as prothrombin or factor IX can be assayed concurrently and a disproportionate lowering of protein C antigen may then be apparent. A few patients have normal protein C antigen and low protein C activity but are not easy to detect as the available assay methods are laborious. Recently, *deficiency of protein S*, which regulates activity of protein C, has been reported to cause a thrombotic tendency. Protein S deficiency is found about as frequently as protein C deficiency in early onset familial thrombosis.

Antithrombin III deficiency The first family with antithrombin III deficiency was recognized 20 years ago. There is an autosomal dominant pattern of inheritance leading to repeated episodes of venous thrombosis starting in early adult life. Arterial thrombosis also occasionally occurs. Plasma concentrations of antithrombin III usually range from 40 to 60 per cent of normal. Homozygotes have not been detected and probably die in infancy. Antithrombin III can be readily assayed using a chromogenic substrate. Antithrombin III concentrate is available to cover surgery and childbirth.

Defects of plasminogen and fibrinogen Plasminogen defects and abnormal fibrinogens are rare causes of a familial thrombotic tendency which can be detected by assays of fibrinolytic potential or of fibrin polymerization, respectively.

Infusion of coagulation factor concentrates
Venous thrombosis commonly occurs after infusion of factor IX concentrate. These preparations contain trace amounts of activated coagulation factors. The complication is particularly prone to occur in patients with liver disease, who have impaired reticulo-endothelial function, and are unable to clear activated clotting proteins normally.

Paroxysmal nocturnal haemoglobinuria
Patients with this rare syndrome (page 19.54) are at increased risk of thrombosis, particularly of the hepatic veins. The reasons are not known: red cell stroma is not strongly procoagulant and complement-mediated platelet damage has been reported.

Effects of venous stasis
There is a high frequency (about 30 per cent) of thrombosis in the veins of paralysed legs. The rate is three times higher in the paralysed than in the unaffected limb in patients with hemiplegia. For unknown reasons the risk declines with time since the onset of weakness. Sluggish venous flow resulting from reduced cardiac output is probably the major factor associated with risk of DVT in heart failure, nephrotic syndrome, and prolonged dehydration. Although experience is anecdotal, there seems a genuine though small risk from prolonged immobility, particularly if associated with partial venous obstruction and dehydration, occurring, for example, during long plane journeys.

Predisposing factors with unknown mechanism
Behçet's syndrome (see Section 24) is an uncommon vasculitic disorder in which there is a recognized risk of DVT (Fig. 14). Vessel wall damage might play a part, particularly as no other obvious mechanism has been identified. In *homocystinuria* (see Section 9) venous and arterial thromboembolism forms part of the symptomatology, the basis for which is unknown: hypotheses include contact activation by homocystine and platelet stimulation by vascular surfaces damaged by homocystine. In patients with the *lupus anticoagulant* (found in 10 per cent of patients with systemic lupus erythematosus, women with recurrent abortions, and others with no recognized illness) venous thrombosis is common. Haemostatic tests show variable prolongation of standard clotting tests (Table 15) and no evidence of hypercoagulability. *Sepsis and inflammation* cause thrombosis of local veins, presumably due mainly to vessel wall damage and release of leucocyte thromboplastins. This is thought to account, for example, for dural sinus thrombosis associated with chronic middle-ear infections, carotid sinus thrombosis complicating facial sepsis, and ileofemoral thrombosis in patients with ulcerative colitis.

Age is the most important of the recognized risk factors. Only 196 of the 3000 fatal cases of pulmonary embolism in England in 1980 occurred in patients less than 55 years old. Many of the other risk associations are commoner in old people, but age is a strong

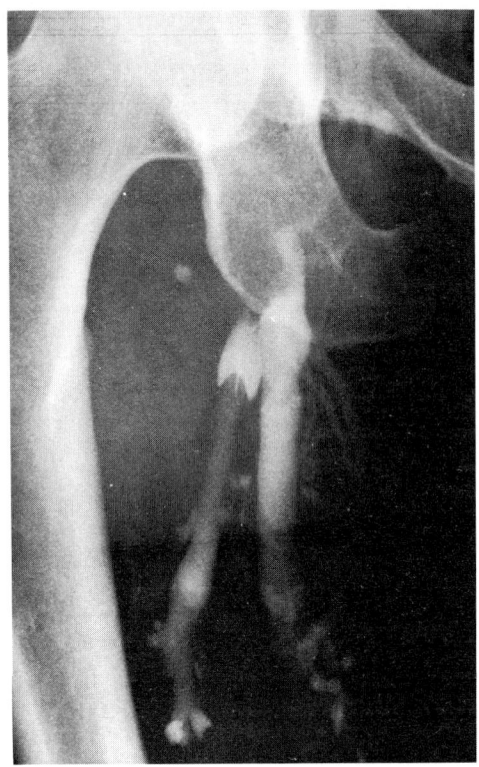

Fig. 14 Ascending venography in a 31-year-old man with Behçet's disease presenting with pain and swelling of the right leg. There is a thrombus originating at the junction of the profunda and superficial femoral veins.

and independent risk factor particularly for postoperative venous thrombosis. The reasons for this are not known.

Presentation and clinical features of deep vein thrombosis
Venous thrombosis involving the lower extremities or pelvis may present in different ways. Not uncommonly the first indication of peripheral venous disease is the onset of symptoms or signs of pulmonary embolism (see Section 13). Non-obstructing ileofemoral or common iliac vein thrombosis is often unsuspected unless pulmonary embolism occurs. Although pelvic veins are frequently suggested as a source of pulmonary emboli, radiographic and post-mortem studies indicate that most arise from leg veins, or external and common iliac veins.

Thrombo-occlusive disease of peripheral veins presents as superficial thrombophlebitis or deep vein thrombosis. Superficial thrombophlebitis is painful and examination reveals a tender cord-like structure immediately under the skin, usually accompanied by surrounding inflammation. It rarely if ever gives rise to significant embolism. Superficial thrombophlebitis commonly occurs as a manifestation of local superficial venous disease co-existing with varicosities or incompetent perforating veins. Rarely it is a manifestation of malignancy.

Deep venous thrombosis can be difficult to recognize and about half of all cases do not produce local symptoms. This is particularly true of loosely adherent thrombi which are not obstructing venous flow. Large thrombi of this type in the ileofemoral segment are especially dangerous because of the risk of sudden massive pulmonary embolism. Typical clinical features when present consist of an aching or cramp-like pain involving the calf or thigh (which can be severe, with a bursting sensation when there is significant obstruction to venous return); mild or moderate tenderness on palpation of the calf or thigh muscles; swelling of the limb which is either obvious or detectable by measuring limb circumference (allowing for a natural difference of at least 1 cm); positive Homans' sign (pain in the calf on dorsiflexion of the foot) though

Table 18 Differential diagnosis of deep vein thrombosis of the leg

Causing swelling

Familial lymphatic incompetence (McIlroy's syndrome)
Lymphatic obstruction
Congestive cardiac failure
Disuse due to paralysis or prolonged immobilization

Causing swelling and inflammation

Erysipelas
Haematoma
Ruptured synovial (Baker's) cyst
Torn muscle fibres

this has no discriminant value and is positive in most other causes of pain in the calf; and more importantly, cyanotic discoloration of the limb, engorged superficial veins, and increased warmth. These signs are usually obvious in severe cases of venous occlusion, the affected leg becoming cyanosed and swollen with marked oedema which extends above the knee. However, absence of signs and symptoms can never be taken to exclude the diagnosis. On rare occasions *venous gangrene* can develop with disappearance of the arterial pulses. This indicates massive venous occlusion involving the deep and superficial veins with total outflow obstruction and almost always indicates the presence of underlying malignant disease.

Significant obstruction from venous thrombosis leads in succeeding months or years to the postphlebitic syndrome. Destruction of deep venous valves with resultant high venous pressures in the leg produces a chronically painful, swollen limb. The pain, aching or bursting in character, comes on with standing and if there is considerable oedema limits mobility. Leakage of red cells induced by high pressure results in brownish pigmentation of the skin and there may be ulceration on the inner aspect of the leg overlying communicating veins.

Diagnosis and management of deep venous thrombosis
Diagnosis of deep venous disease of the legs can be difficult, and if there is the slightest doubt clinically, ascending venography should be carried out unless there are contraindications, e.g. allergy to previous injections of radio-opaque materials. Clinical diagnosis has repeatedly been shown to be unreliable, whereas venography misses only small and probably trivial thrombi in the calf veins. Deep venous thrombosis, particularly confined to the calf, can be confused with several other conditions (Table 18). Some of these may require alternative diagnostic techniques, such as arthrography or ultrasound to detect a ruptured Baker's cyst. Other diagnostic methods for detection of DVT are less sensitive and accurate than venography: isotope venography and thermography are research investigations; impedance plethysmography, Doppler flowmeter examination, and fibrinogen leg scanning are useful as screening methods, usually in combination, but are not as reliable as venography. Tests of haemostatic function are not useful in the diagnosis.

General clinical evaluation should include appraisal of possible risk factors. In patients with recurrent thrombosis, particularly in different sites, more detailed investigation is indicated. However, in most patients with uncomplicated apparently spontaneous thrombosis, laboratory investigation for haemostatic abnormalities and occult malignancy is rarely productive. A few patients in selected categories (see above) should be screened for hereditary haemostatic abnormalities.

Treatment
Acute superficial thrombophlebitis is usually self-limited and responds promptly to analgesics and a short period of rest.

Deep vein thrombosis should be managed in hospital with the aim of preventing progression to a postphlebitic syndrome and the occurrence of a pulmonary embolus. Anticoagulant therapy, analgesia if necessary, and a short period of bed rest are the main lines of treatment. The current practice is to keep patients in bed for a few days until anticoagulation is established, though there is little evidence that this is beneficial. In most cases intravenous heparin should be started immediately and warfarin should be given a minimum of 48 hours before the planned cessation of heparin therapy. Although heparin prolongs the prothrombin time so that oral anticoagulants cannot be precisely controlled, the prothrombin time is lengthened by only a few seconds if heparin treatment is controlled.

Though anticoagulant treatment for symptomatic DVT is almost invariably given there is little objective evidence that it is beneficial. Anticoagulants were introduced before the advent of controlled clinical trials and have not been compared with placebo. Studies done recently have tended to compare the incidence of new cold areas on lung scans, for example, in patients receiving high or low levels of anticoagulation. The results are consistent with a protective effect of anticoagulants against pulmonary embolism.

Anticoagulant treatment does not affect intraluminal thrombus and patients with obstructed venous return are at risk of developing the postphlebitic syndrome. Thrombolytic therapy is sometimes used to prevent this though its use is controversial. Cineradiography has shown that prompt thrombolysis can prevent destruction of the venous valves and there is no doubt that thrombolytic drugs can lyse completely substantial amounts of clot. However, fibrinolytic drugs are more dangerous than standard anticoagulants and thrombolysis occurs in only 30–50 per cent of patients. Long-term follow-up studies have also cast doubt on whether worthwhile clinical improvement is sustained. As thrombolytic drugs are also very expensive it is advisable to consult a physician with practical experience of their use as early as possible after the diagnosis has been made. The dosage regimes are described on page 19.228 *et seq.*

Surgical removal of loosely adherent clot with an embolectomy catheter appears an attractive therapeutic option, but experience has shown that the inevitable damage to the vessel wall leads to prompt rethrombosis in the majority of cases and surgery is hardly ever of benefit.

It is not certain how long patients should be maintained on anticoagulant therapy following a single episode of venous thrombosis. Because recurrent pulmonary emboli are unlikely to occur after six weeks, provided there are no persistent risk factors, it is usual to maintain anticoagulants for 6 to 12 weeks. Warfarin can then be stopped as 'rebound hypercoagulability', if it occurs at all, is not clinically important. If there are persistent risk factors, the patient should probably be maintained indefinitely on anticoagulant therapy.

Once patients are mobilized they should be supplied with properly fitted elastic stockings providing graduated pressure and advised to elevate the leg when sitting. These measures relieve and perhaps partly prevent symptoms of the postphlebitic syndrome. Elastic bandages should never be used as they exert discontinuous pressure which can obstruct venous return. Compression bandaging is only required in the treatment of trophic ulceration.

Prophylaxis of venous thrombosis
Appreciation of the frequency with which symptomless deep venous thrombosis complicates surgery, myocardial infarction, and heart failure, has prompted intensive efforts to provide effective prophylaxis.

Mechanical devices which improve venous blood flow in the legs during surgical operations are effective in preventing formation of calf-vein thrombi. Subcutaneous injection of low-dose heparin and dextran infusions probably both reduce the risk of pulmonary embolism as well as the incidence of radioisotopically detectable venous thrombi postoperatively. A small increase in surgical blood loss occurs and this has limited their use. Some surgeons, particularly in the United Kingdom, also have reservations about whether low-dose heparin prophylaxis prevents lethal pulmonary embolism and large proximal thrombi. The trials required to test the hypothesis would need to be very large, and until and unless results from such studies become available, it is probably sensible to use prophylaxis in patients over the age of 40 years.

Warfarin is a very effective prophylactic drug and significantly reduces the incidence of venous thrombosis and fatal pulmonary embolism following hip surgery, when serious thromboembolic complications are frequent. There is reluctance on the part of most orthopaedic surgeons to use warfarin from fear of major bleeding. One study has shown that aspirin provides effective prophylaxis against deep venous thrombosis following hip surgery. Other antiplatelet agents have not so far been tested in this condition and because of the relatively small platelet component of venous thrombi, seem likely to prove less effective than anticoagulants.

Many medical units employ low-dose heparin routinely to cover the period while patients with cardiac disease are confined to bed. This treatment combined with earlier ambulation probably accounts for much of the reduction in hospital mortality from myocardial infarction in the last 25 years. Doubts amongst physicians about the effectiveness of low-dose heparin are similar to those of their surgical colleagues and there have been no clinical trials to show that death from pulmonary embolism is reduced. However, there is similarly no unequivocal evidence that full anticoagulation with heparin or warfarin protects patients against arterial and venous thromboembolism after myocardial infarction. This has been one of the most contentious issues in therapeutics and it seems unlikely that a consensus will develop soon. There are advocates of full anticoagulation, other physicians who rely on early mobilization, and a majority in the United Kingdom who prescribe low-dose heparin with a variable degree of confidence in its efficacy.

Thrombosis of other veins

Venous thrombotic disease of portal and hepatic veins is considered in Section 12; cerebral sinus thrombosis in Section 21; and renal vein thrombosis in Section 18. Pulmonary embolism and pulmonary venous thrombosis are dealt with in Section 13.

Axillary vein thrombosis (Fig. 15) is uncommon. It is associated with vascular obstruction at the thoracic outlet (by cervical ribs, fascial bands, and malignant lymph glands, for example) insertion of subclavian venous catheters, and vigorous use of the arm as in playing squash or weight lifting. In many cases it apparently occurs spontaneously. Although full recovery often takes place a substantial proportion of cases will be left with residual swelling, discoloration, and pain. Thrombolytic therapy can be highly effective in removing the usually small, localized, thrombus.

Thrombosis and arterial occlusive disease

Few studies have related measurements of haemostatic function prospectively to subsequent development of symptomatic arterial occlusive disease. This is partly because they are difficult to carry out, due to the low event-rate in a normal population even amongst individuals with known risk factors. There is also a general view that abnormalities of haemostasis are not much involved in arterial thrombosis. The changes in coagulation function and platelet behaviour which have been detected are probably largely secondary to damage to the arterial wall from many environmental factors.

Contribution of haemostasis to thrombogenesis in arteries

In addition to the usual difficulties of large-scale epidemiological studies, those involving laboratory measurements of haemostasis

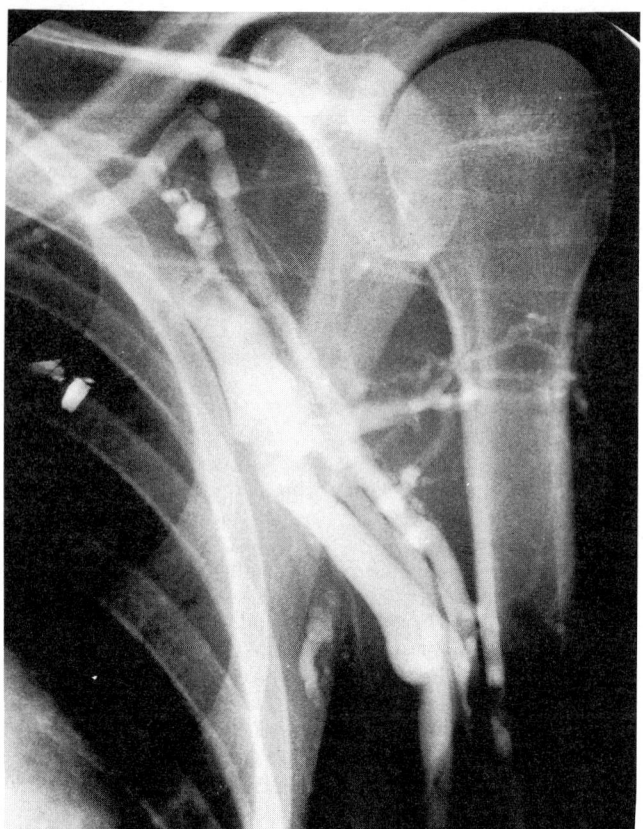

Fig. 15 Venogram of the left arm showing thrombosis of the axillary subclavian vein. The distal section of the axillary vein is dilated and was palpable in the axilla. There had been a minor rugby injury a few weeks previously and some unaccustomed use of the left arm in painting a ceiling. No other aetiological factors were detected.

pose particular technical problems. The Northwick Park Heart Study has shown that high plasma fibrinogen and low fibrinolytic activity are distributed in a pattern similar to that of the recognized risk factors for coronary heart disease. Plasma concentrations of factors VII and VIII, and fibrinogen were found to be significantly higher in an early analysis of individuals who subsequently died from coronary heart disease than in other members of the study population (factory workers in north-west London). A Swedish study has shown that plasma fibrinogen concentration is an important risk factor both for myocardial infarction and more strongly for stroke. Epidemiological association does not prove causality but these results are consistent with the knowledge that myocardial infarction is precipitated by thrombosis occluding a coronary artery. Less directly, they offer support for the hypothesis that thrombotic events might contribute to atherogenesis.

This theory was proposed by Rokitansky in 1852. Recurrent thrombi on the arterial wall were thought to become encrusted, leading to ischaemic damage and ingrowth of abnormal connective tissues. Few would now subscribe to this theory in its original form but pathological and experimental studies suggest that fibrin and platelet deposition might promote atheroma. Histochemistry on post-mortem arterial samples indicates that fibrin and platelet debris are associated with atheromatous plaques. Repetitive arterial injury in animals disrupts normal architecture and leads to smooth-muscle cell proliferation over a period of three to six weeks. Rendering animals thrombocytopenic inhibits development of these lesions, which do not depend on feeding cholesterol. Platelets release a cell mitogen, the platelet-derived growth factor (PDGF), which stimulates smooth-muscle cell proliferation, and release of PDGF at sites of arterial injury could contribute to atherogenesis. Von Willebrand factor contributes to platelet adhesion and pigs with von Willebrand disease are resistant to experimental atheroma; prospective studies to determine whether von Willebrand's disease limits atherosclerosis in patients have not been completed. Hyperlipidaemia, which is the single most powerful risk associaton for coronary heart disease, also affects the haemostatic mechanism. Ingestion of saturated fats tends to shorten blood coagulation times and reduce plasma fibrinolytic activity. Patients with hyperlipidaemias have shorter bleeding times and more active platelets than normolipaemic subjects. Arterial thrombi can be produced more easily in animals fed high-fat diets. Hyperlipidaemia and blood platelets could accordingly have synergistic adverse effects on the vessel wall following intimal trauma.

Acute myocardial infarction

Myocardial infarction is discussed in detail in Section 13. Pathological studies indicate that thrombotic occlusion of a coronary artery occurs in 95 per cent of patients with transmural infarction, though thrombi occur in only about 30 per cent of cases of sudden death. Thrombosis is commonly related to the site of atheromatous narrowing or of plaque rupture. Not surprisingly, blood tests taken at the time of infarction show activation of haemostasis probably as a secondary response. Laboratory tests show the presence of thrombin, increase in plasma fibrinogen, release of platelet proteins, and shortened platelet survival. The coagulation abnormality probably contributes to the increased incidence of arterial and venous thromboembolism in the first week after infarction. The rate of thrombotic complications has declined since treatment has included rapid mobilization. Without prophylaxis, 25 to 30 per cent of patients develop small calf-vein thrombi; and echocardiography has shown that about 35 per cent will develop intraventricular thrombi followed anterior infarction. Whether antithrombotic treatments reduce mortality from acute thromboembolic complications has not been proved. Physicians in the United Kingdom often prescribe low-dose heparin injections subcutaneously as prophylaxis but rarely use full anticoagulation. This is probably a sensible compromise in view of the lack of unequivocal benefit from full anticoagulation, which occasionally causes serious haemorrhage. Deaths from arterial and venous thromboembolism are now rare, so that definitive clinical trials would be extremely difficult to complete.

Fibrinolytic therapy aimed at dissolving coronary artery thrombi, and limiting infarct size by restoring blood flow, has been evaluated over 20 years. There is probably a small reduction in mortality following systemic therapeutic fibrinolysis. Recently this treatment has been modified by infusing fibrinolytic agents directly through a catheter in the coronary artery. Obstructing thrombi can be lysed in about 70 per cent of cases and this probably improves left ventricular function subsequently. Whether this technically demanding therapy improves survival is not yet known. Intravenous injection of human tissue plasminogen activator might prove to be an equally effective and more practicable alternative if the promise of the experimental studies is sustained.

Antithrombotic drugs in the secondary prevention of myocardial infarction

Results from trials of aspirin treatment in the secondary prevention of myocardial infarction are consistent with a reduction of 10 per cent in mortality and 20 per cent in reinfarction rate over the first year. It is not known how aspirin interacts with beta-blockers which are effective prophylactic drugs. Appraisal of the inadequate evidence from clinical trials of anticoagulation is complicated by arguments about the effective dosage level and the difficulty of adequate control. At present, routine prophylaxis with antithrombotic therapy following myocardial infarction cannot be recommended (see Section 21 also).

Cerebrovascular disease

Acute cerebral infarction temporarily disturbs the haemostatic mechanism, but there is little evidence of abnormal blood coagulation a few months later. High plasma fibrinogen concentration is an important risk factor for stroke but the mechanism is not known.

Anticoagulation is not effective in the treatment or prevention of most forms of cerebrovascular disease, partly because of the difficulty of excluding brain haemorrhage. Most physicians believe that anticoagulation suppresses embolization from cardiac thrombi, though large clinical trials have not been carried out. Patients with transient ischaemic attacks pose a more difficult therapeutic choice: in about a third, a stenosing atheroma can be demonstrated in the internal carotid artery and this can be removed surgically, although the procedure has never been evaluated by controlled trial; two randomized trials have shown that treatment with aspirin probably reduces the risk of stroke and death although the results are not unequivocal. The decision over whom to treat and how is accordingly probably best deferred to a specialist (see Section 21 also).

Peripheral vascular disease

Haemostatic function has scarcely been studied in patients with peripheral vascular disease and anticoagulation does not affect its progression. Thrombolytic therapy occasionally restores patency of acutely occluded vessels in patients unfit for surgery.

Atherosclerotic vascular disease is accelerated in patients with diabetes mellitus. There is a great deal of work showing that platelets are more active in patients with diabetes and that the abnormalities can be reversed by intensive insulin therapy. Whether enhanced platelet function is a cause of accelerated atherosclerosis in diabetics is not known, nor is there evidence to indicate that antithrombotic prophylaxis is effective in delaying its onset.

Infusions of prostacyclin (PGI_2) might accelerate healing of ischaemia ulcers in the feet and are symptomatically beneficial in treatment of rest pain. Its effect is likely to be due mainly to vasodilatation rather than platelet inhibition.

Miscellaneous thromboembolic conditions

Synthetic materials cannot be made fully compatible with blood, and as a result thrombosis tends to occur on vascular prostheses, particularly those with a small internal diameter. Platelet consumption occurs in extracorporeal circulations used in cardiac surgery and renal dialysis. Heparin is the standard treatment for preventing thrombosis on by-pass and dialysis circuits; platelet inhibitory drugs reduce platelet consumption but are ineffective used alone. Prostacyclin can be used as a substitute for heparin but is expensive and is most effective when combined with a reduced concentration of heparin.

Disseminated intravascular coagulation has been discussed on page 19.231. In chronic forms, symptoms result largely from thrombosis rather than bleeding, most cases occurring in patients with malignancy or sepsis. Anticoagulation with heparin and warfarin is effective if the underlying condition can be corrected; otherwise thrombosis frequently supervenes even in well-anticoagulated patients.

Thrombotic thrombocytopenic purpura (TTP) (see page 19.150) and *haemolytic uraemic syndrome (HUS)* (see page 19.150) are probably variants of a similar basic process, the latter presenting classically in children. Both conditions are rare and as a result well-controlled trials of therapy are impossible to organize. There is circumstantial evidence that PGI_2 synthesis by the vessel wall is suppressed in some of these patients and treatment with prostacyclin can apparently sometimes interrupt progression of the illness.

Patients with *polycythaemia vera* and *essential thrombocythaemia* (see pages 19.37 and 19.44) are at risk of arterial thrombosis and particularly of stroke. The mechanism is complex, involving increased viscosity and exaggerated platelet function. Treatment with platelet-inhibitory drugs might prevent microvascular thrombosis in patients with thrombocythaemia, but restoration of normal platelet count by treatment with radioactive phosphorus or cytotoxic drugs is the most effective antithrombotic measure.

Treatment with a combination of aspirin and dipyridamole reduces the frequency of graft occlusion in patients with coronary artery by-pass grafts. Anticoagulation inhibits systemic embolization from prosthetic heart valves made of non-biological materials and concurrent administration of aspirin or dipyridamole might have a small additional effect.

References

General

Bloom, A. L. and Thomas, D. P. (1981). *Haemostasis and thrombosis.* Churchill Livingstone, Edinburgh.
Colman, R. W., Hirsh, J., Marder, V. J. and Salzman, E. W. (1982). *Hemostasis and thrombosis: basic principles and clinical practice.* J. B. Lippincott, Philadelphia.

The haemostatic mechanism

Bunting, S., Moncada, S. and Vane, J. R. (1983). The prostacyclin–thromboxane balance: pathophysiological and therapeutic considerations. *Br. Med. Bull.* **39**, 271–276.
Cochrane, C. G. and Griffin, J. H. (1982). The biochemistry and pathophysiology of the contact system of plasma. *Adv. Immunol.* **33**, 241–306.
Collen, D. (1980). On the regulation and control of fibrinolysis. *Thromb. Haemost.* **43**, 77–89.
George, J. N., Nurden, A. T. and Phillips, D. R. (1984). Molecular defects in interactions of platelets with the vessel wall. *N. Engl. J. Med.* **311**, 1084–1098.
Holmsen, H. and Weiss, H. J. (1979). Secretable storage pools in platelets. *Ann. Rev. Med.* **30**, 119–134.
Jackson, C. M. and Nemerson, Y. (1980). Blood coagulation. *Ann. Rev. Biochem.* **49**, 765–811.
Lijnen, H. R. and Collen, D. (1982). Interaction of plasminogen activators and inhibitors with plasminogen and fibrin. *Sem. Thromb. Hemost.* **8**, 2–10.
Ogston, D. (1983). *The physiology of haemostasis.* Croom Helm, London.
Ratnoff, O. D. (1980). A quarter century with Mr. Hageman. *Thromb. Haemost.* **43**, 95–98.

Shatlil, S. J. and Bennett, J. S. (1981). Platelets and their membrane in haemostasis: physiology and pathophysiology. *Ann. Intern. Med.* **94**, 108–118.

Disorders of haemostasis

Hardisty, R. M. (1983). Hereditary disorders of platelet function. *Clin. Haematol.* **12**, 153–173.
Karpatkin, S. (1980). Review: autoimmune thrombocytopenic purpura. *Blood* **56**, 329–343.
McMillan, R. (1981). Chronic idiopathic thrombocytopenic purpura. *N. Engl. J. Med.* **304**, 1135–1147.
Nydegger, U. E. and Miescher, P. A. (1980). Bleeding due to vascular disorders. *Sem. Hemat.* **17**, 178–191.
Ratnoff, O. D. (1980). The psychogenic purpuras: a review of autoerythrocyte sensitization, autosensitization to DNA, 'hysterical' and factitial bleeding and the religious stigmata. *Sem. Hemat.* **17**, 192–213.
Rizza, C. R. (1978). *Treatment of haemophilia A and B and von Willebrand's disease.* Blackwell Scientific Publications, Oxford.
Tuddenham, E. G. D. (1984). The varieties of von Willebrand's disease. *Clin. Lab. Haemat.* **6**, 307–323.

Thrombosis

Hirsh, J. (1981). Blood tests for the diagnosis of venous and arterial thrombosis. *Blood* **57**, 1–8.
Kelton, J. G. (1983). Antiplatelet agents: rationale and results. *Clin. Haemat.* **12**, 311–354.
Kinlough-Rathbone, R. L., Packham, M. A. and Mustard, J. F. (1983). Vessel injury, platelet adherence and platelet survival. *Arteriosclerosis* **3**, 529–546.
Kwaan, H. C. and Bowie, E. J. W. (1982). *Thrombosis.* W. B. Saunders Company, Philadelphia.
Mitchell, J. R. A. (1979). Can we really prevent postoperative pulmonary emboli? *Br. med. J.* **i**, 1523–1524.
Morris G. L. and Mitchell, J. R. A. (1978). Clinical management of venous thromboembolism. *Br. med. Bull.* **34**, 169–175.
Schafer, A. I. and Handin, R. I. (1979). The role of platelets in thrombotic and vascular disease. *Prog. cardiovasc. Dis.* **22**, 31–52.
Sharma, G. V. R. K., Cella, G., Parisi, A. F. and Sasahara, A. A. (1982). Thrombolytic therapy. *N. Engl. J. Med.* **306**, 1268–1276.
Thomas, D. P. (1981). Heparin. *Clin. Haemat.* **10**, 443–458.
Turpie, A. G. G. de Boer, A. C. and Genton, E. (1982). Platelet consumption in cardiovascular disease. *Sem. Thromb. Hemost.* **8**, 161–185.
Wessler, S. and Gitel, S. N. (1984). Warfarin. From bedside to bench. *N. Engl. J. Med.* **311**, 645–652.

THE BLOOD IN SYSTEMIC DISEASE

D. J. WEATHERALL

As mentioned at the beginning of this section, there are few diseases which do not produce some alteration in the blood. Here, some of the haematological changes which accompany and may be the presenting feature of general systemic diseases will be summarized. Many of these topics are discussed elsewhere in this book but they are brought together in order to emphasize how blood changes may give the first indication of the presence of non-haematological disorders.

Malignant disease

By far the commonest haematological finding in malignant disease (Table 1) is the anaemia of chronic disorders which was described on page 19.91. It may occur together with localized or widespread malignancy and is sometimes associated with an elevated ESR. It is found in patients with practically every type of carcinoma or reticulosis, is refractory to haematinics, but may respond to successful removal of a primary tumour.

The anaemia of many patients with carcinoma, particularly of the gastrointestinal tract, may be complicated by chronic blood loss and superimposed iron deficiency. Chronic bleeding of this type is often associated with a mild thrombocytosis.

Disseminated malignancy

The commonest haematological change with disseminated malignancy is a *leucoerythroblastic picture* characterized by the presence in the blood of immature myeloid cells together with some nucleated red cells and, sometimes, a mild reticulocytosis. The red cells often show a moderate degree of anisocytosis and poikilocytosis. This finding is very commonly accompanied by the presence of tumour cells in the bone marrow. Clinically, it can cause confusion with the diagnosis of primary myelosclerosis; splenomegaly is unusual in patients with disseminated carcinoma.

Occasionally, widespread carcinoma leads to a *leukaemoid reaction* with white cell counts in the range seen in chronic myeloid leukaemia. The differentiation between these two conditions was described earlier (page 19.29).

The *microangiopathic haemolytic anaemia* of disseminated malignancy (page 19.149) is most frequently found in association with

Table 1 Principal haematological changes in malignant disorders

Erythrocytes	
Anaemia of chronic disorders	All forms
Iron deficiency anaemia	Gastrointestinal; cervix, uterus
Leucoerythroblastic anaemia	Stomach, breast, thyroid, prostate, bronchus, kidney
Microangiopathic haemolytic anaemia	Mucin-secreting tumours; stomach, bronchus, breast
Secondary myelosclerosis	As for leucoerythroblastic; also reticuloses
Selective red-cell aplasia	Thymus, lymphoma, bronchus
Immune haemolytic anaemia	Ovary; lymphoma; other carcinomas
Megaloblastic anaemia	Myeloma; stomach; rarely others
Sideroblastic anaemia	All forms; myeloproliferative disorders
Polycythaemia	Kidney, liver, posterior fossa, uterus
Leucocytes	
Leucocytosis	All forms
Leukaemoid reactions	As for leucoerythroblastic anaemia
Eosinophilia	Miscellaneous carcinomas and reticuloses
Monocytosis	All forms
Basophilia	Myeloproliferative disease; mastocytosis
Lymphopenia	Carcinoma, reticuloses
Platelets	
Thrombocytosis	Gastrointestinal with bleeding; bronchus and others without bleeding
Thrombocytopenia	As for the microangiopathies
Acquired thrombocytopathy	Macroglobulinaemia; other paraproteinaemias
Coagulation	
Disseminated intravascular coagulation	Prostate, many others
Primary activation of fibrinolysis	Prostate
Selective impairment of coagulation (see Table 2)	
Thrombophlebitis	All forms
Miscellaneous	
Abnormal proteins-cryofibrinogens	Prostate, others
Fetal proteins	Alphafetoprotein—liver and others Carcinoembryonic antigen (CEA)—gastrointestinal neoplasms Fetal haemoglobin—leukaemia, other tumours
Circulating tumour cells	All forms
Effects of cytotoxic drugs	All forms

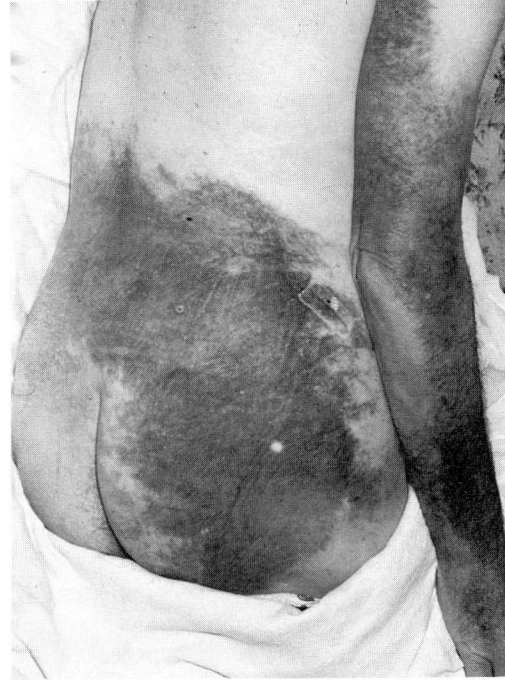

Fig. 1 Disseminated intravascular coagulation in association with carcinoma of the prostate. The patient started to bleed extensively from the iliac crest marrow biopsy site and from venesection sites. Marrow biopsy showed widespread tumour metastases. (Reproduced from *Blood and its disorders*, 2nd edn, 1982, eds R. M. Hardisty and D. J. Weatherall. Blackwell Scientific Publications, Oxford.)

mucin-secreting adenocarcinoma, particularly of the stomach, breast, and lung.

Less common forms of anaemia associated with cancer

Autoimmune haemolytic anaemia is frequently found in patients with an underlying lymphoma. It is much less common in other forms of malignancy except for the association with tumours of the ovary. However, there have been recent reports of autoimmune haemolysis occurring with a wide variety of tumours, including lung, stomach, breast, kidney, colon, and testis.

Pure *red cell aplasia* may occasionally be the presenting feature in a patient with a tumour of the thymus, and there have been occasional reports of this type of anaemia occurring in patients with carcinoma of the bronchus or lymphomas.

Finally, it should be remembered that there is an association between *pernicious anaemia* and carcinoma of the stomach and a patient may present with a megaloblastic anaemia associated with a malignancy of this type. *Sideroblastic anaemias* are occasionally found in patients with carcinoma; in one series of 62 patients who

presented with a sideroblastic anaemia, 10 were found to have an underlying malignancy.

Polycythaemia

The relationship between secondary polycythaemia and an underlying neoplasm was discussed on page 19.155. It has been found in patients with renal tumours, hepatomas, hamartomas of the liver, uterine fibroids, vascular tumours and cystic adenomas of the cerebellum, and carcinoma of the lung.

Changes in the platelets and blood coagulation

An otherwise unexplained thrombocytosis may be the first indication of an underlying malignancy. It is important to remember that this is not always associated with chronic blood loss; bronchial carcinoma may present in this way.

Generalized haemostatic failure associated with disseminated carcinoma was considered in detail on page 19.233 (Figs 1 and 2).

There is an increasing number of examples of bleeding disorders associated with cancer which seem to be due to selective impairment of coagulation. This may result from pathological inhibitors of different parts of the coagulation system or from isolated factor deficiencies. The mechanism is unknown. However, in a patient with a bleeding disorder associated with cancer, which is not characterized by consumption of clotting factors or fibrinolysis, a detailed analysis of the activities of the intrinsic and extrinsic pathways must be carried out in case a correctable lesion is present (Table 2).

White cell abnormalities

Apart from the leukaemoid reaction mentioned earlier, there are several white cell changes which should make the clinician think about an underlying malignancy. For example, a persistent monocytosis or eosinophilia may be associated with Hodgkin's disease or with bronchial carcinoma. Persistent lymphopenia may occur in patients with Hodgkin's disease.

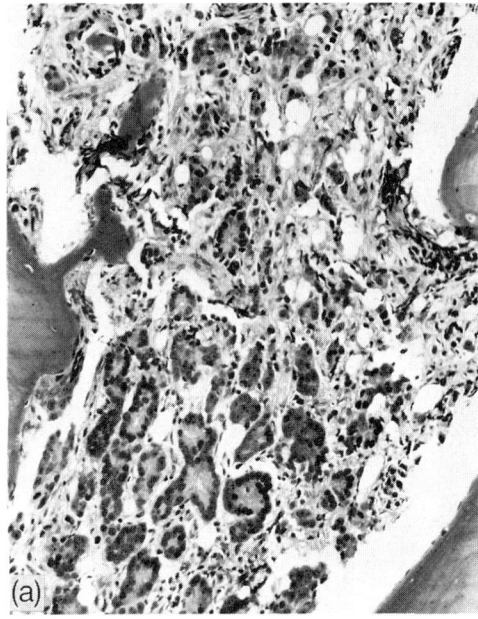

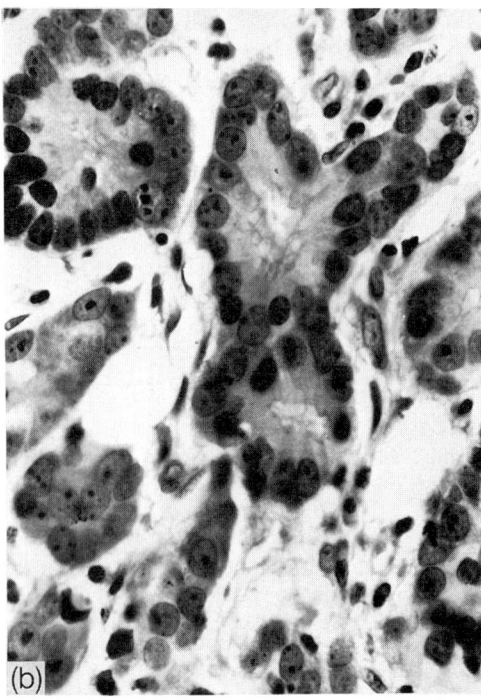

Fig. 2 Sections prepared from Gardner-needle biopsies from bone marrow infiltrated with neoplastic cells; the primary tumour was in the prostate (H and E stain). (a) × 230, (b) × 920. (Reproduced from *Blood and its disorders*, 2nd edn, 1982, eds R. M. Hardisty and D. J. Weatherall. Blackwell Scientific Publications, Oxford.)

Infection

Most of the important haematological changes in association with infection were considered in Section 5. Just a few points of particular haematological relevance are summarized below.

Acute bacterial infection

Most acute bacterial infections are associated with a neutrophil leucocytosis. This may be so marked, and associated with such a 'shift to the left' with production of myelocytes in the blood, that the condition may present a leukaemoid type of reaction. Occasionally, however, patients are encountered severely ill with

Table 2 Selective impairment of coagulation in cancer

Inhibitors	
Paraproteins	Plasma cell disorders
Lupus-like	Hodgkin's disease, lymphoma, myelofibrosis, carcinoma
Factor IX inhibitor	Cancer of colon or prostate
Factor VII inhibitor	Bronchogenic carcinoma
Heparin-like	Bronchogenic carcinoma, myeloma
Isolated factor deficiencies	
Factor XIII	Acute leukaemia, chronic myeloid leukaemia
Factor XII	Chronic myeloid leukaemia
Factor XI	Melanoma
Factor X	Myeloma with amyloid
Factor VIII	Macroglobulinaemia, chronic lymphatic leukaemia, Wilms' tumour
Factor V	Chronic myeloid leukaemia, polycythaemia vera

Modified from Goldsmith (1984).

acute bacterial infection in whom the neutrophil response seems inadequate, or who may be frankly neutropenic. Although some of them will prove to have an underlying haematological disorder or a debilitating condition such as alcoholism, this is not always the case and a proportion of patients who recover from their infection show no such underlying abnormality subsequently. A marrow examination usually reveals a paucity of mature granulocytes. This clinical picture is particularly common in newborn infants, especially those born prematurely.

Other leucocyte changes are less common in acute infection. Monocytosis has been reported in patients with typhoid fever and sometimes in brucellosis or subacute bacterial endocarditis. In the latter condition a monocytosis may be associated with the presence of undifferentiated reticuloendothelial cells in the blood which show erythrophagocytosis.

Some degree of anaemia is found almost invariably in patients with bacterial infection. It usually presents a picture of the anaemia of chronic disorders. Haemolytic anaemia may occur in severe septicaemias and is usually associated with disseminated intravascular coagulation. Some organisms, *Clostridium welchii* for example, produce an alpha toxin which acts as a lecithinase and causes fulminating intravascular haemolysis.

Disseminated intravascular coagulation is a relatively common accompaniment of severe bacterial infection. A number of mechanisms have been suggested including vascular injury with activation of factor XII, or the generation of procoagulants from white cells by the action of endotoxin. Thrombocytopenia is also common in patients with septicaemia. Although this may sometimes reflect disseminated intravascular coagulation the mechanism is probably more complicated. There may be quite dramatic thrombocytopenia without any other evidence of a consumption coagulopathy. Probably several mechanisms are involved including suppression of platelet production by the bone marrow, damage to circulating platelets by immune complexes, endothelial damage, and direct interaction of the platelets with bacteria; phagocytosis of bacteria by platelets may be a factor causing the rapid disappearance of platelets from the circulation.

Chronic bacterial infection

Chronic bacterial infection is usually associated with the anaemia of chronic disorders. There are some particularly interesting haematological changes which are sometimes ascribed to *tuberculosis* (Table 3). While the commonest change is a mild normochromic, normocytic anaemia with a raised ESR, more spectacular blood changes have been reported, particularly in association with disseminated tuberculosis. These clinical pictures include leukaemoid reactions, pancytopenia, myelofibrosis, and even polycythaemia.

Table 3 Haematological changes in tuberculosis

Type of tuberculosis or therapy	Haematological changes
Pulmonary	Anaemia of chronic disorders; iron-deficiency anaemia; Anaemia due to therapy; high ESR
Ileocaecal	Anaemia of chronic disorders; megaloblastic anaemia to vitamin B_{12} or folate deficiency; High ESR
Cryptic miliary (aregenerative)	Leukaemoid reaction; myelosclerosis;* pancytopenia; Polycythaemia,* anaemia of chronic disorders
Antituberculous drugs	
PAS or streptomycin	Fever, lymphadenopathy, eosinophilia
allergy	Sideroblastic anaemia
INAH, cycloserine	Thrombocytopenic purpura
Rifampicin	

* These reports may well represent cases of disseminated tuberculosis in patients with underlying haematological disorders (see text).

The main problem in assessing these associations is whether the reported patients had tuberculous infection or infections due to atypical mycobacteria superimposed on an underlying blood disease, or whether disseminated tuberculosis can occasionally produce a clinical picture similar to leukaemia or a myeloproliferative disease. Unfortunately the answer to this interesting question remains unresolved. In practice any patient who presents with an atypical myeloproliferative disorder, and who is going downhill for no apparent cause, should be investigated for tuberculosis and attempts should be made to grow the organism from bone marrow cultures.

Virus infections

Some of the haematological changes associated with specific viral infections such as infectious mononucleosis were considered in Section 5. However, it is becoming apparent that haematological changes can occur quite commonly in association with many virus illnesses.

Rubella, acquired in childhood or adult life, is often associated with a leucocytosis and an atypical lymphocytosis. A small proportion of patients develop an acute fulminating thrombocytopenic purpura approximately 4 days after the appearance of the rash. This is usually self-limiting but fatalities have been reported. Thrombocytopenia is also common in infants with congenital rubella, and this condition is also characterized by a non-immune haemolytic episode shortly after birth. Thrombocytopenia has also been reported in association with *measles*, and in particularly severe forms of rubella and morbilli severe haemorrhagic states due to disseminated intravascular coagulation have been seen. Similar changes occur occasionally in patients with *varicella* infections.

The haematological changes in infectious mononucleosis were described in Section 5. A very similar picture can occur in patients with *cytomegalovirus (CMV) infection*. In infants with congenital CMV infections there may be striking hepatosplenomegaly with purpura and anaemia. The latter is characterized by a haemolytic picture with the appearances of many normoblasts in the peripheral blood. This form of anaemia may last for several weeks and may be associated with severe thrombocytopenia. There are many well-documented cases of an infectious mononucleosis-like disorder occurring after transfusion with fresh blood or after perfusion for open heart surgery. The syndrome usually occurs 1–3 months after blood transfusion and is self-limiting, resolving within a few weeks. It is characterized by a moderate rise in temperature, with hepatosplenomegaly, lymphadenopathy, and tran-

sient maculopapular rashes. There is a lymphocytosis with a blood picture indistinguishable from that of infectious mononucleosis.

Haematological complications of *infectious hepatitis* are rare but when they occur may be extremely severe. Coombs' positive haemolytic anaemia has been reported, and there is now a considerable literature on the occurrence of aplastic anaemia. This disorder seems predominantly to affect young males, and the onset of the aplasia is usually about 9 weeks after the onset of hepatitis. The condition is associated with a mortality in excess of 90 per cent. In those patients who recover, the period to complete haematological normality ranges between 3 and 20 months.

It is becoming apparent that many viruses are capable of provoking severe bleeding due to intravascular coagulation. Why viruses can fire off the coagulation cascade is far from clear. Activation of factor XII due to vascular injury or damage to platelets with the release of coagulants have been suggested as possible mechanisms.

There is increasing evidence that the *human parvovirus* has a particular affinity for red cell progenitors. It probably causes transient red cell aplasia quite commonly but this only gives rise to a symptomatic anaemia in patients who have a markedly shortened red cell survival. Thus parvovirus infection appears to be responsible for the aplastic crises in patients with sickle cell anaemia, pyruvate kinase deficiency or other congenital haemolytic anaemias. It is also becoming apparent that a variety of viruses can cause acute damage to the bone marrow in immune-suppressed patients as part of the *virus haemophagocytic syndrome* (see page 19.134).

The haematological changes associated with the virus haemorrhagic fevers were described in detail in Section 5.

Parasitic disease

The major haematological accompaniments of the parasitic diseases are described in Section 5. Those which produce important haematological changes will be briefly summarized here.

Toxoplasmosis

Congenital toxoplasmosis can produce a condition identical to erythroblastosis fetalis. The clinical picture is of a pale hydropic infant with a large spleen and liver associated with severe anaemia, thrombocytopenia, and a leucocytosis, often with a marked eosinophilia. In adult life the acquired forms of toxoplasmosis produce a clinical disorder resembling infectious mononucleosis.

Malaria

Malarial infection produces a variety of haematological abnormalities. The most severe changes occur in association with *Plasmodium falciparum* malaria infection. In acute infections in non-immune individuals there is usually minimal anaemia at the onset of the illness, but during the 2–3 weeks after treatment there may be a steady decline in haemoglobin level, the mechanism of which is not yet fully worked out. On the other hand, children or adults with chronic malaria, some degree of immunity, and low level parasitaemias, may be severely anaemic at presentation with an inappropriately low reticulocyte count. The bone marrow is often hyperplastic and shows a marked degree of dyshaemopoiesis (Fig. 3) (see also page 19.134).

In some patients with severe *P. falciparum* infections there may be marked intravascular haemolysis and haemoglobinuria. Again, the mechanism is not certain, and although some of these patients may be glucose-6-phosphate dehydrogenase deficient, this is by no means the whole story. It has been suggested that some patients with fulminating malaria have disseminated intravascular coagulation although this is probably uncommon and plays very little part in the pathophysiology of either the anaemia or haemorrhagic phenomenon which occur in this condition. Thrombocytopenia is extremely common in patients with acute malaria but is only rarely associated with evidence of consumption of blood-clotting factors. In most forms of malarial infection there is a neutropenia, and monocytosis has also been described.

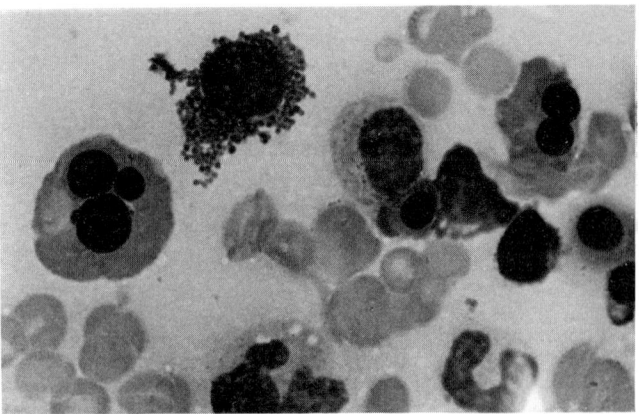

Fig. 3 Bone marrow appearances in *P. falciparum* malaria. There is marked dyserythropoiesis with several multinucleate red cell precursors (Giemsa stain × 800).

Leishmaniasis

Particularly in young children, visceral leishmaniasis, or kala-azar, is associated with hepatosplenomegaly, lymphadenopathy, and a pancytopenia. Early in the course of the disease there is often marked neutropenia and the marrow may be grossly infiltrated with parasitized macrophages. The anaemia is due mainly to a short red cell survival; there is also an inappropriate marrow response and a variable degree of hypersplenism.

Hookworm

The haematological changes of hookworm infestation are described in Section 5. It is one of the commonest causes of iron deficiency anaemia in the world population. During the systemic phase of the illness, when the larvae invade the lungs, there may be a marked eosinophilia. During this phase the bone marrow shows a remarkable increase in the percentage of eosinophilic myelocytes which may be out of proportion to the eosinophilia observed in the peripheral blood.

Visceral larva migrans

This condition is characterized by striking haematological changes including anaemia, a marked leucocytosis with eosinophilia, and changes in the titre of anti-A and anti-B blood group antibodies.

Schistosomiasis

In the chronic phase of mansoni and japonicum infections there may be severe portal hypertension, splenomegaly, and the typical picture of hypersplenism.

Other trematode infestations, including clonorchiasis and paragonamiasis, are associated with eosinophilia and anaemia. Antibodies to the P_1 blood group antigen may be found in grossly elevated titres in the blood of many patients with acute fascioliasis.

Rheumatoid arthritis and related disorders

In patients with rheumatoid arthritis anaemia is extremely common. It usually follows the general pattern of anaemia of chronic disorders. It is occasionally complicated by genuine iron deficiency which may result from a variety of causes including poor diet and chronic blood loss due to the effects of treatment, particularly ingestion of salicylates and non-steroidal anti-inflammatory agents or corticosteroids. Furthermore, it has been found that significant bleeding occurs into actively inflamed joints and it has been estimated that if only two knee joints were affected, the annual blood loss through this mechanism could amount to as much as 2500 ml. It is not certain how much of the iron derived from this blood is available for reutilization for haemoglobin synthesis. The diagnosis of iron deficiency complicating rheumatoid arthritis may not be straightforward; serum iron and iron binding capacity levels may be difficult to interpret because of co-existing inflammation, and determination of marrow stores and estimation of serum ferritin levels may be more helpful. Although the latter are elevated in inflammatory conditions a low level suggests genuine iron deficiency.

There are no particular changes in the neutrophil response in uncomplicated rheumatoid arthritis; a marked leucocytosis may reflect a response to corticosteroid therapy or a superadded infection such as a septic arthritis. The platelet count is elevated in between 20 and 50 per cent of patients with rheumatoid arthritis. The degree of thrombocytosis parallels the degree of activity of the illness and cannot be accounted for on the grounds of associated intestinal blood loss due to drug therapy.

The haematological changes of *Felty's syndrome* are summarized in Section 16. There is anaemia, thrombocytopenia, and marked neutropenia. Although many of these changes are features of hypersplenism, recent studies on the neutropenia in this disorder indicate that it has a complex basis and that immune destruction of neutrophils may play a major role.

The management of the haematological manifestations of rheumatoid arthritis and Felty's syndrome is unsatisfactory. The anaemia generally reflects the activity of the disease. If there is genuine iron deficiency, iron replacement therapy is indicated. The vexed question of whether intramuscular iron administration has some non-specific effect on the anaemia of rheumatoid arthritis, even in the absence of reduced body iron stores, remains unresolved. Similarly, there is considerable controversy about the best way to manage Felty's syndrome. After splenectomy there is sometimes a dramatic rise in the neutrophil and total leucocyte counts, but this is not always associated with a decreased incidence of infection. Furthermore, some patients show no change in the white cell count after surgery. At the present time it is difficult to advise about the best approach to the management of this condition; only if there are recurrent, life-threatening infections should splenectomy be carried out and, because the results are so uncertain, patients require extremely careful surveillance after the operation, and there may be some place for the use of prophylactic antibiotics in those whose neutrophil counts do not respond.

Finally, it should be remembered that there is a variety of haematological changes secondary to drug therapy for rheumatoid arthritis and related disorders. Salicylates may produce chronic blood loss, while drugs containing phenacetin produce methaemoglobinaemia and Heinz body haemolytic anaemia which may sometimes be preceded by a marked eosinophilia. Phenylbutazone produces pancytopenia which may be severe and irreversible; this drug has now been discontinued in the United Kingdom. Oxyphenylbutazone and penicillamine may also cause severe marrow depression.

Systemic lupus erythematosus and other collagen disorders

It is quite common for systemic lupus erythematosus (SLE) to present with a haematological disorder. This is not the case in the other collagen-vascular disorders.

The commonest blood change in SLE is anaemia which occurs in nearly all patients at some stage of the illness. It is usually a mild anaemia of chronic disorders which may be complicated by blood loss from analgesics or anti-inflammatory medication, renal impairment, or haemolysis. Acquired autoimmune haemolytic anaemia may be the sole presenting feature in SLE and may antedate the appearance of other typical features by many years. The incidence of this complication varies in reported series but occurs overall in approximately 5 per cent of cases. The Coombs' test is invariably positive with anticomplementary agents and is positive with anti-IgG during episodes of acute haemolysis. Other forms of anaemia in SLE include those associated with hypersplenism due to splenomegaly, and the occasional occurrence of a hypocellular bone marrow, probably due to involvement of small vessels by the disease process.

The most consistent finding in the white cell count in SLE is leucopenia which occurs in up to half the patients at some time during the illness. This is often a combined neutropenia and lymphopenia. Mild eosinophilia occurs occasionally, particularly in association with skin involvement.

A mild thrombocytopenia occurs in 10–25 per cent of all cases of SLE. More severe thrombocytopenia, producing a picture almost indistinguishable from idiopathic thrombocytopenic purpura, occurs in a small proportion of patients and may be the sole presenting feature in some. Although early reports indicated that splenectomy might be associated with a flare-up of the systemic symptoms of SLE in patients with thrombocytopenia, this has now been shown to be incorrect.

Another potentially important abnormality of coagulation in patients with SLE is the presence of the so-called *lupus anticoagulant*. This is a circulating anticardiolipin which is also responsible for the positive Wassermann reaction, the false-positive serological test for syphilis which occurs in this condition. This antibody, which occurs in conditions other than SLE, interferes with the binding of phospholipid to form prothrombin activator and this affects the intrinsic and extrinsic clotting pathways (see page 19.232). Although it causes a prolonged partial thromboplastin time its presence in patients with SLE seems to produce a clotting rather than a bleeding tendency. A significant number of patients who have the lupus anticoagulant have recurrent thrombotic episodes including cerebral thromboses. It is also associated with recurrent spontaneous abortions and, possibly, with 'idiopathic' pulmonary hypertension.

It has been suggested that the lupus anticoagulant inhibits the production of prostacyclin from vessel walls and it may interfere with the release of arachidonic acid from cell membranes. Even more interestingly it is possible that these antibodies react with complex brain lipids such as sphingomyelin. Early reports of the presence of antibodies of this type in patients with bizarre neurological syndromes such as *Jamaican neuropathy* and Behçet's disease require further confirmation.

The haematological changes in the other collagen-vascular diseases are much less impressive. They are all associated with the anaemia of chronic disorders. Polyarteritis nodosa may be characterized by an eosinophilia.

The interesting syndrome of *polymyalgia rheumatica* and *temporal arteritis* may present to the haematologist (page 19.92 and Section 14). There are usually significant haematological changes characterized by a severe anaemia of chronic disorders with a marked elevation of the ESR. The leucocyte count is usually normal although there may occasionally be a mild eosinophilia. There is a marked increase in the α_2 and γ globulins although this is polyclonal in type. This blood picture can very closely resemble that of multiple myeloma or disseminated malignancy.

Renal disease

Almost all forms of renal disease are associated with haematological changes. However, by far the most important is the severe refractory anaemia which accompanies chronic renal failure.

Anaemia

Anaemia is an important and intractable complication of chronic renal failure. The correlation between the blood urea nitrogen and the haemoglobin level is inconsistent. The anaemia has an extremely complex aetiology which is only partly understood. The red cells of patients with chronic renal disease have a shortened survival although they survive normally when injected into healthy recipients. Similarly, normal red cells have a shortened red cell survival in uraemic recipients. The nature of the intracorpuscular defect has not been determined. Most red cell enzymes are present at normal levels and the intracellular level of ATP is elevated. However, changes in membrane function have been demonstrated, in particular decreased activity of the Na^+–K^+ pumps; the toxic substances which cause these changes have not been identified.

In addition to a shortened red cell survival there is impaired red cell production in the anaemia of chronic renal failure. The lack of marrow activity may be partly due to defective erythropoietin production by damaged kidneys. Furthermore, using *in vitro* assays it has been found that the serum from patients on haemodialysis inhibits the proliferation of erythroid progenitors. The suppressive activity is found in serum fractions containing material of molecular weights ranging from 47 000 to above 150 000. Interestingly, patients on continuous ambulatory peritoneal dialysis (CAPD) have higher haemoglobin levels than those on haemodialysis. It is possible this reflects the more effective removal of middle molecular weight molecules of this type by CAPD. Patients on haemodialysis with low haemoglobin concentrations are more likely to have fibrous replacement of their bone marrow. This has been correlated with secondary hyperparathyroidism, suggesting a role for PTH in the bone marrow unresponsiveness and fibrosis (see page 19.44).

The anaemia of chronic renal failure may be exacerbated by deficiency of iron resulting from excessive blood sampling, blood loss due to incorrect haemodialysis procedures, or bleeding due to defective platelet function (see below). A small proportion of patients with chronic renal failure develop splenomegaly and hypersplenism. Folate deficiency is found occasionally in patients on haemodialysis. There have been a few reports of nephrosis leading to severe urinary loss of transferrin and hence to a low plasma iron-binding capacity. Some patients with renal disease have chronic inflammatory lesions which may lead to a superadded anaemia of chronic disorders (see page 19.91).

The type of renal lesion is also an important factor in determining the severity of anaemia. For example, the renal failure of polycystic disease of the kidneys is associated with a relatively higher haemoglobin level than other forms of renal failure. Interestingly, the shrunken kidneys of some patients on long-term dialysis programmes develop cysts and this phenomenon is also associated with a rise in haemoglobin level. It seems likely that both these conditions are associated with a relative increase in the output of erythropoietin.

The anaemia of chronic renal failure is normochromic and normocytic unless there is associated iron deficiency. The red cells show characteristic deformities with multiple tiny spicules and contracted poikilocytes. The capacity of the red cells for oxygen transport does not seem to be impaired. There is often an increased intracellular concentration of 2,3-diphosphoglycerate (2,3-DPG) in response to anaemia and hyperphosphataemia and the oxygen affinity of haemoglobin is decreased. This right shift in the oxygen dissociation curve may be augmented by uraemic acidosis. However, part of the advantage of the latter is cancelled out by the direct effect of low pH on glycolysis and 2,3-DPG production. Intensive dialysis may cause a reduction in the concentration of intracellular phosphate which has the effect of increasing the oxygen affinity of haemoglobin. This effect may play a role in the so-called dialysis disequilibrium syndrome.

In patients with chronic renal failure who have associated iron deficiency the red cell indices are typical of this condition; the reduced MCH and MCV values are corrected by iron therapy.

The bone marrow in chronic renal failure shows normoblastic erythropoiesis but the degree of erythroid hyperplasia is not compatible with the degree of anaemia, indicating suppression of erythropoiesis.

White cells

The total and differential white cell count is usually normal in patients with chronic renal failure. However, the phagocytic activity of granulocytes may be reduced and complement activation by haemodialysis membranes may cause stasis of white cells in the pulmonary circulation with temporary granulocytopenia. Cell-mediated immunity is also depressed.

Platelets and coagulation

There is a variety of haemostatic defects in different forms of renal disease. Most forms of renal failure are associated with a bleeding tendency which is seen in its most florid form in acute renal failure. The main features are purpura, and mucosal and gastrointestinal bleeding associated with abnormal platelet function and a prolonged bleeding time; these changes are reversible by dialysis. Various mechanisms have been proposed, including a direct action of metabolites on platelet function and a disturbance of prostaglandin balance because of a deficiency of a renal factor which modifies or inhibits vascular production of prostacyclin and/or platelet endoperoxide and thromboxane synthesis. The end result of these changes is an abnormality of the control of platelet cyclic adenosine monophosphate causing the platelets to become refractory to aggregation agents. Many conditions which lead to renal failure are also associated with thrombocytopenia. For example, the circulating immune complexes which are found in patients with acute glomerulonephritis, polyarteritis nodosa or lupus nephritis may be responsible for platelet activation and the release of aggregating agents. Thrombocytopenia may also be aggravated by heparin therapy or the use of immunosuppressant drugs in patients who have received kidney grafts. Mild thrombocytopenia is well recognized in patients with functioning renal allografts. This has also been found to be associated with an inability to clear the immune complexes. Graft rejection is associated with enhanced platelet aggregation and thrombocytopenia.

The nephrotic syndrome is characterized by a marked tendency to thrombosis. This also has a complex pathogenesis. Both platelet aggregation and release reactions have been shown to be enhanced in this condition, and to improve during remission. Protein loss in the urine may also play a role. It has been found that an increased loss of antithrombin III is related to thrombotic episodes. Conversely, coagulation factors IX and XII are also lost in the urine of patients with a nephrotic syndrome; the deficiency of factor IX may be sufficient to induce bleeding.

The haematological changes associated with the *haemolytic uraemic syndrome* and *thrombotic thrombocytopenic purpura* were considered earlier in this section (page 19.150).

Polycythaemia

The polycythaemias associated with renal lesions and following renal transplantation are discussed on pages 19.155 and 19.156.

Treatment of the haematological complications of renal disease

There is no satisfactory form of treatment for the anaemia of chronic renal failure. It is important to determine whether there are any treatable factors which may be contributing to the anaemia such as iron or folate deficiency. Iron deficiency should be corrected by oral iron therapy. In the rare cases where there is splenomegaly with hypersplenism there may be a partial response to splenectomy although it should be emphasized that this is an uncommon complication. Severe anaemia should be treated by blood transfusion. The question of transfusion in patients who are waiting for renal transplantation is considered in Section 18. Although, in the past, attempts to stimulate erythropoiesis by the use of androgens and cobalt have been widely advocated these agents are now seldom used because of side-effects. Recent reports of the production of pure erythropoietin using recombinant DNA technology suggest that erythropoietin replacement therapy may become available for the treatment of the anaemia of renal disease within the forseeable future.

The management of bleeding in patients with acute renal failure is based on correction of uraemia by dialysis and appropriate replacement therapy. Peritoneal dialysis is probably more effec-

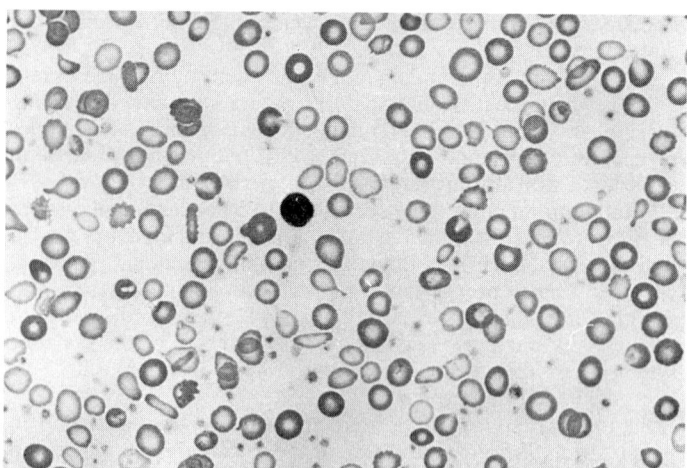

Fig. 4 Peripheral blood picture associated with gastrointestinal bleeding. The red cells show a dimorphic picture with hypochromic and normochromic forms. The platelet count is elevated, a typical finding in bleeding. (Giemsa stain × 600).

tive in reversing abnormalities of platelet function although there is no definite evidence that one form of dialysis is superior to another. If there is severe thrombocytopenia platelet transfusions should be administered.

Gastrointestinal and liver disease

Many of the haematological changes which occur in gastrointestinal and liver disease are described in Section 12. Here we will simply summarize the haematological manifestations of those disorders which present frequently with anaemia or defective haemostasis.

Gastrointestinal blood loss

As mentioned earlier in this section, blood loss in excess of 20 ml per day will always result in a negative iron balance and ultimately in iron deficiency anaemia, the time taken depending on the body stores of iron when the bleeding started.

The haematological picture shows the typical changes of iron deficiency anaemia with hypochromic, microcytic red cell morphology. Occasionally, there are some clues that this blood picture is associated with chronic blood loss. Quite frequently there is a mild to moderate thrombocytosis, and if iron is being taken there may be a dimorphic blood picture (Fig. 4), red cell polychromasia, and a low-grade reticulocytosis. It is always worth examining the peripheral blood film very carefully as it may give some clue as to the site of the blood loss. For example, the presence of target cells may indicate liver disease, whereas the presence of distorted cells and Howell–Jolly bodies suggests malabsorption due to adult coeliac disease complicated by hyposplenism.

The diagnosis of the site of blood loss from the bowel is considered in Section 12.

Inflammatory diseases of the bowel

A mild anaemia of chronic disorders is a common accompaniment of inflammatory disease of the ileum, caecum, and colon. It is observed frequently in patients with *Crohn's disease, ileocaecal tuberculosis, ulcerative colitis*, and other forms of *proctocolitis*. In many of these conditions the anaemia of chronic disorders is often complicated by intermittent blood loss or dietetic iron deficiency. In some cases of extensive Crohn's disease there may be an added factor of malabsorption. Anaemia occurs in about one-third of patients with this condition and occasionally it may be complicated by reduced vitamin B_{12} or folic acid absorption. For example, in one large survey of patients with Crohn's disease, anaemia was present in 79 per cent of the males and 54 per cent of females.

Forty-six out of a total of 63 patients had bone marrow biopsies, and of these 39 per cent were megaloblastic. Of this group, 11 were folate deficient, six vitamin B_{12} deficient, and one had both deficiencies. On the other hand, macrocytic anaemia is unusual in patients with ulcerative colitis and the anaemia is usually hypochromic due to blood loss. Interestingly, there have been occasional reports of autoimmune haemolytic anaemia occurring in association with ulcerative colitis; in several cases the autoantibodies showed rhesus specificity.

The anaemia of intestinal inflammatory disease may be made worse by drugs which are used in its management. Patients who receive salazopyrine for colitis occasionally develop an acute haemolytic anaemia associated with Heinz body formation. Bone marrow depression may occur in patients receiving immunosuppressive treatment for colitis or Crohn's disease. Ileocaecal tuberculosis may be associated with any of the bizarre haematological manifestations of tuberculosis described above, and it may be complicated by the side-effects of antituberculous drug therapy.

Whipple's disease may produce a clinical picture and blood changes which can mimic several primary haematological disorders. The typical clinical triad of diarrhoea, arthropathy, and enlarged lymph nodes is usually associated with a mild normochromic, normocytic anaemia, a raised ESR, and a polymorphonuclear leucocytosis. Quite often there is associated lymphopenia or eosinophilia. Some cases present less typically, and particularly when the spleen is enlarged the condition may closely mimic a primary reticulosis. Malabsorption of vitamin B_{12} or folic acid may occasionally be encountered in this disorder (see Section 5).

Structural disease of the stomach, and small and large bowel

The structural changes and resulting abnormalities of absorption associated with gastritis are described in detail in Section 12. Similarly, the various anatomical abnormalities of the small gut and malabsorption syndromes which lead to vitamin B_{12} and folate deficiency are reviewed earlier in this section (pages 19.99 and 19.100). The relationship between gastric surgery and iron and vitamin B_{12} metabolism is also discussed earlier in this section (pages 19.86 and 19.99).

Most *anatomical lesions of the small bowel* present to the haematologist as a macrocytic anaemia with a megaloblastic bone marrow due to vitamin B_{12} or folate deficiency or as a refractory iron deficiency anaemia. Several abnormalities of the small gut are associated with the production of a relatively profuse bacterial flora with subsequent utilization of vitamin B_{12}. These conditions include surgically produced blind loops, strictures, anastomoses between loops of small bowel, fistulae between various sections of the bowel, diverticulae of the small bowel, malfunctioning gastroenterostomies, interference of gut motility in conditions such as scleroderma, Whipple's disease, post-vagotomy, and after extensive gut resection. In the latter case the disorder may also produce malabsorption. All these conditions are associated with defective vitamin B_{12} absorption which can be partly corrected by the administration of broad spectrum antibiotics but not by intrinsic factor.

Megaloblastic anaemia due to *intestinal malabsorption* is fully reviewed on page 19.100. It should be remembered, however, that the malabsorption syndromes may present to the haematologist in other ways. For example, there is a very high incidence of iron deficiency anaemia in this group and, particularly in childhood, this is the much commoner form of presentation than a megaloblastic anaemia. The peripheral blood changes of hyposplenism are quite frequently associated with an underlying malabsorption syndrome. The latter may also present with a bleeding disorder due to prothrombin deficiency following defective absorption of vitamin K. Patients with malabsorption syndrome frequently have biochemical evidence of vitamin E deficiency; although this may produce a slightly shortened red cell survival, there is no evidence

Table 4 Haematological changes in liver disease

Virus hepatitis
  Haemolytic anaemia, hypoplastic anaemia
Chronic active hepatitis
  Immune haemolytic anaemia, LE cells in blood, hyperglobulinaemia
Chronic liver failure
  Chronic anaemia is often complicated by:
    (*a*) blood loss and iron deficiency
    (*b*) alcohol, direct effect on marrow
    (*c*) folate deficiency
    (*d*) portal hypertension and hypersplenism
    (*e*) acute haemolytic episodes (e.g. Zieve's syndrome, spur-cell syndrome)
  Thrombocytopenia, leucopenia, haemorrhagic diathesis due to:
    (*a*) deficiency of vitamin K-dependent factors
    (*b*) portal hypertension and hypersplenism
    (*c*) increased fibrinolysis
    (*d*) thrombocytopenia
Portal hypertension
  Anaemia, leucopenia, thrombocytopenia, bleeding from varices
Obstructive jaundice
  Mild anaemia, target-cell formation, masking of hereditary spherocytosis
Tumours
  Polycythaemia, leukaemoid reactions, α-feto-protein production
Liver transplantation
  Haemorrhagic and hypercoagulable states

that vitamin E deficiency alone produces a significant degree of anaemia.

Liver disease

There is usually a moderate degree of anaemia in patients with *chronic liver failure* (Table 4). The red cells are normochromic or slightly macrocytic with MCV values ranging from 100 to 115 fl. Target cells and a variable degree of polychromasia with a slightly elevated reticulocyte count are often found. The degree of macrocytosis and target cell formation corresponds reasonably well with the degree of liver failure. The bone marrow tends to be hypercellular with erythroid hyperplasia and macronormoblastic changes.

The actual mechanism of the anaemia of liver failure is uncertain. However, there may be many complicating factors which cause a worsening of the anaemia in this condition. Nutritional folate deficiency is very common in patients with liver disease, particularly the alcoholic form. Secondary iron deficiency is also common and usually results from chronic intestinal blood loss associated with a poor dietetic intake. Interestingly, in patients with severe portal hypertension and cirrhosis, or in those who have undergone portacaval shunt surgery, there may be some increase in iron absorption with marked haemosiderosis of the liver.

A variety of different forms of *haemolytic anaemia* occur in patients with liver disease. In *Zieve's syndrome* there is jaundice, hyperlipidaemia, and haemolytic anaemia which follows an excessive alcohol intake (see page 19.151). Other forms of haemolytic anaemia may occur. Acute haemolysis has been well documented in patients with viral hepatitis, particularly those who are glucose 6-phosphate dehydrogenase deficient. An acquired haemolytic anaemia with a positive Coombs' test may occur occasionally in patients with chronic active hepatitis. Another form of haemolytic anaemia in liver disease, usually alcoholic cirrhosis, has been observed in which there are marked red cell abnormalities with burr and spur-shaped forms predominating (see page 19.151).

The haematological effects of alcohol

Because excessive consumption of alcohol is so common it is important for clinicians to appreciate the remarkably diverse haematological manifestations which it causes.

Anaemia is particularly common in chronic alcoholics. It has an extremely complex aetiology including a deficient diet, chronic blood loss, hepatic dysfunction, and the direct toxic effects of alcohol on the bone marrow.

Macrocytosis is particularly common in chronic alcoholics. An unexplained macrocytic blood picture should always raise the possibility of alcoholism although its absence does not rule out the diagnosis. It may be associated with normoblastic or megaloblastic erythropoiesis. In moderately severe alcoholics who are maintaining a reasonable diet it probably reflects the direct toxic action of alcohol on the bone marrow. The normoblasts may show vacuolation or there may be no specific changes on light microscopy. Megaloblastic anaemia is usually seen in severe alcoholics who are poorly nourished, and is due to folate deficiency. While a folate-poor diet is the major factor there is some evidence that alcohol plays a more direct role in interfering with folate metabolism by an unknown mechanism. It should be remembered that macrocytosis can also occur in alcoholics during a reticulocytosis in response to bleeding or alcohol withdrawal. It may also reflect coexistent liver disease. The occurrence of sideroblastic anaemia in severe alcoholics was mentioned in an earlier chapter (page 19.132). It is often associated with a macrocytosis or a dimorphic blood picture and occurs in severe alcoholics. The sideroblastic changes revert to normal after stopping alcohol.

Simple iron deficiency is also found commonly in alcoholics and probably reflects both a poor diet and chronic blood loss due to gastritis or bleeding varices. It may be associated with folate deficiency; the blood film is then dimorphic with macrocytes, microcytes, and hypersegmented neutrophils. Alcoholics with chronic pancreatitis may develop iron loading due to increased absorption.

As well as these changes, which are specific for alcohol, any of the haematological manifestations of liver disease, as described earlier, may be found in alcoholics.

Alcohol also has deleterious effects on the white cells. Severe alcoholics are prone to infection. The neutropenia of alcoholism may reflect both the toxic effect of alcohol on the marrow and folate deficiency. There is also some evidence that alcohol can interfere with neutrophil locomotion and with their ability to ingest foreign material including micro-organisms.

Thrombocytopenia is commonly seen in chronic alcoholics and may occur without accompanying folate deficiency or splenomegaly. Megakaryocytes may be normal or diminished in number. Following withdrawal of alcohol the platelet count usually returns to normal although it may become markedly elevated for a few days.

Chest disease

(See also carcinoma, page 19.238, tuberculosis, page 19.241, and secondary polycythaemia, page 19.155).

Pneumonia

Most bacterial pneumonias are associated with a neutrophil leucocytosis. There are two relatively common forms of pneumonia which are associated with more specific haematological changes. In mycoplasma pneumonia cold agglutinins can usually be detected in increased amounts towards the end of the first week in up to 80 per cent of cases. The cold antibodies are polyclonal IgM and to the red cell I antigen. Although a positive Coombs' test has been described in these cases, and in most of them there is an increased reticulocyte count, serious haemolysis is rare. Occasionally, the condition is complicated by disseminated intravascular coagulation.

There is increasing evidence that in patients with pneumonia caused by *Legionella pneumophila* (Legionnaires' disease) there may be severe thrombocytopenia and, sometimes, lymphopenia.

Several cases have been reported to be complicated by disseminated intravascular coagulation.

Pulmonary eosinophilia
(See also Sections 15 and 24.)

This term refers to a group of disorders which have in common a raised eosinophil count in the peripheral blood in association with pulmonary infiltrates on the chest X-ray. The exact nature of many of the disorders which constitute this syndrome is uncertain. In its simplest form there may be a brief period of respiratory distress in association with eosinophilia. This condition is sometimes called *Löffler's syndrome*. At the other end of the spectrum there is a severe illness associated with widespread pulmonary infiltrates and eosinophilia which may culminate with the features of polyarteritis nodosa.

The transient disorder described by Löffler probably represents a heterogeneous group of conditions which in many cases are associated with parasitic infection. Many parasitic disorders can cause this type of illness, including ascariasis, ankylostomiasis, trichiuriasis, taeniasis, and fascioliasis. A similar condition has been well described as part of a hypersensitivity reaction to drugs. The commonest is para-aminosalicylic acid but similar reactions have been observed in patients receiving penicillin, sulphonamides, and nitrofurantoin. A similar clinical picture is associated with the syndrome of allergic alveolitis, including farmer's lung, bird fancier's lung, and a variety of other occupational disorders (see Section 15).

Another condition characterized by a marked eosinophilia with pulmonary infiltrates goes under the general term tropical eosinophilia. There is considerable evidence that this disorder is due to occult filarial infection.

Another well-documented cause of pulmonary eosinophilia is hypersensitivity to fungi, particularly *Aspergillus fumigatus*.

Idiopathic pulmonary haemosiderosis and Goodpasture's syndrome
(See Section 18.)

These disorders occasionally present as a refractory anaemia. The latter has the characteristics of the anaemia of chronic disorders although it may become markedly hypochromic and microcytic due to chronic blood loss.

Skin diseases

Megaloblastic anaemia and the skin
The whole relationship between skin disease and megaloblastic anaemia is extremely complex and much of the work in this field is still controversial. The subject is discussed earlier (see page 19.100).

There is no doubt that a proportion of patients with various dermatoses show evidence of folate depletion, at least biochemically, and in some cases, haematologically. This has been reported in patients with erythroderma, psoriasis, or extensive eczema. There is a well-documented association between malabsorption and dermatitis herpetiformis. Although megaloblastic anaemia is not found frequently in association with disorders of the skin, some patients with these conditions do have mild megaloblastic changes. Although earlier reports suggested that a significant proportion of them had abnormalities of small intestinal function and structure, leading to the descriptive term 'dermatogenic enteropathy', this concept has been questioned and it is now agreed that a completely flat small bowel mucosa is rarely seen in these conditions. The relationship between dermatitis herpetiformis and malabsorption of the coeliac type seems to be a special case. Several series have shown a high incidence of small bowel changes of coeliac disease in patients with this condition. Furthermore, there appears to be a high incidence of splenic hypoplasia and many patients show typical haematological changes of defective function of the spleen (see page 19.100).

Systemic mast cell syndrome

Some components of what is called the systemic mast cell syndrome (see also page 19.43) produce striking haematological changes. The syndrome is divided into urticaria pigmentosa of childhood and systemic mastocytosis of adult life. There are rarely changes in the peripheral blood or bone marrow in children with urticaria pigmentosa (see Section 20).

In systemic mastocytosis the clinical manifestations may resemble those of lymphoma or leukaemia; indeed, the disease should probably be classified as reticuloendotheliosis. The skin and mucuous membrane changes are similar to those of childhood urticaria pigmentosa; however, the macules tend to become confluent with persistent telangiectasia. There may be involvement of the mouth, nose, and rectal mucosa associated with progressive cutaneous changes characterized by a chronic lichenified dermatitis. The skin changes are associated with generalized lymphadenopathy, splenomegaly, and hepatomegaly, and the bone marrow contains an abnormal accumulation of mast cells. In addition there may be anaemia, leucopenia, thrombocytopenia, and leukaemoid features. The latter include a monocytosis, lymphocytosis, or eosinophilia. Liver function is impaired and there may be a bleeding tendency from a combination of thrombocythaemia and prothrombin deficiency. Occasionally, mast cells spill into the peripheral blood in large numbers with the picture of *mast cell leukaemia*. Folate deficiency may result from an associated malabsorption. The dermatological aspects of this condition are described in Section 20, and the bone marrow fibrosis which may occur, on page 19.43.

Endocrine disease

Pituitary deficiency

A mild normochromic normocytic anaemia is very common in patients with anterior pituitary deficiency. The mechanism is not absolutely clear although the anaemia has many features in common with that of hypothyroidism and is fully responsive to appropriate replacement therapy.

Thyroid disease

Hypothyroidism is associated with a variety of haematological changes. Anaemia is common and may be normocytic, microcytic, or macrocytic.

Severe microcytic anaemia in hypothyroidism is most commonly seen in women who have menorrhagia which is a frequent complication of this condition. Severe macrocytosis in hypothyroidism usually indicates an associated vitamin B_{12} deficiency; there seems to be a genuine association between pernicious anaemia and myxoedema. It has been suggested that mild macrocytosis may occur in hypothyroidism in the absence of vitamin B_{12} or folate deficiency although published series of studies have shown a remarkable variability in the incidence of this phenomenon. Some patients with severe hypothyroidism have a small proportion of misshapen red cells on their peripheral blood films.

The true anaemia of uncomplicated myxoedema is normochromic and normocytic. The mechanism is still uncertain. However, recent studies have shown that T3, T4, and reverse T3 can all potentiate the effect of erythropoietin on the formation of erythroid colonies *in vitro*. This effect appears to be mediated by receptors with β_2 adrenergic properties. Thus it appears that the thyroid hormones have a direct effect in altering the erythropoietin responsiveness of erythroid progenitors. It has also been suggested that part of the normochromic anaemia of hypothyroidism may be a physiological adaptation to reduced oxygen requirements by the tissues.

Curiously, patients with hyperthyroidism do not have elevated haemoglobin levels. There is some recent evidence that there may be a mild increase in the red cell mass in hyperthyroidism, but that this is compensated for by an increase in plasma volume. In some patients with severe hyperthyroidism there is a mild anaemia associated with abnormal iron utilization.

Adrenal disease

A mild normochromic normocytic anaemia is observed in some patients with Addison's disease. The mechanism is unknown.

Parathyroid disease

Primary hyperparathyroidism is occasionally associated with anaemia which responds to removal of the parathyroid glands. The relationship between parathyroid disease and marrow fibrosis is discussed on page 19.44.

Diabetes mellitus

The structural changes which occur in the haemoglobin of diabetic patients are discussed on page 19.129. There have been recent reports that there may be an increase in the red cell volume of patients with severe diabetes. The mechanism and significance of this observation remains to be clarified. Severe diabetic acidosis is often associated with a marked leucocytosis, even when there is no underlying infection. Hyperosmolarity impairs neutrophil function, and reduced neutrophil migration has been observed in patients with diabetic ketoacidosis or poorly controlled hyperglycaemia. Because of the high incidence of atheroma in patients with diabetes both platelet function and vessel wall metabolism have been studied in considerable detail in this condition. Synthesis of PGI_2 in biopsy specimens of forearm veins is reduced and a variety of changes in platelet reactivity and survival have been observed. The relationship of these changes to the vascular disease of diabetes requires further clarification.

References

Anon (1983). Anaemia of chronic renal failure. *Lancet* **i**, 965–966.

Boxer, H., Ellman, L., Geller, R. and Wang, C.-A. (1977). Anemia in primary hyperparathyroidism. *Arch. Intern. Med.* **137**, 588–590.

Bunch, C. and Weatherall, D. J. (1982). The blood in systemic disease. In *Blood and its disorders* 2nd ed (eds R. M. Hardisty and D. J. Weatherall), pp. 1319–1393 Blackwell Scientific Publications, Oxford.

Caro, J., Brown, S., Moller, O., Murray, T. and Erslev, A. J. (1979). Erythropoietin levels in uremic nephric and anephric patients. *J. Lab. Clin. Med.* **93**, 449–468.

Castaldi, P. A. (1984). Hemostasis and kidney disease. In *Disorders of hemostasis* (eds O. D. Ratnoff and C. D. Forbes), pp. 473–484. Grune and Stratton, Orlando, Florida.

Davidson, R. J. L., Evan-Wong, L. A. and Stowers, J. M. (1981). The mean red cell volume in diabetes mellitus. *Diabetologia* **20**, 583–584.

Erslev, A. J. (1983). Anemia of chronic renal failure. In *Hematology* 3rd edn (eds W. J., Williams, E., Beutler, A. J. Erslev and M. A. Lichtman), pp. 417–424. McGraw Hill Inc., New York.

—— (1983). Anemia of endocrine disorders. In *Hematology* 3rd edn (eds W. J. Williams, E. Beutler, A. J. Erslev and M. A. Lichtman), pp. 425–429. McGraw-Hill, New York.

—— and Shapiro, S. S. (1979). Hematologic aspects of renal failure. In *Diseases of the kidney* (eds L. E. Earley and C. W. Gottshalk), p. 277. Little, Brown, Boston.

Goldsmith, G. H. Jr. (1984). Hemostatic disorders associated with neoplasia. In *Disorders of hemostasis* (eds O. D. Ratnoff and C. D. Forbes), pp. 351–366. Grune and Stratton, Orlando, Florida.

Herbert, E. V. (ed.) (1980). Hematologic complications of anemia in alcoholic patients. *Sem. Hematol.* **17**, nos 1 and 2.

Hughes, G. R. V. (1983). The lupus anticoagulant. *Br. Med. J.* **287**, 1088–1089.

Israels, M. C. G. and Delamore, I. W. (1972). Haematological aspects of systemic disease. *Clin. Haematol.* **1**, 445–670.

McCurdy, P. R. and Rath, C. E. (1980). Vacuolated nucleated bone marrow cells in alcoholism. *Sem. Hematol.* **17**, 100–102.

Oski, F. A. (1983). Anemia related to nutritional deficiencies other than vitamin B_{12} and folic acid. In *Hematology* 3rd edn (eds W. J. Williams, E. Beutler, A. J. Erslev and M. A. Lichtman), pp. 532–537. McGraw-Hill, New York.

Ratnoff, O. D. (1984). Hemostatic defects in liver and biliary tract diseases. In *Disorders of hemostasis* (eds O. D. Ratnoff and C. D. Forbes), pp. 451–472. Grune and Stratton, Orlando, Florida.

Zaroulis, C. G., Kourides, J. A. and Valeri, C. R. (1978). Red cell 2,3-diphosphoglycerate and oxygen affinity of hemoglobin in patients with thyroid disorders. *Blood* **52**, 181–185.

BLOOD REPLACEMENT

Blood transfusion

H. H. GUNSON AND V. J. MARTLEW

Blood transfusion has developed from the early discoveries of antigenic differences between the red cells of human beings. Several hundred blood group antigens have now been defined on red cells, leucocytes, and platelets, and they comprise one of the most complex polymorphisms known in humans. From this base, increasing knowledge of the physicochemical properties of cellular and plasma components acquired during the past two decades has prepared the way for modern transfusion therapy. The ever-increasing pharmacopoeia of chemotherapeutic agents requires the availability of blood components in order that they may be used to their maximum advantage.

The transfusion of blood and its components must not be undertaken lightly. Although this procedure may have benefits to the patient it also carries hazards which must be thoroughly understood. It is not possible in the course of this chapter to discuss all aspects of immunohaematology and blood transfusion, and the reader is referred to texts which will impart knowledge in depth on various aspects of the subject.

Blood group antigens and antibodies

Red cell antigens

Antigens present on the surface membrane of red cells are developed as a result of gene action or interaction. Sets of antigens may show a relationship towards each other, and when their inheritance is independent of other sets are regarded as belonging to a blood group system. Many such systems are known; those encountered most frequently are summarized in Table 1. Some blood group antigens, e.g. Rh, are confined to red cells, whilst others may be present in the tissue or on the surface of other body cells, e.g. A, B, and Lewis. The physiological function of the red cell antigens is not known, although some may serve to maintain the integrity of the membrane.

Red cell antibodies

Antibodies are immunoglobulins, of which there are five classes, IgG, IgM, IgA, IgD, and IgE, each comprising heavy chains which characterize the immunoglobulin and light chains ($\varkappa$ and λ) which are common to each type. Blood group antibodies are principally IgG and/or IgM, although those with IgA specificity have been found. Usually IgA antibodies coexist with molecules which are IgG or IgM. The nature of alloantibodies in the common blood group systems is shown in Table 2. In autoimmune acquired haemolytic anaemia monoclonal autoantibodies with blood group specificity may be found, often with the specificity of anti-I, but more commonly IgG polyclonal autoantibodies are detected; in a few instances specific IgA autoantibodies have been defined.

The presence of an antibody is usually dependent upon stimulation with the appropriate antigen. Thus a person who is Rh-negative can develop anti-Rh if transfused with Rh-positive red cells. The development of such antibodies results from a complex cellular interaction in the reticuloendothelial system (see Section 4). Antibodies are termed 'naturally occurring' when there is no obvious antigenic stimulus. The mechanism for the development of such antibodies is uncertain, but antigens, closely similar to those of blood groups, present in bacteria and foodstuffs may be the antigenic source. The commonest 'naturally occurring' antibodies belong to the ABO blood group systems.

Antibodies have the ability to combine with their corresponding antigen (or possibly closely related antigens when cross-activity occurs). The combination of an antibody with a red cell may result in a change which can be observed *in vitro*. It is in this manner that many of the blood group systems have been discovered, and forms the basis for compatibility testing (see page 19.250). Red cells may also be damaged by the binding of antibodies *in vivo* leading to accelerated destruction. Dependent on the rate and manner of this destruction incompatible transfusion reactions may occur.

Blood group systems

Whilst the detection of antibodies to many of the blood group systems in the serum of a patient may be important in transfusion, two blood group systems, ABO(H) and Rh, have the most clinical importance. A brief review of these systems will be given, with comments on other systems.

The ABO groups

The commonly encountered groups in the ABO system and their corresponding antibodies are shown in Table 3. The frequencies of the different groups varies throughout the world; thus group B diminishes in frequency from east to west. The frequencies given in Table 3 are an average for the United Kingdom.

Anti-A and anti-B combine with their corresponding antigens over a wide range of temperatures *in vitro* and can do so readily *in vitro*. It can be appreciated, therefore, that the transfusion of ABO incompatible blood may lead to the destruction of the transfused cells with, often, serious complications for the patient (see below).

Group O red cells do not bind anti-A or anti-B. It is possible, therefore, to transfuse group O blood to patients of other AB groups. Recourse is taken to this procedure in certain urgent transfusions when time does not permit the determination of the patient's group prior to transfusion. A cautionary word must be given concerning this practice. Certain group O individuals pos-

Table 1 Some examples of blood group systems and their common antigens

Blood group system	Symbols of common antigens
ABO	$A_1 A_2 B H$
Rhesus	C D E c e
MNS	M N S s
P	$P_1 P_2$
Kell	K k
Lewis	$Le^a Le^b$
Lutheran	$Lu^a Lu^b$
Duffy	$Fy^a Fy^b$
Kidd	$Jk^a Jk^b$
Ii	I i

Table 2 The immunoglobulin nature of some common group antibodies

Blood group antibody	Immunoglobulin
Anti–A	IgG + IgM + IgA
Anti–B	
Anti–Rh	IgG + IgM
Anti–K	Usually IgG
Anti–k	
Anti–Fy^a	Usually IgG
Anti–Jk^a	IgM and/or IgG
Anti–P_1	IgM
Anti–Le^a	IgM
Anti–Le^b	

Table 3 The ABO groups, corresponding naturally occurring antibodies and frequencies in the United Kingdom

Group of red cells	Antibody in serum	Approximate frequency in the UK (%)
A_1	Anti–B	32
A_2	Anti–B (+ anti–A_1 in 10%)	10
B	Anti–A	8
O	Anti–A + anti–B	47
A_1B	None	2.3
A_2	None or anti–A_1 (in 25%)	0.7

Table 4 Common Rh phenotypes and genotypes and their frequencies in the United Kingdom

Phenotypes		Commonest genotype	Frequency in the UK (%)
R_1R,	ccDee	CDe/cde	34
R_2r,	ccDEe	cDE/cde	13
R_1R_2,	CcDEe	cDe/cDE	13
R_1R_1,	CCDee	CDe/CDe	18
R_2R_2,	ccDEE	CDE/cDE	3
R_0r,	ccDee	cDe/cde	2
rr,	ccee	cde/cde	15
r'r,	CCee	Cde/cde	1
r''r,	ccEe	cdE/cde	1

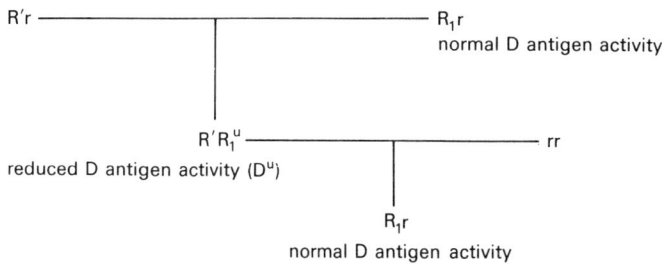

Fig. 1 Suppression of D antigen activity by the R' (Cde) chromosome in the transposition.

sess high concentrations of anti-A (and possibly anti-B). Such antibodies may attain a level which is sufficient to cause destruction of a proportion of the patient's red cells. Laboratory tests (see below) can be carried out to minimize the undesirable effect of such 'dangerous universal donors' but the frequent use of group O blood, particularly in large quantities, for the transfusion of group A, B, and AB patients should be avoided.

Anti-A_1 can be found in group A_2, and more frequently in group A_2B persons. *In vitro*, this antibody is usually reactive only at temperatures considerably lower than 37 °C, and will not cause accelerated red cell destruction *in vitro*; occasional examples have been found to react at 37 °C, and only in these instances appropriate blood lacking the antigen need be selected for transfusion.

The Rh blood groups

Table 4 illustrates the common Rh groups found in the United Kingdom with their approximate frequencies. The five common antigens known are C, D, E, c, and e. Controversy has existed for decades regarding the mechanism for inheritance of the Rh antigens and four nomenclatures have been proposed. The two shown in Table 4 are in common use.

A person who lacks the D antigen is normally referred to as Rh-negative, which comprises about 15 per cent of the Caucasian population, and those possessing the D antigen are called Rh-positive. In order that patients transfused with r'r or r''r blood (which is D negative, Table 4) are not exposed to the C and E antigen, *Rh-negative blood for transfusion* in the United Kingdom also lacks these antigens, although this practice is not uniform in all countries. A variant of the D antigen, D^u, is found in a small proportion of Caucasians, and more frequently in Negroes. A characteristic of the D^u antigen is its poor reactivity *in vitro* and this results from the presence of fewer D antigen sites per red cell than normal, and may be a directly inherited characteristic or arise as a result of suppression of D antigen activity by the r' or Ry chromosomes in the trans position (Fig. 1).

The commonest antibody encountered in the Rh blood group system is anti-D and is found when Rh(D) negative persons are

subjected to stimulation with Rh(D) positive red cells; exposure to red cells is a prerequisite since the Rh antigens are confined to human red cell membranes.

Anti-D can develop in Rh(D) negative mothers during pregnancy as a result of spontaneous transplacental haemorrhage of fetal Rh(D) positive red cells (see page 19.146). Although transplacental haemorrhage can occur at any time during a pregnancy, and anti-D alloimmunization has resulted following spontaneous or induced abortions in the early weeks of gestation, it is commonest at the time of delivery. The administration of anti-D immunoglobulin within 72 hours of transplacental haemorrhage [dosage: 250 i.u. (50 μg) up to 20 weeks gestation and 500 i.u. (100 μg) after 20 weeks or within 72 hours of delivery] has greatly reduced the incidence of anti-D alloimmunization. Failures, however, do occur in approximately 2 per cent of patients; approximately one-half of the failures occur because the anti-D immunoglobulin is not administered and the remainder of the failures are due to inadequate dosage or from too great a delay between the transplacental haemorrhage and the administration of immunoglobulin. The first of the biological causes can be avoided by obtaining an estimate of degree of haemorrhage by means of a Kleihauer test which comprises the washing out of haemoglobin in adult cells on a blood film by an acid solution which leaves those containing fetal haemoglobin intact (Fig. 2). Although the standard dose of 500 i.u. (100 μg) will be sufficient to prevent alloimmunization in over 99 per cent of instances, in the remainder dosage should be increased to 125 i.u. (25 μg) per ml of fetal *red cells* in the maternal circulation. The delay between administration of immunoglobulin and transplacental haemorrhage leading to failure of the prevention of alloimmunization usually occurs due to fetomaternal haemorrhage during gestation. The administration of anti-D immunoglobulin has been recommended to prevent this occurrence but is not universally undertaken.

The inadvertent transfusion of Rh(D) positive red cells to an Rh(D) negative person can also result in anti-D alloimmunization. Since this can lead to serious Rh haemolytic disease of the newborn in subsequent pregnancies, efforts should be made to remove these incompatible red cells in women of child-bearing age by the administration of anti-D immunoglobulin intramuscularly in divided doses over 24 hours at the dosage of 125 i.u. (25 μg) per ml of transfused *red cells*.

Provided clearance occurs within 6–8 days alloimmunization is usually prevented. Intravenous preparations of anti-D immunoglobulin have been used to clear incompatible red cells from the circulation. Care must be exercised with this form of treatment, however, since the rapid removal of a large number of red cells can lead to undesirable effects from the occurrence of a significant rapid haemolysis.

In some female patients anti-D may fall to a low or even indetectable levels during the course of many years, but antibody production will rapidly respond to further stimulation. Thus, females who are Rh-negative or of unknown group should always be given Rh-negative blood; failure to do so may lead to serious, or even fatal, transfusion reactions.

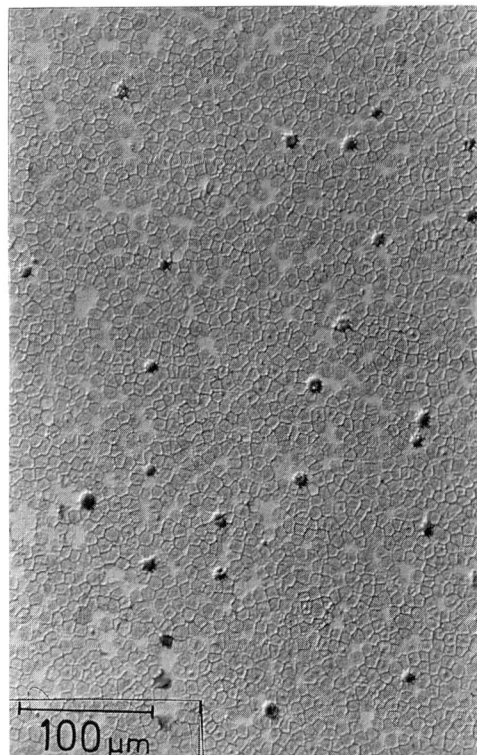

Fig. 2 Appearance of 1 in 100 fetal red cells in the Kleihauer test. The fetal red cells retain their haemoglobin whilst the adult red cells appear as 'ghosts'.

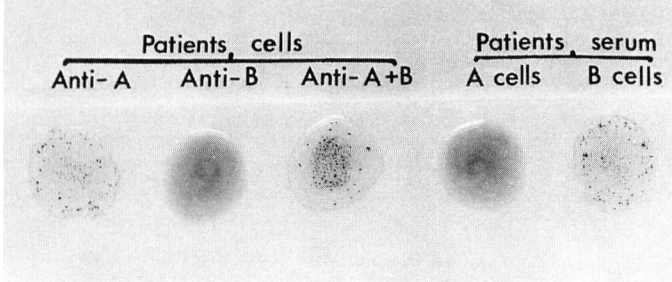

Fig. 3 Agglutination reactions in the determination of ABO blood group: Group A, see Table 3.

Rh(D)-positive individuals may develop Rh antibodies. Anti-E and anti-c are the most commonly encountered. Such patients should be transfused with blood lacking the corresponding antigen. If anti-E is found in an R_1R_1 patient it is advisable to transfuse R_1R_1 blood since such patients also lack c antigen; administration of E-negative, c-positive blood, e.g. R_1r which, although compatible, may stimulate the formation of anti-c.

Other blood groups
Blood group antibodies are found in the sera of patients which belong to systems other than ABO and Rh. Some, e.g. Lewis, Ii, are 'naturally occurring' while others are immune, e.g. Kell, Duffy, Kidd, and in these instances a history will be elicited of previous transfusion or occasionally previous pregnancies. The selection of appropriate blood for transfusion can be carried out in the laboratory, and the difficulty in providing blood will depend on the frequency of donors lacking the appropriate antigen.

Leucocyte and platelet antigens and antibodies
Much work has been carried out on the antigens of leucocytes, and a complex system of antigens (HLA) has been defined. These antigens are expressed on lymphocytes and platelets, and possibly also on other leucocytes. Platelets and neutrophils also possess specific antigens. The antigens of the ABO system are also present on leucocytes and platelets.

Leucocyte antigens have been extensively investigated in connection with organ transplantation, but they also have importance in transfusion. Antibodies to leucocytes and platelets may arise as a result of transfusion and pregnancy, and may cause troublesome pyrexial reactions in patients requiring long-term transfusion (see below).

Compatibility tests
In general, all red cell preparations should be subjected to direct compatibility tests prior to transfusion. The only exception to this rule occurs in severe haemorrhage when time does not permit

their execution. In such emergencies the use of group O, Rh-negative blood is used, and in many hospitals these units of blood are also Kell negative, and have been screened for lower than average levels of anti-A and anti-B.

The compatibility test comprises the determination of the ABO and Rh group of the patient, and a cross-match of the donor red cell sample with the serum of the patient. In many laboratories, prior to the non-urgent transfusion of the patient, antibody screening tests against a panel of typed red cells is also included.

Whilst the tests themselves are performed in the laboratory, compatibility tests *begin with the patient*. Most transfusion accidents result from clerical errors with blood being administered to the wrongly identified patient. It is important that samples for compatibility tests are taken into tubes labelled correctly with the patient's name, and other identification, e.g. address or hospital number, and the date of collection. Multiple numbering systems in use in some hospitals are excellent safety procedures; an individual number is placed on the patient's wrist band, and the same number attached to the specimen bottle, the request form, and any units of blood supplied for the patient. This allows an additional check to be made. Prelabelling specimen tubes for several patients prior to the collection of the samples is extremely dangerous, and must never be practised. The request form is a valuable document and should be completed fully; adequate clinical information is essential for the staff in the laboratory, and lack of information often leads to unnecessary investigations and frustrating delays.

Grouping, cross-matching and tests for antibody activity depend upon the characteristics of the reaction, *in vitro*, between a blood group antibody and its corresponding antigen. A brief review of the principles of these tests is valuable to the understanding of transfusion hazards.

Agglutination tests
Some antibodies have the ability to agglutinate appropriate red cells suspended in saline (0.15 M NaCl) at temperatures up to 37 °C. Many of these antibodies, often referred to as *saline agglutinins*, are IgM, and common examples are anti-A and anti-B. Figure 3 is a photograph of the reactivity of group A red cells with anti-A, anti-B, and group O serum (anti A+B). The serum of this patient agglutinates group B cells and thus contains anti-B; negative reactions can be distinguished by lack of agglutination.

Not all antibodies will agglutinate saline-suspended red cells. However, prior treatment of the red cells with certain proteolytic enzymes, e.g. papain, will effect agglutination. Also, the addition of colloids, e.g. bovine serum albumin, will enable agglutination to occur in some instances. Such antibodies tend to be IgG in nature and common examples are many examples of Rh antibodies, anti-Kell, and anti-Kidd.

During the past few years it has been found that by reducing the ionic strength of the reacting mixture of antibody and red cells, antibody will become attached to the red cells more rapidly, i.e. the rate of association is increased. This principle has been

Table 5 Example of a serological investigation: detection of anti-D and anti-Kell

													Compatibility tests			
Test red cells													Indirect antiglobulin	Agglutination		
														16 °C	37 °C	Albumin
ABO	Rh	MNSs	P$_1$	Le^a	Le^b	K	Lu^a	Lu^b	Fy^a	Fy^b	JK^a	JK^b				
O	R1R1	MMSs	+	+	−	−	−	+	+	−	−	+	++++	−	−	+++
O	R2R2	MMSs	+	−	+	+	−	+	+	+	+	+	++++	−	++	+++
O	R1R2	MNss	−	−	+	−	+	−	−	+	+	+	++++	−	−	+++
O	rr	MNSs	+	−	+	−	+	−	+	−	+	+	−	−	−	−
O	rr	MMSS	+	−	−	+	−	+	−	+	−	+	+++	−	++	++
O	rr	NNSs	−	+	−	−	−	+	+	+	+	−	−	−	−	−
O	r′r	MNSs	+	−	−	+	−	+	+	−	−	+	+++	−	++	++
O	r″r	MMss	+	−	+	−	−	+	+	+	+	+	−	−	−	−

Patient group O Rh negative (rr), KKell negative

employed in both grouping and cross-matching tests in an attempt to reduce the time involved for these procedures.

The antiglobulin test

An antiglobulin serum is raised in animals, usually rabbits, sheep or goats, by injection with human immunoglobulins and complement components. The resultant immune serum is absorbed with normal human red cells to remove species-specific antibodies. Various types of reagents can be prepared. That most commonly used in cross-matching is the broad-spectrum reagent, and contains anti-IgG, anti-IgA, and possibly anti-IgM, together with certain antibodies to complement components, notably antibodies to fragments of the complement components C3 and C4.

When some antibodies bind to red cells suspended in saline, no distinguishable change takes place. If such sensitized cells are washed to remove contaminating proteins, the antibody immunoglobulin on adjacent red cells may combine with the appropriate antibody to the immunoglobulin present in the antiglobulin serum, and agglutination results. Such a reaction occurs most commonly between IgG antibodies and the anti-IgG in the antiglobulin serum.

Some blood group antibodies have the ability to fix complement. Complement comprises a group of nine major components which are present in plasma of all individuals and are activated by certain antigen–antibody complexes to produce an enzyme cascade. If this reaction proceeds to completion, *haemolysis* of the red cells results. Few examples of blood group antibodies will produce haemolysis *in vitro*, and certain examples of anti-A and anti-B are the commonest. More often, the complement-fixing blood group antibodies cause the fixation of C1–4 components. Fragments of C3 (C3b and C3d) are detected readily by anti-C3b and anti-C3d in antiglobulin reagents. It is advantageous to have both antibodies in the antiglobulin reagent since C3b is usually detected with antibody sensitization *in vitro*, whilst the positive direct antiglobulin test due to complement coating of the red cells *in vivo* detects the reaction between C3d and anti-C3d. Some antiglobulin reagents contain anti-C4 but high concentrations are undesirable since they can detect traces of C4 fragments on unsensitized red cells and lead to false-positive results. IgM antibodies almost always fix complement and the presence of an IgM antibody on a red cell is usually more easily detected by reactivity with anticomplement than with anti-IgM, so that the latter component is not essential in the antiglobulin serum. Many IgG antibodies fail to fix complement, e.g. anti-Rh, but others have this ability on occasions, e.g. anti-Kell, anti-Duffy. The ability of an antibody to fix complement has a bearing on the rapidity with which incompatible red cells are removed from the circulation (see below).

Table 6 Complications of blood transfusion

Immune	Non-immune
1. Haemolytic	1. Cardiovascular
(*a*) Immediate, e.g. ABO antibodies	(*a*) Circulatory overload
(*b*) Delayed, e.g. Rhesus antibodies	(*b*) Thrombophlebitis
	(*c*) Venous thrombosis
2. Leucocyte antibodies	(*d*) Air embolism
(*a*) HLA	2. Transfusion haemosiderosis
(*b*) Anti-neutrophil, e.g. anti-NAA′	3. Sequelae of massive transfusion
3. Platelet antibodies	4. Transmission of infection
(*a*) HLA	(*a*) Bacterial
(*b*) Anti-PLA[1]	(*b*) Protozoal, e.g. malaria
4. Plasma allergy	(*c*) Spirochaetal, e.g. syphilis, yaws
5. Pyrogen response, e.g. anti-IgA antibodies	(*d*) Viral
	(i) Hepatitis A; B; non-A non-B
	(ii) Cytomegalovirus
	(iii) Epstein–Barr virus
	(iv) Acquired immune deficiency syndrome (AIDS)

Using a combination of the serological tests described above in combination with a test cell panel, it is usually possible to determine the specificity of blood group antibodies present in the patient's serum, and obtain suitable blood for transfusion. Table 5 illustrates the presence of anti-D + anti-Kell in the serum of a group 0 Rh-negative, Kell-negative patient when tested against such a cell panel; antibodies to the other system which have been defined on these cells have been excluded and cells 4 and 6 would be suitable for transfusion.

Hazards of transfusion

The complications of blood transfusion are often classified by their time of onset into acute and chronic problems, but this results in a degree of overlap. An alternative is to consider possible causes and these fall broadly into two groups, as indicated in Table 6.

Immune hazards

Haemolytic

Increased destruction of red cells gives rise to a haemolytic transfusion reaction which may be immediate or delayed. The usual cause is administration of donor red cells which are incompatible with antibody in the patient's plasma. Avoidance of this complication is the aim of the major cross-match, which should be performed with patient's serum and cells from all units for transfusion. The clinical effect is dependent on several factors:

Dose of antigen administered This is determined by the concentration of antigen per erythrocyte and the amount of blood given. Thus, the consequences of transfusion of group A cells to a group O patient (whose plasma contains anti-A and anti-B) will vary according to the donor's A antigen status. More extensive destruction of A_1 cells would be expected than of A_2 cells, since the latter have less A antigen sites per cell. Rapid transfusion of a large quantity of incompatible blood may produce little haemolysis initially, because the antibody in the recipient's plasma will be absorbed out by the excess transfused red cell antigen and the amount of antibody molecules per cell insufficient to initiate destruction. Within a few days, however, a sharp rise in antibody production gives rise to enough cell binding for a delayed haemolytic reaction.

Quantity and quality of antibody There is a tendency for antibodies present in low concentration to cause less red cell destruction. In certain instances, a recipient may have no detectable antibody prior to transfusion, although previous exposure to an antigen may have initiated the immune response leaving the patient 'primed'. Re-exposure to the appropriate antigen, often in the Rhesus or Kidd system then generates a secondary antibody response and another mechanism for delayed haemolysis in 4–7 days. The binding affinity of antibody for antigen influences the course of the reaction and is dependent on many factors, e.g. pH, temperature etc. In general, those of low avidity evoke less red cell destruction.

The site of lysis The liberation of haemoglobin directly into the circulation is a result of intravascular haemolysis, which usually follows complement-mediated red cell destruction. Extravascular haemolysis occurs over a period of days in the reticuloendothelial system – principally in liver and spleen, but haemoglobinaemia is less common.

Clinical features of haemolytic reactions

Immediate

Rapid intravascular haemolysis of incompatible red cells produces the most severe presentation with fever, rigors, and haemoglobinaemia. The haemoglobin dissociates into dimers for haptoglobin binding prior to removal in the liver. Once haptoglobin carrier molecules are saturated, free plasma haemoglobin is oxidized to methaemoglobin. The globin chain dissociates to form methaemalbumen, which may be detected spectroscopically in the Schumm's test. Another means of haemoglobin excretion is via the renal tract but, unfortunately, the attendant red cell stroma and immune complexes may damage the kidney and contribute to the shock which precipitates renal failure. Skin flushes and chest pain are a consequence of the liberation of vasoactive substance which may also give rise to disseminated intravascular coagulation.

Delayed

The features of extravascular haemolysis often start after the transfusion has been completed when the patient has been 'primed' by previous exposure to an incompatible antigen. There is a failure of the anticipated rise in haemoglobin, often accompanied by post-transfusion jaundice. Haemoglobinaemia and haemosiderinuria occur less frequently. Sometimes the only indication is a progressive anaemia.

It is not possible to match all the red cell antigens of the donor with those of the patient. In practice, ABO and Rhesus compatible blood is prepared for patients and fortunately few transfusions lead to production of alloantibodies. Their incidence increases with exposure to other antigens in pregnancy or repeated blood transfusion. Occasionally red cell antibodies may be formed after

only one unit of blood, and this risk makes it difficult to justify administration of a single unit to an adult.

Leucocyte antibodies

These may give rise to pyrexial episodes about half an hour from the start of their infusion. They are more commonly found in patients receiving repeated transfusions and they may also occur during pregnancy. Two sets of antigens may be involved – the general human leucocyte antigens (HLA), and specific neutrophil systems (e.g. NA^1; NA^2).

Reactions resulting from leucocyte antibodies may be avoided by the administration of leucocyte-poor blood. Should such patients require granulocyte transfusions, the choice of donors who share major HLA antigens as well as ABO and Rhesus groups may then prevent these unpleasant side effects. Rarely anti-NA^1 antibodies produce immune neutropenia about a week after transfusion in the few individuals (2 per cent) who have NA^2 antigens on their neutrophils.

Platelet antibodies

Pyrexial episodes 30 min into a transfusion may also occur as a result of platlet antibodies, similar to leucocyte antibodies, i.e. anti-HLA or platelet specific anti-PLA^1. The HLA antibodies may be boosted by lymphocytes present, but the clinical features are identical with reactions to leucocyte antibodies. Rarely the platelet count may fall about one week after transfusion as the donor platelets are destroyed by platelet antibodies, e.g. anti-PLA^1 occurring in a patient with PLA^2 platelets. This is usually a self-limiting condition as transfused platelets disappear within 10 days.

Plasma reaction

Urticaria may occur as a result of the administration of blood products and is occasionally associated with dyspnoea. These are allergic phenomena, usually relieved by antihistamines in the acute phase.

Certain individuals lack IgA and their introduction to foreign immunoglobulin leads to the development of class specific anti-IgA. Subsequent transfusions may be complicated by a severe allergic response with fever, bronchospasm, colic, and hypertension to be followed by shock. This may be avoided by careful washing of red cells to remove plasma-containing IgA or the choice of IgA-deficient donors to provide appropriate blood products.

Pyrogen response

Pyrogens are produced as a result of metabolic processes within organisms such as bacteria and viruses. They are often heat resistant polysaccharines, capable of producing a febrile reaction in man and must be excluded from all materials used for transfusion.

Non-immune hazards

Cardiovascular

Circulatory overload Rapid infusion of large volumes of fluid increases the workload of the heart. This may precipitate acute left ventricular failure with pulmonary oedema, jugulovenous engorgement, and tachycardia, particularly in the elderly who may already have degenerative vascular disease. This is best avoided by slow transfusion in patients at risk, and diuretic therapy where fluid overload is already established (see page 19.71).

Thrombophlebitis Local inflammation is common at the site of intravenous cannulae for transfusion. It may be averted by an aseptic procedure for cannulation, and regular resiting of peripheral lines to avoid infection. It should rarely be necessary to prescribe antibiotics for this problem in an immunocompetent individual.

Venous thrombosis This is a rare complication of intravenous therapy, more frequently seen where long catheters are *in situ* for some time. Appropriate anticoagulation may be required to prevent susbsequent pulmonary embolism from a large thrombosed vein.

Air embolism A dangerous amount of air (in excess of 10 ml) may be introduced into the circulation when pressure is applied to a bottle with an airway. This risk has largely been eliminated by the collection of blood in plastic packs which collapse as they empty. Some plasma products, e.g. human albumin solution are, however, still contained in bottles.

Transfusion haemosiderosis

Each 500 ml unit of blood contains approximately 250 mg of iron, while the excretion rate in humans is only 1 mg daily. In the absence of bleeding, iron, from repeated transfusions, accumulates in all tissues with a predilection for skin, liver, pancreas, heart, and gonads, and gives rise to symptoms of haemosiderosis. In young people with high transfusion requirements, e.g. thalassaemia major, chelation therapy should be undertaken to prevent iron disposition. Desferrioxamine may be administered intravenously with blood (usually 1 g per unit transfused) and where an iron overload is established regular domiciliary subcutaneous therapy is required most nights to prevent further accumulation (see page 19.87).

Complications of massive transfusion

Massive transfusion is the term used to describe administration of ten or more units of blood to an adult within 24 hours. Such a large volume may give rise to special problems in patients who are usually very ill.

Hypocalcaemia is the consequence of rapid removal of anticoagulant citrate ions from the circulation by circulating cells. A normal adult can withstand 500 ml every 5 min without supplementary calcium, but this facility may be impaired in liver failure or hypothermia.

Under these circumstances, 10 ml of 10 per cent calcium gluconate may be injected intravenously with cardiac monitoring under controlled conditions.

Hypothermia follows rapid infusion of blood straight from refrigeration at 4 °C and may be avoided by the use of a blood warmer and adequate heating of the patient's room.

Prevention of cooling in this way reduces the chances of developing hypocalcaemia, acidosis, and potassium accumulation by providing an optimal temperature for metabolic processes to continue in the patient. Great care must be exercised to ensure that at no time the temperature of fluid infused exceeds 37 °C.

Hyperkalaemia rarely complicates transfusion in the adult unless the rate exceeds 150 ml/min or renal function is impaired. There is, however, a steady loss of potassium from red cells with time to 30 mmol/l after 21 days. This is significant in neonatal therapy where blood older than 5 days should not be administered, and for exchange purposes red cells less than 48 hours old are preferable to avoid potassium toxicity, although for logistic reasons it is often necessary to extend this period by a further 24 hours.

Persistent bleeding may arise from one or more of a variety of causes. Stored blood lacks platelets, is depleted of several coagulation factors and in large volumes has a dilutional effect on the patient's circulation. Furthermore, massive transfusion may itself give rise to disseminated intravascular coagulation with consumption of coagulation factors and platelets. Bleeding postoperatively is a particularly common problem following cardiopulmonary bypass for cardiac surgery, although volumes of blood used may not be truly 'massive'.

In either case, it is advisable to give two units of fresh frozen plasma, and on some occasions platelet concentrate as well, for approximately every five units of stored blood administerd rapidly.

There is a downward trend of *2, 3-diphosphoglycerate* (2, 3-DPG) on storage of blood, which is less marked when citrate phosphate dextrose (CPD) is used as anticoagulant compared with acid citrate dextrose (ACD). 2, 3-DPG is one of the controlling factors in release of oxygen from haemoglobin and the latter is impaired when 2, 3-DPG falls on storage. This is one of the few valid reasons for requesting fresh whole blood in massive transfusion.

Infusion of excess citrate and lactic acid in red cells contributes to acidosis. This impairs erythrocyte metabolism, but it is rarely necessary to correct the fall in pH with bicarbonate infusion.

Transmission of infection

Treponemal

In the United Kingdom, syphilis is the most common organism in this class transmitted by blood. Yaws has similar properties, and may be present in donors from tropical areas. Neither presents a great threat to recipient health, since spirochaetes rarely survive more than 3 days at 4 °C and are sensitive to antibiotic therapy.

All units of blood for transfusion are screened serologically in the United Kingdom, and positive donors are permanently withdrawn.

Viral

Hepatitis Different patterns are recognized clinically and serologically in the transmission of hepatitis (see also Section 12).

Hepatitis A (infectious hepatitis) is a common childhood disease and is spread by the faecal-oral route. The antigen may be recognized serologically. Its course is normally mild and it is not a problem in blood transfusion.

Hepatitis B (homologous serum jaundice) may be transmitted by transfusion of certain blood and blood products. Its incidence in western countries is low, and its spread by blood transfusion has been much reduced by the routine testing of all donations for hepatitis B surface antigen, preferably by the sensitive radioimmunoassay (RIA) or enzyme linked immunosorbent assay (ELISA) techniques. Donors with high levels of hepatitis B surface antibody now contribute specific immunoglobulin for the passive immunization of those at risk. The implications of hepatitis testing are discussed elsewhere, but all carriers of the surface antigen are permanently withdrawn from service as blood donors and should be offered specialist counselling.

Non-A, non-B hepatitis Post-transfusion hepatitis may also be caused by the transfusion of viruses, known collectively as non-A non-B. No specific assay is yet available for these, but evidence of their presence is inferred from a serum transaminitis in the donor. This infection occurs in almost all recipients of large pool coagulation factor concentrates on first exposure, e.g. haemophiliacs treated with factor VIII concentrates. In most cases, there is jaundice with minimal symptoms and a complete recovery, but a few patients go on to develop chronic liver disease. Liver enzymes are not, however, assayed routinely in British blood donors.

Epstein–Barr virus Donors are deferred for 2 years after glandular fever.

Cytomegalovirus Transfusion of blood, platelets or leucocytes may transmit cytomegalovirus to susceptible individuals. In normal recipients there is a mild febrile illness with complete recovery. In immunosuppressed patients, however, the organism may give rise to a severe infection with fever and hepatic impairment. This may be avoided by reserving blood free of cytomegalovirus antibodies (20 per cent) for patients at risk, i.e. neonates, transplant recipients, children with acute leukaemia, and those undergoing open heart surgery.

Acquired immunodeficiency syndrome (AIDS)

(See also Section 5)

AIDS was described in the early part of this decade as the cause of lymphadenopathy, repeated opportunistic infection, e.g. *Pneu-*

mocystis carinii and unusual malignancy, e.g. Kaposi's sarcoma, occurring in young males amongst the homosexual population in San Francisco. The venereal association of the disease was realized from the cluster of patients diagnosed, and the condition was later recognized in the recipients of blood products – in particular haemophiliacs using factor VIII concentrate prepared from large donor pools and in intravenous drug abusers who often share needles.

Recently, the human T cell leukaemia virus (HTLV-3) and the lymphadenopathy associated virus (LAV) have been shown to be the causative agents of AIDS. A significantly high proportion of persons suffering from AIDS have antibodies to HTLV-3/LAV (it is proposed that this should be known as HIV) in their blood. Screening tests for this antibody have been developed and are currently being used to detect those blood donations from donors who have been exposed to the virus. This will significantly increase the safety of transfusion of those cellular and other products which cannot be pasteurized. In addition, the following groups of donors are requested not to give blood.

1. Homosexual or bisexual males
2. Intravenous drug abusers
3. Haemophiliacs
4. Sexual partners of the above groups.

AIDS is a serious disease with considerable morbidity and mortality with no available specific treatment. The implications for those asymptomatic persons who have been exposed to the virus and have anti-HTLV-3/LAV (HIV) in their blood is not yet clear, but up to 20 per cent may subsequently develop AIDS or an AIDS-related condition.

Management of transfusion reactions

Any adverse effects should be thoroughly investigated. The patient must be carefully assessed to determine the specific symptoms and signs of the reaction in relation to the nature and volume of fluid administered. Steps must be taken to institute the necessary laboratory procedure.

Clinical care

All recipients should be carefully observed during their transfusion, with frequent recording of pulse, blood pressure, and temperature, and urine output. These measurements may give the first indication of the event, and associated symptoms may include rigor, backache, central chest pain, and fever. Early jaundice and haemoglobinuria may also indicate incompatible transfusion. It is most important to monitor urine output carefully throughout. Renal failure is one of the most serious complications which is caused by the combination of acute haemolysis, shock, and occasionally a consumptive coagulopathy. The aim of treatment is to maintain the urine output in excess of 100 ml/h and a normal systemic blood pressure until the reaction subsides. A saline (0.9 per cent) or dextrose (5 per cent) infusion is usually adequate for this purpose, but occasionally when urine output declines a forced mannitol diuresis may be carried out to good effect. Fresh frozen plasma may be useful in this situation where coagulation factors are being consumed. In the absence of shock, renal failure should be managed as in acute tubular necrosis (see Section 18). If there is any possibility that the blood was infected, appropriate broad-spectrum antibiotics should be administered with proper regard to their side-effects in view of their nephrotoxicity.

Preparation and uses of blood components

The starting material for the preparation of most cellular components is whole blood. In recent years an increasing requirement for certain products has led to their direct procurement by apheresis techniques. Manual methods are rapidly being superseded by the use of cell separator machines.

Table 7 Methods of preparation of leucocyte-poor blood

Method	Percentage leucocytes removed	Comment
Inverted/differential centrifugation	65–85	Inefficient alone (maybe combined with filtration)
Saline washing	80–90	Red cell loss Slow
Automated batch washing	90–95	Specialized equipment required
Frozen-thawed	95–99	Expensive apparatus Excellent product
Sedimentation { DES / Dextran	90–95	Saline wash extra
Nylon filter	60–70	Unsatisfactory
Cotton wool filter	95–97	Convenient if costly

Red cell preparations

The indications for the transfusion of whole blood are now relatively few: procedures requiring cardiopulmonary bypass, vascular surgery, acute haemorrhage exceeding 30 per cent blood volume, and exchange transfusions. The addition of adenine to the anticoagulant used in collection has increased survival of viable red cells to permit storage up to 35 days at 4 °C.

Red cell concentrates were introduced as a byproduct of the separation of plasma for fractionation, but they have become the treatment of choice in the correction of anaemia and for the first two units administered in acute blood loss. Plasma-reduced blood prepared in England and Wales has a haematocrit of 60–65 per cent after removal of about 180 ml of plasma and passes readily through the standard blood filter of 170 μm.

In order to achieve national self-sufficiency in plasma, means have been sought to obtain more from each donation. Red cells suspended in a nutrient medium, e.g. 'SAG-M' (saline 150 mmol/l, adenine 1.25 mmol/l, glucose 50 mmol/l with added mannitol) exhibit enhanced viability on storage. The use of 100 ml SAG-M as additive allows an extra 90 ml plasma to be removed from the red cells. This increases the plasma yield on each unit by 50 per cent and the remaining cells are resuspended in SAG-M for use in the same situations as plasma-reduced blood.

Leucocyte-poor blood

This should be administered to patients who require regular transfusion over a long period of time in order to prevent febrile reactions to white cell antibodies. It is necessary to remove 90 per cent of the leucocytes and several methods are available to achieve this target (Table 7). Freezing is an expensive exercise, but the introduction of micropore filters ($d = 40$ μm) has proved a convenient option. Once red cells have been rendered leucocyte poor, their pack has been entered and they should be transfused as soon as possible, and not later than 12 hours after preparation.

Leucocytes

Harvest from the buffy layer is a tedious manual technique of poor yield. Filtration though scrubbed nylon produces reasonable numbers of leucocytes with impaired function. The best donations are achieved by cell separation from normal individuals pretreated with corticosteroids to boost their counts. Hydroxyethylstarch in the system minimizes neutrophil trapping in the red cell mass. Patients with chronic granulocytic leukaemia have also been used as a source of neutrophils.

Granulocytes are indicated in the treatment of profoundly neutropenic patterns (0.5×10^9/l) with bacterial infection unresponsive to antibiotics, and who may be expected to recover in the long term. The minimum course should last 4 days and each daily infusion should contain no less than 5×10^9 granulocytes.

Platelet concentrates

These may be obtained by removal *from whole blood* at 20 °C at the earliest opportunity after collection. Separation of most of the platelets from a donation may be performed by gentle centrifugation to sediment the heavier red cells. Using a closed system the supernatant platelet-rich plasma is transfused to a satellite pack, and centrifuged hard to concentrate the platelets. Two hours is allowed for platelets to disaggregate. They should then be stored at 22 °C and agitated until their issue. The shelf life varies according to the choice of their plastic container. Packs have recently been produced which allow sufficient degree of gaseous exchange to allow the survival of functional platelets from 3 to 5 days.

An alternative technique is the collection of platelets from a donor by cell separation. This permits the reinfusion of donor red cells during the procedure and hence the ability to donate more frequently than twice a year. The main advantage is the facility for obtaining a recipient 'dose' from one donor instead of from four to six whole blood donations. This is particularly valuable where the patient exhibits refractoriness to platelet therapy as a result of antibodies, and the pool of suitable donors is small.

The *indications* for platelet transfusion are to control bleeding in thrombocytopenia and/or thrombocytopathia where disorders of function have been demonstrated *in vivo* (bleeding time) or *in vitro* (aggregation; adhesion, etc.). Most clinicans responsible for the care of patients with marrow suppression advocate the use of prophylactic platelet therapy where profound thrombocytopenia is present (platelets less than 20×10^9/l), irrespective of haemorrhage. This practice is directed at the prevention of spontaneous bleeding episodes, e.g. cerebral haemorrhage, but may lead to problems of alloimmunization which then make selected HLA-matched platelets the product of choice.

These trends in platelet therapy, in association with more aggressive regimes in chemotherapy and the advances in bone marrow transplantation have led to marked increases in the use of the concentrate. Objective measurements of therapeutic response are not always helpful, but an increment in the recipient's platelet count is usual in the absence of bleeding, infection or hypersplenism. Control of bleeding is the most important evidence of effective platelet therapy.

Plasma fractions

Plasma is separated from whole blood to provide several different components for clinical use. It is important that a patient is not given cellular components unless these are specifically indicated and this is particularly true in a programme of long-term infusion therapy. Several plasma fractions are in common use.

Fresh frozen plasma

Many coagulation factors are present in this plasma which is separated from red cells as soon as possible after collection and rapidly frozen below −30 °C. It is valuable in the correction of bleeding due to impaired clotting. Its use in association with massive transfusion of whole blood is increasing, particularly since the expansion of facilities for coronary artery bypass grafts which require cardiopulmonary bypass during surgery. It may also be used as a source of protein, particularly effective in replacement therapy for paediatric burns.

Factor VIII preparations

Products vary in their factor VIII content and size of donor pool.

Cryoprecipitate

This is prepared by freezing freshly collected plasma, and rapid thawing to precipitate a concentrate of factor VIII and fibrinogen. It is then frozen and stored as cryoprecipitate at −30 °C containing 70–80 i.u factor VIII in approximately 5–20 ml plasma. As the product of a single donation, it is the treatment of choice in haemophiliac children under 5 years, adult mild haemophiliacs, and von Willebrand's patients because of its lower risk of transmission of viral infection, e.g. hepatitis, AIDS. Cryoprecipitates may be a valuable source of fibrinogen, depending on the method of preparation.

The supernatant residues of cryoprecipitate preparation need not be wasted. Stored at −30 °C it is a valuable source of coagulation factors other than factor VIII, and can replace fresh frozen plasma in the majority of clinical situations.

Lyophilized factor VIII preparations

The raw material for these is cryoprecipitate and further refinements on large donor pools give rise to concentrates of intermediate or high purity stored at 4 °C. The fibrinogen content is inversely proportional to factor VIII concentration. Produced in batches, they are accurately assayed for coagulation activity and the therapeutic dose may thus be accurately determined. Heat-treatment of the dry factor VIII preparations at 70–80 °C for up to 72 hours has been shown to eliminate the anti-HTLV-3/LAV (HIV) virus and such preparations should be free from the danger of AIDS transmission. This is not necessarily true, however, for the transmission of non-A, non-B hepatitis. Heat-treatment of factor VIII causes a significant loss of yield.

Heat-treated factor VIII concentrates are now used in the home therapy of severe haemophiliacs and to prepare such patients for major surgery in a reference centre.

Factor IX complex

This is obtained from cryoprecipitate supernatant by fractionation and purification. The product is lyophilized for the treatment of Christmas disease (haemophilia B).

Albumin solutions

These are hepatitis free after pasteurization by heating to 60 °C for 10 hours.

Human albumin solution

This contains over 90 per cent of the albumin in the plasma, with a final concentration of 45 g/l. It is used to restore blood volume in haemorrhagic shock and burns.

Salt-poor albumin

This is now prepared as a 20 per cent solution in a small volume (100 ml). It is indicated in correction of chronic hypoalbuminaemia in special circumstances of organ failure and fluid overload, e.g. hepatic insufficiency with ascites.

Immunoglobulins

For some years these have been obtained from the plasma known to contain high levels of specific antibodies, e.g. antitetanus; antirubella; antivaricella-zoster; anti-Rh(D) or from fractionation of normal plasma. There is now considerable activity in the pharmaceutical industry in marketing new intravenous immunoglobulins, and many indications for their use have been cited. However, these preparations are expensive and their long-term benefits have yet to be established.

References

Greenwalt, T. J. and Jamieson, G. A. (1978). *The blood platelet in transfusion therapy*. A. R. Liss, Inc., New York.

Issitt, P. D. and Issitt, C. H. (1976). *Applied blood group serology*, 2nd edn. Becton, Dickenson and Co., California.

Mollison, P. L. (1979). *Blood tranfusion in clinical medicine*, 6th edn. Blackwell Scientific Publications, Oxford.

Myhre, B. A. (ed.) (1977). *A seminar on blood components*. American Association of Blood Banks, Washington.

Nusbacher, J. and Berkman, E. M. (1979). *Hemotherapy in trauma and surgery*. American Association of Blood Banks, Washington.

Race, R. R. and Sanger, R. (1975). *Blood groups in man*, 6th edn. Blackwell Scientific Publications, Oxford.

Marrow transplantation

C. BUNCH

Marrow transplantation is a relatively new and in many respects still an experimental approach to the treatment of haematological malignancy, aplastic anaemia, and severe congenital haemopoietic and immune deficiencies. Its foundations lie in studies performed during the 1950s in which it was found that rats and mice exposed to doses of irradiation sufficient to destroy the haemopoietic system could be saved by infusions of marrow cells obtained from either the animal itself prior to irradiation (autologous cells), a genetically identical animal (syngeneic cells) or a genetically non-identical animal (allogeneic cells). Rescue with autologous or syngeneic cells proved relatively straightforward but allogeneic transplanation was found to be complicated by the twin problems of graft rejection by immune competent cells remaining in the host, and graft versus host disease (GVHD) – a progressive and often fatal wasting disease with widespread damage particularly to the skin, liver, gut, and lymphoid system mediated by immune competent cells within the graft itself. These problems could be partially overcome by pretransplant immunosuppressive conditioning to prevent rejection together with posttransplant immunosuppression to modify GVHD. Further progress was made when the importance of the major histocompatibility complex (MHC) became apparent and it was found that allogeneic transplantation can be most reliably performed when donor and recipient are siblings with identical MHC determinants.

Clinical transplantation

Marrow transplantation has been performed with increasing frequency during the past decade. Initially, transplantation was limited to patients with severe aplastic anaemia, which is known to have an otherwise extremely high mortality, and to patients with acute leukaemia in the end stages of their disease who were resistant to chemotherapy and often in poor clinical condition. Marrow was obtained from HLA identical sibling donors by multiple aspirations from the sternum and iliac bones. This procedure can be performed under spinal or general anaesthesia, and 500–1000 ml marrow is collected into heparinized tissue culture medium to be infused intravenously into the recipient after simple filtration to remove bony particles.

For patients with aplastic anaemia, pretransplant conditioning with high doses of cyclophosphamide (200 mg/kg) permitted engraftment in the majority of instances, although subsequent rejection occurred in about one-third of patients. Furthermore, despite sustained engraftment a number of patients developed fatal infections or graft versus host disease. Nevertheless, about 45–50 per cent of patients were successfully transplanted and returned to a normal life, apparently cured.

Patients with acute leukaemia, on the other hand, were treated with high-dose cyclophosphamide (120 mg/kg) and often other cytotoxic agents, together with a single dose of up to 10 Gy total body irradiation (TBI), a dose which would ordinarily be lethal without a subsequent infusion of haemopoietic cells. Graft rejection was not a problem in this series, but the overall results were at first sight much less impressive than in aplastic anaemia (Fig. 1), because a high proportion of patients succumbed within the first three months from infection and GVHD. Despite this intensive approach to therapy, relapse of leukaemia occurred commonly within the first two years. After this time, however, the mortality lessened dramatically, and some 13 per cent of patients became long-term survivors and were perhaps cured of their disease. These patients would otherwise have died within a few days or weeks had transplantation not been available.

Following this favourable experience, various strategies have been adopted in an attempt to improve the overall success rate. It was noted in these early studies that graft rejection occurred more often in patients with aplastic anaemia whose lymphocytes showed

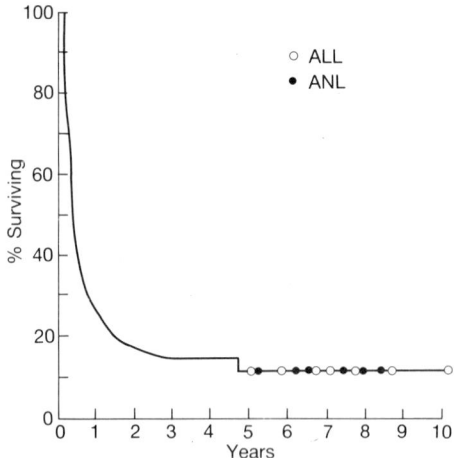

Fig. 1 Marrow transplantation for refractory acute leukaemia in relapse. Kaplan–Meier product–limit estimates of percentage survival for the first 110 patients transplanted in Seattle. (Reproduced from Burchenal, J. H. and Oettgen, H. F., eds, 1980, *Cancer: achievements, challenges and prospects for the 1980s.* Grune and Stratton, by kind permission of Dr E. D. Thomas and the publishers.)

in vitro evidence of sensitization to donor antigens prior to transplantation, or in whom the number of cells transplanted was less than average. In the majority of instances this sensitization was thought to result from previous blood transfusion, making a strong case for transplantation to be undertaken as early as possible in the course of the disease – preferably before transfusion becomes necessary. Indeed, the incidence of rejection in patients who have not previously been transfused is very low. The risk of rejection in other patients can be reduced by more intensive immunosuppression and is virtually eliminated if pretransplant conditioning includes TBI. However, TBI increases the risk of transplantation significantly, and the potential benefit is largely outweighed by a higher mortality from infectious complications and GVHD, although the use of smaller doses of TBI may be equally effective and less toxic.

With available techniques of marrow harvest, it is difficult to envisage how the number of haemopoietic cells transplanted could be increased. However, animal cross-transfusion and transplantation experiments have demonstrated that haemopoietic stem cells circulate in the blood of these species, and it has been shown that the transfusion of peripheral blood mononuclear cells, collected from the marrow donor for several days after marrow transplantation, can effectively reduce the risk of rejection in sensitized patients. It is not absolutely certain whether these supplementary infusions significantly increase the number of haemopoietic cells transplanted, or whether the addition of large numbers of donor lymphocytes actively interferes with the rejection process. The latter seems more probable as the incidence of chronic (but not acute) GVHD is increased somewhat by this manoeuvre.

From the initial clinical studies mentioned above it is clear that acute leukaemia could be cured by marrow transplantation. In many instances failure can be attributed to the patient's poor clinical condition at the time of transplantation or to increased resistance of the leukaemia in the terminal stages of the disease (Fig.1). Consequently, many centres now elect to perform transplantation during periods of haematological remission in patients who are nevertheless considered unlikely to be cured with conventional treatment. In practice this means during the first or subsequent remission in acute myeloid leukaemia (AML) or 'poor risk' acute lymphoblastic leukaemia (ALL), or during the second or subsequent remissions of other patients with ALL.

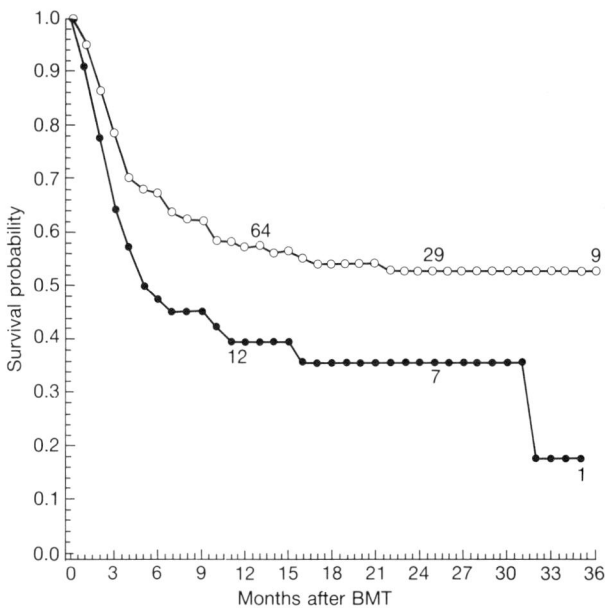

Fig. 2 Marrow transplantation for acute myeloid leukaemia in remission. Probability of survival of 183 patients transplanted in first remission (open circles) and 46 patients transplanted in second remission (closed circles). (Data from the European Bone Marrow Transplant Group, by courtesy of Dr F. E. Zwaan; reproduced from Zwaan and Jansen, 1984, *Sem. Hemat.* **21**, 36–42, by permission.)

Table 1 Principal complications of marrow transplantation

Immediate (days)
    Effects of marrow failure
        Bleeding, infection
    Drug toxicity
        Rashes, cystitis (CY)
        Cardiomyopathy (CY)
        Parotitis (TBI), pancreatitis (TBI)
        Gastrointestinal symptoms (CY, TBI)
Early (weeks)
    Failure of engraftment
    Graft rejection
    Infection: bacterial, fungal, viral
    Acute graft versus host disease (GVHD)
    Interstitial pneumonitis
    Leukaemic relapse
Late (months)
    Chronic GVHD
    Leukaemic relapse
    Infection, particularly herpes viruses and pneumococcal
Long term
    Cataracts
    Sterility and growth retardation
    ? New malignant change

CY = cyclophosphamide; TBI = total body irradiation

The validity of this approach has been amply confirmed by several groups. Patients in remission can be in excellent clinical condition and the transplantation procedure is well tolerated. Indeed, the supportive care required during the immediate post grafting period may be less than that required during intensive remission induction with conventional chemotherapy. Mortality from infectious complications and acute GVHD appears to be less, particularly in younger patients, and the risk of leukaemic relapse is reduced. The results have been most impressive in AML possibly because transplants have generally been performed earlier in the course of this disease, and currently up to half the patients may expect to become long-term survivors (Fig. 2).

Complications
Despite this encouraging progress, results are still short of ideal and clearly many problems remain (Table 1). The most pressing of these are GVHD and relapse of the underlying disease.

Graft versus host disease (GVHD)
Acute GVHD may be seen at any time during the first 2–3 months following transplantation. It usually starts as a non-specific maculopapular rash with or without diarrhoea and biochemical or clinical evidence of liver damage. The rash tends to be generalized, but has a predilection for the face, palms, and soles (Fig.3). In a proportion of patients GVHD progresses to a fulminant form with a severe exfoliative dermatitis, hepatic failure, and debilitating diarrhoea. It is believed that the tissue damage is mediated by cytotoxic T lymphocytes of donor origin.

More recently, with increasing numbers of patients surviving the immediate posttransplantation period, a form of *chronic GVHD* has been recognized which is characterized by a later onset with a progressive sclerodermatous skin reaction (Fig. 3) and, in some patients, liver changes resembling primary biliary cirrhosis. Antibodies may be produced to a variety of tissue antigens, and there are parallels between this form of GVHD and autoimmune disease. It has been suggested that a form of disordered immune

reconstitution with alterations in the proportions of suppressor and helper T cells, may be responsible.

The use of methotrexate (MTX) after transplantation to prevent GVHD was prompted by earlier animal studies, but has been notably less successful in humans with some degree of GVHD occurring in up to two-thirds of patients. Cyclosporin A, a fungal metabolite with activity against T cells, has been more widely used in recent years. In a randomized study it was shown to reduce the incidence and severity of GVHD in comparison to MTX, but overall survival was little affected. Cyclosporin has potentially dangerous side-effects, especially on the kidneys, and must be used with caution. Recent studies indicate that a combination of MTX and cyclosporin may be preferable to either alone.

Appreciation that acute GVHD is mediated by mature cytotoxic T cells within the marrow graft has prompted attempts at removal or depletion of T cells from the donor marrow prior to infusion. Virtually complete T cell depletion can be achieved using a variety of methods, including physicochemical separation, binding to certain plant lectins and lysis by monoclonal anti-T cell antibodies and complement. Recent results show that GVHD can largely be prevented by such techniques but with possibly some increased risk of graft rejection or subsequent leukaemic relapse.

Treatment of established GVHD is generally unsatisfactory, but the administration of large doses of methyl prednisolone at the first sign of GVHD may successfully abrogate the disease and perhaps prevent the later development of the chronic form. An interesting observation that has become more apparent with improved survival is that patients who have had non-fatal GVHD have a much reduced risk of subsequent leukaemic relapse, suggesting that the graft may exert a useful antileukaemic effect. A more desirable long-term goal may thus be to temper GVHD rather than to eliminate it altogether.

Infection
Infectious complications occur commonly after marrow transplantation and are directly related to the profound immunosuppression that results from pretransplant and posttransplant conditioning. Reconstitution of the immune system with cells of donor origin takes many months and is considerably delayed by the presence of GVHD; humoral immunity recovers first, but cell-mediated immunity may never completely return to normal,

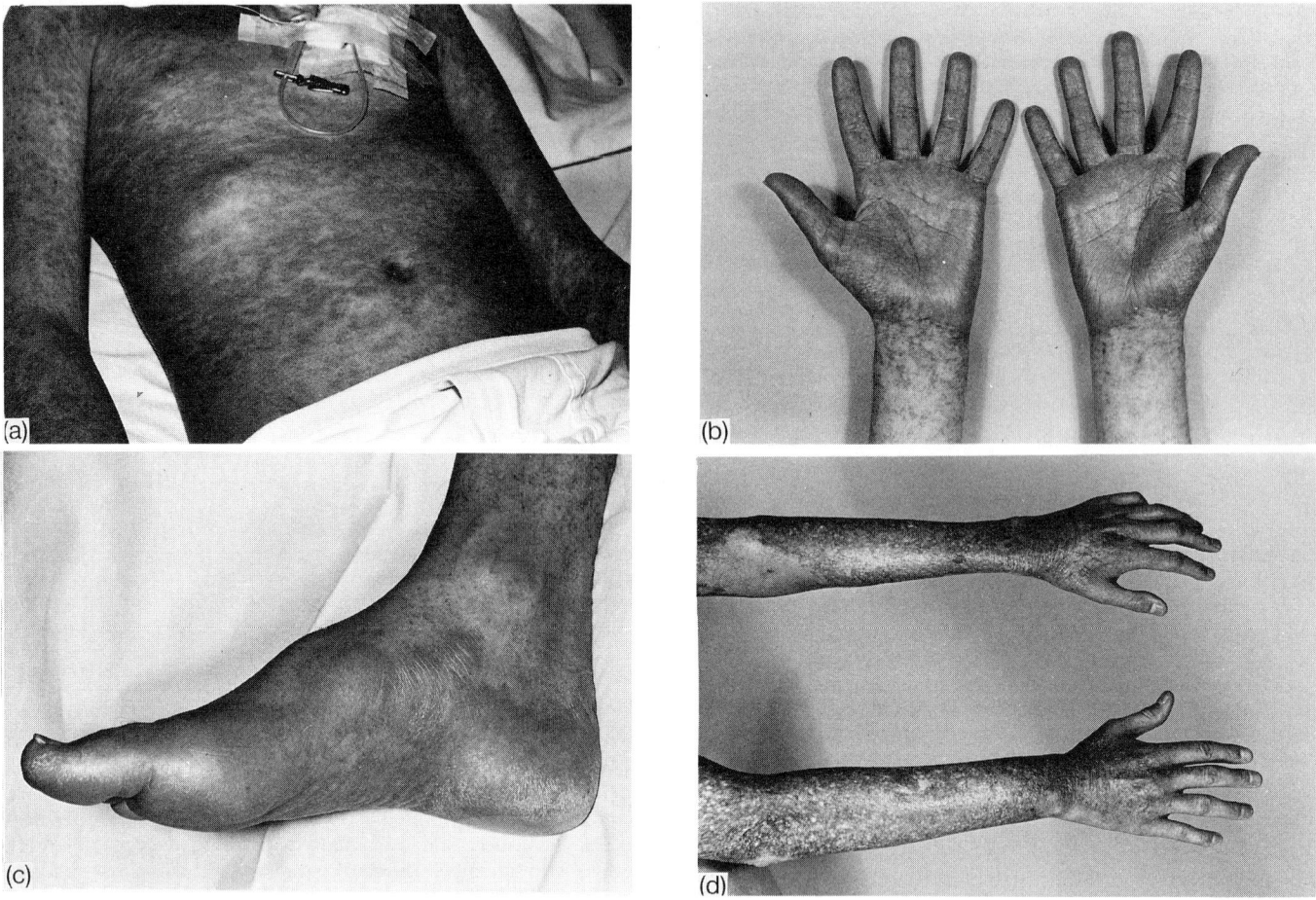

Fig. 3 Graft versus host disease affecting the skin. Early involvement of the trunk, hands, and feet in acute GVHD (a–c). (d) Late changes resembling scleroderma in chronic GVHD.

although in the absence of GVHD the risk of infection is not appreciably increased after the first year. Before this time, both bacterial and viral infections may occur, and pneumococcal, pseudomonal, herpes zoster, and cytomegalovirus (CMV) infections are particularly troublesome.

A common and often fatal complication is *interstitial pneumonitis* which in some centres has developed in 50 per cent or more patients. In many instances CMV infection has been implicated, but in about half the patients a causative organism cannot be found. Other factors, such as radiation or drug damage may be partially responsible for the development of this syndrome. Nevertheless, the association with CMV infection is so strong that vigorous attempts to prevent infection or reactivation of CMV are warranted (page 19.253).

Leukaemic relapse

After infection and GVHD, the major problem encountered in the early series of transplants for leukaemia was subsequent relapse of the disease. As would be expected, in the majority of instances relapse has involved cells of recipient origin, though in a small number of patients, the leukaemic cells have shown the cytogenetic characteristics of donor cells, suggesting perhaps that a transforming agent such as a virus had persisted in the host to cause leukaemic change in the transplanted cells.

Whilst there is good reason to expect that earlier transplantation will reduce the chance of subsequent relapse, the prospects for patients who are already refractory to conventional treatment are less good. Increasing the intensity of chemotherapy prior to transplantation has been generally unrewarding, and 10 Gy is the upper limit of radiation that can be safely administered as a single dose. However, current attempts to increase the effectiveness of

radiotherapy with fractionated TBI at a higher total dose may ultimately prove useful.

Long-term effects

Apart from chronic GVHD, long-term problems following marrow transplantation have been relatively minor or infrequent. Some patients have developed posterior subcapsular cataracts a few years after total body irradiation. An incidence of 80 per cent has been reported for patients given TBI in a single fraction, with a very much lower incidence when fractionation has been used. With careful follow-up a high incidence of obstructive and restrictive defects in pulmonary function have become apparent. Growth velocity is reduced in children receiving TBI, but not cyclophosphamide alone. This is associated with reduction in adrenocortical and growth hormone levels in some. Most patients can expect to be sterile and premature menopause is common.

Of major concern is the potential risk of subsequent malignant change, as has been occasionally noted following renal transplantation or in patients receiving cytotoxic drugs for other conditions. This has not so far been a significant problem in patients transplanted for haemopoietic disorders, but bizarre lymphoproliferative malignancies have developed in some infants who have been transplanted for immunodeficiency diseases, and occasional cases of glioblastoma multiforme have been reported, generally in patients who had received cranial irradiation prior to TBI.

Indications for marrow transplantation

The success of marrow transplantation in the treatment of aplastic anaemia and acute leukaemia has led to its use in the management of an increasing number of conditions (Table 2) although in some, such as thalassaemia, its exact role remains to be defined. Because

Table 2 Indications for marrow transplantation

1 Severe aplastic anaemia
Persistent life-threatening agranulocytosis or thrombocytopenia due to failure of production

2 Acute leukaemia:
Childhood ALL (good prognosis) in relapse or second remission
AML and poor prognosis ALL in relapse or first remission
Blast crisis in CGL

3 CGL in chronic phase

4 Congenital immune deficiency disorders, e.g. SCID

5 Congenital haemopoietic disorders, e.g. chronic granulomatous disease, Wiskott–Aldrich syndrome. Selected patients with thalassaemia for whom long-term transfusion and iron chelation is impracticable

---

AML = acute myelogenous leukaemia; ALL = acute lymphoblastic leukaemia; CML = chronic myeloid leukaemia; SCID = severe combined immune deficiency disease

---

of adverse effects on growth and development, TBI is generally avoided in non-malignant disorders and less-intensive conditioning may fail to eradicate the patient's own, abnormal marrow.

Of particular note are the encouraging results of marrow transplantation in chronic granulocytic leukaemia (CGL). Originally transplantation was confined to patients in blast-cell crisis, in whom results are disappointing, but it has more recently been employed in the chronic phase of the disease. Interestingly the high doses of chemotherapy and TBI employed are able to eliminate the Ph^1 clone – a feat rarely achieved with conventional treatment.

The procedure, and in particular TBI, is poorly tolerated by the elderly, and most leukaemic patients over the age of 45 years are probably best managed by conventional means. The major restriction at the present time is the availability of a suitable donor. The ideal donor would be an identical twin from whom marrow may be transplanted without fear of GVHD and with the prospect of a much more rapid immune reconstitution and correspondingly less risk of infection. More usually, however, transplants are performed between HLA-identical siblings although occasionally a parent may be a suitable donor particularly if, because of an unusual degree of homozygosity within the family, he or she is HLA-identical with the patient. Minor degrees of incompatibility between a patient and a family member donor may be acceptable to some transplant centres, but the risk to the patient is greater.

On rare occasions, transplantation has been successfully undertaken using unrelated donors who are identical at all HLA loci (A, B, C, D). The chance of finding such a donor in the population at large depends upon the specific HLA types involved but is around 1 in 30 000, and the testing and maintenance of a panel of potential donors of sufficient size to guarantee a reasonable chance of finding an HLA-identical donor for the majority of patients is daunting. Nevertheless, several such panels have now been set up, and an increasing number of transplants from unrelated donors may be expected in the future.

Because transplantation is more likely to be successful when performed early in the course of aplastic anaemia or during remission in acute leukaemia, it is important to consider this as a possible therapeutic option when the diagnosis is first made, particularly in patients under the age of 45 years. When possible, patients with leukaemia should have their HLA-A and B types determined before starting chemotherapy, but it is not essential to perform mixed lymphocyte reaction or to do HLA-DR typing at this stage. If a potential donor can be identified by A and B locus typing, further studies can be performed at a convenient time by the transplant centre.

Although marrow transplantation undoubtedly offers the best chance of cure for many patients it is a hazardous undertaking which may impose severe strain on the patient and family. This is particularly the case when the transplant centre is some distance from the patient's home, as it is often desirable for the donor as well as other family members to act as donors of blood products during the immediate posttransplant period. The risks and benefits should obviously be fully discussed with the family before a final decision is reached, but care should be taken to approach potential donors before transplantation is suggested to the patient or other members of the family, as this may otherwise create unexpected tensions and pressures within the family.

Future prospects

Considerable strides have been made in the field of marrow transplantation since clinical studies started in earnest a decade or so ago, and this form of treatment is now becoming available to an increasing number of patients. The problems outlined above are now well defined and much is being learned about the organization of the immune system and its reconstitution with donor cells following successful engraftment that can be expected to help patients in the future.

Of particular interest at the present time are the attempts mentioned above to control GVHD by removing cytotoxic T lymphocytes from the donor marrow prior to transplantation. This approach shows great promise and if, as seems likely, the major immunological barriers can eventually be overcome, transplantation may well become the treatment of choice for a much wider range of conditions.

References

Blume, K. G. and Petz, L. D. (eds) (1983). *Clinical bone marrow transplantation*. Churchill Livingstone, New York.

Buckner, C. D. and Clift, R. A. (1984). Marrow transplantation for acute lymphoblastic leukemia. *Sem. Hemat.* **21**, 43–47.

Gale, R. P. (ed.) (1983). *Recent advances in bone marrow transplantation*. A. R. Liss, New York.

Lucarelli, G., Polchi, P., Galimberti, M., Izzi, T., Delfini, C., Manna, M., Agostinelli, F., Baronciani, D., Giorgi, C., Angelucci, E., Giardini, C., Politi, P. and Manenti, F. (1985). Marrow transplantation for thalassaemia following busulphan and cyclophosphamide. *Lancet* i, 1355–1357.

Storb, R., Thomas, E. D., Buckner, C. D., Appelbaum, F. R., Clift, R.A., Deeg, H. J., Doney, K., Hansen, J. A., Prentice, R. L., Sanders, J. E., Stewart, P., Sullivan, K. M. and Witherspoon, R. P. (1984). Marrow transplantation for aplastic anaemia. *Sem. Hemat.* **21**, 27–35.

Thomas, E. D. (1985). Marrow transplantation for nonmalignant disorders. *N. Engl. J. Med.* **312**, 46–48.

Thomas, E. D. and Storb, R. (1970). Technique for human marrow grafting. *Blood* **36**, 507–515.

Thomas, E. D., Storb, R., Clift, R. A., Fefer, A., Johnson, F. L., Neiman, P. E., Lerner, K. G., Glucksberg, H. and Buckner, C. D. (1975). Bone-marrow transplantation (first of two parts). *N. Engl. J. Med.* **292**, 832–843.

Thomas, E. D., Storb, R., Clift, R. A., Fefer, A., Johnson, F. L., Neiman, P. E., Lerner, K. G., Glucksberg, H. and Buckner, C. D. (1975). Bone-marrow transplantation (second of two parts). *N. Engl. J. Med.* **292**, 895–902.

Zwaan, F. E. and Jansen, J. (1984). Bone marrow transplantation in acute nonlymphoblastic leukaemia. *Sem. Hemat.* **21**, 36–42.

GEOGRAPHICAL VARIATION IN BLOOD DISEASE

Lymphoma and leukaemia

M.S.R. HUTT

Non-Hodgkin's lymphomas (NHL)

Comparison of the incidence of the various subtypes of non-Hodgkin's lymphoma in different regions of the world is complicated by the varied and changing nomenclature applied to this group of tumours, particularly since new immunological methods have been used to identify more precisely the origin and nature of the proliferating neoplastic cells. Nevertheless, it is possible to identify several distinct distribution patterns of NHL in different parts of the world.

Burkitt's lymphoma

The occurrence of a distinct clinico-pathological type of malignant lymphoma in African children, now known as Burkitt's lymphoma, was first described by Denis Burkitt in Uganda in 1958, though surveys of the literature and case records of hospitals in countries of subSaharan Africa show that the condition existed in the region at least since the beginning of this century. Unlike most types of NHL, Burkitt's lymphoma usually presents as an extra-lymphoreticular tumour in a child (see page 19.183). The majority of patients are between 2 and 15 years of age, with a peak about 6 to 7 years. In the younger children the presenting tumour occurs most frequently in one or more quadrants of the jaw. In older children the jaw is less often affected and the ovaries, testes, thyroid, bones, soft tissues, and salivary glands may be involved. Although peripheral lymph-nodes are rarely affected, the retroperitoneal nodes are often involved and this may be associated with the development of a flaccid paraplegia due to spinal cord destruction. Burkitt's lymphoma is now usually classified as a subtype of lymphoblastic lymphoma and is distiguishable by its characteristic histology and cytology. The tumour arises from B-lymphocytes of follicular origin.

Geographical distribution Burkitt's lymphoma is endemic throughout large regions of sub-Saharan Africa and in Papua New Guinea. In these endemic areas it is by far the commonest form of lymphoid malignancy and also the commonest tumour in children. In his original geographical studies in Africa Burkitt was able to delineate the distribution of the tumour within the countries of the subSahara. He showed that the occurrence of the tumour is related to altitude, temperature, and rainfall, features that are also apparent in Papua New Guinea. Essentially, Burkitt's lymphoma occurs in regions where the temperature does not fall below 16 °C or the rainfall below 75 cm. Thus the tumour is common in southern Sudan but almost unknown near Khartoum; it is common everywhere in Uganda except in the mountainous southwest; it is also uncommon in the mountainous regions of Rwanda and eastern Zaire. It is of interest that Burkitt's lymphoma is not seen in the island of Zanzibar though it is common in the coastal regions of neighbouring Tanzania. In Papua New Guinea the majority of cases come from the coastal plains and the tumour is rare in the inhabitants of the central mountain range. It is now known that Burkitt's lymphoma, as defined by cytopathological criteria, occurs sporadically throughout the world. In temperate climates such cases tend to occur in slightly older age-groups and there are differences in the clinical features and reponse to therapy. Some countries of the Middle East, such as Iran, Iraq, and Saudi Arabia, the Far East, such as Malaysia, and South America have incidence rates or proportional frequencies of Burkitt's lymphoma which are higher than in Europe or North America but lower than in subSaharan Africa.

The peculiar geographical distribution of endemic Burkitt's lymphoma and the age distribution of the cases suggest that the responsible environmental factors act on individuals from their first year of life. The association between this tumour and Epstein–Barr virus (EB virus) has been established in all cases from endemic areas and many, but not all cases, seen in other parts of the world. EB virus was first isolated from a tissue culture of tumour cells derived from a childhood case in Uganda. It was later shown that all cases in endemic areas had antibodies to EB virus and that the mean antibody titres in cases were higher than in age-, sex-, and tribe-matched controls. It has also been demonstrated that antibodies to EB virus are present in the serum of children who develop the tumour up to 15 months before there is any clinical evidence of lymphoma, and that in such individuals the antibody titres are often exceptionally high. Further evidence for the oncogenic role of EB virus is provided by the demonstration of EB virus antigens in tumour cells and of EB genomes in the DNA of the malignant lymphoid cells. While this evidence for the involvement of EB virus in the aetiology of Burkitt's lymphoma appears to be convincing this does not explain the geographical distribution of the tumour in Africa or in the world. The association between the occurrence of Burkitt's lymphoma and altitude, temperature, and rainfall is very suggestive of a relationship to an insect vector and corresponds to the distribution of endemic *P. falciparum* malaria; this would also explain the absence of the tumour in Zanzibar where there has been successful eradication of malaria. It is known that repeated attacks of *P. falciparum* malaria in the first few years of life lead to depression of cellular immunity and to B cell cellular stimulation and it is postulated that this provides an appropriate background for EB virus to act as an oncogenic stimulus. The possibility that genetic and other environmental factors play a role has not been excluded.

Adult T cell leukaemia/lymphoma (ATLL)

It has been recognized for some years that the histological pattern of non-Hodgkin's lymphomas in Japan is different from that in Europe and North America. In 1981 an unusual form of lymphoid malignancy was recognized in southern Japan. This condition, now known as adult T cell leukaemia/lymphoma (ATLL) is characterized by an aggressive course with cutaneous and visceral involvement, often with lytic bone lesions and hypercalcaemia.

Geographical distribution Although sporadic cases of ATLL have now been reported from many countries the largest endemic focus is in southern Japan, particularly in the regions of Kyushu and Shoku. ATLL has also been described in the populations of the Caribbean Islands, though many of these cases were first diagnosed in Caribbean immigrants to the USA. Preliminary studies suggest that ATLL also occurs with some frequency in parts of subSaharan Africa and South America.

The clustering of cases in southern Japan especially in the prefecture of Kochi suggested that an infectious agent, probably a virus, was an aetiological factor. In 1980 a new retrovirus was detected in the peripheral blood lymphocytes of a black patient in the USA with an aggressive T cell cutaneous lymphoma. This virus, now known as the human T cell leukaemia/lymphoma virus (HTLV-I) was later isolated from cases of ATLL in southern Japan and the Caribbean. The observation that 70 per cent of new cases of non-Hodgkin's lymphoma in Jamaica have high antibody titres to HTLV-I suggests that this virus may be implicated in many cases of lymphoreticular neoplasia in this region.

Other non-Hodgkin's lymphomas

The study of B and T cell markers in non-Hodgkin's lymphomas helped to unravel the observed differences between the pattern of NHL in Japan, where follicular (nodular), well-differentiated lymphomas are uncommon, and the USA where this type is more frequent – and led to the delineation of ATLL. Further studies of cell markers are necessary to subtype the large-cell lymphomas, formerly called reticulum-cell sarcoma or histiocytic lymphoma (Rappaport), which are relatively, and probably absolutely, more common in the countries of the Middle East from Turkey to Saudi Arabia, subSaharan Africa, parts of Central and South America, than in Europe or North America. It is possible that many of these may turn out to belong to the ATLL group.

Primary upper small intestinal lymphoma (PUSIL–Mediterranean lymphoma) and immunoproliferative disease of the small intestine (IPSID)

PUSIL, associated with IPSID, must be distinguished from the rare primary intestinal lymphomas that occur sporadically throughout the world, usually in the elderly. In endemic regions PUSIL and IPSID usually occur in younger age groups and the patients tend to come from a poor socio-economic background. The pathological lesions are found predominantly in the upper part of the small intestine and are associated with symptoms of malabsorption which often precede the development of the tumour. In the preneoplastic, proliferative phase of the disease (IPSID) there is atrophy of the small intestinal mucosa with a marked increase of lymphocytes and plasma cells in the lamina propria. This may be associated with the production of alpha heavy chains which may be found in the serum and has given rise to the term alpha heavy-chain disease.

Geographical distribution Although this condition is still often known as *Mediterranean lymphoma* the first descriptions of the disease were made in Peru. However, the largest endemic area is in the region of the Mediterranean and the Middle East. Many cases have been reported from Israel, Lebanon, Iraq, Syria, and Iran as well as Greece, Algeria, and Tunisia. In recent years the number of cases seen in Israel has declined. IPSID and PUSIL have also been described in the Cape Coloureds of South Africa and some countries in South America.

The majority of patients who develop this condition come from a poor socio-economic background and many give a history of recurrent attacks of gastroenteritis and of malnutrition in the first years of life. It has been postulated that the lymphocytic and plasma-cell proliferation consequent on recurrent intestinal infections may result in the eventual neoplastic change in IgA-producing cells and to the development of PUSIL. The decline in the incidence of these conditions in Israel has been associated with a marked improvement in the socio-economic status of the immigrant groups from other parts of the Middle East and North Africa. The hypothesis linking IPSID and PUSIL to recurrent gastrointestinal infections does not account for the paucity of this condition in the Indian sub-continent or subSaharan Africa and it is probable that other, as yet unidentified environmental factors are involved in the aetiology.

Histiocytic medullary reticulosis (HMR) and malignant histiocytosis (MH)

The classical form of HMR, first described by Robb Smith, is characterized by the proliferation of malignant histiocytes in the sinusoids of the spleen, liver, lymph-nodes, and marrow. Such patients present with fever, hepatosplenomegaly, haemolytic anaemia, and neutropenia. At a late stage in the disease tumour masses may form in the organs, or these may be present from the start (malignant histiocytosis).

Geographical distribution HMR is a very rare form of lymphoma in Europe and North America, but has been reported with unusual frequency in several countries of subSaharan Africa including Uganda, Kenya, Zambia, and Malawi. The great majority of these patients have been in the second or third decades of life, were diagnosed as having a systemic infection, and were only identified at post-mortem.

The cause of HMR is unknown but the high incidence in the malarious regions of subSaharan Africa suggests that the reactive proliferation of histiocytes in the affected organs, as a result of recurrent parasitaemia, may predispose these cells to the action of other, as yet unidentified, oncogenic agents.

Hodgkin's disease

Comparison of the age-standardized incidence rates for all subtypes of Hodgkin's disease in different countries of the world shows a four-fold variation between those areas with the highest rates (over 3.5 per 100 000 per year in men), and those with the lowest rates (less than 1.4 per 100 000). Higher rates are found in most affluent westernized countries and lower rates in the poorer countries of the tropics. However, low rates are also a feature of Japan and of all three racial groups (Chinese, Indian, and Malaysian) living in Singapore.

If histological subtypes and age of onset are analysed on a geographical basis it becomes apparent that overall rates hide other differences in the pattern of the disease. In most poor countries of the tropics, including subSaharan Africa, Papua New Guinea, and some areas of South America, Hodgkin's disease is unusually common in younger age groups, with nearly half the cases presenting under the age of 25 years and 10 per cent under the age of 10 years – a few being seen under 5 years of age. This unusual age distribution is associated with a much higher frequency of histological subtypes that carry a poor prognosis (mixed cellularity and lymphocyte-depleted types) than is found in the West. Other tropical and subtropical populations also have a relatively high incidence in children but show a higher proportion of the nodular sclerosing subtype. The considerable variations in age distribution and histological subtype in different parts of the world are unexplained. It has been suggested that these are due to the impact of multiple infections affecting the early childhood of children brought up in the poorer countries of the tropics, though this does not explain the relatively low rates in the Japanese.

Acute leukaemia

In North America, Europe, and other westernized populations acute lymphoid leukaemia (ALL) accounts for the high incidence of acute leukaemias in children between the ages of 2 and 5 years and for frequency of leukaemias as childhood malignancies. By contrast ALL is an uncommon malignancy in the tropics, such as subSaharan Africa where Burkitt's lymphoma is the predominant childhood tumour. As a result of this deficiency of ALL in early childhood the overall rates of acute leukaemias are low in the tropics though both acute myeloid leukaemia (AML) and subtypes of ALL are quite common in older children in these regions.

An unusual feature of AML in Africa is the relatively high frequency of the development of chloromatous masses. These may be the presenting feature and often involve the orbit.

The reasons for the differences in the pattern of ALL in the tropics and in Europe and the USA are not known but it is of interest that ALL in the USA is less common in black children during the first 5 years of life than in white children. There also appears to be a significant increase of ALL in black children from higher socio-economic groups, which might be related either to an increased exposure to leukaemogenic agents or to a decrease in childhood infections. Paradoxically, improved social status in black children is associated with a decreased risk of developing Hodgkin's disease in early life. The incidence rates of acute leukaemia in adult life appear to be similar in most parts of the world if allowances are made for diagnostic problems in some regions and specific types such as ATLL are excluded.

Chronic leukaemias

Chronic myeloid (CML) and chronic lymphoid (CLL) leukaemias occur throughout the world though it is difficult to obtain accurate age-standardized incidence rates from many developing countries where cancer registries rely heavily on biopsy-proven diagnoses. The occurrence of lymphoid leukaemoid reactions in some cases of tropical splenomegaly syndrome which is widely distributed in the tropics may give rise to false reporting of cases of CLL at an early age.

Myelomatosis

Myelomatosis occurs throughout the world. The highest rates are recorded in the black populations of the USA (over 6 per 100 000 per year in men and women in the Bay area of San Francisco). Rates of over 4 per 100 000 have also been recorded in Jamaicans and in the Hawaiian and Philippino populations of Hawaii. Low rates (less than 1 per 100 000) are found in Japan, India, and several countries of eastern Europe. It was formerly stated that myelomatosis was uncommon in Africa but with improved facilities more cases are being reported. An unusual feature of myelomatosis in Africa is the frequency with which patients present with a solitary bone tumour rather than with systemic symptoms. The sites of the bone lesions are also different from those seen in temperate climates; over 40 per cent of histologically diagnosed bone myelomas seen in Malawi affect the long bones of the limbs.

Conclusions

There are marked differences in the incidence rates, clinical features, and behaviour of many lymphoreticular and haemopoietic malignancies in different parts of the world. The evidence suggests that these are mainly related to environmental factors, particularly those that affect young children in the first 10 years of life. As new techniques emerge for the subtyping of leukaemias and lymphomas it will be necessary to re-evaluate the geographical distribution in the light of this new knowledge.

References

Malignant lymphoma – general

Correa, P. and O'Conor, G. T. (1973). Geographic pathology of lymphoreticular tumours. *J. Natl. Cancer Inst.* **50**, 1609–1617.

O'Conor, G. T. (1982). Environmental influences on lymphoma incidence. In *Geographical pathology in cancer epidemiology* (eds E. Grundmann, J. Clemmesen, and C. S. Muir), pp. 183–189. Gustav Fischer, Stuttgart, New York.

Human T cell leukaemia/lymphoma.

Blattner, W. A., Blayney, D. W., Robert-Guroff, M., Sarngadharan, M. G., Kalyanaraman, U. S., Saria, P. S., Jaffe, E. S. and Gallo, R. C. (1983). Epidemiology of human T-cell leukaemia/lymhoma virus. *J. Infect. Dis.* **147**, 406–416.

Blattner, W. A., Saxinger, C., Clark, J., Hanchard, B., Gibbs, W. N., Robert-Guroff, M., Lofters, W., Campbell, M. and Gallo, R. C. (1983). Human T-cell neoplasia in Jamaica. *Lancet* **2**, 61–64.

The T and B cell Malignancy Study Group (1981). Statistical analysis of immunologic, clinical and histopathologic data on lymphoid malignancies in Japan. *Jpn J. Clin. Oncol.* **11**, 15–18.

Uchiyama, T., Yoddi, J., Sagawa, K., Takatsuki, K. and Uchino, H. (1977). Adult T cell leukaemia: clinical and haematologic features of 16 cases. *Blood* **50**, 481–491.

Burkitt's lymphoma

Burkitt, D. P. (1958). A sarcoma of the jaw in African children. *Br. J. Surg.* **46**, 126–129.

Burkitt, D. P. (1969). An alternative hypothesis to a vectored virus. *J. natl. Cancer Inst.* **42**, 19–28.

Geser, A., de The, G., Lenoir, G., Day, N. E. and Williams, E. H. (1982). Final case reporting from the Ugandan prospective study of the relationship between EBV and Burkitt's lymphoma. *Int. J. Cancer* **29**, 397–400.

de The, G. (1980). Role of Epstein–Barr virus in human diseases: infectious mononucleosis, Burkitt's lymphoma and nasopharyngeal carcinoma. In *Viral oncology* (ed. G. Klein). Raven Press. New York.

Primary intestinal lymphoma

Ramot, B. and Hulu, N. (1975). Primary intestinal lymphoma and its relation to alpha chain disease. *Br. J. Cancer* **11**, 343–349.

Dutz, W., Borochovitz, D., Kohout, E. and Vessal, K. (1980). The two basic forms of primary intestinal lymphoma. In *Proceedings of the symposium on prevention and detection of cancer*. Marcel Dekker, New York.

Histiocytic medullary reticulosis

Serck-Hanssen, N. and Purohit, G. P. (1968). Histiocytic medullary reticulosis. Report of 14 cases in Uganda. *Br. J. Cancer* **22**, 506–516.

Hodgkin's disease

Burn, C., Davies, J. N. P., Dodge, O. G. and Nias, B. C. (1971). Hodgkin's disease in English and African children. *J. natl. Cancer Inst.* **46**, 37–41.

Vianna, N. J. and Polan, A. K. Immunity in Hodgkin's disease. Importance of age at exposure. **89**, 550–566.

Ziegler, J. L., Morrow, R. H., Fass, L. and Kyalwazi, S. K. (1970). Childhood Hodgkin's disease in Uganda. *East Afr. Med. J.* **47**, 191–192.

Leukaemias

Davies, J. N. P. and Owor, R. (1965) Chloromatous tumours in African children in Uganda. *Br. Med. J.* **2**, 405–407.

Gordis, L., Moyses, S., Thompson, B., Kapaln, A. and Tonaslia, J. A. (1981). An apparent increase of acute non-lymphocytic leukaemia in black children. *Cancer* **47**, 2763–2768.

Kasili, E. G. (1981). Leukaemia in African children. *Postgrad. Dr* **3**, 126–129.

Williams, C. K. O., Folami, A. O., Laditan, A. A. O. and Ukaejiofo, E. O. (1982). Childhood acute leukaemia in a tropical population. *Br. J. Cancer* **46**, 89–94.

Myelomatosis

Talerman, A. (1969). Clinicopathological study of multiple myeloma in Jamaica. *Br. J. Cancer* **23**, 285–293.

Tozer, R. A., Clear, A. S., Davies, D. R. and Hutt, M. S. R. Unusual presentation of patients with myelomatosis in Malawi. *J. Clin. Path.* **33**, 544–546.

Africa

A. F. FLEMING

Introduction

The continent of Africa has an area of over 30 million km^2; nearly 80 per cent lies within the tropics and one-quarter is desert (Fig. 1). To the north of the Sahara are the Mediterranean littoral, scrub, forest, wooded steppe, and the Nile delta (Fig. 2). South of the Sahara are the sahel, woodlands, and savanna (sudan, guinea, and wooded or derived in order of increasing humidity and rainfall): there tend to be wide variations of temperature, both in daily and annual cycles, and the rains are confined to a few months each year, allowing for cattle-raising and seasonal farming, which may be intensive, for example, in northern Nigeria (Fig. 2). In the equatorial rain forest, there are no extremes of heat or cold, humidity remains high and the rains fall during most of the year, permitting continuous farming (Fig. 3); there are no cattle because of tsetse flies (Fig. 4). Within the tropical zone there are the highland areas of (*a*) Ethiopia and Kenya, (*b*) Ruwanda, Burundi, and the Ruwenzori Mountains, and (*c*) Cameroon, where grain may be grown and cattle raised (Figs. 2, 4). To the south are the subtropical and temperate areas of southern Africa, including the highlands of Lesotho and the Rand.

The population of Africa in 1985 is about 450 million: the annual increase is approximately 2.5 per cent, so that a population around 700 million may be predicted in AD 2000. About one-fifth of the population is to the north of the Sahara, centred on the Nile and the Magreb. One-quarter of the population of subsaharan

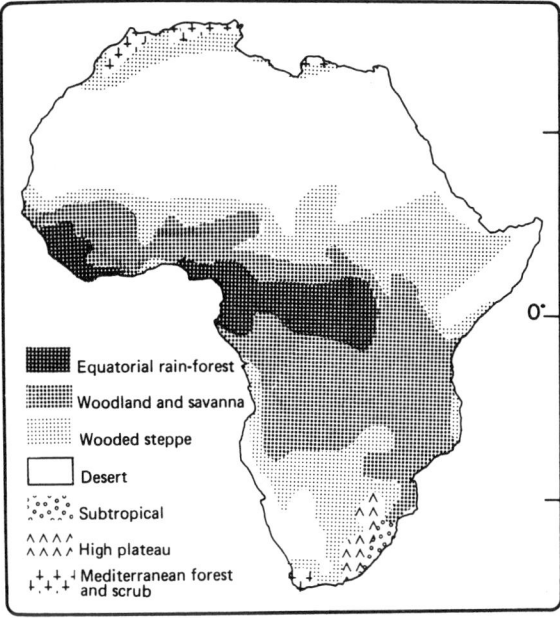

Fig. 1 The major geographical regions of Africa. (Reproduced from Parry, 1984, with permission.)

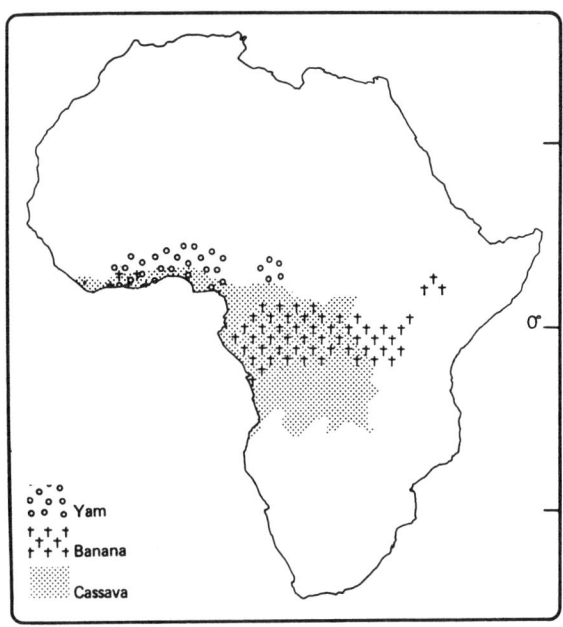

Fig. 3 Root staples and bananas in Africa. (Reproduced from Whittle, H. C., 1984. In Parry, 1984, with permission.)

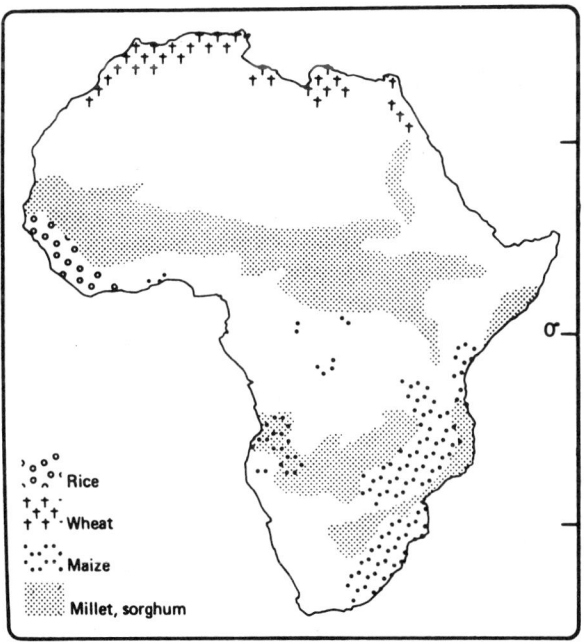

Fig. 2 Cereal staples in Africa. (Reproduced from Whittle, H. C., 1984. In Parry, 1984, with permission.)

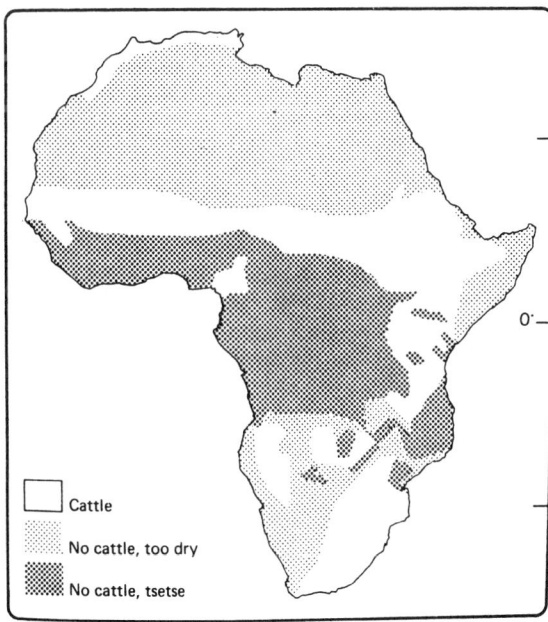

Fig. 4 Distribution of tsetse fly and areas where cattle can survive. (Reproduced from Whittle, H. C., 1984. In Parry, 1984, with permission.)

Africa lives in Nigeria; other areas of dense population are around the lakes of east Africa and in the Republic of South Africa. Eighty per cent of the population are rural, depending largely on the food which is produced locally, but recently there has been a vast increase of importation of wheat-flour and rice, especially by Nigeria.

Mediterranean Africa
The staple of northern Africa is wheat (Fig. 2); animal protein is relatively plentiful from fish and livestock, and is supplemented by protein-rich vegetables such as beans. Nutritional iron deficiency is a common problem. *Schistosoma mansonii* is the most frequent

cause of anaemia in Egypt; the severest iron deficiency anaemias are in farmers with *Ancylostoma duodenale* coinciding with *S. mansonii* and *Schistosoma haematobium*. Malaria has been eradicated, but there remain the inherited adaptations to *Plasmodium falciparum*; β thalassaemia, G6PD deficiency, and, to a lesser extent, sickle cell disease are major health problems (page 19.73).

Tropical savanna and wooded steppe
The main staples of millet and sorghum have 3–4 per cent protein content, while maize has only slightly less (Fig. 2); livestock is generally plentiful (Fig. 4). Protein energy malnutrition (PEM) is relatively uncommon, but is seen towards the end of the dry sea-

Table 1 Prevalence of neonatal jaundice (serum bilirubin >250 μmol/1) and anaemia (haemoglobin less than 11g/dl) in pre-school children and primigravidae in Zaria, in the guinea savanna of Nigeria, and the relative frequency of aetiological factors amongst the anaemic (or jaundiced)

	Neonatal jaundice	Anaemia in childhood	Anaemia in primigravidae
Frequency of anaemia (%)	?	63	43
Number of patients studied	40	59	98
Frequency of aetiological factors (%)			
Malaria	0	62	40
Viral/bacterial infections	85	71	0
Iron deficiency	0	60	49
Folate deficiency	0	40	56
Hypoproteinaemia	0	30	0
Sickle cell disease	0	25	0
G6PD deficiency	33	0	0
Prematurity	40	—	—

From Werblińska *et al.* (1981) *Nigerian J. Paediat.* **8**, 3–10; Fleming and Werblińska (1982) *Ann. trop. Paediat.* **3**, 161–173; and Fleming *et al.* (1985) *Ann. trop. Paediat.* **80**, 211–233.

son and early rains before the new harvest, and at times of drought. The folate content of food is generally low, especially at the end of the dry season. Nutritional iron deficiency is a frequent problem. Hookworm infestation is a common cause of severe anaemia in farmers where the soil is sufficiently moist for transmission in the guinea and wooded savanna. *S. haematobium* is widespread, and makes a significant contribution to anaemia in rural areas, especially along the eastern coastal plain from Somalia to southern Africa: amongst Somalis in north-east Kenya, the highest prevalence of anaemia is in adolescent boys, of whom 46 per cent had haemoglobin values less than 8 g/dl related to *S. haematobium*. *S. mansonii* occurs in small scattered foci, but appears to be increasing rapidly with new irrigation projects.

Malaria is hyperendemic in most of this area, but at the height of the rains, transmission can be even more intense than in holoendemic areas. The prevalence of sickle cell trait (up to 30 per cent) and its survival advantage are apparently greatest where malaria is hyperendemic. GdA⁻ occurs in up to 20 per cent of males.

The pattern of common anaemias of a community in the guinea savanna of northern Nigeria is summarized in Table 1.

Highlands

The highlands of tropical Africa need separate consideration. There is no transmission of malaria: livestock are able to flourish and various cereals of high protein content are grown. However, soils are commonly infertile and erosion is widespread: drought recurs periodically and famine, sometimes of devastating magnitude, follows. The staple of much of Ethiopia is the fine grain of teff (*Eragrostis abyssinica*); traditional methods of threshing lead to contamination, which can raise the iron intake of an adult male to 500 mg per day. Although up to 60 per cent of a rural population may be anaemic, predominantly the result of intercurrent infections, iron deficiency is rare, even in pregnancy, though occurring in children under three years of age.

Equatorial rain forest

The holoendemic transmission of malaria is unaltered throughout equatorial Africa, except in some large cities, and it dominates the picture of anaemia in childhood and pregnancy. The haemoglobin S gene occurs at high frequency throughout the area, reaching more than 0.14 in Nigeria and the Zaire basin (page 19.73). In Nigeria alone, 2 per cent of all infants, or 30 000 subjects are born each year with sickle cell disease (page 19.73). β thalassaemia is centred on Liberia (gene frequency greater than 0.05) and haem-

oglobin C, which is most common in the savanna of Upper Volta and northern Ghana (gene frequency greater than 0.14) spreads into the forest areas of the west coast, notably into the densely populated south west of Nigeria, where 5 per cent carry the gene (page 19.75). The frequency of GdA⁻ (page 19.73) increases from west to east, being reported in 6 per cent of males in the Gambia, 16–18 per cent in Mali, Ghana, and Togo, 22–23 per cent in Nigeria and Cameroon, and 32 per cent among the Luo in the Lake Victoria area of Kenya.

The staples of cassava and plantain (Fig. 3) have a protein content of less than 1 per cent; yams, rice, and maize (which is common as a second staple) are better, but have only 2–3 per cent protein (Figs. 2, 3). As cattle cannot be reared (Fig. 4), the intake of both animal and vegetable protein is low, and PEM is seen commonly.

Iron-status depends on two main factors, the intake of bioavailable iron, and the transmission of hookworm. In western Nigeria, nutritional iron deficiency is uncommon in those who eat the traditional food based on yam and cassava with a 'soup' of oil, vegetables, and some meat or fish. In addition, women do not work in the fields, so that they and small children are not infested heavily by hookworm; severe iron-deficiency anaemia is confined almost entirely to men and older boys who carry heavy hookworm loads. However, there have been changes in eating habits reducing the intake of bioavailable iron, especially in the cities like Ibadan and Lagos in the last 20 years; eggs are eaten commonly and the main staples of many are imported wheat flour and rice: as most urban pregnant women take antimalarial prophylaxis, nutritional iron deficiency is now the commonest cause of moderate anaemia in pregnancy. Nutritional deficiency of iron is common in the rice-growing areas of the Atlantic coast including the Gambia and Sierra Leone (Fig. 2). In Nigeria to the east of the Niger, and throughout equatorial Africa populated by Bantu-speaking peoples, women perform farm work and are accompanied to the fields by small children: severe iron-deficiency anaemia from both hookworm and poor nutrition is a common and serious problem of pregnancy and childhood.

Both plantains and yams are rich sources of folates, but deficiency occurs following seasonal shortages, overcooking, and high demands. The extremely high prevalence of severe megaloblastic anaemia in pregnancy in west Africa (page 19.76) is due to a combination of low intake, malaria, and high rates of multiple pregnancies and sickle cell disease, especially haemoglobin SC disease. Nutritional deficiency of vitamin B₁₂ has been observed in Uganda in people eating exclusively plantain.

Severe neonatal jaundice is common but of unmeasured frequency, caused by sepsis, prematurity, G6PD deficiency, and maternofetal ABO incompatibility. Over 30 per cent of Africans living in the forest with blood group O have strong anti A or anti B haemolysins of IgG type, capable of crossing the placenta. It has been suggested that these follow immunization by red cells carried by mosquitoes making multiple feeds. In over 4 per cent of all pregnancies there are maternal antibodies capable of lysing the infants' red cells.

Southern Africa

The staples of the black inhabitants of southern Africa are maize and sorghum (Fig. 2). Cattle and other livestock do well (Fig. 4), but separation of wage-earning men from their families and conditions in slums allow for high prevalence of PEM, iron deficiency, and folate deficiency in underprivileged children in both rural and peri-urban areas. Anaemia from iron and folate deficiency are common in pregnant Black women. High frequencies of iron deficiency are reported in the vegetarian Indian community of Natal, among whom about 40 per cent of children are anaemic, and in those of mixed race ('coloured') in Cape Town.

Malaria does not occur, except sporadically in Zimbabwe, where it affects children and pregnant women of all parities. Associated with low levels of immunity, malaria in the first trimes-

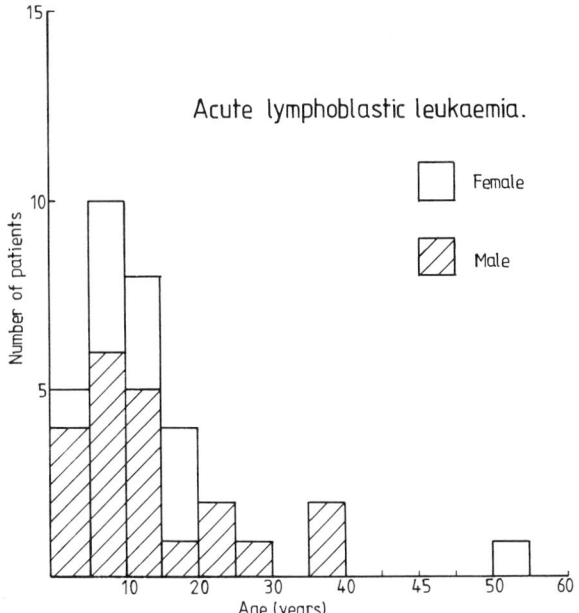

Fig. 5 Age at presentation of 21 males and 12 females with acute lymphoblastic leukaemia, in northern Nigeria. (Reproduced from Fleming and Peters, 1982, with permission.)

ter carries a high risk of abortion, and an overall fetal loss of about 50 per cent.

Sickle cell disease is seen rarely in South Africa and occurs more often in those of Indian descent than in Blacks.

Leukaemias

(See also page 19.261.)

Reliable data on incidence are available from only a few centres, where both the diagnosis of leukaemias is reliable and population statistics are accurate, but there is a large body of information on frequency of the leukaemias seen in hospitals.

Acute lymphoblastic leukaemia (ALL) is seen rarely under the age of five years and the peak of frequency is from 5 to 14 years of age in west and east Africa (Fig. 5). Preliminary reports suggest that 'common' or cALL is in fact uncommon, and that the more frequent type is T-ALL: it is possible that the true incidence of cALL is on the increase in east Africa. Acute myeloid leukaemia (AML) of all types is seen at all ages, but has an exceptionally high prevalence in childhood (Fig. 6); the frequencies of AML and ALL in childhood are equal in tropical Africa, whereas ALL is around four times more common in childhood in the western world. About 25 per cent of patients with AML in east and 10 per cent in west Africa present with chloroma, commonly of the orbit, and especially during childhood.

Chronic granulocytic leukaemia is seen most frequently in the third and fourth decades of life (Fig. 7), as opposed to the fifth decade in the industrialized countries, reflecting the age structures of the two populations. About 10 per cent of patients in Nigeria and 19 per cent in Sudan are below 15 years.

The age frequency and sex distribution of chronic lymphatic leukaemia (CLL) in west Africa suggests strongly that there are two diseases (Fig. 8). About half of patients are seen below the age of 45 years, the youngest recorded being 17 years of age. Below 45 years, women are affected twice as commonly as men, and there is a peak of frequency in women at the end of their period of reproductive life. Above 45 years of age, the male:female ratio is 2:1, as it is in the western world. CLL in younger adults, especially women, seems to be most common in West Africa, but has been reported recently in Uganda and Zambia: it is confined to rural areas, and the poorer social classes. It has been

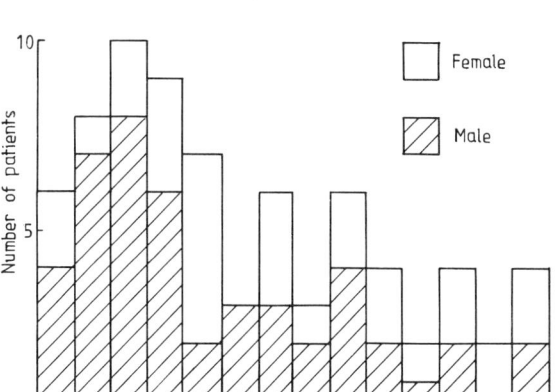

Fig. 6 Age at presentation of 46 males and 28 females with acute myeloid leukaemia in northern Nigeria. (Reproduced from Fleming and Peters, 1982, with permission.)

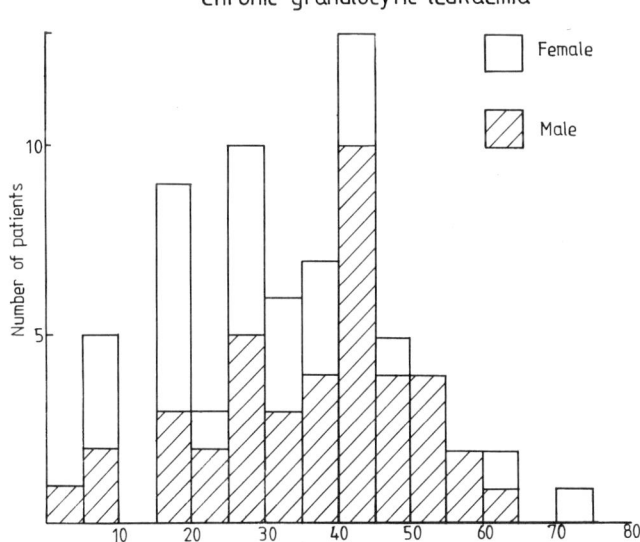

Fig. 7 Age at presentation of 41 males and 27 females with chronic granulocytic leukaemia in northern Nigeria. (Reproduced from Fleming and Peters, 1982, with permission.)

postulated that there is an oncogenic agent being transmitted in the population, to which women are particularly susceptible because of the physiological depression of cell-mediated immunity in normal pregnancies.

Antibodies against the human T cell leukaemia-lymphoma (or lymphotropic) virus type 1 (HTLV-1) is reported in above 2 per cent of symptom-free adults throughout subsaharan Africa, and at a conservative estimate, there are more than 10 million carriers of the virus in Africa, forming the largest reservoir of the infection in the world. A few patients have been identified with adult T cell leukaemia-lymphoma (ATL) in tropical Africa, but it may be predicted that the diagnosis will be made with increasing frequency. HTLV-1 is not associated apparently with CLL in young adults.

The epidemiology of the leukaemias in north Africa and in the Whites of south Africa resembles that of Europe. The pattern in Blacks of south Africa is similar to that of east Africa. Indians in

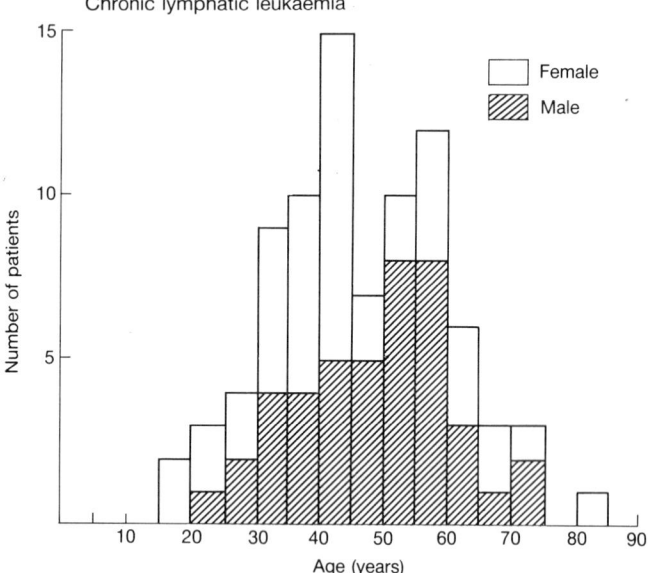

Chronic lymphatic leukaemia

Fig. 8 Age at presentation of 43 males and 42 females with chronic lymphatic leukaemia in northern Nigeria. (Reproduced from Fleming and Peters, 1982, with permission.)

Africa have a high incidence of CGL and a low incidence of CLL, as they do in the Indian subcontinent.

References

(See also References under Anaemia as a World Health Problem.)

Akinkugbe, F. M. (1980). Anaemia in a rural population in Nigeria (Ilora). *Ann. trop. Med. Parasitol.* **74**, 625–633.

Baumslag, N., Edelstein, T. and Metz, J. (1970). Reduction of incidence of prematurity by folic acid supplementation in pregnancy. *Brit. med. J.* **i**, 16–17.

Becker, D., Charlton, R. W. and Bothwell, T. H. (1970). Iron nutrition in pregnant Bantu females. *S. Afr. med. J.* **44**, 414–417.

Domisse, J. and de Toit, E. D. (1969). The incidence and treatment of severe pregnancy anaemia in the Cape Town area. *S. Afr. med. J.* **43**, 244–247.

Fleming, A. F. (1979). Epidemiology of the leukaemias in Africa. *Leuk. Res.* **3**, 51–59.

——, Harrison, K. A., Brigg, N. D., Attai, E. D. E., Ghatoura, G. B. S., Akintunde, E. A. and Shah, N. (1984). Anaemia in young primigravidae in the guinea savanna of Nigeria: sickle-cell trait gives partial protection against malaria. *Ann. trop. Med. Parasitol.* **78**, 395–404.

—— and Peters, B. (1982). The epidemiology of leukaemias in the guinea savanna of Nigeria. *Nigerian med. J.* **12**, 223–233.

Gebre-Medhim, M., Killander, A., Vahlquist, B. and Wuhib, E. (1976). Rarity of anaemia of pregnancy in Ethiopia. *Scand. J. Haemat.* **16**, 168–175.

Greaves, M. F. and Chan, L. C. (eds) (1985). Epidemiology of leukaemia and lymphoma. *Leuk. Res.* **6**, 661–832.

Harrison, K. A. (1982). Anaemia, malaria and sickle cell disease. *Clinics Obstet. Gynaecol.* **9**, 445–477.

Herd, N. and Jordan, T. (1981). An investigation of malaria during pregnancy in Zimbabwe. *Cent. Afr. J. Med.* **27**, 62–68.

Hofvander, Y. (1968). Haematological investigations in Ethiopia, with special reference to a high iron intake. *Act. med. scand.* suppl. 494.

Isah, H. S., Fleming, A. F., Ujah, I. A. O. and Ekwempu, C. C. (1985). Anaemia and iron status of pregnant and non-pregnant women in the guinea savanna of Nigeria. *Ann. trop. Med. Parasitol.* **79**, 485–493.

Kulkarni, A. G., Ibazebo, R. and Fleming, A. F. (1985). High frequency of anti-A and anti-B haemolysins in certain ethnic groups in Nigeria. *Vox Sanguin.* **48**, 39–41.

Margo, G., Baroni, Y., Wells, G., Green, R. and Metz, J. (1978). Protein energy malnutrition and nutritional anaemia in pre-school children in rural KwaZulu. *S. Afr. med. J.* **53**, 21–26.

Mayet, F. G. H. (1976). The prevalence of anaemia and iron deficiency in the Indian community in Natal. *S. Afr. med. J.* **50**, 1889–1892.

Nkrumah, F. K. and Neequaye, J. (1982). Neonatal hyperbilirubinaemia in Ghana. *W. Afr. J. Med.* **1**, 1–6.

Obi, G. O. and Chukudebelu, W. O. (1981). The iron status of anaemic pregnant Igbo women in Nigeria. *Trop. geogr. Med.* **33**, 129–133.

Parry, E. H. O. (ed.) (1984). *Principles of medicine in Africa*, 2nd edn. Oxford University Press, Oxford.

Southeast Asia

P. WASI, A. PIANKIJAGUM, AND S. ISSARAGRISIL

The information in this section is derived mainly from experiences in our unit which is a main haematology centre in Southeast Asia. The types and frequencies of blood and related disorders are illustrated in Table 1. For comparison with western countries, blood diseases in Southeast Asia may be divided into three broad categories, i.e. more, less, and similar in frequency (Table 2).

More frequent

Hereditary blood disorders

Both α and β thalassaemia, haemoglobin E, haemoglobin Constant Spring, and glucose-6-phosphate dehydrogenase (G6PD) deficiency are prevalent in Southeast Asia (see page 19.72 *et seq.*). The frequency of the α thalassaemias reaches 30–40 per cent in Northern Thailand and Laos, and the β thalassaemias occur at a frequency of 3–9 per cent in these regions. Haemoglobin E is the hallmark of Southeast Asia with the highest frequencies, 50–60 per cent, around the junction of Thailand, Laos, and Cambodia. Haemoglobin Constant Spring is detected in up to 8 per cent of the population. These abnormal genes interact to produce over 60 thalassaemia syndromes in this region, more complex than anywhere else in the world. Three thalassaemic diseases are seen more frequently than in other regions, i.e. haemoglobin Bart's hydrops fetalis, haemoglobin H disease, and β thalassaemia/haemoglobin E disease.

G6PD deficiency reaches a frequency of 15 per cent among the people of Northeastern Thailand, Laos, and Cambodia. The most common type is G6PD Mahidol; G6PD Canton is second in prevalence (see page 19.140). Acute haemolysis due to the action of various drugs and acute infections is the major clinical feature of this condition in Thailand.

Table 1 New patients with haematological disorders seen in the Division of Haematology, Department of Medicine, Siriraj Hospital, Bangkok, in 1983

Iron deficiency anaemia	132	Myelofibrosis	16
Megaloblastic anaemia (folate responsive)	2	Non-Hodgkin's lymphoma	106
Thalassaemias	226	Hodgkin's disease	14
G6PD deficiency with acute haemolysis	20	Malignant histiocytosis	16
Paroxysmal nocturnal haemoglobinuria	5	Angioimmunoblastic lymphadenopathy	15
Autoimmune haemolytic anaemia	18	Multiple myeloma	17
		ITP	39
Aplastic anaemia	59	Dengue haemorrhagic fever	31
Polycythaemia vera	6	Haemophilia	7
Acute leukaemia	106	Thrombosis	7
Chronic leukaemia		Systemic lupus erythematosus (SLE)	32
Myeloid	35		
Lymphocytic	5		

Table 2 Geographical variation of blood diseases in Southeast Asia compared to the West

More frequent	Less frequent	Similar
Hereditary blood disorders, i.e. thalassaemia, Hb E, Hb Constant Spring, G6PD deficiency	Megaloblastic anaemia	Acute leukaemia and CML
Aplastic anaemia	Primary haemochromatosis	Lymphoma
Paroxysmal nocturnal haemoglobinuria	Chronic lymphocytic leukaemia	Systemic lupus erythromatosus
Tropical anaemia*	Polycythaemia vera and agnogenic melyoid metaplasia	Immune haemolytic anaemia
Dengue haemorrhagic fever	Infectious mononucleosis	Idiopathic thrombocytopenic purpura (ITP)
Acquired prothrombin complex deficiency	Thromboembolism	Haemophilia
Acquired platelet dysfunction with eosinophilia		

* Defined in text.

Aplastic anaemia

Aplastic anaemia is common throughout the Far East. In our unit alone around 60 new patients are seen each year, over 1000 patients having been diagnosed in the past 20 years. In general, all hospitals with diagnostic facilities see a comparatively large number of patients with this disease.

Paroxysmal nocturnal haemoglobinuria (PNH)

PNH appears to be more frequent in this area. Over 100 patients have been seen in this unit, a large proportion associated with aplastic anaemia. In contrast to patients seen in the West, it occurs in younger people, males more than females, and thromboembolism is rare.

Tropical anaemia

This refers to three types of anaemia common in Southeast Asia, i.e. anaemia due to hookworm infestation, malaria, and rural poverty. Hookworm is so common among the farmers that the finding of chronic severe anaemia without hepatosplenomegaly in rural Thailand should always raise the possibility of this disease. In areas with endemic malaria patients with fever and anaemia will usually have malaria. In rural areas it is common to find mild anaemia with haemoglobin levels of 9–10 g/dl. The frequency of this finding is correlated with the socioeconomic status of the communities. In the poorest, it is observed in over 90 per cent of the villagers. It is probably the result of compound effects of poverty, i.e. poor nutrition, parasites, and infection. It is resistant to treatment. Iron fortification or supplementation alone, although followed by some response, never raises the haemoglobin level to normal. A very recent study in Thailand by Charoenlap, however, indicates that prolonged and intensive oral iron supplementation does raise the haemoglobin level to normal.

Dengue haemorrhagic fever (DHF)

DHF is intermittently epidemic in Southeast Asia. It is a severe febrile disease of children and adolescents. It is characterized by sudden onset of fever, nausea, vomiting, bleeding, and shock. Arboviruses, dengue serotypes 1, 2, 3, and 4 (group B), are responsible for 85–90 per cent of the cases, the rest being due to chikungunya virus. The vector is *Aëdes aegypti* (see Section 5).

Acquired prothrombin complex deficiency (APCD)

APCD is a bleeding disorder observed mainly in infants, one or two months of age, and usually breast fed. The aetiology is not known. It is suspected that the mothers may have ingested substances antagonistic to prothrombin.

Acquired platelet dysfunction with eosinophilia (APDE)

This is manifested in children, who present with ecchymoses. Platelet dysfunction and eosinophilia are observed in the majority. The aetiology is not known. Parasitic infestation may play an important role.

Less frequent

Blood diseases and related disorders seen less frequently than in the West are shown in Table 2.

Megaloblastic anaemia

Pernicious anaemia is almost unknown. Nutritional vitamin B_{12} deficiency is also rare. Nutritional folate deficiency is not encountered frequently, even among pregnant women. This is due to a folate-rich diet.

Primary haemochromatosis

While secondary haemochromatosis due to thalassaemia is common, primary haemochromatosis is never seen, presumably due to the lack of the gene for this defect in Southeast Asia.

Chronic lymphocytic leukaemia (CLL)

Unlike the West, chronic lymphocytic leukaemia is the least commonly encountered leukaemia. As shown in Table 1, while 106 patients with acute leukaemia and 35 with chronic myeloid leukaemia were seen in 1983, only five with CLL were diagnosed. In previous years only two to four patients with CLL were seen annually. CLL is rare throughout the Far East.

Infectious mononucleosis

Typical infectious mononucleosis with heterophil antibody in young adults is extremely rare. This is due to early exposure to Epstein–Barr virus; over 85 per cent of adults have antibody to EB virus.

Thromboembolism

Thromboembolism is infrequent even among pregnant women and postoperative patients. This may be due to dietary factors. The diet in this region contains less lipid but more garlic, onion, and spicy ingredients which may decrease platelet aggregation. Basal plasma fibrinolytic activity is higher than found in Caucasians. After ingestion of chili, fibrinolytic activity increases dramatically!

Similar in frequency

The disorders seen at more or less the same frequency as in western countries include acute and chronic myeloid leukaemias, lymphoma, systemic lupus erythematosus, immune haemolytic anaemia, immune thrombocytopenia, and haemophilia. Of the lymphomas, Hodgkin's disease is seen much less frequently than non-Hodgkin's lymphoma. The latter consists mainly of undifferentiated and histiocytic cell types, formerly known as reticulum cell sarcoma.

References

Isarangkura, P. B. (1979). The pathogenesis of acquired prothrombin complex deficiency syndrome (APCD syndrome) in infants. *Southeast Asian J. trop. Med. Pub. Hlth* **10**, 350–352.

Kruatrachue, M., Wasi, P. and Na-Nakorn, S. (1978). Paroxysmal nocturnal haemoglobinuria in Thailand with special reference to an association with aplastic anaemia. *Br. J. Haematol.* **39**, 267–276.

Mitrakul, C. (1975). Transient, spontaneous bruising with long bleeding time and normal platelet count. *Am. J. Clin. Pathol.* **63**, 81–86.

Na-Nakorn, S. (1979). Deficiency anemia in Thailand. *Proceedings of the fourth meeting of Asian-Pacific Division, International Society of Hematology*, Seoul, pp.147–155.

Panich, V. (1981). Glucose-6-phosphate dehydrogenase deficiency. *Trop. Asia. Clin. Haematol.* **10**, 800–814.

Piankijagum, A., Pacharee, P. and Wasi, P. (1980). Malignant lymphoma in Thailand. *J. Med. Assoc. Thai.* **63**, 181–191.

Suvatte, V., Mahasandana, C., Tanphaichitr, V. and Tuchinda, S. (1979). Acquired platelet dysfunction with eosinophilia: Study of platelet function in 62 cases. *Southeast Asian J. trop. Med. Pub. Hlth* **10**, 358–367.

Suvatte, V. (1981). Haemorrhagic disorders. *Trop. Asia. Clin. Haematol.* **10**, 933–962.

Visudhiphan, S., Poolsuppasit, S., Piboonnukarintr, O. and Tumliang, S. (1982). The relationship between high fibrinolytic activity and daily capsicum ingestions in Thai. *Am. J. Clin. Nutr.* **35**, 1452–1458.

Wasi, P. (1983). Hemoglobinopathies in Southeast Asia. In *Distribution and evolution of hemoglobin and globin loci*, Vol. 4 (ed. J. E. Bowman), pp.179–208. Elsevier, New York.

Latin America

L. SANCHEZ MEDAL AND G. RUIZ REYES

The frequency of haematological disorders in a particular geographical area is influenced by several factors: genetic, climatic, parasitic and infectious diseases endemic in the area, diet, and others. Latin American countries have different genetic compositions. Argentina and Uruguay are populated by European descendants with very little Indian and Negro admixture; a large proportion of their inhabitants are of Italian origin. Their pathology does not differ greatly from other Caucasoid populations. Thus they are excluded in the discussion that follows.

In all Latin American countries two races predominate: Spanish and Indian. The Precolombian Indian component varies from one country to another, being particularly prevalent in Bolivia, Ecuador, Guatemala, Mexico, Paraguay, and Peru. In most of these countries there was no major immigration of Negroes, while in others the admixture of Negro blood is important, Venezuela, Brazil, and Cuba, for example.

Frequency differences due to genetic background

There are many disorders that have a high incidence in particular ethnic groups. Certain diseases are rare among Latin Americans: pernicious anaemia, chronic lymphocytic leukaemia, and haemochromatosis, for example. In Caucasians, chronic lymphatic leukaemia makes up about 40 per cent of all leukaemias. In the Hospital of Nutrition of Mexico, mostly attended by Mexicans, lymphocytic leukaemia makes up only 6.7 per cent of patients with the disorder. This form of leukaemia is also uncommon in American Indians, again reflecting the rarity of this disorder in Mongoloid races. Haemchromatosis and Gaucher's disease are also extremely rare in Latin Americans of Mongoloid stock.

The only haematological disorder seen more frequently in Latin Americans than Caucasoids is aplastic anaemia. In Mexico, Peru, and other Latin American countries with large American Indian populations the ratio of aplastic anaemia to leukaemia is about 1:2, compared with 15:1 in Caucasoid populations.

Analysis of the aetiological basis of aplastic anaemia also indicates a difference between the two racial groups. In Latin America about one-third of cases are probably secondary to the use of insecticides, whereas chloramphenicol has been implicated in only 3–10 per cent of cases. In Caucasoid populations, insecticides have seldom been reported as an aetiological factor.

Sickle cell anaemia and other haemoglobin abnormalities in Latin America

In addition to Spaniards and British, French, Portuguese, and Dutch colonized the Latin American countries. Over three centuries, all these imported black slaves from Africa; the total exceeded 20 million. Other waves of immigration came to Venezuela, Brazil, and Argentina from Germany and Italy; to Brazil and Peru from Japan; and to Guyana from Java, China, and the East Indies. Differences in ethnic compositions and rates of interbreeding, and variation in the selective pressure of malaria from region to region, are responsible for the different frequencies of haemoglobin S and other haemoglobin abnormalities in the Americas. Table 1 summarizes current knowledge about the haemoglobin disorders in American Indians and other Latin American populations.

Frequency differences due to local conditions

A number of Latin Americans, mainly Peruvians, but also Argentinians, Mexicans, and others, live at high altitudes and are polycythaemic. Some Peruvians live and work at 4400 m. They show increased erythropoietin production and high levels of red cell 2,3-diphosphoglycerate. Chronic mountain sickness or Monge's disease is not uncommon in these populations (see Section 6).

For reasons which are still not understood, sprue was common in some Latin American countries, particularly Cuba and Puerto Rico. It occurred mainly among individuals of lower socioeconomic classes. Hygiene and dietary conditions have improved greatly in the past 20 years and, concomitantly, the incidence of sprue has also diminished.

Frequency differences due to parasitic or infectious factors

Hookworm infestation is endemic in many Latin American countries; secondary iron deficiency anaemia is very common. Oroya fever, an acute disorder produced by the infection of *Bartonella bacilliformis*, is restricted to Peru; it causes a severe haemolytic anaemia (see Section 5 and page 19.147).

References

Arends, T. (1984). Epidemiología de las variantes hemoglobínicas en Venezuela. *Gac. Med. de Caracas* **92**, 189–224.

Arends, T., Garlin, G., Pérez-Nández, O. and Anchustegui, M. (1982). Hemoglobin variants in Venezuela. *Hemoglobin* **6**, 243–246.

Colombo, B. and Martínez, G. (1981). Tropical America. *Clin. Hematol.* **10**, 730–756.

Flores Barroeta, F. and Velasco, A. F. V. (1971). Hallazgos en el Hospital General Centro Médico Nacional. *Gac. Med. Mex.* **102**, 208.

Hansen, M. M. (1973). Chronic lymphocytic leukaemia. *Scand. J. Haematol.* **18**, Suppl. 1.

Iparraguirre-de-Weinstein, B., Timpanaro, J. and Chiappe, G. (1985). *Hemoglobinopatías* (to be published).

Lisker, R. (1983). Distribution of abnormal hemoglobins in Latin America. In *Distribution and evolution of hemoglobins and globin loci* (ed. J. E. Bowman), pp. 261–278. Elsevier, Amsterdam.

McMahon, B. and Clark, D. (1956). Incidence of the common forms of human leukemia. *Blood* **11**, 871–881.

Merino, C. (1950). Studies on blood formation and destruction in the polycythemia of high altitude. *Blood* **5**, 1–31.

Monge, C. (1943). High altitude disease. *Physiol. Rev.* **23**, 166.

Prager, D. (1972). An analysis of hematologic disorders presenting in the private practice of hematology. *Blood* **40**, 568.

Reynafarje, C. and Ramos, H. (1961). The hemolytic anemia of human bartonellosis. *Blood* **17**, 562.

Ruiz Reyes, G. (1983). Hemoglobin variants in Mexico. *Hemoglobin* **7**, 601–610.

Sáenz Renauld, G. (1985). *Hemoglobinopathies in Central America and Panama* (in press).

Salzano, F. M. and Tondo, C. V. (1982). Hemoglobin types in Brazilian population. *Hemoglobin* **6**, 85–97.

Sánchez Medal, L. and Arriaga de la, C. L. (1976). La frecuencia de los

Table 1 Distribution of abnormal haemoglobins in Latin America. The haemoglobin variants and thalassaemias are described on page 19.108 *et seq*.

Country	Sickle cell trait				Other types of haemoglobin abnormalities
	American Indians	Positive (%)	Other ethnic groups	Positive (%)	
Argentina	–	–	–	Sporadic	SS, Sβ° or Sβ⁺ thalassaemia, Sα thalassaemia, Hb SC, Hb SD-Los Angeles, β thalassaemia trait, β thalassaemia major, Hb Lepore (Boston), Hb H disease. Other structural variants
Barbados	–	–	912 (various)	7	AC
Belize	260	0	724 (Negro)	22.7	AC
Bolivia	2848	0	378 (various)	0	
Brazil	8538	0	41018 (various)	0–7.9*	SS, SC, S-thalassaemia, many rare structuralvariants
Colombia	1055	0	4039 (various)	1.5–8.7	AC, many rare structural variants
Costa Rica	564	0	17953 (various)	0.8–10.9*	SS, AC, SC, Hb E, Hb Korle Bu
Cuba	108	1.8	31476 (various)	1.1–13.2	SS, SC, AC, CC, many rare structural variants
Curaçao	–	–	1502 (various)	6.5	AC
Chile	998	0		Sporadic	AG
Dominica	–	–	664 (various)	9.5	AC
Dominican Rep.	–	–	4891 (various)	11.8	SS, AC, SC, CC
El Salvador	–	–	Hospital (various)	1.5	
French Guiana	545	0.4–9.8*	–	–	AC
Guadeloupe	266	1.5	46775 (mainly Negro)	7.9	AC
Guatemala	184	0	150 (Negro)	18.0	
Guyana	325	0	–	–	
Haiti	–	–	2761 (various)	11.0	AC
Honduras	141	0	1471(Negro)	10.0	AC
Jamaica	–	–	27501 (various)	10.1	α thalassaemia, β thalassaemia (rare). SS, SC, SO Arabia Sβ° thalassaemia, Sβ⁺ thalassaemia, Many rare structural variants
Martinique	–	–	4559 (various)	7.4	AC
Mexico	3724	0.1	18946 (various)	0–11.2*	SS, AC, SC, Sβ° thalassaemia, Sβ⁺ thalassaemia, Hb H disease, α thalassaemia trait, β thalassaemia trait, β thalassaemia homozygous, δβ thalassaemia, HPFH†, many structural variants
Nicaragua	307	0	–	–	
Panama	681	1.1	7064 (mainly Negro)	4.5–30.0*	AC, SS
Peru	1357	0	–	Sporadic	SS, S-thalassaemia, Hb H disease
Puerto Rico	–	–	13750 (various)	0.8–8.4	AC
St Lucia	–	–	825 (various)	14.0	AC
St Vincent	–	–	748 (various)	8.7	AC
Surinam	–	–	5571 (various)	0–12.8*	AC
Trinidad and Tobago	–	–	379 (Negro)	11.1	AC
Venezuela	5313 (32 groups)	1.7*(5 groups)	37889 (various)	1.9–35.9*	SS, SC, AC, SD, AD, CC, β-thalassaemia intermedia, β-thalassaemia major, Hb H disease, many rare structural variants

* Range of regional variation.
† HPFH = hereditary persistence of fetal haemoglobin.

padecimientos hematológicos en México. *Rev. Invest. Clin. (Méx.)* **28**, 301.

—— and Dorantes, S. (1974). Aplastic anemia. *Paediatrician* **3**, 74.

Wintrobe, M. M. (1974). *Clinical hematology*, p. 1436. Lea and Febiger, Philadelphia.

Japan

S. MIWA

Anaemia and polycythaemia

The incidence of *aplastic anaemia* in Japan is the highest among the developed countries, being between 40 and 50 per million of the population compared to 10 and 20 per million in Europe. A preponderance of males to females has been noted, the ratio being 1:0.85. Among the 1594 cases of aplastic anaemia described in a nationwide survey performed in 1972, 179 patients were found to have received drugs that could induce haematopoietic disorders before and/or at the onset of the disease. Among such drugs, chloramphenicol was administered in 45 per cent of cases, other antibiotics and related agents were given in 16.4 per cent, and antipyretics, analgesics, and sedatives in 13.5 per cent. However, following changes in the regulation of drugs and more strict indication for the use of chloramphenicol issued in December 1975, the number of cases of aplastic anaemia secondary to this drug was markedly reduced, from 14.8 per cent among all aplastic anaemia patients in a survey between 1974 and 1975, to 3.0 per cent in a survey between 1976 and 1977. Age-specific death rates for aplastic anaemia tended to decrease in the younger age group, but increased in older age groups. As a result, the age distribution of aplastic anaemia in Japan is approaching that in western countries.

With regard to *megaloblastic anaemias*, though accurate statistics are lacking, both pernicious anaemia and folate deficiency appear to have a lower incidence among Japanese, compared with Caucasians. The latter may be due to the large amount of fresh green vegetables in the Japanese diet.

The commonest cause of anaemia in Japan is still iron deficiency. However, as in other developed countries, nutrition is not a major factor because the Japanese are eating more meat than before. Hookworm is not endemic in Japan.

According to the results of a nationwide survey performed in 1974, the incidence of *hereditary haemolytic anaemias* among Japanese was estimated to be 5.7–20.2 per million population. Hereditary spherocytosis (HS) comprised 70 per cent of these disorders; the incidence is lower in Japanese than in Caucasian populations. No cases of sickle cell anaemia have been reported in Japan. Unstable-haemoglobin haemolytic anaemia is only rarely reported. The incidence of abnormal haemoglobins among Japanese is estimated to be 1 per 2700. Thalassaemia is also rare in Japan; the incidence of heterozygous thalassaemia is also about 1 in 5000. Glucose-6-phosphate dehydrogenase (G6PD) deficiency is also rare, the incidence being about 0.1 per cent. This figure includes cases with about half normal activity and without signs of drug-induced acute haemolysis. Hence, the incidence of G6PD deficiency which causes acute haemolysis following ingestion of drugs appears to be low.

The incidence of *autoimmune haemolytic anaemia* was estimated to be 3.1–10.8 per million in Japan, while that in Caucasians is about 12.5 per million.

Although statistical studies are lacking, *polycythaemia vera* seems to be uncommon among the Japanese.

Leukaemia, lymphoma and myeloma

Chronic lymphocytic leukaemia is extremely rare in Japan, accounting for only 1.0 per cent of the haematological malignancies recorded. T cell leukaemia is more common than B cell leukaemia in Japanese adults. Adult T cell leukaemia/lymphoma (ATLL) is a unique malignancy first described in Japan by Takatsuki and colleagues. To date more than 500 patients with ATLL have been detected; most of them are from Kyushu, a southern island. More detailed investigation of the patients' birthplaces revealed that they were usually seaside areas or small islands. The predominant physical findings in ATLL patients are peripheral lymph-node enlargement (86 per cent), hepatomegaly (77 per cent), splenomegaly (51 per cent), and skin lesions (49 per cent). However, no mediastinal masses are seen on chest X-rays, and no thymic involvement can be demonstrated histologically at autopsy. The duration of survival ranges from 1 month to more than 6 years. Early reports stated that the course of ATLL is subacute or chronic, but most of the patients studied recently have had a more acute course. Anaemia is relatively mild. The leucocyte count ranges from 9000 to 500 000 × 10^9/1. The percentage of leukaemia cells in the bone marrow is relatively low compared to that in other leukaemias. The leukaemic cells are slightly larger than small lymphocytes and generally exhibit indented or lobulated nuclei, relatively coarsely clumped nuclear chromatin, and scant cytoplasm. The discovery, in 1981, that a type-C retrovirus is the likely aetiological agent of ATLL has attracted much interest. A retrovirus was isolated, characterized, and designated ATLV (adult T cell leukaemia virus) in 1982. Previously, a retrovirus, HTLV (human T cell leukaemia/lymphoma virus) had been isolated from the cultured cells of a patient with an aggressive variant of mycosis fungoides and another patient with Sezary syndrome by Gallo's group in the United States. Although both patients were diagnosed as having cutaneous T cell lymphoma (mycosis fungoides/Sezary syndrome), they had some unusual features which, in retrospect, were similar to those of ATLL. Recent work has shown that HTLV and ATLV are very similair, if not identical, viruses.

The mortality rate for leukaemia among Japanese males in 1975 was 4.27 per 100 000 which is low compared to that of Israel, Greece, Finland, New Zealand, Canada, and Sweden. Females showed the same tendency. It is worth noting, however, that the survivors of the atomic bomb in Hiroshima and Nagasaki developed leukaemia, in particular, chronic myeloid leukaemia, at a higher frequency than that of the general population.

The mortality rate of Hodgkin's disease in Japan is also low compared to that in other countries. The number of patients who died of malignant lymphoma including Hodgkin's disease showed a four-fold increase between 1950 and 1977, and is still increasing. The mortality rate for myeloma is also low, as in other Asian countries.

Haemophilia and other coagulation defects

The incidence of haemophilia in Japan is similar to that in other countries, about 1 to 2 per 10 000 male newborns. The ratio of haemophilia A to B is approximately 5:1. Haemophilia accounts for almost 90 per cent of congenital coagulation defects, the bulk of the remainder being von Willebrand disease.

References

Aoki, K., Ohno, Y., Mizuno, S. and Sasaki, R. (1981). Epidemiological aspects of aplastic anaemia. *Acta haem. Jpn* **44**, 1288–1297.

Takatsuki, K., Yamaguchi, K., Kawano, F., Nishimura, H., Tsuda, H. and Sanada, I. (1984). Adult T cell leukaemia/lymphoma: clincal features and epidemiology and cytogenetic, phenotypic, and functional studies of leukemia cells. In *Human T cell leukemia/lymphoma viruses* (eds R. C. Gallo, M. E. Essex and L. Gross), pp. 261–265. Cold Spring Harbor Laboratory, Cold Spring Harbor, New York.

India

B. C. MEHTA

Anaemia

Anaemia, mainly nutritional, is prevalent in all sections of the Indian population. The incidence is so high that many workers have accepted as 'normal' a level of haemoglobin which is clearly subnormal, namely, 10 g/dl.

Iron-deficiency anaemia

The commonest cause of anaemia, as elsewhere in the world, is iron deficiency. However, unlike western countries, the frequency of iron-deficiency anaemia (IDA) does not differ significantly between the two sexes, between children and adults, and between the pregnant and non-pregnant states – although the severity does differ. The reason for the uniform involvement of the population is the diet consumed by the average Indian. Most of the population is vegetarian because of religious beliefs or economic considerations. The diet is based on cereals from which the bioavailability of iron is of the order of 2–4 per cent. Thus to maintain iron balance, the dietary iron content has to be 25 to 100 mg/day. The daily iron intake of 96 per cent of patients with IDA was found to be less than 20 mg. Marrow iron was absent in almost 50 per cent of apparently normal individuals of both sexes. With such a precarious state of iron balance, even a trivial blood loss can cause severe IDA; it is one of the leading causes of maternal mortality. Parotid enlargement occurs in non-alcoholic patients with IDA who have normal serum protein levels; it regresses with correction of anaemia. Dysphagia as a symptom of iron deficiency shows geographical variation. In Bombay it is uncommon (0.1 per cent of patients with IDA) whereas in Saurashtra (western India) this is a common symptom (1–2 per cent); the incidence of postcricoid carcinoma is also high in the latter population. Abnormalities in electrophysiological response of the myocardium to exercise, nerve conduction velocities in sensory and motor peripheral nerves, gastric acid secretion, D-xylose absorption, volume of salivary secretion, and drug metabolism are observed in IDA. These are corrected within 2–3 days of a total dose of iron dextran therapy, long before a significant elevation of the haemoglobin level. These observations may be related to the effect of iron at tissue level. The incidence of febrile and arthralgic reactions to iron dextran therapy is much higher in India, 40–60 per cent of cases being affected.

The conventional method of preventing iron deficiency by fortification of bread is not applicable in India as most of the population prepares its bread at home. Common salt, which is produced at 3–4 centres in the country, and which is consumed by all sections of the population, is a good vehicle for iron fortification. The National Institute of Nutrition has succeeded in fortifying common salt, and field studies have demonstrated its acceptability and efficacy in improving iron nutrition. This may lead to iron-fortified salt being made available to the whole population.

Megaloblastic anaemia

Addisonian pernicious anaemia is very rare in Indians. The incidence of intrinsic factor antibodies, even amongst individuals with a pattern of vitamin B_{12} malabsorption similar to that which occurs in pernicious anaemia, is lower than that in western countries. However, megaloblastic anaemia due to dietary deficiency and/or malabsorption of vitamin B_{12} or folic acid is common. Vitamin B_{12} deficiency is more common in northeast India while folate deficiency is more frequent in the south. In north and west India vitamin B_{12} and folate deficiencies are equally common. The predominantly vegetarian diet amongst Indians is responsible for poor vitamin B_{12} nutrition; the vitamin is largely derived from bacterial contamination of food and water. Cooking in most parts of India involves boiling of vegetables, and the growing trend is to pressure-cook to save time and fuel. Both these methods destroy folates in the food. Raw green salads are an uncommon constituent of the typical Indian diet. These factors reduce the dietary intake of folate to marginal levels.

Although megaloblastic anaemia is less common than IDA, the serum vitamin B_{12} levels of about 100–150 $\mu g/l$ in apparently healthy non-anaemic Indians indicates borderline vitamin B_{12} nutrition. Anything that causes dietary deprivation or reduces absorption can lead to overt deficiency in a few weeks. Gastrointestinal infections occurring in summer (March–June) are responsible for a number of cases of megaloblastic anaemia seen a couple of months later (June–August). Clusters of cases of megaloblastic anaemia secondary to malabsorption resulting from viral gastroenteritis have been described in south India.

Dimorphic anaemia

Dimorphic anaemia is more common than megaloblastic anaemia. A substantial number of cases of frank megaloblastic anaemia without evidence of iron definiency at the outset (MCV > 100 fl, transferrin saturation > 16 per cent) respond incompletely to vitamin B_{12}/folate therapy. When the haemoglobin level does not rise further, repeat investigations reveal iron deficiency (MCV < 80 fl, transferrin saturation < 16 per cent), and iron therapy restores the haemoglobin level to normal. Most patients with a dimorphic blood picture, particularly those with MCV values in the 80–90 fl range and low transferrin saturation, respond completely to iron therapy alone, while a few need addition of vitamin B_{12}/folic acid for complete response. This suggests that in many cases the deficiency of vitamin B_{12}/folate may be secondary to the adverse effects of iron deficiency on absorption.

Thalassaemias
(See page 19.110.)

Beta thalassaemia
Beta thalassaemia is prevalent all over the Indian subcontinent. Heterozygous β thalassaemia has been observed in 3–5 per cent of apparently normal individuals in different surveys. Though the incidence is much higher (10–15 per cent) in certain communities, e.g. Bhanushali, Lohana, and Sindhi, no community is exempt. Haemoglobin analysis suggests that β° and β^{+} varieties are equally prevalent (see page 19.111). About 15 per cent of heterozygotes have normal Hb A_2 levels and a similar proportion have a normal red cell osmotic red cell fragility. Fetal haemoglobin levels are raised (2–5 per cent) in only about 15 per cent of cases. Investigation of 171 parents of transfusion-dependent cases of thalassaemia major revealed that 1.2 per cent heterozygotes have normal red cell morphology and osmotic fragility, and normal levels of haemoglobin A_2.

The prevalence of β thalassaemia major is 7 per 100 000. Over 90 per cent of these cases are severe and transfusion dependent. A hypertransfusion regimen is available to very few due to economic constraints and therefore these patients show the classical features of Cooley's anaemia (see page 19.112).

Thalassaemia intermedia (see page 19.119) is usually seen in patients who are compound heterozygotes for β and $\delta\beta$ thalassaemia, or β thalassaemia and hereditary persistence of fetal haemoglobin (see page 19.116). A few β thalassaemia heterozygotes show a picture of intermediate severity with moderate to marked splenomegaly, jaundice, chronic non-healing ulcers of the legs, moderately severe anaemia (Hb 5–7 g/dl), and iron overload in the absence of transfusions.

Beta thalassaemia and iron deficiency
The high prevalence of iron deficiency and β thalassaemia on the Indian subcontinent provides a good opportunity to study their interaction. In 95 individuals with β thalassaemia trait, despite the presence of iron deficiency, the haemoglobin A_2 level was still diagnostic, i.e. it was over 3.5 per cent (see page 19.120). In several studies we have demonstrated a negative association between β thalassaemia trait and iron deficiency anaemia, i.e. the incidence of iron deficiency is significantly less amongst carriers of β thalassaemia trait compared to control groups. This might imply an advantage for β thalassaemia trait carriers in maintenance of iron balance, which could confer a survival advantage in a population where the high prevalence of iron deficiency contributes significantly to morbidity and mortality.

Alpha thalassaemia
(See page 19.116.)

Alpha thalassaemia is rare in India. Examination of about 1000 cord blood samples revealed Hb Bart's in 16. However, a high prevalence of α thalassaemia has been detected in tribal populations in western India.

Hereditary spherocytosis
Next to thalassaemia, hereditary spherocytosis is the commonest type of congenital haemolytic anaemia. Affected individuals often attend hospitals for several years and receive non-specific therapy before being correctly diagnosed. This is largely due to the rather cursory attention that a peripheral smear examination receives in the absence of a good haematology department in most parts of the country, including large cities such as Bombay.

Glucose-6-phosphate dehydrogenase (G6PD) and other red cell enzyme deficiencies
G6PD deficiency is widely prevalent in India, affecting about 1 per cent of the population. The occurrence is much higher (10–15 per cent) in certain communities such as Parsees and Bhanushalis. The high incidence in Parsees, who migrated to India from Iran 1300 years ago, has been attributed to selective pressures of malaria to which they were exposed because of their custom of having an open well in the house which provided a breeding place for mosquitoes. Occasional cases of chronic haemolytic anaemia have been reported amongst G6PD-deficient individuals in India. Neonatal jaundice is a common complication attributed to G6PD deficiency. The severity of drug-induced haemolysis suggests that the G6PD deficiency in India is of a Mediterranean type (see page 19.140).

Pyruvate kinase deficiency is rare; other enzyme deficiencies have not been reported.

Haemoglobinopathies
While several abnormal haemoglobins (D, E, J, K, L, M, Q, S) have been reported in India, only three are seen with appreciable frequency in various parts of the country.

Haemoglobin S
The sickle gene is prevalent amongst tribal communities all over the country. Unfortunately, these regions are far removed from large medical institutions and therefore there is no accurate account of the clinical course of the disease in childhood. Most of the reported cases are children over 10 years of age, and adults; their clinical features resemble the mild variety of sickle cell disease described in Middle East countries (see page 19.124). Some of these patients have a palpable spleen even when they have reached the third decade. At least in some of them, the mild course may be the result of the co-existent α thalassaemia.

Haemoglobin E
Haemoglobin E occurs with a high frequency in east India, especially Bengal and Assam, with the result that haemoglobin E-thalassaemia is 2.5 times commoner than homozygous β thalassaemia. Haemoglobin E-thalassaemia subjects have a variable clinical picture, and a number of them reach adult life, and reproduce, although perinatal mortality is high (see page 19.115). They have a significantly higher incidence of intercurrent infection than their unaffected siblings.

Haemoglobin D
Haemoglobin D is encountered mainly in north India though a few cases have been reported from western India.

Haemolytic disease of the newborn
Tetanus toxoid used in pregnant women to prevent tetanus neonatorum has resulted in an increased incidence of haemolytic disease of the newborn due to feto-maternal ABO incompatability. This is related to the increase in the titre of anti A/anti B antibodies in the maternal circulation following the tetanus toxoid injection.

Malaria
With malaria staging a comeback in many parts of India, infection in the first year of life poses diagnostic problems (see Section 5). Anaemia, a palpable spleen, intermittent fever, and a blood picture suggestive of a haemolytic process in the first few months of life point to thalassaemia, which is relatively common. Diagnostic confusion is compounded if malarial parasites go undetected, and if the haemoglobin F level has not yet reached its adult value. Study of the parents helps to exclude thalassaemia, and detection of malarial parasites in the peripheral blood confirms the diagnosis.

Thrombocytopenia and disseminated intravascular clotting (DIC) have been reported in cases of malaria, the presenting features being bleeding and fever. In cases with thrombocytopenia, platelet-associated IgG has been demonstrated, indicating an immune mechanism. During the active phase of malarial infection erythrocyte reduced glutathione, glutathione stability, and glutathione reductase are decreased; these values are restored to normal after antimalarial therapy.

Kala azar
In cases of Kala azar (see Section 5), G6PD activity is decreased; it returns to normal after effective therapy. Red cell survival is decreased and ferrokinetic studies suggest ineffective erythropoieis.

Tropical eosinophilia
Tropical eosinophilia, with or without respiratory manifestations, is so common that any patient with eosinophilia without any obvious cause is treated with diethylcarbamazine (see Section 5). In the absence of any specific tests for tropical eosinophilia, this is the most practical approach.

Leukaemia
Leukaemia accounts for 0.7 to 1.7 per cent of all cases in cancer institutions in India. Amongst childen, it makes up 9 per cent of all cancers. The incidence of leukaemia is 3.0 and 2.5 per 100 000 in males and females, respectively. Chronic myeloid leukaemia (CML) is the commonest type, accounting for 40 per cent of cases. About 80 per cent of CML cases are Philadelphia-chromosome positive. The peak incidence is between 30 and 40 years. Acute lymphoblastic leukaemia (ALL) constitutes about 35 per cent of all cases of leukaemia. The peak age is 5 to 9 years. The incidence of T-ALL is higher (58 per cent in children, 54 per cent in adults) than C-ALL (39 per cent in children and 31 per cent in adults) which may account for the lower rate of complete remission (60–80 per cent) and long-term survival rates (20–30 per cent) observed by Indian workers. Acute myeloblastic leukaemia accounts for about 15 per cent of all cases of leukaemia, with a peak age of 25 to 30 years. Chronic lymphatic leukaemia is the least common variety (10 per cent) with a peak age of 45 to 60 years. Amoebiasis, giardiasis, strongyloidosis, malaria, tuberculosis, and scabies are common complicating infections in cases of acute leukaemia on maintenance therapy.

Lymphoma
Lymphomas account for 3 per cent of all cancers. The proportion of Hodgkin's (HL) to non-Hodgkin's lymphoma is about 7:13. The incidence of HL is 1.0 and 0.6 per 100 000 for males and females, respectively. HL shows a bimodal age distribution with the first peak between 10 and 19 years, and a second between 60 and 69 years for males and a decade later for females. The male to female ratio is 5:1; 25 per cent of cases occur below 14 years of age. Histologically, mixed cellularity, lymphocyte depleted,

lymphocyte predominant, and nodular sclerosis were encountered in 54 per cent, 14 per cent, 23 per cent, and 9 per cent, respectively, in a series of 979 cases.

Idiopathic (autoimmune) thrombocytopenic purpura and anaphylactoid purpura

Chronic idiopathic thrombocytopenic purpura (ITP) is encountered with equal frequency at all ages whereas acute ITP is more common in children than adults. In children there is no sex predilection, whereas among adults, females predominate in both acute and chronic types. Anaphylactoid purpura (Henoch-Schönlein) is slightly less frequent than ITP and is equally common in children and adults. Males predominate in all age groups. In the majority of cases there is no history of preceding infection or drug exposure.

Bleeding disorders and thrombotic states

Inherited coagulation disorders are uncommon, accounting for about 2 per cent of patients attending the haematology clinic of a large teaching hospital in Bombay. Classical haemophilia accounts for about 80 per cent of all inherited coagulation disorders. Although replacement therapy is inadequte and includes only blood or single-unit cryoprecipitate, almost 30 per cent of haemophiliacs in the second decade of life have abnormalities of liver function. This is perhaps due to the higher prevalence of HBSAg in the Indian population. Despite inadequate therapy, about 5 per cent of haemophiliacs have circulating factor VIII:C inhibitors. No cases of AIDS have been reported to date. Christmas disease and von Willebrand's disease each account for about 8 per cent of cases of congenital bleeding disorders.

Liver disease and DIC are the commonest acquired causes of coagulation abnormalities. Apart from the usual causes of DIC, viper bite (*Vipera russelli* and *Echis carinata*) is a common cause in many parts of the country. Investigations of patients with haemorrhagic small-pox have shown evidence of DIC.

Postoperative and postpartum venous thrombosis and thromboembolic complications are rare in India; prophylactic heparin therapy is not necessary. Thrombotic complications during pregnancy and with the use of oral contraceptives are also uncommon compared to western countries.

Aplastic anaemia and agranulocytosis

About 30 per cent of cases of aplastic anaemia follow viral infections, especially hepatitis, measles, and mumps, or ingestion of such drugs as dipyrone, butazolidine, sulphonamides, or chloramphenicol. These drugs are responsible for about 30 cases of agranulocytosis in Bombay every year.

Splenomegaly

Tropical and non-tropical idiopathic splenomegaly (see page 19.189) are encountered with almost equal frequency, in addition to the common causes of an enlarged spleen such as portal hypertension, haemoglobinopathies, and haemolytic anaemias, leukaemias, lymphomas, malaria, and Kala azar. It is unlikely that the tropical splenomegaly syndrome (see page 19.189) that occurs in Africa and other regions occurs frequently in India (see page 19.272). In patients with hepatosplenomegaly, prolonged pyrexia and no other positive findings, tuberculosis and lymphoma are found with almost equal frequency on biopsy, laparotomy or autopsy.

References

Advani, S. H., Jussawalla, D. J., Rao, D. N., Gangadharan, P. and Shetty, P. A. (1979). A study of 1126 leukemia cases – epidemiologic and end result analysis. *Ind. J. Cancer* **16**, 8–17.
Chatterjea, J. B. (1965). Observations on some aspects of iron deficiency anaemia. *J. Assn. Phys. Ind.* **13**, 13–22.
Desai, H. G. and Antia, F. P. (1972). Vitamin B_{12} malabsorption due to intrinsic factor deficiency in Indian subjects. *Blood* **40**, 747–753.
Gupta, S. P., Arya, R. K. and Guliani, R. K. (1977). Latent iron deficiency – prevalence and clinical spectrum. *Ind. J. med. Res.* **65**, 366–371.
Health Statistics of India (1983). Central Bureau of Health Intelligence, Directorate of Health Services, Ministry of Health and Family Welfare, Government of India, Nirman Bhawan, New Delhi, pp. 201, 202, 210.
Mehta, B. C., Doctor, R. G., Purandare, N. M. and Patel, J. C. (1967). Hemorrhagic small-pox: a study of 22 cases to determine the cause of bleeding. *Ind. J. med. Sci.* **21**, 518–523.
——, Dave, V. B., Joshi, S. R., Baxi, A. J., Bhatia, H. M. and Patel, J. C. (1972). Study of hematological and genetical characteristics of Cutchhi Bhanushali community. *Ind. J. med. Res.* **60**, 305–311.
——, Bhatt, P. D. and Patel, J. C. (1973). Aplastic anemia – a study of 37 cases. *Ind. J. med. Sci.* **27**, 440–497.
—— (1981). Inherited coagulation disorders in India. *Ind. J. Pediat.* **48**, 525–531.
—— (1982). Hemoglobinopathies. *J. Assn. Phys. Ind.* **30**, 615–620.
—— (1982). Widespread iron deficiency anemia in India – its causes. *Ind. J. med. Sci.* **36**, 108–112.
—— (1982). Interaction between nutritional anemia and thalassemia. *Ind. J. med. Sci.* **36**, 180–187.
—— (1984). Effects of iron deficiency – an iceberg phenomenon. *J. Assn. Phys. Ind.* **32**, 895–900.
Mukherji, S., Naik, S. R., Srivastava, P. N., Choudhuri, S. N. and Chuttani, H. H. (1982). Salivary secretions in iron deficiency anemia. *J. Oral Med.* **37**, 130–132.
Sukumaran, P. K. (1978). Thalassaemias. *J. Assn Phys. Ind.* **26**, 627–636.
Swarup-Mitra, S. (1983). The clinical and hematological profile of thalassemia and hemoglobinopathies in India. *Ind. Pediat.* **20**, 701–713.
Talwalkar, G. V., Sampat, M. B. and Gangadharan, P. (1982). Hodgkin's disease in Western India. *Cancer* **50**, 353–359.

SECTION 20
DISEASES OF THE SKIN

DISEASES OF THE SKIN

T. J. RYAN

Introduction

What is dermatology?

Dermatology is concerned with the skin and as such it is concerned not only with diseases but with the Greek ideal of beauty manifested in the confident nude typified by the most famous of the sculptures – the Venus de Milo. There is therefore concern with the cosmetic as well as with disease. This in turn causes the dermatologist to look at public attitudes towards disfigurement: parent, school teacher, spouse, employer, beautician, and nurse. Whether it be incipient baldness, the wrinkles of ageing or tattoos, there are cultural factors to be understood and a decision may have to be made about the cost of treatment. When is ugliness illness; how much is disfigurement worth in a court of law, and on what does the quality of life depend.

Throughout this Section, the impairment, disability, and handicap of skin disease will be emphasized and the reader will be thought of as a member of a team of caretakers of the skin. The dermatologist should be the leader but often he or she will be absent and others using the chapter may be the advice givers. I have tried to incorporate into the text the view points of many caretakers of the skin distributed throughout the world.

Dermatology: the scope of this text

When writing a section on dermatology for a general medical textbook it is usual to concentrate on the skin as it is involved coincidently with internal disease processes. This section also aims to help the physician who has no dermatological colleague to help him with the diagnosis and management of what would normally be regarded as purely dermatological conditions.

Dermatology is made difficult by its great variety of physical signs. It is an encyclopaedic subject with more than 1000 named entities. Fortunately, fewer than a dozen diseases represent 70 per cent of dermatological practice – acne; bacteriological, viral, and fungal infections; tumours; dermatitis; psoriasis; leg ulcers; and warts.

Every good physician looks at the skin all the time while he is listening to the patient or eliciting physical signs. Whether he recognizes the minutiae that a dermatologist has been trained to see depends not merely on seeing but knowing their significance. Unfortunately so much of recognition is the naming of physical signs and dermatologists have accumulated an enormous amount of jargon. Not all of this is necessary for management. In this account uncommon signs have been omitted where their recognition results in no benefit to the patient.

A physician should know enough to recognize a physical sign which is a threat to life such as a melanoma, the malignant pustule of anthrax, or the eroded blisters in the mouth in pemphigus vulgaris. Otherwise he should know how to recognize signs which are significant indications of systemic disease such as erythema nodosum, splinter haemorrhages or arsenical keratoses, and the white macules of tuberous sclerosis.

There is no branch of medicine more dependent on clinical acumen and on previous observation and less dependent on the laboratory. However, in no other branch of medicine is there a requirement for the specialist to be so experienced in histopathology. The value of this information is for sorting out that which is unrecognizable to the naked eye: it does not often alter the management of the disease. One advantage of the skin biopsy is that it can be sent away to experts, together with a photograph of the clinical lesion.

Where skin disease is the primary cause of severe handicap in countries where the physician is the only doctor, simple measures to give relief should not be neglected simply because the physician claims not to be specially trained in dermatology and has not learned its language.

In spite of the advances in antibiotics and corticosteroids which have completely altered the nature of skin clinics in technically advanced countries, there is no diminution in the number of patients attending for help with skin problems. There is an increase in skin cancer, in the demand for cosmetic treatment, and in the number of agents in the environment which damage the skin and cause dermatitis. In developing countries the overwhelming demand is for better management of infection of the skin by bacteria and parasites. It does not change for the better because poverty, malnutrition, poor housing, and water shortage are often unsolved.

References

Braverman (1981). *Skin signs of systemic disease* 2nd edn, p. 965. W. B. Saunders, Philadelphia.

Calnan, C. D. and Levene, G. M. (1974). *A colour atlas of dermatology.* Wolfe Medical Books, London.

Fitzpatrick, T. B., Eisen, A. Z., Wolff, K., Freedberg, I. M. and Austen, F. (1979). *Dermatology in general medicine*, p. 1884. McGraw-Hill, New York.

Rook, A., Wilkinson, D. S. and Ebling, F. J. G. (1986). *Textbook of dermatology* 4th edn, p. 2366. Blackwell Scientific Publications, Oxford.

The structure of the skin

The skin consists of the epidermis and its supporting dermis lying on a layer of fat (Fig. 1). In man, unlike most animals, the muscle layer lying beween the dermis and underlying tissues is found only in the scrotum. The epithelium gives rise to eccrine sweat or apocrine glands. In hair-bearing skin, the hair and sebaceous glands are also derived from the epithelial layer. Hair and sweat glands are described in the appropriate sections (see pages 20.52 and 20.56).

The epidermis comprises basal cells adherent to the basal lamina which by division give rise to successive layers of cells (keratinocytes) whose principal function is to synthesize the insoluble protein, keratin. As the cells reach the surface they lose their nucleus and become a dead envelope containing keratin. The epidermis is infiltrated with dendritic cells, melanocytes, and Langerhans cells. Melanocytes feed the basal cells with melanin, a complex polymer which protects the underlying dermis from the damaging effects of sunlight. The Langerhans cells are macrophages which also secrete enzymes which hasten the degeneration and orderly differentiation of the upper dermis. They provide an antigen recognition system expressing Fc, IgG, and C3 receptors as well as 1a antigens. Depletion prevents contact dermatitis mediated by delayed cellular immunity.

The dermis supports the epidermis and its adnexa. The rich vasculature has a generous reserve to meet the requirements of wounding and repair so common at the surface. It is adapted for thermoregulation. The dermis also supports the extremely complex innervation so necessary for touch and for sensing danger.

The main constituents of the dermis are the fibrous matrix collagen and elastic fibres embedded in a mucopolysaccharide ground

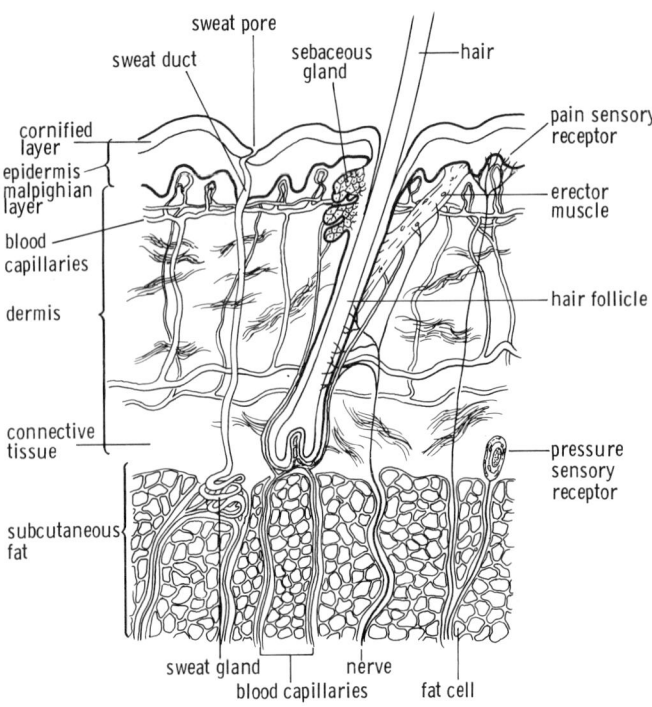

Fig. 1 The structure of human skin.

substance. Fibroblasts, mast cells, and histiocytes are scattered throughout the dermis. The two functions of basal cells, repair or reduplication, and the production of keratin, require that the epidermis should turn over in a controlled way and die in an orderly fashion. The turnover takes about 30 days from the time of reduplication at the basal layer to loss from the surface. The lower layers of the epidermis depend on oxygen for mitosis and migration, but the upper differentiating layers are anaerobic with no mitochondria. The optimum temperature of epidermal metabolism is probably at a lower level than most body cells. The energy of the epidermal cells is derived from both lipid and carbohydrates. Current biochemical interest is in the balance between cyclic AMP and GMP and the role of prostaglandins in the control of epidermal cell turnover.

References

Goldsmith, L. (1982). *Biochemistry and physiology of the skin*, p. 1323. Oxford University Press, Oxford.

Lever, W. E. and Schaunburg-Lever, G. (1975). *Histopathology of the skin* 5th edn. J. B. Lippincott, Philadelphia.

Mier, B. D. and Cotton, D. W. K. (1976). *Molecular biology of the skin*, p. 469. Blackwell Scientific Publications, Oxford.

Functions of the skin

The skin is the largest organ of the body and it is exhibited. It is continuously exposed to injury.

The skin is not only displayed but it is fondled, and together with hair and nails it is a sexual organ of attraction. It has to be both supple and strong because it is bent, stretched, trodden upon, and compressed as well as scratched and prodded. It must have a capacity to repair itself rapidly to form a physical barrier impervious to excessive water loss or to absorption from the environment. It must resist wear and tear. These functions are impaired in skin disease which makes those affected more vulnerable and less able to reconstitute themselves after damage as well as causing them social embarrassment.

The skin contains Langerhans cells. These are macrophages which detect environmental antigens and recognize what is poten-

tially dangerous. The sensation of pain, so finely mediated by the precise innervation of the epidermis, has a similar warning function helping us to recognize the environment and to itch in the presence of smaller invaders and to follow this with an accurate scratch response.

There is increasing evidence that the skin may act as an organ of presystemic metabolism of drugs and other substances applied topically and that it is capable of forming toxic metabolites.

The epidermis is also host to melanocytes which produce the pigment melanin, an absorbent for free radicals released by a variety of inflammatory agents including the injury of ultraviolet irradiation. Vitamin D is synthesized by the epidermis.

The dermis is more than a supporting structure. It determines many of the characteristics of the epidermis and controls regional variations. It is an essential inducer and controller of the adnexal organs such as hair, sweat, and sebaceous glands and provides a selective environment whereby hormones such as oestrogen and testosterone can influence some epithelial organs but not others. The complex anastomoses of the blood supply are there to support all functions, including the need for thermoregulation. Diseases of the dermis result in disorders of growth of the overlying epidermis and changes in responsiveness of the adnexal organs to normal physiological processes as well as in a failure to conserve heat. Sexual attraction is an important function on which the fortunes of the cosmetic industry are founded. It is subject to whim and to advertising. The social anthropologist has done much to draw attention to that which denotes sex appeal. Colouring or decolouring, tattooing, distorting, stretching, and, of course, adorning with jewellery and clothing are part of the appeal. All of which add to the demands for the dermatologist as well as for the beautician, tattooist, trichologist, and a host of fringe activities concerned with health. Sex appeal depends on skin not being too greasy, too matt, or too wrinkled. The white adolescent wants powder to reduce a greasy forehead; the black African wants grease to rid him of any degree of powdery exfoliation. One must have a beauty spot and another must not. The stink of some scents attracts while sweaty feet and rotting shoes repel.

References

Goldsmith, L. (1982). *Biochemistry and physiology of the skin*. Oxford University Press, Oxford.

Jarrett, A. (1973–80). *Physiology and pathophysiology of the skin* Vols 1–7. Academic Press, New York.

Journal of Investigative Dermatology (1980). Analysis of research needs and priorities in dermatology. *J. invest. Derm.* **73**, suppl. 5, 514.

Lancet (1981). The Langerhans cell. **ii**, 672–673.

The influence of the psyche

It is well known that blushing or cold sweats and pallor are skin reflections of the mind. Any group of students shown an acarus under the microscope will laugh at the sudden awareness of itching it induces in one of their number. But such awareness is typical of the relationship of the mind and the skin. There have been many experiments showing that the acute inflammatory process mediating a weal or any exudation is susceptible to enhancement by anxiety or diminution by relaxation. While a 'neurotic' basis for urticaria and prurigo nodularis or lichen simplex are no longer overemphasized by terms such as angioneurotic oedema or neurodermatitis, it is modern western scientific medicine alone which has made such terms unpopular. This is because it cannot be measured, it is mainly subjective, and therefore by some, not to be believed. Pavlovian concepts of the neurovegetative are popular amongst Russian dermatologists. Practitioners of indigenous medicine or fringe medicine, the witch doctor as well as almost every lay person, recognize a link between anxiety and skin disease.

The principal anxieties resulting from skin disease relate to the fear of being infectious, unclean, and ultimately, unwelcome. If one considers what may happen to a patient with leprosy, such fears are well founded. As with venereal disease, often the up-bringing, religious, and social mores of the patient will determine the reaction to skin disease.

It is surprising how few patients will accept that our largest organ can be defective in its own right or that it and it alone can simply wear out or be worn down like the heels of a leather shoe, which after all is only skin. They will, however, believe that their skin disease is due to a malfunction of the liver, an impurity in the blood, or to a dietary indiscretion. Such beliefs have to be met with tactful explanation.

One frustration which is experienced by the skin patient far too often is to ask advice or to seek help and to be told that the problem is trivial. So often a patient sees his problem placed second to an acute emergency and has to accept the correctness of this. However, like all chronic or trivial disease, no one attempts to measure handicap and so the effect it has on the individual is belittled.

The handicap of skin disease

Because patients with skin disease rarely die of it and hardly ever constitute an emergency, the subject of dermatology is a minor specialty. It is not thought essential for medical students to know the subject well and even nursing training may include little of it. As a topic for research it has little glamour and attracts funds less easily than cancer, transplants or CT scanners. Many parts of the world have no dermatological service whatsoever.

Why then should one argue that the need for resources, whether manpower, buildings, or money for research, is greater than previously estimated?

The answer is that the patient with skin disease is at a disadvantage quite as great as most other diseases when consideration is given to a person's capacity to achieve the personal and economic independence of his fellows. This may be due to an inherited or acquired constitutional defect but commonly there is also an environmental factor. Writers of handicap refer to the eastern proverb, 'I wept because I had no shoes, until I met a man who had no feet'.

Dermatologists will know that a man who cannot wear boots because of epidermolysis bullosa or because of a hypersensitivity to agents used in the footwear industry is as disabled as an amputee when the distance he can walk is the measure of his handicap. Personal independence and economic independence constitute the individual's viability as a separate unit.

A human being with skin disease can function like other humans only in respect of his ability to think and communicate. In almost all other respects his functions are threatened.

Common diseases, such as dermatitis and psoriasis, affect the following 'functional specificities' on which personal autonomy depends: (a) to move around in and manipulate the environment; (b) to service oneself; (c) to resist normal stresses and traumas; (d) to groom oneself; and (e) to organize oneself emotionally. Some diseases, such as leprosy, affect other faculties such as sight. To have personal and economic independence it is necessary to perform effectively wherever one finds oneself. Skin diseases which affect the hands and feet prevent the patient from getting out and about or from moving around at home (Figs 2 and 3). Skin disease for a variety of reasons may prevent or threaten the expected care of one's home, self, or family, and it often interferes with education and employment.

The threat to life Before expanding on the subject of handicap, which is the most prominent reason for giving attention to skin disease because it is so common, it is worth considering briefly whether skin disease does sometimes constitute an emergency and whether it may cause death.

Angioedema affecting the upper respiratory tract is the most frightening of dermatological emergencies and it accounts for the deaths of most cases of hereditary angioedema due to C_1 esterase deficiency. Occasionally other causes of urticaria may be responsible.

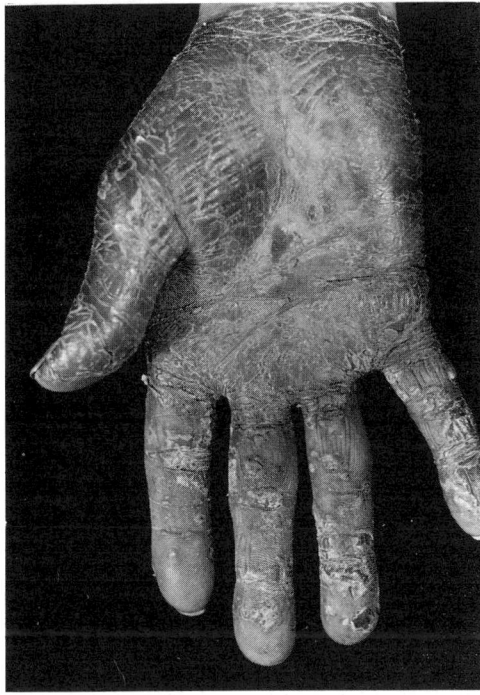

Fig. 2 Psoriasis of the hands interferes with dexterity and makes patients unwelcome in many occupations such as food handling or public relations.

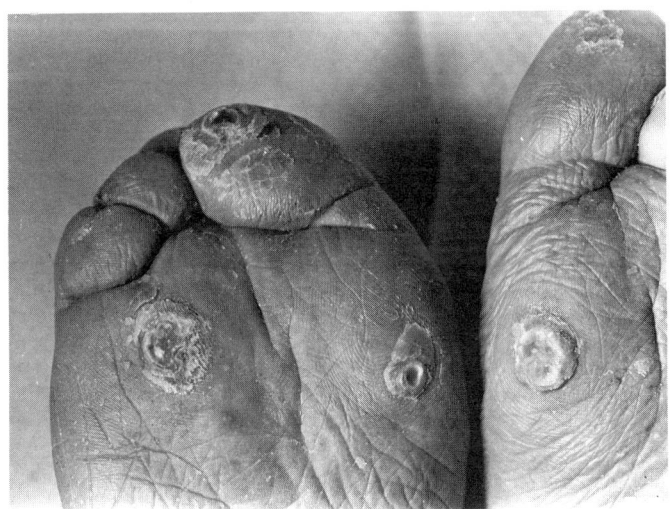

Fig. 3 Callus or corn is common in ageing skin and pain can make walking very difficult. The patient is more handicapped than an amputee with a comfortable prosthesis.

Respiratory obstruction is recorded in other diseases such as epidermolysis bullosa due to inhalation of 'casts' and in Behçet's disease due to ulceration of the larynx.

Because the skin is the largest organ of the body and because it is exposed to the environment, many chronic skin diseases cause death by failure to protect the person from irritants, infective agents, and climate or by loss of fluid or the increased demands on internal organs such as the heart. Blistering disorders, such as pemphigus vulgaris, widespread impetigo, or epidermolysis bullosa, are examples of skin disease which are especially threatening.

Erythroderma due to eczema (Fig. 4), psoriasis, or lymphoma commonly results in failure of body temperature control, heart failure, or more rarely, uncontrollable protein-losing enteropathy.

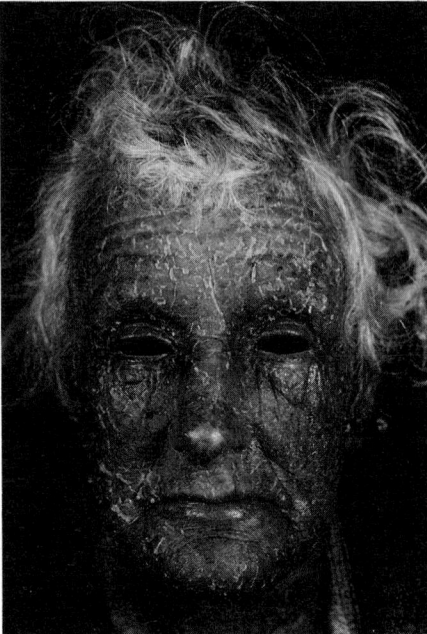

Fig. 4 Some diseases are a threat to life. Exfoliative dermatitis is so because of fluid loss, heart failure, and loss of temperature control. This patient died following perforation of the small intestine while on steroid therapy.

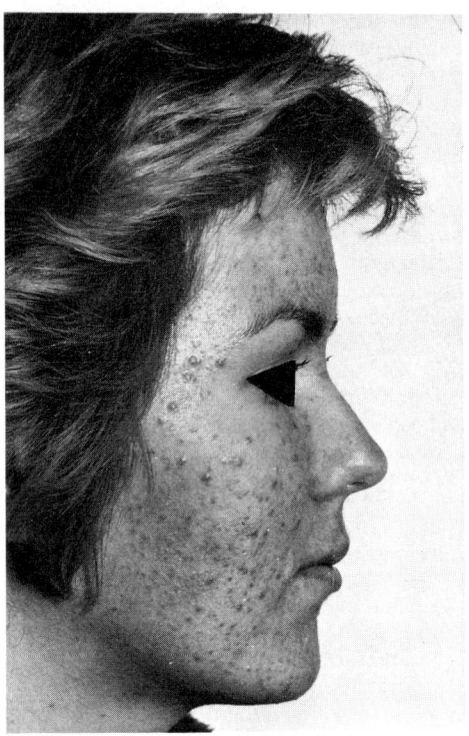

Fig. 5 Acne vulgaris is a cosmetic disability which makes a teenager feel unwelcome and contributes to delinquency.

Fluid loss and prerenal failure are important and particularly relevant in hot countries. In the tropics many die from uncontrolled dermatitis and the superinfections which are often associated with it.

Threatening personal autonomy Not to be able to resist normal stresses and traumas is a common inconvenience. It accounts for the need for sufferers from atopic eczema, even when in remission, to avoid occupations such as hairdressing, nursing, food handling, and mechanical engineering. For those with a lower intelligence quotient unemployment may be the consequence. Wear and tear of the skin is the most common consequence of work and those who have lowered resistance are unable to work. A severe example of such lowered resistance is epidermolysis bullosa. The Koebner phenomenon which is the development of skin disease at sites of injury accounts in part for the common problem of adult psoriasis.

To communicate and to be welcome Because our skin is on the surface it is there for display. Through it we make contact with others. It is observed and touched. If there are defects in it the observer may not like what he sees and will not touch. Many children with such defects experience insults from other children who refuse to hold hands or play with them. Adults experience more subtle signals which may prevent a normal sex life and interfere with employment (Fig. 5).

The greatest handicap of all is to be unwelcome. It matters not whether this is actually so or a belief of the patient without any actual experience of rejection; it is the commonest social effect of skin disease. The whiteness of the skin of vitiligo, the blood on the sheets and scale on clothing and furniture left by the psoriatic are a huge disadvantage. The albino is an outcast in Africa and the severe psoriatic is similarly rejected in the United Kindom.

The patient with skin disease is unemployable in any job in which he or she is in the public eye or involved in food preparation. For the many whose skin is vulnerable to minor wear and tear of quite ordinary living, the list of jobs which should be discouraged is large.

The physician who does nothing to alleviate the handicap of

skin disease is turning his back on an appreciable problem which often only a little knowledge and care can do much to remedy.

Prevalence It is difficult to obtain an estimate of prevalence of skin disease and the extent of the handicap. But an examination of more than 20 000 Americans between the ages of 1 and 74 revealed that 60 per cent had a significant skin condition, actually least frequent amongst children and most common in the old. In about 10 per cent the condition limited activity and was a physical handicap. Often skin complaints persisted for more than five years. Diseases of the hand were the greatest handicap. It has been estimated in the USA that 6.8 million Americans were handicapped in their social relationships because of a skin condition. Diseases of the skin account for almost half of all reported cases of industrial illness in the USA, and the cost of this, estimated by the National Institute of Health, is more than $2542 billion per annum. In a country which is well endowed with dermatologists 60 per cent of the skin conditions are in fact dealt with by general physicians and such conditions are the commonest reason for consultation.

References

Jowett, S. and Ryan, T. (1985). Dermatology patients and their doctors. *Clin. exp. Dermatol.* **10**, 246–254.
—— and —— (1985). Skin disease and handicap: an analysis of the impact of skin conditions. *Soc. Sci. Med.* **20**, 425–429.
Panconesi, E. (1985). Stress and skin diseases. *Psychosomatic dermatology.* J. D. Lippincott, Philadelphia.
Stankler, L. (1981). The effect of psoriasis on the sufferer. *Clin. exp. Dermatol.* **6**, 303–306.
Whitlock, F. A. (1977). *Psychophysiological aspects of skin disease.* Lloyd Luke, London.

The provision of skin care even when the diagnosis is not known

It is not necessary to know the diagnosis – to give a name to the physical signs – in order to treat the skin, but it is a helpful short cut. For the beginner the textbooks listed on page 20.1 are difficult to use. The naming of skin disease is like stamp collecting, and it is helpful to match the physical signs to a picture in a book – there are several excellent catalogues of the skin, listed below.

In this account it is assumed that the reader will be able to diagnose very common disorders like dermatitis, psoriasis, acne, leg ulcers, or warts, and the main purpose of the text will be to guide management.

When the physician is faced with physical signs which are familiar to him, such as pigmentation or purpura, and for which the causes are numerous but not on the tip of his tongue, a checklist is provided often with minimal detail. Intermediate are the large number of specific entities known to dermatologists, but described in no more than a paragraph concerning principal diagnostic features and the best management.

Most patients like to be given a diagnosis but are happy with general terms such as dermatitis, wart, or birth mark. They hope for management in its broadest sense. They want treatment for itch, stink, scale, or disfigurement, and the general principles of the treatment of these are the same whatever the exact diagnosis. They want advice as to whether it is an infection, due to something they have eaten, whether it is hereditary or something missing from their diet, and whether it is a skin cancer or something to which they are allergic. These problems can be approached in general terms and do not need great diagnostic acumen.

When in doubt, a biopsy should be done. This is not difficult and because one can see exactly what one is biopsying it is possible to identify very small areas which are likely to be diagnostic. Biopsies by dermatologists are small compared to those by surgeons, and the morbidity is very slight and scarring negligible.

A biopsy is not necessarily always a certain answer – very often it is the combination of histology and a good clinical description that provides the final diagnosis. No pathologist should be asked to diagnose without good clinical details.

So much of skin disease in the tropics or in the malnourished, the poor, and badly housed is due to or complicated by infection. Bacterial swabs and scrapings for fungus infection should be done even when the suspicion is not high.

As mentioned above, the fear of rejection is great and an important principle of management is a sympathetic hearing. A guide to the questioning which makes such a hearing relevant is listed in the next section. Touch is a signal of acceptance. No dermatologist diagnoses from a distance or even from the end of the bed and the texture of the skin and the depth of the lesion is appreciated by touch. Minor procedures like skin scraping for mycelia or an excision biopsy never fail to convince that the problem is being well managed.

The sympathetic listener

The basis of the interview is optimal communication of information. It should not frustrate or cause anxiety and depression. The doctor should be identified and know who is being interviewed and what has been previously diagnosed or prescribed by reading the patient's notes before the interview. Relevant questioning is important because time is so often limited. The following is a suitable basis for such an interview:

1. How long have you had it; exactly when did it start; have you had it before?

2. Which part of your skin was first affected; where were you when it started; what were you doing?

3. How did it progress, to what sites, and what was there before?

4. Does it come and go; how long does each individual lesion last?

5. Does it itch; is it painful, tender, anaesthetic?

6. Does it develop blisters or clear fluid?

7. Does anything make it better?

8. Does anything make it worse?

9. What ointments, creams, lotions, or bath oils have you used? Have you had any medicine or injections?

10. Has anyone else you know got it; does it run in your family;

do any other diseases like asthma, eczema, or hay fever run in your family?

11. Have you had any previous illnesses?

It should not be forgotten that accurate answers are rare. In rural or tropical climates, particulars about the duration of an ailment are frequently vague.

The examination

Undressing and removal of bandages, and in some countries, even the removal of a hat may be difficult to arrange. One will learn more by looking everywhere and when in doubt, the patient must be undressed. A full examination may include a look at the genitalia and the mouth, but even if the rash is diagnosable at a glance and a history is not obtainable, it is important to speak to the patient. Remember that he has a handicap which responds to a sympathetic hearing as well as to a careful examination.

One should keep looking until something is recognized. Often much of a rash is atypical but somewhere there should be a classical physical sign. Good lighting is essential and of all lighting, the sun is the best. Many hospitals and clinics in the tropics are purposely placed out of the sun and are too dark for accurate observation. One should not be ashamed to use glasses, or even a magnifying glass. This is essential for nailfold telangiectasia or for recognizing an acarus or crab lice.

Touch assures the patient there is no abhorrence and that contagiousness and uncleanliness are insignificant. Papules are palpable, macules are not. This can be important in, for instance, patch testing in which purely macular responses should be ignored. Compression distinguishes between purpura and telangiectasia. It reveals much about the depth of the lesion and its hardness.

Aids

Skin scrapings for fungal mycelia Skin scrapings are best taken from moist areas since mycelia in dried scales or in the nails may be too desiccated. Scrapings should be placed on a slide with 10 per cent potassium hydroxide which helps to clear the keratin of extraneous material which obscures the fungus. Gentle heating is helpful. In hot climates the rate of evaporation from potassium hydroxide is such that crystals form and it is best to renew the bottle regularly.

Finding parasites A microscope is essential for the diagnosis of mycelia, lice, and other parasites. Attempting to find parasites in the skin of patients may be difficult, and is often helped by devices. For instances, vaseline placed over the aperture of a fly bite may encourage the larvae to expose themselves since they cannot survive without oxygen. If onchocerciasis is suspected, a new itchy papule can be picked up on the end of a needle and quickly snipped and placed in saline and examined under the microscope to see whether the microfilaria swims out. The acarus can be picked out of the end of the burrow on the fronts of the wrists and between the fingers.

Wood's light Wood's light is ultraviolet light (UVA, 360 nm) and is used for recognizing white areas in white skin as in tuberous sclerosis. Fluorescence is also helpful for *Microsporum audouini* and *M. canis* which fluoresce green. Erythrasma due to *Corynebacterium minutissimum* fluoresces coral red. Porphyrins in teeth or urine fluoresce pink and anaerobes such as *Bacteroides melanogenicus* in wounds and ulcers fluoresce red.

Biopsy The lesion chosen for biopsy should not be modified by excoriation, therapy, or secondary infection. Small lesions should be totally excised and it is usual to remove skin in the shape of an elipse along lines of stretch known as Langer's lines. On the face this is equivalent to the wrinkles. It is useful to have diagrams on the wall of the operation room (Fig. 6). In subjects prone to keloids it is best to avoid the sides of the face, neck, sternal region, and shoulders. It is often useful to biopsy the edge of the lesion so that it can be compared with adjacent normal-looking skin. Too

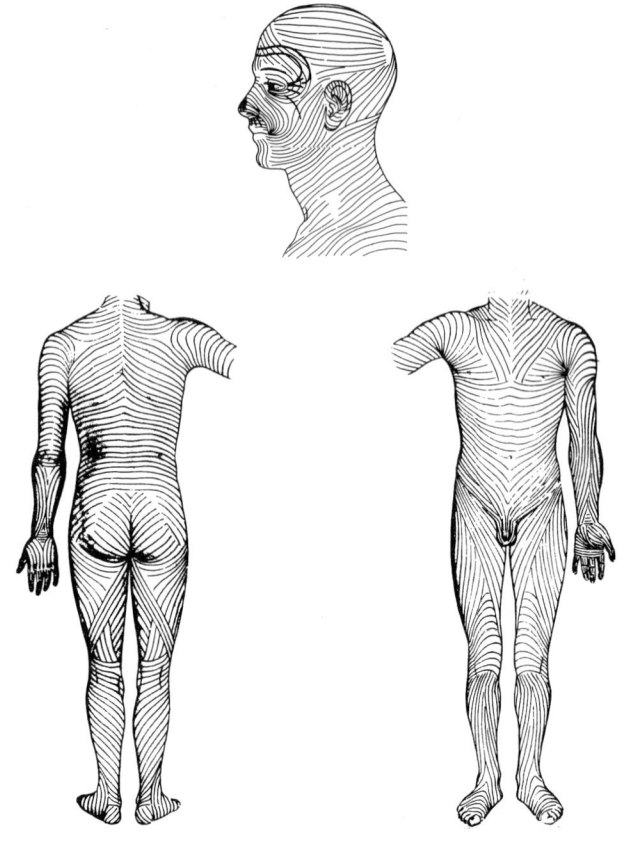

Fig. 6 The lines of tension and elasticity in the skin determine satisfactory healing. Biopsies should be taken with the lines of incision by the knife corresponding with the lines in these figures. They approximately correspond to wrinkles in elderly skin, but there are exceptions, as round the eye, where wrinkles are a safer guide than lines of tension (as indicated by darker lines).

much squeezing of the biopsy by forceps makes it impossible to analyse. An appropriate fixative is 10 per cent formalin for at least 12 hours.

Most bleeding is venous since skin is well endowed with venules. It follows that bleeding can be controlled by elevation and by pressure on the skin surrounding the wound.

Inexpensive transport systems so that biopsies can be posted to experts have been described.

The histological report may include the following terms:

Hyperkeratosis: thickening of the horny layer usually resulting from retention and increased adhesion of epidermal cells.

Parakeratosis: cell nuclei in the horny layer usually resulting from a high rate of cell turnover as in psoriasis.

Spongiosis: separation of prickle cells by oedema fluid, i.e. the epidermis looks like a sponge – a feature of eczema.

Acantholysis: loss of cohesion between prickle cells and isolation, and balloon-like appearance of individual epidermal cells, a feature of pemphigus.

Liquefaction: degeneration and rupture of basal cells – characteristic of lupus erythematosus, lichen planus, and erythema multiforme.

Pigmentary incontinence: the shedding of melanin from the epidermis into the dermis following injury to the basal layer.

Elastotic degeneration: changes in dermal collagen which occur in light-exposed and ageing skin. Whorled masses of disorganized elastin staining fibres replace normal collagen.

Fibrinoid degeneration: deposition of eosinophilic material which resembles fibrin.

Table 1

Disease	Immunofluorescence findings (direct)	Serum (indirect)
Pemphigus	IgG intercellular in the epidermis	Positive in 90%
Pemphigoid	IgG and complement is linear at the dermo-epidermal junction	Positive in 70%
Linear IgA dermatosis	IgA is linear at the dermo-epidermal junction	Negative
Dermatitis herpetiformis	IgA, granular often complement in dermal papillae	None
Lupus erythematosus	Granular band of IgG or IgM or complement at the dermo-epidermal junction	Antinuclear antibodies

Necrobiosis: a type of focal necrosis of collagen which leads to the formation of a palisading granuloma, i.e. macrophages lining up like a fence around the necrotic material.

Lichenoid: a heavy infiltrate of white cells hugs the epidermal interface with the dermis and fills the upper dermis.

Immunofluorescence examination: modern immunofluorescence techniques mostly require frozen biopsies, or storage in special transport media, and they cannot be done on fixed or paraffin embedded material. Immunofluorescence is most useful for bullous disease (Table 1).

References

Ackerman, A. B. (1978). *Histologic diagnosis of inflammatory skin diseases*, p. 863. Lea and Febiger, Philadelphia.

Binford, C. M. and Connor, D. M. (1976). *Pathology of tropical and extraordinary diseases*, Vols 1 and 2. Armed Forces Institute of Pathology.

Jones, R. L. and Ponninghaus, J. M. (1982). *Leprosy Rev.* **53**, 67–68.

Lever, W. E. and Schaunburg-Lever, G. (1975). *Histopathology of the skin*, 5th edn, p. 848. J. B. Lippincott, Philadelphia.

Penneys, N. S. (1984). Immunoperoxidase methods and advances in skin biology. *J. Am. Acad. Dermatol.* **11**, 284–290.

The basis of rashes

The skin is not a homogeneous organ. It varies in thickness, rate of epidermal turnover, amount and quality of hair, sebaceous glands, or sweat, and in many other qualities. Clearly its components have a structure and some rashes affecting only one of these will have the distribution of that constituent, e.g. hair follicles in folliculitis (Fig. 7), sweat glands in prickly heat, sebaceous glands in acne vulgaris, or dermatomal in herpes zoster, or annular and reticulate as in some rashes determined by vascular anatomy.

Inflammation near the surface of the skin usually damages the epidermis so that vesiculation and scaling becomes a feature of the response, whereas deep dermal or subcutaneous inflammation merely produces 'lumps' known as nodules.

The rate of development of the rash often is determined by the type of inflammatory response – oedematous weals or blisters are more acute than white cell infiltration, purpura, or pustules, and ischaemic necrosis and exfoliation are late responses.

The clinician is a detective and in assessing physical signs must know the sequence of events leading up to what he can see. He must look at the distribution of the rash as well as its minutest morphology. Some classic distributions are shown in Fig. 8 while Table 2 illustrates some well-known morphological terms.

The concept of endogenous, constitutional, or host acting as a receptor for an exogenous and noxious trigger is an important explanation of rashes.

The management of skin disease requires elimination of possible agents causing injury and a recognition and treatment of altered host responses. Thus endogenous rashes tend to be symmetrical whereas a biting insect does not know about symmetry, and fleas, for example, will produce groups of bites quite indiscriminately. Unlike the rashes of secondary syphilis the site of the primary chancre is quite uninfluenced by host symmetry (Fig. 11).

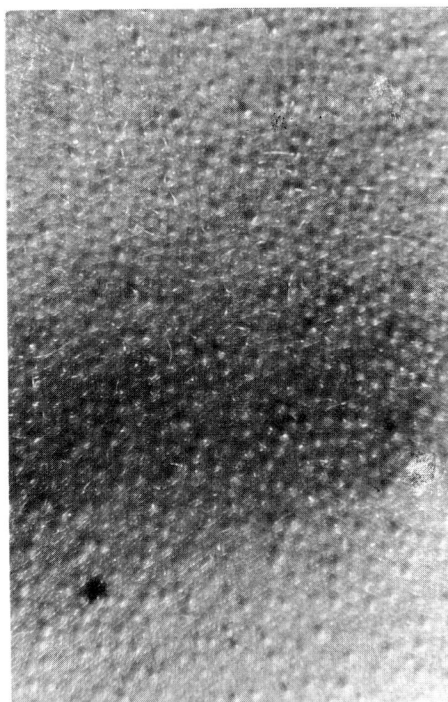

Fig. 7 Perifollicular hyperkeratosis having the distribution of the hair follicle.

Fungus infections such as cattle ringworm or even the human trichophyton rubrum similarly are frequently more obvious on one side of the body than another, whereas psoriasis is usually exactly symmetrical.

Injury to the skin from contact dermatitis usually has the distribution of contact; in cases due, for example, to mascara, gloves, or shoes, there will be symmetry (Fig. 12), but casually brushing against a noxious plant will produce bizarre asymmetrical patterns. Scratching spares the centre of the back, and a completely clear area between the shoulder blades when the rest of the body is covered with scratch marks (Fig. 13a) suggests that the cause of the rash is the injury done by such scratching. *Acarus* seems not to like climbing about in hairy areas so usually spares the head but favours between the fingers, the front of the wrists, or the glans penis.

External irradiation from the sun spares beneath the lobes of the ear and under the chin (Fig. 13b) (page 20.12), whereas an airborne pollen dermatitis will not spare such areas but may have a similar cut off point below the collar. Small islands of normal skin in a generalized erythroderma are characteristic of pityriasis rubra pilaris (Fig. 13c) (page 20.12).

Having recognized signs of exogenous injury, it is clearly more possible to eliminate the cause. Unfortunately much skin disease is due to altered host responses and I will call this 'vulnerability'.

Vulnerability It is a common characteristic in skin disease, and is seen in dermatitis due to the irritants affecting the vulnerable atopic skin. It is seen in the haematogeneous localization of immune complexes or other agents at sites altered by previous injury. It is also seen in the Koebner phenomenon, a term used to describe the development of psoriasis, warts, or lichen planus when the skin is injured to a degree which in most people would not produce more than a temporary wound but in predisposed individuals results in a recognizable skin disease.

Vulnerability is well worth recognizing because it may be possible to treat the predisposition when it may not be possible to eliminate the trigger. Thus, those whose skin breaks down too easily from exposure to solvents they are unable to avoid may be helped and still retain their job by the liberal application of emollients.

Recurrent episodes of vasculitis in the legs due to immune complexes may be reduced by more frequent elevation of the legs, supportive bandages, and avoidance of cold environments. Vulnerability in the legs is due to the chronic stress of blood stasis and venous hypertension which can be shown to cause inhomogeneity of capillary vessel patterns and exhaustion of endothelial secretions such as plasminogen activator.

The ecology of the skin with its integrated, well-balanced interaction between bacteria and surface secretions also determines how the skin shows its interface to the environment. Erythrasma, pityriasis versicolor, and seborrhoeic eczema are partly constitutional and partly due to exogenous organisms. The seborrhoeic diathesis is poorly understood but such persons seem especially vulnerable to infection by more pathogenic organisms.

Factors determining or modifying skin disease

Changes of skin with age, sex, and race

Newborn

Birth marks are usually first noticed in the newborn but some, like cavernous haemangiomas, may not be present on the first day. Certain epidermal or pigmented naevi and some neurofibromas do not appear until puberty. Some birthmarks have important diagnostic significance indicating serious systemic disease. Examples are the hypopigmented lesions of tuberous sclerosis (see Fig. 72, page 20.50) and the telangiectatic lesion of the Sturge–Weber syndrome.

Most Caucasian newborn have a pink skin and the vascular immaturity gives rise to flushing, mottling, reticulate markings, and sometimes segmental or one-sided flushing. This immaturity also prevents adequate cooling or heating in extremes of climate. Skin of the newborn is usually oedematous and often inflammation presents as blistering. Papulo-erythematous lesions of the newborn often contain large numbers of eosinophils. Newborn skin is susceptible to infection both from *Candida* and bacteria such as *Pseudomonas pyocyanea*. See also dermatoses affecting the genitalia (page 20.57), vesicobullous disease in infancy (page 20.72), and Section 5.

Puberty

Secondary sexual characteristics develop at puberty and at the same time an increase in susceptibility to apocrine diseases, sweating, and blushing is characteristic. Acne vulgaris is mainly a problem for the teenager (see page 20.43). Certain diseases such as ichthyosis (see page 20.13) and eczema (see page 20.32) tend to improve while others such as herpes simplex (see page 20.58) and psoriasis (see page 20.37) are more common. Naevi, particularly pigmented ones, tend to become more prominent.

Pregnancy

During pregnancy pigmentation is usually increased, and more hair, spider naevi, and palmar erythema develop. Some naevi, such as neurofibromatosis, become more prominent and certain infections, like perineal warts and candidiasis, are more troublesome. Pruritus, prurigo, blistering disorders such as herpes gestationis (see page 20.72), and the rarer impetigo herpetiformis presenting as pustular psoriasis with hypocalcaemia are associated with pregnancy.

Old age

Skin diseases in old age are common and reduce the quality of life. Most elderly have multiple skin problems including seborrhoeic eczema, intertrigo, and dermatophytosis. Probably the principal characteristic of elderly skin is its inhomogeneity or the increased diversity that develops with age. Some changes are endocrine related such as hirsutism and baldness. Others are more specifically age-related like dryness, decreased sweating, or poor healing of superficial wounds. Dry, scaly, rough skin occurs in about 80 per cent of people over the age of 75 and there are disparities in the size and thickness of the epidermis and in its pigmentation. Seborrhoeic warts, actinic injury, Campbell de Morgan spots, and

Diseases of the skin

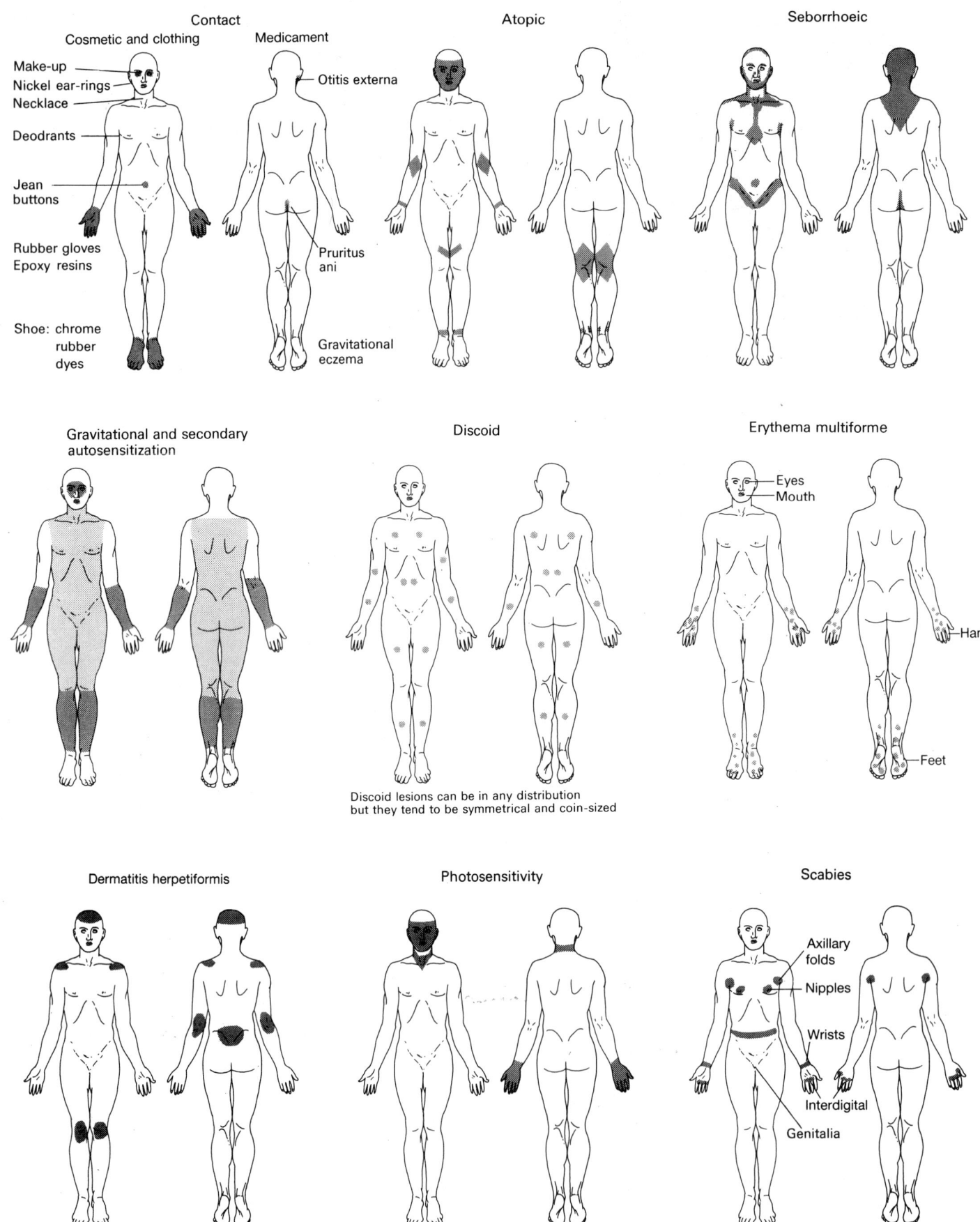

Fig. 8 Distribution of rashes.

dilatation and derangement of superficial venules are common features. Some diseases are age-related for reasons that are obscure. These include pruritus (see page 20.35), pemphigoid (see page 20.71), and lichen sclerosis et atrophicus (see page 20.59).

Degenerative disease and the cumulative exposure to solar radiation explains neoplasia of the skin. Degenerative disease of the vascular system explains venous ulcers and arterial ischaemic diseases.

Race

Differences in populations are partly explained by genetic factors but so much adaptation to environment occurs that customs and diet may determine some attributes. It is frequently reported that certain diseases are absent in tropical climates but this is probably because they have never been looked for or recognized. In dark skins erythema is violaceous and purpura may be difficult to detect; minor skin problems may not be complained of in the tropics where many neoplastic and inflammatory diseases are so florid and attendance for advice is so often delayed. A move to a more temperate climate is often associated with urbanization which can equally influence the skin. The most easily recognized difference from one person to another is skin colour and the consequences of sun exposure are much reduced in dark skins. Vitiligo (see page 20.46) is probably more common in the Caucasian races of the Middle East, North Africa, and India. The Japanese seem to develop rather readily a slatey-blue or ashy discoloration of the trunk following inflammatory disease. On the other hand acne vulgaris is very uncommon in the Japanese and both acne and rosacea seem to be uncommon in the black skin. Another easily recognized factor is hair size and shape. Facial hirsutism is rare in Japanese women and relative sparseness of hair is a feature of mongoloid races. On the other hand Mediterranean and some Indian races seem to be particularly hirsute (Fig. 14). The shininess of black skin is partly due to sebum but also thermal stress encourages increased eccrine sweating. Such skins tend to become rather dry when they move to a temperate climate. Scales show up on dark skins. Blacks like to grease their skin whereas whites prefer to powder it. Keloids (page 20.77) are a considerable problem for the negro and can sometimes be massive. Susceptibility to infection depends on immunological factors and on previous exposure. As with malaria or syphilis, some populations seem to acquire a genetic resistance to tuberculosis and leprosy.

Is it contagious?

One is often asked whether a skin disease is 'infectious'. The questioner means. 'Did I catch it?' 'Can I give it to someone else?' 'Is the treatment of choice a simple antiseptic or antibiotic regimen?' The physician may ask, 'Am I missing something which is a danger to the patients in the rest of the ward or to my nursing staff?'

There are many infections dealt with elsewhere in this *Textbook* in which a highly virulent organism has broken the defences of a normally resistant host, but there are also organisms which are usually harmless but occasionally, because of immunosuppression or other changes in the host produce a rash. Pityriasis versicolor, candidiasis, erythrasma, and trichomycosis axillaris all discussed in Section 5 are examples. More difficult is the relationship with the staphylococcus or streptococcus which for the most part sit in silence on the skin, but are unwelcome in a ward full of more susceptible patients. Psoriasis is not infectious but the massive exfoliation from such a patient is a great source of cross-infection. The bacterial spread by skin scales is considerable. Few would feel bound to treat every psoriatic for bacterial infection but the same degree of infection in atopic eczema is thought of as a contribution to the disease, perhaps through bacterial allergy.

Pathology from skin infection is more common in hot humid climates, and erosions from scratching, prickly heat, and other infections, such as lice or scabies, predispose to boils and other pattern of pyoderma, especially in the groins and axillae.

The primary pathology of infection is often asymmetrical but an immune response attempting to get rid of it is usually exactly symmetrical and takes 5–10 days to develop.

The most difficult diagnostic problem is the viral disease. The hospital doctor is not well placed to recognize its variety. It is the general practitioner called to the patient's home who sees virus disease in its early stages or in its transient phase. It is essential to know what rashes are currently endemic.

Rashes which are due to infection commonly have an associated fever lymphadenopathy, coryza, diarrhoea, vomiting, hepatomegaly, or headache. However, the abrupt sterile pustulation of generalized pustular psoriasis (Fig. 15) or the painful deep swelling of delayed pressure urticaria or vasculitis will also be accompanied by high fever and a neutrophil leucocytosis, but usually in these non-infectious processes there is no lymphadenopathy. Erythema multiforme (see page 20.69), Sweet's disease, and toxic epidermal necrolysis (see page 20.70) similarly show great syste-

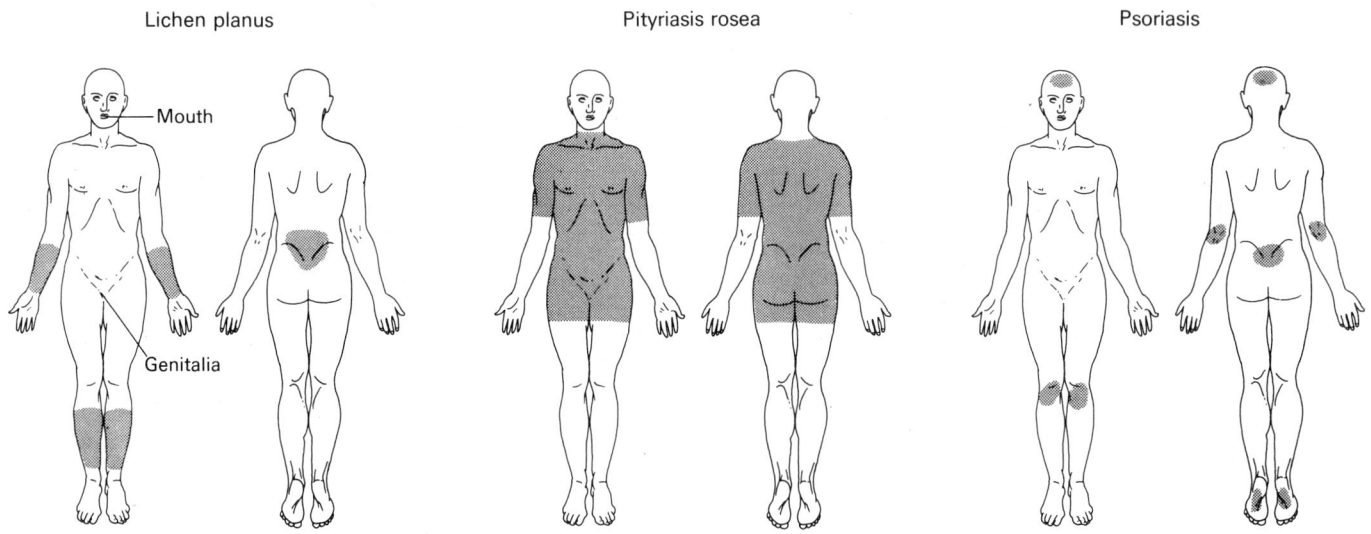

Lichen planus — Mouth — Genitalia

Pityriasis rosea

Psoriasis

Fig. 8 Distribution of rashes – continued.

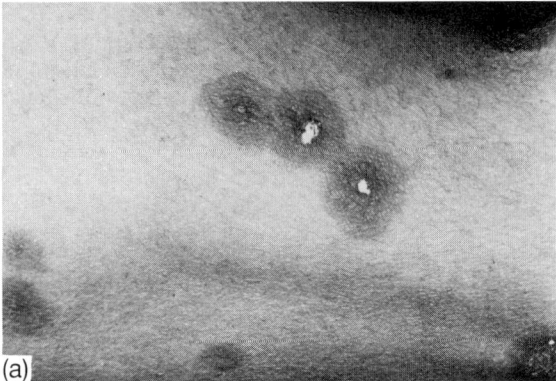

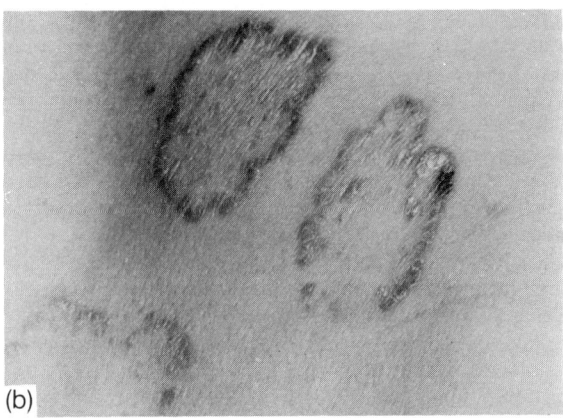

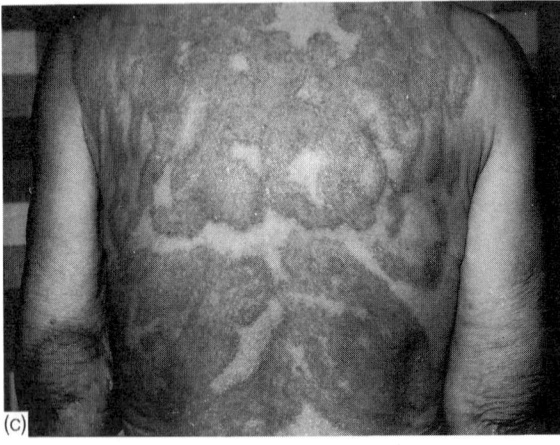

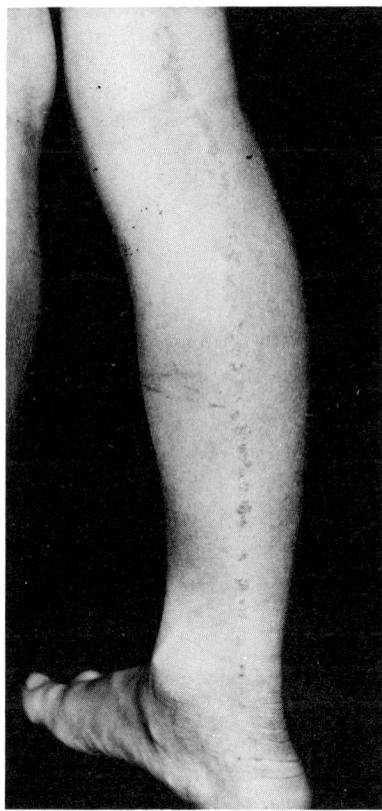

Fig. 10 Example of a linear distribution, in this case lichen planus. The distribution does not conform to a dermatome and the exact cause of linear lesions remains largely unexplained.

Fig. 9 (a) An example of the 'target' lesion of erythema multiforme. (b) Healing of the centre of the lesion is a feature of many skin diseases including fungus infections and in this case, psoriasis. See also Fig. 56. (c) Annular erythema in lupus erythematosus with Ro antibody. This pattern of widespread erythema is also observed in association with underlying malignancy.

Table 2 Some morphological terms

A *macule* is flat without change in surface marking or texture – it may be merely redness, purpura, or melanin

A *papule* is a circumscribed, palpable elevation or a thickening of the epidermis or of the upper dermis by infiltration or oedema

A *plaque* is a disc-shaped lesion often as a result of the coalescence of papules

A *nodule* is a circumscribed palpable mass larger than 1 cm in diameter and usually consisting of oedema, malignant or inflammatory cells filling the dermis or subcutaneous tissue. Some are small and painful (Table 3) others are juxta-articular (Table 4)

Vesicles and *bullae* are visible accumulations of fluid (often the lay person uses the term blister to include wealing in which there are no visible accumulations other than swelling). Vesicles are small, while bullae are larger than 1 cm

Annular lesions result from spreading infiltrations or healing centre often with refractoriness due to such factors as raised tissue pressure or scarring preventing vasodilatation or leakiness in the centre of the lesions. Vascular patterns in the skin have a reticular or annular anatomical distribution (Table 5)

Linear lesions are due to external scratches, developmental or anatomical distribution of lymphatics, blood vessels, or nerves (Table 6)

mic effects. Persons with widespread skin disease may not be able to control their body temperature and high fever in such persons is not necessarily a sign of infection.

Good practice when in doubt is to take adequate swabs and specimens for culture and histological examination as well as to treat and touch the patient as his or her comfort requires. Washing of hands suffices for scabies, fungus, and most bacterial diseases as well as warts and syphilis. The principal care is to protect the practitioner against inoculation of the skin when taking scrapings or

Table 3 Severe pain on compression of a small dermal papule or nodule is a well-recognized symptom of the following lesions. If there is doubt excision is the treatment of choice, so that a definitive histological examination can be made

Glomus	Eccrine spiradenoma
Leiomyoma	Angiolipoma
Neuroma	Chondrodermatitis (of the outer helix)

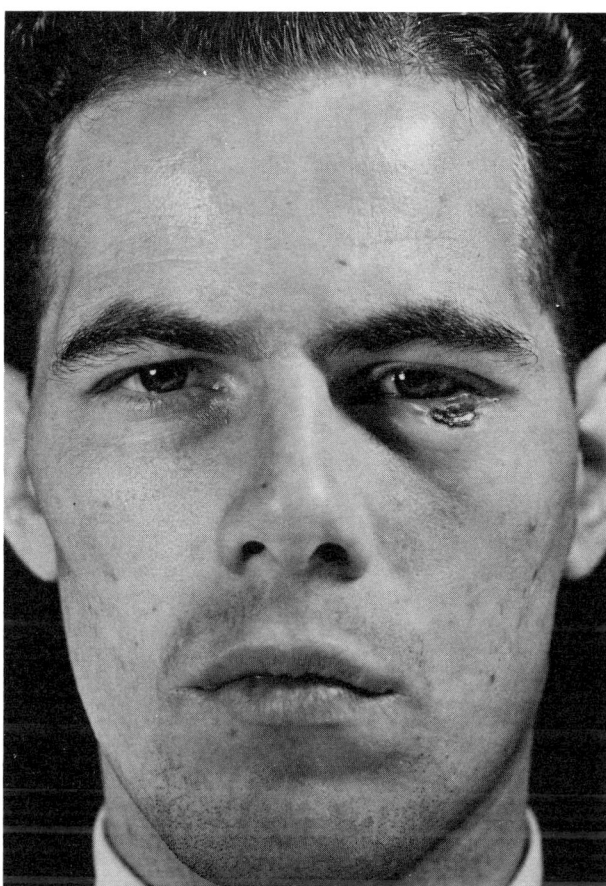

Fig. 11 A primary chancre of the lower left eyelid illustrating how skin diseases due to exogenous causes are often asymmetrical.

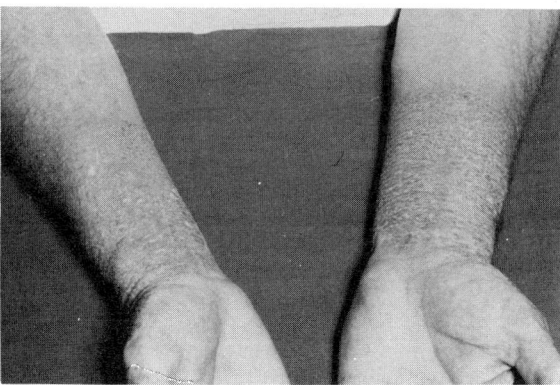

Fig. 12 Occasionally symmetry in the distribution of contact may be due to symmetrical application as in the case of this glove dermatitis.

Table 4 Juxta-articular nodules

Rheumatoid nodules	Granuloma annulare
Gouty tophi	Multicentric reticulo-histiocytosis
Xanthomata	Synovial cysts, ganglia, or Heberden's nodes

doing a biopsy. Patients with much exfoliation should not be nursed on a general ward.

Pustules need not be caused by infection, and in psoriasis or an irritant folliculitis from oils, for instance, the primary lesions are always sterile. Vesicles need not be due to viruses since they are a

Table 5 Some annular lesions

Impetigo	Urticaria
Dermatophytosis	Lichen planus (Fig. 56)
Syphilis	Lupus erythematosus (Ro antibody) (Fig. 9c)
Leprosy	Purpura
Lupus vulgaris	Seborrhoeic eczema
Pityriasis rosea	Sarcoidosis
Erythemas—toxic, urticarial and multiforme (Fig. 9a)	Mycosis fungoides
	Granuloma annulare/multiforme
Psoriasis (Fig. 9b)	Glucagonoma

Table 6 Linear lesions with dermatomal distributions include the well-recognized herpes zoster. Many linear lesions follow a pattern which does not exactly conform to innervation or blood supply especially when it extends the whole way up the leg or arm

Lichen striatus	Artefacta scratching
Lichen planus* (Fig. 10)	Focal dermal hypoplasia
Psoriasis*	Incontinentia pigmenti
Epidermal naevi	Papular mucinosis
Darier's disease*	Sarcoid*
Morphea	Warts*
Porokeratosis of Mibelli	Molluscum contagiosum
Contact dermatitis*	Syringoma
Phytophotodermatitis	

*May be a reaction to a scratch (Koebner phenomenon).
 Note: some linear nodules are determined by lymphatic drainage: mycobacteria, sporotrichosis, neoplasm, coccidioidomycosis.

feature of papular urticaria and vasculitis (see Fig. 94, page 20.65). Dark skins exposed to much oil and cosmetics often have a chronic pustular dermatosis of the lower legs which may be sterile.

Humidity is the principal cause of profuse skin infection, and treatment by cooling and drying has always been a standard therapy for an infected eczema. The fact is that drying is promoted by the use of wet dressings and the consequent evaporation. Wet dressings which are occlusive and changed infrequently encourage infection. Ideally they should be changed every 2–4 hours. Occlusive surfaces such as between the toes, the groins and the breasts need drying agents such as are commonly present in deodorants (aluminium chloride), or the use of powders. Dry mopping of the ear in otitis externa is similarly helpful.

For the rest, the diagnosis of infection is by a process of exclusion. One aspect of this is a thorough inspection of the skin until the lesions are found that are firmly diagnostic, for instance, psoriasis, lichen planus, or vasculitis, or perhaps conclusive of infection such as the burrows between the fingers in scabies (Fig. 16), or the crab louse in the pubic hair.

In some parts of the world skin clinics are overwhelmed by massive numbers of patients suffering from scabies, staphylococcal, and streptococcal infection and dermatophytosis. The doctor's role in Bombay and Calcutta, for instance, can be compared to that of a good administrator or hygienist attempting to control infections in a large family when it is not possible to treat all members of the family (Fig. 17). Control is impossible because reinfection is inevitable. Desai, in Bombay, believes that soap and water does much to reduce the incidence of common dermatoses but water is too valuable to use for washing when there is a drought.

In Mediterranean countries, ringworm of the scalp would be easy to manage (Fig. 18) were it not that the population explosion provides more children for the infection than it is possible to treat and subclinical infections are difficult to recognize. If it is impossible to control head lice in Oxford, the chances of controlling similar infections in Algeria must be very small. Some chronic

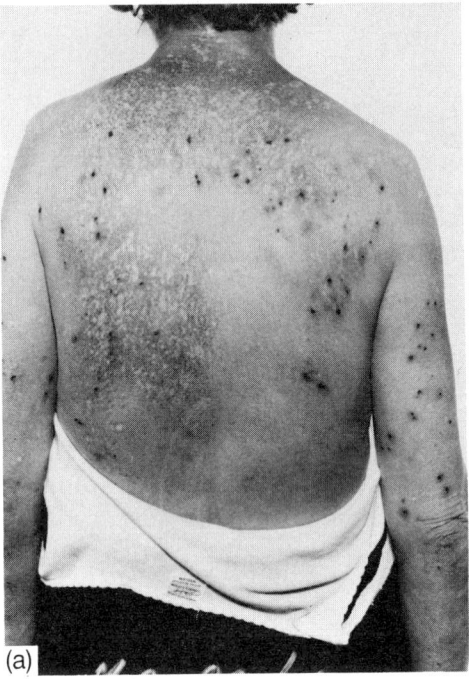
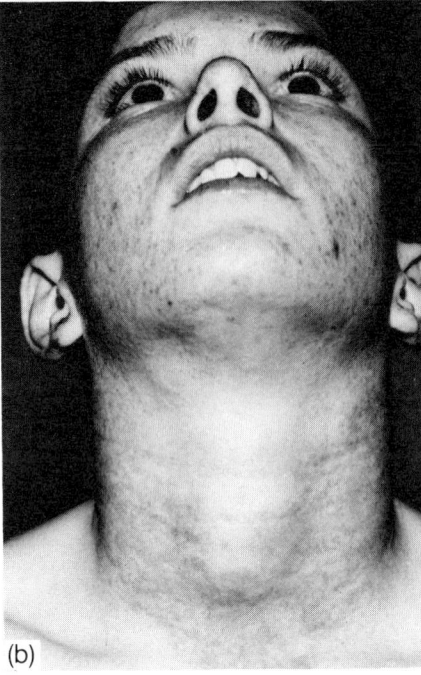
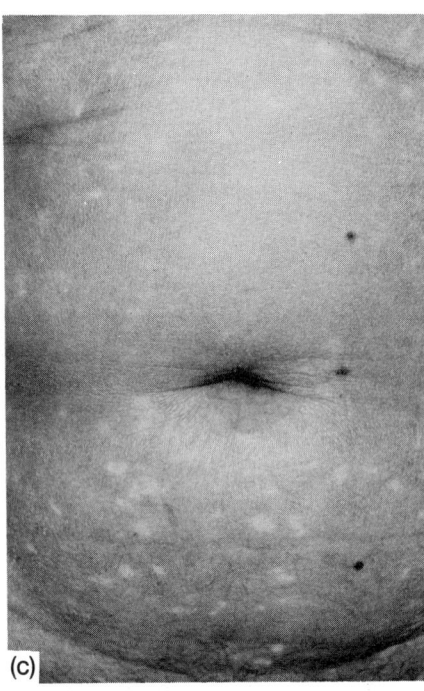

Fig. 13 (a) The central area of the back is spared from this dermatosis induced by scratching for the simple reason that the patient is not able to reach that site. (b) External irradiation from the sun spares the area beneath the lobes of the ear and under the chin in this case of solar dermatitis. (c) Small islands of unaffected skin scattered throughout a generalized redness and keratoderma are characteristic of pityriasis rubra pilaris.

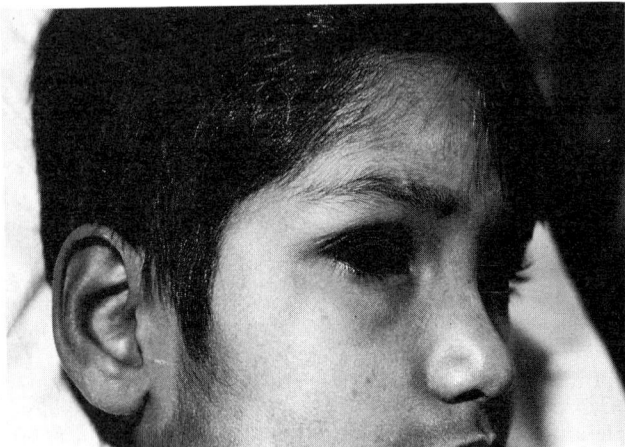

Fig. 14 Hair growth on the forehead of an Indian child. This is entirely within normal limits and is of racial origin.

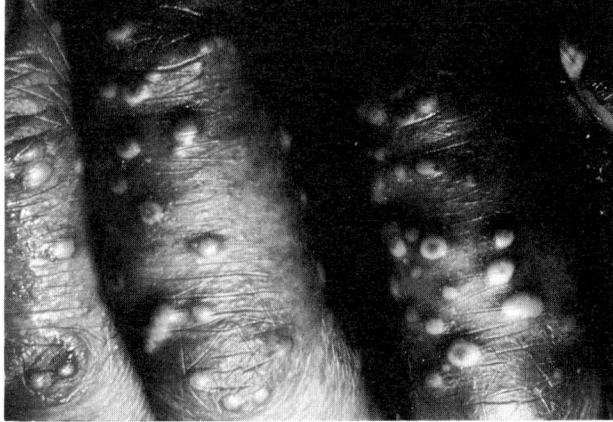

Fig. 15 Pustules are not neccessarily due to infection. These pustules are from pustular psoriasis and they are sterile.

infections presenting as granulomas are discussed and illustrated on page 20.87.

Is it hereditary?

It has long been recognized that many skin disorders, such as eczema and psoriasis, may have a hereditary basis. The concept that some persons have inherent tendencies to develop certain diseases has been supported by the studies of the HLA antigens.

Establishing that there has been a strong family history of the disease, especially if environmental factors such as infection can be ruled out, often helps to make a diagnosis. Thus an intensely itchy eczema in an infant is likely to be due to atopy if there are other members of the family affected by asthma or eczema. Most parents or patients will accept that genetic factors contribute to chronicity and will not expect instant cure.

Each pregnancy carries a 4 per cent risk of congenital malformation and during embryonic life maldevelopment of localized areas of skin can give rise to a variety of developmental defects. Most of the common defects (Table 7) are not inherited but the presence at birth of certain well recognized lesions, like the hypopigmented macule of tuberous sclerosis (see Fig. 72, page 20.50) or extra, fused (see Fig. 120b, page 20.82), or accessory digits, are a feature of some hereditary diseases. Advances in the early recognition of genetic disorders, even *in utero*, and more particularly in the effective use of family planning, have increased the demand for and application of genetic counselling. In the western world fear of transmitting genetic disease is replacing fear of contagion.

With most single gene conditions the risk of having another affected child is substantial – more than one in ten. This is unfortunately not a field for the non-specialist since subtle variations in the distribution or morphology of a skin rash can determine very

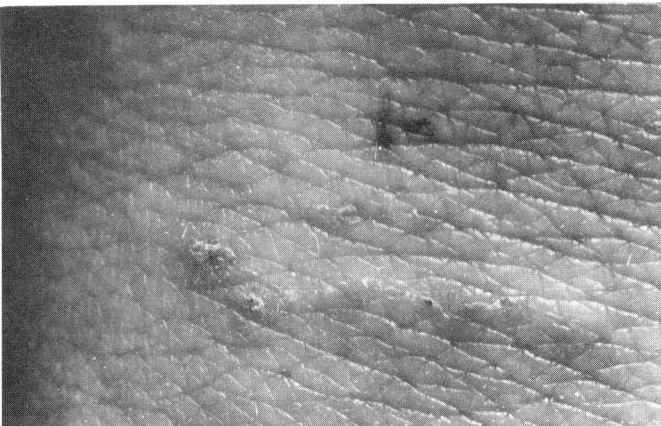

Fig. 16 The diagnostic feature of scabies. The burrow of the mite in the horny layer of the epidermis. The dark spots are the haemoglobin in the belly of the mite.

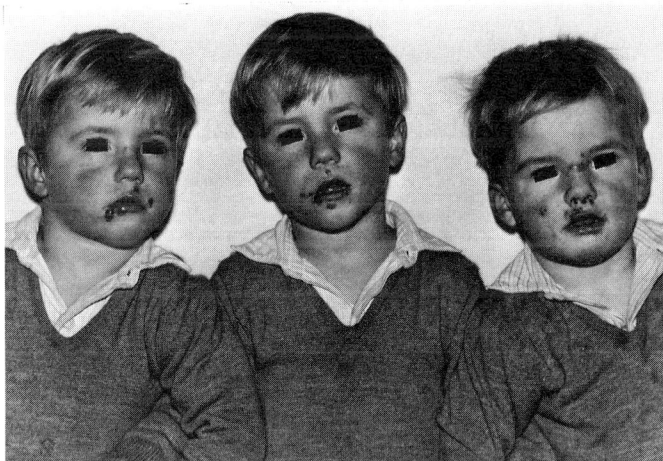

Fig. 17 Infections such as impetigo are highly contagious and tend to be found in more than one member of the family, as in these triplets.

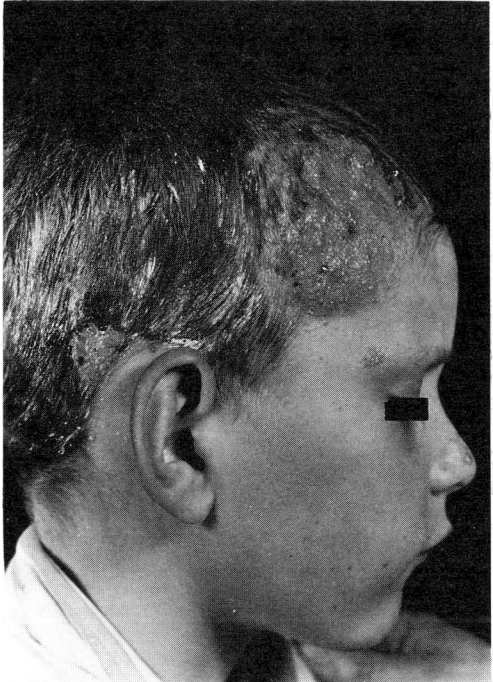

Fig. 18 Multiple exudative lesions due to tinea capitis.

Table 7 Common, minor, non-inherited abnormalities

Accessory nipple
Hypoplastic toenails
Preauricular sinus or skin tag
Overfolded helix
Webbed neck

different advice. Thus, dominant, sex-linked or recessive forms of ichthyosis or epidermolysis bullosa have distinct differences in pattern.

In some countries, first cousin marriages are very common and even encouraged by local customs, law, and religion. One in four of the offspring of recessive heterozygotes will inherit the defect. It can be calculated statistically that in a family of four children born to such parents, one will be affected in 42.2 per cent of cases, two in 21.1 per cent, three in 4.7 per cent, four in 0.4 per cent, and none in 31.6 per cent. About half the subjects of autosomal dominant disorders listed in Table 8 are new mutants. Autosomal recessive inheritance listed in Table 8 is mostly incompatible with normal physical and mental development and some are now more likely to be seen where the standard of nutrition and freedom from infection is high. Xeroderma pigmentosum and albinism, though common in countries such as Africa, rarely survive to old age.

The skin and the nervous system are both ectodermal in origin and hence there are many congenital diseases affecting both systems (Table 9).

Ichthyosis

Ichthyosis is characterized by a dry and scaling skin. Hereditary forms can always be diagnosed before the age of five years and if the disorder is acquired later it usually indicates underlying disease such as carcinoma or Hodgkin's disease. The skin of a severely affected patient is covered by large adherent scales, while fine, white, branny scales characterize mild ichthyosis. Several different types have been described, differentiated by their clinical picture and mode of inheritance.

Ichthyosis vulgaris is the most common type and has a dominant form of inheritance. The lower legs are most affected, involvement becoming progressively less towards the head. The skin is dry and scaling, and most patients show a lozenge-shaped pattern resembling crocodile markings. There is usually very evident sparing of the skin of the popliteal spaces, the antecubital fossae, and the creases of the groin. The skin of the palms and the soles shows increased markings – the so-called fortune teller's nightmare. Perifollicular hyperkeratosis (keratosis pilaris) is also a feature. In some children the ichthyosis is associated with atopic eczema which favours the cubital popliteal fossae and another common problem in children is the appearance of a dirty neck owing to the retention of skin scales. The dryness of the skin is aggravated by the reduced sebaceous and sweat glands secretion; water evaporates from the epidermal cells because those affected lack the thin film of grease present on the surface of normal skin. There is marked seasonal variation in symptoms and many children are in fact better in the summer, possibly because the skin becomes hydrated as a result of sweating. The characteristic histological appearance is a reduced or absent granular layer, and it has been postulated that the condition results from inadequate shedding rather than over-production of the horny layer.

Sex-linked ichthyosis is transmitted by clinically unaffected females and is seen only in males. Parents and children of males with sex-linked ichthyosis have normal skin but their daughters

Table 8 Inherited skin disorders

Autosomal dominant inheritance
  Neurofibromatosis   Peutz–Jeghers syndrome
  Tuberous sclerosis   Hereditary haemorrhagic
  Ehlers–Danlos syndrome   telangiectasia
  Epidermolysis bullosa   Monilethrix
  Ichthyosis vulgaris   Gardner's syndrome
  Tylosis   Pachyonychia congenita
  Benign familial pemphigus   Bullous ichthyosiform
  Darier's disease   hyperkeratosis
  Familial hypercholesterolism   Hidrotic ectodermal dysplasia
Autosomal recessive inheritance
  Albinism oculocutaneous   Mal de Maleda
  Ichthyosiform erythroderma   Xeroderma pigmentosum
  Dystrophic epidermolysis bullosa   Rothmund–Thomson syndrome
  Phenylketonuria   Ataxia telangiectasia
  Werner's syndrome   Lipoid proteinosis
  Acrodermatitis enteropathica   Bloom's syndrome
  Chondroectodermal dysplasia
Sex-linked inheritance
  Ichthyosis   Dyskeratosis congenita
  Anhidrotic ectodermal dysplasia   Menkes' syndrome
  Chronic granulomatous disease   Angiokeratoma corporis diffusa
  Keratosis pilaris atrophica   Aldrich syndrome
Multifactorial, polygenic, and suspected by some as being dominant
  Psoriasis   Alopecia arcata
  Atopic eczema   Acne vulgaris
  Hirsutism   Seborrhoeic dermatitis
Skin manifestations of chromosomal disorders
  47 XXY (Klinefelter): leg ulcers, absent beard
  47 XYY: severe nodular cystic acne
  45 XO (Turner): lymphoedema hands and feet, cystic hygroma
  47 XX (XY) + 21 (Down's): vitiligo, alopecia areata, ichthyosis
  vulgaris

Table 9 Disorders of skin and nervous system

Photosensitivity
  Xeroderma pigmentosum   Retardation, ataxia
  Bloom's syndrome   Sometimes retardation
  Cockayne syndrome   Retardation, deafness, ataxia
  Porphyria   Epilepsy, depression, neuropathy
  Hartnup syndrome   Ataxia, retardation
  Kloepfer syndrome   Retardation
Pigmentary disorder
  Neurofibromatosis   Acoustic neuroma, retardation,
                                epilepsy
  Sneddon's syndrome   Livedo reticularis and arterial stenosis
  Tuberous sclerosis   Epilepsy, retardation
  Sturge–Weber syndrome   Epilepsy, angioma, retardation
  Incontinentia pigmenti   Polymicrogyria, epilepsy, retardation
  Chediak–Higashi syndrome   Deafness
  Laurence–Siep syndrome   Retardation
  Leopard syndrome   Deafness
Hair disorder
  Marinesco–Sjögren syndrome Retardation, ataxia
  Papillon–Lefèvre syndrome   Tremor, retardation
  Menkes' syndrome   Retardation, epilepsy
  Phenylketonuria   Retardation
  Hypoparathyroidism   Epilepsy, retardation
  Argino-succinic aciduria   Epilepsy, retardation
Ichthyosis
  Refsum's disease   Ataxia, deafness, neuritis
  Rud's syndrome   Epilepsy, polyneuritis
  X-linked   Retardation
Linear sebaceous naevus
  Feuerstein syndrome   Retardation and epilepsy

may transmit the condition to their sons. Affected individuals usually have large dark scales. Flexures may be involved but the palms of the hands are spared.

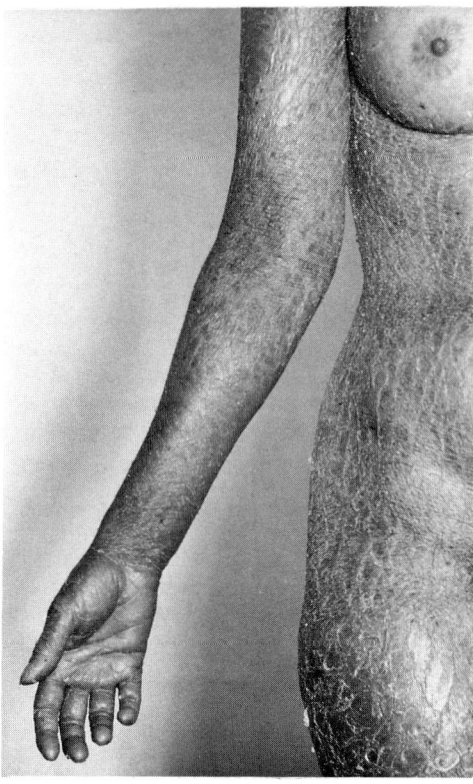

Fig. 19 Subtle variations in the distribution of a rash may determine the nature of genetic counselling. This scaling is typical of the skin changes in icthyosis. The involvement of the flexures rules out the common dominant pattern. The palmar changes make icthyosiform erythroderma (non-bullous) the correct diagnosis. This is a recessive disorder.

Bullous ichthyosiform erythroderma (epidermolytic hyperkeratosis). This rare condition produces a variety of clinical pictures, ranging from local areas of hyperkeratosis of the flexures and peri-umbilical region to gross involvement of the skin (porcupine man). The palms and sole are usually normal.

Ichthyosiform erythroderma is a rare autosomal recessive trait. It may be present at birth as one of the forms of 'collodion fetus' in which the baby seems to be covered by a film of collodion-like material through which it bursts during the first few days of life. There is a widespread involvement of the skin, including the palms and soles, and no improvement with age (Fig. 19). Ectropion is troublesome.

Treatment

There is no known way of stimulating normal sebaceous function in these patients. They should avoid de-greasing their skin by detergents and may be helped by the application of oils and wool fats. Oil or a mixture of emulsifying ointment in hot water (stirred and melted before pouring) may be added to a bath. Creams such as the 10 per cent urea preparation (Calmurid, Aquadrate) have a moisturizing effect through their osmotic activity. Sunbathing and exposure to ultraviolet light is usually of value. Retinoic acid 0.5 mg/kg daily has been life-saving in the neonate and clears the scaling within 2–4 weeks but soreness of the mouth, eyes and genitalia as well as erosions of the skin may be unacceptable.

Epidermolysis bullosa

Epidermolysis bullosa was a name given to a group of inherited diseases characterized by the production of blisters in the skin following trauma. The clinical features of the most common of the 16 recorded patterns are given in Table 10. Epidermolysis bullosa may present for the first time in army recruits who are marching with new boots and develop grotesque blistering. There is a tendency for the condition to improve with age.

The dystrophic forms of epidermolysis bullosa are more often recognized at birth. Severe disability may result, repetitive blistering leading to fusion of the fingers and toes, gross scarring, and dystrophy of the nails; there may also be involvement of the mucosa of the mouth and oesphagus leading to oesophageal stenosis. The cause of the disorder is not known, but there is increasing evidence that these epidermal disorders are caused by a collagen defect in the dermis and in the composition of the basement membrane. The collagen is less well cross linked and collagenase activity is increased. There is an increased tendency to develop neoplasm in the affected scarred areas.

Treatment

There is no specific therapy but much can be done to help these patients by giving them advice on protection and clothing. The very serious blistering that may be seen at birth and which affects the development of the child as a result of the involvement of the oesophageal mucosa can be treated by large doses of prednisolone. Collagenase inhibition by phenytoin or other inhibitors is gaining favour.

Darier's disease and Hailey–Hailey disease

Darier's disease (keratosis follicularis) is an uncommon hereditary disorder, first appearing in young adolescence and fluctuating in intensity throughout life. The condition has an autosomal dominant type of heredity and is characterized by the eruption of small greasy papules, usually on the trunk, extremities, and face which often coalesce to give yellowish-brown scaling sheets. In the groins, perineum, and axillae the lesions may become hypertrophic and liable to secondary infection. Lesions in the mouth are rare but involvement of the fingernails and pitting of the palms and soles is a common accompaniment and the nail change illustrated in Fig. 20 is the commonest.

Pathology

The characteristic change is loosening of the epidermal cells, usually just above the level of the basal cell. This is probably caused by a defect in the tonofibrildesmosome complex. Isolated epidermal cells may appear round (so-called *corps rond*) with a dark-staining nucleus surrounded by a clear zone, the result of tonofilaments aggregating round the nucleus.

Hailey–Hailey disease (familial benign pemphigus)

This is somewhat similar to Darier's disease and is also inherited as a dominant trait. The flexures are eroded and often there are blisters (Fig. 21). Sometimes it is extremely difficult to differentiate between the two conditions.

Treatment

Darier's disease responds to small doses of retinoic acid (page 20.94), but for Hailey–Hailey disease there is no effective treatment; controlling secondary infection when present by antibiotic creams and antiseptic lotions may keep the patient comfortable. Hot weather and exposure to the sun seem to aggravate the condition.

Is it due to malnutrition?

Skin diseases of malnutrition have been termed the dermatoses of the poor. They are common in starving communities but are also seen in those living only on drugs or alcohol, those suffering from malabsorption syndromes, and those debilitated by neoplasia or severe chronic infections. Increasingly elderly patients suffering from dementia are responsible for more cases in Western urban communities. Poor personal hygiene and lack of failure to use water supplies contribute to some aspects of skin diseases in malnutrition as well as to the infections of both skin and mouth which often accompany them.

The skin is 8 per cent of body weight and uses up about one-eighth of the body's protein; hence it is affected early in malnutrition.

In experimental malnutrition and in studies on humans during the Second World War, dryness of the skin and hyperpigmentation were observed as early signs. At birth, malnutrition is seen as loss of vernix and maceration. The skin is wrinkled and peeling with deficient subcutaneous fat.

Older persons proceed to a mild ichthyosis and the associated hyperkeratosis is often a sign of slow turnover. The dry scale is well knit and retains pigment and histologically may be dense and homogenized. The stratum corneum is unsupple and cracks appear in the horny surface, particularly on the front of the legs (Fig. 22, see also Fig. 124, page 20.83). It is known as eczema craquelé and such eczema that develops is often well marginated unlike other forms of endogenous eczema.

Most malnutrition is a consequence of mixed deficiencies including protein loss. There is weight loss, weakness, and emaciation. Anaemia, oedema, sore tongue, and dry thin hair are often featured.

Table 10 Clinical features of the most common patterns of epidermolysis bullosa

	Autosomal inheritance	Pathology	Onset	Course	Distribution	Other features
Epidermolysis bullosa simplex	Dominant	Epidermal; clefts through basal cell layer	Soon after birth; may be delayed	May improve with time; worse in warm weather	Feet and hands, also around mouth and trunk	None, no scars
Epidermolysis bullosa simplex of the hands and feet	Dominant	Epidermal; clefts through basal cell layer	Variable	Improves with time; worse in warm weather	Hands and feet except in babies	None, no scars
Epidermolysis bullosa letalis	Recessive	Junctional; cleft between plasma membrane and basal lamina	At birth	May be mild at onset, usually progressive and fatal; Mild form exists with long-term survivors	Palms soles and vermilion border of lips spared	Nail dystrophy; mouth and oesophagus, also respiratory tract, mild atrophy
Epidermolysis bullosa dystrophica (dermolytic bullous dermatosis)	Dominant	Unknown. Increased sulphated glycosaminoglycans	A few days after birth; may be delayed	Relatively mild; improves with time	Extensor surfaces	Scars; nail dystrophy; milia (common); mucous membrane (uncommon)
Epidermolysis bullosa dystrophica (dermolytic bullous dermatosis)	Recessive	Dermal; cleft under basal lamina; Anchoring fibrils absent Increased collagen degradation	At birth	Often severe with deformity and can be fatal; improves with time	Entire skin; even normal-looking skin has an abnormal texture and blisters easily	Scars; nail dystrophy; milia; mouth and oesophagus

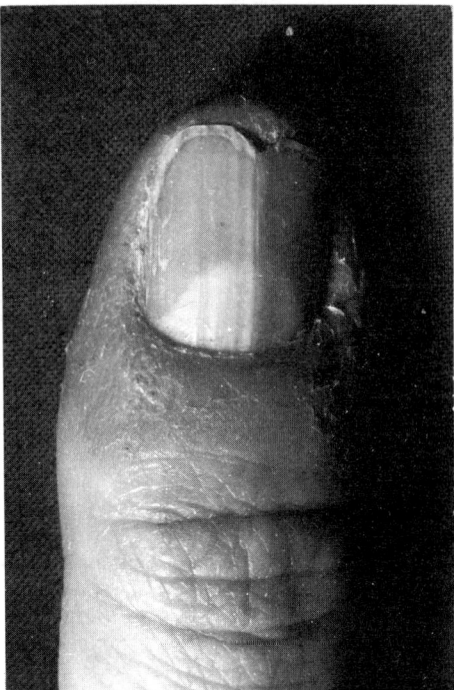

Fig. 20 Minimal signs may be a clue to the diagnosis as in this disease transmitted by a dominant gene. A white line extends from the nailbed to the distal nail plate where there is a 'V' shaped notch. This is the most common finding of all in Darier's disease and is present in most affected persons.

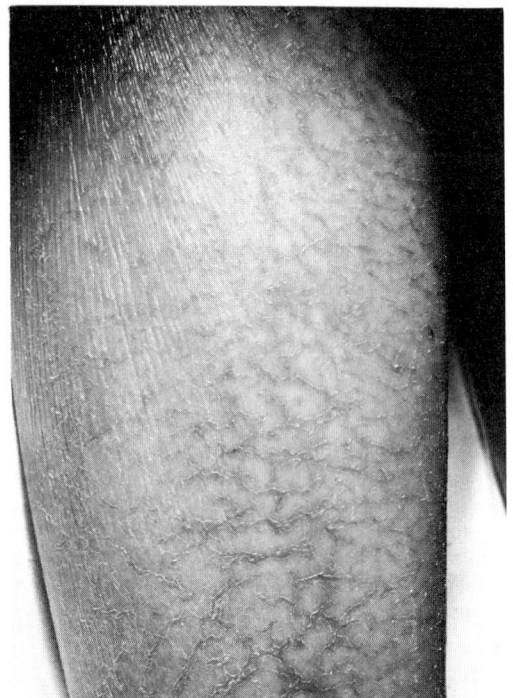

Fig. 22 An early and common sign of malnutrition of the skin especially in the elderly is cracking of a well-made stratum corneum giving a pattern of eczema craquelé.

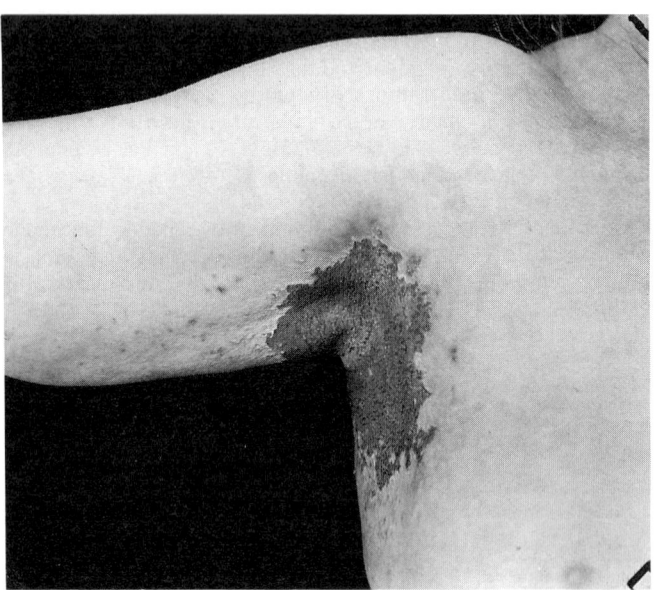

Fig. 21 Erosions of the axilla in Hailey–Hailey disease, a benign hereditary pseudopemphigus.

Vitamin A deficiency should be thought of when there is significant dryness of the eye and perifollicular hyperkeratosis. It is the commonest preventable cause of blindness.

Vitamin B deficiency causes a dermatitis that has a seborrheoic distribution particularly of the nasolabial folds, scrotum, and vulva. The lips are dry, cracked, crusted, or ulcerated; the tongue is sore and smooth.

Nicotinic acid deficiency or pellagra causes the well-known triad of dementia, diarrhoea, and dermatitis. Early signs are prominent

sebaceous follicles of the nose. The light sensitivity dermatosis is also exacerbated by heat, friction, or pressure. The erythema is a characteristic dusky brown and the dermatitis is well marginated. In the dark skin the lesions are relatively depigmented but equally well marginated.

Vitamin C deficiency causes perifollicular haemorrhages, painful bruising, or woody oedema of legs. This means in fact that they look oedematous but are hard to the touch. In the dark skin it may appear that the skin is stretched and shiny. Coiled hairs are an early sign but they are common in the normal population especially in the elderly. Swollen and bleeding gums are an important sign but occur only in those with teeth. It should be considered in any non-healing wound.

Protein deficiency is common in all forms of malnutrition, but where it is supplemented by carbohydrate and there is no active starvation, then a characteristic disease is recognizable. In children this is typified by kwashiorkor. Features of protein deficiency include; (a) erythema as in a second degree burn; (b) dry hyperkeratotic hyperpigmented scales; (c) peeling like enamel paint, cracking like crazy pavement; (d) it is maximal over pressure areas; and (e) there is straightening and reddening of the hair.

In some dark skins, raised annular patches of pigmented scales on the trunk are an early sign of malnutrition. It is known as pityriasis rotunda.

Management includes avoiding secondary deficiencies since, by suddenly providing some but not all the necessary foods, conditions like blindness from vitamin A deficiency, may be precipitated. In malnutrition, zinc may be lacking or poorly absorbed. Some improvement in the rash of kwashiorkor has been described using local zinc ointments, and prescribing other trace elements such as selenium.

Is there an association with gastrointestinal disease?

There is a number of associations of skin disease with disease of the gastrointestinal tract. There is no completely satisfactory system for listing these. Many of the skin diseases are discussed more completely in other sections.

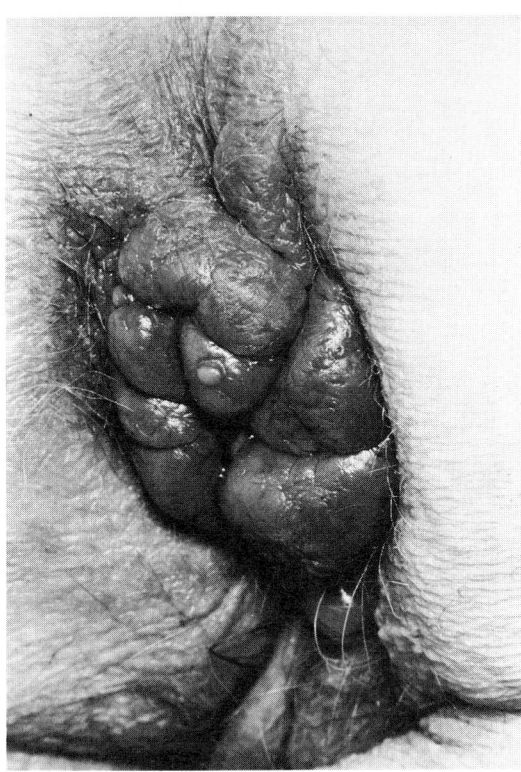

Fig. 23 Perianal granuloma in Crohn's disease.

Oesophagus

In epidermolysis bullosa (see page 20.14) bullae are common and occasionally the entire epithelial lining of the oesophagus may be coughed up as a cast. Bullae also occur in pemphigus. Mucocutaneous pemphigoid and epidermolysis bullosa cause eventual scarring. Erosions also develop in lichen planus.

Stiffness and loss of peristalsis occurs in scleroderma often as an early sign. It is best demonstrated by a prone barium swallow. Carcinoma of the oesophagus has been associated with plantar palmar hyperkeratosis (tylosis) in two families. Webbing of the post-cricoid region with anaemia is associated with dyskeratosis congenita – an atrophy of the skin and nails.

Stomach

Gastric atrophy and the presence of antibody to the parietal cell are associated with vitiligo and alopecia areata. Carcinoma may present with acanthosis nigricans. Gastric polyposis is associated with perioral and finger lentiginoses in the Peutz–Jegher's syndrome as well as with nail dystrophy and alopecia in the Canada–Cronkite syndrome.

Gastrointestinal bleeding is a consequence of telangiectasia in hereditary haemorrhagic telangiectasia as well as in acrosclerosis with telangiectasia, and rarely also in disorders of elastic tissues such as Ehlers–Danlos syndrome or pseudoxanthoma elasticum. Henoch–Schönlein purpura also causes gastrointestinal bleeding.

Small bowel

Regional ileitis may present with granulomatous swelling of the buccal mucosa or lips as well as with perianal granulomata and fistulae (Fig. 23).

Coeliac disease is associated with dermatitis herpetiformis. Pigmentation and malnutrition of the skin is particularly recorded in Whipple's disease.

Colon

Ulcerative colitis is responsible for many disorders of the skin and mouth in affected patients. Aphthous ulcers are more common. Skin rashes include erythema multiforme, erythema nodosum, and pyoderma gangrenosum. Peri-anal abscesses and fistulae are also common associations.

Erythema nodosum sometimes progressing to pyoderma gangrenosum occurs more commonly in Crohn's disease of the colon than from ulcerative colitis.

Pancreas

Migratory thrombophlebitis (Trousseau's sign) is more likely to be associated with carcinoma of the pancreas than with any other carcinoma. Acute fat necrosis of the trunk or limbs is a consequence of acute pancreatitis. There is an increased electrolyte concentration in the sweat of patients with mucoviscoidosis.

The glucagonoma syndrome is a recently recognized eruption of necrolytic migratory erythema due to sometimes quite small tumours of the pancreas. The skin lesions are dusky red, annular, and scaly with a vesicopustular element due to epidermal cell necrosis in the most superficial layers of the epidermis. The associations with diabetes mellitus are carotenaemia, moniliasis and dermatophytosis, necrobiosis lipoidica (see Fig. 137, page 20.91), ulcers and gangrene, insulin lipodystrophy, and xanthoma. Widespread granuloma annulare, pruritus, lichen planus, and psoriasis are probably more common but more data are required to prove this.

Liver

The skin consequences of liver disease includes spider naevi, palmar flush, purpura and bruising, white nails, and clubbing. There is loss of hair in the beard, axillae, and pubic region. Gynaecomastia, acne, Dupuytren's contracture, xanthoma, jaundice, pruritus, and pigmentation are other features.

Is climate responsible?

Climate is responsible for much skin disease although, in the case of pyoderma or through the effects of famine and drought, its influence is indirect. Food and water supply are dependent on the climate and even if the lack or excess of these is not a direct cause, the management of skin disease requires washing, soaking, and adequate nutrition as well as control of body temperature. Children and the newborn, in particular, are susceptible to the influence of climate.

Humidity explained why, in the rainy season, 70 per cent of lost combat man-days in Vietnam were through skin disease. The distribution of water determines the ecology of many organisms that are parasitic on man, biting insects thriving in the rainy season. Wet clothing can cause severe discomfort particularly in a boot or around the waist or between the legs while marching. Even in the Arctic, occlusive clothing can accumulate much sweat and make walking impossible. Immersion foot and paddy foot can bring a military campaign to an end. In Kuwait outbreaks of industrial dermatitis were blamed on the absorption of allergens by the skin that become moisturized in certain seasons, while in Scandinavia a low humidity in some factories accounted for drying of epidermis and consequent irritant dermatitis.

Seasonal variations account not only for increased bacterial injury but also for eczema, as for example in the atopic patient sensitive to pollens or the dermatitis due to plants so common in market gardeners and florists. Sweaty feet in hot weather increase the dermatitis from footwear, and sweat pore occlusion encourages widespread bacterial infections in extreme heat. The incidence of some disease is influenced by height above sea level and by the thickness of the atmosphere. One is unlikely to be sun burned at the low level of the Dead Sea but actinic dermatitis is common in Mexico and in the Andes. Many infections are most exuberant at sea level. At the slightly higher level of 600–1500 m, transmission of leishmaniasis and onchocerciasis by flies is more common. Many of the skin diseases caused by infections that have a unique geographical distinction are discussed in the infectious diseases section, e.g. pinta, buruli ulcer or deep mycoses. In this section they are only mentioned if they are important in differential diagnosis of some physical sign such as depigmentation, wartiness or blisters.

Cold weather and low humidity predispose to irritant dermatitis and the high incidence of dry skin in hospital is explained by central heating and diminished occlusive clothing. Pediculosis is encouraged when people huddle together to keep warm.

Cold

Frostbite and snow blindness will affect every polar explorer if inadequately protected, but individual susceptibility varies so that in more temperate climates where the majority do not die of cold, there is a high incidence of skin disease that can be attributed to it. This is due to inadequate protection against minor degrees of cold injury. Vasoconstriction and increased blood viscosity mediate internal disease.

It is often noted that the resident of the United Kingdom has pink cheeks and blue hands to a degree not seen in, for instance, Australia or the United States. This is because of chronic exposure to cooling. In Canada or Scandinavia where the winters are a danger to the unprotected, there would be no such exposure of the schoolchild or teenager as seen during the winter in the United Kingdom where 10 per cent of the population are affected by chilblains, acrocyanosis, Raynaud's phenomenon, and the various manifestations of perniosis, an incidence never approached in most other parts of the world.

Perniosis

Chronic cold causes thickening of the subcutaneous and dermal tissues as in pigs. During the miniskirt era, thighs of girls regularly became fatter in temperate climates. Fat insulates the surface of the skin from the inside, so cooling of the surface is obvious. Chronic cooling causes telangiectasia, which is often perifollicular, and sometimes even angiokeratoma. Pink cheeks are one consequence but similar changes may be seen over the fat of the calf or upper arm. Cooling causes stasis in the venules so that circulating noxious agents like immune complexes and bacteria are usually localized at such sites.

The anatomy of the skin vasculature is such that cooled skin often shows a pink and blue mottling known as cutis marmorata. If this produces irreversible changes it is then known as livedo reticularis (Fig. 24a). Much disease is localized in the venules of such damaged vasculature. Sneddon's syndrome is livedo reticularis and a non-inflammatory stenosis of cerebral arteries.

Chilblains are essentially an ischaemia induced by cold. Pressure from tight clothing often encourages the damage done by cooling (Fig. 24b).

Ultraviolet radiation and the sun

The sun emits electromagnetic rays comprising a continuous spectrum of short to long waves. Only a narrow range reacts with photocells in the retina and is visible. Heat is due to infrared and this can be felt. Most short wavelengths which can neither be seen nor felt are filtered out by the earth's thick atmosphere which includes ozone and water vapour which screen out these harmful wave bands. As there is less atmosphere on mountain tops the danger of radiation exposure is greater. The content of water vapour in the atmosphere is variable which accounts for protection from sunburn in winter, cloudy days, the early morning, or late evening sun, and the thick atmosphere of the low lying Dead Sea in Israel and Jordan. Glass also protects so that the closed windows of a car will protect even in a tropical desert unless one is sensitive to the longer wave lengths of ultraviolet radiation. Congenital porphyria is, for example, a disease in which it is difficult to protect against sensitivity to long-wave ultraviolet rays.

Ultraviolet rays are classified into three ranges UVB 290–320 nm penetrates and is of high energy and hence damages and produces sunburn. UVA (black light 320–400 nm) is of lower energy but it is penetrating and usually it is only damaging in the presence of sensitizers such as drugs, porphyrins, or plant juices. The short-

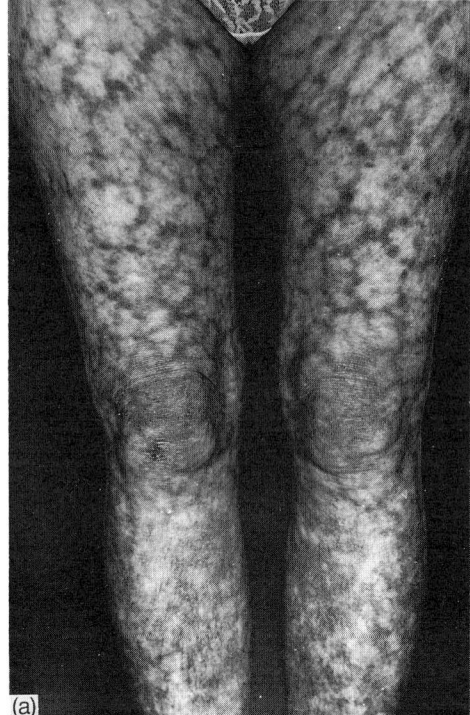

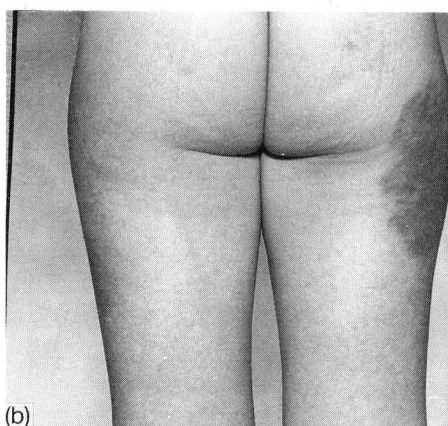

Fig. 24 (a) Chronic vascular disease, especially if inflammatory, summates with the physical effects of cooling to produce livedo reticularis. A non-inflammatory variety associated with cerebrovascular disease is known as Sneddon's syndrome. (b) An equestrian chilblain is due to the combination of the insulating effect of fat and pressure from tight jeans in a young girl riding on a damp and frosty morning.

est is UVC which is non-penetrating 200–290 nm and accounts for the damage to the skin in mountain climbers or from some ultraviolet lamps, especially those used for sterilization.

The diagnosis of ultraviolet damage is determined by recognizing the distribution of the rash as typical of exposure. Thus on the head, nose, and cheeks, which are principally affected, there is often sparing below the eyebrows, under a forelock, beneath and behind the ears, and below the chin (see Fig. 13b). The sides and back of the neck are picked out but there is a sharp border to the sun damage where the collar shields the skin from sunlight. Much, of course, depends on the style of clothing as well as on the direction of irradiation both at work and at play. The backs of the hands and dorsum of the feet are often caught by the sun but there may be some tolerance of such skin previously exposed and tanned so that skin not so tolerant is clearly more damaged. Heat from the sun lowers the itch threshold at sites of vasodilatation. Thus atopic eczema may be aggravated and only partly does such

Table 11 Clinical features of chronic sun exposure

Elastosis	Less elastic, more fragile, yellowish, furrowed
	Telangiectasia, venous lakes, spider angiomas
	Prominent sebaceous glands (Fig. 25)
	Linear and stellate scars
	Idiopathic guttate melanosis
Keratosis	10–25 per cent precancerous
	Yellow-brown hyperkeratosis on a red telangiectatic background—the scale is not laminated as in psoriasis but firmly adherent and removal is painful; unlike lupus erythematosus, it bleeds when the scale is removed
	Cutaneous horn common
	Annular lesions frequent
	Bleed easily when scratched
Solar cheilitis	Lower lip
	Yellow-white thickenings
	Scaling and crusting
	Fissuring
Basal cell epithelioma	Central erosion
	Telangiectasia runs over the edge
	Pearl-like border
	Cystic, pigmented or sclerotic forms
Squamous epithelioma	Indurated beyond the visible margin (Fig. 26)
	Ulcerated, hyperkeratotic, or granulomatous
	Crusted and horny
	Hard, elevated, or undermined edge
Kerato-acanthoma	Rapid growth: 4–6 weeks
	Sharply defined hemispherical
	Central horny core which may leave a crater
	2–12 months disappears spontaneously
	Scarring may be considerable
Bowen's disease	Often single with a well-defined edge
	Usually red scaly or crusted plaques
	Often slightly pigmented
Malignant melanoma	Change in depth of pigmentation (either darkening or loss) irregular notched border
	Growth changes, satellites
	Bleeding, itching, or ulceration
	Family history of atypical multiple pigmented naevi

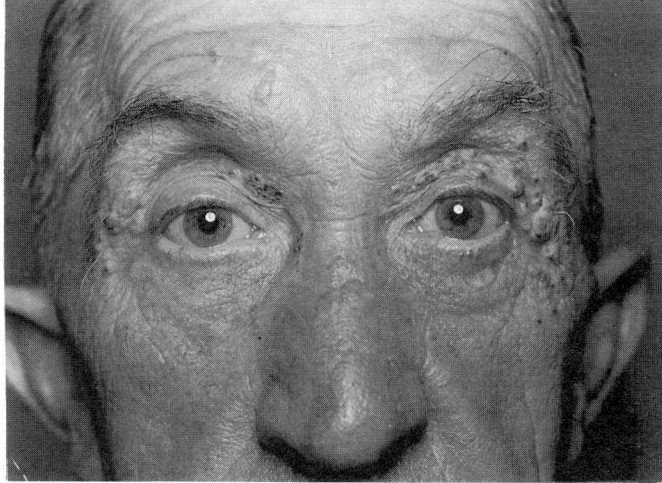

Fig. 25 Prominent sebaceous glands and comedo formation in solar elastosis.

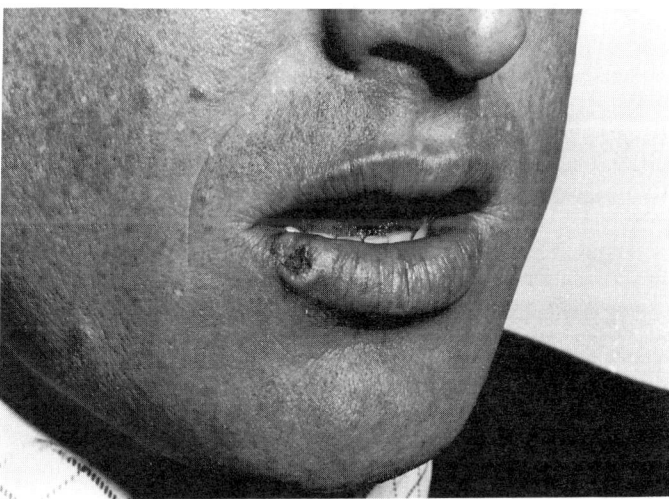

Fig. 26 Squamous epithelioma of lower lip as a consequence of sun exposure.

eczema have a light distribution. It is now recognized that ultraviolet rays may produce a subclinical inflammation which summates with subclinical sensitivity of other forms of injury including cold or airborne allergens. The pharmacological mediation of sunburn erythema is partly from prostaglandin generation. Plant dermatitis often produces a rash in the distribution of sun exposure. The condition phytophoto-dermatitis is a rash in the distribution of actual contact with plant juices on which the sun then acts and produces a burn. The pattern of such casual contact is often streaky and bizarre. Some perfumes containing berloque or musk ambrette are also responsible (see Fig. 60).

White skin and the sun
Hats, parasols, long skirts, and shawls as well as shady verandas have over the last 50 years been replaced by bikinis, solariums, and reckless sun worshipping. Even redheads and blondes attempt to brown themselves.

Exposure to sunlight is a major cause of ageing of the skin and of degenerative diseases of the epidermis and dermis that accompany age. In Australia, South Africa and south-western USA solar keratosis, basal cell epitheliomata, chronic solar cheilitis, and squamous carcinoma are the commonest cause of referral to the dermatologist (Table 11). Even children are not completely immune and persons who burn easily and still persist in exposing themselves regularly to the sun will inevitably suffer gross changes in their skin, even at an early age. Fortunately, malignancy of the skin based on solar degenerative changes has a low potential for metastases.

Malignant melanoma
The incidence of this tumour is increasing. Fortunately, older mutilating surgery has proved less curative than conservative excision and the prognosis has on the whole improved and largely depends on the depth of the lesion at the time of removal. At depths greater than 0.76 mm the prognosis sharply worsens. The role of sun exposure more than two years previously is suggested by geographical distribution, predilection for exposed skin and for depigmented skin. More than half the malignancies arise in a previously recognized mole, lentigo (Fig. 27), or giant hairy naevus. Giant congenital pigmented naevi became malignant in about 10 per cent of cases before the age of five years. Persons with a family history of multiple pigmented naevi and malignant melanoma should practise sun avoidance and use sun screening agents.

Rashes due to sun or artificial light and associated ultraviolet rays
Sunburn is initially an erythema at about 6–8 hours after exposure and may progress to blistering and later peeling; if the exposure is excessive redness may begin as early as 2 hours.

Solar urticaria is an erythema and wealing immediately on exposure to sun often of sites not habitually exposed to the sun.

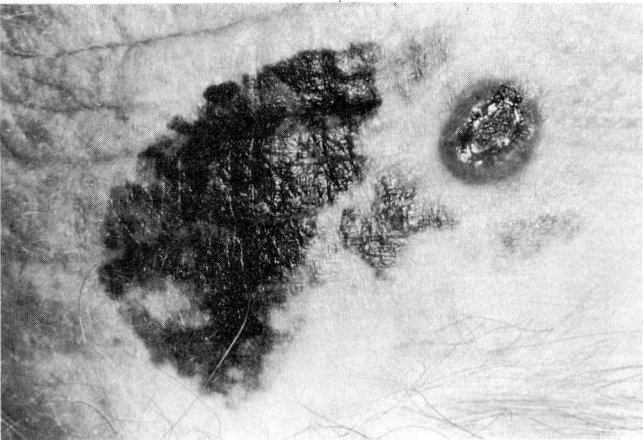

Fig. 27 The features of malignancy in this melanoma are an irregular notched border, variation in colour from red to black, variation in depth or a history of recent change.

Polymorphic light eruption is an altered quality of sunburn. Thus instead of erythema there is itchy papular or eczematous responses about 6–8 hours after exposure which may persist for several days (Fig. 28). There are several variants including a lymphoma-like pattern with heavy lymphocytic infiltrates.

Exacerbation or localization of other dermatoses is characteristic of pellagra, Hartnup's disease, lupus erythematosus, Darier's disease, herpes simplex, rosacea, scleroderma, erythema multiforme, actinic lichen planus (psoriasis) sometimes, and lymphocytoma.

Ultraviolet rays may diminish antigen surveillance by reducing the population of Langerhans cells.

Porphyria The rash of exposed areas is a swelling, bruising, or blistering often noticed immediately after exposure (Fig. 29). There is pitted scarring, scleroderma-like thickening, pigmentation, and hirsutes in the more chronic stages. Fragility of the skin is a feature. Bright sun is not a necessity since it is due to the UVA and blue light. Erythropoetic protoporphyria often presents as a burning sensation shortly after exposure to sun.

Drug eruptions These are acute eruptions of erythema swelling or blistering like severe sunburn but not dependent on bright sun since UVA is often responsible. They are often dose dependent as with psoralens in PUVA therapy. Ingestion of a spinach (*Atriplex*) also causes photosensitivity (see Table 12). Some present only as deep pigmentation.

Xeroderma pigmentosum is the term given to several genetic diseases in which repair of DNA is defective (Fig. 30). Children develop severe redness and swelling up to 72 hours after exposure. Chronic injury results in keratosis, telangiectasia, irregularities of pigmentation, and even, in childhood, the early development of cancers and melanomas.

Severe sunburn in infancy must be investigated by fibroblast DNA repair studies because future protection from sun can much reduce the incidence of subsequent malignancy.

Persistent light eruption is the term given to sensitivity to light induced by agents previously applied to the skin, often years before. Drugs eliciting light sensitivity are listed in Table 12 (see also page 20.26).

Investigations

The questions asked of the patient should include the family history, drug or food ingestion and exposure to perfumes, and the type of occupation as well as how and when exposure took place. It is important to know whether glass or cloud is protective.

Although testing to light may be done with a variety of light sources especially in photobiology units, sunlight is a natural

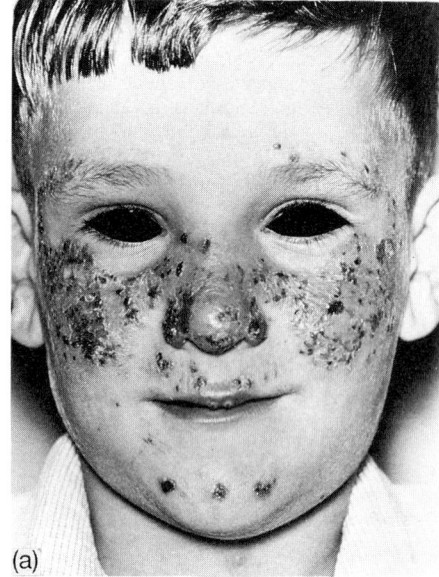

(a)

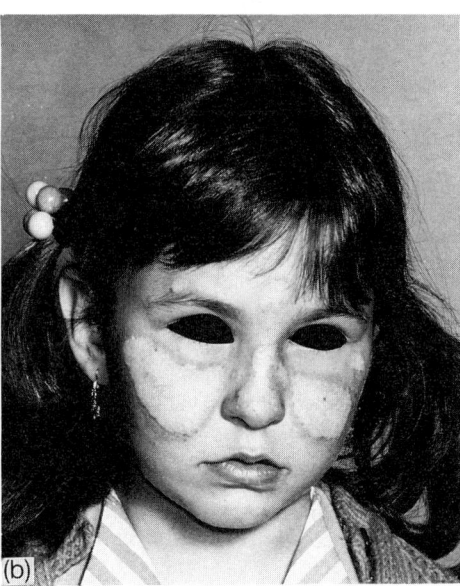

(b)

Fig. 28 Two patterns of altered response to sunburn wave lengths: (a) an eczematous prurigo with excoriations, and (b) a plaque-like form not unlike lupus erythematosus.

source that can be used by blacking out the skin of the back of the trunk and exposing it by opening 'windows' at 5 minute intervals.

Prophylaxis

Health education in schools should emphasize that burning in the sun is not related to heat. It is maximal at mid-day and protection is essential mainly through avoidance by using clothing. Sunscreens are effective if properly used, i.e. they must be applied evenly and thoroughly and well before exposure, but they are not substitute for avoidance. Frequent uninhibited exposure accumulates almost inevitable and irreversible injury which is only apparent some 20 years later.

Management

The ill-effects of a cool sunny and windy noon must be explained as well as the relative safety of a hot sunny evening. Protection from light for those with sensitivity to UVB includes advice on the time of day and season likely to be harmful. Most patients can safely take an early morning or late afternoon bathe. Those with

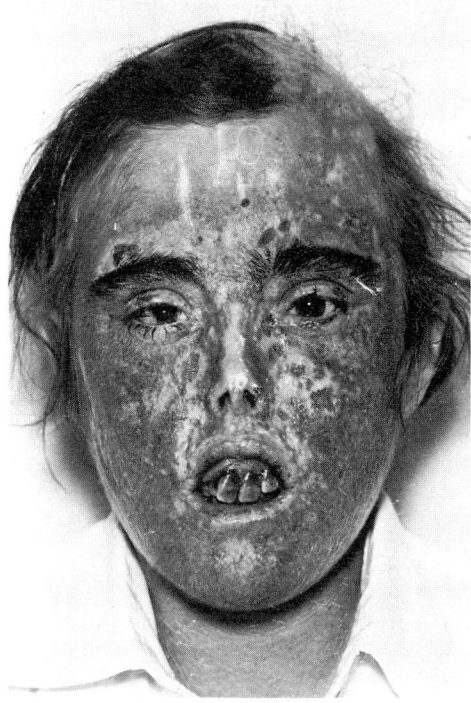

Fig. 29 The congenital erythropoietic form of porphyria. The prinicipal feature is fragility and scarring of the skin. Scleroderma and hirsutes with inequalities of pigmentation are other features seen in this child.

Table 12 Photosensitivity due to drugs

Sulphonamides and related chemicals
   Antibacterial group: sulphathiazole, long-acting sulphonamides
   Diuretics: chlorothiazide, hydrochlorothiazide, quinethazone
   Antidiabetic: sulphonylureas, carbamides
   Rarely: paraphenylenediamine, procaine group of anaesthetics
Antibiotics
   Tetracyclines; tetracycline, dimethylchlortetracycline (Ledermycin)
   Declomycin chlortetracycline (Aureomycin)
   Griseofulvin
Antiarrhythmic
   Amiodarone
Phenothiazines
   Chloropromazine, promazine, trimeprazine, meprazine
romezathine hydrochloride
Other psychotrophic drugs
   Chlordiazepoxide
Antihistamines not of phenothiazine structure
   Diphenhydramine
Antimalarials
   Chloroquine
Occasional, rare or of historical interest
   Isoniazid, psoralens, stilbamidine 9–aminoacridine, eosin,
   trypaflavine, methylene blue, rose bengal, frusemide, nalidixic acid
   (Negram)

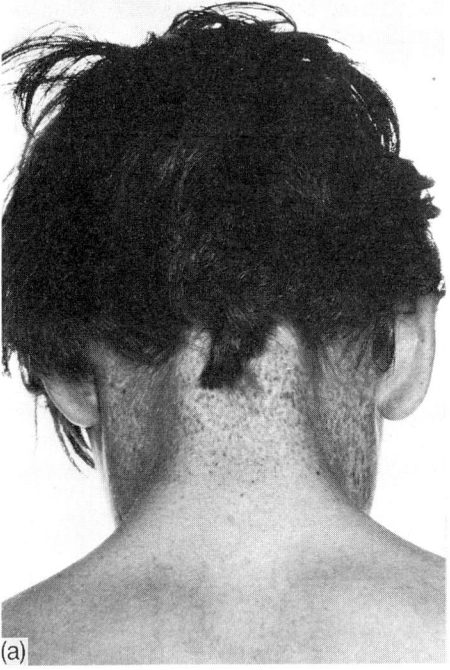

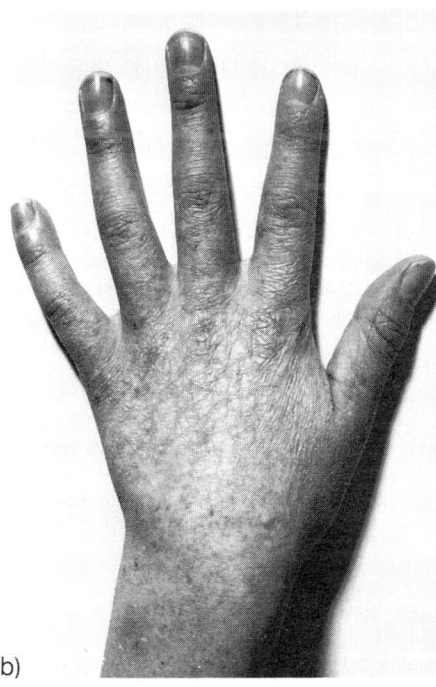

Fig. 30 The ageing effect of the sun is seen on (a) the neck and (b) the hands of this child with xeroderma pigmentosum, a defect of DNA repair in which sun damage is severe. Although only 9 years old, there is atrophy and inhomogeneity of the epidermal and pigment cells.

severe sensitivities such as xeroderma pigmentosum can be saved from all ill-effects by diligent protection including clothing. Indeed, clothing and household shade are the best protections for children sensitive to the sun, but a wet T-shirt can transmit ultraviolet rays; tightly woven silks and cottons are more effective than loose weave yarns or wool. Cold wind and other skin allergies should be avoided at the same time as light exposure, and fluorescent lighting should be kept at a distance. Glass windows and certain plastics are protective against shorter wavelengths. Natural pigment and thickening of the epidermis accounts for normal tolerance.

Sunscreening agents include thick pastes or creams such as titanium dioxide; these are popular with skiers but prevent tanning. They are most useful for lip protection. Some have a number indicating the protection factor; the higher the number the better the protection; above 6 is usually advised but severe sensitivity will require double or treble the degree of protection. Sunscreening agents may reflect light and invisible lotions or creams containing para-aminobenzoic acid in 70 per cent alcohol act in in a more complex way. These preparations absorb ultraviolet rays and allow gradual tanning.

Beta-carotene and mepacrine are pigments which can be taken

by mouth. Mepacrine is probably the most commonly used and can be given 100 mg daily or twice daily. It is chiefly effective against sunburn wave lengths whereas beta-carotene has been used for longer wavelengths. Aspirin, by inhibiting prostaglandin synthetase, reduces the erythema from sunburn.

Ultraviolet light can be cut out by certain somewhat expensive plastic films (UVethon-C or Y), and hospitals concerned with photosensitivity should have at least one area shielded by such films.

Treatment of the long-term effects of sunlight include the destruction and removal of lesions such as epitheliomata. These can be excised with good cosmetic results since they are often based on loose and inelastic skin. Curettage with gentle cautery is also effective. Cryosurgery with adequate freezing using liquid nitrogen is often now used. It is the thawing of intracellular ice crystals which destroys the cells. Swelling and blistering is initially troublesome, but provided secondary infection is avoided, scarring should be minimal. 5-Alpha fluorouracil cream is useful for multiple or widespread keratoses that are not suspected of malignant change. The cream is applied once daily and destroys dysplastic cells. Considerable soreness may result after 2–3 weeks but new healthy cells repopulate the skin as well as stimulate new ground substance in the upper dermis diminishing fine wrinkles and, in a sense, rejuvenating the skin.

X-ray is effective in destroying cancer but eventual inequalities in pigment and atrophy or sclerosis often results in a poorer cosmetic appearance than simple excision.

Is it what I have eaten? Food and drug eruptions

There is a large folklore and a strong belief that skin disorders are induced by what is eaten. The difficulty of proving this by any skin or in vitro test, and the frequency of the idiosyncratic and the rarity of statistical evidence for food hypersensitivity has resulted in swings of the pendulum of medical fashion. Today food allergic disease is taken seriously by many in the medical profession as has always been the case amongst lay people.

It is generally accepted that much of what we eat is antigenic and absorption does occur. Usually allergen is complexed with antibody in the gut wall and tolerance also occurs. It is easy to demonstrate that antibody is made to counteract food allergens and that complexes circulate in the blood as a result of eating. This is not necessarily allergy because resulting inflammation is rare. There is some evidence that the amount of antigen absorbed and complexed is reduced by disodium cromoglycate.

One of the difficulties of interpretation is that hypersensitivity depends on the frequency of ingestion and on the level of tolerance elicited. Infrequent ingestion is more likely to cause allergy than tolerance.

Supporting evidence for food allergic disease comes from the ingestion of medicaments. The public knows well that many drugs taken by mouth can cause a severe generalized eruption, as for instance, sulphonamides at one time commonly elicited.

Both erythema and urticaria can be caused by food. In the atopic, IgE-mediated food allergy is well recognized. It is a contact urticaria (see page 20.28) when eggs or milk touch the lips or it is a generalized urticaria and bowel upset when agents such as fish, nuts, or strawberries are eaten. However, in many patients such eruptions may have little to do with allergy but are pharmacologically induced, or at least they are examples of non-allergic intolerance.

Anaphylactoid reactions are either idiosyncrasies in which an individual reacts abnormally to a substance tolerated by most of the population due to some defect in his physiology, or they result from a direct effect or action of a drug on a mast cell, or other cell, often on first exposure to the eliciting substance. Examples of such non-allergic responses include C1 esterase deficiency and angio-oedema or lactose intolerance and deficiency of lactase, causing diarrhoea.

A high iodine level in a diet induces blistering in dermatitis herpetiformis and exacerbates erythema nodosum leprosum. Sources include iodophors used in dairy cleansing, iodine-containing food supplements and dough improvers in bread, as well as cough mixtures.

Following the development of toxic erythema and purpura in an extensive epidemic amongst eaters of margarine in Holland and Germany, the possibility that food additives could cause a rash has become well recognized. The total number of food additives exceeds 20 000 and an average person eats about 1.5 kg every year. Salicylates and benzoates as well as many colouring agents present in more than 1000 drugs marketed in the USA act in part through the control of prostaglandin metabolism. Ten per cent of persons sensitive to aspirin are also sensitive to the colouring agent tartrazine. The mechanism, though suspected to be related to prostaglandin metabolism, has yet to be clarified. Table 13 lists common foods containing salicylates, benzoates, and tartrazine. It is confusing that some other types of food allergy, perhaps less dependent on IgE and on the release of histamine from the mast cell, are prevented by prostaglandin inhibitors. 'If one takes indomethacin one can eat anything'!

Shellfish and strawberries are well known for not only releasing histamine from mast cells but for causing thrombocytopenic purpura. Usually such agents cause urticaria within hours of ingestion. The response is not consistent since there may be times or forms of presentation of the same food which avoid this effect. Eggs, nuts, chocolate, fish, shellfish, tomatoes, pork, strawberries, milk, cheese, and yeast are common causes of a sudden transient thrombocytopenia, and sensitivity to food in this way is the basis of the thrombo test. A 20 per cent fall in platelet count one hour after ingestion occurs in 70 per cent of persons showing allergy to aspirin, barbiturates, and penicillin. In one series 203 out of 215 cases of urticaria had a prolongation of bleeding time from the ear lobe 2 hours after challenge with a drug, chemical, or food. Bitter lemon or tonic water containing quinine is especially well documented.

In atopic eczema and asthma the problem of food allergy is more complex. These patients seem to be more susceptible to histamine release even from non-allergic sources.

The gut of the newborn with atopy is said to be more immature in its handling of foreign protein, or at least it may be that complexing of IgA is less effective and then IgG is brought into play in a manner not usual for the mature gut. This is the basis for the advocation of breast feeding without cows' milk substitution in all babies of atopic parents. Hypoallergic foods are marketed which contain 'predigested' casein and this is a rapidly developing new industry with a strong following. However, minute amounts of antigens from maternal diet are found in breast milk, so one cannot assume that the first experience of dietary antigen is at the time of weaning. Even the fetus is normally supplied by minute samples of the mother's diet. What matters is how much and when.

Another form of food sensitivity is that occurring in nickel sensitive subjects. Nickel sensitivity is one of the commonest causes of hand dermatitis and there seems little doubt that contamination from metal pots and from some green vegetables can contribute to the eczema in those who are sensitive.

Drug eruptions

The 1975 Boston Collaborative Program of Drug Surveillance observed that 3 per cent of hospital admissions, 14 per cent of medical resources, and 30 per cent of hospital patients developed adverse reactions. This is an epidemic of modern civilization and is partly due to the abuse of free drugs particularly where there are health services. In developing countries cheap drugs such as sulphonamides are the commonest cause of adverse reactions. The drugs known to cause disease in the technically advanced countries are slow to be taken off the market and may even be promoted in countries where the drug industry is poorly supervised.

Table 13A Colouring and preservative free diet (prepared by Karen Ross, John Radcliffe Hospital, Oxford)

Foods allowed	Foods to be avoided
Meat	
All types fresh or plain frozen	Manufactured products, e.g. sausages, burgers, tinned meats, etc.
Fish	
All types, fresh or plain frozen	Manufactured products, e.g. smoked fish, fish fingers, fish in sauces, etc.
Dairy produce	
Eggs, fresh milk, fresh cream, white cheese*, natural yoghurt*	Dried milks, artificial creams, coloured cheese, cheese spreads, flavoured/fruit yoghurt, ice cream
Fruit	
Fresh only	Manufactured products, e.g. fruit pie fillings, some tinned fruits
Vegetables	
Fresh, plain frozen, tinned in salt water only	Manufactured products, e.g. instant potato, tinned vegetable mixes, baked beans, ready mixed salads
Cereals	
Raw cereals, e.g. rice, sago. Flours and homemade flour products, homemade cakes, biscuits, wholemeal bread*, homemade desserts	Manufactured products including cakes, biscuits, bread mixes, etc. Instant puddings, tinned sponges, custards, blancmanges, dessert mixes. Yellow pasta
Beverages	
Tea, coffee, fresh fruit juices*, colour-free squashes* and fizzy drinks, water, soda water	Fruit squashes and fizzy drinks, malted milk drinks
Preserves	
Honey*, homemade jam*, marmalade*, lemon curd	Manufactured jams, marmalades, lemon curd
Soups	
Homemade only	Manufactured tinned and packet soups
Confectionery	
White mints	Sweets and chocolate
Miscellaneous	
Salt, pepper, herbs, fresh spices	Pickles, curry powder, bottled sauces and dressings

* May naturally contain benzoic acid or have an added preservative.

Table 13B

Foods naturally containing benzoic acid

Processed cheese	
Yoghurt: natural and fruit types	Apple juice
Avocado	Grapefruit juice
Cherry	Orange juice
Nectarine	Dried apricot
Papaya	Dried banana
Peach	Dried peach
Strawberry	Dried plum (prune)
Jams: apricot	
blueberry	
cranberry	
strawberry	
Marmalade: grapefruit	
orange	
Honey	

Foods naturally containing salicylates
Salicylate values for foods vary widely and therefore this list may not be exhaustive and should be used as a guide only

Fruit
Dried fruit and all products containing dried fruit, e.g. cake, biscuits, mincemeat, muesli, etc.

Apple	
Banana	Strawberry
Grapes	Raspberry
Rhubarb	Orange
Blackcurrant	Cherry
Blackberry	Prunes
Gooseberry	Plums

Juices based on these fruits
Jams and jellies based on these fruits

Vegetables
Peas
Sweetcorn
Tomato and all products containing tomato, e.g. sauces, tinned spaghetti in tomato sauce, etc.

Miscellaneous
Vinegar and all pickles and sauces containing vinegar
Ice cream
Cake mixes
Liquorice, chewing gum
Almonds
Beer, wine, cider, port, brandy

Diet sheets of this kind are difficult to compile. The DHSS produce a leaflet *Look at the Label* which lists all the additives used in foods, and details their corresponding E numbers, enabling identification of their presence in all manufactured foods.

It is wise to assume that any drug can cause any rash, like syphilis, but until there are simple *in vitro* tests for testing human tissue for hypersensitivity which are both reliable and specific, the diagnosis of drug eruptions will depend entirely on clinical judgement. The physician has to decide whether the rash has some other cause by the recognition of physical signs, ranging from the burrows of the acarus in scabies to the herald patch of pityriasis rosea. Then if a drug seems a likely cause, there must be an attempt to decide which of the medications currently prescribed or taken secretly may be responsible.

Drug rashes are essentially blood borne and therefore often have a symmetrical urticarial, erythematous, or purpuric and ischaemic pattern determined by vascular anatomy. Less likely is a 'primary epithelial' reaction in the initial stages and so scaling or even the vesiculation of eczema as a first manifestation of a drug rash would be unusual. The exceptions are well known and include the intraepidermal immunologically induced 'pemphigus' rash of penicillamine, rifampicin, and captopril, especially when the first of these is used to treat rheumatoid arthritis, and the cell-mediated hypersensitivity to epidermal protein and drug haptens

in a person previously having a contact dermatitis to a local antihistamine or sulphonamide. The psoriasis-like rash of practolol and various other beta-blockers, or the scaly eruption particularly of the scalp from methyldopa, are exceptions.

Nevertheless if a rash looks like eczema, it is probably not caused by a drug. If it is an erythema and urticaria, it may well be. Later stages of the rash are frequently complicated by a secondary epidermal reaction so that diagnosis should be made on the initial manifestation.

Unlikely or likely drugs

It may be helpful to rule out unlikely offenders such as digoxin, paracetamol, steroids, other hormones, and vitamin and electrolyte supplements. In any drug group there are likely and less likely offenders. Thus of antibiotics, oxytetracycline, nystatin, and erythromycin are not under suspicion but dichlortetracycline is a common cause of a photosensitivity rash, and in infectious mononucleosis ampicillin is almost invariably responsible for a characteristic bright pink maculopapular rash.

To be fair to the drug industry, in rating likelihood one also has to take into account the huge amounts of some drugs that are prescribed without any reactions. In this respect, while one occasionally sees rashes from chlordiazepoxide, diazepam, or nitrazepam, it must be an extremely rare event.

Timing

Timing is useful when trying to establish mechanisms such as anaphylaxis or the Arthus phenomenon. The patient should be asked about previous reactions to drugs. In the absence of such history and especially if the drugs were new to the patient it would be unlikely to cause a rash within the first few days of administration. There is an exception to this which may have little to do with recognizing immune mechanisms and that is the way in which drug eruptions develop in combination with infections. A cough mixture given for a sore throat or co-trimoxazole for some infection or other, especially viral, may produce an extremely severe erythema within 2 or 3 days of the intake. Later administrations on another occasion will cause no trouble. Erythema multiforme or Stevens–Johnson syndrome occasionally occurs surprisingly early after a drug's administration and one suspects that the disease for which the drug was given may have prepared the host in some way.

Where there is a known hypersensitivity to the drug such as sulphonamides or penicillin, even when the history of the drug rash was decades earlier, the immunological response can be very rapid.

Slow excretion, genetically determined or due to depot injections, are other reasons for slow recovery from an eruption. It is also helpful to realize that for some drugs taken over many years the likelihood of their being the cause of the rash is small, thus the much prescribed phenylbutazone may produce a drug eruption but it does so usually within months of the first prescription. When examining a list of drugs taken by a patient, drugs added within the previous month are the most likely cause of the rash. However, interference with metabolic pathways by drugs may take many months to produce a rash, as for example, izoniazid and the production of pellagra.

Many patients do not admit to taking a drug, perhaps because it was never prescribed but was borrowed from a neighbour or bought over the counter and therefore considered to be harmless. In general drug rashes do not persist after withdrawal of the drug – exceptions include pemphigus from penicillamine.

Transient susceptibility

The best example of susceptibility is urticaria. Many persons with chronic urticaria are susceptible to it for a period of many months, and during that time the rash may be triggered by prostaglandin synthetase inhibitors, such as aspirin or indomethazine. It is possible that certain acute erythemas require both a drug and an infection to provoke the rash, so the underlying disease of the patient should always be taken into account. One suspects that sometimes immune complex diseases from infective organisms are provoked by interference with immunological mechanisms by certain drugs. The particular set of circumstances, which may not recur, would depend on the formation of antibodies, the nature of the infectious organism, and the taking of the drug at that time. Diseases such as psoriasis or dermatitis herpetiformis may go into spontaneous remission and at such time they are less likely to be provoked by drugs. Psoriasis is expected to be made worse by beta blockers, lithium, or chloroquine but this is unpredictable and not a reason for withholding them. Dermatitis herpetiformis is provoked by iodine so readily that it should be avoided if possible.

Drug allergy is rarely proven but overdosage is a frequent well established fact due to faulty prescribing, attempted suicide, or altered metabolism as in renal or hepatic failure. Drugs may interfere with metabolism, with hormones, they may be deposited, they may react with sunlight, they may modify the ecology of the skin in respect to infective organisms; they may cause reactivity of certain cells such as the mast cell; they may be cytoxic and they can act as allergens in the formation of immune complexes, hapten protein complexes, delayed cellular immunity, and a variety of other mechanisms. Some are not understood such as the effect of

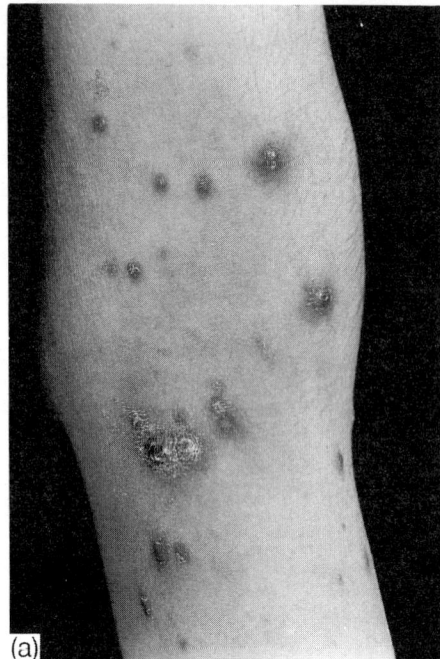

(a)

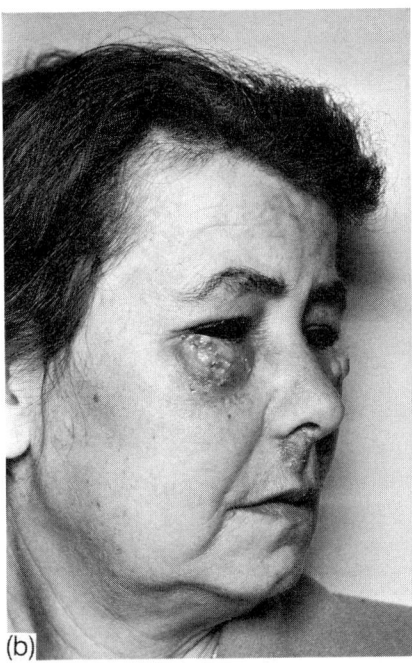

(b)

Fig. 31 (a) Iodides and bromides are occasionally responsible for a granulomatous eruption with pseudo-epitheliomatous hypertrophy. Potassium iodide in a cough mixture was responsible for the eruption in this patient. (b) Prolonged administration of iodides or bromides causes a particularly inflammatory form of acne which, though commonly in the distribution of acne vulgaris, may be more widespread. This eruption was due to an iodide-containing 'tonic' for the blood.

halogens on the formation of granulomata (Fig. 31a) and in the causation of an acneiform eruption (Fig. 31b). This includes the use of fluoride gel preparations applied to the teeth to prevent dental caries.

Specific drug eruptions

The commonest diagnostic problem is a toxic urticated erythema. It begins like measles without the upper respiratory and conjunctival prodromal signs. It usually develops, over a number of hours,

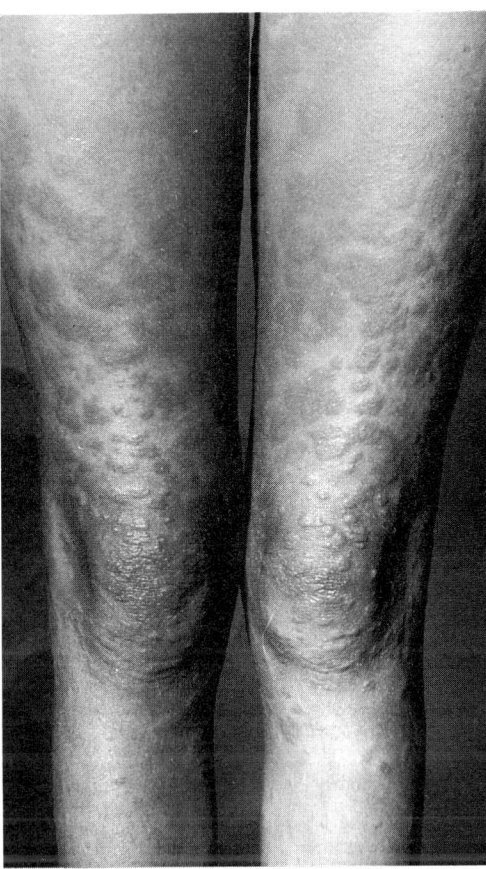

Fig. 32 One of the commonest of drug eruptions, initially a bright pink papular eruption, symmetrical and becoming confluent. This case is due to ampicillin.

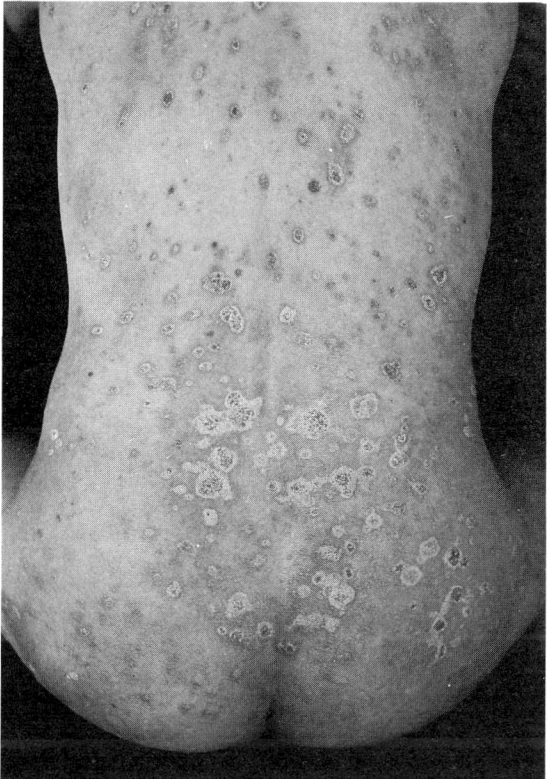

Fig. 33 A later stage of acute drug eruption, in this case due to Myocrisin, in which the epidermis is reacting to the dermal inflammation by hyperplasia spreading centrifugally to produce an annular scaly lesion with the scale exfoliating in the centre of the lesion and attached to the spreading margin.

as a red indurated papular eruption (Fig. 32), and unlike urticaria persists for days, ultimately involving the epidermis and producing scales (Fig. 33). After the first 2–3 days the rash tends to be fixed and the principal changes are due to mild bleeding of the skin with overlying slight peeling. This type of rash is usually not seen before at least 8–10 days after the ingestion of the drug. Fever and arthropathy may be associated. Common causes are ampicillin, phenylbutazone, phenothiazine, co-trimoxazole, diazides, and sulphonylureas. Exfoliative dermatitis is the end result of this type of reaction (Fig. 34). Gold, phenylbutazone, indomethacin, allopurinol, hydantoins, sulphonylureas, and para-amino salicylic acid are causative drugs.

Ampicillin and amoxycillin Ampicillin rash appears 5–14 days after treatment of an infection. Thus the rash is often seen after the course of the drug has been completed. It begins on the extensor aspects of the limbs and has a morbilliform or maculopapular pattern which becomes confluent. It is a bright pink-reddish colour and may become purpuric and desquamate. In the pigmented skin such features are usually recognizable. The rash occurs in 5–7 per cent of all recipients and is the usual consequence of prescribing the drug for infective mononucleosis, cytomegalovirus, or lymphatic leukaemia.

Beta-blockers These cause a psoriasiform scaly eruption that may be modified by basal cell necrosis. The high turnover as in psoriasis, with the slowing down that results from such necrosis, gives rise to a hyperkeratotic scale that is more adherent than in psoriasis and often slightly yellowish. The palms and soles, elbows, and knees are particularly favoured (Fig. 35).

Practolol, labetalol, propranolol, and oxprenolol cause a rash which is partly psoriasiform and partly lichenoid and is most marked over bony prominences. There is hyperkeratosis of the

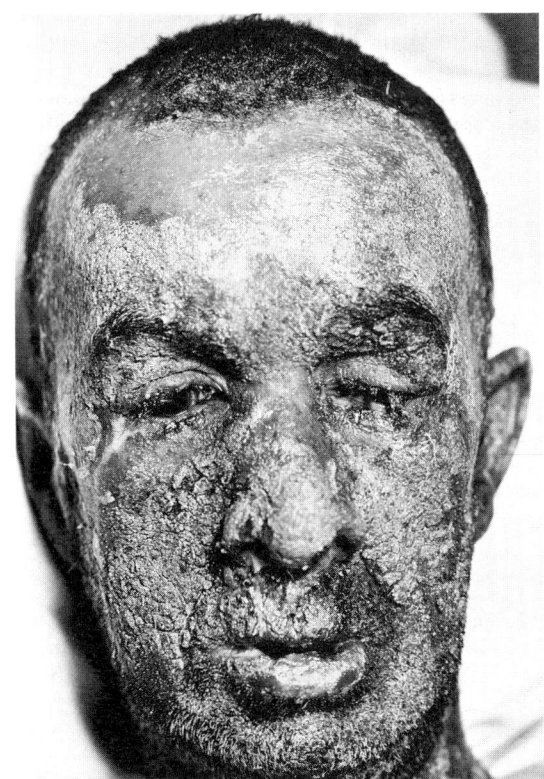

Fig. 34 Severe oedema, crusting, and exfoliation due to dermatitis from arsenicals.

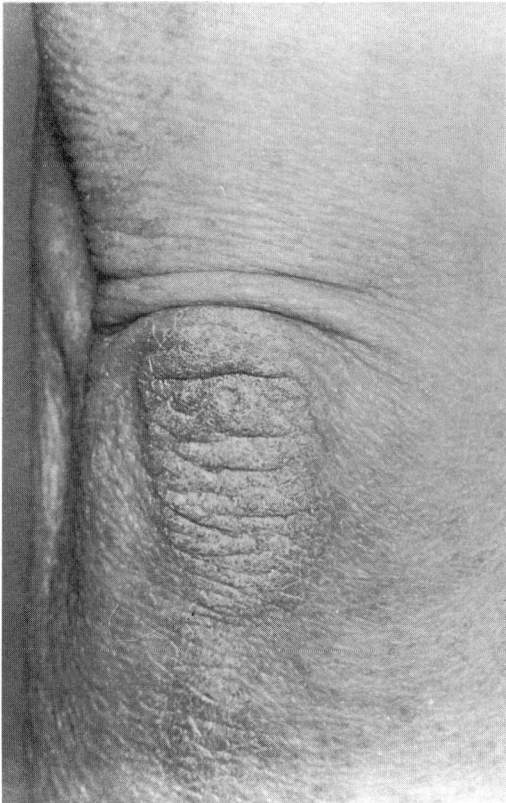

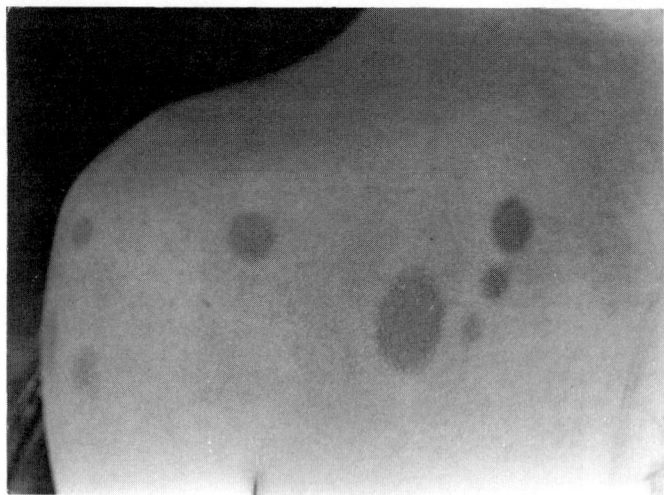

Fig. 36 Fixed drug eruption due to phenolphthalein present in a laxative. Such an eruption characteristically appears within half a day of taking the causative drug and the site affected is the same on every occasion. Violaceous annular lesions are common and may persist for several weeks.

Table 14 Drugs causing fixed drug eruptions

Phenazone (synonym: antipyrine)
Phenolphthalein
Barbiturates
Sulphonamides
Dapsone
Quinine and derivatives
Tetracyclines
Oxyphenbutazone
Chlordiazepoxide

Fig. 35 Hyperkeratosis and slight scaling is a feature of the psoriasiform eruption caused by beta-blockers.

palms and soles which is itchy. The rash of practolol develops over several months and unlike psoriasis there may be antinuclear and antiepithelial antibody resulting in damage to the skin and conjunctiva (initially just hyperaemia but later there is sclerosis with shrinkage). Circulating antibody which binds to the intercellular region of guinea pigs' stratified epithelium can be demonstrated. Eosinophils are sometimes plentiful in the dermis. Most beta-blockers merely exacerbate ordinary psoriasis. Remission results from discontinuation.

Lupus erythematosus
Lupus erythematosus, like erythemas or necrotizing vasculitis are most commonly caused by hydralazine, phenytoin, practolol, penicillamine, and isoniazid. Many other drugs have been incriminated. The drug-induced LE is reversed by withdrawal of the drug but it recurs when it is readministered. The disease is characterized by antinuclear antibody in high titre with normal DNA binding. Inhibition of C4 underlies the immunological disease induced by hydralazine.

Scleroderma
An epidemic originating from denatured rape seed oil in Spain caused facial oedema, exanthems, and ultimately a scleroderma-like syndrome.

Photosensitivity
This occurs in light-exposed areas such as the face, neck, forearms, or the dorsum of the feet. It is usually due to long-wave UVA and so glass and cloud are not necessarily protective. However, photosensitivity does occur more often on a bright spring or summer mid-day. The resulting phototoxic eruption begins as an erythema and, as with severe sunburn can become bullous or as in the case of amiodarone result in blue-grey pigmentation. The problem drugs are listed in Table 12.

Fixed drug eruption
Although the mechanism is unexplained, the eruption is easy to recognize as it is usually annular and erythematous (Fig. 36), it frequently blisters, and after resolution of the acute phase, may be a dull purple-brown colour caused by macrophage transport of melanin to the dermis. It is fixed in site and whenever the subject takes the causative drug the eruption begins within a few hours and is in exactly the same site as on a previous occasion was affected. The tongue and the glans penis are common sites. The affected area can be transplanted without loss of responsiveness in some cases. In pigmented races very dark pigmentation remains between attacks. Purgatives, blood cleansers and tonics, and many other homely remedies may contain phenolphthalein which in most countries is the commonest cause. Causative drugs are listed in Table 14.

The investigation of fixed drug eruption is a little easier than for most other drugs since it is safe to test. Many patients are not aware of the significance of many of the drugs they take as analgesics, laxatives, and tonics, and therefore a very searching history is necessary. Others taking indigenous remedies are complicated by their being largely of unknown content and many of the foods we eat have hundreds of unknown constituents. The mechanism of penicillin reactions is discussed elsewhere.

Management of drug eruptions
The best way is to stop the use of all drugs likely to cause the eruptions. Readministration of the drug is possible for most drug eruptions other than those that cause anaphylactic shock, but it is usually at a risk of considerable morbidity and it should be considered only if essential to the patient. Skin tests are not helpful, as a risk of dangerous anaphylaxis, false negatives, and lack of

knowledge of the antigen, makes skin testing useless. Penicilloyl polylysine has been found useful for testing for penicillin sensitivity. Where there is a medicament dermatitis due from contact, then patch testing is helpful.

Blood tests are of no help in trying to find which drug is causing the problem. Various tests like the reaction of basophil cells or the release of lymphokines from the lymphocyte have not proved of routine value. Eosinophils may suggest that an eruption is due to a drug, and as mentioned above, a fall of platelets within 1 hour or a prolongation of bleeding time 2 hours after injection is helpful for some urticarial rashes.

References

Ackroyd, J. F. (1985). Fixed drug eruptions. *Br. med. J.* 288, 1533–1534.

Alper, J. C. (1981). Principles of genetics as related to the chromosome disorders and congenital malformations with reference to prenatal diagnosis and genetic counseling. *J. Am. Acad. Dermatol.* **4**, 379–394.

Arndt, K. A. and Jick, H. (1976). Rates of cutaneous reaction to drugs. *J. Am. med. Ass.* **235**, 918–923.

Baker, H. (1980). Drug reactions. In *Textbook of dermatology*, 3rd edn. (eds A. Rook, D. S. Wilkinson, and F. J. G. Ebling), pp. 1111–1149. Blackwell Scientific Publications, Oxford.

Bergsma, D. (1979). *Birth defects compendium*. Macmillan, London.

Bleehen, S. S. (1980). Metabolic and nutritional disorders. In *Textbook of dermatology*, 3rd edn. (eds A. Rook, D. S. Wilkinson, and F. J. G. Ebling), pp. 2037–2100. Blackwell Scientific Publications, Oxford.

Bruinsma, W. (1982). *A guide to drug eruptions. A file of adverse reactions to the skin*, p. 124. Distributed by De Zwaluw, PO Box 21, Oosthuizen, The Netherlands.

Dahl, M. V. (1980). HLA-1A and the skin. In *Year book of dermatology* (eds R. L. Dobson and B. H. Thiers), pp. 13–50. Year Book Medical Publishers, Chicago.

Der Kaloustian, V. M. and Kurban, A. K. (1979). *Genetic diseases of the skin*, p. 334. Springer-Verlag, Berlin.

Desai, S. C. (1972). Infections and communicable dermatoses; reflections on the massive morbidity of scabies, pyoderma and mycotic infections. In *Essays on tropical dermatology* Vol. 2 (ed. J. Marshall), pp. 296–300. Excerpta Medica, Amsterdam.

Du Vivier, A. (1982). Spotting the malignant melanoma. *Br. Med. J.* **285**, 671–672.

Ebrahaim, G. J. (1972). The skin in malnutrition. In *Essays on tropical dermatology* Vol. 2 (ed. J. Marshall), pp. 124–128. Excerpta Medica, Amsterdam.

Emmett, E. A. (1984). The skin and occupational diseases. *Arch. Environ. Hlth* **39**, 144–149.

Epstein, J. H. (1979). Systemic disease and light dermatology. In *Dermatology update* (ed. S. L. Moschella), pp. 119–144. Elsevier, New York.

Fitzpatrick, T. B., Eisen, A. Z., Wolff, K., Freedberg, I. M. and Austen, K. F. (1979). *Dermatology in general medicine*, p. 1884. McGraw-Hill, New York.

Gedde-Dahl, T. (1981). Sixteen types of epidermolysis bullosa. *Acta dermatol.* (Suppl. 95), 74–87.

Hanifin, J. M. (1984). Basic and clinical aspects of atopic dermatitis. *Allergy* **52**, 386–394.

Journal of Investigative Dermatology (1979a). Special issue on aging. *J. invest. Dermatol.* 73, Suppl. 1, 134.

—— (1979b). Infections, *J. invest. Dermatol.* **73**, 452–459.

—— (1979c). Birth defects and genetic disorders. *J. invest. Dermatol.* **73**, 460–472.

—— (1979d). Skin reactions to environmental agents. *J. invest. Dermatol.* 73, 501–511.

Lew, R. A., Sober, A. J., Cook, N., Marvell, R. and Fitzpatrick, T. B. (1983). Sun exposure habits in patients with cutaneous melanoma. A case control study. *J. Dermatol. Surg. Oncol.* **9**, 981–986.

Magnus, I. A. (1976). *Dermatological photobiology. Clinical and experimental aspects*. Blackwell Scientific Publications, Oxford.

Miller, K. (1982). Sensitivity to tartrazine. *Br. med. J.* **285**, 1597.

Orkin, M. (1975). Today's scabies. *J. Am. med. Assoc.* **233**, 882–885.

Podell, R. (1985). Unwrapping urticaria. The role of food additives. *Postgrad. Med.* **78**, 83–97.

Rebello, M., Val, T. F., Garijo, F., Quintana, F. and Berciano, J. (1983). Livedo reticularis and cerebrovascular lesions (Sneddon's syndrome), clinical, radiological and pathological features of eight cases. *Brain* **106**, 965–979.

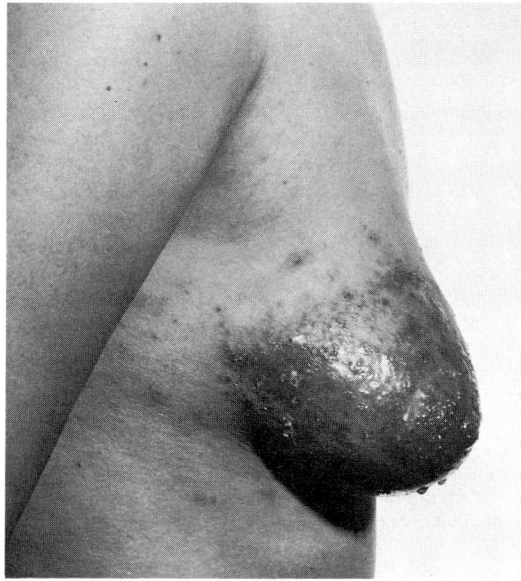

Fig. 37 Acute dermatitis is characterized by an oedematous epidermis in which vesiculation, oozing, and crusting are the principal features. The borders are often ill-defined while the centre of the lesion is confluent.

Rook, A., Wilkinson, D. S., and Ebling, F. J. G. (1979). *Textbook of dermatology* 3rd edn, p. 2366. Blackwell Scientific Publications, Oxford.

Swedlow, A. J. (1979). Incidence of malignant melanoma of the skin in England and Wales and its relationship to sunlight. *Br. med. J.* 282, 1324–1327.

Urbach, F. (1969). *Biologic effects of ultraviolet radiation (with emphasis on skin)*. Pergamon Press, Oxford.

Young, A. W. and Miller, L. (1968). Skin problems in the geriatric and general hospital, incidence, scope cause. *J. Am. Geriat. Soc.* **16**, 1140–1149.

Wall, L. M. and Smith, N. P. (1981). Perniosis: a histopathological review. *Clin. exp. Dermatol.* **6**, 263–272.

Zachary, C. B., Slater, D. N., Holt, D. W., Storey, G. C. A. and MacDonald, D. M. (1984). The pathogenesis of amiodarone-induced pigmentation and photosensitivity. *Br. J. Dermatol.* **10**, 451–456.

Dermatitis

Definition

Dermatitis is the commonest of reaction patterns in the skin. The term is used especially for a reaction of the skin to external injury as in 'industrial' or in 'contact' dermatitis. Eczema has a similar meaning but is used more often for endogenous or constitutional dermatitis.

Clinical features

Dermatitis has both dermal and epidermal components. There are signs confined to the dermis such as swelling, heat, itchiness, tenderness, and redness, but at the same time the epidermis proliferates and therefore thickens and produces scale. The oedema in the dermis extends to the epidermis, swells the cells, and separates them giving the histological appearance of a sponge, known as spongiosis, and frequently this results in vesicles which distinguish dermatitis from other proliferative states of the epidermis such as psoriasis. Acute weeping exudation occurs when the vesicles burst (Fig. 37). In dermatitis itching is usually severe.

The reaction pattern of dermatitis is not homogeneous. It is made up of papular elements of different ages and size sometimes confluent in the centre (Fig. 38) with widely scattered satellite papules or vesicles. The scales are of varied size and broken by excoriation, exudate, and even pinpoint haemorrhages.

A secondary factor prominent in the pigmented skin is loss of melanin or at least failure to retain it in the acute lesion so that the

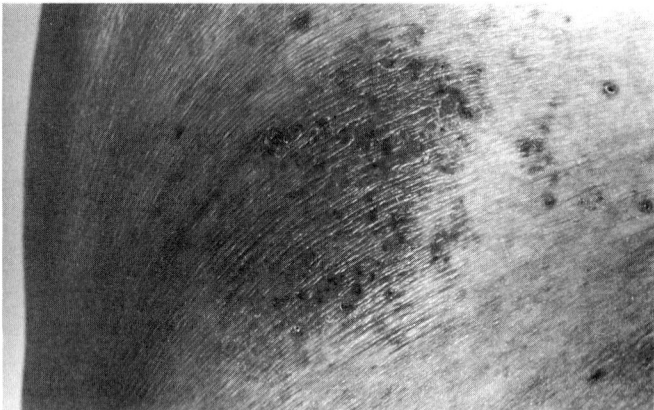

Fig. 38 Dermatitis is comprised of papules which are confluent in the centre and become vesicular or evidently excoriated. Oedema makes the line markings in the skin more prominent. There are satellite lesions beyond an ill-defined border.

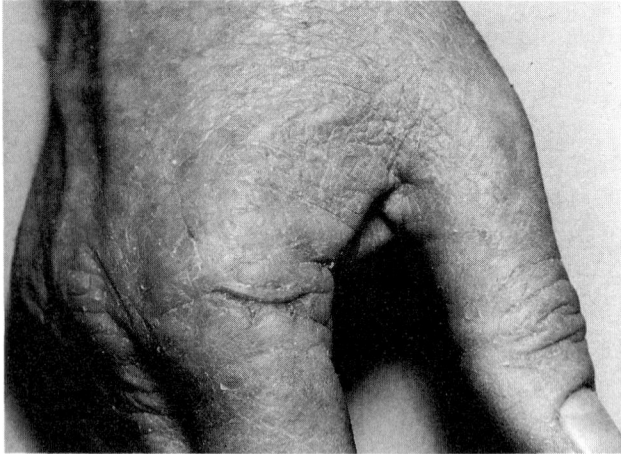

Fig. 39 Chronic dermatitis causes irregular thickening of an inhomogeneous epidermis. The texture of the stratum corneum varies so that it is firmly attached at some points but exfoliates with small scales at others. Loss of moisture causes decreased suppleness, cracking over joints, and exposure of deeper epidermal cells. This causes irritation of the dermis at the bottom of the deep crevasses.

skin is depigmented. In later or more chronic stages the dermis is darkened by 'incontinence' of pigment so that thickened chronic epidermal plaques may contain increased pigment in the underlying dermis. Chronic scratched skin has a brownish violaceous colour due to the combination of pigment, vasodilatation, and epidermal thickening.

For reasons unknown, dermatitis of the hand or foot usually provokes a response at other sites. Thus, vesicular eczema of the hands often follows a fungus infection of the feet, and varicose eczema of the lower legs often spreads to the forearms and face.

Contact dermatitis

Wear and tear or primary irritant

Contact dermatitis is one of the greatest public health problems. It particularly affects the hands. Wear and tear, known as irritant dermatitis, is the commonest cause of hand dermatitis. In other words, simple irritation from external agents accounts for by far the greatest proportion of skin disease (and less than one-fifth of such involvement is due to allergy). Indeed in industry, most outbreaks of dermatitis are not due to allergy but due to the introduction of irritants into the work process or changes in the environment such as humidity or excessive drying. The skin is subjected to and indeed designed to withstand enormous wear and tear. Like leather, to which it may be converted, it can wear out. Industrial or occupational dermatitis are terms which indicate what may happen to the skin through its everyday exposure.

It is important to distinguish between wear and tear, taking into account different degrees of toughness or vulnerability, and allergic contact dermatitis since their aetiology and management are different. A skin that is worn is dry and unsupple. Deep cracks occur through the normally resilient and elastic stratum corneum. Underlying epidermal cells and the dermis are no longer protected and the cracks become secondarily infected (Fig. 39).

An irritant can be defined as a chemical that in most people is capable of producing cell damage if applied for a sufficient time and in a sufficient concentration. Fibreglass spicules rubbed into the skin are a typical example (Fig. 40). Many persons at home or in industry are in daily contact with various chemicals over long periods. They work in wet or extremely dry conditions with skin cleaners, alkalis, acids, cutting fluids, solvents and oxidants, reducing agents, enzymes, and medicaments. The skin is also worn and irritated by cold and heat, sun, pressure, scratching, or friction of various kinds from tools or clothing. There are many variables which influence its toughness or vulnerability. It can be immature in the newborn or worn out in the aged. The most important cause of lowered resistance is constitutional disease such as the ichthyotic skin of old age, atopic eczema (Fig. 41), or

psoriasis. Heredity of mainly polygenic type influences dermatitis by an effect on the constitution of the skin. There is as yet only little evidence in man of a hereditary factor in contact allergic dermatitis, neither HLA studies not twin studies having confirmed such a role in man as compared to animal studies.

Contact urticaria

This is an acute swelling developing within a few minutes to half an hour of contact with certain agents. In atopic eczema there is an especial susceptibility to this phenomenon but it is also well recognized in non-atopic subjects and is particularly common as a result of the application of cosmetics. Many agents commonly applied to the skin will produce irritation in certain sites, such as the eyelids or scrotum, and this is not always an immunological phenomenon. Agents causing contact urticaria are listed in Table 15. It is increasingly well recognized (see page 20.30).

Contact allergic dermatitis

Sensitization can occur 7–10 days after the first contact with a potent allergen. It is more usually, however, a consequence of many months or years of exposure to small amounts of allergen. Once sensitized, contact with allergen can produce dermatitis within 24–48 hours and all areas of the body are equally susceptible. Sensitivity can vary due to the amount of exposure, the degree of penetration of the skin, and the tolerance of the immune system.

It is believed that certain allergens, such a nickel and chrome, have a greater affinity for the skin than others. This is in part the easier recognition and assimilation by the epidermal macrophages known as Langerhans cells. It is uncertain whether the allergen binds to epidermal microsomal protein or to some cell surface marker or even to serum proteins which are plentiful in the epidermis. It is a complex of the allergen with such protein that is recognized as foreign but whether such recognition is peripheral or must be in the lymph node is also not entirely clear. It is the T lymphocyte which ultimately recognizes the complex but the macrophage is a necessary intermediary. Suppression of Langerhan's cells by ultraviolet rays diminishes cell-mediated immunity. Genetic factors play a part in the recognition process. Once recognized, T cell proliferation occurs in the paracortical area of the lymph node. On re-exposure sensitized lymphocytes release lymphokines. The mechanisms of lymphocyte stimulation include some role for suppressor and effector cells but this too is incompletely understood. The role of antibodies, some of which are clearly specific for the

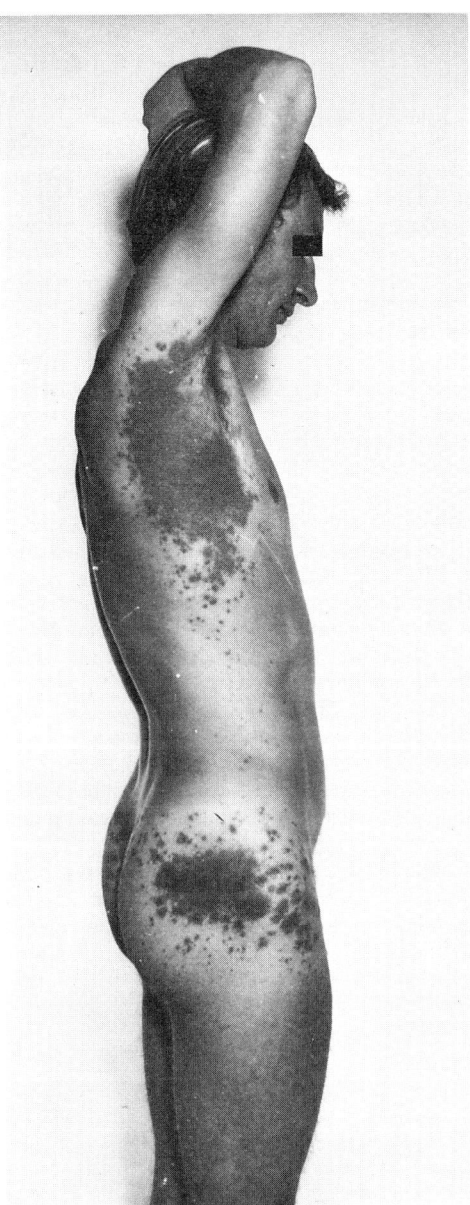

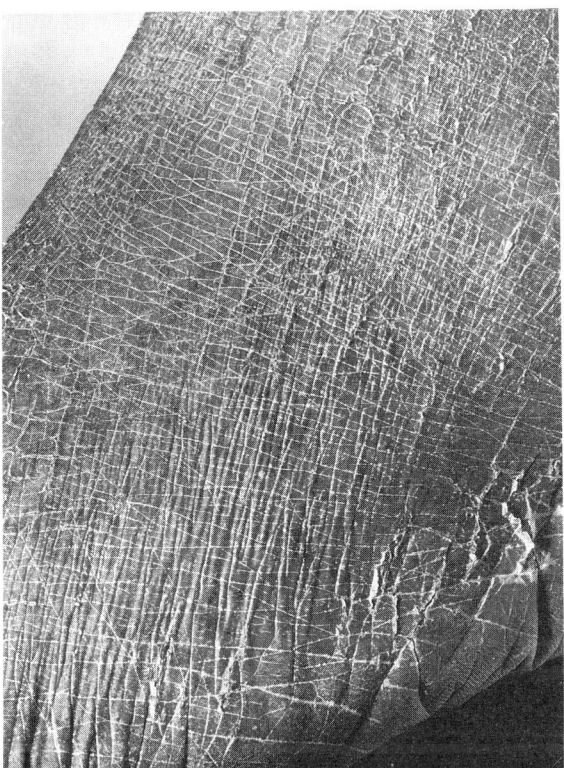

Fig. 41 Chronically thin and slowly turning-over epidermis results in a closely knit stratum corneum which is firmly adherent but cracks excessively. It is characteristic of elderly, malnourished, or ichthyotic skin. Such skin is less resistant to primary irritants.

Vaseline dermatitis in the Bantu is an example. In technically advanced countries deodorants are a common cause of dermatitis, and in the hair industry, hair bleaches such as ammonia persulphate commonly cause immediate non-immune wealing. When in doubt because the constituents are so complex, cosmetics should be tested by direct application to the skin. Hair dyes are now so common that their relative safety can be expected. However, again in developing countries, the dye paraphenylenediamine may produce an acute dermatitis often first affecting the eyelids and other aspects of the face before showing much evidence of dermatitis of the scalp.

2. Clothing and textile dermatitis On the whole this is rare but clips containing metal are a quite common cause of dermatitis (Fig. 42), e.g. jean buttons cause dermatitis of the skin below the umbilicus. There is evidence also that the rubber in elastic of many garments is sometimes the cause of dermatitis. Dyes are usually a problem at sites of friction where there is also moisturization by sweat. The majority are azodyes or paraphenylenediamine. In the textile industry chrome and formaldehyde are important agents causing dermatitis.

Shoe dermatitis is commonly due to chrome but rubber additives such as mercaptobenzothiazole or butyl phenol formaldehyde may also be responsible as may adhesives and dyes. It should be considered in every person with eczema of the feet. It often spares the area between the toes as this is the point at which the shoe is not in contact with the skin. Modern footwear has plasticized toecaps and fails to absorb sweat. Increased sweating encourages shearing strain on the skin particularly in the athletic child. Frictional dermatitis of the foot is common in such children and is known as juvenile plantar dermatosis.

3. Foods In the technically advanced countries the handling of animal feeds including antibiotics gives more trouble than the handling of food for human consumption. Elsewhere plants and fruits such as garlic, cinnamon, onion, and lemon or orange cause

Fig. 40 Primary irritant dermatitis due to small spicules of fibreglass at sites of friction following the insulation of a roof.

same antigen, is also unknown. The inflammatory reaction resulting from recognition is variable and dependent on other pharmacological agents including secretions from the mast cell and on prostaglandins. Some of the variability of response such that persons are consequently labelled as more or less allergic depends on these secondary factors and can be modified by various conditional factors including anxiety and the hormonal status of the monthly menstrual cycle.

Contact dermatitis sensitizers

In the following, I will concentrate on some specific groups of sensitizers and irritants:

1. Cosmetics Cosmetics applied to the skin, though more rarely a cause of dermatitis in technically advanced countries where the industry has worked hard to eliminate allergens, are still a source of much disease in developing countries. Lanolin and parabens are common agents causing contact allergic dermatitis and they are the bases and preservatives of many agents. Perfumes containing tars, formaldehyde and Dowicil are increasingly incriminated.

much trouble, as do shellfish and various species of fish which are sometimes contaminated by algae. This is an important hazard for fisherman and is known as the 'Dogger Bank' itch in the United Kingdom.

4. Plastics A new and increasingly frequent cause of dermatitis is from acrylic and epoxy polymers or resins. Acrylic accounts for dermatitis from adhesive tape, spectacle frames, bonding agents, dentures, hearing aids, bone cement, artificial finger nails, sealants, printing plates, and inks.

Epoxy resins are used as surface coatings for steel pipes and ships, powder paints, electrical insulation adhesives, construction of concrete and steel buildings, and for the surface of roads and bridges. They are amongst the most potent sensitizers and are active in this respect only during their initial handling. Complete polymerization makes the sensitizing monomer non-available. About 90 per cent of contact dermatitis from epoxy resins is from bisphenol A. Protection in industry depends on common sense avoidance of handling and general cleanliness in the workshop.

5. Rubber Natural as well as synthetic rubbers require the addition of several agents that are strong sensitizers. They make the rubber more malleable and supple, prevent perishing by oxidization, and some speed up the processes of manufacture.

Accelerators include thiuram, mercaptobenzothiazole, and guanides; antioxidants include monobenzyl ether of hydroquinone. Most cases of rubber sensitivity are from clothing such as rubber gloves, or in industry they are from tyres or rubber linings in the transport industry. Others include the contraceptive sheath, shoes, fingerstalls, masks, particularly in the motorbike or scuba-diving pursuits, elastic bands, bicycle or golf club handles, and rubber sheets or cushions.

6. Colophony Rosin is made from pine trees and is used worldwide for paper size adhesives, inks, underseal cables, Elastoplast, violin rosin, and cosmetics. Some medicaments like Zambuk, seccaderm salve, or ilonium, also contain colophony, and it explains contact dermatitis from these agents. It is responsible for about

3.5 per cent of eczema patients patch tested in the London contact dermatitis clinics.

7. Plants and wood Sensitivity to plants and woods accounts for enormous worldwide morbidity and occasional mortality. Some plants release their allergen only when bruised, others when lightly touched, and others by airborne pollen. Some produce a contact non-allergic urticaria, i.e. immediate stinging as with the nettle or cowhage; others cause an allergic dermatitis, or even photosensitivity. Many are highly irritant.

In North America the commonest cause is poison ivy. In Europe it is the *Primula obconica*. Both produce a severe streaky blistering eruption from contact allergy mediated by cellular immunity.

The chrysanthemum or ragweed plants, known as the compositae or daisy family, cause a more diffuse redness and oedema of the face from sesquiterpene lactones. This may look like a photosensitivity and be enhanced by sunlight. Avoidance of the plant may be impossible in those persons whose job depends on contact with it and is an especial problem where the environment contains it as a common weed. It accounts for mortality in the region of Poona, India where there is the weed *Partheneum hysterophorus*. There the dermatitis builds up into a severe erythroderma with secondary infection and even pseudolymphoma. In those who are suffering from other diseases it may summate and lead to a very severe illness.

Potentially allergenic plants are most numerous in the cashew family such as poison ivy, poison oak, poison dogweed, elder or sumac, mango, wax, or lacquer trees, and hence in one form or another they are worldwide. Attacks can be aborted by washing within an hour of contact but in some heavily contaminated areas water is in short supply.

When sensitivity is due to the mango or cashew nut, severe oral dermatitis and acute gastrointestinal systems can be troublesome.

Contamination of other agents handled can also cause outbreaks of dermatitis as has been recorded with articles of clothing, mail, and even from voodoo dolls.

Table 15 Causes of contact urticaria

Medicaments	Chemicals	Miscellaneous
Streptomycin	Acrylic monomer and polyacrylic acid	Dander saliva or serum of internal organs of many
Penicillin G	Alcohols (ethyl, cetyl, stearyl)	laboratory animals
Cephalosporins	Aliphatic aldehydes	Egg white or yolk
Neomycin	Aliphatic polyamides	Fish and shell fish
Gentamicin	Aliphatic amine hardeners	Various insects giving rise to cotton seed itch,
Bacitracin	Ammonia	copra itch, grocers' itch, millers' itch, etc.
Chlorpromazine	Amino thiazole	Caterpillars, pteropods, schistosomes
Promazine hydrochloride	Ammonium persulphate and potassium salt	Jelly fish
Aspirin	Benzoic acid and sodium benzoate	Aglycoprotein in human seminal fluid
Oestrogenic cream	Chlorine	Root vegetables
Cod liver oil	Clothing dyes	Nuts
Horse serum	Citrus fruits	Spices
Tetanus antitoxin	Citraconic anhydride (in guinea pigs)	Pollens
Diethyl tolbutamide	Cinnamic aldehyde	Exotic woods
Monoamylamine	DMSO	Numerous common weeds
Mechlorethamine hydrochloride	DNCB	
Benzaphone	Detergents with and without enzymes	
Menthol	Formaldehyde	
Ammoniated mercury	Lindane	
Arsphenamine	Polysorbate 60	
Emetine	Phenylmercuric proprionate	
Aminophenazone	Perlon	
Polyethylene glycol	Platinum salts	
Polysorbate 60	Sodium sulphide	
	Sodium dioxide	
	Sorbic acid	
	Terpinyl acetate	
	'Trafuril'	

From Veronica Kirton, private communication.

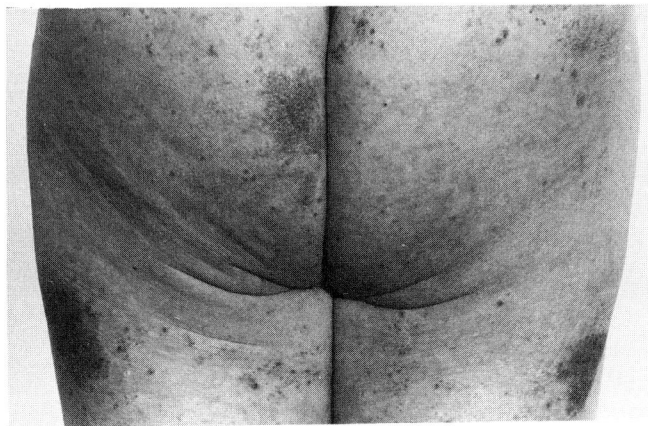

Fig. 42 Contact dermatitis due to garments containing nickel. The diagnosis is made by observing how the distribution of the rash corresponds to the distribution of the contact with the causative agent.

Wood dermatitis is often due to its resins or from lichens, liverworts, and moss, or even its insect parasites are occasionally responsible. It is a severe cause of industrial dermatitis in the furniture industry, but ranges even to mouth dermatitis in children handling wooden toys and it has been noticed also in schools in the music classroom from recorders made of certain woods.

8. *Medicaments* The increasing complexity of our environment includes an enormous number of medicaments. Often the constituents in these are unknown. The problem arises particularly where these have been applied repetitively to the skin over a number of years, and therefore it is found in patients with leg ulcers, pruritus ani, or vulvae, and in those suffering from otitis externa. Local anaesthetics, antibiotics and antiseptics, antifungal compounds, and antihistamines are the most significant groups.

An example of the importance of recognizing such sensitivity is illustrated by ethylene diamine; this is an increasingly common cause of dermatitis and it is present in certain neomycin nystatin ointment mixtures such as triadcortyl. It is also contained in aminophylline suppositories. It is used as a solvent in many industries and is one cause of coolant oil dermatitis. This combination of an industrial use and a medicament may mean that a person may lose his employment as a result of previous use of a medicament. It has serious implications since it is also sometimes used as a preservative of an intravenous medicament aminophylline and deaths have been recorded.

9. *Metal* Beryllium causes skin ulcers, dermatitis, and granulomas in the manufacture of fluorescent lights. Chrome confers hardness to metals and dermatitis from it is also common in the tanning industry. It is a contaminator of cement. In industrial countries it is the commonest sensitizer in men; most obtain their sensitivity from cement but their greatest disability is due to the later inconvenience of not being able to wear leather footwear containing chrome. Ferrous sulphate can be used in cement to convert hexavalent chromium to the less sensitizing trivalent form.

Cobalt sensitivity is commonly found in association with nickel or chrome sensitivity. Jewellery and possibly metal prostheses for hip replacement may be responsible.

Nickel is used in various metal alloys, electroplating, enamels, and glass. It is easily absorbed through the skin and its presence in earrings and in buttons and clips probably accounts for the high incidence of metal dermatitis in women. There is a general trend towards increased nickel sensitivity and it is a worldwide problem. It contributes substantially to hand dermatitis.

While the handling of money or pots and pans seems not to be responsible, abrasive cleaning of such in washing up water releases nickel and is a reason for blaming this occupation or for recommending the use of running water.

10. Employment and contact dermatitis It will be seen from the above that many persons in industry are liable to contact specific types of 'contact dermatitis'. Some industries are particularly susceptible.

Hairdressers During apprenticeship the hands of a hairdresser suffer from the very abnormal wear and tear of frequent shampooing. Atopic subjects almost always break down. Nickel dermatitis is particularly common. When the distribution of the rash affects only the palmar surfaces, contact dermatitis is more likely than irritant dermatitis. The latter commonly affects the more tender dorsa of the hands and between the fingers.

Bakers Dough, sugars, and peels are irritants and in atopic subjects there is often considerable skin damage from these. Many additives are now added to flour and can cause contact urticaria.

Builders Cement is highly irritant but skin quickly hardens. Severe alkaline burns of the lower legs from calcium hydroxide in wet cement is now well recognized especially in the amateur using ready-mixed cement.

Chrome dermatitis may be very similar to constitutional patterns including seborrhoeic and stasis eczema, and for this reason anyone in the building industry who has any pattern of eczema should be patch tested.

Agricultural and horticultural workers Fungicides and pesticides carelessly used are frequent causes of dermatitis. This particularly occurs in isolated farms in developing countries.

Patch testing

The principle of patch testing is to apply to the skin the agent to which the patient may be sensitive, but avoiding irritants, and observe its effect on cell-mediated immunity. It involves: (*a*) applying the agent on a carrier material such as aluminium foil over filter paper covered by adhesive tape; (*b*) using a concentration in white soft paraffin or ethyl alcohol which is non-irritant; for most chemicals 0.1–1 per cent. In the case of cosmetics or medicaments the concentration used in daily life is suitable; (*c*) applying to the back, which is more consistent in its response than arms or legs, and removing the covering adhesive tape and filter paper 2 hours before reading; and (*d*) reading at 2 and 4 days. Most practitioners obtain reagents from Trolab, Karen Trolle-Lassen, Land, Pharm 6B AN, Hansens Alle, 2900 Hellerup, Denmark. These are replaced about every 6 months.

False positives result from sweat gland occlusion, sensitivity to adhesive tape, irritants, and generally increased irritability of the skin usually due to active eczema, but also from exposure to ultraviolet irradiation.

A positive patch test is a papular and a palpable erythema and may be vesicular (Fig. 43). The internationally agreed standard battery of agents is listed in Table 16.

Treatment of contact dermatitis

The level of complaint is often lessened by good industrial relations or a happy home. Those who are well satisfied with life may call their problem merely roughness of the skin; those who are unhappy or dissatisfied may well call their problem dermatitis. Especially in those who have atopic eczema or psoriasis, emotional stress is considered to be a factor worth controlling if possible. Such stresses are often no more than the anxieties and irritations of daily living and employment in a complex society.

Elimination of known irritants or allergens must be attempted but, as in the case of poison ivy in the USA or some of the compositae in Asia, complete avoidance may be impossible. For less severe allergens, such as chrome or nickel, the skin can settle to a tolerable degree merely by removing obvious sources in clothing or jewellery. Dermatologists interested in good relations in industry or local government can encourage cleanliness and ventilation in working environments and substitute less allergenic materials in industrial processes. It is not always advisable to make a worker

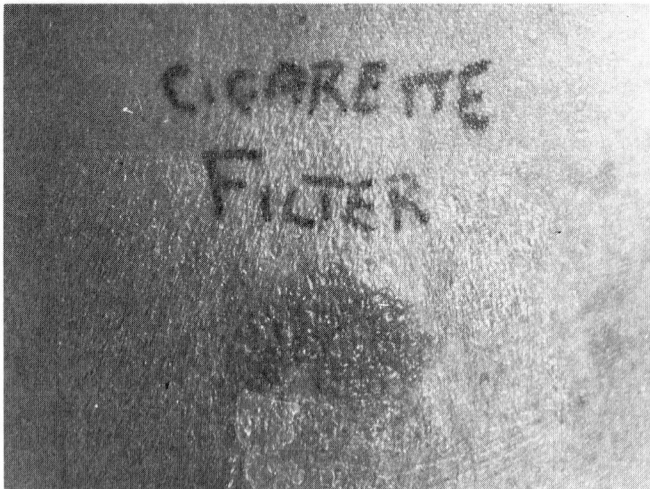

Fig. 43 Contact for about 48 hours with the allergen to which the patient is sensitive can be used as a test at any site on the skin. This is the basis of the patch test reaction. In this case a finger dermatitis due to an allergen in cigarette smoke could be proved by application of the smoked filter paper to the back of the patient.

change his job; this particularly applies to sensitivity to chrome in the building industry since once sensitized, most other jobs are equally difficult and most sufferers can manage with a little more care at work and with the help of emollients. Anti-inflammatory agents such as steroid creams are always of help and can help the affected stay at work, particularly for short periods such as during the training of the hairdresser or nurse.

Severe chronic allergy can be relieved by immunosuppressive drugs such as azathioprine. For nickel dermatitis where life has become intolerable, chelating agents such as Antabuse have been used. Nickel-free diets are complicated but much less unpleasant.

The prognosis for contact dermatitis is often good. Thus 30 per cent of nickel dermatitis of the hands is healed in 6 years. Only 25 per cent of apprentice hairdressers with dermatitis of the hands have to change their job. Only rarely, as with certain plant allergies, is the problem a persistent and intolerable problem affecting many persons in the community.

Photosensitivity is described on page 20.21 and erythroderma on page 20.82.

Atopic eczema

This a constitutional disorder of the skin affecting 1–3 per cent of the population. It is one of the commonest diseases of childhood and one of the main reasons for loss of work in industry. It accounts for about 50 per cent of hand eczema. It is inherited through several genes affecting the capacity to produce reagenic antibody, reactions to the environment as well as the itch and consequent response to scratching.

Allergic respiratory disease affects about 50 per cent of eczema sufferers and 70 per cent of patients are aware of other family members with the disease; for 90 per cent the disorder starts within the first 9 years of life. In the majority, the eczema gradually improves but the skin remains vulnerable to physical and chemical irritants throughout life.

Pathogenesis

There are many theories and most propose that atopic disease is essentially a defect in immunology – possibly most favoured is depressed T-cell function and consequent lack of suppression of some aspects of humoral antibody production.

In normal tissues there is a ratio of 5:1 in beta versus alpha adrenergic activity but in atopics the alpha receptors are increased or

Table 16 European standard battery of patch tests

	Name	Concentration (%)
1	Potassium dichromate	0.5
2	Paraphenylenediamine dihydrochloride	0.5
3	Thiuram mix	1
	Tetramethylthiuram monosulphide	0.25
	Tetramethylthiuram disulphide	0.25
	Tetramethylthiuram disulphide	0.25
	Dipentamethylenthiuram disulphide	0.25
4	Neomycin sulphate	20
5	Cobalt chloride	1
6	Benzocaine	5
7	Nickel sulphate	5
8	Quinoline mix	6
	Clioquinol	3
	Chlorquinaldol	3
9	Colophony	60
10	Parabens	15
	Methyl parahydroxybenzoate	3
	Ethyl parahydroxybenzoate	3
	Propyl parahydroxybenzoate	3
	Butyl parahydroxybenzoate	3
	Benzyl parahydroxybenzoate	3
11	Black rubber mix	0.6
	N-Isopropyl-N′-phenyl paraphenylenediamine	0.1
	N-Cyclohexyl-N′-phenyl paraphenylenediamine	0.25
	N,N′-Diphenyl paraphenylenediamine	0.25
12	Wool alcohols	30
13	Mercapto mix	2
	N-Cyclohexylbenzothiazylsulphenamide	0.5
	Mercaptobenzothiazole	0.5
	Dibenzothiazyl disulphide	0.5
	Morpholinylmercaptobenzothiazole	0.5
14	Epoxy resin	1
15	Balsams of Peru	25
16	Paratertiary butylphenol formaldehyde resin	1
17	Carba mix	3
	1,3-Diphenylguanidine	1
	Bis (diethyldithiocarbamato) zinc	1
	Bis (dibutyldithiocarbamato) zinc	1
18	Formaldehyde (in water)	1
19	Fragrance mix	8
	Cinnamyl alcohol	1
	Cinnamaldehyde	1
	Eugenol	1
	Hydroxycitronellal	1
	Alpha-amylcinnamaldehyde	1
	Geraniol	1
	Isoeugenol	1
	Oak moss absolute	1
20	Ethylenediamine dihydrochloride	1
21	Quaternium 15 (Dowicil 200)	1
22	Primin	0.01

All substances except formaldehyde are incorporated in white petrolatum.

there is beta-adrenergic blockade reducing the capacity to synthesize cyclic AMP and moderating the responses to beta-adrenergic stimulation. This is thought to account both for the eczema and the asthma through an action on lymphocytes. This was first proposed by Szentivanyi in 1968 and he produced experimental models to support the concept. There are blunted responses to beta-adrenergic agents and prostaglandins or histamine but increased responses to alpha-adrenergic agents. More recently changes compatible with adrenergic blockade have been detected in the lymphocytes of patients as well as in those of 1 month-old children born of atopic parents. Some critics believe that beta-adrenergic blockade if it exists is due to therapy with sympathomimetic drugs given to the affected patients. For instance, steroid ointments modify such blockade. Infection too can have such an effect and many affected subjects have considerable secondary infection. House mite antigen is increasingly incriminated.

Immunology

Atopic eczema and asthma have long been thought of as 'allergic'. There is no doubt about the altered reactivity to a variety of irritants including allergens. 'Allergic' rhinitis, asthma, and eczema often fluctuate and even alternate, the one improving as the other worsens.

Skin tests by pricking various antigens into the skin result in weal and flare responses that are often multiple and strongly positive. However, there is a poor correlation between the skin test response and the activity of the eczema which may be even in remission in, for example, the hayfever season in spite of strong reactivity to skin testing with grasses.

The role of food allergy is difficult to test accurately in such a fluctuating and multifactorial disease. Neither prick tests nor allergen specific IgE tests can be used to predict those most likely to benefit from dietary elimination. Exclusive breast feeding is of benefit but not necessarily due to avoidance of factors in the diet. Breast milk contains much IgA. Complete avoidance of cows' milk during the first 6 months of the life of the children of atopic parents is believed to be beneficial but there are nevertheless many who fail to benefit.

Humoral immunity

IgE reagenic antibody is elevated in over 80 per cent of patients with atopic dermatitis often to over 2000 units/ml but the significance of this remains uncertain since atopic eczema can occur in agammaglobulinaemia and normal levels are found in many actively eczematous patients. Of course, serum levels need not reflect the level of activity of the IgE surrounding the mast cell in the skin itself. Complexes with antigen and the mast cell are often after all the basis of the IgE mediated weal and flare. There is an increased frequency of the presence of specific reagin (RAST) to numerous allergens in the sera of atopics.

Reactivity of immune system

About 80 per cent of atopics have an excessive reactivity of the immune system. They react to certain foods and to house dust with immediate itching and swelling of the tissues. The agents to which 90 per cent of atopic patients react differ from those usually encountered in allergic disease. They include a number of animal and vegetable proteins from milk, meat, and corn. Eczema itself is most typically a consequence of delayed or cell-mediated immunity but in the case of the atopic skin there seems to be depression of T-cell function leading to a greater susceptibility to viral, bacterial, and fungal infections. Herpes simplex, vaccinia, warts, *Staphylococcus aureus*, and *Trichophyton rubrum* infections are most favoured; 90 per cent of atopic subjects carry *Staphylococcus aureus* in their skin compared to 10 per cent of normal subjects. Fortunately, the atopic subject is not so susceptible to strains responsible for impetigo, toxic epidermal necrolysis, or furunculosis. There is also decreased reactivity to other common allergens such as poison ivy, *Candida*, or dinitrochlorbenzene (DNCB).

An atopic eczema-like syndrome is also a feature of immune deficiency diseases such as Wiskott–Aldrich syndrome, hyper-IgE syndrome of Buckley, and thymic aplasia, as well as the DiGeorge and Nesselof syndromes which also have high levels of IgE and decreased cell-mediated immunity. It is possible that immaturity of the humoral antibody system results in defective T lymphocyte regulation and IgE production is increased as one consequence.

Characteristics

The principal characteristics of atopic eczema are described below.

A low itch threshold

Indeed a diagnosis should not be made if there is no history of itching. Besides the usual causes of itching, many minor irritants such as wool of clothing or changes in climate cause scratching.

Scratching causes excoriations and ulceration as well as thickening of the epidermis and swelling and redness of the underlying dermis. The broken surface is sore and further irritated by soaps, some ointment bases such as sorbic acid, sea water, or citric fruit juices. It has been found, using intradermal trypsin as a test of itch, that atopics have a prolonged itch reaction though it may be that other patients with other forms of eczema are similarly affected.

Dry and lined skin

In non-excoriated areas the skin is often dry and lined. This is more obvious in hard water areas with temperate climates. The palms are particularly heavily lined and cause embarrassment even to the fortune teller! About 70 per cent of adult patients have a hand dermatitis and such hand dermatitis usually spares the palms. In adults also, nipple eczema may be a problem during breast feeding. It seems that there is a deficiency in sweating and sebum excretion which leads to chapping, wear and tear, particularly from solvents or water. In industry, occupational dermatitis from primary irritants is commonly due to an underlying atopic eczema. Other features of atopic dryness are keratosis pilaris which is a perifollicular hyperkeratosis.

Vasodilation of vasculature

In the popliteal and cubital fossae the vasculature too readily vasodilates, heating the skin and hence inappropriately lowering the itch threshold. When scratched, rubbed, or stretched, the skin blanches for a few minutes beginning 12–15 seconds after injury. This is in part due to upper dermal precapillary shut down and also to persistent inflammatory oedema. Deeper vessels often dilate so that the skin is warm. This combination of hot but pale skin accounts for the itching as well as the atopic pallor.

Clinical features

Itching is the chief feature and becomes apparent during the first 2–6 months of life. The face is usually first affected and scratching begins between the second and third month. Sore lips from licking and chapping as well as conjunctivitis with ectropion are common; 70 per cent of patients have a skin fold or wrinkle just beneath the margin of the lower lid of both eyes (Fig. 44). When the child begins to crawl, the exposed surfaces such as the knees and hands become the most involved. The papules are scratched and become exudative and so secondary infection associated with lymphadenopathy is a common finding. Lymphadenopathy can sometimes be so gross as to lead to suspicion of some dire malignant disease. From 18 months onwards the sites most characteristically involved are the flexures of the elbows, knees, sides of neck, wrists, and ankles (Fig. 45). Local areas of lichenified skin may persist at such sites, and the face too may be heavily lichenified. Rubbing of the eyes is not the whole explanation of why keratoconus and anterior subcapsular cataracts are featured in severe cases. Seasonal influences on the disease are in part climatic due to sunlight and humidity, but probably even more related are seasonal allergies. Pollen is a feature of spring and early summer, while house dust seems to be a feature of late summer.

Associated disorders

Hayfever and asthma occur in 30–50 per cent of patients. Drug reactions of the anaphylactic type are more common and abdominal symptoms due to food allergy are frequently described. Contact urticaria is common. Alopecia areata is associated.

Prognosis

Most children develop their eczema within the first 6 months of life but about one-fifth of patients may have a delayed onset even into adult life. There is in general a tendency for gradual improvement. Complete clearance without breakdown when in contact with skin irritants is unusual but the majority of persons are clear by the time they are teenagers in the absence of major irritants.

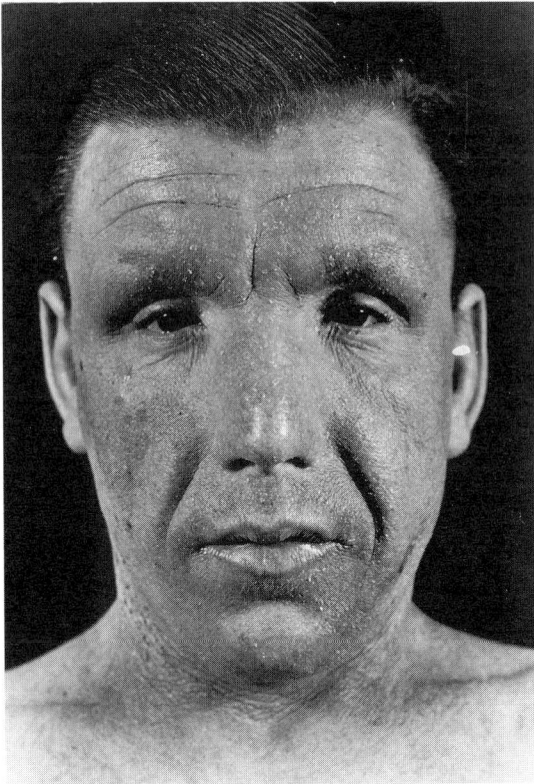

Fig. 44 Atopic eczema in an adult showing the characteristic skin fold of the lower eyelid and the loss of eyebrow hair as well as the thickening of the skin due to rubbing.

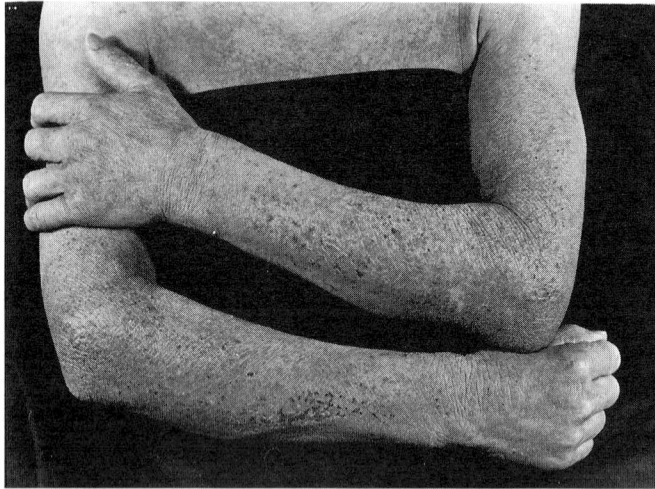

Fig. 45 Typically thickened and excoriated skin of the chronic prurigo of atopic eczema.

Management

The is a multifactorial disease and all factors have to be managed. It is useful for parents to have access both to the doctor and nurse as well as to the literature provided by patient groups such as the Eczema Society. All factors which cause irritation of the skin even in normals, should be even more avoided in the atopic, and these include various primary irritants such as soap, wool, and extremes of climate. Moisturization of the skin is good but evaporation is bad. Washing with liberal soap substitutes based on emulsifying ointments is mostly helpful and these are most effective if applied at least four times a day. The commonsense avoidance of jobs in which there is a large amount of primary irritants should be advised. Fortunately smallpox vaccination is no longer compulsory, but it is difficult to avoid the occasional contact with herpes simplex, molluscum contagiosum, and other viruses affecting the skin. If there is an immunological defect, then it remains difficult to know how to remedy this. The role of food allergy is difficult to determine in such a fluctuating and multifactorial disease. While breast feeding is to be recommended for all infants, it may be especially important for babies with a strong family history of eczema. There is evidence that breast feeding may reduce the incidence of atopic eczema by up to two-thirds, though not all authors agree. It is postulated that there is a period of transient immune vulnerability early in life, during which exposure to food antigens, perhaps by complexing with IgG, IgM, and IgE instead of IgA, as normal, results in allergic sensitization and the subsequent development of atopic eczema. The protection effect of breast feeding may be due to its low antigen load compared to cow's milk. Breast milk is also rich in IgA which may modify the absorption of food antigens. Such breast feeding should be for an extra 3–4 months since any supplement exposes the immature gut to foreign protein. Especially to be avoided is any supplement in hospital during the first week of life. It is not yet certain whether further benefit might be gained by avoiding eggs and cows' milk in the mother's diet since foreign protein can certainly be transmitted through the mother's milk. Where breast feeding is not possible, milk substitutes are second-best since they are expensive and require care to prevent bacterial contamination. Some paediatricians believe cows' milk should be avoided for 1 year and eggs for 18 months but this is an area still much debated.

Some patients appear to benefit from a regime of antigen avoidance, though not all do so. Neither RAST tests nor skin patch tests are reliable in selecting patients who are helped by dietary modification since even those known to benefit from antigen avoidance may not show specifically raised IgE nor positive skin tests.

Elimination diets must be carefully assessed to obtain complete avoidance with at the same time adequate nutrition, and since they are not without risk in this respect, they should be reserved for the most severely affected children. Some authors recommend avoidance of egg, chicken, milk, and artificial colouring agents or preservatives. Goat's milk is not now in favour on nutritional grounds.

It has to be said that while it seems likely that food allergy plays a role, there is as yet no basis on which to match each patient with a diet that takes into account idiosyncrasy.

Other allergens in the environment that can be shown to be important for some children include the house dust mite. Avoidance includes eliminating clothing and furniture that are dust collecting and the use of vacuum cleaning rather than brushing. A cold and dry environment discourages the mite.

Topical therapy

Apart from the liberal use of emollients, steroid creams are effective antipruritics (see Tables 30 and 31, pages 20.93 and 20.94). There has been some fluctuation in the amount they have been prescribed over the past few years. Certainly there was a period in which overprescription resulted in systemic side-effects as well as local atrophy of the skin. Withholding of steroids on the other hand deprives the child of the one effective therapy. Short, sharp bursts of effective therapy with strong steroids may be entirely justified but prolonged daily usage is bound to lead to complications. Topical steroids are stored in the skin and for this reason once daily application may be sufficient. It seems an inexplicable fact of life that ringing the changes with ointments is of benefit and a skilled practitioner will always have an alternative cream on which the worried parents can pin their faith. Secondary infection is so common and bacterial allergy is so important that vigorous treatment of infection is justified and systemic antibiotics should be given according to the sensitivities of the bacteria from time to time. Erythromycin is especially valuable. The matter of climatic therapy remains unpredictable; undoubtedly a change of climate does effect great improvements in some children. It may be exposure to sunlight orto the sea or to a mountain top.

Severe cases of eczema as with asthma may have to be controlled by systemic steroids either in the form of prednisolone or corticosteroid injections. This may be simply to help the patient over an acute period but a small minority of patients may require long-term therapy for several years.

References

Atherton, D. J. (1981). Allergy and atopic eczema. *Clin. exp. Dermatol.* **6**, 317–326.
Emmett, E. A. (1984). The skin and occupational diseases. *Arch. Environ. Hlth* **39**, 144–149.
Epstein, E. (1984). Hand dermatitis: practical management and current concepts. *J. Am. Acad. Dermatol.* **10**, 395–424.
International Symposium on Atopic Dermatitis, Oslo (1979). *Acta dermatol. venereol., Stockh.*, Suppl. 92, p. 137.
Rajka, G. (1975). *Atopic dermatitis*, pp. 149–155. Lloyd Luke, London.
Szentivanyi, A. (1968). The beta adrenergic theory of the atopic abnormality in bronchial asthma. *J. Allergy* **42**, 203–232.

Other patterns of dermatitis

Infected dermatitis

There is increasing evidence that bacterial allergy plays a part in the development of an eczematous response in the skin. The staphylococcus is particularly responsible. This may play a part in all sorts of eczema but occasionally it is the single cause. This is most frequently seen as a rather well demarcated patch of eczema with crusting and scaling on an exposed area. There may be small pustules on an advancing edge; it is seen around discharging wounds, around ulcers, and occasionally around a paronychia or in a flexure, subject to sweating and maceration; it is particularly common around the ear or at sites of occlusion such as under a hat band or between the toes. An underlying pediculosis may be one trigger. Negro skin seems commonly to develop a similar condition principally affecting the shins. Management includes the use of local antiseptics and wet soaks (see page 20.93), or dyes, such as gentian violet, combined with an appropriate systemic antibiotic.

Seborrhoeic dermatitis

This is an unsatisfactory term but it is a recognizable disease affecting mainly the flexures in the distribution of the head, neck, upper chest, axillae, and groin. The aetiology is unknown but the distribution does appear to be in the areas of sebaceous activity. Breakdown of the skin occurs spontaneously but is activated by bacterial infection and by other primary irritants. There is a strong association between neuroleptic-induced parkinsonism and the prevalence of seborrhoeic dermatitis. The most characteristic lesion is a dull or yellowish-red and greasy plaque with a marginated scale. It is most likely to involve hair bearing areas and particularly the scalp that has considerable dandruff; it spreads on to the face and involves the nasolabial folds and eyebrows. It affects the axillae and groins with well-defined brownish-red scaly areas deep into the folds, on the front of the chest, and in the middle of the back there may be small brown follicular papules covered by greasy scales or multiple discrete patches, or rarely a widespread eruption resembles pityriasis rosea with oval lesions with peripheral scale. Severe cases of seborrhoeic dermatitis develop marked crusting and scaling particularly of hair-bearing areas and the genitalia. Otitis externa is one manifestation. The disorder tends to recur and may be chronic.

Management includes an attack on local infection and removal of crusts with wet soaks (see page 20.93). Preparations such as vioform hydrocortisone, sulphur and ichthammol in a variety of water-miscible bases usually in 1–2 per cent concentrations have been traditionally prescribed and are in fact often helpful. Imida-

zoles control pityrosporon over production which is thought to play some part in the diathesis.

Nummular eczema

The main feature of this eczema is that it is discoid or composed of rounded lesions scattered often symmetrically over the body. They are intensely vesicular and intensely itchy. They are undoubtedly endogenous, external influence playing little part in their development although occasionally sensitivity to metals, such as nickel or chrome, may produce a similar picture. Secondary infection is common; sometimes it is as a reaction pattern to a localized primary irritant such as an insect bite.

Asteatotic eczema

This type of eczema is usually associated with drying out of the skin. It is particularly found in the elderly or those suffering from a minor degree of malnutrition (see Figs 22, 41, and 124). It is seen particularly when there is a change of habitat as in admission to a centrally heated hospital and enforced nudity. The essential feature is the drying out and cracking of the skin over certain exposed areas such as the backs of the hands and the fronts of the legs. It gives an appearance of crazy paving with deep fissures. It is aggravated by soaps and other irritants and by scratching. It responds very well to humidifiers and emollients as well as to a weak steroid.

Pityriasis alba

This is a pattern of eczema quite common in children often with darker skins, in which a very low-grade dry eczema with shedding of pigment gives rise to a white patch of skin (see Fig. 71).

PRURITUS

Pruritus is the term used when itching is the primary complaint unaccompanied by visible evidence of lesions predisposing to itch. Of course, itching is the most prominent symptom in skin disease and tends always to evoke scratching or rubbing (insect bites are the commonest cause of pruritic skin lesions). It is subjective and for any one skin disease varies from individual to individual. There are exceptions even to the rule that syphilis never itches. Itch is a sensation largely dependent on superficial nerve endings in an intact upper dermis and epidermis and it is abolished by immersion in water at 40–41 °C. It is common in wound healing. It is induced by a number of agents including histamine, bradykinin, bile salts, and proteases, and is potentiated by prostaglandin E. It can be disassociated from pain in hypoalgesia. Central neurological and emotional psychiatric factors control the threshold to itch or pain. Awareness is a complex attribute modifying or intensifying the response to the itch. The itch itself may cause irritability, depression, or the attitude of the masochist who wears a 'hair shirt'. Thinly myelinated nerves in lateral spinothalamic tracts and secondary neurones to the thalamus relay both pain and itch and the cerebral cortex can modify these responses.

Itching is usually worse when the skin is heated to normal body temperature and when there is little else to distract one – a combination common at night. Vasodilatation in the cubital or popliteal fossae partially accounts for the lower itch threshold at such sites in atopic eczema.

The itch of different dermatoses evokes different types of scratching. Urticaria almost never is scratched and usually it is rubbed or pinched perhaps because the exact site of the itch is difficult to pinpoint. Where intense itching is exactly located it is often persistent and deeply excoriated.

Parasites are an important cause of pruritus but those experienced at examining the skin will usually observe primary urticarial or papular lesions in amongst the scratches. Onchocerciasis, trichinellosis, and schistosomiasis cause severe pruritus usually with marked eosinophilia and well as urticaria, prurigo, and depigmentation. In onchocerciasis loss of elasticity and the development of a leather-like skin hanging in folds is one consequence.

Causes of pruritus (*sine* skin lesions)

A common factor is dryness and desiccation of the stratum corneum, common in the elderly and worse in winter.

The threshold of itching is lowered by isolation, including the common accompaniments of ageing such as blindness, deafness, and loneliness. Endogenous depression is often missed in the elderly and should be treated. Paroxysmal itching may originate in the central nervous system and provoke deep scratching which is pleasurable but injurious. It is a feature of cocaine addiction.

Sweat retention also causes intense pruritus such as prickly heat. The intense pruritus of scabies with much excoriation requires a very careful search for burrows especially in well-groomed persons in the early stages of the disease. Head lice may similarly be elusive and the hair rather than the scalp is the principal hiding place; in the early stages the insect lies very close to the scalp. The classical nit is a relatively late stage. Persons recently engaged in insulating their roof with fibreglass suffer from pruritus due to almost invisible spicules of fibreglass (see Fig. 40).

Generalized pruritus and systemic disease

1. Hepatic disease Obstructive jaundice causes severe pruritus. It is particularly an early feature of biliary cirrhosis and because bile salts rather than bilirubin are responsible for the itch, the degree of jaundice need not to be great. Indeed an oestrogen-induced pruritus of pregnancy or from the contraceptive pill often shows little or no jaundice in spite of intrahepatic biliary obstruction, severe pruritus, and a much raised alkaline phosphatase. Chlorpromazine and testosterone can have the same effect. Bile salts in the skin can achieve a relatively higher concentration than may be indicated by serum levels. Bile salts in a concentration of 1 mmol/l cause itching when applied to a blister base. Dihydroxy salts especially chenodeoxycholate are responsible.

2. Blood disease Iron deficiency also causes itching even when the patient is not anaemic. There is often some thinning of hair. Polycythaemia is frequently associated with itching particularly after a hot bath and it is believed to be related to blood histamine levels and occasionally to iron deficiency and hence the reported response to iron therapy within 2–10 days. Lymphatic leukaemia and Hodgkin's disease are other causes of pruritus often long lasting before it becomes clinically overt.

3. Carcinoma of the internal organs Carcinoma of the bronchus in particular may present with generalized pruritus.

4. Chronic renal failure Itching is not a feature of acute renal failure or even of malignant hypertension, however uraemic. In chronic pyelonephritis and chronic glomerulonephritis, the patients usually suffer greatly from pruritus. Haemodialysis does not necessarily relieve it. Parathyroidectomy, for reasons that remain obscure, relieves itching in those in whom removal is necessitated by secondary hyperparathyroidism. The cause of pruritus in renal failure is unknown but dryness of the skin is one factor, and there are also increased numbers of mast cells in the skin.

5. Endocrine disease Pruritus is sometimes a presenting symptom of diabetes mellitus but mostly this is localized principally to the vulva. About one in ten patients with hyperthyroidism complain of itching. Dry skin in hypothyroidism often itches.

Management of pruritus

Overheating should be avoided as should vasodilators such as alcohol and hot drinks. Calamine lotion is used as a cooling agent. Evaporation is increased by the enhanced surface area provided by the powder. Dryness of the skin should be discouraged by emollients. In hospital a moist microenvironment can be enhanced by the wearing of clothes. Too frequent bathing should be discouraged unless emulsifying ointments are added to the bath as soap

substitutes. Bath salts should be avoided. Proprietary bath oils are more cosmetically acceptable but tend to be expensive for regular daily use. The treatment of the cause of the pruritus is obviously indicated where possible. Antihistamines act principally through their sedative effect and they reduce the awareness. Chlorpromazine may reduce the reactivity to the itch. Plasma exchange has been used to control sweats and pruritus. The anion exchange resin cholestyramine 6–8 g daily or oral activated charcoal helps the pruritus of liver disease and sometimes also its use in chronic renal disease or polycythaemia has been helpful. Suberythema doses of UVB irradiation twice weekly and even natural sunlight help pruritus somewhat unpredictably. They have been used to treat the itching uraemia and of certain acute exanthems such as pityriasis rosea. Hydroxy ethyl rutosides (Paroven) have been advocated in renal failure. The H_2 receptor antagonist cimetidine is sometimes helpful in Hodgkin's disease; 1 per cent menthol and 1 per cent phenol have a mild anaesthetic effect and promote a sensation of cooling. Nails should be kept short and occlusive bandaging may reduce the vicious circle of itch and skin damage.

Are insects biting?

Many a cause of prurigo or papular urticaria is due to insects, especially in the rainy season in hot countries. It is a reaction that is not necessarily immediately preceded by the recognition of insect biting and insects without wings are mainly unseen. Flea bites and such like are grouped and since no insect knows how to bite symmetrically, the pattern of scratched lesions can be identified as exogenous. The human flea is found on the skin only transiently and it is the patient's environment that may need to be treated often by agents which are best not applied to the skin.

Cheyletiella mites from dogs, cats, and other pets are picked up by a strip of transparent sticky tape applied to the pet's skin several times, especially where there is any mange from canine scabies. Birds' nests in the eaves may be one source. Stored cereals, fruits, and other vegetables matter sometimes contain mites as does house dust.

In the case of scabies, most of the rash is a hypersensitive response taking about 3 weeks to develop. The characteristic burrows (see Fig. 16) at the front of the wrist and between the fingers or on the areolae of the breasts are not necessarily themselves a cause of pruritus. Widespread scabies has been reported in renal transplant patients receiving azathioprine and prednisolone. Persistent cutaneous granulomas following treatment for scabies or other parasitic infections are not a sign of persistence of the live insects but may be an immune reaction to the dead parts – mouth parts and other insect antigens may cause persistent lesions for more than 3 months in about 20 per cent of patients.

The use of steroid creams has modified the hypersensitivity response so that the appearances of conditions such as scabies may be atypical.

Irritable papules at sites of contact with insects such as the face, lap, or arms are a feature of infestation from lap dogs and other pets. These may stimulate eczema or dermatitis herpetiformis and, being a hypersensitivity reaction rather than a bite, there are no puncta but necrotic centres may develop.

Delusions of parasitosis are best treated with antipsychotics.

Localized pruritus

Localized intensely itchy areas of skin having no obvious causation are a common problem in the dermatology clinic. The nape of the neck, upper back (Fig. 46), genitalia, lower leg, elbow and outer thigh are easily accessible sites liable to persistent rubbing and scratching. The injury to the skin results in thickening, purple-brown violaceous coloration due to dilatated vessels and post-inflammatory pigmentation. The normal line marks of the skin are exaggerated and excoriations are usually numerous. This is termed lichen simplex or neurodermatitis, and the fairly well defined patches cause paroxysms of itching and emotional upsets with anxiety or irritability which are also promoting factors.

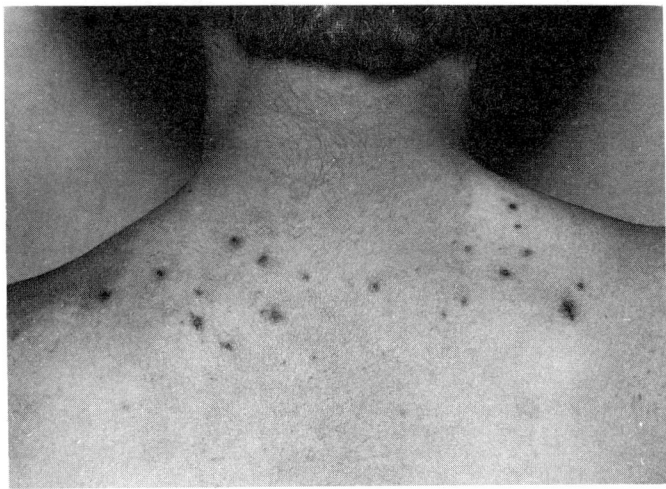

Fig. 46 Prurigo nodularis is a form of scratched lesion which is very exactly localized. The upper back is a common site for such persistent excoriation.

Nodular prurigo is an unexplained reaction to scratching evoking severe very localized pruritus. The nodules are 1–2 cm in diameter and scattered over accessible areas. It is sometimes a consequence of a partially resolved more generalized pruritus from atopic eczema or parasite infestation. Freezing with liquid nitrogen is helpful but depigmentation may result in pigmented races.

Local steroids are helpful and anything which protects the skin from scratching may eventually allow healing. Occlusive tape or bandaging is occasionally helpful but secondary infection is a problem especially in hot countries.

Intralesional injection with triamcinolone causes rapid resolution in some cases but this may be only a temporary response, and where the lesions are large or multiple such inoculation is not without the side-effects of steroid therapy. It is always worth admitting such a patient and treating with traditional dermatological therapies such as tar bandages. A more recent suggestion is that some of these lesions are an immunological response and this has led to therapies as far ranging as azathioprine and thalidomide.

Pruritus ani and pruritus vulvae
Pruritus ani is common in Caucasian adult males. In the negro it is rare except as a manifestation of infestation. An important cause is soiling of the perianal skin. Haemorrhoids, fissures, and fistulae contribute to this. The anal sphincter relaxes in response to anal distension too readily in some sufferers and in others incomplete evacuation of faeces leaves some residual faeces in the folds of the anus. Soft stools are more likely to cause irritation. Diabetes mellitus, trichomoniasis, or candidiasis are amongst the commonest causes of pruritus vulvae. In regions where malnutrition is common pruritus ani and vulvae are rare except as a manifestation of an orogenital syndrome due to vitamin B deficiency. The pruritus is then associated with eczema and angular cheilitis.

Sufferers use a large number of agents to relieve the pruritus some of which cause contact dermatitis. Pruritus vulvae may be caused by sensitivity to the rubber of condoms or spermicidal jelly or even to deodorants. Local anaesthetics and local steroids are much used. The latter encourage secondary infections with fungus or yeasts; these usually spread on to the buttocks and down the thighs.

Management includes a thorough examination to exclude the above and there is a need to recognize skin diseases such as psoriasis, seborrhoeic dermatitis or lichen planus. Lichen sclerosis and atrophicus also usually itches. Threadworm infection is common especially in children.

Perianal soiling often requires cleaning of the area not only immediately after the bowels have been opened but a hour or two later as well. Weak local steroids often mixed with anticandida or antiseptic agents are the mainstay of treatment. Timodine is a safe example.

References
Arnold, H. L. (1984). Paroxysmal pruritus. *J. Am. Acad. Dermatol.* **11**, 322–326.
Cunliffe, W. J. (1980). The skin and the nervous system. In *Textbook of dermatology*, 3rd edn. (eds. A. Rook, D. S. Wilkinson, and F. P. G. Ebling), pp. 1993–2035. Blackwell Scientific Publications, Oxford.
Hampers, C. L., Katz, A. I., Wilson, R. E., and Merrill, J. P. (1968). Disappearance of uraemia itching after sub-total parathyroidectomy. *New Engl. J. Med.* **279**, 695.
Journal of Investigative Dermatology (1979). Pruritis, pain, and sweating disorders, *J. invest. Dermatol.* **73**, 495–500.
Salem, H. H., Van der Weyden, M. B. and Young, I. F. (1982). Pruritus and severe iron deficiency in polycythaemia vera. *Br. med. J.* **285**, 91–92.
Shultz, B. C. and Roenigk, H. H. (1980). Uremic pruritus treated with ultraviolet light. *J. Am. med. Assoc.* **243**, 1836.
Takkunen, H. (1978). Iron deficiency pruritus. *J. Am. med. Assoc.* **239**, 1394.

PSORIASIS

In temperate zones psoriasis affects 2 per cent of the white population. It is less common in sunny climates and in pigmented skins. The mode of inheritance is debated but there is evidence of dominant and polygenic patterns. HLA antigens B13, B17, CW6, and DR7 as well as B27 are associated.

Pathogenesis
The pathogenesis of psoriasis includes a ten-fold increase in the speed of epidermal cell proliferation. The cells pass upwards through the epidermis at a faster rate and seem not to have time to produce a horny layer. The cells remain nucleated even when exfoliated. There are numerous problems which beset the measurement of the cell cycle time in human epidermis. There are the technical difficulties of counting and the exact recognition of different stages of the cell cycle and differentiation. Do all cells in the germinal layer have the potential to divide or is the potential greater in psoriasis? Is the actual cell cycle faster in psoriasis? The answer is probably that the cell cycle is faster and more cells enter the cycle per unit time in psoriasis. The factors inhibiting the cell cycle may be reduced and the factors stimulating are enhanced. Chalones responsible for the former have still to be isolated in sufficient purity. Somatomedins, epidermal growth factor, and fibroblast growth factor are insufficiently studied. Cell surface factors on the immature cell of psoriasis may be different to the normal cell. The exact role of various proteases related to plasmin and complement needs further study. The epidermis in psoriasis contains activated complement C3 and immunoglobulin antibodies to the stratum corneum. There is evidence of depressed T cell number and function.

The biochemical stimulus to the increased cell turnover has variously been attributed to deficiency of sulphur, poor keratohyalin granules, increased activity of certain enzymes in the glycolytic pathways, fatty acid deficiency, increased cyclic GMP, or some localized defect in the availability of cyclic AMP such as prostaglandin regulation. Other candidates include polyamines, putrescine, spermidine, and spermine or a membrane associated enzyme such as aryl sulphatase, B glucosidase, or calmodulin.

Lesion-free skin
The lesion-free skin in persons with psoriasis is not normal. Psoriasis is more readily induced and various medications such as chloroquine and practolol or lithium can produce a flare up. There

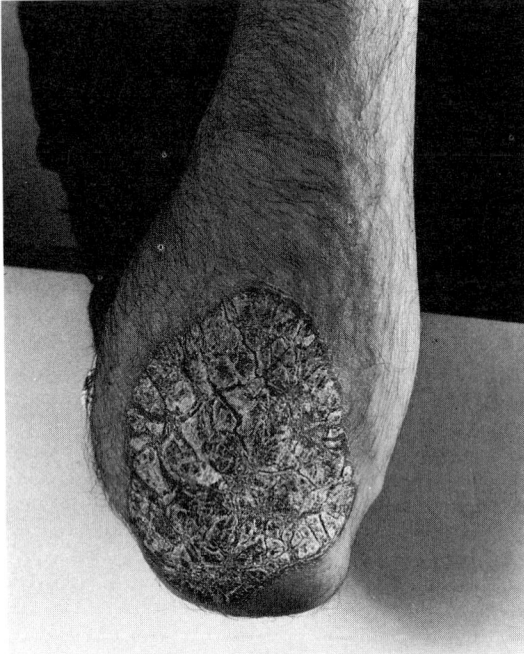

Fig. 47 A plaque of psoriasis showing the silvery scales, well-defined border, and predilection for the elbow.

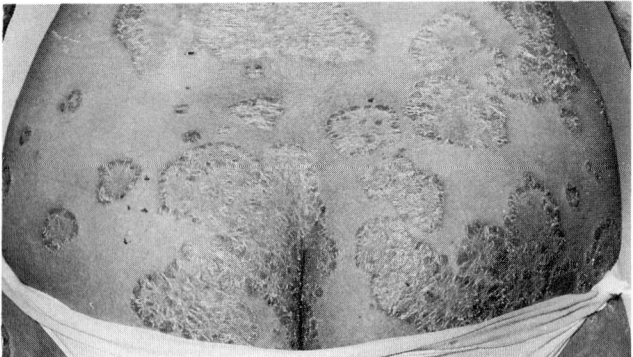

Fig. 48 Psoriasis that is less stable than in Fig. 47. The lesions are erupting and more active at the periphery while healing in the centre.

are more cells available for DNA synthesis but oddly glycogen levels, so high in the psoriatic lesions, may be less than in normal skin. The dermis is not normal and the earliest signs of any abnormality following injury are infiltration with mast cells and macrophages.

The microvasculature in psoriasis is characterized by tortuous and leaky capillaries, generous protein exudation, and poor clearance through immature lymphatics.

Koebner phenomenon

The Koebner phenomenon is a term given to psoriasis developing in traumatized skin. After the initial stimulus to repair, the epidermis gradually thickens and there is accentuation of the papillary interdigitations and the rete ridges. There is an early heavy infiltrate by neutrophils forming microabscesses within the epidermis which is preceded by increased mast cells and macrophages in the dermis. High turnover of the epidermal cells results in a less compact and still partially nucleated scale known as parakeratosis.

Clinical appearance

Psoriasis can affect all age groups but has a peak age of onset in the young adult. The commonest lesion is a sharply marginated plaque with silvery scales (Fig. 47). These mask the underlying redness from tortuous convoluted capillaries which lie close to the surface of the skin. The edges of the lesion are usually the most active and there is commonly clearing in the centre (Fig .48).

Sites most commonly affected are the elbows, knees, and scalp which normally have a higher rate of epidermal turnover. The face is less often affected. Spontaneous fluctuations are common and remissions occur in about one-third of cases per annum. There are several well recognized patterns and it is important to examine the patient thoroughly until a completely recognizable lesion of psoriasis can be detected. Many lesions and some patterns may be quite atypical especially during the development of psoriasis (Fig. 49), or during its resolution.

Guttate psoriasis

This term is derived from *gutta* meaning to drop. The skin looks as though it has been splashed by the psoriasis. It often follows a streptococcal sore throat or vaccination and is especially common

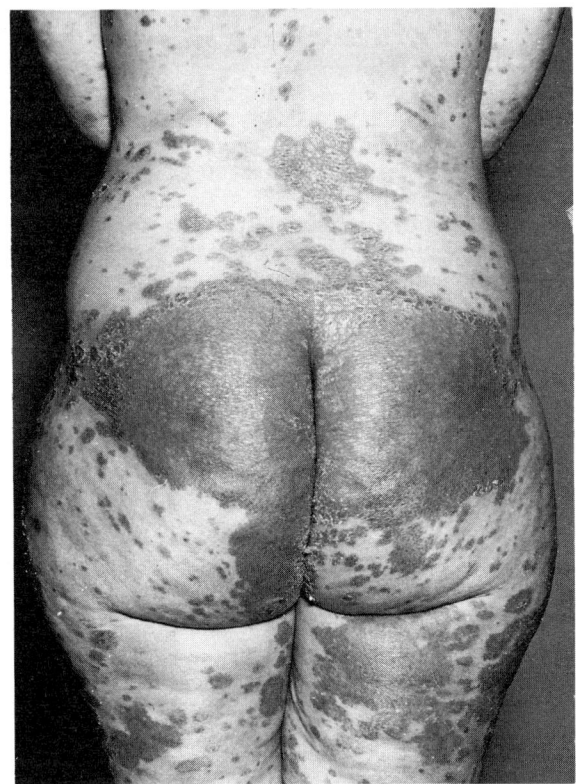

Fig. 49 Still more unstable form of psoriasis tending to be more exudative and exfoliative and not retaining its rapidly produced scale. While tending to be symmetrical, new ill-defined lesions are erupting. There are some linear lesions on the trunk suggestive of the Koebner phenomenon or reaction to injury of the skin, in this case probably from scratching.

in children. The lesions are scattered over the entire body and tend to be no more than a few millimetres in diameter. They may include the face and are often red slightly scaly spots. They appear less well defined and less obviously covered by silvery scales than in classic types of psoriasis. In the absence of a family history the prognosis tends to be good.

Nummular discoid

This is probably the commonest form of psoriasis and coin-shaped lesions of various sizes (Fig. 50) are scattered over the body in a completely symmetrical distribution. Such lesions are usually well-defined and chronic.

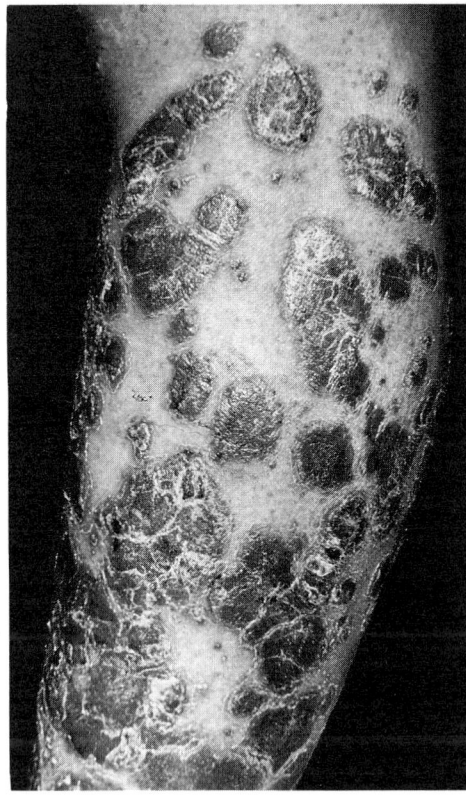

Fig. 50 Discoid lesions still well-defined but almost becoming confluent.

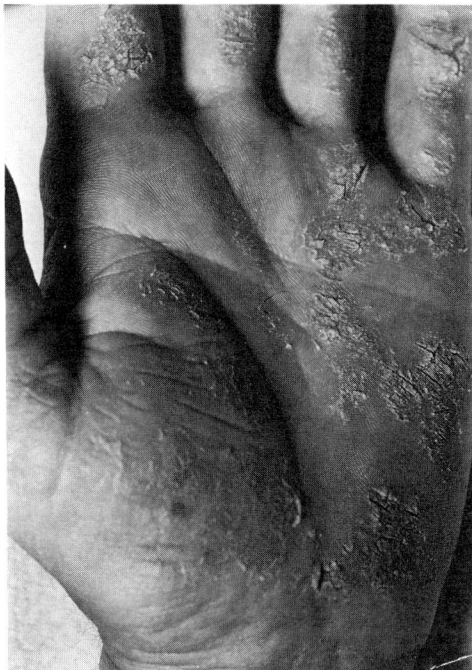

Fig. 51 Psoriasis of the palms may not have the typical scale. It is sometimes pustular or, as in this case, hyperkeratotic with a tendency to form deep cracks. See Fig. 2, page 20.3.

Palmar and plantar psoriasis

This may be typical of lesions elsewhere (see Fig. 2) but there is often a modification of the psoriasis due to the nature of the palmar and plantar skin. The scales tend to be more adherent and less silvery and they are more likely to develop deep cracks because of the thickness of the epidermis at these sites (Fig. 51). Neutrophils tend to collect into larger abscesses trapped by the thicker surface layers of the stratum corneum. The sterile pustules so formed are often the most obvious feature. This pattern may be seen as part of a more generalized disease but in many cases it affects only the hands and feet. There is some evidence that it is a different disease without the above mentioned HLA associations and without obvious increase in the rate of epidermal turnover. It is an occasional and acute response to a form of infection known as pustular bacterid.

Psoriasis of the nails

Pinpoint pitting is usual but can be seen in other disorders affecting nail growth (see Fig. 73). Onycholysis with a salmon-pink discoloration of the base of the uplift of the nail is probably even more characteristic. Sometimes the nail growth is distorted, thickened and friable, and difficult to distinguish from a fungus disorder affecting the nail (see Fig. 76).

Flexural psoriasis

When psoriasis affects the groins, natal cleft or axillae, it is usually less scaly. The bright red plaques are shiny and liable to cracking and maceration. They may be very well defined.

Erythroderma

When psoriasis affects the entire skin the well defined margins are lost and the scales are exfoliated profusely. Generalized redness and loss of normal protective skin function results in the complications listed below. The erythroderma may be indistinguishable from that found in eczema or lymphoma. The skin is the largest organ of the body and when it is inflamed the increase in blood flow can cause high output cardiac failure. When the normal protective function of the skin is lost, bacteraemia is common. The loss of water is difficult to estimate and prerenal failure can develop very rapidly. The vasodilatation and the obstruction to the sweat ducts by the proliferating epidermis results in impaired thermoregulation. Hyperthermia is very common in hot climates; hypothermia can occur in cold climates. Internal organs such as the gut and liver may be impaired and loss of protein both from the skin and the gut is an important complication.

Generalized pustular psoriasis

In this condition, which is relatively rare, waves of bright erythema develop within a few hours with a fever, arthropathy, and leucocytosis. Myriads of pustules (see Fig. 15) quickly develop and equally quickly disappear. This disorder may occur in the absence of a previous history of psoriasis and even occasionally as a viral exanthem. However, most commonly it is only a complication of psoriasis that has been treated by systemic or local steroids. It is an acute rebound phenomenon of steroid withdrawal.

Another rare cause of pustular psoriasis is hypoparathyroidism.

Arthropathic psoriasis

The incidence of polyarthritis in psoriasis is about 7 per cent in hospital series; 4 per cent of all patients with inflammatory polyarthritis have psoriasis. There is a long-standing debate concerning the association of psoriasis with inflammatory polyarthritis; it is not certain whether it is a chance association. Since psoriasis is a common disorder patients with a positive Rose–Waaler test can have coincidental rheumatoid arthritis. Seronegative arthritis in patients with psoriasis is of three types: (a) distal arthritis involving the terminal interphalangeal joints of the hands and the interphalangeal joints of the toes with relative sparing of the metacarpophalangeal and metatarsal phalangeal joints; (b) psoriatic arthritis mutilans which is a severe deforming arthritis involving the multiple small joints of the hands and feet and spine. The hips, cervical, and sacroiliac joints are frequently affected and a complete ankylosing type of spondylitis can occur; and (c) an indistinguishable or rheumatoid-like type very similar to rheumatoid arthritis.

Management

By far the most disabling aspect of psoriasis is its appearance, and patients' lives can be completely taken over by manoeuvres designed to avoid exposing the affected skin to the public eye. Management includes a sympathetic hearing and often admission to an outpatient or inpatient unit where others are being treated.

The aim is to depress epidermal cell turnover without irreversibly damaging the skin or other organs. The physician is faced with a difficult choice of a cosmetically acceptable therapy in the form of a steroid cream, an active mitotic drug taken by mouth, or use of various forms of irradiation. All such therapies have side-effects and the alternatives, which are preferred on grounds of safety, often tend to be tedious and cosmetically unacceptable. The latter include tar and dithranol preparations.

Local steroids

Steroid creams and ointments are often in practice the first line of treatment because they are so easy to use. A few plaques of psoriasis on the elbows, knees, or scalp may be so treated by daily application, and in about one-third of patients the lesions are controlled within 1–2 weeks and remain under control in one-third of those so treated even when the application ceases. The stronger fluorinated steroids or betamethasone valerate are the most effective. One-third of patients need to continue once or twice weekly application and another third show no improvement even with twice daily application. In all those in whom these stronger steroids have to be continued complications gradually develop. These include skin atrophy, gradual extension of the psoriasis, and greater instability of the skin so that psoriasis erupts whenever the therapy is partially or completely withdrawn. Eventual widespread usage and systemic absorption complicates the increasing addiction of the skin for the stronger steroids. Some such patients show no remission until all such therapy is withdrawn and in a few this can be done without any immediate worsening of the psoriasis but in most there is rapid worsening of their skin condition.

Tar

Tar has been known to be effective and safe for more than 50 years. Its smell, colour, and stain make it cosmetically unsatisfactory. Patients should be encouraged to use it because it has no significant side-effects and the clearance of psoriasis is more long lasting. The cruder varieties may be irritant on more vulnerable skin and the more purified varieties of liquor picis carbonis are relatively weak. National Formulary preparations are listed in Table 17.

The preparations are applied twice daily; they are diluted by 50 per cent if they are irritant. Occasionally patients are allergic to one or more of the constituents. The general principle of whether to use a lotion, ointment, or paste are discussed on page 20.93. Acute or inflamed psoriasis responds to ichthammol which has a milder action than coal tar.

Dithranol

Dithranol is more effective than coal tar in the treatment of psoriasis. It is more irritant but by diluting it one can usually find a concentration which is acceptable. Once this is so, the concentration can usually be gradually increased. The dithranol is mixed in zinc oxide and salicylic acid paste (Lassar's paste) in a concentration of 0.1, 0.25, 0.5, 1, or 2 per cent. It is irritant to the eyes and genitalia. Weaker preparations are used in the more sensitive occlusive flexures.

The non-lesional skin may be protected by vaseline and it is usual to apply dithranol paste accurately to the active parts of the skin lesion. Powdering fixes the paste and a gauze or nylon dressing protects the overlying clothing from its staining property. Patients tolerating this regimen are cleared in about 3½ weeks on average. Staining is inevitable and is a sign of effectiveness. It is

Table 17 Preparations for the treatment of psoriasis

Tar preparations
Coal tar solution (liquor picis carbonis)
  20% prepared coal tar ⎫ in 90% alcohol
  10% quillaia   ⎭
Tar bath
  120 ml coal tar solution BP in a 20-gallon bath
Coal tar pomade

Coal tar solution BP	6%
Salicylic acid	2%
Polysorbate 20	1%
Emulsifying ointment to 100%	

Calamine and coal tar ointment

Calamine, finely sifted	12.5 g
Zinc oxide, finely sifted	12.5 g
Strong coal tar solution	2.5 g
Hydrous wood fat	25.0 g
White soft paraffin	47.5 g

Coal tar and salicylic acid ointment

Coal tar	2.0 g
Salicylic acid	2.0 g
Emulsifying wax	11.4 g
White soft paraffin	19.0 kg
Coconut oil	54.0 g
Polysorbate 80	4.0 g
Liquid paraffin	7.6 g

Oil of cade pomade
  10% of cade   ⎫ in spirit soap shampoo
  10% triethanolamine   ⎭
5% to 15% of cade in olive oil for psoriasis of the scalp
Polytar shampoo (contains tar, arachis oil, and   ⎫ cosmetically
  oleyl alcohol)   ⎪ acceptable
Alphosyl lubricating cream; special crude coal   ⎬ but very
  tar extract 5%, allantoin 2%   ⎪ mild
Alphosyl lotion (contains a vanishing cream base)   ⎭

Lassar's paste
Lassar's paste BNF

Zinc oxide	24%
Starch	24%
Salicylic acid	2%
White soft paraffin	50%

'Stiff' Lassar's paste
  Melting point of soft paraffin 46–49 °C with 15% hard paraffin
'Soft' Lassar's paste
  'Stiff' Lassar's paste and emulsifying ointment in equal parts

*Dithranol preparations**
Dithranol pomade

Dithranol	0.4%
Liquid paraffin	75.4%
Cetyl alcohol	21.7%
Sodium lauryl sulphate (finely powdered)	2.5%

Dithranol in 'stiff' Lassar's paste (Stanford)

Dithranol	0.1% to 0.4%	occasionally stronger
Salicylic acid	0.2% to 0.4%	
Hard paraffin	0.5%	
Zinc oxide paste	to 100%	

Dithranol in 'soft' Lassar's paste (Stanford)

Dithranol	0.5%
Salicylic acid	1.0%
Hard paraffin	5.0%

Plain zinc oxide paste in equal parts of soft paraffin

*These now include dithrocreams and sticks which are easy to use but not as effective as pastes.

Modified from Stankler (1976).

short lived. Irritancy like a mild burn is treated by omitting treatment for 1 or 2 days. Various proprietary brands are slightly easier to manage and include vaseline-based preparations and creams or sticks (Table 17). The minute regimen is a system using dithranol 1–5 per cent in vaseline and 2 per cent salicylic acid. It is applied only for about 80 min before removal with an oil. It is suitable for those whose employment requires their skin to be free of ointments for most of the day.

Phototherapy

Natural sunlight is helpful in about 75 per cent of patients and probably accounts for a decreased incidence of psoriasis in sunny climates. Suberythema doses of UVB are a useful substitute and its effectiveness can be increased by prior bathing in or an application of tar which sensitizes the skin to the UVB.

PUVA therapy was introduced for psoriasis 10 years ago. The combination of long-wave ultraviolet rays (UVA or black light) with methoxypsoralen tablets 0.5 mg/kg taken 2 hours before exposure produces effective clearance and a bronze skin in most patients. Exposure of 15–30 minutes twice or thrice weekly succeeds in clearing the psoriasis in a month to 6 weeks. Maintenance therapy is weekly or fortnightly. Recurrences are no less frequent than with other forms of therapy. Dryness, atrophy, and other expected changes of irradiation are a consequence. The risk of skin cancer is as yet difficult to estimate but it is not insignificant. The risk is especially great in those who have arsenical kerotoses or other evidence of previous intake of arsenic.

Climatotherapy is the combination of natural sunlight, or in the case of the Dead Sea, a filtered form of sunlight, with sea salts or other constituents – sulphur, black mud, and bromides – present in different regions. It is effective but no more so than other regimens that provide topical medicaments and mental relaxation. The Dead Sea may be exceptional in the number of its peculiar features such as low humidity, increased atmospheric pressure, filtration of UVB, and minerals in high concentration.

Systemic therapy

ACTH or prednisolone provides short-term control but the incidence of side-effects including irreversible vertebral osteoporosis makes it best avoided if possible. It may be life saving in generalized erythroderma or pustular psoriasis in the elderly. With good nursing in the absence of heart failure or protein-losing enteropathy, most young people do better to avoid steroids. Methotrexate is the most favoured antimitotic or immunosuppressive agent. Carefully monitored and given intermittently the serious side-effects of liver fibrosis are slow to develop and may be justified in the older patient. It can be given weekly or fortnightly in intramuscular intravenous form 0.2–0.4 mg/kg. Most oral regimens are also intermittent:. 0.2–0.4 mg/kg every 1–2 weeks taken as tablets with water. Marrow suppression is rarely a problem but fibrosis of the liver is a late complication.

Retinoic acid given orally as two to three 25 mg tablets daily is helpful in some more difficult cases and it is the treatment of choice in generalized and pustular psoriasis. It is relatively free of serious side-effects but the effective dose is often a cause of annoying dry mouth, sore lips, and conjunctivitis as well as skin irritation and erosions and the high levels of blood lipids induced by the drug are potentially a long-term hazard. It is teratogenic and therefore contraception must be guaranteed for at least a year after discontinuing the drug. Hyperostosis is another long-term side-effect.

References

Baker, H. and Wilkinson, D. S. (1979). Psoriasis. In *Textbook of dermatology*, 3rd edn. (eds A. Rook, D. S. Wilkinson, and F. J. G. Ebling), pp. 1315–1367. Blackwell Scientific Publications, Oxford.

Clinical and Experimental Dermatology (1981). Special symposium on dermatological therapy. *Clin. exp. Dermatol.* **6**, 639–662.

Henseler, T., Honigsmann, H., Wolff, K. and Christophers, E. (1981). Oral methoxypsoralen photochemotherapy of psoriasis. *Lancet* **ii**, 853–857.

Journal of Investigative Dermatology (1979). Psoriasis. *J. invest. Dermatol.* **73**, 402–413.

Stankler, L. (1976). Psoriasis. In *Today's treatment*, pp. 50–55. British Medical Association Publications, London.

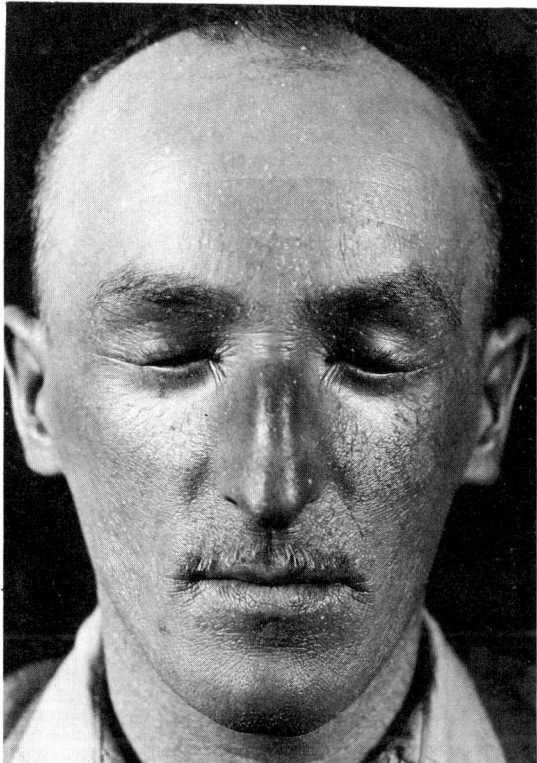

Fig. 52 Pityriasis rubra pilaris, a disorder showing some similarities to psoriasis but differing in its predilection for the face. There is some shrinkage of tissues around the eyes so that ectropion and incomplete closure of the eye lids has developed. This is also a characteristic of the disorder.

Other keratodermas

There are a number of rare scaly disorders of the skin which clinically have a range of patterns lying somewhere between ichthyosis and psoriasis. One of these is pityriasis rubra pilaris; another is ichthyosis hystrix, and others merit the term erythrokeratoderma. The scale is not as silvery or as easily exfoliated as in psoriasis – it is often smaller and more adherent. Most of these disorders are probably inherited, occasionally as a dominant gene but more often as a recessive. Involvement of the face is more characteristic than is the case in psoriasis (Fig. 52). The palms and soles often have a thickened yellow appearance. Nails are less often pitted and quite often show subungual keratosis. A follicular prominence is characteristic of pityriasis rubra pilaris (Fig. 53); the extensor surfaces are favoured and so the knees and elbows are often involved as in psoriasis. Some patterns are present in early childhood while occasionally it may present for the first time in extreme old age. The latter presentation of pityriasis rubra pilaris is probably acquired through influences other than genetic. The management of these conditions is difficult and in the case of the erythrokeratodermas retinoic acid has become the treatment of choice. This is taken by mouth but side-effects of dry mouth and eyes and some soreness of the skin may be sufficiently annoying for the patient to opt for living with his or her disease.

Pityriasis rosea

This not uncommon exanthem is probably due to a virus. The natural history and clustering of cases suggests that it is an infectious disease. It tends to occur in spring and autumn and in any one individual does not recur. Recurrent or prolonged eruptions of similar nature may be a variant of seborrhoeic eczema. The initial lesion or herald patch is usually on the trunk or proximally on the limbs. It is well-defined, oval, erythematous, and scaly. It precedes the generalized eruption by 3–10 days. The rash of pityriasis rosea is characterized by oval lesions orientated in the line

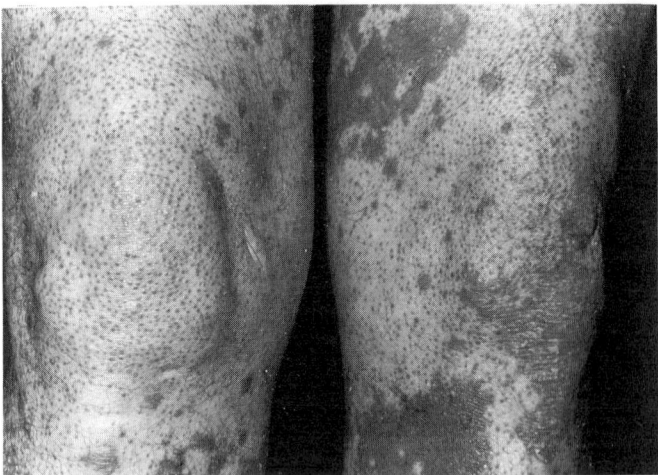

Fig. 53 Pityriasis rubra pilaris is primarily a disorder of the follicular epithelium.

markings of the skin of the trunk. The lesions develop a collarette of scales after 1 week. The rash may spread upwards to the neck and down the arms and legs, usually fading as it reaches below the elbows or knees. It lasts 3–6 weeks. Pruritus may be intense. Slight lymphadenopathy and fever rarely accompany the developing rash.

LICHEN PLANUS AND LICHENOID ERUPTIONS

Lichen planus and lichenoid eruptions are characterized by violaceous papules which are usually flat topped and shiny and heal leaving pigmentation. The histology is highly characteristic and includes damage to the basal layer of the epidermis and an intense infiltration of lymphocytes and a few histiocytes situated immediately below the epidermis (Fig. 54). The disturbances in the growth of the epidermis that result from this damage range from extreme atrophy with ulceration and almost no epidermal cell turnover to considerable hypertrophy and hyperkeratinization giving rise to thick nodules meriting the name hypertrophic lichen planus. Most cases are seen between the ages of 30 and 60 and it is extremely rare in children. More erosive forms are seen in the elderly and pigmented skin tends to develop more hypertrophic varieties.

Aetiology

An immunological basis is probable but it is by no means certain whether the heavy infiltrate with lymphocytes is due to an attack on some altered protein, induced perhaps by a virus, or whether there is a primary biochemical defect. HLA-A3 and A5 occur more often in lichen planus than in controls. Graft versus host reactions in the skin that follow bone marrow transplantation often present with an identical pattern of pathology to that of lichen planus. There is some clinical pathological overlap with the appearance seen in lupus erythematosus. Immunofluorescence studies show heavy deposits of fibrin and immunoglobulin but these could be entirely non-specific. There is some evidence of defective carbohydrate metabolism and abnormal glucose tolerance curves but the basis of this association still has to be explained. Many drugs produce an identical eruption, i.e. gold and organic arsenicals, antituberculous therapy, chlorpromazine and related drugs and, more recently, methyldopa. Lichen planus from contact with colour developers, is well documented, and there is an eczematous form commonly seen on light exposed areas particularly in the Middle East known as tropical or actinic lichen planus.

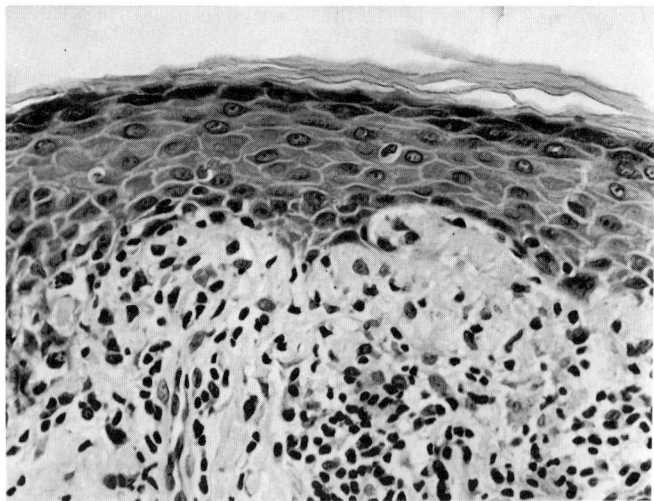

Fig. 54 Lichen planus. There is thickening of the granular layer and necrosis of the basal cell layer. The pale cells at the lower edge of the epidermis are destroyed epidermal cells. The predominant white cell is a lymphocyte. The infiltrate is often confined to the upper dermis.

Clinical features

The classical lesion is a shiny flat-topped papule (Fig. 55) described as polygonal and violaceous. Small white dots or lines in such papules are due to a mixture of oedema, white cell infiltrate, and disturbance of vasculature. They are termed Wickham striae. The papules may become confluent and heal in the centre giving rise to annular (Fig. 56) lesions or plaques with varying degrees of epidermal response. This may result in either atrophic skin or extreme hypertrophy. In lesions of mouth or of the glans penis a lacy-white appearance (Fig. 57) is common. Involvement of the hair follicles may give rise to keratosis pilaris and actual destruction of the hair follicle. Thus, lichen planus is one cause of scarring alopecia. Healing of the lesion is often followed by pigmentation due to melanin in the dermis. Warty hyperkeratotic lesions may be very persistent, as may ulceration, particularly of the peripheries or of the mucosa of the mouth. The initial lesions are commonly on the front of the wrists, in the lumbar region, or around the ankles. The palms and soles may be involved in which case the appearance may even suggest a vesicular eruption. The involvement of the mucosa and tongue which occurs in anything between 30–70 per cent of cases may extend to the genitalia and perianal area, and it has even been described in the rectum, stomach, and larynx. Severe itching is common. Ridging of the nails is essentially due to cessation of nail growth and produces longitudinal linear depressions.

Prognosis

The onset may be very explosive or insidious. Most cases clear slowly but take up to a year so to do; 85 per cent of clearance is in 18 months. Mucuous membrane lesions or extremely hypertrophic lesions on the legs often persist for years, and there is a risk of squamous epitheliomatous changes particularly in ulcerated mucosal lesions.

Treatment

Treatment is mainly aimed at the relief of the itching and local steroid creams are perhaps the most effective. Occasionally for a very severe widespread lichen planus a course of prednisolone or ACTH is justified. Probably it does not influence the course of the disease but merely its intensity. As with all itching conditions of the skin cooling evaporating lotions such as calamine lotion may be helpful. Persistent ulcerated lesions can be excised or grafted. In the mouth local steroid creams, particularly those manufactured for the mouth containing orabase, can be prescribed. A

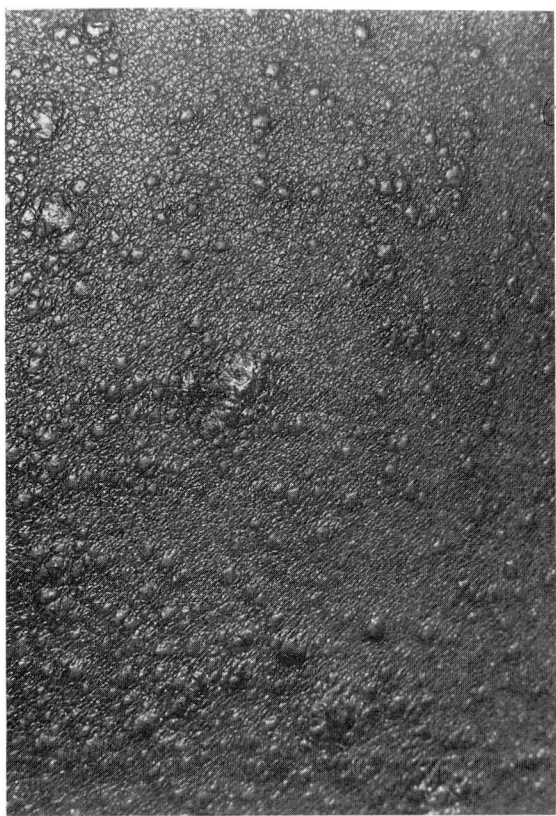

Fig. 55 A black skin affected by the shiny, flat-topped, often polygonal papules of lichen planus.

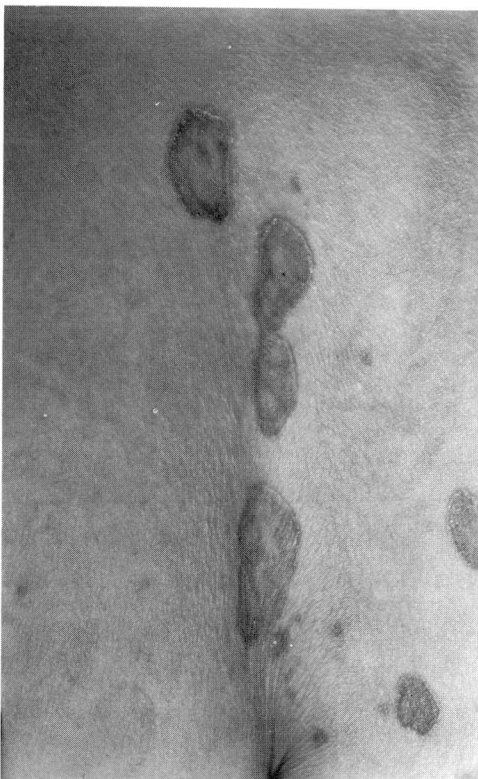

Fig. 56 Lichen planus may heal in the centre leaving atrophy and pigmentation. The edge is slightly raised; this gives rise to the annular form of the condition.

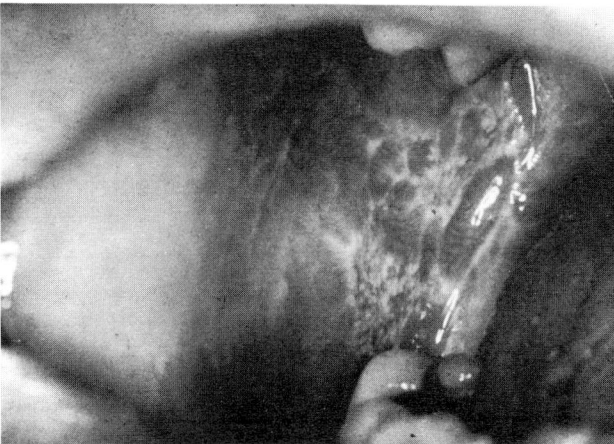

Fig. 57 Lichen planus of the mouth is one cause of mucosal whiteness. Unlike candidiasis the lesions cannot be removed by scraping. They are characteristically 'lacy' in appearance.

spray such as is used in asthma may be a more convenient way of administering steroid to the mucosa of the mouth, emphasizing that its use is without inhalation.

ACNE VULGARIS

Acne vulgaris is the most common disease of the skin affecting teenagers and consequently affecting those who are most conscious of their body image.

Acne is a disorder of the pilosebaceous follicles. These are most numerous on the face and upper trunk, hence the distribution of acne. The lower part of the affected follicle produces an imperfect keratin layer and in the healthy follicle this sloughs and degenerates, thus contributing to the waxy mass of sebaceous lipids which surrounds the small hair enclosed in the follicles. Such debris is normally heavily populated with *Propionibacterium acnes*, an anaerobic diphtheroid. In acne the imperfect keratin layer lining the lower follicles is hyperproliferative and sloughs incompletely. This is probably because the cells are more adhesive. The mouth of the follicle is thus plugged so that sebum and hairs cannot escape. Increased secretion of sebum though characteristic is not thought to be the cause of acne.

Aetiology

The recognition that acne is not so much a disorder of sebum secretion but a disorder of the sebaceous follicle has modified concepts of the aetiology of acne. Sebum consists of triglycerides, wax esters, squalene, and sterolesters. The fatty acids in sebum are inflammatory and are formed by bacteria, even in healthy skin, from unsaturated 14–16 or 18 carbon components of the triglycerides. It is the obstruction to outflow and the build up of wall debris which accounts for acne vulgaris. It is possible that acne in the tropics is due to a secondary response in the rate of turnover of the follicular lining perhaps induced by occlusion under a belt or braces in such a hot environment. The acne of Cushing's disease may also be due to an increased rate of turnover. Chlorinated hydrocarbons also cause acne. Chloracne is an important symptom of poisoning and was present in 168 cases of poisoning in the Seveso disaster. The exact way in which the inflammation is produced is uncertain; the follicle contains fatty acids and bacterial proteases which activate the alternative pathway of complement and attract neutrophils.

Sebaceous gland activity is regulated by hormones and in particular, by androgens from the testes and adrenals which stimulate, and oestrogens which seem to suppress activity. In the adult male the glands are normally maximally stimulated and acne is more severe in boys than in girls. The skin itself is a major site for

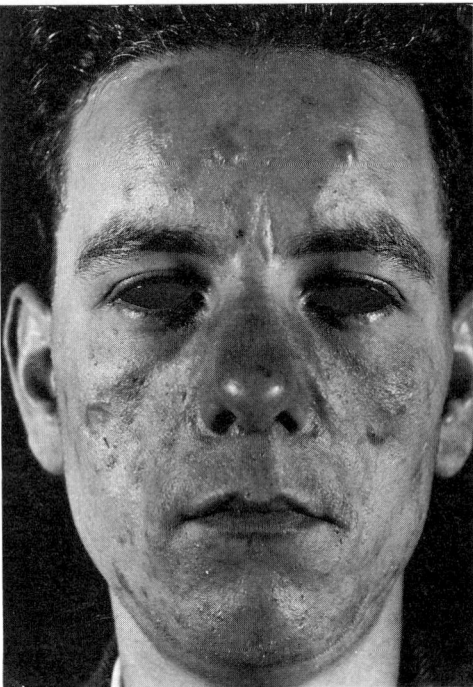

Fig. 58 Greasiness of the skin is a common accompaniment of acne as is comedo formation or 'blackheads' as seen on the forehead of this young man. Whether either are wholly responsible for the consequent inflammation and scarring also seen in this photograph is debatable.

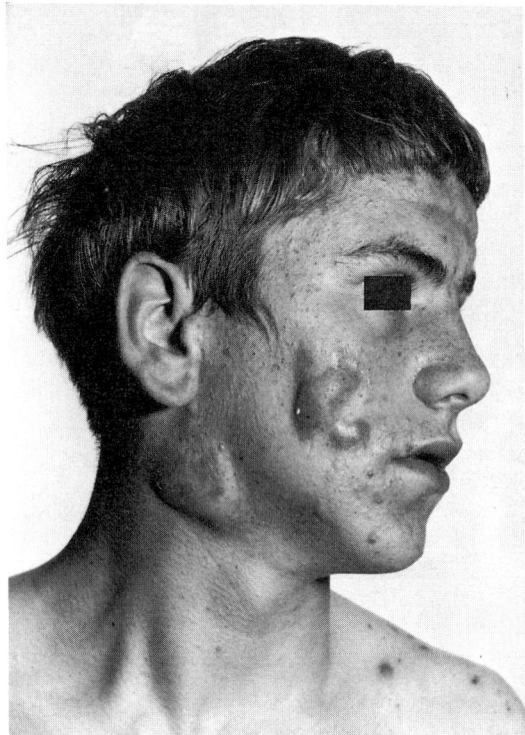

Fig. 59 Large cystic lesions are the most disfiguring aspect of acne vulgaris.

androgenic conversion similar to that observed in the prostate gland and in the male genitalia. Dihydrotestosterone rather than testosterone may be the end organ effector and it is formed within the target cells where it stimulates lipogenesis as well as mitosis. Eunuchs do not develop acne. Oestrogens reduce the size of sebaceous glands and sebum production is diminished.

There is increasing interest in the role of humoral immunity in the inflammatory process. Circulating immune complexes have been detected in severe acne.

Clinical features

The *closed comedo* is the first stage of acne and appears as tiny white nodules below the surface seen especially when the skin is stretched (see Fig. 5). These may rupture giving rise to irritation of the dermis, i.e. inflamed papules, or form the *open comedo* or blackhead by pushing open the mouth of the follicle (Fig. 58). The black material is melanin; blackheads are blacker in dark skins and white in the albino; the melanin is transferred to the keratinocytes before they are shed into the sebaceous follicle. Acne cysts (Fig. 59) occur as the result of ballooning of the distended follicle and often the walls of the cyst and hair and sebaceous apparatus are destroyed. Adjacent cysts often form fistulae and sinuses which rupture displacing epithelium in the dermis, forming irregular channels or foreign-body reactions.

Atrophic or hypertrophic scars of all types may be seen, and often excoriations, picking, and squeezing contribute to the irregularities of pigment and to the epidermal or dermal thickening. Rarely young males develop suppurative and highly inflamed lesions in the skin over the chest with pain, fever, and accompanying polyarthralgia probably mediated by immune mechanisms and the activation of complement.

Acne usually presents before the menarche and clears after a few years. A more persistent form – particularly affecting the chin – may be seen in persons up to middle age, especially in women who have premenstrual exacerbations.

Neonatal acne is of unknown aetiology; it usually clears within 6 months and is probably due to maternal hormones. Acne is induced by iodides (see Fig. 31b) and bromides, steroids, androgens, barbiturates, phenytoin, and phenothiazines.

Cosmetics

In many parts of the world cosmetics contribute to acne and the lesions may be confined to the site of application. Vaseline-type preparations or medicated oil in shampoos in young women with long hair, are a well known cause.

Management

Local preparations

All local preparations produce some erythema and occasional pustulation before the acne comes under control. Sulphur is a time-honoured agent producing local irritation and causing peeling. It is helpful for pustules and may not be so good for comedones which precede pustulation, often by several months. Comedones are reduced by retinoic acid and by 10 per cent salicylic acid in ethanol. Sunlight is a popular therapy and it is undoubtedly helpful for some patients. The tanning effect may be a purely cosmetic form of camouflage. However, there is clinical and experimental evidence that in some patients comedones are increased in number after exposure to sunlight.

Long-acting oxidizing antiseptics such as benzoyl peroxide reduce sebum excretion, reduce comedo production, and inhibit *P. acnes in vitro*. They are the topical treatment of choice, are a mild irritant, and produce peeling after several days' application. It is best to start sparingly with 5 per cent and later to increase the amount applied or the concentration to 10 per cent.

Retinoic acid helps the lining cells of the follicle to slough off without plugging the follicle. It is applied in a cream or a lotion or gel, and is indicated for comedones rather than for pustules or cysts. It is irritant and causes redness and peeling. Its effect is not unlike sunburn and should not be used when there is undue sun exposure either in the summer bather or the winter skier.

Oral therapy

Oral tetracycline is the mainstay of treatment of acne if simple measures have not resulted in clearance. Erythromycin and clindomycin (now usually prescribed as a lotion) are also effective but tetracycline is exceptionally safe. The only side-effect is the discoloration of teeth in the fetus and in children. Anorexia nausea, colic, or vaginal candidiasis are rare. Provided they are taken on an empty stomach, one or two tetracycline tablets taken daily control acne. Rarely Gram-negative folliculitis occurs particularly around the nose or in persistent cysts. This results in suddenly worsening with considerable inflammation and may warrant a course of ampicillin. Severe inflammatory and cystic acne respond to a zinc sulphate citrate complex taken with meals. Acute severe inflammatory disease also responds to prednisolone.

Diet

Studies of the effects of starvation in the obese or the malnourished show little evidence of the effect of diet on acne vulgaris and this is so even in pellagra in which some plugging of the follicles around the nose is an early sign. There may be the individual in whom acne is made worse by chocolate but this has not been shown in trials of larger populations. Nutrition may influence the age of onset of puberty and hence overeating may result in earlier acne.

Acne surgery

Comedo extraction is the expression of a follicle's contents by the application of pressure on the surface often with a special device called a comedo extractor. The benefits of active attack on the lesions counteracting stasis and build up of the contents has to be weighed against the fact that suppression is always incomplete and a tendency to rupture into the dermis may promote inflammation. Cryotherapy destroys the lining of large cysts. Deep sinuses may require externalization. Solitary inflamed lesions benefit from intralesional inoculation of steroids. Persistent acne cysts sometimes resolve with the injection of small amounts of intralesional triamcinolone.

Oestrogen

Oestrogens have to be given in excessive amounts to have an effect in acne and are now used principally in the most physiological form of therapy, the contraceptive pill.

Acne is made worse by 19-nor-testosterone derivatives in the pill. Cyproterone 17 × acetate up to 100 mg for the first 10 days of the cycle plus ethinyl oestradiol 50 μg for 21 days, is used to block the receptor sites for dihydrotestosterone. This antiandrogen effect works only if the drug is given systemically and no topical preparation has so far found to be of help. Small doses of prednisolone suppress androgen activity.

13-*cis*-retinoic acid up to 1 mg/kg is a remarkably effective suppressant of sebum secretion not yet freely available in most countries.

Within 3–6 months the pilosebaceous gland is much reduced. The side-effects are annoying but it is a safe drug in the short term. Contraception is essential for female patients. The Diane contraceptive pill which contains 50 μg ethinyl oestradiol with only 2 mg cyproterone acetate is partially effective if taken for many months. In resistant cases additional cyproterone acetate taken on days 5–14 of the menstrual cycle will improve the effectiveness. Combinations with oxytetracycline show advantages.

References

Crow, K. D. (1981). Chloracne and its potential clinical implications. *Clin. exp. Dermatol.* **6**, 243–57.

Cunliffe, W. J. and Cotterill, W. (1975). *The acnes: clinical features, pathogenesis and treatment.* W. B. Saunders-Lloyd Luke, London.

Darley, M. B. (1984). Recent advances in hormonal aspects of acne vulgaris. *Int. J. Dermatol.* **23**, 539–541.

Dicken, C. H. (1984). Retinoids: a review. *J. Am. Acad. Dermatol.* **10**, 541–551.

Journal of Investigative Dermatology (1979). Acne. *J. Invest. Dermatol.* **73**, 434–42.

Table 18 Localized causes of pigmentation. Light exposed—especially on the face and usually due to increased numbers of normal melanocytes in the epidermis

Actinic or senile lentigo A common grey/brown macule especially of the face and limbs in middle-aged or older persons, usually due to sun exposure in youth. It is without epidermal changes. Spreading pigmented actinic keratoses show slight verrucous changes and can merge into a squamous cell carcinoma or into a lentigo maligna.
Berloque dermatitis Brown often streaky macules often initially inflammatory with redness, blistering, or scaling at sites exposed to perfumes and sunlight. Several plants may be responsible. The streaky pigmentation may persist for years (Fig. 60).
Freckle-ephelis Small brown macules usually numerous in light-exposed skin of genetically fair, blonde, or red-haired and blue-eyed types.
Lentigo maligna Usually a well-defined irregular brown to black mottled macular lesion especially occurring on the face in old persons. The melanocytes are dysplastic, vacuolated in the epidermis and malignant change is common (see Fig. 27).
Melasma or chloasma Usually brown symmetrical macules of the butterfly area of the face or crossbow pattern on the forehead. It is common in pregnancy or in those on the oral contraceptives containing oestrogen (see Fig. 62).
Xeroderma pigmentosum The patchy macular pigmentation is associated with keratoses, telangiectasia, and malignancies. Basal cell and squamous cell carcinomas and even melanoma are common. Intolerance to the sun results in excessive sunburn often 72 hours after exposure. The disorder begins in early childhood, often as a bright erythema and swelling following exposure to the sun. The aetiology is genetic and concerns repair of a defect in DNA, following injury by light (see Fig. 30).

PIGMENTATION

The most immediately recognizable differences between two persons are often related to skin colour. The social consequences of colour extend beyond political implications and may be important in health. The principal pigments in the skin include melanin which is black, phaeomelanin which is reddish-yellow, haemoglobin and its byproducts bilirubin and biliverdin as well as haemosiderin which produce colours of yellow, green, red, and brown. Since the epidermis transmits blue light more effectively than red, pigment in the dermis tends to look blue so a blue naevus is entirely composed of brown melanin deposited in the dermis, whereas the brown discoloration of the junctional naevus is due to pigment at a slightly higher level affecting the epidermal–dermal junction. All discussions of this subject should begin with racial causes of pigmentation because they are so common, but physical causes are important also, since in the white skin visible tanning may occur in the sun. It is known as immediate darkening when it occurs within minutes of the skin being exposed to sunlight. Over a number of days increased pigment production is associated with epidermal thickening and retention of pigment.

Some pigmented lesions are naevi (Tables 18–20), others result from 'incontinence' of pigment which increases the amount of pigment in the dermal macrophages and is commonly post-inflammatory.

Pigmentation as a feature of systemic illness is most significantly due to endocrine dysfunction affecting the melanocyte stimulating hormone. In countries where malnutrition and infections are common, protein and vitamin deficiency as well as cachexia from a variety of causes accounts for disturbances in the colour of the skin.

'Tinea' or pityriasis versicolor is due to a superficial fungus known as *Malassezia furfur*. It usually affects the upper trunk and may spread on to the neck or on to the arms. The lesions are slightly scaly, off-white, pink, and brown. Pityriasis is the term for a bran-like powdery scale and versicolor implies the variation in the colouring (Fig. 65).

In leprosy, hypomelanosis is a feature of tuberculoid and border-line tuberculoid types (Fig. 66). Light touch and later pinprick

Table 19 Pigmentation more commonly on the trunk

Acanthosis nigricans   Pigmentation affects the axillae, groins, and there is a velvety thickening of the skin with skin tags. The condition may be benign when associated with obesity and in the young, but in older persons with oral, facial, or hand pigmentation and thickening, it is more often due to an underlying adenocarcinoma. Pruritus may be associated and indicates underlying carcinoma (see Fig. 125).

Becker's naevus   Large, lightly pigmented, and often hairy macular pigmentation affecting a segment of the trunk such as the shoulder or one flank. It is often noticed after puberty for the first time. It is entirely benign (Fig. 61).

Dermatosis papulosa nigra   This is the commonest dark lesion in the Negro and is a papular variety of seborrhoeic warts producing discrete but multiple dark lesions of the face and neck.

Tinea nigra   A localized asymptomatic fungus infection causing a brown or black macular lesion on the palm; sometimes when there is no scaling it may be taken for a lentigo.

Erythrasma   This is due to a corynebacterial infection of the groins, axillae, and in between the toes. On white skin it is light brown, but in dark skin it may produce a lighter or darker hue. Wood's light shows the coral red fluorescence.

Tinea versicolor   This is a flat to slightly elevated scaly papule or reticulate plaque producing either a brownish coloration or depigmentation. It affects the upper trunk and upper limbs and neck (Fig. 65).

Urticaria pigmentosum   These are pigmented lesions due to nests of mast cells in the skin. In children they may be quite large, palpable lesions about the size of a thumb or they may be lentil-sized and numerous. Occasionally, though, there is a diffuse and velvety texture to the skin. The diagnostic feature of the lesion is the wealing that results from scratching.

Café au lait   These lesions resemble large freckles. They are often as large as the thumb or palm. They tend to be oval in shape. There is a variant known as naevus spilus which is speckled with much darker spots. In neurofibromatosis there is usually at least five *café au lait* spots and generalized freckling extends into the axillae (Fig. 63). Very large pigmented macules being unilateral and having serrated edges are characteristic of Albright's syndrome.

Leopard syndrome   Progressive darkening and very numerous lentigos of the trunk and limbs (Fig. 64) is associated with the following denoted by the letters of the word 'Leopard'. Lentigenoses, ECG abnormalities, ocular defects, pulmonary stenosis, abnormalities of genitalia, retardation of growth, deafness.

Peutz–Jeghers syndrome   This consists of polyposis of the small intestine and is associated with numerous small pigmented macules affecting the perioral buccal areas extending quite far beyond the margins of the lips and affecting also the dorsum of the fingers. Note: Lentigos of the lips and post-inflammatory pigmentation are in themselves quite common and need not be associated with any internal disorder.

Table 20 Disorders of increased pigmentation

Circumscribed brown* hyperpigmentation
  Infection: tinea versicolor: erythrasma
  Café au lait type: Albright's syndrome: neurofibromatosis
  Lentigo type: Leopard syndrome: Peutz–Jeghers syndrome
  Melasma type (chloasma): pregnancy; drugs; idiopathic
  Miscellaneous: acanthosis nigricans; post-inflammatory; stasis; Becker's naevus; fixed drug eruption; urticaria pigmentosa; Minocin-induced (often black)
Generalized brown* hyperpigmentation
  Reticulate: naevoid; poikiloderma; dyskeratosis congenita
  Metabolic: haemochromatosis; porphyria; chronic liver disease
  Endocrine and/or autoimmune: Addison's disease: pregnancy; pernicious anaemia; myxoedema; thyrotoxicosis; Felty's syndrome; ACTH and MSH secreting tumour; scleroderma
  Nutritional: malnutrition; malabsorption
  Drugs: arsenic; busulphan (Myleran); vinca alkaloids; dibromo-mannitol; ACTH; psoralen; atebrin; chlorpromazine (usually reddish brown)
  Other types: post-inflammatory; Whipple's disease; catatonic schizophrenia; Schilder's disease
Generalized slate-grey† hyperpigmentation
  Haemochromatosis
  Nutritional deficiency
  Drugs: chlorpromazine; Minocin; gold; silver

* Brown: increased melanin in epidermal cells.
† Grey, slate or blue: increased melanin in dermis.

sensation is impaired. There is often lack of sweating and there may be loss of hair. An adjacent enlarged peripheral nerve may be palpable; and this may be mistaken for an enlarged lymph node.

Pigmentation of the buccal mucosa tongue or fingernails is significant only in white skin since it is a normal finding in dark races.

Pigmentation by melanin requires the formation of precursor granules known as melanosomes, their melanization, their secretion into keratinocytes and their transport and often their degradation by the keratinocytes.

Depigmentation

Leucoderma is a term used for any whiteness of skin and ranges from a mild hypopigmentation to complete loss of pigment such as characterizes vitiligo. Microbial diseases such as pityriasis versicolor (Fig. 65), leprosy (Fig. 66), and syphilis are important infectious causes of depigmentation. Pinta should be suspected in persons from central or southern America showing a succession of erythematous hyperpigmented lesions progressing to warty or atrophic plaques of depigmented skin. The late stage resembles vitiligo. Naevus anaemicus is a hypovascularity of the skin observed in white skins (Fig. 67). It is not a disorder of melaninization.

Vitiligo

This is a common autoimmune skin disease affecting 1 per cent of the population. The melanocytes are destroyed and the affected skin is totally depigmented. In many parts of the world where skins are deeply pigmented, it is a principal cause of attendance at a dermatology deparment. It affects up to 1 per cent of the population. Except in those persons unable to protect themselves from bright sunlight the disability is purely cosmetic but causes more concern and social handicap than almost any other common disease. However, an association with other autoimmune diseases and a family history of such is found in one-third of cases. The cause is unknown and the melanocyte seems to be damaged by some as yet unidentified antibody or toxin. There is a 20–30 per cent incidence of vitiligo in those who develop melanoma.

Clinical features   The initial depigmentation is often at sites of trauma particularly of the knuckles of the hands and sometimes around a naevus (Figs. 68 and 69). The face and neck are usually affected early. In white skinned persons the first complaint is often in the summer when the unaffected skin is at its darkest from sun exposure. There is usually marked symmetry; the axillary folds and genitalia are commonly affected; the eye is not involved. The depigmentation of the lesion is ultimately total (Fig. 70) and should cause no confusion with the hypopigmentation of diseases such as leprosy. Only in the earlier stages of vitiligo is there hypopigmentation but such areas are never anaesthetic as in leprosy. Pigment may accumulate and be well defined at the borders of the lesion giving a hyperpigmented edge. Melanocytes of hair follicles are usually unaffected and repigmentation, when it occurs, is often from such sites (Fig. 71).

The clinician should be aware of the likely association of diabetes mellitus, pernicious anaemia, Addison's disease, myxoedema, or thyrotoxicosis. Less than one-third of patients show spontaneous repigmentation. In most the loss of pigment gradually extends. Depigmentation of the vulva, penis, and neck is sometimes persistent and of a localized variety, and need not necessarily progress to generalized vitiligo and should be distinguished from the more atrophic lichen sclerosis of those sites.

Management   Patients are usually much distressed by the cosmetic disability. It is helpful to explain that there is a 30 per cent chance of spontaneous cure. Offering advice on camouflage with match-

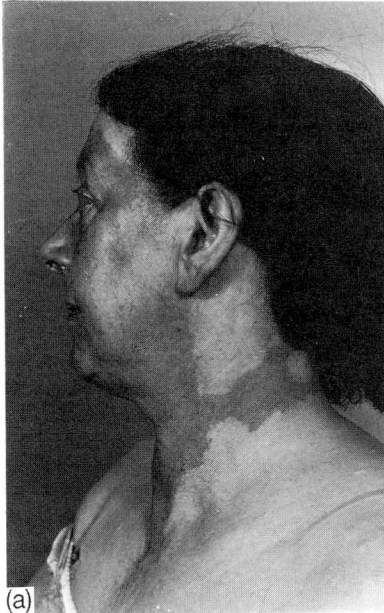

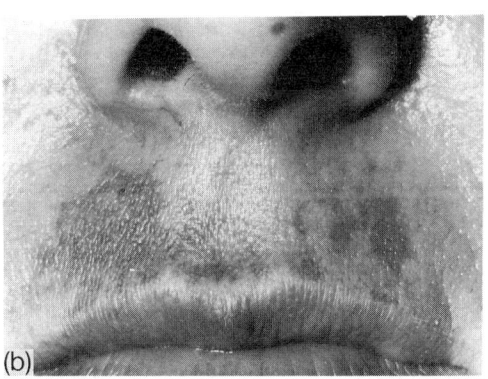

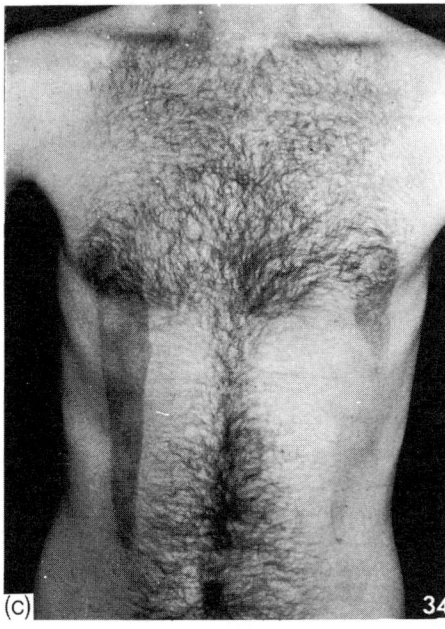

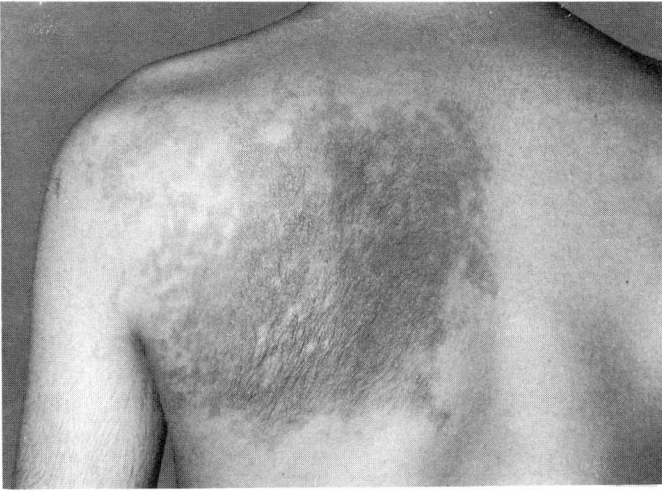

Fig. 61 Becker's naevus is due to melanin in the dermis and it is often segmental and usually hairy. It may become overt only after childhood.

Fig. 60 Pigmentation due to cosmetic agents. Often initially a dermatitis, it is especially induced by exposure to ultraviolet rays. It tends to have the streaky distribution of application. (a) Neck from eau de cologne; (b) lips from lanolin; (c) also from eau de cologne and sun bathing, the bizarre pattern is characteristic of an exogenous cause.

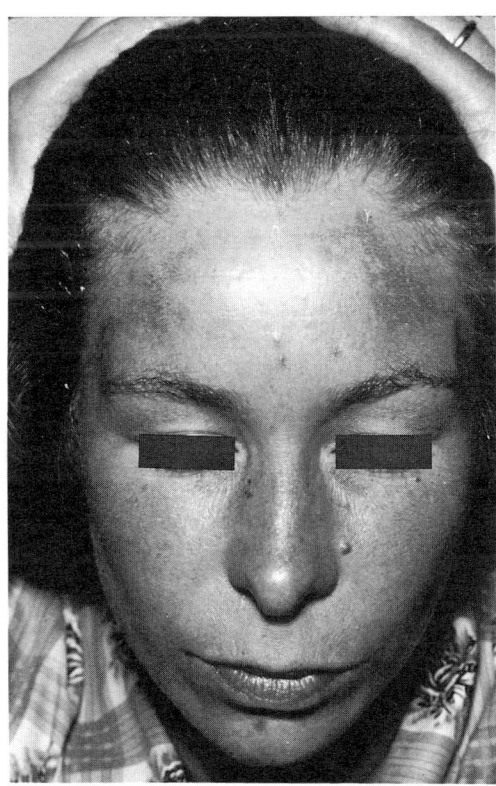

Fig. 62 Crossbow pattern of chloasma in encephalitis, an association that has been described but may be incidental.

ing of the skin with appropriate mixes gives the patients an opportunity to help themselves especially on important social occasions. But such camouflage is tedious and difficult to apply effectively for everyday use. There is no special advantage in the purchase of more expensive cosmetics since the basic constituents are cheap. The best effect is achieved from powder and grease mixtures with a powder finish patted gently into the skin after application. Dihydroxyacetone is the basis of many suntan lotions but again it is difficult to apply satisfactorily without over-pigmenting the adjacent unaffected skin.

Patients should be told to avoid occupations which injure the skin such as playing with animals which scratch. For those whose skin is almost completely depigmented the cosmetic effect of

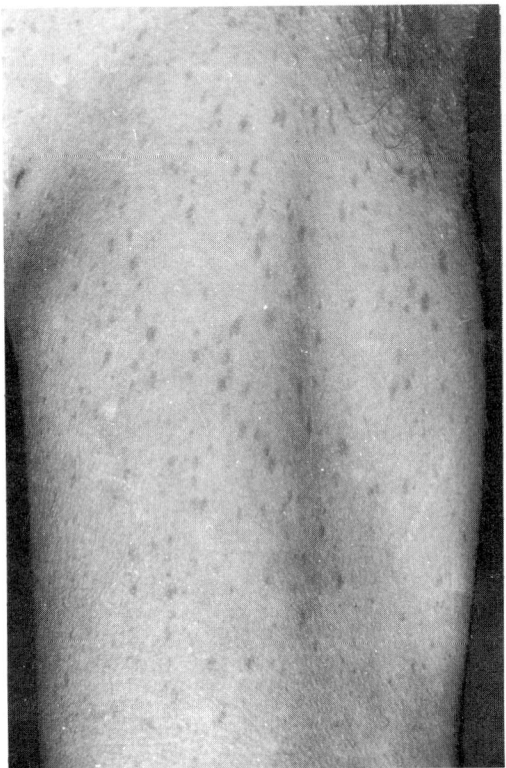

Fig. 63 In neurofibromatosis freckles extend into the axilla. This is a diagnostic feature in incomplete penetrance important in genetic counselling of white persons, but less reliable in black.

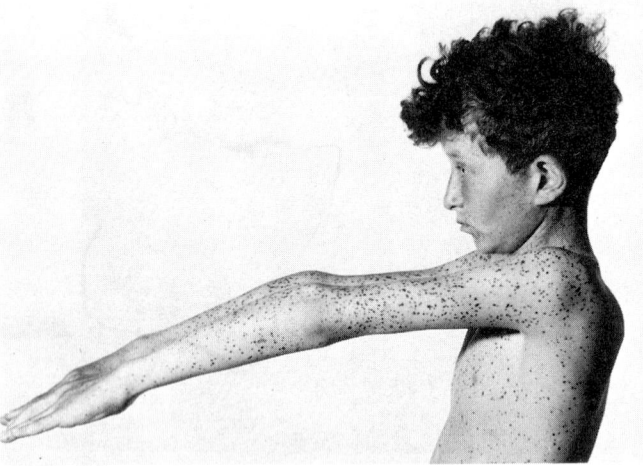

Fig. 64 Syndrome of progressive darkening of numerous lentigos associated with cardiovascular and neurological abnormalities.

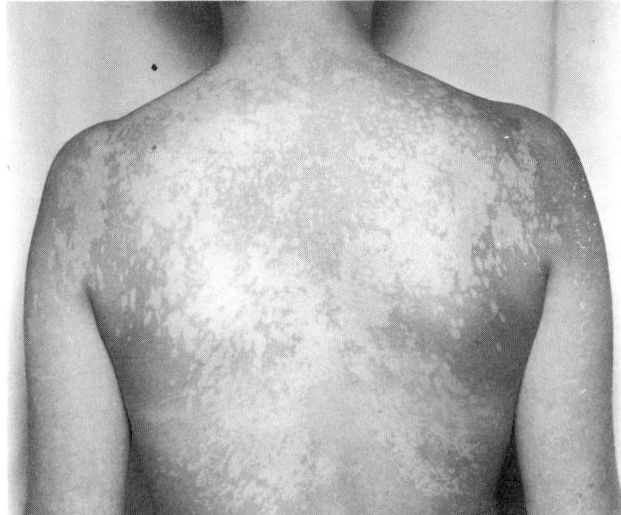

Fig. 65 Pityriasis versicolor due to the organism *Malassezia furfur* causes redness and slight brownish coloration of very pale white skin. In dark or sallow skin it causes depigmentation. It favours the upper trunk.

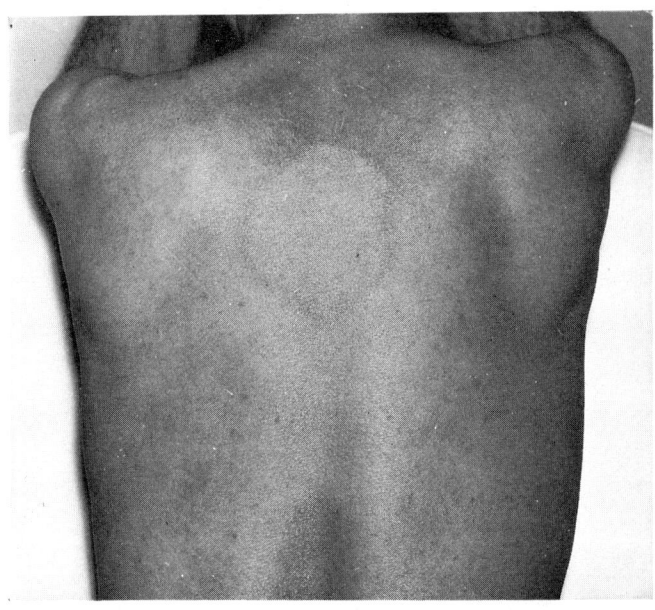

Fig. 66 Hypopigmentation especially with a hyperpigmented border should always be tested for loss of sensation. This lesion is typical of tuberculoid leprosy.

removing the remaining pigment is sometimes preferred. The formulation prepared by Sheffield Royal Infirmary includes the following: hydroquinone 30 g; hydrocortisone BP 6 g; retinoic acid 600 mg; butylated hydroxytoluene 300 mg; and methylated spirit and polyethylene glycol in equal parts to 600 ml.

Psoralens and sunlight are one of the most ancient remedies in medicine and UVA (black light) is a recently developed extension of the older remedy. Psoralens, methoxy- or tri-psoralen, are taken by mouth 2 hours before exposure to light or may be applied topically 30 minutes before exposure. The simplest regimen is a combination of meladinin paint and sunlight. It is necessary to test reactivity with short-time exposure and always to expose the skin at the same time of the day in order not to burn the skin by unex-

pectedly high intensity of UVA. The chances of remission are not much greater than from natural responses and treatment successes may take 2–3 years to complete. As might be expected from an autoimmune disorder local steroid preparations are sometimes helpful. They have been advocated in combination with psoralens but therapeutic triumphs are difficult to assess, and the requirement to use these agents for years rather than days makes side-effects very likely. Local steroids are sometimes used to stabilize a rapidly progressive early stage of the disease. Some Indian practitioners treat cosmetically disabling local patches with light dermabrasion and the application of autologous skin cells from pigmented skin.

Other forms of depigmentation (post-inflammatory)

Chemical depigmentation A complete loss of melanocytes is a well recognized effect of certain chemicals – monobenzyl ether of hydroquinone and butyl phenol. The hands are usually first

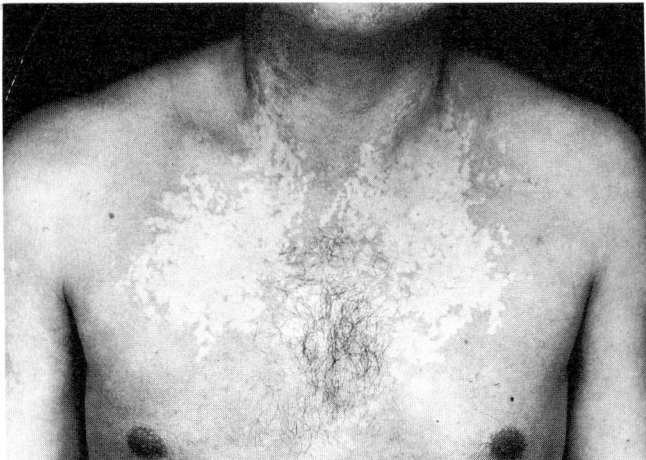

Fig. 67 Not all whiteness is due to loss of pigment. In this case of naevus anaemicus there is decreased vasculature present since birth.

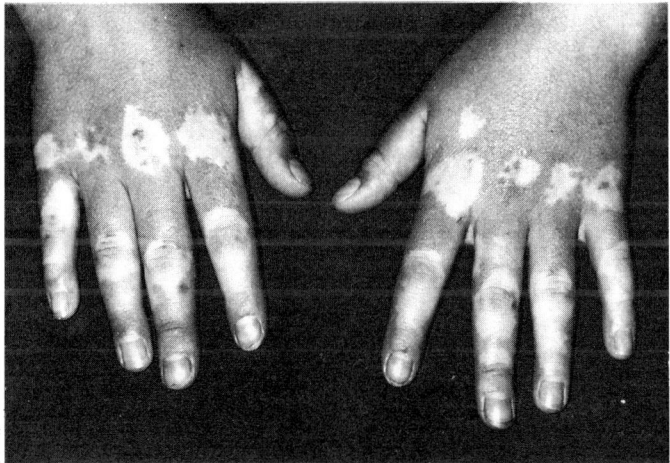

Fig. 68 Vitiligo is complete depigmentation and not merely hypopigmentation; it often begins at sites of minor trauma such as the knuckles. As with all essentially endogenous disorders it is symmetrical.

involved and the rubber industry is the commonest source of this problem.

Albinism This is a group of at least six genetically distinct syndromes determined not by absence of melanocytes but by their inability to synthesize melanin. Since melanin is important not only in the skin but also at such sites as the cochlea and retina, and since also the capacity to transfer organelles other than melanin is sometimes impaired, there are a number of associated defects affecting vision, hearing, and the delivery of lysosomes. In some societies where inbreeding is usual, albinism is common, i.e. San Blas Islands, southern Nigeria. Albinos in many countries are outcast, poor, underfed, and often die from skin cancer.

Complete albinism – autosomal recessive tyrosinase deficiency
Although the melanocytes are in normal numbers, because of a deficiency of tyrosinase no melanin is formed. The hair is white, including the eyebrows and eyelashes, and the iris is pink. There is photophobia, nystagmus, and impaired visual acuity. The principal disadvantage is severe sun damage to the skin so that premature ageing and squamous cell carcinomas are common especially in summer or if social circumstances require a rural outdoor life.

Partial albinism – autosomal recessive melanosomal deficiency
Tyrosinase is present in the melanocytes but transfer of melanin to the keratinocytes is defective. The skin is not usually as pale as

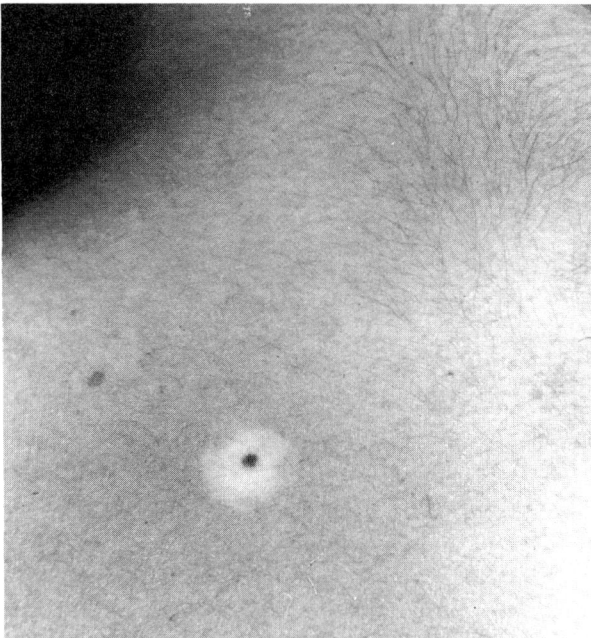

Fig. 69 Vitiligo often begins around a pigmented naevus – a halo naevus.

the complete form and the hair is yellow. Pigment is preserved in some freckles on sun-exposed skin. The eyes are blue but photophobia and nystagmus are usual.

Partial albinism yellow-red mutant variety This is prevalent in the Amish communities in the USA. Phaeomelanin, the pigment of redhead individuals, requires cystine as well as tyrosine.

Phenylketonuria This is a cause of whiteness that should not be forgotten, and it results in elevated levels of phenylalanine which competes for tyrosinase.

Cross syndrome This is an autosomal recessive defect of melanosome formation associated with gingival fibrosis and various maldevelopments of the CNS and eye. Hermansky–Pudlak albinism is associated with an abnormality of platelets which gives rise to bleeding, especially after aspirin.

Chediak–Higashi syndrome This is an autosomal recessive disorder that gives rise to partial albinism and failure of formation of membrane-bound organelles affecting the melanocytes and the white blood cells, the liver, and the brain cells. It is the human equivalent of Aleutian mink disease. The hair is yellow, and photophobia, nystagmus, and eye translucency are not severe. Affected cells produce giant melanosomes and giant lysosomes. The white cell defect predisposes to severe infection causing death in children. Hepatomegaly and lymphadenopathy frequently progress to lymphoma.

Piebaldism This is autosomal dominant absence of melanocytes. It is present at birth and may be difficult to recognize in fair skinned individuals. The hands and feet and centre of the back show normal pigmentation. The hair is normal except for a white forelock. The rest of the body shows loss of pigment with no melanocytes. There are islands of residual pigmentation. The condition is inherited as an autosomal dominant and the offspring should be examined at birth with Wood's light.

Waardenburg's syndrome This is an autosomal dominant disorder in which there is a defect of pigment affecting the cochlea. Deafness is associated with a white forelock as well as bilateral displacement of the medial canthi and fusion of the eyebrows or at least an unusual facial hair distribution.

Tielz's syndrome This is an autosomal dominant deaf mutism with hypoplasia of the eyebrows and absence of pigmentation.

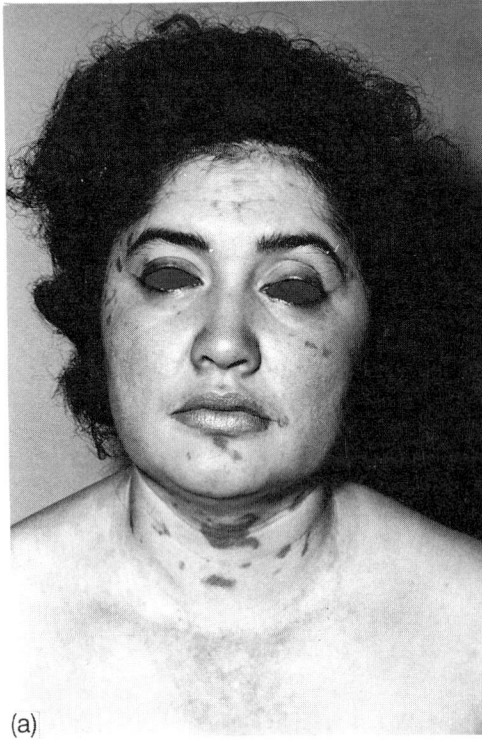

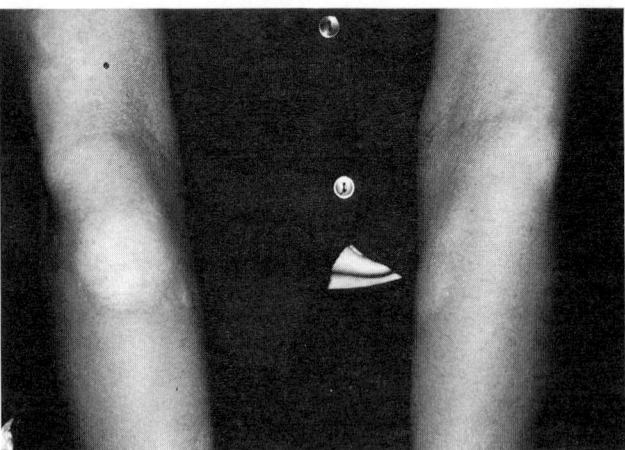

Fig. 71 Pityriasis alba caused by a mild dry eczema. A common cause of discoloration is slightly scaly areas of depigmentation.

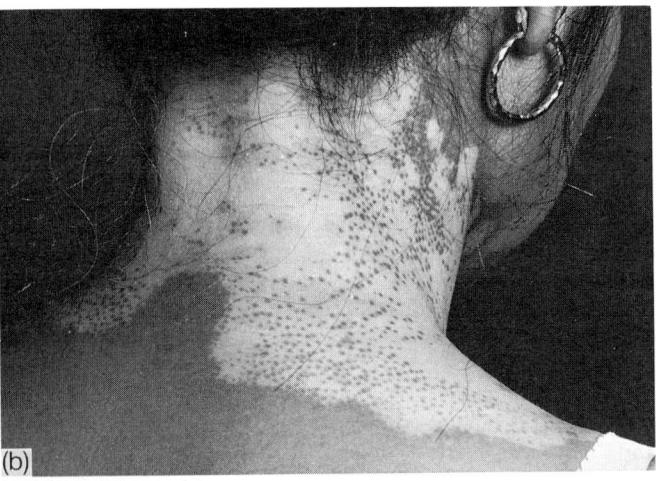

Fig. 70 (a) The pigment loss in this once dark-skinned woman is almost complete. Satisfactory cosmetic management would be depigmentation of the few residual areas of normal skin. (b) Repigmentation of the skin in vitiligo is usually from the follicles. It is slow, unpredictable, and incomplete.

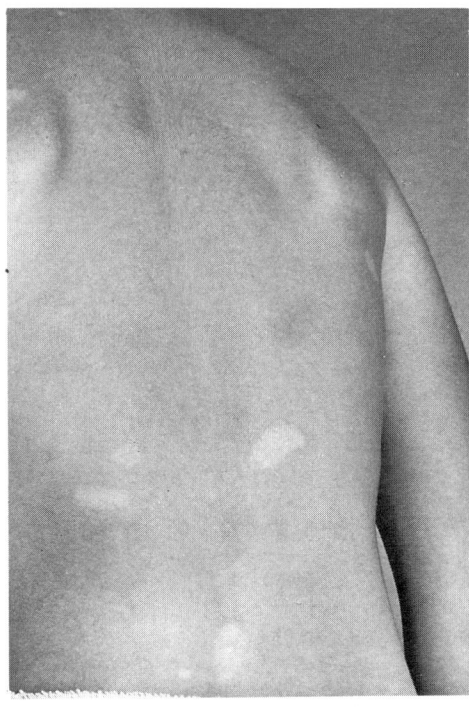

Fig. 72 Typical oval or 'leaf'-like hypopigmented lesions of tuberous sclerosis. They are present at birth.

Vogt–Koyanagi–Harada syndrome This is a vitiligo including white eyelashes and is associated with bilateral uveitis, alopecia areata, tinnitus, and altered host response to viral meningitis.

Halo naevi These are characterized by loss of pigment around benign (see Fig. 69) or very rarely malignant melanocytic naevi. It is a common first sign of vitiligo. Antibodies against the cytoplasm of malignant melanoma cells are found in the serum of patients with halo naevi. The naevus need only be removed if there is a progressive enlargement, bleeding and irregularities of the pigment within the centre of the naevus.

Tuberous sclerosis The oval macules which look like a thumb print and are tapered at one end, sometimes known as leaf-like (Fig. 72), are present in about 90 per cent of affected babies. They are easier to see using Wood's light (UVA).

Idiopathic guttate hypomelanosis This is characterized by small depigmented, sharply defined, often polygonal macules in light-exposed areas. A symmetrical punctate loss of pigment on the shins and extensor surfaces of the arms is described in young adults from Japan and Brazil.

Post-inflammatory depigmentation This is probably the commonest cause of leucoderma. Pigmented skin retains less pigment when there is accelerated epidermal turnover as in wound repair, eczema, or psoriasis. The lesions are not as white as in vitiligo and they are sometimes known as *pityriasis alba* (Fig. 71). This is in fact a variant of a dry eczema and causes mild hypopigmentation. It may be sharply circumscribed and have a halo of surrounding inflammation. It is usually slightly scaly and there is follicular prominence due to hyperkeratosis. The cheeks and upper arms are most commonly affected and atopic children are the most frequent sufferers.

In some parts of the world discoid lupus erythematosus is a common cause of depigmentation. It is preceded by itching, deep violet erythema of light-exposed skin. Hair loss of the scalp is common. This is usually of scarring type.

References

Bleehan, S. S. and Ebling, F. J. G. (1980). Disorders of skin colour. *Textbook of dermatology*, 3rd edn. (eds. A. Rook, D. S. Wilkinson, and D. J. Ebling), 1377. Blackwell Scientific Publications, Oxford.

Bloch, C. A. (1984). Café au lait spots in colored and Indian children. *S. Afr. Med. J.* **65**, 651–652.

Braverman, I. M. (1970). *Skin signs of systemic disease*, ch. 14. W. B. Saunders, Philadelphia.

Fulk, C. S. (1984). Primary disorders of hyperpigmentation. *J. Am. Acad. Dermatol.* **10**, 1–16.

Lerner, A. B. and Nordlund, J. J. (1978). Vitiligo. What is it? Is it important? *J. Am. med. Assoc.* **239**, 1183–1187.

Nordlund, J. J. and Lerner, A. B. (1979). Vitiligo: its relationship to systemic disease. In *Dermatology update* (ed. S. L. Moschella), 411. Elsevier, New York.

Wasserman, H. P. (1974). *Ethnic pigmentation*, Excerpta Medica, Amsterdam.

Diseases of nails, hair, and sweat glands

Nails and hair adorn. In addition, nails aid the picking up of small objects. The handicap of disease of hair or nails is greatest in those who are most conscious of their contribution to the 'body beautiful'. Beauty is not only in the eyes of the beholder but it is also an image in the mind of the subconscious. Hence most consultations concerning hair are about too much or too little in comparison to the norm for a particular population. Excessive sweating and body odour is also a cause of great distress.

Nails

Nails grow continuously throughout life. Normal fingernails grow at the rate of approximately 1 cm in 3 months and toenails take anything from 9 to 24 months. The nails grow more rapidly in psoriasis and more slowly in cold, ischaemia or severe systemic illness.

Koilonychia is a term for a spoon-shaped depression of the nail plate, sometimes brittle, found in iron deficiency or in over-usage of solvents such as nail varnish remover or detergents. It is also a consequence of repetitive trauma such as vibration, or in the case of toenails, from kicking or walking up a hill pushing a trolley, known as rickshaw boy's nail.

Onycholysis is due to premature separation of the nail plate as seen in psoriasis, infection, thyroid disease, and UVA exposure. Trauma from excessive handwashing or keratolytics are other causes.

Clubbing is an increased angle between the nail fold and nail plate and a spongy matrix which is easily depressed. There is also increased curvature of the nail and swelling of the terminal phalanx (see Section 15).

Onychogryphosis is great horny thickening and curving often due to trauma. Sometimes it is a consequence of ischaemia and neglect.

Pits (Fig. 73) are commonest in any quantity due to psoriasis. Lesser degrees are found in eczema. Fine stippling is seen in alopecia areata and longitudinal pits and thinning are seen in lichen planus.

Ridges or grooves are seen in psoriasis, eczema, and fungus infection. Longitudinal central grooves may be due to habit of picking at the base of the thumb but occasionally it is idiopathic (Fig. 74). White lines are a feature of the genetic dyskeratosis Darier's disease (see Fig. 20).

Transverse ridges result from injury to the nail fold from infection as in paronychia or dermatitis (Fig. 75).

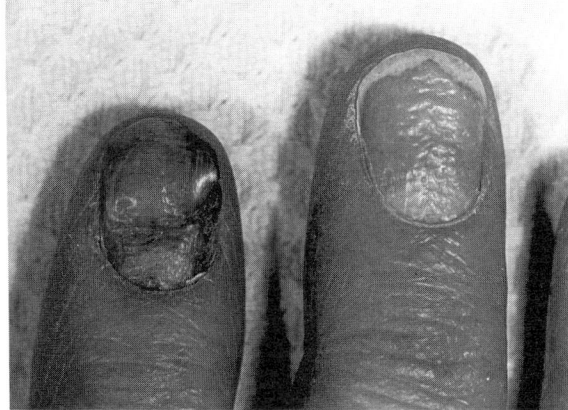

Fig. 73 Pits of the nails are due to very localized accelerations in growth such that the nail keratin is less well knit. In psoriasis such pits are very common.

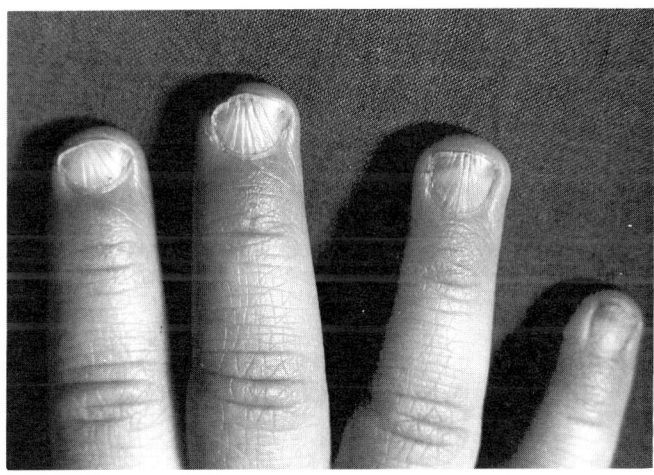

Fig. 74 Longitudinal ridging is usually due to decreased growth and the nails are often thin and poorly made (idiopathic dystrophy).

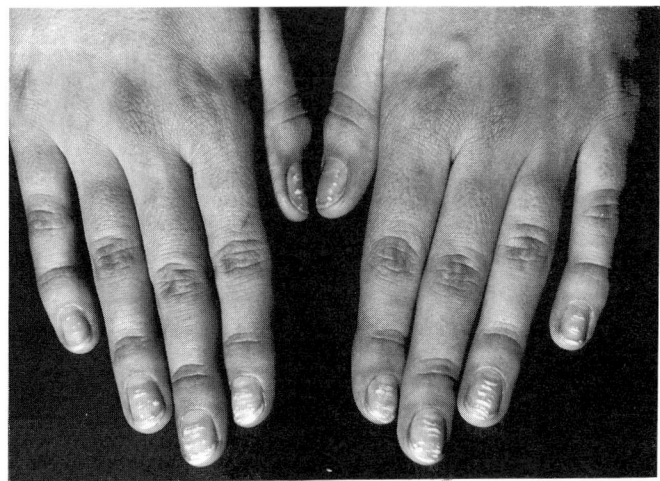

Fig. 75 Transverse white nails, in this case idiopathic, may also indicate arsenical poisoning.

Systemic illness interferes with growth and such furrows are known as Beau's lines.

A common cause of nail deformity producing a longitudinal

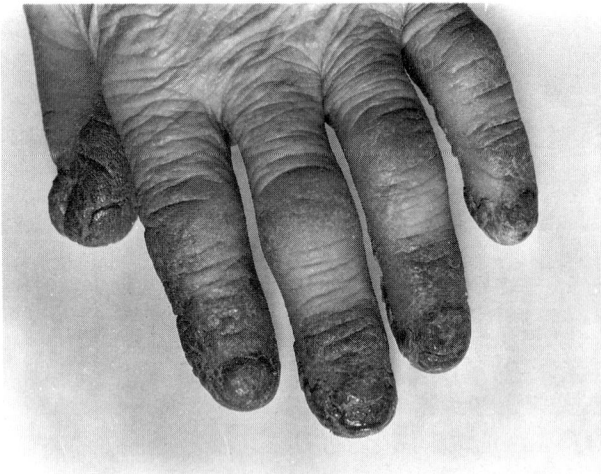

Fig. 76 Severe growth changes of the nail are often a consequence of psoriasis or eczema of the finger tips. The latter may resolve while nail growth disturbance may persist for many months.

Table 21 Colour changes in nails

Colour change	Cause
Blue black	Subungual haematoma, cytoxic drugs, Minocin; pseudomonas infection
	Subungual malignant melanoma
Green	Pseudomonas infection
Brown	Cigarette smoking, potassium permanganate solution, and other dyes
	Chronic renal disease
	Small brown streaks are seen in splinter haemorrhages or thrombi, from trauma, psoriasis, collagen disease, and bacterial endocarditis
	Wider brown streaks are found in pigmented benign naevi; these may be exacerbated by Addison's disease
Yellow nails	Slow or distorted growth may result from ischaemia, psoriasis, and fungus infection. If all nails are affected, this may be due to yellow nail syndrome in which there is increased curvature, thickening, and slow growth associated with defective lymphatics. There may be associated pleural effusions
White nails	Hypoalbuminaemia especially in cirrhosis, sometimes in renal failure or from cytotoxic drugs. Congenital idiopathic whiteness as an autosomal dominant trait is described. Small white spots are of no significance.
	Transverse white spots are seen with arsenic poisoning, but may be idiopathic
Red half moons	Seen in congestive cardiac failure
Blue half moons	Seen in hepatolenticular degeneration or Wilson's disease
Blue nails	Mepacrine

depression is a mucous cyst at the base of the nail. This can be destroyed by cryotherapy or by repeated needling and extrusion of contents over a number of weeks.

Colour changes are listed in Table 21.

Paronychia

This is most commonly due to infection from bacteria and repeated irritation by water and detergents and other agents used by nurses, bar tenders, and bakers. The loss of the natural seal between the nail fold and the nail plate is an important consequence. It is often due to injudicious manicuring. The use of nystatin ointment as a seal applied many times a day before using the hand is an effective therapy, and 3 per cent thymol in chloroform

is a broad spectrum antiseptic used as a paint in this disorder. This is especially useful for discoloration of the nail from *Pseudomonas pyocyanea* which gives rise to a black or green nail. Keeping the hands dry is advisable but difficult to enforce.

Tinea unguium

This is commonly asymmetrical and the toe nails are more involved than the finger nails. Differential diagnosis from psoriasis is often difficult but psoriasis prefers the finger nails and usually it affects them symmetrically and it is associated with terminal phalangeal arthritis. Fungus infection always begins distally unlike the secondary distortion of a paronychia which affects the nail in the nail bed. Softening and fragility or thickening are further consequences of fungus infection. Microscopic examination of the nail after prolonged soaking of the clippings in 5–10 per cent potassium hydroxide should reveal mycelia.

Treatment of toe nails is unsatisfactory and should only be embarked upon if the patient complains of the disorder and is prepared to take griseofulvin 500 mg daily for very many months. Local fungal preparations are only rarely effective.

References

Baran, R. and Dawber, R. P. R. (eds) (1984). *Diseases of the nails and their management.* Blackwell Scientific Publications, Oxford.
Samman, P. D. (1986). *The nails in disease,* 4th edn. Heinemann, London.

Hair

There is no doubt that the majority of hair disorders are associated with changes in other organs and a complaint of hair loss should be treated with the same seriousness as a cough. The management of a hair problem is in part that of making a diagnosis but often it is also important to recognize a personality problem.

Up to about 7 months the fetus is covered by long soft hair. This *lanugo* hair is shed into the amniotic fluid and may be observed in premature babies at which stage loss of scalp hair may cause the mother some anxiety. Postnatal hair ranges from short fine *vellus* hair covering most of the body to the long thick terminal hair of scalp and eyebrows. In the adult most hair is of intermediate type and can become coarser when stimulated by local inflammation or by androgens. Suprapubic and axillary hairs are the most easily stimulated, while hair of the beard area and chest requires higher levels of androgen than are normally found in the female. Genetic and racial factors control the response of the hair to androgen.

The hair cycle

The life of a hair varies up to about 3 years. Unlike some species which moult periodically there is little synchrony in the human. Each hair grows at the rate of about 1 cm per month and this is known as the anagen phase. This is followed fairly abruptly by the catagen stage of involution in which the end of the hair forms a club and is shed. This is followed by telogen which is known as the resting stage during which there is no activity. The number of hairs which are shed from the scalp each day ranges from about 50–300. There are some 300 000 hairs on the scalp and 1 per cent are in catagen at any one time and the rest are completing their 3-year cycle. When there is a systemic illness or 'shock' or a physiological state such as pregnancy, many of the older hairs may pass into catagen earlier so that a partial moult of longer hairs may occur, often a few weeks later. This is known as telogen effluvium. The hair recovers completely within a few months. Cytotoxic drugs, especially cyclophosphamide, inhibit hair growth so that hair loss is a common side-effect. The effect of these drugs can be prevented by cooling the scalp with a tightly fitting ice bag for about 20 minutes while such drugs are given intravenously.

Baldness

Baldness, which for obscure reasons is also called alopecia, has many causes. The most important is physiological sexual maturation. This is due to a shortening of the anagen phase and consequently in an increase of the proportion of hairs in telogen. It is androgen dependent. In its mildest form it is represented by bitemporal recession and occurs in 90 per cent of men and about 80 per cent of women. Frontotemporal loss and thinning of the vertex occurs in 25 per cent of white women by the age of 50 and 60 per cent of men at an earlier age. The commonest pattern is that seen in males and less commonly and severely in females. It begins always as frontal recession exposing the temples and is followed variably by gradual thinning of the vertex or the crown. It is age and sex-related; thus both males and females over 80 are commonly bald but males very usually develop baldness early in adult life. A family history of baldness is so common as to make it very likely that there are genetic factors involved. Most important is the influence of testosterone; it is the relative lack of testosterone in young women that accounts for their lessened tendency to develop baldness. Benign baldness of the forehead is associated with normal or slightly raised serum testosterone and a lowering of sex hormone binding globulin. Males castrated before puberty are similarly protected. Hirsuties and baldness go together, so a very hairy chest is a common accompaniment but sexual potency is non-proven. The baldness is initially due to change from terminal to vellus hair but eventually complete follicular atrophy occurs.

Examination for other causes of hair loss

The scalp should be examined for evidence of disease such as scaliness, redness, injury, or scarring with its associated loss of follicles (Fig. 77). Severe seborrhoeic eczema which produces diffuse and excessive dandruff is often associated with thinning. Psoriasis on the other hand tends to leave some scalp unaffected and mostly the hair grows well. In very thick plaques, hair may get broken off or its growth is occasionally inhibited. Lichen planus and discoid lupus erythematosus both destroy the hair follicles and produce respectively a violaceous or red colour as well as scarring. Tinea capitis (see Fig. 18) is a common cause of hair loss in many parts of the world. The acute, painful, boggy, inflammatory swelling of cattle ringworm known as kerion is sometimes mistaken for a bacterial abscess but closer examination would show satellite lesions which are clearly not abscesses. Kerions of the head often heal with scarring and some permanent loss of hair. Equally classic in presentation are groups of children with discoid patches of slightly scaly red areas of broken hairs due to other forms of animal ringworm. Fortunately most adult scalps are resistant to these. It is particularly a problem with children. In many parts of the world *T. violaceum* is responsible in black children, and *M. canis* in white. White scales and scarring in dark heads is often due to favus. In Africa and the Middle East, favus is due to *T. schöenleini*. Infection of the scalp with streptococcus or staphylococcus is common in parts of the world where generalized impetigo is common. The scalp may carry a persistent staphylococcus in persons who scratch or pick at their scalp, sometimes known as 'tycoon scalp'. The rash of secondary syphilis often causes a patchy pattern of hair loss scattered over the scalp like numerous 'glades in a wood'. Loss of eyebrows is a feature of lepromatous leprosy (Fig. 78).

Scalp hair is damaged by a number of cosmetic procedures including prolonged traction, permanent waving, or hot combs which produce burns at the side of the temple area in the negro attempting to straighten the tightly coiled hair. Scalp massage also damages the hair. Vigorous brushing with old or poor quality nylon brushes or strong selenium-containing shampoos are other causes of hair loss. The hair becomes more fragile and weathered and breaks at various lengths. Fragility and breaking of the hair is a feature of genetic diseases causing sulphur or cysteine deficiency in the hair. The scalp too may be damaged by repetitive hair pulling or twisting or even heating so one may see redness, scaling, and perifollicular inflammation. Hair pulling or twisting with subsequent breaking is a common habit in infants and in the mentally subnormal, or occasionally in the psychotic (Fig. 79). It is not

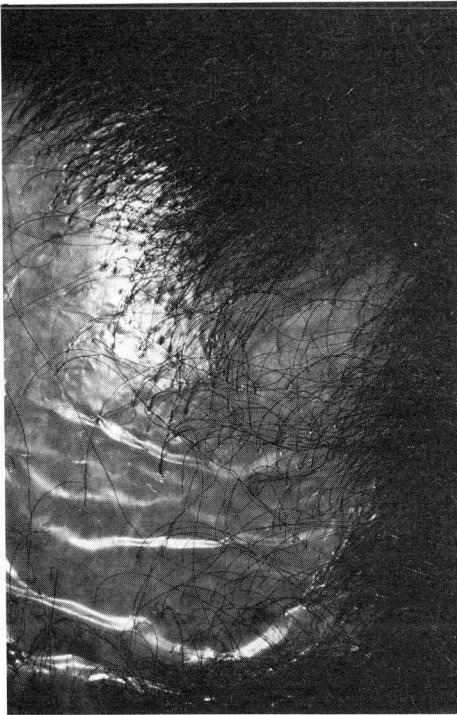

Fig. 77 Scarring is an important prognostic feature because hair loss is irreversible. This pattern of hair loss may be due to a number of chronic inflammatory processes including lichen planus.

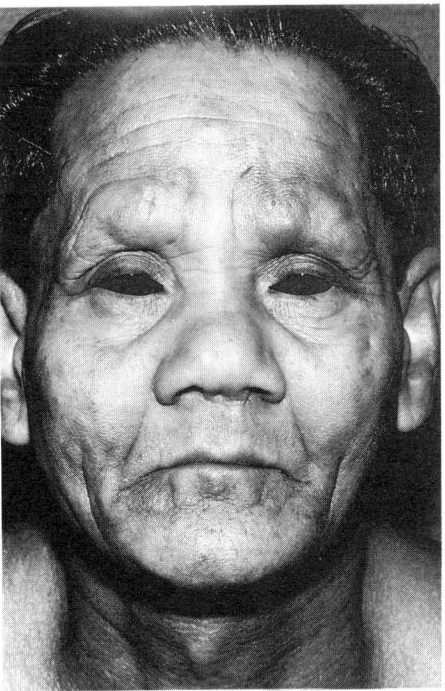

Fig. 78 Loss of eyebrows is a feature of lepromatous leprosy. The skin of the face is thickened but the patient may be unaware of the disease and for this reason the loss of eyebrows could be the first feature about which there is a complaint. Nasal mucosal swelling and erosion is usually obvious.

always consciously done, and if the hair is then eaten there may be little evidence of where the hairs have disappeared to!

Common causes of diffuse hair thinning are iron deficiency,

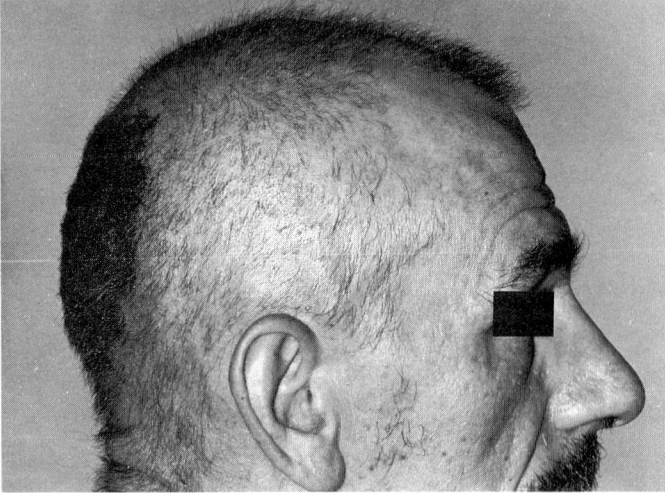

Fig. 79 Trichotillomania or hair pulling gives rise to hair loss and the hair length varies because it is broken irregularly. It is a common habit of children but in the adult it is usually an indication of a personality disorder.

hyperthyroidism, hypopituitarism, severe illness, and drugs such as cyclophosphamide, anticoagulants, and antithyroid drugs, or poisons such as thallium. Temporary thinning is common in those on oral contraceptives.

Rare congenital defects of hair shaft include pili torti which is a flattened and twisted hair reflecting light unevenly. Menkes' syndrome, which is kinky hair associated with retarded mental and physical development, is associated with copper deficiency.

Alopecia areata

The cause is unknown and probably it is multifactorial involving heredity, autoimmunity, stress, infection, and emotional factors in the pathogenesis. It is characterized by localized patches of complete hair loss. In the edges of the lesion there is often a short stubby hair due to abortive hair growth which is similar to an exclamation mark (Fig. 80a). The scalp may be slightly red but scaling is not a feature. The prognosis of a hair growth within 9 months is good for small patches on the vertex in children but hair loss at the temples or occiput is less likely to grow well (Fig. 80b). New growth is often initially white. A strong family history and an association of atopic eczema or recurrent attacks are not encouraging for a good prognosis. There is an association with vitiligo, thyrotoxicosis myxoedema, pernicious anaemia, and it is common in Down's syndrome. There are large numbers of remedies but none more effective than spontaneous remission. Intralesional steroids encourage local regrowth but atrophy of the scalp is an unpredictable side-effect and the hair often falls out again after a few months.

Coalescence of hair loss gives rise to total scalp alopecia or to universal body alopecia.

Dandruff

It is normal to lose small dry scales from the surface of the skin. These tend to be slightly larger in the scalp and show up as white flecks in dark hair or dark clothing. When the skin turns over more rapidly, and in the scalp it normally turns over somewhat faster than in other areas, scales are formed and may even be nucleated. Irritation of the scalp and in particular mild infection with a variety of organisms as in seborrhoeic dermatitis or as with the high rates of turnover in psoriasis results in excessive dandruff or pityriasis capitis. Most cases respond to regular shampooing twice weekly with preparations containing mild antiseptics or tar. Sulphur or mercury have been incorporated to treat infections. Salicylic acid reduces scaling; a common scalp preparation is *lotio acid salicyl et hydrag perchlor*. The imidazoles are also prescribed.

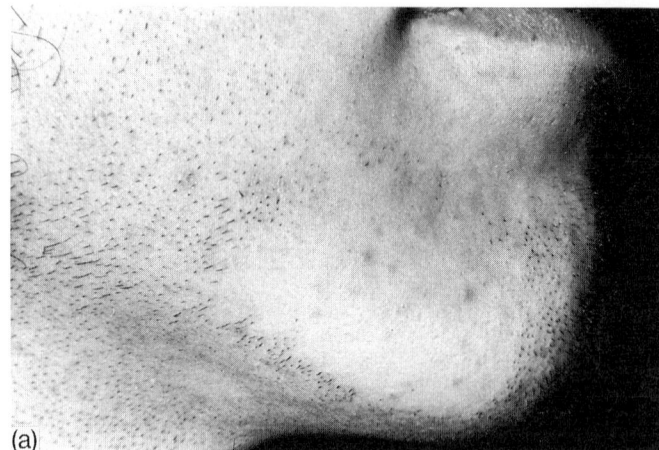

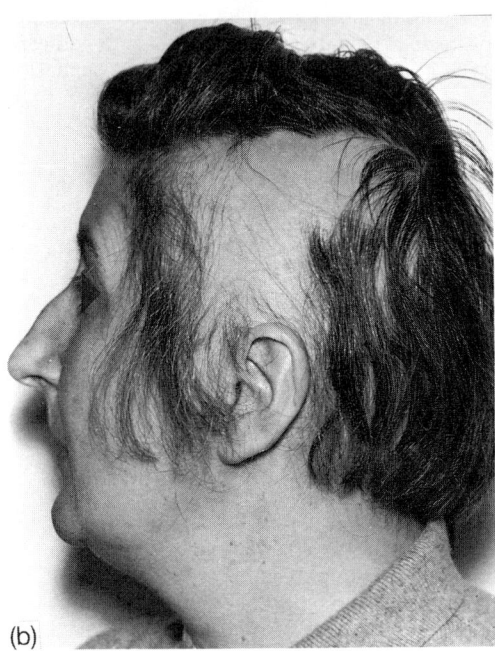

Fig. 80 (a) Alopecia areata is characterized by abortive hair growth and the formation of a short stubby 'exclamation mark' hair at the edge of the area of hair loss. (b) Alopecia of the temple or occiput has a poorer prognosis for regrowth.

The scalp is tolerant to strong steroids and there are several spirit lotions containing anti-inflammatory agents such as Betnovate or Dermovate which are very effective for severe dandruff.

Ingrowing hairs

The tightly coiled hair of the negro frequently has difficulty in clearing the follicle and grows into the epidermis at the mouth of the follicle. Eventually ingrowth into the dermis sets up a foreign body reaction. This is common around the beard area and nape of the neck. Under a hand lens such hairs can be pricked out. Growing a beard often helps to prevent the initial distorted growth pattern.

Wigs and hair transplants

Wigs are made up of either real or artificial hair. The latter have the advantage of being washable and do not lose hair style. However, artificial hair is not as comfortable or as cosmetically satisfactory. For male-pattern baldness hair pieces may suffice.

Hair transplants are the removal of small 'punch' full thickness grafts from the occiput and these are inserted into the bald areas. Fistula formation, scarring, and chronic infection are recorded

Table 22 Hypertrichosis

Malnutrition
Anorexia nervosa
Early
   Dermatomyositis and scleroderma
   Cutaneous porphyria (see Fig. 29)
   Drugs: diazoxide, minoxidil, phenytoin corticosteroids
   Various congenital diseases
   Hypertrichosis lanuginosa either congenital or malignant
Local
   Congenital pigmented naevi
   Spina bifida: faun tail
   Lichen simplex
   Localized chronic inflammation
Endocrine causes of generalized hirsutism
   Sclerocystic ovary syndrome
   Idiopathic
   Cushing's syndrome
   Congenital adrenal hyperplasia
   Androgen-secreting tumours
   Hypothyroidism
   Acromegaly

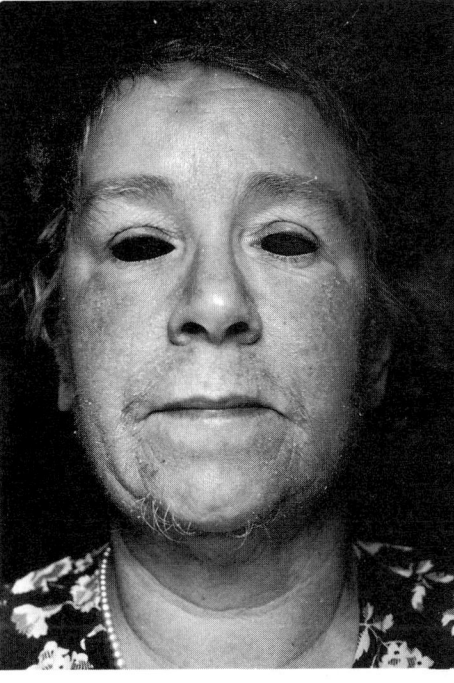

Fig. 81 Many post-menopausal women develop hirsuties due to altered hormonal balance. Nevertheless one should always be aware of other endocrine causes as in this patient who has a pituitary tumour.

complications, but for some persons in the public eye the results are regarded as satisfactory.

Hirsutism

Hirsutism refers to the male pattern of hair growth and baldness is often associated. It should be distinguished from hypertrichosis which is the growth of terminal hair from vellus hair at sites not normally hairy such as the forehead in porphyria (Table 22).

A woman with regular menstruation or normal pregnancy and a family history of hairiness is very unlikely to have endocrine disease. Many dark haired women of India, Wales, and Ireland or of the Mediterranean stock have coarser hair of face, limbs, and trunk than is otherwise observed in Asians or Europeans (see Fig. 14). The Japanese and Chinese are very much less hairy. Many of those who are worried about excess hair are only abnormal because they live amongst persons with an expectation of less hair. Such hirsutism occurs after puberty and can cause great distress in the female and sometimes in the male. After the menopause most women develop coarse hair on the face (Fig. 81). Some normal women may suffer from an enhanced responsiveness of the hair follicles to normal androgen levels in the blood. This is probably due to conversion by the follicle of testosterone into a more active form.

A common cause of hirsutism, also hardly meriting the term disease, is due to the secretion of upper limits of normal amounts of testosterone by the ovary. Such women may suffer from seborrhoea, acne, hidradenitis suppurativa, decreased fertility, and male-pattern baldness.

The adrenal gland produces 75 per cent of plasma testosterone. Hyperplasia or tumours are responsible for Cushing's syndrome and the adrenogenital syndrome. In children pseudohermaphroditism due to male-pattern development of the genitalia in a gonadal female will be a feature. In older women marked hirsutism is usually associated with virilism and failure to menstruate and poor breast development.

Anabolic steroids, anti-oestrogenic drugs, progesterone, and anticonvulsants also cause hirsutism. The polycystic ovary syndrome (Stein–Leventhal) is probably not a single entity and its manifestations vary. Hirsutism is associated with obesity and infertility as well as menstrual disorders. Rarer cause of hirsutism include virilizing tumours of the ovary, gonadal dysgenesis, and Turner's syndrome.

The onset of amenorrhoea, acne, and hirsutism or baldness should merit examination for an enlarged clitoris. This should be followed by plasma testosterone, plasma cortisol, 24-hour urinary

steroid excretion, and an estimate of pituitary size by skull X-ray or scan (Fig. 81).

The development of hypertrichosis or lanugo hair on the face is almost always due to porphyria cutanea tarda or underlying neoplasia.

Treatment

Bleaching with 20 volume hydrogen peroxide makes dark hair on white skin less noticeable. Commercial depilatories are destroyers of hair but not of the hair root. They are highly irritant and many persons find them impossible to use. Various waxes are now available for the legs and arms, some impregnated in gauze which are easy to apply, against the grain, and to pull off with the grain. The abnormally hirsute often require professional electrolysis. The latter is more effective for hairs that have not been repeatedly plucked.

Cyproterone acetate (2 mg daily) is a potent anti-androgen and produces gradual improvement over a period of 6 months to 1 year only if prescribed in the early stages of hair loss. Its long-term effects are not known. It is given as a reversed sequential contraceptive with ethinyloestradiol (50 μg daily).

A combination of prednisone and ethinyloestradiol with progesterone is also helpful. The diameter of the hair is a useful measurement for the assessment of response to therapy. Measurement of plucked hair 1 cm above the root should show thickening within the range 40–120 μm at the end of 3 months and subsequently at 3 monthly intervals.

References

Ginsburg, J. and White, M. C. (1980). Hirsutism and virilism. *Br. med. J.* **i**, 369.

Khun, B. H. (1972). Male pattern alopecia and androgenic hirsutism in females: part 3, definition and aetiology. *J. Am. med. Wom. Assoc.* **27**, 357.

Kvedare, J. C., Gibson, M. and Krusinski, P. A. (1985). Hirsutism: evaluation and treatment. *J. Am. Acad. Dermatol.* **12**, 215–225.

Mitchell, A. J. and Krull, E. A. (1984). Alopecia areata: pathogenesis and treatment. *J. Am. Acad. Dermatol.* **11**, 763–775.

Rook, A. and Dawber, R. P. R. (1982). *Diseases of hair and scalp*. Blackwell Scientific Publications, Oxford.

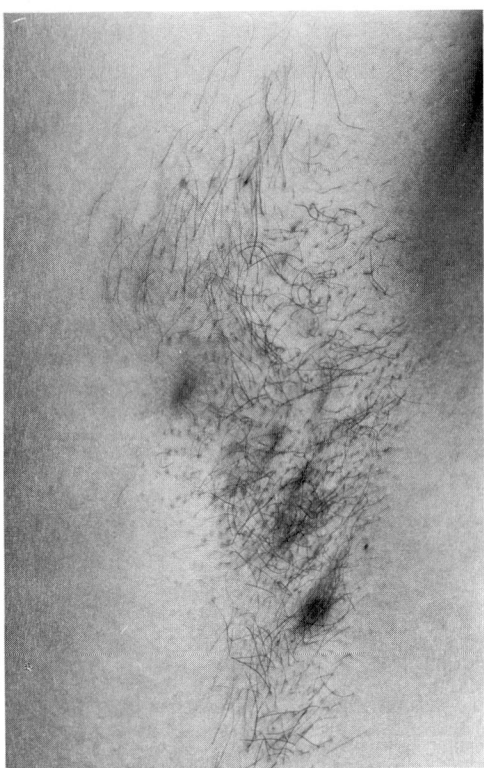

Fig. 82 Axilla showing dusky or violaceous erythema overlying cystic 'blind' boils. The follicular prominent and comedone formation is characteristic of early hydradenitis.

Shuster, S. (1984). The aetiology of dandruff and the mode of action of therapeutic agents. *Br. J. Dermatol.* **111**, 235–242.

Sweating

Apocrine

Apocrine glands occur throughout the skin surface in the embryo but subsequently disappear so that they are found in the adults only in the axillae, areolae, and anogenital region. The secretions are formed by the dissolution of sebaceous gland cells which are discharged in the hair follicles close to the surface of the skin. They are not active until puberty. Bacterial decomposition accounts for body odour and in the animal kingdom the secretions are important for identity and marking out territorial areas. They are also important sexual organs. All such functions are vestigial in man but body odours are sometimes complained of. Washing with soap and water is the first phase of management. Deodorants reduce the bacterial flora. The eating of garlic and betel nuts should be discouraged since these 'perfumes' are excreted in apocrine sweat. Apocrine sweat is sometimes coloured. If staining is severe and uncontrolled by deodorants, then excision of the glands may be necessary. Retention of apocrine sweat and extreme irritation known as Fox–Fordyce disease is similar to prickly heat. Treatment may include use of topical steroids, destruction with cryotherapy, or excision.

Hydradenitis suppurativa

A chronic activity of the apocrine glands in which disturbance of apocrine flow and sometimes secondary infection gives rise to abscesses, sinuses, and scarring especially in the axillae and groin. The age of onset, apocrine gland distribution, high levels of serum testosterone, and the presence of comedones also suggest that an endocrine factor, as in acne vulgaris, is important. The early phase of blind boils (Fig. 82) may be responsive to antiandrogens as for hirsuties (see above). Cryosurgery is helpful; courses of antibiotics such as tetracycline three times daily for several weeks are worth

Table 23 Causes of hyperhidrosis

Hot weather or room
Exercise
Fever: infection or pyrogen
Fear, anxiety, lie detectors
Thyrotoxicosis, acromcgaly, diabetes mellitus
Lymphoma
Cancer
Hypoglycaemia; alcohol intoxication
Nausea
Gustatory
Neurological lesions of the sympathetic nervous system, cortex, basal ganglia, or spinal cord

trying, but wide surgical excision and grafting is often necessary. When there are acute exacerbations steroids by mouth may control the eruption. Overuse of deodorants has been blamed for alterations in bacterial flora.

References

Mortimer, P. S., Dawber, R. P. R., Gales, M. and Moore, R. (1985). Mediation of hidradenitis suppurativa by androgens. *Br. med. J.* **292**, 245–248.

Eccrine sweating

Humans have about 3 to 4 million sweat glands, equivalent in weight to one kidney. They can secrete at a maximum rate of 2–3 litres per hour. The secretory coil produces a plasma-like fluid. Sodium is reabsorbed in the sweat duct.

While eccrine sweat glands occur in all areas, those of the hands, feet, axillae, and face frequently sweat profusely in the absence of general sweating. Man relies on evaporation rather than insulation or panting for protection against a hot environment. Generalized sweating occurs when the body temperature rises and it is a feature of fever as well as thermoregulation in a warm climate, or when the metabolic rate is increased, as in exercise or thyrotoxicosis.

Eccrine sweat glands are largely innervated by unique postganglionic sympathetic fibres that release acetylcholine at the neuroglandular junction. The control centre is in the hypothalamus. It is important to consider whether the sweating is appropriate for the degree of stimulus (Table 23).

Emotional or anxiety-induced sweating is commonly inappropriate for the degree of anxiety. Many teenagers complain of sweating of the hands and feet and the smell which results from bacterial breakdown of skin and clothing. The fear of being unwelcome increases the anxiety and subsequent sweating. It may summate with thermoregulatory sweating and therefore be worse in hot weather or at a dance. Winter clothing is often more troublesome than the loose garments of summer. Sweating of the hands and feet occurs with acrocyanosis and with some forms of keratoderma.

Segmental, unilateral sweatings is often due to irritative lesions of the spine and requires a neurological opinion.

Excessive sweating contributes to tinea pedis and to eczema from footwear.

Treatment of hyperhidrosis

The total daily water loss at rest is about 500 ml but the hyperhidrotic may increase the loss to 12 litres per day or even 3 litres in the first hour. This is faster than it is possible to drink. For this reason it is important to be aware of fluid loss and to restore water and salt in those who are sweating exceptionally.

A sympathetic listener is helpful, as is simple advice on hygiene, washing, keeping cool, and appropriate clothing. The avoidance of obesity; and relaxation if self-conscious are all basic points of management. Clothing such as cotton is more appropriate than non-absorbent fibres, and many shoes are now made with linings which prevent absorption and keep the foot and sock wet. Frequent changes of socks prevents bacterial overgrowth, and readjustment of footwear and the wearing of leather shoes or sandals reduces discomfort. Tranquillizers are sometimes helpful and propantheline 15 mg every few hours may be helpful or can be reserved for a social occasion; abolition of sweating carries a risk of hyperthermia.

Local therapy

A specific inhibitor of sweating is 20 per cent aluminium chloride hexahydrate in absolute alcohol when it is applied as a saturated solution to the skin. It acts by an effect on the cells at the mouth of the sweat duct. The skin should be as dry as possible and the patient as tranquil as possible since dilution of the saturated solution by sweat causes it to become irritant. It is probably most effective for the axillae when applied at night and maintenance therapy need be only once or twice weekly.

Application of 3 per cent formalin soaks to the soles of the feet for 10 minutes or topical glutaraldehyde 10 per cent solution buffered to pH 7.5 are sometimes helpful. Poldine methylsulphate 3–4 per cent in alcohol is another topical agent used on the feet.

Systemic anticholinergic drugs such as propantheline 15 mg three times daily controls sweating in some patients but dry mouth and blurred vision are side-effects which prove too troublesome for others.

Iontophoresis is a method involving a direct current of low voltage and is a somewhat tedious method of reducing sweating. Tap water with or without drugs such as glycopyronium bromide may be used. It is not suitable for hands. Injury to the innervation or to the sweat glands themselves is the aim of several techniques for the management of axillary hyperhidrosis. Freezing with liquid nitrogen, if rigorous enough to produce swelling and blistering, destroys the sweat glands, but the necrosis in the axillae is sometimes quite severe. Undercutting with a scalpel causes denervation since only the glands in the apex of the axillae are responsible for most of the sweating. These can also be removed by snipping away the sweat coils on the undersurface of the skin. Excision of an eclipse of skin 4 × 1.5 cm is also effective after mapping the area with 1 per cent iodine in alcohol followed by starch powder. Excision followed by a 'Z' plasty to avoid a linear scar contraction is also recommended. The transverse arm of the Z lies in the apex of the axillae. Cervical lumbar sympathectomy reduces hyperhidrosis of the hands and feet but the risks and irreversibility of the operation have to be weighed against the expected spontaneous resolution of the problem especially in the teenager.

Hyperhidrosis of the feet is often associated with redness or acrocyanosis and the skin becomes macerated giving rise to a whitening of the keratin as well as to bacterial contamination which produces pits known as pitted keratolysis.

The multiple asymptomatic pits in the keratin have been blamed variously on corynebacteria, streptomyces, and the organism *Dermatophylus congolensis*. It is common in barefoot persons in the rainy season. The treatment is to dry the feet. Antibacterial remedies are not necessary.

Hypohidrosis

This occurs in the newborn and in premature children in the first month of life and it is seen also in infants from occlusion of the sweat ducts especially in the flexures of the folds of the skin of the neck. It may result also from exfoliative dermatitis or erythroderma and it is a feature of *hypohidrotic ectodermal dysplasia* which is a sex-linked recessive disorder. Such patients are usually male and are susceptible to heat stroke and therefore early diagnosis of the affected baby in a hot climate is important. The hair is sparse, dry, fine, and short. The scalp and eyelashes are particularly affected. The skin is smooth and finely wrinkled. The nose is sunken and the teeth conical (Fig. 83). Absence of sweating causes loss of skin moisturization and impaired grip. Examination

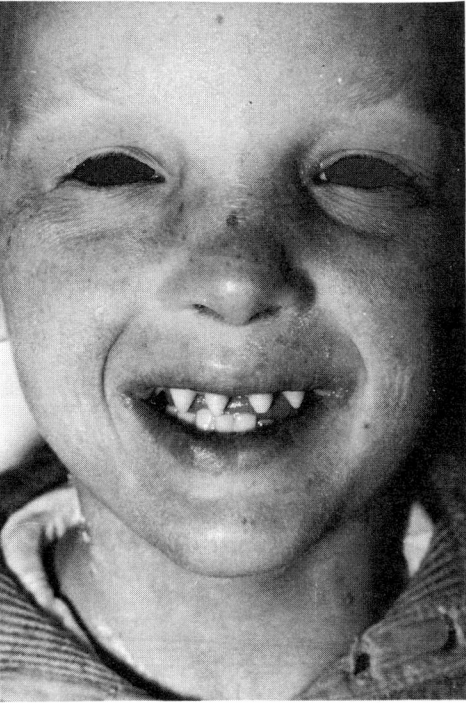

Fig. 83 Conical teeth, sparse eyelashes, and a sunken nose are clues to hyperthermia. This young boy is affected by absence of sweat glands known as hypohidrotic ectodermal dysplasia.

of the palmar surface of the fingers with a magnifying lens will show the absence of duct orifices.

Miliaria

Miliaria crystallina is a superficial obstruction to sweat glands producing clear vesicles. This may occur when the sweat produced by the gland exceeds the ability of the duct to absorb it. It is commonly seen with high fever. Deeper obstruction gives rise to red, itchy papules known as prickly heat. It affects one in three persons exposed to hot climates and while it sometimes begins within a few days of arrival in such a climate it is commonly a problem 2–6 months later. Occlusion of the skin by impermeable clothing aggravates it; bacteria may play some part in its generation as well as in one complication, namely staphylococcal abscesses. It is a contributory factor to extreme thermal stress in the unacclimatized. This is also a feature of workers in hot industries with furnaces or in those underground in mines. Relief from sweating even for a few hours is essential. Loose, non-occlusive clothing and exposure of the skin folds as much as possible is beneficial. Vitamin C 1 g daily was advocated by dermatologists in the British Army in Malaysia. It is important to realize that severe hypohidrosis of the trunk and limbs may be missed as a cause of asthenia if the face is sweating. Shake lotions of calamine powder promote cooling by increasing surface area. Localized loss of sweating may be due to tuberculoid leprosy, syringomyelia, and diabetes mellitus.

Reference

Champion, R. H. (1980). Disorders of sweat glands. In *Textbook of dermatology*, 3rd edn. (eds A. Rook, D. S. Wilkinson, and E. J. G. Ebling), pp. 1675–1689. Blackwell Scientific Publications, Oxford.

Skin disorders affecting the genitalia

A diagnosis of disorders affecting the genitalia cannot be made without looking. Natural shyness on the part of the patient or lack of zeal on the part of the doctor are common. Racial and religious grounds for incomplete examination must be overcome by appropriate selection of the examiner and chaperoning as well as an interpreter.

It may be inappropriate to delve into the sexual, gynaecological, or medical history and so initial questioning may be limited until an examination has indicated the nature of the disease. A contact dermatitis may require the most detailed and searching questioning.

Many skin conditions of the vulva or penis can be best diagnosed by examining the rest of the skin. For example the knees, scalp, and elbows in psoriasis, the front of the wrists and shins in lichen planus, the mouth in pemphigus, or the neck, breasts, or wrists in lichen sclerosis et atrophicus.

Infections

Infections are commonly transmitted by sexual intercourse and tend to be associated with vaginal or urinary meatal symptoms. The sexual partner will require treatment. However, in the female some infections may be asymptomatic and this is so with primary chancre, gonorrhoea, chlamydial infections, or trichomoniasis. Where infection is suspected, swabs for culture should be taken from the cervix, urethra, and rectum.

The pubic region is commonly affected by nits and crablice and viral molluscum contagiosum causes smooth pearly umbilicated papules (see Fig. 131).

Warts

Genital warts commonly begin at the introitus and extend forewards or backwards as filiform pink fleshy lesions often coalescing into velvety or papilliferous masses. They must be distinguished from the moist flat lesions of syphilis.

Perianal warts are commonly confined to that site. Warts are often transmitted by sexual intercourse and other infectious diseases such as syphilis may be masked. Outlying, more scattered warts on the buttocks, shaft of penis, scrotum, or in the genitocrural folds are less commonly venereal as are genital warts in infancy or childhood.

Natural immunity to the wart virus is the only certain cure. The easiest therapy is podophyllin 15–20 per cent solution in compound tincture of benzoin or spirit (see page 20.86). This should be applied to the warts and, depending on the degree of soreness that results in some persons, may be washed off after a few hours. Absorption in the pregnant is recorded as a cause of abortion. An alternative therapy if available is cryotherapy. Local or general anaesthetics followed by curettage and cautery or dissection after lifting up of the wart on a bleb of saline is also effective.

Those who have multiple partners should be examined for other sexually transmitted diseases. Women should have cervical smears at regular intervals because of the increased risk of cervical cancer. Wart destruction for cosmetic reasons is the principal role of the dermatologist.

Candidiasis

Pregnancy, diabetes mellitus, and antibiotics predispose to this infection although a mild degree of non-pathogenic infection is common. White plaques or more diffuse soreness with redness of the vulva of glans penis are common. As part of an intertrigo there is a red flexural rash with a fringe of vesicles, scales, or pustules and more peripheral scattering of satellite lesions. The condition responds to nystatin ointment but clearance of the lower bowel by oral nystatin and treatment of the sexual partner is often necessary. There are now several other effective anticandida agents (see Section 5).

Herpes simplex

Genital infections due to herpes simplex sometimes spread to the adjacent thigh and buttocks. The infection is commonly a recurrent problem unlike herpes zoster. The latter may cause confusion but it is clearly unilateral. Specific treatment is unsatisfactory but

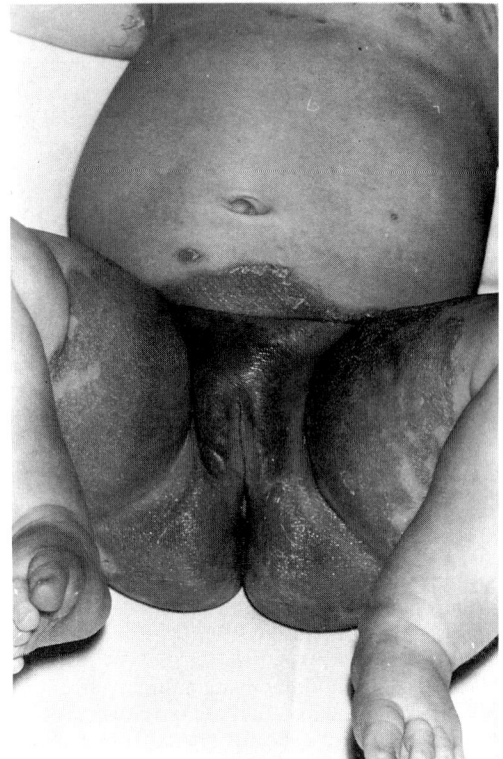

Fig. 84 Flexural nappy rash with involvement of perineum deep into the body folds suggestive of infection, or seborrhoeic eczema.

analgesics and control of secondary infection with antiseptic washes is helpful. Idoxuridine 5 per cent in dimethyl sulphoxide is painful to apply but it is especially useful for aborting recurrences where these are frequent and predictable. Where recurrences are associated with a prior rise in temperature aspirin may be tried to abort the fever as at ovulation or from repeated and recurrent infection (see page 20.72). Oral Acyclovir prevents recurrences only while taking the drug. There are anxieties about viral resistance, long-term side-effects, and rebound infections when the drug is discontinued.

Nappy eruptions

These are inevitable in the infant but vary in their severity and causation. Urine and faeces can cause maceration and irritation especially if left in contact with the skin for several hours so that bacteria and candida have an opportunity to provide ammonia and proteases. The distribution is more nearly that of contact with the nappy so that the genitocrural folds may be spared. The scrotum and labia are often the principally affected site and a variety of irritants produce sharply defined blisters or ulcers. Contact friction with elastic or plastic pants causes well defined linear marks. In the infant red scaly or sore skin in the genitocrural folds is due to primary skin disease such as seborrhoeic eczema or due to secondary bacterial and candida infection (Figs 84 and 85).

All rashes benefit from bathing and frequent changes of nappy. Soap substitutes such as emulsifying ointments or other greases can be used for cleansing the affected areas. The application of an antiseptic with an anticandida agent like nystatin or miconazole and an antipruritic agent such as hydrocortisone considerably shorten the course of the rash but spontaneous remission is usual. The commonly used ointments are timodine or vioform and hydrocortisone. Severe candida infections may require oral ketoconazole if nystatin is unsuccessful.

Children whose families are known to suffer from atopy may present for the first time with red scaly irritated skin in the distribution of the nappy area which is often very persistent and

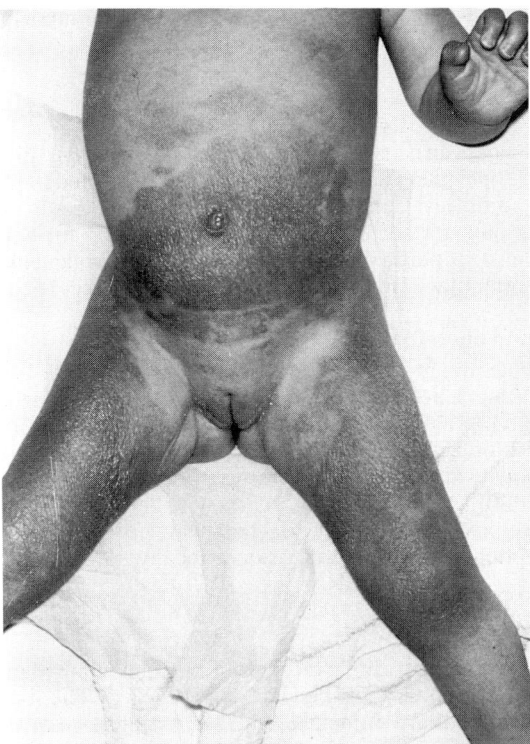

Fig. 85 Sparing of flexures suggests contact with a wet nappy.

Table 24 Causes of contact dermatitis affecting the genitalia

Antiseptics
Fungicides
Ethylene diamine (usually in Triadcortil)
Neomycin
Rubber dermatitis (condoms)
Hexachlorophane
Allergens carried on hands (usually also affect eyelids)
Perfumes, antiseptics in soaps and sprays
Wood dusts, oils, fibreglass; irritants according to occupation

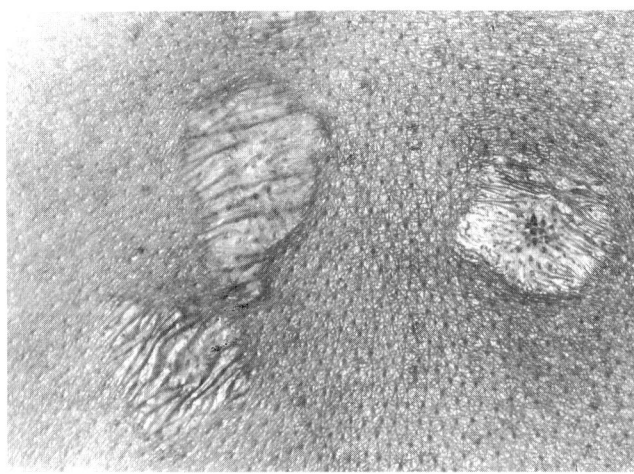

Fig. 86 Lichen sclerosis causes tissue paper-like crinkling or atrophy of the skin. The border is often violaceous but the centre of the lesion is white.

requires much protective grease and sparingly applied steroid creams.

Diseases that are rare but life-threatening include three that present in the nappy area namely, Letterer–Siwe, acrodermatitis enteropathica, and congenital syphilis. Benign seborrhoeic dermatitis often affects the scalp, axillae, and neck as well as in the nappy area. The child is not usually greatly worried by the rash.

Adult intertrigo

Obesity and sweating predispose to mixed irritation and infection in the occluded skin under the breast, axillae, and groins. The affected area is moist, red, fissured, and malodorous. Attempts at keeping the site dry and free of excessive infection have been improved by preparations such as miconazole and hydrocortisone, and Zeosorb powder acting as a drying agent without too much caking. Washing and gentle drying is the most important therapy. Blind boils and comedones are likely to be due to hidradenitis suppurativa.

Psoriasis in the flexures is usually well defined, bright red and, unlike at other sites, is non-scaly. It is worth treating initially for three days with a strong steroid because this sometimes clears the psoriasis. More often the lesions persist and strong steroids are then harmful since they cause so much atrophy. Hydrocortisone can be used but it is only mildly effective. It is important to protect the skin from excessive infection by regular washing.

Dermatitis of the genitalia is commonly due to contact with the agents listed in Table 24. Some to these are added to the bath and inadequately mixed with the water. There may be a considerable immediate contact swelling from certain deodorant sprays. Infection of mixed type may contribute to the problem. Persistent pruritus and scratching is a very common disorder and produces thickening of the skin and a range of colours from white fissured areas to pigmented and violaceous plaques.

In uncircumcized adult males a persistent reddish brown, somewhat fixed balanitis is heavily infiltrated with plasma cells. This benign condition, known as Zoon's balanitis, is cured by circumcision.

Leucoplakia versus atrophy

This is often confusing and it is possible for the skin of the genitalia to be thinned but nevertheless to be covered by a thickened scale. This is so in lichen sclerosis et atrophicus, but close observation and palpation of the skin always indicates its thinness. Thickened plaques of lichen simplex or leucoplakia are composed of a greatly hypertrophied epidermis and usually thickening of the underlying dermis as well. When in doubt, a biopsy should be performed.

Leucoplakia and lichen sclerosis may coexist in as many as 24 per cent of patients. Histologically lichen sclerosis et atrophicus is characterized by an extremely thin epidermis with a thickened scale and an acellular homogenized upper dermis.

Although lichen sclerosis et atrophicus, especially when damaged by scratching, may develop a squamous epithelioma, there is no advantage nor relief of discomfort by prospective vulvectomy. In the case of leucoplakia, vulvectomy is usually advocated as there is a much greater chance of the development of a squamous epithelioma. However, since the skin is predisposed to lichen sclerosis in areas well beyond the genitocrural folds, simple vulvectomy is not a satisfactory treatment for lichen sclerosis itself. The lesion of lichen sclerosis is well defined (Fig. 86), white, but may have a violaceous border and small haemorrhagic blisters are common. The perianal areas are always involved especially in children (Fig. 87). Intractable itching, burning, or soreness of the perineum or genitalia is unfortunately common. In young women it usually slowly improves; in older persons it persists. Attention to hygiene is important as is exclusion of mixed infections or contact dermatitis. Rarely perineal discomfort and eczema may be due to vitamin B_2 deficiency.

Well defined asymmetric plaques of red pigmented skin should be biopsied to exclude intraepidermal carcinoma to which this site is predisposed.

The term Kraurosis vulvae is now obsolete since it does not dif-

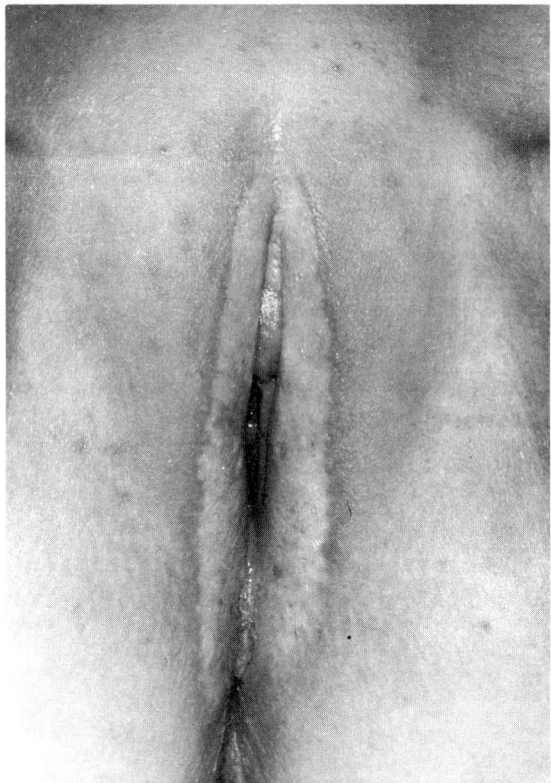

Fig. 87 Lichen sclerosis of the vulva in a child; tends to clear at puberty. In the elderly it is a persistent cause of irritation.

ferentiate senile atrophy from the now well recognized lichen sclerosis.

References

Ridley C. M. (1975). The vulva. In *Major problems in dermatology* (ed. A. Rook), p. 299. Lloyd Luke, London.

Urticaria

Urticaria is a transient swelling and/or flushing of the skin. The underlying vasodilatation and accumulation of tissue fluid in the dermis is due to a succession of mediators of inflammation acting mainly on the small blood vessels. The time taken to bring their effects under control varies and thus the inflammatory response varies from the very transient to more persistent inflammation overlapping with vasculitis.

The knowledge that histamine plays a part in immediate type (anaphylactic) hypersensitivity has caused the widespread misconception that all urticaria must be allergic. A non-immunological pharmacological explanation is more likely in most cases.

Immunology

Allergens of the type commonly incriminated in sufferers from atopic disease are bound to IgE antibodies attached to the surface of the mast cells or basophils whence various mediators are released including histamine, serotonin, and slow-reacting substance (leucotriene) of anaphylaxis. Allergens causing this include egg white, cows' milk, house dust, dandruff, feathers, and tomatoes. It is commonly of contact type affecting the lips during eating or some other parts of the skin when in contact with animals or house dust. Transfusion reactions and some drug rashes are due to complement fixing antibodies attached to blood cells.

The urticaria of serum sickness, penicillin reactions, the acute illness of systemic lupus erythematosus, and many infectious dis-eases are in part due to immune complexes of immunoglobulins, and allergen with complement activation.

Complement activation

While complement is activated by immunological reactions, it is also activated enzymatically by proteases such as plasmin when there are insufficient natural inhibitors of this mediator in the serum and tissues. Congenital or acquired deficiencies in inhibitor levels account for some forms of angioedema and for hereditary angioedema in particular. The activation of complement by the alternative pathway may explain some non-familial cases.

Histamine liberators

Some drugs and foods release histamine from mast cells or at least make such release more likely by inhibiting controlling factors. Inhibition of prostaglandin activity may be one such mechanism. Examples of mast cell stimulators are morphine, codeine, thiamine, polymyxin, and D-tubocurarine. Bee venom, strawberries, and shellfish as well as aspirin, salicylates, benzoates, and tartrazine are enhancers of an urticarial tendency, bringing it to the fore in susceptible subjects as well as occasionally initiating the eruption.

Genetic factors

Familial urticaria is a well recognized phenomenon. Many large families of hereditary angioedema are recorded. The autosomal dominant inheritance is mediated through an absence of C_1 esterase inhibitor. Familial cold urticaria is another autosomal dominant disease described in several families in the USA and others have been described in France and Holland. A low level of chymotrypsin inhibitors was detected in one family. As in atopic eczema studies of HLA antigen have not been very rewarding. BW35 has been associated with acute ordinary urticaria.

Candidiasis has been incriminated in careful studies though it is not so important a factor in the experience of the majority of practitioners.

Types of urticaria

There is variation in the number, size, and depth of weal as well as of the sensation experienced by the patient. The degree of the persistence of the lesion varies. Such features make up named constellations of physical signs.

Contact urticaria

This is a weal and flare reaction occurring for 20–40 minutes after application to the skin of a number of agents listed in Table 15. Some may be IgE mediated such as animal dander, saliva or seminal fluid but most are probably non-immunological as with the nettle or jelly fish sting, or the solar or aquagenic varieties of urticaria. Often there is a consequent or associated dermatitis as in atopic eczema. Many of the ointments used for dermatitis contain bases such as sorbic acid or polyethylene glycol which cause an immediate stinging and slight swelling.

Cholinergic urticaria

This is characterized by numerous, superficial, small swellings which sting, smart, or itch and are surrounded by a blush lasting a few minutes only (Fig. 88). Probably it is mediated by an increase of receptors for acetylcholine from dorsal root nerve endings. The commonest pattern is found in adolescents and young adults and, like blushing, it is brought on by emotion, exercise or hot baths.

Heat urticaria

This is a rare local response to heat in which histamine is released or complement is activated.

Angio-oedema

This is characterized by a few, deep large swellings which may be tender and often itch, sometimes preceded by redness, lasting

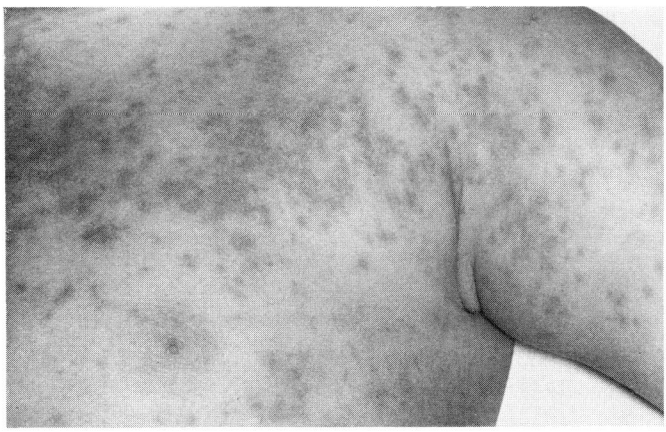

Fig. 88 Cholinergic urticaria is like blushing brought on by emotion, exercise, or heat. It is transient, lasting no more than about 15 minutes and may be associated with small superficial weals with a prominent flush. These tend to sting rather than itch.

several hours or even days. Proteases such as complement, plasmin and kinins are incriminated.

Ordinary urticaria or hives

This is characterized by numerous weals of all sizes, and varying degrees of pallor or redness, which itch and last for one or more hours, but not usually more than a day. Successive lesions may account for long illness. Chronic urticaria is arbitrarily defined as continuous or recurrent lesions of more than 3 months' duration. Histamine is the principal mediator. Current evidence supports the view that skin blood vessels have both H_1 and H_2 receptors.

Time of onset

Cholinergic urticaria is like a blush and develops abruptly and instantaneously within minutes of the triggering event. Ordinary urticaria also develops within minutes of the release of the mediator but not all mediators are released instantaneously. Thus foods and certain allergens or drugs such as aspirin have to be digested and absorbed. Ordinary urticaria is often difficult to relate to events in the life of the patient for this reason. Delayed onset is a well recognized phenomenon of some of the physical urticarias. Thus delayed dermographism is the development of redness and slight wealing several hours after scratching the skin. Delayed pressure urticaria is a tender swelling 2–12 hours after localized pressure injury to the skin. It is possible that the insult localizes noxious agents such as soluble immune complexes or that mechanisms such as transient ischaemia and release of proteases bring to light homeostatic defects such as deficiency of inhibitors of complement or other proteases.

Physical urticaria

Regardless of the exact mediators released by the injury of the skin there are several urticarial eruptions determined only by specific physical insults. These include sunlight, cold, heat, pressure, scratch, or stretch.

Solar urticaria is uncommon. A weal develops within 30 s to 3 min exposure to the sun. Tolerance may develop in sites habitually exposed such as the hands and feet. It is important to recognize it by its history and examination and the differential diagnosis of porphyria, lupus erythematosus, or photosensitivity following drug ingestion has to be considered. In these the urticaria is more persistent, and because the longer, more penetrating ultraviolet rays are responsible, it can occur even on a cloudy day or when the skin is protected from glass, clothing, or sunscreens.

Familial cold urticaria is an autosomal dominant disease in which the rash develops up to several hours after cold exposure from, for example, cold winds, and it usually presents in infancy. Fever and joint pains accompany the rash and there is a leucocyto-

sis. Low levels of a chymotrypsin inhibitor have been demonstrated. It may not be induced by the application of ice to the skin.

Acquired cold urticaria occurs within a few minutes of plunging into cold water or after applying ice to the skin. Mast cells are degranulated and it is one cause of sudden death in young people.

Papular urticaria

This is the only form of urticaria to have a persistent epidermal component. Most often this is due to insect bites and the epidermis is either damaged directly or by mediators in the upper dermis which evoke an eczematous response so that oedema of the epidermis and a proliferative repair effect results in a typical itchy and persistent papule. Such lesions are usually excoriated whereas most urticarias are not deeply scratched but merely rubbed. They often blister (see Fig. 98).

Scaling is not a feature of urticaria and while acute dermatitis and some erythema initially appears to be urticarial the development of scaling immediately excludes such a diagnosis.

The distribution of the rash

Cholinergic urticaria favours the head and upper trunk. Angiooedema most commonly involves mucocutaneous junctions such as the lips, eyes, and penis. The physical urticarias clearly relate to sites of exposure. Thus solar urticaria affects the face and the dorsum of the hands, or if tolerance is developed, it occurs at such sites that are exposed for the first time during the summer. Pressure urticaria favours the soles of the feet when walking or digging, or the backs of the thighs or lumbar region when sitting.

Bizarre patterns

Urticaria evolving and resolving inevitably exhibits changing morphology. The redness of the vasodilatation merges with the veiling pallor of the oedema. Healing in the centre and peripheral spread often produces bizarre gyrate or circinate and serpiginous patterns but they are transient and never scaly, unlike similar patterns in the erythemas or epidermal diseases such as psoriasis.

Investigations

A history is the most effective investigation of urticaria. Intradermal injection of mecholyl (10 μg/0.5 ml saline) reproduces the lesions of cholinergic urticaria. Intradermal histamine 1 μg in 0.1 ml saline produces a weal which should disappear within 1 hour. This disappearance is delayed in pressure urticaria and in immune complex disease. The localization of a noxious agent results in a persistent lesion. In practice, avoidance of cause can be advised only if this is recognized after taking a history and examining the patient. The two most helpful investigations are a full blood count and blood sedimentation rate. An eosinophilia should alert one to parasites such as microfilaria or trichiniasis, and a raised blood sedimentation is due to a systemic illness such as sepsis, malignancy, or 'collagen' disease.

Rubbing or scratching of the skin with the fingernail produces a weal and flare in the dermographic within 2 min.

A weight of 4–6 kg hung for 10 minutes over the shoulder with a bandage or belt, causing a tender swelling 2–8 hours later reveals delayed pressure urticaria. A biopsy at this stage for immunofluorescence may confirm localization of immune complexes. The white count at the time of the biopsy may show neutrophilia especially if there is accompanying fever. Absence of C1 esterase inhibitor in the serum should be looked for in patients with angiooedema especially if initiated by minor surgery, associated with abdominal pains, and having other members of the family affected. Complement levels are not a reliable guide to the participation of proteases and hardly influence the management of urticaria.

Chronic urticaria is a known symptom of filariasis and strongyloidosis, but in ascariasis and enterobiasis it occurs if anything more often in controls. Urticaria is such a difficult disease to assess that possible aetiological factors such as parasitic disease are worth treating in their own right rather than in the expectation of resolution of the eruption.

About 25 per cent of cases of acute hepatitis B present with urticaria.

Foci of infection as a cause of urticaria are statistically difficult to support but dental and sinus infections continue to be described as aetiological factors based on impressive case histories.

Bleeding time and thrombo test

The urticarial reponse to food and drugs where the cause is known can be shown to be correlated with a prolonged bleeding time and a fall in the platelet count. This happens within 1–2 hours of the ingestion of the suspected agent.

Bee stings

The stinging bee injects histamine, serotonin, acetylcholine, and kinins. In addition there are proteins to which the subject becomes allergic and these include phospholipase A and hyaluronidase. IgE is responsible for the immediate hypersensitivity. Symptoms include pain and swelling, pruritus, urticaria, faintness, asthma, vomiting, and diarrhoea. Cardiac arrhythmia is more likely in the elderly. The generalized reaction is preceded by a pulsating feeling in the ears, tightness in the throat, substernal pain, and fear. Acute anxiety causing hyperventilation or coronary thrombosis should be thought of. Death is actually exceedingly rare. Serum sickness or later joint pains and fever are described as well as vasculitis and haematuria. Emergency treatment is 0.5 ml of 1/1000 solution of adrenaline injected deeply subcutaneously and repeated in 10 minutes. Antihistamines and corticosteroids aid recovery (see also page 6.81). The value of desensitization versus its morbidity is not certain.

When should urticaria be taken more seriously?

Urticaria is life threatening when it is part of anaphylaxis, when angio-oedema involves the upper respiratory tract, or when it is part of the systemic immune complex disease and is associated with more dire pathology such as meningococcal septicaemia or lupus erythematosus. The latter type of urticaria is recognized by its more persistent lesion lasting at least 1–2 days and often tender and often ultimately purpuric. It should be remembered that all acute urticaria may be very widespread and be accompanied by joint pains, stomach aches, and fever. However, if the individual lesion lasts for only a few hours it is less likely to be due to a noxious circulating trigger such as immune complex or infective organisms.

Management

Removal of the known physical factor and the known trigger is helpful, but in the majority of cases of chronic urticaria in the adult no cause is found. Food, medicines, and infectious or parasitic diseases are the commonest suspected factors, but in Europe and the USA physical urticaria accounts for more than half of the patients in some series. Cold, heat, and solar urticaria often respond to the induction of tolerance by subthreshold desensitization. It is useful to try antihistamines because of much individual variation in response and in the side effects. Antihistamines are often prescribed in too low a dosage to be effective and patients should be encouraged to rest at home taking rather higher dosage. The evidence that skin blood vessels have both H_1 and H_2 receptors has encouraged trials with their antagonists. At present the financial cost and large number of pills that have to be taken every day is a disadvantage. Most H_1 antihistamines are cheap and free of serious side-effects. Drowsiness is often troublesome but the variations in the response are considerable and they are otherwise effective in the majority if taken regularly to prevent the urticaria rather than to treat the existing weals. Long-acting antihistamines are worth trying when short acting ones fail. The value of combined H_1 and H_2 blockers (4 mg cyproheptadine and 300 mg cimetidine four times daily) remains unproven but like all regimens has

some individual successes. Hydroxazine 100 mg per day in divided doses is often effective in dermographism or cholinergic urticaria. When the urticaria is painful and long-lasting, prednisolone is often effective and need only be given for 2 or 3 days. Avoidance of known triggers of urticaria such as aspirin, tartrazine, benzoate, and other salicylates often requires a rather complex diet (see Table 13).

The acute emergency of upper respiratory obstruction requires the maintenance of the airway, if necessary by intubation or tracheotomy, and administration of oxygen. This should not be delayed while a search is being made for adrenaline and corticosteroids, but if these are quickly available they should be given as nothing is lost and some benefit may be derived. Adrenaline 1/1000 0.5 ml subcutaneously and hydrocortisone 100 mg is given intravenously.

Management of autosomal dominant hereditary angio-oedema

This should be suspected if there is a family history of angio-oedema or a few long-lasting swellings precipitated by trauma. The signs include a transient erythema followed by the oedema. There is often recurring colicky abdominal pain. The diagnosis should be confirmed by looking for low levels in the serum of alpha-neuro-aminoglycoprotein, C_1 esterase inhibitor (normal 18 ± 5 mg/100 ml).

Prophylaxis includes care to protect against trauma especially in the region of the mouth and neck after dental manoeuvres. Methyltestosterone 10 mg as linguets after breakfast and another when there is a suspicion of developing oedema often aborts attacks. Fresh plasma, containing C_1 esterase, therefore, may be given before surgery or at the initiation of an attack. Unlike other forms of chronic urticaria, adrenalin, antihistamines and corticosteroids are of only a little benefit. Trasylol intravenously is an inhibitor of proteases and is sometimes helpful as is epsilon aminocaproic acid 12–18 g daily in divided dosage. The most effective treatment is danazol. This may be supplemented by fresh plasma during attack or if available, C_1 esterase inhibitor concentrate.

References

Czarnetzi, B. M., Meentken, J., Rosenbach, T. and Pokropp, A. (1984). Clinical, pharmacological and immunological aspects of delayed pressure urticaria. *Br. J. Dermatol.* **111**, 315–323.
Kaplan, A. P. (1984). Exercise induced hives. *J. Allergy Clin. Immunol.* **73**, 704–707.
Rubenstein, H. S. (1982). Bee sting diseases, who is at risk? What is the treatment? *Lancet* **i**, 496–499.
Tatnall, F. M., Gaylarde, P. M. and Sarkany, I. (1984). Localized heat urticaria and its management. *Clin. Exp. Dermatol.* **9**, 367–374.
Warin, R. P. and Champion, R. H. (1975). Urticaria. In *Major problems in dermatology* (ed. A. Rook), p. 171. Lloyd Luke, London.

Cutaneous vasculitis

The broadest definition of vasculitis is the response of small blood vessels to injury. No other definition encompasses its great variety which ranges from a transient increase in permeability or wealing, to coagulation and necrosis due to agents ranging from the immune complexes of serum sickness to the physical properties of cold or the ischaemia of gravitational stasis.

The term vasculitis includes many diseases described elsewhere in this *Textbook* such as Henoch–Schönlein purpura, polyarteritis nodosa, nodular vasculitis, Wegener's granulomatosis, hypersensitivity angiitis, and allergic granulomatosis. Examples of diseases that are sometimes included within this term are Behçet's syndrome, pyoderma gangrenosum, purpura fulminans, thromboangiitis obliterans, erythema nodosum, chilblains, atrophie blanche, and livedo reticularis. There are many other named variants, the separate recognition of which is no longer helpful except

FOUR DIFFERENT PATTERNS OF RESPONSE TO IDENTICAL INJURY

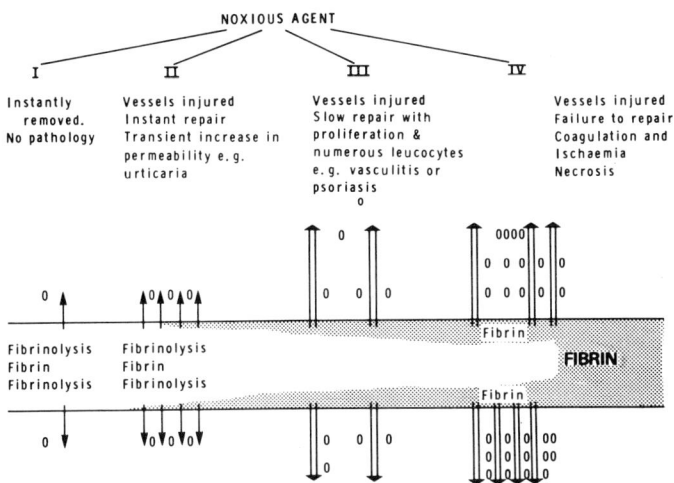

Fig. 89 A spectrum of inflammatory events ranging from a transient wealing or almost physiological permeability through inflammatory neutrophilic infiltration and oedema to complete necrosis of the vessel, due to thrombosis and coagulation or destruction of its wall.

to communicate with people who have already learned such terms and formed an opinion of what they represent.

Vasculitis overlaps with urticaria and with infarction or gangrene. To use some of the older terminology, some authors have described urticaria as the predominant feature of Henoch–Schönlein purpura in children and there have been a number of more recently described vasculitic syndromes in which urticaria is the only skin manifestation. At the other end of the spectrum necrotizing angiitis and polyarteritis nodosa are labels often given to infarctive or more destructive patterns of vasculitis.

The physical signs of skin disease are more or less recognizable as distinct patterns. The names they have been given are of dubious value when it comes to managing the disease. It is possible to explain these patterns and to decide what aspects of the physical signs are the most useful clues to pathogenesis.

Pathology and nomenclature

When a vessel is injured there follows a response which removes or neutralizes the cause of the injury; this is followed by repair. The response depends on the intensity of the injury, on the efficiency of the inflammation, and on the rate and effectiveness of the repair. Herein lies one of the main reasons why a particular injury does not always produce the same rash. The inflammatory response is a very complex sequence of events (Fig. 89) subject to considerable modification by each individual's particular range of mediators. Important factors explaining variability are local tissue architecture and previous experience. Scarring or even temporary exhaustion of mediators by prior injury alters the sequence of events that follow further injury. Formerly authors used to describe sites of lowered resistance: we now know that such sites comprise areas of non-homogeneous blood supply with hypoxia, leakiness, and blood stasis as well as exhausted mast cells and endothelial cells undergoing various stages of repair. Paralysis of the mononuclear phagocytic system is also important.

This variation in the inflammatory response can be superficial or deep and it is modified by the distribution of the injury – gravitational, light exposed, cold exposed, or at sites of pressure or abrasion; this is one explanation of the physical signs that make up classifiable rashes. It is perhaps not surprising that the French used terms like *maladie trisymptome* or *penta symptome* to describe a rash that had urticarial, purpuric, nodular, pigmented, and necrotic lesions; when morphology was all that could be described it was

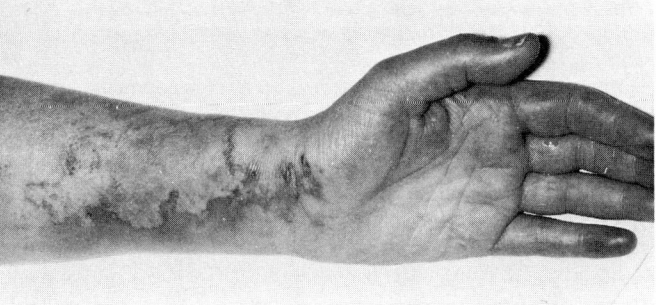

Fig. 90 The white infarct characteristic of embolization or arterial block. Most cutaneous vasculitis that is labelled as arteritis is in fact venular but the white infarct is characteristic of arterial occlusion.

better not to give an eponymous name to any particular combination of physical signs.

Another reason for the later delineation of different syndromes such as Behçet's triad, cutaneous polyarteritis nodosa, or limited Wegener's granulomatosis was the recognition that vasculitis may be confined to either one or more organs. But this too is of dubious value: Behçet described mouth, eye, and genital lesions but the disease is as often more widespread; Wegener's granulomatosis affects the respiratory tract but skin and kidney are frequently affected.

One other point of debate is the value of the term arteritis. Smooth muscle in the arterial wall is damaged by ischaemia and in most small vessels this is due to vasoconstriction, coagulation, and thrombosis or to obstructed flow due to more distal vasculitis. Thus malignant hypertension, coagulation, embolism (Fig. 90), thrombotic thrombocytopenia, or vasculitis are often sufficiently appropriate diagnostic terms and are more helpful when considering prognosis, aetiology, or management. The histological diagnosis of arteritis is similarly unsatisfactory. Damaged venules can themselves look like small arteries and even when an artery is clearly involved it is rarely possible in the same section to see the more distal vasculitis responsible for the obstruction to blood flow and consequent ischaemia.

Harmful agents responsible for vasculitis

Immune complexes, infective agents, drugs, food additives, and circulating particulate matter all injure blood vessels. It is probable that these are present in small amounts in all of us some of the time, but it is likely that the injuries are often so mild as to be imperceptible and quickly repaired.

Immune complexes

The 'defensive' system which clears antigens includes complexing them with antibody and complement to make phagocytosis by macrophages more inevitable. It is a system which is used to remove damaged tissue and it is often difficult to distinguish whether damage preceded or is a consequence of the immune complex. It is the process of complexing that activates complement not the complex itself. Free and poorly complexed antigen may indeed have the greater potential to damage than the well complexed material. Trapping of antigen in a tissue and its exposure to immunoglobulin and complement is determined by local events having little to do with what circulates in the blood stream.

Immune complexes follow the ingestion of food, the presence of a fetus in the pregnant, or invasion of the body by parasites such as scabies or by a neoplasm such as breast cancer, and can be demonstrated in everyone following the most mild of virus infections. For this reason, the mere demonstration of immune complexes is not enough to blame them for coincidental vasculitis.

Immune complexes are mostly harmless but become harmful when they are of certain size and shape or composition. Actual harm is observed only when and as they are localized at a site ill equipped to deal with them and slow to repair the damage done by them.

Often an alteration in host response prevents adequate neutralization of even mildly noxious agents. Recent exposure to similar noxious agents, exhaustion, and insufficient time for recovery of fibrinolytic mechanisms or the phagocytic potential and the secretions of the mononuclear phagocytic system explain why repeated or continuous exposure to harmful agents precipitates vasculitis. Such an explanation most often explains localized recrudescence in the nose, in Wegener's granulomatosis, or in legs affected by gravitational eczema, ulcers, or atrophie blanche. Factors such as severe infection, foods, drugs, diseases promoting coagulation (e.g. hepatitis), and malignancy often alter the inflammatory response and need not act as specific triggers. Immune complexes circulating in a patient known to have disseminated lupus erythematosus may suddenly become damaging when any of these other factors affect the patient. The localization of the defective inflammatory process is often determined by environmental factors: cold exposure, abrasion, or pressure on the skin causing mild stasis and ischaemia are well known examples met clinically; these conditions are also used experimentally to demonstrate the localization of harmful agents from the blood stream.

In recent years the discovery of congenital defects in complement and other protease inhibitors has explained why harmful agents are inadequately neutralized in some people; hereditary angio-oedema is a good example of such a disease. There is a congenital absence of an inhibitor of complement but only in certain circumstances is this important. Trauma or infection sets off the sequence of events which in this case includes the activation of complement by plasmin, dependent in its turn upon the secretion of plasminogen activator by damaged endothelium. Normally this is balanced by other inhibitors and by absorption into small amounts of fibrinogen and fibrin.

Local deficiencies in the sequence of events triggered by injury depend upon blood flow and diffusion not only of activators but also of inhibitors. Injury usually releases activators of fibrinolysis from endothelium and heparin, histamine, and hyaluronidase, amongst other things, from adjacent mast cells. These increase permeability and diffusion but prevent coagulation and the activation of complement. Repeated inoculation of histamine can itself cause vasculitis. It is not always necessary to invoke an immunological mechanism. When the mast cells and endothelium are more or less exhausted and when activating or inhibiting products are released by adjacent epidermal injury the proteases, complement, kinins, and materials like fibrin or C reactive substance occur in sufficient quantities to perpetuate the inflammation and attract white cells in large numbers.

Diagnosis

As Osler (1914) wrote, 'All are exudative, in which the blood elements – either the red blood corpuscles alone, the serum alone, or both combined – pass out of the vessels'. Almost essential to the diagnosis is purpura (Fig. 91), but an urticarial lesion that is tender lasts for more than 12 hours, and leaves a slight bruise on resolution falls within the term vasculitis (Fig. 92). The histology of such a lesion often shows more perivascular neutrophils than the common short-lasting urticarial weal. At the other end of the spectrum is obliterative or sclerosing thromboangiitis in which total occlusion of a small vessel often prevents exudation, and because there is no neutrophilic infiltrate, there may not be such acute destruction of the vessel wall. A similar appearance may be observed in DIC (Fig. 93) and in platelet embolic diseases.

Vasculitis affecting deep dermis or fat and subcutaneous tissues most commonly produces a nodule, sometimes with redness or violaceous skin overlying it. Blistering and pustulation, when they occur as manifestations of vasculitis, are usually part of a superficial polymorphic eruption in which at least some of the lesions are palpable purpura, distinguishing the eruption from other more

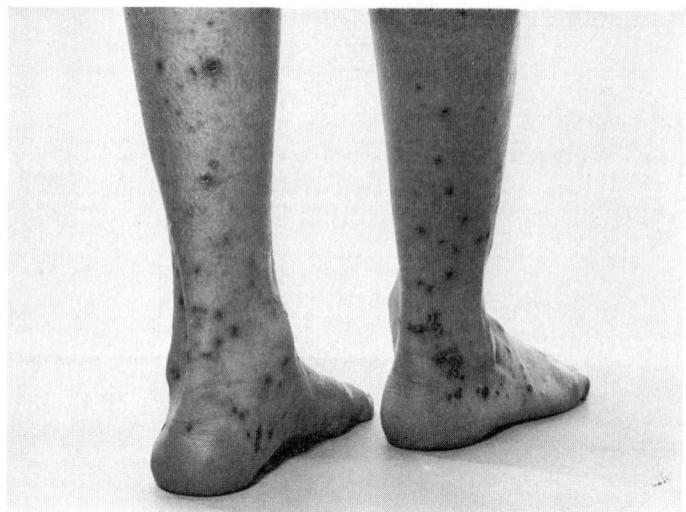

Fig. 91 Typical purpura of the lower leg of adult Henoch–Schönlein purpura. The lesions are palpable and inflammatory.

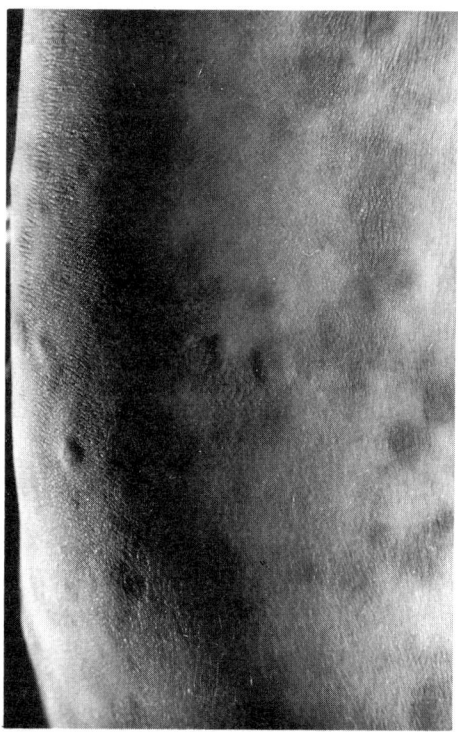

Fig. 92 Typical urticarial initial lesion of vasculitis often proceeding to purpura and later to necrosis. However, in some types, hypocomplementaemic vasculitis, a persistent urticaria, is the only lesion.

monomorphic blistering diseases. These physical signs are illustrated in Fig. 94. Very heavy infiltration with eosinophils is a feature of eosinophilic cellulitis which is sometimes a reaction to arthropod bites.

So far as the diagnosis of purpura is concerned, the traditional classification of thrombocytopenia (Fig. 95) versus non-thrombocytopenia is useful. Vasculitis is included within the latter term.

Vasculitis in which immune complexes have played a causative role is more likely to be leucocytoclastic – a term used to describe numerous disrupted neutrophils at the site of the damaged vessel (Fig. 96). It is now well recognized that a mononuclear variety of vasculitis also occurs which is sometimes termed lymphocytic vasculitis and in which complement activation seems less significant. It is a feature of drug eruptions and also of damage to vessels

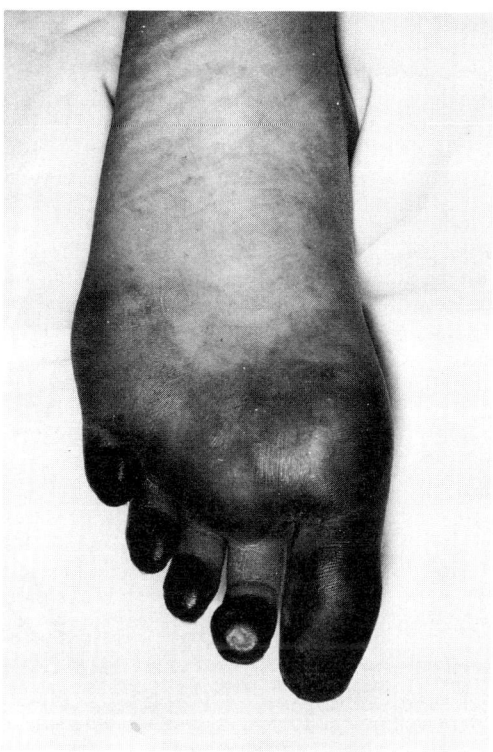

Fig. 93 The blue to black discoloration of the extremities in disseminated intravascular coagulation.

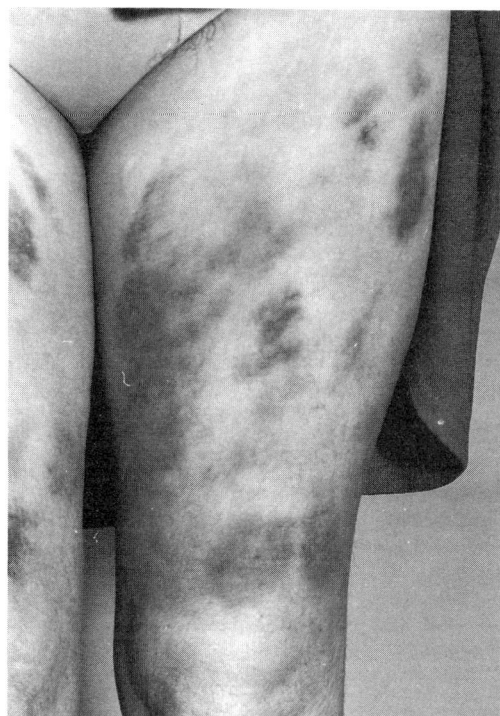

Fig. 95 Bruising or echymosis is most commonly due to thrombocytopenic purpura but it is also a feature of the painful bruising syndrome.

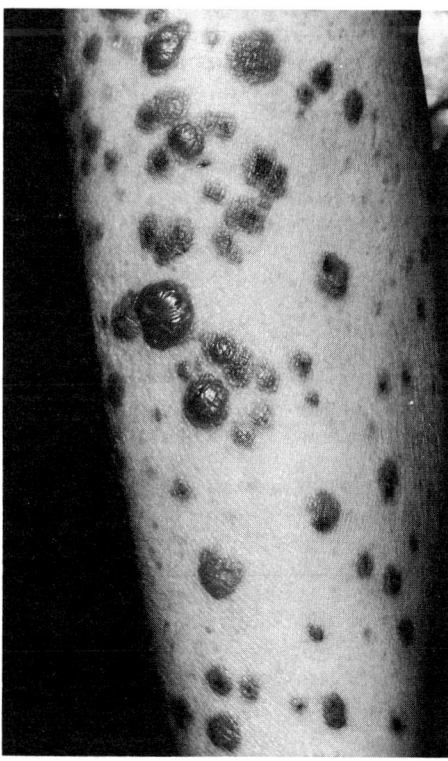

Fig. 94 The presence of blisters in vasculitis is due to the intensity of the oedema in the upper dermis; sometimes it is due to necrosis.

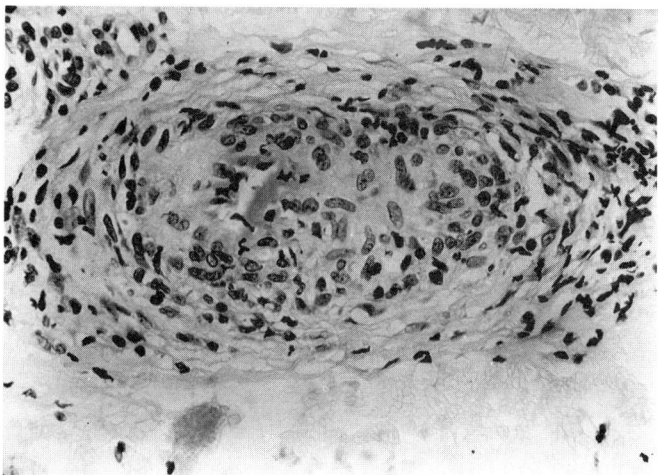

Fig. 96 A damaged vessel surrounded by broken-up neutrophils is typical of the hypocomplementaemic pattern of vasculitis.

Much of the pathology of vasculitis is that of ischaemia. Whatever the cause of the damage to the vessel, there is usually some impairment of blood flow. Hypoxia and infarction are quite capable of causing equally extensive pathology.

The significance of eosinophils in some forms of vasculitis is not known and they are no guide to prognosis or therapy.

Detection of cause

From the patients' point of view the most worthwhile investigation is that which results in improved management. Specialist units have the additional role of exploration to advance understanding. Certain noxious agents should always be looked for in order to eliminate them. Bacteria are the most important of these: the streptococcal sore throat is still the commonest precursor of vasculitis in children and otitis media, dental caries, cystitis, and sinusitis

sometimes prior to the deposition of immune complexes, i.e. within 2 hours of a cutaneous capillary fragility test. In fact macrophages rather than lymphocytes could be the more injurious infiltrate depending on the stage of maturation and their secretion.

occasionally play a role; in many countries tuberculosis or leprosy is the commonest cause; bacterial endocarditis and meningococcal septicaemia are often missed. Other treatable infections occasionally causing vasculitis are syphilis, neisseria, rickettsiae, and mycoplasma. Although viruses usually cannot be eliminated, any history of a recent flu-like illness or vaccination may be relevant. Hepatitis B virus is a well recognized cause.

Lupus erythematosus and rheumatoid arthritis are common causes of immune complex vasculitis. But as mentioned above, it is the exposure of antigen so that its complexing can activate complement that is important, not the complex itself.

Drugs such as penicillin and sulphonamides have often been incriminated but many other drugs appear less likely to be allergens than modifiers of the host response. Similarly some foods may act as allergens and others have a more obscure enhancing action. Enquiries should be directed towards headache pills, throat lozenges, purgatives, health foods, any medicine given for a specific illness, and any recent intake of food or drugs to which the patient is known to be sensitive (see page 20.23).

It is now clear that many patients have cold-precipitated immune complexes and perhaps even more have soluble immune complexes that are localized by blood stasis due to cold, pressure, vasoconstriction, or prior inflammation. The number of patients in whom an antigen has been isolated is small and in still fewer has it been possible to eliminate the antigen, except in the case of bacteria sensitive to antibiotics. It is not particularly helpful to find a cryoglobulin; it does not alter management since every patient should be kept warm in any case. One of the difficulties is that it is often the antibody to the infective agent that in its turn becomes recognized as foreign. Infection may initiate this problem but after elimination of the organism the antibody persists as an autoantigen.

Factors that modify the inflammatory response

These are very numerous and include any known chronic illness such as malnutrition, diabetes mellitus, blood disorders, rheumatoid arthritis or other forms of collagen disease, chronic respiratory disease, disorders of the bowels or liver, and hypertension. Malignancy, whether carcinoma or lymphoma, is a not unusual factor and recent surgery, pregnancy, and unusual anxiety are also included.

The mechanisms involved include coagulation and thrombosis, and since these are treatable, a full blood count should always include a platelet count and other simple relevant tests, especially estimation of prothrombin time, fibrinogen titre, and fibrin degradation products.

Prognosis

The difficulty of naming a constellation of physical signs may force the physician to produce labels which traditionally are linked to a poor prognosis. One example is the term polyarteritis nodosa, another Wegener's granulomatosis.

For all patterns it is useful to use the term vasculitis supplemented by the terms 'limited' or 'local' implying a mild process affecting one locale or organ and 'complicated' meaning severe and affecting many organs. Such adjectives, by describing the severity of the disease, give a lead to its management.

Management

Avoid all further injury

This allows healing to take place and prevents further damage to already inflamed tissue. Rest is essential for all acute inflammation but blood stasis should be counteracted by adequate elevation and movement of the limbs. Cold and direct sunlight should also be avoided since both injure the skin and affect blood flow. Female legs are particularly at risk though, happily, trousers, long skirts, and bobby socks can now be worn; a few years ago the mini-skirt used to be the cause of severe cold injury to the thighs.

Scratching, pinching, pressure, and constriction of the skin by ill-fitting clothing or bandages should not be allowed. Patients lying in bed will develop vasculitis on the buttocks, elbows, and over the greater trochanter unless they shift their position every few minutes. Venepuncture sites become inflamed in some forms of vasculitis, particularly in Behçet's disease and pyoderma gangrenosum but also in severe generalized leucocytoclastic angiitis.

Eliminate circulating noxious agents especially if antigens

Vasculitis following a severe streptococcal sore throat, meningococcal or gonococcal septicaemia, or tuberculosis should be treated with the appropriate antibiotics. Foci of infection, once so popular, are now too rarely thought of; when found they need elimination, sometimes even by surgery. Certain bacterial diseases such as bacterial endocarditis or leprosy are not easily eliminated and require lifelong supervision. Viral diseases are increasingly incriminated but as yet there is no satisfactory way of dealing with them. Immune complex disease, sometimes as a manifestation of rheumatoid arthritis or lupus erythematosus but more often having no particular association, is now the most often suspected cause of vasculitis. Usually there are no specific measures for dealing with the problem but immune complexes become less damaging if the factors localizing them are eliminated. Plasmapheresis is practised by a few specialized units. Drugs and food thought to be responsible can be omitted.

Provide specific treatment

Acute short-lasting itchy weals often respond to antihistamines. Acute tender swelling due to progressive tissue oedema may need steroids. Painful swollen joints, acute optic neuritis, temporal (giant cell) arteritis, erythema nodosum, tender persistent weals, and tense painful swellings at the edge of pyoderma gangrenosum all usually respond to corticosteroids.

Fulminant vasculitis affecting more than one organ and brought about by a known trigger (allergens, drugs), should be covered by steroids once the cause has been eliminated. Immunosuppressive drugs such as azathioprine, cyclophosphamide, and methotrexate are used as a last resort in persistent chronic vasculitis but they are of doubtful value except in granulomatous forms affecting the lung in which they are the treatment of choice. Necrosis and gangrene are usually due to ischaemia. While inflammation alone may account for this in small vessels supplying superficial lesions, hypertension, coagulation, and thrombosis, as well as the cause of cardiac or peripheral vascular disease in general, sometimes underlie large areas of necrosis. The causes of vasculitis are also for the most part the causes of local or disseminated intravascular coagulation. Heparin is probably the drug of choice when fibrinogen, platelets, and prothrombin have been consumed and fibrin degradation products are raised. It is probably the most useful anticoagulant in malignant disease. Aspirin's anti-inflammatory effect is well known and is particularly effective when platelet aggregation is suspected. Dapsone, enhancers of fibrinolysis, and potassium iodide have had their successes and failures in recurrent nodular forms of vasculitis. Good management includes advice on smoking, oral contraception, high blood pressure, and hyperlipidaemia. The prognosis depends on complications: particularly important are those affecting the eyes, central nervous system, and kidneys. Examination of the eyes for papilloedema and of the urine for red cells, protein, and casts is imperative.

Erythema nodosum

It is convenient to include erythema nodosum under the heading vasculitis though some still prefer to call it panniculitis. There is injury to small blood vessels in the deep dermis and subcutaneous tissue but primary injury to the blood vessels from a noxious agent such as soluble immune complexes is difficult to prove: it is characterized by tender red swellings on the front of the shins (Fig. 97) and often also on the thighs and forearms. Bruising is common but necrosis, scarring and atrophy of the tissues is not a feature.

Erythema nodosum is a reaction pattern to infection (viral, bac-

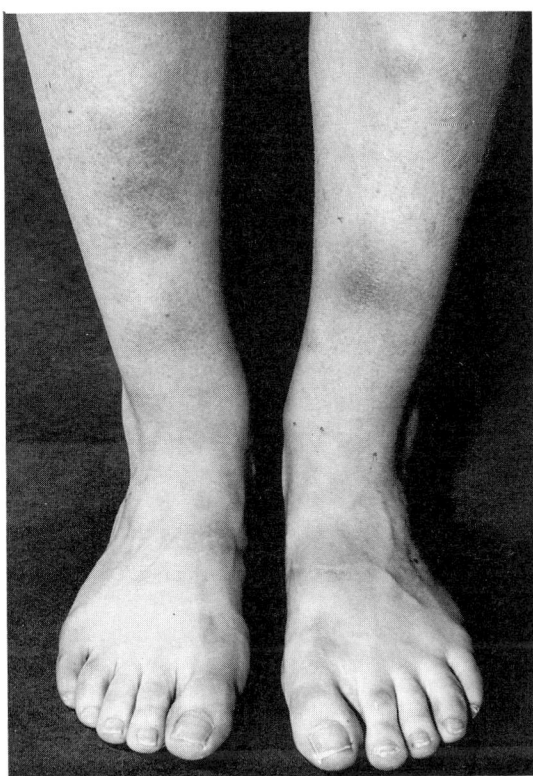

Fig. 97 Tender erythematous swelling on the front of the legs with ill-defined borders is characteristic of erythema nodosum.

terial, and mycotic) and sometimes to drugs. Neoplasia, pregnancy, and sarcoidosis are other causes. The causes are listed in Table 25. By far the commonest is a streptococcal sore throat. Sarcoidosis and tuberculosis are common causes where the incidence of these diseases is high. In teaching hospital practice ulcerative colitis and Crohn's disease are common associations. Worldwide, erythema nodosum is commonly due to lepromatous leprosy. This is a widespread and often very persistent reaction to local antigen and is not typical of erythema nodosum in general. It may become pustular and necrotic. Erythema nodosum is often preceded by or accompanied by fever, malaise, fatigue, loss of weight, and arthralgia. Although it sometimes resolves in 2–3 weeks, persistent and recurrent forms over several months may suggest an alternative diagnosis. It is important not to label the disease as polyarteritis nodosa or rheumatic fever, for instance, merely because it is persistent and the patient is ill for several months, or the blood sedimentation rate is unusually high. The number, size, and chronicity of the lesions is variable. They can be few and as large as the hand or multiple and the size of the thumb nail. They can be acute, tender, and last only a few days, or they can be chronic, less tender and migratory, tending to heal in the centre and spread peripherally as a swollen ring. The more chronic lesions are less red and may be violaceous or any of the colours of a resolving bruise.

Investigations

A chase for the source of infection should include a history of possible contacts at home and abroad, human or other animal. A chest X-ray is essential and the most useful for the diagnosis of sarcoid or tuberculosis. A fall in blood sedimentation rate which is often initially above 100 mm/hour is a useful guide to complete recovery.

Treatment

This is one of the diseases in which ultimate recovery is to be expected. While for the first 2–3 weeks it is possible to keep the

Table 25 Some causes of erythema nodosum

Streptococcus	Blastomycosis
Tuberculosis	Coccidioidomycosis
Sarcoidosis	Trichophyton verrucosum
Lymphogranuloma venereum	Ulcerative colitis
Cat scratch disease	Crohn's disease
Ornithosis	Leukaemia
Epstein–Barr virus	Hodgkin's disease
Tularaemia	Sulphonamides
Histoplasmosis	Bromides
Yersinia	Pregnancy and contraceptive pill
Leprosy	

patient at rest and to prescribe acetyl salicylic acid, the difficult period is often several weeks after the initial illness when the patients have to be mobilized. Firm support bandages or stockings give some relief for persistent aching and swelling of the legs. Steroids reduce swelling and fever but do not affect the length of the illness.

Pyoderma gangrenosum

As the name implies this is a necrosis of the tissues often with a heavy neutrophilic infiltrate but it is not primarily an infection, rather it is a reaction pattern in which venous and capillary engorgement, haemorrhage, and coagulation feature prominently. The exact pathogenesis is uncertain. In many cases there is an associated depression of the immune system demonstrable by *in vitro* and clinical tests. Failure of macrophages to respond to tissue injury or to clear noxious agents is another feature. Its associations are an important guide to its possible causation. These include ulcerative colitis, Crohn's disease, particularly of the colon, rheumatoid arthritis, seronegative arthritis with paraproteinaemia, Wegener's granulomatosis, and plasma cell dyscrasias including myeloma. A bullous variety is associated with leukaemia primary thrombocythaemia and with myelofibrosis. Nevertheless, up to half of the cases seen in dermatology clinics have no significant association. The clinical features are initially varied but all ultimately become turgid and ulcerate. They include a tender red or blue nodule suggestive of erythema nodosum, vesico pustules, or an acneiform folliculitis. The swollen red or blue edge is often acutely tender; blistering may be considerable, especially in the leukaemic variety. The necrosis follows no particular pattern and, like a carbuncle, may have multiple centres. It is usually undermined, and exuberant granulation tissue sprouts from the base of the ulcer. The calves, thighs, buttocks, abdomen, and face are favoured but no site is immune.

There is considerable toxicity associated with the acute varieties. Dermatologists see the chronic variety which is not obviously associated with underlying disease and in which the general health of the patient is not impaired. The ulcerated lesions are not necessarily tender but they are irregular and persistent often for years. Dermatitis artefacta is often suspected and the personality of the patient disabled for many months may be consequently affected and encourage the suspicion. Synergistic gangrene is one cause of very similar acute pathology. Unlike pyoderma gangrenosum which is often multiple, synergistic gangrene is more clearly associated with a recent wound such as an operation on the gastrointestinal tract, and the area of gangrene is solitary and an extension of the wound. From any form of pyoderma gangrenosum, aerobic and anaerobic bacterial culture, amoebiasis, tuberculosis, buruli ulcer, and deep fungus infections such as nocardiosis or blastomycosis should be considered.

The treatment of choice is high-dose corticosteroids by mouth. The management of underlying diseases such as ulcerative colitis or leukaemia is essential. Any suspicion of an infective causation such as amoebiasis requires the appropriate investigations and treatment. For cases responding poorly to steroids, dapsone 100 mg daily or clofazimine is worth a try.

Table 26 Clinical features of Behçet's disease

Aphthous stomatitis	
Ulceration of genitalia	The triad of Behçet
Iritis and uveitis	
Thrombophlebitis	
Erythema nodosum	
Pustules or folliculitis	Common associations
Arthritus	

Thrombosis of large veins including superior and inferior
    vena cava and sagittal sinus
Arterial aneurysms
Orchitis
Ulcerative colitis
Splenomegaly
Glomerulonephritis (very rare)
Sjögren's syndrome

Behçet's disease

The combination of large ulcers in the perineum and mouth with severe iritis and blindness is a distinct syndrome mostly described in Turkey and Israel. In Japan, the ocular manifestations are the most prominent. In many other parts of the world the disease is much less well defined. Even where it is prominent other associated symptoms and signs are common and it is these that seem to present in the United Kingdom. Often in the absence of the full triad of Behçet's description, arthritis and vascular complications such as thrombophlebitis in the legs, are particularly common but there are numerous references to arterial and venous pathology which include large vessels in the thorax or skull (Table 26).

In severe cases ulceration is extensive and deep but mild aphthous ulceration is sufficient to make the diagnosis in the presence of other members of the triad. The classic triad does not always occur together and it is quite common to have to rely on a history of relatively transient mouth, eye, or genital involvement. However, over a number of years it would be unusual for mouth or genital ulceration to be absent if persistent 'vasculitis' or eye signs were due to the disease. The cause of the disease remains unclear but the long held belief that it is in part genetic is supported by the finding of the HLA B5 associated with ocular manifestations. A viral aetiology is unproven but this, as well as environmental pollutants, has its advocates.

With vascular complications so common, the search for a basis of thrombosis or coagulation has not distinguished between cause and effect. Certainly fibrinolysis is often grossly impaired as is platelet aggregation. The finding of circulating soluble immune complexes in Behçet's disease is probably more an indication of tissue damage than of causation.

A peculiar sign shared with pyoderma gangrenosum is the hyper-reactivity of the skin to minor injury such as venepuncture. About one-third of patients develop an inflammatory papule or pustule within 24 hours of trauma sufficient to damage the small vessels in the dermis.

The treatment of this disease is unsatisfactory. Acute and severe ulceration or iritis should be given the chance to respond to systemic steroids. Some respond rapidly whilst others have a persistent and uncontrolled disease. The same is true of fibrinolytic therapy with phenformin 50 mg twice daily and ethyloestrenol 2 mg four times daily, stanozolol 5 mg twice daily, or streptokinase infusions. Colchicine 1–2 mg daily is the latest therapy for which some success is claimed. Minocycline 100 mg daily is worth a trial. It is popular therapy in Japan and South Korea where streptococcal infection is believed to act as an antigen.

References

Couser, W. G. (1981). What are circulating immune complexes doing in glomerulonephritis? *N. Engl. J. Med.* **304**, 1230.

Hickman, J. G. and Lazarus, G. S. (1979). Pyoderma gangrenosum: new concepts, etiology, and treatment. In *Dermatology update* (ed. S. L. Moschella), pp. 325–342. Elsevier, New York.

Osler, W. (1914). The visceral lesions of purpura and allied conditions. *Br. med. J.* **i**, 517.

Ryan, T. J. (1976). *Microvascular injury; vasculitis, stasis and ischaemia.* Lloyd Luke, London.

—— and Wilkinson, D. S. (1986). Cutaneous vasculitis: 'angiitis'. In *Textbook of dermatology* 4th edn (eds A. Rook, D. S. Wilkinson, and F. J. G. Ebling), pp. 993–1058. Blackwell Scientific Publications.

Wiggins, R. C. and Cochrane, C. G. (1981). Current concepts in immunology. Immune complex mediated biologic effects. *N. Eng. J. Med.* **304**.

Wolff, K. and Winkelmann, R. K. (1980). *Vasculitis.* Lloyd Luke, London.

Yankey, K. M. and Lawley, T. J. (1984). Circulating immune complexes and their immunochemistry, biology and detection in selected dermatologic and systemic diseases. *J. Am. Acad. Dermatol.* **10**, 711–731.

VESICO-BLISTERING DISEASES

A vesicle is an elevated circumscribed lesion filled with serum and sometimes blood and pus. It is usually no larger than 0.5 cm in diameter. Above this size a vesicle is called a bulla or blister.

Predisposing factors

These include congenital diseases such as epidermolysis bullosa (see page 20.14) or metabolic disorders such as porphyria.

Causes

Friction or minor knocks can produce blisters in the predisposed or at sites unaccustomed to wear and tear. The hands and feet are most often affected. Friction is increased by damp, sweating skin.

Ischaemia

Prolonged pressure obliterating blood supply for more than 2 hours causes damage to the smooth muscle of small arterioles and underlying fat. The epidermis can survive more than 6 hours of ischaemia and in cool skin with a decreased metabolism much longer periods may be survived. The unconscious or those with sensory loss, especially from barbiturate poisoning are particularly vulnerable but most cases occur from peripheral vascular disease with acute interference of blood supply.

Acute sweat pore occlusion

This occurs especially with fever or in hot climates. Numerous small transparent vesicles especially in the flexures or in parts of the body in which the stratum corneum is unduly thick are usually affected. In the fingers or feet this is called pompholyx.

Burns

Burns can occur from cold (Fig. 98) as in frostbite or from cryotherapy, heat, or ultraviolet irradiation (photosensitivity from plants, porphyria, or pellagra) (Fig. 99). Dermatitis artefacta is often induced by burning the skin; it is clearly self-induced but usually denied and is often a bizarre pattern. Cigarette burns are amongst the commonest induced lesions.

Chemicals

These may be toxic as from mustard gas or cantharidin. Sometimes an allergic dermatitis from contact also produces vesicles due to separation of the epidermal cells by inflammatory oedema. Plant dermatitis is amongst the most common cause; it includes the primula in Europe and poison ivy in the USA.

Fixed drug eruptions

These can cause erythema and blistering and appear and reappear at the same site whenever the causative drug is ingested; usually there is itching within 6 hours of ingestion (see page 20.26).

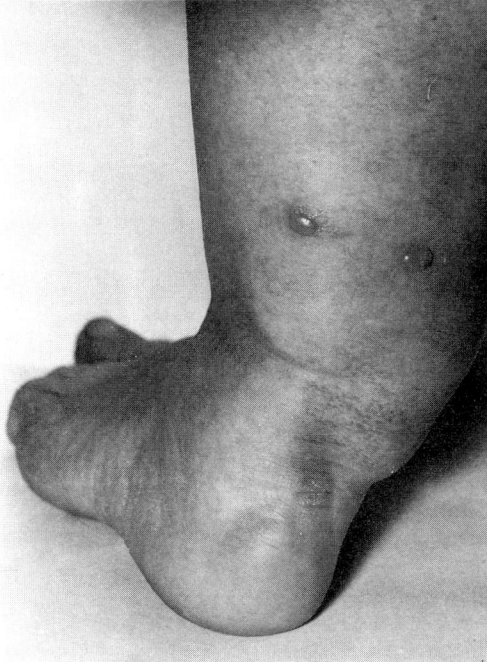

Fig. 98 Urticarial lesions in this case due to cold—they often blister especially on the lower legs.

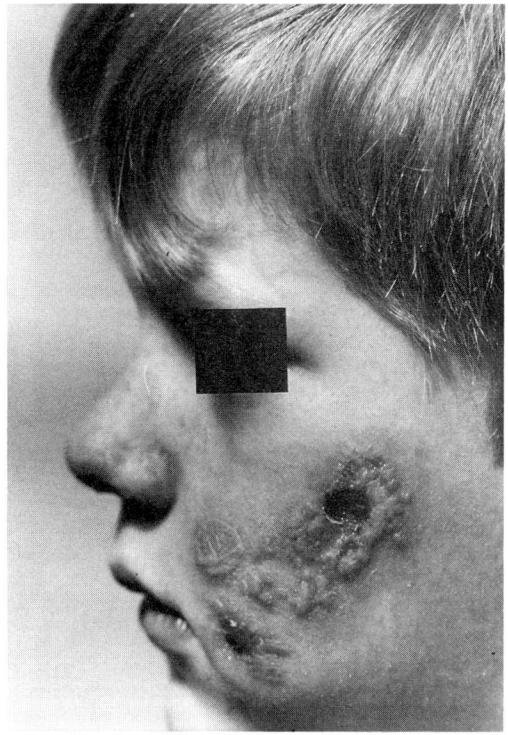

Fig. 100 Blisters on the cheek due to herpes simplex virus.

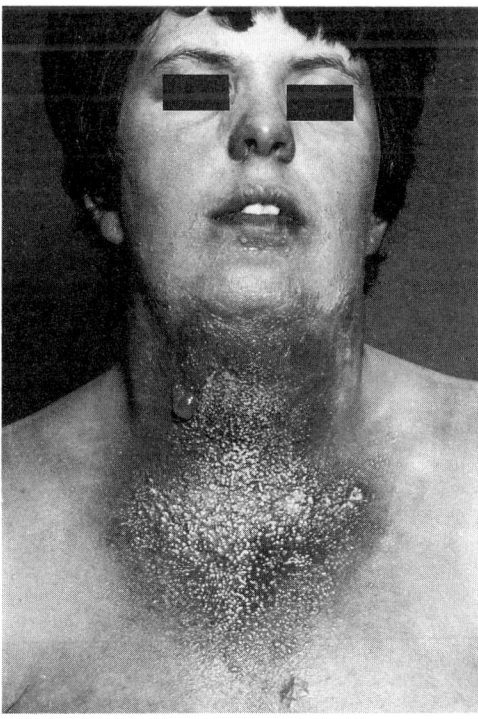

Fig. 99 Blistering on the front of the neck due to an ultraviolet light burn. Self-induced by a home lamp.

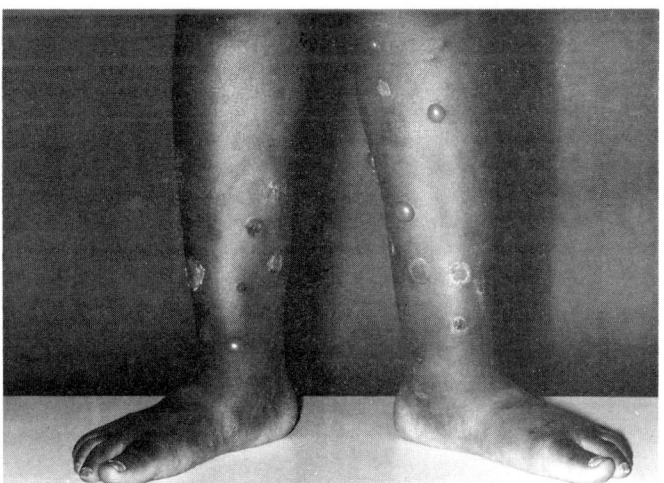

Fig. 101 Typical multiple blisters due to insect bites in the rainy season in India.

Infections

(See under appropriate sections.) Viral disorders including herpes simplex (Fig. 100), zoster, chickenpox, and smallpox, or bacterial diseases most commonly cause blisters particularly the staphyloccus and streptococcus.

Fungus infections commonly present as blistering on the soles of the feet and insect bites give rise to papular urticaria which often blisters on the lower legs (Fig. 101). Blisters, pruritus, and fever have been described in ornithologists bitten by ticks carried by marine birds on the Middle East coast line. Arthropods like the brown recluse spider give rise to necrotic blisters and others like the hairy caterpillar will secrete a toxin in its hairs, which can produce blistering. Some infarctions can produce a vasculitis or disseminated intravascular coagulation which too may present as vesicular or haemorrhagic blisters.

Specific skin disorders

Erythema multiforme

This, as the name implies, can present with a variety of patterns. The classic pattern affects the hands and feet more than the trunk and the lesions have an erythematous and coin-shaped present-

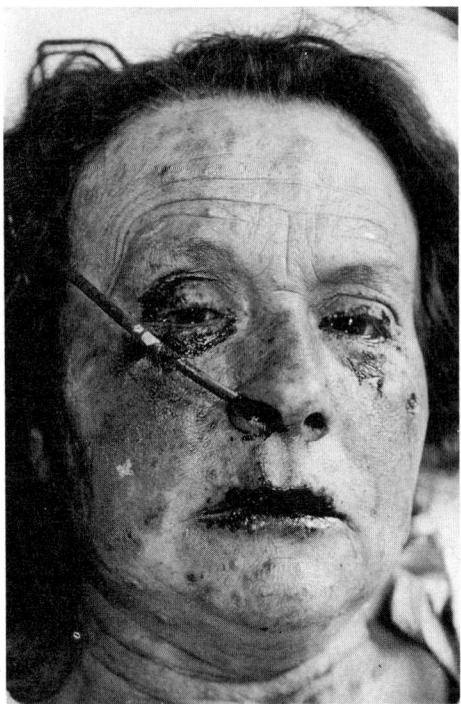

Fig. 102 Stevens–Johnson syndrome or severe erythema multiforme resulting in severe erosions of the mouth and conjunctivitis.

ation which is more intense and blistering in the centre – a target-shaped lesion (see Fig. 9b). Several toxic erythematous eruptions overlap with the classic pattern and sometimes the classic distribution and even the target lesions are missing. Involvement of the mucosa is common so that mouth, eyes, and genitalia may be affected in varying degrees. Where the blistering and mucosal lesions are severe, the disease is termed Stevens–Johnson syndrome (Fig. 102). This is usually associated with high fever and sometimes also anterior uveitis, pneumonia, renal failure, polyarthritis or diarrhoea.

Aetiology
In 50 per cent of these cases the cause is not known. For the rest the commonest causes are herpes simplex, or other viruses such as orf. Infections such as mycoplasma, streptococcus, typhoid, and diphtheria may be incriminated. Drugs also cause this disorder and sulphonamides are amongst the most common. In fact, any infection and any drug can probably give rise to erythema multiforme, usually after a latent period of 1–3 weeks. Other causes include neoplasm and its treatment with drugs or radiotherapy as well as certain other systemic diseases such as rheumatoid arthritis, lupus erythematosus, or ulcerative colitis. One of the difficulties is the overlap with the other patterns of toxic erythema and their causation. The erythema of pregnancy may sometimes be called erythema multiforme.

Pathology
There is vacuolar degeneration of the basal cells of the epidermis; vesicles develop between the cells and the underlying basement membrane. There is vasodilation and a lymphocytic infiltrate around the upper dermal vessels.

Treatment
The cause should be removed if known and systemic steroids should be prescribed if the patient is very uncomfortable and toxic. Recurrent attacks should also be treated by eliminating the cause if known, for instance, treating the earliest stage of the herpes simplex with idoxuridine and avoiding triggers like bright sunlight. Acyclovir is also increasingly recommended but viral resistance and long-term side-effects of frequent usage are causing anxiety.

Toxic epidermal necrolysis
This is a rare variety of erythema with acute epithelial necrosis affecting all areas of the skin. This is sometimes called 'scalded skin syndrome' because of its clinical appearance. It is usually acute in onset and may be preceded by various patterns of toxic erythema or blistering. Pressure and shearing stresses on the skin tend to encourage the extension of the blisters. There are two varieties of the disease: one was originally described by Ritter which is due to a staphylococcus, often phage type 71 and particularly affecting children – the blistering and the resulting erosions are very superficial and they are due to a split at the level of the stratum granulosum; the second is a drug reaction or a toxic consequence of malignant disease or its therapy. The entire epidermis is necrotic. The drugs responsible are sometimes sulphonamides, barbiturates, phenytoin, pyrazolone derivatives, or phenolphthalein, but there are also a number of other drugs more rarely blamed.

Rarer blistering disorders
These include diseases like pemphigus, pemphigoid, and dermatitis herpetiformis. At one time these were all grouped together and their pathogenesis has only recently become clearer. The main distinction is in the level of the blister which determines both clinical and histological features, as pemphigus is an intraepidermal blister whereas the other disorders tend to be subepidermal. The cleavage within the dermis produces dermal inflammation, oedematous papules, infiltration with white cells, as well as bleeding into this blister. The more superficial the blister the more erosive the appearance and the skin lesions may be red and glistening whereas deeper dermal blisters tend to be tense and less easily broken. The type and site of immunoglobulin deposition is a further diagnostic feature (see Table 1).

Pemphigus vulgaris
A blistering condition favouring the mucosa as much as the skin. It is a separation of epidermal cells in the basal layers of the epidermis always in association with an antibody having an affinity with intercellular material in the epidermis. The separated epidermal cell is large, basophilic and rounded and is termed an acantholytic cell.

Aetiology
It is assumed to be an autoimmune disease possibly associated with HLA-A10 and DR4, and is found more commonly in the Jewish race. It is one of the commonest causes of admission to a skin hospital in India. The more superficial variety that affects Brazilians may or may not be a separate genetically determined reaction pattern. The antibody that binds with complement both *in vivo* and *in vitro* is specific for an as yet unidentified intercellular material which activates proteases that lyse intercellular adhesive materials. Several investigators have found that the antibody can frequently cause intraepithelial clefting *in vitro* in human, rabbit, and monkey epithelium. There is an association with thymoma as well as with lymphoma and carcinoma. Not surprisingly, therefore, it occurs with lupus erythematosus and myasthenia gravis.

Penicillamine has been responsible for the development of pemphigus in about 9 per cent of patients treated for rheumatoid arthritis. Captopril and rifampicin as well as meprobamate have also been incriminated.

Clinical features
Erosions of the mucosa of the mouth are the initial problem in more than half the cases. The erosions are often misdiagnosed as

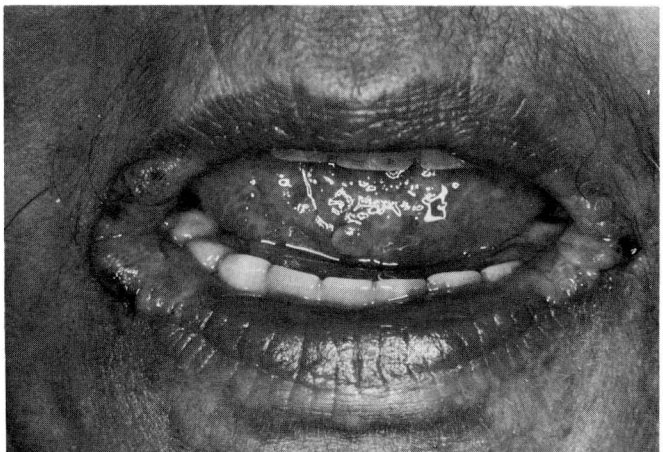

Fig. 103 Pemphigus vegetans showing the typical granulomatous hypertrophy underlying erosions at the angles of the mouth.

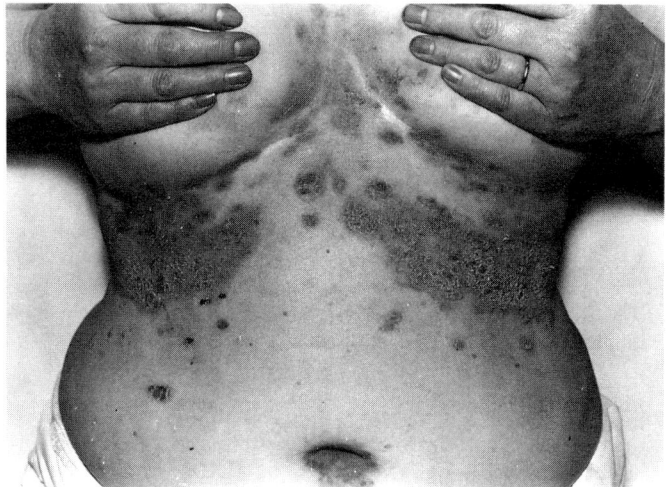

Fig. 104 Pemphigus foliaceous blisters, so superficial that they merely look like crusting of the erosions. In this case it would have to be distinguished from an intertrigo and secondary monilial infection.

mouth ulcers but close examination reveals a friable mucosa with no well defined aphthous ulcers. Actual blisters may be missed because they are so quickly eroded. On the skin the superficial nature of the blisters also determines that the principal lesion is a more painful erosion and the flaccid blisters quickly burst. The base is red and bleeds easily. The epidermis at the edge of the blister is easily dislodged by sliding pressure (Nikolsky sign). There are many reports of clinical and histological overlap with pemphigus foliaceous or pemphigoid. In all such cases pemiphigus vulgaris proves to be the final diagnosis.

Treatment

Corticosteroids are life saving; without them the disease is one of the most dangerous in dermatology. Very high dosage is required. Prednisolone 120 mg daily is a common starting dose and failure to control the eruption within a week merits doubling of even this high dose. As soon as there are no new blisters the steroids are reduced by large increments about every 3 days. Withdrawal is more gradual below 30 mg daily. Most practitioners now add azathioprine, methotrexate, or cyclophosphamide as a steroid sparing immunosuppressant.

In contrast to the presteroid era cure now seems possible and many patients are off all treatment after 2 years. However, the side-effects of the therapy are considerable. Death from gastrointestinal haemorrhage is not infrequent. Thromboembolic disease is probably a consequence of the disease as much as the therapy. Osteoporosis from the steroids with consequent vertebral collapse is a frequent and irreversible side-effect. Bacterial infection of the eroded skin is inevitable and septicaemia is common. The sore mouth and eroded skin require expert nursing – dressings tend to stick to the skin and removal causes further damage to the skin. Fluids given by mouth should not be strongly osmotic and soft diets should not include particles which lodge under blister roofs or in crevices.

Pemphigus vegetans

This is a reaction to the erosions in which the repairing epidermis becomes hypertrophic and the dermal response is granulomatous. It is common in the axillae and groin and the angles of the mouth (Fig. 103). It may be encouraged by steroid suppression. Small pustules surround the vegetations.

Pemphigus foliaceous

This is a more benign variant of pemphigus in which the blisters are more superficial. The bullae are subcorneal and scaling and crusting may be a principal feature (Fig. 104). The face and upper trunk are most often affected. Localized forms may look more like

seborrhoeic warts because of their chronicity and definition. Oral lesions are unusual. Antibodies against intercellular epithelial material are present as in pemphigus vulgaris but basement membrane antibody and antinuclear antibody are also often observed. There is an association with lupus erythematosus and with thymoma and myasthenia gravis.

Fogo selvagem

This is a form of pemphigus foliaceous which is common in Brazil. Many members of one family may be involved. Progression to a generalized erythroderma is usual and the mortality is almost 50 per cent. An immunological reaction to an insect vector has been proposed.

Pemphigoid

The bullae are subepidermal and acantholysis is not a feature. About 80 per cent of patients are over the age of 60. It is about twice as common as pemphigus. There is a specific antibody (usually IgG) for the basement membrane zone of the epidermis and this is present in about 70 per cent of patients. Complement is bound *in vivo*. The basement membrane remains in the floor of the bullae in most cases.

Clinical features

The initial features of pemphigoid are often non-specific and confusing. It can be eczematous or urticarial. The lesions often begin around a site of damage such as a leg ulcer or burn. After 2 or 3 weeks blisters may erupt abruptly. They favour the flexures and are tense and dome-shaped. They often contain blood. Small blisters in the mouth are rare and tend not to erode as in pemphigus. The patients are distressed by itching, and oedema of the skin may be troublesome, but their general health is usually unaffected.

Treatment

The treatment of choice is prednisolone 60–80 mg daily until there are no new blisters. Azathioprine, methotrexate, dapsone or cylophosphamide may be used to allow a lower maintenance dose of the steroid, since morbidity in the elderly is great. Osteoporosis, gastric ulceration, and diabetes mellitus are particularly common complications of steroid therapy. However, complete remission after 1 year is common.

Cicatricial pemphigoid

The cause of this disorder is unknown and the immunology is unclear. It is also called benign mucosal pemphigoid. Although mortality is low, it is responsible for great discomfort. It is a disease of older adults and the subepidermal bullae favour the mucosa of the mouth, conjunctiva, and the perineal orifices. The base of the lesions are heavily infiltrated with lymphocytes and plasma cells and there is eventual fibrosis. The adhesions that occur between the bulbar and palpebral conjunctiva result in eventual shrinkage, and entropion is followed by blindness. The skin is less often involved and the lesions are sparse and often heal by scarring. The scalp is more often affected than other sites.

Treatment
No treatment is very effective but steroids and azathioprine are usually prescribed.

Dermatitis herpetiformis
This is a vesicobullous disorder associated with the granular deposition of IgA in the dermis and a usually symptomless sub-total villus atrophy of the small intestine. The IgA is believed to be derived from plasma cells in the intestine. As in coeliac disease HLA-A8/DRW 3 is associated and may be responsible for a defective Fc receptor status. It is probable that gluten hypersensitivity results in circulating immune complexes that have an affinity for material in the upper dermis; this is possibly reticulin and the Fc receptor dysfunction impairs the removal by macrophages of the immune material. Histology of the skin shows fibrin, neutrophils, and eosinophils in the dermal papillae.

Clinical features
The eruption is characterized by intensely itchy grouped papular or vesicular lesions that lie on an urticarial or erythematous base. The elbows, knees, sacrum, and shoulders are favoured (see Fig. 8) and the face and scalp are more commonly affected than in the case of pemphigus or pemphigoid. The itchy vesicles are quickly excoriated since this relieves the pruritus. The eruption waxes and wanes sometimes being in remission for many months. However, for most it remains a lifelong disorder.

Treatment
Dapsone 100–200 mg daily or sulphapyridine 0.5 g three times daily are remarkably effective and can be used as a diagnostic test since itchiness is relieved within 48 hours. The maintenance dose should be titrated to suit each patient. It may be as low as 50 mg dapsone weekly. Haemolytic anaemia is common on higher dosage and especially when in some cases 400 mg of dapsone is needed daily to control the eruption. A gluten-free diet rapidly adhered to controls some but not all patients; 70 per cent can omit dapsone after 2 years of such dieting.

Steroid therapy is strangely ineffective and heparin oddly effective. Inorganic arsenicals (Fowler's solution) is effective and was once very popular, and it is probably justified in elderly patients much troubled by the disease and unable to tolerate dapsone or sulphapyridine.

Juvenile bullous pemphigoid
This is a bullous disorder characterized by a predilection for the face and perineum. Linear IgA is deposited on the basement membrane of the epidermis. It is not associated with enteropathy nor with HLA-A8. The response to dapsone, sulphapyridine, or steroids is unpredictable.

Herpes gestationis
This differs from the common toxic erythema of pregnancy in having large blisters, often periumbilical, beginning as a degeneration of the epidermal cells. It is associated with HLA-B8/DR3 and with C3 deposition. It is thus a blister above the basement membrane and it is believed to be due to a specific antibody to the basal cell; it is present in the umbilical cord blood. It occurs during or immediately after pregnancy and usually ceases fairly abruptly

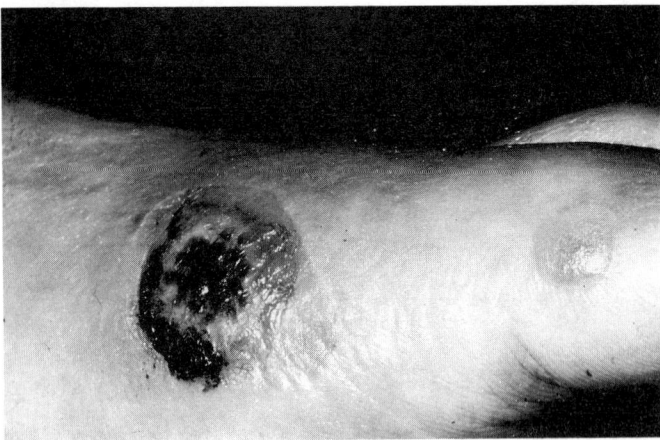

Fig. 105 A haemorrhagic blister on the foot in a patient with diabetes mellitus.

within weeks of parturition. It recurs in subsequent pregnancies or as an effect of oral contraceptives.

Other causes of blistering
Lichen planus and lichen sclerosis et atrophicus both rarely blister. Bullous disease and malignancy are a debated association since so much bullous disease occurs in an age group in which malignancy is common. However, individual case histories of uncontrollable bullous disease with atypical immunofluorescence are impressive.

Trophoneurotic blisters are another debated association. The unconscious patient seems predisposed to produce blisters even at sites not affected by pressure or shearing forces. They are subepidermal. This is an important hazard often causing unjustified accusation of mismanagement in the nursing care of such patients.

Diabetes mellitus is a cause of intraepidermal blisters without immunofluorescent material and showing no acantholysis (Fig. 105).

Vesico-bullous disorders in infancy

Infection
Although infection is the most important cause of bullae in the neonate, such infection is usually contracted during birth. No blisters are seen until at least the second day. However, blisters at birth are described from intrauterine viral infections such as chickenpox or herpes simplex, and it is also seen in congenital syphilis. Blisters at birth are more usually due to genetic disease such as incontinentia pigmenti, mast cell naevi, or epidermolysis bullosa, the latter more often suggesting widespread absence of skin.

From the second-day after birth staphylococcal infections are common and a few days later candidiasis or, in a very sick child, pseudomonas infection may be responsible for blisters. After a few weeks scabies and insect bites should also be considered.

Non-infectious
Milia Forty per cent of full-term infants have scalp, facial, and genital white papules often grouped and not surrounded by erythema. These are inclusions of epithelial products within the epidermis. They are shed after a few days, but they are also seen in adults after any injury causing blistering (Fig. 106).

Erythema toxicum This is an almost inevitable papular red rash of the first five days of life and is characterized by infiltrations of the papules by eosinophils. The trunk is mostly affected.

Transient neonatal pustular melanosis This is commonest in pigmented infants and is initially pustular often at birth, and later develops a scaly collar and thereafter for several weeks there are

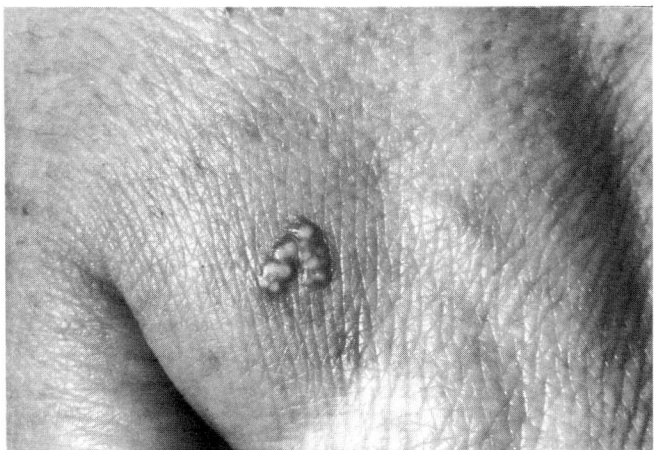

Fig. 106 Milia following a subepidermal blister from a burn.

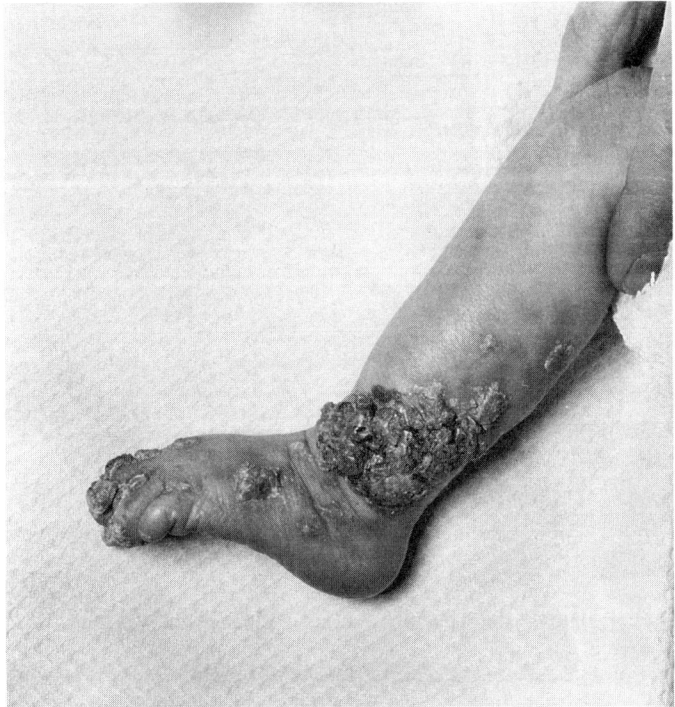

Fig. 107 Incontinentia pigmenti blistering and hyperkeratosis of the leg of a female infant.

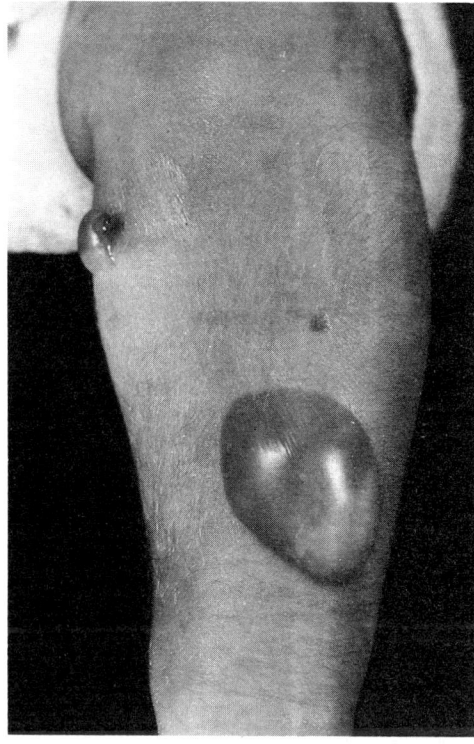

Fig. 108 Blisters on the lower leg of a child with congenital porphyria. Note also the hypertrichosis. The blister occurred following exposure to sunlight.

Epidermolysis bullosa There are several genetic varieties (see elsewhere). Features are widespread areas of absent skin or localized to sites of trauma; blisters may be prominent.

Others Congenital porphyria (Fig. 108), mastocytosis, Letterer–Siwe disease, bullous congenital ichthyosiform erythema, and acrodermatitis enteropathica may all cause blistering.

References

Ahmed, A. R., Graham, J., Jordon, R. E. and Provost, T. T. (1980). Pemiphigus: current concepts. *Ann. intern. Med.* **92**, 396–405.

Alexander, J. O'D. (1975). Dermatitis herpetiformis. In *Major problems in dermatology*, Vol. 4. Lloyd Luke, London.

Journal of Investigative Dermatology (1979). Analysis of research needs and priorities in dermatology. *J. invest. Dermatol.* **73**, Suppl.

Lever, W. F. and Schaumburg-Lever, G. (1984). Treatment of pemphigus vulgaris: results obtained in 84 patients between 1981 and 1982. *Arch. Dermatol.* **120**, 44–47.

Sneddon, I. B. (1980). Bullous eruptions. In *Textbook of dermatology*, 3rd edn (eds A. Rook, D. S. Wilkinson, and F. J. G. Ebling), pp. 1441–1481. Blackwell Scientific Publications, Oxford.

Timlin, D. *et al* (1983). Clues to the aetiology and pathogenesis of herpes gestation. *Br. J. Dermatol.* **109**, 131–139.

hyperpigmented macules. No infectious organism has been isolated.

Infantile acropustulosis Also affects pigmented children and its cause is unknown. It is pruritic and sometimes vesicular and usually affects infants aged 2–10 months. It mostly responds to dapsone 2 mg/kg per day.

Miliaris crystallina There are clear very superficial and small vesicles occurring without inflammation but as a consequence of sweating. They may be seen when the child is overheated from fever or climate, and affect the flexures, face and scalp.

Incontinentia pigmenti This is lethal to males *in utero* amd therefore presents in the neonatal girl. There are crops of inflammatory bullae (Fig. 107), often bizarre in pattern, and accompanied or followed by epidermal hyperplasia and disturbance of pigmentation. Nail, hair, eye, skeletal, and CNS changes are common.

ABNORMAL VASCULARITY OF THE SKIN, ANGIOMA, AND TELANGIECTASIA

Patterns of blood vessel development that are inappropriate for the needs of the skin or for thermoregulation include both overgrowth and atrophy. An excess of capillary and venular vessels is a characteristic of wound healing and of many hyperproliferative conditions of the skin such as psoriasis. These usually present as redness and individual vessels cannot be seen by the naked eye. Proliferation is still more extreme in strawberry haemangioma, granuloma telangiectaticum, also known as pyogenic granuloma, and in certain malignancies such as Kaposi's sarcoma or angio-endothelioma.

On the other hand, telangiectasia is characterized by the dilatation of individual capillaries or venules so that they are visible to the naked eye. There is little evidence that the endothelial cell is at fault and it is more likely that the basic defect is an atrophy or loss of supporting tissue.

Proliferative vasculature is more unstable than that observed in telangiectasia and the natural history is to resolve, often completely. Vessels and wounds or angiomas are vulnerable and the growing phase may be associated with necrosis as a result of thrombosis secondary to injury to the surface of the skin. Telangiectasia on the other hand has no tendency to thrombose and the overlying skin rarely ulcerates. The natural history of such dilated vessels is to persist until extreme old age when they may be partially absorbed.

Strawberry naevi

These are almost never present at birth but may be preceded by a small area of blanching observed at birth. From a few days after birth the lesion consists of nests of granulation tissue which proliferate rapidly. After a few weeks the rate of growth becomes less rapid and some vessels become dilated and cavernous. A stable period of no growth often occurs from about 9 months to about 1 year, after which gradual absorption by fibrosis is to be expected. Management consists of reassurance of the parents and emphasis on satisfactory natural resolution (Fig. 109).

Exceptions to this policy include involvement of the eyelid interfering with sight, in which case plastic surgery may be advised. Some large haemangiomata sequester platelets giving rise to a bleeding tendency (the Kassabach–Merrick syndrome). High-dose steroids (3 mg/kg) are life saving. On withdrawal, rebound overgrowth may be observed, justifying a second or third course. Ulceration of the haemangioma is common especially in the nappy area and when there is a primary irritant rash. Bleeding is easily controlled by light pressure. The ulceration often accelerates resolution.

Sometimes haemangiomata have a deep element in which arteriovenous shunts are a complication. Interference with underlying structures is not common but joint involvement warrants surgical advice and management.

Treatment of haemangiomata has included radiotherapy, more recently systemic steroids, pressure pads, excision and, currently, embolization. The latter requires angiographic control and siting of sclerosing adhesives at the appropriate site.

Port wine naevi

This is a pattern of vascular birth mark present at birth and usually segmental. It is unwise to make a prognosis at birth because pale naevi and segmental patterns of erythema may look similar and often fade. The majority of port wine naevi persist for life. Arteriovenous shunts and gravitational stasis often cause some increase in the vasculature in adult life. The nape of the neck is a site in which a pale plaque of macular telangiectasia is present in the majority of normal babies and persists in more than one half of those affected.

Variants of port wine naevi affecting deeper vasculature range from the Klippel–Trelawney disorder causing enlargement of the limb, to a reticulate and more atrophic pattern associated sometimes with the shortening of the limb. There are developmental patterns of widespread segmental telangiectasia with which asymmetrical gigantisism and disturbances of pigment are associated.

Telangiectasia

Telangiectases are enduring dilatations of blood vessels. They are usually less than 1 mm in length and may be point-like or punctate, linear, starlike, spider, or stellate, forming flat, square,

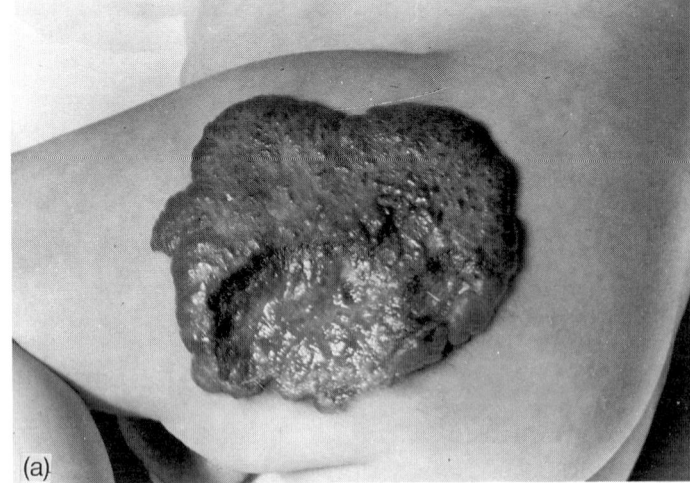

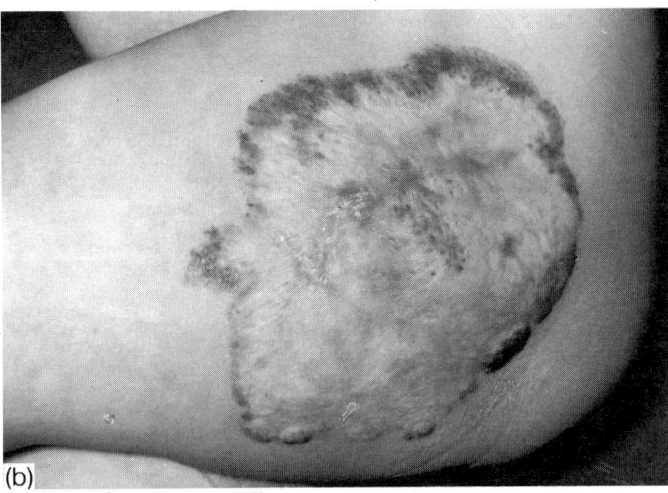

Fig. 109 'Strawberry' naevus; (a) a proliferative but benign neoplasia which after a rapid phase of new growth, stabilizes, and eventually regresses. The lesions often ulcerate if traumatized. In this case ulceration has hastened resolution but the residual scarring (b) is more than usual.

oblong, or oval plaques, or mat-like with an eccentric punctum. They blanch completely when they are compressed. Telangiectasia is not new-vessel formation – indeed new vessels in wounds are not unduly dilated.

Telangiectases are probably always secondary to mesenchymal connective tissue dysplasia but can be congenital and naevoid, acquired and genetic, i.e. familial or hereditary, as well as secondary to 'collagen' disease such as lupus erythematosus, scleroderma, or dermatomyositis, or from radiation damage.

All dilatations of small vessels are made worse by blushing, as is seen in rosacea, carcinoid, or due to oestrogen and related hormonal imbalances as in pregnancy or liver disease. They are also made worse by loss of supporting tissue as in steroid atrophy, solar elastosis, ageing (Fig. 110), or Cushing's syndrome.

Telangiectasia is often associated with increased melanin pigmentation and brown spots may be predominant, even in hereditary haemorrhagic telangiectasia, but poikiloderma is a typical example of atrophy, telangiectasia and pigmentation. Some telangiectasia may be insufficiently dilated to be recognized by the naked eye, and if affecting most of the vessels in an affected area, they may appear as a persistent erythema, for instance, the red cheeks of young children, or some capillary naevi affecting the eyelids, nape of the neck, or forehead known as salmon patches or stork bites. The erythema may be pale pink or deep purple. The darker the lesion the more likely the dilated vessels will be in-high incidence of telangiectasia of up to 40 per cent affecting the trunk is described in aluminium workers. It seems to be associated with the electrolytic processing used in the industry.

Diffuse and acquired patterns of telangiectasia are commonly familial but sporadic cases account for about 20 per cent even in the well known hereditary haemorrhagic telangiectasia. A benign variety of this disease is not associated with severe bleeding and is also probably dominant. Telangiectasia confined to the lips may also present a dominant pattern of inheritance. However, no large scale study has been done to rule out polygenic inheritance in any of these disorders. The haemorrhagic diathesis has been recorded as a dominant gene and many large pedigrees have been described, but even so, 10 per cent of probands with telangiectasia do not bleed. Severe epistaxis and severe bleeding after tooth extraction or cuts and even heavy menstrual bleeding are characteristic of hereditary haemorrhagic telangiectasia. Minor but frequent nose bleeds are common with even the benign forms. Arteriovenous shunts are described commonly in association with hereditary haemorrhagic telangiectasia. They result in pulsating nodules of the skin, and in the lung or brain may have severe consequences. They are occasionally seen in the non-haemorrhagic telangiectatic forms of the disease.

Histology

The dilated vessels are unremarkable but special studies have helped to show that the vessels are venules, i.e. alkaline phosphatase negative, and they secrete generous amounts of plasminogen activator. Supporting tissue and overlying epidermis is usually atrophic.

Treatment

Telangiectases are easy to camouflage with 'covermark' type of preparations but advice may need to be given on its application with respect to the use of cream and powder, blends, and matching of skin colour.

Telangiectases when small and localized can be destroyed by cryotherapy, cautery, electrolysis, or laser therapy. The latter can be endoscopic. The laser specifically burns haemoglobin and it is therefore more successful in the treatment of the larger blood containing dilatations. Sclerotherapy is also possible.

Bleeding should first be treated by the simple first aid measure of elevation and local pressure. Cautery is most effective only on a dry blanched area controlled by compression. Patients can be taught to inflate a lubricated finger cot tied over the end of a small catheter for the immediate control of severe epistaxis.

Oestrogen therapy

Oestrogen therapy is sometimes advocated, e.g. ethinyloestradiol 0.25 mg daily, and increased to 0.5 mg per day at the end of 4 weeks if epistaxis continues. However, its effectiveness is unproven by controlled trials.

Percutaneous embolization

This is increasingly used to close unwanted vasculature but it requires careful angiographic control and skilled surgeons and has not overcome the problem of rapid recanalization and opening up of collaterals. It is nevertheless the treatment of choice for severe uncontrolled bleeding from arteriovenous shunts.

Investigations

Bleeding and clotting times are mostly normal but special studies of factor VIII or local fibrinolysis and of platelet aggregation may show dysfunction. Skin thickness studies may show some thinning. The tourniquet test has been advocated as a useful test of the haemorrhagic variant in persons with telangiectasis.

Prophylaxis

Sun, cold, or gravitational stasis all enhance telangiectasia. Bleeding is often first noted after tooth extraction. Alcoholic excesses

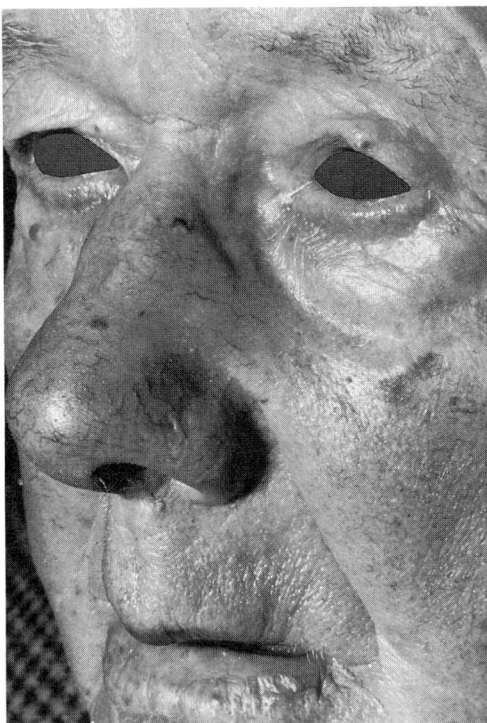

Fig. 110 Ageing is accentuated in light-exposed skins. One feature of ageing is poor collagen support of skin vasculature. Telangiectasia is a common consequence.

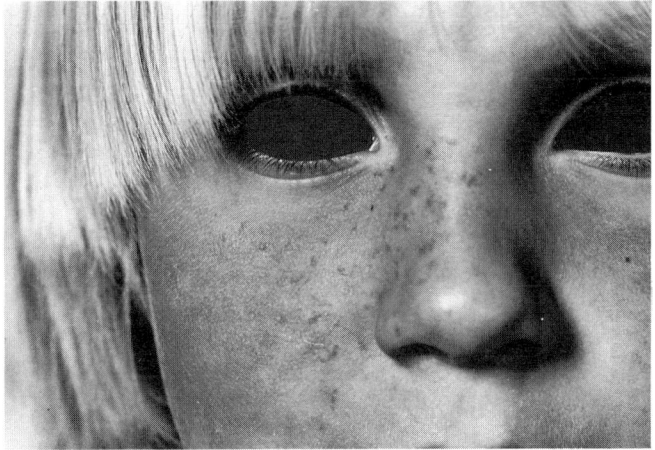

Fig. 111 Segmental telangiectasia of punctate-spider naevoid type.

homogeneous and some will be visible to the naked eye. Naevoid lesions usually affect well defined segments of the skin, though not necessarily dermatomal or unilateral (Fig. 111). The best known are naevi affecting the trigeminal nerve (Sturge–Weber) or sometimes an entire limb.

Diffuse polymorphic patterns that develop in childhood or in young adults favour exposed areas such as the face and forearms, probably because sunlight exaggerates connective tissue dysplasia. However, haemodynamic factors such as gravitational stasis of the venous system also play a part, and the distribution of spider naevi may depend on drainage into the superior vena cava. Gravitational stasis particularly determines the patterns of stellate and arborizing telangiectasia on the legs. Five per cent of the population has two to ten telangiectases on the lip, fingers, palms, and soles, and these sites may be involved by grosser patterns of telangiectasia in disease. Dermatomal or unilateral patterns are rare. A

and the ingestion of aspirin and other prostaglandin inhibitors may precipitate the bleeding problem.

Facial erythema (flushing)

In temperate climates the weather-beaten face of the farmer, or fisherman is largely a reflection of exposure to cold as are the rosy cheeks and shiny morning face of the school child. The 'butterfly' area of the cheeks and bridge of the nose are sites which pick up thermal irradiation whether hot or cold. Marked telangiectasia of the cheeks in adults is a common consequence of rosy cheeks in childhood. It may be associated with thickening of the subcutaneous tissues.

Rosacea is usually associated with acneiform pustulation and lymphoedema. For unknown reasons a keratitis is sometimes associated. A somewhat similar appearance may be seen in sarcoid, especially the lupus pernio variety in which a diffuse granuloma underlies dilated blood vessels filled with slow flowing blue blood. Mitral or pulmonary stenosis also causes a persistent malar flush. In discoid lupus erythematosus, telangiectasia (Fig. 112a) is accompanied by atrophy (Fig. 112b), often with well defined margins and follicular plugging. The borders of the lesions of rosacea and sarcoid tend to be more diffuse. Asymmetry can be a feature of all disorders.

Telangiectasia due to other collagen diseases varies from the redness and oedema of the orbit characteristic of dermatomyositis (Fig. 113) to erythema of the backs of the hands and nailfolds with persistent erythema such that vessels become increasingly inhomogeneous, and quite large dilated forms may be observed.

In scleroderma, especially of the adult acrosclerotic variety, telangiectasia in the form of flat macules often with square or oblong shapes and fairly well-defined margins, are characteristic.

Systemic sclerosis of the face usually causes stiffness and tethering of the skin to deeper structures over the nose and loss of suppleness in the perioral skin. There is of course, the associated Raynaud's phenomenon and digital ischaemia.

A plethoric complexion is a feature of superior vena cava obstruction but also of polycythaemia rubra vera and Cushing's syndrome.

Flushing of the face is a common complaint particularly in the young who may suffer from transient blushing, and in the older age groups it is characterized by persistent rosacea. Carcinoid should be thought of when there is a prolonged blush associated with a bounding pulse, asthma, abdominal pain, and diarrhoea. Frequent applications of steroids to the face for atopic or seborrhoeic eczema produces gross diffuse telangiectasia and there is often rebound eczematous changes on withdrawal (Fig. 114) and the irritation may be severe. The treatment of this condition is complete withdrawal of all steroids until after 3–4 weeks when the condition tends to settle.

DISORDERS OF COLLAGEN AND ELASTIC TISSUE

The metabolism and diseases of collagen are described in Section 16. The fundamental defects are in its chemical structure, its cross linkage between fibres, and its distribution and quantity.

Signs of collagen disease

These include:

1. Diminished skin thickness and increased transparency so that deeper structures such as veins and nerves are visible and the sclerae are blue.

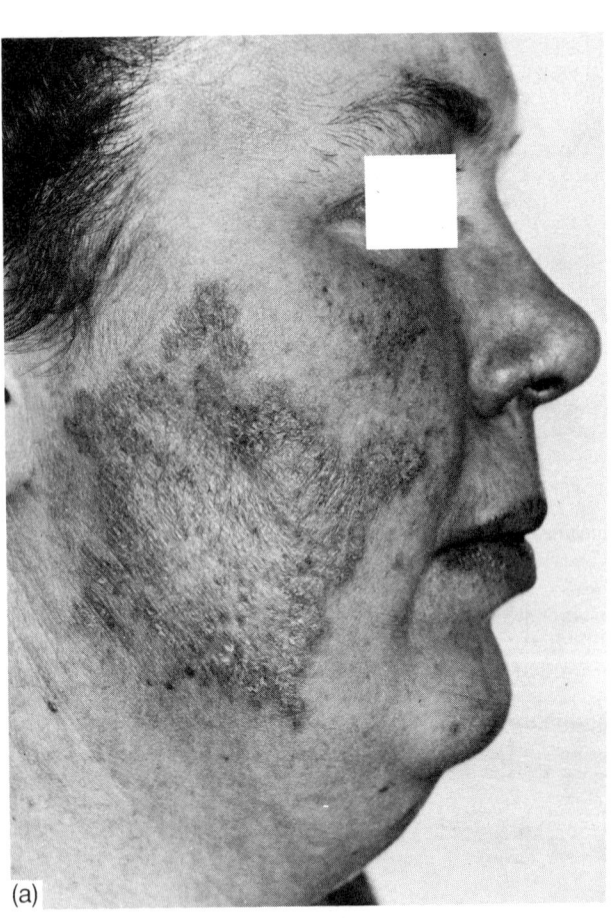 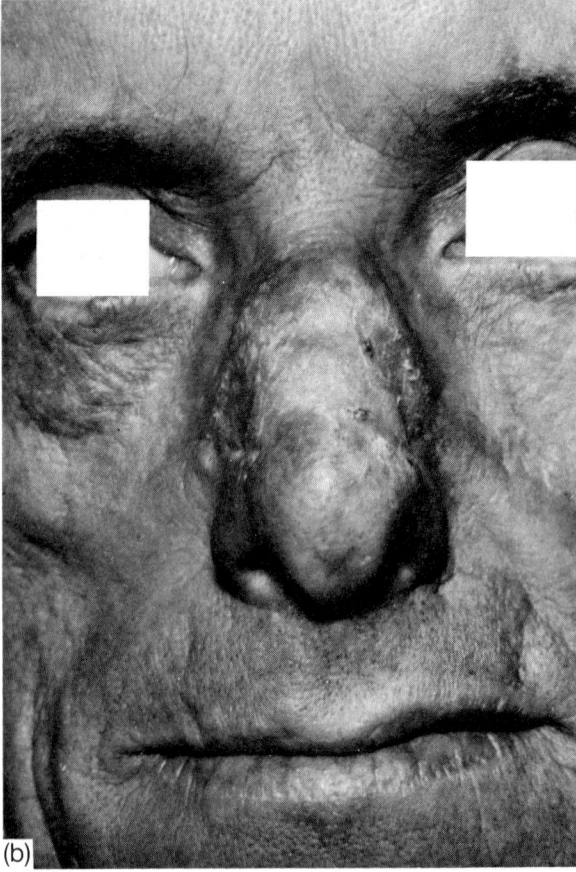

(a) (b)

Fig. 112 In lupus erythematosus – chronic discoid type – (a) telangiectasia and (b) erythema are common. There is follicular plugging and destruction of the skin resulting in pigment loss and scarring.

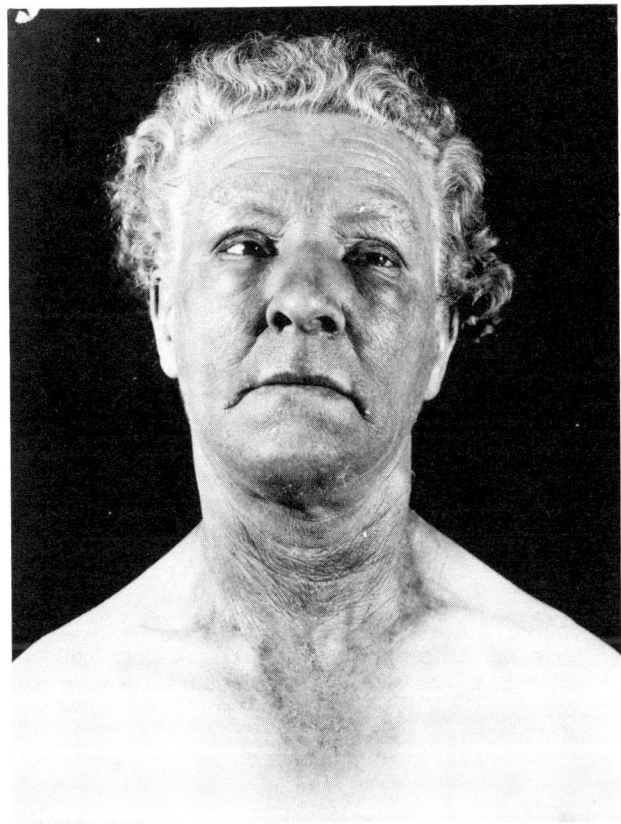

Fig. 113 Bright erythema and oedema of the face, especially periorbitally, is characteristic of dermatomyositis.

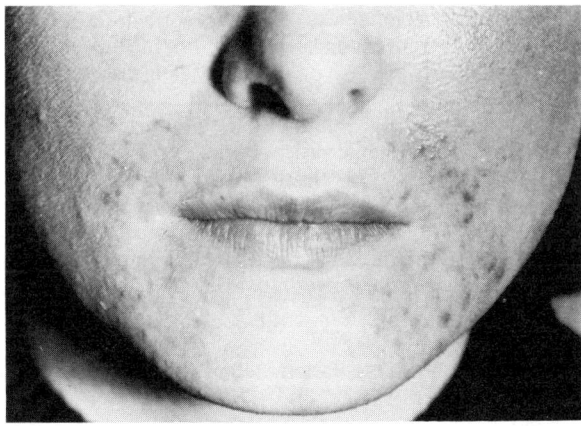

Fig. 114 Perioral dermatitis is a common consequence of the application of fluorinated steroids to the face.

2. Diminished resistance to shear so that the skin splits and tears sometimes even without surface breaks. Purpura is usually associated and healing results in white stellate scars. Cutaneous striae are another pattern of stretching of the skin with separation in this case. Diminished resistance of the skin is a feature of age; osteoporosis and rheumatoid arthritis are other recognized associations. Steroids are responsible for both stellate scars and cutaneous striae and this is the case whether they are endogenously produced, as in Cushing's disease, or prescribed for other diseases. Local application of steroid cream is probably now the commonest cause of these changes.

3. Laxity is the failure of the skin to return rapidly to its former state after distortion by stretch. It is in some way caused by degeneration of elastic tissue but changes in water content and cellularity as well as increased cross-linkage of collagen play some part even when the total collagen is reduced.

Diseases due to defective collagen

Solar and senile elastosis

This affects white races and especially those employed in agricultural or marine work. Chronic exposure to ultraviolet radiation causes abnormal collagen which has the histological staining characteristics of elastic tissue but not its properties. It is broken and aggregated and contributes to a thickened, yellow, wrinkled skin, especially on the exposed areas in old age. The yellow plaques may be sharply marginated on the face. In the neck, deep furrows form a rhomboidal network. The sebaceous glands and ducts are poorly supported, dilated, and patulous forming giant comedones. On the neck the goose pimple or plucked bird appearance is due to the protection provided by hair follicles shading the dermis against ultraviolet rays. Colloid milium is the abnormal production of a scleroprotein by fibroblasts giving rise to yellowish translucent papules or plaque in light-exposed skin. It may begin in childhood.

Striae

These are common but imperfectly understood; stretch is always a factor. The epidermis is thin and elastic fibres are scanty. Striae are seen on the back and thighs of adolescents during growth, especially when there has been a spurt and the child is athletic. It occurs more in girls than in boys. Striae are a feature of pregnancy and affect especially the abdomen and breasts. This is usually due to excessive adrenocortical activity. Incomplete inhibition of fibroblasts causes atrophy of collagen in response to glucocorticoids. When the collagen is ageing or degenerate as follows irradiation or in diseases such as cutis laxa or Ehlers–Danlos syndrome, striae are uncommon and may not appear even in the pregnant or those with Cushing's syndrome. Striae have also been described in chronic infections such as tuberculosis. They are a diagnostic problem only when they are newly formed in which case they may appear to be weal-like and raised. Later they flatten and become bluish-red and still later, white and depressed.

Localized fibrosis, keloids, and hypertrophic scars

The connective tissue response to cutaneous injury exceeds the limits of the needs for repair appropriate to the degree of injury at that site. This is commonly so a few weeks after injury and gives rise to hypertrophic scars. If the scar continues to hypertrophy and extends beyond the limits of the site of the injured skin, especially after a period of 3 months, since the injury, then it is often termed a keloid. Such scars tend to be more tender than hypertrophic scars. Keloids tend to be familial and are commoner in negroes. They are rare in infancy and old age and tend to be less severe after the age of 30. Significant factors are the presence of foreign material in the wound and tension. Preferred areas are the ear lobes, chin, neck shoulders, upper trunk, and lower legs. Keloids in their early stages may respond to strong local steroids applied locally or intralesionally. Compression therapy is sometimes helpful as is cryotherapy in the early stages. Most would now prefer re-excision and radiotherapy to the edges of the wounds.

Ainhum

This is a relatively common disease in negroes and in Africa especially. Recurrent or chronic fissuring of the digitoplantar fold is followed by fibrosis in the form of a constricting band around the base of the digit (Fig. 115). The peak age of incidence is 30–50 years. The most common digit to be affected is the fifth toe.

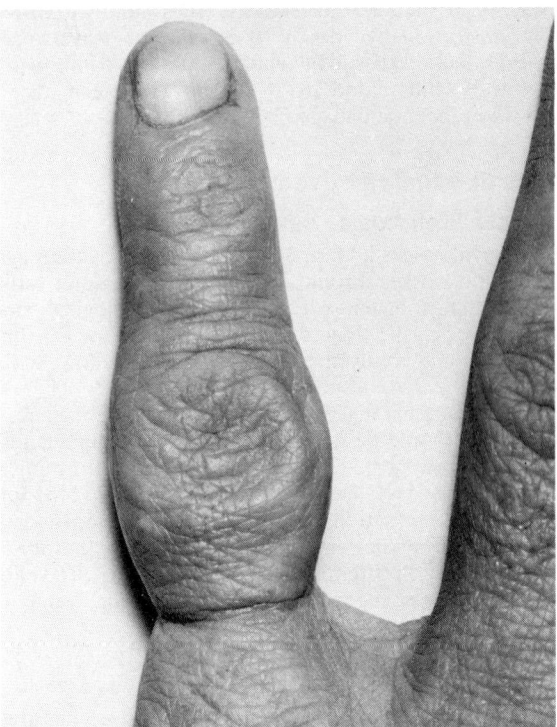

Fig. 115 Constricting band of sclerosis around the finger – Ainhum.

Plastic induration of the penis (Peyronie's disease)

A plaque of firm, fibrous tissue causing painful curvature during erection may be associated with fibrous pads of the hands and feet as well as Dupuytren's contracture.

Werner's disease, Ehlers–Danlos syndrome, cutis laxa, and Marfan's syndrome are described elsewhere.

Pseudoxanthoma elasticum

This is a hereditary disorder of elastic tissue; there are four distinct types:

Dominant type I

Small yellowish papules forming linear or reticulate plaques, which in older persons are soft, lax, and hang in folds, are flexually distributed especially in the groins, axillae and neck (Fig. 116). There is a severe degeneration of Bruch's membrane giving rise to the slate-grey, poorly defined 'angioid' streaks forming an incomplete ring or radiating lesions around the optic disc of the retina. There is early blindness. Vascular complications include intermittent claudication and coronary artery disease.

Dominant type II

The small yellowish papules are fewer and flatter. There is increased extensibility of the skin. The vascular and retinal changes are mild. The sclera is blue and there may be a high arched palate and myopia.

Recessive type I

This resembles dominant type I but the vascular and retinal degeneration is mild. Haematemesis is especially common and women are more often affected than men.

Recessive type II

This is a very rare form but the skin changes are extensive and generalized. There tends to be no systemic complications. The pathology of pseudoxanthoma elasticum includes a deposition of calcium on the elastic fibres. The mid-dermal elastic tissue is fragmented and swollen.

Perforating elastoma

This is a condition of elastic fibres degeneration in the upper dermis with a resulting foreign body reaction and extrusion through the overlying epidermis. This reaction gives rise to papules which develop a central plaque of extruded material. There is a tendency for the formation of annular and serpiginous patterns particularly over the back and neck region. The disorder is associated with mongolism, Marfan syndrome, Ehlers–Danlos syndrome, pseudoxanthoma elasticum, and osteogenesis imperfecta.

Ehlers–Danlos syndrome: cutis hyperelastica

Ehlers–Danlos syndrome (see Section 17) is a rare inherited disorder of connective tissue. Eight varieties are recognized, four are clearly dominant and one is X-chromosome linked. The condition is usually recognized when the child begins to walk since there is hyperextensibility of the joints. Trivial cuts form gaping wounds and heal poorly. The skin feels soft and can be stretched particularly over the knees and elbows. Arterial rupture, aortic dissection, and intestinal perforation have been described in severely affected individuals.

Cutis laxa

This is a rare disease in which the skin hangs in loose folds owing to loss of elastic tissue. Severely affected individuals have associated pulmonary emphysema. There are both dominant and recessive forms of heredity (Fig. 117).

ATROPHY

Atrophy is characterized by thinning, loss of elasticity, loss of hair follicles, and a smooth surface to the skin. When pinched gently the skin produces fine wrinkles and may be compared to tissue paper. The upper dermal atrophy causes poor support to an atrophic vasculature and telangiectasia is often observed. At the same time there tends to be increased pigmentation within the dermis. Atrophy may be a consequence of inflammation following acute bacterial (particularly elastase producing organisms) infection vasculitis or pancreatitis. It may be widespread as in the chronic scarring of leprosy or onchocerciasis. Some circumscribed atrophies follow an urticarial vasculitic process which is probably due to an infection which destroys elastic tissue. Perifollicular atrophy or postacne atrophy is similarly due to strains of staphylococcus which produces elastase. Syphilis is another cause of destruction of elastic tissue. Non-infectious causes include lupus erythematosus and localized scleroderma with its variants.

Poikiloderma

The combination of pigmentation, telangiectasia and atrophy is known as poikiloderma (see Fig. 128). The causes of poikiloderma include irradiation, lymphoma, and collagen diseases such as lupus erythematosus and dermatomyositis. There is a congenital form associated with light sensitivity, skin cancers, and dwarfism. It may follow lichen planus or stasis eczema. It is common on the neck in the light-exposed area and may be aggravated by cosmetics. It is also described in graft-versus-host diseases.

Deep dermal and subcutaneous atrophy

The skin loses its subcutaneous or deep dermal tissue in a number of conditions. Such skin is waxy in colour and may be yellow, pigmented, or bluish with a loss of connective tissue. Deeper vessels may become more obvious so that there is either telangiectasia or obvious cutaneous atrophy and linear stretch marks which are initially red and sometimes protrude above the surface of the skin, but later there is always marked atrophy.

The skin that is atrophic may be tethered to underlying tissue or

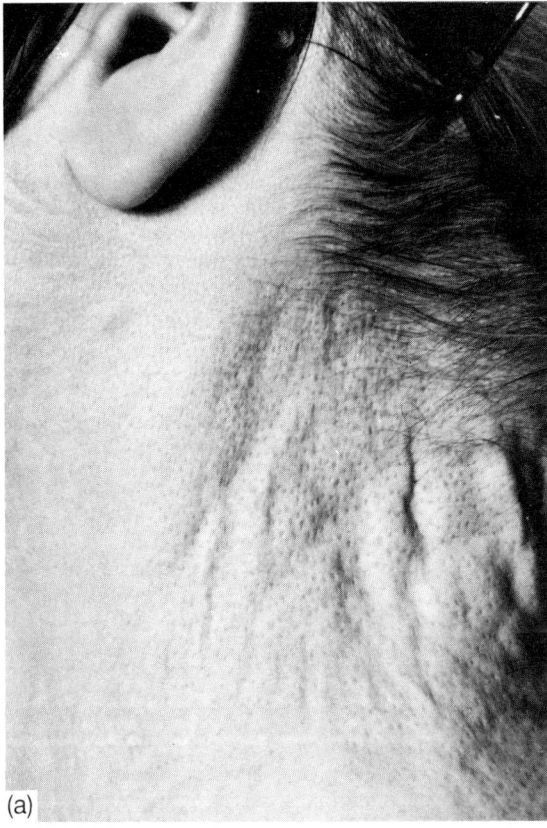
(a)

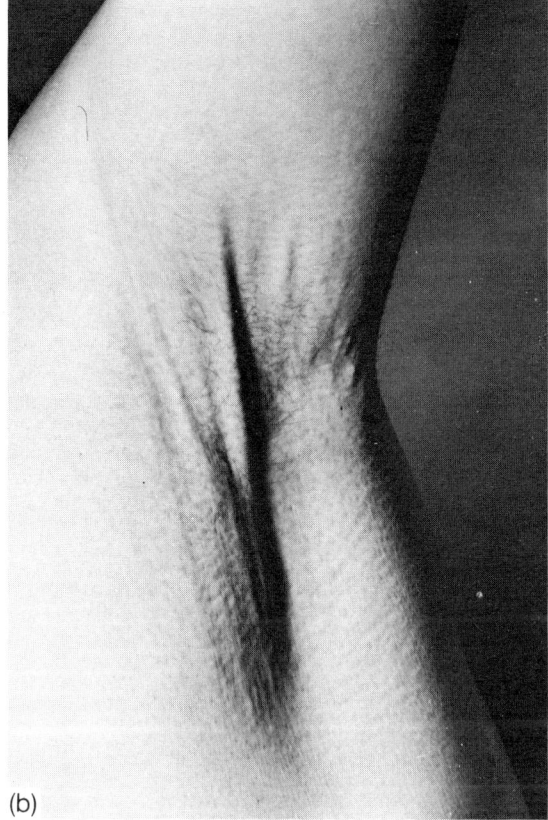
(b)

Fig. 116 (a) and (b) Yellowish papules and loss of elasticity of the skin of the neck and axillae in pseudoxanthoma elasticum. This may be a clue to gastrointestinal bleeding or even blindness.

more obviously scarred. Such skin may feel hard or sclerosed (Table 27).

Morphea

Morphea is a localized form of scleroderma with a good prognosis for complete recovery (Fig. 119). It is not associated with any systemic disease. Occasionally a generalized form produces such tightness of the chest wall that breathing may be impaired. The generalized form of morphea also greatly restricts the limbs and a combination of ischaemia and lymphoedema may result in ulceration of the peripheries.

Other causes of deep dermal atrophy include injection of insulin – this is commonly seen on the thighs or arms of diabetics. Anetoderma is a term used for very discrete round idiopathic losses of dermis. Focal dermal hypoplasia is a rare cause of pitted skin usually observed first at birth and associated with eye and bone defects as well as perioral papillomas (Fig. 120).

Hemi- or generalized atrophy of non-inflammatory origin is mainly of unknown aetiology. Partial lipodystrophy is associated with glomerulonephritis and hypocomplementaemia. The Lawrence–Seip syndrome or total lipoatrophy (with acanthosis nigricans, genital hypertrophy, resistant diabetes, and hepatomegaly) is a condition affecting infants. Atrophie blanche (Fig. 121) is an obliteration of single capillaries in the upper dermis leading to very localized scarring. The causes are listed in Table 28.

MALIGNANT DISEASE

Infiltrations of the skin presenting as papules, *peau d'orange*, nodules, plaques, or ulcerating tumours of the dermis with destruction of overlying epidermis are a common terminal event of malignancy. Such lesions may arise from localized spread as from a carcinoma of the breast and they tend thus to be single or grouped and asymmetrical. More widespread haematogenous spread but with multiple lesions are a still more common terminal event. Certain metastases have diagnostic features and they include the scarring alopecia of breast carcinoma affecting the scalp or the pedunculated tumour of hypernephroma.

In many parts of the world with a high incidence of skin tumours both heredity and environment are determining factors and early diagnosis is rare. Whereas basal cell carcinomas are the predominant skin cancer in the white skin, Africans have a relatively high incidence of squamous carcinoma. Albinism and scarring following burns or other injuries are the main predisposing factors. Malignant melanoma in the African or the black American is especially a tumour of the feet. There is some evidence that a genetic increase in the number of junctional naevi in the lightly pigmented skin of the foot is a factor. In general, sunlight exposure accounts for the incidence of malignant melanoma in white skins and exposed areas of skin are most affected.

Factors favouring malignancy

1. The chronic ingestion of inorganic arsenic. This was at one time given as a tonic for anaemia, often as Fowler's solution. It was combined with bromides for epilepsy or chorea and specifically for psoriasis and blistering disorders. It is still prescribed in many parts of the world although almost obsolete in the UK and USA. Arsenical contamination of water supplies is recorded in Argentina and Taiwan. It has also been used in arsenical fruit sprays or sheep dips in Europe, and there have been descriptions of contamination of dust in the mines of various parts of the world. Keratoses of the palms and soles are usually persistent and are small, 1–3 mm in diameter, round, and hard. Keratoses are one of the few conditions diagnosed by the shaking of the hand. They may progress to squamous carcinoma and should be removed if ulcerated, indurated, or inflamed. Bowen's disease and basal epithelio-

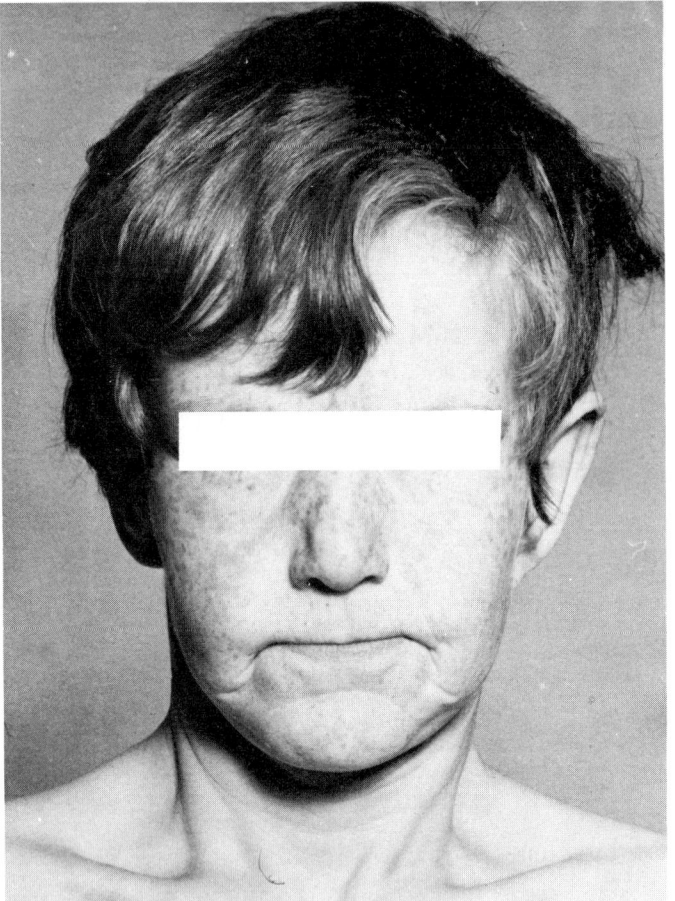

Fig. 117 A 9-year-old boy is showing drooping of the skin of the face due to premature loss of elasticity. The diagnosis is cutis laxa.

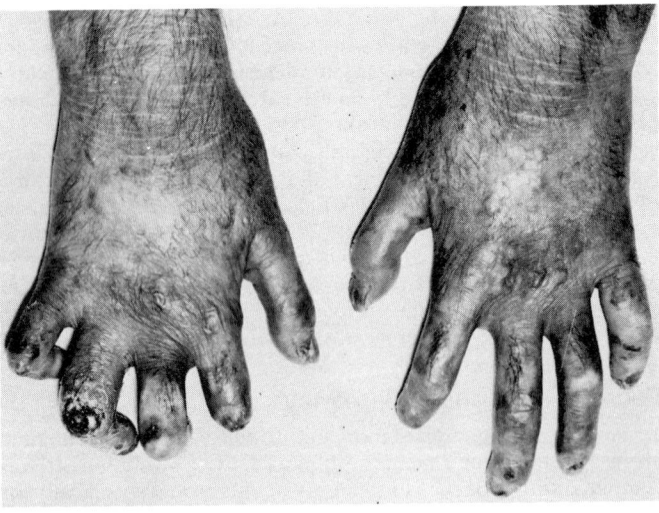

Fig. 118 Scleroderma and loss of finger tissue in porphyria. Hirsuties is also a feature.

mas (Fig. 122) of the trunk are much commoner in chronic arsenically exposed persons. It is a persistent, flat, red, scaly or crusted and pigmented lesion with the features of an intraepidermal carcinoma. Arsenical pigmentation is characterized by a raindrop appearance of areas of paler skin.

2. Skin contact. Prolonged contact on moist skin, such as the scrotum, with coal, soot, and cutting oils may cause malignancy.

Table 27 Conditions causing sclerosis

Scleroderma
Dermatomyositis
Eosinophilic fasciitis (Schulman's syndrome) This resembles scleroderma but the onset of oedema and induration of the extremities is accompanied by eosinophilia
Scleromyxoedema (lichen myxoedematosus) A deposition of mucin associated with a paraprotein, an abnormal lambda light chain affecting face, limbs with thickened skin and exaggeration of natural contours or ridges, and flexion of the fingers. The deposition is papular and often linear
Progeria Associated with alopecia and bird-like facies as well as arteriosclerosis
Porphyria cutanea tarda The scleroderma is associated with hypertrichosis, skin fragility, blistering and scarring in light exposed areas (Figs 29, 108, and 118)
Grafst-versus-host reactions A history of bone marrow or thymus transplant precedes the lichenoid rash and scleroderma
Carcinoid disease and mast cell disorders The release of serotonin and histamine over a prolonged period is sometimes associated with fibroblast proliferation and sclerosis
Pseudoscleroderma This is due to infiltration occurring in amyloid, breast carcinoma, leprosy, lipoid proteinosis, mucopolysaccharide storage disorders, myxoedema. Thickening of the tissues is a feature of acromegaly
Scorbutic pseudoscleroderma In the Bantu this is described as smooth, very dark skin, tightly stretched and hard on the lower aspects of the legs. It has abnormal iron pigment in histological material

3. Radiation. Radiation, especially from ultraviolet B (290–330 nm), is the commonest factor predispoing to skin cancer and explains its high incidence in Australia, Texas, and South Africa. Glass and thick water vapour are protective. Pigmentation by melanin is the natural protective factor. Albinos are more likely to develop carcinoma of the skin. Ionizing radiation explains the high incidence of carcinoma in the skin of the careless practitioner or research worker using irradiated materials. It is a common cause of baldness following X-ray atrophy in persons treated in the past for tinea capitis or ankylosing spondylitis.

4. Radiant heat. Radiant heat sufficient to produce chronic erythema and pigmentation predisposes to squamous epithelioma as from the fire brick of the Kangri cancer of Kashmir or the hot water bottle of the chronically discomforted.

5. Scars. Scars from any chronic disease such as lupus vulgaris (Fig. 123), syphilis, burns, epidermolysis bullosa, or leprosy, or even from common stasis ulcer of the skin may all produce malignant change.

6. Lymphoedema. Lymphoedema predisposes to angiosarcomas, a phenomenon described in post-mastectomy limbs but also in congenital lymphoedema.

7. Genetic syndromes. These are rare but distinctive. *Gorlin's* syndrome results from an autosomal dominant gene and is characterized by dental cysts, hypertelorism, palmar and plantar pits, bifid ribs, and a great tendency to develop basal cell epitheliomata. The palmar pits are flat, being 1–3 mm with a stellate edge. Pseudohypoparathyroidism and medullary blastomas are recorded.

Torre's syndrome This is a condition with multiple sebaceous adenomas and multiple primary malignant tumours of the viscera.

Xeroderma pigmentosum This is a recessively transmitted group of diseases characterized by the progressive development of freckling, telangiectasia, and skin tumours (see page 20.20).

Peutz–Jegher's syndrome This is discussed elsewhere. There is perioral and finger freckling associated with small intestinal polyps and only occasional malignancy.

Gardner's syndrome This is also a condition of polyposis of the gut, combined with osteomas.

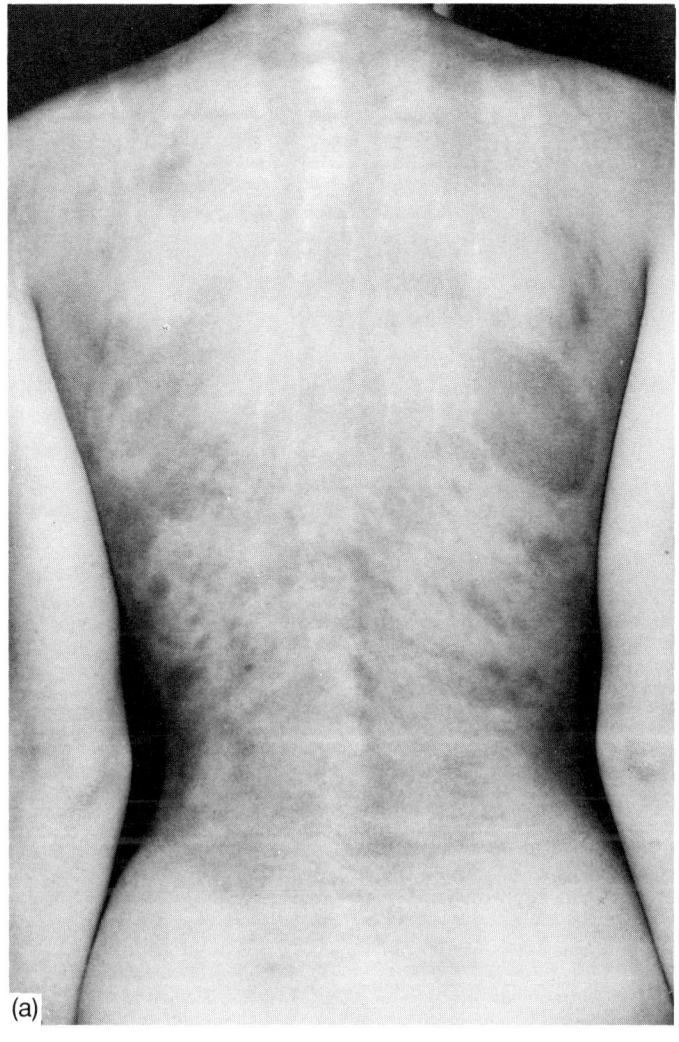

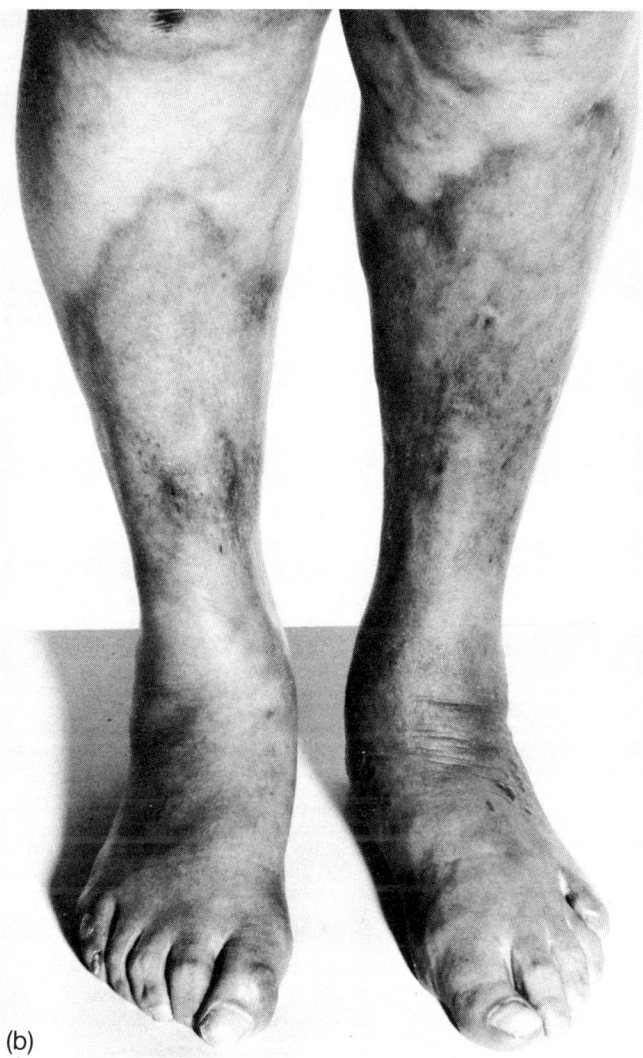

Fig. 119 (a) Widespread hardness of the skin and brownish or violaceous plaques that are often atrophic are features of morphea – a localized form of scleroderma. (b) Pseudoscleroderma, identical to morphea, is also a consequence of post-thrombophlebitic fibrosis of the lower limbs.

Neurocutaneous syndromes These include the acoustic neuromas of neurofibromatosis or phaeochromocytoma in the same disorder.

Tuberous sclerosis Here there is an increased incidence of rhabdomyosarcoma.

8. Immunosuppression. There is an increased incidence of the skin malignancy in the immunosuppressed. After renal transplantation, warts, keratoses, and skin cancer are common especially in light-exposed skin.

Signs of underlying malignancy

The three 'P's of pallor, pigmentation, and pruritus are common terminal events in malignant disease but any one can also be a presenting sign. Defective immunosurveillance predisposes to infections such as candidiasis or herpes simplex and herpes zoster. Disseminated intravascular coagulation is a common terminal event of malignancy but may be a presenting sign of lymphoma, leukaemia, or carcinoma of the pancreas. Rarer diseases associated with malignancy include:

1. Acquired ichthyosis in which the skin becomes progressively drier and more scaly. The surface stratum corneum may crack giving rise to reactive patterns of eczema craquelé (Fig. 124). Increasing scale eventually overlaps with exfoliative dermatitis but unlike the exfoliative dermatitis due to drugs or psoriasis the scale

is more adherent, i.e. less exfoliative. There is usually accompanying atrophy of the skin.

2. Dermatomyositis is commonly caused by malignancy in the white adult. In children or in black Africans it is more often a manifestation of autoimmune (collagen) disease. The muscle weakness is proximal. The skin signs include erythema (see Fig. 113), lichenoid, or psoriaform eruptions, and itching or tenderness may be considerable. Periorbital swelling and redness as well as a streaky erythema in the backs of the fingers and ragged telangiectatic nailfolds are other features.

3. Acanthosis nigricans is pigmentation and wartiness of the axilla and groins. There is a velvety brown thickness of the skin of the hands and at mucocutaneous junctions such as the lips (Fig. 125).

4. Acquired hypertrichosis lanuginosa is a generalized increase in terminal hair and should be distinguished from hirsutes which is an increase in hair in sites normally associated with hair growth such as the chin.

5. Acute onset of multiple irritable seborrhoeic warts is known as the sign of Leser Trélat.

6. Superficial thrombophlebitis or migrating thrombophlebitis is especially associated with carcinoma of the pancreas.

7. Bullous pyoderma gangrenosum is a feature of leukaemia and myeloma.

8. Bullous disease of erythema multiforme type or occasionally more suggestive of pemphigoid, is more likely to be associated

with malignancy if the oral mucosa is involved or if immunofluorescence studies are negative.

9. Erythema gyratum repens (Fig. 126) is one of many patterns of erythema forming repeated concentric rings. The more bizarre and rapidly evolving the process the more likely is it to be associated with malignancy. This is particularly so when it is generalized, oedematous, or scaling (see also Fig. 9c).

10. Palmar keratoses are found in association with cancer of the bladder or lung.

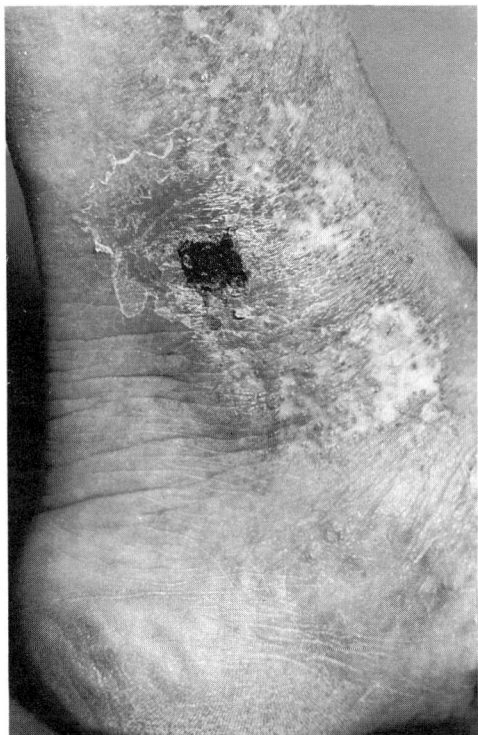

Fig. 121 Atrophie blanche is an obliteration of the capillaries in the upper dermis causing sclerosis. Residual vessels are elongated and coiled. They are liable to thrombosis and overlying ulceration is a consequence.

Table 28 Atrophie blanche: list of associated diseases

Pigmented purpuric eruptions	Rheumatoid arthritis
Gravitational stasis	Hashimoto's disease
Thrombophlebitis	Sickle cell anaemia
Thrombo-angiitis obliterans	Anterior poliomyelitis
Polyarteritis nodosa	Sjögren's syndrome
Diabetes mellitus	Capillary naevi
Scleroderma	Drug eruptions
Lupus erythematosus	Trauma, cuts
Dermatomyositis	Carcinoma

Erythroderma

Erythroderma is considered here because in cases which are difficult to manage other causes such as psoriasis, atopic eczema or drug eruption, can usually be diagnosed and appropriate therapy given. It is the acquired erythroderma in the adult that gives most difficulty with diagnosis and has been named the pre-Sézary syndrome. There may be a short or long history of persistent intermittent dermatitis. often with proven evidence of allergy to several agents with which the skin is in contact. Lymphadenopathy and hepatosplenomegaly may be pronounced. The Sézary syndrome of a leucocytosis of circulating T cells may be intermittent or persistent. Sun may be an aggravating factor; IgE levels may be elevated and either atopic eczema or psoriasis may feature in the past history. The skin is thickened and chronically oedematous with a variable degree of palmar plantar keratoderma and alopecia. The histology is of a severe dermatitis and a frank lymphoma cannot be diagnosed. The partial remissions are only in part due to changes in management, but prednisolone, chlorambucil or azathioprine in low dosage are increasingly prescribed for this syndrome.

Reference

Winkleman, R. K., Buechner, S. A. and Dia-Perez, J. T. (1984). Pre-Sézary syndrome. *J. Am. Acad. Dermatol.* **10**, 992–999.

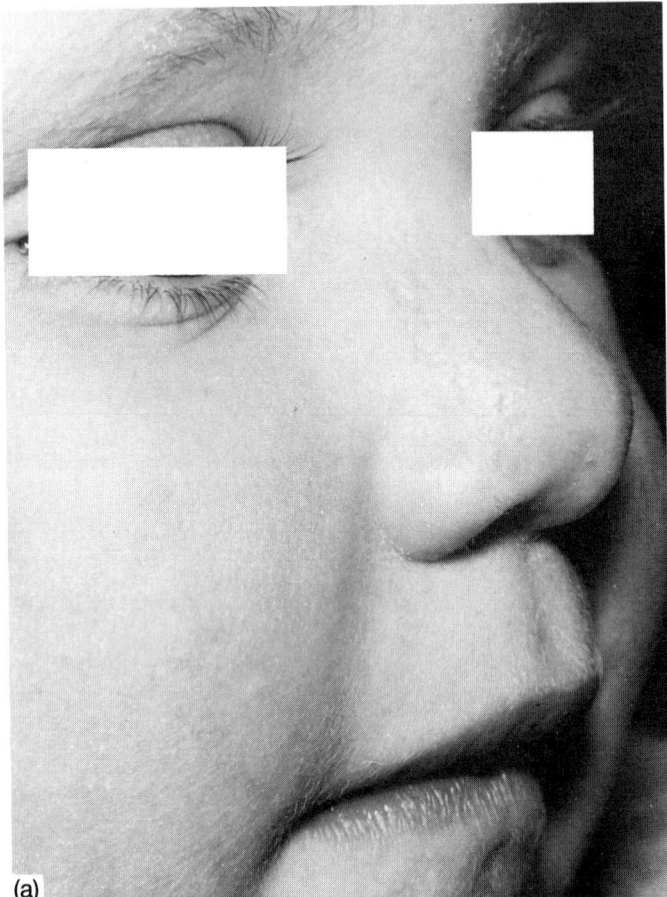

(a)

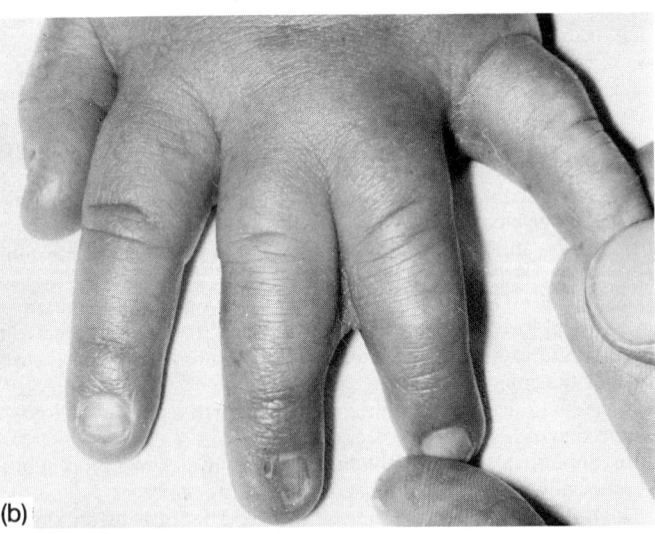

(b)

Fig. 120 Goltz's syndrome (focal dermal atrophy) patchy atrophy and (a) pitting of the skin; (b) with syndactyly.

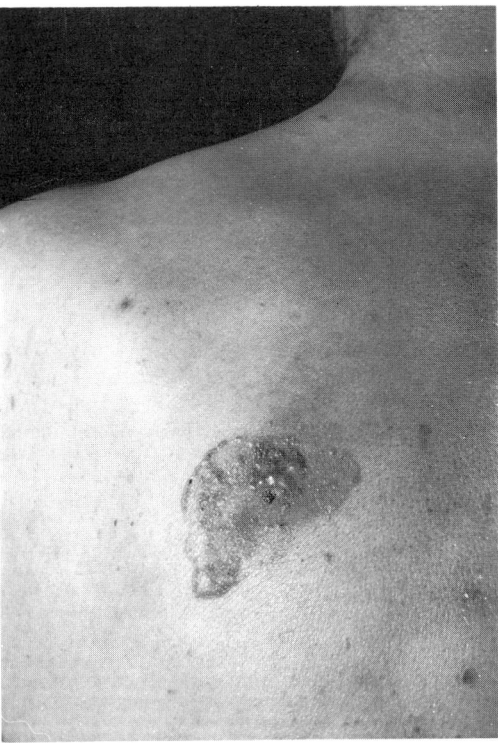

Fig. 122 Multifocal basal cell epitheliomata of the trunk following arsenic ingestion many years previously.

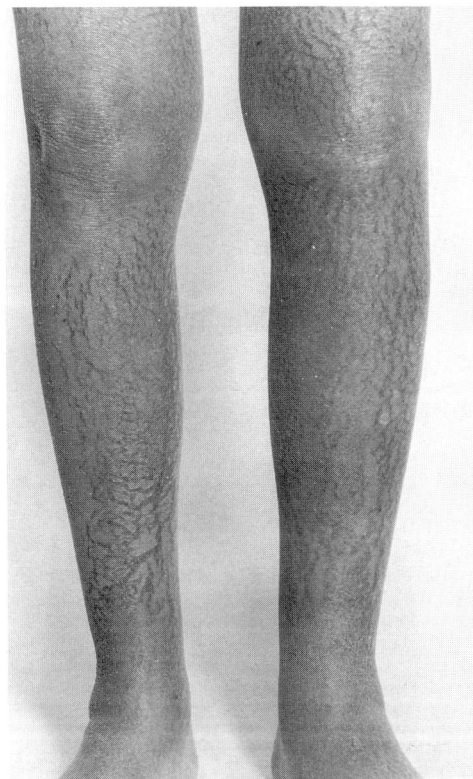

Fig. 124 Eczema craquelé, a consequence of skin malnutrition and an accompaniment and consequence of malignancy.

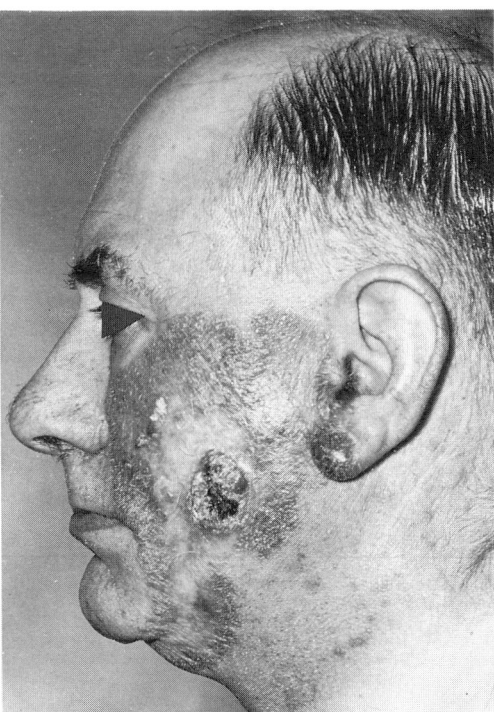

Fig. 123 Lupus vulgaris present for 25 years has resulted in chronic scarring. In this a squamous epithelioma has developed.

Cutaneous lymphoma

Few aspects of dermatology have been more confusing than those concerning lymphoma. In some respects it has been simplified by the recognition and identification of B and T lymphocytes and the realization that terms such as reticulosis, pre-reticulosis, and reti-

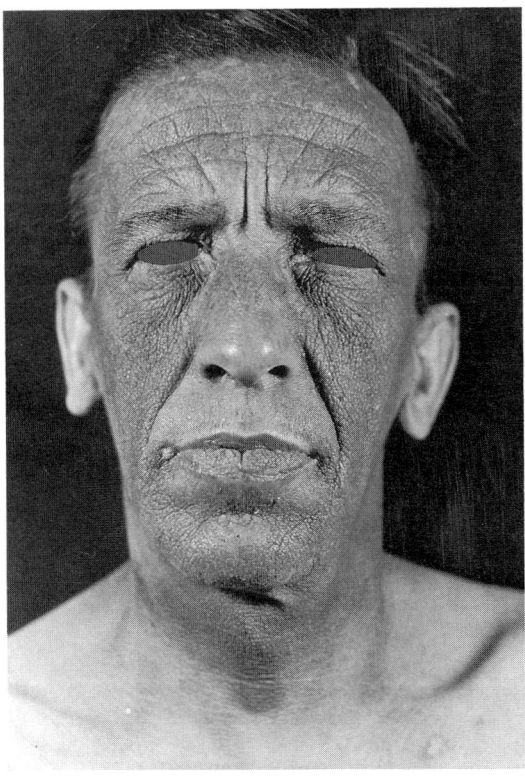

Fig. 125 Acanthosis nigricans; a darkening and thickening of the skin with a tendency to papilloma formation. The angles of the mouth are often involved as in this patient with carcinoma of the lung.

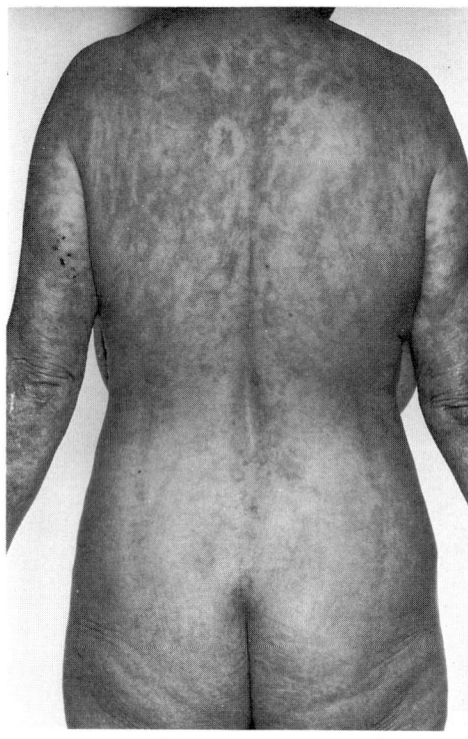

Fig. 126 Erythema gyratum repens in a patient with adenocarcinoma of the colon.

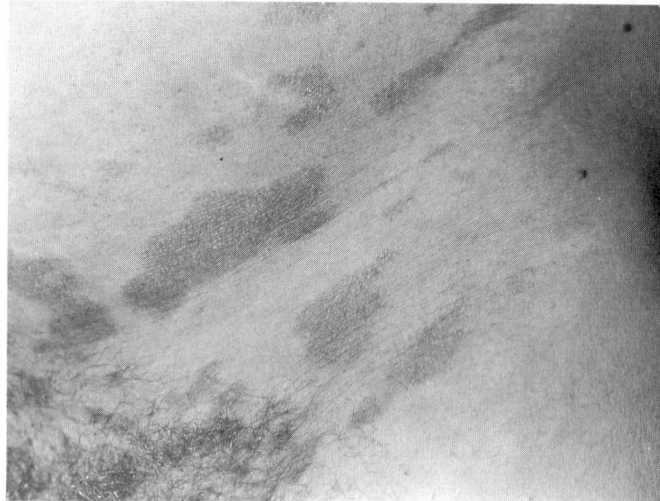

Fig. 127 Lower abdominal, persistent superficial dermatitis (parapsoriasis). These are fixed and persistent digitate (finger-like) patterns, erythematous, and slightly scaly.

culum cell are misapplied. T cells normally traverse through the skin whereas B cells do not. The Hassall's corpuscle in the thymus may have features in common with the cells of the epidermis which explain T cell, Langerhans cell, and epidermal interaction. The simplest classification into B cell, T cell, and non-B and non-T cell lymphoma with a single sub-grouping into small cells, indicating low-grade malignancy, and large cells, indicating high-grade malignancy, is now largely accepted.

Enzymic, cytochemical, immunological, functional and ultrastructural methods applied by research workers are not routinely available, but they indicate that conditions in which the epidermis is eczematous, scaly, or crusting are usually infiltrated with T cells as in mycosis fungoides, Sézary syndrome, and pagetoid reticulosis. Mononuclear phagocytes, including the Langerhans cells and eosinophils, often infiltrate the upper dermis. Most of the purple red tumours showing no involvement of the epidermis and producing sharply demarcated infiltrates in the middle or deep dermis are due to B cell proliferation.

The previously labelled reticulosarcomas starting as solitary tumours, dome-shaped and deep red, are now thought to be lymphoblastic, more often B cell than T cell. Such less differentiated blast cells also give rise to heavy infiltrates in the whole dermis and are less inclined to produce the nest of cells within the epidermis which is a feature of mycosis fungoides. There is destruction of blood vessels and fibrous tissue whereas in mycosis fungoides, blood vessels are well preserved and often characterized by prominent epithelioid endothelial cells as in post-capillary venules of lymph nodes.

All types of lymphoma may affect any organ, including lymph nodes and the blood, but mycosis fungoides, Sézary's syndrome, and pagetoid reticulosis favour the skin and often seem confined to it. The leonine facies is a peculiar feature more often seen in B cell lymphoma as in chronic lymphatic leukaemia.

During the early stage of mycosis fungoides, the behaviour of the T cell cannot be proven to be malignant and some suggest that is is merely hyper-reactive or over-stimulated. The sources of this stimulus could even be the skin macrophage known as the Langer-

hans cell. These are increased in number in mycosis fungoides. Exactly when 'over-stimulus' becomes 'lymphoma' has been debated but no conclusions can be reached.

The distinctive cell found in tissues and blood of the Sézary syndrome and in the epidermis of mycosis fungoides as a T cell with a usually but not invariably hyperconvoluted nucleus. It is also observed in a variety of non-lymphomatous dermatoses and it should be equated more with the 'over-stimulus' concept rather than with malignancy.

Clinical features of lymphoma

Dermatologists have long grappled with the problem of diseases of the skin which are suspected of culminating, often years later, in a malignancy of the lymphoid tissue. These diseases have features of chronic dermatitis and psoriasis (parapsoriasis) because there is a chronic reaction in the dermis and epidermis which is often indistinguishable from other causes of such a reaction. The feature that causes suspicion is lack of symmetry in an atypical distribution. There is also inhomogeneity within the lesion. Infiltration with white cells suggesting tumour formation is one feature. Another is atrophy or thinning of the dermis, telangiectasia, and pigmentation known as poikiloderma. Persistent superficial dermatitis, previously known as parapsoriasis in plaque (benign type), consists of flat, symmetrical slightly scaly, red patches on the trunk or limbs which persist for years. They are round, oval, or finger-like and are sometimes yellowish (Fig. 127). This is now thought to be benign.

Poikiloderma atrophicans vasculare, previously known as parapsoriasis (large plaque or lichenoides), resembles radiodermatitis in that there is atrophy, telangiectasis, and reticulate pigmentation (Fig. 128). It favours areas spared exposure to natural sunlight such as the breasts or buttocks. It may be composed of small papules or large plaques of any shape. The expected outcome often many years later is mycosis fungoides but Hodgkin's disease is also a possibility.

B cell lymphoma when present in the skin forms firm pink-red or skin coloured tumours often in groups coalescing to produce annular or other patterns (Fig. 129).

Lipomelanic reticulosis is a non-specific enlargement of lymph nodes associated with widespread dermatitis or erythroderma.

Mycosis fungoides is initially often no more than a non-specific dermatitis or more commonly poikiloderma atrophicans vasculare. Occasionally it is a tumour from the beginning. The lesions may be symptomless but severe pruritus is common. The affected areas become more infiltrated, scaly and reddened (Fig. 130).

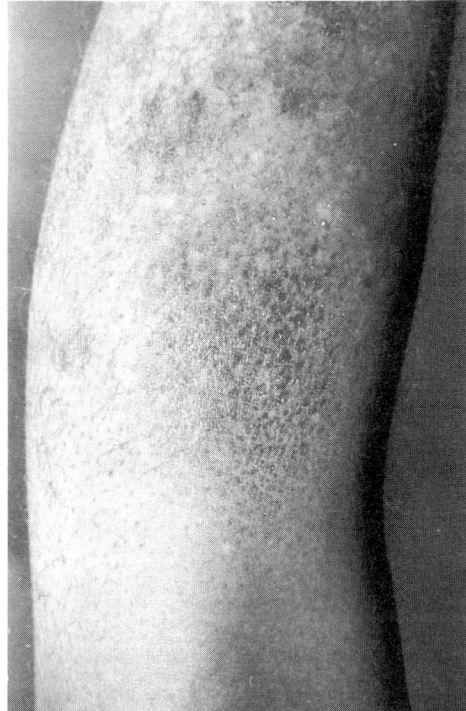

Fig. 128 Poikiloderma; atrophy, pigmentation and telangiectasia, commonly preceding the development of lymphoma in the skin. The clinical appearance is like radiodermatitis.

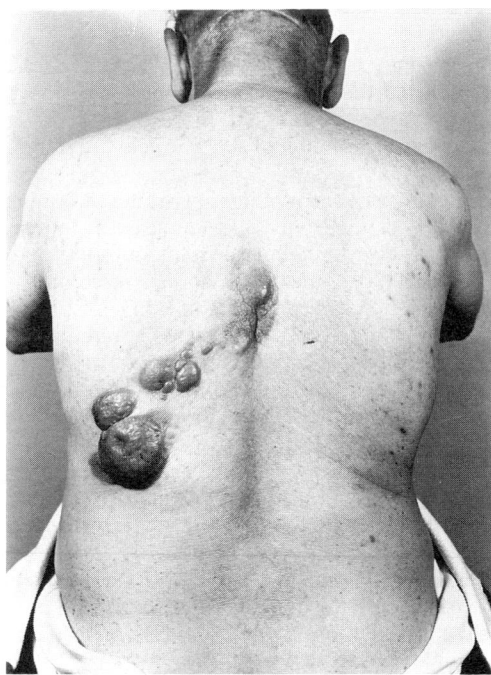

Fig. 129 Fleshy tumours grouped and arising in the dermis without epidermal hyperplasia. This is characteristic of B cell lymphomas.

Often they are annular, serpiginous, or have other bizarre shapes. Erythroderma and widespread ulceration is the final stage of the disease. The diagnostic histological feature is invasion of the epidermis by atypical lymphocytes often in clusters – Pautrier abscesses – and a heavy pleomorphic infiltration of the upper dermis hugging the epidermis but causing less necrosis of individual epidermal cells than in lichen planus.

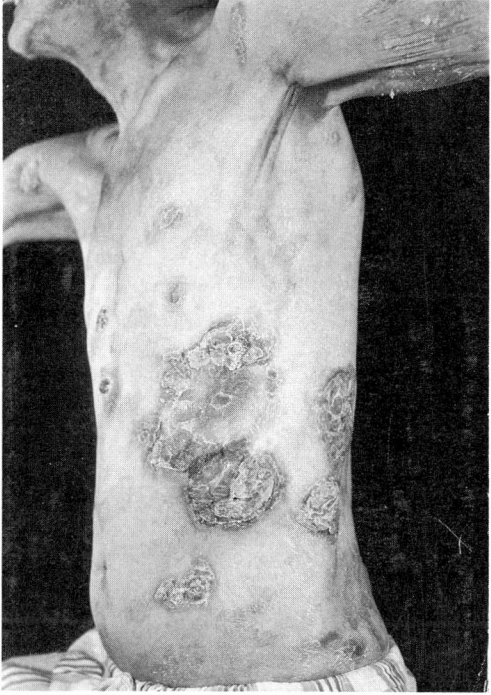

Fig. 130 Marked irregular epidermal reactivity is a characteristic response to T cell lymphoma of the mycosis fungoides type.

Skin manifestations of Hodgkin's disease include infiltration of the skin with nodules of the disease. Pigmentation and pruritus are common. Prurigo with deep excoriations and secondary infection is one of its most distressing manifestations. Ichthyosiform atrophy as part of the terminal wasting disease is common. The scaling is often as severe as an exfoliative dermatitis but shedding of the scale is less than the exfoliation of psoriasis. Hair loss, herpes zoster, and rarely erythema nodosum are other complications.

Management of mycosis fungoides

The rate of progression is highly variable. There is still no clear picture of the natural history of mycosis fungoides. Samman treated a series of patients conservatively and only 45 of 212 cases died of mycosis fungoides. Most of those who died had tumours, skin ulcers or palpable lymph-nodes at the time of presentation, and in the absence of these the prognosis tends to be very good. In patients with benign patterns of the disease it is important not to overtreat.

Radiation therapy

Small field orthovoltage radiation has been standard therapy for many years and it is very useful to control plaques and tumours resistant to other modalities. It is not unusual for patients to require a small dose of radiation to one area only at as little as yearly intervals. Electron beam therapy is recommended for most patients with extensive infiltrated plaques or tumours. A high initial response rate can be expected in a majority of patients but they remain free of disease only for about 3 years.

Topical nitrogen mustard (mechlorethamine, HN$_2$)

This is a useful treatment for patients who have less infiltrated skin lesions. Clinical response may be slow and maintenance therapy may be required for at least 2 years. The chief side-effect is allergic contact dermatitis, occurring in about 30–60 per cent of patients. Desensitization can be attempted but it is difficult to effect. There is some debate as to whether an aqueous or ointment-based preparation is best. It is probable that the ointment-based preparation produces fewer hypersensitivity reactions.

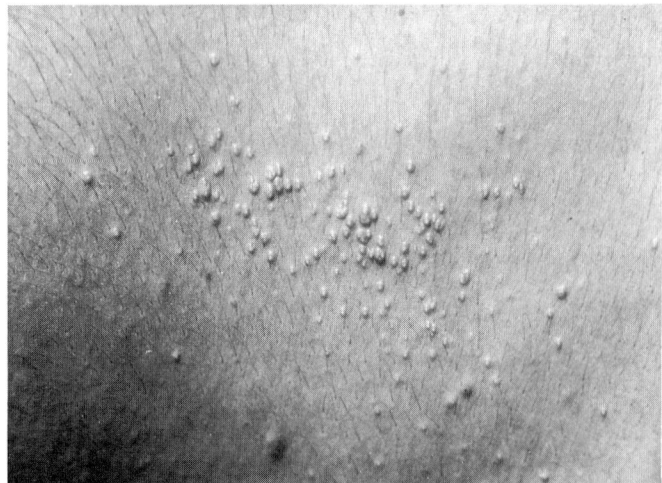

Fig. 131 Molluscum contagiosum: groups of viral induced papules characterized by a central punctum.

PUVA

Several reported series of the good effects of PUVA have resulted in most academic departments using this as a first line of therapy for superficial lesions that are widespread. Penetration of PUVA is limited so that deep tumours are unlikely to be cleared.

Systemic chemotherapy

On the whole this is reserved for palliation in persons with systemic disease and deep tumours. There is usually some initial response. Clearance for more than 1 year is unusual.

References

Abel, E. A. (1981). Photochemotherapy for cutaneous T-cell lymphoma. *J. Am. Acad. Dermatol.* **4**, 423–429.

Du Vivier, A. *et al.* (1978). Mycosis fungoides, nitrogen mustard and skin cancer. *Br. J. Dermatol.* **99**, 61–63.

Hoppe, R. T. *et al.* (1979). Radiation therapy in the management of cutaneous T-cell lymphomas. *Cancer Treat. Rep.* **63**, 625–632.

Minna, J. D. *et al.* (1979). Report of the committee on therapy for MF and Sézary syndrome. *Cancer Treat. Rep.* **63**, 729–736.

Price, N. M. *et al.* (1983). Ointment-based mechlorethamine treatment for MF. *Cancer* **52**, 2214–2219.

Samman, P. (1976). Mycosis fungoides and other cutaneous reticulosis. *Clin. Exp. Dermatol.* **1**, 97–214.

Van Vloten, W. A. *et al.* (1985). Total skin electron beam irradiation for cutaneous T-cell lymphoma (mycosis fungoides). *Br. J. Dermatol.* **112**, 697–702.

VIRAL WARTS

Warts are caused by the papovavirus (see Section 5), which enters the skin through small abrasions, particularly if the skin is moist and warm. Virus is found by electron microscopy in the differentiating cells of the upper epidermis rather than in the proliferating basal cell layer. The incubation period is probably several months. There are a number of strains of wart virus giving rise to different types of warts – common, plantar, mosaic, plane, and anogenital. Molluscum contagiosum is caused by a pox virus (Fig. 131).

The incidence of warts is increased in immunosuppressed patients either from drugs or associated with lymphoma. Cell-mediated immunity is more certainly a factor than humoral immunity. The peak incidence is in children aged 12–16 and in recent years in Europe and the USA there seems to be an increase in infection rate compared to Asia, Australia, or Africa.

Trauma may account for the distribution of warts on the hands and feet. Nail biting in children and shaving in men as well as ill-fitting shoes in adults are all relevant. Twenty per cent of warts

disappear within six months and 65 per cent in two years. Plane warts and mosaic warts are slow to clear.

Common warts are firm papules with a rough horny surface. They occur singly or coalesce into large masses. The knuckles and nail folds are particularly favoured as are the knees and more rarely the shaft of the penis. They should be differentiated from warty tuberculosis which usually is a solitary plaque with an erythematous border. Granuloma annulare of the knuckles does not have a horny surface. A persistent wart on the toes or fingers may be a reaction to a subungual exostosis. Squamous epitheliomata or keratoacanthoma are usually solitary and found in an older population.

Plane warts are smooth, flat or slightly elevated affecting the face or back of hands. They may coalesce or form linear lesions in scratch marks. Lichen planus may be difficult to distinguish from plane warts but is unusual on the face and prefers the flexor surface of the wrists as well as the mucosa of the mouth. The histology of plane warts is unexciting whereas lichen planus shows destruction of the basal cell layer of the epidermis and a heavy infiltrate of mononuclear cells.

Filiform and digitate warts are common in the beard area, on the lips, and in the nasal vestibule.

Plantar warts begin as a small sago grain papule. As it enlarges, paring of the surface with a scalpel distinguishes the wart from the surrounding horny ring of normal epidermis and reveals the small capillaries in the tips of the elongated papillae. Most warts are over pressure points. Clusters of small warts make up a mosaic. A wart which shows numerous thrombosed capillaries and is darker than usual is probably regressing. The fourth interdigital space is a common site for soft corns due to pressure of the little toe on the head of the metatarsal in a tight shoe and in ballet dancers. Soft warts or even condylomata lata have been described at such sites.

Treatment

Spontaneous resolution is to be expected. Overall, 12 weeks is the usual time required to cure warts irrespective of the treatment used and most standard treatments do no better or worse than this. Podophyllin and formalin or salicylic acid are standard therapies.

Podophyllin 10–20 per cent in liquid paraffin or in tincture benzoic compound is painted onto anogenital warts and the area is then powdered. The podophyllin is irritant and some persons need to wash it off in 2 hours. Others have no such discomfort. It should not be used in the pregnant since absorption sufficient to damage the fetus is a possibility. The treatment is repeated at intervals of 1–3 weeks.

Formalin 10 per cent solution can be applied as a soak to multiple warts of the soles of the feet but dryness and fissuring may be troublesome.

Salicylic acid is the most reliable chemical for treating warts. Paints or plasters containing 20–40 per cent salicylic acid are best applied after a 5 minute soak with warm soapy water and preferably after removal of excess surface keratin.

Freezing is with liquid nitrogen either in a special spray or by application from a cotton wool bud on the end of an orange stick. The wart should be whitened for at least 20–30 seconds and blistering is a common consequence.

Local anaesthetic injected into the base of a wart to lift it up from the dermis can be followed by curettage. Compression with the thumb on immediate adjacent tissue prevents bleeding while silver nitrate is applied. The rim of horny tissues around the wart side should be cut away by a pair of scissors.

References

Bunney, M. H. (1980). Viral warts: answering the patients' questions. *Medicine* **31**, 1593–1596.

Gissmann, L., Pfister, H. and zur Hausen, H. (1977). Human papilloma viruses (HPV) characterisation of four different isolates. *Virology* **76**, 569–580.

Von Krogh, G. (1979). Warts. Immunologic factors of prognostic significance. *Int. J. Dermatol.* **18**, 195–205.

GRANULOMATA AND OTHER INFILTRATIONS OF THE SKIN

A granuloma is a compact accumulation of cells, comprised mainly of monocytes or their variants, macrophages, epithelioid cells, and giant cells. Often there is subsequent fibrosis. Lymphocytes are more numerous in granulomata due to allergens to which the host is sensitive. Degeneration or foreign bodies encourage neutrophil and eosinophil participation.

Granulomata are classified as high or low turnover:

High turnover: tissue destructive; induced by toxic irritants or delayed hypersensitivity; continuous recruitment of macrophages and many mitoses; and epithelioid and giant cells frequent.

Low turnover: space occupying but not destructive; induced by inert (bacterial) and non-degradable irritants; no continued recruitment but long survival of macrophages and few mitoses; and few epithelioid and few giant cells.

The clinical features of granulomata are either space-occupying nodules lying in epidermis or, if close to the surface of the skin, they may be seen as yellow or brownish-red and sometimes translucent areas. The chronic changes in blood supply associated with the lesion cause a bluish colour and sometimes telangiectasia. If they are in the upper dermis, then there may be overlying epithelial hyperplasia or ulceration with extrusion of some of the granulomatous material. On the other hand thinning of the epidermis may be considerable. In dark skins, pigmentary changes may include hypo- or hyperpigmentation.

A common cause of granulomata is persistent irritation of the skin by external trauma causing ulceration and pseudo-epitheliomatous hyperplasia. Examples include granuloma fissuratum of the ear or nose due to illfitting spectacles. The ingrowing toenail, the pilonidal sinus, or the presence of extrafollicular but intradermal hair as is seen in the interdigital clefts of barbers, and cattle or horse dealers are other examples.

Granuloma gluteal infantum is seen in the nappy area due to incomplete resolution of an irritant rash in which steroid creams have been too extravagantly applied. Numerous agents acting as a foreign body incompletely degraded and removed are causes of chronic granulomas in the skin. They include sea urchin, silicates, cactus allergen, grit, and various chronic infections such as *Candida albicans*, *Trichophyton verrucosum* (Fig. 132a), coccidioidomycosis, atypical mycobacteria from fish tanks or swimming baths, leprosy (Fig. 132b), tuberculosis (Fig. 132c), leishmaniasis (Fig. 132d), and halogen granulomas (see Fig. 31).

Sarcoidosis

The general features of this disease are discussed in Section 5. Erythema nodosum is the commonest problem and is discussed on page 20.66. The other skin manifestations are present in about 15–25 per cent of cases seen in hospital and are due to accumulations of epithelioid granulomas in the dermis, usually with a free zone sparing the epidermis. It is commoner in blacks than in whites and in women rather than men. The appearance depends on the level in the dermis and the size and confluence of the lesions. Sarcoid favours scars, even the old ones, and these may suggest keloid formation.

Lupus pernio is a pattern mostly seen in women in which bluishred or violaceous swellings present on the nose, cheeks, ears, or hands. The lesions are long-lasting.

The anterior septum and nasal vestibule is commonly involved by granulomatous disease (Table 29 and Fig. 133). It is a site in which

epithelial necrosis may occur secondarily to interference with its blood supply.

Micropapular sarcoid consists of yellowish-brown pin head or pea-sized papules, often grouped and cropping (Fig. 134). Compression with a glass slide removes the reddish vascular dilatation and a translucent yellow lesion, 'the apple jelly', can be observed. This pattern may not be distinguishable from lichen scrofulosorum. In the latter the tuberculin test is strongly positive and the Kveim test is negative. However, in the elderly population of the UK, cases are increasingly described suspected of tubercular aetiology but in the absence of these confirmatory signs, proved to be questionably sarcoid.

The plaque form is a more diffuse sarcoidosis involving the limbs, shoulders, buttocks, and thighs (Fig. 135). The skin is atrophic and the edges may be serpiginous suggesting tertiary lues.

The granuloma of sarcoid is a chronic injury to the skin and may evoke a great variety of responses including scarring alopecia, lupus erythematosus-like epidermal atrophy, ulceration, telangiectasia, hypopigmentation, epidermal hyperplasia, and a psoriasiform plaque or verrucous hypertrophy. Confluence of lesions or healing in the centre gives rise to annular patterns. Histological features of a neat epithelioid granuloma are more diagnostic than the clinical picture.

When sarcoid of the skin presents without other subjective or objective evidence of systemic sarcoidosis, the prognosis is good and the patient is unlikely to develop later systemic disease. This may be because the skin lesion is not a manifestation of the tendency to develop sarcoid but is a localized phenomenon in response to an entirely local event. Chest X-rays and pulmonary function tests as well as slit lamp examination of the eye should nevertheless be done in every case.

Urticaria pigmentosa or mastocytosis

Mast cells are normally present in the skin but the numbers vary greatly with up to 80 per mm^3 in the upper dermis. In mastocytosis they are greatly increased in number and may be found as a single isolated mastocytoma or numerous nests scattered over the entire body, i.e. the classic urticaria pigmentosa, or diffusely throughout the entire skin. Occasionally there is systemic infiltration of all tissues including liver, spleen, and bone marrow. A very rare leukaemic variety is also recognized.

The mast cell releases histamine, leucotrienes, and heparin and these may have systemic effects, but it is increasingly realized that the local contribution is through its secretion of proteases.

In the infant, mastocytosis may present as blisters but more commonly the lightly pigmented swellings in the skin are noted and observed to swell when scratched or after a hot bath or exercise. Rarely there is a generalized flushing and itching. The condition is commonest in the first year of life or at birth and an onset at this age is a good prognosis for eventual complete resolution by adolescence.

In the adult a late onset is associated with diffuse plaques and telangiectasia.

The systemic variety presents in 10 per cent of adult cases causing osteoporosis or osteosclerosis. The spleen may be enlarged and bleeding disorders are the consequence of either thrombocytopenia or from the effects of heparin. Involvement of the gut causes a variety of symptoms including colic and diarrhoea. Rightsided heart failure due to pulmonary hypertension is recorded. Examination of the urine for histamine or PGD_2 may help to confirm the diagnosis when the skin lesions are absent.

Treatment

Treatment is unsatisfactory but the increasing use of H_1 and H_2 antagonists in various combinations is proving beneficial in some cases. The prognosis for eventual resolution is good in children but a solitary or troublesome single lesion in an adult can be excised. The cosmetic appearance of pigmented lesions is helped

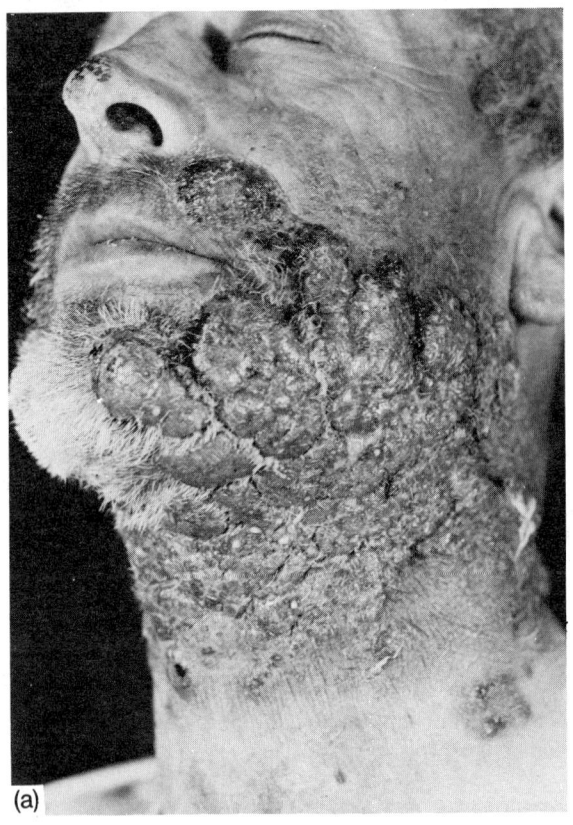

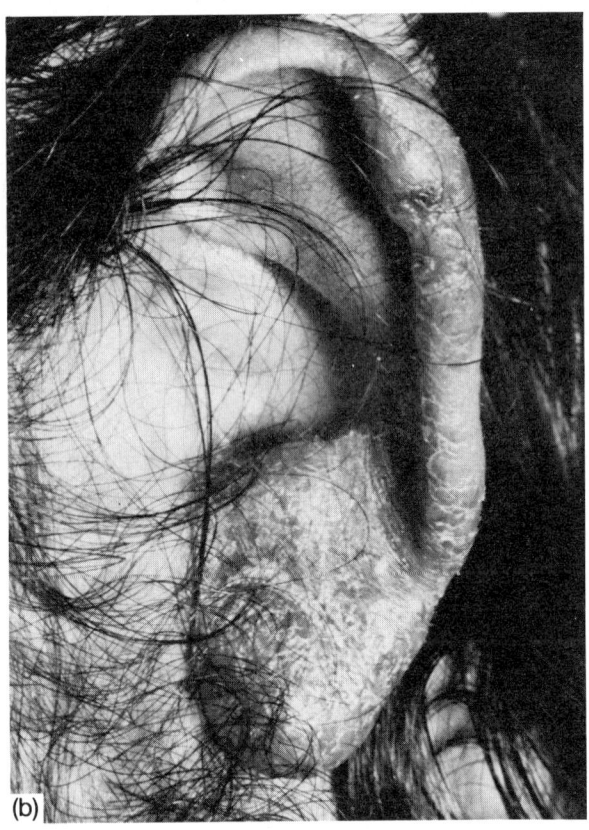

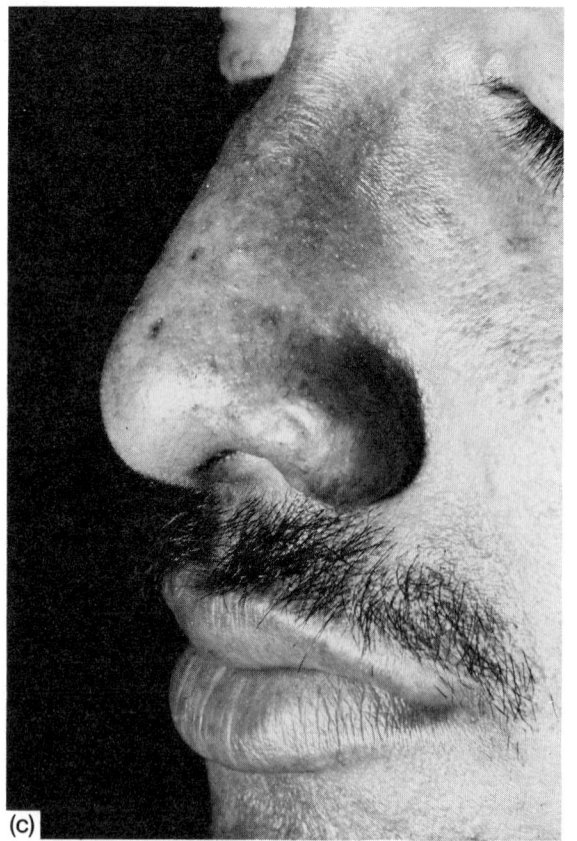

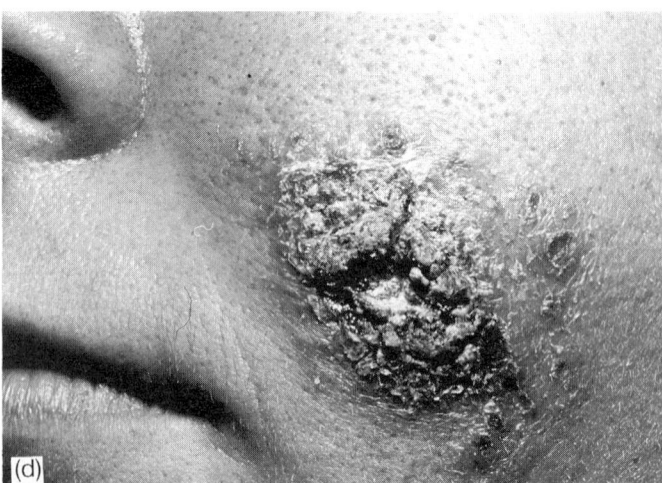

Fig. 132 (a) Chronic granulomas of cattle ringworm: *Trichophyton verrucosum*. (b) The ear involved by lupus vulgaris (tuberculosis); a brownish-red granuloma inducing irritation in the overlying epidermis. (c) The nose is a common site for the granuloma of lepromatous leprosy. (d) Chronic granuloma due to leishmaniasis following a sandfly bite presenting as an ill-defined cresting and wartiness.

by sun exposure or by use of UVA and psoralens, but the number of mast cells is not reduced. Disodium cromoglycate helps some patients with systemic mastocytosis.

Cutaneous manifestations of histiocytosis X

The cutaneous lesions of histiocytosis X are small yellow-brown keratotic scaling papules. These coalesce to form a diffuse seborrhoeic dermatitis which is ulcerative, crusting, and purpuric. Granulomatous eroded plaques that are particularly found in the flexures and in the external auditory meatus cause great discomfort. The hair margins are commonly involved. The common association of diabetes insipidus and hepato-splenomegaly are described in Section 12. The diagnosis is confirmed by demonstrating ultrastructurally the Langerhans cell granule in the histiocyte.

Fibrosis, eosinophils, and giant cells are features of a more benign process.

Melkersson–Rosenthal syndrome

This syndrome can be produced experimentally by ligating all the lymphatics at the head and neck. Granulomas of the lips (Fig. 136) and tongue are a consequence of lymphatic stasis and impaired clearance of protein through the normal channels. The triad of facial palsy, enlarged tongue, and chronically swollen lips is difficult to treat. Current hypothesis supported by some experi-

Table 29 Organisms causing chronic granulomatous disease of the nose; their characteristics, geographical distribution and the animals they infect

Disease and causative organism	Geographical distribution	Susceptible animals	Portal of entry and mode of dissemination
Lupus vulgaris: *Mycobacterium tuberculosis* (2.5–3.5 × 0.3 μm) Acid-fast bacillus; alcohol-fast; stains with Sudan black; Gram positive	Ubiquitous, rare in tropics	Human strain fatal in guinea pigs; rabbits and mice affected less; *M. bovis* virulent to all; chicken not affected by both strains	Inhalation, ingestion and skin inoculation; lymph and blood-borne spread
Leprosy: *Mycobacterium leprae* (1–8 × 0.2–0.5μm) AFB less alcohol-fast; not stained by Sudan black; Gram positive; uncultivatable	Tropics, sub-tropics and endemic in Malta, Cyprus, and countries on the Adriatic, Mediterranean, and Black seas	Ear of hamster, mouse footpad, and armadillo	Undecided; cutaneous? dissemination by blood and nerves
Rhinoscleroma: *Klebsiella rhinoscleromatis* (1.6–2.4 × 0.8 μm) Gram negative	Central Europe, Russia, China, India, Indonesia, North Africa, Central and South America	Mice	Unknown ?inhalation (upper respiratory tract); localized extension
Venereal syphilis: *Treponema pallidum* (6–15 × 0.09–0.18 μm) Close, rigid (8–20 coils spirochaete); rotar and flexion movements; uncultivatable	Ubiquitous in urban communities	Apes, rabbits, and hamsters	Genital and extragenital, skin and mucosa; transplacental; blood-borne dissemination
Non-venereal endemic syphilis (bejel): same as venereal syphilis; uncultivatable	Arid deserts of Asia and Africa	Apes, rabbits, and hamsters	Mouth (communal drinking, food utensils, and kissing)
Yaws: same as venereal syphilis; uncultivatable	Tropical, humid jungles of Central Africa, Asia, Australia and South and Central America	Monkeys, rabbits, and hamsters	Abrasions or bite in skin by direct contact by vector (hippelates fly); blood-borne dissemination
Mucocutaneous leishmaniasis: *Leishmania brasiliensis* (2–4 × 0.5–2.5 μm)	Endemic in Central and South America (damp forests)	Monkey, dog, guinea pigs, bat, white rat, squirrel, and hamster	Through a bite by local sandfly (phlebotomus) in skin; dissemination by lymph and blood
Lutz's mycosis: *Paracoccidioides brasiliensis* (10–60 μm diameter); spherical and budding	Brazil, South and Central America, occasionally USA, Italy, Portugal, Morocco, and Bulgaria	Inoculated into guinea pigs, specific orchitis. In hamsters and mice, dissemination	Undecided? lungs, skin, GI tract, and buccopharyngeal mucosa; blood-borne and lymphatic dissemination
Rhinosporidiosis: *Rhinosporidium seeberi* Dimorphic fungus; sporangium = 2.5 mm diameter; endospores 6–7 μm diameter; uncultivatable	Endemic in India and Ceylon; sporadic elsewhere	Natural infection in nose of cattle and horses; experimental inoculation failed	Unknown.? Direct inoculation in nose; dissemination only 2 cases (blood-borne)
Rhinophycomycosis: *Entomophthora coronata* (5–25 μm diameter) PAS positive; grows better at 25 °C	Tropics and sub-tropics	Inoculation experiments in young animals failed	Portal of entry unknown? by inhalation
Glanders: *Actinobacillus mallei* Short coccoid, rod-shaped bacillus; Gram negative	Eastern Europe, Asia Minor, Asia, and North Africa	Natural disease of solipeds; horse, mule, donkey, and occasionally sheep; accidental in man by contact with animals or laboratory material	In animals through the intestinal wall by contaminated fodder with nasal discharge and sputum; dissemination blood-borne

From Kanan and Ryan (1976).

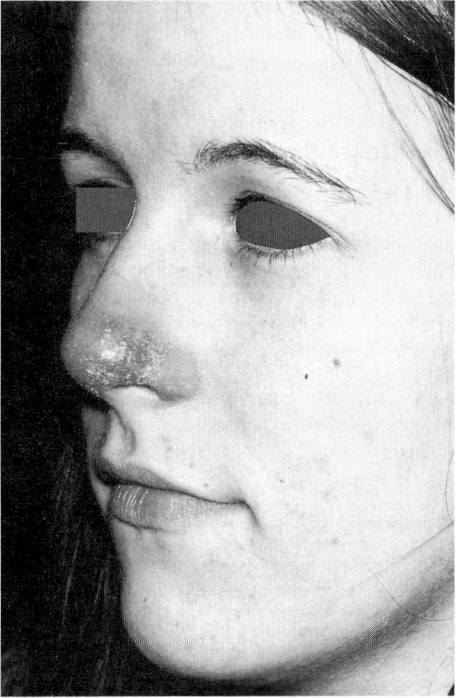

Fig. 133 Chronic granuloma of the nose due to sarcoid.

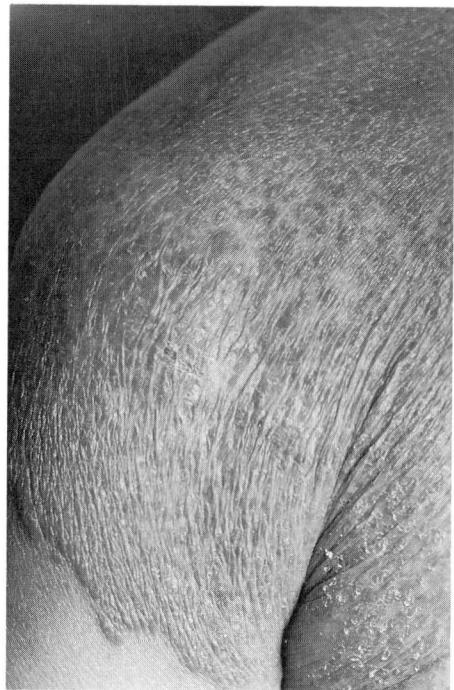

Fig. 135 Plaque of sarcoid affecting the skin of the shoulder and causing a brownish-red infiltration with atrophy of the overlying dermis. Unlike lupus vulgaris there is less irritation of the overlying epidermis; it is merely thinned and the scale is due to retention of a well-knit, dried-out stratum corneum.

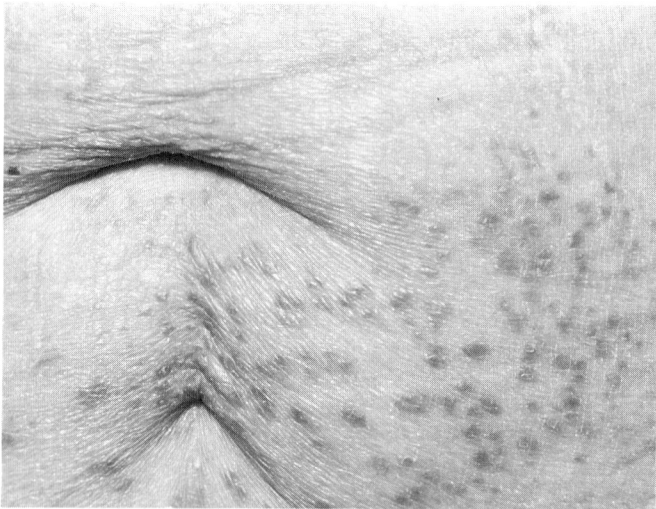

Fig. 134 Grouped brownish-red nodules in the dermis: micropapular sarcoid. This appearance is also compatible with tuberculosis, lichen scrofulosorum variety.

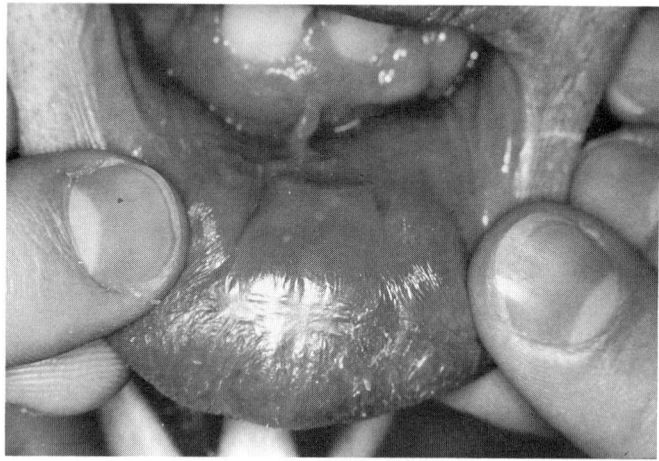

Fig. 136 Granuloma of the lip in which sarcoid and Crohn's disease were part of the differential diagnosis of the Melkersson–Rosenthal syndrome of lymphostasis.

mental work in rats suggest that stimulation of macrophages by hydroxyethylrutoside, Paroven, 200 mg three times daily, may help to clear the protein but penicillin V is often also prescribed to reduce current episodes of cellulitis.

Granuloma annulare and necrobiosis lipoidica

A partial necrosis of the collagen and the connective tissue cells associated with immunoglobulin and complement deposition results in a lymphocytic and histiocytic response that is known as a palisading granuloma. This is entirely reversible over many months and years in granuloma annulare, but in necrobiosis lipoidica it tends to result in fibrosis and scarring. The association with insulin-dependent diabetes mellitus is unpredictable and is to be expected in more widespread forms or in older age groups of granuloma annulare and in about 75 per cent of necrobiosis lipoidica.

In children, granuloma annulare are commonly on the knuckles (Fig. 137), fingers, and dorsum of the feet. Ears and elbows are quite frequently affected. They may be mistaken for warts but the overlying epidermis if closely inspected is rarely papilliferous. The tendency to heal in the centre and spread centrifugally over many weeks gives rise to an annular appearance.

Necrobiosis lipoidica is commonly to be found on both shins (Fig. 138). Widespread forms of granuloma annulare may be often of giant type, forming large violaceous plaques or rings. No treatment is necessary since eventual resolution of granuloma annulare is expected in 75 per cent in two years, but intralesional steroids probably speed resolution, particularly sometimes aborting necrobiosis lipoidica.

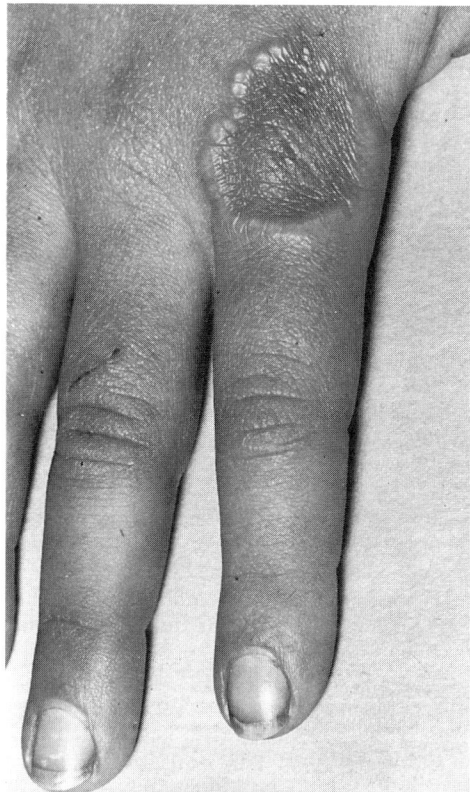

Fig. 137 Papules of granuloma annulare forming a ring around a now healed but previously affected area on the knuckle.

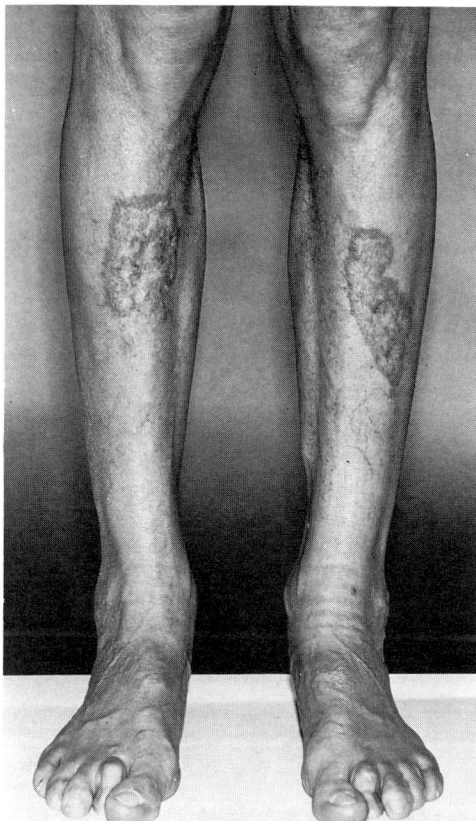

Fig. 138 Necrobiosis lipoidica usually affects the skin of the shins. The yellowish atrophic plaques are associated with diabetes mellitus.

Pretibial myxoedema

Pretibial myxoedema may present acutely as a slightly tender erythema nodosum-like swelling, but more often it is a shiny red and non-tender infiltration of the front of the shins. Chronic forms have the appearance of a local elephantiasis. Classically it is associated with clubbing and exophthalmus and a history and signs of a previous thyroidectomy. Intralesional steroids often encourage resolution of the more acute varieties.

Cutaneous amyloidosis

Systemic amyloidosis is described elsewhere. The features that should suggest the diagnosis in the skin are its waxy appearance and the ease with which purpura develops within the lesions on slight trauma.

Lichen amyloidosis consists of discrete, firm, hemispheroidal papules. Hyperkeratosis and pigmentation is common suggesting a waxy infiltrated lichen simplex. The lower legs and outer thighs are involved (Fig. 139). There is no systemic implication.

Macular amyloid is a common pigmented variant affecting the shoulders and back of Asians. It is often in a rippled pattern (Fig. 139b).

Lipoid proteinosis

Yellowish papules contain hyaline material and are found especially in the eyelids and elbows. The involvement of the vocal cords causing hoarseness from birth is a distinctive feature. Intracranial calcification and epilepsy are associated complications.

Multicentric reticulohistiocytosis

Granulomata are juxta-articular especially on the fingers but they also affect the lips, nostrils, and ears. There is an associated polyarthritis and underlying neoplastic disease is frequently associated. The diagnostic features are numerous multinucleated giant cells in the granuloma.

Crohn's disease

This is a well-recognized cause of chronic granulomatous infiltration perianally (see Fig. 23) or in the buccal mucosa.

References

Fitzpatrick, R., Rapaport, M. J. and Silva, D. G. (1981). Histiocytosis X. *Arch. dermatol.* **117**, 253–257.

Kanan, M. W. and Ryan, T. J. (1976). The localization of granulomatous diseases. In *Microvascular diseases*, pp. 195–220. Lloyd Luke, London.

Kendall, M. E., Fields, J. P. and King, L. E. Jr (1984). Cutaneous mastocytosis without clinically obvious skin lesions *J. Am. Acad. Dermatol.* **10** (Part 2), 903–905.

Kerdal, F. A. and Moschella, S. M. (1984). Sarcoidosis. *J. Am. Acad. Dermatol.* **11**, 1–19.

Muhlemann, M. F. and Williams, D. R. R. (1984). Localized granuloma annulare is associated with insulin-dependent diabetes mellitus. *Br. J. Dermatol.* **111**, 322–329.

Roper, S. S. and Spraker, M. K. (1985). Cutaneous histiocytosis syndromes. *Pediatr. Dermatol.* **3**, 19–30.

Ryan, T. J. (1978). Lymphatics of the skin. In *Physiology and pathophysiology of the skin* Vol. 5 (ed. A. Jarrett), pp. 1755–1808. Academic Press, New York.

Management of skin disease

General principles

There are several general principles that can be applied to diseases of skin whatsoever their causes.

Acute skin lesions require rest. Limbs should be elevated because this reduces swelling. Dressings should be applied lightly

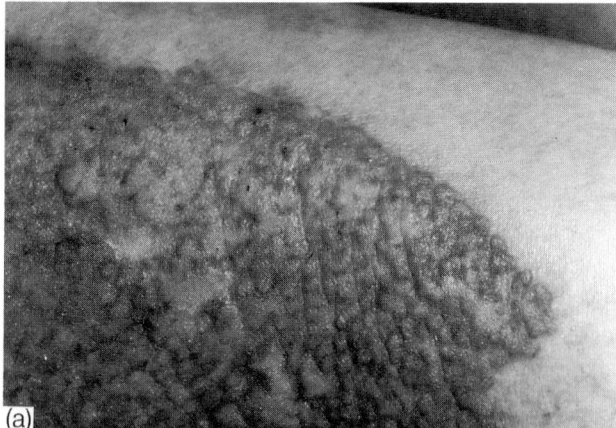

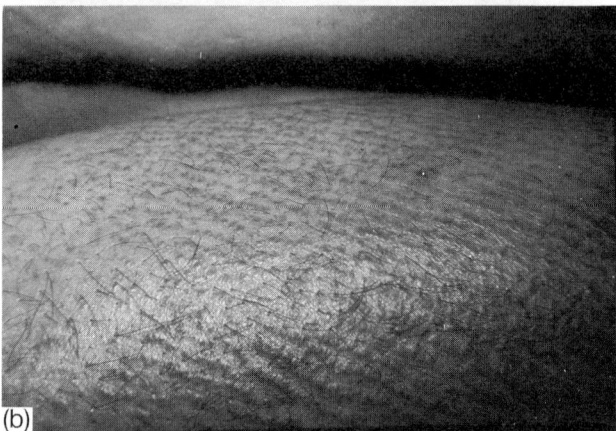

Fig. 139 (a) Lichen amyloidosis commonly affects the shins or outer aspects of the thighs. The brownish, waxy, lichenified skin is pruritic. (b) Rippled pigmentation of macular amyloid.

and evenly to the surface and should support the inflamed area without drag or compression. All agents applied to the skin should be no stronger than necessary. It is very easy for instance, to make a potassium permanganate solution too strong or to use poorly mixed and inhomogeneous medicaments. Never apply to the skin any substance the components of which are unknown. This is particularly relevant to indigenous medicine. There is no need for complex mixtures and most agents applied to the skin need contain a base and only two to three active ingredients. Anyway a simple agent used well and familiar to the prescriber is always safer than the haphazard prescription of a range of new and poorly tested agents.

Elimination of cause of the skin lesion is essential. This applies particularly to dermatitis from primary irritants or allergens, but it is also important to know and eliminate infection if possible but this does not mean attempting to make a chronic ulcer sterile.

Damaged skin is vulnerable skin and every effort should be made to protect it from further injury. Scratching, rubbing, wrongly applied dressings, and unsuitable local medicaments are reasons for worsening of the skin condition and for the impairment of natural defences and repair mechanisms.

Chronic skin conditions are obviously more difficult to cure, and correct diagnosis is even more important than in acute skin conditions which are likely to heal spontaneously if the cause is eliminated. A biopsy for histological analysis is often helpful and where chronic infection is a possibility, bacterial or mycological analysis is clearly indicated.

The handicap of the chronic lesion includes a feeling of being unwelcome, often leading to the accusation of 'unclean' and leading to being 'outcaste'. The physician and nurse can sometimes do more to alleviate the skin condition by attention to this aspect of the handicap than by using more specific measures. Sympathetic questioning along the lines indicated on page 20.5 will help to relieve the patient's suspicion that one is not interested in the problem. Touching the skin during examination often does more to make the patient feel that the physician cares than any other manoeuvre.

When treating any skin disease, the overall objective is to create the body image which the patient hopes for, and when this fails, to help him to live with his problem and expect less. Every effort should be made to ensure that children remain willing to go to school, adults stay at work, and the old are kept comfortable. Remedies should be convenient and cosmetically acceptable, and if this is not possible, the social support should be that much more intensive. Attention to diet, camouflage measures, and regular careful attention to the skin can be very irksome for the patient, but can be made less so through co-operating with the doctor, nurse, or patient association, for example the obesity clinic supported by a weightwatchers group.

It is essential that the skin be protected from further injury: short-term gains from the use of powerful remedies must be weighed against possible long-term side effects. Often the risk is worth taking but it should at least be taken into account. Homely advice such as 'keep warm and out of the sun' and 'rest as much as possible with your feet up' is appropriate for much acute or severe skin disease. Some of the oldest remedies such as calamine lotion and British National Formulary preparations of tar (see Table 17) do least harm, but in chronic skin disease the patient is unlikely to persevere with these unless he is educated and encouraged. This takes time. Remember, patients spend more time listening to other patients in the waiting room than they do with the doctor – and are often in a more receptive frame of mind then. Make sure that the advice given in the waiting room is correct by handing out leaflets and teaching groups of patients, for example with audiovisual aids. Many patients do best with printed sheets of instructions so that they can read at their own pace quietly without anxiety of the presence of the physician. If appropriate, they should be told that their disease is neither catching nor cancer.

Some skin diseases which are chronic and incurable become easier to tolerate when better understood. Time given to the education of the patient may not reduce morbidity but it increases patient satisfaction and makes them demand less from the service.

The priorities of the patient with skin disease differ from those of the doctor who is treating him. Thus the patient equates severity with social ostracism or the subjective itch rather than with the percentages of body involved or systemic complications. Other people who should be drawn into the management of the patient with skin disease include parents, school teachers, employers, hairdressers, and the sporting fraternity – for example swimming-bath attendants. A school report which refers to weeping sores and scratching which interfere with the work of other children should be a thing of the past.

Patients can be told to live with their disease if given the tools to do so and if people are helpful and understanding. Unfortunately, only too often skin patients find that doctors admit to ignorance and show as little evidence of knowing how to manage their problem as the average doctor at a road accident. Moreover, just as with first aid, the management of common skin ailments is often better understood by the layman – more a reflection on the poor quality of medical education than on public interest in this case.

There are a number of paramedical aids to the management of skin disease which can be of immense value. A high proportion of skin patients are found to be suffering from the stresses of their domestic environment, confused elderly relatives or delinquent teenage children, for example. For these patients the help of a medical social worker is often very successful. The British Red Cross Society in the UK now provide a 'beauty care' service which has been extended to the provision of camouflage. Patients' associations often provide a great deal of education and support.

In hospital practice inpatient treatment is only occasionally

Table 30 Bases and their properties

Base	Site for application	Effect	Disadvantage	Examples
Watery and shake lotions (powder in water)	Acutely inflamed, wet and oozing	Drying, soothing, and cooling	Tedious to apply; frequent changes (lessened by polyethylene occlusion); powder in shake lotions may clump	Fuller's earth solution Lotio Terra silica Saline solution BPC Potassium permanganate 1/8000– 1/18 000 0.5 acetic acid in water Eusol in chlorinated lime and boric acid solution
Creams	Both moist and dry	Cooling, emollient, and moisturizing	Short bench life; fungal and bacterial growth in base; sensitivities to preservatives and emulsifying agents	Oily cream BP Aqueous cream BP, i.e. variants on water oil, and water mixes
Fatty acid, propylene, glycol	Both moist and dry	Emollient and moisturizing	May sting when applied; occasional sensitivity to propylene glycol	FAPG base
Ointments	Dry and scaly	Occlusive and emollient	Messy to apply and soils clothing; removed with an oil	Soft white paraffin Vaseline Hydrous wool fat (lanolin) Emulsifying ointment BP
Pastes; powder/ointment mixture	Dry, lichenified, and scaly	Protective and emollient; delays absorption of grease	Messy and tedious to apply (linen or calico needed)	Zinc compound paste BP Lassar's paste BP
Dusting powders	Flexures; may be slightly moist	Lessens friction	If too wet, clumps and irritates	Talc, dusting powder BPC Zinc, starch, and talc dusting powder BPC

necessary and can be greatly reduced by adequate provision of a good outpatient treatment service. Some departments link this to their inpatient department in order to provide a service outside of the normal convenient department's working hours – it is clearly more convenient for a working man to attend a department which is open in the evening.

Many chronic skin conditions are either hypertrophic or atrophic. Hypertrophic conditions require suppression as is described in the section on psoriasis. Common suppressants are corticosteroids or radiotherapy. On the other hand these are unsuitable for atrophy.

Management of skin disease in technically developed countries usually assumes regular follow-up. In developing countries in Africa or India, or with the Nomads of the Middle East, there is almost no possibility of follow-up. Treatments with a high risk of side-effects or exacerbations on withdrawal are not therefore ideal. Because malnutrition and infection is so common, dietary supplements and antibiotics are of value in almost any disease in which the host or constitutional vulnerability is a factor. Health education is always difficult but the mother with children is usually the most receptive pupil.

Local topical treatment

Drugs are dissolved or suspended in bases which have properties of their own quite independent of the active ingredient. As in Table 30 bases were originally either powder, water, or grease. However, modern processes have prepared bases which are essentially much more complex than this, although still retaining the objectives of the primary agents. Powder may repel water or absorb it and allow further evaporation. Modern powders tend not to cake and abrade the skin as much as the original talc or starch. Watery lotions evaporate and cool as well as wet and dissolve. Various agents such as alcohol or glycerine may be added to increase any one of these properties. Creams and emulsions of oil and water (aqueous or milky) or water in oil (butter or oily) are cooling, moisturising, and emollient. Penetration of active agents through the skin is aided by the aqueous (vanishing) oil and water creams. Ointments based on vaseline or paraffin are more occlusive and less quickly absorbed. They are better at softening dry surface scales.

There are various other preparations which are also water soluble, such as macrogels or emulsifying ointment in which a wax or animal fat is mixed with mineral oil. Pastes are powder and oil mixtures, such as talc and vaseline. They are more occlusive and protective. They are useful for slow release at the surface of agents such as dithranol. The addition of an active ingredient to a base often makes it unstable and hence various other agents are added as a preservative or to control pH. Further dilution usually makes the preparation still more unstable and, in other words, shortens its shelf life. Much of the skill in preparing an ointment or cream or paste is in the use of the homogenizer by the pharmacist.

The actions and side-effects of topical steroids are illustrated in Table 31. Tar and dithranol preparations are discussed in the section on psoriasis (page 20.37).

Skin cleaning

It is naive to attempt to sterilize the skin and the consequences of obsessive washing or the use of local antibiotics in the long-term are always worse than original state of the skin. Antibiotic regimens are essential for acute complications such as cellulitis or specific infections such as erysipelas. Washing is important for reducing smell and for removing debris but this is best done by soaking rather than scrubbing. Soaking is in fact one of the most effective of skin treatments for oozing exudative condition. Soaps irritate because they are alkaline and degrease. Some patients are sensitive to perfumes and other additives in the soaps. Most skin will tolerate some soaping but in hard water areas the amounts needed to degrease can cause considerable dryness and cracking of the skin. Soft rainwater or boiled milk should not be despised. Bran is an ancient and harmless water softener. About a pound of bran or oatmeal is tied into a muslin bag and soaked in boiling water. A very thin, starchy emulsion results. The stratum corneum drys, shrinks, and cracks in the cold. Cold water is not good for the skin. The skin that is dry is best treated at body temperature.

Emulsifying ointment is a useful soap substitute; it can be made into 'cakes' of soap or spooned out of a pot and mixed with hot water to soften it. Liberally applied it is a useful softener of crusts.

Bathing in water often for prolonged periods several times a day is an effective remedy for generalized soreness of the skin. The skin tends to dry excessively when all grease is removed and this

Table 31 Topical steroids

Active constituents Include hydrocortisone and synthetic halogenated derivatives of prednisolone such as betamethasone 17-valerate, triamcinolone acetonide, and fluocinolone acetonide. Halogenation increases topical activity
Bases Available in lotions, creams, fatty acid propylene glycol base, and ointments. Over 100 preparations listed in MIMS
Penetration Readily penetrate skin via the horny layer and appendages. Form a reservoir in the horny layer. Polyethylene occlusion and the use of higher concentrations increase penetration
Metabolism Some, though probably minor, metabolism in epidermis and dermis (for example, hydrocortisone conversion and other metabolites). Leave skin via dermal vascular plexus and enter general metabolic pool of steroids. Further metabolism in liver
Excretion As sulphate esters and glucuronides
Action Anti-inflammatory
　　Vasoconstrict
　　Decrease permeability of dermal vessels
　　Decrease phagocytic migration and activity
　　Decrease fibrin deposition
　　Decrease kinin formation
　　Decrease prostaglandin synthesis
　　Depress fibroblastic activity
　　Stabilize lysosomal membranes
　　Immunosuppressive: antigen–antibody interaction unaffected but inflammatory consequences lessened (above mechanisms)
　　Decrease rate of epidermal turnover
Side-effects
　Thinning of epidermis
　Thinning of dermis
　Telangiectasia and striae (due to thinning of epidermis and dermis)
　Bruising (due to thinning of dermis and vascular wall fragility)
　Hirsutism
　Folliculitis and acneiform eruptions
　May worsen or disguise infection (bacterial, viral, and fungal)
　Systemic absorption (rare but, for example, occurs in infants, when applied in large quantities under polyethylene pants)
Uses Eczema. Psoriasis in a few instances (facial, flexural, and palms/soles). Many non-infective pruritic dermatoses

Currently there are at least 60 different topical corticosteroids available in the UK which can be classified into four groups: mild, moderate, potent, and very potent. When treating skin disease, the doctor should select one from each group and test its efficacy and limitations; this should cover all contingencies. The least potent corticosteroids that gives good control should be used, starting with a mild preparation and increasing potency as required. With experience more potent corticosteroids can be used appropriately from the outset. If a very potent agent is required, it should be remembered that more than 50 g/week leads to measurable adrenal suppression. Because of the reservoir once daily application is recommended, supplemented by frequent emollients.
Modified from Hunter (1976).

can enhance pruritus. For this reason emulsifying ointments and proprietary (oilatum) oils are usually added to the bath.

The use of antiseptics in the bath is of dubious value but weak solutions of potassium permanganate 1/8000 to 1/16000 are often used. The patient often uses these agents too extravagantly. High concentrations of antiseptics poured into a bath may lie on the bottom and burn the skin, especially in sensitive areas such as the scrotum.

Bacteria are best dealt with by removing crusts and other debris – soaking does this even without the addition of antiseptics. In intertriginous areas soaking should be followed by drying. Under the breasts and in the groins or between the toes, organisms thrive in moist crevasses. At such sites powders which do not cake are helpful. Many proprietary brands of powders such as Zeosorb can be recommended.

The softening of crusts and exudate

Crusts and exudate, such as may be observed in impetigo, fungus infection, acute dermatitis, and psoriasis, require softening by prolonged contact with a wetting or greasing agent. The problem with wetness is that it quickly evaporates and dries. Wet soaks require absorbent dressings. Modern hospitals often supply only

gauze which is not particularly wettable. Old-fashioned linen or cotton sheets are ideal for wet dressings; usually these are applied in several layers and covered with a light ventilated dressing such as a hand towel or tubular gauze. Occlusive dressings are too heating. Polythene occlusion should not be used. Less rapidly drying agents include the ancient boric and starch poultice. The principle is 30 g of starch and 4 g of boric acid mixed in a pint of water and cooled and smeared onto linen strips which it should thickly impregnate. This wet dressing is applied to the crusted area and changed 4 hourly. Vaseline ointments are also suitable for softening scales as in psoriasis. Where the skin is dry and non-exudative, scaling is best softened with a paste made of 50 per cent vaseline and 50 per cent talc. Talc releases the vaseline slowly over a number of hours.

Smell

Malodorous necrotic skin is always very difficult to deal with. Removal of debris and dead tissues is essential. Antibiotics and local antiseptics cut down bacterial degradation which is a cause of smell. Metronidazole 400 mg three times daily is sometimes used to reduce the smell of tumours and it is effective against various anaerobic bacteria. Charcoal dressings (Johnson and Johnson) are also helpful.

Itching

Itching is described in the section on pruritus (page 20.35). Elimination of the causes are discussed therein and are always an important beginning to management. Management includes cooling, or at least, not over-heating. Excessive cooling is drying and this can cause pruritis. Water-miscible creams are cooling whereas vaseline-based ointments are heating. Antipruritic agents include ichthammol, tar, menthol, camphor, phenol, local anaesthetics and steroids (Table 31). Most of these are used in a 1 per cent concentration.

Protection of the skin from obsessional rubbing is helped by occlusive dressings in those who will tolerate them. In young children or in the adult who prefers to scratch, it is difficult to impose an occlusive regime. Cutting nails and encouraging gentle rubbing rather than scratching reduces the damage done to the skin.

Diet

Widespread skin disease is a cause of water and protein loss. The tongue and thirst are a good guide to water loss as is the specific gravity of the urine. High protein diets are necessary especially when there is great exfoliation.

Retinoids

The greatest advance in dermatological therapeutics of the last decade has been the introduction of systemic retinoids. The main retinoids available are Ro-accutane (CIS retinoic acid) and etretinate (retinoic acid). These modulate cell differentiation and growth, inhibit polymorphonuclear cell chemotaxis, inhibit polyamine formation, and inhibit eicosanoid formation. They are effective in acne, psoriasis, and genetic dyskeratoses. Their side-effects include teratogenesis, hyperostosis, lipidaemia, hepatitis, and various minor skin, bowel, and neurological problems previously recorded with vitamin A prescribing. They are prescribed in combination with other topical therapies or psoralen UVA therapy in an attempt to reduce their dosage and consequent side-effects.

Mood controlling drugs

Apart from the value of psychotherapeutic drugs to control the secondary emotional reactions to skin disease (many such drugs are used to control skin symptoms) antipruritics are often sedative but hydroxyzine and trimeprazine are favoured. Delusions of parasitosis and obsessive concern with pruritus is relieved by pimozide.

The placebo

For many skin conditions such as alopecia areata there is no specific treatment, and for some patients the available effective remedies are inappropriate, such as the painful treatments for warts in very young children. Nevertheless to do nothing at all is to encourage despair. Placebos such as mild lotions for the alopecia areata or warts should be harmless, cheap and given knowingly without self-deception.

Subjective symptoms such as itchiness are intolerable for some patients and sometimes can be relieved by inert agents such as calcium lactate or vitamin B pills given with assurance and confidence.

Bed rest

It is hard for the patient with skin disease to play the sick role especially when otherwise he is well. When told to rest at home sitting on a couch and pottering is often only a partial acceptance of the sick role. Admission to hospital and complete bed rest often switches off skin disease such as atopic eczema within 2 or 3 days. For psoriasis, 2 or 3 weeks is often required.

Irritable and distraught, the patient and his family may need rest from each other as well as acceptance that the illness is genuine and severe enough to take to bed. The bed of the skin patients should be placed where he is not a danger to other patients from cross infection (exfoliative skin disease is a rich source of staphylococcal infection), and this means that the neighbouring patient should be selected both for their likely resistance to infection but also for their likely good companionship. Modern hospitals include a high proportion of single cubicles for patients with skin disease together with a day room for social mixing once the dressings of the skin have been completed.

Intertrigo

The treatment of intertrigo is essentially to protect the area from chafing and secondary infection and to encourage dryness. Underlying disorders such as diabetes mellitus or obesity must be managed along traditional lines. Infection from bacteria, candida, or fungus requires monitoring by appropriate swabs and scrapings. Bed rest and nudity are helpful. In hot climates a fan encourages evaporation and drying. The folds of the skin should be kept apart by ventilated loose weave dressings. Acute eczema requires bland wet lotions, steroid creams, and simple antibacterial agents such as gentian violet or vioform cream. When dry, powdering is to be encouraged. Frequent bathing is always helpful.

Hand dermatitis

To provide healing and prevent relapse of dermatitis of the hands patients should use lukewarm water and emulsifying ointments when washing. If possible, running water is better than a prolonged soak in a bowl of detergent soap. Soap should be used sparingly and the hands thoroughly rinsed and dried carefully with a clean towel. As far as possible there should be no direct contact with detergents and other strong cleansing agents, shampoos, polishes, and stain removers. Oranges, lemons, grapefruit juices, and various other irritant vegetables should be avoided. Rings should not be worn during housework or other work even when the dermatitis has healed. This is because irritants often collect under them. Rings should be cleaned on the inside frequently with a brush and left in ammonia (one tablespoon to 500 ml of water) overnight and rinsed thoroughly. If gloves are used for washing dishes and clothes, they should be plastic and not rubber since the latter often causes dermatitis. They should not be worn for more than 15–20 minutes at a time. If water happens to enter a glove, it must immediately be taken off. The gloves should be turned inside out and rinsed several times a week. Sprinkling with talc before they are used helps to dry them. Cotton gloves can be used under the plastic ones. They should only be worn a few times before they are washed.

Table 32 Patients' associations (self-help groups) in the United Kingdom

The Psoriasis Association
7 Milton Street
Northampton NN2 7JG

National Eczema Society
5–7 Tavistock Place
London WC1H 9SR

Dystrophic Epidermolysis Bullosa Research Association
Secretary: Mrs Winnie Foster
38 Cornwall Avenue
Clayton
Newcastle-under-Lyme
Staffordshire

Vulnerability

The skin in many diseases is vulnerable. This is manifested as the tendency to produce disease even from minor trauma. It is seen in the primary irritant dermatitis of the atopic eczema sufferer, the Koebner phenomenon of psoriasis, or lichen planus. The hyperreactivity of the skin to needle puncture or pressure localization in vasculitis and in the ulceration that results from minor knocks of the skin of the legs in gravitational stasis. The skin's vulnerability is severe in epidermolysis bullosa.

In all these diseases advice has to be given about protection of the skin. It can be given in the form of information sheets about the care of the hands or legs or in booklet form for mothers of children with epidermolysis bullosa. The various patient associations produce excellent literature in this respect (Table 32).

Management of leg ulceration

The cause of ulceration should be identified and if possible eliminated. However, the aetiology of an ulcer in elderly women living in a city is likely to be different to that of a young man in a rural area in Central Africa. The causes of ulceration are listed in Table 33.

Elevation

The general management of ulceration is otherwise quite simple whatsoever the cause. The leg being below the level of the heart, there is always a tendency to develop venous hypertension and stasis. Deep vein thrombosis, absence of valves in the deep veins, and shunting of blood from the deep veins to the superficial veins via perforators are a significant cause of congestive changes in the microcirculation supplying the epidermis.

Healing of leg ulceration is always helped by elevation. If there is a major degree of arterial disease so that there are absent peripheral pulses then it should not be raised more than about 23 cm above the level of the heart. In every other case emptying of the distended veins and superficial venules is helped by lying the patient in a prone position and elevating the legs to an angle of at least 45°. This is best done by placing an object such as a chair under a mattress (Fig. 140). It is also best during the day because the patient cannot sustain such a position when asleep, but will curl up into a bundle at the top of the bed.

When stiff hips, heart failure, and obesity are factors preventing elevation of the legs a compromise includes compression bandages (see below) and attempts to make the most of any muscle pump in the lower leg. Intermittent positive pressure inflatable bags are marketed. These are leggings that blow up and squeeze the legs at a pressure and rate that can be regulated.

Elevation is also a requirement for lymphoedema but the protein collecting in the tissues of a swollen leg usually fails to clear satisfactorily via the lymphatics. To hasten its passage out of the tissues into the lymphatics, movement such as massage, vibration, or ankle exercise are necessary. Provided the solid elements of the skin, i.e. collagen fibres, are moved, the massage or vibration need not be very sophisticated. In the absence of lymphatics the

Table 33 Causes of leg ulceration

Trauma	External injuries, burns, scalds, chemical, self-inflicted, artefacts, contact dermatitis
Infections	
Viral	
Bacterial	Acute: 'desert sore', gas gangrene
	Chronic: buruli ulcer, tuberculosis, leprosy, swimming pool granuloma
Anaerobic	Meleney's ulcer, synergistic gangrene
Streptococcal	
Mycotic	Superficial or deep fungus
Spirochaetal	Syphilis, yaws
Leishmaniasis	
Infestations, bites	Spiders, scorpions, snakes
Metabolic	Diabetes
Vasculitis	Collagen disease, immune complex disease
Pyoderma gangrenosum	
Perniosis erythrocyanosis	
Venous	Stasis, congenital absence of veins, post-thrombotic
Atrophie blanche	
Necrobiosis lipoidica	
Neoplastic	Epithelioma, Kaposi's sarcoma, leukaemia, reticulosis, melanoma
Arteriovenous anastomoses	
Ischaemic	Scars, fibrosis, radiodermatitis
Arterial	Hypertension, temporal arteritis, atherosclerosis
Thrombosis, embolism, platelet agglutination	
Blood diseases	Coagulation, platelet disorders; impaired fibrinolysis
	Thrombocythaemia, polycythaemia
	Dysglobulinaemia, spherocytosis, sickle cell anaemia
Neuropathic ('trophic')	Diabetes mellitus, leprosy
	Tabes dorsalis, syringomyelia, alcoholic neuropathy

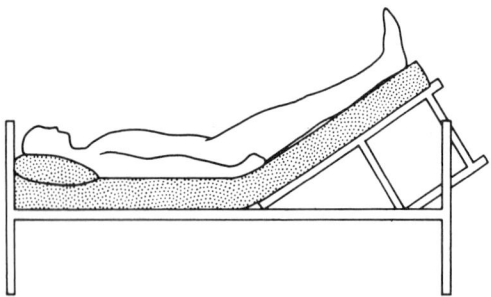

Fig. 140 Elevation of legs above the heart, necessary in the treatment of leg ulcers. A chair can be used to prop up the end of the mattress.

only other way protein can be removed from the tissues is by macrophages. There is some evidence that macrophage stimulators such as hydroxyethylrutoside (Paroven) is helpful in this respect and it is certainly otherwise harmless.

Movement
Inflammation is aimed at removing injurious agents and promoting healing. In acute infection or injury there is often a need for immobilization. However, such immobilization should be localized to the site of injury. Gentle passive movement of the joints and active movement of the main muscles of the leg are encouraged by wriggling the toes or ankles, or by quadriceps exercises.

Unfortunately many persons with ulceration continue to be immobile and to dread any movement which causes pain long after any need for immobilization to contain the inflammation. Stiffness of the ankle and contractures at the joints are common and delay healing as well as considerably add to crippling.

Deep vein thrombosis is a consequence of immobilization and this too contributes to morbidity as well as mortality. Thus in general terms the maintenance of mobility is essential in the management of leg ulcers.

Exercises in bed can be followed by exercises in the standing position aimed at maintaining an upright posture and ankle mobility as well as to strengthen the muscles of the calves which are so important in pumping blood through and away from the deep veins. For those who are able, walking should be encouraged. Especial instruction should be given concerning the harm done by sitting with the legs dependent or crossed, or standing without movement at the ankle. Even a soldier standing to attention needs to maintain venous return by imperceptible but nevertheless effective wriggling of the toes. For the housewife 'march at the sink' is a suitable war cry.

Dressings and bandages
The objective of bandaging is to hold the dressing in position to protect the leg from further injury and to provide a sleeve against which movement of the underlying muscles can compress and empty the superficial veins.

The superficial vessels of the skin of the leg are often distorted and congested from chronic inflammation and gravitational stasis. Such vessels are often damaged and cause ischaemic ulceration as a result of external injury which includes the kinks, wrinkles, and inequalities of an ill-fitting bandage. It should be remembered that a leg that swells can develop severe ischaemia beneath a constricting bandage which was quite loose when applied before the leg became swollen. Large swollen legs as in lymphoedema or after deep vein thrombosis can tolerate unskilled bandaging and tight compressive bandages. By contrast a thin, ischaemic or ageing skin suffers greatly from carelessly applied bandages. The secret is never to encircle the leg completely and to avoid any twists or kinks. The leg is an awkward shape, particularly around the ankle, and many of the twists and the bulk of the bandage tends to be over the bony prominences where the skin is thin and ulcers are common. One system of bandaging is to use two layers – the one as a dressing and the other as a cover. The bandage which is used as a dressing is virtually strips of material no longer than one and a half the circumference of the leg. These may be applied from a bandage which is cut repeatedly whenever the direction of the bandage requires a change (Fig. 141). Above the ankle the bandage is folded at the side of the leg and reversed so as not completely encircle the leg (Fig. 142). Most bandages used in this way are no more than a cotton bandage dipped in a powder, water, or cream mixture. As the water evaporates or is absorbed, the residual powder sets and a more solid and splinting sleeve is produced. Where such bandages are not available any strips of materials such as calico or linen similarly impregnated (spreads) will do as well. The overlying covering bandage should be more stretchable than cotton – plasticity rather than the elasticity is necessary in a thin leg. Large lymphoedematous legs may be covered by a stronger elastic material. The tendency for too much bandage to collect around the ankle can be prevented by cutting a strip of bandage and placing it first of all around the ankle (Fig. 143). Thereafter this strip can be avoided by subsequent bandages (Fig. 144). In this way usually two or three turns of the bandage succeeds in covering the entire foot.

The control of infection—what should be put on the ulcer?
If the cause of ulceration is eliminated then healing should take place. However, healing depends on healthy epidermis at the edge of the ulcer. Often this is damaged by proteolytic enzymes from slough and infection. Unhappily common is the damage done by irritation or sensitivity to medicaments. For this reason, simple

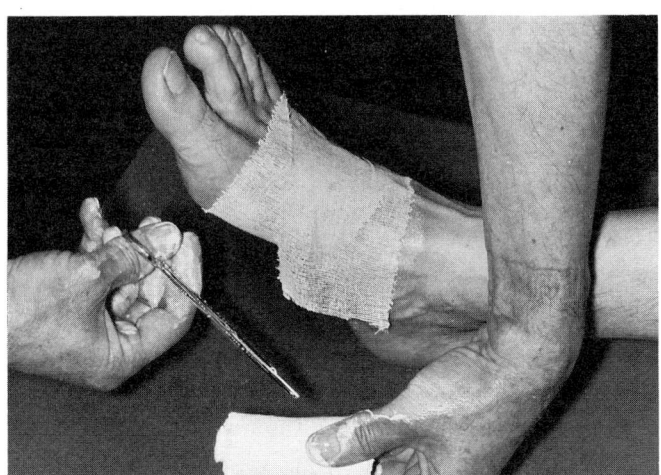

Fig. 141 Cotton bandages soaked in various pastes can be used as a firm comfortable and closely applied supportive dressing of a limb. By repeated cutting of the bandage, awkward wrinkles and folds can be eliminated and if swelling of the limb occurs, the bandage can expand and so avoid becoming a constricting band.

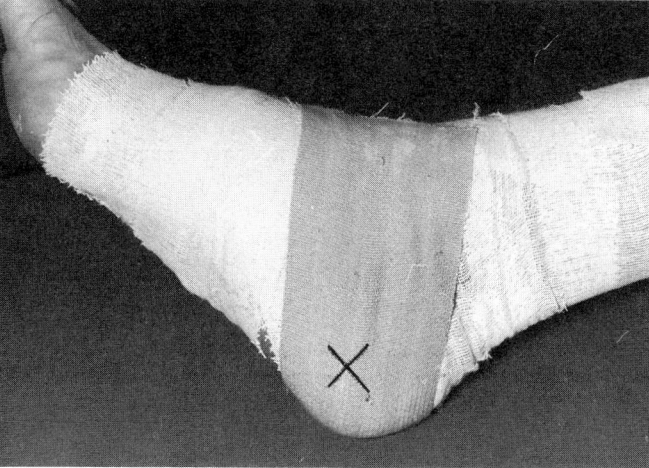

Fig. 143 The ankle is a very awkward shape for bandaging. To avoid having too much bandage for easy accommodation within a shoe, a strip placed over the heel before applying the rest of the bandage allows for complete coverage of the area using only three turns around the foot and lower leg.

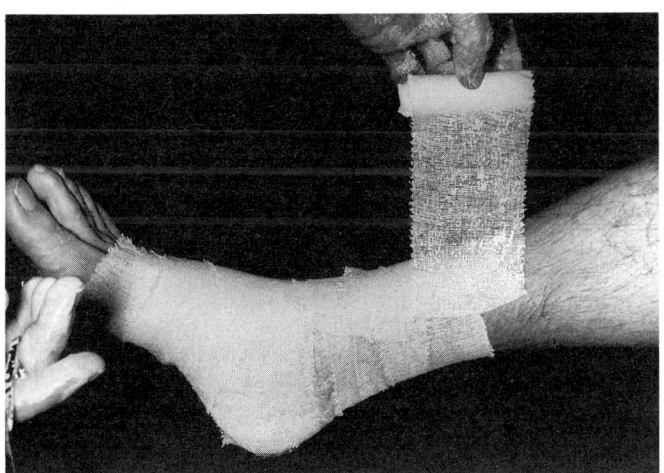

Fig. 142 Folding the bandage back also prevents it acting as a circumferential constricting band.

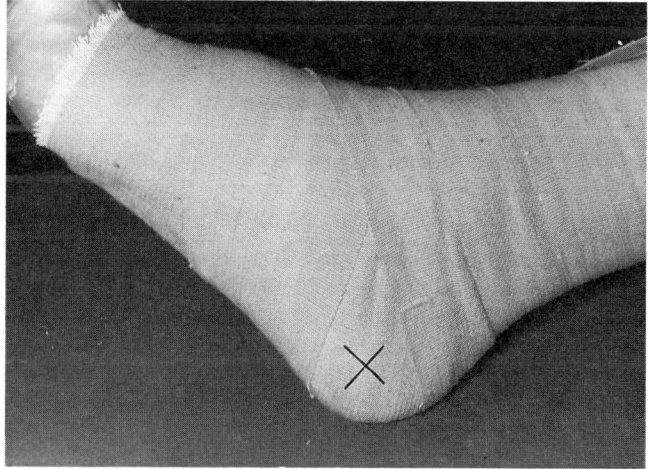

Fig. 144 The strip in Fig. 143 can then be avoided by subsequent bandages.

bland therapy aimed at reducing debris should be used. Debris will float off if softened. Hard adherent crusts are usually dry. The most effective remedy is wetness and saline is sufficient to give this provided it is applied very frequently as a wet dressing. Surgical debridement should be removed with a scalpel or scissors if there is any non-viable tissue. This is not difficult provided one remembers that dead tissue has no sensation. In other words, trim away anything the patient is unaware of, provided the diseases causing neuropathy like leprosy and diabetes mellitus have been excluded, in which case only that which is necrotic and non-adherent should be removed. Antiseptics such as eusol, 0.5 per cent acetic acid (a teaspoon of vinegar in a pint of water), or 0.5 per cent silver nitrate in aqueous solutions are other wetting agents. While helpful to remove slough they inhibit granulation tissue and are less often recommended.

Many antibiotics are applied to ulcers and they rarely control infection. It is naive to believe that an ulcer can be made sterile. It is common for antibiotics to be inhibited rapidly by serum and debris under a bandage. It is common also for such agents to do damage to the epidermis. In this respect it is sometimes forgotten that the health of the surrounding epidermis is more important for healing than the state of the ulcer bed. Tropical phagedenic ulcers

often follow trauma and relative avascularity encourages invasion by fusospirochetal organisms.

Contact dermatitis

Healing is often delayed and ulcers may be enlarged by damage to the surrounding epidermis by medicaments. Such dermatitis as is seen so often around the ulcer occurs either because of the medicament or due to bacterial toxins or allergy. Table 34 is a list of common causes of contact dermatitis.

Toe nails

Poor sight, apathy, stiff hips, and obesity are all reasons why toenails are uncut. It is surprising how the western world has come to expect 'professionals' to deal with this problem when in fact toe nail cutting is something any good neighbour can do. Clippers rather than scissors are to be recommended because they cut hard thickened nail more effectively. The nails should be softened by soaking them in warm water for 10 minutes. Only the distal part of the nail protruding beyond the toe need be cut. Good positioning of the cutter and patient is adequate light is essential. Only very distorted nails or the foot with arteriosclerosis and the conse-

Table 34 Common causes of contact dermatitis in leg ulcers

Ointment bases and preservatives	Additives in bandages
Wool alcohols (lanolin)	Ester gum resin
Parabens	Azo disperse yellow No. 3
Propylene glycol	Colophony
Chlorocresol	Mercaptobcnzothiazolc thiuram
Ethylene diamine	(rubber)
Antibacterial agents	Self-medication
Sodium fusidate	Caine mix (local anaesthetics)
Gentamicin sulphate	Antihistamine creams
Neomycin	Dettol
Soframycin	Germolene
Quinoline mix (Vioform)	

quences of diabetes mellitus need the attention of a chiropodist where such is available.

Corns

These are due to thickening of the epidermis due to pressure from without or from pressure from underlying bony prominences. It should be possible to avoid pressure from without by adjustment to footwear and skilful padding so that the weight is taken on less bony areas of the foot. Surgery is sometimes necessary to remove bony prominences. The thickening of the skin is self-perpetuated and is greatly helped by careful paring away of excess keratin, avoiding damage to underlying blood capillaries which often project upwards to near the surface.

Carcinoma

Carcinoma develops in the hypopigmented margin of ulcers that have persisted for many years. Such ulcers often invade bone but rarely metastasize. Local excision and grafting is often preferable to amputation.

Surgery

Whereas in technically developed countries, amputation and a good prothesis may convert a cripple into an active and otherwise normal person, amputation is objected to by certain races, such as the Bantu, or by certain religions, such as the Hindu. It inevitably causes them to be dejected and rejected so that they are unemployable and outcast.

Injection of superficial veins with sclerosants or their removal, is indicated only when the deep veins are patent. If the deep veins are blocked, then the superficial veins are the only venous drainage of the legs and they should be preserved. The assessment of the proportion of flow returned through the superficial veins is greatly facilitated by the Doppler flowmeter. Surgical debridement and skin grafting is often a means of quickly healing ulceration but it is outside the scope of this textbook. Consideration of amputation must take into account social circumstances and the degree of subsequent aftercare.

Elephantiasis – the swollen limb

The handicap of a large swollen limb is considerable. The causes include congenital absence of lymphatics, malignancy and its removal, filariasis, and the poisoning of macrophages by silica. The problem of elephantiasis is discussed on page 6.165 but in this section some general measures for large swollen limbs will be discussed.

All patients should avoid further injury and infections, such as insect bites. Extremes of climate such as sunburn or chilblains, indeed any factor which produces inflammation, severely exacerbate the problem of lymphoedema. The patients need to be instructed in the simplest details of hygiene and chiropody. While in some academic departments surgical attempts to produce lymphatic venous anastomoses has produced some remarkable cures, many of the operations also produce considerable mutilation. Conservative therapy should always be tried; this includes gentle manual massage, particularly at the junction of the lymphoedematous tissue with normal tissue where collaterals can often be developed. Elevation and exercise of a limb which has been well-bandaged or fitted with a tight sleeve can often produce a great reduction in limb circumference and volume. Even severe fibrosis may be eliminated. Modern therapy can produce socially acceptable limbs with restored function and a greatly decreased incidence of cellulitis. There is some evidence that benzopyrones such as coumarin encourage the removal of protein by macrophages and thus reduce protein-containing oedema and consequent fibrosis.

References

Baker, H. and Wilkinson, D. S. (1979). In *Textbook of dermatology* (eds A. Roth, D. S. Wilkinson, and F. J. G. Ebling), ch. 67–70. Blackwell Scientific Publications, Oxford.

Foldi, M. and Caseley-Smith, J. R. (1983). *Lymph angiology*, p. 832. Schattauer Verlag, Stuttgart, New York.

Hunter, J. A. A. (1976). *Today's treatment*, 7. Blackwell Scientific Publications, Oxford.

Sheard, C. (1978). *Treatment of skin diseases*, p. 404. Year Book Medical Publishers, Chicago.

The decubitus ulcer

The decubitus ulcer is a consequence of distortion of the tissues, often due to pressure which obstructs blood flow. It occurs especially in neurological disease in which painful stimuli from tissue distortion or ischaemia is not recognized. Because the pathogenesis includes impaired perfusion by blood, anything which affects blood supply can contribute to the problem. Thus, in general, old patients who are ill or dying, and especially if they have vascular disease, are most likely to develop sores. Such sores are unusual in purely motor neurological disease with no sensory loss or in the very old who tend to have a healthy vascular system.

Because it is distortion of the tissues rather than simply pressure that induces sores shearing forces on the sacral area and heels are also to be taken into account. Such forces are increased by moisture from sweating or incontinence. Distortion of the tissues is enhanced by deformities such as kyphoscoliosis or contractures.

While the basis of management is relief of tissue distortion by frequent relaxation of stress and strains on the tissues, best brought about by movement, factors contributing to poor perfusion must also be attended to. These include intercurrent illness causing hypoxia, hypotension, immobility, dehydration, impairment of consciousness or peripheral sensation. Most acute illnesses requiring admission to hospital provide the necessary criteria for the development of a decubitus ulcer within the first hours or days. The chronic sickness which determines prolonged bed rest at home rarely produces this degree of tissue ischaemia and thus the hospital nurse gets blamed for what has never occurred at home. The blame is partly misdirected because, for example, an old woman with a fractured hip may develop the decubitus ulcers from immobility in the ambulance, on a hard trolley waiting for a bed or on the operating table. Education concerning the causes of decubitus ulcer should be widely dispersed amongst all attendants.

All ill patients are best put to bed. Some of the worst pressure sores can occur while sitting in a collapsed state in a day room or during the postoperative phase of 'mobilization'. The basis of management is regular 2 hourly turning. Heavy and unco-operative patients, together with inadequate staffing, especially at night, are a constellation of factors that frequently combine so that the resources are not enough to prevent pressure sores. Good equipment to modify pressure on a bed surface is important and may include a fleece under the heels, a bed cradle to take the weight of the bed clothes, a variety of soft surfaces, and alternating pressure as in a ripple bed preferably with large ripples.

In countries where such equipment is not available, there is often a large contingent of relatives at the bed side whose attentiveness can be mobilized to assist in turning and passive movements at frequent intervals.

A long severe illness is difficult to manage outside an intensive care unit because as implied by the word intensive, there is a requirement for vigilance of all aspects of the physical, conscious state and activity of the patient. It is for this reason that some nursing schools demand that a check list known as the Norton pressure sore score is regularly noted. But even this becomes less accurate each day as a long illness drags on. Once an ulcer has developed it becomes the problem of wound healing. Removal of dead tissue is essential, often by surgical debridement. The development of granulation tissue and re-epithelialization will follow only if general health improves and blood supply is adequate. There are so many agents advocated for the healing of wounds that it is important to realize that none are essential and many are harmful to healthy tissue. Those which will remove slough may inhibit living cells. Granulation tissue is the best protection against infection and it is discouraged by many of the strongest antiseptics. All wound dressings should aim to reduce debris, to keep the wound moist, and to promote granulation tissue perfused by an adequate supply of normal blood.

z

SECTION 21
NEUROLOGY

INTRODUCTION

C. D. MARSDEN

Neurological diseases contribute a major burden on health care resources. It has been estimated that cerebrovascular disease alone is responsible for 4.4 per cent of inpatient days, and 10.9 per cent of loss of life expectancy in the United Kingdom. Neurological illness accounts for 9.8 per cent of outpatient referrals to hospital. On average, all neurological disease is estimated to be responsible for 7.8 per cent of the total burden on the National Health Service.

Some neurological problems are particularly common. About 20 per cent of women and 12 per cent of men have migraine, of which about half consult a doctor, and a fifth see a neurologist. Stroke is one of the commonest causes of death and morbidity in most countries, being responsible for something like one in five of deaths. It has been estimated that some 50 per cent of stroke victims die within 30 days of the acute event. Of those who survive, some 10 per cent are left with little disability, 40 per cent have mild residual disability, another 40 per cent have sufficient disability to require specialized care, and 10 per cent need institutional care because of severe neurological impairment. It has been

Table 1 Approximate average annual incidence and point prevalence per 100 000 population for neurological disorders

Disorder	Annual incidence	Point prevalence
Migraine	—	20 000
Cerebrovascular disease	200	500
Epilepsy	40	500
Parkinson's disease	20	200
Cerebral palsy	—	60
Bell's palsy	20	—
Primary brain tumour	10	40
Trigeminal neuralgia	4	—
Multiple sclerosis	2	50
Guillain-Barré neuropathy	1	—
Charcot-Marie-Tooth disease	—	2
Friedreich's ataxia	—	1
Motor neurone diseases	1	5
Huntington's chorea	0.5	6
Wilson's disease	0.2	1
Syringomyelia	0.3	8
Myaesthenia gravis	0.4	4
Polymyositis	0.5	6
Muscular dystrophy	—	6
Myotonic dystrophy	—	2

Modified from Kurland (1980).

estimated that head injuries account for 1 per cent of all deaths, 20 per cent of accidental deaths, and about 50 per cent of road traffic accident deaths in the United Kingdom. Head injuries are responsible for about 3 per cent of all acute admissions to hospital. Some 1 in 200 of the population have epilepsy, 1 in 1000 have Parkinson's disease (rising to over 1 in 200 in those aged over 60 years), and 1 in 2000 have multiple sclerosis. For every 1000 total births (live plus stillborn), about 13 infants will have a major malformation, of which about 25 per cent will be of the CNS. Some 2.5 per 1000 children of school age have cerebral palsy. Most other neurological illnesses are less frequent or rare (Table 1), but there are many of them; perhaps there are more than 400 different neurological diseases.

With far fewer than 200 specialist neurologists in the United Kingdom, it is inevitable that a major proportion of patients with neurological diseases must be cared for by other practitioners. This is the case for most of the developed countries, and certainly for the Third World. In a past era, neurology was much to do with diagnosis, but little was on offer for treatment. Now this is different. Many of the major neurological illnesses (migraine, epilepsy, and Parkinson's disease, for example) pose major therapeutic challenges. Neurosurgery can attack a range of brain and spinal tumours and malformations. Furthermore, developments in rehabilitation have revolutionized the lot of those with neurological disability. Neurology today comprises the triad of diagnosis, treatment, and rehabilitation, with the added continual challenge of discovery prompted by dramatic developments in basic neuroscience.

References

Alberman, E. M. (1980). Cerebral palsy. In *Clinical neuroepidemiology* (ed. F. C. Rose), pp. 312–317. Pitman, London.

Black, D. A. K. and Pole, J. D. (1975). Priorities in biomedical research: indices of burden. *Br. J. Prevent. Soc. Med.* **29**, 222–227.

Jennett, B. (1980). Epidemiology of head injuries. In *Clinical neuroepidemiology* (ed. F. C. Ross), pp. 356–360. Pitman, London.

Kurland, L. T. (1980). The contribution of the Mayo Clinic centralised diagnostic index to neuroepidemiology in the United States. In *Clinical neuroepidemiology* (ed. F. C. Rose), pp. 37–46. Pitman, London.

Kurtzke, J. F. (1980). An overview of congenital malformations of the nervous system. In *Clinical neuroepidemiology* (ed. F. C. Rose), pp. 170–195. Pitman, London.

Waters, W. E. (1980). Migraine. In *Clinical neuroepidemiology* (ed. F. C. Rose), pp. 384–390. Pitman, London.

INVESTIGATIONS USED IN NEUROLOGICAL DISEASE

Electroencephalography

B. MACGILLIVRAY

The EEG record

The electroencephalogram (EEG) relates to the brain roughly as the ECG relates to the heart. Whereas the generation of the ECG is well understood, the EEG is much more complex and there is a less satisfactory model. The electrical activity on the scalp is rather like the waves and ripples on the surface of the sea. Each pen or channel records the amplitude of the waves and their shapes and rates of change with time. There are usually 8 or 16 channels of recording derived from combinations of linkages (montages) between 20 and 22 electrodes placed on the scalp in a standardized regular grid pattern which relates the recording to the anatomical regions of the brain. The electrodes are about 6–8 cm apart. The voltages are very small, 10–100 μV normally, but up to 500 μV in epilepsy.

The routine EEG record consists of a fan-folded sheaf of some 20–30 pages bound at the left-hand edge to be read as a book. It is annotated with relevant patient data and observations, the montages in use, sensitivity of recording, and other technical information. The actual recording time is 10–15 min, although the procedure takes 30–45 min in all, and usually includes a three-minute period of hyperventilation which has the effect of activating latent EEG abnormalities (hypocapnic alkalosis). The equipment requires a fair skill and knowledge to achieve satisfactory artefact-free records. Interpretation of the record requires a familarity with the technology involved, the ability to identify artefacts, and the effects of age and changes in conscious state, as well as sound clinical knowledge. It is not a matter for the inexperienced.

Generation of the EEG

In practice the EEG may be assumed to be generated directly only by the neurones of the cerebral cortex. Non-neuronal elements, tumours, blood clots, infarcts, cysts, and abscesses, are intrinsically silent although often very active in EEG terms because of the effects they may have on the functioning of adjacent and distant neurones and their connections. The functional behaviour of cortical neurones as reflected in the EEG is affected by local circumstances, glial scarring, infiltrations, infections, anoxic or metabolic effects, for example, as well as, and very profoundly, by excitatory and inhibitory influences from connections with deeper structures, the thalamus, and the brainstem. Some of the most dramatic EEG changes occur in normal physiological sleep when they often exceed those seen in many pathological conditions.

Abnormalities in the EEG are either due to disconnections, and here the long connections from deep structures in the brainstem are particularly significant in producing abnormalities distant from the site of the lesion, in the frontal regions, for example, or result from 'active' synchronized discharge of neurones of which the prime example is in epilepsy. The reader should conclude that the presence of an EEG abnormality at some location on the head does not necessarily indicate local pathology; the subjacent cortex may be quite normal. All EEG abnormalities must be related to the anatomical connections within the brain.

Each electrode 'sees' the co-ordinated or synchronized activity of the neurones in about a 2–3 cm diameter subjacent volume of cortex. This represents the mean activity of large populations of neurones, at least tens of thousands and most often millions depending on circumstances. If the activity of these neurones is desynchronized, as, for example, is normally the case when the cortex is actively processing information, the EEG trace is of low voltage, shows no waves and resembles noise. This is shown in Fig. 1a, where the normal 10 c/s occipital rhythm is abolished on eye opening, an alerting response. This simple manoeuvre, and the response, allows incidentally, the very important conclusion that the alerting systems of the brainstem are functional and operative on the cortex at the relevant electrode and that the anatomical pathways must be intact.

Note also that the EEG waves represent the statistical mean or average behaviour from moment to moment of large populations of neurones (strictly, the average of the postsynaptic potentials of the large pyramidal neurones of the cortex). Despite the natural impression that because very sensitive equipment is being used to record minute electrical potentials and must therefore detect very small changes in the brain, the opposite is true. At the neuronal level, the EEG is a relatively crude measure of change, the behaviour of individual neurones being of no consequence. On the other hand, because EEG changes represent statistical shifts in the mean behaviour of large populations, they can be expected to have high intrinsic validity. Note also that cortex in the depths of sulci, or buried beneath operculae as in the insula, or on the mesial or basal aspects of the brain is generally inaccessible to

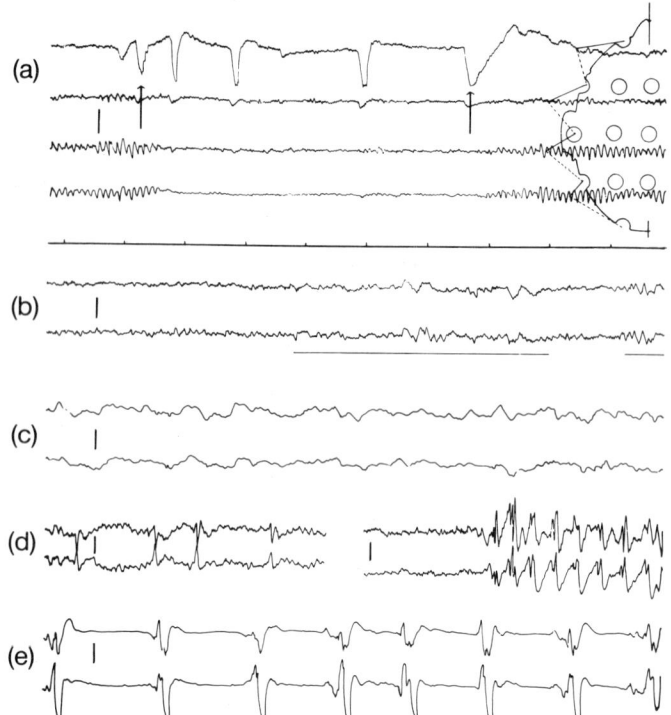

Fig. 1 Samples of EEG traces. (a) Normal record and effects of attention on eye opening, between arrows. Montage on right. (b) Modest intermittent abnormality in cerebro-vascular disease. (c) Irregular pattern in encephalitis. (d) Local epileptic spikes on left, onset of generalized epileptic discharge on right. (e) Repetitive high voltage discharges following global cerebral anoxia predicting fatal outcome. Marker indicates seconds for all traces, vertical bar = 100 μV.

direct EEG recording. This amounts to one-third of the entire cortex. Active lesions in this inaccessible cortex may however be inferred from changes elsewhere, but this gap in coverage needs to be remembered when relating the EEG to clinical circumstances.

The EEG report

In interpreting the EEG, one takes into account such aspects as the shape and distribution of waves, rhythms, and complexes, incidence of normal and abnormal features, symmetry and paroxysmal events, and many other features the details of which may be found in the texts cited. It is customary for the EEG report to begin with some factual synopsis of the record, the purpose of which is, firstly, to act as an *aide-mémoire* from which some mental picture of the trace can be reconstructed as a point of reference, and, secondly, to indicate to the reader the salient points on which the interpretation has been based. For the initiated the factual report carries a useful indication of the degree of abnormality and may even allow reinterpretation of the trace in changed clinical circumstanes. It is, however, never fully comprehensive.

Most of the terms used in reports have fairly ordinary meanings although the reader may not be fully aware of their implications. *Alpha rhythm* refers to a normal near-sinusoidal sequence of waves at between 8 and <13 c/s which is seen in the occipital area when the eyes are closed in the resting state (Fig. 1a). It may be slowed in a variety of metabolic and toxic conditions and with some lesions locally. *Beta rhythms* are fast frequencies above 13 c/s seen normally in anterior regions and about the vertex. They may be abnormal locally with superficial and usually chronic lesions and are often enhanced by sedative drugs. There is a genetic predisposition. *Delta waves* or *rhythms* if they are repetitive, are slow waves, <4 c/s. They are always abnormal in the alert adult and commonly associated with pathology, but are normal in sleep, and in infants and youngsters. They become increasingly unacceptable from adolescence onwards. *Theta waves*, or intermediate slow frequencies, 4 – <8 c/s, are very variable, occur·commonly in the temporal regions, and decline with maturity. They are frequently of pathological significance.

Following on the factual observations the report will have a short conclusion or interpretation. At this point it is important to note that the reporter will generally offer a limited, best interpretation of the record, based on experience and the clinical information available. The majority of EEG abnormalities are non-specific and the differential possibilities are likely to be quite large. If germane clinical information is omitted, inadequate or incorrect, then the report may likewise be inappropriate or wrong. It is good practice to discuss inappropriate conclusions with the reporter if maximum use is to be made of the EEG. The interpretation must always be related to context.

Use of the EEG – general principles

Like the history and physical examination, neurophysiological investigations reflect the functional state of neurones. Therein lies their value and their weakness; they rarely carry intrinsic aetiological significance. In general, the effects of pathology are most stable in the peripheral nervous system, less so in the spinal cord, and least in the brain. Fluctuating EEG observations quite correctly reflect changing states, the observations themselves are accurate even if their significance is not clear.

The routine EEG is but a 10 min sample in a continuum of the brain's reaction to pathology. Repeated and extended recordings may often be appropriate, in epilepsy, for example. As indicated below, the EEG may quite often be negative in the presence of clearly identifiable pathology and a negative result carries little weight in some circumstances. A positive result, however, has the validity of a clinical sign and always needs an explanation.

In general terms, the EEG is likely to be of greatest value in detecting and monitoring changes of state in cerebral activity, irrespective of pathology. As a further generalization, acute or rapidly changing conditions produce much more dramatic EEG abnormalities than slowly changing or chronic states. There is a strong tendency for the EEG to return to normal with the recovery from acute cerebral insults despite the continued existence of quite substantial pathology.

Specific applications

Paediatrics

The infant brain is highly reactive in EEG terms, becoming less so with age. The principles of interpreting adult EEGs apply, but it may often be impossible to say more than that something is wrong. Repeated observations are often necessary. The condition of hypsarrhythmia (q.v.) is an important diagnostic entity. The EEG is useful in all forms of epilepsy and paroxysmal disorders of the nervous system, the encephalitides and encephalopathies, and the metabolic degenerative disorders.

Tumours

The EEG is of limited value, being too imprecise as to location. The investigations of choice are imaging techniques. The EEG has value when these are negative or equivocal. It often shows abnormalities which antedate the development of a clear image particularly in the slowly evolving infiltrating gliomas. It is sometimes quite helpful in identifying secondaries when only one lesion has been visualized. It may be helpful in detecting recurrence. Sometimes it is useful in pathological differentiation and it often shows the secondary neurological effects of neoplasia elsewhere.

Vascular lesions

Very helpful when there are ischaemic changes rather than infarction. May be helpful with transient ischaemic attacks and often indicates permanent effects (Fig. 1). Completed and resolved infarcts are often quite silent. Superficial frontal infarcts and infarction of the caudate, putamen, and occasionally of the thalamus, can be silent. In classical acute hemiplegia which is clinically a stroke, a near normal EEG is virtually diagnostic of capsular infarction. Intracerebral haemorrhage usually produces marked abnormalities. The EEG is often helpful in determining the site and vessel involved in subarachnoid haemorrhage. Subdural haematomas are often fortuitously found but can be quite silent and missed especially if small, bilateral, and chronic. Cerebrovascular malformations can be silent unless they produce infarction, haemorrhage, or epilepsy. The EEG is often helpful in defining vascular dementia. Migraine can produce quite marked EEG abnormalities even between attacks, sometimes of an epileptiform appearance.

Head injury

Very useful. In early stages of closed head injury the EEG will provide evidence of the degree of cerebral commotio. Useful follow-up for resolution and indications of potential epilepsy.

Metabolic and toxic disorders and the encephalopathies

Often diagnostic. Useful monitor especially in the hepatic encephalopathies and in dialysis problems. Hypoglycaemia has marked effects. A normal EEG generally excludes a severe metabolic toxic or encephalopathic disorder.

Encephalitis

Usually diagnostic (Fig. 1c). May be helpful in identifying herpes simplex encephalitis. Often clinching in subacute sclerosing panencephalitis (SSPE) and in Creutzfeld-Jacob disease, when characteristic EEG patterns occur. Little change in meningitis but shows degree of associated encephalitis. (Good in cerebral abscess.)

Epilepsy

Epilepsy is a clinical phenonemon and a clinical diagnosis. The presence of epileptic activity (characteristically paroxysmal and containing very sharp short duration 'spikes', Fig. 1d) is helpful in determining the type of epilepsy, localized or generalized, particular forms, such as spike and wave, and in general, indicating stability or otherwise and giving some indication as to the likelihood of clinical attacks. It should be a routine investigation in undiagnosed episodic loss of consciousness. Long-term monitoring may be of diagnostic value in indeterminate cases as sometimes may special recording techniques, sleep deprivation, induced sleep (methohexitone, pentobarbital) with sphenoidal leads. About 20–30 per cent of known epileptics may have normal EEGs on occasions.

Psychiatry and behaviour disorders

The classic psychiatric syndromes, personality disorders, and neuroses show little helpful in the way of changes in the EEG which is often normal. Primary value lies in a warning of organic disease and epilepsy as aetiological factors. Helpful screen, but negative results not necessarily as reassuring as sometimes thought. Abnormalities frequently occur in behavioural disorders and are often of unknown significance. Psychotropic drugs may produce or aggravate EEG abnormalities.

Coma

Very useful in assisting with diagnosis. Good monitor. Absent EEG activity is not required to demonstrate cerebral death in the United Kingdom but may be used elsewhere. There are special recording requirements. The EEG in some circumstances, brain stem infarction and global anoxia, for example, is a reliable predictor of a fatal outcome (Fig. 1e). Useful monitor in cardiac bypass surgery.

Concluding comments

The emphasis in this section has been on general principles in the hope of providing some understanding of the nature of the EEG as an investigatory tool. Used with discrimination and a clear brief it can be invaluable. It provides a unique insight into cerebral activity for which there is no substitute.

References

Kiloh, L. G., McComas, A. J., Osselton, J. W. and Upton, A. R. M. (1981). *Clinical electroencephalography*, 4th edn. Butterworths, London.

Niedermeyer, E. and Lopes da Silva, F. (eds) (1982). *Electroencephalography. Basic principles, clinical applications and related fields*. Urban and Scharzenberg, Baltimore and Munich.

Principles of neuroradiology

I. ISHERWOOD

Progress in neuroradiology during the last decade has been rapid, and the impact of new imaging methods on clinical practice profound. The quest for a method to demonstrate neural tissue directly *in vivo* has, to a large extent, been realized in computerized tomography (CT) and magnetic resonance imaging (MRI). The neuroradiological armamentarium is nevertheless considerable and an awareness of the value, limitations, and potential role in clinical management of the various available methods is important.

Intracranial disorders

Plain films

The ready availability of CT in some neuroradiological units has led to a re-evaluation of the role of conventional skull radiographs, though their importance in studies of the skull base and pituitary fossa remains undiminished.

The basic radiographic projections include a lateral, a postero-anterior with 20° caudal tube tilt, a semi-axial with 30° caudal tube tilt (Towne's), and a submento-vertical (basal), though additional radiographic projections including tomography may be necessary to demonstrate specific features.

Tomography is a method of presenting a plane of tissue whilst blurring structures above and below. The image is achieved by equal and opposite movements of X-ray tube and film. Such movement is commonly linear but can be complex, namely circular, elliptical or hypocycloidal. The extent of movement influences the thickness of the focal plane which may be reduced to 1–2 mm. Tomography is especially valuable where fine detail of bone or calcification is required.

Computed tomography

In CT, film is replaced by sensitive detectors which move synchronously with a collimated X-ray beam directed at the edge of a narrow slice of tissue. The precise measurements of transmitted X-radiation are processed by computer to produce information about very small elements of tissue in the cross-section of head or body. Each element has a numerical value which represents the ability of this small volume of tissue to attenuate X-rays. The thickness of the slice is usually 2–13 mm and the cross-sectional area of each element less than 1 mm by 1 mm. The smaller the element the higher the resolution. The numerical values (Hounsfield numbers) range from − 1000 (air) to + 1000 (bone) with water as zero.

The image is viewed on a television monitor as a grey scaled analog version of the digital data. High numbers are white and low numbers are black. The digital nature of the image enables the observer to interrogate the whole range of tissues contained within the uniformly thin slice of tissue. The high sensitivity of the method enables very small differences in X-ray attenuation which accompany disease to be detected. In the brain, discrimination is possible between white and grey matter, cerebral ventricles, and the CSF pathways (Fig. 1). In the orbit the optic nerve, orbital muscles, and other retrobulbar structures are identifiable due to surrounding low-density fat (Fig. 2). Coronal sections (Fig. 3) can be achieved by positioning of the head but reformatting of the

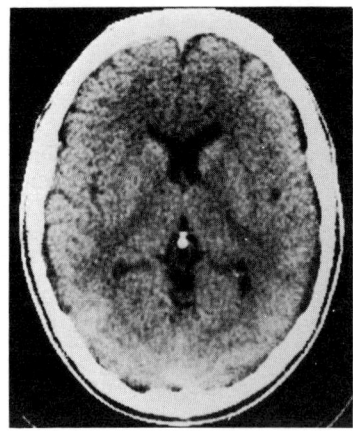

Fig. 1 CT scan of normal brain, midventricular section. Note grey/white matter discrimination and calcification in pineal.

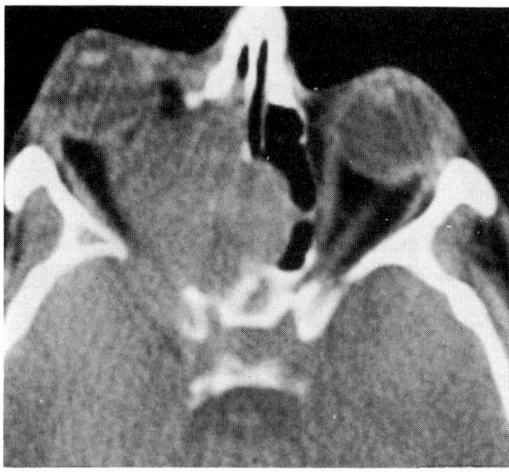

Fig. 2 CT scan of post-nasal carcinoma with orbital and intracranial extension, orbital section. Note extraconal position of tumour and bone erosion.

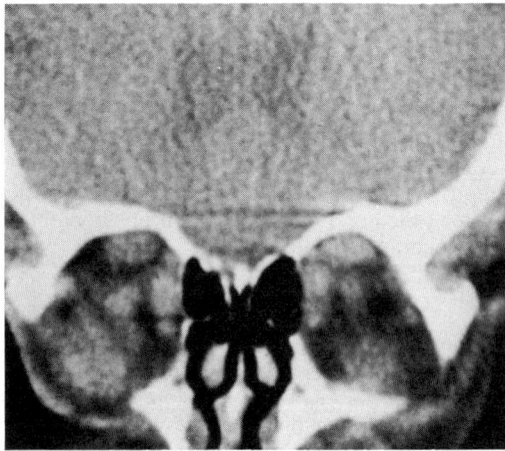

Fig. 3 CT scan of thyroid exophthalmos, coronal section. Note symmetrical thickening of orbital muscles.

digital data from multiple slices will permit reconstruction in any plane (Fig. 5).

The sensitivity of CT in the brain can be enhanced by intravenous injection of an iodine-containing contrast medium. Increased vascularity or defects in the blood–brain barrier result in retention of high-density iodine. The diagnostic accuracy of CT in the inves-

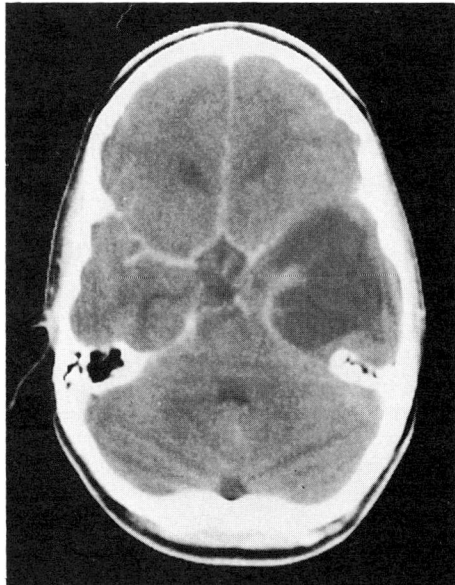

Fig. 4 CT scan with contrast enhancement of cystic astrocytoma in the left temporal lobe. A tumour nodule is present on the medial aspect and the left middle cerebral artery is displaced.

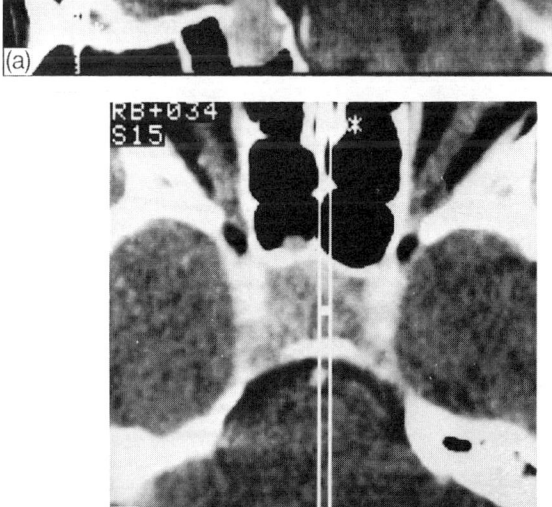

Fig. 5 (a) Sagittal reformatted image of enhancing pituitary tumour expanding the pituitary fossa and extending into the suprasellar cistern. (b) CT transverse section of the same tumour.

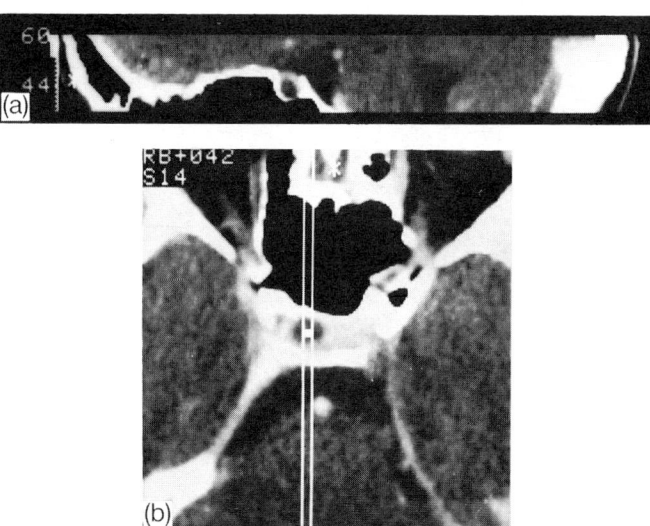

Fig. 6 (a) Sagittal reformatted image of a non-enhancing pituitary microadenoma in a normal sized pituitary fossa. The rim of enhancing normal pituitary gland is present above the tumour. (b) CT transverse section of the same tumour.

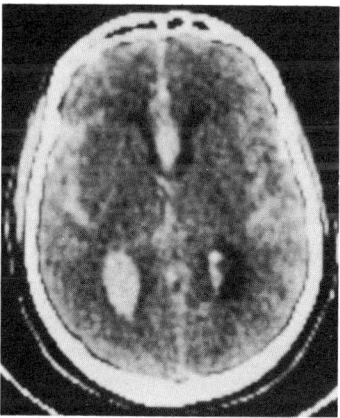

Fig. 7 CT scan of subarachnoid haemorrhage from anterior cerebral artery aneurysm. Note blood in the ventricles, subarachnoid space, and at the site of the aneurysm.

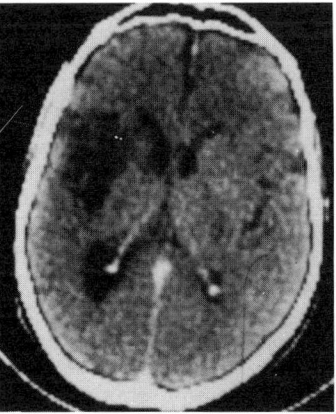

Fig. 8 CT scan of cerebral infarction.

tigation of brain disorders is significantly improved by such contrast enhancement: 99 per cent of supratentorial mass lesions are detectable. Whilst certain patterns of enhancement are recognizable (Fig. 4), precise tissue characterization is not possible. The use of intravenous contrast in conjunction with reformatting in alternative planes has particular value in the study of pituitary lesions. The normal pituitary gland enhances with intravenous contrast. Tumours of the gland may also enhance (Fig. 5) or, in the case of microadenomas, may be represented by non-enhancing zones (Fig. 6).

Recent intracranial hematomata, whether intra- or extracerebral, have a high density due to the presence of haemoglobin (Fig. 7). Absorption of haemoglobin results in a reduction of this density which on the basis of a normal haematocrit at the outset is likely to be isodense with brain in two to four weeks and of lower density later if no further bleeding occurs. Conversely infarcted brain has a low density (Fig. 8) but may enchance for a period when the blood–brain barrier is disrupted and there is luxury perfusion.

CT, because of its non-invasive nature, its availability as an out-

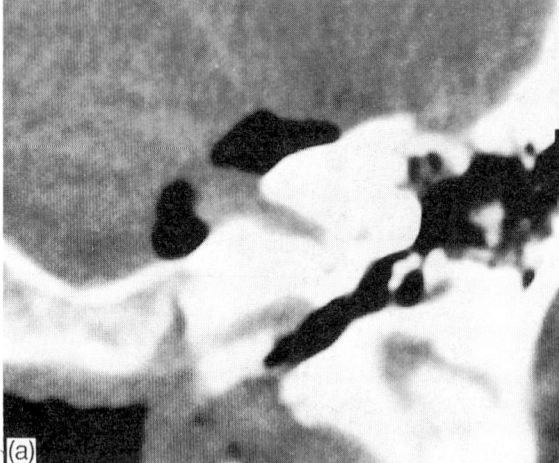

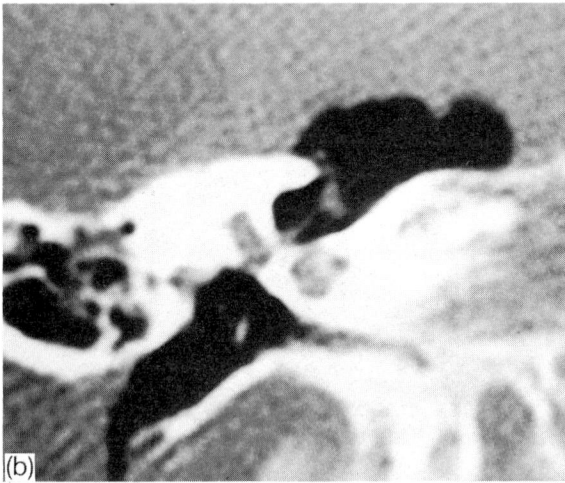

Fig. 9 CT air cisternography of (a) small intrameatal acoustic neuroma and (b) normal auditory nerve complex.

patient procedure, and its ability to image brain directly is now the primary investigative method in many neurological disorders.

The increased sensitivity of CT to tissue density differences can be exploited further to demonstrate very low concentrations of water-soluble contrast medium in the CSF spaces in the absence of raised intracranial pressure. CT cisternography following intrathecal injection of isotonic, non-ionic, low osmolality, water-soluble contrast medium with low neurotoxicity, permits detailed investigation of the CSF pathways and circulation.

CT cisternography with very small (5 ml) quantities of air and selective positioning of the head is a valuable technique for the investigation of the internal auditory canal and cerebello-pontine angle (Fig. 9).

Cerebral angiography

Visualization of the intracranial circulation can be achieved either by percutaneous puncture or selective catheterization of the appropriate carotid or vertebral artery and injection of iodinated contrast. In these circumstances selective catheterization is performed by the Seldinger technique, a percutaneous method of introducing a catheter and flexible guide wire into a peripheral artery. The femoral artery is the most commonly employed and is the safest. Cerebral angiography is a well established technique in departments of neuroradiology for the demonstration of topographical vascular anatomy. Improvement in vascular detail can be achieved by rapid serial film studies with subtraction and radiographic magnification. Subtraction is a photographic or electronic

technique whereby the distracting background to a contrast procedure can be removed.

Local and distant displacement of cerebral vessels may permit an anatomical diagnosis whilst the demonstration of an abnormal circulation can enable a pathological diagnosis to be achieved (Fig. 10). Precise delineation of vascular anomalies and occlusive diseases can only be achieved by angiography. The disposition of the anterior cerebral artery and the thalamo-striate veins can be used to indicate the size of the cerebral ventricles, but the role of cerebral angiography as a screening method has now been replaced by CT.

Digital fluorography

Digital fluorography is a technique providing digitization of the video output of an image intensifier. Whilst spatial resolution is not yet as good as conventional film, electronic subtraction of video frames together with other image processing techniques allows demonstration of intra- and extracerebral vessels by simple intravenous injection of contrast medium. The intravenous technique has particular merit in those circumstances where direct invasion of the arterial system would be hazardous, in the monitoring of intracerebral disease and in the exclusion of large aneur-

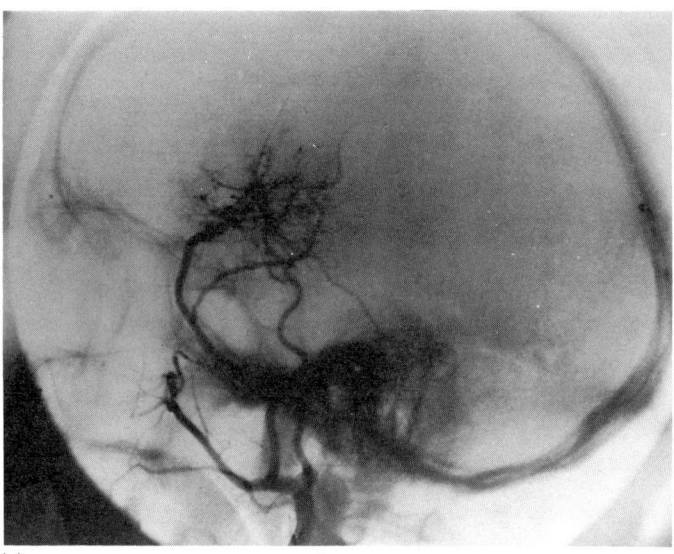

(a)

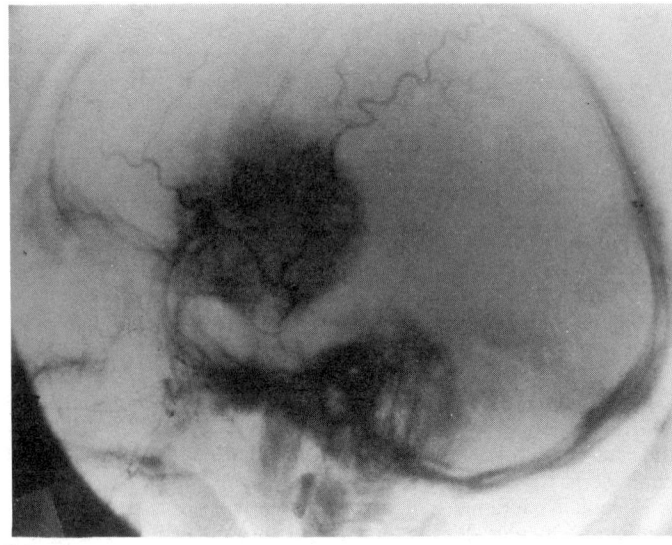

(b)

Fig. 10 Carotid angiography, with subtraction, of sphenoidal meningioma: (a) arterial phase; (b) capillary phase.

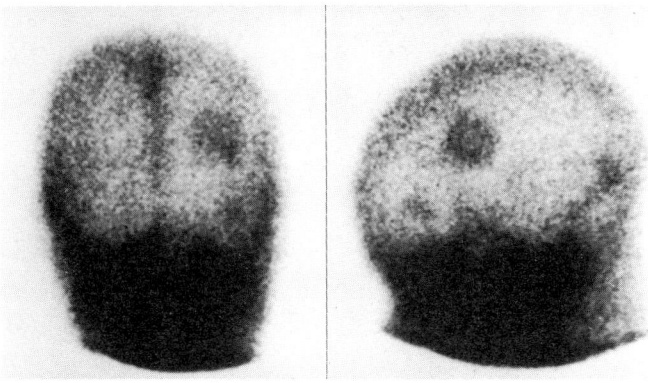

Fig. 11 Radionuclide scan with $^{99}Tc^m$ of multiple metastases: left: antero-posterior projection; right: left lateral.

ysms. It is simple to perform and can be carried out on an outpatient basis. A disadvantage is the non-selective nature of the vascular display. Digital fluorography, in association with arterial injection of contrast medium, permits smaller volumes of contrast medium to be used than are necessary in conventional arteriography. It has the added attraction of immediate television viewing. Both factors are of importance in interventional procedures.

Isotope brain scanning

Radiopharmaceuticals administered intravenously equilibrate with extracellular fluid and do not normally penetrate the blood-brain barrier. Technetium as $^{99}Tc^m$ in its pertechnetate form is the agent most commonly used intravenously for static brain studies. Detectors in a rectilinear scanner or gamma camera register activity for normal soft tissue, the major venous sinuses and some pathological processes within the brain. The normal structures of brain are not visualized. Only those abnormalities which are vascular or destroy the blood–brain barrier are demonstrated. Radio-nuclide imaging of the brain is safe, carries little radiation dose, and can be carried out as an outpatient procedure. Its sensitivity depends not only upon the location and size but also on the nature of the abnormality (Fig. 11). A high false negative rate can be anticipated in the posterior fossa and skull base, irrespective of size or histological character, due to overlying activity. Conventional radionuclide imaging suffers significantly from lack of tissue characterization. Zones of cerebral infarction, for example, may, in the first two weeks, mimic tumour activity due to uptake of isotope. A number of methods for the measurement of blood flow have been proposed using non-diffusable tracers, e.g. ^{133}Xe, by inhalation or intracarotid injection though they are rarely a routine of clinical management. A minicomputer linked to a gamma camera enables rapid dynamic images (one per second or faster) to be obtained, stored in digital form, and later processed. Such radionuclide 'angiography' can have value in demonstrating variations in abnormal vascularity.

Images depicting the distribution of radioactivity in tomographic section are available. Emission computed tomography (ECT) provides a new dimension in the assessment of brain function. A new class of cerebral agent labelled with single photon short-lived gamma emitters (IMP, iodo-isopropyl amphetamine, and HM-PAO, hexa-methyl-propoline-amine) which cross the blood–brain barrier rapidly, should enable quantitative assessment of regional cerebral blood flow to be made. Positron emission tomography (PET) enables short-lived radioactive isotopes, namely, ^{11}C, ^{13}N and ^{15}O to be detected, but requires a cyclotron in close proximity. Studies of glucose metabolism and protein synthesis as functions of brain activity are encouraging, particularly in the study of the cognitive disorders.

Radionuclide cisternography can be performed with non-lipid-soluble materials injected intrathecally. A labelled protein, eg RISA, or inorganic chelate, e.g. ^{169}Yb, is usually used. CT with a non-ionic water-soluble contrast medium as described earlier, however, now provides a more attractive method of visualizing both the morphology and dynamics of the CSF circulation.

Ventriculography

Demonstration of the cerebral ventricular system by the introduction of air, iodized oil, or water-soluble iodinated contrast material through a burr hole requires neurosurgical intervention and will only be considered after appropriate consultation. Ventriculography has now been almost completely replaced by CT.

Pneumoencephalography

Demonstration of the ventricular system and subarachnoid spaces by air is a technique appropriate to specialized departments of neuroradiology. The accepted procedure is fractional introduction of 25–30 ml of air by the lumbar route with selective positioning of the patient's head to outline the appropriate structures. Tomography is necessary to depict detailed structure. Where CT is available, pneumoencephalography is now rarely performed but can be of value in the demonstration of midline lesions. It should not, except under exceptional circumstances, be performed in the presence of raised intracranial pressure.

Ultrasound

Ultrasonic vibrations are produced by passing an electric current through a suitable crystal. The soundwaves thus generated pass directly through homogeneous matter but are reflected back by certain interfaces and detected by the same crystal. This procedure is known as an 'A' scan. A 'B' scan is designed to produce a display of internal structures by controlled movement of the probe and can be obtained in real time. Ultrasound does not employ ionizing radiation and has no hazard but does require considerable operator skill.

An 'A' scan can demonstrate midline intracranial structures and may also reveal the ventricular walls and subdural collections. 'B' and 'real time' scanning procedures can be used effectively in the cranial cavity through the 'window' of the open fontanelle in infants. In this age group it can have an effective role in the demonstration of ventricular size and the detection of intracerebral haemorrhage in the new born. The technique can also be employed peroperatively in the adult.

Nuclear magnetic resonance

Nuclear magnetic resonance (NMR) employs radiofrequency radiation in the presence of a magnetic field to produce images. The information in magnetic resonance imaging (MRI) is derived from the signals emitted when certain naturally occurring magnetic elements in the brain or body are caused to resonate in the magnetic field. Hydrogen is the most abundant of these elements and can be detected at relatively low magnetic field strengths (0·02 Tesla upwards). In proton imaging the MR signal depends not only on the proton density and relaxation times, T_1 and T_2 of those protons following radiofrequency disturbance, but also on the timing parameters of the radiofrequency pulse sequences used. Image contrast depends on the interaction between all these factors, and not simply, as in CT, on the attenuating properties of tissue to X-rays. An understanding, therefore, of both the imaging process and the neuropathology under investigation, are important in the proper use of MRI (Fig. 12). Magnetic resonance does not employ ionizing radiation. Furthermore, it can provide sections in any anatomical plane. Compact bone and calcium do not produce a signal. Posterior fossa images are therefore free of the obtrusive artifacts which may be produced during CT (Fig. 13) but the inability to display calcium can be a disadvantage. Magnetic resonance is more sensitive in the detection of demyelinating plaques than CT (Fig. 12), but its role in the clinical management of multiple sclerosis has yet to be determined.

Recent advances in tissue discrimination include the use of paramagnetic tracers such as Gadolinium-DTPA, which crosses the

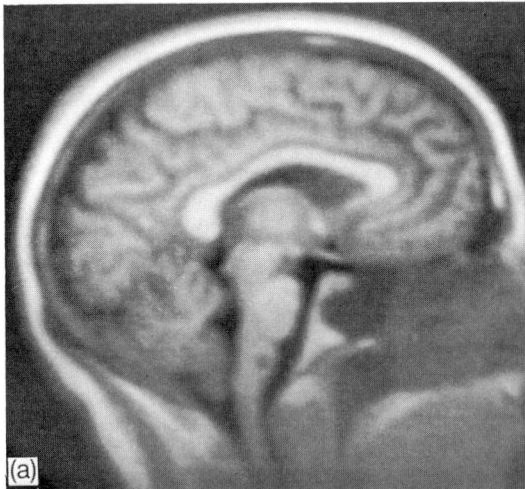

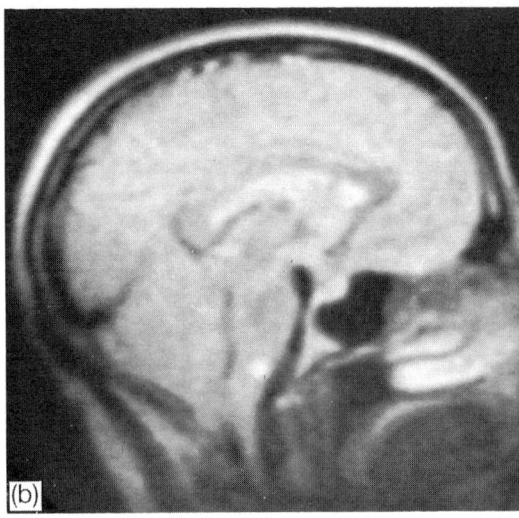

Fig. 12 Magnetic resonance imaging in the sagittal plane of a demyelinating plaque in the brain stem. (a) T_1-weighted RF sequence. (b) T_2-weighted RF sequence. A second plaque adjacent to the frontal horn of the lateral ventricle is detectable on this sequence.

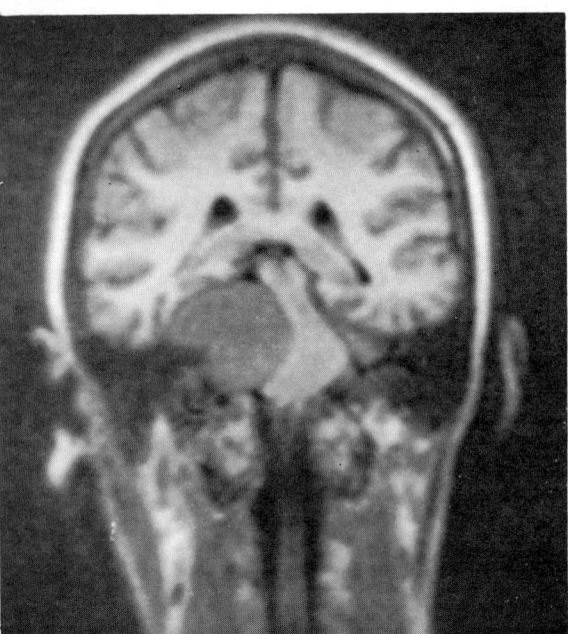

Fig. 13 Magnetic resonance imaging in the coronal plane of bilateral acoustic neuroma. The brain stem is displaced by the larger lesion on the right. T_1-weighted RF sequence.

damaged blood–brain barrier and produces contrast enhancement by a shortening of T_1 and T_2 relaxation times at the target site. Improvements in spatial resolution and image quality can be achieved by the use of small radiofrequency surface coils.

At higher field strengths (over 1.5 Tesla) the study of iron metabolism in the brain is possible by virtue of its natural paramagnetic effect on surrounding protons. It is possible, by NMR spectroscopy, to study the metabolism of naturally occurring phosphorus and to monitor inorganic phosphorus, ATP, and phospho-creatinine. A number of muscle disorders, including McArdle's syndrome, have been studied by this method. ^{13}C has a very low natural abundance but can be added as a label and used to study the glucolytic reactions by which glucose is metabolised inside the living cell.

Spinal disorders

Plain films

Conventional radiography may reveal congenital and acquired bone abnormalities together with indirect evidence of intervertebral disc disease. In the case of tumour erosion a significant proportion of a vertebral body must be destroyed before a lesion is detectable. Demonstration of neural or soft tissue involvement requires more sophisticated techniques.

Isotope bone scanning

The vertebrae are the most frequent sites of skeletal metastases in common cancers. Their detection forms the widest application of skeletal scanning. Several radiopharmaceuticals are available, and their uptake is influenced by the blood supply and mineral turnover of bone. One of the most commonly employed is a technetium-labelled phosphate complex (methanine diphosphonate).

The role of radioisotope bone scanning as a primary screening method in the study of metastatic bone disease in the spine is well established. A number of non-malignant conditions, notably degenerative disease of axial synovial joints, can, however, also give rise to increased isotope activity and plain films together with CT may then be necessary as further investigations.

Myelography

Investigation of neural tissue within the spinal canal requires the introduction of contrast medium into the subarachnoid space. Negative (air) and positive (iodinated) contrast media are used. Air myelography requires tomography in addition. Iodized oil (Myodil) has been widely used in the spinal subarachnoid space though it is now recognized that arachnoiditis is a frequent complication. The preferred medium is now a non-ionic, low-osmolarity contrast which, because of its water-solubility and lower density, permits good demonstration of nerve roots. When confined to the lumbar spine, the technique is referred to as radiculography (Fig. 14).

The role of myelography is to obtain accurate anatomical localization of pathological processes in the spinal canal, particularly their relationship to the dura, i.e. extra- or intradural, and to the spinal cord, i.e. extra- or intramedullary. Contrast can be introduced by the lumbar or cisternal route.

Computerized tomography (CT) and computer-assisted myelography (CAM)

CT as described above is a non-invasive procedure providing an axial projection of spinal topographical anatomy against a detailed background of paravertebral muscles, vascular structures, and body cavity organs. In particular it provides a more precise identification of the articular configuration of the apophyseal joints and

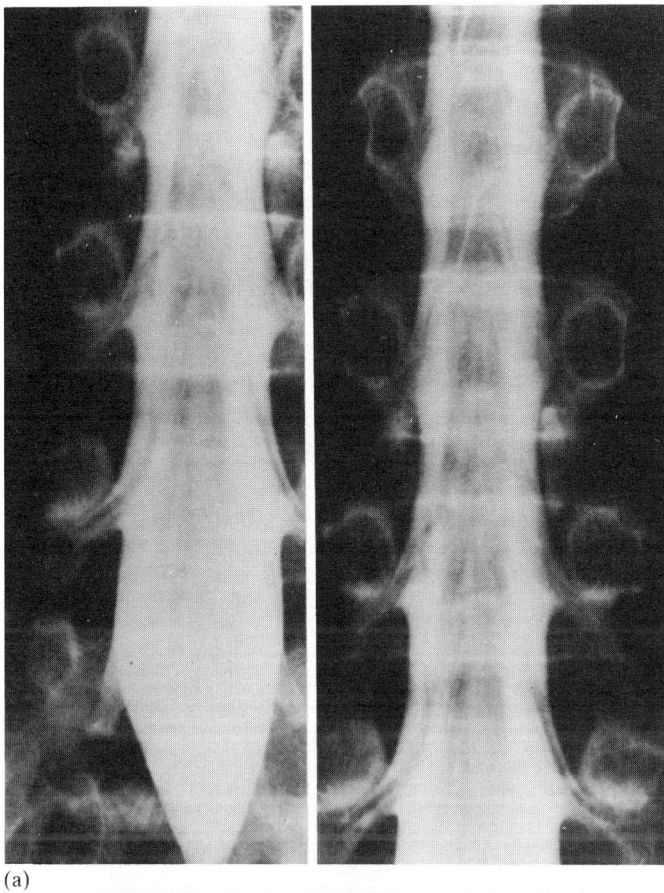

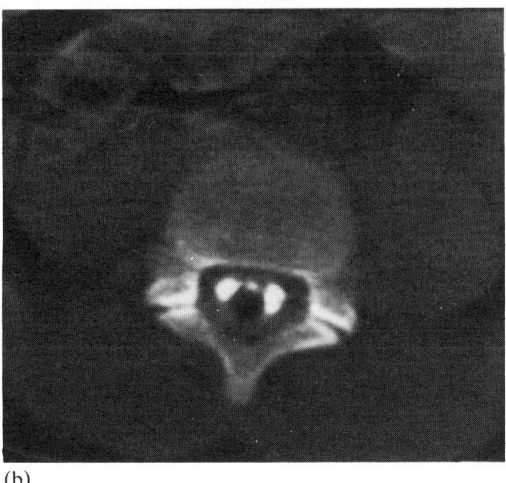

Fig. 14 Spinal dysraphism. Note tethered cord and intramedullary fat. (a) Water-soluble contrast myelography. (b) Computer assisted myelography.

their relation to the spinal canal and intervertebral foramina. By its quantitative nature it also has a role in the direct estimation of bone mineral in the axial skeleton.

CAM refers to the study of water-soluble contrast medium in the spinal subarachnoid space by CT. The increased sensitivity of CT enables water-soluble contrast medium to be detected in much lower concentrations than would be possible by conventional radiology. When injected by the lumbar route, contrast medium appears in the thoracic spine in one hour and in the cervical and intracerebral subarachnoid space in one to two hours (Fig. 14).

It seems likely that the role of CT and CAM in the evaluation of

spinal disorders will be increasingly challenged by magnetic resonance imaging.

Spinal angiography

The main blood supply to the spinal cord is the midline anterior spinal artery complex which receives multiple feeding vessels from radicular arteries. The main feeding vessel of a vascular abnormality may arise at a distance. Selective catheterization of many segmental vessels, usually via the femoral artery with subtraction techniques, is therefore necessary in this procedure.

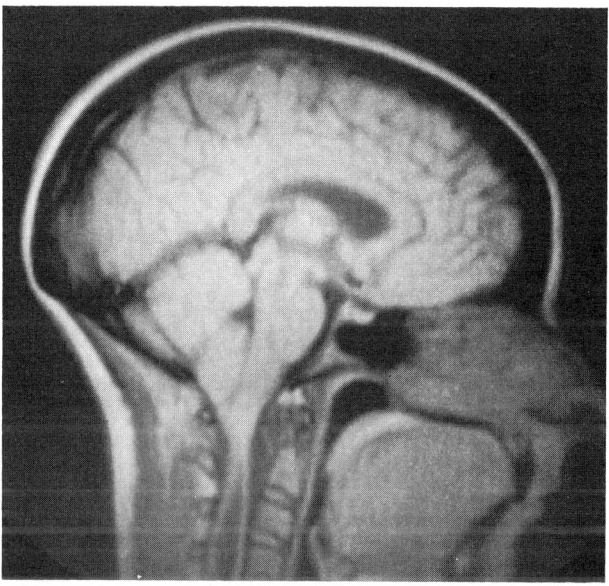

Fig. 15 Magnetic resonance imaging. A sagittal section of Chiari malformation with herniation of hindbrain and cavitation of the cervical cord.

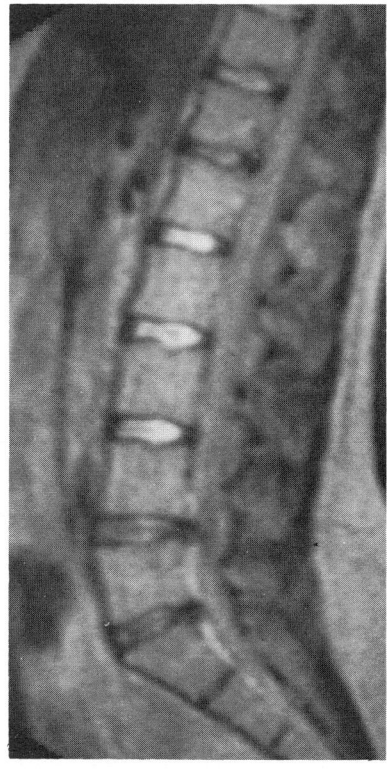

Fig. 16 Magnetic resonance imaging of lumbar spine, sagittal section. Degenerate discs at L4/5 and L5/S1 with loss of the normal nucleus signal and herniation of the annulus.

Spinal angiography has proved valuable in the diagnosis of spinal vascular malformations but has only a limited role in the investigation of spinal tumours. The method is obviously of importance in the radiological management of embolization procedures.

Nuclear magnetic resonance

Magnetic resonance imaging can be used to demonstrate the spinal cord throughout its length, employing sagittal or coronal sections. It has proved of particular value at the craniocervical junction in the demonstration of syringomyelic cavities and associated herniations of the hindbrain (Fig. 15). Neurofibromas, unlike meningiomas, usually have a high signal.

The nucleus of a normal intervertebral disc has a high signal on T_2-weighted sequences. This signal is lost in degenerative disc disease (Fig. 16). The use of appropriate radiofrequency sequences enables cerebrospinal fluid to be displayed white, producing in effect an 'MR myelogram'. Herniation of the annulus can then be demonstrated (Fig. 16).

It seems likely that magnetic resonance imaging will play an increasingly important role in the evaluation of spinal disorders.

Lumbar puncture

R. A. FISHMAN

Indications

Changes in the composition of the cerebrospinal fluid (CSF) serve as guides to neurological diagnosis and management. Lumbar puncture (LP) should be performed only after clinical evaluation of the patient and consideration of the potential value and hazards of the procedure. LP is needed urgently if meningitis is suspected. In many patients with a fever of unknown origin, even in the absence of meningeal signs, LP is essential. CSF cytological studies are also particularly useful in the diagnosis of leukaemic and carcinomatous meningitis, as well as some brain or spinal cord tumours. CSF examination is usually necessary in patients with suspected intracranial bleeding to establish the diagnosis although computerized tomography (CT), when available, may be more valuable. For example, primary intracerebral haemorrhage or post-traumatic haemorrhage is often readily observed with CT making lumbar puncture an unnecessary hazard. However, in primary subarachnoid haemorrhage LP may establish the diagnosis when CT is falsely negative. CSF findings prove invaluable in the evaluation of many other clinical problems, e.g. in the differential diagnosis of confusional states due to viral encephalitis, tuberculous meningitis, or neurosyphilis. CSF should be examined in patients acutely ill with unexplained seizures. LP is valuable in establishing the diagnosis of multiple sclerosis, the vasculitides, and other inflammatory disorders of the central nervous system (CNS) and meninges. LP is often used to ascertain that the CSF is free of blood before anticoagulant therapy for stroke is begun. (However, extensive subarachnoid bleeding is a rare complication of heparin anticoagulation, begun as long as 4 hours after a traumatic bloody tap. Therefore heparin therapy should not begin for at least 4 hours after a bloody tap.) LP has limited therapeutic usefulness, e.g. intrathecal therapy has a role in some cases of CNS lymphoma and fungal meningitis.

Contraindications

Lumbar puncture in contraindicated in the presence of suppuration in the skin overlying the spinal canal. A serious complication of LP is the possibility of aggravating a pre-existing, often unrecognized *brain herniation syndrome* (e.g. uncal, cerebellar, or cingulate herniation) associated with intracranial hypertension. This hazard is the basis for considering papilloedema to be a relative contraindication to lumbar puncture. The availability of CT has simplified the management of patients with papilloedema. If CT reveals no evidence of a mass lesion, specifically displacement of the ventricular system, then LP is appropriate in the presence of papilloedema to document the presence of intracranial hypertension or to find evidence of inflammatory or neoplastic disease.

Hazards of bleeding diatheses

Thrombocytopenia and other bleeding diatheses predispose patients to needle-induced subarachnoid, subdural, and epidural haemorrhage. Prothrombin, bleeding and clotting times, and platelet count should be evaluated before LP in vulnerable patients; it should be undertaken only for urgent clinical indications when the platelet count is depressed to about 50 000/μl or below. Platelet transfusion just before the puncture is recommended if the count is below 20 000/μl or dropping rapidly. The administration of protamine to patients on heparin, and vitamin K or fresh frozen plasma to those receiving coumadin, is recommended before LP to minimize the hazard of the procedure (see Section 19).

Complications

Lumbar puncture is usually well tolerated although there are several potential complications of the procedure. These include worsening of brain herniation or spinal cord compression, headache, subarachnoid bleeding, diplopia, backache, and radicular symptoms.

Post-LP headache is the most common complication occurring in about 10–15 per cent of patients usually lasting 2–8 days. It results from low CSF pressures due to persistent fluid leakage through the dural hole. Characteristically, pain is present in the upright position and promptly relieved with the supine position. Aching of the neck and low back are common. The headache is aggravated by cough or strain. Occasionally it is associated with nausea, vomiting or tinnitus. It is avoided when a small styletted needle is used and if multiple puncture holes are not made. The management of postspinal headache depends upon strict bed rest in the horizontal position, adequate hydration, and simple analgesics. If conservative measures fail, the use of a 'blood patch' is indicated. The technique utilizes the epidural injection of autologous blood at the site of the dural puncture to form a thrombotic tamponade which seals the dural hole. The technique is widely used by anaesthetists to treat postanaesthetic spinal headache.

CSF pressure

The CSF pressure should be measured routinely. The pressure level within the right atrium is the reference level with the patient in the lateral decubitus position. The normal lumbar CSF pressure ranges between 50 and 200 mm (and as high as 250 mm in very obese subjects). With the use of the clinical manometer the arterially derived pulsatile pressures are obscured but respiratory pressure waves reflecting changes in central venous pressures are visible. Low pressures are seen in dehydration, spinal subarachnoid block, following previous LP or other CSF leaks, or may be technical in origin when the needle is not in the subarachnoid space. Increased pressures occur with brain oedema, intracranial mass lesions, infections, acute stroke, cerebral venous occlusions, congestive heart failure, pulmonary insufficiency, and benign intracranial hypertension (pseudotumour cerebri) of diverse aetiology.

CSF cells

Normal CSF contains no more than five lymphocytes or mononuclear cells per μl. A higher white cell count is pathognomonic of disease in the CNS or meninges. A stained smear of the sediment must be prepared to allow an accurate differential cell count. A variety of sedimentation and centrifugal techniques have been applied; the cytocentrifuge is quite useful in this regard. A pleocytosis occurs with the gamut of inflammatory disorders; the changes characteristic of the various meningitides are listed in Table 1. Other disorders associated with a pleocytosis include brain infarction, subarachnoid bleeding, previous intrathecal infections, acute

Table 1 Cerebrospinal fluid findings in meningitis

Meningitis	Pressure (mm H$_2$O)	Leukocytes/μl	Protein (g/l)	Glucose (mmol/l)
Acute bacterial	Usually elevated	Several hundred to more than 60 000; usually a few thousand; occasionally less than 100 (especially meningococcal or early in disease) polymorphonuclear cells predominate	Usually 1 to 5, occasionally more than 10	0.2 to 2.2 in most cases (in absence of hyperglycaemia)
Tuberculous	Usually elevated; may be low with dynamic block in advanced stages	Usually 25 to 100; rarely more than 500; lymphocytes predominate except in early stages when polymorphonuclear cells may account for 80 per cent of cells	Nearly always elevated, usually 1 to 2; may be much higher if dynamic block	Usually reduced; less than 2.5 in 3/4 cases
Cryptococcal	Usually elevated	0 to 800; average, 50; lymphocytes predominate	Usually 0.2 to 5; average 1	Reduced in most cases; average 1.7 (in absence of hyperglycaemia)
Viral	Normal to moderately elevated	5 to few hundred; but may be more than 1000, particularly with lymphocytic choriomeningitis; lymphocytes predominate but may be more than 80 per cent polymorphonuclear cells in first few days	Frequently normal or slightly elevated; less than 1; may show greater elevation in severe cases	Normal (reduced in 1/4 cases of mumps and herpes simplex)
Syphilitic (acute)	Usually elevated	Average 500; usually lymphocytes; rarely polymorphonuclear cells	Average, 1	Normal (rarely reduced)
Cysticercosis	Often increased; low with dynamic block	Increased mononuclear cells and polymorphonuclear cells with 2 to 7 per cent eosinophilia in about 1/2 cases	Usually 0.5 to 2	Reduced in 1/5 cases
Sarcoid	Normal to considerably elevated	0 to less than 100 mononuclear cells	Slight to moderate elevation	Reduced in 1/2 cases
Tumour	Normal or elevated	0 to several hundred mononuclear cells plus malignant cells	Elevated often to high levels	Normal or greatly reduced (low in 3/4 carcinomatous meningitis cases)

CSF immunoglubulins are commonly increased in all of the above (including carcinomatous meningitis) as well as in multiple sclerosis. CSF immunoglobulins are assessed by the IgG index: $\dfrac{\text{IgG (CSF)} \times \text{albumin (serum)}}{\text{IgG (serum)} \times \text{albumin (CSF)}}$; the normal index is less than 0.65. The presence of oligoclonal bands (with gel electrophoresis) is also a measure of abnormally increased CSF immunoglobulins.

demyelination, and brain tumours. Eosinophilia most often accompanies parasitic infections, e.g. cysticercosis. Cytologic studies for malignant cells are often rewarding with primary and metastatic tumours.

In cases of bloody CSF due to a traumatic puncture the white count is elevated by the cells contributed by the blood. A useful approximation of a true white cell count can be obtained by using the following correction for the presence of the added blood: if the patient has a normal peripheral blood count, subtract from the total white blood cell (WBC) count (per μl) one white cell for each 1000 red blood cells (RBC) present. Thus, if bloody fluid contains 10 000 red cells and 100 white cells per μl, 10 white cells would be accounted for by the added blood and the corrected leukocyte count would be 90 per μl. If the patient's blood count reveals significant anaemia or leukocytosis, the following formula may be used to determine more accurately the number of white cells (W) in the spinal fluid before the blood was added:

$$W = \frac{\text{Blood WBC} \times \text{CSF RBC}}{\text{Blood RBC}} \times 100$$

The presence of blood in the subarachnoid space produces a secondary inflammatory response which leads to a disproportionate increase in the number of white cells. Following an acute subarachnoid haemorrhage, this elevation in the white cell count is most marked about 48 hours after the ictus, at a time when meningeal signs are most striking.

To correct CSF protein values for the presence of added blood due to needle trauma, subtract 1 mg for every 100 red blood cells. Thus, if the red cell count is 10 000 per μl and the total protein is 1.1 g/l, the corrected protein level would be about 1.0 g/l. The corrections are reliable only if the cell count and total protein are both made on the same tube of fluid.

Blood in the CSF: differential diagnosis and the three-tube test

Several observations are required to differentiate between a traumatic spinal puncture and pre-existing subarachnoid haemorrhage. At the time of puncture, the fluid should be collected in at least three separate tubes (the 'three-tube test'). In traumatic punctures, the fluid generally clears between the first and the third collections. This is detectable by the naked eye and should be confirmed by cell count. In subarachnoid bleeding, the blood is generally evenly admixed in the three tubes. A sample of the bloody fluid should be centrifuged and the supernatant fluid compared with tap water to exclude the presence of pigment.

The supernatant fluid is crystal clear if the red count is less than about 100 000 cells/μl. With bloody contamination of greater magnitude, plasma proteins are present sufficient to cause minimal xanthochromia; this requires enough serum to raise the protein concentration about 1.0 g/l above the initial level. Following subarachnoid bleeding the supernatant fluid becomes pigmented, indicating the blood has been present for sufficient time to permit lysis of red cells. This probably requires at least 2–4 hours (even though the average life of the red cell in the peripheral blood is about 120 days). Crenation of the red blood cells is of no value in differentiating between traumatic and subarachnoid bleeding, for it occurs in both circumstances.

It should be noted that the supernatant fluid usually remains clear for 2–4 hours and even longer after the onset of subarachnoid bleeding. The clear supernatant may mislead the physician to conclude erroneously that the observed blood is due to needle trauma in patients who have received a lumbar puncture within 4 hours of aneurysmal rupture. After an especially traumatic puncture, some blood and xanthochromia may be present for as long as 2–5 days following the initial puncture. In pathological states associated with a CSF protein greater than 1.5 g/l and in the absence of bleeding, a faint degree of xanthochromia may be detected. When the protein is elevated to much higher levels, as in spinal block, polyneuritis, and meningitis, the xanthochromia may be considerable. A xanthochromic fluid with a normal protein level or a minor elevation to less than 1.5 g/l usually indicates a previous subarachnoid or intracerebral haemorrhage (although rarely the xanthochromia is due to severe jaundice).

Pigments

Two major pigments derived from red cells may be observed in the fluid, oxyhaemoglobin and bilirubin. Methaemoglobin is only seen spectrophotometrically. Oxyhaemoglobin is released with lysis of red cells and may be detected in the supernatant fluid within 2 hours after the release of blood in the subarachnoid space. It reaches a maximum in about the first 36 hours and gradually disappears over the next 7–10 days.

Bilirubin is produced *in vivo* by leptomeningeal cells following the haemolysis of red cells. With severe jaundice, both free and conjugated bilirubin are detected in the CSF, and the degree of bilirubin pigmentation is increased when the CSF protein is elevated. Bilirubin is first detected about 10 hours after the onset of subarachnoid bleeding. It reaches a maximum at 48 hours and may persist for 2–4 weeks after extensive bleeding. The severity of the meningeal signs associated with subarachnoid bleeding correlates with the inflammatory response, i.e. the maximal pleocytosis. It may be roughly correlated with the level of bilirubin in the spinal fluid, although bilirubin itself does not cause meningeal irritation (in severe jaundice, the CSF is bilirubin stained without a pleocytosis). Bilirubin is also the major pigment responsible for the xanthochromia associated with a high spinal fluid protein level.

It is useful to note the degree of pigmentation in relation to the protein level. The presence of xanthochromic spinal fluid out of proportion to the total protein content (under 1.5 g/l), and in the absence of jaundice is a reliable index of previous bleeding into the CSF, the brain or spinal cord adjacent to the CSF.

Total protein

The total protein level of CSF ranges between 0.15 and 0.5 g/l. While an elevated protein level lacks specificity, it is a useful index of neurological disease reflecting a pathological increase in endothelial cell permeability. It is often a more sensitive measure than contrast enhancement with computed tomography. Greatly increased protein levels, 5.0 g/l and above, are seen chiefly in meningitis, bloody fluids or cord tumour with spinal block. Inflammatory polyneuritis (Guillain–Barré syndrome), diabetic radiculoneuropathy, myxedoema also may increase the level to 1.0–3.0 g/l. Low protein levels, below 0.15 g/l occur most often with CSF leaks due to a previous LP or traumatic dural leaks.

Immunoglobulins

Although a vast number of proteins may be measured in CSF only an increase in immunoglobulins is of diagnostic importance. Such increases are indicative of an inflammatory response in the CNS and occur with bacterial, viral, spirochaetal, and fungal diseases. However, immunoglobulin assays are most useful in the diagnosis of multiple sclerosis, other demyelinating diseases and CNS vasculitis. The CSF level is corrected for the entry of immunoglobulins from the serum by calculating the IgG index (see Table 1). The presence of more than one oligoclonal band with gel electrophoresis is also abnormal, occurring in 90 per cent of multiple sclerosis cases, as well as the gamut of inflammatory diseases.

Glucose

The CSF glucose concentration is dependent upon the blood-level. The normal range of CSF is between 2.5 and 4.5 mmol/l in patients with a blood glucose between 4 and 7 mmol/l; i.e. 60–80 per cent of the normal blood level. CSF values between 2.2 and 2.5 mmol/l are usually abnormal, and values below 2.2 mmol/l

invariably so. Hyperglycaemia during the 4 hours prior to lumbar puncture results in a parallel increase in CSF glucose. The latter approaches a maximum and the CSF/blood ratio may be as low as 0.35 in the presence of a greatly elevated blood glucose level and in the absence of any neurological disease. An increase in CSF glucose is of no diagnostic significance apart from reflecting hyperglycaemia within the 4 hours prior to lumbar puncture. The CSF glucose level is abnormally low (hypoglycorrhachia) in several diseases of the nervous system apart from hypoglycaemia. It is characteristic of acute purulent meningitis, and a usual finding in tuberculous and fungal meningitis. It is usually normal in viral meningitis, although reduced in about 25 per cent of mumps cases, and in some cases of herpes simplex and zoster meningoencephalitis. The CSF glucose is also reduced in other inflammatory meningitides including cysticercosis, amoebic meningitis (*Naegleria*), acute syphilitic meningitis, sarcoidosis, granulomatous arteritis, and other vasculitides. The glucose level is also reduced in the chemical meningitis that follows intrathecal injections, and in subarachnoid haemorrhage, usually 4–8 days after the bleed. The major factor responsible for the depressed glucose levels is increased anaerobic glycolysis in adjacent neural tissues and to a lesser degree by polymorphonuclear leukocytes. Thus, the decrease in CSF glucose level is accompanied by an inverse increase in CSF lactic acid level.

Microbiological and serological reactions

The use of appropriate stains and cultures are essential in cases of suspected infection. Tests for specific bacterial and fungal antigens, countercurrent immunoelectrophoresis (CIE tests), are useful in establishing a specific aetiology. Serological tests on CSF for syphilis include (1) reagin antibody tests, and (2) specific treponemal antibody tests. The former are particularly useful in evaluating CSF because positive results occur even in the absence of a negative blood serology. There seems to be no basis for applying to CSF the specific treponemal antibody tests (such as the FTA-ABS test) because these CSF antibodies are derived from the plasma where they are present in greater concentration.

References

Fishman, R. A. (1980). *Cerebrospinal fluid in diseases of the nervous system*. W. B. Saunders, Philadelphia.

Henry, J. B. (1984). *Clinical diagnosis and management by laboratory methods*, 17th ed. W. B. Saunders, Philadelphia.

Electrophysiological investigation of the peripheral nervous system

J. PAYAN

When a patient's symptoms include weakness or wasting, undue fatiguability, sensory impairment or paraesthesiae, it is usually desirable, and often essential, to supplement clinical examination by the study of electrical activity in nerve and muscle. This form of investigation is known as clinical electromyography and has its origins in late eighteenth-century Italian speculation and experiment concerning the nature of 'animal electricity'. Early electrodiagnosis was based upon the use of galvanic and faradic currents, and the 'strength–duration curve', reflecting the diminished excitability of denervated muscle, was the test most commonly used until advances in electrical recording allowed electromyography to develop as a clinical method.

Clinical electromyography (EMG)

The conventional use of this term embraces the study both of the motor unit, an individual motor nerve cell and the muscle fibres it activates, and of peripheral conduction of the nerve impulse. It

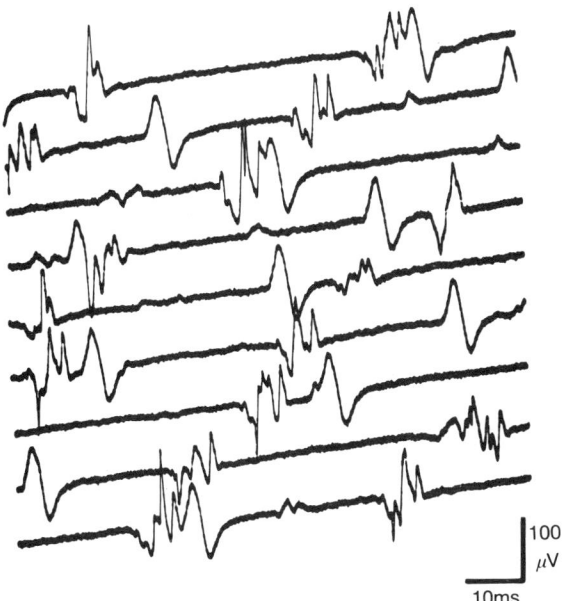

Fig. 1 Motor unit potentials as they appear on the oscilloscope screen on weak effort. Measurements are made of their amplitude in microvolts (μV), duration in milliseconds (ms), and number of phases. Note that some are of simple form, others polyphasic. In this record, which is from the 1st dorsal interosseous muscle of a patient with a chronic lesion of the ulnar nerve at the elbow, an increased incidence of polyphasic potentials indicates that denervated muscle fibres have been incorporated into surviving units by collateral sprouting of healthy nerve fibres.

aims to detect, and distinguish between, disorders of anterior horn cell, root, plexus, peripheral nerve, neuromuscular junction, and muscle, to determine their extent and severity, and to relate neurophysiological abnormality to the clinical context in which it is found. Specific pathological changes such as inflammation in muscle or demyelination of nerve can be inferred, but electromyography will not by itself furnish the diagnosis. It is rarely of value when clinical examination gives complete normal results, especially when the only complaint is of pain. EMG can neither prove nor disprove the existence of an upper motor neurone lesion.

The motor unit

This is studied by inserting a concentric needle electrode into muscle and recording its voluntary or spontaneous electrical activity. A platinum wire is exposed at the bevelled tip of a stainless steel needle, from which it is insulated, and differences in electrical potential between the two are amplified, displayed on an oscilloscope screen, and monitored aurally by means of a loudspeaker. A so-called motor unit potential (MUP) is the sum of action potentials from only those muscle fibres belonging to the unit which happen to lie near the needle tip, but by sampling from many electrode positions average characteristics are obtained which provide information concerning the motor unit as a whole and reflect the anatomical level and pathological kind of damage and repair (Fig. 1). Subtle changes in the reorganization of the motor unit can be analysed by means of the complementary technique of single fibre electromyography, which employs a special needle with a very small recording surface.

The study of MUPs is necessarily made during weak effort, when they can be seen separately. With stronger degrees of effort overlapping potentials from a large number of motor units create an 'interference pattern' whose characteristics vary according to the kind of weakness – functional or organic, lower or upper motor neurone, nerve or primary muscle. Attempts at automatic quantification of EMG data have centred upon the interference pattern, with no generally acceptable result.

Spontaneous activity

Fibrillation

When a motor nerve degenerates, the membrane properties of muscle fibres it supplies undergo changes which result after a few days or weeks in spontaneous activity called fibrillation. This may also be seen in muscle disease, especially acute polymyositis and severe muscular dystrophy, and its appearance in botulism and nerve block suggests that interruption of the flow of nerve impulses alone can sometimes be the cause. Since fibrillation is the contraction of single muscle fibres it can be seen with the naked eye only in the denervated tongue and not through the skin.

Fasciculation

This is the random spontaneous contraction of a whole or part of a motor unit and is visible through the skin unless it occurs deep in the muscle. A very important diagnostic feature of motor neurone disease, it is seen infrequently in peripheral nerve and rarely in muscle disease. It is a well-known source of anxiety to healthy subjects, who can be reassured that their fasciculation is benign by the demonstration of normal motor units.

Myokymia

This is a continuous, slow undulating or quivering movement of overlying skin imparted by spontaneously occurring rhythmic motor unit discharges. Myokymia in the face may denote a brainstem tumour or a plaque of multiple sclerosis. Elsewhere it has followed plexus irradiation and peripheral nerve injury. The term has been loosely applied to benign fasciculation and even to the flickering around the eye common in stress and fatigue. In the contrasting condition of hemifacial spasm sudden bursts of motor unit activity occur synchronously in several muscles on the same side.

Sustained muscle activity

EMG is important in the study of conditions characterized by muscle cramp or failure of relaxation, including common muscle cramps, tetany, the myotonias, neuromyotonia ('continuous muscle fibre activity'), and the very rare 'stiff man syndrome'.

Nerve conduction

When brief electrical pulses are applied to a nerve the resulting action potentials in nerve or in muscle can be recorded and measured. The stimuli are usually delivered through small surface pad electrodes soaked in saline, but a needle can be used if the nerve lies deeply. The response is picked up either by a pair of surface electrodes or by a concentric needle electrode, and is characterized by amplitude, form, and stimulus–response interval.

Conduction velocity

The principle will be illustrated by reference to the median nerve. A supramaximal stimulus (capable of exciting all underlying fibres) applied to the nerve at the wrist crease will be followed by a thenar muscle potential after, say, 3 ms, an interval called the distal motor latency. If the nerve is now stimulated at the level of the elbow and the response follows after 7 ms, conduction from elbow to wrist has taken 4 ms and the conduction velocity, given a distance between the two points of 240 mm, will be 60 mm/ms, or 60 m/s.

Slowing of conduction may be focal, as when an increase in distal motor latency in the median nerve at the wrist enables a carpal tunnel syndrome to be diagnosed, or general, as in polyneuropathy. The velocity in fastest conducting fibres is normally 50–70 m/s in the upper limb and 40–60 m/s in the lower limb. The broad division of the polyneuropathies into axonal and demyelinating types is based upon the degree of slowing.

Nerve action potentials

These may be purely sensory or mixed, and since their amplitude reflects the number of medium to large myelinated fibres lying near the recording electrode they are of great importance in the study of nerve lesions of all kinds. Small myelinated and unmyelinated fibres are accessible only to a research technique called microneurography.

The amplitude of sensory action potentials is a very sensitive indicator of the presence of a polyneuropathy, and may be reduced before the patient is aware of any sensory disturbance. By contrast, it is unaffected by lesions of the sensory pathway proximal to the dorsal root ganglion, such as root avulsion or syringomyelia.

Weakness

Acute, general
When general weakness develops rapidly the differential diagnosis will include anterior poliomyelitis, acute postinfective polyradiculoneuropathy (Guillain-Barré), porphyria, toxic polyneuropathy, myasthenia gravis, and acute polymyositis. The distinction between nerve, end-plate, and muscle disease is usually made without difficulty by means of appropriate EMG studies, which by exclusion may point to a functional or a pyramidal disorder.

Acute, focal
Sudden isolated lower motor neurone weakness, when not immediately reversible and hence due to transient nerve ischaemia, is nearly always caused by the block of nerve conduction which occurs when compression or stretching results in demyelination of a small segment of nerve (neurapraxia). In conditions such as Saturday night palsy of radial nerve, Bell's facial palsy, and the 'strawberry pickers' palsy' of the common peroneal nerve which follows prolonged squatting, stimulation of the nerve distal to the lesion results in normal movement, although later axonal degeneration (axonotmesis) in severe lesions sometimes makes this impossible. EMG also helps in the diagnosis of acutely painful conditions associated with weakness and later wasting, such as neuralgic amyotrophy and diabetic radiculopathy.

Chronic, general
The clinical diagnosis of chronic painless weakness without sensory loss can be difficult if not impossible, especially in children, and EMG is indispensable in deciding between the two principal alternatives, anterior horn cell and primary muscle disease. Each affects the MUP in a very different and characteristic way, whether genetically determined or acquired. In anterior horn cell disease there is a great increase in amplitude, duration, and instability, and in primary muscle disease a preponderance of small, complex, mainly stable potentials. Adequate sampling and statistical comparison with the normal should leave few cases in doubt, but secondary pathological changes occasionally lead to confusion, and even disagreement with the histologist. Thus in spinal muscular atrophy MUPs typical of a myopathy may be encountered, while in long-standing collagen muscle disease amplitudes suggestive of chronic partial denervation can occur. A further, sometimes insoluble, problem associated with the latter group of muscle disorders is that of deciding whether increased weakness is due to the condition itself or to an added steroid-induced myopathy.

The cause of weakness may be a clinically evident upper motor neurone disorder but when a lower motor neurone lesion develops in a spastic limb it is often missed until EMG is performed. Such a combination in a lower limb will confirm a suspected diagnosis of amyotrophic lateral sclerosis.

Chronic, focal
Diagnosis depends on the distribution and kind of EMG abnormality, and tends to rely more on nerve conduction studies, as when a greatly increased distal motor latency to adductor pollicis shows that small hand muscle wasting is due not to motor neurone disease but to a lesion of the deep palmar branch of the ulnar nerve.

Functional
Psychologically determined weakness shows itself electromyographically in two main forms, the irregularly fluctuating activation of normal motor units which parallels the findings on clinical testing, and the complete paralysis of a muscle group or limb which moves quite normally when the appropriate nerve is stimulated electrically. Foot drop, more often on the non-dominant side, is perhaps the commonest example: an apparently flail and useless foot rises strongly into full dorsiflexion when the common peroneal nerve is stimulated, an event to which the patient's response may be revealing. Conversely, a patient judged to be malingering, hysterical or merely lazy is sometimes shown by the electromyographer to be suffering from an unrecognized disorder which, if not wholly responsible for the indisposition, may have decided the form it has taken. The forensic importance of such an objective test needs no emphasis.

When all EMG findings are normal the cause of apparent weakness may lie outside the nervous system, as when a tendon is ruptured or of the wrong length, or movement is limited by pain or joint disease.

Wasting
The bulk and strength of muscle may remain normal even when its nerve is undergoing progressive damage, provided that by collateral sprouting the surviving axons can reinnervate and thus preserve the function of denervated muscle fibres. When this compensatory process proves inadequate the muscle will atrophy. Failure to appreciate this point sometimes leads to the erroneous belief that denervation cannot be present because there is no wasting.

EMG differentiates wasting due to a lesion of the motor unit, in which MUP abnormality occurs, from disuse atrophy, parietal wasting, and congenital absence of muscle (e.g. abductor pollicis brevis or pectoralis major), in which it does not. Thus, a bed-ridden patient with wasted shin muscles may be thought to have disuse atrophy until EMG reveals compression of the common peroneal nerve which should have been prevented. An unsuspected focal nerve lesion, sometimes responsible for discomfort or distress, may be detected in a limb whose incapacity was thought to be wholly due to a condition such as a stroke.

Wasting near an inflamed joint often has multiple causes: taking the example of the metacarpophalangeal joint in rheumatoid arthritis, thenar wasting may be due to a combination of disuse atrophy associated with pain, inflammatory myopathy, rheumatoid polyneuropathy, and carpal tunnel compression. Since only the last is readily remediable, its recognition by EMG may be of great benefit.

Frail elderly people are sometimes unnecessarily referred for EMG merely because they are thin, but in weight loss due, for example, to thyrotoxicosis, malignant disease or anorexia nervosa a myopathy may be detected.

Fatiguability
When a patient complains of tiring easily rather than of being continuously weak, repetitive nerve stimulation may result in progressive reduction in the amplitude of the evoked muscle potential, signifying myasthenia gravis. In mild cases this test is insufficiently sensitive and an increase in 'jitter' is sought with the single fibre needle (see page 21.13). Jitter is the variability in time interval between action potentials from single muscle fibres at consecutive discharges of their parent motor unit. An increase occurs in any condition in which neuromuscular transmission is impaired, and over 80 per cent of cases of generalized myasthenia can be diagnosed in this way, considerably fewer of the purely ocular form. Needle EMG is in any case required in order to exclude conditions which may co-exist with myasthenia gravis such as polymyositis and thyrotoxic myopathy. The 'Tensilon' (edrophonium

chloride) test is useful, but both false negative and false positive results occur.

In the myasthenic syndrome of Eaton and Lambert (see Section 22) repetitive nerve stimulation is the diagnostically decisive test. An initially small evoked muscle potential increases in amplitude by several hundred per cent at rapid stimulation rates.

Entrapment neuropathies

Acute nerve compression has already been referred to (see 'Acute weakness'). When chronic compression occurs EMG must determine not only its level, but how much of the clinical picture is due to block of conduction and how much to axonal degeneration. The higher the proportion of block the better the prospect of spontaneous recovery. Surgery to relieve compression should ideally be preceded by electromyography in order that a baseline be established by which to judge its results. Failure to relieve symptoms of carpal tunnel compression, for example, may be due to faulty technique or to impaired recovery in the presence of a generalized neuropathy, but if surgery can be shown to have reversed the diagnostic abnormality of nerve conduction the source of symptoms may lie elsewhere. Anomalous innervation is a rare source of difficulty which EMG should resolve.

Polyneuropathy

The commonest difficulty, especially where medical services are readily available and patients present early, is that of assessing the significance of relatively minor sensory symptoms. Patients are referred, for example, because paraesthesiae in the ulnar distribution which used to be negligible or intermittent have become more troublesome or persistent, making it necessary to determine (a) whether there is a lesion of the nerve itself, the lower brachial plexus or the C8 root, and (b) whether this is the first expression of a subclinical polyneuropathy. The diagnosis of diabetes is not infrequently made for the first time when a patient sent for confirmation of carpal tunnel compression on one side proves to have not only subclinical compression on the other, but also bilateral subclinical ulnar lesions at the elbows. Such lesions, for which the term 'mononeuritis multiplex' is inappropriate, are simply drawing attention to a symmetrical polyneuropathy which is unsuspected and perhaps even clinically undetectable.

EMG is indispensable in the early diagnosis of a polyneuropathy and in monitoring its natural course or response to treatment. Nerve conduction studies require essentially no cooperation, indeed can be performed when the patient is unconscious. This makes them of especial value at the extremes of life, when the history may be poor or unobtainable and physical examination difficult or misleading. Polyneuropathy discovered when there is coma, confusion or spasticity may raise the possibility of Wernicke's encephalopathy, vitamin B_{12} deficiency, porphyria or metachromatic leucodystrophy. The important matter of distinguishing axonal from demyelinating polyneuropathies by means of the degree of slowing of conduction has already been mentioned. This is crucial in the identification of the various hereditary neuropathies and their differentiation from such conditions as Friedreich's ataxia and the spinal muscular atrophies.

When systematic nerve conduction studies in upper and lower limbs give normal results in a patient with symptoms suggestive of a polyneuropathy there are several possible explanations. A neuropathy may indeed be present but is not yet severe enough to give abnormal results with the methods available, or the fibres affected are inaccessible by reason of their small diameter or extremely peripheral situation. Symptoms may, however, be due to an unrecognized pathological process at a proximal level such as rheumatoid disintegration of the cervical spine, tabes dorsalis or multiple sclerosis. A patient's fear that she has the latter condition may even induce hyperventilation and further complicate the picture. Finally, it may have to be assumed that there is no organic basis for the sensory symptoms.

EMG and the surgeon

Apart from its role in the investigation of certain highly specialized organs such as the eye, larynx, bladder, and rectum, there are two main areas of usefulness, the diagnosis and management of nerve compression, already mentioned, and in cases of nerve trauma. When clinical examination suggests that complete nerve degeneration has taken place, such as in the flail arm of the infant with obstetric palsy or the youth injured by a motor cycle accident, EMG may detect surviving motor units and thus change the prognosis. The electromyographer is often asked whether nerve regeneration is occurring spontaneously, or after nerve repair.

Non-diagnostic uses of EMG

EMG techniques have found application outside the purely clinical sphere, for example, in the study of toxic and environmental hazards, of abnormal voluntary and involuntary movements, and of the posture of those engaged in heavy static work. The development of aids to rehabilitation is a particularly active field.

References

Ludin, H.-P. (1980). *Electromyography in practice.* Georg Thieme Verlag, Stuttgart, New York.
Stålberg, E. and Young, R. R. (1981). *Clinical neurophysiology.* Butterworths, London.

Evoked potentials

A. M. HALLIDAY

Introduction

Electrophysiological investigation of the peripheral nerve action potential can be extended to the potentials generated by the afferent volley within the central nervous system by the use of the averaging technique, introduced by Dawson in 1951. Because these potentials are recorded from scalp or neck electrodes at a considerable distance from their generators in the spinal cord, brainstem or cerebral hemispheres, the voltages generated are extremely small, generally of the order of 0.25 and 25.00 μV. Such small responses are easily obscured by the much larger potentials produced by coincidental muscular or EEG activity and can only be clearly detected by summing the responses to a large number of repeated stimuli. This is conveniently done with a small digital computer (an 'averager'). The interfering background activity ('noise') has no systematic relationship in time with the stimulus and tends to cancel itself out as the averaging trials are accumulated, while the sum of the consistent responses evoked by each stimulus ('signal') grows steadily within the computer store in proportion to the number of trials added together. This averaging technique allows clear recordings to be obtained of the evoked potentials to repeated visual, auditory, and somatosensory stimuli, a prerequisite being that the stimulus shall be sharp-fronted, accurately timed, and synchronized with the averager.

Evoked potential recording has in this way proved useful in the investigation of disorders affecting the central sensory pathways. The somatosensory evoked potential (SEP), for instance, can helpfully complement studies of the peripheral nerve action potential in severe neuropathy, as the cortical response to electrical stimulation of a peripheral nerve is often preserved long after the peripheral nerve action potential is unrecordable by ordinary techniques. Moreover, the combined recording of peripheral and central responses often allows the exact site of the lesion along the pathway to be much more accurately determined in those cases of sensory disturbance where this is in doubt. The method thus has a well-established place in the investigation of unexplained cases of visual failure, hearing loss, and impaired sensation.

Since it provides an objective method of testing sensory func-

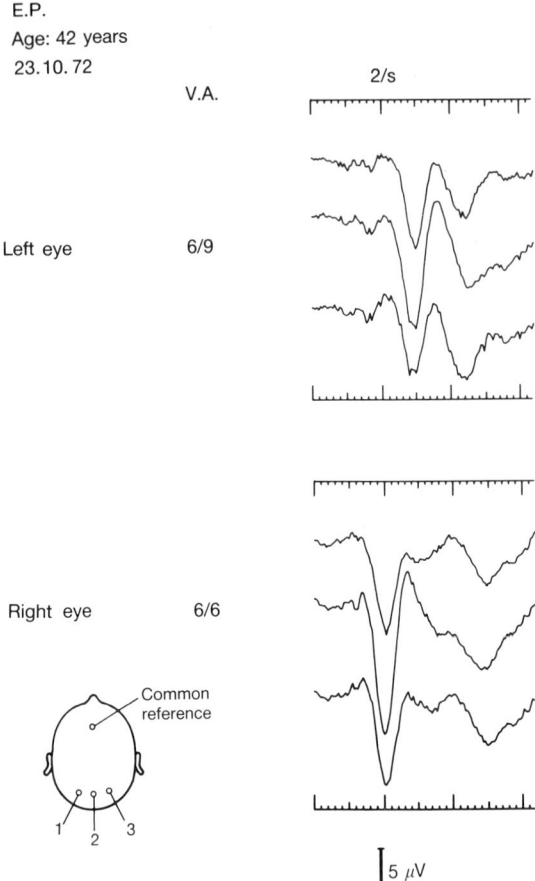

E.P.
Age: 42 years
23.10.72

V.A.

2/s

Left eye   6/9

Right eye   6/6

Common reference

1   2   3

5 μV

Fig. 1 Pattern reversal responses from each eye of a patient recorded one month after an attack of left optic neuritis. The response from the right eye is of normal waveform and latency, the major positive component (P100) being clearly seen preceded and followed by the smaller negative components (N75 and N145). The response from the affected left eye is delayed by 45 ms. Time scale 10, 50, and 100 ms.

tion, it can be used to investigate patients unable or unwilling to co-operate. Hence the auditory evoked response has found an important application in testing for hearing disorders in infancy, where subjective audiometry is impossible, and where the differentiation of organic deafness from mental deficiency, autism, and the sequelae of minimal brain damage poses a major problem. For the same reason, it may be useful in distinguishing functional and organic sensory loss in older subjects in suspected malingering or hysteria. Perhaps the most clinically valuable feature of the method, however, is its great sensitivity to demyelinating or compressive lesions, which often allows it to reveal very marked abnormalities at a time when the lesion may be clinically 'silent' or exhibiting only minimal signs or symptoms.

Visual evoked potential (VEP)

The visual stimulus most commonly used in clinical testing is the sudden reversal of the black and white squares in a checkerboard display ('pattern reversal') (Fig. 1). VEPs can also be evoked by a repetitive, unpatterned flash stimulus from a stroboscope (gas discharge tube). In general, the flash response is much less sensitive to minor lesions of the visual pathways than the pattern reversal response, but, being more robust, it may still be obtained when the pattern response has been abolished (as in cases of severely impaired visual acuity). The flash stimulus is also more effective when studying the electroretinogram (ERG). Conversely the response to pattern reversal is particularly sensitive to early or clinically unmanifest lesions, whether demyelinating or compres-

sive, and its amplitude shows a much closer correlation with changes in acuity level.

VEP abnormalities in demyelinating disease
Optic neuritis
Following an attack of optic neuritis about 95 per cent of patients will be found to have a pattern reversal VEP from the affected eye with a latency delayed beyond the upper limit of the normal range (Fig. 1). Even in the 5 per cent of patients whose responses fall within the normal latency range, some will be found to have a latency difference between the response from each eye which exceeds the small normal interocular latency difference. Once they have occurred, these latency increases are usually persistent, although, in up to 10 per cent of adult patients, the responses may have reverted to normal or near-normal latencies when recorded some months or years later.

Amplitude changes are, by comparison, much more labile, tending to follow the changes in visual acuity level associated with the acute attack and the recovery of vision, which commonly occurs quickly and dramatically within a few days thereafter. The mean delay in the latency of the major positivity after the acute optic neuritis is of the order of 35–45 ms, but delays of up to 100 ms may be encountered. These values are for the pattern reversal response. The flash response is invariably less delayed and also shows less marked amplitude changes than the pattern reversal response in line with its lower sensitivity to the effect of lesions.

Multiple sclerosis
Similarly, delayed pattern reversal evoked potentials (EPs) are also found in patients with multiple sclerosis who have no history of optic neuritis and even in some patients with normal fundi, colour vision, and perimetry. Such clinically 'silent' VEP abnormalities are found in over half such patients with definite multiple sclerosis (MS) and well over a third of those with possible or probable MS. The exact percentage has varied from study to study and is largely dependent on unrecognized differences in patient selection and the particular testing technique used.

VEP abnormalities in undiagnosed spastic paraparesis
About a third of patients presenting with progressive spastic paraparesis of unknown aetiology have an abnormally delayed pattern reversal VEP.

Compressive lesions
Delayed VEPs are not specific to demyelinating disease and may be encountered also in compressive lesions affecting the visual pathways, although the shape of the normal waveform of the response tends to be more markedly altered by compression than by primary demyelinating disease and the magnitude of the delays encountered is significantly smaller in most cases. The pattern reversal VEP is very sensitive to early compression and may show gross changes at a time when clinical signs and symptoms are still minimal. Like retrobulbar neuritis optic nerve compression is associated with abnormalities of the response from the affected eye and these are particularly easy to detect in comparison with the response from the unaffected eye. Chiasmal compression, frequently encountered in patients with a pituitary adenoma or craniopharyngioma, is associated with abnormalities of the response from both eyes, the so-called 'crossed asymmetry', resulting from the depression of the response from the temporal half field in each eye (Fig. 2). More posteriorly placed lesions involving the optic tract or intrahemispheric visual pathways affect the response from the homonymous contralateral half fields, producing 'uncrossed asymmetries' of the VEP, showing a similar abnormality for the response from both left and right eyes (Fig. 3). Limits of normal asymmetry can be calculated from control observations on the healthy population and will allow each laboratory to set up a criterion by which to recognize an unequivocally abnormal response.

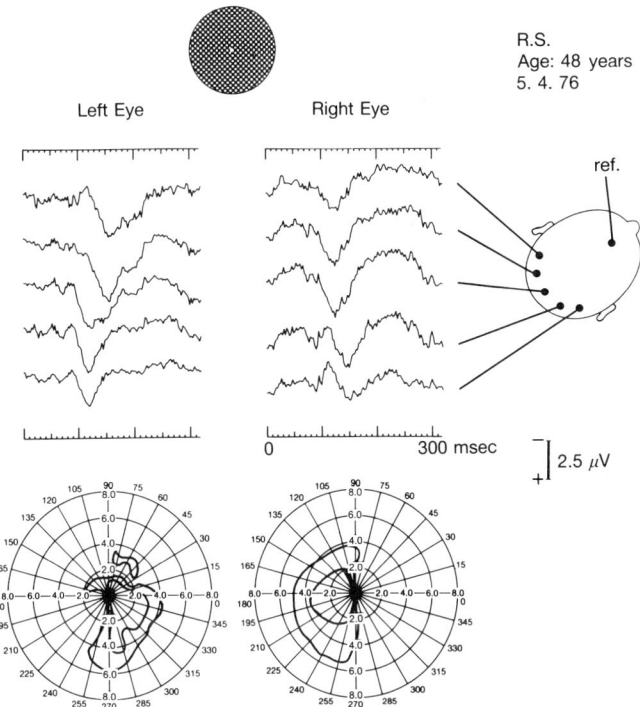

Fig. 2 Pattern reversal responses to a full field checkerboard stimulus from each eye of a 48-year-old man with a craniopharyngioma, associated with a bitemporal hemianopia. The responses show a 'crossed asymmetry', the P100 component being seen at the electrodes in the midline and ipsilateral to the preserved half field (i.e. on the right side for the left eye and on the left side for the right eye). (Reproduced from Blumhardt et al., 1977, with permission.)

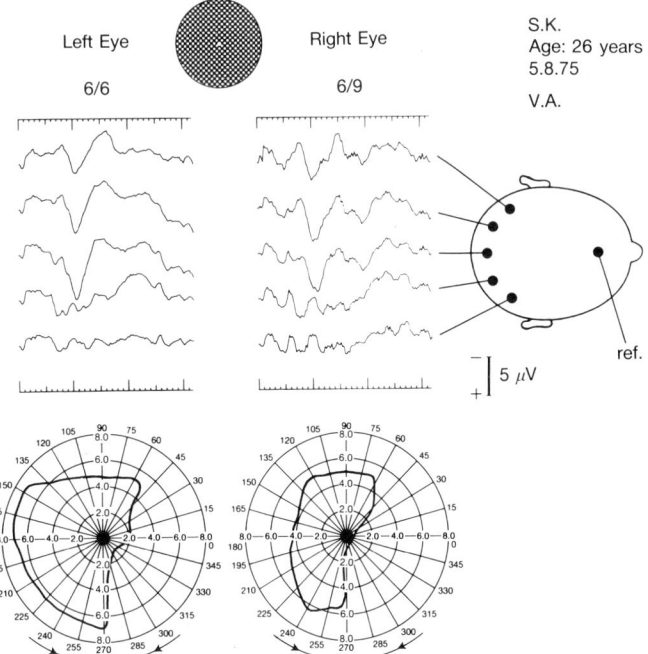

Fig. 3 Pattern reversal responses to a full field checkerboard stimulus for each eye from a 26-year-old man with an incomplete homonymous hemianopia, associated with a vascular lesion of the posterior cerebral circulation in the left hemisphere. The responses show an 'uncrossed asymmetry', the P100 component being seen at the electrodes in the midline and ipsilateral to the preserved left half field. (Reproduced from Halliday, 1982, with permission.)

The detection of chiasmal and retro-chiasmal lesions may be greatly improved by the use of pattern reversal stimulation applied in each half field separately.

Hereditary degenerative disorders
The VEP may also show minor abnormalities in a variety of other conditions, particularly those associated with optic atrophy, such as Friedreich's ataxia, Leber's optic atrophy, dominant optic atrophy, cerebro-macular degeneration, Parkinsonism, hereditary spastic paraplegia, and Huntington's chorea.

Nutritional disorders
VEP abnormalities may also be encountered in vitamin B_{12} deficiency, whether or not associated with pernicious anaemia and subacute combined degeneration. A very characteristic change in the waveform of the response, in which the major positivity (P100) is replaced by a negative peak, is also seen in association with dense central scotomata, as in untreated cases of tobacco/alcohol amblyopia or West Indian amblyopia.

Somatosensory evoked response
Technique
The somatosensory evoked potential (SEP) is usually evoked by an electrical stimulus applied transcutaneously to a peripheral nerve either in the upper limb (the median or ulnar nerve at the wrist or elbow are commonly used), the lower limb (posterior tibial nerve at the ankle or lateral popliteal at the knee) or, less commonly, the face (trigeminal nerve). In the normal response to stimulation of the median nerve at the wrist (Fig. 4) a series of subcortical and cortical components can be identified, originating in the region of the brachial plexus (N9), spinal roots or dorsal columns (N11), dorsal horns near the site of entry to the cord (N13), medial lemniscus (N14), and sensory cortex (N20). Alterations of one or other of these components will often provide information of localizing value in the case of a focal lesion, particularly if this is unilateral and the response from the two sides can be compared.

Demyelinating disease
Upper limb SEPs are found to be abnormal in 75–80 per cent of patients with clinically definite multiple sclerosis and in 40–50 per cent of arms in which there is no history of sensory symptoms or signs. The percentage of abnormal responses is slightly higher for stimulation of the lower limb than for the upper limb, presumably because of the longer pathway involved. The method is thus capable of providing evidence of clinically 'silent' disseminated lesions and may be very helpful in establishing the diagnosis of multiple sclerosis. However, cases of isolated optic neuritis seldom have abnormal SEPs (less than 10 per cent in our own data) and the incidence of abnormalities in early and doubtful cases is not nearly so high as in the established disease. The commonest abnormality consists of a delay in the initial negativity of the cortical response and the preceding lemniscal component with preservation of a normal latency for the earlier potentials (Fig. 4). However, abnormalities of the earlier components in isolation (N13/P13) are also seen.

Degenerative diseases
The SEP shows alteration in many diseases affecting the peripheral or central somatosensory pathways. While the abnormalities are in no sense diagnostic, the combination of abnormal findings is in some cases highly characteristic of a particular disease. In general, the abnormalities seen in hereditary degenerative conditions are bilateral and symmetrical, in contradistinction to those encountered in multiple sclerosis which are often unilateral or markedly different on the two sides. In Friedreich's ataxia, the peripheral component (N9) is absent or very much reduced in amplitude, consistent with an axonal type of degeneration in the peripheral nerves, while the initial cortical negativity (N20) shows a peculiar prolongation, so that its duration from onset to peak

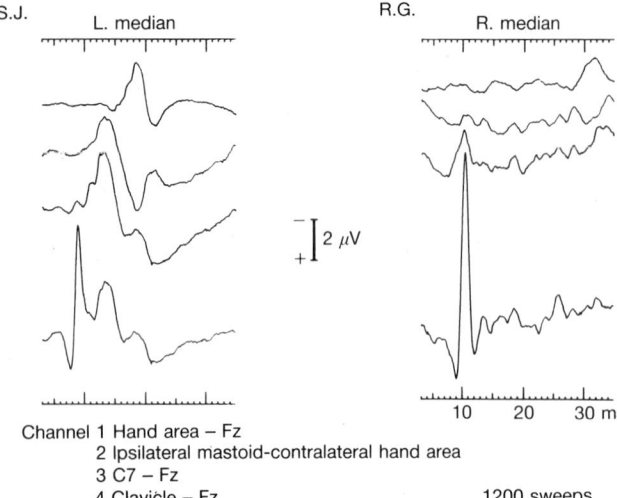

Channel 1 Hand area – Fz
          2 Ipsilateral mastoid-contralateral hand area
          3 C7 – Fz
          4 Clavicle – Fz   1200 sweeps

Fig. 4 Somatosensory responses to electrical stimulation of the median nerve at the wrist in a healthy subject (left-hand record) and in a patient suffering from multiple sclerosis (right-hand record). The contralateral Rolandic response (channel 1) shows a well marked early cortical component (N20) in the normal record. This component is very greatly delayed in the MS patient, occurring with a latency of about 32 ms. The peripheral N9 component from the brachial plexus, recorded over the clavicle (channel 4), is within normal limits for both records. The cervical response (channel 3) shows a prominent N13 component preceded by a smaller N11 and an even smaller N9. The N14 component is best seen in the mastoid recording (channel 2) where it appears as a prolongation of the N13 component. Apart from N9 none of the components of the 'electrospinogram' are seen in the record from the MS patient. (Reproduced from Halliday, 1978a, with permission.)

may be increased four-fold. In type I hereditary motor sensory neuropathy (Charcot–Marie–Tooth disease) the peripheral nerve action potential (NAP) is again often unidentifiable, but the initial cortical negativity shows no marked prolongation, although both subcortical and cortical components are delayed in peak latency.

Abnormalities have also been reported in a minority of patients with hereditary cerebellar ataxia and hereditary spastic paraplegia. In Huntington's chorea, the initial cortical component has been reported to be only slightly delayed, but of markedly reduced amplitude. In Parkinson's disease, on the other hand, the SEP has been found to be essentially normal. Greatly enhanced cortical responses are encountered in progressive myoclonic epilepsy, whether associated pathologically with Lafora bodies, lipid inclusions or a system degeneration of the grey matter (Unverricht–Lundborg disease). In this condition the early cortical potentials may be increased up to five or ten times the normal amplitude, particularly when patients are exhibiting marked myoclonic jerking. Control of the latter by medication is associated with a diminution in the size of the cortical SEP, often to within normal limits.

Trauma

The SEP has proved useful in the investigation and monitoring of traumatic injuries to the peripheral nerves or the cord, and also in the detection of lesions secondary to nerve entrapment, as in the carpal tunnel syndrome. In brachial plexus traction injuries, for instance, it may be possible to provide firm evidence of a preserved central response to peripheral stimulation where the continuity of possibly avulsed spinal roots is in question, while a preserved N9 shows that the peripheral fibres are still intact at least as far as the posterior root ganglion. The SEP to lower limb stimulation can be continuously monitored during orthopaedic surgery for scoliosis to control for any adverse effects of traction.

Tumours and infarcts of brainstem, thalamus, and cerebral hemispheres

The SEP can provide useful localizing information on the level of a vascular or neoplastic lesion affecting the central somatosensory pathways. Preservation of the earlier components combined with delay, conduction or loss of the later components often enables the site of the lesion to be localized to cord, brainstem, thalamic or cortical level, while the comparison of the responses on the two sides indicates whether the lesion is unilateral or bilateral. Even extrinsic compression, as by a meningioma or a subarachnoid haemorrhage, may be associated with abnormalities of the SEP.

Coma and brain death

In contrast to the brainstem auditory EP (BAEP), where some brain dead patients do not have even eighth nerve action potentials (wave I) present, due to trauma at the base of the skull or in the middle or inner ear, the early central somatosensory components P13/N13 are usually preserved. Since these early components indicate that the stimulus volley has reached the CNS, the absence of later components then becomes highly significant. Under these circumstances, preservation of the cortical SEP carries a relatively good prognosis. In patients with coma, prolongation of the central conduction time may provide a useful warning of incipient ischaemic damage.

Auditory evoked potential

Brainstem auditory evoked potentials (BAEP) have been applied clinically in two major fields: in testing hearing in infants and older children or adults who are unable or unwilling to co-operate in conventional audiometry (evoked response audiometry, ERA); and in the investigation of patients with suspected demyelinating disease or neurological lesions of the auditory pathways. In both contexts, the recording of the central responses can be usefully combined with electrocochleography in appropriate cases.

The response has been particularly useful in the detection of clinically 'silent' demyelinating lesions in multiple sclerosis and in detecting tumours of the cerebello-pontine angle. In interpreting the results, a useful rough correlation has emerged between the site of the lesion and the character of the abnormality. The normal response consists of seven components occurring within the first 10 ms following a click or brief tone burst stimulus (Fig. 5). These

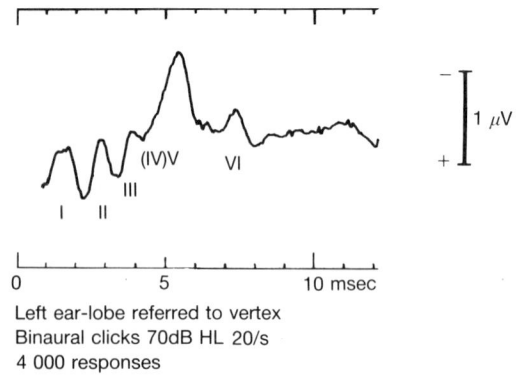

Left ear-lobe referred to vertex
Binaural clicks 70dB HL 20/s
4 000 responses

Fig. 5 Average response to 4000 click stimuli, 70 dBHL, at 20 a second recorded between the left ear lobe and the vertex in a healthy individual, showing 5 of the 7 components of the BAEP. As in many normal subjects, component IV is not separately distinguishable from component V, and component VII is not seen in this record. Studies of the effect of localized lesions in both animals and humans have suggested that the generators of the individual components are situated in or near the following structures: I (N1.5) auditory nerve; II (N3.0) cochlear nucleus; III (N4.0) superior olives; IV (N5.0) nuclei of lateral lemniscus; V (N5.8) inferior colliculi; VI (N7.4) ? medial geniculate; VII (N9.5) ? geniculocortical radiation. (Reproduced from Halliday, 1978b, with permission.)

components appear to be generated by the arrival of the afferent sensory volley at or near the following points on the auditory pathway: the auditory nerve (wave I), the cochlear nucleus (wave II), the superior olivary complex (wave III), the lateral lemniscus (wave IV), the inferior colliculus (wave V), the medial geniculate (wave VI), and the geniculo-cortical fibres (wave VII). The origins of the last two components are the least securely established, and little clinical use is made of them, the most important and useful components clinically being waves I and V.

Demyelinating disease
A high percentage of BAEP abnormalities is found in patients with clinically definite MS, ranging from 70 to 90 per cent, but the rate of abnormality is considerably lower in patients with probable, possible or suspected MS (abnormal in roughly a third overall, but with values ranging from 12 to 69 per cent in different studies). In terms of clinically 'silent' cases, without signs or symptoms to suggest a brainstem lesion, the rate drops to about 1 in 5 or even lower. These values are certainly lower than the corresponding ones for the SEP. All EP tests, however, were able to detect lesions in patients who proved normal on tests for the EPs in the other two modalities. There is thus a value in doing more than one test if the diagnostic information available from EP testing is to be maximized.

Posterior fossa tumours
The brainstem response has been shown to be useful in the early detection of acoustic neuromas although care has to be taken with the interpretation of the records if false positive and false negative results are to be minimized. The response is invariably abnormal in brainstem gliomas and often gives a clear indication of the level of the lesion, but the method is seldom important diagnostically in this context. Vascular lesions of the vertebro-basilar circulation are associated with abnormal responses only if the lesion encroaches on the auditory pathways themselves, and the BAEP is usually normal in patients with transient ischaemic attacks, although not invariably so.

Coma and brain death
The brainstem responses may be well preserved in association with cortical necrosis and the apallic syndrome, so that the presence of the response, while indicative of preserved brainstem function, is not necessarily a good prognostic sign. Conversely, the complete absence of all BAEP components can occur secondarily to a peripheral lesion of the auditory system, particularly in cases of head injury associated with a fracture of the base of the skull. Such absence, is therefore not inconsistent with a normal functioning of the nervous pathways themselves. For these reasons, the BAEP has little place in the determination of brain death. The preservation of the normal BAEP may, however, be a valuable sign in patients who have taken an overdose of barbiturates or other drugs, as the response may still be preserved and normal in the absence of all the conventional brainstem reflexes.

Other conditions
The BAEP has been investigated in a variety of other conditions and abnormalities have been noted in some progressive degenerative disorders such as the leucodystrophies, spino-cerebellar ataxia, Charcot–Marie–Tooth disease, hereditary spastic paraplegia, chronic alcoholism, uraemia, and mental retardation.

Evoked response audiometry
The use of the click-evoked BAEP in detecting severe deafness in infants is now well established, but with the conventional click or brief tone burst stimulus the test does not provide the same frequency specific information as conventional audiometry. Several attempts have been made to get over this limitation, including the use of narrow band filtering for the stimulus combined with masking noise from which a corresponding window of the frequency range has been cleared (the so called 'notched noise' technique). Galambos has recently reported an alternative technique using 40 Hz auditory stimulation which provides a response with more adequate sensitivity to low-frequency hearing deficits. These techniques are, however, still being explored.

Longer latency components of the auditory EP, have been used in the investigation of higher function (e.g. as an objective substitute for speech audiometry or in testing 'cognitive' abilities). The later components have also been used in testing for dementia, as some of them appear to be increased in latency when the processes of comprehension or recognition are prolonged.

References
Blumhardt, L. D., Barrett, G. and Halliday, A. M. (1977). The asymmetrical visual evoked potential to pattern reversal in one half-field and its significance for the analysis of visual field defects. *Br. J. Ophthal.* **61**, 456–461.
Bodis Wollner, I. (ed.) (1982). *Evoked potentials. Ann. NY Acad. Sci.* **388**, 1–738.
Chiappa, K. (1984). *Evoked potentials in clinical medicine*, p. 340. Raven Press, New York.
Courjon, J., Maugière, F. and Revol, M. (eds) (1982). *Clinical applications of evoked potentials in neurology*, pp. 1–577. Raven Press, New York.
Halliday, A. M. (1978a). Clinical applications of evoked potentials. In *Recent advances in clinical neurology* (eds W. B. Matthews and G. H. Glaser), pp. 47–73. Churchill Livingstone, Edinburgh.
—— (1978b). New developments in clinical application of evoked potentials. In *Contemporary clinical neurophysiology* (eds W. A. Cobb and H. van Duijn), pp. 105–121. Elsevier, Amsterdam.
—— (ed.) (1982). *Evoked potentials in clinical testing*, pp. 1–575. Churchill Livingstone, Edinburgh.

PAIN

The pathogenesis of pain

P.W. NATHAN

Introduction
It might be thought that defining pain is unnecessary as everyone knows what it is; and when we do try to define it, we realize that it is difficult to draw the boundaries. Even to label it as unpleasant is not fully true. A masochist would no doubt say that there are pains pleasant and pains unpleasant. The International Association for the Study of Pain (1979, 1982) defined pain as 'An unpleasant sensory and emotional experience associated with actual or potential tissue damage, or described in terms of such damage'.

Most tissues of the body can give rise to pain when they are stimulated appropriately. As the skin is the tissue most in touch with the external environment, it can be stimulated in many ways that cause pain. Hollow viscera, such as the bowel, give rise to pain when the onward passage of their contents is obstructed; this pain is due to strong contraction or stretching of the visceral musculature. Traction on the mesentery also causes pain. Muscles and tendons, fascia, joint capsules, periosteum, the parietal peritoneum and pleura, blood vessels, the pelvis of the kidney, the ureter and the bladder, the gonads, all produce pain with appropriate stimulation; so does the dentine of the teeth. The lung, liver, and spleen do not give rise to pain, even when inflamed or being destroyed by neoplastic tissue. Stimulation of the brain by pulling, pushing, cutting or burning is painless except for a few regions; this is so even though there is pain arising spontaneously in the central nervous system.

Nociception and feeling pain are not equivalent. Being consciously aware of pain is only a part of the total response. If there is a sudden stimulation of the skin of a noxious kind, there is reflex removal of the region. The autonomic nervous system is alerted and responds, and the animal is likely to signal to others that it has pain by squeaking or shrieking.

Afferent nerve fibres

In 1967, Hagbarth and Vallbo demonstrated that it was possible to record signals from nerve fibres of human peripheral nerves by using a needle electrode passed through the skin. With this technique, three kinds of investigations have been carried out. One approach has been to stimulate tissues in natural ways and record the action potentials in nerve fibres. Another is to excite single nerve fibres by using an intraneural recording electrode as a stimulating electrode. A third method consists of stimulating single nerve fibres peripherally, recording from them above the site of stimulation, and correlating the findings with the subject's sensations.

The essential groups of fibres concerned with nociception are the small delta myelinated and the C non-myelinated fibres. The kinds of natural stimuli that activate C fibres are strong mechanical stimulation, pinching the skin, pinprick, warmth, cold or noxious heat, and chemical substances such as histamine, naphthalene, papain injected subepidermally, and stinging nettles. There are different C fibres for reporting hot pain, and dull aching pain; some only report stimulation that causes itch.

Electrical stimulation of the large myelinated fibres causes the feeling that the skin is being tapped or pressed on, or it causes a feeling of buzzing or vibration. Electrical stimulation of delta fibres can cause a stinging sensation. Delta fibres are active when the stimulus to the skin is pressure, a high temperature or a chemical irritant.

Sensation, including pain, is not just a result of what comes in from the peripheral nerves, and particularly not from single isolated nerve fibres. C fibres may be firing off impulses at a rate of 10 Hz when the stimulus is mechanical and the sensation is one of pressure with no pain; they can be firing at rates of 2–6 Hz with a noxious stimulus that causes pain. Further, the threshold for experiencing pain does not correspond with the onset of C fibre activity; and pain can increase while the discharge in the peripheral nerves decreases.

Afferents from the viscera serve their reflex organization; only occasionally does this input invade the private world of consciousness. The afferents of the vagus go to the nucleus solitarius and do not give rise to pain. The visceral afferents that can give rise to pain run with the sympathetic fibres, in the sympathetic chains, and then into the posterior roots, along with all other afferent fibres. The fibres from the heart run with the sympathetic fibres and then enter the upper five posterior thoracic roots. These myelinated and non-myelinated fibres are constantly discharging, reporting normal and specific haemodynamic events. Their tonic discharge is increased with damage to the tissue and this faster rate gives rise to pain. Afferents from the rectum and the bladder run in the 2nd and 3rd sacral nerves and less commonly in the 1st and 4th nerves. In some animals, there are also vesical afferents from the trigonal area, running in the hypogastric nerves. In the bladder, rectum, and colon, the same afferent nerve fibres are activated by substances that cause pain, such as potassium chloride and bradykinin, and by distension and contraction of the viscus,

and by ischaemia. This means that the very same peripheral nerve fibres are used to signal that the bladder or rectum is full, to subserve the desire to micturate or defaecate, and to convey impulses interpreted as severe pain in the viscera. Thus, in the case of the viscera and the heart, pain appears to be due to a summation of impulses arriving in the same nerve fibres that are used when other sensations are evoked, and not in a special group of fibres reserved for impulses caused by noxious events. Not everyone accepts these conclusions, however.

Teeth are innervated only by delta and non-myelinated fibres. Electrical stimulation of the pulp of the teeth causes a sensation that some people call pain or warmth and tingling, and others call burning. These feelings are all due to impulses in the delta fibres. When the C fibres are brought into activity, the pain is very severe.

Transmisson and modulation

Messages from the periphery to the spinal cord are relayed by transmitters and modulators. The first and immediate report is signalled by the transmitters; modulators are more slowly acting with prolonged and varied effects. Most of the work on this subject so far has been on small animals and not on humans. The transmitters and modulators of large afferent nerve fibres have not yet been identified, and without doubt there are many more to be discovered for the smaller fibres; the list of neuropeptides grows day by day.

Substance P is emitted at both ends of 10–15 per cent of non-myelinated afferent fibres; it is found in 50 per cent of visceral afferents but in none of the non-myelinated fibres from the somatic musculature. At the periphery, it is probable that substance P is responsible for the flare and possibly the wheal of the triple response. At the central ends of these fibres, it is emitted in the neighbourhood of short-axoned inhibitory neurones that emit encephalin (see Section 10). It may be that the encephalinergic neurones counteract the input from the non-myelinated fibres. *Somatostatin* is emitted by 5–10 per cent of non-myelinated afferent fibres; it is inhibitory. *VIP* (see Section 12) occurs in the largest amounts in the small afferents from the pelvic viscera.

Modulators and transmitters are made in the same neurones, so that, for instance, a monoaminergic neuron puts out noradrenalin and a peptide, and cholinergic neurones acetylcholine and a peptide modulator. Many neurones emit two modulators with an amine transmitter. These same peptides are emitted by interneurones of the posterior horns and by fibres descending from the brain to the posterior horns. There is no relationship between the kind of modulator and transmitter of a posterior root fibre and the sensory modality of the fibre.

Neurones of the posterior horns and sensory cranial nerve nuclei

The anatomy of the nervous system is not completely static like a road or railway line. Although the lines are laid down, the terminals at both ends are constantly changing; they are altered by use, disuse, experience and learning, injury, and by disease. A continual input can alter the responsiveness of posterior horn neurones. This change spreads from the neurones receiving the input to neighbouring neurones so that eventually the state of a local region of posterior horns has become different. The changing peripheral fields of neurones or laminae I, II, and III have been studied in cats. During an experiment in which the peripheral field of neurones of these laminae was being examined, the field of a neurone could change from being only the foot and toes to being the whole of the caudal surface of the hindlimb. In some experiments it was found that damage to the skin made neurones of lamina I more excitable, with a lower threshold to mechanical stimulation of the skin. Even more remarkable, the peripheral fields of neighbouring posterior horn neurones expanded towards the damaged region of skin. This occurs with a continual discharge of the non-myelinated afferent fibres; they may be emitting peptides and not the classical transmitters.

Compared with the soma, there are very few afferent visceral fibres. There are also only a few neurones of the posterior horns receiving an exclusively noxious input. Most neurones subserving pain receive a noxious and an innocuous mechanical input as well. Most of these neurones are organized on the basis of surround inhibition. Further, the kinds of stimulation that excite or inhibit the neurone are not the same. A common pattern of organization is for the central field of a posterior horn neurone to be nociceptive and the surrounding field to be non-noxious and mechanoreceptive. Thus light brushing on the surrounding skin tends to inhibit the cell that is excited by noxious stimuli.

Unexpectedly, there are no neurones of the posterior horns with an exclusive visceral input; neurones receiving an input from the viscera also receive inputs from the skin and in many cases from the somatic musculature. The neurones with an input from the heart also have somatic receptive fields. Those receiving an input from the colon also have an input from the bladder; these neurones also receive an input from the soma, which may or may not include a nociceptive input; some of them receive an input reporting noxious events in the skin.

Centrifugal nerve fibres to the posterior horns and sensory cranial nerve nuclei

Sensation is not merely the reproduction in consciousness of everything that strikes the central nervous system; the brain selects. By means of descending facilitation and inhibition, the brain increases or decreases the efficacy of different inputs, thus providing a mechanism for focussing attention on what is important.

This subject has been studied in rats and cats; how far it applies to humans has not yet been worked out. The first step in organizing the input to the central nervous system is carried out locally, by neurones of the substania gelatinosa. They can both inhibit and facilitate the input. Their short axons run cranio-caudally in Lissauer's tract, which lies at the tip of the posterior horns. The presynaptic inhibition that they deliver can block some branches of the incoming posterior root fibres, leaving impulses to arrive in others. This mechanism might direct impulses into one lot of branches so that they would reach one lamina rather than another. It can also totally block the input so that it is not relayed in the spinal cord.

One of the important discoveries of the past 25 years has been that nerve fibres descending from various parts of the brain stem can completely block a noxious input, so that it is not relayed in the spinal cord. Inhibition is also applied to the cells of origin of the spinothalamic and spinoreticular tracts. The source of the centrifugal inhibition is the periaqueductal gray of the midbrain, the nuclei coeruleus and subcoeruleus, certain of the midline raphe nuclei, and other nuclei of the reticular formation.

The effect of descending control of posterior horn neurones is shown in Fig. 1. From this study we learnt that there was tonic inhibition coming from the lower levels of the brain, which decreased excitation. This allowed the posterior horn neurones to respond only to a small area of stimulation and to respond only to the input of certain afferent fibres and not to that of others. Descending control affects the excitability of posterior horn neurones, both differentially and totally. For example, the input to a posterior horn neurone arriving in large myelinated fibres can be enhanced whilst that in non-myelinated fibres is reduced or blocked. The size of a receptive field of a posterior horn neurone, or any neurone on an afferent pathway, can be altered by descending facilitation or inhibition. Descending inhibition can be organized to stop the noxious input that causes pain. Excitation of the ventral part of the periaqueductal gray matter of the midbrain produces such inhibition of a noxious input to the spinal cord that an animal can be operated on without an anaesthetic. It is probable that the nerve impulses from the noxious stimulation are not getting into the spinal cord.

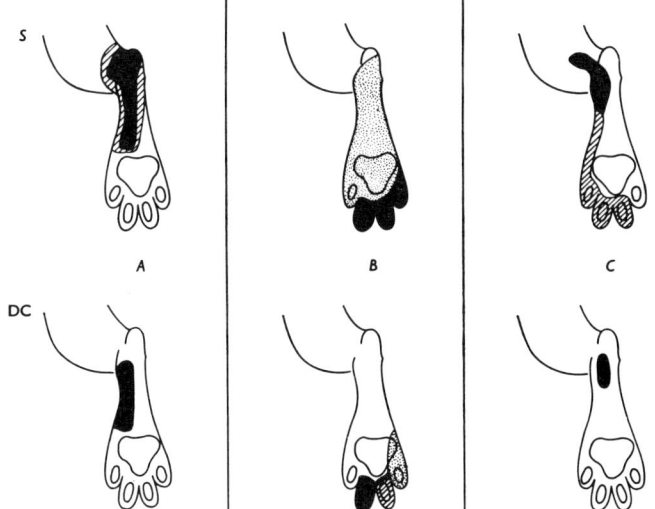

Fig. 1 Receptive fields of three cells in lamina VI of the cat. S shows the receptive fields in the spinal animal; DC shows the receptive fields of the same cells in the decerebrate animal. The black areas indicate the regions in which brushing produced firing of the cell; hatching indicates the region that required touch; and stippling, the region that required pressure. (Reproduced from *J. Physiol.* **188**, 403–423, with permission.)

When inhibition is applied to the convergent neurones which are the neurones of origin of the spinothalmic and spinoreticular tracts, it reduces their excitability. This could have the effect of stopping mechanoreceptive and slight noxious input from affecting them, leaving a stronger noxious input still able to excite them. The neurones that receive only a noxious input are not subjected to descending inhibition, and so they would continue to fire with a noxious input. It may be that this is the mechanism of feeling pain given that the main input to the brain comes from convergent neurones, that is, neurones reporting non-noxious mechanical and noxious stimuli.

Descending inhibition can be brought into action by pain. A strong pain can cause inhibition of vast numbers of wide dynamic range posterior horn neurones, via a spino-bulbo-spinal pathway. In experiments on many species, including humans, it has been shown that a larger, more extensive and more intense pain can suppress a lesser pain. In rats, it was found that this suppression of pain was due to a diffuse inhibition of all convergent neurones. This inhibition can be brought into activity by Pavlovian conditioning. If experiments are carried out on rats in which a pain is induced on repeated occasions by an identical procedure, the animal soon learns to raise its pain threshold before it is placed in the apparatus. This phenomenon is mediated by descending inhibitory fibres originating in the raphe nuclei.

In rats and mice stress brings in this inhibition, and so it is called *stress analgesia*. It is activated by many forms of stress, including fighting and sexual activity.

When it was understood that there were regions of the brain that prevented a noxious input reaching neurones of the posterior horn, and which thus completely blocked pain, neurosurgeons implanted electrodes in the brains of patients with chronic pain. It was found that, while electrical stimulation stopped constant chronic pain, it had no effect in blocking the input of any new stimulus – just the opposite to what was found in experiments on animals in the laboratory. The sites where electrodes have been implanted permanently are the caudate nucleus, the sensory part of the internal capsule, the ventrobasal part of the thalamus, the periventricular region near the IIIrd ventricle, and the periaqueductal gray.

But there is a way of stopping the pain from new noxious stimuli: acupuncture, electroacupuncture or low frequency (10 Hz) electric stimulation. This hypoalgesia or analgesia has a prolonged time course, in terms of most physiological mechanisms. It takes

20 min to induce and it lasts for more than 20 min after cessation of stimulation. The stimulation has to activate the delta and C fibres from deep structures, such as the muscles. Slow rate stimulation produces endorphins and fast rate stimulation metencephalin in the cerebrospinal fluid. Electroacupuncture is one of the mechanisms of analgesia used in China for surgery. The other mechanism is local segmental inhibition, induced by a faster rate of stimulation. When the method is most successful, the patient says that the knife making the skin incision feels like a blunt pencil being dragged along the skin. But the analgesia is not complete: pulling on the mesentery and strong stimulation of blood vessels can still cause pain.

The brain

The ascending pathways from the cord and the afferent cranial nerve nuclei that transmit impulses essential for feeling pain are spino-reticulo-thalamic, spino-mesencephalic, spino-tectal, and spino-thalamic; there are similar pathways from the nucleus caudalis of the 5th cranial nerve, but it is usual to talk only of the quinto-thalamic tract. It is possible that there is a subsidiary pathway that can be used consisting of intrinsic fibres of the grey matter.

The spino-thalamic and quinto-thalamic fibres run to the ventro-basal complex of the thalamus (the nuclei ventro-postero-lateralis and ventro-postero-medialis), to the medial and intralaminar nuclei and to the zona incerta. The spino-reticular fibres run to many relays of the reticular formation. Spino-reticular and spino-thalamic fibres in humans are shown in Fig. 2.

Some fibres reaching the brain among spino-thalamic and spino-reticular fibres terminate in the nucleus raphe magnus and the neighbouring lateral reticular formation; others terminate throughout the periaqueductal gray and adjacent nuclei. The latter form a feedback pathway to the parts of the brainstem that control the input to the spinal cord. After a relay in the reticular formation, fibres continue to the medial or intralaminar nuclei of the thalmus, to the ventro-basal complex, to the subthalamic region and to the posterior hypothalamus.

Anatomically and physiologically the nociceptive regions of the *thalamus* are separable into two regions a lateral part consisting of the ventro-basal complex and a medial part made up of several medial thalamic nuclei. In addition, there is an area of the ventro-basal complex lying near the medial geniculate body called PO. The lateral part of the thalamus receives afferents coming from the posterior column nuclei in the medial lemniscus as well as the spinothalamic tract. This input is arranged in a topographical, point-to-point manner, with the neurones having small peripheral fields. The input to the medial nuclei and to PO is arranged with neurones receiving an input from a very large peripheral field, some receiving from both sides of the body. The input to PO may be only tactile. Neurones of the intralaminar nucleus, in the monkey, are activated by any stimulus that alerts the animal and makes it move. This region has been examined in conscious humans. In the medial nuclei of the centrum medianum-parafascicular complex, neurones respond to pinprick and some to heat. Most of the parafascicular neurones respond to stimuli on both sides of the body. Electric stimulation of these nuclei causes a burning pain felt in extensive areas of the body, more contralateral than bilateral. Although there are these large fields, lesions made in these nuclei cause no loss of any kind of sensibility. In general, the lateral part is concerned with accurate temporal and spatial localization of all pain and thermal sense, while the medial part is concerned with the emotional and affective aspects of sensation; and the connections to the hypothalamus provide the autonomic responses to the input.

The fibres from the nuclei postero-ventro-lateralis run to SI of the postcentral gyrus and to SII of the parietal operculum. SI provides information of intensity and exact localization of the pain. The fibres from the medial thalamic nuclei go to SII and to the orbital cortex of the frontal lobe and to the septal area, to the tem-

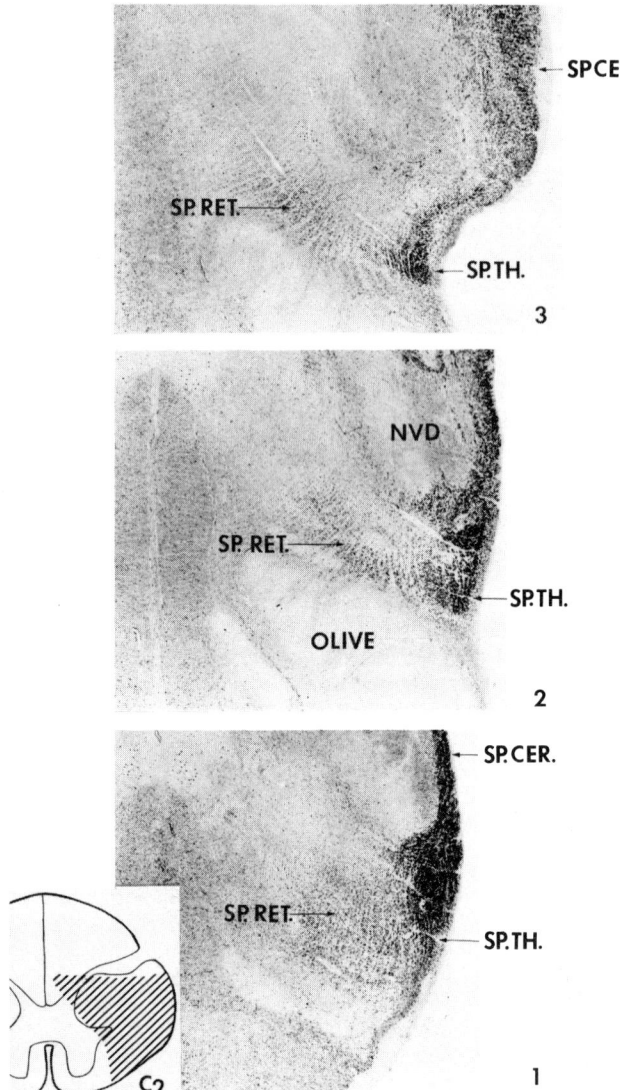

Fig. 2 Three sections of the medulla oblongata of humans showing degeneration of ascending fibres following an antero-lateral cordotomy at the 2nd cervical segment. At these levesl the separation of the spinothalamic and spinoreticular tract is clearly seen. Degenerating fibres are stained black in these Marchi preparations.

poral and occipital lobes, and to the amygdala and putamen. Investigations of the parietal cortex of the monkey have shown that there is no area with neurons devoted only to noxious events; nociceptive neurones lie intermingled with non-nociceptive neurones. Further, the input from the ventrobasal complex and the zona incerta does not go only to the primary somatic areas but also to other sensory areas, such as the auditory cortex.

The spinothalamic tract is mainly concerned with conduction of impulses giving rise to pain, warmth, and cold; it also conveys impulses originating in mechanoreceptors. A bilateral antero-lateral cordotomy, cutting all the fibres of this complex, renders all parts of the body below the lesion totally analgesic.

Referred pain

The site of a pain is not necessarily the place from which it is originating. The term 'referred pain' has been used more widely in recent years; though it always means the wrong localization of pain arising in deep tissues. It used to be used to mean pain referred from a hollow viscus to the soma. Currently is is also used to describe pain from proximal joints and ligaments that is experienced as running down a limb. Other examples include pain referred to the opposite kidney; pain referred from the diaphragm to the tip of the shoulder; and the pain of myocardial ischaemia being felt in the chest wall or running down the left upper limb or up into the neck.

Referred pain is in one direction only; it is from the deep to the superficial tissues; a burn on the hand does not cause abdominal colic! Thus referred pain is not merely false localization; it is a particular type of false localization. It is referred from an unknown or imperceived part to a known part of the body. It is more commonly from hollow viscera.

As well as referred pain, there is referred sensitivity. The deep tissue of the somatic wall may be painful when pressed upon if there is an acute pathological state of a viscus; and the skin may be abnormally sensitive to stroking or light pinching.

Noxious input from all tissues, skin, muscle, and viscera, summates at the spinal level and causes a local state of hyperexcitability. If the region to which the pain is referred is rendered completely analgesic, the pain may or may not be referred to that area. In patients in whom the cervical nerves have been divided so that the skin over the shoulder and clavicular region is totally insensitive, stimulation of the phrenic nerve coming from the diaphragm can still cause pain in the shoulder-tip area. In this case, summation of impulses from the skin and the diaphragm is not essential for producing pain referred to the shoulder; a large input from the diaphragm is enough. On the other hand, the pain of angina pectoris can be abolished by injecting local anaesthetic into tender points in the muscles of the chest wall; or by infiltrating all the subcutaneous tissues of the overlying skin, rendering this skin analgesic.

In the cat some neurones of lamina V receive fine myelinated fibres from the skin and from the viscera and others from the skin and somatic muscles. This applies also to cardiac muscle: spinal neurones receiving afferents from the heart also receive them from the body wall. There is the same convergence in neurones of the thalamus: there are neurones receiving both from the viscera and the skin. However, the demonstration that impulses from viscera, muscles, and skin converge on to the same groups of neurones in the posterior horns does not alone account for the false localization of visceral pain.

The relation between the two inputs in the spinal gray matter is not one of summation. Volleys in the visceral afferent fibres presynaptically inhibit those in the cutaneous fibres, and vice versa; and volleys in one lot of visceral afferents presynaptically inhibit those in another. Similar and more complicated relationships are likely to exist in the thalamus and hypothalamus. Thus our knowledge of the anatomy cannot account for referrred pain until the physiological events have been made clear.

It is probable that the skin is provided with a large number of neurones in the sensory regions of the brain, the muscles with fewer, and the viscera with least. If this is so, then good localization for the skin and poor localization for the viscera might follow; though this still would not entail a reference of pain.

Chronic pain

In recent years the mechanism of chronic pain has been investigated by producing chronic arthritis in rats or by injecting substances into an animal's paw that cause chronic inflammation and pain. The peripheral endings of non-myelinated and other fibres become sensitized by the inflammatory exudates. The threshold to the lightest touches is lowered. There is also an increased sensitivity of delta nociceptors of the joint capsules. When these receptors are strongly excited, they respond abnormally. Many of the afferent C fibres have a lower threshold than normal and also have an enhanced response to stimulation. This change in behaviour of the receptors causes an abnormal state in the related neurones of the central nervous system. In the posterior horns, there may be continuous firing of some neurones. Many more neurones respond to tactile stimulation than normal, and neurones that are normally fired maximally by noxious stimuli now respond in the same way

to light touch. In the thalamus and sensory cortex, there is continuous neuronal activity in neurones related to the affected joints, and in the thalamus neurones become unusually responsive to joint movements; brushing the skin over the inflamed joints causes prolonged after-discharge. Neurones of the superficial layers of the parietal cortex respond to pinching the inflamed joints. These central effects are due to sensitization of nerve fibres in the joint capsules. All of these effects are reduced by aspirin.

The peripheral nerves as a source of pain

When peripheral nerves or posterior nerve roots are constantly stretched or compressed or when they have been partially or completely divided, there is not necessarily an absence of messages to the spinal cord. So, cutting nerves in order to stop an input that is causing pain seldom removes pain associated with damage to peripheral nerves. After a major input has been cut off from the spinal cord or corresponding region of the brain, anatomical and physiological reorganization follows; and part of this process consists of increased activity in the neurones previously receiving the input.

Damaged peripheral nerve fibres tend to fire off impulses spontaneously. It is probable that the same thing takes place among damaged nerve fibres within the central nervous system; and it could occur in multiple sclerosis, where the nerve fibres have been damaged by a plaque. Spontaneous firing causes paraesthesiae, dyasthesiae, and, in the peripheral nerves, pain. This spontaneous firing occurs in the neuromata that form at the peripheral end of a cut nerve and also in the course of a peripheral nerve being chafed or constricted.

Not only do impulses arise spontaneously in the peripheral nerve fibres but also in the posterior root ganglion cells of damaged nerves. These ganglia become sensitive to pressure, pulling, and constriction. Outgrowing nerve fibres at the site of damage are very sensitive to mechanical stimulation, and some are sensitive to adrenalin and noradrenalin. This is a feature of some outgrowing fibres: the axonic membrane has changed characteristics and it is now sensitive to transmitter substances that normally do not excite it. Whether damaged nerve fibres within the central nervous system are also sensitive to noradrenalin is not yet known.

Spontaneous activity can be recorded in humans in the constricted nerve giving rise to *meralgia paraesthetica*; and it has been seen in other nerves in entrapment syndromes. The spontaneous firing is occurring in both myelinated and non-myelinated fibres. Traction lesions of the bracial plexus often produce severe pain and it can continue for years. Trauma to the cauda equina causes damage to the posterior and sacral roots that make up the cauda. Pain occurs far more commonly with multiple root lesions than with lesions of the spinal cord itself. Usually there is severe pain immediately after the traumatic lesion; it is likely to increase for the first few weeks after which it slowly subsides and usually disappears. Another very painful posterior root lesion is intercostal neuralgia. It either comes on spontaneously or is the result of surgery on the thoracic wall. When it occurs spontaneously, the pain may come on suddenly, during the course of one day.

An abnormal state in the peripheral nerves induces a similar state in the posterior horns which spreads from the neurones receiving the input to neighbouring neurones. This phenomenon accounts for the hyperalgesia that follows many kinds of peripheral nerve injuries and also for the spreading of abnormal cutaneous and deep sensitivity that occurs with some peripheral injuries, particularly *causalgia*. A causalgic state starting in the territory of the median nerve and may eventually spread up the arm.

The central nervous system as a source of pain

Pain is due not only to impulses arriving at the central nervous system; it may also arise within the central nervous system itself and is then called *central pain*.

The commonest and worst of central pains is the *thalamic syndrome* first described by Déjerine and Roussy (1906). It is prob-

21.24   **Neurology**

able that this pain occurs when the nuclei postero-ventro-lateralis and medialis are destroyed or large parts of them are damaged. In the cat neurones of the ventro-basal complex inhibit neurones of the intralaminar nuclei and the posterior hypothalamus; the removal of this inhibition may be the cause of thalamic pain. In this condition, pain comes on gradually, sometimes over several years. The same pattern follows a thrombosis of the posterior inferior cerebellar artery, another cause of central pain. In both of these conditions, the pain is on the side of the body contralateral to the lesion. It does not always involve the entire half of the body but may occur only in a forequarter or hindquarter or be restricted to one limb. When the pain involves the face, there is usually a severe pain in the eye, which the patient may describe as feeling as though an eye is being torn out. In a few cases, the pain is restricted to one side of the mouth and lateral side of the hand which corresponds to the thalamic and the cortical representation of these parts of the body. In addition to constant pain, there is an increase in pain with every sort of stimulation in the effected region. With central lesions, there can be any sort of pain; burning, soreness, aching, or a sensation of sitting or lying on rocks.

Although the lesion causing the pain is, by definition, in the central nervous system, an input from the periphery is necessary. This can be shown by blocking the input from the lower limb by a spinal or epidural anaesthetic or from the upper limb by a brachial plexus block. During the time of effectiveness of the block, there is no pain in the limb. But treatment by measures designed to make such peripheral blocks permanent does not work. Central pain can occur with pathological conditions of the spinal cord. It is common in syringomyelia and with tumours of the cord. In syringomyelia, it is usually a deep pain, and it can also be a deep burning pain; it comes into the differential diagnosis of pains in the shoulder, neck, and face. As the split in the spinal cord is commonly in the posterior horn and extends many segments from the upper cervical region to the upper thoracic region, these pains may extend unilaterally from the lower face, through the neck and shoulders and into the limb. So pain in the shoulder or the face may be the presenting and only manifestation of the disorder, for clinical signs may be absent or minimal. It is surprising to find that the pain of these conditions, given the morbid anatomical basis for them, may not be constant. It may last for a few weeks and then not return for years; it then recurs in the same place. The onset or the return of the pain may be precipitated by a physical strain. In addition to deep pain, there may be lightning pain, similar to those of tabes. Central pains can occur in multiple sclerosis; they may be aching, burning or girdle pains.

Pain occurs with spinal paraplegia and paraparesis. This can be burning, constricting, and shooting, a deep boring pain, and dysaesthesiae, felt below and up to the level of the transverse lesion. In paraplegia, patients may also have pain associated with spastic muscles. This is either constant, when the muscles are strongly contracting, and/or more severe when there is muscle spasm. Exactly the same kind of spasticity and involuntary muscular spasm is seen in patients without pain and in those with pain, and it is unknown why there is pain in one case and not in another.

References

Adriaensen, H., Gybels, J., Handwerker, H. O. and Van Hees, J. (1983). Response properties of thin myelinated (A-delta) fibres in human skin. *J. Neurophysiol.* **49**, 111–122.
Cassinari, V. and Pagni, C. A. (1969). *Central pain.* Harvard University Press, Cambridge, Mass.
Déjerine, J. and Roussy, G. (1906). Le syndrome thalamique. *Rev. neurol.* **14**, 521–532.
Dubuisson, D., Fitzgerald, M. and Wall, P. D. (1979). Amoeboid receptive fields of cells in laminae 1, 2, and 3. *Brain Res.* **177**, 376–378.
Dubuisson, D. and Wall, P. D. (1980). Descending influences on receptive fields and activity of single units recorded in laminae 1, 2, and 3 of cat spinal cord. *Brain Res.* **199**, 283–298.

Hagbarth, K.-E. and Vallbo, A. B. (1967). Mechanoreceptor activity recorded percutaneously with semi-microelectrodes in human peripheral nerves. *Acta physiol. Scand.* **69**, 121–122.
IASP (1979). Pain terms: a list with definitions and notes on usage. *Pain* **6**, 249–252.
IASP (1982). Pain terms: a supplementary note. *Pain* **14**, 205–206.
McMahon, S. B. and Wall, P. D. (1984). Receptive fields of rat lamina I projection cells move to incorporate a nearby region of injury. *Pain* **19**, 235–247.
Pomeranz, B., Wall, P. D. and Weber, W. V. (1968). Cord cells responding to fine myelinated afferents from viscera, muscle, and skin. *J. Physiol. (Lond.)* **199**, 511–532.
Torebjörk, H. E. and Hallin, R. G. (1973). Perceptual changes accompanying controlled preferential blocking of A and C fibre responses in human skin nerve. *Exp. Brain Res.* **16**, 321–332.
Torebjörk, H. E. and Hallin, R. G. (1974). Responses in A and C fibres to repeated electrical intradermal stimulation. *J. Neurol. Neurosurg. Psychiat.* **37**, 653–664.
Van Hees, J. and Gybels, J. M. (1972). Pain related to single afferent C fibres from human skin. *Brain Res.* **48**, 397–400.
Van Hees, J. and Gybels, J. M. (1981). C nociceptor activity in human nerve during painful and non-painful skin stimulation. *J. Neurol. Neurosurg. Psychiat.* **44**, 600–607.
Wall, P. D. (1967). The laminar organization of dorsal horn and effects of descending impulses. *J. Physiol.* **88**, 403–423.
Wynn-Parry, C. B. (1980). Pain in avulsion lesions of the brachial plexus. *Pain* **9**, 41–53.

The management of chronic pain

J. W. LLOYD

Advances in medicine today have brought us to the stage where many painful diseases are amenable to treatment. One condition, however, still defies the rule books; that is, intractable pain. It is defined as pain that has been present for over a month and unremitting despite treatment. It has therefore become a useless pain and has lost any alerting function as to its underlying pathology.

This type of pain is often equated with cancer and this is unfortunate because many patients with cancer do not have pain and certainly in the standard United Kingdom pain centre they constitute perhaps only 25 per cent of the total admissions. The remainder are made up of patients with non-malignant pain perhaps condemned to a life-time of pain and misery.

The Hospice movement is now accelerating and performing a very useful function in caring for the terminal cancer patients. They are also fortunate in avoiding the therapeutic restrictions which apply to the non-malignant group.

Any involvement in pain management demands an appreciation of the vast difference between acute and chronic pain. The former is self-limiting in the majority of cases: the latter is not. Many of the disappointments in managing chronic pain are due to failure in understanding this difference. Acute pain, if not properly managed in the first instance, will slowly merge into the insidious descending spiral of chronic pain with its diminution of response to treatment until the final stage of no return is reached.

In the mid-1960s a 'pain explosion' took place. From being closeted in a cupboard with morphia chronic pain became something of interest. Physicians not only talked about it but more importantly thought about it. The gate theory of pain may be in some way responsible for this and even if it is not wholly acceptable in its present form it must take much credit for the interest it stimulated.

Gaps in scientific knowledge were filled by experience gained largely in pain clinics which appeared at the same time. There are now some 200 pain clinics in the United Kingdom and they make a valuable contribution, not only in exposing our ignorance but also in providing a haven which the chronic pain sufferer has been in need of for so long.

It must be understood that these patients have been treated in many hospitals and clinics unsuccessfully, and their morale is at a very low ebb. There is also resentment, not only of their plight but of previous failures to cure them. These are factors which have a considerable bearing on the successful outcome of treatment. In this context it can be argued that these patients can only be satisfactorily treated as in patients where they can be exposed to a multidisciplinary team of specialists in a properly equipped, and staffed, Pain Unit. Unfortunately there are too few such units in the United Kingdom, but one would like to envisage in the future a Pain Unit in each region which would take the more complicated referrals from less well-endowed satellite pain clinics.

The corner stones of chronic pain relief are the use of drugs and interruption of pain pathways by various means. Pain may be the only symptom that is preventing the patient leading a normal life and it is felt that in such cases treatment by some form of nerve block is indicated. Many patients in the Oxford Unit say that they prefer to have nerve blocks rather than drug therapy, as the latter may make them confused and drowsy, and if they stop taking the drugs the pain returns and they can never forget about it.

Methods of interrupting pain pathways

Chemical methods

Intrathecal phenol and chlorocresol (neurolytic)

This method introduced by Maher in 1955 is still widely used. A spinal needle is introduced into the cerebro-spinal fluid at the required dermatome level. With the patients lying on their affected sides a hyperbaric bolus of 5 per cent phenol in glycerine is then deposited on the appropriate nerve roots. The concentration of phenol, although causing some demyelination of posterior columns, does not appear to have an adverse affect on function, unless there is severe wasting already present.

Dosage
    Cervical : 1 ml
    Thoracic : 1–2 ml
    Lumbar : 0.6–0.8 ml

Complications Bladder dysfunction is more likely in lower lumbar and lumbo-sacral areas. Even judicious posturing may not be successful in avoiding this.

Duration of effect This may be up to 14 months.

Contraindications Non-malignancy.

Sympathetic blocks

For a stellate ganglion block for the upper extremity a No. 1 gauge needle is inserted between carotid sheath and sternomastoid to strike the body of C7. The needle is withdrawn to clear the periosteum and 8 ml of local anaesthetic without adrenaline are injected.

For permanent block it is advisable to refer the patients to a neurosurgeon who can extirpate the 4th, 3rd, and 2nd sympathetic ganglia and easily avoid a permanent Horner's syndrome which can be cosmetically upsetting.

Lumbar sympathetic blocks

Under X-ray control a 6 inch needle is inserted at four fingers breadth from mid-line to strike the body of L2 vertebra. The angle of the needle is then altered to slide over the convexity of the body of the vertebra until the sympathetic chain, lying in its plane on the antero-lateral surface of the vertebra, is reached.

Dose Local anaesthetic (diagnostic); 10 ml of 1 per cent lignocaine. Phenol (permanent); 3 ml of 6 per cent phenol in water.

Complications High incidence of groin neuralgia, which responds to transcutaneous nerve stimulation.

Coeliac plexus block

As for lumbar sympathetic block except that proximity of the pleural membrane limits the lateral placement of the needle. It is perhaps noteworthy that the final position of the needle is almost 90° to skin.

Hypophysectomy

This technique was introduced by Moricca in 1974 and is performed under image intensification. It involves the placement of a needle into the pituitary gland and injection of 1 ml of absolute alcohol.

Immediate complications If visual defects occur the injection should be stopped. Bleeding may also occur and is stopped by nasal packs.

Trigeminal ganglion block

This is performed under X-ray control and can be effected by the injection of alcohol (only for malignant disorders). More recently refined techniques have been introduced which involve the use of radio-frequency lesion generation, cryoanalgesia, injection of glycerine into Meckel's cave, and injection of the peripheral divisions of the nerve where they emerge onto the face and mouth.

Hip block

This is the block of the obturator nerve and the nerve to quadratus femoris with 0.5 per cent bupivacaine (James, 1976). It is a perfect example of the breaking of the vicious cycle of pain, as some of these patients exist happily without pain for up to one year, although there is no improvement in mobility.

Intercostal block

This technique blocks conduction in the intercostal nerve, lying in the intercostal groove. It can be accomplished using local anaesthetic, 6 per cent phenol in water (not recommended), radio-frequency lesion or cryotherapy.

Physical methods

Cerebro-spinal fluid (CSF) replacement with hypothermic saline

This is a method introduced by Hitchcock (1967), where 60–80 ml of CSF were withdrawn and replaced by 20 ml of saline at 0 °C. It has the advantage that one injection in the lumbar area can relieve multiple foci of pain, but is very painful and thus requires a general anaesthetic. It frequently causes headache.

Barbotage

This method, introduced by Lloyd (1980), consists of the alternate withdrawal and injection of 20 ml of CSF to and fro from the subarachnoid space. Sixty per cent of patients have relief of pain varying from three to seven months.

Cordotomy (percutaneous or surgical)

Both procedures aim at destroying conduction in the spinothalamic tract subserving pain and temperature. They are not used in non-malignant pain.

Interspinous hypertonic saline injection

This is a method introduced by Whitty and Hockaday (1967) to control pain by injecting 6 per cent saline into the interspinous ligament. This in itself produces pain in the root distribution but can be dispelled by an injection of lignocaine through the same needle. In approximately 45 per cent of patients the original pain is also relieved for weeks or months.

Cryoanalgesia

This procedure was introduced by Lloyd et al. (1976) and involves the destruction of nerves by application of extreme cold. It is unique in that it is a percutaneous technique seeking the nerve by electrical stimulation. Scar tissue is minimal and the whole process is reversible. Recovery of function takes place in 8–12 weeks.

Radiofrequency (RF) lesions

This is the opposite to cryoanalgesia in that it heats the nerve to temperatures of 70°C and above to provide a long-term result.

Acupuncture

Whether the practice of inserting a fine needle into a trigger point is called acupuncture or something else, there is no doubt that in certain situations it can be effective. This may also be said for injections of local anaesthetic.

The practice of acupuncture varies from the complicated and mystical approach to the lay and totally untrained practice of placing needles where it hurts. Reversal of acupuncture analgesia by naloxone involved encephalins and gave the technique respectability, but it should be emphasized that this is not a constant finding. Mann (1983), who has a very considerable experience, discounts the meridian theory but believes in the existence of focal points which can give pain relief if needled.

Other authorities believe that the insertion of a needle achieves pain relief by stimulating mechano-receptors to produce presynaptic inhibition at spinal cord level. Whatever the mechanism the practice has become very popular but its place in the management of chronic pain has yet to be evaluated.

Transcutaneous nerve stimulators (TNS)

These were developed as a result of the gate theory: they are simple, high output impedance generators providing a spiked or square wave form in repetitive firing rate. The malleable carbon electrodes are strapped on to the painful area and by controlling the variables (output, pulse, width, and frequency) a pleasant warm tingling sensation may be achieved which overrides the pain. In a smaller number of cases the pain relief may last for some hours after the instrument has been turned off.

The technique seems to have more success when the pain is manifested cutaneously, as with neuralgias, phantom limbs, and stump pains. It is not so effective in chronic back pain, and of no benefit in cancer pain. Perhaps one of its principal advantages is that it is non-invasive, but it should not be used in patients with cardiac pacemakers. The price range is enormous and is difficult to correlate with effectiveness.

Hypnotherapy

Hypnotherapy has sometimes been thought of as being useful in the management of chronic pain. Any procedure involving suggestion will relieve moderate pain at least to an extent, but it is clear that with hypnosis the relief is far from being complete when there is an important physical cause for the pain, as with the pain of cancer.

In the light of available evidence, summarized by Merskey (1971), reports of the effective relief of severe pain by hypnotism must be treated cautiously.

The management of clinical pain

Cancer pain

Patients in this category form 28 per cent of admissions to the Oxford Regional Pain Relief Unit. In general they are the easiest group to treat as they can be exposed to the whole gamut of pain therapy without adverse comment. High-dose opium can be used as also can neurolytic agents for nerve blocking. Both of these methods would not be permitted in non-malignant pain.

Intrathecal phenol is a useful technique where pain is the predominant symptom. Intercostal cryotherapy is also used for lung cancer and if the cryoprobe is inserted through the sacral hiatus to freeze the fourth sacral nerve root, excellent analgesia is obtained where there is pain in the perineum due, for instance, to rectal carcinoma.

For multiple soft tissue secondaries hypothermic irrigation of the CSF or barbotage is indicated. When pain is unilateral either percutaneous or surgical cordotomy gives excellent results.

When the disease becomes generalized opiates by mouth are the treatment of choice. Many patients express their misery and anxiety as pain, and in these circumstances antidepressants are most valuable.

The discovery of opiate receptors in the dorsal horn of the spinal cord (Yaksh and Rudy, 1976) has led to the administration of extradural and intrathecal opiates. In theory this should be the ideal method but the occasional late onset of respiratory depression has made it a technique to be used with caution. In some continental countries extradural catheters are left *in situ* for up to one year. The catheter is 'topped up' daily by nursing staff or by the patient's relatives at home. The intrathecal route would probably be the most effective if it were not for the difficulty of leaving an indwelling catheter in the CSF. It is likely that an implantable pump will overcome this problem in the near future and extremely small doses will then be used with maximum effect.

Skeletal pain

Back pain is responsible for the loss of 19 million work days per year and it is estimated that 10 per cent of the population have a chronic back disorder.

Because many back injuries are work related, the possibility of compensation may be an important factor. Approximately 50 per cent of patients with a compensation-related back injury remain off work longer than six months, whilst 31 per cent remain unemployed for over two years. Ghia *et al.* (1979) consider that, with chronic back pain below the waist 55 per cent of patients had pain of central or psychogenic origin, 30 per cent of patients had sympathetically mediated pain and only 15 per cent was somatic pain due to a demonstrable pathological lesion.

Extradural block with local anaesthetic and a long acting steroid may be helpful, but the likelihood of improvement falls sharply if the patient has previously had one or more laminectomies.

When there is degenerative disease of the facet joints a good result can be expected by blocking the facetal nerve with a cryoprobe or radio-frequency lesion generator.

Arachnoiditis often follows a neuroradiological procedure and is extremely refractory to treatment. If the pain is felt predominantly in the legs some relief may be obtained from a lumbar sympathetic block.

The most useful analgesic for this condition is sublingual buprenorphine.

Neuralgias

Into this category fall trigeminal neuralgia, atypical facial neuralgia, posttraumatic neuralgia, postherpetic neuralgia, occipital neuralgia, and the rare glosso-pharyngeal neuralgia.

Where the trigeminal nerve is involved a good result is obtained by the application of cryoanalgesia to the respective branch of the 5th nerve as it emerges from the skull. The same can be said for occipital neuralgia.

Postherpetic neuralgia can be treated successfully by sympathetic blockade if given within three weeks of the acute attack. After this period the pain gradually assumes a central quality so that in a year no treatment is likely to be effective. Tricyclic antidepressants are then the most useful drug.

The occipital nerve can be cut, frozen or destroyed by a radio-frequency current in the troublesome complaint of occipital neuralgia.

Glosso-pharyngeal neuralgia is very uncommon but can be treated by application of a cryoprobe to the tonsillar bed and thereby freezing the glossopharyngeal nerve as it passes underneath. The most useful drugs are carbamazepine, sodium valproate or clonazepam.

Non-skeletal pain

Postoperative wound pain syndromes

Three surgical operations are associated with a postoperative pain in or around the scar which may persist for years: thoracotomy, nephrectomy and inguinal herniorrhaphy. There is commonly a psychological component and analgesic drugs are often ineffective.

Blocking the respective nerves with local anaesthetic followed by cryoanalgesia or R. F. lesion is usually helpful. Tricyclic antidepressants, and mild analgesics are also useful.

Abdominal pain

Pain of *cancer of the pancreas* responds well to a coeliac plexus block but surprisingly the pain of chronic pancreatitis does not. Pain of *chronic renal colic* is abolished by extradural block at L1 and was followed by the passage of a stone within a week in one series.

Myofascial pain

This can be treated by injecting the focal point with local anaesthesia. Alternatively acupuncture is often used with success.

Neurological disorders

Spinal cord injuries

The burning dysaesthesia of this complaint may respond to sympathetic blockade, barbotage of the CSF or interspinous hypertonic saline one segment above the damaged level. The success rate is not high and best results are probably obtained from the anticonvulsant group of drugs.

Multiple sclerosis

Pain in this condition is commonly associated with muscle spasm and can be controlled by intrathecal phenol or intramuscular alcohol (40 per cent). Intrathecal buprenorphine has also been very effective and also in other conditions where pain and spasm are related. Occasionally pain occurs without spasm and a sympathetic block is then indicated, but for some unknown reason pain in the leg is much more likely to be relieved than pain in the trunk. The most useful drugs are mild analgesics, dantrolene sodium, and diazepam.

Syringomyelia

This may respond to interspinous hypertonic saline, barbotage or hypothermic irrigation of the CSF.

Spinal cord tumours

Von Recklinghausen's disease, and vascular malformation of the spinal vessels. Intrathecal manipulations are contraindicated in these conditions.

Deafferentation pain

This is pain, usually burning in character, which is felt in areas which are insensitive. It may occur after peripheral nerve section or sensory root rhizotomy. Thalamic pain may also be included in this group.

Treatment by sympathetic blockade may be helpful. Success has been reported in a few cases with the use of naloxone and physostigmine, but results are inconsistent. Clonazepam may be helpful. In recent years a new surgical technique has been introduced whereby the entry zone of the dorsal horn of the spinal cord is destroyed using a fine electrode. Although early results are encouraging, time will prove the place of the technique.

Sympathetic dystrophies

These include causalgia, Sudeck's atrophy, Raynaud's disease, shoulder/hand syndrome, and phantom pain.

These conditions all respond well to sympathetic blockade but success is inversely proportional to the time that elapses before treatment. The most useful drugs are benzodiazepines and L-tryptophan.

Ischaemic pain

Included in this group are ischaemic rest pain, gangrene, and Paget's disease. In a series of 148 patients with rest pain who received a phenol (6 per cent) injection of the lumbar sympathetic chain, 59 per cent were free of pain until follow-up or death (Reid *et al.*, 1970). Where gangrene is confined to the toes a phenol sympathetic block frequently relieves pain and allows demarcation

and separation of tissue. Paget's disease of bone can be very painful and phenol injections of the sympathetic chain at appropriate levels have relieved pain for 6–8 years (Reid, 1960).

Drugs (see also Section 27)

Whereas most pain occurring immediately after trauma or operation responds to conventional analgesics that is not necessarily true in chronic pain. The simplest clinical guideline is that where pain occurs in a numb area (e.g. dysaesthesia) or in non-existent areas (phantom limb pain) conventional analgesics are unlikely to be helpful. In the Oxford Regional Pain Relief Unit, approximately one-third of patients with either malignant or non-malignant pain show a poor response to conventional analgesia.

Table 1

Conventional analgesics			
Mild	Acetyl salicylic acid (aspirin)		
	Paracetamol		
	Dihydrocodeine		
	Non-steroidal anti-inflammatory drugs		
	Levorphanol (dromoran)		
	Phenazocine		
Strong	Morphine		
	Other agonist opioids		
	Buprenorphine		
	Other partial agonist opioids		
	Phenazocine		
Unconventional analgesics			
Antidepressants			
	Tricyclics		Amitriptyline
			Dothiepin
	Benzodiazepines	Clobazam	
	Other		Nomifensine
			Mianserin
Anticonvulsants			
	Sodium valproate		
	Clonazepam		
	Phenytoin		

As in other branches of medicine the concept of a ladder, with the mild peripherally acting analgesics as the bottom rungs and strong narcotic agents as the top, is helpful (Table 1). The major limitation in implementing the ladder for non-malignant pain is the problem of using strong opiate analgesics with their potential for dependence.

The use of antidepressants in chronic pain management is widespread, but with little support from controlled studies. The dosages used (e.g. amitriptyline 25 mg *nocte*) do not result in plasma concentrations required for treatment of depression: any benefit is unlikely to be from measurable antidepressant effect. Despite the uncertainties over mode of action, in postherpetic neuralgia this is the single most effective treatment.

The use of anticonvulsants is best known from the prescribing of carbamazepine in trigeminal neuralgia. Sodium valproate and clonazepam are probably the commonest anticonvulsants used in the management of chronic pain, and it is encouraging that this unconventional approach is now being recognized by the major pharmaceutical companies as it is likely that the breakthrough will come in this group.

References

Beals, R. K. and Hickman, N. W. (1972). Industrial injuries of the back and extremities. *J. Bone Joint Surg.* **54A, 8**, 1593–1599.

Ghia, J. N., Duncan, G., Toomey, T. C., Mao, W. and Geff, J. M. (1979). The pharmacologic approach in differential diagnosis of chronic pain. *Spine* 4, 54–58.

Glynn, C. J., McQuay, H. J., Lloyd, J. W., Moore, R. A. and Teddy, P. J. (1984). Intrathecal buprenorphine for painful muscle spasms in paraplegic patients. *Pain* Suppl. 2, S341.

Hitchcock, E. (1967). Hypothermic subarachnoid injection for intractable pain. *Lancet* i, 1133.

James, C. D. T. and Little, T. F. (1976). Regional hip blockade. *Anaesthesia* 31, 1060–1067.

Lloyd, J. W. (1980). The anaesthetist and the pain clinic. *Br. Med. J.* ii, 432–434.

——, Barnard, J. D. W. and Glynn, C. J. (1976). Cryoanalgesia. A new approach to pain relief. *Lancet* ii, 932–934.

——, and Carrie, L. E. S. (1965). A method of treating renal colic. *Proc. R. Soc. Med.* 58, 634.

——, Hughes, J. T. and Davies Jones, G. A. B. (1972). The relief of severe intractable pain by barbotage of the cerebrospinal fluid. *Lancet* i, 354–355.

Maher, R. M. (1955). Relief of pain in incurable cancer. *Lancet* i, 18.

Mann, F. (1983). *Scientific aspects of acupuncture*, pp. 27–49. William Heinemann Medical Books, London.

Melzack, R. and Wall, P. D. (1969). Pain mechanisms a new theory. *Science* 150, 971.

Merskey, H. (1971). An appraisal of hypnosis. *Postgrad. Med. J.* 47, 572.

Moricca, G. (1974). Chemical hypophysectomy for cancer pain. In *Advances in neurology*, Vol. 4 (ed. J. J. Bonica), p. 707. Raven Press, New York.

Nashold, B. S. Jr and Brill, H. E. (1979). Dorsal root entry zone lesions for pain relief. *J. Neurosurg.* 51, 59–69.

Reid, W. (1960). The relief of pain in osteitis deformans (Paget's disease of bone) by phenol injection of the sympathetic chain. *Scot. Med. J.* 5, 71–75.

Reid, W., Kennedy, J., Watt, J. and Gray, T. G. (1970). Phenol injection of the sympathetic chain. *Br. J. Surg.* 57, 45–50.

Smith, M. C. (1964). Histological findings following intrathecal injections of phenol for the relief of pain. *Br. J. Anaesth.* 36, 387–390.

Whitty, C. W. M. and Hockaday, D. (1967). Patterns of referred pain in the normal subject. *Brain* 90, 481–484.

Yaksh, T. L. and Rudy, T. A. (1976) Narcotic analgesia produced by a direct action on the spinal cord. *Science* 192, 1357–1358.

HEADACHE

J. M. S. PEARCE

Headache is the most common symptom demanding a physician's attention. If we know what makes the head ache we may understand both the nature of the complaint and how its many causes disturb normal physiology and thus alert us to their presence.

Mechanisms

Much of the arachnoid membrane, the ependyma lining the ventricles and the brain parenchyma are *insensitive* to pain. Direct pressure or traction on those cranial nerves bearing somatic afferent fibres will evoke pain. The cerebral arterial trunks, large veins and venous sinuses and parts of the dura are the main pain-sensitive structures. Pain is produced if they are displaced by a lump (tumour, abscess or haematoma), or by a low-pressure state, e.g. following lumbar puncture. A throbbing, pulsatile headache is thus common in many intracranial lesions and is mediated via the afferent nerve fibres to the thalamus and its cortical connections. Migraine is the commonest vascular pain.

Pain arising from the dura or vessels is referred by trigeminal branches to the ipsilateral forehead and eye if the causal lesion is in the anterior or middle cranial fossae. Pain arising in the upper cervical spine is often referred by the C_2 root to the occiput. Infratentorial lesions in the posterior fossa cause referred pain in the occiput and neck via the upper three cervical nerves. Posterior fossa tumours may cause frontal headache by causing obstructive hydrocephalus which distends the lateral ventricles, displacing outwards the vessels adjacent to their walls.

Referred pain and muscle contraction headache

The orbits, paranasal sinuses, and teeth cause pain referred via branches of the trigeminal nerve to the forehead and temple. Sinusitis and toothache are commonplace examples, but glaucoma, orbital cellulitis, and cavernous sinus thrombosis may produce frontal pain beyond their immediate locality. Secondary involuntary contraction of scalp and facial muscles further complicate the clinical picture, causing a secondary 'tension headache' which may obscure the primary source.

Primary tension headache is psychogenic; its mechanisms are not wholly understood. Stretching of pain sensitive nerve endings within muscle fascicles and compression and traction of scalp blood vessels are considered important. Infiltration of lignocaine temporarily relieves the pain which is transmitted in the trigeminal and upper cervical nerves.

Cranial neuralgias

'Idiopathic' trigeminal and glossopharyngeal neuralgias are thought to be due to an irritative lesion of these nerves, causing strictly anatomical localization of the pain (see page 21.93). In those instances where the neuralgia results from extrinsic compression (e.g. tumour or aberrant vessels in the posterior fossa) the mechanism and quality of pain are similar. Postherpetic neuralgia is a classic example of pain secondary to an inflammatory irritative lesion, though its prolonged course is thought to be due to a 'central component' related to facilitation in the reticular formation and its input to the thalamus.

Apart from these localized cranial neuralgias, the position of headache is not a reliable indicator of its site of origin. Vascular, throbbing pain is aggravated by vasodilators, alcohol, exertion, and by coughing or straining. Typical of migraine, these factors are not specific since a vascular element operates in other lesions.

Few headaches fail to evoke some anxiety, which can distort and magnify the clinical features as well as complicating problems of management. Table 1 shows the more common causes of headache at different ages.

Migraine

Definition

Classic migraine

This is a paroxysmal disorder with headaches, often unilateral at the onset, associated with nausea, anorexia, and often vomiting; it

Table 1 Common causes of headache at different ages

Children	Adults (18–65 yrs)	Elderly 65
Migraine	Tension	Persisting
Psychogenic/fatigue	Migraine	
Post-traumatic	Cluster headache	Cranial arteritis
	Post-traumatic	Glaucoma
	Tumours	Tumour
	Subdural haematoma	Paget's disease
	Referred from cervical spine	Referred from cervical spine
	Paget's disease of skull	
	Glaucoma	

is preceded or accompanied by visual, sensory, motor or mood disturbances and is often familial.

Common migraine

This refers to similar paroxysmal headaches without the aura. Both types of attack may occur at various times in the same patient, and it is common for migraine sufferers to have tension headaches between their migraines: these should be identified to prevent misdirected treatment.

Prevalence

Migraine is common, affecting approximately 20 per cent of women and 15 per cent of men at some time in their lives. However, many attacks are not incapacitating, and half the sufferers may never seek medical attention. It is thus disproportionately overreported in the anxiety-prone and health-conscious.

Clinical features

The earliest attacks are before the age of 10 years in a third of patients. These may be missed if the child is unable to describe clearly headaches and strange visual and sensory experiences; or may be concealed by labels of 'bilious attacks', 'periodic syndrome' or 'acidosis'. Affected children may simply appear pale, ill, limp, and inert, complaining of ill-localized abdominal pain. Headache is usually present, vomiting is common, and there may be a fever of up to 38.5 °C. Mesenteric adenitis and appendicitis are important considerations, though a past history of self-limiting episodes is a helpful pointer to *abdominal migraine*. Over 80 per cent of migraineurs have their first attacks before the age of 30 years, and the diagnosis should be viewed with suspicion in anyone over 40 years. Some subjects have only a few attacks in a lifetime; most have several attacks each year. Promises of remission at the menopause are often ill-founded, though attacks tend to lessen after the age of 50 years, when headache may disappear leaving attacks of aura alone. Remission occurs in 70 per cent of pregnancies; exacerbation or complicated migraine with infarction may follow the use of oral contraceptives.

Prodrome

For several hours before an attack some patients describe tiredness, unexplained depression or elation. Yawning, craving for food or sugar may similarly forewarn of a headache the next day. These cerebral symptoms are a clue to the essentially neural origin of the attack.

Aura

Warning symptoms are most commonly visual. Flashing zig-zag lights (teichopsiae), complex figures, fragmentation like a jig-saw puzzle or homonymous hemianopia or scotomata are common. Shimmering 'heat-haze' or 'looking through frosted glass or water' are often observed. These symptoms spread slowly across the visual fields, often from centre to periphery, disappearing in 20 to 40 min. Sensory symptoms include characteristic tingling and numbness round the lips, or pins and needles in one or both hands spreading slowly over minutes to the arm, face, and rarely the leg. Bilateral teichopsiae and tingling with dysarthria and vertigo characterize *basilar artery migraine*. Hemiparesis and dysphasia are less common but provoke the fear of a stroke, especially when newly experienced. Resolution within 20 to 40 min is the rule. Headaches, typically contralateral, and vomiting follow or overlap these focal symptoms. The aura is reflected in oligaemia shown in regional cerebral blood flow, but the pattern and spread of oligaemia does not conform to territories of major cerebral vessels. A neural initiation with depression of cortical neuronal function is probably responsible for a secondary oligaemia of the microcirculation.

Headache

This is almost invariable. It can be sited anywhere in the head, but is most commonly located in the temple or forehead. Character-

Table 2 Common migraine precipitants

Anxiety
Relaxation after stress
Exercise (esp. football)
Change in sleep pattern
Bright lights
Fasting (missing a meal)
Alcohol
Specific food intolerance
Oral contraceptives
Menstruation

istically unilateral at the onset, it may spread to the whole cranium and neck. Some 30–40 per cent of patients have generalized headache. The side may vary from one attack to the next, but pain felt on the same side in all attacks rarely signifies sinister pathology. The pain is throbbing, aching or pounding, but tightness, heaviness, and pressure more typical of tension headache may be the main complaint. Headache is worsened by exertion, jarring, light (photophobia), and noise (phonophobia), and is eased by quiet, darkness, and sleep. Migraine headache builds up in an hour or two to its crescendo which may be very severe and prostrating. Rarely it may be so abrupt in onset as to simulate subarachnoid bleeding or meningitis. Headache usually lasts 12 to 48 hours, but is briefer in children.

Accompanying symptoms

Nausea and anorexia are the most commonly associated symptoms and over half the victims will vomit in most attacks. Distaste for food, light and noise, and worsening by exertion are frequent. Rest lessens the pain, and sleep – uncommon in other acute painful maladies – forms an integral part of the attack, heralding recovery. Changed perceptions of shape, size, and distortions of vision are features of *complicated migraine* resulting from dysfunction of the parietal and occipital lobes. Similarly, hemiplegia or hemisensory symptoms outlasting the headache (as opposed to the brief symptoms seen in the aura phase) are features of *hemiplegic migraine*. Hemiparesis, hemianopia, and dysphasia occasionally persist for hours or days, with pleocytosis and raised protein in the CSF and may be accompanied by low-density infarcts on CT. Permanent clinical sequelae are exceptional but are predisposed to by use of oral contraceptives and by hypertension.

Treatment

Assessment of the patient's habits, work, personality, and stresses is important. Known precipitants should be elicited, if necessary with the aid of a diary and should when possible be eliminated (Table 2). The recognition of stressful patterns and the patient's acceptance of an essentially benign disorder will achieve some benefit. Good rapport enhances reassurance and also facilitates the marked placebo effect of all therapy, often confounding objective analysis of drug trials.

Symptomatic treatment

This is offered for individual attacks (Table 3). Rest, dark, and quiet, where practicable are supplemented by simple analgesics – paracetamol 1 g, or aspirin 0.6 g. The addition of caffeine and spasmolytics add to expense but not to benefit. Codeine 15–30 mg may enhance pain relief. Analgesics should be taken as soon as the attack begins and should be repeated four to six hourly as needed. Absorption is improved by taking aspirin or paracetamol with, or 10 min after, metoclopramide 10 mg or domperidone 10–20 mg. These drugs are useful both in relieving gastric stasis and as antiemetics. If vomiting is severe, suppositories of prochlorperazine or chlorpromazine are valuable. Ergotamine is effective in 50 per cent of cases, but is badly absorbed orally and should be given by suppository (Cafergot) or by inhalation (Medihaler Ergotamine

Table 3 Treatment of migraine

Avoid	Prophylactic*	Symptomatic

Physical factors
  Bright light
  Fasting
  Fatigue
  Irregular sleep
Dietary
  Individual precipitants
  ?Tyramine (e.g cheese)
  ?Phenylethylamine
    (e.g. chocolate)
  Alcohol
  Sodium nitrate
  Monosodium
    glutamate
	Cyproheptadine,
	  pizotifen,
	  propranolol,
	  methysergide,
	  ?nifedipine/
	  nimodipine
		Oral
		  Aspirin or
		  paracetamol with
		  metaclopramide
		Rectal
		  Suppository
		  ergotamine,
		  Suppository
		  chlorpromazine
		Inhalation
		  'Medihaler'
		  ergotamine
		Intramuscular†
		  Codeine,
		  chlorpromazine or
		  prochlorperazine

* If migraine frequency is greater than twice a month.

† Very rarely needed.

0.36 mg/puff). If a single dose does not work, it should not be repeated. Ergotamine has no place as a prophylactic and when overused leads to habituation with Ergot-induced headache. This can be confused with migraine status; if suspected, total withdrawal is necessary.

Such symptomatic measures abort or improve most attacks; demands for strong analgesics should be resisted.

Prophylaxis

Prophylaxis should be attempted if attacks occur more often than twice each month. Acupuncture, hypnosis, and biofeedback techniques are successful in certain subjects, but claims for their general application should be viewed with scepticism. Many drugs are used to reduce the frequency, but none is a panacea. In patients with exacerbation clearly related to stress or anxiety, Amitriptyline 50–100 mg *nocte* introduced gradually is often effective. Which of its actions – sedative, antidepressant, and calcium channel blockade – is implicated is not known. Benzodiazepines are useful in short courses of 4–8 weeks. Propranolol, atenolol, and metoprolol give adequate reduction in about 60 per cent of cases, and are most helpful in the hypertensive subject with tachycardia or in those with overt physical signs of autonomic 'overdrive'. Their action is presumably central.

Serotonin inhibitors are valuable in 60–70 per cent of patients. Cyproheptadine 4 mg t.d.s. produces calcium channel blockade as well as serotonin inhibitory action. Pizotifen 0.5 mg t.d.s. or 1.5 mg *nocte* is moderately effective and free of hazards other than weight gain. Methysergide 1–2 mg t.d.s. is the most potent of this group but should be used only under hospital supervision in courses not exceeding 3–4 months. Pleural, pericardial, and retroperitoneal fibrosis are rare but serious side effects which may result from more prolonged use; they usually regress when the drug is stopped. Calcium antagonists (Nifedipine; Nimodipine*) have been established as prophylactics in recent trials.

Migraine occurring exclusively with menstruation is uncommon, but worsening before or during menstruation is common and usually resistant to diuretics and hormonal manipulation, though occasional benefit follows oestrogen implants.

Aetiology

The phasic pattern and diversity of precipitating (Table 2) agents support the notion of a cerebral rather than a primary vascular disorder. Genetic factors operate in 70 per cent of patients but there is no simple Mendelian pattern. Distended scalp arteries with increased pulsation and the release of vasoactive pain producing

*Marketed in the United States.

peptides are related to the pain. Cerebral symptoms of the aura may be caused by depression of neuronal activity with secondary regional oligaemia. Food idiosyncrasies, rarely allergies, specific dietary amines (e.g. tyramine) and omission of food are precipitants but not causes. Remissions in 70 per cent of pregnancies and aggravation by oral contraceptives tell of the ill-understood but important role of hormonal factors. Worsening by emotional stress and fatigue is commonplace but not causal. Biochemical anomalies of serotonin, platelet function, prostaglandins, and diverse peptides have been reported, but provide no general explanation for migraine. It appears to be a non-specific symptom complex based on a variable cerebral threshold: individual attacks being determined by a variety of external and endogenous trigger factors.

Cluster headache

(Synonyms: migrainous neuralgia, Harris's syndrome, Horton's syndrome.)

This is a distinctive clinical syndrome separable from migraine, which predominantly affects men. It begins at any age, most often 20 to 50 years, and is manifest as daily bouts of unilateral headache of great severity lasting 30–120 min. The brevity, severity, lack of aura, and vomiting occurring daily in clusters lasting usually for 4–16 weeks clearly separate it from migraine. The pain is boring, aching or stabbing and is centred on one orbit with radiation to the forehead, temple or cheek and jaws ('lower-half headache'). It characteristically strikes at night, an hour or so after sleep, and may recur during the day, often at the same time ('alarm-clock headache').

In many cases the ipsilateral eye becomes red and bloodshot, watering profusely. The nostril may be blocked or run. A transient Horner's syndrome is seen in 25 per cent of cases and occasionally this persists. Restlessness betrays the frightening severity of the pain, and in contrast to migraine most patients get out of bed and pace the floor, even taking nocturnal walks. Alcohol and other vasodilators are important precipitating factors; nitroglycerine has been used as a provocative test – a typical attack following within an hour of a sublingual tablet. Clusters last for one to four months though occasionally the condition continues for a year or more – *chronic migrainous neuralgia*. Remissions are complete but the clusters usually recur every year or two.

The aetiology is unknown, and elevated blood histamine levels during attacks are of uncertain significance. Autonomic involvement is shown by the Horner's syndrome, and segmental mural oedema of the carotid syphon has been shown at angiography.

Investigation is not necessary, nor is cluster headache in typical form symptomatic of other cranial lesions. The quality, timing, duration, and distribution of pain separate it from trigeminal neuralgia, migraine, and other cephalgias. It is surprisingly uncommon for a patient to have both migraine and cluster headache, but these patients have an unexplained high incidence of peptic ulcer.

The essence of treatment is prevention. During clusters Ergotamine is given one hour in *anticipation* of daytime attacks, and just before getting into bed for nocturnal attacks. Suppositories are the most useful preparation. Control is excellent in most patients and the drug is stopped each Sunday to see if the cluster re-emerges; if so, Ergotamine is continued for a further week, until the cluster ends. If ergot is unsuccessful Methysergide 1–2 mg t.d.s. is a useful alternative. Pizotifen is less effective, and lithium can be used in the chronic variant if other methods fail. In intractable cases, oxygen and steroids meet with occasional dramatic results.

Tension headache

(Synonym: muscle contraction headache.)

Tension headache is the most common human complaint causing a patient to consult a doctor. It constitutes 70 per cent of referrals to a 'Headache Clinic' and in random samples of healthy subjects over 90 per cent volunteer one or more previous attacks of recognizable tension headache. In most instances it is a short-lived complaint with obvious preceding cause: overwork, lack of sleep or an emotional crisis. This is entirely benign and is recognized by patients as 'normal headaches'. Rarely it can present in *acute form* as an emergency; the headache has usually built up over a few hours, but has become very severe. The patient looks ill, anxious and pallid with tachycardia and may simulate subarachnoid bleeding, especially if photophobic with a stiff neck. There are no other signs, the victim is afebrile, but lumbar puncture is occasionally necessary to exclude meningeal irritation by blood or infection. More often the emotional basis is obvious and recovery ensues quickly with reassurance, analgesia, and a brief period of sedation.

Chronic tension headache

The chronic is very much more common than the acute syndrome. Chronic tension headache is encountered widely by physicians in almost all branches of clinical practice. The pain is usually diffusely felt all over the head. It is, however, often located on the vertex, or may start in the forehead or in the neck. Some patients describe several points of pain which they describe with a single finger, usually in both parietal regions or over the crown. It may radiate over the glabella on to the bridge of the nose, or from the temples into the jaws. It is commonly felt bilaterally, but there are cases where the pain is apparently localized to one side. In all other respects of its description, however, it resembles the more classic diffuse or vertex pain; the unilaterality has no obvious explanation.

The quality of the pain is highly characteristic. It is experienced as a sense of pressure, a feeling of tightness or as if a heavy weight were pressing down on the crown. 'A tight band like a skullcap' or 'as if a clamp or vice was squeezing my head' are common descriptions. Some are at pains to relate 'it is not really a pain, but a pressure'. The symptoms may also seem to derive from inside the cranium as witnessed by the descriptions 'as if my head is bursting' or 'about to explode'. A 'creepy' sensation (formication) may be felt under the scalp, or a sense of sharp knives or needles driven in, burning hot, may be related by other patients.

Tension headache of this sort is a daily occurrence, in contrast to the periodic and paroxysmal attacks of migraine. It is worse as the day goes by, whereas migraine is commonly present on waking. Visual disturbance and vomiting do not occur, though nausea may accompany the pain.

Most patients continue to carry on their normal work with tension headache, and photophobia and confinement to bed in a darkened room – so common in migraine – are not features of this syndrome. Symptoms continue for months or years without evident deterioration of general health. They are worse when the victim is tired or under pressure at work, and they are more troublesome in the face of personal or domestic stresses. Most sufferers have insight into these relationships so that a carefully taken history usually clarifies both the diagnosis and the relevant aggravating circumstances.

Clinical examination may appear to be superfluous in the face of such distinctive symptoms, but it is of great importance. Most such patients are frightened, emotional and anxious. They harbour fears of brain tumours, or hypertension and of 'clots in the brain'. A thorough examination including a full neurological assessment is of the utmost therapeutic value as well as providing a rational basis for effective reassurance. It is my practice to enquire specifically about fears of serious brain disease, whether the fears are voiced by the patient or not. 'Television illnesses' are not infrequently 'contagious', as are those suffered by relatives and acquaintances; these too need careful appraisal.

Treatment is most effective when the history is short; to cure such headaches after ten or more years is a daunting and often unsuccessful task. The main step is to try hard to ascertain the events which determined the onset. These are often forgotten, or perhaps suppressed, yet repeated enquiry at subsequent consultations will often unravel the apparent mystery, the consequent knowledge being sufficient to explain the cause to the patient. No amount of superficial reassurance will eradicate tension headache if its origins are obscure and the complex psychological mechanisms deriving from the source are untreated. Similarly, sedatives, tranquillisers and tension-relieving drugs will be of limited value unless the psychological aberration is adequately handled*. When the history is short and if a cause is exposed drugs are unnecessary if reassurance is adequate. In the common situation where daily pain has persisted for years, the prognosis is less predictable, but short courses of benzodiazepines for four to eight weeks or amitryptilene may be helpful and will secure the occasional 'cure'.

Latent depression presenting as tension headache is easy to overlook. Early morning insomnia, negativism, guilt, and diurnal mood swings are suggestive. The headache is worse in the morning (resembling that of raised pressure), and a cause for the misery is often inapparent. Full doses of tricyclic antidepressants, if necessary administered on an inpatient basis are needed. When beginning in the fifties or sixties in a patient free of previous psychiatric morbidity, the outlook is excellent.

Headaches as a symptom of intracranial disease

Confronted by a patient with headaches, the major clinical decision is to exclude a structural or dynamic cause. Although any expanding mass can cause cranial pain (page 21.175) the mechanisms of raised intracranial pressure and traction/displacement of cranial structures produce similar pain. Its location is non-specific, but it is: (*a*) worse in the morning; (*b*) aggravated by sitting up or standing and relieved by lying down; (*c*) aggravated by coughing, straining, and vomiting; (*d*) relieved by aspirin or paracetamol in the early stages (in contrast to psychogenic headache); (*e*) associated with vomiting and eventually by papilloedema and progressing focal signs. By the stage of stupor and hemiplegia with a dilated pupil, diagnosis has been delayed too long.

Headaches caused by *acute meningeal irritation* result from subarachnoid haemorrhage, pyogenic or viral meningitis, trauma or rarely migraine. An abrupt onset, fever, neck stiffness, and Kernig's sign accompany the obvious severe pain, vomiting, and photophobia. CSF examination is mandatory if infection is considered, provided that an abscess mass or haematoma have been first excluded by clinical assessment and computerized tomography.

Atypical facial pain

This label conceals a number of cases with chronic faceache whose cause we do not understand. One major group present a characteristic and clinically recognizable pattern. This is a group of patients, mostly women aged 30 to 50 years with a dull constant aching pain in one, or both cheeks. It has no trigger factors, but is worse with fatigue and under mental duress. It is continuous, though often sparing sleep, and may radiate into the ear, forehead, and jaw. There are no physical signs, and often there is no overt evidence of depression. Occasionally the onset can be related to some grave personal hurt or Freudian 'slap in the face'. With reassurance and a prolonged course of tricyclics or MAOI drugs many patients obtain lasting relief.

Temporo-mandibular pain

Although patients with rheumatoid and osteoarthritic changes on radiographs of their temporo-mandibular (T-M) joints seldom have pain, myofascial pain dysfunction is a common cause of complaint in young adults. Modern views of overclosure of the joint or malocclusion tend to discount these mechanisms, but favour a 'neuromuscular dysfunction causing spasm and fatigue' of masticatory muscles. The syndrome is of aching pain in front of the ear, worse with jaw opening and accompanied by clicks and clunks –

*Taken from Pearce (1985) *The neurobiology of pain*, pp. 13–15. Manchester University Press, Manchester.

signs not uncommon in asymptomatic people. The quality and relation of pain to chewing and jaw opening distinguish it from trigeminal neuralgia (page 21.93); radiographs exclude sinus disease and neoplasm. Anxiety and latent depression are important factors, but despite extensive investigation, treatment is based on reassurance and symptomatic non-invasive analgesia. After a decade of study, one expert's view is 'the best therapy . . . in most cases appears to be the least.' Nonetheless, correction of any gross disorder of dental bite is worthwhile, and a trial injection of lignocaine 2 per cent into the joint will afford striking relief in some patients. A trial of amitryptilene can also provide substantial benefit in some sufferers.

Headache in the elderly

In addition to the causes of headache already discussed, certain syndromes feature more prominently in the middle aged and elderly, although age is not a diagnostic barrier. Masked depression is a common cause of somewhat atypical 'psychogenic headache'. Physical signs are absent, investigations are unrewarding, and suitable antidepressant treatment will sometimes reverse the symptoms.

Cervicogenic headache

Cervicogenic headache refers to head pain referred from cervical spondylosis. It is undoubtedly common, with pain on one or both sides of the neck radiating to the occiput, but also to the temples and frontal region. It may be a dull 'toothache' pain, worse in the morning when the neck has been badly positioned at an angle on a misplaced high pillow during sleep. It may last throughout the day and be aggravated by neck movement. It is a rather non-descript pain, with no accompanying vomiting and no physical signs other than marked restriction of lateral flexion and rotation of the neck. Such signs are common, however, in those without headache, and thus are of limited value. Vague and intermittent symptoms of tinnitus, dizziness, and visual disturbance are sometimes attributed to compression of the vertebral arteries traversing the foramina transversaria, but in most instances this is unproven speculation. It is probable that the symptoms arise from the posterior zygapophyseal joints and related ligaments as the result of osteophytes; irritation of the C_2 nerve root or of the greater occipital nerves are important contributory factors which may respond well to local injection of lignocaine and hydrocortisone. Immobilization in a collar is an alternative empirical treatment, often used but of unconvincing efficacy in the majority. Manipulation endangers the vertebral arteries and is contraindicated.

Giant cell arteritis

(Synonyms: cranial, temporal.)

This condition, dealt with in Section 16 is important neurologically as an eminently treatable cause of headache in the over 60s; but also as a preventable cause of blindness and strokes. Headache is generalized or may be sited over an engorged, reddened tender superficial temporal, or, occipital artery. It is aching, throbbing or felt as sharp stabs of pain, often worse at night. The history is usually short, i.e. of a few weeks duration; the patient is unwell with muscle aches and pains in the shoulders and pelvic girdle muscles (polymyalgia rheumatica) and there may be fever, sweats, and masseter claudication. Visual involvement is due to an ischaemic optic neuropathy which presents with unilateral blindness or with a branch retinal occlusion. It is irreversible. Ophthalmoplegia is due to ischaemic lesions in the third, fourth or sixth cranial nerves, and either of these symptoms may be the presenting sign, before the onset of headache and malaise: hence the importance of early diagnosis. The disease also affects the vertebral arteries and less often the carotids, and may present as a stroke or transient ischaemic attack (TIA).

Every elderly subject with these manifestations should be suspected of harbouring this condition, and serial ESRs supple-

mented by an adequate biopsy of the clinically involved scalp vessel which should be serially sectioned will prove the diagnosis. Biopsy is indicated in the uncertain case with a borderline ESR of 30–50. Steroid therapy will avert blindness in almost every case, and should be started immediately the patient is seen and the ESR taken. It does not affect biopsy changes for at least 48 hours. The initial dose of 60 mg prednisolone is quickly reduced as symptoms abate and the ESR falls; a maintenance dose of 5 to 10 mg/day is usually reached within a month or two and is governed by clinical progress and ESR measurements. Late relapses are common and treatment is continued for many years with very gradual reductions by 1 mg per month only when the patient and the ESR have been normal for over three years. In many subjects, small doses are necessary for life, as indicated by relapse when attempts are made to reduce the dose of prednisolone.

Atypical presentations which should prompt assiduous investigation include: (a) patients with minimal headache; (b) an initially normal ESR; (c) fever of unknown origin; (d) psychiatric symptoms of hallucinations, depression, and 'confusional states.'

Post-traumatic headache (see also page 21.189)

Headache following injury is a common complaint. In most circumstances a knock on the head will cause local bruising and abrasions no different from those resulting from a kick on the shin; local pain subsides in a few days without sequelae. The emotional vulnerability of the head and the common recourse to medicolegal compensation complicate both symptoms and mechanisms. Many victims of *severe* head injury, with post-traumatic amnesia of 24 hours or more wake up with no headache. Similarly, the headache of patients after major craniotomy seldom lasts more than 3 to 7 days. The commonest complaints are heard from those with minor injury, often without loss of consciousness. Minor head injuries are those with: (1) loss of consciousness less than 20 min; (2) Glasgow coma scale (GCS) 13–18 (see page 21.46); (3) stay in hospital less than 48 hours.

The crucial importance of strict definition is emphasized by the vague and often subjective complaints of plaintiffs. Their genuine nature has been supported by claims of cognitive deficits present in even the mildly injured with brief unconsciousness and Post-Traumatic Amnesia (PTA). In contrast, there is clear evidence that the majority of such cases leave hospital within a few days, have no organic signs, recover quickly, and return to work without further complaints. This is particularly true of those suffering injury during contact sports, many victims continuing the game, or returning to normal activities the next day without ill effect.

Assessment of symptoms and disability

The main concern of physicians is the assessment of the significance of symptoms and disability (Table 4). Headaches persist without accompanying neurological signs, but often with a collection of intrinsically subjective symptoms often referred to as the *Post-traumatic syndrome*. The commonest are: forgetfulness, irritability, slowness, poor concentration, fatigue, dizziness (usually not vertigo), somnolence, intolerance of light and noise, loss of initiative, depression, anxiety, loss of interests, and impaired libido. The number of complaints is not related to the severity of the injury (see also page 21.189).

Table 4 Symptoms and disability following head injury

1 Initial pain, suffering, loss of work
2 Estimate of severity: hospital attendance and treatment
3 Persisting organic symptoms
4 Persisting psychological symptoms
5 Disability related to (a) Work prospects and capability
　　　　　　　　　　　(b) Domestic activities
　　　　　　　　　　　(c) Quality of life
　　　　　　　　　　　(d) Loss of earnings

The failure of doctors to provide complete reassurance shortly after injury is important in determining patients' fears of brain damage or subdural haematoma; it may also delay return to work and induce morbid anxiety. Headaches are either localized to the site of trauma, often with local scalp tenderness, or like tension headaches are diffuse, aching or tight and heavy. They are often resistant to analgesics and investigations in these patients are unwarranted and unrevealing. Anxieties, phobias, loss of self esteem, resentment, and depression are genuine accompanying features in some cases, and serve to induce or to aggravate headache. Deliberate exaggeration or malingering are present in other cases with the aim of financial gain. In litigants there is great pressure from Union officials and legal advisers, which together with the common delay in legal settlement contrive to prolong and exaggerate the symptoms. Headaches generally improve when the patient returns to normal work, and often though not invariably disappear when satisfactory settlement is attained.

References

Cawson, R. A. (1984). Pain in the temporomandibular joint. *Br. Med. J.* **2**, 1857–1858.

Dalessio, D. J. (ed.) (1980). *Wolff's headache and other head pains*, 4th edn. Oxford University Press, Oxford.

Hall, S., Lie, J. T., Kurland, L. T. *et al.* (1983). The therapeutic impact of temporal artery biopsy. *Lancet* **2**, 1217–1220.

Lance J. W. (1982). *Mechanism and management of headache*, 4th edn. Butterworths, London.

Lascelles, R. G. (1966). Atypical facial pain and depression. *Br. J. Psychiat.* **112**, 651–659.

Merskey, H. (1982). Pain and emotion: their correlation in headache. *Advances in Neurology*, Vol. 33 (ed. M. Critchley), pp. 135–143. Raven Press, New York.

Pearce, J. M. S. (1975). *Modern topics in migraine*. William Heinemann, London.

—— (1984). Migraine: a cerebral disorder. *Lancet* **2**, 86–89.

Sacks, O. (1970). *Migraine, evolution of a common disorder*. Faber and Faber, London.

DISTURBANCES OF HIGHER CEREBRAL FUNCTION

J. OXBURY AND MARIA A. WYKE

The pathology underlying disturbances of higher cerebral function may be diffuse, as in Alzheimer's disease, or focal as in cerebral infarction and small tumours. Diffuse pathology produces *dementia* with a global impairment of intellect, personality, and memory. The personality change may lead to, for instance, social withdrawal, slovenliness, alcohol abuse, sexual aberration, and ultimately to gross personal neglect and wandering. The associated mood change may be apathy, depression, or euphoria. There may be fear and anxiety, particularly when insight is retained. Forgetfulness is especially common, and indeed a diagnosis of dementia should be questioned if memory function is normal. Disorders of cognition appear as any combination of those described below.

Focal pathology produces more restricted cognitive impairment. The nature of the impairment depends upon the situation of the pathology in the brain. Often there is no change of personality or loss of memory. However, the pathology responsible for a focal disturbance sometimes produces generalized secondary effects as well. For instance, focal tumours can grow to such a size that the intracranial pressure is raised and blood vessels remote from the tumour are distorted. The result is that generalized effects are superimposed on an initially specific disturbance of higher cerebral function, and if consciousness is well preserved, the mental picture may be mistaken for a general dementia.

Localization of cognitive function

The concept that higher mental functions (e.g. language, auditory and visual perception, control of voluntary movement) are subserved by specific areas of the brain has a long and contentious history. The notion of localization began with Franz Gall (1758–1828), founder of phrenology, and grew in stature with contributions from many subsequent workers. The pioneers of the concept tended to overlook facts, both anatomical and clinical, which did not fit with their theories, but their work was of great importance in the development of neuropsychology.

The 19th century also witnessed strong criticisms developed in opposition to localization theories. These were voiced particularly by Hughlings Jackson, Henry Head – who branded the localizationists with the contemptuous title of 'Diagram Makers' – and Kurt Goldstein. During the early part of the 20th century antilocalizationist views also developed from animal experimentation, particularly that of Lashley who proposed the principle of 'Mass Action', i.e. the generalization that areas of cortex function as a whole during learning; he added that the most important factor in disrupting learning after a cortical lesion was the extent of the destruction, not its locus.

Recent research on the breakdown of cognitive function in patients with focal cerebral pathology has swung the pendulum back towards a localizationist view and there is now extensive evidence against the concepts of unification of the mind or notions that different regions of the brain are equipotential for the control of cognitive function. The introduction of radiological imaging techniques, especially computerized tomography, has been a particularly important stimulus to the increased attention to issues of localization in neuropsychology during the last decade. A special emphasis in this research has been to explore the differential function of the left and right hemispheres, demonstrating asymmetries. This is in addition to the time honoured separation of function in parallel with anatomical division of the brain into lobes (frontal, temporal, parietal, occipital). These anatomical divisions are somewhat arbitrary, but a simplified list of the major cognitive deficits that traditionally have been associated with the different regions of the brain (Table 1) may be helpful to the student as an introduction to the field of clinical neuropsychology.

Cerebral dominance and the asymmetry of cerebral function

First Dax and then Broca, both in the middle of the 19th century, noted the relationship between aphasia, right hemiplegia, and left hemisphere pathology. These observations led to the concept of cerebral dominance which in its original form implied that the anatomical bases of language are vested exclusively in one 'major' cerebral hemisphere – usually the left. It has subsequently become clear that the 'minor' hemisphere – usually the right – also has some capacity to subserve language function. Furthermore, it has also become clear that the hemisphere which is 'minor' for language may be 'major' for other non-linguistic abilities such as visuospatial perception. Some cognitive functions seem to be particularly affected by damage to the left hemisphere and others by damage on the right; some seem equally affected by damage to *either* side, and yet others seem to be only markedly affected when there is damage to both sides. Table 1 gives a simplified scheme. There is a complex relationship between cognitive function, laterality of damage, and handedness. Furthermore, a particular skill, for instance the ability to construct three-dimensional models,

Table 1 Relationship between behavioural impairment and site of brain pathology

Lobe	Behaviour effected or syndrome	Main hemisphere involved			
		Left	Right	Left = Right	Bilateral
Frontal	Language–aphasia, verbal fluency ↓	+			
	Speech–dysarthria			+	
	Memory for recency impaired			+	
	Movement control ↓			+	
	Planning ability ↓			+ <	+ +
	Disinhibition–social and motor			+ <	+ +
Temporal	Memory–verbal aspects ↓	+			
	Non-verbal aspects ↓		+		
	Severe amnesia				+
	Music perception ↓		+		
	Language comprehension ↓	+			
	Kluver–Bucy syndrome				+
	Aggression, rage, depression	+			
	Indifference, euphoria		+		
Parietal and occipital	Primary visual/tactile sensation ↓			+	
	Visual discrimination ↓		+		
	Gaze deviation		+		
	Gaze apraxia				+
	Visual disorientation				+
	Visual agnosia				+
	Prosopagnosia				+
	Hemi-neglect–visuospatial and body		+		
	Topographical disorientation – Major				+
	Minor		+		
	Dressing apraxia		+		
	Constructional apraxia			+	
	Ideomotor apraxia	+			
	Acalculia – Spatial		+		
	Anarithmia	+			
	Finger agnosia	+			
	Right–left disorientation	+			
	Alexia and agraphia	+			

may be affected in different ways according to the laterality of the brain damage; similarly it may be affected by damage situated diffusely, more or less regardless of location, in one hemisphere, whereas it is only affected by damage at a particular locus in the other hemisphere.

The recent keen interest in establishing differential specialization of the two hemispheres is largely due to the development of techniques which permit a behavioural analysis of the two halves of the brain independently in normal individuals. Previously, the only way to obtain information about the dual functional asymmetry of the human brain had been experimental investigations of patients with unilateral brain damage. Much of the new evidence of cerebral specialization in normal individuals has been derived from the use of three main techniques; comparing differences in performance between the right and left side of the visual field (tachistoscopic studies); analysis of responses to stimuli presented to the left and right ear (dichotic listening studies); and assessing the performance of voluntary movements with the left and right arm. As a result, the concept of left cerebral dominance has been abandoned, to be replaced by one of complementary specialization with the left mostly subserving language functions and the right mostly organizing visuospatial abilities.

Aphasia

Aphasia is a defect of language function due to brain damage. It is usually manifest in all four language 'modalities' – speech production, speech comprehension, reading, and writing. Aphasia must be distinguished from motor disturbances of voice production such as *dysarthria** and *stuttering†*, from poverty of speech due to intellectual impairment, from language abnormalities as in schizophre-

nia, and from hysterical mutism. A distinction between the terms 'aphasia' and 'dysphasia' is not useful – the former will be used throughout.

Laterality of language representation

More than 90 per cent of normal right-handed people have language represented on the left in the sense that left hemisphere damage could make them overtly aphasic but right-sided damage would not do so. Nevertheless, it seems that the right hemisphere of such a person does have some capacity for language. The evidence is derived from a number of sources. Firstly, some degree of language expression and comprehension may return, as may a rudimentary ability to read and write, after complete left hemispherectomy which has occasionally been carried out in adult life as a treatment for tumour. Secondly, sodium amytal injected into one internal carotid artery, and on a subsequent occasion into the other (the Wada test), may produce aphasic responses from both injections even though the amytal is delivered only unilaterally.

* *Dysarthria* is a disorder of speech production arising from dysfunction of the muscles of articulation. The dysfunction can be secondary to damage in the system at any point from the cerebral cortex (and then the dysarthria may be associated with aphasia) to the muscles themselves. The precise quality of the dysarthria depends on the site of the pathology and various forms are recognized, e.g. spastic dysarthria, ataxic dysarthria.
† *Stuttering (stammering)* is an abnormality of speech production characterized by hesitancy and repetitions of speech sounds such that the next expected sound is delayed or not produced. The disruption of the proper sequence of activity in the muscles responsible for articulation may be accompanied by grimaces and other tic-like movements of the head, neck, and limbs. The condition may have a psychogenic basis, it is sometimes considered to be associated with incomplete language dominance, and it very occasionally occurs (usually transiently) in association with aphasia.

Thirdly, electrical stimulation of the right cerebral hemisphere in a conscious subject may produce or inhibit vocalization, or may cause distortion of words and vowels. Fourthly, the most important source of information regarding the role of the non-dominant cerebral hemisphere in language function has emerged from the studies of patients in whom the interhemispheric connections have been severed surgically for the relief of epilepsy (Fig. 1). These individuals offer a unique opportunity to examine left and right cerebral functions independently in the same patients, for after the operation the interhemispheric transfer of complex information is abolished, so that each cerebral hemisphere is restricted to using information gained through its primary pathways (Fig. 2). For instance, if the patient's eyes are closed, an object which is actively explored by the left hand cannot be recognized by the right and vice versa. Similarly, if these patients are shown printed words for a short time in the left visual half field (thereby restricting the visual input to the non-dominant hemisphere) they can identify, by touching with their left hand, objects corresponding to the words presented, although they cannot as a rule describe them in speech or writing. Until recently the scope of investigation carried out in patients with commissurotomies has been restricted by the method of testing (i.e. tachistoscopic presentation of stimuli lasting less than 100 ms). However, a novel technique of presentation has now been introduced allowing long exposures of the stimuli and free ocular scanning. With this method virtually any type of test may be used enabling quantitative comparisons between the two hemispheres in the same patient.

The studies in the split brain patients have largely confirmed the functional asymmetries of the left and right hemisphere and also the findings which indicate that the right hemisphere does exhibit some degree of linguistic capacity. Recent work has indicated that the vocabulary of the right hemisphere corresponds approximately to that of a child aged 11–12 years, but the question of whether the

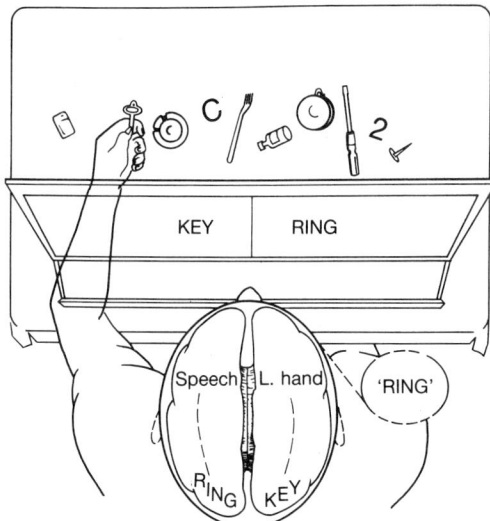

Fig. 2 Sample split-brain responses: Subject reports (through speaking hemisphere) having seen only the visual stimulus flashed to right half of screen and denies having seen left-field stimulus or recognizing objects presented to left hand. At the same time, left hand correctly retrieves objects named left field for which subject verbally denies having any knowledge. When asked to name object selected by left hand, speaking hemisphere refers it to stimulus shown in right field. (Based on Sperry, 1974, Lateral specialization in the surgically separated hemispheres. In *Neurosciences 3rd Study Program* (eds F. O. Schmitt and F. G. Warden). MIT Press, Cambridge, Mass.)

right hemisphere possesses some latent ability for verbal expression still remains unanswered.

Handedness, cerebral dominance, and aphasia

Early concepts of cerebral dominance held that the dominant hemisphere is contralateral to the preferred hand. This does apply to 95–98 per cent of right-handers without early childhood cerebral pathology. However, the left hemisphere is also dominant in about 70 per cent of left-handers without such cerebral pathology. About 20 per cent of the others have right hemisphere dominance, and in 10 per cent language function is more or less equally distributed between the two hemispheres (bilateral representation). The incidence of left hemisphere dominance may be considerably less than 70 per cent in left-handers who sustained early childhood left hemisphere damage, the precise figure depending upon the nature and extent of the pathology. These figures have been derived from various sources including studies of the incidence of aphasia according to handedness and laterality of brain pathology, aphasia during intracarotid amytal (Wada) testing, and language defects in the period immediately after unilateral electroconvulsive therapy.

Left-handers as a group are more likely to develop aphasia than right-handers, presumably because a greater proportion of them have bilateral language representation making them liable to the condition regardless of which hemisphere is damaged. However, the left-handers' aphasia tends to be less severe and to recover more rapidly than that of right-handers, and there is some suggestion that language function is more diffusely represented in the left-handers' brain irrespective of which hemisphere is dominant.

Localization within the left hemisphere

The areas most important for language are: the posterior part of the inferior frontal gyrus (Broca's area) situated immediately anterior to the primary motor cortical representation for the face, mouth, and tongue; the posterior part of the superior temporal gyrus (Wernicke's area); the inferior parietal lobule including the supramarginal and angular gyri; and the cortex of the frontoparietal operculum. Although these are pre-eminent, sensitive tech-

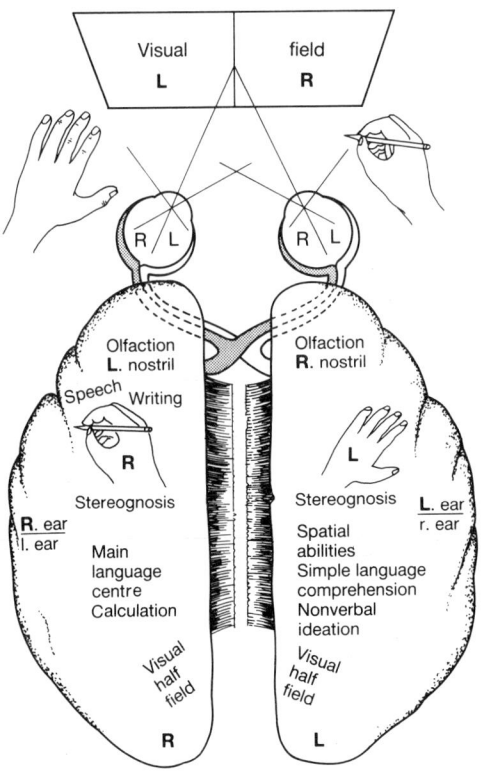

Fig. 1 Functions separated by surgery: a simplified summary combined from known neuroanatomy, cortical lesion data, and postoperative testing. (Based on Sperry, 1974, Lateral specialization in the surgically separated hemispheres. In *Neurosciences 3rd Study Program* (eds F. O. Schmitt and F. G. Warden). MIT Press, Cambridge, Mass.)

niques can often detect some linguistic abnormality after damage to other parts of the left hemisphere, including subcortical areas.

Characteristics of aphasia

Word finding difficulty is a major deficit lying at the root of aphasia and is responsible for many of the characteristic hesitancies and/or circumlocutions.

Spontaneous speech

The patient's spontaneous speech may be described as 'fluent' or 'non-fluent'.

Non-fluent aphasia, at its most severe, consists of complete loss of speech and phonation. This is nearly always associated with inability to comprehend anything but the simplest spoken language, and with complete inability to read or write. Often there is a *bucco-facial apraxia* (a defect of voluntary tongue/palatal movements and of voluntary facial movements, as in whistling or imitating actions such as laughing or blowing, even though all these movements are normal when performed automatically; in the acute phase there may also be an impairment of voluntary swallowing). With some recovery the patient may make phonated but inarticulate utterances or may develop a recurring utterance that is recognizable. The latter is a word, often 'yes' or 'no', or sometimes a phrase. It is produced indiscriminately whenever speech seems necessary; so it has no meaning nor any propositional sense for the listener. Sometimes propositional speech may break through for a brief period especially in very emotional situations. Occasionally the patient can speak only in an automatic fashion such as swearing.

When the aphasia is less severe, the speech is agrammatic. The style is telegraphic, the language being reduced to a bare minimum by the omission of all those auxiliary and relational words, especially prepositions, which normally enrich it. Nevertheless, the information content is often high and adequate meaning can often be conveyed to a patient listener despite the hesitancies and distorted articulation. Greetings and simple every day social interactions may be produced quite normally. The quality of writing is similar to that of the spoken language.

Fluent aphasia is characterized by spontaneous speech which is abnormal or even completely incomprehensible, not because it is reduced in amount or articulated badly but because it contains non-existent words, wrong words, and words arranged in an inappropriate order so that meaning is lost. Wrong words have been called *paraphasias* and various types have been described. These include:

Semantic paraphasia The substitution of a word related in meaning to the correct one (e.g. cat for dog)

Phonemic paraphasia The substitution of a word that sounds similar (e.g. tip for top)

Neologism The substitution of a non-existent word (e.g. broomstruck for broomstick).

In some classifications words containing only one or few inappropriate syllables are labelled as *literal paraphasias* if the original word is still recognizable, and the term neologism is then restricted to words that neither exist nor are recognizable. Wrong words can also be simply perseverations of previously used words or random in the sense of having no determinable relationship to the other words in the phrase or sentence. *Jargon aphasia* is the condition where words put together in the wrong order are mixed with non-existent words, and phrases and sentences with no or very little meaning are produced quite uncritically, usually with entirely normal and quick articulation. Patients with jargon aphasia may be misdiagnosed as suffering from confusion or an acute psychosis. Careful examination often reveals a right homonomous visual field defect and/or sensory diminution down the right side of the body in addition to the aphasia. *Echolalia* is a seemingly com-

pulsive repetition of words without any apparent understanding of their meaning. *Palilalia* is a similar repetition reiterated with increasing frequency. Echolalia and palilalia are usually manifestations of diffuse brain disease such as Alzheimer's disease or encephalitis.

Ability to name objects

Most aphasics have some defect of the ability to name objects, although mild aphasia may cause difficulty only with less common objects. This *anomia* is sometimes the first manifestation of aphasia. It has certain characteristics making it distinguishable from anomia due to other causes such as agnosia. Aphasic anomia is usually independent of the sensory modality through which the object to be named is perceived. Thus a bunch of keys will be equally difficult to name regardless of whether it is shown to the patient, felt tactually, or jangled so that he or she hears them but does not touch or see them. In contrast, the anomia of *visual agnosia* is restricted to objects presented visually. All but the severest aphasics can describe or mime the use of objects which they cannot name. Likewise, they usually accept the correct name when it is suggested, rejecting incorrect suggestions, and they can point to the correct object from amongst an array when its name is offered. When an aphasic offers an incorrect name, it is most frequently that of a semantically related object (e.g. table for chair, or hat for coat), or a phonetically related name (e.g. bat for cat, or band for hand). Unusual objects are more difficult to name than common ones.

Understanding speech

Impaired ability to comprehend speech is perhaps the most important functional defect in aphasia. There is little doubt that difficulty in comprehending a statement increases as a function of its linguistic complexity and its length. As with naming, confusions tend to be both semantic and phonetic. The bedside analysis of comprehension disturbances is difficult, and a common error is to overestimate the extent to which an aphasic patient can understand what is said.

Writing

Disturbances of writing – *agraphia* – can be due to a number of causes including aphasia, apraxia, and spatial disorder secondary to parietal lobe damage. Occasionally agraphia occurs in isolation but this is rare. The writing of aphasics usually contains the same linguistic abnormalities as their speech. Letters and words may be omitted. There are grammatical errors, paraphasias, and other wrong words. Misspelling is particularly common. Copying is usually least impaired, writing to dictation more so, and spontaneous writing most of all. Parietal lobe damage, either left or right, produces additional non-aphasic disturbances of writing. The calligraphic form is poor, the lines may be oblique or intersecting, there may be excessive margins and poor positioning on the page, and single letters or groups of letters may be situated in isolation. Redundant looping is common, particularly on the letters m, n, and l. These abnormalities may be due to visuospatial disturbances. With right parietal lobe damage all the writing may be situated on the right side of the page, the left being neglected.

Reading

As with writing, so abnormalities of reading are usually proportional to the aphasia. There are hesitancies, word substitutions, omissions, and impaired comprehension. The ability to read aloud is sometimes better preserved than the ability to comprehend the material, but the reverse may happen. Occasionally the *alexia* is disproportionately severe in comparison to the abnormality of speaking or comprehending speech, and rarely severe alexia exists without other manifestations of aphasia.

Non-linguistic cognitive defects

These are often associated with aphasia. They may considerably influence the aphasic's ability to compensate for the disability and

Table 2 Examination of the aphasic patient

History must be obtained in full including from a relative/friend (essential if the aphasia is more than minimal)

Spontaneous speech must be assessed in conversation if possible. Note: articulation and rhythm, hesitancies and word-finding difficulties, circumlocutions, grammatical errors, paraphasias and neologisms

Examine patient's ability to:

1 *Name objects* and note frequency/nature of errors (visual presentation as standard, but also auditory/tactile presentation if there is a possibility of agnosia). Use clearly identifiable pictures or three-dimensional objects. Request patient to use gesture/mime to establish that the object is recognized. Ask patient to point to named objects

2 *Recite series* e.g days of week/months of year, forwards and backwards – errors tend to occur especially on backwards series

3 *Generate words* by saying as many words of a defined character (e.g. beginning with C or names of towns) in a limited time e.g. one minute

4 *Repeat* sentences of varying complexity

5 *Write* sentences spontaneously and to dictation. Note spelling errors, word omissions, caligraphy

6 *Read* a prose passage. Note nature and frequency of errors

Comprehension should be assessed as far as possible (see text)

Other cognitive abilities such as visuo-spatial, praxis, and memory should be examined at least briefly

Physical examination of other aspects of neurological function (especially for visual field defect, hemiparesis, and localized sensory change) is very important because aphasia is often associated with other features of left pathology

to benefit from therapeutic endeavours, so they must be recognized.

Examination of the aphasic patient (Table 2)

A full history must be taken from the patient in so far as the aphasia allows. This provides an excellent opportunity to assess the patient's spontaneous speech, particularly if the aphasia is only mild when it may provide the only abnormalities detectable on clinical as opposed to laboratory examination. It is also essential to take a history from a relative or close friend particularly if the aphasia is more than mild.

Any previous disturbances such as stuttering or difficulty in learning to read and write should be noted. The language background must be explored. What was the patient's native language? Did he speak foreign languages? Was he a fluent talker or was he always hesitant? Was he a fluent fast reader or slow and laborious? His education and occupational background must be recorded. Even a mild aphasia cripples some, such as a barrister, whereas others do their jobs well despite quite marked aphasia. Hand preferences must be noted, remembering that some people write with the right hand but nevertheless prefer the left, or are ambidextrous, for other activities. A family history of left-handedness should be noted.

A scheme for examination is given in Table 2. Much of this consists of looking for abnormalities of the sort described in the preceding section. Comprehension is particularly difficult to assess at the bedside. Some measure can be obtained by assessing the ability to respond correctly to commands of increasing complexity. Thus, with a collection of common objects on a table, the patient may be instructed to carry out commands varying between, for instance, 'close the book' (very simple) and 'close the book, touch the cup, and give me the button' (more complex). With this sort of testing, errors only occur when the aphasia is moderate or severe, and even then they may be due to other factors such as apraxia and memory disorder. A standard test such as the Token Test should be used for milder cases. Here chips of two different shapes (square and circle), two different sizes (large and small), and five different colours are placed before the patient who is given a series of 36 questions which progressively increase in complexity, e.g. 'pick up the yellow square' (simple), 'together with the yellow circle, take the blue circle' (complex). Performance is not much affected by mild generalized intellectual deterioration. A quantitative score is obtained (number of correct responses) and the test can be repeated at intervals to assess improvement or deterioration.

Classification and localization of aphasic syndromes

Classification and localization studies have been closely linked to each other in that categories of language disability must be defined with some precision if their production is to be related to disturbances of specific anatomical structures within the brain. According to current ideas, a rigid doctrine of precisely localized cerebral lesions giving rise to pure forms of aphasia is untenable. Nevertheless, it is generally accepted that abnormalities of the major components of language function, that is, comprehension, expression, reading, and writing, are significantly related to the occurrence of lesions involving relatively circumscribed regions in the cerebral cortex and their subadjacent connections.

At present the most widely used classification of aphasia is that proposed by Geschwind in 1972 (Fig. 3). He viewed disorders of language as belonging to two main groups: those resulting from lesions anterior to the lateral fissure and those related to lesions posterior to the lateral fissure. Each of these two groups were subdivided thus:

Anterior aphasias which are characteristically non-fluent – aphemia, Broca's and transcortical motor;

Posterior aphasias Wernicke's, pure word deafness, transcortical sensory, conduction, and nominal.

In addition the term '*global aphasia*' was employed to describe a severe impairment of all aspects of language function. The validity of this classification, which is based on a clinico-anatomical correlation, has gained ground from recent studies which have shown a good correlation between the site of lesions seen on cranial computed tomography (CT scan) and the type of aphasia.

Aphemia

This is considered to be a rare type of aphasia. It presents in the form of mutism or *cortical dysarthria*. There may be a *dysprosody*

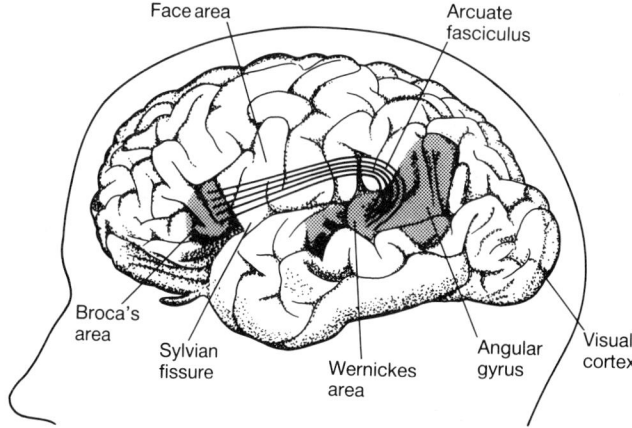

Fig. 3 Primary language areas of the human brain are thought to be located in the left hemisphere, because only rarely does damage to the right hemisphere cause language disorders. Broca's area, which is adjacent to the region of the motor cortex that controls the movement of the muscles of the lips, the jaw, the tongue, the soft palate and the vocal cords, apparently incorporates programs for the coordination of these muscles in speech. Damage to Broca's area results in slow and labored speech, but comprehension of language remains intact. Wernicke's area lies between Heschl's gyrus, which is the primary receiver of auditory stimuli, and the angular gyrus, which acts as a way station between the auditory and the visual regions. When Wernicke's area is damaged, speech is fluent but has little content and comprehension is usually lost. Wernicke and Broca areas are joined by a nerve bundle called the arcuate fasciculus. When it is damaged, speech is fluent but abnormal, and patient can comprehend words but cannot repeat them. (Based on Geschwind, 1972, *Scientific American* **226**, 76–83.)

of speech which is an abnormality of rhythm and intonation giving a 'foreign' sound. The patients show no defect in grammar or in other aspects of language function, including reading and writing. On the whole it is difficult to distinguish aphemia from a pure Broca's aphasia. The possibility of hysteria should always be considered when there is mutism without any specifically aphasic features (i.e. no abnormality of comprehension, reading or writing).

Broca's (expressive) aphasia

This is the most common type of aphasia other than global. Typically the patients lose verbal fluency, and there is cortical dysarthria and agrammatism. The speech has a telegraphic quality, and connecting words such as articles, prepositions, and conjunctions, are missing. The patient's verbal comprehension is adequate. The site of the lesion is most frequently at the foot of the third frontal convolution but usually also involves cortex of the insula and the lower part of the motor strip and/or deep structures such as the caudate nucleus and internal capsule.

Transcortical motor aphasia

This is also a rare type of aphasia which resembles Broca's aphasia in that there is a marked loss of fluency with no severe deficit of verbal comprehension. It differs from Broca's aphasia in that the verbal repetition is significantly less impaired. It has been thought that it arises from the isolation of Broca's area from the remainder of the frontal lobe.

Wernicke's aphasia (sensory receptive)

This is characterized by a profound loss of the ability to comprehend language. Usually the patients have a fluent speech with a marked logorrhoea or press of speech and paraphasias. Not infrequently there are frank neologisms and a jargon-type of speech. Reading and writing are usually impaired. The lesion is usually found in the posterior aspect of the superior temporal gyrus.

Pure word deafness

This condition is characterized by the inability to understand spoken language or repeat it although there are no primary auditory defects. The patients can, however, understand written material and are able to write. The brain damage usually affects either the primary acoustic area in each hemisphere, or that area on the left along with the connecting fibres from the right.

Transcortical sensory aphasia (isolation of the speech area)

In this type of disorder, unlike transcortical motor aphasia, there is a significant comprehension deficit for both spoken and written language. The patient can, however, repeat isolated words and sentences without difficulty. Spontaneous speech is fluent and frequently the patients show marked echolalia. They cannot name objects shown to them and cannot write to dictation. The lesions are usually situated in the posterior part of the temporoparietal lobe.

Conduction aphasia

This is characterized by a striking difficulty in repeating words and phrases. Speech is usually fluent although marked by frequent paraphasias. Verbal comprehension is on the whole adequate. The lesions associated with conduction aphasia usually involve the perisylvian region, including the arcuate fasciculus which connects the cortex of Wernicke's area to that of Broca's area.

Nominal aphasia (amnestic, anomic)

The main feature of this disorder is the inability to find the correct name for objects, colours, letters, and numbers. The naming errors are of three main types: circumlocutions (e.g. 'use in door' instead of key); phonetic errors; and semantic errors. Spontaneous speech is fluent although there are frequent word-finding difficulties. There are no comprehension deficits. Most frequently the site of the lesion is in the region of the posterior superior temporal gyrus bordering on the angular gyrus whose involvement may add other deficits, such as reading and spelling difficulties, to the basic pattern. Anomic deficits can also arise from lesions in other parts of the brain and it is generally agreed that nominal aphasia does not have firm localizing value.

Global aphasia (central)

Many moderately severe aphasics cannot easily be classified as either Broca's or Wernicke's in type. They have the expressive disturbance characteristic of Broca's aphasia with the comprehension loss characteristic of Wernicke's and without disproportion between the two. When the aphasia is severe, speech may be limited to phonated inarticulate or recurrent utterances. Then there is almost always a marked disturbance of comprehension and inability to read or write. This is the characteristic situation after infarction of the territory supplied by the left middle cerebral artery such that there is involvement of both the cortical area whose damage causes Broca's aphasia and that responsible for Wernicke's aphasia. The outlook for adequate recovery is poor.

Language and subcortical nuclei

In recent years, evidence has been amassed indicating that damage to subcortical structures may cause aphasia. This evidence has come primarily from the analysis of patients with subcortical haemorrhages and other naturally occurring lesions, from the observation of speech disturbances following stereotactic surgery, and from studies of electrical stimulation of various subcortical nuclei.

Thalamus

The aphasia after thalamic haemorrhage or infarction seems very similar to transcortical motor aphasia. There is a significant left laterality effect but aphasia only occurs in a proportion of cases. One explanation is that aphasia is not related to the destruction of a specific nucleus but depends on damage to a particular constellation of nuclei; when this occurs the deficits are likely to be long-lasting. The evidence derived from observations during stereotactic surgery suggests that damage to the left ventrolateral nucleus of the thalamus may be important in the genesis of both receptive and expressive defects. The expressive disorders include alterations of fluency, general hesitation and blocking of language, and naming disturbances.

Basal ganglia

Aphasia has also been reported after ischaemic infarction in the basal ganglia of the dominant hemisphere. The precise pattern of impairment after infarction in the caudate and/or lenticular nucleus is not fully established, but at least some patients have features of Broca's aphasia combined with some features of transcortical or nominal aphasia. Stereotactic surgery on the globus pallidus may be followed by reduced accuracy and completeness of oral language formulation and expression; there may also be a reduction of fluency and some impairments in reading and comprehension.

Disturbances closely allied to aphasia

There are a number of disturbances, some of them rare, which are usually regarded as features of damage in the posterior part of the left hemisphere. They are allied to aphasia either because of common underlying neuropsychological mechanisms or because of geographical proximity between their anatomical substrates.

Alexia with agraphia (cortical, parietal)

The underlying brain damage involves the left angular gyrus. The alexia is severe so that only an occasional word can be read and the patient makes many errors identifying single letters. The ability to read numbers and music is sometimes preserved. The identification of letters is not aided by tracing them with a finger, which is one way that alexia with agraphia differs from pure alexia. Oral spelling is poor and the patient has great difficulty identifying words spelt out letter by letter. The agraphia usually matches the alexia so that the patient may even be unable to write some single letters spontaneously or to command. Copying is less impaired but not normal.

Pure alexia (pure word-blindness)

This syndrome is thought to be due to pathology situated in the pathway between the primary visual cortex and the left angular gyrus, which is of major importance for reading, such that there is a 'disconnection' between the two areas. The characteristics of the alexia are as in alexia with agraphia except that the letters can usually be recognized if traced with a finger, and indeed whole words or phrases can be recognized using this strategy. The ability to read numbers and music may or may not be preserved. Oral spelling and the recognition of words spelt aloud are normal. Similarly, writing is normal except for those errors due to the patients' inability to read back what they have written. Most patients have a right homonomous hemianopia and some also have colour anomia. *Developmental dyslexia* is a condition where the ability to read is significantly retarded in comparison to the other aspects of general intellectual development. It is usually detected in childhood or early adolescence. Some children with reading backwardness have unsuspected mental retardation, some have as yet undetected visual or auditory deficit, some have a cerebral pathology, some have emotional disturbance, and some simply lack the necessary academic motivation or have been badly taught. A small proportion, more boys than girls, have idiopathic developmental dyslexia for which no cause can be established. They may have a high-normal IQ despite their reading disability, and even if their reading ability becomes adequate with increasing age they may continue to be very poor at spelling.

Colour anomia

This is a bizarre disorder in which patients do not name colours correctly and make errors pointing to named colours, even though they match colours normally and have normal colour vision assessed by the Ishihara pseudo-isochromatic plates. Occasional patients have features of visual agnosia, and acalculia is common.

The syndromes of pure alexia and/or colour anomia are usually due to occlusion of the left posterior cerebral artery causing infarction of the left occipital lobe and the splenium of the corpus callosum. However, it occasionally occurs with a glioma of the splenium spreading into the left occipital lobe; then there is often severe amnesia as well.

Pure agraphia (motor)

Agraphia more or less uncontaminated by other features of aphasia has been reported as a manifestation of damage in the parasaggital portion of the left parietal lobe. It may also occur as part of a Gerstmann's syndrome in damage to the left supramarginal gyrus. It has also been reported after damage to the posterior portion of the left middle (second) frontal gyrus immediately anterior to the motor cortical representation of the right hand.

Gerstmann syndrome

This consists of finger agnosia, right–left disorientation, agraphia, and acalculia. With *finger agnosia* the patients are unable to name their fingers and can neither indicate nor identify their own or other people's fingers or fingers demonstrated on models. There is not necessarily any impairment of skilled hand movement. In mild cases the thumb and little finger are spared. Severe cases not only have involvement of all the fingers and both thumbs, but they may be unable to name or identify their toes and other parts of the body as well. The abnormality is almost invariably bilateral and due to left hemisphere damage involving the supramarginal gyrus. The *right–left disorientation* applies to body parts (of both patient and other people) more than to inanimate objects in extracorporeal space. The pathological significance of Gerstmann syndrome is not clear because the features can be found in various combinations with or without other disturbances such as constructional apraxia, aphasia, and alexia. Indeed, the isolated and complete syndrome is rare.

Acalculia

Impaired ability to calculate can be due to a number of underlying disorders. It is a common early sign of memory failure, as in general dementia, because interference with calculation arises from forgetting the results of the intermediate steps. Also, aphasia interferes with the ability to calculate because the patient may fail to comprehend exactly what is required, or may express the results of the calculation in the wrong symbols. *Asymbolic acalculia* is a disturbance of calculating due to inability to appreciate the meaning of the digit signs or other symbols (e.g. × and +) used in arithmetic. This form of acalculia is closely related to aphasia but may exist without any other manifestation of it. *Anarithmia* is a primary failure of the ability to calculate even though the meaning of the relevant signs and symbols is understood. Anarithmia and asymbolic acalculia commonly result from damage to the extrastriate cortex of the left occipital lobe. *Spatial acalculia* can arise from damage to either parietal lobe and produces difficulty particularly with written calculation. The difficulty is secondary to failure to organize the spatial components involved in the calculations. Certain figures or columns of figures may be ignored, or they may be positioned incorrectly and the horizontal and vertical directions may be interchanged with inevitable confusion.

Apraxia

Apraxia is defined as a condition where there is a high level disturbance of voluntary purposeful movements, not attributable to weakness, inco-ordination or sensory loss, as usually understood, and not attributable to an aphasic comprehension disorder. Learned skilled movements are performed incorrectly. A rather large number of apraxias has been described. Here only ideomotor (and ideational) apraxia and constructional apraxia will be considered. Buccofacial apraxia has been mentioned in the section on aphasia and dressing apraxia will be mentioned in the section on disorders of body perception.

Ideomotor apraxia is a defect of the ability to mime actions, to imitate how a tool or object would be used, and to make symbolic gestures. Performance improves when using an actual object or tool, to demonstrate its use, but even then movement sequences and spatial orientation may be abnormal. Thus, the patient may be very defective when, for instance, imitating the action of lighting a cigarette – pretending to take out a packet of cigarettes, putting one in the mouth, taking out a match, striking it on the box, lighting the cigarette, and extinguishing the match; the sequence of movements contributing to the whole action is performed more normally, even if not completely so, when a cigarette is actually lit. The disorder is almost invariably due to posterior left hemisphere pathology and many apraxic patients are also aphasic. The apraxia can be confined to the left limbs when there is damage to transcallosal fibres crossing to the right hemisphere. Heilmann has suggested that the disorder occurs either when the cerebral pathology destroys movement engrams or when it interrupts pathways between the site of those engrams and the motor cortex controlling the limb involved. He further suggests that movement engrams are located exclusively in the left hemisphere in some people and bilaterally in others (but rarely if ever exclusively in the right hemisphere of right-handers). This would explain why apraxia does not occur as often as aphasia with left hemisphere damage even though it rarely occurs in right-handers with damage on the right.

Ideational apraxia is a more severe disorder in that actual use of objects and tools is markedly disturbed, but it is probably not qualitatively distinct from ideomotor apraxia. Many of the patients regarded as having ideational apraxia also have a generalized intellectual deterioration.

Constructional apraxia is manifest in formative activities such as building, arranging, and drawing. There is difficulty putting units together to form two- or three-dimensional figures or patterns.

Occasionally patients complain of symptoms arising from their constructional apraxia. Thus they may no longer be able to do simple mechanical tasks such as modelling, embroidery, or laying the dinner table. More often the disorder is demonstrated only on clinical examination. Spontaneous drawing and copying is poor. The patients are unable to copy simple designs with, for instance, matchsticks. Drawings tend to be smaller than the model and may be crowded into one corner of the page. The lines may be wavy, they may not meet accurately, and they may even be superimposed on the model. There is a tendency to make horizontal and vertical lines oblique. One dimension of the drawing may be unduly prolonged, and large parts may be omitted, particularly by patients with right hemisphere damage who leave off the left side. There is a general lack of perspective and mirror reversals sometimes occur. Attempts to copy simple designs with matchsticks result in similar abnormalities.

Unlike ideomotor apraxia, constructional apraxia can arise from either right or left cerebral hemisphere damage. The right hemisphere damage is usually situated focally in the parieto-temporo-occipital junction area and may also cause left-sided visuospatial neglect, left hemianopia, severe sensory loss down the left side of the body, a tendency to ignore the left side of the body, and sometimes dressing apraxia. The left-sided damage tends to be more diffusely distributed in the posterior part of the hemisphere. There have been many attempts to demonstrate that constructional apraxia from right-sided damage is primarily due to a visuospatial disturbance and that with left damage it is primarily an executive disorder, akin to ideomotor apraxia. As yet, however, this differentiation has not been established.

Disorders of visual, spatial, and body perception

These disorders arise very predominantly in association with damage to cortex in the parieto-temporo-occipital junction area of the right hemisphere, or bilaterally, and only rarely with unilateral left hemisphere pathology.

Disorders of visuospatial perception and space exploration

The extent of the right hemisphere 'dominance' in the control of behaviour concerned with visuospatial perception and space exploration is not as great as that of the left hemisphere in relation to language, but it tends in that direction. Vision is a highly developed sense in humans, much used in the exploration of environmental space, and it is not surprising that spatial disorders are closely related to high level visual system disorders, particularly of eye movement control and attention.

Unilateral visuospatial neglect

This is a disregard of, and a failure to attend to, one half of external space, almost invariably the left. Patients tend to collide with objects situated on the left and have a marked preference for taking right rather than left turns, so that they may get lost taking routes from one place to another. They tend to leave the left side off drawings, although the right side can be drawn very well. Writing may be crowded over to the right side of the page, the left remaining blank. They may have great difficulty reading because they neglect the left side of lines or of individual words. The disorder is usually associated with a left hemianopia and left-sided sensory loss. Neither of these can be wholly responsible, however, and certainly most patients with one or both do not have clinically detectable neglect. The patients may be fully aware of their disability but nevertheless unable to overcome it. Damage to the right inferior parietal lobule seems to be the anatomical substrate. When right-sided neglect occurs, associated with left parietal damage, it is only in a minor form.

Gaze apraxia

This is an inability to direct the eyes towards, and then maintain fixation upon, an object appearing in an intact visual field even though there is no oculomotor palsy and both random eye movements and oculocephalic reflexes seem normal. It is usually associated with biparietal damage and most patients also have visual disorientation.

Visual disorientation

As described by Gordon Holmes, visual disorientation is an inability to orient towards and accurately locate objects in space, using vision alone, even though the visual acuity and field seems adequate. It is usually associated with gaze apraxia and damage to both parietal lobes. Judgements of distance, length, and size are faulty. The patients misreach. Their groping and inability to fixate an object gives the impression that they are blind, but they may recognize objects correctly and they may point accurately at sources of sound.

Defective topographical memory or topographical disorientation

This is usually due to bilateral cerebral damage which may not be restricted to the parietal cortex. The patients are unable to remember or describe routes even though they may have been very familiar. For instance, they may lose themselves in their own homes or in villages where they have spent all their lives. The disorder is usually associated with other features of cognitive impairment but very occasionally it exists in relative isolation, in which case it may be due to damage restricted to the right posterior parietal and occipital cortex. Such unilateral damage can cause milder disturbances of topographical relationships resulting, for instance, in failure to orientate correctly on plans with preserved ability to find and describe routes. Route finding difficulty sometimes arises as part of an agnosic disturbance, such that the patient no longer recognizes the specific features of landmarks and so cannot use them for guidance. This is usually associated with prosopagnosia.

Disorders of visual perception

Laboratory studies suggest that patients with posterior right hemisphere damage have more difficulty with complex visual discrimination tasks than do those with similar left-sided damage. However, the majority of patients with clinically recognizable visual perceptual disorders have either focal damage in both hemispheres or diffuse damage.

Visual agnosia

Visual agnosia is a failure to identify objects by sight alone, sufficient acuity of vision and cerebral function being present, and the patient being still able to recognize the objects in question through some other sensory modality such as touch or audition. The recognition failure results in an anomia which can be mistaken for aphasia. However, the characteristics of the naming failure in visual agnosia are quite different to those of aphasia. The anomia is restricted to objects presented visually, the errors are often bizarre (e.g. 'a coal scuttle' for a telephone) rather than semantic or phonetic confusions, as occur in aphasia, and the correct use of the object is not described or indicated by mime. Furthermore, the patient often fails to point correctly to named objects. These features of visual agnosia are also different from those of *optic aphasia* – the anomia of the latter is more or less restricted to the visual modality but within those confines the abnormalities are typically aphasic. Even in every day life the recognition failure of visual agnosia leads to abnormal behaviour such as putting jam rather than sugar in the tea. Features of visual agnosia are of course common in patients with dementia but visual agnosia with well-preserved intellect is rare.

Prosopagnosia

Prosopagnosia is the inability to recognize people from their facial appearances or from pictures. It may be so severe that even close relatives and old acquaintances are not recognized until they speak or until some characteristic item of their clothing is seen. The disorder can be very disabling and may make employment difficult. The underlying pathology seems to be situated more or less symmetrically in the posterior temporal and inferior parietal regions of both hemispheres, and it is usually possible to demonstrate bilateral homonomous visual field defects.

Disorders of body perception

The higher order disturbances of body perception, except for Gerstmann syndrome, affect predominantly the left limbs just as visuospatial neglect is a predominantly left-sided phenomenon.

Hemiasomatognosia is a loss of appreciation of one side of the body, usually the left, resulting from disturbed function of the contralateral parietal lobe. Patients may spontaneously complain that one side of their body, or one limb, feels as if it is not there or does not belong to them. The symptom is usually short lasting and due to epilepsy, migraine, or a transient ischaemic episode. When there is a pathological basis, it is usually situated in the right parieto-temporo-occipital region.

Neglect of one side is a less transient disturbance. In its most exaggerated form, where there appears to be an almost complete unawareness and occasionally even denial of the existence of one side of the body, it almost invariably affects the left and is due to extensive right hemisphere damage with superadded confusion. The disturbance is usually combined with a dense hemiplegia. There may be *anosognosia* which is a denial that there is any paralysis of the affected limbs. Patients seem convinced thay they can and do move these limbs normally and may even seem to think that they had just demonstrated this capacity. The lack of awareness is one factor making rehabilitation of some left hemiplegics very difficult. Severe somatosensory loss, hemianopia, constructional and dressing apraxias, and unilateral visuospatial neglect are often associated with unilateral somatic neglect and anosognosia.

Dressing apraxia is a severe and bizarre disturbance of the ability to put on clothes. It arises virtually always from right parietal lobe damage. Most patients also have constructional apraxia, left visuospatial neglect, and left hemiasomatagnosia. The patients have great difficulty orienting individual items of clothing with their bodies. This is not only a left–right and back–front disorientation. There may be great uncertainty about which article goes where, for instance, patients may attempt to step into their shirt sleeves or put trousers over their heads.

Frontal lobe damage

Damage to the frontal lobes classically produces a combination of personality change and intellectual deterioration. But it is not unusual for even extensive damage to be present without detectable symptoms or signs, and this is why slow-growing frontal tumours may remain silent until they have reached a very considerable size. Changes in mood and character include euphoria, impulsiveness, and facetiousness with apparently decreased anxiety and little concern about consequences of any actions that are undertaken. Such disinhibition may occur without any evidence of intellectual impairment. The patient may be fully aware of the disinhibition but nevertheless unable to control it. On the other hand, the personality change may produce depression with decreased initiative and spontaneity.

The intellectual deterioration has been difficult to characterize, especially in the laboratory. There seems to be a decreased ability for abstract thought and for planning behaviour taking into account past experience and future consequences. Perseveration of various types is common. The patients may be very distractable and unable to concentrate or keep their attention focused on one topic for more than a short time. This produces an apparent interference with memory. However, frontal damage does not produce amnesia in the strict sense, except perhaps during the acute phase after damage to the cingulate cortex. Patients with large frontal meningiomas may be disorientated, hypokinetic, and apathetic; they usually have raised intracranial pressure in addition to damage which probably extends well beyond the frontal lobes.

Damage restricted to the prefrontal areas of the left hemisphere can produce what really amounts to a mild aphasia without articulation defect of paraphasias; it appears as a loss of spontaneity and fluency in speaking without a definite difficulty in selecting appropriate words and without impaired comprehension.

Amnesia

Memory impairment is a common early feature of many brain diseases, especially Alzheimer's disease and slowly rising intracranial pressure as from obstructive hydrocephalus. The ability to remember information from the past, and to lay down new memories, depends to some extent upon the proper working of many cerebral structures. There are certain structures, however, which are of major importance. These include the medial parts of the temporal lobe, especially the hippocampus and amygdala; the fornix system; certain thalamic and hypothalamic nuclei especially the dorsomedial nuclei and possibly the mammillary bodies; and parts of the frontal lobes. Pathology involving these structures is particularly liable to cause memory impairment which is generalized if the damage is bilateral and can amount to severe amnesia. Pathology that is restricted to one side of the brain tends to produce a predominantly verbal memory deficit if it is on the left and a nonverbal memory deficit if it is on the right.

A verbal memory deficit makes it difficult for patients to remember what has been said to them, or what they have read; they forget messages, names, and the content of conversations; and reading may cease to be a pleasure because they cannot remember back beyond a few lines or paragraphs. The deficit occurs especially with damage to the left hippocampus and amygdala and it may be the presenting feature of a left temporal lobe tumour.

The non-veral memory deficit from right medial temporal lobe damage is much more intangible. Often the symptoms are only minimal but the defect appears in the laboratory as difficulty remembering material which cannot be easily verbalized, such as relative spatial location and facial features.

Severe amnesia is usually the consequence of bilateral damage to structures mentioned above and some of the causes are listed in Table 3. New material can be remembered for a few seconds, or few minutes at most, and then only if there is no distraction. Usually there is also a *retrograde amnesia*, that is, a loss of memory for events which occurred during the period immediately before the onset of the brain disorder, which may extend back over a few months or even years.

Trauma (see also page 21.189)
Amnesia is common after head injuries severe enough to cause unconsciousness. The duration of the *posttraumatic amnesia* is the period between the injury and the resumption of normal continuous memory. It includes the period of unconsciousness and the subsequent period of confusion; it can also include a further

Table 3 Causes of severe amnesia

ALCOHOL–Korsakoff psychosis
Other causes of thiamine deficiency–inadequate feeding, hyperemesis gravidarum, stomach cancer
TUMOURS around IIIrd ventricle
VASCULAR–bilateral thalamic infarcts, posterior cerebral artery territory infarcts (especially left)
METABOLIC damage to hippocampi consequent upon anoxia, hypoglycaemia, severe convulsions
Meningitis–especially tuberculous, sarcoid
Encephalitis predominantly affecting temporal lobes–especially herpes simplex virus encephalitis, limbic encephalitis
ALZHEIMER'S DISEASE–occasionally presents as very severe memory failure with only minor general deterioration

---

Major causes in capitals.

period in which the behaviour seems to be normal, but which cannot be remembered in detail afterwards. The length of the posttraumatic amnesia is one of the better indices of the severity of head injuries. When it lasts longer than 24 hours, the injury was probably severe and there may be permanent brain damage. The duration of the *retrograde amnesia* is the period between the injury and the last clear memory before it happened. Characteristically it shrinks slowly, becoming shorter as time since the injury increases. The process of shrinking may take several months but most cases have a final retrograde amnesia of no more than a few seconds and it is only longer in those with very severe injuries. Occasionally the retrograde amnesia contains an 'island' of memory for events immediately prior to the injury. Likewise, the posttraumatic amnesia may contain periods which are partially remembered.

Transient global amnesia (see page 21.158)

This is a condition of dense amnesia lasting usually for several hours, but occasionally only 0–60 min, during which the patient behaves like somebody with severe amnesia. New memories cannot be laid down, and as in severe amnesia new material can only be retained for a few seconds, or, at the most minutes, provided there are no distractions. The attack is usually followed by an apparently complete recovery of memory function, except that events which occurred during it cannot be recalled; (laboratory examination within two or three weeks of an attack may reveal evidence of a mild verbal or non-verbal memory deficit, but this only occasionally persists beyond six months). At the onset of an attack there is a retrograde amnesia which may be for a period as long as several years; this shrinks during the course of the attack and is said to be only short immediately before recovery. The patient is fully conscious throughout the attack and may carry out complex acts, such as driving long distances, quite normally. They usually seem mildly confused and agitated, frequently repeating the same questions. Most patients have no further neurological abnormality, but sometimes there are signs suggestive of ischaemia in the territory supplied by the vertebrobasilar system. These transient global amnesic attacks must be differentiated from the automatisms of temporal lobe epilepsy and from hysterical amnesia; an almost identical phenomenon is sometimes seen as part of a migraine attack.

References

Benson, D. F. (1979). *Aphasia, alexia and agraphia*. Churchill Livingstone, Edinburgh.

De Renzi, E. (1982). *Disorders of space exploration and cognition*. John Wiley and Sons, Chichester.

Heilman, K. M., Rothi, L. J. G. and Watson, R. T (1987). Apraxia: disorders of skilled movement. In *Clinical neurology* (eds M. Swash and J. Oxbury), Churchill Livingstone, Edinburgh.

Kolb, B. and Whitshaw, W. H. (1980). *Fundamentals of neuropsychology*. Freeman and Co., San Francisco.

Mayes, A. and Mendell, P. (1983). Amnesia in humans and other animals. In *Memory in animals and humans* (ed. A. Mayes). Van Nostrand Reinhold (UK), Wokingham.

Springer, S. P. and Deutch, V. W. (1981). *Left brain, right brain*. Freeman and Co, San Francisco.

Wyke, M. A. (1983). Disorders of language. In *Handbook of psychiatry* (eds M. Shepherd and O. L. Zangwill). Cambridge University Press, Cambridge.

DEMENTIA

W. B. MATTHEWS

Dementia is the term used to describe progressive intellectual deterioration. The psychiatric aspects of this common and important problem and its diagnosis and distinction from specific psychiatric disorders are discussed in detail in Section 25. The differential diagnosis, the important reversible causes, and some of the degenerative disorders which give rise to this condition are considered here.

Differential diagnosis of dementia and its causes

In selected hospital series of patients suspected of being demented approximately 10 per cent are found not to have any cognitive defect but to be suffering from psychiatric illness, depression or occasionally schizophrenia. The distinction of mild dementia from depression can be difficult, as simple tests of memory and intellect may be poorly performed from apathy or preoccupation with matters more important to the patient. More sophisticated psychological testing will usually allow the distinction to be made but it is not unknown for a frontal meningioma to be treated with electroconvulsant therapy.

Dementia was originally held to be, by definition, irreversible, but this view has been abandoned and the most important reason for investigation is the detection of potentially treatable causes. It is also highly desirable to reach a positive diagnosis, even of an intractable condition, as knowledge will not be advanced by the use of the category of 'simple dementia' still encountered in mental hospital notes, and there may also be important genetic implications.

Potentially reversible causes

If dementia is confirmed potentially reversible causes can be found in approximately 10 per cent of cases.

Chronic intoxication with barbiturates, chloral or, in former times, bromide, may be suspected from the fluctuation of the symptoms and the frequent association with slurred speech and nystagmus. Alcoholic addiction can lead to the amnesic syndrome of Wernicke's encephalopathy, but its role in dementia is still controversial, particularly the question of recovery on abstinence.

The severity of the mental retardation of myxoedema may sometimes be out of proportion to other signs of the disease and tests of thyroid function should be routinely performed.

The classical clinical picture of general paresis is now rare, but neurosyphilis can cause progressive dementia without distinctive features although particular attention should always be paid to the pupillary reactions. Physicians with great experience held that neurosyphilis could not be excluded on the grounds of negative serology and this is still a reason for examining the CSF. Tuberculous meningitis should be remembered as a cause of relatively rapid intellectual failure.

Metabolic causes include vitamin B_{12} deficiency, hepatic, and renal failure, for which clinical evidence may be found and which can be confirmed by routine blood tests. The EEG is often severely disturbed with a great excess of high-voltage slow activity. Dementia due to poor cerebral perfusion in heart block may be reversed by the insertion of a pacemaker.

An intracranial tumour involving the right frontal lobe, such as an olfactory groove meningioma, may present as mild dementia without focal signs, apart, perhaps, from unilateral anosmia, which could escape detection. The location of the tumour is not, however, critical, as large intracranial masses involving any part of the cerebral hemispheres may also cause intellectual failure although often with more obvious focal signs. Any tumour resulting in hydrocephalus may present in the same way, for example, an VIIIth nerve tumour may indirectly cause memory failure.

Computerized tomography (CT) is therefore an essential investigation which will not only reveal tumours but also demonstrate dilation of the cerebral ventricles and cortical atrophy. It is important to recognize that the correlation between observed atrophy and intellectual loss is remarkably poor. However, if the patient is severely demented and no focal lesion or significant ventricular dilation or cortical atrophy are seen a reversible metabolic cause is probable. In the context of revealing potentially reversible causes of dementia the presence of marked hydrocephalus with little cortical atrophy will suggest the condition of *normal pressure hydrocephalus*.

This title merely implies the presence of hydrocephalus with no evidence of raised intracranial pressure at the time of investigation, although pressure monitoring will reveal intermittent waves of greatly increased pressure. The hydrocephalus is *communicating*, that is to say the CSF can pass from the ventricles to the subarachnoid space but its absorption is prevented either by obstruction at the tentorial opening or at the arachnoid villi in the superior longitudinal sinus. There may be a past history of meningitis or subarachnoid haemorrhage but usually no antecedent cause can be suggested.

The characteristic triad of symptoms is that of dementia, an ataxic gait, and incontinence of urine, but any of these features may predominate. The gait disturbance appears to be due to weakness of the legs but without signs of upper motor neurone involvement. The CT scan appearances are usually characteristic and diagnostic methods involving the flow of radioisotopes through the CSF pathways are now seldom used. The importance of establishing the diagnosis lies in the hope of circumventing the failure of CSF absorption by means of a valved shunt between a lateral ventricle and the left atrium.

The response to such treatment is often initially most impressive but cannot easily be predicted. Improvement in gait following the removal of a large volume of CSF at lumbar puncture is regarded as a good prognostic sign. Unfortunately the collapse of the dilated ventricles following shunting often leads to the vacant space being occupied by subdural haematomas and other dangerous complications are intraventricular haemorrhage and infection of the valve. Initial enthusiasm has waned.

Irreversible causes

Dementia may form a part of the clinical syndrome of inoperable cerebral tumours, especially multiple metastases.

Alzheimer's and Pick's disease are described in detail later; the former accounts for the dementia in the great majority of cases where a definite cause is established. Creutzfeldt-Jakob disease soon declares itself as a rapidly fatal condition. In Huntington's chorea (page 21.232) dementia may be present before the onset of involuntary movements and the diagnosis will be of the utmost importance to the family. The family history itself is the most revealing feature. The CT scan, in advanced disease, may show specific atrophy of the caudate nucleus but not with merely early dementia.

Multiple sclerosis (page 21.211) may present with dementia and if there is gait ataxia and urinary incontinence a mistaken diagnosis of normal pressure hydrocephalus may be reached.

Arteriosclerotic or multiple infarct dementia can usually be distinguished from Alzheimer's disease by such features as abrupt onset, steplike deterioration, a history of strokes, emotional lability, hypertension, evidence of atheroma, and focal neurological symptoms and signs.

Dementia may develop in a variety of forms of progressive neurological disease in addition to those already mentioned, but in such circumstances the diagnosis is seldom difficult. Patients with Parkinson's disease, progressive supranuclear palsy, olivopontocerebellar atrophy, Friedreich's ataxia, and occasionally with motor neurone disease, may become demented. Dementia may also occur as a non-metastatic effect of carcinoma, but probably always accompanied by widespread evidence of neurological disease.

ALZHEIMER'S DISEASE

This is the commonest cause of progressive presenile dementia and of severe dementia in old age, and is defined by characteristic histological changes.

Occurrence

Precise figures for incidence and prevalence are difficult to obtain because of problems of clinical diagnosis, case ascertainment, and histological interpretation. It has been estimated that about 15 per cent of those who are over 65 years are demented to a significant degree and at least half of these have what is often referred to in life as 'senile dementia of Alzheimer's type', in fact, Alzheimer's disease. The prevalence of presenile dementia has never been determined, but it is a distressingly common clinical problem and most such patients will be found to have Alzheimer's disease. Sex incidence is probably equal in the presenium with female preponderance with advancing age. Occasional cases are encountered in the fourth decade but there is a steep rise in incidence in the next two decades. Familial Alzheimer's disease is described below.

Pathology

The brain of a patient who has died with advanced Alzheimer's disease is severely atrophied, shown by narrowed gyri, widened sulci, and enlarged lateral ventricles (Fig. 1). Histological examination shows severe loss of cortical neurones, maximal in frontal, occipital, and temporal lobes. Histologically many neurones are seen to contain neurofibrillary tangles, shown on electron microscopy to consist of paired helical fibrils. A second characteristic change is the presence of large numbers of amyloid plaques averaging 50 μm in diameter throughout the cerebral cortex, and more

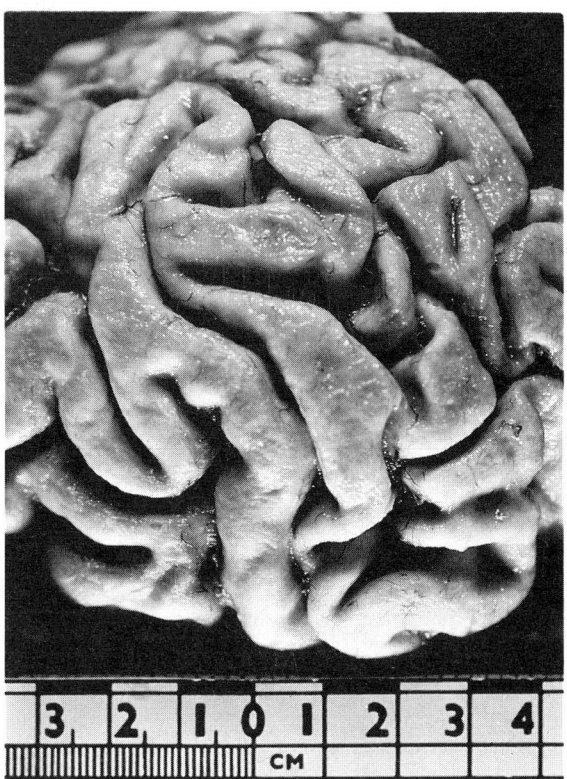

Fig. 1 Alzheimer's disease. Cortical atrophy. The gyri are narrowed and sulci unduly wide.

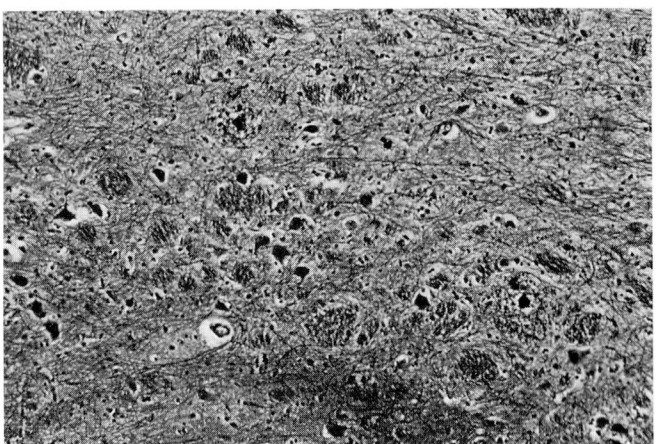

Fig. 2 Alzheimer's disease. Numerous 'senile' plaques in the thalamus, seen as rounded structures.

sparsely in the basal ganglia and cerebellum (Fig. 2). These changes may be regarded as the hallmarks of Alzheimer's disease but histological appearances in aged demented subjects do not differ from those in presenile dementia. Clear definition of Alzheimer's disease on histological grounds is, however, obscured by the presence of smaller numbers of identical 'senile' plaques and occasional tangles in the brains of old people who have not been demented.

Clinical features

The initial complaint is of failing memory and difficulty in concentration. There are many causes for such symptoms and the differential diagnosis is discussed on page 21.42. In Alzheimer's disease the patient's complaint will be confirmed by relatives and associates at work. The defect is plainly more severe than the commonplace inability to recall the names of acquaintances that affects most people with advancing years. Even at an early stage it is often quite possible to detect abnormalities in speech function or in spatial orientation. Dysphasic errors occur in spontaneous speech or writing or may be elicited on testing. Inability to find the way in familiar surroundings is an ominous symptom. In other patients vocabulary is relatively well preserved so that an effective conversational facade may be maintained, concealing severe cognitive defects.

As the disease progresses, ability to follow a printed page or the plot of a television soap opera is lost and interest also fails. Speech becomes repetitive. Assistance is required with dressing, washing, and in the lavatory, and urinary incontinence is common. Vision is not affected and locomotion remains normal until a late stage. Intermittent aggression, a tendency to wander, and nocturnal confusion are distressing symptoms. Epileptic fits may occur and also myoclonus, particularly in rapidly advancing disease.

In Alzheimer's disease with onset between 45 and 65 years life expectancy is reduced by about two-thirds and in older subjects by a half. The mean duration is between five and seven years but much more acute forms with death within a year have been recognized. There is an interesting link with Down's syndrome as over the age of 40 years the clinical and pathological features of Alzheimer's disease usually develop.

Ischaemic or haemorrhagic cerebrovascular disease may result from congophilic angiopathy that is relatively common in Alzheimer's disease.

Investigation

Apart from cerebral biopsy, which should not be undertaken, there is no specific diagnostic test for Alzheimer's disease. In advanced disease cortical atrophy and ventricular dilation are seen on the CT scan. The EEG contains diffuse slow activity. The CSF is normal on routine examination.

Pathophysiology

There is now considerable evidence that degeneration of specific cholinergic neurones in the nucleus basalis of Meynert and neighbouring structures is an essential feature of Alzheimer's disease. These neurones relay extensively to the cerebral cortex. In Alzheimer's disease the appropriate muscarinic receptors are initially preserved but choline acetyl transferase, concerned in the synthesis of acetyl choline, is deficient. Lack of this activity has been directly correlated with the degree of dementia and with the number of cells showing fibrillary degeneration. Other transmitter systems are, however, also affected and the cause of neuronal degeneration in the basal ganglia and cortex has not been determined.

Aetiology

A genetic theory is difficult to maintain as definite familial Alzheimer's disease is uncommon. There are obvious difficulties in tracing pedigrees in a disease of late onset. Families in which Alzheimer's disease is transmitted as an autosomal dominant are, however, fully documented. No specific link with the chromosome abnormality of Down's syndrome has been suggested. Among possible toxic causes aluminium deposition in the brain was suspected but this is not present in excess in all cases. The original claim that animals injected with brain extracts from familial Alzheimer's disease developed spongiform encephalopathy has not been sustained but there are recent suggestions that the amyloid plaques may be arrays of proteinaceous infectious agents (prions).

Treatment

The discovery of a defect in production of the neurotransmitter acetyl choline led to attempts at symptomatic treatment. Precursors of acetyl choline, choline, and lecithin, have proved ineffective. There are conflicting reports on the effects of physostigmine, an anticholinesterase with a central action, in improving memory in Alzheimer's disease. Any effect is temporary and certainly far less effective than the manipulation of neurotransmitters in Parkinson's disease. Vasopressin and naloxone have also been given on the basis of animal experiments on memory but have proved valueless.

Management

Alzheimer's disease has a disastrous effect on family life and much social support is needed. The physician's role is that of explanation, advice and, when required, sedation. Habit training, regular routines, and the preservation of interests are admirable aims, often thwarted by advancing disease. The degree of insight is difficult to assess, but often mercifully appears to be limited.

PICK'S DISEASE

This is a rare cause of presenile dementia, difficult to distinguish on clinical grounds from Alzheimer's disease. The cortical atrophy is more often localized, particularly to the frontal and temporal lobes. Histologically there is intense subcortical gliosis. Cortical neuronal loss may be accompanied by changes indistinguishable from those of Alzheimer's disease and indeed the two diseases may co-exist. The supposedly characteristic swollen neurones containing silver-staining inclusions – the Pick cells – were rather confusingly first described by Alzheimer.

The clinical features are those of progressive dementia with severe loss of speech function. A surprising feature is that the EEG may remain normal in the presence of severe dementia. The CT scan may indicate the lobar distribution of the cortical atrophy. Nothing is known of the causation except that dominant inheritance is found more often than in Alzheimer's disease.

Other forms of 'primary dementia' have been described, being distinguished on histological grounds and classification is imprecise.

CREUTZFELDT–JAKOB DISEASE

This rare degenerative disease suddenly assumed importance when it was shown that it was transmissible to laboratory animals.

Incidence

The annual incidence in England is 0.45 per million. Onset in the great majority of cases is between 50 and 65 years with extremes from the second decade to old age. Females are affected more than males in a ratio of 1.5:1. A positive family history is found in 6 per cent of cases, the pedigrees suggesting dominant autosomal inheritance.

Clinical features

Vague prodromal symptoms of dizziness, fatigue, difficulty in concentration, insomnia or nocturnal myoclonus, are present in 25 per cent of cases, but often the onset is abrupt. Focal neurological symptoms such as aphasia, limb weakness, cerebellar ataxia, hemianopia or cortical blindness are accompanied or immediately followed by rapidly advancing dementia. Focal or generalized fits are common. Speech functions are soon severely affected so that patients become entirely mute. Walking is soon impossible and within a few weeks the patient is helpless in the decerebrate or decorticate posture. Myoclonus is common and may affect any group of muscles and a generalized myoclonic response to startle is often present. Death may occur as soon as three weeks from the onset and only a small proportion survive for a year. It is probable that Creutzfeldt–Jakob disease is invariably fatal.

Diagnosis in the early stages is difficult and the advanced disease may be confused with the acute form of Alzheimer's disease and with many causes of rapidly advancing brain disease, including glioma, metastases, and progressive multifocal leucoencephalopathy. A particular variety in which dementia is accompanied by evidence of extensive wasting of lower motor neurone origin may resemble motor neurone disease.

The CSF protein may be slightly raised but there is no pleocytosis. The EEG usually shows at some stage diffuse periodic discharges of slow waves and spikes. Liver function tests are sometimes abnormal but there is no other evidence of systemic disease. The CT scan is usually normal, reflecting the rapid course of the disease with little time for atrophy.

Pathology

The grey matter is predominantly affected, with neuronal loss and severe astrocytic gliosis. A characteristic feature is spongiform degeneration with cytoplasmic and nuclear vacuoles in both neurones and glia. There is no inflammatory reaction.

Aetiology

Creutzfeldt–Jakob disease can be transmitted to laboratory animals. This was first achieved by intracerebral injection of brain material into chimpanzees. Other modes of transmission have succeeded including injecting peripheral tissue by a peripheral route and certain laboratory rodents have proved susceptible. The incubation period is always prolonged. The nature of the transmissible agent is uncertain, as it cannot be cultured or identified microscopically. It is similar in properties, including resistance to heat, disinfectants, formalin, and boiling, to the agent of scrapie, a natural disease of sheep, and to that of kuru, an epidemic disease in certain people in New Guinea. At first labelled 'slow virus' diseases, there have been recent indications that the agent is a proteinaceous structure for which the term prion has been coined. In this group of diseases, but not in Alzheimer's disease, ultramicroscopic fibrils, labelled scrapie associated fibrils (SAF), can be identified in brain extracts. These resemble amyloid fibrils but it is now thought unlikely that SAF are accumulations of infective particles and are more probably an epiphenomenon.

Creutzfeldt–Jakob disease is certainly transmissible in humans by means of neurosurgical operations or corneal transplants, and recently injections of human growth hormone have been incriminated. These findings naturally caused great alarm and the fear of an undetectable agent, very difficult to destroy, causing a fatal disease, led to reluctance to conduct post-mortem examinations in cases of dementia. However, no accidental transmission from the laboratory has occurred and in nursing patients with Creutzfeldt–Jakob disease it is a sufficient precaution to use rubber gloves when handling any material contaminated by blood. The disinfection of contaminated instruments presents obvious difficulties. Prolonged autoclaving under increased pressure should be used where possible. Domestic bleach in a 1 in 10 dilution will also destroy the agent.

There are a few suggestions of case-to-case transmissions of the familial form of the disease and this may explain the apparently dominant pedigree in these families.

Treatment

No treatment has been of proven benefit. Temporary improvement has been claimed with amantadine and vidarabin but this is not consistent.

KURU

As far as it is known, kuru is confined to the Fore people of New Guinea. It is a progressive disease presenting with cerebellar ataxia and leading to a fatal outcome within a year. Kuru is transmissible in the laboratory and the pathology closely resembles that of Creutzfeldt–Jakob disease but amyloid plaques are often present and it has been suggested that these may contain or consist of the infective agent. The route of natural transmission appeared to be ritual cannibalism. Fresh cases still occur many years after cannibalism was abolished but children are no longer affected.

GERSTMANN–STRÄUSSLER SYNDROME

Repeated attempts have been made to transmit other degenerative diseases of the nervous system but with little success. Spongiform encephalopathy has, however, been induced in animals by injection of cerebral material from a small number of patients considered to have had the Gerstmann–Sträussler syndrome. This is a form of progressive cerebellar ataxia with dementia and pyramidal signs, with an earlier age of onset than classical Creutzfeldt–Jakob disease and a longer course. The pathological findings include spongy degeneration and unusual parenchymal accumulations of amyloid. A family history characteristic of dominant inheritance may be found. The disease is probably a variant of Creutzfeldt–Jakob disease.

References

Davis, K. L. and Mohs, R. C. (1982). Enhancement of memory processes in Alzheimer's disease with multiple dose intravenous physostigmine. *Am. J. Psychiat.* **139**, 1421–1424.

Hachinski, V., Iliffe, L. D., Zilkha, E., Du Boulay, G. H., McAllister, V. L., Marshall, J., Russell, R. W. R. and Symon, L. (1975). Cerebral blood flow in dementia. *Arch. Neurol.* **32**, 632–637.

Katzman, R. (1976). The prevalence and malignancy of Alzheimer disease. *Arch. Neurol.* **33**, 217–218.

Kokmen, E. (1984). Dementia – Alzheimer type. *Mayo Clin. Proc.* **59**, 35–42.

Marsden, C. D. and Harrison, M. J. G. (1972). Outcome of investigation of patients with presenile dementia. *Brit. Med. J.* **2**, 249–252.

Masse, G., Mikol, J. and Brion, S. (1981). Atypical presenile dementia. *J. Neurol. Sci.* **52**, 245–267.

Masters, D. L., Gajdusek, D. C. and Gibbs, C. J. (1981). Creutzfeldt–Jakob disease virus isolations from the Gerstmann–Sträussler syndrome: with an analysis of the various forms of amyloid plaque deposition in the virus-induced spongiform encephalopathies. *Brain* **104**, 559–588.

Matthews, W. B. (1982). Spongiform virus encephalopathy. *Recent advances in clinical neurology*, Vol. III (eds W. B. Matthews and G. H. Glaser), pp. 229–238. Churchill Livingstone, Edinburgh.

Olson, M. I. and Shaw, C.-M. (1969). Presenile dementia and Alzheimer's disease in mongolism. *Brain* **92**, 147–156.

Prusiner, S. B. (1984). Some speculations about prions, amyloid and Alzheimer's disease. *N. Eng. J. Med.* **310**, 661–663.

Smith, J. S. and Kiloh, L. G. (1981). The investigation of dementia: results in 200 consecutive admissions. *Lancet* **i**, 824–827.

Soininen, H., Puranen, M. and Riekkinen, P. J. (1982). Computed tomography findings in senile dementia and normal aging. *J. Neurol. Neurosurg. Psychiat.* **45**, 50–54.

Strachan, R. W. and Henderson, J. G. (1965). Psychiatric syndromes due to avitaminosis B$_{12}$ with normal blood and bone marrow. *Q. J. Med.* **34**, 303–317.

Tissot, R., Constantinidis, J. and Richard, J. (1975). *La Maladie de Pick*. Masson et Cie, Paris.

Whitehouse, P. J., Price, D. L., Clark, A. W., Coyle, J. T. and DeLong, M. R. (1981). Alzheimer disease: evidence for selective loss of cholinergic neurons in the nucleus basalis. *Ann. Neurol.* **10**, 122–126.

Wilcock, G. K., Esiri, M. M., Bowen, D. M. and Smith, C. C. T. (1982). Alzheimer's disease: correlation of cortical choline acetyltransferase activity with the severity of dementia and histological abnormalities. *J. Neurol. Sci.* **57**, 407–417.

COMA

M. J. G. HARRISON

The emergency measures to be instigated when a patient presents in coma are considered in detail in Section 14. Here are described the subsequent neurological assessment and how a diagnosis is arrived at.

Consciousness is maintained by activity of the reticular formation of the brain stem (Fig. 1). It follows that coma may be due to the global suppression of neuronal function or to the presence of a focal lesion in the brain stem. The latter may be an intrinsic lesion such as an infarct, or may be secondary to the compressive effects of an enlarging mass (Fig. 2). After the essential first steps in the care of the unconscious patient – maintenance of an airway, assessment of life threatening injuries or cardiopulmonary problems, etc. (see Section 14), the neurological history taking and examination must be geared to the task of distinguishing global and 'metabolic' causes of coma from those of brain stem origin. It is particularly important to detect those whose declining conscious level is due to secondary compression of the brain stem since they may need neurosurgical relief of the expanding mass in the supratentorial compartment.

History

The history may provide important clues. A fit may have been witnessed and the coma prove to be only that transiently seen after a grand mal attack, or the patient may have fallen to the ground holding his head as though struck down by severe headache, suggesting subarachnoid haemorrhage. An empty pill bottle or a history of depression may suggest a drug overdose, and a history of diabetes prompts consideration of ketotic or hypoglycaemic coma. Vague mental symptoms and headaches over the previous weeks should raise suspicions of a tumour that is now causing coma by brain stem compression.

Clinical assessment

Level of coma

Documentation of the level of coma is important since progressive deterioration suggests brain stem compression. By contrast most patients with metabolic causes of coma or an intrinsic brain stem lesion have a stable or improving level of awareness. To detect subtle changes in the level of consciousness requires careful description of the patient's response to specific stimuli. Words like semicoma are to be avoided as they are inexact and mean different things to different observers. The coma scale of Jennett and Teasdale is in general use and overcomes these difficulties (Table 1). It records the best level of response of eyelids, speech, and limb movement to verbal request, shouts, and painful stimuli. Deterioration can be detected readily, even when different observers are responsible for the sequential examinations. For example, a patient whose eyes opened when she was spoken to and replied in a confused way has obviously deteriorated when her eyes only open to a painful stimulus, and the verbal response consists only of a groan.

Focal signs

The presence of a hemiparesis suggests the possibility of a cerebral hemisphere mass lesion as the cause of the coma. Its presence must be inferred in the unconscious patient from observation of asymmetries: of the face during expiration, of spontaneous limb movements or tone, and of responses to painful stimuli. If a decor-

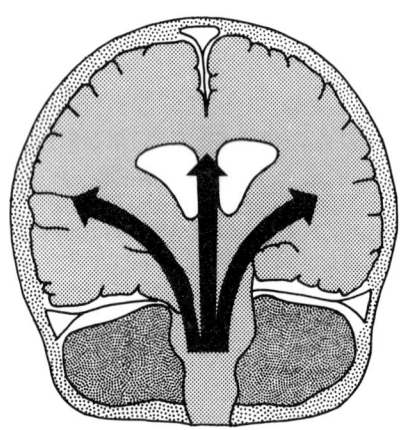

Fig. 1 Schematic representation of the role of reticular formation in the brain stem in maintenance of an aroused state of the cerebral hemispheres.

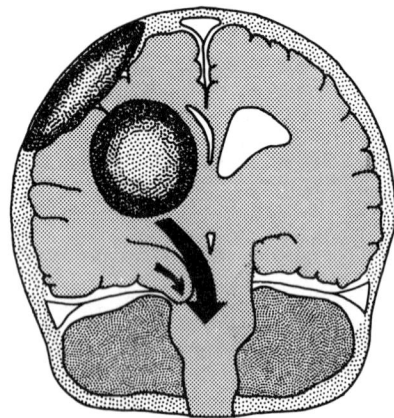

Fig. 2 Illustration of herniation of the temporal lobe (small arrow) and displacement of the upper brain stem (large arrow) resulting from an intracranial mass whether extra or intracerebral.

Table 1 Glasgow coma scale

Eyes open	Spontaneously To speech To pain Never
Best verbal response	Orientated Confused Inappropriate words Incomprehensible sounds None
Best motor response	Obeys commands Localizes pain Flexion to pain Extension to pain None

ticate or decerebrate posture develops symmetrically in response to painful stimuli, no localizing significance is implied. If, however, the responses are asymmetrical, e.g. flexion of one arm and extension of the other, then the latter side showing the more primitive reaction is 'hemiparetic'. Rarely asymmetries result from hypoglycaemia, hyponatremia or hepatic failure. Most will prove to reflect structural lesions in the cerebral hemisphere.

Eye signs (see also Section 14)
A key part of the examination concerns the assessment of the pupillary responses and eye movements. If these brain stem functions are normal the cause of coma is likely to be metabolic or due to a diffuse disease. Structural damage to the brain stem, on the other hand, whether local or secondarily provoked, manifests itself by loss of pupil reflexes and abnormalities of eye movement. Herniation of the temporal lobe over the free edge of the tentorial opening causes compression of the third cranial nerve so a unilaterally dilated fixed pupil is indicative of the presence of a compressing mass lesion. Central herniation of the brain stem through the tentorial hiatus reflects a pressure gradient between a supratentorial mass-containing compartment and the posterior fossa. Such a pressure gradient is dramatically and dangerously increased by ill-advised lumbar puncture. Central herniation causes progressive brain stem compression with sequential loss of pupil responses, and abnormalities of eye movements passing from a stage of readily elicitable symmetrical horizontal eye movements to a stage of dysconjugate eye movements or unilateral paralysis of gaze, and finally to total immobility of the eyes. Eye movements in the unconscious patient are tested by counter rolling of the head or by cold water syringing of the external auditory meati to cause a unilateral suppression of tonic vestibular input to the brain stem gaze centres. Patients in deep metabolic coma may show total loss of eye movement but in them the pupil reflexes will be retained. With central herniation pupil reflexes are lost as the eye movements become abnormal or are lost. Anoxia may cause large fixed pupils with coma due to diffuse neuronal damage. Its occurrence has usually been documented however.

Respiration
Little has been said about respiratory patterns since these are of limited value. Deep breathing suggests acidosis as in diabetic coma, regular but shallow breathing suggests depression by drug overdose, and Cheyne Stokes breathing has no diagnostic significance. All other departures from a normal pattern, if not due to respiratory disease, suggest some brain stem compromise.

Diagnosis of type of coma and cause
The distinction between the three broad categories of coma can thus be made by bedside observations (Table 2). Associated clinical features, and special investigations such as the EEG and CT scans are then needed to make specific diagnoses (Table 3). If the coma appears metabolic in type but no systemic disorder or drug

Table 2 Diagnosis of coma

Diagnostic category	Diagnostic features
A 'Metabolic'	Normal pupil responses Normal or absent eye movements depending on depth of coma Suppressed or Cheyne Stokes respiration Symmetrical limb signs usually hypotonic
B Brain stem: intrinsic	From outset: Abnormal pupil responses Abnormal eye movements Abnormal respiratory pattern Cranial nerve signs Bilateral long tract signs
C Brain stem: compression	Papilloedema Hemiparesis Progressive: Loss of pupillary responses Loss of eye movements Abnormal respiratory pattern Long tract signs and/or Appearance of 3rd nerve palsy

Table 3 Causes of coma

Metabolic	Drug overdose Ischaemia/hypoxia Diabetic Hypoglycaemia Cardiac failure Respiratory failure Renal failure Hepatic failure Hyponatremia Hypercalcaemia
Diffuse intracranial disease	Head injury Meningitis Subarachnoid haemorrhage Encephalitis Epilepsy Hypertensive encephalopathy Cerebral malaria
Cerebral hemisphere lesions (with brain stem compression)	Cerebral infarct Cerebral haemorrhage Subdural haematoma Extradural haematoma Abscess Tumour
Brain stem lesion	Brain stem infarct Brain stem haemorrhage Tumour/abscess Cerebellar infarct/haemorrhage

overdose has been diagnosed the CSF should be examined. Both meningitis and subarachnoid haemorrhage may cause coma, and neck stiffness is often missing when the conscious level is depressed. (If there are focal signs or papilloedema is detected a lumbar puncture is contraindicated until after CT scan or EEG and angiography have excluded a mass lesion.) Other investigations that may be needed when the diagnosis is in doubt include arterial blood gases, urea, electrolytes, liver function tests, osmolarity, cortisol, and thyroid studies. The blood sugar should always be measured as delayed correction of hypoglycaemia can cause severe permanent neurological disability. The EEG can be helpful in detecting encephalitis especially that due to herpes hominis, some kinds of metabolic coma such as that due to hepatic encephalopathy, and status epilepticus.

If a focal lesion is suspected a CT scan is needed to see if there is a surgically accessible problem such as a subdural haematoma or meningioma. In the posterior fossa, cerebellar haemorrhage may cause a rapidly evolving coma due to local pontine compression. This may cause unilateral ataxia at an early stage but may have to be recognized by the presence of a unilateral paralysis of horizontal eye movement in the absence of a matching hemiparesis, in a patient whose conscious level is declining. Surgery is indicated for all but the smallest haematomas. Pontine haemorrhage causes coma with loss of horizontal eye movements and pin point pupils that may still just react to a bright light. There are bilateral long tract signs and the patients often develop hyperpyrexia. Surgery is rarely possible. Massive cerebral haemorrhage causing coma is also usually inoperable.

Related conditions

Confusional state

Patients suffering from an acute confusional state have a short attention span and are distractable. They often appear perplexed or bewildered and have difficulty in following questions and commands. Their memory is poor and they have some problems with orientation. They tend to misinterpret what they see. The acute onset of such a state with some variable drowsiness and inattentiveness is usually due to toxic metabolic conditions and the diagnosis depends on defining the underlying physical condition. Purely psychiatric causes of confusion, and dementia in its early stages, do not affect the level of awareness, so identification of drowsiness is all important in the distinction.

Delirium

This too is usually due to toxic/metabolic problems such as alcohol or barbiturate withdrawal and hepatic failure, or encephalitis. It may be seen during recovery from head injury. There is disorientation, confusion, and reduced attention as in confusion but the picture is more florid with agitation, irritability, and fear, and the disorientation is more profound. Complex delusions are often seen with prominent visual hallucinations (auditory hallucinations are more often seen in psychoses).

Locked-in syndrome

If patients have a paralysis of vocalization and speech, and of movement of the face and limbs they may appear unconscious when in fact they are not. Often the patients have had damage to the pontine base or medulla, for example, due to multiple sclerosis or a stroke. Communication can usually be established. They can blink or perhaps make some vertical eye movement which can be coded as 'yes' and 'no' in order that they may signal their wishes and converse in a limited way. A similar incapacity may occur with myasthenia gravis or the Guillain–Barré syndrome but its evolution does not give rise to the same problems of knowing that the patient is alert and of undiminished intellect. An EEG can help show an alert state reactive to external stimuli.

Akinetic mutism

This superficially resembles the locked-in state with a patient who is mute and immobile, though apparently alert. No communication can be established, however, and the patient is doubly incontinent. The usual cause is bilateral frontal lobe damage or diffuse anoxic damage, or a small lesion in the reticular formation.

Psychogenic unresponsiveness

Mutism and a lack of response to the environment may also be seen in primarily psychiatric conditions such as catatonia, depression, and hysteria. In these situations the pupil responses are normal, and caloric stimulation of the ears provokes nystagmus as in the normal subject. The EEG shows a responsive wakeful pattern. (By contrast patients with akinetic mutism of organic origin have an EEG dominated by slow wave activity.)

Chronic vegetative state (see page 21.50)

Prolonged survival after severe injury may lead to the development of this state. There is no evidence of recovery of higher function but cycles of wakefulness appear. Some patients are akinetic but some are not. Their eyes may open to verbal stimuli. Spontaneous respiration and maintenance of blood pressure ensures continuation of life, until death from complications such as bronchopneumonia. At post-mortem the brain stem is relatively spared, the forebrain showing extensive damage. The cortex usually shows laminar necrosis.

References

Plum, F. and Posner, J. B. (1980). *Diagnosis of stupor and coma*, 3rd edn. F. A. Davis Co, Philadelphia.
Harrison, M. J. G. (1984). Coma. In *Contemporary neurology* (ed. M. J. G. Harrison). Butterworths, Guildford.

BRAIN DEATH AND THE VEGETATIVE STATE

B. JENNETT

Cardiopulmonary resuscitation and intensive care are now commonplace in acute hospitals in developed countries and when used to avert a temporary threat to life they can result in complete recovery and long survival. But the price paid for these successes can be to prolong the process of dying from a few minutes to many days in a large number of other patients; and to leave a few to survive for months or years in the vegetative state, which some have described as a living death. This price can be too high unless there is wider recognition of when it is appropriate to initiate, to continue or to withdraw technological interventions that will not save worthwhile life. The problem is not a small one. The American hospital that pioneered 'Do not resuscitate' orders found ten years later that no less than a third of patients who died there had had one or more attempts at cardiopulmonary resuscitation. In the United Kingdom, where intensive care beds are much fewer than in the United States, there are estimated to be at least 4000 cases of brain death each year; there must be many more that have prolonged attempts at resuscitation without being formally recognized as brain dead. There are likely to be more patients in these states in the future unless clear rules are established for withholding resuscitation from certain patients and in others for abandoning it once it is recognized that brain failure is irreversible. Fortunately there is no longer any dearth of data from which to derive reliable criteria for recognizing brain death and the vegetative state. Society is now sending clear signals to its doctors in both the United Kingdom and the United States that it expects them to try to avoid undignified persistence with technology when no benefit can come from it. We may not be able to anticipate the occurrence of these artefacts of nature that are the by-products of technological innovation; but we can at least take steps to see that they do not persist any longer than necessary once they have been reliably recognized.

Much of the controversy about brain death, now largely resolved, arose from misconceptions about the nature of death (Pallis, 1983). Only when concepts of death are clarified can criteria consonant with them be accepted with confidence. The first concept is that death is a process and not an event, that organs cease to function in several sequences and that what is regarded as the time of death is arbitrary rather than actual. Death is when the body as a whole ceases irreversibly to function, but this does not imply that all organs (let alone all cells) have already 'died'. Consider the common sequences by which the process of death can occur. Most often the heart fails first and within minutes hypoxia causes brain stem failure; the respiratory drive then stops and breathing ceases. Much less often respiratory failure is primary; the brain stem then fails but the heart can go on beating for 15–30 min. Although resuscitation from cardiac or respiratory arrest may be completely successful it is sometimes too late to save the cerebral cortex, which is more vulnerable to hypoxia than the brain stem; the patient then survives in a vegetative state. This may also result from severe head injury without cardiorespiratory arrest having occurred. Sometimes resuscitaton is too late for even the brain stem to survive yet the heart continues to beat, because the myocardium is more resistant to hypoxia than the brain stem. Much more often this combination of a dead brain, mechanically maintained ventilation, and a spontaneously beating heart (the syndrome of brain death) results from a primary intracranial catastrophe. Breathing stops from brain stem dysfunction but mechanical ventilation is established in the hope that the intracranial crises will be reversible. On occasions it is and prompt respiratory resuscitation is then rightly recognized as having been lifesaving. It is when the brain failure cannot be reversed that the outcome of these worthy efforts is brain death.

Brain death

The crucial lesion is irreversible loss of function of the brain stem with subsequent lack of downward drive to maintain respiration, and of upward activation of the cerebral cortex by the ascending reticular pathways. Except when systemic hypoxia has been the initial insult the cerebral cortex may be structurally intact and islands of electrical activity may be detected on EEG. However, this makes no difference to the inevitability of spontaneous cardiac asystole within a few days of death of the brain stem. Early definitions of brain death (e.g. in the Harvard criteria of 1968) implied that the whole nervous system was dead with a flat EEG and absence of all motor activity. But the spinal cord is more resistant to hypoxia and is unaffected by intracranial catastrophes that wreck the brain stem – so spinal reflexes often persist after brain death. Indeed reflex limb movements frequently become more active if ventilation is maintained for more than 24 hours after the brain stem has ceased to function. It has been suggested that uncertainties might be dispelled if the nomenclature were changed to brain *stem* death; but the term brain death is difficult to displace after a quarter of a century.

What matters for practical purposes is that if the brain stem is dead, the brain is dead. And if the brain is dead, the person is dead. It was as long ago as 1970 that the State of Kansas enacted the first brain death law and Finland led the Europeans a year later. By 1983 all but 16 American States had such a law and six of the exceptions had legal precedents for accepting death of the brain as indicating legal death. Britain is less liable to look to lawyers for leadership in such matters and it was the Medical Royal Colleges' Memorandum in 1979 that stated that death should be declared when brain death is diagnosed, not at the later time when the heart stops. This removes any ambiguity about the action of the doctor who discontinues ventilation after diagnosing brain death. He is simply stopping doing something useless to someone who is already dead; that is different from withdrawing support from someone who is hopelessly ill so as to allow death to occur.

Causes and frequency of brain death

About half the cases of brain death in the United Kingdom follow head injury, respiratory failure occurring after hours or days of intensive treatment. This may be due to brain stem distortion from a compressing intracranial haematoma that can be surgically evacuated, but more often it results from a combination of brain swelling and reduced cerebral perfusion. About a third of cases of brain death are associated with spontaneous intracranial haemorrhage, either ruptured aneurysm in a younger person or hypertensive haemorrhage in older patients. Brain death is particularly likely when a recurrent subarachnoid haemorrhage occurs in a patient who is waiting in hospital for investigation or for surgery, for it is then that a ventilator is at hand. The remaining cases of brain death follow failure to control a variety of intracranial conditions (e.g. tumour or infection), or from cardiopulmonary resuscitation necessitated by extracranial events. Systematic study of brain death in the United Kingdom has revealed that three-quarters of the cases occur in non-teaching hospitals that do not have a neurosurgical unit (Jennett and Hessett, 1981). The criteria for diagnosing brain death therefore need to be widely applicable; they should not depend on neurosurgeons or neurologists, nor on investigations that are available only in specialist regional centres.

Criteria for diagnosis

Undue emphasis on the final confirmation that no residual brain function persists has sometimes distracted attention from the step-wise process of diagnosing brain death, in which these tests are only the last stage. Indeed the most important step is the first one, satisfying the *preconditions*. These require that the patient be apnoeic and in deep coma due to irreversible structural damage to the brain, and this implies that reversible causes of brain stem depression have been adequately excluded. It is usually obvious that structural brain damage has occurred – there has been a recent head injury or a classical history of spontaneous intracranial haemorrhage or of some less acute intracranial condition. Establishing the irreversibility of such brain damage depends on failure to improve with the passage of time and after the correction of factors such as systemic hypotension and hypoxia, and raised intracranial pressure. Other factors that can cause temporary absence of brain stem function are depressant drugs (including alcohol), neuromuscular relaxant drugs, and physiological factors such as hypothermia and gross metabolic imbalance. The first two of these may complicate cases of structural brain damage but it is only in a minority of cases that serious doubts arise about confusing factors. For example, when a patient is found unconscious and no satisfactory history can be discovered it may be necessary to undertake formal screening for drugs; also to delay the diagnosis of brain death until sufficient time has passed for the exclusion of all temporary causes of brain stem depression.

The tests applied to indicate lack of brain stem function are simple to carry out and to interpret. There should be no response of the pupils to light, of the eyelids to corneal touching, of the facial muscles to pain, of the throat muscles to movement of the endotracheal tube, or of the eyes to syringing of each external auditory meatus with ice-cold water (the caloric or vestibulo-ocular reflex). Only when there has been a negative response to all of these is the final crucial test applied – to verify that there is still apnoea. There must be no respiratory movement after disconnection from the ventilator for long enough to allow the $PaCO_2$ to rise to 60 mmHg, oxygenation being maintained by delivering 6 l/min of oxygen down the endotracheal tube. It is usual to require that all these tests are repeated to exclude any possibility of observer error; the interval before repeating the two tests need be no more than half an hour, provided that the preconditions were fully satisfied before undertaking tests for the first time.

The validity of these criteria has now been tested in thousands of cases. For it was several years before clinicians were confident enough to disconnect the ventilator once brain death had been diagnosed and experience from many places is that the heart always stops within 14 days, usually within 2–4 days. However, the concept of brain death is still not readily grasped even by all doctors and nurses, only a tiny minority of whom ever encounter it. Moreover, the notion that the beat of the heart is the signal of life, which took root when the stethoscope was invented 150 years ago, dies hard. Taken together with a certain public disquiet about organ transplantation, particularly of the heart, this led during the 1970s to the suspicion that doctors might sometimes be tempted to diagnose brain death prematurely, in their eagerness to secure donor organs. The fact is that few brain death cases lead to organ donation, as transplant surgeons frequently complain. If transplantation were superseded as a means of treating organ failure there would still be decisions to make about discontinuing ventilators in brain dead patients in every acute hospital in the land. However, during the 1970s sporadic reports appeared in the lay press of patients who had recovered after supposedly having been brain dead, and this reached a climax on BBC television in 1980. In the event this led to a reaffirmation of the brain death criteria that the Royal Colleges had originally published in 1976 and to clarification of the situation in a second edition of the Code of Practice of the Health Departments in the United Kingdom. Since then there has been much wider acceptance of the concept of brain death and of the propriety of making an early diagnosis and of then withdrawing ventilation.

Nonetheless, it remains important to be sensitive to the misunderstandings that can arise in what is still a delicate area of decision-making in medicine. Perhaps the commonest situation is when a family is told soon after an acute episode of brain damage that the outcome is 'almost hopeless'. Resuscitation of such patients is sometimes successful, otherwise it would not be undertaken; but by that time relatives may themselves have raised the matter of organ donation. Rather than replying that such an offer is welcome but premature, doctors or nurses may be drawn into discussing the procedures that would be involved if brain death did occur. It is easy to see how it may then appear as though 'they nearly took his kidneys'. The same can happen when depressant drugs are not at first suspected but with the passage of time brain stem depression proves to have been temporary. Occasionally doctors unfamiliar with brain death consider it as a possible explanation for other unresponsive states, such as the vegetative state. But the activity of the brain stem should rule out any serious question of confusion. Sometimes a brain dead patient is suspected by naive bystanders of being still alive, because of the persistence of spinal reflexes – a misunderstanding to anticipate by ensuring that all witnesses of this phenomenon have it explained to them.

The best safeguard against such embarrassment is a well-written set of guidelines in the hands of experienced doctors – two of whom should always be involved in the diagnosis. Experience is more important in assessing the preconditions than in applying the brain stem tests. Time is the other safeguard – time to satisfy the preconditions, to establish the diagnosis and to ensure that the state is not reversible. This time varies widely according to the circumstances, at least six hours is needed to satisfy the preconditions and 12–24 hours is more usual. Least time is required when a patient with a known lesion develops a crisis (e.g. recurrent subarachnoid haemorrhage after angiography has already disclosed the lesion); most time is needed for the patient found in coma with no history but a suspicion of drug ingestion.

In the past some clinicians have sought diagnostic support from laboratory investigations designed to show either arrest of the cerebral circulation or the absence of cerebral electrical activity. Circulatory tests are complex and not without risk, whilst EEG is more often available and involves no hazard. But critics maintain that EEG is irrelevant and potentially misleading because it reflects activity in the cerebral cortex and not in the brain stem; and because securing an isoelectric recording can be technically difficult in the electronically active environment of an intensive care unit. Criteria used in the United Kingdom for the diagnosis of brain death specifically state that EEG is not required, whilst more recent American recommendations emphasize that its use there is optional.

Action after diagnosis of brain death

There is now wide acceptance of the concept that when the brain is dead the person is dead. It can help to clarify the situation for nurses and relatives if a death certificate can be issued before discontinuing the ventilator. Some doctors are still reluctant to make this diagnosis explicitly and then to act logically and legally by disconnecting the ventilator. The useless ventilation of brain dead patients wastes resources for intensive care, deprives the patient of death with dignity, needlessly prolongs the distress of relatives, and is bad for the morale of nursing staff. Moreover, the opportunity to offer organs for transplantation is lost because gradual circulatory failure makes such organs useless for donation. It would be of benefit to bereaved families, nurses, and other patients if doctors shared a greater readiness to recognize brain death and then to act appropriately.

The vegetative state

Unlike brain death, which results from permanent brain stem failure and is always the precursor of early cardiac asystole, the vegetative state is the consequence of permanent inaction of the cerebral cortex and is compatible with survival for several years. When the underlying lesion is neocortical necrosis from delayed cardiopulmonary resuscitation microscopy shows total absence of cortical neurones. The other common cause is diffuse axonal injury due to shearing forces sustained at impact by acceleration/deceleration injury to the head. Extensive tearing of fibres in the subcortical white matter and brain stem leaves the structurally intact cerebral cortex functionally inactive and isolated. Microscopy some weeks after such an injury shows extensive degeneration in the cortical descending fibres in the brain stem and spinal cord. Features of the type of injury that causes extensive shearing lesions in the white matter are that the patient is deeply unconscious from the moment of impact, that the skull is seldom fractured and that cerebral contusions are usually very limited. Less common causes of the vegetative state are stroke (especially when a second episode affects the opposite cerebral hemisphere to that first affected), meningitis or encephalitis, and some congenital abnormalities of the brain.

When the vegetative state follows an acute insult such as cardiorespiratory failure, head injury or stroke, the patient is initially in coma, and there may be a period of apnoea requiring ventilator support. After traumatic coma it is usually a week or two before the eyes open (indicating emergence from coma), because the whole reticular activating system has been out of action. But after non-traumatic coma eye opening may occur within a day or so. But although awake for long periods the vegetative patient shows no sign of awareness, no evidence of any activity or response that is psychologically meaningful as judged behaviourally. There is a range of reflex movements in the spastic limbs, the patient may grimace and even groan when a stimulus is applied and there may be grasping responses in the hands and fingers. These may be interpreted as voluntary squeezing of a relative's hand, or when evoked by contact with a nasogastric tube as a voluntary attempt to remove this. The eyes may deviate towards a sound or light and may follow a moving object. It is important to realize that this repertoire of reflex activity does not require the involvement of the cerebral cortex and does not therefore imply sentience.

Before Jennett and Plum proposed in 1972 the term vegetative state, which has now been widely accepted, this condition was variously described as persisting, permanent or prolonged coma; as severe post-traumatic dementia; or as the apallic syndrome. The latter is still espoused by some continental Europeans and their occasional use of the term 'partial apallic syndrome' is particularly unfortunate. The criteria for definition of the vegetative state should be strict; patients who do occasionally but unequivocally obey commands or utter even the occasional word should be categorized as severely disabled and dependent, and not as vegetative.

Prognosis

When a patient is suspected of being vegetative, say two or three weeks after an acute episode of brain damage, two questions arise: what are the chances of improvement, and if they are poor, how long is survival in this state likely? How soon a patient can be considered to be permanently vegetative depends partly on the cause of the brain damage and partly on the experience of the observers. One month after head injury even experienced clinicians can still have doubts as to whether a patient is vegetative or is very severely disabled; of those in one series in whom there was such doubt 13 per cent eventually became independent though still disabled (Jennett and Teasdale, 1981), but this occurred also in 7 per cent of those confidently diagnosed as vegetative. However, no patient considered vegetative three months after injury ever became independent and almost all who survived remained vegetative. After non-traumatic coma it is easier to make a confident diagnosis sooner, perhaps because there is not the confusion of concussion or of complex pathological lesions; the chances of regaining independence if vegetative one month after a non-traumatic ictus are virtually nil.

Survival in the vegetative state can be prolonged, given adequate nutrition and nursing care. The longest recorded in Britain is 18 years but many vegetative patients are still alive five years after head injury; after non-traumatic coma patients are older and often affected by progressive disease so that prolonged survival is unusual. The question of whether it is appropriate to provide the nutrition and nursing care required to ensure survival once the persistent vegetative state has been diagnosed is now a topic of debate. There is good evidence that many people consider survival in the vegetative state to be an outcome worse than death (Jennett, 1976); it is therefore now commonplace for it to be agreed between doctors, nurses, and the patient's family that no antibiotics should be given in the event of intercurrent infection. Even with such limited treatment these patients are remarkably robust, once the first few months have passed. It is for this reason that there are now tentative proposals that it might be proper to withdraw nutrition whilst maintaining fluid intake. In this regard it is important to note that the propriety of withdrawing support from patients who are either terminally ill or whose quality of life is unacceptable has been explicitly stated both by the United States President's Commission of 1983 and by the Canadian Law Reform Report of 1984.

References

Anonymous (1981). Brain death. *Lancet* i, 362–364.
Campbell, A. G. M. (1984). Children in a persistent vegetative state. *Br. Med. J.* **289**, 1022–1023.
Conference of Medical Royal Colleges and their Faculties in the United Kingdom (1976). Diagnosis of brain death. *Br. Med. J.* **2**, 1187–1188.
Conference of the Medical Royal Colleges and their Faculties in the United Kingdom (1979). Diagnosis of death. *Br. Med. J.* **1**, 322.
Curran, W. J. (1984). Quality of life and treatment decisions: the Canadian Law Reform Report. *New Engl. J. Med.* **310**, 297–298.
Health Departments of Great Britain and Northern Ireland (1983). *Cadaveric organs for transplantation: a code of practice, including the diagnosis of brain death.* HMSO, London.
Jennett, B. (1976). Resource allocation for the severely brain damaged. *Arch. Neurol.* **33**, 595–597.
——, Gleave, J. and Wilson, P. (1981). Brain death in three neurosurgical units. *Br. Med. J.* **281**, 533–539.
—— and Hessett, C. (1981). Brain death in Britain as reflected in renal donors. *Br. Med. J.* **283**, 359.
—— and Plum, F. (1972). Persistent vegetative state after brain damage. *Lancet* i, 734–737.
—— and Teasdale, G. (1981). *Management of head injuries.* F. A. Davis, Philadelphia.
President's Commission for the Studies of Ethical Problems in Medicine (1981). Guidelines for the determination of death. *J. Am. Med. Assoc.* **246**, 2184–2186.
President's Commission for the Study of Ethical Problems in Medicine and Biomedical and Behavioral Research (1983). *Deciding to forego life-sustaining treatment: ethical, medical and legal issues in treatment decisions.* US Government Printing Office, Washington.
Report of the Ad Hoc Committee of the Harvard Medical School to examine the definition of brain death (1968). *JAMA* **205**, 85–88.

DISORDERS CHARACTERIZED BY EPISODIC CHANGES IN CONSCIOUSNESS

Syncope

R. W. GILLIATT

Syncope may be defined as 'transient loss of consciousness due to an acute decrease in cerebral blood-flow' (Sharpey-Schafer, 1956). Some aetiological factors are shown in Table 1.

Vasovagal Syncope is the name given by Sir Thomas Lewis to the common type of fainting which occurs in young people. His original description of a personally observed case cannot be bettered and is given below.

The patient was sitting and a few cubic centimetres of blood had been withdrawn from a vein in the arm and the needle removed. He was watching the operation and began to feel queer, 'as though his stomach had turned upside down'. He complained of dizziness, facial pallor was noticed, and his head fell forward to his knees. He was placed at once in a long easy-chair and further observed. By this time the pallor was intense and he was restless. The pulse was imperceptible; the heart sounds distant, and its rate of beating 50 per min. The patient was limp, mentally confused, or actually unconscious, for several minutes; a heavy sweat broke out over his forehead, spreading over chest and body, the pallor remained extreme. Respiration was slow and sighing. The pulse was imperceptible for several minutes; as it returned, the systolic blood pressure was registered at 60 mm; the pulse rate varied between 50 and 60. Five minutes after the onset some recovery was observed; the pulse rate had risen to 64 and the blood pressure to 80. Nine minutes after the onset the patient was able to respond to questions. The pulse rate was 88 and the blood pressure was 105; the blood pressure gradually rose to 110 (Lewis, 1932).

The term vasovagal syncope implies that both vagal slowing of the heart and decreased vasomotor tone contribute to the fall in blood pressure during the faint. Lewis had noted that when atropine was given to abolish the vagal bradycardia, it did not wholly reverse the fall in blood pressure. Since the skin remained pale, he suspected that vasodilation was occurring in the splanchnic region, but subsequent work has shown that the most marked changes in peripheral resistance and in blood flow are in striated muscle. While the skin vessels remain constricted, there is a marked

Table 1 Causes of syncope

Reflex, (vasovagal)	Cardiac
Haemorrhage	Dysrhythmias
Fear or pain	Ventricular outflow obstruction
Anoxia	
Upright posture	Areflexic or paralytic postural
Carotid sinus syndrome	hypotension
	Tabes
Respiratory	Diabetes
Trumpeting	Polyneuropathy
Weight lifting	Shy–Drager syndrome
Coughing	Traumatic quadriplegia
	Alcohol and drugs
Micturition	Old age (particularly with drugs)

increase in muscle blood flow before consciousness is lost. The early studies of forearm blood flow by Professor Barcroft and his collaborators showed that in these circumstances peak muscle blood flow was higher than that recorded from a sympathectomized or nerve-blocked limb, and it was concluded that sympathetic vasodilator fibres were involved. However, direct recording from muscle nerves in recent years has not so far confirmed the presence of sympathetic vasodilator fibres. Wallin and his colleagues in Sweden, who have carried out much of this work, using fine tungsten electrodes inserted into human peripheral nerves, have observed the sudden cessation of tonic activity in vasoconstrictor fibres during fainting, but have not been able to identify other sympathetic efferent fibres showing a pattern of activity which might be responsible for active vasodilation.

In the present context the most interesting feature of vasovagal syncope is the constancy of the physiological changes, regardless of the cause of the attack. An episode induced by venesection is shown in Fig. 1 but similar changes have been demonstrated in attacks due to fear, anoxia, and the upright posture. In the example shown in Fig. 1 there was an increase in heart rate and in peripheral resistance as the circulating blood volume was reduced by venesection, until a point was reached at which these changes were abruptly reversed, just before consciousness was lost. The sudden fall in peripheral resistance appeared to be the critical factor in causing unconsciousness, as the cardiac output, which had fallen steadily during the venesection, actually increased slightly during the faint itself.

Sudden increases in forearm blood flow associated with mental perturbation are shown in Fig. 2, and illustrate the importance of this type of stimulus in triggering a faint. Vasovagal syncope during dental anaesthesia was originally attributed to the combined effects of sitting upright in a dental chair, plus anoxia during the inhalation of pure nitrous oxide, but subsequent work suggested that fear of the procedure was a more important factor in triggering the attack. In vasovagal syncope associated with the upright posture it seems that a lordotic posture can obstruct flow in the inferior vena cava at the level of the diaphragm and thus exaggerate the effect of gravity in reducing venous return to the heart. This mechanism has been put forward to explain the common occurrence of fainting in soldiers standing stiffly to attention during parades and inspections.

What has been said above should not give the impression that a fall in peripheral resistance is always the critical factor in vasovagal syncope. In some patients vagal hyperactivity is sufficient to cause complete cardiac arrest, in which case the state of the peripheral resistance becomes irrelevant. This is sometimes called *cardio-inhibitory syncope* and it is particularly likely to occur in response to painful stimuli to the head and neck. Pressure on the eyeball is a potent stimulus (the oculo-cardiac reflex). Vagal cardiac arrest also occurs in *carotid sinus syncope*, a relatively rare condition in which atheroma in the region of the carotid bifurcation is associated with excessive sensitivity of the carotid sinus baroceptors. In such cases neck movement or mild pressure over

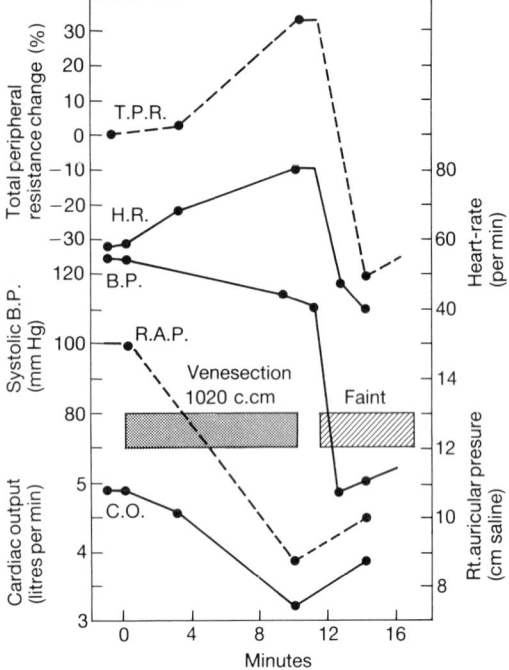

Fig. 1 Vasovagal syncope during venesection. As blood volume was reduced, right auricular pressure (RAP) and cardiac output (C.O.) fell. Systolic blood pressure (B.P.) fell slightly in spite of an increase in total peripheral resistance (T.P.R.) and heart rate (H.R.). Just before consciousness was lost there was an abrupt decrease in T.P.R. and H.R.; and systolic B.P. fell to approximately 40 mmHg, from which level it only slowly recovered in spite of an increase in C.O. (From Barcroft *et al.*, 1944, by courtesy of the *Lancet*.)

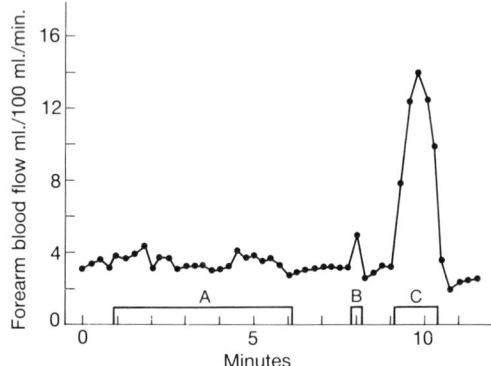

Fig. 2 Vasodilation in the forearm induced by mental perturbation. The subject, a healthy volunteer, was asked to do mental arithmetic in A, was threatened with boiling water in B, and was told that the laboratory was on fire in C. (From Roddie, 1963, by courtesy of the *Annals of the Royal College of Surgeons*.)

the sinus may cause prolonged cardiac arrest with unconsciousness. If the diagnosis is confirmed by carotid massage under ECG control, treatment with atropine should be started, followed by a pacemaker or surgical denervation of the carotid sinus.

In most cases of vasovagal syncope the patient is limp and motionless while unconscious, with pallor and sweating that persist after recovery of consciousness. Slight stiffening or a few muscle jerks are not uncommon; with deep anoxia convulsions which are violent enough to suggest epilepsy can occur (*convulsive syncope*). This is particularly likely when there is complete cardiac arrest, as in the carotid sinus syndrome.

In *respiratory syncope* the attack is triggered by a sustained rise in intrathoracic pressure, sufficient to obstruct venous return to the heart. This can occur in healthy subjects during breath-holding (the Valsalva and Weber manoeuvres, the mess-trick, the fainting lark) and in singers or those playing wind instruments when a prolonged expiratory effort is required. The trumpet is the instrument which appears to cause the greatest increase in intrathoracic pressure, and Faulkner and Sharpey-Schafer have written that Wagner is the composer 'with least consideration for the feelings of the trumpet player'.

The physiological changes during competitive weight-lifting may also lead to syncope. Some subjects hyperventilate beforehand in order to eliminate the desire to breathe during the lift itself. They then maintain a high intrathoracic and intraabdominal pressure during the process of lifting. It should be noted that hyperventilation itself has only a mild hypotensive effect, but it can contribute to syncope in this situation and in others in which multiple factors operate.

In medical clinics the most important form of respiratory syncope is that due to coughing (cough syncope; the laryngeal vertigo of Charcot). This is usually seen in men with chronic bronchitis and emphysema, in whom the intrathoracic pressure may reach peaks of more than 250 mmHg during violent coughs. These high-pressure transients are communicated directly to arterial baroceptors outside the thoracic cavity, initiating muscle vasodilation which exaggerates the effect of the reduced cardiac output. In addition the rise in intrathoracic pressure is communicated to the CSF via the lumbar veins, so that cerebral arterial perfusion is further reduced. Convulsive movements commonly occur during cough syncope, and the distinction from true epilepsy becomes particularly important, since treatment should be directed towards improving the chest condition. Some patients have a degree of amnesia for their attacks and deny that violent coughing took place before they lost consciousness. In such cases an independent history from a witness is needed to establish the true state of affairs.

Syncope during defaecation or micturition is sometimes included in this group, on the assumption that there is impairment of venous return to the heart during straining. While this may be true of syncope during defaecation (which is in any case a rare phenomenon), micturition syncope requires separate consideration. There is no evidence that raised intrathoracic pressure contributes to this syndrome which is better categorized as a form of postural syncope. In its typical form it occurs in men who get up at night to pass urine. Thermoregulatory vasodilation during sleep may contribute to the postural hypotension but the critical factor is bladder-emptying itself. Distension of the bladder is a strong pressor stimulus which can in spinal man raise systolic blood pressure to the region of 250 mmHg. In intact man there are compensatory mechanisms which prevent a marked rise in blood pressure, but the sudden withdrawal of pressor drive from a distended bladder is likely to exaggerate any postural hypotension already present. That the upright posture does contribute to micturition syncope is clear from the fact that attacks can usually be prevented by micturating in the sitting position.

Attacks of cardiac syncope can be subdivided into those associated with cardiac dysrhythmias (paroxysmal tachycardia, fibrillation, heart-block leading to asystole) and those associated with ventricular outflow obstruction. In patients with dysrhythmias there is often no history of cardiac disease, and correct assessment of the syncopal attack itself is essential if the patient is to receive treatment by pacing or drugs. While the identification and subsequent treatment of such cases has been greatly helped by the widespread use of ambulant ECG monitoring, the seriousness of the threat to life from the underlying cardiac pathology should not be underestimated. In a recent American follow-up study of patients with cardiac syncope, sudden death occurred within one year in approximately 20 per cent of cases (Kapoor et al., 1983). In this group intracardiac electrophysiological studies may be needed in some cases to establish the nature of the dysrhythmia and to allow effective treatment (Morady et al., 1983).

The term areflexic or paralytic syncope is used to distinguish that form of postural syncope which occurs in patients with depressed or absent autonomic reflexes due to neurological disease, ganglion blockers or other drugs. Unlike those with vasovagal syncope, patients with autonomic failure lose consciousness without a change in pulse rate, and without skin vasoconstriction or sweating. Syncopal attacks of this type can occur in tabes dorsalis, diabetic neuropathy, inflammatory polyneuritis (Guillain–Barré syndrome), traumatic paraplegia, and multisystem atrophy (Shy–Drager syndrome). Simple bedside tests of skin temperature and sweating in the extremities, the effect of deep breathing on the pulse rate, and the effect of standing on the blood pressure, may be sufficient to suggest the diagnosis. It is important to remember that in many cases the causes are multiple, for example, dehydration due to diarrhoea or fever combined with depressed autonomic reflexes. This is particularly important in the elderly; in a study of old people living at home Caird et al. (1973) showed that it was possible to demonstrate a fall in systolic blood pressure (of more than 20 mmHg) on standing in 20 per cent of those over 65 years, and 30 per cent of those over 75 years. Drugs which were thought to contribute to the postural hypotension included ganglion blockers, oral diuretics, phenothiazines, antihistamines, tricyclic antidepressants, benzodiazepines, barbiturates, and antiParkinsonian drugs. In this age group drug withdrawal is likely to be more helpful than the use of additional preparations designed to expand plasma volume and increase cardiac output. In younger patients fludrocortisone may be tried. Sleeping in the semi-upright position may prevent the normal nocturnal fall in plasma volume; this measure has proved helpful in some neurological patients with postural hypotension. In selected cases an antigravity suit may be useful.

For the differential diagnosis of syncopy and its distinction from other transient attacks, see the chapter on page 21.69.

References

Caird, F. I., Andrews, G. R. and Kennedy, R. D. (1973). Effect of posture on blood pressure in the elderly. Br. Heart J. **35**, 527–530.
Kapoor, W. N., Karpf, M., Wieand, S., Peterson, J. R. and Levey, G. S. (1983). A prospective evaluation and follow-up of patients with syncope. N. Engl. J. Med. **309**, 197–204.
Lewis, T. (1932). Vasovagal syncope and the carotid sinus mechanism. Br. med. J. **1**, 873–876.
Morady, F., Shen, E., Schwartz, A., Hess, D., Bhandari, A., Sung, R. and Scheinman, M. (1983). Long-term follow-up of patients with recurrent syncope of unknown origin evaluated by electrophysiologic testing. J. Am. Coll. Cardiol. **2**, 1053–1059.
Roddie, I. C. (1977). Human responses to emotional stress. Irish. J. Med. Sci. **146**, 395–417.
Sharpey-Scafer, E. P. (1956). Syncope. Br. med. J. **1**, 506–509.
Schatz, I. J. (1984). Orthostatic hypotension: I & II. Arch. Intern. Med. **144**, 773–777., 1037–1041.
Wallin, G. (1983). Intraneural recording and autonomic function in man. In Autonomic failure: a textbook of clinical disorders of the autonomic nervous system (ed. Sir R. Bannister), pp. 36–51. Oxford University Press, Oxford.

Epilepsy

A. HOPKINS

Definitions

An epileptic seizure

Throughout life neurones interact in an orderly and organized way, as can be revealed by micro-electrode recordings within or adjacent to cells, or by cortical or scalp electrodes of relatively large diameter integrating the changes in voltage generated by large populations of cells. The basic event common to all seizures is a paroxysmal discharge of cerebral neurones. Not all paroxysmal discharges result in overt events. For example, the electroencephalogram (EEG) of a man with epilepsy between seizures may well show spikes over one temporal lobe which represent the paroxysmal discharges of neurones. Such events, unaccompanied by any clinical phenomenon, are not generally considered to be seizures. For the definition of a seizure, therefore, it is necessary to add that the paroxysmal discharge of cerebral neurones must be apparent to either an external observer, as for example in the case of a grand mal seizure, or as an abnormal perceptual experience suffered by the subject.

Synonyms of seizure in everyday use include the words attack, fit, turn, spell, or, if resulting in jactitation, convulsions. In conversation with patients the word chosen by them can be used, but for the general usage it is best to stick to the word 'seizure', qualified by adjectives describing the type of seizure, preferably using the classification recommended by the World Health Organization. The various types of seizure are discussed on page 21.55.

In older literature, a sudden cerebrovascular event such as an intracerebral haemorrhage was called an apoplectic seizure, but the word 'seizure' now implies a paroxysmal discharge of cerebral neurones, usually but not necessarily epileptic in type. For example, a seizure induced by anoxia during some anaesthetic accident would not be regarded as epileptic in nature.

Epilepsy

For practical purposes epilepsy may be defined as a continuing tendency to epileptic seizures. For epidemiological purposes an operational definition of epilepsy is more than one non-febrile seizure of any type. The question of febrile convulsions, and their relation to epilepsy, is discussed on page 21.59.

It can immediately be seen from these definitions that confusions and inconsistencies arise. For example, a common reason for referral to neurological clinics is for assessment after the initial seizure. As is discussed on page 21.62, a significant minority do not have further seizures. These individuals should not, by definition, be described as having epilepsy until the second seizure occurs. But what of a person who has one seizure at the age of 18, and another at the age of 50? What has the diagnosis been in the intervening 32 years? Or what of a young woman aged 21 who had many seizures during her early teens, but none for the last five years? Do we say that she still has epilepsy, or that her epilepsy is in remission, or that her epilepsy has stopped? Certainly, it is known that her chances of having further seizures are greater than someone who has never had a seizure at all, and it cannot, therefore, be said that her epilepsy has definitely stopped.

Some of these inconsistencies are removed if it is realized that an epileptic seizure is just one of the very limited ways that the brain has of expressing that it is in trouble. It is a symptom, exactly as breathlessness is a symptom of various types of pulmonary insufficiency. A neuro-epidemiologist trying to make sense of the causes and prognosis of epilepsy is in exactly the same position as a respiratory epidemiologist might be if he were trying to assess the prevalence, causes, and prognosis of breathlessness, without accurate diagnostic classifications of the cause of the breathlessness. Unfortunately, most published work does not acknowledge this difficulty, and many papers on the treatment and prognosis of epilepsy group together patients of different ages, with different genetic constitutions, and seizures of different types due to a multitude of different causes.

The second point which may clarify the semantic confusion is to appreciate that any individual can be made to convulse if the stimulus is adequate. Anoxia has been mentioned above, but this is not a reliable producer of seizures. A volatile substance known as pentylene tetrazol will induce seizures in virtually 100 per cent of those who inhale it. It would clearly be non-sensical to call such people epileptics. This substance is sufficient to cause everyone to cross the threshold to convulsions. However, the threshold is of different levels for different people, and a stimulus which might be sufficient to cause a seizure in one person will leave another unscathed. Anyone can have a seizure if sufficiently provoked, but the vast majority never do. Those with a low threshold will have a

Table 1 Prevalence (per 100 000) of epileptic seizures of different types and of different degrees of activity

Activity	Seizure in last six months*	Seizure in last two years*	No siezure for two years but still on drugs*	Seizure any time in life†
Typical absences	7	7	20	240
Partial seizures	130	150	40	2100
Tonic-clonic seizures	90	160	160	1300
Any type of seizure	170	230	100	3400

* Based on sample of those with epilepsy aged over 16 (Hopkins and Scambler 1977).

† Based on Mayo Clinic study (Hauser and Kurland 1975, Table V-7).

greater tendency to seizures throughout life, a variety of stimuli at different times being sufficient to trigger the seizures.

Epileptic

People with epilepsy are understandably reluctant to be called epileptics, and the word is best avoided. Other words to avoid are epileptoid and epileptiform. The use of these words suggests that the doctor is skating round the subject and is unwilling to face the patient with the fact that he has had an epileptic seizure. If there remains doubt about the type of event witnessed, then it is best to say so.

The approach used by some psychiatrists is useful in elaborating a diagnosis of epilepsy. The diagnosis should be expanded to a short diagnostic formulation, describing the patient's present age, the age of onset of seizures, the types of seizures suffered, the present frequency of seizures of each type, the presumed causation, the associated features such as mental retardation, and the patient's present social and economic position. For example, it is not much help knowing that 'John Brown is an epileptic'; it is much more useful to know that 'John Brown, a school teacher aged 33, had his first of three generalized tonic-clonic seizures at the age of 12, the last being at the age of 31. He has, however, also continued to have frequent complex partial seizures (see page 21.56), beginning at the age of 15. These now occur about once a week. His employing education authority does not know of his seizures. The cause of his seizures is not known, but may be related to a presumed meningitic illness at the age of nine.'

Prevalence and incidence of epilepsy

There have been numerous studies in different countries of the prevalence of epilepsy in the population. The rates vary widely according to the definition chosen. Associations for patients with epilepsy usually quote a rate of about 0.5 per cent, or 500 per 100 000. However, if active epilepsy is defined as including those who have had more than one non-febrile seizure within the previous two years, and those who are on continuing anti-convulsant medication for more than one non-febrile seizure in the past, the prevalence of active epilepsy is about 700 per 100 000 in children under the age of 16 years and about 330 per 100 000 in adults (Table 1).

Figure 1 illustrates the incidence rates for new cases of epilepsy at different ages. It can be seen that the incidence of new cases is highest in infancy and in old age, but new cases can occur at any age. The average annual incidence rate for all types of seizures over a period of more than 30 years in this study was found to be 49 per 100 000 per year. It follows that, if an average lifespan is considered to be 70 years, the chances of developing epilepsy is at least $49 \times 70/100\,000$ or about 3.4 per cent. A figure in this range is supported by the findings of a study in Tonbridge, UK, in which all the medical records of a population of 6000 registered with one general practitioner were inspected. A lifetime incidence of recorded non-febrile seizures of nearly 2 per cent was found. Bearing in mind that some records are likely to have been incomplete, and the study population was made up of widely different

Table 2 Classification of epileptic seizures

Generalized seizures: more or less symmetrical, no evidence of focal onset
1 Absence seizures

    (a) Typical absences: abrupt onset and cessation of impairment of consciousness with or without automatisms, myoclonic jerks, tonic, or autonomic components. A 3 Hz spike and wave discharge is the only acceptable EEG abnormality for this diagnosis.

    (b) Atypical absences: less abrupt onset and/or cessation of consciousness, more prolonged changes in tone, EEG abnormality other than 3 Hz spike and wave discharge

2 Myoclonic seizures

    (a) Myoclonic jerks, single or multiple
    (b) Clonic seizures

3 Tonic-clonic seizures: synonyms: grand mal, major convulsion
4 Tonic seizures
5 Atonic or akinetic seizures

Partial seizures: seizures which start by activation of a group of neurones limited to one part of one hemisphere
1 Simple, without impairment of consciousness. Depending upon anatomical site of origin of seizure discharge, initial sympton may be motor, sensory, aphasic, cognitive, affective, dysmnesic, illusional, olfactory, or psychic. Synonyms include Jacksonian, temporal lobe, or psychomotor seizures according to type
2 Complex partial, with impairment of consciousness

    (a) Simple partial onset, followed by impairment of consciousness
    (b) Impairment of consciousness at onset: symptoms as in simple, above

3 Partial seizures, either simple or complex, evolving to generalized tonic-clonic seizures; synonym: secondarily generalized seizures
4 Generalized tonic-clonic seizures, with EEG but not clinical evidence of focal onset; synonym: secondarily generalized seizures

Unclassified seizures – as yet undefined

The different types of epileptic seizure

An international classification of epileptic seizures was agreed by a Commission of The International League against Epilepsy in 1969, and has now been adopted by the World Health Organization. This classification is now used in most scientific communications, but many clinicians regret the passing of the easily understood terms such as temporal lobe seizure, and psychomotor seizure. These have now become complex partial seizures. Recently modifications have been proposed to this classification. Table 2 shows these new proposals, although they have not been finally accepted.

Classification of seizure types depends upon an analysis of clinical phenomena observed during the seizure, the changes in the EEG between the seizures, the presumed anatomical substrate and aetiology, and the age of onset.

Figure 2 illustrates the two main classes of origin of seizure. In the top left of the figure, the hatched area indicates a number of neurones which are in some way abnormal, tending to discharge in paroxysms. They have the facility of driving other neurones to follow their abnormal patterns of discharge. The paths of influence of these abnormal neurones are indicated by the arrows. As long as the discharge remains in one part of the brain, the seizure is said to be a partial seizure. What happens during such a seizure depends upon the site and pattern of discharge of abnormal neurones. In Fig. 2, the abnormal focus is shown in the temporal lobe, by far the commonest site of origin of partial seizures. Clinically observed features of these and other types of partial seizures are described on page 21.56.

The abnormal discharge may spread, as is shown in the top right section of Fig. 2, through connections linking the two halves of the brain, or, by affecting poorly identified central collections of cells, initiate a generalized seizure discharge. In this case the seizure is said to be a partial seizure with secondary generalization. Some tonic-clonic (grand mal seizures) are of this type.

The lower section of Fig. 2 illustrates the second main class of seizure. In this, central collections of cells are themselves in some way abnormal in their behaviour, even though they may seem structurally sound by histological examination. Because of their central position, and the direction and power of their transmissions, a seizure discharge generated within them spreads more or less simultaneously to all parts of the brain. Such a seizure, generalized at onset, is a primary generalized seizure. Typical

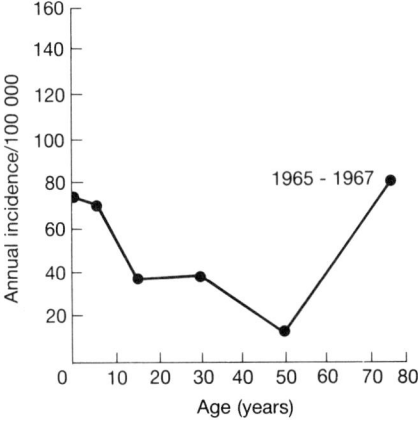

Fig. 1 The incidence of epileptic seizures at different ages. Note the relatively high incidence towards the end of life. (Redrawn from Hauser W. A. and Kurland L. T. (1975), *Epilepsia* **16**, 1.)

ages, it can be seen that epilepsy is not a rare or unusual disorder, but one which at some time in life may afflict about 1 in 30 of the population.

Another way of expressing the frequency of epilepsy is to consider that on each day in the United Kingdom 65 people suffer their first seizure. A typical British general practitioner will have under his care about four adults and three or four children who have had a seizure in the last two years, and about two adults and two children who remain on anti-convulsants for seizures in the past. In the United Kingdom there are about 136 000 adults and 90 000 children on anti-convulsants at any one time.

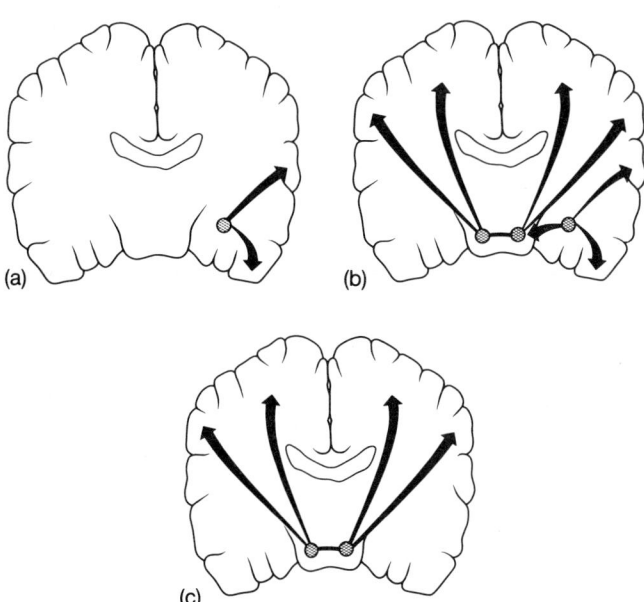

Fig. 2 Origins of different types of epileptic seizure. See text for further details.

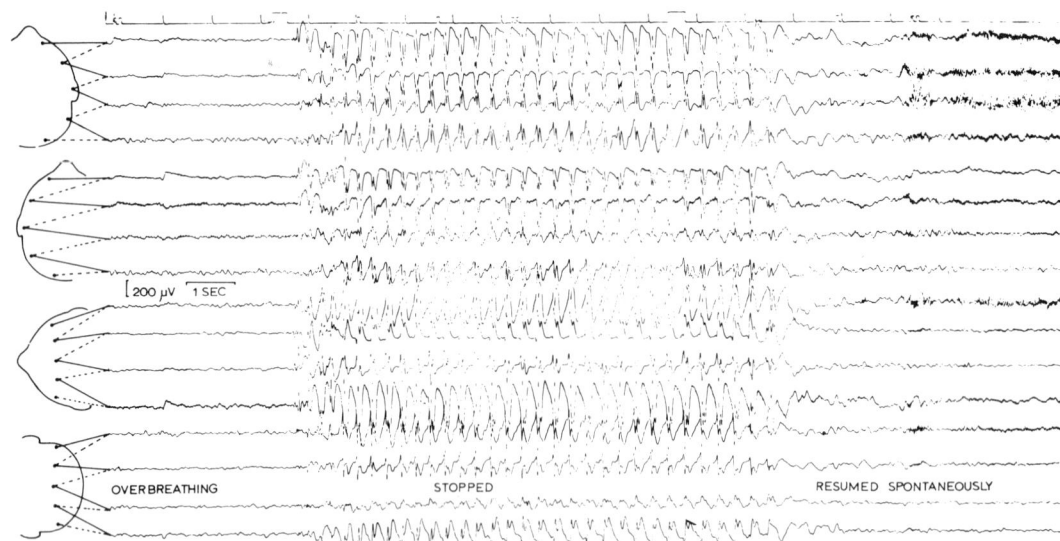

Fig. 3 Electro-encephalogram (EEG) of child during typical absences.

absences (petit mal absences) and some tonic-clonic seizures (grand mal seizures) are of this type.

Tonic-clonic seizures (grand mal seizures, generalized convulsions)
Whether the paroxysmal discharge be primary, or secondarily generalized from a cortical focus, the hallmark of a grand mal seizure is disordered muscular contraction. The first phase is known as the tonic phase. The body becomes rigid, and, as it is incapable of maintaining a normal co-ordinated posture, the subject will, if standing, fall to the ground. The chest muscles also contract, forcing the air out through the larynx in an involuntary grunt or cry. The jaw muscles also contract, and the tongue may be bitten. The absence of ventilatory movements and the high oxygen consumption of the vigorously contracting muscles result in the rapid onset of cyanosis. The face becomes suffused by desaturated blood, which is prevented from draining into the thorax by the raised intrathoracic pressure. The normal movements of swallowing are lost, so that saliva may dribble from the mouth. The disordered contraction of abdominal and sphincter muscles may result in incontinence of urine, and occasionally faeces.

After a brief time in the tonic phase, which may vary from a few seconds to a minute, the seizure passes into a clonic or convulsive phase, with rhythmic contractions of limbs and trunk muscles. The amplitude of these contractions is very variable. They continue for a few seconds to a few minutes, after which the subject lies in a deep stupor, which gradually lightens through a stage of confusion into full consciousness. After the seizure the subject may have a headache, and feel generally bruised and battered by the vigorous muscular contractions. Post-ictal confusion must be distinguished from the automatic behaviour of a seizure arising in the temporal lobe (see page 21.57).

No bystander behaves very sensibly when he first witnesses a seizure. Relatives of those with epilepsy understandably want to know what they should do during such an attack. If the origin of the tonic-clonic seizure is a partial seizure, there may be sufficient warning for the subject to be helped to a place of safety during the partial phase of the attack, or at least the relative may be able to break the subject's fall. Once on the ground the subject should be turned into the 'coma position' – that is to say into a semi-prone position – so that secretions drain from the subject's mouth, rather than into the larynx. Any vomiting that occurs will also find easy egress this way. There is no point in trying to force an object between tightly clenched teeth. The tongue is usually bitten at the onset of the seizure, the airway is not significantly improved by opening the mouth, and damage to the teeth may result from mis-

guided attempts to force a passage. It is, however, useful to give the subject a sharp clap on the back, to drive the tongue forwards. The post-ictal confusion can be minimized by acting calmly, explaining clearly to the subject what has happened, and avoiding calling an ambulance, unless injury has occurred.

Typical absences (petit mal seizures)
This description should only be given to absence attacks associated with classical 3 Hz spike and wave activity in the electro-encephalogram (see Fig. 3).

Petit mal is a disorder with onset in childhood, and attacks continuing into adult life are rare. A typical absence attack is very brief, lasting only a few seconds. The onset and termination are abrupt. The child ceases what he is doing, stares, looks a little pale, and may flutter the eyelids. Sometimes more extensive bodily movements occur, such as dropping the head forwards, and there may be a few clonic movements of the arms. Attacks are very commonly provoked by hyperventilation for three minutes or so, and this is well worth doing in the outpatient clinic or during electroencephalography.

The interruption of the normal stream of consciousness is very brief, and the child may be unaware of the attacks, as indeed may be the parents for some time after onset, assuming that the child is just daydreaming.

It is in this type of disorder that the distinction between an EEG abnormality and an overt attack becomes least clear. For example, during the EEG the child may have frequent short bursts of spike and wave activity, without any overt clinical concomitant. However, it can be shown that, if tests of abstract reasoning are administered during the course of the recording, the rate of intellectual processing is slower during the time at which the spike and wave discharges occur.

About one-third of all children with petit mal will have one or more tonic-clonic convulsions. This inter-relationship is illustrated in Fig. 4.

Partial seizures (focal seizures)
Partial seizures reflect a neuronal discharge more or less localized to one part of the brain. The exact internal perception or external manifestation depends upon the site of origin of discharge of the abnormal neurones. If these are in the motor cortex, the initial manifestation will be a contraction of the muscles in the opposite side of the body. Partial motor seizures are most likely to begin at the angle of the mouth, the index finger and thumb, or the big toe. If the seizure discharge then spreads through contiguous layers of

TYPES OF EPILEPSY
a + b = Symptomatic epilepsy
c + d = Cryptogenic epilepsy
d + e = Idiopathic epilepsy (primary generalised or constitutional epilepsy)

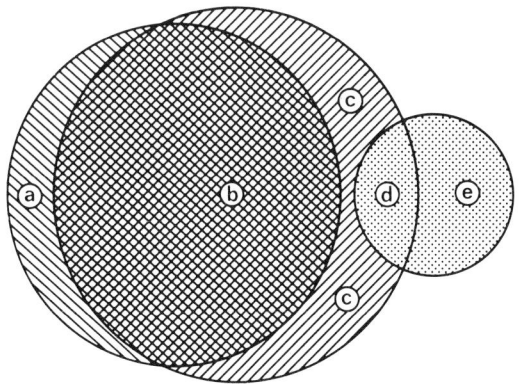

a) Partial seizures alone
b) Partial seizures evolving to tonic-clonic seizures
c) Tonic-clonic seizures of uncertain origin
d) Tonic-clonic seizures in association with typical absences
e) Typical absences alone

Fig. 4 The relationship between different types of epileptic seizure and different types of epilepsy. See text for explanation.

cortex, the clinical manifestations march into the homologous parts of the body. A seizure of this type is called a *Jacksonian seizure*, after one of the neurologists who first described them. The reason for these parts of the body being the sites at which seizures most commonly begin is partly because there are many cortical cells assigned to controlling these muscles, which are concerned with the fine tuning of manual skills and facial expression, and partly because their thresholds of excitation are lowest, as judged by direct cortical stimulation.

Another type of partial seizure associated with movement is the *versive seizure*. Version is usually away from the hemisphere in which the abnormal cells lie, so these seizures are often called *adversive*. In such an attack the eyes are deviated, followed by the head, and sometimes the whole body may turn on its own axis, often with elevation and abduction of the arm. The site of origin of such seizures is in the posterior frontal region, or, occasionally, the responsible lesion may be in the posterior part of the temporal lobe.

In the partial seizures so far described, there is an overt motor expression of the seizure. However, other groups of abnormal neurones may cause only an abnormal internal event. For example, a somatosensory seizure may result in the subject experiencing only a warmth or tingling in the limbs contralateral to the collection of abnormal neurones in the parietal cortex.

However, by far the most common type of partial seizure is that arising from a discharge of abnormal neurones in the temporal lobe. Such seizures are often called *temporal lobe seizures*, but more recently have become called *complex partial seizures*. The newly proposed classification refers to them as *partial seizures with psychic symptoms*, or with *autonomic symptoms*, or with *special-sensory symptoms*.

The seizure discharge in complex partial seizures is manifested by distortions of consciousness which range from partial loss of awareness, such that the subject is dimly aware of what is going on around him although he may be unable to reply, through to complete inaccessibility, with amnesia for events occurring during the seizure. Even in these, it may be possible to superimpose normal behaviour on the seizure, for example, the subject may be led passively to a chair, so that he can complete the seizure sitting down.

Partial seizures arising in the temporal lobe are often accompa-

nied by stereotyped motor behaviour involving the lower part of the face. Grimacing and sucking movements are quite common, and there may be rotation of the head and eyes as the seizure discharge spreads forwards. Sometimes complex stereotyped behaviour such as undressing may occur, or the patient may be able to continue walking along the road, and indeed crossing streets making appropriate judgements with regard to oncoming traffic, even though he is in the midst of a seizure.

Distorted perceptions during a partial seizure arising in the temporal lobe may give the clue to the correct diagnosis. The subject may say he is aware of a sense of unreality, even if partially aware of his surroundings. The phrase '*déjà vu*' is used to describe a sensation that what is happening around him has already occurred at some previous time. The phrase '*jamais vu*' is used to describe a perception that what is seen is so unreal that it bears no relation to the subject's previous life events. There may be a pervasive feeling of fear and dizziness; olfactory, and visual hallucinations are not uncommon. The visual hallucinations are well-formed, so that the subject may recount complex scenes, almost analogous to a film. For example, one 12-year-old boy told me that during some of his partial seizures he was aware of another boy, who was familiar in some way, although he did not know him. He saw this other boy standing the other side of a shower, and the other boy appeared to put his leg under the running water, and then the subject put his leg under the running water alternately. Such hallucinations are quite different from the ill-formed visual flashes and scotomata that may arise from migrainous phenomena, which usually affect the occipital lobe.

A very common initial symptom of a partial seizure arising in the temporal lobe is a vague feeling of discomfort in the upper abdomen, which may be accompanied by borborygmi, the discomfort rising to the chest, this then being followed by a sensation of fullness in the head as the seizure continues. Vertigo may be another symptom that occurs during a complex partial seizure arising in the temporal lobe.

The term 'aura' is often used to describe the epigastric sensation, or distorted perception. It must be realized, however, that these symptoms are the initial symptoms of the seizure itself.

As already indicated in Fig. 2, the seizure discharge of any partial seizure may become generalized. For example, a brief olfactory hallucination may be an initial symptom immediately preceding a generalized seizure. This indicates that the seizure discharge was briefly confined to one or other temporal lobe before becoming generalized. All patterns may occur. For example, on some days the patient may have a partial seizure alone, on other days a generalized tonic-clonic convulsion preceded by a partial seizure, and yet on other days the secondary generalization may be so rapid that the initial symptom is not experienced. In yet other patients, the only evidence of focal onset of a seizure may be electroencephalographic (Fig. 5).

Relationship between seizure type and types of epilepsy

Figure 4 indicates the relationship between seizure types and types of epilepsy. The term 'idiopathic' epilepsy is often used when there is no apparent cause for the seizure. More prolonged EEG recordings, using various activating techniques (see page 21.1), and the advent of cranial computed scanning have shown that many tonic-clonic seizures previously considered to be idiopathic arise from a structural lesion. Partial seizures always arise from some focal area of structural abnormality in the brain, and if such exists, the epilepsy is clearly symptomatic of such structural lesion, even though the lesion may be clinically unimportant, such as a small area of atrophy in one temporal lobe. The term idiopathic epilepsy has been replaced by primary generalized epilepsy. In this type, the epileptic seizures are generalized from the onset, either taking the form of tonic-clonic seizures, or typical absences, or just the myoclonus associated with absences. The characteristic 3 Hz spike and wave activity, illustrated in Fig. 3, is the hallmark of this type of epilepsy.

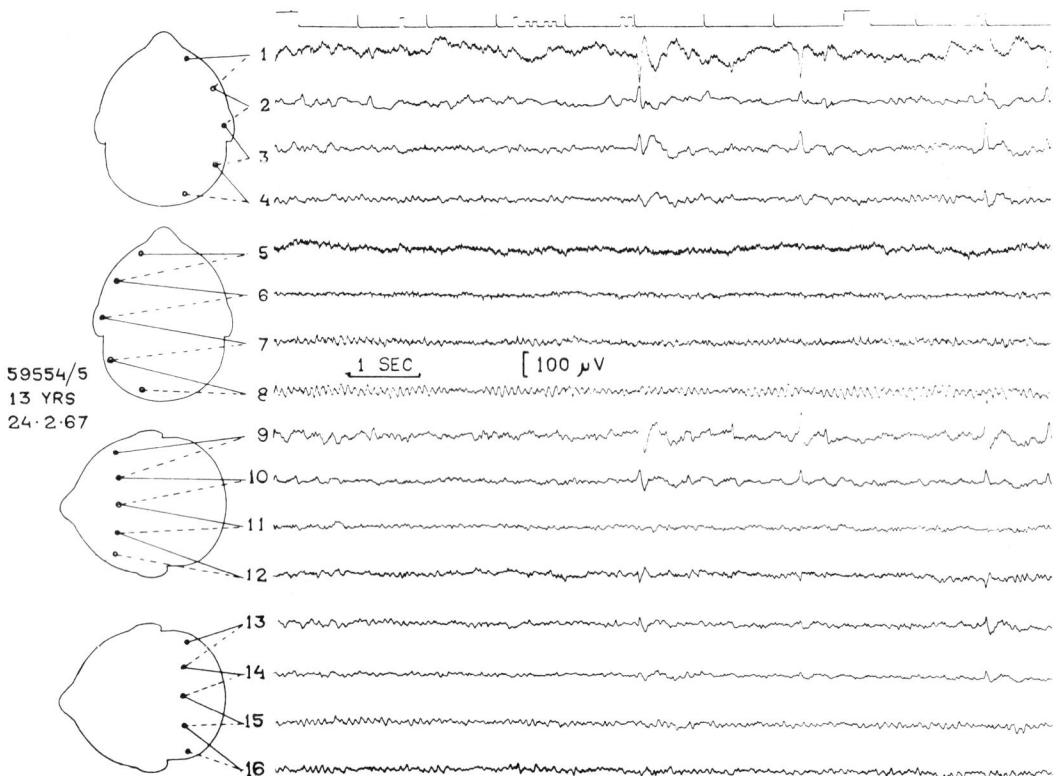

Fig. 5 Interictal EEG on a child with temporal lobe epilepsy. Note the sharp spike followed by a slow wave recorded focally from the right anterior temporal region.

Sometimes it is not possible to be certain whether generalized tonic-clonic seizures are on the basis of primary generalized epilepsy, in which the EEG happens not to have shown any seizure discharge at the time of the recording, or alternatively the tonic-clonic seizures are very rapidly generalized from a focus which is clinically silent. Such 'cryptogenic' cases should not, however, be called idiopathic.

Table 1 shows the prevalence of seizures of different types in a sample of adults drawn from the lists of general practitioners in Metropolitan London. In this study, 56 per cent of the sample had had partial seizures at some time. In a further 12 per cent, even though partial seizures by themselves had not occurred, there was clear clinical evidence of partial onset, or EEG evidence of focal onset to the generalized tonic-clonic seizure. Even without the benefit of CT scanning there was, therefore, evidence of a focal and presumably structural origin for the attacks in nearly 70 per cent of the subjects. It is clear from this that in an adult sample true idiopathic epilepsy, as defined above, is rare. Even if a survey is confined to children of school age, only 12 per cent are found to have had petit mal seizures.

Rarer types of seizures

Atypical absences occur. They may be clinically indistinguishable from a typical absence, but show EEG discharges that are different from the 3 Hz spike and wave discharge illustrated in Fig. 3. A common associated feature with an atypical absence is known as a 'recruiting epileptic rhythm', which is initially rapid and of low amplitude, but then gradually becomes slower and of higher amplitude. Another variant is disordered spike and wave complexes at a rate slower than the classical frequency of 3 Hz. Such petit mal variant absences are often associated with mental retardation, and evidence of cerebral atrophy, and a much worse prognosis for seizure control. This is sometimes known as the *Lennox–Gastaut* syndrome (see page 21.235).

Sometimes *tonic* seizures occur. In these there is a tonic posturing of all limbs, or just the limbs on one side of the body. Such

seizures occur in multiple sclerosis on rare occasions, and in some of the lipidoses of childhood.

In *infantile spasms*, there is a brief sudden flexion of the head, trunk, and limbs, as if the infant is bowing a 'salaam'. These are, therefore, sometimes known as salaam seizures. These seizures are often accompanied by failure of development and progressive retardation. The EEG is characteristic, distinguished by irregular high-voltage, diffuse, slow spike and wave complexes that are repeated at brief intervals on high-voltage slow background rhythms. *Myoclonic epilepsy* is considered on pages 21.210 and 21.235.

Causes of epilepsy

Inheritance

Until about 30 years ago, it was believed that inheritance was a major factor in causing epilepsy. This belief is still strong amongst patients, who often express surprise when told of the diagnosis of epilepsy because 'there is nothing like that in the family'. The strength of the belief that inheritance was a major factor caused some of the States of America and some Scandinavian countries to promulgate laws forbidding those with epilepsy to marry.

It is certainly true that inheritance does play some part. For example, seizures may be a feature of some of the recessively inherited lipidoses such as the ceroid lipofuscinoses, and Tay–Sachs disease. These seizures are often myoclonic in character.

Epileptic seizures may also be a manifestation of dominantly inherited disorders such as neurofibromatosis, tuberose sclerosis, and Lafora body disease. In these disorders, and in the recessively inherited disorders listed above, the seizures are only one manifestation of a diffuse cerebral dysfunction, in which retardation with progressive dementia are major features. Of perhaps greater interest for epilepsy as a whole is the good evidence that primary generalized epilepsy is also probably inherited as an autosomal dominant disorder. It has been shown that the characteristic EEG with spike-wave discharges occurring at 3 Hz is seen in about 40

Table 3 Identified causes of epilepsy in three studies

Cause	Study 1* (%)	Study 2† (%)	Study 3‡ (%)
Birth trauma and anoxia	2.5	6.3	
Cranial injury; post-operative	3.6	7.0	
Infections	2.9	3.2	
Vascular	5.2	3.2	
Tumours	4.1	3.2	
Congenital	2.3	1.1	
'Uncomplicated epilepsy'			74
'Epilepsy in association with structural brain disorder'			26
Total	20.6	24.0	

* Hauser and Kurland. Rochester, Minnesota. 516 cases of epilepsy presenting 1935–67. All ages.
† Hopkins and Scambler. London. 94 cases of epilepsy prevalent in 1973 on the lists of 17 general practitioners. Age over 16.
‡ Rutter and colleagues. Isle of Wight. 86 cases of epilepsy prevalent in 1965. Aged 5–14.

per cent of siblings of children with primary generalized epilepsy, even if they have not had any overt seizures. A smaller proportion of the parents of children with primary generalized epilepsy will also show the characteristic EEG seizure discharge. From sequential studies of children with 3 Hz spike and wave discharges it is clear that these become much less frequent with age, so the absence of discharges in adult life does not mean that the parent did not have unrecorded and unapparent discharges in childhood.

If a sibling of a child with primary generalized epilepsy has 3 Hz spike and wave discharges, it does not necessarily follow that overt seizures will occur.

This variability in clinical expression of the inherited EEG discharge accounts for the occurrence of primary generalized epilepsy in a child of parents neither of whom has ever had an overt seizure. The trait is expressed by seizures in only about one-third of the children to whom it is transmitted.

Genetic factors are also important in the causation of *febrile convulsions*. Twin studies have shown that if one of identical twins has a febrile convulsion, then the other has an 80 per cent chance of having a similar episode. A non-identical twin or sibling of a child who has had a febrile convulsion has about a 25 per cent chance of having one, a likelihood several times higher than that for the population as a whole. In so far as severe and prolonged febrile convulsions may lead to hippocampal sclerosis, which then forms a focus of origin for seizures in later life, it can be seen that temporal lobe seizures may have a genetic basis in part, even though their cause is due to structural brain damage. It has also been shown that those suffering severe head injuries are more likely to develop post-traumatic epilepsy if there is a family history of epilepsy.

It is possible that there is a 'convulsive threshold', the level of which is genetically determined, probably by the interaction of a number of genes. If this is the case, it is difficult to be dogmatic about assigning 'causes' for epilepsy. There are, however, some events which are so typically followed by the development of epilepsy, that it is clear that the event is playing a major role in the genesis of seizures (Table 3). These are now discussed.

Trauma

Penetrating injuries such as those caused by shrapnel or rifle bullets in wartime are a potent cause of epilepsy. However, in civilian life most head injuries are caused by road traffic accidents and industrial accidents, and result from some deceleration injury to the brain transmitted through the skull without any penetration of the skull itself. Trivial head injuries are one of the commonest causes for attendance at Accident and Emergency Departments, but very few result in the later development of epilepsy.

W. B. Jennett has done a great deal to separate out those factors in a head injury that are most likely to be associated with the subsequent development of epilepsy. His findings are summarized in Fig. 6. Important factors are listed underneath the bar chart. Post-traumatic amnesia is that period for which the patient, albeit possibly conscious, is not recording in his memory on-going events, even though he may appear to be behaving rationally at that time. The duration of post-traumatic amnesia may vary from a few seconds or minutes, when the term concussion is often applied, to many weeks or even months. Obviously, the longer durations of post-traumatic amnesia are usually associated with significant impairment of consciousness in the early stages. However, it should be realized that substantial head injuries may occur without any major interruption in consciousness. It can be seen from the bar chart that, even if the other factors were not present, long post-traumatic amnesia was followed by the development of epilepsy in a substantial proportion of cases. If local cortical damage is added to the head injury, as may occur if there is a depressed fracture with a dural tear, or if the head injury is sufficiently severe that focal neurological signs develop, then the addition of these two other factors increases the risk of the later development of post-traumatic epilepsy to approximately 40 per cent. If there was no dural tear, no focal neurological signs, and the post-traumatic amnesia had lasted less than 24 hours, the risk of the subsequent development of epilepsy was about 2 per cent in the follow up period, probably not different from that of the risk of the general population.

Another factor that Jennett defined as being of considerable importance was the occurrence of a seizure in the first week after a head injury. It may be that such an early seizure is just the marker of an inherited low convulsive threshold. In any event it proved to be a potent predictor of late post-traumatic epilepsy, as is shown in the bar chart.

There are, of course, other types of cranial trauma apart from that caused by road traffic and industrial accidents. Trauma may occur at the time of birth, either through direct cerebral compression as the head is moulded through the birth canal, or there may be significant intra-cranial haemorrhage, resulting in the development of a glial scar, the edge of which is capable of generating seizures. Alternatively, the cause of the cerebral injury in the perinatal period may be anoxia. Perinatal injury, whatever the cause, is one of the commonest reasons for the association of cerebral palsy and epilepsy, or mental retardation and epilepsy. It is probably this association which had led, at least in part, to popular misconceptions about those with epilepsy, though fortunately improvements in obstetric care have made these events less frequent.

Tumours

Older textbooks of medicine stress the need for intensive investigation of patients with 'epilepsy of late onset'. The implication is

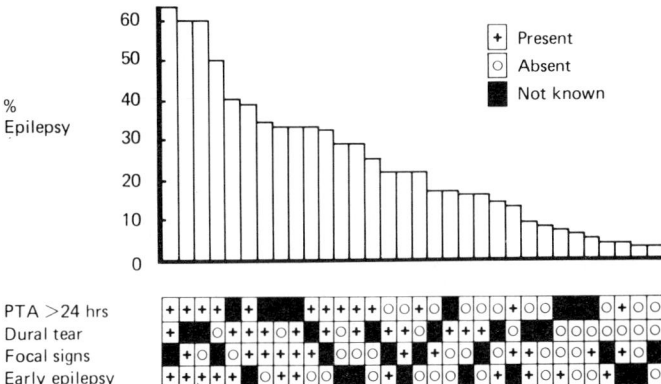

Fig. 6 Incidence of late epilepsy after compound depressed fracture of the skull when three or four factors were known. (Redrawn from Jennett, W. B. (1970), *Epilepsy after non-missile head injuries*. Heinemann, London.) PTA = post-traumatic amnesia.

that epilepsy of late onset is unusual, and frequently due to a tumour, which should not be missed. However, it is now realized, and demonstrated in Fig. 1, that the age specific incidence curve is more or less flat between the ages of 10 and 59, rising sharply thereafter. The cause of the steep increase in older age is the increasing proportion of patients with seizures due to neuronal degenerations and cerebrovascular disease. Tumours play only a comparatively small part (see Table 3). Furthermore, in practice 'missing' a primary cerebral tumour is not quite so devastating as most non-neurologists would believe. Many cerebral tumours are metastatic, usually from bronchus or breast, and as such are clearly a manifestation of disseminated malignant disease for which treatment is largely ineffective even if early diagnosis of dissemination is made. Furthermore, the results of surgical removal or irradiation of astrocytomas is disappointing, and in many cases a neurologist will advise against operation even if the epilepsy has clearly been demonstrated to be due to tumour. Benign epileptogenic tumours such as meningiomas make up less than 10 per cent of all intracerebral tumours.

Infectious diseases

Bacterial meningitis may scar the cortical mantle, resulting in the subsequent development of seizures. Acute bacterial infections in the form of a cerebral abscess may also cause seizures in association with the abscess. Even if the abscess is drained and heals, the thick-walled gliotic scar may well cause seizures subsequently. It is for this reason that cerebral abscesses are often excised after they have been drained.

Viral encephalitis may cause seizures during the acute illness, and subsequent seizures after the initial infection has passed. In England the commonest identified cause is the herpes simplex virus. Persistent viral infection such as occurs in subacute sclerosing pan-encephalitis, in which the measles virus persists after an initial infection, may also be accompanied by generalized seizures and myoclonus.

Echinococcal cysts, cysticercosis, toxocariasis, and toxoplasmosis are, in the United Kingdom, rarer causes of seizures, though some consider that widespread contamination of children's playing fields by *Toxocara canis* is an important cause of epilepsy in childhood.

Degenerative disorders

As already noted, the incidence of seizures increases in old age. They occur in Alzheimer's disease, although usually they are overshadowed by the social and intellectual deterioration.

Vascular disease

Seizures may certainly result from embolic infarcts. For example, in mitral valve disease, cerebral emboli may be the result of thrombus formation in the left atrium. Furthermore, after replacement of a diseased valve by some types of prosthesis, cerebral embolism may occur after thrombus formation on the new valve. Seizures may also result from emboli following myocardial infarction, or from atheromatous emboli in association with carotid artery disease.

Presumably all these vascular causes have in common their ability to damage the brain by anoxia. Occasionally diffuse cerebral anoxia, such as may follow a transient cardiac arrest, may result in subsequent epilepsy.

CT scanning shows a considerable excess of infarcts in the brains of those whose epilepsy starts later in life compared to scans of controls matched for age. These infarcts are often deep-seated lacunes, sometimes clinically silent except for the epilepsy. Deep lacunar infarction (page 21.162) probably does not in itself cause the seizures, but is merely a marker of more widespread vascular disease.

Alcohol

Chronic abuse of alcohol may result in seizures which then continue even if the subject abstains. Seizures also occur sometimes in acute alcohol intoxication.

Reversible causes of seizures

Apart from the example of acute alcohol intoxication noted above, it is well recognized that some drugs may precipitate seizures. The drugs in everyday use that have been most often incriminated include phenothiazines and tricyclic antidepressants. Other reversible metabolic causes of seizures include hypoglycaemia, most usually induced by exogenous insulin used in the treatment of diabetes, hypocalcaemia, particularly in neonates, and uraemia. Hyperglycaemia has also been reported recently as a cause of partial seizures.

Table 3 illustrates the causes of seizures suffered by 516 consecutive patients investigated at a large American hospital. Note that an identifiable cause could only be discovered in approximately one-fifth of all cases. A very similar distribution of causes was found in London.

Precipitants of seizures

Distinct from the causes of a continuing tendency to seizures are those factors which may precipitate an attack. For example, many patients with epilepsy say that they have more seizures when they are upset or worried; conversely some, particularly those with complex seizures, if they are relaxed, and their mind is not concentrating on any particular task. Other precipitants include alcohol and drugs as already mentioned above, menstruation, lack of sleep, and intercurrent illness. All these precipitants may prove very 'personal'. That is to say although staying up late may precipitate seizures the following day in one child, this is not true of every child, and the remote possibility of seizures being caused by everyday events should not be used by parents as an excuse to cocoon their child in a protective web of inaction.

Although lack of sleep may precipitate seizures the following day, drowsiness and sleep may allow seizures to 'escape'. Indeed drowsiness is such a potent activator of abnormal discharges in the EEG that the recordist will often encourage the subject to try to go to sleep during the recording. In some patients with epilepsy, seizures are virtually confined to the hours of sleep. However, one follow-up study of those who said that they had always had nocturnal grand mal showed that approximately one-third of them had an attack during waking hours within the next five years.

In some subjects, precipitants of the seizures are so potent and so stereotyped as to warrant the name 'reflex epilepsy'. Many such cases are amongst the curiosities of medicine, for example, the subject who has a seizure only when he hears church bells, or on reading, or on looking at repetitive patterns such as squares of linoleum tiling. It may be presumed that the perception of such external stimuli results in a particular pattern of neuronal discharge—indeed this is presumably in part how we recognize patterns, tunes, and words. One can only imagine that this particular set of neuronal discharge in susceptible people acts as a specific template which, like a key in a lock, unlooses a seizure.

The commonest type of reflex epilepsy is *television epilepsy*. This is not due to any malfunction of the set, but susceptible children may have seizures induced by the normal traverse of the spot down the face of the tube. Such children are most at risk when the screen occupies a considerable proportion of the visual field, as will occur if the size of the screen is large, and the child sits close to it. It has been shown that observing the set with one eye covered prevents the occurrence of these seizures.

Differential diagnosis of seizures

A considerable part of the work-load of a neurologist is sorting out 'funny turns' or 'blackouts' of some sort. Before embarking upon anticonvulsant treatment, it is therefore essential to ensure that such complaints are due to a paroxysmal discharge of cerebral neurones – a seizure – and not some other event. What other events have to be considered?

Syncopal attacks (see page 21.51)

Syncope is distinguished from a seizure principally by the circumstances in which the event occurs. Syncope never occurs in bed and rarely in the horizontal position. Micturition syncope can be diagnosed by its characteristic history. It occurs when a man gets out of bed at night to pass urine, and, usually just after completing the act of micturition, he suddenly loses consciousness. It has been shown that not only is there the postural fall of blood-pressure resulting from the assumption of the erect posture, but at the onset of micturition there is a reflex vasodilatation in the legs. Loss of consciousness occurring in crowded trains, waiting at bus stops, or in school assembly, should always be presumed to be syncopal in nature unless there is clearcut evidence to the contrary. These are circumstances in which many of us have felt unwell, and may indeed lose consciousness, particularly during adolescence.

The type of symptoms experienced before loss of consciousness may help in reaching the correct diagnosis. For a minute or two before fainting, the subject will usually feel nauseated, cold, and clammy. It should be noted that a sensation of 'voices being distant' or 'feeling far away' often occurs before syncope, although such phrases may suggest the distorted consciousness sometimes found with complex partial seizures.

Cardiac arrhythmia

A falling cardiac output due to a bradycardia or paroxysmal tachycardia may lead to a disturbance of consciousness with symptoms similar to syncope, but occurring in circumstances when syncope is unlikely, such as whilst reading quietly in a chair. Distinction between such cases and epileptic seizures may be singularly difficult, especially if no bystander observes the pulse during the attack. Holter monitoring may detect transient disturbances of cardiac rhythm with or without associated neurological disturbances.

The frequency with which such cases are diagnosed depends on the clinic from which the cases are reported, but in at least one series disturbances of cardiac rhythm were shown to account for about one-fifth of all cases of transiently disturbed consciousness originally believed to be neurological in nature.

Transient ischaemic attacks

Transient ischaemic attacks, although causing a focal disturbance of neurological function, are essentially 'negative' phenomena. That is to say they are manifest by an absence of function, usually with little disturbance of consciousness. Jactitation is not seen (see page 21.157).

Migraine

Migraine (see page 21.28) is another type of transient disturbance of cerebral function in which positive phenomena such as visual hallucinations may occur. However, such hallucinations are virtually always ill-formed, classically scintillating scotomata rather than the formed visual hallucination which may be part of a complex partial seizure. If the area of cortical ischaemia is further forward in the hemisphere, then the symptomatology is like that of a transient ischaemic attack with weakness, numbness, or disturbance of the functions of language.

Narcolepsy and cataplexy

The relationship, if any, between these fascinating conditions (see page 21.67) and epileptic seizures is obscure, and the diagnosis is seldom missed once it is thought of. A narcoleptic episode is usually preceded by an intense desire to sleep, however short-lived, against which the subject fights. This is not an initial symptom of any type of epileptic attack.

Furthermore, the association of narcolepsy with cataplexy – the sudden loss of postural tone precipitated by anger or laughter – is so characteristic that little doubt remains. It is also worth enquiring about the other rarer associated symptoms of sleep paralysis and hypnagogic hallucinations.

Drop attacks

Drop attacks are not infrequent in middle-aged women. They say that whilst walking they suddenly fall to their knees, without any

disturbance of consciousness. There is no warning of the event, and they are able to get up as soon as they recover their composure. Although many textbooks suggest that vertebro-basilar ischaemia is a cause of these episodes, the distribution of ages and sex affected is so different from that in which arterial disease is found that it is hard to believe that this is really an important factor. Whatever the cause, the attacks usually disappear after a year or two, and it is clear that they have no relation to epilepsy.

Night terrors

Night terrors in children may sometimes be mistaken for epileptic attacks. These affect children aged between about six and eight, who, while sleeping soundly, suddenly awaken wide-eyed, screaming, and inconsolable. They are amnesic for the events the following morning. They seem to occur just as often in happy children as in children who are not doing well at school or in the family. Fortunately they, too, pass quickly, and once thought of, the diagnosis is quite straightforward.

Breath-holding attacks

Breath-holding attacks affect much younger children, aged between one and two years. A typical story is of a child who has some minor injury, or who is crossed in some way so that he becomes suddenly angry, upset, or frightened. He cries vigorously once or twice, and then holds his breath at the end of one expiration. After a few seconds he becomes cyanosed, and then loses consciousness, lying limply. One or two jerks may occur, and then normal respiration and consciousness resume. The association with frustration, rage, or a sudden injury is the most useful pointer to the correct diagnosis. Again, such attacks terminate spontaneously without treatment.

Tics, habits, and ritualistic movements

These usually begin at about the age of seven or eight, and affect principally the upper part of the face, are bilateral, and are not associated with any disturbance of consciousness. Although the child has a compulsion to undertake such movements, they can be controlled, at least for a brief interval, by command. Sometimes infants indulge in repetitive rocking movements of the trunk which are believed to be masturbatory.

Vertigo

Vertigo, especially if profound, as may be experienced in the course of a paroxysm of Menière's disease, may be mistaken for a seizure. It is true that vertigo may rarely be an initial symptom in a seizure arising from the posterior temporal lobe, but a competent otological examination will usually reveal peripheral labyrinthine causes for vertigo.

Overbreathing (hyperventilation)

Anxiety or stress may result, particularly in adolescent girls, in hyperventilation with resulting respiratory alkalosis, decline in the proportion of ionized calcium, and tetanic posturing of the hands and clouding of consciousness. Such symptoms are rapidly relieved by asking the subject to rebreath his expired air in and out of a paper or polythene bag.

Simulated seizures

Simulated seizures are often a problem in differential diagnosis, especially in those who undoubtedly have some true seizures. Simulated attacks may be used as an attention-seeking device by those with epilepsy, or by siblings or school-friends of those with epilepsy. It can be surprisingly difficult to distinguish true from simulated seizures. Perhaps the best guide is that the simulator tends to overplay the seizure, and the temporal coincidence of seizures whenever there is a suitable observer. Features such as injury, tongue-biting, and incontinence can be, and often are, simulated. If serum can be obtained about 20 min after a true seizure, serum prolactins of four or five times the normal level will be found; the level returns to normal within 24 hours. Elevated serum prolactins will be found shortly after true tonic-clonic seizures and complex partial seizures, but not after simulated seizures, nor after true partial seizures arising in parts of the brain other than the temporal lobe.

The investigation of seizures

Once a clinical diagnosis of a seizure has been made, it is reasonable to consider whether any further investigation will be useful. There are three principal reasons for such investigation: (a) to improve the certainty with which the diagnosis of a seizure is correct (rather than some other event, as considered above); (b) to ascertain the type of seizure, which is important when considering appropriate medication; and (c) to ascertain the cause of seizures, in case treatment of the underlying cause is necessary. It is important to bear these three entirely separate concepts in mind. There is no point whatsoever in undertaking a ritual EEG in the case of a man of 35 who has had his first grand mal seizure approximately seven months after a major head injury. In this clearcut example, the EEG is almost certain to be abnormal in some way, and the recording will not aid either diagnosis of the cause, or future management. Electro-encephalography is, however, a useful tool for distinguishing the various types of seizure. Sometimes there may be some confusion between disturbances of consciousness due to typical absences, and disturbances due to complex partial seizures. If abnormalities are seen during the recordings from two patients with such seizure types, and there almost certainly will be a recorded spike and wave discharge in someone with frequent typical absences, then a clearcut distinction between the two types of seizures can be made. This is important not only for the correct choice of therapy (see page 21.63) but also for prognosis (see page 21.65).

Figure 3 shows the EEG for a girl aged eight with typical absences. The complexes of spikes and slow waves occurred during overbreathing at a frequency of 3 Hz. Consciousness was disturbed during this episode which lasted for about ten seconds, in so far as she spontaneously stopped overbreathing during the discharge, and resumed thereafter. Figure 5 shows the EEG of a girl aged thirteen who had experienced brief blank spells lasting two to three seconds during the previous two years. Channels 1, 2, 3, 9, and 10 all show the occurrence of the spike followed by a slow-wave occurring three times in the ten seconds of recording. From the positions of the electrodes shown diagrammatically on the left of the record, it can be seen that all the channels that show the spike are derived from electrodes on the right side of the head, from the scalp overlying the anterior temporal lobe. The spikes in channels 1 and 2 are virtually mirror images. This reversal of phase between the two channels indicates that the abnormal discharges are propagated from a group of neurones in close proximity to the electrode common to both channels.

Both the records illustrated show unequivocal abnormalities. A great majority of records from those with epilepsy, however, show changes which are much less open to easy interpretation. There is a danger of over-reporting records such that minor asymmetries in temporal rhythms are considered to be 'diagnostic'.

There is seldom any indication for serial EEG records. Improvement in seizure control is not necessarily accompanied by improvement in any underlying abnormality in the EEG. Furthermore, abnormalities on the EEG in adults have proved to be no predictor of subsequent relapse on stopping anticonvulsant therapy, though in children relapse is more likely if the EEG is abnormal when the anticonvulsants are discontinued.

It must be clearly understood that the EEG does not prove, nor disprove the diagnosis of epilepsy. The record can be normal in someone with undoubted epilepsy. There is always the danger that a doctor, hovering on the brink of making a diagnosis of epilepsy, may be tipped into making a 'definite' diagnosis of epilepsy by the presence of marginal abnormalities on the EEG. If the record does show clearcut paroxysmal activity, then this does lend considerable support to the diagnosis. If the record shows only a minor excess of slower rhythms, and the report reads that the

record is 'compatible with epilepsy', then the doctor and his patient are no further forward in establishing any diagnosis.

Whatever its limitations, the EEG is the best current available method of recording cerebral function. Recent studies using cyclotron generated radioactive oxygen are of great theoretical interest in so far as they can provide images and direct measurements of local areas of abnormal cerebral metabolism. However, the lack of ready availability of this technique due to the need for a cyclotron is clearly going to confine the method to a few research centres.

Computerized axial tomography (see page 21.4) is the best current method of detecting abnormalities of cerebral structure. As scanners become more readily available, it will be difficult to decide which patients should be scanned, and which should not. Clearly anyone with recent onset of seizures in association with physical signs warrants a CT scan as the seizures must be a manifestation of some abnormality of cerebral structure. A subject whose seizures seem difficult to control, or whose seizures change in pattern also should have a CT scan. As already pointed out on page 21.59, a large proportion of those with epilepsy have seizures arising from a structural abnormality of the brain, and it follows that some of these will be sufficiently large to be shown up on the scan.

Other radiological investigations are still occasionally employed in the management of epilepsy. Plain films of the skull seldom give any information more relevant than that obtained by scanning. Air encephalography is now seldom indicated. Arteriography may be indicated if scanning has shown evidence of an angioma or a tumour for which operation is being considered.

It is unusual for any test on the blood to be helpful in elucidating the cause of epilepsy in adults. Occasionally, a blood alcohol estimation without warning may be fruitful, or a serological test for syphilis. However, abnormalities of glucose, calcium, magnesium, or amine metabolism in young children may be revealed by appropriate tests.

Lumbar puncture is only very rarely required in the investigation of epilepsy per se, although it may of course be needed if seizures occur on a background in which meningitis or some other acute illness is suspected.

Direct histological examination of cerebral tissue is not usually undertaken, although it may be justified in exceptional circumstances. However, biopsy of the skin abnormalities associated with tuberose sclerosis or neurofibromatosis may confirm a previously suspected diagnosis. Rectal biopsy may be useful, in so far as abnormal lipids may be deposited in the neurones in the submucosal plexus.

Treatment of epilepsy

Prescription of anticonvulsant drugs

Seven useful principles of anticonvulsant therapy are listed in Table 4.

The first point is to reconsider the decision as to whether anticonvulsants should be given. It is not unusual to meet subjects with rare seizures occurring at intervals of three to seven years, and in these circumstances many patients quite reasonably prefer to take no medication at all. Clearly, the likely social effects of subsequent seizures, on employment and on eligibility to hold a driving licence may influence the subjects in this regard.

Most patients will go to their doctor after their first tonic-clonic seizure, and the doctor will then have to decide whether it is worth advising anticonvulsant treatment at this stage. In a report of US Navy personnel who had had one seizure, follow-up study showed that about two-thirds had a subsequent seizure within the next three years. In spite of this, the usual practice is to treat the first seizure only if a second would have serious effects upon the subject's life and work.

Choice of anticonvulsant drug

The first factor to consider is the type of seizure. It is well-worth

Table 4 The seven principles of anticonvulsant therapy

1 Consider decision: should anticonvulsants be given anyway?
2 Choose a drug, considering the following factors:
    The seizure type(s)
    Age
    The possibility of pregnancy
    Interaction with other drugs
    Price
3 Give only one drug, except in unusual circumstances
4 Begin chosen drug in modest dosage
5 Give full information to the patient about:
    The names and alternative names of the drug supplied
    The initial dosage schedule with dates of planned changes in dosage
    The need for compliance with instructions
    Adverse effects of the drugs
6 Monitor progress
    Inform subject of date and place of next review
    Monitor seizure frequency
    Monitor unwanted side-effects of drugs
    Monitor blood level of drug
7 Determine policy for termination of treatment

Table 5 Anticonvulsant drugs of choice for seizure types

Seizure type	Anticonvulsant drugs of choice	Therapeutic levels in serum (μmol/l)*	Typical adult dose per day (mg)
Typical absences (petit mal)	Sodium valproate		1500
	Ethosuximide	285–850	1000
	Clonazepam		2–4
Myoclonic and akinetic seizures	Sodium valproate		1500
	Nitrazepam		
	Clonazepam		2–4
Tonic-clonic seizures (grand mal) in association with typical absences (petit mal)	Sodium valproate		1800
	Phenytoin	28–100	300
	Phenobarbitone	65–170	90
Tonic-clonic seizures (grand mal) in association with partial seizures, or partial seizures alone	Carbamazepine	17–42	600
	Phenytoin	40–100	300
	Phenobarbitone	65–170	90
	Primidone		750
Infantile spasms	ACTH		
	Nitrazepam		

* The level below which therapeutic effects are unlikely to occur and above which toxic effects are likely to occur.

categorizing the type as accurately as possible, using a combination of clinical history and electroencephalography. Table 5 shows the anticonvulsant drugs of choice for seizures of different types, typical adult dosage per day, and therapeutic levels which represent a reasonable target.

Carbamazepine (Tegretol) This drug was introduced in the early 1960s and has gained increasingly wide acceptance for the treatment of partial seizures, and for tonic-clonic seizures with partial onset. It is reasonably free of side effects. A few patients develop a skin rash within a few days of starting the drug. Very rare cases of marrow depression have occurred. Sedation is relatively slight. There is a roughly linear relationship between oral dose and serum level. This means that it is a comparatively simple matter to increase the oral dose based upon a knowledge of past serum levels, without significant danger of intoxication.

Phenytoin (Epanutin, Dilantin) This is a successful drug for the treatment of tonic-clonic seizures, and to a lesser extent for partial seizures. Because the enzymes responsible for hydroxylating phenytoin may become saturated, a small increment in phenytoin dosage may result in a large increase in serum level. For this

reason it is relatively difficult to predict an appropriate increase in oral dosage towards a target serum level, although, now that experience has increased, this can usually be accomplished without major difficulty. Nomograms have been published to aid these calculations.

Phenytoin has significant drawbacks in young people. It causes hirsuties, coarsening of the facies, hypertrophy of the gums, and acne. More unusual side-effects result from the increased hepatic levels of hydroxylating enzymes induced by phenytoin. These enzymes not only hydroxylate phenytoin, but also steroid hormones, including vitamin D. Osteomalacia and rickets may result in rare circumstances, if the subject has a relatively low exposure to sunlight, or a pigmented skin. Oestrogens in contraceptive pills may also be hydroxylated in excess, resulting in inadequate contraception.

Skin rashes may also occur with phenytoin. Overdosage may result in marked sedation, but sometimes a cerebellar syndrome is seen before significant sedation occurs. Tremor, ataxia, and nystagmus are features of this. Another unusual manifestation of intoxication is chorea. Prolonged phenytoin medication may result in a neuropathy, a cerebellar degeneration, and induction of Dupuytren's contracture.

In spite of this rather alarming list, a great deal is known about this drug, serum levels are relatively easily measured, and many patients have their epilepsy successfully controlled by modest doses.

Sodium valproate (Epilim, Depakine) This is the most successful recently introduced anticonvulsant. It was widely used in France and Italy in the 1960s but only became available in England in the middle 1970s. Since then it has become the drug of choice for primary generalized epilepsy (typical absences and tonic-clonic seizures associated with typical absences). It is also worth trying if carbamazepine and phenytoin have failed in the management of partial seizures.

The drug should be introduced, like all anticonvulsant drugs, in a relatively low dosage and increased to a maximum of 2.5 g daily. Many patients are controlled on less than this. There is now good evidence that the clinical effect does not bear any relationship to the serum level, which in any event fluctuates markedly after the ingestion of each tablet. Presumably the drug is bound to an intracellular component, as the anticonvulsant effect may long outlast its administration.

Sodium valproate is usually relatively trouble-free, but a small number of patients develop an acute hepatitis. It is impossible to predict who will develop this, but it is clear that the drug should be avoided in those with a history of liver disease, and the manufacturers recommend that tests of liver function should be carried out as the dosage is increased. In high dosage the drug may cause tremor, but this is rapidly relieved by reducing the dose. Even at average doses, however, a significant side-effect is some thinning of the hair. Fortunately the hair regrows even if the drug is continued, but the newly produced hair may be unusually curly.

Phenobarbitone Phenobarbitone is undoubtedly an effective anticonvulsant, and may be worth a trial if the newer drugs have failed to control seizures. However, it is certainly not a drug of first choice as older people may become depressed and confused, and children excitable and irritable on this drug. Those in middle-age often state that they feel unpleasantly sedated even on moderate dosage.

Primidone (Mysoline) Primidone is an effective anticonvulsant. This is probably largely because it is metabolized to phenobarbitone, although another metabolite (phenyl-ethyl malonamide) also has anticonvulsant activity. If primidone is chosen, it should be commenced at a low dosage, and increased gradually, or else sedation may be severe. Even a quarter of a 250 mg tablet twice a day is not too cautious a beginning for an adult.

Clonazepam (Rivotril) Clonazepam is a benzodiazepine which is sometimes used in the management of severe childhood epilepsy, although it is unpleasantly sedative. It may be effective in myoclonic epilepsy when other drugs have failed.

Nitrazepam (Mogadon) This is a simple benzodiazepine which may be effective in controlling myoclonic jerks if these are the only remaining epileptic manifestation of primary generalized epilepsy.

Diazepam (Valium) Although effective in the treatment of status epilepticus (see page 21.65), this is not an effective anticonvulsant for daily use.

Other drugs are still advertised, though now seldom used. These include ethosuximide (Zarontin, Emeside).

A greater knowledge of the pharmacokinetics of the various anticonvulsant drugs has allowed more rational use. The half-life of phenobarbitone, phenytoin, and primidone is such that the total daily requirements can be given in one dosage on going to bed at night. The half life of carbamazepine is significantly shorter, so that the total daily dose should be divided in three fractions. The mid-day dose is often forgotten by schoolchildren and working adults, so this in itself may be sufficient reason to use one of the longer acting drugs. Sodium valproate has a short half-life as judged by serum levels, but, as already noted above, its biological half-life is much longer.

Table 4 shows some of the other factors, apart from seizure type, that should be considered when choosing an appropriate anticonvulsant drug. Fortunately price is not, in general, a significant problem with any of the drugs, though sodium valproate is by far the most expensive. Even so a year's treatment with 1500 mg a day will only cost £160, compared to about £3 for phenytoin given in a dosage of 300 mg per day.

The possibility of pregnancy must certainly be considered when prescribing an anticonvulsant drug. Sodium valproate causes teratogenic effects in animals, and valproate should be used only if the likely benefits in severe epilepsy resistant to other drugs outweigh the risks of teratogenicity. However, it has been shown that an epileptic woman taking both phenobarbitone and phenytoin is between two or three times more likely to have an abnormal baby than other women. The risk of congenital heart disease is increased by a factor of about four, and of harelip and cleft palate by a factor of about eight. The risks of fetal maldevelopment must be weighed against the risks to the fetus and to the mother of uncontrolled epilepsy. As any fetal damage due to drugs occurs in in the first few weeks of pregnancy, perhaps even before the mother realizes that she is pregnant, the decision whether to stop drugs or not has, by default, often already been taken. In this case the mother might as well continue anticonvulsant therapy in modest dosage, and protect herself and the baby against the risks of epilepsy.

There is no clear evidence that pregnancy itself increases the frequency of epileptic seizures, although the hormonal changes may have some influence on serum binding of anticonvulsants. Epilepsy is therefore virtually never an indicator for termination of pregnancy on medical grounds, although there may be social indications if it is considered that the mother has so many seizures that she is likely to have trouble in caring for the child.

Only one anticonvulsant should be given initially, and that anticonvulsant increased until appropriate levels are found in the serum, or until control of the seizures occurs. Only if this drug fails should another drug be tried, and that preferably in isolation rather than in combination. The interactions between anticonvulsant drugs are complex. For example, the introduction of sulthiam may result in an extraordinary elevation of phenytoin, resulting in intoxication. There are also interactions between anticonvulsant drugs and other drugs, notably steroid hormones and anticoagulants. Of these the most important is that the contraceptive effect of the Pill is partly counteracted by phenytoin.

Table 4 stresses the need to give full information to the patient about the names and alternative names of the drugs supplied, and the initial dosage given. Confusion so easily arises that it is well worthwhile taking the trouble to write out the schedule with the dates of changes planned, and to stress that seizure control is much more likely to occur if the patient understands and follows the instructions given. It is always difficult to know how much to say about the unwanted effects of the drugs. A full list of the unwanted effects of phenytoin would be so alarming that many patients might refuse to take it if they did not realize how rare many of the unwanted effects are. However, it is certainly worth mentioning the possibility of a skin rash in the early days, and explaining that sedation, if present even on the small doses with which medication is started, usually disappears as the tablets are continued.

As so many patients with epilepsy are referred to hospital clinics, it is important that the patient, the neurologist, and the general practitioner all realize who is responsible for what aspects of treatment. Failure of compliance is often due to failure of communication, rather than to 'disobedience' of the patient. However, it is worth pointing out to the patient that there is no need to panic if one or two doses of the longer acting anticonvulsants are omitted. The drug is so slowly metabolized that the omission can be easily made up the next day.

Although it is easy to accumulate a mass of redundant data, it is worthwhile asking the patient to record the frequency, type, and severity of his seizures, so that any improvement resulting from changes in medication can be observed. As seizures often appear to occur on a random basis, without any obvious precipitant, though sometimes in clusters, there are no adequate statistical methods of handling changes in seizure frequency. Probably the best available method is that of the cumulative sum technique.

One question that patients will undoubtedly want to ask is when they will be able to stop treatment. Clearly this depends upon seizure control, but even if immediate control of seizures results, most clinicians will advise continuing anticonvulsants for approximately three years thereafter. Most people whose seizures have stopped view cessation of therapy as the final hallmark of cure, and others are very reasonably concerned about the possible long-term effects of medication, though trouble on this score is most unlikely. Unfortunately, apart from clinical control of seizures, there is no observation or investigation that can be used to judge whether remission is likely to continue without anticonvulsant therapy. It has been shown that the EEG is not a successful predictor in adults. A Medical Research Council trial is underway in an attempt to identify factors that will predict relapse on withdrawal of drugs.

There may be factors which encourage a patient to continue drugs, rather than to try withdrawing them. For example, a trial of managing without therapy may be disastrous if it results in the loss of a driving licence only recently regained. If a decision to withdraw drugs is made, then it seems good sense to reduce the drug gradually over a period of many months. Unfortunately, the occasional subject relapses shortly after the very last tablet was stopped, suggesting that his seizures were controlled by a tiny dose of anticonvulsants that would not normally be considered adequate for the control of epilepsy.

The management of infantile spasms requires special mention. Although the benzodiazepines and sodium valproate may have some benefit, there is no doubt that ACTH or prednisone is more effective. The dose by adult standards is very high – about 2 mg/kg of prednisone a day, or 40 units of ACTH a day for one or two weeks followed by a smaller dosage for a longer period. Seizures will be controlled in about 50 per cent of the children on such a regime but the longer term prognosis for normal intellectual development and the cessation of seizures is much less certain.

Status epilepticus

Occasionally seizures may follow each other without remission. If they are generalized tonic-clonic seizures, with major convulsions occurring in sequence without remission, the patient is very much at risk from death through cardiorespiratory failure. Immediate control of the seizures is necessary. Although diazepam (Valium) is ineffective in the management of epilepsy on a day-to-day basis, it is a highly effective treatment for the management of status epilepticus. It, or the similar drugs lorazepam or clonazepam, should be given as a bolus intravenous injection as soon as it is clear that the subject is having continuous seizures without remission. A suitable dose of diazepam is 10 mg in 2 ml given over two to five minutes. If given more rapidly than this respiratory depression may occur. A bolus injection of this type is often sufficient to abort the episode, but if not an intravenous infusion containing 200 mg of diazepam per litre should be set up. The flow rate should be adjusted to control the seizures. It is often not realized what large quantities of diazepam may be necessary; it is not unusual to give 500 to 600 mg in a 24-hour period.

If diazepam fails to control the seizures, then admission to an Intensive Care Unit is required, and an alternative drug should be tried. Thiopentone or chlormethiazole are two commonly used alternatives. Both may suppress ventilation, so means for ventilatory support should be readily available.

If facilities for measuring serum anticonvulsants are readily available, then infusion wih phenytoin may prove to be a successful treatment for status epilepticus. If the patient has had no previous treatment, 15–20 mg/kg body weight will rapidly establish therapeutic levels of phenytoin. Very often, of course, the admitting physician is in some doubt as to the patient's previous anticonvulsant medication, so unless there are good reasons to the contrary, diazepam remains the drug of choice for the management of tonic-clonic status epilepticus.

Absence status or temporal lobe status may also occur, in which the presentation is not with overt convulsive seizures but with a confusional state, the origin of which may not be readily recognized. The principles of treatment are much the same as recorded above, though in this case electro-encephalographic control is useful. Continual focal motor epilepsy is known as *epilepsia partialis continua*, and is often exceedingly difficult to control, continuing for many days without significant disturbance of consciousness.

Other forms of treatment

There are other methods of treating epilepsy apart from the use of anticonvulsant drugs. Patients should, of course, be advised to avoid known precipitants, such as television, in cases in which it has clearly been established that the seizures are precipitated in this way. There are, however, comparatively few occasions in which the precipitant is quite so clearcut.

Children with epilepsy unresponsive to moderate doses of anticonvulsant drugs may benefit from a ketogenic diet. The diet first described by Wilder at the Mayo Clinic in 1921 was very rich in fat, and relatively unpalatable, and expensive to buy. Medium chain triglyceride oils may be used in place of ordinary dietary fat. About 70 per cent of the total daily calorie requirement is given as medium chain triglyceride oil, the remainder as protein and carbohydrate with vitamin supplements. The drawbacks to this diet include the frequent occurrence of smelly diarrhoea, and sometimes apparent reduction in the rate of growth. There is no evidence that these large quantities of oils increase the serum cholesterol or lipoproteins believed to be factors in the genesis of coronary artery disease.

Surgery may occasionally benefit refractory cases of epilepsy. It is most usually undertaken for refractory temporal lobe epilepsy. Prolonged and repeated EEG recordings are necessary to show that the epileptogenic lesion is confined to one or other temporal lobe, as bilateral temporal lobectomy is not possible because of the severe amnesic syndrome that results. No attempt is made to identify the local area of the temporal lobe that is abnormal. The anterior 5 cm are amputated as a single block, containing the uncus, amygdala, and anterior hippocampus. Histological studies of such amputated blocks has furthered our understanding of the genesis of temporal lobe epilepsy. *Mesial temporal sclerosis* is the

commonest lesion found, but occasionally small previously unidentified tumours or hamartomas or aggregates of abnormal looking giant neurones are found.

There are types of focal epilepsy arising from other parts of the brain, and occasionally cortical excision of an epileptogenic focus such as an angioma or scar following a penetrating head injury may result in control of previously refractory seizures.

Another surgical approach is to place stereotactic lesions in white matter which is believed to carry epileptic discharges from the diencephalon. Lesions have been placed with moderate success in the lateral thalamus or in the sub-thalamic field of Forel in an attempt to prevent generalization of paroxysmal discharges from focal lesions.

Another method being explored is to employ the inhibitory functions of the cerebellum from the cortex. Techniques have been developed by Cooper in New York whereby electrodes are placed on the inferior surface of the cerebellum and activated by electro-magnetic coupling through an antenna placed subcutaneously on the chest. Initial reports of this procedure suggested striking benefit in a few patients, but controlled studies have largely failed to substantiate the earlier claims.

In the last decade extensive studies have been carried out upon the effects of *biofeedback* in 'normalizing' the EEG. Although there is no doubt that subjects can learn to increase the amount of alpha rhythm generated, the question of whether they modify seizure frequency is much less certain. Although further research in this field is clearly justified, the present consensus is that EEG biofeedback is an unpredictable treatment which is costly in terms of time and equipment used.

Prognosis and complications of epilepsy

Prognosis

Pessimism about the prognosis of epilepsy derives from hospital and special clinic surveys. The prognosis of epilepsy as judged from the outcome in community based samples is very much more favourable. The top curve in Fig. 7 indicates the probability of completing a period of five consecutive years without seizures. For example, six years after diagnosis 42 per cent of subjects have been seizure free for five years. It is necessary to talk in terms of five-year remission rates rather than cure, because, analogous to the survival of cases of carcinoma of the breast, subsequent relapse many years after the onset is always possible. The curves in Fig. 7 flatten off with the passage of time. This means that if remission of seizures is not accomplished within the first few years of the onset, subsequent worthwhile remission becomes less likely. For example, although the net probability of achieving a five-year remission within ten years after diagnosis was 65 per cent, for patients not in remission five years after diagnosis the probability of achieving remission within the next ten years was only 33 per cent, the same proportion as based on the older surveys of established epilepsy in hospital practice.

Some factors are known to be particularly unfavourable: the combination of complex partial seizures with tonic-clonic seizures, clustering of seizures, injury occurring during tonic-clonic seizures, associated physical signs, and associated mental retardation are all factors known to be associated with failure to remit.

Complications

Clearly there are circumstances in which epilepsy is based upon an underlying and progressive disorder, which gradually assumes more importance than the epilepsy itself. However, there are certain complications which seem to be associated with epilepsy *per se*. First amongst these must be considered the psychiatric disorders associated with epilepsy. Someone with frequent seizures has a significant reduction in his chances in life. Furthermore, he has to act as his own public relations officer in deciding how much of his epilepsy to reveal, and to whom. Limitations in employment, and usually in driving, reduce his earning power, social status, and long-term financial security. Personal relationships with

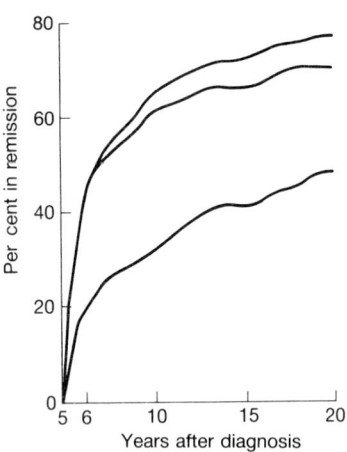

Fig. 7 Remission of epilepsy. *Top curve:* probability of completing a period of five consecutive years without seizure. For example, six years after diagnosis 42 per cent of subjects have been seizure-free for five years. *Middle curve:* the probability of being in remission, at any time, for at least the past five years. The difference between the top and middle curve is due to relapse after achievement of a five-year remission. For example, at 20 years after diagnosis 70 per cent are currently free from seizures and have been for five years and a further 6 per cent have had at least one seizure-free period of at least five years duration, but have subsequently relapsed. *Lowest curve:* the probability of being free of seizures for at least five years whilst not taking anticonvulsant drugs. In summary, 20 years after diagnosis 50 per cent have been free from seizures without anticonvulsant drugs for at least five years. A further 20 per cent continue to take anticonvulsant medication and are also free from seizures. Seizures continue, in spite of medication, in 30 per cent. (Redrawn from Anneger, J. F., Hauser, W. H., and Elveback, L. R. (1979). *Epilepsia* **29**, 729.)

the opposite sex may be spoilt by the fact of epilepsy. Not surprisingly, therefore, many people with epilepsy become unhappy and depressed. Suicide is approximately five times commoner in those with epilepsy than in the general population.

If the cause of the epilepsy is perinatal damage, there may be associated psychological defects in learning, or the epilepsy may be associated with hyperkinesis.

A psychotic illness with symptoms similar to those of paranoid schizophrenia may arise in those with temporal lobe epilepsy.

Some patients with temporal lobe epilepsy complain of loss of libido and impotence, which may respond to treatment with anticonvulsant drugs.

There is no good evidence that continuing seizures result in a dementing illness. However, prolonged and repeated episodes of status epilepticus may result in cerebral damage occurring through repeated episodes of hypoxia.

Social aspects of epilepsy

Children with epilepsy should, as far as possible, be educated alongside their siblings in normal schools. Clearly, if there are difficulties in learning due to associated cerebral injury in the perinatal period, this would not be appropriate and the child would be better placed at a special school. Occasionally, children with frequent seizures, but with normal intelligence, will do best at a special school for epileptic children, where all members of the staff are trained in and competent to cope with the various manifestations of seizures.

Restrictions on activities of children with epilepsy should be few. It is clearly not sensible to allow them to swim alone, nor to climb ropes in the school gym. If bathing alone at home, the depth of the water should be limited. No danger will result from the usual sports of football or similar games.

Restrictions on adults with epilepsy should also be few. Epileptic mothers with very young children should not bath infants

alone, in case they have a seizure during the bath and the baby drowns. Problems will certainly arise about employment. Obviously it is not safe to work with heavy moving machinery, or at heights. Unfortunately, problems more often arise because of the inability of the employer to realize that the vast majority of people with epilepsy have only occasional seizures, and then not often at work. Nevertheless the employer is not willing to accept the 'responsibility' of employing someone with epilepsy, even in a straightforward commercial or office job. For this reason many people with reasonably well-controlled seizures conceal their epilepsy from their employers. Someone with epilepsy may consider becoming registered as a disabled person, in order to benefit from the provisions of the Disabled Persons (Employment) Acts of 1944 and 1958 by which employers in the United Kingdom of more than 20 people have a statutory requirement to employ a quota of 3 per cent of their employees from those on the Disablement Register though it is present government policy to repeal this requirement.

The eligibility of those with epilepsy to hold a driving licence varies from country to country, but in the United Kingdom it is governed by the Motor Vehicles (Driving Licences) Regulations of 1982. The Regulations in the relevant paragraph read in full:

> (2) Epilepsy is prescribed for the purposes of section 87 (3) (b) of the Act of 1972 and an applicant for a licence suffering from epilepsy shall satisfy the conditions that:
>
> (a) he shall have been free from any epileptic attack during the period of two years immediately preceding the date when the licence is to have effect; or
>
> (b) in the case of an applicant who has had such attacks whilst asleep during that period, he shall have had such attacks only whilst asleep during a period of at least three years immediately preceding the date when the licence is to have effect; and
>
> (c) the driving of a vehicle by him in pursuance of the licence is not likely to be a source of danger to the public.

The concession to those with seizures whilst asleep is generous, as a considerable proportion of these are subsequently shown by follow-up to have seizures whilst awake.

Although not stated in the Regulations, it is understood that the practice of the Department of Transport is to allow an applicant for a driving licence who has had one seizure, without physical signs, and without any obvious cause for the seizure apparent, to drive after an interval of one year.

The restrictions on those who wish to drive heavy goods vehicles are even more rigorous. The appropriate regulation reads that the applicant 'shall not at any time since he attained the age of five years have had an epileptic attack'.

Life insurance can be obtained, without excessive difficulty, although the premium is obviously dependent upon the frequency and control of seizures, and the underlying cause.

Special provisions are necessary for those with the worst epilepsy. Occasionally someone with frequent seizures, especially if there are associated social behavioural and psychological problems, may benefit from living in a community for people with epilepsy. This is most likely to be necessary when the death occurs of the last surviving parent of someone with bad epilepsy who has been cared for all his life at home.

References

Editorial (1985). First year fits. *Br. Med. J.* **290**, 1095–1096

Editorial (1985). New drugs for epilepsy. *Lancet* i, 198–200.

Elwes, R. D. L., Johnson, A. L., Shorvon, S. and Reynolds, E. H. (1984). The prognosis for seizure control in newly diagnosed epilepsy. *New Engl. J. Med.* **311**, 944–947.

Hauser, W. A. and Kurland, L. T. (1975). The epidemiology of epilepsy in Rochester, Minnesota, 1935 through 1967. *Epilepsia* **16**, 1–66.

Hopkins, A. and Scambler, G. (1977). How doctors deal with epilepsy. *Lancet* i, 183–186.

Hrachovy, R. A., Frost, J. D. and Kellaway, P. (1979). A controlled study of prednisone therapy in infantile spasms. *Epilepsia* **20**, 403–413.

Juel-Jensen, P. (1968). Frequency of recurrence after discontinuance of anticonvulsant therapy in patients with epileptic seizures. *Epilepsia* **9**, 11–16.

Hopkins, A. (1987). *Epilepsy.* Chapman and Hall, London.

Laxer, K. D., Mullooly, J. P. and Howell, B. (1985). Prolactin changes after seizures classified by EEG monitoring. *Neurology* **35**, 31–35.

Shorvon, S. D. (1984). The temporal aspects of prognosis in epilepsy. *J. Neurol. Neurosurg. Psychiatry* **47**, 1157–1165.

——, Gilliatt, R. W., Lax T. C. S. and Yu, Y. C. (1984). Evidence of vascular disease from CT scanning in late onset epilepsy. *J. Neurol. Neurosurg. Psychiatry* **47**, 225–230.

Verity, C. M., Butler, N. R. and Golding, J. (1985). Febrile convulsions in a national cohort followed up from birth. *Br. Med. J.* **290**, 1307–1315.

Narcolepsy and related sleep disorders

C. D. MARSDEN

Definition

Described by Gelineau in 1880, narcolepsy is defined as 'a syndrome of unknown origin that is characterized by abnormal sleep tendencies, including excessive daytime sleepiness and often disturbed nocturnal sleep, and pathological manifestations of REM [rapid eye movements] sleep. The REM sleep abnormalities include sleep-onset REM periods and the dissociated REM sleep inhibitory processes, cataplexy, and sleep paralysis. Excessive daytime sleepiness, cataplexy, and less often sleep paralysis and hypnagogic hallucinations are the major symptoms of the disease'. (Definition drafted by the First International Symposium on Narcolepsy, 1975.)

Pathophysiology

The cause of narcolepsy is unknown. It is no longer considered to be a rare disease, for it has been estimated to occur in between 20–50 per 100 000 of the population. Between 10 and 40 per cent of patients with narcolepsy give a history of a similar disorder amongst other family members, and about a quarter describe a parent as affected. However, genetic analysis does not suggest a simple dominant mode of transmission of the disorder, nor do the data support a recessive hypothesis.

No convincing pathological or biochemical abnormality has been found as yet in patients suffering from narcolepsy, but neurophysiological studies have revealed a disturbance of sleep mechanisms. Normal sleep begins with a change in the electroencephalogram (EEG) from the fast activity characteristic of wakefulness to increasingly slower frequencies. After about 90 minutes or so of early sleep, short (10–15 minutes) periods occur in which REM take place, accompanied by cessation of bodily movement, loss of all muscle tone, and a tendency to dream. Between three and six periods of REM sleep occur during the average night, each period becoming progressively longer, so that the total duration of REM sleep corresponds to about 20–25 per cent of total sleep time. Light sleep in patients with narcolepsy very commonly commences with a period of REM sleep and this abnormality is believed to be responsible for sleep paralysis, due to inhibition of movement and loss of muscle tone, and hypnagogic hallucinations. Daytime sleep attacks also commonly commence with a period of REM activity, and the sudden falling attacks characteristic of cataplexy also may be associated with bursts of REM activity. These neurophysiological abnormalities point towards an abnormal dissociation between the brainstem mechanisms responsible for maintaining wakefulness due to activation of the cerebral cortex, and other parallel brainstem mechanisms responsible for generating REM activity and maintaining muscle tone. Why there should be disordered control of REM sleep in narcolepsy is not known, but animal experiments suggest that sleep mechanisms are under the control of brainstem reticular formation pathways utilizing monoaminergic neurotransmitters. This may explain why drugs influencing cerebral monoamines, such as amphetamines and tricyclic antidepressants, are used to treat the disorder. A remarkable finding is that all patients with narcolepsy studied so far express the major histocompatibility antigen HLA DR2, compared with about a quarter of normal controls. This confirms the genetic origin of this disease and links it with the short arm of chromosome 6.

Clinical symptoms

The narcoleptic tetrad consists of excessive daytime sleepiness with sleep attacks (narcolepsy), episodes of sudden falling associated with emotion (cataplexy), sleep paralysis, and hypnagogic hallucinations. Virtually every patient develops excessive daytime sleepiness and sleep attacks, about two-thirds experience cataplexy, about a third suffer hypnagogic hallucinations, and about a sixth have sleep paralysis. Approximately 15 per cent of patients experience all four symptoms.

Excessive daytime sleepiness and sleep attacks are the hallmark of narcolepsy. On average, patients will report between two to six attacks of falling asleep each day, but some may experience up to 20 or 30 episodes. Each attack lasts, on average, around 10 or 20 minutes, but sometimes they may be as brief as a minute or as long as two hours. Attacks are common after heavy meals, alcohol, and monotony, and in warm rooms or while driving. Of course, the normal person may fall asleep in these circumstances, but the hallmark of narcolepsy is the bizarreness of the situations in which the patient may drop off to sleep. Thus, narcoleptics may fall asleep over their meals dropping into the soup, may nod off while standing, during intercourse, and even while driving a car or flying an aeroplane. Patients describe such episodes as irresistible and are quite overwhelmed by their sleepiness. Many have to give up going out in the evenings to friends, and find it pointless to watch a film or television. Night-time sleep frequently is disturbed in narcolepsy. Apart from the problems of sleep paralysis and hypnagogic hallucinations, excessive sleep during the day frequently leads to shorter deep sleep at night, although the total time spent in REM sleep usually is normal. Overall, most narcoleptics do not sleep excessively throughout the whole 24 hour period.

Cataplexy

This describes an abrupt but reversible paralysis into which a narcoleptic patient may be precipitated by emotional events. The severity of cataplectic attacks can vary from total paralysis with collapse to the ground, to lesser degrees in which the jaw sags and the head drops. Consciousness is preserved throughout the attack, but the patient may see double. Attacks last from a few seconds to as long as 30 minutes. They occur more frequently at times of stress, fatigue, or after heavy meals. Laughter and anger are the commonest triggers, but elation or any other intense emotion may be sufficient to precipitate an episode. A stimulus may come from something heard or seen, or may arise while listening to music, reading a book, or even just remembering a happy or emotional event. The excitement of a successful athletic activity, such as a fine stroke at cricket or tennis, or even the thrill of sexual intercourse may prompt an episode. Cataplectic attacks occur at least daily in over three-quarters of those with narcolepsy and some patients may have many attacks each day.

Sleep paralysis

In this state the patient becomes totally unable to perform a voluntary movement despite remaining alert and aware. It may occur either on falling asleep (hypnagogic) or on awakening (hypnapomic). During an episode the patient is powerless to move, speak or even open his eyes although he is fully aware of his condition and can recall it completely afterwards. Naturally, such episodes may cause extreme terror particularly if they are accompanied by vivid and frightening hallucinations. The patient may feel as though he is dying, and since he cannot move, is terrified of being buried alive. An episode rarely lasts more than 10 minutes, and usually much less.

Hypnagogic hallucinations almost always involve visions, which may consist merely of simple coloured forms, still or in motion, or may take the shape of animals or persons. Frightening or erotic scenes are quite common. Noises, voices, or melodies occur less frequently. Psychic hallucinations taking the form of an impression that somebody is present can be particularly distressing. The narcoleptic frequently experiences these hallucinations as vivid and real, making them all the more terrifying.

While sleep attacks, cataplexy, sleep paralysis, and hypnagogic hallucinations form the core of the narcoleptic tetrad, these patients also experience other symptoms. Particularly distressing are periods of automatic behaviour, lapses of memory, and 'blackouts'. In such episodes, for which the patient has little or no memory, he may continue activity which does not require extensive skill, but may make frequent mistakes. Many patients have experienced such episodes while driving, and most have developed automatic behaviour in social situations. Simple questions are answered appropriately, but if the conversation requires more thought, the patient may respond with inappropriate or meaningless sentences. Such episodes may occur daily and cause great difficulties. In almost every respect they represent the automatic behaviour with amnesia characteristic of nocturnal sleepwalking. In view of the many and bizarre symptoms encountered in narcolepsy, a proportion of patients may become considerably disturbed by their illness. A secondary reactive depression or anxiety state is not uncommon, and may add to the symptomatology. In evaluating psychiatric symptoms, the effects of drug treatment also must be taken into account.

Course

Narcolepsy begins in adolescence or in early adulthood, and is lifelong. Around 60 per cent of cases commence between 15 and 30 years of age, but a few start before the age of 10 years or up to the age of about 50 years. Sleep attacks are the first symptom in 90 per cent of cases, but a few patients begin with cataplexy or hypnagogic hallucinations. Once established, excessive daytime sleepiness and sleep attacks never cease completely during the patient's lifetime, but cataplexy tends to become less of a problem as the patient becomes older.

Differential diagnosis

The excessive daytime sleepiness and sleep attacks characteristic of narcolepsy are difficult, on occasion, to distinguish from the range of normal. The best index of pathological sleepiness is an unambiguous history of inappropriate daytime sleep episodes. The bizarre situations in which narcoleptics fall asleep are diagnostic, and most patients will give a history of blackouts and automatic behaviour if questioned carefully. If there is any doubt, a history of cataplexy settles the issue.

Problems in diagnosis arise in separating narcolepsy and its associated features from epilepsy, in distinguishing cataplexy from other causes of drop attacks, and in separating excessive daytime sleepiness and sleep attacks from other causes of pathological sleep.

Sleep attacks may be mistaken for minor fits, hypnagogic hallucinations and night terrors for nocturnal seizures or temporal lobe partial complex seizures, and cataplectic drop attacks for akinetic seizures. Periods of automatism in narcolepsy also may be indistinguishable from post-epileptic automatic behaviour; in both situations the patient is in a state of being able to move around in a relatively normal manner, but is at the same time lacking in understanding or purpose, and subsequently cannot clearly recall what occurred during that period. A similar state is characteristic of transient global amnesia due to ischaemia in posterior cerebral arterial territories.

Symptomatic narcolepsy is exceedingly rare. Encephalitis lethargica was said to cause narcolepsy and cataplexy, but the association was uncommon. Many structural lesions of the central nervous system may cause pathological drowsiness, but this seldom resembles narcolepsy and the other features of this illness do not occur. Drugs are not known to cause true narcolepsy. Structural lesions in the hypothalamus may cause periodic somnolence and hormonal disturbances, but they do not cause classical narcolepsy.

Narcolepsy may be distinguished from other conditions causing excessive daytime sleepiness (hypersomnia) by its characteristically short duration (one to five minutes), irresistible sleep attacks, and by the presence of cataplexy, sleep paralysis, and hypnagogic hallucinations, which do not occur in the other hypersomniac states. The latter cause longer (hours to days or even weeks) periods of sleep without the other features of the narcoleptic tetrad.

Symptomatic hypersomnia occurs in a range of organic brain diseases including encephalitis, toxic or metabolic encephalopathies, tumour, vascular or traumatic brain damage. Sleep, as distinct from coma from which the patient cannot be awakened, frequently is more or less continuous in these conditions.

Functional hypersomnias are periodic. The sleep attacks may last one to several hours, with attacks occurring most days (short cycle), or may last a day to several weeks, with attacks occurring at intervals of a month to several years (long cycle). Patients with either short cycle or long cycle hypersomnias are normal between attacks. Other functional hypersomnias are associated with respiratory disorders during sleep, so-called sleep apnoea.

Four short-cycle periodic functional hypersomnias are recognized.

Idiopathic hypersomnia is characterized by excessive prolonged night-time sleep, extreme difficulty in awakening, signs of 'sleep drunkenness' on awakening, and prolonged periods of sleep during the day. Such patients may sleep 15 or even 20 hours a day if not disturbed. The condition is hereditary in as many as a third to a half of patients.

Neurotic hypersomnia may occur in some hysterics or 'faint hearted' neuraesthenic individuals, and a complaint of excessive tiredness is common in depression.

Nocturnal myoclonus syndrome is characterized by short bouts of muscle jerking at night, which disturb night sleep. This is accompanied by extreme restlessness of the legs, and is often associated with daytime sleepiness. A nocturnal dose of clonazepam (Rivotril) may help.

Sleep apnoea is characterized by extreme restlessness with frequent respiratory pauses and snoring during night sleep, and by daytime drowsiness and irritability. Such a syndrome may occur (a) in those with severe obesity, chronic alveolar hypoventilation, right heart failure, and polycythaemia (*Pickwickian syndrome*); (b) in those with upper respiratory tract obstruction due, for example, to prognathism, acromegaly, goitre, tonsillar and adenoidal hypertrophy, or laryngeal stenosis; or (c) in those with primary alveolar hypoventilation ('Ondine's curse'). The diagnosis is established by polygraphic recording of sleep which shows fragment periods (at least 30 of 10 or more seconds duration in 7 hours of sleep) of apnoea. Such patients are chronically timid during the day, have fragment periods of daytime sleep and of automation behaviour. Untreated it can lead to pulmonary and systemic hypertension, cardiac arrhythmias and sudden death. Weight loss, surgical correction, and nocturnal continuous transnasal positive airways pressure may help. This condition is considered further in Section 15. Tracheostomy may be required to restore normal sleep.

Long cycle periodic functional hypersomnia is rare, and may or may not be accompanied by excessive eating (*Kleine–Levin syndrome*). Such patients, most commonly young adult males, begin to overeat prodigiously (bulimia), become irritable and restless, and then fall into a deep sleep for a day to a few weeks, during which time they awake to attend to toilet needs and can be aroused to eat. On awakening they are amnesic for that period, but rapidly return to normal behaviour and sleep patterns, and remain free of attacks for months or years. Another cause of recurrent hypersomnia at intervals longer than a day is periodic disruption of the normal sleep–wake cycle, as may occur in flying crews and shift workers.

Treatment

Narcoleptic sleep attacks and excessive daytime sleepiness are in many cases greatly improved by the regular use of amphetamine (5–120 mg daily), methylphenidate (10–100 mg daily), or mazindol (2–10 mg daily). Despite the possible misuse and unwanted effects of such stimulants on chronic use, at present they are the only effective drugs available. In fact, although some patients develop tolerance, and require progressively higher dosage, addiction in narcoleptics is very uncommon. These drugs do not affect cataplexy, but tricyclic antidepressants such as chlormipramine (10–25 mg nightly) may abolish both cataplexy and sleep paralysis. Chlormipramine can be used safely with amphetamines or other stimulants, but blood pressure should be monitored.

References

Guilleminault, C., Dement, W. C. and Passouant, P. (eds.) (1976). *Narcolepsy.* Spectrum Publications, New York.

Langdon, N., Welsh, K. I., van Dam, M., Vaughan, R. W. and Parkes, D. (1984). Genetic markers in narcolepsy. *Lancet* **ii**, 1178.

Parkes, J. D. (1981). Daytime drowsiness. *Lancet* **ii**, 1213.

An approach to transient loss of consciousness

R. W. GILLIATT

While there are many different causes of stupor and coma, *recurrent* attacks of unconsciousness in patients who are otherwise well are likely to be due to either epilepsy or syncope. Other causes include spontaneous hypoglycaemia, vertebrobasilar migraine, and transient ischaemic attacks affecting the vertebrobasilar territory. Raised intracranial pressure may cause recurrent episodes of depressed consciousness, characteristically associated with headache and vomiting. Alcohol or drug abuse must be considered in any patient with unexplained attacks of confusion or depressed consciousness, particularly if the onset is gradual and the unconsciousness is of relatively long duration. Hysterical or simulated seizures can prove extremely difficult to distinguish from true epilepsy and may require inpatient observation, including closed-circuit television and EEG monitoring.

History

The first step in the diagnosis of epilepsy or syncope is to obtain a good clinical history. Patients are often unaware of how much they can contribute ('I passed out, Doctor, so I can't tell you much about it'). In fact, there are few of the questions listed below which require to be answered by a relative or other witness of the attack.

Time of day or night

Most nocturnal attacks are epileptic but these have to be distinguished from nightmares, sleepwalking, night terrors, sleep apnoea, and nocturnal confusion in the elderly. Cardiac arrhythmias can occasionally cause convulsive syncope during the night.

Was the patient standing, sitting or lying?

Vasovagal syncope is unlikely if the patient was lying down at the time of the attack, but it must be remembered that complete cardiac arrest will produce syncope with convulsive movements, regardless of a patient's posture.

Did anything set off the attack?

While tension or excitement can occasionally precipitate epilepsy in children, and other forms of reflex epilepsy are known (e.g. television epilepsy due to photic stimulation), a story of attacks of unconsciousness occurring in response to anxiety or pain usually indicates syncope. Into this category come 'habitual fainters' in whom attacks can be triggered not only by the sight of blood but by discussion of accidents or operations.

Was there a warning? If so what form did it take?

The distinction between the prodromal symptoms of a faint and the prodromata of temporal lobe epilepsy (epigastric sensation rising to head, flushing, sense of unreality or fear) can be difficult. Other more typical features of temporal lobe attacks (abnormal taste or smell, *déjà vu* experience) are easily recognized. Attacks which occur without warning are more likely to be epileptic than syncopal but this is not a certain guide. Cardiac arrest can produce unconsciousness and convulsive movements without warning.

Could the patient have aborted the attack by bending down or any other manoeuvre?

Some patients with postural syncope learn to sit down or crouch in time to prevent unconsciousness. It is rare for an epileptic to be able to 'fight off' an attack but this can occur; in such cases the attack usually has a focal onset and a tendency to spread slowly.

Was there a fall? If so, was there bruising or injury?

Patients are much more likely to injure themselves in epilepsy than in syncope but the distinction is not absolute.

Was the patient completely unconscious or still dimly aware?

Partial preservation of consciousness can occur in either epilepsy or syncope. If, however, consciousness is preserved at a time when the patient has generalized paraesthesiae, stiffening or jerky movements, the attack is more likely to be due to anxiety with hyperventilation, or to a hysterical or simulated seizure.

How long was the period of unconsciousness or amnesia?

The duration of the attack is one of the most reliable criteria by which epilepsy can be distinguished from syncope. The patient who collapses unconscious and remembers nothing more until he or she is in the ambulance or in hospital is much more likely to have epilepsy than syncope. While the duration of stiffening and movements may be short in some epileptic attacks, they are usually followed by a period of coma and then by confusion. The patient subsequently has amnesia for all these phases.

What was the patient like while unconscious?

While the patient may be able to answer this from hearsay, details should be confirmed by a witness. Questions should be asked about facial colour, whether the eyes were open, and whether stiffening, jerky movements or altered breathing occurred. Pallor during and after the attack would favour syncope whereas cyanosis and altered breathing would suggest epilepsy. While stiffening and some myoclonic jerks are allowed in syncope, a classical tonic–clonic sequence is much more likely to indicate epilepsy. Clenching of the jaw can occur in syncope but rhythmic jaw movements with foaming at the mouth are only seen in epilepsy.

Was the pulse recorded?

Information about the rate and volume of the pulse during an attack is sometimes available but is not usually helpful unless a trained observer such as a doctor or nurse was present. Changes in pulse rate can occur in temporal lobe epilepsy but absence of pulsation at the onset of unconsciousness is good evidence of syncope.

Was there incontinence or tongue-biting?

In the absence of a witness, the patient can nearly always recall this. Incontinence of urine can occur in syncope but faecal incontinence is strongly suggestive of epilepsy. Tongue-biting is diagnostic of epilepsy.

Was there sleepiness or confusion after the attack?

Both of these features suggest epilepsy. A patient who speaks to the doctor after regaining consciousness, but who subsequently remembers nothing of it, is likely to suffer from epilepsy. Headache and drowsiness for several hours after an attack also favour epilepsy.

Investigations

In distinguishing epilepsy from syncope, laboratory investigations should include an EEG, ECG, and, if a local intracranial lesion is suspected, a CT scan. While EEG abnormalities can occur in patients with syncope, they are not usually of an epileptic kind, and the presence of paroxysmal activity with spikes or sharp waves would favour epilepsy. If the EEG is recorded during a syncopal attack it is likely to show flattening or bilateral slow wave activity, but spikes and sharp waves are not seen.

The EEG is normal between attacks in a significant proportion of epileptic patients; in some focal seizures, including temporal lobe attacks, the EEG does not even show epileptic activity during the attack, at least on the scalp. However, in a generalized attack with unconsciousness, stiffening and rhythmic jerking, a normal or near-normal EEG is suspicious of a hysterical or simulated seizure. The presence of a normal alpha rhythm during 'unconsciousness' is highly suggestive, and if the alpha rhythm is blocked by attempts to rouse the patient, the diagnosis of hysteria or simulation is confirmed.

The likelihood of observing an actual attack is greatly increased by a system incorporating closed-circuit television and EEG monitoring. Before these were available, admission of a patient to hospital for observation usually meant that attacks were witnessed by another patient in the ward, rather than by a nurse or a doctor; routine EEGs with recording for 20–30 min sometimes revealed interseizure abnormalities but were unlikely to catch an attack. With modern monitoring systems, ambulant EEG recording can be continued for several days. If closed-circuit television is being used as well, the patient needs to be in a side-room on the ward where he or she can remain in view of the TV camera (Fig. 1). Recording at night presents no problem provided an infrared light source and sensitive camera are used.

Monitoring of the ECG alone is usually sufficient to distinguish cardiac syncope from epilepsy of late onset. Brief episodes of cardiac dysrhythmia can occur without producing symptoms, so that it is important to continue monitoring long enough to include a cli-

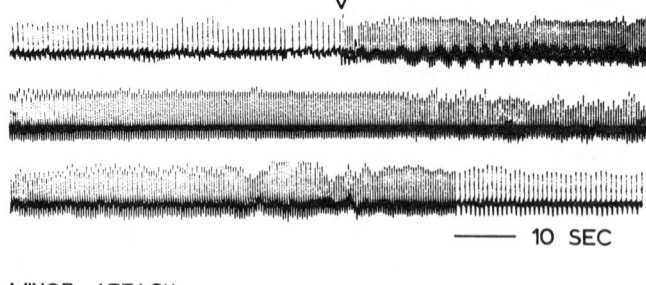

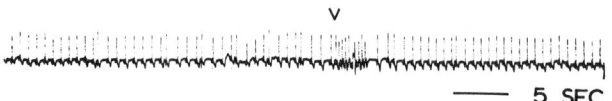

Fig. 2 (Top) Paroxysmal atrial tachycardia accompanied by syncope in a patient with the Lown–Ganong–Levine syndrome*. (Bottom) A brief episode observed during the same recording, which did not give rise to symptoms.   *Short PR interval.

nical attack. In the example shown in Fig. 2 the patient, a man of 64 years, had suffered from infrequent attacks of unconsciousness without involuntary movements for several years. Since these were preceded by a sensation in one leg, they had been regarded as epileptic but anticonvulsants had not altered their frequency. Several EEGs had been normal but, during a 72-hour period of ECG monitoring in hospital, the patient had an episode of unconsciousness associated with a paroxysm of supraventricular tachycardia lasting 3–4 min. A much briefer asymptomatic paroxysm was also found on the tape. During the longer episode a nurse was summoned and found the pulse to be normal although the patient had not fully recovered consciousness. This gave rise to a report that the pulse was normal *during* the attack, a misstatement which could have had serious clinical implications if a taped record of the ECG had not also been available.

When episodes of cardiac dysrhythmia are thought to be the cause of attacks of unconsciousness, but ambulant ECG monitoring is negative, intracardiac recording may reveal evidence of a conduction defect; in some cases programmed stimulation has been used to provoke an attack. These special techniques are likely to be particularly helpful in establishing the nature of attacks associated with ischaemic heart disease, in which the mortality is known to be high.

In distinguishing true epilepsy from a hysterical or simulated seizure, the estimation of serum prolactin in the postictal period is a useful additional test. The level is nearly always raised after a grand mal or complex partial seizure; this is in contrast to a non-epileptic seizure, which does not cause a significant rise in serum level.

References

Cull, R., Gilliatt, R. W., Willison, R. G. and Quy, R. (1982). Prolonged observation and EEG monitoring of epileptic patients. In *A textbook of epilepsy* (eds J. Laidlaw and A. Richens), pp. 211–226. Churchill Livingstone, London.

Dana-Haeri, J., Trimble, M. R. and Oxley, J. (1983). Prolactin and gonadotrophin changes following generalised and partial seizures. *J. Neurol. Neurosurg. Psychiat.* **46**, 331–335.

Gilliatt, R. W. and Roberts, R. C. (1986). Syncope and non-epileptic seizures. In *Diseases of the nervous system* Vol. 2 (eds A. Asbury, G. M. McKhann and W. I. McDonald), pp. 1033–1043. W. B. Saunders Company, Philadelphia.

Roberts, R. C. and Fitch, P. (1985). Monitoring at the National Hospital, Queen Square, London. In *Longterm monitoring in epilepsy*, *EEG Clin. Neurophysiol.* Suppl. 37, 423–436.

Sharma, A. D., Klein, G. J. and Milstein, S. (1984). Diagnostic assessment of recurrent syncope. *PACE* **7**, 749–759.

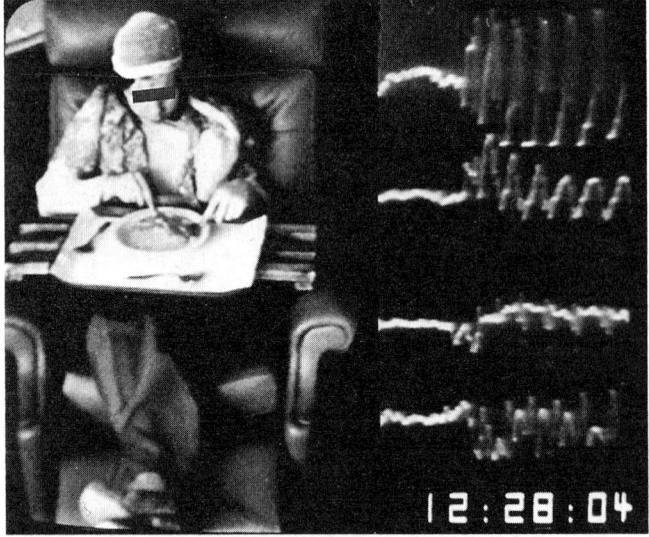

Fig. 1 Seizure monitoring with a TV camera and EEG telemetry. A photograph of the split-screen television display shows a patient at the onset of a petit mal attack while eating. (Reproduced from Bowden *et al.*, 1975, by courtesy of the *Proceedings of the Royal Society of Medicine*.)

THE MOTOR AND SENSORY SYSTEMS AND EFFECTS OF SUBCORTICAL BRAIN LESIONS

W. B. MATTHEWS

The motor system

The lower motor neurone

The motor unit consists of a number of muscle fibres, ranging from 100 in the facial muscles to 2000 in the quadriceps, supplied by a single fast-conducting alpha motor fibre. These originate from large cells in the anterior horns of the grey matter of the spinal cord and in the somatic motor nuclei of the cranial nerves, and are known as the lower motor neurones. Loss of function of the anterior horn cells, or interruption of their axons, causes weakness or paralysis of the muscles they supply, with loss of stretch reflex activity, shown by flaccidity and loss of tendon jerks, and if paralysis persists, wasting of the muscle due to loss of excitable tissue. The extent and severity of these signs vary with the distribution and speed of onset and duration of the lower motor neurone lesion. Acute destruction of the anterior horn cells causes paralysis of the muscles wholly supplied by the segments involved, but many muscles receive motor fibres from two or more segments. Gradual progressive reduction in the number of anterior horn cells or of their axons does not at first cause weakness or wasting, as surviving axons sprout and supply muscle fibres deprived of their nerve supply. The resulting giant motor units are unstable and may fire spontaneously, resulting in fasciculation. This can be seen as irregular, brief, flickering contraction of parts of the muscle. This is quite distinct from fibrillation which occurs in denervated muscle, but which can be detected only by using needle electrodes and an electromyograph, and, as its name implies, is due to the contraction of single muscle fibres, probably as the result of denervation hypersensitivity to circulating acetylcholine. Fibrillation does not occur unless the motor nerve supply is anatomically interrupted, and is indeed a sign that this has occurred. In peripheral nerves, however, a state of reversible conduction block without axonal disruption is a common event. This results in paralysis in the distribution of the nerve, but wasting does not develop.

The upper motor neurone

The main descending motor pathway is derived from the upper motor neurones in the precentral gyrus. Movements of the foot are controlled by neurones in the upper part of the gyrus on the medial surface of the hemisphere, and from above downwards on the lateral surface are the areas for the leg, trunk, arm, hand, face, and tongue. These must not be thought of as rigidly demarcated centres, but the distribution of function within the motor cortex is of practical importance. Descending axons converge in the genu and posterior limb of the internal capsule, with fibres destined for the motor nuclei of the cranial nerves lying anteriorly. The corticospinal tract occupies the middle third of the cerebral peduncle. In the pons the fibres are more dispersed and become concentrated again in the prominent pyramid, from which the name pyramidal tract is derived, seen on the anterior surface of the medulla. At the lower end of the medulla, most of the fibres cross and descend in the lateral columns of the spinal cord. The small uncrossed tract lies anteriorly, but its functional importance is unknown. Probably only a small proportion of corticospinal axons synapse directly on anterior horn cells, and most terminate on interneurones.

An acute complete lesion of the corticospinal and corticobulbar tract results in flaccid paralysis with loss of tendon reflexes. With the passage of time or with a partial or progressive lesion, the characteristic effect is spastic weakness or paralysis. This implies that the loss of power is accompanied by an increase in stretch reflex activity elicited by passive movement of the limb. The weakness, the negative symptom, is usually most obvious in distal muscles of the upper limb, but movements at the hip joint may be affected when no other loss of power can be found in the lower limb. Selective lesions, particularly of the motor cortex, can produce localized weakness and loss of function. Loss of fine movement of the hand and to a less obvious extent of the foot, is often more prominent than loss of strength. Individual finger movements may be impossible even when the grip is normal. In many complex movements, such as walking, the normal precise sequence of contraction and relaxation of opposing muscles is lost.

The increased resistance to passive movements is more marked in the flexor muscles of the arm and the extensor muscles of the leg. It often has a 'clasp knife' character, in that the initial resistance suddenly lapses, owing to a reflex lengthening reaction. These positive symptoms are due to release of spinal reflex activity from some inhibitory effect of the corticospinal pathway, although details of the effect are still controversial. The tendon reflexes are exaggerated. Those normally elicited in the upper limb, the biceps, supinator and triceps jerks, are increased, and reflexes can be obtained from other muscles, in particular the finger flexors and pectorals. *Hoffmann's sign*, elicited by flexing and suddenly releasing the terminal phalanx of the middle finger, consists of reflex flexion of all the digits. It is a sign merely of reflex activity and is not specific for an upper motor neurone lesion. Sometimes any sharp movement of the arm will produce reflex contraction of muscles not obviously stretched. This is not due to abnormal spread of excitation but to minute and inapparent stretch acting as an adequate stimulus. In the lower limb, the knee and ankle jerks may be increased to the point of clonus, where maintained stretch produces an inexhaustible repetitive response. Stretch reflexes may also be elicited from the adductors and hamstring muscles.

The normal plantar reflex consists of plantar flexion of all the digits on firm stroking of the lateral side of the sole of the foot. In the extensor or *Babinski reflex*, the big toe dorsiflexes and the other toes fan. This response can be elicited by a number of other stimuli, but the only one of much value is the Oppenheim sign induced by firm pressure of the thumb sliding down the shin and anterior tibial muscles. A Babinski reflex is reliably found when a upper motor neurone lesion or loss of function is undeniably present, but is far less useful as a diagnostic test in cases of doubt, when it is usually recorded as 'equivocal'. The increase in tone in the extensor muscles results in the lower limb being an effective prop on standing and walking provided some voluntary movement is retained. In severe progressive spinal cord disease, an increase in flexor tone often supervenes. Spasm in the flexor muscles, often painful, leads to permanent flexion at the hip and knee, a posture of great discomfort, in which any residual voluntary action cannot be usefully exerted. The posture of a spastic upper limb is usually that of flexion at the elbow, wrist and finger joints, and adduction at the shoulder. To what extent spasticity interferes with the effective use of residual muscular power is uncertain.

A curious feature of upper motor neurone lesions is loss of certain cutaneous reflexes. The superficial abdominal reflexes elicited from each quadrant by light stroking are normally a variable finding, particularly after middle age, but asymmetrical loss is occasionally a valuable sign. Loss of the cremasteric reflex in which the testicle is withdrawn on stroking the thigh and the gluteal contraction on stroking the skin of the buttock are less reliable signs.

Upper motor neurone lesions also affect the function of muscles supplied by the cranial nerves. An acute unilateral lesion usually causes dysphagia and dysarthria for a few days only. Bilateral lesions cause similar but persistent symptoms with slow and clumsy movements of the tongue and sometimes an exaggerated jaw jerk. This is elicited by a tap on the chin with the mouth half open and is normally just detectable. It is, however, not a reliable sign. A bilateral upper movement neurone or supranuclear disturbance of function of the lower cranial nerves is known as pseudobulbar palsy, in distinction from the lower motor neurone bulbar palsy. It is often accompanied by minor degrees of spasticity of the limbs, usually a shuffling gait, and great lability of the expression of emotion with inappropriate laughter and ready tears evoked by trivial misfortunes. An upper motor neurone facial palsy differs in a number of respects from a nuclear or peripheral lesion. The muscles of the upper face are relatively or entirely spared, apparently because of bilateral cortical control. There may be dissociation between forced voluntary movement such as showing the teeth to order, which may be satisfactorily performed, while smiling induced by emotion is obviously asymmetrical.

Symptoms

The patient's complaints of weakness and wasting arising from lower neurone lesions are seldom difficult to interpret. Weakness confined to the pelvic girdle may give rise to a complaint of unsteadiness and the gait may indeed be ataxic. The initial complaint in a progressive upper motor neurone lesion may be of loss of use rather than of weakness. If spasticity is prominent, the toes may be scraped on walking, or there may be sudden falls due to loss of extensor tone. In all forms of weakness, the complaint may confusingly be of numbness, reflecting the very real difficulty of subjective distinction between loss of feeling and loss of strength.

The sensory system

The afferent inflow from skin, muscles, tendons, and joints arises from end organs specifically adapted to respond to appropriate stimuli and also probably from a non-specific network of cutaneous nerve endings. To what degree the sensations actually aroused by such stimuli as enter consciousness depend on the nature of the receptor organ or on the central pathways is still to some extent uncertain, but in the clinical context it is the anatomy of the sensory tracts that is of obvious relevance. The afferents from muscle spindles and other proprioceptive organs are not consciously perceived, except in the sense that we are aware of the posture of our limbs and can tell with great precision when they are moved and in what direction. We are not aware of the reflex activity that controls our posture and many aspects of voluntary and automatic movement in which the muscle spindles and their control through the fusimotor fibres play so large a part.

The afferent fibres from the limbs are formed by one branch of the axons of the neurones of the posterior root ganglia, the other branch of which enters the spinal cord. The somatic sensory cranial nerves are similarly organized with equivalent ganglia on the fifth and ninth nerves. The posterior spinal roots enter the grey matter, where many, apparently concerned with reflex activity, form synapses with interneurones or with anterior horn cells. The main afferent stream divides; some axons pass into the posterior columns of the spinal cord and ascend to the dorsal column nuclei at the junction with the medulla where they synapse with a second neural relay from which axons cross and ascend as the medial lemniscus to the thalamus. These fibres serve the functions of postural sense and to some extent that of the appreciation of touch. The other main sensory pathway is concerned with pain, thermal sensibility, and also touch. These fibres ascend on the same side of the spinal cord for several segments and then synapse with cells in the posterior grey matter. The axons of the secondary neurones cross in the centre of the cord and ascend in the anterior and lateral columns as the spinothalamic tracts. These are laterally placed in the medulla, but eventually join the medial lemniscus and synapse in the thalamus. The sensory relay is continued to the post-central gyrus and to a wide area of the posterior part of the cerebral hemisphere. The afferent fibres of the trigeminal nerve, with cells of origin in the Gasserian ganglion, synapse in the nucleus within the pons and also in the descending nucleus that extends into the upper cervical spinal cord. Secondary neurones cross the midline and ascend in association with the spinal tracts.

Sensory loss from interruption of a peripheral nerve or posterior nerve root affects all modalities, the extent and severity depending on the nature of the lesion. Thus, cutting a single posterior root may result in no detectable sensory loss, because of overlap from neighbouring roots. Similarly, the area of sensory loss resulting from a peripheral nerve lesion will be much less extensive than the full distribution of the nerve. Within the central nervous system, the separation of the sensory tracts in the spinal cord allows selective loss of different sensory modalities. Pain and thermal sensation will be impaired when the spinothalamic tracts are damaged, while lesions of the posterior columns result in loss of postural sense. Sense of touch is distributed between both pathways, the element involved in tickle passing through the spinothalamic tracts. Vibration sense, so useful to the neurologist, is thought to be conveyed in the posterior columns but is so often impaired in isolation that there is some room for doubt.

Lesions of the parietal cortex may result in loss of all forms of sensation including that of pain, but sometimes there is severe loss of discriminatory forms of sensation with retention of appreciation of crude modalties.

Symptoms

Patients' complaints arising from disorders of the sensory system are often difficult to interpret. Loss of cutaneous sensation may be sufficiently obvious, as with a complaint of being unable to feel the feet on the floor or to judge the temperature of the bath water, but other sensory symptoms are less easy to attribute to disturbance of a particular modality and the distinction of positive from negative symptoms is also difficult. The familiar paraesthesiae, 'pins and needles', may apparently result from lesions in the sensory pathways at any level. A complaint that the affected limbs feel too large or that they 'do not belong to me' usually, but not invariably, indicates loss of postural sense, but when the hand is involved, the complaint may be merely that of 'uselessness'. A sensation of a tight bandage round the leg is commonly complained of by patients with a lesion of the posterior columns of the spinal cord.

Loss of proprioceptive sensation results in sensory ataxia. Difficulty in maintaining balance is greatly increased when information derived from vision is also lost, leading, on examination, to Romberg's sign, consisting of falling when standing with feet together and eyes closed, and to the complaint of inability to walk outside after dusk.

Pain may result from disease of the peripheral and, less commonly, of the central nervous system. Compression of a peripheral nerve, or more particularly of a dorsal root, may cause paraesthesiae and pain in the distribution of the sensory fibres. Pain of a peculiarly distressing burning character can arise from lesions of the spinothalamic tract and in the spinal cord or brain stem, and similar and even more persistent pain and dysaesthesia, or unpleasantly altered cutaneous sensation on stimulation, from thalamic lesions. Pain from cortical lesions is usually episodic and a symptom of focal sensory epilepsy.

Signs of subcortical brain lesions

The cerebellum

The cerebellum receives an afferent supply from all somatic sensory systems and from those of the special senses and yet the symptoms of cerebellar disease are exclusively motor. This is because the inflow does not reach consciousness but modifies the cortical control of movement. In the clinical context, evidence of localization of function within the cerebellum is limited. A lesion of one cerebellar hemisphere causes dysfunction of the limbs on the same side. If midline cerebellar structures are affected, disability predominantly affects equilibrium in the upright posture.

An acute lesion of one cerebellar hemisphere causes inco-ordination, hypotonia, and some loss of power in the limbs on the side of the lesion. In cerebellar ataxia, voluntary movements are performed inaccurately with misjudgments of the appropriate effort (dysmetria). This is usually tested by the patient touching his own nose and the examiner's finger alternately and, in the lower limb, running the heel of one leg down the opposite shin. There is particular difficulty in rapid alternation such as turning the hand (adiadochokinesia). If the outstretched arm is displaced, it sways back beyond its original posture. If the arm is pushed down against resistance and suddenly released, it will fly up without the normal reflex arrest. A similar failure of reflex inhibition is shown by the 'pendular' nature of the knee jerk in which the leg swings repeatedly after a single contraction of the quadriceps. The pointing test involves the patient touching the examiner's finger with his eyes open and attempting to repeat this with eyes closed, when the hand will deviate to the side of the cerebellar lesion. The weakness resulting from an acute cerebellar lesion is seldom pronounced and usually transitory. Skew deviation of the eyes in which the ipsilateral eye is deviated downwards and inwards and the contralateral upwards and outwards is occasionally seen but nystagmus is the more usual ocular sign.

Chronic bilateral cerebellar disease is more commonly encountered. In addition to the ataxia of the limbs, there will usually be nystagmus. This does not have specific characteristics and the direction and other features are not of localizing value. Nystagmus is sometimes absent even when other signs of cerebellar disease are pronounced. Dysarthria with slurred and jerky speech is common. The gait is disturbed in unilateral cerebellar disease when the patient will deviate to the side of the lesion. A more severe test that may disclose slight abnormalities is for the patient to walk a few paces with eyes closed. A lesion involving the vermis may cause ataxia for walking with little or no abnormality of the limbs when tested separately. The gait is waddling with the feet widely placed. In severe examples the patient may be unable to stand or even sit upright, the so-called trunkal ataxia. Tremor is often described but rhythmic contraction of opposing groups of muscles either at rest or when sustaining a posture is most unusual. Many patients with other evidence of cerebellar dysfunction have intention tremor in which the hand oscillates with increasing amplitude as it nears its objective, but this may be due to associated lesions of the brain stem. Episodic vertigo, as opposed to sensations of unsteadiness, can seldom be attributed to cerebellar disease.

The ataxia of cerebellar disorders must be distinguished from the effect of weakness of proximal limb muscles and from sensory ataxia. This distinction cannot be made on the patient's description of the symptoms and must depend on characteristic findings on examination.

The internal capsule

In the internal capsule the descending motor fibres are condensed into a small space, immediately anterior to the similarly narrowly localized ascending sensory fibres. Even relatively small lesions in this area can therefore produce severe hemiplegia of the opposite limbs, accompanied by sensory loss and, if the destruction extends more posteriorly, by hemianopia. This is in contrast to the more restricted effects of a lesion of comparable size in the cerebral cortex.

The basal ganglia

With few exceptions focal lesions of the basal ganglia are not associated with specific symptoms or signs. Involuntary movements of many kinds are often attributed to such lesions, for example chorea, but on insufficient evidence. Diseases involving these structures are described in a later section.

The thalamus

The symptom most common associated with a lesion of the thalamus is that of spontaneous pain in the opposite side of the body. This *thalamic syndrome* is usually of sudden onset, due to a stroke, and is accompanied by hemiplegia which rapidly recovers. The patient is left with persistent peculiarly unpleasant pain in the affected limbs and trunk, usually sparing the face. The pain is greatly aggravated by almost any stimulus applied to that side of the body. It is usually possible to detect some loss of sense of position but cutaneous sensation cannot easily be examined.

The exact relationship of this syndrome to lesions of the thalamus is doubtful and it may certainly occur both with lesions of the parietal cortex and of the sensory pathways caudal to the thalamus. The distressing symptoms are probably related more to the pattern of involvement of the sensory tracts and other structures than to any precise localization.

The hypothalamus (see page 21.75)

As the main regulating centre of the autonomic system it might be supposed that clearcut syndromes due to lesions of the separate hypothalamic nuclei would easily identifiable. These nuclei are, however, small and closely aligned, so that while disorders of such functions as sleep, nutrition, and temperature regulation may be suspected as being of hypothalamic origin this is often difficult to demonstrate. The anatomical and functional relationships to the posterior and anterior lobes of the pituitary are close. Many expanding lesions in this region will necessarily encroach on the third ventricle and interfere with the flow of cerebrospinal fluid, thus further complicating the symptomatology. Pure hypothalamic syndromes are, therefore, difficult to define, particularly as pathological evidence is usually lacking. Symptoms that may be encountered include diabetes insipidus, obesity, marasmus in the child, hypo- and hyperthermia, and somnolence.

The midbrain

Among the crowded tracts and nuclei of the midbrain, those that can most readily be identified as contributing to the symptomatology of lesions in this area are the descending corticospinal and corticobulbar tracts; the red nucleus; the nuclei of the third and fourth cranial nerves; and the reticular formation. The contiguous superior cerebellar peduncles may also be involved. A number of syndromes have been awarded eponymous titles that serve some purpose in the cause of brevity.

In *Weber's syndrome* the lesion involves the cerebral peduncle containing descending motor fibres, and the third nerve just before it leaves the brain. The result is an ipsilateral third nerve palsy and hemiplegia on the opposite side. *Benedikt's syndrome*, of a variety of involuntary movements on the side opposite to a third nerve palsy is thought to arise from involvement of the red nucleus. *Nothnagel's syndrome* consists of cerebellar ataxia which may be bilateral combined with a variety of ocular palsies. It results from a posteriorly placed lesion involving oculomotor nuclei and cerebellar peduncles.

The nuclei of the third and fourth cranial nerves are arranged in columns of cells so that nuclear lesions are unlikely to cause complete isolated palsies. A characteristic sign of midbrain involvement, either by an intrinsic lesion or from external pressure, is *Parinaud's syndrome*. In its fully developed form this consists of failure of conjugate upward gaze, of convergence and of pupillary reflexes. In vestigial forms loss of upward gaze is a common feature of increasing intracranial pressure with downward displacement of the midbrain.

Lesions involving the reticular formation have been held responsible for disturbances of conscious level and also for the condition of akinetic mutism in which the patient makes no voluntary movement except of the eyes.

The pons and medulla

The pons and medulla contain nuclei of the fifth to the twelfth cranial nerves, important connections with the cerebellum and motor, sensory, and autonomic fibre tracts. Precise localization of lesions is sometimes possible from a close study of physical signs and an intimate knowledge of anatomy. Pathological processes do not often, however, involve the sharply delineated areas depicted in many diagrams and bilateral, asymmetrical, and discontinuous lesions produce bewildering signs.

Two syndromes can be identified as caused by medullary lesions of which the *lateral medullary syndrome of Wallenberg* is by far the more common. It causes dysphagia and dysarthria (ninth and tenth nerve nuclei), vomiting (nucleus ambiguus), hiccough (reticular formation) and vertigo (vestibular nuclei) combined with cerebellar ataxia of the limbs on the side of the lesion (inferior cerebellar peduncle), ipsilateral Horner's syndrome (descending autonomic fibres), loss of pain and thermal sensation on the face on the side of the lesion (fifth nerve nucleus) and in the opposite limbs (lateral lemniscus). There is usually no weakness as the pyramidal tracts are spared. Diplopia may be complained of but no ocular palsy can be detected.

The rare *medial medullary syndrome* consists of weakness and loss of postural sense in the limbs on the side opposite to the lesion (pyramidal tract and medial lemniscus) and ipsilateral paralysis of the tongue (twelfth nerve nucleus).

Lateralized lesions of the pons similarly give rise to ipsilateral cranial nerve involvement with crossed paralysis or sensory loss from destruction of long tracts. The syndrome most easily recognised is that of *Millard–Gubler* with sixth and seventh nerve palsies and crossed hemiplegia. This may be combined with damage to supranuclear fibres controlling eye movements so that conjugate gaze towards the side of the lesion may be paralysed (*Foville*). If the cerebellum is also affected, a complex syndrome of ipsilateral ataxia and Horner's syndrome with crossed loss of pain and thermal sensation may result. An acute centrally placed pontine lesion will cause coma with characteristically extremely contracted pupils.

Certain signs indicative of brainstem pathology may be encountered in isolation or combined with more widespread evidence of disease. An internuclear ophthalmoplegia of the only form commonly seen consists of failure of adduction of the eye in lateral conjugate gaze to one or both sides but with preservation of convergence. This implies that the medial rectus muscle is not paralysed but that it cannot act in conjunction with the opposite lateral rectus. This is thought to be due to a lesion in the medial longitudinal bundle connecting the sixth and third nerve nuclei.

The strange condition of *palatal myoclonus* is associated with degeneration of the ipsilateral dentate nucleus in the cerebellum and the contralateral inferior medullary olive. The palate contracts almost rhythmically at a rate of 1–2 per second sometimes producing an audible click. This may become bilateral or spread to the facial muscles, the upper limb, diaphragm, or rarely the ocular muscles. It is said to be the only involuntary movement to persist during sleep.

The *'locked in' syndrome* results from interruption of the descending and ascending long tracts in the brain stem below the oculomotor nuclei and without disturbing consciousness. As patients cannot talk or move, it is easy to presume that they cannot understand but this is not so. Eye movement is maintained and such patients readily learn to communicate by means of signalling, looking right for 'yes' and so on. This syndrome differs from akinetic mutism where, although the eyes are moved, no communication can be established (see page 21.48).

References

Bickerstaff, E. R. (1980). *Neurological examination in clinical practice*, 4th edn. Blackwell Scientific Publications, Oxford.

Brodal, A. (1981) *Neurological anatomy in relation to clinical medicine*, 3rd edn. Oxford University Press, London.

Currier, R. D. (1969). Syndromes of the medulla oblongata. In *Handbook of clinical neurology* (eds. P. J. Vinken and G. W. Bruyn), vol. 2. North Holland, Amsterdam.

Gardner, E. (1968). *Fundamentals of neurology,* 5th edn. W. B. Saunders, Philadelphia.

Loeb, C. and Meyer, J. S. (1969). Pontine syndromes. In *Handbook of clinical neurology* (eds. P. J. Vinken and G. W. Bruyn), vol. 2. North Holland, Amsterdam.

Matthews, W. B. (1975). *Practical neurology*, 3rd edn. Blackwell Scientific Publications, Oxford.

THE AUTONOMIC NERVOUS SYSTEM AND HYPOTHALAMUS

R. BANNISTER

Introduction

The autonomic nervous system innervates every visceral organ in the body. It has as complex a neural organization in the brain, spinal cord, and periphery as the somatic nervous system, but remains largely involuntary or automatic. As Claude Bernard put it 'nature thought it provident to remove these important phenomena from the caprice of an ignorant will'. Langley, who in 1898 first proposed the term 'autonomic nervous system', based his experiments on the blocking action of nicotine at synapses in ganglia. In 1921 Loewi discovered 'Vagusstoff' which was released by stimulation of the vagus nerve and proved to be acetylcholine. In the same year Cannon discovered that 'sympathin', later shown to be noradrenaline, was produced by stimulation of the sympathetic trunk. The basis was therefore laid for Dale's distinction between cholinergic and adrenergic transmission in the autonomic nervous system.

Anatomy and physiology

The peripheral autonomic nervous system, an efferent system, is made up of neurones which lie outside the CNS which are concerned with visceral innervation. Both sympathetic and parasympathetic systems have preganglionic neurones in the brain and spinal cord arranged as shown in Fig. 1. The afferent limbs of autonomic reflexes may lie in any afferent nerve. The preganglionic sympathetic fibres are myelinated and leave the spinal roots as white rami communicantes and synapse in the ganglia. Unmyelinated postganglionic fibres rejoin the anterior spinal roots by the arrangement shown in Fig. 2, although some sympathetic fibres traverse the ganglia and synapse in more peripheral ganglia, following the arrangement of the parasympathetic fibres.

The transmitter at all preganglionic terminals is acetylcholine which is not paralysed by atropine (the nicotinic effect) whereas the action of acetylcholine at the distal end of the cholinergic postganglionic fibres is paralysed by atropine (the muscarinic effect). Noradrenaline is the principal transmitter for postganglionic sympathetic nerves, the exceptions being sudomotor nerves, which are cholinergic in humans, some vasodilator fibres to muscle, and the adrenal medulla which is innervated by preganglionic (cholinergic fibres) and itself secretes mainly adrenaline. Noradrenaline is stored in the terminals and is released by nerve activity or by sym-

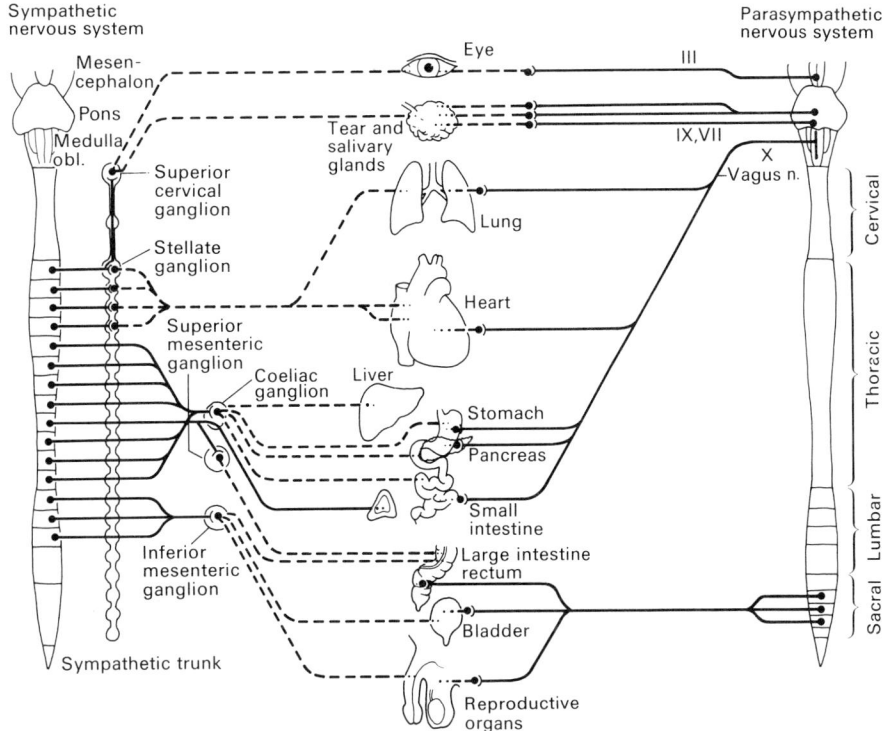

Fig. 1 Peripheral autonomic nervous system. The sympathetic innervation of vessels, sweat glands, and piloerector muscles is not shown. Solid lines, preganglionic axons, dashed lines, postganglionic axons. (Reproduced from Bannister, *Brain's clinical neurology*, Oxford University Press, with permission.)

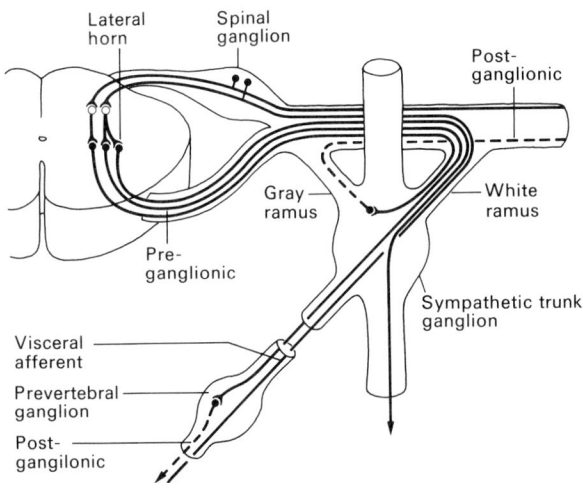

Fig. 2 The autonomic spinal reflex arc. (Reproduced from Bannister, *Brain's clinical neurology*, Oxford University Press.)

pathomimetic drugs, which may act partly indirectly on the ganglia or more centrally, such as ephedrine and amphetamine or on the terminals such as phenylephrine or tyramine. The different actions of noradrenaline and adrenaline are caused by relative effects on different receptors. Alpha receptors mediate vasoconstriction, intestinal relaxation, and dilation of the pupil (and are blocked by thymoxamine). Alpha receptors may be either postsynaptic (alpha 1) or presynaptic (alpha 2), which, when stimulated, decrease the release of the transmitter. Beta receptors mediate vasodilation, especially in muscles, increase the rate and force of the heart with a tendency to arrhythmias, and cause bronchial relaxation. They are further subdivided into beta 1 receptors, mediating the chronotropic cardiac action of isoprenaline, whereas beta 2 receptors are responsible for most of the peripheral effects of beta adrenergic stimulation.

The cells of the autonomic nervous system tend to act in conjunction and this is achieved mainly by specialized intercellular junctions at the ganglion cells which have been demonstrated by electron microscopy and freeze fracture techniques. The autonomic ganglia also contain small intensely fluorescent cells (SIF cells) which contain many peptides, and are thought to act as modulators and transmitters at synaptic sites. Substance P, vasoactive intestinal peptide (VIP), encephalins, and somatostatin have all been identified in autonomic ganglia although their precise role in control of nerve transmission is not yet known.

The old-fashioned notion of a simple duality of a sympathetic–adrenergic system causing a rather unselective 'fight or flight' response and a parasympathetic–cholinergic system providing tonic activity, has now given way to a new view of a highly selective autonomic nervous system. Though the two systems in general have antagonistic functions there is a subtlety of integrative action at least as complex as that of the somatic nervous system. New transmitters and modulators have been discovered, many still putative, and receptors, both presynaptic or postsynaptic, can be blocked, activated or modified in their numbers and affinities. New general biological principles have emerged with 'up and down' regulation, by agonists of receptor numbers and affinities, and with the manipulation pharmacologically of presynaptic and postsynaptic receptors by transmitter release, depletion or blockade.

The hypothalamus

Introduction

The hypothalamus can be considered the 'highest' level of integration of autonomic function. It remains under the influence of the cortex and the group of structures known as the 'limbic system' which includes the olfactory areas, the hippocampus and amygdaloid complex, the cingulate cortex, and the septal area. These regions of the brain regulate the hypothalamus and are critical for emotional and affective expression. In phylogenetic development the limbic system represents the older or palaeomammalian cortex as opposed to the neomammalian cortex. Its function is thought to be concerned with levels below cognitive behaviour, and inductive and deductive reasoning, though it nevertheless is concerned with a feeling of individuality and identity. It analyses the significance of the input of sensation to the organism in relation to the instinctive drives which promote the perpetuation of the individual by satisfying hunger, thirst, and sexual needs. It is also concerned with maintaining homeostasis against a changing environment and ensures the perpetuation of the species by sexual and parental drives which can at times override more selfish self-perpetuating drives of the individual. The essence of its function is choice, based on sensory information, of patterns of behaviour. As it overlaps both with the sensory and motor systems it is essential for many aspects of memory and learning. The autonomic nervous system and many metabolic functions are under the control of the limbic system by means of nerve centres, many of which are situated in the hypothalamus, lying ventrally to the thalamus and constituting the floor of the third ventricle. The hypothalamus contains a large number of scattered ganglion cells, which have been differentiated into a number of nuclei. The projections of the hypothalamus are not yet completely known.

Anatomy and physiology

The hypothalamus controls the autonomic nervous system in two ways, by means of the pituitary and hence other endocrine glands (see Section 10) and by direct descending nervous pathways. Although the latter exist some regions of the brain stem are to some extent autonomous and function in animals after pontine section of the brain stem. These include cardiac and respiratory function and 'centres' for 'vomiting' and 'micturition', but under natural circumstances cardiovascular responses never occur in isolation but accompany the processes of exercise, digestion, sexual function, and temperature regulation. The integration of these changes takes place in the hypothalamus. The course taken by descending sympathetic fibres from the hypothalamus is uncrossed and by way of the lateral tegmentum of the brain stem and lateral medullary formation. Some fibres end directly on the intermediolateral column cells, while others synapse in the reticular formation.

It is incorrect to use the term 'centre' except as representing an area which if damaged results in a disturbance of these functions and so is in some way essential for the proper performances of these functions. Heat loss responses in animals are elicited by local heating of the anterior hypothalamus suggesting the presence of cells which act as 'thermoreceptors'. Conversely, after destructive lesions of the posterior hypothalamus shivering and peripheral vasoconstriction do not occur on exposure to cold. Postoperative hyperthermia occurs in humans after injury to the anterior hypothalamus. Also in the hypothalamus a lateral 'feeding centre' and medial 'satiety centre' have been identified by ablation experiments in animals.

Hypothalamic lesions

The principal disturbances which may follow hypothalamic lesions in humans are those of sleep, sexual function, pituitary function, food and water balance, and temperature and blood pressure regulation (see Section 13). The neurological lesions may be tumours, such as craniopharyngioma, chronic basal meningitis, such as sarcoidosis, or a vascular lesion, particularly rupture of an aneurysm on the circle of Willis. Investigation follows the usual lines for an intracerebral lesion with a range of endocrine tests added. The commonest cause of a hypothalamic lesion is a severe head injury, after which diabetes insipidus may follow.

Classification of autonomic disorders

A convenient clinical classification of progressive autonomic failure is as follows (see Table 1 and page 21.226).

1. Patients with 'pure' progressive autonomic failure, without associated neurological disorders.
2. Patients with progressive autonomic failure and a variety of neurological disturbances (commonly but not always including parkinsonism). This in general corresponds to the Shy–Drager syndrome.
3. Patients with progressive autonomic failure and Parkinson's disease.

Progressive autonomic failure (PAF) occurs alone or as an additional feature in two distinct and well-recognized types of primary neurological degenerative disease, namely, Parkinson's disease (PD) and multiple system atrophy (MSA) (see page 21.226). In its pure form progressive autonomic failure was first reported by Bradbury and Eggleston (1925) and was known as 'idiopathic orthostatic hypotension' (IOH). Shy and Drager (1960) described the more complex neurological syndrome, that bears their name, now called progressive autonomic failure (PAF) with multiple system atrophy (MSA), in which postural hypotension may be accompanied by pyramidal, extrapyramidal and cerebellar signs (see page 21.227). Later the variant was recognized in which autonomic failure was associated with apparent typical idiopathic Parkinsonism. Cases of clinically 'pure' progressive autonomic failure examined at post-mortem show either Lewy intranuclear inclusion bodies, linking these cases to PD, or minor changes of MSA (see page 21.227). Unnecessary confusion results when the term 'idiopathic orthostatic hypotension' (IOH), is used by some as a similar name for the Shy–Drager syndrome, while others use the same term exclusively for cases of 'pure' progressive autonomic failure. The remedy for this confusion would be to drop the use of the term IOH altogether. The cases of PAF with PD are therefore distinct from cases of MSA in which striatonigral degeneration (SND) or olivopontocerebellar atrophy (OPCA) or both may be present (see page 21.227).

Clinical features of progressive autonomic failure

When the effects of drugs and adrenal insufficiency have been excluded, persistent postural hypotension is almost certainly due to a neurological lesion, and the commonest presenting symptoms of postural hypotension are postural dizziness and fatigue or attacks of loss of consciousness on exercise. However, the first symptoms of progressive autonomic failure are mild, insidious, and frequently overlooked or misdiagnosed. The patients are

Table 1 Classification of autonomic disorders

1 Central, primary
  (a) Progressive autonomic failure (PAF)
  (b) Progressive autonomic failure with multiple system (MSA)
  (c) Progressive autonomic failure with Parkinson's disease
2 Central, secondary
  (a) Central brain lesions: craniopharyngioma, vascular lesions
  (b) Infections of the nervous system: tabes dorsalis, Chagas' disease
  (c) Spinal cord lesions
  (d) Familial dysautonomia
3 Distal autonomic neuropathies
  (a) General medical disorders: diabetes, amyloid, porphyria, Tangier disease, Fabry's disease
  (b) Autoimmune disease: acute and subacute pandysautonomia; Guillain-Barré syndrome, myasthenia, rheumatoid arthritis
4 Drugs
  (a) Selective neurotoxic drugs; alcoholism; Wernicke's encephalopathy
  (b) Tranquillizers: phenothiazines, barbiturates
  (c) Antidepressants: tricyclics; monoamine oxidase inhibitors
  (d) Vasodilator hypotensive drugs: prazosin, hydralazine
  (e) Centrally acting hypotensive drugs: methyldopa, clonidine
  (f) Adrenergic neurone blocking drugs: phenoxybenzamine, labetalol
  (h) Ganglion blocking drugs: hexamethonium, mecamylamine
  (i) Angiotensin converting enzyme inhibitors: captopril

middle aged, or elderly and males are affected about twice as often as females. In men, impotence and loss of libido are commonly the first symptoms. Patients living in a hot climate may complain of an inability to sweat. Later, the first symptoms of postural dizziness or syncope occur, followed by bladder symptoms including incontinence. The postural attacks may be 'drop' attacks resembling sudden brain stem vascular dysfunction but more commonly there is a gradual fading of consciousness over half a minute or so while the patient is standing or walking. A transient ache in the neck radiating to the occipital region of the skull and shoulders often precedes actual loss of consciousness. Sometimes there are transient visual disturbances, scotomata or positive hallucinations or tunnel vision, suggesting occipital lobe ischaemia. The patient may then fall to his knees. Experience teaches him that after lying flat, recovery and loss of all symptoms including the neckache will occur within a few minutes. The recovery from such transient neurological symptoms is usually complete and (possibly because the patients have virtually continuous cerebrovasodilation due to years of postural hypotension) occlusive cerebrovascular incidents are rare. The attack differs from the usual 'faint' in that the patient cannot sweat and there is no vagal cardiac slowing. The disease is likely to be progressive for five or more years before significant incapacity occurs. Some rarer non-neurological presentations occur. A few patients if treated by bed rest for hypotensive symptoms develop persistent recumbent hypertension of such severity that they may develop papilloedema with retinal haemorrhages.

The neurological as opposed to the cardiovascular features are equally insidious (see page 21.227). The commonest early features are an extrapyramidal disorder in which rigidity is more obvious than akinesis or tremor. The true diagnosis is sometimes dramatically revealed when mild postural hypotension becomes severe on treatment with levodopa or there is unexpected lack of response to levodopa in what appears at first to be a case of Parkinson's disease. In some patients a cerebellar tremor often with a marked truncal component is the earliest sign of cerebellar system involvement. The extrapyramidal syndrome may progress and additional symptoms and signs may emerge including pyramidal signs, muscle wasting, pupillary inequalities, and respiratory abnormalities including sleep apnoea and laryngeal stridor. The order of the development of neurological symptoms is variable.

Testing autonomic function

Introduction

Testing autonomic function (Table 2) is complicated by the fact that within each part of the output from the autonomic system fractionation occurs and any defects whether central of peripheral, may be partially corrected by other neuronal, chemical or hormonal mechanisms. When we add that the lesions caused by disease are often multiple and variable, the task of correlating reflex defects and pathology in humans might seem daunting. However, the cardiovascular system has proved suitable for an analysis of the principles used in testing for autonomic dysfunction and analysing cardiovascular control is doubly relevant because postural hypotension is one of the commonest symptoms of defective autonomic function. The homeostatic control of blood pressure may be disturbed by lesions at several levels from the hypothalamus to the periphery. Figure 3 shows a much simplified diagram of some of the neurological pathways involved in the regulation of blood pressure. There are cortical, limbic, anterior and posterior hypothalamic and medullary 'centres' at which the input from the carotid sinus and other afferents can be integrated and the output through the vagus and sympathetic system to the heart and blood vessels may be co-ordinated. In autonomic failure the baroreceptors, as feedback transducers in cybernetic terms, do not produce the required responses in the effectors, the resistance and capacity vessels, the heart and the kidneys. This causes both a change in the 'set point' pressure and an instability in the response to various stresses.

Table 2 Some useful clinical tests of autonomic failure

A *Cardiovascular reflexes*
Tests performed and responses:
1 Change of posture: BP and pulse rate monitored while subject is supine and then repeated measurements are made at 60° head-up tilt position. Pulse rate and plasma noradrenaline responses to standing. Lower body negative pressure is an alternative to standing
2 Deep breathing: presence or absence of sinus arrhythmia; test of vagal efferent pathway
3 Carotid massage: right and left sides, in turn monitoring cardiac rate and blood pressure; test of vagal efferent pathway. Caution in case of supersensitivity
4 Hyperventilation: for 30 s, causing hypocapnia and fall in blood pressure; response suggests afferent lesion, if baroreflex block
5 Inspiratory gasp: causing reflex vasoconstriction of hands; spinal-cord reflex
6 Stress: causing hypertension and tachycardia; tests of sympathetic efferent pathway
    (*a*) Hand grip, submaximal sustained for 90 s
    (*b*) Sudden cortical arousal by unexpected noise
    (*c*) Mental arithmetic (rapid serial subtraction of 7 from 100)
    (*d*) Cold pressor test-hand immersed in water at 4 °C for 90 s
7 Breath holding: test of central breathing control; prolonged if vagal afferent dysfunction
8 Valsalva manoeuvre: After a deep inspiration the patient performs a forced expiration for 12 s through a tube connected to mercury manometer. Most subjects can maintain a pressure of 30 mmHg. In normal subjects there is an increasing tachycardia for the 10 s of sustained forced expiration. Blood pressure falls initially but should cease to fall after the first few seconds if peripheral sympathetic vasoconstriction is normal. On release from blowing there is normally a BP overshoot and a compensatory reflex bradycardia
9 Pharmacological tests:
    (*a*) Plasma noradrenaline at rest and after 30 min standing or tilt
    (*b*) Pressor response and cardiac slowing to infusion of noradrenaline (or phenylephrine) test of baroreflex sensitivity
    (*c*) Pressor response and noradrenaline response to infusion of tyramine; test of cytoplasmic stores of noradrenaline
    (*d*) Cardiac slowing to atropine; test of vagal function

B *Sweating*
1 Response to body heating in order to cause a rise of 1 °C oral or rectal temperature in the course of 90 min. Record sweating and measure hand blood-flow. Test of sympathetic pathway from hypothalamus to periphery
2 Response to brief trunk heating with electric lamp source for 90 s; a reflex response, without involving change of blood temperature, utilizing same efferent pathway as response to body heating
3 Responses to intramuscular pilocarpine; acts directly on sweat glands
4 Pilomotor and sudomotor response to intradermal methacholine; absent with complete postganglionic lesion

C *Pupillary responses*
1 Instillation of 1:1000 adrenaline. Response: dilation after sympathetic postganglionic denervation; no effect on normal pupil
2 Instillation of fresh 2.5 per cent cocaine. Response: dilation of normal pupil; no effect after sympathetic denervation
3 Instillation of fresh 2.5 per cent methacholine. Response: constriction after parasympathetic denervation; no effect on normal pupil

D *Skin response*
Intracutaneous injection of 0.05 ml of 1 per cent 1000 histamine phosphate causes a wheal surrounded by erythema and erythematous flare. The flare of this triple response is an axon reflex mediated by antidromic transmission along sensory fibres

Clinical testing of autonomic function

When a fall of more than some 20 points systolic on standing is found in a patient with symptoms, further investigation is justified and a battery of tests is now available and summarized in Table 2. Radial or brachial artery catheterization will show precisely the postural fall and the fluctuations with various manoeuvres. On tilt the blood pressure falls due to lack of constriction in resistance and capacity vessels in muscles and in the splanchnic area

(Fig. 4). There is also a lack of the overshoot in phase IV of the Valsalva which normally occurs as a result of reflex peripheral vasoconstriction (Fig. 5). The instability of blood pressure in autonomic failure is due partly to lack of baroreflex control but also to supersensitivity of partially denervated vessels to the transmitter noradrenaline and this may cause recumbent hypertension.

Cardiovascular reflexes, like somatic reflexes, have efferent, central, and afferent connections and the next stage in the investigation of postural hypotension and a 'blocked' Valsalva manoeuvre is to try to show whether the lesion is afferent or efferent. If the vasoconstrictor response to stress, a reflex arising from the hypothalamus, is lost, as it is in almost all cases of progressive autonomic failure, then the lesion is presumed to be efferent. There is no simple way of testing the afferent pathway in the presence of an efferent lesion. Recently techniques of investigation have been used combining lower body suction to simulate the effect of posture with neck pressure to 'unload' the carotid baroreceptors and so isolate the contribution of other afferents, including those from low-pressure areas. Further evidence of the lack of sympathetic activity has also been provided by assay of plasma noradrenaline, which is low in patients with autonomic failure and fails to rise on standing (Fig. 6). There is some uncertainty whether patients with 'pure' progressive autonomic failure have a lower resting plasma noradrenaline than autonomic failure with multiple system atrophy, though in neither is there a rise on standing.

A major difficulty is to decide whether the sympathetic efferent lesion is preganglionic or postganglionic or both. This is of practical importance because it affects the degree of denervation supersensitivity and the response to pressor drugs. Following complete postganglionic sympathetic denervation, supersensitivity of vessels to the transmitter noradrenaline occurs, with loss of the response to tyramine. Tyramine acts by releasing noradrenaline from the cytoplasmic pool but not the granular pool, which is accessible to the nerve impulse. All patients with progressive autonomic failure show some supersensitivity to intravenous noradrenaline and there is evidence that this is greater in pure progressive autonomic failure than in autonomic failure with multiple system atrophy. Recently it has been shown that alpha and beta receptor binding on platelets and lymphocytes is increased in

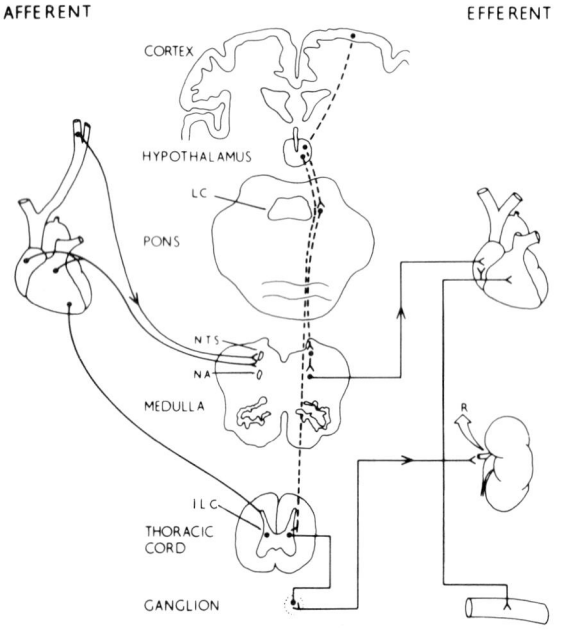

Fig. 3 Diagram of cardiovascular control mechanisms. L. C. – locus coeruleus; N.T.S. – nucleus tractus solitarius; I.L.C. – intermediolateral column; R. – renin. (Reproduced from Bannister, 1983, *Autonomic failure*, Oxford University Press, with permission.)

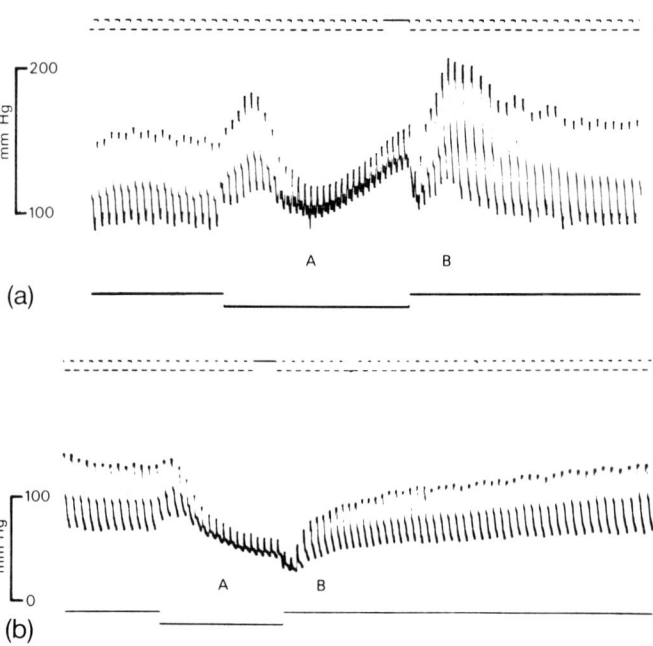

Fig. 4 (a) Valsalva response in a normal subject showing blood pressure (upper trace), cardiac beat-to-beat record (lower trace). (b) Valsalva manoeuvre showing very abnormal response in progressive autonomic failure. (Records reproduced from Bannister, 1983, *Autonomic failure*, Oxford University Press, with permission.)

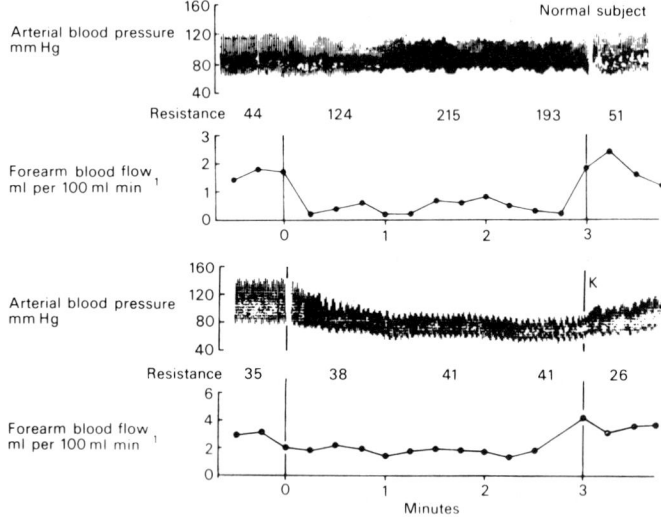

Fig. 5 The effect of suction on arterial blood pressure, forearm resistance, and forearm blood flow in a normal subject (upper part), and in a patient with progressive autonomic failure (lower part). (Reproduced from Bannister, 1983, *Autonomic failure*, Oxford University Press, with permission.)

autonomic failure and there may be similar changes in alpha and beta receptors in the myocardial and limb blood vessels.

Such studies in cases of progressive autonomic failure have provided good evidence of an efferent sympathetic lesion which is more postganglionic in 'pure' progressive autonomic failure. This sympathetic efferent lesion, affecting resistance and capacity vessels and the heart, is usually more severe than the vagal lesion, shown by lack of sinus arrhythmia. This makes an interesting contrast with the distal diabetic autonomic neuropathy in which the vagal efferent lesion is usually more severe than the sympathetic efferent lesion.

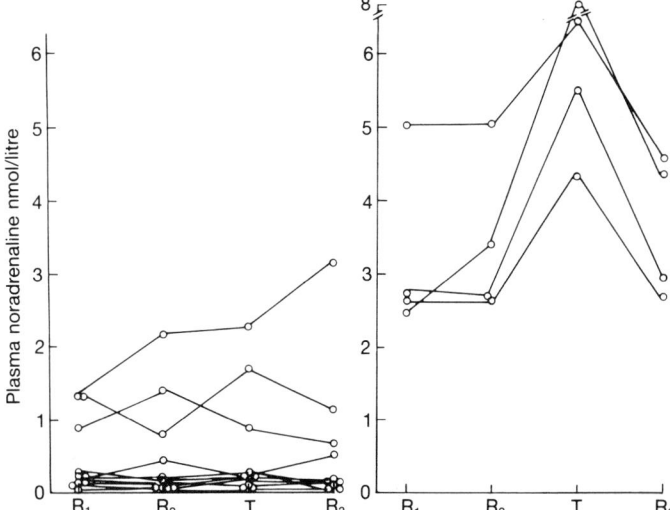

Fig. 6 Effect of tilt on plasma noradrenaline concentration (nmol/1) in patients with autonomic failure (left) and in control subjects (right). R1 and R2 denote recordings following 1 and 2 h of recumbency, respectively. The T recording following a 10 min 60° tilt, and the R3 recording a further 1 h of recumbency. (Reproduced from Bannister *et al.*, 1977, with permission.)

Neuropathology of progressive autonomic failure

In almost all patients carefully studied there has been a reduction by up to 80 per cent in the number of sympathetic preganglionic neurones in the intermediolateral columns of the spinal cord. There have also been brain stem abnormalities with loss of pigment in the melanin-containing nuclei which are derived from the basal plate of the primitive neural tube, including the substantia nigra, dorsal nucleus of the vagus, the locus coeruleus, and the nucleus tractus solitarius. In patients with progressive autonomic failure (PAF) with idiopathic Parkinsonism, Lewy bodies are found. These are inclusion bodies which contain remnants of melanin from the oxidation of catecholamines. The neurochemical defects in progressive autonomic failure with multiple system atrophy can be distinguished from those of Parkinson's disease (PD). At the limbic-hypothalamic level in PAF with MSA there is a marked reduction in noradrenaline involving also the septal nuclei, which is not present in PD. This is supported by the observation of very marked reduction in tyrosine hydroxylase, the rate-limiting enzyme for noradrenaline synthesis, in the hypothalamus, again not present in PD. This observation also correlates with the low CSF noradrenaline levels in the MSA with PAF. The associated NA depletion in MSA is likely to be the explanation for poor response to the extrapyramidal features of MS to dopaminergic agents which is in marked contrast to PD. In all patients with PAF there is, as might be expected, a reduction of the catecholamine fluorescence of sympathetic nerve endings on muscle blood vessels, and on electron microscopy of the endings there is a reduction in the number of small dense-core noradrenergic vesicles.

The pathogenesis of chronic autonomic failure

The pathogenesis of progressive autonomic failure remains unknown but there are some interesting clues to possible genetic influences. In addition to the rare familial cases of PAF and olivopontocerebellar atrophy, itself sometimes familial, there are a few cases with a family history of Parkinson's disease. Recently it has been shown that the histocompatibility antigen HLA AW32 is 13 times more common in PAF than in controls giving a relative risk rate of 28.7. Certain individuals with PAF therefore have clear genetic features in common but obviously other factors determine whether PAF occurs, possibly exposure to a neurotropic virus,

against a background of altered immunity. The hypothesis that several different chronic neuronal degenerations have features in common accords well with the current view of PAF and also provides hope that, apart from increasing our understanding about aetiology, early and effective replacement treatment of neurotransmitters might delay secondary anterograde or retrograde cell loss.

Distal autonomic neuropathies

In contrast to progressive autonomic failure there are also true distal autonomic neuropathies (see Table 1) in which the clinical features resulting from interruption of the efferent autonomic pathways produce certain symptoms and signs which resemble those of progressive autonomic failure. The onset may be more acute, however, and partial or complete recovery may occur, whereas recovery never occurs in progressive autonomic failure. The distal neuropathies with autonomic involvement are mainly described elsewhere in this book (see Table 1 and page 21.124) but the methods of investigation and treatment are similar to those of progressive autonomic failure. There is, however, one distal neuropathy which requires special mention. This is the rare *acute or subacute pandysautonomia* which mayy involve either sympathetic or parasympathetic fibres or both. The autonomic defects can be identified as in progressive autonomic failure. This disease appears to have an autoimmune basis with a tendency to gradual recovery which may be incomplete. It may be thought of as a variant of the type of autonomic neuropathy which occurs as a feature of the Guillain–Barré syndrome, where autonomic features are often present but rather obscured by the somatic neuropathy (see page 21.126).

Treatment of autonomic failure

There are several methods of varying complexity which can be used to counteract the postural hypotension but all are in various ways unsatisfactory. Obviously, if the volume into which the pooling of blood takes place on standing is reduced, this will help the patients; or if the volume of blood is increased, then this will also reduce the severity of the postural hypotension. However, because of lack of baroreflexes all patients have a very labile blood pressure, high when lying and low when standing, and relatively low in the morning and after meals and rising towards evening. It is therefore difficult, unless systematic observations are made, to know what blood pressure should be recorded when attempting to compare one form of treatment with another. The most impressive feature of the blood pressure regulation of these patients is their extreme sensitivity to changes in posture.

In PAF it is important not be overconcerned with a low-standing blood pressure if the patient is without symptoms. Patients can sometimes tolerate a standing systolic blood pressure as low as 80 mmHg without dizziness or syncope probably because their capacity for cerebral autoregulation is better than normal subjects. On lying flat overnight, patients with autonomic failure lose more sodium and fluid than a normal individual. Some are able to release renin normally on head-up tilt and these observations led to the successful introduction of postural treatment by head-up tilt at night. When the patient is made to sleep in a semierect position, therefore having a lower blood pressure at night and retaining more fluid and sodium, there is an increase in the body weight, which on a short-term basis can be attributed to an increase in extracellular fluid volume, and the standing blood pressure improves (Fig. 7). Almost all patients with postural hypotension due to any form of autonomic failure can be helped by the head-up bed tilt at night. Once patients have experienced the benefits they will usually be ready to tolerate the degree of discomfort this may entail. With certain precautions to avoid hyponatraemia, intranasal nocturnal DDAVP can be used to prevent nocturnal fluid loss in these patients.

A second line of treatment which is usually helpful is the use of fludrocortisone. In a smaller dose (0.1 mg) than necessary to

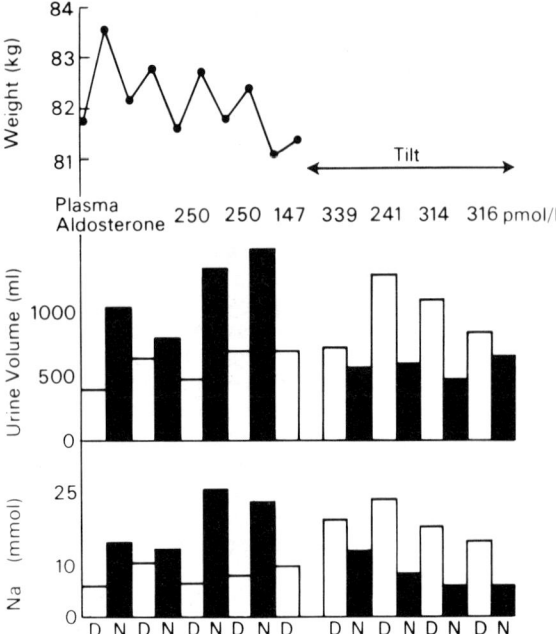

Fig. 7 Diurnal changes in water and sodium excretion in a patient with progressive autonomic failure and multiple system atrophy during five days lying flat at night and five days of head-up tilt at night. D = day, N = night. (Reproduced from Bannister, 1983, *Autonomic failure*, Oxford University Press, with permission.)

increase blood volume, fludrocortisone appears to increase the sensitivity of blood vessels to very small amounts of noradrenaline which may still be capable of being released in autonomic failure. There is no reason to believe that effects of this low dose are the result and effect of an increase in blood volume. Larger doses of fludrocortisone do of course increase blood volume but there appears to be an 'escape' effect which occurs after two or three weeks and so the effect on the blood volume is not as satisfactory as relying on increasing sensitivity to noradrenaline caused by a smaller dose. The use of the external support of the leg and trunk with elastic support garments or an 'anti-gravity suit' is unphysiological in that it reduces intrinsic myogenic tone and is rarely of much long-term benefit.

There have been many pressor drugs studied in autonomic failure. These include phenylephrine which acts directly on sympathetic vascular endings and ephedrine which acts indirectly, and there have also been trials of combinations of tyramine and monoamine oxidase inhibitors. More recently, the beta-blockers such as propanolol and selective blockers with some direct agonist action such as pindolol have been used and there have also been attempts to increase the vasoconstrictor response using the prosta-

glandin inhibitor, indomethacin. All these drugs tend to have the disadvantage of causing greater relative recumbent hypertension. This is because there are no normal baroreflex mechanisms damping down the rise in blood pressure when the patient is recumbent. These pressor drug mixtures rarely improve the patient's standing blood pressure. When the patient is exposed to recumbent hypertension, this probably induces some cerebrovascular constriction. The patients are then less able to adapt to the low blood pressure which they continue to face on standing. Some patients with autonomic failure have continued relatively symptom free with this treatment for many years. Recumbency due to hypotension or an intercurrent illness is always serious because this causes recumbent hypertension and probably induces some cerebrovascular constriction. The patients are then less able to adapt to the low blood pressure which they continue to face on standing. Some patients with autonomic failure have continued relatively symptom free with standing systolic pressures in the region of 80 mmHg for many years. The important fact in treating postural hypotension is therefore to remember that it is the patient's symptoms, if any, that require treatment rather than the mere observation that the standing blood pressure appears to be unusually low.

Course of progressive autonomic failure
Though the natural history of progressive autonomic failure of the pure type is of a slow progression over some 10 to 15 years, patients with multiple system atrophy rarely survive longer than five years from the diagnosis of the disease. Their downhill course is marked by increasing rigidity, urinary incontinence, and sometimes marked stridor which may require tracheostomy. In some the central disturbance of respiratory control and sleep apnoea may be the final cause of death. Alternatively the denervation supersensitivity of sympathetic alpha and beta receptors of the heart may render patients more liable to cardiac arrhythmias from which they may die. The extrapyramidal features rarely respond to levodopa (in the form of levodopa with a dopamine decarboxylase inhibitor) probably because the central defect of noradrenaline as well as dopamine prevents effective levels of dopamine being achieved (see page 21.227).

References
Appenzeller, O. (1982). *The autonomic nervous system, an introduction to basic and clinical concepts*, 3rd edn. Elsevier, North Holland, Amsterdam.
Bannister, R. (ed.) (1983). *Autonomic failure, a textbook of diseases of the autonomic nervous system*. Oxford University Press, Oxford.
——, Sever, P. and Gross, M. (1977). Cardiovascular reflexes and biochemical responses in progressive autonomic failure. *Brain* **100**, 327–344.
Bradbury, S. and Eggleston, C. (1925). Postural hypotension; a report of three cases. *Am. Heart J.* **1**, 73–86.
Johnson, R. H., Lambie, D. G. and Spalding, J. M. K. (1984). *Neurocardiology*. W. B. Saunders, London.
Shy, G. M. and Drager, G. A. (1960). A neurological syndrome associated with orthostatic hypotension. *Arch. Neurol.* **2**. 511–527.

THE CRANIAL NERVES

The visual pathways: structure and function

R. W. ROSS RUSSELL

The visual pathways

Composed of 1.2 million medullated axons derived from retinal ganglion cells, each optic nerve extends from the optic disc to the chiasma, a distance of 4.5 cm. It traverses the funnel-shaped optic

foramen in the sphenoid bone and the last part of its course is intracranial. The majority of fibres originate in small ganglion cells in the foveal region which subserve the central parts of the visual field and respond to stimulation by cone photoreceptors.

The optic nerve is enclosed in a tough dural sheath and the pia arachnoid is continuous with the intracranial subarachnoid space. The substance of the optic nerve is unlike other tracts in the central nervous system in having abundant fibrous tissue septa. Optic nerve axons have no neurilemmal sheaths.

The blood supply to the orbital portion of the optic nerve is derived from the ophthalmic and short ciliary arteries with branches from the central retinal artery. The intracranial portion of the optic nerve is supplied by numerous small branches from the anterior cerebral and ophthalmic arteries.

As the optic nerves approach the chiasma the axons from each nasal retina (medial to the fovea), comprising 60 per cent of the total optic nerve fibres, separate from the remainder and cross to the other side of the chiasma to join the optic tract. The lower

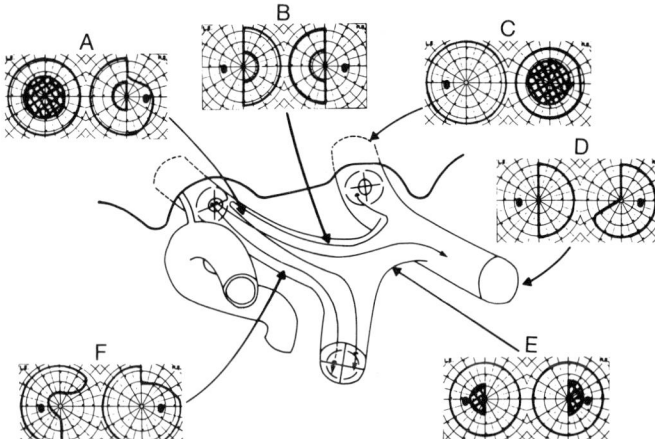

Fig. 1 Optic chiasma and left internal carotid artery viewed from behind to show the arrangement of nerve fibres and the effect of lesions at various points. (a) Lesion at junction of left optic nerve and chiasma (e.g. meningioma) left central scotoma and right upper quadrantic defect. (Note route taken by lower crossing fibres from right optice nerve.) (b) Central chiasmal lesion interrupting all crossing fibres (e.g. pituitary tumour). Bitemporal hemianopia. (c) Lesion of right optic nerve (e.g. meningioma, optic neuritis). Central scotoma and peripheral constriction. (d) Lesion of right optic tract, e.g. craniopharyngioma. Left homonymous hemianopic (incongrous). (e) Lesion affecting posterior aspect of chiasm (crossing fibres from central field), e.g. craniopharyngioma. Scotomatous bitemporal hemianopia. (f) Lesion affecting lateral aspect of chiasm, e.g. carotid aneurysm. Central and nasal field defect left eye with early upper quadrantanopia right eye.

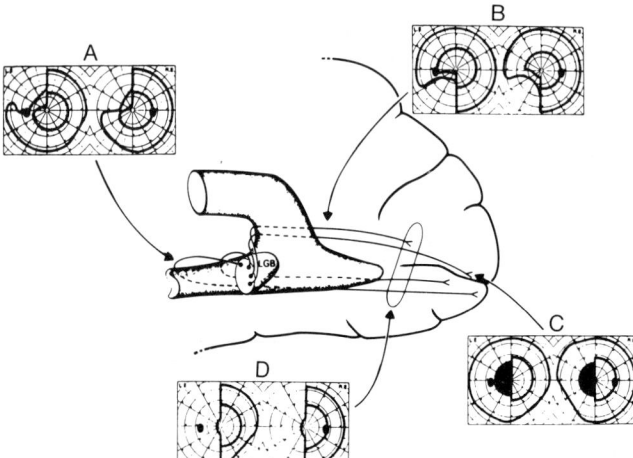

Fig. 2 Right cerebral hemisphere viewed from its medial aspect to show visual radiation from lateral geniculate body (LGB) to calcarine cortex, and visual field defects produced by lesion at various points. (a) Lesion involving lower fibres of radiation which loop around temporal horn of right lateral ventricle (e.g. glioma, abscess of temporal lobe). Left upper quadrantanopia. (b) Lesion involving upper fibres of radiation in posterior parietal lobe (e.g. glioma, haemorrhage). Left lower quadrantanopia. (c) Lesion involving occipital pole and projection of 'macular' fibres (small vascular occlusion). Left homonymous hemianopic scotomas. (d) Lesion involving posterior radiation and visual cortex (e.g. posterior cerebral artery occlusion). Complete left homonymous hemianopia.

fibres take a slightly different course from the upper fibres (Fig. 1). 'Macular' fibres cross in the posterior portion of the chiasma. The optic chiasma is situated just above the sella and pituitary gland and lies in the chiasmatic cistern. Its most important relation is the carotid artery (Fig. 2). The chiasmal blood supply comes from small arteries derived from the Circle of Willis, especially the anterior cerebral and anterior communicating arteries and the terminal carotid artery.

The optic tracts extend from the chiasma to the lateral geniculate bodies arching round the cerebral peduncles. Macular fibres lie on the medial aspect of the tract anteriorly, but further back occupy a dorsal position. In the lateral geniculate body fibres from corresponding parts of the two retinae are inserted into vertical columns of cells. The majority of axons synapse in the lateral geniculate body, but some fibres or branches bypass the nucleus and proceed to the superior colliculus and midbrain tectum. These are concerned with the pupillary light reflex and with reflex eye movements which orientate the axis of the eyes towards the object of interest.

From the lateral geniculate body the fibres of the optic radiation pass laterally toward the trigone of the lateral ventricle. They then spread over a wider area, superior fibres passing directly backwards to the occipital cortex and ending in the upper bank of the calcarine fissure. The lower fibres take a longer looping course through the temporal lobe before terminating in the lower bank of the calcarine fissure (Fig. 2).

The blood supply to this region is complex. The first part of the geniculo-calcarine pathway is supplied by the posterior choroidal artery, the remainder of the radiation by the middle cerebral artery in its upper part and the posterior cerebral artery in its lower part.

The visual cortex is situated on the medial surface of the occipital lobe partly buried in the calcarine fissure. Connections from corresponding half retinae project in a point-to-point fashion on to columns of cells precisely arranged in a retinotopic map. Central parts of the field have a relatively large cortical representation situated near the occipital poles.

The visual cortex is adapted to the detection and localization of visual stimuli and to elementary contour perception. Further relays occur to cortex and to parietal and temporal lobes. These secondary prestriate projections deal with parallel steps of visual processing such as colour perception, appreciation of movement, shape discrimination, visual recognition, and memory. Localization is less precise than in the calcarine cortex and some areas receive projections from both half fields.

Lesions of the visual pathways

Optic nerve

In the optic nerve (see also Section 23) uniocular defects are the rule except in the hereditary and toxic neuropathies. Lesions of the optic nerve produce a general depression of visual function in one eye which is most pronounced in the central part of the field producing a relative or absolute central scotoma (Fig. 1). However, fibre bundle (arcuate) defects may also occur. Visual acuity and colour vision are usually severely affected. The speed and amplitude of the pupillary light reflex is reduced (afferent pupillary defect). In long-standing cases pallor of the optic disc develops and in acute lesions the disc may be swollen.

Swelling of the optic disc has a number of causes (Table 1). The term papilloedema is reserved by convention for swelling resulting from raised intracranial pressure. This is usually bilateral, causes little interference with visual acuity, and is accompanied by other features of raised pressure such as headache, vomiting, and diminished conscious level. The visual fields show enlargement of the blind spots and usually some peripheral constriction. An important symptom in papilloedema are attacks of visual obscuration,

Table 1 Optic disc swelling

	Congenital anomaly (pseudopapilloedema)	Papilloedema	Papillitis	Ischaemic neuropathy	Posterior uveitis
Laterality	Either or both eyes	Bilateral	Unilateral	Unilateral	One or both eyes
Acuity	Variable, usually normal	Normal until late stage	Early loss	Usually affected	Usually affected from macular oedema
Colour vision	Usually normal	Normal	Early loss	Early loss	Normal
Pupils	Usually normal	Normal	RAPD*	RAPD*	Normal
Visual fields	Normal / variable loss	Normal except enlargement of blind spots until terminal stages then constriction	Central scotoma	Inferior altitudinal defect	Normal
Disc	Abnormal size, shape, vessels, refraction, etc.	Swollen	Swollen	Pale, asymmetrical swelling	Swollen
Fundus	May have abnormal vessels, choroidal pigmentation, etc.	Normal	Normal	Vessels may have arterio-sclerotic or hypertensive changes	Vitreous cellular infiltrate
Common causes	—	Intracerebral or orbital tumour, haematoma, abscess, benign intracranial hypertension, venous sinus obstruction, retinal vein occlusion, CO_2 retention	Retrobulbar neuritis, infarction of disc, primary or metastatic tumour	Vascular disease	See Section 23

* RAPD = relative afferent pupillary defect.

brief episodes of visual loss related to stooping or sudden standing. If untreated these may progress to complete visual loss from optic disc ischaemia.

Pseudo papilloedema refers to congenital abnormalities which resemble papilloedema but occur without raised intracranial pressure. Drusen of the disc is such a condition; it may be dominantly inherited and may cause visual field loss. Pearly excrescences can usually be discerned in the substance of the nerve head.

Swelling of the disc from demyelination, inflammation or ischaemia is referred to as papillitis (see below). The appearances are similar to papilloedema but the amount of visual loss, both of acuity and fields, is much greater. Optic atrophy may follow a variety of optic nerve disorders. The disc becomes pale or white from gliosis, loss of axons, and reduced vascularity. The edges of the disc remain clear cut and the vessels are normal. If the disc has previously been swollen before optic atrophy supervenes the edges may be indistinct and the retinal arteries may be sheathed (consecutive optic atrophy). For further discussion of optic nerve disease see also Section 23.

Demyelinating disease (multiple sclerosis)
This is the commonest cause of an optic nerve lesion. The part of the optic nerve undergoing demyelination may be close to the disc, causing disc swelling (papillitis) or may be located more posteriorly (retrobulbar neuritis). Ocular pain occurs and is characteristically worse on eye movement. Any degree of visual loss may occur, even loss of light perception, but most patients make a full functional recovery. An increased latency and a reduced amplitude of the cortical potential evoked by a visual stimulus can be detected in the majority of patients with demyelinating optic neuritis and in many patients with multiple sclerosis including those who have no visual symptoms.

Compression of the optic nerve
Compression may be extrinsic or intrinsic. Within the orbit and optic foramen, tumours such as meningioma of the nerve sheath, lymphoma, haemangioma or secondary carcinoma are the commonest types. Compression by swollen ocular muscles may occur in dysthyroid eye disease. In its intracranial portion the optic nerve may be compressed by tumour such as meningioma (Fig. 3a) or pituitary adenoma, or by aneurysms or by ectatic carotid arteries. Intrinsic compression is caused by optic nerve glioma, a rare tumour of childhood, often associated with neurofibromatosis (Fig. 3b).

Inflammatory lesions
Lesions spreading from contiguous sinus infection in the ethmoid or sphenoid sinus are a rare cause of optic neuritis affecting one or both nerves. Chronic meningeal infiltration (e.g. syphilis, tuberculosis) may involve the intracranial portion. Granulomas such as sarcoidosis may also occur. The optic nerves may be involved in specific virus infections (e.g. herpes zoster) or as part of a generalized post-infective immunological disorder following virus infection or vaccination.

Vascular lesions (ischaemic optic neuropathy)
This condition (see also Section 23) occurs most often in elderly patients with atherosclerosis. The optic disc is a likely site for ischaemia because of its tenuous blood supply from the posterior ciliary arteries. Haemorrhagic hypotension or anaemia may provoke disc infarction in patients with normal vessels, but in most cases there is widespread narrowing of many small arteries such as occurs in hypertension, diabetes or cranial arteritis. The field defect is altitudinal in type due to involvement of bundles of nerve fibres within the nerve. Some central vision is often preserved.

Hereditary optic atrophy
Atrophy is usually progressive, bilateral, and symmetrical. It may form part of a known syndrome (e.g. Friedreich's ataxia), may occur in association with diabetes or may occur in isolation. In some types the loss of optic nerve fibres is secondary to retinal disease (e.g. retinitis pigmentosa). Various patterns of inheritance are described. The best known type is *Leber's disease*, which predominantly affects males, causes uniocular visual loss in the second or third decade followed after an interval by involvement of the second eye. In some cases visual loss is rapid with disc swelling. The end result is bilateral optic atrophy with dense central scotomas. The suggested metabolic defect is failure to detoxify cyanide.

Toxic and nutritional amblyopias

Amblyopias are characterized by painless slowly progressive bilateral visual loss with diminished acuity, central or centro-caecal scotomas and a variable degree of optic atrophy. They may occur in generalized malnutrition or in specific deficiency states (e.g. thiamine or vitamin B_{12} deficiency). The syndrome may also follow a variety of toxic substances or drugs such as alcohol (usually in combination with tobacco), ethambutol, clioquinol, isoniazid, chlorpropamide, ergotamine, streptomycin, digitalis, heavy metal).

Chiasma

Although both nasal and temporal fibres may be affected, the crossing fibres from the nasal retina are particularly at risk in compressive lesions of the chiasm. The resulting loss of the temporal fields with an abrupt break at the vertical axis of the visual field is a sure indication of a lesion at or behind the chiasma. Central chiasmal lesions produce symmetrical bitemporal field loss (see Fig. 1). Optic atrophy usually occurs and central visual acuity is often reduced.

Two important variations occur in eccentrically placed lesions: an ipsilateral central scotoma and contralateral upper temporal field loss is caused by a lesion at the junction of nerve and chiasma, an ipsilateral central and nasal field loss with contralateral upper temporal loss is caused by a lesion affecting the lateral side of the chiasm (Fig. 1). The more important lesions affecting this region are compressive and the principal features of the four main types are shown in Table 2.

Diagnosis and management of chiasmal lesions

Because most of the causes of chiasmal compression are benign and treatable, early and accurate diagnosis is essential. Plain X-rays of the skull and optic foramina may show expansion and destruction of the sella indicating a pituitary tumour but tomography may be necessary to show small tumours (microadenomas). Optic nerve glioma expands the optic foramen.

Computerized tomography (CT) scan with enhancement reliably shows a pituitary tumour which extends upwards from the sella (Fig. 3d) or meningioma arising from the planum of the sphenoid bone (Fig. 3c). Carotid angiography is usually necessary to exclude an aneurysm.

Tests of pituitary function may show excessive secretion, e.g. of growth hormone, prolactin or ACTH in functioning adenomas. Various degrees of hypopituitarism with diminished secretion of

ACTH, TSH or gonadotrophins may be found in destructive lesions of the pituitary from any cause.

Treatment of chiasmal lesions

A variety of surgical and medical treatments are available for chiasmal compression, depending on the size and type of tumour, the severity of visual loss and the variety of endocrine disorder. Intracranial surgical removal by subfrontal craniotomy is indicated for meningiomas and for some pituitary tumours with substantial upward extension. Craniopharyngioma (Fig. 3e) may be accessible to radical excision via a subtemporal approach or to a more conservative measure such as aspiration of a cyst or relief of hydrocephalus by ventriculo-peritoneal shunting.

A large aneurysm of the terminal carotid artery (Fig. 3f) may sometimes be excised or evacuated and reduced in size if a clip can be placed on the neck connecting it to the parent artery.

Trans-sphenoidal surgical removal is increasingly practised for pituitary tumours, especially those expanding downwards into the sphenoid sinus. This approach carries less morbidity than craniotomy and is especially suitable for elderly patients. Postoperative radiotherapy is advisable for pituitary adenoma whatever the type of operation. Medical treatment with bromocriptine is a valuable method of treating pituitary tumour, especially prolactinomas, and can cause regression of tumour size and of visual field defect. The response of non-prolactin-secreting tumours is less marked, but is currently being evaluated. Bromocriptine must be continued for life and the dose necessary to suppress excess prolactin may cause nausea. It may be combined with radiotherapy treatment.

Optic tract

Lesions of the optic tract are rare. The usual causes are pituitary adenoma or craniopharyngioma. The visual field defect is noncongruous and homonymous, i.e. affects the two eyes to different extents. Optic atrophy is often present and the pupils may be unequal.

Optic radiation: parietal lobe

Cerebral tumours are the commonest type of lesion to involve the visual radiation. They are usually malignant gliomas in the posterior parietal region (Fig. 3h), but other types (metastases, meningioma etc.) and spontaneous intracerebral haemorrhage may also occur. At an early stage tumours damage the upper fibres of the radiation, causing a lower quadrantic homonymous hemianopia which gradually extends to become complete. Optokinetic nys-

Table 2 Lesions of the optic chiasma

	Occurrence	Visual field defect	Optic disc	Associated features	Radiological features	Treatment
Pituitary adenoma	Adults	Bitemporal hemianopia	Atrophy	Endocrine excess secretion GH, ACTH, prolactin	Expansion of fossa	Surgery, transnasal or transcranial Bromocriptine Radiotherapy
Parasellar meningioma	Adults F > M	Central scotoma or bitemporal hemianopia	Atrophy	None	Hyperostosis	Surgery
Craniopharyngioma	Any age	Bitemporal hemianopia, homonymous hemianopia	Papilloedema (children) atrophy	Retarded growth and sexual development (children), mental change, diabetes insipidus	Suprasellar calcification	Surgery (radical or palliative), Radiotherapy if incomplete removal
Optic nerve/chiasmal glioma	Children	Central scotoma, bitemporal hemianopia	Atrophy	Neurofibromatosis	Expansion of optic foramen	Very slow growing possibly radiosensitive
Carotid aneurysm	Elderly F > M	Central and nasal loss (ipsilateral): later contralateral temporal loss	Atrophy (late)	Pain (face or orbit) rarely subarachnoid haemorrhage	Calcification in wall	Usually conservative, carotid ligation: rarely excision of wall

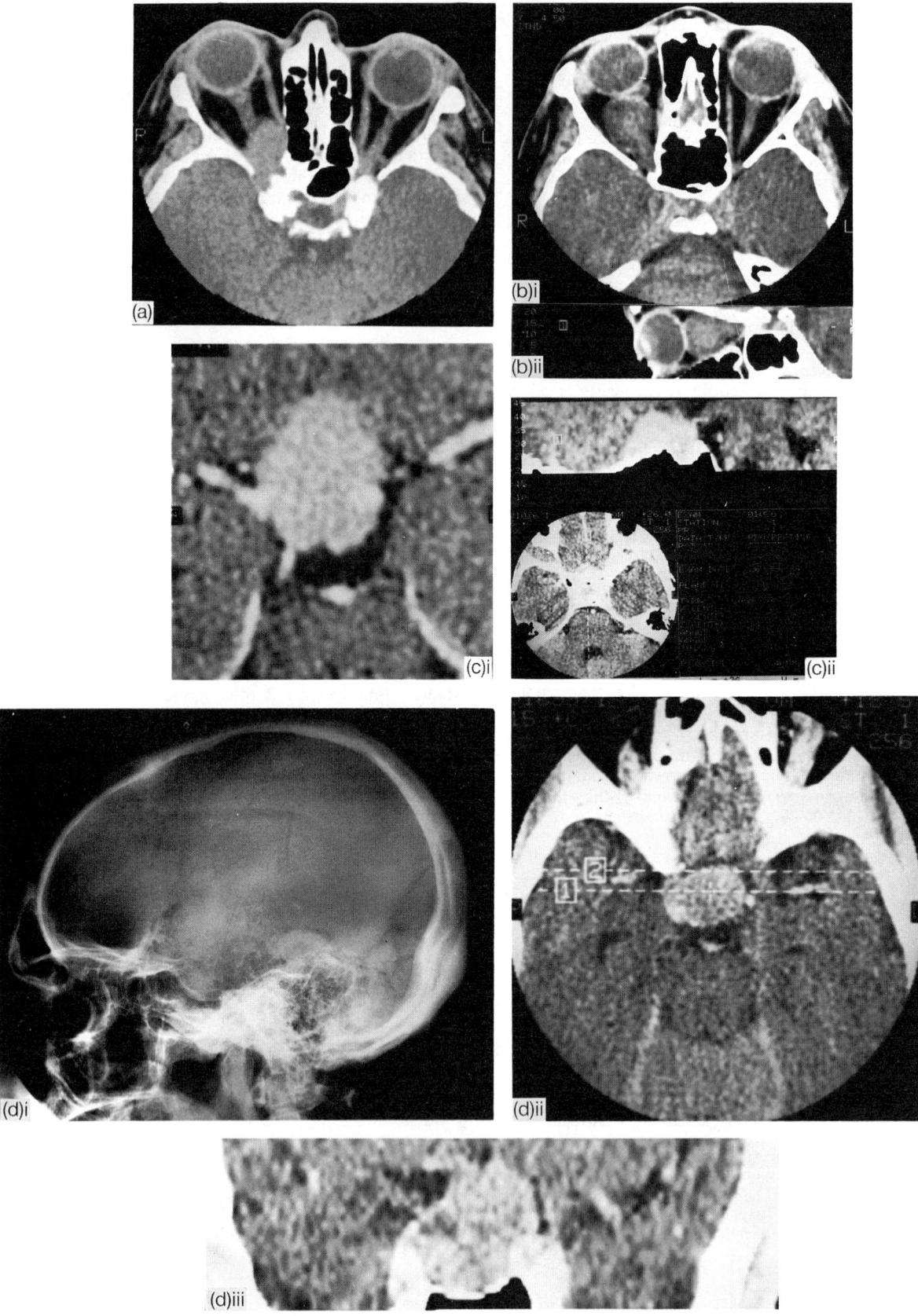

Fig. 3 Lesions of the visual pathways. (a) Orbital meningioma: CT scan of a 45-year-old female patient with left proptosis and progressive visual loss in the right eye; meningioma of orbital apex. (b) Optic nerve glioma: CT scan of a 14-year-old child with progressive visual loss in the left eye caused by glioma of the optic nerve. i. Horizontal plane mid orbit. ii. Sagittal plane through optic nerve. (c) Meningioma (parasellar): High-resolution CT scan (after contrast enhancement) of pituitary region in a 35-year-old male patient with meningioma of planum sphenoidale causing chiasmal compression. i. Horizontal plane. ii. Sagittal plane. The tumour is extending forwards and upwards from the anterior clinoid processes. (d) Pituitary tumour: A 50-year-old male patient with chromophobe adenoma of pituitary causing bitemporal hemianopia. i. Lateral skull X-ray showing expansion of the pituitary fossa. ii. CT scan in horizontal plane above pituitary fossa. iii. Reconstruction in coronal plane through tumour.

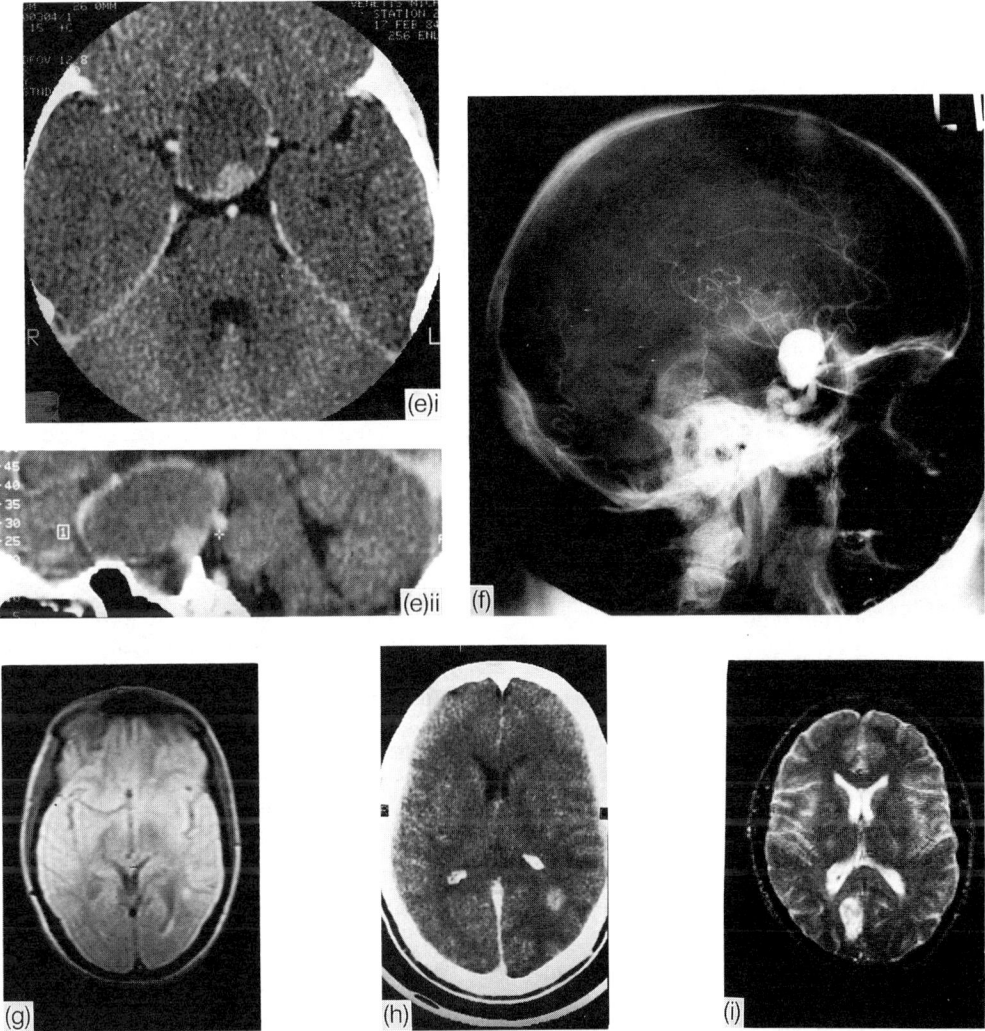

Fig. 3 Continued (e) Craniopharyngioma: CT scan of a 25-year-old man presenting with retardation of growth and sexual development, optic atrophy, and bitemporal hemianopia. Craniopharyngioma. i. Horizontal plane. ii. Sagittal reconstruction. (f) Carotid aneurysm: carotid angiogram in a 65-year-old female patient with progressive visual loss caused by chiasmal compression from a giant carotid aneurysm. (g) Multiple sclerosis: Magnetic resonance scan of a 25-year-old female patient with left homonymous quadrantanopia caused by plaque of multiple sclerosis in right visual radiation. (h) Glioma: CT scan of a 45-year-old patient with epileptic seizures, left homonymous hemianopia and dressing dyspraxia; malignant glioma involving right visual radiation. (i) Infarction of left occipital cortex: magnetic resonance scan in horizontal plane of cerebral hemispheres in a 56-year-old female to show occipital infarction. This followed occlusion of left posterior cerebral artery by embolism from left atrium.

tagmus is disturbed and visual pursuit is defective toward the side of the lesion. In addition to the visual field defect epilepsy and features of raised intracranial pressure may occur. Patients may show associated defects which reflect the different function of the two hemispheres. Lesions of the dominant hemisphere (usually left sided) produce dyslexia, dysgraphia, acalculia, right/left disorientation, and finger agnosia. On the non-dominant hemisphere patients show unilateral neglect, spatial disorientation with difficulties in route finding and dressing in addition to a left-sided homonymous hemianopia.

Optic radiation: temporal lobe
The lower fibres of the visual radiation sweep around the temporal horn of the lateral ventricle. Lesions of the posterior part of the temporal lobe may interrupt this pathway, giving rise to an upper quadrantanopia. In the dominant hemisphere dysphasia and memory loss may be present in addition. Lesions may also cause temporal lobe (psychomotor) epilepsy in which the patient may experience distortion of vision, or formed visual hallucinations often accompanied by *déjà vu*.

Intrinsic tumours (gliomas) are the most frequent lesions in this site. They may be of any grade of malignancy from low-grade astrocytoma to haemorrhagic glioblastoma. Temporal lobe abscess may follow chronic suppuration in the inner ear, but is now rare. Extrinsic compressive lesions include meningioma, aneurysm, and pituitary tumour. Multiple sclerosis may also involve the visual radiation (Fig. 3g).

Visual cortex: occipital lobe
Lesions of the occipital lobe give rise to a homonymous hemianopia, often complete, but with preserved visual acuity. Characteristically this is an isolated visual defect without motor or sensory loss. Optokinetic nystagmus is preserved and pupils are normal. Limited lesions may produce scotomatous defects showing congruity (i.e. exactly similar in the two eyes). The field defect may extend up to the fixation point. Epilepsy may occur in occipital lesions and may be accompanied by unformed visual hallucinations consisting of patterns, lines, or colours, or by flickerinng scintillating scotomas.

The majority of occipital lesions are vascular (Fig. 3j). The blood supply to the area is from the posterior cerebral artery and the border zone between this and the middle cerebral territory runs close to the posterior pole. The area near the posterior pole on which is represented the central part of the visual field, may escape damage in vascular lesions because of the alternative route of blood supply. This may be responsible for 'macular sparing' seen in such cases. Gliomas, abscesses, and meningiomas also occur; aneurysms are rare, but angiomas and other vascular malformations including the Sturge–Weber syndrome may arise in this region.

Simultaneous or successive occlusion of both posterior cerebral arteries may cause bilateral homonymous hemianopia. There may be total visual loss (cerebral blindness) but more commonly a small island of central vision is retained. The pupillary light reactions remain normal. These patients frequently show other cortical defects such as hallucinations and memory loss and may deny that they are blind (Anton's syndrome).

Other rare defects which may be found in patients with partial bilateral hemianopia include loss of colour vision (achromatopsia) and loss of recognition of faces (prosopagnosia), loss of visual orientation and localization. These defects usually indicate damage to visual association cortex or to connecting tracts.

Visual object agnosia in which the patient retains normal visual perception but fails to recognize objects is a very rare defect but may be found with an extensive lesion of the posterior part of the dominant hemisphere. It is usually transient.

References

Glaser, J. S. (1978). *Neuro ophthalmology*. Harper and Row, Maryland.
Walsh, F. B. and Hoyt, W. F. (1969). *Clinical neuro ophthalmology*. Williams and Wilkins, Baltimore.

The eighth cranial nerve

P. RUDGE

Introduction

The VIIIth cranial nerve has two components, namely, the auditory and vestibular parts. The auditory part of the VIIIth nerve innervates the cochlear sensory receptors; all the nerve fibres are myelinated and the myelin surrounds the cell bodies as well as the axons. The central auditory pathways are complex with multiple decussations; synapses occur in the cochlear nuclei, superior olivary complex, lateral lemnisci, inferior colliculi, and medial geniculate bodies. There are several cortical areas associated with hearing including Heschl's gyrus and a precise tonotopic organization is maintained to this level.

The vestibular nerve innervates two types of receptor, namely, the semicircular canals and otolith organs (saccule and utricle). Angular acceleration in the three cardinal planes is detected by the semicircular canals which partially integrate the signal to one of velocity. Linear acceleration (gravity) is detected in the sagittal and coronal planes by the otolith-bearing structures. Exceedingly complex connections between the second-order neurons of the vestibular nuclei pass to the somatic musculature, extra-ocular muscles, cerebellum, and cerebral cortex. In clinical medicine, connections to the extra-ocular muscles are most important as they are concerned with the vestibulo-ocular reflex (VOR) which maintains the eye position relative to space and derangement of which gives clues to the site of pathology.

Symptoms and signs due to dysfunction of the VIIIth nerve

Auditory system

Symptoms

Deafness is the cardinal feature of damage to the cochlea or its afferent pathways. Loss of hearing can be unilateral only if the dis-

ease process affects the end organ, VIIIth nerve or cochlear nucleus. More central lesions cause symmetrical hearing loss but significant deafness from such lesions is rare. Distortion of hearing is a frequent accompaniment of cochlear loss as is tinnitus but neither symptom is confined to such lesions.

Tests of auditory function

The first step in the investigation of a patient who complains of hearing loss is to determine if such a loss exists. This is done by means of pure tone air conduction audiometry in which pulsed pure tones at octave intervals (approximately 250–8000 Hz) are administered via earphones and the sound pressure level varied. The level at which a tone is just heard is the threshold of hearing for that frequency.

Having determined that the patient does have a hearing loss it is vital to ascertain by tuning fork tests whether the deafness is conductive or sensorineural. In the normal subject the cochlear hair cells can be stimulated via two routes: air conduction or bone conduction. The first can be tested by placing a tuning fork of 256 or 512 Hz adjacent to the external auditory meatus. The pressure waves set up in the air contained within the external auditory canal causes the tympanic membrane and ossicles to vibrate and transmit the sound waves to the cochlea. Bone conduction can be tested by placing a vibrating tuning fork against the skull which then transmits the signal directly to the hair cells. Since air conduction is much more efficient than bone conduction in normal individuals a vibrating tuning fork placed adjacent to the external meatus until the sound is no longer detected cannot be heard if it is then placed on the skull. A similar situation exists if a sensorineural hearing loss is present; the abnormality involves the cochlea or its nerve fibres and this does not alter the relative efficiency of transduction of sound waves via the two routes to the cochlea. Conversely, if there is an abnormality of the external canal, e.g. wax, or of the ossicles, e.g. otosclerosis, the efficiency of only the air conducting route will be impaired. In these circumstances sound will be transmitted more efficiently by bone conduction. To detect this phenomenon clinically a vibrating tuning fork is placed adjacent to the external meatus until the sound is no longer heard; it is then placed on the mastoid process. The sound will again be detected if a conductive loss is present. This is known as the *Rinne test*. Similarly, if a vibrating tuning fork is placed on the teeth or forehead in a normal subject, the sound is located at the mid line. On the other hand in a unilateral sensorineural hearing loss the sound is appreciated towards the unimpaired side and with a conductive loss to the impaired side. This is the *Weber test*.

Having performed these basic clinical tests it should be clear whether the patient has a conductive or sensorineural hearing loss. Conductive deafness will not be discussed further as this is the province of the otologist. If sensorineural hearing loss is present, tests of loudness function, adaptation, and speech audiometry will help to differentiate that due to hair cell loss, e.g. Ménière's disease, from that due to retro-cochlear lesions e.g. VIIIth nerve tumours. The following account is a brief summary of the more commonly used tests; the reader is referred to the monograph by Katz (1972) for detailed discussion.

Tests of recruitment (alternate loudness balance test, loudness discomfort level)

Loudness is a perception; it is partly dependent upon the intensity of the stimulus. In normal subjects a tone of given intensity applied to one ear can be matched for loudness to a tone of similar intensity applied to the other. It might be thought that if a subject has a unilateral hearing loss a tone would appear to be of similar loudness in the two ears (one normal, the other impaired) if the intensity applied to the impaired ear was greater than that applied to the normal ear by an amount equal to the hearing loss. This is indeed the case in all conductive and some retrocochlear losses, but does not hold for cochlear impairment where growth of loudness with intensity is greater than anticipated. This phenomenon is known as recruitment and is the reason why older subjects suffering presbyacusis ask one to speak up because of their hearing loss only to complain, when their instruction is obeyed, that there is no reason to shout!

Recruitment can be assessed by two methods. The first is the alternate loudness balance test. This can only be used in cases of unilateral hearing loss. A tone of given intensity is applied to the normal ear and the patient attempts to match its loudness to a tone of the same frequency applied to the impaired ear. This is repeated at several intensities and frequencies. In cochlear hearing loss, recruitment occurs; indeed in some cases at high intensities the tone appears louder in the impaired ear, so-called overrecruitment. Conversely, in some cases of retrocochlear loss there is no recruitment; there may even be reversal of it, i.e. the rate of growth of loudness with increasing intensity declines. The second method applicable to all cases of hearing loss, including those that are bilateral, is to use loudness discomfort levels. In this technique the intensity of a tone is increased until it is unpleasantly loud. This level is remarkably constant in normal subjects and in those with hair cell loss; it occurs at about 100 dB. Loudness discomfort levels are elevated in many patients with retrocochlear lesions.

Tests of tone decay

If a tone is applied to a normal ear at an intensity just above threshold it will continue to be heard indefinitely. In general this also applies to cochlear hearing loss. On the other hand, some patients with a retrocochlear hearing loss are only able to perceive the tone for a short time and its intensity has to be progressively increased for them to regain and maintain perception of the tone. This is known as tone decay and the amount by which the intensity has to be increased is a measure of it. Tone decay can be marked in some, but not all, retrocochlear lesions.

Speech audiometry

The ability to discriminate phonetically balanced words can be determined by routine speech audiometry in which lists of words are presented at different intensities. From this it is possible to see if there is an intensity at which all the words are correctly identified and to plot an intensity–score graph, i.e. speech audiogram. Although speech discrimination is frequently impaired in cochlear lesions the impairment is disproportionately greater in retrocochlear disorders. Indeed with retrocochlear lesions speech discrimination sometimes declines rather than improves at high intensity. This is known as the 'roll-over' phenomenon.

Stapedius reflex

If a high-intensity tone is applied to one ear the stapedius muscle contracts bilaterally, thereby tensing the tympanic membrane and altering its conductance. The reflex depends upon the cochlea and VIIIth nerve for the afferent input and the VIIth nerve for the efferent component, with connections between the two within the brain stem. In normal subjects a reflex is usually obtained at frequencies of 4 kHz or less at intensities of 85 to 100 dB. If the tone is maintained for 10 s the reflex contraction shows little attenuation for frequencies of 500 and 1000 Hz, but there is some 'decay' at 2000 and 4000 Hz.

Cochlear hearing loss causes little alteration in the stapedius reflex threshold because of recruitment and it does not show abnormal attenuation over 10 s. On the other hand, retrocochlear lesions such as acoustic neuromas characteristically raise the threshold of the reflex and cause its pathological 'decay'.

Brain stem auditory evoked potentials

It is possible to record, via scalp electrodes, neural activity generated in response to a click stimulus by stimulus-locked averaging techniques. A series of components occurring within the first 10 ms arises from the VIIIth nerve and brain stem auditory pathways. These are conventionally labelled I (auditory nerve), II (cochlear nuclei), III (superior olivary complex), IV (nuclei of the lateral lemnisci), V (inferior colliculus) (Fig. 1). Components VI

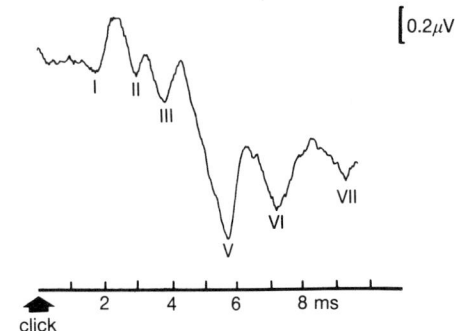

Fig. 1 Brain stem auditory evoked potential from a normal subject. Stimulus given at arrow. Downward deflection indicates that the vertex electrode is positive relative to the ipsilateral mastoid electrode. The high pass filter is arranged to accentuate component V. Components I–V arise from VIIIth nerve and brain stem structures (see text).

and VII and later waves arise from diencephalic and cortical structures. Those arising after wave VII are classified by latency into middle and late components.

Brain stem evoked potentials have proved to be of diagnostic value in two groups of disorders, namely, deafness and certain neurological conditions such as multiple sclerosis and coma. We shall confine our discussion to the former. If a click of high intensity is used as the stimulus the effect of any recruiting hearing loss should be minimized. This is the case in cochlear lesions, e.g. Ménière's disease, where there is little alteration in any of the components of the brain stem auditory evoked potentials (BSAEP) unless the hearing loss is severe (greater than 70 dB). On the other hand, non-recruiting hearing loss due to retrocochlear lesions, e.g. acoustic neuromas, causes marked changes in the BSAEP: this may take the form of a loss of all components from the affected ear except component I, a marked delay of component V or a greatly increased I–V interval compared with the normal side. Of considerable interest, however, is the fact that the BSAEP is frequently abnormal in retrocochlear lesions even if the hearing loss is a recruiting one, suggesting that the initial concept that it is the degree of recruitment that separates peripheral from retrocochlear lesions on BSAEP recording is wrong. Be that as it may the test is extremely valuable (see page 21.90).

Electrocochleography

The VIIIth nerve action potential (AP) is small and can be difficult to detect using scalp electrodes. By placing a needle electrode against the medial wall of the middle ear via the tympanic membrane it is possible to record a large VIIIth nerve action potential as well as the cochlear microphonic and summating potentials (SP). This technique is useful for identifying component I of the BSAEP and also in studying the morphology of component I in a number of conditions including acoustic neuromata and Ménière's disease. As the technique is invasive, although quite safe, its main uses are in the diagnosis of Ménière's disease and hearing loss in children. In Ménière's disease the summating potential is large relative to the action potential (SP/AP > 0.3) whereas in other causes of deafness this is not the case.

Vestibular system

Symptoms

Damage to the vestibular receptors or their neural connections results in a mismatch of input between them (so-called tonus imbalance) and also with the other receptors signalling orientation in space such as vision, proprioception, and joint position. This results in an unpleasant sensation of imbalance and vertigo which, in extreme cases, causes nausea and vomiting; the patient is reluctant to move and prefers to be in bed. Lesions are usually destructive and their effects are rapidly compensated centrally such that

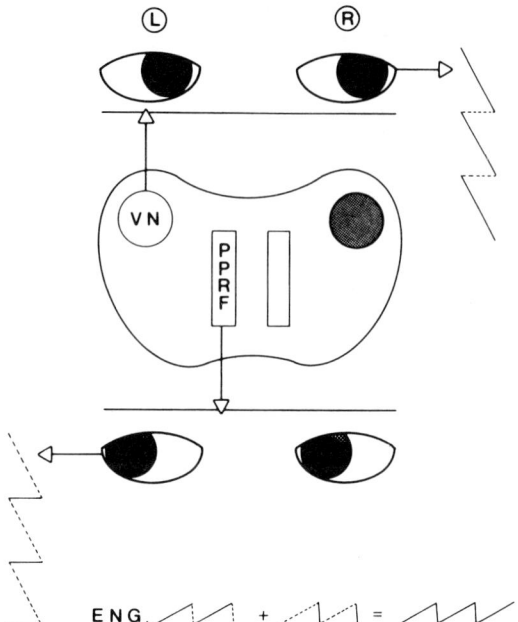

Fig. 2 Diagrammatic explanation of vestibular nystagmus due to destruction of the right vestibular apparatus, nerve or nucleus. Slow phase represented at right, fast phase at left and summation of two revealed in electronystagmogram (ENG) below. VN, vestibular nucleus; PPRF, paramedian pontine reticular formation.

the patient becomes asymptomatic over a period of a few weeks. Exceptionally, compensation, which depends upon brain stem structures including the olivary nuclei and cerebellum, is incomplete and the symptoms persist.

Signs of vestibular dysfunction

Nystagmus

Spontaneous nystagmus, which comes in many forms, confuses all clinicians and yet is an extremely useful sign of vestibular dysfunction. We shall begin our discussion with nystagmus in the horizontal plane. Conventionally the direction of nystagmus is specified by the *fast* phase.

Vestibular nystagmus

The vestibular apparatus and nuclei are paired, one set on each side of the brain stem. The horizontal canals, and the vestibular nuclei with which they connect, drive the eyes as a slow movement towards the opposite side. Thus in the normal subject equal and opposite forces act on the eye muscles and the eyes remain central. Destruction of one set of vestibular end organs, their nerves or nuclei results in the eyes drifting towards that side as a slow movement (Fig. 2). This phenomenon arises because of the unopposed activity of the intact vestibular apparatus. It is rapidly detected and a counter movement is generated by another system, the saccadic (fast) generator lying in the paramedian pontine reticular formation (PPRF). This saccadic movement to one side is generated by the ipsilateral PPFR. Thus in a right-sided vestibular lesion the eyes are pushed slowly to the right by the intact left vestibular system and then rapidly returned towards the mid line under the influence of the left PPRF. Repetition of this results in vestibular nystagmus, with its characteristic saw-toothed wave form and fast phase to side opposite the lesion.

Gaze-paretic nystagmus

Not all nystagmus has the saw-toothed form. In some cases the slow component has an exponential shape on electronystagmographic (ENG) recording and is known as gaze-paretic nystagmus. This is thought to be due to an impairment of the gaze maintenance mechanism and can be seen in a variety of conditions includ-

ing myopathies, especially myasthenia gravis, and lesions in the pons or the cerebellum. These CNS lesions are thought to impair the function of the PPRF and imply that the fundamental abnormality is in the generation of the fast phase.

Significance of horizontal nystagmus

Unilateral horizontal nystagmus, especially if its magnitude increases as the eyes are deviated in the direction of the fast phase (Alexander's law), is most commonly due to a peripheral lesion but can occur with lesions of the VIIIth nerve or vestibular nucleus. On the other hand, horizontal nystagmus that occurs to both sides at the same time is invariably due to a central lesion.

Removal of optic fixation and recording the eye movements, either with ENG or observing the eyes with an infrared viewer, also helps to differentiate between peripheral and central lesions. Characteristically, nystagmus due to a lesion of the end organ is enhanced by removal of fixation (Fig. 3), whereas that due to a central lesion, including vestibular nuclear lesions, is slowed or abolished. The pathway for this fixation suppression passes from the retina, especially the fovea, via the accessory olivary tract to the cerebellum and thence to the vestibular nuclei. Disruption of this central pathway means that vestibular nystagmus cannot be inhibited fully by fixation, i.e. the nystagmus is little affected by removal of fixation. In contrast, if the pathway is intact fixation inhibition can occur, as in normal subjects, and removal of fixation results in enhancement of the nystagmus which in some cases is only apparent in darkness.

Disease processes usually damage all three semicircular canals on one side and the effect of this is identical to that of destruction of the horizontal canal alone since the vertical vectors of the posterior and anterior canals are cancelled leaving only the horizontal one. Selective damage to part of the semicircular canal system can result in oblique or rotatory nystagmus. In all the above discussion it has been assumed that a lesion is a destructive one. If in fact it is irritative the nystagmus is in the opposite sense.

Vertical nystagmus

Although acquired spontaneous nystagmus in the vertical plane is virtually never due to an VIIIth cranial nerve disturbance, brief mention of it will be made here.

Up beat nystagmus i.e. the fast phase is upwards, occurs in patients with lesions in the floor of the fourth ventricle, pontine tegmentum, and perhaps anterior cerebellum. It rarely occurs in isolation but is not infrequent in patients with an internuclear ophthalmoplegia.

Down beat nystagmus i.e. the fast phase is downwards, is also uncommon. It indicates either a structural abnormality at the level of the foramen magnum, for example, cerebellar tonsillar herniation or cerebellar dysfunction especially an atrophic process.

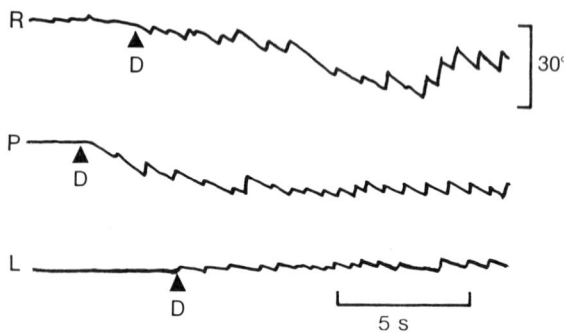

Fig. 3 Nystagmogram following left labyrinthectomy. Note the accentuation of the nystagmus as the gaze is directed towards the fast phase (Alexander's law) and the enhancement of the nystagmus and drift towards the damaged side with removal of fixation at D. R, L eyes deviated to right or left. P eyes in primary position.

Characteristically, down beat nystagmus is accentuated when the eyes are moved horizontally 30° to one side or the other. It is also sensitive to the position of the patient; for example, it may only be apparent in the supine position and disappear when the patient is upright or prone. The importance of this type of nystagmus is that it may indicate the presence of a correctable abnormality.

Positional and positioning nystagmus

Nystagmus induced by altering the position of the head with respect to the gravitational field is known as positioning nystagmus, while that induced by maintenance of such a position is positional nystagmus.

The best way to examine patients in the clinic is to have them sit on the couch in an upright position with the eyes open and the head rotated to the left or right. The head is grasped by the examiner and the patient instructed to fixate the examiner's forehead while the head is rapidly lowered below the horizontal over the end of the couch. Any nystagmus is noted and the patient then returned to the upright position. This is repeated with the head turned to the opposite shoulder. Basically two types of responses occur, one of which is due to a peripheral defect, the other to a central problem (Table 1).

Benign positional nystagmus

In this form there is a rotatory nystagmus with the fast phase towards the dependent ear, i.e. counterclockwise if the right ear is dependent, clockwise if the left ear is dependent. This nystagmus occurs after a latent interval of a few seconds and lasts 10–20 s. It is accompanied by vertigo. On returning to the upright position a lesser nystagmus of opposite sense occurs. Repetition of the test results in an attenuation of the response, this adaptation lasting a number of hours. Classically there is no nystagmus when the other ear is dependent.

Dix and Hallpike (1952) showed that this type of nystagmus is associated with utricular damage and Schucknecht (1969) has proposed, on the basis of limited pathological studies, that debris from the damaged utricle collects on the cupula of the posterior semicircular canal, the lowermost part of the vestibular apparatus, such that its mass is greater than normal. The cupula is then sensitive to gravitational pull. When the head is in the inverted position the cupula moves under the influence of gravity and induces nystagmus. The debris rapidly falls from the underside of the cupula which then returns to its normal position and the nystagmus ceases. Repetition of this manoeuvre does not induce further nystagmus since the debris has not had time to reaccumulate on the cupula. Section of the posterior semicircular canal nerve cures the patient supporting the concept of cupulolithiasis. In most cases, however, conservative therapy with vestibular sedatives and advice about head positioning are all that is necessary for this self-limiting condition.

Central position nystagmus

This form of nystagmus differs from the above in that its direction is not towards the dependent ear; it may be in any direction and is persistent and often unassociated with vertigo. It is commonly produced by positioning on either side. It is thought that this form of nystagmus signifies a central lesion, especially one involving the vestibulo-cerebellum.

Table 1 Characteristics of positional nystagmus

	Benign	Central
Direction	Towards lower ear	Any
Vertigo	++	±
Latent interval	+	0
Adaptation	+	0
Fatigue	+	0

++ Severe. + Moderate. ± Slight. 0 Absent.

Harrison and Ozsahinoglu (1972) reviewed a number of patients with different forms of positional nystagmus and observed that in the majority no cause could be found. In practice, the vast majority of patients with benign positional nystagmus of classical type have a peripheral and benign lesion (often following head injury, or associated with hypertension or cervical spondylosis), while central positional nystagmus requires investigation to exclude a central nervous system disorder (e.g. multiple sclerosis, tumour) although in a substantial proportion no cause will be found.

Gait and stance

Damage to the vestibular apparatus results in an abnormality of stance and gait since the vestibulo-spinal tracts carry inadequate information. The patient tends to fall towards the side of the lesion if it is destructive and veers to that side when walking. These abnormalities are most marked if the eyes are closed and if the lesion is a peripheral one.

Tests of vestibular function

Nystagmus induced by either visual or vestibular stimuli can help the clinician decide the anatomical site of a lesion. Two vestibular investigations are commonly employed, namely, the caloric test and various rotational tests. Both these techniques examine the integrity of the semicircular canals and their connections. There are no tests that are routinely available with which to study otolith function.

The caloric test

The bithermal binaural caloric test is the only way to assess the function of one horizontal semicircular canal system independently of the other. The head is placed such that the horizontal canal is vertical with the ampulla uppermost (the head is elevated 30° when the patent is lying supine). Irrigation with cold water (30 °C for 40 s) results in a movement of the endolymph away from the ampulla, while hot water (44 °C for 40 s) causes the reverse. Since the afferent nerves of the horizontal canal increase their firing rate with ampullo-petal movement, hot water causes nystagmus towards the ipsilateral side and cold water nystagmus to the contralateral side. The duration of the nystagmic response to irrigation is assessed either visually or with electronystagmography; the latter technique enables other variables, e.g. slow phase velocity, to be determined.

Two sorts of abnormality occur. The first is reduced function from one side, known as a canal paresis, and implies unilateral damage to the vestibular apparatus, VIIIth nerve or vestibular nucleus. The other type of abnormality is characterized by greater nystagmus in one direction than the other. This is known as a directional preponderance. It occurs with lesions in a wide variety of sites within the CNS as well as with nerve or end organ dysfunction. In the case of an acute destructive unilateral vestibular lesion the directional preponderance is to the side opposite the lesion, i.e. in the same direction as any spontaneous nystagmus. The presence of a directional preponderance in these circumstances implies incomplete compensation from such a lesion.

Rotational tests

Rotational tests are conducted by impulsively spinning patients, gradually accelerating them or sinusoidally rotating them. The advantage of the technique compared with the caloric test is that it is possible to quantify the stimulus and therefore assess the sensitivity of the semicircular canals. The disadvantage is that both horizontal canals are tested simultaneously, one increasing and the other decreasing its firing rate. It is thus not possible to detect unilateral failure.

The effect of fixation upon nystagmus induced by either the caloric test or rotational stimuli can give important clues as to the likely site of a lesion in the same way as it does in the case of spontaneous nystagmus (see above). An easy way of assessing clinically the effect of fixation on nystagmus induced by rotational stimuli is to ask the patient to fixate a target which is clenched in the mouth and then to rotate the head horizontally in a sinusoidal motion at a fairly low velocity. In normal subjects nystagmus does not occur until the head velocity is 40 or 50 °/s, whereas in patients with a CNS lesion fixation suppression may be entirely abolished and nystagmus readily elicited even at low velocities.

Optokinetic nystagmus
If a small striped drum is rotated in front of the patient nystagmus is induced. The fast phase is in the direction opposite to that of the drum rotation. This task is basically pursuit, and is foveally dependent. In the laboratory the patient can be surrounded by a striped curtain and full-field stimulation admininstered. This type of nystagmus depends upon the whole retina and is less dependent upon pursuit. Characteristically, optokinetic nystagmus is normal in peripheral compensated lesions although there may be a directional preponderance if compensation is incomplete. On the other hand, it is frequently abnormal in central lesions, particularly those involving the cerebellum.

Specific disorders of the VIIIth nerve system

There are numerous affections of the VIIIth nerve and we can only cover one or two important ones.

CEREBELLO-PONTINE ANGLE TUMOURS
Although all tumours of the cerebello-pontine angle are rare early diagnosis is important since the majority are benign and morbidity of surgical removal less if attempted when the tumours are small. About 70 per cent of the tumours are schwannomas, the remainder being meningiomas, epidermoids, neuromas of nerves other than the VIIIth, and a host of other rare lesions.

Acoustic schwannomas and neurofibromas
Pathology and incidence
Acoustic schwannomas usually arise on the vestibular nerves, especially the superior component. Exceptionally the tumours are bilateral; in a proportion of these the patient has neurofibromatosis and the tumours have a complex histology, i.e. they are neurofibromas. No age is exempt but the maximum incidence at presentation is in the fourth and fifth decades except in the case of neurofibromatosis where the onset is earlier. The sex incidence is approximately equal.

Symptoms
The presenting symptom is typically a progressive deafness with unsteadiness. When the tumours protrude beyond the internal acoustic porus, or arise more centrally, other cranial nerves are involved. The Vth nerve is particularly vulnerable; its involvement causes numbness on the face on the appropriate side. Larger tumours, which compress the brain stem, cause increasing unsteadiness and ultimately, in untreated cases, hydrocephalus. Occipital headache is a frequent symptom of acoustic tumours even before hydrocephalus develops.

Signs
The deafness is sensorineural, and in many patients with small tumours it has the features of a cochlear rather than a retrocochlear origin, i.e. there is recruitment and reasonably preserved speech reception. Later, as the tumour enlarges, the classical signs of a retrocochlear deafness occur. The stapedius reflex is abnormal with elevated thresholds and abnormal decay of the response in a high proportion of cases.

Brain stem evoked potentials are the best non-invasive auditory test for the detection of cerebello-pontine angle tumours, especially acoustic schwannomas. Abnormalities, which are found in over 90 per cent of cases, include a total absence of all compo-

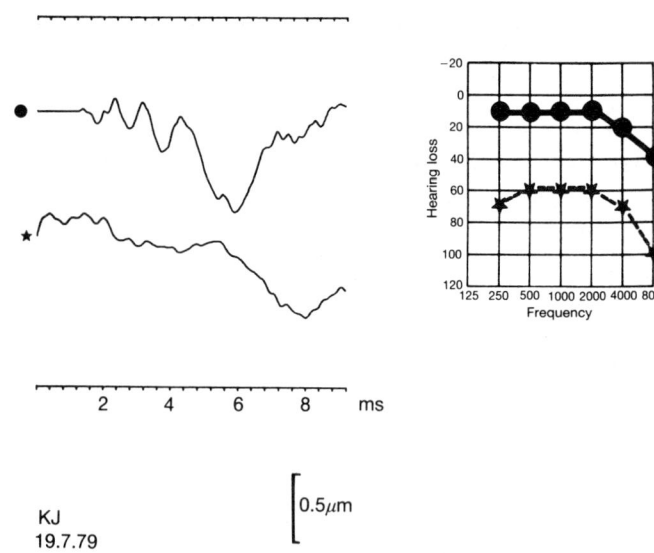

Fig. 4 Brain stem auditory evoked potential (BSAEP) from patient with left-sided cerebello-pontine angle tumour. Audiogram inset. Note the abnormal morphology of the BSAEP obtained from stimulation of the left ear with marked delay of component V and the normal response obtained on stimulation of the right ear, i.e. ITV markedly increased.

nents beyond wave I or an increased delay of component V on stimulation of the 'tumour' ear, and an abnormally large difference between components V (ITV) or of the I–V intervals (IT I–V) obtained on stimulation of the 'tumour' and 'non-tumour' ears, respectively (Fig. 4). Abnormal brain stem evoked potentials on stimulation of the normal ear occur with large tumours. Since in Ménière's disease there is little alteration of the BSAEP until the deafness is severe (>70 dB), this test has considerable specificity and can be used to separate many peripheral hearing losses from that due to cerebello-pontine angle tumours.

Vestibular function is also abnormal in a high proportion of patients. The majority have a canal paresis on caloric testing by the time they present to the clinician. They veer to the side of the lesion and Romberg's test is often positive. Nystagmus develops in all patients at some time during their illness. Initially there is vestibular nystagmus to the side opposite the tumour; later when the tumour is large and impinges upon the brain stem a gaze-paretic nystagmus towards the side of the lesion is found.

Fifth nerve signs, especially loss of the corneal reflex, are found with large tumours but, surprisingly, facial weakness is not a prominent sign in many cases. Long tract signs, especially mild ipsilateral pyramidal features such as hyperreflexia, are found when the tumours impinge upon the brain stem.

Other tumours
Meningiomas, which are more common in females, and epidermoids are much rarer than acoustic schwannomas but can mimic the latter. Deafness is in general less severe and the caloric responses are more frequently normal. The brain stem evoked potentials from the unimpaired ear are usually normal even in large tumours.

Imaging and treatment
Nuclear magnetic resonance scanning is the best non-invasive way to demonstrate cerebello-pontine angle tumours especially intracanalicular acoustic tumours. If this technique is not available computerized tomography (CT) scanning with iodine enhancement is reasonably good at detecting large tumours protruding through the porus but in the case of small intracanalicular tumours intracisternal air or metrizamide injection is required to detect them. Tomograms of the internal auditory meati, which are

widened in about 70 per cent of acoustic tumours, are rapidly joining the list of historical investigations.

Surgical removal is the only curative therapy. Morbidity is directly related to the size of the tumour. It is very rare to save hearing although the VIIth nerve can be preserved with modern techniques. If the tumours are bilateral it is important to teach the patient to lip read before operating upon the tumour if possible.

MÉNIÈRE'S DISEASE

Pathology

Ménière's disease is an uncommon condition associated with endolymphatic hydrops involving the pars inferior of the otic capsule. Its cause is unknown. No age is immune but the peak incidence of the onset of vertigo is in the fourth and fifth decades. Although it is the impression that females are more commonly affected, there is probably no sexual preference if only definite cases are considered.

Symptoms

The triad of episodic vertigo, tinnitus, and fluctuating deafness are the classical features of Ménière's disease. There is often a premonitory symptom of fullness of the appropriate ear. Initially the hearing loss recovers between attacks but later becomes permanent and progressive. Tinnitus is a constant feature which typically increases during the attacks. Vertigo is the most distressing symptom and the patient is usually prostrated with nausea and vomiting. It lasts less than 24 hours. The attacks occur in clusters with weeks or months free; the remissions are longer as the disease progresses.

Signs

The hearing loss in Ménière's disease is characteristically of low frequency initially, but later severe loss (about 60 dB) at all frequencies occurs. Loudness function studies indicate that the hearing loss is peripheral in origin, and in some cases the recruitment can be extremely marked, such that at high intensity the sound seems louder in the impaired than in the good ear, so-called over-recruitment. The deafness becomes bilateral in 10–25 per cent of patients.

Loss of vestibular function is frequently bilateral. A canal paresis on one or both sides is typical. Nystagmus is seen in all patients during the acute episode and tends to be towards the affected ear at the time of an attack. During the quiescent phase of the disease the nystagmus is often present when fixation is removed but its direction is variable even in apparently unilateral disease.

Some authors believe that electrocochleography is useful in the diagnosis of Ménière's disease, the summating potential being large relative to the action potential (> 30 per cent) (Fig. 5). This certainly seems to be the case provided the deafness exceeds 40 dB. Brain stem auditory evoked potentials are classically normal until the deafness is severe when there is an increase in latency of the later components. Dehydration tests, e.g. giving glycerol, are useful in diagnosis, the pure tone audiogram typically improving during the test in Ménière's disease but not in other causes of sensori-neural hearing loss.

Treatment

A low salt diet and administration of diuretics is of value in reducing the severity and frequency of attacks of vertigo. Beta-histine 8–16 mg three times daily may also reduce attacks, probably from its action on the stria-vascularis. Surgical therapy in the form of saccus decompression has its advocates although there is no good evidence as to its efficacy.

Other vestibular disturbances

Episodic vertigo

Many systemic conditions, e.g. arteritis, diabetes, hypertension, system degenerations, can cause vestibular or auditory failure. Space does not permit a discussion of these but the reader is referred to the monographs by Konigsmark and Gorlin (1976), and Rudge (1983) for a detailed discussion of many such disorders.

Mention must be made, however, of that common clinical problem, the patient with *episodic vertigo* not usually accompanied by deafness. Not all patients with episodic vertigo have Ménière's disease. Indeed the majority do not. An occasional patient has *syphilis*; Morrison (1975) has pointed out that syphilis can mimic Ménière's disease completely. An interesting feature of syphilis confined to the VIIIth nerve system is that the deafness is often progressive in spite of treatment with penicillin. It is mandatory to do fluorescent treponemal antibody tests in anyone presenting with a Ménière's syndrome. *Migraine* is a disorder that profoundly affects the vestibular system and, to a lesser extent, hearing. Acute attacks of migraine may frequently be associated with vestibular abnormalities (vertigo, nausea, and vomiting) and auditory dysfunction (phonophobia), both in the basilar artery form as well as classical migraine. In addition, patients who have had migraine in the past occasionally develop sporadic vertigo unaccompanied by headache; the cause is unknown.

Vestibular neuronitis is a syndrome of paroxysmal vertigo first described by Dix and Hallpike (1952). They thought the abnormality was in Scarpa's ganglion and indeed the evidence for this has been found at autopsy. The syndrome is, however, common and found particularly in patients with hypertension, and following systemic viral infections where the term 'neuronitis' implies an unwarranted precision of diagnosis. The symptoms result from an episode of vestibular failure of which neuronitis is but one cause.

Finally we should mention vestibular failure as an uncommon complication of *aminoglycoside* toxicity usually in elderly patients with renal impairment. These patients classically complain initially of a visual disturbance with oscillopsia due to loss of the vestibulo-ocular reflex (VOR) rather than vertigo or aural symptoms; there is no mechanism that can substitute for the VOR in stabilizing the eyes at high frequencies of head movement, i.e. > 1 Hz. Auditory function is usually preserved with the aminoglycosides that are now in clinical use, e.g. gentamicin. There is no way of detecting incipient vestibular failure due to these agents: careful prescribing and measurement of blood levels of gentamicin is the best precaution, and therapy should be stopped if vertigo occurs, provided alternative antibiotics are available.

Treatment of the vertiginous patient

During an episode of acute vestibular failure patients are understandably terrified and fear that they are about to die. They require reassurance that they will recover, and should be put to bed and told not to move their heads. Vestibular sedatives such a prochlorperazine 12.5 mg i.m. will be required if the patient is vomiting. Oral therapy can be given as soon as vomiting ceases. There is a wide variety of such sedatives available, none of which

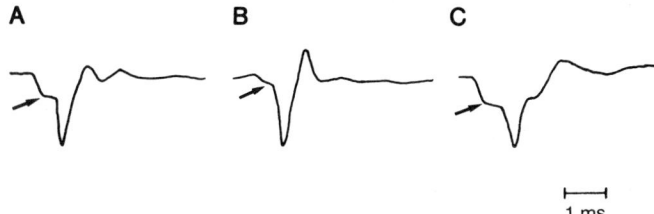

Fig. 5 Electrocochleogram from normal subject (A), cochlear hearing loss not due to Ménière's disease (B), and Ménière's disease (C). Arrow indicates summating potential on the down slope of the nerve action potential. Note large size of summating potential *relative* to action potential in Ménière's disease.

is ideal; in general a combination of sympathomimetic and anti-parasympathomimetic drugs is the most efficient way of lessening symptoms, although in clinical practice anticholinergic drugs alone are usually given. Cinnarizine 15 mg t.d.s or flunarizine 1 tablet in the morning are the most commonly prescribed agents and are moderately effective. Usually the drugs can be discontinued after 2–4 weeks and most patients have recovered completely by this time.

Occasionally symptoms persist. Sometimes this may take the form of benign positional vertigo for which vestibular sedatives and advice about lying down are all that is required. Other patients are frightened to walk and need vestibular exercises to retrain their vestibular system using input from other sensory modalities. Some patients are helped by clonazepam, partly because of its sedative properties but also by its central action on the vestibular system. Such patients may require psychiatric help even though they have a good organic cause for their vertigo.

Conclusion

The VIIIth nerve innervates the two most important sensory organs. Complete loss of the auditory component is a major disaster for any patient while loss of the vestibular element can be socially and physically crippling. Careful assessment of these two elements is an essential prerequisite for adequate management of the patient who complains of deafness, distortion of hearing, imbalance or vertigo.

References

Borg, E. (1973). On the neuronal organisation of the acoustic middle ear reflex. A physiological and anatomical study. *Brain Res.* **49**, 101–123.

Chambers, B. R. and Gresty, M. A. (1982). Effects of fixation and optokinetic stimulation on vestibulo-ocular reflex suppression. *J. Neurol. Neurosurg. Psychiat.* **45**, 998–1004.

Chiveralls, K. and Fitzsimmons, R. (1973). Stapedial reflex action in normal subjects. *Br. J. Audiol.* **7**, 105–110.

Chiveralls, K. (1977). A further examination of the use of the stapedius reflex in the diagnosis of acoustic neuroma. *Audiology* **16**, 331–337.

Dix, M. R. and Hallpike, C. S. (1952). The pathology, symptomatology and diagnosis of certain disorders of the vestibular system. *Proc. R. Soc. Med. Lond.* **45**, 341–354.

Eggermont, J. J., Don, M. and Brackmann, D. E. (1980). Electro-cochleography and auditory brain stem electric response in patients with pontine angle tumours. *Ann. Otol. Rhinol. Laryngol.* **89** (Suppl. 75), 1–19.

Fisher, A., Gresty, M., Chambers, B. and Rudge, P. (1983). Primary position upbeating nystagmus: a variety of central positional nystagmus. *Brain* **106**, 949–964.

Fitzgerald, G. and Hallpike, C. S. (1942). Studies in human vestibular function. Observations on the directional preponderance of caloric nystagmus resulting from cerebral lesions. *Brain* **65**, 115–137.

Gacek, R. R. (1974). Transection of the posterior auditory nerve for relief of benign paroxysmal positional vertigo. *Ann. Otol. Rhinol. Laryngol.* **83**, 596–605.

Gibson, W. P. R., Prasher, D. K. and Kilkenny, G. P. (1983). The diagnostic significance of transtympanic electro-cochleography in Ménière's disease. *Ann. Otol. Rhinol. Laryngol.* **92**, 155–159.

Hallpike, C. S. and Cairns, B. J. (1938). Observations of the pathology of Ménière's syndrome. *J. Otol. Rhinol. Laryngol.* **53**, 625–654.

Halmagyi, G. M., Rudge, P., Gresty, M. A. and Sanders, M. D. (1983). Downbeating nystagmus: A review of 62 cases. *Arch. Neurol.* **40**, 777–784.

Harrison, M. S. and Ozsahinoglu, C. (1972). Positional vertigo: Aetiology and clinical significance. *Brain* **95**, 369–372.

Johnson, E. W. (1977). Auditory test results in 500 cases of acoustic neuroma. *Arch. Otolaryngol.* **103**, 152–158.

Katz, J. (1972). *Handbook of clinical audiology.* Williams and Wilkins, Baltimore.

Kayan, A. and Hood, J. D. (1984). Neuro-otological manifestations of migraine. *Brain* **107**, 1123–1142.

Konigsmark, B. W. and Gorlin, R. J. (1976). *Genetic and metabolic deafness.* W. B. Saunders, Philadelphia.

Korres, S. (1978a). Electro-nystagmographic criteria in neuro-otological diagnosis 1: Peripheral lesions. *J. Neurol. Neurosurg. Psychiat.* **41**, 249–253.

Korres, S. (1978b). Electro-nystagmographic criteria in neuro-otological diagnosis 2: Central nervous system lesion. *J. Neurol. Neurosurg. Psychiat.* **41**, 214–264.

Morrison, A. W. (1975). *Management of sensorineural deafness.* Butterworths, London.

Oosterveld, W. J. (1983). *Ménière's disease.* John Wiley and Sons, Chichester.

Robinson, K. and Rudge, P. (1983). The differential diagnosis of cerebello-pontine angle lesions. *J. Neurol. Sci.* **60**, 1–21.

Rudge, P. (1983). *Clinical neuro-otology.* Churchill Livingstone, Edinburgh.

Schuknecht, H. F. (1969). Cupulolithiasis. *Arch. Otolaryngol.* **90**, 765–778.

Selters, W. A. and Brackmann, D. E. (1977). Acoustic tumour detection with brainstem electric response audiometry. *Arch. Otolaryngol.* **103**, 181–187.

Thomas, K. and Harrison, M. S. (1971). Long term follow up of 610 cases of Ménière's disease. *Proc. R. Soc. Med. Lond.* **64**, 853–866.

Other cranial nerves

P. K. THOMAS

The olfactory nerve

Loss of the sense of smell (anosmia) is most commonly encountered as a sequel to head injury and is probably related to severance of the central processes of the neurones of the olfactory mucosa as they pass through the cribriform plate to the olfactory bulb. It is usually permanent. Distortion of olfaction (parosmia) may occur and may be persistent. The sense of smell is occasionally congenitally absent or may be acutely and permanently lost after a coryzal infection. Bilateral anosmia is frequently accompanied by impairment of taste related to reduced detection of the volatile substances that impart flavours to foods. Unilateral anosmia may occur in olfactory groove meningiomas or other subfrontal tumours. This is usually not detected by the patient.

The central connections of the olfactory pathways are complex and include projections to the temporal lobes, hypothalamus, the septal region, and the amygdaloid nuclei. Olfactory hallucinations are well known to occur as a manifestation of temporal lobe epilepsy. Identification of odours may be impaired after bilateral medial temporal lesions and may be defective in multiple sclerosis, possibly as the result of demyelination in the olfactory tracts. Complaints of hypersensitivity of the sense of smell commonly have a psychoneurotic basis and persistent olfactory hallucinations may be reported by psychotic patients. Persistent parosmia is sometimes produced by temporal lobe lesions.

Third, fourth, and sixth cranial nerves

The third or oculomotor nerve supplies all the external ocular muscles with the exception of the superior oblique and lateral rectus. It also carries the parasympathetic innervation of the pupilloconstrictor fibres of the iris. A complete third nerve lesion produces a dilated and unreactive pupil, complete ptosis, and loss of upward, downward, and medial movement of the eye. The eye becomes deviated downwards and laterally. Diplopia is only experienced when the lid is held up.

The fourth or trochlear nerve supplies the superior oblique muscle. Following a lesion of this nerve, there is extorsion of the eye when the patient looks outwards. When the patient looks downwards and medially, diplopia is experienced. This is particularly disturbing because of its occurrence on looking downwards and produces difficulty in walking and in descending stairs. The patient may compensate for this by tilting the head to the opposite side.

The sixth or abducens nerve supplies the lateral rectus. A lesion of this nerve causes convergent strabismus, and inability to abduct the affected eye, and diplopia which is maximal on lateral gaze to the affected side.

The third, fourth, and sixth nerves may be affected singly or in combination and the paralysis may be complete or partial. In some instances, the lesion is within the brainstem where it may affect either the nuclei or intramedullary portion of the nerve fibres. In a young adult, the commonest cause is multiple sclerosis, and in an older patient, brainstem vascular disease and neoplasms.

Extramedullary lesions of the third, fourth, and sixth nerves are more frequent and may occur at any point along their course, either intracranially or within the orbit. A third nerve palsy may develop in the region of the tentorial hiatus as a false localizing sign related to brainstem displacement produced by supratentorial space-occupying conditions. Unilateral or bilateral sixth nerve palsies may also arise as a consequence of raised intracranial pressure, probably caused by traction, again secondary to brainstem displacement. These nerves can be involved singly or together in conditions such as chronic basal meningitis or carcinomas of the skull base. *Gradenigo's syndrome* comprises a sixth nerve palsy and pain of trigeminal distribution. It is produced by a lesion at the apex of the petrous temporal bone. As this syndrome was most commonly infective in origin and related to chronic middle ear disease, it is now encountered considerably less frequently.

The third, fourth, and sixth nerves traverse the cavernous sinus, as do the first and second divisions of the trigeminal nerve. In this situation, they are most commonly damaged by an intracavernous aneurysm of the internal carotid artery. The third nerve is affected more often than the fourth and sixth. The consequent internal and external ophthalmoplegia is frequently accompanied by pain, and sometimes sensory loss and paraesthesiae, in the corresponding frontal region related to compression of the first division of the trigeminal nerve, and occasionally in the cheek from damage to the maxillary division. In the superior orbital fissure syndrome, caused for example by a tumour invading the fissure, a total ophthalmoplegia may result, associated with pain and sensory loss in the distribution of the first division of the trigeminal nerve. The eye is often proptosed because of obstruction of the ophthalmic vein. The *Tolosa–Hunt syndrome* consists of a painful external ophthalmoplegia related to a granulomatous angiitis. Within the orbit, the third, fourth, and sixth nerves may be affected by conditions such as tumours and granulomas. They may be damaged as a result of trauma at any point along their course and may be affected singly or in combination as part of a cranial neuropathy of which diabetes and sarcoidosis are the most important examples.

Internal and external ophthalmoplegias are common and this list of causes is by no means exhaustive.

Pupillary abnormalities

Constriction of the pupil (miosis) occurs as a result of paralysis of the sympathetic innervation of the pupillo-dilator fibres of the iris and may be accompanied by the other features of *Horner's syndrome*, namely a mild ptosis, and vasodilatation and anhidrosis of the face on the same side. The ocular manifestations may be encountered alone if the damage is restricted to the intracranial portion of the sympathetic plexus around the carotid artery. *Raeder's syndrome* consists of these components of Horner's syndrome together with involvement of the first division of the trigeminal nerve. It may be caused by tumours of the skull base. Miosis may also be produced by the local action of eserine and by morphine and related compounds.

Pupillary dilatation may be caused by lesions of the third nerve, although it is of interest that the isolated third nerve palsies of presumed vascular origin that may occur in diabetes mellitus, in contradistinction to compressive lesions of the nerve, characteristically spare the pupil. Anticholinergic drugs such as atropine and related substances give rise to pupillary dilatation, as does cocaine.

The Argyll Robertson pupil is small, fails to react to light, but constricts on ocular convergence, and if bilateral the pupils are frequently unequal in size (anisocoria). The pupil may be irregular in outline and it does not dilate fully in response to mydriatics. Argyll Robertson pupils are almost always related to neurosyphilis but are occasionally encountered in diabetic neuropathy and in some hereditary neuropathies.

The myotonic pupil (*Holmes–Adie syndrome*) reacts abnormally slowly both to light and on convergence, but particularly so for the response to illumination. A very bright light may be required to demonstrate any pupillary constriction, or if the patient remains in a dark room for some minutes, the pupil slowly dilates. The condition may be unilateral or bilateral and is commoner in women than men. Myotonic pupils may be associated with absence or depression of the tendon reflexes and occasionally with anhidrosis in the limbs.

Trigeminal nerve

The fifth cranial nerve is predominantly sensory in function, but also innervates the muscles of mastication. It emerges from the pons and runs forward to the Gasserian ganglion which is situated in Meckel's cave near the apex of the petrous temporal bone. The three sensory divisions of the nerve run anteriorly from the ganglion. The first or frontal division passes through the cavernous sinus and the superior orbital fissure. Its branches supply sensation to the anterior part of the scalp, the forehead, and the eye, including the conjunctiva and cornea. The second or maxillary division leaves the skull through the foramen rotundum, traverses the infraorbital canal and supplies the cheek. The mandibular division emerges from the skull through the foramen ovale to reach the infratemporal fossa with the motor root with which it unites to form a single trunk. It is distributed to the lower lip, chin, and the lower part of the cheek, and its auriculotemporal branch supplies part of the ear and temporal area. It also supplies the inner aspect of the cheek and the anterior two-thirds of the tongue, and its lingual branch carries taste fibres from the anterior two-thirds of the tongue which leave it in the chorda tympani to join the facial nerve. It is important that the skin over the angle of the jaw is supplied from the second cervical nerve root, and the absence of this 'trigeminal notch' may be useful in distinguishing hysterical loss of sensation on the face which usually follows the angle of the jaw. The motor root innervates the temporalis muscle, the masseter, the pterygoids, mylohyoid, the anterior belly of the digastric, and also tensor tympani and tensor palati. With unilateral paralysis of the masticatory muscles, the jaw deviates towards the affected side on opening because of the action of the unopposed external pterygoid on the unaffected side.

The trigeminal nerve may be affected by intramedullary lesions, it may be damaged during the intracranial part of its course, or its branches may be compromised extracranially. An acoustic neurinoma may compress the nerve in the posterior fossa or the nucleus of the descending root may be affected by direct compression of the brainstem by this tumour. Loss of corneal sensation is usually the earliest feature. Reference has already been made to involvement of the nerve in association with damage to the sixth nerve at the apex of the petrous temporal bone (*Gradenigo's syndrome*), as has involvement of the first and second divisions in the cavernous sinus, or the first division in the superior orbital fissure.

Trigeminal neuralgia

Symptoms

This condition is characterized by paroxysms of intense pain strictly confined to the distribution of the trigeminal nerve. In most cases the cause is unknown. It is generally encountered in individuals over the age of 50. In younger patients it may be due to multiple sclerosis. Rarely, compression of the nerve, for example by tumours in the cerebellopontine angle, is responsible.

The salient feature of the disorder is pain which is usually unilateral and is felt either within the territory of one division of the nerve only, or may involve two adjacent divisions or affect the whole territory of the nerve. Less commonly it is bilateral.

The pain occurs in brief searing paroxysms, each attack lasting only a matter of seconds. The pain is often described as piercing or knife-like. Its intense quality may cause the patient to screw up his face in agony, hence the use of the term *tic douloureux* to describe the condition. The paroxysms may be spontaneous or provoked by movements of the face and jaw, by touching the skin, or by draughts of cold air on the face. Eating and speaking may become extremely difficult. 'Trigger spots' on the skin of the face may be present, the touching of which provokes the paroxysms. The attacks may be followed by less severe pain of a dull, boring character and by tenderness of the skin in the affected area. Fortunately the attacks usually cease at night.

The quality of the pain is characteristic, and when trigeminal neuralgia is present, the diagnosis is not usually missed, especially if a paroxysm is witnessed. The usual mistake is to regard as trigeminal neuralgia pain that is due to some other cause, and since there are many conditions that give rise to facial pain, the opportunities for error are numerous. Pain that is of a continuous character is not trigeminal neuralgia and some other cause must be sought. Absence of provocation by eating, talking, or the touching of trigger spots also makes the diagnosis unlikely. Once the diagnosis is accepted, it is essential to exclude compressive lesions affecting the nerve.

In the early stages, remissions lasting for months or years are usual, but in older patients remissions, if they occur, are likely to be brief. In all cases the remissions tend to become shorter as time goes on, and without treatment the condition persists for the rest of the patient's life.

The distribution of the pain is usually in one or two divisions of the nerve. The first division is rarely affected primarily, but pain may spread into it from the second division. If the pain begins in the second division it may, after a time, affect the third, and vice versa.

Treatment

The introduction of carbamazepine revolutionized treatment of this distressing condition. In a high proportion of cases, the paroxysms can be abolished or reduced. A dosage of 200 mg three to five times per day is employed. Ataxia and drowsiness may be troublesome side-effects with higher dosages, and aggravation of ataxia even with modest dosages may impede treatment in cases of multiple sclerosis. Hypersensitivity reactions producing skin rashes or rarely bone marrow depression may develop but are fortunately uncommon.

If carbamazepine is not successful, or it the patients fail to tolerate it, thermocoagulation of the ganglion may have to be considered. This should be undertaken only if the disorder is established so that a prolonged natural remission is unlikely to occur. It should also not be undertaken unless the patient is completely unable to tolerate the disorder, despite analgesics and sedation, and if he is fully aware of the consequences. The persistent analgesia and sometimes dysaesthesiae may subsequently be troublesome, and when the first division is made anaesthetic, damage to the conjunctiva leading to corneal scarring has to be avoided. It may be possible to limit the anaesthesia to the affected area, sparing for instance the eye if the first division is not involved in the pain. If thermocoagulation fails, section of the sensory root by a posterior fossa approach employing a microsurgical technique is indicated.

Ophthalmic herpes zoster

In elderly individuals, the fifth nerve is prone to involvement in herpes zoster, the first division being most vulnerable, giving rise to the distressing condition of ophthalmic herpes. The clinical features and treatment of herpes zoster are considered elsewhere (see Section 5). An unfortunate sequel may be visual impairment from residual corneal scarring. Particularly in older subjects, postherpetic neuralgia may also be a sequel. This gives rise to persistent and unremitting spontaneous pain associated with cutaneous hyperaesthesia in the affected area. Treatment is difficult. Analgesics, sedation, and antidepressive preparations to combat the secondary depression that is frequently present may be of some assistance.

Isolated trigeminal neuropathy

Rarely, a chronic isolated unilateral or bilateral affection of the trigeminal nerve may occur as a manifestation of *Sjögren's syndrome* or systemic lupus erythematosus, although most cases are idiopathic. Extensive nasal scarring and tissue loss may occur secondary to repeated injury from picking and scratching.

Facial nerve

The seventh cranial nerve is largely motor. The nerve traverses the facial canal in the petrous temporal bone in close relationship to the middle ear and emerges at the stylomastoid foramen. Its branches pass forward through the parotid gland to be distributed to the muscles of the face, including the platysma. Within the petrous bone, a branch is given to the stapedius muscle. The chorda tympani, carrying the taste fibres from the anterior two-thirds of the tongue joins the nerve within the facial canal and a small branch supplies cutaneous sensation to the region of the external auditory meatus. The nerve also carries preganglionic parasympathetic fibres destined for the lachrymal gland.

The distinction between upper and lower motor neurone lesions of the facial muscles is usually easy. In general, with upper motor neurone lesions there is a relative preservation of power in the upper facial muscles, because these have a bilateral innervation from the cerebral hemispheres. There is no loss of tone with upper motor neurone lesions, so that the sagging of the face that is an unsightly feature of lower motor neurone palsy does not occur.

In common with the trigeminal nerve, the facial nerve may be affected by tumours in the cerebellopontine angle. In the past, it was often involved from middle ear infections. It may be involved in cephalic herpes zoster, but the most common lesion by far is Bell's palsy. More peripherally, the nerve may be implicated in tumours of the parotid gland.

Bell's palsy

This term describes a usually unilateral facial paralysis of relatively rapid onset related to a lesion of the nerve within the facial canal. Taste may also be affected. It may develop at any age, most commonly between 20 and 50 years, and affects both sexes equally. Its causation is unknown. In the acute stage, the nerve is swollen and compression within the facial canal may contribute to the nerve fibre damage.

The onset is rapid and is frequently heralded or accompanied by aching pain below the ear or in the mastoid region. This clears within a few days and is not present in every case. The paralysis usually reaches its maximum severity after one or two days but occasionally progresses over the course of several days. Complete paralysis may occur. In the lower face, this may cause a mild dysarthria and some difficulty in eating because of food collecting between the gums and the inner sides of the cheek and the escape of fluid when drinking. The face sags and on smiling is drawn across to the unaffected side. Paralysis of orbicularis oculi renders voluntary eye closure impossible and, particularly in the older subject, ectropion develops. This can result in conjunctival injury from foreign bodies or conjunctivitis. If the paralysis is partial, the lower face is usually affected to a greater extent than the upper.

In the more severe cases, loss of taste over the anterior two-thirds of the tongue is often present, and paralysis of the stapedius muscle may result in a lack of tolerance for high-pitched or loud sounds.

Bell's palsy has to be distinguished from selective lesions of the facial nerve within the brainstem, in which instance taste will not be affected. A facial paralysis superficially resembling Bell's palsy may occur in multiple sclerosis, in which event evidence of more widespread neurological disease may well be detected on examination, or the history may indicate episodes of neurological disturbance in the past. With respect to peripheral lesions, middle ear disease requires exclusion. Facial paralysis related to cephalic herpes zoster is discussed below. A lesion of the facial nerve may represent a mononeuropathy from some generalized disorder of which diabetes and sarcoidosis are the most important. Bell's palsy is rarely bilateral and the occurrence of bilateral facial paralysis would raise the possibility of the *Guillain–Barré syndrome*. This may begin with facial weakness, or the weakness may remain restricted to the facial musculature. The occurrence of bilateral facial weakness would also raise the possibility of sarcoidosis.

In approximately 85 per cent of cases of Bell's palsy, the paralysis is the result of a local conduction block within the facial canal without axonal degeneration and this is effectively the situation in all instances of mild weakness. The conduction block is presumably the consequence of segmental demyelination. Providing that such cases do not progress to more severe weakness, all recover fully within a few weeks. In cases where there is total paralysis, a proportion of these will be the result of a conduction block, but in about 15 per cent, axonal degeneration will have occurred. Those with a conduction block will again recover satisfactorily within a few weeks. In patients with a degenerative lesion, recovery has to take place by axonal regeneration. Evidence of re-innervation does not appear in under three months and the ultimate recovery is often incomplete or may fail to occur altogether. Synkinesis is frequent after re-innervation so that blinking, for example, results in a simultaneous contraction of the angle of the mouth. Aberrant parasympathetic re-innervation may also occur, leading for instance to gustatory lachrymation ('crocodile tears').

Axons remain excitable distal to the lesion for three or four days after interruption. It is therefore not possible to be certain from electrodiagnostic tests whether axonal degeneration has taken place until after this time. At that stage, electrical stimulation of the facial nerve at the stylomastoid foramen with brief pulses will still elicit a muscle contraction if the paralysis is due to conduction block, whereas none will be obtained if axonal degeneration has taken place.

In the early stages, the main endeavour of treatment should be to prevent either a partial lesion, or complete paralysis related to a conduction block, progressing to a degenerative lesion. There is some evidence that corticosteroids may be advantageous by reducing oedema in the nerve. Thus it is justifiable to treat all cases with corticosteroids or ACTH if seen within a few days of onset, providing no contra-indication to such treatment exists. A course of a week's duration with an initially high dosage is recommended.

Surgical decompression of the nerve has been advised. To be effective, this would have to be performed at the outset, which is not justifiable as 85 per cent of cases will recover satisfactorily without treatment. So far there are no means of predicting which cases will progress to a degenerative lesion. If this were available, decompression could be undertaken selectively in such cases.

It is helpful to perform electrodiagnostic studies at about one week after the onset. If this reveals a degenerative lesion, it is then known that recovery will be delayed. A prosthesis attached to the teeth to elevate the angle of the mouth to reduce facial deformity may be helpful. In patients with severe ectropion, a lateral tarsorrhaphy to protect the eye may be required. Electrical stimulation of the paralysed facial muscles has no effect on the ultimate prognosis.

In those cases in which regeneration fails to occur, operation may be desirable for cosmetic reasons to counteract the facial deformity. The angle of the mouth may be elevated by a fascial sling attached to the temporalis fascia, but the result is never highly satisfactory. Restoration of facial tone may be achieved by anastomosis of the hypoglossal nerve to the facial, but at the expense of denervation of the tongue on that side. Any operation should not be contemplated before an adequate length of time has been allowed for regeneration. This should be of the order of nine months.

Facial paralysis related to 'geniculate' herpes zoster (Ramsay Hunt syndrome)

Facial paralysis of rapid onset accompanied by severe pain in and around the external auditory meatus and in the throat may accompany 'cephalic zoster'. Vesicles may be detectable in the ear and ulceration in the fauces, or anywhere on the head. Occasionally there is concomitant vertigo, tinnitus, and some deafness with involvement of the eighth nerve ('otic herpes zoster'). Prognosis for recovery of the facial paralysis is less good than in Bell's palsy.

Hemifacial spasm

This consists of a unilateral disturbance affecting the facial muscles producing irregular clonic or twitching movements of the facial muscles, usually of insidious onset. It most commonly occurs in middle-aged women. There may be a mild degree of facial weakness, but severe paralysis does not occur. Usually no underlying cause is demonstrable. The condition selectively affects the facial nerve, possibly within the brainstem.

It begins with intermittent twitching of the facial muscles such as around the eye or at the angle of the mouth. These movements gradually become more frequent and extend to involve the rest of the facial muscles, often gradually advancing over the course of some years. If they become severe, the face is contorted by irregular clonic spasms which may keep the eye closed for prolonged periods. The facial distortion is often a considerable embarrassment to the patient, who finds that the spasms tend to be aggravated by emotional stress.

The condition requires to be distinguished from benign fasciculation of the face ('live blood'), which usually occurs around the eyes, related to fatigue or emotional tension, and from the myokymic twitching that is occasionally encountered as a manifestation of multiple sclerosis. The latter consists of a persisting irregular rippling movement of the facial muscles that usually subsides after a week or two. These conditions can be distinguished by electromyography (see page 21.22).

No satisfactory treatment is available. If exaggeration by emotional factors is evident, the administration of diazepam or similar preparation may produce a marginal improvement. In severe cases, selective division or alcohol injection into branches of the facial nerve may be advisable, although re-innervation with recurrence of the twitching usually occurs. Neurosurgical intervention to relieve compression of the nerve by aberrant vessels in its intracranial course has been advocated.

Glossopharyngeal nerve

The ninth cranial nerve leaves the skull through the jugular foramen, closely related to the tenth nerve. It supplies the stylopharyngeus muscle and the constrictor muscles of the pharynx. Parasympathetic fibres are supplied to the parotid gland. Sensory fibres are carried from the posterior third of the tongue, the ear, the fauces, and the nasopharynx, and chemoreceptor and baroreceptor afferents from the carotid sinus.

The glossopharyngeal nerve is rarely affected in isolation. Lesions usually occur in conjunction with involvement of the vagus and give rise to some dysphagia, impaired pharyngeal sensation, and loss of taste over the posterior third of the tongue. It may be affected in the jugular foramen syndrome (*Vernet's syndrome*), along with the tenth and eleventh nerves, of which glomus tumours or metastatic carcinoma are the commonest causes. The nerve may also be involved in diphtheritic neuropathy and in a polyneuritis cranialis.

Glossopharyngeal neuralgia is a rare form of neuralgia within the distribution of the glossopharyngeal nerve. Its features are otherwise strictly comparable to those of trigeminal neuralgia in the quality and severity of the pain, its occurrence in brief paroxysms, its provocation by actions such as speaking or swallowing, and the remissions in its course. As with trigeminal neuralgia, it is most often encountered in elderly subjects, and the pain may initially be confined to individual branches. Thus it may be felt deep in the ear, related to the tympanic branch, or in the throat, related to the pharyngeal branches.

In treatment, carbamazepine may be effective. In instances of severe pain unrelieved by this preparation, surgical treatment, usually avulsion of the nerve, may be required.

Vagus nerve

The tenth cranial nerve is structurally complex. Within the skull it is joined by the cranial division of the eleventh nerve. It leaves the skull through the jugular foramen. Cutaneous sensory fibres are carried from the external ear and visceral afferent fibres are carried from the pharynx, larynx, trachea, oesophagus, and the thoracic and abdominal viscera. Motor fibres are supplied to the striated musculature of the palate and pharynx and, through the external and recurrent laryngeal nerves, to the muscles of the larynx. Parasympathetic fibres are provided to innervate the parotid gland (through the glossopharyngeal nerve), the heart and the abdominal viscera.

The important symptoms of vagal nerve damage are those relating to pharyngeal and laryngeal innervation. The cells of origin in the nucleus ambiguus of the medulla may be damaged in the lateral medullary syndrome, in motor neurone disease, and in acute bulbar poliomyelitis, leading to dysphagia and dysphonia. Involvement along with the glossopharyngeal nerve in the jugular foramen syndrome has already been mentioned. The recurrent laryngeal nerve may be damaged during operations on the thyroid gland or by tumours within the neck, or within the thorax, usually by carcinoma of the bronchus. The nerve on the left is vulnerable to damage from aneurysm of the aortic arch. Isolated and unexplained lesions of the recurrent laryngeal nerve are not uncommon.

Nuclear or high vagal lesions, as well as involving the larynx, cause palatal and pharyngeal paralysis. If unilateral, there are no symptoms from palatopharyngeal paralysis. The uvula is pulled up to the opposite side on phonation and pharyngeal sensation is impaired on the affected side. With bilateral paralysis, the palate is paretic leading to nasality of the voice and nasal regurgitation of liquids on attempts at swallowing. Bilateral palatopharyngeal paralysis may be encountered in motor neurone disease, bulbar poliomyelitis, diphtheritic neuropathy, and polyneuritis cranialis.

Unilateral intrinsic laryngeal paralysis from lesions of the recurrent nerve may be asymptomatic or give rise to hoarseness of the voice. If the superior laryngeal nerve is also involved leading to paralysis of the cricothyroid muscle, the affected cord lies in a paramedian or cadaveric position. The effects of bilateral lesions of the recurrent laryngeal nerves depend upon the degree of approximation of the vocal cords. Lesions of insidious onset tend to give rise to dysphonia and also to stridor on exertion. In partial lesions, close approximation of the cords may result from selective paralysis of the abductor muscles giving rise to limitation of the airway and sometimes necessitating tracheostomy. With bilateral lesions involving both the recurrent and superior laryngeal nerves, both

cords are paralysed and in the cadaveric position. Phonation is impossible.

Spinal accessory nerve

The spinal accessory portion of the eleventh cranial nerve arises from the upper cervical cord and the lower medulla. The nerve passes through the foramen magnum and joins the cranial portion of the nerve before emerging from the skull through the jugular foramen. The spinal accessory nerve then separates and supplies the sternomastoid and trapezius muscles, the latter also receiving an innervation from the cervical plexus.

The nerve may be affected by lesions in the region of the jugular foramen, but more commonly it is damaged by injuries to the neck or by operations for removal of cervical glands, particularly as it crosses the posterior triangle of the neck. Isolated and unexplained lesions of the nerve are occasionally encountered.

Unilateral paralysis of the sternomastoid usually passes unnoticed by the patient. The muscle does not stand out when the head is turned to the opposite side. Paralysis of the trapezius, on the other hand, causes difficulty in lifting the arm above the horizontal, in shrugging the shoulder and in approximating the scapula to the midline and therefore also in carrying the extended arm backwards. The shoulder droops when the arm is hanging at the side and there is moderate winging of the scapula which is accentuated when the patient attempts to elevate the arm laterally.

The hypoglossal nerve

The twelfth cranial nerve supplies all the muscles of the tongue, both intrinsic and extrinsic. It leaves the skull through the anterior condyloid foramen. A unilateral lesion of the hypoglossal nerve causes weakness and atrophy of the tongue on the affected side. When protruded, the tongue deviates to the affected side. Articulation is unaffected. The nerve may be affected by tumours in the region of the anterior condyloid foramen, or by tumours or penetrating injuries in the neck. If the lesion is the result of a unilateral lower brainstem lesion, it may be combined with a crossed hemiplegia.

Bilateral lesions give rise to generalized atrophy of the tongue. Protrusion becomes impossible and articulation is disturbed. The commonest cause is motor neurone disease (progressive bulbar palsy). The wasting of the tongue is usually accompanied by fasciculation.

References

Asbury, A. K., Aldredge, H., Hershberg, R. and Fisher, C. M. (1970). Oculomotor palsy in diabetes mellitus: a clinicopathological study. *Brain* **93**, 555–566.

Brodal, A. (1965). *The cranial nerves*, 2nd edn. Blackwell Scientific Publications, Oxford.

Cogan, D. G. (1956). *Neurology of the ocular muscles*, 2nd edn. C. C. Thomas, Springfield.

—— (1966) *Neurology of the visual system*. C. C. Thomas, Springfield.

Dyck, P. J., Thomas, P. K., Lambert, E. H. and Bunge, R. (eds.) (1984). *Peripheral neuropathy*, 2nd edn. W. B. Saunders, Philadelphia.

Matthews, W. B. (1982). Treatment of Bell's palsy. In *Recent advances in clinical neurology*, vol. 3 (eds. W. B. Matthews and G. H. Glaser), 239. Churchill Livingstone, Edinburgh.

Penman, J. (1968). Trigeminal neuralgia. In *Handbook of clinical neurology* (ed. P. J. Vinken and G. W. Bruyn), vol. 5. North Holland, Amsterdam.

Rushton, J. G. and Olafson, R. A. (1965). Trigeminal neuralgia associated with multiple sclerosis: Report of 35 cases. *Archs Neurol.* **13**, 383–386.

Spillane, J. D. and Wells, C. E. C. (1959). Isolated trigeminal neuropathy: a report of 16 cases. *Brain* **82**, 391–416.

Sumner, D. (1964). Post-traumatic anosmia. *Brain* **87**, 107–120.

—— (1967). Post-traumatic ageusia. *Brain* **90**, 187–202.

THE SPINAL CORD AND ROOTS

Spinal cord disease

W. B. MATTHEWS

The spinal cord is involved in many diffuse conditions, notably multiple sclerosis and motor neurone disease, but may also be the primary or sole site of disease.

Anatomy

The diagnosis and management of lesions of the spinal cord depend to a large degree on knowledge of its functional anatomy. The spinal cord extends from the foramen magnum to the lower border of the first lumbar vertebra, being enclosed by the arachnoid membrane and by the dura mater, both of which extend below the termination of the cord into the sacral canal. The cord is anchored throughout its length by the denticulate ligament on each side, extending from the pia on the surface of the cord to the dura. The blood supply of the spinal cord is complex and consists essentially of a posterior system supplying the posterior columns and posterior grey matter, and an anterior system supplying the remainder, including the descending corticospinal tracts, spinothalamic tracts, and anterior horns of grey matter, separate branches supplying the right and left sides. Both the posterior and anterior spinal arteries receive feeding vessels at many levels and blood flow may be in a rostral or caudal direction at different levels. The most constant contributions to the anterior spinal artery are from the vertebral arteries and the arteria magna of Adamkiewicz that arises from the tenth left intercostal artery, but even these are subject to much variation and radicular arteries may enter the spinal system at any level.

The sensory inflow to the spinal cord through the posterior roots divides into two streams of obvious clinical importance. Fibres concerned mainly with postural sensation and with some aspects of touch, and possibly with vibration, proceed in the posterior column of the same side of the spinal cord to the dorsal column nuclei in the medulla, from which arise the secondary sensory neurones whose axons decussate and pass upwards in the medial lemniscus. Fibres concerned with pain, thermal sensation, and partly with touch, synapse in the posterior horns and the axons of the secondary neurones proceed upwards for a few segments before decussating and passing up in the lateral and anterior columns forming the spinothalamic tracts. In the posterior columns the fibres most laterally placed are those entering the cord in the cervical region, while in the spinothalamic tracts the decussation places these fibres medially. This description is an extreme simplification and takes no account of the many fibres concerned with reflex activity or with carrying the afferent supply to the cerebellum and which do not convey sensations into consciousness.

The main descending motor pathway is the lateral corticospinal or pyramidal tract conveying fibres that have decussated at the lower end of the medulla and which eventually synapse with the anterior horn cells, the lower motor neurones. These cells provide the large-diameter axons to the motor units but the grey matter contains many smaller motor cells supplying the intrafusal muscle fibres that are so important in the regulation of voluntary and reflex activity.

The spinal cord also mediates most important functions concerned with the sphincters and sexual activity. Both ascending pathways conveying sensation from bladder and bowel to consciousness and descending fibres exercising some degree of voluntary initiation and restraint lie in close proximity to the lateral spinothalamic tracts.

Knowledge of the spinal segments concerned in the reflex arcs of the tendon jerks and cutaneous reflexes commonly elicited in clinical practice is of some assistance in the localization of spinal cord lesions. Some individual variation and spread beyond a single segment must be expected, but in general the pattern is as follows:

C_6 Biceps and supinator
C_7 Triceps
L_4 Knee jerk
S_1 Ankle jerk
D_{7-12} Superficial abdominal reflexes
L_2 Cremasteric
S_1 Plantar reflex

A reflex cannot be obtained if the arc is interrupted by disease of the relevant segment of the spinal cord.

The relationship of the spinal cord segments to the vertebral bodies and palpable spinous processes is of practical importance. In the cervical cord, each segment is at the level of the spinous process immediately above; for example, the sixth segment is opposite the fifth spinous process. In the upper thoracic region, the fifth segment is at the level of the third thoracic spinous process, while below this level the interval widens, the first lumbar segment being at the tenth vertebral level. The spinal cord terminates at the lower border of the first lumbar vertebra.

From such anatomical approximations, it is possible to identify the level and extent of spinal cord lesions. Beginning at the lower end, a lesion within the conus medullaris will cause weakness and wasting only of those muscles supplied by the lower sacral segments, mainly the glutei. Sensory loss will involve the buttocks and perineum. The anus will be patulous and the anal reflex, the contraction of the sphincter normally induced by pricking the neighbouring skin, will be absent. There is no sensation of fullness of the bladder or desire to empty the rectum, and reflex emptying is also impaired, resulting in a large atonic bladder with overflow incontinence. Sexual function in the male is lost.

A complete transverse lesion of the dorsal cord results in spastic paralysis and loss of all forms of sensation below the level of the segment involved. With partial lesions both motor and sensory deficits will be incomplete and, in particular, it is often possible to detect that the major impact is on one-half of the cord, producing some elements of the *Brown-Séquard syndrome*. The fully developed effects of hemisection of the spinal cord are, of course, seldom seen, and in practice the syndrome encountered is that of spastic weakness of the leg on the side of the lesion, with some impairment of postural sense, and blunting of pain and thermal sensation on the opposite side, due to damage to the spinothalamic tract containing crossed fibres, while light touch is little disturbed. It is important to realize that a unilateral level below which some modes of sensation are lost provides no accurate indication of the level at which the cord is damaged. A motor level can sometimes be established in the mid-dorsal region, for if the lower abdominal muscles are paralysed, the normal muscles of the upper abdomen will pull the umbilicus upwards when an attempt is made to raise the shoulders from the bed. This test is of most use, however, in the distinction of organic from hysterical paraplegia. The superficial abdominal reflexes may be lost below the level of an obvious lesion, but are too inconstant to be of much diagnostic use.

In the cervical cord the clinical picture is further complicated by involvement of the upper limbs. A lesion involving the lower part of the cervical enlargement will cause wasting of the hand muscles, while a discrete lesion at the sixth cervical segment will result in lower motor neurone paralysis of flexion at the elbow and abolition of the flexor tendon reflexes, the biceps and supinator jerks, with spastic paralysis and increased reflexes, including the triceps jerks, below this level. It is often found that striking the biceps tendon, while not resulting in any contraction of that muscle, causes flexion of the fingers, the so-called 'inverted' reflex. This is not due to any aberrant reflex arc within the cord, but simply to the minute stretch imparted to the finger flexor muscles by the movement of the arm, indicating heightened reflex activity. A similar phenomenon accounts for crossed reflexes sometimes encountered in the lower limbs, when, for example, adduction of both thighs occurs when one patellar tendon is tapped. A complete lesion of the lower cervical cord will cause respiratory embarrassment from paralysis of the muscles of the chest wall and abdomen. A similar lesion above the fourth cervical segment, the main origin of the phrenic nerves, results in respiratory paralysis and is incompatible with life without artificial respiration. A complete lesion of the spinal cord at any level will cause retention of urine with eventual overflow. Incomplete lesions of the spinal cord may result in a small hyperactive bladder with resulting urgency and incontinence.

Not all clinical phenomena are readily explicable in simple anatomical terms. For example, reflex activity often appears to be enchanced *above* the level of a cervical cord lesion, and conversely a lesion at the foramen magnum may be accompanied by wasting of the hand muscles. This latter effect is the result of infarction resulting from obstruction of venous return, and there is no doubt that interference with the somewhat precarious and anatomically inconstant arterial supply is responsible for a number of apparently anomalous clinical features of spinal cord lesions.

Non-traumatic paraplegia

Acute and subacute

The patient with rapidly advancing weakness of the lower limbs presents an urgent problem of diagnosis and management. The presumption is that there is a localized lesion of the spinal cord and it must not be forgotten that in spinal shock the limbs are flaccid, tendon reflexes may be absent, and plantar reflexes unobtainable. Confusion with acute polyneuritis, the Guillain-Barré syndrome (page 21.126), is possible and the distinction is not always immediately obvious. A sensory level on the trunk must be carefully sought as, if present, it is strong evidence of a spinal cord lesion.

The further distinction must then be made, as quickly as possible, between spinal cord compression, perhaps demanding surgical relief, and an intrinsic lesion of the cord requiring quite different management. Pain and tenderness over the spinal column or pain of obviously root distribution are of little diagnostic value and certainly occur with many non-compressive lesions. Retention of urine is usual and may even distract attention from the weakness of the legs.

Intrinsic lesions

Acute paraplegia may occur in multiple sclerosis, even as the first attack, but there are often preceding relevant events or more diffuse signs. Minor or dubious abnormalities – temporal pallor of the optic discs, nystagmus at the extremes of gaze or paraesthesiae in the hands, for example, must not be accepted as evidence of multiple lesions.

Myelitis may follow infections or inoculations or occur for no detectable reason. It is an occasional complication of systemic disease, including Behcet's disease and systemic lupus erythematosus. Syphilitic myelitis is now a rarity. Acute necrosis of the spinal cord may be a remote effect of carcinoma.

The spinal arteries are not subject to atheroma and, apart from their occasional involvement in polyarteritis nodosa or sarcoidosis, vascular disease affecting the spinal cord has more remote origins. Infarction may result from atheroma of the aorta, dissecting aortic aneurysm or severe hypotensive shock. The infarcted territory is often that of the anterior spinal artery, with preservation of the posterior columns. Emboli may cause infarction of the cord in bacterial endocarditis. Spontaneous haemorrhage within the spinal cord is very rare but may occur in systemic lupus. Spinal subarachnoid haemorrhage from rupture of an arterio-venous malformation may cause acute paraplegia.

Spinal cord compression

Causes of spinal cord compression are conventionally divided into extradural, intradural but extramedullary, and intramedullary categories. These distinctions are indeed important in management and prognosis but less so in the diagnosis of the cause of acute paraplegia.

Such causes may have been present for a long time before the rapid onset of symptoms is precipitated by a fall or other minor trauma. A benign tumour, a neurofibroma or meningioma, for example, may cause acute symptoms in this way and patients with a narrowed cervical canal from spondylosis, but without neurological symptoms, are vulnerable to minor injuries causing neck extension. The man who falls when drunk and is unable to rise again, though fully conscious, has probably injured his cervical spinal cord (see page 21.103). In rheumatoid arthritis spontaneous dislocation of the cervical vertebrae may cause acute spinal cord damage.

Patients with coagulation dcfccts, either from disease or iatrogenic, are at risk to spontaneous epidural haemorrhage and paraplegia.

Unfortunately most tumours causing acute or subacute paraplegia are malignant, usually metastatic vertebral deposits or invasion of the meninges by carcinoma, leukaemia or reticulosis. Staphylococcal epidural abscess may closely mimic a malignant lesion. Acute paraplegia is now uncommon in spinal tuberculosis.

Management

Urinary retention must be relieved. The level of the lesion should be determined by clinical means, and this may present no difficulty as there is often a sharp sensory level. A unilateral level is not clearly localizing except as indicating the lowest possible site of the lesion. A common error is to fail to test the sacral dermatomes in patients with urinary retention. As the vertebral column is longer than the spinal cord the vertebral level will be two or three segments higher than the neurological level in the thoracic region and the conus medullaris is opposite the body of the first lumbar vertebra.

The principles of spinal localization are as described for chronic progressive paraparesis (page 21.99), with the exception that in acute lesions there is no focal wasting.

The examination must naturally include a search for possible sources of metastatic lesions or infection.

The spine must be X-rayed at the appropriate level, and a chest film and blood count obtained. These investigations may reveal metastatic disease with or without a collapsed vertebra. Benign tumours and vertebral infection may also show radiological changes.

If there is any suspicion that the spinal cord is compressed a lumbar puncture with a view to examining the CSF must *not* be done. A moderate increase in cells and total protein may be found in many conditions, from multiple sclerosis to epidural abscess, and is of no immediate diagnostic help. A greatly raised protein will suggest compression but lumbar puncture has no part to play in this diagnosis. Queckenstedt's test in which failure of the CSF pressure to rise on jugular compression indicates spinal block, has been abandoned because of frequent false negative results. If compression is present lumbar puncture may precipitate severe aggravation.

If bone changes identify the level of the lesion CT scanning is probably the best subsequent investigation. If there are no bone changes and no fever or other evidence to suggest an abscess a myelogram should be done despite the risk of causing clinical deterioration. CT scanning alone, even if the clinical level is precise, cannot exclude spinal cord compression, but will demonstrate an epidural abscess. If there is a coagulation defect this must be corrected before the myelogram as the lumbar puncture may cause further haemorrhage.

The treatment of the causes of acute non-traumatic paraplegia is described under the relevant diseases. Most surgeons aim now to avoid laminectomy in maligant disease although other surgical approaches may be less hazardous. A biopsy may be needed to identify tumours that may be hormone sensitive. If the patient is still ambulant, steroids and radiotherapy may induce substantial relief.

Chronic progressive paraparesis

Here again the most important distinction is between spinal cord compression and intrinsic lesions. Among the latter the progressive spinal form of multiple sclerosis is the commonest cause, but motor neurone disease can present with spastic weakness of the lower limbs. Hereditary spastic paraplegia is an occasional cause. The distinctive features of subacute combined degeneration (page 21.101) and syringomyelia (page 21.100) should prevent diagnostic confusion.

A spinal arteriovenous malformation may cause paraparesis with a fluctuating or stepwise course, easily confused with multiple sclerosis. Intramedullary spinal cord tumours are rare. Diagnosis is often difficult because of the elongated cyst that may form with an ependymoma, resulting in unusual physical signs.

Chronic spinal cord compression is commonly due to benign causes – cervical spondylotic myelopathy, prolapsed dorsal disc, neurofibroma, meningioma or Paget's disease of the bone. Malignant causes include myeloma, chordoma, and intrinsic gliomata.

Clinical features of cord compression

Sensory symptomas usually precede weakness and may be misinterpreted. Root pain is easily recognizable in the cervical region, but when thoracic roots are involved visceral pain may be mimicked. The characteristic pain on movement or coughing may be thought to arise in the chest. Compression of the sensory pathways may cause paraesthesiae or pain in the lower limbs. Cutaneous sensory loss due to involvement of the spinothalamic tract may show 'sacral sparing' as lamination of fibres in the tract allows those from lower sacral segments to escape. This sign is not, however, diagnostic of cord compression.

Motor involvement is usually asymmetrical and, with a cervical cord lesion, classically affects the arm on the side of the lesion, then the ipsilateral leg, the other leg, and eventually the contralateral arm. The degree of sphincter involvement is highly variable.

The diagnosis of the level of the responsible lesion must often be approximate. Lesions may involve several segments asymmetrically and, in life, physical signs do not always accord with the conventional diagrams. This is well exemplified by the wasting of the intrinsic hand muscles often seen with lesions in the region of the foramen magnum.

At all levels below the lumbar enlargement there will be weakness and hyperreflexia below the level of the lesion. With cervical cord lesions, particularly at C4 and above, there is risk of respiratory paralysis. Intrinsic lesions at this level may cause a Horner's syndrome. Sensory levels are shown in Fig. 1 on pages 21.110 and 21.111. A unilateral sensory level is usually several segments lower than the lesion. In early or partial lesions signs may be slight and syndromes incomplete. Lesions at any level may cause urinary incontinence or retention.

Particular features at certain levels may be emphasized.

C2   The root distribution of sensory loss is on the back of the scalp. Hand muscles may be wasted.

C5–6   Weakness and wasting of deltoid, elbow flexors, and spinati. Loss or inversion of biceps and supinator reflexes.

C7   Triceps muscle, and extensors of wrist and fingers involved.

C8   Hand muscles wasted.

T1   Hand muscles wasted. Horner's syndrome.

T10   Upper abdominal muscles spared so that the umbilicus moves upwards on attempting to sit up.

Lumbar enlargement

More rostral lesions cause weakness of hip flexion and knee extension. The knee jerk is absent if L3/4 segment is involved, with preservation of the ankle jerk. More distal lesions cause loss of the ankle jerks, wasting of the glutei and distal leg muscles.

Lower sacral segments

Painless bladder distension occurs with lesions of the sacral segments and cauda equina, sometimes without obvious motor involvement. Sensory loss involves the saddle area. Anal and bulbo-cavernosus reflexes are lost.

Management

If multiple sclerosis is suspected abnormal visual evoked potentials may obviate the need for invasive radiology. Plain radiographs should not be neglected, including oblique views of the cervical spine when relevant.

The relative values of myelography, CT scanning, NMR or combined techniques are discussed on page 21.8 *et seq.* Any CSF obtained should be sent for analysis, including examination for IgG banding, characteristically present in multiple sclerosis.

Cervical myelopathy

Spondylosis and cord lesions due to disc prolapse are considered on pages 21.109 to 21.115.

Spinal cord tumours

In contrast to the brain, the majority of tumours involving the spinal cord are extrinsic, and many are benign. The neurofibroma arises from the Schwann cells of the spinal roots at any level. It may be part of generalized neurofibromatosis but is usually single. Because of its site of origin, pain of root distribution is a common early symptom and in the thoracic region in particular this may give rise to diagnostic confusion with visceral disease. The effects of spinal cord compression often progress very slowly, but may be exacerbated by minor trauma. The cerebrospinal fluid protein is greatly increased except in cervical lesions where it may be normal, and myelography shows distinctive changes. The results of surgical removal, even when spinal cord damage appears to be severe, are remarkably successful and complete recovery is often achieved. The spinal meningioma arising from the dura cannot with certainty be distinguished on clinical or radiological grounds from a neurofibroma, and the results of removal are equally good.

The common malignant tumour compressing the spinal cord is secondary carcinoma, either involving the vertebrae or forming a dense band of meningeal infiltration.

Precise diagnosis may be important as with hormone-responsive or radiosensitive tumours good results may be obtained by prompt treatment. The results of surgical decompression of, for example, a spinal secondary from lung cancer are, however, uniformly bad.

Paraplegia is often rapid with much local pain.

In young patients, Hodgkin's disease may present in the same way. A *chordoma*, a malignant tumour, arising from remnants of the notochord, may arise in the sacral area, causing compression of the cauda equina, or more rarely, in the cervical region.

Intrinsic tumours of the spinal cord are usually malignant but seldom expand rapidly. The most common forms are the *astrocytoma* and the technically benign *ependymoma*, both of which cause progressive paraplegia. The latter may be associated with a cyst within the spinal cord that may extend over many segments, resulting in sensory loss resembling that of syringomyelia. If the tumour is confined to a small nodule within the cyst surgery may be successful.

An ependymoma of the filum terminale which may be accessible to surgery, causes a cauda equina syndrome with early sphincter involvement and sensory loss over the perineum, but may also most confusingly cause papilloedema, attributed unconvincingly to the high cerebrospinal fluid protein content. Intrinsic tumours are difficult to diagnose even with myelography or direct inspection at operation, particularly as biopsy of the spinal cord is not to be recommended. Radiotherapy from evidence that might in other sites be regarded as inadequate is often followed by prolonged remission that may cast doubt on the original diagnosis. Multiple sclerosis can also cause swelling of the spinal cord visible on myelography.

Arteriovenous malformations

At the time of diagnosis these important lesions appear to consist of a tangled mass of hypertrophied veins containing arterial blood, nearly always situated on the dorsal surface of the spinal cord beneath the arachnoid. This appearance results from the presence of one or more arteriovenous shunts, presumably congenital in origin.

The clinical presentation is varied. A spinal subarachnoid haemorrhage causes sudden severe pain in the back – the coup de poignard – followed by signs of neck rigidity and even by loss of consciousness. The spinal origin may be shown by evidence of damage to the cord, but this is not invariable.

More commonly the onset is with weakness of the legs, with varying degrees of sensory loss and sphincter disturbance. A focal spinal cord lesion may not be suspected, however, because of the tendency of the symptons to fluctuate leading to confusion with multiple sclerosis. Relapse during pregnancy in particular may be followed by complete recovery. A cutaneous angiomatous lesion is sometimes an important clue and occasionally a pulsatile bruit may be heard over the lesion. The thoracic region is most commonly involved but the lesion may be very extensive and involve the whole length of the spinal cord.

Even if the diagnosis is suspected confirmation may prove difficult as on myelography it is not easy to interpret the significance of possibly dilated blood vessels. CT scanning may be helpful but angiography via the intercostal vessels is the most reliable method. If an arteriovenous malformation is present and treatment is contemplated, angiography is essential, as modern treatment involves the excision or embolization of the shunts that can only be identified in this way.

The mechanism of the production of symptoms is not fully understood. Some element of cord compression may be present but it is also likely that blood is diverted or 'stolen' from the cord by the shunt. Unfortunately treatment is not always followed by improvement of existing symptoms, no doubt because of infarction of the cord, but further deterioration and the risk of haemorrhage may be avoided.

Spinal arachnoiditis

Chronic arachnoiditis of the spinal cord may occur many years after acute meningitis or may accompany ankylosing spondylitis. Myelography, even with modern contrast media, can cause arachnoiditis and other identifiable causes are intrathecal steroids, spinal anaesthesia, and subarachnoid haemorrhage. Usually no cause can be found. The presentation is again that of slowly progressive spastic paraparesis without a clear sensory level. Myelography, essential for diagnosis, shows partial obstruction to the flow of the dye at many levels. Neither surgical treatment nor steroids locally or systemically have proved effective. Spinal arachnoiditis is sometimes a cause of syringomyelia.

Pott's paraplegia (see page 21.105 and Section 5)

In areas of the world where tuberculosis is now relatively uncommon, spinal cord compression resulting from a cold abscess of the vertebral column is seldom seen, but where tuberculosis is rife,

this is still a common cause of paraplegia. Systemic symptoms of chronic infection are usually present and the distinctive bone lesion can be seen on radiographs of the spine. Treatment, apart from the essential antituberculous drugs, is largely a matter for the orthopaedic surgeon. Paraparesis may sometimes occur as a late result of spinal tuberculosis, apparently due to the severe angular deformity of the vertebral column.

Epidural abscess

An acute abscess in the epidural space is usually the result of staphylococcal infection, either metastatic or more rarely by spread from some contiguous site of sepsis. The clinical picture is that of rapidly advancing paraplegia and local tenderness at the site of the abscess; signs of constitutional illness and an inflammatory reaction in the cerebrospinal fluid are to be expected, but are not always present. This renders the distinction from other causes of acute or subacute paraplegia impossible on clinical grounds alone, and the possibility that an abscess may be the cause is an imperative indication for myelography or preferably computerized tomographic scanning if the level can be identified. Following evacuation of the abscess and intensive antibiotic therapy, complete recovery may occur, but the prognosis is unfortunately not always so good, even with prompt diagnosis and treatment, and permanent cord damage may result.

Epidural haemorrhage

Haemorrhage into the epidural space is rare and is usually a complication of anticoagulant therapy. The cervical spine is the usual site and haemorrhage should be suspected as the cause of rapidly progressive quadriplegia in a patient on anticoagulants. Recovery following evacuation of the haemorrhage is usually complete.

Myelitis (see also page 21.105)

A diagnosis of myelitis is often made, without any clear idea of the underlying pathology, in the context of acute or sub-acute paraplegia, demonstrably not due to any cause of spinal cord compression. An acute transverse spinal cord lesion may occur as an isolated event in post-infective encephalomyelitis, and in multiple sclerosis, but in other patients with an identical clinical course, no evidence of either condition is found, even on prolonged observation. An acute transverse cord lesion may occur in systemic lupus, polyarteritis nodosa and Behçet's disease. In some patients the lesion appears to be based on a pre-existing vascular anomaly, leading to venous thrombosis and infarction, and here the lesion may not be transverse, in the sense of involving one or two segments only, but may result in necrosis of the spinal cord below an upper level—sub-acute necrotizing myelitis. The paraplegia remains flaccid, as reflex activity cannot return. It is also probable that thrombophlebitis in the pelvis may lead to spreading venous occlusion and spinal cord damage.

It is naturally extremely important not to overlook some cause of spinal cord compression, but in the great majority of patients with acute paraplegia the myelogram will be normal and no cause for the disastrous illness will be found. It is also natural to give a course of corticotrophin in the hope of influencing the pathological process, but except in demyelinating disease, the prognosis for recovery is poor and many patients are left with severe or total paraplegia.

Syringomyelia

Syringomyelia, for long regarded as due to some ill-defined degeneration of the spinal cord, has recently been the subject of considerable advances in knowledge. The essential lesion implied by the name is a cavity within the spinal cord. Such a cavity may form a part of a cystic tumour, in particular an ependymoma, but the term syringomyelia has been restricted to non-tumorous conditions, until recently without adequate explanation.

Pathology

The pathology, insofar as it affects the spinal cord, comprises an irregular asymmetrical fluid-filled cavity extending over many segments of the cord, or even its entire length. This cavity, at least when examined after death in a necessarily advanced stage of the disease, is not the vestigial central canal of the spinal cord abnormally dilated. The cavity is usually most extensive in the cervical enlargement. Contiguous structures are destroyed, in particular the anterior horn cells, the sensory fibres decussating within the spinal cord and concerned with pain and thermal sensation, and the lateral corticospinal tracts. Sometimes the syrinx extends into the medulla where the nuclei of the lower cranial nerves may be involved.

Clinical features and course

There is a wide range of age of onset of symptoms but this is most common in early adult life. Symptoms usually develop in one upper limb, with a combination of wasting, particularly of the hand muscles, weakness, and loss of sensation, often resulting in painless burns, either from cigarettes or from cooking. Examination at this early stage will show wasting more extensive than could be accounted for by any single peripheral nerve lesion, accompanied by loss of tendon jerks in the arm, even when proximal muscles do not appear to be otherwise involved. Sensory loss, classically of 'dissociated' type with preservation of light touch and of proprioception, but loss of pain and thermal sensation, extends over the whole arm and upper thorax, or may be bilateral over the whole 'cape' area, even when symptoms are only present on one side. Scars of painless burns and cuts may provide a diagnostic clue in unsuspected cases. A Horner's syndrome, or more commonly, unilateral hyperidrosis on the face, may indicate involvement of the cervical sympathetic. A dorsal scoliosis, usually of mild degree, is almost invariable.

There are many deviations from this classical mode of onset. Pain in the arm can be severe and of the peculiarly unpleasant character associated with 'irritative' lesions of the spinothalamic tract. The pyramidal tracts may be involved at an early stage, resulting in spastic weakness of the legs, but some abnormal signs will be present in the arms. The formerly popular diagnosis of lumbar syringomyelia, with symptoms supposedly originating from a syrinx in the lower cord, has now been shown to be erroneous, such cases being examples of chronic sensory neuropathy. Although the onset of symptoms of syringomyelia is usually insidious, sudden exacerbations are common, particularly after exertion, coughing, or sneezing.

Although in some fortunate patients the symptons and signs remain unchanged for many years, syringomyelia is usually progressive. Wasting spreads in the upper limbs and sensory loss becomes increasingly dense, involving all modalities and extending to the trunk and legs, but retains some elements of a suspended distribution in that normal sensation is present in segments below and often above the areas of analgesia. One or both hands may become swollen and painless trophic ulcers may destroy the digits. Charcot's painless destructive arthropathy is not uncommon in the shoulder joints.

Involvement of the medulla, syringobulbia, may occur from the onset without evidence of spinal cord involvement or, more commonly, as an extension of syringomyelia. The extension of sensory loss on to the face does not imply a medullary lesion as the sensory nucleus of the trigeminal nerve extends into the cervical spinal cord. The usual pattern of sensory loss does not follow the distribution of the branches of the trigeminal nerve, but involves the more peripheral areas of the face with sparing of the nose and mouth ('Balaclava helmet' distribution). Syringobulbia involves the nuclei of the tenth, eleventh, and twelfth cranial nerves, usually asymmetrically, causing wasting of the tongue, dysphagia, vocal cord paralysis, and weakness of the sternomastoids and trapezius muscles. Rotatory nystagmus, no doubt due to destruction of cerebellar connections, is a common finding.

Diagnosis

In the early stages syringomyelia must be distinguished from the many other causes of wasting of the hand muscles and, while this may be a difficult matter, the pattern of sensory loss and of absent tendon jerks is usually distinctive. An intrinsic tumour of the spinal cord, particularly when resulting in a long cyst, will produce an indistinguishable clinical syndrome, except that the presence of scoliosis is more suggestive of syringomyelia.

A diagnosis of syringomyelia is, however, no longer adequate. It is now claimed that in the great majority of cases the cause lies in some interference with the normal flow of cerebrospinal fluid. The manner in which this results in an expanding destructive syrinx is still to some extent controversial. A factor common to most cases is partial obstruction of the outflow of cerebrospinal fluid from the foramina in the roof of the fourth ventricle. The commonest cause is the congenital abnormality known as the Chiari or Arnold-Chiari malformation, in which aberrant cerebellar tissue extends through the foramen magnum into the cervical spinal canal. To some extent this impedes the flow of cerebrospinal fluid into the spinal arachnoid but the fourth ventricle foramina are also partially obstructed. A probable course of events in the production of syringomyelia is that cerebrospinal fluid distends the central canal of the spinal cord and eventually ruptures into the substance of the cord. This may occur suddenly as the result of a rapid rise in venous pressure, and accounts for the immediate exacerbations that may follow sneezing. Other causes are more rarely encountered. Arachnoiditis following meningitis or without known cause can result in syringomyelia, and the clinical picture of this condition may accompany primary basilar impression or platybasia (see page 21.197) although a syrinx may not be present. The fluid that fills the syrinx in all these conditions is cerebrospinal fluid of normal constitution, in communication with the ventricular and subarachnoid cerebrospinal fluid—communicating syringomyelia. Less is known about the forms of syrinx, apart from those associated with spinal tumour, that do not communicate with the cerebrospinal fluid. The syrinx that sometimes develops from the site of spinal cord injury may fall into this category.

The practical importance of this new knowledge is that it leads to at least partially successful treatment. This must be based on accurate anatomical diagnosis. X-rays of the cervical spine may show an increase in the diameter of the spinal canal in either plane but this is not essential for diagnosis. The Chiari malformation can be demonstrated by myelography with opaque dye or air which shows the cerebellar extension through the foramen magnum. Arachnoiditis breaks up the column of dye and causes partial obstruction to its flow at many levels. In a small proportion of patients with the clinical picture of syringomyelia, the myelogram shows no abnormality.

Treatment

If the Chiari malformation is present, surgical treatment directed to the decompression of the foramen magnum and allowing free flow of cerebrospinal fluid from the fourth ventricle is indicated unless symptoms are mild and non-progressive, or alternatively, the patient has been so severely incapacitated for many years that irreversible damage must be assumed. The results of such treatment are unpredictable, but significant improvement in both sensory and motor symptoms and signs may occur, and, in particular, pain may be immediately relieved. In other patients the disease appears to be arrested, but even this degree of success cannot be counted on. Operative treatment for arachnoiditis is not possible.

Sub-acute combined degeneration of the spinal cord (see also Section 19)

Definition

Degeneration of the lateral and posterior columns of the spinal cord due to deficiency of vitamin B$_{12}$.

Aetiology

Sub-acute combined degeneration is the commonest and most serious neurological complication of the deficiency of vitamin B_{12} which also results in Addisonian pernicious anaemia. The existence of spinal cord lesions, as opposed to those confined to the peripheral nerves, in other causes of B_{12} deficiency is problematical.

Pathology

The name is derived from the combined degeneration observed in the lateral and posterior columns of the spinal cord. Demyelination is marked and appears to precede loss of axons. This is of some practical importance with regard to recovery of function if the deficiency is corrected before the disease has become too advanced. The pathological process probably always also involves the peripheral nerves. Small areas of necrosis in the spinal cord and brain have also been described.

Clinical features

The patients are in the age range of pernicious anaemia, that is to say, predominantly middle aged or older. The initial symptom is always symmetrical paraesthesiae of the feet or very occasionally of the hands. The sensations experienced vary from mild tingling to severe burning. Increasing difficulty in walking soon develops due to a combination of weakness and loss of postural sense.

The sensory symptoms also involve the upper limbs but cause little or no disability. Examination at this stage shows variable combinations of the signs of peripheral nerve and spinal cord involvement. Weakness is accompanied by extensor plantar reflexes. The tendon reflexes may be increased, but it is more usual for the ankle jerks to be absent. Loss of postural sense is often severe and there is distal cutaneous sensory blunting. The signs are almost invariably symmetrical.

If the disease is unrecognized and untreated it progresses, so that within a few weeks of the onset the patient is unable to walk. Before treatment was available, severe paraplegia proved fatal within a year in nearly all patients.

More widespread signs of vitamin B_{12} deficiency may be present, in particular a mild dementia. Sometimes this is indeed the presenting or only feature, but accounts for a disappointingly small proportion of demented patients.

The optic nerves may also be involved, again usually as an isolated symptom. Visual loss results from a scotoma extending from the fixation point to the blind spot. The condition greatly resembles tobacco amblyopia induced by pipe-smoking and may be due to the lack of the detoxifying effect of vitamin B_{12} on cyanide derived from tobacco smoke.

Clinical evidence of anaemia may be obvious or entirely lacking. The peripheral blood may be normal and the bone marrow does not always show a megaloblastic reaction. Achlorhydria is present. If suspected, the diagnosis can readily be confirmed by the low level of vitamin B_{12} in the blood. The serum vitamin B_{12} level is commonly lower in sub-acute combined degeneration of the spinal cord than in uncomplicated pernicious anaemia. In one series the mean figures for the first were 30 ng/l and the second 75 ng/l: the normal range being 160–925 ng/l. If vitamin B_{12} injections have been given it may be necessary to carry out tests of vitamin B_{12} absorption. The differential diagnosis includes peripheral neuropathy from other causes, tabes dorsalis, spinal cord tumours, and, in younger patients, multiple sclerosis. A more common error, however, is simply to regard the paraesthesiae and stumbling gait as the inevitable consequences of advancing age.

Treatment

As soon as the diagnosis is established treatment must be urgent and energetic: hydroxocobalamine 1 mg should be injected immediately and repeated twice daily for a week and thereafter at weekly intervals for several weeks before going on to a monthly schedule. This is almost certainly enormously more than is needed but the neurological complications require higher doses than those necessary to restore the blood picture, and it is vital that the damage to the spinal cord be reversed as quickly as possible. The results of treatment are in general excellent. Even if the patient is bedridden, normal walking can be restored and extensor plantar reflexes become flexor. Beyond a certain point of disability, however, treatment is unavailing, presumably because of axonal loss, but this is now quite exceptional. The sensory symptoms are usually extremely persistent and a patient rescued from severe disability will continue to complain bitterly of the paraesthesiae. Mental symptoms also respond excellently but restoration of normal vision in B_{12} deficiency amblyopia is less predictable.

Vascular disease

The small arteries that supply the spinal cord are not involved in atherosclerosis and only rarely in any form of arteritis, and ischaemic disease, therefore, results from more remote causes. *Infarction of the spinal cord* may result from atheroma of the aorta, dissecting aneurysm of the aorta, aortic, thoracic or spinal surgery, and severe hypotension from such causes as cardiac infarction or arrest, and occasionally from embolism arising from endocarditis. The clinical syndrome is usually that of a lesion in the distribution of the anterior spinal artery, more commonly affecting both sides of the spinal cord. Acute pain at the level of the lesion often occurs at the onset. Paraplegia develops within minutes or even instantaneously, and characteristically the sensory loss is confined to those modalities conveyed in the spinothalamic tract, pain and thermal sensibility, with sparing of postural sense. The signs naturally vary with the site of the lesion, usually mid-dorsal or lower cervical. Occasionally the entire cord may be infarcted below an upper segmental level. Recovery from incomplete lesions is often remarkably good, but it is in such cases that opportunity to confirm the diagnosis does not arise. Other patients may have severe residual disability. Transient ischaemic attacks of the spinal cord, resulting in paraplegia for an hour or less, with complete recovery, may occur in arteriopathic patients.

The existence of chronic progressive *ischaemic myelopathy* due solely to arterial disease is much more difficult to establish. Patients in whom this may be suspected are elderly, with advanced atherosclerosis of the abdominal aorta and slowly progressive weakness and wasting of the lower limbs with extensor plantar reflexes and variable incomplete sensory loss.

Haemorrhage within the spinal cord is rare. It may occur with rupture of an arteriovenous malformation, as the result of trauma, disturbances of clotting mechanisms, or for no detectable reason. *Haematomyelia* is usually abrupt in onset but, particularly in patients in whom no trauma or other cause can be incriminated, there may be an ingravescent course. The symptomatology does not differ significantly from that of other acute or sub-acute spinal cord lesions, except that the central site and elongated shape of the haemorrhage may be indicated by the dissociated sensory loss of the type seen in syringomyelia, extending over many segments.

Much less is known about disease of the spinal venous system. *Thrombophlebitis* is thought to be the cause of the rapidly progressive paraplegia that occurs in sub-acute necrotic myelitis. It is possible that this originates from infection, either pelvic or in the lower limbs, but this is not always evident. The spinal cord lesion is usually not complete. Clinically the condition is difficult to distinguish from acute demyelination of the spinal cord or other causes of myelitis. The cerebrospinal fluid is abnormal, containing an increased level of protein, and often a slight pleocytosis. The prognosis is poor and the condition may spread up the spinal cord in successive episodes. Obstruction of flow in the veins of the spinal cord may play an important part in the production of symptoms from compressive lesions. There is experimental evidence that the otherwise inexplicable signs of involvement of the lower cervical cord seen in lesions at the cisterna magna are due to venous obstruction and infarction of the grey matter at a distance from the lesion.

Radiation myelopathy

The spinal cord is vulnerable to damage from X-irradiation directed to structures in the neck. The incidence is low and is clearly dose-related. The commonest form is benign and consists of mainly sensory symptoms in the limbs, often accompanied by Lhermitte's sign of an electric shock sensation down the spine on flexing the neck. These symptoms develop during or immediately following treatment and remit completely after a few weeks. Much more serious is delayed myelopathy developing from six months to five years after exposure. Initial sensory symptoms herald a progressive transverse cord lesion with resulting severe disability. The cord may be swollen and infarcted. The prolonged latent period has not been adequately explained.

References

Baker, A. S., Ojemann, R. G., Swartz, M. N. and Richardson, E. P. (1975). Spinal epidural abscess. *N. Engl. J. Med.* **293**, 464–468.

Barnett, H. J. M., Foster, J. B. and Hudgson, P. (1973). *Syringomyelia*. W. B. Saunders, London.

British Medical Journal (1978). Cauda equina tumours. **1**, 808.

Esses, S. I. and Morley, T. P. (1983). Spinal arachnoiditis. *Can. J. Neurol. Sci.* **10**, 2–10.

Findlay, G. F. G. (1984). Adverse effects of the management of malignant spinal cord compression. *J. Neurol. Neurosurg. Psychiat.* **47**, 761–768.

Garland, H., Greenberg, J. and Harriman, D. G. F. (1966). Infarction of the spinal cord. *Brain* **89**, 645–662.

Godwin-Austen, R. B., Howell, D. A. and Worthington, B. (1975). Observations on radiation myelopathy. *Brain* **98**, 557–568.

Henson, R. A. and Parsons, M. (1967). Ischaemic lesions of the spinal cord: an illustrated review. *Q. J. Med.* **36**, 205–222.

Hughes, J. T. (1978). *Pathology of the spinal cord*, 2nd edn. Blackwell, Oxford.

Leys, D., Lesoin, F., Viaud, C., Pasquier, F., Rousseaux, M., Jomin, M. and Petit, H. (1984). Decreased morbidity from acute bacterial epidural abscesses using computed tomography and nonsurgical treatment in selected patients. *Ann. Neurol.* **17**, 350–355.

Lipton, H. L. and Teasdale, R. D. (1973). Acute transverse myelopathy in adults. *Arch. Neurol.* **28**, 252–257.

Logue, V. (1979). Angiomas of the spinal cord: review of the pathogenesis, clinical features and results of surgery. *J. Neurol. Neurosurg. Psychiat.* **42**, 1–11.

Martin, N. S. (1971). Pott's paraplegia. *J. Bone Joint Surg.* **53B**, 596–608.

Northfield, D. W. C. (1973). *The surgery of the central nervous system*, Chaps 21 and 22. Blackwell, Oxford.

Palmer, J. J. (1972). Radiation myelopathy. *Brain* **95**, 109–122.

Paty, D. W., Blume, W. T., Brown, W. F., Jaatoul, N., Kertesz, A. and McInnis, W. (1979). Chronic progressive myelopathy: investigation with CSF electrophoresis, evoked potentials and CT scan. *Ann. Neurol.* **6**, 419–424.

Russell, J. S. R., Batten, F. E. and Collier, J. (1900). Subacute combined degeneration of the spinal cord. *Brain* **23**, 39–110.

Ungar-Sargon, J. Y., Lovelace, R. E. and Brust, J. C. M. (1980). Spastic paraparesis: a reappraisal. *J. Neurol. Sci.* **46**, 1–12.

Wilkinson, M. (1971). *Cervical spondylosis: its early diagnosis and treatment*. Heinemann, London.

Williams, B. (1980). On the pathogenesis of syringomyelia: a review. *J. R. Soc. Med.* **73**, 798–806.

Injury of the spinal cord and the management of paraplegia

J. R. SILVER AND S. WILLIAMS

Introduction

Traumatic injuries of the spinal cord have been recognized since ancient times. Until quite recently they usually resulted in death from the effects of pressure sores and urinary tract infection (Fig. 1). The situation remained unchanged until the Second World War when specialist units were set up throughout the United Kingdom to deal with injured servicemen. The coincidental development of blood transfusion and antibiotic therapy, and the prevention and management of pressure sores, combined with a better understanding and management of the urinary tract has led to a much improved life expectancy for these paralysed patients. There are now approximately 350 new traumatic spinal injury patients per year in the United Kingdom, mainly as the result of road traffic accidents. There are many thousands of chronic paraplegic patients.

Patients with acute spinal injuries are initially admitted under the care of the accident department or the neurosurgeon and the successful outcome of their management is based on the treatment of any life-threatening associated injuries, the establishment of the correct diagnosis, the exclusion of any remediable surgical conditions of the cord or spinal column, and the transfer of the patient to a specialist centre without undue delay.

Although the management of paraplegia has become highly specialized, there are several reasons why any clinician should have some knowledge of this increasingly important topic.

First, serious neurological damage may be done by mishandling the patient immediately after an injury. Second, the spinal injury may be misdiagnosed; the patient may be thought to be suffering from hysteria, the effects of drink or drugs, hypothermia, or head injury, for example. Third, correct diagnosis may be made and the patient admitted initially to an intensive care unit where the physician will be responsible for resuscitation and ventilation; important medical complications may be encountered at this stage

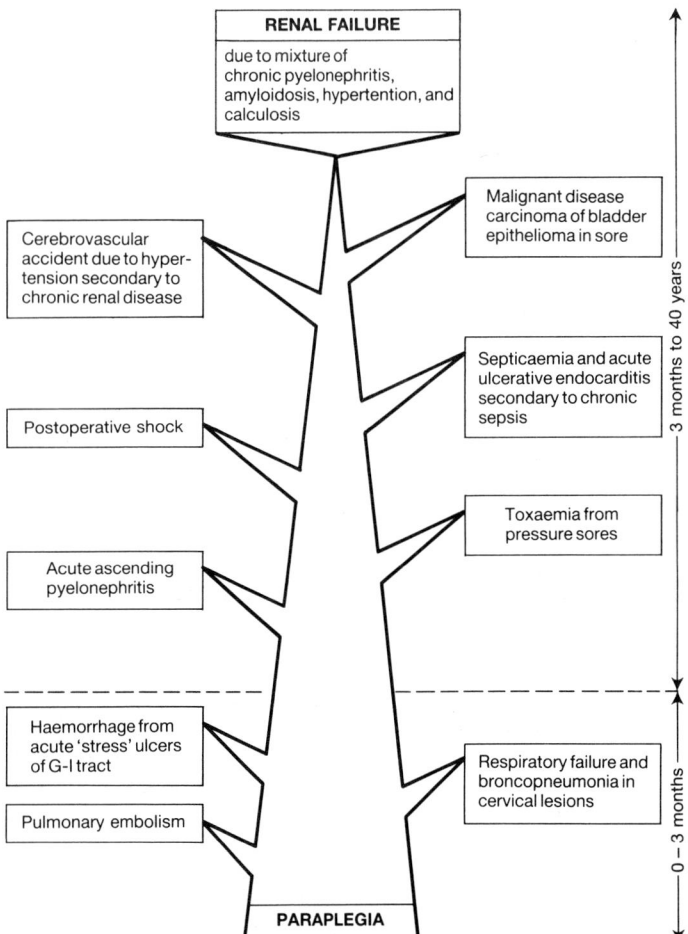

Fig. 1 Causes of death in paraplegia. (Reproduced with permission from Tribe and Silver, 1969, *Renal failure in paraplegia*, Fig. 2.2.)

including pressure sores, urinary tract infections and renal failure. Finally, the principles of the management of spinal injuries can be applied to any disorder in which there is damage to the spinal cord.

The immediate management of suspected spinal injury

Spinal injuries seldom happen in isolation; three-quarters of them are associated with damage to other organs, particularly head injuries, which may mask the injury to the spine. In patients with head injuries the possibility of a fractured cervical spine should always be borne in mind and particular care should be taken when moving the head. Similarly, if a patient presents with a stove-in chest an injury to the thoracic spine should be suspected and great care should be taken when moving the patient.

It is essential to avoid movements of the arms or legs that could jeopardize the injured spine. Any damage to the skin caused during the initial management of these patients may lead to serious pressure sores. Hard objects, such as keys, pens, and match boxes should be removed from the patient's pockets; they should not be sat up but should be rolled gently and any clothing cut away. Nursing staff or orderlies should remove rings or watches to avoid traumatizing the skin. Any movement should be carried out by four or five persons and must be slow and ordered so that the patient is turned and lifted in one piece.

The position in which patients with spinal injuries are treated initially is a matter of controversy. In general, those who are conscious should be placed on their backs. If they are brought into hospital in another position they should be gently turned onto their backs. The prone position is sometimes advocated but is hazardous in patients with cervical injuries and in those with associated damage to the chest or abdomen. Only those who are unconscious should be placed in the lateral or semilateral position to avoid obstruction by the tongue and secretions draining into the lungs. This is particularly important in patients with severe facio-maxillary injuries with bleeding into the upper respiratory tract.

The head should be kept within a straight line to the axis of the body. An improvized roll such as a jacket can be placed under the suspected site of the injury to restore the normal curvature of the spine and thus relieve pressure on the cord. During this phase of management patients may become shocked from intercurrent injuries and considerable damage may be done to the skin, thus leading to severe pressure sores later. Pads of soft material should be placed between the knees and, in particular, the ankles; they should be loosely bound together and a soft support placed between the calves to prevent pressure sores from developing on the heels. It is also extremely important to avoid prolonged pressure on the calves in order to reduce the likelihood of deep vein thromboses. The patient should be kept warm at this stage as they may easily develop hypothermia. They should be transported to X-ray departments on a rigid trolley; stretchers should not be used because of the danger of sagging of the spine. They must be accompanied by a medical attendant to ensure that these precautions are maintained while they are being X-rayed.

In patients who have sustained extensive injuries certain investigations should be carried out while they are being examined and X-rayed. These include a haemoglobin level and PVC, blood gas analysis and, where possible, a baseline vital capacity to assess respiratory function together with X-rays of the chest and any other sites of suspected injury. Blood should be taken for grouping and cross-matching. Particular care should be taken over the use of morphia in patients with high cervical or chest injuries because of the danger of respiratory depression.

Diagnostic difficulties

Missed injuries of the spinal cord

Patients may be sent away from casualty departments with missed fractures of their spinal column (Fig. 2). In one British regional

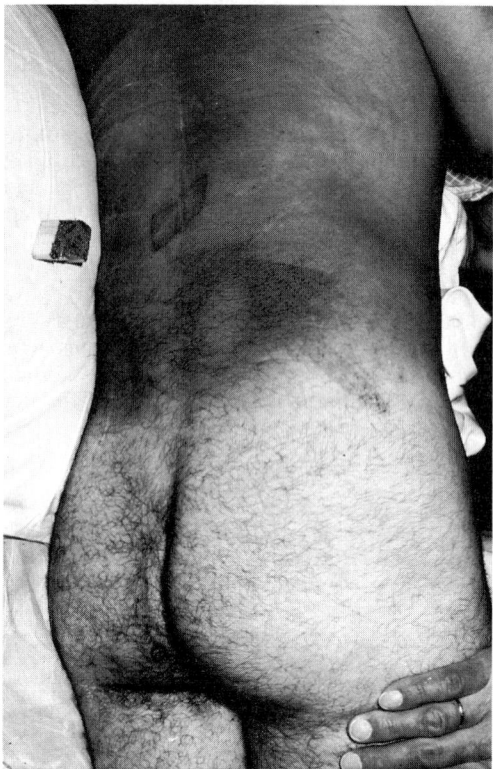

Fig. 2 Patient injured two days previously in the docks. State on arrival at at Stoke Mandeville Hospital: Note bizarre sore with piece of wood still present beneath the patient. He had obviously not been turned nor had his back examined throughout his stay. It is hardly surprising that this patient developed a sore, or clearly in view of the inadequate examination, could have had a missed fracture. (Reproduced from *Geriatric Medicine*, with permission.)

spinal injuries centre it was found that, of 70 tetraplegic patients, half were referred without the bony lesion being identified. A systematic study of a consecutive series of 353 traumatic spinal injury patients admitted under the care of one consultant at the National Spinal Injuries Centre showed that the injury of the spinal cord had not been recognized at the receiving hospital in 15 cases. In at least 10 cases the missed diagnosis of the cord caused significant neurological deterioration. The contributory factors were the circumstances surrounding the accident, the initial absence of any neurological deficit, head injury or suppression of consciousness by drugs, multiple injuries, radiographic or radiodiagnostic errors, and failure to appreciate the mechanism of injury and the forces involved.

Ambience

The emergency room is not the best place to make a careful and studied diagnosis. The staff are hurried by the pressure of work, patients are frequently drunk when involved in road traffic accidents, and tempers are short; a history of being chased by the police on a suspected charge of theft, a strong smell of alcohol, or a previous diagnosis of progressive neurological or orthopaedic disorder can colour the opinion of the medical staff.

Minimal or no neurological deficit on admission

Many patients can suffer an injury to the spine which is unstable and initially causes no damage to the spinal cord, but injudicious handling can give rise to pressure on the cord or nerve roots, leading to severe paralysis. Unfortunately, patients may have a minimal neurological deficit and the clinician may not appreciate the significance of absent reflexes, extensor plantar responses, impaired sensation combined with localized pain, or tenderness and bruising of the spinal column.

Severe head injury or drugs masking the level of consciousness

Because of the nature of car accidents, it is almost invariable that patients have severe associated injuries, of which a head injury is particularly common, so that they are admitted either dazed or deeply unconscious and the attention of the doctor is directed to the management of the head injury. Spinal cord paralysis due to a spinal lesion may be missed in deeply unconscious patients but routine X-rays of the entire spine in all cases of severe head injury with detailed and repeated neurological assessment should prevent this common mistake.

Multiple injuries

In addition to injuries of the spinal cord, multiple skeletal and soft tissue injuries are often present; these include multiple rib fractures and haemothoraces in the case of mid-thoracic fractures, fractured skull, and profound shock. In these severely ill patients the medical teams may be devoting all their attention to resuscitation and miss the spinal injury; it is sad to reflect that in many cases it is the relatives who first record that the legs are paralysed.

Radiological misdiagnosis

Although the diagnosis of cord injuries should be suspected from the clinical history, the diagnosis is often missed if it is associated with fractures of the cervical or dorsal spines. In the majority of cases it is the poor quality of the X-rays that make early recognition of the bony injury difficult. An X-ray of the spine is not complete unless the whole spine, including the odontoid peg and the C7 vertebra, are visualized. Particular care must be taken in looking for minor chip fractures and extension injuries of the cervical vertebrae. In elderly patients with cervical spondylosis radiographic demonstration of the fractures may be difficult, but any undue widening of a disc space, separation of osteophytes, avulsion of the anterior margins of the body or fracture of the spinous process should alert the clinician to the possibility of a major ligamentous disruption. Sometimes, unexplained widening of the prevertebral soft tissue may be the only radiological sign of an injury to the cervical spine. However, there are patients in whom no bony injury can be demonstrated even after the most careful radiological assessment and the clinician must be guided by the clinical findings alone.

Mechanism of injury

Most injuries are the result of considerable violence, and by understanding the mechanism of injury the outcome of a fractured spine can be predicted. For example, when a rugby player has dived or driven his head into the ground or a diver strikes the bottom of a pool, far less force is required to dislocate the spine than when the head is free. When patients with a history of severe violence to the head present in the casualty department with pain in their neck, tingling in their arms, and partial paralysis, they should be carefully examined and assumed to have a spinal injury until proved otherwise, and not sent home or to the police station. A careful history and examination with particular reference to local tenderness of the spine and the motor and reflex changes is of particular importance. When paralysis follows initial mismanagement or when it is observed by the victim or relatives and is ignored by the medical staff, litigation against the hospital is inevitable.

Extension injury of the cervical spine

An important condition that frequently comes under the care of physicians and is often misdiagnosed is an extension injury of the cervical spine. A typical story is of an elderly relative who is visiting their children. They get out of bed in the middle of the night to go to the toilet, but because of the unfamiliar surroundings they become confused and tumble down the stairs and are found the next morning, partially paralysed. Such a fall can also be caused by alcohol. A similar type of accident may occur in old people who

are living on their own; they may lie exposed to a low temperature for a long period and may be admitted to a geriatric ward thought to be suffering from hypothermia. Alternatively, patients who have suffered this type of injury may be thought to be drunk and either lifted or dragged on to a bed to 'sleep it off', until retention of urine directs attention to a more serious diagnosis. An abrasion on the head can mask the more serious spinal injury. The physical signs may be merely a bruise on the head and an incomplete tetraplegia with preservation of power in the legs, loss of power in the arms, and loss of appreciation of pin prick below the appropriate segment with preservation of the posterior columns. X-rays may merely reveal damage to an osteophyte.

There is controversy about how the spinal cord is damaged after this type of injury. It has been suggested that during hyperextension there is backward dislocation of one cervical vertebra on another at a disc space, the cord being carried backwards against the sharp leading edge of the lamina of the lower vertebra. On the other hand many of these patients may not have dislocations and the lesion may be caused by compression of the cord when the spinal canal is narrowed by felted thickening of the ligamentum flavum in the presence of cervical spondylosis, a common finding in the elderly (see page 21.114). It has been found that in patients with chronic myelopathy the size of the spinal canal is reduced and this may well be an important factor in causing this syndrome in patients with acute hyperextension injuries; the author has seen examples of both types of pathology at post-mortem.

Infection of the vertebra

Pyogenic disease of the vertebra is a rare but very important cause of paraplegia. The diagnosis is often made late, frequently after the paraplegia has developed, with confusion with tuberculous or malignant disease so that the wrong treatment (or no treatment) is instituted. However, if diagnosed early and correctly managed it is eminently treatable. In a recent series 37 per cent of cases presented to general physicians; the main features were back pain, febrile episodes preceding the pain, and a delay in diagnosis averaging 13 weeks. There were two incidence peaks, age 10–20 and 40–60 years. ESR and blood cultures were not helpful in making the diagnosis and X-rays were very difficult to interpret; there was sometimes narrowing of the disc spaces, best seen on the lateral view. Positive cultures were only obtained in 60 per cent of the patients; the organisms included staphyloccoci, coliforms, and proteus. A common cause was urinary tract infection. Five of the cases were misdiagnosed as tuberculosis. This condition requires aggressive treatment with appropriate antibiotics; once neurological signs develop urgent decompression is required (see Section 5).

Tuberculous disease of the spine is now uncommon in western countries except in immigrant populations, but is still a major problem in many parts of the world. It frequently has an insidious onset and, because the paraplegic symptoms may occur suddenly, may be confused with a spinal injury if not thought of. The diagnosis and management of this condition is discussed in detail in Section 5.

Management problems

Respiratory problems after spinal injuries

Respiratory complications are common causes of morbidity and mortality in patients with spinal cord injuries, especially those with cervical lesions. The mortality of acute spinal injury has fallen dramatically in recent years, due largely to better respiratory care and improved intensive care facilities and management.

The spinal injury may result in impaired respiratory function by a number of mechanisms: (*a*) weakness or paralysis of the muscles primarily involved in ventilation, (*b*) reduced tone in some respiratory muscles, (*c*) other associated injuries, and (*d*) pulmonary embolism.

Table 1 Groups of muscles involved in respiration

Muscle group	Nerve supply	Main respiratory function
Abdominals	T2–L1	Expiration
Intercostals	T1–T11	Inspiration and expiration
Diaphragm	C3–C5	Inspiration
Accessory muscles	C1–C8	Inspiration

Weakness or paralysis of the respiratory muscles

Injury to the spine may impair or abolish the function of muscles innervated at and below that level. There are four main groups of muscles involved in respiration (Table 1).

Lesions of the upper thoracic spinal cord and above affect the abdominal and intercostal muscles. During quiet breathing, expiration is usually a passive process achieved by relaxation of the muscles of inspiration. At greater levels of ventilation and in forced expiration such as coughing, the abdominal muscles (recti, internal and external oblique, and transversus) contract powerfully. In high thoracic or cervical cord injuries the ability to cough is severely impaired. This may result in sputum retention and, together with a reduced vital capacity, may cause microatelectasis, major segmental, lobar or lung collapse and an increased susceptibility to respiratory infections. Microatelectasis results in ventilation and perfusion mismatch causing hypoxia with a normal or low arterial carbon dioxide. Significant hypoxia occurs in about half such patients with an acute cervical cord injury and is not closely correlated with the impairment of vital capacity. Arterial blood gases should be monitored closely in all acute thoracic and cervical injuries and inspired oxygen given if necessary. Hypoxia is especially dangerous in these patients as it may cause further damage to the spinal cord and, especially in patients with head injuries, increases confusion and makes nursing and management more difficult.

Sputum retention may result in major segmental, lobar or lung collapse. Frequent chest physiotherapy with regular change of position should be instituted early in patients with an acute spinal injury to avoid these complications. It is important to nurse the patients on both sides even if there are rib fractures. Patients with a chronic injury may develop similar problems secondary to a viral chest infection. It is not uncommon for a patient with a vital capacity as low as 600 ml to remain well for long periods only to develop severe problems with sputum retention secondary to a relatively minor chest infection. Such patients may require a tracheostomy to provide access to the trachea for suction. When a major collapse has occurred, bronchoscopy is frequently necessary. It is our practice to anaesthetize these patients and use a fibreoptic bronchoscope through an indwelling endotracheal tube. When the major airways have been cleared of visible secretions, 5–10 ml of warm saline is instilled into the affected bronchus, the bronchoscope withdrawn, and the patient ventilated by vigorous 'bagging' for several breaths together with external shaking of the chest. This frequently loosens more secretions which can then be removed. Most spinal patients who have collapsed a lobe or a lung require ventilation for a short period and should not be immediately extubated after the bronchscopy. The retained secretions may become infected and should be sent regularly for culture. However, antibiotics are best reserved for definite episodes of infection and are not given prophylactically.

The intercostal muscles are inspiratory in action at low lung volumes and expiratory at high volumes. If their function is impaired the muscles available for inspiration and expiration are reduced. Just as we change hands with increasing frequency when we carry a heavy suitcase, there is evidence that the body rotates the use of respiratory muscles when they are under stress. The ability to do this is severely impaired if the intercostals are paralysed and this reduces the respiratory muscle reserve, making it far more liable to fail due to fatigue.

The main muscle of inspiration is the diaphragm. Its function can be assessed at the bedside by inspection or palpation of the upper abdomen during a full inspiration. Normally both the chest and abdominal walls move outward during inspiration. If the diaphragm is paralysed or weak the negative intrathoracic pressure during inspiration will suck the diaphragm up into the thorax and the upper abdomen will move in during inspiration.

In a complete lesion above C3 the diaphragm is paralysed leaving only the accessory muscles, in particular sternocleidomastoid (C1–3) and trapezius (C1–4) available for inspiration. Although these muscles can sometimes produce a vital capacity of several hundred millilitres they are usually incapable of providing adequate long-term ventilation. A few patients can be taught glossopharyngeal breathing, where contraction of the muscles of the cheeks and pharynx with the mouth closed forces air into the trachea. This rarely provides adequate ventilation for a significant period and cannot be used during sleep. Such patients need long-term ventilation. A battery driven ventilator may be fitted to an electrically driven wheelchair to enable them to have some mobility and independence during the day. They may be able to speak using a non-cuffed tracheostomy tube with a slight air leak or using a Pitts tracheostomy tube which directs a small amount of external gas up through the vocal cords when a valve is closed.

Diaphragmatic pacing is sometimes useful in these patients. A paralysed diaphragm may be electrically stimulated if the lower motor neurones in the phrenic nerve are intact and the cell bodies in C3, 4, and 5 segments of the spinal cord are viable. The viability of the phrenic nerve and diaphragm must first be established by percutaneous stimulation. The movement of the diaphragm on stimulation can be estimated by palpation, X-ray screening or ultrasound. Phrenic nerve conduction time is measured using surface electrodes in a lower intercostal space. If the results are satisfactory, electrodes are placed on the phrenic nerve, either in the neck or thorax, and connected to receivers embedded in the skin of the anterior chest wall. A radiotransmitter can then be placed on the skin surface over the receiver and the phrenic nerve stimulated.

Reduced tone in the respiratory muscles

The abdominal and intercostal muscles have other important functions in ventilation. Contraction of the abdominal muscles is important in maintaining the efficiency of the diaphragm. The latter is normally shaped like a dome above the lower ribs. It is maintained in this position in the erect posture because of the effect of increased abdominal muscle tone on the incompressible abdominal contents. If the abdominal muscles are paralysed the abdominal contents fall downwards and forwards when the patient is erect. The diaphragm then descends lower into the abdominal cavity and may lie at right angles or below the lower ribs at the start of inspiration. When the diaphragm contracts in this position the lower ribs are pulled inwards reducing the diameter of the lower chest. The force of contraction of any muscle is greater if it is stretched (within certain limits). The intra-abdominal pressure caused by abdominal muscle contraction maintains a degree of stretch in the diaphragm. Because these beneficial effects of abdominal muscle contraction are lost in patients with high spinal injury their vital capacity may fall by as much as 45 per cent when they are tipped vertical. This effect may be reduced by applying abdominal binders although care must be taken that they are not applied too tightly and that they do not compress the lower ribs.

When the patient is tilted head down the abdominal contents push the diaphragm up and increase the vital capacity but also make it more difficult to breathe as the diaphragm has to push the abdominal contents against gravity.

If one leaf of the diaphragm is paralysed there may be dramatic differences in the vital capacity when the patient is tilted from side to side. The intercostal muscles normally contract during a full inspiration to prevent the intercostal spaces being sucked in by the negative intrathoracic pressure produced by contraction of the diaphragm. If they are paralysed this may not happen and the

Table 2 Simple observation and investigations for patients with potential respiratory failure due to spinal injury

Inspection of chest wall movements for inequality and degree of paradox
Inspection or palpation of the upper abdomen to assess diaphragm function
Observation of the efficiency of the cough mechanism
Auscultation for retained secretions, collapse or pleural fluid
Vital capacity in all positions in which patient is going to be nursed
Arterial blood gases

chest wall may move in paradoxically on inspiration. It has been shown recently that in some spinal patients this paradoxical movement may be very great; two thirds of the movement of the diaphragm on inspiration may be wasted by paradox. It has also been found that there is considerable variation in degree of paradox between patients with similar vital capacities. Therefore, monitoring these patients by vital capacity alone may be misleading.

The commonest site for a cervical injury is C5, 6. In this case the vital capacity will be reduced because of paralysis of some inspiratory muscles, paradoxical movement of the chest wall, and possibly an abnormal, inefficient position of the diaphragm. The vital capacity usually falls to about 30 per cent predicted immediately after injury. In the first few days respiratory function may deteriorate even further due to fatigue, collapse of part of the lung, or an ascending neurological lesion. If the diaphragm is involved the vital capacity may be as low as 200–300 ml. In our series of spinal patients who required ventilation, it was started between the second and seventh day after injury in two-thirds of the cases. All were hypoxic, but over 80 per cent had a normal or low arterial carbon dioxide indicating major ventilation perfusion mismatch. In patients with unstable cervical injuries, extreme care must be taken during intubation to reduce movement of the neck to a minimum. In difficult cases it may be useful to use the fibreoptic bronchoscope as an introducer for the endotracheal tube.

Usually the vital capacity gradually improves. By the fifth month it is stable at about 50 per cent predicted, most of the improvement occurring in the first five or six weeks. This may be due to resolution of oedema in the spinal cord, increased tone in paralysed intercostal muscles reducing the degree of paradox, and possibly some reinnervation of partly paralysed muscle.

Considerable help in managing these patients can be obtained from very simple observations and tests of respiratory function (Table 2). These observations should be performed and recorded frequently in all patients with high spinal injuries and at regular intervals thereafter.

Associated injuries

A high proportion of patients have major trauma in addition to the spinal injury sustained at the time of the initial accident. These injuries may affect respiratory performance. For example, patients with cervical injuries may have head injuries which can depress respiration, as may the use of strong analgesics. Thoracic spine injuries may be complicated by rib fractures with a haemothorax and/or pneumothorax and *flail segment of chest wall*. Blood or air in the pleural space should be drained by an underwater drain and a patient with a flail chest wall segment should be ventilated before they develop respiratory failure. A common X-ray finding in patients with an upper thoracic vertebral fracture is widening of the mediastinum. This is due to haematoma around the site of the bony injury. It often disappears after a few days as the blood tracks into the pleural space. Spinal patients with multiple long-bone fractures and who have required many blood transfusions may develop the adult respiratory distress syndrome. This is treated in the usual way (see Section 15) with fluid restrictions and by increasing the inspired oxygen, and may require ventilation and positive end expiratory pressure (PEEP).

Pulmonary embolism

There is a high risk of phlebothrombosis and subsequent pulmonary embolism in patients with traumatic spinal injuries. Consequently, prophylactic anticoagulant therapy has been adopted at main spinal injuries centres. It is vital that this be established as quickly as possible, since if the anticoagulation is delayed deep vein thrombosis may already have occurred. Later anticoagulation will not prevent a pulmonary embolism or deep vein thrombosis but it may prevent a fatality.

Autonomic dysfunction

Vascular

Patients who have damaged their spinal cord above the sympathetic outflow frequently have autonomic dysfunction affecting a variety of systems. Because of reduced vascular tone combined with blood loss from the associated injuries, the blood pressure is frequently low and may fall even further if positive pressure ventilation is used. Before ventilation, the circulatory volume should be fully restored to avoid a severe drop in cardiac output. The vasculature does not respond normally to a change in posture and the blood pressure may fall precipitously when the patient is tipped up. The lack of sympathetic venous tone in these patients make interpretation of the central venous pressure even more difficult than usual. It may not rise during a rapid intravenous infusion and yet the patient may develop acute pulmonary oedema. Conversely, at a later stage there may be a sudden increase in vascular tone and severe hypertension, often precipitated by a bladder washout or a blocked catheter. Because of autonomic dysfunction there may be defective vasodilation, vasoconstriction or sweating in response to changes in environmental temperature. This may lead to hypothermia or hyperpyrexia. Patients with high cord transections may develop drenching sweats in response to irritation of the bladder or rectum. On the other hand there may be no sweating in response to hypoglycaemia and the treatment of a tetraplegic who has diabetes is extremely difficult.

Heart

Suction of the pharynx and manipulation of the larynx may cause increased vagal activity, and its unopposed action due to the paralysis of the sympathetic in these patients may result in profound bradycardia or even asystole. Atropine should always be readily available and the pulse should be monitored when any procedures are performed.

Bowels

These patients frequently develop gastric dilations and paralytic ileus in the early days after injury. There is a high incidence of gastrointestinal bleeding due to acute stress ulcers, reflux oesophagitis, and flare-up of pre-existing peptic ulceration in the early days after injury. The introduction of oral fluids should be delayed to prevent vomiting and possible aspiration.

Pressure sores

Pathogenesis

Pressure sores occur because the weight of the body is not evenly transmitted throughout its whole surface area, but through the feet on standing, the scapula, sacrum, and heels on lying, and the lateral malleoli, trochanters, and shoulder girdle when turned on one side. Consequently, in these critical areas greater pressure is generated than over other parts of the body. In order to nourish the tissues, the blood pressure has to be greater than the pressure generated in the tissues. When the patient is lying on these areas the blood pressure is insufficient, and, if left unrelieved, blistering, bruising, and infarction of the tissues occurs. The damage can be aggravated by shearing strains caused by injudicious dragging or the use of inadequate equipment such as a drawsheet or a hard chair. The length of time that the pressure is generated is critical; a

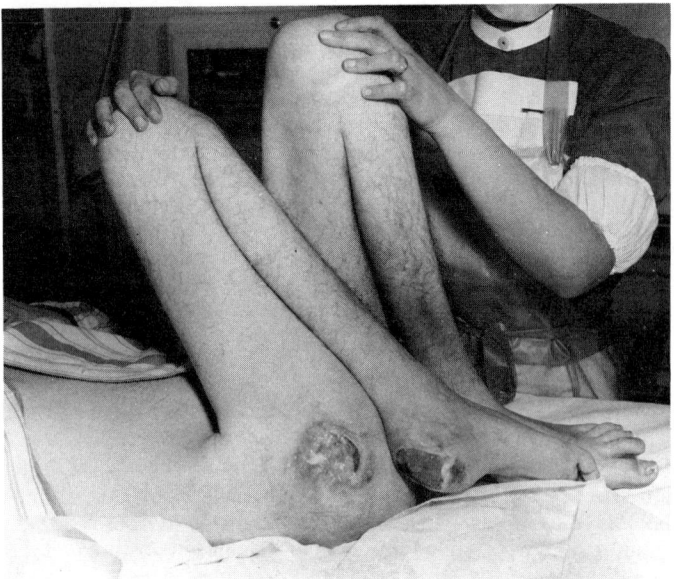

Fig. 3 Severe spasticity makes it difficult to turn the patient. The constant movement due to spasms will prevent healing. The contractures make it impossible to get the legs straight.

short bout of very high pressure can be just as injurious as long, continued low pressure. The process is aggravated if the tissues are macerated by urine or faeces. It has been shown in a United Kingdom survey of some 737 wards, in which 14 448 patients were studied, that 961 had pressure sores, a prevalence of 6.65 per cent; the highest incidence (9.22 per cent) was in geriatric units. In general surgical units there was a 4.1 per cent incidence.

Paraplegic patients are particulary liable to develop pressure sores. Mechanisms include hypotension, sympathetic paralysis, hypoxia, loss of sensation, maceration of skin, and difficulty in turning due to paralysis, spasms or contractures (Fig. 3).

The natural history of fatal pressure sores is a large lesion that heals and breaks down, and then involves bone, particularly the femoral head, with persistent sequestrum and sinus formation. There is a mistaken belief that pressure sores are sterile. This is not the case; they are infected and can give rise to septicaemia and, in the long term, amyloidosis.

Amyloidosis
Studies of post-mortems on spinal patients at Stoke Mandeville Hospital who died later than six weeks after injury have suggested that there is an association between pressure sores and the devel-

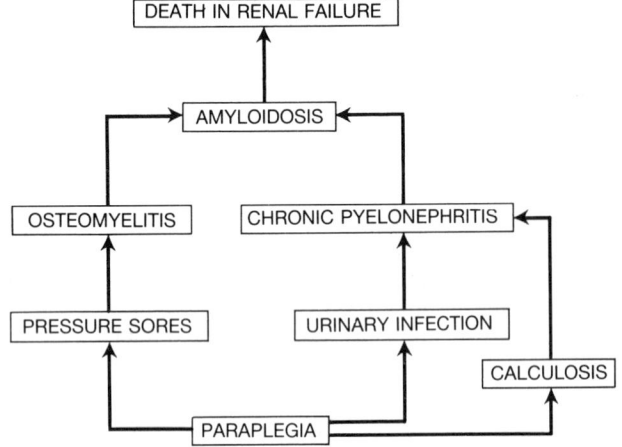

Fig. 4 Relationship between the complications of paraplegia. (Reproduced from Tribe and Silver, 1969, *Renal failure in paraplegia*, Fig. 6.1.)

opment of amyloidosis. In the majority of cases there was gross renal sepsis in addition to the pressure sores (Fig. 4). Attempts to establish a diagnosis in life from biopsy material were not successful. The single consistent pointer to the development of amyloidosis is a urinary protein excretion of more than 5 g in 24 hours. Amyloid is found in the kidney, liver, spleen, bowel, and heart muscle, the classical sites of secondary amyloidosis. The kidney is the most important site from the point of view of the prognosis. The mean survival time is 10 years, compared with a near normal life expectancy for a paraplegic patient without this complication. Death is due to severe hypoproteinaemia, septicaemia which is commonly complicated by subacute or acute endocarditis, fungal endocarditis, haematemesis, pancreatitis, and renal failure due to a combination of amyloid, pyelonephritis, and calculus formation. Early deaths are due to infection, later to renal failure.

Prevention and treatment
Unless the patient is turned regularly, sores will develop. It is not sufficient simply to request regular turning; correct equipment, including specialized pillows and mechanized beds, is required. If pillows are used alone, provision must be made to maintain the position of the patient when they are on their sides by the additional use of sandbags to support the back, and pillows must be placed between the knees. It is possible to maintain skull traction while turning the patient adequately if specialized beds are used. Although ripple-cell mattresses have their advocates, unless the patient is turned regularly in addition sores will develop. In short, the equipment and the method used is as good as the staff who are involved.

Once pressure sores have developed there are certain principles which underlie their management. First, pressure should be removed from the site by regular turning. A good standard of nutrition should be maintained, particularly with respect to protein intake. Great care should be taken to avoid soiling with urine or faeces. Necrotic tissue should be removed, careful bacteriological surveillance of the wound maintained by regular culture, and closed pockets opened up to provide free drainage. The sore should be inspected daily with frequent dressings which should attempt to seal the wounds to prevent further colonization of the skin with bacteria from the wound. Ideally, patients with severe bed sores should be barrier nursed to prevent spread of infection to other patients. More specialized surgical management includes skin grafting and the concurrent management of flexor spasms by alcohol nerve block of anterior rhizotomy; both procedures may reduce constant movement and hence aid healing. Similarly, underlying bony prominences should be removed if healing cannot be achieved.

Bladder and renal complications
Pathogenesis
Immediately after a spinal injury, unless it is very mild, there is retention of urine due to inadequate detrusor contractions which are insufficient to overcome resistance in the urethra. These may return, depending on the patient's age and the way in which the initial retention of urine has been managed. If there is interruption in lower motor neurone pathways, detruser contraction cannot occur. Severe stretching of muscle fibres due to overdistension of the bladder may result in secondary hypotonia. This may be made worse by infection.

Unskilled and traumatic catheterization introduces infection. Combined with inadequate emptying this leads to severe ascending infection. Although more skilled management has now largely eliminated this complication renal complications are still a major cause of long-term damage to the urinary tract. The main pathological processes are: pyelonephritis, amyloidosis, hypertension, and calculus formation.

At post-mortem it is usual to find evidence of chronic urinary tract infection. The bladder is thick-walled with areas of perivesicular fibrosis and there is a high incidence of carcinoma. The ureters are dilated with thickened walls and the kidneys show pyelonephritic changes and may be hydronephrotic.

The paraplegic patient is particularly liable to form renal calculi which consist of calcium and magnesium phosphate; oxalate stones occur occasionally. The main aetiological factors are immobilization, stasis, and chronic infection. Immobilization, together with multiple fractures, leads to a demineralization of bone and hypercalcinuria. Hypercalcaemia can also occur, particularly in children and tetraplegics. These patients are at particular risk of calculus formation during this stage, particulary if the fluid intake is restricted. In addition, urinary infection, particularly if caused by urea splitting organisms, results in an alkaline urine which encourages the formation of calculi. There is a strong association between calculi, renal infection, and amyloidosis.

Prevention and management

Immediately after injury the patient will usually be unable to pass urine because of the absence of detrusor contractions. Hence, the bladder must be drained. Methods include manual expression, continuous drainage, or intermittent catheterization. Although there has been some recent interest in the use of manual expression this requires expert monitoring and is not recommended for general use. The most satisfactory form of drainage is the use of intermittent catheterization. The distension serves to stimulate the return of detrusor contraction. This form of treatment should only be carried out by trained staff under expert supervision. The urethra should be filled with lubricant combined with local antiseptic and each urine sample should be monitored bacteriologically. Intermittent catheterization has now been successfully applied in spinal injury centres in many countries and, in expert hands, appears to be the method of choice but it requires very close monitoring, particularly with regard to infection and overdistension. If an indwelling catheter is used it must be strapped to the anterior abdominal wall to prevent angulation with subsequent damage to the urethra. It should be changed weekly and the bladder gently washed out with saline. If it becomes blocked it should be removed; no attempt should be made to unblock it. In females, the use of fine bore suprapubic catheters may be helpful, but they have the disadvantage of easy blocking.

Apart from expert attention to the bladder, the factors in preventing renal damage in paraplegic patients are the maintenance of adequate hydration and the early treatment of urinary tract infection with appropriate antibiotics.

References

Bauze, R. J. and Ardran, G. M. (1978). Experimental production of forward dislocation in the human cervical spine. *J. Bone Joint Surg.* **60B**, 239–245.

Bors, E. and Comarr, A. E. (1971). *Neurological urology. Physiology of micturition – its neurological disorders and sequelae.* S. Karger AG, Basel.

Cameron, G. S., Scott, J. W., Jousse, A. T. and Botterell, E. H. (1955). Diaphragmatic respiration in the quadriplegic patient and the effect of position on his vital capacity. *Ann. Surg.* **141**, 451–456.

Claus-Walker, J., Carter, R. E., Campos, R.J. and Spencer, W. A. (1975). Hypercalcaemia in early traumatic quadriplegia. *J. Chron. Dis.* **28**, 81–90.

Crooks, F. and Birkett, A. N. (1944). Fractures and dislocations of the cervical spine. *Br. J. Surg.* **31**, 252–265.

Digby, M. and Kersley, J. B. (1979). Pyogenic non-tuberculous spinal infection. *J. Bone Joint Surg.* **61B**, 47–55.

Dollfus, P. and Frankel, H. (1965). Cardiovascular reflexes in tracheostomised tetraplegics. *Paraplegia* **2**, 227–231.

El Masri, W. S. and Fellows, G. (1981). Bladder cancer after spinal cord injury. *Paraplegia* **19**, 265–270.

—— and Silver, J. R. (1981). Prophylactic anticoagulant therapy in patients with spinal cord injury. *Paraplegia* **19**, 334–342.

Forsyth, H. F. (1964). Extension injuries of the cervical spine. *J. Bone Joint Surg.* **46** 1792– 1797.

Geisler, W. O., Jousse, A. T. and Wynne-Jones, M. (1977). Survival in traumatic transverse myelitis. *Paraplegia* **14**, 262–275.

——, ——, —— and Breithaupt, D. (1983). Survival in traumatic spinal cord injury. *Paraplegia* **21**, 364–373.

Guttmann, L. (1976). *Spinal cord injuries, comprehensive management and research*, 2nd edn. Blackwell Scientific Publications, Oxford.

——, Silver, J. R. and Wyndham, C. (1958). Thermoregulation in the spinal man. *J. Physiol* **142**, 406–418.

—— and Whitteridge, D. (1947). Effects of bladder distension on autonomic mechanisms after spinal cord injuries. *Brain* **70**, 361–404.

Hachen, H. J. (1974). Anticoagulation therapy in patients with spinal cord injury. *Paraplegia* **12**, 176–187.

Hardy, A. G. (1976). Survival periods in traumatic tetraplegia. *Paraplegia* **14**, 41–46.

Marar, B. C. (1974). Hyperextension injuries of the cervical spine. The pathogenesis of damage to the spinal cord. *J. Bone Joint Surg.* **56**, 1655–1662.

Melzak, J. (1966). The incidence of bladder cancer in paraplegia. *Paraplegia* **4**, 85–96.

Moulton, A. and Silver, J. R. (1970). Chest movements in patients with traumatic injuries of the cervical cord. *Clin. Sci.* **39**, 407–422.

Ohry, A., Brooks, M. E. and Rozin, R. (1980). Misdiagnosis of spinal cord injuries – the psychiatrist's point of view. *Paraplegia* **18**, 15–20.

Ravichandran, G. and Silver, J. R. (1982). Missed injuries of the spinal cord. *Br. Med. J.* **284**, 953– 960.

—— and —— (1982). Survival following traumatic tetraplegia. *Paraplegia* **20**, 264–269.

Silver, J. R. (1974). The prophylactic use of anticoagulants in the prevention of pulmonary emboli in 100 consecutive spinal injury patients. *Paraplegia* **12**, 188–196.

—— (1975). Pressure sores 2. Management of complications. *Mod. Ger.* **5**, 6–16.

—— (1980). *Rehabilitation medicine. The management of physical disabilities*, 2nd edn (ed. P. J. R. Nichols), pp. 223–250. Butterworth, London.

—— and Gibbon, N. O. K. (1968). Prognosis in tetraplegia. *Br. Med. J.* **4**. 79–83.

——, Morris, W. R. and Otfinowski, J. S. (1980). Associated injuries in patients with spinal injury. *Injury* **12**, 219–224.

—— and Moulton, A. (1970). Prophylatic anticoagulant therapy against pulmonary emboli in acute paraplegia. *Br. Med. J.* **2**, 338–340.

Talbot, H. S. (1966). Renal disease and hypertension in paraplegics and quadriplegics. *Med. Serv. J. Canada* **22**, 570–575.

Taor, W. S. (1984). *Progress in rehabilitation paraplegia*, (eds R. Capildeo and A. Maxwell), pp. 25–30. MacMillan Press, London.

Thorburn, W. (1887). Cases of injury to the cervical region of the spinal cord. *Brain* **9**, 510–543.

Tribe, C. R. and Silver, J. R. (1969). *Renal failure in paraplegia*, pp. 3–11. Pitman, London.

Thompson Walker, J. (1937). Treatment of bladder in spinal injuries in war. *Br. J. Urol.* **9**, 217–230.

Watson, N. (1978). Anticoagulant therapy in the prevention of venous thrombosis and pulmonary embolism in the spinal cord injury. *Paraplegia* **16**, 265–269.

Disorders of the spinal nerve roots

R. S. MAURICE-WILLIAMS

Anatomy

Each segment of the spinal cord gives off a ventral (motor) and dorsal (sensory) root on each side. These unite in the intervertebral foramina to leave the spinal canal as mixed spinal roots. As the spinal cord ends at the lower border of the Ll vertebra, the lower spinal roots originate from the cord above their corresponding skeletal levels and run an increasingly oblique course before they reach their foramina. The spinal dura, enclosing the spinal subarachnoid space, extends to the middle of the sacral canal, and the leash of roots within it, together with the fibrous band (the filum terminale) which is the continuation of the tip of the cord, form the cauda equina.

There are 8 cervical, 12 dorsal, 5 sacral, and 1 coccygeal pairs of roots. Each root has motor and sensory fibres which at some levels

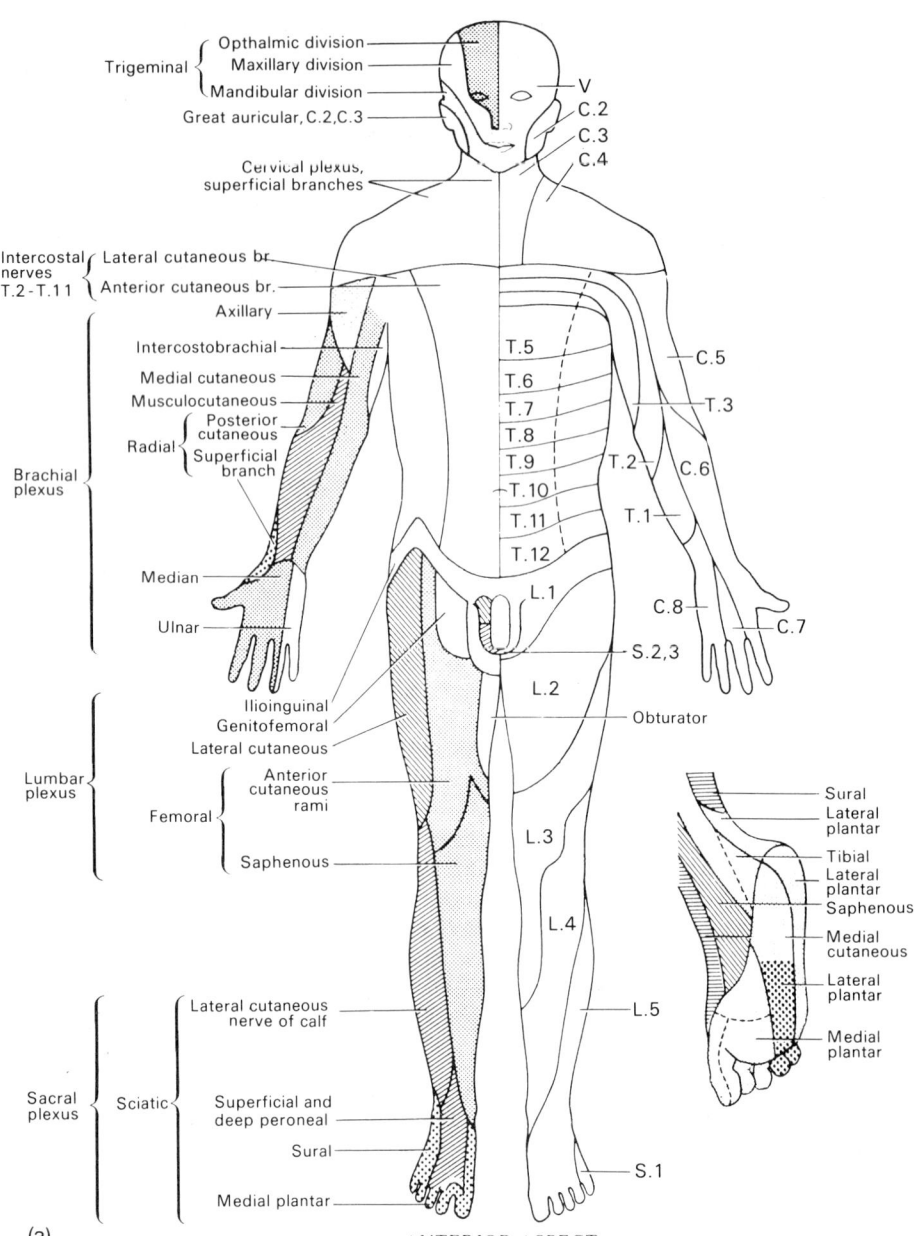

Fig. 1 Cutaneous areas of distribution of spinal segments and the peripheral nerves. (a) Anterior aspect. (b) Posterior aspect. (Reproduced from Bannister, *Brain's clinical neurology*, Oxford University Press, with permission.)

(a)   ANTERIOR ASPECT

subserve clinically important tendon reflexes. The roots supplying these are shown in Table 1. The sympathetic outflow leaves the cord via roots Dl–L1, while the caudal parasympathetic outflow is via roots S2–S4. The area of skin whose sensation is supplied by a single root is known as a dermatome and the corresponding block of deep tissues is called a sclerotome. Figure 1 shows a dermatome map of the body. The first cervical root contains no cutaneous sensory fibres, so the C2 dermatome adjoins the area of skin supplied by the trigeminal nerve. The overlap of dermatomes and anatomi-

cal variation between individuals means that loss of a single root may give rise to a variable sensory loss which may not be detectable clinically. The main motor supply of the different roots is given in Table 2 in terms of movements. Again there is some variation in anatomy between individuals so that precise localization of a root lesion on the basis of the pattern of motor loss, may be difficult. This is especially so for roots C5–8.

The effect of root lesions

In addition to motor, sensory, and reflex loss, irritation or compression of a root may give to rise to pain and paraesthesiae in the sensory distribution of that root. Root pain is characteristically made worse by movement of the spine and by actions which cause sudden pulses of pressure in the spinal subarachnoid space, such as coughing or sneezing. Root pain in a limb often has two components – a dull deep ill-defined ache thought to correspond to the sensory supply to muscle and bone (the sclerotome) and a sharp, superficial better defined pain related to the dermatome of that root.

    On a few roots there are important arterial feeders reinforcing

Table 1 Roots involved in tendon reflexes

Reflex	Roots
Biceps jerk	Cervical 5–6
Supinator jerk	Cervical 5–6
Triceps jerk	Cervical 6–7
Finger jerk	Cervical 7–8
Knee jerk	Lumbar 2–4
Ankle jerk	Sacral 1–2

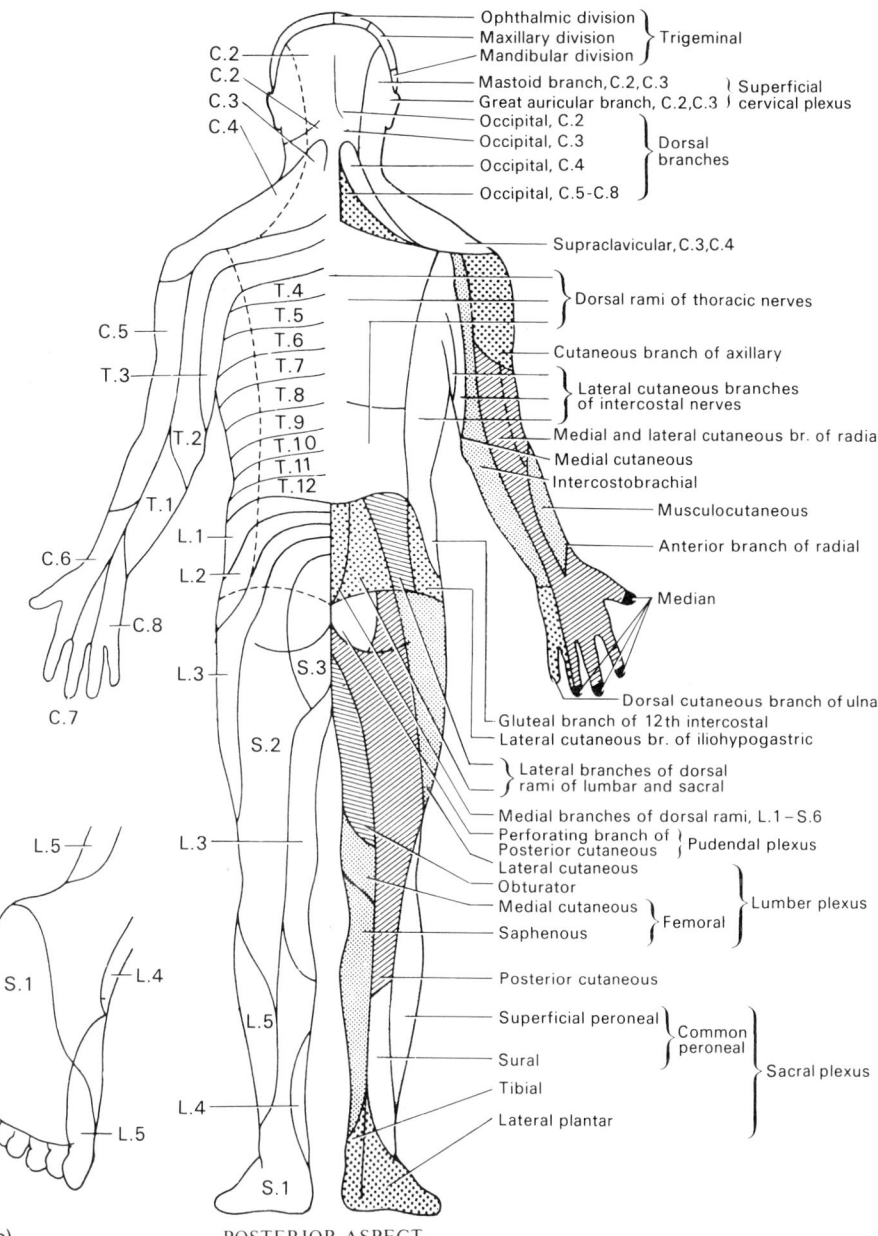

Ophthalmic division	Trigeminal
Maxillary division	
Mandibular division	
Mastoid branch, C.2, C.3	Superficial cervical plexus
Great auricular branch, C.2, C.3	
Occipital, C.2	Dorsal branches
Occipital, C.3	
Occipital, C.4	
Occipital, C.5-C.8	

Supraclavicular, C.3, C.4

Dorsal rami of thoracic nerves

Cutaneous branch of axillary

Lateral cutaneous branches of intercostal nerves

Medial and lateral cutaneous br. of radial

Medial cutaneous

Intercostobrachial

Musculocutaneous

Anterior branch of radial

Median

Dorsal cutaneous branch of ulnar

Gluteal branch of 12th intercostal

Lateral cutaneous br. of iliohypogastric

Lateral branches of dorsal rami of lumbar and sacral

Medial branches of dorsal rami, L.1 – S.6

Perforating branch of Posterior cutaneous } Pudendal plexus

Lateral cutaneous

Obturator

Medial cutaneous } Femoral } Lumber plexus

Saphenous

Posterior cutaneous

Superficial peroneal } Common peroneal

Sural

Tibial } Sacral plexus

Lateral plantar

(b)   POSTERIOR ASPECT

---

the longitudinally running arteries of the spinal cord, mainly the anterior spinal artery; damage to one of these roots may lead to cord ischaemia. A major feeder is usually present on one of the lower cervical roots and on one of the roots of the dorso-lumbar junction (the great artery of Adamkiewicz).

Causes of root lesions

Spinal degenerative disease
This is the commonest cause of a root lesion, usually in the lower lumbar or lower cervical region. It is discussed in detail below.

Tumours
Spinal extradural tumours, such as metastatic carcinoma or lymphomas, lying either in the bone of a vertebra or in the fibro-fatty epidural space, often produce root compression and root pain. Of the spinal intradural tumours, root pain is most often associated with a neurofibroma, which usually originates from a dorsal root. Carcinoma of the lung apex may involve the first dorsal root, producing pain and numbness down the inner surface of the arm, weakness of the small muscles of the hand, and a Horner's syn-

drome. This clinical picture is known as a *Pancoast syndrome*. Pelvic or retroperitoneal tumours may involve roots after they have left the spinal canal.

Trauma
Rarely, stab and bullet wounds may damage spinal roots. Violent upward or downward movements of the shoulder girdle on the trunk can damage roots contributing to the upper or lower parts of the brachial plexus. The so-called *Erb-Duchenne palsy*, due to avulsion of the C5 and C6 roots, is caused by forcible depression of the shoulder, as may occur in a difficult delivery or nowadays more commonly when a person is flung off a motor cycle and lands on the point of his shoulder. Avulsion of the C8 and D1 roots (*Klumpke palsy*) may follow a fall in which the arm catches on a projection and is jerked upwards violently (see page 21.119).

Cervical rib syndrome
The C8 and D1 roots run over the surface of the first rib, together with the subclavian artery. All these structures may be compressed if they are elevated at this point by the presence of a *cervi-*

Table 2 Main motor supply of roots

C1–4	Neck muscles (apart from spinal accessory supply to sternomastoid and trapezius)
	Longitudinal spinal muscles
	Diaphragm (C3–5, mainly C4)
C5	Shoulder abductors
C6	Elbow flexors
C7	Elbow extensors
	Wrist flexors/extensors
C8	Finger flexors and extensors
D1	Small hand muscles
D2–D12	Trunk muscles
	Longitudinal spinal muscles
L1	Hip flexors
L2	Hip flexors
	Hip adductors
	Knee extensors
L3	Knee extensors
	Hip flexors
	Hip adductors
L4	Knee extensors
	Ankle dorsiflexors
	Knee flexors
	Hip extensors
L5	Ankle dorsiflexors
	Dorsiflexor of hallux
	Hip extensors
	Knee flexors
S1	Ankle plantar flexors
	Hip extensors
	Knee flexors

cal rib or a *congenital fibrous band* running from the tip of a prominent C7 transverse process to the first rib beneath them. Root symptoms from this cause are usually associated with signs of vascular insufficiency in the hand from compression of the subclavian artery. The hand symptoms may be of a Raynaud phenomenon type or multiple lesions due to emboli thrown off from a patch of thrombus within the compressed subclavian artery. A true cervical rib syndrome is rare. In the past it was probably overdiagnosed and confused with root lesions caused by cervical disc protrusions.

Neuralgic amyotrophy

This is believed to be an inflammatory involvement of C5, C6, and sometimes the C7 roots. It may occur spontaneously or may follow either an infective illness or an immunization injection into the deltoid muscle. Over the course of a few days, pain around the shoulder is followed by weakness and wasting of the muscles supplied by the affected roots. In most cases a good spontaneous recovery occurs over a matter of months. Like the cervical rib syndrome, this may have often been misdiagnosed in the past in cases of root compression caused by cervical disc protrusions.

Arachnoiditis

Progressive fibrosis of the arachnoid membrane is a rare condition which may involve roots, especially those of the cauda equina. In most cases there has been some clear-cut insult to the arachnoid, perhaps years before, such as a spinal infection, radiotherapy, trauma or surgery. The irritant effects of the oil-based contrast media which were used for myelography until recently are thought to have contributed to many cases, especially if the lumbar puncture for the original myelogram was difficult and caused bleeding into the subarachnoid space.

Herpes zoster

(See Section 5)

The inflammatory process of herpes zoster is based in the dorsal root ganglion and the first symptoms are pain and hyperalgesia in the area supplied by the affected root(s), to be followed a few days later by a skin rash in the corresponding dermatomes. Spread of infection into the anterior horn cells of the cord may produce motor loss in the same segments.

Degenerative disease of the spine

This condition is the principal cause of lesions of the spinal nerve roots. The term disease is rather misleading for by the age of 60 years the great majority of the population show some radiological evidence of degeneration of the spine. The condition is not necessarily symptomatic and it is perhaps best regarded as a normal ageing process which advances at different rates in different individuals.

The pathological basis of the condition lies in degeneration of the intervertebral discs. These structures act as buffers and fulcra between the vertebral bodies. They permit movement between the vertebrae while cushioning longitudinally acting stress. The discs are thickest at those parts of the spine which are most mobile and which abut fixed sections, namely, the lower cervical spine and the lower lumbar spine. In these regions the discs are subjected to the greatest stress and are most prone to symptomatic degenerative change.

In the young adult the nucleus of the intervertebral disc is a tense well-hydrated structure which holds apart the adjacent intervertebral bodies. Degeneration begins to appear in the third decade and consists of a progressive desiccation and collapse of the nucleus which may begin to fissure and break up into fragments. By old age the process of fibrosis may lead to what amounts to a fibrous ankylosis between the vertebral bodies. Disc degeneration appears to be a normal wear and tear phenomenon and bears only a limited relationship to heavy occupational stress.

Collapse of the disc space leads to a number of secondary phenomena. The annulus of the disc bulges outwards, lifting the periosteum off the vertebral bodies and giving rise to the deposition of marginal osteophytes. The narrowing of the disc space leads to a misalignment of the posterior facet joints which may accordingly show hypertrophic, osteoarthritic change. As the vertebral bodies come closer to each other, the posterior longitudinal ligament and the ligamenta flava buckle up. Finally the disc narrowing and facet joint misalignment may permit some degree of forward or backwards subluxation of one vertebra upon another. This happens most often at the L4/5 level, where the axes of the facet joints in some individuals may permit the development of a forward spondylolisthesis.

All the above changes, osteophytic ridges, swollen facet joints, and concertinaed ligaments, may intrude into the spinal canal and intervertebral foramina and cause cord or root compression. Collectively these chronic degenerative changes are known as spinal spondylosis. Cervical spondylosis is most marked at the C4/5, C5/6, and C6/7 levels. It may be associated with the development of a myelopathy (see below) or with root compression. The latter occurs in the intervertebral foramina which may be narrowed anteriorly by osteophytes originating from the sides of the intervertebral disc and uncovertebral joints and posteriorly by hypertrophied facet joints. Lumbar spondylosis may lead to narrowing of the lumbar canal and compression of the cauda equina (see below) or to compression of individual nerve roots where they lie in the lateral recesses of the spinal canal before they reach their foramina. This so-called lateral recess stenosis results from bulging of the discs in front and the facet joints and yellow ligament behind.

Disc protrusions

In addition to the insidious neural compression caused by spondylosis, a more sudden root or cord compression may follow protrusion of an intervertebral disc. A disc protrusion consists of an acute or subacute backwards dislocation of disc substance. It may take the form of a bulge of disc material within an intact annulus or the annulus may tear at one point, permitting extrusion of a free fragment of nuclear material into the spinal canal. The latter event is known as sequestration of a disc. Disc protrusions may occur in any direction, but only the backward protrusions produce symptoms, either by causing root or cord compression or by stretching the highly innervated posterior longitudinal ligament and posterior annulus. The posterior longitudinal ligament tends to reinforce the central part of the posterior annulus and deflects protrusions postero-laterally. Disc protrusions often follow an episode of sudden or unusual exertion, but the underlying degeneration and fissuring of the disc will have been developing silently for some time as a result of normal wear and tear strains.

Cervical disc protrusions

These are commonest at the C4/5, C5/6, and C6/7 levels, compressing the C5, C6, and C7 roots, respectively. A symptomatic protrusion occurs most often between the ages of 25 and 50 years. The onset of symptoms is generally over the course of a few days and may occur spontaneously or follow some unusual strain. The first symptom is pain and stiffness in the neck usually extending into the shoulder or proximal arm on one side in a rather ill-defined fashion. This may be referred pain resulting from stretching of the annulus. As root compression develops there appears a better defined severe lancinating pain in the territory of that root. With worsening root compression there may be paraesthesiae and numbness in the dermatome of the root and reduction or loss of any tendon reflexes subserved by the root. Marked motor loss is unusual and usually indicates very severe root compression. Painful limitation of some neck movements is almost invariably found.

The main differential diagnoses are median and ulnar nerve palsies, lesions of the rotator cuff of the shoulder joint, and involvement of the lower part of the brachial plexus by an apical carcinoma of the lung (Pancoast's syndrome). The peripheral nerve palsies will not be accompanied by neck and proximal arm pain and they can be confirmed by conduction studies. Shoulder capsule lesions give rise to limitation of passive movements of the shoulder. An apical lung carcinoma causes a Horner's syndrome from involvement of the sympathetic outflow in the first dorsal root. Many patients diagnosed in the past as suffering from either neuralgic amyotophy or compression of the lower brachial plexus by cervical ribs or bands may have had root compression from cervical disc protrusions.

In the great majority of cases the symptoms abate within a few weeks with conservative measures – a collar, bedrest if necessary, and mild analgesia. Recurrent attacks are much less common than in the case of lumbar disc protrusions. Surgery is reserved for the small number of patients with an incapacitating degree of pain which persists or recurs or where severe root compression has led to disabling motor or sensory loss. Before operation the level of the root compression should be confirmed by myelography which also serves to exclude unexpected pathology causing root compression within the spinal canal, such as a tumour. Surgical decompression of the root may be carried out from behind (facetectomy or foraminotomy) or from in front. In the latter approach the anterior longitudinal ligament is incised permitting opening up of the disc space and direct removal of extruding disc material from anterior to the root. On the whole, the results of surgery are extremely good.

A central cervical disc protrusion may give rise to acute or subacute compression of the spinal cord. Young adults are usually affected and an onset after trauma is common. Urgent removal by the anterior route is indicated. A posterior approach via laminectomy is usually more hazardous as it requires mobilization and retraction of the compressed cord.

Dorsal disc protrusions

As the dorsal spine is relatively immobile and is splinted by the rib cage, symptomatic disc protrusions are extremely rare. Root compression is unusual. In most cases a dorsal disc protrusion presents as cord compression. This may be of insidious onset. The protruded material is often hard and calcified and may gradually erode through the anterior dura to become embedded in the spinal cord. Surgical treatment is difficult and hazardous and there is a real risk of catastrophic neurological worsening after surgery, especially if removal is attempted from behind via a standard laminectomy. The preferred approaches are those which give access to the protruded disc from the side or in front without any need for cord retraction, such as a costotransversectomy or the transthoracic route.

Lumbar disc protrusions

Most symptomatic disc protrusions are lumbar and 95 per cent of these occur at the two lowest levels, L4/5 and L5/S1. Lumbar disc protrusions are thought to account for many and perhaps most attacks of acute low back pain and sciatica, although in only a small proportion of cases is the diagnosis confirmed by myelography and surgery.

The characteristic course of a lumbar disc protrusion is of recurrent attacks of low back pain radiating into one or other leg. The peak incidence is between the ages of 25 and 50 years. Relapses often follow exertion but heavy manual workers are no more liable to the condition than are those in sedentary occupations. Relapses often occur abruptly and protective spasm of the erector spinae muscles may cause 'locking' of the lumbar spine with severe pain. Initial attacks consist of low back pain spreading into the region of the sacro-iliac joint and buttock in an ill-defined fashion. These symptoms are thought to reflect distension of the sensitive posterior annulus and posterior longitudinal ligament. Many patients never progress beyond this stage, but in some patients root compression occurs. If this happens, the low back pain lessens and is replaced by severe well-localized pain in the territory of the root, made worse by coughing or straining. An L4/5 disc protrusion compresses the L5 root some way above its intervertebral foramen causing pain down the outside of the leg and radiating to the top of the foot, which may become numb. An L5/S1 disc protrusion compresses the S1 root causing posterior leg pain radiating to the sole. The outer edge of the foot may become numb.

On examination signs of root compression will be found. In the case of the lower 3 lumbar discs, affecting roots L4–S1, there will be limited straight leg raising with a positive stretch test (*Lasegue's test*). Compression of roots L1 to 3 which run anterior to the hip joint, gives rise to a positive femoral stretch test. The neurological changes correspond to the root affected and vary according to how severely it is compressed. L5 root involvement leads to weakness of dorsiflexion and eversion of the ankle, numbness on the dorsum of the foot and lateral shin, but no reflex loss. S1 root involvement causes numbness of the outer border of the foot and little toe, weakness of plantar flexion at the ankle and a reduced or absent ankle jerk.

Most patients recover within a matter of two to three weeks with bedrest alone. Surgery is only indicated if there is prolonged or recurrent incapacitating root compression or in those cases where serious motor loss appears, especially if an L4/5 disc protrusion leads to marked weakness of dorsiflexion of the ankle. The one absolute indication for surgery is a central protrusion compressing the cauda equina (see below). Patients with clear signs of root compression do well after operation. Those with back pain as the dominant symptom fare much less well.

Plain X-rays of the lumbar spine are of little value in predicting the level of asymptomatic protrusion but plain X-rays of the lumbar spine and pelvis should be taken to make sure that an unsuspected tumour is not producing bone destruction. Surgery should be preceded by myelography to confirm the level of root compression, to exclude any element of canal stenosis as a contributing factor, and to make sure that there is not an unexpected spinal tumour present.

At operation the root is exposed from behind by a laminectomy or by more limited excision of the yellow ligament and the adjacent bone (fenestration) on one side. The root is then retracted to permit removal of any extruded disc material beneath it. The point where the annulus has given way allows instruments to be inserted into the disc space which is cleared of any loose degenerate material which might protrude in the future. The outcome of surgery depends on case selection but in approximately 80 per cent of cases the patient is able to resume a normal life with little disability.

Cauda equina lesions

Compression of the cauda equina produces bilateral leg weakness and numbness, loss of sphincter control and loss of sexual potency. The upper level of the motor and sensory disturbance will be determined by the level of the compressing lesion but weakness is usually most marked at the ankles and sensory loss is generally most prominent over the lower sacral dermatomes – the 'saddle' area of the buttocks and perineum. The ankle jerks and anal reflexes are always lost and, depending on the level of the compression, the knee jerks may also be reduced. Any sphincter disturbance is of a lower motor neurone type with a patulous anus and an 'atonic' bladder which dribbles urine.

The common causes of cauda equina compression are a central lumbar disc protrusion, degenerative spondylolisthesis (most often at the L4/5 level) and a tumour. A mild intermittent compression caused by degenerative stenosis of the lumbar canal leads to a syndrome known as *claudication of the cauda equina* (see below). Neoplastic compression of the cauda equina is most often due to an extradural malignant tumour such as a metastasis or a lymphoma. Intradural tumours are much rarer but are important clinically because they are often benign. They include neurofibromas, meningiomas, and ependymomas. The latter arise from ependymal cells within the filum terminale. The symptoms of a benign tumour of the cauda equina are generally insidious in onset and have often been present for a long time before the diagnosis is made. A characteristic feature is back or root pain which is worse on lying down and is relieved by getting up and walking around. This 'night pain' has a relationship to physical activity which is the reverse of that produced by disc protrusion.

The cauda equina compression produced by a lumbar disc protrusion is often fairly abrupt in onset. The sudden onset usually reflects complete extrusion of a nuclear fragment through a tear in the annulus into the spinal canal. A past history of attacks of low back pain or sciatica may give a clue to the diagnosis. The cauda equina compression is generally accompanied by excruciating bilateral sciatica in addition to motor and sensory loss below the affected level. Surgery is a matter of great urgency if there is to be any chance of neurological recovery.

Claudication of the cauda equina

In this condition symptoms of dysfunction of the cauda equina appear on walking or prolonged standing and are relieved by rest. The underlying cause is almost always a *congenital stenosis of the lumbar canal* which has been made worse in middle age by the development of degenerative change. Bulges of the lumbar discs, infolded yellow ligament and enlarged facet joints intrude into the constitutionally narrow lumbar spinal canal so that the contained neural structures suffer mild chronic compression. Stenosis may be over several segments of the lumbar spine or at a single level. If the latter, the L4/5 level is most commonly involved. This is normally the narrowest part of the lumbar canal and is also the level most often affected by spondylolisthesis caused by degenerative arthritis of the facet joints.

Symptoms are generally absent at rest and only appear on walking or prolonged standing. On walking there is friction between the nerve roots and the walls of the tight lumbar canal, whilst standing leads to increased extension of the lumbar spine which has the effect of narrowing the lumbar canal further. The irritation of the cauda equina gives rise to pain which spreads from the lumbar spine to the buttocks and down the back of the legs to the feet.

Often the pain is accompanied by paraesthesiae and numbness which 'marches' over the sacral dermatomes if the patient continues walking or standing. Motor impairment may become manifest as floppiness of the ankles. The differential diagnosis from vascular claudication may be difficult. Both conditions afflict the middle-aged and elderly and may co-exist in the same person. Features suggesting claudication of the cauda equina are the 'march' of the pain, its paraesthetic quality and the fact that on rest the symptoms may take 5–10 min to go away, a much longer period than is required for the symptoms of vascular claudication to evaporate. Sometimes the symptoms disappear more quickly if the patient adopts a position which flexes the lumbar spine such as crouching down on the heels or sitting forward in a chair. The reason for this is that flexion tends to widen the lumbar canal.

There are few physical signs at rest. Root tension signs such as limited straight leg raising or a positive femoral stretch test, are absent and usually the only neurological deficit to be found is absence of the ankle jerks. However, if the patient exercises until symptoms are produced root tension signs and a more extensive neurological disturbance may appear. The only treatment is surgery which should be advised if the symptoms are incapacitating. A complete laminectomy with thorough posterior decompression of the compressed neural structures relieves symptoms in the great majority of cases.

Cervical spondylotic myelopathy

In some elderly people the features of a cervical cord disturbance are found to be associated with the changes of cervical spondylosis. These spondylotic changes include chronic disc bulges with posterior osteophyte formation, infolding of the yellow ligament, facet joint hypertrophy, and minor forward or backward slips of one vertebra on the next. All of these changes may impinge on the cervical spinal canal and it is natural enough to suppose that the myelopathy is caused by chronic spinal cord compression especially as the affected patients tend to have rather narrow cervical canals in addition to the superimposed spondylotic changes. However, at operation the degree of spinal cord compression is often found to be relatively slight in relation to the neurological disturbance and a thorough surgical decompression seldom leads to much neurological recovery. This is in marked contrast to the situation found when the cervical canal is compressed by a longstanding tumour, where cord compression may be very marked before serious neurological disturbance develops and where surgical removal of the compression generally leads to dramatic neurological recovery. To explain this disparity it has been suggested that production of a myelopathy by spondylosis involves more than simple compression. Amongst the other mechanisms that have been postulated are compression of radicular feeding arteries or the anterior spinal artery, and intermittent tractional or frictional stresses from restriction of the normal upward and downward movement of the cervical cord with neck movement.

None of these explanations is entirely satisfactory and it is possible that in many cases the association between the myelopathy and the spondylosis is based on nothing more than coincidence. It has long been recognized that there is a group of middle-aged and elderly patients with a cervical cord disturbance of obscure origin. Inevitably many of these patients will have cervical spondylosis which is common enough in that age group.

Two related conditions, in both of which there is an undoubted relationship between degenerative change of the spine and cord damage, must be differentiated from cervical spondylotic myelopathy. One is acute compression of the cervical cord by a soft disc protrusion. Here compression is indisputably the mechanism involved and surgical removal of the disc protrusion may lead to a gratifying degree of neurological recovery. The other condition is focal spinal cord damage caused by a combination of cervical spondylosis and a hyperextension injury (see page 21.105). Extension of the neck as may happen with a fall forwards onto the face or intubation for anaesthesia, leads to a narrowing of the cervical spinal canal. If the canal is already narrowed by cervical spondylosis, sudden hyperextension may lead to a focal cord contusion. An apparently mild hyperextension injury in an elderly person with cervical spondylosis may lead to severe cord damage in the absence of any cervical fracture or dislocation.

The natural course of cervical spondylotic myelopathy is variable. In a few patients there is progression to severe disability over the course of two or three years, while in others the disorder advances more insidiously, sometimes with episodes of sudden worsening. The most common course is for an initial period of progression, over a matter of a few months or so, followed by a plateau phase of stabilization which may last indefinitely or even be followed by a phase of spontaneous improvement. The unpredictable natural history makes assessment of the results of treatment difficult to say the least.

The predominant symptoms are tingling and weakness of the hands and stiffness and clumsiness of the legs. Any sphincter disturbance is usually slight and sphincter control may be preserved even in advanced cases. Physical examination reveals spasticity of the legs with brisk reflexes and extensor plantar responses. There may be slight weakness of hip flexion and ankle dorsiflexion but interference with gait seems to be caused more by spasticity than by weakness. Sensory loss in the legs is generally minimal or absent. Vibration sense may be impaired but loss of joint position sense is unusual. Any loss of light touch or pinprick sensation is usually patchy and ill defined. In the arms wasting and weakness of the arm muscles is often marked. Again sensory loss is often mild and may be confined to a patchy paraesthetic numbness of the hands and fingers. The arm tendon reflexes are brisk below the level of the spondylosis and are lost at the level of the apparent cord involvement either from interruption of the reflex arc within the cord itself or from associated root compression by osteophytes.

The first treatment to be offered the patient is a cervical collar. It is doubtful if this alters the course of the condition but at least it can do no harm. Few patients wear the collar consistently or tightly enough to limit movements of the neck to any great extent. A few surgeons have argued that surgery in the earlier stages of the disorder produces the best results, as well it may, as such a course means operating on many patients whose natural history would be mild and self-limiting. Most neurosurgeons reserve surgery for those patients where serious progression occurs despite a collar. Even in such patients caution should be exercised when surgery is offered. Neurological worsening after operation is by no means uncommon and there can be few neurosurgeons who have not experienced catastrophes in treating this condition. Two surgical approaches are available. Where the cord disorder seems to be related to spondylosis at multiple levels, and if there is evidence of some generalized stenosis of the spinal canal, then laminectomy over as many segments as is necessary to decompress the cord is carried out. As an addition to this the dura may be opened and the dentate ligaments divided to allow the cord to fall away from anterior osteophytes. If the spondylotic change impinging on the cord is confined to anterior osteophytes at one or two levels, then an anterior cervical decompression and fusion (Cloward operation) is best. The front of the vertebral column is exposed and a cylinder of the affected disc and adjacent bone is drilled out with a special drill. This exposes a circular area of the anterior dura so that disc material and osteophytes can be removed under direct vision. This space is then fused with a bone graft taken from the iliac crest.

There is a wide variation in the reported results of surgery, which may well reflect differences in the selection of patients for operation. On the whole the results of the anterior operation appear best. This may be because patients selected for such operartions are likely to show the best correlation between the level of the spondylotic change and the level of the cord disturbance. In rough terms, 25 per cent of patients improve after surgery while in about a further 50 per cent operation is followed by stabilization of the condition. In the remaining patients the disease continues to progress or the patients are actually worse after operation.

References

Fearnside, M. R. and Adams, C. B. T. (1978). Tumours of the cauda equina, *J. Neurol. Neurosurg. Psychiat.* **41**, 24–31.

Jennett, W. B. (1956). A study of 25 cases of compression of the cauda equina by prolapsed intervertebral discs, *J. Neurol. Neurosurg. Psychiat.* **19**, 109–116.

Kavanagh, G. J., Svien, H. J., Holman, C. B. *et al.* (1968). Pseudoclaudication syndrome produced by compression of the cauda equina, *JAMA*, **206**, 2477–2481.

Marshall, J. (1955). Spastic paraplegia of middle age, *Lancet* **i**, 643–646.

Maurice-Williams, R. S. (1981). *Spinal degenerative disease*. John Wright and Sons, Bristol.

Monro, P. (1984). What has surgery to offer in cervical spondylosis? In *Dilemmas in the management of the neurological patient* (eds C. Warlow and J. Garfield), pp. 168–187. Churchill Livingstone, Edinburgh.

Murphey, F. (1968). Sources and patterns of pain in disc disease, *Clin. Neurosurg.* **15**, 343–351.

——, Simmons, J. C. H. and Brunson, B. (1973). Ruptured cervical discs 1939–1972, *Clin. Neurosurg.* **20**, 9–17.

O'Connell, J. E. A. (1951). Protrusions of the lumbar intervertebral discs. *J. Bone Joint Surg.* **33** B, 8–30.

Shaw. M. D. M., Russell, J. A. and Grossart, K. W. (1978). The changing pattern of spinal arachnoiditis, *J. Neurol. Neurosurg. Psychiat.* **41**, 97–107.

MOTOR NEURONE DISEASE

W. B. MATTHEWS

Synonyms amyotrophic lateral sclerosis – ALS; progressive spinal muscular atrophy; progressive bulbar palsy.

Motor neurone disease (MND) is a degenerative disease of unknown cause that affects predominantly or, in most cases, exclusively, the motor neurones of the spinal cord, the cranial nerve nuclei, and the motor cortex.

Occurrence

Motor neurone disease occurs worldwide, with an incidence of approximately 1:100 000 and a prevalence of 4:100 000. Although occasionally seen in younger patients the disease is rare under the age of 50 years, incidence reaches a peak at age 70 years, with a fall after this age in most studies. Males are more frequently affected in a ratio of 1.5:1, except in progressive bulbar palsy when the sex incidence is equal. About 5 per cent of cases are familial, with a pattern of autosomal dominant inheritance and with a rather earlier age of onset. Areas of much higher incidence are known in Guam and in parts of Japan and New Guinea (but it is not certain that this is the same disease).

Pathology

The impact of the disease is on the anterior horn cells in the spinal cord, the equivalent cells in the lower cranial nerve nuclei, and the neurones of the motor cortex. The affected cells degenerate, first showing chromatolysis and eventually disappearing. The process is gradual and initially focal, but becoming widespread. The oculomotor nuclei are seldom involved and a small island of anterior horn cells in the second sacral segment, the nucleus of Onufrowicz, is also spared. There is no inflammatory reaction. The corticospinal tracts show secondary degeneration, the 'lateral sclerosis' of Charcot's title. Changes beyond the motor system are inconstant and it is not certain that the mild axonal loss in the posterior columns occasionally seen is beyond that encountered in elderly people. The muscles show neurogenic atrophy, with preservation of the muscle spindles, as the fusimotor neurones are not affected.

Clinical features

The commonest presentation is with weakness and wasting of the muscles of one hand. Some more generalized weakness of the arm may be found and, characteristically, fasciculation is present in the muscles of the upper arm and shoulder girdle, often bilaterally. This is seen as irregular rapid contraction of segments of muscle, not moving the limb. Most people experience this as a transient phenomenon, particularly in the calves of the legs, and members of the medical profession may fear that they have MND. Pathological fasciculation, however, is persistent and shifts irregularly from one muscle to another. It may occur in any condition where there has been partial loss of motor neurones but is commonly seen in MND. The pathophysiology is considered in Section 22.

Early in the disease painful cramps are common, particularly in the forearm muscles. Complaints of paraesthesiae or pain are not rare but there are few credible reports of sensory loss. The obvious evidence of lower motor neurone involvement is usually accompanied by a paradoxical increase in tendon reflexes, indicating loss of cortical motor neurones.

A much more difficult diagnostic problem is presented by weakness or wasting involving one lower limb, often with loss of tendon reflexes and suggesting spinal root compression. It is particularly in such cases also that the effect of fatigue on the development of symptoms is most obvious, weakness rapidly increasing on exertion.

Progressive bulbar palsy presents with dysarthria and, a little later, dysphagia. Speech is at first only slightly slurred and there is occasional choking on fluids. These are, however, ominous symptoms, being followed by progressive disability and obvious wasting and fasciculation of the tongue. Flickering of the protruded tongue should not be accepted as fasciculation unless also present when the tongue is lying in the floor of the mouth. Upper motor neurone involvement may be shown by a brisk jaw jerk and the emotional lability of pseudobulbar palsy.

Course

MND is progressive and deterioration is usually obvious to both patient and physician at every visit. The different forms of presentation tend to merge as the disease evolves. The patient with the wasted arm will develop spastic weakness of the legs – the classical amyotrophic lateral sclerosis. Bulbar palsy may be accompanied by widespread fasciculation, first seen in the shoulder girdle. In the form at first recognized as progressive spinal muscular atrophy signs of lower motor neurone disease may predominate throughout the entire course. Increasing weakness of the limbs leads to severe disability. Facial weakness is common but ocular palsy is distinctly rare. Sphincter function is not affected, perhaps because the nucleus of Onufrowicz is spared. Respiratory weakness is a source of particular distress, especially at night. Speech may become unintelligible and mealtimes a misery of choking attacks. Although dementia may occasionally develop the intellect is usually fully preserved to the end.

Apart from a few unconvincing claims of recovery MND is a mortal disease, with a mean duration of between two and four years in different series. Some 20 per cent, however, live for more than five years, and 5 per cent for over ten years. The cases with long duration surprisingly include some presenting with bulbar symptoms which usually carry a particularly bad prognosis. The course in the progressive spinal atrophy form is apt to be relatively prolonged. A variant of MND is sometimes encountered in young adults with very slowly progressive and markedly asymmetrical wasting of the limbs. Familial MND often progresses very rapidly.

Differential diagnosis

In advanced disease the diagnosis is usually all too plain, but some difficulties are encountered in early cases. Dysarthria without wasting of the tongue, or limb weakness developing with fatigue may suggest myasthenia gravis. Dysphagia and dysarthria in this age group are often due to the pseudobulbar palsy of cerebrovascular disease. Wasting and fasciculation of the upper limbs, without sensory loss, can occur in cervical myelopathy but a radicular pattern may be detected. Thyrotoxic myopathy also causes weakness and wasting of the upper limbs and fasciculation may occur although there is no denervation. Asymmetrical weakness and wasting of lower limb muscles without sensory loss can be due to diabetic amyotrophy, a form of peripheral neuropathy. Motor peripheral neuropathy should be suspected with a symmetrical pattern of weakness and persistent absence of signs of upper motor neurone involvement.

MND may occasionally present with progressive spastic weakness of the legs, but in such cases fasciculation can be seen in the arms. The syndrome of dementia and neurogenic muscle wasting occurs in one form of Creutzfeldt-Jakob disease.

Investigation

The results of investigation are sometimes misleading. The serum CK is increased in over 40 per cent of cases, sometimes to very high levels, leading to a mistaken diagnosis of polymyositis. The CSF total protein is significantly raised in about 20 per cent of patients, but there is no cellular reaction. Motor nerve conduction velocity should theoretically be normal in surviving axons, but is sometimes somewhat reduced. Loss of the sensory action potential from the sural nerve, when found in MND, is usually attributed to trauma to the nerve. EMG and muscle biopsy merely confirm the evident neurogenic atrophy.

Pathophysiology

As the α–motor neurones degenerate the muscle fibres they previously supplied are reinnervated by axonal sprouting from surviving motor units. Muscle power can be preserved by reinnervation until some 50 per cent of motor neurones have been lost and sprouting can continue until no more than 5 per cent survive. In MND sprouting is apparently effective but in some patients a serum factor has been found that inhibits sprouting in an animal model of partial denervation. Reduction in muscarinic and glycine receptors in the anterior horn cell layer probably only indicates loss of motor neurones, but the recent report of temporary gain in strength following intravenous thyrotropin-releasing hormone is of greater interest. This hormone is found in nerve endings in the anterior horns and has been considered to be a 'trophic' factor or, presumably, a transmitter between upper and lower motor neurones.

Aetiology

Despite intensive search there are no convincing indications of the cause of this relentless and depressing disease, although many have been suggested. There is no consistent relationship with any systemic disease. Heredity does not play a part in the great majority of cases and no HLA tissue type association has been confirmed. Retrospective case/control studies have shown an increased incidence of physical trauma to the limbs, and a particular relation to electric shock has been claimed in individual cases. The use of vibrating tools at some period in the past is unduly common and there is an increased risk in leather workers, but not in all series. Toxic factors such as lead or selenium are not constantly present. An increased incidence of antecedent paralytic poliomyelitis has been reported, but in most such patients the progressive disease that subsequently develops is much more benign than MND. Attempts to transmit MND to animals have failed and if a 'slow virus' is present it has not been detected.

Treatment

There is no curative or palliative treatment and it is useless to catalogue the failures. Management presents formidable problems. The patient is soon aware of the prognosis and many, but certainly not all, will wish to discuss the future. The isolation resulting from dysarthria may be helped by small electronic printers and similar devices. The diet must be adapted to assist swallowing but eventually dysphagia becomes the major cause of distress. A nasogastric tube is difficult to introduce and a gastrostomy is preferable. Inhalation is the common immediate cause of death. Cricopharyngeal myotomy has been tried with limited success. This muscle is normally in tonic contraction and its section enlarges the pharyngeal opening. Nocturnal respiratory weakness can sometimes be helped by a cuirass respirator in the home. I have never used assisted ventilation by tracheostomy or endotracheal tube as this can only lead to prolongation of an intolerable life, and the final stages demand the use of diamorphine.

References

Brownell, B., Oppenheimer D. R. and Hughes, J. T. (1970). The central nervous system in motor neurone disease. *J. Neurol. Neurosurg. Psychiat.* **33**, 338–357.

Engel, W. K., Siddique, T. and Nicoloff, J. T. (1983). Effect on weakness and spasticity in amyotrophic lateral sclerosis of thyrotropin-releasing hormone. *Lancet* **2**, 73–75.

Kondo, K. and Tsubaki, T. (1981). Case-control studies of motor neuron disease. *Arch. Neurol.* **38**, 220–226.

Kurtzke, J. F. (1982). Epidemiology of amyotrophic lateral sclerosis. *Adv. Neurol.* **36**, 281–300.

Lebo, C. P., Ü, K. S. and Norris, F. H. (1976). Cricopharyngeal myotomy in amyotrophic lateral sclerosis. *Laryngoscope* **86**, 862–868.

Ståhlberg, E. (1982). Electrophysiological studies of reinnervation in ALS. *Adv. Neurol.* **36**, 47–57.

Vejjajiva A., Foster, J. B. and Miller, H. (1967). Motor neuron disease: a clinical study. *J. Neurol. Sci.* **4**, 299–314.

PERIPHERAL NEUROPATHY

P. K. THOMAS

Pathophysiological considerations

The peripheral nerves consist of bundles (fascicles) of unmyelinated and myelinated axons that have their cell bodies in the anterior horns, dorsal root ganglia, or autonomic ganglia. The fascicles are surrounded by a lamellated sheath, the perineurium, which provides a diffusion barrier that separates the intrafascicular or endoneurial compartment from the extracellular tissues. Peripheral nerve trunks usually consist of several fascicles bound together by the mainly collagenous epineurial connective tissue. The nutrient vessels connect with a longitudinal anastomotic network of arterioles and venules in the epineurium. This in turn communicates through the perforating vessels with a longitudinal intrafascicular capillary anastomotic network. This anastomotic system is extremely efficient: experimentally it is very difficult to produce ischaemia of nerve trunks by ligation of nutrient vessels. The occurrence of an ischaemic neuropathy, therefore, implies widespread vascular insufficiency. A blood–nerve barrier comparable to the blood–brain barrier, exists in peripheral nerve (except in the sensory and autonomic ganglia). This, in conjunction with the diffusion barrier provided by the perineurium, probably regulates the composition of the endoneurial connective tissue fluid and thus the ionic environment of the nerve fibres.

All nerve fibres, whether myelinated or unmyelinated, are closely related to satellite cells, the cells of Schwann. There is evidence that they may provide metabolic support for the axons, which often extend for very considerable distances from their perikarya. In myelinated fibres the myelin segments are derived by the spiralling of Schwann cell surface membrane around the axons. The axon is exposed at the nodes of Ranvier, which represent the gaps between adjacent myelin segments. Conduction in unmyelinated axons takes place by the spread of a continuous wave of depolarization, the action potential, that migrates along the axolemma. In myelinated fibres, because of the high electrical resistance of the lipid in the myelin lamellae, the generation of the action potential is restricted to the region of the nodes of Ranvier. Conduction is therefore saltatory, jumping from one node to the next by local currents that traverse the axon and the extracellular tissue fluid. By this means, conduction velocity is increased from about 1 metre per second in unmyelinated axons to 60–70 metres per second in the largest myelinated fibres in human nerve.

The majority of the synthetic mechanisms in neurones are sited in the cell bodies. Synthesized materials are then transported down the axons to the termination of the fibres by an active transport system. This involves a fast system with a rate of about 400 mm per day, and a slow system, in which the structural proteins travel, at 1–2 mm per day. The system is bidirectional: apart from the two anterograde fluxes, there is a retrograde system transporting materials back from the periphery to the cell body. The retrograde system may be involved in the regulation of protein synthesis in the cell body and probably carries the signal for chromatolysis which ensues on transection.

Disorders of peripheral nerve function can be categorized in terms of the site of the primary disturbance. Conditions that lead to the death of the neurone as a whole, with the loss of the cell body and the axon, are categorized as *neuronopathies*. Conditions that have a selective effect on axons are termed *axonopathies*. A selective effect on axonal conduction is seen in poisoning with tetrodotoxin, which blocks the sodium channels at the nodes. Axonopathies may be focal or generalized. Focal axonopathies occur as a result of insults such as trauma or ischaemia. Axonal interruption leads to Wallerian degeneration below the site of the injury. Recovery has to take place by axonal regeneration which is a slow process: the rate of axonal regeneration is about 1–2 mm per day.

Generalized axonopathies often lead to a selective degeneration of the distal portion of the fibres which then extends proximally. The axons are said to 'die back' towards the cell bodies. This pattern is seen in many toxic neuropathies and neuropathies due to nutritional deficiency. It has been suggested that in these conditions, the axonal breakdown may result either from interference with enzymes involved in glycolysis and which provide the metabolic energy for axonal transport mechanisms, or to cofactor deficiency or inactivation. As the enzymes are synthesized in the cell body and then transported down the axons, the further the distance from the cell body the greater will be the likelihood of the occurrence of metabolic insufficiency. This probably accounts for the distal distribution of many such neuropathies, as longer axons will be more vulnerable. Recovery again has to take place by axonal regeneration. In many distal axonopathies that involve the peripheral nervous system, not only does the degeneration affect the distal parts of the motor and sensory axons in the periphery, but the terminal parts of the centrally directed axons derived from the dorsal root ganglion cells also degenerate. Thus degeneration may be found in the rostral portions of the posterior columns. This process has been referred to as *central-peripheral distal axonopathy*. Neuropathy from iminodipropionitrile (IDPN) blocks the slow axonal transport system and leads to large swellings in the proximal parts of the axons that contain aggregations of neurofilaments (proximal axonopathy).

Other neuropathies primarily affect the myelin, either directly, or through an interference with Schwann cell function. The consequence is a selective demyelination with relative preservation of axonal integrity. This may be restricted to the region of the nodes of Ranvier (paranodal demyelination) or involve whole internodal segments (segmental demyelination) with consequent conduction block. The selective myelin damage may occur, for example, as the result of a cell-mediated attack on myelin by sensitized mononuclear cells, which is the likely explanation of the Guillain–Barré syndrome. Another instance is in diphtheritic neuropathy where the demyelination is considered to be secondary to an interference with Schwann cell protein metabolism. Local compression by a tourniquet also gives rise to selective damage to myelin through mechanical effects, although more severe pressure also causes axonal interruption. In diffuse demyelinating neuropathies, the distribution of the clinical effects, as for distal axonopathies, is often maximal peripherally. Presumably, this is a statistical effect: the longer the nerve fibre, the more likely will it be that it develops a region of demyelinating conduction block.

Recovery after paranodal or segmental demyelination occurs by remyelination. Initially, the newly-formed myelin is thin, which results in abnormally slow conduction velocity. Such reductions in conduction velocity may be focal, for example in relation to localized myelin damage in entrapment neuropathies, or widespread as in the Guillain–Barré syndrome or the inherited demyelinating neuropathies. In the latter, motor nerve conduction velocity is sometimes reduced to 10 metres per second or less.

Finally, in other neuropathies the nerve fibres may be secondarily damaged by processes that primarily affect the connective tissues of nerve or the vasa nervorum. Usually a combination of demyelination and axonal loss occurs.

Clinical categories of neuropathy

Mononeuropathy, multiple mononeuropathy, and polyneuropathy
Peripheral neuropathies may be divided into two broad categories depending upon the distribution of the involvement. The first category comprises lesions of isolated peripheral nerves or nerve roots termed *mononeuropathy* or multiple isolated lesions termed *multiple mononeuropathy* ('mononeuritis multiplex'). The lesions in a widespread multiple mononeuropathy may summate to produce a symmetrical disturbance, but the history or a careful examination may indicate the involvement of individual nerves. Isolated or multiple isolated peripheral nerve lesions arise from conditions that produce localized damage, such as mechanical injury, nerve entrapment, thermal, electrical, or radiation injury, vascular causes, granulomatous, neoplastic, or other other infiltrations, and nerve tumours.

Secondly, there may be a diffuse and bilaterally symmetrical disturbance of function which can be designated *polyneuropathy*. When such a process affects the spinal roots, or affects the roots and the peripheral nerve trunks, the terms polyradiculopathy and polyradiculoneuropathy are sometimes employed. In general terms, polyneuropathies result from causes that act diffusely on the peripheral nervous system, such as metabolic disturbances, toxic agents, deficiency states, and certain instances of immune reaction. Isolated nerve lesions may sometimes be superimposed upon a symmetrical polyneuropathy, as a consequence, for example, of pressure lesions in a patient confined to bed. In certain polyneuropathies, there is an abnormal susceptibility to pressure lesions.

Symptomatology
Weakness or paralysis may be due either to a conduction block in the motor nerve fibres or to axonal degeneration. Conduction block is related to demyelination with preservation of axonal continuity (neurapraxia). Recovery may occur by remyelination and may be rapid and complete. This can be the situation in localized nerve lesions, for example, 'Saturday night' paralysis of the radial nerve, or in more widespread polyneuropathies such as in acute idiopathic polyneuropathy (Guillain–Barré syndrome). If axonal interruption takes place, axonal degeneration occurs below the site of interruption. The muscle weakness is accompanied by denervation atrophy, and electromyographic signs of denervation. In a reversible process, recovery has to take place by axonal regeneration which is often slow and incomplete. An important recovery mechanism in conditions in which muscles become partially denervated is re-innervation of denervated muscle fibres by collateral sprouting from the remaining intact axons.

In generalized symmetrical polyneuropathies, the muscle weakness and wasting are commonly peripheral in distribution with an onset in the lower limbs. This results in bilateral footdroop and a 'steppage' gait in which the affected individual lifts his feet to an abnormal extent to avoid catching his toes against the ground. Involvement of the upper limbs begins with weakness and wasting of the small hand muscles and usually weakness of the finger and wrist extensors before the forearm flexor muscles are affected. At times, a symmetrical involvement of the proximal musculature in the limbs occurs in polyneuropathies, for example in the Guillain–Barré syndrome or porphyric neuropathy. Fasciculation due to spontaneous contraction of isolated motor units is most often a feature of anterior horn cell disease but may be encountered in peripheral neuropathies, as may muscle cramps. A rare manifestation of peripheral neuropathy is the occurrence of continuous repetitive discharges in motor nerve fibres leading to generalized muscular rigidity or 'neuromyotonia' (*Isaacs' syndrome*, continuous motor unit activity syndrome). This represents one form of the *'stiff man' syndrome.*

Loss of the tendon reflexes is a frequent accompaniment of a peripheral neuropathy, and usually first affects the ankle jerks. In assessing the clinical findings, it is important to remember that the ankle jerks may be lost in later life, probably as a result of senile changes in the peripheral nerves.

Sensory symptoms and sensory loss in symmetrical polyneuropathies are usually distal in distributiuon, giving rise to the 'glove and stocking' pattern of involvement. Only rarely is a proximal pattern encountered. The sensory loss may affect all modalities or be restricted to certain forms of sensation. If the loss is restricted, two broad patterns are discernible. In the first, the impairment predominantly affects joint position sense, and vibration and touch-pressure sensibility, corresponding to a predominant loss of function in the larger myelinated nerve fibres. Loss of postural sensibility may lead to sensory ataxia in the limbs and to 'pseudo-athetosis', that is, involuntary movements most often of the fingers and hands, that occur for example, when the patient holds his arms outstretched with his eyes closed. In the second pattern of selective sensory loss, pain and temperature sensibility are predominantly affected, often associated with loss of autonomic function, corresponding to a predominant loss of small myelinated and unmyelinated axons. 'Trophic changes' may complicate peripheral neuropathies. The most important factor in their genesis is the loss of the protective effect of pain sensation with the consequent development of persistent ulceration or more extensive tissue loss, most commonly in the feet, and neuropathic joint degeneration.

Paraesthesiae are a frequent feature in peripheral neuropathy. These are usually of a tingling nature ('pins and needles'), but may involve thermal sensations, most often with a burning quality. The paraesthesiae may be aggravated by touching or rubbing the skin. Stimuli that are normally not painful may acquire an unpleasant quality and painful stimuli may give rise to an excessive or hyperpathic response, in which the stimulus, for example a pin prick, is abnormally intense. With repeated stimulation at the same site, the pain that is felt may spread widely and reach an intolerable intensity. An unusual symptom encountered most often in uraemic neuropathy is that of 'restless legs' (*Ekbom's syndrome*). The affected individuals experience sensations in the feet and legs that they find difficult to describe but which are temporarily relieved by movement of the feet and legs. Ekbom's syndrome may also occur in the absence of any detectable disease process.

Spontaneous pains of an aching or lancinating character may complicate a number of generalized polyneuropathies. Severe paroxysms of lancinating pain occur in trigeminal neuralgia, but here the responsible lesion may well lie within the central nervous system. *Causalgia* constitutes a particularly troublesome painful syndrome, most often following gunshot wounds injuring the median nerve, the lower trunk of the brachial plexus, or the tibial nerve. It is a severe persistent pain, often with a burning quality that is characteristically aggravated by emotional factors. Sympathectomy relieves a high proportion of such cases.

Disturbances of autonomic function are occasionally the salient abnormality in a peripheral neuropathy, as in the Riley–Day syndrome, or they may accompany other manifestations, and can be observed both with localized peripheral nerve lesions and in generalized neuropathies.

Diagnosis and investigation

The history and physical examination frequently indicate that the disturbance has affected the peripheral nerves. If confirmation is required, this may usually be obtained by nerve conduction studies. Conduction may be examined in motor and sensory nerve fibres, and can give evidence of both localized and generalized neuropathies. Severely reduced conduction velocity may occur as a result of segmental demyelination or because of conduction in regenerating axons of small calibre after axonal degeneration.

Examination of the cerebrospinal fluid is not commonly of value in the diagnosis of peripheral neuropathies, although the substantially elevated protein content that often occurs in the Guillain–Barré syndrome may be helpful.

Nerve biopsy is rarely required in establishing the existence of a peripheral neuropathy, but may be of diagnostic value in establishing the cause of the neuropathy, particularly in conditions that affect the vasa nervorum or neural connective tissues, or in 'storage' disorders.

Individual nerves

Phrenic nerve (C_{2-4})

This nerve innervates the diaphragm. When the diaphragm is totally paralysed, the normal protrusion of the upper abdomen during inspiration is lost, or is replaced by retraction. Radiographically, paralysis may be detected by unilateral or bilateral elevation of the diaphragm in a chest radiograph and its failure to descend on inspiration. The phrenic nerve may be involved in its course through the neck or thorax by wounds, or tumours such as bronchial carcinoma, and it is sometimes affected in idiopathic brachial plexus neuropathy (neuralgic amyotrophy).

Nerve to serratus anterior (C_{5-7})

The serratus anterior acts as a fixator of the scapula, holding the scapula against the chest wall when forward pressure is exerted by the arm. It is involved in forward movement of the shoulder as in a rapier thrust and in elevation of the arm, when it rotates the scapula. When serratus anterior is paralysed in isolation, the position of the scapula is normal at rest but if the extended arm is pushed forwards against resistance, 'winging' of the scapula becomes evident. The vertebral border, particularly in its lower portion, stands away from the chest wall. The nerve to serratus anterior may be involved in penetrating wounds, but usually in association with damage to the brachial plexus. It may be injured by forcible depression of the shoulder. Serratus anterior weakness is a com-

mon component of idiopathic brachial plexus neuropathy (neuralgic amyotrophy) and it is not infrequently encountered as an isolated and unexplained lesion.

Brachial plexus

The brachial plexus may be affected by penetrating wounds of the neck, in fractures and dislocations of the shoulder and clavicle, as a result of traction on the arm, by pressure from an aneurysm or a cervical rib, and by neoplastic involvement.

Traction lesions

Traction on the arm may result in damage to the plexus itself or may lead to avulsion of the spinal roots from the cord. If the roots are avulsed, sensory nerve action potentials will be preserved if recorded from affected fingers despite total anaesthesia, and the histamine flare response will be preserved in anaesthetic skin. This follows from the fact that the nerve fibres are interrupted proximal to the dorsal root ganglia and therefore the peripheral sensory axons do not degenerate.

In severe traction lesions, commonly encountered in current medical practice as a result of motorcycle accidents, the whole of the plexus may be damaged. With forcible downward displacement of the shoulder, as when someone is thrown forwards and the shoulder strikes against an obstacle, only the upper part of the plexus, involving the contribution from the fifth and sixth cervical nerve roots, may be damaged. This may also be encountered as a birth injury from traction on the head, or on the trunk in a breech presentation (*Erb's palsy*), and rarely in anaesthetized patients during operation or in individuals carrying heavy rucksacks. Selective injury to the lower part of the plexus involving the contributions from the eighth cervical and first thoracic nerve roots occurs as a result of traction with the arm extended, as when an individual falls from a height and tries to save himself by hanging on to a ledge. It may also occur as a birth injury following traction with the arm extended (*Klumpke's paralysis*), but is less common than upper plexus damage.

Selective damage to the upper portion of the plexus (C_5 and C_6 roots or upper trunk) results in paralysis of deltoid, biceps, brachialis, brachioradialis, and sometimes supraspinatus, infraspinatus, and subscapularis. If the roots are avulsed from the cord, the rhomboids, serratus anterior, levator scapulae, and the scalene muscles will be affected. The arm hangs at the side, internally rotated at the shoulder, with the elbow extended and the forearm pronated in the 'waiter's tip' position. Abduction at the shoulder and flexion at the elbow are not possible. The biceps and brachioradialis jerks are lost. Sensory loss affects the lateral aspect of the shoulder and upper arm and the radial border of the forearm. Selective paralysis of the lower brachial plexus ($C_8 T_1$) results in paralysis of all the intrinsic hand muscles and a consequent claw-hand deformity, weakness of the medial finger and wrist flexors, and sensory loss along the medial border of the forearm and hand and over the medial two fingers. Cervical sympathetic paralysis, giving rise to Horner's syndrome, is frequently associated.

When the spinal roots are avulsed from the cord, regeneration is impossible. With total brachial plexus lesions, amputation of the limb may be advisable. Where the injury is distal to the dorsal root ganglia, lesions of the upper portion of the brachial plexus recover more satisfactorily than lower plexus lesions. The value of surgical repair is still a controversial issue. In the Erb's form of birth injury, weakness of abduction at the shoulder and flexion at the elbow often persist although there may be little residual sensory loss. Full recovery takes place in about a third of the cases. It is less likely to occur with lower plexus injuries or if the whole plexus is involved. Early recognition and the application of measures to reduce the risk of joint contractures are important. Surgical treatment is of no value.

Cervical rib

The contribution of the eighth cervical and first thoracic roots to the brachial plexus may be damaged by angulation over an abnormal rib or fibrous band arising from the seventh cervical vertebra and attached to the first rib. Although local structures such as the tendon of scalenus anterior may be involved in the production of symptoms, the isolation of a separate 'scalenus anterior syndrome' or of 'costoclavicular compression' is not justified. The subclavian artery may be affected by cervical ribs giving rise to aneurysmal dilatation and vascular symptoms such as Raynaud's syndrome and embolic phenomena, but the simultaneous occurrence of both neural and vascular phenomena is rare.

Damage to the lower part of the brachial plexus leads to weakness and wasting of the small hand muscles, and of the medial forearm wrist and finger flexors. Occasionally, there is selective wasting of the thenar pad in the hand, mimicking to some extent the appearances of the carpal tunnel syndrome. Numbness, pain, and paraesthesiae occur along the inner border of the forearm and hand, extending into the medial two fingers. The pain tends to be provoked by carrying heavy articles in the hand on the affected side. Horner's syndrome may be a feature. Nerve conduction studies are helpful when there are difficulties in distinguishing a cervical rib syndrome from a lesion of the ulnar or median nerves on clinical grounds. Surgical removal of the rib or fibrous band often leads to abolition of the pain and paraesthesiae, but recovery of power in the small hand muscles is frequently disappointing.

Neoplastic involvement

Tumours may arise locally in the brachial plexus, such as neurofibromata in von Recklinghausen's disease or a solitary neurinoma, or the plexus may be invaded by tumours arising in other structures. In the latter eventuality the commonest situation is involvement of the lower part of the plexus by an apical carcinoma of the lung (*Pancoast's syndrome*), which gives rise to wasting and weakness of the small hand muscles and of the medial forearm wrist and finger flexors, pain and sensory loss affecting the medial border of the forearm and hand, and cervical sympathetic paralysis. Other tumours that may invade the brachial plexus include carcinoma of the breast and malignant lymphomas affecting the lymph glands in the root of the neck.

Idiopathic brachial plexus neuropathy

This condition was not clearly differentiated from the other painful paralytic disorders of the shoulder and upper arm, such as root compression from disc prolapse, until the Second World War. It has been described in a variety of terms, including 'neuralgic amyotrophy' and 'paralytic brachial neuritis'. It may follow immunizing procedures, in particular the administration of antitetanus serum, or operations, or occur without recognizable antecedent event. Occasionally brachial plexus neuropathy is encountered in several members of a family suggesting a genetic predisposition.

The disorder develops acutely with intense pain in the shoulder region which may take some weeks before it subsides completely although generally it ceases after a few days. Paralysis of the muscles of the shoulder girdle becomes evident within a day or two of the onset of the pain, sometimes also of the arms or of the diaphragm. It may be unilateral or bilateral and may be associated with sensory loss. The cerebrospinal fluid is consistently normal. The affected muscles show electromyographic evidence of denervation, but recovery is usually ultimately satisfactory. Not all cases recover fully and recurrences may occur.

The pattern of muscle involvement and sensory disturbances suggests that the condition affects the brachial plexus in a patchy manner. An immune reaction is assumed but not established. The condition takes the same course whether or not it follows an immunizing procedure. Corticosteroids do not influence either the initial pain or the ultimate outcome.

Post-irradiation brachial plexus neuropathy

Brachial plexus damage may occur as a sequel to radiotherapy from breast carcinoma or other tumours in the neck. The onset of symptoms is usually several years after treatment, but may be within months. It can be difficult to distinguish from tumour recurrence but is less likely to be painful.

Radial nerve (C$_{5-8}$)

The long course of the radial nerve and its position in relation to the humerus make this nerve unusually susceptible to external compression. It is a continuation of the posterior cord of the brachial plexus. In the upper arm it supplies triceps and anconeus and the skin on the back of the arm through the posterior brachial cutaneous nerve. The lateral aspect of the lower part of the upper arm is supplied by the lower lateral brachial cutaneous branch and the dorsal aspect of the forearm by the posterior antebrachial cutaneous nerve. Muscular branches of the radial nerve innervate brachioradialis and extensor carpi radialis longus and brevis. The superficial branch of the nerve is its continuation. It descends along the radial border of the forearm and supplies the skin over the dorsum of the hand and the thumb, index, and middle fingers. The deep branch winds around the lateral aspect of the radius, passes through the supinator which it supplies and innervates the extensor digitorum, extensor digiti minimi, extensor carpi ulnaris, and often extensor carpi radialis brevis. Its continuation is the posterior interosseus nerve which supplies the abductor pollicis longus, extensor pollicis longus and brevis, and extensor indicis.

The nerve may be injured in wounds of the axilla so that the paralysis includes triceps, resulting in loss of extension at the elbow. The most frequent type of injury is compression of the nerve in the middle third of the arm against the humerus. This is encountered as '*Saturday night paralysis*' in which an individual falls asleep when intoxicated with his upper arm over the arm of a chair. Triceps is spared, but brachioradialis, supinator, and all the forearm extensor muscles are paralysed. Sensory impairment is limited to the dorsum of the hand. Commonly the lesion consists of a localized conduction block (neurapraxia) so that muscle wasting does not occur and a muscle response can be obtained on stimulation of the nerve below the level of the lesion. Recovery is complete within a matter of weeks. A cock-up wrist splint may be helpful while recovery is awaited. At times, there is some associated axonal degeneration so that electromyographic evidence of denervation is detectable and recovery is correspondingly delayed.

Many muscles supplied by the radial nerve work at a disadvantage when the wrist and finger extensors are paralysed. These defects must not be mistaken for signs of injury to other nerves. Owing to the flexed position of the wrist, gripping is impaired, but if the power of the wrist and finger flexors is tested with the wrist extended, it can be shown to be normal. The action of the interossei in abducting and adducting the fingers is also feeble when the wrist is flexed, but full power is demonstrable if these muscles are tested with the hand resting flat on a table.

The deep branch of the nerve may be injured distal to the supinator muscle. This muscle is, of course, spared, together with brachioradialis and the radial wrist extensors, and there is no sensory loss. A lesion of the posterior interosseus nerve gives rise to weakness confined to abduction and extension of the thumb and extension of the index finger.

Axillary nerve (C$_{5,6}$)

This is a branch of the posterior cord of the brachial plexus. It supplies deltoid and teres minor and the skin over deltoid through the upper lateral brachial cutaneous nerve. It may be damaged in injuries to the shoulder and the chief symptom is an almost complete inability to raise the arm at the shoulder. In the past, it was sometimes injured by pressure from a crutch ('crutch palsy').

Musculocutaneous nerve (C$_{5,6}$)

This nerve is rarely damaged alone, but may be involved in injuries to the brachial plexus. It supplies coracobrachialis, biceps, and brachialis and the skin over the lateral aspect of the forearm through the lateral antebrachial cutaneous nerve. Flexion at the elbow is still possible by brachioradialis, but is weak, and sensation may be impaired along the radial border of the forearm.

Median nerve (C$_{6-8}$ T$_1$)

The median nerve arises from the medial and lateral cords of the brachial plexus and descends with the brachial artery through the upper arm entering the forearm deep to the bicipital aponeurosis. It has no muscular branches above the elbow. It supplies all the muscles in the anterior aspect of the forearm except flexor carpi ulnaris and the medial half of flexor digitorum profundus. The main trunk of the nerve supplies pronator teres, flexor carpi radialis, palmaris longus, and flexor digitorum superficialis. Through the anterior interosseus branch, it also supplies flexor pollicis longus, the lateral aspect of flexor digitorum profundus, and pronator quadratus. The main trunk passes deep to the flexor retinaculum of the wrist and its recurrent muscular branch supplies abductor pollicis brevis, opponens pollicis, and contributes to the innervation of flexor pollicis brevis. It also supplies the lateral two lumbrical muscles and the skin of the lateral aspect of the palm and the lateral three and a half digits over their palmar aspects and terminal parts of their dorsal aspects.

Lesions of the forearm

The median nerve may be injured in the region of the elbow or compressed at the level of the pronator teres muscle. Entrapment neuropathies in the upper forearm, however, are uncommon. Occasionally the anterior interosseus branch is involved in isolation.

Complete lesions of the median nerve at the elbow give rise to paralysis of pronator teres, the radial flexor of the wrist, the long finger flexors except the ulnar half of the deep flexor, most of the muscles of the thenar eminence, and the two radial lumbricals. In brief, there is an inability to flex the index finger and the distal phalanx of the thumb, flexion of the middle finger is weak, and opposition of the thumb is defective. The appearance of the hand has been described as simian; it shows ulnar deviation, the index and middle fingers are more extended than normal, and the thumb lies in the same plane as the fingers.

In more detail, pronation is incomplete and defective. The patient attempts to overcome this by rotating the whole limb at the shoulder. Paralysis of the wrist flexors is evident when attempts are made to flex against resistance. The tendon of flexor carpi ulnaris stands out alone and the hand goes into ulnar deviation. Flexion of the fingers is good in the ulnar two fingers, although weaker than normal. The index finger cannot be flexed, and the middle finger only incompletely. Flexion at the metacarpophalangeal joints is possible in all fingers, including the index, and flexion at these joints with extension at the interphalangeal joints is accomplished by the interossei and lumbricals. If the proximal phalanx of the thumb is immobilized, it will be found that flexion of the terminal phalanx is abolished because of paralysis of flexor pollicis longus. Paralysis of the thenar muscles gives rise to defective abduction and opposition of the thumb. By means of the abductor, the thumb can be drawn into the palm, but as the radial fingers cannot be flexed or the thumb opposed, it is impossible to place the tip of the thumb on the fingers.

Sensory loss is evident over the lateral three and a half digits and the lateral aspect of the palm, although individual variations occur. There is almost complete anaesthesia over the two terminal phalanges of the index and middle fingers. This degree of sensory loss, combined with the motor deficit, renders the thumb and index fingers almost useless and makes paralysis of the median the most serious single nerve lesion in the upper limb.

Vasomotor and trophic changes often ensue. The skin in the distribution of the median nerve tends to become reddened, dry, and atrophic. The pulp of the affected fingers becomes atrophic and ulceration occasionally develops in the tip of the index finger. The nails may become white and atrophic.

After a total transection of the nerve in the region of the elbow,

even with a satisfactory surgical repair, recovery is slow and rarely complete, particularly with respect to the innervation of the hand.

With partial lesions of the median nerve in the arm or forearm, causalgia may be a troublesome consequence. This most often follows gunshot wounds. The pain develops at any time from a few hours to 45 days after the injury. The pain is severe and unremitting, frequently of a burning or smarting quality. Upon this may be superimposed severe paroxysms of pain provoked by touching or jarring the limb or by emotional factors. Vasomotor and sudomotor changes may be associated. The skin usually becomes dry and scaly, but excessive sweating may be a feature. The patient adopts a protective attitude towards the limb, so that fixation of the joints of the fingers and wrist may develop, together with atrophic changes in the skin and subcutaneous tissue. About 80 per cent of cases of true causalgia are relieved by sympathectomy. Untreated, the pain gradually subsides over months or years.

Lesions at the wrist

The superficial situation of the median nerve at the wrist renders it liable to injury in lacerations sustained by falling against a window with the hand outstretched or in suicidal attempts. It may also be damaged as an occupational hazard by individuals who exert repeated pressure on the butt of the hand.

Much the most common lesion at this site is the *carpal tunnel syndrome*, in which the median nerve is compressed as it passes deep to the flexor retinaculum. The usual presentation is with acroparaesthesiae. These consist of numbness, tingling, and burning sensations felt in the hand and fingers, the pain sometimes radiating up the forearm as far as the elbow or even as high as the shoulder or root of the neck. The paraesthesiae are sometimes restricted to the radial fingers, but may affect all the digits as some fibres from the median nerve are distributed to the fifth finger through a communication with the ulnar nerve in the palm. The attacks of pain and paraesthesiae are most common at night and often wake the patient from sleep. They are then relieved by shaking the hand. The hand tends to feel numb and useless on waking in the morning but recovers after it has been used for some minutes. The symptoms may recur during the day following use, or at times if the patient sits with the hands immobile. Such symptoms of acroparaesthesiae may persist for many years without the appearance of symptoms of median nerve damage. In other patients, weakness of the thenar muscles develops, particularly of abduction of the thumb, and is associated with atrophy of the lateral aspect of the thenar eminence (Fig. 1). Sensory loss may appear over the tips of the median innervated fingers. Occasionally patients present with symptoms of median nerve deficit in the hand without attacks of acroparaesthesiae having occurred, or motor and sensory signs may be discovered incidentally in the absence of symptoms, particularly in older individuals.

The symptoms are usually characteristic. If confirmation is required in atypical cases, this can generally be obtained by nerve conduction studies. In patients who are experiencing frequent attacks of acroparaesthesiae, the symptoms may be reproduced by inflating a sphygmomanometer cuff around the arm above arterial pressure for two minutes. At times percussion over the carpal tunnel may elicit a Tinel's sign, or symptoms may be provoked by hyperextension of the wrist.

The majority of cases occur in middle-aged and often obese housewives. In younger women it is commonly associated with excessive use of the hands, and it may develop in males after unaccustomed use of the hands, such as in house-painting. In these instances, tenosynovitis of the flexor tendons is responsible. It may also be caused by tuberculous tenosynovitis at the wrist or involvement of the wrist joint in rheumatoid arthritis. It may develop as a consequence of osteoarthritis of the carpus, perhaps related to an old fracture. Other predisposing causes are pregnancy, myxoedema, acromegaly, and infiltration of the flexor retinaculum in primary amyloidosis.

In cases in which muscle weakness and wasting, or sensory loss,

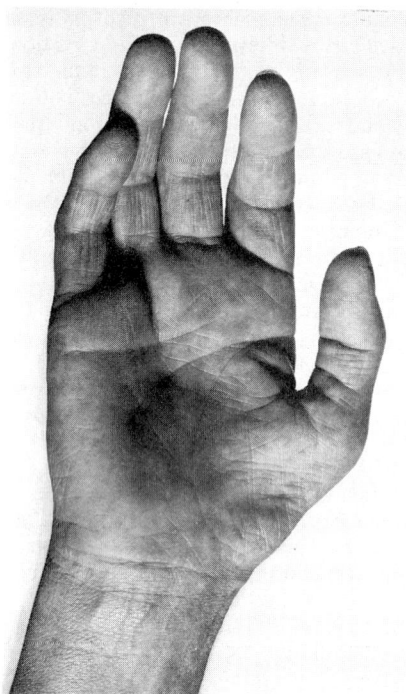

Fig. 1 Thenar wasting in a patient with the carpal tunnel syndrome.

are present when the patient is first seen, treatment should be decompression of the nerve by section of the flexor retinaculum. In patients with acroparaesthesiae alone and in which the cause is probably tenosynovitis at the wrist, reduction in the amount of activity engaged in with the hands may be sufficient to allow the symptoms to subside. Injection of the carpal tunnel with a long-acting hydrocortisone preparation may give temporary relief. Splinting of the wrist to reduce movement during the day may also be useful. If the symptoms persist despite conservative measures, decompression is then advisable.

The majority of patients with acroparaesthesiae are relieved by decompression. In patients with sensory impairment and cutaneous hyperaesthesia, such symptoms may persist for prolonged periods and if denervation of the thenar muscles has been present for any length of time, recovery may not occur.

Ulnar nerve (C$_{7,8}$ T$_1$)
This nerve arises from the medial cord of the plexus, usually with a contribution from the lateral cord. It descends in the medial side of the upper arm, passes around the elbow in the ulnar groove and enters the forearm under an aponeurotic band between the humeral and ulnar heads of flexor carpi ulnaris. It then runs superficial to flexor digitorum profundus to the wrist and enters the hand between the pisiform bone and the hook of the hamate, superficial to the flexor retinaculum. After penetrating the hypothenar muscles, its deep branch crosses the palm and ends in the flexor pollicis brevis.

In the upper arm, branches arise that supply flexor carpi ulnaris and the medial part of flexor digitorum profundus. In the forearm, the dorsal branch arises that winds around the ulna and supplies the skin over the dorsal aspect of the hand and the medial one and a half fingers. In the hand, a superficial branch supplies palmaris brevis and the skin over the medial aspect of the palm and the medial one and half fingers. The deep branch, after supplying the hypothenar muscles, innervates the interossei, the third and fourth lumbricals, the adductor pollicis, and part of flexor pollicis brevis.

Lesions at the elbow
Total paralysis from lesions at this level, including the branches to flexor carpi ulnaris and flexor digitorum profundus, gives rise to

wasting along the medial side of the forearm flexor mass. There is weakness of flexion of the fourth and fifth fingers. If the proximal portions of these fingers are held immobilized, flexion of the terminal phalanges is not possible. When the hand is flexed to the ulnar side against resistance, the tendon of flexor carpi ulnaris is not palpable. Paralysis of the hypothenar muscles abolishes abduction of the fifth finger. Paralysis of the interossei and the medial two lumbricals gives rise to the 'claw-hand' deformity (Fig. 2). The action of these muscles is to flex the fingers at the metacarpophalangeal joints with the fingers extended at the interphalangeal joints. In the claw hand, the posture of the fingers is opposite to this, namely, extension of the metacarpophalangeal joints with flexion at the interphalangeal joints. Although all the interossei are paralysed, the defect is seen mainly in the ulnar fingers since the radial lumbricals supplied by the median nerve are still active. The long extensors of the fingers, being unopposed, overextend the proximal joints, and the flexor digitorum superficialis flexes the proximal interphalangeal joints.

In the hand, there is wasting of the hypothenar muscles, of the interossei, and the medial part of the thenar eminence. Movements of abduction and adduction of the fingers are weak, as is adduction to the extended thumb against the palm. Sensory loss affects the dorsal and palmar aspects of the medial side of the hand and the medial one and a half fingers.

The ulnar nerve may be damaged by dislocations or fracture dislocations at the elbow and is sometimes compressed in individuals who habitually lean on their elbows. Entrapment may occur in the cubital tunnel as the nerve underlies the aponeurotic band between the two heads of the flexor carpi ulnaris. This is most likely to occur in heavy manual workers or if there is an excessive carrying angle at the elbow, as may occur following a previous malunited supracondylar fracture of the humerus ('tardy ulnar palsy'). The medial wall of the cubital tunnel is formed by the elbow joint; osteoarthritis of the elbow can lead to osteophytic encroachment on the tunnel and compression of the ulnar nerve. In the cubital tunnel syndrome, the ulnar nerve is often palpably enlarged in the ulnar groove and for a short distance proximally. Ulnar nerve lesions are not infrequent in leprosy. Here the

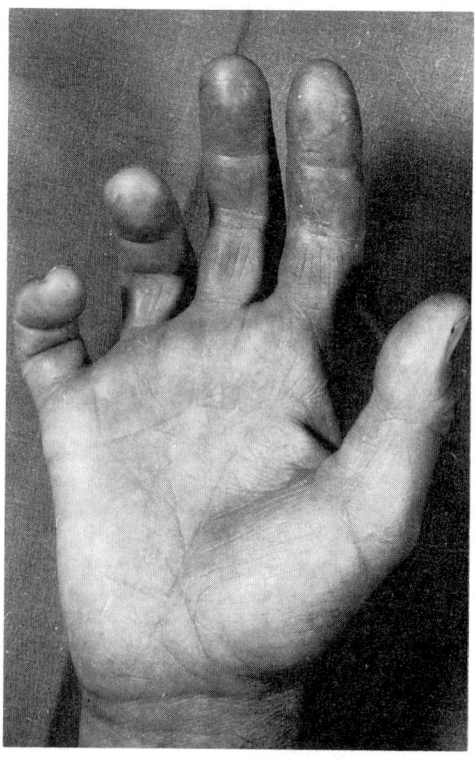

Fig. 2 Claw-hand deformity in a patient with an ulnar nerve lesion.

enlargement of the nerve tends to be maximal at a little distance above the elbow.

When it is suspected that the nerve has been subjected to repeated compression at the elbow, surgical transposition to the front of the medial epicondyle should be considered. If the nerve is compressed in the cubital tunnel, decompression by slitting the aponeurosis may suffice.

Lesions at the wrist or in the hand

Damage to the nerve at the wrist will spare the dorsal branch, so that cutaneous sensation over the dorsum of the hand and fingers is spared. A lesion just proximal to the wrist will give rise to sensory impairment on the palmar aspect of the hand and fingers alone, and weakness of all the ulnar-innervated intrinsic hand muscles. A slightly more distal lesion spares the superficial branch of the nerve and therefore produces no sensory deficit. Finally, damage to the deep palmar branch spares the hypothenar muscles, but causes weakness of the other ulnar-innervated small hand muscles. Lesions at the wrist or in the hand are usually the result of compression by ganglia or by repeated occupational trauma. Damage to the deep palmar branch, for example, may be caused by firm pressure from a screwdriver or drill. If occupational pressure is the cause, recovery follows cessation of the precipitating cause. Should improvement fail to occur after an appropriate interval, surgical exploration to establish whether a ganglion is present is merited.

It is not always easy on clinical grounds to decide whether the lesion is at the elbow or the wrist. Compression of the nerve in the cubital tunnel, for example, may spare the branches of the flexor carpi ulnaris and flexor digitorum profundus. In these circumstances, nerve conduction studies may be helpful, as they may in distinguishing between lesions of the ulnar nerve and damage to the eighth cervical and first thoracic spinal roots.

Lumbosacral plexus

Lesions of the lumbosacral plexus are not common. The plexus may be involved in pelvic malignancy, such as from carcinoma of the cervix, bladder, prostate, or rectum, or be the site of a local neural tumour. It may be compressed by a haematoma in patients receiving anticoagulant therapy or suffering from haemophilia, or be involved in fractures of the pelvis. The lumbosacral cord may be compressed against the rim of the pelvis by the fetal head during parturition, with consequent weakness of the anterior tibial and peroneal muscles, and sensory impairment in the distribution of the fourth and fifth lumbar dermatomes. The superior gluteal nerve may also be affected. Recovery is initially good but may not be complete. Rare instances of idiopathic lumbosacral plexus neuropathy are encountered, comparable to the corresponding disorder that affects the brachial plexus.

Femoral nerve (L$_{2-4}$)

This nerve arises from the lumbar plexus, crosses the iliac fossa between the psoas and iliacus muscles, and enters the thigh deep to the middle of the inguinal ligament. In the iliac fossa it supplies the iliacus, and in the thigh, pectineus, sartorius, and quadriceps femoris, and anterior cutaneous branches to the front of the thigh. The continuation of the femoral nerve is the saphenous which supplies the skin over the medial aspect of the lower leg as far as the medial malleolus.

Damage to the femoral nerve causes weakness of knee extension, wasting of the quadriceps, loss of the knee jerk, and sensory impairment over the front of the thigh and in the distribution of the saphenous nerve. With a proximal lesion, there may also be weakness of hip flexion from paralysis of iliacus.

The femoral nerve may be injured in fractures of the pelvis or femur, in dislocations of the hip, and at times during operations on the hip. It may be involved by psoas abscesses, tumours, or implicated in wounds of the thigh. It is commonly involved in large psoas muscle haematomas in haemophiliacs (see Section 19).

Owing to the rapid dispersion of the branches in the thigh, partial lesions are common from wounds at this site. The nerve to quadriceps is most often injured. The resulting paralysis causes considerable difficulty in walking as the knee cannot be locked in extension and gives way, especially when descending stairs. The saphenous nerve is sometimes damaged in operations for the treatment of varicose veins.

Obturator nerve (L$_{2-4}$)

The nerve emerges from the lateral border of psoas, crosses the lateral wall of the pelvis, and enters the thigh through the obturator foramen where it supplies gracilis, adductor longus and brevis, adductor magnus, obturator externus, and sometimes also pectineus, and the skin over the lower medial aspect of the thigh.

Damage to the obturator nerve results in weakness of adduction and internal rotation at the hip, pain in the groin, and sensory impairment on the medial part of the thigh. The nerve may be involved in neoplastic infiltration in the pelvis and can be damaged by the fetal head or by forceps during parturition.

Lateral cutaneous nerve of the thigh (L$_{2,3}$)

This nerve arises from the lumbar plexus, passes obliquely across iliacus and enters the thigh under the lateral part of the inguinal ligament. It supplies the skin over the anterolateral aspect of the thigh.

Meralgia paraesthetica is an entrapment neuropathy resulting from compression of this nerve as it passes under the inguinal ligament. It is more common in men, who are often obese, and may be unilateral or bilateral. The symptoms consist of numbness in the territory of the nerve combined with tingling or burning paraesthesiae provoked by prolonged standing, or following excessive walking. Weight reduction may be helpful and in many instances the condition subsides spontaneously. Decompression of the nerve is rarely necessary.

Sciatic nerve (L$_{4,5}$ S$_{1-3}$)

The sciatic nerve enters the thigh through the sciatic notch. It is composed of the tibial and peroneal divisions which are usually bound together within a common sheath. It descends the posterior aspect of the thigh, initially deep to gluteus maximus and supplies semitendinosus, semimembranosus, and the long head of biceps through its peroneal division. It separates into the tibial and common peroneal nerves in the lower thigh, which supply all the muscles below the knee, and both nerves contribute to the formation of the sural nerve.

Total interruption of the sciatic nerve gives rise to foot drop. Walking is possible, but the patient cannot stand on the toes or the heel of the affected foot and the ankle is unstable. All movement below the knee is paralysed. If the injury is in the upper thigh, flexion of the knee is also weak. The skin is completely anaesthetic over the entire foot except for the medial border which is supplied by the saphenous nerve. Pressure sores may develop. The anaesthesia extends upwards on the posterolateral aspect of the calf in its lower two-thirds. Joint position sense is abolished in the foot and toes. Beyond this area of complete anaesthesia, there is a wide zone in which sensibility may be diminished. Sweating is absent on the sole and dorsum of the foot, but is preserved on the medial side. The ankle jerk is lost but the knee jerk is retained.

The sciatic nerve may be involved in pelvic tumours or injured by fractures of the pelvis or femur. After the radial and ulnar, it is implicated in gunshot wounds more frequently than any other nerve. Partial injury of the tibial division may be followed by causalgia. Incomplete lesions of the nerve may be caused by pressure of the nerve against the hard edge of a chair in individuals who fall asleep while intoxicated. Similar lesions may occur in diabetic subjects, in whom the peripheral nerves are more susceptible to pressure neuropathy.

The syndrome of root pain and sciatica is considered on page 21.113.

Tibial nerve (L$_{4,5}$ S$_{1-3}$)

After separating from the peroneal division of the sciatic nerve in the lower thigh, this nerve passes through the popliteal fossa and enters the calf deep to gastrocnemius through the fibrous arch of soleus. It descends through the calf to the medial side of the ankle, passes beneath the flexor retinaculum, and divides into the medial and lateral plantar nerves. It supplies the popliteus, all the muscles of the calf, and through the plantar nerves, the small muscles of the sole of the foot and sensation to the sole.

When the nerve is interrupted, the patient is unable to plantar-flex or invert the foot, or flex the toes. He cannot stand on the ball of the foot. Paralysis of the interossei leads to a claw-like deformity of the toes. Sensation is lost over the sole. Causalgia may arise after partial lesions. Injury to the distal portion of the nerve by a penetrating injury or deep wound of the calf gives rise to paralysis of the intrinsic muscles of the foot but spares the muscles acting at the ankle. Sensation is lost on the sole of the foot and this may be accompanied by pain. If the injury is distal to the origin of the branches to flexor hallucis longus and flexor digitorum longus, the lesion may escape detection since paralysis of the small foot muscles and sensory loss over the sole may be overlooked.

The tibial nerve is occasionally compressed under the flexor retinaculum (*tarsal tunnel syndrome*), usually precipitated by osteoarthritis or post-traumatic deformities at the ankle or by tenosynovitis. Burning pain and tingling paraesthesiae occur in the sole, usually following prolonged standing or walking. The condition is generally unilateral. Careful examination may demonstrate wasting of the intrinsic muscles in the medial aspect of the foot, and sensory impairment over the sole. Nerve conduction studies may be diagnostically helpful. Treatment is by surgical section of the flexor retinaculum.

Painful neuromas sometimes develop on the digital branches of the plantar nerves. These give rise to the syndrome of *Morton's metatarsalgia* in which pain occurs in the anterior part of the foot on standing. A localized area of tenderness is detectable on palpation. The condition is relieved by excision of the neuroma.

Common peroneal nerve (L$_{4,5}$ S$_{1,2}$)

After separating from the tibial division of the sciatic nerve in the lower part of the thigh, this nerve descends through the popliteal fossa, winds around the neck of the fibula, and divides into its superficial and deep branches. The superficial peroneal nerve passes down in front of the fibula, supplies peroneus longus and brevis, and emerges in the lower leg. It crosses the extensor retinaculum and supplies the skin on the dorsum of the foot and the second to the fifth toes. The deep peroneal branch continues to wind around the fibula, pierces the anterior intermuscular septum, and descends on the anterior interosseous membrane. It innervates tibialis anterior, extensor hallucis longus, extensor digitorum longus, and peroneus tertius. It passes deep to the extensor retinaculum where it supplies the extensor digitorum brevis and the skin of the adjacent sides of the first and second toes.

Damage to the common peroneal nerve is more frequent than injury to its two branches because of its vulnerable superficial position at the neck of the fibula. It gives rise to foot drop with paralysis of dorsiflexion and eversion at the ankle and of toe extension. Cutaneous sensation is impaired over the lateral aspect of the lower leg and ankle and on the dorsum of the foot.

The common peroneal nerve may be compressed at the neck of the fibula by habitual sitting with the legs crossed, prolonged squatting, pressure during sleep or while anaesthetized, and various other events. It can be damaged by traction caused by fractures of the tibia and fibula and is sometimes damaged by ischaemia in the anterior tibial syndrome. Paralysis caused by external pressure frequently gives rise to a local conduction block (neurapraxia) with satisfactory recovery within a few weeks. If electromyography indicates that nerve degeneration has taken place a foot drop support should be provided while axonal regeneration is awaited.

Sural nerve (L$_5$ S$_{1-2}$)

This arises from the sciatic nerve and descends to the back of the calf, winds around to the lateral side of the ankle and reaches the lateral border of the foot. It supplies the skin in this distribution. Sensory impairment occasionally results from pressure on the nerve as it lies in a superficial situation in the back of the calf.

Generalized neuropathies

Neuropathies related to metabolic and endocrine disorders

Diabetes mellitus

A significant degree of peripheral neuropathy develops in about 15 per cent of patients with diabetes, although a substantially greater number either have minor symptoms without signs, or evidence of a subclinical neuropathy either on clinical examination or on the basis of abnormalities of nerve conduction. In general, the neuropathies that appear can be divided into symmetrical sensory polyneuropathies and autonomic neuropathies on the one hand, and isolated peripheral nerve lesions or multiple mononeuropathies on the other. Mixed syndromes are common.

The commonest form is a mild symmetrical *sensory polyneuropathy*, giving rise to numbness and tingling paraesthesiae in the toes and feet and less often in the fingers. Aching or lancinating pains in the feet and legs, particularly at night, may be a troublesome feature. Examination reveals loss of vibration sense in the feet, depression of the ankle jerks, and mild distal cutaneous sensory impairment. More rarely a more severe sensory neuropathy develops, sometimes referred to as 'diabetic pseudotabes'. Loss of pain sense results in perforating ulcers on the feet and neuropathic joint degeneration, particularly in the toes and in the tarsal joints; impaired postural sense gives rise to an ataxic gait. An acute painful diabetic neuropathy also occurs that predominantly affects the lower limbs. The onset is often associated with poor diabetic control and precipitate weight loss ('diabetic neuropathic cachexia').

Autonomic neuropathy frequently accompanies the sensory neuropathy and may be the salient manifestation. It rarely occurs in isolation. Pupillary disturbances usually take the form of a reduced response to light, but changes of Argyll Robertson type may be present. Gustatory sweating on the face is probably due to aberrant regeneration. Anhidrosis may occur distally in the limbs; if it is extensive and also affects the trunk, heat intolerance may result. Symptoms referable to the alimentary tract include dysphagia from oesophageal involvement, episodes of vomiting related to gastric atony, and episodic nocturnal diarrhoea, often alternating with periods of constipation. Those related to the genito-urinary system include impotence, retrograde ejaculation, and bladder atony with difficulty in voiding and urinary retention with overflow. Vascular denervation sometimes results in postural hypotension, and cardiac denervation may be demonstrable by an elevated resting heart rate and the absence of beat-to-beat variation with respiration.

Isolated nerve lesions tend to occur more commonly in elderly diabetic subjects. At times they develop insidiously, at others they have an abrupt onset with pain. Of the cranial nerves, the nerves to the external ocular muscles, particularly the third, and also the facial nerve, are the most often affected. In contradistinction to the effects of compression of the third nerve by a carotid aneurysm, the pupillary innervation is often spared. In the limbs, the lesions tend to occur at the common sites of compression or entrapment. It seems likely that diabetic nerve exhibits an excessive vulnerability to damage from pressure.

Diabetic amyotrophy represents a particular example of a multiple mononeuropathy that develops usually in elderly obese diabetics. It consists of an asymmetrical proximal motor syndrome that affects the anterior thigh muscles and hip flexors, and sometimes also the anterolateral muscles of the lower leg. Less commonly it is symmetrical. Its onset may be acute or insidious and is often accompanied by pain, particularly at night. There is generally little or no associated sensory loss. The knee jerks are usually depressed or absent.

The causation of diabetic neuropathy is uncertain. It tends to occur more often in poorly controlled diabetics, but the correlation is not close. It may occur for the first time on initiation of treatment with insulin, or be the presenting symptom in maturity onset diabetes. There is evidence to suggest that diabetic microangiopathy is important in the genesis of isolated nerve lesions. Probably metabolic factors are more important in the origin of the symmetrical polyneuropathies, but their nature is uncertain. An increased concentration of sorbitol and a reduced concentration of myoinositol, both secondary to hyperglycaemia, may be involved in causing nerve fibre dysfunction.

Focal peripheral nerve lesions and diabetic amyotrophy, if of acute onset, often recover adequately, as does acute painful neuropathy when satisfactory control is achieved. The symmetrical sensory and autonomic neuropathy, once established, recovers less satisfactorily, even with good diabetic control, including the use of insulin pumps. Trials of aldose reductase inhibitors to reduce sorbitol accumulation, or of dietary myoinositol supplementation, have so far not given clear evidence of improvement in neuropathy. Pain may sometimes be helped by carbamazepine or by a combination of a tricyclic antidepressant and a phenothiazine.

Amyloidosis

The various forms of amyloid disease are described in Section 9. The peripheral nerves may be involved in primary amyloidosis and in amyloidosis related to myeloma. There are also several dominantly inherited forms of amyloid neuropathy, the most important being the Portuguese type. Isolated lesions may occur from the infiltration of amyloid into nerves or from compression of the median nerve in the carpal tunnel because of deposits in the flexor retinaculum. More strikingly, a generalized neuropathy may develop. It begins with selective loss of pain and temperature sensation in the feet and later in the hands. Motor involvement, loss of tendon reflexes, and impairment of other sensory modalities occur later. Autonomic involvement is an early feature, causing impotence, postural hypotension, bladder atony, and disturbances of alimentary function. Amyloid deposits are present in the peripheral nerve trunks, which may be enlarged, and in the dorsal root and sympathetic ganglia.

No treatment influences the progress of the neuropathy. The spontaneous pains are sometimes improved by carbamazepine. Care must be taken to prevent damage to the anaesthetic feet, lower legs, and hands.

Uraemia

Uraemic neuropathy did not become a clinical problem until the advent of treatment of endstage renal failure by haemodialysis. It occurs in patients with severe chronic renal failure, and is most often seen in patients under treatment with periodic haemodialysis. The symptoms are usually predominantly sensory, with numbness and tingling paraesthesiae in the feet. 'Restless legs' (*Ekbom's syndrome*) are often a conspicuous feature (see Section 22). A distal motor neuropathy may be associated and occasional cases are purely motor. The condition is improved by increased haemodialysis and more dramatically by renal transplantation. A retained metabolite is assumed to be the cause, but this has not so far been identified.

Myxoedema (see Section 10)

Compression of the median nerve in the carpal tunnel in myxoedema has already been discussed. Rarely a generalized mixed motor and sensory neuropathy develops. This improves on treatment of the hypothyroidism.

The slow contraction and relaxation observed in the tendon reflexes is not due to a disturbance of peripheral nerve function, but to an alteration in the contractile mechanism of the muscle fibres.

Acromegaly (see Section 10)

The occurrence of the carpal tunnel syndrome in acromegaly has also been mentioned. A rare manifestation of this condition is a sensorimotor polyneuropathy in which the peripheral nerves are thickened because of an overgrowth of the neural connective tissues. A similar neuropathy is occasionally observed in pituitary gigantism.

Other metabolic disorders

It has been claimed that a generalized peripheral neuropathy may be caused by either acute or chronic hepatic failure, but this is probably uncommon. A mild painful sensory neuropathy is occasionally encountered in primary biliary cirrhosis, sometimes related to xanthomatous deposits in the cutaneous nerve trunks. A motor neuropathy is a rare sequel to severe recurrent hypoglycaemia.

Toxic neuropathies
Industrial and environmental subtances

Acrylamide This substance is now widely employed industrially. The monomer is neurotoxic and causes peripheral neuropathy with mixed motor and sensory features. Ataxia is prominent and is possibly the result of concomitant cerebellar damage. Axonal degeneration affecting the periphery of the fibres occurs and slow recovery takes place on cessation of exposure.

Arsenic Arsenical poisoning is occasionally seen as a result of accidental or homicidal ingestion of insecticides containing arsenic, or from indigenous medicines in India. Gastrointestinal symptoms develop after acute ingestion, followed by a mixed sensory and motor neuropathy after one to three weeks. Desquamation of the skin of the feet and hands takes place after about six weeks and white lines (Mees' lines) appear in the nails. With ingestion of smaller quantities on a chronic basis, gastrointestinal symptoms are less obtrusive and a slowly progressive neuropathy makes its appearance. The skin may become generally pigmented or show focal 'raindrop' pigmentation, and hyperkeratosis of the palms of the hands and soles of the feet may appear.

Slow recovery in the neuropathy occurs with removal from exposure. Chelating agents are of value in treating the non-neurological complications, but it is uncertain whether they are effective for the neuropathy.

Lead Lead neuropathy is now a rare occurrence in Britain, although it is encountered as a consequence of the contamination of drinking water by lead pipes in old buildings. Subclinical neuropathy may be detectable in lead workers. It remains a hazard in certain parts of the world from the use of lead glazes in pottery. Lead neuropathy is predominantly motor, typically giving rise to wrist and foot drop. The 'lead colic' that may occur is probably a manifestation of autonomic involvement. Other features of lead poisoning that may be associated include a sideroblastic anaemia and a 'lead line' on carious teeth. The neuropathy improves on cessation of lead intake; the utility of treatment with BAL, edetate, or penicillamine is uncertain.

Mercury Exposure to inorganic mercury salts and to organic mercurial compounds may lead to neurological damage, as in 'Minamata disease' which was related to consumption of fish contaminated by organic mercury. Dementia, cortical blindness, and ataxia occur, together with sensory changes in the limbs attributed to a sensory neuropathy, although how far these have a peripheral origin is uncertain. Historically, a peripheral neuropathy was an important component of 'pink disease' which was caused by the administration of mercury-containing purgatives.

Thallium This is present in certain pesticides and rodent poisons and was formerly used as a depilatory agent. Accidental or homicidal poisoning is occasionally encountered. Abdominal pain and diarrhoea are followed after two or five days by the development of a mixed motor and sensory neuropathy which is often painful.

Evidence of central nervous system damage may be present with behaviour disorder, optic neuropathy, and choreiform movements. Alopecia develops later, after about two or three weeks, and renal damage may be produced. Diethyldithiocarbamate, which binds thallium, has been employed in treatment.

Triorthocresyl phosphate (TOCP) This substance is used industrially as a high-temperature lubricant. Outbreaks of a sensori-motor neuropathy, often accompanied by evidence of CNS damage, occur periodically, usually as a consequence of the contamination of cooking ingredients or utensils. The original description was in relation to illegal liquor distillation (ginger jake paralysis) in the USA during the prohibition era. In more recent years, a large outbreak occurred in Morocco from the use of contaminated cooking oil. Recovery is slow and often incomplete.

Other industrial substances Carbon disulphide, used in the manufacture of rayon, occasionally gives rise to a mild sensory neuropathy. Neuropathy may occur as a result of industrial exposure to the organic solvents *n*-hexane and methyl *n*-butyl ketone. The former is also encountered as a consequence of 'glue-sniffing'; *n*-hexane, which has an intoxicant action, has been used as a solvent in certain glues. An extensive outbreak of a multisystem disorder in which neuropathy was the main manifestation recently occurred in Spain, related to the consumption of adulterated rapeseed oil. The precise toxic substance was not identified.

Iatrogenic

Isoniazid A mixed motor and sensory neuropathy may be produced by isoniazid and is more likely to occur in individuals who acetylate the drug slowly. The neuropathy is related to an interference with pyridoxine metabolism. Axonal degeneration occurs in the peripheral nerves. The neuropathy recovers slowly on cessation of administration of the drug and may be prevented by giving pyridoxine, which does not interfere with the antituberculous action of the isoniazid.

Nitrofurantoin Excessively high blood levels of this preparation, as may occur in patients with reduced renal function, can cause a mixed motor and sensory neuropathy.

Vincristine A neuropathy will occur in all subjects if sufficient amounts of this cytotoxic agent are administered. Mild sensory symptoms and loss of tendon reflexes may have to be accepted if a satisfactory therapeutic effect of the drug is to be achieved. If the neuropathy advances, bilateral weakness of the extensors of the wrist and fingers develops, followed by more widespread weakness. The neuropathy improves satisfactorily if the drug is withdrawn or if the dosage is reduced.

Other substances Less important drugs that may give rise to neuropathy are metronidazole, misonidazole, cisplatinum, perhexilene, disulphiram, gold, nitrous oxide (with a myelopathy) and tricyclic antidepressant drugs. A mild sensory neuropathy may develop after prolonged administration of phenytoin and neuropathy was one of the complications produced by thalidomide. Pyridoxine, if taken in large doses, as 'megavitamin therapy', causes a sensory neuropathy.

Deficiency neuropathies
Beri beri neuropathy (see also Section 8)
This disorder is predominantly encountered in populations subsisting on diets composed largely of polished rice, but a similar neuropathy may be observed in other malnourished communities. Thiamine deficiency is probably involved, but a deficiency of other vitamins of the B group may also be implicated. A distal motor and sensory neuropathy develops which is frequently accompanied by spontaneous aching pain in the extremities, cutaneous hyperaesthesia, and tenderness of the soles of the feet and calves. Involvement of the recurrent laryngeal nerves may lead to hoarseness of the voice. The neuropathy may be associated with a cardio-

myopathy ('wet beri beri'). Thiamine deficiency is established by the finding of reduced erythrocyte transketolase activity. This enzyme requires thiamine as a cofactor.

Axonal degeneration occurs in the peripheral nerves and slow recovery ensues with vitamin replacement.

Strachan's syndrome
Strachan's syndrome, originally described in Jamaica but also observed in other parts of the world under conditions of nutritional deficiency, is characterized by the combination of a painful sensory neuropathy with amblyopia and at times deafness, in association with an orogenital dermatitis. It is assumed to be due to B vitamin deficiency, but the precise deficit has not been identified.

Alcoholic neuropathy
This always occurs on a background of nutritional deficiency. The dietary intake of the alcoholic is high in carbohydrates and low in vitamins. Moreover, alcoholics are known to have a reduced capacity to absorb thiamine. A direct toxic effect of alcohol on peripheral nerve may also be involved. The clinical features of alcoholic neuropathy are similar to those of beri beri. Other deficiency states may coexist, such as the Wernicke–Korsakoff syndrome. Improvement may take place with vitamin replacement, but it is beset with the usual difficulties met in treating alcoholic patients.

Pyridoxine deficiency
Attention has already been drawn to the fact that isoniazid neuropathy is related to an interference with pyridoxine metabolism. Pyridoxine deficiency may contribute to the neuropathy that occurs in nutritional deficiency states, and possibly accounts for the mild neuropathy of pellagra.

Pantothenic acid deficiency
Experimental deficiency of pantothenic acid in human volunteers is known to give rise to a sensory neuropathy, and the administration of pantothenic acid has been reported to alleviate the *'burning feet' syndrome* which sometimes develops in deficiency states.

Vitamin B$_{12}$ deficiency
Vitamin B$_{12}$ deficiency from whatever cause, may be responsible for the development of a distal sensory neuropathy, with 'glove and stocking' sensory loss and paraesthesiae, and areflexia, either in isolation or in association with a myelopathy or other central nervous system manifestations. Haematological changes are not always present. The peripheral neuropathy improves more satisfactorily with treatment than the central disturbances. This condition is considered in detail on page 21.101.

A peripheral neuropathy is one component of *Nigerian ataxic neuropathy*, in which the other features are posterior column degeneration, sensorineural deafness, and optic atrophy. It has been suggested that an interference with vitamin B$_{12}$ metabolism by cyanide derived from cassava in the diet, combined with nutritional deficiency, may be responsible. This condition is considered further on page 21.274.

Chronic severe vitamin E deficiency has recently been established as a cause for peripheral neuropathy in combination with a spinocerebellar degeneration. This may occur in abetalipoproteinaemia, congenital biliary atresia, cystic fibrosis, and occasional adults with chronic intestinal malabsorption.

Inflammatory and post-infective neuropathies
Leprous neuropathy
Peripheral nerve involvement in leprosy is considered in Section 5.

Acute idiopathic inflammatory polyneuropathy (Guillain–Barré syndrome)
This disorder is characterized by a polyneuropathy which develops acutely over the course of a few days, or sometimes more insi-

diously over several weeks. An identifiable infection may precede the onset of the neuropathy by one to three weeks. This is commonly an upper respiratory infection or an infection with an enterovirus, mycoplasma, or with one of the psittacosis group of organisms. Other cases follow surgical operations, but in approximately half of the cases, no antecedent event is recognizable. The neuropathy that may follow infectious mononucleosis is possibly distinct.

The neuropathy may be ushered in by severe lumbar or interscapular pain. Motor involvement usually predominates over sensory loss and may be of a proximal, distal, or generalized distribution, and in severe cases affects the respiratory musculature. Distal paraesthesiae in the limbs are common and if sensory loss occurs, it tends to affect tactile, vibratory, and postural sensibility. The cranial nerves may be affected, in particular the facial nerves, but bulbar involvement also sometimes occurs. Autonomic disturbances may be associated, including bladder atony, and also hypertension, possibly the result of denervation of the carotid sinus. Associated central nervous system involvement is occasionally encountered, particularly after infectious mononucleosis and such cases are sometimes excluded from the Guillain–Barré syndrome as such. Papilloedema occasionally develops, possibly related to impaired cerebrospinal fluid resorption because of the elevated protein content. Further variants are a combination of an external ophthalmoplegia, ataxia and areflexia (*Miller Fisher syndrome*), or a diffuse cranial nerve involvement (*polyneuritis cranialis*), as possibly are instances of acute sensory neuropathy or pandysautonomia.

The cerebrospinal fluid protein content in the Guillain–Barré syndrome is usually raised, often to a substantial degree, but may be normal, particularly in the early stages. The cell content is usually normal but there may be a mild lymphocytic pleocytosis. A greater pleocytosis tends to occur in those cases that follow infectious mononucleosis. Histologically, the abnormalities are maximal in the spinal roots, but also occur diffusely throughout the peripheral nerves. Focal perivascular collections of inflammatory cells are associated with segmental demyelination of the nerve fibres and relative preservation of axonal continuity. The disease probably represents a cell-mediated delayed hypersensitivity reaction in which myelin is stripped off the axons by mononuclear cells. Whether antibody-mediated demyelination is also involved has not yet been established. Recovery occurs by remyelination.

Most cases of the Guillain–Barré syndrome recover satisfactorily within weeks or months. Severely affected patients, particularly those that require assisted respiration and in whom extensive axonal degeneration occurs recover more slowly and often show residual muscle weakness. Occasional patients have recurrences, which are sometimes multiple.

Corticosteroids have been widely employed in the treatment of acute inflammatory polyneuropathy as have to a lesser extent cytotoxic drugs such as azathioprine. The present evidence is that corticosteroids have no beneficial effect in the acute stage and may retard recovery. Recently the use of plasma exchange has been demonstrated to be beneficial. Its use is best reserved for the severer cases.

Chronic relapsing and chronic progressive idiopathic inflammatory polyneuropathy

Instances of peripheral neuropathy occur that resemble the Guillain–Barré syndrome in that the neurological involvement is predominantly motor and the CSF protein level is elevated, but which pursue either a chronic relapsing or chronic progressive course. They are also associated with widespread demyelination in the spinal roots and peripheral nerves and with inflammatory infiltrates. Some of the relapsing cases respond to corticosteroid treatment whereas others fail to do so. Plasma exchange may be beneficial on a temporary basis. The response is less satisfactory in the chronic progressive cases.

Bannwarth's syndrome (lymphocytic meningoradiculitis)

This follows a tick bite and consists of weakness particularly affecting the facial muscles, pain, and hyperaesthesia, and may be accompanied by a skin rash (erythema chronica migrans). A similar condition occurs in the New England area of the United States (Lyme disease) where it is also associated with a polyarthropathy.

Acquired immunodeficiency syndrome

A subacute polyneuropathy with painful dysaesthesiae may be encountered in this condition. The explanation is uncertain. Some cases resemble the Guillain–Barré syndrome or its chronic progressive variant. Focal cranial neuropathies may be related to fungal meningitis (or to lymphomatous infiltration).

Sarcoid neuropathy

Sarcoidosis (see Section 5) may give rise to a multiple mononeuropathy with a particular tendency to involve the facial nerves or to a generalized neuropathy. The neuropathy may be restricted to the cranial nerves (polyneuritis cranialis). Evidence of involvement of other systems is not always present and sarcoid tissue may or may not be detectable on nerve biopsy.

Diphtheritic neuropathy

The neuropathy of diphtheria (Section 5) is caused by the exotoxin which produces segmental demyelination by interfering with Schwann cell function, probably by affecting protein synthesis. The nerves are not invaded by the bacteria.

Palatal weakness tends to develop after two or three weeks following pharyngeal diphtheria and local muscle paralysis after a similar interval following cutaneous diphtheria. Paralysis of accommodation and sometimes of the external ocular muscles appears after an interval of four to five weeks. A generalized predominantly motor neuropathy of distal distribution may develop after five to seven weeks. In severe cases the respiratory muscles are affected, but if death occurs it is usually as a result of an associated myocarditis.

Neuropathy in autoimmune connective tissue disorders

Peripheral nerve involvement may be encountered in a wide range of the 'collagen-vascular' disorders. Polyarteritis nodosa characteristically gives rise to a multiple mononeuropathy, often with considerable pain. Wegener's granulomatosis may similarly be associated with such a florid neuropathy and in both instances, the peripheral nerve damage is related to a necrotizing angiitis of the vasa nervorum. Such changes may also occur in rheumatoid arthritis in association with a florid multiple mononeuropathy. At other times, a less aggressive neuropathy is observed, either in the form of a distal sensory neuropathy or restricted to the digital nerves. Entrapment neuropathies also occur in rheumatoid arthritis, for example median nerve compression in the carpal tunnel, related to articular or tendon sheath changes.

A multiple mononeuropathy, presumably of vascular origin, may be a feature in systemic lupus erythematosus, Sjögren's syndrome, and occasionally in systemic sclerosis. In the former two conditions, a symmetrical distal sensory neuropathy may also appear, as may an isolated trigeminal neuropathy.

The neuropathy of polyarteritis nodosa and rheumatoid arthritis may be alleviated by corticosteroids although large dosages may be required. It is unlikely that neuropathy is precipitated by corticosteroids in rheumatoid arthritis, as has been suggested at times.

Neoplastic neuropathy

Peripheral neuropathy may develop as a non-metastatic complication of carcinoma, most often bronchial or gastric, or lymphoreticular proliferative disorders. The precise mechanism of production of the neuropathy is uncertain. The neuropathy may antedate the discovery of the carcinoma by as much as two or three years. In relation to carcinoma of the bronchus, the neuropathy may be purely sensory, either subacute or chronic, often with troublesome distal dysaesthesiae, or mixed sensory and motor. That associated with multiple myeloma may consist of a demyelinating motor neuropathy sometimes associated with a dermatoendocrine syndrome (pigmentation, oedema, hypertrichosis, gynaecomastia) and papilloedema. A neuropathy identical or closely similar to acute idiopathic inflammatory polyneuropathy (Guillain–Barré syndrome) may be encountered in Hodgkin's disease and in chronic lymphocyctic leukaemia, and a subacute mainly motor neuropathy in relation to lymphoma.

Non-metastatic carcinomatous neuropathies may regress following removal of the underlying tumour or may remain unaffected. Direct invasion of cranial nerves or spinal roots may occur in cases of malignant infiltration of the meninges. Infiltration of peripheral nerve trunks is seen most commonly from malignant lymphomas.

Paraproteinaemic neuropathy

A peripheral neuropathy taking the form of either a multifocal neuropathy or a symmetrical mixed motor and sensory polyneuropathy may occur in association with either monoclonal or mixed gammopathies. It may be due to a vasculitis of the vasa nervorum produced by the deposition of immune complexes, or to a diffuse demyelinating process. A demyelinating neuropathy related to a benign monoclonal IgM paraproteinaemia has recently been recognized; the paraprotein can be demonstrated to be attached to peripheral nerve myelin. Otherwise the neuropathy may be related to single or mixed cryoglobulins in myelomatosis, lymphoma, systemic lupus erythematosus, rheumatoid arthritis, or Waldenström's macroglobulinaemia. These neuropathies occasionally respond to treatment either with immunosuppressive or cytotoxic drugs, or repeated plasma exchange.

Genetic neuropathies

Porphyria (see also Section 9)

A predominantly motor neuropathy may complicate acute attacks of acute intermittent and variegate porphyria and hereditary coproporphyria. It tends to affect the proximal muscles to a greater extent. There may be associated sensory loss which, although sometimes distal in distribution, can affect the trunk and the proximal portions of the limbs. The tendon reflexes are lost, with occasional paradoxical sparing of the ankle jerks. Accompanying autonomic features include abdominal pain and vomiting, tachycardia and hypertension; mental confusion, psychotic behaviour, and epilepsy may be associated.

The explanation of the neurological damage has not been established. Axonal degeneration occurs in the peripheral nerves so that recovery is slow and often incomplete.

Attacks may be provoked by a variety of drugs including barbiturates, sulphonamides, and the contraceptive pill, and by alcohol, probably by enzyme induction in the liver (see Section 12).

Treatment with oral or intravenous glucose, or by infusions of laevulose or haematin, has been shown to reduce the urinary excretion of porphyrin precursors, but a beneficial effect on the neurological disturbances has not been established.

Hereditary motor and sensory neuropathy, types I and II (peroneal muscular atrophy, Charcot–Marie–Tooth disease)

Hereditary motor and sensory neuropathy (HMSN) types I and II usually present during childhood or adolescence with difficulty in walking or because of foot deformity. The deformity is most commonly pes cavus associated with clawing of the toes and sometimes with an equinovarus position of the foot. Muscle weakness tends to affect the lower leg muscles and may give rise to a bilateral foot drop with a 'steppage' gait. The muscle wasting is often restricted to below the knees producing a 'stork leg' appearance (Fig. 3). Weakness and wasting of the small hand muscles may appear later. The tendon reflexes become depressed or lost and there is a variable degree of distal sensory loss. Tremor in the upper limbs

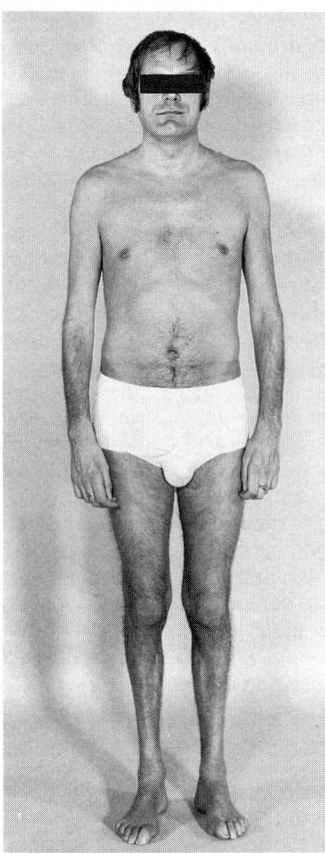

Fig. 3 Patient with type I hereditary motor and sensory neuropathy (Charcot–Marie–Tooth disease) showing symmetrical distal lower limb muscle wasting.

may be a feature in some cases. Progress of the disorder is slow and abortive cases are common.

In the commoner type I families there is a diffuse demyelinating neuropathy. The onset is most frequently in the first decade. Foot deformity and scoliosis occur more often than in HMSN type II. Sensory loss and ataxia tend to be greater and generalized tendon areflexia is usual. Weakness in the hands appears earlier. The peripheral nerves may be thickened. Cases with ataxia are sometimes referred to as the *Roussy–Lévy syndrome*. They are not genetically distinct. The onset in the type II form is most often in the second decade but it may be delayed until middle or even late adult life. Some families with HMSN type I show genetic linkage with the Duffy blood group.

Nerve conduction velocity is severely reduced in type I cases but is either normal or only slightly reduced in the type II form.

Affected individuals may be helped by the use of orthotic appliances and sometimes by surgical correction of foot deformity or tendon transfer.

Hereditary motor and sensory neuropathy, type III (Dejerine–Sottas disease)

Although the term Dejerine–Sottas disease has been used more widely in the past, it should now be restricted to a disorder that produces a slowly progressive mixed motor and sensory polyneuropathy with an onset in childhood, often accompanied by ataxia. The inheritance is autosomal recessive. There is hypomyelination and extensive segmental demyelination in the peripheral nerves with accompanying hypertrophic changes (concentric Schwann cell proliferation), a type of pathological change that was formerly termed *hypertrophic interstitial neuropathy*. Striking enlargement of the peripheral nerve trunks is detectable on palpation or even may be visibly evident.

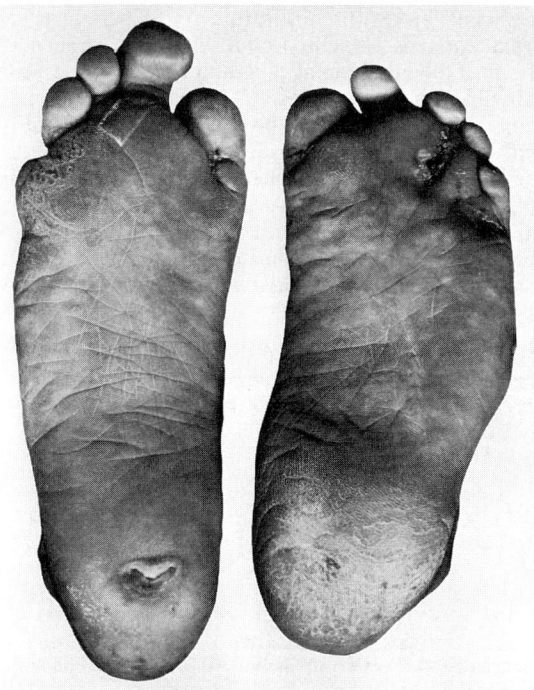

Fig. 4 Chronic foot ulceration and deformity in a case of hereditary sensory neuropathy.

Refsum's disease

This is a rare disorder inherited as an autosomal recessive trait that gives rise to a mixed motor and sensory polyneuropathy accompanied by a variety of other clinical features including ataxia, pigmentary retinal degeneration, pupillary abnormalities, deafness, cardiomyopathy, and ichthyosis. The presentation is usually during adolescence or early adult life and the course may be steadily progressive or relapsing. The peripheral nerves become thickened and display hypertrophic changes. Nerve conduction velocity is usually severely reduced.

The disorder is due to an inability to metabolize phytanic acid, a long-chain fatty acid, which accumulates in the blood and tissues. It is largely derived from dietary phytol, and clinical improvement may be achieved with diets low in phytol. For acute episodes of deterioration, plasma exchange is effective.

Hereditary sensory neuropathies

Predominantly sensory neuropathies may occur with either an autosomal dominant or recessive inheritance. The symptoms in the latter instance are usually present from birth; in the former they generally develop during the second or third decades. In both, the sensory loss often leads to a mutilating acropathy with neuropathic joint degeneration and chronic cutaneous ulceration, particularly in the feet (Fig. 4). A further rare recessive neuro-

pathy combines congenital insensitivity to pain and anhidrosis. Cases of 'congenital insensitivity to pain' are probably examples of small fibre neuropathies.

Familial dysautonomia

Otherwise known as the *Riley–Day syndrome*, this recessively inherited disorder is encountered most often in Jewish populations. There is an aplasia of peripheral autonomic neurones that leads to a variety of symptoms including absence of tears, unexplained pyrexia, cutaneous blotching, and episodic sweating attacks. These symptoms are present at birth and are accompanied by a congenital insensitivity to pain related to an associated sensory neuropathy. In early infancy there is usually difficulty in feeding because of poor sucking, and repeated episodes of pneumonia. Later stunted growth and often kyphoscoliosis become evident.

Other hereditary neuropathies (see also page 21.206 and Section 9)
Peripheral nerve involvement occurs in both metachromatic and globoid cell leucodystrophy, in Fabry's disease, and in hereditary lipoprotein deficiency (Tangier disease and hereditary abetalipoproteinaemia). Certain families show an inherited liability to pressure palsies. Giant axonal neuropathy is a rare disorder with an onset in childhood, characterized by segmental axonal enlargements containing accumulations of neurofilaments. Affected children usually have abnormally curly hair.

Cryptogenic neuropathy

Despite extensive investigation, the cause of a substantial number of peripheral neuropathies remains unknown. This applies in particular to examples of chronic progressive neuropathy, some of which may be instances of type II hereditary motor and sensory neuropathy. A careful family history in such cases may reveal evidence of undetected neuropathy in relatives.

References

Asbury, A. K. and Gilliatt, R. W. (1984). *Peripheral nerve disorders. A practical approach.* Butterworths, London.
—— and Johnson, P. C. (1978). *Pathology of peripheral nerve.* W. B. Saunders, Philadelphia.
Downie, A. (1982). Peripheral nerve compression syndromes. In *Recent advances in clinical neurology*, vol. 3 (eds W. B. Matthews and G. H. Glaser), p. 47. Churchill Livingstone, Edinburgh.
Dyck, P. J., Thomas, P. K., Lambert, E. H. and Bunge, R. (1984). *Peripheral neuropathy*, 2nd edn. W. B. Saunders, Philadelphia.
Henson, R. A. and Urich, H. (1982). *Cancer and the nervous system.* Blackwell, Oxford.
Schaumburg, H. H., Spencer, P. S. and Thomas, P. K. (1983). *Disorders of peripheral nerves.* F. A. Davis, Philadelphia.
Spencer, P. S. and Schaumburg, H. H. (1980). *Experimental and clinical neurotoxicology.* Williams and Wilkins, Baltimore.
Sunderland, S. (1978). *Nerves and nerve injuries*, 2nd edn. Churchill Livingstone, Edinburgh.
Thomas, P. K. and Harding, A. E. (1982). Peripheral neuropathies. In *The principles and practice of medical genetics* (eds A. E. H. Emery and D. L. Rimoin). Churchill Livingstone, Edinburgh.

INFECTIONS OF THE NERVOUS SYSTEM

Bacterial meningitis

B. E. JUEL-JENSEN, PRIDA PHUAPRADIT, AND D. A. WARRELL

Bacterial meningitis, also known as pyogenic, purulent or cerebrospinal meningitis, is an inflammation of the leptomeninges with infection of the cerebrospinal fluid within the subarachnoid space of the brain and spinal cord, and the ventricular system.

Anatomy of the subarachnoid space

In the absence of pathological blockages, bacteria entering the subarachnoid space at any point can spread over the surface of the brain and into the perivascular spaces of Virchow Robin. After reaching the basal cisterns they can pass through the foramina of Luschka and Magendie into the fourth ventricle, and thence through the cerebral aqueduct of Sylvius to reach the third ventricle, and though the interventricular foramina of Monro to the lateral ventricles. Subdural empyema (pachymeningitis interna) or effusion complicating leptomeningitis can also spread freely because the arachnoid membrane and dura mater are almost entirely separated. By contrast, because of the tight application of the dura mater to the periosteum of the skull, epidural collections of pus are localized. In the spinal column, however, the epidural space is loose and contains fat, permitting the extension of a posterior spinal epidural abscess over several vertebral segments. Within the subarachnoid space and intraventricular system, infection may produce blockages of CSF circulation, especially at the various foramina or in the aqueduct, causing obstructive hydroce-phalus or spinal block. If reabsorption of CSF across the subarachnoid granulations is prevented by a subarachnoid haematoma or thrombosis of the intracranial veins and venous sinuses, communicating hydrocephalus will result. In patients with meningitis, intracranial hypertension may be the result of cerebral oedema, the ventricular dilatation of hydrocephalus, or subdural or epidural collections of pus. Obstructive hydrocephalus and intracranial collections of pus carry a special risk of producing brain herniation after lumbar puncture.

Because they cross the inflamed basal meninges, the cranial nerves and cerebral arteries may be damaged. Cranial nerves may

Table 1 Less common causes of bacterial meningitis

Organism	Special clinical association	Antimicrobial for initial treatment*
Acinetobacter calcoaceticus (anitratus)	Hospital	Ticarcillin or co-trimoxazole
Actinobacillus actinomycetemcomitans	Endocarditis, brain abscess	A
Actinobacillus lignieresii	Endocarditis, animal bites	A
Aerococcus viridans	Children	P
Aeromonas hydrophila	Diarrhoea, trauma, fish and reptile contact	C
Alcaligenes faecalis	Trauma	3rd generation cephalosporin
Bacillus anthracis	Septicaemia	P
B. cereus	Trauma, brain abscess	C
Bordetella bronchiseptica	Trauma, animal contact	Co-trimoxazole
Branhamella catarrhalis	Chronic respiratory disease, immunodeficiency	Cefuroxime or 3rd generation cephalosporin
Brucella species		C, A
Campylobacter jejuni	Endocarditis	C
Campylobacter fetus	Neonates	C
Citrobacter koseri	Neonates, brain abscess	β-l+a
Clostridium perfringens	Trauma, septicaemia	P
Corynebacteria species (JK, bovis etc.)	Trauma, atrioventricular shunt	P, rifampicin, vancomycin
DF-2	Dog bite, splenectomy	P
Edwardsiella tarda	Trauma, fish and reptile contact	β-l+a
Eikenella corrodens	Trauma, human bite	P
Enterobacter species	Hospital, neonates	3rd generation cephalosporin or ticarcillin + aminoglycoside or co-trimoxazole
Escherichia coli	Neonates	See Table 3, 'Gram negative'
Flavobacterium meningosepticum	Neonates, adults trauma	Rifampicin, C, co-trimoxazole, or 3rd generation cephalosporin
Francisella tularensis (tularaemia)	Septicaemia, rodent tick contact, fleas from other small mammals, hares and lemmings	C, tetracycline
Fusobacterium necrophorum	Vincent's angina	P, metronidazole
Gemella haemolysans	Trauma	P
Haemophilus aphrophilus	Trauma, dog and human bites	A
Haemophilus parainfluenzae	Trauma (commensal in normal upper respiratory tract)	C
Kingella kingae		P
Klebsiella species	Neonates	See Table 3
Lactobacillus species	Neonates	P
Moraxella		P
Neisseria species		P
Nocardia asteroides	Immunosuppression	Sulphonamides
Pasteurella multocida, pneumotropica etc.	Dog, cat, rodent bites	P
Proteus species	Neonates	See Table 3
Plesiomonas shigelloides	Fish and reptile contact, neonates	C, co-trimoxazole
Propionibacterium acnes	Trauma	P
Pseudomonas cepacia	Hospital	Co-trimoxazole
Pseudomonas pickettii		Co-trimoxazole, 3rd generation cephalosporin
Pseudomonas putrefaciens		C, 3rd generation cephalosporin
Pseudomonas pseudomallei (melioidosis)	Pneumonia, septicaemia (endemic in parts of southeast Asia)	Co-trimoxazole
Pseudomonas maltophilia		C, co-trimoxazole
Pseudomonas mallei (glanders)	Horse contact	Co-trimoxazole
Salmonella species		C or co-trimoxazole
Serratia marcescens	Humidifiers, neonates	β-l+a or co-trimoxazole
Streptococcus pyogenes	Trauma	P
Streptococcus viridans group	Endocarditis, frontal sinusitis	P
Yersinia enterocolitica		C
Yersinia pestis (plague)	Septicaemia	C, tetracycline

A = ampicillin, C = chloramphenicol, G = gentamicin, P = penicillin, β-l+a = β-lactam + aminoglycoside, '3rd generation cephalosporin' = cefotaxime or latamoxef.
* To be changed, if necessary, as soon as precise sensitivity pattern is known. Where co-trimoxazole is recommended as drug of first choice, substitute trimethoprim in patients who are known to be hypersensitive to sulphonamides.
(For further information see page 5.376.)

be compressed by intracranial hypertension (VI) or brain herniation (III) or suffer ischaemic damage from vasculitis.

Acute bacterial meningitis

Bacteriology and susceptibility

Overall, *Neisseria meningitidis*, *Streptococcus pneumoniae*, and *Haemophilus influenzae* remain the most important causes of acute bacterial meningitis. The incidence of infections by the various organisms and their serotypes varies geographically and with the age and immunocompetence of the patient. There are also changing trends in incidence over the years.

In neonates, meningitis is most commonly caused by group B_{III} streptococci, *Escherichia coli K1* and *Listeria monocytogenes* acquired during birth from the mother's vagina or, post-partum, from the hands of the mother or nursing staff. In the age group from 2–3 months to 3–6 years, *H. influenzae* is the commonest cause of bacterial meningitis in most countries with *N. meningitidis* and *S. pneumoniae* second and third. In the United States there has been a relative and absolute increase in the incidence of *H. influenzae* meningitis in adults over the past 40 years. In older children and adults *N. meningitidis* is the commonest cause in Europe and savanna Africa ('meningitis belt'), *H. influenzae* is commonest in the United States and Australia, and *S. pneumoniae* in south western Nigeria. In recent years there have been epidemics of *N. meningitidis* type A in parts of India and in valleys of Nepal.

Some of the changes in importance of bacteria and their strains over the years have been attributed to the use of antimicrobials and vaccines. Thus, in the United States, *N. meningitidis* type B replaced type A as the predominant organism as a result of sulphonamide resistance. Type C later gave way to type Y in places where type C vaccine had been used. The increasing importance of *H. influenzae* as a cause of meningitis in adults has been attributed to the more widespread use in childhood infections of antimicrobials active against Gram-negative organisms, thus reducing the chances of acquiring natural immunity.

The highest incidence of bacterial meningitis is found in the age group 6–12 months. In the case of *N. meningitidis* it is the period when serum neutralizing antibody is at its lowest.

Susceptibility to bacterial meningitis may be determined by race, by congenital deficiencies in the complement system, and by chronic illness and malignancies. This is seen most dramatically with pneumococcal meningitis. Irrespective of socio-economic status, American negroes have a more than five-fold greater risk of infection than whites. Perhaps as a result of autosplenectomy, those with homozygous sickle cell disease have a 36 times greater risk than other negroes and a 314 times greater risk than whites. One in 24 children with this condition will develop pneumococcal meningitis. Other predisposing conditions include alcoholism, hypogammaglobulinaemia, splenectomy, splenosis, congenital asplenia, pregnancy, nephrotic syndrome, cirrhosis, and diabetes mellitus. *H. influenzae* meningitis is also commoner in negroes, Navajo Indians, and in Eskimos, than in whites; but poor white people are at greater risk than their more affluent countrymen.

Immunocompromised patients are vulnerable to meningeal infections by some unusual bacteria. In those with defective cell-mediated immunity (transplant recipients, those with lymphomas, especially Hodgkin's disease, and any patient on corticosteroids and other immunosuppressant drugs), *Listeria monocytogenes*, *M. tuberculosis*, and atypical mycobacteria may cause meningitis. In those with defective humoral immunity (chronic lymphocytic leukaemia, myelomatosis, and Hodgkin's disease) there is an increased risk of infection by the usual meningitis-producing organisms. Neutropenia and neutrophil abnormalities predispose to infection with *Pseudomonas aeruginosa* and *Enterobacteriaceae*. Effects of splenectomy have been mentioned above.

Meningeal infection by many of the unusual organisms listed in Table 1 is secondary to septicaemia, often associated with infective endocarditis, especially in patients with reduced resistance to infection. Infection may also spread directly from septic foci adjacent to the brain and spinal cord: e.g. osteomyelitis of the skull and vertebrae, suppurative intracranial phlebitis, infection of the paranasal sinuses (particularly with *S. milleri* and anaerobes), middle ear and mastoid air sinuses, and intracranial abscesses. Infection may spread via lymphatics from retropharyngeal, posterior mediastinal, retroperitoneal, and psoas abscesses to the spinal cord. Injuries may allow bacteria (Table 2) access to the meninges, e.g. compound fractures of the skull, minor fractures of the base of the skull especially those associated with CSF rhinorrhoea or otorrhoea, insertion of atrioventricular shunts for the relief of hydrocephalus, other neurosurgical procedures, lumbar puncture, and spinal anaesthesia. Finally, congenital abnormalities such as dermoid sinus tracks and meningomyeloceles may also provide a route of infection.

Epidemiology

Meningococcal, pneumococcal, and *H. influenzae* meningitides follow nasopharyngeal colonization by these pathogens. In the case of meningococcal meningitis (page 5.200) attempts have been made to relate epidemics to a preceding increase in carrier rate. However, in the meningitis belt of Africa, other factors related to climate are also necessary to initiate the epidemic. The highest risk of infection is amongst family contacts of a case of meningitis, especially siblings. Epidemics do arise in institutions, but there is no simple relationship to crowding. Factors predisposing to pneumococcal meningitis have already been discussed. Up to 50 per cent of the population carry pneumococci in their upper respiratory tract, but pneumococcal meningitis is usually associated with infection by certain virulent strains. Eighteen serotypes, including 1, 3, 6, 7, 14, 17, 18, 19, 21, and 23, are responsible for 90 per cent of cases of meningitis. *H. influenzae* meningitis is usually associated with nasopharyngeal carriage of the virulent capsulated type b, but some untypable unencapsulated strains are also involved. The risk of infection is highest in young household contacts, as in the case of meningococcal meningitis.

Pathogenesis and pathophysiology

Work with animal models of bacterial meningitis has shown that, at least in the case of *H. influenzae*, bacteria pass from the nasopharynx into the blood stream and then invade the subarachnoid space through the walls of the large intracranial venous sinuses. There is inflammation of meningeal blood vessels with escape of neutrophil leucocytes and exudation of plasma. Bacteria multiply rapidly in the CSF which is deficient in some elements of the immunological defence system, such as complement. Attempts have been made to define the characteristics of those bacteria which are most often successful in invading the CSF. The first step of infection, adhesion to the oro- and nasopharyngeal mucosae, probably involves the specific interaction of bacterial pili and mucosal receptors. Encapsulated bacteria such as *H. influenzae* b, *E. coli* Kl, *Streptococcus* B_{III}, and *L. monocytogenes* 46 may be protected from phagocytosis. Epidemics of meningococcal meningitis in the African meningitis belt arise when atmospheric humidity is at its lowest, suggesting that drying of the nasopharyngeal

Table 2 Common causes of bacterial meningitis in patients with traumatic or congenital access to the subarachnoid space

Closed fractures of the skull with CSF leak	*Streptococcus pneumoniae*, *Haemophilus influenzae* and *parainfluenzae*
Surgery including drainage of CSF in hydrocephalus (shunts)	*Staphylococcus epidermidis*, *Staphylococcus aureus*, *Corynebacteria*, *Pseudomonas*
Congenital dermal sinuses etc. Lumbar puncture and spinal anaesthesia	*Staphylococcus epidermidis*, *Corynebacteria*, *Escherichia coli*, *Pseudomonas*, *Bacillus cereus*

membranes and perhaps deficiency in secretory IgA may allow invasion by meningococci at this season.

The importance of the polyribose phosphate capsule of *H. influenzae* b has been demonstrated in animals and humans. Anti-polyribose phosphate antibodies are protective. Recent work in an animal model of pneumococcal meningitis has suggested that the cell wall rather than the capsule is responsible for the inflammatory response in the meninges. An effect of β-lactam antimicrobials would be to release cell wall constituents into the CSF. This might produce a deleterious increase in the inflammatory reaction. Neutrophil leucocytes may migrate into the superficial layer of the brain and spinal cord, but, however intense the inflammation, the pia mater is a barrier to bacteria. Metabolic disturbances associated with bacterial meningitis include inhibition of the facilitated membrane transport of glucose in and out of the CSF, a switch from aerobic to anaerobic cerebral carbohydrate metabolism with increased consumption of glucose and production of lactate. Increased cerebral glucose consumption is now thought to be the main cause of the low CSF glucose concentration in this condition. In patients comatose with pneumococcal meningitis, total cerebral blood flow and cerebral oxygen consumption were reduced, cerebral glucose consumption was normal or increased, and there was marked CSF lactic acidosis. Autoregulation of cerebral blood flow was lost in some patients but response to carbon dioxide was intact. Intracranial hypertension is indicated by an elevated CSF opening pressure in more than 90 per cent of patients. In one study, the pressure was between 200 and 500 mm in 75 per cent, and between 500 and 1000 mm in 15 per cent of patients. This is attributable to cerebral oedema, hydrocephalus or intracranial collections of pus.

Pathology

There is diffuse acute inflammation of the pia-arachnoid, with migration of neutrophil leucocytes and exudation of fibrin into the CSF. Pus accumulates over the surface of the brain, especially around its base and the emerging cranial nerves, and round the spinal cord. The meningeal vessels are dilated and congested and may also be surrounded by pus. Pus and fibrin are also found in the ventricles and there is ventriculitis, with loss of ependymal lining and subependymal gliosis. Dilatation of the ventricular system may result from obstructive or communicating hydrocephalus. Other abnormalities include subdural effusion or empyema, septic thrombosis of the cerebral venous sinuses, subarachnoid haematomas, compression of intracranial structures as a result of intracranial hypertension, and herniation of the temporal lobes or cerebellum. Gross changes, such as pressure coning, which would provide an obvious cause of death, are rarely found. In some cases death may be attributable to related septicaemia (Fig. 1), although the familiar finding of bilateral adrenal haemorrhage (Waterhouse–Friderichsen syndrome) may well be a terminal phenomenon rather than a cause of fatal adrenal insufficiency as was once imagined. Patients with meningococcal septicaemia may develop acute pulmonary oedema. Myocarditis was a common finding in some series of patients. Histological appearances were of an acute interstitial myocarditis, occasionally with myocardial necrosis and thrombosis of small arterioles. Pericarditis and pericardial effusion is a feature, particularly of group C meningococcal infections. Myocarditis and Waterhouse–Friderichsen syndrome also occur, less frequently than in meningococcal septicaemia, in septicaemia caused by *H. influenzae*, pneumococcal, streptococcal, and staphylococcal infections.

Clinical features

Acute bacterial meningitis carries a mortality in untreated patients of between 70 and 100 per cent. Delay in treatment greatly increases the risk of permanent neurological sequelae. The early diagnosis of this condition is, therefore, a formidable challenge to clinical acumen, but it is clear from our own experience and from the medical literature that early clinical suspicion of meningitis

may be impossible in many cases, especially in neonates and small children. When meningitis is secondary to infection elsewhere, such as pneumococcal pneumonia or *H. influenzae* otitis media, the presenting symptoms may be those of the original infection. The incubation period is only a few days. Progression is occasionally so rapid (*N. meningitidis*) that the patient becomes comatose within a few hours after the first symptoms. Early manifestations include non-specific malaise, apprehension or irritability, followed by fever usually without rigors, headache, myalgias, and vomiting. Convulsions occur in infants and children, and meningitis must always enter into the differential diagnosis of childhood febrile convulsions. Photophobia, drowsiness or more severe impairment of consciousness usually develops later. Headache quickly becomes more severe and is the dominant symptom. In older children and adults the symptoms most suggestive of meningitis are irritability, severe headache, and vomiting. An early symptom of meningococcal septicaemia is pain in the calves.

There is rarely any doubt that the child or adult with meningitis is severely ill and distressed. Meningism is best elicited by gentle passive flexion or rotation of the neck with the patient lying supine. To elicit Kernig's sign the lower limb is flexed at the hip. The patient with meningism will resist extension of the knee by contracting the hamstring muscles. Brudzinski's neck sign is best elicited while the patient sits up in bed with the legs stretched out. Gentle flexion of the neck will induce a sympathetic flexion of the hips, knees, and sometimes the upper limbs. Later, the patient with marked meningism lies in a characteristic position with the neck and back fully extended (Fig. 2) as in tetanic opisthotonos (Fig. 3). Local causes of neck stiffness, such as local sepsis, cervical spondylitis (particularly common in the elderly), and pharyngeal lesions should be considered. The optic fundi should be examined as a prelude to lumbar puncture. Papilloedema is suggestive of cerebral oedema or an intracranial space-occupying lesion such as a cerebral abscess or a subdural or epidural collection of pus. The absence of papilloedema does not, however, exclude cerebral oedema, and if in doubt, and computer-assisted

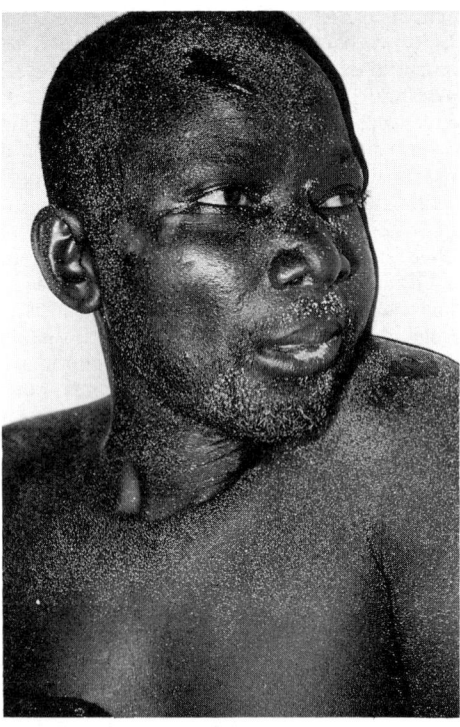

Fig. 1 Nigerian patient with pneumococcal meningitis and septicaemia who developed 'urea frost' and later died of renal failure. This illustrates the importance of septicaemic complications outside the central nervous system in determining mortality. (Copyright D. A. Warrell.)

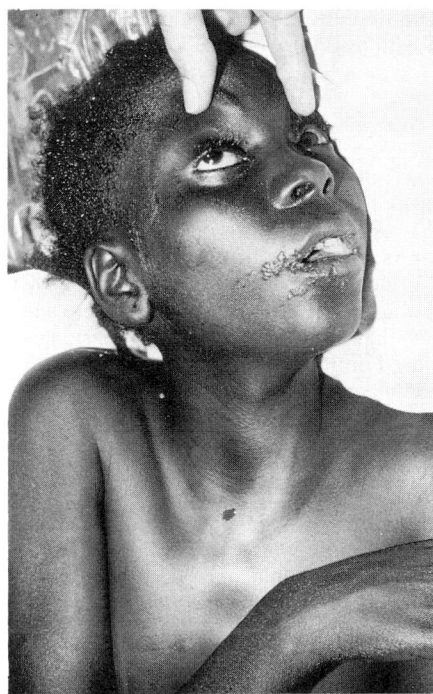

Fig. 2 Nigerian girl in coma with severe meningococcal meningoencephalitis. Note head retraction, dysconjugate gaze, and herpes labialis. (Copyright D. A. Warrell.)

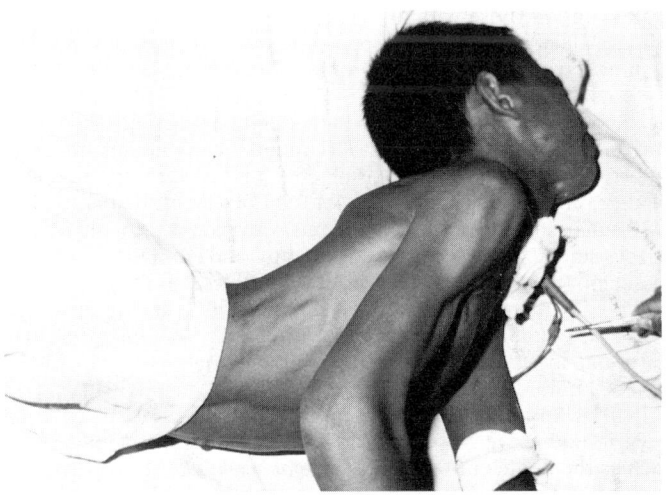

Fig. 3 Thai man with tetanus showing opisthotonos mimicking meningism, but note muscle spasm. (Copyright D. A. Warrell.)

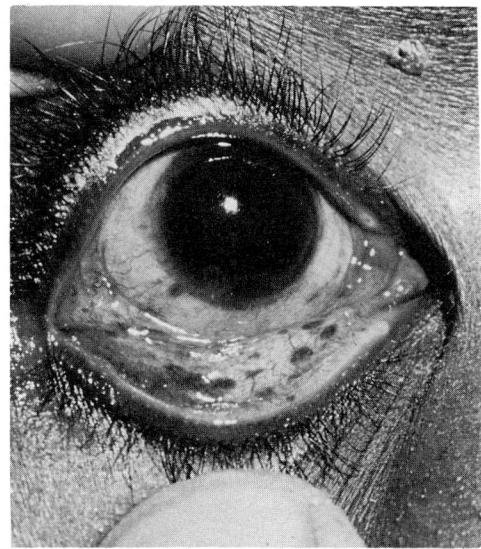

Fig. 4 Conjunctival petechiae in a Nigerian boy with meningococcal meningitis. (Copyright D. A. Warrell.)

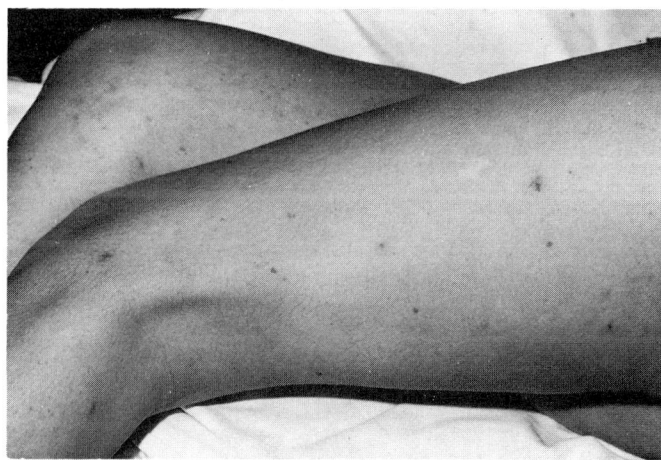

Fig. 5 Cutaneous petechiae in an English woman with meningococcal meningitis. (Copyright D. A. Warrell.)

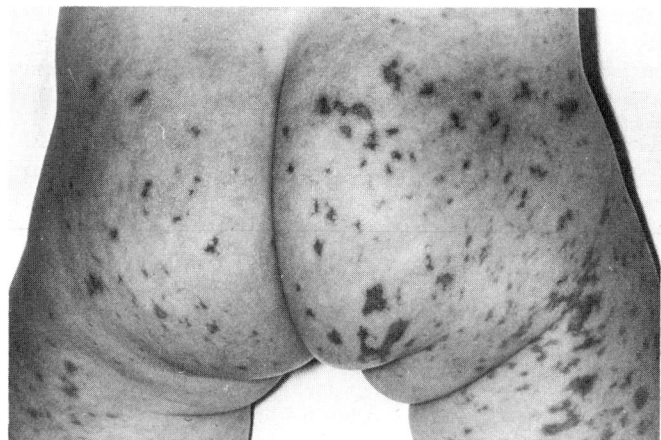

Fig. 6 The rash of meningococcal septicaemia in an English child.

tomography is available, that investigation must precede a lumbar puncture. Hypertensive retinopathy will suggest hypertensive encephalopathy, and subhyaloid haemorrhages a subarachnoid haemorrhage. Patients with meningococcal meningitis associated with meningococcal antigenaemia have a petechial rash best seen on the bulbar or tarsal conjunctivae (Fig. 4), but sometimes visible on the palate and skin (Fig. 5). An identical rash is occasionally seen in patients with echovirus type 9, leptospiral, *Staphylococcus aureus*, pneumonoccal, *H. influenzae*, *Salmonella typhi*, and other infections, especially in those associated with infective endocarditis. The brownish or reddish geometrical, vasculitic rash of fulminant meningococcaemia is unmistakable (Fig. 6) and, characteristically, the toes and fingers become necrotic (Fig. 7). There is associated profound hypotension, shock with peripheral cyanosis and spontaneous systemic bleeding. Herpes labialis is commonly seen in all forms of bacterial meningitis, because a fever is the rule, and recurrences are provoked by any fever in most herpetics (see Figs. 2 and 8). Physical examination must exclude otitis media, sinusitis, mastoiditis, and nasopharyngeal sepsis. In patients with recurrent bacterial meningitis, a search should be made for a congenital dermal sinus, which is usually in

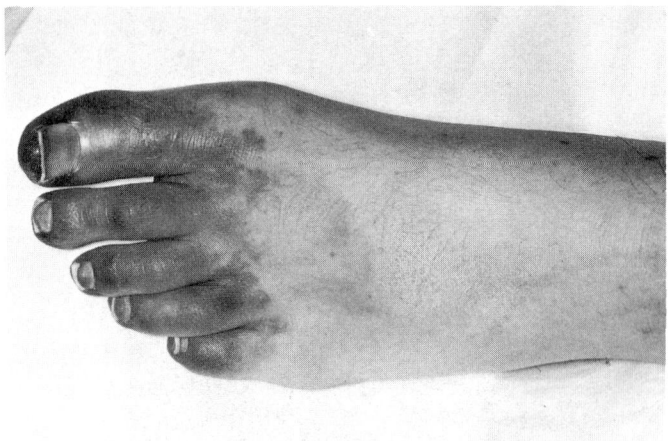

Fig. 7 Necrosis of toes in young student with meningococcal septicaemia.

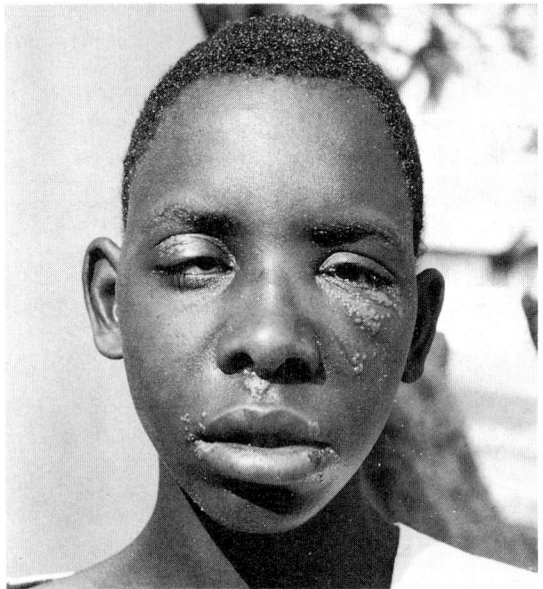

Fig. 8 Nigerian man recovering from meningococcal meningitis. Note right VI nerve lesion and herpes labialis. (Copyright D. A. Warrell.)

the midline between head and coccyx, and is often marked by a tuft of long hairs. Watery discharge from the nose or ears should be collected and tested for glucose; the possibility of a basal skull fracture with cerebrospinal fluid leak should be excluded.

Cranial nerve lesions may become evident as the disease progresses. The commonest are VI (Fig. 8), III, VII, VIII, and II. Patients who become unconscious (meningo-encephalomyelitis) may lose all signs of meningism and develop focal neurological signs, focal epileptiform convulsions, dysconjugate gaze, upper motor neurone signs, and involuntary movements. Vascular lesions may produce hemiparesis or quadriparesis, speech disorders, and visual field defects.

Papilloedema, with or without other symptoms and signs of intracranial hypertension (vomiting, coma, high blood pressure, bradycardia, etc.) and localizing neurological signs, suggests a subdural effusion or empyema. This is particularly common in children under 2 years old with *H. influenzae* meningitis.

Neonates and infants
Meningitis is particularly difficult to diagnose in this age group. Infants may become irritable or lethargic, stop feeding, and are found to have a bulging fontanelle, separation of the cranial sutures, meningism, and opisthotonos, and they may develop con-

vulsions. These findings are uncommon in neonates, who sometimes present with respiratory distress, diarrhoea or jaundice.

Diagnosis
The dangers of diagnostic lumbar puncture (fatal pressure coning, introduction of infection, and conversion of bacteraemia into meningitis) are real, but can be greatly reduced by taking the normal precautions, and are in any case completely outweighed by the importance of making a diagnosis of this potentially fatal but treatable condition (see page 21.10). Lumbar puncture is contraindicated if there is local skin sepsis or any clinical suspicion of spinal cord compression. Patients with papilloedema or focal neurological signs (other than the common III nerve lesion) should not be lumbar punctured until an intracranial space-occupying lesion has been excluded by computer-assisted tomography. The appearance of a turbid, yellowish or greenish CSF is virtually diagnostic of acute bacterial meningitis. A Gram stain and cell count should be done immediately. The CSF should be plated for bacterial culture and sensitivity tests set up, especially to detect ampicillin resistance in *H. influenzae* and penicillin resistance in *S. pneumoniae*. CSF glucose and protein concentrations must be measured and a blood sample should be taken simultaneously for glucose estimation and culture. The combination of more than 1000 neutrophils per μl of CSF, a CSF glucose concentration less than 40 per cent of the simultaneous blood level (normal 66 per cent) or less than 1.7 mmol/l (30 mg/dl) and a protein concentration in excess of 1.5 g/l is strongly suggestive of bacterial meningitis. A Gram stain should produce a specific diagnosis in more than 75 per cent of untreated cases. However, CSF findings may be confusing. Leucocytes may be scanty in the CSF of some patients with early bacterial meningitis, and in those with overwhelming pneumococcal meningitis with a defective leucocyte response. *L. canicola* may mimic a viral meningitis and may be missed unless thought of. Ten per cent of patients with bacterial meningitis have a predominantly lymphocytic pleocytosis. Some viral meningitides may, especially in the early stages, be associated with a predominantly neutrophil pleocytosis (e.g. lymphocytic choriomeningitis, eastern equine encephalitis, enterovirus meningitis, and St Louis encephalitis). A low CSF glucose may be found in patients with viral meningitides (e.g. herpes simplex, varicella, zoster, mumps, and lymphocytic choriomeningitis) but in most instances the low glucose is caused by starvation. In malignant hypertension, meningism and a very high leucocyte count may be associated with a very low glucose. It may be found in sarcoidosis and other granulomatous meningitides, subarachnoid haemorrhage, carcinomatous meningitis, and in patients who for other reasons are hypoglycaemic (e.g. cerebral malaria and Reye's syndrome). Some rare causes of meningitis such as the penicillin-resistant *Acinetobacter calcoaceticus* may be mistaken for meningococci because they are Gram negative. Countercurrent immunoelectrophoresis is a rapid technique for detecting bacterial antigens in CSF and serum but latex agglutination may be more sensitive. These tests remain positive even after patients have started antimicrobial treatment. The *Limulus lysate* assay may be useful in detecting endotoxin in CSF as evidence of a Gram-negative meningitis. The finding of red cells in an atraumatic tap or xanthochromia suggests subarachnoid haemorrhage or a haemorrhagic encephalitis, very occasionally seen in herpes simplex. CSF lactate and lactic dehydrogenase concentrations are much higher in bacterial than in viral meningitis. CSF lactate is also elevated in cerebral malaria.

Repeated lumbar puncture is indicated if there is failure of clinical response (and that includes persistent fever) to antimicrobial treatment. In patients whose initial CSF contained neutrophils but no culturable bacteria (aseptic meningitis) the second sample of CSF may show the change to lymphocytic pleocytosis characteristic of viral meningitides. In those cases in which the initial CSF was 'aseptic' because of prior antimicrobial treatment, an increase in cell count and protein and fall in glucose concentration in the second CSF specimen suggests that the wrong antimicrobial drug has been used. If the second CSF specimen is completely normal, antimicrobial therapy can safely be stopped, even if fever persists, *provided* that other foci of infection have been eliminated (e.g. ethmoid sinusitis). One of the most useful investigations for monitoring the course of the infection is the C reactive protein which when the infection is overcome by appropriate treatment returns to normal (<0.8 mg/dl) more rapidly than the sedimentation rate. In pneumococcal meningitis it is particularly important to keep up adequate *intravenous* doses of benzylpenicillin until all evidence of activity has disappeared. Organisms are often embedded in a near impenetrable exudate and debris and only prolonged chemotherapy will cure this. In two-thirds of cases the pneumococcus comes from a focus elsewhere such as lung and mastoids. Whereas pneumococcal pneumonia may be cured with small doses of benzylpenicillin, much higher and prolonged doses are required to eradicate infection in bone.

Other useful investigations include radiographs of the skull (with special views of the paranasal sinuses, middle ear, and mastoids), vertebral column, and chest for evidence of septic foci or trauma; computer-assisted tomography to detect intracranial, intraspinal subdural or epidural abscesses and ventricular dilatation indicating hydrocephalus; angiograms; myelograms; and isotope studies to detect CSF leaks.

Differential diagnosis

Meningeal irritation is seen in many acute febrile conditions, especially in children. Local infections of the nasopharynx, cervical lymph-nodes, muscles, and spine may produce convincing neck stiffness. Tetanus may be easily confused with meningitis if the persisting rigidity and recurrent spasms are not noticed. In all these conditions the CSF will be normal. Subarachnoid haemorrhage can present with sudden headache, neck stiffness, and deteriorating consciousness, and a less dramatic progression of symptoms is seen in patients with some intracranial tumours. Tuberculous and cryptococcal and other fungal meningitides usually develop more slowly than acute bacterial meningitis. They may be distinguished by examining CSF. Cryptococci and free-living amoebae may be mistaken for lymphocytes in the CSF unless an Indian ink preparation is examined to reveal the capsule of cryptococcus and the characteristic movements of amoebae. Aseptic meningitis comprises a large number of conditions many of them caused by viruses (see page 21.148) in which there are clinical signs of meningism and the CSF is found to be abnormal. This group includes partially treated bacterial meningitis and the chemical meningitides, resulting from the introduction of irritants into the subarachnoid space (contrast media, antimicrobial agents, and contaminants of lumbar puncture and spinal anaesthesia). The CSF glucose concentration may be very low. Discharge of a tuberculoma may produce a sterile tuberculin reaction and the discharge of the contents of a craniopharyngioma or epidermoid cyst into the CSF may also cause chemical meningitis. Lead encephalopathy may present with meningism, lymphocyte pleocytosis, and an increase in CSF protein.

Recurrent purulent meningitis

This suggests congenital or traumatic access to the subarachnoid space, such as a fracture of the base of the skull, particularly involving the cribriform plate or following surgery (e.g. hypophysectomy), or recurrent sepsis close to the meninges (e.g. otitis media, sinusitis). In about half the traumatic cases there is a history of chronic CSF leakage, which stops just before development of meningitic symptoms. Such patients must be investigated by radiographs, radioisotope techniques, and computer-assisted tomography with contrast cisternography. The organisms responsible for recurrent bacterial meningitis are listed in Table 2. *S. pneumoniae*, *H. influenzae*, and Gram-negative bacilli are the commonest causes.

Mollaret's meningitis (benign recurrent aseptic meningitis) is mentioned here because it is an important differential diagnosis of

recurrent bacterial meningitis. It is a sporadic condition presenting between the ages of 5 and 60 years. The symptoms are typical of acute bacterial meningitis – malaise, fever, vomiting, neck stiffness, convulsions, and coma. There is complete spontaneous recovery, usually within a few days, and symptom-free intervals lasting from a few days to years. About half the patients develop other neurological disturbances including hallucinations, diplopia, cranial nerve lesions, and signs of an upper motor neurone lesion. Pleocytosis is usually less than 3000/μl, with a predominance of lymphocytes, monocytes, and large endothelial ('Mollaret's') cells, but occasionally neutrophils are in the majority. The CSF protein is mildly increased, with increased gammaglobulin. CSF glucose concentration may be decreased. Other causes of recurrent meningitis include Behçet's syndrome, Vogt–Koyanagi–Harada syndrome, sarcoidosis, and systemic lupus erythematosus, and undiagnosed viral meningitis (e.g. that due to encephalomyocarditis virus).

Management

Bacterial meningitis progresses rapidly and has a high mortality. Antimicrobial treatment must therefore be started as soon as possible after the diagnosis is suspected clinically. This is vitally important in meningococcal meningitis. If this condition is suspected by the practitioner (and in Britain the first doctor the patient meets is usually the general practitioner) the patient should without delay be given benzylpenicillin (say three million units intramuscularly) preferably after a blood culture has been taken. Antigen may still be found in the CSF later in hospital. Patients with no papilloedema or lateralizing neurological signs that suggest a space-occupying lesion, and with no other contraindications (see above), should be lumbar punctured immediately. Antimicrobial treatment should then be started, based on clinical assessment, *before* the results of the CSF examination are known. Chloramphenicol is probably the best choice for 'blind' treatment of suspected bacterial meningitis, for it is effective against all four major bacterial pathogens (*N. meningitidis*, *S. pneumoniae*, *H. influenzae*, and *L. monocytogenes*) and many other Gram-negative organisms. However, it should not be used in neonates and infants unless serum concentrations can be monitored as there is a risk of severe toxicity with neutropenia, circulatory collapse, and 'grey baby' syndrome (because the neonate is deficient in glucuronyl transferase and very high levels of the drug rapidly occur, and the unconjugated drug is toxic to both bone marrow and kidney). Patients with liver disease or those taking drugs such as phenytoin which compete with chloramphenicol for hepatic metabolism will have higher plasma concentrations, while those taking phenobarbitone which induces hepatic inactivation of chloramphenicol will have lower concentrations than are normally expected. In Europe, bacterial meningitis between the ages of 6 months and 3 years is most likely to be caused by *H. influenzae* and so chloramphenicol should be used. In the United States, ampicillin is combined with chloramphenicol for the initial treatment of meningitis in this age group: chloramphenicol is stopped if the organism proves not to produce β-lactamase. In Europe and North America, bacterial meningitis above the age of 6 years is more likely to be pneumococcal or meningococcal, making benzylpenicillin the drug of choice. These recommendations assume that the patient shows no evidence of a chronic debilitating illness or immunosuppression in which case broader spectrum treatment would be needed to deal with the wider range of possible pathogens, for example, a third generation cephalosporin, such as cefotaxime or cefuroxime in combination with ampicillin or an aminoglycoside.

Antimicrobial drugs must be given by intravenous injection or infusion, until it is clear the patient is afebrile and well on the way to recovery. Intrathecal injection of penicillin is not necessary and is potentially dangerous. Although we agree with Christie that theoretically there might be no harm in instilling penicillin once only at the end of a diagnostic lumbar puncture, provided a non-irritant preparation is used in the correct dosage (not more than

10 000 units of benzylpenicillin in adults, and 5000 units or less in children) the advantage in practice is highly problematical, for a higher level of penicillin will have been achieved in the CSF about a quarter of an hour after systemic administration of adequate doses of benzylpenicillin than would ever be reached by the intrathecal route. We have twice seen instant death caused because a young doctor got his decimal point wrong. There is in our view no longer any justification for administration of intrathecal penicillin.

Once a specific diagnosis has been made by Gram stain, immunodiagnosis or culture, antimicrobial treatment may be changed to the drug of choice (Tables 1 and 3). The duration of antimicrobial treatment is difficult to decide. Most authorities recommend 7–10 days, assuming a satisfactory clinical response. However, the excellent results of single-dose treatment with a long-acting chloramphenicol preparation (Tifomycine) during meningitis epidemics in Africa (see page 5.206) suggest that much shorter therapy might be effective, provided there is no extrameningeal focus of infection. It is important to remember that antagonism between antimicrobial agents has been demonstrated in the treatment of bacterial meningitis. Penicillin with tetracycline was less effective than penicillin alone and ampicillin was more effective than a combination of ampicillin, chloramphenicol, and streptomycin. In an animal model of pneumococcal meningitis, penicillin was more effective than a combination of penicillin and chloramphenicol.

The treatment of neonatal Gram-negative bacillary meningitis is particularly difficult because 70 per cent have ventriculitis. Aminoglycosides, until recently the most effective drugs, can be delivered to this site only by intraventricular injection or through an indwelling reservoir. Using this technique the mortality has been reduced to 6 per cent. However, third generation cephalosporins have proved effective when given by intravenous injection and are now the treatment of choice where they can be afforded.

Many clinicians reduce the dose of the antimicrobial drug when the patient shows improvement. That may be illogical, for as the meningitis subsides, the blood–brain barrier is re-established and it may be that one in fact ought to *increase* the dose as the patient gets better (e.g. in small children with *H. influenzae* meningitis).

General management

Patients with bacterial meningitis should be nursed as other patients with impaired consciousness, bearing in mind the risk of convulsions and aspiration pneumonia. They should be laid on their side, and the position changed every 2 hours. The airway must be kept patent and convulsions prevented with intramuscular phenobarbitone sodium (7 mg/kg, maximum 600 mg daily: remember its effect on chloramphenicol metabolism) or treated with intravenous diazepam (1 mg for each year of age to a maximum of 10 mg by slow intravenous injection, repeat after 4 hours if necessary; it is painful and may depress respiration). Phenytoin sodium (diphenyl hydantoin USP) (5 mg/kg/day in two doses) has the advantages of inhibiting antidiuretic hormone secretion and not causing drowsiness or respiratory depression but the disadvantage of competing with chloramphenicol for hepatic metabolism. Hyperpyrexia must be prevented by fanning, sponging, and antipyretic drugs. The headache is so severe that parenteral pethidine

Table 3 Antimicrobial chemotherapy of some of the common causes of acute bacterial meningitis

Organism	First choice	Second choice
Neisseria meningitidis / *Streptococcus pneumoniae*	Benzylpenicillin i.v.: *adults* 4 mega units (2.4 g) 4 hourly; *children* 50 000 units/kg (30 mg) 4 hourly. In *S. pneumoniae*: if no response double dose	Chloramphenicol i.v.: *adults* 20–25 mg/kg 6 hourly, up to 4 g/d; *children* 12.5 mg/kg 6–8 hourly. Cave: dangerous in neonates and infants
Haemophilus influenzae 'Gram negative'	Chloramphenicol i.v. (dose, see above). Cefuroxime (or 3rd generation cephalosporin*) i.v.: *adults* 3 g, 8 hourly; *children* 200–240 mg/kg/d initially	Ampicillin i.v. 50 mg/kg 4 hourly. Co-trimoxazole i.v.: *adults* 160 mg trimethoprim + 800 mg sulphamethoxazole 12 hourly; *children* 6 + 30 mg/kg/d. cave: hypersensitivity to sulphonamide
Pseudomonas aeruginosa	Piperacillin i.v.: *adults* 4 g, 6–8 hourly; *children* 100–300 mg/kg/d or ceftazidime i.v.: *adults* 2 g, 8–12 hourly; *children* 30–100 mg/kg/d + tobramycin i.v.: *adults* 3–5 mg/kg/d; *children* 6–7.5 mg/kg/daily or netilmicin 4–6 mg/kg/daily in divided doses (8 hourly)	Ticarcillin or mezlocillin + gentamicin 5 mg/kg/d
Staphylococcus aureus	Flucloxacillin (or oxacillin or nafcillin USP): *adults* 3 g 6 hourly; *children* 300 mg/kg/d	Vancomycin i.v.[†]: *adults* 500 mg 6 hourly; *children* 40 mg/kg/d
Staphylococcus epidermidis	Vancomycin i.v.[†] + gentamicin 5 mg/kg/d + rifampicin: *adults* 1.2 g/d; *children* 20 mg/kg/d (penicillin-sensitive organism should be treated with benzylpenicillin i.v., dose as above)	
Listeria monocytogenes	Ampicillin i.v. (dose see above) (+ gentamicin i.v. for immunocompromised patients)	Chloramphenicol i.v. or co-trimoxazole i.v. (dose as above)
Streptococcus agalactiae (Group B)	Benzylpenicillin i.v.: *neonates* 150 000–250 000 units/kg/d (90–150 mg/kg/d)	

Note: In all cases, normal renal function is assumed. In renal failure dose must be reduced after the initial dose; as a rough guide:

$$\frac{\text{normal plasma creatinine}}{\text{patient's plasma creatinine}} \times \text{normal dose may be used}$$

* 3rd generation cephalosporins such as cefotaxime or latamoxef.
† Intrathecal, intraventricular or intrashunt injection of vancomycin or gentamicin may be used (contact manufacturers for special preparation and dosage).

or morphine are frequently required. It is interesting, in view of early descriptions of bacterial meningitis as 'water on the brain' or 'dropsy of the brain' that cerebral oedema, hydrocephalus, and intracranial effusions should now be recognized as important consequences of this condition. No treatment is required for cerebral oedema, unless the patient develops papilloedema or other signs of cerebral compression or incipient herniation of the brain. Intracranial pressure can be lowered by hyperventilating the patient with a mechanical ventilator to reduce the arterial P_{CO_2} below 4.7 kPa (35 mmHg). An intravenous infusion of 20 per cent mannitol (1 g/kg body weight in the first 10 minutes, then 2 g/kg for the next 2 hours) is also effective but may cause fluid and electrolyte disturbances and acute pulmonary oedema. The efficacy of corticosteroids in bacterial meningitis, and in particular their action on the associated cerebral oedema, is unproved. In a rabbit model of pneumococcal meningitis, dexamethasone in a dose of 1 mg/kg produced a rapid resolution of cerebral oedema, and reductions in CSF lactate concentration and CSF pressure. A properly controlled clinical study is urgently needed.

Urethral catheterization may be required. Fluid balance is important. Dehydration and hypovolaemia may contribute to hypotension, whereas cerebral oedema may be a problem in some patients. Meningitis and cerebral abscess like other intracranial lesions, may give rise to inappropriate secretion of antidiuretic hormone, resulting in fluid retention and profound hyponatraemia. This abnormality has been found in the majority of children with bacterial meningitis. It may be exaggerated by mannitol therapy for cerebral oedema. If hyponatraemia is thought to be contributing to coma (serum sodium concentration less than 110 m Eq/l) hypertonic (5 per cent) saline in a dose calculated to restore a serum sodium concentration of 125 mEq/l can be cautiously infused, together with a diuretic such as frusemide. Dimethylchlortetracycline can be given to antagonize the action of ADH on the distal tubule, provided there is no evidence of renal failure. If there is the drug must be used with extreme caution. Sudden death during convalescence, as described so distressingly by Aldous Huxley in *Point Counter Point* (1928), is probably attributable to an intracranial bleed or rupture of a collection of pus.

In children under the age of 18 months, subdural effusion is a common complication of *H. influenzae* and *S. pneumoniae* meningitides. This may be detected by measuring the head circumference and transilluminating the skull. Subdural paracentesis may be performed through the anterior fontanelle. Obstructive and communicating hydrocephalus may respond to antimicrobial treatment, but about 2 per cent of cases require surgical intervention. Cerebral arteries, veins, and venous sinuses may be occluded. Cerebral venous thrombosis is associated particularly with *H. influenzae* meningitis. There is a late deterioration in consciousness, often heralded by a Jacksonian seizure and then generalized convulsions and postictal paralysis. In children and adults, suspicion of intracranial collections of pus should prompt computer-assisted tomography and drainage through a burr hole if an abscess is found.

Management of associated septicaemias

Effects of infection outside the central nervous system may be seen in patients with septicaemia. Infective endocarditis may be the cause of meningitis through embolisation and mycotic aneurysm formation in the brain. In meningococcal septicaemia, disseminated intravascular coagulation, spontaneous bleeding, hypotension, and myocarditis contribute to the severe cardiovascular dysfunction. Corticosteroids are of doubtful value in this syndrome and heparin is likely to lead to rapid death from cerebrovascular haemorrhage and is absolutely contraindicated; but rapid digitalization, isoprenaline or dopamine and the use of clotting factors and platelet concentrates may be effective.

Immunological complications of meningococcal infection should be treated with anti-inflammatory drugs, such as salicylates. If there is associated septicaemia (particularly in meningococcal sep-

ticaemia), shock lung may require positive end expiratory pressure ventilation. The outlook is grave if this stage has been reached.

Prognosis and sequelae

In Europe and North America the overall mortality of meningitis caused by *N. meningitidis* is about 7–14 per cent; for *H. influenzae*, 3–10 per cent; *S. pneumoniae*, 15–60 per cent; and for group B streptococci and *L. monocytogenes* meningitis, above 20 per cent. The mortality is much higher in the very young and old and in patients with debilitating illnesses.

Permanent neurological sequelae include mental retardation, deafness, and other cranial nerve deficits and hydrocephalus. The reported incidence of sensorineural deafness after meningitis ranges from 5 to 40 per cent. A large proportion recover within a few months. *Neisseria meningitidis* and *H. influenzae* are the main causes of this complication. *Streptococcus suis* meningitis is frequently followed by deafness. *H. influenzae* appears to be the major cause of acquired mental retardation in the United States. This complication is found in 30–50 per cent of children who have suffered from *H. influenzae* meningitis.

Prevention

Monovalent and polyvalent capsular polysaccharide vaccines are now available for meningococcal meningitis (sero groups A, C. Y, and W –135). These can be used to protect people with a high risk of infection in institutions and for vaccination of family contacts during epidemics or for people when work (e.g. relief missions) takes them to areas with an epidemic outbreak (page 5.207). A polyvalent pneumococcal vaccine against 23 serotypes is available. It is indicated in people at special risk (e.g. postsplenectomy, sickle cell disease, chronic debilitating illnesses, and severe cardiorespiratory disease). The patient must be vaccinated *before* splenectomy is undertaken (for instance in Hodgkin's disease).

Chemoprophylaxis is indicated for close household and other intimate contacts of patients with *N. meningitidis* and *H. influenzae* meningitis.

Hospital staff are often very anxious, especially if a patient has died of meningitis on the ward. Prophylaxis is not needed in this case, except for those involved in mouth-to-mouth resuscitation or close inspection of the patient's upper respiratory tract. *N. meningitidis* is hardly ever isolated from the throats of patients with meningococcal meningitis. Sulphadiazine (3 g daily for adults, 1.5 g for children) is still effective in a majority of cases in some countries (e.g. in Britain). Minocycline is effective but contraindicated because of vertigo and other side-effects. Rifampicin is effective for prophylaxis against meningococci (600 mg twice a day for adults, 20 mg/kg/day for children for 2 days), and against *H. influenzae* (in the same dose for 4 days).

Tuberculous meningitis

Epidemiology

In western countries, the incidence of tuberculous meningitis has fallen in parallel with tuberculosis as a whole. For example, in the late 1940s there were 2000 cases per year in England and Wales, accounting for 10–20 per cent of cases of bacterial meningitis, but by the early 1970s this had fallen to less than 4 per cent. However, it remains a major problem and cause of death in developing countries. In India, 2–5 per cent of patients admitted to paediatric hospitals are suffering from tuberculous meningitis and in Africa and Southeast Asia, tuberculous meningitis accounts for 1–12 per cent of all neurological admissions. Human *Mycobacterium tuberculosis* is now responsible for most cases of tuberculous meningitis. Bovine organisms, which formerly caused more than 40 per cent, are now implicated in only 4–8 per cent. Avian and atypical organisms (e.g. *M. kansasii* and *M. scrofulaceum*) are rarely involved. In debilitated or immunocompromised patients, such as those with the acquired immune deficiency syndrome (AIDS), disseminated *M. avium-intracellulare* has been reported.

In Britain now, immigrants from Pakistan, India, Africa, and the West Indies are the most likely to contract the disease. Most cases of tuberculous meningitis are in young children between the ages of 3 months and 3 years, but, in recent years, in both western and developing countries, primary infection has been acquired at a later age and, as a result, a larger proportion of patients with tuberculous meningitis are now adults. The disease is very uncommon, but severe, in pregnant women.

Pathogenesis

Small caseous microtubercles develop in the brain, meninges or, less commonly, in the bones of the skull and vertebrae close to the meninges. This infection has seeded through the blood stream from the primary lesion or a site of chronic infection. Many patients develop miliary tuberculosis at the stage of haematogenous spread. Infection of the meninges results from rupture of a microtubercle with discharge of tuberculoprotein and mycobacteria into the subarachnoid space. In the sensitized (tuberculin-positive) patient, this event will be marked by an episode of fever and meningeal irritation caused by the intrathecal tuberculin reaction. Subacute inflammation, especially of the basal meninges, then develops producing cranial nerve lesions, cerebral arteritis causing infarction, impairment of CSF absorption or obstruction to the CSF circulation causing hydrocephalus and, in the spinal cord, spinal arachnoiditis, producing multiple radiculopathy or myelopathy.

Pathology

Meningeal miliary tubercles may be found on the surfaces of the brains of most victims of miliary tuberculosis. They are usually few in number and occur in the region of the Sylvian fissure, while there may be larger caseous plaques deeper in the sulci. The brains of patients dying of tuberculous meningitis are usually oedematous. A mass of thick greyish exudate encases the base of the brain, filling the basal cisterns. Within the ventricular system there is ependymitis with a similar exudate choking the choroid plexus. The exudate consists of lymphocytes, plasma cells, giant cells, and foci of caseation, but mycobacteria are usually scanty. At the base of the brain the cranial nerves and the internal carotid artery and its branches are trapped and damaged by the exudate. Arteries are obliterated by an endarteritis, with resulting ischaemia and infarction of superficial areas of the brain, basal ganglia, hypothalamus, brain stem, and spinal cord. There is congestion and phlebitis of the meningeal veins. Both the inflammatory exudate and the arteritis are probably a delayed hypersensitivity reaction to the tuberculoprotein. Some degree of hydrocephalus develops in most cases. Usually the hydrocephalus is communicating in type and is caused by obliteration of the basal cisterns. Less commonly compression or blockage of the aqueduct of Sylvius or, more commonly, the foramina of Luschka and Magendie in the fourth ventricle, causes obstructive hydrocephalus. A detailed review of these changes is given by Tandon (1978).

Clinical features

Typically, symptoms of meningitis and central nervous system involvement are preceded by 2–8 weeks of non-specific prodromal symptoms unlikely to raise the suspicion of tuberculous meningitis. This phase of vague malaise, irritability, insomnia, lethargy, anorexia, headache, abdominal pain, vomiting, and behavioural changes may develop after a head injury, surgical operation or common childhood infection such as measles, influenza or otitis media. The implication is that meningeal infection is precipitated by these conditions. By the time patients have developed obvious symptoms and signs of meningitis, the disease is well advanced. Patients usually have low grade fever, but severe pyrexia can occur. Up to three-quarters of the patients will have symptoms and signs of tuberculosis in the lungs or elsewhere. Rarely, tuberculous meningitis presents dramatically with an acute encephalopathy with severe headache, neck stiffness, vomiting, and seizures, suggesting subarachnoid haemorrhage, acute bacterial meningitis or cerebrovascular accident.

During the second stage there is obvious meningeal irritation (headache, vomiting, neck stiffness) and evidence of cranial nerve damage, cerebral endarteritis, and developing hydrocephalus. Infants are irritable with opisthotonos and a tense fontanelle. Cranial nerve lesions, seen in 25 per cent of cases, involve one or more of the following: II, III, IV, VI, VII, VIII (Figs 9 and 10). The pupils may be dilated, unequal, and unresponsive, and many patients develop a squint from abducens nerve palsy. Fundal examination reveals papilloedema in 40 per cent and sometimes evidence of optic atrophy. Choroid tubercles are occasionally seen (Fig. 11). Vascular lesions result in a wide variety of abnormalities including aphasia, hemianopia, hemiparesis, and paraplegia. Various types of convulsive disorders are common, especially in children (10–15 per cent). If the disease is allowed to progress to a third stage of coma with signs of more severe damage to the brain and spinal cord, less than half can be expected to survive despite active treatment. Severe intracranial hypertension, a common complication of tuberculous meningitis, results from cerebral oedema, hydrocephalus, and less commonly from various space-taking lesions, such as tuberculomas, and tuberculous abscesses. Hydrocephalus should be suspected in all patients with tuberculous meningitis who develop an impaired level of consciousness. They often have severe headache, ocular palsy, pyramidal signs in the lower limbs, incontinence of urine and persistent elevation of the intracranial pressure. If left untreated the patients become stuporous or comatose and develop signs of brain stem damage, such as decerebrate rigidity, irregular breathing, and loss of brain stem reflexes. The syndrome of inappropriate secretion of antidiuretic hormone (SIADH) is also common in patients with severe tuberculous meningitis. It produces impairment of consciousness, but

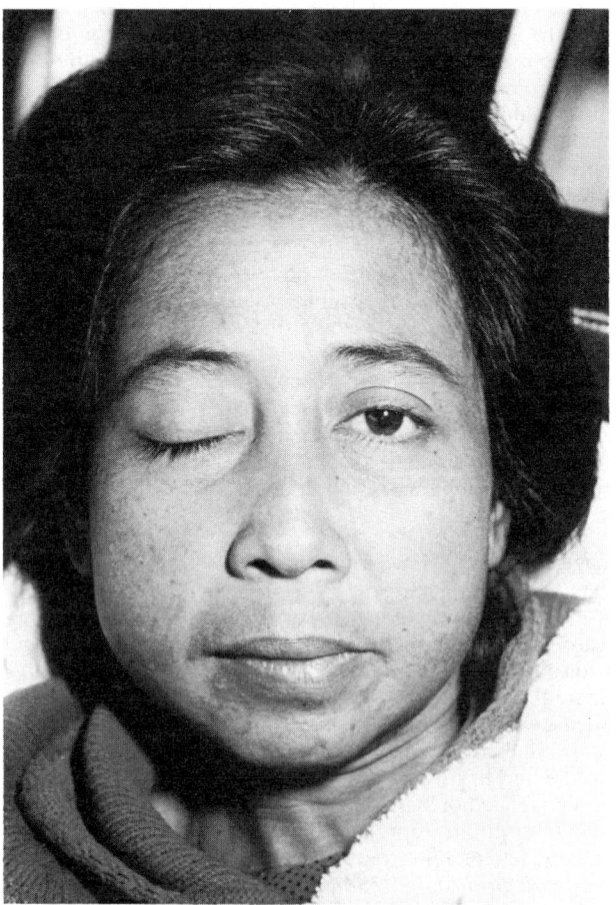

Fig. 9 Right III nerve palsy in a Thai woman with tuberculous meningitis.

decerebrate rigidity or other signs of brain stem damage are not found. Other uncommon neurological abnormalities include cerebellar signs, involuntary movements such as chorea, hemiballismus, and myoclonus, hypothalamic disorders leading to loss of control of blood pressure and body temperature and abnormal patterns of respiration, and various spinal cord syndromes (tuberculous spinal arachnoiditis) (see Fig. 12).

Diagnosis

Examination of CSF is crucial. Lumbar puncture does not seem to be subject to the same dangers as in acute bacterial meningitis and, apparently, lumbar puncture has been repeated safely in patients with tuberculous meningitis even when there is papilloedema. CSF opening pressure is raised in the majority of patients, but it is low or falls in those developing spinal block. The CSF is usually macroscopically clear, but may form a spider's web clot on standing. The mechnism of the cobweb formation is unclear, but it does not appear to be caused by the high protein concentration. In patients with spinal block the fluid may be xanthochromic with a very high protein concentration and may quickly form a jelly (Froin's syndrome). Total cell counts range between 50 and 500/μl with an initial preponderance of neutrophils, but a later increase in lymphocytes up to 400/μl – the result of an intrathecal tuberculin reaction. Occasionally the cell count may exceed 1000/μl. The CSF glucose concentration of the intial CSF sample is low in about 90 per cent of the patients. Although non-specific, this finding is of great practical use, because it differentiates tuberculous meningitis presumptively from most cases of viral meningitis. Indeed tuberculous meningitis must be strongly suspected in any patient who presents with lymphocytic meningitis and a low CSF glucose concentration. CSF chloride concentration is low in tuberculous meningitis, in parallel with the degree of hypochloraemia, result-

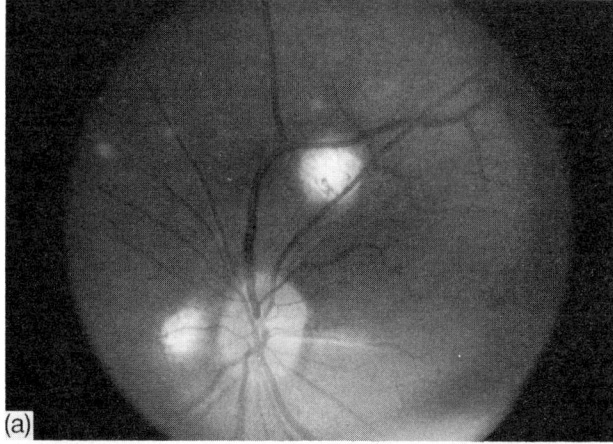
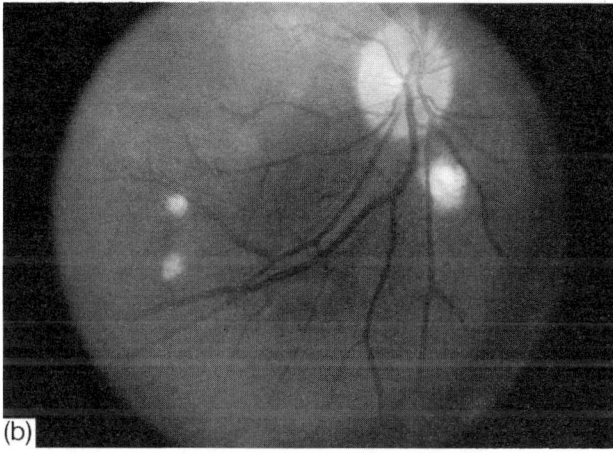

Fig. 11 (a, b) Tuberculous choroiditis in a 23-year-old Thai girl.

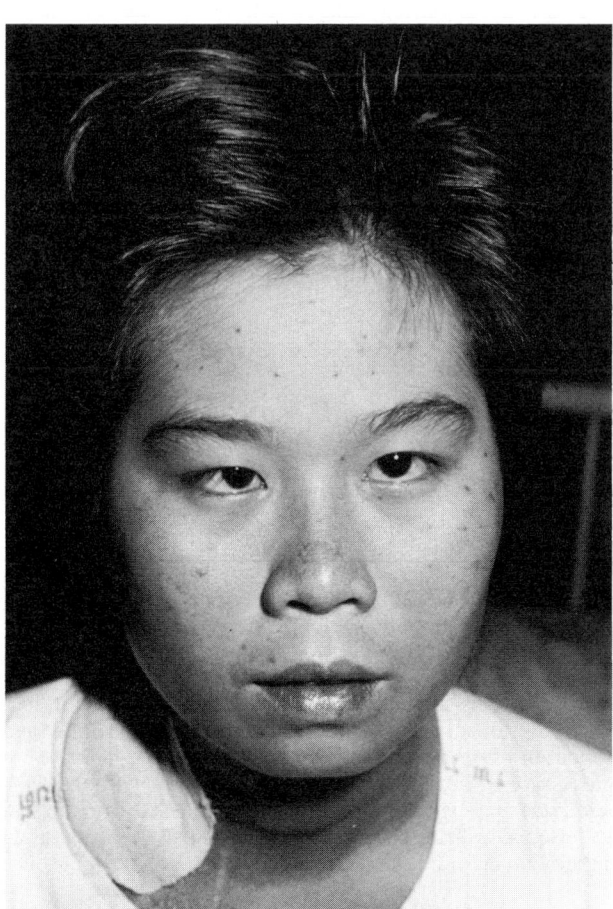

Fig. 10 Bilateral VI nerve palsies in a Thai girl with tuberculous meningitis. The cervical node biopsy was positive for acid fast bacilli.

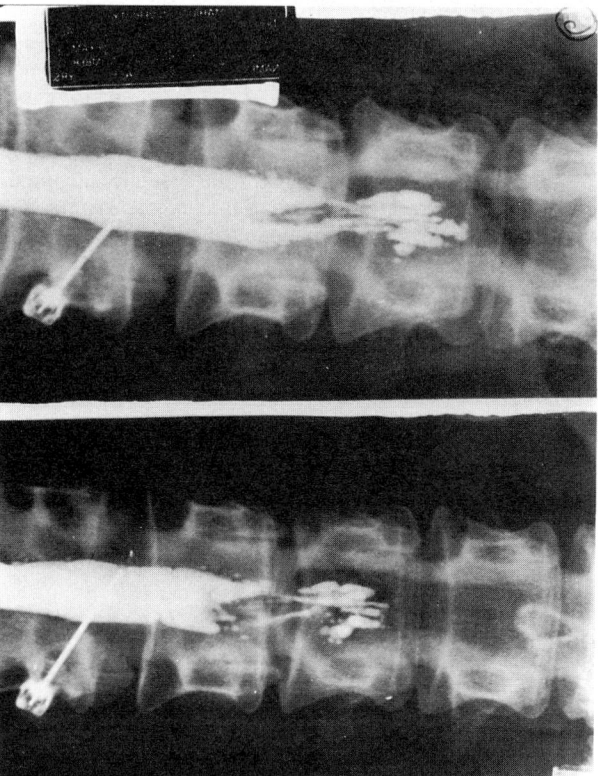

Fig. 12 Spinal tuberculoma and spinal arachnoiditis revealed by myelography in a Thai patient with tuberculous meningitis.

ing from repeated vomiting and perhaps inappropriate ADH secretion. It has no special diagnostic value. Very rarely the CSF may be misleadingly normal in some patients who present with features of cerebral tumour or a spinal cord lesion. In these cases, the tuberculous focus is presumably not communicating with the lumbar CSF. Sudden rupture of a large caseous lesion may produce symptoms, signs, and a marked neutrophil pleocytosis suggesting acute bacterial meningitis. Success in detecting tubercle bacilli in CSF by acid-fast, auramine or fluorescent staining can, in some hands, be increased from the usual average of 10–20 per cent to almost 100 per cent of cases. The secret is to start with a large volume of CSF (10–20 ml), to centrifuge it long and hard, and to examine the sediment under a microscope for 30 to 90 minutes. Repeated lumbar punctures increase the chance of finding tubercle bacilli and of observing the characteristic changes in CSF composition. Culture of myobacteria is successful in 10–90 per cent of cases. Specimens other than CSF (e.g. sputum, gastric washings in children, urine, etc.) should also be cultured in order to establish the sensitivity of the infecting organism. The bromide partition test, although still having its advocates, is not of practical use, because it lacks specificity. It is abnormal in other types of meningitis and even in cerebral malaria. The test is time consuming and is no more sensitive than the CSF glucose levels. A rapid test for detecting plasma membrane antigen of tubercle bacilli in CSF has been developed using slide agglutination of sensitised latex particles and enzyme-linked immunosorbent assay. Preliminary results have been very encouraging. The tuberculin test is positive in 50–95 per cent of patients with tuberculous meningitis, but this reactivity may be suppressed in debilitated or immunosuppressed patients. A search for evidence of tuberculosis elsewhere in the body is useful, but the chest radiograph is normal in up to half the patients and miliary mottling is seen only in a minority. CT scans are useful to support the diagnosis and detection of the complications of tuberculous meningitis. Communicating hydrocephalus and its characteristically enhanced basal exudates can be demonstrated by CT scans in about 80 per cent of the patients. They may also reveal associated tuberculomas or cerebral infarct secondary to the arteritis.

Differential diagnosis

Although a few patients with tuberculous meningitis present acutely, the majority show a subacute or chronic progression. Clinically, the differential diagnosis should include cryptococcal meningitis, and various subacute or chronic aseptic meningitides including partially treated bacterial meningitis, parameningial infections, neoplastic and granulomatous infiltrations of the meninges (e.g. carcinomas, leukaemias, lymphomas, sarcoidosis) and cerebral tumours. Fungal meningitides (*Cryptococcus, Coccidioides, Histoplasma, Candida*) may present like tuberculous meningitis. Other conditions which have caused confusion in particular clinical or geographical settings are meningovascular syphi-

lis, toxoplasmal meningitis in immunosuppressed patients, notably in AIDS, cysticercosis, African trypanosomiasis, and schistosomal myelopathy. In most of these cases, CSF examination including cytology, India ink preparation, immunodiagnostic tests (e.g. cryptococcal latex agglutination), serological tests and microbial culture will allow differentiation.

Treatment

The untreated mortality of tuberculous meningitis is close to 100 per cent. As with acute bacterial meningitis, chemotherapy must be started on the basis of clinical suspicion immediately after adequate samples have been taken for microscopy, immunodiagnosis, culture, and animal inoculation. Isoniazid, pyrazinamide, ethionamide, and cycloserine are freely distributed into the CSF. Penetration is limited, but still adequate during the first few months of the meningitis, in the case of rifampicin, ethambutol and streptomycin. Para-aminosalisylic acid should not be used because it does not enter the CSF. At least two drugs to which the organism is sensitive should be used. The combination of isoniazid and rifampicin for 18 to 24 months is currently the most popular (Table 4). In severe cases pyrazinamide and streptomycin are added for the first few months. There is some evidence that streptomycin is more effective when given intrathecally, but this is probably not necessary, because CSF levels during the active stage of the meningitis are adequate.

In countries where rifampicin cannot be afforded, triple therapy with isoniazid, streptomycin, and pyrazinamide should be tried. Treatment of tuberculous meningitis during an initial 2-month intensive phase with isoniazid, rifampicin, pyrazinamide, and streptomycin, followed by isoniazid plus rifampicin for 7 months, has been investigated recently. Preliminary results of this trial have been encouraging. Adverse drug reactions such as drug rashes and hepatotoxicity may occur during the treatment. In adults daily single doses of 300 mg of isoniazid, 600 mg of rifampicin, and 1500 mg of pyrazinamide provide adequate levels in the sera and CSF of patients with active tuberculous meningitis. Higher doses of these drugs are not necessary and may result in a higher incidence of hepatotoxicity.

Response to antituberculosis chemotherapy is slow. Particularly in patients who are not given corticosteroids (see below), there may be an increase in temperature and CSF protein concentration, and transient neutrophil pleocytosis during the first two to three weeks after starting optimal chemotherapy. However, some sign of clinical improvement is usually seen within the first two weeks. Usually the first clinical evidence of response is an improvement of the headache, sense of general well-being, and settling of the temperature. A rapid return to normal in CSF composition (e.g. in 1–2 weeks) virtually excludes the diagnosis of tuberculous meningitis, in which case antituberculosis treatment should be stopped. Usually it would take at least a few weeks to a few months for the cells, CSF glucose, and protein to return to normal. In some patients the high protein concentration persists.

'Trial' of chemotherapy is justified when there is clinical suspicion of tuberculous meningitis and is widely used where diagnostic facilities are limited. Treatment should be continued for 18 months unless there is very rapid improvement in the patient's condition and CSF composition, suggesting another cause of aseptic meningitis. In some severely ill patients who present acutely with features of acute bacterial meningitis (e.g. neutrophil pleocytosis) but in whom initial laboratory results are not helpful, it may be necessary to initiate 'blind' treatment for acute bacterial and tuberculous meningitis simultaneously. In these, fortunately rare, cases, isoniazid, rifampicin and streptomycin or ethambutol, together with chloramphenicol (see Tables 3 and 4) can be given.

Treatment of complications

The complications of tuberculous meningitis are common and some often are serious enough to cause severe morbidity and

Table 4 Treatment of tuberculous meningitis

Drug	Dose (frequency, route)	Length of treatment (months)
1 Isoniazid + pyridoxine	10 mg*/kg/d max 300 mg* (o.d., oral) adult 10 mg, child 5 mg (b.d., oral)	18–24
2 Rifampicin	10 mg*/kg/d max 600 mg (o.d., oral)	5–6
3 Streptomycin	20 mg/kg/d max 1 g (o.d., i.m.)	2–3
4 Ethambutol	15 mg*/kg/d (o.d., oral)	18–24
5 Thiacetazone	4 mg/kg/d max 150 mg (o.d., oral)	18–24
6 Pyrazinamide	20–30 mg/kg/d max 1500 mg (o.d., oral)	18–24

* Dose can be doubled initially.
First choice: 1 + 2 + 3 (add 4 *or* 6 in severe cases)
Second choice: 1 + 3 + 4
Economical regimens: 1 + 3 + 5, 1 + 3 + 6

death in spite of active treatment with antituberculosis drugs. Increased intracranial pressure, found in about 90 per cent of the patients, is often associated with communicating hydrocephalus and basal arachnoiditis. Less commonly it is caused by diffuse cerebral oedema with small lateral ventricles. In these patients conservative treatment with repeated lumbar punctures and corticosteroid should be tried. If these measures fail, surgical treatment will be needed for the hydrocephalus. However in patients who are very ill with impaired consciousness, ventricular drainage or insertion of a shunt should be performed without delay.

Costicosteroids might be expected to reduce the inflammatory reaction and the fibrotic organization of exudate in the brain and spinal cord but their value remains controversial. No controlled trial has demonstrated that corticosteroids increase survival or reduce sequelae. Despite their familiar side effects, they are still recommended empirically for patients with threatened or established spinal block, evidence of hydrocephalus or cerebral oedema, visual failure from optochiasmic arachnoiditis, those who develop focal neurological signs caused by arteritis, young children, and the severely ill. The usual regimen is oral prednisolone, 60–80 mg per day for adults, 1–3 mg/kg/day for children, given in a tapering course over 4–6 weeks. Intrathecal injection of corticosteroids is unnecessary.

Fluid, electrolyte, and acid–base disturbances are common, the result of vomiting, inadequate intake, and inappropriate secretion of ADH. Inappropriate secretion of ADH can be treated as in acute bacterial meningitis (see above). Progressive loss of vision caused by fibrosing exudate around the optic chiasma may respond to surgical decompression. Cerebral tuberculomas may occasionally develop during the course of the treatment of tuberculous meningitis. They should be treated conservatively, and the response to the treatment assessed by CT scan. Biopsy or surgical intervention is not necessary and may be harmful. Nursing care is very important during the acute illness when there are the usual problems presented by unconscious patients (see above) and during the prolonged phase of convalescence and rehabilitation. Anticonvulsants are often needed, especially in children.

Prognosis and sequelae

In western industrialized countries, the mortality of tuberculous meningitis is still rather high at about 15 to 30 per cent, and in developing countries it remains between 30 and 50 per cent. The prognosis is worst and the risk of sequelae highest in those admitted in coma with signs of brain stem damage, in the very young and very old, pregnant women and those with malnutrition or other diseases, those who develop hydrocephalus and in those with the most abnormal CSF composition before treatment. There are permanent sequelae in 10 to 30 per cent of survivors. Intellectual impairment is especially common in infants and young children. As many as 60 per cent of patients who have seizures during the illness will suffer recurrences. Up to 25 per cent of survivors will have cranial nerve deficits including blindness, deafness, and squints. 10 to 25 per cent of survivors have some residual weakness after hemiplegia or paraplegia (tuberculous spinal arachnoiditis). Patients with pituitary and hypothalmic abnormalities such as hypogonadism and diabetes insipidus may have calcification of the pituitary fossa. 10 to 40 per cent of patients develop CSF spinal block at some stage of the illness, but this will recover completely in at least half of them. Neurological deficits may progress or appear months or years after the illness as the subarachnoid exudate becomes fibrotic and calcified.

Prevention (see page 5.284)

BCG vaccination at birth reduces the risk of infection by at least 80 per cent, but this seems to vary in different countries. It is recommended for all infants born into communities where tuberculosis is prevalent including Asians living in Britain and expa-

triates living in tropical countries. To prevent the development of tuberculous meningitis in household contacts of newly diagnosed cases of pulmonary tuberculosis, prophylaxis with isoniazid 5–10 mg/kg daily for 6–12 months is recommended for all Mantoux positive children under the age of 5 years.

References
Acute bacterial meningitis
Adams, R. D., Kubik, C. S. and Bonner, F. J. (1948). The clinical and pathological aspects of influenzal meningitis. *Arch. Pediatr.* **65**, 354–351.

Christie, A. B. (1980). *Infectious diseases: epidemiology and clinical practice* 3rd edn, pp. 605–646. Churchill Livingstone, Edinburgh.

Feigin, R. D. (1981). Bacterial meningitis beyond the neonatal period. In *Textbook of pediatric infectious diseases* (eds R. D. Feigin and J. O. Cherry), pp. 293–308. W. B. Saunders, Philadelphia.

Hardman, J. M. and Earle, K. M. (1969). Myocarditis in 200 fatal meningococcal infections. *Arch. Pathol.* **87**, 318–325.

Levin, S., Harris, A. A. and Sokalski, S. J. (1978), Bacterial meningitis. In *Handbook of clinical neurology* Vol. 33 (eds P. J. Vinken and G. W. Bruyn), pp. 1–19. North-Holland, Amsterdam.

—— and Painter, M. B. (1966). The treatment of acute meningococcal infection in adults. *Ann. intern. Med.* **64**, 1049–1056.

Molavi, A. and Le Frock, J. L. (eds) (1985). Infections of the central nervous system. *Med. Clin. N. Am.* **69**, 1–434.

Mollaret, P. (1977). La meningite endothelio-leucocytaire multirecurrente benigne. *Rev. Neurol.* **133**, 225–244.

Moxon, E. R., Smith, A. L., Averill, D. R., *et al.* (1974). *Hemophilus influenzae* meningitis in infant rats after intranasal inoculation. *J. infect. Dis.* **129**, 154–162.

Tauber, M. G., Khayam-Bashi, H. and Sande, M. A. (1985). Effects of ampicillin and corticosteroids on brain water content, cerebrospinal fluid pressure, and cerebrospinal fluid lactate levels in experimental pneumococcal meningitis. *J. infect. Dis.* **151**, 528–534.

Tugwell, P., Greenwood, B. M. and Warrell, D. A. (1976). Pneumococcal meningitis: a clinical and laboratory study. *Q. J. Med.* **45**, 583–601.

Tuomanen, E., Tomasz, A., Hengstler, B, and Zak, O. (1985). The relative role of bacterial cell wall and capsule in the induction of inflammation in pneumococcal meningitis. *J. infect. Dis.* **151**, 535–540.

Tuberculous meningitis
(The reviews by Parsons and Tandon are particularly helpful.)

Bateman, D. E., Newman, P. K. and Foster, J. B. (1983). A restrospective survey of proven cases of tuberculous meningitis in the Northern Region, 1970–1980. *J. R. Coll. Physns.* **17**, 106–110.

Kennedy, D. H. and Fallon, R. J. (1979). Tuberculous meningitis. *J. Am. Med. Assn.* **241**, 264–268.

Kocen, R. S. and Parsons, M. (1970). Neurological complications of tuberculous meningitis. Some unusual manifestations. *Quart. J. Med.* **39**, 17–30.

Krambovitis, E., McIllmurray, M. B., Lock, P. E., Hendrickse, W. and Holzel, H. (1984). Rapid diagnosis of tuberculous meningitis by latex particle agglutination. *Lancet* **ii**, 1229–1231.

Parsons, M. (1979). *Tuberculous meningitis. A handbook for clinicians.* Oxford University Press, Oxford.

Rich, A. R. and McCordock, H. A. (1933). The pathogenesis of tuberculous meningitis. *Bull. Johns Hopkins Hosp.* **52**, 5–37.

Smith, H. V. (1964). Tuberculous meningitis. *Int. J. Neurol.* **4**, 134–157.

Tandon, P. N. (1978). Tuberculous meningitis (cranial and spinal). In *Handbook of clinical neurology* Vol. 33 (eds P. J. Vinken and G. W. Bruyn), pp. 195–262. North-Holland, Amsterdam.

Traub, M., Colchester, A. C. F., Kingsley, D. P. E. and Swash, M. (1984). Tuberculosis of the central nervous system. *Q. J. Med.* **53**, 81–100.

Neurosyphilis

J. B. FOSTER

Despite a dramatic decline in the incidence of neurosyphilis in the last three decades, invasion of the human nervous system by *Treponema pallidum* is still occurring and, frequently, the clinical presentation does not follow the traditional course of the preantibiotic era (see also Section 5).

General features

The biological characteristics of *T. pallidum* are described in Section 5. The organism reaches the central nervous system during the first few weeks or months after introduction into the body. The initial invasion of the CNS produces meningitis in about 25 per cent of cases. This may occasionally induce a frank clinical meningitic illness, or the patients may remain asymptomatic. About 10 per cent of patients will later develop what is described as tertiary or late neurosyphilis. In asymptomatic cases of syphilitic meningitis there may be abnormalities in the spinal fluid, and in those in whom the meningitis is more intense there may be cranial nerve palsies or convulsions similar to those occurring following invasion by a pyogenic organism. All cases of acute and subacute meningitis should have a serological examination for syphilis.

Chronic meningitis accompanies all forms of neurospecific disease and indeed, *T. pallidum* is the organism producing the most chronic form of meningitis in the human. Most of the pathological changes peculiar to syphilis are due to this chronicity with resulting arteritis and luminal thrombosis, meningo-encephalitis, ependymitis, and meningomyelitis. Thus the late forms of syphilis – general paralysis of the insane, tabes dorsalis, and optic atrophy – have a common origin in chronic syphilitic meningitis. Examination of spinal fluid in all such cases will reveal the presence of meningeal inflammation with pleocytosis and increase in the protein content of the fluid with positive serological tests. Thus, in so-called 'active neurosyphilis' there will be a pleocytosis of 200–300 mononuclear cells (mainly lymphocytes with a few plasma cells), and a protein level raised to about 2 g/l (200 mg/100 ml), with a high gammaglobulin content. A high colloidal gold curve (e.g. 5554311000) and positive serological test are diagnostic.

Serological tests for neurosyphilis depend upon the demonstration of non-specific antibodies and also of specific treponemal antibodies, for during infection with the organism a variety of antibodies are produced, only some of which are specific (see section 5). The Wasserman reaction (WR) was the first serological test used for this disease and, indeed, is still widely used. It depends on complement fixation of lipoidal antibody in the presence of a non-specific antigen. A more sophisticated test using purified antigen, cardiolipin, has refined the WR test. Kilmer's test is another test widely used in the USA. The most extensively used and important of the flocculation tests, i.e. the demonstration of reagin causing aggregation of a colloidal suspension of lipoidal particles, is the Venereal Disease Research Laboratory slide test (VDRL) which, in the United Kingdom, has largely replaced the WR.

Tests for group-reactive antitreponemal antibody include the Reiter protein complement fixation (RPCF) test. More recently, specific treponemal immobilization testing has been possible, i.e. the TPI test. This is still the most specific method for the diagnosis of syphilis. In active neurosyphilis, serology shows a positive VDRL in about 75 per cent of cases and a positive TPI or treponemal haemagglutination test and fluorescent treponemal antibody absorption test in nearly all cases. (For further discussion see Section 5.)

Examination of the cerebrospinal fluid monitors the activity and successful treatment of neurosyphilis. Specific tests for syphilis are virtually always positive in active disease but frequently remain positive even after adequate treatment. Thus a positive CSF test does not necessarily indicate active disease. Active neurosyphilis of any type produces a pleocytosis with rise of protein and high gammaglobulin concentration.

Clinical and pathological types

While accepting that so-called parenchymatous neurosyphilis results from a chronic inflammation of the meninges, certain clinical and pathological types of the disease can be described, although none exists in pure form.

Asymptomatic neurosyphilis

When the CSF examination indicates syphilitic involvement of the nervous system and there are no clinical symptoms and no abnormal physical signs, the condition is termed 'asymptomatic'. This situation may obtain at any time after the first few weeks of infection: all patients with positive results of serological tests should therefore have their CSF examined for any evidence of early invasion of the nervous system. Specific tests are positive in almost all asymptomatic cases, and especially in the CSF.

Meningovascular neurosyphilis

Clinically evident involvement of the meninges and meningeal vessels occurs within 12 years of primary infection. Thus, in any young adult presenting with a stroke, isolated cranial nerve palsy, or papillitis, serological tests for syphilis are obligatory. The underlying pathology is a chronic leptomeningitis as described, with subintimal fibroblastic proliferation (so-called Heubner's endarteritis obliterans). The commonest symptoms of meningeal involvement are headache and neck stiffness, with cranial nerve palsies of the oculomotor nerves in particular. Convulsions and mental confusion may occur. Occasionally the symptoms are more florid, with headache, papilloedema, nausea, and vomiting suggesting raised intracranial pressure. Fever does not usually accompany the neurological symptoms, which is a useful clue to the differentiation of neurovascular syphilis from tuberculous and the other chronic forms of meningitis. With adequate treatment, the prognosis at this stage is good. With the involvement of the arachnoid and pial blood vessels, sudden cerebrovascular accidents are common and cause focal neurological deficits such as hemiparesis, aphasia, sensory abnormalities, or visual disturbances. In such cases the CSF is almost always abnormal and specific tests are positive. The vascular complications tend to occur later in the course of this disease than in pure syphilitic meningitis.

Parenchymatous neurosyphilis

Approximately 15–20 years after the inoculation of *Treponema pallidum*, patients may develop one or another form of so-called 'parenchymatous neurosyphilis'. Although all these forms are based on chronic meningitis, the different types of the disease are usually considered separately as *general paralysis of the insane* (GPI) or *dementia paralytica*, *syphilitic meningo-encephalitis*, and *tabes dorsalis*. The classic review of this condition was published by Kraepelin in 1913; at that time the disease constituted one of the major causes of insanity.

Pathology

This chronic form of meningo-encephalitis is more frequent in men than in women, and shows specific neuropathological changes with cortical atrophy and ventricular dilatation. The meninges become thickened and opacified, and the ventricular walls are studded with ependymal granulations. There is a gross degree of gyral or convolutional atrophy, and histological examination of the cortex shows severe reduction in the number of neurones with secondary demyelination and proliferation of astrocytes with gliosis in both the grey and white matter. Glial stars are seen and iron deposition occurs in large amounts in the microglia and in the perivascular spaces. The infiltration of the leptomeninges extends into the Virchow–Robin spaces and the subglial and cortical vessels show a characteristic syphilitic endarteritis. The cytoarchitecture of the cortex is disrupted and, in these areas, special fluorescent techniques will demonstrate *Treponema pallidum* in about 50 per cent of the cases.

Clinical picture

Such diffuse changes in the cerebral cortex are reflected in the clinical picture, which is one of progressive intellectual deterioration with memory disturbance, lack of concentration, and lack of

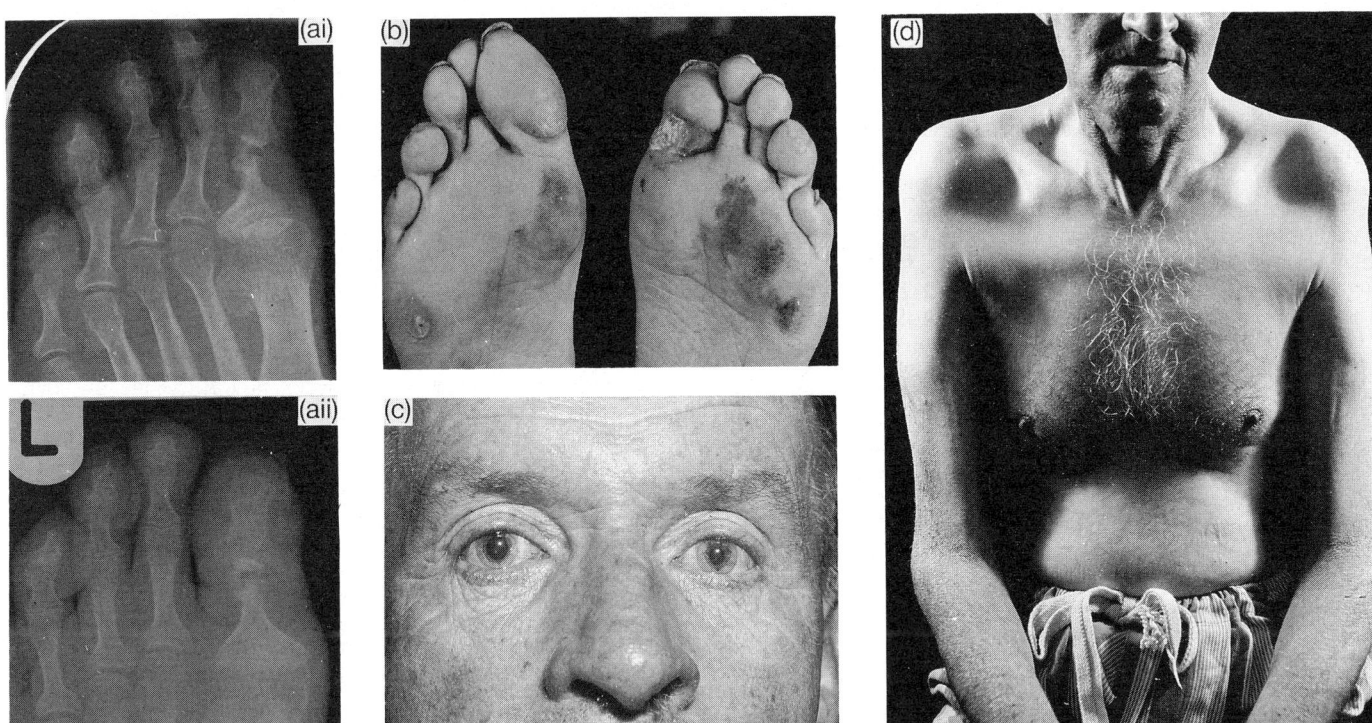

Fig. 1 Tables dorsalis with syphilitic amyotrophy. This patient has (*a*) Charcot toe joints; (*b*) ulcers of the feet; (*c*) unequal but not constricted pupils that do not react to light; and (*d*) amyotrophy affecting the shoulder girdle.

insight. The patient becomes ineffective, inefficient, lacking in judgement, untidy, and shows general and progressive mental disintegration. In addition to the dementia, he suffers from dysarthria, various forms of tremor and seizures, and has hyperactive reflexes with extensor plantar responses and accompanying Argyll Robertson pupils (see below). The grandiose megalomaniacal delusional picture is now rarely seen; more commonly the patient becomes depressed and morbidly delusional. The disease now appears to be less florid in its presentation than former descriptions would imply and the patient typically presents with simple dementia. Thus any patient with a dementing illness at any age must be tested for syphilis, which cannot be entirely excluded as the cause without examination of the CSF.

As the disease progresses the characteristic tremor of the hands is seen, with the so-called trombone tongue. The unsteadiness eventually forces the patient to take to his bed permanently, and it may then be apparent that he has notable focal neurological signs, in addition to the global dementia. In GPI, serological tests are almost invariably positive. The state of the spinal fluid reflects the presence of chronic meningitis, with cellular pleocytosis, increased protein level and positive tests for syphilis. The prognosis in cases diagnosed early may be quite good, with about 30 per cent making a recovery sufficient to enable them to carry on their previous occupation. Without treatment, the patient dies within three to four years of the onset of symptoms.

Differential diagnosis

Conditions to be considered in patients suspected to be suffering from general paralysis are psychotic states such as schizophrenia, and other forms of presenile dementia such as Alzheimer's disease, in addition to the effects of small vessel vascular disease. Frontal tumours, chronic abscess and other forms of chronic inflammatory disease of the brain, alcoholism, drug addiction, and renal and hepatic failure may mimic GPI; occasionally B_{12} encephalopathy will present with progressive dementia. Chronic intractable epilepsy, severe head injury, subdural haematoma, Huntington's chorea, and carcinomatosis, may also be mistaken for parenchymatous neurosyphilis.

Tabes dorsalis

Clinical picture

About 10–25 years after infection, the syphilitic patient may present with the features of *locomotor ataxia* or *tabes dorsalis*. The clinical picture (Fig. 1) is characterized by lightning pains in the limbs, and progressive ataxia with accompanying sphincter disturbance. Although new cases are not commonly seen, tabes was at one time said to occur in 10 per cent of all cases of syphilis. Men are much more commonly affected than women. The first symptoms of the disease usually appear in the fourth and fifth decade. Occasionally, tabes dorsalis complicates congenital syphilis and appears in adolescence or early adult life. The disease derives its name from the involvement of the posterior columns of the spinal cord which, on histological examination, show gross demyelination secondary to destruction of the posterior roots, possibly by a constrictive meningitis, or possibly a direct toxic radiculopathy. In addition to the spinal cord changes, Argyll Robertson pupils, i.e. small pupils not reacting to light but reacting on convergence, are almost invariably present. It is suggested that the responsible lesion lies either in the periaqueductal grey matter of the midbrain or in the ciliary ganglion.

The possible presentations of this disease are legion, from an acute presentation with lightning pains in the thighs, to a more chronic disturbance of bladder function. The ataxia may be early and evolving. The high-stepping gait consequent upon the proprioceptive loss is characteristic, and failing vision, impotence, double vision, deafness, a neurogenic arthropathy, or perforating trophic ulcers on the feet may all be the presenting clinical phenomena. The lightning pains which occur in about 90 per cent of cases may be localized or move from place to place: these pains are severe, and pass through, rather than down, the lower limbs. The ataxia due to proprioceptive loss is much worse with the eyes closed, or in the dark, and the loss of muscular tone contributes to the disability induced by the ataxia. The patient may complain that his feet feel numb and that he has the sensation of walking on cotton wool. Paroxysmal pains may affect parts other than the limbs; for example, acute abdominal pain of a 'gastric crisis', often associated with severe vomiting and anorexia, may mimic an 'acute abdomen'. Occasionally, severe rectal pain with tenesmus is noted, and there may be pain in the larynx, associated with breathlessness or stridor.

Examination of such patients may reveal Argyll Robertson pupils, optic atrophy, absence of deep tendon reflexes, proprioceptive loss in the lower limbs with loss of joint position sense, flaccid wasting of muscles, a characteristic facial appearance with bilateral ptosis, and impaired appreciation of pinprick sensation which is marked over the centre of the face and the chest and has a glove and stocking distribution in the periphery of the limbs. The patient may develop a perceptive, or sensory neural, deafness. Deep sensibility is lost in the Achilles tendon and, later in the disease, testicular pain is lost. A characteristic Charcot joint or neurogenic arthropathy develops more frequently in the lower than in the upper limbs (cf. syringomyelia and diabetic polyneuropathy). The joint becomes swollen and disorganized, without an inflammatory reaction and without pain. The loss of sense of joint pain, together with osteophyte formation, destroy the articular surfaces: the joint becomes hypermobile and crepitus can readily be elicited. The radiological changes are quite characteristic. Perforating ulcers, painful and indolent, may be seen on the plantar surface of the feet. General examination may well reveal more extensive CNS involvement, such as early dementia, and there may be evidence of syphilitic aortitis on cardiological examination.

Modified cases of tabes are now the rule, the fully developed picture being rare. Lightning pains, Charcot knee joints, and absent ankle jerks may persist unchanged for many years, the more severe manifestations apparently being arrested.

The CSF in tabes dorsalis shows a mild pleocytosis of lymphocytes up to about $100/\mu l$ and a slight increase in protein (page 21.11). The colloidal gold curve may be luetic, with a high mid zone (e.g. 1233321000); the specific tests are usually positive.

Differential diagnosis
The differential diagnosis of tabes dorsalis must include all those chronic disorders which involve the spinal cord, and the disease may mimic sensory peripheral neuropathies, i.e. those associated with diabetes, those having an infective origin, alcoholism, vitamin deficiency, or heavy metal poisoning. Tabes dorsalis must be distinguished from hypertrophic polyneuropathy and from diseases of the spinal cord such as subacute combined degeneration, multiple sclerosis, and the hereditary ataxias. In addition, intrinsic and extrinsic cord tumours and syringomyelia must be ruled out. Syphilitic optic atrophy must be differentiated from those disorders causing optic nerve compression, such as pituitary tumour or craniopharyngioma. The lightning pains must be differentiated from other causes of acute abdomen, and the arthropathy must be differentiated from other chronic diseases of the joints. The Argyll Robertson pupil is of diagnostic value but may cause confusion when patients are admitted with unrelated conditions, for example, head injury.

Prognosis
Unfortunately, the treatment of tabes dorsalis is, as a rule, unsatisfactory. By the time the patient comes to diagnosis, too much destruction of the neuraxis has occurred and the patient continues to complain of his lightning pains and symptoms stemming from his posterior column loss, in particular progressive ataxia.

Spinal syphilis
There are other forms of cord involvement in neurosyphilis. A syphilitic meningomyelitis, traditionally termed Erb's spastic paraplegia, has been recognized, as has spinal meningovascular syphilis. In the latter, involvement of the anterior spinal artery may result in its occlusion and also produce a syndrome of radicular pain and wasting of the small muscles of the hand.

Congenital neurosyphilis
The features of neurosyphilis affecting the nervous system after a congenitally acquired infection differ very little from those seen in the adult. Basically, the condition pathologically is meningo-encephalitis, with meningovascular disease seen during the first few years after birth. During school years, GPI may present with progressive dementia and seizures. Tabes is much less common, but a mixture of tabes and GPI, so-called taboparesis is seen. An optic atrophy develops secondary to choroidoretinitis.

Treatment (see also Section 5)
Penicillin is still the most effective remedy and the antibiotic of choice in the treatment of all forms of neurosyphilis. Although other antibiotics, such as erythromycin and tetracycline, are sometimes used in the treatment of neurosyphilis, none are as effective as penicillin. Heavy metals such as mercury, bismuth, and arsenic are ineffective, and so is potassium iodide and the malarial treatment of GPI. The most effective form of penicillin is benzylpenicillin G, best given by injection, 1 megaunit/day for 10 days or alternatively, 3 megaunits, given at intervals of 7 days to a total of 12 megaunits. In the absence of overt meningeal inflammation it is considered better to administer benzylpenicillin intravenously. The so-called Jarisch–Herxheimer reaction which so disturbed clinicians after the advent of penicillin, is a rare complication of penicillin usage and of little importance in the management of neurosyphilis, although some would recommend the prophylactic use of steroids, (30–50 mg of prednisone/day by mouth). It is said that some 50 per cent of patients with primary syphilis may show a generalized reaction of this type, i.e. a fever followed by headache, malaise, flushing, and sweating, perhaps with rigors and generalized arthralgia lasting a few hours. Full examination of the patient before treatment should include careful cardiological screening.

The spinal fluid should be examined six weeks after the course of penicillin treatment and again three months later. If the pleocytosis persists, then a further course of high-dosage treatment should be given. The CSF should be examined each year for several years after the completion of treatment. Symptomatic treatment is often required, for example anticonvulsants for any seizure disorder. Lightning pains may be controlled by simple analgesics but occasionally relief may be given by 200 mg carbamazepine (Tegretol) three or four times daily. Phenytoin may also be useful, and the patient may benefit from an infusion of 500 mg of procaine hydrochloride in 500 ml saline, infused intravenously over the course of one hour on four successive days. Physiotherapy may subsequently help the ataxia. Urinary tract infections must be diagnosed at an early stage and treated with effective antibiotics. Patients with severe bladder disturbances should be taught to empty the hypotonic bladder regularly, perhaps with the help of carbachol or a synthetic cholinergic drug. With regard to the neurogenic arthropathy, the disorganized joints require splinting and support, but surgery should be avoided. Perforating foot ulcers require specialized attention but amputation is rarely required, in contrast to cases of acrodystrophic neuropathy.

References
Adams, R. D., Solomon, H. C. and Merritt, H. H. (1946). *Neurosyphilis.* Oxford University Press, New York.
Brown, W. J. (1971). Status and control of syphilis in the United States. *J. infect. Dis.* **124**, 428–433.
Clark, E. G. and Danbolt, N. (1964). The Oslo study of the natural course of untreated syphilis. *Med. Clin. N. Amer.* **48**, 613–623.
Dattner, B., Thomas, E. W. and Wexler, G. (1944). *The management of neurosyphilis.* Grune and Stratton, New York.
Ekbom, K. (1972). Carbamazepine in the treatment of tabetic lightning pain. *Arch. Neurol. (Chic.)* **26**, 374–378.
Hahn, R. D., Webster, B., Weickhardt, G., Thomas, E., Tiberlake, W., Solomon, H., Stokes, J. H., Heyman, A., Gammon, G., Gleeson, G. A., Curtis, A. C. and Cutler, J. C. (1958). The results of treatment in

1,086 general paralytics the majority of whom were followed for more than five years. *J. chron. Dis.* **7**, 209–227.

Hooshimand, H., Escober, M. R. and Kopf, S. W. (1972). Neurosyphilis: A study of 241 patients. *J. Am. Med. Ass.* **219**, 726–729.

Joffe, R., Black, M. M. and Floyd, M. (1968). Changing clinical picture of neurosyphilis; report of seven unusual cases. *Brit. med. J.* **1**, 211–212.

Rose, A. S. and Carmen, L. R. (1951). Clinical follow-up studies of 130 cases of long-standing paretic neurosyphilis treated with penicillin. *Amer. J. Syph.* **35**, 278–283.

Sparling, P. F. (1971). Diagnosis and treatment of syphilis. *New Eng. J. Med.* **284**, 642–653.

Storm-Mathisen, A. (1978). Syphilis. In *Handbook of clinical neurology*, vol. 33 (eds. P. J. Vinken and G. W. Bruyn), 337. North Holland, Amsterdam.

Thomas, E. W. (1964). Some aspects of neurosyphilis. *Med. Clin. N. Amer.* **48**, 699–705.

Wetherill, J. H., Webb, H. E. and Catterall, R. D. (1965). Syphilis presenting as an acute neurological illness. *Brit. med. J.* **1**, 1157–1158.

Wilner, E. and Brody, J. A. (1968). Prognosis of general paresis after treatment. *Lancet* ii, 1370–1371.

Acute viral infections of the central nervous system

D. A. WARRELL AND W. B. MATTHEWS

Viruses invade and damage the central nervous system in two ways; directly, by infecting the leptomeninges, brain, and spinal cord, and indirectly, by inducing an immunological reaction resulting in para- and postinfectious syndromes (see page 21.216). In both cases, the terms meningitis, encephalitis, and myelitis are used alone or in combination. Meningitis implies inflammation of the meninges without alteration of consciousness; in encephalitis there is impairment of cerebral function, usually with an altered state of consciousness, while myelitis indicates involvement of the spinal cord. Chronic and 'slow' viral infections of the central nervous system are dealt with elsewhere (see Section 5 and pages 21.45 and 5.160).

Virology

There is considerable geographical and seasonal variation in the kinds of viruses causing meningitis, myelitis, and encephalitis; but, compared with bacterial infections of the central nervous system, there is less variation with age and immunocompetence.

Enteroviruses are responsible for 80 to 90 per cent of diagnosed cases of *viral meningitis*. Almost all the serotypes have been implicated in sporadic cases, and outbreaks have been associated with Coxsackie viruses A7 and 9, all the Coxsackie B types, and many of the echoviruses, especially 4, 6, 9, 11, 14, 16, and 30. Mumps is responsible for about 10 to 20 per cent of cases of viral meningitis. Other less common causes include herpes zoster (VZV), herpes simplex (HSV) (predominantly type 2), measles, adenoviruses, Epstein–Barr virus (EBV), and in the United States, togaviruses, such as St Louis, eastern and western equine encephalitides (SLE, EEE, WEE), and bunyaviruses such as California (La Crosse) encephalitis (CE) viruses.

Polioviruses are almost the only cause of *viral 'paralytic' myelitis* through out the world, but Coxsackie A7 (AB IV) has caused occasional small outbreaks and other Coxsackie A and B viruses, echoviruses, and enterovirus 70 have caused sporadic cases. VZV, paralytic rabies, EBV, and *Herpes simiae* B virus can cause myelitis or ascending paralysis and HSV-2 can cause lumbo-sacral myeloradiculitis.

Viruses causing *encephalitis* vary from country to country. Japanese B encephalitis (JE) virus is the most widespread human togavirus infection in the world and is the major cause of encephalitis throughout Asia. In Thailand there are an average of 1500 cases each year with 370 deaths. In North America, HSV is the commonest cause of viral encephalitis, followed by CE group,

SLE, VZV, enteroviruses, mumps, and measles. In the United States HSE has an estimated incidence of 2.3/million population each year. HSV-1 accounts for 95 per cent of cases. In the United Kingdom, mumps is the most frequently diagnosed viral cause of encephalitis, followed by echoviruses, Coxsackie viruses, measles, HSV, VZV, EBV virus, and adenoviruses. Louping ill (pronounced to rhyme with 'shouting') is the only indigenous arthropod-borne virus infection in Britain and has caused a few cases of encephalitis (see Section 5). In many tropical countries rabies is an important cause of viral encephalitis. Other regional causes are Rift Valley fever virus, arenaviruses (Junin, Lassa, and Machupo), Marburg and Ebola viruses, and Colorado tick fever virus.

Postinfectious encephalomyelitis most commonly follows measles, vaccinia, varicella, rubella, mumps, and influenza. Guillain-Barré syndrome, a sensori-motor polyneuropathy (page 21.126) is associated with infections by EBV, CMV, Coxsackie B, and VZV. Nervous tissue vaccines against rabies may give rise to postvaccinal encephalitis (page 5.113) while vaccination against rabies, influenza, and smallpox has been complicated by Guillain-Barré syndrome.

Immunodeficient patients are particularly vulnerable to some viral infections. Those with depressed cell-mediated immunity (Hodgkin's disease) may develop VZV encephalitis, and CMV may cause a subacute encephalitis in patients with AIDS. In children or adults with hypogammaglobulinaemia, enteroviruses, including live attenuated polio vaccine, may produce a progressive and fatal meningo-encephalitis. Progressive multifocal leucoencephalopathy, a chronic and fatal papovavirus infection in patients with impaired cell-mediated immunity is described below (see Section 5 also). HIV infection of the brain and meninges may be responsible for acute meningo-encephalitis at the time of seroconversion and subacute and for chronic encephalopathies and dementia in patients with AIDS.

Epidemiology

Many viral infections of the central nervous system occur in seasonal peaks or as epidemics, while others, such as herpes simplex encephalitis (HSE), are sporadic. Epidemics of JE occur in the summer or rainy season because of the abundance of the vector mosquitoes (principally *Culex tritaeniorhynchus*) which have been infected by first feeding on the bird or mammal reservoir species. Tick-borne encephalitides occur in spring and early summer when the ticks are most active. Mumps encephalitis is commonest in the spring, while enterovirus infections occur most often in the summer and autumn. Rodent-related encephalitides, such as the arenaviruses are most common when the rodent population is at its peak, either in the fields (Machupo and Junin viruses) or in the home (lymphocytic choriomeningitis virus, LCM). The zoonotic viral infections survive periods of cold weather, during which the invertebrate–vertebrate cycle is suspended by 'over-wintering' in their arthropod vectors or hibernating vertebrate reservoirs.

Invasion of the central nervous system seems to be a rare event in most viral infections. In the case of some togavirus infections such as JE, there may be only one case of encephalitis for every 500 to 1000 asymptomatic infections. EEE produces a much higher proportion of encephalitic cases than other togaviruses.

Infections by many neurotropic viruses are most frequent and severe in children or in the elderly. HSE affects all age groups but shows peaks of incidence in those aged 5–30 years and above 50 years. When HSV-2 invades the central nervous system it is likely to cause a benign lymphocytic meningitis in adults, but in neonates it usually produces a severe encephalitis. Among mosquito-borne epidemic encephalitides, CE is most common in children, SLE encephalitis in the elderly, while EEE, WEE, and JE affect both the very young and the elderly. Postinfectious encephalitis is most frequent in children, for it complicates the common childhood exanthematous infections. It is the most common demyelinating disease in the world.

Pathogenesis

This subject has been reviewed thoroughly by Johnson (1982) and Mims and White (1984). Most viral infections reach the central nervous system from the primary site of infection and multiplication via the blood stream. Viruses inoculated through the skin include those transmitted by arthropods, rabies, HSV, herpes simiae B, and LCM. Arthropod-borne viruses are presumed to replicate in local lymph-nodes, vascular endothelium, and circulating and fixed macrophages, in order to sustain viraemia. Rabies virus multiplies locally in the cytoplasm of muscle cells before entering peripheral nerves. Viruses which enter through the respiratory tract (e.g. measles, mumps, varicella) or gut (enteroviruses) multiply in local lymphoid tissue before they enter the blood stream. Viraemia is a feature of most viral infections, yet invasion of the central nervous system is rare in most of them. The explanation for this is not known. In the case of rabies, HSV, and VZV, the virus enters the central nervous system through the peripheral nerves. Although the subarachnoid space surrounding the olfactory nerves projects through the cribriform plate and is directly beneath the nasal mucosa, this route of infection seems to be extremely rare in humans and has been proven only in a few cases of inhaled rabies virus infection, and HSE. Virus has been inoculated directly into the central nervous system by infected corneal transplant grafts (rabies) and infected brain surface electrodes (Creutzfeld–Jakob disease). HSE may complicate primary HSV infection in children and young adults, but in most adult cases of HSE the cause is thought to be reactivation of latent virus (HSV-1) in the trigeminal nerve, autonomic nerve roots or brain.

Some viruses, such as the enteroviruses and mumps, usually infect the meninges rather than the parenchyma of the central nervous system, whereas others, such as the togaviruses, usually cause encephalitis. Johnson (1980) has emphasized the selective vulnerability of different neural cells to different neurotropic viruses. Examples are the predilection of polioviruses for motor neurones of the anterior horns of the spinal cord, and rabies for neurones of the limbic system and cerebellar Purkinje cells. The pathological effects of viral infections on the central nervous system include: (1) the destruction and phagocytosis of neurones (neuronophagia) either as a result of viral invasion *per se* or immune lysis, (2) demyelination, (3) inflammatory oedema with the compressive effects of raised intracranial pressure, and, in some cases, (4) vascular lesions. In rabies, a universally fatal encephalitis, the relatively mild degree of neuronolysis has always puzzled neuropathologists. However, recent work suggests that rabies virus may produce its devastating effects by interfering with neurotransmission at central as well as peripheral cholinergic junctions. This virus also produces severe systemic effects, perhaps as a result of its centrifugal spread (e.g. in the case of myocarditis and cardiac arrhythmias) or its focal effects on vasomotor and respiratory centres in the brain stem (page 5.107).

Postinfectious encephalitis and Guillain–Barré syndrome are thought to result from sensitization to central and peripheral myelin, respectively. The experimental model is allergic encephalomyelitis induced by immunization with myelin basic protein. It is uncertain how the preceding viral infection induces this autoimmune response. In the case of postvaccinal encephalomyelitis resulting from nervous tissue antirabies vaccines, the explanation is more obvious, as these vaccines contain myelin from the animal in which the virus was grown.

Pathology

Poliomyelitis

Virus is distributed widely throughout the brain and spinal cord, possibly even in non-paralytic cases, but, usually, the only cells to suffer chromatolysis and phagocytosis are motor neurones in the anterior horns of the spinal cord, medulla, and grey matter of the precentral gyrus.

Encephalitis

Most viral encephalitides are characterized by lymphocytic infiltration of the meninges, perivascular cuffing in the cortex, and underlying white matter, consisting of lymphocytes, plasma cells, histiocytes, and some neutrophils and proliferation of microglia with formation of glial nodules. Neuronolysis and demyelination are variable in their degree and location. Infected neurones may show characteristic inclusion bodies in their nuclei (measles, HSV, and adenoviruses) or cytoplasm (the rabies Negri body).

Herpes simplex encephalitis The special features of this condition are gross cerebral oedema and severe haemorrhagic and necrotizing encephalitis which is often asymmetrically localized to the inferior and medial parts of the temporal lobe, the insula, and the orbital part of the frontal lobe. Histological sections show eosinophilic Cowdry type A intranuclear inclusions with margination of chromatin in neurones, oligodendrocytes, and astrocytes, inflammatory and haemorrhagic perivascular reactions, but no demyelination. Cowdry type A inclusions are also found in VZV and CMV encephalitides. Latency of HSV-1 in trigeminal, superior cervical, and vagal ganglia has been confirmed. The unique cerebral localization of HSE may be explained by spread of reactivated virus from the trigeminal ganglia through sensory fibres innervating the dura near these regions.

Japanese B encephalitis Microscopical appearances are typical of other viral encephalitides: there is oedema, congestion, and focal haemorrhages of the brain and meninges. However, histological examination shows unusually widespread neuronolysis and neuronophagia involving the cerebral cortex, cerebellum (where there is marked destruction of Purkinje cells), and the spinal cord. Viral antigen is localized to neurones, especially in the brain stem and thalamus.

Postinfectious encephalomyelitis This is a perivenous microglial encephalitis with demyelination. Fibrinoid necrosis of arterioles is an associated lesion in a more severe form designated acute haemorrhagic leucoencephalitis.

Clinical features

Meningitis

A prodromal influenza-like illness, followed by a brief remission of symptoms is typical of LCM and some outbreaks of enteroviral meningitis (e.g. echo 9) but in most cases of viral meningitis, symptoms start suddenly. As with bacterial meningitis, there is fever, headache, a stiff neck, and vomiting, especially in children. Compared with bacterial meningitis, headache is less severe and tends to be frontal or retrobulbar (eye movements may be painful) and neck stiffness is less marked. Nausea, anorexia, abdominal pain, myalgias, and sore throat are particularly common in enteroviral meningitis. Myalgia is particularly severe with Coxsackie B infections. As in acute bacterial meningitis, infants usually present with vague irritability and a tense fontanelle and young children with fever and irritability or lethargy. Conjunctival injection, pharyngitis, and cervical lymphadenopathy may be found. Macular or petechial exanthems or enanthems are seen with Coxsackie A and B and echovirus infections (especially echo 9). Vesicles on the hands, feet, and mouth have been reported, with Coxsackie A16 and enterovirus 71 infections. By definition the level of consciousness is normal in simple meningitis. Neurological features include vertigo, nystagmus, cerebellar ataxia, facial spasms, and involuntary movements.

The specific cause of viral meningitis may be suggested by characteristic signs outside the nervous system such as genital or rectal vesicles in the sexually active age group (HSV-2), herpes zoster skin lesions, swelling in the parotid region (mumps and occasionally Coxsackie, LCM, and EBV), orchitis (mumps and LCM), and arthritis (LCM). However, potentially helpful features such as gastrointestinal symptoms associated with enteroviral

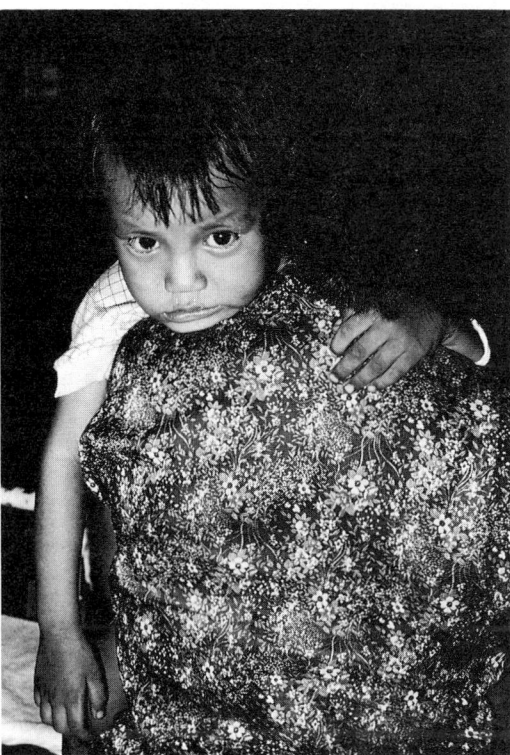

Fig. 1 Paralytic poliomyelitis in a 3-year-old Thai child. Note systemic illness and paralysis of right arm. (Copyright D. A. Warrell.)

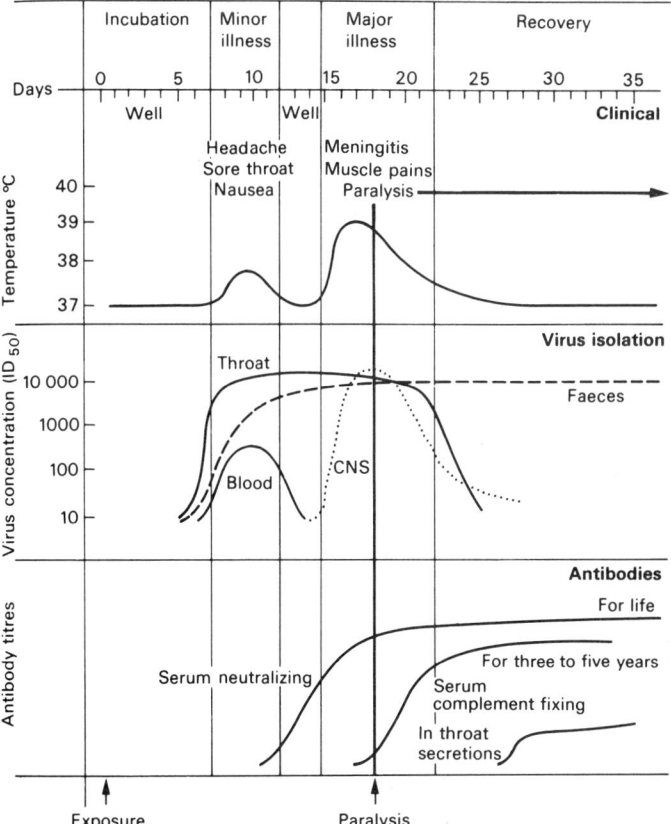

Fig. 2 The course of a paralytic poliomyelitis infection. (Reproduced from Christie, 1981, *Medicine International*, **1**, 139. Adapted from Bodian, D., 1957. Mechanisms of infection with polio viruses. In *Cellular biology, nucleic acids, and viruses*. New York Academy of Sciences, by permission.)

infections, and parotitis associated with mumps, may be completely absent in patients with meningitis.

Paralytic poliomyelitis

The infection (see page 5.96 also) is acquired by droplet spread from the respiratory tract or by the faecal–oral route. The 'minor illness', coinciding with viraemia, is a non-specific episode of influenza-like symptoms – fever, headache, sore throat, malaise, and mild gastrointestinal symptoms – which resolves in a few days. Most of those infected have no further symptoms, but in a minority, the 'major illness' follows, sometimes after a few days' remission of symptoms. The features are those of viral meningitis: muscle pain, spasms and sensory disturbances may precede or accompany the development of lower motor neurone (flaccid) paralysis. Any combination of motor unit deficits may be seen (Fig. 1). It is most unusual for paralysis to extend after the first three days or after the temperature has fallen (Fig. 2). Respiratory and bulbar paralysis is life-threatening. Encephalitis is rare. The commonest causes of death are aspiration and airway obstruction, resulting from bulbar paralysis, and paralysis of respiratory muscles. Disturbances of respiratory and cardiac rhythm, thought to be the result of damage to medullary vasomotor and respiratory centres, are extremely uncommon. Other complications include impaired control of body temperature and blood pressure, gastrointestinal haemorrhage, aspiration pneumonia, and paralysis of the bladder and bowel.

Encephalitis

Most patients with viral encephalitis present with the symptoms of meningitis (fever, headache, neck stiffness, vomiting) together with altered consciousness, convulsions, and sometimes focal neurological signs or psychiatric symptoms. Patients with JE develop a prodromal illness consisting of sudden fever, headache, and respiratory or gastrointestinal symptoms lasting two to three days. Meningism, unconsciousness, and convulsions are the principal features. Muscle tone may be increased or decreased, there are mask-like facies, ataxia, involuntary movements, cogwheel rigidity, cranial nerve lesions, bulbar paralysis, upper motor neurone defects or a myelitic pattern. In survivors, fever lasts for 6 to 7 days, while neurological symptoms persist for 1 to 2 weeks. Fatal cases show persistent fever, progressive neurological abnormalities, cardiorespiratory complications, and death in 7–10 days.

Herpes simplex encephalitis This is a relatively common sporadic encephalitis that may occur in any age group. The origin of the virus is almost always unknown. The majority of cases are presumed to be due to reactivation of latent virus, possibly HSV-1 from the trigeminal ganglion. In neonates HSE is caused by HSV-2.

As well as the usual clinical features of a severe viral encephalitis, patients with HSE have symptoms related to the focal nature of the encephalitis (frontal and temporal cortex and limbic system). These include behavioural abnormalities, olfactory and gustatory hallucinations, anosmia, amnesia, expressive aphasia, and temporal lobe seizures. Herpetic skin or mucosal lesions are rarely found. Effects of cerebral oedema are unusually severe. Patients usually lapse into coma towards the end of the first week and most die within the first two weeks. This condition is considered in detail on page 5.64.

Postinfectious encephalomyelitis Sudden convulsions, coma, fever or pareses appear 10 to 14 days after the start of vaccination (vaccinia or nervous tissue rabies vaccine) or after infection with measles, varicella, rubella, mumps or influenza. In the case of measles, varicella, and rubella, encephalitic symptoms develop 2–12 days after the rash has appeared, and in mumps before or after parotid swelling. Involuntary movements, cranial nerve lesions (VII, III), pupillary abnormalities, nystagmus, ataxia, and upper motor neurone signs are common.

Diagnosis

Epidemiological factors such as the time of year, known current epidemics, the patient's age, occupation, and countries or states visited recently may help to narrow down the possibilities. A specific diagnosis may be suggested by distinctive clinical features of the encephalitis itself (e.g. hydrophobia in rabies, temporal lobe features in HSE), or of the associated infection (e.g. mumps parotitis, measles rash, skin, mucosal lesions of herpes viruses, and gastrointestinal symptoms associated with enteroviral infections).

Investigations should aim to demonstrate a specific viral agent (particularly important for the potentially treatable herpes virus infections) or exclude potentially treatable non-viral causes of meningitis or encephalomyelitis (Table 1). The most important investigation is examination of the CSF. Contraindications to lumbar puncture are the same as in acute bacterial meningitis (see pages 21.20 and 21.134). CSF pressure is increased especially in HSE where there is intense cerebral oedema. Pleocytosis ranges from tens to thousands of cells/μl. Lymphocytes and other mononuclear cells predominate, except in the early stages of some infections (e.g. enteroviruses, HSE).

CSF contains erythrocytes or is xanthochromic in haemorrhagic encephalitides such as HSE and acute necrotic leucoencephalitis. Protein concentration is usually increased in the range 50 to 150 mg/dl with an increasing proportion of IgG as the disease progresses. Leakage of serum IgG into the CSF and intrathecal IgG synthesis, indicated by a monoclonal band, are responsible. CSF glucose concentration is usually normal or increased towards the level in a blood sample taken simultaneously, but low levels are occasionally reported, especially in mumps and LCM infections. CSF lactate concentrations are normal in most patients with viral infections of the CNS in contrast to bacterial infections and cere-

Table 1 Causes of aseptic meningitis*, with or without encephalitis or myelitis, other than viruses and postinfectious/postvaccinal syndromes

Cause	Diagnostic clinical feature or investigation
Bacteria	
Acute bacterial meningitis (partially treated)	CSF antigen detection (CIE, LA), repeated CSF examination
Intracranial/spinal abscess or empyema	Physical examination (exclude otitis media, trauma, dermoid sinus, etc.) radiographs, CT scans, myelogram
Mycobacteria	CSF microscopy, LA, culture; Mantoux test, chest radiograph
Spirochaetes	
Leptospira	Serology
Relapsing fevers	Blood smear, mouse inoculation
Lyme disease	Serology (ELISA, IFA), culture, skin biopsy, CSF IgG (ELISA, IFT)
Syphilis	Serology (FTA–ABS) serum and CSF
Spirillum minor	Microscopy of wound or lymph-node aspirates, mouse inoculation
Rickettsiae	
(Rocky Mountain spotted fever, murine, epidemic, scrub typhus)	Serology (Weil-Felix), skin biopsy IFT (RMSF)
Mycoplasma	CSF + serum IgM (IFA)
Cat scratch disease bacillus	Warthin–Starry stain skin and lymph-node, skin test
Fungi	
Cryptococcus	CSF India ink, LA – beware false-positive with agar syneresis fluid, culture
Histoplasma	CSF culture (repeated), demonstration at other sites, serum, urine, CSF antigen detection (RIA)
Coccidioidomycosis	CSF–CFT, culture, microscopy
Candida	CSF culture (repeated)
Protozoa	
Cerebral malaria	Blood smear (try bone marrow aspirate or intradermal puncture if negative)
Trypanosomiasis (African and South American)	Blood smear (buffy coat), lymph node aspirate, CSF microscopy, and IgM, serology, xenodiagnosis
Amoebae (Acanthamoeba, Naegleria)	CSF microscopy (fresh wet preparation + India ink), culture
Toxoplasma	(Immunocompromised patients–AIDS) CSF animal inoculation, serology, brain biopsy
Helminths	
Strongyloides stercoralis	(Immunocompromised patients) larvae, ova in stool, duodenal fluid, etc.
Angiostrongylus cantonensis	CSF larvae, eosinophils
Gnathostoma spinigerum	Cutaneous migratory swelling, CSF eosinophils
Cysticercosis	CT scan, radiographs, examination for subcutaneous cysts, CSF–CFT, histology
Hydatid disease	Casoni test, serology, CT scan, radiographs
Sparganosis	Histology, CT scan
Schistosomiasis	Low transverse myelitis (*S. mansoni*), ova in stool, CT scan, CSF eosinophils, myelogram, histology
Paragonimus	CSF ova, eosinophils, serology, CT scan or skull radiograph, histology
Sarcoidosis	Histology, Kveim test, Mantoux test
Whipple's disease	Clinical features, jejunal histology
Mollaret's meningitis	Recurrence, CSF 'Mollaret's' cells
Behçet's syndrome	Clinical syndrome
Vogt-Koyanagi-Harada syndrome	Clinical syndrome
Systemic lupus erythematosus	Antinuclear antibodies, DNA antibodies, LEcells
Carcinomas, leukaemias, lymphomas	CSF cytology, evidence of condition elsewhere
Lead encephalopathy	Blood lead, blood smear, urinary coproporphyrins
Chemical	Recent lumbar puncture, spinal anaesthesia, etc.

* *Aseptic meningitis* – CSF pleocytosis but no bacteria stained by Gram's method and no growth on standard bacterial culture media.

CIE	= counter current immunoelectrophoresis.
FTA–ABS	= fixed Treponema antigen–antibody slide test.
IFA	= immunofluorescent antibody.
LA	= latex agglutination.
RIA	= radioimmunoassay.

bral malaria where they are increased. CSF examination may be misleading if it is normal, as it is at the first examination in 10 to 15 per cent of patients with HSE, if there is a predominantly neutrophil pleocytosis, or if the glucose concentration is low.

A specific virus can be identified in 70 to 75 per cent of cases of lymphocytic meningitis and 30 to 40 per cent of patients with meningoencephalitis. At appropriate stages of the illness, a rapid diagnosis by direct immunofluorescence may be made of HSV (skin and brain), VZV (skin lesion scrapings), rabies (skin sections and brain), measles (nasopharyngeal aspirate), and some non-viral causes such as Rocky Mountain spotted fever (skin). Electron microscopy (EM) of skin lesions will identify a herpes virus. Some viruses can be isolated from the CSF (e.g. mumps, enteroviruses, LCM, Central European encephalitides, Louping ill, and HIV). Virus cultured from a distant site may help with the diagnosis (e.g. polio and other enteroviruses from stool, or arthropod-borne viruses from blood culture), but they may not be related to the neurological symptoms (e.g. CMV from the pharynx or urine, HSV from skin or mucosa, or adenovirus seen in stool by EM). Specific viral IgM can be detected in serum for mumps, EBV, CMV or measles, or using a μ-capture technique, in the CSF for JE. The method is being used increasingly for IgM to other viruses. A viral diagnosis is often delayed until a rising convalescent antibody titre is found by an appropriate technique. This is usually the case for mumps, Coxsackie, and most arthropod-borne viruses.

For the rapid confirmation of HSE there is at present no substitute for brain biopsy. Electroencephalography, computerized tomographic (CT) scan, angiography or technetium scans can help to direct the surgeon towards the affected area of brain. Failing this, a biopsy of the medial or inferior surface of the temporal lobe is most likely to yield the diagnosis. Opinion is divided about the safety and importance of this procedure.

Differential diagnosis

Viral infections of the CNS must be distinguished from the many other conditions which produce similar clinical features and CSF abnormalities (Table 1). The differential diagnosis of *viral meningitis* includes the other causes of aseptic meningitis, such as partially treated bacterial meningitis, tuberculous meningitis, spirochaetal infections (leptospirosis, borreliosis, Lyme disease, and syphilis), fungal, amoebic, neoplastic, granulomatous, and idiopathic meningitides. *Viral myelitides* must be distinguished from other causes of transverse myelitis and Brown–Séquard syndrome. These include spinal compression by tumours, abscesses, helminths or their ova, or vertebral disease.

The differential diagnosis of *paralytic poliomyelitis* includes postinfectious and other immunopathic polyneuroradiculopathies such as Guillain–Barré syndrome and Landry's ascending paralysis, metabolic neuropathies such as acute porphyria, paralytic rabies, neoplastic polyradiculoneuropathies and rarities, such as tick paralysis and herpes simiae B virus infection. The lack of objective sensory loss in poliomyelitis usually distinguishes it from these other entities.

The differential diagnosis of *viral encephalitis* includes other infective encephalopathies – bacterial, fungal, protozoal, and parasitic; intracranial abscesses and neoplasms, toxic and metabolic encephalopathies, and heat stroke. The diagnosis of 'viral encephalitis' should not be made too hastily, as it may condemn the patient with concealed cerebral malaria or some other curable encephalopathy to delayed treatment or even death.

Treatment

Antiviral chemotherapy with acyclovir ('Zovirax') and, to a lesser extent, vidarabine (ara-A) has proved effective in HSE. This subject is discussed on page 5.66. Since acyclovir is free of serious toxicity, treatment can be started as soon as HSE is suspected clinically: it is not necessary to confirm the diagnosis by brain biopsy. Acyclovir and vidarabine are also used for VZV encepha-

litis, but have not produced convincing evidence of benefit in CMV infections of the CNS. The rare but very dangerous encephalomyelitis caused by *Herpes simiae* B virus should be treated with acyclovir (see page 5.75). Ribavirin is effective in Lassa fever, and possibly in other arenavirus infections associated with encephalitis.

Interferons have been used by intravenous, intrathecal or intraventricular routes in the treatment of rabies, VZV, and other herpes virus encephalitides, but have not proved effective.

Hyperimmune plasma given within 8 days of the start of symptoms has reduced the mortality of Argentinian haemorrhagic fever (Junin virus) from 20–30 to 1–3 per cent but is not effective in Lassa fever.

Corticosteroids have been used in most of the viral encephalomyelitides, both in an attempt to combat cerebral oedema (especially in HSE) and for their other anti-inflammatory effects. Convincing evidence of benefit, from controlled trials, is lacking, but the immunosuppressive effects of corticosteroids have not led to obvious clinical deterioration except perhaps in some cases of diffuse myelitis. Corticosteroids or ACTH have also been used for postinfectious and postvaccinal encephalomyelitides, but the evidence for their efficacy is not convincing. Nursing and general care are the same as for acute bacterial meningitis (page 21.136) and tuberculous meningitis (page 21.140).

Paralytic poliomyelitis

Most authorities recommend rest and even mild sedation during the preparalytic stage of the 'major illness', because of the suspicion that exercise increases paralysis. The severe muscle pains and spasms reported from some parts of the world are treated with mild analgesics such as salicylates and with hot-water bottles. During the phase of developing paralysis, patients must be observed closely and if possible assessed objectively for the development of life-threatening bulbar and respiratory paralysis. Those with weakness of swallowing should be nursed on their sides to prevent aspiration. The need for a cuffed tracheostomy tube may be avoided by careful positioning, frequent observations, and suction. Indications for mechanical ventilation are a progressive decline in ventilatory capacity to less than 30 to 50 per cent of normal, hypoxaemia or gross disturbances of respiratory rhythm (Cheyne–Stokes respiration, long apnoeic intervals, etc.) suggesting damage to the respiratory centres. Respiratory weakness without bulbar paralysis may be treated in a tank respirator or rocking bed, which do not require tracheostomy. However, patients with severe or rapidly progressing respiratory paralysis need urgent tracheostomy and intermittent positive pressure ventilation. Overventilation must be avoided. Assisted ventilation may be required for long periods, but attempts should be made to wean patients off the ventilator as soon as their condition becomes stable. Severe fluctuations in body temperature and blood pressure, reminiscent of those in severe tetanus and rabies, may require intensive care. The paralysed patient may have to lie in bed for many months and will develop complications of this prolonged immobilization. These include bed sores, osteomalacia, hypercalciuria leading to renal calculi, recurrent urinary tract infections resulting from chronic urethral catheterization, respiratory infections, and contractures of muscles and tendons leading to severe musculoskeletal deformities which will require orthopaedic correction. Some can be prevented by passive movement of joints and splinting. Physiotherapy and psychological support are needed during the prolonged phase of rehabilitation.

Prognosis and sequelae

Viral meningitis has an excellent prognosis, but some patients with HSV-2 infection have recurrent attacks with spinal cord or nerve root involvement. Mortalities of some viral encephalomyelitides are as follows: rabies 100 per cent; HSE (untreated) 40 to more than 75 per cent (highest in neonates and those over 30 years old); EEE 50 per cent; JE 10–40 per cent; measles 10–20 per cent; varicella 10–30 per cent; WEE 8 per cent; SLE 3 per cent; CE, Venezuelan encephalitis (VEE), and mumps less than 1 per cent. The mortality of paralytic poliomyelitis increases from 5 per cent in young children to more than 20 per cent in adults. Postinfectious and postvaccinal encephalomyelitides carry mortalities of 15 to 40 per cent.

Neurological sequelae are found in 5–75 per cent of survivors of JE and HSE and are especially common in infants. They include mental retardation, loss of memory, speech abnormalities (including subtle expressive aphasias), hemiparesis, ataxia, dystonic brain stem and cranial nerve lesions, recurrent convulsions, and various behavioural and personality disturbances. Sequelae are common with postinfectious encephalomyelitis. An unusual sequel to paralytic poliomyelitis is a form of progressive motor neurone disease (see page 21.116).

Prevention

Prophylactic vaccination against poliomyelitis and measles has virtually eradicated encephalitides caused by these viruses in many communities. Postexposure rabies vaccination has also proved effective in preventing rabies encephalitis and human diploid cell strain vaccine is used increasingly for pre-exposure prophylaxis. A formalin-inactivated adult mouse brain vaccine is manufactured in Osaka for JE. It appears to be effective and carries a very low risk of objective neurological complications (one in a million courses). Vaccines for use in humans have been prepared against a number of other arthropod-borne viruses (e.g. European tick-borne encephalitis).

Hyperimmune immunoglobulin has been used for prophylaxis (and in some cases attempted treatment) of measles, VZV, HSV-2, vaccinia, rabies, and some other infections in high-risk groups. Immunocompromised patients, such as those with leukaemia, who are household contacts of a case of VZV infection, should be given prophylactic hyperimmune globulin, and if they develop skin lesions they should be treated with acyclovir to prevent development of severe disease.

Interferons have been used with some success to prevent herpes virus infections, such as CMV in high-risk groups such as renal transplant recipients. However, the evidence does not yet justify their recommendation.

Caesarean section before rupture of the membranes in a full-term pregnant woman with genital herpes may prevent HSV-2 encephalitis in the neonate. If the herpetic lesions are discovered during or after vaginal delivery, topical acyclovir should be applied to the eyes of the neonate, as they are the most likely portal of entry.

Control of animal vectors and reservoirs Arthropod-borne viral encephalitides can be prevented by avoiding or controlling the arthropod vectors (e.g. by the use of mosquito nets, insect repellents, insecticides, etc.), by attempting to control the numbers of wild vertebrate reservoir species, or by immunizing domestic animals, such as horses (EEE and VEE) and pigs (JE). To control rabies, the principal wild mammalian vectors can be reduced in numbers or they can be immunized (e.g. wild foxes have been immunized by distributing oral vaccine in bait). Domestic dogs and cats can be vaccinated. To prevent the viral encephalitides transmissable from laboratory animals (e.g. LCM from mice and rats, *Herpes simiae* B from monkeys) their quarantine, handling, and housing should be strictly controlled.

Reye's syndrome

Reye's syndrome (pronounced rye not ray) is an acute encephalopathy affecting children between the ages of 2 and 16 years (see also page 12.265). It is rapidly fatal in 10–40 per cent of cases. The defining characteristics are sudden impairment of consciousness, increase in serum aminotransferase concentrations (or, if a biopsy is done, a fatty liver), and the exclusion of other diseases. Symptoms develop a few days after varicella or an upper respiratory tract or gastrointestinal illness. Clusters of cases (median age 11 years) have been associated with influenza B epidemics, while sporadic cases (median age 6 years) have followed varicella, Coxsackie, dengue, and other viral infections. Recent studies in the United States have suggested an association between Reye's syndrome and the use of salicylates, but not to paracetamol, during the preceding viral illness. This has led the Committee on Safety of Medicines to recommend that aspirin should not be given to children under 12 years of age, unless specifically indicated for childhood rheumatic conditions. Aflatoxin has been implicated in Thailand. In the United States, the annual incidence of Reye's syndrome in those under 18 years old is 0.42 per 100 000 urban dwellers and 1.8 per 100 000 rural and suburban dwellers.

The child is nauseated and retches or vomits for one or two days before becoming confused or comatose and requiring admission to hospital. Most are afebrile and have hepatomegaly but no jaundice at presentation. Fever develops later. The CSF is usually normal or contains a few mononuclear cells. Irritability, extreme agitation, aggression, and delirium are succeeded by coma and death in 2–3 days. Decorticate and decerebrate posturing and convulsions may be partly attributable to hypoglycaemia which occurs in the majority of cases. There is rapid neurological deterioration with loss of pupillary and oculovestibular reflexes, evidence of increased intracranial pressure, deepening coma, and death. Neurological sequelae are common in survivors. Blood ammonia is increased above the normal limit of 48 μg/dl in almost all cases. The characteristic histological abnormality is fatty droplets in the liver cells. Mitochondrial abnormalities but no inflammatory changes have also been seen in neurones and hepatocytes.

The differential diagnosis includes acute hepatic encephalopathy, especially associated with poisoning, infective encephalopathies such as cerebral malaria (usually distinguishable by positive blood smear) or bacterial, viral, and fungal meningoencephalitides (distinguished by characteristic CSF abnormalities).

There is no specific treatment, but mortality can be reduced by treating hypoglycaemia, cerebral oedema, respiratory failure, fluid and electrolyte disturbances, and other complications. These measures are considered further in Section 12.

Other viral infections or disorders in which viruses may play a role in the pathogenesis of neurological disease

Subacute sclerosing panencephalitis

This disorder (see also Section 5) is a form of subacute encephalitis affecting children and young adults due to persistent infection with the measles virus. The cumbersome title, usually abbreviated to SSPE, is derived from the conditions formerly known as subacute sclerosing leucoencephalitis and inclusion-body encephalitis, now known to be the same disease.

Aetiology

An infective cause was long suspected and there is now conclusive evidence to incriminate the measles virus. Measles virus antibody titres are extremely high in blood and CSF, measles antigen has been demonstrated in the brain and the virus has sometimes been isolated, but only with difficulty. Most affected children have had measles at an unusually early age and there is a mean interval of some six years between infection and the onset of encephalitis. The disease can occur in children vaccinated with live measles virus but the risk is much lower than that following the natural disease.

The measles virus in SSPE appears to be incomplete as the matrix (M) protein required to attach the nucleocapsid to the cytoplasmic membrane prior to budding is deficient or absent. It is not known whether the absence of M protein from the brain is the result of an abnormality of the virus or of the host, and, if the latter, whether inborn or acquired. It is thought that during the long symptom-free interval between infection and appearance of disease, viral material accumulates, eventually leading to cell damage. The paradox of high antimeasles antibodies, except against M protein, and persistent virus has not been fully explained. The comparatively early age of clinical measles in affected children, often below the age of 2 years, may indicate that the immature immune system permits entry and persistence of the virus in the brain.

Pathology

As its name implies both grey and white matter show the changes of encephalitis, with perivascular cuffing and more diffuse cellular infiltration, neuronal loss, and myelin destruction, with variable glial scarring or sclerosis. Acidophilic nuclear inclusion bodies are never profuse and may not be detected. No visceral lesions are found.

Clinical features

In the great majority, the onset is in the first two decades but young adults may also be affected. The disease is twice as common in boys as in girls. Incidence has fallen sharply in countries where measles vaccination is at a high level; the annual incidence in England and Wales has fallen from 20 to around 5. SSPE remains relatively common in parts of Eastern Europe, Egypt, and the Lebanon. No convincing predisposing factors have been identified and, in particular, immunosuppressed children are not at special risk but may occasionally develop acute measles inclusion-body encephalitis.

The speed of onset is extremely variable, but there is usually a prolonged period of altered behaviour, mild intellectual deterioration, and loss of energy and interest, often misinterpreted as sloth or neurosis. After some weeks or months increasing clumsiness or the appearance of focal neurological symptoms draws attention to the organic nature of the disease. Periodic involuntary movements then appear, the commonest form being myoclonus, consisting of a stereotyped jerk or lapse of posture involving the limbs, often asymmetrically, occurring every 3 to 6 s. The myoclonus may result in sudden falls which are occasionally the presenting symptom. Visual signs may be prominent, with papilloedema, retinitis, optic atrophy or cortical blindness. Choroidoretinal scarring is present in 30 per cent of cases. In other cases the onset is relatively abrupt with no recognizable prodromal stage. There is no fever or other evidence of systemic infection.

Further progression is marked by intellectual deterioration, rigidity, and spasticity, and increasing helplessness. Some 40 per cent die within a year but a similar proportion survive for more than 2 years. A period of apparent arrest is common and in some patients, particularly at the upper end of the age range, substantial remission and prolonged survival occur. Even in such cases there may be radiological evidence of continued cerebral damage and it is probable that the disease is always eventually fatal.

Investigation

There is no significant pleocytosis in the cerebrospinal fluid and total protein is not increased but there is evidence of intrathecal synthesis of immunoglobulin and oligoclonal bands of IgG. The measles antibody titres in blood and CSF are usually raised to high figures, but occasionally overlap control values. In established disease the EEG shows highly characteristic periodic discharges, synchronous with the myoclonus, but persisting in the absence of the movements. Computerized tomographic (CT) scan shows low density white matter lesions and cerebral atrophy.

Treatment

The antiviral agent inosiplex, 100 mg/kg daily by mouth in divided doses, probably prolongs survival, particularly in older patients with disease of slow onset, but adequately controlled trials are naturally difficult to mount. Interferon given by intraventricular catheter has been reported to induce partial remission.

Progressive multifocal leucoencephalopathy (PML)

This disease (see also Section 5) is caused by opportunist infection by papovaviruses, most commonly JC virus and SV40. A high proportion of normal adults have antibodies to the former and the agent appears to be ubiquitous. The reservoir of SV40 is in monkeys and the agent was apparently transmitted in early types of poliomyelitis vaccine, without evident ill effects. These viruses are potentially oncogenic but non-pathogenic for humans unless the immune system has been compromised.

PML thus occurs in patients already affected by such conditions as lymphoproliferative diseases, sarcoidosis or, more recently, AIDS, and also in those therapeutically immunosuppressed. Most patients are over 50 years old but, with the spread of AIDS, younger people are being affected, with a male preponderance. There are no reliable incidence figures but PML is rare.

Pathology

The virus particularly invades the nuclei of the oligodendroglia and, as a result, there is demyelination of the white matter of the cerebral hemispheres, spreading from numerous foci. The cerebellum and brain stem are less often involved and the spinal cord is spared. Abnormal giant forms of oligodendrocytes are seen microscopically and arrays of intranuclear virus particles can often be identified by electron microscopy.

Clinical features

The onset is usually with progressive signs of a focal lesion of one cerebral hemisphere; limb weakness, aphasia or visual field defect. More widespread signs gradually develop, leading to intellectual deterioration, dysarthria, and bilateral weakness. Fits are rare. There is no systemic evidence of infection. Spontaneous temporary arrest or partial remission are common but eventual progression causes death within a few months, although much more chronic cases are on record.

Investigation

The CSF is normal and is not under increased pressure. The EEG shows a bilateral excess of slow activity. The CT scan may at first show little abnormality but eventually large low density lesions appear in the cerebral white matter. Serum antibodies are of no diagnostic help but the response in the CSF has not been fully evaluated. The diagnosis can be confirmed only by cerebral biopsy, but it is essential that white matter is included in the specimen.

Treatment

No treatment is of proven value, but cytosine arabinoside has sometimes appeared to induce partial remission.

Progressive rubella panencephalitis

This extremely rare disorder (see also Section 5) may follow congenital rubella or rubella in early childhood. It evolves insidiously some 10 years after the original illness and is characterized by progressive mental retardation with behaviour changes, fits, ataxia, spasticity, optic atrophy, and macular degeneration. Pathological changes are those of encephalitis with perivascular infiltration. The CSF may show a slight rise in white cell and protein content, elevation of gamma globulin, and of antirubella antibodies to an extent greater than the rise in the serum level, suggesting local production of antibody within the CNS. The EEG may show changes similar to those seen in subacute sclerosing panencephalitis due to measles virus. The mechanism responsible for the appearance of this disorder is unknown and there is no effective treatment.

Vogt–Koyanagi–Harada syndrome

The cause of this rare syndrome is thought to be an inflammatory auto-immune reaction to an unidentified viral infection. The disorder affects tissues having a common embryological origin, the uvea and leptomeninges, and the melanoblasts, ocular pigments, and auditory labyrinth pigments originating from the neural crest. The dermatological features consist of patchy whitening of eyelashes, eyebrows, and scalp hair, alopecia, and vitiligo. Neurological manifestations include meningo-encephalitis, raised intracranial pressure, neurosensory deafness, tinnitus, nystagmus, ataxia, ocular palsies, and focal cerebral deficits. Ocular features are those of uveitis with pain and photophobia, more generalized inflammation of the eye, retinopathy, and impaired visual acuity. The condition tends to be self-limiting but may result in serious permanent ocular and neurological deficits. Steroids and immunosuppressive drugs have been used and are said to arrest the progression of at least some features of the disorder.

Epidemic neuromyasthenia

The existence of this disorder (see Section 5) sometimes known as epidemic or benign myalgic encephalomyelitis, is denied by some. Its main features are said to be headache, fever, muscle pains, and psychiatric disturbances such as lassitude, depression, and possibly hysterical reactions. Symptoms of upper respiratory infection and lymphadenopathy may occur. Transient oculomotor palsies, peripheral weakness, altered reflexes, and altered sensation have been recorded in some patients said to be suffering from this disorder. The cerebrospinal fluid is normal. Abnormal lymphocytes have been seen in the peripheral blood films in some patients but no specific infective agent has been isolated.

Viral causes of psychiatric illness

Mental changes are common in patients with encephalitis. Influenza, infectious mononucleosis, and infectious hepatitis are sometimes followed by psychiatric sequelae, in particular a depressive reaction. Psychosis following encephalitis lethargica was reported on occasions.

Other possible virus infections in which the nervous system is involved

Acute disseminated encephalomyelitis is considered on page 21.216. *Reye's syndrome* is further described in Section 12 and *Behçet's syndrome* in Section 24. *Mollaret's meningitis* is discussed on page 21.135.

References

Brown, F. and Wilson, G. (eds) (1984). *Topley and Wilson's principles of bacteriology, virology and immunity* 7th edn, Vol. 4. Edward Arnold, London.

Christie, A. B. (1980). *Infectious diseases: epidemiology and clinical practice* 3rd edn. Churchill Livingstone, Edinburgh.

Corey, L. and Spear, P. G. (1986). Infections with herpes simplex viruses. *N. Engl. J. Med.* **314**, 686–691, 749–757.

Davies, J. A., Hughes, J. T. and Oppenheimer, D. R. (1973). Richardson's disease progressive multifocal leucoencephalopathy. *Q.J. Med.* **42**, 481–501.

Feigin, R. D. and Cherry, J. D. (eds) (1981). *Textbook of pediatric infectious diseases*. W. B. Saunders, Philadelphia.

Fiddian, A. P. and Grant, D. M. (1985). Developments in anti-herpes agents: progress and prospects. *Abs. Hyg. Comm. Dis.* **60**, RI–R22.

Griffiths, J. F. (1985). SSPE and lymphocytes. *N. Eng. J. Med.* **313**, 952–953.

Ho, D. D., Rota, T. R., Schooley, R. T., *et al.* (1985). Isolation of HTLV-III from cerebrospinal fluid and neural tissues of patients with neurologic syndromes related to the acquired immunodeficiency syndrome. *N. Engl. J. Med* **313**, 1493–1497.

Johnson, R. T. (1982). *Viral infections of the nervous system*. Raven Press, New York.

——, Burke, D. S., Elwell, M. *et al.* (1985). Japanese encephalitis: immunocytochemical studies of viral antigen and inflammatory cells in fatal cases. *Ann. Neurol.* **18**, 567–573.

—— and Mims, C. A. (1968). Pathogenesis of viral infection of the nervous system. *N. Engl. J. Med.* **278**, 23–30, 84–92.

Jones, C. E., Dyken, P. R., Huttenlocher, P. R., Jabbour, J. Y. and Maxwell, K. W. (1982). Inosiplex therapy in subacute sclerosing panencephalitis. A multicentre, non-randomised study in 98 patients. *Lancet* i, 1034–1036.

Krupp, L. B., Lipton, R. B., Swerdlow, M. L., Leeds, N. E. and Llena, J. (1985). Progressive multifocal leukoencephalopathy: clinical and radiological features. *Ann. Neurol.* **17**, 344–349.

Meyer, H. M., Johnson, R. T., Crawford, I. P., Dascomb, H. E. and Rogers, N. G. (1960). Central nervous system syndromes of 'viral' etiology. A study of 713 cases. *Am. J. Med.* **29**, 334–347.

Mims, C. A. and White, D. O. (1984). *Viral pathogenesis and immunology*. Blackwell Scientific Publications, Oxford.

Molavi, A. and LeFrock, J. L. (eds) (1985). Infections of the central nervous system. *Med. Clin. N. Am.* **69**, 1–435.

Oxman, M. N. (1981). Herpes simplex encephalitis and meningitis. In *Medical microbiology and infectious diseases* (ed. A. I. Braude), pp. 1309–1328. W. B. Saunders, Philadelphia.

Panitch, H. S., Gomez-Plascencia, J., Norris, F. H., Cantell, K. and Smith, R. A. (1986). Subacute sclerosing panencephalitis. Remission after treatment with intraventricular interferon. *Neurology* **36**, 562–566.

Pattison, E. M. (1965). Uveomeningoencephalitic syndrome (Vogt–Koyanagi–Harada). *Archs Neurol.* **12**, 197–205.

Price, R. W. and Plum, F. (1978). Poliomyelitis. In *Handbook of clinical neurology*, Vol. 34, p. 93. North Holland, Amsterdam.

Resnick, L., di Marzo-Veronese, F. and Schupbach, J. (1985). Intrablood–brain barrier synthesis of HTLV-III-specific IgG in patients with neurologic symptoms associated with AIDS or AIDS-related complex. *N. Engl. J. Med.* **313**, 1498–1504.

Townsend, J. J., Baringer, J. R., Wolinsky, J. S., Malamud, N., Mednick, J. P., Panitch, H. S., Scott, R. A. T., Oshiro, L. S. and Cremer, N. E. (1975). Progressive rubella panencephalitis – late onset after congenital rubella. *New Engl. J. Med.* **292**, 990–993.

Vinken, P. J. and Bruyn, G. W. (eds) (1978). Infections of the nervous system, Part II. *Handbook of clinical neurology*, Vol. 34. North Holland, Amsterdam.

Walker, D. L. (1978). Progressive multifocal leukoencephalopathy: an opportunistic viral infection of the central nervous system. In *Handbook of clinical neurology* Vol. 34 (eds G. Bruyn and P. J. Vinken), pp. 307–329. North Holland, Amsterdam.

Whitley, R. J., Alford, C. A., Hirsch, M. S. *et al.* (1986). Vidarabine versus Acyclovir therapy in herpes simplex encephalitis. *N. Engl. J. Med.* **314**, 144–149.

Wolinsky, J. S., Johnson, K. P., Rand, K. and Merrigan, T. E. (1976). Progressive multifocal leucoencephalopathy: clinical pathological correlates and failure of a drug trial in two patients. *Trans. Am. Neurol. Assoc.* **101**, 81–82.

Intracranial abscess

P. J. TEDDY

Intracranial abscesses may occur within the extradural or subdural space or may be intracerebral. Occasionally abscesses exist in more than one tissue plane. Intracerebral abscesses and subdural abscesses may rupture into the subarachnoid space and be accompanied by meningitis and intracerebral pus may rupture into the ventricular system and produce ventriculitis.

Incidence

A neurosurgical unit in the United Kingdom serving a population of about 3 million would expect to treat about 12 cases of cerebral abscess a year and about five cases of subdural empyema unrelated to trauma or previous surgery. Extradural abscesses are rather less common.

Aetiology

Extradural abscesses are usually related to focal osteomyelitis of the skull, mastoiditis and nasal sinusitis, penetrating injuries of the skull, and are a rare complication of craniotomy. They are occasionally found in combination with subdural empyema and as a complication of infected dermal sinuses of the scalp.

Subdural empyema is related most commonly to infection of the paranasal sinuses and middle ear. Other causes include septicaemia related to cyanotic congenital heart disease, lung abscess, trauma, and intracranial surgery.

The commonest intracranial abscess is found within the intracerebral compartment, with about 60 per cent related to middle-ear infection and 20 per cent to frontal sinusitis. Other established causes are septicaemia related to congenital heart disease with a right-to-left shunt, lung abscess, bronchiectasis, penetrating injuries of the head, and bacteraemia following tooth extraction. In about 10 per cent of cases no primary source of infection can be identified. Owing to their strong connection with sinus and middle-ear disease most intracerebral abscesses are found within the frontal or temporal lobes, or within the cerebellum. Infection disseminated through the blood stream from more distant sites may result in multiple abscesses in any part of the brain. Cerebellar abscess is almost exclusively related to middle-ear infection but about 60 per cent of abscesses associated with middle-ear disease are found within the temporal lobe. Frontal sinusitis is most commonly related to frontal-lobe abscess or subdural empyema. In infants, subdural empyema most commonly occurs as a secondary infection following bacterial meningitis.

Indirect spread of infection from distant sites is probably venous, either by embolic spread through venous pathways or by extension of venous thrombosis with pyogenic infections.

Microbiology

Some 15 years ago up to 30 per cent of cultures of pus from intracranial abscesses might have been expected to show no growth. This percentage has dropped considerably owing to better methods of culture and identification of obligate anaerobic microorganisms. The demonstration of such anaerobes in intracranial abscesses and the institution of appropriate therapy has probably been a major factor in the decline in mortality from cerebral abscess during this period.

The commonest organisms associated with subdural empyema are aerobic, anaerobic, and microaerophilic streptococci, *Staphylococcus aureus*, and Bacteroides species. In infants with subdural empyema secondary to bacterial meningitis the principal organisms are *Haemophilus influenzae*, *Neisseria meningitidis*, and *Streptococcus pneumoniae*. Even in these cases anaerobic organisms may yet be shown to be present in apparently sterile cultures.

Cerebral abscesses associated with otitis media, mastoiditis, and nasal sinusitis usually show a mixed growth of anaerobes and aerobic organisms including anaerobic and microaerophilic streptococci and bacteroides. *Streptococcus viridans* and *Staph. aureus* are frequently seen. Infections from distant sources also show mixed growths and usually include anaerobic and microaerophilic streptococci, staphylococci, Klebsiella, and sometimes actinomycosis and pseudomonas.

Pathology

Infection within an accessory air sinus or the petrous bone may cause an area of localized osteitis just above the dura, which can then spread intracranially. Initially it may be entirely confined to the extradural space, but will eventually penetrate the dura and spread subdurally or, if the adjacent arachnoid is stuck to the inflamed patch of dura, then it will spread into the subarachnoid space to give meningitis. If the subarachnoid space has been obliterated it may penetrate the brain to produce initially a focal cerebritis. Usually after about 10 days the area of cerebritis becomes enclosed within an area of gliotic brain, and after about three weeks a firm capsule forms around the pus. Large intracerebral abscesses may rupture into the ventricular system, thus producing a ventriculitis. Thick-walled abscesses are most commonly associated with penetrating injuries of the skull and with middle-ear or mastoid disease, whereas infection from the frontal sinuses, and those associated with congenital heart disease and haematogenous spread from distant foci, are more often thin-walled.

Cerebral abscesses are usually surrounded by considerable areas of oedematous brain, which may exert a considerable mass effect. An extradural empyema is seldom large, but subdural abscesses may be extremely extensive with the pus flowing over the convexity of the brain to reach the space between the falx cerebri and the medial surface of the hemisphere. This is a feature which is important in terms of treatment. Cerebral abscesses may be either single or multiple and the single abscess is often multilocular.

Clinical features

The clinical features of intracranial abscess will depend upon the site, size, and number of lesions, and involvement of neighbouring structures such as the cerebral ventricles and the venous sinuses. The signs are therefore legion, but the diagnosis should be considered in any case where there is an obvious primary source of infection associated with evidence of either raised intracranial pressure, focal neurological signs, epileptic seizures, or meningeal irritation, or any combination of these.

Extradural abscess may be difficult to detect clinically, but is sometimes manifest by severe unremitting localized headache in association with sinusitis or mastoiditis. Patients with subdural empyema most commonly appear toxic with a swinging pyrexia, severe headache, a depressed level of consciousness, contralateral hemiparesis, papilloedema, meningeal irritation, and seizures. There is usually an accompanying frontal sinusitis with tenderness of the forehead and redness and swelling of the eyelids, or mastoiditis or scalp infection. Of patients with intracerebral abscess about 70 per cent will present with headache, 60 per cent with impaired consciousness, 40 per cent with a hemiparesis, and 30 per cent with seizures. The focal neurological signs will depend upon the site of the abscess, with temporal-lobe lesions producing an early superior homonymous quadrantanopia together with dysphasia if the dominant temporal lobe is involved. There may also be a brachiofacial weakness. Cerebellar abscesses are accompanied by ipsilateral limb ataxia and hypotonia, and by nystagmus. Blood-borne abscesses often seed to the parietal region and produce little in the way of early focal neurological signs.

As with any mass lesion the most pressing symptoms and signs associated with intracranial abscesses are those of raised intracranial pressure, namely, headache, vomiting, and impaired conscious level, often, but not invariably, accompanied by papilloedema.

Diagnosis

Despite advances in antimicrobial therapy and radiological investigations intracranial abscess remains a disease with a high mortality and morbidity. Outcome is closely related to the conscious level prior to operative treatment, and one major factor contributing to morbidity is late diagnosis. The development of massive cerebral oedema with brain-stem compression, secondary ventriculitis or meningitis, and missed multiple lesions also contribute to a high morbidity.

If a brain abscess is suspected, predisposing sources of infection, including possible distant sites, should be carefully sought, as intracranial abscesses derived by haematogenous spread are often more fulminating in their course than those associated with local cranial disease. Initial investigations should include plain X-rays of the skull (and sinuses where indicated) and the chest.

The investigation of choice for all forms of suspected intracranial abscess is a computerized tomographic (CT) scan, both with and without contrast. This will normally demonstrate both extradural and subdural empyema, may demonstrate diffuse cerebritis

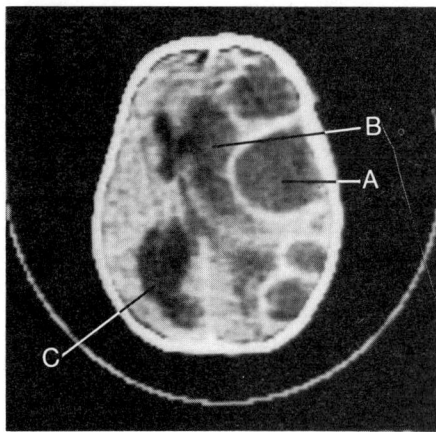

Fig. 1 Contrast scan showing massive right-sided multilocular subdural empyema secondary to a pansinusitis (arrow A). Note cerebral oedema (B) and displacement of ventricular system (C). The child made a complete recovery after evacuation of the pus and antimicrobial therapy.

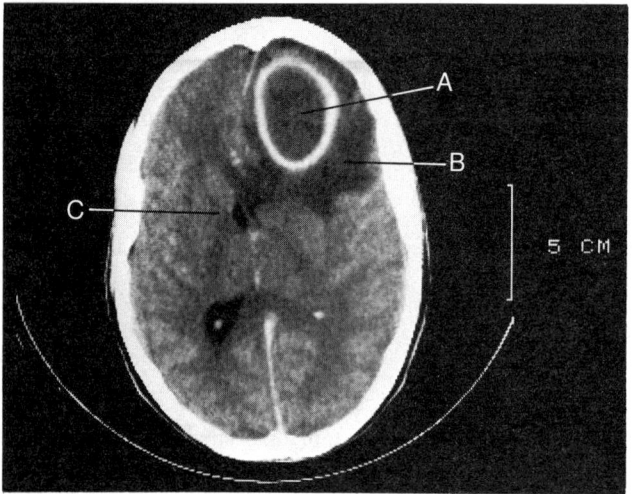

Fig. 2 Contrast CT scan showing large right frontal cerebral abscess (A) with surrounding oedema (B) and ventricular compression (C).

in early cases, and will normally show intracerebral abscesses as ring-enhancing lesions with low attenuation centres (see Figs 1 and 2). Nevertheless, there are pitfalls, particularly in the early stages both of subdural empyema and of cerebral abscess. Subdural empyema may initially be fairly thinly spread over the cerebral cortex and produce relatively little midline shift and be virtually isodense with brain. Under such circumstances the skull and sinus X-rays are of particular importance. If the patient is not too ill the CT scan may be repeated after a few days. If the scan appearances are doubtful, cerebral angiography may demonstrate displacement of peripheral vessels. In acute cases, if there is a high index of suspicion of subdural empyema, exploratory burr holes should be performed even in the presence of an apparently normal scan. Patients suspected on CT scan as having an area of cerebritis adjacent to sinus or middle-ear disease should have a scan repeated after a few days. Both plain skull X-ray and CT scan may demonstrate free gas when gas-forming organisms are present.

The principal differential diagnoses in intracranial abscess are meningitis, subdural haematoma, and intracranial tumour. It is not always possible to differentiate between intracerebral abscess and tumour on CT scan, particularly when there is an appearance of ring enhancement. It is largely for this reason that biopsy of suspected cerebral tumour is advocated in nearly all such cases.

One obvious concern is to differentiate between bacterial meningitis and intracerebral abscess. Both may present with pyrexia, neck stiffness, and with some focal signs, but if there is any evidence whatever of raised intracranial pressure, or any other supportive evidence of cerebral abscess a lumbar puncture should be strictly avoided until a neurosurgical opinion has been sought. Lumbar puncture in the presence of cerebral abscess can lead to tonsillar or tentorial herniation, and in any event, the CSF can be entirely normal.

Management

Management of intracranial abscess is essentially treatment of the abscess itself and treatment of the underlying cause. Except in a few cases of multiple or inaccessible abscess, and the occasional patient whose general medical condition is such that surgery is precluded, treatment of the intracranial infection requires evacuation of pus and high-dose intravenous antibiotic therapy.

Although there is evidence that serial CT scanning and more effective antimicrobial therapy has reduced the mortality and morbidity of intracranial abscesses over the past decade, the single main factor in securing a good outcome is early diagnosis. Early management includes taking specimens for blood culture and culture of any extracranial infective lesion, setting up an intravenous infusion, administration of anticonvulsant agents and, in cases of grossly depressed level of consciousness and massive cerebral oedema seen on CT scan, giving intravenous dexamethasone.

Pus from the suspected primary site of infection should be collected immediately and both aerobic and anaerobic cultures obtained. The intracranial pus must be similarly cultured. Antimicrobial treatment, using massive intravenous doses, should be commenced immediately without waiting for the culture report, and subsequently changed in the light of the sensitivity findings. The antimicrobial regime should include penicillin (4 megaunits four-hourly), metronidazole, ampicillin, and either gentamicin or chloramphenicol depending on the likely source of infection and infective agent. Intravenous antimicrobials should be continued for at least one week before reverting to oral medication.

Most supratentorial abscesses can be sterilized by aspiration through a burr hole, and the direct instillation of antibiotics is sometimes employed. Aspiration must usually be repeated several times, but in about 30 per cent of cases a single aspiration will suffice. Once the abscess is sterile, the capsule will shrink and finally form an irregular gliotic scar within the brain. Shrinkage of the abscess must be checked by serial CT scan. Subdural empyema should be evacuated through a craniotomy rather than burr holes, as very often the pus can spread widely, and particularly alongside the falx cerebri. Extradural empyema is evacuated through a burr hole or through a craniotomy for larger collections.

Cerebellar abscess, when diagnosed early, may be aspirated through a burr hole, but immediate total excision is often recommended because the small volume of the posterior cranial fossa leaves little latitude in terms of tonsillar herniation and death. Some superficial supratentorial abscesses with thickened capsules may be excised rather than aspirated, and in a few cases in which there is extensive brain swelling and continuing tentorial herniation, excision through a craniotomy might similarly be advised. In cases of otitis media and frontal sinusitis, mastoidectomy or drainage of the frontal sinus should be performed in conjunction with a neurosurgical procedure. Where there is osteitis the infected skull bone should also be removed.

Prognosis

Until fairly recently the mortality figure for intracranial abscess stood between 30 and 50 per cent. The use of serial CT scanning to localize the lesion and to show that surgical treatment has been successful, improved microbiological investigation, and antimicrobial therapy have all combined to reduce the mortality rate to around 10 per cent, but the main problems remain those of late diagnosis and resistant bacteria. Even with an otherwise good outcome, epilepsy may continue in about 30 per cent of cases, particularly in patients with temporal-lobe abscess and subdural empyema.

References

Alderson, D., Strong, A. J., Ingham, H. R. and Selkon, J. B. (1981). Fifteen year review of the mortality of brain abscess. *Neurosurgery* **8**, 1–6.

Bannister, G., Williams, B. and Smith S. (1981). Treatment of subdural empyema. *J. Neurosurg.* **55**, 82–88.

De Louvois, J., Gortvai, P. and Hurley, R. (1977). Bacteriology of abscesses of the central nervous system : a multicentre prospective study. *Br. Med. J.* **ii**, 981.

Garfield, J. (1978). Brain abscesses and focal suppurative infections. In *Infections of the nervous system. Part 1. Handbook of clinical neurology*, Vol. 33 (eds P. J. Vinken and G. W. Bruyn), pp. 107–147. North Holland, Amsterdam.

Jefferson, A. A. and Keogh, A. J. (1977). Intracranial abscesses : A review of treated patients over 20 years. *Q. J. Med.* **46**, 389.

Youmans, J. R. (ed.) (1982). *Neurological surgery*, 2nd edn (6 vols). W. B. Saunders, Philadelphia.

CEREBROVASCULAR DISEASE

C. P. WARLOW

Cerebrovascular disease includes any disorder of the vascular system which causes ischaemia, infarction, or haemorrhage within the brain. In developed countries it is the third commonest cause of death, after ischaemic heart disease and cancer, and is responsible for much of the physical and mental disability in the elderly. Many terms used to describe the various forms of cerebrovascular disease are confusing and imprecise, but there are two generally accepted definitions: a *transient ischaemic attack* (TIA) is an acute loss of focal cerebral or ocular function with symptoms lasting less than 24 hours and which, after adequate investigation, is presumed to be due to embolic or thrombotic vascular disease, while a *stroke* (or cerebrovascular accident) is a rapidly developing episode of focal and at times global (applied to patients in deep coma and to those with subarachnoid haemorrhage) loss of cerebral function, with symptoms lasting more than 24 hours or leading to death, with no apparent cause other than that of vascular origin. The main subcategories of stroke are cerebral infarction, primary intracerebral haemorrhage, and subarachnoid haemorrhage. These two rather rigid definitions have somewhat indistinct boundaries in clinical practice, particularly because the 24-hour time limit separating stroke from TIA is entirely arbitrary. There are many patients whose symptoms resolve in a matter of days and who therefore have had, by definition, a stroke even though there is no persisting neurological disability; along with TIA such episodes are sometimes referred to as 'reversible ischaemic attacks' and their pathogenesis, management, and treatment are probably the same as for TIA.

Epidemiology

The annual incidence of stroke in North America and Europe is between one and two per 1000 population, but the exact figure depends on the age structure of the population under consideration since the incidence rises steeply with increasing age (Fig. 1). In the United Kingdom, where approximately 100 000 people have a first stroke every year, cerebrovascular disease causes only approximately 10 deaths per 100 000 population at the age of 40 years, but 1000 deaths per 100 000 population at the age of 75 years. Other causes for variation in published incidence rates between and within countries are differences in diagnostic criteria, whether first ever strokes or all strokes are being analysed, and perhaps the year of the study since the incidence of both cerebral infarction and primary intracerebral haemorrhage may be falling in several countries, particularly in the United States.

The incidence and prevalence of TIA are uncertain since transient neurological symptoms are frequently forgotten or simply not reported to doctors and questionnaires are inaccurate. The annual incidence of TIA may be in the region of 0.5 per 1000 population and a total of about 25 000 new cases per annum occur in the United Kingdom.

Until the recent introduction of computerized tomography (CT

scanning), the epidemiology of cerebrovascular disease was hampered by the almost impossible task of differentiating intracranial haemorrhage, with the exception of subarachnoid haemorrhage, from cerebral infarction on the basis of clinical symptoms and signs. This differentiation must have an important bearing on stroke epidemiology since these two main causes of stroke have a different pathogenesis. A further problem is that stroke is essentially a disorder of the elderly and the majority do not come to necropsy. As a rough estimate about 80 per cent of strokes are due to cerebral infarction, 10 per cent to subarachnoid haemorrhage, and 10 per cent to primary intracerebral haemorrhage.

Cross-sectional and prospective epidemiological studies have identified various risk factors for stroke and the most important, both for cerebral infarction and primary intracerebral haemorrhage, is hypertension. The risk of cerebral infarction increases with increasing levels of blood pressure (the systolic being more predictive than the diastolic) in both sexes and at all ages. Interestingly, there is much less difference in the incidence of cerebral infarction between males and females (Fig. 1) than there is for myocardial infarction. Other risk factors for cerebral infarction include heart disease of any kind, atrial fibrillation, transient ischaemic attack, peripheral vascular disease, diabetes mellitus, a cervical arterial bruit, and a high haematocrit. Less definite risk factors include cigarette smoking, obesity, high plasma fibrinogen, excessive alcohol consumption, and hyperlipidaemia. In young and middle-aged women the contraceptive pill increases the risk of stroke by about three times. The effect of racial and genetic factors is not fully known. It has been claimed that by identifying the

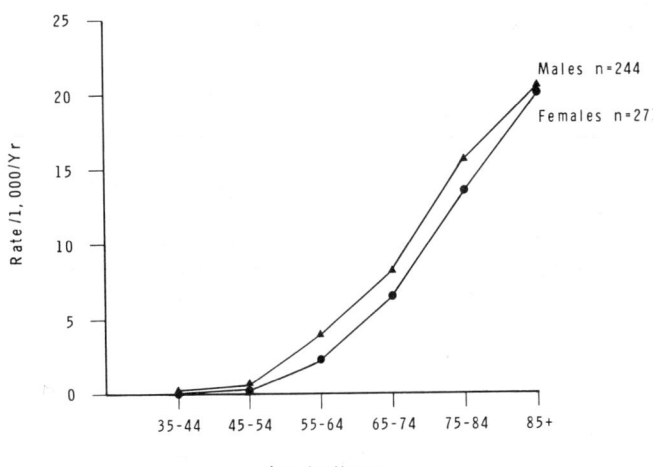

Fig. 1 Incidence of first stroke by increasing age in males and females taken from the Oxfordshire Community Stroke Project, 1981–84.

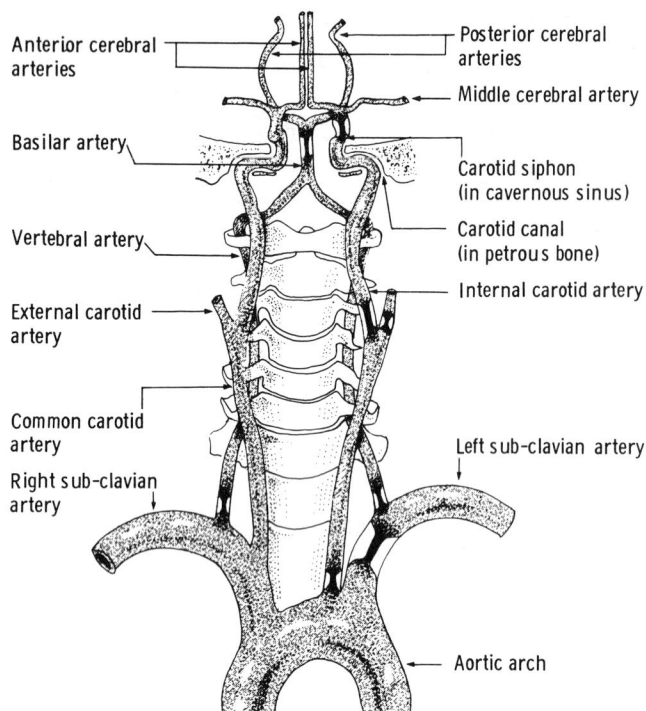

Fig. 2 The arterial blood supply to the brain. Places most often affected by atherothrombosis are shown as white indentations into the arterial lumen.

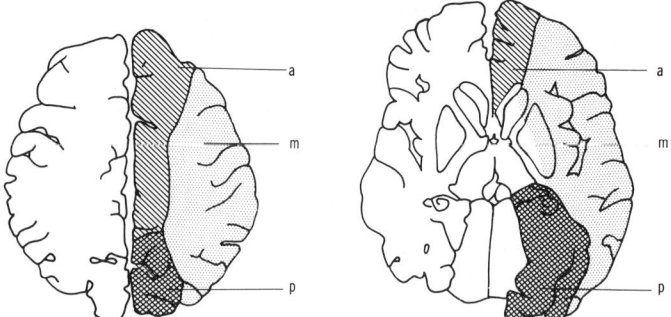

Fig. 3 The distribution of supply of the anterior (a), middle (m), and posterior (p) cerebral arteries. These distributions are a composite derived from six normal brains sliced parallel to the orbito-meatal line to simulate CT scan slices. On the left the slice is above the lateral ventricles and on the right through the internal capsules. (Reproduced by courtesy of Dr Nigel Hyman).

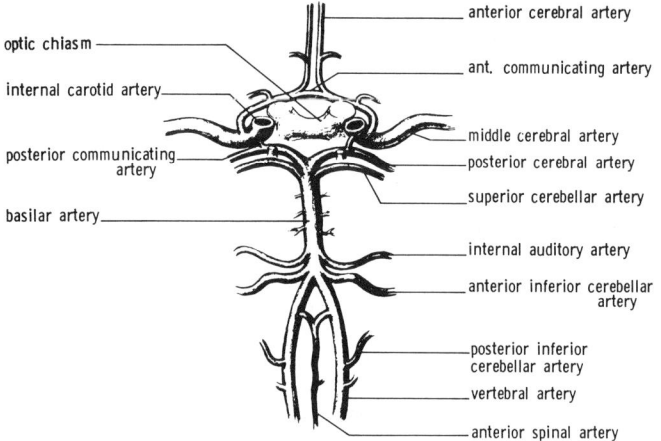

Fig. 4 Diagram of the Circle of Willis as seen at the base of the brain.

important risk factors for stroke in an asymptomatic population it is possible to identify the 10 per cent from which 50 per cent of the subsequent cases of stroke will emerge. Indeed, stroke is distinctly unusual in an individual without one or more risk factors for vascular disease.

The blood supply to the brain

Since most strokes are the result of cerebral infarction, caused by an impaired blood supply to the brain, it is important to be familiar with the anatomy of both the extracranial and intracranial arterial supply and the way in which it is affected by atheroma, the commonest disorder of arteries in the Western World. The brain has a particularly rich blood supply which is derived from four main arteries; the left and right internal carotid and vertebral arteries (Fig. 2). The internal carotid artery (ICA) supplies the eye through the ophthalmic artery and then divides into the anterior and middle cerebral arteries which supply the anterior two-thirds of the cerebral hemisphere, the basal ganglia, and the internal capsule regions (Fig. 3). The vertebral arteries unite to form the basilar artery, whose branches supply the brain stem and cerebellum, which then divides into the two posterior cerebral arteries supplying the posterior one-third of the cerebral hemisphere (Fig. 3). The carotid arterial systems are interconnected by the anterior communicating artery and are linked to the vertebrobasilar system by the posterior communicating arteries so forming the circle of Willis at the base of the brain (Fig. 4). In many individuals parts of this arterial ring are hypoplastic and less than half are of the standard pattern. Nonetheless, it can form, unless affected by disease, an excellent collateral channel for blood supply to the brain if one or more of the four main extracranial arteries become occluded. Other potential collateral channels may also become functionally important; branches of the ICA and external carotid artery (ECA) anastomose with each other around and within the orbit, leptomeningeal anastomoses between cortical arterial branches since the dura is supplied by the ICA, ECA, and vertebral arteries, and there are various anastomoses between the major arteries in the neck.

Cerebral blood flow (CBF) is 'autoregulated' to ensure a constant supply of blood to the brain between a mean systemic blood pressure of approximately 60 and 160 mmHg. Within this range a rise in blood pressure is met by intracranial vasoconstriction, and a fall by vasodilation. However, outside these limits CBF follows perfusion pressure and, therefore, ischaemia occurs if the systemic blood pressure falls, and vasogenic oedema and ultimately hypertensive encephalopathy if it rises. These limits within which autoregulation is effective are 'set' higher in patients with chronic hypertension who will, therefore, experience ischaemia at a higher level of systemic blood pressure than normotensive individuals. However, a patient with sustained hypertension and whose autoregulation is 'set' higher, is less likely to sustain cerebral damage and 'hypertensive encephalopathy' than a normotensive patient under circumstances of an acute increase in blood pressure.

When the brain is damaged as a result of stroke and other diseases, focal areas may no longer autoregulate normally and blood flow will follow fluctuations in systemic blood pressure while the reactivity to arterial $PaCO_2$ is often impaired as well (under normal circumstances a rise of 1 mmHg in $PaCO_2$ increases CBF by 5 per cent). These changes are extremely unpredictable and presumably depend on the age of the lesion and exactly where flow is being considered in relation to that lesion.

CBF is also influenced by haematocrit since it falls with increasing levels of haematocrit even through the commonly accepted 'normal' range. However, this is not so much because the high haematocrit increases whole blood viscosity, but because the higher oxygen carrying capacity of the high haematocrit blood allows a lower CBF for the same oxygen delivery.

The pattern of atheroma

Atheroma is a generalized disorder of large and medium-sized arteries affecting, either clinically or subclinically, the blood supply to many organs and parts of the body. It tends to occur at points of arterial branching and tortuosity which are sites of maximal haemodynamic stress on the arterial wall. It is more extensive in hypertensive than normotensive individuals. The common sites of atheroma in the arterial supply to the brain are indicated in Fig. 2 and the most important are the bifurcation of the common carotid artery (CCA) into the ICA and ECA, the carotid siphon within the cavernous sinus, the origin and terminations of the vertebral arteries, the basilar artery, the circle of Willis, the proximal portions of the three cerebral arteries and the origins of the major arteries from the aorta. It is remarkable how free of atheroma certain areas can be, particularly the ICA between its origin and the siphon.

Atheroma itself may not have become more common in the last 100 years but its complications of arterial thrombosis and embolism have since the frequency of both cerebral infarction and myocardial infarction has risen so much, at least until the last decade or two. Thrombosis occurs on atheromatous plaques which have ulcerated as a result of plaque fracture, necrosis or intraplaque haemorrhage, and also in areas of turbulent or sluggish blood flow in relation to atheromatous stenotic areas which are severe enough to have an important haemodynamic effect. Thrombi may occlude arteries, embolize to distal sites, be lysed, become incorporated into the plaques themselves, or propagate proximally and/or distally. The whole process of 'athero-thrombo-embolism' may be at different stages in different arteries, or even within one artery of a single individual. It is this underlying pathology which is the single most common cause of cerebral ischaemia and infarction. It is important to stress the close relationship between atheroma in arteries supplying the brain, coronary artery atheroma, and arterial disease in the periphery; a patient with clinically manifest disease in one area will almost certainly have subclinical or clinically manifest disease in other areas.

Transient ischaemic attacks

Transient ischaemia of the eye and brain is normally presumed to be due to embolism from proximal sites of atherothrombosis or the heart, and occasionally to thrombotic occlusion of the arteries supplying the eye or brain. The causes of ischaemia and infarction are probably identical and the difference is quantitative rather than qualitative; on the whole any cause of ischaemia will, if prolonged, cause infarction particularly if the collateral supply to the ischaemic area is inadequate. Although a TIA is defined as causing symptoms for less than 24 hours, it is exceedingly unlikely that the brain or eye is actually ischaemic for such a long period. One is presumably observing the effect of reversible impairment of neuronal function (lasting for some hours) which has resulted from a short period of ischaemia, perhaps lasting only a few minutes.

TIA are due to athero-thrombo-embolism more often than anything else and in patients with episodes in the distribution of a carotid artery the prevalence of angiographically demonstrated disease of that artery is about 50 per cent. However, the heart is a particularly potent source of emboli to the brain, eye, and elsewhere, and about 30 per cent of TIA patients have a potential, if not a definite, cardiac source of embolism; in perhaps 5–10 per cent of patients embolism from the heart is the *actual* cause of TIA. The various sources of cardiac emboli are listed in Table 1. A small proportion of patients have rare forms of arterial disease (Table 2) and some patients have a haematological disorder which causes ischaemia (Table 3). 'Hypercoagulability states' or 'prethrombotic' changes in the blood are much discussed but are probably not relevant to the aetiology of TIA. The possibility that vasospasm can cause transient ischaemia is very difficult to prove and such a phenomenon has only actually been observed in

humans after subarachnoid haemorrhage or direct stimulation of vessels during neurosurgery. During the aura of classical migraine there are focal neurological symptoms, associated with or caused by ischaemia of part of the brain, but this normally has the obvious features of migraine and is clinically quite different from TIA.

It has been suggested that a transient fall in blood pressure (e.g. due to postural hypotension, vasodilators, cardiac arrhythmia, hot bath, heavy meal etc.) can cause TIA but this must be a very rare explanation unless one or more arteries to the brain are extremely stenotic or occluded, or there is a focal area of defective autoregulation as a result of previous ischaemic damage. A fall in blood pressure usually causes non-focal neurological symptoms such as faintness, vertigo, bilateral dimming of vision, and generalized weakness. The pathogenesis of TIA in the vertebrobasilar distribution has been less well studied but is probably similar to that in the carotid distribution although haemodynamic rather than embolic causes may be more common, and very occasionally dis-

Table 1 Cardiac sources of embolism (in anatomical sequence)

Paradoxical embolism from the venous system	Left ventricle mural thrombus
Atrial septal defect	Myocardial infarction
Patent foramen ovale	Left ventricular aneurysm
Pulmonary AVM	Myxoma
Left atrium	Cardiomyopathy
Thrombus (particularly if there is atrial fibrillation)	Aortic valve
	Infective endocarditis
Myxoma	Rheumatic endocarditis
Sino-atrial disease	Marantic endocarditis
Mitral valve	Sclerosis and/or calcification
Infective endocarditis	Syphilis
Rheumatic endocarditis	Prosthetic valve
Marantic endocarditis	Congenital cardiac disorders
Mitral annulus calcification	Cardiac surgery
Prosthetic valve	Air embolism
Mitral leaflet prolapse	Platelet/fibrin embolism

Table 2 Causes of arterial disease

Atheroma	Dissection
Arteritis	Cystic medial necrosis
Giant cell arteritis	Trauma
Systemic lupus erythematosus	Atheroma
Granulomatous angiitis	Marfan's syndrome
Polyarteritis nodosa	Fibromuscular dysplasia
Wegener's granulomatosis	Inflammatory arterial disease
Sarcoid angiitis	Ehlers Danlos syndrome
Behcet's disease	Pseudo-xanthoma elasticum
Scleroderma	Congenital
Rheumatoid disease	Fibromuscular dysplasia
Sjogren syndrome	Loops, coils, etc.
Relapsing polychondritis	Aneurysms
Rheumatic fever	Infections
Takayasu's disease	Tonsilitis, pharyngitis
Malignant atrophic papulosis	Cervical lymphadentis
(Köhlmeier-Degos disease)	Endarteritis obliterans due to
Necrotizing angiitis associated	TB, syphilis, bacterial or fungal
with drug abuse	meningitis, etc
Trauma	Herpes zoster
Penetrating injuries of the neck	Mucormycosis
Blow to the neck	Miscellaneous
Cervical manipulation	Homocystinaemia
Yoga	Angioendotheliosis
Cervical rib	Neoplastic invasion of the
'Whiplash' injury	arterial wall
Tonsillectomy	Irradiation
Strangulation	Embolism from extra or
Atlanto-axial dislocation	intracranial aneurysm sacs
Fractured clavicle	Fabry's disease
Angiography	Inflammatory bowel disease
	Mitochondrial cytopathy

Table 3 Haematological causes of cerebral ischaemia or infarction (see Section 19)

Sickle cell disease
Polycythaemia rubra vera
Acute or chronic leukaemia
Essential thrombocythaemia
Thrombotic thrombocytopaenic purpura
Paroxysmal nocturnal haemoglobinuria
'Hyperviscosity' syndromes
  Multiple myeloma
  Waldenstrom's macroglobulinaemia
Severe anaemia (probably causes only transient symptoms)

Table 4 Causes of transient monocular blindness (i.e. amaurosis fugax)

Retinal ischaemia
Papilloedema
Glaucoma
Migraine
Uhtoff's phenomenon in retrobulbar neuritis
Retinal haemorrhage
Retinal detachment
Orbital tumours
Macular degeneration
Carotico-cavernous fistula
Intracranial arteriovenous malformation

---

tortion of the vertebral arteries by cervical spondylosis can be relevant. It is important to emphasize that the pathogenesis of TIA is heterogeneous and even though the majority of episodes may well be due to embolism, the emboli themselves can consist of platelet aggregates, fibrin, calcific debri from heart valves, cholesterol arising from atheromatous plaques, or any combination of these constituents. A proportion of TIA patients, perhaps 25 per cent, do not seem to have any serious or identifiable disease.

Clinical features

TIA start abruptly and are not normally related to any particular activity. In *rare* cases, movement of the neck or standing up precipitates an attack by temporary obstruction of arterial blood flow in a neck artery (particularly the vertebral in cervical spondylosis) or a postural fall in blood pressure, respectively; this explanation can probably only be correct if there is very severe arterial disease in the neck which is usually obvious (arterial bruits, absent arterial pulsation).

TIA may be single and infrequent or repetitive, and involve one or more parts of the brain. On occasions they can be remarkably stereotyped. The symptoms usually all appear within a matter of seconds, with no 'spread' from one part of the body to another, and depend on where in the brain the ischaemia occurs. The exact location of ischaemia in an individual patient, depending as it almost always does on a history taken after recovery, is often difficult to elucidate but it is useful to attempt to divide TIA into carotid and vertebrobasilar distribution events. Ischaemia in the carotid territory may cause weakness in the contralateral arm, hand, leg or face in isolation or in various combinations; numbness or paraesthesiae but rarely pain in a similar distribution; language disturbance if the dominant hemisphere is affected; dysarthria but usually only in association with facial weakness; and amaurosis fugax (AFx) in the ipsilateral eye. Ischaemic AFx may involve the whole visual field of one eye or only the top or bottom half of the field and often appears like a 'blind', 'curtain', or 'shutter' obscuring vision over a matter of seconds. It is important to realize that amaurosis fugax (i.e. transient *monocular* blindness) is a symptom, and not a disease, which has several causes (Table 4). Symptoms during a TIA may, by definition, last up to 24 hours but are normally over in a matter of a few minutes or perhaps an hour, and ischaemic AFx rarely lasts more than 5 min. The rate of recovery is usually slower than the onset of the symptoms. Ischaemia in the vertebrobasilar territory may cause hemiparesis or hemisensory disturbance, cortical blindness or a homonymous hemianopia, diplopia, vertigo, nausea, vomiting, deafness, tinnitus, dysarthria, dysphagia, ataxia, a bilateral motor deficit, or a bilateral sensory deficit. Thus, in patients with only unilateral motor or sensory symptoms it can be impossible to determine in which arterial distribution ischaemia has occurred unless there is some other symptom which definitely suggests carotid or vertebrobasilar ischaemia.

Some patients develop headache during a TIA and there may be chest pain or palpitations at the onset of an attack in the rare case precipitated by a cardiac arrhythmia. It is extremely unusual for consciousness to be lost and, if it is, then to make the diagnosis there must also be some additional *focal* neurological feature. Vertigo, dizziness, or faintness as isolated symptoms *can* be to due to thrombo-embolism in the vertebrobasilar territory but are much more often caused by something else such as a drop in blood pressure, sudden head movement, and labyrinthine disorders. TIA should not be diagnosed if there are only non-focal neurological symptoms.

Drop attacks

Drop attacks are sometimes due to vertebrobasilar TIA. The patient, usually a middle-aged or elderly woman, suddenly falls to the ground while walking or standing. Consciousness may be lost for a fraction of a second so that the patient does not remember the actual fall. Considerable injury can result from such attacks. However, in most patients no cause is found and there is no particular evidence of vascular disease.

Transient global amnesia

Transient global amnesia is occasionally caused by vertebrobasilar ischaemia affecting the temporal lobes or thalamus bilaterally through the posterior cerebral arterial supply. For a matter of a few hours there is a profound loss of ability to remember any new information and there is usually a retrograde amnesia as well, sometimes stretching back many years. The patient is fully conscious and able to continue normal activities such as eating, walking, or even driving. He or she is confused about what they have just done and often repetitively question any observer about such matters. There is no loss of personal identity. Recovery is normally complete but memory for the duration of the attack itself is not regained. Repeated attacks are said to be unusual. Occasional cases are caused by epilepsy but usually the cause is completely obscure. In most patients the prognosis is very good, certainly much better than after a TIA.

Subclavian steal

Subclavian steal is a rare syndrome in which, as a result of stenosis or occlusion of the subclavian artery proximal to the origin of the vertebral artery, the increased metabolic demand of the arm musculature during ipsilateral arm exercise is met by retrograde blood flow down the vertebral artery to cause symptoms of basilar ischaemia, particularly dizziness. There is always a difference between the two radial pulses and unequal systolic blood pressure between the two arms, usually greater than 30 mmHg. There is often a bruit in the supraclavicular fossa over the affected subclavian artery. Similar 'steal' phenomena may occur between cerebral arteries but are impossible to recognize clinically.

Differential diagnosis

TIA may be caused by any kind of arterial (Table 2), cardiac embolic (Table 1), haematological (Table 3), or other disease leading to transient ischaemia or anoxia of the brain. They must be differentiated from migraine and focal epilepsy on the basis of an adequate history, if necessary from a witness as well as the patient. The aura of migraine is a 'spreading' and slowly intensifying phenomenon and the symptoms are usually 'positive', (e.g. scintillating scotomata). The aura characteristically lasts 20–30 min and is usually, but not always, followed by severe headache, often with nausea and vomiting. Focal epilepsy also normally causes positive symptoms which 'spread' or 'march' up one limb and from one limb to another on the same side, particularly twitching, jerking, or dysaesthesiae. Rare causes of transient focal neurological disturbances include structural brain disorders such as tumours, subdural haematoma, angioma, and giant aneurysm, but these are very unusual effects of such lesions; malignant hypertension; hypoglycaemia; severe anaemia; the paroxysmal symptoms which sometimes occur in multiple sclerosis; peripheral nerve lesions; and hysteria.

Physical signs

If the patient happens to be examined during an attack, then the signs appropriate to damage in the relevant part of the nervous system will be found. However, usually the patient is examined after the attack and at that stage there should be no abnormal neurological signs and if there are then that is an indication that some, perhaps only trivial, neurological damage has occurred. Whether or not abnormal physical signs are found also depends on the length of time from the last attack and on the competence of the examiner; 'soft' neurological signs have very poor inter-observer reliability. It is also important to examine carefully the arterioles in the retina in case there is any evidence of embolization (Fig. 5). Emboli appear as white bodies passing through the circulation if they consist of platelets, dense white deposits which often obstruct the retinal circulation near the disc margin if they

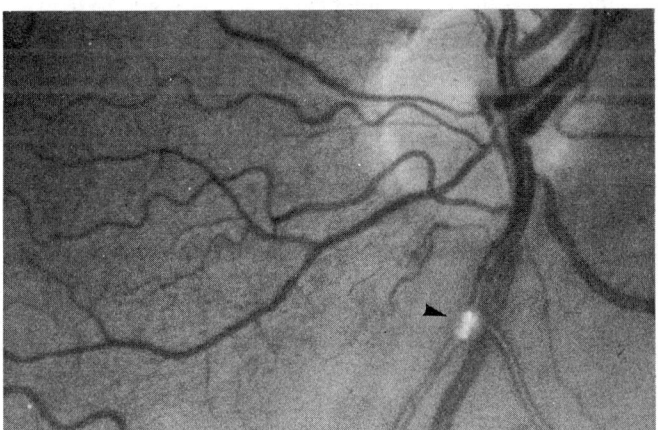

Fig. 5 A cholesterol embolus (black arrow) at the bifurcation of a retinal arteriole. Cholesterol emboli are yellow refractile bodies which usually impact at arteriolar branching points without necessarily obstructing blood flow.

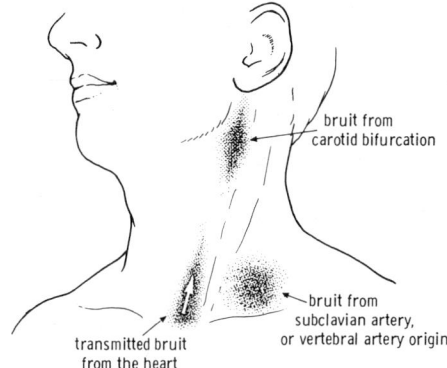

Fig. 6 Diagram to show the sites of maximum intensity of arterial bruits in the neck. Bruits behind the angle of the jaw may be due to either internal or external carotid origin stenosis, while bruits in the supraclavicular region may be due to stenosis of the subclavian or vertebral arteries.

Table 5 Causes of cervical bruits

Arterial disease
Internal carotid artery origin stenosis
External carotid artery origin stenosis
Subclavian stenosis
Vertebral artery origin stenosis
Transmitted bruit from arch of aorta, or heart
Increased blood flow
Anaemia
Thyrotoxicosis
Fever
Intracranial AVM
Haemodialysis arteriovenous fistula in the AVM
Occlusion of contralateral ICA
Goitre
Venous 'hums' in the supraclavicular region
Benign arterial bruits in young adults

are calcific fragments of heart valve, or refractile yellow particles more peripherally, particularly at arteriolar branching points, if they consist of cholesterol crystals. Of considerable importance is a full examination of the vascular system with a search for bruits over the carotid and subclavian arteries, absent or diminished foot pulses, femoral bruits, the pulses and blood pressure in both arms, and any sign of ischaemic or valvular heart disease. The site of various bruits in the neck is shown in Fig. 6, and their causes in Table 5.

Investigations

Investigation should be directed towards establishing the diagnosis of TIA and excluding other causes of transient focal neurological attacks, finding the cause of the TIA, defining risk factors for vascular disease in general, and the management of any associated vascular disease. In all patients this should include a haemoglobin, haematocrit, white cell count, platelet count, erythrocyte sedimentation rate, blood urea, blood glucose, syphilis serology, urine examination, chest X-ray, and ECG. Computerized tomography, if it is available, will exclude most structural intracranial disorders, but these are found unexpectedly in very few cases (less than 5 per cent). If there is any reason to believe that there is a cardiac source of embolism then echocardiography followed by further appropriate cardiological investigation is required; i.e. clinical signs of a potential cardiac source of embolism, ischaemia in more than one arterial territory, a young patient with no risk factors for or evidence of arterial disease. If one of the rare causes of ischaemia is suspected, then naturally the appropriate tests should be carried out. Plasma lipids may be important in young patients who might benefit from dietary or drug correction of hyperlipidaemia. On the whole, 24-hour monitoring of the ECG is unnecessary unless the patient is also complaining of transient non-focal neurological symptoms such as a faintness or giddiness, or the transient focal neurological symptoms are associated with chest pain or palpitations. Electroencephalography is not usually particularly helpful.

Angiography

The diagnosis of TIA is clinical and does not depend on the result of angiography which is done only to delineate the anatomy of arterial lesions which are appropriate to the symptoms and potentially amenable to surgery. If there are no CT scanning facilities angiography will also help exclude structural intracranial lesions such as tumours. Since the surgical possibilities are limited in patients with vertebrobasilar ischaemia, angiography is seldom required unless there are symptoms and signs of subclavian steal, in which case arch aortography is needed. For carotid distribution TIA selective intra-arterial carotid angiography (by conventional or digital techniques) is undertaken to demonstrate the anatomy of the symptomatic ICA in the neck and the intracranial circulation, but only if the patient is fit enough for subsequent carotid

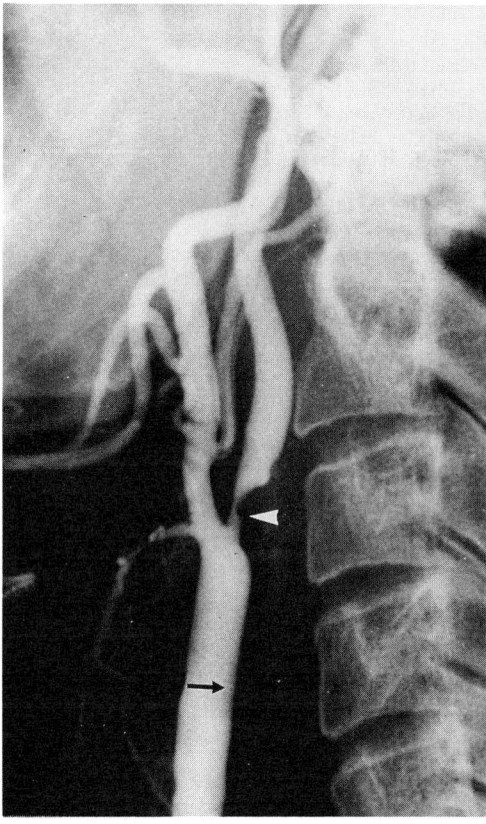

Fig. 7 Lateral view of a selective carotid angiogram to show stenosis of the origin of the internal carotid artery (white arrow) just past the bifurcation of the common carotid artery (black arrow).

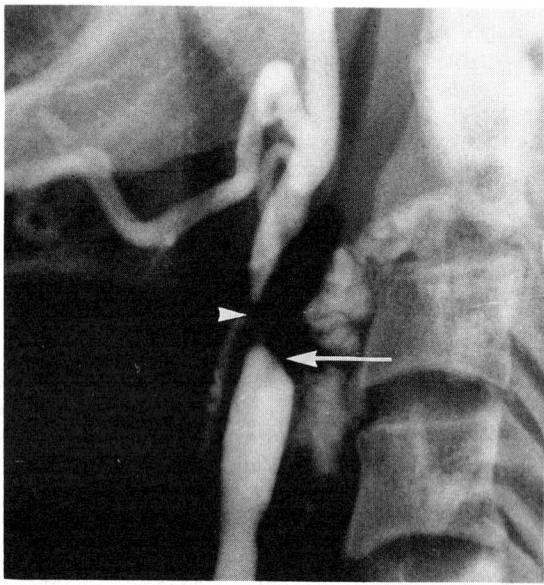

Fig. 8 Lateral view of a selective carotid angiogram to show occlusion of the internal carotid artery at its origin (arrow with tail). The external carotid artery is stenosed (arrow). It is always possible to distinguish the internal from external carotid artery since the latter has several branches in the neck, whilst the former does not.

endarterectomy. Stenosing and/or ulcerating lesions at the origin of the ICA (Fig. 7) are operable whereas intracranial lesions and ICA occlusion (Fig. 8) cannot be operated on directly. In patients with carotid TIAs, about 40 per cent have ipsilateral internal carotid stenosis at the origin, and 10 per cent ICA occlusion. The pres-

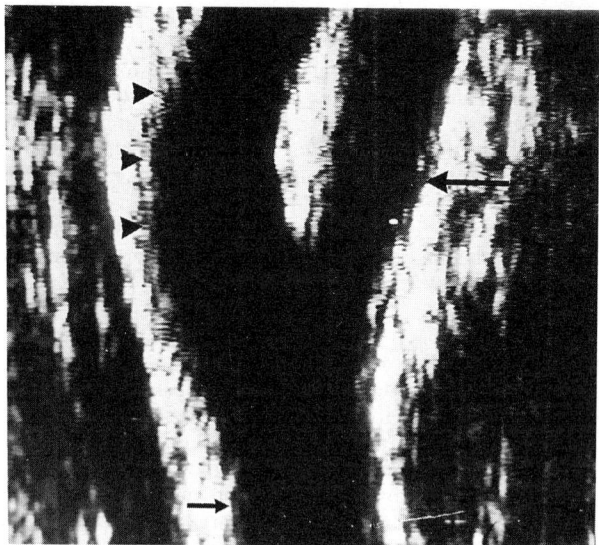

Fig. 9 Real-time ultrasound (lateral image) of a normal carotid bifurcation. The common carotid artery (small arrow with tail) bifurcates into the internal (arrows without tails) and external (large arrow) carotid arteries. (Reproduced by courtesy of Dr Pierre-Jean Touboul.)

ence of a carotid bruit makes the likelihood of ICA stenosis very high but even without a bruit there may be ulceration without stenosis, extreme stenosis with very low blood flow, or complete occlusion. Conversely there can be a bruit, even in the presence of a normal or occluded ICA, due to ECA stenosis or transmitted from the aortic valve or aortic arch. The absence of a carotid bruit should not, therefore, discourage one from angiography if it is thought that subsequent surgical intervention for carotid disease could be helpful. Palpating the carotid artery in the neck is not very useful since it is usually the common or external carotid pulsation that is being felt; if there is no pulsation at all then the common carotid artery is occluded. There are various non-invasive tests which have been suggested as screening procedures to detect carotid stenosis and occlusion and thus to avoid the risks of angiography if the artery is normal. However, only real-time ultrasound is sufficiently reliable and sensitive enough (in the right hands) to be helpful (Fig. 9); unfortunately, it is not widely available.

Medical treatment

TIA are, by definition, short lasting and they are seldom frequent or worrying enough to require treatment in their own right. Unfortunately the prognosis in an individual TIA patient is unpredictable but, on average, the risk of stroke is approximately 5 per cent per annum, that of stroke and/or death about 10 per cent per annum, and the commonest cause of death is not stroke but myocardial infarction (MI) and sudden, presumed cardiac, death. The risk of non-fatal and fatal MI is about the same as the risk of stroke (Fig. 10). The age-standardized mortality ratio for TIA patients compared with a TIA-free population is about three and the excess risk of stroke perhaps five times. The risk of stroke and other serious vascular events increases with age, blood pressure, the presence of clinically apparent ischaemic heart disease, and probably with the degree of disease found at cerebral angiography.

The most important issue in management is, therefore, reduction in the risk of stroke and MI which can occur hours, days, weeks, or years after the first or the most recent transient episode. It is, therefore, logical to start any treatment as soon as the diagnosis of TIA is made, even if there has only been one attack.

The most important treatment in patients with athero-thromboembolism is the control of risk factors for stroke and MI, particularly hypertension and cigarette smoking. The phase V diastolic blood pressure should be lowered to between 100 and 110 mmHg.

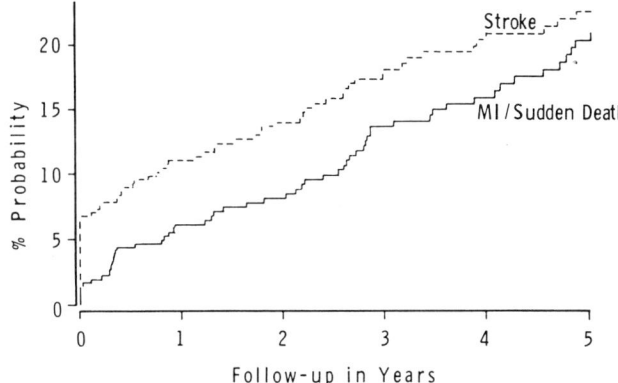

Fig. 10 The probability of stroke and myocardial infarction/sudden death over a five-year period in a population of 390 TIA patients admitted to Duke University Hospital, North Carolina. The high early risk of stroke is mostly due to medical intervention (carotid angiography and carotid endarterectomy). (Reproduced from Heyman et al., 1984, *Neurology* **34**, 626–630, by permission from Dr A. Heyman and the publishers of *Neurology*.)

In elderly patients it is important to do this extremely cautiously because of the possibility of side effects, particularly postural hypotension. It is probably helpful to control very abnormal glucose tolerance even if there are no symptoms of diabetes, to normalize excessive weight if possible, encourage exercise, and possibly to attempt to normalize abnormal lipid patterns in young patients.

Whether long-term antithrombotic drugs are useful is still uncertain. Conventional anticoagulation with warfarin, or one of the other oral anticoagulants, was once fashionable but there is no evidence that it is useful, and no evidence that it is not. However, since anticoagulation is difficult to control, time consuming, expensive, and sometimes dangerous it is probably not worth using particularly in elderly patients. Antiplatelet drugs are more likely to be effective since arterial thrombi are composed largely of platelets rather than fibrin. However, sulphinpyrazone (Anturan) and dipyridamole (Persantin) are ineffective and dipyridamole in combination with aspirin is no more effective than aspirin alone. Long-term aspirin reduces the risk of non-fatal stroke or non-fatal myocardial infarction by about 25 per cent, and of vascular deaths by about 15 per cent or so. Probably the best dose to use is 300 mg daily, provided there are no contraindications such as peptic ulceration. But if this dose causes indigestion then either enteric-coated preparations should be used or a lower dose, but no lower than 75 mg daily. It is conceivable that antiplatelet drugs (like anticoagulants) increase the risk of intracranial haemorrhage and this may counteract any beneficial effect in reducing the risk of cerebral infarction. If, as is sometimes the case, aspirin does not control very frequent TIA then it is reasonable to try formal oral anticoagulation which can be tailed off and replaced by aspirin a few weeks after the attacks stop. If the TIA do not stop either the diagnosis is wrong, or the treatment is ineffective in which case it should be reconsidered and perhaps stopped.

Patients with a definite major cardiac valvular source of embolism, such as mitral stenosis or a prosthetic valve, should probably be anticoagulated indefinitely to prevent further intracardiac fibrin formation, particularly if atrial fibrillation is also present. Some authorities recommend anticoagulation if there is atrial fibrillation and no other cardiac disorder, apart from ischaemic heart disease, but this is probably unwise and certainly lacks any evidence for efficacy. If TIA occur within days or weeks of an acute MI, anticoagulation is usually only required for a matter of three to six months.

In patients who have neither cardiac nor arterial disease, or in whom any disease is only very minor, it is sensible to limit treatment to the reversal of any important risk factors for stroke and MI; in such patients the prognosis is probably very good.

Surgery

In patients who have recovered from a carotid ischaemic event, the removal of a stenosing or ulcerating atheromatous lesion at the origin of the ICA by carotid endarterectomy is logical since it is likely to cause thrombosis and potential embolism, or a reduction in blood flow if the stenosis is extreme. In fact total volume flow and blood pressure distal to a single stenotic lesion are not affected until the residual lumen is reduced to between 2 and 5 mm which is equivalent to stenosis, on diameter measurements, of approximately 65 per cent. Carotid endarterectomy should only be done in centres with adequate experience and only in patients with carotid distribution TIA or mild ischaemic strokes. The operative risk of stroke and/or death should be less than 5 per cent to make the operation worthwhile in the prevention of stroke in the ipsilateral cerebral hemisphere. However, there is still considerable controversy surrounding this operation and randomized trials are being done. Some authorities would not consider operating unless the frequency of the TIA become quite unacceptable.

Subclavian stenosis or occlusion causing subclavian steal can be dealt with by a variety of vascular surgical procedures which are usually highly effective in abolishing the symptoms. Frequent vertebrobasilar TIA due to vertebral stenosis or occlusion can occasionally be reduced in frequency by vascular surgical procedures in the neck.

Using microsurgical techniques it is possible to anastamose the superficial temporal artery, a branch of the ECA, to a distal branch of the middle cerebral artery and thus bypass ICA occlusion, or inaccessible and severe intracranial carotid or proximal middle cerebral artery disease; the so-called 'extracranial to intracranial bypass'. This procedure does not appear to reduce the risk of stroke but, in very occasional patients with severe arterial disease in the neck and head, may possibly improve symptoms directly due to low blood flow such as focal neurological signs or even syncope occurring on standing up (but with no fall in systemic blood pressure).

Cerebral infarction

Cerebral infarction usually causes the clinical picture of stroke but occasionally there may only be a transient neurological deficit for less than 24 hours (e.g. a TIA), or even no symptoms at all. The underlying pathogenesis is, like TIA, usually either atherothrombo-embolism, or embolism from the heart and any difference between ischaemia and infarction is one of degree; a process which causes ischaemia must, if prolonged, eventually cause infarction particularly if the potential collateral blood supply is compromised by pre-existing disease. A fall in systemic blood pressure does not normally cause *focal* cerebral infarction unless a focal area of brain is already ischaemic, is supplied by an extremely stenotic artery, or is critically dependent on a collateral blood supply from a stenotic artery. Prolonged hypotension or anoxia normally causes widespread cerebral infarction and, if the patient survives the circulatory catastrophe, this infarction is often found to have occurred in the boundary zones between arterial territories.

Cerebral infarcts are pale at first but may become haemorrhagic particularly if the necrotic brain and damaged vascular endothelium is exposed to blood under arterial pressure before the infarct has become organized into a gliotic scar. This can happen in embolic infarction if the emboli fragment, and also if blood reflows into the periphery of an infarct from a collateral arterial supply. Cerebral infarction is associated with surrounding cerebral oedema, and in large supratentorial infarcts the amount of 'swelling' and thus occupation of space, is extensive enough to cause

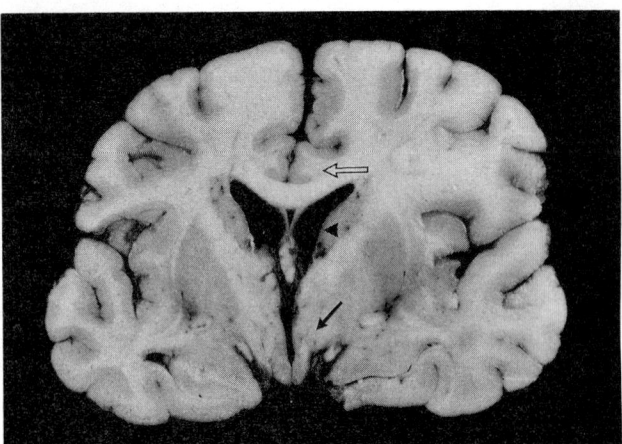

Fig. 11 Coronal section of brain to show a large infarct in the distribution of the right middle cerebral artery. The whole of the right cerebral hemisphere is swollen with oedema and there is downward herniation of the thalamus and mamillary bodies (closed arrow) and herniation of the cingulate gyrus across the midline (open arrow) below the falx. The right lateral ventricle is compressed and distorted (arrow without tail). Note the loss of demarcation between the cortical grey and underlying white matter in the swollen hemisphere. (Reproduced by courtesy of Dr Richard Greenhall.)

transtentorial herniation of the medial part of the temporal lobe (Fig. 11). This leads to secondary midbrain haemorrhage due to distortion and rupture of small penetrating vessels and sometimes to occipital infarction due to compression of the posterior cerebral artery against the edge of the tentorium. Cerebral oedema associated with an infarct usually takes a few days to develop to its maximum extent and then gradually resolves in three to four weeks.

Clinical features

The symptoms, signs, duration, and severity of stroke due to cerebral infarction are very varied and depend on the location and extent of the lesion. It is often difficult to relate the clinical picture very exactly to thrombosis or embolism in one particular artery since the state of the collateral blood supply is of very particular importance in determining whether arterial occlusion causes infarction rather than ischaemia, and if so, how extensive it is. At one extreme it is possible to occlude the ICA without any symptoms but, at the other extreme, if the circle of Willis is compromised by arterial disease, the whole ipsilateral cerebral hemisphere can undergo infarction. The proportion of patients in different subcategories of cerebral infarction is shown in Table 6.

The onset of symptoms is normally quite sudden, or occurs during sleep, but there may be progression in a subacute or 'step-wise' fashion over a few hours; occasionally the clinical picture develops over a matter of several days but very rarely over a few weeks. An increase in the neurological deficit over a few hours is sometimes referred to as a 'stroke-in-evolution' but the cause may not only be propogating thrombosis, but further embolization, haemorrhage into infarcted brain, or cerebral oedema and these possibilities are

Table 6 The distribution of cerebral infarction in 515 first ever strokes (unpublished from the Oxfordshire Community Stroke Project)

	per cent
Infarction in the distribution of part of the internal carotid artery	30
Lacunar infarction	26
Infarction in the distribution of the vertebrobasilar system, including the posterior cerebral arteries	23
Infarction in the distribution of the entire internal carotid artery	17
Unknown	4

difficult, if not impossible, to diagnose clinically with any degree of certainty.

Cerebral hemisphere infarcts

Infarction in a cerebral hemisphere may cause contralateral hemiparesis or hemiplegia, hemisensory loss, or homonymous hemianopia. The motor and/or sensory disturbance may involve the entire side of the body, the upper limb, the face, and the upper limb, both limbs, occasionally the leg alone, and rarely just the face. A small cortical infarct may cause clumsiness of the hand, or only of some of the fingers of one hand. To begin with any hemiplegia tends to be of the flaccid type with diminished deep tendon reflexes, albeit with an extensor plantar response, but within days or weeks spasticity and increased reflexes gradually appear. Lesions in the dominant hemisphere are likely to impair language function (speaking, reading or writing) while in the non-dominant hemisphere may cause visuo-spatial problems such as constructional apraxia or dressing apraxia. If the parietal lobe is affected there is a tendency for the patient to ignore the contralateral side of the body, astereognosis, sensory inattention, sensory loss to all modalities, or just isolated loss of joint position sense. To begin with the head and eyes may be turned towards the side of the lesion but this usually resolves in a few days. Dysarthria tends to be in proportion to the extent of any facial weakness. Initially there is often some contralateral palatal weakness and dysphagia. Headache is quite common, but not usually very severe. Epilepsy is unusual but can be an early or more often late complication of cerebral infarction (less than 5 per cent of patients). If the infarct is extensive, and particularly if transtentorial herniation occurs, consciousness becomes impaired and Cheyne–Stokes or some other abnormality of the respiratory pattern develops. Occlusion of the ICA, particularly if it is traumatic or due to arterial dissection, can cause an ipsilateral Horner's syndrome due, it is thought, to damage to the sympathetic nerves in the carotid sheath.

Lacunar syndromes

Small deep infarcts (usually less than 1.5 cm in diameter) in the region of the basal ganglia, thalamus, internal capsule, and pons are called 'lacunes'. They can often be recognized by the development of a number of characteristic clinical syndromes. Higher cortical function is normal and the patient is conscious. Many remain asymptomatic.

Pure motor stroke Complete or incomplete weakness of the whole of one side of the body, the face, and the upper limb, or the arm and the leg. Sensory symptoms, but not signs, may be present transiently and there may be dysarthria and sometimes dysphagia. The lesion is in the contralateral internal capsule or pons.

Pure sensory stroke Sensory symptoms and/or sensory signs (but not impaired joint position sense alone) occur in the same distribution as pure motor stroke. The lesion is usually in the contralateral thalamus.

Sensori-motor stroke is a combination of pure motor and pure sensory stroke. The lesion is in the basal ganglia/internal capsule region and is often rather larger than that causing pure motor or pure sensory stroke.

Ataxic hemiparesis is a combination of hemiparesis and ipsilateral 'cerebellar' ataxia, often with marked dysarthria, clumsiness of the hand, and unsteadiness. The lesion is in the contralateral pons, or internal capsule area.

Hemichorea, hemiballismus, and 'thalamic' pain are usually caused by lacunar infarction in the contralateral basal ganglia region.

Most lacunar infarcts are thought to be caused by hypertensive changes in the small perforating vessels within the brain substance. There is tortuosity, lipohyalinosis, and disorganization of the vessel wall. It is these damaged vessels which form microaneurysms (Charcot–Bouchard aneurysms) which rupture to produce either small localized haematomas or massive intracerebral haematomas (see below). Therefore, lacunar syndromes are *usually* caused by small vessel disease leading to small deep infarcts, but they can be caused by embolism to the same vessels or to small intracerebral haematomas in the same part of the brain.

Brain stem infarction

Infarction in the brain stem tends to cause a rather complicated neurological deficit which is hardly surprising given the fact that all the ascending and descending pathways are close together at this point. Hemiparesis, hemiplegia, tetraparesis, tetraplegia, and unilateral or bilateral sensory loss can all occur. In addition there may be a disturbance of gaze or extra-ocular muscle palsies, dysphagia, dysarthria, hiccups, ataxia, Horner's syndrome due to lesions involving the descending sympathetic pathways, deafness, tinnitus, vertigo, nausea, vomiting, periodic breathing, and respiratory arrest particularly during sleep. An extensive brain stem infarct can result in the 'locked-in' syndrome in which, despite being conscious, the patient is unable to move anything except perhaps the eyelids or the eyes in the vertical plane, and can neither speak nor swallow. It is important to remember that thrombo-embolism within the vertebro-basilar arterial system may cause not only brain stem infarction but also occipital infarction, with a homonymous hemianopia or even cortical blindness, due to ischaemia in the posterior cerebral arterial supply.

Cortical venous and/or dural sinus thrombosis

Thrombosis of the cortical veins or dural sinuses is a much less common cause of cerebral infarction than arterial disease and occurs as a result of local conditions affecting the cortical veins or dural sinus, or of systemic disorders (Table 7). Venous infarcts are commonly haemorrhagic. The clinical picture can be similar to cerebral hemisphere infarction caused by arterial occlusion but epilepsy and impaired consciousness are more common and raised intracranial pressure develops rapidly if the dural sinuses become obstructed. Cortical venous and sinus thrombosis may propagate widely to produce a catastrophic 'encephalopathic' illness with very similar features to severe viral encephalitis. Isolated sagittal or transverse dural sinus thrombosis is one cause of 'benign intracranial hypertension'. Thrombosis of the cavernous sinus is rare but is usually due to pyogenic infection spreading from the face, sinuses, or nasal space. The symptoms include orbital pain and swelling with the development of visual loss and papilloedema, and often palsies of the third, fourth, fifth, and sixth cranial nerves.

Table 7 Causes of cortical venous and/or dural sinus thrombosis

Local conditions affecting the veins and sinuses directly
  Head injury
  Intracranial surgery
  Local sepsis (sinuses, ears, scalp, nasopharynx)
  Neurosyphilis
  Bacterial meningitis
  Tumour invasion of dural sinuses
  Catheterization of jugular veins for parenteral nutrition etc.
Systemic disorders
  Dehydration
  Septicaemia
  Pregnancy and the puerperium
  Contraceptive pill effects
  Haematological disorders (Table 3)
  Hyperviscosity syndromes (Table 3)
  Inflammatory arterial disease (Table 2)
  Diabetes mellitus
  Congestive cardiac failure
  Inflammatory bowel disease
  Androgen therapy
  Non-metastatic effect of extracranial malignancy

Boundary zone or 'watershed' infarction

A profound but transient fall in systemic blood pressure usually causes syncope, faintness, vertigo, or generalized weakness, and if it continues for some minutes, an epileptic seizure can occur. More prolonged hypotension of the sort that occurs after cardiac arrest, massive blood loss, or the overenthusiastic use of hypotensive drugs can cause massive cerebral infarction leading to a persistent vegetative state or death, or sometimes infarction between arterial territories, particularly in the parieto-occipital region which is the boundary zone between the middle, anterior, and posterior cerebral arteries. Boundary zone infarction in this area is commonly bilateral and the symptoms include cortical blindness or visual disorientation, associated with a visual field defect and often memory impairment.

Cerebral infarction and migraine

Occasionally cerebral infarction and a persistent neurological deficit occur during a migranious episode. This is possibly due to arterial narrowing caused by oedema of the vessel wall rather than 'vasospasm'. Such an event probably only occurs in patients with classical migraine and the neurological deficit has a similar clinical pattern to the transient neurological symptoms during the previously experienced migrainous auras.

Stroke and pregnancy

Stroke occurs most often in the last trimester of pregnancy or in the puerperium. However, this is very rare; about 5 cases/10 000 deliveries in the United Kingdom. It is usually due to arterial rather than venous thrombosis. The middle cerebral artery is the most frequently occluded vessel, but the cause is unknown since there appears to be no underlying arterial disease. Some cases might be due to paradoxical embolism from thrombosis in the venous system of the legs or pelvis.

Moya Moya syndrome

This is not a disease but a characteristic angiographic appearance of bilateral occlusion or stenosis of the distal internal carotid arteries, often with involvement of the circle of Willis, and the development of net-like collaterals at the base of the brain. Usually no cause can be found, although a congenital vascular anomaly has been suggested as also have infections at the base of the brain. The syndrome was first described in the Japanese but is not entirely confined to this race.

Differential diagnosis of cerebral infarction

The clinical picture of stroke, either due to cerebral infarction or indeed to primary intracerebral haemorrhage, is characteristic and the diagnosis depends not so much on where the lesion is thought to be, but on the sudden or subacute onset in a previously well patient with no history of head injury. It is important to consider the possibility of a chronic subdural haematoma (page 21.184), or drug overdose, in an unconscious patient with few or no focal signs, and without a good history of a sudden onset. Encephalitis, cerebral abscess, sudden deterioration in a patient with a cerebral tumour, multiple sclerosis, peripheral nerve lesion, hypoglycaemia, and hysteria can usually be excluded after an adequate history, clinical examination, and straightforward investigations. In acute stroke, like in other severe acute illnesses, there is often transient hyperglycaemia, glycosuria, and a neutrophil leucocytosis. Sometimes there are ischaemic changes (but not the classical development of Q waves) and arrhythmias on the electrocardiogram making it difficult to know if cerebral infarction has occurred as a result of embolism from left ventricular mural thrombus overlying an acute myocardial infarct. In any stroke patient it is important to remember that there are rare but often treatable underlying causes (Tables 1, 2, and 3) although usually the cause is athero-thrombo-embolism or hypertension.

Complications

The most important local complication of cerebral infarction is the development of cerebral oedema which will impair, possibly only

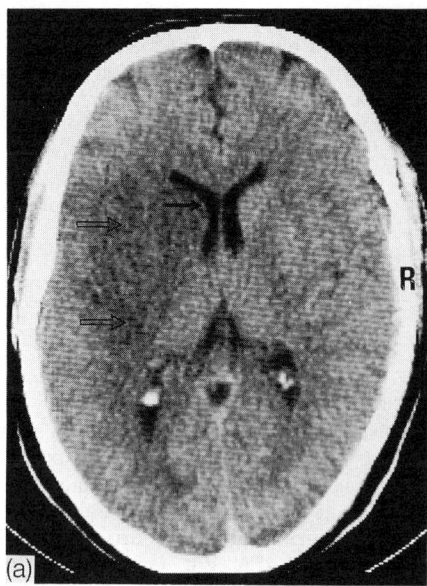 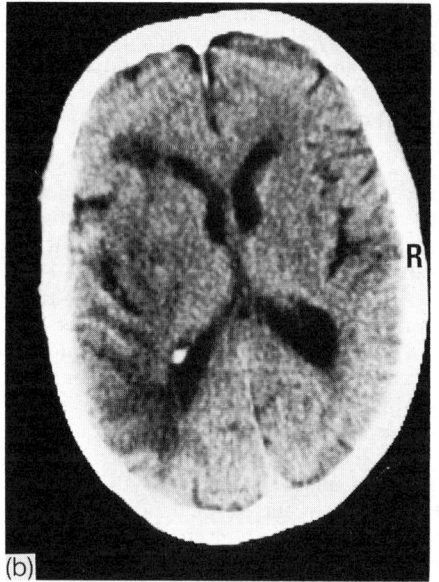

Fig. 12 CT scan of cerebral infarction due to left middle cerebral artery occlusion. (a) The scan has been taken at 24 hours poststroke and shows a vague low density throughout most of the left cerebral hemisphere (open arrows) with possible compression of the anterior horn of the left lateral ventricle (closed arrow). (b) Three weeks poststroke, the low-density area of infarction is sharply defined and the ventricles slightly dilated.

temporarily, local blood flow and neuronal function over a wider area than just the infarct and, if extensive, cause transtentorial herniation. There are a number of general complications of acute paralysis which include bronchopneumonia, particularly if consciousness or swallowing mechanisms are impaired; venous thrombo-embolism; pressure sores and septicaemia; urinary infection, particularly if catheterization is necessary, and eventually uraemia; contractures in spastic limbs; frozen shoulder; cardiac rhythm disturbances; and depression (Table 8). Death in the first week is almost always due to the infarct itself and the effects of cerebral oedema but later is more often due to one of the above general complications, particularly pneumonia.

Table 8 General complications of stroke

Respiratory:	Pneumonia
	Inhalation
	Pulmonary embolism
Cardiovascular:	Myocardial infarction
	Cardiac failure
	Cardiac arrhythmia
	Neurogenic pulmonary oedema
Infections:	Pneumonia
	Urinary
	Skin
	Septicaemia
Metabolic:	Dehydration
	Electrolyte imbalance
	Hyperglycaemia
	Renal failure
'Mechanical':	Spasticity
	Contractures
	Subluxation of the shoulder
	'Frozen' shoulder
	Falls and fractures
Others:	Depression, anxiety, apathy
	Epilepsy
	Pressure sores
	Deep venous thrombosis
	Dependent oedema
	Acute peptic ulceration
	Incontinence of urine/faeces
	Pressure palsies of peripheral nerves
	Unemployment
	Financial loss

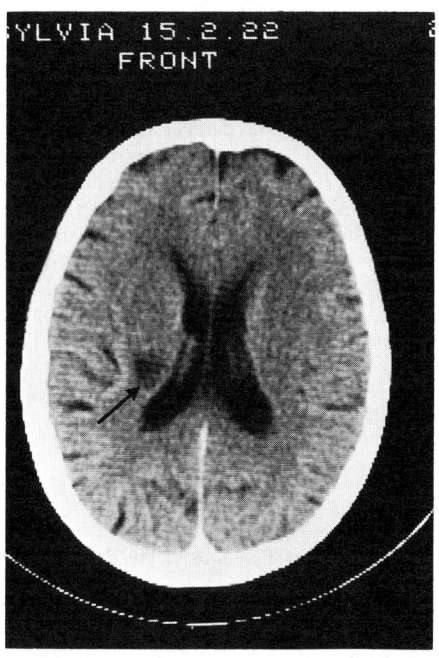

Fig. 13 CT scan of a lacunar infarct in the region of the posterior limb of the left internal capsule (arrow). This scan was done three days after the onset of stroke. If it had been done four weeks after the stroke the appearances would have been consistent with *either* an old haemorrhage, *or* an old infarct.

Investigations

These are the same as in TIA patients but should be tempered by the age of the patient, the likelihood of recovery, and the chance that they will influence the patients' immediate and long-term management. Computerized tomographic scanning, angiography, and the examination of the CSF merit special discussion.

The most reliable way in which primary intracerebral haemorrhage can be differentiated from cerebral infarction is by an unenhanced CT scan within two or three weeks of the onset, since the clinical picture and the absence of blood in the CSF can be most misleading. Small haemorrhages or infarcts, particularly in the

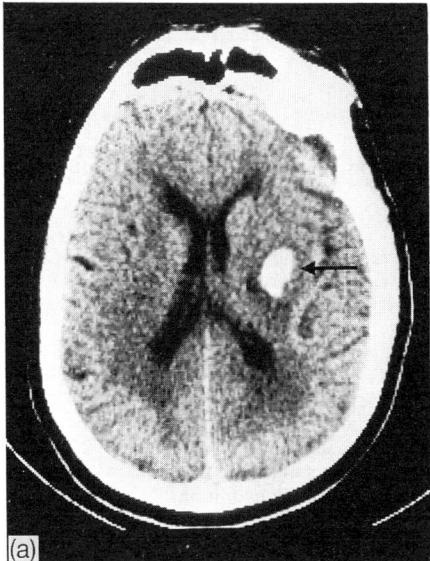 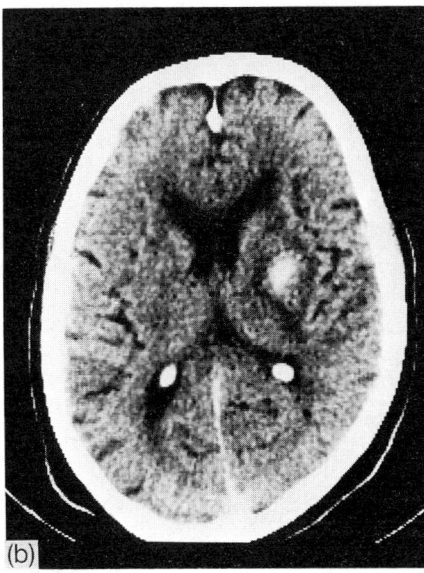 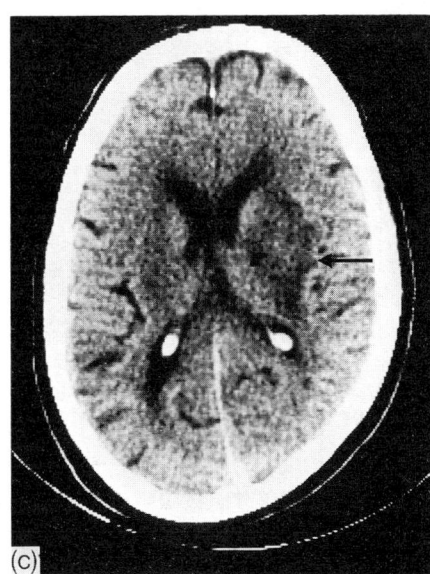

Fig. 14 CT scan of intracerebral haemorrhage. (a) Four days poststroke. The haematoma is clearly shown as a high-density area in the right basal ganglia region (arrow). (b) Twelve days poststroke. The high-density area is less obvious. (c) Eighteen days poststroke. The high-density area has been replaced by a low-density area (arrow) which, without knowledge of the previous scan, might easily be mistaken for infarction.

posterior fossa, can be missed by CT scanning. The characteristic low-density appearance of infarction usually takes a day or two to appear (Figs. 12 and 13) while the high density of an intracerebral haematoma appears at once although after it has resolved (in a matter of a few weeks and possibly only two weeks if the haematoma is small) the scan may become normal or show only a low-density area very similar to that appearing after cerebral infarction (Fig. 14). If the haemorrhage versus infarct distinction is academic, which it almost always is unless surgical intervention or antithrombotic and thus inevitably antihaemostatic drugs are being or are going to be used, then a CT scan is not strictly necessary unless there is a reasonable possibility of an intracranial lesion other than stroke. Examination of the CSF is not an adequate way to exclude primary intracerebral haemorrhage since blood often does not escape into the CSF. Furthermore, lumbar puncture can be dangerous if the cerebral infarct is behaving like a space occupying lesion, or if the diagnosis is incorrect and a space occupying lesion is actually present. The CSF may, however, need to be examined if there is a possibility of encephalitis, neurosyphilis, or multiple sclerosis. Ideally stroke patients should never be anticoagulated nor even exposed to antiplatelet drugs unless a CT scan has been done to exclude primary intracerebral haemorrhage or haemorrhagic infarction as far as it is possible to do so. An isotope brain scan can be useful in the diagnosis of subdural haematoma

Table 9 Indications for CT scan in acute stroke

1 Uncertain diagnosis with the possibility of non-stroke intracranial pathology, particularly cerebral tumour or subdural haematoma. This situation usually only arises if there is uncertainty over the details of the onset and time course of the neurological deficit
2 The patient is taking or may need antihaemostatic drugs (anticoagulants, antiplatelet drugs). To distinguish reliably between primary intracerebral haemorrhage and cerebral infarction, the scan should be done as soon as possible, preferably within one or two weeks of the onset. A normal scan or hypodense lesion more than four weeks poststroke does not exclude a haemorrhagic origin
3 Cerebellar stroke
4 Subarachnoid haemorrhage
5 Uncharacteristic deterioration after the first 24 hours making non-stroke intracranial pathology rather more likely
6 Mild stroke possibly suitable for carotid endarterectomy
7 Young patient

but has largely been superseded by CT scanning. Indications for CT scanning are summarized in Table 9.

Cerebral angiography is not usually indicated during the acute phase of cerebral infarction since the result is unlikely to influence the immediate management, and the procedure itself can make the patient worse. In a young patient there is an argument for urgent angiography if there is a possibility of a congenital arterial anomaly, neck trauma, angioma, or perhaps an aneurysm but usually it is best left until recovery is well under way. Early angiography can be useful to confirm the diagnosis of dural sinus thrombosis. There are no reliable angiographic criteria for distinguishing between arterial embolism and thrombosis and even at necropsy there can still be considerable uncertainty. If there is complete recovery or only minimal residual disability after a cerebral infarct, then the indications for carotid angiography and possible endarterectomy are the same as in TIA patients (see page 21.159).

Prognosis and treatment
Recovery to some extent is the rule after cerebral infarction unless the infarct and cerebral oedema are severe enough to cause death within a few days. Sudden death, (i.e. within one hour of the onset of symptoms), is very rarely due to cerebral infarction or any other form of cerebrovascular disease except for spontaneous subarachnoid haemorrhage. Most of any recovery occurs in the first three months but may not be absolutely complete for something like one or two years. The immediate prognosis is particularly poor if there is hemiplegia, unconsciousness, or sustained lateral deviation of gaze. Case fatality is about 20 per cent at one month for stroke in general but is much higher as a result of primary intracerebral haemorrhage than of cerebral infarction (Fig. 15). Of the survivors from stroke about a half recover completely or more or less completely, while the rest are disabled to some degree. The long-term death rate is about 5–10 per cent per annum, these late deaths being mostly due to recurrent stroke or myocardial infarction (Fig. 16). The risk of recurrent stroke is no more than 10 per cent per annum.

There is probably little that medical treatment and nothing that vascular surgery can do to alter the immediate outcome after cerebral infarction. In theory the reduction of cerebral oedema, if it is actually present, by the use of mannitol, glycerol, or dexamethazone should be useful. Unfortunately there have been no adequate clinical trials of these treatments. Dextran, vasodilators,

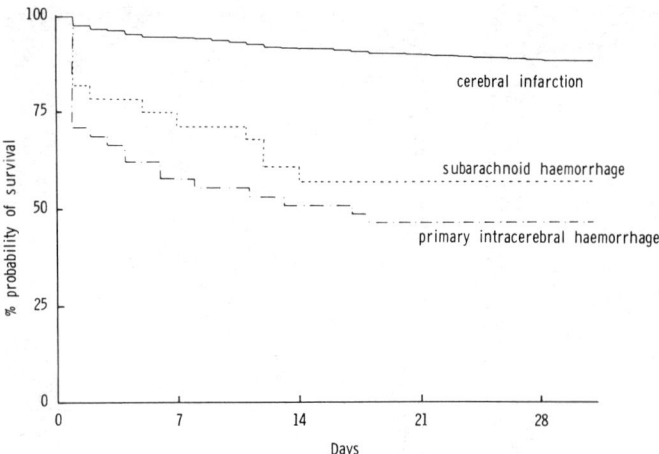

Fig. 15 Probability of survival in the first month after first ever stroke by pathological subtype in 515 consecutive patients in the Oxfordshire Community Stroke Project, 1981–84.

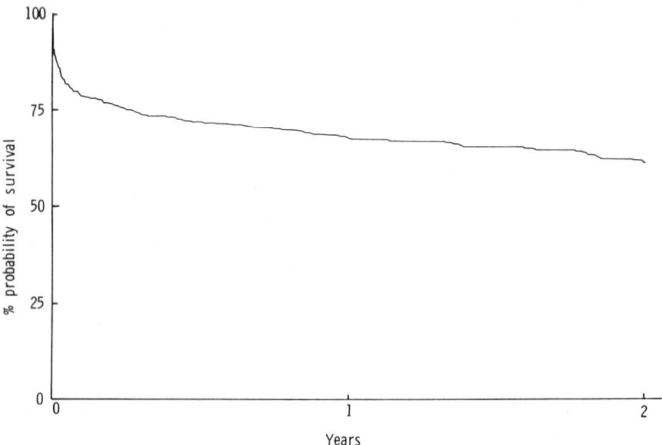

Fig. 16 Probability of survival over two years in the 515 first ever stroke patients in the Oxfordshire Community Stroke Project, 1981–84.

Table 10 Causes of neurological deterioration after stroke

Local:	Extension of thrombus
	Recurrent embolism
	Recurrent haemorrhage
	Haemorrhagic infarction
	Cerebral oedema
	Brain shift and herniation
	Hydrocephalus
	Epilepsy
General:	Hypoxia (pneumonia, pulmonary embolism, inhalation, cardiac failure)
	Infection (chest, urine, septicaemia)
	Cardiac failure (myocardial infarction, arrhythmia, neurogenic pulmonary oedema)
	Pulmonary embolism
	Dehydration, hyponatraemia
	Hyper, or hypoglycaemia
	Hypotension (cardiac failure, septicaemia, pulmonary embolism, dehydration, pneumonia, drugs, bleeding or perforated peptic ulcer)

hypercapnia, hypocapnia, hyperbaric oxygen, and stellate ganglion block seem to have no very useful effect, and although barbiturate anaesthesia has been suggested there are no clinical trials to support such an impractical treatment. Fibrinolytic drugs and anticoagulation increase the risk of intracranial bleeding and should not be used. Heparin has been recommended for 'stroke-in-evolution' although there have been no convincing trials and, since some cases may be due to haemorrhage into infarcted brain or even to primary intracerebral haemorrhage from the beginning, this treatment is not normally to be recommended. It is important to remember that there are several reasons for stroke patients to deteriorate, and some are potentially reversible (Table 10). Haemodilution, usually by venesection and volume replacement by dextran, to reduce whole blood viscosity and increase blood flow and oxygen delivery to ischaemic brain has been suggested and clinical trials are in progress.

If there is a definite major cardiac source of embolism the patient should probably be anticoagulated in an attempt to restrict thrombogenesis and further embolization provided of course that there is no CT scan evidence of intracranial haemorrhage (see discussion of this issue in TIA patients on page 21.160). Anticoagulants are contraindicated in bacterial endocarditis because of the very real risk of haemorrhage from mycotic aneurysms which form when the arterial wall is weakened by bacterial infection spreading from an infected embolus. Anticoagulation in acute embolic stroke always carries some risk because of the possibility of haem-

orrhage into infarcted brain so there is a dilemma between anticoagulating too early and causing cerebral haemorrhage and too late after further embolization has occurred. It is probably advisable to use an oral anticoagulant and achieve full anticoagulation (a prothrombin time two to three times the control value) over a matter of a few days.

Cerebral infarction often causes transient hypertension which settles without treatment. However, if there is evidence of long-standing hypertension such as left ventricular hypertrophy or characteristic changes in the retina, then the blood pressure should probably be gently lowered so that the phase V diastolic pressure is below 110 mmHg. Any such reduction must be done slowly over a matter of days, and with extreme caution because not only is there loss of normal cerebral autoregulation in and around infarcts, but in chronic hypertension autoregulation is 'set' higher so that rapid and extreme reduction of blood pressure can lead to a catastrophic fall in cerebral blood flow and more extensive cerebral infarction. Surprisingly, no trials of the speed and extent to which hypertension should be controlled have yet been done.

Naturally, if a reversible underlying cause for cerebral infarction can be found the appropriate treatment should be used; for example, corticosteroids for giant cell arteritis, antibiotics for bacterial endocarditis etc. Analgesics, tranquillizers, anti-emetics, laxatives, and antispastic drugs all have their place in the relief of the appropriate symptoms.

The complications of cerebral infarction are often preventable and treatable (Table 8). Chest physiotherapy and care of the airway, particularly in unconscious patients and those with difficulty swallowing, will reduce the risk of pneumonia which, if it occurs, can be treated with antibiotics Occasionally, intubation and tracheostomy are needed in patients who cannot protect their airways due to impaired brain stem reflexes, but who are otherwise expected to have a reasonably good prognosis. Nasogastric tube feeding must be used for adequate hydration and electrolyte balance in patients who cannot swallow, and later for feeding if necessary. Good nursing should prevent pressure sores. Early physiotherapy will reduce the risk of contractures, pain, and stiffness in hemiplegic limbs and leads on naturally into active physical rehabilitation. Urinary catheterization is often avoidable in males for whom an appliance is a better alternative, but in females it may be necessary so that the skin can be kept dry to reduce the chance of pressure sores. Cardiac arrhythmias should be treated on their merits but are not normally a problem. Since cerebral infarcts can become haemorrhagic, it is uncertain whether deep venous thrombosis in the legs and pulmonary emoblism can be prevented or even treated satisfactorily with drugs but the benefit of high-dose heparin followed by oral anticoagulation for major pulmonary embolism probably outweighs its risks. Epilepsy, if it occurs, should be treated in the normal way.

Vigorous rehabilitation is essential from as early in the illness as is reasonable and may include physiotherapy, occupational therapy, and probably speech therapy if there is dysphasia. Stroke clubs, day centre care, health visitors, district nurses, and help from enthusiastic volunteers all have their place. In some patients there may be a need for specific retraining for work and also advice concerning sexual activity which can normally be resumed without any particular danger. For secondary prevention risk factors for vascular disease should be minimized in a similar way as in TIA patients (page 21.160). There is little doubt that the adequate treatment of hypertension after stroke will reduce the risk of recurrence and fears that any such treatment will, by causing low pressure, lead to cerebral infarction are unfounded provided drugs are used carefully and overt postural hypotension avoided.

In the United Kingdom about 50 per cent of stroke patients are treated at home by their general practitioners and it is uncertain whether hospital treatment in a non-specialist unit confers any particular benefit unless the domestic circumstances are such that home nursing is impossible. However, units specifically designed for the acute care and subsequent rehabilitation of stroke patients may reduce both case fatality and morbidity and would undoubtedly increase the understanding of stroke and make the running of adequate clinical trials to assess potential treatments easier than it is now. It is astonishing how many treatments have been suggested for cerebral infarction and yet how few adequate trials have been undertaken. Any hospital-based stroke service should extend into the community and include an early diagnostic component with appropriate neuroradiological backup, and a nursing and rehabilitation component. With good organization it should be possible to manage more stroke patients at home provided there is adequate support from the family and good domiciliary nursing.

Multi-infarct dementia

Multi-infarct dementia is defined as a deterioration in mental function due to cerebrovascular disease. It is a much less common cause of dementia than Alzheimer's disease. The main distinction between the two conditions is that in multi-infarct dementia the progression tends to be in a series of more or less sudden 'steps' since it is due to repeated episodes of ischaemia, infarction, or possibly even haemorrhage, some of which may cause overt strokes. It is more likely to be the cause of dementia than Alzheimer's disease if there is hypertension, focal neurological symptoms or signs, focal or lateralizing features on the electroencephalogram, vascular bruits, and reduced regional cerebral blood flow. It is, however, impossible to delineate these two main causes of dementia precisely during life and it could be argued that, since there is no specific treatment for either, there is no particular advantage in distinguishing one from the other in routine clinical practice.

Some believe that *Binswanger's disease* is a distinct nosological entity causing slowly progressive dementia in late middle age, punctuated by TIA and stroke-like episodes. The patients are usually hypertensive and there is patchy or diffuse loss of cerebral white matter which is shown as low attenuation on CT scan. The underlying pathology may be the same as hypertensive vascular disease.

Cerebrovascular disease seldom causes a well-defined *Parkinsonian syndrome* but, when widespread, is one of the common causes of *pseudo-bulbar palsy*. In this condition there are bilateral lesions in the cortico-bulbar pathways causing dysfunction of the lower cranial nerves with dysarthria, dysphagia, and slow tongue movements. In addition there are bilateral cortico-spinal tract signs in the arms and legs and the patient often has a characteristic gait with rapid short steps, so-called *marche a petits pas*. There is commonly emotional lability and dementia in addition.

Spontaneous intracranial haemorrhage

About 20 per cent of strokes are due to intracranial haemorrhage which usually occurs as a result of rupture of an intracranial aneurysm, an arteriovenous malformation (AVM), or hypertensive vascular disease. Rare causes include thrombocytopaenia, leukaemia, hypocoaguability as a result of disease such as haemophilia or anticoagulation, sickle cell disease, cortical venous thrombosis, thrombotic thrombocytopenic purpura, mycotic aneurysms, intracranial vasculitis, congophilic angiography, and richly vascularized tumours. The site of bleeding may be destroyed as a result of the haemorrhage which is usually into the subarachnoid space from intracranial aneurysm and AVM and directly into the brain (primary intracerebral haemorrhage) from hypertensive vascular disease. There can be blood in both sites after intracranial haemorrhage from any cause.

Primary intracerebral haemorrhage

Not every patient with primary intracerebral haemorrhage has hypertension and hypertensive vascular disease affecting the small arteries perforating the brain substance; sometimes the rupture of very small AVMs or other rare disorders may be responsible. However, Charcot–Bouchard aneurysms do tend to occur where haemorrhage is common (the basal ganglia, thalamus, cerebellar hemispheres, pons, and subcortical areas) and their rupture is thought to explain the majority. Haemorrhage in the cerebral hemispheres outside the basal ganglia region (so-called lobar haemorrhage) is less likely to be due to hypertensive vascular disease than to one of the other causes mentioned above. A haematoma may cause transtentorial herniation in the same way as cerebral infarction.

Clinical features

Clinically, it is difficult if not impossible to distinguish reliably between primary intracerebral haemorrhage and cerebral infarction unless a substantial amount of blood has entered the CSF, via the ventricles and/or the surface of the brain, in which case meningism usually develops. Headache and coma occur in both cerebral haemorrhage and infarction and are not very reliable differentiating features. However, *severe* headache and coma within a few hours is very unusual in cerebral infarction, while TIA are very rare preceding intracerebral haemorrhage. The symptoms, signs, investigations, differential diagnosis, and general management of both infarction and haemorrhage are similar but with some important exceptions which need to be discussed separately.

Cerebellar haematoma

This condition, although rare, is important since surgical treatment can be life-saving and survivors may have remarkably little neurological disability. The patient usually presents with occipital headache, 'dizziness', truncal ataxia, rapid reduction in consciousness, a gaze palsy to the side of the lesion, ipsilateral facial weakness, and often raised intracranial pressure due to acute obstruction of CSF flow. Cerebellar signs cannot normally be elicited unless the patient is conscious. Any hemiparesis is mild although bilateral extensor plantars are common. Sensory signs are also unusual. The diagnosis is confirmed by CT scan (Fig. 17).

Angiography

Cerebral angiography is unnecessary if a haematoma has been demonstrated by CT scanning and the patient is extremely ill or very seriously disabled. However, if the patient has recovered useful function, is normotensive, and not particularly elderly or com-

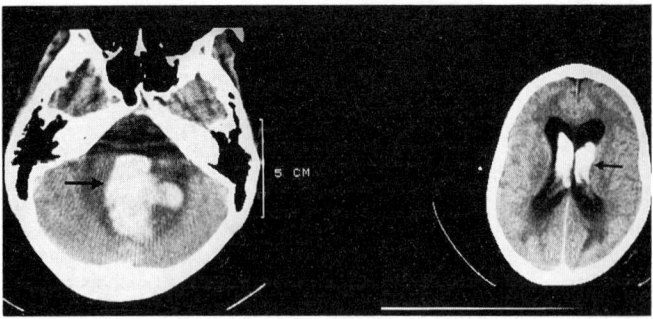

Fig. 17 Cerebellar haematoma. On the left the CT scan through the posterior fossa shows the haemorrhage as a large white area (arrow) more on the right than on the left. On the right, the CT scan is through the lateral ventricles to show their enlargement due to obstruction of CSF flow from the ventricular system by the haematoma in the cerebellum, and blood has spread from the haematoma through the ventricular system into the lateral ventricles (arrow).

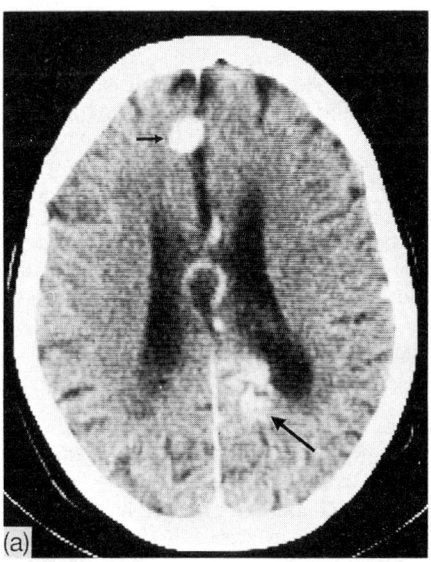

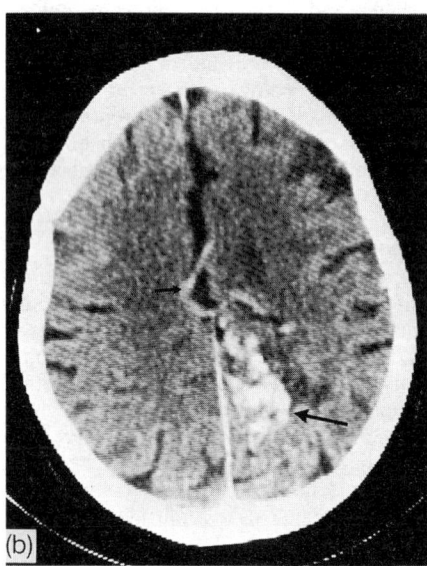

Fig. 18 (a, b) CT scans after intravenous contrast injection to show the typical appearance of a large intracerebral arteriovenous malformation. The abnormal vasculature in the right occipital lobe is enhanced (large arrow) and a large draining vein can be seen (small arrow).

promised by some other disease, angiography may reveal a cause for the haemorrhage which is potentially surgically treatable; for example, an AVM, or an aneurysm which has bled directly into the brain substance rather than into the subarachnoid space. Both these lesions, if large, may be suspected on CT scanning if contrast material is used to reveal the abnormal vascularity (Fig. 18). An AVM may cause a cranial bruit which is usually best heard by auscultation over the orbits and often there is a past history of epilepsy.

Medical treatment

Naturally, anticoagulants are contraindicated. It is not certain whether aspirin also increases the risk of cerebral haemorrhage but, since it undoubtedly leads to a haemostatic defect, it is probably best avoided. If a patient's course is complicated by pulmonary embolism, the possible benefits of anticoagulation may be not much more than the risks. The medical treatment and rehabilitation is otherwise the same as for patients with cerebral infarction. If a patient survives, the recovery and long-term prognosis are often remarkably good.

Surgical treatment

The evacuation of a haematoma, particularly if it is superficial, is a tempting surgical possibility but whether this increases the chance of recovery is uncertain. Some surgeons operate on haematomas acutely but there have been no clinical trials to support such a policy. A more widely accepted indication is in the patient whose conscious level is deteriorating, usually because of brain shift and transtentorial herniation. Surgery will not improve the situation in a deeply unconscious patient nor in one who is improving and has only a mild neurological deficit. Surgical evacuation and/or ventricular drainage is the treatment for cerebellar haemorrhage unless spontaneous recovery is already occurring.

Spontaneous subarachnoid haemorrhage

The majority of patients with this condition have ruptured an intracranial berry aneurysm; about 5 per cent have bled from an AVM, and a few have rare causes of intracranial haemorrhage as described earlier. In about 15 per cent of patients no cause can be identified and in this group the prognosis is particularly good.

The clinical picture is distinctive and not easily confused with that of stroke due to cerebral infarction or primary intracerebral haemorrhage. The onset is very sudden with headache, usually but not always severe, which is often occipital and radiates over the head and down the neck, sometimes down as far as the back or legs as blood tracks down the spinal canal. Consciousness is often impaired or lost transiently at the onset and if the haemorrhage is extensive the patient remains comatose. Vomiting is quite common and occasionally epilepsy is an early feature. Meningism develops, but sometimes not for several hours, and there are not usually signs of focal neurological damage unless bleeding has also occurred into the brain substance, or unless there is an oculomotor palsy due to the presence of a posterior communicating artery or distal internal carotid artery aneurysm. The patient is very often irritable, confused, and drowsy for several days, and headache may persist for weeks. AVMs may occasionally be diagnosed clinically if there is a cranial bruit, or a carotid bruit due to the greatly increased blood flow secondary to a large lesion. A rapid rise in the intracranial pressure at the onset of subarachnoid haemorrhage is the probable cause of the subhyaloid haemorrhages which are often observed in the fundus.

The diagnosis can now usually be most easily confirmed by CT scanning which shows blood in the CSF pathways (Fig. 19) and often a collection of blood in relation to the aneurysm or AVM; the latter will be more easily visualized after intravenous injection of iodinated contrast material provided it is fairly large (Fig. 18). If a CT scan is not easily available or is normal, then lumbar puncture is mandatory and the CSF will be blood stained. If the

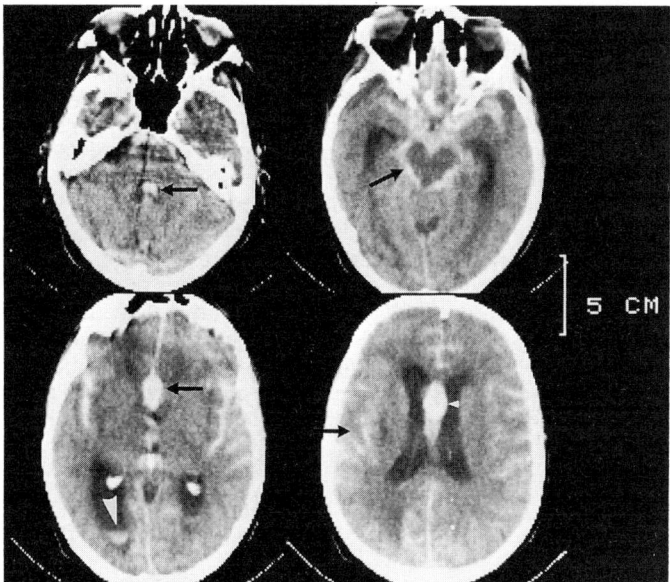

Fig. 19 CT scan 24 hours after subarachnoid haemorrhage. Top left panel shows blood in the fourth ventricle (arrow); top right panel shows blood (high density) outlining the brain stem (arrow); bottom left panel shows blood around the ruptured anterior communicating artery aneurysm (black arrow) and in the occipital horn of the left lateral ventricle (white arrow); bottom right panel shows blood tracking back from the ruptured aneurysm into the septum pellucidum (white arrow). There is also blood in the cortical sulci (black arrow).

haemorrhage is more than a day or two old, the CSF is xanthochromic due to altered blood pigment. Clearly, if there is any clinical difficulty distinguishing between subarachnoid haemorrhage and acute meningitis, then the CSF should be examined at once.

The complications of subarachnoid haemorrhage are similar to those of cerebral infarction and primary intracerebral haemorrhage. In addition organized blood clot in the subarachnoid space may cause obstruction to CSF flow and acute hydrocephalus. This is common and often asymptomatic, but may lead to a deterioration in the patient's conscious level a few days or weeks after the onset of the haemorrhage when progress has otherwise been satisfactory. This complication can be easily diagnosed by CT scanning and then treated with a ventricular drainage procedure. Occasionally the disturbance of CSF flow may not present until some years after the subarachnoid haemorrhage and the clinical picture is then of 'normal' pressure hydrocephalus. Vasospasm is discussed below.

Intracranial aneurysms

These develop on the medium-sized arteries at the base of the brain and the common sites are at the distal internal carotid and posterior communicating artery origin (25 per cent), the anterior communicating artery complex (30 per cent), and at the bifurcation of the middle cerebral artery (25 per cent). The basilar artery is a less common site (5 per cent). About 15 per cent of cases have multiple aneurysms. The aneurysms vary from a few millimetres to several centimetres in diameter. Some aneurysms may be congenital but others develop in adult life, probably as a result of arteriosclerosis and hypertension. Their rupture may be caused by sudden increases in blood pressure during strenuous exercise, lifting, defaecation, and coitus. Many aneurysms remain asymptomatic and are found in 1–4 per cent of routine necropsies. A few grow to a large size and present as a space-occupying lesion.

Arterio-venous malformations (AVMs)

AVMs are congenital vascular anomalies which vary greatly in size from a few millimetres to several centimetres in diameter. They consist of a convoluted mass of blood vessels which are fed by

large arteries and drained by increasingly large veins as time goes by. They result in an arterio-venous shunt. They may present with epilepsy, subarachnoid haemorrhage, primary intracerebral haemorrhage, and rarely as a space-occupying lesion or headache. In infants they may very occasionally cause high output cardiac failure. Early death (about 10 per cent) and risk of rebleeding is much less common than after rupture of an intracranial aneurysm but neurological damage is usually more extensive. However, even after several recurrent haemorrhages, patients may survive for many years with remarkably little disability.

There are other less common vascular anomalies which involve the brain and which may occasionally bleed. Telangiectases, or capillary angiomas, are made up of groups of dilated capillaries. They may be associated with the Osler–Rendu–Weber syndrome (see Section 19) and may occasionally rupture although this is very unusual. *Cavernous haemangiomas* form lobulated masses, usually above the tentorium, which consist of small and large blood-filled spaces. They may be associated with similar lesions elsewhere in the body. *Haemangioblastomas* are true tumours of angioblastic origin. They consist of vascular channels and spaces and tend to form cysts. They are usually found subtentorially, often in the cerebellum, medulla or even the spinal cord. They are often associated with anomalies elsewhere in the body. For example, there may be an associated haemangioblastoma of the retina (*von Hippel's disease*). Similar lesions may occur in the spinal cord and there may be associated cysts of the pancreas and kidneys, hypernephromas or tumours of the suprarenal glands. The association of these lesions is known as *Lindau's disease* and is familial in approximately 25 per cent of cases. Bleeding is unusual although polycythaemia may occur. Finally, in the *Sturge–Weber syndrome* there may be extensive capillary–venous malformations affecting one hemisphere, particularly the parieto-occipital region associated with a characteristic wavy pattern of subcortical calcification. There is usually an associated 'port-wine' stain on the face on the affected side and there may be associated buphthalmos with contralateral hemiparesis and epilepsy.

Management

About 25 per cent of patients die within 24 hours of aneurysmal subarachnoid haemorrhage and cannot be treated. About another 25 per cent die in the first month (this is usually due to recurrent haemorrhage or infarction as a consequence of vasospasm) and 50 per cent survive for longer but still with a risk of rebleeding (about 2 per cent per annum) (Fig. 20). The first week is the time of maximum

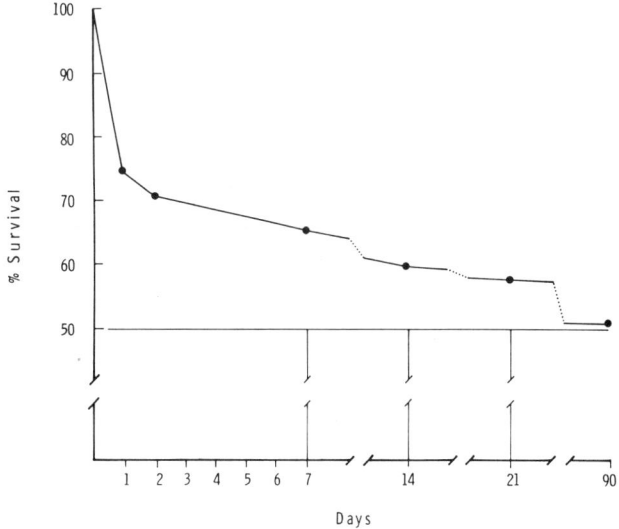

Fig. 20 Probability of survival after subarachnoid haemorrhage during the first three months in 146 patients. (Reproduced from Fogelholm, 1981, *Stroke* **12**, 296–301, by permission of Dr Fogelholm and the publishers of *Stroke*.)

risk of rebleeding so, if possible, neurosurgical intervention should be as soon as possible after the first bleed to reduce this risk. However, the risk of surgery is unacceptably high if the patient is unconscious or has a severe neurological deficit. If the patient is conscious with little or no deficit, then four-vessel angiography should be undertaken to delineate the site of the aneurysm and surgery carried out soon afterwards. The rationale of surgery is to clip the aneurysm if it is accessible, but if it is not, then carotid ligation in the neck will reduce the risk of early rebleeding in the case of aneurysms in the region of the termination of the ICA. Angiography in very sick patients is, therefore, unnecessary unless CT scanning is unavailable to show any intracerebral haematoma which might usefully be evacuated. Vasospasm and secondary cerebral infarction may occur in relation to, and even at a distance from, the aneurysm-bearing artery and is one explanation for the high risks of surgery in ill patients. The cause of vasospasm is unknown but is probably to do with some constituent of the blood entering the subarachnoid space.

If an AVM has bled and is surgically accessible it should probably be removed. Ligation of the feeding vessels has little or nothing to offer since the AVM will be revascularized by vessels too small to be seen on the preoperative angiogram. Embolization and radiotherapy have been suggested but, like even surgical removal, there have been no adequate clinical trials.

From the medical point of view cautious control of severe hypertension is wise and occasionally cardiac rhythm disturbances or even acute neurogenic pulmonary oedema require appropriate treatment. Naturally, analgesia for the headache and sedation if the patient is very irritable are useful. Antifibrinolytic drugs such as epsilonaminocaproic acid or tranexamic acid reduce the risk of rebleeding by reducing the lysis of the fibrin clot plugging the ruptured aneurysm but do not improve the overall prognosis, probably because the risk of vasospasm is increased. Bedrest for four to six weeks is usually recommended but there is an increasing tendency gently to mobilize patients when the headache has resolved.

The prevention of stroke

Since the medical and surgical treatment of stroke is usually so unrewarding, it is sensible to concentrate considerable effort on stroke prevention. There are two ways in which this may be achieved: primary prevention in asymptomatic individuals, and secondary prevention in patients who have already experienced a TIA or stroke. Primary prevention must at the moment depend largely on the detection and adequate treatment of hypertension and perhaps also on the reduction of cigarette smoking. Manipulation of diet on a large-scale population basis is likely to be exceptionally difficult to achieve, and if the effect in the prevention of MI is uncertain, any effect in the primary prevention of cerebral infarction where hyperlipidaemia is a less obvious risk factor will be even more controversial. The use of antithrombotic drugs such as aspirin in asymptomatic individuals has been suggested and clinical trials, notably among many thousand British and American doctors, are under way. The secondary prevention of ischaemic stroke has already been dealt with under the management of TIA.

Asymptomatic cervical bruits are fairly common in the elderly and do not require specific treatment. They are a marker for ischaemic heart disease as well as for cerebrovascular disease and, as such, point to the need to control vascular risk factors in such patients.

References

Harrison, M. J. G. and Dyken, M. L. (1983). *Cerebral vascular disease.* Butterworths, London.
Kapp, J. P. and Schmidek, H. H. (1984). *The cerebral venous system and its disorders.* Grune and Stratton, Orlando.
Marquardsen, J. (1969). *The natural history of acute cerebrovascular disease.* Munksgaard, Copenhagen.
Ross Russell, R. W. (1983). *Vascular disease of the central nervous system.* Churchill Livingstone, Edinburgh.
Wade, D. T., Langton Hewer, R., Skilbeck, C. E. and David, R. M. (1985). *Stroke, a critical approach to diagnosis, treatment, and management.* Chapman and Hall, London.
Warlow, C. P. and Morris, P. J. (1982). *Transient ischaemic attacks.* Marcel Dekker, New York.
—— (1984). Carotid endarterectomy: does it work? *Stroke* **15**, 1068–1076.

INTRACRANIAL TUMOURS

P. J. TEDDY

Introduction

As in all other parts of the body, intracranial tumours may be benign or malignant, primary or secondary. However, perhaps more than at any other site, management of tumours within the cranial cavity is influenced as much by their exact location and by the potential adverse effects of treatment on surrounding normal tissue as by the degree of malignancy of the neoplasm itself. Most primary tumours of the brain in adults occur above the tentorium cerebelli and must be considered generally to be malignant. The intracranial tumours of childhood differ considerably from the adult forms in terms of distribution within the brain, histological characteristics, and prognosis.

Incidence and distribution

Autopsy findings suggest that intracranial tumours comprise approximately 8 per cent of all primary neoplasms. The annual incidence in the United Kingdom is about 5 per 100 000 of population. Metastatic lesions account for about 25 per cent of all intracranial tumours found at autopsy. In children the central nervous system is the second most common site for primary tumours and about 70 per cent of childhood intracranial neoplasms are infra-

tentorial. Intracranial tumours represent the sixth most common form of neoplasm in adults, of which 70 per cent occur above the tentorium. Cerebral gliomas rarely occur in the first two decades of life but the incidence then steadily increases. They are twice as common in males as in females. Meningiomas and Schwannomas occur mainly in women and are rare in childhood. Medulloblastoma, cerebellar astrocytoma, and true pineal tumours occur mainly in childhood. There appears to be an increased incidence of craniopharyngioma and pineal germinoma in Japan, ependymoma in India, and medulloblastoma in Europe and North America. Otherwise, geographical distribution of intracranial tumours is probably even throughout the world.

Aetiology and associated lesions

It has been estimated that the risk of developing an intracranial tumour of any type is marginally greater in close relatives of patients with known cerebral gliomas. There have also been occasional reports of families having a high incidence of various intracranial tumours but no clear-cut pattern of inheritance of the development of isolated intracranial neoplasm has been demonstrated. Von Recklinghausen's disease (neurofibromatosis) is

Table 1 Classification of intracranial tumours

Tumour type	Cells/site of origin	Cellular precursor	Site of predilection
Astrocytoma	Astrocytes	Neural tube	Cerebral hemisphere, cerebellum, brain stem, optic pathways
Glioblastoma	Astrocytes		Cerebral hemisphere
Oligodendroglioma	Oligodenrocytes		Cerebral hemisphere
Ependymoma	Ependymal cells	Neural tube	Lateral and IV ventricle
Colloid cyst			III ventricle
Choroid plexus papilloma			Lateral and IV ventricle
Medulloblastoma	Neurones	Neural tube	IV ventricle, cerebellar vermis
Ganglioneuroma			
Ganglioglioma			
Pinealoma	Pinealcytes	Neural tube	Pineal gland
Pineoblastoma			
Neurofibroma		Neural crest	Cranial nerves
Schwannoma	Schwann cells		VIII and V nerves
Meningioma	Arachnoid		Dural surface, ventricles
Craniopharyngioma	Epithelial cells	Ectoderm	Hypothalamus, III ventricle
Cholesteatoma			
Chordoma		Notochord	Clivus
Germinoma	Germ cells		Pineal gland
Teratoma		Germinal layers	Pineal gland
Microglia	Uncertain		Cerebral hemisphere
Sarcoma	Connective tissue		Meninges
Glomus tumour	Glomus jugulare		Glomus jugulare
Pituitary adenoma	Adenphyophyseal cells		Pituitary gland
Haemangioblastoma	Uncertain	? Vascular	Cerebellum
Secondary tumours	Bronchus, breast, kidney, thyroid, melanoma, large bowel, leukaemia, lymphoma		Cerebral hemisphere, cerebellum, meninges
Tumours of the skull	Cholesteatoma, osteoma, chordoma, osteoblastoma, bone cysts, myeloma, osteosarcoma		
	Secondary tumours	Nasopharynx, breast, prostate, bronchus, thyroid	

associated with optic and hypothalamic glioma, Schwannomas of various cranial nerves, most commonly the eighth, and intracranial meningiomas. Tuberose sclerosis is associated with periventricular glioma, and von Hippel–Lindau disease with cerebellar haemangioblastoma which have a tendency to recur. Earlier beliefs that head injury or glial scarring increased the risk of glioma have not been substantiated but meningiomas have occasionally been reported as occurring directly below the site of focal injury to the skull. Transplant and other patients receiving immunosuppressive therapy have been shown to have an increased risk of intracranial lymphoreticular neoplasms. Some patients have been shown to develop local meningiosarcoma or glioma following local irradiation of the scalp for ringworm or high-dose irradiation for pituitary neoplasms.

Pathology

Primary intracranial tumours may be derived from the skull itself, from any of the structures lying within it or from their tissue precursors. They may be divided into tumours of neurectodermal origin (derived from the neural tube, neural crest, and ectoderm) and those of other cell types (see Table 1). It is better to avoid assessing malignancy of primary intracranial tumours on histological grounds alone or on their propensity to metastasize outside the CNS. Primary tumours may involve almost all parts of the brain, are not limited by sulci, and may cross the mid line in corpus callosum, hypothalamic or thalamic regions. Equally, however, histologically benign lesions may involve vital structures, rendering tumour management much more difficult than some of their more malignant counterparts. Histologically low-grade gliomas may undergo rapid and frank malignant change after many years of slow progression. Metastases outside the CNS from primary tumours are rare but do occur, particularly with medulloblastoma. Widespread dissemination through the brain and spinal cord is seen in cases of medulloblastoma, ependymoma, and pineal germinoma. The spread occurs along the pial or ependymal surfaces or through the cerebrospinal fluid. Leukaemic or carcinomatous

Table 2 Incidence of commoner intracranial tumours

Tumour	Overall percentage incidence	Commonest ages of presentation
Astrocytoma and glioblastoma (adults)	38	40–60 years
Astrocytoma (childhood)	Approximately 50 per cent of childhood primary intracranial tumours	6–12 years
Oligodendroglioma	3	30–60 years
Ependymoma	3	6–12 years, occasional in adults
Medulloblastoma	3	5–15 years, occasional in adults
Schwannoma	8	40–70 years
Meningioma	18.5	40–60 years
Craniopharyngioma	2	5–60 years, about half in children
Haemangioblastoma	9	10–20 years
Pituitary adenoma	10	Adult life
Metastatic	4, but 25 per cent of all intracranial tumours at autopsy	
Miscellaneous	1.5	

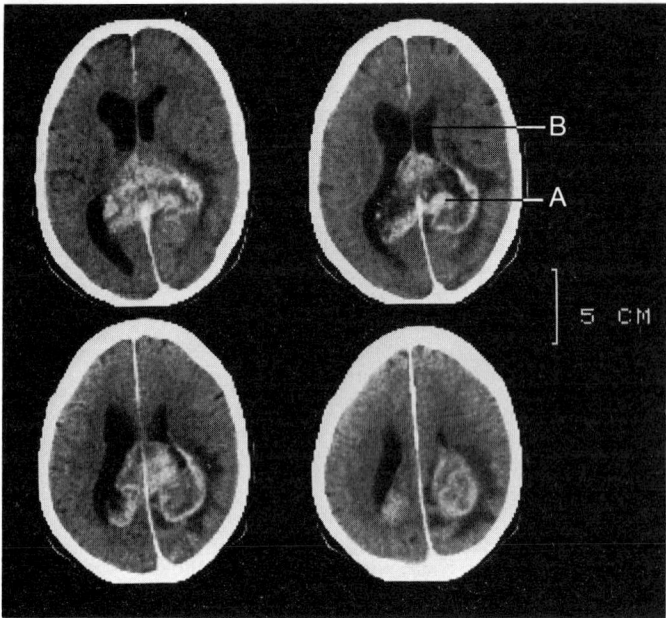

Fig. 1 Contrast CT scan showing typical 'butterfly' malignant glioma (arrow A) spreading across midline in posterior corpus callosum. Note compression and displacement of lateral ventricle (B).

deposits on the meninges may also disseminate widely through the cerebrospinal fluid pathways (see Section 19).

An estimate of degree of malignancy of neurectodermal tumours is often made by histological grading such as in the Kernohan scale (see below). This differentiation is at best an approximation as the tumours may be extremely heterogeneous and tissue sampling made by very limited biopsy. An estimate of malignant propensity and growth rate of the tumour may often be made more accurately by observing the clinical progress of the patient. A comprehensive list of intracranial tumours together with their cells of origin is given in Table 1 and the classification and frequency of occurrence of the more common intracranial tumours in Table 2. Note that whilst the term glioma may loosely be used to describe all tumours derived from neural tube and particularly those of glial cell origin (astrocytes, oligodendrocytes, and ependyma), its everyday use is usually confined to tumours of astrocytic origin, i.e. astrocytoma and glioblastoma.

Astrocytomas

These are the commonest primary intracranial tumours. They are derived from the supportive astrocytic framework of the brain and graded between I and IV with grades I and II being of relatively low malignancy and III and IV being frankly malignant. The distinction between grades is not always clear and individual tumours may be quite heterogeneous. Supratentorial astrocytomas in children have been thought to be more benign than their adult counterparts, but recent evidence suggests that this is not the case. The benign astrocytomas of childhood arise in either the optic nerve or chiasm, the hypothalamus, or the cerebellum. Within the cerebellum they are generally cystic and the cyst wall contains a well-circumscribed solid component of variable size. The solid part of the tumour secretes a yellowish glairy cyst fluid. Such lesions are usually very slow growing and curable by complete removal although some are frankly malignant and show a tendency to recur. The so-called *piloid astrocytomas* which involve the optic pathways and hypothalamus are slowly growing but because of their position are difficult to remove.

Low-grade astrocytomas in the cerebral hemispheres in both adults and children may remain well circumscribed for many years or show only slowly progressive infiltration accompanied by few clinical symptoms. Some undergo patchy calcification but others undergo change to a more malignant form after long periods of apparent quiescence.

Malignant astrocytomas are seen in the brain stem, usually of children and adolescents, and produce enlargement of the brain stem itself ('megapons'). Disturbances of gait, conjugate gaze, and lower cranial nerves are common but, interestingly, obstructive hydrocephalus is usually a late complication.

In adults, malignant astrocytomas are most frequently found in the cerebral hemispheres. They are rapidly growing, diffusely infiltrating, and commonly undergo central necrosis. The most malignant forms are often designated *glioblastoma multiforme*. Malignant gliomas commonly induce considerable oedema in the surrounding 'reactive' brain (see Fig. 1).

Oligodendroglioma

These are usually slow growing tumours with a very long history (10 to 15 years) and occur almost invariably in adults. They may show patchy calcification. Eventually they tend to undergo differentiation to become indistinguishable from malignant astrocytoma. When the tumour abuts the ventricle it has a tendency to seed throughout the ventricular system and when adjacent to the surface of the brain may spread over the pia.

Ependymomas

These are predominantly tumours of children or young adults and arise in the walls of the fourth or less commonly the lateral ventricle. They are usually malignant and tend to disseminate widely through the CSF pathways.

Medulloblastomas

These are highly malignant tumours usually arising in the roof of the fourth ventricle and infiltrating locally into the cerebellar vermis. They occur most commonly in the first decade of life and rarely beyond the mid-teens. They have a tendency to metastasize, not only through the CSF pathways but also outside the CNS to involve bone, bone marrow, and lymph-nodes. Theories have been advanced that widespread dissemination of ependymoma and medulloblastoma may occur after posterior fossa surgery and ventricular shunting but the evidence for this is dubious.

Pineal tumours

Pineal and parapineal tumours are a mixed group and the natural history of the individual components is uncertain since surgical access to them is often limited or hazardous and many have therefore been treated by a shunt procedure and irradiation without biopsy. The group includes teratomas, so-called pineal gliomas, true pinealomas, and germinomas, the latter being the commonest form. Some teratomas are ectopic in that they develop in the floor of the third ventricle and spread to the parapineal region. Pineal tumours quite often spread within CSF pathways including the spinal canal. Histologically, germinomas resemble ovarian dysgerminoma and seminoma and have a marked preponderence in males.

Schwannomas

These lesions are derived from Schwann cells of the neural sheaths and are known as neurilemmomas and neurinomas as well as by the common misnomer of neuroma. They are benign and usually arise on the vestibular branch of the eighth nerve or less commonly on the trigeminal nerve, and rarely on the vagal group. They are usually very slow growing but can reach an enormous size with consequent pressure effects on surrounding structures. Bilateral eighth nerve Schwannomas have been found in association with von Recklinghausen's neurofibromatosis.

Meningiomas

These tumours arise from the arachnoid covering the brain, particularly from the arachnoid villi, and are thus commonly found close to the major dural venous sinuses. They arise most often from the dura of the falx (parasaggital), the sphenoid wing, the convexity of the cerebral hemispheres, and from the olfactory groove in the anterior fossa. However, they derive from any dural compartment and may be found on the tentorium, in the suprasellar region and even within the lateral ventricle. They are mainly adult tumours, occurring between the ages of 40 and 50 years, and are occasionally multiple. Most are benign but, incompletely removed, have a tendency to recur. Some are frankly malignant and recur rapidly even after apparently complete removal. Meningosarcomas may form pulmonary metastases. Rare cases of meningioma occurring entirely outside the skull have been reported.

Meningiomas tend to involve the skull close to the site of dural origin invoking a focal endostosis or occasionally an exostosis. Sometimes there will be osteal hypertrophy and sclerosis overlying the tumour and this is generally seen in the meningioma *en plaque* of the sphenoid wing. The form and consistency of meningiomas varies considerably. Microscopically they may be endotheliomatous masses comprising epithelial-like cells arranged in sheets or islands separated by vascular connective tissue trabeculae and forming whorls which are often hyalinized and calcified to form so-called psammoma bodies. Some present a more fibroblastic appearance. Richly vascularized meningiomas are described as angioblastic. The more vascular tumours may produce erosion of the skull at the point of tumour attachment to the dura. Meningiomas are usually benign and slow growing but may reach an enormous size before presentation, particularly when adjacent to relatively silent parts of the brain, (Fig. 2). They tend to form a nest in the brain and have a relatively clear arachnoid plane between tumour capsule and surrounding cortex. The more indolent lesions may calcify or even ossify. Even when entirely benign the position of some meningiomas makes them either inoperable or amenable only to partial excision. This is particularly true of those which involve the cavernous and saggital sinuses or surround the proximal part of the internal carotid artery.

Craniopharyngiomas

These tumours, which are found both in adults and children, are formed of epithelial cell remnants in the region of the pituitary

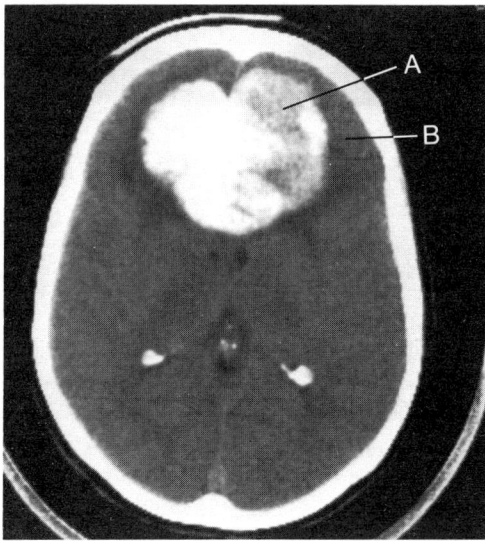

Fig. 2 Contrast CT scan. Large bifrontal meningioma (A) with surrounding oedema (B).

stalk. It was thought that they represented a persistent form of Rathke's pouch but this theory has been questioned. Although considered to be a congenital anomaly they may grow extensively, causing compression of the optic nerves and chiasm, obstruction of the third ventricle with subsequent hydrocephalus, and may expand into the pituitary fossa with resultant hypopituitarism. They may even grow in a far more widespread manner towards the cavernous sinus, under the frontal and temporal lobes, and occasionally into the posterior fossa. About 50 per cent of craniopharyngiomas are calcified and may be identified on skull X-ray as speckled areas of calcification above the posterior clinoid process. A few tumours may be confined within the pituitary fossa itself. They may be wholly or partially cystic and the cyst contains fluid with many cholesterol crystals which have a typical shimmering appearance.

Pituitary adenomas
(See also Section 10.)

These are the commonest neoplasm of the pituitary gland and although usually benign they range in size from small growths entirely limited to the adenohypophysis to giant forms. They may have large suprasellar components, or extend laterally to involve the cavernous sinus or beyond into the basal cisterns and under the frontal and temporal lobes (invasive adenoma). Adenocarcinomas of the pituitary are extremely rare and resemble metastatic lesions.

Pituitary adenomas are divided into secreting and non-secreting tumours and, although the differentation into chromophil and chromophobe adenomas still pertains, immunofluorescent techniques and electron microscopic studies are progressively changing classification in simple histological terms. The non-secretory adenomas comprise cells of variable size and morphology ranged as simple masses or in a trabecular pattern. The secretory adenomas contain many types of cell dependent upon the cellular precursor from which they are derived. They may produce prolactin, growth hormone, and adrenocorticotrophic hormone. The abnormalities produced by the secretory tumours include Cushing's syndrome, acromegaly or gigantism, and hyperprolactinaemia. The non-secretory tumours may compress normal pituitary tissue and produce hypopituitarism.

Both non-secretory and secretory tumours may also produce effects through space occupation, the commonest sequel being compression of the optic chiasm from below. Occasionally the tumours can become big enough to occlude the third ventricle and produce an obstructive hydrocephalus.

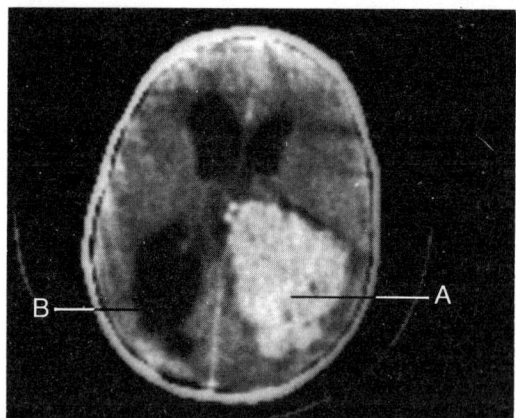

Fig. 3 Contrast CT scan showing large choroid plexus papilloma in right lateral ventricle (A). Associated hydrocephalus (B).

Colloid cysts

Colloid cysts occur in the third ventricle, always at its anterior end. They are rare tumours and occur predominantly in young adults. They are benign, probably arising from ependyma in the region of the tela choroidea. They comprise a capsule with an epithelial lining and usually contain glairy mucoid material with debris of desquamation. The cells lining the cyst sometimes have cilia. Although these masses may present slowly with evidence of progressive dementia or mental changes, they more often present with acute episodes of loss of consciousness. This is thought to be related to their acting intermittently as a ball valve with obstruction of the foramen of Munro. Occasionally they may be large enough to completely fill the third ventricle and even obstruct the entrance to the aqueduct.

Choroid plexus papillomas

These frond-like tumours are usually benign and arise, predominantly in the first decade of life, in the lateral and fourth ventricles. Very occasionally they arise in the third ventricle. They may reach an enormous size (see Fig. 3) and produce symptoms by mass effect through obstructive hydrocephalus or by excessive secretion of cerebrospinal fluid. Occasionally they are malignant and may seed through the CSF pathways. Even when benign their rich vascularity may make surgical treatment extremely hazardous. Histologically they are papillary outgrowths identical with normal choroid plexus.

Ganglioneuromas and gangliogliomas

These are rare, well-circumscribed tumours occurring mainly in children and found predominantly in the floor of the third ventricle. They may contain a mixture of two cell types derived from both neuronal and astrocytic components surrounded by fibrous connective tissue and they are often partially cystic. They are fairly indolent and tend not to recur if removal is complete.

Cholesteatomas

These are developmental inclusion lesions in which epithelial remnants are incorporated into deeper layers. They include epidermoid and dermoid cysts. The epidermoid cysts have a thin connective tissue capsule and contain material rich in cholesterol from the breakdown of keratin which is shed by the desquamating epithelial cells. Dermoid cysts may also contain follicles, sebaceous glands, and sweat glands. These rare tumours are found predominantly in the cerebellopontine angle and in the parasellar region. They have a tendency to recur, for whereas the contents of the cyst (pearly-white degenerative material) is easy enough to remove, the capsule is thin and adherent to many of the surrounding structures. Failure to remove the whole capsule results in further desquamation of cells and a gradual accumulation of the contents of the cyst.

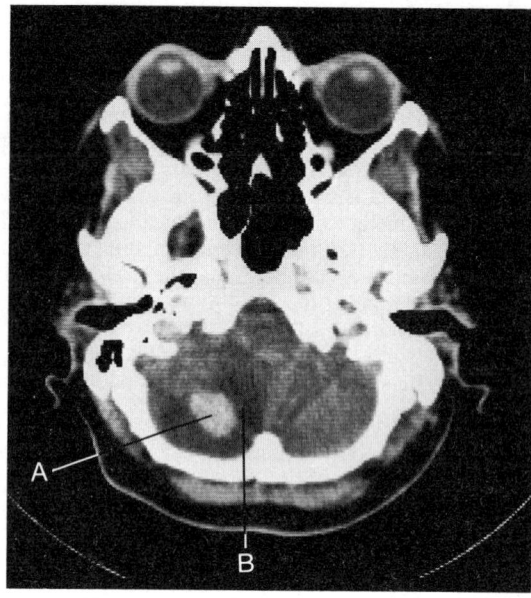

Fig. 4 Contrast CT scan of posterior fossa. Solid nodule (A) within typical cyst cavity (B) of haemangioblastoma.

Chordomas

Chordomas arise from remnants of the primitive notochord. Intracranial chordomas arise therefore from the clivus and sella turcica. They contain clear cells surrounded by connective tissue trabeculae and are usually lobulated tumours. They may be locally invasive with bony erosion despite usually being benign. One of the chief problems in their treatment is their inaccessibility.

Haemangioblastomas

These tumours are seen in older children and young adults and are most commonly found in the cerebellum. They constitute about 2 per cent of all intracranial tumours. Rarely, they are found within the medulla or above the tentorium. Most are single but they may be associated with retinal and renal or pancreatic cysts and occur in families – von Hippel–Lindau disease. Haemangioblastomas are occasionally solid but much more commonly cystic and contain a small mural nodule attached to the inner wall of the cyst (see Fig. 4). The cyst fluid is a golden-yellow colour and the solid nodule cherry red. The nodule contains multiple small capillaries, reticulin fibres, and clear cells. Their true origin is uncertain but they are commonly regarded as being vascular tumours. They are usually benign and the solitary lesions generally do not recur if complete removal is effected. The familial forms tend to recur more frequently. Occasionally, they are associated with ectopic erythropoietin production and polycythaemia (see Section 19).

Glomus jugulare tumours

These are very rare neoplasms arising from the jugular body in the adventitia of the jugular bulb. The mass grows into the middle ear and may present as a pulsating vascular lesion at the external auditory meatus. In about half the cases growth is into the posterior fossa and presents as a cerebellopontine angle mass. The tumours are similar to those of the cartoid body with large clear cells in a connective tissue framework and a very rich vascular supply. They may secrete serotonin.

Sarcomas

Intracranial sarcomas are uncommon and are of two general types. Fibrosarcomas arise chiefly from the meninges and are diffuse tumours which may include the surrounding brain. Microgliomas (reticulum cell sarcomas) occur in older adults, chiefly involving the cerebral hemispheres near the midline. They contain

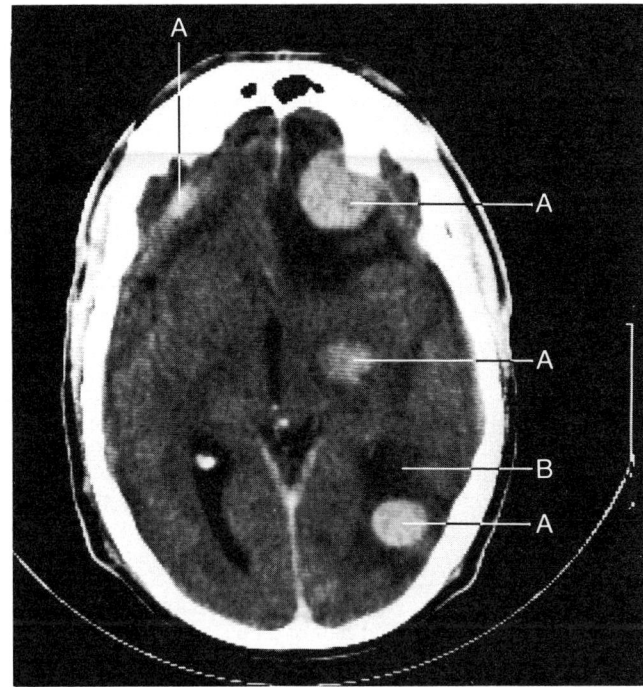

Fig. 5 Contrast CT scan. Multiple metastatic deposits (arrows A) each surrounded by area of cerebral oedema (B).

masses of reticulum cells and small cells resembling lymphocytes. They are diffusely infiltrating and rarely amenable to treatment.

Intracranial metastases

Although the incidence of secondary intracranial neoplasm is only about 4.5 per cent of all intracranial tumours in neurosurgical practice these secondary tumours represent about 25 per cent of the total in autopsy studies. They may occur in the skull or involve any structure within the cranium. Although they most commonly occur in the cerebral hemispheres or cerebellum, the brain stem, meninges or cranial nerves may be involved. They are usually multiple (see Fig. 5), variable in size, and well circumscribed, but the differentiation between tumour and surrounding brain is not always clear. They are variable in consistency and the greater use of computerized tomographic (CT) scanning has demonstrated that haemorrhage into these tumours occurs more frequently than was once thought. The cellular appearance is usually that of the primary source, but the origin of the more anaplastic tumours and those exhibiting severe necrosis can be difficult to determine. The most common primary tumours are those of bronchus and breast, followed by malignant melanoma, renal carcinoma, and various carcinomas of the alimentary tract. Thyroid carcinoma, although rare, also metastasizes to brain. Retinoblastomas of childhood may infiltrate the subarachnoid space, as may leukaemic and lymphomatous deposits. Malignant lymphoma and melanoma may be seen as primary neoplasms within the intracranial cavity. Infiltration of the meninges by carcinoma, leukaemia, and lymphoma may produce a malignant meningitis often associated with lower cranial nerve palsies owing to infiltration around the brain stem.

Pathophysiology

The pathological effects of any enlarging intracranial neoplasm and the speed with which they progress will depend upon the morphological characteristics of the mass, its rate of growth, its anatomical location, the neural tissues which it compresses, distorts or invades, its capacity to induce oedema of the surrounding brain, and the displacement or obstruction of fluid components (blood and CSF) within the cranium. The effects may be local or generalized or both.

By infiltrating or compressing normal structures close to the site

of the mass, tumours produce focal neurological deficits. Irritation of the cerebral hemisphere may result in epilepsy, and infiltration of the dura may lead to local pain and to meningeal irritation. Increase in the size of the mass within the effectively fixed volume of the skull will lead to a rise in intracranial pressure. Of all these effects the latter is usually the most important in terms of precipitating rapid irreversible deterioration.

For practical purposes the skull may be considered as a closed rigid box containing three principal elements, the brain, CSF, and blood. Any increase of the volume of these elements will lead to a rise in intracranial pressure but this may be offset initially by compensating mechanisms. For instance, a slowly enlarging tumour may increase the volume of the cerebral contents but be compensated for by a reduction in the volume of CSF which becomes squeezed out of the compressed lateral ventricles and the basal cisterns. Clearly, the compensatory mechanisms will be more effective if the factors increasing pressure are only slowly progressive. The pressure–volume curve relating to intracranial pressure is not linear but exponential so that the effects of increased volume due to a slowly growing tumour may be compensated for over a long time without undue rise in pressure. A point is then reached at which reduction in CSF volume, brain displacement, and perhaps reduction in cerebral perfusion can no longer be compensated for as efficiently. At this point even small rises in volume will produce substantial rises in intracranial pressure.

As intracranial masses increase in size other phenomena occur which are of great significance in terms of brain function and which may prelude rapid clinical deterioration (see Figs. 6 and 7). Axial displacement of the brain at the foramen magnum, when the cerebellar tonsils are driven through this aperture, is commonly seen with masses in the posterior fossa. This cerebellar tonsillar herniation is known as coning. The term has been extended to include axial and lateral displacement of the brain at the level of the hiatus. A unilateral hemisphere mass may displace towards the unaffected side causing the medial part of the temporal lobe (the uncus) to be pushed into the tentorial hiatus. Lateral displacement of the brain combines with the uncal herniation to force the contralateral cerebral peduncle against the free edge of the tentorium. Conduction in the fibres traversing the compressed peduncle becomes impaired leading to a false localizing sign with ipsilateral hemiparesis (Kernohan's notch phenomenon). Lateral displacement producing tentorial herniation may also press the oculomotor nerve against the petroclinoid ligament and stretch it by virtue of downward displacement of the posterior cerebral artery around which it hooks. This will result in pupillary dilatation and fixation which may be reversible in the early stages but which may become irreversible if the blood supply to the nerve is impaired.

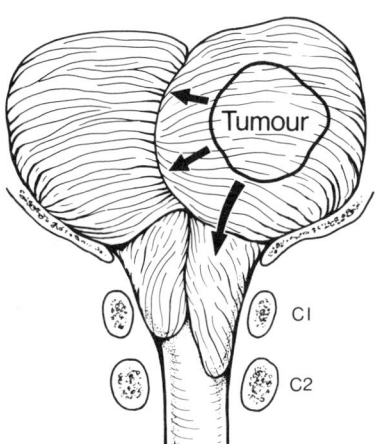

Fig. 6 Herniation of cerebellar tonsils. (Reproduced from Jefferson, *Oxford textbook of medicine*, 1st edn.)

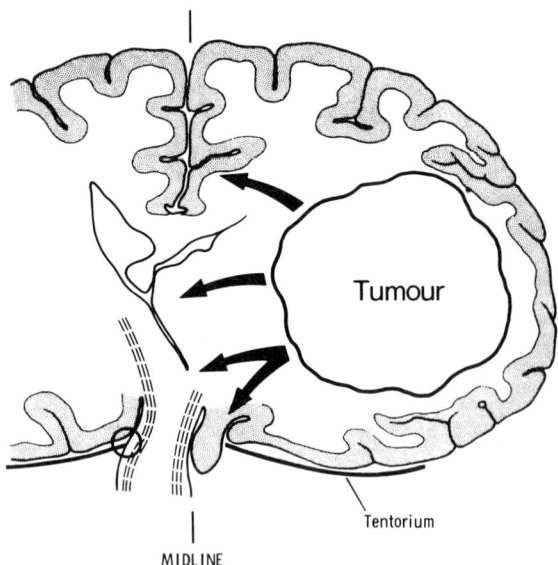

Fig. 7 Diagram of inferior aspect of the brain with left temporal tumour. The arrow shows the uncus compressing the oculomotor nerve. Note also how descent of the posterior cerebral artery stretches the nerve. (Reproduced from Jefferson, *Oxford textbook of medicine*, 1st edn.)

Supratentorial masses may also depress the tentorium and displace the contents of the posterior fossa downwards so that the cerebellar tonsils herniate through the foramen magnum. Deformation of the brain-stem distorts arteries which penetrate it and with severe brain-stem distortion infarcts and haemorrhages may occur which may be fatal. With incipient tentorial and tonsillar herniation a further change in pressure differential between the supratentorial and infratentorial or infratentorial and spinal compartments may be catastrophic. Lumbar puncture must therefore be strictly avoided until a suspected intracranial mass lesion has been excluded.

Papilloedema is most probably caused by the effects of increased intracranial pressure transmitted to the CSF in the optic nerve sheath. However, even very large slowly growing intracranial masses can present without demonstrable papilloedema. This may relate anatomically to differing degrees of patency of the optic nerve sheaths. Papilloedema will be absent in cases in which optic atrophy has already supervened.

Prolonged raised intracranial pressure may result in erosion of the base of the skull so that patients present with CSF rhinorrhoea or meningitis. Extensive erosion of the pituitary fossa can occur, especially in cases of severe hydrocephalus, and the posterior clinoid process will be eroded. Chronic raised pressure may also cause focal erosions of the inner table of the skull and lead to a 'thumb-printing' pattern on skull X-ray.

Clinical features

Despite their adverse nature, all intracranial tumours will present in one of (or in a combination of) three ways: raised intracranial pressure, focal neurological deficits, or epilepsy.

Focal epileptic seizures may, in their own right, be of localizing value. The neurological deficit will depend to a large extent upon the site of the tumour, and raised intracranial pressure may be a function of the tumour mass itself, of reactive oedema in the surrounding brain, and of obstructive hydrocephalus. More generalized systemic disturbances may be evident, particularly in cases of hormone-secreting tumours of the pituitary and in metastatic disease. Neck stiffness and pain in patients with intracranial tumour can be caused either by local filtration of the meninges or by tonsillar herniation.

Raised intracranial pressure

Evidence of raised intracranial pressure is, perhaps, the most ominous feature of intracranial mass lesions and should prompt urgent investigation. The cardinal symptoms are those of headache, vomiting, and drowsiness. The headaches may come on at any time of day but characteristically occur early in the morning or wake the patient from sleep. This is due, in part, to relative CO_2 retention during sleep with cerebrovascular dilatation and further increase in intracranial pressure. The headaches may be increased by stooping or coughing and are generally recognized as being different in character from headaches suffered previously even in patients who have a past history of migraine. The headache may be accompanied by vomiting which may partially relieve the headache. Headaches are seldom of localizing value although tumours of the posterior fossa may produce occipital and upper cervical pain. Evidence of neck stiffness in conjunction with nuchal pain in the patient with a suspected intracranial mass lesion requires immediate investigation.

Vomiting sometimes occurs as an isolated symptom or precedes headache by many months, particularly in cases of fourth ventricular tumour.

Two sinister symptoms of raised intracranial pressure are failing vision and deterioration of the level of consciousness. Papilloedema is present in only about half of all patients with intracranial tumours. However, chronic papilloedema may result in enlargement of the blind spot and defects of central vision, and ultimately leads to episodes of transient blindness (visual obscurations). These attacks are often exacerbated by coughing, straining or stooping. Prolonged raised intracranial pressure may produce complete visual failure when optic atrophy supervenes.

In the early stages, alteration of the level of consciousness may be noticed by relatives and friends simply by increased lethargy, tiredness, and somnolence. More severe degrees of raised pressure associated with brain-stem distortion and tentorial or tonsillar herniation may lead to dramatic deterioration in conscious level and require prompt attention.

In infants raised intracranial pressure can present with failure to thrive, lethargy, head clutching, and vomiting, and be associated with an increasing head circumference and a tense bulging fontanelle. In older children there may be separation of the sutures of the skull vault and on percussion the skull may give a 'cracked pot' note.

Focal neurological deficits

These are legion owing to the variability of type and site of intracranial tumours and only a few specific syndromes associated with the more common tumours can be described here.

In general, lesions involving the cerebral hemisphere produce mental and behavioural changes when the frontal lobes are involved, contralateral hemiparesis when the posterior frontal motor cortex is involved, contralateral cortical sensory impairment and homonymous hemianopia with parietal lesions, disturbance of memory, mood, and sometimes hemianopia or quadrantanopia with temporal lesions, and dysphasia with lesions of the temporofrontal or temporoparietal areas of the dominant hemisphere. Tumours of the brain stem commonly present with disorders of ocular movement, balance, and motor impairment. Cerebellar hemisphere lesions produce limb ataxia and central cerebellar lesions produce gait ataxia. Tumours compressing or invading the visual pathways may produce visual failure or field defects. Masses within the cerebellopontine angle produce evidence of brain-stem and cerebellar compression and affect specifically the cranial nerves V, VII, VIII, and sometimes the vagal group. Tumours of the non-dominant frontal and anterior temporal lobe and those within the anterior one-third of the corpus callosum or within a ventricle may be manifest purely by symptoms and signs of raised intracranial pressure without focal deficit. Bifrontal lesions may result in intellectual deterioration with memory loss and urinary incontinence, and those involving the third ventricle and hypothalamus can cause hormonal and metabolic changes together with raised intracranial pressure through obstructive hydrocephalus.

Two facets of neurological examination are frequently overlooked or improperly performed by inexperienced clinicians; testing the sense of smell and assessing visual fields. There are probably many patients who have been diagnosed as having simple dementia whose large olfactory groove meningiomas have been missed for want of simple tests of sense of smell. Smell may also be lost in cases of extrinsic tumours invading through the floor of the anterior cranial fossa.

Apart from the effects of papilloedema, vision will be impaired when masses stretch or compress the optic nerves and chiasm or when tumours interrupt some or all of the optic radiations in one hemisphere. Chiasmal lesions are classically regarded as producing a bitemporal hemianopia, and whilst this is very commonly the case, the deficit is often asymmetric, producing obvious symptoms in one eye whilst the other eye shows changes demonstratable only by refined field testing. When the optic radiations are involved either the right or left halves of both visual fields are affected (homonymous hemianopia). Temporal lesions affect chiefly the contralateral upper quadrants, and parietal lesions the contralateral lower quadrants. A surprising degree of visual loss may occur without the patient being aware of the deficit; for example, unilateral visual loss may remain unnoticed until the healthy eye is obscured for some reason, or road traffic accidents may occur through loss of peripheral vision. Visual field and acuity deterioration is particularly hard to demonstrate in children.

Tumours of the midbrain may produce complex disorders of eye movement (internuclear ocular palsies). Isolated third nerve palsy may be nuclear in origin but is more likely to be peripheral and associated with uncal herniation. Unilateral or bilateral sixth nerve palsy may occur and is rarely of localizing value. It is usually a secondary effect of raised intracranial pressure when displacement of the brain presses the nerve against the anterior inferior cerebellar artery. Tumours in the pineal region compress the dorsal midbrain, resulting in failure of upward gaze and abnormal pupillary reactions (*Parinaud's syndrome*).

Disorders of fifth nerve function are usually manifest as either numbness or pain in the face in one or more divisions of the sensory root. The commonest site for tumours to affect fifth nerve function is in the region of the pons, most particularly meningiomas or Schwannomas in the cerebellopontine angle. Occasionally both sensory and motor impairment of the trigeminal nerve is seen with intrinsic pontine lesions.

Peripheral facial nerve lesions are sometimes associated with tumours in the base of the skull, but facial weakness is more commonly seen with tumours of the cerebral hemispheres which extend deeply into the brain and involve the internal capsule. Acoustic Schwannomas may greatly stretch the facial nerve but facial weakness is usually a very late sign.

The vast majority of Schwannomas of the eighth nerve arise on the vestibular division and present with unilateral sensorineural hearing loss (see also page 21.90). This is accompanied by diminished or absent caloric responses (cold water applied to the external ear will normally stimulate the lateral semicircular canal and produce nystagmus with the fast component away from the irrigated ear). Downward enlargement of the tumour may impair ninth and tenth cranial nerve function, posterior enlargement affects the cerebellum and produces truncal and limb ataxia, and medial enlargement may encroach upon fifth nerve and brain stem producing sensory impairment in the face and long tract signs. Acoustic nerve tumours are often seen in late middle age and elderly patients, in whom the significance of dementia, deafness, and ataxia is not always appreciated.

Eleventh and twelfth cranial nerves are affected by tumours of the base of the skull such as chordomas or by other large tumours of the posterior fossa which project towards the foramen magnum.

Epilepsy
(See also page 21.59.)

Only some 10 per cent of adults presenting with late onset epilepsy (after age 25 years) will prove to have an intracranial supratentorial neoplasm. However, the diagnosis should at least be suspected, particularly in cases of focal epilepsy in which the character of the attacks changes. Epilepsy occurs in about 30 per cent of cases of supratentorial tumour and the type of fit may give some idea as to the site and nature of the tumour. Gustatory or olfactory attacks imply an intrinsic tumour within the medial temporal lobe, whilst focal attacks, particularly of sensory type starting in the foot or lower limb are strongly indicative of a falcine or parasaggital meningioma. Sometimes apparently idiopathic attacks may precede other symptoms suggestive of intracranial tumours by many years and give a clue as to the true natural history of the tumour. This is particularly the case in oligodendrogliomas, but with the faster growing malignant astrocytomas there may be only a few weeks between the onset of fits and the appearance of other neurological abnormalities.

Other symptoms and signs

It is important when dealing with cases of suspected behavioral change or memory impairment to obtain a full history from relatives or close friends of the patients and not to rely on the patients for an accurate description of their symptoms. The changes may be subtle and go unrecognized or ignored by the patient. Relatives can comment more accurately on increased aggression, lethargy or neglect, failure to cope at work, and memory disorder. Expressive dysphasia may sometimes be mistakenly described as confusion and receptive dysphasia as deafness and it is important to distinguish these by simple clinical testing.

More generalized systemic disturbances may be seen in patients with intracranial metastases when the systemic signs relate to the primary neoplasm. Non-secretory pituitary adenomas and craniopharyngiomas may produce hypopituitarism whereas secretory tumours may give rise to acromegaly and gigantism, or hyperprolactinaemia with infertility, galactorrhoea, and amenorrhoea. Pinealomas are sometimes associated with precocious puberty and lesions affecting the hypothalamus (e.g. craniopharyngioma) may produce diabetes insipidus, hyperphagia, and disorders of temperature regulation.

Differential diagnosis

The symptoms associated with intracranial tumours are usually of gradual onset so that the major differential diagnoses are other causes of raised intracranial pressure or progressive neurological signs and fits rather than causes of abrupt deterioration such as stroke. However, one catch is that of meningioma presenting in a stuttering fashion suggestive of transient ischaemic attacks or incomplete stroke. The differential diagnosis of intracranial neoplasm includes chronic subdural haematoma which is not always associated with known head injury and is often attended by a fluctuating level of consciousness; cerebral infarction; cortical venous thrombosis; benign intracranial hypertension which normally presents in young women and although headache, papilloedema and sixth nerve palsy may be seen is not associated with drowsiness; cerebral abscess which is usually associated with infection of the sinuses and middle ear or with congenital heart disease; herpes simplex encephalitis; granulomatous disease including syphilitic gumma and tuberculoma; and causes of hydrocephalus other than those associated with neoplasm (e.g. aqueduct stenosis). Patients who are already known to have malignant disease elsewhere who present with neurological symptoms should not be assumed necessarily to have intracranial metastases.

Investigations

The speed of progression of symptoms with particular reference to the presence of raised intracranial pressure will determine the urgency of investigation and whether hospital admission is required. Non-radiological investigation may include formal plotting of visual fields in cases of suspected optic nerve or chiasmal compression, caloric testing, audiometry, and measurement of brain-stem evoked potentials in cases of possible acoustic tumour, full endocrine assessment for cases of suspected pituitary adenoma, and serological and haematological investigation to help exclude syphilis and other bacterial infection.

Electroencephalography has a limited role to play in the diagnosis of cerebral tumour. It may be useful in certain cases of focal epilepsy and, together with sphenoidal recordings, may be of particular value in temporal lobe seizures in children. In these cases it may demonstrate a single focus for the fits in the mesial temporal lobe and indicate whether temporal lobectomy or hippocampectomy would be beneficial.

Chest X-ray is mandatory in all cases of suspected intracranial tumour to exclude primary neoplasm or tuberculosis.

Skull radiographs

Plain X-rays of the skull may show evidence of raised intracranial pressure in both adults and children (erosion of the dorsum sellae, 'copper beating' of the skull vault, and separation of the sutures). Calcification is commonly seen in oligodendroglioma and in virtually all cases of craniopharyngioma of childhood and about half the adult cases with this particular neoplasm. Calcification of the pineal in children is highly suggestive of pineal tumour. Unilateral tumours of the cerebral hemispheres may displace a calcified pineal gland.

Hyperostosis or bony erosion of the skull can occur immediately adjacent to meningiomas, and acoustic Schwannomas commonly erode the internal auditory meatus. In such cases tomography of the petrous bones may be indicated.

Radioisotope brain scan

This investigation is of some use in that it may reveal between 50 and 75 per cent of supratentorial neoplasms. It is of little value in detecting posterior fossa masses.

Nuclear magnetic resonance (NMR) scanning

NMR is unlikely to replace CT scanning completely in the investigation of intracranial mass lesions but it has so far been found useful for demonstrating small multiple metastases, basal intracranial tumours, and particularly for showing cerebral demyelination.

Computerized tomographic scanning

This is now the investigation of choice for all suspected intracranial tumours. With contrast enhancement over 95 per cent of intracranial tumours can be demonstrated with a resolution of around 2 mm depending on the density of the tumour compared with the surrounding brain. CT scanning will also show whether the tumour is solid or partially cystic and show the amount of lateral shift produced by the tumour mass and surrounding oedema. Tumour size may not always be accurately assessed as there may be difficulty in differentiating between solid components of low-grade infiltrative gliomas and the surrounding reactive oedema of the brain itself. Tumours often have peripheral reactive hyperaemia and when the neoplasms are partially necrotic they show up as ring enhancing lesions with low-density centres. Under these circumstances it may be impossible to differentiate a tumour from a cerebral abscess. It is therefore important to consider the clinical history and to have good quality plain skull X-rays to demonstrate opacity of the sinuses and osteitis of the skull which may accompany cerebral abscess. Finally, the CT scan will also demonstrate the presence of obstructive hydrocephalus associated with intracranial tumour.

Cerebral angiography

Prior to CT scanning this was the investigation of choice for confirming the diagnosis of cerebral tumour. It is now mainly used as an adjunct to scanning to exclude anteriovenous malformations, to differentiate between possible menigioma and intrinsic tumour,

and as a preoperative investigation to demonstrate the blood supply of tumours and their relationship to important vascular structures. Study of the venous phase of angiography is important in planning operations on parasaggital meningiomas in which the saggital sinus may be involved.

Management

Except for cases in which age or general medical condition preclude operation most intracranial tumours will require some form of surgery either to obtain a histological diagnosis, to palliate and help to control fits or neurological symptoms, or to achieve total removal. With malignant tumours radiotherapy is often used in conjunction with a surgical procedure (see Table 3). Medical treatment is largely supportive and symptomatic in the absence of any specific antitumour agent.

Immediate treatment

The principal features associated with intracranial neoplasms which require urgent investigation and treatment are raised intracranial pressure particularly when associated with deteriorating level of consciousness and/or failing vision, and epileptic fits. Fits should be aborted promptly with 10 mg i.v. diazepam, or if this fails, 10 ml of i.m. paraldehyde (adult doses). It is important to establish the cause of raised intracranial pressure and the only certain way of doing this is by carrying out a CT scan. Raised pressure associated with tumour mass and surrounding reactive oedema may be reduced by giving intravenous frusemide or 20 per cent w/v solution of mannitol (200 ml over about 15 min). Intravenous dexamethasone (12 to 16 mg) may also be used in extreme cases.

Corticosteroids may also be used in rather less urgent cases when, for example, an intracranial mass has been shown on CT scan to be associated with cerebral oedema and there has been slow progression of neurological signs. Dexamethasone (4 mg six-hourly) may produce symptomatic relief by reducing brain swelling and may make subsequent surgery safer. If there is doubt as to whether a mass lesion may be an abscess or neoplasm steroids should be avoided until a diagnosis has been firmly established.

Raised intracranial pressure from obstructive hydrocephalus requires some form of ventricular drainage procedure or ventricular shunting. Once this has been done fuller investigation may be undertaken rather less urgently and elective surgery planned as required.

Severe headaches should be treated with codeine or dihydrocodeine but other opiate analgesics are generally contraindicated owing to their tendency to depress respiration, conscious level, and pupillary responses. Vomiting may be controlled with metaclopramide or cyclizine.

Surgical treatment

Surgery is aimed, whenever possible, at obtaining as complete a removal as is feasible without producing neurological deficit. Benign tumours which are surgically accessible and not involving important structures such as brain stem, basal ganglia or major vessels are curable by complete surgical excision. At operation, however, a balance might have to be struck between potential cure from a risky complete excision, and accepting the possibility of recurrence over many years by leaving small fragments of tumour and preserving vital structures. Tumours in which complete excision is most commonly attempted include meningiomas, colloid cysts, neurofibromas, Schwannomas, and pituitary adenomas. Most supratentorial tumours are removed at craniotomy, the exact approach being dictated by the site of the tumour. Pituitary adenomas are removed transsphenoidally, transethmoidally, or transcranially. Adenomas with a large suprasellar component, particularly when associated with compression of the chiasm or optic nerves have traditionally been removed at craniotomy. However, even very large pituitary adenomas may now be removed effectively by the transsphenoidal route, with better preservation of functioning pituitary tissue and minimal risk of postoperative epilepsy.

Gliomas of the frontal, temporal, and occipital poles might seem curable by lobectomy with a line of excision well behind the apparent limits of the tumour as judged on the CT scan. However, even in these circumstances histological examination often shows tumour cells to be present right up to the line of excision implying that removal has not been complete. The benefit of this procedure is a good internal decompression and, with the more slowly growing neoplasms, a considerable remission of symptoms. Lobectomy is most appropriate to polar tumours in patients with evidence of raised intracranial pressure but few focal neurological signs.

Complete removal of single metastatic lesions is often well worth while. Even in those cases in which prolongation of life cannot be achieved the quality of the survival time is often improved, sometimes remarkably so. For instance, patients who are completely incapacitated by vomiting and ataxia related to a metastasis in the cerebellum can achieve almost complete alleviation of these symptoms by excision of the mass.

The decision to attempt complete surgical removal is particularly difficult in some cases of craniopharyngioma. These tumours have a great tendency to recur if incompletely removed and the best chance of cure is to obtain as complete a removal as possible followed by radiotherapy. However, radical removal is often attended by severe hypothalamic and pituitary dysfunction and the endocrine deficits may be so debilitating as to make life intolerable for the patient.

Similarly, the best chance of long-term survival in cases of medulloblastoma and ependymoma is as complete a macroscopic removal as possible followed by radiotherapy. Attempts at complete excision in these cases are usually limited by risk of damage to structures in the floor of the fourth ventricle. Nevertheless, complete excision should be the aim whenever possible.

Malignant gliomas infiltrate diffusely and it is rarely possible to excise them completely. The aim of surgery is to remove the maximum amount of tumour possible without producing or adding to neurological deficit. At operation a good internal decompression can often be obtained and at the same time provide the theoretical advantage of reducing tumour bulk to make for more effective radiotherapy. The decision to embark upon subtotal resection depends upon the age and general medical condition of the patient, the consistency of the tumour as judged by CT scan

Table 3 Treatment and prognosis of commoner intracranial tumours

Tumour	Commonest surgical procedure	Effect of radiotherapy	Prognosis
Glioblastoma	Biopsy or partial removal	Minimal	Less than 20 per cent one-year survival rate
Astrocytoma	Biopsy or subtotal removal, decompression	Variable, average of 10 per cent increase in survival	Up to 50 per cent five-year survival rate reported
Oligodendroglioma	Biopsy or subtotal removal	Given for 'recurrent' tumour; marginal effect	55 per cent 10-year survival rate. Tend to undergo malignant change
Cerebellar cystic astrocytoma	Complete removal	Not generally used	Over 70 per cent recurrence-free
Ependymoma	Radical removal, possibly with shunt	Variable, probably sensitive	30–40 per cent five year survival rate
Medulloblastoma	Radical removal, possibly with shunt	Whole neuraxis irradiation improves survival	Average survival about one year, recent reports much more favourable
Haemangioblastoma	Complete removal, possibly with shunt	Not generally used	15 per cent recurrence; excellent prognosis if totally removed
Meningioma	Complete removal	Minimal effect	10 per cent recurrence after 'total' removal. Occasionally frankly malignant
Acoustic Schwannoma (neuroma)	Complete removal	Not used	Excellent prognosis if totally removed; high rate of recurrence with subcapsular removal
Craniopharyngioma	Complete removal or subtotal removal	Given after subtotal removal; claims of less than 10 per cent five-year recurrence	10 per cent five-year recurrence after total removal, but high risk of endocrine dysfunction
Pituitary adenoma	Transnasal microadenectomy. Transfrontal craniotomy for mainly suprasellar tumours Total removal by transsphenoidal or transethmoidal routes	Given for invasive or recurrent tumour. Variable response, probably beneficial	About 12 per cent recurrence after surgery and radiotherapy

Tables 2 and 3 are derived from tables published in *Medicine International* and reproduced with kind permission of Medical Education (International) Ltd.

(tumours with small solid components and large cysts may be readily decompressed), and the site of the lesion itself. Superficial tumours in the non-dominant hemisphere may be amenable to more radical surgery than those deeply placed within the dominant hemisphere.

With the advent of CT scanning it was thought that sufficient definition could be achieved to recognize with total confidence intracranial neoplasms and to distinguish them from other pathology. Despite advances in scan technology there may still be difficulty in differentiating abscess, benign tumour or malignant neoplasm. For these reasons it is preferable in almost all cases to obtain a tissue diagnosis by biopsy. This may be carried out through a burr hole with needle biopsy, by a stereotaxic procedure or by craniotomy. However, the mass may be lying in the basal ganglia, thalamus, or brain stem in which case even needle biopsy could be detrimental. One may then elect (as is commonly the case with suspected brain-stem gliomas) to give radiotherapy without a tissue diagnosis, or simply to follow up the patient by serial CT scanning and to operate only if raised intracranial pressure supervenes or if the risk of producing surgical neurological deficit becomes more balanced in the face of progressive neurological signs. Both burr hole and stereotaxic biopsy provide small specimens of tumour from within a possibly heterogeneous mass so that histological grading is potentially inaccurate and prognosis improperly assessed.

Other surgical procedures include ventriculoatrial and ventriculoperitoneal shunting or the insertion of a temporary ventricular drain in cases of obstructive hydrocephalus associated with posterior fossa or third ventricular tumours. This may be carried out as a prelude to definitive surgery or used as a palliative procedure in cases which are deemed inoperable. Large tumour cysts are sometimes drained by burr hole aspiration or by the insertion of a drain and reservoir system which allows frequent tapping of the cyst fluid and administration of local chemotherapy.

Radiotherapy

The usual method of irradiating intracranial tumours is to give external irradiation to the site of the tumour in fractionated doses over a period of about six weeks. Improved techniques over the past few years reduced many of the unwanted side effects of cranial irradiation although lethargy, hair loss, and minor radiation damage to the scalp are almost invariably seen.

Benign tumours are generally insensitive to irradiation and histologically benign mengiomas which have been treated only by partial excision are not influenced by postoperative radiotherapy. Irradiation is frequently given in cases of malignant meningioma which have a tendency to recur rapidly even after complete excision but such treatment has yet to be shown to be of any great value.

The tumours showing the greatest sensitivity to radiotherapy are medulloblastoma and pineal germinoma. Ependymomas and cystic astrocytomas of the cerebellum show variable sensitivity but postoperative radiotherapy is generally advised particularly if surgical excision is judged not to have been complete. Medulloblastoma, ependymoma, and pineal germinoma are treated by whole neuraxis irradiation (brain and spinal cord) because of their tendency to disseminate through CSF pathways. Even with complete removal and high-dose irradiation the prognosis with medulloblastoma has always been considered poor (about 30 per cent two-year survival) but more recent reports suggest that up to 80 per cent five-year survival rates can be achieved in this manner.

Craniopharyngioma, optic glioma, and hypothalamic gliomas are usually irradiated, most frequently following some form of surgery. Potential radiation damage due to the visual pathways, pituitary, and hypothalamus, however, has to be balanced against a low risk of recurrence in cases in which there has been complete surgical excision. Cases of pituitary invasive adenoma which have been treated by partial surgical excision are generally given postoperative radiotherapy. Similarly, certain forms of metastatic tumour may be given postoperative irradiation when the primary tumour is known to be radiosensitive.

The role of radiotherapy in the treatment of malignant gliomas is uncertain. Many trials have been carried out comparing the role of radiotherapy, chemotherapy, and surgery in their treatment but despite claims to the contrary there is no definite evidence that radiotherapy significantly extends or improves the quality of life in patients with high-grade glioma. In patients whose general condition is good and who are shown to have a tumour which is amenable to some form of surgery and to be histologically grade I or II, the treatment of choice is (subtotal) resection with postoperative external radiotherapy. There have been reports of a mean increase in survival time of up to 10 per cent using postoperative irradiation. The prognosis with higher grade tumours is much less favourable (see Table 3).

Despite the available evidence there is a natural tendency to submit patients with known malignant gliomas to radiotherapy on the basis that they are young, are in otherwise good health, and have a family to support. Nevertheless, one must consider that if life expectancy is very short it is often preferable for the patient to spend this time in family surroundings rather than attending hospital appointments. It is under these circumstances that frank, honest discussion with the patients and their relatives is essential and a policy of management decided as a result of a combined and agreed decision by both physicians and family.

Neuroradiotherapeutic techniques which hold some promise for the future include stereotaxic radiosurgery (which has been found to be of some benefit in the early treatment of small deep-seated gliomas and arteriovenous malformations) and boron/neutron capture irradiation. This latter method involves subtotal tumour resection and systemic administration of boron which is preferentially taken up by tumour tissue. The primed tumour remnant is then bombarded with neutrons.

Chemotherapy

Various forms of chemotherapy may have a place in the treatment of secondary deposits within the brain (e.g. cis-platinum in the treatment of seminoma; the nitrosoureas, vincristine, and procarbazine in secondary lymphoma) but there is no real evidence as yet to suggest that chemotherapy has any significant role to play in the treatment of primary intracranial tumours. The management of cerebral leukaemia and lymphomia is considered further in Section 19.

Prognosis and long-term management

The prognosis relating to most of the common intracranial tumours is given in Table 3. Patients with glioblastomas have a mean survival time of only 6 to 12 weeks from presentation. Patients with low-grade tumours have a mean survival of about nine months following surgery and radiotherapy although there have been reports of up to 50 per cent five-year survival in grade I cases.

Meningiomas, apparently completely resected, are still associated with a 5 to 10 per cent recurrence rate within 10 years and this rises to over 20 per cent symptomatic recurrence if fragments of tumour are known to have been left behind. Cerebellar astrocytomas and haemangioblastomas are associated with a good prognosis after complete removal although occasionally cerebellar astrocytoma may act in a more malignant fashion. Fourth ventricular ependymoma has a poor prognosis if incompletely removed; the prognosis of medulloblastoma has already been described. The generally accepted recurrence rate of craniopharyngioma following radical surgery and irradiation is about 25 per cent within five years but some reports suggest a less than 10 per cent recurrence rate. Radical treatment, however, may lead to severe morbidity despite increased survival time. Acoustic Schwannomas will recur if incompletely removed but their growth rate is usually slow and in a few elderly patients with large tumours it may be preferable to accept this risk of slow recurrence and opt for a subcapsular resection. In all other instances radical removal should be attempted.

Patients with intracranial tumours, particularly those associated with large amounts of cerebral oedema, are generally kept on steroid medication throughout their course of surgery and on a lower dose during their course of radiotherapy. They will need to be warned about the potential side-effects of steroids. Some patients with malignant gliomas or with inoperable recurrent tumour who have some evidence of raised intracranial pressure but without rapidly progressive focal deficit may also be treated with dexamethasone. However, the long-term use of steroids in these instances should be avoided as they certainly become less effective after a few weeks.

Patients should also be warned of the possible social consequences of their tumour and its treatment with particular reference to driving. Patients with benign supratentorial lesions who have undergone major surgery will normally be banned from driving in the United Kingdom for one year following operation even if they have suffered no fits. Drivers of heavy goods vehicles may well have their licence withdrawn permanently. Patients who have suffered fits will normally have their licence revoked for a period of two years following the last seizure. Those patients who have malignant intracranial tumours may have to have these general rules appled more cautiously. Following major supratentorial craniotomy most surgeons will advise continuing treatment with anticonvulsant agents for one to two years.

References

Blackwood, W. and Corsellis, J. A. N. (eds) (1976). *Greenfield's neuropathology*. Edward Arnold, London.

Courville, C. B. (1967). Intracranial tumours. Notes upon a series of three thousand verified cases with some current observations obtaining to their mortality. *Bull. Los Angeles Neurol. Soc.* **32**. Suppl. 2.

Northfield, D. W. C. (1973). *The surgery of the central nervous system*. Blackwell Scientific Publications, Oxford.

Teddy, P. J. (1983). Intracranial tumours. *Med. Internat.* **31**, 1456–1460.

Weller, R. O., Swash, M., McLelland, D. L. and Scholtz, C. L. (1982). *Clinical neuropathology*. Springer Verlag, Berlin.

Youmans, J. R. (ed.) (1982). *Neurological surgery*. 2nd edn (6 vols). W. B. Saunders, Philadelphia.

BENIGN INTRACRANIAL HYPERTENSION

N. F. LAWTON

Synonym

Pseudotumour cerebri.

Definition

Benign intracranial hypertension (BIH) is a syndrome of raised intracranial pressure occurring in the absence of a mass lesion or enlargement of the cerebral ventricles due to hydrocephalus. The term *pseudotumour cerebri* is sometimes preferred because the outcome is not invariably benign. Although rarely life-threatening, the rise in intracranial pressure may result in permanent visual loss due to optic-nerve damage.

Incidence

BIH is a rare disease. The precise incidence is unknown but a study of cases admitted to a neurological unit in the United Kingdom yielded 124 patients in a 30-year period and a review of the experience in a North American centre 120 patients in a decade.

The disease is certainly more common in females, the preponderance over males ranging from 3:1 to 8:1 in large series. Although BIH may occur in infants and the elderly it is primarily a disease of young women between the ages of 17 and 40 years. Very rarely BIH is familial and may occur in more than one generation.

Clinical features

It is the hallmark of BIH that presenting symptoms and signs are those of raised intracranial pressure alone. The diagnosis should not be entertained in the presence of neurological features which suggest a focal lesion. Furthermore, there is a remarkable preservation of consciousness and intellectual function rarely encountered in patients with mass lesions or hydrocephalus. A history of epilepsy, either generalized or focal, virtually excludes the diagnosis of BIH, though seizures may occur in the small group of patients with massive venous thrombosis (*vide infra*). Preservation of cerebral function also distinguishes BIH from toxic and metabolic encephalopathies as well as from viral or bacterial meningoencephalitis. Patients with BIH routinely present to out-patient departments and not as medical emergencies.

Headache

This is the commonest symptom and is present to some degree in virtually every case. Characteristically the headache is typical of raised intracranial pressure. It is then generalized, throbbing, worse on waking, and aggravated by factors which temporarily increase CSF pressure such as straining, coughing, or changing posture. Not infrequently, however, headache is mild and non-specific, so that the distinction from common tension headaches may be difficult. At presentation headache has usually been present for weeks, though sometimes for months. Occasionally the diagnosis of BIH is made at lumbar puncture in asymptomatic patients. Although up to 50 per cent of patients complain of nausea, typical early morning projectile vomiting is rare.

Obesity

Amongst the medical conditions associated with BIH, obesity is sufficiently common to be a characteristic feature. Up to 90 per cent of patients in reported series are overweight, though a history of rapid weight gain immediately prior to the onset is most unusual.

Papilloedema

This is a virtually universal finding and the importance of fundus examination in every patient with headache cannot be over emphasized. Papilloedema is usually moderate and may be unilateral. Occasionally the appearance of the optic discs may be equivocal, and fluorescein angiography is indicated to demonstrate the characteristic leakage of dye in true papilloedema.

The classical symptom of papilloedema, which is not specific to BIH, is a transient obscuration of vision often described as a fleeting greyness, a halo, or a more vivid episode of 'catherine wheels' lasting for a few seconds. Obscurations may be provoked by straining or a change in posture, but may also occur spontaneously. Persistent blurring of vision may also occur and patients may describe scotomata in the field of vision associated with optic nerve damage. Occasionally sudden and permanent loss of vision results from infarction of the optic nerve.

Visual obscurations, persistent blurring or scotomata are reported by 30–70 per cent of patients.

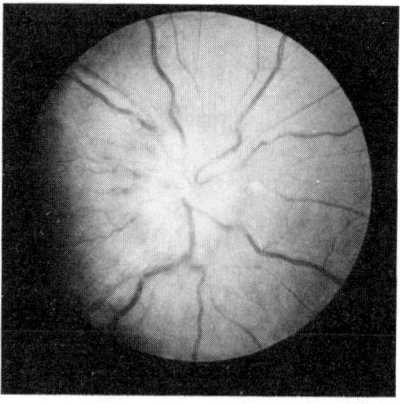

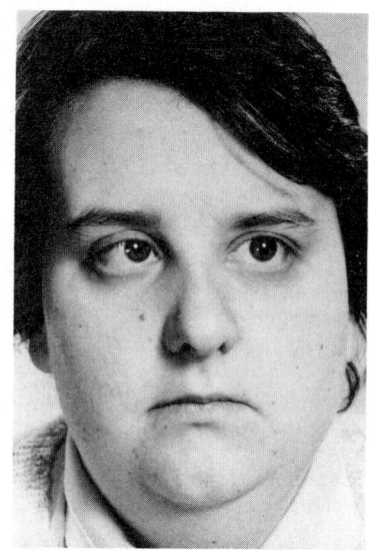

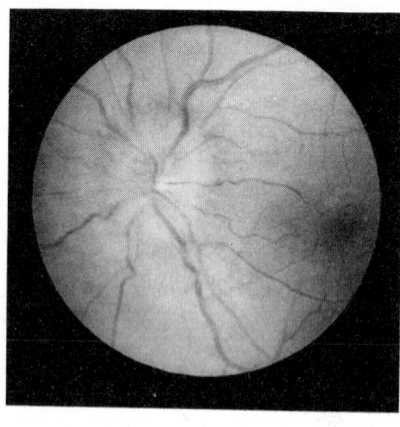

Right fundus   Left fundus

Fig. 1 Bilateral papilloedema and left VIth nerve palsy in benign intracranial hypertension. (Patient looking to the left.) (Reproduced with permission.)

Visual field defects

Visual field analysis should form part of the examination in every patient with suspected BIH. The most common defects are enlargement of the blind spots, generalized constriction of the fields and scotomata caused by optic nerve damage. Colour vision is affected at an early stage.

Diplopia

About 30 per cent of patients complain of horizontal diplopia due to VIth nerve palsy which may be bilateral. It is due to VIth nerve compression and is a false localizing sign of raised intracranial pressure.

Figure 1 shows a typical patient with BIH who presented with a six-week history of headache, visual obscurations, and diplopia, but without any disturbance of consciousness.

Investigations

The diagnosis of BIH can only be confirmed by measurement of CSF pressure but in suspected cases it is essential to exclude a mass lesion or hydrocephalus before proceeding to lumbar puncture.

Radiology

The plain skull X-ray is usually normal, but in 5 per cent of cases shows the changes of raised pressure, including erosion of the dorsum sellae and widening of the sutures in children. The pituitary fossa may be enlarged, reflecting an association with the empty sella syndrome.

Prior to computerized tomography (CT) scanning, angiography, and air encephalography were required to establish ventricular size. Air encephalograms characteristically showed ventricles which were small and slit-like. Although this is less easily demonstrated by CT scanning, careful measurements confirm that the ventricles are small and that ventricular volume increases as BIH resolves. An associated empty sella is usually shown by the CT scan. Dural sinus thrombosis may also be visualized but angiography is required to exclude this with certainty in the small group of patients in whom it is the predisposing cause.

CSF pressure

It is a criterion for the diagnosis that mean CSF pressure is raised. In the majority of patients this is confirmed at lumbar puncture by an opening pressure of >200 mm CSF. In a few patients the opening pressure is normal, but continuous monitoring demonstrates intermittent peaks of raised pressure.

CSF analysis

The composition of the CSF in typical BIH is entirely normal, and the presence of white cells or a raised protein concentration cast serious doubt on the diagnosis. An exception to this rule is a rare syndrome resembling BIH which occurs in association with post-infective polyneuropathy and with spinal tumours. Both conditions may lead to raised intracranial pressure with papilloedema and normal-sized ventricles but a marked rise in CSF protein.

Aetiology

In the majority of patients with BIH no cause can be identified. A wide variety of clinical associations have been reported, but in many instances may have occurred by chance. Preceding minor head injury and intercurrent infections come into this category. Furthermore, the known associations are rare, with the exceptions of obesity and the predilection for females. Heredity, vitamin deficiency, and drugs are each a factor in less than 2 per cent of cases.

Dural sinus thrombosis

Prior to the advent of antibiotics, BIH was frequently associated with chronic middle ear disease. It is probable that BIH in these cases was secondary to dural sinus thrombosis as a result of intracranial spread of infection. The term 'otitic hydrocephalus' was coined in the belief that middle ear disease was the primary cause and on the erroneous assumption that ventricular enlargement was present.

Although true 'otitic hydrocephalus' is now rare, BIH may still occur following venous thrombosis in dural sinuses or in the extracranial jugular system. Thrombosis may complicate pregnancy, the use of oral contraceptives or venous occlusive disease such as mediastinal malignancy. In the majority of patients, however, venous obstruction is not the predisposing cause and the cerebral venous system is normally patent.

Menstrual disorders

Apart from the complication of venous thrombosis, BIH is associated with pregnancy *per se*. It is not clear whether an association with menstrual irregularity is more than would occur by chance in obese young women. An association with menarche has been reported.

Deficiency states

A rare cause of BIH in children is hypovitaminosis A due to generalized nutritional deficiency or a malabsorption syndrome. In such cases BIH responds specifically to vitamin A supplements.

Interestingly, poisoning with vitamin A due to excessive consumption of fish or animal liver may cause BIH. Iron deficiency anaemia due to nutritional deficiency or chronic blood loss may be a further predisposing cause.

Iatrogenic causes
Although nalidixic acid, nitrofurantoin, tetracycline, and corticosteroids may cause BIH it is an extremely rare complication of treatment with any of these drugs. Corticosteroids usually lead to BIH during their withdrawal after chronic treatment.

Empty sella
It has been suggested that this association in about 4 per cent of cases is caused by raised intracranial pressure in combination with incompetence of the diaphragma sellae. The theory is supported by the finding of raised pressure at lumbar puncture in some patients with empty sella, suggesting chronic BIH as the underlying cause. Hypopituitarism does not occur, but occasionally the empty sella may harbour a prolactinoma.

Pathogenesis
The mechanism by which intracranial pressure rises is poorly understood and the contribution of various factors controversial. Since the intracranial contents are housed in a rigid container an increase in CSF pressure may result from an increase in blood volume, swelling of the brain parenchyma or an increase in CSF volume due to overproduction or malabsorption.

Increase in blood volume
A disorder of autoregulation leading to an increase in blood volume was originally proposed as the important factor. Measurements of cerebral blood volume (CBV) based on the clearance rate of injected isotope certainly indicate an increase in CBV which reverts to normal as BIH remits. However, the increase in CBV would only account for a volume increase in intracranial content of approximately 1 per cent and would not be sufficient to produce a sustained rise in CSF pressure. It is generally held, therefore, that an increased blood volume plays a minor role, and may indeed be secondary to the rise in intracranial pressure.

Swelling of the brain parenchyma
Direct evidence for swelling due to cerebral oedema is slight. An early report of oedematous changes in biopsied brain has not been confirmed since neither biopsy nor surgical decompression are indicated in current management. However, the tendency for the ventricles to be small may indicate an increase in cerebral volume.

If cerebral oedema is a significant factor it is almost certainly due to leakage from the cerebral vascular bed rather than transudation of CSF from the ventricular system. The CT scan in BIH does not show the periventricular leakage of CSF which occurs in hydrocephalus. Although there is currently no direct evidence for vasogenic cerebral oedema, this factor cannot be ignored because it is the only mechanism for raised pressure which does not anticipate some degree of hydrocephalus.

Increased production of CSF
Indirect measurements do not suggest that this is a significant factor. Furthermore, tripling the volume of CSF by saline infusion into the subarachnoid space of normal subjects produces only a small rise in CSF pressure.

Decreased absorption of CSF
A defect of CSF absorption is widely regarded as the important factor in the pathogenesis of BIH. Apart from those cases in which there is dural sinus thrombosis, it is assumed that the defect lies in the arachnoid villi of the superior saggital sinus where the bulk of CSF absorption normally takes place. The delayed clearance of radioiodinated human serum albumin (RISA) from the ventricular system after injection into the lumbar subarachnoid space is indirect evidence of reduced CSF absorption. In a recent study,

simultaneous cannulation of the superior saggital sinus and the subarachnoid space showed increased resistance to CSF absorption in the majority of cases. Finally, vitamin A deficiency in rats and cows produces a rise in intracranial pressure associated with diminished absorption of CSF and histological changes in the arachnoid villi which are reversible with vitamin A supplements.

The major objection to the theory of reduced absorption is the absence of hydrocephalus. Even though the obstruction to CSF flow is unusually sited, a degree of ventricular enlargement might be expected. Protagonists of the theory argue, however, that hydrocephalus should not occur when the rise in intracranial pressure is equally distributed between the subarachnoid space and the cerebral ventricles.

Endocrine investigations
In spite of the clinical associations which suggest an underlying disorder of female endocrinology, hormonal studies have not shown a consistent abnormality. The pituitary–adrenal axis is intact and occasional abnormal responses may be due to obesity rather than BIH. There have been few studies of thyroid function or prolactin secretion but both appear to be normal. CSF vasopressin levels are raised, but this is not specific and may occur in a variety of neurological diseases. A recent report of a specific increase in CSF oestrone, which might link BIH with obesity because adipocytes are the major source of oestrone, awaits confirmation.

Management
Except in rare cases due to vitamin deficiency or drugs, management of BIH is aimed at reducing intracranial pressure in order to abolish headache and protect vision. The methods advocated are difficult to evaluate because of the high spontaneous remission rate and the lack of controlled trials to compare different treatments.

The first approach is to carry out repeated therapeutic lumbar punctures every 2 to 5 days, withdrawing up to 30 ml CSF. Although pressure monitoring has shown that this procedure lowers CSF pressure for only 1.5 hours, a number of patients improve for some days. In about 20 per cent of cases, a spontaneous remission occurs after only two lumbar punctures. Although it is possible to continue with repeated punctures, corticosteroids are usually given if CSF pressure remains high on two or three occasions. A majority of patients respond to prednisolone 40–60 mg daily within two weeks and do not relapse after withdrawal. Longer steroid treatment does not significantly increase the remission rate and surgical drainage by a shunt should then be considered. Because of the technical difficulty of tapping small ventricles, a lumbo-peritoneal shunt is usually favoured. The timing of repeated lumbar punctures, the use of steroids, and the insertion of a shunt, depends on the severity of visual loss and whether it is progressive. In the small minority of patients whose vision continues to worsen despite a shunt, surgical incision of the optic nerve sheath should be considered, although there is a risk of further visual loss postoperatively.

Although it is not established that weight loss *per se* is effective, a reducing diet is recommended for all obese patients.

Thiazide diuretics and carbonic anhydrase inhibitors produce a modest fall in CSF pressure but have little place in management when vision is threatened.

Pregnancy
The major threat is to the fetus and the rate of spontaneous abortion is increased. Spontaneous remission of BIH during pregnancy has been the rule, although the number of reported cases is small. It would seem reasonable to raise the clinical threshold for the use of steroids and rely upon repeated lumbar punctures during the early weeks, though steroids and shunt operations may occasionally be required.

Prognosis

Rarely, symptoms and progressive visual loss continue for years, temporarily relieved by medical or surgical treatment. Spontaneous remission is the rule, however, though there is evidence that remissions are clinical and that raised intracranial pressure may be found at follow-up lumbar puncture several years later. Clinical recurrence occurs in about 10 per cent of cases, often within a year, but sometimes several years later.

Mortality from BIH is nil in most recent series, though an underlying sagittal sinus thrombosis may lead to a fatal outcome. Permanent visual loss occurs in up to 50 per cent of patients and is a significant disability in 10 per cent. Apart from the fact that patients with permanent disability have visual symptoms and severe papilloedema at presentation, there are no known risk factors for visual loss. The height of the CSF pressure is not relevant. Because treatment is determined primarily by progression of optic nerve damage, serial visual field analysis is the important yardstick of clinical progress.

References

Ahlskog, J. E. (1982). Pseudotumor cerebri. *Ann. Intern. Med.* **97**, 249–256.
Janny, P., Chazal, J., Colnet, G., Irthum, B. and Georget, A. (1981). Benign instracranial hypertension and disorders of CSF absorption. *Surg. Neurol.* **15**, 168–174.
Johnston, I. and Paterson, A. (1974). Benign intracranial hypertension. *Brain* **97**, 289–312.
McComb, J. G. (1983). Recent research into the nature of cerebrospinal fluid formation and absorption. *J. Neurosurg.* **59**, 369–383.
Rush, J. A. (1980). Pseudotumour cerebri: clinical profile and visual outcome in 63 patients. *Mayo Clin. Proc.* **55**, 541–546.
Weisberg, L. A. (1975). Benign intracranial hypertension. *Medicine* (Balt.) **54**, 197–207.

HEAD INJURIES

G. M. TEASDALE

Each year in the United Kingdom one million head-injured patients attend hospital. Fortunately most injuries prove to be mild: 80 per cent of patients have not even been 'knocked out', only one in five is admitted to hospital and most of these stay for less than 48 hours. Nevertheless, some 5000 patients die each year and many others survive with mental disability. In a proportion of these cases outcome could have been improved by either more prompt or more effective recognition and treatment of secondary complications of the injury.

Many head-injury victims are young adult males and head injury is a leading cause of death and long-lasting mental disablement in the productive years of life. More than half of the more severe injuries are caused by road traffic accidents; other frequent causes are falls and assaults, often also related to alcohol intake.

The pathology of head injury

Scalp and skull injury

A scalp laceration is present in about 40 per cent of patients who attend hospital but a skull fracture is found in only 1.5 per cent. Although each feature can indicate the location and severity of impact on the head, this is less important diagnostically than the contribution they make to establishing that a head injury has occurred – if a history is not available – and the clue they provide to the risk of subsequent complications. The excellent healing of the scalp after surgical toilet and closure reflects its generous blood supply, but this can sometimes result in a laceration bleeding so profusely that shock ensues. This risk is highest in children or elderly people with extensive scalp injuries.

A skull fracture is described by several features. (*a*) *Location*: the vault of the cranial cavity; the posterior fossa; or the base of the skull. (*b*) *Shape*: linear (fissure) or comminuted into fragments. (*c*) If the fragments are *depressed* inwards. (*d*) If it is *open*, or compound, i.e. associated with a local wound which creates a passage between the exterior and the interior of the cranial cavity.

Traumatic brain damage (Table 1)

A certain amount of brain damage is sustained at the time of injury and in a closed, non-missile injury is the result of shear strains occurring within the head at the moment of impact. More important than such primary damage, at least from the point of view of early management, are the complications which lead to secondary brain damage. In a severe injury it is common for more than one disorder to be present; indeed the interactions between the various pathophysiological processes illustrated in Fig. 1 can pose the greatest threat to the brain, with ischaemia being the most important final mechanism in most cases.

Primary traumatic brain damage

Diffuse axonal injury results when the shear strains between different parts of the brain cause distortion, stretching, and even tearing of the axons in the white matter of the cerebral hemispheres and brain stem. The tiny neuronal lesions that result are distributed widely and diffusely and it is now believed that the number of these lesions and whether or not they are reversible or permanent, are the main determinants of the initial severity of a head injury. Clinically their characteristic feature is an immediate impairment of consciousness. In its most mild form, this may be

Table 1 Traumatic brain damage

Primary (impact) damage
Diffuse: axonal injury
Focal: cortical contusion and lacerations

Secondary complications
Extracranial: hypoxia, hypotension
Intracranial: haematoma, infection

Consequences of complications
Brain swelling, raised intracranial pressure
Brain shift
Hypoxic/ischaemic brain damage

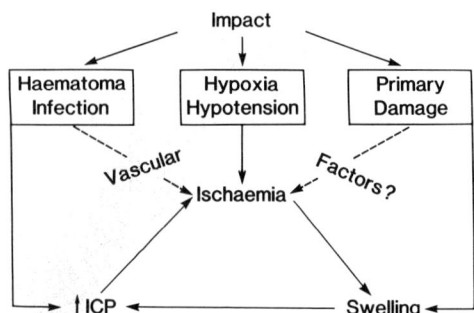

Fig. 1 Interactions between impact brain damage and the complications leading to secondary ischaemic brain damage.

restricted to a transient loss of awareness and memory for a few minutes classically referred to as 'concussion'. At the other extreme the patient may be in profound and prolonged coma. Diffuse white matter lesions are also thought to underlie many of the symptoms and much of the disability that follows when consciousness is ultimately recovered.

Contusions and lacerations are found focally, predominantly in the cerebral cortex. Whatever the site of blow on the head, the subsequent contusions are located maximally on the undersurfaces of the frontal and temporal lobes, and are due to displacement of the brain and contact with the sharp bony ridges at the base of the skull. The concept of a 'contrecoup' distribution of injury, i.e. maximal opposite to the point of impact on the skull, is now thought to be invalid. A blow struck violently with a sharp instrument may produce a compound depressed fracture with a contusion directly underlying the wound.

When contusions occur in an eloquent area of the cortex there may be focal neurological signs in the acute stage. Contusions in the frontal and temporal lobes also may contribute to the changes in personality and mental state and the epilepsy that can follow a head injury.

Secondary brain damage

Secondary brain damage develops after a delay and should be treatable or preventable. The damage to the brain is ultimately the result of ischaemia, secondary to inadequate delivery of oxygen, and is usually either a consequence of impaired oxygenation of the blood or an inadequate cerebral blood flow. The difference between the systemic arterial pressure and the intracranial pressure (ICP) is termed the cerebral perfusion pressure. Either a low blood pressure or a high ICP may threaten cerebral blood flow, and a combination is particularly dangerous.

Normally the brain copes with reductions in blood oxygenation or in cerebral perfusion pressure by adjusting the cerebral circulation to maintain adequate blood flow and oxygenation. Primary brain damage interferes with this autoregulatory mechanism so that flow may become dependent on the perfusion pressure, therefore, the brain is even more vulnerable after a head injury.

Extracranial complications

The most important complication of the immediate loss of consciousness characteristic of a head injury is airway obstruction and/or inadequate ventilation. So long as consciousness is impaired, and especially if a patient has other serious injuries, several factors may lead to hypoxia or hypotension (Table 2). Hypoxia and hypotension are particularly likely to occur during the transport of a patient between different departments in a hospital or between two hospitals.

Table 2 Causes of hypoxia or hypotension after a head injury

Hypoxia
Airway obstruction
Chest injuries (fractures, flail chest, haemo/pneumo/thorax)
Chest infection and pulmonary collapse
Lung shunting
Fat emboli
Adult respiratory distress syndrome
Neurogenic pulmonary oedema (rare)

Hypotension
Multiple injuries with blood loss
Associated spinal cord injury
Excessive bleeding from scalp, from a base of skull fracture, or, in an infant, with an extradural clot
Myocardial injury or infarct

Table 3 Risks of an intracranial haematoma in adult head injured. Patients assessed at the time of first hospital attendance

	Percentage of head injuries	Risk of a haematoma
No skull fracture		
Fully oriented	91	1 in 6000
Not oriented	7	1 in 120
Skull fractured		
Fully oriented	1	1 in 30
Not oriented	1	1 in 4

Data derived from Mendelow et al, 1983.

Intracranial complications

Traumatic intracranial haematoma

Although only 1 in 500 patients attending hospital develops intracranial bleeding, the supposed unpredictability of this complication is responsible for the treacherous reputation of head injuries.

An extradural haematoma is usually associated with a skull fracture and is the result of bleeding between the site of the fracture and the underlying dura.

Intradural haematomas are more common (three out of four cases). The bleed may be into the subdural space or within the brain itself (intracerebral haematoma); in a third of cases there is a combination of subdural bleeding, cortical laceration, and intracerebral haemorrhage, the so-called 'burst' frontal or temporal lobes. Many patients have a skull fracture but intradural clots often are not closely related to the fracture as are the extradural clots.

Blood vessels giving rise to a traumatic intracranial haematoma probably are damaged at the time of injury, but some time is needed before the size of the haematoma is sufficient to exhaust the brain's capacity to compensate for a space-occupying lesion. There then ensues a combination of shift and mechanical distortion of the brain and also an impairment of cerebral blood flow secondary to the rise in intracranial pressure. The most important clinical characteristic of the resulting cerebral ischaemia is a deteriorating level of consciousness.

The interval between injury and deterioration is usually measured in hours, or days, but may be as short as a few minutes, or occasionally as long as a few weeks. During this period the patient is rarely completely well, most have persisting confusion or altered consciousness as a result of a degree of primary damage.

Risk of a haematoma During this 'silent' interval information about the presence or absence of a skull fracture and whether or not the patient is fully conscious can be used to estimate the risk of the patient later developing a haematoma (Table 3). More profound degrees of impairment of consciousness carry much greater risks. Even without a fracture, persisting coma carries a risk of a haemotoma of 1 in 4.

Infection

Meningitis and brain abscess are complications of either a compound depressed fracture of the vault of the skull, or an open fracture of the base of the skull. In the latter case, where the fracture runs into the paranasal air spaces, the clue to the risk of infection is the presence of a leak of CSF from the nose (rhinorrhea) or from the ears (otorrhea). Other signs of a basal fracture are corneal or conjunctival haemorrhage without a posterior limit, a black eye on both sides, and bruising developing behind the ear (Battle's sign). Sixty per cent of cases are due to the pneumococcus but a wide variety of organisms can be responsible. Infection may develop several days, weeks or sometimes years after the injury.

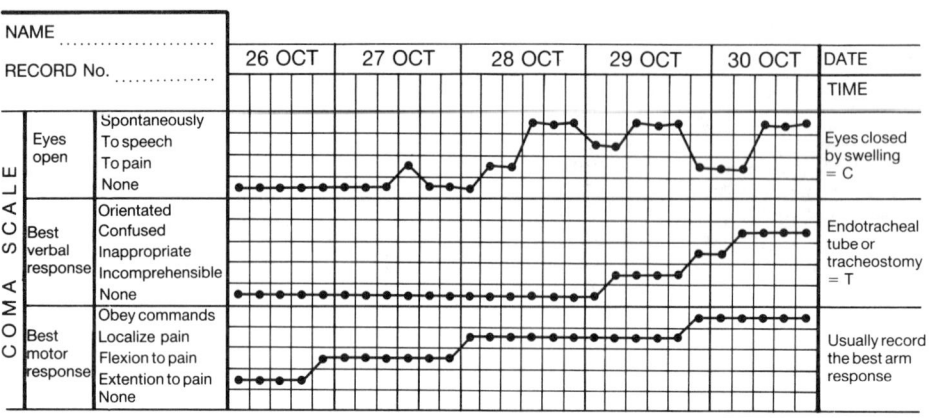

Fig. 2 Chart showing Glasgow Coma Scale recorded on a patient progressively recovering from a diffuse primary head injury. (Reproduced by kind permission of the *Journal of the Royal College of Physicians*.)

Brain swelling

The damaged brain around a contusion or underneath a blood clot may become progressively swollen; this can also occur diffusely in one or both cerebral hemispheres. The cause may be a vascular engorgement or true oedema, i.e. an accumulation of water. Oedema and engorgement may be less common than previously believed. They seem to occur often as a response to an injury, rather than being a primary mechanism in producing damage.

Other neurological complications

Other structures that may be injured in a head injury include the cranial nerves (especially the olfactory, optic, occulomotor, facial, and auditory nerves), and, in severe injuries, the pituitary gland and hypothalamus. Deafness and dizziness may also be caused by damage to the structures of the middle and inner ear, either as a result of the initial forces of the injury or a fracture of the base of the skull.

Management in the acute stage

Resuscitation

(See also Section 14.)

The ABC of resuscitation is the priority in those patients who arrive at hospital in coma, or who have multiple injuries. The *airway* must be cleared and maintained free from the earliest possible moment. As a temporary measure this may be achieved by placing the patient in the semiprone position; later the use of oropharyngeal or endotracheal tubes may be necessary. If *breathing* proves inadequate, particularly as judged by abnormal blood gas values, mechanical ventilation may be necessary. Restoration of an adequate *circulation* is essential; hypotension is rarely the result of a head injury alone and should be a signal to search for serious extracranial injuries.

Diagnosis

In a patient with impaired consciousness an accurate initial diagnosis can be difficult but it is important to discover the answers to two questions. Has the patient had a head injury? Has the patient had only a head injury? Common errors include the misdiagnosis of a head-injured patient as being 'drunk' or suffering from a stroke, or the overlooking of major injuries elsewhere in the body in a patient with an obvious head injury.

Assessing brain damage and its evolution

Changes in the level of consciousness are more important than focal neurological signs and provide an overall index of brain dysfunction and damage. Repeated assessments of the degree of altered consciousness provide a guide to the initial severity of brain damage and to the pattern of recovery. When a patient has suffered only primary damage, a steady improvement can be anticipated; if the patient's consciousness does not improve, and particularly if there is deterioration, the occurrence of secondary damage should be suspected.

It is therefore important to learn as much as possible about the immediate effects of the injury on conscious level and to reassess consciousness frequently. Communication of such information between nurses and doctors, and with doctors in other hospitals is an essential part of management and this task has been made simpler by the use of the Glasgow Coma Scale (see page 21.47).

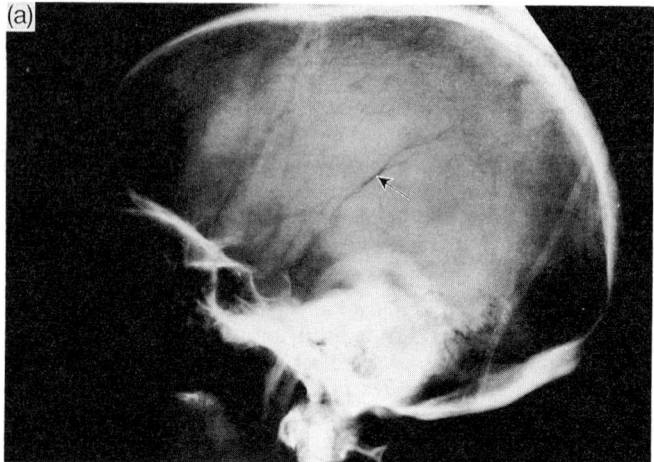

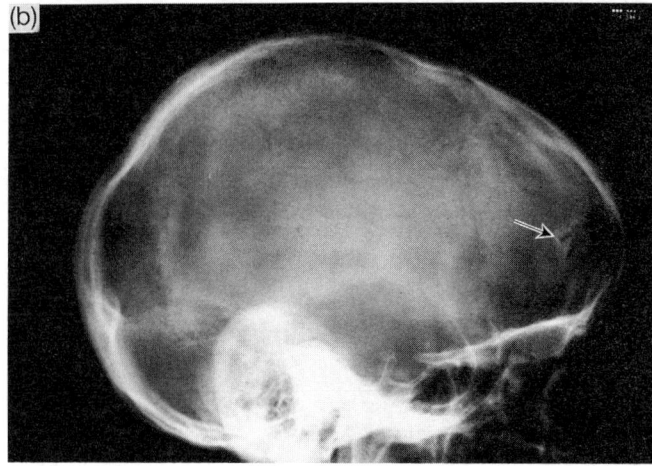

Fig. 3 Examples of X-rays of head-injured patients showing (a) Linear, fissure, fracture crossing the course of the posterior branches of the middle meningeal vessels. (b) A depressed comminuted fracture of the skull vault.

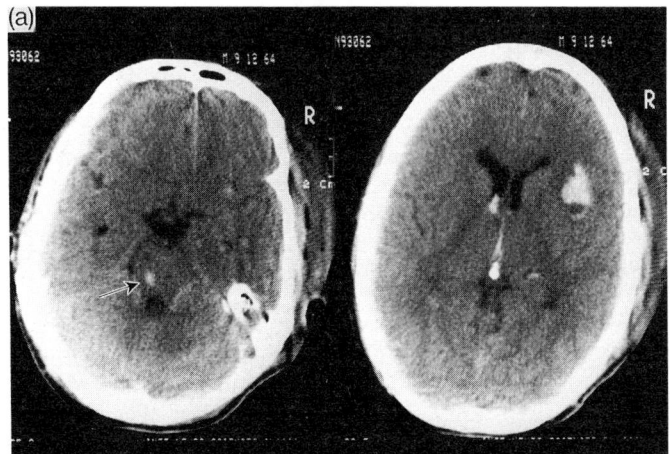

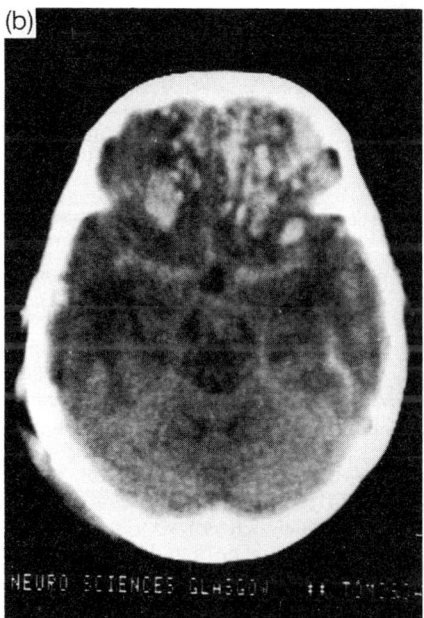
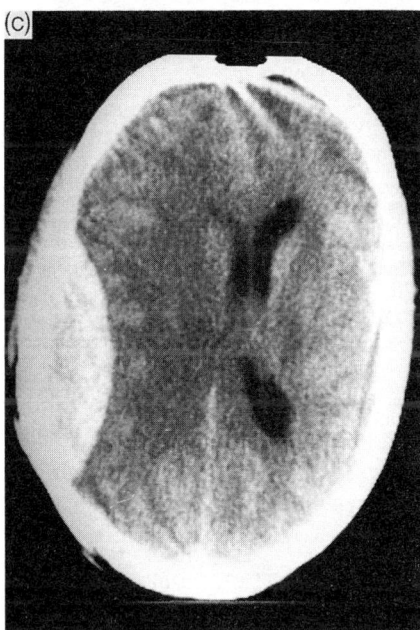
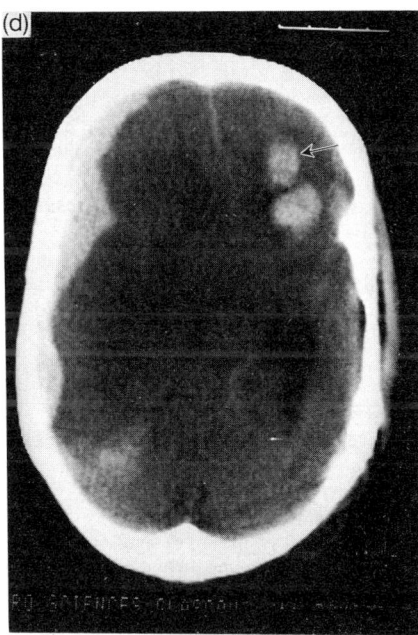

Fig. 4 Computed tomographic images of head injury. (a) Small areas of bleeding (white lesions) in the basal ganglia and brain stem (arrowed) of a patient with severe diffuse axonal injury. (b) Contusions in the cortex of frontal and temporal lobes. (c) An extradural haematoma. (d) Subdural and intracerebral (arrowed) bleeding.

This assesses three aspects of consciousness: eye opening, verbal, and motor responses, and can be readily and clearly charted (Fig. 2). Its use in coma is described in more detail on page 21.47 and Section 14. Comparisons of the movements and power of the limbs can be useful clues to focal damage, but tendon and plantar reflexes are rarely helpful. Changes in the response of the pupil to light are an important sign of dysfunction of the IIIrd cranial nerve and of developing intracranial shift and brain stem compression.

Radiological investigations (Fig. 3)
A skull X-ray can provide helpful information because the finding of a fracture greatly increases the risk of intracranial complications. Fractures of the vault are readily shown in X-rays but fractures in the base of the skull can be difficult to detect because some bones are paper thin and others extremely thick and dense. Suspicion should be raised by the finding of intracranial air or fluid levels in the paranasal air sinuses.

A skull X-ray is not needed for all head injuries, and clinical criteria that help to select patients for radiography are shown in Table 4. Whenever there is a question of multiple injuries, additional plain X-rays of the cervical spine, chest, and pelvis should be taken.

Table 4 Guidelines for the performance of a skull X-ray in a recently head-injured patient

Clinical judgement is necessary but the following criteria are helpful:

1 Loss of consciousness or amnesia at any time
2 Neurological symptoms or signs
3 Cerebrospinal fluid or blood from the nose or ear
4 Suspected penetrating injury
5 Scalp bruising or swelling
6 Difficulty in assessing the patient (i.e. alcohol intoxication, epilepsy, children)

Computerized tomography (CT) scanning
CT scanning (Fig. 4) can detect only the more severe forms of primary brain damage but its ability to show very clearly the presence of a haematoma has transformed the management of head injuries. Selection of patients for CT scanning is discussed below.

Intracranial pressure (ICP) monitoring
ICP monitoring is used in some units in the management of more severe injuries. Many of the complications of head injury cause a

rise in ICP and monitoring can provide early warning of their development and so direct appropriate management.

Management of intracranial complications

Intracranial haematoma

Until recently the diagnosis of an intracranial haemorrhage rested mainly upon finding evidence of deteriorating responsiveness. This led to the admission of many patients for observation in hospital for 1–2 days, most of whom proved not to have a haematoma. In practice there is not a characteristic sequence of changes in consciousness, and delayed recognition of deterioration allows secondary degree brain damage to develop. The capacity of CT scanning to enable diagnosis before deterioration becomes advanced and before cerebral compression becomes irreversible has provided the opportunity for more effective intervention. CT scanning often involves transfer to a neurosurgical unit and it is therefore necessary to select patients most likely to benefit.

The data about a skull fracture, the patient's initial conscious level, and the risk of a haematoma (Table 3) provide a basis for guidelines about which patients may merit admission for observation, which adults can be sent home, and those for whom CT scanning should be arranged without delay. Tables 5 and 6 show the guidelines used in the West of Scotland; essentially similar criteria have been put forward by a national group of neurosurgeons and accepted by a Government working party and it is expected that their use will improve the results of management of head injuries.

The outcome of operation for an extradural haematoma is usually good, with a mortality of 10–15 per cent. Although an intradural clot is more often associated with primary brain damage and mortality is 30–40 per cent, prompt evacuation is also usually followed by recovery.

Table 5 Guidelines for admission of adult head-injured patients to hospital

1 Confusion or any other depression of the level of consciousness at the time of examination
2 Skull fracture
3 Neurological symptoms or signs
4 Difficulty in assessing the patient, e.g. alcohol, epilepsy
5 Other medical conditions, e.g. haemophilia
6 The patient's social conditions or lack of a responsible adult/relative

Post-traumatic amnesia or unconsciousness with full recovery is not necessarily an indication for admission

Patients sent home should receive advice to return immediately if there is any deterioration

Table 6 Guidelines for consultation with a neurosurgeon about a head injured patient

1 Fractured skull
   with confusion or worse impairment of consciousness or
   with focal neurological signs or
   with fits, or
   with any other neurological symptoms or signs
2 Coma continuing after resuscitation – even if no skull fracture
3 Deterioration in level of consciousness or other neurological signs
4 Confusion or other neurological disturbances persisting for more than 6–8 hours, even if there is no skull fracture
5 Compound depressed fracture of the vault of the skull
6 Suspected fracture of base of skull (CSF rhinorrhoea or otorrhoea, bilateral orbital haematoma, mastoid haematoma) or other penetrating injury (gunshot etc.)
   Patients in categories 1–3 should be referred urgently

NOTE: In all cases the diagnosis and initial treatment of serious extracranial injuries takes priority over transfer to the neurosurgical unit

Depressed skull fracture

Open fractures of the vault of the skull require surgical debridement and closure both of the skin and of the dura. The latter forms a very good barrier to subsequent infection. If the operation is carried out within the first 24 hours the risk of infection is minimal, but heavily contaminated wounds are treated with prophylactic antibiotics.

CSF leakage and basal fracture

Such injuries are often associated with substantial primary damage to the brain but many of these fractures heal spontaneously. Therefore it is usual to delay operation and to close the fistula only in patients whose CSF leak persists for more than a week. Although there is controversy about their value, most British neurosurgeons recommend prophylactic antibiotic treatment during this period. Penicillin is administered because of its efficacy against pneumococcus, and sulphadimidine because of its ability to penetrate into the CSF

Multiple injuries

It is vital to diagnose and treat these injuries in order to stabilize the general condition of the head-injured patient. This takes priority over investigation and operation on intracranial injuries and is particularly important in victims of high-speed road traffic accidents. On the other hand, it is best to avoid extensive definitive surgery, e.g. for internal fixation of major limb fractures, which can often be postponed for some days, during which time simple external fixation suffices. Prolonged anaesthesia and major general surgery interfere with the monitoring of the patient's condition. If there is extensive bleeding with hypotension or if the anaesthetic agent raises the intracranial pressure, additional brain damage may be incurred. Table 7 shows the recommendations given to hospitals in the West of Scotland for the assessment and management of patients in coma or with multiple injuries prior to transfer to the neurosurgical unit.

Persisting coma

This carries risks of respiratory dysfunction and infection, fluid and electrolyte imbalance, nutritional deficiency, joint contractures, bedsores, and urinary infection. The avoidance of these usually entails management in a well-staffed and equipped intensive care unit (see Section 14).

Ventilation

This is necessary in patients whose respiratory dysfunction threatens adequate oxygenation. In some departments prolonged artificial ventilation is employed routinely in order to lower the patient's CO_2 level, and hence to reduce intracranial pressure. Evidence that this treatment actually benefits recovery from brain damage is lacking.

Osmotic agents

Agents such as mannitol or frusemide are given intravenously to remove water from the brain and effectively lower intracranial

Table 7 Guidelines for patients in coma or with possible multiple injuries

1 Assess for respiratory insufficiency, for shock, and for internal injuries, especially after a high-velocity injury, e.g. a road traffic accident
2 Perform: (*a*) chest X-ray; (*b*) blood gas estimation; (*c*) cervical spine X-ray; (*d*) other investigations as relevant
3 Appropriate treatment may include:
   Intubate (e.g. if airway obstructed or threatened)
   Ventilate (e.g. cyanosis, PaO_2 <60 mmHg, $PaCO_2$ >45 mmHg
   Commence IV infusion (1500 ml/24 hours)
   Mannitol, only after consultation with neurosurgeon
   Application of cervical collar or cervical traction
   Immobilization of fractures, treatment of internal injuries
4 If accepted for transfer the patient should be accompanied by personnel able to insert or to reposition an endotracheal tube, and to initiate or to maintain ventilation

pressure. They can be useful in producing a temporary improvement, e.g. to buy sufficient time to allow definitive intracranial investigation, but repeated doses lose efficacy and may result in hypovolemia with reduced cerebral perfusion pressure, as well as leading to electrolyte imbalance.

Drugs

Drugs that have been used with the aim of preventing or ameliorating brain damage include corticosteroids (in the expectation of reducing cerebral oedema) and barbiturates (to depress cerebral metabolism). Although experimentally effective when given before an injury, recent clinical studies have shown conclusively that these treatments are not of value and they carry risks of increased infection and hypotension.

Late sequelae and disability after head injury

Amnesia

Recovery from altered consciousness is usually followed by a period of confusion and loss of memory. The time from the injury to the restoration of on-going memory is referred to as *post-traumatic amnesia (PTA)* and its duration provides a good index, albeit in retrospect, of the severity of brain damage. Some loss of memory for events immediately prior to the injury is common but such *retrograde amnesia* is usually relatively brief and shrinks as time passes.

Postconcussional symptoms

Even an apparently mild injury can be followed by a variety of symptoms, including headache, dizziness, failure of concentration, and impairment of memory. Because physical signs may be lacking, and any abnormalites are often subtle, the basis of these symptoms has been in debate. There is now evidence that periods of loss of consciousness of even as little as 5 min can result in diffuse axonal brain damage. This has provided a valid basis for many complaints, especially when they develop within the first few days after an injury. In many patients the symptoms resolve spontaneously, if sometimes slowly, but they can be perpetuated by premature return to 'stressful' work or by other causes of anxiety or depression. When there is a gap of some weeks between the injury and the onset of 'postconcussional' symptoms, it is likely that psychological factors are prominent in their generation.

Disability after severe injury

Prolonged loss of consciousness in the early stage increases the risk of persisting disabilities, and these are almost invariable when post-traumatic amnesia has been longer than a month. Obvious physical deficits, such as hemiparesis and ataxia, are less common and much less important than changes in mental function, and particularly in memory and personality. Assessment of outcome after head injury should therefore be directed to overall social reintegration as shown in Table 8.

Post-traumatic epilepsy

(See also page 21.59.)

Epilepsy occurring within one week of a head injury is distinguished from that developing later, which is more likely to recur. The main pointers to the risk of late epilepsy are the presence, in the acute stage, of an intracranial haematoma, a compound depressed skull fracture, particularly with dural laceration, and amnesia for more than 24 hours. The treatment of post-traumatic epilepsy should be with conventional anticonvulsant drugs. Prophylactic treatment may be considered appropriate if the risk is judged to be very high but compliance is often poor unless or until a seizure occurs.

Chronic subdural haematoma

A fluid collection of blood between the dura and the brain can follow even a relatively mild head injury, particularly in the elderly,

Table 8 Glasgow scale of outcome after severe head injury

Death	Most occur in the first week but may be
Vegetative state	delayed several months. Spontaneous breathing and eye opening and 'sleep–wake' cycles present but no sign of psychologically mediated responses; do not speak; do not obey commands
Severe disability	Conscious, speaking, some have no physical disabilities but mental changes predominate in making a person dependent for survival in society, e.g. cannot shop, cannot go on public transport
Moderate disability	Independent, but are unable to resume fully preinjury activities; may work but in a reduced capacity
Good recovery	Able to resume preinjury life-style, even if mild residual neurological deficits are present

alcoholics, or those with impaired coagulation function. In about half of cases no injury is recalled. Symptoms may occur hours or even months after the injury. If the condition follows a severe head injury with unconsciousness, the patient may recover consciousness only to lapse into coma again. In more chronic cases the course is typically fluctuating. Particularly in the elderly, however, the trivial injury is frequently forgotten. The commonest symptom is headache and, as the condition worsens, vomiting. The condition may cause considerable diagnostic difficulty in the elderly, particularly if it presents with mood changes, irritability, urinary incontinence, or drowsiness, all of which may be mistakenly attributed to senescence. The commonest neurological signs are pupillary inequality, and long track signs with motor limb asymmetry and, occasionally, an extensor plantar response. Dysphasia occurs in about a fifth of patients. Fits are less common although they occurred in approximately 5–10 per cent of cases in one large series.

This condition should be suspected in any patient who deteriorates after an initial period of improvement after a head injury or who presents with an unusual neurological picture at any age. In the majority of cases the condition can be diagnosed by CT scanning although, because the subdural collection may be isodense at some stage during its evolution, the interpretation can be difficult. Isotope scanning is also accurate in about 90 per cent of cases. The treatment of choice is to evacuate the haematoma through burr holes. It is possible that very small collections can be allowed to resolve under careful surveillance. It has also been suggested that corticosteroids may have a place to play in mild cases although this remains uncertain; subdural haematoma should never be treated without expert neurosurgical advice. A review of recent results showed that the overall mortality was 6 per cent which seems to have changed little following the advent of CT scanning. Another 5 per cent showed severe disability while the outcome was good in 89 per cent of cases. Importantly, the prognosis was not related to age and therefore this condition should be sought for and treated actively in all age groups.

Hydrocephalus

Hydrocephalus very occasionally results from an obstruction of the CSF pathways and should not be confused with the passive *ex vacuo* ventricular enlargement which occurs with cerebral atrophy after a severe head injury. This can be brought about by fibrosis, a sequel to bleeding in the early stages, and such patients may be greatly benefited by insertion of a ventriculoperitoneal shunt in order to divert the CSF flow.

Brain damage after boxing, post-traumatic encephalopathy

It has been recognized for many years that certain boxers developed a syndrome characterized by forgetfulness, irritability, dysarthria, pyramidal damage, and ataxia. This occurred particularly after a long but unsuccessful career – prompting the term 'punch drunk'. Although in some cases the deterioration appeared to be simply an acceleration of normal aging processes, in others it progressed more rapidly. In such cases a specific accentuation of damage in the hippocampus and mamillary bodies has been suggested by post-mortem studies.

There is clinical evidence that repeated minor head injuries in many other sports (e.g. riding) may also cause cumulative brain damage, and there is now great concern that sports' participants should be warned of this risk. Although it is customary to advise a person who has been 'knocked out' to refrain from sport for some time, it is not known for how long this should be, or indeed if it will ever be 'safe' again.

References

Adams, J. H., Graham, D. I., Scott, G., Parker, L. S. and Doyle, D. (1980) Brain damage after fatal non-missile head injury. *J. Clin. Pathol.* **33**, 1132–1145.

Anon (1984). Guidelines for initial management after head injuries in adults *Br. Med. J.* **288**, 983–985.

Brooks, N. *et al.* (1984). *Closed head injury. Psychological, social and family consequences.* Oxford University Press, Oxford.

Fenton Lewis, A. (1983). *The management of acute head injury.* Harrogate Seminar Report 8, Department of Health and Social Security, London.

Jennett, B. and Teasdale, G. (1981). *Management of head injuries.* F. A. Davies, Philadelphia.

Mendelow, A. D., Teasdale, G., Jennett, B., Bryden, J., Hessett, C. and Murray, G. (1983). Risks of intracranial haematoma in head-injured adults. *Br. Med. J.* **287**, 1173–1176.

Teasdale, G. and Jennett, B. (1974). Assessment of impaired consciousness and coma. *Lancet* **ii**, 81–84.

DEVELOPMENTAL ABNORMALITIES OF THE NERVOUS SYSTEM

D. GARDNER-MEDWIN

Introduction

In about 1 per cent of all births the baby has a malformation of the nervous system. About 2 per cent of school children are mentally retarded, and at least 3 per cent of school leavers have some form of neurological handicap.

Developmental disorders are defined by the coexistence and mutual effects of a pathological lesion or function and continued growth and development. Primary agenesis or early destruction of a structure is followed by abnormal development or dysgenesis of related ones. The extent to which this happens is greatest during embryogenesis, but it occurs in an anatomical sense at least to the age of 2 years, and all neurological lesions in early life have effects on the functional and social development of children for as long as their personalities and the patterns of their lives continue to grow.

Down syndrome, spina bifida and probably the fragile X syndrome are the commonest entities, but several hundred different anomalies and syndromes contribute to the remainder and a variety of noxious agents and accidents, most of them poorly understood, may interfere with the complex development of the nervous system before or after birth. Ideally it should be equally possible to classify the developmental disorders according to the clinical features, or the pathology, or the developmental processes involved, or the causation. In practice, none of these is wholly feasible. A variety of causes may give the same clinical or pathological effect, and the timing of an insult is usually more important than its nature in determining its outcome. In most developmental malformations the cause is unknown, and while the origin of some may be dated to a particular stage of embryogenesis the defects in others clearly span long periods of development. Tables 1 and 2 illustrate some known associations but classification in this chapter is arranged on a clinical and anatomical basis.

Neurological assessment of a patient with a developmental disorder of the nervous system should be designed to identify

1. the site of the lesion(s);
2. the nature of the pathology;
3. the nature and degree of the handicapping effect on the patient and his family;
4. the genetic recurrence risk for other members of the family; and
5. any opportunity for specific treatment.

Therapy to alleviate or circumvent handicap is possible in all cases whether it is aimed at developing the skills of the patient or, in the most profoundly handicapping disorders, at providing relief for the parents and family who are the principal sufferers in such a situation.

Mental retardation

Mental retardation or subnormality is defined as permanent impairment of intelligence necessitating special care or training; in severe subnormality the person is incapable of independent life or of protecting himself from exploitation. For educational purposes children are classified as educationally subnormal whether moderately (ESN(M)) or severely (ESN(S)). The IQ lies in the range 50–69 or below 50 respectively. Profound retardation implies an IQ below 30. Among school children the prevalence rates for ESN(M) lie between 15 and 25 per 1000, for ESN(S) between three and four per 1000. In addition many children suffer from lesser degrees, and often specific patterns, of learning difficulties requiring special help at normal schools.

Severe subnormality occurs almost equally frequently at all socioeconomic groups. It is usually associated with identifiable cerebral pathology (Table 3). Moderate handicap is more rarely so; some cases represent the lowest part of the range of normal human intelligence, others have minimal pathology. To polygenic hereditary factors in families of low intelligence are added the effects of deprivation of intellectual stimulation or training, the inculcation of maladaptive patterns of behaviour, and in some families, the effects of poor nutrition, emotional deprivation or frank non-accidental injury.

The responsibilities of the doctor to this major section of our society lie in three main areas:

1. the early diagnosis of mental retardation and its differential diagnosis from other causes of delayed or deviant development;
2. the recognition of specific causes of mental retardation and the provision of genetic counselling and, if possible, treatment;
3. the recognition and management of associated handicaps involving impaired vision, hearing, behaviour, motor skills or epilepsy.

Retardation may be predicted at birth if a major associated malformation syndrome or microcephaly are recognized. However, certain abnormal-looking babies, for example with the Treacher–Collins syndrome, Moebius syndrome or certain craniofacial dysostoses may be expected to have normal intelligence. Other children 'at risk' of handicap because of adverse factors in their

Table 1 Brain development and malformations

Postovulatory stage	Developmental process	Some related malformations
Preconception	Gametogenesis	Chromosome anomalies
Preconception to 3 days	Gametogenesis, early cell division	Mutant genetic disorders
	Embryogenesis	
15–17 Days	Neural plate	None, or lethal
18–30 Days	Notochord present	Induction disorders— vertebral clefts; ? chordomas; ? teratomas; ? holoprosencephaly
22–24 to 40+ Days	Forebrain and optic vesicles appear	Holoprosencephaly
24–26 Days	Anterior neuropore closes	Anencephaly
26–32+ Days	Neural crest cells proliferate	? Neurocutaneous syndromes; ? Sturge–Weber syndrome
26–28 Days	Posterior neuropore closes	Spina bifida
28–32 Days	Spinal nerve roots form	Thalidomide intoxication
30 Days to 25 weeks (especially 10–18 weeks)	Neuronal proliferation	Primary microcephaly; ? megalencephalies; ? embryonal cell tumours
7–20+ Weeks	Neuronal migration	Lissencephaly, 3rd–6th month; Zellweger syndrome; ? fetal alcohol syndrome; ? agenesis of corpus callosum, 10–15 weeks ? Craniopharyngiomas *Destruction* causes hydranencephaly and polymicrogyria
4–8 Weeks	Cerebellar vermis forms	Dandy–Walker syndrome Joubert syndrome
	Later fetal development	
20 Weeks to 4 years	Glial proliferation	Fetal malnutrition; 2° microcephaly
18 Weeks to 2nd decade (mainly 32 weeks to 2 years)	Myelin formation	Amino acid disorders and leucodystrophies
18+ Weeks to 4+ years	Synapse formation	? Phenylketonuria; secondary 'deprivation' syndromes

gestation or birth, or severe cerebral symptoms in the newborn period, must be assessed at intervals and given special stimulation and support until their developmental status declares itself. These children, and those others who come to attention because of delay in the attainment of normal motor, language and behaviour skills, must not be judged to be intellectually retarded until alternatives, especially deafness, specific motor or language handicaps, infantile autism, emotional deprivation, and chronic illness have been excluded. Developmental assessment techniques may be used to screen the population for children who are delayed; the analysis of the nature and degree of their handicaps requires repeated assessment by a skilled team over a prolonged period of infancy, coupled always with stimulation, provision of opportunities for learning, and repeated assessment of the response to this intervention.

Once mental handicap is identified or suspected, its cause should be sought. In most large-scale reviews 20–40 per cent of cases are of unknown cause, and of the remainder about two-thirds originate before birth and one-third are acquired in the perinatal period or later. A detailed history of the gestation and birth (preferably from the obstetric notes) may reveal 'risk factors'; a search for dysmorphic features may provide clues, not only to specific syndromes but sometimes to the timing of a lesion in relation to embryogenesis. Abnormalties of stature and of head growth are further clues in many cases. At this stage a search of one of several books on dysmorphic syndromes may prevent the

Table 2 Some causes of prenatal malformations

Cause	Effects or examples
Parental balanced translocation	Chromosome disorders
Single gene defects	For example, Crouzon, Meckel, Aicardi, Zellweger syndromes
Low maternal age	? Septo-optic dysplasia; predisposes to cerebral palsy
High maternal age	Down syndrome
High paternal age	Genetic mutations
Radiation	Microcephaly, retardation, cerebellar defects
Trauma	For example, amniocentesis, failed abortion, maternal hypotension
Maternal fever	Retardation + dysmorphism
Exogenous toxins	For example, thalidomide, alcohol, organic mercury
Endogenous toxins	
Maternal	Maternal phenylketonuria or diabetes
Fetal	For example, Zellweger syndrome
General nutritional deficiency or placental insufficiency	Microcephaly, retardation; predisposes to perinatal asphyxia
Specific nutritional deficiency	Iodine deficiency (endemic); ? vitamins and neural tube defects
Intrauterine infection	Cytomegalovirus, rubella, etc.
Death of a twin	Microcephaly, encephalomalacia in the survivor

Table 3 Causes of severe mental retardation*

	Moser and Wolf (1971) IQ < 70†	Turner (1975) IQ < 50‡
Metabolic and genetic disorders	4.2	11.6
Down syndrome	17.0	[18]
Other chromosome anomalies	1.7	1.1
Multiple anomaly syndromes	5.9	2.7
Congenital CNS malformations	4.7	3.9
Prenatal infections	2.8	1.9
Postnatal infections	3.9	5.3
Perinatal encephalopathies	17.4	11.9
Postnatal trauma, etc.	1.9	1.9
Unknown, with neurological signs	20.2 ⎫	
with fits but no signs	3.0 ⎬ 39.3 (63% male)	41.7
without fits or neurological signs	16.1 ⎭	
Others	1.3	—

* Figures (per cent) adapted from original data.
† 1378 residents of a state institution (IQ < 50 in 78%); all ages.
‡ 1000 children assessed for IQ < 51; Down syndrome separately estimated.

need for extensive investigation. Otherwise the depth of investigation of a child with mental handicap will depend on the clinical findings but is usually designed to identify congenital infections, chromosome anomalies, and those of the inborn errors of metabolism that are compatible with the clinical picture. Some of the amino acid disorders and mucopolysaccharidoses may present with featureless retardation. Clinical features necessitating wider investigation for metabolic errors include:

1. regression in development;
2. progressive microcephaly or megalencephaly;
3. deteriorating epilepsy;
4. progressively abnormal neurological signs;
5. intermittent neurological deterioration, especially during infections or fasting;
6. suggestive ocular, skeletal, abdominal, skin or hair abnormalities;
7. a suggestive family history.

In males with featureless and unexplained mental retardation, the fragile X syndrome and preclinical Duchenne muscular dystrophy should be excluded.

Treatable (or partially treatable) causes of mental retardation are few and are usually indicated by progressive or fluctuating symptoms. Examples are congenital hypothyroidism, phenylketonuria, galactosaemia and some of the vitamin-responsive neurometabolic disorders (see Section 9), compressive disorders, especially hydrocephalus, bilateral subdural haematomas or craniosynostosis, and some epileptic syndromes in which chronic minor status may occur.

Specific learning disorders

Mild or subtle handicaps are common, are recognized late and are often managed less well than severe ones. A child with intelligence 'within the normal range' but well below the rest of the family, and the child with normal overall intelligence but a specific learning disorder, mild motor handicap or behavioural disorder may suffer the impatience and misunderstanding of parents and teachers. If they come to medical attention at all such symptoms as *dyslexia*, *clumsiness* or *hyperkinesis* may be falsely elevated to the status of diagnoses. In such circumstances the search for physical signs of neurological dysfunction must be extended beyond the routine of the neurologist by a clinical psychologist willing to analyse defects of perception or concentration, disconnection of sensorimotor function, etc. This provides a starting point for a search for the underlying pathology, and for planning remedial education. The aetiology of specific learning disorders is rarely identifiable with certainty. Genetic factors and prenatal or perinatal risk factors should be critically examined before being accepted as relevant.

Epilepsy or a past history of cerebral trauma, encephalitis or meningitis are found in a minority. Cognitive problems are occasionally the presenting symptom of subacute sclerosing panencephalitis (SSPE) or of adrenoleucodystrophy, Huntington's chorea, or other progressive genetic encephalopathies, so in unusual cases follow-up to rule out progressive disorders is wise. There is an increased incidence of congenital apraxia in sex chromosome reduplication disorders.

Infantile autism

This is a particular form of deviant and delayed development characterized in 1943 by Kanner. Autistic children look normal, even graceful, but their severe language disorder and lack of emotional rapport or even eye contact, are major barriers to communication. Solitary and orderly, they treat people as objects, sometimes favourite objects, and words as meaningless sounds. Speech and gesture are absent at first or at best echoes and stereotypies. About half develop useful speech by the age of 5 years. Play is repetitive, joyless and ritualistic but sometimes mechanically skilful. Spinning objects and toe-walking are common habits. Adaptive behaviour is often seriously retarded though sometimes nearly normal; 40 per cent have IQs below 50 and 30 per cent above 70. About 25 per cent develop epilepsy, usually in adolescence.

Most autistic children are abnormal from birth, in a few language and behavioural regression occur in the second year after an initial normal period of development. In such children, neurodegenerative disease, Rett syndrome, the epileptic aphasia syndrome, minor status epilepticus, and psychosis enter the differential diagnosis.

Autistic features are often seen in the behaviour of deaf children or those with other severe language disorders, yet a disorder *sui generis* does seem to exist. Special education as 'maladjusted' children requiring individual teaching offers some improvement in the generally poor social prognosis. The incidence is 0.2–0.4 per 1000; sibs, except monozygotic twins, are rarely affected. The aetiology is unknown; no consistent neuropathological changes have been discovered.

CHROMOSOME ANOMALIES

Down syndrome (trisomy 21)*

This is the most frequent single cause of mental retardation. It contributes 20–30 per cent of the total population prevalence and in most large mental retardation hospitals about 15–20 per cent of the patients have Down syndrome. The familiar facies can be recognized in renaissance paintings, yet the first case description was in 1846 by Seguin, 20 years before the account by Langdon Down. In 1959, 3 years after the normal number of human chromosomes had been established as 46, an extra G chromosome was discovered in Down syndrome by Lejeune and by Jacobs and their colleagues.

Trisomy 21 due to non-disjunction (see Section 4) accounts for all but 8 per cent of cases. The rest are the result of translocations, usually group F or G chromosomes, or rarely of parental mosaicism. The resulting neuropathology is not very obvious, but the brain weight is low with relative hypoplasia of the superior temporal gyri and the cerebellum. There is a simple gyral pattern, and the density of cortical neurones and the number of synapses are reduced.

The natural incidence is about 1.5 per 1000 live births in most races. It rises exponentially with increasing maternal age (0.38 per cent at age 35 years, 3.75 per cent at age 46 years). There is some evidence that maternal hypothyroidism is an occasional predisposing factor. Studies of spontaneous abortuses suggest that two-thirds of trisomy 21 fetuses fail to survive to term. The increasing use of amniocentesis to screen for chromosome anomalies in mothers over the age of 35 has resulted in a decline in the incidence.

*The nomenclature of chromosome abnormalities is described in Section 4.

Clinical features

The major clinical features are a round flat face with slightly up-slanting palpebral fissures, Brushfield spots on the iris, epicanthus, brachycephaly, short stature especially affecting the limbs, small hands and fingers, small 5th middle phalanges, clinodactyly, transverse palmar creases, a prominent fissured tongue, hypoplastic ears, and infantile hypotonia. Certain dermatoglyphic anomalies (more than eight digital ulnar loops, and distal axial triradii) are characteristic. Redundant skin folds over the nape, and hypotonia may be prominent at birth. The development of walking is delayed and throughout life the gait remains broad-based; the speech is usually dysarthric and hoarse. Strabismus, nystagmus and myopia are common.

The usual range of IQ in Down syndrome is 20–80, in most cases being between 35 and 55. The rare mosaic cases are often brighter.

Practical self-help skills, personal affection, a sense of humour, mimicry, and musical appreciation are relatively well-preserved while abstract thought and number sense are very poor. A decline in IQ is sometimes observed in late childhood or subsequently. Institutionalization or hypothyroidism are sometimes responsible, but dementia associated with the pathology of Alzheimer disease is also a frequent and specific complication even in childhood but more often after the age of 30 years. Few adults survive beyond 50 years.

Complications

Neurological complications in childhood include centrencephalic epilepsy in up to 10 per cent of cases, infantile spasms being particularly associated with subsequent profound handicap. Occasionally spinal cord compression, due to atlantoaxial dislocation, causes a progressive tetraparesis.

Severe complications may occur in infancy as a result of some common associated malformations especially congenital heart disease (in nearly 40 per cent of cases) duodenal atresia (2.5 per cent) or imperforate anus (0.7 per cent). The cardiac defects in decreasing order of frequency are atrial and ventricular septal defects, tetralogy of Fallot and patent ductus. Respiratory obstruction by adenoids in a hypoplastic pharynx, and aspiration pneumonitis are common. Acute myeloblastic leukaemia in the newborn and lymphoblastic leukaemia in older children are both relatively frequent but transient leukaemoid responses are a common source of error; together they affect 1 per cent of all cases of Down syndrome. Acquired autoimmune hypothyroidism is a frequent association. Most girls are subfertile, but pregnancy can occur; males are sterile. A distressing complication in adult life is corneal clouding consequent upon keratoconus.

Difficult decisions about treating life-threatening complications must often be made in early life. However, a half-hearted approach to the management of heart disease or epilepsy, for example, often results in more disabling and difficult symptoms later. Problems which are not likely to be fatal are best treated promptly and effectively both to avoid distress to the child and to support the parents in their attempts at an unequivocal approach to making his life as worthwhile as possible. Most children with Down syndrome are brought up by their families, in later life their relatively good social skills often make hostel accommodation and sheltered employment successful.

Prevention depends upon the screening of 'elderly' mothers by amniocentesis, and genetic counselling after checking both parents, and if necessary other relatives for balanced translocations. A low level of maternal serum alphafetoprotein is a potentially useful marker for Down syndrome and a normal level may reduce the need for amniocentesis in lower-risk pregnancies.

Other trisomies

Trisomy 13 and trisomy 18

Trisomy 13 and trisomy 18 are not infrequent malformation syndromes at birth, but are almost always lethal. The following rarer trisomies are compatible with survival into adult life (see also Section 4).

Trisomy 22

Intelligence may be normal, though most cases are mentally handicapped. The usual features are cleft palate, iris colobomas, preauricular appendages and sinuses, anal atresia, and congenital heart disease but there is much variation. Many survive to adult life. Affected relatives are common, so karyotyping and counselling the family is important.

Normal/trisomy 8 mosaic

Intelligence varies from normal to severe subnormality. Extra vertebrae, dolichocephaly, hypertelorism, bulbous nose, high-arched palate, joint contractures, absent patellae, deep palmar and plantar creases, thick skin and congenital heart disease occur. Agenesis of the corpus callosum is common.

Trisomy 9p

This disorder is characterized by retardation, short stature, microcephaly, hypertelorism, prominent nasal bridge and globular tip, simple ears, small fingers especially the fifth and hypoplastic nails.

Neurological aspects of the sex chromosome aneuploidies

Mental retardation occurs in a few cases of *Klinefelter's syndrome* (XXY syndrome), in which the average IQ is less than 10 points below controls, and with increasing frequency and severity in the XXXY and XXXXY syndromes. Apathy, lack of emotion and fatigue are common, and hypotonia, specific learning difficulties, tremor and congenital apraxia have been associated with these disorders, though not consistently. Men with XYY or XYYY are usually only mildly retarded if at all, but these anomalies have been associated with antisocial behaviour. Girls with *Turner's syndrome* (45X) are generally of average intelligence without neurological symptoms, but a rather consistent impairment of performance skills compared with normal verbal skills is found, together with defective number sense, and right–left disorientation (see also Section 4).

Deletion syndromes and other structural chromosomal defects

Major deletions of parts of chromosomes are generally fatal before birth or in infancy. Small deletions, while presumably more often compatible with survival, are more difficult to demonstrate. Grouchy in 1963 described a patient with 18p-. Shortly afterwards Lejeune and his colleagues described the first patients with the *cri du chat syndrome*, in which quite large deletions of the short arm of chromosome 5 (5p-) are compatible with survival at least into the sixth decade. The syndromes associated with the deletions 4p-, 13p-, 18q- and 21p- were identified in the 1960s. With improved banding techniques, quite small deletions, duplications, and chromosomal structural defects have been found to be associated with previously well-known syndromes such as the Prader–Willi syndrome and most importantly with certain cases of X-linked mental retardation which were not identified as comprising a recognizable entity until the discovery of the fragile site on the X chromosome which now gives the syndrome its name. It is certain that more of these small defects remain to be discovered and they may well hold the key to the pathogenesis of more retardation syndromes with which we are already familiar. The examples that follow are some of the deletion syndromes with implications beyond the period of early childhood.

Cri du chat syndrome (5p-)

This occurs in about one in 50 000 births. Some cases are familial with a balanced translocation of the deleted fragment in one

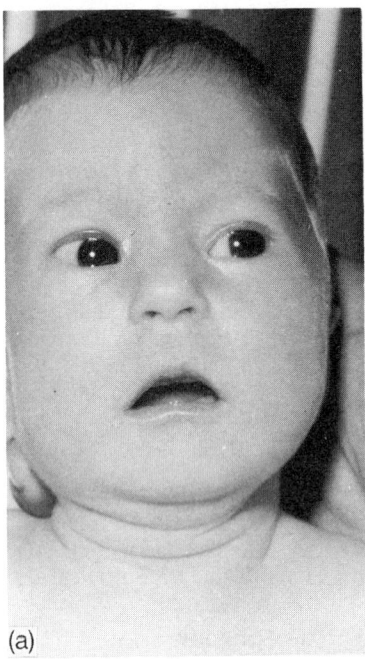
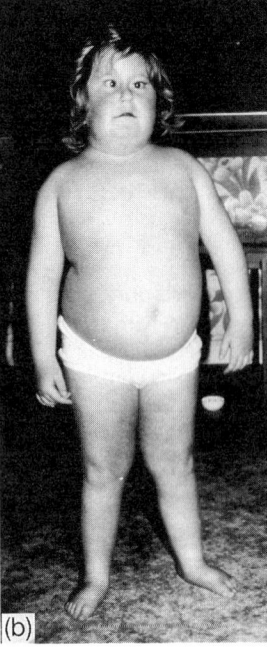

Fig. 1 Prader–Willi syndrome. The same patient aged (a) 3 weeks (b) 5 years; severe infantile hypotonia, later moderate retardation and obesity.

parent. Mental retardation is usually profound, but may be so mild as to comprise a selective learning disorder, the degree of retardation correlating broadly with the size of the deletion. The other cardinal features are remarkably constant: short stature, a mewing cry in the early years of life and distorted laryngeal anatomy, microcephaly, a wide nasal bridge, epicanthus, sometimes hypertelorism and micrognathia. Neonatal feeding and respiratory difficulties are frequent. About 30 per cent of cases have congenital heart defects. Many cases reach adulthood.

18p- Deletion

This is a rare disorder. Severe retardation, short stature, epicanthus, abnormal teeth, short neck, ptosis, etc. are usual. Some cases have arhinencephaly.

18q- Deletion

This is also rare. Severe infantile hypotonia, midface hypoplasia, eye anomalies, malformed ears, and genital hypoplasia in both sexes are associated with moderate or severe retardation and often with long survival.

The Prader–Willi syndrome

This syndrome is frequently associated with a small deletion at the q11 site on chromosome 15; possibly improved cytogenetic techniques will make the relationship more consistent. The presenting problem is severe neonatal hypotonia with swallowing difficulties usually requiring tube-feeding for several days or weeks. The typical facies may be recognizable in infancy with experience, and the ulnar border of the hand is abnormally straight (Fig. 1a). The genitalia are hypoplastic, often with cryptorchidism. Despite the hypotonia, muscle paralysis is not a feature and muscle biopsy reveals only immature muscle development. In later life short stature, small hands and feet, severe obesity (evident from about 9 to 15 months) and retardation (in the IQ range 20–90, usually 50–80) are the major features (Fig. 1b). The severe hyperphagia requires stringent calorie restriction for its control. Non-insulin-dependent diabetes is a frequent complication. Other minor endocrine anomalies are probably secondary to the obesity rather than causal. A defect in lipolysis has been suggested. Most cases arise *de novo*, and the risk of recurrence in sibs is under 2 per cent. A population incidence of one in 20 000 is possibly an underestimate.

The fragile X syndrome

This major cause of mental retardation, possibly accounting for 10–15 per cent of all cases, was identified as recently as 1969 (see also Section 4). The fragile site at Xq28 (near the tip of the long arm of the X chromosome) can be demonstrated only with difficulty, using special conditions of low concentrations of calf serum, thymidine and folate in the culture medium. Routine karyotyping, even with banding techniques, is of no value in excluding it. Further research is needed to allow easier routine diagnosis. At present the fragile site can not always be found even in affected siblings of proven cases, and occasionally it is found in normal males. The use of recombinant DNA techniques may prove helpful in the future.

The clinical diagnosis is no easier. The IQ is in the range 20–80, usually 50–60. Affected adult males are of normal stature but typically have high foreheads, large mandibles, prominent ears and, most characteristically, large testes, but these findings are not consistent (Fig. 2). Neurological examination is usually normal but tremor, apraxia and a broad-based gait are occasionally recorded. Stuttering repetitive speech is common. Affected young boys are even less easy to recognize. Macro-orchidism is often absent; the average birthweight and head circumference are slightly increased. Female carriers of the gene may themselves be retarded though most are normal. Turner found that 7 per cent of non-specific retardation among females in the IQ range 55–75 was associated with heterozygosity for the 'fragile X'.

The neuropathology and complications of the fragile X syndrome are not yet known.

Haemoglobin H disease and mental retardation

A *de novo* deletion which includes the site of one of the α-globin genes on chromosome 16 is probably responsible for the occurrence of several cases in which haemoglobin H disease has been associated with a syndrome of mental retardation (see also Section 19). Manifestation of α-thalassaemia (Hb H formation) depends in most cases upon inheritance from one parent of an abnormal α-globin gene on the other chromosome of the pair. Moderate or severe retardation, hypotonia, impaired co-ordination, talipes and mild anaemia with red cell inclusions were reported in the original cases. Whether an isolated deletion at this site, without the associ-

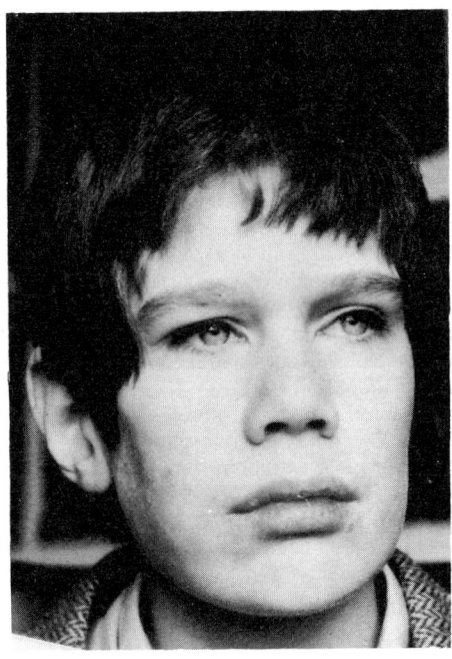

Fig. 2 Fragile X syndrome: a boy with severe mental subnormality and macro-orchidism. (Courtesy of Dr M. Bhate.)

ated 'marker' Hb H disease, occurs more frequently as a cause of mental retardation is not known.

Infections and teratogens

Congenital infections
The congenital infections are discussed in detail in Section 5. The principal agents which may cause congenital cerebral abnormalities are the viruses of rubella, cytomegalovirus (CMV), herpes simplex, acquired immune deficiency syndrome (AIDS), and rarely varicella or vaccinia, and various other organisms especially those of syphilis and toxoplasmosis, and occasionally listeriosis, tuberculosis, or malaria. Hamsters, for example, may develop aqueduct stenosis following mumps infection during gestation; and the association has been suspected but not proven in human beings.

Mental retardation is particularly associated with congenital rubella, CMV and toxoplasmosis. Microcephaly, hydrocephalus, and intracranial calcification can occur in CMV, herpes simplex, and toxoplasmosis. In all of these conditions an active meningoencephalitis may be present at birth; the infection may persist and in some cases cause progressive symptoms. Deafness may occur in any of these infections but is most prominent in rubella and CMV, while epilepsy is uncommon only in congenital rubella and is particularly frequent after perinatal herpes simplex infection.

Congenital CMV infection is probably the most important handicapping prenatal infection in the United Kingdom with a possible combined incidence of deafness and mental handicap of one in 2000–3000 live births (inapparent congenital infection is probably ten times as frequent). However, retrospective diagnosis is rarely possible if proof of infection (throat swab or urine culture or CMV-specific IgM antibody in the blood) has not been obtained within 3 weeks of birth. Primary maternal infection (not reinfection) at widely varying stages of pregnancy may lead to CNS handicaps, hence no simple clinically identifiable 'syndrome' can be defined.

Fetal damage by alcohol
Overt alcoholism during pregnancy causes a fairly uniform group of anomalies. The principal features are growth failure before and after birth, mental retardation (mean IQ 60–70), irritable behaviour in infancy and later hyperkinesis, microcephaly, short palpebral fissures, a short nose, small philtrum and thin upper lips, joint contractures, abnormal palmar creases and cardiac septal defects. A few cases have cervical vertebral anomalies, neural tube defects or hydrocephalus. The neuropathological features include microcephaly, defects of neuronal migration and, in some cases, callosal agenesis or cerebellar hypoplasia. Mild cerebral atrophy and cerebellar hypoplasia may be shown by CT scanning. Hepatic fibrosis is seen in some cases. Lesser alcohol consumption is associated with milder anomalies, but a measurable effect upon growth and a high fetal loss rate may occur when the maternal intake is the equivalent of two drinks daily (100 g alcohol per week); no 'safe' level has yet been established. The effect of publicity has been to stop many women drinking any alcohol in pregnancy. Nevertheless surveys, especially in Sweden, New York and Glasgow have shown a continued high incidence of the overt syndrome in some populations (one in 600 to one in 1000 live births).

Other teratogens
Direct evidence that a particular agent causes a CNS anomaly in a human fetus is uncommon. That the timing of a noxious stimulus is as important as its nature is clear from the graded series of different CNS malformations that result from experimental exposure of fetal rats at various stages of gestation to X-rays or vitamin A. The importance of the timing of exposure to thalidomide, or to rubella virus are parallel human examples. The effects of dosage,

duration of exposure, individual susceptibility or of variation in maternal metabolism or diet are not understood.

There are relatively consistent associations between maternal thalidomide ingestion at 24–40 days after conception and limb reduction defects secondary to embryonic sensory neuropathy, or earlier exposure causing microtia and deafness. Less consistent, but very frequent, are the occurrence of CNS malformations (hydrocephalus, anencephaly) and dysmorphism after ingestion of aminopterin or methotrexate at 4–10 weeks' gestation; microcephaly, mental retardation, and optic atrophy after warfarin ingestion in the second or third trimester (earlier exposure causes an embryopathy resembling Conradi syndrome, a dominantly inherited form of chondrodysplasia punctuata); retardation, microcephaly, blindness, and deafness after maternal methyl mercury intoxication; and microtia, deafness, and microcephaly with or without aqueduct stenosis and hydrocephalus and microphthalmos after the ingestion of high-dose vitamin A or the treatment of acne with retinoic acid derivatives.

The effect of other toxins upon the fetus has been less uniform, and occasional effects may require very large population surveys to distinguish them from chance associations. Such has been the fetal alcohol syndrome (see above) and the fetal phenytoin syndrome. The latter consists of short stature, hypertelorism, wide flat nasal bridge, short nose, cupid lip, cleft lip or palate, distal digital hypoplasia and various skeletal anomalies, and hirsutism. There is often retardation and microcephaly. As in the fetal alcohol syndrome only a minority of exposed fetuses manifest the syndrome and no clear dose effect or 'safe dose' is established. Other drugs in which there appears to be an increased risk of fetal CNS malformations, but which need further study, are valproate, troxidone, bromides, and organic solvents.

High fever in the mother at 4–14 weeks' gestation may cause an increased incidence of neural tube defects, central hypotonia, seizures, microcephaly, heterotopia or polymicrogyria, microphthalmos and various dysmorphisms.

Maternal iodine deficiency may cause mental retardation, spastic diplegia, deafness and cerebellar defects as well as growth retardation in the fetus. Uncontrolled maternal phenylketonuria (PKU) results in severe mental retardation and microcephaly often with spasticity and seizures.

References will be found in Emery and Rimoin (1983), and Smith (1982).

Complex malformation syndromes

Numerous rather specific syndromes are recognized, mostly of unknown aetiology, but some representing single gene defects and together contributing about 5 per cent of cases of mental retardation. The following are a few of the most frequent ones.

Aicardi syndrome
Here the main features are mental retardation, infantile spasms and later epilepsy, multiple lacunar retinal defects, agenesis of the corpus callosum, and independent electrical activity of the two hemispheres in the EEG. The disorder is confined to girls (probably X-linked dominant lethal in males).

Angelman syndrome
Also called the 'happy puppet' syndrome, this consists of moderate retardation without speech, microcephaly, flat occiput, jerky ataxic movements, smiling face, and gales of inappropriate laughter, protruded tongue, usually epilepsy and severe EEG polyspike and slow wave activity. It is non-progressive; the aetiology is unknown, and sibs are rarely affected.

Cockayne syndrome
The features are mental retardation, short stature, deep set orbits, microcephaly, retinal pigmentation, sensorineural deafness,

photosensitive rash, later peripheral neuropathy and ataxia. Cerebral calcification and leucodystrophy may be seen on CT scan. The disorder is of autosomal recessive inheritance.

Coffin–Lowry syndrome

In this disorder there is severe retardation, moderate growth retardation, downslanting eyes, hypertelorism, small maxilla, wide nose, short sternum, scoliosis and vertebral anomalies (on X-ray), large soft hands, tapering fingers, tufted distal phalanges (also on X-ray), and lax ligaments. It is of X-linked recessive inheritance; mothers may have scoliosis and the finger anomalies.

De Lange syndrome

This disorder is distinguished by severe retardation, short stature, low-pitched cry, microcephaly, hirsutism, synophrys, long eyelashes, small anteverted nose, small hands and feet and various minor skeletal anomalies. It is usually sporadic, and the aetiology is unknown. Many predict that a chromosomal deletion will be found.

Rubinstein–Taybi syndrome

Here there is retardation (usually severe), short stature, retarded bone growth, microcephaly, high arched palate, beaked nose, low set ears, broad thumbs and toes, and various other less constant anomalies including agenesis of the corpus callosum. It is a sporadic disorder, of unknown aetiology.

Smith–Lemli–Opitz syndrome

This comprises mental retardation, low birth weight, failure to thrive, irritability, microcephaly, severe hypotonia (central), anteverted nose, ptosis, broad maxillary alveolar ridges, cryptorchidism and hypospadias in males. It is of autosomal recessive inheritance. There are multiple anomalies of cerebrum, cerebellum and spinal cord.

Sotos syndrome (cerebral gigantism)

This is shown by mild to moderate retardation, high birthweight, macrosomia in childhood but advanced bone age and early epiphyseal fusion, megalencephaly, large hands and feet, high forehead, slight downslant of eyes, characterisitic facies, impaired coordination, increased incidence of febrile convulsions, and often scoliosis. It is sporadic, and probably of autosomal dominant inheritance confined to new mutants.

Williams syndrome (severe infantile idiopathic hypercalcaemia)

Here there is moderate or mild retardation, 'elfin facies', and supravalvular aortic stenosis. Hypercalcaemia may be severe in infancy but does not persist. There is early failure to thrive and vomiting. The retardation affects speech less than perceptual and motor skills. The disorder is sporadic and the aetiology and significance of the hypercalcaemia are unknown. Absorption of calcium is increased and sensitivity to vitamin D may be a factor. Restriction of calcium and vitamin D intake is useful in the hypercalcaemic phase of the disease, but not curative.

Zellweger (cerebrohepatorenal) syndrome

Features of this disorder are profound retardation, severe central hypotonia, areflexia, feeding difficulties, high forehead, flat facies, hepatomegaly, cirrhosis and sometimes liver failure, multiple small renal cysts, and often early seizures. Survival is usually under 6 months. The neuropathological features are micropolygyria, pachygyria, and defects of neuronal migration. Biochemical defects include excessive iron storage, excretion of pipecolic acid and failure to metabolize very long-chain fatty acids (carbon chains of 24–26 carbon atoms). Though uncommon, this disorder deserves mention as a rare example of cerebral malformation associated with a known biochemical defect. It is of autosomal recessive inheritance.

Non-specific defects of embryogenesis

Many malformations of the nervous system occur in such varied circumstances that they are plainly of multiple aetiology, yet they involve one or more particular embryonic processes so that their origin may be dated to before the completion of that process (see Table 1). The following examples involve the brain and cranial nerves, but spina bifida is another important example (see page 21.200).

Holoprosencephaly

This is complex malformation of the telencephalon and diencephalon in which a single forebrain ventricle may imitate hydranencephaly. Failure of the prosencephalon to form normal telencephalic, olfactory, optic and hypophyseal diverticula may reflect a failure of induction by adjacent mesodermal or neural crest tissue. The hemispheres fail to form, partially or completely, the olfactory system is often absent (arhinencephaly) and there may be malformation or aplasia of the optic nerves, the eyes and the pituitary. Associated facial malformations reflect the severity of the brain anomaly and range from anophthalmia or cyclopia with a proboscis, through various nasal malformations, hypertelorism and cleft lip, to mild anomalies of the midline of the face. Microcephaly and severe retardation are usual but their degree depends on the severity of the cerebral malformation. The most severe forms are fatal in infancy.

Chromosome anomalies (especially trisomy 13, trisomy 18 and 13q-; see page 21.193) are frequent causes of holoprosencephaly; various single gene disorders can also cause this malformation and many cases are of unknown cause. The milder forms can be seen in adults and may carry a high risk of dominant or X-linked transmission, so recognition of the anomaly must be followed by more precise diagnosis of its basis.

Agenesis of the corpus callosum

The characteristic appearence in ultrasound or CT scans makes this malformation easy to diagnose. With other anomalies it may be seen in the Dandy–Walker syndrome, holoprosencephaly, Aicardi syndrome, Rubinstein–Taybi syndrome, trisomy 13 or in rubella embryopathy (see pages 21.195) but as an apparently isolated finding it is usually but not always associated with mental retardation. Partial agenesis usually affects the posterior part of the corpus callosum. Dissociation of hemisphere functions is not as consistent a feature as one might expect probably because of sparing of other interhemispheric fibre tracts. Rarely, otherwise asymptomatic agenesis of the corpus callosum is associated later with episodic severe hyperhidrosis and hypothermia. The corpus callosum forms at 70–100 days gestation, so agenesis must date from this period or earlier.

Lissencephaly

This is a malformation in which the cerebral gyri are diminished or absent (agyria) or crudely thickened (pachygyria) and the cortical mantle lacks its normal six-layer structure. The pyramidal tracts are hypoplastic and there are often other cerebral anomalies. Defective neuronal migration at 8–16 weeks' gestation seems to be a fundamental feature, but not necessarily the primary cause. Microcephaly, mental retardation, spasticity and seizures (often infantile spasms) are the main clinical features. An autosomal recessive form (the Miller–Dieker syndrome) is characterized by a high, vertically furrowed forehead and short nose, low set ears and congenital cardiac, renal and genital anomalies; small deletions of chromosome 17p have been seen in some cases. An excess of fast rhythms is seen in the EEG. Other familial forms are reported and many cases are sporadic and of unknown aetiology. CT scanning effectively demonstrates agyria.

Septo-optic dysplasia

This is a syndrome of unilateral or bilateral optic nerve hypoplasia with variable dysplasia of the septum pellucidum and diencephalon. A characteristic small optic disc surrounded by a peripapillary halo ('double ring sign') distinguishes this condition from the rather vague entity '*Leber's congenital optic atrophy*' which also is frequently associated with cerebral malformation. Both of these disorders present with development delay, impaired vision and searching eye movements. The main features of septo-optic dysplasia are sporadic occurrence, a striking association with *low* maternal age, often neonatal jaundice and hypoglycaemia. Perinatal problems often apparently cause secondary additional brain damage, otherwise there is mild to moderate primary mental retardation (or none) and often hypothalamic or pituitary insufficiency. Most cases have seizures. The aetiology is not understood and may be multifactorial, probably acting in the first 40 days of gestation.

Cerebellar malformations

Various types of cerebellar agenesis or hypoplasia may be combined with other brain anomalies.

Joubert syndrome

Agenesis of the vermis or at least of its posteroinferior part is associated with severe mental retardation, inco-ordination, pendular eye movements and, characteristically, in the neonatal period, with periods of very rapid breathing (120–180/min) alternating with apnoea. Inheritance is autosomal recessive. Other associated defects such as meningomyelocele or tapetoretinal degeneration occur in some cases.

Chiari malformations

Herniation into the spinal canal of the cerebellar tonsils (in type I) or of parts of the hind-brain, vermis and IVth ventricle (in type II) was described by Chiari in cases of hydrocephalus. Type II is commonly associated with meningomyeloceles, but otherwise it may present in infancy with hydrocephalus or with brain-stem dysfunction (stridor and poor swallowing). It has its origin at the time of closure of the neuropores in the 4th week of embryonic development.

When hydrocephalus is slight or absent the type I or II anomaly may present much later in adult life, usually with the symptoms of associated syringomyelia (see page 21.100) or syringobulbia, but sometimes with neck pain, occipital headache, vertigo, drop attacks, ataxia or spasticity of gait. The symptoms are usually insidious but coughing or straining may precipitate them suddenly. Typical findings are vertical nystagmus and spastic paraparesis often with an obviously short neck and low hair-line, with or without dissociated anaesthesia, atrophy of the hand muscles, or lower cranial nerve palsies. Myelography in the supine position, CT scanning or, ideally, MRI scanning will demonstrate the anomaly. A skull X-ray may show basilar impression (*platybasia* – upward displacement of the base of the skull and the odontoid process) and cervical vertebral anomalies. Surgical decompression of the foramen magnum is helpful when compression is demonstrably contributing to the symptoms, but prior shunting of the hydrocephalus, if present, is essential.

The Dandy–Walker syndrome

In this anomaly hypoplasia of the vermis of the cerebellum is associated with cystic dilation of the IVth ventricle. The posterior fossa is expanded, often palpably, and usually there is secondary hydrocephalus. Atresia of the foramen of Magendie is possibly a factor, but it is not the primary defect. Multiple malformations of the brain and cord are often present probably dating from before the 7th week of gestation. The symptoms are usually obvious at birth but hydrocephalus may develop later and imitate the presentation of a posterior fossa tumour in late childhood or even in

adult life. CT scanning shows the wedge-shaped posterior fossa cyst and aplasia of the vermis. Hydrocephalus should be shunted on its own merits, but sometimes the cyst itself requires shunting.

Cranial nerve anomalies

Moebius syndrome

Congenital bilateral facial paralysis is associated in the great majority of cases with bilateral VIth nerve palsies, and less often with a total horizontal gaze palsy or with lesions of the IIIrd, IVth, motor Vth, Xth or XIIth nerves. Sometimes the lesions are asymmetrical. Talipes or widespread arthrogryposis, and mental retardation (in 10–15 per cent of cases only) are occasional features. Deafness is rare. The baby has difficulty in sucking, and later suffers from dysarthria and the social and emotional consequences of his expressionless face. Almost all cases are sporadic but occasionally dominant inheritance is reported. Controversy has persisted for almost 100 years as to whether aplasia or degeneration of the cranial nerve nuclei is responsible; convincing pathological evidence of each is found in various reports and the syndrome probably has more than one cause. Bilateral facial paresis is seen also in the congenital forms of myotonic dystrophy and facioscapulohumeral muscular dystrophy.

Other anomalies of the cranial nerves and eye movements

Isolated unilateral congenital pareses of the IIIrd, VIIth, XIIth or sometimes other cranial nerves are not uncommon. Two congenital disorders of eye movement which often cause clinical confusion are Duane syndrome and congenital oculomotor apraxia.

Duane syndrome

In this disorder, fibrosis of the lateral rectus muscle causes paresis of abduction, and retraction of the eye and ptosis on adduction. It may be unilateral or bilateral, is sometimes inherited as a dominant trait, and is occasionally associated with pseudopapilloedema and the Klippel–Feil syndrome.

Congenital oculomotor apraxia

This is a disorder of voluntary lateral conjugate eye movement with preservation of reflex movements. Slow pursuit movements may be possible but rapid saccadic movements are not, and the patient blinks and jerks his head to achieve rapid alterations of gaze by the 'doll's eye' reflex. This anomaly is a common feature of ataxia telangiectasia.

Abnormal enlargement of the head in infancy

Measuring the head circumference in infancy and plotting its growth on standard percentile charts provide a valuable guide to normal cerebral development or to excessive or defective growth. By the age of 2 years 66 per cent, and by 12 years 90 per cent of the normal postnatal growth in head circumference have occurred; between these ages space-occupying lesions increasingly tend to cause raised intracranial pressure instead of expanding the head. Papilloedema is rare before 2 years. Spreading of the sutures may persist but it rarely begins after the age of 12 years when their fusion usually is complete; thus the head circumference in adult hydrocephalus is a guide to its chronicity.

In infancy a steeply rising head circumference may indicate an excess of cerebrospinal fluid (in hydrocephalus, hydranencephaly or an arachnoid cyst), subdural haematomas, occasionally the direct effect of a very large tumour, or diffusely abnormal brain growth (megalencephaly).

Megalencephaly

A large non-hydrocephalic head growing parallel to the centile lines is often the result of simple benign familial megalencephaly; but tuberose sclerosis (see Section 24), neurofibromatosis (see page 21.208) and Sotos syndrome (see page 21.196) are the commonest cerebral disorders associated with megalencephaly.

Progressive megalencephaly

This is rarer and suggests a metabolic disease such as Hurler's (see Section 9), Tay–Sachs' (see Section 9), Canavan's (see Section 21) or Alexander's disease (in which the presence of refractile bodies in the astrocytes is associated with epilepsy megalencephaly and spastic quadriplegia). Unilateral megalencephaly often causes severe retardation and intractable epilepsy in infancy, but may be asymptomatic throughout life.

Hydranencephaly

This is the absence of the greater part of both cerebral hemispheres within a normal skull and with intact meninges. The child may appear to be normal at birth and may even survive for many months. Failure of development and often excessive head growth lead to the discovery (by transillumination or ultrasonography) that only the diencephalon and some variable parts of the occipital or temporal lobes are present, the remainder of the hemispheres being replaced by cerebrospinal fluid. Either agenesis or destructive processes arising in the 3rd month of gestation or later may be involved in different cases, but evidence for inflammatory, vascular, or genetic mechanisms is rarely convincing. Why the skull continues to grow in the absence of an expanding brain remains obscure.

Hydrocephalus

Hydrocephalus is dilation of the cerebral ventricles resulting from obstructed flow or impaired absorption of the CSF, or rarely from its excessive production. Enlarged ventricles also occur in cerebral atrophy which may be distinguished from hydrocephalus by the absence of raised intracranial pressure and usually by its association, in childhood, with microcephaly. In *communicating hydrocephalus* the obstruction to CSF flow is in the basal cisterns or in the cerebral subarachnoid space (thus allowing flow or 'communication' from the lateral ventricles to the lumbar subarachnoid space but preventing CSF absorption from the arachnoid villi). In *non-communicating hydrocephalus* the obstruction is in the ventricular system or at the exit foramina of the IVth ventricle.

In early childhood communicating hydrocephalus is usually the consequence of intraventricular haemorrhage (often in preterm infants), subarachnoid haemorrhage (due to birth trauma), or meningitis. Less often congenital infections, especially toxoplasmosis or cytomegalovirus, are responsible. It may occur in the course of tuberculous meningitis in infancy. It may rarely result from excessive production of protein-containing CSF by a choroid plexus papilloma. Often it is of unknown cause. Non-communicating hydrocephalus occurs in aqueduct stenosis, in obstruction of the foramina of Monro, the aqueduct or the IVth ventricle by tumours, and in various malformations especially the Chiari malformation and the Dandy–Walker syndrome (see page 21.196).

The incidence of congenital hydrocephalus, excluding cases of spina bifida, is about 0.4 per 1000 live births.

The normal CSF volume increases from 50 ml at birth to 120–150 ml in the adult; its rate of active secretion by the choroid plexuses is 0.3–0.4 ml/min and the arachnoid granulations are capable of absorbing it (passively) into the venous sinuses at up to four times this rate under an increased pressure gradient. The normal CSF pressure (in the lying position) varies between about 20 and 80 mmH$_2$O in infants and up to 150–200 mmH$_2$O (10–15 mmHg) in adults. Small fluctuations occur with the pulse and respiration. In raised intracranial pressure, monitored with an intraventricular device, a normal or high background pressure may be punctuated by plateau waves of 70 mmHg or more for periods of 10–20 min, or by briefer spikes of high pressure. The former may be accompanied, when severe, by clinical 'hydroce-

phalic attacks'. Eventually very high pressure approaches the arterial pressure and diminishes cerebral blood flow, a rapidly fatal situation.

Diagnosis

In infancy, rapid enlargement of the head and a tense fontanelle are accompanied by drowsiness, irritability and vomiting. Lid retraction with impaired upgaze ('sunsetting') and the enlarged forehead give a diagnostic appearance (imitated, however, by some cases of bilateral subdural haematoma). Large heads of a normal or atypical shape are rarely hydrocephalic. Squints, spasticity and opisthotonos may develop.

In older children with closed fontanelles, papilloedema may occur in acute cases, but this is not usual when the onset is gradual. Headache, ataxia, incontinence and spasticity are the usual features together with selective intellectual impairment involving verbal less than performance skills (on the Wechsler intelligence scales). Fine motor skills and concentration are often poor. Third ventricular dilation may impair growth and rarely cause other endocrine defects. Squints, especially VIth nerve palsies, often accompany sudden increases in pressure.

Very acute or severe hydrocephalus may lead rapidly to coma with preceding severe headache and nausea, and with arterial hypertension, bradycardia, opisthotonos, impaired upgaze, constricted or less often dilated pupils and Cheyne Stokes respiration. Such 'hydrocephalic attacks' require lifesaving emergency ventricular drainage.

Ultrasonography is helpful in infants, especially for repeated ventricular measurement. Skull X-ray may reveal spread sutures in infancy, erosion of the sella after about the age of 9 years, expansion of the sella in chronic aqueduct stenosis, and calcification in toxoplasmosis or cytomegalovirus infection, longstanding tuberculosis or in certain tumours. CT scanning will show dilated ventricles (sparing the IVth ventricle in aqueduct stenosis), a posterior fossa cyst in the Dandy–Walker syndrome, and obliteration of the cerebral sulci and interhemisphere fissure, contrasting with their prominence in cerebral atrophy. Hydrocephalus causing raised intracranial pressure may occur in a microcephalic brain in infancy, and as a new feature in adults presenting with dementia, and the differential diagnosis from atrophy may then be subtle. Radioisotope cisternography is still occasionally helpful in making this distinction. Magnetic resonance imaging gives clear images of brain-stem malformation. Ventriculography is obsolete except in occasional diagnostic difficulty between stenosis and obstruction of the aqueduct where CT scans may be unhelpful. Early prenatal diagnosis of hydrocephalus by ultrasonography is sometimes possible but has not yet led to useful therapy.

Management

All cases should be investigated to exclude a treatable underlying disorder and identify the site of the obstruction. In the neonate who has had an intraventricular haemorrhage, repeated lumbar or ventricular taps may remove enough blood and CSF to avoid the need for further treatment. Hydrocephalus which does not cause rapid head growth or symptoms of raised pressure should be left untreated, unless it becomes clear that it is impairing motor or intellectual function when shunting should be given a trial. When the decision is difficult, a period of monitoring the intracranial pressure may be helpful, but the results should rarely take precedence over the evidence provided by the head growth chart or repeated psychological testing.

Shunts and their complications

Symptomatic hydrocephalus not due to a remediable cause requires shunting. A Torkildsen shunt (from the lateral ventricle to the posterior fossa) may be used in aqueduct stenosis but is not satisfactory in growing children. Ventriculoperitoneal shunts are now used in preference to ventriculoatrial shunts in the great majority of cases. Both are subject to a number of important complications.

1. *Overdrainage* leading to abnormally low intracranial pressure with consequences varying from postural headache to severe secondary subdural haemorrhage. This is a particular risk when very chronic hydrocephalus is first treated in adolescents or adults and is best prevented by careful valve selection.

2. *Blockage or detachment* leading to a sudden or intermittent return of raised pressure and requiring revision of the shunt. Most children require several revisions, fewer with ventriculoperitoneal shunts. 'Prophylactic' revision as the child grows is generally recommended, especially for ventriculoatrial shunts.

3. *Infection*. The shunt acts as a privileged site and once colonized by bacteria, it cannot be sterilized by antibiotic treatment. Removal, and external ventricular drainage must therefore be used whenever meningitis or ventriculitis complicate shunted hydrocephalus. Staphylococci are commonly responsible. This situation should be suspected whenever unexplained pyrexia, anaemia or splenomegaly occurs. Infection of ventriculoatrial shunts particularly may give rise to chronic mild septicaemia, subacute bacterial endocarditis or glomerular nephritis.

4. *Thrombosis* at the tip of ventriculoatrial shunts may lead to chronic pulmonary microembolism, pulmonary hypertension and heart failure, or to thrombosis of the superior vena cava. Thrombosis may occur with or without shunt infection and is more likely when growth pulls the shunt tip out of the right atrium into the vena cava.

Medical treatment of hydrocephalus with acetazolamide or isosorbide is of little value except as an aid to procrastination in marginal cases.

Genetic counselling

This is important in cases associated with spina bifida (see page 21.200) and when there are associated malformations which may be due to single gene defects. Laurence gives the recurrence risk in uncomplicated hydrocephalus as one in 40 after an affected boy, one in 80 after an affected girl. After a case of aqueduct stenosis the risk to a brother of an affected boy is one in 22 and to a sister one in 50.

Aqueduct stenosis

About one-third of all childhood hydrocephalus (excluding spina bifida) results from stenosis of the Sylvian aqueduct, normally only 0.2–1.8 mm in diameter at birth. The stenosis may follow intraventricular haemorrhage or ependymitis, for example in bacterial meningitis, prenatal toxoplasmosis, and probably either fetal or postnatal mumps encephalitis. In such cases there is gliosis around the aqueduct. It is also associated with some cases of neurofibromatosis and occurs as an X-linked genetic disorder characterized by severe mental retardation, spasticity, and hypoplasia of the first metacarpals with adduction of the thumbs. It is often seen in the Chiari malformation in addition to the IVth ventricular outlet obstruction. As an isolated defect, in which forking and blind passages of the aqueduct are seen at post-mortem, aqueduct stenosis may present with insidiously progressive symptoms at any age, though commonly enlargement of the head provides evidence for its origin in childhood. The features in later life are ataxia of gait (without signs of cerebellar involvement), incontinence and dementia with mild pyramidal signs in addition to the symptoms and signs of raised intracranial pressure. Epilepsy and hypopituitarism are less frequent. Typically, palpation of the skull, and X-rays, reveal a small posterior fossa.

Other developmental abnormalities involving the skull and brain

Encephaloceles

Cranial fusion defects are rarer than spina bifida (about one in 2000–5000 births). Probably only occipital encephaloceles, and not those in other sites, are actually neural tube defects. A meningeal sac containing a variable amount of cerebral or cerebellar tissue bulges through a cranial defect usually without a defect in the scalp. About 75 per cent are occipital, and CT scanning will define the contents and often show associated hydrocephalus. Occipital meningoceles and small encephaloceles should be corrected early, and partial removal of herniated brain tissue may be necessary; large encephaloceles may be inoperable. Even small lesions may later be found to be associated with a disappointing degree of mental retardation. Midline frontal or nasal lesions and orbital lesions are less frequently associated with retardation but they may pose formidable problems in surgical closure and facial reconstruction. Transsphenoidal lesions may be associated with hypopituitarism. *Meckel's syndrome* (occipital encephalocele and polycystic kidneys) is of autosomal recessive inheritance; other occipital cases carry a recurrence risk equivalent to that in spina bifida. For other sites the recurrence risk is low.

Microcephaly

A brain weight or head circumference more than 1 s.d. below the mean may arise for numerous reasons. Microcephaly is a physical sign of cerebral malformation and not a diagnosis. Broadly it may result from hypoplasia or destruction but in early prenatal development the two may be inseparable. When the head circumference falls gradually away below the 3rd growth centile a recent destructive ('encephaloclastic') lesion (often hypoxic or inflammatory), or a progressive degenerative disorder is likely. Most early prenatal causes lead to microcephaly at birth with subsequent growth parallel to the centiles. Chromosome anomalies, complex malformation syndromes, intrauterine infections or intoxication, and variety of single gene disorders may cause microcephaly. As an isolated feature in autosomal recessive microcephaly it is associated with severe intellectual retardation but relatively normal function in other respects. In intrauterine growth retardation due to placental insufficiency, the growth of the brain is generally relatively spared; so in dwarfed children with relative microcephaly another cause should be sought.

Craniosynostosis

Premature fusion which involves all of the cranial sutures is almost always the result of impaired brain growth, not its cause. The rare exceptions present with raised intracranial pressure. Selective premature fusion gives rise to an obviously deformed skull which is not usually microcephalic. With the exception of pure sagittal synostosis, selective craniosynostosis is usually seen in one of several genetically determined craniofacial dysostoses (such as Crouzon's syndrome, which also includes midface hypoplasia, shallow orbits, and proptosis). Precise diagnosis and genetic counselling are important. In severe cases, surgical treatment in the first few months of life may improve the ultimate skull shape, or it may be required to protect the optic nerves when papilloedema develops.

Intracranial cysts

Arachnoid cysts

It is difficult to distinguish developmental cysts of the arachnoid from those that follow meningitis or trauma, unless extensive arachnoiditis is present.

Intracranial arachnoid cysts may occur between the hemispheres, in the suprasellar region or in the posterior fossa causing local compressive symptoms and raised intracranial pressure. They are most frequently found, however, in the middle cranial fossa which they expand and where they compress or displace the anterior part of the temporal lobe and adjacent frontal lobe. Epilepsy and the symptoms of raised intracranial pressure are the usual presenting features and the diagnosis may be suspected from the expanded appearance of the middle fossa in a skull X-ray. Surgical decompression is useful but often fails to improve the epilepsy. The origin and nature of these cysts remains controversial.

Various other meningeal cysts secondary to hydrocephalus, trauma or meningitis may cause similar symptoms. Anomalies like the Dandy–Walker syndrome or encephaloceles produce large cysts. Intracerebral developmental ('glial') cysts are usually found in more widespread developmental disorders such as neurofibromatosis.

Other cysts

Porencephaly This is a pseudocyst secondary to an infarct or other destructive cerebral lesion.

Schizencephaly This is a form of local cystic symmetrical agenesis of the cerebral hemispheres, not vascular in origin and usually associated with severe mental retardation. It is probably more akin to hydranencephaly than porencephaly.

Cystic tumours Cystic tumours such as craniopharyngiomas and cerebellar astrocytomas, though developmental in origin, are discussed on pages 21.171–21.174.

Cerebrovascular malformations

Arteriovenous malformations (AVMs) and aneurysms are discussed on page 21.169. Large congenital arteriovenous malformations of the great vein of Galen present with high output cardiac failure in the neonatal period. Surgical management is hazardous. When the early fetal vascular anastomoses between the carotid and vertebral systems fail to involute a persistent trigeminal, acoustic or hypoglossal artery results and may compress neural structures. The trigeminal artery, for example, may damage the IIIrd, IVth or VIth cranial nerves in the middle fossa.

The Sturge–Weber syndrome

This is characterized by a facial 'portwine stain' naevus associated with meningeal angiomatosis on the surface of the ipsilateral hemisphere, and contralateral focal (and generalized) seizures, often with a hemiparesis and hemianopia. The hemiparesis may deteriorate and the fits are often difficult to control. Mental retardation is a frequent feature. Often there is congenital glaucoma on the side of the naevus. The angioma is usually parietal or occipital and there is calcification in the underlying cortex which shows as characteristic 'tramline markings' on X-ray. Virtually all cases are sporadic although the dominant inheritance of similar uncomplicated naevi has led to a popular misconception that the Sturge–Weber syndrome is genetic in origin.

Developmental abnormalities of the spine

Spina bifida far outnumbers other spinal abnormalities.

Klippel–Feil syndrome

Fusion of two or more cervical vertebrae in this syndrome is associated with a short neck and restricted movement. 'Mirror movements' of the hands may result from an associated cord anomaly, and secondary spastic tetraparesis due to subluxation is an occasional complication. A defect of segmentation of the cervical somites before the 7th week of gestation seems to be responsible. Several patterns of defect occur with various associated anomalies. One syndrome, with Duane's anomaly (see page 21.197), facial asymmetry and deafness, occurs only in females.

Sacral agenesis

Sacral agenesis with reduction defects of the lower limbs (the caudal regression syndrome) is often associated with maternal diabetes. In another syndrome an anterior meningocele accompanies partial sacral agenesis. This may present as a pelvic mass but occasionally also causes denervation of the bladder.

Spinal arachnoid cysts

These may cause back pain or minor cord or root compression; often the symptoms vary with posture. The most troublesome cause disturbances of sphincter or sexual function. Myelographic demonstration may require 'late' films to be taken several hours after injection of the dye. Surgical results are variable. These cysts must be distinguished from anterior meningoceles. A radiological anomaly of the sacrum occurs with the latter, and often a symptomatic mass in the pelvis.

Spina bifida

During the 1980s and 1990s there will be a 'bulge' in the frequency of cases of spina bifida cystica reaching adult life, the consequence of surgical advances in the 1960s outpacing our understanding of their effects. They will bring with them unfamiliar problems in medical care.

Definitions

Neural tube defects (NTD) comprise spina bifida and anencephaly. *Spina bifida* means the defective fusion of the posterior vertebral arches. This may be isolated to one vertebra and insignificant (in 5 per cent of the population) or, in symptomatic *spina bifida occulta*, may be more extensive and associated with an overlying tuft of hair or haemangioma, intraspinal or extraspinal lipoma, a low conus, diastematomyelia or dermal sinuses or cysts. In *spina bifida cystica* the meninges protrude through the defect, either without any neural tissue (in a *meningocele*) or with nerve roots or dysplastic cord (in a *meningomyelocele*, or in the widely open lesion *rachischisis*). Meningoceles are usually covered with epithelium, meningomyeloceles only occasionally so. *Anencephaly* is the absence of the cerebral hemispheres and overlying tissues, leaving the diencephalon exposed to the surface. It is incompatible with survival but, as part of the continuum of neural tube defects is of epidemiological importance.

Embryogenesis and incidence

The neural tube differentiates from ectoderm overlying the notochord at 18 days. Closure begins at 22 days and extends upwards and downwards, the caudal neuropore closing at 26 days. Neural tissue caudal to the neuropore arises from the caudal cell mass (anomalies of which may be responsible for sacral agenesis and teratomas) by 28 days; the meninges differentiate at 40–50 days and closure of the vertebral arches continues from then until term. Thus, while simple spinal fusion defects may arise much later, cystic lesions result from defects of neural tube closure before 26 days. Defects at the cranial neuropore result in anencephaly, and slightly lower defects in occipital encephaloceles. Known rare causes of spina bifida include fetal exposure to aminopterin, various chromosomal anomalies including trisomy 13 or 18, and especially Meckel syndrome, an autosomal recessive disorder. However, the primary cause of spina bifida is unknown; notochord dysfunction is possibly involved as it may be in such other vertebral anomalies as diastematomyelia, hemivertebrae, and also neurenteric cysts in which endodermal (bowel) tissue is found in prevertebral cysts, in the spinal canal, or even exposed dorsally at the surface. Anterior meningoceles are also probably different in their pathogenesis.

The incidence of spina bifida cystica has changed over the last century and varies geographically. It is higher in females. The incidence in Great Britain in the 1960s and 1970s was ten times higher than in Southeast Asia or Africa, and varied from 4.0 to 4.5 per 1000 total births in Ireland and South Wales, to 1.5 per 1000 in Southeast England. When anencephaly is included these figures are approximately doubled. The racial incidence varies and tends to take precedence over geographical factors in multiracial communities. Monozygous twins are often discordant for spina bifida ruling out a simple genetic cause, yet the recurrence risk to sibs is one in 20 after one and one in 10 after two cases of spina bifida or anencephaly. Symptomatic spina bifida occulta carries nearly the same recurrence risk. Affected adults have a 4 per cent risk of having an affected child.

The incidence in Boston, United States rose to a peak between 1925 and 1945 and has fallen since. In South Wales, Liverpool, Sheffield and Newcastle the birth incidence has fallen sharply, but perhaps not permanently, since the 1960s, by as much as 50 per cent. Therapeutic abortions contributed only a small proportion to this decline. There is widespread speculation that nutritional factors are responsible, and trials are in progress of the preventive effect of taking added vitamins, especially folic acid, at the time of conception.

Prenatal diagnosis is possible in 90 per cent of serious neural tube defects by fetal ultrasound scanning, and by amniocentesis with measurement of the amniotic fluid levels of alphafetoprotein (AFP) and acetylcholinesterase. Effective prevention depends on selection of cases for amniocentesis. Women with a family history of neural tube defects should be offered this, and maternal *serum* alphafetoprotein levels are a helpful guide to other high-risk pregnancies.

Spina bifida cystica

In addition to the cystic defect itself most cases have extensive abnormalities of the cord and of the hind-brain. Meningomyeloceles are almost invariably associated with the Chiari type II malformation (see page 21.197). Hydrocephalus occurs in 95 per cent of cases; usually it is attributable to the IVth ventricle outlet obstruction caused by the Chiari malformation, but aqueduct stenosis may also be present. Reduplication of the spinal cord both proximal and distal to the plaque, posterior column defects, lipomas of the filum or dura, syringomyelia and hydromyelia are present in various combinations in most cases. The plaques themselves may occur at any level, but thoracolumbar, lumbar and lumbosacral lesions are the most frequent. Anomalies of the ribs and vertebral bodies and paraspinal muscle denervation combine to cause kyphoscoliosis. An association with renal anomalies and microphthalmia suggests the autosomal recessive Meckel syndrome (page 21.194).

Management of neonatal problems

The child born with spina bifida cystica needs urgent skilled assessment. The major complications of meningomyeloceles are paralysis of the legs, anaesthesia, urinary and faecal incontinence, hydronephrosis and hydrocephalus. Assessment on day one is designed to predict the quality of life to be expected from the size and position of the defect, the degree of disability already present and the degree of hydrocephalus. Delay in treatment leads to drying of the membranes and nerve roots, a deterioration in the function of the legs and sphincters and an increasing risk of meningitis. Treatment of epithelialized meningoceles is less urgent. Once primary surgical closure of the plaque is performed, the survival rate is greatly increased, shunting of hydrocephalus is soon required in most cases, and a sequence of events is thereby set in motion which involves a lifetime of multiple operations and medical surveillance. Withholding surgery leads to fatal complications, usually meningitis, in about 90 per cent of cases, but in the rest spontaneous epithelialization of the plaque may permit prolonged survival with very severe and increasing disabilities. The situation may then demand late closure of the spinal lesion and late shunting of the hydrocephalus. In practice, in the last 10 years some of the criteria commonly used to select infants for treatment have been the absence of

1. severe paralysis with a motor level above L3;
2. kyphosis or severe scoliosis;
3. severe hydrocephalus with a head circumference above about 39 cm at birth or a cortical mantle of less than about 1 cm in depth;
4. associated heart disease or other severe defects;
5. other individual major factors.

Depending on their approach various units treat between 25 and 75 per cent of cases, and of those treated about 70–85 per cent survive.

Meningoceles require only simple excision, but hydrocephalus may develop in about 20 per cent of cases.

Management in childhood and adolescence

The complex problems of severe spina bifida are managed in childhood and adolescence by teams often involving a paediatrician, neurosurgeon, urological surgeon, orthopaedic surgeon, psychiatrist, psychologist, physiotherapist, and social worker as well as the family doctor, and community nurse. Equivalent teams to manage adult cases have rarely been developed. Yet most of the problems in this disorder are lifelong and many patients report increasing disability in adult life. The permanent problems include the following.

Hydrocephalus

Ventriculoperitoneal shunts are commonly used now, but in the 1960s and 1970s ventriculoatrial shunts were the rule. Ventriculitis and meningitis after shunting are potent causes of additional neurological handicap. The shunts need frequent revision in childhood. The problems are discussed in the section on hydrocephalus (page 21.198).

Paralysis

The level of the lesion will determine whether there is a pure lower motor neurone paresis, or a combination of this with spasticity of the muscles innervated by an isolated section of the spinal cord below the lesion. These factors in turn will determine the pattern of paralysis and deformity of the lower limbs to be found in each case. A few patients with lesions above L1 can walk in full-length calipers attached to a spinal brace, but most are confined to wheelchairs. Patients with lesions from L2 to L3 have a higher success rate but they are likely to need below-knee calipers while those with lesions below S2 usually need no appliances to help them to walk. Much depends however on the patient's intelligence, and the presence or absence of deformity as well as the severity of the paralysis. Early passive stretching and splinting of joints are followed by orthopaedic procedures in childhood to correct such frequent complications as dislocation of the hips, hyperextension or flexion deformity at the knees, or a wide variety of foot deformities, which depend on the site of the lesion. Treatment of these deformities should have a specific functional objective, usually the achievement of walking or comfortable seating, or a very obvious cosmetic benefit. Spastic adduction of the hips sometimes requires corrective tenotomy to improve hygiene and bladder management. In adolescence, walking may become increasingly difficult and many teenagers resort to wheelchairs.

Sensory loss and pressure sores

Children need to learn early the dangers of painless burns, of sitting on surfaces causing local pressure, and of neglecting early skin lesions. They should learn to inspect their pressure points using a mirror. Scrupulous attention to footwear and appliances is essential. It is likely that the complications of anaesthesia will increase with age especially if parental care declines. Vigorous treatment of incipient sores by relief of pressure, control of infection and later, if necessary, surgical excision is important. In adolescents and adults increasing pressure and declining standards of vigilance may worsen pressure sores. Charcot joints sometimes develop. Painless fractures occurring in paralysed limbs should be treated in the simplest possible way; to plaster the limb is to risk causing pressure sores and displacement is uncommon. Existing calipers form effective splints, and normal wheelchair activities can often be resumed at once.

Spinal deformity

Kyphosis at birth carries a poor prognosis for severe persistent deformity. Congenital scoliosis may result from vertebral anomalies but more often paralytic scoliosis develops and progresses during childhood. Effective bracing is difficult, especially when there is sensory loss. Milwaukee braces are effective but moulded braces are more comfortable and less restricting. Early local spinal fusion is sometimes required in congenital curvatures. More often fusion is undertaken in early adolescence when increasing spinal curvature is a common cause of loss of the ability to walk. However, complications due to skin anaesthesia, hip deformity, respiratory impairment, or poor co-operation in retarded children are common.

Neuropathic bladder
Most children with meningomyeloceles have neuropathic bladders, with the usual consequences of urinary incontinence, infection and reflux with dilation of the upper urinary tracts. A few develop normal continence. For most adults the control of continence remains a major problem. Early assessment is designed to identify dribbling overflow or failure of the sphincter to relax during detrusor activity, and to check renal function. A combined micturating cystogram and cystometrogram can be performed even in a neonate. If there is no significant reflux or bladder neck obstruction, intermittent manual expression every 2 hours will prevent residual urine accumulating and becoming infected. Temporary catheterization may be required if ureteric reflux occurs. Treatment with propantheline is valuable for decreasing excessive detrusor contractility, and with ephedrine to increase the bladder neck resistance. Less often phenoxybenzamine is used to diminish alpha-adrenergic (internal sphincter) bladder neck resistance. These measures usually suffice until intermittent catheterization, using a clean but not sterile technique, can be introduced. The control of incontinence by the use of this method by the parents and later, whenever possible, by the child has been a major recent advance in the management of spina bifida and is the method of choice in over 70 per cent of cases, sometimes combined with drug therapy. However, it may not be feasible in the presence of severe deformity, and may be very awkward when full-length calipers are worn. Transurethral sphincterotomy, sphincter plication, penile drainage appliances, incontinence pads and urinary diversion to ileal loops are now second-line methods though useful in some cases. Urinary diversion was once almost routine and many young adults have ileostomies *in situ*. Late complications such as ureteric reflux, and the loss of ileal tone may require reimplantation of the ureters into the bladder, and the reintroduction of regular catheterization. Infection of the disused bladder may require surgical drainage. Late deterioration of bladder function may result from hydromyelia or diastematomyelia (see below). Whichever techniques are used to control bladder function, regular checks for reflux, urinary infection, renal dysfunction and arterial hypertension are important.

Bowel incontinence
Defective bowel sensation and impaired sphincter tone combine to cause constipation and overflow incontinence. Regular toileting, laxatives, teaching active abdominal muscle contraction, manual evacuation and regular enemas may all play a part in management. Most patients become 'socially continent', except when they suffer diarrhoea, but few manage without active control measures.

Intelligence and education
Large series of cases of meningomyelocele who have not required shunting tend to have IQ levels about 10 points below matched controls. Those with shunts are about 30 points below. As in other children with hydrocephalus the WISC (Wechsler) performance scale levels are lower than the verbal scales. Visual perception, body-image awareness and comprehension skills are often impaired. Manual dexterity, especially handwriting, may be affected by minor spinal cord anomalies as well as by hydrocephalus. The education of children with spina bifida has generally, and very successfully, been undertaken in schools for the physically handicapped where they form one of the largest diagnostic categories. But reintegration into society is a major hurdle for school leavers.

Intensive residential courses in domestic and social independence for teenagers organized by the Association for Spina Bifida and Hydrocephalus (ASBAH) are a valuable stepping stone. Active measures to provide suitable accommodation, transport and employment are vital if true independence is to become possible.

Spina bifida occulta (spinal dysraphism)
Symptomatic spina bifida occulta almost never occurs without some external sign, an area of atrophic skin, a tuft of hair, a haemangioma, a visible sinus or a subcutaneous lipoma overlying the lesion. The cervical and lumbosacral regions are the commonest sites. Sinuses may provide access for bacteria causing recurrent meningitis and should be excised. Otherwise most visible lesions are asymptomatic. Some children develop a syndrome of pes cavus and growth failure of the foot or leg, usually asymmetrical, with or without sensory loss, and muscle weakness in root distribution, and loss of the ankle jerk. Some develop a neuropathic bladder. These signs are uncommon at birth but may appear at any age, the bladder problems occasionally manifesting in late adult life. The foot deformity of spinal dysraphism may be confused with that of congenital talipes, familial pes cavus, hereditary sensorimotor neuropathy, the hereditary ataxias or compressive cord lesions. Myelography combined with CT scanning may reveal an intradural lipoma, a central bony or cartilaginous spur tethering a split cord (diastematomyelia), or merely translucencies representing tethering fibrous bands between the cord and the dura, abnormally angulated nerve roots, a wide filum terminale or, most controversially, a low-placed conus (below L3). The normal adult level of the conus at T12–L3 (almost always at L1–L2) is reached by the age of 5 months, the average level at 30 weeks gestation being L3 and at term L2. So the concept that tethering of the conus might cause increasing traction on the cord in later childhood is dubious. The indications for myelography and surgery are controversial, but all cases with sphincter disturbance merit myelography, all those with bony spurs visible on spine X-rays, and also cases of demonstrably progressive deformity or weakness of the lower limbs. Surgery is directed at removing fibrous or bony spurs, dermoid cysts or compressive lipomas when possible, and at cutting abnormal fibrous bands and often the filum. It is generally agreed at best to prevent further neurological deterioration and, rarely, to give much improvement.

Lipomeningoceles
Lipomeningoceles lie on the border between cystic and occult spina bifida. Small meningoceles are found on CT scanning to be adjacent to the lipoma and the latter extends from a visible, often asymmetrical, subcutaneous mass to be attached to and buried within the split dorsal surface of the spinal cord where the dura is deficient. The cord may be compressed by a fibrous band just above the lipoma and surgical treatment is usually necessary.

The cerebral palsies
The term cerebral palsy describes the general situation in which a non-progressive lesion occurring in the developing brain before, during, or after birth leaves the child with a predominantly motor handicap. It is an unsatisfactory concept in the early stages when the emphasis is on the care of an ill baby, and when years of assessment of the nature and degree of a potentially multiple handicap lie ahead. It is more useful as a diagnosis in retrospect when its differentiation from other motor disorders, progressive or acquired, may be the issue. The motor deficit is very variable in its distribution, nature and degree and the relationship between aetiology and pathology is far from consistent. The simple classification in Table 4 is adequate for most purposes, but mixed forms are common.

The age-specific prevalence of cerebral palsy varies between 1.3 and about 5 per 1000 in different communities and represents the

Table 4 Classification of cerebral palsies

Spastic	Hemiplegia
	Bilateral hemiplegia (tetraplegia)
	Diplegia
Dyskinetic	Athetosis
	Dystonia
Ataxic	Pure ataxia
	Spastic-ataxic diplegia
Mixed	

difference between the prevention of death and of handicap in babies exposed to different standards of care. In most developed countries it is currently about 2.0 per 1000 liveborn children ascertained at school entry.

Aetiology and pathology

The earlier prenatal cerebral damage occurs the more likely it is to be accompanied by deviant development of the damaged brain amounting to a malformation. Hydranencephaly may be an extreme example. Prenatal cerebral infarction has been associated with the death of a twin fetus, and with maternal hypotension, hypoxia, trauma or intoxication, but it is frequently unexplained. Often when the cause is not clear-cut the best that can be done is to list statistically associated 'risk factors' such as multiparity, twin pregnancy, toxaemia, poor fetal growth, and low standards of maternal health and antenatal care.

Infants born before term have always been vulnerable; with modern neonatal care they may survive at 24 weeks gestation weighing as little as 500 g. Cerebral ischaemia and haemorrhage, hypoxia secondary to respiratory distress, acidosis, hypothermia, hypoglycaemia due to liver immaturity, lack of autoregulation of cerebral blood flow in relation to blood pressure, and trauma even of mild degree are some of the interrelated factors predisposing to cerebral damage in such preterm infants. Neonatal intensive care has improved the mortality and cerebral palsy rates in babies under 2000 g at birth, but of those under 1000 g more are surviving both with and without cerebral palsy.

In the preterm infant ischaemic necrosis of the white matter (periventricular leucomalacia, PVL) and haemorrhage arising from the germinal matrix (GMH) are the principal pathological findings. The germinal matrices are the local subependymal centres of neuronal multiplication which degenerate at 24–35 weeks of gestation; before 20 weeks more active neuronal multiplication extends throughout the subependymal tissue. Ultrasound scanning shows that about half of all babies under 1500 g develop matrix haemorrhage in the first few hours after birth. Correlation with cerebral palsy depends upon its extent and association with periventricular leucomalacia.

At any stage of gestation birth asphyxia (due to precipitate, prolonged or difficult deliveries, antepartum haemorrhages, etc.), birth trauma which tears subdural bridging veins or dural sinuses, neonatal meningitis, rhesus incompatibility causing kernicterus, or hypoglycaemia are all well-established causes of cerebral palsy. Subdural bleeding is the principal pathological finding in damaged children surviving traumatic deliveries, and in those with later non-accidental injury. Subarachnoid and intraventricular bleeding may lead to later hydrocephalus.

Perinatal hypoxia and ischaemia may produce white matter lesions (PVL) in term as well as in preterm infants, but cortical infarction is also present in babies asphyxiated at term. Cortical laminar necrosis, worst in the depths of the sulci, and necrosis of the thalamus, hippocampus, brain-stem and cerebellum are characteristic. The duration of neonatal asphyxia (with its attendant apnoea, bradycardia and acidosis) correlates well with subsequent cerebral palsy. With an Apgar score of 3 or less for 5 minutes the proportion with later cerebral palsy is 1 per cent, after 15 minutes 9 per cent, and thereafter the rate rises steeply. Pro-

longed neonatal seizures are another poor prognostic feature. Episodes of hypotension may be responsible for cases of infarction in arterial boundary zones. In long-term survivors cystic degeneration is combined with micropolygyria and in the basal ganglia loss of neurones and gliosis are combined with aberrant myelinated fibres (status marmoratus).

Important postnatal causes of cerebral palsy are encephalitis, meningitis, trauma (perhaps especially non-accidental injury), and hypoxia or impaired cerebral perfusion during major operations especially for severe congenital heart defects.

Diagnosis

The effects of an insult occurring during a continuous process of cerebral development may not be evident until long afterwards when the full function of the damaged neuronal system comes into play. Furthermore, the plasticity of early development permits some functions to be taken over by alternative neurones if damage occurs sufficiently early. So the early diagnosis of cerebral palsy should always be tentative. After a major episode of hypoxia, trauma or infection causing severe hypotonia, unresponsiveness or coma, the degree of cerebral palsy will emerge during a period of follow-up for assessment and supportive therapy. Any impairment of mental, linguistic, visual, auditory and sensory function is also assessed so that a comprehensive diagnosis of the handicap can be made at the time of school entry. Children subject to risk factors but without obvious initial handicap should be assessed at intervals in the same way. Unrecognized prenatal damage may be evident at birth if the child is microcephalic or has a disorder of tone or movement. However, in many cases delayed motor development or the premature development of 'handedness', or the appearance of involuntary movements or abnormal gait patterns may be the first symptoms. A detailed history of the acquisition and loss of motor skills will usually distinguish clearly between cerebral palsy and progressive disorders such as Friedreich's ataxia, hereditary spastic paraparesis or intracranial tumours. Athetoid and dystonic movements always develop over the first few years of life, but from a background of previous hypotonia and lack of movement; the loss of previously acquired motor skills requires investigation for alternative causes. Impaired growth of the affected limbs is a useful clue to the early onset of a hemiparesis encountered in adult life. Serial measurement of the head may reveal hydrocephalus as a potentially treatable component in the cause of cerebral palsy.

Baraitser (1982) reviewed the genetic risks for sibs in cerebral palsy. For cases with an obvious cause or with asymmetrical signs the risk is 1–2 per cent, but for unexplained spastic diplegia, athetosis or ataxia, about 10 per cent.

Spastic diplegia

William Little in 1861 described the association of spastic rigidity of the limbs with abnormal and premature births. The legs are more severely affected than the arms, in spastic adduction and extension. There is an initial hypotonic phase followed by dystonia before the spasticity is evident. Infants develop 'scissoring' of the legs in vertical suspension, later the gait is laboured and jerky with severe plantiflexion and adduction. Leg growth may be limited. Spastic dysarthria is frequent, often with drooling. The arms, though relatively spared, are at the least hyperreflexic with impaired dexterity. Sensation and intelligence are usually relatively well preserved. Internal strabismus is very frequent and should be surgically corrected. About a quarter of all cases have major seizures.

There is a strong association with short gestation and with periventricular leucomalacia. The incidence of spastic diplegia fell sharply in the 1950s to 1970s with improvements in the care of preterm infants but it has risen recently, perhaps because of the survival of even smaller infants. Cases born at term without an obvious cause may require investigation; some are probably genetic in origin.

Spastic hemiplegia

This is the commonest form of cerebral palsy and there has been little recent change in its incidence. For some reason in about 55 per cent of cases the right limbs are affected. Almost always the lesion involves the cortex so epilepsy and learning disorders are frequent. About 40 per cent of cases are retarded. The severity of the disability depends not only on the degree of paralysis but on the associated cortical sensory loss which may amount to almost total unawareness of the affected side. Hemianopia is a common additional handicap. Cerebral dominance for handedness and speech may develop in the opposite hemisphere if the lesion occurs early enough, but unfortunately cases arising at birth often have bilateral though asymmetrical lesions which may prevent this. Speech delay and global retardation are more frequent than clear-cut aphasia if the onset is before the age of 2 years.

Between a third and half of cases are prenatal, and about 40 per cent perinatal in origin. Often poor fetal growth and perinatal asphyxia are associated factors. The asymmetry of posture and use of the hands may not be noticed until 3–12 months of age. But this is the most frequent pattern of cerebral palsy to develop after birth, especially in meningitis, encephalitis, prolonged febrile or other convulsions, trauma, migraine, sickle cell disease, congenital heart disease, the moya-moya syndrome, and other vascular disorders. When the lesion is not a simple arterial occlusion the incidence of later epilepsy is very high. Early postnatal hemiplegia often develops a dystonic element which becomes increasingly troublesome in adolescence and may sometimes justify stereotactic surgery for its relief.

Bilateral hemiplegia and tetraplegia

Bilateral hemisphere damage makes this the most severe of all the cerebral palsies. Mental retardation is invariable and usually severe, epilepsy is very common and severe bulbar involvement causes major feeding difficulties. Bilateral spasticity, worse in the arms, blindness due to optic atrophy or cortical damage and strabismus are the usual features. Where the origin is prenatal microcephaly is usually obvious at birth, but sometimes there is hydrocephalus (in prenatal infections) or hydranencephaly. The most severe perinatal hypoxia or anaesthetic disasters often result in such cases. In unexplained cases metabolic disorders or Alper's disease (a genetic cortical degeneration) should be considered, and if no metabolic disorder is found and progressive deterioration is confirmed by follow-up, brain biopsy may be justified to permit genetic counselling. The mortality rate is high among severely tetraplegic children, at school entry they represent only 5 per cent of cerebral palsy.

Dyskinetic cerebral palsies

Athetosis

Kernicterus and perinatal asphyxia are the principal causes of this form of cerebral palsy (see also page 21.203). In the former, defective upgaze and deafness are the other cardinal features. Typically the baby is initially hypotonic, irritable, and later lethargic. After several months tongue-thrusting movements develop and may make feeding very difficult, but choreic and later slow writhing athetoid movements of the limbs and trunk are not usually seen till the second or third year, or even later. All aspects of motor development are very delayed. Intelligence may be normal, but speech is often extremely dysarthric with the same character of variable 'mobile spasm' as the limbs; drooling and dysphagia may be troublesome. Seizures are uncommon. Of all the cerebral palsies this is the one most likely to result in a mistaken diagnosis of mental retardation. Kernicterus due to rhesus incompatibility, once very frequent, is now rare in developed countries. However, severe neonatal jaundice still may be seen in ABO incompatibility (see Section 19), the Crigler–Najjar syndrome (see Section 12) or glucose-6 phosphate dehydrogenase (G6PD) deficiency (see Section 19), and requires phototherapy or exchange transfusion to prevent kernicterus.

Dystonia

A dystonic stage often intervenes between the hypotonic and spastic stages of diplegic cerebral palsy. Rarely dystonia or rigidity may remain the dominant features often with an element of tremor or myoclonus. Such cases should be carefully investigated for metabolic genetic disorders.

Ataxic 'cerebral' palsy

Although hypoglycaemia and hypothyroidism may predominantly affect the cerebellum in the neonatal period, ataxic 'cerebral' palsy is usually the result of cerebellar malformations determined early in embryonal development (see page 21.191). Hypotonia in an alert infant long precedes identifiable tremor and may be mistaken for neuromuscular disease, but associated mental retardation is also quite common. The disequilibrium syndrome is a separate form often, if not always, genetic in origin (autosomal recessive) in which early hypotonia and feeding difficulties are followed by the very late development of standing balance (at 7–9 years). The patients have very poor righting reflexes and tend to fall 'like a log'.

Spastic ataxic diplegia

This frequent combination is sometimes allied to spastic diplegia. Often it is associated with hydrocephalus for which probably intraventricular haemorrhage in the preterm infant may be responsible, but which results from a cerebellar malformation in some cases. Ventricular dilation itself may contribute largely to both the spasticity and the ataxia. Very similar signs occur in a number of genetic disorders, and it is particularly important to look out for progressive disability in unexplained cases.

Other types

Monoplegias less often represent localized lesions than incompletely identified hemipareses. Tripareses are common, often they represent the combination of a hemiplegia and diplegia. Combinations of spastic and dyskinetic signs are very frequent. 'Hypotonic cerebral palsy' is usually the early phase of diplegic or especially the athetoid or ataxic forms. Persistently floppy children with evidence of cerebral dysfunction may turn out to have a chromosome anomaly, the Prader–Willi syndrome (see page 21.194) or one of the complex malformation syndromes such as the Smith–Lemli–Opitz syndrome (see page 21.196). Children with severe congenital hypotonia for any reason are, however, especially liable to suffer perinatal asphyxia. Hypotonic cerebral palsy is not an acceptable diagnosis in its own right.

Management of cerebral palsy

A full understanding of an individual child's skills and handicaps is impossible until at least the age of 5–10 years. In the meantime some aspects of the handicap may be greatly modified by active management. So the child 'at risk' is treated before the diagnostic process is complete. Comprehensive treatment requires assessment by a wide variety of doctors and therapists, and active intervention by some of them. Its aims are:

1. the identification and treatment of associated handicaps and complications;
2. the prevention of secondary 'deprivation' handicaps;
3. the education and support of the family in the child's care;
4. the removal of as many as possible of the obstacles to the child's development and education and the promotion of independence.

Treatable associated handicaps include strabismus, refractive errors, deafness, contractures and deformities, and epilepsy. Deafness is particularly frequent in low birthweight babies and after kernicterus. Congenital and secondary dislocation of the hip is often overlooked in severely spastic children, and windswept deformities of the hips and scoliosis may develop. Many other deformities and contractures occur and orthopaedic surgery has much to contribute to correcting deformity and improving function by judicious tenotomy, tendon transplantation or arthrodesis in various situations.

Loss of opportunity may prevent the normal development of function in parts of the brain undamaged by the original lesion. Examples include failure to develop tactile discrimination in an unused paretic hand, visual perceptual problems in the child with no experience of the vertical position or with no chance to explore his surroundings, and developmental language disorder in the deaf child, or more controversially the child with disabling dysarthria. Much of therapy is designed to circumvent these problems, and at the same time to capitalize on the child's best residual functions to develop skills for the future.

Regular contact with skilled therapists provides the parents with a source of advice and a chance to learn techniques of feeding, handling and communicating with the child at home. The lack of convincing evidence of the efficacy of physical therapy techniques, and indeed the wide variety of 'methods' available and the highly theoretical justifications which are put forward to support them are discouraging. Nevertheless it is common experience that skilled manipulation can alleviate unwanted reflexes and capitalize on others; that stretching muscles promotes their growth and prevents contractures; that repeated passive movements may be followed by active ones; that good seating support can inhibit dystonic posturing and provide a stable basis for the child to perform otherwise impossible tasks; that guided practice improves function, and that well-chosen specialized equipment can permit many new activities and promote independence. Two of the most important items that may be needed are the right wheelchair for the individual's needs, and special switching equipment to allow a severely handicapped but intelligent child to use a typewriter, symbol board, electronic communicator, environmental control system, or computer by the use of any adequately controlled movement such as with either the head or one foot. Many aspects of treatment including speech therapy and remedial education can often be combined in schools practising 'conductive education'. Ingram (1964) found 20 years ago that of his surviving cases of cerebral palsy who had left school, 35 per cent of males and 12 per cent of females were in open employment, and 48 per cent and 61 per cent were unemployed. Today – *plus ça change*!

Miscellaneous disorders of development

Congenital apraxia and the clumsy child

Troublesome clumsiness may affect 2–5 per cent of the population, more often boys than girls, and in a few of them is severely disabling. The problem usually escapes notice on mere social acquaintance or standard neurological examination, but is obvious in the classroom or on the sportsfield. Apraxia or agnosia can be detected in some cases. Clumsiness is sometimes due to 'minimal cerebral palsy' with some of the same epidemiological risk factors and minor neurological signs but it is not always so, and various disconnection syndromes, specific cortical sensory defects, disorders of cerebral dominance, and defective registration of new memories for sensorimotor patterns may all play a part in different individuals. Sometimes the defect is genetic. In addition to the primary defect of late development of fine motor skills (feeding, dressing, tying laces, and buttoning clothes, handwriting, playing ball games, etc.), there are often secondary emotional symptoms. Skilled neuropsychological analysis may be necessary to identify the nature of the defect in severe cases, but the large majority must be content with more homely solutions. Therapy consists of a judicious combination of intensive practice, diversion to activities where the child is more competent, and detailed explanation of the nature of the problem to the child, the parents, and the teachers.

Developmental speech disorders

Some 5 per cent of children are unintelligible to strangers when they start at school, and 1 per cent have seriously delayed language development. Mental retardation and deafness are the most important reasons, together with cerebral palsy, cleft palate and autism. Many have mild articulatory defects or immaturity with a good prognosis. But there is a small group (about 0.8 per 1000) who have a severe dysarthria or specific language delay.

Pseudobulbar palsy

Pseudobulbar palsy is a localized bilateral upper motor neurone disorder, characterized by dysphagia, drooling, palatal palsy and a brisk jaw jerk.

Articulatory dyspraxia

Articulatory dyspraxia is indicated by impaired voluntary movements of the lips and tongue with preservation of such reflexes as licking jam from the lips.

Specific language disorders

Specific language disorders may be identifiable as predominantly expressive or predominantly receptive ('word deafness') but are often complex; they are much commoner in boys and are often profoundly handicapping, pervading all aspects of education and social contact. The prognosis for the development of intelligible speech is poor, but intensive training may develop an overall system of communication. Speech therapy is augmented by the use of Bliss symbol boards (Blissymbolics), signing systems and electronic communicators. A few children with specific language delay also have chromosome anomalies.

References

Apley, J. (ed.) (1978). *Care of the handicapped child*. Spastics International Medical Publications, Heinemann, London.

Baraitser, M. (1982). *The genetics of neurological disorders*. Oxford University Press, Oxford.

Beattie, J. O., Day, R. E. and Cockburn, F. (1983). Alcohol and the fetus in the West of Scotland. *Br. Med. J.* **287**, 17–20.

Brett, E. M. (ed.) (1983), *Paediatric neurology*. Churchill Livingstone, Edinburgh.

Brocklehurst, G. (1976). *Spina bifida for the clinician*. Spastics International Medical Publications, Heinemann, London.

Editorial (1985). Vitamin A and teratogenesis. *Lancet* i, 319–320.

Emery, A. E. H. and Rimoin, D. L. (1983). *Principles and practice of medical genetics*. Churchill Livingstone, Edinburgh.

Gordon, N. and McKinlay, I. (1980). *Helping clumsy children*. Churchill Livingstone, Edinburgh.

Gubbay, S. S., Ellis, E., Walton, J. N. and Court, S. D. M. (1965). Clumsy children: a study of apraxic and agnostic defects in 21 children. *Brain* **88**, 295–312.

Ingram, T. T. S. (1964). *Paediatric aspects of cerebral palsy*. Livingstone, Edinburgh.

Larroche, J.-C. (1984). Malformations of the nervous system; *and* Perinatal brain damage. In *Greenfield's neuropathology* (eds J. Hume Adams, J. A. N. Corsellis and L. W. Duchen) pp. 385–450, and 451–489. Arnold, London.

LeWitt, P. A., Newman, R. P., Greenberg, H. S., Rocher, L. L., Calne, D. B. and Ehrenkranz, J. R. L. (1983). Episodic hyperhidrosis, hypothermia and agenesis of corpus callosum. *Neurology* **33**, 1122–1129.

Margalith, D., Jan, J. E., McCormick, A. Q., Tze, W. J. and Lapointe, J. (1984). Clinical spectrum of congenital optic nerve hypoplasia: review of 51 patients. *Dev. Med. Child Neurol.* **26**, 311–322.

McCarthy, G. T. (ed.) (1984). *The physically handicapped child: an interdisciplinary approach to management*. Faber and Faber, London.

Menkes, J. H. (1985). *Textbook of child neurology*, 3rd edn. Lea and Febiger, Philadelphia.

Moser, H. W. and Wolf, P. E. (1971). The nosology of mental retardation. In *Birth defects: original article series* **VII**, no. 1, 117–134.

Nelson, K. B. and Ellenberg, J. H. (1981) Apgar scores as predictors of chronic neurologic disability. *Pediatrics* **68**, 36–44.

Owens, J. R., Harris, F., McAllister, E. and West, L. (1981) 19-Year incidence of neural tube defects in area under constant surveillance. *Lancet* **ii**, 1032–1035.

Pape, K. E. and Wigglesworth, J. S. (1979). *Haemorrhage, ischaemia and the perinatal brain*. Spastics International Medical Publications, Heinemann, London.

Rutter, M. and Martin, J. A. (eds) (1972). *The child with delayed speech*. Spastics International Medical Publications, Heinemann, London.

Samilson, R. L. (ed.) (1975). Orthopaedic aspects of cerebral palsy. Spastics International Medical Publications, Heinemann, London.

Smith, D. W. (1982) *Recognisable patterns of human malformation*, 3rd edn. Saunders, Philadelphia.

Stanley, F. and Alberman, E. (eds.) (1984). *The epidemiology of the cerebral palsies*. Spastics International Medical Publications, Blackwell, Oxford.

Turner, G. (1975). An aetiological study of 1,000 patients with an I.Q. assessment below 51. *Med. J. Aust.* **2**, 927–931.

Vinken, P. J., Bruyn, G. W. and Myrianthopoulos, N. C. (eds) (1977–78). *Congenital malformations of the brain and skull* and *Congenital malformations of the spine and spinal cord*, volumes 30–32 in *Handbook of clinical neurology*, North-Holland, Amsterdam.

Warkany, J., Lemire, R. J. Cohen, M. M. (1981). *Mental retardation and congenital malformations of the central nervous system*. Year Book Medical Publishers, Chicago.

Weatherall, D. J. and 12 other authors (1981). Haemoglobin H disease and mental retardation, *N. Engl. J. Med.* **305**, 607–612.

Zellweger, H. and Simpson, J. (1977). *Chromosomes of man*. Spastics International Medical Publications, Heinemann, London.

INHERITED DISORDERS

P. K. THOMAS

There exists a large number of neurological disorders that are genetically determined, and others in which a genetic predisposition can be detected. Inherited disorders of the extrapyramidal system, peripheral nerves and muscle, and those aminoacidurias that are associated with neurological involvement are considered elsewhere, as is the question of genetic predisposition in the aetiology of conditions such as developmental abnormalities of the nervous system, epilepsy, migraine, Alzheimer's disease, and multiple sclerosis. The genetic neuropathies are considered on page 21.128.

Hereditary ataxias

The classification of the hereditary ataxias remains a matter of controversy. A spinocerebellar degeneration may develop in disorders with a known metabolic basis. This category includes abetalipoproteinaemia (see Section 9), ataxia telangiectasia (see section 4) and xeroderma pigmentosum (see Sections 4 and 20). The majority of the inherited cerebellar and spinocerebellar degenerations are at present of unknown causation. In general these can be divided into examples of early onset (under the age of 20 years), which are usually of autosomal recessive inheritance and of which Friedreich's ataxia is the commonest example, and the later onset cases of cerebellar degeneration that are most often dominantly inherited.

Early onset hereditary ataxis

Friedreich's ataxia This disorder is an example of a spinocerebellar degeneration and is dominated by progressive ataxia with an onset in childhood or adolesence. The condition is inherited as an autosomal recessive trait and affects males and females approximately equally. Degeneration of the larger dorsal root ganglion cells occurs with consequent loss of the larger myelinated fibres in the peripheral nerves and degeneration of the dorsal columns. Degeneration is also evident in Clarke's column, in the spinocerebellar tracts, and in the corticospinal pathways. There is variable loss of Purkinje cells in the cerebellum.

The average age of onset is 11-12 years. The initial symptom is almost invariably ataxia of gait, although foot or spinal deformity may antedate this. At first it is noted that the child walks awkwardly with a tendency to stumble and fall readily; in cases of early onset, walking may never have been normal. As the disease progresses, the gait slowly becomes more irregular and clumsy. The patient walks on a broad base and tends to lurch from side to side. Involvement of the upper limbs develops later, at first giving rise to clumsiness of fine movements, subsequently for all movements. A coarse intention tremor becomes obvious. The trunk is also affected, leading to oscillation of the body when standing or sitting unsupported. A regular tremor of the head (titubation)

occasionally appears. Phasic nystagmus is present in about a quarter of the cases. Dysarthria of cerebellar type develops and may become severe enough to make speech almost unintelligible.

Initially weakness is not obtrusive, but this develops as the disease advances, beginning in the legs and later involving the upper limbs. It results from degeneration in the corticospinal pathways and tends to vary in severity between cases. The plantar responses become extensor, but tone is not usually increased because of the accompanying disturbance of the afferent fibres from muscle spindles. There may be mild wasting of the anterior tibial and small hand muscles related to loss of anterior horn cells. Bladder and bowel function is usually unaffected.

Loss of the larger dorsal root ganglion cells leads to impairment of joint position sense, vibration sense, and to some extent of touch-pressure sensibility, initially distally in the legs. The impairment of proprioception superimposes a sensory element in the cerebellar ataxia. The tendon reflexes are depressed or absent.

Apart from nystagmus, the ocular movements are usually intact. The pupils are unaffected. Optic atrophy is present in about one third of cases and 10 per cent develop sensorineural deafness.

Associated skeletal deformities are common, in particular foot deformities (pes cavus and pes equinovarus) and kyphoscoliosis. Contractures of the knees may develop in the later stages. Electrocardiography demonstrates widespread T-wave inversion and ventricular hypertrophy in nearly 70 per cent of patients. Echocardiography may suggest the presence of hypertrophic obstructive cardiomyopathy, but these findings are not specific and the ECG is a more sensitive investigation for the detection of cardiomyopathy. The ECG changes are present early in the disease and tend not to be associated with symptoms. Cardiac failure occurs late and is usually precipitated by supraventricular arrhythmias.

Although progressive dementia is not a feature of the disease, reduced intelligence is present in some cases. There is an increased incidence of diabetes mellitus in Friedreich's ataxia (10 per cent).

The disease is slowly progressive, the average age of death being in the latter part of the fourth decade. The foot and spinal deformities may require orthopaedic correction. Ultimately patients become bed-ridden. Death is usually from an intercurrent infection with associated cardiac failure.

Other early onset hereditary ataxis A genetically distinct disorder that resembles Friedreich's ataxia is recognizable but which has a more benign prognosis. The condition has a similar age of onset, is also of autosomal recessive inheritance, but exhibits preserved tendon reflexes and is unassociated with cardiac abnormalities or diabetes. Further rare autosomal recessive disorders in this category include *dyssynergia cerebellaris myoclonica* (Ramsey Hunt) in which a spinocerebellar degeneration is associated with myoclonic epilepsy, and a cerebellar degeneration that is accompanied by hypogonadism. The former condition is rather poorly delineated at present.

Later onset hereditary ataxis

The category of *Marie's delayed cerebellar atrophy* was introduced to describe cases of hereditary ataxia with a later onset than Friedreich's ataxia in which the symptoms develop during the third or fourth decades of life or later. It is clear that Marie collected together a heterogeneous group of disorders, but his description served to emphasize the broad subdivision of the hereditary ataxias into the early and later onset groups.

Autosomal dominant cerebellar ataxia This comprises the main disorder within the adult onset hereditary ataxias. The age of onset ranges from the third to the fifth decades and represents the area in which there is most diagnostic confusion. Much of this stems from the fact that the clinical manifestions vary considerably between individuals within families, and between families, so that the existence of a wide range of separate disorders has been claimed. Until adequate genetic markers or linkage studies have shown that different main genes are responsible, at the present state of knowledge it is more satisfactory to group these families together. The occurrence of a slowly progressive cerebellar ataxia with dysarthria, intention tremor in the upper limbs, and an ataxic gait is the salient clinical feature. However, most of these patients show additional clinical manifestations that include dementia, optic atrophy, ophthalmoplegia, and extrapyramidal rigidity which occur in varying combinations. This disorder includes the families described by Sanger Brown, Ferguson and Critchley, and Schut and Haymaker. It probably also encompasses *Machado-Joseph disease*, the dominantly inherited cerebellar degeneration associated with ophthalmoplegia and other features in Portuguese families originating in the Azores that has been described in recent years. Pathologically these dominantly inherited cerebellar ataxias have been equated with olivopontocerebellar atrophy, although it is clear that the neuropathological changes are more widespread than this, and that the pattern of the neuropathological change also varies between individuals within the same family. Some patients with late onset cerebellar ataxia have recently been shown to have glutamate dehydrogenase deficiency.

Other late onset cerebellar degenerations A *late cortical cerebellar degeneration* that develops at around the fifth decade of life was defined by Marie, Foix, and Alajouanine. It is typified by a predominantly gait and truncal ataxia related to degeneration of the cerebellar vermis. Rare late onset dominantly inherited cerebellar degenerations, such as one associated with deafness and myoclonus, have been described. Many instances of late onset cerebellar ataxia, particularly those without ophthalmoplegia or optic atrophy, are probably non-genetic.

Hereditary spastic paraplegia

Hereditary spastic paraplegia can be subdivided into a 'pure' form (Strümpell's disease) and others in which a variety of other features coexist. Strümpell's disease may display either an autosomal dominant or autosomal recessive inheritance. It may present during childhood or even with delayed motor development in infancy; in other cases the onset is retarded until adult life. It gives rise to difficulty in walkihg because of weakness and spasticity in the legs. The tendon reflexes are exaggerated and the plantar responses are extensor. In cases of early onset, foot deformity may be present. Some patients show a mild degree of cerebellar ataxia and sensory impairment in the legs of posterior column type. The disease progresses slowly and may later affect the upper limbs. Precipitancy of micturition or urinary incontinence may occur. Pathologically there is degeneration of the corticospinal pathways

in the lateral columns of the spinal cord and some fibre loss in the gracile fasciculi.

With regard to treatment, if there is severe spasticity, this may be alleviated to some extent by baclofen at dosages of 5–20 mg three times daily or dantrolene at a dosage of 75–100 mg daily in divided doses. The precipitancy of micturition may be improved by propantheline 15 mg three times daily. Surgical correction of foot deformities is sometimes required.

Genetically distinct disorders in which a spastic paraplegia is associated with other clinical features include the *Sjögren–Larsson syndrome*, a recessively inherited condition which combines congenital ichthyosis and oligophrenia with a childhood onset spastic paraplegia, and the dominantly inherited disorder in which the paraplegia is associated with distal amyotrophy in the limbs resembling peroneal muscular atrophy.

Disorders of lipid metabolism
(See also Section 9.)

Neurolipidoses
The lipidoses constitute a group of disorders characterized by the intracellular accumulation of a variety of different lipids. Some predominantly involve the nervous system; others primarily affect the reticulo-endothelial system but may also involve nervous tissue. They may be classified in terms of the particular lipid that is stored.

Sphingomyelin lipidoses (Niemann–Pick disease) These consist of a group of recessively inherited disorders in which there is an accumulation of sphingomyelin in characteristic foam cells in the reticulo-endothelial system related in the first three types to a deficiency of sphingomyelinase. Five types exist. The most common is type A in which progressive mental deterioration and hypotonic paralysis in association with hepatosplenomegaly appear in the first six months of life leading to death before the age of three years. Cherry-red spots are present at the maculae in 50 per cent. Other more chronic variants exist.

Glucosyl ceramide lipidosis (Gaucher's disease) Three variants exist, all recessively inherited, characterized by hepatosplenomegaly related to the accumulation of glucosyl ceramide in histiocytes as a consequence of a deficiency of the enzyme glucocerebrosidase. The type 1 adult onset form does not affect the nervous system but types 2 and 3, with an infantile and juvenile onset respectively, and a more rapid progression, display widespread cerebral involvement.

Gangliosidoses These comprise a group of recessively inherited disorders in which there is a combination of progressive dementia, epilepsy, and visual failure. They were formely termed familial amaurotic idiocy and are related to defective ganglioside degradation. Several GM_1 gangliosidoses exist and are the result of an inherited deficiency of acid β-galactosidase. In the infantile form there is a generalized storage of GM_1 ganglioside affecting the brain, the viscera, and the skeleton. The onset is at birth or in early infancy, and initially is manifested by a failure to thrive and by hepatosplenomegaly. Later, mental and motor deterioration become evident, and a cherry-red spot may be present at the macula, related to retinal degeneration. Skeletal abnormalities including abnormal facial features have led to the condition being referred to as the 'pseudo-Hurler syndrome'. Death takes place before the age of three years. A juvenile onset variant also exists.

The GM_2 gangliosidoses involve the storage of GM_2 gangliosides, which are largely confined to the nervous system. In the type 1 variety (Tay-Sachs disease), the disorder usually begins within the first six months of life. It is encountered most frequently in Ashkenazi Jews. Initially there is retardation of development which is followed by progressive dementia, hypotonic weakness, and blindness. There is a cherry-red spot at the macula. Later, seizures occur and terminally generalized spasticity develops. Death generally takes place in the fourth year of life. The disorder is related to an inherited deficiency of hexosaminidase A. Carrier detection is possible by a serum assay and mass screening programmes have been undertaken in some countries. Antenatal diagnosis by amniocentesis is also possible. There is no specific therapy. The type 2 form (*Sandhoff's disease*) is similar clinically but involves a combined deficiency of hexosaminidase A and B. A form with juvenile onset also exists, as do phenotypes presenting as spinal muscular atrophy, spinocerebellar degeneration or as a dystonic syndrome.

Neuronal ceroid lipofuscinosis Under this heading are grouped a number of rare disorders in which retinal degeneration, progressive dementia, epilepsy, spasticity, and ataxia occur in various combinations. The age of onset may be infantile (Santavuori), late infantile (Jansky–Bielschowsky), juvenile (Spielmeyer–Vogt) or adult (Kufs). Eponyms abound: the late infantile and juvenile cases are often collectively termed Batten's disease. There is neuronal storage of lipopigment.

Leucodystrophies

These disorders are characterized by a diffuse disintegration of white matter in the central nervous system and sometimes also by segmental demyelination in the peripheral nerves. The cell bodies of the neurones are generally spared, although both myelin sheaths and axons show destruction in the white matter lesions.

Metachromatic leucodystrophy (sulphatide lipidosis) The most common variant is the late infantile type which usually begins in the third year of life with weakness and ataxia in the limbs. Subsequently a progressive dementia supervenes, seizures may occur, and in some instances optic atrophy develops. The tendon reflexes may be depressed or absent in those patients in whom peripheral nerve involvement is prominent. Nerve conduction velocity is reduced. Death sometimes occurs after a course of a few months, sometimes of as much as five or six years. Terminally the affected children are demented, with a spastic tetraplegia, and are often blind.

The term metachromatic leucodystrophy is derived from the presence of galactosyl sulphatide in the affected tissues. This stains metachromatically with dyes such as cresyl violet and toluidine blue. It may be demonstrated within cells in fresh specimens of urine and also within Schwann cells and macrophages in biopsies of the peripheral nerves or rectal wall. The disorder is inherited in an autosomal recessive manner, and is due to a deficiency of aryl sulphatase A. This can be demonstrated by assay on leucocytes.

Juvenile and adult onset forms of metachromatic leucodystrophy are also encountered but are rare. Prenatal diagnosis by amniocentesis and assay of aryl sulphatase activity on cultured amniotic fibroblasts is possible in both the late infantile and juvenile forms. Variants related to multiple sulphatase deficiency and to deficiency of activator protein also occur.

Globoid cell leucodystrophy (Krabbe's disease) This derives its title from the presence of large multinucleate cells containing galactosylceramide in areas of white matter damage. The condition begins at the age of three or four months as a failure to thrive. Developmental regression then becomes evident and the tendon reflexes are lost. As the disease advances, generalized hypertonus appears, together with various types of seizure, and optic atrophy. Death often occurs in the first year of life or may be delayed into the second year. There are also rare late onset cases.

The peripheral nerves are affected, biopsies showing segmental demyelination and inclusions within Schwann cells. Nerve conduction velocity is reduced.

The disorder is inherited in an autosomal recessive manner and is due to a deficiency of galactosylceramide β-galactosidase. This may be demonstrated by assays in leucocytes or serum.

Adrenoleucodystrophy (X-linked Schilder's disease) Amongst a group of conditions that give rise to widespread demyelination in the brain with an onset during childhood, cases of adrenoleucodystrophy can be separated by virtue of X-linked inheritance and associated adrenal insufficiency with features resembling Addison's disease. The affected boys exhibit a progressive illness characterized by the development of dementia. cortical blindness, ataxia, and spastic weakness in the limbs. A myeloneuropathy is sometimes the presenting deficit. Manifesting female carriers may show a mild spastic paraparesis or adrenal insufficiency.

Other rare demyelinating conditions Pelizaeus–Merzbacher disease is an X-linked recessive disease that appears in early infancy. Affected males develop ataxia and spasticity. *Canavan's disease* also develops in early infancy, is of autosomal recessive inheritance, and gives rise to progressive mental deterioration and megalencephaly associated with spongy degeneration of the white matter. The metabolic basis is not known for either of these disorders.

Fabry's disease (α-galactosidase A deficiency) (see also Section 9) This condition, otherwise known as *angiokeratoma corporis diffusum*, is an inborn error of glycosphingolipid metabolism. Neutral glycosphingolipids are deposited in various tissues as a consequence of a deficiency of the enzyme *α*-galactosidase A. The disorder is inherited in an X-linked recessive manner. Affected hemizygous males develop a mild peripheral neuropathy which is manifested by the occurrence of severe pains in the extremities, often beginning in childhood. Cerebrovascular lesions also occur, either cerebral infarction or haemorrhage. Non-neurological features include corneal opacification, punctate angiectatic lesions over the lower trunk, buttocks and upper legs, and cardiac and renal lesions. Heterozygous females may display mild manifestations, most usually corneal opacification.

Hereditary lipoprotein deficiency (see also Section 9) The occurrence of peripheral neuropathy in *hereditary high density lipoprotein deficiency (Tangier disease)* is discussed on page 21.129. *Hereditary abetalipoproteinaemia (Bassen–Kornzweig disease)* is a recessively inherited disorder in which a spinocerebellar degeneration may develop with features that bear some resemblance to Friedreich's ataxia. Other manifestations of this uncommon disorder include intestinal malabsorption, pigmentary retinal degeneration. and the presence of acanthocytes in the peripheral blood (see Section 9). In addition to the absence of serum low density lipoproteins, the serum cholesterol level is substantially reduced. There is evidence that the development of the neurological lesions may be prevented by the administration of vitamin E, the absorption of which from the gut is impaired. A spinocerebellar degeneration has also been described with hereditary hypobetalipoproteinaemia, a genetically separate condition.

Neurocutaneous syndromes

This category encompasses a number of disorders in which a variety of neurological disturbances is associated with congenital defects of the skin and retina, possibly related to their common ectodermal origin.

Neurofibromatosis (von Recklinghausen's disease)

Neurofibromatosis is inherited as an autosomal dominant trait and may display a wide range of abnormalities of which the most constant are focal areas of cutaneous hyperpigmentation (café-au-lait spots) and multiple neurofibromas. For reasons that are not clear, the disease tends to be more severe when transmitted by a male. The tumours arise from the peripheral nerves, spinal roots, and cranial nerves and frequently have a subcutaneous position. They are composed of proliferated Schwann cells and fibroblasts in a collagenous matrix, through which course nerve fibres in an irregular manner.

The disorder may be limited to the presence of a few cutaneous pigmented areas. Such areas may be encountered in normal individuals, but then they are usually smaller in size and do not exceed

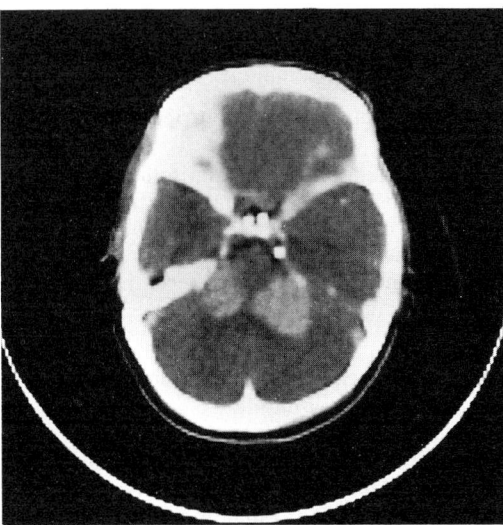

Fig. 1 CT scan showing bilateral acoustic neurinomas in a patient with central neurofibromatosis. She also had an astrocytoma of the thoracic spinal cord.

five in number. In neurofibromatosis they vary in dimensions and can be extremely numerous. They are most commonly found over the trunk and in particular in the axillae. The neurofibromas also vary considerably in number between individuals. Sessile or pedunculated cutaneous fibromas occur, or neurofibromas may be present as soft or firm single lobulated mobile subcutaneous lumps, or be felt as nodules along the course of a peripheral nerve. They are usually asymptomatic. Those on spinal roots may develop intraspinally or extend into the spinal canal through the intervertebral foramina in a 'dumb-bell' manner and lead to compression of the spinal cord or cauda equina, and tumours on peripheral nerve trunks may similarly give rise to pressure effects. Neurinomas, unilateral or bilateral, may develop on the eighth cranial nerve. At times, giant plexiform neuromas in which there is a diffuse subcutaneous overgrowth of neurofibromatous tissue may cause grotesque deformities. Mental retardation and epilepsy, related to a diffuse cortical dysgenesis, occurs in at least 10 per cent of affected individuals.

Other tumours may be associated. There is an increased incidence of gliomas and meningiomas in neurofibromatosis and also of ganglioneuromas and phaeochromocytomas. Orbital haemangiomas may occur. The neurofibromas occasionally undergo sarcomatous change. Skeletal abnormalities may coexist of which the most frequent is kyphoscoliosis. Pathological fractures with nonunion and the formation of pseudoarthrosis also may occur. Local gigantism of a limb is sometimes a feature.

In general there is a broad subdivision into a peripheral form with prominence of the cutaneous manifestations and of neurofibromas on peripheral nerves and spinal roots, and a central form with cranial nerve tumours (Fig.1), mental retardation, and a tendency to the development of gliomas or meningiomas.

Most cases require no treatment. Neurofibromas causing pressure may necessitate excision and others may merit removal for cosmetic reasons. Cases with kyphoscoliosis may require orthopaedic attention.

Tuberous sclerosis (Bourneville's disease, epiloia)

The features of this condition are mental subnormality, epilepsy, and the occurrence of characteristic skin lesions. The disorder is dominantly inherited, but may be transmitted by individuals who are asymptomatic and who show only minimal clinical evidence of the disease. Isolated cases are frequent, comprising as many as 80 or 90 per cent of index cases. Many of them probably represent new mutations; others are transmitted by gene carriers with trivial manifestions.

The earliest cutaneous lesions are irregular foliate areas of depigmentation over the trunk. These patches are readily identified when viewed under ultraviolet illumination using a Wood's lamp. Adenoma sebaceum is a second type of skin lesion which develops over the cheeks in a 'butterfly' distribution and on the forehead (Fig. 2). Multiple small warty elevations appear which histologically are fibromatous and not adenomatous. Finally, a 'shagreen patch' may be present over the lower back. This consists of an area of elevated roughened skin with a yellowish tinge which has been likened to shark skin.

The cerebral changes give rise to mental retardation evident in early life which may be static or involve a slowly progressive dementia, often complicated by behaviour disorder. Epilepsy with recurrent generalized or focal seizures may occur in association with mental retardation or in individuals of normal intelligence. The cerebral lesions, which are demonstrable by CT scanning, are typified by nodular or tuberous masses composed of proliferated glial cells and enlarged distorted neurones. They may become calcified. They are found scattered throughout the cerebral cortex and also extend into the ventricles to produce an appearance that was considered to resemble 'candle guttering' when seen in pneumo-encephalograms. Gliomas sometimes arise in these lesions.

Retinal tumours, termed phakomas, may be present, and cardiac rhabdomyomas occasionally arise as well as hamartomas of the lungs and kidneys. Polycystic disease of the kidneys may also be associated.

Treatment consists of control of the epilepsy and the management of the mental retardation and behaviour disorder. Many of the more severe cases require institutionalization.

Cerebelloretinal haemangioblastosis (von Hippel–Lindau disease)

This condition comprises the occurrence of vascular tumours in the retina and within the central nervous system, most commonly in the cerebellum and spinal cord. The inheritance is autosomal dominant in pattern.

The retinal lesions consists of angiomatous vascular malformations. The cerebellar lesion is a haemangioblastoma, often cystic, which may slowly expand and present with features of a cerebellar tumour. It may require surgical treatment. Such tumours may be

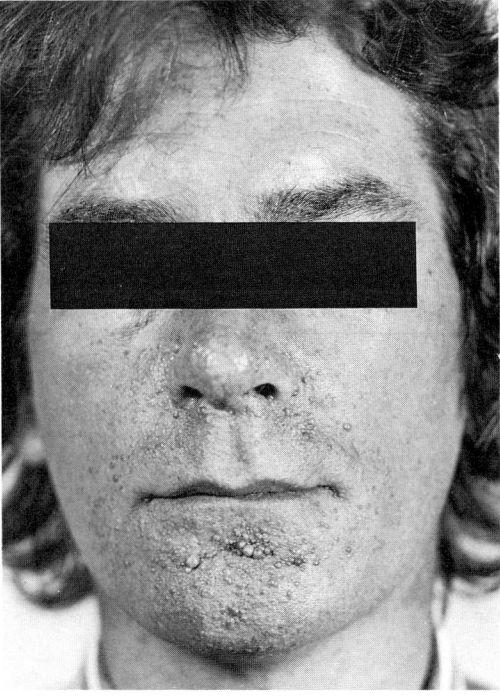

Fig. 2 Adenoma sebaceum in a patient with tuberous sclerosis.

associated with polycythaemia, possibly related to the production of erythropoietin by the tumour. Haemangioblastomas may occur in the spinal cord and rarely in the cerebral hemispheres.

The skin is not involved but other tissues outside the nervous system may be implicated, including the development of haemangioblastomas of the pancreas, kidney, and adrenal glands which may be associated with the presence of multiple cysts. Hypernephromas can occur.

It should be emphasized that the majority of cerebellar haemangioblastomas are non-genetic.

Ataxia telangiectasia (Louis–Bar syndrome)
(See also page 21.229 and Section 19.)

The inclusion of this disorder with the neurocutaneous syndromes depends upon the coincidence of a progressive cerebellar degeneration with cutaneous vascular lesions. The inheritance is of autosomal recessive type. Ataxia begins in early childhood and choreoathetosis may appear later. Telangiectasia of the conjunctivae is present as a relatively early feature and later becomes evident in the pinnae, over the face, and in the limb flexures. Some patients show an immunoglobulin deficiency and recurrent infections, or the development of malignancies may complicate the clinical picture. Defective DNA repair after X-irradiation is demonstrable in cultured skin fibroblasts. Affected children usually become unable to walk by the age of 12 years and death occurs during the second or sometimes third decade of life.

Hereditary myoclonic epilepsies
(See also page 21.230.)

A number of conditions exist in which generalized epileptic seizures and myoclonus are associated with a progressive degenerative neurological disorder occurring on a genetic basis. Their classification is still a matter of considerable uncertainty.

Lafora body disease
This is the most clearly defined form of progressive myoclonic epilepsy. It consists of a combination of major seizures, myoclonus and progressive dementia with an onset in late childhood or early adolescence, and death usually before adult life is reached. Cerebellar signs may appear later in the illness. The condition is characterized by the presence of intracellular inclusion bodies found most consistently in neurones of the cerebral cortex and in the cerebellar dentate nuclei. They are also detectable in the liver and in skeletal muscles, both of which are convenient sites for biopsy in order to establish the diagnosis. These Lafora bodies are composed of a polyglucosan. The disorder is caused by an autosomal recessive gene. Treatment is directed towards control of the epilepsy.

Less well-characterized disorders with a more prolonged time course in which epilepsy and myoclonus are associated with the features of a spinocerebellar degeneration have been described under the titles of dyssynergia cerebellaris myoclonica of Ramsey Hunt and progressive familial myoclonic epilepsy of Unverricht–Lundborg type (Baltic myoclonus). Lafora bodies are not present and their pathological basis and identity are less certain.

Cherry-red spot–myoclonus syndrome (sialidosis 1)
This is a recently described autosomal recessive disorder with onset during childhood, adolescence or early adult life of a cerebellar ataxia with intention myoclonus, cherry-red spots at the maculae, and cataracts. It is due to a deficiency an α-neuraminidase.

The myoclonus in these inherited conditions may respond to treatment with clonazepam at dosages of 1 mg three times daily, although drowsiness may be a troublesome side-effect. 5-hydroxy tryptophan is less effective than for postanoxic action myoclonus.

Hereditary spinal muscular atrophies
The hereditary spinal muscular atrophies constitute a group of disorders that involve a selective degeneration of the anterior horn cells and sometimes also the lower cranial nerve motor nuclei. They can be classified in terms of the pattern of involvement and the age of onset. Only the commoner varieties will be described.

Hereditary infantile spinal muscular atrophy (Werdnig–Hoffman disease)
This condition is inherited as an autosomal recessive trait and almost always begins within the first year of life. It may have a prenatal onset and is one cause for the 'rag-doll' child syndrome of hypotonic muscle weakness in infancy. Progressive proximal muscular weakness and wasting later becoming generalized and involving the bulbar musculature, usually lead to death before the age of four years.

Hereditary juvenile proximal spinal muscular atrophy (Kugelberg–Welander disease)
The onset is during childhood after the age of two years or as late as adolescence. The involvement of the proximal limb and trunk musculature mimics limb girdle muscular dystrophy, but fasciculation may be observed. The course is relatively benign, but progressive disability in adult life occurs in some cases; others remain relatively mildly affected. Both autosomal dominant and autosomal recessive inheritance has been described.

Hereditary distal spinal muscular atrophy
This variety presents with foot deformity, commonly pes cavus, sometimes combined with an equinovarus deformity, or with distal weakness in the legs, usually during the first decade of life. It is slowly progressive, with weakness of the hands appearing later in the disease. The ankle jerks may be lost. The condition represents one form of peroneal muscular atrophy, but in contradistinction to types I and II hereditary motor and sensory neuropathy (see page 21.128), there is no sensory disturbance. The usual pattern of inheritance is autosomal dominant.

X-linked bulbospinal neuronopathy
This recently characterized disorder consists of the development, commonly in the third or fourth decades, of progressive limb weakness, and, later, a bulbar palsy. Contraction fasciculation of the facial muscles is usually present. Muscle cramps and upper limb postural tremor are often evident from early adult life. About 50 per cent of cases show gynaecomastia and some have diabetes mellitus.

Other miscellaneous disorders
A wide variety of other rare inherited conditions that affect the nervous system exist, of which the following deserve brief mention.

Hereditary optic atrophy
Dominantly inherited juvenile optic atrophy This disorder gives rise to the insidious bilateral onset of optic atrophy during childhood with either mild or severe loss of vision. A central or centrocaecal scotoma may be detectable. Electroretinography and visual evoked potentials demonstrate no loss of retinal receptors and suggest that the lesion affects retinal neuronal elements. There are no associated neurological abnormalities.

Leber's disease This disorder consists of the occurrence of bilateral optic atrophy of relatively rapid onset in early adult life. It may begin unilaterally. A spastic paraparesis and posterior column sensory loss may develop as a late sequel. The inheritance is not clearly understood. Males are affected six times as commonly as females, but the pattern of inheritance is not typical of an X-linked recessive trait or of any other form of Mendelian inheritance. Cytoplasmic inheritance has been suggested.

Mucopolysaccharidoses
(See Section 9.)

The mucopolysaccharidoses, which are described in more detail in Section 9, constitute a group of disorders related to deficiencies of specific lysosomal enzymes and which involve an accumulation in various tissues of acid mucopolysaccharides and gangliosides, and by the presence of mucopolysaccharides in the urine. In both the recessively inherited Hurler's syndrome and the X-linked recessive Hunter's syndrome, the skeletal and other manifestations may be accompanied by mental retardation and pigmentary retinal degeneration. A spastic weakness in the limbs may develop in Hurler's syndrome. Mental retardation is also seen in the recessively inherited Sanfillipo's syndrome. Entrapment neuropathies are a feature in some forms, related to the skeletal changes.

Subacute necrotizing encephalopathy of infancy (Leigh's disease)
With an onset during the first two years of life, a fatal encephalopathy develops, mainly characterized by necrotic lesions in the brain stem and a prominence of small blood vessels. Haemorrhage does not occur. The distribution of the lesions bears some resemblance to Wernicke's encephalopathy and defective activation of the pyruvate dehydrogenase complex may underlie the disorder. The inheritance is probably of autosomal recessive pattern, but the clinical features are non-specific and the condition may well be heterogeneous. Cases with a later onset have been described.

Infantile neuroaxonal dystrophy (Seitelberger's disease)
This is a rare, probably recessive condition that develops between the ages of one and three years and gives rise to progressive motor weakness from both upper and lower motor neurone deficits. Optic atrophy also occurs and death usually ensues before the end of the first decade. Degenerative changes are present in the brain and the spinal cord, the most striking feature of which is the occurrence of large axonal swellings in the grey matter of the brain and spinal cord.

Menkes' syndrome ('kinky' or 'steely' hair)
Menkes' syndrome is an X-linked recessive disorder in which developmental regression begins within a few months of birth. Muscle hypotonus or hypertonus and seizures appear and are associated with abnormal hair. The scalp hair is sparse, stubbly and greyish in colour. When examined under magnification, the hairs are seen to be twisted and display partial breaks. The serum copper and caeruloplasmin levels are low and the condition prob-ably results from defective copper absorption from the gut. Prenatal diagnosis is possible.

Lesch–Nyhan syndrome
This is an X-linked recessive disorder (see also page 21.229 and Section 9) related to the absence of an enzyme of purine metabolism, hypoxanthine-guanine phosphoribosyl transferase. The salient features are overproduction of uric acid and consequent hyperuricaemia which are associated with various behavioural and neurological manifestations including mental retardation, self-mutilation, choreoathetosis, pyramidal signs, and spasticity in the limbs. The neurological abnormalities develop in childhood and death usually occurs in the second or third decade from renal failure. Allopurinol may reduce some of the non-neurological consequences of the hyperuricaemia, but no treatment influences the neurological abnormalities, the mechanism of which is not understood. Prenatal diagnosis and carrier detection are available.

Cockayne's syndrome
This is of autosomal recessive inheritance and consists of the development in childhood of dwarfism, microcephaly, mental retardation, cataract, pigmentary retinopathy, and ataxia. There is cutaneous sensitivity to ultraviolet light. The cerebral changes are those of a leucodystrophy. A demyelinating neuropathy coexists.

References
Baraitser, M. (1982). *Genetics of neurological disorders*. Oxford University Press, Oxford.
Bundey, S. (1985). *Genetics and neurology*. Churchill Livingstone, Edingburgh.
Gomez, M. R. (ed.) (1979). *Tuberous sclerosis*. Raven Press, New York.
Harding, A. E. (1984). *The hereditary ataxias and related disorders*. Churchill Livingstone, Edinburgh.
Harper, P. S. (1980). *Practical genetic counselling*. Wright, Bristol.
Kark, R. A. P., Rosenberg, R. N. and Schut, L. J. (eds) (1978). *Advances in neurology*. Vol. 21, *Inherited ataxias*. Raven Press, New York.
Riccardi, V. M. (1981). Von Recklinghausen neurofibromatosis. *New Engl. J.Med.* **305**, 1617.
Stanbury, J. B., Wyngaarden, J. B., and Fredrickson, D. S. (eds) (1982). *Metabolic basis of inherited metabolic disorders*, 5th edn. McGraw-Hill, New York.

DEMYELINATING DISEASE
W. B. MATTHEWS

Definition
The concept of primary demyelinating disease implies a pathological process that destroys the myelin sheaths while sparing the neurones and their axonal processes.

Within the central nervous system, myelin is formed by the oligodendrocytes and surrounds the axons in a spiral formation. The sheath is not continuous but, as in peripheral nerves, is divided into short segments, each segment being maintained by a single oligodendrocyte which, however, also maintains myelin segments on neighbouring axons. Destruction of myelin could, therefore, result either from a disease process selectively involving the oligodendroglia or from biochemical or immunological attack on the proteolipid of myelin. If an axon is divided or otherwise destroyed, the myelin sheath is involved in the resulting Wallerian degeneration, and in this sense demyelination is therefore encountered in all forms of organic nervous disease. Loss of myelin with anatomical preservation of axons characteristically occurs in the early lesions of a distinctive group of diseases, of which multiple sclerosis is by far the most important.

MULTIPLE SCLEROSIS (disseminated sclerosis)
Prevalence
Because of difficulties of case ascertainment and precise diagnosis the prevalence of multiple sclerosis is difficult to determine. There is, however, general agreement that there are wide and apparently systematized variations. Regions of low prevalence (less than 5/100 000), medium (up to 30/100 000), and high prevalence (up to about 300/100 000) can be identified although naturally these do not have sharp boundaries. With the notable exception of Japan, where prevalence is low, the general rule is that high prevalence is positively correlated with distance from the equator, in both hemispheres. In England prevalence is around 60/100 000 but is higher in Scotland, particularly in Shetland and Orkney, where the high-

est known prevalence has been recorded. Recent surveys indicate that the prevalence gradient between northern Europe and the Mediterranean is less marked than had been thought.

Incidence

Annual incidence naturally shows similar variations, from 0.4/100 000 for those born in South Africa to 9.5/100 000 for Orkney.

Age incidence shows a similar pattern in all geographical areas, with very few cases in the first decade, a steep rise later in the second decade to a peak around the age of 30 years, followed by a decline, with new cases after the age of 50 years being increasingly rare.

Sex incidence shows a variable female preponderance around 3:2.

Incidence is increased in the relatives of known cases, but no distinctive pattern of inheritance can be discerned. The risk of multiple sclerosis in the offspring of a known case is about 1 per cent and there is an approximately ten-fold risk in first degree relatives. Concordance is higher in mono- than in dizygotic twins, but most pairs are non-concordant.

Pathology

The name of the disease implies that there are scattered areas of scarring in the nervous system, but the initial lesion is the plaque of demyelination (Figs 1–3). These may occur anywhere within the central nervous system including the optic nerves, but the peripheral nervous system is not involved. Plaques range in size from a few millimetres in diameter to confluent areas involving most of the cross section of the spinal cord or brain stem, or large areas of the cerebral hemispheres. They can be identified at autopsy as grey shrunken areas on the surface and in sections can be seen to involve mainly the white matter, but also to extend into the cerebral cortex, the basal ganglia, and the grey matter of the spinal cord. The distribution of plaques is never precisely symmetrical or systematized, but there are certain sites of predilection, notably the optic nerves, the periventricular areas of the cerebral hemispheres, the brain stem, and the cervical spinal cord. In early lesions, which often form around small veins (Fig. 2), microscopy shows that myelin has been destroyed, but axons appear to be intact, although even at this stage there is glial proliferation. Normal oligodendrocytes cannot be identified within the plaque, but aberrant forms may be present in the periphery. There is a mild degree of lymphocytic perivascular cuffing. Areas in which myelin sheaths are present, but unduly thin – shadow plaques – , often seem to form extensions of the fully developed lesions. In later stages glial scarring, the sclerosis of the title, is prominent, and a small proportion of axons are also destroyed, leading to considerable atrophy. Indisputable evidence of multiple sclerosis may

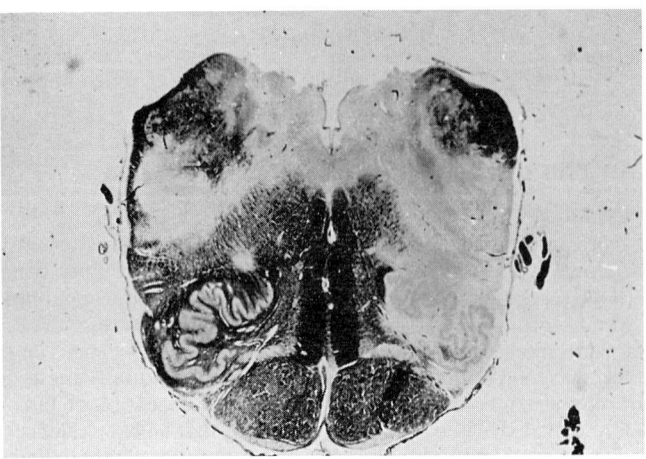

Fig. 1 Multiple sclerosis. Cross section of medulla showing characteristic plaques.

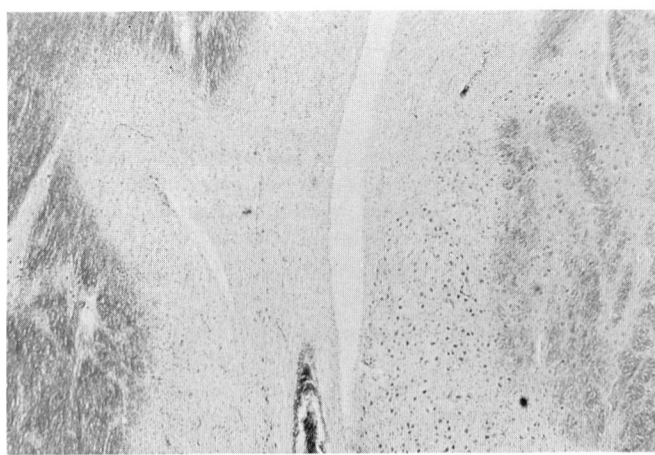

Fig. 2 A plaque extending along a small vein.

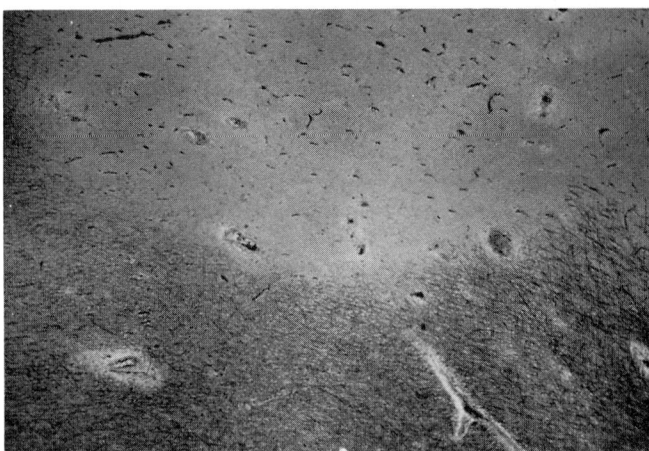

Fig. 3 The sharp edge of a chronic plaque, showing abrupt transition to normal white matter.

occasionally be found at routine autopsy in patients who have never had symptoms of the disease.

Clinical features

The onset of the disease is monosymptomatic with evidence of a single lesion of the central nervous system in 55 per cent of cases, or there may be symptoms of multiple lesions from the beginning. As any part of the central nervous system may be involved, the symptoms are naturally extremely diverse, but the common clinical presentations reflect the selective distribution of plaques already described. Presenting symptoms are therefore usually due to lesions in the optic nerves, the brainstem, or spinal cord.

A plaque in the optic nerve causes retrobulbar neuritis if posteriorly situated, or optic neuritis if the nerve head is visibly involved. The first symptom is usually pain in or around the eye, rapidly followed by blurred vision, which may continue to deteriorate for a week, during which the pain persists, being worse on moving the eye. The degree of visual loss varies from slight dulling of colour vision to complete monocular blindness, but typically central vision is reduced to 6/60 with retention of peripheral vision. This central scotoma is due to predominant involvement of fibres coming from the macula. The optic disc usually appears normal but is sometimes swollen. Fine haemorrhages radiating from the disc may be seen. The severe central visual loss distinguishes this appearance from papilloedema. Vision nearly always begins to improve within a week or two and progresses over several months. Acuity often returns to normal and severe residual loss is most unusual after an initial attack. Even with normal vision, the temporal half of the optic disc, containing fibres from the macula, often becomes pale and this temporal pallor is commonly found in patients with multiple sclerosis with no history of retrobulbar neuritis. Uncommon variations in clinical course include bilateral simultaneous optic neuritis, visual field changes other than central scotomata, and progressive visual failure. Optic neuritis can occur in sarcoidosis, systemic lupus, neurosyphilis, and in other inflammatory conditions, or may occur as an isolated event, but multiple sclerosis is by far the most common cause, particularly of retrobulbar neuritis.

Initial symptoms due to involvement of the brain stem include double vision and vertigo. The former may be due to a VIth nerve palsy or to internuclear palsy (see page 21.92), and nystagmus is also often present. Vertigo can be severe and prostrating and characteristically persists for a week or longer and does not occur in brief paroxysms, and hearing is usually preserved. The distinction from vestibular neuronitis (see page 21.91) is difficult. Remission of brain stem symptoms of this type is usually complete.

Plaques within the spinal cord may present with either motor or sensory symptoms. Weakness of one or both legs is a common mode of onset. Typically, dragging of one leg is at first only noticed after prolonged exertion, but soon becomes obvious during ordinary activities and may affect the other leg. Sensory symptoms often take the form of numbness, beginning in the feet and spreading in the course of a few days up to the waist. Sensation over the buttocks and perineum is altered, but there is usually no loss of sphincter control. As there is no weakness and reflex activity is not altered, the patient's claim that she feels something between her skin and the examiner's pin may not be believed. Tingling paraesthesiae may accompany numbness or occur independently, usually persisting for about six weeks. Hysteria is also sometimes diagnosed when the complaint is of a useless hand, rendered so by loss of postural sense, again without weakness or reflex signs.

Many other symptoms encountered in the course of the disease may occasionally be the presenting feature, and may cause diagnostic difficulty. Mental symptoms, amounting to mild dementia, may occur early, often accompanied by dysarthria. Urinary incontinence or retention may occur in isolation, but impotence in the male without other symptoms or signs is unlikely to be due to multiple sclerosis. Of grave prognostic significance is onset with an acute brain stem syndrome which may advance with such rapidity as to arouse suspicion of a stroke. Complex ocular palsies are combined with bulbar palsy, facial weakness, and sensory loss, and extensive paralysis, ataxia, and sensory loss in the limbs. Hemiplegia due to multiple sclerosis may even more closely resemble a stroke, sometimes developing overnight. Onset with a transverse lesion of the spinal cord producing paraplegia, with a sensory level, is fortunately rare, as recovery is often slight.

Course

The course of the disease is that of repeated relapse and remission in 80 per cent of patients and of steadily progressive disability in the remainder. In the remitting form it is usual for complete recovery to follow the initial attack, but for increasing residual disability to persist after later relapses. Thus, a young woman may have retrobulbar neuritis with complete recovery within two months, followed three months later by numbness of the legs, again with recovery within a few weeks. The next relapse might follow after a similar interval, and if this involved weakness of the legs it might not be followed by complete remission but by persistent slight difficulty in walking. Significant improvement after relapse cannot be expected after about six months. In a severe case further relapses are followed by a stage of progressive deterioration without recognizable acute episodes. Particularly in older patients the disease may be progressive from the outset, most frequently with signs of spinal cord disease. There is a remarkable contrast between the patient in whom, after perhaps one or two clearly recognizable episodes of multiple sclerosis, the disease becomes entirely quies-

cent and the severe case where crippling disability persists after the first attack.

A patient with established disease may therefore have only minor disability due to, for example, slight spastic weakness and ataxia of the legs, but despite much initial variation, patients with more severe forms of multiple sclerosis eventually develop a characteristic clinical state. A typical patient at the ambulant stage will show pallor of the temporal halves of both optic discs but visual acuity will be normal. Nystagmus will be present and often this takes a characteristic so-called ataxic form in which on lateral gaze the abducting eye develops nystagmus, while the adducting eye does not. Speech may be slightly slurred. Strength of the upper limbs is likely to be normal, but function of one or both hands may be disturbed by cerebellar ataxia or intention tremor. The gait will be spastic and ataxic, and even when only one leg is complained of, both plantar reflexes will be extensor and tendon reflexes increased. The abdominal reflexes are usually absent. The confidence sometimes expressed in this sign is misplaced. Persistent cutaneous sensory loss is most unusual, but vibration sense is lost in the legs and postural sense often impaired. Bladder symptoms are often peculiarly distressing, at first urgency of micturition and later incontinence due to frequent uncontrolled emptying of a small-capacity bladder. A few patients have repeated attacks of urinary retention. Erectile impotence in the male is usual and there may be loss of genital sensation in women. The mental condition may appear quite normal, but precise testing often reveals mild dementia which may later become more obvious and be expressed in the classical euphoria. Depression is, however, not uncommon.

Brief paroxysmal symptoms bearing little resemblance to the familiar effects of loss of neuronal function may occur either at the onset or in the established disease but are uncommon. Of these, trigeminal neuralgia, indistinguishable from the idiopathic form, except for onset at an early age, is the best known. Unilateral, usually painful, spasms of the limbs, which adopt the tetanic posture, are highly characteristic. These begin suddenly and occur up to 50 times a day, being precipitated by movement or overbreathing. Each tonic seizure lasts less than 2 min and, even if not painful, is extremely unpleasant. Paroxysmal dysarthria also occurs in very frequent, equally brief episodes, usually accompanied by sharply localized paraesthesiae in the face or arm, or by ataxia. Pain in the limbs is not uncommon, but only rarely presents in typical paroxysmal form comparable to trigeminal neuralgia. These symptoms have an important feature in common, in that they can be abolished by small doses of carbamazepine, and eventually remit completely. They do not appear to be related to epilepsy, which is a rare symptom of multiple sclerosis, and are probably the result of abnormal spread of excitation between demyelinated axons within plaques in the spinal cord or brain stem.

Another symptom that is often misinterpreted is facial myokymia. This consists of constant flickering contraction of all the muscles on one side of the face resulting in slight closure of the eye and retraction of the angle of the mouth. This should not be confused with the commonplace twitching of the eyelids apparently related to fatigue.

Many patients notice apparently random fluctuations of their symptoms in the course of the day, but more obviously related to the demyelinating process is the specific effect of heat and exertion. Patients may have to give up having hot baths because of the severe but temporary increase in weakness of the legs induced. Visual acuity may also be reduced at the same time and is particularly influenced by severe physical exertion.

As the disease progresses, walking becomes more difficult and a wheelchair life is reluctantly adopted, and eventually the patient becomes helpless. At this stage vision may be affected by optic atrophy, dysarthria is severe, and dementia often obvious. The arms are incapable of use because of ataxia and the legs are paralysed, at first in extension, but increasingly becoming fixed in flexion by spasm and contracture. Complete incontinence is now the rule and survival depends on nursing care. Death results from respiratory paralysis, bedsores, urinary infection, status epilepticus or terminal coma of undetermined nature.

Prognosis

In some 20 per cent of patients multiple sclerosis may be said to have followed a benign course when there is no disability after 10 or 15 years. Such patients are not, however, free from risk of severe relapse. In 5 per cent the disease follows a malignant course with death within five years. Prognostic indicators would obviously be of great value but unfortunately it has proved far easier to foretell a grave outcome than mild disease. Adverse factors include advanced age at onset, progressive course or incomplete recovery from the initial attack, early cerebellar ataxia or persistent weakness and early loss of mental acuity. Onset with sensory symptoms or optic neuritis has a relatively good prognosis on a statistical basis but this is of no value in the individual patient.

The average duration of life from onset of symptoms has been between 20 and 30 years in recent series. Probably 15 per cent die within ten years and one-third within 15 years. The prognosis as to remaining at work, however, is very much less favourable.

Diagnosis

When there is a history of relapsing disease, and symptoms and signs of multiple lesions in characteristic sites, there is seldom any diagnostic difficulty. It is true that meningovascular syphilis, Behcet's disease, neurological sarcoid, and systemic lupus can also cause lesions scattered in time and site within the central nervous system, but all are rare and are seldom mistaken for multiple sclerosis, as all have distinctive diagnostic features. Difficulty more often arises from the presentation of chronic progressive multiple sclerosis with symptoms confined to those attributable to a single lesion. The classical error is to diagnose spinal cord compression from a neurofibroma as spinal multiple sclerosis. A persistent cutaneous sensory level is most unusual in multiple sclerosis and root pain should also throw doubt on this diagnosis. Many patients with multiple sclerosis are now submitted to myelography in a somewhat exaggerated determination not to overlook a tumour. This is an unpleasant investigation, not to be lightly undertaken, and is certainly not indicated if there is firm evidence of multiple lesions. Doubful pallor of the optic discs, a few jerks of nystagmus on lateral gaze or pins and needles in the hands should not, however, be accepted as proof of dissemination. Distinction from cervical myelopathy due to spondylosis is exceptionally difficult, particularly as the two conditions may co-exist. Localized muscular wasting, following the pattern of root distribution, that may occur in myelopathy, is not a feature of multiple sclerosis although some diffuse wasting of the hand muscles may be seen. Loss of tendon reflexes in the upper limbs is also rare in multiple sclerosis. Often only unequivocal cranial nerve involvement enables the distinction to be made. Subacute combined degeneration of the spinal cord occurs in older people, and is a symmetrical systematized condition. Progressive bilateral visual failure with optic atrophy can occur in multiple sclerosis, but this diagnosis should be accepted with great reluctance in the absence of other signs of the disease, as compression of the optic chiasma is a more probable cause. The clinical course of a pontine glioma may sometimes be inexplicably marked by remission and relapse, and, particularly in view of its situation, confusion with multiple sclerosis is understandable, but the brain stem angioma often advanced as a cause for similar symptoms is seldom diagnostically credible.

As a contribution to positive diagnosis, it has been claimed that the retinal veins show a characteristic sheathing in a high proportion of cases of multiple sclerosis, but most observers have not found this a useful or consistent finding. Further positive diagnostic aid, as opposed to the exclusion of other conditions, can be derived from the examination of the cerebrospinal fluid. In about one-third of cases, the lymphocyte count is raised but seldom

above $0.05 \times 10^9/l$. The total protein is raised in a rather smaller proportion of patients, but not above 1.2 g/l. These changes, which do not necessarily run in parallel, are non-specific and are not obviously related to the clinical activity of the disease. The Lange colloidal gold curve is of the 'paretic' type – 55432100 – in about 25 per cent of cases. This reaction depends on an increase in globulin relative to albumin and may be positive when the total protein is normal. Gamma globulin forms 25 per cent or more of the total protein in 60 per cent of cases, and does not reach this proportion in other diseases likely to be confused on clinical grounds, except neurosyphilis. Slightly more specific is the level of IgG which is over 15 per cent of the total protein in about 66 per cent of cases of multiple sclerosis. The interpretation of these results obviously depends on the reliability of the estimations which, with regard to the total protein, are notoriously based on an outmoded subjective test of turbidity. Immuno-electrophoresis, a technique not yet generally available, demonstrates oligoclonal gamma globulin bands in the cerebrospinal fluid in over 90 per cent of cases and is of great diagnostic value, but is not specific.

Using electronic averaging techniques it is now possible to record from the surface of the scalp or neck the response evoked within the central nervous system by a variety of stimuli: visual, sensory or auditory. Abnormalities in these evoked potentials are often present in patients with multiple sclerosis (Fig. 4). The diagnostic value of this finding lies in the demonstration of abnormalities thought to be due to slowed or blocked conduction in areas of the central nervous system not clinically involved in the disease. By this means the presence of multiple lesions can be detected. For example, a delayed response to a visual stimulus presented to one or both eyes may be found in a patient with clinical evidence only of progressive spinal cord disease. These changes are not, however, specific as delayed or otherwise abnormal evoked responses may be found in, for example, the hereditary ataxias, and abnormal results are not commonly found in the early stages of multiple sclerosis when the diagnosis is most often in doubt.

The computerized tomography (CT) scan may show a number of abnormalities in multiple sclerosis, the most common being dilation of the lateral ventricles and cortical atrophy. Low-density areas in the white matter of the cerebral hemispheres, presumably indicating chronic plaques are less common. In acute relapse multiple focal lesions, often enhancing with iodine-containing contrast, may be visible.

Nuclear magnetic resonance (NMR) scanning is capable of demonstrating many more lesions than can be seen by CT, but the diagnostic potential of this technique has not been fully explored.

Great interest has surrounded the highly controversial diagnos-

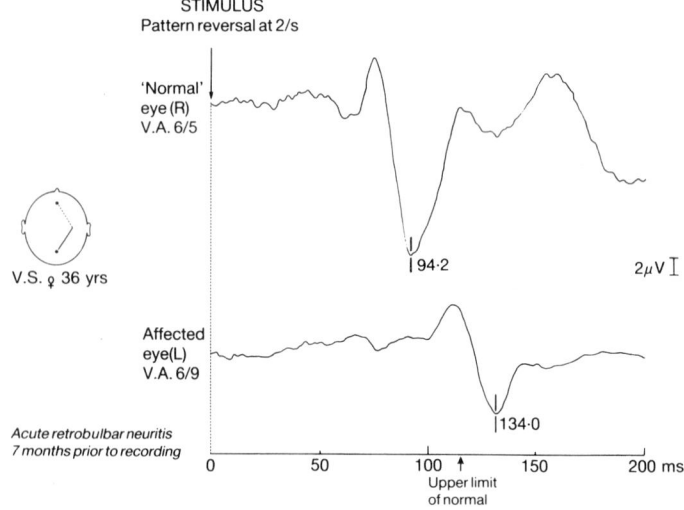

Fig. 4 Visual evoked potential showing persistent abnormality seven months after an attack of optic neuritis.

tic test based on the effects of polyunsaturated fatty acids on the motility of the patient's red cells in an electrical field. Much appears to depend on precise details of technique. The merits of the claim that children liable to develop the disease as adults can be identified by this test clearly cannot be decided until the children have passed the peak age of onset, still many years ahead.

Pathophysiology

The relation of the lesions of multiple sclerosis to the symptoms is unexpectedly complex. There are well-documented examples of normal function in, for example, the spinal cord, in spite of chronic extensive demyelination found soon afterwards post-mortem. There is little evidence of effective remyelination and yet complete clinical recovery can occur from apparently devastating paralysis or blindness. However, even with complete restoration of function, it is possible to demonstrate by electrical means that axonal conduction is slow or blocked. Demyelination by whatever means can block conduction in the intact axons. It is thought that with the passage of time changes in the bared axonal membrane occur permitting conduction, but not of the normal rapid saltatory type. Conduction in such axons is vulnerable to minute changes in temperature, an increase leading to blocking of conduction, and no doubt other unknown agents may be operating. The restored slow conduction through the plaques does, however, seem to be capable of sustaining normal function although of course often failing to do so.

Inability to conduct faithfully rapid trains of impulses, demonstrable in demyelinated single fibres in animal experiments, may account for the fatigue that is often such a prominent feature.

These observations on the lack of correlation between the state of the myelin and the clinical symptoms throw considerable doubt on the value of purely clinical observations in establishing the time of onset of the disease and the state of activity of the disease process.

Other mechanisms have been involved to explain, at least in part, the causation of symptoms. In an acute plaque the blood–brain barrier is opened and there is considerable oedema. Resolution of the swelling has been proposed as the basis of rapid remission of symptoms. Circulating agents with the property of blocking synaptic transmission have been found in a proportion of patients with multiple sclerosis but also in other diseases, and their role is doubtful.

The strange paroxysmal symptoms of multiple sclerosis may arise from ephaptic transmission between axons stripped of their myelin. A sensory impulse, ascending the spinothalamic tract, may be blocked by a plaque, but spread laterally to the descending corticospinal pathway in the same plaque and cause a paroxysm of tonic muscular contraction.

Paraesthesiae, and also possibly myokymia, probably originate from spontaneous abnormal discharge from demyelinated axons such as has been found in experimental demyelination.

Aetiology and pathogenesis

The cause of multiple sclerosis is unknown, but this is not because of any failure to accumulate clinical and experimental data from which some support can now be extracted for virtually any theory propounded. Attention has recently centred on three possibly interrelated factors: lipid metabolism, autoimmunity, and infection.

The idea of a generalized disorder of lipid metabolism has always seemed attractive in view of the lipid content of myelin and has appeared to receive some support from a reported relative deficiency of unsaturated fatty acids in histologically normal areas of multiple sclerosis brain and a reduced level of linoleic acid in the serum. In common with most of the experimental observations in this disease there is no general agreement on these findings and attention has recently been more directed to the lipid content of the cell membrane. There is a possible correlation between high prevalence and consumption of saturated animal fats but no theory of causation based on dietary factors has yet proved convincing.

A chronic, spontaneously relapsing, and remitting demyelinating disease can be produced in a number of animal species by the injection of extracts of central nervous system tissue plus adjuvant. The histopathology is indistinguishable from that of multiple sclerosis; oligoclonal bands of IgG are present in the CSF, and visual and other evoked potentials are abnormal. The pathogenesis of this autoimmune disease, experimental allergic encephalomyelitis (EAE), may be accepted, at least provisionally, as being the same as that of multiple sclerosis. The aetiology, however, is clearly distinct, as patients with multiple sclerosis have not been injected with myelin basic protein, the encephalitogenic agent of EAE. If multiple sclerosis is a form of autoimmune disease the responsible antigen has not been determined.

It was naturally hoped that the oligoclonal bands of IgG, being presumably antibodies, could be used to identify relevant antigens, but this is not so. In multiple sclerosis the bands are not absorbed by any virus tested or by any component of nervous tissues. It is now thought that they are 'nonsense' antibodies, affording no clue to aetiology.

Further evidence of an autoimmune process is provided by the intrathecal synthesis of IgG and the fall in circulating suppressor T cells that accompanies clinical relapse. As with many phenomena in multiple sclerosis it is not known whether these changes are an indication of the disease process or an effect of the lesions.

There have been repeated claims to have isolated an infective agent from the nervous system in multiple sclerosis or to have detected the notoriously fallible 'virus-like particles'. These claims have not been substantiated but, particularly since the appreciation of the role of temperate or slow viruses in certain other diseases of the nervous system, the theory of infection remains attractive. An increase in measles antibodies in the serum and CSF has repeatedly been confirmed and specific antimeasles IgG antibody has been found in the CSF. The measles antigen has not, however, been found in the nervous system, and there is as yet no serious support for a theory of slow measles encephalomyelitis in the adult as the cause of the disease. The related canine distemper virus has been suggested on epidemiological grounds. A number of animal models have been developed where disseminated inflammatory demyelination is induced by viral infection. An infection or acquired agent would explain some of the epidemiological data which indicate that to migrate from a high-risk to a low-risk area before the age of 15 years is to acquire the low risk of the new country, whereas migrants older than 15 years carry their high risk with them. Further inferences from studies of families with information on duration of common exposure to a hypothetical agent also suggest that if infection is indeed the cause, it takes place around the age of 14 years. An environmental factor is strongly suggested by the geographical distribution.

There is an obvious influence from genetic factors, shown by the relative preponderance of HLA tissue types DR2 and B7 in northern Europe, although other types predominate in different geographical areas. There have been suggestions that multiple sclerosis has been spread throughout the world by people of British descent.

An attractive theory, for which evidence is far from conclusive, is that multiple sclerosis is a virus-induced autoimmune disease, favoured by certain HLA tissue types.

Patchy inflammatory demyelination may be a response to a variety of noxious agents and a unitary 'cause' of multiple sclerosis may not exist.

Treatment

In many diseases the lack of any coherent explanation of causation has not proved an insuperable obstacle to effective treatment, at least on a symptomatic level. In multiple sclerosis, however, ignorance of the aetiology of the disease, of the immediate causes of the relapses, and of the mechanism of remission has effectively prevented any rational approach to treatment, and both the empirical approach and informed guesswork have proved unavailing. The stage of glial scarring may well be beyond the reach of therapy, but the earlier stages in which patients may remain symptom-free for many years or may recover spontaneously from severe paralysis should provide opportunities for both preventive and curative treatment. There is no evidence that effective remyelination takes place, the shadow plaques being probably areas of spreading destruction rather than of repair. An understanding of how, for example, visual acuity can return to normal, although the optic nerve head remains pale, and presumably persistently demyelinated, might go far to resolve the enigma. In default of knowledge, treatment is singularly ineffective.

There are peculiar difficulties in establishing the efficacy of any treatment in multiple sclerosis. The course of the disease is subject to unpredictable fluctuations. There is intense emotional involvement of patients and investigators. There is no means of monitoring the course of the disease or the activity of the disease process except by clinical examination. There may even be uncertainty of diagnosis. Criteria laid down for the conduct of therapeutic trials in multiple sclerosis are necessarily stringent – so stringent that they have probably never been fully adopted.

There is reasonable evidence that a course of corticotrophin will speed recovery from acute relapse although without improving the final outcome. Corticotrophin gel 40 units twice a day may be given for a week, with half this dose for a further week, and gradual reduction for a third week. The dose should be reduced if fluid retention or acne prove troublesome. Many neurologists would also prescribe such a course in an attempt to arrest progressive deterioration. Chronic administration of corticotrophin or steroids does not prevent relapse or improve prognosis, and such treatment should not be given.

The beneficial effect of corticotrophin and steroids is probably that of reduction of oedema and inflammation in acute plaques rather than any effect on immune mechanisms but many attempts have been made to alter the immune state. Transfer factor has been given on the assumption that there is an immunodeficiency, perhaps specifically towards the measles virus. In a well-conducted trial monthly injections appeared to slow the progress of the disease.

There have been extensive trials of many forms of immunosuppression. Relatively few have been controlled in any way and double-blind randomized controlled trials are very difficult to organize. It is clear that no method so far employed completely arrests the disease. It is possible that either long-term azathioprine or short courses of intravenous cyclophosphamide may have a beneficial effect on the course but extended trials are still in progress. Other methods employed have included plasmapheresis, lymphocytopheresis, thymectomy, and high-dose bolus steroids.

Interferon has been given both intravenously and by intrathecal injection, in the hope of overcoming a presumed viral infection. The side effects may prove prohibitive.

Hyperbaric oxygen has been used in the United States by a few enthusiasts for many years and this method has recently become popular in the United Kingdom. As with many forms of attempted treatment of multiple sclerosis the theoretical basis has shifted sharply and it is now held that oxygen will counteract the effects of fat embolism proposed as the cause of the disease. Results are disappointing, particularly to the patients.

Linoleic acid dietary supplements have been claimed to reduce the severity of relapse, but the regular consumption of sunflower seed oil containing unsaturated fatty acid is not an effective therapeutic measure. Avoidance of animal fats has also been claimed to be beneficial, but without controlled supporting evidence.

Symptomatic treatment is often important. Physiotherapy may improve the ability to walk but is of little value in advanced disease. Spasticity in the ambulant patient can be reduced by baclofen or diazepam, but sometimes at the cost of increased weakness. In bedridden patients, baclofen is the best drug for preventing flexor spasm, but is not always successful. Intrathecal injection of phenol in glycerine may be needed to allow the paient to sit in a chair. Urgency of micturition is often helped by ephedrine, 15 mg thrice daily or emepromium bromide. Clean intermittent self-catheterization should be more widely used. Severe incontinence, particularly in the female, is a formidable and unsolved problem. Permanent catheterization should be used only if there is no other way of protecting the skin from constant exposure to urine. It is to be hoped that methods of electrical stimulation of the sphincters or partial interruption of the hyperexcitable reflex activity responsible for incontinence in the spastic patient will eventually prove to be successful. Spinal cord stimulation through epidural electrodes, for which exaggerated claims have been made in the symptomatic treatment of multiple sclerosis, may find a place in improving function of the neurogenic bladder. In the meantime, recourse has to be made to a rubber urinal in the male and to padding and waterproof pants in the female.

Management

It is unwise to inform a patient that multiple sclerosis is suspected after an initial episode, however apparently typical. The diagnosis may be wrong, or if correct, there may be prolonged remission. An incapacitating hysterical reaction often follows such ill-judged pronouncements. If asked directly it seems best to say that this is one of the diagnoses being considered but that it is impossible to be sure after a single attack. Difficult and indeed insoluble problems arise when a patient suspected of having the disease announces an intention to get married. Once persistent symptoms are established, it is best to reveal the diagnosis. This does not have the adverse effect on morale that results from continued prevarication and patients are often relieved to be told that their medical attendants know what is wrong with them.

Advice may be required on specific aspects. There is a slightly increased risk of relapse in the puerperium, the odds against relapse in one year in a non-pregnant woman being 6 to 1 compared with 4 to 1 during a pregnancy year in a woman of the same age, but evidence suggests that pregnancy does not affect the eventual outcome. Multiple sclerosis is not, therefore, an absolute bar to bearing children, but clearly a large family is undesirable. Surgical operations have not been shown to cause relapse. It is usual to advise that exceptional care should be taken to avoid fatigue, particularly during infections, but there is no serious evidence that relapse is thereby avoided. Necessary inoculations may be given as these have been shown not to be dangerous.

In this bald account of the disease it has been impossible to convey the human aspects of multiple sclerosis. Previously healthy young adults experience strange symptoms, mild or severe but always threatening. Diagnosis may be easy or difficult but is often inexcusably concealed. There is little sensible advice that can be given on what the future holds or how to avoid further relapse. Sexual difficulties, often ignored by doctors, and increasing disability lead to broken homes. The care of young disabled patients, either at home or institutional, is often lamentably inadequate. These burdens are nearly always borne with admirable stoicism.

OTHER DEMYELINATING DISEASES

Acute disseminated encephalomyelitis

In acute disseminated encephalomyelitis there is a far more pronounced inflammatory reaction accompanied by perivenous demyelination. The disorder originally described as acute haemorrhagic leuco-encephalitis is probably a more severe form of the same condition. The disease may occur in obvious relationship to an acute specific infection, most commonly measles, chickenpox, and smallpox vaccination, but also apparently in isolation or following an unidentified febrile illness.

Children between the ages of three and ten years are most commonly affected, but adults are also susceptible, particularly after primary smallpox vaccination. Postvaccinial encephalomyelitis was rare, estimates varying from one in 5000 to one in 80 000 vaccinations.

The onset is usually abrupt, a few days after the appearance of the exanthem, although the timing is variable, or up to ten days after vaccination. Fever, headache, vomiting, and increased drowsiness may be accompanied by focal or diffuse signs of brain or spinal cord disease, most commonly hemiparesis or cerebellar ataxia. Convulsions are common. Acute optic neuritis may cause temporary complete loss of vision. Paraplegia may result from myelitis and, in distinction from multiple sclerosis, there may be evidence of peripheral nerve involvement. In severe cases, the child becomes comatose and there is a mortality of around 20 per cent. Recovery is, however, often unexpectedly rapid and complete, but in other children there may be residual hemiparesis, epilepsy or mental defects. In the acute stages the cerebrospinal fluid usually contains a moderate excess of protein and mononuclear cells, but may be normal.

There is an obvious resemblance between acute disseminated encephalomyelitis in the human and experimental allergic encephalomyelitis in the animal, particularly in the acute perivenous demyelination in response to some effect of a foreign antigen. Opinion is divided as to whether there is any parallel with multiple sclerosis. Certainly in the great majority of cases there is no question of relapsing disease, but in the adult it is naturally sometimes difficult to distinguish encephalomyelitis from a severe initial attack of multiple sclerosis. A further difficulty is in the clinical distinction from encephalitis due to viral invasion of the brain. This is of some importance as it is usual to treat disseminated encephalomyelitis with corticotrophin which might be contraindicated in active viral infection. It is difficult to be certain of any therapeutic effect and certainly the disease may be fatal in spite of early treatment or recovery may be complete without treatment.

Encephalomyelitis clinically resembling acute multiple sclerosis, but sometimes combined with evidence of peripheral nerve involvement, may follow vaccination against rabies. The pathological changes are thought to differ in some respects from those of acute disseminated encephalomyelitis. Modern vaccines have proved to be less 'neuroparalytic'.

Neuromyelitis optica
Synonym Devic's syndrome.

The combination of visual failure due to optic neuritis with spinal cord disease, either simultaneously or as separate events has been described in a separate category of neuromyelitis optica. Varieties of this syndrome are obviously common in multiple sclerosis, but the title is usually restricted without much justification to bilateral severe visual loss accompanied by a transverse spinal cord lesion. Patients who present with rapidly developing blindness and paraplegia, with a pleocytosis of several hundred cells in the CSF, certainly do not appear at the time to have multiple sclerosis, but the subsequent course may be that of remission and relapse, with features typical of this disease. In other patients the visual and spinal symptoms may be separated by a long interval. There may be complete remission or persistent symptoms but no subsequent relapse. It is doubtful whether a specific *disease* exists. The syndrome can result from multiple sclerosis, acute disseminated encephalomyelitis, systemic lupus, and possibly from other infections or intoxications.

Diffuse sclerosis
Synonyms Schilder's disease; encephalitis periaxalis diffusa.

The concept of diffuse sclerosis has been confused from the outset and the name has been used to include a great variety of unrelated conditions. From these it is possible to isolate a condition characterized by massive destruction of the myelin in the white matter of the cerebral hemispheres not due to any recognizable noxious agent and initially with sparing of the axons. This demyelinating process is distinct from the dysmyelinating diseases in which there is failure to form normal myelin. The pathology of what for convenience may be called Schilder's disease overlaps in many respects with that of multiple sclerosis, but the disease occurs in children.

The extensive bilateral lesions result in a progressive disorder, often with unrecognized minor symptoms for several months, but leading to intellectual deterioration, central blindness, and deafness, generalized or focal fits and spastic paralysis. Cerebral swelling may result in raised intracranial pressure and papilloedema. The CSF may be normal on routine examination. Most examples of this form of diffuse sclerosis are fatal within 12 months. The disease is exceedingly rare and familial incidence of this type of Schilder's disease has not been conclusively demonstrated. It is now generally regarded as a form of multiple sclerosis occurring in the young child.

Among the diseases described by Schilder one has now been identified as adrenoleucodystrophy, described on page 21.208.

Other rare genetic dysmyelinating disorders are described on page 21.208.

Concentric sclerosis
This extremely rare condition has never been diagnosed in life. The name is descriptive of the remarkable alternating rings or bands of normal and demyelinated tissue in the cerebral hemispheres and cerebellum. Young adults are affected, presenting with psychotic symptoms followed by rapidly progressive signs of generalized and focal cerebral disease, to a fatal outcome in a few weeks or months. It is probably a variant of multiple sclerosis.

Central pontine myelinolysis
This disease was first described in malnourished alcoholics, but may also occur in patients with carcinoma or in association with other forms of organic nervous disease, even in children.

As the name implies, there is demyelination centrally in the pons but also sometimes in the thalamus and basal ganglia. In contrast to multiple sclerosis there is no inflammatory reaction and the disease process is clearly distinct.

The pontine lesion causes progressive quadriparesis and bulbar palsy, usually with a subacute course. There are often additional confusing features of Wernicke's encephalopathy in alcoholics, with ocular palsies and mental changes. The diagnosis can often be established by CT scanning which shows a low-density pontine lesion.

The disease is often fatal but with better understanding of its causation and management survival and even complete recovery are possible. In nearly every case it is possible to detect a preceding episode of hyponatraemia, precipitated by water intoxication from beer drinking, diuretics or other drugs. It is probable, however, that it is the overenthusiastic correction of the sodium deficit that precipitates the myelinolysis. In vulnerable patients the serum sodium should be restored to a level that ensures consciousness and freedom from fits, that is to say around 130 mEq/l, but hypernatraemia must be avoided.

It has been suggested that the electrolyte imbalance causes cerebral oedema affecting mainly the grey matter. In the pons the myelinated tracts traverse grey matter and might be exposed to damage from pressure. This is unlikely to be the whole explanation.

Marchiafava–Bignami disease
This is another form of non-inflammatory demyelination affecting mainly alcoholics. The corpus callosum and the white matter of the cerebral hemispheres are predominantly affected.

The onset is often sudden, with increasing stupor and coma and focal or generalized fits. The white matter lesions in the hemispheres can be seen on CT scanning. Nothing is known of the causation of this condition, except that it affects those who drink too much red wine. There is an isolated report of recovery following treatment with thiamine.

References

Blairas, J. G. (1980). Management of bladder dysfunction in multiple sclerosis. *Br. J. Urol.* **48**, 193–198.

Courville, C. B. (1970). Concentric sclerosis. In *Handbook of clinical neurology*, Vol. 9, (eds P. J. Vinken and G. W. Bruyn), p. 437. North-Holland, Amsterdam.

Ebers, G. C. and Paty, D. W. (1980). CSF electrophoresis in one thousand patients. *Can. J. Neurol. Sci.* **7**, 275–280.

Gonsette, R. E. (1984). Immunological treatments in multiple sclerosis. In *Multiple sclerosis, present and future* (eds G. Scarlato and W. B. Matthews), pp. 215–257.

Johnson, R. T. (1982). *Viral infections of the nervous system*, pp. 169–200. Raven Press, New York.

Kinney, E. L., Beidoff, R. L., Rao, N. S. and Fox, L. M. (1979). Devic's syndrome and systemic lupus erythematosus. *Arch. Neurol.* **36**, 643–644.

Koeppen, A. H. and Barron, K. D. (1978). Marchiafava-Bignami disease. *Neurology* **28**, 290–294.

Matthews, W. B. (1975). Paroxysmal symptoms in multiple sclerosis. *J. Neurol. Neurosurg. Psychiat.* **38**, 617–623.

Matthews, W. B., Small, D. G., Small, M. and Pountney, E. (1977). Pattern reversal visual potential in the diagnosis of multiple sclerosis. *J. Neurol. Neurosurg. Psychiat.* **40**, 1009–1014.

Matthews, W. B., Acheson, E. D., Batchelor, J. R. and Weller, R. D. (1984). *McAlpine's multiple sclerosis.* Churchill Livingstone, Edinburgh.

Millar, J. H. D., Zilkha, K. J., Langman, M. J. S., Wright, H. P., Smith, A. D., Belin, J. and Thompson, R. H. S. (1973). Double blind trial of linoleate supplementation of the diet in multiple sclerosis. *Br. Med. J.* **1**, 765–768.

Miller, H. G., Stanton, J. B. and Gibbons, J. L. (1956). Para-infectious encephalomyelitis. *Q. J. Med.* **25**, 427–505.

Norenberg, M. D. (1983). A hypothesis of osmotic endothelial injury: a pathogenetic mechanism in central pontine myelinolysis. *Arch. Neurol.* **40**, 66–69.

Poser, C. M. (1970). Myeloclastic diffuse and transitional sclerosis. In *Handbook of clinical neurology*, Vol. 9 (eds P. J. Vinken and G. W. Bruyn), pp. 469–484.

Telfer, R. B. and Miller, E. M. (1979). Central pontine myelinolysis following hyponatremia, demonstrated by computerised tomography. *Ann. Neurol.* **6**, 455–456.

Tourtellotte, W. W. and Ma, B. I. (1978). Multiple sclerosis: the blood brain barrier and measurement of *de novo* central nervous system IgG synthesis. *Neurology* **28**, 76–83.

Vas, C. J. (1969). Sexual impotence and some anatomical disturbances in men with multiple sclerosis. *Acta Neurol. Scand.* **45**, 166–183.

Weinstein, M. A., Lederman, R. J., Rothner, A. D., Duchesnan, P. M. and Norman, D. (1978). Interval computed tomography in multiple sclerosis. *Radiology* **129**, 689–694.

MOVEMENT DISORDERS

C. D. MARSDEN

Diseases of the extrapyramidal motor system cause either a loss of movement (akinesia) accompanied by an increase in muscle tone (rigidity), or abnormal involuntary movements (dyskinesias) often accompanied by a reduction in muscle tone. The akinetic-rigid syndrome, sometimes called Parkinsonism, and the dyskinesias represent opposite ends of the spectrum of extrapyramidal disease.

AKINETIC–RIGID SYNDROMES

Parkinson's disease

Definition

This is a disease with insidious onset usually in the second half of life, characterized by slowly progressive akinesia, rigidity, postural abnormality, and tremor (Fig. 1). Described by James Parkinson, a Hoxton practitioner, in 1817, as the 'shaking palsy', the symptoms of Parkinson's disease have now been established as due to striatal dopamine deficiency consequent on death of the substantia nigra.

Aetiology

The cause of Parkinson's disease is unknown. A similar akinetic-rigid syndrome with characteristic tremor (Parkinsonism) was a common aftermath of the worldwide epidemic of encephalitis lethargica that occurred fifty years ago (1918–30) (post-encephalitic Parkinsonism). Neuroleptic drugs (such as reserpine, phenothiazines, and butyrophenones) also may produce the same clinical picture (drug-induced Parkinsonism) by blockade of striatal dopamine receptors (Table 1).

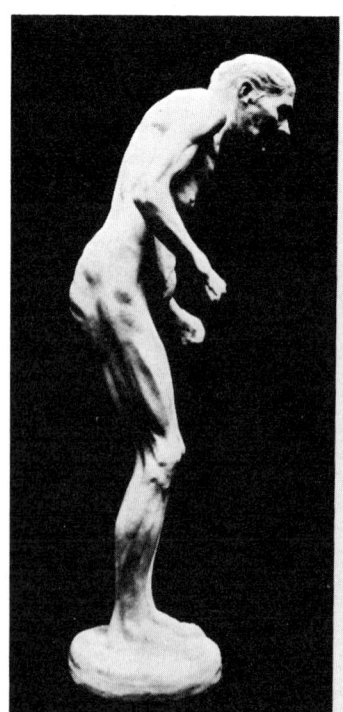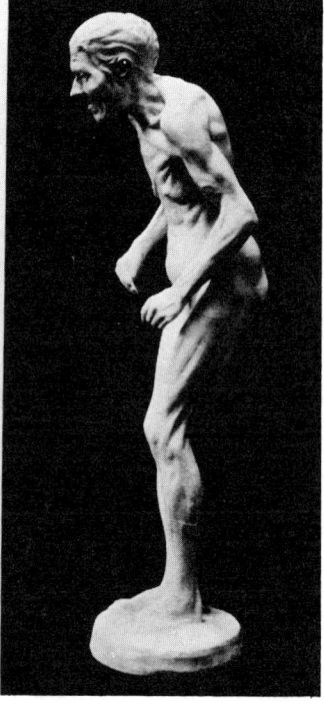

Fig. 1 Reproduction of a photograph showing Paul Richer's '*statuette pathologique*' of a patient with Parkinson's disease.

Table 1 Causes of akinetic-rigid syndrome in adults

Pure Parkinsonism	Parkinsonism-plus
Parkinson's disease	Progressive supranuclear palsy
Drug-induced Parkinsonism	Multiple system atrophy
Post-encephalitic Parkinsonism	olivo-ponto-cerebellar degeneration
MTP toxicity	strio-nigral degeneration
Other toxins	progressive autonomic failure
	(Shy–Drager)
	Basal ganglia calcification

Table 2 Diffuse brain diseases causing multifocal dementia in adults, in which elements of Parkinsonism also may occur

Common	Rare
Alzheimer's disease (including senile dementia)	Cortico-basal degeneration
	Pick's disease
Multi-infarct dementia	Creutzfeldt–Jakob disease
Binswanger's disease	Manganese poisoning
Congophilic angiopathy	Neurosyphilis
Head injury (e.g. boxers)	Cysticercosis
Cerebral anoxia	Communicating hydrocephalus

Parkinsonism also may be the main feature of a number of other degenerative diseases of the central nervous system, but other abnormalities point to the diagnosis of these various syndromes of 'Parkinsonism-plus' (Table 1). They include progressive supranuclear palsy and multiple system atrophy, which are discussed later.

Parkinsonism also may be apparent in any diffuse brain disease causing generalized cerebral damage. In addition to dementia, paralysis and other signs of widespread brain damage, an akinetic-rigid syndrome occurs in many such cases. Parkinsonism is common in Alzheimer's disease and cerebrovascular disease, but also occurs in many other such conditions (Table 2). Much has been written about 'arteriosclerotic Parkinsonism', a term which has created confusion. That Parkinsonism occurs as a part of the symptomatology of cerebrovascular disease is not in doubt, but vascular brain damage is not a cause of pure Parkinson's disease, for the substantia nigra is strikingly resistant to stroke. Isolated focal lesions of the substantia nigra, due to trauma, tuberculoma, and tumours, do cause contralateral hemi-Parkinsonism, but such cases are exceedingly rare.

Parkinson's disease is a common disorder with a prevalence of about 1 in 1000, rising exponentially after the age of 50 years to 1 in 200 in the elderly. It occurs worldwide in all ethnic groups (although perhaps less frequently amongst the Chinese and Japanese), in all social classes, and is slightly more common in men than women. Hereditary factors are not evident in the majority of cases, but about 5–10 per cent of patients give a history of the same illness in other family members. Recent studies of identical twins, however, have failed to find concordance when one twin is affected with Parkinson's disease. This suggests that heredity plays little or no role in the condition.

The only general epidemiological clue to the aetiology of Parkinson's disease relates to smoking. Patients with Parkinson's disease smoke less, and die less frequently from carcinoma of the lung, than the normal population. The significance of this observation is unknown. It may be a reflection of the Parkinsonian's premorbid personality; it is even possible that tobacco contains some protective agent.

Extensive viral studies have failed to identify any viral agent responsible for Parkinson's disease, and attempts to suggest that all cases are due to residual effects of encephalitis lethargica have been discredited. Parkinson's disease neither occurs in nor can be transmitted to animals, which perhaps do not usually live long enough to be at risk of such an illness.

A recent exciting observation is that a toxin can provoke human Parkinsonism. Certain drug addicts in California, in the course of synthesizing a heroin substitute meperidine, inadvertently produced a contaminant, known as MPTP. Within a few days of injecting this compound intravenously, they developed acute severe Parkinsonism similar in nearly all clinical, pathological, and biochemical features to the idiopathic disease. This has led to an intensive search for similar environmental toxins, but none have been identified as yet. However, MPTP resembles structurally a number of naturally occurring pyridines and is similar to some synthetic herbicides (e.g. Paraquat). MPTP induces Parkinsonism in primates but not in lower animal species. Its mode of toxicity is

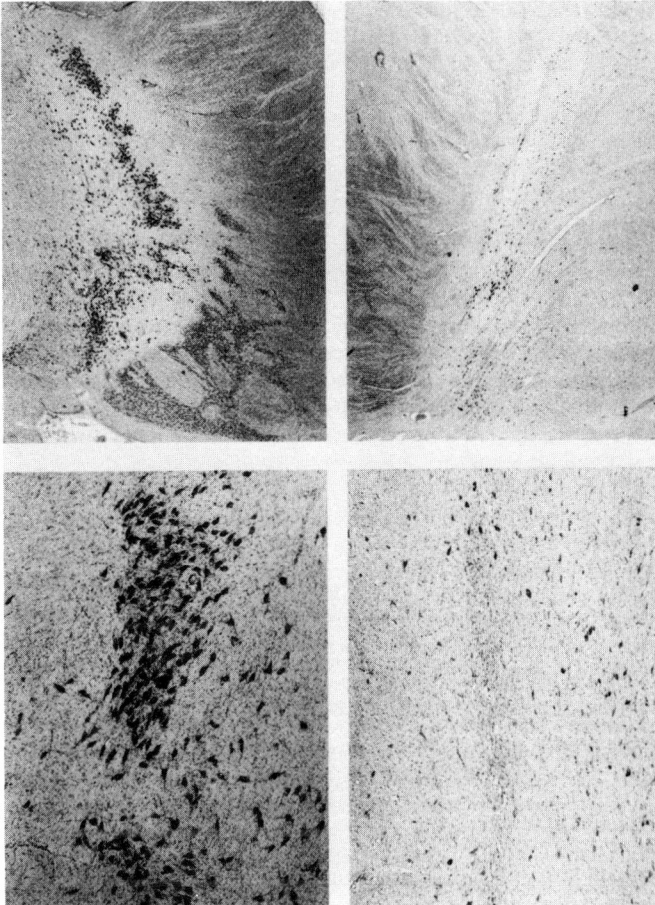

Fig. 2 The pathology of Parkinson's disease. Top, medium power and bottom, low power photomicrographs of midbrain from a normal subject (left) and from the brain of a patient with Parkinson's disease (right). The normal substantia nigra contains many densely staining dark pigmented nerve cells, running as a vertical band deep to the cerebral peduncle. Few pigmented cells are left in the Parkinsonian substantia nigra. (Haemotoxylin and eosin.)

complex. MPTP is converted in the brain, probably in glia, to the active neurotoxin MPP^+, by the action of the enzyme monoamine oxidase B. MPP^+ is then trapped in dopamine (more than noradrenaline) neurones by the normal dopamine re-uptake system. Once inside the dopamine neurones, MPP^+ binds to neuromelanin, which is present in large amounts in the primate substantia nigra pars compacta (but not in lower species). MPP^+ then generates toxic free radical species to destroy selectively the dopaminergic nigro-striatal system. MPTP toxicity can, therefore, be prevented in the experimental animal by monoamine oxidase B inhibitors (e.g. deprenyl), dopamine re-uptake blockers (e.g. mazindole), and antioxidants and free radical scavengers (e.g. vitamins C and E). These findings have implications for the treatment of the cause of Parkinson's disease (if it is true that it may be due to exposure to something like MPTP in the environment).

Pathology

Anatomical

The essential pathological abnormality is cell degeneration and loss of pigmented neurones in the pars compacta of the substantia nigra (Fig. 2). The pigmented cells of the nigra, which contain neuromelanin, project to the caudate nucleus and putamen (neostriatum), and employ dopamine as their neurotransmitter. The adjacent pigmented ventral segmental areas, which project dopaminergic axons to mesolimbic and mesocortical regions also degenerate. Other pigmented brainstem nuclei are also affected in

Parkinson's disease, including the noradrenergic locus coeruleus. Non-pigmented cholingeric neurones in the substantia innominata, including those of the nucleus basalis of Meynert, are also involved.

In all cases of Parkinson's disease the degenerating pigmented brainstem neurones contain eosinophilic inclusions and non-pigmented Lewy bodies, which are characteristic of the disease. Lewy bodies are found also in about 4 per cent of brains from patients without Parkinsonism dying of other causes; these may be patients with subclinical Parkinson's disease, for 80 per cent of the zona compacta must degenerate before clinical symptoms appear. Lewy bodies are composed of protein, but they do not have the electron-microscopic appearances of any known viral or other infective agent. They contain accumulations of normal neurofilaments, but their origin is unexplained. Lewy bodies are found not only in pigmented neurones, but also in other areas including the substantia innominata, the lateral grey horns of the thoracic cord, and even in sympathetic ganglia.

Degeneration of brainstem pigmented nuclei is the crucial feature of the pathology of Parkinson's disease, but often there are other changes, some of which may reflect the typical pathology found in the brains of many of the elderly. However, there also may be other more specific changes in many cases of Parkinson's disease, such as loss of neurones and degeneration of their dendrites in the striatum and globus pallidus. Such changes may be of importance in those treated successfully with levodopa for long periods, but careful quantitative estimates of cell populations are required to confirm these observations. Such changes, if verified, may reflect transsynaptic degeneration due to long-standing and severe loss of the dopaminergic nigrostriatal pathway.

Biochemical

The original discovery in 1960 by Ehringer and Hornykiewicz of profound loss of dopamine in the striatum (putamen more than caudate) and substantia nigra of patients with Parkinson's disease has been amply confirmed by many subsequent studies (Table 3). Loss of dopamine in the caudate nucleus and putamen correlates with the extensive cell loss, atrophy, and glial scarring in the substantia nigra, the damage being more severe and diffuse in post-

encephalitic patients than in those with idiopathic Parkinson's disease. Indeed, there is a close correlation between the extent of nigral cell loss, the degree of depletion of striatal dopamine, and the severity of akinesia.

It is necessary to lose something of the order of 80–85 per cent of nigral neurones, and to deplete the striatum of about 80–85 per cent of its dopamine content, for frank motor symptoms of Parkinson's disease to appear. The pathology of the illness, focusing on nigral cell loss in the zona compacta, is progressive. It is assumed that there must be a prolonged period of asymptomatic striatal dopamine depletion until the critical level for appearance of symptoms is reached. During this asymptomatic period, a variety of mechanisms attempt to compensate for the loss of the nigrostriatal dopamine pathway. The concentration of the dopamine metabolite, homovanillic acid, falls less than that of the transmitter itself; the ratio of homovanillic acid to dopamine increases, suggesting that the turnover rate of dopamine has increased. Those nigral neurones remaining appear to operate harder in an attempt to overcome the dopamine deficiency. A second compensatory mechanism involves changes in the sensitivity of the post-synaptic receptor on which dopamine acts in the striatum. Lesions of the nigrostriatal system in animals lead to denervation supersensitivity of the post-synaptic striatal dopamine receptors. This is evidenced by both an enhanced pharmacological response to dopamine agonists, and an increase in the number of receptors measured by tritiated ligand binding techniques. The latter have been applied to the brains of patients with Parkinson's disease and the results suggest that a similar post-synaptic dopamine receptor supersensitivity may exist at least initially in such patients.

Recently, Hornykiewicz has also reported the results of analysing dopamine content in other brain areas in patients with Parkinson's disease. In the nucleus accumbens (which in man forms an inferior part of the head of the caudate nucleus identified by a high noradrenaline content), there was a marked decrease in both dopamine and homovanillic acid concentrations to some 42 per cent of normal, in comparison to a reduction of caudate nucleus dopamine to 36 per cent and putamen dopamine to 9 per cent of control values respectively. The concentration of homovanillic acid in the nucleus accumbens fell less than that of dopamine, indicating an increased turnover of dopamine in the remaining functional neurones in this region, as well as in the striatum. Current pharmacological evidence suggests that the nucleus accumbens is involved with locomotor control in animals, so dopamine depletion in this brain area may contribute to the motor deficits in patients with Parkinson's disease. In the same study a search was made for evidence of dopamine in human cerebral cortex. Of all the areas examined, only the parolfactory gyrus (Brodmann area 25) contained appreciable concentrations of dopamine, and there was a severe dopamine reduction in this area of limbic cortex. It is tempting to associate this change in the cortical dopamine systems with the affective disturbances and psychic changes that can be seen in some patients with Parkinson's disease.

Since the striatal dopamine depletion is due to degeneration of dopaminergic nigrostriatal pathway, the intraneuronal enzymes required for dopamine synthesis also are markedly diminished. Thus, L-aromatic amino acid decarboxylase (dopa decarboxylase), an intraneuronal enzyme responsible for the conversion of dopa to dopamine, is strikingly low in the nigrostriatal regions of the Parkinsonian brain. Likewise, the rate-limiting enzyme, tyrosine hydroxylase, responsible for conversion of tyrosine to dopa, is also depleted in dopamine-containing brain regions.

In addition to the crucial changes in brain dopamine in Parkinson's disease described above, less marked depletion of noradrenaline and 5-hydroxytryptamine has been noted in this illness. Studies on acetylcholine activity of post-mortem brain samples suggest that cholinergic neurones in the basal ganglia system are relatively well preserved in Parkinson's disease. However, a reduction in cerebral cortical choline acetyltransferase, a marker of cholinergic neurones, has been described recently, particularly

Table 3 Neurotransmitters and their enzymes in the striatum in Parkinson's disease

	Control	Parkinson's disease	
Dopamine (μg/g)	5.37	0.50	9%
Homovanillic acid (μg/g)	11.40	2.06	18%
DA/HVA ratio	2.1	4.1	
Dopa decarboxylase (nmol/100 mg protein/h)	432	32	7%
Tyrosine hydroxylase (nmol/100 mg protein/h)	36	8	22%
Monoamine oxidase (nmol/100 mg protein/h)	1520	1650	Normal
Catechol-0-methyl transferase (nmol/100 mg protein/h)	24	20	Normal
5-hydroxytryptamine (μg/g)	0.32	0.14	44%
Noradrenaline (μg/g)	1.29	0.52	40%
Choline acetyltransferase (mol/kg protein/h)	49	37	75%
Glutamic acid decarboxylase (μmol/100 mg protein/h)	4.7	3.9	Normal

Mean values are shown for putamen, except for noradrenaline which was measured in nucleus accumbens.

All differences were statistically significant at $p < 0.05$ or less, except where indicated by 'normal'.

Data from Hornykiewicz et al., McGeer and McGeer (see Marsden, 1981).

in those with dementia. This is believed to reflect loss of neurones in substantia innominata which project to cerebral cortex. In this respect the demented Parkinsonian resembles the patient with Alzheimer's disease biochemically. In addition, dementia patients with Parkinson's disease and those with Alzheimer's disease exhibit a loss of somatostatin neurones in the cortical cortex. Changes in the enzyme glutamic acid decarboxylase (GAD) responsible for synthesis of γ-aminobutyric acid (GABA) have been demonstrated in Parkinson's disease; GAD concentration is reduced in the substantia nigra and cerebral cortex. One of the major strionigral pathways utilizes GABA as its neurotransmitter, and the changes in nigral GAD may represent some functional reduction in activity of this pathway, for levodopa therapy restores glutamic acid decarboxylase levels back towards normal. Specific binding of ^{3}H-GABA also is altered in Parkinson's disease; there is a striking reduction in the number of GABA binding sites in the substantia nigra, with normal levels in the caudate nucleus, putamen, and cerebral cortex. Since the GABA strionigral pathway synapses, at least in part, on dopaminergic nigral neurones, this loss of nigral GABA binding is interpreted as due to loss of nigral dopamine nerve cells containing the GABA receptors. There is also loss of certain peptide neuronal systems in the basal ganglia, particularly those containing encephalins and substance P.

Symptoms

The onset is insidious and in 70 per cent of patients the presenting feature is *tremor*, which usually commences unilaterally. Parkinsonian tremor is present at rest, decreased by action, is increased by emotion or stress, and disappears during sleep. The arms are most often affected initially, but tremor may spread to involve the head, jaw, and legs. It is due to rhythmical alternating contraction in opposing muscles at a frequency of 4–6 Hz (Fig. 3). In the arm it characteristically causes rhythmic pronation/supination and 'pill-rolling' of the opposed thumb and fingers. Occasionally tremor may be more evident on posture and movement, particularly in the initial stages of the illness, when it is at a faster frequency of 6–7 Hz. *Rigidity* is appreciated by the patient as stiff muscles, and by the examiner as a plastic resistance to passive movement, equal in opposing muscle groups and constant throughout the range of manipulation. Rigidity affects all muscles, but is most marked in the neck and trunk, and in proximal muscles at the shoulder or hip. When tremor coexists, the smooth plastic nature of rigidity may be broken up by rhythmic catches (cogwheel phenomenon). *Akinesia* refers to the poverty (hypokinesia) and slowness (bradykinesia) of movement so characteristic of Parkinson's disease. It is not merely the effect of rigidity, for stereotaxic thalamotomy (see below) can abolish limb rigidity without improving

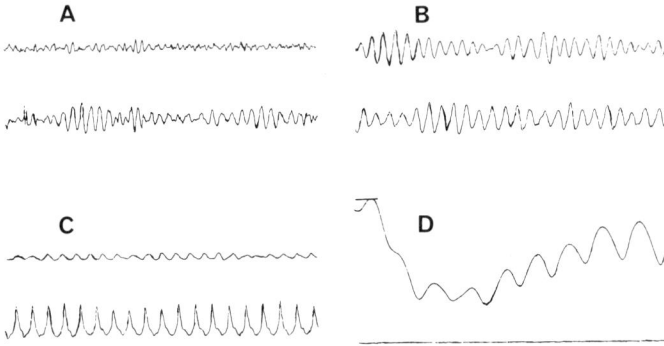

Fig. 3 Recordings of tremor with accelerometers placed on the right arm (above) and the left arm (below) in: (A) a patient with enhanced physiological tremor of the outstretched arms (frequency 9–10 Hz); (B) a patient with benign essential tremor with the arms outstretched (frequency 7 Hz); (C) a patient with left-sided Parkinson's disease at rest (frequency 5 Hz); and (D) a patient with severe cerebellar disease and marked intention tremor attempting to touch his nose with the right hand (frequency 2–3 Hz). All recordings are of 4 s duration. (By courtesy of Dr M. Gresty.)

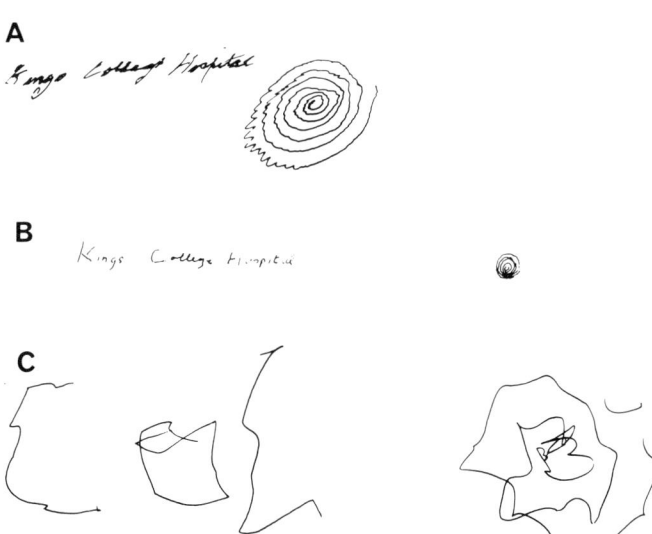

Fig. 4 Samples of handwriting and spiral drawings from: (A) a 50-year-old woman with benign essential tremor; (B) a 38-year-old man with Parkinson's disease; and (C) a 20-year-old boy with torsion dystonia (who attempts to write COLLEGE).

akinesia. There is a delay in initiation of movement, a slowness in execution of voluntary movement, and a loss of normal automatic movements such as those of emotional expression and blinking. *Postural changes* include generalized flexion of the limbs, neck, and trunk, and postural instability causing falls.

These four cardinal signs of Parkinson's disease – tremor, rigidity, akinesia and postural change – contribute to the many typical features and disabilities of the illness (Fig. 1). The face is strikingly blank and mask-like. The voice loses volume and normal modulation of tone to become soft and monotonous. The bent flexed patient walks with slow, small steps, without swinging the arms; it may be difficult to start walking ('freezing'), but once in motion the pace may quicken and the patient may be unable to stop ('festination'). He may 'freeze' into immobility when passing through a door or around furniture. While standing, a push may lead to falling or tottering in the direction of displacement until the patient falls, or comes into contact with a solid object. He sits immobile and flexed like a statue. Getting out of a chair and turning over in bed may be impossible. The handwriting becomes small (micrographia), tremulous, and untidy (Fig. 4). Rapid movements of the hands and feet are impaired. Eating, washing, and toilet demands become increasingly difficult.

While objective sensibility is unimpaired, patients often complain of fatigue, pain, and discomfort, and of hot or cold sensations. Vision, hearing, taste, and smell are normal. Eye movements are unaffected, except for paralysis of convergence, some limitation of up-gaze, loss of speed of voluntary saccades, and break-up of smooth pursuit movements, which become jerky or saccadic. All these defects in eye movement are most marked in horizontal and vertical up-gaze; down-gaze is spared. The pupils are normal. The eyelids may be tremulous (blepharoclonus) and spasms of eye closure (blepharospasm) may occur. Drooling of saliva is common, due to failure to swallow, and dysphagia may occur. Constipation is universal; urinary frequency and incontinence is a frequent complaint. Excessive sweating and a greasy skin (seborrhoea) contribute to the facial appearance. Some patients develop progressive autonomic failure (see pages 21.76–21.79), but the majority do not have postural hypotension. The tendon reflexes and plantar responses are normal.

Most patients have normal intellectual and cognitive function initially, but drug therapy commonly provokes mental disturbances and with the passage of time and progression of the disease, a proportion of patients develop organic mental changes.

Depression is very common, affecting 30 per cent or more, and often antedates the appearance of obvious physical symptoms. The commonest mental consequence of drug therapy is a toxic confusional state, but other behavioural disturbances such as a schizophreniform psychosis or isolated hallucinosis with insight can occur. Many patients complain of slowness of thought (bradyphrenia) and defects of memory in the later stages of the illness, and a proportion (perhaps 20 per cent) finally develop a frank global dementia. The latter may sometimes be due to the coexistence of Alzheimer's disease in this elderly population, but the appearance of dementia in a patient with Parkinson's disease warrants full investigation to exclude other treatable causes. The pathology of Parkinson's disease itself, particularly in the cholinergic substatia innominata, may predispose to dementia if other causes are excluded.

Natural history

The mean age of onset of Parkinson's disease is about 55 years. Onset under 40 years is rare, but thereafter the incidence rises exponentially with increasing age. Most patients localize the onset of symptoms to one or other side, but progression to bilateral signs and disability is the rule. Symptoms and signs confined to one side (hemi-Parkinsonism) is uncommon. In most patients the untreated disease progresses inexorably with increasing difficulty in speaking, eating, washing, dressing, standing, and walking. Eventually, in those most severely affected, the patient becomes chair- or bed-bound and anarthric. Many patients, however, remain reasonably active, but with increasing restrictions, until they die from other causes. The rate of progression is very variable. Prior to the advent of levodopa therapy, death occurred on average about 9 years after the onset of symptoms (Fig. 5); the range varied from benign Parkinsonism with little or no progression over 30 years or more, to malignant Parkinsonism with death in 1 or 2 years from onset. Mortality was some three times that expected in a general population of the same age and sex. Death was usually from vascular diseases, bronchopneumonia, or intercurrent neoplasia. Older treatments did not influence the prognosis of idiopathic Parkinson's disease, but it is likely that levodopa therapy has prolonged life expectancy. Indeed, a number of studies have now shown that with present-day treatment the patient with Parkinson's disease is likely on average, to live as long as unaffected people of the same age.

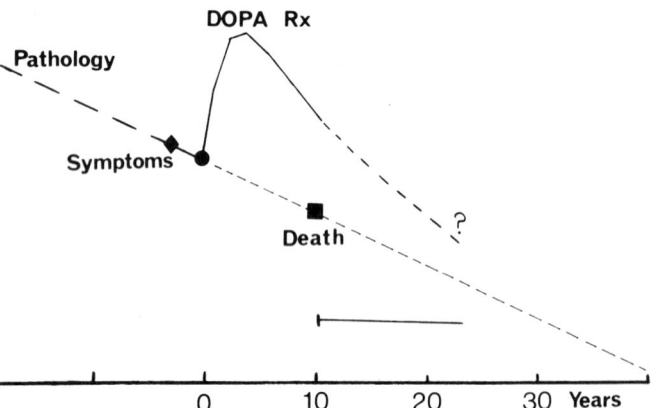

Fig. 5 The impact of levodopa therapy on Parkinson's disesae. A hypothetical concept of the effects of chronic levodopa treatment. The underlying pathology (of unknown cause) is believed to progress over many years irrespective of therapy. After an initial period it becomes severe enough to cause symptoms. Before levodopa, pathological changes and disability progressed to cause death on average about 9 years after onset. Levodopa therapy results in considerable initial symptomatic improvement, but no change in pathology. Despite some loss of benefit after a few years of treatment, life expectancy is prolonged, but this means that new aspects and consequences of the progression of the disease are likely to emerge. (Reproduced with permission from Marsden and Parkes, *Lancet*, 1977, **i**, 349.)

Diagnosis

The combination of tremor, rigidity, akinesia, and postural abnormality constitutes the syndrome of Parkinsonism (see Tables 1 and 2). A history of encephalitis lethargica in the 1920s or 1930s (the epidemic then ceased, although sporadic cases still occur today), plus additional features characteristic of the sequelae of encephalitis lethargica, indicate the diagnosis of *post-encephalitic Parkinsonism*. These include spasms of eye deviation, often with compulsive thought (oculogyric crises), pupillary abnormalities, and dyskinesias such as torsion dystonia. About 80 per cent of patients with post-encephalitic Parkinsonism developed their symptoms within 10 years of infection. Post-encephalitic Parkinsonism was a more benign disease, and only about 25 per cent of patients were severely disabled after 20 years of illness.

A history of intake of neuroleptic drugs indicates *drug-induced Parkinsonism*, which remits in 95 per cent of cases slowly over weeks or months when the offending drug is withdrawn.

A number of other degenerative diseases affecting the basal ganglia may produce a Parkinsonian syndrome, but other distinctive features give the clue to the true diagnosis. A gaze palsy for voluntary and following eye movements, particularly when downgaze is affected, with preserved vestibulo-ocular reflex eye movements indicates *progressive supranuclear palsy* (see below). A cerebellar ataxia or cerebellar atrophy on CT scan, and orthostatic hypotension with other features of an autonomic neuropathy, point to *multiple system atrophy* (see below).

The presence of frank dementia and pyramidal signs indicate a diffuse disease such as *Alzheimer's disease*, or cerebrovascular disease such as *multi-infarct dementia*. The latter most commonly occurs in long-standing sufferers of poorly controlled hypertension and often is characterized by the additional presence of a pseudobulbar palsy with emotional incontinence and a distinctive gait which is upright, short-stepped and military (*marche à petit pas*). Diffuse brain disease with an akinetic-rigid syndrome as part of the clinical picture is also caused by a single severe head injury, or by repeated head injury ('*punch drunk*' *syndrome*, see page 21.189), and by cerebral anoxia due either to cardiac arrest or secondary to carbon monoxide poisoning. Occasionally, calcification of the basal ganglia may be associated with Parkinsonism (see below).

Parkinson's disease is the diagnosis when the syndrome appears in middle or late life without other evidence of neurological damage, and in the absence of any history of provoking drugs or encephalitis lethargica.

Hemi-Parkinsonism may be confused with hemiplegia, but in the latter the tendon reflexes will be pathologically brisk, the abdominal reflexes absent, and the plantar response extensor on the affected side. True hemi-Parkinsonism may very rarely be due to a cerebral tumour or other focal lesion affecting the opposite hemisphere.

The condition of *benign essential tremor* is commonly mistaken for Parkinson's disease. However, in benign essential tremor, which is often inherited, the tremor is postural and other signs of Parkinsonism are absent, for there is no true rigidity or akinesia. However, postural tremor of the outstretched hands may be the initial or only feature of Parkinson's disease, and in some patients it is exceedingly difficult to decide initially on the true diagnosis. In general, such patients will have developed obvious other signs of Parkinson's disease within about a year of the onset of their tremor.

Depression also poses diagnostic problems. Patients with profound psychomotor retardation due to severe depression often exhibit a superficial resemblance to those with Parkinson's disease, particularly with their sad expressionless face, bowed posture, and immobility. Indeed, it seems quite likely that many of these physical manifestations of depression may be due to mild and reversible biochemical abnormality of basal ganglia function. Many patients with the earliest symptoms of Parkinson's disease are misdiagnosed as depressed, which indeed they may well be.

Finally, a proportion of patients with Parkinson's disease present with generalized ill-health, fatigue, restlessness, sleep difficulties, bizarre sensory symptoms, or non-specific neurasthenia. The diagnosis may be exceedingly difficult in such patients unless the impassive face, the stooped posture, and the short-stepped gait with failure to swing the arms are spotted early on in the interview.

Treatment

The treatment of Parkinson's disease involves the use of drugs, physical therapy, and occasionally surgery.

Drug treatment

Introduction Until 1967, when oral levodopa was introduced generally, treatment was with anticholinergic drugs and stereotaxic surgery. Levodopa is now the best therapy available, and stereotaxic surgery is only rarely indicated. Levodopa is converted into dopamine in the brain by the enzyme dopa decarboxylase, thereby restoring striatal dopamine action. Less than 5 per cent of an oral dose of levodopa reaches the brain; the rest is metabolized by dopa decarboxylase in gut wall, liver, kidney, and cerebral capillaries. This peripheral decarboxylation can be prevented by the addition of a selective extracerebral decarboxylase inhibitor, such as carbidopa or benserazide, which themselves do not penetrate into the brain. Levodopa combined with carbidopa (Sinemet) or benserazide (Madopar) is now the treatment of choice when levodopa is indicated. Such combined therapy requires a lower dose of levodopa for optimal benefit, and results in a quicker therapeutic response and a lower incidence of those side-effects that are due to the formation of levodopa metabolites outside the blood–brain barrier. These include nausea and vomiting, cardiac dysrhythmias, and, at least in part, postural hypotension. The main side-effects of combined therapy are dyskinesias and psychiatric disturbances. Both are dose-dependent and remit when drug dosage is reduced. There are few contraindications of levodopa therapy, but it should never be given with a monoamine oxidase inhibitor.

Initiation Sinemet or Madopar, which appear similar in potency and side-effects, do not improve the underlying pathology or cause of Parkinson's disease; they are equivalent to a substitution therapy for striatal dopamine deficiency. It is not necessary to use such drugs in every patient on diagnosis. Either Sinemet or Madopar is indicated if disability is severe, or if it fails to respond to simple therapy. In the mild case, an anticholinergic such as benzhexol (Artane) 2 or 5 mg tablets and 5 mg sustained release capsules, or orphenadrine (Disipal) 50 mg tablets, three to eight times daily may be sufficient. Anticholinergics cause peripheral parasympathetic blockade with a dry mouth, blurred vision, and constipation, and a toxic confusional state. Mental side-effects of anticholinergics are particularly common in the elderly, and this group of drugs should be avoided in those with Parkinson's disease in later life. They may also precipitate glaucoma and urinary retention. Small doses should be used initially and gradually increased. Alternatively, in a mild case, amantadine hydrochloride (Symmetrel) 100 mg twice or three times daily may be effective. Amantadine, originally introduced as an antiviral agent, is slightly more powerful than anticholinergics, but less effective than levodopa. However, it causes few side-effects, mainly ankle oedema and the skin rash, livedo reticularis. In high dosage it can provoke a toxic confusional state or fits.

If levodopa is indicated, Sinemet or Madopar should be started in small dosage and gradually increased over a period of weeks to the maximum tolerated, or until adequate therapeutic benefit has been obtained. Nausea and vomiting are less common with these combined preparations than with plain levodopa, and if it occurs it can usually be prevented by taking the drug after meals, prefaced by an antiemetic such as domperidone. The commonest dose-limiting side-effects are dyskinesias and mental disturbances and the aim should be to keep the patient free of these complications.

The usual starting dose of Sinemet (each tablet of Sinemet 275 contains 250 mg levodopa and 25 mg carbidopa) is half a tablet twice or three times daily. The average optimum dose is three to four tablets daily. The elderly are particularly sensitive to levodopa, and Sinemet 110 (containing 100 mg levodopa and 10 mg carbidopa) may be used. Sinemet Plus (containing 100 mg levodopa and 25 mg carbidopa) has also been introduced to provide adequate carbidopa intake for those on low doses of levodopa. For Madopar the starting dose is 1 capsule twice or three times daily of Madopar 125 (which contains 100 mg levodopa and 25 mg benserazide). The average optimum dose is two to four capsules daily of Madopar 250 (which contains 200 mg levodopa and 50 mg benserazide). Maximum dosage of Sinemet 275 is about six to eight tablets daily, and of Madopar 250 about five to eight capsules daily but some patients require even more than this.

Maintenance The initial response to levodopa therapy is dramatic (restitution of mormal function) in about one-third of patients, good (considerable improvement, but some residual handicap) in another third, and moderate (some response, but residual disabling handicap) or nil in the remaining third. In those who fail to obtain adequate benefit, the addition of an anticholinergic drug or/and amantadine may give added improvement. Failure to respond to levodopa at all should prompt a review of the diagnosis, for such patients are unlikely to have Parkinson's disease.

In those who do respond, approximately two-thirds will experience some loss of benefit after 2–5 years treatment (Fig. 5). Those patients who do deteriorate while on long-term levodopa therapy do so in one of two ways. Some experience a progressive recurrence of their Parkinsonian disability, particularly akinesia and postural instability with freezing and falls. Such patients usually are elderly and frequently show signs of dementia as well. Such a progressive loss of benefit and deterioration is very difficult to reverse. Increasing the daily dose of levodopa often causes toxic confusional states without added benefit. A few such patients may gain renewed relief by switching to a directly acting dopamine agonist such as bromocriptine (see below), but mental side-effects are common with this drug. As indicated above, if dementia supervenes, all treatable causes should be excluded by appropriate investigation.

A number of patients with Parkinson's disease deteriorate rapidly in the face of an intercurrent infection, particularly urinary tract infections which are common, or incidental surgery, which should be avoided unless absolutely necessary. Following such a dramatic relapse, it may be a matter of weeks or months before such a patient regains their previous response to levodopa and their usual mobility.

Other patients on long-term levodopa therapy develop fluctuations in mobility throughout the day. Initially these usually take the form of end-of-dose deterioration or the 'wearing-off' effect. When levodopa is first started, each dose usually lasts for a matter of 6 hours or so. With the passage of years, the duration of action of each dose of the drug shortens to as little as 1 or 2 hours. On the usual three or four times daily regimen, this means that patients begin to experience a recurrence of disability, particularly immobility, prior to the next dose. At this stage, the correct management is to divide the daily levodopa dose into smaller but more frequent portions. Such patients may require to take levodopa every 2 hours or so.

Unfortunately, many of those with end-of-dose deterioration cannot be controlled adequately by such dose adjustments, or go on to develop other types of fluctuation in response. Typically, levodopa-induced dyskinesias become more severe, either at the peak time of levodopa action or biphasically prior to and at the end of action of each dose. In addition, the swings from mobility (with dyskinesias) to immobility (with distress and sometimes tremor and rigidity) become more frequent and abrupt, hence the description of this problem as the 'on–off' effect for it can be like switching a light on and off. Such swings also become increasingly unpredictable and variable, quite unrelated to the timing of levodopa dosage, so that the patient may 'yo-yo' from mobility to immobility many times a day.

The management of severe 'on–off' problems, which usually occur in the younger patient with preserved intellect, is exceedingly difficult. Once stabilized on optimum timing of levodopa dosage, it may be helpful to add the drug deprenyl, a selective monoamine oxidase B inhibitor. Human brain dopamine is catabolized by the iso-enzyme monoamine oxidase B, whereas extracerebral monoamine oxidase activity responsible for catabolizing endogenous monoamines and exogenous amines such as tyramine in cheese is of the A type isoenzyme. Conventional monoamine oxidase inhibitors inhibit monoamine oxidase A, so cannot be given with levodopa, for the combination provokes severe hypertension. But deprenyl, now known as selegiline (Eldepryl), can be used safely and does prolong the therapeutic action of levodopa.

If levodopa plus deprenyl fails to control the problems of 'on–off' effects, then consideration should be given to switching to a directly acting dopamine agonist such as bromocriptine. The latter is employed widely as a dopamine agonist in endocrinological practice, but much larger doses are required in Parkinson's disease. Bromocriptine is about as effective therapeutically as levodopa, and has a similar range of unwanted effects, although psychiatric complications may be most common, and it is much more expensive. However, bromocriptine can be of some value in those experiencing 'on–off' problems. It is introduced in a dose of 2.5 mg nightly and gradually built up by 2.5 mg increments to a three or four times daily regime normally totalling about 20–40 mg daily, although doses of up to about 100 mg/day can be used. Levodopa dosage must be reduced concomitantly, for the effects of the two drugs are additive. There is some evidence to suggest that the emergence of disabling fluctuations in response to long-term levodopa therapy may be due to the drug treatment itself. Accordingly, there is now a move towards introduction of bromocriptine earlier in the course of the disease in order to reduce the dosage of levodopa. If the patient cannot be maintained on Sinemet or Madopar in doses of four Sinemet 275 tablets or four Madopar 250 capsules, then this may be the time to add bromocriptine.

Unfortunately, some patients who develop severe 'on–off' phenomena during chronic levodopa therapy eventually become resistant to all form of treatment. Current developments in an attempt to help such patients include the use of 'drug holidays', the introduction of new dopamine agonist drugs, and the use of intravenous Itrodopa or subcutaneous lisuride infusions, but these manoeuvres are restricted to special centres evaluating such new therapy. Transplantation of fetal substantia nigra tissue, while successful in rodents, cannot yet be applied to humans.

Based on the MPTP story (see above) there are now suggestions as to how to treat the cause of Parkinson's disease. Clinical trials of deprenyl, mazindole, and vitamin C and E therapy, initiated on diagnosis, are underway to see if these approaches can halt or slow progression of the illness.

Surgery
In the 1950s and early 1960s, stereotaxic surgery was employed widely to treat Parkinson's disease. The initial target was the globus pallidus, but subsequent experience showed that the most favourable site was in the ventrolateral nucleus of the thalamus. A small lesion at that site was created mechanically, electrolytically, or thermally. Such a stereotaxic thalamotomy could abolish rigidity and tremor in the opposite limbs, but unfortunately did not relieve the disabling akinesia and postural instability. Both were found subsequently to respond to levodopa, at least initially, so by the early 1970s most centres were doing few or no stereotaxic operations for Parkinson's disease. Today, the operation is reserved for the uncommon patient with early Parkinson's disease, whose tremor is severe, resistant to drug therapy and so disabling as to prevent work.

Physical therapy and aids
Parkinson's disease produces a wide range of functional locomotor disabilities, many of which can be helped by sensible aids. An initial assessment by the physiotherapist and occupational therapist will identify each individual patient's particular problems. Special training can then be given to help eating, washing, dressing, and walking. Intensive training may aid equilibrium and restore effective gait patterns, and the physiotherapist can teach a simple sequence of useful exercises for use at home. Advice on shoes ('slip-on' with sliding soles, not rubber), the use of 'Velcro' rather than zips, feeding utensils with built-up handles, and other aids is invaluable. A visit to the patient's home will allow assessment of the need for structural alterations such as hand rails in the bathroom and lavatory, raising the toilet seat, removal of door sills, provision of high chairs (patients with Parkinson's disease find great difficulty in getting out of the usual low soft chair or sofa), removal of scatter rugs which slip, and provision of rubber mats. Sticks and other walking aids often are not very useful to patients with Parkinson's disease, but can be tried. Regular physiotherapy is not warranted, but reassessment if circumstances change or disability increases is essential.

Management of specific problems
Many particular problems arise in the treatment of Parkinson's disease and pose difficult management decisions.

Psychiatric illness Toxic confusional states are common in Parkinson's disease, and may be due to drug overdosage or intercurrent acute illness such as infection with fever. In practice, if no obvious other condition is apparent, it is wise to assume that drugs are the cause, for any of those employed to treat Parkinson's disease may provoke delirium. In those taking multiple drug therapy, amantadine may be stopped first, then the dose of anticholinergics can be halved and subsequently these drugs can be withdrawn. Finally, if confusion persists, it is reasonable to decrease gradually levodopa intake until either the mental state clears, or immobility gets worse. For reasons that are not clear, it may take some days or even weeks for such a patient to regain mental clarity. Some never do, and it is apparent that this acute toxic confusional state was superimposed upon an underlying dementia, which should be investigated in its own right.

Psychotic behaviour, disrupting home life or ward routine, can occur in such patients. Conventional neuroleptic drugs are best avoided in Parkinson's disease, because they antagonize dopamine action, but may have to be used. In fact, the noisy disruptive Parkinsonian may be calmed without deterioration in their mobility by a judiciously chosen dose of thioridazine (Melleril) or other neuroleptic. Such drugs also may be of value for night sedation of those with reversed sleep rhythm, but must be used with considerable caution, for they may provoke a severe deterioration in the severity of the Parkinsonism. A limited 'drug holiday' may help some of those with otherwise uncontrollable mental toxicity from levodopa or bromocriptine. The drugs are withdrawn for one day a week. Longer periods of drug withdrawal may cause drastic worsening of the Parkinsonism.

Depression has been noted as very common in Parkinson's disease, often demanding treatment. Conventional monoamine oxidase inhibitors are quite contraindicated for they interact with levodopa to cause severe hypertension. However, tricyclics such as amitryptiline (Tryptizol) can be used in the usual way, and their anticholinergic properties may add a little anti-Parkinsonian action. A large nocturnal dose of a sedative antidepressant such as amitryptiline (50–150 mg) often gives a gratifying night's sleep, and may prove of more value than benzodiazepine hypnotics in patients with Parkinson's disease. Newer, less sedative antidepressants with little peripheral anticholinergic action, such as mianserin (Bolvidon) may also be used. If severe depression does not respond to adequate antidepressant drug therapy, electroconvulsive treatment (ECT) may be used without fear of complications.

Indeed, ECT by itself may provoke considerable, but transient, improvement in the physical symptoms of Parkinson's disease.

Levodopa treatment has been associated with provocation of a wide range of other psychiatric symptoms. Enhanced sexual desire and prowess was overestimated and exaggerated by the press, but levodopa can occasionally unmask latent sexual deviant behaviour; such tendencies disappear when the dose of the drug is reduced. Likewise, reversible mania may appear. A very distinctive acute, but reversible, visual hallucinosis often with delusions, in the setting of clear consciousness, preserved insight, and intact thought also is not uncommon. In general, all such side effects remit if levodopa dosage is reduced.

Intercurrent physical illness Patients with Parkinson's disease are of an age when other illness may strike, to pose a number of difficulties.

The mobility of patients with Parkinson's disease may deteriorate dramatically if they get influenza, a chest infection, or urinary tract infection. Indeed, any sudden unexplained deterioration in such patients should prompt a careful search for some such infective illness. Levodopa replacement therapy should be continued, via a nasogastric tube if necessary, throughout any intercurrent illness. Stopping levodopa will soon provoke a severe loss of mobility, with respiratory restriction and risk of deep vein thrombosis.

Many of the warning symptoms of other illness already are present in patients with Parkinson's disease. Constipation, for example, is universal; it is due to a combination of immobility, dietary restriction, neglecting roughage and liquid, and anticholinergic drug therapy. However, a definite change in bowel habit should be investigated as usual. Likewise, urinary hesitancy with frequency and urgency may occur in Parkinson's disease, but also may be due to infection, prostatic hypertrophy, or prolapse. In general, it is best to undertake appropriate investigation for such symptoms rather than blame them on Parkinson's disease, although this may turn out to be the case. This is particularly true of weight loss, which may be frightening in some individuals with rapidly progressive Parkinson's disease.

A recent myocardial infarct poses a problem in a patient with Parkinson's disease, for levodopa can provoke cardiac arrhythmias due mainly to metabolism to vasoactive amines. Combination of levodopa with a selective extracerebral decarboxylase inhibitor, as in Sinemet and Madopar, goes some way to avoiding this problem, by preventing levodopa metabolism. However, it is unwise to commence levodopa therapy in the month after a new myocardial infarct, particularly as the increased mobility may provoke extra strain. Levodopa, in combined form, can be continued in those already on treatment who have a myocardial infarct, but the dose can be reduced during any period of bed-rest.

A few other symptoms occur sufficiently often in Parkinson's disease to warrant mention. Ankle oedema due to immobility (and amantadine) is unsightly but not usually serious. Postural hypotension, sometimes exacerbated by drug therapy, rarely causes symptoms, and requires no treatment unless it does. However, some patients do develop progressive autonomic failure requiring symptomatic treatment (see page 21.79). Seborrhoea may be severe, causing dandruff and dermatitis, and conjuctivitis leading to sore red eyes and crusted lids may require local therapy. Salivation is particularly unpleasant, leading to dribbling. Anticholinergic drugs may help, and improved swallowing produced by levodopa therapy may avoid the problem, but occasionally continuous dribbling is so distressing the irradiation of the parotids is justified.

Drug interaction Patients with Parkinson's disease often require other drugs to control other illnesses. No interactions between anti-Parkinsonian drugs and the following have been noted: anticoagulants, benzodiazepines, tricyclic antidepressants, digoxin, diuretics, trinitrin, propranolol, anti-arrhythmic drugs, antibiotics, thyroxine, and hypoglycaemic agents.

Diabetic control is not altered usually. Hypotensive therapy with α-methyldopa (Aldomet) leads to an increase in levodopa-induced side effects, for α-methyldopa inhibits dopa decarboxylase. Propranolol (Inderal) or other beta-adrenergic antagonists probably are the drugs of choice to treat hypertension for they also slightly benefit Parkinsonian tremor.

Levodopa should never be given with a conventional mono-amine oxidase inhibitor, and the directly acting sympathomimetic amines contained in bronchodilators and some cold remedies are best avoided due to the risks of paroxysmal hypertension.

The fact that neuroleptics, all of which are dopamine antagonists, may cause deterioration in Parkinson's disease and may reverse the beneficial actions of levodopa, has already been noted. Phenothiazines, butyrophenones, and thioxanthines are best avoided if possible, as is papaverine, included in many so-called cerebral vasodilators, for it too is a dopamine antagonist.

Pyridoxine (vitamin B_6) is a co-factor for decarboxylase, so enhances metabolism of plain levodopa. Many combined vitamin preparations contain pyridoxine and may reverse the beneficial actions of plain levodopa. However, pyridoxine can be given with Sinemet or Madopar.

Surgery

Patients with Parkinson's disease may require surgery for other illnesses, but the need should always be balanced against the risks. Some patients deteriorate severely after anaesthesia and enforced bed-rest, and may never make up the lost ground. If surgery is essential, then levodopa therapy should be continued up to the night of the operation. The morning dose is omitted, but treatment is re-started as soon as the patient can swallow. In those with prolonged post-operative difficulties, levodopa can be given via a nasogastric tube, or as a rectal infusion if necessary.

OTHER AKINETIC–RIGID SYNDROMES IN ADULTS

Progressive supranuclear palsy

Definition

In 1964 Steele, Richardson, and Olszewski described a syndrome with similarities to Parkinsonism, but with an additional characteristic and diagnostic abnormality of voluntary eye movement. The illness is characterized by a progressive supranuclear paralysis of voluntary vertical eye movements (especially for down-gaze), dysarthria, and axial rigidity, along with other signs of Parkinsonism and slowing of mental processes with onset in middle or late life.

Aetiology

The cause of progressive supranuclear palsy is not known. It is a rare disease. Males are affected more than females, and no familial cases have been described. Onset usually is in the fifth to seventh decades.

Pathology

There is widespread neuronal loss and gliosis in the brainstem, affecting particularly the globus pallidus, substantia nigra, subthalamus, red nucleus, tectum and peri-aqueductal grey matter, and dentate nucleus. Such affected nerve cells show neurofibrillary tangles. The cerebral cortex, however, is unaffected and senile plaques do not occur.

Symptoms

The illness most commonly presents either with imbalance or visual symptoms. The latter consist of difficulty with reading or coming down stairs, because both demand voluntary downward gaze, and vertical gaze characteristically is impaired. The patient cannot voluntarily look up and down, nor follow an object moved in the vertical plane (Fig. 6). But a full range of vertical eye movements can be elicited reflexly by rapid posturing of the head (the

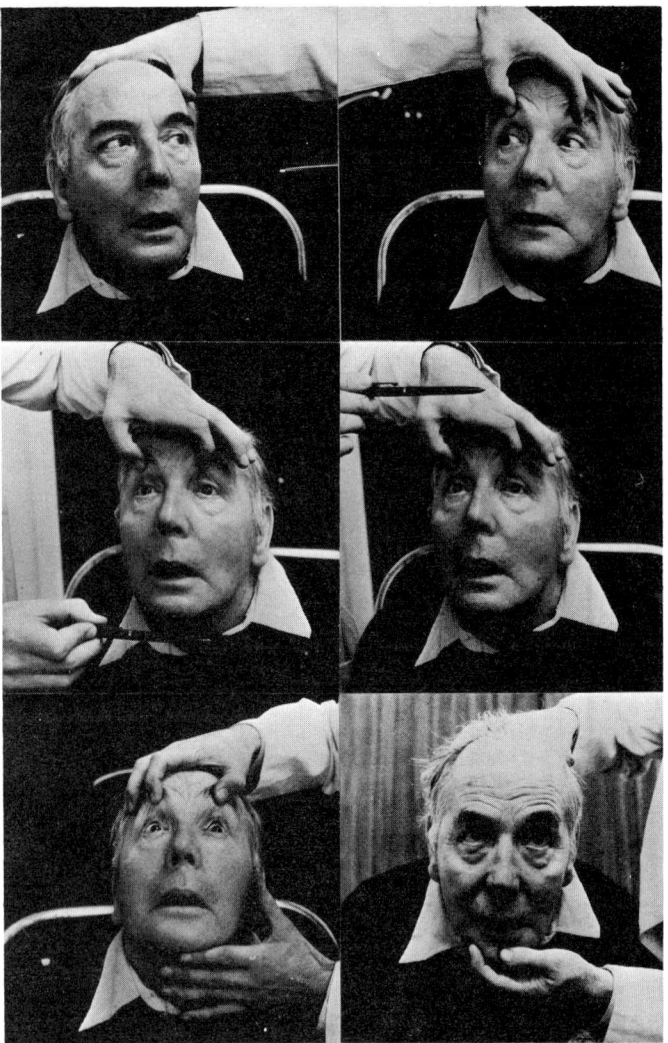

Fig. 6 Defective ocular movements in progressive supranuclear palsy. The patient, a 67-year-old man, can voluntarily look to left and right (upper panels), but cannot voluntarily look down or up, or follow a moving object (a pen) down or up (middle panels). However, when the head is passively extended or flexed, a full range of reflex vertical eye movement is achieved (lower panels).

doll's eye manoeuvre), or by activation of brainstem reflex eye movement by injection of water into the ears to elicit the caloric vestibulo-ocular reflexes. Horizontal eye movement also is similarly affected, but usually later than vertical eye movement. The earliest signs of impairment of eye movement is a breakdown of swift, smooth, rapid voluntary movement into short jerky repetitive saccades. The characteristic profound and early involvement of vertical gaze is accompanied by a typical dystonic extension of the neck, and a fixed wide-eyed stare. The patient looks around by moving the head, rather than eyes.

Imbalance and unexplained falls are a common early complaint. At this stage the patient also will exhibit characteristic axial rigidity of neck, trunk, and proximal limb muscles, and poverty of movement, particularly of whole body movement. Speech is dysarthric as in a pseudobulbar palsy, and swallowing may be impaired. Dystonic postures and other abnormal movements, including tremor, may occur. Akinesia and rigidity are evident, but power is preserved as is sensation; the tendon reflexes are brisk and the plantar responses may be extensor.

Mental function is impaired. The patient may give an impression of dementia, with difficulty in memory and loss of intellectual power. Careful examination, however, reveals that memory and

intellect are better than is apparent at first sight, provided the patient is given adequate time to formulate answers. This severe slowness of mental processes has been termed 'subcortical dementia', but this term has fallen into disrepute.

Natural history
The disease is relentlessly progressive, the patient becoming bed-ridden and anarthric, leading to death in 5–7 years.

Diagnosis
The crucial diagnostic feature is the supranuclear gaze palsy. However, eye movements also may be abnormal in patients with Parkinson's disease, who are superficially similar in other respects to those with progressive supranuclear palsy. The characteristic abnormality of eye movement in Parkinson's disease is a restriction of up-gaze and convergence; in addition, horizontal eye movements may become slow and broken up. Progressive supranuclear palsy is diagnosed with confidence only when down-gaze is affected. However, involvement of down-gaze may only appear later in the illness, making early diagnosis difficult. In addition, there are other causes of an akinetic rigid syndrome with a supranuclear vertical gaze palsy (e.g. some cases of olivo-ponto-cerebellar degeneration and cortico-basal degeneration).

Treatment
There is no effective treatment for this condition, which does not respond to levodopa or other dopamine agonists. Such drugs, and amantadine, may cause a slight but useful alerting effect, but usually have little other action.

Multiple system atrophy
(See also pages 21.75–21.80).

Definition
Three separate conditions are included in this category, olivopontocerebellar atrophy, strionigral degeneration, and progressive autonomic failure (Shy–Drager syndrome).

The term olivopontocerebellar degeneration was given by Thomas and Dejerine to an isolated case of ataxia in middle life, with widespread degeneration affecting particularly the cerebellar cortex, inferior olives, and pontine nuclei. In fact, Thomas and Dejerine had described a sporadic case of the familial cerebellar ataxia originally described by Menzel in 1891. Such patients also may exhibit an akinetic-rigid Parkinsonian syndrome, and have additional degeneration in the striatum and substantia nigra.

In 1961 Adams, van Bogaert, and Van der Eeken described a group of middle-aged patients indistinguishable clinically from those with Parkinson's disease, but with severe cell loss and gliosis in the striatum (especially the putamen) and substantia nigra. Many such patients, however, also exhibit the pathological changes of olivopontocerebellar atrophy.

In 1960 Shy and Drager drew attention to a syndrome characterized by autonomic failure with severe postural hypotension, and often akinesia and rigidity. Pathologically such cases exhibited extensive loss of cells in the intermediolateral nuclei of the lateral horns in the spinal cord; these cells are the pre-ganglionic sympathetic neurones. In addition, there often was severe cell loss and gliosis in the olivopontocerebellar and strionigral regions.

Thus three clinical syndromes, cerebellar ataxia due to olivopontocerebellar degeneration, Parkinsonism due to strionigral degeneration, and progressive autonomic failure overlap, and share a common widespread pathology, which Oppenheimer has named multiple system atrophy (see also page 21.76).

Aetiology
The cause of this disease, which is rare, is unknown. Most cases presenting with the syndromes of strionigral degeneration and autonomic failure are sporadic, but some of those with cerebellar

ataxia have a family history, often with inheritance through many generations as an autosomal dominant trait. Both sexes are affected and symptoms begin in early adult or middle age in most cases. Recently a partial deficiency of the enzyme glutamate dehydrogenase in lymphocytes has been identified in some patients with olivopontocerebellar degeneration.

Pathology
(See Table 4.)

Anatomical
The most striking abnormality to the naked eye in *olivopontocerebellar degeneration* is gross shrinkage of the pons and middle cerebellar peduncles due to loss of pontine nuclei and of their transverse fibres. In the medulla there is loss of neurones in the inferior olives and of their olivocerebellar fibres. The cerebellar cortex has lost Purkinje cells, but the deep cerebellar nuclei are preserved.

In *strionigral degeneration* there is gliosis and extensive loss of neurones in the caudate and especially in the putamen, and in the substantia nigra.

In progressive *autonomic failure* there is widespread neuronal loss in caudate nucleus, substantia nigra, locus coeruleus, inferior olives, Purkinje cells, dorsal vagal nucleus, and intermediolateral column of the thoracic cord, the latter being held responsible for the sympathetic failure (see pages 21.75–21.80).

Biochemical
The main neurochemical findings described in multiple system atrophy are a considerable loss of dopamine in the caudate and putamen, nucleus accumbens, and substantia nigra (to between 5 and 50 per cent of normal), a profound reduction of noradrenaline particularly in the nucleus accumbens, septal nuclei, hypothalamus and locus coeruleus (to between 10 and 27 per cent of normal), a general reduction in glutamic acid decarboxylase in cerebral cortex, brainstem, and cerebellum (to between 1 and 48 per cent of normal), and a similar generalized reduction in choline acetyltransferase in most brain areas examined (to between 10 and 47 per cent of normal). The changes in dopamine and noradrenaline reflect degeneration in the substantia nigra and locus coeruleus, but the changes in glutamic acid decarboxylase probably were due to the prolonged anoxic mode of death. In contrast, choline acetyltransferase is largely unaffected by antemortem factors and probably reflects extensive loss of cholinergic neurones.

Table 4 Sites of pathology in different basal ganglia degenerations

	Parkinson's disease	Progressive supranuclear palsy	Multiple system atrophy
Cerebral cortex	(+)	−	(+)
Striatum	(+)	(+)	+
Globus pallidus	(+)	++	−
Subthalamus	(+)	++	−
Pigmented nuclei	++	++	+
Pontine nuclei	−	(+)	+
Inferior olives	−	(+)	+
Purkinje cells	−	(+)	+
Dentate nucleus	−	++	−
Intermediolateral columns	(+)	(+)	+
Sympathetic ganglia	+	?	−
Pyramidal tracts	−	+	+
Cellular change	Lewy body	Neurofibrillary tangle	

++ always or nearly always affected.
+ commonly affected.
(+) occasionally affected.
− seldom if ever affected.
After Oppenheimer (1976).

Clinical features
Olivopontocerebellar degeneration presents as a progressive cerebellar ataxia of gait and arms, accompanied by dysarthria and, often, nystagmus. In addition, pyramidal signs, akinesia, and rigidity, and optic atrophy often develop.

Strionigral degeneration presents a Parkinsonian syndrome indistinguishable from that of Parkinson's disease, although cerebellar atrophy may be evident on CT scan.

Progressive *autonomic failure* (Shy–Drager syndrome) presents as postural (orthostatic) hypotension, urinary incontinence, loss of sweating, sexual impotence, akinesia and rigidity, and sometimes tremor and severe dysarthria. Serious respiratory stridor and sleep apnoea may develop.

Diagnosis
Multiple system atrophy may be confused with any of the other causes of a progressive cerebellar syndrome, including cerebellar tumour, other spinocerebellar degenerations, multiple sclerosis, and the cerebellar ataxia that may be associated with myxoedema, a remote neoplasm, or alcoholism.

Strionigral degeneration usually is misdiagnosed as Parkinson's disease, but does not respond to treatment.

Orthostatic hypotension may be due to drugs, diabetes, or other causes of an autonomic neuropathy including amyloid. Most difficult is to separate orthostatic hypotension due to multiple system atrophy from Parkinson's disease due to Lewy body degeneration with postural hypotension. Other features of an autonomic neuropathy, however, do not occur in Parkinson's disease.

Treatment
Unfortunately, there is no effective therapy for multiple system atrophy. The akinetic-rigid Parkinsonian features do not usually respond to levodopa replacement therapy as well as they do in Parkinson's disease. Indeed, many patients with multiple system atrophy are quite resistant to dopamine agonists or anticholinergic drugs.

Postural hypotension may be helped by elastic stockings, a G-suit, and fludrocortisone combined with head-up tilt at night.

The diagnosis and management of progressive autonomic failure with particular regard to postural hypotension is considered on page 21.79.

Cerebral anoxia
Aetiology and pathology
Severe cerebral anoxia, whether its cause be cardiac arrest, carbon monoxide poisoning, or pure anoxic anoxia, may cause disproportionate damage to the basal ganglia leading to bilateral necrosis of the striatum or globus pallidus. While the effects of damage to the cerebral cortex are apparent immediately, those resulting from basal ganglia destruction may appear days or up to about a month after the insult, and thereafter for reasons that are not clear, the syndrome may progress.

Symptoms
After the episode of cerebral anoxia, the patient may recover from the initial coma, only to relapse over the next few weeks into an increasingly severe akinetic-rigid state with profound dysarthria and dysphagia. The arms characteristically are flexed while the legs are extended, all limbs showing dystonic posturing and athetoid movements of the fingers and toes.

Progression to death may occur, but the condition can arrest or even improve and levodopa sometimes helps (see also page 21.252).

Basal ganglia calcification
Many elderly brains at necropsy show a mild degree of calcification in the striopallidal structures, most evident in the globus palli-

dus, without symptoms in life. Such asymptomatic brain calcification is found in about 0.5 per cent of CT scans of elderly subjects.

About 20–30 per cent of those with widespread calcification of the basal ganglia and other structures, including the dentate nucleus, exhibit neurological symptoms and signs, which include an akinetic-rigid Parkinsonian syndrome, dyskinesias such as chorea or dystonia, and sometimes epilepsy, ataxia, and dementia.

Some patients with symptomatic basal ganglia calcification previously have had radical thyroid surgery, and others have idiopathic hypoparathyroidism or pseudohypoparathyroidism. Many such patients, however, including some familial cases, have no demonstrable endocrine or metabolic disorder.

AKINETIC–RIGID SYNDROMES IN CHILDHOOD

The causes of an akinetic-rigid syndrome in childhood or adolescence are quite different from those responsible for a similar syndrome in middle or late life (Table 5).

A number of diseases of childhood may produce a variety of different symptoms in different patients. Many children with Huntington's disease present with the Westphal variant of the disease, namely an akinetic-rigid syndrome. So too may other hereditary diseases such as Wilson's disease, Hallervorden–Spatz disease, progressive pallidal degeneration, and Pelizaeus–Merzbacher's disease.

Wilson's disease will be described in detail, for it is a treatable and preventable cause of extrapyramidal (and liver) disease in childhood, adolescence, and young adult life. Brief notes follow on the other rare disorders. All these conditions may present not only with a Parkinsonian clinical picture in some children, but also in others with a range of abnormal involuntary movements such as chorea or torsion spasms. Certain other rare diseases of childhood also may be present with such extrapyramidal disorders, and brief notes on these conditions, such as ataxia telangectasia, the Lesch–Nyhan syndrome, also are included at this point for they enter into any differential diagnosis of a movement disorder in a child.

Wilson's disease

The pathophysiology, clinical features, and treatment of this condition are considered in Section 9. Here we shall review briefly the main neurological aspects.

Wilson's disease presents to neurologists as a behaviour disturbance, an akinetic-rigid syndrome and with a variety of dyskinesias: or it presents to hepatologists with the complication of acute hepatitis or chronic cirrhosis. Onset is usually in childhood or adolescence, but may be delayed as late as the fifth decade of life. The first symptoms of the disease frequently lead to psychiatric referral with conduct disorders, personality change, or frank psychotic disturbance. Common initial neurological symptoms include tremor of any type, dysarthria and drooling (Fig. 7), chorea, dystonic spasms and posturing, or akinesia and rigidity. Without treatment, progression is inevitable, with dementia, increasingly severe dysarthria, and dysphagia, and increasing akinesia and rigidity leading to contractures and immobility. Vision, hearing, and sen-

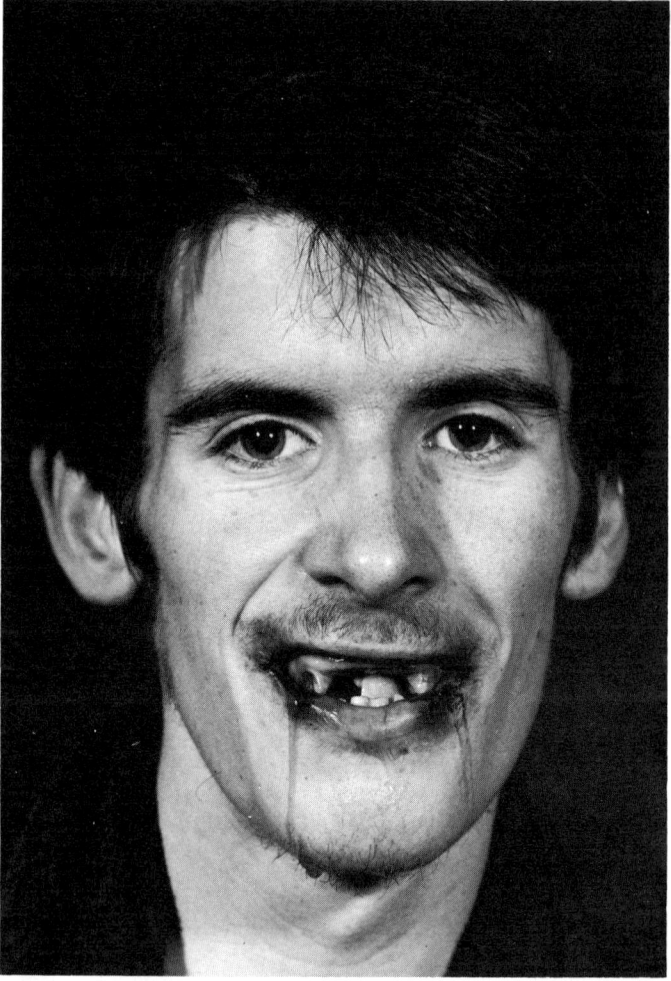

Fig. 7 The facies of a 20-year-old man with severe Wilson's disease, causing a severe pseudobulbar palsy with marked dysarthria and dysphagia, as well as a generalized akinetic-rigid syndrome. A Kayser-Fleischer ring is just evident around the periphery of the cornea, especially on the right.

sation are not affected, and the tendon reflexes and plantar responses are usually normal. Fits may occur in a minority of cases.

A Kayser–Fleischer ring may be seen in the cornea with the naked eye and is always present in those with neurological symptoms when looked for with a slit-lamp. It consists of a ring of greenish-brown copper pigment deposited around the margin of the cornea in Descemet's membrane. A 'sunflower' cataract, due to copper deposition in the lens, also may be seen. Copper deposition in the nailbeds produces blue lunalae, while copper deposits in the kidney may produce selective proteinuria and aminoaciduria.

Clinical evidence of liver disease may occur without neurological symptoms and signs. In those with neurological deficit, there can be no clinical evidence of liver damage, but a history of hepatitis or jaundice may be obtained and the liver often will be found to be damaged on investigation. Hepatic coma and gastrointestinal haemorrhage due to varices may occur.

Without treatment the disease is usually fatal in 5–14 years from the onset.

The diagnosis and management are described in Section 9.

Hallervorden–Spatz disease

In 1922, Hallervorden and Spatz described a very rare, often familial condition of childhood in which iron-containing pigment is deposited particularly in the globus pallidus and zona reticulata of

Table 5 Causes of akinetic-rigid syndrome in childhood

Hereditary	Other
Wilson's disease	Drugs
Hallervorden–Spatz disease	Athetoid cerebral palsy
Progressive pallidal atrophy	
Juvenile Huntington's disease	
Pelizaeus–Merzbacher disease	
Ataxia telangiectasia	
Lesch–Nyhan disease	

All the hereditary diseases of childhood affecting the basal ganglia may also cause abnormal involuntary movements such as torsion spasms and, sometimes, chorea.

the substantia nigra. Large oval spheroids, probably containing mucoprotein, are found in these pigmented areas, and are thought to be degenerating axons.

A family history is obtained in less than a quarter of cases, usually affected siblings, indicating autosomal recessive inheritance. Similar neuroaxonal dystrophic changes also can be caused by exogenous agents in animals, such as vitamin E deficiency.

Clinically, the condition presents as progressive rigidity, initially in the legs with a characteristic equinovarus foot deformity (club foot), later of the arms. Dystonic movements of the affected limbs are common, as is dysarthria and dementia. The illness does not respond to treatment and most children die by early adult life.

Progressive pallidal atrophy

In 1917, Ramsay Hunt described a very rare syndrome of progressive Parkinsonism with onset in childhood or adolescence ('juvenile Parkinsonism'). One such patient came to necropsy and showed severe degeneration of the globus pallidus, with other changes in the striatum. Subsequently, similar cases have been reported with variable degeneration of the globus pallidus, subthalamic nuclei (pallido-Luysian degeneration), and pyramidal pathways (pallidopyramidal degeneration).

Many patients have a family history suggesting inheritance usually as an autosomal dominant trait, but sometimes the illness only appears in siblings.

Clinically, the conditions presents in childhood or adolescence with a progressive Parkinsonian syndrome, including akinesia, rigidity with rest tremor, with preserved intellect and sensation, but often with pyramidal signs and sometimes with dystonia and torsion spasms. The Parkinsonian features may respond to levodopa therapy.

Pelizaeus–Merzbacher disease

A rare demyelinating leucodystrophy of unknown cause, histologically distinct from Krabbe's disease, metachromatic leucodystrophy and adrenoleucodystrophy, inherited as an autosomal recessive or sex-linked recessive trait. The illness characteristically presents in the first decade of life with progressive dementia, gross nystagmus, and ataxia, and sometimes optic atrophy and spasticity, often with fits. Extrapyramidal features also may be prominent, particularly dystonic postures and torsion spasms, and finally an akinetic rigid state. Most patients with childhood onset die before the age of 20 years, but a few cases with onset in adult life and slower progression have been recorded.

Ataxia telangiectasia

(See also page 21.210 and Section 4.)

Madame Louis-Bar in 1941 described an illness, apparently inherited as an autosomal recessive trait, characterized by the gradual appearance in early childhood of ataxia, Parkinsonian features, and abnormal movements such as chorea or torsion spasms. In addition, dysarthria, nystagmus, a supranuclear gaze palsy and ocolomotor apraxia evolve, associated with hypotonia and areflexia. Intelligence is preserved until later in the illness, which is slowly progressive. Telangiectasia develops in the conjunctiva, pinna of the ear, face, and limb flexures, but may not appear until after the age of 5 years. Such children are very prone to infection, particularly respiratory infection, for they also exhibit immunological deficiencies, characteristically hypogammaglobulinaemia with gross loss or absence of IgA.

Lesch–Nyhan syndrome

(See also page 21.211 and Section 4.)

A rare condition, apparently inherited as a sex-linked recessive trait, with onset in infancy or early childhood with progressive abnormal movements such as chorea and torsion spasms, mental retardation, spasticity, and characteristically a tendency to self-

Table 6 Causes of tremor

Rest tremor
  Parkinson's disease
  Post-encephalitic Parkinsonism
  Drug-induced Parkinsonism
  Other extrapyramidal diseases

Postural tremor
  Physiological tremor
  Exaggerated physiological tremor, i.e.
    Thyrotoxicosis
    Anxiety states
    Alcohol
    Drugs (sympathomimetics, antidepressants, lithium)
    Heavy metal poisoning (i.e. mercury – the 'hatter's shakes')
  Structural brain disease, i.e.
    Severe cerebellar lesions ('red nucleus tremor')
    Wilson's disease
    Neurosyphilis
  Benign essential (familial) tremor

Intention tremor
  Brainstem or cerebellar disease, i.e.
    Multiple sclerosis
    Spinocerebellar degenerations
    Vascular disease
    Tumour

mutilation as the child grows older. Diagnosis is established by the finding of a raised serum uric acid, due to deficiency of hypoxanthine-guanine phosphoribosyl-transferase. Uric acid renal calculi may develop, so treatment with allopurinol is justified, although the reduction in serum uric acid levels does not prevent neurological deterioration.

THE DYSKINESIAS

Most abnormal involuntary movements may be classified into one of five main categories: tremor, chorea, myoclonus, tics, and torsion dystonia. Each type of dyskinesia may be caused by a variety of diseases. In some patients the dyskinesia is accompanied by other neurological deficits or some other clue as to the cause; in others, the involuntary movements occur in isolation and constitute the illness. Nearly all dyskinesias disappear in sleep, are made worse by anxiety and stress, and are improved by relaxation.

Tremor is a rhythmic sinusoidal movement of a body part, due to regular rhythmic muscle contractions. The common causes of tremor are shown in Table 6.

Chorea consists of a continuous flow of irregular, jerky, and explosive movements, that flit from one portion of the body to another in random sequence. Each muscle contraction is brief, often appearing as a fragment of what might have been a normal movement, and quite unpredictable in timing or site (Fig. 8). The common causes of chorea are shown in Table 7.

Myoclonus consists of rapid shock-like muscle jerks, often repetitive and sometimes rhythmic. The common causes of myoclonus are shown in Table 8.

Tics are similar to myoclonic jerks in appearance, but are repetitive, stereotyped movements that can be mimicked voluntarily and can be held in check by an effort of will at the expense of mounting inner tension. The common causes of tics are shown in Table 9.

Torsion dystonia consists of sustained torsion spasms of muscle contraction which distort the limbs and trunk into characteristic dystonic postures – the twisted neck (torticollis), flexed (antecollis) or extended neck (retrocollis), the arched back (lordosis) or twisted back (scoliosis), the hyperpronated arm, and plantarflexed inverted foot. Such dystonic spasms typically occur on willed action (action dystonia); they may be repetitive to give a rhythmic character, or sustained to hold a fixed dystonic posture. The common causes of torsion dystonia are shown in Table 10.

There is confusion between the use of the terms dystonia and athetosis, which are employed interchangeably. Dystonia literally means any abnormality of muscle tone, but most neurologists employ it to describe postures instantly recognized as dystonic. The term dystonia is frequently qualified as torsion dystonia, to emphasize the twisted nature of the abnormal postures. Many patients with torsion dystonia, whatever its cause, not only have abnormal postures, but also abnormal involuntary movements. The latter are either called dystonic movements (torsion spasms), particularly if they affect proximal joints (axial torsion dystonia), or athetoid movements, particularly if they affect the fingers and toes (distal athetosis). The term athetosis originally was introduced to describe the sinuous, writhing digital movements that may follow a stroke. Subsequently, athetosis became synonymous with one type of cerebral palsy, happily fast disappearing due to improved perinatal care, resulting from brain damage due to anoxia or kernicterus at birth. Such babies typically were floppy, exhibited delayed motor milestones, and sometime before the age of 5 years developed athetoid abnormal movements. The whole syndrome is known as athetoid cerebral palsy, or simply athetosis.

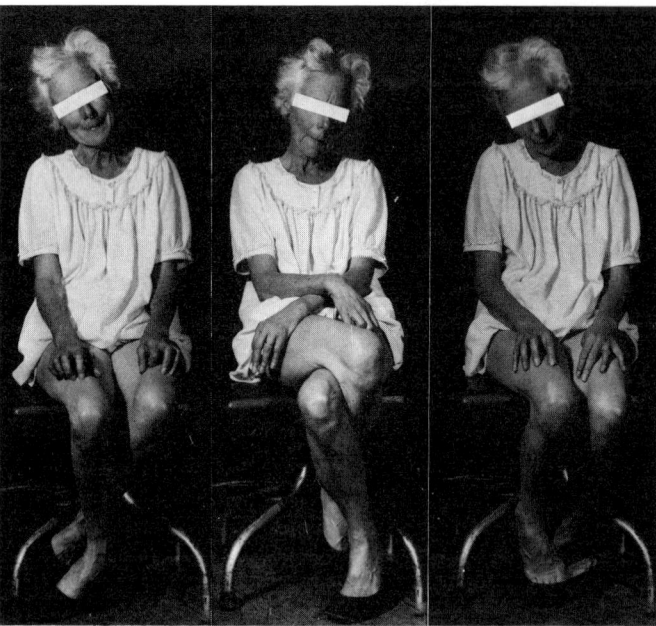

Fig. 8 Chorea due to polycythaemia rubra vera in a 57-year-old woman. The characteristic fleeting choreic movements are captured in these three sequential frames.

Table 7 Causes of chorea

Sydenham's chorea
    Variants include: chorea gravidarum, chorea caused by contraceptive pill

Huntington's disease
    Variants include: senile chorea, juvenile chorea, Westphal variant

Benign hereditary chorea

Hereditary chorea with acanthocytosis (neuroacanthocytosis)

Symptomatic chorea
    Thyrotoxicosis
    Systemic lupus erythematosus
    Polycythaemia rubra vera
    Encephalitis lethargica
    Hypernatraemia
    Hypoparathyroidism
    Subdural haematoma

Drug-induced chorea
    Neuroleptic drugs
    Phenytoin
    Alcohol

Hemiballism (hemichorea)
    Stroke
    Tumour
    Trauma
    Post-thalamotomy

Table 8 Causes of myoclonus

Generalized myoclonus
Progressive myoclonic encephalopathies*
    With demonstrable metabolic cause:
        Lafora body disease
        GM_2 gangliosidosis (Tay–Sachs disease) (hexosaminidase)
        Gaucher's disease (juvenile) (glucocerebrosidase)
        Ceroid lipofuscinosis (Batten's disease) (? peroxidase)
        Sialidosis (cherry-red spot-myoclonus syndrome)
    Hereditary myoclonus with no known metabolic cause:
        Familial myoclonic epilepsy (Unverricht–Lundborg disease)
        Myoclonus associated with spinocerebellar degenerations (Ramsay Hunt syndrome)
        Myoclonus, ataxia, and deafness syndrome
        Juvenile neuroaxonal dystrophy
        Infantile poliodystrophies (Alper's disease)
    Other sporadic diseases:
        Encephalitis lethargica
        Subacute sclerosing leucoencephalitis
        Creutzfeldt–Jakob disease
        Alzheimer's disease
        Metabolic myoclonus
            Uraemia
            Hyponatraemia
            Hypocalcaemia
            Hepatic failure
            CO_2 narcosis
            Drug-induced myoclonus
            Alcohol and drug withdrawal

Static myoclonic encephalopathies†
    Infantile perinatal myoclonic encephalopathy
    Post-anoxic action myoclonus (Lance–Adams syndrome)
    Post-traumatic myoclonus

Myoclonic epilepsies‡
    First year of life
        Infantile spasms
        Benign infantile myoclonus
        'Dancing eyes' syndrome
    Two or six years
        Lennox–Gastaut syndrome
        Cryptogenic myoclonic epilepsy (Aicardi syndrome)
    Older children and adolescents (and adults)
        Photosensitive epileptic myoclonus
        Myoclonic absences
        Morning myoclonus – primary generalized epilepsy

Benign essential (familial) myoclonus
    Paramyoclonus multiplex (Friedreich)
    Nocturnal myoclonus (restless legs syndrome)

Focal myoclonus (segmental)
    Spinal
    Tumour
    Infarct
    Trauma
  Palatal myoclonus
  Hemifacial spasm
  Cortical reflex myoclonus
  Epilepsia partialis continua

  * Obvious myoclonus (with or without fits) clearly as part of a progressive encephalopathy.
    † Obvious myoclonus after some acute and now static cerebral insult.
    ‡ Obvious epilepsy as the main problem, with myoclonus.

Many of the diseases known to cause the various dyskinesias shown in Tables 6–10 are discussed elsewhere. However, a number of conditions in which the dyskinesia is the major feature of the illness will be described here.

Table 9 Causes of tics

Simple tics
    Transient tic of childhood
    Chronic simple tic
Complex multiple tics
    Chronic multiple tics
    Gilles de la Tourette syndrome
Symptomatic tics
    Encephalitis lethargica
    Drug-induced tics
Post-traumatic
Neuroacanthocytosis

Table 10 Causes of torsion dystonia

Generalized dystonia
Idiopathic dystonia musculorum deformans
    Autosomal recessive
    Sex-linked recessive
    Autosomal dominant
    Sporadic
Drug-induced dystonia
    Acute dystonic reactions
    Chronic tardive dystonia
Symptomatic dystonia
    GM1 gangliosidosis
    GM2 gangliosidosis
    Metachromatic leucodystrophy
    Homocystinuria
    Acidosis*
    Ceroid lipofuscinosis
    Sea blue histiocytosis
    Ataxia telangectasia
    Leigh's distase*
    Mitochondrial encephalopathies
    Athetoid cerebral palsy*
    Encephalitis lethargica
    Wilson's disease*
    Lesch–Nyhan disease
    Juvenile Huntington's disease
    Hallervorden–Spatz disease
    Progressive pallidal atrophy
    Pelizaeus–Merzbacher disease
    Spino-cerebellar degenerations
    Toxic*
    Post-anoxic
Paroxysmal dystonia (paroxysmal choreoathetosis)
    Paroxysmal kinesogenic choreoathetosis
    Paroxysmal dystonic choreoathetosis
    Dystonia with marked diurnal fluctuations

Focal dystonia
Spasmodic torticollis
Axial (truncal) dystonica
Dystonic writer's cramp (and other occupational cramps)
Oromandibular dystonia ⎫
                    ⎬ Cranial dystonia
Blepharospasm ⎭

Hemiplegic dystonia (hemidystonia)
Hemiplegic dystonia G
    Stroke*
    Tumour*
    A-V malformation
    Trauma*
    Encephalitis
    Post-thalamotomy

* May cause low-density lesions in basal ganglia on CT scan.

Benign essential (familial) tremor

Definition
An illness characterized by postural tremor of the arms and head, often inherited as an autosomal dominant trait, which presents at any age and is usually only slowly progressive causing mild disability.

Aetiology
The cause of benign essential tremor, which may appear in childhood, adolescence (juvenile tremor), early adult life, or old age (senile tremor), is unknown. A positive family history is obtained in over half of such patients and the pattern of inheritance in such families indicates an autosomal dominant trait.

Pathophysiology
No pathological or biochemical abnormality has been identified in benign essential tremor, but few cases have come to necropsy. The condition may well represent some instability in the many feedback neuronal loops that control the posture of the hands, head, and other parts of the body.

Everyone has a physiological tremor of the outstretched hands, at about 8–12 Hz (see Fig. 3), due to summation of many factors which combine to generate an oscillation at this frequency. Such factors include (a) the tendency for motor units to start firing at about 8 Hz, which is below the natural tetanic fusion frequency of human muscle (about 12 Hz); (b) the natural movement frequency of the outstretched arms is about 8–12 Hz; and (c) loop delay in operation of the stretch reflex arc is such as to cause a tendency to oscillate at 10 Hz.

Essential tremor usually is of a somewhat slower frequency at about 5–8 Hz (see Fig. 3). It is probably due to an oscillation in one of three brain or spinal servo loops controlling muscle contraction. Another characteristic of essential tremor is that it is very susceptible to the impact of emotional stress, and this is partly due to activation of β-adrenergic receptors in muscle and perhaps in the central nervous system also. Alcohol suppresses essential tremor, but the mechanism responsible is unknown.

Symptoms
Tremor is present in one or both hands on maintaining a posture, as when holding a cup or glass. Handwriting becomes untidy and tremulous (see Fig. 4). There is no tremor at rest, but a rhythmic oscillation develops when the patient holds the arms outstretched. On movement, as in finger–nose testing, the tremor continues but does not get strikingly worse as is the case with cerebellar intention tremor. Tremor of the head (titubation) and jaw is present in about 50 per cent of cases, and tremor of the legs occurs in about a third. Despite the tremor, tests of coordination usually are performed normally, walking is unaffected, and there are no other neurological abnormalities. In particular, there are no signs of cerebellar ataxia or of Parkinsonism (patients with essential tremor often show 'cog-wheeling' on passive manipulation of the arms, but this does not indicate a diagnosis of Parkinson's disease).

Two other factors are characteristic of this disorder. First, a family history (see above) and secondly, the observation that small or moderate doses of alcohol may suppress the tremor. A large sherry, or gin and tonic, may be sufficient to 'steady the hands'. The illness is static or only slowly progressive in most patients, causing predominantly a social disability, but individuals dependent upon manual skill, for example surgeons, watchmakers, and violinists, may be severely disabled by such tremor. The condition may become more severe and progressive in a small minority of patients, producing increasing severe disability so that eventually such individuals cannot hold a cup or plate securely enough to drink or eat, and speech may become tremulous and dysarthric in such cases.

Some other variants of the syndrome are encountered occasionally. Thus isolated, inherited, head tremor may occur, with either 'yes-yes' or 'no-no' movements, and tremulous 'writer's cramp' (primary writing tremor) is recognized.

Treatment

Although alcohol may suppress the tremor effectively, and can be of value if used wisely, there is a risk of patients with benign essential tremor becoming alcoholics. Benzodiazepines, such as diazepam (Valium), may give some relief at times of stress, but have no major effect on the tremor. A proportion of patients, perhaps 30–40 per cent, respond satisfactorily to a beta-adrenergic receptor antagonist such as propranolol (Inderal). This appears to be due mainly to inhibition of peripheral β-2 adrenoceptors. Provided there is no contraindication such as asthma, it is usual to start patients on 20 mg three or four times daily increasing gradually up to a daily intake sufficient to control the tremor, or about 240 mg a day; higher doses give no added benefit. Unfortunately, many patients gain only slight or even no relief from propranolol, and most other drugs are of little value. Anti-Parkinsonian drugs have no effect. Recently, primidone (Mysoline), in standard anticonvulsant dosages, has been reported to help some patients. Stereotaxic thalamotomy may be required in the very small number of patients whose tremor is so severe that it warrants the risks of such surgery.

Chorea

Sydenham's chorea

Definition

This is development of chorea (St Vitus' dance) and often psychological disturbance due to rheumatic fever (rheumatic chorea) in childhood and adolescence. Thomas Sydenham described the condition in 1686. Rheumatic fever is discussed in Section 5.

Aetiology and pathology

Sydenham's chorea is now a rare disease, for the incidence of rheumatic fever has declined dramatically. It affects children and adolescents between the ages of 3 and 20 years, most often in spring months. In about a third of cases is appears up to 3 months after a bout of rheumatic fever due to group A streptococcal infection, but the remainder give no such history. It may recur in adult life, particularly in pregnant women (chorea gravidarum) or in those taking the contraceptive pill. Pathologically the brain shows a diffuse inflammatory encephalitis. Vascular changes are not conspicuous, and the cerebral complications of rheumatic fever may be due to deposition of immune complexes, as in disseminated lupus erythematosus, although this is not proven.

Symptoms

Most cases (75 per cent or so) occur between the ages of 7 and 12 years. The onset usually is gradual, but may be abrupt. The initial symptoms are often psychological, with irritability, agitation, disobedience, and inattentiveness. A frank organic confusional state occurs in about 10 per cent of patients. Generalized chorea then appears and may get worse for a few weeks, causing difficulty in holding objects and walking. Speech is impaired in about a third of patients, but headaches, fits, and sensory changes are not features of the illness. The chorea may be predominantly unilateral in about 20 per cent of patients, and in severe cases is accompanied by flaccidity and subjective weakness (chorea mollis). Although cardiac disease may be found, the child usually has no fever or other manifestations of rheumatic fever; the erythrocyte sedimentation rate characteristically is normal and the antistreptolysin titre is not raised.

The chorea and psychological disturbance slowly recover over 1–3 months, rarely up to 6 months, but recurrences occur in about a quarter of patients in the next 2 years. About a third of patients will show evidence of rheumatic cardiac involvement at the time of the illness, and about the same proportion later develop chronic rheumatic heart disease. Those who have suffered one or more attacks of Sydenham's chorea are at particular risk of developing chorea in adult life during pregnancy (chorea gravidarum), or when exposed to drugs such as oral contraceptives or phenytoin.

Treatment

Treatment as for rheumatic fever is necessary, with bed-rest and sedation. The chorea may be controlled with diazepam (Valium), a phenothiazine, or tetrabenazine (Nitoman). A course of penicillin should be given, and prophylactic oral penicillin should be continued until about the age of 20 years to prevent further streptococcal infection (see Section 5).

Huntington's disease

Definition

A rare, dominantly inherited, relentlessly progressive disease, usually of middle life, characterized by chorea and dementia, first described in 1872 by George Huntington, a year after he had qualified in medicine.

Aetiology

The prevalence of the disease is about 1 in 20 000, but it occurs worldwide and in all ethnic groups. The cause is unknown. The illness is inherited as an autosomal dominant trait with full penetrance, so that the children of an affected parent have a 50 per cent risk of the disease, which never skips a generation. The risk of a grandchild of a sufferer, when the child's parent is free of symptoms, is roughly half the parent's risk. The father is more likely to transmit the disease than the mother in those in whom symptoms begin in childhood. New mutations are almost unknown, but relatives frequently conceal the family history.

Recent linkage studies have shown the abnormal gene to lie on the short arm of the 4th chromosome. The DNA probe G8 identifies a restriction fragment length polymorphism linked to the Huntington's disease gene (see Section 4).

Pathology

Anatomical

The brain is generally atrophic, with conspicuous damage to the cerebral cortex and corpus striatum, where there is loss of nerve cells and reactive gliosis without inflammatory changes.

The characteristic feature on a coronal section of the brain is dilation of the lateral ventricle, whose floor become concave rather than convex, due to marked caudate atrophy (Fig. 9); a degree of cortical atrophy is also commonly evident. The main histological abnormality is found in the caudate and putamen, where there is extensive loss of small neurones leading to shrinkage, and a false impression of gliosis. Small neurones elsewhere also are lost, particularly in the thalamus, zona reticulata of substantia nigra (but not the pigmented zona compacta), the superior olive, the hypothalamus, and deep cerebellar nuclei. Neuronal loss and gliosis also is found in the third and, to a lesser extent, in the fourth and fifth layers of the cerebral cortex, particularly of the frontal lobes.

Biochemical

There has been an extensive biochemical study of neurotransmitter changes in the brain in Huntington's disease in recent years (Table 11). There is a profound reduction in the enzymes synthesizing GABA* (glutamic acid decarboxylase), and acetylcholine (choline acetyltransferase) in the striatum, reflecting the extensive loss of GABA-ergic and cholinergic striatal neurones. However, some striatal neurones, particularly those containing somatostatin, are spared. Similarly there is a depletion of GABA and GAD, and of angiotensin-converting enzyme and metenkephalin in the zona reticulata of the substantia nigra, reflecting loss of all types of

---

*γ-aminobutyric acid (page 21.221).

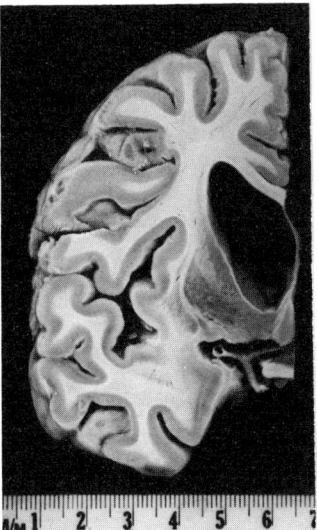
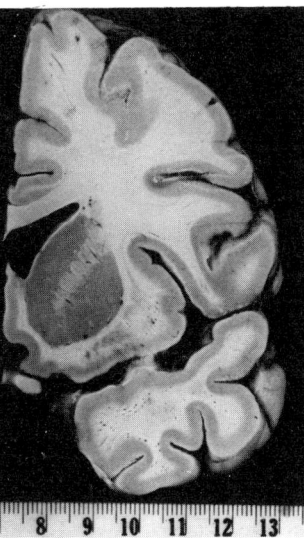

Fig. 9 Coronal section of the brain, on the left, of a patient with Huntington's disease (a woman aged 49 years; brain weight 1065 g) compared, on the right, with a normal brain (a woman aged 69; brain weight 1415 g). Note (a) the gross loss of substance in the caudate nucleus and putamen, and (b) the thinning of the cortical mantle and widening of the sulci. (Reproduced from Corsellis, (1976). In *Greenfield's Neuropathology*, 3rd ed. Arnold, London, with permission.)

Table 11 Neurotransmitters and their enzymes in the striatum in Huntington's disease

	Control	Huntington's disease	
Dopamine (µg/g)	1.6	1.6	Normal
Tyrosine hydroxylase (nmol/g/h)	1.5	1.3	Normal
Choline acetyltransferase (µmol/g/h)	21.6	9.5	44%
GABA (µmol/g)	2.2	1.3	59%
Glutamic acid decarboxylase (µmol/g/h)	4.4	0.8	18%
Angiotensin-converting enzyme (pmol His-Leu/min/mg)	205	98	49%
Substance P (pmol/mg)	42.9	29.1	68%
Metenkephalin (pg/mg)	661	230	35%

Mean values are shown for putamen, except for substance P and metenkephalin which were meausred in the pars reticulata of substantia nigra to which the strionigral pathway projects.

All differences were statistically significant at $p < 0.05$ or less, except when indicated by 'normal'.

Data from Bird and Iversen, Kanazawa *et al.*, and Arregui *et al.* (see Marsden, 1981).

(Differences between Tables 3 and 11 in absolute values reflect different dissection and analytical techniques.)

strionigral pathways. Dopamine and tyrosine hydroxylase activity, however, are not altered in most cases, as is to be expected since the pigmented cells of the zona compacta of the substantia nigra are preserved.

The chorea of Huntington's disease appears to result from relative overactivity of dopamine mechanisms in the brain, perhaps because the intact dopaminergic nigrostriatal pathway is releasing approximately normal quantities of dopamine on to only a few remaining striatal neurones.

All these biochemical changes are likely to be markers of cell loss in the disease, rather than to be clues as to its cause. Tentative reports of alteration in membrane structures and growth rates of fibroblasts in tissue culture may point to a generalized defect of membrane structure in Huntington's disease, but such evidence at present is no more than suggestive. However, recent positron emission tomographic studies using [18]FDG have revealed a profound reduction of glucose metabolism in the striatum, even in those with no atrophy on CT scan.

Symptoms

The onset, which is insidious, is in middle life, usually between the ages of 30 and 50 years. The initial symptoms are frequently those of a change in personality and behaviour, but chorea may be the first sign of the illness. The initial mental disturbances often are subtle. The family, who, if aware of the situation, are constantly looking for early signs of the disease, notice a change in personality, a coarsening of sensitivities, a blunting of drive and depth of feeling, an irritability and truculence, a tendency to uncontrolled aggressive or sexual behaviour. At this stage the patient often retains distressing insight, fully aware of what is in store. Serious depression is common and suicide is a risk. Erratic behaviour at work or in society may lead to psychiatric referral, or a frank schizophreniform psychosis may develop. As the disease progresses, dementia becomes more pronounced and chorea more severe and grotesque. Walking, speech, and use of the hands become impaired. A continual flow of choreiform movements distorts all normal action. Attempts to pick up a cup or wield a pen lead to sudden uncontrolled lunges, while walking assumes a curious deformed dancing air, with abrupt lurches, staggers, and thrusts. The face assumes a curiously provocative look with sudden, irregular lifts of an eyebrow, puckering of the lips, and tilts of the head. As the disease progresses, many patients develop increasing rigidity and akinesia, leading to slowing and reduction of the chorea. Finally the patient becomes bed-ridden and emaciated. Death occurs on average about 14 years from the onset.

Huntington's chorea does not always present in this fashion, and a number of variants are recognized. About 6 per cent of patients present, not with chorea, but with an akinetic-rigid Parkinsonian syndrome (the Westphal variant), which is commonest in children (see below).

While most patients with Huntington's disease first develop symptoms in middle life, some (about 8 per cent) present in childhood (juvenile Huntington's disease). Huntington's disease with onset in childhood (usually between 10–20 years of age) differs in certain aspects from the commoner adult-onset form of the illness. Epilepsy is common, occurring in up to half of those with juvenile-onset, as against in 2 per cent or so of those with adult-onset. Dementia is profound and early in those with juvenile-onset. About a half of juvenile cases present with, or rapidly develop, the akinetic-rigid Westphal variant. Finally, as noted above, children presenting with Huntington's disease commonly have inherited the condition from their father.

Huntington's disease also may present in old age, but if a family history is not available and chorea is the only manifestation (senile chorea), the diagnosis may be very difficult. The pathology in those cases of senile chorea that have come to necropsy has been that of Huntington's disease.

Diagnosis

Despite the wide spectrum of clinical manifestations of Huntington's disease, the diagnosis is not difficult if the characteristic and unique family history is available. Problems arise when no family history is known, or is hidden. In children, Huntington's disease must be differentiated from Sydenham's chorea, from 'juvenile Parkinsonism', and athetoid cerebral palsy, and from the many other degenerative conditions affecting the basal ganglia in childhood (see Table 5).

There is another rare form of chorea, known as benign hereditary chorea, which also is inherited as an autosomal dominant trait. This illness presents in childhood, but with no intellectual change, and such patients have only mild disability and show no progression throughout life.

In adults, it is important to exclude thyrotoxicosis, drugs including neuroleptics and the contraceptive pill, polycythaemia rubra vera and systemic lupus erythematosus as causes of sporadic chorea. Senile chorea must be differentiated from hemiplegic chorea that may follow stroke.

Treatment

There is no cure for the disease. The chorea may be controlled by a phenothiazine such as thiopropazate (Dartalan), chlorpromazine (Largactil), or perphenazine (Fentazin), or by drugs such as haloperidol (Serenace), pimozide (Orap), flupenthixol (Depixol), reserpine (Serpasil), or tetrabenazine (Nitoman). Such drugs are administered in increasing dosage until chorea is controlled, or drug-induced Parkinsonism causes disabling symptoms. These drugs also help to control the mental complications of the illness, but not depression which often is so distressing. Sooner or later chronic hospital care is required. Increasing nursing problems may require admission to hospital, but commonly it is the insupportable psychological stress on the family that finally demands residential care.

Particular attention should be directed towards supporting the family, for the nature of the diseases poses great ethical and emotional problems.

Genetic counselling

The spouse or close relative bears the brunt of the patient's anger, frustration, and mental disintegration, and the hereditary nature of the illness raises agonizing issues. Children of a parent with Huntington's disease inevitably have a 1 in 2 risk of developing the illness themselves, and their children have a 1 in 4 risk. These predictions begin to decrease a little as age advances over middle life (exact risk factors for a given age are available), but the maximum risk is still operative at the time when the genetic advice is most needed, namely when a child at risk reaches adult procreative life. A past tendency to hide the problems from such an individual, to protect him or her from distress, has been replaced by realism and a natural request by those in such a situation to be apprised of the facts. A truthful explanation has to be handled with great compassion and knowledge of the illness and its impact. Inevitably, those at risk, once aware of the facts, ask whether there is some means of predicting whether they have inherited the disease. The discovery of a marker for the Huntington's disease gene, the G8 probe, means that predictive testing will soon be available. However, this probe is not close enough to the gene to be of value to a single individual at risk, but it may well be informative if sufficient members of the family are available for testing. Advances in this area of research are likely to be rapid, so families should be prepared for genetic testing and blood stored for DNA extraction (see also Section 4).

Hemiballism (hemichorea)

Hemiballism refers to wild flinging or throwing movements of one arm and leg. These movements, like those of chorea, are irregular in timing and force, but predominantly involve the large proximal muscles of the shoulder and pelvic girdle.

The occasional child or adolescent with Sydenham's chorea may present with hemiballism, but the syndrome usually is seen in elderly hypertensive diabetic patients as a result of a stroke. Hemiballism may appear as the hemiplegic weakness improves, when it is often accompanied by thalamic pain. In other patients the hemiballism appears abruptly without weakness or sensory deficit. The intensity of the movements varies from mild to such a severity as to cause injury and to require treatment. Acute hemiballism usually, but not always, is due to a vascular lesion in the region of contralateral subthalamic nucleus (corpus Luysi).

Tumour at the same site rarely may produce progressive hemiballism.

Hemiballism due to stroke usually gradually remits spontaneously over 3–6 months. Treatment with a phenothiazine or tetrabenazine (Nitoman) will usually control hemiballism until recovery occurs, but stereotaxic surgery is occasionally required.

Myoclonus

Unexpected, involuntary muscle jerks occur in many neurological diseases (see Table 8). Generalized myoclonus occurs in four clinical settings: (a) as a dominant feature of a progressive brain disease (progressive myoclonic encephalopathy); (b) as a residual feature of some transient brain insult (static myoclonic encephalopathy); (c) as a feature of obvious epilepsy (myoclonic epilepsy); or (d) as the solitary feature of the illness (essential myoclonus).

Myoclonic encephalopathies

Most of these diseases causing a progressive myoclonic encephalopathy are described in detail elsewhere, particularly the lysosomal storage enzyme defects and other metabolic disorders (see Section 9) and the spinocerebellar degenerations (see page 21.206 et seq.).

Familial myoclonic epilepsy

Originally described by Unverricht and Lundborg, it appears to be inherited as an autosomal recessive trait. As it is common in Nordic races, this condition has been called Baltic myoclonus. Fits and myoclonus commence in childhood, accompanied by slowly progressive ataxia and dysarthria. Spasticity eventually develops and the affected individual eventually becomes chair-bound, but progression is slow and dementia is mild or absent. The myoclonus is strikingly stimulus sensitive and occurs also on willed movement. At necropsy the brain shows Purkinje cell loss but no inclusion bodies. Familial myoclonus epilepsy must be distinguished from dyssynergia cerebellaris myoclonica and Lafora body disease (see below and page 21.210).

Dyssynergia cerebellaris myoclonica (Ramsay Hunt syndrome)

This also describes progressive cerebellar ataxia with nystagmus and dysarthria, but without dementia, accompanied by stimulus-sensitive and action myoclonus and occasional fits. The original cases described were sporadic, and onset could be in adult life.

Lafora body disease

This disease, in which the brain at necropsy is found to contain mucopolysaccharide inclusions in nerve cells, also commences with myoclonus and fits in childhood or adolescence, and frequently is familial with autosomal recessive inheritance. However, there is a progressive dementia, blindness, ataxia, and spasticity so that death occurs within 5–10 years of onset. Lafora bodies also are found outside the brain, for example in liver and intestinal mucosa (see also page 21.210).

Postanoxic action myoclonus

This is a distinct entity that may appear after a period of cerebral anoxia due to cardiac arrest or any other anoxic insult. After recovery of consciousness, such patients exhibit muscle jerks affecting face, trunk, and limbs, often provoked by sensory stimuli, and strikingly excited by willed voluntary action. A cerebellar ataxia also may be evident, as may dementia, spasticity, and incontinence. But action myoclonus may be the only evident residual deficit after anoxia in some patients. Treatment with clonazepam (Rivotril) or 5-hydroxytryptophan may be dramatically effective in some cases.

Myoclonic epilepsies

In the myoclonic epilepsies, epileptic seizures are the obvious and dominant feature of the illness. There is some confusion in separating the many conditions that may cause this syndrome, which occurs particularly in children. A convenient, if arbitrary, distinction is based on the age of onset.

In the first year of life, infantile spasms (West's syndrome) poses a particular problem. The peculiar seizures characteristic of infantile spasm (salaam attacks) commence usually between the ages of 3–9 months. Many hereditary, antenatal and postnatal brain insults may cause infantile spasms, which are associated with mental retardation in over 80 per cent of cases.

In older children, up to the age of about 6 years, there is a group who develop an epileptic syndrome of tonic fits, head nods ('cornflakes fits') and falls. These unfortunate children may repeatedly damage themselves due to unexpected drop attacks and may require to wear protective helmets. Many are found to show atypical spike and wave activity in the electroencephalogram (EEG), reminiscent of the classical 3 Hz spike and wave seen in true petit mal, but at a slower frequency. Lennox and Gastaut termed this syndrome 'a petit mal variant', an unfortunate choice for it differs greatly from true petit mal in which absence attacks are the dominant feature of the seizure disorder and the prognosis is good. Unfortunately, the outlook for those with the Lennox–Gastaut syndrome may be gloomy, with a large proportion of such children (90 per cent or more) suffering from severe uncontrolled epilepsy with many falls, and mental deterioration. Such children show irregular spike-wave complexes at 1.5–2.5 Hz in the EEG. This syndrome, like infantile spasms at younger age, indicates a severe disorder of cerebral function. There are, however, other children of this age with tonic fits, head nods and falls, who exhibit spike-wave complexes at or above 2.5 Hz in the EEG, in whom the prognosis is not as gloomy as in those with the Lennox–Gastaut syndrome.

In children over the age of 7 years, and in adolescents, myoclonus in epilepsy takes different forms of epilepsy. Many such children with idiopathic epilepsy experience early morning myoclonic jerks of the arms ('the flying saucer' syndrome describes how they throw away the teacup at breakfast). Also there is the syndrome of photosensitive myoclonus and epilepsy, in which children are provoked to periocular and facial myoclonus, often progressing to a generalized seizure, by a flickering television set. Such photosensitive children, who frequently give a family history of similar disorder, sometimes learn to provoke their own fits by shaking the hand with open fingers in front of their eyes while gazing at the sun.

Benign essential myoclonus

Friedreich originally described, as paramyoclonus multiplex, a condition of myoclonus producing widespread, random muscle jerks affecting all four limbs, trunk, neck, and face, occurring at about 10–50/min, enhanced by action and sensory stimuli. Since then many families inheriting the condition as an autosomal dominant trait have been described. Onset usually is in childhood or adolescence, but disability is strikingly mild, there is no progression, intellect is normal, fits do not occur, and no other deficit appears. Some patients report that alcohol helps their jerks, and many respond to a beta-adrenergic antagonist such as propranolol (Inderal).

Focal myoclonus

There are a number of conditions in which myoclonic muscle jerking may be restricted to one part of the body. Some pathological processes may cause focal myoclonus limited to those segments innervated by the part of the brainstem or spinal cord affected (segmental myoclonus). Similar pathologies causing cerebral damage, particularly to the cerebral cortex, may cause rhythmic repetitive focal muscle jerking associated with electrical evidence of epileptic cortical discharge in the EEG (epilepsia partialis continua).

Spinal myoclonus

Repetitive, often rhythmical myoclonic jerking restricted to a limb, or even to a few muscles of an arm or leg, may occur in local viral myelitis, spinal cord tumour or angioma, or after spinal cord trauma. Rarely, similar focal myoclonus may be caused by pathology affecting spinal roots or plexi. Similar segmental myoclonus may occur in bulbar muscles when such pathology affects the brainstem. The rhythmic muscle jerking occurs spontaneously, at 20–180/min, is not affected by peripheral stimuli, often persists in sleep, and is not associated with any change in the EEG. Anticonvulsants may help, but such spinal myoclonus is often very difficult to control.

Epilepsia partialis continua (page 21.65)

Encephalitis, tumour, abscess, infarct, haemorrhage, or trauma to the cerebral cortex rarely may cause repetitive, rhythmic jerking once or twice a second, confined to one collection of muscles, persisting even in sleep for days, weeks, or months, Usually the damage involves not only the cerebral cortex, but also deeper structures including the thalamus. Because of its large cortical representations, the hand most commonly is the site of epilepsia partialis continua. Many of these patients exhibit stimulus sensitivity, such that touch or muscle stretch, as well as action, can trigger muscle jerks in the affected part (cortical reflex myoclonus). Typical Jacksonian focal motor fits, and grand mal seizures also may occur in such patients. The surface EEG usually shows a spike discharge over the opposite motor cortex preceding each jerk by a short interval. Treatment is with anticonvulsants, but may be very difficult.

Hemifacial spasm

Hemifacial spasm most commonly affects middle-aged or elderly women, and usually appears without obvious cause. Rarely, it may be symptomatic of obvious facial nerve compression due to a cerebellopontine angle tumour or angioma, when it can be accompanied by trigeminal neuralgia. Some patients with Paget's disease may develop hemifacial spasm, presumably because of compression of the seventh nerve by bony overgrowth, and it may appear after incomplete recovery from a Bell's palsy. However, in most cases the cause is not obvious. Possibly it is due to compression of the facial nerve in the posterior fossa by aberrant or ectatic blood vessel (as appears to be the cause of trigemminal neuralgia).

The condition consists of irregular, but repetitive clonic twitching of the muscles of one side of the face. Usually those around the eyes are first involved, producing a feeling identical to the benign myokymia of the lower eyelid which occurs in normal people when fatigued. However, the repetitive twitching spreads slowly to involve the whole face, each spasm closing the eye and drawing up the corner of the mouth. At this stage, a mild facial weakness and contraction becomes evident, but a frank facial palsy never develops. Facial sensation is normal and there are no other physical signs in idiopathic hemifacial spasm.

The disorder is so distinctive and unilateral that it is rarely confused with other conditions. The similarity in the early stages to benign myokymia has been noted. True facial myokymia, due to brainstem tumour or demyelination, consists of a continuous rippling contraction of the facial muscles, giving the typical appearance of a 'bag of worms'.

Treatment with drugs is usually unrewarding, and partial section of the facial nerve only gives relief for between 6–12 months. Recently, it has been found that posterior fossa exploration, with careful mobilization of the seventh nerve throughout its course with separation from adjacent blood vessels, will give long-lasting relief. Another recent approach is to inject botulinum toxin into the affected facial muscles to produce local (although temporary) paralysis.

Palatal myoclonus
An infarct involving the brainstem, or more rarely demyelination or a tumour in the same region, may produce the curious syndrome of palatal myoclonus. In some cases, the cause is not evident, but degeneration in the region of the olivo-dentato-rubral pathways is found.

Rhythmic contraction of the soft palate occurs, at 60–180 times per minute, and persists throughout the day and night. Such contractions interfere with speech, to cause a tremulous dysarthria, and swallowing. Sometimes the rhythmic myoclonus spreads to involve the pharynx and larynx, which can be seen to bob up and down in time with the palate, the intercostal muscles and diaphragms, and even the eyes to cause ocular myoclonus. A particularly annoying symptom is rhythmic clicking in the ear due to contraction of stapedius.

Drug therapy usually does not help, but occasional responses to 5-hydroxytryptophan or benzhexol (Artane) have been reported.

Tics

The concept of tics has changed. *A simple tic* is a sudden rapid twitch-like movement always of the same nature and at the same site. Such tics are part of our motor personality, such as an eye twitch, a grimace, a sniff, or a hand gesture. Simple motor tics occur in about a quarter of all children and often disapear within a year or so (*transient tic of childhood*). Sometimes, however, they persist into adult life, but are rarely considered as abnormal (*chronic simple tic*). Simple tics in a minority of people become so marked as to lead to a request for medical help. Frequently the request is for psychiatric assistance, for the tics are an expression of an underlying psychological disorder. The tics themselves do not indicate neurological abnormality, but are a motor expression of emotional disturbance. They must be distinguished from other dyskinesias, particularly chorea and myoclonus, which do indicate a cerebral disease.

Sometimes tics are more widespread and severe, and take the form of complicated stereotyped patterns of motor action (*complex tics*). Characteristically, complex and simple tics can be suppressed voluntarily. However, this causes mounting inner tension which is relieved by letting the tics come out. Complex multiple tics may be accompanied by vocal utterances, particularly swear-words (copralalia) and compulsive thoughts. This constitutes the syndrome of Gilles de la Tourette. Evidence is accumulating to suggest that this is an organic cerebral disease, but its nature is quite obscure. *Chronic complex multiple tics* without vocalization is also likely to be a manifestation of Gilles de la Tourette syndrome. Finally, the psychiatrist may apply the term tic to a sudden, but repetitive, thought or impulsive acts (*psychical tics*), although the use of the word is disappearing.

Gilles de la Tourette syndrome

Aetiology
George Gilles de la Tourette published the first comprehensive description of this bizarre illness in 1885, although Itard had described the first case much earlier in 1825. Its cause is quite unknown, and no pathological or pathophysiological abnormality has been identified. Indeed, although originally considered to be due to degenerative changes in the brain, when psychodynamic theory became fashionable in the early part of the present century, such tics were ascribed and treated as the consequence of unresolved sexual or other conflicts. However, such notions are not now considered appropriate, and Gilles de la Tourette syndrome is viewed as an unexplained disease of the central nervous system, probably of the basal ganglia. The latter are believed to be involved because similar symptoms occurred in encephalitis leth-

argica, and because drugs acting on the basal ganglia, for example haloperidol (Serenace), are used to control the symptoms of the disease.

Symptoms
The illness begins between the ages of 5 and 15 years, with multiple involuntary repetitive muscular tics. These affect particularly the upper part of the body, especially the face, neck and shoulders, more than the limbs and trunk. Typical initial symptoms are eye blinking, head nodding, sniffing, or stuttering. With time other more complex tics appear affecting other parts of the body. The individual tics are brief and variable, but are repetitive and reproducible. Their severity and frequency waxes and wanes, being worse while relaxed, and often disappearing while under scrutiny or attending to a demanding task.

Sooner or later, many patients with multiple tics begin to make involuntary noises, such as grunting, squealing, yelping, sniffing, or barking. Indeed, the coexistence of such noises with multiple tics is essential for the diagnosis of Gilles de la Tourette's syndrome. In about 60 per cent of cases such noises become transformed into swear-words of which the commonest are 'fuck' or 'shit' (coprolalia). Coprolalia usually occurs first in childhood but may not appear until middle or adult life. About a third of patients also exhibit echolalia—an involuntary tendency to repeat words or sentences just spoken to them. A smaller proportion of patients also exhibit copropraxia (involuntary obscene gesturing) and echopraxia (involuntary imitation of the movements of others), as well as palilalia (involuntary repetition of their own words or sounds). It should be noted that echolalia and palilalia were also encountered as symptoms following encephalitis lethargica.

A larger proportion of those with Gilles de la Tourette syndrome also exhibit typical features of an obsessive-compulsive nature. These psychic manifestations of the illness may be even more disabling than the tics.

Once established, Gilles de la Tourette's syndrome usually is life-long, although its severity waxes and wanes. A small proportion of cases, probably less than one in 20, experience spontaneous remission of symptoms after adolescence, but in most both the multiple tics and the coprolalia, if present, persist. However, no other neurological abnormality develops; intellect and motor co-ordination are normal.

Diagnosis
Patients with tics and vocal utterances, which are essential for the diagnosis of Gilles de la Tourette's syndrome, often are labelled as suffering a psychiatric disorder, or if organic disease is considered, they are thought to have chorea or dystonia. Once coprolalia is evident there is no difficulty in establishing the correct diagnosis, but even in its absence, the character of the tics is quite distinctive, and the vocal utterances are characteristic. Thus, tics are short, brief muscle jerks, not the prolonged spasms of muscle contraction that occur in torsion dystonia. Likewise, tics, although irregular, are repetitive in time, site, and character, unlike the chaotic random nature of chorea.

Treatment
Both the multiple tics, and the vocalizations of coprolalia cause considerable distress, social isolation, and psychological harm. Neuroleptic drugs such as haloperidol (Serenace) or pimozide (Orap) may satisfactorily control tics, noises, and coprolalia. The effective dose requires careful and gradual titration of each individual patient, and side-effects from large doses are common. Most serious is the emergence of a tardive dyskinesia after months or years of therapy (see below). Since treatment must usually be for life, the risk must be carefully balanced against the real need for any form of therapy. Alternative therapy which is effective in some patients includes clonidine (Catapres) and tetrabenazine (Nitoman). Since the severity of the illness waxes and wanes, intermittent treatment may be used to cover bad periods.

Idiopathic torsion dystonia

Definition

This is a group of illnesses characterized by dyskinesias consisting of prolonged spasms of muscle contraction affecting various parts of the body, without evident cause or other neurological deficit. Torsion dystonia may affect the whole body (generalized dystonia or *dystonia musculorum deformans*), may affect adjacent parts such as an arm and the neck (segmental dystonia), or may be restricted to one part (focal dystonia) as in *spasmodic torticollis, dystonic writer's cramp, blepharospasm,* and *oromandibular dystonia.*

Aetiology

No pathological or biochemical abnormality has been identified in any of these diseases. However, similar clinical syndromes may be caused by a variety of cerebral insults (symptomatic dystonia) (see Table 10, page 21.231), or by drugs. Since the characteristic feature of such symptomatic dystonias is damage to the basal ganglia, it is presumed, by inference, that idiopathic torsion dystonia is due to some unidentified functional basal ganglia abnormality.

Dystonia musculorum deformans often is inherited (see below), but the focal dystonias of spasmodic torticollis, writer's cramp, blepharospasm and oromandibular dystonia usually occur as sporadic cases with onset in middle life. Such focal dystonias, however, appear to be isolated fragments of the syndrome of idiopathic torsion dystonia, for (*a*) they may occur in families inheriting generalized torsion dystonia as an autosomal dominant trait, (*b*) they are often the presenting feature of childhood dystonia musculorum deformans, and (*c*) not infrequently they are accompanied in adults by other signs of torsion dystonia.

Dystonia musculorum deformans

Symptoms

This is a rare disease, usually with onset in childhood when it is frequently inherited, most commonly in Ashkenazi Jews who are particularly prone to the illness. Inheritance is usually as an autosomal dominant trait, although rarer autosomal recessive and even sex-linked recessive inheritance is sometimes seen. The illness usually presents in children with dystonic spasms of the legs on walking, or sometimes of the arms, trunk, or neck. The affected child often begins to walk on the toes with the foot plantar-flexed and inverted. Typically, such an action dystonia only appears on walking at this stage. Indeed, the child may only exhibit the dystonic posture of the legs and feet on walking forwards, while walking backwards and running may be normal. Initial dystonic abnormalities of the arm involve writing, such that the fingers grip the pen excessively and the arm contorts, often with the elbow rising, as the sufferer tries to execute legible script. At this stage, other manual actions may be performed normally. Other common early symptoms are torticollis or truncal dystonia.

The illness is usually progressive when it commences in childhood; the spasms spread to all body parts leading to severe disability within about 10 years. The intellect is preserved and there are no signs of pyramidal or sensory deficit. Speech is often spared, allowing such patients to pursue intellectual employment despite severe physical disability. A spontaneous remission of symptoms occurs in about one in 20 of patients, usually in the first 5 years of the illness. There is no way of predicting who will remit or when such a remission will occur. Most remissions are transitory, lasting a matter of weeks or months, but occasionally they may appear to be permanent.

A similar disease occurs in adults, but in this case there is usually no evidence of inheritance, the arms and neck are affected and the legs are spared, and progression is slow. Such adults with segmental dystonia most commonly exhibit a combination of a dystonic arm, with typical dystonic writer's cramp, plus torticollis.

Treatment

Dystonia musculorum deformans is distressing and difficult to treat. A few patients, mostly children, have been reported to respond dramatically to treatment with carbamazepine (Tegretol) or levodopa. Some of the therapeutic successes claimed for such treatment were probably spontaneous remissions, or in the case of levodopa, the disease may not have been dystonia musculorum deformans but the closely related condition of dystonia with marked diurnal variation which does respond dramatically to levodopa. However, both drugs are worth a trial, in conventional dosage, in all patients with disabling dystonia musculorum deformans.

The drugs which most patients find helpful, and continue to take to suppress their muscle spasm, are a benzodiazepine such as diazepam (Valium) often in a large dose of 20–50 mg daily, and an anticholinergic such as benzhexol (Artane), again in large doses. Indeed, recent experience with very high doses of benzhexol up to as much as 120 mg/day, shows that some 50 per cent of patients will gain great benefit. Benzhexol is now the treatment of choice; it is started at a low dose, then very slowly increased over many months to avoid unwanted effects. Phenothiazines and other neuroleptics such as haloperidol (Serenace) may also help some patients, as may tetrabenazine (Nitoman), but usually at the expense of drug-induced Parkinsonism. Unfortunately, dystonia is far less responsive to neuroleptics than is chorea, and the margin between benefit and side-effects is very small. The patient often will obtain relief from the dystonia only at the expense of a degree of drug-induced Parkinsonism or depression that is more disabling than the original illness. Many other drugs have been tried in dystonia musculorum deformans, but none has gained wide acceptance.

When advanced, the disease may be so disabling that stereotaxic surgery seems warranted. A unilateral thalamotomy may suppress dystonia of the contralateral limbs, with a risk of hemiplegia of about 1 per cent. Unfortunately, however, severe dystonia usually is bilateral and involves axial structures. Bilateral thalamotomy is required in such cases, with the additional risk of severe impairment of speech in 15 per cent or more patients, and axial dystonia responds far less favourably to thalamotomy than does limb dystonia. Often the decision is between taking the risk of imperilling speech in an intelligent but severely physically disabled individual, for a chance of some benefits that cannot be more than 50:50.

Spasmodic torticollis

Symptoms

Spasmodic torticollis may be the presenting feature of dystonia musculorum deformans in childhood, but isolated spasmodic torticollis usually occurs in the middle-aged or elderly. A similar condition was produced by encephalitis lethargica, but no cause is evident in most patients now. Attempts to attribute the illness to hysteria or depression are not supported by careful psychiatric assessment, which reveals no excess psychiatric morbidity in patients with spasmodic torticollis. The onset is usually insidious, often with initial pain, and sometimes appears to be precipitated by trauma. The dystonic spasms, affect sternomastoid and other neck muscles to cause the head to turn to one side (torticollis) (Fig. 10), or occasionally to extend (retrocollis) or to flex (antecollis). The spasms may be repetitive to cause tremulous torticollis, or sustained to hold the posture fixed. The trunk commonly shows a compensatory lordosis.

The illness is usually lifelong, but remissions of a year or more occur in about a fifth of cases. Most patients are otherwise normal apart from their torticollis, although some way may exhibit a postural tremor similar to that of benign essential tremor, and a minority of patients may go on to develop dystonia elsewhere, usually in the form of a dystonic arm, to produce a syndrome of segmental dystonia. As with all types of dystonia, the frequency

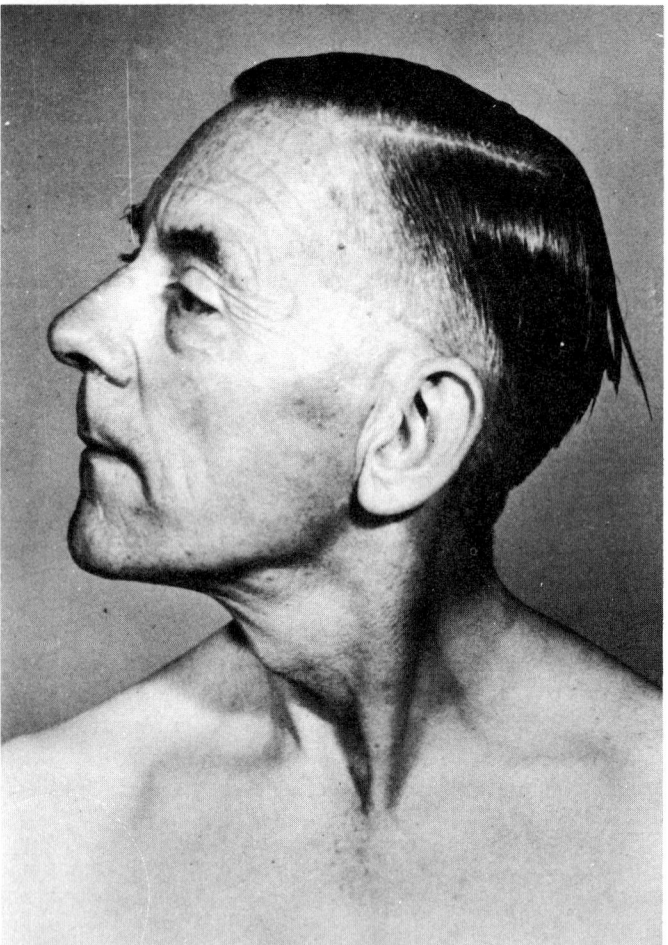

Fig. 10 Spasmodic torticollis in a 57-year-old man. The hypertrophy of the sternomastoid muscle is evident.

and intensity of the muscle spasms vary considerably, being particularly worse in conditions of mental or emotional stress. A feature characteristic of spasmodic torticollis is the '*geste antagonistique*', in which the patient discovers some particular manual act which controls the deviation of the head. A touch of the forefinger to the jaw may suffice, but other more complex and bizarre actions are common.

Treatment

Spasmodic torticollis, like other types of torsion dystonia, is difficult to treat, and about 50 per cent of patients find no relief from therapy. The problem is that it is impossible to predict which patients will respond to which drugs. Levodopa and other dopamine agonists have been reported to help in a very few patients. Phenothiazines and other neuroleptics such as haloperidol (Serenace) also may give some relief, but side-effects are common and long-term complications such as tardive dyskinesias (see below) may occur. Tetrabenazine (Nitoman) also may help, but often causes depression. Many find that a benzodiazepine such as diazepam (Valium) with or without an anticholinergic such as benzhexol (Artane) is the only drug of value.

Stereotaxic thalamotomy was used once, but the results were unreliable and the bilateral lesions required often caused speech defects, so this form of surgery now has been discarded. An alternative surgical approach is to divide the nerve supply to the neck muscles. Local section of the eleventh nerve in the neck is always inadequate. More radical denervation is required, in the form of section of the upper three or four cervical motor roots bilaterally, with intrathecal section of the eleventh nerves. This may reduce torticollis, but at the expense initially of a floppy neck

and frequently later on of severe, painful, and disabling cervical spondylosis. Recently this operation has been modified by undertaking posterior primary ramicectomy of upper cervical roots, without the need for laminectomy. Surgery should be avoided, unless demanded after careful counselling.

Dystonic writer's cramp

Symptoms

A specific complaint of inability to write (or to type, to play a musical instrument, or to wield any manual instrument) may be due to a variety of causes, including joint disease, a carpal tunnel syndrome, a spastic or ataxic hand, Parkinson's disease, or benign essential tremor. However, no objective neurological deficit is found in many patients, other than abnormal posturing of the hand and arm on writing. Typically the pen is gripped with great force and driven into the paper (Fig. 11). However, in some patients the arm adopts a typical dystonic posture and in such cases of *dystonic writer's cramp*, other manual acts such as wielding a knife or screwdriver are similarly affected. Such dystonic writer's cramp may be the initial symptom of generalized torsion dystonia, but in adults it often remains as an isolated disability. In other patients it is only the act of writing that is impaired and this remains an isolated disability (*simple writer's cramp*). However, a small proportion of such patients subsequently develop dystonic writer's cramp and even obvious dystonia elsewhere, so simple writer's cramp also may be an isolated initial manifestation of torsion dystonia.

The same considerations apply to other occupational cramps such as pianist's cramp, drummer's cramp, violinist's cramp, typist's cramp, morse-code operator's (telegraphist's) cramp, and the wide range of other such disabilities described in association with specific repetitive manual activities. The alternative view is that these occupational cramps are primarily psychological or neurotic reactions to an unsatisfactory work situation. However, it is remarkable how many of these patients laboriously teach themselves to write with the opposite hand or devise other means to ensure continued employment, and how many of them show no evidence of psychiatric disability. The similarity of these disabilities to the action dystonia that characterizes generalized torsion dystonia, and their frequent occurrence in the latter disease points to their origin as an ill-understood, but very real disease of the motor system.

Treatment

Writer's cramp, and other similar conditions, are usually permanent disabilities which do not respond satisfactorily to psychiatric, behavioural, or drug therapy. In an era when large sections of the population earned their living by wielding a pen, rest was advised and apparently many recovered. Today, such instruction rarely helps. Advice to write with the opposite hand allows most to cope with everyday events, such as signature or brief correspondence, but approximately one in 20 then develops the same problem in the non-dominant hand. Drugs rarely are of benefit, frequently because unwanted effects are more troublesome than the original disability. Benzhexol (Artane) and diazepam (Valium) are worth a try, but more potent drugs rarely are indicated. Advice to adjust to the disability is often the best that can be offered.

Blepharospasm and oromandibular dystonia (cranial dystonia)

Symptoms

Blepharospasm refers to recurrent spasms of eye closure. The orbicularis oculi forcibly contracts for seconds or minutes, often repetitively and sometimes so frequently as to render the patient functionally blind (Fig. 12). Spasms of eye closure commonly occur while reading or watching television, or in bright light; they often decrease or disappear when the subject is alerted or under

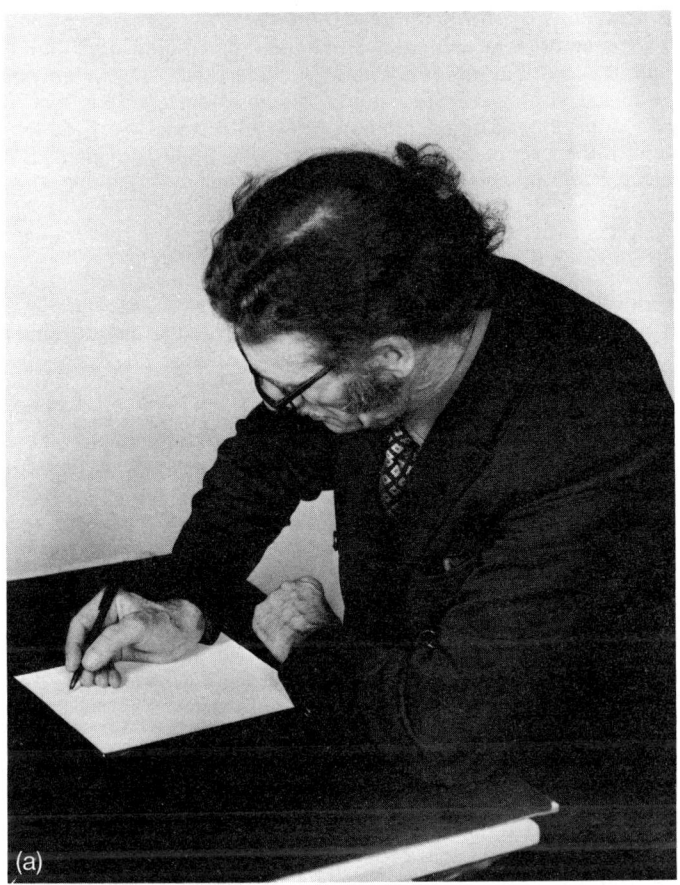

scrutiny. Oromandibular dystonia refers to recurrent spasms of muscle contraction affecting the mouth, tongue, jaw, larynx and pharynx, causing spasms of lip protrusion or retraction, jaw closure or opening (Fig. 13), and difficulty in speech and swallowing. Such patients may lacerate their lips and tongue or even dislocate their jaw, and usually are unable to cope with dentures. Speech may take on a characteristic, forced strained quality, referred to as spastic dysphonia, perhaps due to dystonic spasms of the larynx closing off the glottis. Spastic dysphonia also may occur in isolation in some otherwise normal middle-aged individuals.

These two conditions are closely related, for the patient with blepharospasm may develop oromandibular dystonia and vice versa. Both conditions may occur in generalized torsion dystonia, or be produced by drugs, but also appear in isolation in late life without evident cause. Other dystonic phenomena are rare, but a few patients go on to develop features such as torticollis, dystonic writer's cramp, or spasms of the diaphragm and trunk muscles. Psychiatric abnormality is unusual at the onset but the condition is usually permanent and an understandable depression reactive to the physical disability and social distress commonly develops.

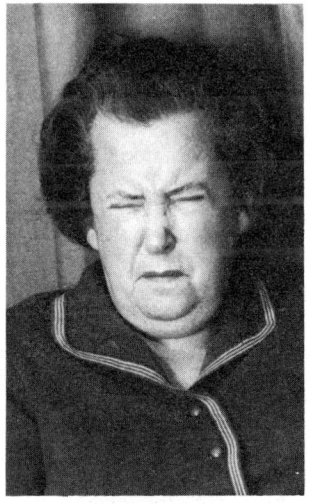

Fig. 12 Blepharospasm in a 57-year-old woman. Her jaw also is forcibly clamped shut, biting her gums, and some spasm of orbicularis oris is evident, in addition to the obvious spasm of orbicularis oculi.

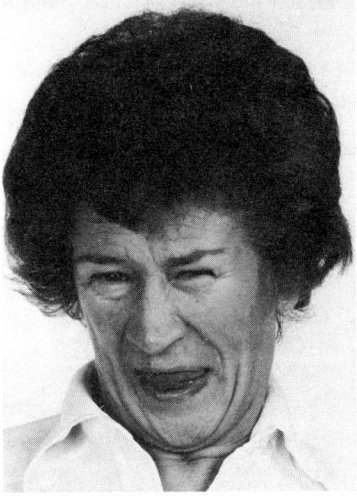

Fig. 11 Dystonic writer's cramp in a 52-year-old man, whose right elbow rises and whose fingers grip the pen so tightly that they slide off (a), making writing and spiral drawing well-nigh impossible (b).

Fig. 13 Oromandibular dystonia in a 42-year-old woman. The spasm of forced jaw opening with tongue protrusion is evident.

Treatment

Unfortunately, both blepharospasm and oromandibular dystonia are notoriously difficult to control with drugs. Some (approximately a third) patients may be helped by agents such as benzhexol (Artane), and may take a benzodiazepine such as diazepam (Valium) to relieve anxiety. Some find that a neuroleptic, such as phenothiazine or haloperidol (Serenace), of value, while others gain relief from tetrabenazine (Nitoman). However, the drug-induced Parkinsonism and depression provoked by such drugs are frequently too disabling to justify their continuation. Treatment of any associated depressive illness often is necessary.

Surgery has nothing to offer those with oromandibular dystonia, but can relieve blepharospasm. Effective surgery requires isolation and division of all branches of the facial nerve supplying the orbicularis oculi so as to paralyse eye closure. The operation must be bilateral to preserve facial symmetry, and the branches to the upper lip also must be divided to prevent reinnervation and recurrence. Such drastic surgery prevents blepharospasm, without paralysing the eyelids, but leaves the face blank and expressionless. However, it is justified in those rendered functionally blind by their blepharospasm. A newer technique, which avoids widespread facial paralysis, is to inject botulinum toxin into orbicularis oculi. This gives relief from blepharospasm in about 70–80 per cent of cases, thereby restoring normal vision for about 3 months. The injections can be repeated as necessary.

Paroxysmal dystonia

Dystonia musculorum deformans or focal dystonias often commence with the appearance of a dystonic posture or spasm only on one motor act (action dystonia), but there are three, rare, usually familial disorders in which dramatic dystonia occurs intermittently.

Paroxysmal kinesigenic choreoathetosis

This is a rare condition, inherited as an autosomal dominant trait in 70 per cent or more of cases, with onset in childhood or adolescence of brief attacks of abnormal involuntary movements provoked by sudden movements. Typically, the patient finds that getting up from a chair quickly, stepping out briskly, or gesturing suddenly, may cause the abrupt onset of dystonic posturing, torsion spasms, or ballistic movements. Some patients fall heavily, but consciousness is preserved. The attack lasts less than 5 minutes, usually only a minute or so, but attacks may occur frequently, even up to 100 per day.

Such patients have no other neurological abnormality, and are quite normal between attacks. Epileptic fits usually do not occur, the EEG is normal, but the attacks can be abolished by treatment with anticonvulsants.

Paroxysmal dystonic choreoathetosis

This is another rare condition, inherited as an autosomal dominant trait, with onset in childhood or adolescence, of spontaneous attacks of dystonic posturing and torsion spasms, without loss of consciousness, lasting 5 minutes or up to 4 hours. Such attacks tend to be infrequent. No immediate precipitant is evident, but alcohol and fatigue may increase the tendency to such episodes. Between attacks such patients are normal, as is the EEG.

Anticonvulsants in general are of no value, but clonazepam (Rivotril) may help to decrease the frequency of attacks.

Dystonia with marked diurnal variation

This is another rare familial condition, inherited as an autosomal dominant trait, characterized by the onset of typical dystonic posturing and torsion spasms of the legs in childhood and adolescence, but usually with marked diurnal variation in the severity of symptoms. Such patients may have little or no dystonia on waking from sleep, but as the day goes on, dystonia gets worse, particularly with exercise, so that by the afternoon or evening they exhibit their worst symptoms. Rest without sleep does not help, but sleep relieves their dystonia. Many of these patients also exhibit features of Parkinsonism.

The other feature characteristic of this curious syndrome is its dramatic response to treatment with levodopa which may completely abolish all signs of the illness. Small doses are effective, and a stable therapeutic response continues for a decade or more.

Drug-induced extrapyramidal disease

The extensive use of antipsychotic neuroleptic drugs (which include the phenothiazines, butyrophenones, thioxanthenes, and dibutylpiperidines) has led to much iatrogenic extrapyramidal disease. These drugs are used widely to control acute psychotic behaviour, whatever its cause, and to prevent relapse of schizophrenia. They also are employed as antiemetics, as are other similar drugs such as metoclopramide, and in vertigo. The major neurological complications of such drug therapy are summarized in Table 12. No more needs to be said about *drug-induced tremor* or *Parkinsonism*. *Akathisia* refers to an irresistible and unpleasant sensation of motor restlessness, and the inability to sit or stand still, all of which may be mistaken for a recurrence of psychotic behaviour. *Acute dystonic reactions* commonly consist of trismus, neck retraction, or torticollis, and may be mistaken for tetanus or meningitis. Although uncommon, acute dystonic reactions pose a repeated diagnostic problem in casualty departments. Those unfamiliar with their bizarre characteristics often dismiss such behaviour as 'hysterical'. The acute dystonia rapidly disappears after an intravenous injection of an anticholinergic drug. *Chronic tardive dyskinesias* are the most serious complications, for they may be

Table 12 Drug-induced extrapyramidal disease

Disorder	Drugs responsible	Susceptible age group	Incidence	Onset after initiation of therapy	Effect of withdrawal of drug	Treatment
Tremor	Bronchodilators Tricyclics Lithium carbonate Caffeine	Any	Dose-dependent about 35 per cent	Rapid	Disappears	Withdraw drug
Parkinsonism	Reserpine Tetrabenazine Neuroleptics	Any but increases with age	Dose-dependent about 50 per cent	Gradual, within first months	Disappears slowly, may take a year	Anticholinergics
Acute dystonia	Neuroleptics Diazoxide	Children, young adults	2–5 per cent	Acute, within first few hours or days	Disappears	Anticholinergics Diazepam
Akathisia	Neuroleptics	Any	About 30 per cent	Gradual, within first months	Disappears	Anticholinergics
Tardive dyskinesia	Neuroleptics	Increases with age	20–40 per cent	Delayed, but increases	May get worse; persists in about 40 per cent	Withdraw drug Tetrabenazine

permanent despite drug withdrawal. The characteristic syndrome is one of orofacial mouthing, with lip smacking and tongue protrusion (orobuccolingual dyskinesia), accompanied by trunk rocking and distal chorea of hands and feet. In younger patients the picture may be dominated by axial and cranial dystonia (tardive dystonia). The crucial factor is the duration of neuroleptic treatment. Tardive dyskinesias appear after at least 6 months' neuroleptic drug therapy, and their incidence increases with exposure to the drugs; and also with the age of the patients exposed to such drugs. Tardive dyskinesias often get worse in the weeks immediately after stopping the offending drug, or may appear then for the first time. After drug withdrawal, tardive dyskinesias disappear in about 60 per cent or more of patients over the next 3 years, but continue unaltered in the remainder.

That many other drugs may cause dyskinesias has been noted (Tables 2–5), and the fact that levodopa may provoke any form of dyskinesia in patients with Parkinson's disease has been discussed. It seems likely that all such drug-induced dyskinesias are due to pharmacological effects on dopamine receptors in the basal ganglia, resulting in dopaminergic overactivity, in contrast to the akinetic-rigid syndrome produced by dopamine depletion or blockade.

References

General

Denny-Brown, D. (1960). Diseases of the basal ganglia. *Lancet* ii, 1099–1105, 1155–1162.

—— (1962). *The basal ganglia and their relation to disorders of movement*. Oxford University Press, London.

Jankovic, J. (ed.) (1984). Movement disorders. *Neurologic clinics* Vol. 2. W. B. Saunders, Philadelphia.

Marsden, C. D. (1981). Extrapyramidal diseases. In *The molecular basis of neuropathology* (eds A. N. Davison and R. H. S. Thompson), pp. 345–383. Arnold, London.

—— (1982). Neurotransmitters and CNS disease. *Lancet* ii, 1141–1146.

—— and Fahn, S. (eds.) (1982). *Movement disorders*. Butterworth, London.

——, —— (1986). *Movement disorders II*. Butterworth, London.

Martin, J. P. (1968). *The basal ganglia and posture*. Pitman Medical, London.

Oppenheimer, D. R. (1976). Diseases of the basal ganglia, cerebellum and motor neurons. In *Greenfield's neuropathology*, 3rd edn. (eds W. Blackwood and J. A. N. Corsellis). Arnold, London.

Vinken, P. J. and Bruyn, G. W. (eds) (1968). Diseases of the basal ganglia. In *Handbook of clinical neurology*, vol. 6. North-Holland. Amsterdam.

Yahr, M. D. (ed.) (1976). The basal ganglia. *Ass. Res. Nerv. Ment. Dis.* **55**.

Parkinson's disease

Brown, R. and Marsden, C. D. (1986). Cognitive function in Parkinson's disease. In *Movement Disorders* II (eds C. D. Marsden and S. Fahn). Butterworths, London.

Calne, D. B. (1970). *Parkinsonism: physiology, pharmacology, and treatment*. Butterworths, London.

—— (1971). Parkinsonism: physiology and pharmacology. *Br. Med. J.* **iii**, 693–697.

Cooper, I. S. (1965). The surgical treatment of Parkinsonism. *Ann. Rev. Med.* **16**, 309–330.

Cotzias, G. C., van Woert, M. H., and Schiffer, L. M. (1967). Aromatic amino acids and modification of Parkinsonism. *N. Engl. J. Med.* **276**, 374–379.

Duvoisin, R. C. (1982). The cause of Parkinson's disease. In *Movement Disorders* (eds C. D. Marsden and S. Fahn). Butterworths, London.

Greenfield, J. G. and Bosanquet, F. D. (1953). The brain-stem lesions in Parkinsonism. *J. Neurol. Neurosurg. Psychiat.* **16**, 213–226.

Hoehn, M. M. and Yahr, M. D. (1967). Parkinsonism: onset, progression, and mortality. *Neurology, Minneap.* **17**, 427–442.

Hornykiewicz, O. (1973). Dopamine in the basal ganglia: its role and therapeutic implications (including the clinical use of L-dopa). *Br. Med. Bull.* **29**, 172–178.

—— (1982). Brain neurotransmitter changes in Parkinson's disease. In *Movement disorders* (eds C. D. Marsden and S. Fahn), pp. 41–58. Butterworths, London.

Jellinger, K. (1986). Pathology of Parkinson's disease. In *Movement Disorders* II (eds C. D. Marsden and S. Fahn). Butterworths, London.

Langston, J. W., Ballard, P., Tetrud, J. W. and Irwin, I. (1983). Chronic Parkinsonism in humans due to a product of meperidine-analog synthesis. *Science* **219**, 979–980.

——, (1986). MPTP and Parkinsonism. In *Movement Disorders* II (eds C. D. Marsden and S. Fahn). pp. 41–58 Butterworths, London.

Marsden, C. D. and Parkes, J. D. (1976). 'On-off' effects in patients with Parkinson's disease on chronic levodopa therapy. *Lancet* i, 292–299.

——, —— (1977). Success and problems of long-term levodopa therapy in Parkinson's disease. *Lancet* ii, 345–349.

——, ——, and Quinn, N. (1982). Fluctuations of disability in Parkinson's disease: clinical aspects. In *Movement disorders* (eds C. D. Marsden and S. Fahn), pp. 96–123. Butterworths, London.

Mayeux, R. (1982). Depression and dementia in Parkinson's disease. In *Movement disorders* (eds C. D. Marsden and S. Fahn), pp. 75–95. Butterworths, London.

Pallis, C. A. (1971). Parkinsonism: natural history and clinical features. *Br. Med. J.* **iii**, 683–690.

Yahr, M. D., Duvoisin, R. C., Schear, M. J., Barrett, R. E. and Hoehn, M. M. (1969). Treatment of Parkinsonism with levodopa. *Arch. Neurol.* **21**, 343–354.

Other akinetic–rigid syndromes

Bannister, R. and Oppenheimer, D. R. (1982). Parkinsonism, system degenerations, and autonomic failure. In *Movement disorders* (eds C. D. Marsden and S. Fahn), pp. 174–190. Butterworths, London.

Critchley, M. (1929). Arteriosclerotic Parkinsonism. *Brain* **52**, 23.

Duvoisin, R. C., Chokroverty, S., Lepore, F. and Nicklas, W. (1983). Glutamane dehydrogenase deficiency in patients with olivopontocerebellar atrophy. *Neurology* **33**, 1322–1331.

Duvoisin, R. C. (1986). Olivopontocerebellar degeneration. In *Movement Disorders* II (eds C. D. Marsden and S. Fahn). Butterworths, London.

Hall, A. J. (1931). Chronic epidemic encephalitis, with special reference to the ocular attacks. *Br. Med. J.* **ii**, 833–837.

Lees, A. J. (1986). Progressive supranuclear palsy. In *Movement Disorders* II (eds C. D. Marsden and S. Fahn). Butterworths, London.

Steele, J. C., Richardson, J. C., and Olzewski, J. (1964). Progressive supranuclear palsy. *Arch. Neurol.* **10**, 333–359.

Strickland, G. T., Frommer, D., Leu, M. L., Pollard, R., Sherlock, S., and Cumings, J. N. (1973). Wilson's disease in the United Kingdom and Taiwan, I. General characteristics of 142 cases and prognosis. II. A genetic analysis of 88 cases. *Q. J. Med.* **42**, 619–638.

Walshe, J. M. (1956). Penicillamine: a new oral therapy for Wilson's disease. *Am. J. Med.* **21**, 487–495.

—— (1973). Copper chelation in patients with Wilson's disease. A comparison of penicillamine and triethylene tetra-amine dihydrochloride. *Q. J. Med.* **42**, 441–452.

Tremor

Critchley, E. (1949). Observations on essential (heredofamilial) tremor. *Brain* **72**, 113–139.

Desmedt, J. E. (ed.) (1978). Physiological tremor, pathological tremors and clonus. *Progress in clinical neurophysiology*, vol. 5. Karger, Basel.

Findlay, L. (1986). The pharmacology of essential tremor. In *Movement Disorders* II (eds C. D. Marsden and S. Fahn). Butterworths, London.

Growdon, J. H., Shahani, B. T., and Young, R. R. (1975). The effect of alcohol on essential tremor. *Neurology, Minneap.* **25**, 259–262.

Larsen, T. A. and Calne, D. B. (1983). Essential tremor. *Clin. Neuropharmacol.* **6**, 185–206.

Lee, R. (1986). The pathophysiology of essential tremor. In *Movement Disorders* II (eds C. D. Marsden and S. Fahn). Butterworths, London.

Chorea

Aron, A. M., Freeman, J. M., and Carter, S. (1965). The natural history of Sydenham's chorea. *Am. J. Med.* **38**, 83–95.

Barbeau, A., Chase, T. N., and Paulson, G. W. (eds.) (1972). Huntington's chorea, 1872–1972. *Advances in neurology*, vol. 1. Raven Press, New York.

Chase, T. N., Wexler, N. S., and Barbeau, A. (eds.) (1979). Huntington's disease. *Advances in neurology*, vol. 23. Raven Press, New York.

Gusella, J. F., Wexler, N. S., Conneally, P. M., Naylor, S. L., Anderson, M. A., Tanzi, R. E., Watkins, P. C., Ottina, K., Wallace, M. R., Sakaguchi, A. Y., Young, R. R., Shoulson, I., Bonilla, E. and Martin, J. B. (1983). Polymorphic DNA marker genetically linked to Huntington's disease. *Nature* **306**, 234–238.

Hayden, M. R. (1981). *Huntington's chorea*. Springer-Verlag, Berlin.

Kuhl, D. E., Phelps, M. E., Markham, C. H., Metter, E. J., Riege, W. H. and Winter, J. (1982). Cerebral metabolism and atrophy in Huntington's disease determined by [18]FDG and computed tomographic scan. *Ann. Neurol.* **12**, 425–434.

Myers, R., Sweeney, D. B., and Schwidde, J. T. (1950). Hemiballismus. Aetiology and surgical treatment. *J. Neurosurg. Psychiat.* **13**, 115–126.

Myoclonus and tics

Aigner, B. R. and Mulder, D. W. (1960). Myoclonus, *Arch. Neurol.* **2**, 600–615.

Chadwick, D., Hallett, M., Harris, R., Jenner, P., Reynolds, E. H., and Marsden, C. D. (1977). Clinical, biochemical, and physiological features distinguishing myoclonus responsive to 5-hydroxytryptophan, tryptophan with a monoamine oxidase inhibitor, and clonazepam. *Brain* **100**, 455–487.

Gastaut, H. and Villeneuve, A. (1967). The startle disease or hyperekplexia. *J. Neurol. Sci.* **5**, 523–542.

Fahn, S., Marsden, C. D. and Van Woert, M. (1986). Myoclonus Advances in Neurology Vol. 32. Raven Press, New York.

Hermann, C. and Brown, J. N. (1967). Palatal myoclonus: a reappraisal. *J. Neurol. Sci.* **5**, 473–492.

Hopkins, A. P. and Michael, W. F. (1974). Spinal myoclonus. *J. Neurol. Neurosurg. Psychiat.* **37**, 1112–1115.

Jankovic, J. (1986). The neurology of tics. In *Movement Disorders* II (eds C. D. Marsden and S. Fahn). Butterworths, London.

Lance, J. W. and Adams, R. D. (1963). The syndrome of intention or action myoclonus as a sequel to hypoxic encephalopathy. *Brain* **86**, 111–136.

Lees, A. J. (1986). *Tics*. Churchill Livingstone, London.

Mahloudji, M. and Pikielny, R. J. (1967). Hereditary essential myoclonus. *Brain* **90**, 669–674.

Marsden, C. D., Hallett, M. and Fahn, S. (1982). The nosology and pathophysiology of myoclonus. In *Movement disorders* (eds C. D. Marsden and S. Fahn), pp. 196–248. Butterworths, London.

Shapiro, A. K., Shapiro, E. S., Bruun, R. D. and Sweet, R. D. (1978). *Gilles de la Tourette syndrome*. Raven Press, New York.

Trimble, M. (1986). The psychiatry of tics. In *Movement Disorders* II (eds C. D. Marsden and S. Fahn). Butterworths, London.

Dystonia

Andrew, J., Fowler, C. J. and Harrison, M. J. G. (1983). Stereotaxic thalamotomy in 55 cases of dystonia. *Brain* **106**, 981–1000.

Bucy, P. C. and Buchanan, D. N. (1932). Athetosis, *Brain* **55**, 479–492.

Cooper, I. S. (1970). Neurosurgical treatment of dystonia. *Neurology, Minneap.* **20**, pt 2, 133–148.

Eldridge, R. (1970). The torsion dystonias: literature review and genetic and clinical studies. *Neurology, Minneap.* **20**, pt 2, 1–78.

—— and Fahn, S. (eds) (1976). Dystonia, *Advances in neurology*, vol. 14. Raven Press, New York.

Fahn, S., Marsden, C. D. and Calne, D. B. (1986). Dystonia II. Advances in Neurology. Raven Press, New York.

——, ——. The treatment of torsion dystonia. In *Movement Disorders* II (eds C. D. Marsden and S. Fahn). Butterworths, London.

Marsden, C. D. (1976). Dystonia: the spectrum of the disease. In *The basal ganglia* (ed. M. D. Yahr), pp. 351–367. Raven Press, New York.

——, Marion, M-H. and Quinn, N. (1984). The treatment of severe dystonia in children and adults. *J. Neurol. Neurosurg. Psychiat.* **47**, 1166.

Sheehy, M. P. and Marsden, C. D. (1982). Writer's cramp—a focal dystonia. *Brain* **105**, 461–480.

Zeman, W. and Dyken, P. (1968). Dystonia musculorum deformans. In *Handbook of clinical neurology*, Vol. 6 (eds P. J. Vinken and G. W. Bruyn), pp. 517–543, North-Holland, Amsterdam.

NEUROLOGICAL COMPLICATIONS OF SYSTEMIC DISEASES

M. J. G. HARRISON

Many multisystem diseases and neoplastic conditions produce striking neurological complications. In some the cause is attributable to a vasculitis (collagenoses), in others to granulomatous infiltration (sarcoidosis), or to metastatic invasion (neoplasm). Often the mechanism of neurological damage is poorly understood, for example, in the case of some of the so-called non-metastitic complications of malignancies.

In most situations diagnosis depends on the identification of a well-established systemic disorder, but the neurological involvement can sometimes be the presenting feature, or even be the only clinical manifestation. Some understanding of the likely and unlikely syndromes that may be encountered is thus important.

CONNECTIVE TISSUE DISEASES (COLLAGENOSES)

These may affect the central or the peripheral nervous system, the underlying damage often being from microinfarction due to a vasculitis affecting small vessels. A combination of neurological signs implicating both the central nervous system and the peripheral nervous system in the same patient at the same time should raise suspicions of one of these disorders. In the CNS the combination of signs of a diffuse disorder or encephalopathy plus some focal signs is suggestive, and in the peripheral nervous system a patchy neuropathy or mononeuritis multiplex is equally suspicious (of a vasculitis).

Systemic lupus erythematosus (SLE) (see also Section 16)

This is probably the commonest of the so-called connective tissue diseases and most often affects women of child-bearing age. It is especially common in North American and West Indian negro women. From one-third to one-half of the patients have neurological problems mostly due to involvement of the CNS by a vasculitis affecting small vessels ($> 100 \mu m$ in diameter). Such vessels show fibrinoid necrosis and proliferative wall thickening. Microinfarcts are sometimes found at post-mortem without an associated vasculitis, however. The role of deposition of antigen antibody complexes, for example in the choroid plexus, is uncertain.

Osler described recurrent attacks of hemiplegia in a young physician who later developed nephritis, and such stroke-like episodes in the cerebral hemispheres or brain stem are not uncommon. More usual, however, and perhaps affecting 40 per cent of victims, are mental changes. These may take the form of depression, mania, or a schizophrenic-like psychosis with hallucinations, paranoia, and even catatonia. The mental state may be difficult to distinguish from a steroid psychosis if the patient is on steroids for systemic features of the disease. Focal electroencephalogram (EEG) changes and an abnormal CSF are helpful pointers to CNS lupus. Seizures occur in up to 1 in 7 cases, probably due to microinfarcts. They may respond to steroids. Confusion is possible when an epileptic patient develops a drug-induced SLE syndrome due to anticonvulsants. Chorea is also well described and is indistinguishable from that due to rheumatic fever or associated with the use of an oral contraceptive agent. It usually remits in 2 to 3 months. Microinfarction in the cord may produce a rapidly evolving paraplegia with sensory level and sphincter involvement. The CSF sugar content may be low. There is usually little recovery. The tendency for microinfarction to occur in the brain stem, spinal cord, and optic nerve sometimes produces a multiple sclerosis-like picture, and the CSF may contain oligoclonal IgG. The systemic features of the disease with arthritis, skin lesions, alopecia, pleurisy, Raynaud's phenomenon, and nephritis make the distinction.

Rarer involvement of the peripheral nervous system may pro-

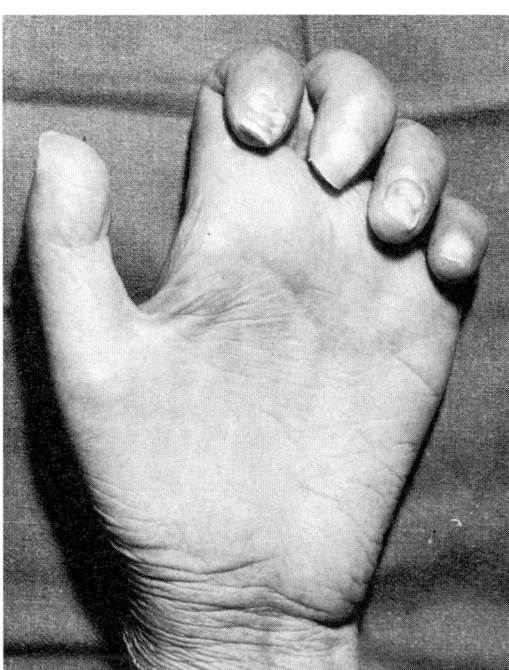

Fig. 1 Claw hand deformity due to combined median and ulnar nerve lesion in a case of vasculitis ? SLE.

duce a neuropathy that may take one of several forms (Fig. 1). Microinfarction of peripheral nerves can produce a mononeuritis multiplex or cause a diffuse neuropathy. Rarely a rapid onset is reminiscent of a Guillain–Barré neuropathy. Polymyositis may need to be distinguished from a steroid myopathy by electromyography (EMG), CK assay, and biopsy. A more than chance association with myasthenia gravis has been described.

Diagnosis

EEGs are commonly though non-specifically abnormal, and the CSF often has an excess of cells and an elevated protein content even when there is no clinical evidence of meningism. CSF levels of complement may be depressed but the hope that they would be an accurate marker of disease activity has not been substantiated. Computerized tomography (CT) scans may show infarcts or haemorrhage or more commonly simple atrophy. Regional oxygen metabolism measured by positron tomography has been reported to show patchy disturbances in cerebral lupus but this has yet to be confirmed. The diagnosis remains essentially a clinical one with multisystem involvement and antidouble-stranded DNA and cardiolipid antibodies. It should be suspected if a patient shows signs of both peripheral and central nervous system disturbances. The prognosis for CNS involvement, which is usually seen in the first year of the disease, is initially good. Conservative measures are advised for all but the severest complications. In severe cases corticosteroids are usually combined with cytotoxic agents and plasmapheresis may be tried.

Complications of SLE

These may affect the CNS. Thus renal failure may cause headache, confusion, drowsiness, tremor, myoclonic jerking, and fits. Hypertension may be responsible for focal signs, or headache, fits and coma due to hypertensive encephalopathy. A tendency to infection includes the possibility of meningitis and emboli may occur from the heart affected by Libman–Sacks endocarditis. Two haematolgical complications have important neurological sequelae.

Lupus anticoagulant

This is an antibody that is misnamed since its presence, usually in SLE but occasionally with other collagenoses, causes thrombotic complications. There is evidence that it affects the prothrombin complex, and it may also inhibit prostacyclin formation by the vessel wall (see Sections 16 and 19). It can be responsible for recurrent thrombotic episodes, deep vein thromboses, pulmonary embolism, and cerebral infarction being the commonest.

Thrombotic thrombocytopenic purpura (see also Section 19)

This rare condition, which may complicate SLE, is probably due to immune complex formation. It causes a thrombocytopenic purpura, haemolytic anaemia, neurological abnormalities, fever, and evidence of renal disease. Ninety per cent of cases have neurological symptoms and signs though these are often fleeting in nature. Frequent seizures, fever, and coma occur terminally, when the autopsy reveals widespread small vessel occlusions in the brain. The course of the disease is usually aggressive though some patients have been kept alive for a few years by the use of immunosuppression, antiplatelet agents, and plasmapheresis.

Polyarteritis nodosa (see also Section 16)

This rare but serious disease is characterized by fibrinoid necrosis of the media extending to involve the adventitia and intima. The intense inflammatory response that is also seen in all three layers of the walls of small and medium-sized arteries may be secondary. Weakened areas of the necrotic wall may lead to aneurysm formation (hence 'nodosa'). The vasculitis causes thromboses, infarctions, and haemorrhage. Most patients are male and have fever, malaise, arthritis, abdominal pain, renal disease, hypertension, and pulmonary involvement in some combination or other.

Neurological complications are common. Some 50 per cent of patients have a peripheral neuropathy, and at autopsy as many as 75 per cent may show signs of involvement of the vasa nervorum. A mononeuritis multiplex, often presenting with a peroneal nerve palsy causing a foot drop, may be the first sign of the disease. Individual nerve lesions may come on over a few hours and follow a relapsing and remitting course. The neuropathy is commonly more motor than sensory in its manifestations and affects the legs more than the arms. Less commonly a diffuse and symmetrical mixed polyneuropathy may develop which is often accompanied by weight loss and anorexia. A subclinical neuropathy may be detected by nerve conduction studies or biopsy.

Muscle pain is reported by many patients, due either to a polymyalgia rheumatica-like syndrome or to polymyositis, with elevated CK levels and a biopsy finding of arteritis and microinfarcts. Some biopsies prove normal, however, due to the patchy nature of the changes.

Central nervous system manifestations are protean and tend to wax and wane. Organic psychoses, seizures, and focal lesions may result from vessel occlusions and subarachnoid or cerebral haemorrhage may be seen. A meningeal illness with or without cranial nerve palsies can occur with a cellular CSF.

The diagnosis of polyarteritis nodosa may be suggested by fever, weight loss, purpura, arthritis, proteinuria, red cell urinary casts, abdominal pain from bowel ischaemia, and renal failure. The ESR may be raised and there is usually a leucocytosis. Biopsy confirmation may be obtained from muscle, nerve or kidney. Polymyositis and the mononeuritis multiplex may respond to steroids but the response is unpredictable. Involvement of the CNS implies a poor outlook, but is uncommon.

Progressive systemic sclerosis (diffuse scleroderma) (see also Section 16)

This collagenosis mainly affects females. It is rare, with something like 2.7 per million per year new cases appearing in the United Kingdom. It is often more severe in negroes. There is a widespread and progressive sclerosis affecting the skin, lungs, kidneys, upper gastrointestinal tract, and myocardium. Raynaud's disease and painful stiffness of the hands are frequent early features together with fatigue and headache. Over 5 per cent develop oesophageal motility disturbances and many have reticular shadowing on chest X-ray. Progressive pulmonary hypertension and right heart failure may develop late in the disease. Renal involvement is common and carries a poor prognosis.

Many patients have an insidious onset of proximal muscle weakness, and wasting and weakness of neck muscles is often striking. EMG studies usually suggest that this is due to a simple myopathy. In a few cases, however, CK levels are elevated and the EMG suggests a myositis, and in this subgroup steroids are indicated.

Cranial nerve lesions may also develop, with trigeminal sensory loss being the commonest finding. This develops insidiously and may be accompanied by a facial nerve lesion mimicking a Bell's palsy. Trigeminal neuropathy may even be the presenting feature before skin changes are obvious. These cranial nerve lesions may be due to perineural sclerosis or a microangiopathy. A peripheral neuropathy like that seen in rheumatoid arthritis, and a stroke due to progressive narrowing of the cervical carotid artery are rare complications. Dementia, and a pseudotabetic picture due to posterior column degeneration have also been described.

Rheumatoid arthritis (see also Section 16)

Assessment of neurological complications is made difficult by pain and deformity due to joint disease. Muscle wasting and weakness may be due to disuse as well as to neuropathy and EMG studies may be needed to make such distinctions.

As many as one in three patients develop true muscle weakness. In some cases this is due to steroid myopathy with type II fibre atrophy though the same histological appearance may be found in patients who have never been given steroids ('rheumatic myopathy'). Less commonly biopsies show an inflammatory myositis. Commonest of all is a minimal histological change whose pathogenesis is not fully understood.

Occasional patients, especially those with the cutaneous stigmata of vasculitis, develop a peripheral neuropathy. This is usually predominantly sensory in nature and most obvious in the legs but it occasionally produces distal weakness and wasting as well as impairment of all modalities of sensation. Victims have usually had long-standing arthritis and have skin nodules, vasculitic skin lesions, weight loss, and fever, and high titres of rheumatoid factor. Many more patients manifest nerve compression syndromes, for example, of the median nerve in a carpal tunnel compromised by rheumatoid changes in the carpus and flexor tendons, or the ulnar nerve at a disorganized elbow. Muscle wasting in the hand may thus be due to disuse associated with destructive joint changes, median or ulnar neuropathy, or peripheral neuropathy, the distinction being aided by EMG and nerve conduction studies. Pallis and Scott brought to general attention an unusual digital neuropathy in victims of rheumatoid arthritis. Sensory testing may reveal loss to pinprick restricted to one side of a finger.

The prognosis for peripheral nerve involvement tends to be good for those with solitary nerve lesions though surgical decompression may be required. Some recovery of the predominantly sensory neuropathy can occur but the severe mixed neuropathy or a mononeuritis multiplex appears to be a reflection of an aggressive vasculitic form of the disease. Such patients commonly succumb to septicaemia or the effects of coronary or mesenteric arteritis.

Serial X-rays of the cervical spine show that patients seropositive for IgM rheumatoid factor, especially females on steroids, tend to develop atlanto-axial or subaxial subluxation (Fig. 2). These changes and vertical movement of the odontoid peg result from disruption of ligaments and decalcification of the bones (e.g. of the occiput). Such involvement of the cervical spine may only cause the appearance of brisk reflexes in the upper limbs but in the late stages of the disease a dangerous myelopathy may develop. The patients may then present with a paraplegia or with atrophy of hand muscles and painless sensory loss in hands. Root pain over the occipital region (C2) is also common. If the odontoid is dis-

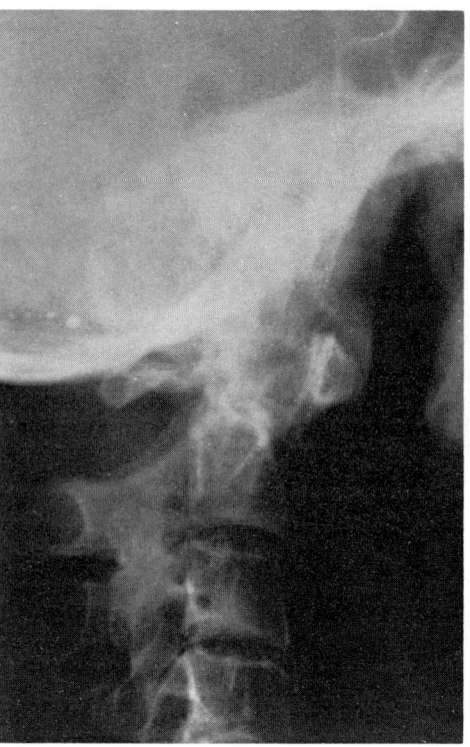

Fig. 2 Lateral X-ray view of the cervical spine of a patient with long-standing rheumatoid arthritis showing atlantoaxial dislocation with wide separation of the arch of the atlas and the odontoid peg (courtesy of Dr M. Chapman).

placed upwards nystagmus and dysarthria may be added to the picture of high cord compression. Immobilization externally or internally is essential, but is difficult and often hazardous.

Sjögren's syndrome

Lymphocytic infiltration may develop in the lacrimal and salivary glands of patients with a connective tissue disorder, usually rheumatoid arthritis or SLE. Keratoconjunctivitis sicca (dry eyes) may be accompanied by xerostoma (dry mouth) and salivary gland enlargement. An associated arteritis may cause an isolated trigeminal neuropathy as seen in progressive systemic sclerosis and some 10 per cent develop a mild distal sensory neuropathy.

SARCOIDOSIS (see also Section 5)

This systemic disease is defined pathologically by granuloma formation in many organs. A granulomatous meningoencephalitis underlies most of the neurological features though confluent granulomas may rarely produce a mass lesion in the CNS.

Early in the course of the disease there may be cranial nerve lesions or a neuropathy. The second and seventh nerves are most often affected, and sarcoidosis should always be suspected in cases of bilateral Bell's palsy and optic neuritis. These individual nerve lesions tend to be transient. The diagnosis is suggested by the presence of concurrent intrathoracic or ocular disease, e.g. uveitis or lacrimal gland swelling. Because of the granulomatous changes in the meninges, root lesions may also be seen. The CSF is commonly abnormal with a lymphocytic pleocytosis, elevated protein, and, in about a third, a reduced glucose level. Oligoclonal IgG may be found, raising suspicions of multiple sclerosis.

Late in the disease the CNS may be involved, especially in the hypothalamic-pituitary areas with diabetes insipidus, amenorrhoea, and somnolence. Hemisphere masses may be indistinguishable before biopsy from a glioma. Such CNS involvement is usually chronic. When it occurs without systemic disease the diagnosis depends on the CT scan appearances, CSF changes, and a Kveim test which is positive in 75 per cent of cases. Biopsy of the liver, lymph-nodes, or muscle, even though the latter is usually asymptomatic, can also be diagnostic.

Steroids are always worth trying but their effects are unpredictable. As suggested the prognosis for peripheral nerve lesions is better than for involvement of the cord or brain.

Systemic sarcoidosis may also cause neurological symptoms by causing hypercalcaemia. Confusion, irritability or proximal muscle weakness may occur which must be distinguished from the effects of neurosarcoidosis *per se*.

BEHÇET'S SYNDROME (see also Section 24)

Behçet, a Turkish dermatologist, described the triad of relapsing oral and genital ulcers with uveitis. Arthritis and skin changes such as erythema nodosum are also frequent and the nervous system is involved in 10–25 per cent of patients. The neurological complications also tend to relapse and remit so that the differential diagnosis is often between Behçet's syndrome and multiple sclerosis (MS). Behçet's is more likely than MS to produce a hemiplegia or pseudobulbar palsy, and to be associated with an elevated ESR and occasionally with a slight lymphocyte pleocytosis in the CSF. There are also likely to be systemic symptoms with a fresh crop of mouth and genital ulcers, joint pains, uveitis, and vascular thrombosis at the time of each neurological relapse. Recurrent brainstem episodes may also be confused with recurrent strokes. The pathological changes responsible for focal neurological changes include necrosis and demyelination with scarring (Fig. 3). Some vessels also show an inflammatory cell infiltration. Other presentations with, for example, headache and papilloedema, reflect the occurrence of a meningoencephalitis or cerebral venous thrombosis.

There are no specific tests, the cornerstone of diagnosis being a long history of mouth and genital ulcers and uveitis, as neurological complications are usually a late feature of the syndrome. Patients may have to be asked directly about ulcers as many have become accustomed to them as part of their normal lives. CT scans may show non-specific low-density lesions or masses. Once the diagnosis of the neurological type of Behçet's syndrome is

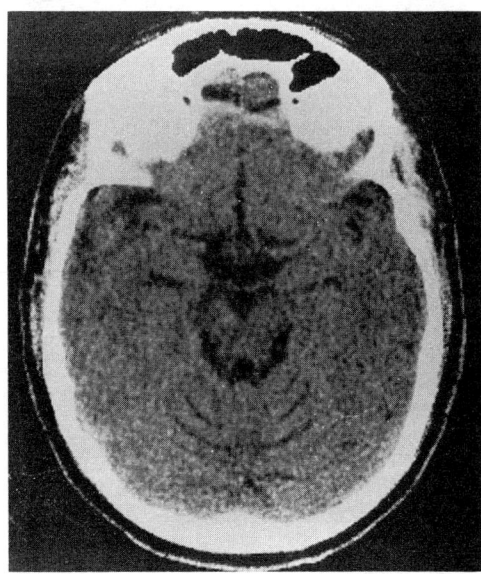

Fig. 3 CT scan showing prominence of cerebellar folii and CSF spaces around the brain stem due to atrophy after an episode of brain stem disturbance in a case of Behçet's syndrome (courtesy of Dr R. Kocen).

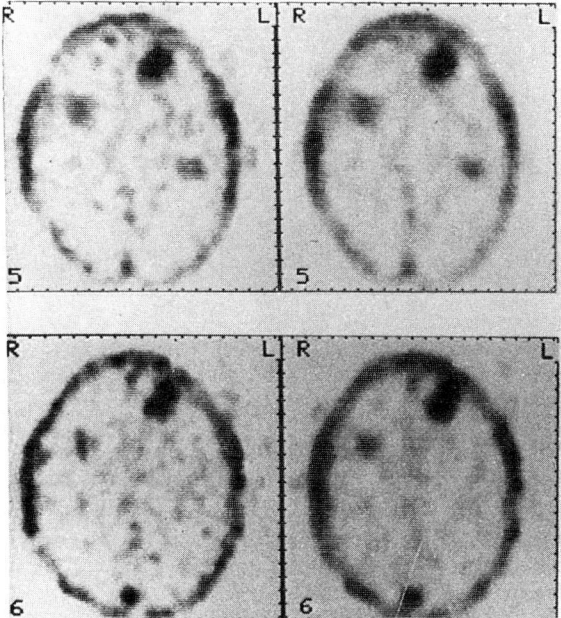

Fig. 4 Radionuclide brain scan after an injection of 99 Tc^{m} glucoheptonate showing multiple metastases from carcinoma of the breast (courtesy of Dr P. Ell).

made, treatment with steroids should be tried. Few patients die of their neurological involvement.

WEGENER'S GRANULOMATOSIS (see also Section 16)

This is a rare form of necrotizing vasculitis of the upper and lower respiratory tract with granuloma formation, usually accompanied by glomerulonephritis. Ulceration of the nasal mucosa often occurs and patients present with haemorrhagic sinusitis or pulmonary infiltration. The chest X-ray shows diffuse infiltrates or nodular opacities often mimicking metastases. The diagnosis can be made by biopsying the nasal mucosa, lung and kidney. The nervous system is affected in some 25 per cent of cases . The vasculitis causes damage to cranial nerves or peripheral nerves when it produces the picture of a mononeuritis multiplex. Less commonly direct spread from the nasopharynx may affect the orbit or cause cranial nerve lesions. Modern treatment combines steroids with cytotoxic agents.

Malignancy

As many as 1 in 5 patients with generalized cancer develop evidence of involvement of the nervous system. Metastases often develop in the brain or in the epidural space and at death some 10–20 per cent of cancer victims have a cerebral metastasis (Fig. 4). Other patients develop neurological problems as a result of their antineoplastic treatment whether this is by radiation or chemotherapy. In a third group neurological features are unrelated to spread of malignant tissue. In these the mechanism is poorly understood though some are due to opportunistic infections in the immunodeficient patient. Others are known as 'non-metastatic' complications or the 'remote effects' of cancer on the nervous system. Both lymphomas and cancers produce these manifestations but there are important differences.

Lymphoma (see also Section 19)

Generalized lymphomas rarely cause intracerebral deposits but spinal cord compression from epidural masses arises in up to 5 per

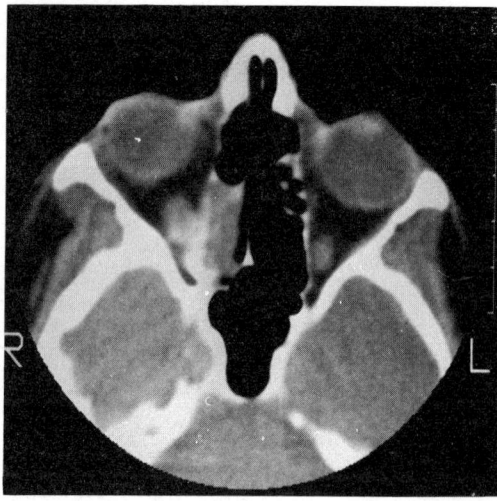

Fig. 5 CT scan showing a soft tissue mass in the left side of the naso-pharynx obliterating the air passages. The patient had presented with a sixth nerve palsy. Biopsy confirmed that the nasopharyngeal tumour was a non-Hodgkin's lymphoma.

cent of cases. Local back pain is usual, often accompanied by root pain. Most patients have a deposit between mid-cervical and mid-thoracic levels. At first the only signs may be of lost abdominal re-flexes and extensor plantars and the diagnosis needs to be made by myelography at this early stage to obtain the best results from treatment by steroids and radiotherapy. Later, sensory loss, weak-ness, and sphincter damage develop, sometimes acutely with flac-cidity and areflexia from spinal shock. Once paralysis is marked there is little chance of recovery.

Although cerebral masses are rare nasopharyngeal or orbital deposits are not uncommon especially in non-Hodgkin's lym-phoma (Fig. 5). Patients present with a proptosis or with nerve palsies. A local mass must be demonstrated clinically or radiologi-cally to distinguish an extracranial lesion from a lymphomatous meningitis which may also cause cranial nerve palsies. In the latter case headache and vomiting are usually prominent and cytology of the CSF is diagnostic. If no diagnostic cells are seen, myelography sometimes shows nodules. Such patients need radiotherapy and intrathecal chemotherapy. A CT scan should precede the lumbar puncture if at all possible.

Opportunistic infections are common in the lymphomata caus-ing meningitis with or without hydrocephalus or brain abscess. Listeria, herpes zoster, cryptococcus, toxoplasma, coccidiomyco-sis, and aspergillus all need consideration with appropriate bac-teriological or virological study of the CSF and search for antibodies. A peculiar invasion of the white matter with papova-like virus may cause a progressive unilateral then bilateral hemi-sphere disorder with visual disturbance, hemiparesis, and mental change. CT scans show non-enhancing low-density changes in the white matter. The condition (progressive multifocal leucoence-phalopathy or PML) is rapidly fatal in most instances (Fig. 6) (see also page 21.151). Alternatively, an encephalitic illness with men-tal changes sometimes amounting to dementia or a severe amnesic state may occur. Although there are inflammatory changes some-times concentrated on the limbic area no infective agent has yet been identified in these patients. Fits suggest the rare alternative possibility of an intracerebral lymphomatous mass.

Several other non-metastatic complications may be seen in patients with a lymphoma. A subacute cerebellar ataxia may cause severe disability within a few months. Various types of peripheral neuropathy are encountered ranging from an acute Guillain–Barré-like illness to a mixed neuropathy indistinguishable from that due to diabetes mellitus. Asymmetrical wasting with weak-ness and fasciculation is particularly associated with lymphoma;

anterior horn cell loss is responsible and there is some associated dorsal column change though sensory loss is slight. A subacute sensory neuropathy with disabling loss of position sense can also occur and is due to mononuclear cell infiltration and cell loss in the dorsal root ganglia.

Carcinoma

Metastases

In the case of carcinoma intracerebral metastases (Fig. 4) predo-minate, affecting as many as 20–40 per cent of patients with carci-noma of the bronchus, for example. Almost any primary tumour may metastasize to the brain, and as survival lengthens with modern treatment more unusual tumours are appearing as causes of cerebral secondaries. The commonest sources of cerebral metastases are tumours of the lung, breast, testes, and skin (mela-noma). The presentation is indistinguishable from a primary intra-cerebral tumour until scans show a second or third lesion. Multiple deposits are more common than single ones, and the brain is rarely the only site of metastatic spread. Isotope scanning is reliable in detecting over 80 per cent of cerebral metastases and is the first investigation of choice. Surgery may be indicated for a solitary posterior fossa deposit to relieve vertigo and vomiting, and radiotherapy and steroids may add several months good qual-ity life in other selected cases.

Occasionally the deposits are in the skull base with cranial nerve palsies or in vertebrae with secondary spinal cord compression. In the latter case plain spine films will often show an eroded pedicle. Radiotherapy and steroids are indicated for such a patient if the tumour is radiosensitive though a laminectomy may be needed, especially if signs progress under treatment or there is no tissue diagnosis. A carcinomatous meningitis causing multiple cranial nerve palsies may also occur as described for lymphomas. Oppor-tunistic infections also occur though PML is rare.

Non-metastatic complications

Non-metastatic complications are more common. For example, a subacute progressive ataxia, which often causes severe disability, may develop particularly in cases of carcinoma of the bronchus, breast, and ovary. A *peripheral neuropathy* not infrequently develops terminally, especially in patients with carcinoma of the bronchus. Limb weakness can be due to cachexia or a neuropathy or a mixed picture may develop in which some of the features look

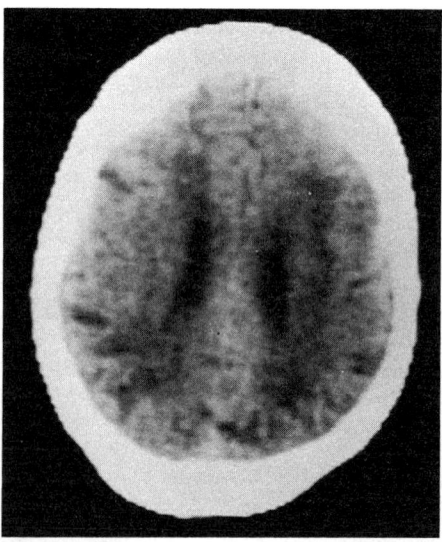

Fig. 6 CT scan showing low density in the white matter particularly of the right hemisphere. The patient demented rapidly with a left homonymous hemianopia, left hemiparesis, and dysphasia (right handed). Changes due to progressive multifocal leukoencephalopathy associated with a lymphoma.

myopathic (proximal weakness) and some neuropathic (absent ankle jerks). The fact that a particular syndrome is due to an underlying neoplasm may be suggested by combinations of neurological features such as lost ankle jerks from a neuropathy, and extensor plantar responses all in a patient with a cerebellar syndrome.

Polymyositis, with or without dermatological changes, sometimes proves to be associated with a neoplasm particularly in males over the age of 50 years. Proximal muscle weakness is accompanied by pain and muscle tenderness though these latter diagnostic features may be missing. EMG changes, an elevated CK, and a high ESR may be confirmatory but the diagnosis is finally dependent upon a muscle biopsy which reveals muscle cell damage and inflammatory cell infiltration. Corticosteroids may be indicated, the prognosis being good in the short term for suppression of the myositis but dominated in the longer term by the underlying malignancy.

Rarely a syndrome of fatiguable weakness is seen. This is the *Eaton Lambert syndrome*, in which an autoimmune process affects the release of acetycholine quanta at the neuromuscular junction. Patients have a myasthenic-like weakness, usually affecting limb rather than eye muscles, in contrast to most cases of myasthenia gravis. The diagnosis may be suggested clinically by the finding that depressed or absent reflexes are enhanced by prior voluntary contraction of the muscle. This effect is best demonstrated, however, by repetitive nerve stimulation with recordings of the evoked muscle action potential which may increase two- to six-fold. Power may be improved by oral doses of guanidine (see Section 22).

Some cancer patients develop an *encephalomyelitis* which affects the limbic areas (with amnesia, hallucinations, and epilepsy), the spinal cord, or dorsal root ganglia with a sensory ataxia as described with lymphomas. These syndromes may be accompanied by a cellular response in the CSF. There is no specific treatment. Antibodies to dorsal root ganglia and Purkinje cells have been identified in individual cases and these encephalitic complications may well prove to be due to immunological processes.

Multiple myelomatosis (see also Section 19)

This disorder very commonly involves vertebrae with back pain and cord compression usually with a sensory level. The diagnosis is made by an elevated ESR and alkaline phosphatase, and by protein electrophoresis and bone marrow biospy. Hypercalcaemia from myeloma, or from multiple carcinomatous bony metastases may itself cause symptoms either of muscle weakness or of lethargy, drowsiness, confusion or delirium. Symptoms are likely with a corrected calcium level of 3.5 mM and almost universal at 4.0 mM. Myeloma patients also develop a peripheral neuropathy even when the myeloma is restricted to a solitary bone. Amyloidosis may complicate myeloma and cause a painful small fibre neuropathy with autonomic changes, and distal pain and temperature loss. If the myeloma proteins cause a hyperviscosity syndrome, mental confusion and clouding of consciousness may be accompanied by visual disturbance due to retinal haemorrhages and exudates.

Brachial plexus lesions

Carcinoma of the breast also affects the brachial plexus by local infiltration. A painful progessive paralysis of the arm develops. It has to be distinguished from radiation damage to the plexus after radiotherapy to axillary nodes. The latter may be painless but the distinction often requires surgical exploration.

Leukaemia (see also Section 19)

As treatment of leukaemia increases survival more patients develop involvement of the nervous system. Leukaemic cells may

be found in the walls of veins, the arachnoid and in the brain parenchyma. Some patients have multiple episodes of neurological involvement and relapses may occur when the patient is in complete systemic remission. The brain is a sanctuary for leukaemic cells as chemotherapy may fail to cross the blood–brain barrier. This problem has led to prophylactic treatment of the asymptomatic CNS, for example, in children with acute lymphatic leukaemia, when a combination of radiotherapy and intrathecal cytotoxic drugs is often employed.

Involvement of the CNS by leukaemia represents a serious advance in the disease and carries a poor prognosis. A meningeal picture is commonest with headache, drowsiness, vomiting, papilloedema, and neck stiffness. The CSF pressure is elevated as is the cell count and the glucose level may be low. It is important that the nature of the CSF cells be identified. A leukaemic patient may have leukaemic cells in the CSF with infiltration of the arachnoid and dura, but equally might be suffering from a superadded viral meningitis, e.g. due to herpes zoster, in which case the cells are mature lymphocytes. CT scans may show hydrocephalus due to meningeal block.

Cerebral haemorrhage is a common terminal event and is associated with high blood white cell counts and, sometimes, with the presence of intracerebral leukaemic nodules. Multiple haemorrhages tend to occur in the cerebral white matter often associated with a general bleeding tendency due to thrombocytopenia.

Infiltration can cause cranial nerve or peripheral nerve lesions and a 'non-metastatic' neuropathy can occur. There is a common problem of an encephalopathy with lethargy, confusion, and drowsiness which may have a variety of causes. Intracranial hypertension from meningeal infiltration and hydrocephalus, subdural haematoma from a bleeding tendency, diffuse intravascular coagulation with multiple infarcts, and progressive multifocal leukoencephalopathy are all possible and best distinguished by CT scanning.

Finally patients with leukaemia are vulnerable to opportunistic infections especially fungal meningitis and brain abscess.

Complications of treatment

Damage to the brachial plexus during radiotherapy to the axilla in patients with cancer of the breast has already been mentioned. Similar damage to the pelvic plexus may develop after treatment of the cervix or lower bowel.

Radiotherapy can also damage the spinal cord either transiently in the few weeks after a course of treatment or rarely a progressive

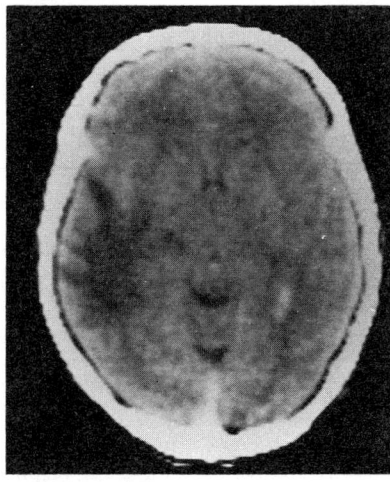

Fig. 7 CT scan showing low-density area in the left hemisphere due to radionecrosis after radiotherapy to the parotid bed. The patient presented with temporal lobe epilepsy.

cord syndrome may develop six months or even years after irradiation. Such radiation necrosis of the cord can be fatal and is resistant to treatment though steroids may be tried. Aggressive treatment of carcinoma of the larynx or bronchus is often responsible.

Radiation necrosis can also occur in the brain (Fig. 7). Sometimes this causes a swollen mass that behaves clinically like a tumour and may be indistinguishable from a new tumour or tumour recurrence before biopsy. If it produces a mass effect surgical excision is needed. Other patients develop an atrophic lesion which may cause epilepsy, memory loss or somnolence. The risk of radionecrosis depends on the total dose and fraction size, it being unwise to exceed 200 cGy to the brain per treatment.

Of the *drugs used in cancer patients*, several cause a peripheral neuropathy, e.g. cisplatinum and vincristine. The latter regularly causes areflexia after as little as 5 mg and after about three injections the patients complain of paraesthesiae in the fingers. Weakness is often prominent in finger extensors and autonomic fibre damage may produce postural hypotension. The changes are reversible if the drug is stopped early in the development of the symptomatic phase. Methotrexate is neurotoxic, causing cerebellar ataxia, epilepsy, and impaired intellectual development when given intrathecally in combination with radiotherapy in the prophylaxis against CNS involvement in childhood leukaemia.

References

Systemic lupus erythematosus
Feinglass, E. J., Arrett, F. G., Dorsch, C. A., Zizic, T. M. and Stevens, M. B. (1976). Neuropsychiatric manifestations of systemic lupus erythematosus diagnosis, clinical spectrum and relationship to other features of the disease. *Medicine* **55**, 323–339.

Polyarteritis nodosa
Cohen, R. D., Conn, D. L. and Ilstrup, D. M. (1980). Clinical features, prognosis and response to treatment in polyarteritis. *Mayo Clin. Proc.* **55**, 146–155.

Scleroderma
Clements, P. J., Furst, D. E., Campion, D. S., Bohan, A., Harris, R., Levy, J. and Paulus, M. E. (1978). Muscle disease in progressive systemic sclerosis. *Arthr. Rheum.* **21**, 62–71.
Teasdell, R. D., Frayhan, R. A. and Schulman, L. E. (1980). Cranial nerve involvement in systemic sclerosis (scleroderma). A report of 10 cases. *Medicine* **59**, 149–159.

Rheumatoid arthritis
Pallis, C. A. and Scott, J. T. (1965). Peripheral neuropathy in rheumatoid arthritis. *Br. Med. J.* **1** 1141–1147.
Nabaro, K. K., Schoena, W. C., Baker, R. A. and Dawson, D. M. (1978). The cervical myelopathy associated with rheumatoid arthritis: analysis of 32 patients – with 2 post-mortem cases. *Ann. Neurol.* **3**, 144–151.

Neoplasms
Henson, R. A. and Urich, H. (1982). *Cancer and the nervous system.* Blackwell Scientific Publications, Oxford.

Sarcoidosis
Matthews, W. B. (1965). Sarcoidosis of the nervous system. *J. Neurol. Neurosurg. Psychiat.* **28** 23–29.
Delaney, P. (1977). Neurologic manifestations in sarcoidosis. *Ann. Int. Med.* **87**, 336–345.

Behçet's syndrome
Lehner, T. and Barnes, C. G. (eds) (1979). *Behçet's disease.* Academic Press, London.
O'Duffy, J. D. and Goldstein, N. P. (1976). Neurologic involvement in seven patients with Behçet's disease. *Am. J. Med.* **61**, 170–178.

Wegener's granulomatosis
Wolff, S. M., Fauci, A. S., Horn, R. G. and Dale, D. C. (1974). Wegener's granulomatosis. *Ann. Int. Med.* **81**, 513–525.

RESPIRATORY PROBLEMS IN NEUROLOGICAL DISEASE

J. NEWSOM-DAVIS

Introduction
Disorders of breathing may arise from disease affecting the central or peripheral nervous system. Knowing how breathing is organized is essential for their diagnosis and management. It is of special importance to recognize that the respiratory muscles are under the control of two major systems – the automatic (chemosensitive) and the behavioural (willed) – that are anatomically distinct and whose descending projections compete for control over spinal respiratory motoneurone activity. This section therefore outlines the central control mechanisms and the role of the peripheral respiratory muscles before describing specific disorders and their management. The progressive nature of the disease processes has sometimes led to a pessimistic approach but, as will be seen, in those with chronic peripheral ventilatory failure, therapy can often be effective and rewarding.

Central neural mechanisms controlling respiration

The localization of structures generating the respiratory drive is more important to clinicians than a knowledge of their detailed interaction, which is in any case poorly understood. Figure 1 sets out the broad outline.

The automatic system

This system depends primarily on brain stem structures. It is responsive to chemoreceptive and vagal inputs.

Brain stem nuclei
Two columns of neurones in the medulla appear essential for rhythm genesis in humans, namely, the nucleus retroambigualis (NRA) and nucleus tractus solitarius (NTS) (Fig. 1). NRA lies ventrolateral to the nucleus ambiguus, extending from the vagal rootlets rostrally to the upper cervical root caudally. NTS lies ventrolateral to the tractus solitarius. It is largely composed of inspiratory neurones which receive a strong vagal (Hering-Breuer) input.

Nucleus parabrachialis medialis (NPBM) in the rostral pons, sometimes known as the pneumotaxic region, is concerned with switching between respiratory phases.

The integration of the neural activity of these nuclei that provides the normally smooth respiratory pattern is not understood.

Chemoreceptor inputs
The carotid and aortic bodies served by the carotid sinus nerve provide the main hypoxic drive in humans. The hypercapnic drive is mediated mainly by chemoreceptors close to the ventral surface of the medulla which respond to changes in CO_2 via pH changes in the CSF.

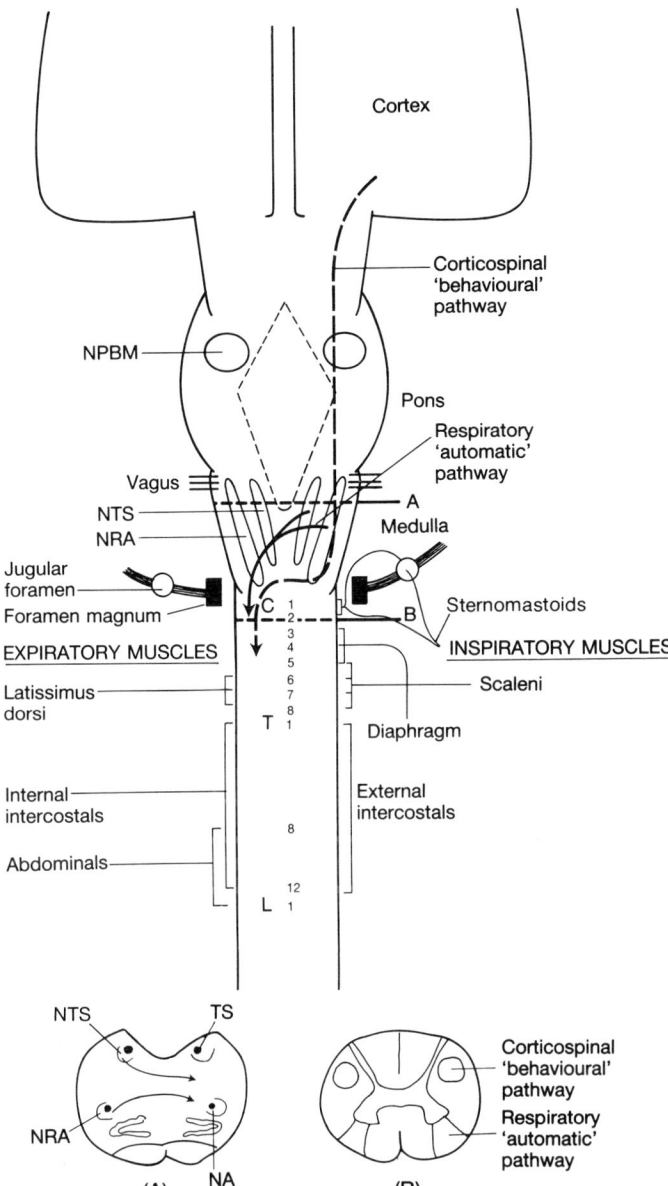

Fig. 1 Neural organization of breathing (schematic). TS, tractus solitarius; NTS, nucleus tractus solitarius; NA, nucleus ambiguus; NRA, nucleus retroambigualis. Transverse sections are shown for levels A (mid-medulla) and B (upper cervical cord).

Descending respiratory pathway

The descending projections from NRA and NTS cross over a relatively wide area in the medulla and descend in the ventrolateral region of the spinal cord (Fig. 1). Bilateral interruption of this pathway above C3 disconnects the automatic system from the respiratory muscles, and spontaneous breathing stops.

The behavioural system

Cerebral cortex

Inhibitory and excitatory effects on breathing can be produced by electrical stimulation of different areas of cortex, notably the anterior cingulate region and the ventromedial aspects of the temporal lobe. The behavioural system subserves all willed activities involving respiratory muscles including breath-holding and voluntary deep breathing (e.g. vital capacity).

Descending behavioural pathway

This is presumed to lie with the main corticospinal and corticobulbar projections. The former decussates in the lower medulla and descends in the dorsolateral columns of the spinal cord (Fig. 1), entirely separate from the descending automatic respiratory pathways.

Interaction between automatic and behavioural systems

These two systems interact both at medullary and spinal cord level. In non-REM ('rapid eye movement') sleep, the behavioural system is quiescent; under these conditions the automatic system operates in functional isolation and breathing is characteristically regular. During wakefulness, the automatic system can be transiently overridden by the behavioural system, most strikingly during breath-holding. The respiratory distress ('breathlessness') occurring at the break point appears to depend on a normally functioning automatic system.

In extreme cases, lesions of either the behavioural or automatic system may leave the other functioning in anatomical isolation. Destruction of the ventral pons, which results in the 'locked-in' syndrome, disconnects the behavioural system, and breathing becomes 'supernormal' in its regularity. Conversely, disconnection of the automatic system (e.g. destruction of respiratory nuclei) results in very irregular ('behavioural') breathing during wakefulness and cessation of breathing during drowsiness or sleep ('Ondine's curse').

Major peripheral ventilatory apparatus

The principal inspiratory muscle is the diaphragm. Other inspiratory and expiratory muscles are shown in Fig. 1. Accessory inspiratory activity (sternomastoids and scaleni) is particularly evident when other inspiratory muscles are paralysed or when the level of respiratory drive is high.

Diaphragm

Downward (inspiratory) movement of the diaphragm is accompanied by outward movement of the abdominal wall, i.e. the two structures operate in series; this is because the floor and posterior wall of the abdomen are rigid and its contents non-compressible.

Central disorders of breathing

Central respiratory failure

Causes

Lesions affecting NTS, NRA or the descending automatic respiratory pathways in the upper cervical cord cause central respiratory failure. The most common pathologies are listed in Table 1.

Clinical features

Patients may report a sense of respiratory unease and may be (justifiably) fearful of sleep. Breathlessness, which requires an intact automatic system, is not a feature. Signs of hypoventilation may be present (see below). There is virtually always evidence of brain stem dysfunction, particularly dysphagia and dysphonia (CN X) loss of glossopharyngeal sensation (CN IX) and hiccup. Reflex coughing (e.g. during tracheal stimulation) is depressed. The breathing pattern is abnormal. During wakefulness, tidal volume and frequency are abnormally variable, and variability increases during drowsiness and sleep, perhaps leading to apnoea. Breath hold may be prolonged, but voluntary control is unaffected (e.g. vital capacity).

Assessment

Monitoring the breathing pattern and blood gases (indwelling arterial line or oxymeter) during drowsiness or sleep is crucial.

Table 1 Main neurological causes of respiratory failure

	Acute	Chronic
Central		
Medulla	Infarct	Tumour
	Haemorrhage	Encephalitis
	Abscess	Leigh's disease
	Encephalitis	Motor neurone disease
	(e.g. poliomyelitis)	Demyelination
	Compression	
	Trauma	
	Hypoxia	
	Drugs	
Cervical cord (C1–3)	Compression	Tumour
	Trauma	Compression
		Demyelination
Peripheral		
Anterior horn	Poliomyelitis	Motor neurone disease (ALS)
		Spinal muscular atrophy
Peripheral nerve	Guillain–Barré	Progressive inflammatory
	Diphtheria	polyneuropathy
	Toxins	Paraneoplastic neuropathy
	Porphyria	
Neuromuscular junction	Myasthenia gravis	
	Congenital myasthenia	
	Botulism	
Muscle	Polymyositis	Acid maltase deficiency
	Periodic paralysis	Limb girdle dystrophy
	Metabolic	Dystrophia myotonica
		Polymyositis
		Nemaline myopathy

Blood gas measurements during wakefulness are often unhelpful because the contribution of the behavioural system cannot be evaluated. Similarly, the vital capacity (a behavioural manoeuvre) provides no index of the integrity of the automatic system, and even the breathing pattern in wakefulness can be misleading if the subject is trying to breathe 'normally'. Ventilatory response to CO_2 or O_2 will be decreased.

Management

Immediate intubation and assisted ventilation is usually required while the underlying pathology (Table 1) is identified and appropriate measures taken. Tracheostomy may be needed later, and the possibility of indefinite assisted ventilation has to be accepted. Patient triggered ventilation is clearly inappropriate. If patients are allowed to breathe spontaneously during wakefulness, a breathing monitor should be used with a suitable alarm system. Phrenic nerve stimulation is potentially usable in these patients, but has not gained general acceptance. Associated dysphagia will require nasogastric intubation. The impaired cough response makes physiotherapy and tracheal toilet particularly important.

Central respiratory insufficiency

Persistent hypoventilation ('central alveolar hypoventilation') may be due to occult brain stem disease (e.g. encephalitis), previous hypoxia or nocturnal obstructive apnoea (see Section 15). Features of hypoventilation are present. These include morning headache, poor sleep, nightmares, daytime somnolence, fatigue, decreased exercise tolerance, cyanosis, polycythaemia, pulmonary hypertension, right heart failure, seizures, confusion, and coma. Management may require assisted nocturnal ventilation by cuirass or correction of nocturnal obstruction (continuous positive airway pressure via nasal mask, or tracheostomy).

Disorders of the breathing pattern

This section will deal with disorders of the breathng pattern other than the irregular breathing of central respiratory failure already described (Fig. 2). These disorders are not normally associated with hypoventilation. They may help in localizing lesions of the CNS. For the majority, no treatment specifically for the dysrhythmia is indicated (or indeed available).

Cheyne–Stokes respiration

This is characterized by a smoothly incremental and decremental pattern that has a cycle time lasting a minute or more, sometimes with brief intercycle apnoea (Fig. 2). Hyperventilation occurs throughout the cycle. The disorder is a sign of cardiac and/or cerebral cortex dysfunction, not of brain stem disorder. The two commonest causes are cerebrovascular disease (e.g. multiple infarcts) and prolonged circulation time (as in heart failure). The mechanisms contributing to the periodicity are complex but include interference with the 'damping' influence of the cerebral cortex (a behavioural effect) on the automatic system, the effects of pulmonary congestion and hypoxaemia, and the consequences of prolongation in the lung to chemoreceptor transit time.

Neurogenic hyperventilation

This very rare condition is characterized by rapid deep breathing (Fig. 2) a low $PaCO_2$ and normal PaO_2. Neurogenic hyperventilation may follow damage to the midbrain, particularly the periaqueductal grey matter, and has been described in association with brain stem tumour. It should not be confused with the much commoner hyperpnoea occurring in obtunded patients which arises from pulmonary congestion and vagal reflex stimulation of the automatic system. These patients may also have a low $PaCO_2$ but, by contrast with neurogenic hyperventilation, the PaO_2 is reduced because of pulmonary shunting.

Apneustic breathing

Inspiratory or, less commonly, expiratory breath-holding occurs which may be prolonged and followed by the breakthrough of rapid rhythmic breathing (Fig. 2). The disorder associates with damage to the dorsolateral rostral pons involving NPBM.

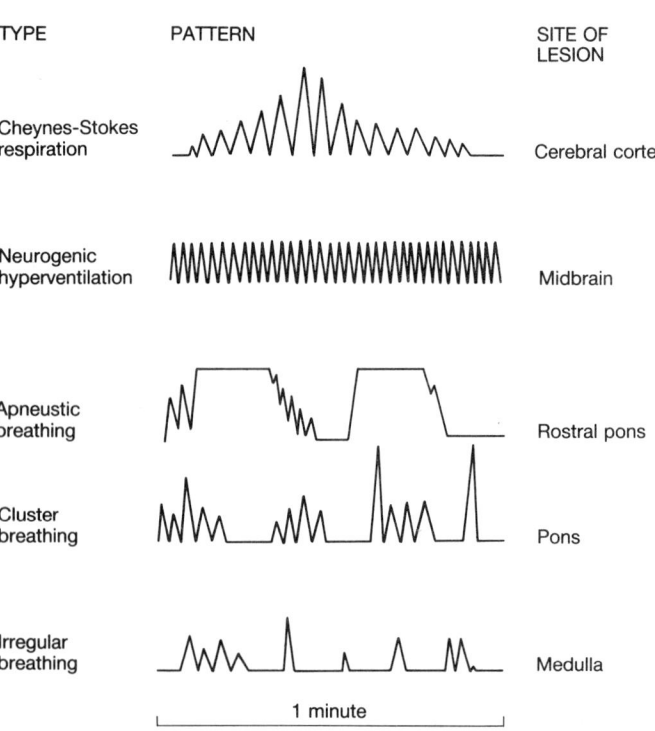

Fig. 2 Disorders of respiratory rhythm (schematic). Note that irregular breathing associated with a medullary lesion indicates failure of automatic breathing.

Cluster breathing

This irregular breathing pattern lacks the smooth incremental/decremental pattern of Cheyne–Stokes respiration (Fig. 2). Involuntary sighs may be frequent. It occurs with damage to the rostral pontine tegmentum.

Epileptic apnoea

In view of the strong inhibitory projections from the temporal lobe to respiratory motoneurones, it is not surprising that apnoea occurs in epilepsy and indeed can be a cause of death. In rare instances, apnoea may be the sole manifestation of temporal lobe seizures. Diagnosis and management are as for other forms of epilepsy (see page 21.62).

Spinal cord lesions

The higher the lesion, the greater is the mortality, and automatic breathing is lost completely with transection above C3. Lower cervical cord lesions allow spontaneous inspiration to continue (via the diaphragm); expiration is largely passive, through the elastic recoil of the ribcage and lungs, but preserved accessory muscle expiratory activity may also be used (see also page 21.105 *et seq.*).

Hiccup

A hiccup consists of an intense synchronous diaphragmatic and inspiratory intercostal muscle contraction lasting about 500 ms, followed 30 ms after its onset by glottal closure, which generates the characteristic inspiratory sound and the discomfort. Mean frequency of hiccup is usually less than 30/min. Increasing $PaCO_2$, and breath-holding, reduce hiccup frequency (and may eliminate it); a low $PaCO_2$ increases the amplitude but not frequency. Hiccup occurs in late fetal life and is frequent in the newborn. It seems to be served by a supraspinal mechanism largely distinct from the automatic respiratory system. Its characteristics suggest a gastrointestinal nature; its function (if any) is unknown.

Persistent or frequently recurrent hiccup may occur with neurological disease affecting the medulla in the region of NTS (Table 1), particularly brain stem tumour, infarction, encephalitis, and occasionally meningitis. It also occurs with metabolic disease such as uraemia and in a variety of thoracic, cardiac, and abdominal conditions, probably mediated via the vagus nerves. 'Pathological' hiccup may continue during sleep, being one of the few involuntary movements to do so. Emotional stimuli (e.g. shock, sexual intercourse) may end a bout of hiccup.

Management

Post-prandial hiccup either resolves spontaneously or responds to measures that stimulate the pharynx (e.g. drinking iced water) or increase in $PaCO_2$ (e.g. rebreathing). Nasal mucosal stimulation sufficient to provoke sneezing may also abort hiccup, as first reported by Plato (The Symposium, 416 BC) whose observations have not always been acknowledged by later authors. Nasopharyngeal stimulation stops hiccup in a high proportion of postoperative cases. When hiccup is secondary to neurological or metabolic disease, none of these methods is likely to provide sustained relief. The wide range of remedies proposed for chronic hiccup implies that none are pre-eminently effective. Chlorpromazine, haloperidol, and diazepam are commonly prescribed. Phrenic nerve section, although sometimes undertaken, seems inadvisable because hiccup will continue in other inspiratory muscles and ventilatory capacity may be compromised by the diaphragm paralysis.

Peripheral ventilatory failure

Causes

Peripheral ventilatory failure is much more common than central failure. It occurs terminally in many patients with progressive neuromuscular disorders, and may be a presenting or prominent early feature in others (see Table 1).

Clinical features

Acute ventilatory failure is characterized by anxiety, shortness of breath, tachycardia, and poor sleep leading to hypoxic confusion, seizure, and coma. Chronic ventilatory failure develops more insidiously and is often overlooked initially. Clinical features of hypoventilation occur (see above). Dyspnoea is often absent at rest and patients may tolerate markedly abnormal blood gases without distress. Seizures may occur during exacerbations of chronic hypoxia.

Clinical assessment

There is accessory muscle activity and often flaring of the ala nasi, particularly in acute failure. Weakness or paralysis of the diaphragm, which can be relatively selective in some disorders (e.g. acid maltase deficiency) causes breathlessness in the supine posture (orthopnoea); such patients may thus elect to sleep upright. Diaphragm fatigue may contribute to its impaired function.

An important (and often overlooked) physical sign of diaphragm weakness or paralysis is paradoxical (inward) movement of the abdominal wall during inspiration in the supine posture, which comes about because of the in-series coupling between diaphragm and abdominal wall (see above). Gravitational forces increase this effect in the head down posture (which is usually intolerable for such patients) but decrease it in the upright posture. A further sign of a paralysed diaphragm is the apparently excessive movement of the ribcage during inspiration in the supine posture, which is sometimes misinterpreted as being due to anxiety or as 'functional'. This increased ribcage movement is required to compensate for the passive upward displacement of the diaphragm in inspiration.

Laboratory assessment

Vital capacity will be reduced. The earliest change in blood gases is a fall in $PaCO_2$ with a normal or reduced PaO_2 probably because micro-atelectasis leads to shunting and a reflex increase in respiratory drive. In chronic ventilatory failure, hypoxia and hypercapnia may increase considerably during sleep. Blood gas monitoring (indwelling arterial catheter or by percutaneous oxymeter) is necessary.

Diaphragm function is most readily assessed by measuring the vital capacity in the erect and supine postures. A decline when moving from the upright to the supine posture implies selective diaphragm weakness. A 50 per cent reduction is usual when the diaphragm is totally paralysed. Screening (fluoroscopy), particularly in the upright posture, is unreliable in cases where both halves of the diaphragm are paralysed because it cannot readily distinguish between active and passive downward movement of the diaphragm, but it is valuable in the diagnosis of unilateral diaphragm paralysis. Transdiaphragmatic pressure is the best index of diaphragm function, but the measurement is available in only a few special centres. Peak inspiratory pressure provides an index of overall inspiratory force. Measurement of phrenic nerve conduction may occasionally be useful.

Management

Chest infection is common and can be life-threatening. It requires vigorous physiotherapy and early antibiotic treatment (see also page 21.105 *et seq.*).

In acute ventilatory failure, control of the airway (e.g. intubation) and assisted ventilation should be immediately undertaken before treatment (when available) is directed to the underlying pathology. If this is unlikely to be corrected within a few days, tracheostomy will be needed.

In chronic ventilatory failure, initial treatment by continuous assisted ventilation corrects daytime blood gases and the systemic consequences of chronic hypoventilation. Improvement can later usually be maintained by assisted ventilation solely at night. This is best achieved by a cuirass jacket attached to a pump, which can be used at home. In cases who require tracheostomy (e.g. because of nocturnal obstructive apnoea while in the cuirass), intermittent positive pressure ventilation may be used. Treatment in this way not only improves or fully corrects daytime blood gases, but also greatly increases the quality of life by reducing fatigue and somnolence. Progressive muscle disease often affects young adults who may have families dependent on them. Nocturnal cuirass ventilation usually enables patients to return to work or to take up their previous household activities. It may also greatly relieve the respiratory distress observed in more severely affected patients particularly those cases of motoneurone disease in whom the respiratory muscles are early and severely involved. The commitment to assisted ventilation is not indefinite because progressive bulbar and respiratory muscle weakness ultimately leads to a terminal chest infection.

Nocturnal obstructive apnoea

(See Section 15.)

References

Beal, M. F., Richardson, E. P., Brandstetter, R., Hedley-Whyte, E. T. and Hochberg, F. H. (1983). Localised brainstem ischemic damage and Ondine's curse after near-drowning. *Neurology (Cleveland)* **33**, 717–721.

Cherniack, N. S. and Longobardo, G. S. (1973). Cheyne–Stokes breathing. *N. Engl. J. Med.* **288**, 952–957.

Harrison, B. D. W., Collins, J. V., Brown, K. G. E. and Hughes, T. J. H. (1971). Respiratory failure in neuromuscular disease. *Thorax* **26**, 579–584.

Kalia, M. P. (1981). Anatomical organisation of central respiratory neurons. *Ann. Rev. Physiol.* **43**, 105–120.

Loh, L., Goldman, M. and Newsom-Davis J. (1977). The assessment of diaphragm function. *Medicine (Baltimore.)* **56**, 165–169.

Nelson, D. A. and Ray, C. D. (1968). Respiratory arrest from seizure discharges in limbic system. *Arch. Neurol.* **19**, 199–207.

Newsom-Davis, J. (1970). An experimental study of hiccup. *Brain* **93**, 851–872.

—— (1980). The respiratory system in muscular dystrophy. *Br. Med. Bull.* **36**, 135–138.

—— (1985). The neural control of respiratory function. In *Neurosurgery: the scientific basis of clinical practice* (eds H. A. Crockard, R. D. Hayward and J. T. Hoff). Blackwell Scientific Publications, Oxford.

——, Goldman, M., Loh, L. and Casson, M. (1976). Diaphragm function and alveolar hypoventilation. *Q. J. Med.* **45**, 87–100.

Plum, F. and Alvord, E. C. (1964). Apneustic breathing in man. *Arch. Neurol. (Chicago)* **10**, 101–112.

Plum, F. and Posner J. B. (1980). *The diagnosis of stupor and coma* 3rd edn, pp. 32–41. F. A. Davis, Philadelphia.

Roussos, C. and Macklem, P. T. (1982). The respiratory muscles. *New Engl. J. Med.* **307**, 786–797.

Sullivan, C. E., Berthon-Jones, M. and Issa, F. G. (1983). Remission of severe obesity-hypoventilation syndrome after short-term treatment during sleep with nasal continuous positive airway pressure. *Am. Rev. Respir. Dis.* **128**, 177–181.

METABOLIC AND DEFICIENCY DISORDERS OF THE NERVOUS SYSTEM

C. D. MARSDEN

The brain depends entirely on glycolysis and respiration to synthesize its energy needs. An adequate supply of glucose and oxygen depends upon cerebral blood flow which, under normal resting conditions, is about 55 cm^3 per 100 g/minute, an amount equal to 15–20 per cent of the resting cardiac output. Each 100 g of brain of the normal human utilizes about 0.31 μmol (5·5 mg) of glucose per minute. In the basal fasting state the brain's consumption of glucose almost equals the total amount the liver produces. Under normal conditions, glucose consumption varies enormously from region to region of the brain depending upon local functional changes. The brain contains only minute stores of glucose and glycogen such that if blood supply is abruptly cut off, normal function can only continue for two to three minutes. If the brain is deprived of both glucose and oxygen, as occurs in cardiac arrest, normal energy metabolism can only continue for about 10–15 seconds.

General metabolic disorders

Hypoglycaemia

Hypoglycaemic coma is frequent, difficult to diagnose, and dangerous. In any case of coma or stupor of unknown cause, blood should be drawn for glucose analysis, and then 25 g of glucose should be administered intravenously. Such an injection can do no harm and may save life.

The commonest cause of hypoglycaemia is insulin overdose, or excessive hypoglycaemic drug intake. Hyperinsulinism due to an adenoma of islets of Langerhans in the pancreas is uncommon, as is hypoglycaemia due to a retroperitoneal sarcoma. Hypoglycaemia may also occur in alcoholism and liver disease, and after gastric surgery.

Hypoglycaemia usually presents in one of four manners: (*a*) as an organic toxic confusional state, sleepy confusion, or mania; (*b*) as unexplained coma with brainstem dysfunction including decerebrate spasms and neurogenic hyperventilation, but with preserved oculocephalic reflexes and pupillary responses; (*c*) as a stroke-like illness with focal deficit; and (*d*) as epilepsy. Hyperinsulinism, very rarely, also causes predominantly motor peripheral neuropathy.

Hypoglycaemia is established by measurement of blood glucose concentration, and by clinical response to intravenous glucose replacement. Hyperinsulinism is difficult to diagnose on occasion, but can be established by satisfying the criteria for Whipple's triad, namely symptoms of hypoglycaemia, associated with a low blood sugar and a disproportionately high serum insulin, and clinical response to glucose replacement. A 72-hour fast, measuring morning blood sugar and insulin levels, will detect nearly all pancreatic islet cell adenomas (see Section 9).

Anoxia

Acute cerebral anoxia is commonly due to cardiac arrest, either resulting from heart disease, cardiac surgery, or anaesthetic catastrophe. Carbon monoxide poisoning, usually suicidal, also damages the brain by anoxia.

Acute anoxia rapidly leads to loss of consciousness, generalized fits, dilated pupils, and bilateral extensor plantar responses. If tissue oxygenation is restored quickly, consciousness returns in seconds or minutes. However, if oxygen deprivation lasts longer than a few minutes, permanent or prolonged but reversible brain damage occurs. Severe anoxia may lead to irreversible coma with flaccidity and loss of all reflex function except heart beat and tendon jerks. Pupils remain fixed and dilated and the EEG is flat on repeated examination. (Drugs and hypothermia may cause a flat EEG, but recovery is possible.) Such patients may be said to have suffered irreversible brain death if all signs of brainstem function are absent on repeated examination over 12–24 hours (see page 21.48). Other, less severely affected, patients show partial recovery of reflex function, such as pupillary responses, reflex eye movements, and muscle tone, and may breathe spontaneously. However, no sign of consciousness or intelligent response to the external world occurs, and they may remain in such a 'persistent vegetative state' for months or years. Lesser degrees of anoxia may cause transient coma with recovery of consciousness but with residual dementia, amnesic syndrome, pseudobulbar palsy and other pyramidal signs, gait ataxia, and incontinence. Some of these patients may be severely disabled by action myoclonus, that is dramatic muscle jerking on attempted movement. These residual deficits following prolonged cerebral anoxia with survival may be permanent, but in other patients they gradually recover. In general, the potential for recovery following cerebral anoxia is considerable over months or years. An optimistic prognosis is justifiable in the early stages, and the final outcome can never be predicted with certainty, except in those with unequivocal evidence of cerebral death.

In a small number of patients apparent recovery from an acute anoxic insult is followed some weeks or months later by delayed post-anoxic encephalopathy. The patient recovers, but days or weeks later relapses with increasing irritability, apathy, and confusion. An akinetic-rigid syndrome with or without spasticity then emerges and the condition may progress to coma or death over a matter of some weeks or months. Often, these neurological changes are first mistaken for psychological disorder, until frank neurological signs clarify the diagnosis. The cause of delayed post-anoxic deterioraton is not clear, but pathologically there is a diffuse, severe, bilateral white matter degeneration in the hemispheres.

Subacute or gradual anoxia may occur in severe anaemia, heart failure, pulmonary disease, or exposure to high altitude. It produces inattentiveness, fatigue, and intellectual deterioration, followed by memory difficulties and ataxia.

Cerebral anoxia also is the main cause of neurological symptoms in a number of other systemic conditions. *Disseminated intravascular coagulation* (see Section 19) resulting from platelet aggregation and fibrin formation, can be produced by a number of illnesses, including sepsis, and malignancy. Patients complain of headache and difficulty in concentration, vertigo, blurred vision, and speech difficulties. Such confusion and disorientation may progress to stupor and coma with focal or generalized signs of brain disturbance. Spontaneous bleeding is common, in the form of petechiae in the skin or optic fundus, purpura, and even intracranial haemorrhage. *Cerebral malaria* (see Section 5) is a complication of infection with *Plasmodium falciparum*, and should always be borne in mind as a cause of unexplained coma in patients recently returning from an infective area. Most patients describe chills and fever for a few days prior to the onset of lethargy, stupor, and finally coma. The diagnosis is established by finding the parasite in fixed smears of the blood.

Fat embolism follows severe trauma, particularly to the limbs, but may also be a complication of burns and other severe system disturbance. Multiple pulmonary micro-emboli of fat may lead to progressive hypoxia and respiratory failure. Multiple cerebral micro-emboli produce confusion, lethargy, stupor, and finally coma. Symptoms often begin hours to days after the original injury, and are accompanied by fever and hyperventilation. A characteristic petechial rash usually develops over the upper half of the body on the second to third day after injury. There may also be fundal haemorrhages. The respiratory features range from the appearance of linear streaks radiating from the hilar region or patchy opacities on the chest X-ray to the fully developed adult distress syndrome (see Section 15). Clotting abnormalities range from mild thrombocytopenia to acute disseminated intravascular coagulation (see Section 19). Management consists of correcting hypoxia, in severe cases with positive end-expiratory pressure (PEEP), and correction of the coagulation disorder (see Section 19). There have been anecdotal reports of the value of high doses of methylprednisolone (30 mg/kg given eight-hourly).

Cardiac surgery, at least in the earlier days of bypass pump oxygenation, produced frequent transient neurological damage in many patients. Improvements in technique, such as the introduction of filters in blood perfusion lines to remove debris, have greatly reduced neurological complications of the procedure. However, some patients still come round from the anaesthetic with signs of diffuse or focal brain damage. If they survive the acute episode, prognosis usually is good.

Metabolic complications of organ failure

Hepatic failure

Patients with liver disease of whatever cause (see Section 12) may develop acute hepatic coma or a more chronic form of hepatic encephalopathy with behavioural disturbance and other neurological symptoms.

Acute hepatic coma occurs with massive liver necrosis due to severe hepatitis or poisons such as paracetamol. In other patients, who may have relatively well preserved liver function but extensive portal-systemic shunts, coma may be precipitated by a sudden intake of nitrogenous substances as occurs with gastrointestinal bleeding, infections, or high protein diets. Confusion, apathy, and lack of concentration, or occasionally excitement requiring sedation, are rapidly followed by stupor and coma in the matter of a few hours or days. Characteristic findings are asterixis ('liver flap'), in which the outstretched hands show postural lapses, and hepatic foetor. Chorea and pyramidal signs may appear as the patient lapses into coma. Decerebrate posturing is common at this stage, and focal deficits such as hemiplegia may occur. Nystagmus, conjugate deviation of the eyes, skew deviation, and even disconjugate eye movements may be evident, but reflex eye movements and pupillary responses are preserved, until the patient becomes totally unresponsive and dies. Paroxysmal and later persistent high-voltage triphasic slow waves are present in the EEG until death is imminent. Many metabolic abnormalities may contribute to the cause of hepatic coma. Hyperammonaemia (more than 145 μmol/l or 200 mg/dl), which results from the products of intestinal digestion bypassing the urea-synthesizing mechanisms of the liver, has most often been held to be the main cause. However, hypoglycaemia and hyperventilation producing a respiratory alkalosis also are almost always present, and excessive amino acid release, absorption, or formation of toxic amines such as octopamine, and impaired uptake in the brain of short-chain monocarboxylic fatty acids such as acetate, butyrate, and pyruvate, also have been incriminated. Intravascular coagulation occurs, as do other coagulation defects leading to secondary vascular damage to the brain. Hepatic coma carries a high mortality, but if the patient can be kept alive, liver regeneration and recovery may occur. Treatment includes sterilizing the bowel, correction of metabolic and bleeding abnormalities, and haemoperfusion or other techniques to remove toxins.

Chronic hepatic encephalopathy refers to the development of changes in intellect, cognitive function, and consciousness, often accompanied by other neurological signs (such as tremor or chorea, an akinetic-rigid syndrome, ataxia, or even spastic paraparesis) occurring in those with chronic liver failure, and particularly in those with extensive portal-system anastomoses. The latter result in a large shunt of portal blood containing toxins absorbed from the gut direct to the brain, but the exact nature of the substances responsible for chronic hepatic encephalopathy has not been established. Characteristically the disorder fluctuates with episodes of marked confusion, excitement, or frank hepatic coma. In addition, intellectual changes, Parkinsonism, ataxia, or spasticity may gradually progress. Treatment consists of a low-protein diet and antibiotics to sterilize the gut. The place of other measures such as lactulose, levodopa, and liver transplantation remains to be established.

Renal failure

Renal failure (see Section 18) is associated with a variety of neurological complications. *Uraemic encephalopathy* was common before the use of dialysis. Patients become progressively drowsy, stuporose, and finally lapse into coma. Hyperventilation, multifocal myoclonus, tremor, asterixis, tetany, and generalized fits are common. Eye movements and pupillary reactions are not affected. Uraemia, metabolic acidosis, hyperkalaemia, hypocalcaemia, water intoxication, and hypertensive encephalopathy all contribute to the clinical picture. Dialysis rapidly reverses the metabolic abnormalitics of uraemia, but the encephalopathy may take days to clear. Many patients develop the *dialysis disequilibrium syndrome* during correction of their uraemic abnormalities. Rapid correction of the metabolic changes leads to the emergence of asterixis, myoclonus, delirium, generalized convulsions, stupor, and even coma. The blood–brain barrier is only slowly permeable to urea and other biological molecules, so that rapid correction of serum hyperosmolarity leaves the brain hyperosmolar relative to blood, resulting in a shift of water from plasma to brain. *Dialysis dementia* occurred in a proportion of those dialysed for years with water having a high aluminium content. The additional use of aluminium hydroxide gels to bind intestinal phosphate also may have contributed to excess aluminium intake. Such patients, after three to seven years of dialysis, begin to develop speech disturbance, intellectual and cognitive abnormalities, convulsions, myoclonus, and sometimes focal neurological abnormalities. Other complications of chronic renal failure include myopathy due to chronic hypocalcaemia, a peripheral neuropathy which may be resistant to dialysis, and Wernicke's encephalopathy due to chronic dialysis without vitamin supplements. Patients with renal disease are particularly prone to develop toxic complications of drugs normally excreted in the urine, as for example a peripheral neuropathy due to nitrofurantoin, labyrinthine damage due to streptomycin, or optic atrophy due to ethambutol.

Respiratory failure

Hypoventilation due to lung disease (see Section 15) or neurological disorders (page 21.248) can lead to encephalopathy or coma. Hypoxaemia, hypercapnia, congestive heart failure, systemic infection, fatigue due to laboured respiration, and nocturnal sleep apnoea all contribute to the syndrome. Serum acidosis by itself probably is not the important factor, since alkali infusions without ventilatory support do not improve cerebral function in these patients. They develop dull, diffuse headache, accompanied by progressive drowsiness, stupor, and coma. Eye movements and pupillary reactions are normal. However, a small proportion of such patients develop ophthalmic venous distension and papilloedema. Most exhibit asterixis and multifocal myoclonus but epileptic fits are unusual. Respiratory encephalopathy may begin gradually, or may be precipitated by infection or sedative drugs. All such patients hypoventilate, and those with obstructive emphysema gasp and puff. Oxygen therapy in these circumstances may be dangerous, for by removing the hypoxaemic drive to respiration, it may lead to lethal hypercapnia. If low concentrations of oxygen cause respiratory depression, assisted ventilation may be necessary.

Metabolic disorders due to endocrine disease

(See Sections 9 and 10.)

Diabetes mellitus

Diabetes causes a wide variety of neurological disturbances. Stupor or coma may be produced by hyperosmolality, ketoacidosis, lactic acidosis, hypoglycaemia due to treatment, uraemia, or hypertensive encephalopathy. Stroke due to cerebral arteriosclerosis is common in diabetics. Peripheral nerve damage may occur in established diabetics, or may be the presenting feature of the illness (see Section 9). Single nerve lesions (mononeuritis) such as isolated ocular nerve palsies, Bell's palsy, or a lateral popliteal nerve palsy, are common, and may result from haemorrhage or infarction of the nerve. A carpal tunnel syndrome or an ulnar nerve palsy may result from the undue susceptibility of peripheral nerves in diabetes to pressure palsies. Mononeuritis multiplex may

occur. Diabetic amyotrophy refers to the subacute weakness and wasting, often with pain, affecting quadriceps muscles usually asymmetrically. It is probably due to ischaemia or haemorrhage in the femoral nerve or lumbosacral plexus. Symmetrical peripheral neuropathy in diabetes may take the form of a mild or asymptomatic sensory neuropathy with loss of vibration sense in the feet and absent ankle jerks. Less commonly there is a severe and progressive predominantly sensory neuropathy affecting the legs before the arms. Autonomic neuropathy is common, producing impotence, diarrhoea, loss of sweating, and abnormal pupils. The latter may be irregular, and unreactive to light, mimicking Argyll Robertson pupils. Autonomic neuropathy causes orthostatic hypotension, syncope, and sometimes abrupt cardiac arrest in diabetics.

Cushing's syndrome

Spontaneous hyperadrenalism is most often due to adrenal tumour, but occasionally occurs with with a basophil pituitary adenoma as after adrenalectomy for breast cancer. Iatrogenic hyperadrenalism due to prolonged excessive steroid administration causes similar neurological symptoms. Cushing's syndrome frequently leads to an encephalopathy often manifest by behavioural changes such as elation or depression. Frank psychotic disturbance occasionally may be accompanied by headache and papilloedema, and may progress to stupor or coma. Cushing's syndrome also may be associated with proximal myopathy, which can be severe and painful.

Addison's disease

Hypoadrenalism due to adrenal failure causes hypotension, hyponatraemia, hyperkalaemia, and often hypoglycaemia as well. Patients with untreated Addison's disease complain of weakness and lassitude, and stupor or coma may be precipitated by surgical procedures or other acute illlness. Addisonian crisis may be accompanied by generalized convulsions, which are attributed to hyponatraemia and water intoxication. Benign intracranial hypertension with papilloedema and a proximal myopathy also may occur.

Myxoedema

Hypothyroidism may present as a toxic confusional state or frank dementing illness. Infection, trauma, exposure to cold, or sedation may provoke hypothermic coma. Episodic encephalopathy has been reported in patients with thyroiditis. Myxoedema is associated with the peculiar failure of relaxation of muscle (pseudomyotonia) which produces prolonged tendon jerks. The carpal tunnel syndrome may occur due to deposits of myxoedematous tissue around the median nerve of the wrist. Occasionally myxoedema may present as an ataxic syndrome suggesting cerebellar disease.

Thyrotoxicosis

Thyroid overactivity usually present with signs of nervous overactivity including anxiety, tremor, tachycardia, and fever. Chorea or mania may occur. A severe proximal myopathy is common. Dysthyroid eye disease may occur in hyperthyroid or euthyroid patients. Diplopia due to superior rectus weakness is the commonest initial symptom, but the condition may progress to external ophthalmoplegia with proptosis and chemosis.

Metabolic disorders due to ionic or acid–base abnormalities

Hyponatraemia or 'water intoxication'

Sodium is the most abundant serum cation, so that hyponatraemia (see Section 18) is almost always the cause of hypo-osmolality. Serum osmolality is approximately equal to double the serum sodium concentration plus 10, provided glucose and urea levels are normal. Normal serum osmolality is 290 ± 5 mosmol/kg;

serum osmolality below about 260 or above about 330 mosmol/kg is likely to produce cerebral changes. Hyponatraemia means that body water is increased relative to solute, resulting in water excess in the brain. Rapid changes in serum sodium osmolality produce much greater neurological effects than does slowly developing chronic hyponatraemia. Hyponatraemia occurs in renal disease as a result of excessive intravenous water infusions, or may result from inappropriate secretion of antidiuretic hormone that occurs in bronchial carcinoma, diffuse brain disease resulting from head injury, meningitis or encephalitis, or subarachnoid haemorrhage, or focal hypothalamic damage due to neoplasm or infection. Patients with hyponatraemia become confused and restless, and develop asterixis, multifocal myoclonus, generalized convulsions, stupor, and coma. Symptoms may appear when the plasma sodium drops below about 120 mmol/l, and fits and coma usually are associated with plasma sodium values below 110 mmol/l. A few patients with chronic hyponatraemia may develop the syndrome of central pontine myelinolysis (page 21.217). Treatment is by water restriction; infusions of hypertonic saline are rarely required.

Hypernatraemia
The common cause of hyperosmolality is diabetes, producing severe hyperglycaemia. Hyperosmolality due to hypernatraemia is rare. Chronic uncompensated water loss in untreated diabetes insipidus may result in mild hypernatraemia, but such patients only develop severe hypernatraemia if they fail to drink. Patients with simple diabetes insipidus usually maintain thirst, but if intercurrent illness leads to excessive water loss and restricted water intake, they may become dehydrated, drowsy, stuporose, and unconscious. Simple diabetes insipidus may be due to pituitary surgery, trauma, or pituitary tumours. If pathology extends into the hypothalamic region, not only may secretion of antidiuretic hormone be deficient, but thirst regulation also may be abolished. Hypothalamic damage causing severe hypernatraemia may occur in large pituitary tumours, craniopharyngiomas, hypothalamic tumours, sarcoidosis, or Hand–Schüller–Christian disease. Loss of thirst in such patients often precipitates hypernatraemic coma with serum sodium rising above 160–170 mmol/l. Hypernatraemia also may occur as a result of severe water depletion, particularly in children with intense diarrhoea.

Hypercalcaemia
A high serum calcium concentration may be due to primary hyperparathyroidism, immobilization, sarcoidosis, vitamin D intoxication, or multiple bony metastases. Symptoms include anorexia, nausea, vomiting, intense thirst, polyuria, and polydipsia. Muscle weakness, lassitude, and a mild encephalopathy are common. The latter may produce delusions and changes in mood so that many such patients are initially treated for a psychiatric condition. A toxic confusional state with generalized or focal seizures and papilloedema also may occur.

Hypocalcaemia
Reduced serum calcium concentration may be caused by parathyroid or thyroid surgery, chronic renal failure, or chronic anticonvulsant drug treatment. It also occurs in primary idiopathic hypoparathyroidism, and in Albright's syndrome of pseudohypoparathyroidism (in which there is no response to parathyroid hormone and skeletal deformities are present). Pseudopseudohypoparathyroidism refers to this syndrome with similar skeletal abnormalities but normal serum calcium. In all these conditions hypocalcaemia causes neuromuscular irritability, tetany with a positive Chvostek's sign, and a mild encephalopathy. Severe degrees of hypocalcaemia produce generalized convulsions, psychotic behavioural disturbances, stupor, and coma. Raised intracranial pressure with papilloedema may occur. Hypocalcaemia commonly is misdiagnosed as mental retardation, dementia, or epilepsy. Skin changes and cataracts are characteristic. Calcification in basal ganglia on skull X-ray or CT scan may be evident. Rarely, basal ganglia calcification may be associated with extra-pyramidal disorders.

Acid–base disturbances
Systemic acidosis and alkalosis (see Section 18) occur in many diseases causing metabolic coma, but of the four disorders of acid–base balance (respiratory acidosis and alkalosis, and metabolic acidosis and alkalosis) only respiratory acidosis acts as a direct cause of stupor and coma. Hypoxia associated with respiratory acidosis may be important in producing neurological abnormalities. Metabolic acidosis may be important in producing neurological abnormalities. Metabolic acidosis, by itself, usually only causes delirium or, at most, drowsiness. The reason why even severe disorders of systemic acid–base balance usually do not interfere with the function of the brain is that it possesses powerful mechanisms for protecting its own acid–base balance, including respiratory compensation, changes in cerebral blood flow, and cellular buffering in nervous tissue. Coma in metabolic acidosis due to diabetic ketosis or hyperosmolality, lactic acidosis, uraemia, alcohol poisoning, or intake of ethylene glycol, methyl alcohol, or paraldehyde is usually due to associated metabolic abnormalities or direct effects of other toxins in these conditions. Severe respiratory acidosis produces a reduction in alertness parallel to the degree of acidosis. Respiratory alkalosis, although constricting cerebral arterioles and decreasing cerebral blood flow, rarely interferes with cerebral function. A patient in coma with respiratory alkalosis due to hyperventilation, has some other condition such as sepsis, hepatic disease, pulmonary infarction, or salicylate overdose. Even severe metabolic alkalosis only produces a confusional state rather than stupor or coma.

Alcohol

Alcohol hits the nervous system in many ways. Some are the result of acute or chronic poisoning, while others are a consequence of associated vitamin deficiency. We are not concerned here with the acute effects of alcohol, such as drunkenness and delirium tremens, but with the neurological consequences of chronic, excessive alcohol intake.

The Wernicke–Korsakow syndrome
Aetiology
Inadequate intake of thiamine, of whatever cause, may lead to foci of marked hyperaemia with multiple small haemorrhages effecting particularly the upper brainstem, hypothalamus, and thalamus adjacent to the third ventricle, and the mamillary bodies. Histologically there is a proliferation of dilated capillaries with perivascular haemorrhage in these areas. The extent of such pathology can vary considerably from case to case, and may be associated with evidence of alcohol-induced damage to the cerebral cortex, cerebellum, and peripheral nerves.

Such pathology can be produced in animals by a diet deficient in thiamine. Thiamine deficiency can be demonstrated in patients with the Wernicke–Korsakow syndrome, and administration of thiamine can reverse many of the symptoms and signs of the Wernicke–Korsakow syndrome. Thiamine and its pyrophosphate is a cofactor to at least four enzymes, pyruvate decarboxylate, alpha-ketoglutarate dehydrogenase, the branched-chain ketoacid decarboxylase system, and transketolase. Thiamine deficiency results in reduced conversion of pyruvate to acetylCoA, causing elevated plasma and tissue pyruvate levels, with decreased flux through the Krebs cycle, reducing ATP production, and impairing energy supply. In addition, there is a shortage of acetyl groups for biosynthesis leading, amongst other effects, to reduced formation of acetylcholine. Other neurotransmitters also are affected, including glutamate and noradrenaline.

Alcoholism with an inadequate diet is the commonest cause

today. Malnutrition in prisoners of war, or at times of famine, also may be responsible. Chronic vomiting, for example, during pregnancy or due to gastrointestinal disease, is a rare cause.

Clinical features

The onset may be insidious or subacute with increasing lethargy and inattentiveness, which develops into a typical confusional state with disorientation in time and place, loss of memory, and altered consciousness. Ophthalmoplegia develops with diplopia. The commonest eye signs are nystagmus on lateral or vertical gaze, sixth nerve palsies, or defects of conjugate gaze. Retinal haemorrhages may occur. Most alcoholic patients will also have signs of a peripheral neuropathy, and many exhibit ataxia. Untreated, the patient lapses into stupor and then coma, and dies. Hypothermia may appear.

In less acute cases, or in those recovering from the acute confusional phase, the characteristic features of the Korsakow psychosis or amnesic syndrome will appear. The patient has a gross defect of memory for recent events, such that new information cannot be retained for more than a matter of minutes or hours. The patient is disorientated in time and place, but alert. Despite the severe defect of recent money, he or she can recall events in the remote past. Gaps in memory are filled by giving imaginary and often graphic accounts of events (confabulation). Many patients who recover from a severe episode of Wernicke–Korsakow syndrome are left with such an impaired recent memory that they can only function by writing all essential information into a book to replace their defective memory.

Diagnosis

Diagnosis is essentially clinical. Examination of the CSF is usually normal, although the protein may be slightly raised. A computerized tomography (CT) brain scan is normal, but it is worth remembering that alcoholics who fall are a common source of subdural haematomas. Demonstration of reduced red cell transketolase activity, or of raised plasma pyruvate levels, are often invalidated by intake of food as soon as the patient comes under supervision.

Treatment

The Wernicke–Korsakow syndrome must be considered in any individual with unexplained confusion, stupor or coma, particularly in the presence of eye signs, a peripheral neuropathy, or a history of alcoholism or excessive vomiting. Thiamine should be given to all such patients. Usually this is in the form of combined vitamin B and C by an injection containing 250 mg of thiamine. Such high potency vitamin injections should be given daily until oral vitamin B complex preparations can be taken.

A particular problem arises commonly in the Emergency Department when cases of stupor or coma of unknown cause are admitted. All such patients should be given high-dose thiamine and glucose parenterally. The risk is if glucose is given *without* thiamine to a patient with the Wernicke–Korsakow syndrome, for this leads to rapid deterioration and death. Those who are thiamine deficient cannot handle the glucose load. The emergency-room doctor always needs two syringes in this situation, one with glucose, the other with thiamine.

Effective treatment will restore consciousness and reverse eye signs, but unfortunately the Korsakow amnesic syndrome frequently does not resolve. The earlier the treatment, the better the chances of recovery, so suspicion or possibility of diagnosis is a medical emergency.

Alcoholic peripheral neuropathy

(See also page 21.126.)

Aetiology

As with the Wernicke–Korsakow syndrome, thiamine deficiency is thought to play an important role in the production of the peripheral neuropathy associated with chronic alcoholism. Pathologically the picture of peripheral nerve damage is very similar to that seen in beri-beri. There is a predominantly axonal neuropathy of the 'dying back' type, affecting the somatic and sometimes the autonomic nerves. However, pure thiamine deficiency may not be the sole cause of such a neuropathy. Other vitamin deficiencies may contribute, and a direct toxic effect of alcohol on peripheral nerves may occur.

Clinical features

Alcoholic peripheral neuropathy predominantly involves sensory nerves, producing distal paraesthesiae in feet followed by the hands, and characteristic pain. The latter may be intense and agonizing. Squeezing the calves or scratching the soles of the feet may cause severe discomfort. At a later stage, weakness and wasting of the distal muscles of the legs and arms follows. Tendon reflexes are lost. Evidence of autonomic neuropathy may be seen in abnormal pupillary reactions and tachycardia, although postural hypotension is rare and the sphincters are usually spared.

Treatment

Alcohol must be proscribed and high-potency vitamin B given parenterally for some 10 days and then orally. Prognosis depends on how early treatment is commenced. Symptoms may take a few weeks to recover, but in more severe cases recovery may take many months or may be incomplete.

Alcoholic cerebellar degeneration

Some alcoholics may develop a relatively pure syndrome of ataxia, with a progressive unsteadiness of gait and of leg movements, with little or no involvement of the arms. Speech is not affected, and nystagmus is not present. Many such patients also have evidence of alcoholic peripheral neuropathy. Pathologically there is degeneration of the cerebellar cortex, particularly of the Purkinje cells, and also of the olivary nuclei. Changes in the cerebellum characteristically affect the anterior and superior parts of the vermis and hemispheres. This complication of alcoholism does not seem to be due to thiamine deficiency. However, withdrawal of alcohol and vitamin replacement can lead to recovery.

Alcoholic dementia

(See also page 21.42 and Section 25.)

In the past, there has been much debate over whether alcoholism produces dementia. However, it is now clear that a large proportion of those who habitually take excessive alcohol develop cognitive deficits. These can vary from mild changes to severe diffuse global dementia. They are associated with evidence of atrophy of the cerebral cortex and enlargement of the cerebral ventricles on CT brain scan.

The dementia has the usual features of change of personality, loss of memory, impairment of intellectual capacity, and emotional instability. Such patients commonly fail at work or in marriage. The gradual drift into destitution is only too well described in the literature and recognized on the streets. Head injuries in alcoholic bouts and epilepsy may occur and contribute to the overall final picture. The fully developed case of the 'down and out' is an antisocial demented individual, with dysarthric speech, tremor, an ataxic gait, and a peripheral neuropathy, who still clutches to the bottle and a bag of residual belongings.

The dementia of alcoholism is not directly related to thiamine deficiency alone. Treatment by withdrawal of alcohol, if possible, and vitamin replacement can lead to improvement. Indeed, some degree of reversal of evidence of cerebral atrophy on CT brain scan can be seen after drying out. However, the prognosis is generally poor, not least because of the difficulties of persuading such people to stop drinking.

Marchiafava–Bignami disease

This rare disease was first described in Italian drinkers of crude red wine, but occurs in other alcoholics. It presents as a subacute dementing illness, which progresses rapidly to fits, rigidity, and paralysis, culminating in coma and death within a few months. Pathologically there is widespread demyelination and axonal damage in the corpus callosum and the central white matter of the cerebral hemispheres, as well as in the optic chiasma and middle cerebellar peduncles.

Central pontine myelinolysis (page 21.217)

This is another rare disease, occurring in alcoholics and a number of other illnesses including severe liver and renal disease, and other metabolic disturbances. A common association is with hyponatraemia, and rapid attempts to correct serum sodium by parenteral fluids. The disease is characterized by a rapidly progressive flaccid or spastic quadriplegia, with involvement of bulbar muscles to produce dysarthria and dysphagia. Consciousness and eye movement may remain intact. At worst the patient may be unable to speak or swallow, or to move any muscle except those of the eyes. Death is common, but remarkable recovery may occur.

Alcoholic myopathy

Acute alcohol poisoning can produce a dramatic toxic myopathy. There is severe pain, muscle tenderness, and oedema, and weakness, which may be associated with myoglobinuria, renal damage and hyperkalaemia. A subacute painless myopathy resolving after withdrawal of alcohol also has been described.

Tobacco–alcohol amblyopia

Another uncommon complication of alcohol occurs in combination with strong tobacco. The patient develops sudden or subacute bilateral visual failure, associated with bilateral centrocaecal scotomas. The condition has been attributed to cyanide in tobacco causing a disorder of vitamin B_{12} metabolism. Visual failure and optic atrophy may occur in patients with pernicious anaemia, particularly those who smoke. A related condition is tropical amblyopia, occurring in Africa. This has been related to excessive consumption of cassava root containing cyanide. Treatment of these conditions is with hydroxycobalamine injections.

Other deficiency states

Vitamin B_{12} and folic acid deficiencies are considered on page 21.101 and in Section 19. Other B group vitamins are discussed in Section 8.

References

Metabolic diseases

Arieff, A. I., Cooper, J. D., Armstrong, D. and Lazarowitz, V. C. (1979). Dementia, renal failure, and brain aluminium. *Ann. Intern. Med*, **90**, 741–747.

Bulens, C. (1981). Neurologic complication of hyperthyroidism. *Arch. Neurol.* **38**, 669–670.

Cogan, M. G., Covey, C. M., Arieff, A. I., Wisniewski, A. and Clark, O. H. (1978). Central nervous system manifestations of hyperparathyroidism. *Am. J. Med.* **65**, 563–630.

Drake, F. R. (1957). Neuropsychiatric-like symptomatology of Addison's disease: A review of the literature. *Am. J. Med.* **234**, 106–113.

Glaser, G. H. (1960). Metabolic encephalopathy in hepatic, adrenal or pulmonary disorders. *Postgrad. Med. J.* **27**, 611–628.

Haussain, M. (1970). Neurological and psychiatric manifestations of idiopathic hypoparathyroidism: Response to treatment. *J. Neurol. Neurosurg. Psychiat.* **33**, 153–156.

Jellinek, E. H. and Kelly, R. E. (1960). Cerebellar syndrome in myxoedema. *Lancet* **ii**, 225–227.

Krieger, D. T. (1972). The central nervous system in Cushing's syndrome. *Mt Sinai J. Med*, **39**, 416–428.

Lester, M. C. and Nelson, P. B. (1981). Neurological aspects of vasopressin release and the syndrome of inappropriate secretion of antidiuretic hormone. *Neurosurgery* **8**, 735–740.

Locke, S., Merrill, J. T. and Tyler, H. R. (1961). Neurologic complications of acute uraemia. *Arch. Intern. Med*, **108**, 519–525.

Raskin, N. H. and Fishman, R. A. (1976). Neurologic disorders in renal failure. *N. Engl. J. Med.* **294**, 143–148, 204–210.

Richardson, J. C., Chambers, R. A. and Haywood, P. M. (1959). Encephalopathies of anoxia and hypoglycaemia. *Arch. Neurol.* **1**, 178–190.

Resnick, M. E. and Patterson, C. (1969). Coma and convulsions due to compulsive water drinking. *Neurology Minn*, **19**, 1125–1126.

Sanders, V. (1962). Neurologic manifestations of myxoedema *N. Engl. J. Med*, **266**, 547–552, 559.

Summerskill, W. H. J., Davidson, E. A., Sherlock, S. and Steiner, R. E. (1956). The neuropsychiatric syndrome associated with hepatic cirrhosis and an extensive portal collateral circulation. *Q. J. Med*, **25**, 245–266.

Wilkinson, D. S. and Prockop, L. D. (1976). Hypoglycaemia: effects on the nervous system. In *Handbook of clinical neurology* Vol. 27 (eds P. J. Vinken and G. W. Bruyn) pp. 53–78. Elsevier North Holland, New York.

Alcohol

Harper, C. (1983). The incidence of Wernicke's encephalopathy in Australia – A neuropathological study of 131 cases. *J. Neurol. Neurosurg. Psychiat.* **46**, 593–598.

Lishman, W. A. (1981). Cerebral disorder in alcoholism: Syndromes of impairment. *Brain* **104**, 1–20.

Ron, M. A. (1977). Brain damage in chronic alcoholism: Neuropathological, neuroradiological and psychological review. *Psychol. Med.* **7**, 103–112.

Ron, M. A., Acker, W., Shaw, G. K. and Lishman, W. A. (1982). Computerized tomography of the brain in chronic alcoholism. *Brain* **105**, 497–514.

Victor, M. and Adams, R. D. (1953). The effect of alcohol on the nervous system. *Res. Publ. Assoc. Res. Nerve Ment. Dis.* **32**, 526–573.

Victor, M., Adams, R. D. and Mancall, E. L. (1959). A restricted form of cerebellar cortical degeneration occurring in alcoholic patients. *Arch. Neurol.* **1**, 579–688.

Victor, M. and Dreyfus, P. M. (1965). Tobacco–alcohol amblyopia. Further comments on its pathology. *Arch. Ophthalmol.* **74**, 649–657.

Victor, M., Adams, R. D. and Collins G. H. (1971). *Wernicke–Korsakoff syndrome.* F. A. Davis, Philadelphia.

NEUROLOGICAL DISORDERS DUE TO PHYSICAL AGENTS

C. D. MARSDEN

More detailed accounts of the conditions described here can be found in Section 6. The discussion below summarizes the main neurological features.

Heat stroke

Heat stroke occurs in both young people undertaking excessive exercise in unaccustomed heat, and in older people or those taking anticholinergic drugs (for instance, those with Parkinson's disease) exposed to high temperatures. Anything that interferes with sweating may provoke heat stroke. Usually, such patients become agitated and confused, before passing into stupor or coma, often with generalized convulsions. The patient's skin usually is hot and dry, and there is tachycardia and hypotension. Death due to circulatory collapse occurs unless the patient is rapidly cooled. Some patients who survive heat stroke are left with permanant neurological complications, including amnesia, dysarthria, ataxia, dementia, and hemiparesis. Occasionally, polyneuropathy may complicate hyperthermia.

Malignant hyperthermia is a rare disorder of muscle metabolism characterized by a sudden fulminating unexpected increase in body metabolism amd temperature in patients exposed to anaesthetics. High fever, respiratory and metabolic acidosis, and diffuse muscular rigidity occur in susceptible individuals given anaesthetic agents such as halothane or succinylcholine. Malignant hyperthermia occurs as a result of an abnormality of muscle metabolism which is inherited as an autosomal dominant trait. It affects approximately one in 20 000 of patients exposed to anaesthesia (see Section 7).

Hypothermia

Accidental hypothermia follows prolonged exposure to cold on mountains or in water. Hypothermia may also occur in the elderly without food and heating, and in myxoedema or hypopituitarism. A low body temperature also occurs in metabolic coma due to hypoglycaemia and drug overdose, particularly with barbiturates, phenothiazines, or alcohol. The hypothermic patient gradually lapses into confusion, stupor, then coma. Respirations are slow and shallow, shivering is usually absent, the pulse is very slow, and blood pressure may be unmeasurable. Such patients are sometimes thought to be dead when first seen. Body temperature is usually less than 32.2° C.

Decompression sickness

This condition ('the bends') affects deep-sea divers, tunnel workers operating in a pressurized atmosphere, and amateur scuba divers unaccustomed to depth. It is due to release of bubbles of nitrogen into the blood during a too-rapid decompression, causing gas emboli and micro-infarction in the nervous system. That a sudden reduction in pressure may cause liberation of gas bubbles is familiar to all who remove the top of a carbonated drink. Since nitrogen is especially soluble in body fat, it is liberated in large amounts in the nervous system, and fat men are more liable to decompression sickness than those of thinner habitus. Neurological symptoms include hemiplegia, paraplegia, visual disturbance, and vertigo. Any neurological symptoms indicate the need for urgent recompression in a compressed air chamber, with subsequent controlled slow decompression. Neurological recovery usually is slow, but may be complete.

Electrical injury

Electrocution may be immediately fatal due to cardiac arrest. Less severe electrical shocks cause local burns and tissue necrosis. Changes in the nervous system are most likely to occur when the current has been applied to the skull. A severe electric shock causes immediate coma. Lesser shocks may lead to severe pain associated with hemiplegia, a flaccid paraplegia or tetraplegia, or peripheral nerve damage. Such acute neurological complications of electrical injury may disappear after about 12 hours, but some are permanent. Delayed effects of electric shock have been recorded, including a delayed myelopathy and neuropathy, not unlike motor neurone disease.

Radiation injury

Damage to the nervous system may be produced by radiotherapy directed at cerebral or spinal tumours, or may occur incidentally as a result of radiation employed to treat tumours elsewhere, such as those of the neck, ear or breast. *Radiation myelopathy* may develop acutely during radiotherapy concentrated in the region of the cord, or may appear much later. Acute radiation myelopathy usually is transient and recovers within a matter of weeks. However, a slowly progressive paraparesis or tetraparesis may occur within one to four years after a course of radiation in the region of the cord. Weakness, spasticity, and sensory loss gradually develop, usually with sphincter impairment, and progress inexorably. The dose of radiation nearly always exceeds 4000 rad and usually is of the order of 6000–8000 rad. *Radiation encephalopathy* follows similar large doses applied to the head, as for example have been employed in the treatment of pituitary tumours. Radiation necrosis may cause swelling, producing the appearances of a temporal lobe tumour, or multifocal white matter degeneration. Irradiation in the region of the optic nerves or brachial plexus very occasionally may cause delayed optic atrophy or brachial neuropathy. Delayed radiation necrosis appears to be mainly the result of vascular damage with ischaemic change. There is no known treatment. This topic is discussed in Section 19.

References

Burns, R. A., Jones, A. N. and Robertson, J. S. (1972). Pathology of radiation myelopathy. *J. Neurol, Neurosurg. Psychiat.* **35**, 888–898.

Davis, J. C., Tager, R., Polkovitz, H. T. and Workman, R. D. (1971). Neurological decompression sickness. *Aerospace Med.* **42**, 85–94.

Jellinger, K. and Sturm, K. W. (1971). Delayed radiation myelopathy in man. *J. neurol. Sci.* **14**, 389–393.

Mehta, A. C. and Baker, R. N. (1970). Persistent neurological deficits in heat stroke. *Neurology, Minneap.* **20**, 336–340.

GEOGRAPHICAL VARIATIONS IN NEUROLOGICAL DISEASE

Subacute myelo-optico-neuropathy (SMON) in Japan

K. NAKAE

Clinical features

Subacute myelo-optico neuropathy (SMON) is a condition characterized clinically by an acute or subacute onset of dysaesthesiae in the lower extremities accompanied by a variable degree of weakness and visual loss, preceded by abdominal symptoms such as diarrhoea, constipation, and pain, and pathologically by the presence of symmetrical degeneration of the peripheral nerves, spinal cord, particularly posterior column and corticospinal tract, and in many cases, the optic nerve and tract.

Table 1 shows the clinical diagnostic guidelines of this disease

set up by the SMON Research Committee of Japan in 1969 when the aetiological agent had not yet been revealed. Table 2 shows the frequencies of symptoms and signs in the patients with SMON which were obtained by a nationwide survey in Japan. In typical cases the abdominal pain is so severe that it is only relieved by narcotics or corticosteroids. The dysaesthesiae may be so marked as to disturb patients' sleep. It often begins in the soles and rapidly spreads to more proximal parts of lower extremities, and in severe cases further up the trunk and to the distal ends of upper extremities. It is usually described as an unpleasant numbness, rather like sponge or rubber adhering to the soles, tightness or squeezing sensation around the ankles or feet, or a sensation of scrubbing, tingling, thrusting or stabbing. Greenish discoloration of the dorsum of tongue, which is the only specific feature of SMON outside the nervous system, is observed in more than a half of cases in the

Table 1 Clinical diagnostic guideline of SMON (SMON Research Commission of Japan)

Cardinal signs
1 Abdominal symptoms (abdominal pain, diarrhoea, etc.) before the onset of neurological symptoms
2 Acute or subacute onset of bilateral ascending paresthesia and dysesthesia of the lower extremities
Other major signs
1 Impairment of deep sensation and weakness in the lower limbs, with or without pyramidal signs
2 Less commonly, sensorimotor disturbances in the upper limbs.
3 Occasionally, one or more of the following: (a) bilateral impairment of vision; (b) disturbances of consciousness, convulsions, psychic symptoms, and other cerebral symptoms; (c) greenish discoloration of the tongue and faeces; (d) sphincter disturbances
4 Protracted course with occasional relapses
5 No significant laboratory findings in the blood and cerebrospinal fluid
6 Rare occurrence in children

Table 3 Criteria for histological diagnosis of SMON (Pathological section of SMON Research Commission)

1 Bilateral and almost symmetrical degeneration is confined to the long tracts of the spinal cord and to the peripheral nerves. Degeneration is severer towards the termination of the neuron
   Spinal cord
   (a) Fasciculus gracilis (Goll) shows most evident degeneration
   (b) The lateral pyramidal tracts are affected
   (c) The anterior horn neurons in the lumbar cord show central chromatolysis
   Peripheral nerves
   (a) Degeneration in the lower extremities is more severe than in the upper
   (b) Degeneration in the posterior roots is more severe than in the anterior
   (c) Neurons of the dorsal root ganglia are affected
   (d) The autonomic nervous system is affected
2 Other parts of the nervous system may also be affected in some cases
   (a) The optic tract, chiasma and occasionally the ganglion cells of the retina are affected
   (b) The olivary nucleus is affected
3 Such definite changes seen above are not usually found in the cerebrum and cerebellum

acute stage. The fatality rate of SMON was about 3–4 per cent in the period of an endemic outbreak but decreased to about 1 per cent after a marked decline of the occurrence of the disease. About a half of the patients returned to a normal life within 1–2 years, but with some residual sensory disorder, and 10–15 per cent were completely incapacitated.

Pathological features
Table 3 shows the criteria for the histological diagnosis of SMON. The most important pathological findings are restricted to the central and/or peripheral nervous tissues and the optic nerve. The histopathological findings have the following characteristics: (a) symmetrical axonal degeneration and demyelination in Goll's and pyramidal tracts of the spinal cord, the optic nerve, and the peripheral nerves of the lower extremities; (b) the absence of inflammatory changes in nervous tissues; (c) similarity of the changes to those of subacute combined degeneration of the spinal cord (see page 21.101).

Epidemiological features
SMON is rare outside Japan, although some reports suggest that a clioquinol-induced neurological disorder indistinguishable from SMON has occurred in Asia outside Japan, and in Europe, and the United States. The nationwide epidemiologic survey of Japan

Table 2 Frequencies of clinical symptoms and signs in 5839 patients with SMON (Toyokura and Takasu, 1975)

Symptoms and signs	Frequencies (%)	Recoveries (%)
Abdominal symptoms	99	42.5
Abdominal pain	75	
Diarrhoea	68	
Other	9	
Onset of neurologic symptoms		40.0
Gradual	20	
Acute or subacute	80	
Sensory disturbances	98	43.0
Bilateral	75	
Predominant in lower limbs	86	
Upper level obscure	33	
Dysesthesiae	95	94.9
Adhering	18	
Squeezed or tightened up	15	
Scrubbed, thrust, or stabbed	24	
Deep sensation disturbance in lower limbs	68	37.0
Muscular weakness in lower limbs	73	92.0
Pyramidal signs	67	39.0
Hyperreflexia in lower limbs	52	
Babinski sign	17	
Other	3	
Motor disturbances in upper limbs	7	41.0
Sensory disturbances in upper limbs	16	40.3
Bilateral visual disturbances	25	93.0
Cerebral or psychic symptoms	8	40.3
Green tongue	15	36.3
Green faeces	8	33.5
Bladder or rectal disturbances	19	88.0
Protracted course	76	36.9
Relapses	26	34.9
Blood abnormalities	7	31.1
CSF abnormalities	3	18.5

revealed that, at the end of 1975, there have been 11 127 patients with SMON. It disclosed that 80 per cent of cases occurred from January 1966 to August 1970, i.e. 924 in 1966, 1616 in 1967, 2002 in 1968, 2778 in 1969, and 1540 prior to August 1970. A steep reduction in new cases was observed after September 1970, i.e. 85 from September to December in 1970, 58 in 1971, 11 in 1972, 1 in 1973, and none after 1974. Children under 10 years of age are rarely affected (0.22 per cent); the peak incidence is at the age of 34–44 years in males and 50–64 years in females. The female/male ratio is 2.04 after the age of 20 years.

Morbidity rates classified by occupation of SMON patients were 10.4 per 100 000 population in clerical workers, and 7.7 in medical and paramedical personnel, and 7.5 in housewives, whereas the rates were only 2.1 in farmers, 1.8 in fishermen, 2.2 in mine industry workers, and 2.6 in traffic services workers. The geographical distribution of SMON in Japan does not follow any particular pattern. Other epidemiological features are as follows: (a) a seasonal outbreak in the summer was observed in 1967–69 when the SMON epidemic was at its peak in Japan; (b) familial aggregation of occurrence was sometimes observed in endemic areas, although it was recognized in only 3 per cent of the patients (c) clustering of the patients to some medical institutions or doctors, who were not always neurologists; (d) an endemic in a small city or town continued for several years, although the disease was usually sporadic in most other areas of Japan; (e) a previous history of pulmonary tuberculosis or abdominal operation were positively related with the occurrence of SMON.

Aetiology

Extensive efforts were directed to find any causative microbial agent, as infection seemed to be the most plausible basis for the disease from the epidemiological findings. Several cytopathic (CP) agents, i.e. echovirus type 21, coxsackie A group viruses, herpes-like virus, and enterovirus-like agent were isolated from the spinal cord, spinal fluid, blood, and faeces. However, they are unlikely to be the aetiological agents because these findings were not consistent. Furthermore, the marked decrease of SMON after September 1970 is not adequately explained on an infective basis.

On the contrary, clioquinol (Enterovioform) intoxication can explain most of epidemiological and neuropathological findings of SMON; the evidence can be summarized as follows: (a) The proportion of SMON patients who took clioquinol during the six months before the onset of the neurological symptoms was in the range 63–100 per cent. The best estimate is 82 per cent. This figure is much higher for patients who developed SMON than those without SMON but with abnormal symptoms (10–25 per cent). (b) In almost all areas with SMON outbreaks during 1955–69, a close relationship between clioquinol intake and the occurrence of SMON was disclosed. (c) The decrease of the occurrence of SMON after September 1970 could be ascribed to the Japanese Government banning the scale of clioquinol on 7 September 1970.

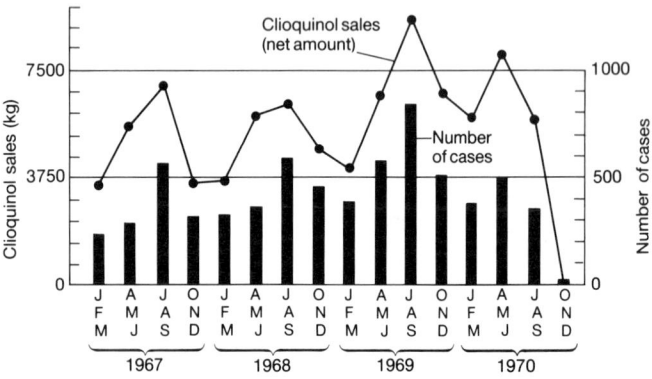

Fig. 1 Relationship between quarterly amount of clioquinol sale and number of SMON occurrences. (Reproduced by courtesy of Dr R. Kono.)

Figure 1 shows the relation between net weight of clioquinol sold and the number of SMON occurrences from 1967 to 1970. (d) A dose–response relationship exists between the amount of clioquinol taken and the incidence of SMON (Figs 2–4). Figure 2 shows the probability density function obtained by the differential of the sigmoid curve in Fig. 3. This function takes the shape of a normal logarithmic curve coinciding with the dose–response curve obtained from experiments in animals. Figure 4 suggests that, even in cases with the same total clioquinol intake, the higher the daily dose, the higher the incidence rate of SMON. It was also found by autopsy examination that a close relation was observed between the severity of pathological changes in the nervous system and the total dose administered. (e) Neuropathological changes extremely similar to SMON in humans can be produced in experimental animals. (f) At the cellular level, clioquinol exerts a hazardous effect on the electron transport system in mitochondria. In vitro experiments suggest that a minimum toxic dose of clioquinol is about 6–8 μg/ml in the medium.

Thus although many other toxic agents have been suggested as candidates for causing SMON, there is overwhelming epidemiolo-

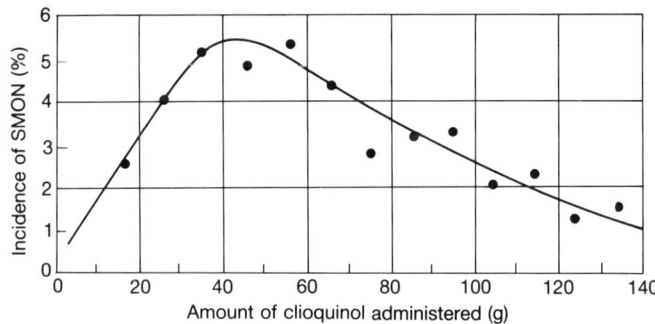

Fig. 2 Probability density distribution of dose–response relationship between clioquinol intake and incidence of SMON. (Reproduced from Nakae and Shibata, 1978, with permission.)

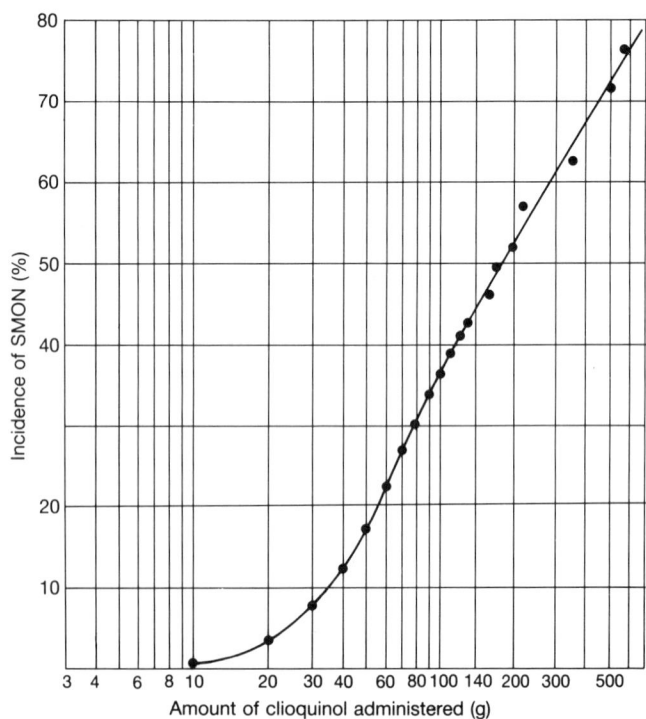

Fig. 3 Corrected dose–response relationship between clioquinol intake and incidence of SMON. (Reproduced from Nakae and Shibata, 1978, with permission.)

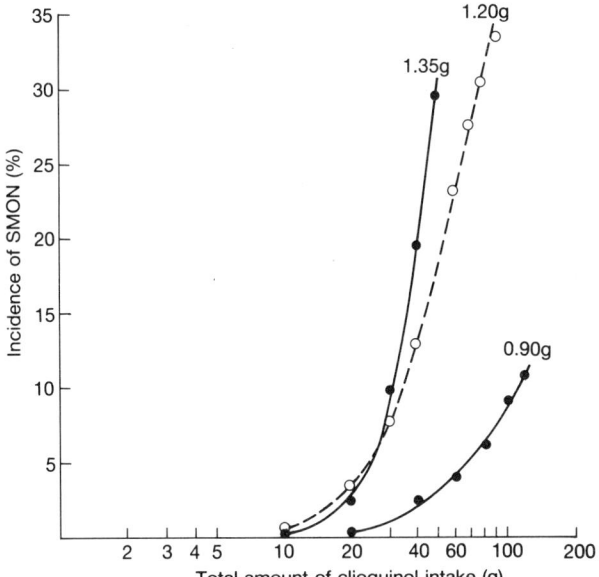

Fig. 4 Corrected dose–response relationship between clioquinol intake and incidence of SMON by daily dose. (Reproduced from Nakae and Shibata, 1978, with permission.)

gical evidence that clioquinol was the major cause of the disease in Japan.

References

Inoue, Y. K. Nishibe, Y. and Nakamura, Y. (1971). Virus associated with SMON in Japan. *Lancet* **i**, 853.

Kodama, H., Egarashi, Y., Otani, S. and Ohkawa, T. (1973). Experiments to reproduce human neuropathology of SMON in monkeys and dogs by oral administration of clioquinol. *Tr. Soc. Path. Jpn.* **62**, 122 (in Japanese).

Kono, R. (1975). Introductory review of subacute myelo-optico-neuropathy (SMON) and its studies done by the SMON Research Commission. *Jpn. J. Med. Sci. Biol.* **28**, Suppl., 1.

Nakae, K., Yamamoto, S. and Igata, A. (1971). Subacute myelo-optico-neuropathy (SMON) in Japan: a community survey. *Lancet*, **ii**, 510.

Nakae, K., Yamamoto, S., Shigematsu, I. and Kono R. (1973). Relation between subacute myelo-optico-neuropathy (SMON) and clioquinol; nationwide survey. *Lancet*, **i**, 171.

Nakae, K. and Shibata, T. (1978). *A hospital survey on SMON in the Japanese town of Yubara. Epidemiological issues in reported drug-induced illnesses; SMON and other examples*, p. 216. McMaster University Library Press, Hamilton, Ontario.

Shigematsu, I., Yanagawa, H., Yamamoto, S. and Nakae, K. (1975). Epidemiological approach to SMON (subacute myelo-optico-neuropathy). *Jpn. J. Med. Sci. Biol.* **28**, Suppl. 23.

SMON Research Commission (1971). Survey of chinoform administration in SMON patients. *Reports of SMON Research Commission*, No. 8, p. 81 (in Japanese).

SMON Research Commission, Section of Pathology (1975). A short history of autopsy of SMON in Japan and peripheral lesions of the spinal cord in 113 autopsy cases. *Jpn. J. Med. Sci. Biol.* **28**, Suppl. 63.

Sobue, I., Aoki, K. and Otani M. (1975). Prognosis of SMON patients. *Jpn. J. Med. Sci. Biol.* **28**, Suppl. 203.

Tamura, Z. (1975). Clinical chemistry clioquinol. *Jpn. J. Med. Sci. Biol.* **28**, Suppl. 69.

Tagaya, I. (1975). Summarized report of research works by the members of the virology subsection, the Microbiology Section. *Jpn. J. Med. Sci. Biol.* **28**, Suppl. 197.

Tateishi, J. and Otsuki, S. (1975). Experimental reproduction of SMON in animals by prolonged administration of clioquinol; clinico-pathological findings. *Jpn. J. Med. Sci. Biol.* **28**, Suppl. 165.

Toyokura, Y. and Takasu, T. (1975). Clinical features of SMON. *Jpn. J. Med. Sci. Biol.* **28**, Suppl. 87.

Toyokura, Y., Takasu, T. and Mitsuoka, O. (1975). Experimental studies utilizing radio-nuclides of clioquinol as tracer *in vivo*. *Jpn. J. Med. Sci. Biol.* **28**, Suppl. 79.

Yanagawa, H. (1978). *Observations on the decrease in SMON cases in Japan before the suspension of clioquinol sales. Epidemiological issues in reported drug-induced illnesses; SMON and other examples*. McMaster University Library Press, p. 196.

South America

J.O. TRELLES AND L. TRELLES

The prevalence and incidence of neurological disease has not been studied in all the countries of South America. The remarkable racial heterogeneity of the population, the tropical climate, and the extremely high birth rate and low mean age of the population, may all contribute to the difference in the spectrum of neurological disease between Latin American and other populations. There is a general agreement that multiple sclerosis and cerebrovascular disease are much less common than in European or North American populations. On the other hand, epilepsy and the neurological complications of certain parasitic conditions such as cysticercosis, Chagas disease, Bartonellosis, and hydatid disease are very common.

Multiple sclerosis

The incidence of this condition is not known although it appears to be higher in Argentina and Chile. Overall, however, it is much less common than in European populations. Preliminary studies suggest that the disease is seen in an older age group than in European populations and that the pattern of neurological involvement may be different.

Bartonellosis

The clinical and diagnostic features of this condition are described in detail in Section 5. Neurological complications are frequently seen in South America. During the acute phase of the illness the central nervous system may be involved, giving rise to meningoencephalitis or meningomyelitis. The former is characterized by a reduced level of consciousness, generalized convulsions, and cerebellar or pyramidal syndromes. A spinal form is well recognized and is characterized by paraplegia or quadriplegia. Recently, a variety of this condition has been described under the term *pseudopoliomyelitis*; it appears to result from an occlusion of the branches of the anterior spinal artery. These neurological complications result from direct invasion of the nervous system and proliferation of the vascular endothelium of arteries and capillaries. There is a breakdown in the blood–brain barrier and the organism enters the brain, producing microglial nodules. The neuropathology of this condition is shown in Fig. 1.

Neurocysticercosis

The clinical features of cysticercosis are described in detail in Section 5. The neurological disorders, which are seen frequently in South America, are classified into cerebral and spinal forms. The former is associated with signs of raised intracranial pressure, epilepsy, and an organic psychiatric syndrome characterized by progressive dementia. In the spinal form the majority of cases, though not all, involve the cervical region. The neurological picture is that of a compressive lesion of the cord. These conditions can be best diagnosed by demonstration of the lesions directly by CAT scanning.

Pathology

There are two main pathological varieties, cystic and racemose. In the former, the vesicles are located principally in the cerebral cortex and the meninges, and occasionally in the brain stem and cervical cord. Racemose cysticercosis is characterized by the presence, mainly in the optic cistern, of large vesicles of variable morphology in which the vesicular membrane develops enor-

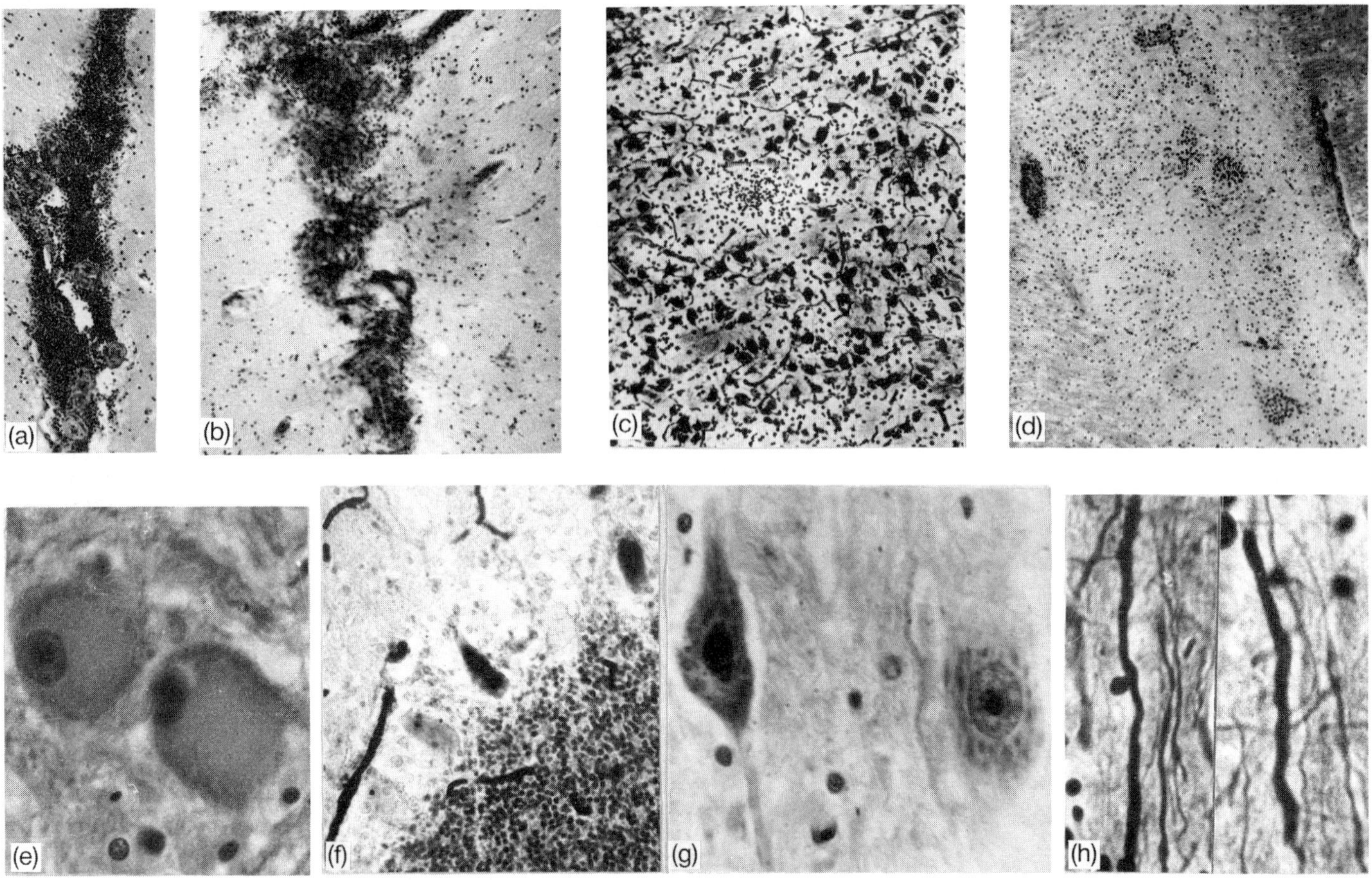

Fig. 1 Bartonellosis involving the nervous system. (a) and (b) Meningocortical lesions. (c) Marked glial proliferation with the formation of microglial nodules. (d) Perivascular infiltration with the formation of microglial nodules in the hippocampus. (e) Ischaemic cells in the nucleus of Bechterew. (f) Dilated capillaries with thrombotic lesions. (g) Purkinje cells showing hyperchromia and ischaemic changes. (h) Axonal lesions.

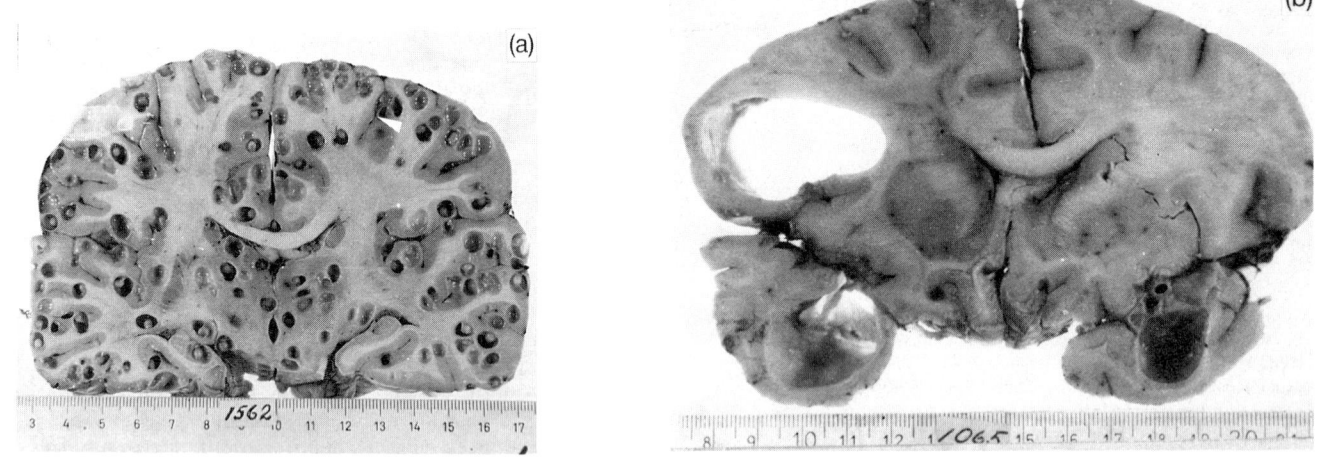

Fig. 2 Cysticercosis of the nervous system. (a) Massive invasion of the cortex and central grey nucleus. (b) A large cystic lesion page 21.262. (c) Macroscopic and microscopic changes showing intramedullary cysticercosis. (d) Hydatic cyst located in pariet-occipital areas.

mously. This membrane has ciliary and conciliary structure, through which the parasite is in contact with the surrounding tissue. The neuropathology of this condition is shown in Fig. 2a–d on pages 21.262 and 21.263.

Chagas disease

The pathogenesis and clinical features of this condition are described in Section 5. Neurological complications are common in South America. *Trypanosoma cruzi* can affect the central nervous system, the autonomic system or the peripheral nerves. Both acute and chronic forms of neurological involvement are observed. In the acute phase, associated with fever, lymphadenopathy and hepatosplenomegaly, there is often a meningoencephalitis. The chronic manifestations involve mainly the autonomic nervous system and are responsible for many of the common abnormalities of cardiac, oesophageal, and intestinal function.

Hydatid disease

Intracerebral hydatid disease is seen very frequently in South America, both in children and adults. Cerebral hydatid disease

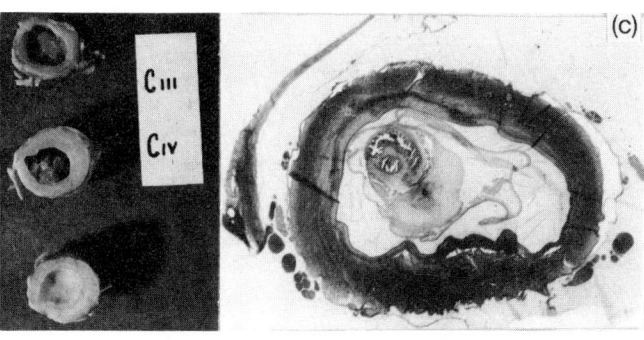

(c)

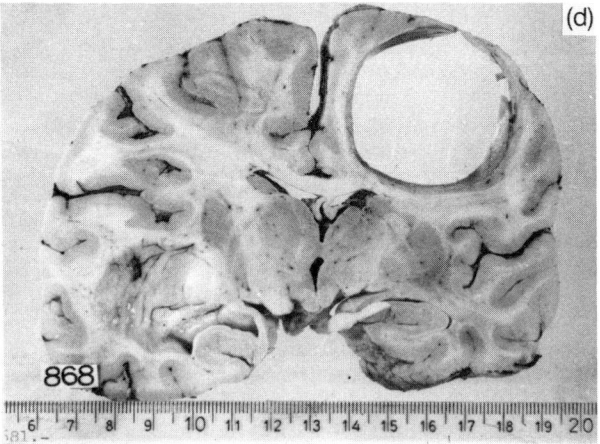

(d)

Fig. 2 Cysticercosis of the nervous system (*cont.*).

usually presents with a syndrome of raised intracranial pressure with a wide variety of focal signs depending on the location of the lesions. However, vertebral hydatid disease is much more common; the condition usually presents with the picture of spinal cord compression.

Tropical spastic paraparesis

Recent publications have reported, in Western Colombia, a progressive spastic paraparesia with mild sensory disturbances in the legs. Recently, we have studied a patient with similar motor findings, but with minimal sensory involvement. He came from an area located in Northeast Peru, where it seems there are patients with similar pathology. A prospective study will be carried out in the near future to establish the clinical and epidemiological profiles of this syndrome.

References

Arana-Iñiguez, R. (1973). Hydatid echinococcosis of the nervous system. In *Tropical neurology* (ed. J. D. Spillane). Oxford University Press, Oxford.

Arana-Iñiguez, R. (1978). Echinococcoccosis of the nervous system. In *Handbook of clinical neurology*, Vol. 35 (eds P. J. Vinken and G. W. Bruyn) pp. 175–208. Elsevier, Amsterdam.

Escalante, S. (1973). *Cisticercosis. I. Epidemiología y clínica. II. Cisticercosis*. Tesis, Lima.

Franco, P. J. (1971) *Patogenia y Tratamiento de la Neurocisticercosis*. Tesis, Lima.

Roman, G.C., Roman, L.N., Spencer, P. S. and Schoemberg, B. S. (1985). Tropical spastic paraparesis: a neuroepidemiological study in Colombia. *Ann. Neurol.* **17**, 361–365.

Spillane, J. D. (1973). *Tropical neurology*, Vol. 1. Oxford University Press, Oxford.

Spina-Franca, A. and Mattosinho-Franca, L. C. (1973). Chagas' disease and the nervous system. In *Tropical neurology* (ed. J. D. Spillane). Oxford University Press, Oxford.

—— and —— (1973). American trypanosomiasis (Chagas disease). In *Tropical neurology*, (ed. J. D. Spillane). Oxford University Press, Oxford.

Trelles, L. (1969). *Contribucion a la histopatología de la Neurobartonelosis*. Tesis, Lima.

Trelles, J. O. (1978). Parasitic diseases and tropical neurology. In *Handbook of clinical neurology* (eds P. J. Vinken and G. W. Bruyn), pp. 1–23. Elsevier, Amsterdam.

—— and Lazarte, H. (1941). La cisticercosis cerebral. La Prensa, Lima.

——, Palomino, L. and Caceres, A. (1967). Histopathologie de la cysticercose cérébrale. *Acta neuropath.* **8**, 115–132.

——, Trelles, L. and Palomino, L. (1969). Formas neurológicas de la Enfermedad de Carrión. *Rev. de Neuropsiq.* **xxxii**, 245–306.

—— and Chia, P. (1962). Epidemiología de las enfermedades cerebro-vasculares en el Perú. *World Neurol.* **3**, 475–484.

—— and Trelles, L. (1978). Cysticercosis of the Nervous System. In *Handbook of clinical neurology* (eds P. J. Vinken and G. W. Bruyn), pp. 291–320. Elsevier, Amsterdam.

India

N. H. WADIA

Although accurate epidemiological and statistical data on neurological disease are not available in India, the collective experience of established Indian neurologists indicates that the broad range of nervous diseases is the same as elsewhere in the world. Yet, disease is often the result of one's environment and genes and, hence, there is a greater or lesser prevalence of certain nervous diseases in India compared with the West. This account is intended to highlight these differences.

In an economically underprivileged environment infection and malnutrition still prevail and absence of easy communication and widespread education makes the prevention of spread of resultant disease difficult. Hence, infectious diseases of the nervous system and those resulting from malnutrition are much more often seen than in the West.

The environment includes the local soil, climate, and flora and fauna. Neurological diseases unique to particular regions can be related to these factors. Lathyriasis, neurological complications of fluorosis (fluorine intoxication), heat stroke, and the paralytic effects of snake bites, to name a few conditions, are seen by neurologists in some parts of India.

Conversely, technical advance and affluence are not an unmixed blessing. Two examples suffice. Although age-matched cerebrovascular diseases are probably no less common in India, the brevity of life expectation (54 years) prevents the overall population from reaching an age when the greatest impact of 'stroke' is felt. The problems arising from the vast morbidity and mortality of strokes or senility seen in the West have just begun to appear in the more affluent and senescent part of the population of India. The remainder of the people simply do not live long enough. Similarly, excluding a few large urban medical centres, the residual effects of cardiorespiratory arrest and cerebral anoxia and the neurological complications of dialysis, major cardiac surgery, prolonged immunosuppressant therapy, anticoagulants, sedatives, hypnotics, etc. are not seen, as the 'advances' of modern medicine have not universally arrived.

Ethnic and genetic differences may explain why craniovertebral anomaly and its neurological complications, an indigenous variety of heredofamilial spinocerebellar degeneration, some types of chronic anterior horn cell disease (motor neurone disease) especially in the young and 'hot-water' epilepsy are more prevalent in India. Similarly, it may explain why multiple sclerosis and perhaps congenital berry aneurysms are less commonly seen.

Table 1 lists the disorders a Western physician does not usually see, but which form a part of Indian practice. The list will grow as neurologists spread throughout the country to expose hitherto unrecognized diseases especially amongst children.

Infections

(See Section 5 for a detailed description of the following infections.)

Table 1 Neurological diseases prevalent in India

Infections	Environmental	Ethnic and genetic	Miscellaneous
Leprosy	Malnutrition	Hereditary ataxia with	Aortic arch – syndrome
Tuberculosis	B-complex	supranuclear –	Infantile tremor –
Basal meningitis	deficiency	ophthalmoplegia	syndrome
Spinal meningitis	especially pellagra	Craniovertebral anoma-	Painful ophthalmo-
Tuberculomas of brain	Vitamin-D deficiency	lies; myelopathy due	plegia
and spinal cord	– osteomalacic	to atlanto-axial	Tropical spastic
Tetanus	myopathy	dislocation	paraplegia
Rabies	Kwashiorkor and	Motor neurone	Eale's disease
Encephalitis	marasmus	disease (MND)	
Japanese B	Lathyriasis	Hot water epilepsy	
Kyasanur forest disease	Fluorosis		
Enterovirus 70 disease	Heat stroke		
(Acute haemorrhagic			
conjunctivitis with			
'poliomyelitis')			
Cerebral malaria			
Neurocysticercosis			

Leprosy

This commonest peripheral neuropathy (neuritis), endemic in India since 1400 BC, is believed to affect 3.2 million Indians, though this may be an underestimate.

The prevalence rate varies from less than 2 to as high as 30 (per thousand population) in certain parts of South India. Cases are classified depending on the host response to the infection as 'tuberculoid' or 'lepromatous' with at least three borderline shades in between. The borderline tuberculoid variety predominates and in India 80 per cent of the cases are of the 'non-lepromatous' variety. In the tuberculoid variety in which the hypergic state prevents the bacilli from multiplying, the patient often presents with mononeuritis or polyneuritis (mononeuritis multiplex). It is important to look for a related dermal lesion which may have escaped the patient's notice. In some borderline cases even this may be absent and careful examination should be made for thickened or tender nerves. At other times the patient may come with a single skin patch or area of numbness and detecting even slight sensory loss and a thickened subcutaneous nerve 'leaving' the lesion establishes early diagnosis. In lepromatous leprosy with low host resistance and bacillaemia the dermal lesions are usually obvious when the neurological signs appear.

The available drugs would have had a vast impact if constant examination of contacts, arousing general awareness, or simply training paramedics or even intelligent village elders in heavily infected areas had led to early diagnosis. However, drug resistance, expense, and poor compliance with prolonged therapy have led to failure of leprosy control. With this in mind the WHO has recommended multidrug, shorter regimes. Full details are provided in Section 5.

Tuberculosis

Among 3646 consecutive autopsies performed in a paediatric hospital in Bombay, 9.8 per cent showed tuberculosis somewhere in the body, and in 65.5 per cent of these the nervous system was involved. Among Indian children it is the second most frequent neurological disease after epilepsy, and adults up to the age of 30 years and sometimes much older are also affected.

Nearly 80 per cent of all those who have tuberculosis of the nervous system present with signs of basal meningitis. Intracranial tuberculoma, spinal tuberculous meningitis, and tuberculoma of the spinal cord follow in that order of frequency. Compressive myelopathy resulting from vertebral tuberculosis still remains common.

Tuberculous basal meningitis

Between 2 and 5 per cent of all admissions in Indian paediatric departments are for tuberculous basal meningitis and four or five

adults under treatment are found at any time in a neurology ward. It must be realized that it may manifest in many ways besides the classical syndrome. For example, it may present (a) in early childhood with progressive enlargement of the head, occasional vomiting, and blindness (chronic hydrocephalus); (b) with single or multiple cranial nerve palsies of acute onset or with slowly progressive course; or (c) with acute, often unilateral, neurological symptoms such as hemiplegia, speech disorder, or predominating psychiatric symptoms. All this can happen without fever, vomiting, headache, or neck stiffness, because, with varying grades of infection and immune response, sometimes altered by blunderbuss use of chemotherapy, the meningeal reaction may be mild, but the sequelae such as blockage of CSF flow or entrapment of nerves or arteries at the base of the brain may be more predominant.

Early diagnosis and treatment give the best results, and this is only achieved by developing a fine clinical sense. Even in cities where good laboratory facilities are available the demonstration of acid fast bacilli in CSF (the surest means of diagnosis) is possible in less than 30 per cent of cases and positive cultures are reported only after an unacceptable delay. A variety of tests, including those devised to detect specific antibodies or antigens have as yet failed to reach the strict criteria of reliability for early diagnosis.

Relatively newer drugs like rifampicin have yet to make an impact on the morbidity and mortality rates, especially as the length and expense of the conventional 18-month, three or four drug regime makes compliance difficult. Controlled trials to rationalize and shorten treatment would have immense value. Ventriculo-peritoneal shunts, judiciously used to correct the complicating hydrocephalus, give good results and the computerized tomography (CT) scan wherever available has helped in its early detection.

Tuberculous spinal meningitis

Whereas spinal extension of the basal meningitis causing paraplegia has long been recognized, reports from India have stressed the not uncommon presentation of meningitis with spinal symptoms alone. It is usually seen in adults and it may present (a) with single or multiple root pains and an acute paraplegia mimicking ascending myelitis which, if unchecked by therapy, often ends with symptoms of basal meningitis; fever and spinal pain may be present, or (b) as a subacute or even chronic progressive paraplegia with a sensory level which may be clinically inseparable from spinal cord compression. The complaint of root pains often below or above the level of the spinal cord lesion suggests the diagnosis, but myelography or surgery may be required for confirmation.

The detection of tuberculosis elsewhere in the body hints at the diagnosis. The cerebrospinal fluid shows a cellular response and increased protein, often with xanthochromia and a spinal block. Myelography reveals typical filling defects in the dye column and/ or a ragged-edged block which may not coincide with the clinical level. Prolonged treatment with antituberculous drugs is only beneficial when begun early.

Tuberculoma

Tuberculomas are far commoner in the brain than in the spinal cord. Approximately 20 per cent of intracranial tumours in India are tuberculomas, more than half occurring in children and 75 per cent below the age of 25 years. Between 40 and 50 per cent of posterior fossa tumours in children are tuberculomas. These figures have been compiled from earlier surgical and autopsy series of patients with well-developed signs of focal lesion and/or those of raised intracranial pressure. But with the advent of the CT scan these may need revision as early diagnosis and medical treatment have become increasingly possible. It is now not uncommon to diagnose tuberculoma when the patient has had only one or more focal fits and a lesion on the CT scan. The diagnosis is based on clinical and circumstantial evidence, CT scan appearance and therapeutic response to antituberculous drugs.

The treatment of choice is no longer surgical, and medical treatment has cured surgically inaccessible tumours. In fact, unless there is evidence to the contrary, most patients with a parenchymatous brain tumour are given a trial of treatment with antituberculous drugs under careful serial CT monitoring assuming it to be a tuberculoma. There is no standardized approach to this problem based on controlled trials; the choice of drugs or duration of therapy reflects individual clinician's fancies! Usually a three-drug regime is recommended.

The selection (at times depending on toxicity and financial considerations) is from rifampicin, isonicotinic acid hydrazide (INH), streptomycin, pyrazinamide, and ethambutol, with the first two most preferred. The duration is the conventional 18-month period with ethambutol replacing streptomycin, rifampicin or pyrazinamide during the second half of the course. INH is given throughout the treatment. Surgery is reserved only for a tuberculoma which is resistant to drugs or if there is a marked rise of intracranial pressure; even then many prefer to give medical therapy with anti-oedema drugs after inserting a ventriculo-peritoneal shunt.

Tetanus

The approximate incidence of tetanus in India is 1 in 20 000 population. Large teaching hospitals in Bombay admit from 300 to 700 cases each year, 30–50 per cent of whom still die. In some parts of India the annual mortality rate is as high as 90 per 100 000 population. Despite advances in prophylactic immunization and intensive therapy, these benefits have not percolated through to the populations who need them most. Except in a few advanced centres, curarization and intermittent positive pressure respiration, which have yielded good results elsewhere, are still not used.

Rabies

This variety of meningoencephalitis still prevails in India. Its incidence is not known. The 'hydrophobic' or 'spastic' form of the disease is easy to diagnose, but the 'tranquil' or 'paralytic' (rabies without hydrophobia) which presents as an ascending paralysis of the Landry-type often goes unrecognized even when bulbar, respiratory, and terminal encephalitic symptoms appear. Pain and paraesthesiae at the site of the animal bite often precede the paralysis. There is often no objective sensory loss.

The history of dog bite may remain unrevealed especially if it has occurred some months earlier. The animal may be alive at the time of the patient's illness. At times the differential diagnosis from postvaccinal encephalomyelitis may not be easy, if the patient has received some rabies vaccine. Treatment has, so far, failed.

Encephalitis

Viral encephalitis is not infrequently seen in India and the agent is not easy to identify. However, of local concern are Japanese encephalitis and Kyasanur forest disease which occur in both epidemic and endemic forms. Recurrent epidemics of Japanese encephalitis with high mortality have occurred in north eastern and southern India since 1955. The presentation is typical with headache, high fever, convulsions, disorders of consciousness, paralysis, and involuntary movements. The mosquito is the main vector for transmission, and the pig, cattle, and certain birds are the main hosts for the viral cycle though they do not manifest the disease. Humans are tangential hosts and do not participate in the cycles of viral propagation. Epidemics occur in humans only when the population of infected virus is vastly increased.

Kyasanur forest disease is caused by an arbovirus in the same group B as the virus of Japanese encephalitis. It is the only tick-borne virus disease of any significance in India. The disease was first detected amongst the monkeys and men of Kyasanur forest of South India. Overt encephalitis in humans was uncommon though autopsies in monkies showed its presence. The disease has now spread over a wider area and more human cases of encephalitis are being reported. The nervous system is affected in the second phase of a biundulant fever which begins with headache, sore throat, myalgia, abdominal pain, and diarrhoea.

Enterovirus 70 disease

In 1971 and 1981 two epidemics of acute haemorrhagic conjunctivitis spread across India. The former was part of a pandemic which spanned an area from Ghana to Japan. Since then no continent has been spared except Australia. In 1971, we recognized that in a very small proportion of these patients and even contacts, the disease, though mainly manifest in the eyes, also affected the nervous system. They developed an acute, asymmetrical, mainly proximal, hypotonic, areflexic paralysis of the limbs. The upper limbs were less affected and rarely alone. Motor cranial nerve palsies, alone or with the spinal disease, were also seen; unilateral facial nerve palsy was most common. Fever and malaise followed by muscle and root pains often preceded the paralysis and in a few cases transitory retention of urine, sensory disturbance, pyramidal signs, and vertigo were seen at onset. All this closely mimicked poliomyelitis, except that male adults were most affected. The latent interval between the eye and CNS disease was usually short, but extended up to two months. The CSF showed pleocytosis and raised protein. Predictably, a new enterovirus (EV 70) was isolated from the conjunctivae of Japanese patients and its neurovirulence demonstrated in monkeys. Though no virus has been isolated from the CSF or CNS in India, collaboratively we have shown significantly high antibody titres to EV 70 both in the serum and CSF of Indian patients. This confirms the clinical impression that, like the polio viruses, this virus can actually invade the nervous system and does not merely cause the disease by an autoimmune CNS response. Similar confirmatory clinical and serological observations have also been made in Thailand, Taiwan, and Senegal. Although death has been reported from acute bulbar and respiratory muscle paralysis, no pathological information is available. Wasted limbs and paralysis remained in over a third of the patients. Though other viruses can cause epidemic and sporadic conjunctivitis and similar paralysis independently, the combination of the two is caused by EV 70 alone, hence the suggested label of Enterovirus 70 disease for this entity. Public health measures at the first sign of the epidemic are required. Several thousand persons have been paralysed already in this last decade and many more will follow if the virus turns more neurovirulent.

Cerebral malaria

Despite efforts since 1976 to control the resurgence of malaria in India, latest estimates still show an incidence of 2 million cases a year and this may be an underestimate. The most disturbing fact has been the relative increase in the number of chloroquine-resistant cases of *Plasmodium falciparum* malaria which can cause rapidly fatal cerebral disease if not treated properly. See Section 5 for details of treatment.

Neurocysticercosis

The known prevalence of neurocysticercosis in India has become more evident with the availability of the CT scan to show small parenchymatous brain lesions which were impossible to detect by all other investigative methods available earlier. It occurs not only in those who eat infected pork, but also in strict vegetarians, through vegetables contaminated with the ova of taenia solium. It manifests with focal or generalized convulsions or symptoms of raised intracranial tension with or without focal signs and papilloedema. It can also present with chronic headache or subacute progressive dementia or less commonly with symptoms simulating meningoencephalitis. Spinal cord lesions are rare. Many cases of enlarged muscles (*pseudohypertrophic myopathy*) due to the presence of an enormous number of cystic larvae have been reported from India. Bilateral symmetrical enlargement usually of the lower limbs and shoulder girdle have been described. My experience (unpublished) has been that this happens in a more specific 'miliary' form of the disease which we have now come to recognize clinically and especially more clearly through the CT scan. The patient presents with progressive dementia, repeated convulsions, and obviously enlarged muscles, with or without overt signs of raised intracranial pressure. The CT scan shows hundreds of small calcified cysticerci in the unenhanced brain scan (like 'a starry night') and the CT scan of the muscles shows widespread largely uncalcified or finely calcified cysts throughout the body which are not seen on routine X-ray examination (Figs 1 and 2).

Corticosteroid therapy reduces brain swelling and is effective even over a long period. Surgical removal of the large cystic forms may become necessary. The new drug Praziquantel (50 mg/kg body weight a day in three divided doses for 15 days) seems to offer a healthier future for these patients, but more long-term results are awaited and not all cases, which have to be carefully selected, respond. The drug may cause a further rise in intracranial pressure or increase the frequency of fits, which require careful management. More than one course may be necessary.

Environmental diseases

Nutritional disorders of the nervous system

Although malnutrition is widespread, particularly in children in rural India, systematic surveys of its impact on the nervous system are not available. Data gathered in urban hospitals do not truly reflect the correct position, and do not include any accounts of Wernicke–Korsakoff's syndrome, central pontine myelinolysis, Marchiafava–Bignami disease, and cerebellar cortical degeneration which form the main parts of chapters on 'nutritional disorders of the nervous system' written in many Western textbooks. Sheer deprivation seems to affect the nervous system in a different way than malnutrition in Western alcoholics.

Pellagra causing dementia, dermatitis, peripheral neuropathy, and myelopathy is still abundant in certain parts of rural India. Peripheral neuropathy and myelopathy from multiple B-vitamin deficiency, neuromyelopathy due to vitamin B_{12} deficiency resulting from intestinal malabsorption (not from pernicious anaemia), and predominant proximal muscle weakness in patients with osteomalacia are constantly seen.

Kwashiorkor and marasmus in children are common and cause mental dulling, apathy, and irritability. Proximal muscle weakness with a waddling gait, wasting, hypotonia, and hyporeflexia believed to result mostly from the direct effect of the protein energy deprivation on the muscles have been described.

Evidence, though debatable, has also been produced to show that protein energy malnutrition in infancy can impair the normal growth of the developing brain, leading to subtle pathological changes and a permanent lowering of the mental performance in those who survive to adulthood. At a conservative estimate 20 per cent of Indian children between the age of one and five years are believed to be suffering from frank protein energy malnutrition.

Lathyriasis

This age-old disease is still endemic in certain parts of Central India. It results from excessive consumption of *Lathyrus sativus*, especially during a lean monsoon season when the drought-resistant pea is consumed as a major part of the diet for several months and the disease may then appear in epidemic proportions. The usually acute onset of severe cramps and spastic paralysis of the lower limbs is often precipitated by undue exertion or exposure to inclement weather, though a more chronic form is also known. The paralysis may lead to total incapacity, but it is not uncommon to see patients of all ages walking with a spastic gait with the help of a stick in an affected village. Spasticity is a greater handicap than weakness. The upper limbs usually escape or merely show brisk reflexes.

It is now believed that possibly the toxic agent is B-(*N*)-oxalyl aminoalanine (BOAA) which can be removed by parboiling the pulse before cooking. Educating the farmer to plant alternative crops has only been successful where water has been provided to do so.

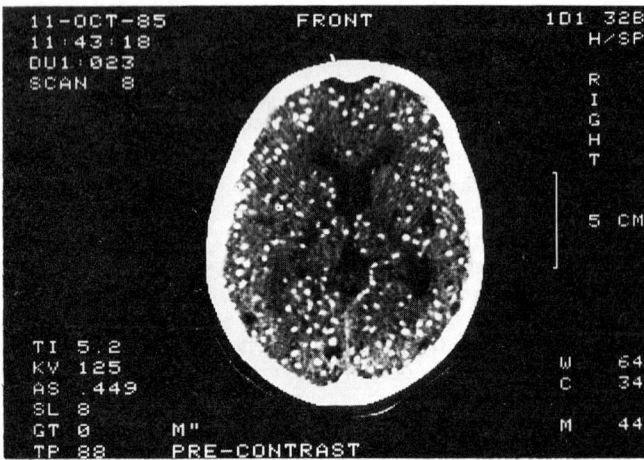

Fig. 1 Pre-contrast CT scan of the brain of a patient with disseminated (miliary) cysticercosis showing lesions with high attenuation, probably caused by the calcifying scolax of innumerable cysticercii. No enhancement was seen on contrast administration.

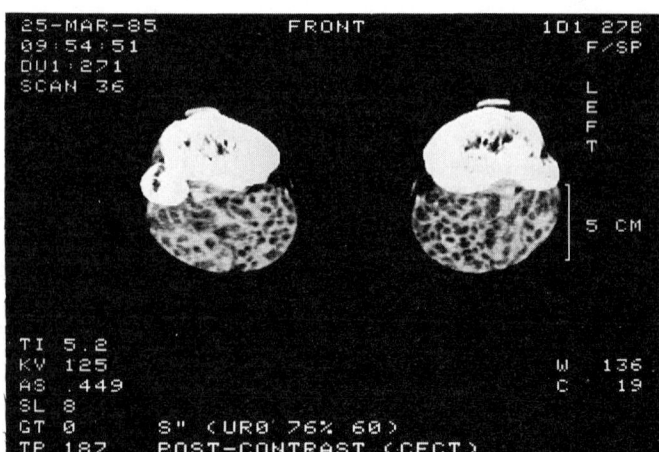

Fig. 2 Post-contrast CT scan of muscles behind both knees showing rounded areas with low attenuation caused by disseminated cysticercii. No calcification is seen. No contrast enhancement is seen.

Fluorosis

Endemic fluorosis is prevalent in South India, particularly in part of Andhra Pradesh, and in the Punjab where the fluoride content of the drinking-water is high. About 10 per cent of these patients develop neurological signs at an advanced stage of the bone disease as a result of compression of the spinal cord or roots, or less commonly the peripheral nerves. Progressive, disabling spastic or atrophic weakness of limbs, or a combination of both, predominate, at times simulating motor neurone disease, but root pains, paraesthesiae, patchy sensory loss, sphincter disturbance, and occasionally deafness, combined with radiological evidence of fluorosis in bones makes the diagnosis obvious. Decompressive surgery has met with little success.

Heat stroke (Section 6)

In its usual form this condition is still prevalent in India in certain regions in the summer, especially amongst children. It can be mistaken for encephalitis.

Ethnic and genetic diseases

Heredito-familial spinocerebellar degeneration

This condition probably occurs at a similar level to other populations, but an autosomal dominant variety, initially described in Bombay and rarely noted outside India, is the most frequent. It is distinguished by a supranuclear ophthalmoplegia which is remarkable in that there is progressive reduction in the velocity of the saccadic eye movements without limitation of range until an advanced stage of the disease. The 'viscous' eye movements are compensated by the patient by quick jerking of the head to scan the surroundings. The patient is unaware of this disability and presents with symptoms of a progressive cerebellar ataxia usually in the second and third decade, leading to increasing disability and to death within 15 years from the onset.

The deep reflexes are often suppressed and deep sensations are impaired indicating peripheral nerve or spinal cord involvement. Autopsy has confirmed this to be a variety of olivopontocerebellar degeneration with some degeneration of the posterior columns, anterior horn cells, and peripheral nerves.

Craniovertebral anomalies – myelopathy complicating congenital atlanto-axial dislocation

Neurological manifestations of craniovertebral anomalies, notably dislocation of the atlanto-axial joints and basilar invagination, have been widely reported. The former seems to be commoner and has distinguishing clinical and radiological features. Atlanto-axial dislocation may present with pain and stiffness of the neck, but the congenital variety more often causes symptoms of medullospinal junction or upper cervical cord compression. The symptoms may be transitory on sudden flexion of the neck, lasting for a few hours or days. Such episodes of quadriparesis, paraesthesia below the neck, or sudden unconsciousness alone or in combination may recur, leaving behind increasing signs of a high cervical cord lesion. However, some patients simply present with signs of progressive, often asymmetrical, upper cervical cord compression, indistinguishable from that due to any other cause.

Almost all patients have various degrees of pyramidal tract signs, often an asymmetrical quadriparesis. Loss of appreciation of postural sensibility and vibration particularly in the upper limbs, causing clumsiness of hands, is common. All limb reflexes are almost invariably exaggerated. Wasting of the upper limbs, especially the hands, forequarter dissociated sensory loss, cerebellar signs, and Horner's syndrome are less often seen. In many patients a short neck helps to make the diagnosis.

Radiologically several varieties of anomaly of the odontoid and atlas leading to the dislocation have been described. Surgical correction in skilled hands has yielded good results, but unfortunately many patients come too late.

Basilar invagination more often presents with lower cranial nerve signs, diminished corneal reflexes, cerebellar ataxia, dissociated sensory loss in the upper limbs, and pyramidal and posterior column signs. A short neck is invariably present.

It is usually easy with the aid of tomography and CT scan to distinguish the two conditions, though they may be associated at times in the same patient. Surgical decompression is rewarding.

Motor neurone diseases (MND)

The classical motor neurone disease of middle age and spinal muscular atrophy are seen in India as elsewhere, but more benign forms in young adults (10 to 30 years) seem to be more frequent. Three varieties have been reported: Madras motor neurone disease, monomelic amyotrophy (juvenile MND), and 'wasted leg syndrome'. In the slowly progressive but disabling Madras variety there is ultimately weakness and wasting of all limbs with spasticity especially in the lower limbs. The distal muscles are most affected. Dysarthria, dysphagia, and facial weakness are seen in two out of three patients, and deafness in a third. The disease appears to be largely confined to South India. In the monomelic amyotrophy, weakness and wasting are confined to one limb, more often an upper one and progress is very slow occurring over years. It has been seen all over India for a long time, but improperly reported. The wasted leg syndrome described an accidently discovered non-progressive wasting of one leg without any substantial weakness. Electromyography and muscle biopsy have indicated the lesions in all disorders to be in the anterior horn cells. No autopsy confirmation is available. The aetiology of these conditions is unknown.

Epilepsy ('hot water epilepsy')

The only survey from South India shows the incidence of epilepsy as 9 per 1000 population, comparable to that elsewhere in the world. All types are recorded, but of indigenous interest and especially in South India, is a reflex excitation form designated as 'hot-water' epilepsy and commonly seen in children. The attacks are precipitated when hot water from a vessel is poured over the head as is the common bathing practice. The attacks are usually of the 'temporal lobe' or grand mal variety. Electroencephalographic dysrhythmia has been recorded during such attacks and interictally; 20 per cent of these patients have epileptic attacks without reflex excitation.

Miscellaneous diseases

Cerebrovascular disease (aortic arch syndrome)

Cerebrovascular diseases (CVD) predominate in neurological practice as anywhere else. Although initial impressions were that in India's poorer population the incidence of CVD was less than in the affluent West, more methodical data from clinicians and pathologists indicate that atherosclerosis and hypertension and the concomitant CVD are equally prevalent in all socio-economic groups. It was also thought that the incidence of stroke in the young (those below 40–45 years) was higher than elsewhere. This too has been found to be largely untrue. The percentage population at risk from 'stroke' is smaller in India as the average life span of 54 years falls below the peak years at which stroke occurs. This in turn swells the percentage incidence of stroke in the young, thus conveying a false impression.

As elsewhere, ischaemic vascular disease and intracranial haemorrhage account for approximately 80 per cent and 20 per cent, respectively, of all strokes. The percentage of intracranial and extracranial arterial lesions causing cerebral infarction is the same as reported in the West, but interestingly the incidence of cerebral infarction from embolism seems to be higher, notably in young Indians.

Cerebral infarction due to obliterative disease of the aortic arch and its major branches – the aortic arch syndrome – and cortical venous thrombosis appear to be common amongst Indians, both usually occurring below the age of 45 years. The aortic arch disease is believed to be due to two different pathological conditions: that occurring in young females and causing obliteration of the pulses (pulseless disease, Takayasu's disease) from an inflammatory arteritis of uncertain aetiology, and the other as a juvenile or premature form of atherosclerosis in males between 35 and 55 years. Consequent to the progressive obliteration of the major arteries supplying the brain, an extensive opening of collateral circulation occurs, and depending on its efficacy, the patient may have either a minor transient focal neurological deficit, an acute severe stroke, or symptoms of chronic progressive brain and optic nerve damage, all resulting from large or small, single or multiple ischaemic infarction of the brain. We even see patients with no palpable pulses in the neck and arms, with no neurological disorder.

The reason for the considerably higher incidence of cortical venous thrombosis amongst Indians, especially pregnant women, has not been clarified although puerperal infection has been ruled out.

For many years reports from India indicated that subarachnoid haemorrhage and congenital aneurysms were uncommonly seen and whereas this is still true in clinical practice, carefully conducted autopsies record a higher incidence. Our impression is that these patients remain undetected and do not reach centres where angiography or special autopsy examinations would reveal their presence. The greatest incidence of subarachnoid haemorrhage has been reported from Kerala, South India, where aneurysms and angiomas are frequently seen.

Infantile tremor syndrome

The recognition of the infantile tremor syndrome in 1960 as a not uncommon indigenous disease illustrates the need for further exploration of the vast untapped field of paediatric neurology in India. Occurring in the first 30 months of life, this striking, coarse, high-frequency tremor appears acutely after a period of mental apathy, developmental retardation, and in some instances, fever. The child belongs to the lower socio-economic group. Pallor, vacant expression, and open mouth, light coloured silky hair, and a plump face are usually the identifying marks accompanying the tremor. The disease runs a self-limiting course with slow regression of all symptoms, but in the majority mental retardation persists.

The aetiology is uncertain. Trephine biopsy of the brain has shown changes of meningo-encephalitis, but equally strong evidence of vitamin B_{12} deficiency in the child and in the mother's milk has been presented.

Painful ophthalmoplegia

This is a relatively common disease; over 100 cases have been reported from our departments in 18 years. It presents with an acute unilateral paralysis of one or more oculomotor nerves, often with sparing of the pupil, and preceded by severe peri-orbital pain and occasional malaise. The condition is self-limiting and often mistaken for an intracranial aneurysm, though in the latter the pupil is most often paralysed. Recurrent attacks of paralysis and sometimes involvement of other cranial nerves has given it the alternate title of polyneuritis cranialis. In some cases the CSF shows pleocytosis and raised proteins. The ESR may be elevated. The aetiology is not known, but the current belief that immuno-allergic reactions cause the disease has led to the use of corticosteroids, which rapidly relieve the pain.

Tropical spastic paraplegia

This appears to be a well-defined syndrome first described from South India. Most patients are affected in late adulthood. The disease progresses over several weeks or months and the dominant signs are of spastic disabling paraplegia with more occasional milder involvement of the upper limbs, distal paraethesiae, and sensory loss and disorder of micturition. Various degrees of disability persist and a large proportion die of complications of decubitus.

In a few patients the CSF shows a slight rise of protein and very occasionally of cells. All other investigations have been negative.

The disease differs from lathyriasis. Similar patients have been reported in clusters from other equitorial regions in Africa, South America, Jamaica, and the Seychelles, but no common clues as to aetiology have been found even after autopsy. Patients with a less well-defined picture of chronic progressive or occasionally relapsing myelopathy of unknown aetiology affecting essentially the thoracic cord are not uncommon all over India, but it is uncertain whether they belong to the same nosological group.

Eale's disease

Attention has been drawn to the prevalence, though infrequent, of the neurological manifestations of Eale's disease which usually affects only the eyes, with periphlebitis, retinal haemorrhages, and neovascular formation. The patients, usually male, present with acute or subacute paraplegia, urinary retention, and sensory loss from a lesion in the upper dorsal cord, a few weeks to years after the eye symptoms. Occasionally, signs of cervical cord, brain stem, and cerebral involvement have been seen. Slight remissions and relapses occur but on the whole the disability is permanent and death occurs from complications of decubitus and urinary infection. In the acute phase a remarkable increase in cells and protein in the CSF are reported. Differential diagnosis includes multiple sclerosis and chronic spinal, mostly tuberculous, meningitis, but the preceding eye disease is tell-tale.

Pathological examination reveals various stages of venous changes from proliferation to dilation and haemorrhage, or thickening with hylinization. Perivenular demyelination with axon preservation is seen.

Multiple sclerosis

This disorder is seen infrequently in India, though prevalence in the Parsi (Zoroastrian) community appears to be clearly greater. On an average 2 or 3 new cases in a year would be encountered in a large neurological practice. This contrast with the West has been variously and inconsistently explained on the basis of the colour of the skin, the climate related to temperature and latitude, and socio-economic factors and general hygiene, but with the emergence of the data on histocompatibility antigens, it now appears that a greater or lesser genetic predilection to the disease acquired through environmental factors or an infective agent such as a virus exists in certain persons and populations. The histocompatibility antigens associated with multiple sclerosis in Indians are different from those in Caucasians and the causative agent may also be different.

References

Bharucha, E. P. and Pavri, K. M. (1979). Encephalitis in India. In *Progress in clinical medicine* (ed. M. M. S. Ahuja), pp. 511–531. Arnold-Heinemann Publishers, New Delhi.
Chopra, J. S., Banerjee, A. K., Murthy, J. M. K. and Pal, S. R. (1980). Paralytic rabies – a clinico-pathological study. *Brain* **103**, 789–802.
Dalal, P. M. (1973). The aortic arch syndrome – an idiopathic form of non-inflammatory occlusive vascular disease. In *Tropical neurology* (ed. J. D. Spillane), pp. 92–98. Oxford University Press, London.
—— (1979). Strokes in the young in West Central India. In *Advances in neurology* (eds M. Goldstein *et al.*), pp. 339–348. Raven Press, New York.
Dastur, F. D. and D'Sa J. (1979). Tetanus – present knowledge and experiences in India. In *Progress in clinical medicine* (ed. M. M. S. Ahuja) pp. 68–87. Arnold-Heinemann Publishers, New Delhi.
Dastur, H. M. (1975). Tuberculoma. In *Handbook of clinical neurology*, Vol. 18 (eds P. J. Vinken and G. W. Bruyn), pp. 413–426. North-Holland, Amsterdam.
Dharmendra (1978). The present distribution and general considerations of leprosy. In *Leprosy* (ed. Dharmendra), pp. 22–32. Kothari Publishing House, Bombay.
Editorial (1982). Neurovirulence of Enterovirus 70. *Lancet* i, 373.
Editorial (1982). Chemotherapy of leprosy. *Lancet* ii, 77–78.
Gopalan, C. (1970). Some recent studies in the nutrition research laboratories, Hyderabad. *Am. J. clin. Nutr.* **23**, 35–42.
Gourie-Devi, M., Suresh, T. G. and Shankar, S. K. (1984). Monomelic amyotrophy. *Arch. Neurol.* **41**, 388–394.
Jagannathan, K. (1973). Juvenile motor neurone disease. In *Tropical neurology* (ed. J. D. Spillane), pp. 127–130. Oxford University Press, London.

Mani, K. S. (1973). Neurological diseases in South India. In *Tropical neurology* (ed. J. D. Spillane), pp. 78–85. Oxford University Press, London.

Mathew, N. T. and Chandy, J. (1970). Painful ophthalmoplegia. *J. Neurol. Sci.* **11**, 243–256.

Prabhakar, S., Chopra, J. S., Banerjee, A. K. and Rana, P. V. S. (1981). Wasted leg syndrome: A clinical, electrophysiological and histopathological study. *Clin. Neurol. Neurosurg.* **83**, 19–28.

Raja Reddy, D. (1979). Skeletal fluorosis. In *Handbook of clinical neurology*, Vol. 36 (eds P. J. Vinken and G. W. Bruyn), pp. 465–504. North-Holland, Amsterdam.

Sharma, V. P. (1984). Drug resistant *Plasmodium Falciparum* malaria in India. In *Proceedings of the Indo-UK Workshop on Malaria* (ed. V. P. Sharma), pp. 169–184. Malaria Research Centre (ICMR), Delhi.

Singhal, B. S. and Dastur, D. K. (1976). Eale's disease with neurological involvement. *J. Neurol. Sci.* **27**, 313–321.

Tandon, P. N. (1978). Tuberculous meningitis (cranial and spinal). In *Handbook of clinical neurology*, Vol. 33 (eds P. J. Vinken and G. W. Bruyn), pp. 195–262. North-Holland, Amsterdam.

—— (1983). Cerebral cysticercosis. *Neurosurg. Rev.* **6**, 119–127.

—— and Bajpai, P. C. (1973). The infantile tremor syndrome. In *Tropical neurology* (ed. J. D. Spillane), pp. 114–119. Oxford University Press, London.

Wadia, N. H. (1967). Myelopathy complicating congenital atlanto-axial dislocation (a study of 28 cases). *Brain* **90**, 449–472.

—— (1973). An introduction to neurology in India. In *Tropical neurology* (ed. J. D. Spillane), pp. 25–36. Oxford University Press, London.

—— (1977). Heredo-familial spinocerebellar degeneration with slow eye movements – another variety of olivopontocerebellar degeneration. *Neurol. India* **25**, 147–160.

—— (1979). Nutritional disorders of the nervous system. In *Progress in clinical medicine* (ed. M. M. S. Ahuja), pp. 487–510. Arnold-Heinemann Publishers, New Delhi.

—— (1984). A variety of olivopontocerebellar atrophy distinguished by slow eye movements and peripheral neuropathy. In *The olivopontocerebellar atrophies* (eds R. C. Duvoisin and A. Plaitakis), pp. 149–177. Raven Press, New York.

—— and Dastur, D. K. (1969). Spinal meningitis with radiculopathy – clinical and radiological features. *J. Neurol. Sci.* **8**, 239–260.

—— and Swami, R. K. (1971). A new form of heredo-familial spinocerebellar degeneration with slow eye movements (nine families) *Brain* **94**, 359–374.

——, Trikannad, V. S. and Krishnaswamy, P. R. (1981). HLA antigens in multiple sclerosis amongst Indians. *J. Neurol. Neurosurg. Psychiat.* **44**, 849–851.

——, Wadia, P. N., Katrak, S. M. and Misra, V. P. (1983). A study of the neurological disorders associated with acute haemorrhagic conjunctivitis due to Enterovirus 70. *J. Neurol. Neurosurg. Psychiat.* **46**, 599–610.

Southeast Asia

A. VEJJAJIVA

The pattern of neurological disease

Despite a high standard of living of a number of people in big cities, poverty and illiteracy are still the main factors responsible for major health problems among the rural people and the urban underprivileged who comprise the majority of the population in Southeast Asia. In addition, local customs and dietary habits help to contribute to a distinctive pattern of neurological disease in the region. When compared with that seen in a developed country in the West, there are some similarities and differences which can be summarized as follows:–

1. There is probably no significant difference in the prevalence and clinical presentation of cerebrovascular diseases, cerebral and spinal tumour, migraine, Parkinson's disease, myasthenia gravis, and motor neurone disease.

2. Multiple sclerosis, a highly prevalent disease in the temperate zone, is much less common in Southeast Asia, and pernicious anaemia with accompanying neurological features is virtually non-existent.

3. Certain disorders that are rarely seen in the West are much more prevalent in Southeast Asia. Included in this category are tuberculous and pyogenic meningitides, rabies, Japanese B encephalitis, cysticercosis, tetanus, recurrent painful ophthalmoplegia, beriberi, non-familial periodic paralysis, and neurological sequelae of vaccination against rabies.

4. Two parasitic diseases are unique to the region, namely, an eosinophilic meningitis due to *Angiostrongylus cantonensis* and nervous system invasion by *Gnathostoma spinigerum*.

Neurological complication of acute haemorrhagic conjunctivitis caused by enterovirus (EV70), as seen in India during the 1971 and 1981 epidemics, was also encountered in Thailand during the 1974 and 1981 outbreaks (page 21.265).

Multiple sclerosis

The disease is uncommon among the population of Southeast Asia and only one autopsy-proved case has been reported from Thailand. Usual presenting features are optic neuritis, and spinal cord involvement, i.e. the clinical picture of neuromyelitis optica. Brainstem lesions are sometimes seen in subsequent attacks and they are presenting features only in a minority of patients. Tonic seizure is commoner in Asian patients with multiple sclerosis. Brief, frequent, painful tonic spasms of one or more limbs often occur during the recovery phase after paralysis. The attacks may last weeks or months and are successfully controlled by carbamazepine. On the whole, the illness is clinically indistinguishable from multiple sclerosis seen in the West, but the course in some patients tends to be shorter with death ensuing in a few years from superimposed infection.

Non-familial periodic paralysis

Recurrent attacks of muscular weakness and paralysis associated with hypokalaemia are commonly seen in Chinese and Thai adults but only rarely in Malay or Indian adults in the region. Usually, they are encountered either in patients with thyrotoxicosis, with an incidence said to be of about 5 per cent in Chinese, or in apparently healthy individuals with no family history of the disorder. Occasionally, they are seen in patients with renal disorders, in particular renal tubular acidosis, in which severe loss of potassium in the urine occurs. In the thyrotoxic variety, the age of onset is usually between 20 and 30 years and males predominate. Attacks vary both in frequency and severity. In the idiopathic group, there are some patients who suffer one or two attacks then remain symptom-free for years. In the thyrotoxic group, although the occurrence of paralytic attacks is not related to the duration and severity of hyperthyroidism, they subside when patients become euthyroid.

A mild attack may consist of transient weakness of a group of limb muscles, while in a severe attack patients may wake up in the early hours finding themselves unable to move their legs, trunk, and arms. Involvement of bulbar or respiratory muscles is very rare. Attacks may last a few hours to a few days. A heavy meal of rice and a long rest after vigorous exercise are important predisposing factors. An attack of paralysis is successfully terminated with oral or intravenous potassium chloride. The salt is given prophylactically to those non-thyrotoxic patients with frequent attacks.

Neurological sequelae of antirabic vaccination

Since it can be produced locally in great quantity and at low cost, vaccine containing animal neural tissue is still widely used as treatment after exposure to animals suspected of having rabies. Neurological complication from the use of Semple vaccine occurs in about 1 in 1000 cases. A course of 14 injections is usually given, though daily injections extended to three weeks are administered to patients with facial wounds.

Neurological symptoms often occur during the second week of vaccination. Rarely, they manifest during the first week or they are delayed for as long as three weeks after the course of 14 daily injections of the vaccine has been completed. Four main clinical types are recognized; namely, meningoencephalomyelitis, meningoencephalitis, transverse myelitis, and polyradiculoneuritis. The first three types are common, while paralysis from nerve root involvement is rare, being encountered in only 1 among the 35 patients in a reported series.

The usual presenting symptoms are headache, fever, drowsiness, lower limb paralysis, and urinary retention. Severe cases may become comatose soon after the onset. Optic neuritis and cranial nerve palsy are rare.

In almost all patients the CSF is abnormal with mild lymphocytic pleocytosis, slight to moderately increased protein often not exceeding 150 mg/100 ml but invariably with high immunoglobulin content. The pressure of the CSF is abnormally raised in less than one-third of the cases, while the glucose is almost always normal.

The illness may last from a few days to several months. Recovery is complete in over half of the cases, while about one in five patients has residual disability. The mortality rate in a reported series was 17 per cent. Spontaneous recurrence of symptoms has not been observed in any patient who has completely recovered from the neuroparalytic accident, although some instances of rabies postvaccinal encephalomyelitis with chronic symptoms and signs and with pathological appearances strikingly reminiscent of multiple sclerosis were reported from Japan.

Cysticercosis

(See also Section 5.)
Cysticercosis is an infestation of humans with *Cysticercus cellulosae*, the encysted larvae of the tape worm, *Taenia solium*. Cysts are most commonly present in the brain and muscles, and in the latter tend to become calcified.

Aetiology

Humans acquire the disease from eating food contaminated with the ova of *Taenia solium*. This could be due to auto-infection, the patient harbouring the adult worm in the intestine and accidentally ingesting food contaminated with the ova he or she excreted. More commonly, perhaps, infestation is acquired from unhygienic food handlers who are *Taenia* carriers. Rarely, in the latter, massive intestinal infestation by reverse peristalsis may deposit ova in the stomach where the gastric juice releases the embryos. Among the Bantu in South Africa, herbalists frequently employ tapeworm proglottides in the preparation of certain medicines. The embryos liberated from the ingested ova by the gastric juice in the stomach penetrate the intestinal mucosa, enter the blood stream, and are disseminated throughout the body. Their chief clinical importance, however, lies in their invasion of the nervous system. In the brain, the cysts usually measure about 1 cm in diameter but, occasionally, a giant cyst measuring a few centimetres in size and producing a tumour-like effect is seen. A racemose form, a cluster of grape-like cystic bodies with thin, translucent walls containing colourless fluid is not uncommonly encountered in the fourth ventricle and basal cisterns.

Signs and symptoms

The onset of symptoms varies from less than one year to 30 years since the infestation, with an average interval of about five years. Epilepsy, focal or generalized, is the commonest presenting symptom. Cysticercosis is indeed the commonest cause of epilepsy of late onset among the population of Southeast Asia. Intracranial hypertension may be due to cysts in the third or fourth ventricle causing intermittent obstructive hydrocephalus with paroxysmal severe headache, vomiting, papilloedema, and postural vertigo. Equally common are patients who have communicating hydrocephalus and who present with chronic headache, dementia, and gait disturbance. Less commonly seen are patients with attacks of meningoencephalitis, subacute meningitis, or spinal cord or cauda equina lesions. Attacks of meningoencephalitis are usually self-limiting but, occasionally, an initial event can be severe and causes problems in diagnosis and treatment.

Diagnosis

Due to its varied manifestations, cysticercosis has to be included among the differential diagnosis of various neurological problems in the endemic area. Collateral evidence of infestation should always be sought. Subcutaneous nodules are found in less than half of all cases. When available, biopsy should be carried out to confirm the diagnosis. X-rays of the limbs and trunk may demonstrate calcified cysts in the muscles but X-rays of the skull are usually unhelpful. Computerized tomography (CT) of the brain has been found to be a very helpful diagnostic aid. Calcified cysticercus cysts in the cerebral parenchyma often show up on tomography as high-density spots and their presence with evidence of dilated ventricles in patients with intracranial hypertension helps to make the diagnosis. Less commonly, CT scan shows multiple cysts of differing size with low attenuation values and with or without peripheral enhancement. In acute lesions which are multiple, precontrast CT studies often show severe cerebral oedema, compressed ventricles, poorly visualized cisterns, and cortical sulci. Scanning after contrast injection reveals enhancement of numerous small ring-like areas. In the acute single lesion, the precontrast image shows an area of decreased attentuation due to focal oedema whilst a small ring-like area is visualized in the centre of the area of decreased attentuation after contrast injection. Occasionally, in patients with spinal cord or cauda equina lesions, the presence of more than one round movable filling defect of the contrast medium on myelography is strongly suggestive of the diagnosis of cysticercosis.

The CSF is often under increased pressure with slight increase of cells, usually not exceeding 100 and consisting mostly of mononuclear cells. Eosinophils are present in about one-third of cases and tend to be found in patients with acute meningoencephalitis, and subacute or chronic meningitis. They are usually absent in the CSF of patients presenting with epileptic attacks. Eosinophilic pleocytosis is usually mild, being mostly less than 10 per cent of the total cell count. Very rarely, a figure of up to 30 per cent of eosinophils has been recorded. The CSF total protein is usually normal or slightly increased unless there is subarachnoid block. A level of 100 mg/100 ml is rare; but the immunoglobulin content is often disproportionately high. Cerebrospinal fluid glucose is decreased in about half the cases and levels of less than 10 mg/100 ml have been encountered.

Cysticercosis complement fixation test on the CSF is often helpful and diagnostic, being positive in about 80 per cent of cases, particularly in those with intraventricular, cisternal or meningeal lesions. The yield is much less in calcified lesions.

Treatment

Until recently, there was no specific treatment for cysticercosis. In 1978, successful treatment of porcine cysticercosis with praziquantel was reported. The drug was subsequently tried on patients with cerebral cysticercosis. The dosage given was 50 mg per kg of body weight daily for 15 days. During treatment, a stong inflammatory reaction sometimes occurred, as evidenced by increase in CSF protein and cells. This finding correlated with headache, exacerbation of neurological symptoms, and presence of oedema around cystic lesions as seen in CT scans of the brain. It is, therefore, advisable to give corticosteroid concurrently with praziquantel to minimize those undesirable effects. Clinical improvement is seen after three months of treatment. The mean diameter and total number of cysts decrease significantly.

In addition to praziquantel, long-term anticonvulsant therapy is still necessary for the control of epilepsy. Cysts causing intraventricular obstruction, or spinal cord or cauda equina compression should be surgically treated. In patients with communicating hydrocephalus, shunting procedures not infrequently relieve symptoms temporarily and should thus be considered.

Prognosis is often poor in patients with heavy infestation of the cerebral parenchyma, giving rise to dementia and increased intracranial pressure. The outcome is better in those with isolated intraventricular or subarachnoid cysts that are amendable to surgery. Patients with epileptic attacks often have a normal life-span although they may need life-long anticonvulsant treatment. The role of praziquantel in altering the outcome of the disease needs further elucidation.

Eosinophilic meningitis due to *Angiostrongylus cantonensis*

The rat lung worm, *Angiostrongylus cantonensis*, primarily a parasite of rodents, is largely responsible for human cases of eosinophilic meningitis in Southeast Asia.

Aetiology

The disease is produced by invasion of the central nervous system by larvae of *A. cantonensis*. The adult worms live in the pulmonary arteries of different species of rat. First-stage larvae develop from eggs in the pulmonary arterioles, migrate through the respiratory passages of the rat into the pharynx, are swallowed, and subsequently are excreted in the faeces. They further develop in one of several species of snails or slugs which serve as intermediate hosts. The larvae may enter the mollusc by actively penetrating the cuticle, or the mollusc may ingest the larvae with the faeces of the rat. In the mollusc, the larvae become encapsulated by fibrous tissue of the host. They grow and undergo two moults. The second-stage larva is immobile. The third-stage larva is infective for the mammalian host. Humans acquire the infection mostly from eating raw or undercooked infected snails or slugs and occasionally from invertebrate transport hosts such as fresh water prawns and land crabs. In Thailand, the disease is particularly prevalent in the north-eastern and central regions and appears to be confined to traditional Thai people of the lower socio-economic groups. The rarity among the resident Chinese and their first-generation descendants is noteworthy. The disease often has seasonal occurrence and is frequently seen in epidemic extent. A large number of cases are encountered during the rainy season when *Pila* snails breed and are readily available. It is not uncommon that several adults and children are affected, a week or two after they have enjoyed a common meal consisting of raw *Pila* snails which are considered to be a great delicacy.

Clinical manifestations

The incubation period ranges from three days to five weeks with an average of about two weeks. The commonest presenting symptom is headache which occurs in almost all patients either abruptly or insidiously. It usually begins in and is localized to the occipital region, although bitemporal and retrobulbar headaches often occur. When severe, it tends to be generalized. It is often throbbing or bursting in nature. usually intermittent in the beginning, but soon becomes persistent and is often associated with nausea and vomiting. Stabbing pains in the head and paraesthesia of the scalp are occasionally present. Fever is recorded in less than half the cases and is of low grade, rarely exceeding 38 °C and lasting only a few days. Rarely, mental confusion and generalized convulsions occur, and a few patients complain of generalized weakness of the extremities. Examination reveals neck stiffness and Kernig's sign in practically all cases. In the majority of cases, no other abnormal neurological signs are noted. Impairment of vision and swelling of optic discs are found in about 15 per cent of patients. Occasionally, slight swelling of both eyelids, paresis of the abducens nerve, and facial palsy are seen. In another type with purely ocular involvement, young adult worms have been found in the anterior chamber of the eye or in the vitreous substance. Blepharospasm, ciliary injection, iritis, and increased ocular tension were noted in the affected eye. A patient with the parasite in the eye two weeks after a mild attack of meningitis has also been reported. Hyperaesthesia of a limb or the trunk is detected in about a third of cases and may be the result of migration of worms in the nerve roots. Spinal cord symptoms and signs are rare in this disease.

Laboratory findings

Blood leucocytosis of over $10 \times 10^9/1$ is found in about 50 per cent of cases and eosinophilia of over 10 per cent is present in the majority of patients. The latter tends to increase during the first few days of the disease, then slowly decreases, and may persist for several weeks. The CSF is always abnormal except in patients with ocular angiostrongyliasis. Pressure is often increased and the fluid is usually turbid, likened to water after washing rice grains. The white cell count is over 500/mm^3 in 75 per cent of cases and may be as high as 5000. Eosinophils ranging from 20 to 70 per cent of the total cells are common, and over 90 per cent have been recorded; the remaining cells are neutrophils and lymphocytes. There seems to be no connection between the level of blood and CSF eosinophils. Spinal fluid eosinophils tend to be high between the second and fourth weeks after the onset of clinical symptoms, then decline, only to increase again during the sixth and eighth week, usually disappearing at the end of the third month. The CSF protein is often elevated but is usually less than 100 mg/100 ml. The immunoglobulin content is always disproportionately high and remains so for some time. This is a helpful diagnostic point in cases with suggestive clinical features and in whom the CSF is examined at a stage when eosinophil count is low. The CSF glucose content is normal, although a slight decrease has been observed in a few cases. Exceptionally, a living fifth stage *A. cantonensis*, measuring about 0.5–1.5 cm in length has been isolated from CSF at lumbar puncture. Other investigations including chest and skull X-rays are normal and the electroencephalogram often shows generalized, non-specific abnormalities.

Clinical course

The duration of the disease ranges from a few days to a month. Most patients recover completely. Permanent impairment of vision is occasionally seen in patients with optic nerve involvement and in those with ocular form of angiostrongyliasis after surgical removal of the worm from the eye. Long-term follow-up of patients is necessary, since late-onset epilepsy and impaired mental function may develop. The mortality rate of the disease is about 11 per cent.

Treatment

There is no specific treatment for the disease. Prompt and dramatic relief of headache occurs following the release of CSF and repeated tappings are often necessary. In severe cases, corticosteroid treatment has been tried, but efficacy is doubtful. Prevention of the disease rests on the control of rodents and molluscs and proper cooking of snails and prawns to destroy the infective larvae of *A. cantonensis* before they are eaten.

Gnathostomiasis

Gnathostomiasis is an infestation of humans by the nematode, *Gnathostoma spinigerum*.

Aetiology

The adult worms are parasites inhabiting the stomach walls of cats, dogs, and tigers. Fertilized ova excreted with the host's faeces are flushed by rain into ponds, canals, and rivers where they hatch into first-stage larvae which are then ingested by small crustaceans of genus *Cyclops*, the first intermediate host. There the larvae develop into the second stage. Infected *Cyclops* are eaten by fish, frogs, and eels, and the larvae penetrate the intestines of these second intermediate hosts to become encysted in their flesh or viscera and develop into third-stage larvae which are infective. Humans acquire the infection from eating raw or undercooked freshwater fish. The third-stage larvae that are ingested migrate and soon transform into immature worms, each of about 1 cm in length.

Signs and symptoms

Most of the clinical manifestations of human gnathostomiasis are due to the high motility of the immature worms. These commonly cause painless migratory subcutaneous swellings which usually last for a few days and subside spontaneously. The swelling may recur several times a year and the disease may last several years. Occasionally, the worms migrate into the eye, the lung, and pleura, the intestine, the urinary tract, and the uterus; but it is due to invasion of the nervous system that a severe, incapacitating, and occasionally fatal illness develops.

The neurological onset is acute and may or may not be preceded by migratory subcutaneous swellings. The presenting symptom is usually severe, sharp, agonizing radicular pain in the trunk or a limb, often followed within a few days by sudden paraplegia and urinary retention. Less commonly paralysis ascends to involve the upper extremities and respiratory muscles. In some patients, the brain stem is affected resulting in cranial nerve palsies with dysphagia, dysarthria, facial weakness, and diplopia. Impairment of consciousness and respiratory failure follow and the mortality rate is high in these cases. Occasionally, patients present with headache, disturbance of consciousness, and cranial nerve palsies without clinical evidence of radiculomyelitis while others have classical features of primary subarachnoid haemorrhage without any neurological deficit.

Diagnosis

The CSF of patients with gnathostomiasis is unlike that seen in eosinophilic meningitis due to *A. cantonesis* in that it is usually bloodstained or xanthochromic. At least a few red blood cells are usually present while eosinophils from 5 to over 90 per cent are found among the total white cells that range from 20 up to almost 1500/μl. The CSF protein is increased, but is seldom over 100 mg/100 ml, while the sugar level is normal.

The peripheral blood picture often shows slight to moderate leucocytosis with an eosinophilia of up to almost 40 per cent during the nervous system manifestations. A higher figure is sometimes encountered during the migration of worms in other parts of the body.

The diagnosis of gnathostomiasis is confirmed in some patients when the worms, after causing neurological symptoms and signs, appear beneath the skin and are removed via small surgical incisions. In those who die, living immature parasites are occasionally isolated from the brain and spinal cord at autopsy and sections of the brain stem and spinal cord always show multiple haemorrhagic tracks. In others who survive and from whom the worms cannot be isolated, the diagnosis of the disease rests on the clinical features, the CSF changes, and the history of eating raw or undercooked freshwater fish. The mortality rate is higher than that of eosinophilic meningitis due to *A. cantonensis* and neurological morbidity is much commoner.

Treatment

No specific antihelminthic drug is available. Isolation of the immature worm through surgical skin incision when subcutaneous swelling occurs usually results in a cure unless there is re-infection. Potent analgesics are often needed for the severe radicular pain, and corticosteroids are commonly administered although their efficacy is not well proven. Endotracheal intubation and assisted respiration are often life-saving in patients with respiratory failure.

References
Boongird, P., Phuapradit, P., Siridej, N., Chirachariyavej, T., Chauhiran, S. and Vejjajiva, A. (1977). Neurological manifestations of gnathostomiasis. *J. Neurol. Sci.* **31**, 279–291.
Daengsvang, S. (1980). *A monograph on the genus gnathostoma and gnathostomiasis in Thailand.* Southeast Asian Medical Information Center, Tokyo.
Jindrak, K. (1975). *Angiostrongyliasis cantonensis* (eosinophilic meningitis, Alicata's disease). In *Topics on tropical neurology* (ed. R. W. Hornabrook), p. 133. F. A. Davis, Philadelphia.
Kuroiwa, Y., Hung, T-P., Landsborough, D., Park, C. S., Singhal, B. S., Soemargo, S., Vejjajiva, A. and Shibasaki, H. (1977). Multiple sclerosis in Asia. *Neurology (Minneap.)* **27**, 188–192.
Minguetti, G. and Ferreira, M.V.C. (1983). Computed tomography in neurocysticercosis. *J. Neurol. Neurosurg. Psychiatr.* **46**, 936–942.
Phuapradit, P., Roongwithu, N., Limsukon, P., Boongird, P. and Vejjajiva, A. (1976). Radiculomyelitis complicating acute haemorrhagic conjunctivitis: A clinical study. *J. Neurol. Sci.* **27**, 117–122.
Sotelo, J., Escobedo, F., Rodriguez-Carbajal, J., Torres, B. and Rubio-Donnadieu, F. (1984). Therapy of parenchymal brain cysticercosis with praziquantel. *N. Engl. J. Med.* **310**, 1001–1007.
Vejjajiva, A. (1968). Neurological sequelae of anti-rabic inoculation. *Proc. Aust. Ass. Neurol.* **5**, 367–370.
Vejjajiva, A. (1973). Neurology in Thailand. In *Tropical neurology* (ed. J.D. Spillane), p. 335. Oxford University Press, London.

Africa

O. BADEMOSI

The impact of geography on general medicine and neurology in particular has become increasingly appreciated within the last decade. It is difficult to obtain a true picture of neurology in Africa for various obvious reasons. There is a dearth of trained personnel in the neurosciences, technical expertise, and resources for investigations; definitive diagnosis of neurological disorders are either non-existent or grossly inadequate and the accuracy of data from most developing countries is questionable.

In this context Africa is restricted to all parts of Africa excluding 'White' South Africa. It includes the following regions: North Africa extending from Morocco to Egypt, inhabited by people of Hamito-Semitic origin; West Africa extending from Senegal in the West to the Camerouns, peopled mainly by 'West African' Negroes; Central and East African countries occupying the main central hinterland and extending eastwards to Ethiopia and Eritrea with people of mixed origin namely the scattered central pygmy lands, the Nilotes, and Nilo-Hamites in the northern and eastern regions, and the Bantus in the south. The diversity in Africa includes not only its peoples but also the climate, vegetation, resources, culture, socioeconomic characteristics, and standard of medical practice amongst other features; and these factors modify both the pattern of disease and accuracy of any data collected.

There is paucity of accurate epidemiological data on neurological diseases in most parts of Africa. Most of the data and information available are based on hospital population studies and anecdotal reports, and many of the community-based surveys have inherent flaws in methodology. These factors make it impossible to obtain the true picture of the prevalence of neurological disorders in various communities, and to make meaningful comparisons with patterns in other environments difficult. Despite these constraints, there is an identifiable trend in the pattern of neurological diseases in Africa, even though the aetiological factors responsible for the same clinical syndrome often vary from one environment to another.

Infections of the nervous system

Infectious disorders of the nervous system constitute the commonest neurological problem in Africa, accounting for 20–40 per cent of all neurological diseases seen.

Meningitis

The commonest forms are meningococcal, pneumococcal, tuberculous, and *Haemophilus influenzae* meningitis.

Meningococcal meningitis

This is endemic in tropical Africa and has a tendency towards 2- to 10-yearly epidemics. The epidemics are restricted to the savannah belt between latitudes 8° and 16°N stretching across the Sahel region from Senegal, Mali, Burkina Fasso (formerly Upper Volta), Ghana, the northern part of Nigeria, southern regions of Sudan, and northern parts of Uganda to Ethiopia. These regions fall within an annual rainfall belt of 300–1100 mm and have long, dry, hot seasons from November to April. The carrier rate in the community rises from 5 per 1000 in the non-epidemic years to about 20 and 80 per 1000 at the beginning and peak of the epidemic, respectively. Although sero-groups A, B, C, and Y are the main causes of disease in humans, the major epidemics in Africa have been due mainly to groups A and C.

It is a disease of young adults, usually under the age of 50 years, with a peak incidence between 5 and 15 years during epidemics. The prognosis is good with a mortality rate of less than 2 per cent although this rises to between 5 and 15 per cent during epidemics. The major complications encountered are cutaneous vasculitis in the form of punched-out skin ulcers in the extremities, episcleritis, polyarthritis, and rarely peripheral vascular collapse ('endotoxic shock', Waterhouse syndrome) (see Section 5). These complications are immune-mediated. Clinical awareness and early diagnosis, particularly in the population at risk, are essential in forestalling disastrous outbreaks of epidemics. Apart from reducing factors which favour transmission, prophylactic drug treatment of high-risk groups with broad-spectrum antibiotics like ampicillin is preferred because of the emergence of sulphonamide-resistant strains. In addition, vaccination of the community with antigen of the serotype responsible for the epidemic dramatically alters the course of the epidemic. Group A, B, and C meningococcal vaccines are currently available.

Pneumococcal meningitis

This is 4–10 times more frequent in developing than in the developed countries. The infection is endemic in the tropical rain forest belt of Africa and epidemics are unknown. The majority of cases occur during the dry season reaching a peak during February and March. It afflicts mainly young adults and shows a male to female ratio of 3:2; 9 per cent of the cases are under 40 years old with a peak incidence in the second decade. In up to 40 per cent of cases no obvious primary focus is encountered, although lobar pneumonia is present in 20 per cent. Sickle cell disease and pregnancy are important predisposing factors in Nigerians; others include cirrhosis of the liver, nephrotic syndrome, and gastrointestinal malignancies.

Crystalline penicillin remains the antibiotic of choice, best given intravenously for the first 96 hours and continued for at least a week after resolution of the clinical signs of meningeal irritation to prevent recrudescence and minimize complications. Steroids have not proved effective in Nigerians. Despite advances in treatment and management, mortality and morbidity remain high. The mortality rate reported from most studies in Africa range from 10 to 60 per cent. Neurological sequelae encountered in about 10–20 per cent of cases include encephalopathy in form of personality and intellectual changes, cranial neuropathy especially perceptive deafness, focal deficits such as hemiparesis, cerebellar incoordination, choreoathetosis, Parkinsonism, and epilepsy.

Tuberculous meningitis

Although its true incidence is difficult to determine in most developing countries where tuberculosis is endemic, meningitis has been reported in 5–10 per cent of patients with pulmonary tuberculosis. It is more frequent in young people, especially in the first decade; 90 per cent of the cases are under 50 years old. The presentation is of a subacute infection with an insiduous onset although in 20 per cent the onset is acute. Signs of meningeal irritation and alteration in level of consciousness are found in 80 per cent of adult cases; in children, generalized convulsions are the presenting feature in about a third of the cases and about 40 per cent are admitted in coma.

However, an acute onset with polymorphonuclear CSF leucocytosis and markedly reduced sugar (< 0.5 mmol/l) is seen in 10–15 per cent of the cases. The occurrence of neurological complications and sequelae is more frequent than with pneumococcal meningitis. Delay in diagnosis and institution of specific therapy or associated miliary spread, and coma worsen prognosis. Treatment is by the current standard antituberculous drug regimen. The effectiveness of empirical steroid therapy is questionable.

Haemophilus influenza

This is the commonest organism responsible for bacterial meningitis in children under 5 years old particularly between the ages of 3 months and 3 years. The clinical picture and prognosis are similar to those of pneumococcal meningitis. In Senegal, the disease occurs mainly during the wet season.

Viral meningitis

This occurs mainly in children, and is commonly associated with Coxsackie and echo viruses. In some cases, poliomyelitis or influenza virus may be incriminated. The CSF shows a lymphocytosis and normal sugar content. Treatment is essentially symptomatic. Complete recovery occurs in the majority of cases within 3 weeks except when there is associated encephalitis.

Other forms of meningitis

These are relatively uncommon. Some of the organisms identified include Salmonella species, especially *S. typhi, Candida albicans*, pseudomonas, proteus, and *Cryptococcus neoformans*.

Encephalitis

This may arise as a primary disease or a complication of an underlying local or generalized infective process. Viruses are the commonest cause; the most frequently isolated are the arboviruses, enteroviruses, the herpes group, influenza, rabies, and measles virus, respectively (see page 21.145). Other common causes include trypanosome infection (*T. gambiense* and *T. rhodesiense*) and typhoid fever (see Section 5). There are three clinical forms:

Acute This occurs mainly in children and presents with continuous fever and impaired consciousness. In children, vomiting, restlessness, delirium, and general convulsions are more uncommon. Complications include hemiparesis, choreoathetosis, Parkinsonian features, personality changes, and epilepsy.

Subacute This presents mainly with impaired consciousness and progressive mental deterioration. The common causes are trypanosomiasis and syphilis. Occasionally, subacute sclerosing panencephalitis (SSPE) associated with measles is seen. It is difficult to explain the relatively low incidence of SSPE despite the high prevalence rate of measles in most parts of tropical Africa.

Chronic This has been associated with a group of clinical syndromes characterized by a progressive deterioration of mental function associated with chronic infection of a transmissible virus. It includes the clinical entities of Creutzfeldt–Jakob disease (see page 21.45), Kuru (see Section 5), and Pick's disease (page 21.44) in humans. These disorders are rare in tropical Africa.

Rabies

This is not common in most parts of Africa. It has an annual hospital incidence rate of 1–2 cases per year at Ibadan, Nigeria. The clinical course is similar to the pattern in other environments (see Section 5).

Poliomyelitis

This is endemic in Africa and its incidence tends to rise before, during, and just after the rainy season. It occurs mainly in children with a peak between 2 and 3 years and is rare before the age of 3 months and above 7 years; 90 per cent of children in tropical Africa show serological evidence of contact with the virus by the age of 5 years. Involvement of the lumbar segments of the spinal cord with asymmetrical weakness of the lower limbs is the most frequent presentation of its paralytic form. Contractures of the lower limbs, flail limbs, and skeletal deformities are the usual late sequelae, although complete recovery is observed in 90–95 per cent of cases.

Trypanosomiasis (sleeping sickness)

Trypanosomiasis in humans is caused by trypanosome species *T. gambiense* and *T. rhodesiense* in Africa (see Section 5). It is limited to latitudes 10°N and 25°S and transmitted by the tse-tse fly, Glossina species. *Trypanosoma gambiense*, more widely distributed than *T. rhodesiense*, occurs mainly in West and Central Africa but is seen in East Africa, especially in the northern parts of Uganda. It is transmitted by *G. palpalis*, *G. pollides*, *G. tachinoides*, and *G. morsitans*. *Trypanosoma rhodesiense* is limited to East and Central Africa with *G. morsitans* as its main vector. The clinical features of the two diseases are similar: the illness due to *T. gambiense* is usually mild but tends to have acute exacerbations, while that due to *T. rhodesiense* has a shorter incubation period and runs a more fulminant course. The early phase of the disease is characterized by a tender swelling over the site of insect bite followed by fever, headache, and non-tender firm enlargement of the superficial lymph-nodes. Central nervous system involvement, which occurs between 4 and 6 months of the initial symptoms, presents as progressive personality disintegration, impairment of consciousness with increased somnolence, psychosis simulating schizophrenia and dementia. If undiagnosed and untreated, coma develops, and death results from internment infection and cardiac failure. Diagnosis is made by the demonstration of trypanosomes in blood, aspirate from the enlarged lymph-nodes, or CSF; sometimes animal innoculation and culture on special media is required to establish the diagnosis.

Neurosyphilis

This is not uncommon in Africa, although it is restricted to the urban areas. Meningovascular neurosyphilis and general paralysis of the insane are the commoner forms of the disease and tabes dorsalis is relatively rare (see page 21.141). The relative absence of neurosyphilis in some areas such as southern Nigeria and Ghana has been related to the protection of cross-immunity induced by yaws (caused by *Treponema pertenue*) which was at one time endemic in those areas.

Tetanus

Tetanus is prevalent in children and adults in most parts of Africa (see Section 5). Its incidence appears to be diminishing probably as a result of increased medical awareness and mass immunization. The major predisposing factors or portals of entry in adults are traumas which occur on farms and highways, genital sepsis particularly following delivery, chronic otitis media, and following surgical procedures such as scarifications by 'traditional' surgeons. The majority of cases present with generalized tetanus; cephalic or localized forms are exceedingly rare. In about 30 per cent of the cases, either the portal of entry is unidentified or the time of innoculation undetermined, making calculation of the incubation period difficult. The features which carry a poor prognosis are a short period of onset (interval between first symptom and onset of muscle spasms), severity of disease as determined by frequency and appearance of spontaneous spasms, laryngeal spasms, apnoeic spells, tachycardia, as well as elevated serum glutamic oxalate transaminase and blood urea on admission. The mortality rate in adults reported from most studies range from 10 to 50 per cent and may be as high as 90 per cent. The common causes of death include pulmonary embolism, intercurrent chest infection, aspiration pneumonia, cardiac complications, especially ventricular fibrillation, and acute respiratory failure. Other unusual complications encountered are painless fracture of the body of the vertebrae and myositis ossificans especially in large muscle groups such as the quadriceps femoris or around the elbow and knee joints. Apart from the use of human immunoglobulin when available, management should include adequate fluid and caloric replacement, sedation with parenteral diazepam, basic care to prevent decubitus ulcers, aspiration pneumonia, and pulmonary embolism (see Section 3). Therapeutic antitetanus serum (ATS), 20 000 i.u. intravenously, after a test dose, is still advised. Any wound should be appropriately treated, with debridement when indicated, routine dressing, and specific antibiotic therapy dictated by identification of organisms. In some cases tracheostomy with or without assisted respiration would be life-saving. The efficacy of intrathecal heterologous ATS still needs to be proven.

Helminthic infestations

Experience of cysticercosis in Africa is limited to isolated case reports. Most of the cases present with epilepsy although spinal forms have been described. The relative rarity of the disease in most parts of Africa is probably due to the influence of Islam which prohibits ingestion of pork.

Schistosomiasis

This is endemic in most parts of Africa. *Schistosoma mansoni* infects the gastrointestinal and genitourinary tracts, *S. japonicum* the gastrointestinal tract, and *S. haematobium* the genitourinary tract. Involvement of the nervous system is rare, although its incidence may be rising in Central Africa especially Zimbabwe. It may present as an acute or subacute encephalitis, intracranial or intracerebral granuloma, or as a spinal cord lesion.

Vascular disorders of the nervous system

Recent studies suggest that cerebrovascular disorders (CVD) are becoming a major cause of morbidity and mortality in Africa, contrary to previously held views. CVD is commoner in males, its incidence rises with age, and is uncommon in the young. It appears that the pathology and pathogenesis of CVD in the African is different from that in Caucasians and Black Americans. The overall incidence from the only available community survey of 26 per 100 000 is markedly lower than the values of 50 to 400/100 000 in developed countries; the age-specific rates for those under 45 years old is markedly lower, 4/100 000 compared with 10–20/100 000 in Europe and Japan, but comparable for the 45–65 age group with values of 2.5–5.4/100 000 and 0.7–6.7/100 000, respectively; the drop of the age-specific rates in individuals above 65 years old has been related to low frequency of cerebral atherosclerosis in Africans.

Non-embolic CVD constitutes 60–70 per cent of all CVD, and the mortality rate is about 20 per cent. The lesions involve mainly the middle cerebral artery although precerebral occlusive disease especially of the carotid artery is sometimes encountered. Cerebral haemorrhage, responsible for 20–30 per cent of the cases, carries a poor prognosis with a case fatality rate of 60 per cent. The most important predisposing factor for these forms of CVD are hypertension and diabetes mellitus; others include pregnancy, meningitis, and sickle cell disease.

Primary subarachnoid haemorrhage accounts for 10 per cent of the cases, shows a male to female ratio of 3:1, and has a mortality rate of 50–60 per cent. It is caused mainly by vascular malformations (aneurysms being more frequent than arteriovenous malformations), and is occasionally encountered in sickle cell disease particularly in children and adolescents. Embolic CVD is encountered in about 10 per cent; the main sources of emboli are cardiac diseases especially infective endocarditis, rheumatic heart disease, congestive cardiomyopathy, endomyocardial fibrosis, and atrial fibrillation. The emboli arise from the intramural thrombi or vegetations.

Hypertensive encephalopathy is relatively uncommon, accounting for less than 5 per cent of cases. It is encountered in eclampsia, chronic renal failure, usually with an acute decompensation, and occasionally in patients with severe accelerating hypertension. The mortality rate is high in these patients.

Transient ischaemic attacks (TIAs) are not uncommon but apparently have a worse prognosis in Africans than Caucasians. The low incidence of TIAs in Black Africans has been ascribed to the rarity of severe atherosclerosis of the large arterial vessels.

Spinal cord lesions

The common causes of spinal cord syndromes are trauma, tuberculosis of the spine with compression of the cord, transverse myelitis, tropical ataxic nutritional neuropathy, and tumour masses which are most frequently sited extradurally. Malignant lymphomas including Hodgkin's disease and Burkitt's lymphoma, and metastatic deposits mainly from the prostate and thyroid gland constitute most of these cases. Meningiomas and neurofibromas are the main types of primary neurogenous cord lesions seen. Intraspinal astrocytoma and ependymoma are uncommon. Less common causes include *Histoplasma duboisii* infection (African histoplasmosis) and other pyogenic osteomyelitis of the vertebrae, cervical spondylosis, and canal stenosis.

In about 20 per cent of the cases, no definite aetiological factor is identified. This group of obscure myelopathies apparently shows no sex predilection, tends to affect individuals under 40 years old, presents primarily with spastic paresis in most of the cases, and runs a non-fatal course. Normal myelographic findings suggest that arachnoiditis and granulomata are unlikely causes. The pattern and distribution of the cord involvement suggest a demyelinating process related to an autoimmune mechanism in the majority of cases.

Tropical ataxic nutritional neuropathy

This is characterized by symmetrical peripheral neuropathy, bilateral primary optic atrophy, bilateral sensorineural deafness, and posterior column deficit. In about 5–10 per cent, there may be associated spastic paraparesis. Epidemiological studies show that it is common in parts of Nigeria, Senegal, Uganda, and Ghana. It is due to chronic cyanide intoxication resulting from ingesting cassava and other tubers rich in cyanide, and inadequate protein supplements. The majority of patients have evidence of malnutrition and other vitamin B group deficiency states such as mucocutaneous lesions, angular stomatitis, and glossitis. The characteristic biochemical changes are raised plasma cyanide and thiocyanate as well as urinary thiocyanate. There is no biochemical evidence of vitamin B_{12} deficiency as shown by plasma levels and urinary methylmalonic acid concentrations. Recent clinical impressions suggest that its incidence is reduced probably due to better standards of living.

Peripheral nerve disease

Peripheral nerve disease (PND) excluding primary neoplastic lesions is common, and affects mainly adults; only 10 per cent of cases are under 20 years old. Autonomic neuropathy as the initial presentation is rare. Symmetrical peripheral neuropathy as a group is the commonest form of PND seen: sensorimotor type (50 per cent) pure sensory (10 per cent), and motor peripheral neuropathy (5 per cent). The common causes are Guillain–Barré syndrome (GBS), nutritional deficiency states related to the vitamin B group, and diabetes mellitus; no cause is found in one-third of cases. Females appear more prone to nutritional peripheral neuropathy than males, with pregnancy and lactation acting as the precipitating factors. PND due to vitamin B_{12} deficiency and subacute combined degeneration are rare in the African.

The individual peripheral nerves commonly involved in mononeuritis simplex and multiplex are the median, ulnar, common peroneal, and radial nerves. Hansen's disease (leprosy) affecting mainly the ulnar and common peroneal nerves is the commonest cause. Direct trauma and pressure (entrapment neuropathy) are the other main causes. Carpal tunnel syndrome, the most frequent form of mononeuritis simplex is associated with pregnancy, acromegaly, nephrotic syndrome, hypothyroidism, and rheumatoid arthritis. Sciatica and slipped disc syndromes are rarely encountered in peasant farmers. Lumbosacral plexus injury with foot drop is the usual presenting feature of obstetric neuropraxia. It is associated with spontaneous vertex delivery especially in short primiparous women (height < 1.58 m), and prolonged or obstructed labour is the major precipitating factor. The prognosis is good however, as complete recovery occurs in 80 per cent of the cases within six weeks of onset.

Cranial neuropathy excluding isolated peripheral facial nerve paresis is uncommon (10–12 per cent); malignancies related to structures around the head and neck especially the sinuses, and metastatic deposits from tumours such as Burkitt's lymphoma or choriocarcinoma are the commonest causes; others include migraine and GBS. Peripheral facial nerve paresis (facial palsy) is common and its incidence is markedly lower in the western than in northern parts of Africa. Bell's palsy is the commonest cause (60–95 per cent). Other causes are GBS and Hansen's disease, and following pyogenic meningitis, chronic otitis media and trauma. Metastatic deposits from choriocarcinoma, primary liver cell, and ovarian carcinoma are unusual causes.

Basal ganglia disorders

Recent studies suggest that Parkinsonism is as common in Africans as in Caucasians, contrary to previous observations. It has a male to female ratio of 3:1, with the peak frequency in the sixth decade. The mean ages of onset of paralysis agitans (idiopathic), atherosclerotic (vascular), and postencephalitic Parkinsonism are 55.6, 55.8, and 20.7 years, respectively, in Nigeria. Other causes include drugs, typhoid fever, and chronic liver disease, especially cirrhosis of the liver. Drug-induced Parkinsonism was associated with psychotropic drugs especially chlorpromazine and haloperidol, but symptoms tend to persist on withdrawal of the offending drug in a third of cases. Parkinsonism occurs occasionally during the acute phase of typhoid fever and clears on recovery. Wilson's disease, Huntington's chorea, and Parkinsonism related to long-term professional pugilism ('punch drunk' syndrome) are rare in Black Africans.

Paroxysmal disorders

Epilepsy

Epilepsy remains one of the commonest neurological conditions in developing countries and has a prevalence rate of between 10 and 49 per 1000. In most parts of Africa, it still attracts myths and is socially unacceptable. Partial, with or without secondarily generalized tonic-clonic seizures, are the commonest type seen (50–70 per cent), of which complex partial seizures are the most frequent clinical variant. Primary generalized tonic-clonic seizures account for only 10–15 per cent. Absence seizures (petit mal) and other forms of childhood epilepsies (akinetic 'salam' fit, myoclonic epilepsy, Lennox Gastaut syndrome) are relatively rare. No cause is found in the majority of cases (60–80 per cent). Symptomatic epilepsy is associated with infections (meningitis and encephalitis), vascular lesions such as arteriovenous malformations and CVD, head injury, cerebral tumours, and birth injuries. Parasitic infections such as toxoplasmosis, toxocariasis, and schistosomiasis are unusual, although in the Bantus cysticercosis is observed in 6–16 per cent of cases. In a recent survey in Nigeria, febrile convulsions were identified as a major cause of epilepsy.

Headache syndromes

Headache is a common presenting symptom. It accounts for up to 20 per cent of neurological outpatient attendance, and 10 per cent of the rural community suffer from it. Tension headache is the commonest variant (60–70 per cent) and associated features of anxiety are present in the majority. Migraine has a female to male ratio of 3:1. In a rural community survey in Nigeria, its point prevalence was 69/1000, and a positive family history was present in 80 per cent. The relative distribution of the clinical variants of migraine is common migraine (52 per cent), classical migraine (27 per cent), complicated migraine (16 per cent), and cluster headache of Horton's type (5 per cent). In Nigeria, the sickle cell trait is significantly more frequent in complicated than other clinical types of migraine. The main feature of complicated migraine, apart from headache, is ophthalmoplegia usually involving the oculomotor nerve; less common features are hemiparesis, ipsilateral amaurosis, vertigo, loss of consciousness, and, rarely, segmental visual field defects. In these patients, no structural intracranial lesions are demonstrable.

Headache following trivial or severe head injuries is frequently encountered. The majority of patients with posttraumatic headache (anxiety/accident neurosis) have often had a trivial head injury, and have associated anxiety features; objective neurological deficits are absent and the electroencephalograms (EEG) are normal. There is paucity of medico-legal awareness in respect of accidents in the general population in most parts of Africa. Thus, it is unlikely that compensation claims play a major role in these patients. However, persistence of the symptoms, unwillingness to return to work, and perennial visits to hospitals suggest that some motivation operates in a proportion.

Disease of muscle

The muscular dystrophies including myotonic disorders are not rare. The main clinical forms seen are Duchenne, limb-girdle, facioscapulohumeral types of muscular dystrophy, and dystrophia myotonica. Other forms are exceedingly rare.

Polymyositis is occasionally encountered, and is commoner in females. The disease often presents without other associated disorders. Cutaneous changes of dermatomyositis are not unusual. The main associated conditions seen are lymphomas and mixed connective tissue disease especially rheumatoid arthritis.

Myaesthenia gravis Its incidence is similar to that in Caucasians, it affects females more than males, and only 10–15 per cent of the cases are over 40 years of age at presentation. Severe muscle wasting is present. Limitations of the disease to ocular muscles and spontaneous remission are uncommon. It is associated with squamous and bronchogenic carcinoma in patients in Nigeria but none had features for the Eaton–Lambert type (see Section 22). Associated thyroid disease and thymoma have not been reported so far. Although medication is the mainstay of therapy, thymectomy is effective in Nigeria.

Proximal myopathy has been encountered in patients with connective tissue disease (polyarteritis nodosa, systemic lupus erythematosus), acromegaly, thyrotoxocosis, and chronic renal failure.

Pyomyositis An acute suppurative disease of muscle, is the commonest type of primary muscle disease in the tropics (see Section 5). Eighty per cent are under 30 years old and males outnumber females. Staphylococcus and coliforms are the organisms most commonly incriminated. The muscle groups usually involved are the quadriceps femoris, hamstrings, gastronemius, erector spinae, latissimus dorsi, and trapezius. Surgical drainage and appropriate antibiotic therapy are the mainstays of management.

Congenital and hereditary neurodegenerative disorders

Congenital malformations of the neural axis are uncommon in tropical Africa unlike the clinical impression in North Africa. The major types seen in tropical Africa are spina bifida, hydrocephalus, meningocoele, and meningomyelocoele. Craniostenosis is frequent in North Africa especially in Algeria, Morocco, and Tunisia, but has also been reported from Kenya.

The rarity of hereditary neurodegenerative disorders has been related to numerous factors: consanguinity is exceptional, a slowly progressive disability may be culturally acceptable, and limited facilities in the neurosciences. Familial essential tremor, the most frequent type seen, shows a male to female ratio of 9:1. Other forms seen are Huntington's chorea, hereditary ataxia of either predominant cerebellar or spinal type, Charcot–Marie–Tooth disease, and ataxia telangiectasia.

Writer's cramp is occasionally seen. The hospital incidence ranges from 4 to 7 per 100 000, and males are predominantly affected (male:female ratio 10:1). It seems restricted to occupations associated with much writing such as teachers, civil servants, students, and court registrars.

References

Adeloye, A., Olumide, A. O., Bademosi, O. and Kolawole, T. M. (1981). Intracranial vascular anomalies in Nigerians. *Trop. geogr. Med.* **33**, 263–267.

Aiyesimoju, A. B., Osuntokun, B. O., Bademosi, O. and Adeuja, A. O. (1984). Hereditary neurodegenerative disorders in Nigerian Africans. *Neurology (Cleveland)* **34**, 361–362.

Bademosi, O. and Osuntokun, B. O. (1979). Prednisolone in the treatment of pneumococcal meningitis: a clinical study in Ibadan. *Trop. geogr. Med.* **31**, 53–56.

—— and —— (1982). Obscure myelopathy in the Nigerian African: a prospective study of 74 patients. *E. Afr. Med. J.* **56**, 586–597.

——, ——, Bademosi, O. and Adebonojo, S. A. (1982). Myaesthenia gravis: its clinical course and management in the African. *Nig. Med. J.* **12**, 329–336.

El-Ebiary, H. M. (1971). Facial paralysis: a clinical study of 580 cases. *Rheum. Phys. Med.* **11**, 100–119.

Kelly, G. (1981). The posttraumatic syndrome. *Proc. R. Soc. Med.* **74**, 242–245.

Miller, H. (1961). Accident neurosis. *Br. Med. J.* **1**, 919–925.

Mohammed, I. (1983). Prophylaxis and management of meningitis in the tropical meningitis belt. *Postgrad. Doc.* **5**, 46–52.

Osuntokun, B. O. (1977). Stroke in the African. *Afr. J. Med. Sci.* **6**, 39–53.

—— (1981). Cassava diet, chronic cyanide intoxication and neuropathy in Nigerian Africans. *Wld Rev. Nutr. Dietet.* **36**, 141–173.

—— and Bademosi, O. (1979). Parkinsonism in the Nigerian African: a prospective study of 217 patients. *E. Afr. Med. J.* **56**, 597–607.

Spillane, J. D. (ed.) (1973). *Tropical neurology* Part 2, pp. 133–334. Oxford University Press, Oxford.

Tugwell, P., Greenwood, B. M. and Warrel, D. A. (1976). Pneumococcal meningitis: a clinical and laboratory study. *Q. J. Med.* **55**, 583–601.

Williams, A. O., Loewenson, R. B., Lippert, D. M. and Resch, J. A. (1975). Cerebral atherosclerosis and its relationship to selected diseases in Nigerians: A pathological study. *Stroke* **6**, 395–401.

SECTION 22
DISEASES OF VOLUNTARY MUSCLE

DISEASES OF VOLUNTARY MUSCLE

J. WALTON

The anatomy and physiology of muscle

A voluntary muscle is composed of muscle fibres, each of which is a multinucleate cell containing myofibrils, sarcoplasm, and discrete intracellular organelles including mitochondria, ribosomes, and the sarcotubular system. Each fibre is enclosed within a sarcolemmal sheath beneath which the muscle nuclei are situated and each has a motor end-plate in which the nerve fibre terminates. Electron microscopy has shown that the sarcolemma consists of three layers, of which the innermost is the plasma membrane, the middle layer the basement membrane, and the outer layer is collagen. The amorphous basement membrane, about 50 nm thick, acts as a microskeleton for the muscle fibre and in the motor end-plate region is more specialized, containing the enzyme acetylcholinesterase which degrades acetylcholine (ACh). The plasma membrane, which is 10 nm thick, is a more specialized lipoprotein bilayer. It is differentially permeable to various ions and this helps to maintain the marked contrast in ionic composition of the intracellular and extracellular fluids which is in turn responsible for the resting membrane potential of the muscle fibre (see below). The permeability of this membrane is altered in a number of diseases.

Under normal conditions muscle fibres never contract singly, but the functional unit of muscle activity is the motor unit, namely that group of muscle fibres supplied by a single anterior horn cell and its axon. Discharge of such an anterior horn cell causes simultaneous contraction of all of its muscle fibres. While most or all of the fibres of a motor unit may be located within a single bundle or fasciculus, recent evidence suggests that the various fasciculi, and indeed the individual muscle fibres which make up the motor unit, may be widely separated anatomically within the muscle. The electrical activity which accompanies contraction of a motor unit and which can be recorded electromyographically, depends upon many physical factors including the characteristics of the recording electrode and special features of the muscle examined. In the biceps brachii of a healthy young adult, a single motor unit action potential usually appears as a di- or triphasic wave with a duration of 5–8 ms and an amplitude of not less than 250 μV, but there is considerable normal variation in form, amplitude, and duration. Probably these so-called motor unit potentials are often produced not by the electrical activity of the muscle fibres of the entire unit but by the summated electrical activity of a proportion of its component fibres which can be thought of as constituting a subunit.

In 1934 Dale first demonstrated that ACh is the humoral element responsible for transmission of the nerve impulse at the myoneural junction. Synaptic vesicles in the motor nerve terminal contain packets of ACh and these are continually released spontaneously to give small depolarizations (miniature end-plate potentials) which can be recorded with a micro-electrode inserted in the region of the end-plate. When a nerve action potential reaches the nerve terminal, Ca_2^+ ions enter the axon terminal and many packets of ACh are released synchronously. Once released, the ACh diffuses through the synaptic clefts to combine with receptors on the muscle fibre membrane. These receptors (AChR) are highly concentrated in the terminal expansions of the postsynaptic junctional folds of the plasma membrane of the muscle fibre, with a packing density of $10^4/\mu m^2$ (see Engel, 1984). The AChR molecule is about 11 nm long and 8.5 nm in diameter, spans the lipid bilayer of the membrane and protrudes 5.5 nm above its surface. It has a molecular weight of about 250 000 and is composed of five glycosylated polypeptide subunits. In normal mature muscle the ACh receptors are localized to the end-plate but after denervation of a muscle fibre extra-junctional receptors are formed. When the arrival of the nerve action potential initiates the process described above, this causes a localized depolarization of the muscle fibre membrane, giving rise to an end-plate potential. When the latter reaches a critical size, an action potential is induced which travels from the end-plate along the surface membrane of the fibre. At rest, the inside of the fibre membrane is some 80 mV negative with respect to the outside, but as the action potential passes, the polarization of the membrane reverses so that the inside of the fibre becomes transiently positive. This reversal of electrical polarity is caused by increased sodium permeability of the membrane. The wave of excitation spreads into the substance of the fibre along the transverse system of tubules (T-system) and the resulting release of calcium ions in the sarcoplasmic recticulum initiates contraction of the fibrils.

The unit of structure of the individual myofibril is the sarcomere, extending from one Z-line (situated in the midst of the I-band) to the next (Fig. 1). Attached to each Z-line are a series of thin filaments of actin which interdigitate with thicker myosin filaments, the latter corresponding to the dark (birefringent) A-bands of the myofibrils (Fig. 2). In cross-section, each filament of myosin is surrounded by a hexagonal array of actin filaments and the actin and myosin filaments are joined by molecular cross-bridges. During contraction these cross-bridges repeatedly disengage and re-engage at successive sites on the actin filaments and as a result the actin and myosin filaments slide upon one another so that the myofibril shortens. The biochemical changes which accompany this process are very complex, but creatine phosphate is certainly broken down in the presence of calcium to creatine and phosphate, and adenosine triphosphate (ATP) is broken down to adenosine diphosphate (ADP). This release of high-energy phosphate bonds provides much of the necessary energy.

It is now recognized that skeletal muscles are not homogeneous and contain at least two main types of muscle fibre which are morphologically and histochemically distinct and the second type (Type 2) can in turn be further subdivided (Table 1). The so-called Type 1 fibre is slightly smaller than the Type 2 and contains myofibrils which are generally somewhat slender, and a large number of mitochondria. Histochemical staining shows that these fibres contain a high concentration of oxidative enzymes and a higher concentration of fat than do the second type. In the larger Type 2 fibres, which generally have slightly coarser and broader and more widely dispersed myofibrils, there are fewer mitochondria and less fat is present, but there is a higher concentration of glycogen and a greater concentration of enzymes such as phosphorylase which are concerned with anaerobic metabolism. In man, all skeletal muscles contain an admixture of Type 1 and Type 2 fibres, so that in sections stained histochemically a typical checkerboard pattern is seen. Physiologically, it is now apparent that the Type 1 fibres are concerned largely with the maintenance of posture and upon stimulation are found to contract and relax relatively slowly. Type 2 fibres, by contrast, are more rapidly contracting (fast-twitch muscles). Subdivision of Type 2 fibres into Types 2a and 2b is also possible on the basis of their intensity of staining with the myofibrillar ATPase reaction at different acid pHs and their oxidative enzyme content, the Type 2a fibres showing inhibition of ATPase activity at pH 4.6 and a relatively higher content of

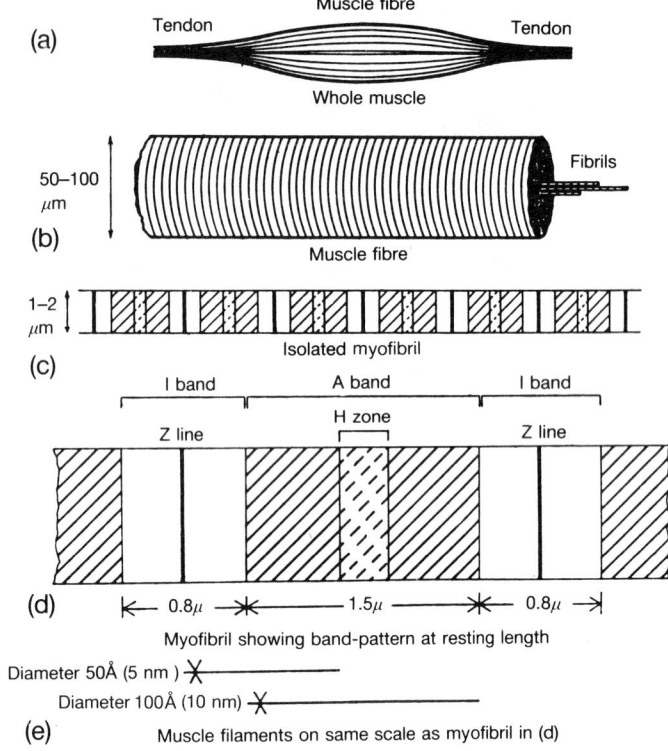

(a) Tendon — Muscle fibre — Tendon
Whole muscle

(b) 50–100 μm — Fibrils
Muscle fibre

(c) 1–2 μm
Isolated myofibril

(d)
I band | A band | I band
Z line | H zone | Z line
← 0.8μ → ← 1.5μ → ← 0.8μ →
Myofibril showing band-pattern at resting length

Diameter 50Å (5 nm) ✕ ————
Diameter 100Å (10 nm) ✕ ————

(e) Muscle filaments on same scale as myofibril in (d)

Fig. 1 Diagram illustrating the dimensions and arrangement of the contractile components in a muscle. The whole muscle (a) is made up of fibres (b) which contain cross-striated myofibrils (c, d). These are constructed of two types of protein filaments (e), put together as shown in Fig. 2. (Reproduced from Huxley and Hanson, 1960, in *The structure and function of muscle* Vol. 1 (ed. G. H. Bourne). Academic Press, New York.)

oxidative enzymes than the Type 2b fibres in which the ATPase activity is only inhibited at pH 4.3 (Fig. 3). Both subtypes are physiologically fast-twitch fibres, but because of their greater oxidative metabolic activity the Type 2a fibres are more fatigue-resistant than are those of Type 2b.

The two major fibre types are also distinguishable through the properties of their myosin light chains and through the tropomyo-

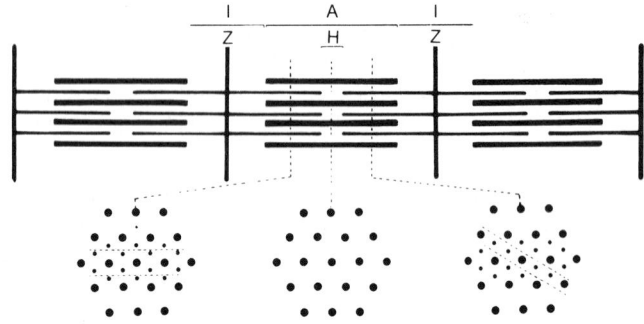

Fig. 2 Diagram illustrating the arrangement of the kinds of protein filaments (thick filaments – myosin, thin filaments – actin) in a myofibril. At the top are three sarcomeres drawn as they would appear in longitudinal section. Below are transverse sections taken through the H-zone and through the other parts of the A-band where the thick and thin filaments interdigitate. The plane of section determines whether, in electron micrographs, there seem to be one or two thin (actin) filaments between two thick (myosin) ones. (Reproduced from Huxley and Hanson, 1960, in *The structure and function of muscle* Vol. 1 (ed. G. H. Bourne). Academic Press, New York.)

sin and troponin which they contain, the respective proteins in Type 1 and Type 2 fibres being immunochemically distinct. Clearly the motor nerve controls not only the physiological behaviour, but also the histochemical structure of the muscle fibres in that transposition of the motor nerve supply from a group of 'fast' fibres to a group of 'slow' ones in animals may reverse the physiological and histochemical characteristics of the fibres. It follows that all muscle fibres being supplied by a single motor neurone are of the same histochemical type and that in a sense, therefore, we can talk of Type 1 and Type 2 neurones. Hence, when a muscle has been partially denervated, say in a form of spinal muscular atrophy (see below), surviving neurones may sprout, grow out into the muscle, and then adopt denervated muscle fibres which, on being re-innervated, form groups of muscle fibres which are all of the same histochemical fibre type (fibre type grouping – see Fig. 7).

Finally, certain drugs which act at the neuromuscular junction may be mentioned. ACh is normally broken down by cholinesterase which is present in the subneural apparatus of the end-plate and can be demonstrated histochemically. Curare acts on the postjunctional membrane and reduces or prevents the depolarizing effect of the ACh released by the nerve impulse. Drugs such as neostigmine destroy cholinesterase and allow ACh to accumulate. Guanidine hydrochloride and 4-amidopyrine act by increasing the output of ACh. Initially the accumulation of ACh produces muscular contraction as a result of depolarization of the fibre membrane, but if it accumulates in excess, depolarization persists and may then block the muscle action potential (depolarization block). Whereas drugs like curare and gallamine compete with ACh for the end-plate chemical receptors and are thus known as competitive inhibitors, drugs such as decamethonium and suxamethonium produce muscle paralysis first as a result of depolarization block, but later also cause competitive block so that they are said to have a 'dual' action.

General comments on muscle disorders

Since conditions which affect muscle through disease of the spinal cord, anterior horn cells and peripheral nerves have been dealt with in preceding pages, this commentary will deal only with those disorders which primarily affect voluntary muscle and the myoneural junction. The term 'myopathy' can reasonably be used to define any disease or syndrome in which the patient's symptoms and/or physical signs can be attributed to pathological, biochemical, or electrophysiological changes which are occurring in the muscle fibres or in the muscular interstitial tissues and in which there is no evidence that the symptoms are wholly secondary to disordered function of the central or peripheral nervous system. This group of diseases includes many disorders which are genetically determined, as well as others of metabolic origin, and yet others in which the disease process is inflammatory.

Clinical nosology

Pain, muscular weakness, and fatiguability are the most important symptoms of muscle disease. Muscle *cramps* occurring in the elderly particularly in bed at night, are common and may be relieved by a nocturnal dose of quinine or phenytoin; in younger individuals cramp may follow unaccustomed exertion but is sometimes a manifestation of metabolic muscle disease. Spontaneous muscle *pain* at rest can occur in inflammatory disorders of muscle, but pain experienced on exertion generally implies either muscle ischaemia or a metabolic disorder such as hypothyroidism, deficiency of phosphorylase or of one of the many other enzymes concerned with the degradation of glycogen, carnitine palmityl transferase deficiency or one of the other rare metabolic disorders of muscle, such as AMP deaminase deficiency, to be mentioned below. There is also an uncommon syndrome of *benign exertional muscle pain* for which no cause has been identified, while it is also important to recall that pain in the calf muscles following effort

Table 1 Histochemical and physiological characteristics of the three major muscle fibre types

	Fibre type		
	1	2A	2B
Enzyme reactions			
NADH-tetrazolium reductase and SDH	+++	++	+
Myofibrillar ATPase			
pH 9.4	+	+++	+++
pH 4.6	+++	—	+++
pH 4.3	+++	—	—
Phosphorylase	+	+++	+++
Physiological properties			
Twitch speed	Slow	Fast	Fast
Fatigue resistance	+++	++	+
Nomenclature			
Peter *et al.* (1972)	Slow-twitch Oxidative	Fast-twitch Oxidative-glycolytic	Fast-twitch Glycolytic
Burke *et al.* (1971)	S (slow contracting)	FR (fast contracting, fatigue resistant)	FF (fast contracting, fast fatigue)

From Walton and Mastaglia (1980b).

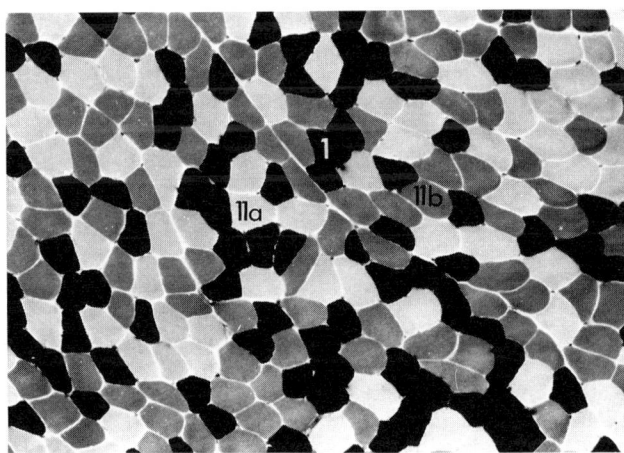

Fig. 3 A transverse section of normal human skeletal muscle stained for the myofibrillar ATPase reaction after preincubation at pH 4.6, × 150. The Type 1 and 2a and 2b fibres are labelled. In the more usual myofibrillar ATPase reaction at pH 9.4, the Type 1 fibres stain light and the Type 2 fibres dark. In this so-called reverse ATPase reaction, however, at pH 4.6, the 2a and 2b fibres are easier to distinguish. (Kindly supplied by Dr Margaret Johnson.)

may be an early manifestation of increased muscle tone (spasticity), occurring, for example, in early multiple sclerosis. In addition, every physician with an interest in muscle disease is familiar with patients who complain bitterly of diffuse muscular pain induced by effort which greatly restricts their activity but for which no physical or biochemical cause can at present be demonstrated. Some such individuals are of obsessional and introspective temperament, and it is likely that their symptoms may be of emotional origin although treatment with tranquillizing drugs is only rarely helpful. But in other similar cases one can only conclude that the patient is probably suffering from an as yet unidentified metabolic disorder of muscle; unfortunately symptomatic treatment with analgesic and relaxant drugs is often of little if any benefit and the symptoms may prove to be both persistent and disabling. For reasons which are as yet obscure, a few such patients find that their pain is relieved by verapamil (Walton, 1981).

Muscle *weakness* is the predominant symptom of most forms of myopathy. It is important to judge its distribution and tempo of development. Thus proximal muscle weakness in the upper limbs gives difficulty in lifting the arms above the head, and in the lower limbs difficulty in climbing the stairs and in rising from the floor or a low chair. In most of the genetically determined disorders of muscle, weakness develops gradually over many months or years; a more rapid onset of weakness suggests that the patient is more probably suffering from an inflammatory or metabolic myopathy. Periodic attacks of weakness with complete recovery in between strongly suggest that the patient may be suffering from one of the periodic paralyses. *Fatiguability* is characteristic of myasthenia gravis and myasthenic syndromes. The term implies that muscle weakness increases with continuing exercise; many patients mention that the more they exert themselves the weaker they become, or that weakness increases towards the end of the day. The *family history* is also of great importance in that if blood relatives are affected, a genetically determined disorder of muscle is probable.

On *physical examination*, the importance of general examination must be stressed as there may be changes in the eyes, skin, lymph nodes, or viscera indicating that the patient's muscular weakness is but one manifestation of a systemic multisystem disease. On examining the muscular system itself, the presence of *atrophy*, *hypertrophy*, or *fasciculation* may be of diagnostic value, and so too may the presence of muscular *contractures* with consequent skeletal deformity. *Fibrillation* (the spontaneous contraction of single muscle fibres) is an electrical phenomenon which can be recorded electromyographically from denervated muscle, but cannot be seen through the intact skin. *Fasciculation* (the spontaneous contraction of individual muscle fasciculi) is a phenomenon seen most often in patients with anterior horn cell disease; it is uncommon in primary muscle disease but is rarely seen in polymyositis or thyrotoxic myopathy. Coarse fasciculation, occurring particularly in the calf muscles, is a benign phenomenon which may be seen in normal individuals. When such coarse benign fasciculation is widespread and is accompanied by hyperhidrosis, this syndrome is often called *myokymia*. However, this term has been applied to an intermittent twitch of the lower eyelid often observed in normal individuals when fatigued ('benign myokymia of the lower eyelid'); to a curious continuous rippling movement of the muscles of one side of the face ('facial myokymia', usually of unknown aetiology but occasionally a manifestation of multiple sclerosis); and also to a rare syndrome (also called 'neuromyotonia' or 'continuous muscle fibre activity and spasm') in which a form of coarse fasciculation is often associated with muscular spasms, with delayed relaxation resembling myotonia (see below) and with continuous activity, which can be recorded electromyographically, in affected muscles.

Delayed muscular relaxation after voluntary contraction or following percussion of a muscle is the most prominent feature of *myotonia*, a diagnosis which can be confirmed electromyographically (see Section 21), but in hypothyroidism both muscular contraction and relaxation are often greatly slowed and the time-course of the tendon reflexes is typically slower than normal. *Myoidema* is a name given to the formation of a localized ridge, lasting a few seconds after local percussion of a muscle; this type of ridge is electrically silent and the phenomenon tends to occur particularly in patients with malnutrition or cachexia due to malignant disease, though it is also seen rarely in hypothyroidism. Physiological *contracture*, which differs from pathological contracture with permanent shortening of muscles and tendons due to fibrosis in chronic muscle disease, in that it is a reversible shortening of muscle lasting for some minutes after exercise, may be seen particularly in muscle phosphorylase deficiency (McArdle's disease) and in related disorders of glycogen breakdown. Direct *myotatic irritability* is the name attached to the reflex contraction which occurs in the belly of a muscle when it is percussed or stimulated directly by mechanical means. As with the tendon reflexes, this direct reflex response can be accentuated by anxiety but is particularly striking in patients with tetany and hypocalcaemia.

The response of muscle to stretch, i.e. *muscle tone*, is also of diagnostic value. Increased tone (*spasticity* or *rigidity*) implies disease in the central nervous system, but there are many primary disorders of muscle which cause reduced tone (limpness or *hypotonia*); differential diagnosis of these disorders may be particularly difficult in infancy. *Palpation* of muscles can also be helpful. Tenderness can imply inflammation, an abnormally firm consistency infiltration with fat, connective tissue, calcium, or even the presence of a primary neoplasm, but muscle tumours are rare and localized swellings usually imply either haematoma formation, rupture of a tendon, herniation of muscle tissue through its covering fascia or, much more rarely, a muscle infarct (as in polyarteritis nodosa) or severe local inflammation (as in tropical or pyogenic myositis or localized nodular myositis).

The examination of *muscle power* is sufficiently important almost to warrant a chapter to itself. Certainly careful testing of the power of individual muscles, combined with an attempt at quantitative assessment, is a most important facet of the clinical examination. Different diseases show different *patterns of muscular involvement* and selective atrophy and weakness of certain muscles with sparing of others may give an important clue to the nature of the patient's illness. The *tendon reflexes* in muscle disease are usually diminished or lost when the muscles subserving the reflex being examined are involved in the disease process. In general, however, in muscular dystrophy the tendon reflexes tend to disappear early, in myasthenia gravis and in polymyositis they often remain unexpectedly brisk even in the presence of substantial weakness, and in the myopathy of metabolic bone disease they are often exaggerated, even in very weak muscles.

Diagnostic methods

When involvement of the voluntary muscles is but one part of a systemic inflammatory or metabolic affliction, many investigations, including differential white cell counts, erythrocyte sedimentation rate, serum electrophoresis, and estimations of the serum electrolytes and of calcium and phosphorus, may be relevant and, where considered individually of importance, will be mentioned in relation to specific disease entities. In any patient suffering from muscular weakness it is first necessary to determine whether the weakness is secondary to disease primarily involving other tissues or organs. If such a process can be excluded, the next step is to determine whether the pathological process responsible lies in the lower motor neurone, at the myoneural junction, or in

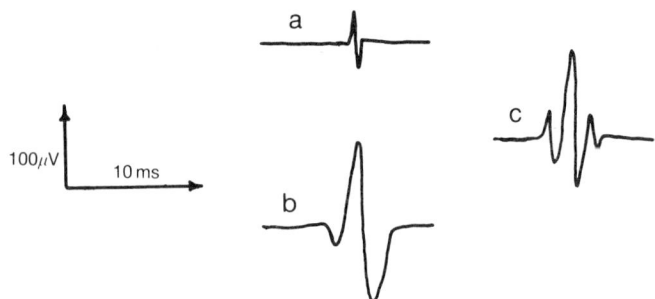

Fig. 4 Diagrammatic representation of muscle action potentials recorded in the electromyogram: a = fibrillation (single fibre) potential; b = triphasic motor unit action potential; c = polyphasic motor unit potential.

the muscle itself. The techniques of most value in providing this information, in distinguishing between neuropathic and myopathic disorders on the one hand and between specific myopathic conditions on the other, are respectively electromyography, biochemical techniques, of which serum enzyme studies are among the most important, and finally muscle biopsy.

Electromyography (EMG) (see also Section 21)

In neuropathic disorders, spontaneous fibrillation potentials may be recorded from a relaxed and resting muscle undergoing an active process of denervation; these potentials, usually diphasic or triphasic spikes of about 1 ms duration and 100 μV in amplitude, are generally easy to distinguish from motor unit action potentials (Fig. 4). The potentials of spontaneous fasciculation, by contrast, are morphologically indistinguishable from normal motor unit potentials, although in myokymia 'doublets' or 'triplets' (multiple potentials) are often recorded. The pattern of motor unit activity on volition is reduced by partial denervation (Fig. 5), but the surviving motor unit potentials are either normal or increased in size. In the myopathies, spontaneous fibrillation is uncommon though it can be seen in polymyositis and less often in muscular dystrophy. Myotonia is accompanied by a discharge of high-frequency activity evoked by movement of the exploring electrode; it waxes and wanes repeatedly to give a characteristic appearance on the cathode ray oscilloscope and a typical sound in the loudspeaker, the so-called 'dive-bomber' note. Volitional activity in all myopathies, including fatigued muscle in patients with myasthenia, demonstrates a breakdown of motor unit action potentials with a consequent increase in the proportion of short-duration and polyphasic potentials (Fig. 5). Measurement shows that the mean action potential duration and amplitude are decreased and that the motor unit territory is diminished. In chronic neuropathic disorders, by contrast, in which sprouting neurones have adopted denervated muscle fibres, the mean action potential duration, and amplitude are increased and motor unit territory is larger than normal. The introduction of single fibre EMG, utilizing very fine microelectrodes which are inserted into the muscle, with the measurement of 'jitter' (a variable interval between the recordings of activity derived from two adjacent muscle fibres) has added considerable precision to diagnosis, especially in the recognition of disorders of neuromuscular transmission such as myasthenia gravis.

Nerve conduction velocity measurements, which are of great value in identifying and localizing lesions of peripheral nerves, and in distinguishing the various forms of polyneuropathy, are normal in all primary myopathies. In myasthenia gravis, supramaximal stimulation of the motor nerve supply to a myasthenic muscle at a rate of 3–5 Hz may give a progressive diminution in the amplitude of the evoked action potential (Fig. 6) (the myasthenic response). This is only seen, however, in clinically affected muscles. At tetanic rates of stimulation (50 Hz) the amplitude of the evoked action potential may actually increase markedly in cases of the myasthenic-myopathic (Lambert-Eaton) syndrome (Fig. 6). However,

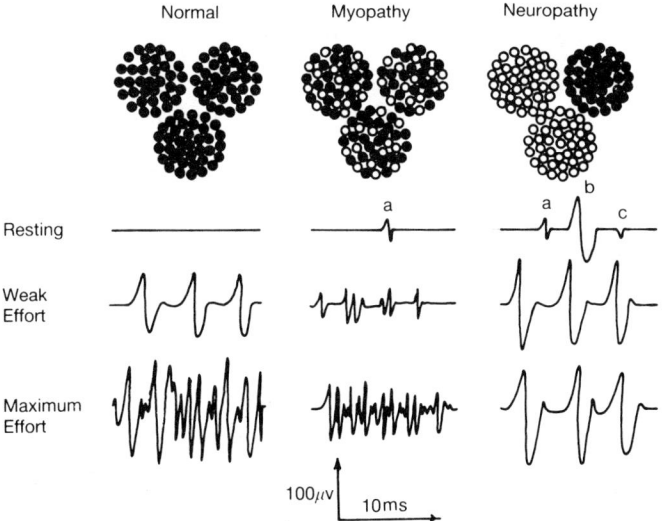

Resting

Weak Effort

Maximum Effort

100μv 10ms

Fig. 5 Diagrammatic representation of electromyographic recordings from normal muscle, from myopathic muscle and from partially denervated muscle (redrawn from an illustration from R. J. Johns). a = spontaneous fibrillation; b = fasciculation potential; c = positive sharp wave ('saw-tooth potential').

Normal muscle is silent at rest, shows discrete motor unit action potentials during weak effort, and a full 'interference pattern' of motor unit action potentials during maximum effort. In myopathy, spontaneous fibrillation is occasionally recorded, while during volition the motor unit action potentials are of short duration and of low amplitude, or else polyphasic; the interference pattern is full but of low amplitude and 'spiky' or complex. In partially denervated muscle, spontaneous fibrillation, fasciculation, and positive sharp waves may be recorded, while on weak effort the surviving motor units are either normal or larger than normal in size, and on maximum effort the interference pattern is reduced and made up sometimes of discrete motor unit action potentials.

these electrophysiological tests for myasthenia and myasthenic syndromes are imprecise and have been largely supplanted by single fibre EMG and by immunological tests (see below).

Biochemical diagnosis

In the various endocrine myopathies to be described below, many tests related to the diagnosis of individual endocrine disorders may be required. In the periodic paralysis syndromes, in addition to serial estimations of serum potassium and measures designed to precipitate attacks for diagnostic purposes, there are cases in which sodium and potassium output in the urine, and even sodium and potassium balance, may need to be measured. In patients with generalized muscle pain and weakness, myoglobin must be sought in the urine, while in individuals suffering muscle pain after effort, it may be necessary to exclude some forms of glycogen storage disease by measuring lactate in venous blood distal to a tourniquet before and after a period of ischaemic work. In such cases estimations of phosphorylase, of other glycolytic enzymes and of AMP deaminase in muscle biopsy samples may also be needed. The identification of other disorders of glycogen storage involving muscle which do not cause exertional pain may necessitate estimations of the total glycogen content of a muscle biopsy specimen, and of other enzymes such as acid maltase. Similarly, in a lipid storage myopathy it may be necessary to measure total muscle lipids, individual fatty acids, carnitine or specific enzymes such as carnitine palmityl transferase. And the mitochondrial myopathies are now known to be so complex that many sophisticated and complex biochemical methods may prove to be necessary when a muscle disorder is found to be associated with a mitochondrial abnormality (see below).

In cases of muscle disease in general, there may be an excessive urinary output of creatine and diminished creatininuria, but these

findings are non-specific, as is the amino aciduria which occurs in some cases. The serum aldolase and transaminases (aminotransferases) may be substantially raised in various forms of myopathy including the more rapidly progressive varieties of muscular dystrophy and polymyositis, but the most useful serum enzyme in the diagnosis of muscle disease is unquestionably creatine kinase (CK) (normal <75 i.u./l). In early or preclinical cases of muscular dystrophy of the Duchenne type, a 300-fold increase in the serum activity of CK is often found and changes of similar magnitude occur in some cases of acute and subacute polymyositis. Less striking rises may be observed in patients with other more indolent forms of myopathy and the more benign varieties of muscular dystrophy. In some endocrine and metabolic myopathies and in the benign congenital myopathies, serum CK activity is not infrequently normal, as it often is in patients suffering from muscular weakness secondary to disease of the anterior horn cell or motor nerve. However, in the chronic spinal muscular atrophies (such as the Kugelberg–Welander syndrome), and in some cases of motor neurone disease the continual and recurrent process of denervation and reinnervation of muscle fibres, combined with the trauma to which weakened muscles are subjected through use, appears to produce a secondary myopathic change in affected muscles so that often in such cases serum CK activity is considerably increased. Indeed these changes may also produce myopathic potentials in the EMG in some areas of partially denervated muscle and appearances suggesting myopathy in some parts of muscle biopsy sections; these findings may lead the unwary erroneously to diagnose a primary myopathy in some such cases.

Muscle biopsy

While it is generally possible from the findings observed in sections of muscle obtained by biopsy to distinguish with reasonable confidence between muscular atrophy secondary to denervation on the one hand and that resulting from primary myopathic processes on the other, differential diagnosis between the various

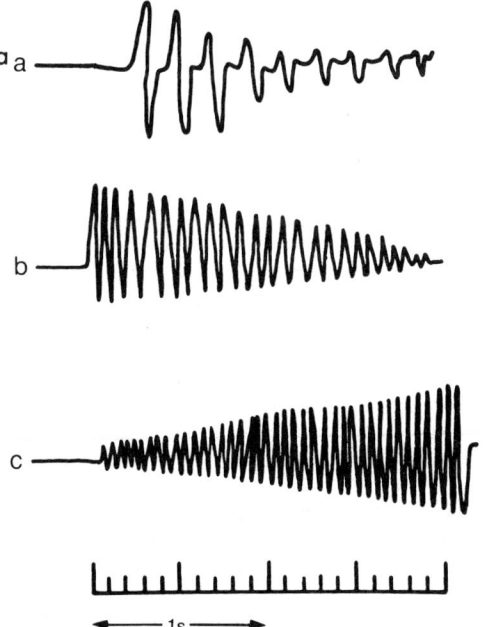

Fig. 6 Diagrammatic representation of recording of evoked muscle action potentials from one hypothenar eminence during supramaximal stimulation of the ulnar nerve. (a) Myasthenia gravis; stimulation at 5 Hz demonstrating a progressive decrement in the amplitude of the evoked potential. (b) Myasthenia gravis; a similar decrement is observed at tetanic (30 Hz) rates of stimulation. (c) Myasthenic-myopathic syndrome; during stimulation at 50 Hz there is an increment in the amplitude of the evoked potential.

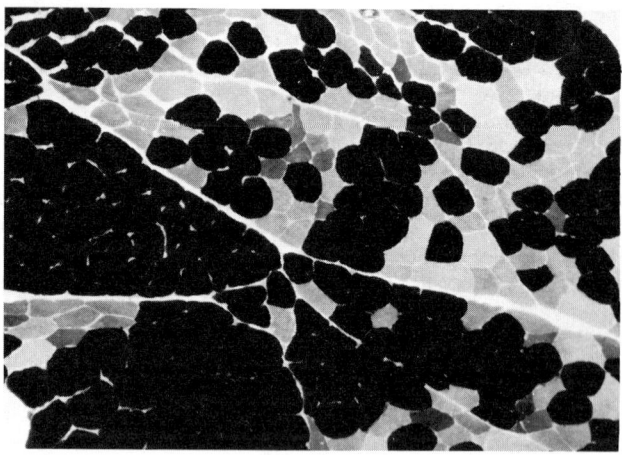

Fig. 7 A transverse section of human skeletal muscle obtained by biopsy from a patient with peripheral neuropathy, stained for the myofibrillar ATPase reaction after preincubation at pH 4.6, × 150. There is extensive evidence of fibre type grouping, particularly of the Type 1 fibres, resulting from reinnervation. (Kindly supplied by Dr Margaret Johnson.)

forms of myopathy is much less exact. Modern techniques, including intravital staining of the motor end-plate, histochemistry, immunochemistry and electron microscopy, have yielded much valuable research information but only in a few disorders have they added precision to histological diagnosis. Thus 'fibre type grouping' (large groups of fibres of uniform histochemical type) is usually diagnostic of chronic denervation atrophy (Fig. 7). The histological features noted in cases of muscular dystrophy are similar in all varieties of the disease, though varying considerably in severity. The most common changes are marked variations in fibre size, fibre-splitting, central migration of sarcolemmal nuclei, patchy atrophy of individual muscle fibres, the formation of nuclear chains, the presence of segmental areas of necrosis within fibres with phagocytosis of necrotic sarcoplasm, and basophilia of sarcoplasm with enlargement of sarcolemmal nuclei showing prominent nucleoli (changes construed as being regenerative in character); there is also progressive infiltration by fat cells and connective tissue. In subacute or chronic polymyositis, the changes may be similar, but evidence of muscle fibre destruction and repair (necrosis, phagocytosis, and regeneration) is usually more striking and widespread; in addition, there are often interstitial or perivascular infiltrations of inflammatory cells such as lymphocytes or plasma cells, usually in perifascicular distribution and associated with perifascicular fibre atrophy; the absence of inflammatory cells does not, however, exclude polymyositis. There are cases in which distinction between muscular dystrophy on the one hand and polymyositis on the other is difficult or impossible on histological grounds alone. In some cases of myasthenia gravis and in thyrotoxic and other endocrine myopathies, focal collections of lymphocytes (lymphorrhages) may be seen, either around blood vessels or between fibres, but in many patients with thyrotoxic and other endocrine myopathies, and in the myasthenic-myopathic (Lambert–Eaton) syndrome, histological changes are often mild and non-specific. Striated annulets (*ringbinden*), in which striated myofibrils encircle muscle fibres cut in transverse section, are often seen in biopsies from patients with myotonic dystrophy but also in other forms of muscle disease; in myotonic dystrophy, chains of nuclei within muscle fibres are particularly prominent and there may also be peripheral masses of palely staining homogeneous sarcoplasm (sarcoplasmic masses) but these, too, are non-specific and have been noted in some patients with muscular symptoms in myxoedema.

Vacuolar change within muscle fibres, if striking and widespread, usually indicates the storage of abnormal metabolites within the cells and is particularly prominent in cases of glycogen storage disease. In such cases specific stains for glycogen (e.g. PAS), before and after diastase digestion, are helpful in identifying the stored material as glycogen. Similarly, stains for neutral lipid such as Oil Red O or Sudan Black B will usually identify the abnormal storage of fat which is seen, for example, in lipid storage myopathy due to carnitine deficiency (see Fig. 12). In frozen sections stained for oxidative enzymes such as NADH diaphorase, dark rings or clumps around the periphery of the Type 1 muscle fibres indicate accumulations of abnormal mitochondria and in such cases the internal architecture of the fibres is often deranged ('ragged-red fibres') (Fig. 8): the abnormal mitochondria can then be seen more clearly in sections examined in the electron microscope (see Fig. 13).

Widespread vacuolar change less striking than that seen in the storage diseases is often seen in muscle biopsies taken from patients with periodic paralysis during the attacks and rarely in systemic lupus erythematosus or in the myopathy resulting from long-continued chloroquine administration. In some rare benign congenital and non-progressive myopathies described in recent years, special stains of muscle biopsy sections may be needed to demonstrate the specific morphological abnormalities of the muscle fibre which have been described and which will be mentioned in the appropriate sections.

THE MUSCULAR DYSTROPHIES

While muscular dystrophy can reasonably be defined as genetically determined primary degenerative myopathy, there are several other rare myopathies to be referred to later which are also genetically determined but which are not normally regarded as being muscular dystrophies in the accepted sense of the term.

Classification

Classification of a case of muscular dystrophy is the only safe guide to prognosis and genetic counselling and the most satisfactory clinico-genetic classification of the 'pure' muscular dystrophies based upon current knowledge is as follows:

1. X-linked muscular dystrophy.
   Severe (Duchenne type)
   Benign (Becker type)

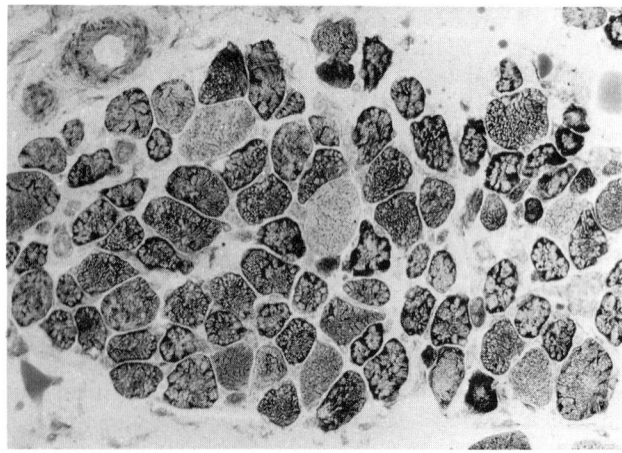

Fig. 8 A transverse section of skeletal muscle obtained from a patient with a mitochondrial myopathy, stained for the NADH-TR reaction, × 384. The Type 1 fibres are darkly stained and show the typical reticulated appearance of so-called 'ragged-red fibres' with massive clumping of mitochondria, particularly in many fibres just deep to the sarcolemma. (Kindly supplied by Dr Margaret Johnson.)

2. Autosomal recessive muscular dystrophy.
    Limb-girdle type
    Childhood muscular dystrophy (resembling Duchenne)
    Congenital muscular dystrophies
3. Autosomal dominant muscular dystrophy.
    Facioscapulohumeral
    Scapuloperoneal
    Late-onset proximal
    Distal
    Ocular
    Oculopharyngeal

Although this classification seems to be the most satisfactory at the present time, there are still some cases which are difficult to fit into any of the groups described.

Aetiology

Though all forms of muscular dystrophy are genetically determined, the exact nature of the process causing the muscles to waste is still unknown. No deficiency of a single enzyme nor any specific abnormality of a single muscle protein has yet been identified in any of form of muscular dystrophy and hypotheses, suggesting that a disorder of muscle blood supply or of its innervation have been discarded. There is some evidence that the primary abnormality may lie within the plasma membrane of the muscle cell, and that this may allow the uncontrolled entry of extracellular Ca^{2+}, activating calcium-activated neutral proteases which then digest the contents of the muscle fibre. This so-called 'membrane theory' is undoubtedly an over-simplification; however, it receives some support from work utilizing biochemical, biophysical, and ultrastructural techniques which has suggested that in the muscular dystrophies there may be membrane defects in other tissues including red and white blood cells and fibroblasts. While no precise and specific marker for any dystrophy gene or genes has yet been identified, work in progress seems likely in the near future to locate and characterize the Duchenne gene (see below). Such a discovery will first give a precise method of identifying carriers of the gene, secondly a method of identifying the affected male fetus *in utero* through amniocentesis and amniotic cell culture or chorionic biopsy, and thirdly it should represent a major step towards identifying the nature of the pathogenetic process responsible for muscle cell breakdown.

The muscular dystrophies are comparatively rare, but appear to be worldwide, affecting all races; the Duchenne type is the commonest, with an incidence of between 13 and 33 per 100 000 live births, but it has been estimated that there are probably 5–6000 cases of muscular dystrophy of all kinds in the United Kingdom at any one time.

Pathology

Although the nature of the pathological process which causes the muscular weakness and wasting is similar in character if different in tempo in the various clinical and genetic types, there are certain other features, including differences in the pattern of muscular involvement and in the degree to which enzymes such as CK leak into the serum in the different forms of the disease, which strongly suggest that they may eventually prove to be different diseases aetiologically. While fibre necrosis and phagocytosis and abortive regenerative activity are commonly seen in muscle biopsy samples obtained in the early stages of all forms of the disease, and particularly in the more rapidly progressive varieties, in the later stages infiltration with fat and connective tissue, marked variation in fibre size and central nucleation of many muscle fibres are predominant. The histological hallmark of early Duchenne dystrophy is that in transverse frozen sections stained with haematoxylin and eosin, scattered opaque hyalinized fibres are numerous. Figure 9 gives an outline of what are believed to be the successive changes of muscle fibre breakdown in such cases, as observed with the electron microscope.

Electromyography

Electromyography reveals volitional activity characteristic of any form of myopathy, and spontaneous activity is usually absent on recording from relaxed, resting muscle, although spontaneous fibrillation and positive sharp waves are occasionally recorded, especially in more rapidly progressive cases.

Symptoms and signs

These depend upon the muscles which are first involved by the disease process and upon its rate of progress. Weakness of pelvic girdle muscles gives slowness in walking, inability to run, frequent falling, difficulty in climbing stairs or in rising from the floor, and eventually accentuation of the lumbar lordosis with a characteristic waddling gait. Climbing up the legs on rising from the floor (Gower's sign) is characteristic but not specific for muscular dystrophy as it occurs in any disorder in which pelvic girdle muscles are weakened. Involvement of the shoulder girdles gives a sloping appearance of the shoulders with a tendency for the scapulae to rise prominently when the patient tries to abduct the arms. Many use trick movements by placing one hand beneath the other elbow in order to lift the hand to the face or head. Facial weakness, as seen in facioscapulohumeral dystrophy, causes inability to whistle and difficulty in pouting the lips or in closing the eyes, while distal weakness in the extremities (as seen in the distal variety) causes weakness of grip and of fine finger movement, and foot-drop. Contractures are a common feature of all forms of dystrophy in the later stages, but are seen especially in the Duchenne type. They may be due to weakness developing in muscles whose antagonists remain powerful (this accounts for the equinovarus deformity of the feet seen in advancing cases of the Duchenne type which causes the children to walk on their toes; it is due to weakness of anterior tibial muscles while those of the calf remain powerful). Contractures are also accentuated by postural factors in patients confined to a wheelchair when biceps and hamstrings usually shorten. The most important clinical characteristic of all forms of muscular dystrophy is that muscles are picked out by the disease in a selective manner. Though there are certain differences in the patterns of weakness and no wasting seen in the various subvarieties, it is common in the upper limbs to find that the serrati and pectoral muscles are weak and atrophic, as are biceps and brachioradialis, while deltoid and triceps remain relatively unaffected. In the lower limbs, quadriceps and anterior tibials are usually involved first, and the calf muscles are spared, but in limb-girdle cases the hamstrings and quadriceps are often affected equally.

The severe X-linked Duchenne type

Though there is ample evidence to confirm that this condition is due to an X-linked recessive gene, about half of the affected boys seem to be isolated cases and in about one-third the disease is presumed to have resulted from a new mutation occurring in the ovarian cells of the mother or maternal grandmother.

The condition usually first becomes apparent towards the end of the third year of life with slowness in walking, frequent falling and difficulty in climbing stairs. However, muscle biopsies obtained within the first few weeks of life in preclinical cases (younger brothers of affected boys, identified at birth by serum CK estimation) clearly show that the pathological process is active even at birth and many affected boys walk late (at 18 months of age or later). Nevertheless early symptoms and signs (even though readily recognizable to parents who have seen them before in an older child) are very difficult for the doctor to detect. It is important to think of this possibility in young boys who walk late or develop walking difficulty in early life, when estimation of the serum CK will always be wise. Enlargement of the calf muscles and sometimes of quadriceps and deltoids occurs in about 90 per cent of cases at some stage, but later disappears. The latter phenomenon, often referred to in the past as pseudohypertrophy, is more often due to true compensatory hypertrophy of unaffected

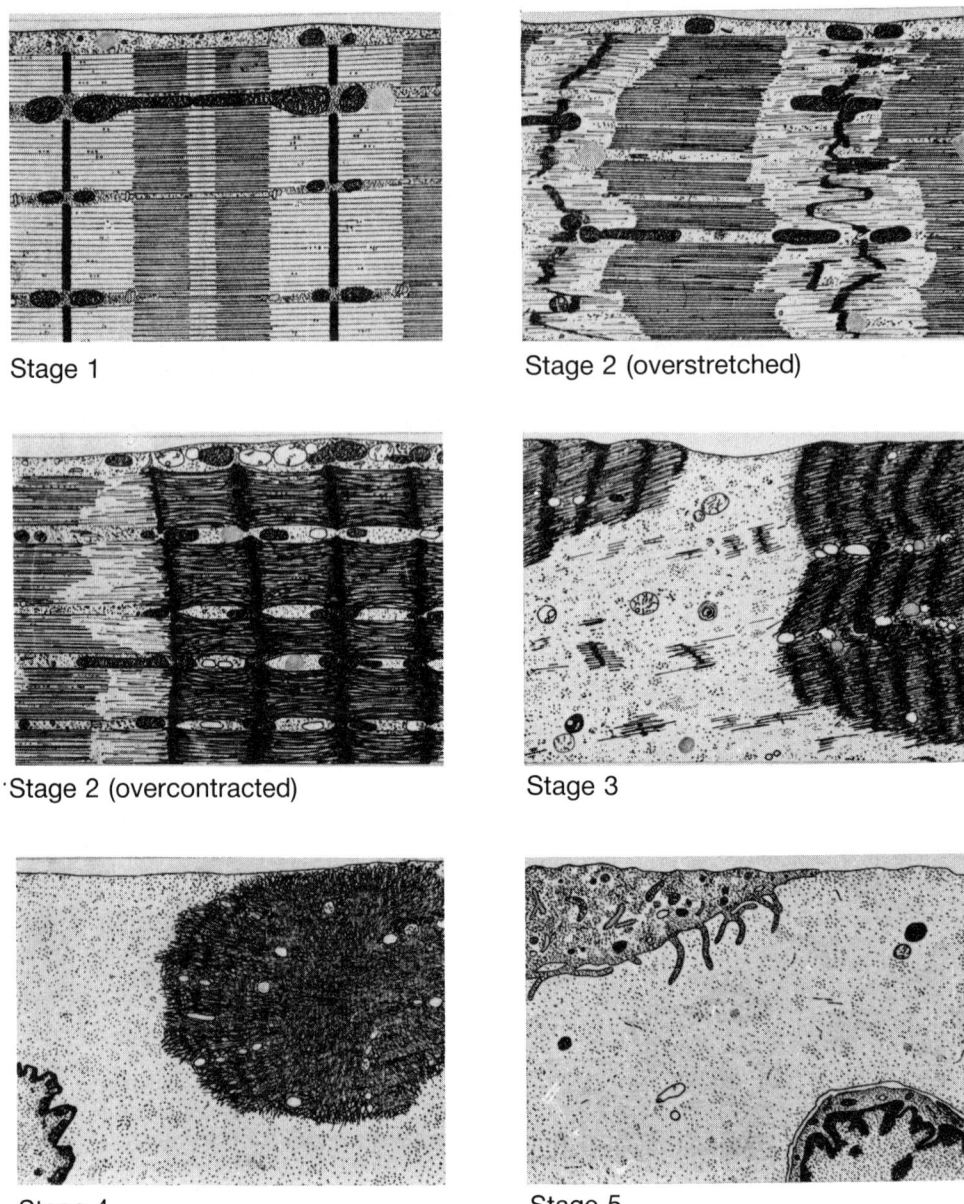

Stage 1

Stage 2 (overstretched)

Stage 2 (overcontracted)

Stage 3

Stage 4

Stage 5

Fig. 9 A diagrammatic representation of the successive stages of muscle fibre breakdown seen in biopsy material obtained from patients with muscular dystrophy of the Duchenne type, as studied with the electron microscope. (From Cullen and Fulthorpe (1975), reproduced by kind permission of the authors and publishers.)

muscle fibres. Most patients deteriorate steadily and become unable to walk by about the age of 10 years, but apparent improvement may occur between the ages of five and eight when the rate of deterioration is outstripped by the processes of normal development. When the child is confined to a wheelchair, progressive deformity with skeletal distortion and atrophy occur and death usually results from inanition, respiratory infection or cardiac failure towards the end of the second decade, although with improved management including the prevention of scoliosis and early treatment of complications, some now survive much longer than was usual in the past. Some affected boys waste progressively, but others become obese; macroglossia and absence of certain incisor teeth are occasionally seen. The intelligence quotient is 10 per cent or more lower than in a group of control children of comparable age and sex. Skeletal atrophy may so affect the shafts of long bones that they fracture on minimal trauma. Involvement of cardiac muscle is invariable, though not clinically detectable in the early stages; the ECG typically shows tall R waves in the right precordial leads and deep Q waves in the limb and left precordial leads.

The benign X-linked (Becker) type

This disorder differs from the severe Duchenne variety in that the onset of the disease is usually between five and 25 years, the disorder may be transmitted by affected males through carrier daughters to their grandsons, there is often an initial phase of generalized muscular hypertrophy before weakness and wasting of pelvic and later of shoulder-girdle muscles develops, so that most patients become unable to walk 25 years or more after the onset. Cardiac involvement is usually absent, contractures and skeletal deformity occur late, and many patients, though severely disabled, survive to a normal age.

Neonatal screening

By means of the luciferase technique for serum CK estimation and using a single drop of blood on a filter paper it is possible to identify at birth (with subsequent confirmation from a venous blood sample) those newborn male infants who will subsequently develop Duchenne muscular dystrophy. Since there is no means of preventing the clinical features of the disease from developing and progressing, many authorities have opposed the proposal that all newborn males should be screened, but others have pointed out, first, that parents when consulted have almost invariably wished they had been told when their son was an infant what they had to face; and secondly, more importantly, many families have been reported in which a second or even a third affected boy had been born before the disease was diagnosed in the firstborn. While, therefore, in the light of inadequate resources as well as the medical implications, neonatal screening has only been introduced on a very limited scale in a few localities, it is now evident that estimation of the serum CK should be considered in every male infant with walking difficulty and certainly in all of those not walking by 18 months of age.

Developments in molecular genetics

The new techniques of DNA recombinant technology have resulted in exciting developments in relation to the mapping of individual genes upon the X chromosome and there is reason to hope that the mutant gene responsible for Duchenne muscular dystrophy will soon be isolated and characterized. Two principal methods of study are being pursued. First, there are now several well-authenticated reports of girls suffering clinically from Duchenne muscular dystrophy in whom chromosomal translocations between the X chromosome and various autosomes have been identified. Most breaks of the X chromosome have occurred close to the Xp21 locus near where the Duchenne gene is known to lie; use of material from such patients is making it possible to isolate cloned DNA sequences at or close to the breakpoint and consequently close to the gene (see Roses, 1984; Rosenberg, 1984; Steel, 1984). In parallel, other studies are utilizing synthesized nucleic acid segments known as complementary DNA probes, and a series of flanking probes identifying DNA segments coming closer and closer to the Duchenne gene have been and still are being identified. Recently it became clear that the gene lies between the C7 and M2C probe loci on one side and the OTC locus on the other (Davies, 1985). More recently still, even closer flanking markers have been defined (Bakker *et al.*, 1985) and the part 87 marker (Monaco *et al.*, 1985) may even lie at the edge of the gene; deletions in the region of the gene have also been identified. Isolation and characterization of the gene will give, first, an infallible method of carrier detection and antenatal diagnosis (see below) and, secondly, will represent a first step along the road towards identifying the precise effects of the mutant gene with ultimately, perhaps, the prospect of modifying, or even reversing, its effects. As yet there is no evidence as to the chromosomal location of any of the other forms of muscular dystrophy (see below) except for dystrophia myotonica, now located on chromosome 19. Similar laborious methods of chromosomal mapping will ultimately be applied with the objective of gene isolation (see Section 4).

Carrier detection

The sisters of males suffering from the two X-linked forms of muscular dystrophy are clearly at risk of being carriers and of passing on the disease; half the sons of a female carrier will be affected and half her daughters will themselves be carriers. In fact, as many cases result from spontaneous mutation, the risk of being a carrier is less than 50:50 for any sister of a dystrophic boy. Even in a family with no past history of the disease in previous generations, it is difficult to be certain whether the mutation occurred in the ovarian cells of the mother or maternal grandmother: if it occurred in the grandmother the mother would be a carrier, if in the cells of a segment of the mother's ovary she would not. For practical purposes it is reasonable to assume that about half the sisters of Duchenne sufferers will probably be carriers. An important advance was the discovery that female carriers of the gene responsible for the severe X-linked Duchenne type could often be detected by serum CK estimation and by other methods, which included, in various centres, quantitative electromyography, muscle biopsy, electrocardiography, manual muscle testing, biochemical studies of red blood cell membranes, and many more techniques. Bayesian probability calculations based upon serum CK activity (the mean of three estimations) in both the mother and maternal grandmother is still the single most reliable test, although some workers have found serum pyruvate kinase and radioimmunoassay of serum myoglobin helpful. Since increased serum enzyme activity in carriers is presumed to depend upon the operation of the Lyon hypothesis (see Section 4), so that some muscle cell nuclei in carrier women express the dystrophic gene, and since these nuclei die off as the carrier grows older, it now seems that carrier detection with these methods is more reliable if carried out in young girls between the ages of 12 and 16 years. To date, a smaller proportion of carriers of the benign Becker type are detectable by these methods.

Carrier detection has been shown to be a major practical advance; where vigorously pursued, it has been shown to reduce the incidence of new cases of Duchenne dystrophy by one-third. However, this method can only be applied in families with a known history of the disease and nothing can at present be done to reduce the incidence of new cases resulting from mutation. Selective abortion of male fetuses after sex determination by amniocentesis has the advantage of allowing carriers to have female children but the disadvantage of increasing the potential carrier population. Isolation and characterization of the Duchenne gene will improve the position as it will offer a precise technique of carrier identification. Probes already available are more than 90 per cent accurate (Williamson, 1983; Bakker *et al.*, 1985; Monaco *et al.*, 1985). Ultimately it might in consequence be feasible (though the cost and medical justification would require careful consideration) to screen young females in order to identify carriers in families with no past history of the disease. It should also be possible to achieve the same result in Becker families, though it is still uncertain as to whether the Duchenne and Becker genes are at the same or different loci.

Prenatal diagnosis

In recent years attempts have been made in known female carriers not only to identify the sex of the unborn fetus but, using fetal blood sampling through fetoscopy and estimation of serum CK and other enzymes, to identify, with a view to subsequent abortion, only the affected males. Gene isolation should soon lead to a precise technique of prenatal diagnosis, hopefully in fragments of chorion obtained *per vaginam* or cultured amniotic cells, so that selective abortion of affected males and possibly also of female carriers will become feasible.

Limb-girdle muscular dystrophy

This form of the disease occurs equally in the two sexes and usually begins in the second or third decade of life, but occasionally first appears in middle life. Though it is usually inherited as an autosomal recessive trait, many cases appear to be sporadic and some may be due to manifestation in the heterozygote. In about half the cases muscle weakness begins in the shoulder-girdle muscles and may not spread to involve the pelvic girdle for many years, but in the remainder the pelvic-girdle muscles are first involved and weakness affects the shoulders within about 10 years. Enlargement of calf muscles is not uncommon. Sometimes muscular weakness and wasting are asymmetrical initially and occasionally the disease process arrests temporarily, but most patients are severely disabled within 20 years of the onset. A scapuloperoneal distribution of muscular weakness and wasting with involvement of serrati, pectorals, and biceps in the upper limbs and of the anterior tibial and peroneal group in the lower limbs is occasionally seen. This so-called 'scapuloperoneal muscular dystrophy' is probably a variant of limb-girdle dystrophy; it is much less common than scapuloperoneal muscular atrophy which is a form of spinal muscular atrophy.

The course of the disease is generally more benign in those in whom upper limb muscles are first involved. Contractures and skeletal deformity occur late but progress more rapidly when the patient is confined to a wheelchair. Most sufferers are severely disabled in middle life and many die before the normal age. Many patients thought in the past to suffer from this condition have been shown to be cases of spinal muscular atrophy (the Kugelberg–Welander syndrome), and others have proved to have one of the metabolic myopathies to be discussed below. It is now generally accepted first that the limb-girdle muscular dystrophy syndrome is a disorder of multiple aetiology and secondly that true cases of muscular dystrophy of the limb-girdle type are much less common than was once believed.

Childhood muscular dystrophy with autosomal recessive inheritance

The existence of this comparatively rare form of the disease has been demonstrated by the occasional occurrence of muscular dystrophy superficially resembling the Duchenne type in young girls and occurring in a few families in which parental consanguinity made autosomal recessive inheritance likely. This form of the disease is clinically similar to the Duchenne type, but more benign. It is also, as a rule, more benign than the true Duchenne muscular dystrophy which occurs in girls with X/21 chromosomal translocation as mentioned above (Gomez et al., 1977). This variety of the disease, though rare in the United Kingdom and North America, is much more common in the Middle East and North Africa (Ben Hamida et al., 1983). The onset may be in the second year or as late as the fourteenth, but is most often in the second half of the first decade. Progression is comparatively slow and patients usually become unable to walk in their early twenties, but sometimes as early as 15 years or as late as 40 years. The pattern of weakness is similar to that found in typical Duchenne dystrophy and most patients die in middle life. Recent evidence suggests that many cases so diagnosed in the past were probably suffering from spinal muscular atrophy, but there is general agreement that some such patients, especially in the Middle East, are suffering from a true dystrophic process.

Congenital muscular dystrophy

This rare disorder presents with severe, generalized muscular hypotonia which is noted from birth and is followed by the subsequent development of progressive muscular wasting and weakness. In many affected children there are widespread contractures suggesting arthrogryposis multiplex congenita. Occasionally the weakness increases rapidly after birth and the disease terminates fatally within the first year of life, but there are other cases in which it seems relatively non-progressive. Few affected patients are ever able, however, to sit or stand unsupported and the prognosis is uniformly unfavourable. Diagnosis from spinal muscular atrophy of infancy can only be made with confidence by EMG, serum enzyme studies, and muscle biopsy. The occasional involvement of sibs supports the suggestion that this rare disorder may be due to an autosomal recessive gene. It can be distinguished from the benign congenital myopathies to be discussed below, first by its severity and secondly by the fact that the histological changes in muscle biopsy specimens are similar to those observed in other forms of muscular dystrophy.

Facioscapulohumeral muscular dystrophy

This variety inherited by an autosomal dominant mechanism, occurs equally in the two sexes and can begin at any age from childhood until adult life but is usually first recognized in adolescence. Facial involvement, with a typical pouting appearance of the lips and difficulty in closing the eyes, is apparent early and is accompanied by weakness of the shoulder-girdle muscles with bilateral winging of the scapulae and wasting of the pectorals. Muscular enlargement is uncommon; in the lower limbs the anterior tibial muscles are often first involved, causing bilateral footdrop. In many patients the disease is benign and runs a prolonged course with periods of apparent arrest, so that contractures and skeletal deformity are late in developing. However, in some patients the condition progresses more rapidly and severe accentuation of the lumbar lordosis is seen early; by contrast, in others the disease process is abortive and after certain muscles have been affected, the spread of weakness seems to cease. Most affected individuals survive and remain active to a normal age. Heart muscle is not involved and the range of intelligence is normal. As in limb-girdle muscular dystrophy, it is now clear that in some cases presenting with the typical clinical syndrome the disease process is neuropathic (spinal muscular atrophy) rather than myopathic. Even in some myopathic cases, inflammatory cell infiltrates in muscle biopsy sections are unexpectedly common, but there is no clinical improvement on treatment with steroids.

Distal muscular dystrophy

This variety is rare in Britain and in the United States, but not uncommon in Sweden. It is generally inherited as an autosomal dominant character, beginning usually between the ages of 40 and 60 years and involving both sexes. Weakness begins in the small hand muscles and in the anterior tibials and calves, but eventually spreads to proximal muscles, unlike the pattern seen in peroneal muscular atrophy with which it is most often confused. In Sweden the condition is comparatively benign, but sporadic cases observed in other countries tend to be more severe and rapidly progressive.

Ocular myopathy

This disorder usually begins with bilateral ptosis and goes on to give progressive bilateral external ophthalmoplegia. In the past it was referred to in the literature as 'progressive nuclear ophthalmoplegia', but pathological studies have shown that the muscular involvement is usually myopathic. Many patients also have some weakness of upper facial muscles (particularly orbicularis oculi) and often the neck and shoulder-girdle muscles are slender and slightly weak. Most cases are sporadic, but the condition is sometimes inherited by an autosomal dominant mechanism.

Oculopharyngeal muscular dystrophy

Whereas ocular myopathy, as described above, often begins in early adult life, this condition usually develops first in middle life but otherwise differs only from ocular myopathy in that dysphagia is invariable due to pharyngeal muscular involvement. The condition is slow to progress and the prognosis in general is good as disability usually remains slight for many years. Many reported cases were of French-Canadian ancestry and Huguenot origin. Abnormal mitochondria have been a prominent feature in muscle biopsy specimens obtained from many such cases. Indeed, evidence continues to emerge to suggest that this condition and many cases of ocular myopathy may well ultimately be classified with the mitochondrial myopathies (see below).

Diagnosis

In the typical case of muscular dystrophy showing the usual slowly progressive pattern of increasing muscular weakness and selective atrophy of proximal limb muscles, the diagnosis is often self-evident especially in a case of the Duchenne type. If the pattern of weakness and wasting is obscured by subcutaneous fat, or when involvement is predominantly distal, it is not always easy to distinguish muscular dystrophy from neuropathic disorders; here the EMG may be of particular value. This is particularly true in distinguishing between the limb-girdle and facioscapulohumeral types of muscular dystrophy on the one hand and benign spinal muscular atrophy (the Kugelberg–Welander syndrome) on the other, as these two conditions may be readily confused. Polymyositis may also resemble limb-girdle muscular dystrophy; in polymyositis, however, the onset is often more rapid, muscular weakness and wasting are less selective, neck muscles are frequently involved and dysphagia is common, while the family history is negative; associated phenomena such as skin changes and the Raynaud syndrome may be conclusive.

Estimation of the serum CK activity is of particular value in diagnosing Duchenne muscular dystrophy since in early cases it may be increased almost 300-fold (up to 200 000 i.u./l). Less striking increases up to 10 or 20 times the normal upper limit may be found in the other more benign varieties of muscular dystrophy, and surprisingly in congenital muscular dystrophy its activity is often little increased.

The value of muscle biopsy has already been described. However, it should be stressed again that in long-standing denervation due to spinal muscular atrophy, secondary myopathic change in muscle biopsy sections may lead the unwary to diagnose a primary myopathy unless histochemical studies (which may demonstrate fibre type grouping in such cases) are also carried out.

Treatment

Unfortunately no drug has any influence upon the course of the disease, though complications such as respiratory and urinary infections may demand antibiotics. Physical exercise appears to delay the march of the weakness and the onset of contractures, and a regular programme of such activities may be started under the supervision of a skilled physiotherapist and subsequently continued at home by the patients and their relatives. Passive stretching of those tendons which show a tendency to shorten should also be carried out regularly. In some cases, light spinal supports may help to delay the development of skeletal deformity and the Luque or other similar operative procedure for the control of scoliosis may well be justified, while in some cases, too, calipers are valuable; surgical lengthening of shortened tendons is only to be advised if this can be followed by immediate mobilization of the patient in walking plasters or calipers. Immobilization or prolonged bed-rest must be avoided as these inevitably cause rapid deterioration. Psychological management demands considerable reserves of patience and understanding on the part of parents, doctors, nurses, and social workers. Optimism and encouragement, however unjustifiable in the face of continuing deterioration, are of great importance.

Course and prognosis

This has been mentioned in relation to the individual subvarieties of the disease.

MYOTONIC DISORDERS

Myotonia is the continued act of contraction of a muscle which persists after the cessation of voluntary effort or stimulation; an electrical after-discharge can be seen to accompany the phenomenon in the EMG. Clinically it is best demonstrated as slowness in relaxation of the grip or by persistent dimpling after a sharp blow on a muscle belly, e.g. in the thenar eminence or tongue. It is due to an abnormality of the muscle fibre, as it persists after section or blocking of the motor nerve and after curarization. It is associated with an abnormality of chloride conductance in the muscle fibre membrane.

Myotonia appears in three hereditary syndromes, all of autosomal dominant inheritance, namely myotonia congenita, dystrophia myotonica and paramyotonia. The three conditions breed true and they are plainly different diseases. While dystrophic changes occur in certain muscles in one of them, namely dystro-

phia myotonica, these disorders are more closely related to each other than they are to the muscular dystrophies. There is an obvious relationship between paramyotonia on the one hand and the periodic paralyses on the other.

In a rare syndrome mentioned briefly above, variously called 'one form of myokymia', 'pseudomyotonia', 'neuromyotonia', 'the myotonia–myokymia–hyperhidrosis syndrome' and 'a syndrome of continuous muscle fibre activity and spasm', a phenomenon similar clinically but electrically different from myotonia is associated with myokymia (benign coarse fasciculation), cramps, hyperhidrosis, and sometimes muscle wasting. Its nature is little understood, but the impaired relaxation in these cases, like that of myotonia, seems to be relieved by phenytoin and related remedies.

Myotonia congenita

Synonym Thomsen's disease (the dominant form)
This condition is usually present from birth. Myotonia is generalized, accentuated by rest and by cold, and gradually relieved by exercise. In infancy, these children are often difficult to feed and have a peculiarly strangled cry. Later, myotonia of the tongue may cause difficulty in speaking. Diffuse hypertrophy of muscles usually persists throughout life, though the myotonia tends to improve with increasing age; rarely, it increases during exertion (myotonia paradoxa) but must then be distinguished from the cramping stiffness of McArdle's disease. Hypertrophia musculorum vera may well be a variant of this condition. A recessively inherited variant of myotonia congenita, clinically milder and significantly more common than Thomsen's disease, often first becomes apparent later in childhood, usually during the first decade.

Dystrophia myotonica

Dystrophia myotonica (myotonica atrophica or Steinert's disease) is a diffuse systemic disorder in which myotonia, facial myopathy, and distal muscular atrophy are accompanied by cataracts, frontal baldness in the male (Fig. 10), gonadal atrophy, cardiomyopathy, impaired pulmonary ventilation, mild endocrine anomalies, bone changes, mental defect or dementia, and abnormalities of the serum immunoglobulins. The affected families show progressive social decline in successive generations, diminished fertility, and an increased infantile mortality rate. The condition is about as common as muscular dystrophy of the Duchenne type. The gene responsible for the disease has now been located on chromosome 19 and seems to lie within 10 centimorgans of the complement C3 polymorphism locus. The latter marker can thus be applied to linkage analysis with a 10 per cent error (Roses, 1984). It is hoped that even closer flanking marker haplotypes will soon be identified which could then be used in the detection of preclinical cases and/ or antenatal diagnosis of the affected fetus with a view to selective therapeutic abortion.

The presenting symptoms are usually weakness of the hands and difficulty in walking, and myotonia is rarely obtrusive. Poor vision, weight-loss, impotence, ptosis, and increased sweating are common. The condition may present in infancy and childhood with severe muscular weakness and hypotonia or delay in walking, and these children may be erroneously regarded as examples of benign congenital myopathy or hypotonia unless the existence of myotonic dystrophy in one parent, almost invariably the mother, is recognized. More often the condition becomes clinically overt between the ages of 20 and 50 years.

The facial appearance is typically long and haggard; ptosis is usual and rarely there is external ophthalmoplegia. Wasting of the masseters, temporal muscles, and sternomastoids is invariable and in the extremities weakness and wasting involves particularly forearm muscles (sparing the small muscles of the hands), the anterior

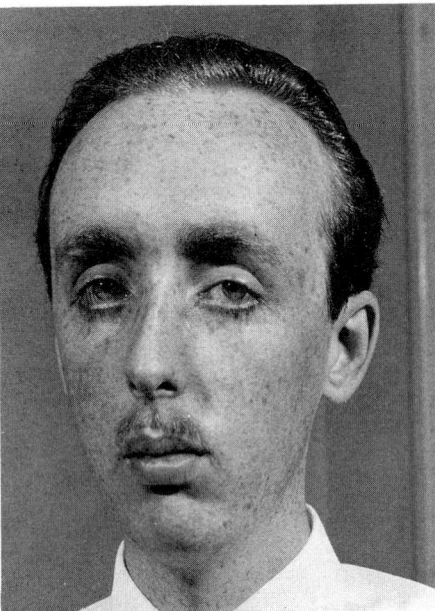

Fig. 10 The typical facial appearance of myotonic dystrophy (dystrophia myotonica).

tibial group and the calves and peronei. Slit-lamp examination reveals cataracts in most cases. Cardiac conduction defects and/or cardiomyopathy are common and the pulmonary vital capacity and maximum expiratory pressure are often impaired, so that many patients tolerate barbiturate anaesthesia poorly. Drowsiness and hypersomnolence are common. Dysphagia can be shown to be due to disordered oesophageal contraction. The testes are usually small and histologically the changes are like those of Klinefelter's syndrome. Females often show irregular menstruation, infertility, and prolonged parturition. Pituitary function is usually normal, but there may be a selective failure of adrenal androgenic function and occasionally thyroid activity and glucose utilization are impaired. Hyperostosis of the skull vault and a small sella turcica are often found radiologically, while both mental defect and progressive dementia occur. There is a high incidence of abnormal EEGs in such cases, and CT scanning or pneumoencephalography may demonstrate cerebral cortical atrophy, or more often progressive ventricular enlargement. Excessive catabolism of immunoglobulin-G, abnormalities of insulin secretion, in the sensitivity of blood platelets to adrenaline and of erythrocyte membranes, have been demonstrated in some cases.

Paramyotonia

This condition is characterized by myotonia appearing only on exposure to cold. In addition, patients experience attacks of generalized muscular weakness like those of familial hyperkalaemic periodic paralysis. Myotonia in the upper lids on looking upwards may be particularly prominent in these cases which are sometimes called myotonic periodic paralysis.

Chondrodystrophic myotonia

In this rare condition, also called the Schwartz–Jampel syndrome, choking on cold drinks with hip contractures or dislocations are noted in infancy and are followed by progressive hip deformities and other skeletal abnormalities. Growth fails progressively, the muscles becomes stiff and hypertrophied and the affected children show tense puckering of the mouth, blepharospasm, small palpebral fissures, and irregular eyelashes. Myotonia is widespread and muscular atrophy often develops in later childhood.

Diagnosis

Myotonia must be distinguished from the slowness of muscular contraction and relaxation which may occur in hypothyroidism and from the similar clinical phenomenon of delayed relaxation with prolonged dimpling on percussion of muscle which is rarely seen in patients with polymyositis, polyneuropathy, and spinal muscular atrophy. The painful and physiological (reversible) contracture which may follow exertion in patients with myophosphorylase deficiency (McArdle's disease) and related diseases may also give rise to diagnostic difficulty, but these various disorders may be distinguished with confidence electromyographically. The distal muscular wasting and areflexia seen in dystrophia myotonica, and the diffuse muscular hypotonia occurring in affected infants, are readily confused with the similar phenomena which can occur in other neuromuscular diseases unless the presence of myotonia is recognized either clinically or electromyographically in the patient or in his relatives. In dystrophia myotonica, the EMG demonstrates not only myotonic discharges evoked by movement of the exploring electrode, but myopathic potentials are recorded from weakened and wasted muscles during volition. The serum CK activity is normal in myotonia congenita and paramyotonia, but may be raised to between two and 10 times the normal upper limit in myotonic dystrophy. In muscle biopsy samples, cases of myotonia congenita and paramyotonia may show nothing more than hypertrophy of muscle fibres and perhaps occasional *ringbinden*, but in myotonic dystrophy changes similar to those of muscular dystrophy are seen in addition to frequent long chains of nuclei in the centre of muscle fibres, combined sometimes with ringed annulets and peripheral sarcoplasmic masses. The latter changes are much less striking in biopsy samples taken during life than they are in muscle examined post-mortem. In frozen sections studied histochemically, selective atrophy of type I fibres is characteristic.

Treatment

In dystrophia myotonica, no treatment influences the progressive muscular wasting and weakness which eventually develops. In paramyotonia, treatment and prevention of the attacks of paralysis is that which is appropriate in familial periodic paralysis. Myotonia itself can, however, be relieved by drugs; this is particularly helpful in myotonia congenita and in some patients with myotonic dystrophy in whom myotonia is severe. Quinine and prednisone help in some cases, but procainamide in a dosage of 250–500 mg three or four times daily is superior, and sodium phenytoin in a dosage of 100 mg three or four times daily is the most effective remedy in some cases, though others do not respond.

Course and prognosis

Myotonia congenita is essentially a benign disorder which does not shorten life, and the same is true of paramyotonia. Most patients with dystrophia myotonica, however, show progressive deterioration and become severely disabled and unable to walk within 15–20 years of the onset. Death from respiratory infection or cardiac failure usually occurs well before the normal age.

INFLAMMATORY DISEASES OF MUSCLE (see Table 2)
Myopathies due to microbial agents and parasites
Viral myositis
Influenza

While diffuse myalgia commonly precedes or accompanies the other manifestations of influenza, a post-influenzal variety of myositis is well documented. This syndrome is seen in the week after an attack of influenza and is characterized by severe pain, tenderness, and sometimes swelling, usually of calf muscles but sometimes also involving those of the thigh; it usually resolves spontaneously within about a week. The serum CK activity is

Table 2 Classification of inflammatory myopathies

Due to identified infective agents	Idiopathic inflammatory myopathies
Viral	
Influenza	Myositis in collagen disease and sarcoidosis
Coxsackie A and B	Polymyositis
	Dermatomyositis
Bacterial	Inclusion-body myositis
Pyomyositis (*Staph. aureus*;	Granulomatous myositis
Strep. pyogenes)	Eosinophilic myositis
Clostridial myositis	Localized nodular myositis
	Polymyalgia rheumatica
Parasitic	
Trichinosis	
Cysticercosis	
Toxoplasmosis	
Sarcosporidiosis	
Echinococcosis	
Trypanosomiasis	
Actinomycosis	

Modified from Mastaglia and Walton (1982).

usually increased. Pathological evidence of a necrotizing inflammatory myopathy is found in some cases, and the condition has been observed particularly in children with influenza B, A2 Hong Kong virus, and influenza A virus, but can also occur in adults. Influenza virus was isolated from muscle in a case of acute polymyositis with myoglobinuria.

Enteroviruses

The Coxsackie B virus, particularly B5, is typically associated with epidemic pleurodynia (Bornholm disease), a self-limiting disorder occurring usually in childhood and characterized by acute and severe pain with tenderness of the chest, back, shoulders or abdomen. A fulminant acute form of polymyositis with myoglobinuria has been linked with Coxsackie B6 virus infection. Cases of acute myositis and acute rhabdomyolysis associated with Echo 9 virus infection have also been reported. There is also evidence to suggest that Coxsackie and Echo viruses may sometimes precipitate the autoimmune process presumed to account for polymyositis and/or dermatomyositis.

Other viruses

There have also been reports of human inflammatory myopathy in patients harbouring hepatitis B virus, the herpes group, rubella virus, and respiratory syncytial virus, but the evidence that the virus in question caused the myositis in each of these circumstances is somewhat indefinite.

Bacterial myositis

Acute suppurative (tropical) myositis

While suppurative myositis may complicate penetrating or crush injuries or pressure sores and is occasionally seen in patients with pyococcal arthritis, suppurative myositis is uncommon in developed countries. In tropical and subtropical countries, however, pyomyositis with suppurative staphyloccal inflammation involving the skeletal muscles is common and is seen more often in men than in women, usually without any specific antecedent illness (see Section 5). The muscles most often affected are the glutei and quadriceps. Single or multiple muscle abscesses may occur and treatment consists of high doses of penicillin with surgical drainage. Functional recovery is usually good.

Clostridial myositis

Clostridium welchii produces a toxin and enzymes including collagenase and hyaluronidase which cause necrosis of muscle fibres and interstitial tissues, with vascular congestion, fibrin exudation, intense polymorphonuclear leucocytic infiltration, and haemorrhage. Clostridial toxin may cause discrete defects in the muscle fibre plasma membrane leading to fibre necrosis. This condition

(gas gangrene) usually follows septic wounds involving extensive areas of skeletal muscle; if the infection is controlled by antibiotics and necrotic muscle tissue is entirely removed, regeneration may be effective, but marked fibrosis and muscular atrophy usually result.

Other forms of bacterial myositis

Tuberculous and syphilitic myositis are now virtually unknown, though very occasionally tuberculous granulomas still occur in skeletal muscle in tropical countries. Leprous inflammation of muscle is also occasionally seen, especially when there is associated evidence of denervation atrophy with granulomatous lesions in intramuscular nerves.

Parasitic myositis

Trichinosis

This is the commonest parasitic infection of muscle. The causative agent, *Trichinella spiralis*, is a nematode usually acquired by humans as the result of eating incompletely cooked pork, bear meat or horse meat. The larvae penetrate the mucosa of the small intestine, enter the lymphatics and the blood-stream and are then disseminated widely. Muscles are invaded at about the end of the first week and there is severe myalgia and tenderness, often associated with weakness, which may be generalized or limited to certain groups such as the ocular muscles. Periorbital and conjunctival oedema is common and a skin eruption often occurs. There is often eosinophilia, and muscle biopsy may demonstrate the parasites in various stages of development and encystment. Except in very severe infestations, recovery is usual.

Cysticercosis

This condition is common in India and Eastern Europe, being less frequent in other parts of the world, and results from infestation with the encysted larval stage of the pork tapeworm *Taenia solium*. The larval parasites invade the intestine and are disseminated by the blood to all parts of the body, particularly muscle and brain. In the acute stage there is often muscle tenderness, fever, and eosinophilia, but often there is no such illness and evidence of involvement of the muscle and of the central nervous system is only found many years later when the patient presents with a hypertrophic myopathy or with epilepsy. Nodules are sometimes palpable in the tongue and other muscles, but in the hypertrophic form gross enlargement of multiple limb muscles may occur. Spindle-shaped cysts may be found in the interstitial connective tissue in muscle biopsy specimens.

Echinococcosis

This is very rare, even in countries in which hydatid disease is common. The cysts forming in muscle are usually solitary, large, and surrounded by granulomatous inflammation with prominent eosinophils, but on occasions individual cysts may rupture leading to the formation of daughter cysts. When muscles are involved, those most commonly affected are the posterior trunk, inner thigh, neck, and upper arm muscles.

Toxoplasmosis

Toxoplasma gondii can give a multifocal disseminated myositis and the organism may be revealed by muscle biopsy. In the foci of myositis, the necrotic fibres are surrounded and infiltrated by neutrophil leucocytes, lymphocytes, and plasma cells. Pseudocysts, which are round or oval and often about 20–60 μm in diameter, containing multiple parasites, are occasionally found in otherwise healthy muscle fibres.

Sarcosporidiosis

Sarcocystis lindemanni rarely invades skeletal muscles in humans; when it does so, the condition is usually asymptomatic and the parasite may be found unexpectedly in a muscle biopsy. Rarely, the parasite cysts, which are filled with many sporozoites and which may be 1–5 mm in length, are associated with muscle aching, slight weakness, and loss of tendon reflexes.

Trypanosomiasis cruzi (Chagas' disease)

This condition, indigenous to South America, is characterized by disseminated focal polymyositis, myocarditis, and encephalomyelitis. In muscle, parasites are localized within individual fibres and form small thin-walled cysts loaded with trypanosomes which may be difficult to distinguish from toxoplasma pseudocysts.

Fungal myositis

Actinomycosis may invoke skeletal muscle through direct extension from a neighbouring infective focus in pleura or skin, when abscesses and fistulae discharging purulent material and containing the characteristic yellow granules composed of colonies of the fungus are often seen.

Muscular involvement in collagen or connective tissue diseases and in sarcoidosis

In rheumatoid arthritis, muscle biopsy sections may demonstrate foci of inflammatory cell infiltration, but this *focal nodular myositis* is not usually accompanied by specific muscular wasting and weakness, save for that resulting secondarily from joint disease. This pathological finding must be distinguished from the clinical syndrome of *localized nodular myositis*, a rare condition in which localized painful and tender swellings may develop in one or more skeletal muscles (such as quadriceps, or rarely even masseter) and are shown on biopsy to demonstrate massive muscle fibre necrosis and cellular infiltration. This condition appears to be related to polymyositis (see below) and some sufferers go on to develop evidence of more diffuse inflammatory muscle disease.

In *sarcoidosis*, muscle involvement may cause a subacute weakness and wasting of proximal muscles and typical sarcoid granulomas may be observed on muscle biopsy. Localized muscle pain, subcutaneous oedema, and tenderness can also occur as a result of muscle infarction in polyarteritis nodosa and in Wegener's granulomatosis. In systemic lupus erythematosus, muscular involvement is sometimes severe and diffuse and is then indistinguishable from polymyositis, although in occasional such cases muscle biopsies demonstrate a vacuolar myopathy.

Polymyositis

This term is generally used to identify a group of cases in which muscular weakness and wasting may be associated with muscle pain and tenderness or with evidence of some form of connective tissue or collagen disease. The term is commonly used to embrace cases with florid skin change which are more properly called dermatomyositis; it is usually taken to identify the so-called idiopathic syndrome and excludes disorders such as polymyalgia rheumatica (see Section 16) and also the infective and parasitic myositides described above. With the exception of the specific myasthenic–myopathic syndrome (see page 22.17) which has been observed in patients with lung cancer, many cases of so-called carcinomatous myopathy probably belong to the syndrome of polymyositis.

Aetiology

Work demonstrating that experimental allergic myositis may be produced in animals by the injection of muscle homogenates with Freund's adjuvant and that lymphocytes from patients with polymyositis are cytotoxic to muscle in tissue culture supports the view that this syndrome in the human is due to lymphocyte-mediated delayed hypersensitivity or cell-mediated immunity. Recent work has suggested that sensitized T-cells, mostly $T8^+$ with associated macrophages, which can be identified in muscle sections using specific monoclonal antibodies, may invade and destroy muscle in such cases. However, there is also evidence of a disorder of complement formation and utilization in many such patients, and of immunoglobulin deposition in vessel walls within muscle, so that a

humoral factor may also be involved. A Jo-1 antigen has recently been characterized and preliminary work suggests that a circulating Jo-1 antibody may be specific for polymyositis; previous attempts to identify circulating antibodies against muscle in the serum were uniformly unsuccessful. As yet no consistent relationship between this disease in any of its clinical subvarieties on the one hand and any components of the HLA antigen system on the other has been found. At present it may simply be suggested that polymyositis in which clinical evidence suggests that the disease process is limited to muscle, may be regarded as an organ-specific autoimmune disease, while in cases showing involvement of skin or joints, it can be accepted as being the muscular manifestation of non-organ specific autoimmune disease. The well-recognized relationship between polymyositis and dermatomyositis on the one hand and malignant disease in patients over 45 years of age on the other suggests that the condition may also on occasion be the result of a conditioned autoimmune response in patients suffering from cancer. The close relationship of the condition to other disorders of the connective tissue group is underlined by the occurrence of certain cases which may successively present manifestations of polymyositis, systemic lupus erythematosus and/or scleroderma or systemic sclerosis.

Polymyositis is worldwide, occurs in many races and in both sexes. It is more common in adult life than muscular dystrophy, but less common than the latter in childhood. About 15 per cent of cases occur under the age of 15 years, another 15 per cent between the ages of 16 and 30, about a quarter between 31 and 45, and a third between the ages of 45 and 60. It usually develops spontaneously but can follow febrile illness or the administration of various drugs including sulphonamides.

Classification

The following four clinical categories of polymyositis have been arbitrarily defined:

Group I:

$$\text{Polymyositis} \begin{cases} \text{Acute, with myoglobinuria} \\ \text{Subacute or chronic} \begin{cases} \text{in childhood} \\ \text{in early adult life} \\ \text{in middle or late life} \end{cases} \end{cases}$$

Group II: Polymyositis with dominant muscular weakness but with some evidence of an associated collagen disease *or* dermatomyositis with severe muscular disability and with minimal or transient skin changes.

Group III: Polymyositis complicating severe collagen disease, e.g. rheumatoid arthritis or systemic lupus, *or* dermatomyositis with florid skin changes and minor muscle weakness.

Group IV: Polymyositis and dermatomyositis complicating malignant disease.

Symptoms and signs

Apart from occasional acute cases in which widespread muscle pain, fever, constitutional upset, and rapidly progressive paralysis, often with respiratory weakness, may develop, the condition usually runs a subacute or chronic course. Muscle pain and tenderness occur in approximately 50 per cent of cases, as does dysphagia. Cutaneous manifestations are seen in about two-thirds of all patients and may take the form of widespread erythema with desquamation seen particularly on the face and on other exposed areas of the trunk, but occasionally involving the whole body. Heliotrope erythema around the eyes and periorbital oedema are particularly characteristic and so, too, is congestion of the nail beds. Sometimes the skin changes are slight in the form of a faint butterfly-type rash on the face, while in others, particularly in childhood, there may be ulceration over bony prominences with subcutaneous calcification. Raynaud's syndrome is a common association and many younger patients develop loss of elasticity of the skin over the fingers, face, and anterior chest wall, indistinguishable from the appearances of scleroderma or acrosclerosis.

In about a quarter of the patients joint pain and stiffness occur at some stage. Proximal limb muscles are almost invariably involved and the neck muscles are characteristically affected in about one-third of all cases so that some patients may have difficulty in holding up the head. Involvement of distal limb muscles is less common, but weakness may be generalized in about a third of all cases, and when the condition runs a subacute or chronic course contractures sometimes develop (*chronic fibrosing myositis*). Facial weakness and involvement of the external ocular muscles are rare. Occasionally fatiguability like that of myasthenia is striking and is partially responsive to edrophonium or neostigmine, but treatment with these or related drugs usually produces only temporary improvement. The deep tendon reflexes may be depressed in the affected muscles but are often surprisingly brisk despite the severe weakness.

Diagnosis
In many cases the clinical picture is entirely characteristic, but when involvement of the skin and joints is unobtrusive and the course of the illness is subacute, it may be mistaken for muscular dystrophy or for various forms of metabolic myopathy.

The pattern of muscular involvement does not show the selectivity characteristic of muscular dystrophy, the serum potassium, calcium, and phosphorus are normal, and signs of associated endocrine disease are absent. The serum CK activity is often greatly raised in acute or subacute cases; the erythrocyte sedimentation rate is often, though not invariably, increased, and there may be a rise in the serum γ-globulin with a particularly striking increase in serum IgG in some cases. Electromyography demonstrates a myopathic pattern of volitional activity, but in addition there may be spontaneous fibrillation, positive sharp waves, and occasional pseudomyotonic discharges recorded from resting muscle. Muscle biopsy specimens often demonstrate widespread necrosis and phagocytosis of muscle fibres and interstitial and perivascular infiltrations of inflammatory cells, mainly lymphocytes and plasma cells; in transverse sections these changes and fibre atrophy are often seen in perifascicular distribution and aggressive lymphocytes can be seen, especially with the electron microscope, emerging from the interfascicular blood vessels and invading muscle. However, in some clinically active cases inflammatory cells are surprisingly absent and the picture is that of a necrotizing myopathy; the absence of such infiltrates in a single muscle biopsy section does not, therefore, exclude the diagnosis of polymyositis. In occasional cases where the clinical picture is typical but the exact diagnosis remains in doubt after full investigation, a therapeutic trial of steroid drugs is indicated.

Treatment
The condition should usually be treated with 60 mg of prednisone daily, given for 4 or 5 days, thereafter reducing the dose to 50 mg daily when clinical improvement appears, and subsequently regulating the maintenance dose according to the level of serum CK activity and the clinical response. Occasionally even higher doses of prednisone may be required for short periods, even as much as 120 mg daily. Alternate-day treatment with prednisone, begun when the disease has been brought under control by daily treatment, may have the advantage in childhood of causing less growth suppression. Maintenance therapy may have to be continued for several years before the drug can eventually be withdrawn. Respiratory and urinary infections should be treated with appropriate antibiotics and in occasional acute cases, intermittent positive-pressure respiration is necessary. Most authorities now give an immunosuppressive drug such as azathioprine, methotrexate, or cyclophosphamide in an appropriate level of dosage depending upon age and body weight, along with prednisone from the beginning. Thus it is usual to give, say, in an adult, azathioprine 100 mg daily from the onset, for 6 months, followed by 50 mg daily for up to a total of 12–18 months. Even though the evidence of disordered humoral immunity in such cases is limited, some authorities find plasmapheresis of temporary or even lasting benefit in steroid-resistant cases. Also in intractable cases it has been found that total body irradiation is sometimes successful and cyclosporin is now under test. Following the acute stage, active and passive movements carried out under the supervision of a skilled physiotherapist help to speed recovery.

Clinical variants of polymyositis
Sarcoid myopathy, localized nodular myositis, polymyalgia rheumatica, and focal nodular myositis have been mentioned above. Other related disorders include the following.

Neuromyositis
This term has been used to identify cases in which there is clinical or other evidence suggestive of concomitant involvement of peripheral nerves. Combined manifestations of an inflammatory myopathy and of a demyelinating polyneuropathy sometimes occur in patients with connective tissue disease or malignancy. It is not surprising that an autoimmune disorder involving muscle does from time to time also damage peripheral nerves, and there is no benefit in regarding neuromyositis as an independent clinical or pathological entity.

Inclusion body myositis
This condition appears to be a distinctive variety of idiopathic inflammatory myopathy. It is a relatively benign and chronic myopathy not associated with connective tissue disease or with malignant disease. It occurs particularly in men in their sixties, though it occasionally occurs in younger patients. Slowly progressive painless weakness involves distal as well as proximal muscle groups and there is often associated dysphagia. The rate of progression is variable and some patients are severely handicapped even within two years; treatment with corticosteroids and other immunosuppressive agents is usually ineffective.

The distinctive pathological features of this condition are, first, that bluish granular inclusions are found around the edges of slit-like vacuoles within muscle fibres stained with haematoxylin and eosin. These granules are removed by lipid solvents; they often show acid phosphatase activity and ultrastructurally are composed of polymorphic whorls of membrane. There are also interstitial inflammatory cell infiltrates, but the other most distinctive feature is that under the electron microscope there are masses of filaments or filamentous microtubules, 15–18 nm in diameter, within the nuclei and cytoplasm of muscle fibres. Attempts to isolate a virus from muscle in such patients have been unsuccessful to date and the nature of the inclusions remains uncertain.

Eosinophilic polymyositis
This rare form of inflammatory myopathy occurs as a part of the systemic hypereosinophilic syndrome characterized by eosinophilia, anaemia, hypergammaglobulinaemia, cardiac and pulmonary involvement, skin changes, peripheral neuropathy, and encephalopathy. The myositis usually presents with a localized tender swelling in a muscle in one calf or thigh, like localized nodular myositis. There is an increase in the serum CK and often a more extensive proximal myopathy develops. The relationship of this condition to eosinophilic fasciitis is somewhat uncertain, though the fact that in many cases of the latter type skeletal muscle is also involved makes it probable that the two conditions are closely related. Most such cases show a satisfactory response to steroids.

Granulomatous myositis
Granulomatous lesions similar to those of sarcoid, developing in the absence of any clinical or pathological evidence of sarcoidosis involving other tissues and organs, occurring in patients with a clinical picture suggesting polymyositis, identify the syndrome of granulomatous myositis. These patients show a response to steroid therapy which is generally as satisfactory as that demonstrated by patients with subacute polymyositis.

Course and prognosis

Even without treatment, the course of the illness is variable. Sometimes it runs a fluctuating course with spontaneous exacerbations and remissions. Progressive deterioration with a fatal termination within a few weeks or months of the onset is seen particularly in acute dermatomyositis, but spontaneous arrest occasionally occurs. Slow insidious progression is seen particularly in middle age, but spontaneous recovery may occur in childhood; nevertheless, before the introduction of steroid drugs, the overall mortality of the disease was about 50 per cent.

The high incidence of malignant disease in such cases indicates that all patients developing this syndrome in middle or late life should be investigated with the possibility of occult neoplasia in mind. In general, the prognosis is best in children and in young adults; after the age of 30, some patients go on to develop evidence of diffuse connective tissue disease (systemic lupus erythematosus or systemic sclerosis) unresponsive to treatment, while after the age of 50 the presence of malignant disease, especially in men with dermatomyositis, is the single factor most likely to affect the prognosis adversely.

MYASTHENIA GRAVIS

This is a disease with a tendency to remit and to relapse, characterized by abnormal muscular fatiguability sometimes confined to, or predominant in, an isolated group of muscles and later associated in many cases with permanent weakness of some muscles. There is a disorder of conduction at the myoneural junction which can be temporarily relieved by neostigmine and similar drugs and some patients benefit from removal of the thymus gland.

Aetiology and incidence

Myasthenia occurs in all races and affects both sexes, but occurs in women twice as often as in men. Only rarely does it affect more than one member of the same family. While usually beginning in early adult life, it sometimes develops in childhood and occasionally as late as the ninth decade. Most remissions occur within the first five years of the disease process and most deaths also occur within this period. Neonatal myasthenia is seen in about one in seven of the children born to myasthenic mothers, but usually recovers within a few weeks. Myasthenia is closely related to thyrotoxicosis and the two diseases occur in the same individual more often than can be accounted for by chance. In occasional cases there is an association with diabetes mellitus, rheumatoid arthritis, systemic lupus erythematosus, and sarcoidosis. This clinical observation suggested to Simpson (1950) that myasthenia might be an autoimmune disorder and this suggestion has been amply confirmed by immunological studies. There is now clear evidence that in myasthenic patients there are circulating antibodies to the ACh receptor (AChR). There is also evidence that T lymphocytes (derived from the thymus) play an important role, in collaboration with B lymphocytes, in producing these antibodies. Immune complexes (IgG and complement) can be demonstrated on the postsynaptic membrane. A syndrome resembling human myasthenia can be induced in animals injected with AChR and Freund's adjuvant and passive transfer to the mouse can be achieved with human myasthenic IgG. The fact that the clinical severity of the human disease does not always correlate with the titre of circulating antibodies against AChR is probably explained by the fact that the receptor itself has been shown to demonstrate heterogeneity and different subvarieties of AChR may therefore be involved in different cases. However, it seems clear that these circulating antibodies, through binding to receptor sites, cause depletion of functional receptor sites on the postsynaptic membrane and that this mechanism is largely responsible for the clinical features of the disease. That genetic susceptibility is also involved is supported by the finding of an association with the

HLA determinants A2 and B8 in some groups of myasthenic patients. There is also some evidence to suggest that there may be fundamental pathophysiological and aetiological differences between various clinical forms of myasthenia: thus acute and severe myasthenia in young women is somewhat different immunologically and in its response to treatment from that occurring in a middle-aged man with a thymoma.

Classification

The symptom of muscular fatiguability or myasthenia is not peculiar to one disease, as similar weakness, increasing after exercise, is sometimes seen in muscles of patients suffering from polymyositis, systemic lupus erythematosus, dermatomyositis and in the myasthenic-myopathic syndrome (see below). However, a therapeutic response to anticholinesterase drugs is usually striking in true myasthenia gravis and although some response may be found in the symptomatic myasthenias, this is rarely dramatic and often fails within a few weeks. In myasthenia gravis, by contrast, the response to such treatment is usually sustained and the disease has an individual natural history and pathology. True myasthenia of autoimmune origin is also fundamentally different from several rare forms of congenital myasthenia in which there is no evidence of disordered immunity (see below).

Pathology

Muscle sections obtained by biopsy may in early cases show no significant abnormality, but in some patients areas of focal necrosis and phagocytosis of muscle fibres are seen and sometimes collections of lymphocytes (lymphorrhages) are found around blood vessels or between the fibres. These changes are, however, nonspecific and the same is true of changes which have been described in the terminal intramuscular motor nerves.

Thymic enlargement is often observed, particularly in younger patients, and histological examination of the thymus shows prominent germinal centres and Hassall's corpuscles. Thymic enlargement may, however, be due to a thymoma and some thymomas are malignant.

Symptoms and signs

The muscles most often affected are the external ocular, bulbar, neck, and shoulder-girdle muscles in this descending order, but not infrequently those of respiration and the proximal lower-limb muscles are also involved early. Ptosis of one or both upper lids, developing gradually, is often the first symptom and is soon associated with diplopia due to paralysis of one or more of the external ocular muscles. These symptoms typically appear in the evening when the patient is tired and disappear after a night's rest. When bulbar muscles are first involved, difficulty in swallowing and/or in chewing is described, developing during the course of a meal, and speech may become indistinct.

On examination, there may be unilateral or bilateral ptosis accentuated by upward gaze. External ocular muscle weakness is usually asymmetrical, though it may progress to complete external ophthalmoplegia. Rarely a single ocular muscle such as the external rectus is involved, thus mimicking the effects of a sixth-nerve palsy. The pupillary reflexes are usually normal. The facial muscles are almost always affected with weakness of the orbicularis oculi and of the retractors of the angles of the mouth, giving a characteristic 'myasthenic snarl'. Weakness of jaw muscles leads to difficulty in chewing and weakness of the muscles of the soft palate, pharynx, tongue, and larynx to difficulty in swallowing and in articulation. If the patient is asked to count aloud, speech becomes progressively less distinct and more nasal, and fluids may regurgitate through the nose when he tries to swallow. Neck muscle weakness may cause the head to fall forwards, a sign seen most often in myasthenia but sometimes in polymyositis. In severe cases, upper limb weakness is such that the hands cannot be lifted to the mouth; typically muscle power may initially be satisfactory but after testing a movement several times, strength rapidly declines. Breathlessness is always a sinister symptom as respiratory weakness can develop rapidly and may even cause sudden death.

Muscular wasting is unusual in the early stages, but in long-standing cases there may be permanent myopathic change, irreversible by drugs, in the external ocular muscles and in certain limb muscles, particularly triceps brachii. In some cases the disease remains limited to most external ocular muscles, but in most those of the head and neck, trunk, and limbs are eventually involved. The tendon reflexes are almost always brisk even in the presence of severe weakness.

Diagnosis

Clinical diagnosis depends not only upon the typical clinical picture and upon fatiguability, which may be demonstrated electrically by repetitive supramaximal stimulation of a peripheral nerve while recording the evoked muscle potential from a suitable group of muscles, or by demonstrating increased 'jitter' in the course of single-fibre EMG studies, but also upon the clinical response to an injection of neostigmine or edrophonium chloride. The quick-acting edrophonium is given initially in a dosage of 2 mg intravenously, followed immediately by a further 8 mg if there is no severe reaction. The increased muscle power following the injection lasts for only a few minutes but is usually diagnostic. In ocular myasthenia, measurement of intraocular pressure by tonometry before and after edrophonium may be helpful. Provocative tests designed to accentuate myasthenic symptoms, utilizing such drugs as curare and quinine are dangerous and now outdated. Much precision has now been added to diagnosis by measuring the titre in the serum of circulating AChR antibodies, which are increased in well over 90 per cent of cases; this test is now obligatory when the diagnosis is suspected.

Treatment

The standard treatment for myasthenia gravis in the past was neostigmine or the closely related drug pyridostigmine. The usual initial dose of neostigmine is a 15 mg tablet three or four times a day, and it may to necessary also to give atropine, 0.6 mg or, preferably, propantheline hydrochloride 15 mg twice daily, to overcome muscarinic side-effects. Pyridostigmine, with its longer action, became preferable as the standard medication; the initial dosage is 60 mg three or four times a day, again with atropine or propantheline. The dosage is steadily increased until maximum benefit is obtained. Some patients require to take the drugs every two, three, or four hours, but this is an individual matter. Another drug of value in some cases is ambenonium hydrochloride in which the usual dosage is 10–25 mg three or four times daily. While opinions differ and some authorities (see Engel, 1984) still recommend the use of anticholinesterase drugs as the preferred treatment in ocular myasthenia, there is now a reasonable consensus that corticosteroid drugs (usually prednisone or prednisolone) given with or without immunosuppressive drugs such as azathioprine (in a regimen comparable to that described above for polymyositis) are probably the initial treatment of choice in all cases and that when significant clinical improvement has occurred, except in restricted ocular cases, thymectomy should be the next step unless there are powerful contraindications such as age, poor general condition, etc. Even in some acute and severe cases, the response to steroids and immunosuppressants is occasionally disappointing, when plasmapheresis (a means of removing circulating antibodies) or the use of anticholinesterase drugs must then be considered. Former controversies about thymectomy are slowly being resolved. It is certainly indicated in all patients with thymoma. It was once thought that in other cases the results were better in women than in men, especially in young women with a short history and severe generalized disease. Increasingly it has become apparent that while the results are still not totally predictable, all cases of generalized disease, irrespective of sex, who are

fit to withstand the operation and wish to have it, should be given the benefit, though many patients need to continue medication afterwards and less than a quarter to one-third are able to stop all treatment.

Plasmapheresis is certainly dramatically successful in the short term in many cases. This technique is particularly valuable in myasthenic crises, in patients with respiratory failure (see below), or for use as an emergency measure while awaiting a response to prednisone or thymectomy. Most authorities only use this method in such emergency situations, but some still recommend regular plasma exchange every few weeks and believe that it may produce sustained benefit.

In the diminishing number of patients now being treated with anticholinesterase drugs, differential diagnosis between myasthenic and cholinergic crises can be very difficult and is important as respiratory weakness in such crises may threaten life. The most useful test is to give intravenous edrophonium. If this increases muscle power, then the weakness is likely to be myasthenic and requires more treatment, while if weakness increases it is probably cholinergic and treatment must be reduced. Any hint of impending respiratory insufficiency may indicate that all drugs should be withdrawn and that assisted respiration with positive-pressure apparatus and tracheostomy should be used. Unfortunately some patients show a differential sensitivity of different muscles to various drugs, so that a dose of pyridostigmine which improves power in the limb muscles may be sufficient to cause cholinergic paralysis of the diaphragm.

Course and prognosis

Despite all forms of treatment, there are some patients in whom death occurs in the first two to three years. Spontaneous remission may occur and is sometimes complete and long-lasting, but is more often temporary and followed by relapse after an interval of months or years. After five to 10 years the disease in many patients seems to enter a static phase with only a moderate response to treatment and a varying degree of residual disability. Even after thymectomy, two out of three patients with thymomas die within five years, but the survivors may benefit to the same extent as those without a tumour.

THE MYASTHENIC–MYOPATHIC (LAMBERT–EATON) SYNDROME

This syndrome is generally associated with oat-cell carcinoma of the bronchus, though it is occasionally seen in patients with carcinoma elsewhere and even rarely in some with no evidence of malignant disease, even after prolonged observation. Muscular weakness, wasting, and fatiguability usually affect the proximal part of the limbs and trunk and the patient often complains of increased enfeeblement after exertion, but in many cases muscle power may in fact be increased by brief exercise, a so-called reversed myasthenic effect. In contrast to the findings in true myasthenia, the tendon reflexes in this condition are almost always depressed or absent; muscle power is only slightly improved by treatment with neostigmine, even though definite improvement may follow an injection of edrophonium. Neurophysiological evidence based upon microelectrode recordings from intercostal muscle biopsies derived from such patients suggests that there is a defect in release of ACh at the nerve terminals in such cases. Weakness and fatiguability may be improved in such cases by the oral administration of guanidine hydrochloride in a dosage of 20–50 mg per kg body weight daily. Recently it has become apparent that this condition, like true myasthenia, is autoimmune (its electrophysiological features can be transferred to mice using IgG obtained from human cases) and it responds to treatment with prednisone and/or plasmapheresis whether the condition is neoplastic or non-neoplastic (see Engel, 1984).

Congenital myasthenia

In recent years no fewer than four, rare, genetically determined, non-autoimmune varieties of congenital myasthenia, variably responsive to anticholinesterase medication, have been described (see Engel, 1984). All result from developmental abnormalities at the neuromuscular junction. They include a putative defect in ACh synthesis or packaging (familial infantile myasthenia); congenital end-plate acetylcholinesterase deficiency (a single reported case to date); the 'slow-channel' syndrome (with selective weakness and fatiguability of limb, bulbar and ocular muscles); and congenital end-plate AChR deficiency.

ENDOCRINE MYOPATHIES

See Section 10 also.

Disorders of the thyroid gland

Thyrotoxic myopathy

In severe cases of thyrotoxicosis, weakness and wasting of proximal limb muscles may occur, particularly in the upper extremities, and may resolve when the thyroid disease is effectively treated. Quantitative electromyographic studies have shown that in thyrotoxicosis there is almost always a reversible abnormality of muscle function which may be readily overlooked, but that recovery is almost always complete following adequate treatment of the thyrotoxicosis. The cause of the weakness is unclear. Mitochondrial respiratory control is normal; an abnormally active plasma membrane sodium pump has been postulated and it has been suggested that the membrane contains increased catecholamine receptor sites, but no single causative factor has been identified. Acute bulbar muscle weakness developing in thyrotoxic patients is usually the result of associated myasthenia gravis.

Ophthalmic Graves' disease (exophthalmic ophthalmoplegia)

The principal effect of this disorder is upon the external ocular muscles which are greatly increased in bulk, as are the entire orbital contents. The main symptoms are exophthalmos, pain in the eyes, and diplopia. Papilloedema and even corneal ulceration may occur in the presence of severe exophthalmos and, if not relieved, the patient may go on to develop optic atrophy and blindness. Surgical decompression of the orbit is occasionally required, even as an emergency measure. Guanethidine eye drops may reduce lid retraction and high-dose steroid treatment or plasmapheresis may reduce exophthalmos quickly, as may cyclosporin.

Thyrotoxicosis and myasthenia gravis

About 5 per cent of myasthenic patients have thyrotoxicosis and the myasthenia may become worse when hyperthyroidism increases. Both conditions must be treated in the standard way, but the risks of thyroidectomy are greatly increased in patients with myasthenia.

Thyrotoxic periodic paralysis

An association between thyrotoxicosis and periodic paralysis has been observed particularly in the Japanese and Chinese. Adequate treatment of the hyperthyroidism results in disappearance of the periodic attacks of weakness or in a marked decrease of their number and severity; the attacks of paralysis are usually hypokalaemic.

Myopathy in hypothyroidism

Muscular hypertrophy with weakness and slowness of muscular contraction and relaxation has been described in children suffering from sporadic cretinism (the *Debré-Semelaigne syndrome*). A similar condition in adults, causing pain and aching in the hyper-

trophied muscles after exertion, is known as *Hoffman's syndrome* and may superficially resemble myotonia, though electromyographically no myotonic discharges are found in this condition. Rarely, too, myxoedema may be associated with a true girdle myopathy causing mild proximal weakness and wasting which responds to treatment with thyroxin.

Disorders of the pituitary and adrenal glands

In acromegaly and pituitary gigantism, and conversely in hypopituitarism, widespread muscular weakness with some degree of atrophy has been observed but is non-specific clinically, electromyographically, and pathologically. General weakness may also be seen in Addison's disease and probably results from changes in plasma and muscle water and electrolytes.

Myopathy in Cushing's syndrome

Weakness of the muscles of the pelvic girdle and thighs, sometimes with pain in the quadriceps, is now well recognized as an occasional complication of Cushing's syndrome. Both electromyography and muscle biopsy may demonstrate relatively non-specific myopathic changes in such cases. However, in transverse sections stained histochemically there is selective atrophy of Type 2 fibres. Similar changes occur in patients under treatment with steroid drugs and particularly with those, such as triamcinolone, which have a fluorine atom in the 9α-position. The myopathy of Cushing's disease improves after treatment of the condition, and steroid myopathy generally recovers completely when steroid drugs are withdrawn; the latter condition is less common in patients receiving prednisone than it is in those treated with other related drugs.

Corticotrophin myopathy

Proximal muscle weakness, fatiguability, and minor degrees of muscle wasting may also occur in pigmented patients who had previously undergone adrenalectomy for Cushing's disease. Electromyography confirms that this weakness is myopathic and muscle biopsy sections show an accumulation of fat within the muscle fibres; this disorder appears to be due to increased circulating corticotrophin.

METABOLIC MYOPATHIES

Myopathy in metabolic bone disease

Non-selective weakness (with less overt wasting) of proximal limb muscles with pain and discomfort on movement, hypotonia and brisk tendon reflexes are the main features of this myopathy which may be seen in patients with hyperparathyroidism, but more often in those suffering from osteomalacia. The condition may be due to interference with excitation–contraction coupling involving the entry of calcium into the muscle fibre and may be related to abnormalities of vitamin D metabolism. It can occur in the malabsorption syndrome without gross rarefaction of bone when it responds dramatically to treatment with vitamin D. A somewhat similar myopathy may occur in patients with chronic renal failure and associated bone disease. In uraemic hyperparathyroidism, metabolic calcification in vessel walls can cause focal cutaneous necrosis, visceral infarcts and a necrotizing myopathy with myoglobinuria.

Alcoholic myopathy

An acute myopathy with widespread muscular pain, tenderness and myoglobinuria may occur in chronic alcoholic subjects after a debauch and is associated pathologically with necrosis of muscle fibres and a deficiency of muscle phosphorylase similar to that occurring in McArdle's disease. A subacute proximal myopathy has also been described as an uncommon complication of chronic alcoholism; in most such patients muscular weakness and wasting are neuropathic.

Drug-induced myopathies

Increasing attention has been paid of late to the many forms of myopathy and disorders of neuromuscular transmission which may follow the administration of various drugs or exposure to toxic agents. Thus myasthenic fatiguability with impaired neuromuscular transmission is an occasional and transient effect of various antibiotics including streptomycin, penicillin and their derivatives, while D-penicillamine, given for instance as treatment for rheumatoid arthritis, may rarely produce a more severe and persistent myasthenic disorder, associated with a significant increase in the titre of circulating antibodies to AChR. This neuromuscular syndrome becomes self-perpetuating and only rarely resolves when the drug is withdrawn.

Drugs such as vincristine sulphate and chloroquine can damage both peripheral nerve and skeletal muscle, causing neuromyopathy which may improve slowly after drug withdrawal. Among the many drugs which have been shown to cause subacute myopathy are emetine, beta-adrenergic blocking agents, and epsilon-amino-caproic acid; the latter remedy, used as an anti-fibrinolytic agent in the treatment of subarachnoid haemorrhage, rarely causes a severe and widespread acute necrotizing myopathy. It is also well-recognized that myotonia may be produced by various diazo-cholesterol preparations, including some of the earlier remedies introduced in an attempt to lower blood cholesterol.

Malignant hyperpyrexia

Widespread muscular rigidity and hyperpyrexia, developing as a complication of general anaesthesia, seems to be due to an as yet unidentified metabolic abnormality of skeletal muscle. The reaction is associated with a sudden increase in free sarcoplasmic Ca^{2+} in the muscle fibres and this in turn seems to be due to defective calcium uptake by the sarcoplasmic reticulum. The condition is most often precipitated by inhalational anaesthetics such as halothane and by relaxant drugs like succinylcholine. Local, regional, and spinal anaesthesia are probably safe in susceptible individuals and, for general anaesthesia, a combination of diazepam, thiopentone, fentanyl citrate, and nitrous oxide and oxygen are advised. The disorder is fortunately rare and is often dominantly inherited. A family history of death during anaesthesia should alert anaesthetists to the possibility of this disorder. The only effective screening procedure is an *in vitro* study of the halothane-induced contracture in a sample of muscle obtained by open biopsy under local anaesthesia; in affected families estimation of serum CK activity has been found to be helpful in detecting the trait.

The most effective drug to be used in treatment and in prevention of this condition is dantrolene sodium given intravenously (1–2 mg/kg body weight) and repeated every 5–10 min up to 10 mg/kg.

Xanthinuria

Symptomatic myopathy has been described in a patient with xanthinuria due to inherited xanthine oxidase deficiency; crystals of xanthine were demonstrated in muscle by electron microscopy. Similar crystals not producing clinical manifestations of muscle disease may be found in patients with gout treated with allopurinol.

Disorders of lipid metabolism

Two primary disorders of muscle lipid metabolism have been identified. The first is due to a deficiency of the enzyme carnitine pal-

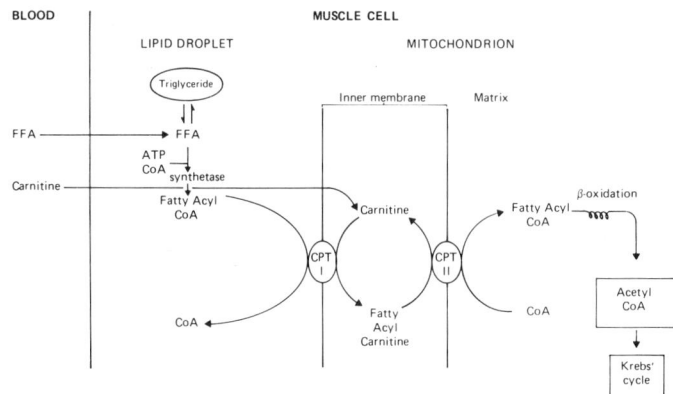

Fig. 11 A diagrammatic representation of fatty acid metabolism as it occurs in skeletal muscle with particular reference to the role of carnitine. (From Walton and Mastaglia (1980b), reproduced by kind permission of the editors and publisher.)

mityl transferase (CPT) which controls the entry of long-chain fatty acids into the mitochondria, and the second to a deficiency of carnitine which is the obligatory carrier for the entry of such fatty acids (Fig. 11).

Carnitine palmityl transferase deficiency

This condition is characterized by recurrent episodes of muscle pain, cramps, and myoglobinuria (see below) precipitated by prolonged exercise (such as long-distance running or mountain climbing), fasting, or particularly by a combination of both, or by exposure to severe cold. Rarely the myoglobinuria is severe enough to cause renal failure. After severe attacks there may be painful swelling and weakness of muscles, due to acute muscle necrosis. The enzyme defect is present in white blood cells or cultured fibroblasts and can be confirmed by a biochemical assay performed on a muscle sample or peripheral blood. The prognosis is good if precipitants can be avoided. As yet no effective treatment or prophylaxis is available.

Carnitine deficiency

This disorder, of autosomal recessive inheritance, may, when confined to skeletal muscle, give rise to a lipid storage myopathy with marked accumulation of neutral lipid (both diglyceride and triglyceride) in the muscle fibres, especially those of Type 1 (Fig. 12). The clinical picture is that of a slowly progressive myopathy, often with severe involvement of neck muscles and sometimes with facial and pharyngeal muscle weakness, and with depressed or absent deep tendon reflexes. Muscle carnitine levels are usually reduced to 10–20 per cent of normal and the mitochondria often show abnormal inclusions under the electron microscope. In some cases muscle strength has improved markedly with oral carnitine given along with a diet rich in medium-chain triglycerides. Other patients have shown some improvement on treatment with prednisone.

The less common systemic carnitine deficiency which involves the liver as well as skeletal muscle has a much less favourable outlook and is usually fatal in infancy, childhood or early adult life. Lactic acidosis is a common feature of such cases.

Disorders of pyruvate metabolism

While inborn errors of pyruvate dehydrogenase have been described and certainly affect muscle structure and function, they are usually characterized by evidence of CNS dysfunction. However, some cases of progressive external ophthalmoplegia with mitochondrial myopathy may be associated with a defect of pyruvate oxidation.

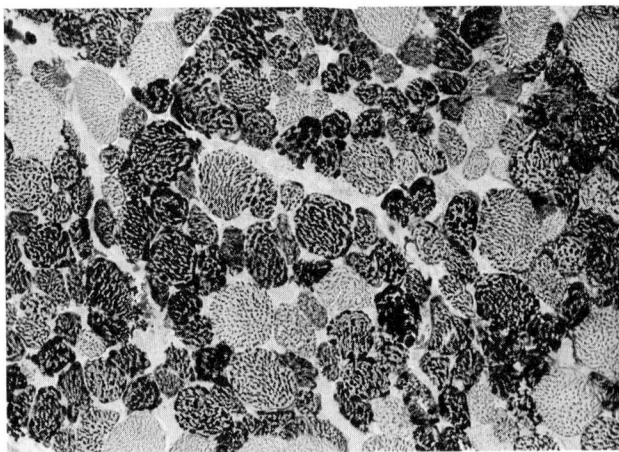

Fig. 12 A transverse section of human skeletal muscle obtained from a patient with carnitine deficiency and stained with Sudan black B, × 196. The massive accumulation of neutral fat, especially within the Type 1 fibres, is evident.

Table 3 Neuromuscular disorders associated with defective mitochondrial metabolism

---

1 Defects in transport or enzymatic processes essential for substrate utilization
   (*a*) Carnitine deficiency
   (*b*) CPT deficiency
   (*c*) Pyruvate dehydrogenase complex defects
2 Defects of mitochondrial energy conservation
   (*a*) Luft's hypermetabolic myopathy
   (*b*) Mitochondrial ATPase deficiency
3 Defects of respiratory chain
   (*a*) Cytochrome b deficiency
   (*b*) Cytochrome aa$_3$ deficiency
   (*c*) Cytochrome aa$_3$ and b deficiency
   (*d*) Cytochrome c deficiency
   (*e*) NADH-coenzyme Q reductase complex

Modified from Morgan-Hughes *et al*. (1979).

Other mitochondrial myopathies

These are a group of myopathies (Table 3) in each of which structural changes in mitochondria have been identified ultrastructurally and have been shown to be associated with a variety of abnormalities of mitochondrial function. The clinical manifestations of these disorders are wide and varied and for practical purposes can be classified into four syndromes described below.

Hypermetabolic state with myopathy

This rare disorder presents with severe heat intolerance, fever, profuse sweating, and diffuse muscle weakness with evidence of mitochondrial abnormalities on histochemical and ultrastructural examination of muscle. There is a marked increase in basal metabolic rate without evidence of thyrotoxicosis, and biochemical examination of mitochondrial function reveals 'loosely coupled' oxidative phosphorylation. Chloramphenicol was found to be helpful in one case.

Progressive external ophthalmoplegia

As already mentioned, the syndrome of ocular or oculopharyngeal myopathy may be associated with mitochondrial abnormalities in the external ocular muscles. However, in some cases there is also involvement of bulbar and limb muscles, heart block, retinal pigmentation and cerebellar ataxia, and abnormal mitochondria may also be found in liver and brain (the 'oculo-cranio-somatic' or Kearnes–Sayre syndrome). The mitochondria often show typical

rectangular paracrystalline inclusions (Fig. 13). No single specific biochemical abnormality has yet been identified in such cases although, as mentioned above, there may be a defect of pyruvate oxidation.

Myopathy with paralytic attacks provoked by exercise, alcohol or cold

In two cases presenting with these clinical features a defect in NADH-coenzyme Q reductase was identified by Morgan-Hughes *et al*. (1979). Subsequent reports have shown that marked muscle weakness (also, in children who survive sufficiently long for it to be noted, increased by exertion and associated with lactic acidaemia) can be due to cytochrome b or c deficiency. Cytochrome c deficiency in particular can cause a severe disorder with death in infancy.

Cytochrome aa$_3$ deficiency (see Table 3) is not apparently associated with clinically overt muscle involvement but with the Fanconi syndrome and with Menkes' syndrome (trichopoliodystrophy) due to an inborn error of copper metabolism.

Facioscapulohumeral or limb-girdle syndrome

Many cases are now on record of patients presenting with a subacute myopathy resembling clinically the facioscapulohumeral or limb-girdle muscular dystrophies but in which 'ragged-red' fibres were found in muscle biopsy sections examined histochemically; under the electron microscope the muscle fibres were found to contain large numbers of abnormal mitochondria, many with large inclusions. In many families the myopathy has proved to be of autosomal dominant inheritance and in some there has been associated evidence of cardiomyopathy, diabetes mellitus, lactic acidaemia (occasionally resulting in fatal lactic acidosis) and rarely cerebral degeneration. In one syndrome of mitochondrial myopathy, encephalopathy, lactic acidosis, and stroke-like episodes, the biochemical defect could not be demonstrated (Pavlakis *et al*., 1984). In many cases mitochondrial respiration has been shown to be abnormal, and phosphorylation to be loosely coupled. In at

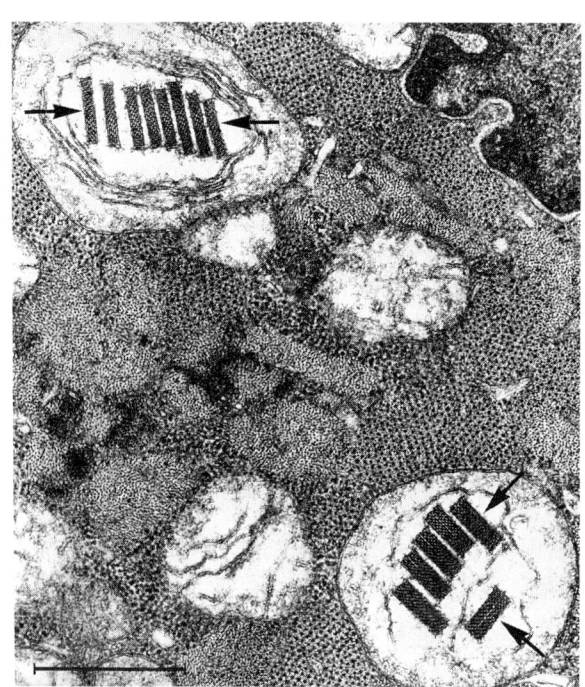

Fig. 13 A transverse section of a biopsy specimen obtained from one quadriceps muscle in a patient with mitochondrial myopathy showing arrays of paracrystalline inclusions in the damaged mitochondria. Bar = 1 μm. (Illustration kindly provided by Dr Michael Cullen.)

least one case a deficiency of cytochrome b has been identified but it seems likely that many different biochemical defects in the electron transport chain can produce such a syndrome. Apart from methods designed to control the lactic acidosis when present, no form of treatment is effective.

Muscle adenylate deaminase deficiency

This rare disorder can give rise to muscle weakness, pain, cramps and fatigue induced by exercise. The enzyme defect can be demonstrated histochemically and confirmed by enzymatic assay. Doubt has recently been cast upon the specificity of this defect. It is also well recognized that there exists a group of patients suffering from benign but troublesome exercise-induced muscle pain (sometimes with cramps) in whom no convincing biochemical defect can be identified. In a few such patients, pain is dramatically relieved by verapamil (Walton, 1981) for reasons which are still obscure.

Glycogen storage disease of muscle (see Section 9)

McArdle's disease

In 1951 McArdle described the case of a man of 30 who had developed generalized muscular pain and stiffness which increased during exertion. He showed that the blood lactate and pyruvate levels failed to rise after exercise and suggested that the disorder was due to a defect of glucose utilization. Subsequently it was shown that this condition is a disorder of glycogen storage due to absence or deficiency of myophosphorylase in muscle fibres; myoglobinuria is observed after exertion in some cases, and after repeated contraction the muscles may go into a state of physiological contracture. The condition runs a benign course, though some degree of permanent muscular weakness and wasting develops in some cases. There is evidence now that a total absence of myophosphorylase may give rise to a disorder which is severe and disabling in infancy or early childhood (a 'floppy infant' syndrome with death in the first few months, see below), a less marked or partial deficiency to a more benign condition (either a subacute proximal myopathy or troublesome cramps of late onset) presenting in adult life. The condition is usually due to an autosomal recessive gene but dominant inheritance has been described. No treatment has any influence upon the symptoms.

Other forms of glycogen storage disease

A myopathic disorder resembling McArdle's disease clinically has been shown to be due to *phosphofructokinase deficiency*. Deficiency of *phosphoglycerate mutase*, lactate dehydrogenase, and of *phosphoglycerate kinase* have also been identified in adult life in patients suffering from cramps and pigmenturia since adolescence. *Pompe's disease*, due to a deficiency of amylo-1,4-glucosidase (acid maltase), usually gives glycogen storage in the heart, skeletal muscles, and central nervous system and was once thought to be incompatible with survival beyond the first few weeks of life. However, it is now evident that certain patients with acid maltase deficiency may present with an apparently progressive myopathy of girdle muscles in late childhood or adult life. This diagnosis must be considered in all cases of suspected limb-girdle muscular dystrophy arising in middle life; muscle biopsy may be diagnostic as striking vacuolation of muscle fibres is usually demonstrated easily and the vacuoles contain large quantities of glycogen. Unfortunately this condition, too, does not appear to be amenable to treatment.

The rare inherited deficiencies of *amylo-1,6-glucosidase (debrancher enzyme)* and of *amylo-(1,4-1,6)-transglycosylase (brancher enzyme)* (Table 4) also give rise to glycogen storage in skeletal muscle with weakness but in both cases the clinical picture is dominated by other clinical manifestations (growth retardation and hepatic dysfunction). The former runs an unexpectedly benign course in many cases, whereas the latter is usually fatal in early adult life as a result of hepatic failure.

PERIODIC PARALYSIS SYNDROMES

These familial disorders, which are usually dominantly inherited, are characterized by episodic attacks of flaccid muscular weakness, accompanied by alterations in the serum potassium and by associated fluxes of K^+ in and out of muscle cells. The clinical features of the two principal types are summarized in Table 5.

Although it is often possible to distinguish the two main forms on the basis of the frequency and duration of attacks, the factors which precipitate them and by measuring the serum K^+ in the early stages of an attack, this is not always possible and it may be necessary to provoke an attack in order to establish the diagnosis. In the hypokalaemic form this can often be done by giving glucose and insulin intravenously to induce hypokalaemia (perhaps after an initial saline load and a period of exercise), while in the hyperkalaemic variety, oral potassium salts may provoke an episode of weakness.

Hypokalaemic periodic paralysis

This condition gives attacks of generalized weakness of the voluntary muscles, but those of speech, swallowing and respiration are usually spared. Attacks usually begin in the second decade and are commonest in early adult life. Often they start on waking, after a period of rest following exertion or after a heavy carbohydrate meal, and usually they last for several hours. During attacks the plasma potassium level is found to be low (usually less than 3 mmol/l); there is positive balance of potassium and some or all of the retained potassium seems to pass into the muscle cell. Muscle biopsy specimens taken during an attack usually show that many muscle fibres are vacuolated as a result of dilatation of the sarcoplasmic reticulum.

The suggestion that this form of periodic paralysis may be due to intermittent aldosteronism has been disproved; aldosteronism can be distinguished from periodic paralysis by the associated hypertension, alkalosis, and hypernatraemia and by the persistent hypokalaemia between the attacks. Administration of potassium chloride 4–6 g daily, may be helpful in attacks. Spironolactone, 25 mg four times a day, and other similar aldosterone antagonists were found greatly to reduce the frequency and severity of the attacks, but have been supplanted by acetazolamide or thiazide diuretics, also effective in the hyperkalaemic variety (see below) but which, paradoxically, are of striking prophylactic value in hypokalaemic cases. Rarely in such cases muscle weakness is localized to one or more muscle groups and sometimes permanent atrophy of selected muscles develops after frequent episodes of weakness, but most patients improve spontaneously with age.

Hyperkalaemic periodic paralysis (adynamia episodica hereditaria)

In this condition, which, like the hypokalaemic variety, is inherited as an autosomal dominant trait, the attacks are usually much shorter in duration, lasting on average 30–40 minutes and they may be precipitated immediately by exercise. In the attacks the serum potassium usually rises, though some patients have severe weakness when the level is no higher than 4 mmol/l. Some patients show definite myotonia, but in others this phenomenon seems curiously limited to the muscles around the eyes. The attacks may be cut short by the intravenous administration of calcium gluconate, while acetazolamide (250 mg two or three times daily), and dichlorphenamide have all been used successfully for prophylaxis.

Sodium-responsive normokalaemic periodic paralysis

This is probably a variant of the hyperkalaemic type, except that the attacks may occasionally last for days or weeks and often develop at night. The paralysis is always increased by the administration of potassium and is improved by large doses of sodium chloride. Acetazolamide combined with 9-α-fluorohydrocorti-sone, 0.1 mg daily, usually prevents the attacks.

Plainly full investigation of every case of periodic paralysis is necessary to establish the nature of the patient's illness. Attempts to demonstrate a specific disorder or carbohydrate metabolism in such cases have been unsuccessful, but treatment given either prophylactically or in order to shorten the attacks has proved successful in most cases once the character of the attacks has been defined by investigation.

MYOGLOBINURIA (see also Sections 18 and 26)

Myoglobin may appear in the urine as a result of widespread crush injury to muscle, in acute polymyositis and in localized ischaemic muscular necrosis. In a specific syndrome of *paroxysmal myoglobinuria* or *rhabdomyolysis* of unknown aetiology, patients suffer acute attacks of severe cramp-like muscle pain and tenderness associated with weakness or paralysis and accompanied by profuse myoglobinuria. In some cases occurring predominantly in adolescent or young adult males, pain and myoglobinuria follow exercise and recurrent attacks may lead to permanent muscular weakness and wasting. Probably many cases of this type are due to carnitine palmityl transferase deficiency. In a second type which is commonest in childhood, the attacks are severe, often follow acute infection, are accompanied by fever and leucocytosis, but occur at progressively longer intervals and usually clear up eventually. The cause of this syndrome is unknown and no treatment has any influence upon it.

THE FLOPPY INFANT SYNDROME

Generalized muscular hypotonia in infancy may be due to many causes, including cerebral palsy, mental retardation, cerebral degenerative disease and a number of neuromuscular disorders. Spinal muscular atrophy (Werdnig–Hoffman disease) is an important cause and in such cases the hypotonia is usually pro-

Table 4 Major features of the glycogen storage diseases in which skeletal muscle is involved

Enzyme deficiency	Eponym	Inheritance	Clinical syndrome	Other tissues	Ischaemic lactate test	Diagnosis	Glycogen structure
a-1,4 and 1,6-Glucosidase (acid maltase)	Pompe's disease (infantile form)	AR	(a) *Infantile* cardiomegaly, hepatomegaly, hypotonia, weakness; death in first year of life	All tissues, especially muscle heart, CNS, PNS	Not possible	Enzyme assay on muscle tissue, cultured fibroblasts or amniotic cells; reduced urinary excretion of acid maltase in late-onset forms	Normal
			(b) *Late-onset* progressive proximal myopathy; respiratory muscle involvement	Liver	Normal		
Myophosphorylase	McArdle's disease	AR in most; AD in some	(a) Rapidly progressive fatal infantile form (b) Exercise-induced muscle pain, contracture, myoglobinuria; onset in adolescence or adult life (most frequent form)	—	Abnormal	Muscle histochemistry or enzyme assay	Normal
Muscle phosphofructokinase	Tarui's disease	Usually AR; AD in one family	Exercise-induced muscle pain, cramps, and myoglobinuria; progressive myopathy in one family	Red blood cells	Abnormal	Muscle histochemistry or enzyme assay. Red blood cell PFK activity reduced	Normal
Muscle phosphoglycerate mutase	Di Mauro's disease	Probably AR	Exercise-induced muscle pain, cramps, myoglobinuria	—	Abnormal	Muscle histochemistry or enzyme assay	Normal
Muscle phosphoglycerate kinase	Di Mauro's disease	Probably AR	Exercise-indiced muscle pain, cramps, myoglobinuria	—	Abnormal	Muscle histochemistry or enzyme assay	Normal
Muscle lactate dehydrogenase	—	Probably AR	Exercise-induced, muscle pain, cramps, myoglobinuria	—	Abnormal	Muscle histochemistry or enzyme assay	Normal
Amylo-1,6-glucosidase (debrancher) enzyme	Cori–Forbes disease	AR	Hepatomegaly, fasting hypoglycaemia up to puberty; later, progressive muscle weakness and atrophy; distal muscles may be affected	Liver, red blood cells, fibroblasts	Abnormal	Enzyme assay on muscle tissue or liver	Phosphorylase limit dextrin—short outer chains
Amylo-(1,4–1,6)-transglycosylase (brancher enzyme)	Andersen's disease	AR	Hepatosplenomegaly, cirrhosis; hypotonia, muscle atrophy, weakness, depressed reflexes in some cases; onset in early childhood	Liver, heart, kidney, leucocytes, CNS, PNS, spleen	—	Enzyme assay on leucocytes	Abnormal; longer outer chains with fewer branching points

AR = autosomal recessive; AD = autosomal dominant. Modified from Walton and Mastaglia (1980b).

Table 5 Classification of the periodic paralyses

Hypokalaemic periodic paralysis
familial
thyrotoxic
acquired hypokalaemia
Hyperkalaemic periodic paralysis
familial
paramyotonia congenita
acquired hyperkalaemia

From Walton and Mastaglia (1980b).

found and widespread, there is generalized areflexia, respiratory muscle weakness, and often fasciculation of the tongue. The diagnosis can be confirmed by EMG and muscle biopsy; this condition, of grave prognosis, may be mimicked by congenital muscular dystrophy as described above.

Benign congenital hypotonia

This term is often used to identify those floppy infants in whom hypotonia is not shown to be the result of any specific metabolic disorder, nor secondary to mental defect, or disease in the central or peripheral nervous system; in such cases full investigation, including EMG and muscle biopsy, may fail to demonstrate any specific abnormality of the muscle fibres other than, in some cases, an overall decrease in their diameter. Sometimes all the muscle fibres seem to be of one uniform histochemical type, suggesting a disorder of muscle differentiation, but these cases are rare. In yet others there is a marked disproportion in number and size between the fibres of different histochemical types (*congenital fibre type disproportion*). The aetiology of the latter condition is unknown but it improves progressively with increasing age. Undoubtedly the syndrome of benign congenital hypotonia is one of multiple aetiology. In some patients demonstrating similar diffuse hypotonia in early infancy, improvement occurs but yet the muscles remain weak, slender, and hypotonic throughout life, and these cases may be regarded as examples of 'benign congenital myopathy' even though the EMG and muscle biopsy findings in such individuals are often non-specific. In recent years it has been shown that some such patients are suffering from apparently specific though benign disorders of muscle which will now be described.

Central core disease

In 1956 Shy and Magee described a family in which affected children did not walk until the age of four years. There was widespread muscular hypotonia and muscle biopsy revealed large muscle fibres, most of which showed one or sometimes two central cores which had different staining properties from the other fibrils. The central core was shown to be devoid of oxidative enzymes and of phosphorylase activity and seemed to be non-functioning. The condition is probably due to an autosomal recessive gene and runs a benign course, but its pathogenesis is obscure. In one syndrome which is similar clinically, multiple cores (multicore disease) can be found in the affected muscle fibres.

Nemaline myopathy

This is another congenital and relatively non-progressive myopathy in which collections of rod-shaped bodies are found within the muscle fibres, lying usually beneath the sarcolemma. These patients often show evidence of diffuse myopathy, but also facial weakness, a high arched palate, prognathism of the lower jaw, and skeletal changes resembling those of arachnodactyly, though none of the other stigmata of Marfan's syndrome are present. Examination of muscle from such cases with the electron microscope has shown that the subsarcolemmal rods appear to be due to a selective swelling and degeneration of Z-bands with consequent destruction of myofilaments in the adjacent part of the muscle fibre.

Fingerprint body myopathy and tubular aggregates

Other forms of myopathy associated with non-progressive muscular weakness in infancy and early childhood have also been described in recent years, one showing hypertrophy of Type 2 fibres with finger-print-like inclusions demonstrated with the electron microscope in the Type 2 fibres, another demonstrating widespread tubular aggregates in all fibres. The nature and specificity of these ultrastructural changes remain in doubt.

Myotubular or centronuclear myopathy

In 1966 Spiro, Shy and Gonatas reported the case of a nine-year-old child suffering from a form of Möbius syndrome characterized by facial diplegia, external ocular palsies, a decrease in muscle mass, moderate symmetrical muscle weakness, and poor development of all limb muscles. Most muscle fibres contained central nuclei, often lying in chains; the appearances in the muscle were similar to those of the myotubes seen in normal fetal muscle in the early months of intrauterine life. These fibres are in several respects different from fetal myotubes, but nevertheless the condition seems to represent an example of cellular developmental arrest. It usually runs a benign course with progressive improvement, but occasional very severe cases with death in early infancy have been reported.

While it cannot be concluded that all of the syndromes mentioned represent specific disease entities, within the difficult field of 'benign congenital myopathy' advances are occurring rapidly and many new and apparently specific structural abnormalities of the muscle fibre are being demonstrated by modern techniques.

SOME MISCELLANEOUS MUSCULAR DISORDERS

Restless legs

The aetiology of this syndrome (Ekbom's syndrome) is unknown; it gives rise to unpleasant aching in the muscles of the lower limbs when the patient rests in a chair or on lying in bed. This aching, accompanied by a sense of intolerable restlessness, may be accompanied by muscular cramps which interfere with sleep. There are no abnormal physical signs on examination and in the EMG, nerve conduction velocity measurements and muscle biopsy all give normal findings. Some patients are helped by treatment with chkklorpromazine and/or by diazepam and phenytoin (see Section 21 also).

Tibialis anterior syndrome

Severe boring pain in the tibialis anterior muscle may occur on one or both sides after unaccustomed exercise; the condition is due to ischaemic swelling of the muscle within its tight fascial compartment. Rarely the pain is intense and widespread necrosis of the muscles occurs. In mild chronic cases recurrent pain occurs after any exertion and relief can only then be obtained by surgical decompression of the anterior crural compartment.

Progressive myositis ossificans

Localized ossification in voluntary muscle may occur as a result of its repeated involvement in the trauma of certain exercises or occupations (as in horse-riders) and is occasionally seen in muscles around the hip joint following spastic paraparesis. Progressive myositis ossificans is, however, a genetically determined disorder in which there is widespread ossification of the muscles which seems to be preceded by sclerosis of the intramuscular connective tissue. Most cases present in childhood and affected individuals often have associated anomalies of their great toes or other digits. The condition is probably due to a dominant gene showing incomplete penetrance; it begins usually with swelling or swellings in the neck mimicking congenital torticollis and eventually the muscles of the back, shoulder and pelvic girdles, particularly, become ossified. The overlying skin may ulcerate and terminal aspiration pneumonia is common, but the condition may run a benign course over many decades.

The stiff-man syndrome

This syndrome of so called progressive fluctuating muscular rigidity and spasm predominantly affects male adults who, after a prodromal phase of aching and tightness of the axial muscles, go on to develop a symmetrical continuous stiffness of the skeletal muscles upon which painful muscular spasms are superimposed and may be precipitated by movement. The aetiology of the condition is unknown but it may be a disorder of interneurones in the spinal cord; it is usually successfully controlled by treatment with diazepam.

References

Aberfeld, D. C., Hinterbuchner, L. P. and Schneider, M. (1965). Myotonia, dwarfism, diffuse bone disease and unusual ocular and facial abnormalities (a new syndrome). *Brain* **88**, 313–322.
—— and Astrom, K. (1981). Pathological reactions of the skeletal muscle fibre in man. In *Disorders of voluntary muscle*, 4th edn (ed. J. N. Walton), pp. 151–208. Churchill Livingstone, Edinburgh.
Angelini, C. (1976). Lipid storage myopathies. A review of metabolic defect and of treatment. *J. Neurol.* **214**, 1–11.
Appel, S. H., Elias, S. B. and Chauvin, P. (1979). The role of acetylcholine receptor antibodies in myasthenia gravis. *Fed. Proc.* **38**, 2381–2385.
Arahata, K. and Engel, A. G. (1984). Monoclonal antibody analysis of mononuclear cells in myopathies. I. Quantitation of subsets according to diagnosis and sites of accumulation and demonstration and counts of muscle fibers invaded by T cells. *Ann. Neurol.* **16**, 193–208.
Argov, Z. and Mastaglia, F. L. (1979). Disorders of neuromuscular transmission caused by drugs. *New Engl. J. Med.* **301**, 409–413.
Ashby, B., Frieden, C. and Bischoff, R. (1979). Immunofluorescent and histochemical localization of AMP deaminase in skeletal muscle. *J. Cell Biol.* **81**, 361–373.
Astrom, K. E., Kugelberg, E. and Müller, R. (1961). Hypothyroid myopathy. *Arch. Neurol., Chicago* **5**, 472–482.
Austin, K. L. and Denborough, M. A. (1977). Drug treatment of malignant hyperpyrexia. *Anesth. Intens. Care* **5**, 207–213.
Bakker, E. *et al.* (1985). Prenatal diagnosis and carrier detection of Duchenne muscular dystrophy with closely linked RFLPs. Lancet i, 655–658.
Bank, J. W., DiMauro, S., Bonilla, E, Capuzzi, D. M. and Rowland, L. P. (1975). A disorder of muscle lipid metabolism and myoglobinuria. Absence of carnitine palmityltransferase. *N. Engl. J. Med.* **292**, 443–449.
Barwick, D. D. (1981). Clinical electromyography. In *Disorders of voluntary muscle*, 4th edn (ed. J. N. Walton), pp. 952–975. Churchill Livingstone, Edinburgh.
Ben Hamida, M., Fardeau, M. and Attia, N. (1983). Severe childhood muscular dystrophy affecting both sexes and frequent in Tunisia. *Muscle Nerve* **6**, 469–480.
Blass, J. P. (1979). Disorders of pyruvate metabolism. *Neurology, Minneap.* **29**, 280–286.
Bosch, E. P. and Munsat, T. L. (1979). Metabolic myopathies. *Med. Clin. N. Am.* **63**, 759–782.
Bradley, W. G., Hudgson, P., Gardner-Medwin, D., and Walton, J. N. (1969). Myopathy associated with abnormal lipid metabolism in skeletal muscle. *Lancet* i, 495–498.
Bresolin, N., Miranda, A., Chang, H. W., Shanske, S. and DiMauro, S. (1984). Phosphoglycerate kinase deficiency myopathy: biochemical and immunological studies of the mutant enzyme. *Muscle Nerve* **7**, 542–551.
Campbell, M. J., Rebeiz, J. J. and Walton, J. N. (1969). Myotubular, centronuclear or pericentronuclear myopathy? *J. neurol. Sci.* **8**, 425–433.
Coomes, E. N. (1965). Corticosteroid myopathy. *Ann. rheum. Dis.* **24**, 465.
Cornelio, F., Di Donato, S., Peluchetti, D., Bizzi, A., Bertagnolio, B., D'Angelo, A. and Wiesmann, U. (1977). Fatal cases of lipid storage myopathy with carnitine deficiency. *J. Neurol. Neurosurg. Psychiat.* **40**, 170–178.
Cullen, M. J. and Fulthorpe, J. J. (1975). Stages in fibre breakdown in Duchenne muscular dystrophy. *J. neurol. Sci.* **24**, 179–200.

Cumming, W. J. K., Hardy, M., Hudgson, P., and Walls, J. (1976). Carnitine-palmityl-transferase deficiency. *J. neurol. Sci.* **30**, 247–258.
Currie, S. (1981). Inflammatory disorders of muscle. Polymyositis and related disorders. In *Disorders of voluntary muscle*, 4th edn (ed. J. N. Walton), pp. 525–568. Churchill Livingstone, Edinburgh.
——, Saunders, M., Knowles, M. and Brown, A. E. (1971). Immunological aspects of polymyositis. *Q. J. Med.* **40**, 63–84.
Dale, H. (1934). Chemical transmission of the effects of nerve impulses. *Br. med. J.* **ii**, 835.
Davies, K. (1985). Personal communication.
DiMauro, S., Bonilla, E., Lee, C. P., Schotland, D. L., Scarpa, A., Conn, H. and Chance, B. (1976). Luft's disease. Further biochemical and ultrastructural studies of skeletal muscle in the second case. *J. neurol. Sci.* **27**, 217–232.
——, Miranda, A. F., Olarte, M., Friedman, R. and Hays, A. P. (1982). Muscle phosphoglycerate mutase deficiency. *Neurology, Minneap.* **32**, 584–591.
——, Schotland, D. L., Bonilla, E., Chau-Pu, L., Gambetti, P. and Rowland, L. P. (1973). Progressive ophthalmoplegia, glycogen storage and abnormal mitochondria. *Arch. Neurol., Chicago* **29**, 170–179.
Dubowitz, V. (1968). *Developing and diseased muscle.* Heinemann. London.
—— and Brooke, M. H. (1973). *Muscle biopsy: a modern approach.* W. B. Saunders, London, Philadelphia, Toronto.
Ekbom, K. A. (1960). Restless legs syndrome. *Neurology, Minneap.* **10**, 868–873.
——, Hed, R., Kirstein, L. and Astrom, K. E. (1964). Muscular affections in chronic alcoholism. *Arch. Neurol., Chicago,* **10**, 449–458.
Ellis. F. R., Harriman, D. G. F., Currie, S. and Cain. P. A. (1978). Screening for malignant hyperthermia in susceptible patients. In *Malignant hyperthermia* (eds J. A. Aldrete and B. A. Britt). Grune and Stratton, New York.
Emery, A. E. H. (1980). Duchenne muscular dystrophy: genetic aspects, carrier detection and antenatal diagnosis. *Br. med Bull.* **36**, 117–122.
—— and Walton. J. N. (1967). The genetics of muscular dystrophy. In *Progress in medical genetics* (eds A. G. Steinberg and A. G. Bearn). vol. V, pp. 116–145. Grune and Stratton. New York.
—— (1981). Metabolic and endocrine myopathies. In *Disorders of voluntary muscle*, 4th edn (ed. J. N. Walton), pp. 664–711. Churchill Livingstone. Edinburgh.
Engel, A. G. (1984). Myasthenia gravis and myasthenic syndromes. *Ann. Neurol.* **16**, 519–534.
—— and Angelini. C. (1973). Carnitine deficiency of human skeletal muscle with associated lipid storage myopathy: a new syndrome. *Science* **173**, 899–902.
—— and Arahata, K. (1984). Monoclonal antibody analysis of mononuclear cells in myopathies. II. Phenotypes of autoinvasive cells in polymyositis and inclusion body myositis. *Ann. Neurol.* **16**, 209–215.
Fishbein, W. N., Armbrustmacher, V. W. and Griffin, J. L. (1978). Myoadenylate deaminase dficiency: a new disease of muscle. *Science* **200**, 545–548.
Gomez, M. R., Engel, A. G., Dewald, G. and Peterson, H. A. (1977). Failure of inactivation of Duchenne dystrophy X-chromosome in one of female identical twins. *Neurology, Minneap.* **27**, 537–541.
Harper, P. S. (1979). *Myotonic dystrophy.* W. B. Saunders, Philadelphia.
Howard, F. M. (1963). A new and effective drug in the treatment of stiff-man syndrome. *Proc. Mayo Clin.* **38**, 203–212.
Hudgson, P., Gardner-Medwin, D., Fulthorpe, J. J. and Walton, J. N. (1967). Nemaline myopathy. *Neurology, Minneap.* **17**, 1125–1142.
——, ——, Worsfold, M., Pennington, R. J. T. and Walton. J. N. (1968). Adult myopathy from glycogen storage disease due to acid maltase deficiency. *Brain* **91**, 435–462.
Huxley, H. E. and Hanson, J. (1960). The molecular basis of contraction. In *Structure and function of muscle* (ed. G. H. Bourne), vol. 1. Academic Press, New York.
Isaacs, H. (1961). A syndrome of continuous muscle fibre activity. *J. Neurol. Neurosurg. Psychiat.* **24**, 319–325.
Kakulas, B. A. and Adams, R. D. (1985). *Diseases of muscle*, 4th edn. Harper and Row, New York.
Kalow, W., Britt, B. A., Terreau, M. E. and Haist, C. (1970). Metabolic error of muscle metabolism after recovery from malignant hyperthermia. *Lancet* **ii**, 895–898.
Kanno, T., Sudo, K. and Takeuchi, I. (1980). Hereditary deficiency of lactate dehydrogenase M-subunit. *Clin. Chim. Acta* **108**, 267–276.
Keaney, N. P. and Ellis, F. R. (1971). Malignant hyperpyrexia. *Br. med. J.* **iv**, 49.

Kilburn, K. H., Eagan, J. T., Sieker, H. O. and Heyman, A. (1959). Cardiopulmonary insufficiency in myotonic and progressive muscular dystrophy. *New Engl. J. Med.* **261**, 1089–1096.

Kiloh, L. G. and Nevin, S. (1951). Progressive dystrophy of external ocular muscles (ocular myopathy). *Brain* **74**, 115–143.

Korein, J., Coddon, D. R. and Mowrey, F. H. (1959). The clinical syndrome of paroxysmal paralytic myoglobinuria. *Neurology, Minneap.* **9**, 767–785.

Land, J. M. and Clark, J. B. (1979). Mitochondrial myopathies. *Biochem. Soc. Trans.* **7**, 231–245.

Lane, R. J. M., Maskrey, P., Nicholson, G. A., Siddiqui, P. Q. R., Nicholson, M., Gascoigne, P., Pennington, R. J. T., Gardner-Medwin, D. and Walton, J. N. (1979). An evaluation of some carrier detection techniques in Duchenne muscular dystrophy. *J. neurol. Sci.* **43**, 377–394.

Layzer, R. B., Rowland, L. P., and Ranney, H. M. (1967). Muscle phosphofructokinase deficiency. *Arch. Neurol., Chicago* **17**, 512–523.

Lindstrom, J. and Lambert, E. H. (1978). Content of acetylcholine receptor and antibodies bound to receptor in myasthenia gravis, experimental autoimmune myasthenia gravis, and Eaton–Lambert syndrome. *Neurology, Minneap.* **28**, 130–138.

Luft, R., Ikkos, D., Palmieri, G., Ernster, L., and Afzelius, B. (1962). A case of severe hypermetabolism of nonthyroid origin with a defect in the maintenance of mitochondrial respiratory control: a correlated clinical, biochemical, and morphological study. *J. clin. Invest.* **41**, 1776–1804.

Mahoney, M. J., Haseltine, F. P., Hobbins, J. C., Banker, B. Q., Caskey, C. T. and Globus. M. S. (1977). Prenatal diagnosis of Duchenne's muscular dystrophy. *N. Engl. J. Med.* **297**, 968–973.

Mastaglia, F. L. and Argov, Z. (1980). Drug-induced neuromuscular disorders in man. In *Disorders of voluntary muscle*, 4th edn (ed. J. N. Walton), pp. 873–906. Churchill Livingstone, Edinburgh.

—— and Walton, J. N. (1982). *Skeletal muscle pathology*. Churchill Livingstone, Edinburgh.

McKusick, V. (1956). *Heritable disorders of connective tissue.* p. 184. Mosby, St. Louis.

McQuillen, M. P. and Johns, R. J. (1966). The nature of the defect in the Eaton–Lambert syndrome. *Neurology. Minneap.* **17**, 527–536.

Moersch, F. P. and Woltman, H. W. (1956). Progressive fluctuating muscular rigidity and spasm (stiff-man syndrome). *Proc. Mayo Clin.* **31**, 421–427.

Mokri, B. and Engel, A. G. (1975). Duchenne dystrophy: electron microscopic findings pointing to a basic or early abnormality in the plasma membrane of the muscle fibre. *Neurology, Minneap.* **25**, 1111–1120.

Monaco *et al.* (1985). Detection of deletions spanning the Duchenne muscular dystrophy locus using a tightly linked DNA segment. *Nature* **316**, 842–845.

Morgan-Hughes, J. A., Darveniza, P., Kahn, S. N., Landon, D. N., Sherratt, R. M., Land, J. M. and Clark, J. B. (1977). A mitochondrial myopathy characterised by deficiency in reducible cytochrome b. *Brain* **100**, 617–640.

——, Landon, D. N., Land, J. M. and Clark, J. B. (1979). A mitochondrial myopathy with a deficiency of respiratory chain NADH-CoQ reductase activity. *J. neurol. Sci.* **43**, 27–46.

Müller, R. and Kugelberg, E. (1959). Myopathy in Cushing's syndrome. *J. Neurol. Neurosurg. Psychiat.* **22**, 314–319.

Nicholson, G. A., Gardner-Medwin, D., Pennington, R. J. T. and Walton, J. N. (1979). Carrier detection in Duchenne muscular dystrophy: assessment of the effect of age on detection-rate with serum-creatine-kinase activity. *Lancet* i, 692–694.

Paine, R. S. (1963). The future of the 'floppy infant'. *Develop. Med. Child Neurol.* **5**, 115–124.

Pallis, C. and Lewis, P. D. (1981). Inflammatory myopathies. Part II: Involvement of human muscle by parasites. In *Disorders of voluntary muscle*, 4th edn (ed. J. N. Walton), pp. 569–584. Churchill Livingstone, Edinburgh.

Pavlakis, S. G., Phillips, P. C., DiMauro, S., De Vivo, D. C. and Rowland, L. P. (1984). Mitochondrial myopathy, encephalopathy, lactic acidosis, and strokelike episodes: a distinctive clinical syndrome. *Ann. Neurol.* **16**, 481–488.

Pennington, R. J. T. (1980). Clinical biochemistry of muscular dystrophy. *Br. med. Bull.* **36**, 123–126.

Perkoff, G. T., Hardy, P., and Velez-Garcia, E. (1966). Reversible acute muscular syndrome in chronic alcoholism. *N. Engl. J. Med.* **274**, 1277–1285.

Plishker, G. A., Gitelman, H. J. and Appel, S. H. (1978). Myotonic muscular dystrophy: altered calcium transport in erythrocytes. *Science* **200**, 323–325.

Poskanzer, D. C. and Kerr, D. N. S. (1961). A third type of periodic paralysis with normokalaemia and favourable response to sodium chloride. *Am. J. Med.* **31**, 328–342.

Prineas, J. W., Hall, R., Barwick, D. D. and Watson, A. J. (1968). Myopathy associated with pigmentation following adrenalectomy for Cushing's syndrome. *Q. J. Med.* **37**, 63–77.

Rose, A. L. and Walton, J. N. (1966). Polymyosits: a survey of 89 cases with particular reference to treatment and prognosis. *Brain* **89**, 747–768.

Rosenberg, R. N. (1984). Molecular genetics, recombinant DNA techniques, and genetic neurological disease. *Ann. Neurol.* **15**, 511–520.

Roses, A. D. (1984). Molecular genetics of myotonic and Duchenne muscular dystrophy. *TINS* **7**, 190–193.

Schwartz, O. and Jampel, R. S. (1962). Congenital blepharophimosis associated with a unique generalized myopathy. *Arch. Ophthal.* **68**, 52–57.

Shy, G. M., Engel, W. K., Somers, J. E. and Wanko, T. (1963). Nemaline myopathy, a new congenital myopathy. *Brain* **86**, 793–810.

—— and Magee, K. R. (1956). A new congenital non-progressive myopathy. *Brain* **79**, 610–620.

Simpson, J. A. (1960). Myasthenia gravis: a new hypothesis. *Scott. med. J.* **5**, 419–436.

—— (1981). Myasthenia gravis and myasthenic syndromes. In *Disorders of voluntary muscle*, 4th edn (ed. J. N. Walton), pp. 585–624. Churchill Livingstone, Edinburgh.

Smith, R. and Stern, G. M. (1967). Myopathy, osteomalacia, and hyperparathyroidism. *Brain* **90**, 593–602.

Spiro, A. J., Shy, G. M. and Gonatas, N. K. (1966). Myotubular myopathy. *Arch. Neurol., Chicago*, **14**, 1–14.

Steel, C. M. (1984). DNA in medicine: the tools. *Lancet* ii, 908, 966–968.

Takagi, A., Schotland, D. L., DiMauro, S. and Rowland, L. P. (1973). Thyrotoxic periodic paralysis. Function of sarcoplasmic reticulum and muscle glycogen. *Neurology, Minneap.* **23**, 1008–1016.

Tarui, S., Okuno, G., Ikura, Y., Tanaka, T., Suda, M. and Nishikawa, M. (1965). Phosphofructokinase deficiency in skeletal muscle. *Biochem. Biophys. Res. Comm.* **19**, 517–523.

Van't Hoff, W. (1962). Familial myotonic periodic paralysis. *Q.J. Med.* **31**, 385–402.

Walton, J. N. (1981) (ed.). *Disorders of voluntary muscle*, 4th edn. Churchill Livingstone, Edinburgh.

—— (1981). The clinical examination of the voluntary muscles. In *Disorders of voluntary muscle*, 4th edn (ed. J. N. Walton), pp. 448–480. Churchill Livingstone. Edinburgh.

—— (1981). Diffuse exercise-induced muscle pain of undetermined cause relieved by verapamil. *Lancet* i, 993.

—— (1983). The inflammatory myopathies. *J. Roy. Soc. Med.* **76**, 998–1010.

—— and Gardner-Medwin, D. (1981). Progressive muscular dystrophy, the myotonic disorders and other genetically-determined myopathies. In *Disorders of voluntary muscle*, 4th edn (ed. J. N. Walton), pp. 481–524. Churchill Livingstone, Edinburgh.

—— and Mastaglia, F. L. (eds) (1980a). The muscular dystrophies. *Br. med. Bull.* **36**, no. 2.

—— and —— (1980b). The molecular basis of muscle disease. In *The molecular basis of neuropathology* (eds R. H. S. Thompson and A. N. Davison), pp. 442–520. Arnold, London.

—— and Nattrass, F. J. (1954). On the classification, natural history and treatment of the myopathies. *Brain* **77**, 169–231.

Williamson, R. (1983). Cloned gene probes and the study of human inherited disease. *Hosp. Update* **9**, 25–32.

Zellweger, H., Afifi, A., McCormick, W. F. and Mergner, W. (1967). Severe congenital muscular dystrophy. *Am. J. Dis. Child.* **114**, 191–602.

SECTION 23
DISORDERS OF THE EYE IN GENERAL MEDICINE

DISORDERS OF THE EYE IN GENERAL MEDICINE

D. J. SPALTON

Retinopathies

Introduction

An appreciation of the normal ocular vascular anatomy is essential to the understanding of retinal disease. The eye has a dual blood supply from the retinal and choroidal circulations, both being derived from the ophthalmic artery, the first branch of the internal carotid artery above the carotid siphon, which runs forwards under the dura to enter the orbit through the optic canal with the optic nerve. In the posterior orbit it gives rise to 10–20 posterior ciliary arteries which run forwards to pierce the globe circumferentially to the optic disc and supply the optic disc itself and the choroid. The choroid is responsible for the vascular supply of the outer retina (the photoreceptors), and to reach this region the metabolic products must pass through the outer blood–retinal barrier (the retinal pigment epithelial cells) by active transport.

The central retinal artery leaves the ophthalmic artery more anteriorly in the orbit and pierces the optic nerve about 1 cm posterior to the optic disc. It may supply some of the retrobulbar optic nerve but does not contribute to the supply of the optic disc or choroid which is entirely derived from the posterior ciliary circulation. The central retinal artery divides into four branches on the optic disc and these end arteries supply the neuroretina in a quadrantic manner. The macula is avascular and receives its blood supply through the retinal pigment epithelial cells from the choroid. The choroidal capillaries have fenestrations in their wall so that plasma readily leaks out of the circulation whereas the retinal vessels have tight endothelial junctions (the inner blood–retinal barrier). Venous return from the retina is by the central retinal vein and from the choroid by four vortex veins to the orbital venous plexus.

Functionally, the retina can be divided into the outer retina where the metabolic processes in the photoreceptors and retinal pigment epithelial cells initiate photochemical changes, and the inner or neuroretina where neurological processing of visual information begins.

Diagnosis of retinal pathology is made on fundoscopy through a well-dilated pupil and can be supplemented by fundus photography and fluorescein angiography. This involves the intravenous injection of fluorescein dye and observation of its transit through both the choroidal and retinal circulations which is usually photographed for later study. The diagnosis of a retinopathy depends on an accurate interpretation of the physical signs. The retina has only a limited number of ways of reacting to a disease process and therefore a fundus appearance may be the end result of a number of dissimilar disease processes. The common physical signs are described below and illustrated in the colour plates.

Cotton wool spots (Plate 1)

These used to be known as soft exudates or cytoid bodies. They represent infarcts of the retinal nerve fibre layer and hold-up of axoplasmic flow, both orthograde and retrograde, and are, therefore, a sign of microvascular ischaemia. They are initially seen as soft fluffy superficial lesions which absorb over 6–8 weeks, leaving a defect in the retinal nerve fibre layer. In diabetic retinopathy cotton wool spots may persist for a longer time.

Hard exudates

These represent accumulation of lipid and lipoproteins in the retina and are a sign of vascular leakage. The lipid is deposited in the retina some distance from the leaking vascular defect and in the posterior pole take the form of complete or incomplete rings known as circinate exudates (Plate 2). The macula is particularly susceptible to oedema and lipid exudation which is seen in linear radial lines surrounding the macula in the nerve fibre layer of Henlé as a macular star (Plate 16). These are often incomplete being more prominent on the side adjacent to the leaking focus e.g. the optic disc. Further leakage into a circinate exudate or macular star leads to plaque formation. If the leakage is stopped, for example, by laser photocoagulation, hard exudates eventually absorb. Lipid exudate may also be found in the subretinal space with some retinopathies.

Haemorrhages

The morphology of haemorrhages indicates their localization within the retina, and to some extent their aetiology. Preretinal haemorrhages lie between the posterior vitreous face and retina. They have a fluid level and are the result of bleeding from preretinal neovascularization or haemorrhage with rupture through the internal limiting membrane of the retina. These haemorrhages are also sometimes known as subhyaloid or retrogel haemorrhages. Rupture of the superficial retinal capillary plexus produces flame-shaped haemorrhages tracking along the nerve fibres in the posterior pole where the nerve fibre layer is thickest; they absorb without permanent sequelae. Blotchy haemorrhages are found deeper in the retina in the posterior pole or in equatorial retina where the nerve fibres have a vertical course, restricting spread of the bleeding. Full thickness retinal haemorrhages have a widespread dark brown blotchy appearance which indicates gross retinal ischaemia and a risk of neovascularization. Subretinal haemorrhages occur from choroidal pathology and have a dark brown or greenish appearance from blocking of the transmission of red light by the retinal pigment epithelial cells.

Roth spots

These are haemorrhages with white centres sometimes due to infarction or septic emboli. They are also seen in the posterior pole in a variety of anaemic retinopathies and are not restricted to subacute bacterial endocarditis.

Drusen (colloid bodies)

These are yellowish, deep retinal lesions, lying at the level of the retinal pigment epithelium (Plate 3). They are a sign of deranged photoreceptor-retinal pigment epithelial-cell metabolism and are usually seen in the macular area as a sign of senile macular degeneration but occasionally can be more widespread in the retina. They are often associated with atrophy and hypertrophy of the retinal pigment epithelium and sometimes become invaded by neovascularization from the choroid to produce a disciform senile macular degeneration. They may also have a glinting, calcified appearance and occasionally produce a flat confluent subretinal mass with sinister implications for central vision.

Microaneurysms

Microaneurysms are outpouchings of the capillary circulation and are seen as 'dots' in the posterior pole, sometimes only distinguishable from 'blots' or small haemorrhages by fluorescein angiography. Whilst they occur in other retinopathies they are the hallmark of diabetic retinopathy.

Macroaneurysms

These are found on the retinal arteries. They are outpouchings of the vessel wall and are an unusual sign, usually seen where the vessel wall has been damaged by an embolus and systemic hypertension.

Neovascularization

This is discussed more fully in conjunction with diabetic retinopathy but new vessels can be produced by a wide variety of conditions. They may be found on the retina and optic disc, under the retina or on the iris. All new vessels in the eye have similar properties. They have loose endothelial cell junctions in contrast to the normal tight junctions which constitute the blood–retinal barrier of normal vessels. They leak fluorescein dye intensively, they are fragile and bleed or leak fluid to produce visual loss from haemorrhage, lipid exudation or fibrosis with traction on the retina leading to detachment.

Pigmentation

Pigmentation may be seen in the retina as intraretinal pigmentation which has a bone corpuscular morphology. This is a reflection of long-standing disease in the photoreceptor–retinal pigment epithelial-cell area, usually as a result of an inherited retinal dystrophy such as retinitis pigmentosa. Focal pigmentation is seen around areas of old choroiditis and scattered pigmentation is seen in the macular area with atrophy and hyperpigmentation as a feature of senile macular degeneration.

Arterial occlusion of the retina

Central retinal artery occlusion produces dramatic and sudden unilateral visual loss, although the affected eye occasionally retains a peripheral rim of visual field because the peripheral retina is thin and can be supplied from the choroid. Cloudy white intracellular oedema of the retina in the posterior pole (where the retina is thickest) is seen within a few hours of the occlusion and this whiteness is contrasted to the 'cherry red spot' appearance at the macula. Here the retina is avascular and only one cell thick so that the normal and unaffected choroidal vasculature can be seen through this window producing the redness to contrast with the surrounding white and infarcted retina (Plate 4). In the acute stage, the retinal vessels may be attenuated and show slowing of the blood flow with 'cattle trucking' in the vascular columns. Emboli may be seen within the arterial tree and sometimes there is mild optic disc swelling from hold-up of retrograde axoplasmic flow. The acute retinal appearances are not always very apparent, being more easily seen in pigmented eyes and less easily seen in those with hypopigmentation or thin retinas such as myopes. The acute changes resolve within a few days to a week or two leaving a normally appearing retina, frequently with normal retinal vessels. Optic atrophy appears 6–8 weeks later.

Central retinal artery occlusion occurs from localized thrombosis within the artery as it lies within the optic nerve or from occlusion by emboli, usually from an atheromatous plaque at the carotid bifurcation but occasionally from fragments of a calcific aortic valve. Vascular spasm is a controversial concept which probably only occurs in conditions such as ergot poisoning. In younger patients an inflammatory arteritis is an unusual cause of occlusion which may suggest underlying aetiologies such as systemic lupus erythematosus, syphilis or polyarteritis nodosa. Central retinal artery occlusion is a relatively uncommon presentation of temporal arteritis, being responsible for visual loss in only about 4 per cent of patients, an anterior ischaemic optic neuropathy being much more common.

Occasionally, eyes with a central retinal artery occlusion may regain some vision. This may be due to the presence of an unaffected cilio-retinal artery (a branch of the posterior ciliary circulation) or fragmentation of an impacted embolus. One or more cilio-retinal arteries are present to some degree in about 20 per cent of eyes and occasionally these may provide a substantial retinal supply. A cilio-retinal artery will be spared in the presence of a central retinal artery occlusion and vice versa, because of its origin from the posterior ciliary circulation. If a patient is seen within a few hours of a central retinal artery occlusion it is worthwhile presuming that the aetiology is embolic and attempting to dislodge the embolus by massaging the eye to lower the intraocular pressure. Visual improvement is unusual however and the prognosis in most cases extremely poor. All patients require thorough investigation to exclude an embolic source, underlying atheroma or arteritic disease, as appropriate.

Branch retinal artery occlusion is virtually always due to retinal emboli. The most common causes are cholesterol crystals from an atheromatous plaque, platelet, and fibrin emboli, or fragments from a calcific aortic valve (Plate 5). Cholesterol crystals (sometimes known as *Hollenhorst plaques*) are seen as yellowish glinting plaques, usually at the bifurcation of a retinal artery (Plate 6). They have a planar morphology and may not completely occlude the artery; they may be seen as they glint with tilting of the ophthalmoscope beam. A large and long-standing embolus may damage the vascular wall leading to lipid deposition within the wall producing a characteristic 'trouser leg' sheathing at a bifurcation. Platelet emboli are frequently associated with *amaurosis fugax*, (transient uniocular visual loss lasting from minutes to 3 or 4 hours with vision returning to normal) (see Section 21). They originate from atheromatous plaques and can sometimes be seen slowly traversing the retinal circulation as a porridgy intravascular mass as the attack evolves (Plate 7). Calcific cardiac fragments are readily distinguished from other types of emboli by their pearly white globular appearance and their tendency to lodge within the major retinal arteries on or adjacent to the optic disc with complete occlusion of the affected vessel. An embolus within the retina is an important physical sign, even if asymptomatic, as it is an indication that the patient is at risk of further embolism with possible permanent visual or neurological loss from obstruction within the intracranial distribution of the internal carotid artery. All patients require investigation to elicit the embolic source, with appropriate medical or surgical treatment (see Section 21).

Venous occlusion in the retina

Venous occlusion within the retina can affect either the central retinal vein or its tributary branches. The physical signs of venous occlusion are confined to the territory drained by the affected vessel and in the acute stage consist of scattered retinal haemorrhages and venous dilation with variable amounts of retinal oedema and retinal ischaemia, depending on the severity of the occlusion. Concomitant retinal ischaemia is diagnosed by the features of cotton wool spots, dense blotchy dark haemorrhage, and retinal capillary closure, which is sometimes difficult to identify without fluorescein angiography. Venous occlusions vary from the mild to the severe.

Central retinal vein occlusion

Within the optic nerve, posterior to the globe, the retinal artery and vein share a common fascial sheath. It is thought that arteriosclerotic thickening of the artery compromizes this space and the central retinal vein to produce venous obstruction. Central retinal vein occlusion is, therefore, a disease of the arteriosclerotic, hypertensive or diabetic individual. There is also an important association with chronic simple glaucoma, and all patients require measurement of their intraocular pressures, particularly as there may be asymptomatic glaucoma in the other eye which may be the better eye for the future. Central retinal vein occlusion in young people has sometimes been attributed to a vasculitis of the vein but these patients rarely have any other evidence of an immunological disease and atherosclerosis is a much more likely cause.

Symptoms are often present on waking, the patient's vision having been normal the night before and it has been shown that many of these patients have labile blood and intraocular pressure. Visual loss varies from mild transient blurring to severe; mild central retinal vein occlusion may be asymptomatic. Severe occlusion produces structural damage and severe visual loss.

The physical signs vary from patient to patient and depend on the acuteness and severity of the occlusion. Some patients have marked swelling of the optic disc; in others it is normal or even glaucomatous (Plates 8 and 9). The pathognomonic sign is of venous dilation with retinal haemorrhages spreading throughout the fundus to the equatorial retina in contrast to papilloedema where the haemorrhages are confined to the vicinity of the optic disc. The haemorrhages may vary from superficial flame-shaped lesions to blotchy deeper haemorrhages in the posterior pole: extensive brownish haemorrhages indicate gross retinal ischaemia, capillary closure, and structural retinal damage. Cotton wool spots are a sign of infarction of the retinal axons and microvascular ischaemia. Retinal oedema is often difficult to diagnose without specialist equipment but is present with most central retinal venous occlusions in the early stage and persists in those with severe disease.

In milder cases, recanalization of the central retinal vein leads to resolution of the retinopathy over a period of weeks, with visual improvement. Collateral or shunt vessels are commonly seen on the optic disc following marked venous congestion; these are mature vessels which shunt blood from the obstructed retinal circulation to the lower pressure choroidal circulation and must not be confused with neovascularization of the optic disc.

Retinal capillary closure with retinal hypoxia is seen in severely affected eyes. This is similar to that found in diabetic and other vascular retinopathies and can be diagnosed from the clinical signs or by fluorescein angiography. Retinal hypoxia leads to neovascularization but with central vein occlusion this rarely occurs on the optic disc or retina and instead these patients develop neovascularization on the anterior surface of the iris, typically about 90 days after the initial occlusion (*rubiosis iridis*). This neovascular membrane frequently progresses to occlude the angle of the anterior chamber and obstruct the aqueous humour outflow. This dreaded complication is known as *thrombotic glaucoma* and leads to a blind, painful eye which sometimes has to be removed.

No medical therapy has been shown to be beneficial in improving the visual prognosis. Anticoagulants or fibrinolytics often lead to devastating vitreous haemorrhage and are contraindicated. Panretinal photocoagulation can forestall or control rubiosis in severely affected eyes, retaining what little residual vision is present or producing a quiescent painless blind eye. Once a thrombotic glaucoma is established, topical atropine and steroids are helpful in keeping the eye asymptomatic but failure of this therapy leads to enucleation.

Branch retinal vein occlusion

This is a common vascular retinopathy and is usually due to occlusion of a branch retinal vein at an arteriovenous crossing where the artery and vein share the fascial sheath and the artery passes superficial to the vein. These arteriovenous crossings are found in the retina temporal to the optic disc and are comparatively rare in the nasal fundus where the blood vessels have a more radial distribution. Arteriosclerotic changes compromize the venous return at these points leading to venous occlusion and therefore branch retinal vein occlusions are seen in hypertensive, diabetic or arteriosclerotic individuals. Occasionally, an inflammatory phlebitis leads to occlusion along a segment of a vein in diseases such as sarcoidosis, with similar retinal signs in the presence of posterior uveitis. If the affected vein drains the macular region, the patient will present with blurring of vision, other venous occlusions may present as field defects, vitreous floaters from rupture of haemorrhage into the vitreous gel, or may be asymptomatic. The physical signs are of venous dilation and haemorrhage within the affected

venous territory; retinal oedema may be present and there may be variable amounts of retinal ischaemia shown by the presence of cotton wool spots or blotchy dark brown haemorrhage (Plate 10).

The retinopathy of mild venous occlusion resolves over a few weeks with improvement of vision and the formation of venous collateral shunts on the retina. The visual prognosis is poor if the vascular arcade surrounding the macula is ruptured. Occasionally, a severely ischaemic branch retinal vein occlusion will lead to neovascularization on the adjacent sector of the optic disc or at the junction with normal retina, but in contrast to central retinal vein occlusion, rubiosis of the iris is uncommon. The neovascularization can be destroyed by photocoagulation if required. A few patients lose more vision some time after a venous occlusion from lipid exudation into the retina and this can also be controlled by photocoagulation.

Hyperviscosity and slow-flow retinopathy

Hyperviscosity produces a retinopathy which has similar appearances to that of a central retinal vein occlusion, but which, in contrast, is bilateral. Retinopathy from hyperviscosity is seen in conditions such as Waldenstrom's macroglobulaemia and polycythaemia or occasionally with a very high leucocyte count in leukaemia. The associated retinopathy is frequently quite mild. Venous engorgement is often noticeable and some peripheral retinal haemorrhages may be present but it is uncommon to see marked retinal haemorrhages and ischaemia. Many patients with these conditions are also anaemic and this may counterbalance the tendency to hyperviscosity (see Section 19).

A slow-flow retinopathy from carotid occlusive disease produces a similar picture, but sometimes more gross changes of retinal venous engorgement, retinal oedema, and haemorrhage occur, but with the important and additional sign of low central retinal artery pressure. This can be diagnosed by the ease with which the central retinal artery can be made to pulsate by digital pressure on the eye during ophthalmoscopy. Most patients have a unilateral retinopathy from atheromatous disease in the carotid artery, but severe and bilateral cases can be seen with Takayasu's disease (Section 13), and the hypoxia may be severe enough to produce neovascularization in the eye. Some patients complain of a strange transient blurring of vision in which they have the sensation of things going white or pale or the sensation of looking through a watery car windscreen, which is thought to be due to poor perfusion of the neuroretina and is sometimes precipitated by bright light.

Diabetic retinopathy

Diabetics lose vision from cataracts (page 23.18) or retinopathy. Diabetic retinopathy is the commonest cause of blindness in the working population and is still the commonest preventable cause of blindness in the Western World. The cause of the retinopathy is unknown but it is clear that the presence of retinopathy correlates with the duration of diabetes although there is a difference between early and late onset diabetics. Retinopathy will be present to some extent in early onset juvenile diabetics in 25 per cent of cases by ten years of disease duration whereas adult non-insulin-dependent patients appear to be more susceptible, and they have an incidence of about 50 per cent at this stage. Some patients present with a retinopathy as the first sign of their diabetes.

The influence of blood sugar control on the prevention of retinopathy is controversial. Early studies appear to indicate that good control retards the onset of retinopathy and large-scale controlled trials are at present underway to confirm this. Once a retinopathy is established it is more doubtful whether good control has any beneficial influence and there are, as yet, no large studies available that carefully correlate grades of retinopathy with progression. The retinopathy in some patients with *Mauriac's syndrome* (poorly controlled diabetes, growth retardation, delayed puberty) rapidly deteriorates when good control is established. Hormonal influences seem to be important as retinopathy is not usually seen in diabetics prior to puberty. Pregnancy can have a markedly adverse effect and all diabetics require careful ophthalmic monitoring during pregnancy; the disease can usually be controlled until delivery when there is a tendency for the retinopathy to improve. Abortion is not required or justified on ophthalmic grounds. Systemic hypertension and renal failure also probably exacerbate the retinopathy whereas optic atrophy, high myopia, glaucoma or degenerative retinal disease seem to protect the eye, possibly by reduction in the metabolic demands. Thus a grossly asymmetrical diabetic retinopathy should prompt investigation for an underlying cause.

The earliest changes in the retina are found in the microvascular circulation and changes in the major retinal arteries or veins are only found late in the course of the disease or in the presence of additional factors such as systemic hypertension. The characteristic lesion is the microaneurysm and whilst this may be seen in other retinopathies it never occurs in the same profusion as in diabetes. Microaneurysms are an outpouching of the retinal capillary wall. They have a dark red appearance and are about the same diameter as a retinal branch arteriole is in calibre. They rupture to produce haemorrhages (dot and blot retinopathy) or leak plasma and lipid into the retina to produce retinal oedema and hard exudates. The other typical feature of diabetic retinopathy is closure of areas of the retinal capillary bed leading to retinal hypoxia and the subsequent risk of neovascularization.

The understanding of diabetic retinopathy and the management of patients has been greatly clarified by classification of the retinal disease (Fig. 1). From absence of diabetic retinopathy a background retinopathy appears and progresses to the stage of microaneurysms, dot and blot haemorrhages, hard exudates, and small areas of retinal capillary closure but, by definition, visual activity remains normal at 6/6 or better. Further progression leads to visual loss from either maculopathy or retinal neovascularization. This classification is broadly applicable although maculopathy and neovascularization may co-exist in some patients. Background retinopathy is seen in the posterior pole of the eye but especially in the area temporal to the macula where there is a watershed zone between the superior and inferior temporal retinal vessels (Plate 11). With maculopathy, visual activity is lost due to deposition of hard exudate, retinal oedema or ischaemia in the macula area (Plates 12a, b). This is the most common cause of visual loss in diabetics, accounting for 70 per cent of legal blindness and whilst these patients lose central visual acuity they still retain the peripheral field of vision so that they can lead independent lives. In the remaining patients increasing retinal ischaemia leads to retinal or optic disc neovascularization with the sequelae of vitreous heamorrhage, fibrosis causing retinal traction, and detachment producing complete blindness. Neovascularization is therefore much more serious in its visual effects than a maculopathy and about 70 per cent of eyes with neovascularization of the optic disc or retina will be completely blind within 5 years unless the eye is treated. These patients also tend to have severe systemic disease and a limited life expectancy.

The sequence of events in the development of neovascularization appears to be that increasing areas of retinal capillary closure lead to retinal hypoxia and there is now good clinical and experimental evidence to show that a hypoxic retina secretes a neovascular factor which stimulates revascularization from the adjacent retina at the junction of hypoxic and normal retina or on the optic disc which is itself an area of junctional blood supply. The new vessels appear as fine, flat thready vessels from either side of the capillary circulation. Like any neovascular tissue within the eye, they have loose endothelial cell junctions, and are leaky and fragile (Fig. 2). Initially, the new vessels lie flat on the retina or optic disc but changes in the overlying vitreous gel occur which detaches from the retinal surface pulling the neovascular tissue forwards so that it proliferates on the posterior vitreous face; the vessels do not penetrate the gel itself which is thought to contain a neovascular inhibitory factor. Minor trauma causes the vessels to rupture

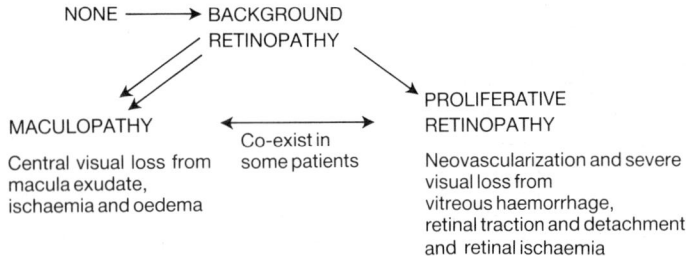

Fig. 1 Flow chart of diabetic retinopathy. From a background retinopathy patients progress in two broad groups. Most lose vision from maculopathy with lipid exudation, ischaemia or oedema; others develop neovascularization of the retina or optic disc with subsequent blindness. Both types of pathology co-exist in some patients.

and bleed producing vitreous or retinal haemorrhage. Fibrosis develops and the combination of retinal neovascularization and fibrosis is known as *retinitis proliferans*. Contraction leads to retinal traction and detachment and a blind eye.

Pathogenesis

The pathogenesis of diabetic retinopathy is unknown but the earliest structural changes in the retina are seen in the capillaries as loss of the intramural pericytes, endothelial cells and thickening of capillary basement membrane. Whilst microaneurysms may occur in other vascular retinopathies, they do not occur to the same extent as in diabetes, and studies of other systemic circulations in diabetics show that they are a relatively uncommon finding elsewhere. Basement membrane thickening is common in many other diabetic organs. Claims have been made that loss of the intramural pericytes is the essential lesion in the diabetic retina; selective loss does not occur in other types of vascular retinopathy. These cells appear to be phagocytic and contractile and may control autoregulation in the retina. Capillary endothelial cells appear to be less metabolically active but are lost as the disease progresses. Local weakness of the vessel wall may lead to the formation of microaneurysms, and avascular capillaries are not perfused by blood, possibly leading to retinal ischaemia. Other authorities believe that capillary closure is the primary event. The biochemical basis of these events is speculative but present evidence speculates that both aldose reductase pathways and the influence of growth hormone or its variants are important mechanisms. Aldose reductase metabolism leading to sorbitol accumulation might induce the primary cellular damage whilst growth hormone may promote neovascularization.

Treatment

All diabetics require to have their visual acuity checked with spectacles plus a pinhole to exclude refractive error at each outpatient visit. Those with background retinopathy (normal vision) need to be watched at intervals until vision deteriorates or neovascularization develops.

Maculopathy from hard exudation can be controlled providing the patient is referred early enough. If the acuity has fallen below 6/12, permanent retinal damage occurs and although photocoagulation produces a morphological improvement, vision does not recover. Thus maculopathies must be referred early for ophthalmological assessment. The principle of treatment is to destroy the leaking vascular abnormalities adjacent to the macula which produce the hard exudation; therefore, photocoagulation is focal. Whilst control of exudative maculopathy is reasonably successful maculopathy due to retinal oedema or ischaemia cannot be helped or prevented by photocoagulation and patients with these changes lose central vision.

Retinal neovascularization is often preceded by signs of retinal ischaemia such as cotton wool spots (microinfarcts), focal dilation or pouching of retinal veins and capillary closure which can be

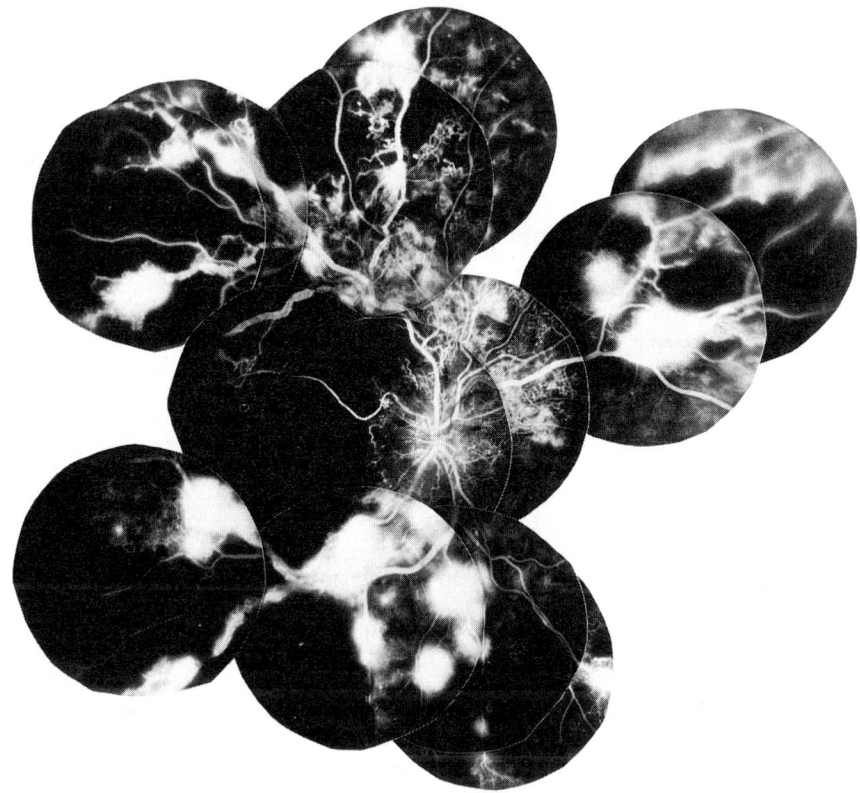

Fig. 2 Diabetic retinopathy. A composite fluorescein angiogram shows gross areas of peripheral capillary closure (dense black regions). Tufts of neovascularization have developed at the junctional areas of perfused and non-perfused retina which leak fluorescein intensively (white areas).

seen as a subtle colour change in the retina. These patients are often described as having a *preproliferative retinopathy*. This is a useful term because although they do not require treatment at this stage, they are in imminent danger of developing neovascularization and need careful observation. Neovascularization does not, of course, affect visual acuity until complications develop and it is important to emphasize that diabetics cannot be screened by visual acuity without fundoscopy. The development of neovascularization on the optic disc or retina is an absolute indication for panretinal photocoagulation. The technique of panretinal photocoagulation is carried out using an argon laser or xenon arc to ablate the peripheral retina outside the temporal retinal vessels. The rationale of this therapy is to convert hypoxic retina to anoxic, and halt secretion of the mysterious neovascular factor. Retinal neovascularization atrophies within 3–4 weeks of successful treatment. As the macula area is not photocoagulated, visual acuity remains normal but patients often notice some constriction of visual field and poor night vision (Plates 13a, b).

Pituitary ablation, although it has a beneficial effect on retinal neovascularization has now been completely superseded by photocoagulation. No drug therapy has been shown to have any therapeutic effect on any type of diabetic retinopathy.

Hypertensive retinopathy

The eye is the only organ where blood vessels can be directly inspected and the effects of hypertension seen. Systemic hypertension produces changes in the retinal, choroidal, and optic disc circulations which depend on the acuteness of the blood pressure change, its severity, and its duration as well as on the age of the patient. Retinal 'arteries' are in reality arterioles by histological criteria. Attempts to classify and grade systemic hypertension by the retinal appearances are confused by the difficulty of distinguishing early hypertensive changes from arteriolar sclerosis with ageing. Both diseases will produce arteriolar constriction,

changes in the light reflex of the vessel wall, and arteriovenous crossing changes.

Animal work has shown that the initial response to an increase in blood pressure is constriction of the retinal arteries from autoregulation. This is followed by ischaemic damage or necrosis of the vascular endothelium and smooth muscle cells of the media. This stage is followed by vasodilation. Autoregulation fails and the capillary bed is exposed to high vascular pressures leading to disruption of the blood–retinal barrier and leakage of plasma into the retina. Haemorrhages occur together with fibrinoid necrosis due to exudation of plasma into the arteriolar wall leading to vascular obstruction and infarction. If the elevation of blood pressure is not severe, an exudative phase may not take place and sclerotic changes develop which are seen clinically as changes in the light reflex of the vessel wall. Pathologically, these vessels show hyperplastic sclerosis with thickening of the tunica media and hyperplasia of muscle cells.

The fundoscopic appearances will depend on how long the hypertension has been present and hence whether protective sclerotic changes have had time to develop. The signs of hypertensive changes in the retina are constriction of the arteries with areas of focal narrowing and dilation and a heightened light reflex from the vessel wall (silver or copper wiring) (Plate 14). At the sites of arteriovenous crossing, where the arteries pass superficially to the veins, the underlying vein becomes compressed by thickened arterial wall which may be severe enough to lead to a branch vein occlusion (page 23.3). Further generalized decompression produces splinter or blotchy haemorrhages and cotton wool spots (Plate 15). Hard exudates indicate breakdown of the blood–retinal barrier which tend to be seen in the macular area as a star; this is particularly common in the resolving phases of hypertensive optic disc swelling (Plate 16) or with localized retinal pathology such as an arterial macroaneurysm.

These signs of hypertensive retinopathy have been recognized since the 19th century. The first major attempt to classify them was made in 1939 by Keith, Wagner, and Barker who tried to relate the retinopathy to the severity of hypertension and patient survival. They proposed four grades of retinopathy:

1. Mild to moderate narrowing or sclerosis of the retinal arteries.
2. Moderate to marked sclerosis, exaggeration of the light reflex, A–V crossing changes.
3. In addition, the appearance of cotton wool spots and haemorrhages.
4. The appearance of optic disc swelling.

This classification has formed the basis of much clinical work but it is apparent that there is great difficulty in distinguishing stages 1 and 2 from arteriolar sclerosis. Controlled studies performed by the examination of fundus photographs by different physicians on repeated occasions have shown that correct diagnosis can be very subjective. Focal arterial constriction and dilation and A–V changes can be helpful but in reality the early retinal changes must be interpreted in the light of the clinical picture. A–V changes are more significant when found in the eye of a 20-year-old than in a 70-year-old person. The presence of haemorrhage, cotton wool spots, and optic disc oedema indicate acute decompensation. For these reasons stages 1 and 2 cannot be easily distinguished from arteriolar sclerosis with ageing, and stages 3 and 4 are sometimes grouped together as accelerated hypertensive retinopathy. It is important to remember that localized retinal pathology such as a branch vein occlusion may be present and that associated haemorrhages and cotton wool spots do not necessarily imply an accelerated hypertensive retinopathy.

Careful retinal examination provides useful clues to the severity and duration of the disease. If haemorrhages and infarcts are seen without compensatory retinal arterial changes, this suggests the onset of the hypertension has been acute and severe, whereas the presence of sclerotic arterial changes indicates decompensation during the course of established disease. Other factors influence the appearance of the retinopathy such as diabetes, systemic lupus erythematosus, and anaemia. With renal failure, very much more hard exudation may be seen whereas with a phaechromacytoma florid retinal changes can occur from the swings in blood pressure.

Interesting changes are also found in the choroidal and optic disc circulations. *Hypertensive choroidopathy* is often seen in acutely hypertensive patients where there has been vascular decompensation. Anatomically, the choroidal arteries are short and of large diameter so that the pressure is directly transmitted to the choriocapillaries. In the acute stages, bullous retinal detachment may be seen from breakdown of the outer blood–retinal barrier. Choroidal infarcts can be seen as *Elschnig's spots* in the posterior pole, or *Siegrist streaks* in the peripheral retina (Fig. 3). The former are small pigmented spots surrounded by a halo of retinal pigment epithelial atrophy in the posterior pole of the eye which correspond to infarcts of the choroidal lobules, whilst the latter are linear pigmented wedge-shaped areas of infarction in the retinal periphery from occlusion of a peripheral choroidal artery. Choroidopathy is common in pre-eclamptic toxaemia and other types of acute hypertension. Optic disc swelling (Plate 17) has a time-honoured place in the assessment of systemic hypertension and yet the pathology is not understood. The optic disc appearances cannot be distinguished from other types of optic swelling except by the other retinal signs. Not all patients have raised intracranial pressure and it is likely that local vascular or mechanical changes in the optic disc are an important mechanism in producing swelling.

Sickle cell retinopathy

This is a neovascular retinopathy of the peripheral retina which is seen predominantly in patients with haemoglobin (Hb) SC disease but also occurs with other sickle cell disorders such as sickle cell anaemia or sickle cell β-thalassaemia (see Section 19). The patho-

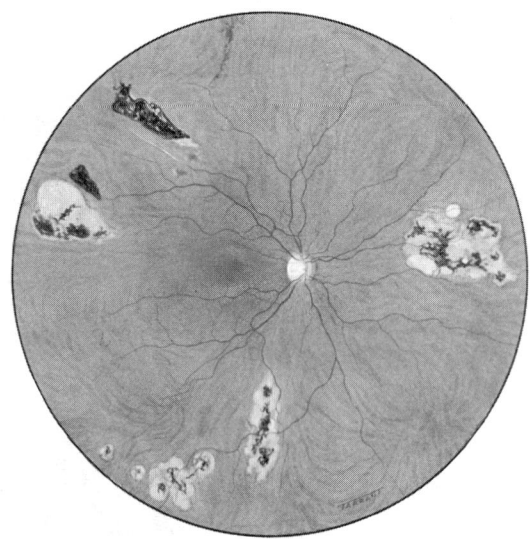

Fig. 3 A fundus painting showing peripheral choroidal infarcts (Siegrist streaks) in a hypertensive patient with SLE.

genesis of the retinopathy is thought to be localized thromboses from sickling in the peripheral retinal arterioles where decreasing vascular calibre and falling pH coincide. The predominance of retinopathy in HbSC disease may be accounted for by the fact that these patients are less anaemic than those with other sickle cell disorders who are protected by anaemia and lower blood viscosity. The closure of the peripheral retinal arterioles leads to capillary non-perfusion of the peripheral retina. At this junction abnormal vascular shunts develop and neovascularization appears as fans of new vessels often projecting forwards and attached to the posterior vitreous face (Plate 18). The appearance of these fans has been likened to that of coral and for this reason they are known colloquially as 'seafans'. Peripheral to the normal retina there is closure of the retinal capillary bed and as the major retinal arteries and veins pass into this area they become white and sclerosed. Choroidal infarcts can be sometimes found as a feature of sickle cell retinopathy. In the acute stages they have a reddish yellow appearance, lying deep to the retina in the peripheral fundus. At this stage they are known as 'salmon patches'; later they become pigmented scars and are called 'sunbursts'. Their presence causes no visual symptoms.

Neovascularization in sickle cell retinopathy can progress to vitreous haemorrhage, localized fibrosis, and retinitis proliferans or retinal tears and detachment but the prognosis for vision is very much better than with other types of neovascularization as the neovascular tissue has a tendency to autoinfarction. Laser photocoagulation can be used to destroy the neovascularization but controlled studies have shown that it is of no benefit to the patient; instead it can induce the retinopathy to move centrally with potentially serious consequences. For this reason, patients are best observed and active treatment restricted to those who develop complications.

Sickling may be seen in the conjunctival vessels, the '*comma*' *sign*. These are numerous small obstructed vessels which are curved and purplish in colour and represent localized thromboses.

Anaemia

Severe anaemia may produce a retinopathy with blotchy retinal haemorrhages in the equatorial and peripheral retina. These are of no visual significance and absorb spontaneously. These peripheral retinal haemorrhages must be distinguished from those seen with a retinal vein occlusion or slow-flow retinopathy and this distinction is easily made by the absence of other features of venous obstruction. *Roth spots* (haemorrhage with white centres) can be seen in some patients.

Systemic lupus erythematosus (SLE)

The retinopathy of SLE is a combination of localized arteritic lesions from vasculitis, hypertension, and anaemia. Cotton wool spots may be seen in the fundus in the absence of systemic hypertension and are probably due to direct involvement of the retinal microvasculature by the arteritic process (Plate 19). More rarely, patients with SLE may develop occlusions of the branch retinal arteries with localized infarction of the retina and appropriate field defects. Scleritis, or dry eyes, are also a feature of SLE but anterior or posterior uveitis is not seen.

Retinitis pigmentosa (RP)

This is the triad of night blindness, peripheral visual field constriction, and a pigmentary retinopathy. The disease is due to metabolic disturbance of the photoreceptor and retinal pigment epithelial (RPE) cells. In this region, known as the outer retina, the photoreceptors convert light in photochemical reactions, photochemical pigments are regenerated, and the outer segments of the photoreceptors are removed by the RPE cells, the mostly highly phagocytic cells in the body. The fundus appearance of retinitis pigmentosa probably reflects a number of different metabolic faults in these processes; the same retinopathy represents a number of different but similar diseases.

The early fundus appearance is of patchy RPE atrophy in the equatorial retina giving the fundus a dappled appearance. This requires experience to identify, and diagnosis can be aided by fluorescein angiography and electrodiagnostic tests. Over a period of years there is a progressive attenuation of the retinal arteries, pallor of the optic disc, and increasing field loss. Intraretinal bone corpuscular pigmentation of the peripheral retina is a comparatively late feature appearing several years after the onset (Plate 20). Affected patients usually have good visual acuity but grossly constricted visual fields, most have been night blind for many years.

In the majority of patients retinitis pigmentosa is only an ocular disease and about 50 per cent of patients have a family history of the disease, inherited in a dominant, recessive or X-linked pattern. Diagnosis of the inherited pattern provides a visual and occupational prognosis and is essential for genetic counselling. The gene locus for X-linked retinitis pigmentosa has recently been defined. The remainder of the patients either have an inadequate family history, or their disease is due to a new mutation or pseudoretinitis pigmentosa from a large number of conditions which can simulate RP such as syphilitic choroiditis or ocular trauma. No treatment has been shown to effect the natural history of the disease.

A pigmentary retinopathy can be associated with systemic disease in a range of rare syndromes. The commonest of these are chronic progressive external ophthalmoplegia (*Kearns–Sayre syndrome*), *Usher's syndrome (congenital nerve deafness and RP)*, *Lawrence–Moon syndrome (RP, polydactyly, mental retardation, obesity, and hypogonadism)*, *Refsum's disease (phytanic acid storage)*, *abetalipoproteinaemia, Batten's disease*, etc. Most of these syndromes are excessively rare but abetalipoproteinaemia is important as early treatment will prevent visual deterioration (see Sections 9 and 19).

Inflammatory eye disease

Uveitis

Introduction

Despite much experimental work, the immunology of human uveitis is still not understood; no animal model produces the characteristic relapsing and remitting course of human disease. The eye has a number of unique features which affect the immune response. There is a dual blood supply from the retina and choroid and no lymphatic drainage so that antigens must either be removed by the blood or processed locally to elicit an immune reaction. The blood–ocular barriers protect the ocular tissues and the avascularity of tissues such as the cornea, lens or vitreous gel retards removal of antigen or antibody, forming a reservoir which may prolong an inflammatory response. Other factors which play a significant role in some diseases are the tissue type (anterior uveitis, Behcet's disease), racial origin (e.g. Vogt–Koyanagi–Harada syndrome) or sex (Reiter's disease is common in men, Still's disease in girls).

Classification of uveitis

Uveitis is a generic term given to inflammation within the uveal tract which compromizes the iris, ciliary body, and choroid. This process may affect the whole uveal tract or only part of it, but since the iris, ciliary body, and choroid lie in continuity with each other it is not surprising that severe inflammation in one region may spill over to affect an adjacent area. Thus a severe iritis may be accompanied by a cellular infiltration of the anterior vitreous gel ('iridocyclitis') or choroiditis by an anterior uveitis. Uveitis is a common sequelae of many ocular diseases and occurs as either a primary idiopathic event or secondary to disease processes associated with intraocular infection, surgery or trauma. Uveitis may also occur secondary to an adjacent inflammatory focus such as scleritis, keratitis or retinal vasculitis.

There is no single classification of uveitis which is free from confusion. Endogenous uveitis has been used to describe inflammation from a source within the body, usually reaching the eye by the blood, whilst exogenous uveitis is preceded by perforation of the globe. Either can be divided into infectious or non-infectious types but usage of these terms is becoming redundant as a better understanding of immunology blurs their distinction. Another classification divides anterior uveitis by the clinical appearances into granulomatous or non-granulomatous types with the implication that granulomatous uveitis reflects a similar systemic aetiology (tuberculosis, sarcoid, etc.). Whilst this is sometimes true, the distinction is not always helpful as some conditions (such as sarcoidosis) may present in either way; it can be difficult to decide whether the clinical picture is granulomatous or not; in many eyes with granulomatous uveitis, no underlying systemic aetiology is found. Another clinical distinction that has been used is whether the inflammation presents acutely or chronically. However, some patients present with acute uveitis which becomes chronic and others may have chronic disease with acute exacerbations. In view of these difficulties, an attempt at international definitions has been made which classifies the disease anatomically.

1. Anterior uveitis to include inflammation extending posteriorly and as far as the pars plana of the ciliary body. This term now includes iritis, iridocyclitis, anterior cyclitis, etc.
2. Intermediate uveitis – inflammation of the pars plana and peripheral retina to include such terms as pars planitis, peripheral uveitis, peripheral retinitis, etc.
3. Posterior uveitis is located behind the posterior hyaloid face and may be focal, multifocal or diffuse.
4. Panuveitis, to imply involvement of the whole uveal tract.

Other suggested criteria are the onset to be classified as sudden or insidious, the duration as short if less than 3 months, the pattern as single or repeated, and the severity as none, mild or severe.

The most useful information in the management of uveitis is to determine the major anatomical location of the inflammation as this will predict the clinical signs and the likely visual consequences. Apart from this, perhaps the most useful method is to describe the patient as completely as possible: 'a 55-year-old woman with chronic anterior uveitis and a mild acute relapse and secondary glaucoma presenting initially with herpes zoster ophthalmicus nine months previously'.

Clinical presentation of uveitis

The presentation of uveitis depends on the severity of the inflammation, the site within the eye, and its rapidity of onset.

Acute anterior uveitis (AAU) is one of the causes of a red, painful eye. Patients usually present with a history of a few days of redness, pain, and photophobia, and, as with any inflamed eye, there may be watery discharge which can be confused with a conjunctivitis. Pain from uveitis has an aching or boring character behind or around the eye, whereas that from conjunctivitis produces a gritty, foreign-body sensation. The pain from uveitis originates in the iris and ciliary body and is eased by paralysis of these muscles with atropine. The conjunctival hyperaemia that is seen with AAU typically has a circumlimbal or 'ciliary' distribution (around the cornea) whereas that from conjunctivitis produces a diffuse reaction. This hyperaemia is caused by the anastamosis of the conjunctival and uveal circulations around the cornea with overspill of intraocular inflammation producing vasodilation.

Whilst the distinction of ciliary or conjunctival hyperaemia is useful, a severe anterior uveitis may produce such an intense hyperaemia that the whole conjunctiva becomes inflamed. Photophobia is often a prominent symptom. Visual acuity in AAU is affected only if the inflammation within the anterior chamber is sufficient to obscure the media so that patients with mild uveitis will not usually complain of blurred vision. With a less acute or more indolent anterior uveitis there is correspondingly less pain and redness of the eye. The most extreme example of this is seen in the chronic anterior uveitis of childhood associated with *Still's disease*, in which there is a complete absence of pain or redness of the eye and the affected child presents with visual loss from band keratopathy, glaucoma or cataract in a totally white eye.

Commonly, posterior uveitis does not produce a red eye unless there is overspill of inflammation into the anterior chamber producing a panuveitis. Patients usually present with floaters from debris in the vitreous gel or blurred vision from cellular infiltration of the vitreous gel or macular oedema. Occasionally, an intense chorioretinitis involves the macula or the overlying retinal nerve fibre layer to produce a noticeable field defect.

The classical signs of inflammation within the anterior chamber are keratitic precipitations (KP), flare, cells, and posterior synecheiae (Fig. 4). These can only be seen satisfactorily by slit lamp examination. With inflammation of the ocular blood vessels the blood–ocular barrier breaks down causing leakage of leucocytes and protein into the ocular media. Leucocytes ('cells') can be seen within the aqueous humour by an intense narrow slit lamp beam and appear as spots similar to dust in a sunbeam. The increased exudation of protein produces a 'flare' within the aqueous humour which defines the slit beam in a similar way to a car headlight cutting into a foggy night. Cells circulate within the anterior chamber by convection currents to become deposited on the corneal endothelium, frequently in the inferior quadrant where they are seen as KP. With a granulomatous type of uveitis these have a large, pale white globular appearance known as 'mutton fat' KP. The presence of cells correlates with the degree of inflammation within the eye, appearing and disappearing accordingly. Severe inflammation within the eye, however, can produce permanent damage of the blood–ocular barrier and a flare may persist indefinitely as evidence of this process, even after the uveitis has resolved. Severe inflammation within the anterior chamber can lead to leakage of fibrinogen to produce a fibrin clot in the aqueous humour ('plastic uveitis') or such gross leucocyte exudation that a hypopyon is formed by the precipitation of the leucocytes. A hypopyon is a particularly common feature of Behcet's disease.

Posterior synechiae are adhesions between the pupil margin and anterior lens capsule, (Plate 21) which may progress to surround and seclude the pupil preventing dilation and leading to glaucoma

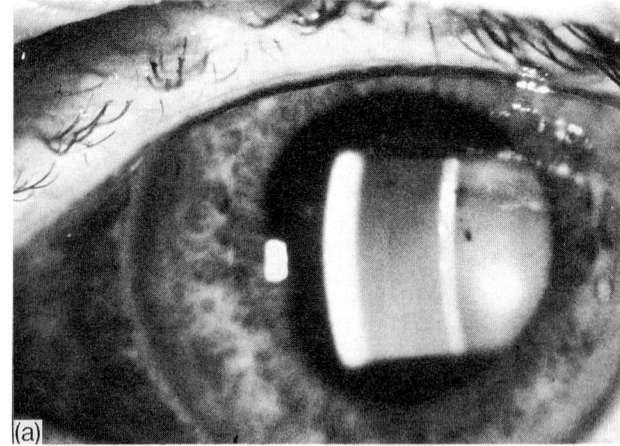

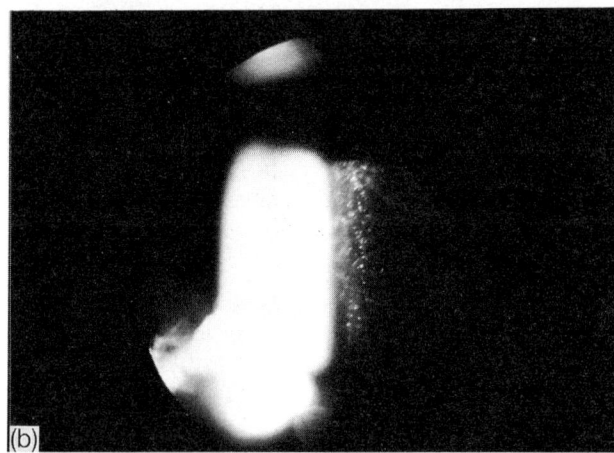

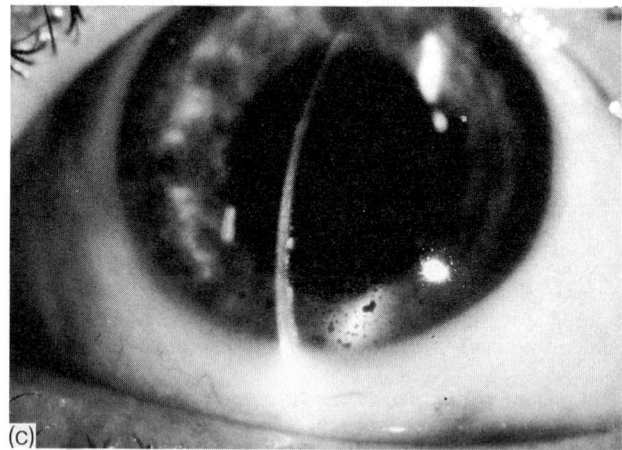

Fig. 4 Inflammatory changes in the anterior chamber. (a) Protein exudation into the aqueous humour indicates breakdown of the blood–ocular barrier and is seen as a 'flare' in the slit-lamp beam. (b) Leucocytes in the aqueous humour seen as particles in a slit-lamp beam. (c) Keratitic precipitates (KPs) are deposits of leucocytes on the corneal epithelium. This patient shows large mutton fat KP in a white eye which is a sign of granulomatous uveitis.

from the restriction of aqueous humour circulation. Their prevention by mydriasis is one of the cornerstones of the treatment of uveitis. Accumulation of cells can sometimes be seen on the iris itself. These are known as *Koeppé nodules* when they appear on the pupillary margin, or *Busacca nodules* when they are seen on the anterior stromal surface of the iris; both types of cellular accumulation are considered to be signs of granulomatous uveitis and disappear without trace on successful control of the inflammation. Discrete swellings within the iris stroma are occasionally seen in 'granulomatous' disease. Vasculitic disease of the radial iris blood vessels can produce sectorial iris atrophy with pupillary spiralling, such iris damage is a particularly common finding in anterior uveitis associated with herpes zoster.

With posterior uveitis the cellular infiltration is limited to the vitreous cavity. This process is the equivalent of that in the anterior chamber but because the circulation is restricted by the viscosity of the gel it is often localized to the area of inflammation, for example, over an area of toxoplasmic chorioretinitis or over the pars plana with an intermediate uveitis. When this cellular debris is located near the retina, the patient notices floaters as it crosses the visual axis, casting a shadow on the retina. Vitreous infiltration can last for a prolonged time and in chronic cases there may be some opacification of the gel by protein exudation and cellular debris. In all cases of posterior uveitis fluorescein angiography shows leakage from the retinal vessels. Further evidence of retinal vascular involvement includes haemorrhages and whitish fluffy perivascular sheathing, occasionally causing vascular occlusion leading to capillary closure with neovascularization and retinal or macular oedema. Vascular involvement almost always affects retinal veins rather than arteries.

Macular oedema can be difficult to diagnose without specialist equipment. It is a common finding associated with many retinal diseases apart from inflammation (e.g. diabetes, venous occlusion). Mild degrees are seen as a blurring of the macular light reflex; in more severe cases cystic spaces can be seen within the macular area. Fluorescein angiography is very useful in demonstrating the clinical severity of leakage as visual acuity correlates poorly with macular oedema.

Visual loss in uveitis

An attack of acute anterior uveitis rarely produces any ocular morbidity but prolonged inflammation, particularly with posterior uveitis or chronic anterior uveitis, is associated with visual loss from cataract, glaucoma or retinal damage due to inflammatory scarring, macular oedema or vascular occlusion and subsequent neovascularization. Visual loss from corneal band keratopathy sometimes occurs in chronically inflamed eyes and this is a well-recognized feature of the chronic uveitis associated with Still's disease.

Some degree of cataract formation occurs in most patients after about two years of chronic inflammation. The earliest changes occur in the posterior subcapsular zone of the lens and eventually progress to maturity with increasing visual loss. Similar morphological cataractous changes are seen as a result of topical or systemic steroid therapy and in many patients this is a contributing factor, although of course, either condition occurs in isolation and this side-effect of steroid therapy does not influence its usage; the risk of visual loss due to uncontrolled intraocular inflammation is greater. Pupillary miosis and posterior synechiae (adhesions of the iris to the anterior lens capsule) enhance the effects of lens opacities by restricting pupillary dilation. Cataract surgery in uveitis calls for careful clinical judgement as there are risks of exacerbating both the uveitis and producing postoperative glaucoma. It is important to control both the inflammation and intraocular pressure as completely as possible prior to surgery and the results are better if the uveitis has 'burnt out'. Glaucoma is a common problem in uveitis, occurring either as a result of the inflammation or its treatment with topical steroids which may induce a chronic glaucoma in genetically susceptible individuals. Neovascularization of the iris with secondary angle closure is an occasional, but devastating complication of severe uveitis, and severe and prolonged intraocular inflammation can result in ocular hypotony from destruction of the ciliary body.

Retinal damage from posterior uveitis can result from direct retinal destruction as part of the primary inflammatory process such as with a retinochoroiditis but the most common cause of

visual loss from uveitis is macular oedema. This is a frequent finding in the presence of posterior uveitis, but the susceptibility of individual patients varies enormously. Some patients develop marked severe macular oedema with even mild inflammation, and occasionally macular oedema is seen with an anterior uveitis although careful examination will always show some degree of vitreous infiltration; others seem to be able to tolerate much more severe inflammation without macular damage.

Specific types of uveitis

Acute anterior uveitis

There are numerous diseases associated with acute anterior uveitis (AAU) but in the absence of other clinical evidence the most common associations in Britain are sarcoidosis, Reiter's syndrome, and ankylosing spondylitis; these diseases only account for about 5 per cent of the total number of cases however. Other entities which present as anterior uveitis are panuveitis or an 'overspill' anterior uveitis from primary posterior segment, corneal or scleral disease. AAU with herpes simplex or zoster is usually diagnosed from the history and findings of associated corneal or cutaneous disease. The routine investigation of a new patient is dictated by the clinical history and findings, and can usually be restricted, in the absence of other clinical indications, to screening by X-rays of the chest and sacro-iliac joints, a blood count, and sedimentation rate. Both tuberculosis and syphilis are rare causes of uveitis these days, but it is important not to forget them. Otherwise, more detailed or sophisticated investigations should be reserved for unusual or atypical cases.

An acute attack of AAU usually starts over a day or two with pain, redness, lacrimation, and photophobia. Uniocular disease is more common than bilateral but the other eye may be the one to be affected in subsequent episodes. The severity of the attack is indicated by the clinical symptoms and signs; very severe attacks may produce a fibrin clot in the anterior chamber which is sometimes known as a 'plastic' uveitis or a hypopyon although this is rare in AAU without associated systemic disease. The fundus should be examined under mydriasis in all patients. A mild cellular reaction in the anterior vitreous gel is not uncommon and is sometimes termed an iridocyclitis; otherwise the examination should be normal, although macular oedema may occasionally be found.

Prompt treatment of AAU with topical atropine and steroids produces relief, the atropine preventing the formation of posterior synechiae and relaxing the painful spasm of the ciliary muscle. An uncomplicated attack of AAU can be expected to resolve over 4–6 weeks of treatment, with a very low risk of visual morbidity, and patients can almost invariably be controlled by topical or subconjunctival steroids without recourse to systemic therapy.

Reiter's disease is the triad of non-specific urethritis or bacillary dysentery with arthritis and ocular involvement either as a conjunctivitis or anterior uveitis. Patients are usually HLA B27 positive and typically young males. The urogenital form of the disease seems to be associated with chlamydial infection and the dysenteric form with shigella, salmonella or yersinia infection. Patients develop acute arthritis and eye signs 1–4 weeks later. Rheumatoid factor is negative and in the majority the disease is a self-limiting acute illness. Approximately 20 per cent of patients with ankylosing spondylitis will suffer an attack of AAU which may be the presenting sign of the disease and the uveitis does not differ in any way to that seen from other causes. Most patients will have up to six to eight attacks in either eye before the disease burns out in later life, which do not correlate with exacerbations of the joint disease.

Definite evidence of the importance of genetic factors in AAU was established when the high association of the HLA B27 tissue antigen with the disease was demonstrated. About 50 per cent of patients with AAU will be positive for B27, whereas the incidence in a control population is in the region of 10 per cent. AAU has an incidence of about 12 per 100 000 in a Caucasian population per year but in B27 individuals the incidence is 1:1300 a year. There is no major difference in acute anterior uveitis between patients with B27 and those without. Other factors must be important: not all B27 people develop uveitis or the other B27 associated arthritides. Conversely, a patient may develop ankylosing spondylitis in association with B27 and may or may not ever suffer an attack of uveitis. No other immunological or serological marker apart from HLA B27 has been specifically identified in patients with AAU. Studies of auto-antibodies, immunoglobulin fractions, immune complexes or T cell subsets show no significant difference from control populations.

Chronic anterior uveitis with Still's disease

About 10 per cent of arthritis in children is indistinguishable from adult rheumatoid arthritis or ankylosing spondylitis, but in the other 90 per cent the disease differs both clinically and pathologically (see Section 16). Juvenile chronic arthritis (Still's disease) can be divided into three main subtypes based on the presentation and pattern of joint disease: systemic, polyarticular or pauciarticular. Ocular involvement is almost always restricted to the pauciarticular type which is the most common form. Both sexes are equally involved, with arthritis limited to less than five joints, usually large joints such as the knee, ankle or elbow.

The pauciarticular type can be divided into early (less than 8 years of age) or late onset and chronic iridocyclitis is most commonly seen in girls with the early onset form. Typically rheumatoid factor is negative in all types but ocular involvement correlates strongly with the presence of antinuclear antibodies (ANA). In a series of 160 patients with juvenile arthritis and uveitis, 95 per cent had a pauciarticular type of disease and 82 per cent were ANA positive. There is no definite correlation with HLA type, but HLA DR5 appears to be associated with an increased risk of ocular involvement.

Affected children usually present with visual loss and chronic anterior uveitis and occasionally the uveitis may precede the joint symptoms. The uveitis may be found at presentation and usually develops within a year of onset of the arthritis, but it is essential that all children with the pauciarticular form, and particularly those with positive antinuclear antibodies, are kept under ophthalmic supervision. Development of uveitis after 5 years of joint disease is unusual. Typically, the uveitis is bilateral and the eye is completely white and painless (Plate 22). Unless the iridocyclitis is picked up by routine examination children present with visual loss from band keratopathy, glaucoma, cataract or macular oedema. Pathology shows that there is an intense inflammation of the iris and ciliary body with plasmacytes and it is likely the other features of the ocular disease are secondary to this process.

The treatment of chronic anterior uveitis is difficult. Most cases are controlled by topical or systemic steroids, but in a few, cytotoxic therapy may be needed. If cataract surgery is required, conventional methods are inadequate and it appears that a lensectomy with partial or total vitrectomy is the treatment of choice, although there is a high incidence of visual loss from macular oedema. Secondary glaucoma is a devastating complication that responds poorly to standard medical or surgical therapy. It is important to remember that sarcoidosis in children can present in an almost identical way to Still's disease, both in the ocular and systemic manifestations.

Herpes zoster

The ophthalmic division of the fifth cranial nerve is particularly susceptible to involvement with herpes zoster (see also Section 5). Attacks of herpes zoster (shingles) can be precipitated by malaise, immunosuppression, or malignant disease, although most patients have no underlying disease. Recurrent attacks or multiple cutaneous nerve involvement are exceptionally rare. *Herpes zoster ophthalmicus* is frequently preceded by pain in the dermatome, which can be severe, followed by cutaneous erythema and vesicles a few days later. Ocular involvement is said to be more common if

the nasociliary branch of the trigeminal nerve is involved as this has an intraocular distribution, but this is not invariable. The cutaneous vesicles are anaesthetic, they appear together in a crop with erythema, oedema, and a toxic reaction, and are sometimes followed by secondary infection. The rash lasts for 10–14 days and heals by scabbing. The patient usually feels very ill and debilitated. Postherpetic neuralgia in the cutaneous distribution of the affected nerve occurs to some extent in most patients but in a few is a permanent and disabling complication.

Ocular involvement tends to be more common and severe with gross cutaneous involvement but this is not always the case and the eye can be affected with mild cases and vice versa. Some degree of conjunctivitis is extremely common and in the first few days may be followed by a corneal stromal keratitis which may persist to become visually disabling. An anterior uveitis is found within a few days in the affected eye in about 40 per cent of patients and can persist for up to 2 years. The initial presentation is usually of a subacute anterior uveitis, frequently with some degree of corneal anaesthesia and the presence of a stromal keratitis, but anterior uveitis is seen in the absence of this. Apart from optic neuritis involvement of the posterior segment is very rare. Pathological material shows that the underlying process in the eye varies from patient to patient and can be a vasculitis with ischaemia, chronic neuritis, arteritis or direct virus invasion of the structures involved.

During the course of the illness, the uveitis tends to become chronic with acute exacerbations. Glaucoma may be a management problem and the intraocular pressure must be monitored. Other occasional ocular findings, apart from the corneal disease and uveitis, are III, IV or VI nerve palsies, scleritis, and late cataract. Optic neuritis is a rare but well-documented association and a contralateral hemiplegia is occasionally seen from vasculitis of the internal carotid artery due to contiguous spread of inflammation within the cavernous sinus.

The conventional treatment of herpes zoster anterior uveitis has been to use topical steroids and atropine which often has to be continued for 1–2 years. It has been suggested, however, that treatment with Acyclovir, orally, in the acute vesicular stage of the rash reduces the risks of subsequent ocular complications and that a mild uveitis is best treated with topical Acyclovir rather than steroids as the inflammation resolves more rapidly with fewer recurrences. These observations await confirmation (see Section 5).

Toxoplasmosis

Toxoplasmosis (see also Section 5) is one of the few uveitic syndromes which can usually be diagnosed from the morphology of the fundus lesion. The reservoir for *Toxoplasma gondii* is in the cat and in humans the parasite has a predilection for neural tissue. Infection is usually caused by transplacental infection of the fetus from a primary infection of a non-immunized mother. In the worst cases the fetus is severely affected with intracranial infection producing mental retardation, hydrocephalus, characteristic intracranial calcification, and retinochoroiditis. More commonly the ocular lesions are the only manifestation of congenital infection and these are circumscribed chorioretinal scars in the posterior pole of one or both eyes (Plate 23). They are usually densely pigmented with areas of atrophy and well-defined edges and vary from a quarter to about three to four disc diameters in size; they may be isolated or multiple in the same eye. Acuity is affected if the macula or its fibres are involved, but otherwise the scars produce an arcuate field defect of which the patient is usually unaware. These quiescent lesions are signs of previous retinochoroiditis and need no active treatment.

Further disability from the disease is caused by the reactivation of retinochoroiditis at these sites. This usually occurs in or adjacent to a previous congenital scar and is seen as a white exudative area with overlying vitreous cellular infiltration, sometimes with considerable exudative retinal periphlebitis. Reactivation in a

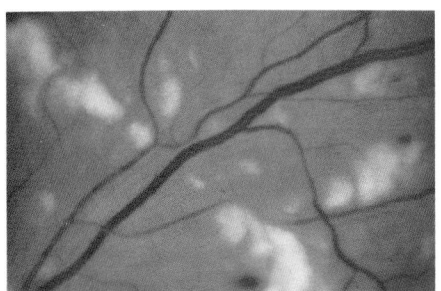

1 Fresh cotton wool spots are seen in the retinal nerve fibre layer. They represent micro-infarcts with blockage of axoplasmic transport.

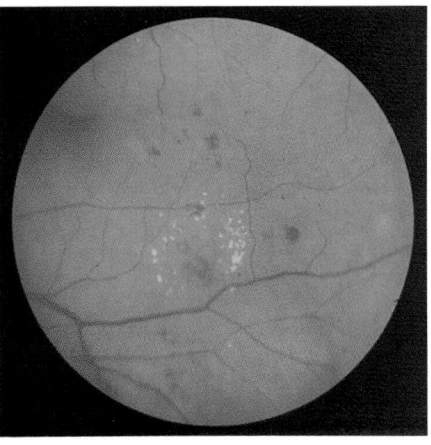

2 Lipid exudates are seen surrounding a microvascular abnormality in a diabetic eye with a typical circumferential or circinate pattern, further accumulation leads to plaque formation.

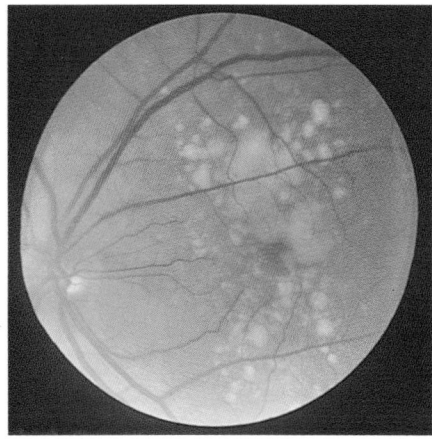

3 Drusen are a common finding in the aging Caucasian eye. They lie at the level of the retinal pigment epithelium and lead to senile macular degeneration from either atrophic changes or subretinal neovascularization (disciform macular degeneration).

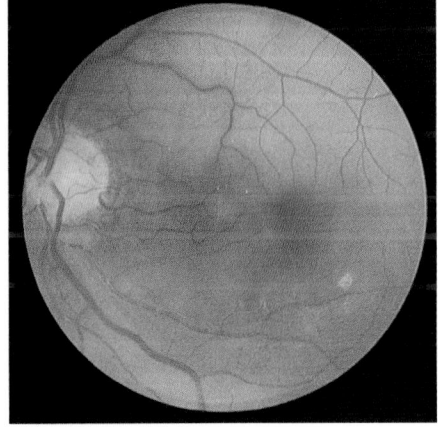

4 Acute central retinal artery occlusion. Multiple cholesterol emboli are seen in the retinal circulation. A patch of retina temporal to the disc is spared from infarction by its cilioretinal arterial supply.

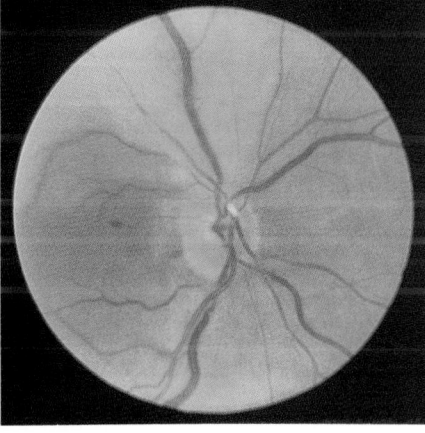

5 Superior temporal branch retinal arterial occlusion by a globular white calcific aortic valve fragment, seen in the vessel on the optic disc.

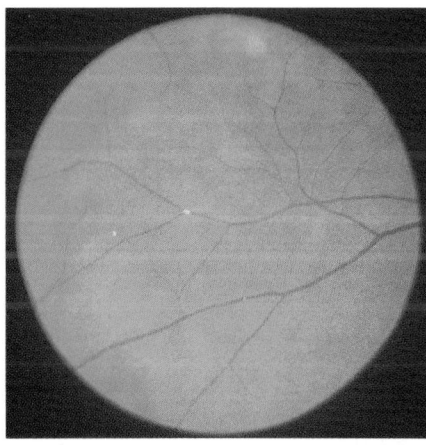

6 A cholesterol embolus lying at the bifurcation of a retinal artery. Such crystals have a planar morphology and may not completely occlude the vessel.

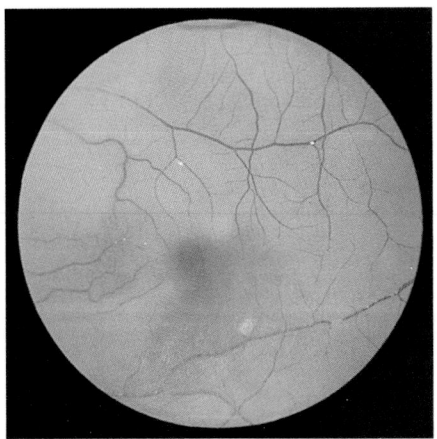

7 Platelet emboli are seen in the inferior temporal artery in another view of Plate 4. They have a whitish broken linear morphology and pass slowly through the vessel. A cholesterol embolus can be seen in the superior temporal artery.

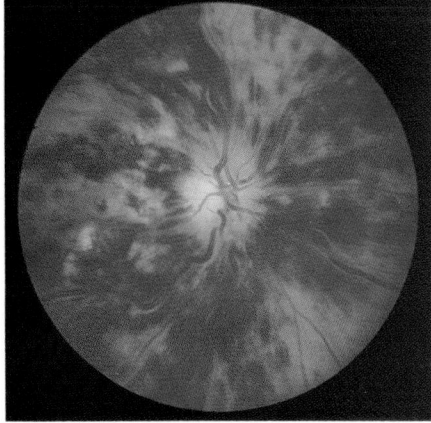

8 Recent central retinal vein occlusion with marked nerve fibre layer and deeper retinal haemorrhages. Cotton wool spots temporal to the disc indicate retinal ischaemia.

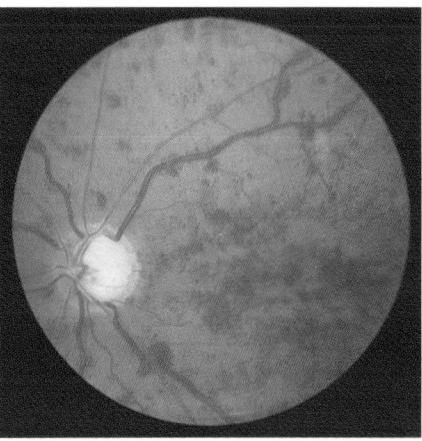

9 Central retinal vein occlusion with glaucomatous cupping of the optic disc.

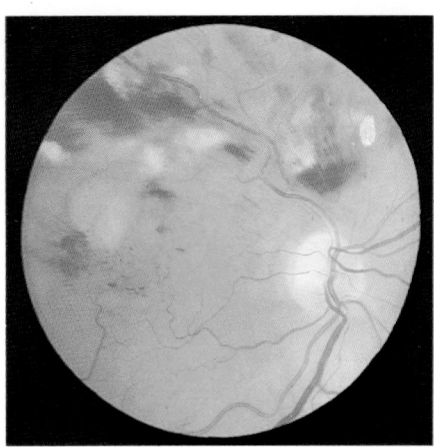

10 Occlusion of the superior temporal vein at an arterio-venous crossing just above the optic disc. Blotchy brown haemorrhage and cotton wool spots indicate retinal ischaemia. Fluorescein angiography demonstrated marked capillary closure.

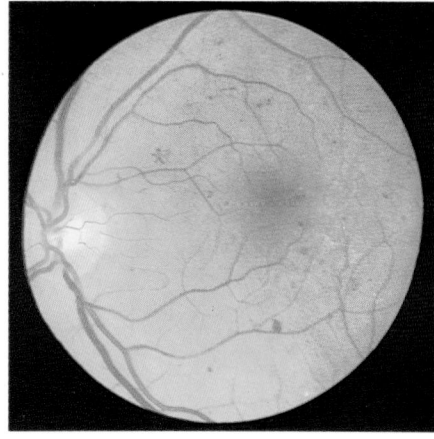

11 This fundus shows an early 'dot and blot' background diabetic retinopathy.

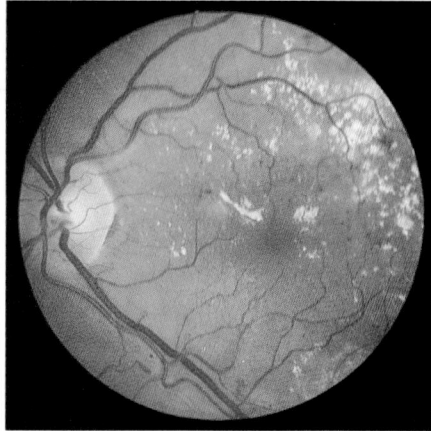

12 (a) This fundus shows an exudative background retinopathy with early macular improvement.

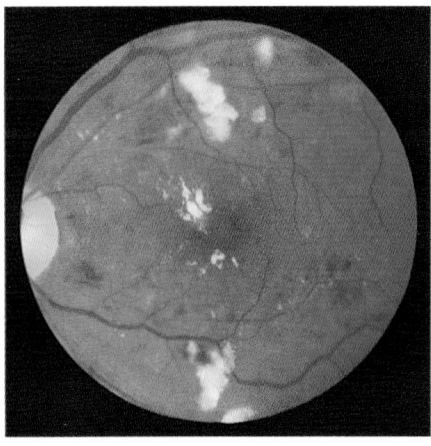

12 (b) This patient shows early exudative changes into the macula area but the presence of cotton wool spots indicates retinal ischaemia as well.

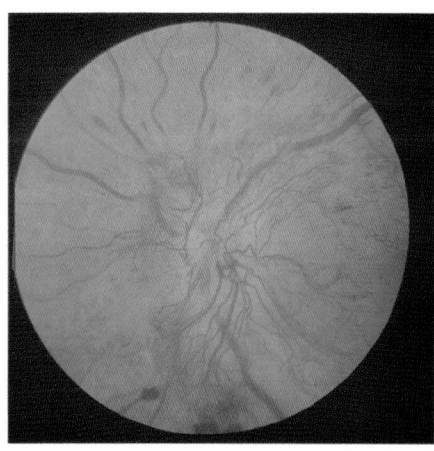

13 (a) Florid neovascularization of the optic disc indicates a very poor prognosis.

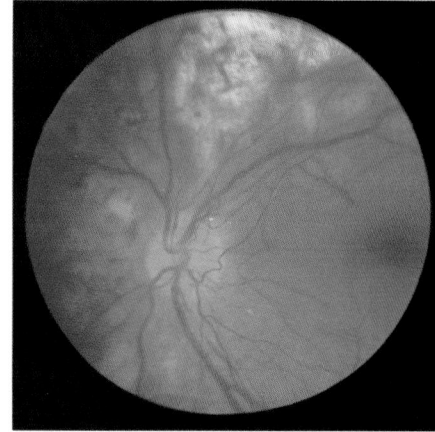

13 (b) Following heavy photocoagulation neovascularization has regressed although abnormal but mature vessels remain on the disc.

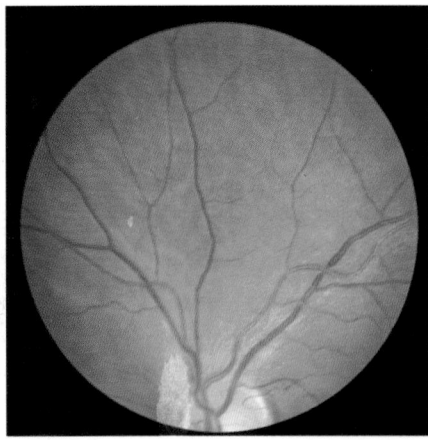

14 Early hypertensive changes in the fundus of a 40-year-old man show a heightened light reflex of the superior temporal artery, some irregularity of vessel calibre and changes where the artery crosses over the vein.

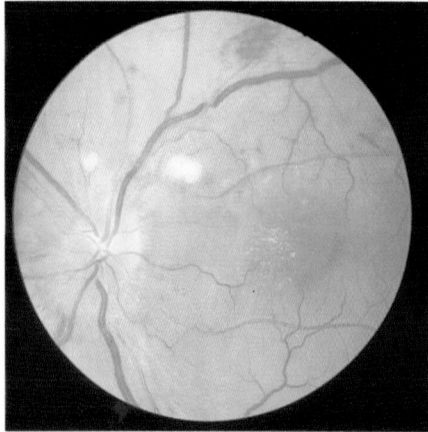

15 This fundus shows marked arterial hypertensive changes, (constriction, irregular calibre, crossing changes), cotton wool spots, flame-shaped haemorrhages, with hard exudate in the macula and early swelling of the optic disc, compatible with accelerated hypertension.,

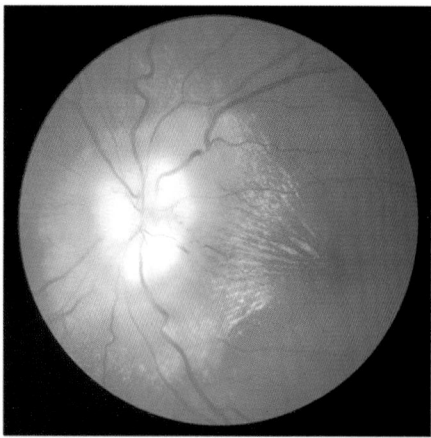

16 A pale infarcted optic disc in a Negro eye with a pronounced macular star.

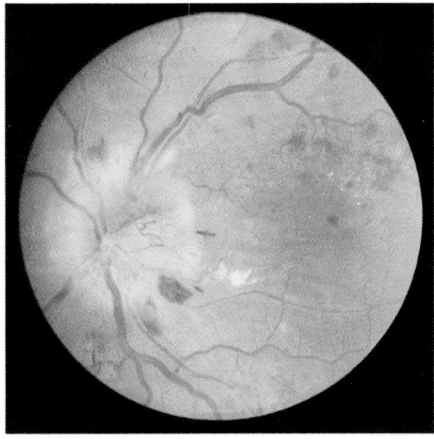

17 Florid optic disc swelling and hypertensive retinopathy. Choroidal folds indicate the disc has been swollen for some time.

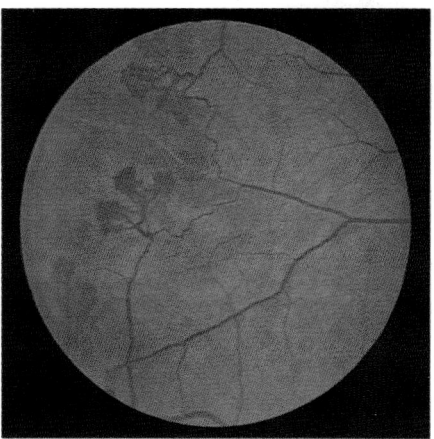

18 Sickle cell retinopathy. Early neovascularization of the peripheral retina has the appearance of 'seafans'. Abnormal shunts are present and beyond the neovascularization a large artery is white and sclerosed.

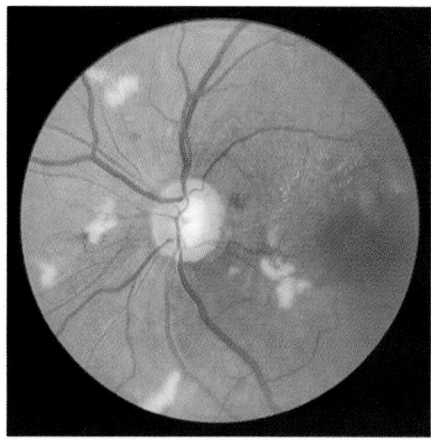

19 Multiple cotton wool spots in a Negro with systemic lupus erythematosis.

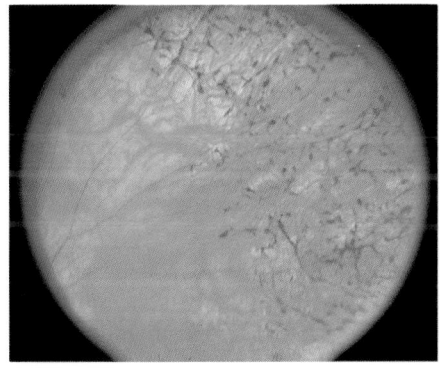

20 Peripheral intraretinal bone corpuscular pigmentation with retinitis pigmentosa. This is a classic example but the morphology of the pigmentation can vary widely.

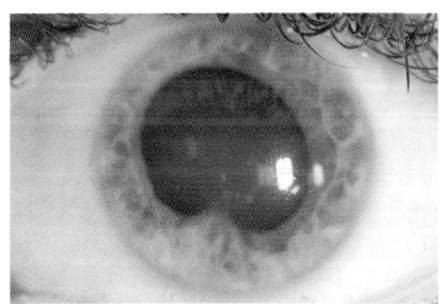

21 Posterior synechiae are adhesions between the iris and anterior lens surface which festoon the pupil on dilation. Ring adhesions are a serious complication of uveitis which are prevented by adequate pupillary dilation.

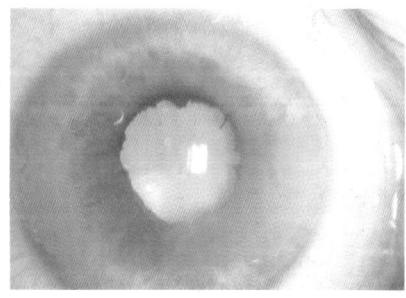

22 Cataract and early corneal band keratopathy in a patient with Still's disease. Note the eye is white and the presence of circumferential posterior synechiae. (Patient of Mr J Kanski.)

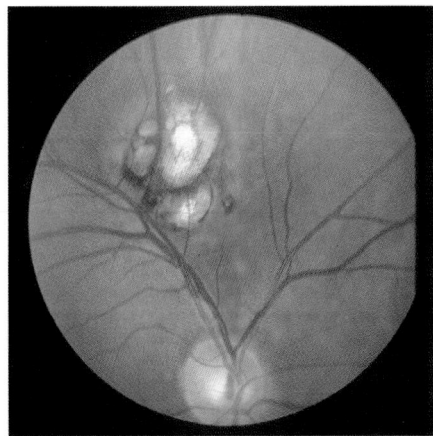

23 Inactive chorio-retinal scarring from congenital ocular toxoplasmosis.

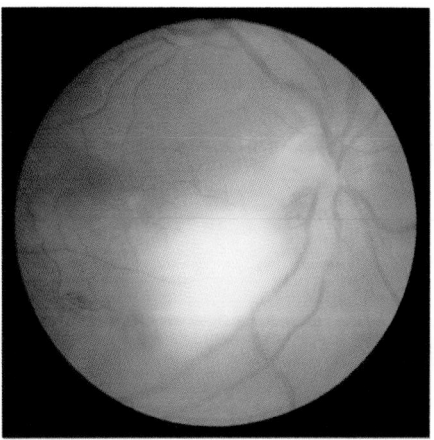

24 Active toxoplasmic chorio-retinitis, more commonly reactivation occurs in an area with marked pigmentary scarring.

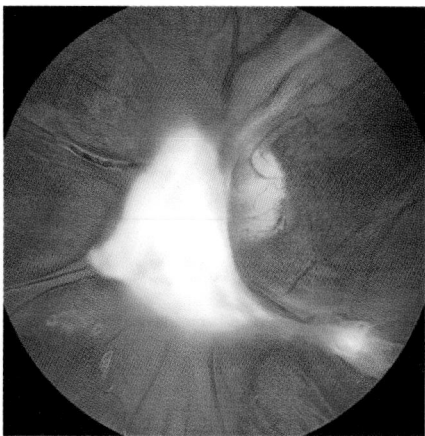

25 A preretinal granuloma with retinal traction in a 12-year-old girl with ocular toxocariasis.

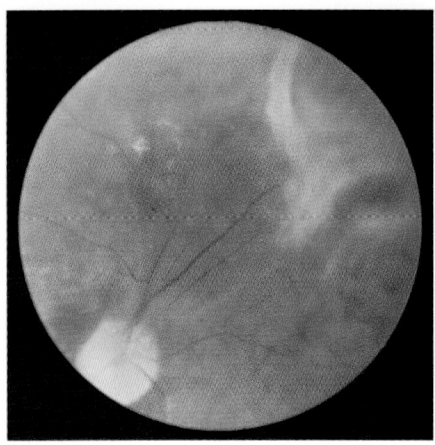

26 Long-standing chorio-retinal scarring from congenital syphilitic retinopathy.

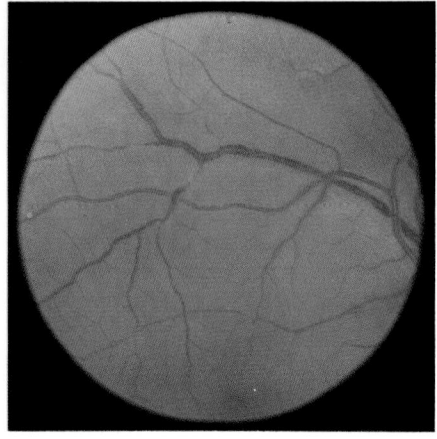

27 An inflammatory periphlebitis in a patient with sarcoidosis. The superior temporal vein has an irregular calibre with areas of fluffy white periphlebitis.

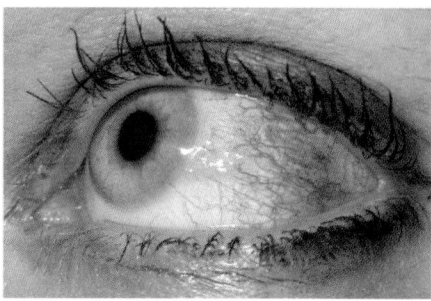

28 Episcleritis is seen as a localized red and slightly tender area on the bulbar surface.

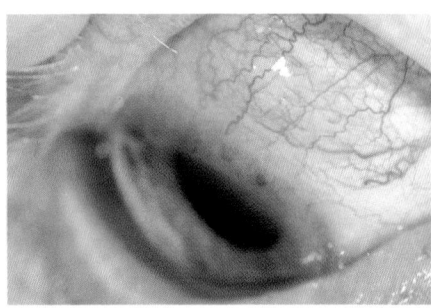

29 Scleritis produces localized redness and oedema of the sclera. Pain is a useful diagnostic sign but differentiation from episcleritis can be difficult without slit lamp examination.

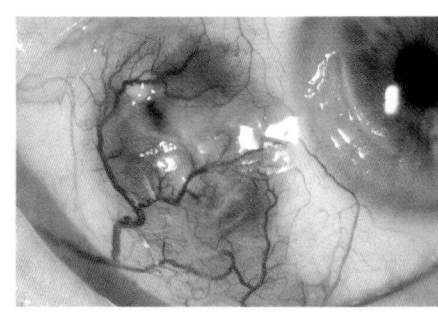

30 Scleromalacia perforans in a long-standing seropositive rheumatoid patient. Note the lack of inflammation, the scleral melting to expose the choroid, and guttering of the adjacent cornea.

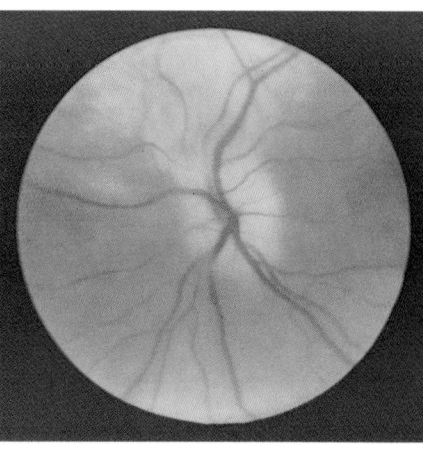

31 Anterior ischaemic optic neuropathy is the most common cause of visual loss in temporal arteritis. This optic disc shows the acute changes of a pale, mildly swollen disc in a blind eye from infarction of the disc by arteritis in the short posterior ciliary arteries.

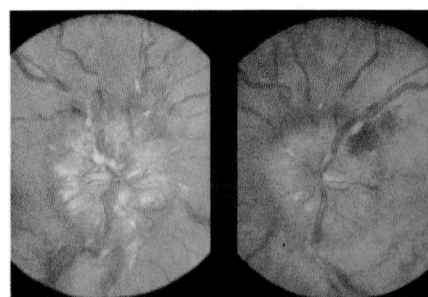

32 Acute decompensated papilloedema. The marked disc oedema with florid haemorrhages and cotton wool spots demonstrate that the patient has suffered a rapid and severe rise in intracranial pressure, probably within the last few weeks. Visual acuity and fields are normal.

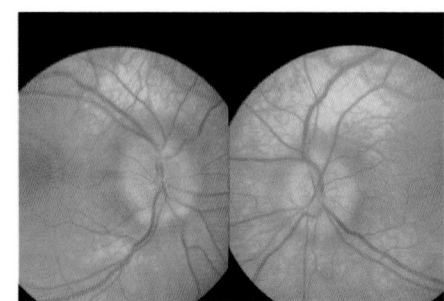

33 These discs are swollen and pale and the absence of haemorrhages and cotton wool spots suggests that the intracranial pressure has been raised for several months. Pallor indicates that nerve fibre loss and therefore field loss is occurring but acuity remains normal at this stage.

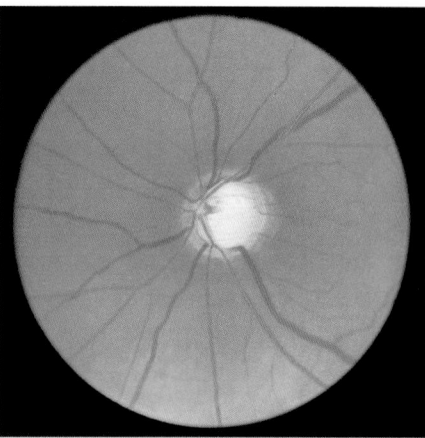

34 Severe glaucomatous cupping in chronic simple glaucoma. There is vertical enlargement of the optic cup and hooking of the superior and inferior temporal vessels as they cross over the disc margin.

lesion leads to further retinal damage from direct invasion by the parasite with a secondary inflammatory response. Toxoplasmosis does not appear to be associated with posterior or anterior uveitis in the absence of focal retinal lesions but occasionally an area of active retinochoroiditis occurs in the absence of previous retinal scarring and this is presumed to be due to reactivation at the site in the retina of a previous subclinical lesion (Plate 24). Reactivation can occur at any site and a common place is adjacent to the optic disc. This characteristic lesion was known as juxtapapillary choroiditis and in the older literature was ascribed to a tubercular origin: toxoplasmosis is now recognized to be the most common cause.

Acquired toxoplasmosis in the non-immunized adult can be associated with a febrile illness, lymphadenopathy, and hepatosplenomegaly, and serological testing of the adult population indicates a high incidence of previous toxoplasmic infection, most of which must be due to subclinical disease. Retinal involvement with acquired toxoplasmosis is very rare but has been proven to occur.

The diagnosis of toxoplasmic eye disease is made on the findings of characteristic fundus lesions and positive serology indicating previous toxoplasmic infection (see Section 5). The toxoplasma dye test is specific but results of serological titres do not correspond to the level of activity of ocular disease. Thus low serological titres are compatible with active retinochoroiditis and there is a documented case where titres of 1:1 were found in the serum and yet histological examination of the eye confirmed the presence of *Toxoplasma gondii*. Thus any level of positivity in the serum demonstrates that the patient has been exposed to toxoplasmosis in the past. In a prospective study of the incidence of congenital toxoplasmosis in non-immunized mothers, a serum dye test conversion rate of 1 per cent was found during pregnancy. Eighty per cent of these pregnancies produced children with ocular lesions and of these affected children 40 per cent had visual loss in one eye attributable to toxoplasmosis. However, no child had bilateral visual loss nor did any child have neurological sequelae. These findings indicate the high degree of infection of the fetus but the relatively low risk of visual or neurological morbidity.

Toxoplasma gondii is sensitive to sulphonamides (sulphadiazine) and pyrimethazine but early trials of treatment with these drugs did not seem to confer any advantage. The disease usually runs a self-limiting course, resolving over a period of months with further retinal scarring. Some authorities suggest that if the macula is threatened systemic steroids are indicated to reduce the destructive inflammatory response. Whilst this is often helpful, a few cases deteriorate while on steroids and some untreated patients develop a severe endophthalmitis. *Toxoplasma gondii* is sensitive to clindamycin and it would appear from animal work that treatment for 3–4 weeks with this drug alone or in combination with sulphadiazine is more effective in limiting retinal damage and speeding recovery.

Toxocara

The life cycle and mode of transmission of this nematode is described in detail in Section 5.

In humans, *Toxocara canis* produces either a systemic illness (visceral larva migrans) or ocular disease. Both are uncommon. Visceral larva migrans is seen in young children usually of 1–4 years of age who present with a systemic illness. Ocular involvement is very uncommon with this illness but is seen in older children (4–8 years of age) without a history of systemic disease. Ocular disease is unilateral. In the eye the larva produces either preretinal or subretinal granulomas which lie at the posterior pole or periphery (Plate 25). Posterior uveitis is usually low grade although some patients develop a chronic endophthalmitis. Vision is lost from direct macular involvement with the granuloma, or from retinal traction or posterior uveitis. Diagnosis of toxocara infestation is made by an enzyme-linked immunosorbent assay (ELISA) test which can be performed on the serum or aqueous humour. Serum tests have to be interpreted with caution as a sig-

nificant number of the normal population have positive titres and these may not correlate with ocular findings (cf. toxoplasmosis): a case has been reported of a 4-year-old child presenting with leucocoria and a low ELISA titre of 1:4 in whom a typical larva was found on histological examination of the eye.

Most cases of ocular toxocarasis settle to leave an inactive granuloma in a quiet eye. Systemic steroids have been advocated for chronic endophthalmitis. Antihelmintic drugs do not appear to be helpful, but there has been recent interest in the role of virectomy in cases with chronic endophthalmitis or visual loss from retinal traction. The most important differential diagnosis of leucocoria, other than toxocara, in this age group is retinoblastoma.

Syphilis

Syphilis (see also Section 5) was once considered to be a common cause of uveitis, but since the Second World War the incidence has declined and the disease is now comparatively rare. In recent years, however, an increase has been seen again particularly in the homosexual population and the disease must always be borne in mind because of its potentially serious complications. Ocular disease is seen with early and late congenital syphilis and secondary syphilis; optic atrophy and pupillary abnormalities are features of late neurological disease.

Congenital syphilis is rare. Infected children can present with fulminant congenital syphilis at birth or signs of early secondary syphilis. A diffuse chorioretinitis can occur at this stage but this is rarely seen in the active phases by an ophthalmologist and the diagnosis is made later in life by the appearance of the fundus, together with the history and serology. The retinal changes are characteristically bilateral and show diffuse patchy atrophy and hypertrophy of the retinal pigment epithelium, sometimes known as the 'pepper and salt' fundus. The severity of the fundus appearance varies widely and can stimulate retinitis pigmentosa with optic atrophy and retinal vascular attenuation (Plate 26). The differential diagnosis is usually easy to make by the association of other stigmata of congenital infection such as nerve deafness, nasal and dental deformities with positive serology. Visual function is normally very much better than would be expected with a similar degree of fundus change from retinitis pigmentosa. Late congenital syphilis develops in an apparently normal child in the 5–30 year age group. The ophthalmic hallmark is active interstitial keratitis and iritis, chorioretinitis appears to be less common at this stage.

Syphilitic uveitis is seen as a feature of acquired secondary syphilis, either accompanying the skin rash or independently preceding or succeeding it. It is particularly important to think of the diagnosis in an atypical or indolent anterior uveitis, especially in homosexuals or those with a military, naval or travelling background. Secondary syphilis also produces changes in the posterior segment which can vary widely. There is usually a mild cellular reaction in the vitreous and signs of optic nerve involvement such as papillitis or ischaemic anterior optic neuropathy are common. Frequently, there is evidence of subretinal inflammation at the same time with small discrete palish yellow lesions at the level of the retinal pigment epithelium and serous retinal detachment with subretinal fluid in the posterior pole. Syphilitic uveitis readily responds to standard treatment with penicillin and systemic steroids.

Tuberculosis

Ocular involvement with tuberculosis occurs as a result of direct infection of the uveal tract or as an immunological reaction to the infection elsewhere in the body (see also Section 5).

Choroidal tubercles are a feature of miliary tuberculosis. The acute lesions are subretinal, slightly elevated yellowish lesions about a quarter of a disc diameter in size and are not often seen by the ophthalmologist at this stage as the patient is usually moribund. In the healed phase the chorioretinal lesions become atrophic pigmented scars which are not distinguishable from other causes of multiple foci of choroiditis.

Hypersensitivity to tuberculosis has a special place in the history of uveitis. At one time syphilis and tuberculosis were thought to be responsible for a substantial number of cases of uveitis, but over the years tuberculosis has become a much less recognized association. This is due to the decreased prevalence of the condition in the western world, a better appreciation of the role of skin testing with PPD, and a more critical appraisal of the natural history of the disease and its treatment. Tuberculosis is, however, associated with a granulomatous chronic iridocyclitis or occasionally a retinal vasculitis. In the United States the concept of testing patients with a chronic iridocyclitis by a Mantoux test has been popularized. Those with a strong reaction are given a 'therapeutic trial' of a three-month course of isoniazid; some patients' eyes undoubtedly improve and they are then assumed to have a tuberculous uveitis and given formal chemotherapy. There are both practical and theoretical problems with this approach which cannot be applied to the British population where the vast majority have already been vaccinated with BCG and will therefore already have a positive Mantoux test. There is also a possible risk that short courses of treatment with only one chemotherapeutic agent might lead to the development of a resistant bacteria with potentially grave implications.

Tuberculosis can occasionally be associated with a retinal vasculitis, presumably due to some type of hypersensitivity mechanism; genetic factors appear to be important as many of these patients are of Asiatic origin. Retinal veins are affected and florid changes can lead to vascular occlusion and later retinal neovascularization which may present after the inflammatory signs have subsided.

Peripheral neovascular retinopathy (Eales' disease) is especially common in India and it is possible that some racial or genetic hypersensitivity to tuberculosis exists to account for this (see Section 21).

Intermediate uveitis

This is a common ocular disease which occurs in children and young adults. The diagnosis is made on the clinical findings and it is probably the most common type of posterior uveitis. The name is synonymous with *pars planitis*, *peripheral uveitis*, *chronic cyclitis* or other pseudonyms, and recently '*intermediate uveitis*' has become the approved term in an attempt to standardize the uveitis terminology.

Patients present with an insidious onset of floaters from vitreous debris or blurred vision from macular oedema. The disease is usually bilateral, but may be asymmetrical or unilateral. The eye is white with a quiet anterior chamber or a few cells and flare, though a few patients have a more marked anterior uveitis. The vitreous gel shows a cellular infiltrate. In some patients accumulation of cells known as 'snowballs' are seen in the inferior vitreous gel and others have a 'snowbank' of white cellular exudate overlying the inferior pars plana. There may be low-grade vascular sheathing of the peripheral retinal veins or small pigmented scars in the peripheral retina and there may be mild swelling of the optic disc consistent with a posterior uveitis. Most patients have a good visual prognosis, the disease burning out after a number of years. Visual loss occurs in the minority from macular oedema, haziness of the vitreous gel or cataracts with long-standing disease, and occasionally from vitreous haemorrhage or retinal detachment. In the majority of patients, there is no systemically associated disease but a few patients are found to have sarcoidosis or multiple sclerosis.

Behçet's disease

The classical signs of this disease are the triad of oral ulceration, genital ulceration, and uveitis but the disease has a multisystem spectrum and skin changes, arthritis, venous thrombosis, bowel, and neurological involvement can be found (see Section 24).

Ocular movement is seen in 75 per cent of patients and is the most serious feature of the disease. Anterior uveitis is the most widely recognized feature but involvement of the posterior segment is almost universal and is responsible for the blinding complications. Patients present with posterior uveitis or panuveitis. Hypopyon formation is a noticeable feature of the anterior uveitis in some patients. It tends to occur repeatedly throughout the illness and, in contrast to HLA B27 associated disorders, the hypopyon often appears in a relatively white eye. The posterior uveitis is severe and diffuse. Macular oedema is a common cause of visual loss but the disease is distinguished from other causes of posterior uveitis by the retinal features which can be so characteristic as to suggest the systemic diagnosis. In acute exacerbations, patches of infiltration are seen in the superficial retina. These occur as creamy white polymorphic leucocytic infiltrates in the superficial layers of viable retina, either in the posterior pole or equatorial areas, and not directly related to large retinal vessels. These lesions evolve and resolve over a period of several weeks, leaving apparently normal retina, with little retinal pigment epithelial scarring. Branch vein occlusion is common and in the presence of posterior uveitis should suggest the diagnosis of Behçet's disease. It is frequently followed by capillary closure and the devastating complications of neovascularization, vitreous haemorrhage or retinal detachment. Progressive retinal destruction is seen with time, and in the terminal stages the fundus appearance is of optic atrophy and gross attenuation of retinal arteries and veins with comparatively mild retinal pigmentary scarring.

If the ocular complications are untreated the visual prognosis is not good, most patients becoming blind within 3–4 years of the onset. Men are said to have a worse outlook than women. Systemic steroids may be helpful in controlling the inflammation but most patients require cytotoxic therapy as well. Azathiaprine, colchicine or chlorambucil appear to be the drugs of choice and careful management of the steroid and cytotoxic therapy improves the visual prognosis although the side-effects of treatment can be severe. More recently cyclosporin A has been used successfully in the management of Beçhet's disease and may offer great future potential.

Ocular involvement is associated with the HLA B5 antigen and in particular the BW51 subtype and patients with this tissue type have a × 6 relative risk factor. The racial distribution of this antigen and the disease has been attributed to the spread to the antigen by the nomadic tribes along the old silk routes. No virus has been identified consistently in the oral or cutaneous lesions but there is indirect evidence that herpes simplex virus may play a role. High levels of circulating immune complexes are also found in the serum of patients and probably play some part in the pathogenesis.

Sarcoidosis (see Section 5)

Ocular involvement occurs in about 25 per cent of patients and is seen as either infiltration of the ocular adnexa, intraocular inflammation or infiltration of the retrobulbar visual pathways. Most ocular disease presents in the early phases of acute systemic sarcoidosis and new ocular manifestations become less common two years after the onset or in the chronic stages of the disease.

Involvement of the adnexa is most frequently seen as cutaneous infiltration of the lids, conjunctivae or lacrimal glands. Circumscribed and discrete granulomas within the orbit are very rare, as is myositis of the external ocular muscles. Orbital signs can occasionally be seen as an orbital apex or superior orbital fissure syndrome due to involvement of the apex by granuloma.

Lacrimal gland involvement is probably more common than is recognized. With acute disease the gland can be bilaterally infiltrated, enlarged and palpated through the skin although it is usually asymptomatic. Biopsy of the gland can be performed to confirm the diagnosis, but if necessary this should be performed through the skin rather than the conjunctiva as this can damage the lacrimal ductules and potentially cause a dry eye in a situation where this is already a risk. Gallium scanning shows lacrimal uptake in up to 75 per cent of patients with acute sarcoidosis and in most of these patients the gland is not palpable. Lacrimal infiltration may also occur with salivary gland infiltration (*Mikulizc's syndrome*) or uveo-parotid fever (*Heerfordt's syndrome*). Dry eyes are unusual in the acute phase, presumably because the accessary glands maintain tear secretion, but a few patients develop dryness with the chronic fibrotic stages of the disease.

Cutaneous involvement of the lids can be seen as discrete skin granulomas, lupus pernio, or sometimes as pearly 'millet seed' granulomas along the lid margin which provide an opportunity to obtain a biopsy. Conjunctival involvement more commonly affects the inferior fornix where it produces a chronic follicular type of change. Biopsy of apparently normal conjunctiva sometimes shows histological changes and 'blind conjunctival biopsy' has its advocates as a useful test in patients where the diagnosis of sarcoidosis is in doubt.

Sarcoidosis may produce either an anterior or posterior uveitis. Anterior uveitis is usually a feature of the acute stage of the disease associated with erythema nodosum, and most patients will have a uveitis of sufficient activity and severity to produce symptoms, but a chronic anterior uveitis of the type seen with Still's disease can rarely occur. The anterior uveitis may be acute or chronic, granulomatous or non-granulomatous. Most patients will have bilateral disease, but unilateral or asymmetrical involvement is well recognized. An anterior uveitis with granulomatous KP, nodules on the iris, or iris stromal infiltration should suggest the possibility of sarcoidosis. Involvement of the angle of the anterior chamber by granulomas on the trabecular meshwork has been said to be common and diagnostic of sarcoidosis; glaucoma may present in these patients but usually intraocular pressure is normal.

Posterior uveitis may occur in the absence of anterior uveitis. It is responsible for most of the visual morbidity and may take on a variety of patterns such as intermediate uveitis, retinal vasculitis or localized infiltration of the choroid or optic disc. The classical pattern is of retinal periphlebitis (Plate 27). Small vessel involvement is reflected by a retinopathy characterized by retinal haemorrhages and cotton wool spots but most patients show some signs of larger retinal venous disease as well. This typically involves the small equatorial veins and in its most marked form is seen as a focal fluffy white perivascular cuffing (candle wax dripping) which can progress to venous occlusion, peripheral closure, and retinal neovascularization. Involvement of the central retinal vein or retinal arteries is uncommon. Some degree of vitreous infiltration is always found on careful examination of patients with retinal vasculitis but the degree of vascular involvement can be difficult to identify and in these patients fluorescein angiography is of great help in demonstrating subclinical foci of retinal phlebitis.

Optic disc swelling can be a common feature of any posterior uveitis and with sarcoidosis can be due to local tissue oedema, local infiltration by granulomatous tissue in the disc or papilloedema from neurosarcoid with raised intracranial pressure. In most patients it is a reflection of posterior uveitis and resolves; sarcoidosis is an important differential diagnosis of bilateral or unilateral optic disc swelling of unknown aetiology. All such patients require careful examination of the vitreous for cells which will provide evidence of an inflammatory aetiology.

Aquired immune deficiency syndrome (AIDS)

The acquired immune deficiency syndrome was first recognized in promiscuous American homosexuals in the early 1980s when outbreaks of *Pneumocystis carinii* pneumonia, Kaposi's sarcoma, and other opportunistic infections occurred in the homosexual population of California and New York. With the identification of the clinical syndrome, it became immediately apparent that patients suffered a severe and widespread defect of cellular immunity with cutaneous anergy, lymphopenia, depletion of T helper cells, and an increased ratio of T suppressor to helper cells. In 1984, Gallo and colleagues identified the virus HTLV-3 as the cause of the syndrome (now also known as human immunodeficiency virus, HIV). Transmission of the disease is through sexual or haematogenous contact and the disease has now reached epidemic proportions in homosexuals, drug addicts, and haemophiliacs, although it appears to have been endemic in Central Africa in the heterosexual population for many years. The incubation period appears to be from a few months to two years but only a minority of infected persons appear to develop the clinical disease of AIDS.

Patients are susceptible to a limited range of viral, bacterial, and fungal infections such as herpes zoster and simplex, mycobacteria, *Pneumocystis carinii*, toxoplasma, candidiasis, cryptococci, cytomegalovirus infections as well as Kaposi's sarcoma. Some patients develop a dementia during the illness due to HTLV-3 viral encephalopathy. Persistent generalized lymphadenopathy affecting lymph-nodes in more than one extra-inguinal site for over 3 months in the absence of any other cause occurs in some patients. Patients develop fatigue, weight loss, malaise, and fever, and once the disease is clinically manifest the outcome appears to be fatal.

Ocular complications of AIDS are well recognized. The HTLV-3 virus can be identified in tears and corneal tissue which has marked implications for sterilization of ophthalmic equipment or corneal transplantation. So far, however, there is no evidence of infection through tear secretions and the chances of infection by this route appears to be low. Kaposi sarcoma lesions can be seen in the conjunctiva. Herpes zoster ophthalmicus has become a well-recognized feature.

A retinopathy is a frequent occurrence at some stage in the illness. Patients may develop cotton wool spots which do not differ in any way from those seen in other conditions. Histological examination has failed so far to show evidence of viral infection in these lesions and it has been postulated that they are microinfarcts from high levels of circulating immune complexes. Cotton wool spots appear to be a poor prognostic sign both for further ocular problems and for the life expectancy of patients. Cytomegalovirus retinitis is the most common ocular infection although ocular infections such as herpes simplex retinitis, toxoplasmosis, cryptococcus, and mycobacterium avium intracellulare have been reported. In a study of autopsy eyes from 75 patients with AIDS, Holland and colleagues found cotton wool spots in 65 per cent of the eyes, no micro-organisms or viral particles could be found in these lesions. Cytomegalovirus retinitis was the only common infection found and 28 per cent of the cases had a cytomegalovirus retinopathy. They hypothesized that the retinal microvascular changes predisposed to cytomegalovirus infection by allowing access of viral particles to the retina from breakdown of the blood–ocular barrier during viraemia.

Treatment of cytomegaloviral infection with AIDS is unsatisfactory. The infection responds to dihydroxy propoxymethyl guanine (DHPG) but the retinopathy relapses after treatment with further retinal destruction. Maintenance chemotherapy has been used to prevent relapse but the logistics of arranging daily treatment are often insurmountable and the efficiency is unproven.

Vogt–Koyanagi–Harada syndrome

This is rare in the West but represents about 8 per cent of endogenous uveitis in Japan. The racial incidence is related to tissue type antigens HLA BW54, DWa, DR4, and MT3. BW54 and DWa are specific Japanese antigens and MT3 carries a 75 per cent increase in relative risk. It has been suggested that non-oriental patients frequently have some oriental ancestry and this appears to be borne out by the fact that many American patients with the disease have some American Indian blood. The disease has seasonal peaks of incidence in the spring and autumn.

The clinical picture is of acute bilateral granulomatous panuveitis in patients in the 20–50 year old age range, sometimes preceded by a few days of prodromal illness with nausea, headache, orbital pain, and meningism. In some patients the uveitis is less marked and retinal pigment epithelial changes predominate. In the acute phase, serous retinal detachments or pigment epithelial detach-

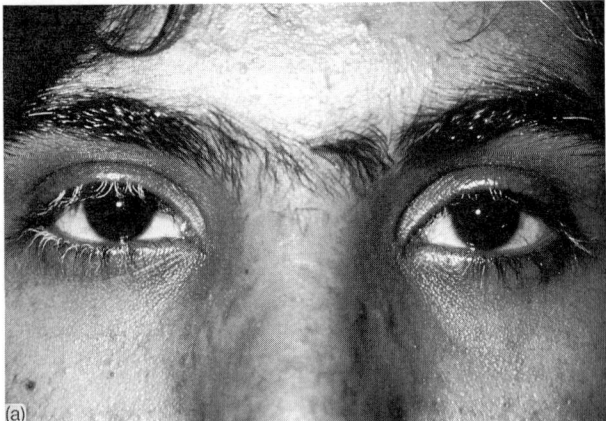

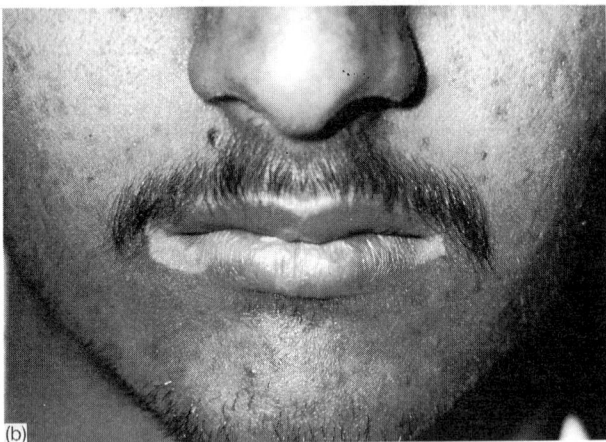

Fig. 5 Vogt–Koyanagi–Harada syndrome. (a) Poliosis of the eyelashes. (b) Vitiligo of the lips.

ments are common and a spotty yellowish disturbance of the retinal pigment epithelium can often be seen in the posterior pole. The disease has clinical and pathological similarities to sympathetic ophthalmitis which is seen after perforating injuries of the eye.

In the acute stages, patients may have dysacousia, which is usually mild, meningism, and a lymphocyte pleocytosis of the CSF. In the recovery phase vitiligo and poliosis (white eye lashes, brows or patches of hair) can be found as well as localized areas of alopecia (Fig. 5). Patients respond to systemic steroids and the disease has a better visual prognosis than sympathetic ophthalmitis, usually subsiding over a period of months although relapses can occur.

Uveitis with neurological disease

Neurological symptoms with inflammatory eye disease are seen with neurosarcoidosis, Behçet's disease, Vogt–Koyanagi–Harada syndrome, Whipple's disease, and multiple sclerosis (MS) as well as with the recognized bacterial, parasitic, and viral infections which affect the nervous system (see Section 21 also.)

Peripheral periphlebitis in the eyes of MS patients with 'snow balls' in the vitreous overlaying the retina was first described by Rucker at the Mayo Clinic. Further studies have confirmed that this occurs in about 10 per cent of patients, probably being under-diagnosed as the peripheral retina is not frequently carefully examined by neurologists. Intermediate uveitis and granulomatous iridocyclitis are also found in a few patients with MS. Characteristically, the retinal periphlebitis is peripheral, low grade, and asymptomatic with a mild cellular reaction in the vitreous; vascular occlusion and obliteration are not seen.

Bowel disease with uveitis

Various types of inflammatory eye disease have been reported in association with bowel disease (see also Section 12); the dysenteric form of Reiter's disease has already been mentioned. Ocular complications of ulcerative colitis appear to be extremely uncommon and in some reports it is possible that the diagnosis of ulcerative colitis and Crohn's disease have been confused, with the ocular disease being wrongly attributed to the former. Crohn's disease is associated with a wide range of ocular manifestations and it has been estimated that up to 10 per cent of patients will have some eye manifestation. Episcleritis is the most common sign, scleritis is less common, and a destructive subepithelial keratitis has been described which has preceded overt abdominal disease and led to the diagnosis of the bowel disease being made. Both iridocyclitis and choroiditis can occur and the inflammatory signs fluctuate with the activity of bowel disease and clear up with its surgical excision. Whipple's disease is an exceptionally rare bowel disease due to infiltration by an unknown bacterial species. Papillitis or choroiditis may occur with or without associated neurological involvement. Ocular disease clears up when the bowel disease is treated with the appropriate broad-spectrum antibiotic. The parasite *Giardia lamblia* has been found in the faeces of a few patients with retinal arteritis and iridocyclitis which has been unresponsive to steroid treatment but has improved on treatment with antiparasitic drugs.

Retinal vasculitis

This is diagnosed by the presence of a posterior uveitis with signs of retinal vascular involvement indicated by fluffy white perivascular sheathing of retinal vessels and retinal haemorrhages. In the eye a vasculitis almost always affects the retinal veins and retinal arterial involvement is uncommon and usually a sign of diseases such as syphilis, systemic lupus erythematosus, polyarteritis nodosa or toxoplasmosis. Severe periphlebitis may lead to venous occlusion, peripheral vascular closure, and retinal neovascularization. The most common associations of retinal vasculitis in clinical practice are sarcoidosis and Behçet's disease, but in the majority of cases no systemic disease is found. These patients are sometimes described as having *Eales' disease* – retinal vasculitis of unknown aetiology. Inflammatory retinal vasculitis with neovascularization must be differentiated from neovascularization associated with metabolic disease (diabetes), haemoglobinopathy or severe ocular ischaemia from carotid artery disease.

Episcleritis and scleritis

Both of these conditions cause localized redness on the bulbar conjunctiva. Episcleritis is a benign self-limiting condition seen in young adults which may be bilateral. The patient presents with ocular discomfort, soreness or a gritty feeling, and a watery discharge; the pain is not severe and there is no photophobia. Examination shows a localized patch of redness on the globe which may have a nodular or diffuse pattern and is slightly tender to pressure over the eyelids (Plate 28). Slit lamp examination shows that the inflammation lies in the connective tissue underlying the conjunctiva and over the sclera (in Tenon's capsule). Episcleritis is not associated with serious systemic disease and responds readily to treatment with topical phenylbutazone ointment or steroids.

In contrast, scleritis is painful, and has serious ocular and systemic associations. The condition is usually much more painful than episcleritis and this is a helpful diagnostic feature. Severe inflammation may be accompanied by keratitis, photophobia or uveitis. The disease is seen in four basic patterns: diffuse, nodular or necrotizing anterior scleritis, and posterior scleritis. Examination of the globe shows a deep localized redness with oedema of the sclera and overlying episcleritis and conjunctival injection (Plate 29). This can be blanched by a drop of 1:1000 adrenalin to demonstrate the deeper scleral changes more clearly. Scleritis is due to vasculitis and is associated with collagen disorders such as systemic lupus erythematosus, Wegener's granuloma, polyarteritis nodosa or 'vasculitic' rheumatoid arthritis, and may sometimes be seen in association with other conditions such as Crohn's disease, herpes zoster or localized trauma. Posterior scleritis is located behind the equator of the globe and the patient usually presents with a unilateral intensively painful eye with a variable amount of conjunctival oedema, redness, proptosis, and limitation of ocular movement. Vision may be affected if the optic nerve is involved or if the inflammation spreads forwards into the eye to produce an exudative retinal or choroidal detachment. Scleritis usually requires systemic treatment to control the inflammation which resolves with thinning of the sclera to produce a greyish area from increased visualization of the underlying choroidal pigmentation.

Sclero-malacia perforans is a necrotizing anterior scleritis without overlying inflammation which is an unusual feature of longstanding seropositive rheumatoid arthritis and is due to an occlusive vasculitis with infarction and melting of the sclera (Plate 30). The appearances are dramatic but perforation of the globe is rare although most patients lose vision from ocular complications.

The optic disc

The optic disc is 1.5 mm in diameter and contains about 1.2 million nerve fibres passing from the retinal ganglion cells to their synapses in the lateral geniculate body (approximately 30 per cent of the afferent input to the brain). Retinal axons are unmyelinated but become myelinated at the cribriform plate; the absence of photoreceptors at the disc produces the blind spot lying in the temporal visual field 10–15° from fixation. Optic disc swelling can be produced by a large number of causes such as congenital abnormalities, raised intracranial pressure, infiltration, ischaemia or inflammation, and an accurate diagnosis can only be made from the history and physical signs. Similarly, optic atrophy can be produced by a wide variety of causes such as genetic disease, demyelination, compression or ischaemia and it is impossible to diagnose the cause of a pale disc by the morphology alone. The only instance when this is possible is when the optic atrophy is secondary to other retinal disease (e.g. retinitis pigmentosa) and therefore the previous classifications of primary or secondary optic atrophy have no relevance in present neuro-ophthalmology.

Ischaemic optic neuropathy

This is usually a disease of the 50–70 year old age group presenting as unilateral painless visual loss of sudden onset in a white eye. The condition is due to infarction of the short posterior ciliary arteries which supply the optic disc (see above) and although patients often have evidence of other atherosclerotic disease it frequently occurs in otherwise apparently healthy people. Visual loss is usually partial. Acuity is lost if macular fibres are involved. The superior hemisphere of the disc is usually affected, producing has an inferior attitudinal field defect. Other physical signs are reduction in colour and brightness sensation and a relative afferent pupillary defect. In the acute stages there is asymmetrical pallid swelling of the disc, frequently being paler superiorly with greater hyperaemia, and swelling and haemorrhage inferiorly where the remaining viable nerve fibres are compromized. Swelling subsides over 6–8 weeks leaving asymmetrical atrophy of the disc; the predilection of the superior part of the optic disc to the inferior is unexplained. The fellow eye is subsequently affected in a substantial number of patients. In the elderly patient, all systemic investigations are invariably normal and non-contributory but in younger patients, infarction of the disc may be associated with migraine, syphilis, collagen disorders etc. and full investigation is essential.

The systemic manifestations of temporal arteritis are discussed in Section 16. The posterior ciliary arteries are very susceptible to involvement and infarction of the optic disc is the most common ocular presentation of the disease, central retinal artery occlusion being comparatively unusual. Arteritic infarction of the disc is frequently the presenting sign of temporal arteritis. These discs are pale and mildly swollen with few haemorrhages. (Plate 31) and the eye is usually completely blind, in contrast to the non-arteritic

type. Visual loss is permanent but the condition should be treated as a medical emergency with high-dose steroids as there is a grave risk of the second eye becoming involved and blind within hours of the first. Temporal arteritis may also present to the ophthalmologist as an isolated third or sixth nerve palsy.

Papilloedema

Optic disc swelling can be due to a wide variety of causes and papilloedema is now used to imply optic disc swelling from raised intracranial pressure and therefore excludes other causes of a swollen disc so that the term has important implications in the neuroradiological investigation and management of the patient. Some patients with well-developed papilloedema are asymptomatic but others complain of headache, particularly on waking in the mornings, which vary in severity and localization. Nausea may be present. Obscurations of vision are fleeting episodes of visual loss in one or both eyes lasting a few seconds before the vision returns to normal and when present are pathognomic of established papilloedema with serious visual implications if untreated. Sixth nerve palsy can occur as a false localizing sign and other symptoms and signs depend on the cause of the raised intracranial pressure. It is important to appreciate that papilloedema does not produce either loss of visual acuity or field until it has been present for many months and atrophic changes have begun to develop. Enlargement of the blind spot is seen in established papilloedema and is due to the disc swelling masking surrounding photoreceptors.

The primary pathology in papilloedema is of hold up of orthograde oxoplasmin transport, producing dilation of the axons with secondary effects from venous stasis and oedema.

The optic disc appearances reflect the acuteness, severity, and duration of raised intracranial pressure. Papilloedema may be classified into early, acute, chronic or atrophic types. The earliest changes are seen as thickening of the retinal nerve fibres, particularly on the superior, inferior, and nasal aspects of the disc, which is due to hold up of axoplasmic transport. Venous pulsation can be seen on 80 per cent of normal discs and its absence is a useful but soft sign of raised intracranial pressure. The early nerve fibre changes are followed by increasing elevation, venous engorgement, and flame-shaped haemorrhages, which are restricted to the vicinity of the disc (cf. central retinal vein occlusion). In acute established papilloedema there is obvious disc swelling with surrounding flame-shaped haemorrhage, cotton wool spots, and dilation of the superficial capillary plexus. The retinal veins are engorged and often disappear into the swollen nerve fibres as they leave the disc. As the raised intracranial pressure becomes chronic the disc changes show less haemorrhage and cotton wool spots (Plates 32 and 33). Choroidal folds and optic ciliary shunt vessels may appear and small white glistening and refractable bodies can be seen on the disc surface. This is sometimes called 'vintage' papilloedema. Finally, and after many months duration disc pallor begins to appear, there is progressive field constriction eventually leaving the patient with tunnel vision. Visual acuity remains good until the terminal stages. At this time the disc is pale, optico-ciliary vessels shunt the venous return to the lower pressure choroidal circulation and the disc swelling decreases. This is because the disc swelling is due to axons engorged by axoplasmic material; optic atrophy implies axonal loss and therefore there are fewer axons remaining to swell. Following control of raised intracranial pressure, the disc changes resolve over 6–8 weeks.

Early papilloedema is difficult to diagnose and serial observation of the disc aided by fundus photography and fluorescein angiography is of great use in demonstrating progressive changes. CT scanning has removed much of the morbidity from the neuroradiological investigation of papilloedema and high resolution CT scanners now demonstrate tortuosity and enlargement of the optic nerve sheath distended by the CSF.

It is important to be aware that a number of benign ophthalmic conditions can simulate papilloedema and ophthalmic advice is important in the assessment of difficult or unusual cases of disc swelling.

Congenital abnormalities such as glial remnants, hypoplasia or asymmetry of the disc and hypermetropia can all simulate disc swelling. Many of these produce characteristic changes in size and shape of the disc with anomalous vascular patterns and absence of a physiological cup. Drusen of the disc (a condition unrelated to retinal drusen) is characterized by elevation of the disc, anomalous vascular pattern, absence of a physiological cup, and exposed hyaline bodies on the disc surface. It is a benign ocular condition, sometimes dominantly inherited, which is occasionally associated with a field defect and frequently produces a difficult diagnostic problem. CT scans or ultrasound show the diagnostic presence of calcification in the nerve head. Other causes of pseudopapilloedema are infarction of the disc, infiltration, and inflammatory disorders with posterior uveitis.

Papillitis

Inflammation of the optic nerve head produces optic disc swelling and this distinguishes papillitis from retrobulbar neuritis. Papillitis is usually unilateral and is characterized by rapid visual loss usually over 1–3 days with visual acuity often reduced to levels of 6/60 or to counting fingers. The typical patient is a young adult and papillitis is more common in females. Pain on ocular movement and tenderness of the globe to retropulsion are useful signs but may not be as marked as with retrobulbar neuritis. Other physical signs are loss of brightness and colour sensation and a relative afferent pupillary defect. Visual field examination shows a central scotoma which is often most easily identified by a confrontation field test with a red target. Disc swelling is usually mild and cannot be distinguished ophthalmoscopically from that due to papilloedema (except that it is unilateral). Visual recovery takes place over 2–4 weeks to give virtually normal function, although there is often considerable pallor of the optic disc with loss of retinal nerve fibres ophthalmoscopically and subtle tests show a residual visual deficit.

In adults the most common cause of papillitis is demyelination. Retrobulbar neuritis is a more common presentation of this and carries a risk of 50–70 per cent of developing multiple sclerosis on long-term follow-up. Some authorities suggest that if a patient presents with papillitis there is a lesser risk of subsequent multiple sclerosis, but papillitis is less common than retrobulbar neuritis and no long-term studies are available. No treatment influences the visual recovery or eventual prognosis although systemic steroids are often prescribed. In the individual case there is no means of forecasting the long-term prognosis but tissue typing, oligoclonal bands in the CSF, and nuclear magnetic resonance scanning seem likely to indicate prognostic factors in the future. As no treatment is of any help there is little need to investigate the typical case extensively, although a neurological examination and visual and auditory evoked potentials are useful in diagnosing subclinical demyelination. CSF examination can be helpful. In other patients papillitis can be associated with an upper respiratory viral type of illness. Patients, however, who do not make a full visual recovery require complete investigation to diagnose more unusual causes of papillitis such as syphilis, collagen disorders, local orbital or sinus disease or compressive lesions of the optic nerve.

In children, papillitis may present as an unusual manifestation of the exanthemata. It is usually bilateral and visual loss may be marked but the condition is benign. Visual recovery is usually excellent and there is no long-term risk of multiple sclerosis.

Other eye diseases of general medical importance

Dry eyes

Mild tear deficiency produces symptoms of a gritty sensation, redness, and soreness, and many patients have associated blepharitis from staphylococcal infection of the eyelash follicles; more severe disease renders the patient unable to cry (e.g when peeling onions). Severe dryness is a most distressing and blinding disease as the corneal epithelium loses its integrity and transparency and the eye is at risk of being lost from corneal ulceration and secondary infection which is often exacerbated by conjunctival scarring leading to upper or lower lid entropion.

Mild tear deficiency is most commonly associated with *Sjögren's syndrome*, typically seen in elderly ladies with rheumatoid arthritis. Other collagen diseases may be associated with dryness but the most common cause of dry eyes with untreatable blindness worldwide is conjunctival scarring from *trachoma*. Chronic staphylococcal conjunctivitis and blepharitis may sometimes lead to severe dryness as do chemical burns of the eye from ammonia. Other causes are drugs such as practolol, cyclophosphamide or prolonged idoxuridine therapy for herpes simplex keratitis. Severe conjunctival scarring and dryness may result from previous mucous membrane ulceration with Stevens–Johnson syndrome. 'Benign' mucus membrane pemphigoid produces progressive conjunctival ulceration and scarring in the elderly, systemic features are often comparatively minor and overlooked being restricted to the mouth and anus. Sarcoidosis may occasionally destroy the lacrimal glands but this is not common. Thyroid eye disease produces alterations in the composition of the tear film and its mucus and symptoms of ocular irritation are common in these patients which are exacerbated by corneal exposure with proptosis.

Traditionally, *Schirmer's test* (saturation of blotting paper strips inserted under the lids) has been used by physicians to diagnose tear deficiency but it is a very poor test. Many patients will have symptoms of dryness with an apparently adequate Schirmer's test and this is because the tear film is a complex tripartite structure of fluid providing nutrition, mucus as a wetting agent, and oily secretions which reduce evaporation from the eye. Any disturbance in this balance may produce symptoms and the best way to assess the adequacy of tear production is to observe the tear film on the slit lamp and stain the conjunctiva with rose bengal dye which stains desiccated epithelium and mucus. Excessive mucus may become attached to the corneal epithelium producing long filaments which are intensely irritating (filamentary keratitis).

Simple treatment of dryness is by tear film replacement with a substitute drop. There are many proprietary types and it is worth trying a number to find the most suitable for each patient. More severe symptoms can be greatly alleviated by cautery of lacrimal puncta to retain the residual secretions, and treatment within the conjunctival sac. G Acetyl cysteine is often helpful in breaking down excessive mucus in the tear film.

Thyroid eye disease (ophthalmic Graves' disease)

Thyroid eye disease (see also Section 10) is the commonest cause of unilateral or bilateral proptosis. The primary pathology lies in the external ocular muscles which become enlarged by lymphocytic infiltration and oedema; the signs of the disease are a direct result of this process and its effects on the surrounding soft tissues and optic nerve. Thyroid eye disease can occur in euthyroid, hypothroid, and hyperthyroid patients and the severity of the eye signs do not correlate with the degree of hormonal abnormality or bear any temporal relationship to other aspects of the disease. Patients may present with eye signs and develop hormonal problems later or not at all, other patients develop orbital disease many years after thyroidectomy or radio-iodine treatment. About 70 per cent of patients with orbital disease will have a biochemical abnormality, an abnormal TRH test being the most consistent finding. Autoantibodies to thyroid constituents are found in many patients but do not correlate with orbital disease. Muscular enlargement can be readily seen on orbital CT scans (Fig. 6) and this is now the diagnostic technique of choice, allowing a firm diagnosis to be made and excluding other causes of proptosis. External ocular muscle is different from skeletal muscle and recently monoclonal antibody techniques have demonstrated a circulating soluble IgG

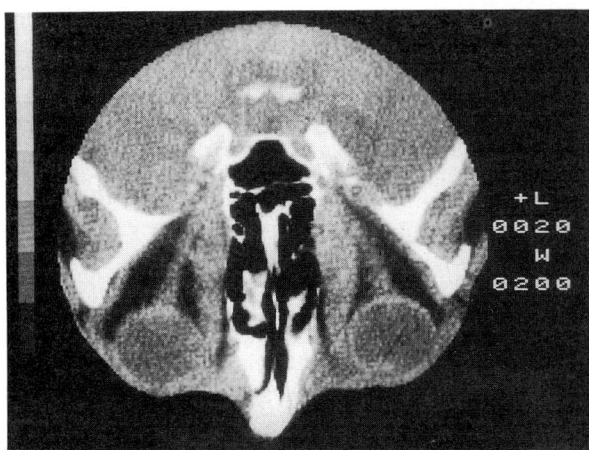

Fig. 6 Thyroid ophthalmopathy. Marked hypertrophy of the medial rectus muscle can be seen in each orbit. Optic nerve compression is produced by muscular hypertrophy within the tight orbital apex.

antibody to ocular muscle which seems likely to have a pathogenetic role, though the significance of this is not understood as cellular immune mechanisms are probably important as well.

The clinical signs of thyroid eye disease are proptosis which is axial (i.e. along the visual axis) and which is often asymmetrical and occasionally unilateral. The degree of proptosis is easily measured clinically with an exophthalmometer. Lid-lag and lid retraction are consistent clinical signs although both may be seen in anxious normal patients. Lid retraction is due to overaction of Müller's muscle in the upper and lower lids and is demonstrated by exposure of the sclera above and below the cornea on forward gaze. Swelling and oedema of the lids is often noticeable and this is probably due to inflammation and increased orbital pressure interfering with drainage of extracellular fluid. In the acute case lid oedema may be pronounced and associated with conjunctival hyperaemia and oedema as well. Orbital tension can be assessed by ballotting the globes under closed lids into the orbit. Normally the globe can be retropulsed against a soft orbital fat pad with ease but marked resistance to retropulsion is found with thyroid eye disease. In a congested orbit dilated blood vessels can be seen over the external ocular muscle insertions. The clinical problems are due to cosmetic effects from the proptosis and lid retraction and corneal, muscular, and optic nerve involvement. These may be graded but such systems are artificial as they tend to imply a continuity of orbital disease from the trivial to the severe which is not found in clinical practice: severe optic nerve compression, for example, is often found in the presence of mild proptosis. *Malignant exophthalmos* is a term given to the rare situation of acute proptosis and chemosis where there is a risk of losing sight from corneal ulceration or optic nerve compression and these patients may require an urgent orbital decompression to control their disease.

Many patients are young females and the cosmetic problems associated with the disease should not be underestimated. Lid retraction may be alleviated by guanethidine drops but these are often irritating for the patient. Lateral tarsorraphy can help and other surgical procedures are available to lower the lids, particularly the upper lid, very satisfactorily. In the United States orbital decompression is sometimes performed for cosmetic reasons alone.

Corneal exposure is usually seen in those patients with acute onset of disease with marked proptosis and chemosis as in most long-standing cases, the lids compensate to cover the cornea adequately. Mild corneal exposure can be demonstrated by staining with fluorescein and can be treated with lubricating ointment or drops, marked proptosis can progress to ulceration and loss of the eye, and in these patients the cornea should be protected by tarsorraphy, lid surgery or orbital decompression.

Many patients with mild orbital disease complain of ocular irritation and this is not always due to corneal exposure as alteration in tear film metabolism occurs which produces abnormal wetting of the eye. Staining with Rose Bengal dye sometimes produces a characteristic pattern on the conjunctiva superior to the cornea known as superior limbic keratitis. These patients are usually helped by a lubricating eye drop.

Double vision is common. The inferior recti are the most commonly affected muscles and fibrotic changes here can tether the globe, limiting up-gaze, and causing vertical diplopia. The fibrotic muscle indents the globe on up-gaze producing a transient rise in intraocular pressure which is a helpful confirmatory sign. CT scanning shows that involvement of all other external ocular muscles is common and management of the resulting diplopia is a difficult problem. Some patients can be managed with Fresnel prisms in their spectacles, others require surgery after the double vision has stabilized over several months.

Optic nerve compression is one of the most serious and poorly diagnosed complications which often occurs in patients with comparatively mild proptosis (those with marked proptosis tend to decompress their own orbit). The swollen ocular muscles crowd the optic nerve at the orbital apex. Patients lose visual acuity in association with a field defect (usually central), relative afferent pupillary defect, and colour loss; the optic disc may be normal, swollen or atrophic. Because of the insidious nature of the visual loss it is important to enquire whether a patient with thyroid eye disease has noted any visual deterioration at each consultation. Systemic steroids will control the optic nerve compression in many patients, but failure to respond at acceptable dosages is an indication for orbital decompression, the operation of choice being a medio-inferior approach to decompress the orbit into the ethmoidal, sphenoidal, and maxillary sinuses. Results of this type of surgery are good although diplopia can be produced or exacerbated. Orbital radiotherapy, cytotoxic agents, and plasmaphoresis have been used for thyroid eye disease with dubious results.

Strabismus (squint)

Concomitant squints are those seen in childhood which develop from a failure to establish and maintain the normal binocular reflexes. Typically, the deviation between the two eyes remains constant and does not vary with the direction of gaze. The child does not complain of diplopia, has no binocular visual reflexes, and frequently has an associated amblyopia of one eye (poor visual acuity in a structurally normal eye with normal visual field, colour vision, and pupillary reflexes). Treatment is concerned with preventing amblyopia, cosmetically realigning the visual axes and trying to establish binocular vision, although this latter aspect is rarely achieved. In contrast, a paralytic or incomitant squint is due to a III, IV, or VI palsy, restrictive tethering of an ocular muscle, myasthenia gravis, etc. (see Section 21). The angle of deviation between the two eyes varies with the direction of gaze (i.e. if a patient has a left VI palsy the angle of deviation and symptoms of diplopia are most pronounced on left gaze and will be normal on right gaze). If a squint develops after maturation of the binocular reflexes at 6–7 years of age, the patient complains of diplopia. Paralytic squints are unusual in childhood and tend to result from serious acquired disease; ophthalmic assessment is directed at identifying the affected muscles with the appropriate neurological investigations.

Occasionally, a patient will present with a decompensated concomitant squint. These patients are usually teenagers or older and usually complain of diplopia. Helpful symptoms will be a history of childhood treatment or surgery for squint or an associated head posture that has developed to compensate for the ocular deviation. Ophthalmic investigations will demonstrate abnormally weak binocular reflexes, amblyopia or sometimes an excessive binocular fusional range that has been used to control a deviation between the two eyes that can no longer be maintained.

It is important to realize that many paediatric ocular diseases will present initially as a squint and any patient with a suspected squint should be referred for ophthalmic examination to exclude serious intraocular defects.

Glaucoma

Glaucoma implies a raised intraocular pressure above the normal level of 22 mm Hg. Congenital glaucoma (buphthalmos) is rare and is seen as a result of an isolated ocular developmental defect or sometimes as a feature of neurofibromatosis or the Sturge–Weber syndrome.

Acquired glaucoma is divided into three basic categories: acute closed angle glaucoma, chronic simple glaucoma or glaucoma secondary to other ocular problems. *Acute closed angle glaucoma* is an ocular emergency and it is essential to start hypotensive treatment within the first 24–48 hours if a satisfactory visual outcome is to be achieved. It is typically a disease of the elderly female and only occurs in younger people with structurally abnormal eyes. The disease is caused by physical obstruction of the trabecular meshwork by the peripheral iris and typically occurs in hypermetrophic eyes with shallow anterior chambers and a 'narrow' drainage angle. When the pupil dilates the symptoms are of visual loss, pain, redness, polychromatic haloes, and photophobia, and the signs are a very hard eye with conjunctival hyperaemia, typically in a ciliary distribution, corneal oedema, and a semidilated pupil fixed to light and accommodation. Patients frequently have had prodromal symptoms leading up to the attack of episodes of rainbow coloured haloes around polychromatic white lights and redness or pain. Treatment lies in rapidly lowering the intraocular pressure medically and then performing an iridectomy to relieve the pupil block which is the cause of the condition. There is a substantial risk of the same disease developing in the fellow eye and a prophylactic iridectomy is usually performed on that eye during the acute illness.

Chronic simple glaucoma presents very differently but is, too, a disease which occurs most commonly in the elderly. The disease is a triad of raised intraocular pressure, cupping of the optic disc and typical patterns of visual field loss. It is caused by chronic obstruction to outflow of aqueous humour within the trabecular meshwork. It is a very common cause of blindness in the elderly and occurs in a completely asymptomatic white eye. The effects are insidious and only in the late stages does the patient notice loss of visual field and acuity. Intraocular pressures are raised but at lower levels than with acute glaucoma (20–30 mm Hg as against 50–70 mm Hg). This produces glaucomatous cupping of the optic disc and typical patterns of visual field loss. Visual field loss is insidious over many years and visual acuity tends to remain normal until the terminal stages. Glaucomatous cupping of the optic disc is diagnosed by observing the disc under mydriasis to look for the early signs of enlargement of the normal physiological cup along the vertical axis, an asymmetrical neuroretinal rim with sectorial pallor, and the more advanced signs when retinal blood vessels hook under the disc margin as they cross to enter or leave the eye (Plate 34). Treatment relies on reducing the intraocular pressure to normal levels by topical or systemic medication, laser trabeculoplasty or surgery.

Secondary glaucoma is a feature of a wide variety of intraocular conditions which produce an increase in intraocular pressure by numerous mechanisms such as inflammation, haemorrhage, iris neovascularization or seclusion of the pupil with inflammatory adhesions.

Cataracts

Cataract is a generic term for denaturation of the lens proteins producing an opacity within the lens which may vary in severity from insignificance to severe visual loss. With a mature cataract the lens becomes completely opacified and is seen as a white mass behind the iris. The location of early lens opacities may be anywhere within the lens and the visual effects depend on their encroachment on the visual axis and proximity to the nodal point, (the optical centre of the eye just posterior to the lens). For this reason, an opacity in the posterior subcapsular area (a very common site for cataract formation seen, for example, in steroid-induced cataracts) has a particularly devastating effect on vision whereas a similar opacity placed more anteriorly in the lens will have a less marked visual effect. In the majority of patients cataracts are slowly progressive over a number of years. There is no effective treatment apart from surgery and the indication for this is when the visual requirements of the patient fall below that required to manage his normal daily life. Congenital cataracts are rare. Maternal rubella infection in the first trimester is the most common cause. Other causes are hereditary cataract, chromosome aberrations, intrauterine infection, associated intraocular disease, and metabolic causes of which galactosaemia is the most common. Treatment of congenital cataract requires specialized facilities and is best carried out by ophthalmologists with a special interest in the subject.

The most common cause of acquired cataract is aging and all other causes apart from diabetes are comparatively rare. Cataract is, however, a feature of metabolic disease (diabetes mellitus, hypoparathyroidism, Wilson's disease), trauma (blunt injury, surgery, radiation), drugs (topical or systemic steroid treatment), associated intraocular disease (high myopia, uveitis, retinal dystrophy etc.), and systemic diseases such as dystrophia myotonica, severe eczema or anorexia nervosa. The morphology of the cataractous changes gives very limited information on their aetiology. Cataracts in diabetes cannot be distinguished from senile changes except that they occur at an earlier age as the disease appears to enhance the aging process of the lens (page 23.3). This is the only disease in which the biochemical defect is known and this is the result of aldose reductase in the lens epithelium converting fructose to sorbitol. This cannot diffuse from the lens with consequent osmotic changes. Acute refractive changes are common in poorly controlled diabetes due to this process, and may rarely lead to the sudden dramatic development of cataract. Prolonged hypocalcaemia from any cause is a very rare but well-known association of cataract. Wilson's disease is associated with a brown discoloration of the anterior lens surface that does not cause visual loss. Cataracts are an important manifestation of dystrophia myotonica as they have a characteristic polychromatic morphology in the earliest stages which is a useful genetic marker of the condition that can be found before neurological involvement is apparent. They usually progress to cause significant visual loss in early middle age. Cataractous changes are seen in many patients on prolonged systemic or topical steroid therapy. The earliest changes are found in the posterior subcapsular zone and some degree of change can be found in many patients after 2 years of treatment. Cataract is very much more common in tropical countries and recently work has shown that this prevalence may be related to gastroenteritis producing dehydration and cyanides in the bowel which interfere with lens metabolism. Treatment is surgical removal of the opaque lens with insertion of a plastic implant if the eye is otherwise normal.

Dislocated lens

Dislocated lenses are a feature of Marfan's syndrome and homocystinuria as well as occurring in isolation of systemic disease. For some unknown reason the lens in Marfan's patients tends to subluxate superiorly whereas in homocystinuria it subluxates inferiorly. Preoperative diagnosis of homocystinuria is important as these patients have an increased risk of vascular thrombosis.

Blindness as a world health problem

In the Western World the commonest causes of blindness are genetic defects in the young, diabetic retinopathy in the middle aged, and glaucoma, cataract or macular degeneration in the elderly. This distribution is different in the developing countries where blindness is much more common and is a major economic factor. Here the major causes are cataract, glaucoma, trachoma, onchocerciasis, vitamin A deficiency, and leprosy, together with trauma. Blindness in these countries can affect from 0.3 to 5.0 per cent of the population, often with a wide variation between urban and rural communities. Poor hygiene and nutrition play a major role in these diseases.

It is estimated that there are 45 million people in the world with visual acuities of less than 6/60, and these are classified as 'economically blind'. Of these, 28 million have acuities of less than 3/60; these people need assistance and are classified as 'socially blind'. When averaged these statistics imply that 1 per cent of the world's population has acuities of less than 6/60 and with expansion of world population these figures are increasing. Whilst these statistics are horrifying they must be interpreted with care as they only concern distance acuity and no figures are available for near acuity which is often much better: a myope will have poor acuity in the distance but still be able to read and see clearly near to, and as near vision is more important in underdeveloped countries to the patient's daily lives the amount of real visual handicap is probably less than indicated, although still of immense proportions. It is estimated that 80 per cent of the socially blind population have a preventable form of blindness.

Cataract

Cataract is probably the greatest cause of blindness in the world and is the biggest surgical workload of all ophthalmic services. The high prevalence in the underdeveloped world is probably related to high sunlight levels resulting in ultraviolet light-induced lens damage and to severe dehydration from infection and diarrhoea. In a recent study patients who had two or more episodes of severe dehydration had a 21 times normal risk of developing cataract and the study suggested that this alone may account for up to 40 per cent of cases of cataract in India. The biochemical mechanism appears to be cynanate-induced carbamylation of lens protein, together with osmotic pressure changes. In the long-term better social conditions may reduce the incidence of cataract but for the foreseeable future treatment will be surgical. In the underdeveloped countries this is often carried out by paramedical teams in eye camps, with reasonable visual results in view of the scale of the problem and the lower visual requirements of a rural population.

Trachoma (see Section 5)

This is a form of conjunctivitis caused by chlamydial infection. The same infection occurs in the Western World where the disease is seen as an isolated conjunctivitis (with distinctive pathological appearances), in association with urogenital infection. The ocular disease usually occurs as a secondary cross-infection from this. This isolated conjunctivitis responds to tetracyclines and heals without scarring or further sequelae.

Trachoma is a disease of hot, dry climates and is prevalent in the Middle East, India, and Australia. Infection is spread by eye-to-eye contact (hyperendemic trachoma) from contact with ocular secretions due to poor hygiene or flies. Initial infection occurs in infants and childhood as a follicular conjunctivitis and is followed by repeated cycles of infection and secondary bacterial intercurrent infection. Over a period of years this leads to conjunctival scarring and the sequelae of a dry eye, contraction, and shrinkage of the conjunctiva and lids with trichiasis (ingrowing lashes) and visual loss from mechanical corneal abrasion, secondary infection, vascularization, and perhaps perforation. If the disease is less severe the patient will be left with variable amounts of conjunctival and corneal scarring which is characterized by a typical pattern of horizontal linear scars on the upper tarsal plate and pannus (superficial fibrovascular membrane) on the superior corneal limbus. The disease is extremely common in the Middle East and most adults show signs of infection to some extent and, although these patients have inactive disease, they frequently complain of intermittent ocular irritation and redness.

Active trachoma responds to tetracyclines but the public control

of disease lies in better hygiene facilities. A recent epidemiological survey found that the severity of ocular disease was directly and inversely related to the frequency of face washing. Treatment of the later cicatricial effects lies in symptomatic relief of irritation by artificial tear substitutes, surgical correction of lid deformities cannot be overemphasized, and replacement of the opacified cornea by a corneal graft. It is estimated that 100 million people show signs of trachoma and 7 million of these are blind from the disease.

Vitamin A deficiency (xerophthalmia) (see Section 8)

This affects children after the cessation of breast feeding in the age range 6 months to 4 years and is prevalent in the Far East where for social and economic reasons there is a deficiency of green vegetables in the diet. Many children are also protein and calorie deficient and the disease carries a high morbidity and mortality from intercurrent bowel and respiratory infections as well as measles. In some areas the disease is particularly related to the eating of polished rice as western influence has made brown rice unfashionable and in these communities the disease may be more common in the middle classes as the poor cannot afford polished rice.

About 800 000 children go blind from vitamin A deficiency each year and many of these will die. The earliest signs are bilateral and are found in the epithelium of the conjunctiva and cornea where patchy epithelial breakdown occurs; tear film deficiency is not seen until the later stages. Affected children have a lack lustre appearance to the cornea and conjunctiva. Bitot's spots are an early feature. These are triangular patches lateral to the cornea on the exposed conjunctiva in the palpebral aperture. They have a white 'foamy' appearance, about 4–5 mm in diameter and represent areas of keratinized non-wettable conjunctiva. Further epithelial erosion of the cornea leads to loss from secondary bacterial infection and endophthalmitis or from continued melting of the corneal stroma which can be rapidly progressive to perforation (keratomalacia). In the conjunctiva loss of goblet cells produces a deficiency of mucus in the tear film so that the tears do not wet the eye which leads to keratinization of the cornea and conjunctiva or secondary infection and ulceration. Treatment lies in systemic therapy to replace vitamin A and protein. Night blindness is a feature of vitamin A deficiency but the symptoms of this are usually overshadowed by the anterior segment disease.

Leprosy (see Section 5)

It has only recently been appreciated that leprosy has blinding complications. The worldwide incidence is thought to be 15 million patients and perhaps 1 million of these are blind. The ocular sequelae vary widely between racial groups and geographical locations and are related to the predominance of lepromatous leprosy, temperate climate, the availability of health care, and compliance with drug therapy. Damage to the eye occurs either from direct invasion of the anterior segment by the bacillus in lepromatous leprosy or from the impaired lid closure and corneal sensation which result from VII and V nerve palsies or facial deformity from nodules or loss of tissue. These lead to corneal complications from exposure and secondary infection.

Loss of eyelashes is a sign of lepromatous leprosy which marks out the sufferer to other people as an infected person. A variety of lid deformities occur of which ectropion (eversion of the lower eyelid) from VII nerve palsy is the most common. Entropion and trichiasis (ingrowing lashes) are less common. Anterior chamber temperature is lower than body temperature and this provides a favourable environment for invasion of the cornea and anterior segment in lepromatous disease. Involvement of corneal nerves can be seen as beading along their course in some patients. Reduced corneal sensation produces less tendency to blink and this exacerbates the corneal exposure from lid complications.

Inflammatory signs may be seen as episcleritis, scleritis or scleral nodules. Acute iritis may occur but a peculiar feature of lepromatous leprosy is a chronic iritis with low-grade inflammation in the eye that eventually destroys the iris tissue and causes a cataract. A typical feature of this is the development of a minute pin-point pupil which enhances the deleterious effects of corneal or lens opacity and this miosis is possibly the result of a neuropathy of the autonomic and sensory nerves in the iris. Retinal signs of leprosy are extremely rare and are not usually of any importance.

Much of the ocular morbidity from leprosy can be minimized by recognition of the risks of corneal exposure and simple surgical procedures to the eyelids to protect the globe. Lepromatous eyes respond well to cataract surgery with a broad iridectomy to restore sight.

Onchocerciasis (river blindness) (see Section 5)

This disease is seen in West Africa and Central and Southern America where it was probably introduced by the slave trade. It is an infestation caused by the parasite *Onchocerca volvulus* and humans are the host. The disease is characterized by relatively few subcutaneous nodules containing adult worms which produce millions of microfilariae. These are transmitted by a black fly of Simulus genus to infect the next host. The major effects of the disease are in the eye where blindness is produced from corneal scarring, chorio-retinal atrophy, optic nerve disease or the effects of anterior uveitis.

Viable organisms appear to be relatively well tolerated and the damage to the eye is produced by chronic inflammation from the dead microfilariae. Infestation of the eye probably occurs from contiguous subcutaneous spread from adjacent skin although the parasite can be found in the blood in heavily infested patients. Conjunctivitis is common. Viable microfilariae can be seen in the cornea, anterior chamber or vitreous gel in heavily infected patients. Ocular damage occurs over many years. In the cornea dead microfilariae produce a fluffy snowflake appearance in the anterior stroma. Progressive disease produces a corneal haze in the interpalpebral fissure which is then followed by a sclerosing keratitis when the cornea becomes totally opaque. The anterior uveitis is low grade and chronic, the inferior iris is particularly susceptible which becomes atrophic with the pupil distorted inferiorly and adhesions between the iris and lens enhance the effect of any corneal or cataractous changes and may cause glaucoma. Chorio-retinal atrophy is common and this is the result of a low-grade chorio-retinitis. The posterior pole of the eye is affected particularly temporal to the macula where the early changes are seen as atrophy of the retinal pigment epithelium. These areas become confluent areas of chorio-retinal atrophy so that the outer retina and choriocapillaries are lost revealing the larger choroidal vessels, subretinal fibrosis, and pigmentary changes. The changes in the retina are heterogenous and asymmetrical and it has been suggested they result from invasion of microfilariae along the course of the posterior ciliary arteries as they penetrate the sclera. The macula is often spared until late in the disease and the susceptibility of the temporal retina has been explained by its proximity to subcutaneous nodules on the temples – a common site for the adult worms. Optic nerve disease is common and results in visual field constriction which may occur in the absence of chorio-retinal changes. Oedema of the optic disc may be found in the acute stages of optic nerve disease.

Onchocerciasis affects 8–10 million people in Africa and South America of which 1 million are blind. As the ocular changes are produced by death of the parasite, treatment is fraught with problems and visual function can deteriorate acutely with treatment. Nodules of adult worms may be excised surgically. Suramin is the only drug available to destroy the adult worms, but must be given intravenously and causes severe systemic reaction as well as optic nerve toxicity. Diethylcarbamazine (DEC) destroys the microfilariae but causes systemic reactions and carries the risk of producing further visual loss. During treatment increased numbers of microfilariae can be seen within the eye, as DEC appears to activate and mobilize the parasite, 'driving' them into the eye. Anterior uveitis may be exacerbated and visual acuity or field can be lost acutely from optic nerve damage. Heavily infested patients present a major therapeutic problem and there is doubt whether any of the present drugs offer an improvement in the visual prognosis in these cases.

Recently a new drug, ivermectin, has been introduced for the treatment of onchocerciasis and initial results indicate that this is likely to be a major therapeutic advance.

References

Slow flow retinopathy
Ross Russell, R. W. and Page, N. G. R. (1983). Critical perfusion of brain and retina. *Brain* **106**, 419–434.

Diabetic retinopathy
British Multicentre Study Group (1983). Photocoagulation for diabetic maculopathy – a randomized controlled clinical trial using the xenon arc. *Diabetes* **32**, 1010–1016.

British Multicentre Study Group (1984). Photocoagulation for proliferative diabetic retinopathy – a randomized controlled clinical trial using the xenon arc. *Diabetologica* **26**, 109–115.

Frank, R. N. (1984). On the pathogenesis of diabetic retinopathy. *Ophthalmology* **91**, 626–634.

Klein, R., Klein, B. E. K. and Moss, S. (1984). Visual impairment in diabetes. *Ophthalmology* **91**, 1–8.

Pavan, P. R. (ed.) (1984). Ocular manifestations of diabetes. *Int. Ophthalmol. Clin.* **24**, no. 4.

Hypertensive retinopathy
Garner, A., Ashton, N. Tripathi, R. *et al.* (1975). Pathogenesis of hypertensive retinopathy. An experimental study in the monkey. *Br. J. Ophthalmol.* **59**, 3–44.

Keith, N. M., Wagner, H. P. and Barker, N. W. (1939). Some different types of essential hypertension – their course and prognosis. *Am. J. Med. Sci.* **197**, 332–343.

Tso, M. O. M. and Lee Jampol (1982). Pathophysiology of hypertensive retinopathy. *Ophthalmology* **89**, 1132–1145.

Sickle cell retinopathy
Condon, P. I. and Serjeant, G. R. (1980). Behaviour of untreated proliferative sickle retinopathy. *Br. J. Ophthalmol.* **64**, 404–411.

Hayes, R. J., Condon, P. I. and Serjeant, G. R. (1981). Haematological factors associated with proliferative retinopathy in sickle cell haemoglobin C disease. *Br. J. Ophthalmol.* **65**, 712–717.

——, —— and —— (1981). Haematological factors associated with proliferative retinopathy in homozygous sickle cell disease. *Br. J. Ophthalmol.* **65**, 29–35.

Serjeant, B. E. and Mason, K. P. *et al.* Blood rheology and proliferative retinopathy in sickle cell haemoglobin C disease. *Br. J. Ophthalmol.* **68**, 325–328.

Systemic lupus erythematosus
Graham, E. M., Spalton, D. J., Barnard, R. O., Garner, A. and Ross Russell, R. W. (1985). Cerebral and retinal vascular changes in systemic lupus erythematosus. *Ophthalmology* **92**, 444–448.

Retinitis pigmentosa
Fishman, G. (1980). Hereditary retinal and choroidal diseases. Principles and practice of ophthalmology (eds G. A. Peyman, D. R. Saunders and M. F. Goldberg). W. B. Saunders, Philadelphia.

Spalton, D. J. (1985). Pigmentary retinopathies. In *The eye in general medicine* (ed. C. Rose). Chapman and Hall, London.

Uveitis
Arnold A. C. *et al.* (1984). Retinal periphlebitis and retinitis in multiple sclerosis. *Ophthalmology* **91**, 255–262.

Brewerton, D. A. *et al.* (1973). Acute anterior uveitis in HLA. B27. *Lancet* **ii**, 994–996.

Culbertson, W. W., Tabbara, K. F. and O'Connor, G. R. (1982). Experimental ocular toxoplasmosis in primates. *Arch. Ophthalmol.* **100**, 321–323.

Hedges, T. R. and Albert, D. M. (1982). The progression of the ocular abnormalities of herpes zoster. Histopathological observations in 9 cases. *Opthalmology* **89**, 165–177.

Kanski, J. J. and Shun-Shin, G. A. (1984). Systemic uveitis syndromes in childhood: an analysis of 340 cases. *Ophthalmology* **91**, 1247–1252.

Knox, D. L., Schachat, A. P. and Mustonen E. (1984). Primary, secondary and coincidental complications of Crohn's disease. *Ophthalmology* **91**, 163–173.

Loewer-Sieger, D. H., Rothova, A., Koppe, J. G. (1984). Congenital toxoplasmosis – a prospective study based on 1821 pregnant women. *Prac. 1st International Symposium on Uveitis*. Excerpta Medica, Amsterdam.

Magill, J., Chapman C. and Makasingam M. (1983). Acyclovir therapy in herpes zoster infection, a practical guide. *Trans. Ophthal. Soc. UK.* **103**, 111–114.

Nussenblatt, R. B., Palestine, A. G. and Chan C. C. (1983). Cyclosporin A therapy in the treatment of intraocular inflammatory disease resistant to systemic corticosteroids and cytotoxic agents. *Am. J. Ophthalmol.* **96**, 275–282.

Obenauf, C. D. *et al.* (1978). Sarcoidosis and its ophthalmic manifestations. *Am. J. Ophthalmol.* **86**, 648–655.

O'Connor, G. R. (1983). Factors related to the initiation and recurrence of uveitis. *Am. J. Ophthalmol.* **96**, 577–599.

Palestine A. G. *et al.* (1984). Ophthalmic involvement in acquired immunodeficiency syndrome. *Ophthalmology* **91**, 1092–1099.

Royal Society of Medicine (1985). *Proceedings of the International Conference on Behcet's Disease*. London.

Spalton, D. J. and Sanders, M. D. (1981). Fundus changes in histologically confirmed sarcoidosis. *Br. J. Ophthalmol.* **51**, 348–358.

Watzke, R. C., Oaks, J. A. and Folk, J. C. (1984). Toxocara canis infection of the eye. Correlation of clinical observations with developing pathology in a primate model. *Arch. Ophthalmol.* **102**, 282–291.

Womack, L. W. and Liesegang, T. J. (1983). Complications of herpes zoster ophthalmicus. *Arch. Ophthalmol.* **101**, 42–45.

Acquired immune deficiency syndrome

Gallo, R. C. *et al.* (1984). Frequent detection and isolation of cytopathic retro-virus (HTLV3) from patients with AIDS and at risk of AIDS. *Science* **224**, 500.

Humphry, R. C., Weber, J. N. and Marsh, R. J. (1986). The ophthalmic findings of a group of ambulatory patients infected by human T cell. Lymphotrophic virus type III – a prospective study. *Br. J. Ophthalm.* (in press).

Holland, G. N. *et al.* (1986). Ocular disease in acquired immune deficiency syndrome: clinicopathological correlations. *Proceedings of the 4th International Symposium of the Immunology and Immunopathology of the Eye* (in press).

Pepose, J. *et al.* (1985). Acquired immune deficiency syndrome, pathogenic mechanisms of ocular disease. *Ophthalm.* **92**, 472–484.

Scleritis

Watson, P. G. (1982). The nature and the treatment of scleral inflammation. *Trans. Ophthalmol. Soc. UK.* **102**, 257–281.

—— and Hazleman, B. L. (1976). The sclera and systemic disorders. W. B. Saunders, London.

Optic disc

Glaser J. S. (1978). Neuro-ophthalmology. Harper and Row, New York.

Walsh, F. B. and Hoyt, W. F. (1969). *Clinical neuro-ophthalmology* 3rd edn Williams and Wilkins, 4th edn N. R. Miller, Philadelphia.

Dry eyes

Bron A. J. (1985). Prospects for the dry eye. *Trans. Ophthalmol. Soc. UK* (in press).

Wright P. (1985). Cicatrizing conjunctivitis. *Trans. Ophthalmol. Soc. UK* (in press).

Thyroid

Kodama, K., Sikorska, H., Bandy-Defoe, P. *et al.* (1982) Demonstration of a circulating autoantibody against a soluble eye muscle antigen in Graves' ophthalmopathy. *Lancet* ii, 1353–1355.

McCord, C. D. (1985). Current trends in orbital decompression. *Ophthalmology* **92**, 21–33.

Trobe, J. D., Glaser, J. S. and Laflamme P. (1978). Dysthyroid optic neuropathy, clinical profile and rationale for management. *Arch. Ophthalmol.* **96**, 1199–1209.

Trokel, S. L. and Jakobiec F.A. (1981). Correlation of CT scanning and pathological features of ophthalmic Graves' disease. *Ophthalmology* **88**, 553–564.

Werner, S. C. (1977). Modification of the classification of the eye changes of Graves' disease. *J. Clin. Endocrinol. Met.* **44**, 203–204.

World health

Bird, A. C. *et al.* (1976). Morphology of posterior segment lesions of the eye in patients with onchocerciasis. *Br. J. Ophthalmol.* **60**, 2–20.

—— *et al.* (1980). Changes in visual function and in the posterior segment of the eye during treatment of onchocerciasis with diethylcarbamazine citrate. *Br. J. Ophthalmol.* **64**, 191–200.

ffytche, T. J. (1985). Ocular leprosy. *Trop. Doc.* **15**, 118–125.

Minassian, D. C., Mehten, U. and Jones, B. R. (1984). Dehydrational crises from severe diarrhoea or heat stroke and risk of cataract. *Lancet* i, 751–753.

Smith, R. S., Farrell, T. and Bailey, T. (1975). Keratomalacia. *Surg. Ophthalmol.* **20**, 213.

Taylor, H. R. and Greene, B. M. (1981). Ocular changes with oral and transepidermal diethylcarbamazine therapy of onchocerciasis. *Br. J. Ophthalmol.* **65**, 194–502.

SECTION 24
DISORDERS OF UNCERTAIN AETIOLOGY

DISORDERS OF UNCERTAIN AETIOLOGY

Kawasaki disease

T. KAWASAKI

Synonyms

MCLS: Infantile acute febrile mucocutaneous lymph-node syndrome

Introduction

Kawasaki disease (KD) is an acute febrile eruptive disease commonly occurring in infants and young children under 5 years of age. It was first described by Kawasaki in 1967. Originally, the prognosis was believed to be favourable. However, as more studies were carried out, the fatality rate was found to be 0.3–0.5 per cent, and autopsy findings revealed unique pathological features such as coronary artery aneurysms with thrombosis in many cases. Since this disease cannot be differentiated histopathologically from infantile periarteritis nodosa, which has rarely been reported in American and European literature, it is still unclear whether it is a new entity or a disease which has previously been overlooked. This problem will remain unsolved until the pathogenesis is determined.

The disease has attracted much attention recently because asymptomatic coronary artery lesions (mainly aneurysms) have remained as sequelae in 5 to 10 per cent of the patients. These lesions are considered to cause sudden death, myocardial infarction or mitral insufficiency, probably due to the papillary muscle dysfunction syndrome.

Kawasaki disease is a clear-cut clinical entity which can be diagnosed after recognition and analysis of six principal symptoms.

Clinical manifestations

The clinical features of KD can be classified into two categories: principal and subsidiary. At least five of the six principal features should be present for the diagnosis of KD. However, patients with four features can also be diagnosed as having the condition provided that coronary aneurysms are identified by echo-cardiography or coronary angiography.

Principal features

Fever of unknown aetiology lasting five days or more In general, the onset of KD is usually with abrupt high fever but without prodromal symptoms such as coughing, sneezing or rhinorrhoea. Sometimes, however, lymphadenopathy is felt, particularly if the patient complains of neck pain. At times, these symptoms precede the abrupt high fever by a day. Usually there is remittent or continuous fever ranging from 38 to 40 °C for one to two weeks. High fever lasting more than two weeks is seen in 14 to 20 per cent of cases. Fever lasting 30 days is rarely seen, while high fever lasting any longer suggests another disease. There is no response to antibiotics. The mean temperature reached is between 39.0 and 39.9 °C. It is believed that the longer the fever continues, the greater the possibility of coronary artery aneurysm.

Bilateral congestion of ocular conjunctiva Two to four days after the onset, conjunctival injection occurs. On close examination each capillary vessel is dilated. There is no purulent discharge so the term 'conjunctivitis' is not appropriate. In most cases redness of the eyes is obvious, but in some cases it can be seen only upon very close examination. Pseudomembrane formation, iris adhesion or visual disturbance has not been reported. With careful slit-lamp examination early in the course of the disease, anterior uveitis can be observed in some cases. Conjunctival injection usually subsides within one week and rarely continues for more than several weeks. It is seen in nearly 90 per cent of confirmed cases.

Changes of lips and oral cavity Three to five days after the onset, dryness, redness, and fissuring of lips is present. In some cases there is bleeding and crust formation; it seems as if there is lipstick on the lips. The membranes of the oral cavity and pharyngeal mucosa are diffusely red. There is no vesicle, aphtha or pseudo-membrane formation. Frequently there is prominence of the tongue papillae, referred to as a strawberry tongue and similar to that seen in scarlet fever. These changes subside two weeks after the onset, but often the reddening of the lips continues for three to four weeks.

Acute non-purulent swelling of cervical lymph-nodes From the day before the onset of fever, or together with fever, there is swelling of the cervical lymph-nodes. The patient complains of pain and often suffers a wryneck. In some cases the swelling occurs several days after the onset of fever. The nodes range from 1.5 to 5 cm and form a firm, non-fluctuant mass. Sometimes there is bilateral swelling leading to a misdiagnosis of mumps. Cervical lymph-adenopathy is seen in about two-thirds of cases in Japan. Significant lymph-node enlargement is the least important of the criteria for diagnosis. Usually it disappears with defervescence.

Polymorphous exanthema From the first to the fifth day after the onset of fever, a polymorphic rash appears on the trunk or extremeties. It is variously morbilliform, scarlatiniform, urticariform, or erythema multiform-like. In each case the rash is a different combination of these forms. The individual lesions measure 5 to 30 mm in diameter and spread over the trunk and extremeties within two days. Each lesion becomes increasingly large, and they often coalesce. They are not accompanied by vesicles or crusts but sometimes there are small aseptic pustules on the knees, buttocks or other sites. The eruptions usually disappear in less than a week. There may also be localized redness at the sites of BCG inoculations in the acute stage.

Changes of the extremeties Approximately two to five days after the onset of the disease, when the rash on the trunk has appeared, there is reddening of the palms and soles. Simultaneously, there is an indurative oedema. Sometimes the degree of swelling is considerable and the skin is shiny and appears to be about to burst (Fig. 1). When the fever goes down the swelling usually disappears. From 10 to 15 days after the onset of the illness, desquamation begins from the tip of the fingers and membranous desquamation spreads over the palms up to the wrist. From a month and a half to two months after onset, transverse furrows frequently appear in the nails of both fingers and toes.

Other clinical manifestations and complications

Cardiovascular changes The most important complications of KD are changes in the cardiovascular system. In the acute stage, pancarditis and coronary arteritis frequently occur. Auscultation reveals gallop rhythms and distant heart sounds, and in some cases the ECG shows variable PQ and QT prolongation, low-voltage, ST and T wave changes, and arrythmias.

Two-dimensional echo-cardiography or selective angiography (Fig. 2) reveals that coronary artery aneurysms or dilation occur in about 40 per cent of cases, 10 to 12 days from the onset of the illness. However, about 30 days after the onset, the incidence

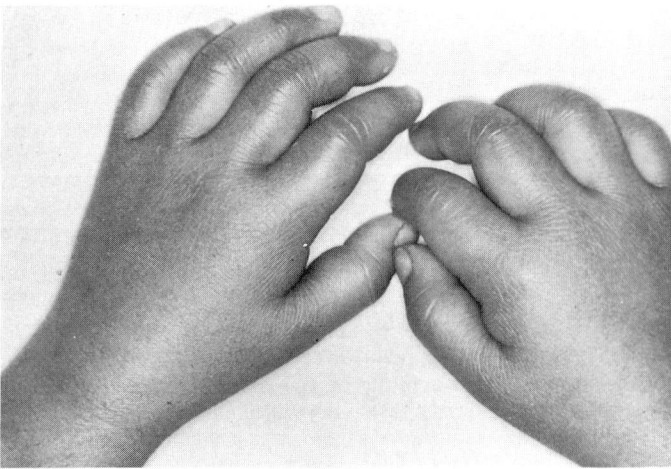

Fig. 1 Indurative oedema of the hands in Kawasaki's disease.

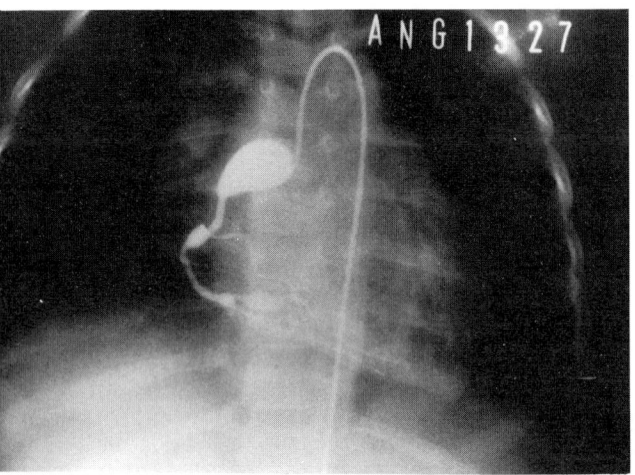

Fig. 2 Multiple aneurysms of the coronary artery in Kawasaki's disease.

decreases to about 20 per cent of all cases; by 60 days, the incidence is reduced to about 10 per cent of cases.

Kato (1974) first reported regression of aneurysms, and it has been confirmed subsequently that aneurysms in KD regress with time. In general, stenosis and obstruction do not occur in aneurysms which quickly regress; regression depends upon the shape (saccular, cylindrical, or fusiform) and diameter of the aneurysm.

If the diameter is more than 8 mm, there is little possibility of regression and often stenosis or occlusion occur. If the diameter is less than 4 mm, almost all cases show regressiuon. In cases in which the diameter is between 4 and 8 mm, the prognosis is usually favourable. In general, stenosis or occlusion is liable to occur in large saccular and cylindrical aneurysms. Consequently, cases with aneurysms or dilation larger than 4 mm should have selective angiography carried out from 1 to 3 months after onset to determine accurately the shape and diameter of the aneurysm. According to recent Japanese literature, stenosis or occlusion occurs in 3 to 5 per cent of all cases studied with coronary artery angiography.

Gastrointestinal tract Diarrhoea occurs in about 35 per cent of patients. Patients with gall bladder involvement often suffer severe abdominal pain, especially in the upper right quadrant. Ultrasound examination is useful in the diagnosis. Mild jaundice occurs in about 5 per cent of cases. The total serum bilirubin level is almost always lower than 10 mg/dl. In the acute phase, serum transaminase levels are often increased. Serum GOT and GPT

increase from 60 to 200 iu and LDH increases from 600 to 900 iu. Paralytic ileus has been reported.

Blood In almost all cases there is a leucocytosis with a shift to the left, an increased ESR, positive C reactive protein and an increased α_2-globulin level. The platelet count increases from the second week and may reach $1000-1500 \times 10^9$ per litre. Hypoalbuminaemia and slight anaemia frequently occur.

Urinary tract Albuminuria is frequently seen in the acute phase, with aseptic microscopic pyuria. These findings disappear in the convalescent phase.

Respiratory system Cough and rhinorrhoea may be present at the onset. Abnormal infiltrates on the chest X-ray are occasionally seen.

Joints Arthralgia or arthritis are seen in about 25 per cent of cases. These symptoms disappear within 30 days after onset in most cases.

Nervous system Aseptic meningitis occurs in 20 to 50 per cent of cases. Aseptic meningitis in KD, compared to mumps meningitis, shows higher numbers of macrophages, ependymal cells and pia-arachnoid cells. Other neurological complications such as facial palsy, hemiplegia, and encephalopathy have been reported.

Pathological findings

KD is an acute inflammatory disease with systemic angiitis which is distinguishable from classic periarteritis nodosa of Kussmaul–Maier type. Coronary aneurysms are usually present at autopsy (Fig. 3). The angiitis is characterized by acute inflammation with mild fibrinoid necrosis. The course of the angiitis can be classified into four stages according to the duration of the illness.

Stage 1 (1–2 weeks from onset) shows perivasculitis and vasculitis of microvessels, small arteries, and veins. There is inflammation of the intima, externa, and perivascular areas in the medium- and large-sized arteries. Oedema and infiltration with leucocytes and lymphocytes is also present.

Stage 2 (2–4 weeks from onset) shows less inflammation in the vessels than in stage 1. Aneurysms with thrombus and stenosis in the middle-sized arteries, especially in the coronary arteries, are present.

Stage 3 (4–7 weeks from onset) shows subsidence of inflammation in the vessels. Granulation may occur in the medium-sized arteries.

Stage 4 (more than 7 weeks from onset) reveals scar formation and intimal thickening with aneurysms, thrombus and stenosis in the medium-sized arteries.

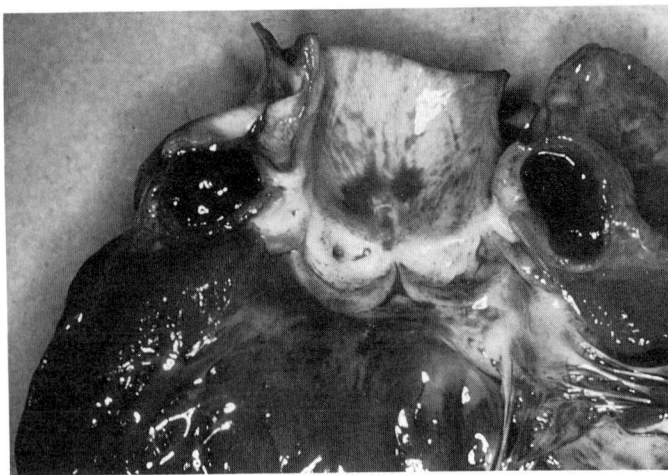

Fig. 3 Postmortem findings in Kawasaki's disease. This 9-month-old boy died suddenly at 49 days after the onset of the illness. A large aneurysm of the coronary vessels is shown.

Other lesions include myocarditis involving conduction systems, pericarditis, endocarditis, and inflammation of almost all organs. All these lesions are frequently seen in Stages 1 and 2, but rarely in Stage 4.

Ischaemic heart disease usually occurs in Stages 2–4. The major cause of death in Stage 1 is myocarditis including inflammation of conduction systems. In Stages 2 and 3, the causes are ischaemic heart disease, rupture of an aneurysm (rare), and myocarditis. In Stage 4, there may be ischaemic heart disease and, in rare cases, heart failure due to mitral insufficiency.

Epidemiology

In 1970 the first nationwide survey was conducted by the Japanese KD Research Committee. Since then, eight surveys have been carried out at two-year intervals up to December 1984. A total of 63 399 cases (36 891 males and 26 508 females, M/F = 1.4) has been reported, including 321 (0.5 per cent) deaths. The number of cases reported has been steadily increasing since 1971. A high incidence of the disease was recognized in the early or late spring of 1979 and 1982 throughout Japan. A shift of the epidemic wave from warm to cool geographical areas was observed in 1979, but not in 1982. The male:female rate was 1.3–1.5:1. The age distribution of the cases showed monomodal curves reaching a peak at 6–11 months. Eighty-five per cent of cases were less than five years of age. The sex ratio tended to be lower and the age of incidence tended to be younger in epidemic years.

Since 1974, outside of Japan, a number of cases have been reported from Korea, the United States, Canada, West Germany, France, the United Kingdom, and other countries. However, reports from the developing countries are still rare.

Aetiology

Many agents such as rickettsia, viruses, bacteria (streptococcus, staphylococcus, propionibacterium, etc.), chemical substances (detergents, mercury, drugs etc.), and mite antigens have been suggested as the cause of KD. Other possible factors such as an abnormal host reaction to a variety of agents or a unique genetic susceptibility (HLA-BW 22 J 2) and circulating immune complexes have been proposed. Another hypothesis is that KD may be triggered or initiated in a susceptible child by an infection with a variety of common viruses prevalent among children in the community. KD, therefore, may be a unique clinical reaction pattern to several agents, just as a variety of agents may trigger such disorders as Reye's, Guillian-Barré or Stevens-Johnson syndromes.

Treatment

For the acute phase of Kawasaki disease, aspirin treatment is recommended because of its anti-inflammatory and anti-platelet effects. In Japan, high dose of aspirin, 100 mg/kg/day, has been used. However, even at this dose, coronary artery aneurysms could not be prevented and frequently there were side effects including abnormal liver function. Because of these problems, it is current practice to administer 30–50 mg/kg/day of aspirin in the initial stage.

From July 1981 to October 1982 the Research Committee on Kawasaki Disease carried out a randomized, prospective, controlled study of three forms of treatment: aspirin, flurbiprofen, and prednisolone plus dipyridamole. Several criteria for selection of patients were required: seven days from the onset of disease, under five years of age, and no previous administration of aspirin or steroids. The aspirin dosage (101 cases) was 50 mg/kg/day until the 30th day from onset, the flurbiprofen dosage (104 cases) was 4 mg/kg/day until the 30th day from onset, and the predisolone plus dipyridamole dosage (101 cases) was 2 mg/kg/day of prednisolone for seven days and 5 mg/kg/day of dipyridamole for 30 days from onset. If coronary aneurysms remained after 30 days from onset, 10 mg/kg/day of aspirin were given to patients in all three groups until regression of aneurysms.

One year from onset, only one case of coronary aneurysm occurred in the aspirin group. The flurbiprofen group and the prednisolone plus dipyridamole groups each had seven cases of coronary aneurysms. All three groups showed significant regression of coronary aneurysms over the period of one year.

These data are considered to be a useful guide to treatment, but they are not absolutely clear-cut because there was variation in the reported percentages of remaining coronary aneurysms in the aspirin-treated group.

Recently, Furusho and colleagues have published their findings on 'high-dose intravenous gammaglobulin for Kawasaki disease' and have found that this treatment is more effective than aspirin therapy. This has been confirmed by a study in the USA but further work is required to define which patients require this expensive therapy.

Management

KD patients should be hospitalized and closly monitored for coronary artery changes by two-dimensional echo-cardiography. If there are no changes, drug treatment can be discontinued. For those patients with persistent coronary artery aneurysms, low dose aspirin, 10 mg/kg/day, should be administered until the aneurysms disappear. As mentioned earlier, patients with large aneurysms should have selective coronary angiography performed from one to three months after the onset; this should be repeated after one or two years.

If myocardial infarction or myocardial insufficiency due to mitral regurgitation occurs, bypass surgery should be considered; this complication is more likely in younger patients.

References

Bell, D. M., Brink, E. W., Nitzkin, J. L., Hall, C. B., Wulff, H., Berkowitzl, D., Feorino, P. M., Holman, R. C., Meade, R. H., Gilfillan, R. F., Keim, D. E. and Modlin, J. F. (1981). Kawasaki syndrome: description of two outbreaks in the United States. *N. Engl. J. Med.* **304**, 1568–1575.

Cremer, H.J. (1981). Das Kawasaki-syndrome in der bundesrepublik. *Padiat. prax.* **25**, 243–260.

Feigen, R. D. and Barron, K. S. (1986). Treatment of Kawasaki syndrome. *N. Engl. J. Med.* **315**, 388–390.

Fujiwara, H. and Hamashima, Y. (1978). Pathology of the heart in Kawasaki disease. *Pediatrics* **61**, 100–107.

Fukushige, J., Nihill, M. R. and Mcnamara, D. G. (1980). Spectrum of cardiovascular lesions in mucocutaneous lymph node syndrome: analysis of eight cases. *Am. J. Cardiol.* **45**, 98–107.

Furusho, K., Ohba, T., Soeda, T., Kimoto, K., Okabe, T. and Hirota, T. (1981). Possible role for mite antigen in KD. *Lancet* **ii**, 194–195.

Furusho, K., Kamiya, T., Nakano, H., Kiyosawa, N., Shinomiya, K., Hayashidera, T., Tamura, T., Hirose, O., Manabe, Y., Yokoyama, T., Kawarano, M., Baba K. and Mori, C. (1984). High-dose intraveneous gammaglobulin for KD. *Lancet* **ii**, 1055–1058.

Germain, B. F., Moroney, J. D., Guggino, G. S., Cimino, L., Rodriguex, C. and Bocanegra, T. S. (1980). Anterior uveitis in KD. *J. Pediatr.* **97**, 780.

Gray, J. A. and Welsby, P. D. (1984). KD, a report of 26 patients. *J. Infect.* **9**, 17–21.

Hamashima, Y., Kishi, K. and Tasaka, K. (1973). Richettsia like bodies in infantile acute febrile mucocutaneous lymph node syndrome. *Lancet* **ii**, 42.

Kato, H., Koike, S. and Yokoyama, T. (1979). Kawasaki disease: effect of treatment on coronary artery involvement. *Pediatrics* **63**, 175–179.

——, Ichinose, E., Yoshioka, F., Takechi, T., Matsunaga, S., Suzuki, K. and Rikitake, N. (1982). Fate of coronary aneurysms in Kawasaki disease: serial coronary angiography and long-term follow-up study. *Am. J. Cardiol.* **49**, 1758–1766.

——, Fujimoto, T., Inoue, O., Kondo, M., Koga, Y., Yamamoto, S., Shingu, M., Tominaga, K. and Sasaguri, Y. (1983). Variant strain of propionibacterium acnes: A clue to the aetiology of Kawasaki disease. *Lancet* **ii**, 1383–1387.

——, Kimura, M., Tsuji, K., Kusakawa, S., Asai, T., Juji, T. and Kawasaki, T. (1978). HLA antigens in Kawasaki disease. *Pediatrics* **61**, 252–255.

Kawasaki, T., Kosaki, F., Okawa, S., Shigematsu, I. and Yanagawa, H.

(1974). A new infantile acute febrile mucocutaneous lymph node syndrome prevailing in Japan. *Pediatrics* **54**, 273–276.

Kikuta, H., Mizuno, F., Osato, T., Konno, M., Ishikawa, N., Noro, S. and Sakurada, N. (1984). Kawasaki disease and an unusual primary infection with Epstein-Barr virus. *Pediatrics* **73**, 413–414.

Kitamura, S., Kawashima, Y., Kawachi, K., Harima, R., Ihara, K., Nakano, S., Shimazaki, Y. and Mori, T. (1980). Severe mitral regurgitation due to coronary arteritis of mucocutaneous lymph node syndrome: A new surgical entity. *J. Thorac. Cardiovasc. Surg.* **80**, 629–636.

Krensky, A. M., Berenberg, W., Shanley, K. and Yunis, E. J. (1981). HLA antigens in mucocutaneous lymph node syndrome in New England. *Pediatrics* **67**, 741–743.

Landing, B. H. and Larson, E. J. (1977). Are infantile periarteritis nodosa with coronary artery involvement and fatal mucocutaneous lymph node syndrome the same? Comparison of 20 patients from North America with patients from Hawaii and Japan. *Pediatrics* **59**, 651–662.

Magilavy, D. B., Speert, D. P., Silever, T. M. and Sullivan, D. B. (1978). Mucocutaneous lymph node syndrome: report of two cases complicated by gallbladder mydrops and diagnosed by ultrasound. *Pediatrics* **61**, 699–702.

Melish, M. E., Hicks, R. V. and Larson, E. J. (1976). Mucocutaneous lymph node syndrome in the United States. *Am. J. Dis. Child.* **130**, 599–607.

Morens, D. M., Anderson, L. J. and Hurwitz, E. S. (1980). National surveillance of Kawasaki disease. *Pediatrics* **65**, 21–25.

Shigematsu, I., Tamashiro, H., Shibata, S., Kawasaki, T. and Kusakawa, S. (1980). World wide survey on Kawasaki disease. *Lancet* **i**, 976.

Tanaka, N., Sekimoto, K. and Naoe, S. (1976). Kawasaki disease: relationship with infantile periarteritis nodosa. *Arch. pathol. Lab. Med.* **100**, 81–86.

Yanagawa, H. and Shigematsu, I. (1983). Epidemiological features of Kawasaki disease in Japan. *Acta paediatr. Jpn* **25**, 94–107.

Yoshikawa, J., Yanagihara, K., Owaki, T., Kato, H., Takagi, Y., Okumachi, F., Fukaya, T., Tomita, Y. and Baba, K. (1979). Cross-sectional echo-cardiographic diagnosis of coronary artery aneurysms in patients with the mucocutaneous lymph node syndrome. *Circulation* **59**, 133–139.

Recurrent polyserositis (familial Mediterranean fever, periodic disease)

M. ELIAKIM AND M. RACHMILEWITZ†

Recurrent polyserositis is a genetic disorder characterized by bouts of abdominal pain and fever. Pleurisy and arthritis, affecting one or more joints, occur in more than half the cases. The disease exhibits a preference for Jews, Arabs, Armenians, and Turks but may affect subjects of any ethnic group. It is frequently familial and is inherited by recessive autosomal transmission. Prognosis is generally good, but some patients develop amyloidosis with nephropathy which is usually fatal.

History

The first thorough description of recurrent polyserositis was provided by Siegal in 1945. Rachmilewitz and Ehrenfeld described the first cases in Israel in 1946. In 1948, Reimann, Cattan, and Mamou published additional cases under the designation 'periodic disease'. In 1952, Mamou identified the renal lesion as amyloidosis. Extensive studies on various aspects of the disease were reported later by Heller and his co-workers. The effect of colchicine on the symptoms was reported independently by Goldfinder in 1972 and Eliakim and Licht in 1973. Large series of patients have been published from Israel, France, the United States, and Russia.

Nomenclature

The nomenclature of recurrent polyserositis is subject to controversy. The term 'familial Mediterranean fever' has been used widely, although it fails to convey the recurrent character of the disorder and the symptoms due to serosal inflammation. The disease is not limited to the Mediterranean region any more than are thalassaemia and brucellosis, the latter also known as Mediterranean fever. The term 'familial' is inadequate, since many other hereditary disorders with familial clustering are not referred to as 'familial'. Periodic disease implies recurrence at regular intervals and a close relationship to other periodic disorders. In fact, the paroxysms of recurrent polyserositis occur usually at irregular intervals. The term '*Recurrent polyserositis*' is preferable and will be employed herein, because it seems to convey most closely the main characteristics of the disease.

Racial and ethnic distribution

Recurrent polyserositis occurs predominantly in Jews, Armenians, Arabs, and Turks. However, it has been reported in subjects of many other nationalities and races. More than 90 per cent of the Jewish patients are of either Sepharadic or Iraqi origin. Sepharadic Jews are those whose ancestors left Spain in the fifteenth century and were dispersed over various North African, Middle Eastern, and South American countries, while Iraqi Jews are descendants of the Babylonian Jews exiled to Mesopotamia about 2600 years ago. Most of the Sepharadic patients originate from North African countries.

Mode of inheritance

Recurrent polyserositis is inherited by recessive autosomal transmission. The incidence of multiple familial occurrence varies between 20 and 40 per cent in families reported in different series. The disease usually occurs in several members of one generation. The actual incidence in families with healthy parents has been reported to be 18 per cent, and that in families with one affected parent, 36 per cent. With full penetrance, the expected figures would have to be 25 and 50 per cent respectively. The lower figures observed can be explained by incomplete penetrance of the gene, or alternatively, by later appearance of the disease in some of the children. The disease is slightly more prevalent in males (1.7 to 1.0). The male predominance has not been explained adequately, but may be accounted for by the milder form of disease leading to undiagnosed cases in females. Partial penetrance in females is an alternative explanation. The frequency of the gene in Sepharadic and Iraqi Jews has been calculated to be 1 in 45 and the homozygous incidence 1 in 2000. The respective figures for the Armenian population in Lebanon are 1 in 32 and 1 in 1000. The HLA system has been studied in a smaller number of subjects but no associations have been found.

Pathology

The underlying pathological lesion in recurrent polyserositis is hyperaemia and an acute non-bacterial inflammatory reaction, affecting mainly the serous membranes. Adhesions, when present, are thin and mechanical ileus is extremely rare. Microscopically, the picture is that of non-specific inflammation. The most striking finding is marked hyperaemia and a cellular infiltrate consisting of varying proportions of neutrophils, lymphocytes, monocytes, and sometimes, plasma cells and eosinophils. The picture is different from the ordinary inflammation observed in appendicitis and cholecystitis in that it is not as purulent. The reaction seems to originate in the serosa and may not reach the mucosa. The inflammatory exudate concentrates around the venules and arterioles, some of which have thickened walls. In the synovia, pannus formation and extensive intra-articular damage may occur. Ultrastructural studies of synovial biopsies have shown that the most prominent vascular change is thickening of the basement membrane, which is organized in many concentric, closely arranged layers, separated by a less dense ground substance (Fig. 1). It has been suggested that reduplication of the basement membrane is due to repeated episodes of cell death and regeneration, each lamina representing the residue of one cell generation.

† Deceased.

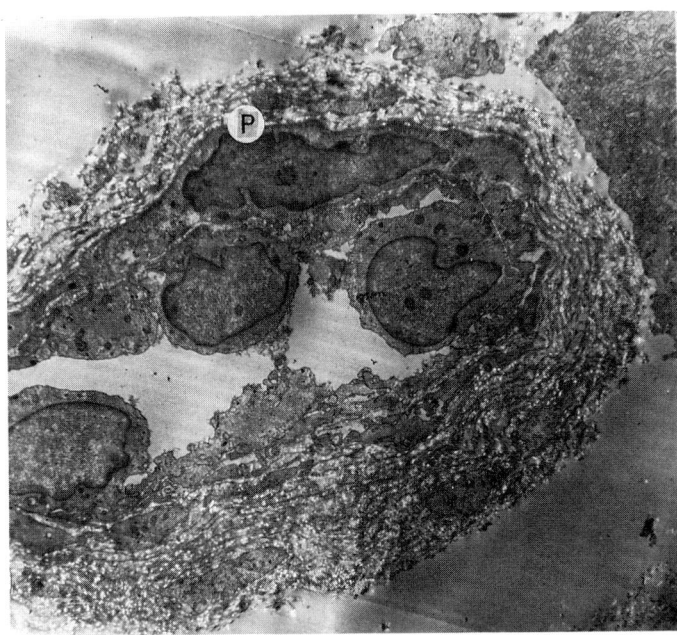

Fig. 1 Electron microscopic picture of a synovial blood vessel with a pericyte (P) and cell processes in between the many basement membrane layers. [Reproduced from Eliakim *et al.*, 1981, *Recurrent polyserositis (familial Mediterranean fever, periodic disease)*. Elsevier/North Holland Biomedical Press, Amsterdam, by permission.]

Aetiology and pathogenesis

The aetiology of recurrent polyserositis is unknown. The blood vessels seem to be the primary target organ of the disease process. This is indicated by the ultrastructural changes in the vessels, as well as by the systemic manifestations of the disease, the fleeting character of the symptoms, the appearance of transient haematuria, electrocardiographic and electroencephalographic abnormalities, and the occasional development of permanent vascular damage. The pathogenesis of the vascular lesion is, however, obscure. Most authors tend to relate recurrent polyserositis to the 'collagen' disorders. The similarity between the former and systemic lupus erythematosus is sometimes striking. The incidence of atopic allergy, rheumatic fever, glomerulonephritis, Schönlein–Henoch purpura, and periarteritis nodosa is higher in recurrent polyserositis than in the general population. High serum immunoglobulin levels, circulating immune complexes, and lymphocytotoxins have been demonstrated in patients suffering from the disease. Results of additional immunologic studies are still controversial. Although the pathogenesis of recurrent polyserositis is not clear, several facts seem to be established: the genetic nature of the disease, the involvement of the vascular system, and the presence of immunological disturbances.

Recently, it has been suggested that C5a-inhibitor deficiency in joint and peritoneal fluids from patients with recurrent polyserositis may have a role in the pathogenesis of the attacks. This inhibitor antagonizes the chemotactic activity of C5a and its deficiency may result in severe inflammatory attacks following the accidental release of C5a.

Clinical manifestations

The symptoms start in the first decade of life in about 50 per cent of the cases and before the age of 20 years in at least 80 per cent. Only 1 per cent of the patients may manifest the first symptoms after the age of 40 years, a fact of importance in the differential diagnosis. Almost all patients have attacks of abdominal pain, often originating in one area, but spreading over the whole abdomen within a few hours. The temperature rises to 38–40 °C with tachycardia, and about one quarter of the patients report a chill.

The attack usually reaches its peak in 12 hours. The clinical picture is that of acute peritonitis, manifested by exquisite abdominal tenderness, involuntary rigidity, rebound tenderness, and diminished peristalsis. Constipation is the rule and vomiting is frequent. The patients frequently flex their thighs and lie motionless to relieve the pain. Surprisingly, however, instead of developing into classical peritonitis which terminates in shock and death, the crisis resolves spontaneously and is usually over within 24 to 48 hours. The temperature returns to normal after a variable period of 12 hours to three days and the pain subsides gradually. The attacks recur, usually at irregular periods of several days to several months. Spontaneous remissions may last years. The severity of the pain varies from mild discomfort to that in severe generalized peritonitis. Mild attacks may be afebrile. In pregnant women, the attacks usually abate spontaneously after the second trimester. After the first attacks, many patients avoid visits to the emergency wards because they fear aggressive treatment. In fact, they learn to caution their physicians against performing unnecessary surgery and request symptomatic relief of pain.

Pleurisy

More than 50 per cent have chest pain due to pleurisy. Pain in the chest is sharp and stabbing, localized in the lower part, more frequently on the right than on the left, and radiating to the abdomen and the shoulders. Patients with stethalgia splint their respiratory excursions, deeper breath sounds causing much pain. Suppression of breath sounds over the affected side is usual but pleural friction is exceptional. A small effusion is occasionally detected in the costophrenic angle.

Arthritis

Arthritis is another common manifestation of the disease, its incidence varying between 24 and 84 per cent in various reported series (mean 55 per cent). Sepharadic Jews seem to be affected more frequently than patients of other ethnic origins. Several clinical forms have been identified. Rheumatic fever is more common in patients with recurrent polyserositis and has to be differentiated from the clinical forms typical of the disease. Most patients manifest an *asymmetric, non-destructive mono- or oligoarthritis* affecting the large joints. The knees and ankles are affected about three times more often than the hips, shoulders, feet, and wrists. Involvement of small joints is very rare. The affected joint becomes painful and swollen but local redness and heat are not pronounced and may be absent. The synovial fluid is usually turbid but it forms a good mucin clot. The white count ranges between 15 000 and 30 000 polymorphonuclears per mm^3 and the fluid is always sterile. The symptoms intensify during the first 24 to 48 hours but may last as long as a week. Usually, one or mostly two large joints are affected at a time. However, when the attacks are frequent, involvement of one joint may start before the symptoms from the previous joint have subsided, and the impression of migratory arthritis is created. The clue to the differential diagnosis may lie in the temperature curve which shows high peaks lasting one to three days. In about 5 per cent of the cases, the acute attack fails to resolve and the symptoms may persist several weeks or even months before they abate with no residual damage. About 2 per cent of the patients develop a *chronic destructive mono- or oligoarthritis* affecting most frequently the hip or the knee. Permanent organic damage results from one protracted attack or from repeated short attacks. Marked X-ray abnormalities and functional disability may result and surgical treatment may be necessary. Recently, *sacroiliitis*, frequently asymptomatic, has been described in a considerable number of patients. The radiographic changes include loss of cortical definition, sclerosis with or without bone erosion and fusion of the joints.

Skin rash

Skin rash occurs in 10–20 per cent of the cases. The typical lesion resembles erysipelas, which appears invariably over the extensor surfaces of the legs below the knees, over the ankle joints, or the dorsum of the foot. The skin becomes bright-red, hot, swollen, and painful. The rash is usually unilateral and its border may or may not be sharply defined. It resembles cellulitis and frequently prompts initiation of antibiotic therapy. Fever and arthralgia or arthritis are frequently present. The symptoms intensify rapidly and then fade within two to three days without any therapy. On biopsy the epidermis shows mild acanthosis and hyperkeratosis, while the dermis contains an inflammatory exudate consisting of polymorphonuclear cells, lymphocytes, and some histiocytes contentrated mainly around the blood vessels. Nodular rashes, Schoenlein–Henoch purpura, and urticaria are also encountered.

Other manifestations

Attacks of pericarditis appear occasionally and severe headache may occur during attacks. Transient electrocardiographic signs of myo-pericarditis and non-specific electroencephalographic abnormalities have been observed during paroxysms. Severe myalgia has been reported and muscle atrophy adjacent to affected joints is not infrequent. Numerous attacks in children may lead to growth retardation. Colloid bodies are often found in the eye grounds and the spleen is palpable in more than one third of the patients.

Laboratory investigations

There are no specific laboratory criteria for the diagnosis of recurrent polyserositis. The urine may show transient microscopic haematuria during attacks. Persistent albuminuria is due to renal amyloidosis or, more rarely, glomerulonephritis. The white blood count usually rises to 12 000–18 000 per mm³ during attacks and the differential count remains normal or shows mild neutrophilia. Persistent leucocytosis is frequent in the presence of amyloidosis. The red cell count is normal but mild anaemia may occur. The erythrocyte sedimentation rate rises during attacks, usually to between 40 and 60 mm after one hour and the plasma fibrinogen level to more than 5 g/l. Other serum protein changes include inversion of the albumin–globulin ratio, a rise in alpha 2 and, less consistently, gamma globulin and a rise in IgG, IgA, and IgM. Liver function tests are normal, although a mild and transient hyperbilirubinaemia has been reported. Bacteriological and serological examinations of blood, throat, urine, stool, peritoneal and joint exudates reveal no abnormal findings. The Rose–Waaler and latex globulin fixation tests are negative, and antinuclear factor and LE cells are not found.

Amyloidosis

This is the most important complication of recurrent polyserositis and its incidence varies between 0 and 27 per cent in various reported series. Amyloidosis occurs more frequently in Sepharadic Jews and Turks and is rare in non-Sepharadic Jews and Armenians. Patients who develop amyloidosis have a higher familial incidence, more frequent joint involvement, and skin rashes. The first sign of amyloidosis is massive albuminuria. Within several years, the clinical picture of complete nephrotic syndrome and advancing renal failure develops. Renal vein thrombosis is a frequent complication, signalled by a rapid decline of renal function. Unless treated, the patients will die within three to thirteen years. Most patients are subjected to haemodialysis and renal transplantation. Rectal biopsy will confirm the diagnosis in 70 per cent of the cases. On autopsy, amyloid deposits are found in the kidneys, intestines, adrenals, heart, ovaries, pancreas, and muscles. In most organs the deposition is perivascular. Recently, the complete amino acid sequence of the amyloid has been identified as the A component characteristic of amyloidosis secondary to chronic inflammatory diseases. A marked decrease in new cases of amyloidosis seems to have occurred since the advent of colchicine therapy. Genetic factors probably explain the greater incidence of amyloidosis in Sepharadic Jews. In fact a form of familial amyloidosis occurs in this ethnic group in the absence of symptoms of recurrent polyserositis.

Differential diagnosis

During the initial attacks, most patients are erroneously diagnosed as suffering from *appendicitis* or *cholecystitis*. Explorative laparotomy is performed so frequently as to constitute a characteristic anamnestic detail. It is important that cholecystitis, diverticulitis, pancreatitis, and perforation of peptic ulcer are unlikely to occur before the age of 30. Helpful hints in the differential diagnosis are the early fall of the temperature, the history of previous attacks, a positive family history, and the ethnic origin of the patient. A high plasma fibrinogen and a normal amylase are of additional help. Recurrent pleurisy may occasionally simulate *pulmonary embolism*. Joint attacks are frequently misdiagnosed as *septic arthritis*. The main feature of the arthritic attacks in recurrent polyserositis is their episodic occurrence starting during childhood or adolescence. The temperature curve is typical, the leucocyte count in the synovial fluid rarely exceeds 30 000 per mm³, and the fluid is always sterile. The destructive form of arthritis may be mistaken for *juvenile rheumatoid arthritis* or *tuberculous arthritis* but the diagnosis should present no difficulties. The association of fever, arthritis, splenomegaly, and skin rashes may suggest the diagnosis of *systemic lupus erythematosus*. However, accepted criteria for this disease will not be met, in particular, the LE cell and antinuclear factor tests are always negative and the leucocyte count is usually high. In cases of doubt, a therapeutic trial with colchicine is indicated. Indeed, suppression of attacks is the only reliable diagnostic test.

Treatment

Since 1972, colchicine has been established as the only effective treatment of recurrent polyserositis. A daily dose of 1.0–1.5 mg will prevent the attacks in 95 per cent of the cases. Short courses of colchicine taken at the onset of attacks have been reported to suppress the symptoms but continuous therapy is more reliable. The mechanism of the action of colchicine is not definitively established. Patients on colchicine manifest diminished polymorphonuclear chemotaxis both *in vitro* and *in vivo*. It seems, therefore, that a failure to amplify the inflammatory reaction and to generate a normal response to inflammation may account for the suppression of attacks. Chromosome studies have revealed no abnormalities after four years of treatment. Cessation of therapy three months before a contemplated pregnancy is recommended and, before more knowledge is accumulated, caution should be exercised in the treatment of children.

Prognosis

Most authors regard recurrent polyserositis as a relatively benign disease which does not affect the life expectancy of the patients, unless amyloidosis appears. Children are frequently physically underdeveloped because of the recurrent fever, nausea, and vomiting. Colchicine therapy seems to provide, for the first time, relief of much suffering for many patients, and opens a new horizon as a potential drug for the prevention of amyloidosis. The prognosis of patients with amyloidosis on chronic dialysis seems to be similar to that of patients with renal failure due to other causes.

References

Eliakim, M., Levy, M. and Ehrenfeld, M. (1981). *Recurrent polyserositis (familial Mediterranean fever, periodic disease)*. Elsevier/North Holland Biomedical Press, Amsterdam.

Levy, M. and Eliakim, M. (1977). Long-term colchicine prophylaxis in familial Mediterranean fever. *Br. med. J.* **ii**, 808.

Mazner, Y. and Brzezinski, A. (1984). C5a-inhibitor deficiency in peritoneal fluids from patients with familial Mediterranean fever. *N. Engl. J. Med.* **311**, 287–290.

Reimann, H. A. (1963). *Periodic diseases*. Blackwell Scientific Publications, Oxford.

Schwabe, A. D. and Peters, R. (1974). *Medicine* **53**, 453–462.

Siegal, S. (1964). Familial paroxysmal polyserositis. *Am. J. Med.* **36**, 893–918.

Sohar, E., Gafni, J. and Heller, H. (1967). Familial Mediterranean fever. *Am. J. Med.* **43**, 227–253.

Fibrosing syndromes (multicentric fibrosclerosis)

P. B. BEESON

This chapter deals with a group of poorly understood diseases characterized by proliferation of dense connective tissue in body spaces where loose aveolar tissue is usually present. At times the fibrosing process is confined to one anatomic site, but frequently there is simultaneous involvement of other areas with the result that a substantial number of combinations of fibrosing processes has been recorded. A peculiar feature is the tendency of the process to affect locations in the midline of the body.

In some instances an explanation of the aetiology of pathogenesis can be suggested, but in the majority this is not possible. In a few there seems to have been a genetic predisposition; in others, the process is related to ingestion of a drug; in still others, there is an antecedent infection in the area, or an association with neoplastic disease. In at least two-thirds of the cases, however, no clue to the pathogenetic mechanism is apparent, and it has been postulated that some kind of autoimmune phenomenon is responsible.

Retroperitoneal fibrosis

The commonest and best described fibrosing syndrome is one in which a dense plaque of fibrous tissue forms in the middle of the lower abdomen, over the aorta and vena cava. It tends to progress laterally, and downwards from about the level of the renal arteries, forming an apron-like structure extending to the level of the promontory of the sacrum. The oldest and most central portion of the plaque contains only bundles of dense scar tissue, but at the growing margins there is histological evidence of chronic inflammation with mononuclear cells, a few giant cells, and occasional eosinophils. Vasculitis may also be observed. Peculiarly, this scarring process usually fails to penetrate nearby hollow structures. Although adherent to the overlying peritonium, it does not really incorporate that structure, nor does it grow into the large midline blood vessels, or the ureters. Nevertheless, the ureters may become so encased in the plaque that peristalsis is prevented, and this can lead to serious obstructive nephropathy.

Recognized predisposing factors include ingestion of the drug methysergide in treatment of migraine; various tumours, particularly carcinoid tumours, but also occasionally carcinomas of the breast, colon, or prostate, where there are retroperitoneal metastases. Severe and longstanding urinary tract infection seems to have initiated the process in rare instances, usually when there is extravasation of infected urine from the kidney or upper ureter. Haemorrhage, due to trauma or bleeding tendency, may be the initiating factor. There are at least a score of case reports of retroperitoneal fibrosis in association with aortic aneurysm.

The idiopathic variety is encountered most commonly in males in the fifth and sixth decades of life, whereas there is no particular sex or age predilection in those cases where an aetiologic association is evident.

The early clinical manifestations are not distinctive. Most commonly there is pain in a girdle-like distribution, from the low back to the lower abdomen. The only helpful laboratory finding is elevation of the erythrocyte sedimentation rate.

The principal hazard lies in its tendency to cause unilateral or bilateral obstruction of urine flow. When this happens the patient begins to exhibit the clinical manifestations of renal insufficiency, and by then the biochemical signs of renal failure are present.

Because of the great danger of serious renal damage, retroperitoneal fibrosis should be thought of in patients with otherwise unexplained vague lower abdominal, or low back discomfort, especially if there is an accompanying increase in erythrocyte sedimentation rate. Usually the first clue to the diagnosis is given by intravenous pyelography, which shows upper urinary tract obstruction and a tendency for the ureters to be displaced medially. Sonographic examination is called for, and this may provide a firm diagnosis. The fibrous plaque appears as a relatively echo-free mass, with smooth borders, thickest in the region of the sacral promontory. Computerized tomography is sometimes superior to sonography in delineating the plaque.

Retroperitoneal fibrosis demands surgical treatment, and the results can be very good. If there is anuria and the patient's condition does not permit surgery immediately, it is sometimes possible to temporize, by passing catheters into both upper ureters, permitting the kidneys to resume their excretory function. At surgery it is recommended that a long midline incision be made so that careful search can be made for evidence of tumour. For that reason also, it is prudent to remove several full-thickness samples of the tissue for histologic study. The ureters can usually be dissected free of encasing fibrous tissue, and brought out on to the surface of the plaque, and peritoneum or mesentery can then be interposed between them. This procedure can be expected to relieve pain, and result in recovery of renal function. The fibrous mass may resolve gradually over time, but in a small number of cases studied thus far, sonography indicates that the plaque often remains more or less unchanged for years. Nevertheless, prognosis is relatively good if the obstructive nephropathy can be relieved early enough.

Some case reports indicate benefit from steroid therapy, in association with surgery, but steroids should seldom if ever be relied upon as the sole method of management.

Mediastinal fibrosis

The pathologic process just described in connection with retroperitoneal fibrosis can also develop in the upper mediastinum. There it tends to be located around the bronchi, the cardiac atria, the pulmonary arteries and veins, the superior vena cava, and the azygos vein; rarely, it also envelops the oesophagus. Symptoms vary according to the structures principally affected. There may be cardiopulmonary manifestations because of scar tissue about the atria, pulmonary vessels, or bronchi, and dysphagia can result from oesophageal constriction. One of the commonest clinical manifestations is due to obstruction of the superior vena cava with distension of veins in the neck and upper extremities.

Mediastinal fibrosis sometimes appears without discernible cause, and at times is associated with fibrosclerosing processes elsewhere in the body. The condition is encountered most commonly in people who reside in localities where histoplasmosis is endemic, notably in the central part of the United States. Hence, most of the case reports have come from clinics located in the Mississippi river valley. Studies of some of these patients have revealed the existence of large granulomata due to histoplasmosis, with eventual rupture into the superior mediastinum and subsequent growth of the dense masses of scar tissue characteristic of the fibrosing syndromes. A curious anomaly is that tuberculosis rarely, if ever, causes this syndrome.

The diagnosis is suggested by radiographic demonstration of large granulomata of the fibrous tissue in the affected areas. Histological verification of the diagnosis can be made by biopsy, most easily by employing the technique of mediastinoscopy.

Surgical treatment of mediastinal fibrosis is much more hazardous and much less likely to be beneficial than in the case of retroperitoneal fibrosis. There is risk of injury to the vascular structures in the mediastinum during attempts to remove the fibrous tissue; furthermore, serious bleeding may be encountered because of the variable location of enlarged collateral veins. Despite this, some experienced thoracic surgeons recommend that attempts be made to remove large granulomatous masses of histoplasmosis where possible. Also, attempts have been made to free the oesophagus from constricting scar tissue when dysphagia is a special problem.

Chemotherapy for histoplasmosis (or tuberculosis) has not been very effective. In view of the tendency of the fibrosing process to burn out eventually, it may be possible to ameliorate the manifestations by steroid therapy, and thus gain time for collateral circulation to develop.

Sclerosing cholangitis (see also Section 12)
This comparatively rare disorder results from extensive proliferation of scar tissue around the extrahepatic and intrahepatic bile ducts, and is usually discovered during surgical attempts to relieve biliary obstruction. The clinical and laboratory manifestations are those of gradually worsening obstructive jaundice. A fairly certain diagnosis can be made by endoscopic retrograde cholangiography, although this may not differentiate between sclerosing cholangitis and sclerosing neoplastic disorders. Treatment is not satisfactory. Shunting of the bile flow by way of a cholecyst-enterostomy is not usually feasible because the process can affect the cystic duct and intrahepatic bile passages. Some palliation may be achieved by the use of corticosteroid therapy.

There is an unexplained association of sclerosing cholangitis with inflammatory bowel disease, especially chronic ulcerative colitis. This rare complication is encountered in about 1 per cent of patients with ulcerative colitis.

Rare fibrosing syndromes
In association with some of the fibrosing syndromes already mentioned, other varieties of this process have been reported involving the thyroid gland (*Riedel's thyroiditis*), the *pancreas*, the *salivary glands*, and *orbital tissue*. The last-mentioned can cause severe proptosis and damage to the optic nerve, leading to loss of vision.

Peyronie's disease is characterized by the deposition of fibrous plaques in the corpora cavernosa of the penis. These plaques, which can be detected by palpation, may cause discomfort and angulation during penile erection.

References
Dines, D. E., Payne, W. S., Bernatz, P. E. and Pairolero, P. C. (1979). Medistinal granuloma and fibrosing mediastinis. *Chest* **75**, 320–324.

Feinstein, R. S., Baghdassarian Gatewood, O. M., Goldman, S. M., *et al.* (1981). Computerized tomography in the diagnosis of retroperitoneal fibrosis. *J. Urol.* **126**, 255–259.

Früh, D., Jaeger, W. and Käfer, O. (1975). Orbital involvement in retroperitoneal fibrosis (morbus Ormond). *Mod. Probl. Opthal.* **14**, 651–656.

Lepor, H. and Walsh, P. C. (1979). Idiopathic retroperitoneal fibrosis. *J. Urol.* **122**, 1–6.

Schowengerdt, C. G., Suyemoto, R., and Main, F. B. (1969). Granulomatous and fibrous mediastinitis: A review and analysis of 180 cases. *J. thorac. cardiovasc. Surg.* **57**, 365–379.

Eosinophilia and the hypereosinophilic syndromes

P. B. BEESON

The eosinophil
Although the recognition of eosinophils (see also Section 19) has been relatively easy since Ehrlich's discovery of their peculiar staining property, and although tens of thousands of publications have described their behaviour, contents, and other characteristics, their role in the intact animal remains conjectural. Their presence in all animals above the most primitive vertebrates suggests that they do serve some physiological function or functions. Among the total complement of leucocytes, their proportion is roughly the same in all species. They are formed in the bone marrow and, generally speaking, the number present in the blood reflects the rate of bone marrow production. This rate can vary substantially, resulting in wide differences in the number of circulating cells.

Despite similarities between neutrophils and eosinophils, in morphology, motility, and phagocytic activity, as well as certain lysosomal contents, these two kinds of leucocytes exhibit striking differences in behaviour. In some respects eosinophils appear to act as a component of the immune system. For example, T lymphocytes can stimulate their rate of production and eosinophilia commonly accompanies certain immunological reactions. In contrast with the behaviour of neutrophils, eosinophils decrease in number during most bacterial infections, and also decrease in response to injection of adrenal glucocorticoids.

Several hypotheses have been offered regarding possible functions of eosinophils. Their behaviour in allergic conditions such as seasonal rhinitis, atopic asthma, and drug allergies, has prompted the suggestion that they serve to modulate the intensity of IgE-mediated reactions. In support of this, it is known that eosinophil products can antagonize the pharmacological effects of such mast cell components as histamine and the slow reacting substance of anaphylaxis. Currently there is also much interest in the possibility that eosinophils protect against certain metazoan parasites by enhancing host resistance to re-infection, as for example, in schistosomiasis. In a wholly different functional realm, it is known that eosinophils react with such hormones as glucocorticoids, oestrogens, and adrenaline. Possibly, therefore, they may serve as carriers, or mediators, of the actions of these or other hormones.

Although it seems likely that eosinophils serve some useful functions in the host, there is also some evidence that their presence in excess over long periods of time can result in tissue injury, especially to the heart, possibly also to the nervous system.

Evaluation of eosinophilia in clinical practice
In normal circumstances the number of eosinophils in the blood is less than 350 per mm^3 (or up to 4 per cent of the total circulating white blood cells). Counts above this level are encountered from time to time in a considerable number and variety of disorders. In these infrequent events, the eosinophilia is probably not integral, but may instead merely indicate a peculiar response to some stimulus, analogous to the production of an ectopic hormone. For example, eosinophilia is encountered occasionally in *neoplastic diseases* (usually when the process is extensive, with massive metastic depositions.) Among the lymphomas, Hodgkin's disease is fairly often accompanied by a modest eosinophil elevation. Certain syndromes involving *congenital defects* have been associated with eosinophilia. A mild increase may be found in patients with *inflammatory bowel diseases*. Patients recovering from acute haemorrhagic *pancreatitis* may exhibit eosinophilia, and it has also been observed in some patients with *chronic active hepatitis*. Generally speaking, the eosinophilia is not a striking or regular association in these conditions and is probably of little consequence in the outcome of the diseases.

Diseases commonly associated with eosinophilia
The outstanding example is *infection by metazoan parasites*, during the stage of tissue invasion or migration. Thus, one expects to find substantial eosinophilia in the active phase of trichinosis, schistosomiasis, filariasis, and toxocariasis. The discovery of a marked and persisting eosinophilia always calls for careful search for tissue invasion by metazoan parasites.

Some *skin diseases*, notably pemphigus and pemphigoid, may be associated with marked eosinophilia.

As already mentioned, *atopic states*, with IgE-mediated allergic reactions, are usually accompanied by modest eosinophilia, although the level seldom exceeds 1500 per mm^3 of blood. The same is true of *drug allergies*.

There are unquestionably cases of true *eosinophilic leukaemia*, in which the circulating cells are immature, and leukaemia markers such as the Philadelphia chromosome can be found. The clinical course is similar to other granulocytic leukaemias, except for a greater tendency to cardiac and cerebral injury.

A number of different kinds of *pulmonary disease with eosinophilia* have been recognized. One of the mildest clinical forms is the so-called *Löffler's syndrome*, i.e. transient pulmonary infiltrations with eosinophilia. A more severe kind of pulmonary eosinophilia, the *PIE syndrome*, may last for months and is associated with persistent pulmonary infiltrations, fever, and severe disability. This disease is usually ameliorated by steroid therapy. *Tropical pulmonary eosinophilia*, a disease seen in India, Southeast Asia, and some of the southern Pacific islands, is now thought to be a human manifestation of a form of filariasis (not *Wuchereria bancrofti*). Demonstration of the filaria in pulmonary tissue has only been accomplished a few times, but strong evidence of that aetiology lies in the fact that clinical improvement usually follows therapy with the anti-filarial drug diethylcarbamazine. Patients with *asthma* who develop pulmonary infiltrates may also have an impressive elevation of the eosinophil count. Such states are thought to be due to the presence in pulmonary tissue of some organism capable of producing a low-grade chronic inflammation; the best known of these is aspergillus.

The hypereosinophilic syndromes

This imprecise term has been applied to a wide spectrum of disorders characterized by prolonged eosinophilia and evidence of disease in one or more organs. As introduced in 1968, it referred to a continuum ranging from the benign self-limited Löffler's syndrome through the PIE syndrome, disseminated eosinophilic collagen disease, Löffler's endomyocarditis, and eosinophilic leukaemia. The term should be regarded, therefore, only as referring to a large group of different disorders. Several of the entities included in this spectrum have already been mentioned here and are also discussed in other sections of this textbook. At present, the tendency is to use the term to refer to prolonged and life-threatening states, more serious than the Löffler's syndrome. Chusid *et al.* proposed the following diagnostic criteria for the label: (*a*) an eosinophil count greater than 1500 per cent per mm^3 persisting for six months or more; (*b*) lack of evidence of allergic or parasitic disease to account for eosinophilia; (*c*) manifestations of organ involvement. The organs most often affected are the heart, lung, brain, liver, spleen, and the skin. This is clearly a 'mixed bag' of diseases; for instance, cases of the PIE syndrome would satisfy the criteria, as would eosinophilic leukaemia. There remains, however, a slightly more uniform group, with features suggestive of an eosinophilic myeloproliferative syndrome. Numerous mature eosinophils are present in blood and bone marrow, and in various tissues. The affected persons often have hepatomegaly and splenomegaly. They are subject to a wide variety of neurologic manifestations, but especially are subject to development of Löffler's eosinophilic endomyocarditis, which is to be described subsequently. Nevertheless, even within this group there appear to be differences, both in natural course and in response to the therapeutic agents. Some patients eventually experience spontaneous remissions without any therapy. Some greatly benefit from steroid treatment, whereas most do not. Others appear to improve under the influence of cytotoxic or immunosuppressive agents such as hydroxyurea and cyclophosphamide. Therapy with hydroxyurea has seemed especially beneficial in some serious and life-threatening forms, even when there is evidence of severe cardiac involvement.

Löffler's eosinophilic endomyocarditis

There are scores of case reports of a form of hypereosinophilic syndrome in which the most serious injury is to the heart. It is by far more common in the male sex. The clinical features resemble those of a restrictive cardiomyopathy, because of endocardial fibrosis, mural thrombi, and degeneration of subendocardial myocardium. The diagnosis can sometimes be made by echocardiography. According to the observations of Spry, an important lead to the recognition of this kind of cardiac injury can be obtained by careful examination of the circulating eosinophils. The key finding is vacuolization. The suggestion is that lysosomal contents are being liberated from circulating eosinophils, injuring the lining of the heart and producing the pathologic changes just described.

As mentioned previously, treatment with hydroxyurea may be beneficial. A few patients have been treated by cardiac surgery: with debridement of the ventricular cavities and insertion of prosthetic valves.

References

Beeson, P. B. and Bass, D. A. (1977). *The Eosinophil* (ed. L. H. Smith, Jr). W. B. Saunders, Philadelphia.

Davies, J., Spry, C. J. F., Sapsford, R., Olsen, E. G. J., Perez, G. du, Oakley, C. M. and Goodwin, J. F. (1983). Cardiovascular features of eleven patients with eosinophilic endomyocardial disease. *Q. J. Med.* **52**, 23–39.

Fauci, A. S., Harley, J. B., Roberts, W. C., Ferrana, V. J., Gralnick, H. R. and Bjornson, B. H. (1982). The idiopathic hypereosinophilic syndrome. Clinical, pathophysiologic and therapeutic considerations. *Ann. Intern. Med.* **97**, 78–92.

Hardy, W. R. and Anderson, R. E. (1968). The hypereosinophilic syndromes. *Ann. Intern. Med.* **68**, 1220–1229.

Kim, C. H., Vlietstra, R. E., Edwards, W. D., Reeder, G. S. and Gleich, G. J. (1984). Steroid-responsive eosinophilic myocarditis. Diagnosis by endomyocardial biopsy. *Am. J. Cardiol.* **53**, 1472–1473.

Slungard, A., Ascensao, J., Zanjani, E. and Jacob, H. S. (1983). Pulmonary carcinoma with eosinophilia. Demonstration of a tumor-derived eosinophilopoietic factor. *N. Engl. J. Med.* **309**, 778–781.

Spry, C. J. F. (1983). Lung diseases associated with eosinophils. In *Current perspectives in allergy* (eds E. J. Goetzl and A. B. Kay), Vol. 1, pp. 67–77. Churchill Livingstone, Edinburgh.

——, Davies, J., Tai, P-C., Olsen, E. G. J., Oakley, C. M. and Goodwin, J. F. (1983). Clinical features of fifteen patients with the hypereosinophilic syndrome. *Q. J. Med.* **52**, 1–2.

Laurence–Moon–Biedl syndrome

J. G. G. LEDINGHAM

This very rare congenital disorder is inherited by an autosomal recessive mechanism. The usual manifestations consist of obesity, hypogonadism, polydactyly or syndactyly, mental retardation and retinitis pigmentosa. Some patients diagnosed to suffer from the syndrome are spared one or more of the manifestations which may be variable within families. Others have been reported to have various congenital cardiac malformations, or abnormalities of skull morphology. Renal involvement has been described and may be the commonest cause of death. Manifestations include mesangial glomerulonephritis, glomerulosclerosis, obstructive uropathy and cortical cysts, but the commonest renal abnormality is ductal ectasia of the renal tubules with medullary cysts close to the calyces, an appearance resembling the changes of medullary sponge kidney. Diabetes mellitus has been described in association.

Obesity which affects the majority is apparent in early childhood, but retinal degeneration with or without the classical appearances of retinitis pigmentosa may not be evident early, although it causes blindness in many affected patients by the age of 30.

Hypogonadism has been reported in relation to gonadotrophin deficiency in some patients, but to primary gonadal failure in others.

Mental retardation is usual but not invariable.

There is no specific investigation which proves the diagnosis, which must be made on clinical grounds.

References

Bluett, N. H., Chantler, C., Singer, J. D. and Saxton, H. M. (1977). Congenital renal abnormalities in the Laurence–Moon–Biedl syndrome. *Archs Dis. Childh.* **52**, 968–970.

Churchill, D. N., McManamon, P. and Hurley, R. M. (1981). Renal disease–a sixth cardinal feature of Laurence–Moon–Biedl syndrome. *Clin. Neurol.* **16**, 151–154.

Oettle. A. G., Rabinowitz, D. and Seftel, H. C. (1960). The Laurence–Moon syndrome with germinal aplasia of the testis. *J. clin. Endocr.* **20**, 683–699.

Schachat, A. P. and Maumenee, I. H. (1982). Bardet–Biedl syndrome and related disorders. *Arch. Ophthalmol.* **100**, 285–288.

Adenoma sebaceum, tuberous sclerosis, renal, lung, and other hamartomata, and the 'formes fruste'

F. W. WRIGHT

This is a condition in which multiple hamartomas occur in various parts of the body and in single or multiple tissue systems. Usually they are benign and multiple, but rarely malignant forms may occur, with distant metastases. They commonly occur in the 'butterfly' position on the face, as *adenoma sebaceum* or '*epiloia*' affecting the sebacous glands (Fig. 1), dermal, subungual, and periungual fibromas, pigmented naevi, *café au lait* spots, and may be seen in the retina as 'phakomata'. In the brain multiple masses or tubers, particularly occurring in the basal ganglia, give rise to the condition known as *tuberous sclerosis* which causes mental retardation, epilepsy, and hydrocephalus (Fig. 2). There may also be dense areas in bone, e.g. in the lumbar spine or pelvis, and similar to the common innocent dense bone islands, though more numerous. In the hands and feet small cysts, sclerotic lesions, and periosteal thickening may be present, especially in the phalanges (Fig. 3). In the brain the tubers often calcify and hence may be seen in plain radiographs, but they may also be shown by computer tomography or air encephalography. Sometimes the condition is associated with hyperteliorism, when there is overgrowth of the basisphenoid and the orbits become abnormally separated. Not all hamartomas are associated with adenoma sebaceum or tuberous sclerosis, and many individuals have one or two small such lesions in their skin or other organs. Some have a 'forme fruste' with facial, bony, renal, pulmonary, or brain lesions and no disability.

Hamartomas in the lungs may give rise to a variety of manifestations. Solitary lesions are not uncommon and may be seen on chest X-rays as rounded smooth nodules, the cartilage element of

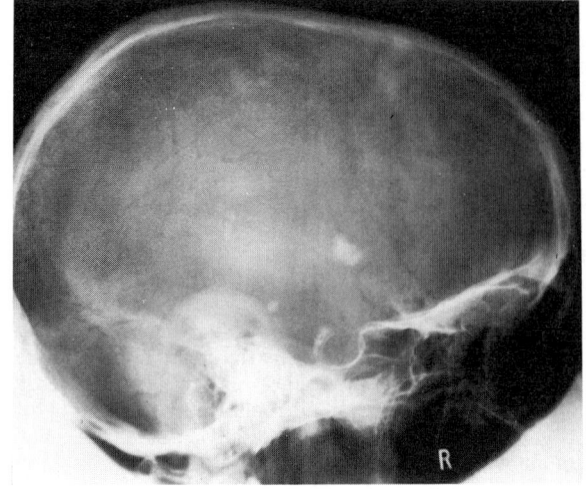

Fig. 2 Calcification in tubers in the brain.

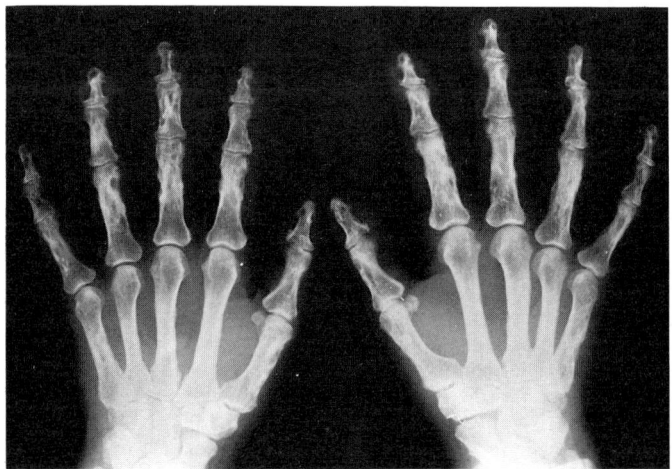

Fig. 3 Calcified nodules and 'cystic changes' in phalanges and metacarpals.

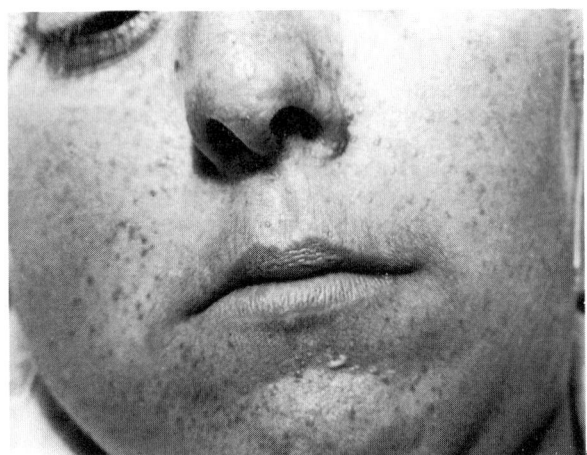

Fig. 1 Adenoma sebaceum on face. (Photograph reproduced by kind permission of Dr T. J. Ryan.)

which may calcify giving a central 'popcorn' appearance, especially when they become large. In tuberous sclerosis, multiple small nodules or a fine honeycomb appearance with bullae are more common, and may be the cause of a spontaneous pneumothorax. In an emergency case with honeycomb lung and a spontaneous pneumothorax, always think of the possibility of tuberous sclerosis or histiocytosis – in the former the patient is likely to be mentally deficient and in the latter to have diabetes insipidus! Such pulmonary cases usually have a bad prognosis from the time of presentation, usually no more than one or two years, because of the lung destruction caused by the nodules and small cysts. Pulmonary tuberous sclerosis (sometimes also termed 'muscular hyperplasia of the lung) may give a pathological appearance, with haemosiderin laden macrophages on broncho-alveolar lavage, identical to that seen in pulmonary lymphangiomyomatosis (see Section 12), which may be regarded as a 'forme fruste'.

Occasionally patients with multiple hamartomas of the lungs may present with multiple pulmonary nodules on a chest X-ray, mimicking pulmonary metastases (Fig. 4). Some may have calcified centres. Such should always be considered if, for example, a young, healthy woman has this finding on a routine chest radiograph – the author has seen this three or four times. When present it is usually a 'forme fruste' without any other stigmata of aden-

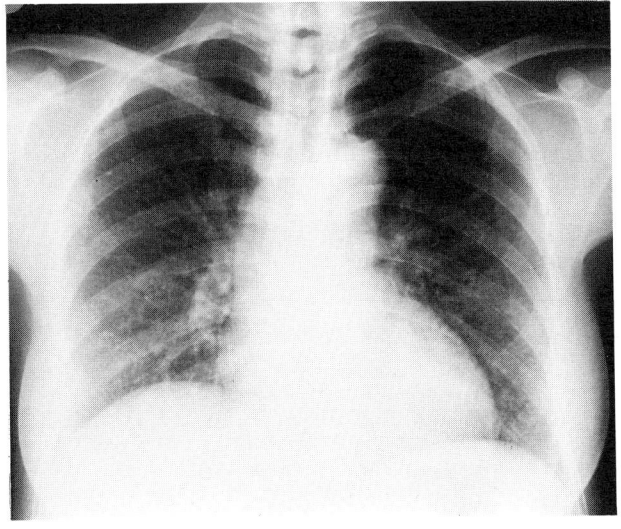

Fig. 4 Small nodules in the lungs.

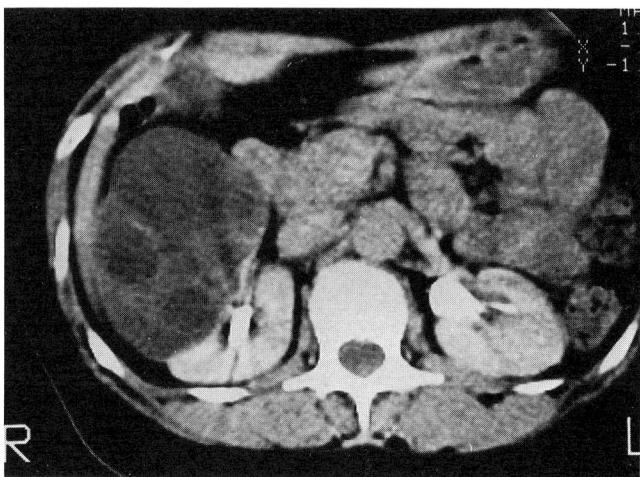

Fig. 5 Fatty masses in a renal hamartoma, shown by CT scan.

oma sebaceum. However, note the Carney syndrome described below. Computed tomography (CT) may be particularly helpful in demonstrating pulmonary chondromas in this condition. Solitary pulmonary hamartomata have often been removed, but when they are calcified they may confidently be ignored–the differential diagnosis being a calcified tuberculoma or possibly a secondary deposit from a previously diagnosed osteogenic sarcoma. The calcification with the 'pop corn' centre should be clearly shown by tomography. CT may also show increased density in nodules which do not have overt calcification. When muscle tissue predominates the nodules may more properly be termed fibro-leiomyomas or myomas, and may resemble metastasizing low-grade leiomyosarcomas.

Hamartomas in the kidneys have to be considered in the differential diagnosis of renal masses, which may be small and multiple, or larger and contain fat which may be seen on plain films, conventional tomograms or CT (Fig. 5). Such hamartomas may give rise to haematuria or bleeding within the kidney or perirenal tissues. When multiple they may mimic polycystic disease with a similar pyelographic appearance, i.e. large kidneys and 'spider calyces' (Fig. 6). At angiography, vessels in hamartomas often show multiple-beaded aneurysms (2–3 mm in diameter and larger than those of polyarteritis nodosa), which will distinguish them from true neoplasms (Fig. 7). In some cases there may even be a mixture of polycystic disease and hamartomas, and it has even been questioned if polycystic disease is a form of hamartoma.

Hamartomatous masses may also occur in other organs, e.g. heart, gastrointestinal tract, liver, vaginal wall, etc. Heart tumours are virtually otherwise unknown but in this condition may cause an obstructive cardiomyopathy, fatal pericardial haemorrhage, or even given rise to metastases, and one recorded case presented with multiple cavitating pulmonary secondary deposits.

The author has personally seen a case of a gastric hamartoma in a young woman in which the primary tumour was calcified and calcification was also present in subsequent secondary deposits in the liver, peritoneum, and lungs (Fig. 8). This has subsequently been termed the *Carney syndrome*. Hamartomatous enlargement of abdominal lymph-nodes, mimicking lymphoma, is sometimes referred to as the *Castleman tumour*. Like renal hamartomas, myomas arising in the alimentary tract are often very vascular.

Mesenchymal hamartomas of a diffuse soft tissue and vascular type, often with serious malformation of lymphatic trunks, may also be found in the limbs or in the chest and/or abdominal wall. They may look and behave like locally malignant tissue with erosion of ribs, soft tissue masses, spread into the chest or abdomen, and with exudation of lymph into the pleura, peritoneum or externally. On CT the lesions may be even more extensive than

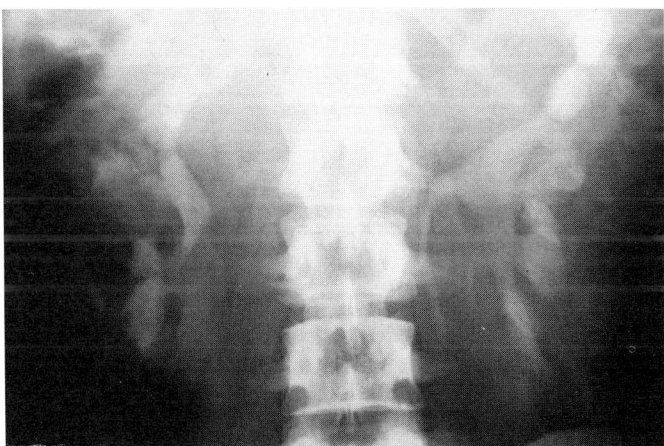

Fig. 6 Enlarged kidneys bilaterally due to renal hamartomas – a similar appearance to polycystic kidney.

appeared at first sight. Polyposis of the small bowel, i.e. the Peutz–Jaeger syndrome, may be an allied condition.

In considering the question of hamartomas and malignant disease, one should consider the term hamartoma. This word was first used by Albrecht in 1904. He derived it from the Greek word ἁμαρτανειν (to 'go wrong' or 'err') and the suffix ὠμα (a 'mass'). He used the term to describe a mass formed by mixed mesodermal rests, which occur in the soft tissue elements of the body. No malignant nature of the 'formations' (only somewhat distorted caricatures of normal tissue) was implied by the term. Albrecht did not specifically exclude the possibility of the development of neoplasm, though more recent writers have suggested that hamartomas never become malignant (but if this is so they must be one of the few tissues that cannot undergo malignant change.) If a mesenchymal or other tumour is present, then such authors would state that it could not have been derived from a hamartoma and it must have been a malignant tumour *ab initio*. It would, however, seem more likely that both benign masses (hamartomas) and others of varying grades of malignancy (mesenchymomas or sarcomas) may occur. Pathologically, hamartomas have been given various labels depending on the relative amounts of adipose, muscular, fibrous, or vascular tissue present in them. The muscular elements are always smooth muscle and the abnormal blood vessels are typically tortuous thick-walled structures (which give the beaded vessels or tiny aneurysms on angiograms). Terms which have been used to describe these masses have been angiolipomas, angiomyolipomas, lipofibrosarcoma, angiomyoliposarcoma, and haemangiopericytomas, etc. They probably also include 'simpler' lesions termed fibromas, lipomas, and myomas; in these masses the morphological configuration being more clearly defined. Evidence of malignancy is not often seen.

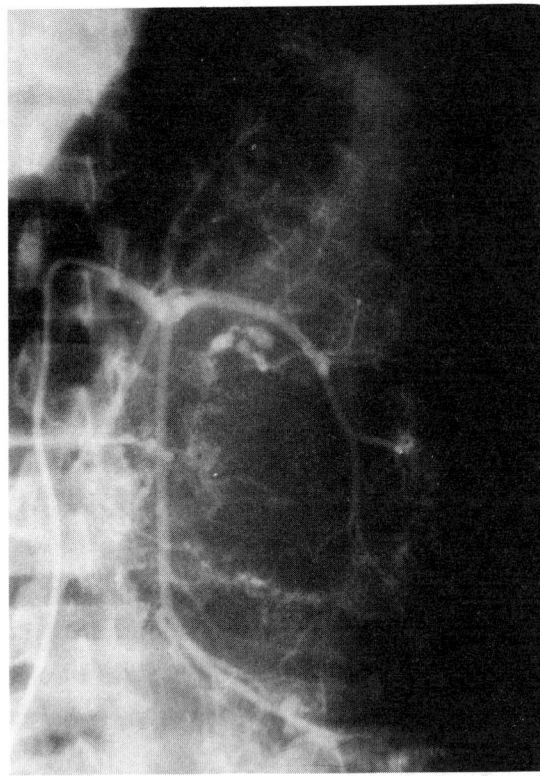

Fig. 7 Renal hamartoma showing multisacculated aneurysmal dilations within the renal vessels.

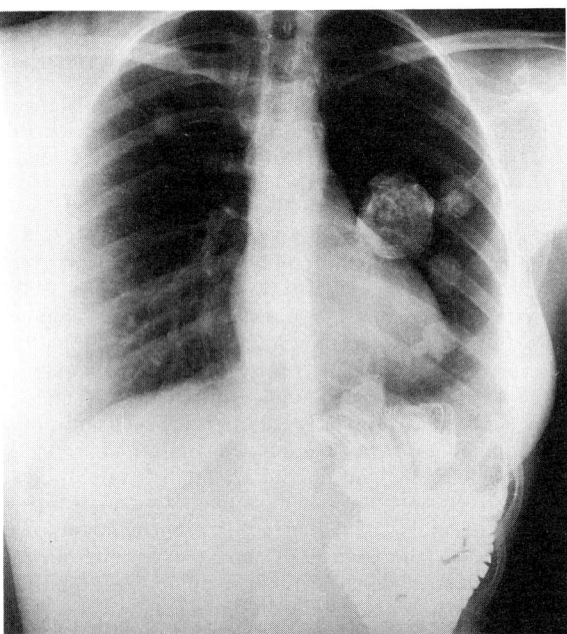

Fig. 8 Calcifying pulmonary hamartomatous metastases in a case of the Carney syndrome (note the previous gastrectomy).

Prognosis

Life expectancy and morbidity depend upon the site, multiplicity, and complications. Pulmonary cases have already been discussed. Neurological cases cannot be helped, except for some with obstructive hydrocephalus. Renal cases may die from torrential renal haemorrhage (which is usually outside the kidney and not into the renal tract), or present with enlarged kidneys and renal failure, but more commonly are found as a result of hypertension or the chance finding of a renal mass or masses, which are commonly mistaken for neoplasms and are often excised as such.

References

Albrecht, E. (1904). Ueber hamartome. *Verhandlungen der Deutschen Pathologischen Gesellschaft* **7**, 153.

Bret, P. M., Bretagnolle, M., Gaillard, D., Plauchu, H., Labadie, M., Lapray, J-F., Roullard, Y. and Cooperberg, P. (1985). Small, asymptomatic angiomyolipomas of the kidney. *Radiology* **154**, 7–10.

Carney, J. A. (1979). The triad of gastric epithelioid leiomyosarcoma, functioning extra-adrenal paraganglioma and pulmonary chondroma. *Cancer* **43**, 374–382.

Chew, F. S., Hudson, T. M. and Hawkins, T. F. (1980). Radiology of infiltrating angiolipoma. *Am. J. Roentgenol.* **135**, 781–787.

Gentry, L. R., Gould, H. R., Alter, A. J., Wegenke, J. D. and Atwell, D. T. (1981). Haemorrhagic angiomyolipoma: Demonstration by computed tomography. *J. Comp. Assist. Tom.* **5**, 861–865.

Iida, E., Kohno, A., Mikami, T., Kumekawa, H., Akimoto, S. and Hamano, K. (1983). Mesenteric Castleman tumour. *J. Comp. Assist. Tom.* **7**, 338–340.

Liberman, B. A., Chamberlain, D. W. and Goldstein, R. S. (1984). Tuberose sclerosis with pulmonary involvement. *J. Can. Med. Assoc.* **130**. 287–289.

Martin, E. (1983). Leiomyomatous lung lesions: a proposed classification. *Am. J. Roentgenol.* **141**, 269–272.

McGahan, J. P. (1983). Carney syndrome: usefulness of computer tomography in demonstrating pulmonary chondromas. *J. Comp. Assist. Tom.* **7**, 137–139.

Meiisel, P. and Apitzsch, D. E. (1978). *Atlas der nierenangiographie.* Springer Verlag, Berlin.

Ovenfors, C-O., Dahlgren, S. E., Ripe, I. and Ost, A. (1980). Muscular hyperplasia of the lung. Clinical radiographic and histopathologic studies. *Am. J. Roentgenol.* **135**, 703–712.

Silverstein, E. F., Ellis, K., Wolff, M. and Jaretzki, A. (1974). Pulmonary lymphangiomyomatosis. *Am. J. Roentgenol.* **120**, 832–849.

Steinberg, H., Chait, R., Sciubba, J., Aftalion, B. and Pillini, G. (1980). Metastasing fibro-leioma. *NY Stat. J. Med.* **81**, 372–375.

Uflacker, R., Amaral, N. M., Lima, S., Wholey, M., Pereira, E. C., Nobrega, M. and Tavaras, T. (1981). Angiography in primary myomas of the alimentary tract. *Radiology* **139**, 361–369.

Vera-Rōman, J. M., Sobonya, R. E., Gomez-Garcia, J. L., Sanz-Bondia, J. R. and Paris-Romeu, F. (1983). Leiomyoma of the lung: Literature review and case report. *Cancer* **52**, 936–941.

Wright, F. W., Ledingham, J. G. G., Dunnill, M. S. and Grieve, N.W.T. (1974). Polycystic kidneys, renal hamartomas, their variants and complications. *Clin. Radiol.* **25**, 27–43.

Werner's syndrome

J. G. G. LEDINGHAM

The major feature of this autosomal recessively inherited disorder is premature aging. Fifty per cent of patients develop maturity onset diabetes often described as 'insulin resistant'. There is usually some retardation of growth and ultimate shortness of stature. An elderly appearance is characterized by thin atrophic skin, which may resemble scleroderma, early greying of the hair, cataracts, and peripheral vascular disease, often with arterial calcification. Vascular ulcers develop in the feet and ankles. Some degree of hypogonadism is common, particularly in the male. In women periods are scanty and irregular. The menopause is usually early. Premature osteoporosis and hyperlipidaemia are also described.

References

Epstein, C. J., Martin, G. M., Schultz, A. L. and Motulsky, A. G. (1966). Werner's syndrome: a review of its symptomatology, natural history, pathologic features, genetics, and relationship to the natural aging process. *Medicine (Balt.)* **45**, 177–221.

Salk, D. (1982). Werner's syndrome: a review of recent research with an analysis of connective tissue metabolism, growth control of cultured cells, and chromosomal aberrations. *Human Gen.* **62**, 1–5.

Behçet's syndrome

T. LEHNER

Introduction

This is a recurrent, multifocal disorder which usually persists over many years and decades. The syndrome was first described by Hippocrates in ancient Greece. Initially Behçet's syndrome (BS) consisted of oral and genital ulcers and uveitis but later a number of other clinical features were added, notably skin, joint, neurological, and vascular manifestations. This creates considerable difficulties in diagnosis and a multidisciplinary approach is often required.

Epidemiology

The striking feature of BS is the relatively high prevalence in Japan (1:10 000). Indeed, in 1977 there was an estimated total of 11 000 patients with BS in Japan. The prevalence of BS is also high in countries bordering the Mediterranean: Italy, Greece, Turkey, Israel, Egypt, Lebanon, Syria, Jordan, Saudi Arabia, as well as Algeria and Tunisia. An epidemiological study in the United Kingdom has shown a prevalence of 1:170 000 which compares with 1:800 000 in a study in the United States.

Although BS may develop at any age, the most common onset is in the third decade. However, the disease can start in childhood with orogenital ulcers, followed by the other manifestations years or decades later. Male predominance is found in most reported series, but this may vary from 2:1 in Japan to 9:1 in the Middle East. Increased familial prevalence of the syndrome has been frequently recorded and there is an immunogenetic basis for the disease.

Aetiology

The cause of BS is unknown but an immunogenetic basis of the disease has now been established. HLA-B51 is significantly associated with Behçet's syndrome in Japan, Turkey, Israel, France, and England. Furthermore, HLA-B51, B12, DR7, and DR2 might in some way be associated with tissue localization of disease. Whereas B51 is the most discriminating marker of the ocular type of BS, DR7 also shows a significant increase in the ocular and neurological types. Indeed, most if not all patients with the ocular type have B51 and/or DR7. B12 and/or DR2 is significantly increased at the less severe end of the spectrum, the mucocutaneous and arthritic types. A significant relationship was also reported between the DRw52(MT2) alloantigen in the neurological type and DRw53(MT3) in the ocular type of BS. As with other HLA disease associations, there are at least two interpretations of these findings: (*a*) the HLA antigens might function as specific receptors for viruses (or pathogens); or (*b*) the antigenic determinants of some pathogens might mimic the HLA antigens.

A viral aetiology for BS has often been claimed, but attempts to isolate viruses from patients have failed. An indirect approach to the study of a viral aetiology in autoimmune diseases has been the finding that herpes simplex virus failed to replicate in activated cultures of mononuclear cells from patients with BS. The interference with growth of the virus was considered to be consistent with a viral aetiology of BS. However, a direct approach, using herpes simplex virus DNA probes and *in situ* hybridization with the complementary RNA in mononuclear cells revealed a significant increase in hybridization in those with BS. The results suggest that at least part of the herpes simplex virus genome is transcribed in circulating mononuclear cells of these patients. The role of the virus in the immunopathogenesis of BS, however, has not been elucidated; it may induce some defect in immunoregulation or invoke an autoimmune response.

Immunopathology

An early lymphomonocytic infiltration is usually found at the onset of ulceration in the lamina propria, the adjacent epithelium and around small blood vessels. The latter may show endothelial cell proliferation and some obliteration of the lumen. Though the early stages are suggestive of the type IV cell-mediated immune reaction, this is followed later by a polymorphonuclear infiltration and fibrinoid necrosis in the blood vessels, consistent with type III Arthus reaction.

Cell-mediated immune responses can be induced *in vitro* by homogenates of oral mucosa; these elicit lymphoproliferative responses, leucocyte migration inhibition, and cytotoxicity. The proportion of T4 cells may be decreased but that of T8 cells remains within the normal range.

Circulating immune complexes have been detected by a variety of assays in 40–60 per cent of patients with BS. The amount of immune complexes is associated with the disease activity. Although the concentration of serum C3 and C4 is normal, careful sequential studies revealed that C3, C4, and C2 were significantly reduced before an attack of uveitis, suggesting complement consumption by the classical pathway. Electron microscopical examination of centrifuged pellets of serum revealed the presence of small membrane fragments, some of which showed complement dependent holes. These findings suggest that the soluble immune complex may generate C5b-9 complexes which may bind to the surface of cells and result in cell lysis.

Acute phase proteins are increased in BS and this applies especially to serum C-reactive protein and C9; α_1-acid glycoprotein is significantly increased in the ocular type and factor B in the neurological type of BS. Serum C9 is a good marker of disease activity and can be useful in monitoring treatment.

An increased serum chemotactic activity is found with normal polymorphonuclear leucocytes and this might be due to IgG complexes releasing chemotactic factors. However, leucocytes from patients with BS may show a depressed response to chemotactic stimuli and this might be ascribed to IgA complexes. It should be noted that serum IgA is often increased but IgG and IgM are variable in BS.

Unlike most autoimmune diseases, nuclear, thyroid, and gastric autoantibodies are not found in greater proportion in BS than in the normal population. Rheumatoid factor is also negative, even with joint involvement.

Clinical features

The patients often appear to be generally well and complain only of the localized lesions. However, occasionally they present with acute exacerbation of malaise, fever, dysphagia, and loss of weight. In view of the widespread manifestations of BS, these are presented in Table 1.

Recurrent oral ulcers (ROU)

These are the presenting feature in most but not all patients with BS. ROU can be of the minor or major aphthous or herpetiform type (see Section 12). However, since ROU are rather common (found in 10–34 per cent of the population) and often trivial in relation to some of the serious manifestations of BS, they may be missed in the patient's history. Indeed, the least severe minor aphthous ulcers are found in 67 per cent of the neurological and 76 per cent of ocular types of BS, whereas the most severe type of major aphthous ulcers are found in 40 and 64 per cent of the mucocutaneous and arthritic types of BS. Herpetiform ulcers are found mostly in the mucocutaneous type of BS (45 per cent). The essen-

Table 1 Clinical manifestations of Behçet's syndrome

1 *Mucocutaneous*
    Recurrent oral ulcers: aphthous or herpetiform
    Recurrent genital ulcers: vulval, vaginal, penile or scrotal
    Skin lesions: pustules, erythema nodosum, perianal ulceration,
        erythema multiforme
2 *Arthritic*
    Polyarthritis of predominantly large joints
    Polyarthralgia of large joints
3 *Neurological*
    Brain stem syndrome, resembling minor strokes
    Meningomyelitis or meningoencephalitis
    Organic confusional syndromes
    Multiple sclerosis-like disorder
4 *Ocular*
    Uveitis with or without hypopyon
    Iridocyclitis
    Retinal vascular lesions
    Optic atrophy
5 *Vascular*
    Venous thrombosis
    Aneurysms
6 *Gastrointestinal*
    Abdominal pain, diarrhoea, distension, nausea and anorexia
7 *Others*
    Pulmonary: haemoptysis
    Renal: asymptomatic proteinuria and haematuria

tial feature of ROU is that the ulcers recur frequently, at intervals of weeks or months, and this varies from one patient to another. The long cherished view that oral ulcers in BS are rather severe and associated with scarring is no longer tenable. The clinical manifestations can be readily recognized and differentiated from other diseases (see Section 12). The pharynx can also be the site of aphthous ulcers which tend to be rather large, shallow, and covered with a fibrinopurulent exudate.

Genital ulcers

These are found in most but not all patients and can be of the three types described for oral ulcers. The ulcers affect females more commonly than males and scars may follow healing of ulcers in either sex. Females develop recurrent ulcers on their labia or vagina and they suffer from dysuria and dyspareunia which can ruin their marriage. Males develop recurrent ulcers on the penis or scrotum, again with dysuria and pain on sexual intercourse; some patients develop epididymo-orchitis.

Skin lesions

These vary but diffuse pustular lesions on the face and particularly the back are most common. Erythema nodosum may affect the limbs or other parts of the body. Occasionally erythema multiforme is found. Both females and males may develop perianal ulcers and curiously these may present in the young, well before genital ulcers have appeared.

Ocular lesions

These are the most serious developments in Behçet's syndrome. Relapsing uveitis, with or without hypopyon, iridocyclitis, retinal vascular lesions and optic atrophy are common findings. Relapsing conjunctivitis, keratitis, and choroiditis are also features of BS. Gross retinal vessel changes affect both arteries and veins, and fluorescein angiography is particularly helpful. Both eyes tend to be involved in 90 per cent of patients within a period of two years of onset of symptoms in one eye. Visual prognosis is poor, as useful vision (less than 6/60) is lost in about half the patients within four years of onset of the ocular symptoms.

Neurological features

These are found in 10–25 per cent of patients with BS (see also Section 21). The patients develop transient or persistent brain stem syndrome, resembling minor strokes. Transient focal cere-

bral syndrome and spinal cord involvement are also found. Others may present with meningomyelitis or meningoencephalitis and some with organic confusional syndromes. Multiple sclerosis-like features have also been described. The cerebrospinal fluid sometimes shows pleocytosis and raised protein level but more often is normal. CT scan does not usually reveal abnormalities but EEG can show slowing of basic rhythm. The prognosis of BS with neurological features was poor, with mortality of about 40 per cent in the literature before 1970. However, recently the prognosis has been markedly improved, with greatly reduced mortality, though whether this can be attributed to steroid and/or cytotoxic agents remains uncertain.

Arthritis or arthralgia

One of these is found in about half the patients with BS, at irregular intervals and in more than one joint. Usually, the knees, ankles, wrists, and elbows are involved and less frequently the joints of hands, feet, shoulders, and hips. Effusions, especially in the knee joint cause considerable disability. X-rays of the joints do not demonstrate erosive or destructive changes, but a number of exceptions have now been recorded, with erosive changes in the hips, wrists, and elbows. The test for rheumatoid factor is negative.

Vascular lesions

Recurrent thrombophlebitis of the leg veins is a significant feature of BS. This has been ascribed to a decreased plasma fibrinolytic activity. Less frequently, superior or inferior vena cava thrombosis may develop. Arterial aneurysms have also been reported.

Gastrointestinal manifestations

These are ill-defined. The Japanese literature records diarrhoea, distension, nausea, and anorexia in more than half the patients. Radiological examination revealed abnormalities affecting predominantly the small intestine; dilation, gas and fluid retention, segmentation and thickening of intestinal folds. However, a recent British series failed to identify consistent gastrointestinal manifestations, though transient symptoms were noted in 13 of 70 patients; two of these had rectal ulcers and one each had an anal ulcer, small intestinal ulcer, perianal fistula, and coeliac disease. It should be noted that patients with inflammatory bowel disease are excluded from the diagnosis of BS by the Mayo Clinic, although they may fulfil the criteria for BS.

Renal involvement

This has not been established in BS. A small number of patients were reported with BS and amyloidosis affecting the kidneys and a small number with glomerulonephritis. It is doubtful if these renal changes can be considered as primary manifestations of BS and they might be coincidental findings. Asymptomatic proteinuria and haematuria, without evidence of either amyloidosis or nephritis were also reported in a small number of patients. In a prospective British study two out of 38 patients with BS showed evidence of renal disease. One patient showed on percutaneous renal biopsy focal proliferative glomerulonephritis which, over a five-year follow up period, has not caused any clinical symptoms and the glomerular filtration rate has remained normal.

Pulmonary manifestations

These have been occasionally reported, usually as haemoptysis. In some of these patients pulmonary tuberculosis was suspected.

Diagnosis

There are no definitive criteria for the diagnosis of BS and the various schemes suggested rely on the association between two, three or four clinical features. Accordingly, the terms incomplete and complete BS are often used. However, in view of the multifocal involvement, we have grouped BS into a spectrum of four types which appear to have an immunogenetic basis: (*a*) Mucocutaneous type which involves oral and genital ulcers, with or without skin manifestations; HLA-B12 and/or DR2 is significantly raised. (*b*) Arthritic type which involves the joints, with some or all of the mucocutaneous manifestations; again HLA-B12 and/or DR2 is raised. (*c*) Neurological type which involves the central nervous system and some or all of the features in (*a*) and (*b*); here HLA-DR7 or DRw52 (MT2) is raised. (*d*) Ocular type which affects the eyes with some or all of the features described in (*a*), (*b*), and (*c*); HLA-B51 and/or DR7 is raised. Thrombosis of blood vessels can be found in any one of the four types of BS, as can be some of the other inconsistent features of BS.

HLA-B51, B12, DR2, DR7, and DRw52 are significantly associated with the four types of BS but are not diagnostic of the disease. The presence of immune complexes is consistent with BS and so are the raised levels of acute phase proteins; C9 is particularly useful in monitoring the course of the disease. The 'prick test' (pathergy test) whereby a subcutaneous puncture alone may develop into erythema 24 or 48 hours later has been found useful in the Middle Eastern countries.

Patients with rheumatoid arthritis, osteoarthritis or Reiter's syndrome are excluded from the diagnosis of BS, as are patients with a firm diagnosis of ulcerative colitis or Crohn's disease. Stevens–Johnson syndrome may mimic BS, but the recurrences are less frequent and tend to be seasonal, the ulcers are large and shallow, the lips are often covered with haemorrhagic crusts and the skin may show the typical lesions of erythema multiforme.

Treatment

The management of patients with BS can be difficult, as it requires close liaison between different specialties. Whenever possible topical treatment of local lesions should be attempted before embarking on systemic anti-inflammatory or immunosuppressive therapy. Oral and genital ulcers often respond to topical application of steroids or tetracycline or both, as described elsewhere (see Section 12). Uveitis is also initially treated with local steroids. However, at some stage systemic prednisolone is usually administered, with a starting daily dose of 20–60 mg which is rapidly brought down to a minimum effective maintenance dose of about 10 mg. There is usually a prompt response, though a small core of patients are resistant to steroids. Azathioprine is often used with prednisolone (2–3 mg/kg body weight daily). It is uncertain if azathioprine has additional beneficial effects, though it probably acts as a steroid sparing agent. Colchicine has been particularly advocated by Japanese and Turkish physicians for the treatment of BS (recommended dose is 0.5 mg bd). The rationale is that the drug inhibits the motility of polymorphonuclear leukocytes, which is increased in BS. Subjective assessment suggests that colchicine can be helpful, though it is not certain whether the drug may not have a selective beneficial effect on some lesions. There is general consensus that chlorambucil should be used in patients with unresponsive uveitis, in spite of the possible serious side effects. Recently cyclosporin has been applied successfully in the treatment of uveitis in BS but the side effects may limit its applications. Among the immunopotentiating agents, levamisole is helpful, especially with the orogenital ulcers. Unfortunately, levamisole can cause neutropenia in some patients, so that the use of this drug has been largely discontinued. Thalidomide has recently been found to be effective in the treatment of orogenital ulcers, but the teratogenic effect of this drug may severely restrict its use.

References

Inaba G., (ed.) (1982). Behçet's disease. *Proceedings of the international conference on Behçet's disease.* University of Tokyo Press.
Lehner, T. and Barnes, C. G. (eds) (1979). *Behçet's syndrome.* Academic Press, London.
—— and —— (eds) (1986). *Behçet's disease.* Royal Society of Medicine, London (in press).

The POEMS syndrome

C. R. W. EDWARDS

In 1968 Shimpo discovered a multisystem disorder in which a plasmacytoma was associated with a severe sensorimotor peripheral neuropathy. In 1980 Bardwick detailed two further cases and reviewed the 42 cases published since Shimpo's original description. He coined the acronym POEMS to describe the syndrome (P, polyneuropathy; O, organomegaly; E, endocrinopathy; M, M protein band; S, skin changes). The majority of cases reported have been in Japanese males.

Associated with the polyneuropathy there is a raised CSF protein in 95 per cent of cases and papilloedema in 63 per cent. The organomegaly includes hepatomegaly (68 per cent), splenomegaly (39 per cent), and lymphadenopathy (64 per cent).

The endocrinopathy is of particular interest in that primary thyroid, gonadal, and adrenal failure have been described without a compensatory rise in trophic hormones, suggesting that there is an associated hypothalamic or pituitary dysfunction. Glucose tolerance has been impaired in 50 per cent of patients. Gynaecomastia is common (69 per cent).

A monoclonal gammopathy has been found in the majority of cases, more commonly IgG than IgA. About half the cases have an increase in plasma cells in the marrow.

The skin changes include pigmentation (98 per cent), thickening or tethering, and hirsutism.

Peripheral oedema is a common feature and many patients have ascites or pleural effusion. A pyrexia is present in about half the patients.

The aetiology of the syndrome is unknown. There are no specific diagnostic tests but the fullblown syndrome is unmistakable.

Treatment with corticosteroids usually combined with cytotoxic drugs has been of benefit. Occasional cases have improved after plasmapheresis. If a solitary plasmacytoma can be found, this can be irradiated, leading in some patients to remarkable improvement including resolution of insulin-dependent diabetes. The prognosis relates to the peripheral neuropathy and no patient has developed the myeloma syndrome.

References

Bardwick, P. A. and Evaifler, N. J. (1980). Plasma cell dyscrasia with polyneuropathy, organomegaly, endocrinopathy, M protein and skin changes – the POEMS syndrome. *Medicine (Balt.)* **59**, 211.
Shimpo, S. (1968). Solitary plasmacytoma with polyneuritis and endocrine disturbances. *Jpn J. Clin. Med.* **26**, 2444.

SECTION 25
PSYCHIATRY AND MEDICINE

PSYCHIATRIC DISORDERS AS THEY CONCERN THE PHYSICIAN

Introduction

M. G. GELDER

Unlike most other sections of this textbook, this section on psychiatry makes no attempt to provide a detailed and comprehensive account of its subject. This limitation is necessary because the subject-matter of psychiatry is too wide to be covered adequately in a brief account. The present section is therefore selective, focussing on topics likely to be of practical value to the physician. Child psychiatry and mental handicap are excluded, since this Textbook does not deal systematically with diseases of children. Readers who require a more comprehensive account of psychiatry as a whole, and this applies particularly to medical students and general practitioners, are referred to the *Oxford textbook of psychiatry* or other texts listed below. In particular it should be noted that in this book anorexia nervosa and bulimia nervosa are considered in Section 8 (Nutrition) and not in this section on psychiatry.

This section is in four parts. The first describes common psychiatric disorders, focussing on aspects important to the physician. The second part deals with the interplay of psychiatric and physical disorders: how physical illness can lead to psychiatric disorder, and how psychiatric factors can influence the onset and course of physical illness. The third part outlines aspects of psychiatric treatment that may be of practical value to the physician. The account here is limited to simple measures that can be adopted whilst patients are receiving treatment for physical illness; wider aspects of treatment are considered in the *Oxford textbook of psychiatry*. The final part briefly reviews cultural factors that may influence the manifestations of psychiatric illness and their recognition.

In all four parts the emphasis is on psychiatry in relation to physical illness because surveys have clearly shown that psychiatric disorders are common amongst patients in medical wards. For example, in a large teaching hospital in England 230 medical inpatients were systematically screened for psychiatric disorders. On the strict criteria of a standardized psychiatric interview, 45 patients were found to be psychiatrically ill, of whom 25 were rated as mildly, 13 as moderately and seven as severely so. Most of these patients (80 per cent) were suffering from emotional disorders. Similar levels of morbidity have been reported in the USA and elsewhere.

In the same investigation it was found that as many as 22 of the 45 patients were not identified as psychiatrically disturbed by the ward staff. These unrecognized patients were generally unobtrusive and compliant, whilst the 23 whose disorder was detected were conspicuous because of the signs such as tearfulness or agitation, or behaviour interfering with treatment. Again this finding has been replicated elsewhere.

There are good reasons why physicians should be alert to detect psychiatric disorder in their patients. The severe conditions are likely to need psychiatric treatment, and some carry the risk of suicide. Disorders of moderate severity, thought less hazardous, may also need specific treatment, and if persistent may seriously interfere with recovery from physical illness. Mild disorders are a cause of distress which could be remedied. For these reasons physicians should include in their care of patients, the diagnosis and treatment of accompanying psychiatric disorders.

If the physician is to detect and assess psychiatric disorders, he or she needs a sound basic knowledge of psychiatric symptoms and signs, and of the procedures for taking a psychiatric history and examining the mental state. In common with other sections of the *Oxford textbook of medicine*, this section on psychiatry assumes that the reader already has such basic knowledge, and no systematic account of these topics will be given here. Readers seeking further information are referred to the *Oxford textbook of psychiatry* or the monograph by Leff and Isaacs (1978). However, attention will now be drawn to some aspects of psychiatric assessment that require emphasis.

The first point concerns the willingness of some physicians to ask about psychiatric symptoms. These clinicians hesitate to enquire about symptoms such as tearfulness or pessimism, because they are concerned that they may alarm patients or make them feel worse. These reservations are particularly common when the patient has a malignant physical condition. Whilst the patient's feelings should of course always be treated sympathetically, there is seldom any justification for withholding enquiry about them. Questions about feelings may induce an immediate reaction of weeping and other signs of distress, but this is not harmful provided that the doctor leaves time to listen sympathetically to the patient. Indeed, patients generally feel relieved when they can express their feelings and share their concerns.

The second point is that it is often valuable to interview another informant, such as a relative or close friend of the patient. This is because some patients do not recognize the nature or extent of their own psychiatric disorder, and the full picture is revealed only by the other informant.

The next point concerns the detection of psychiatric disorder in those patients who, as mentioned above, remain inconspicuous in a busy medical ward because they are quiet and compliant. It is particularly easy to miss depressive disorder in such patients, unless it is routine to ask a few questions about anxiety and depressive symptoms. For example, questions should be asked tactfully about low spirits, worries and tension; loss of interest in activities, and energy level; and difficulty in sleeping. If these screening questions reveal emotional disorder, a more systematic mental state enquiry should be made.

An alternative to the inclusion of simple screening questions in the medical history taking, is the use of a standardized screening questionnaire completed by the patient. These questionnaires can be used not only to detect psychiatric symptoms but also to measure their severity. Several valid and reliable questionnaires are available, of which the *General health questionnaire* (Goldberg, 1970) is particularly useful for medical patients. Such questionnaires have been used widely in medical and surgical clinics, and have proved generally acceptable to patients.

The next point about clinical assessment is that certain symptoms and signs may be difficult to evaluate in medical wards or clinics because they can result from physical as well as psychiatric illness. For example, tiredness, poor concentration, forgetfulness, and sleep disturbance are all useful in making the diagnosis of psychiatric disorder in a physically healthy person but are much less valuable in medical patients because they arise as a direct result of physical illness. When there is doubt about the significance of such symptoms, the uncertainty can usually be resolved by enquiring about other more discriminating symptoms of psychiatric syndromes (described in the subsequent sections).

As mentioned above, about 80 per cent of the psychiatric disorders detected in medical wards are emotional disorders. If the physician detects emotional symptoms in a patient, the next step is to decide whether they represent a normal reaction to physical illness, or a morbid psychiatric state. Normal emotional reactions can be understood as appropriate responses to the physical adverse circumstances of the condition and its treatment. A degree of dejection or fear is a normal response in a person who is physically ill, experiencing pain or other physical discomfort, in unfamiliar surroundings, and uncertain about the future. Such a normal reaction is recognized partly by making a commonsense judgement of what is appropriate, and partly by enquiring about and failing to find symptoms characteristic of a depressive syndrome or anxiety neurosis. The physician who sees many patients with the particular illnesses that fall within his specialty is often better placed than a psychiatrist to judge what is a normal psychological reaction to an uncommon physical illness.

When a morbid psychiatric state has been diagnosed, the physician should next assess its severity. In general, severity can be judged in terms of the intensity of the patient's distress; the duration and course of the disorder; and the kind of symptoms present (for example, in severe depressive disorders the patient may have delusions and hallucinations). These points are considered further when the various psychiatric syndromes are reviewed in subsequent sections.

Estimates vary, but probably 5 to 10 per cent of patients admitted to medical wards need to be referred to a psychiatrist because of a psychiatric disorder. The main indications for psychiatric referral are: uncertainty about the psychiatric diagnosis; failure of the psychiatric disorder to respond to treatment prescribed by the physician; a disorder of great severity and particularly one in which there may be a risk of suicide or harm to other people; and behaviour that is disruptive and cannot be brought under control by reassurance or simple sedation. These points are taken up in subsequent sections.

References

Gelder, M. G., Gath, D. H. and Mayou, R. (1983). *Oxford textbook of psychiatry*. Oxford University Press, Oxford.
Goldberg, D., Cooper, B., Eastwood, M., Kedward, H. and Shepherd, M. (1970). A psychiatric interview suitable for use in community surveys. *Br. J. Soc. Prev. Med.* **24**, 18–26.
Kaplan, H. I. and Sadock, B. J. (1985). *Comprehensive textbook of psychiatry*, 3 Vols, 4th ed. Williams and Wilkins, Baltimore.
Leff, J. P. and Isaacs, A. D. (1978). *Psychiatric examination in clinical practice*. Blackwell Scientific Publications, Oxford.
Shepherd, M. (ed.) (1983). *Handbook of psychiatry*, Vols 1–5. Cambridge University Press, Cambridge.

Neurosis

M. G. GELDER

Anxiety neurosis

Many patients who are being treated by physicians feel anxious at some time during their illness. This section is concerned not with these normal reactions but with the syndrome of anxiety neurosis in which anxiety is out of proportion to the stress which the patient is experiencing, either in its severity or its duration. Anxiety neurosis is mainly important to physicians because its symptoms can resemble those of certain kinds of physical illness.

Anxiety neuroses are common conditions. Their prevalence in the population is about 3 per cent among women and about half this among men.

Clinical features

The symptoms of anxiety neurosis are psychological and physical. *Psychological symptoms* include a feeling of fearful anticipation, irritability, sensitivity to noise, and poor concentration. Some patients complain of poor memory secondary to this failure of concentration but true memory disorder does not occur in anxiety disorders (if found a careful search should be made for an organic disorder). Many anxious patients worry repeatedly about their

physical health and some are very hard to reassure. Some patients also have minor depressive symptoms. Anxious people have difficulty in falling asleep and wake frequently during the night. However, they do not usually show the early morning wakening that is so frequent in depressive disorders.

The *physical symptoms* of anxiety neurosis are of three kinds: those due to autonomic overactivity, those due to increased tension in skeletal muscles; and those due to hyperventilation. The symptoms of *autonomic overactivity* include sweating and tremor; palpitations and a feeling of precordial discomfort; dry mouth, difficulty in swallowing, epigastric discomfort, and frequent or loose motions; frequency and urgency to micturition, failure of erection, and lack of libido. *Increased tone in skeletal muscles* may account for the frequent complaint of 'tension' headache, which is usually experienced as a bilateral feeling of constriction or pressure in the frontal or occipital regions. Pain in the neck, back, and shoulders has the same cause. *Hyperventilation* may cause dizziness, faintness, tinnitus, palpitations, precordial discomfort, and (a characteristic symptom) numbness and tingling in the hands, feet, and face; in severe cases there may be carpopedal spasm.

Some anxious patients experience sudden severe and unexplained exacerbations of their symptoms ('panic attacks'). Others report that anxiety is confined to particular situations which they tend to avoid ('phobic anxiety'). The episodic symptoms of these patients may resemble episodic medical disorders such as paroxysmal tachycardia or partial complex seizures.

Aetiology

Genetic factors contribute to the predisposition to anxiety neurosis. It is generally agreed that insecurity in childhood can predispose, though there is less agreement about the significance of particular experiences such as rivalry between siblings. The precipitating factors of an anxiety neurosis are generally events of a threatening kind. The physiological mechanisms through which the symptoms are expressed involve adrenergic systems controlling arousal in the central nervous system, processes of conditioning and learning which contribute to the generalization and persistence of the disorder, and peripheral adrenergic mechanisms.

Differential diagnosis

The physical symptoms of anxiety neurosis may be mistaken for those of physical illness, and unnecessary investigations performed. This mistake is most likely to happen when a patient complains of a single severe physical symptom without mentioning the anxious mood which accompanies it. When this happens the correct diagnosis can usually be made by asking about the full range of symptoms of an anxiety neurosis. Thus if the patient complains only of palpitations, the doctor should ask questions about anxious mood, dry mouth, sweating, tremor, frequency of micturition.

The second kind of diagnostic problem is to overlook a physical illness causing symptoms resembling an anxiety neurosis. The most important of these illnesses are thyrotoxicosis, hypoglycaemia, and phaeochromocytoma. The third kind of difficulty occurs when a psychiatric disorder other than anxiety neurosis presents with anxiety symptoms. Depressive disorder, dementia, schizophrenia, or the withdrawal syndrome of alcohol or anxiolytic drugs (e.g. benzodiazepines) can all present in this way. In the differential diagnosis of anxiety neurosis and *depressive disorder* particular attention should be paid to typical depressive symptoms of low mood, early morning waking, and depressive thinking. In the least severe cases it is not always possible to make a clear distinction between anxiety and depressive disorders, and the non-committal term 'minor affective disorder' is often used. With *senile or presenile dementia* the important diagnostic point is the presence of definite disorder of memory (present in dementia but not in anxiety neurosis). Rarely, *schizophrenia* presents with anxiety symptoms and when this happens, diagnosis may be difficult. Questions concerning the patient's ideas about the causes of the symptoms may uncover persecutory delusions or other symptoms such as ideas of reference which point to the correct diagnosis.

Prognosis

About three-quarters of anxiety disorders of recent onset recover within a few months. Of cases lasting more than six months, about three-quarters persist for three years. Generally, anxiety neuroses provoked by short-lived stressful events recover quickly, and those associated with prolonged problems or with personality disorder persist.

Treatment

Before starting treatment it is important to consider why the patient has chosen to consult a doctor. Some anxious patients seek advice not because their symptoms are severe, but because they have a special reason to be concerned about them. For example, a patient with tension headaches may have a relative whose headaches were caused by a cerebral tumour. In such cases it may be more important to deal with the patient's concerns than with the symptoms.

When anxiety is not severe, satisfactory relief of symptoms can be achieved without drugs by using brief supportive interviews which need take no longer than the proper supervision of drug treatment. This supportive treatment should include an explanation that physical symptoms of anxiety neurosis are merely an exaggeration of the normal reaction to stressful events. At the same time patients should be encouraged to resolve any relevant problems in their lives, or if they cannot do this come to terms with them.

In more severe cases anxiolytic drugs are needed though they should be prescribed for as short a period as possible, and rarely more than six weeks. Benzodiazepines are the safest of the effective anxiolytic drugs (see page 25.51). Of the many benzodiazepines, diazepam is a suitable drug given in a dosage from 5 mg twice a day to 10 mg three times a day according to the severity of the symptoms. If, for some special reason, the drugs have to be prescribed for more than a few weeks, they should be stopped gradually to avoid withdrawal effects.

If symptoms of anxiety neurosis persist for more than about two months, a psychiatric opinion should be obtained. The options at this stage are further psychological treatment or an alternative kind of drug treatment. Psychological treatment may be behavioural (directed mainly to the control of symptoms) or psychotherapeutic (directed mainly to the patient's way of reacting to problems). The appropriate behavioural treatment is either relaxation training or anxiety management (see page 25.53). There are three alternative kinds of drug treatment. Beta-adrenergic blockers have a small place in the treatment of persistent anxiety neuroses in which the predominant symptoms are tachycardia or tremor. There are important contraindications for the use of beta-blockers, notably heart block, a history of bronchospasm, metabolic alkalosis, and prolonged fasting; and the drugs should be used with great caution when there is evidence of poor cardiac reserve. The second alternative drug treatment is a tricyclic antidepressant (see page 25.48). There is some evidence that imipramine is effective in suppressing anxiety in cases with frequent panic attacks. The third alternative is with a monoamine oxidase inhibitor (see page 25.49). Phenelzine reduces symptoms particularly in phobic anxiety neuroses.

Phobic neuroses

In phobic neuroses there is an abnormally intense dread of, and a tendency to avoid, an object or situation. Three main phobic syndromes are generally recognized: simple phobia, agoraphobia, and social phobia. The prevalence of phobic disorders in the community is about 6 per 1000. Physicians are most likely to encounter the condition when the patient complains not of dread or anxiety in the situation but of palpitations, faintness, or breathlessness.

Simple phobic neuroses

These disorders are grossly exaggerated versions of common fears (e.g. fear of heights, thunderstorms, spiders). Although the fears may be very intense and cause considerable suffering they seldom present a serious medical problem. Treatment is by behaviour therapy (see page 25.53).

Agoraphobia

Agoraphobic patients become severely anxious when they leave home, enter crowded places, or are in situations that they cannot easily leave. In addition to the physical symptoms of any severe anxiety neurosis these patients characteristically fear that they will faint or suffer a heart attack. For this reason many consult a physician in the early stage of the illness seeking reassurance about their physical health. These patients generally restrict their activities in an attempt to avoid situations that provoke anxiety but this avoidance actually increases the symptoms which appear in new situations. As a result some seriously affected patients become virtually housebound. Treatment by behaviour therapy (exposure) is usually effective.

Social phobic neuroses

These patients experience severe anxiety in situations in which they may be observed by others, for example, in canteens, buses, business meetings, and social gatherings. The symptoms resemble those of other anxiety neuroses although blushing, trembling, nausea, and frequency of micturition are common. Patients are occupied with the idea that others are observing them in a critical way. They are less likely than agoraphobics to ascribe their symptoms to physical illness and less likely to consult physicians. However, some seek advice about urinary frequency or urgency of defaecation which they experience when anxious. Treatment is by behaviour therapy using a suitably modified version of the exposure techniques developed for agoraphobia.

Hysteria

Hysterical symptoms are symptoms which resemble those of physical illness but occur in the absence of corresponding physical pathology. Hysterical symptoms can occur in organic disease of the central nervous system (in which although there is pathology it is not in the site to which the symptoms draw attention), and in anxiety and depressive disorders. In these cases the hysterical symptoms are secondary to another condition. In the syndrome of hysteria the symptoms are primary and result from unconscious mental processes.

Nowadays the syndrome is less common in developed countries than in developing ones. Hysteria is more frequent among younger people, first cases being unusual after the age of 40 years.

Clinical features

The variety of the symptoms of hysteria is great but there are several common features. The first two have been mentioned already: the symptoms suggest physical illness but occur in the absence of physical pathology; and these symptoms and signs are produced unconsciously. In practice it is seldom possible to exclude a pathological lesion in the early stages of an illness that may be hysteria. For this reason the diagnosis of hysteria is usually provisional at first, to be confirmed when appropriate follow-up strengthens the evidence that there is no physical pathology. This important point is considered further under 'Differential diagnosis' below.

The symptoms of hysteria are often divided into two groups: dissociative symptoms and conversion symptoms. The term *dissociative* describes an apparent failure of the integration of mental activity; it refers to amnesia, fugue (amnesia and wandering), multiple personality, and somnambulism. The term *conversion* originates in the largely abandoned theory that in hysteria mental problems become converted into physical symptoms; the term refers, for example, to fits, blindness, and anaesthesia. Although these terms are still employed widely it is more useful to classify symptoms as physical and mental.

Many of the *physical symptoms* of hysteria resemble those of disease of the *nervous system*. Motor symptoms include seizures, paralysis of voluntary muscles, aphonia and mutism, tremor, tics, and disorders of gait. The sensory symptoms include anaesthesia, paraesthesia, pain, deafness, and blindness. In organic disease of the nervous system there is, of course, a rather precise relationship between the site of a lesion and the occurrence of physical signs. In hysteria physical signs differ in important ways from the signs in organic disease. Sometimes the differences are gross, for example, extensor and flexor muscles are both active in a limb that cannot be moved. Sometimes the differences are less obvious, for example, minor discrepancies in the distribution of sensory impairment demonstrated only after careful examination. Hysterical *seizures* differ from epilepsy in several ways. Although the patient may seem inaccessible he or she does not lose consciousness; the convulsive movements lack the regular and stereotyped form of those seen in epilepsy; there is no incontinence, cyanosis or injury; and the tongue is not bitten. These criteria distinguish most cases but it is sometimes difficult to make the distinction between complex partial seizures and hysteria. For these difficult problems ambulatory monitoring of the electroencephalogram (EEG) during an 'attack' may help to reveal the cause.

Symptoms related to *other systems* of the body include abdominal discomfort or pain, difficulty in swallowing, and vomiting. Each of these symptoms requires particularly careful physical investigation, for although each can occasionally occur in hysteria there is more often an undiscovered physical cause. This is particularly true of the difficulty in swallowing called *globus hystericus* which is often due to an undiscovered tumour, another disease of the oesophagus, or an abnormality of the mechanism of swallowing. *Torticollis* and *writer's cramp* are sometimes considered to be forms of hysteria but the reasons for this are not convincing and they are better regarded as neurological disorders of unknown cause (see Section 21).

The *mental symptoms* of hysteria include amnesia, fugue, 'hysterical psychosis', and multiple personality. Of these symptoms physicians are most likely to encounter amnesias. Hysterical amnesia generally differs from amnesia caused by organic disease in starting abruptly in relation to a definite stress and affecting the recall of distant as well as recent events, sometimes with denial of knowledge about personal identity. It is important to note that hysterical amnesia can occur in patients with pre-existing disorder of the central nervous system including epilepsy, multiple sclerosis, or the late effects of head injury.

Two other features of hysteria have been described: 'belle indifference'; and secondary gain. *Belle indifference* refers to the characteristic lack of concern about their disability, shown by patients with hysteria. Although characteristic of hysteria, such lack of concern is not confined to this syndrome; therefore is not a useful pointer to diagnosis. *Secondary gain* refers to the advantage conferred by hysterical symptoms – usually by excusing the patient from some activity that he or she would rather avoid. (The term 'primary gain' refers to the advantage of avoiding the anxiety that might have been provoked by the stressful events had no hysterical symptoms appeared.) Although secondary gain is invariable in hysteria, it is not confined to this disorder; people with physical illness sometimes succeed in obtaining advantage from their symptoms. Therefore this feature is not a good guide to diagnosis.

Variants of hysteria

In *hysterical pseudodementia*, the patient replies to questions devised to test intellectual function, by giving answers which, while wrong, strongly suggest awareness of the correct response in

that they are systematically related to this response (e.g. 2+2=5; 3+3=7). The condition is rare and when it occurs it is often uncertain whether the symptoms are being produced deliberately or by hysterical mechanisms. Consequently some writers classify the condition as a factitious disorder (see page 25.5). Since patients with parietal lobe lesions may behave in a similar way, the diagnosis of hysterical pseudodementia should only be made after the most careful neurological examination. In the rare *Ganser syndrome* hysterical pseudodementia is accompanied by narrowing of consciousness and hallucinations.

Epidemic hysteria usually begins in a closed social group, for example, a school or hostel often of girls or young women, though cases have been described among young males. The epidemic generally starts with a single case of real or apparent physical illness which alarms the other members of the group. Next a few predisposed individuals develop hysteria, and the anxiety of the group rises further. As this happens more people become affected. The epidemic often begins at a time when an unrelated problem within the institution has already increased the anxiety of its members.

In *compensation neurosis* symptoms are related to a claim for compensation after an injury or to the payment of a disability pension. Because such cases are usually seen after accidents, many are seen by orthopaedic surgeons. Among physicians they are seen most often by neurologists. It is often difficult in these cases to decide how far the symptoms have arisen through unconscious mechanisms, and how far from conscious exaggeration. Whatever the mechanism, several features suggest that the symptoms are related to the potential for compensation rather than the injury as such. Thus compensation neurosis is more frequent after accidents at work or on the road than after accidents during sporting events or in the house; and the more severe the injury, the *less* the likelihood of neurosis afterwards. Symptoms usually persist despite treatment until the claim for compensation is settled. After a settlement most cases remit unless payment has been made conditional upon the results of periodic medical reviews.

Aetiology

Hysteria like other neuroses develops when a predisposed person experiences stressful events. It is not certain what causes this predisposition. The few *genetic* studies are inconclusive, and theories implicating *experiences in childhood* (of which Freud's are the best known) are unsubstantiated. The predisposition seems to be increased, in a way that is not understood, by organic *disease of the nervous system*.

Differential diagnosis

Many of the important points have been referred to already. The difficulties of distinguishing hysteria from *undiagnosed organic disease* are so great that the diagnosis of hysteria should generally be regarded as provisional until adequate follow-up information has been obtained. It has been explained already that when symptoms point to disease of the nervous system, a confident diagnosis can sometimes be made after careful physical examination. When there is doubt it is helpful to consider four points. First hysteria, like other neuroses, occurs in response to stress; if no stressors can be identified the condition is less likely to be hysteria. Evidence of stressful circumstances does not, however, strengthen the diagnosis of hysteria because these circumstances may be associated by chance with the onset of organic illness. Second, secondary gain is invariable in hysteria and its absence argues against the diagnosis. However, the presence of secondary gain does not strengthen the diagnosis of hysteria since advantages can be obtained from physical illness as well. Third, belle indifference is not a reliable indicator of hysteria. Fourth, hysteria seldom occurs for the first time in patients over the age of 40 years. By paying attention to these points many errors of diagnosis can be avoided.

Hysteria has to be distinguished from *malingering* in which symptoms are produced by deliberate deception and for obvious gain. Malingering cannot be sustained consistently for long periods, while the unconsciously produced symptoms and signs of hysteria persist indefinitely. However, the distinction is often less than straightforward because some patients with hysteria deliberately exaggerate symptoms which have arisen unconsciously. In practice malingering is not common outside the special circumstances of prison, the armed services, or legal claims for compensation.

Prognosis

Most of the cases of hysteria of recent onset seen in general practice or hospital emergency departments recover quickly. Cases lasting for one year usually persist for several more. Any discussion of prognosis has to take account of the frequency with which physical disease is missed in patients with chronic hysteria. In one series from a specialist neurological hospital, a third of patients originally diagnosed as hysteria had developed a definite organic disease within the follow-up period which varied from seven to eleven years.

Treatment

Treatment should be along simple practical lines. The first step is to give a clear, unhurried explanation to the patient, indicating not only the steps which have been taken to exclude physical pathology but also what *is* thought to be wrong. It is not enough to leave patients with a list of conditions from which they are not suffering; a well thought out explanation is needed of the way in which the symptoms have arisen from emotional causes. This explanation requires a special interview, it cannot be done hurriedly in the course of a ward round.

It is important not to encourage the persistence of symptoms by paying too much attention to them. Instead the doctor should show concern about the problems which provoked the symptoms and encourage the patient to resolve them, if necessary with help from a social worker. Once this process has begun, strong suggestion should be given that the physical symptoms will improve. It is often helpful to accompany this suggestion by some form of physiotherapy. Throughout treatment physicians should remember that the diagnosis of hysteria is provisional until confirmed by follow-up. However, they should keep any doubts to themselves, watching unobtrusively for anything which might call for a review of the physical investigations.

Although patients with hysteria readily produce material for psychological exploration, they seldom benefit from intensive psychotherapy. Psychological treatment should be directed instead to ways in which patients could deal wih future problems more effectively than they have done with those in the past.

Factitious disorders

This term, taken from the diagnostic scheme used in the United States (DSM III), is used to describe a condition in which a person deliberately produces physical or psychological symptoms without the obvious motive which is present in cases of malingering. The most florid example is Munchausen's syndrome. Less extreme disorders involve a variety of individual physical symptoms. Some authors classify the Ganser syndrome as a factitious disorder; in this book it is considered under 'variants of hysteria' (page 25.4).

Munchausen's syndrome is a rare disorder, named by Asher in 1951, in which patients present repeatedly with dramatic symptoms suggesting the need for urgent surgical treatment or the administration of powerful analgesics. Patients are more often men and the commonest symptoms include acute abdominal or loin pain, haematemesis, and haemoptysis. The symptoms and signs appear to have been produced deliberately and there is usually other evidence that patients are trying to deceive their doctors; for example, their accounts of previous hospital admissions and even their names and addresses are often incorrect. The

extreme lengths to which these patients go to imitate illness strongly suggest a profound disorder of personality. How this disorder has arisen can seldom be decided because patients generally evade efforts to obtain accurate information about their past lives. Psychiatric treatment is seldom effective, and in any case patients seldom remain long enough to take part in it.

In *dermatitis artefacta* skin lesions are deliberately produced by patients who conceal this fact from their doctors. The condition is usually one episode in a long history of emotional difficulties arising from a disorder of personality. (It is possible that some cases of the painful bruising syndrome have a similar origin, see Section 19.) In another (unnamed) factitious disorder patients produce spurious evidence of a febrile illness by falsifying thermometer readings.

Obsessive compulsive neurosis

In obsessive compulsive neurosis the outstanding symptoms are thoughts which intrude insistently into patients' awareness and are recognized by them as inappropriate or nonsensical. Physicians are most likely to encounter obsessional neuroses when patients' preoccupations are about physical illness; such thoughts do not respond to ordinary investigation and reassurance.

Obsessional neuroses are considerably less common than anxiety neuroses or depressive disorders. The one-year prevalence is about 1 per 1000. Men and women are affected equally.

Clinical features

The syndrome of obsessional neurosis includes obsessional thoughts and rituals, anxiety, depression, and depersonalization. Obsessional *thoughts* are usually about unpleasant themes and patients try hard but unsuccessfully to exclude them from their minds. One common theme is the idea that the person is spreading disease by contaminating objects. Other obsessional thoughts take the form of fearful preoccupations about illness ('disease phobias'), for example, thoughts about cancer or venereal disease. Symptoms of this kind may lead to repeated requests for 'second opinions'. Other kinds of obsessional thoughts include *ruminations* (repeated internal debates), and *impulses* to perform dangerous or embarrassing acts (e.g. to jump from a height or shout blasphemies in church). Obsessional *rituals* (also known as compulsive rituals) include mental activities such as repeated counting, and behaviours such as repeated handwashing.

Aetiology

Obsessional neurosis begins when a predisposed person is subjected to stress though it often persists long after the stress has disappeared. Often, but not invariably, the predisposition is evident as an *obsessional personality* disorder. The cause of this predisposition is uncertain. It is likely that there is a *genetic* aetiology though the evidence for this is incomplete. Psychological theories, including those of Freud, which implicate events in childhood have not been confirmed.

Differential diagnosis

Obsessional neurosis may be mistaken for *anxiety neurosis* if the characteristic thoughts are not elicited. Some patients with a depressive disorder have prominent obsessional symptoms; and so occasionally do schizophrenics. In either case, careful examination of the mental state should reveal the other characteristic symptoms of the primary disorder. The differential diagnosis of obsessional neurosis can be difficult and a psychiatric opinion should usually be obtained.

Prognosis

About two-thirds of cases of recent onset improve within a year. The remainder usually run a fluctuating course over many years often with long periods of partial or complete remission.

Treatment

Mild cases of recent onset require no more than supportive treatment and encouragement not to give way to rituals. Associated depressive disorder should be treated because improvement in depression is often followed by improvement in the obsessions. More persistent disorders often improve with a special form of behaviour therapy known as 'response prevention'. Intensive psychotherapy is rarely beneficial. A few intractable cases have been treated by psychosurgery but the long-term value of this procedure is uncertain. Unless the disorder is mild and of recent onset, psychiatric advice should be obtained.

Hypochondriasis

Hypochondriasis is a persistent preoccupation with ill-health or concerns about appearance, out of proportion to any physical justification. Minor hypochondriacal symptoms are encountered frequently in medical practice when they may occur in the absence of any psychiatric disorder. Severe and persistent hypochondriasis is generally associated with a psychiatric illness or personality disorder.

Clinical features

Hypochondriacal concerns take many forms, of which the most common is repeated complaining about pain. The common sites of this pain are the head, the lower lumbar region, and the right iliac fossa. The distribution of this pain is usually diffuse and the description of its quality seldom precise. Gastrointestinal complaints are also common. They include indigestion, nausea, dysphagia, regurgitation of acid, flatulence, and abdominal pain. Preoccupations with cardiovascular symptoms include palpitations, missed beats, left-sided chest pain, dyspnoea on inspiration, and worries about blood pressure. Concerns about bladder function are also quite frequent. Some patients are inappropriately preoccupied with their appearance especially the shape of the nose and ears and, among women, the breasts; sometimes the preoccupations are concerned with supposed body odours caused by sweating, bad breath, or flatus.

Aetiology

Mild and transient cases may be provoked by everyday problems. The commonest disorders causing more severe and persistent hypochondriacal symptoms are depressive illness, anxiety neurosis, and obsessional neurosis. In a small minority, hypochondriacal symptoms are the first evidence of schizophrenia or dementia. Most of the remaining severe and persistent cases are associated with a personality disorder. There is no single personality type, although obsessional and paranoid traits are quite common.

Treatment

Minor hypochondriacal symptoms generally respond to reassurance based on appropriate physical investigation. More severe problems associated with psychiatric disorder require treatment of the primary condition. Hypochondriacal complaints secondary to depressive disorder or anxiety neurosis are likely to improve when the primary condition is treated. Hypochondriacal symptoms forming part of an obsessional neurosis are less easy to modify in a lasting way, though they often run a phasic course. When symptoms are secondary to schizophrenia or dementia treatment is difficult.

Some hypochondriacal patients cannot be reassured easily and may be very demanding. Once the appropriate physical investigations have been carried out, demands for repeated specialist opinions should be resisted. The doctor should avoid repeated fruitless discussions of the physical complaints and instead try to encourage patients to talk about the other problems in their lives – or arrange for a social worker to do so. While it is important to show sympathy and indicate that the patient's distress is understood, firm rules are needed about the amount of time that can be given to the patient.

Hypochondriacal symptoms associated with an abnormal personality require particularly skilled management. This is especially necessary in cases in which the patient believes that the supposed physical illness is the cause of some major failure in life. If the doctor tries to remove this psychological defence against accepting personal shortcomings, a patient may be left in a state of despair which is more serious than the original hypochondriasis. Partly for this reason, patients with persistent hypochondriasis who appear to have personality problems should be reviewed by a psychiatrist, even though he or she is unlikely to be able to offer effective treatment to more than a few. Since hypochondriasis confers no protection against actual physical illness, sooner or later most of these patients will seek help for a serious condition. The physician should never forget this obvious point however demanding the patient has been in the past.

Psychogenic pain

Pain with mainly psychological rather than physical causes can arise in the course of any of the psychiatric disorders considered in this section. It is sufficiently frequent to merit a brief separate consideration. Psychogenic pain can be experienced in any part of the body, but the head, neck, and lower back are common sites. Psychogenic pain is most often associated with depressive disorders and anxiety neuroses (in the latter the symptom is often associated with increased muscle tension). Though pain is a recognized symptom of hysteria, follow-up enquiries show that this diagnosis is made too often, for in many cases organic causes are discovered later. Patients with long-standing psychogenic pain often have disorders of personality.

Diagnosis

This depends on a careful description of the site, radiation, and timing of the pain which allows a comparison with the features of pain with organic causes. At the same time questions should be asked about symptoms of each of the relevant psychiatric disorders. Although descriptions of psychogenic pain are often vague and dramatic, this is not a sound basis for diagnosis since these aspects of the description depend more on the personality of the patient than on the cause of the pain.

Attempts have been made to identify *pain prone patients* but none is convincing. There seems to be no single reason why some people complain of pain when emotionally disturbed; and no one type of personality among those who do this. Among patients with psychiatric disorders, pain is rather more common among those who are older and possibly among people of lower intelligence. Suggestions that pent-up anger or guilt provoke pain are not convincing as general explanations though they have some truth in particular cases.

Prognosis

The *prognosis* of psychogenic pain is that of the associated psychiatric disorder.

Treatment

Treatment depends on the cause.

Disorders of appetite

Anorexia nervosa and *bulimia nervosa* are often considered to be psychiatric disorders. However, in this book these disorders are considered in Section 8.

References

Asher, R. (1951). Munchausen's syndrome. *Lancet* **i**, 339–340.
Gelder, M. G., Gath, D. H. and Mayou, R. (1983). *Oxford textbook of psychiatry*, chaps 7 and 8. Oxford University Press, Oxford.

Mersky, H. and Spear, F. G. (1967). *Pain: psychological and psychiatric aspects.* Balliere Tyndall, London.

Miller, H. (1961). Accident neurosis. *Br. Med. J.* **i**, 919–925, 992–998.

Personality disorder

M. G. GELDER

Personality refers to enduring qualities of an individual shown in the ways of behaving in a wide variety of circumstances. Personality disorder refers to a degree of abnormality of personality that causes suffering to the patient or to other people. This criterion though imprecise is more useful in clinical practice than more exact criteria depending on psychological tests. Personality determines the way in which a patient reacts to illness and its treatment.

Clinical features

Many kinds of abnormal personality are recognized. The brief descriptions that follow are directed to the requirements of physicians; fuller information will be found in the *Oxford textbook of psychiatry.*

People with *hysterical* (histrionic) *personality disorder* cause particular difficulties to physicians because of their demonstrative and demanding behaviour. The central features are self-dramatization, craving for novelty, and a self-centred approach to relationships. When ill, and particularly when required to comply with the routines of a hospital ward, these people are often inconsiderate, demanding, and selfish. Symptoms are described in a demonstrative way, often with an excessive display of emotion. These people are impatient and difficult to please, and may engage in tantrums of rage or exaggerated expressions of despair which exhaust those who are attempting to care for them, although quickly forgotten by the patient. The behaviour of such people may antagonize doctors to the point that investigations are curtailed and genuine disease is overlooked. If this error is to be avoided it is essential not to become involved in the patient's emotional displays.

People with *paranoid personality disorder* are markedly sensitive, touchy, and suspicious. They distrust other people, are secretive, argumentative, and ungrateful. Such people readily feel humiliated and take offence easily and yet their behaviour invites rebuffs. People of this kind make difficult patients, who seem constantly ungrateful for the help that is given. Some make unreasonable complaints about their treatment and continue to pursue these long after other people would have agreed to settle the case.

People with *obsessional* (anankastic) *personality disorder* are rigid in their views, adapt badly to change, and expect unreasonable standards of performance from themselves and other people. They are guilt-ridden, moralistic, and lack the capacity for enjoyment. Obsessional personalities are indecisive, asking for more and more advice, and after making a decision worrying that it is wrong. Although outwardly polite and eager to please, these people are given to unexpressed feelings of anger. They respond badly to the changes imposed by illness and find difficulty in making choices about treatment. In the ward they are irritated by small deviations from the planned routine, and although outwardly polite to the point of subservience may seethe with unexpressed resentment at what they see as failure to reach their own unrealistic standards.

People with *schizoid personality disorders* are emotionally cold, introspective, and self-sufficient to a fault. They appear aloof and ill at ease in company. In extreme cases are callous, seclusive, and friendless. When ill, such people are likely to underplay their suffering and fail to express their concerns. Their lack of warmth and awkwardness in company makes it difficult for the doctor to empathize with them or discover their real concerns.

Antisocial personality disorder is also called *psychopathic personality*. There are four important features: failure to make loving relationships, impulsive actions, lack of guilt, and failure to learn from experience. Such people are heartless, cruel, and often violent. In some these aggressive qualities are obvious, in others they are masked by a superficial and deceptive charm. The pattern of life of these people lacks consistent goals, and they prefer immediate gratification to long-term achievement. Many offend repeatedly against the law, and some engage in callous acts of violence. Often their behaviour is made more extreme by indulgence in alcohol or drugs. These people make inadequate parents, neglecting or abusing their children, so that the family may be well known to the general practitioner, to paediatricians, and to the social services. When unwell these people are difficult, demanding, and aggressive patients. They expect immediate help from others but generally avoid taking responsibility for themselves, and fail to comply with long-term plans for treatment. When frustrated they become angry, and at times their violent behaviour is dangerous. Doctors often have to be content to do what the patient will allow at the time, keeping in touch with him or her and the family over a longer period so that if the patient cannot be helped, at least the harm caused to others can be minimized.

Several other kinds of personality disorder are recognized but as they are of less concern to physicians they will not be described at length. *Affective personality disorder* is characterized by persistently low or, less often, persistently elevated mood, or by alternations between the two. *Explosive personality disorder* shares the readiness to anger and aggressive acts of the antisocial personality without the other difficulties of that group. People with *asthenic personality disorder* are weak-willed, easily led, and lack vigour. They complain about their situations and often about their health, but do little to help themselves.

Aetiology

The cause of personality disorder is not understood. The substantial literature on the subject is reviewed in textbooks of psychiatry and will not be considered here.

Differential diagnosis

Personality disorder is diagnosed when there is a continuous history of abnormal behaviour originating in the teenage years. Usually the distinction from mental illness can be made of the history, but two circumstances give rise to difficulty. First, when a chronic illness begins in adolescence: this illness is usually schizophrenia or an organic disorder such as encephalitis or the effects of serious head injury. Second, when an abnormal personality experiences acute stress, the reaction may resemble mental illness: in practice this problem usually arises with paranoid or antisocial personalities whose reactions may resemble schizophrenia. Doubtful cases require a psychiatric opinion.

Prognosis

Personality disorders change little with time (or treatment) but patients often present fewer problems for their doctors as they and their families come to recognize their limitations and adapt their lives accordingly.

Treatment

Even with intensive psychological treatment only small changes can be brought about in most personality disorders, and it is usually more realistic to help the patient adapt life in a way that leads to fewer problems. This is a lengthy business usually taking years, but as it requires a common sense approach rather than specialized training in psychiatry it can be done by whichever doctor the patient trusts most. This doctor may be the general practitioner, or a physician who is caring for a chronic medical disorder. However, a psychiatric assessment may be useful to make sure that the patient is not one of the few who are likely to benefit from psychotherapy.

References

Gelder, M. G., Gath, D. H. and Mayou, R. (1983). Personality disorder. *Oxford textbook of psychiatry*, ch. 5. Oxford University Press, Oxford.

Vaillant, G. E. and Perry, J. C. (1980). Personality disorders. In *Comprehensive textbook of psychiatry*, 3rd edn, Vol. 3. (eds H. I. Kaplan, A. M. Freedman and B. J. Sadock), Ch. 22. Williams and Wilkins, Baltimore.

Affective disorders

M. G. GELDER

Depressive disorders

It is, of course, normal to feel sad at times of adversity. It is not surprising therefore that depressive symptoms are reported commonly by people who are physically ill. This section is concerned with more profound disorders of mood, in which the prominent symptom of depression is associated with other symptoms in a characteristic syndrome. Physicians encounter depressive disorders in two main circumstances. First, when a depressive disorder is provoked by physical illness. Second, when a depressive disorder presents with symptoms resembling those of physical illness.

Depressive disorders are quite common in the population: the reported point prevalence is about 3 per cent for men and about 7 per cent for women. Several surveys have shown that depressive disorders are also common among patients in medical wards, and that not all these disorders are identified by physicians.

Clinical features

The clinical features of depressive disorders are very varied and it is useful to consider separately the symptoms of mild, moderate, and severe cases. For the purposes of description it is convenient to begin with cases of moderate severity, treating the others as variants on this basic pattern.

The central features of a *depressive disorder of moderate severity* are summarized in Table 1. They consist of complaints of low mood, lack of the capacity to feel pleasure, and reduced energy. The patient appears sad with vertical furrows in the brow, down-turned corners of the mouth, and a stooped posture. Movement and speech are slow, and the tone of voice is monotonous. The dominant mood is one of intense sadness, although the person may also be irritable and anxious. The patient withdraws from other people, loses interest in work and hobbies, and finds everyday tasks a burden. Thoughts are dominated by guilty recollections and by pessimistic ideas which may include ruminations about death. Some depressed patients are convinced that they have a mortal physical illness; some wish for death and make plans for suicide. Careful enquiries about suicide should be made in every case (see page 25.20). The depressed patient has difficulty in concentrating, and through inattention may fail to register what is happening, thus giving an impression of poor memory. (True disorder of memory does not occur in a depressive disorder and if found should always prompt a search for organic disorder.)

A particularly important group of features are often called 'biological'. These features are: sleep disorder characterized by early morning waking, symptoms that are worse in the morning than later in the day, loss of appetite and weight, complaints of constipation, diminished libido and, among women, amenorrhoea. Of these symptoms, early morning waking and worsening of mood in the morning are particularly important since they help to distinguish depressive disorders from an anxiety neurosis. In the latter condition patients often describe difficulty in falling asleep but do not generally wake early, and they feel worse in the later part of the day.

There are several important variations of this typical clinical picture. Not all patients with a depressive disorder appear sad, and their smiling faces and denial of sadness can mislead a doctor who

Table 1 Central features of depressive disorders

Low mood
Reduced energy and activities
Loss of enjoyment

Pessimistic thoughts
Guilty recollections
Suicidal ideas

Early morning waking
Duirnal mood variation
Loss of appetite and weight
Complaints of constipation
Loss of libido
Amenorrhoea

does not ask about the other characteristic symptoms of the disorder. Other depressed patients are restless and agitated rather than retarded; their behaviour may suggest an anxiety neurosis unless appropriate questions are asked about sleep, mood, and thinking. Finally some patients overeat when depressed and gain weight instead of losing it; and a few sleep more rather than less.

In *depressive disorders of a severe degree* all the features of a case of moderate severity are present in greater intensity and there are some additional features as well. These features are delusions and hallucinations, and when they are present the disorder is sometimes called a *psychotic* depression. These delusions and hallucinations are concerned with guilt, worthlessness, ill health, and (more rarely) poverty. Some depressed patients have persecutory delusions but unlike the schizophrenic, depressed patients regard the supposed persecution as something they have brought on themselves. When hallucinations occur they usually take the form of words or phrases that appear to confirm the patient's ideas of worthlessness (e.g. 'he is wicked'). These symptoms are an indication for urgent referral to a psychiatrist, and the most careful assessment of suicide risk (see page 25.20).

The symptoms of *mild depressive disorders* fall into two groups. The first group resembles the symptoms of a depressive disorder of moderate degree, except that they are less intense. These symptoms are low mood, lack of energy, and interest, irritability, and sleep disturbance. The latter may resemble either the early waking that is typical of more severe cases, or the difficulty in falling asleep and fitful sleep in the middle of the night seen in anxiety neuroses. The second group of symptoms are not generally found in moderate or severe depressive disorders. These symptoms are anxiety, phobias, and obsessions. The presence of these additional ('neurotic') symptoms has led to the suggestion that these mild depressive disorders are distinct from the moderate and severe ones, and the term neurotic depression has been used to describe them. This is still a controversial matter because there is insufficient evidence to decide the issue.

The dexamethasone suppression test is abnormal in about a third of patients with moderate or severe depression. These patients do not show the suppression of cortisol secretion normally induced by a standard dose of dexamethasone given at midnight on the previous day. It has been suggested that this endocrine abnormality is indicative of a hypothalamic disorder and may be a marker of cases requiring drug treatment. However, similar abnormalities are found among patients who do not have a depressive disorder and there are other reasons for thinking that a simple view of the significance of abnormal test findings is unlikely to be correct.

Depressive disorder presenting with somatic symptoms

Physicians are particularly likely to encounter depressive disorders in which the patient's main complaint is of symptoms suggesting physical disease rather than low mood. These symptoms include malaise, lack of appetite, constipation, and discomfort or pain in various parts of the body. These symptoms are viewed in a pessimistic way and often interpreted by the patient as evidence of serious illness, and the patient does not respond to reassurance after appropriate investigation. Cases of this kind are sometimes called 'masked depression' because mood disorder and depressive thinking – although present – are not obvious. There are two other ways in which depressive disorders can appear in a masked form. In the first, the depressive disorder reduces the patient's tolerance for an established chronic physical condition and the complaints increase. In the second, the depressive disorder leads to changes in behaviour that lead to physical ill health. These two modes of presentation will now be considered in a little more detail.

Increased complaining about pre-existing illness occurs when low mood caused by a depressive disorder makes a patient unable to tolerate a degree of discomfort that was previously endured. Increased complaints about low back pain, osteoarthritis, and chronic bronchitis should suggest a depressive disorder when there is no evidence that the physical condition has worsened.

Depressed patients may act in a way that worsens their physical condition. Some take alcohol in excessive amounts in an attempt to improve their mood. Others smoke or eat more than usual. Still others fail to take the treatment prescribed to control a pre-existing physical illness such as diabetes either because they lack initiative or because they think their situation hopeless. In this way they present with an exacerbation of the disorder rather than with complaints of depression.

Aetiology

Genetic factors have been shown to be important determinants of severe depressive disorders but their role in other cases is less certain. Adverse *experiences in childhood*, especially separation from the mother, appear to predispose to depression in later life, probably by affecting the way in which the person responds to adverse circumstances. Depressive disorders are precipitated directly by some *physical illnesses* and certain treatments for such illnesses, as described on pages 25.32–25.40. *Stressful events* may also provoke a depressive disorder, generally those involving some kind of loss – especially bereavement, but also loss of a job or separation from a loved person, both of which may be an indirect consequence of physical illness. *Personality* plays a part in determining this response to stress. Among women certain *longstanding social difficulties* seem to increase vulnerability to depression; these include the lack of a person to confide in, and having to care for small children. These genetic and environmental factors appear to act partly through *biochemical mechanisms*. These mechanisms probably involve mono-amine pathways in the brain but it is uncertain whether the main disorder is of serotonergic or adrenergic transmission.

Differential diagnosis

In cases seen by a physician there are usually four main issues: (*a*) when depressive symptoms are obvious, distinguishing between a depressive disorder and normal feelings of depression associated with physical ill health; (*b*) when the presenting complaints suggest physical illness, detecting the underlying depressive disorder; (*c*) when it has been established that there is a depressive disorder, deciding whether it is secondary to physical illness or arising from another cause; (*d*) distinguishing depressive disorder from another psychiatric disorder especially dementia.

Depressive disorders can be distinguished from normal feelings of depression associated with ill health by enquiring carefully about symptoms: a normal reaction does not have the pattern of symptoms that characterizes a depressive disorder, the finding of 'biological' symptoms being particularly significant while the (uncommon) presence of psychotic symptoms is even more important. In the absence of such symptoms, doubtful cases require a commonsense appraisal of the severity of the depressive mood change, comparing it with what would seem to be a normal reaction to physical illness given all the patient's circumstances. In

doubtful cases an interview with a relative will often reveal evidence of features of the depressive syndrome such as loss of energy and interests, disturbed sleep and gloomy preoccupations. The second criterion concerns the course of the disorder. A careful enquiry about whether the physical symptoms or the psychological and behavioural symptoms came first will often settle the matter. If doubt remains, the opinion of a psychiatrist should be obtained.

In deciding whether a depressive disorder is directly due to physical illness it is necessary to consider the known association between particular illnesses and their treatment and depressive disorder (reviewed on pages 25.32–25.40). General practitioners should remember that depressive symptoms may be the first evidence of physical illness including dementia. This possibility should be considered particularly in middle-aged or elderly patients developing a depressive disorder for the first time.

The third diagnostic problem is the detection of a depressive disorder when the presenting symptoms suggest physical illness. The diagnosis of these '*masked*' *depressive disorders* is not usually difficult to make once the possibility has been considered. Correct diagnosis usually requires only a few questions about the characteristic symptoms of a depressive disorder: low mood, loss of interest in work and hobbies, a subjective feeling of slowing of mental activities, early morning waking, diurnal mood variation, and gloomy preoccupations.

Prognosis

The untreated course of depressive disorders varies between the extremes of a few weeks and several years, but most cases last for between three and nine months. Almost all young and middle-aged patients eventually make a complete recovery, but incomplete recovery is more frequent in elderly patients. Recurrences are common, particularly among patients who also have episodes of mania (see below). Depressive disorders carry an increased risk of suicide: of people who have suffered a severe (bipolar) depressive disorder, between 10 and 15 per cent eventually die by suicide.

Treatment

This section should be read in conjunction with the sections on drug treatment (page 25.47) and on psychological treatment (page 25.52). All cases require simple psychological management, and most cases of moderate to severe depressive disorder also require an antidepressant drug.

Physicians will begin by assessing whether the case is one that they can reasonably treat themselves or whether the advice of a psychiatrist should be obtained. Indications for a specialist opinion include: severe cases especially those with psychotic or marked 'biological' symptoms; any patient who has definite suicidal ideas or in whom the assessment of suicide is difficult (see page 25.20 for the assessment of suicidal intent); and cases in which the diagnosis is uncertain.

Psychological treatment begins with reassurance intended to sustain the patient until spontaneous recovery has taken place or antidepressant drugs have started to exert their therapeutic effects (usually seven to ten days after the first dose). A simple clear explanation should be given of the nature of the disorder, its likely response to treatment, and the side effects of any drugs which have been prescribed. The patient should be helped to reveal concerns about the illness and the future, and talk about problems. However, if the depressive disorder is severe it is often best to defer detailed plans for solving problems until the patient's mood has improved a little. When this is the case, an assurance should be given that the doctor will provide appropriate help when the time comes for the patient to deal with the problems.

In many cases the physician can arrange the necessary *drug treatment* without the advice of a specialist. Drug treatment should generally be limited to an antidepressant – the addition of anxiolytic or hypnotic drugs is seldom required because antidepressant drugs are available with substantial anxiolytic and sedative properties. Because antidepressant drugs have a long half-life they can be given as a single dose at night unless the dose is very large. The *tricyclic antidepressant* amitriptyline is a well-tried drug which can be used unless its anticholinergic side effects are likely to cause difficulties (e.g. for a patient with prostatic enlargement). In these circumstances another antidepressant drug such as mianserin should be chosen (see page 25.49). Although *monoamine oxidase inhibitors* have been claimed to be particularly suitable for mild depressive disorders with anxiety symptoms, the evidence is not strong and the interactions of these drugs with other drugs and with foodstuffs make them generally unsuitable as a first line of treatment (see page 25.49). Further information about antidepressant drugs is given on pages 25.48–25.50.

It is important to explain to the patient that although side effects are likely to appear early, the therapeutic effect will be delayed for up to 10–14 days. Unless this is done many patients feel discouraged by the apparent lack of response and stop taking the drugs. The patient should also be warned about the effects of taking alcohol while receiving antidepressants, and of driving if sedative side-effects are experienced. If no improvement has taken place after three weeks, or if the patient's condition worsens significantly before this, a psychiatrist should be consulted. However, in most cases of mild to moderate severity treatment will be straightforward and the result will be good.

Electroconvulsive therapy (ECT) is required only for the most severe and urgent cases, especially those in which the patient is refusing to eat or drink. ECT is a specialist procedure which will not be described here.

Mania and manic depressive disorder

Mania is characterized by elevated mood, increased activity, and self-important ideas. People who experience mania at one time in their lives usually have severe depressive disorders at other times. This combination is called manic-depressive disorder or *bipolar affective disorder* (bipolar referring to the opposite 'poles' of mania and depression). As well as this sequence of mania and depressive disorder, a few patients show features of both conditions at the same time (e.g. increased activity with depressive ideas). Such patients are said to have a *mixed affective disorder*.

States of mania are much less common than depressive disorders. Estimates of the annual incidence of manic-depressive (bipolar) disorders in the population vary from about 10 to 15 per 100 000 among men and 10 to 30 per 100 000 among women.

Clinical features

The principal features of the syndrome of mania are summarized in Table 2. As noted above they are elevated mood, increased activity, and self-important ideas. The mood is usually one of cheerfulness and optimism but some patients are irritable instead. Sleep is reduced and patients wake early; at this early hour they feel energetic and refreshed, and may behave in a noisy or interfering way. Behaviour is uninhibited, and the patient may engage in extravagant purchases or unsound business schemes. In a medical ward interfering, noisy or restless behaviour is likely to draw attention to the problem at an early stage. Appetite for food is increased and so are sexual desires. Speech is rapid and the patient's conversation moves quickly from one topic to another as one idea crowds out another, or patients are distracted either by things around them or by the opportunities for puns and rhymes in what they are saying ('flight of ideas'). There are grandiose ideas or in some cases delusions of grandeur, patients believing firmly that they are, for example, a religious prophet or a person destined to lead the nation. Because manic patients seldom have insight into the morbid nature of these experiences, it is difficult to obtain their collaboration with treatment.

Table 2 Central features of manic disorders

Elevated mood
Increased energy and activity
Expansive ideas
Impaired insight
Reduced sleep
Increased appetite
Increased libido

Aetiology

The causes of mania are closely related to those already described for depressive disorders, except that genetic factors play a larger, and environmental factors a smaller part, in mania than in depressive disorders.

Differential diagnosis

The physician is most likely to mistake mania for restless behaviour of a patient with an acute organic psychiatric disorder; more rarely the condition may be confused with schizophrenia. When the behaviour of a physically ill patient becomes disturbed, an important differential diagnosis is between mania and an *acute organic disorder*; the distinction can usually be made by the presence of clouding of consciousness (characteristic of the latter). (The many causes of acute organic disorders are reviewed on page 25.13). *Schizophrenia* is differentiated from mania by the characteristic features of the mental state (see page 25.11). Although it is sometimes difficult to distinguish mania and acute schizophrenia, this need seldom cause problems for the physician since the emergency treatment of the two kinds of state of excitement is the same (see page 25.54).

Prognosis

Without treatment, mania usually lasts for a few months, though some mild cases recover more quickly. Almost all patients recover eventually, but may have further episodes of mania and/or depressive disorder after a period of ill health.

Treatment

Treatment is mainly with drugs, though appropriate psychological management is also important. It is especially important to avoid responding to the patient's uninhibited behaviour or irritable mood as if it were directed at the doctor, rather than a symptom of illness. A major tranquillizer will usually control symptoms, haloperidol being a drug of choice. Such treatment usually suppresses symptoms quickly. Treatment may need to be continued with a smaller dose for weeks or months and the advice of a psychiatrist should be obtained. Further information on treatment is given in the section on the treatment of emergencies (page 25.54) and the section on drug treatment (page 25.48). The use of lithium in the prophylaxis of mania is discussed briefly on page 25.49.

References

Gelder, M. G., Gath, D. H. and Mayou, R. (1983). *Oxford textbook of psychiatry*, chap. 8. Oxford University Press, Oxford.

Hawton, K. E. (1981). The long-term outcome of psychiatric morbidity detected in general medical patients. *J. Psychosomat. Res.* **25**, 237–243.

Maguire, G. P., Julier, D. L., Hawton, K. E. and Bancroft, J. H. J. (1974). Psychiatric morbidity and referral on two general medical wards. *Br. Med. J.* **1**, 268–270.

Paykel, E. S. (ed.) (1982). *Handbook of affective disorders*. Churchill Livingstone, Edinburgh.

Schizophrenia and paranoid states

M. G. GELDER

Schizophrenia

Schizophrenia has an acute and a chronic form. Some patients have a single acute illness; some have recurrent acute episodes with varying degrees of recovery between episodes; others develop a chronic illness after either the first or subsequent acute episodes. Once the chronic form is established few patients recover. Physicians may encounter cases of acute schizophrenia in patients treated for physical illness, and they may be asked to treat a chronic schizophrenic patient who is physically ill.

The annual incidence of schizophrenia is difficult to determine but probably lies between 0.1 and 0.2 per 1000. Because many cases persist the one year prevalence is about 3 per 1000 of the population.

Clinical features

The *acute syndrome* will be described first (see Table 1). The predominant features are delusions, hallucinations, and abnormal thinking. In some cases behaviour is disordered as well. (These features are sometimes called positive symptoms.) *Delusions* in schizophrenia are commonly persecutory ('paranoid') or grandiose. These kinds of delusion, though frequent in schizophrenia, are found in other conditions as well so they are not helpful in diagnosis. Certain other delusions though less common are seldom seen in other conditions and are therefore more valuable in diagnosis. These 'first rank' symptoms (listed in Table 2) are: the delusion that the patient's thoughts are being transmitted to other people ('thought broadcasting'); the delusion that thoughts are being taken out of the patient's head ('thought withdrawal'); the delusion that some of a person's thoughts have been implanted by an outside agency ('thought insertion'); the delusion that the patient's actions are being controlled by an outside agency; and 'delusional perception'. The latter term refers to the attaching of a particularly odd or unusual significance to a normal percept; for example, that the positioning of a chair indicates to the patient that he or she is about to be harmed by persecutors. In schizophrenia *hallucinations* are of several kinds. Auditory hallucinations are among the most frequent symptoms of schizophrenia. According to the degree of complexity they can be experienced as noises, or as voices uttering words, phrases or conversations. The voices may appear to speak to the patient or to discuss him with each other, and it is this latter kind of hallucination (known as a 'third person' hallucination because the voices refer to the patient as 'he' or 'she') that has the most value in diagnosis. Other kinds of hallucination that are particularly characteristic of schizophrenia (though not found frequently) are those in which patients hear their own thoughts spoken aloud as if by another person, and hallucinations involving bodily sensations. Visual hallucinations and those involving taste and smell also occur.

The *disorders of thinking* in schizophrenia which are varied and

Table 1 Common symptoms of schizophrenia

Acute syndrome
Persecutory and grandiose delusions
Auditory hallucinations
Thought disorder
Abnormal affective responses
Disordered behaviour

Chronic syndrome
Apathy
Slowness
Social withdrawal
Any of the symptoms listed above

Table 2 Diagnostic ('first-rank') symptoms of schizophrenia

Hearing thoughts spoken aloud
'Third person' hallucinations
Hallucinations in the form of a commentary
Somatic hallucinations
Thought withdrawal or insertion
Thought broadcasting
Delusional perception
Feelings or actions experienced as made or influenced by others

complicated need not be described in detail because they are not a reliable guide to diagnosis. The common feature is a persistent lack of logical connection between ideas. The thought disorder is reflected in the patient's speech which is vague, difficult to follow, becoming more obscure as the doctor seeks further points of clarification. *Emotional responses* may be abnormal in several ways. The most common abnormalities are a lack of emotional response ('flattened affect') and inappropriate responses (e.g. laughing in response to sad news). The *behaviour disorder* in schizophrenia more often takes the form of withdrawal from social situations or oddity of manner than noisy or disruptive acts, though doctors are more likely to be called to deal with the latter.

In *chronic schizophrenia* the main features are apathy, slowness, and social withdrawal. (These features are sometimes called *negative symptoms*.) Delusions, hallucinations, and disordered thinking are also present to a varying degree but are generally less prominent than in the acute form of the illness. Depressive symptoms are also frequent in chronic schizophrenia, and may be exacerbated by treatment with antipsychotic drugs.

In both forms of schizophrenia, memory and consciousness are unimpaired and the finding of any disorder of these functions should prompt a search for an organic cause of the mental disorder.

Occasionally the first evidence of schizophrenia is a complaint about *physical symptoms*. In the early stages of the disorder, patients occasionally experience somatic hallucinations in the form of uncomfortable feelings in the chest, abdomen, or genital regions. These hallucinatory sensations are often interpreted in a delusional way. For example, sensations in the vagina may be ascribed to the actions of unknown people who are having intercourse with the patient during her sleep; or hallucinatory sensations in the abdomen ascribed to food that has been poisoned by malefactors. In most cases the true nature of the problem is revealed when patients are questioned tactfully but firmly about their ideas concerning the cause of the symptoms. Also a relative or other informant should be asked about abnormal behaviour or ideas. For cases of this kind the opinion of a psychiatrist is usually required.

Aetiology

There is strong evidence that the predisposition to develop schizophrenia is determined to a substantial degree by *genetic causes* presumably acting through biochemical mechanisms. There is some evidence that this inherited predisposition can be increased by *minor neurological disorder* in childhood. Some acute episodes of schizophrenia are precipitated by *stressful life events*, but others start gradually without any obvious precipitant. Occasionally schizophrenia is provoked by *physical illness* (see page 25.16), though a minority, these cases are of obvious importance to the physician. The *biochemical disorder* in schizophrenia has not been identified. Drugs that control schizophrenia block dopamine receptors but it has not been established that overactivity of dopamine systems is the central disorder in the disease (there may be a parallel with Parkinsonism in which anticholinergic drugs control symptoms but the primary disorder is not of cholinergic transmission). Once the disease is established, events that lead to increased *CNS arousal* increase the risk of relapse. Intense relationships within the family are important examples of such events.

Differential diagnosis

In established cases diagnosis is usually obvious but the early diagnosis of first episodes of illness can be difficult and generally requires the advice of a psychiatrist. When schizophrenia presents as a state of excitement it has to be distinguished from *mania*; when the patient is withdrawn it may resemble a *depressive disorder*. In either case diagnosis depends on eliciting the characteristic delusions, hallucinations, and other mental phenomena of the schizophrenic syndrome. In some cases these are obvious, in others great skill in interviewing is required to uncover these symptoms. For the physician, it is particularly important to distinguish schizophrenia from *acute organic psychiatric disorders* especially drug-induced states, complex partial seizures, and (rarely now, but more often in the past) general paralysis of the insane (see Section 21). Of the *drug-induced states* (page 25.38), that caused by amphetamine abuse most closely resembles schizophrenia, but the effects of abuse of LSD or, less commonly, large amounts of cannabis can cause diagnostic problems. Some patients with long-standing complex partial seizures arising in the temporal lobe develop a mental illness with persecutory delusions that is indistinguishable from schizophrenia (see pages 25.34–25.35). Finally, it is often difficult to distinguish between *personality disorder* and schizophrenia starting insidiously in a young person. The physician will usually need the advice of a psychiatrist in making these difficult diagnostic distinctions.

Prognosis

Schizophrenia has a variable outcome and it is difficult to predict this during the first episode of illness. As a broad generalization, about a quarter of patients with a first illness make a good and lasting recovery, another quarter develop a chronic illness, 10 per cent die by suicide, and the rest have repeated illnesses with varying degrees of recovery between episodes. Prognosis tends to be better in cases with sudden onset, a definite precipitant, and prominent affective symptoms. A prompt response to immediate treatment also suggests a favourable long-term outcome. There is some evidence from international comparisons that prognosis is better in developing than in developed countries, but this finding could have arisen because in the developing countries cases of insidious onset (and worse prognosis) are less likely to reach the medical services than acute cases (of better prognosis) whose behaviour is less easily tolerated by families.

Treatment

The long-term care of schizophrenic patients is a complicated matter involving rehabilitation and work with families. It is described in textbooks of psychiatry. The physician is more likely to be concerned with two specific aspects of treatment: the control of symptoms in an emergency, and the continuation of drug treatment of chronic patients admitted to hospital for the treatment of intercurrent medical illness. The treatment of acute symptoms is described in the section of psychiatric emergencies, and only maintenance drug treatment will be discussed here.

Clinical trials have demonstrated that relapse rate is reduced if patients with chronic schizophrenia receive continued treatment with an antipsychotic drug. Because many schizophrenic patients fail to take oral medication regularly, the drugs are often given by the intramuscular injection of a long-acting preparation. Fluphenazine decanoate is a commonly used preparation which is given once every two to four weeks in a schedule and dosage that is established for each patient. The physician may need to arrange a continuation of this treatment while the patient is in hospital. If there is reason to consider doing otherwise the advice of a psychiatrist should be obtained. Antiparkinsonian medication should not be given routinely, but may be needed to reduce the side effects of the antipsychotic drugs. If the stress of physical illness causes an exacerbation of symptoms it is usually better to give additional oral rather than intramuscular medication. Suitable drugs include chlorpromazine if a sedating effect is required, and trifluoperazine if it is not. (See page 25.50 for further information about antipsychotic drugs.)

Paranoid states

The physician will occasionally encounter patients who have prominent paranoid delusions without any evidence of schizophrenia, depressive disorder or organic disease of the brain. These 'paranoid states' sometimes turn out to be an early stage of one of these other conditions, and the true diagnosis becomes apparent when other symptoms emerge. However, others do not run this course. Some are transient reactions to stressful events or physical illness ('acute paranoid reactions'). Others run a prolonged course without the appearance of any of the symptoms of another disorder. Among the latter, several rare syndromes can be defined. Physicians are more likely to see the acute paranoid reactions.

The principal symptoms of an acute or chronic paranoid reaction are paranoid delusions and hallucinations. The term paranoid refers to ideas concerned with some change in the relationship between the patient and other people: commonly the ideas are to do with persecution (and paranoid is often used, wrongly, as if synonymous with 'persecutory'), but they may also centre round love or jealousy, or be concerned with litigation or with the supernatural. Often the ideas remain hidden at first so that the patient is not noticed to be mentally ill, until a sudden unexpected act draws attention to the problem. Thus patients may suddenly appear terrified and attempt to run away from a medical ward or attack another person who they believe to be a persecutor; or they may simply demand to leave hospital before the appointed time.

Acute paranoid reactions are more likely to appear in people with a touchy, suspicious personality, and in circumstances in which the patients are in some way cut off from a full awareness of their surroundings, e.g. because they are deaf, or their eyes have been bandaged, or they are isolated from visitors. However, a small minority of people can develop a paranoid reaction in the course of ordinary medical treatment.

Acute paranoid reactions are usually short-lived, often lasting only a few days and rarely more than a few weeks. To restore contact with reality is an important step in treatment. The acute symptoms can generally be controlled quickly with an antipsychotic drug, used as for acute schizophrenia. With this medication, treatment of the medical illness can usually be continued on a general ward, but occasionally a brief admission to a psychiatric ward is necessary.

Persistent paranoid states are much more difficult to treat. They are rare conditions that will seldom be encountered by physicians. Some persistent paranoid states centre round ideas of persecution, others round jealousy ('pathological jealousy'), erotic ideas (de Clerambault's syndrome) or litigation. Each type is described further in the Oxford Textbook of Psychiatry. The physician should discuss all patients with chronic paranoid delusions with the family doctor, and arrange for referral to a psychiatrist if this has not been done already. Treatment is difficult and in some cases there is a serious risk that violent behaviour will be directed to the person who is the object of the delusional ideas. It is particularly important to be aware of this risk in cases of pathological jealousy.

References

Fish, F.J. (1962). *Schizophrenia*. John Wright, Bristol.
Watts, F.N. and Bennett, D.H. (1983). *Theory and practice of psychiatric rehabilitation*. John Wiley, Chichester.

Organic mental states

G. STORES

Psychiatry and general medicine are closely related in several ways. First, any ill person is likely to experience emotional upset. Secondly, some basically psychiatric disorders, especially anxiety and depressive states, include physical symptoms and signs (see pages 25.2 and 25.8). Thirdly, physical pathology (especially that involving the central nervous system directly) often leads to alteration of behaviour which initially may be the only sign of the disorder. Lishman (see pages 25.32–25.40) describes the specific conditions which may give rise to mental disorders in this way. Such disorders commonly lead to emergency situations as discussed by Mayou (see page 25.54). The present account is confined to a general review of the behavioural states which can be produced by physical illness.

Types of organic mental state

Although individual differences in personality and background may provide the 'colouring' in each case, behavioural reactions to any kind of organic illness show enough consistency for certain types of reactions or syndromes to have been described. Therefore although in the new American psychiatric classification of organic mental states (DSM III) more emphasis is given to the diversity of psychiatric manifestations of cerebral disorders, the present account draws attention to the similarities.

Before describing the principal organic syndromes it is necessary to explain the meaning of two sets of commonly used terms. The first set of terms refers to symptoms. *Confusion* refers to difficulty in thinking clearly and coherently which can occur both in organic and non-organic conditions. (Confusional state is another name for the syndrome also known as an acute or subacute organic reaction – see below.) Several terms are used to describe impairment of consciousness, an important symptom which usually signifies organic pathology. The term *clouding of consciousness* is sometimes used to describe the symptom in its mildest form, when there is slight impairment of cognitive function and reduced awareness of the environment. *Coma* describes the most extreme form of impaired consciousness with little evidence of responsiveness. *Stupor* refers to a state characterized by lack of responsiveness but with some evidence that conscious awareness is preserved.

The second set of terms refer to syndromes. The broadest distinction in organic psychiatric illness is between *acute reactions* also called *acute brain syndromes* and *chronic reactions* also called *chronic brain syndromes*. In general, acute conditions are of abrupt onset and short duration; chronic disorders develop gradually and persist. The clinical features of both may be combined in the *subacute reactions* (or brain syndromes). The term *delirium* is ambiguous. It is used to describe an acute organic syndrome in which impairment of consciousness is accompanied by marked distortion of the perception of the world in the form of illusions, hallucinations, and delusions, as well as striking changes of mood and activity. However, other writers use delirium as a synonym for acute organic syndrome. The term *twilight state* is particularly ambiguous and best avoided: one meaning is a prolonged state in which the patient although not asleep experiences vivid images with the quality of a dream.

There are two chronic syndromes: *dementia* and the *amnesic syndrome*. The syndrome of *dementia* is an acquired global impairment of intellect, memory, and personality without impairment of consciousness. It is usually of long duration, progressive, and irreversible. Dementia is the most common form of chronic organic syndrome. A less common form is the *chronic amnesic syndrome* which consists of a circumscribed defect of short-term memory with little or no other type of cognitive impairment.

In addition to these syndromes of a general type, characteristic constellations of symptoms and signs have been ascribed to organic lesions in particular parts of the brain. These changes may have valuable localizing value. Tumours provide the best examples and are discussed by Lishman (see page 25.33). It is important to realize that any form of disturbed behaviour, including personality change and psychosis, may have an organic base.

Acute organic reactions

Synonyms: acute brain syndrome, acute confusional state, delirium.

The most common form of psychiatric disorder encountered on medical or surgical wards is probably the acute reaction to any of the numerous pathological processes which can compromise brain function.

Causes

The many conditions which may act this way include respiratory or cardiac failure and other systemic causes of cerebral hypoxia. Myocardial infarction can produce acute behavioural disturbance without any other obvious early sign ('silent coronary') as can a cerebrovascular accident or acute chest infection. Other causes include metabolic and endocrine disorders, toxic states (such as alcohol or drug abuse and withdrawal), vitamin deficiencies, and intracranial infections or space-occupying lesions. Some forms of epileptic seizure take the form of acute behavioural disturbance without convulsive features.

The elderly are at special risk, as several physical causes may act together to impair cerebral function. Although postoperative reactions can occur at any age, older people are less tolerant of general anaesthesia, surgery, or other causes of metabolic upset. The elderly are also particularly vulnerable to the adverse behavioural effects of drugs, and special care is needed in deciding the dosage, combinations, and administration of their treatment. Finally, older patients may very readily become disorientated by being removed from the familiar surroundings of home and placed in a strange hospital environment. This is especially likely if stimulation is either too restricted or too varied. Alarming effects of sensory deprivation are sometimes seen even in younger patients after eye surgery, when immobilized for long periods in special care units, or in other situations where sensory stimulation is reduced. Chronic loss of sleep because of pain or any other cause can produce a similar disturbance.

Clinical features

Acute organic reactions are characterized by recent and abrupt onset with evidence (in many cases) of a physical illness. Other important diagnostic features are fluctuation in the clinical picture with worsening in the evening or at night. Some patients are only disturbed nocturnally and are lucid during the day. The condition is usually self-limiting or reversible with treatment of the underlying cause, although interim measures are important. Recovery is often sharp with patchy or incomplete amnesia for the episode.

Impaired consciousness is the most salient feature from which many of the other behavioural disturbances follow. Mild clouding of consciousness may be largely subjective in nature with vague feelings of malaise and difficulty in focusing attention or thinking coherently. Time perception is affected early in the process producing disorientation in time. More severe impairment of consciousness is obvious to others. Patients may appear drowsy and slow to respond. They may be distractable and unable to sustain a logical line of reasoning or to grasp even fundamental aspects of the situation, such as their own whereabouts or identities. Their speech may be slurred and perseverative.

In the early stages emotional and perceptual processes are likely to be blunted to produce a picture of indifference or mild perplexity with aimless and restless movements such as picking at the bedclothes. Later a state of delirium often develops (or alternates with the stage of apathy). In this state there are visual illusions and hallucinations, and delusions of a persecutory type into which medical and nursing staff are likely to be incorporated. Understandably, these experiences can terrify patients who may try to escape or aggressively resist attempts to restrain them. At other times their extreme restlessness is less well-directed. Delirium tremens (following complete withdrawal of alcohol in the alcohol-dependent person, see page 25.23) exemplifies this florid type of reaction which is likely to cause severe disruption on a medical ward.

Diagnosis and assessment

In acute organic reactions attention has to be directed to identifying the nature of the underlying physical disorder. As far as a psychiatric diagnosis is concerned, a history of recent and acute onset of disturbed behaviour and physical illness should present no problems of recognition if the patient is disorientated or shows other evidence of impaired consciousness. The latter feature is not seen in other patients with acutely disturbed behaviour such as those with acute anxiety states, and manic or other psychotic outbursts.

The main diagnostic difficulties arise with subacute reactions in which consciousness is impaired without florid behavioural accompaniments, producing a picture of bewilderment or perplexity which may be prolonged for days or even weeks, e.g. in older patients with undiagnosed infections or following a series of convulsions. This clinical picture can be mistaken for dementia, a depressive disorder, or a withdrawn psychotic state. The problems are intensified if no history of the onset is available, in old people (who may have shown a degree of dementia before the onset of additional acute or subacute symptoms), and in the subnormal or the very young whose powers of communication are limited. The patient's level of consciousness should be ascertained by assessing as far as possible alertness, orientation, and ability to focus and sustain attention. There should be no such impairment in dementia unless far advanced, or depressive disorder or schizophrenia. The EEG is very sensitive to changes in level of consciousness and should be used in difficult cases. Widespread slow activity can be expected in both acute and subacute reactions. Occasionally focal features in the EEG will be seen suggesting a localized lesion.

Management

While the underlying physical illness is being investigated and treated, the acutely disturbed patient usually needs sedation and nursing care. Sedation may obscure important physical or mental signs but if it is considered necessary, it must be adequate. An undersedated patient will become more confused and disturbed. Barbiturates are particularly likely to have this effect. Chlorpromazine is an appropriate drug, given orally (preferably as syrup) or parenterally if necessary in doses of 200–300 mg per day in four-to six-hourly doses; haloperidol is a suitable alternative. The largest dose should be given at night if the degree of disturbance is greatest then. Patients' confusion will be reduced if they can be nursed in a side room by the same nurse or as few nurses as possible. In this way they can be repeatedly reassured by a familiar person who should also try to reorientate them during their lucid periods. Physical force should be avoided if possible; understandably, it increases the patient's fear and suspicion. If forceful restraint has to be used, it should be effective and quick. Sedation can often be withdrawn after 24–48 hours.

Chronic organic reactions: dementia

Gradually increasing inability to concentrate, forgetfulness, and other feelings of inability to cope with the intellectual demands of work or everyday life are commonplace. In the majority of cases these symptoms form part of an anxiety state, depressive disorder, or other primarily psychiatric condition. At other times, however, such symptoms (or, more usually, the observation by relatives or workmates of a concurrent decline in competence) are the first features of a dementing illness. Dementia is a large-scale problem in the elderly. It has been estimated that 10 per cent of old people are demented but that the majority of these are not recognized until a crisis occurs in the patient's life such as a stroke, loss of a spouse, or change within the family such that usual coping methods are no longer adequate.

Causes

There are many causes of dementia and these vary somewhat with the age of onset. Although most consist of some form of irreversible degenerative process, some causes are treatable such as vitamin B_{12} deficiency, hypothyroidism, and normal pressure hydrocephalus (see Section 21). Other therapeutic possibilities often exist in elderly people whose intellectual deterioration can be exaggerated by chronic chest or urinary tract infection, heart failure, nutritional deficiencies, or medication, especially barbiturates. It is likely that in the past senile and arterio-sclerotic dementia have been diagnosed too readily in some cases and chances of successful treatment overlooked.

Senile dementia (sometimes known as senile dementia of the Alzheimer type, abbreviated SDAT) occurs after the age of 70 years, predominantly in women, and consists of a gradual and progressive decline without specific causal factors, although possibly complicated by treatable physical illness or neglect as just described. Only in comparatively recent times has this condition been clearly separated from the other psychiatric illnesses of old age such as affective disorders or psychotic states which often respond to treatment. True senile dementia usually advances rapidly. The pathological changes in senile dementia resemble those of Alzheimer's disease (see Section 21).

Multi-infarct dementia (arterio-sclerotic dementia) is somewhat more common in late middle or old age. It occurs rather more commonly in men than in women. There may be clinical evidence of arterial disease or hypertension, but a history of repeated cerebrovascular accidents provides a firmer basis for the diagnosis. Repeated episodes of clouding of consciousness characteristically occur producing a fluctuating course of deterioration. Cerebral atheroma is not a common cause of dementia; recent estimates suggest that it accounts for only about 15 per cent of cases.

Presenile dementias are a group of conditions in which there is usually a familial tendency for cerebral atrophy to occur below the age of about 60 years, without any apparent cause (as distinct from the many other causes of dementia which may occur in the 'presenile' period). These conditions are slowly progressive. Alzheimer's disease (see Section 21) is the most common, and affects the cortex and subcortex diffusely to produce a variety of signs. Pick's disease (see Section 21) is said mainly to affect the frontal and temporal cortex to produce the 'frontal lobe syndrome' consisting of personality change in the direction of apathy, disinhibition, insensitivity, and fatuous euphoria, as well as neurological signs of frontal lobe involvement. In Huntington's chorea (see Section 21) dementia is commonly combined with other psychiatric disorders from personality change to paranoid psychosis. Creutzfeld–Jacob's disease (see Section 21) does not show familial features and seems to be caused by a transmissable agent.

Dementia may be caused by cerebral infections such as neurosyphilis, herpes simplex encephalitis, or by the measles virus which is thought to be responsible for subacute sclerosing panencephalitis in children. Cerebral tumours may have the same effect especially if slow growing and in frontal or temporal regions or in the midline. Dementia can result from cerebral metastases, and is also a non-metastatic complication particularly of carcinoma of the bronchus.

Other causal factors include head injury (resulting in gross brain damage, subdural haematoma, or cerebral degeneration as in boxers from repeated blows to the head); prolonged nutritional, metabolic, endocrine disorders; toxic states (such as alcohol or drug abuse); cerebral anoxia (including carbon monoxide poisoning); and normal pressure hydrocephalus. More detailed discussion of these conditions will be found in Section 21. Frequently, no cause can be found.

Clinical features
Because of the diffuse nature of many of the diseases resulting in dementia, the clinical picture shows basic similarities from one patient to another, although variation is seen depending on the age of onset of the illness, premorbid personality, and intelligence, as well as the location, nature, and rate of progression of the lesion. The patient's social circumstances and amount of environmental stimulation are also important. Predisposition to other psychiatric illness may be reactivated to produce a mixed clinical picture.

The early, non-specific features of intellectual decline have already been mentioned. Sometimes patients conceal these first changes by using memory aids or by keeping to rigid routines to minimize mistakes in the hope of allaying their own anxieties or preserving their jobs. In time such strategies become inadequate. The memory deficits, which initially affect recent events, gradually extend to include remote memories and orientation. The ability to think abstractly is lost, patients cannot understand new ideas and no longer learn from past experience. Eventually their thoughts are few, perseverative, and disconnected.

Personality is likely to show a similar disintegration. Less attractive traits may be accentuated initially, but more serious changes often occur which make it impossible for relatives to cope. Sometimes the patient gets into trouble because of impropriety including sexual indiscretions. In general, demented patients become more selfish, quarrelsome, and rigid. Incontinence and serious self-neglect are likely to develop later. While insight is retained, patients may react to their plight by becoming anxious, agitated, and depressed even to the point of attempts at suicide. As contact with reality is lost, emotions become shallow, flattened, or labile. Perplexity easily gives rise to paranoid ideas and unpredictable behaviour. Apart from these psychiatric changes there may be neurological evidence of brain damage such as motor or sensory deficits, aphasia, apraxia, agnosia, or seizures.

Diagnosis and assessment
Certain basic questions need to be answered about patients showing signs of intellectual decline.

The first is whether there is evidence of an organic process rather than another cause for the mental state. Particularly in the elderly, the clinical features of dementia and other psychiatric states (especially depression) can be very similar. Depressed patients may have an identifiable cause for their distress or a family history of a similar disorder. Although slowness and poor concentration and memory are common to the two conditions, the depressed patient's difficulties are caused by lack of interest, anxiety, or a preoccupation with morbid thoughts. With encouragement, a coherent account can be given in which the patient's sense of distress is likely to be communicated. Demented patients, in contrast, have difficulty in formulating their thoughts, and their emotions are likely to be impoverished or unpredictable.

The finding of neurological or other physical abnormalities on examination support the diagnosis of an organic syndrome, as will the demonstration of organic changes in the EEG, although a normal EEG is compatible with dementia. Clinical assessment should be adequate in most cases to demonstrate the global intellectual impairment of dementia, but formal psychological testing can be important in providing confirmatory evidence of intellectual loss (especially in relation to past educational and work records), or, by serial assessment, measuring the rate of decline. Tests of overall intelligence, such as the Wechsler scales, are appropriate for these purposes, but other tests of more specific functions, such as new learning ability, memory (in its different phases), verbal or perceptual skills, can sometimes indicate localized lesions. Depressed or otherwise psychiatrically disturbed patients will not

show such patterns of impairment, and their overall performance can usually be shown to be influenced by poor motivation rather than intrinsic intellectual loss. Such distinctions are not always easy in elderly patients, however, although there is some evidence that the type of error made in learning tests is different in the two conditions.

Another non-organic psychiatric disorder sometimes confused with dementia is schizophrenia, especially those forms with emotional flattening, apathy, and impaired thought processes, other forms of schizophrenia being usually recognizable by the presence of well-formed delusional systems and auditory hallucinations. In both types of schizophrenia general intellectual function and memory are preserved. Some hysterical reactions ('hysterical pseudo-dementia'), are characterized by inconsistent or unconvincing intellectual impairment and a motive of gain. Great care should be taken before making the diagnosis of hysteria in these circumstances, not least because even gross attention-seeking behaviour or conversion symptoms can occur as part of the organic disease. Full physical investigation should be arranged in doubtful cases.

If convincing evidence of organic illness is present, the second question concerns the distinction between dementia and other organic reactions. The comparison with acute and subacute reactions was made in the last section with emphasis on the presence in the latter conditions of acute onset and alteration of consciousness as well as preservation of intellect in lucid intervals. The chronic amnesic syndrome (see below) may simulate dementia, but assessment will reveal that the general intelligence and long-term memory of patients with this condition are intact. Mild dysphasia can also seem like a dementing illness but, again, intelligence is usually intact and the patient is often distressed, in contrast to the emotional indifference or unpredictability of dementia. The restrictions on movement imposed by Parkinsonism, especially the lack of facial expression, may also give the mistaken impression of dementia, although actual intellectual impairment may accompany this condition (see page 25.35).

Given that a patient really is demented, the question then arises: what is the cause? Important points include a family history of dementing illness and a past personal history of alcohol or drug abuse, head injury, or transient neurological disorder. Recent illnesses and current treatment must also be ascertained. A full physical examination should be carried out in view of the many possible underlying conditions. The findings will suggest appropriate special investigations (such as tests of thyroid function or vitamin B_{12} levels), in addition to the routine of haemoglobin estimation, ESR, urinalysis, and serological tests for syphilis. Skull and chest X-rays should also be carried out routinely. Computerized tomography (CT) scanning is important because of its ability to demonstrate clearly the degree and distribution of cerebral atrophy as well as many of the focal lesions that can be associated with dementia. Other neuro-radiological investigations may be required in special cases. The value of EEG studies has already been discussed.

Finally, the patient's social and family circumstances need to be known, mainly to assess the prospects of continued management or rehabilitation in the community.

Assessment is not a once and for all exercise and repeated investigation may be required to settle the issues discussed above.

Management
Medical management of a demented patient consists of treating the basic cause (in the relatively few cases where this is possible) or treating associated conditions such as depression or the effects of physical neglect.

In all patients, physical health must be maintained by means of adequate diet and appropriate physical activity, as well as regular medical examinations. Promazine is probably the most suitable tranquillizer and lorazepam an appropriate hypnotic. The claims that have been made for various treatments (including cerebral vasodilators) that they can reverse intellectual decline remain unconvincing. Indeed cerebral vasodilators can be hazardous if they produce postural hypotension.

Psychological support in the early stages can reduce patients' distress about their own limitations. Ideally employment should be continued as long as this is feasible. For patients at home various practical measures can reduce difficulties in everyday living, such as keeping change to a minimum and arranging as simple and familiar a daily routine as possible. Relatives need to know the nature of the patient's condition, its prognosis, and the ways in which they can help. They may need support in their own right, especially spouses. Welfare services, such as a home help or meals-on-wheels, are important particularly for patients with no family support. Social contact with family and friends should be encouraged. As the condition worsens, day hospital attendance or holiday admissions to relieve relatives are required and, ultimately, admission to a hospital or hostel where skilled nursing care is available in the long term. The impact this change necessarily imposes should be minimized and activities promoted to slow the process of decline as much as possible.

Chronic brain reactions: the chronic amnesic syndrome

The chronic amnesic syndrome is an uncommon form of chronic organic reaction. It consists of an impairment of short-term memory without altered consciousness, general intellectual deterioration, or perceptual abnormality to account for the memorizing failure. Confabulation is a usual accompaniment. The syndrome is usually associated with thiamine deficiency from chronic alcoholism (Korsakoff's syndrome, see Section 21) but also occurs in association with prolonged and severe vomiting, starvation, pernicious anaemia, and chronic haemodialysis. The main neuropathological accompaniment in such cases is damage to the mamillary bodies. The same effects can follow encroachment of pituitary tumours on the floor of the third ventricle or when the hypothalamus is damaged by infiltration of the basal meninges. Alternatively, the amnesic syndrome can be produced by hippocampal damage, usually bilateral. This can occur selectively in herpes simplex encephalitis or may result from cerebral hypoxia as in carbon monoxide poisoning, cardiac arrest, and even unsuccessful attempts at hanging. The common factor throughout all cases of the chronic amnesic syndrome is damage to the limbic system. The degree of memory impairment varies but can be incapacitating. As mentioned earlier, the syndrome can be mistaken for dementia.

Personality change

Personality implies the enduring, characteristic forms of social behaviour which allow prediction of how a person will act in certain circumstances. Uncharacteristic behaviour, without obvious cause, can be an important sign of cerebral disease. The nature of this change, which can vary greatly from one person to another, includes unpredictable alterations of mood, loss of drive or initiative in a normally decisive person, or the onset of attention-seeking behaviour in someone not normally given to histrionic display. Aggression, irritability, and improper or otherwise disinhibited behaviour may be an early feature of organic involvement.

It is important, therefore, to assess the patient's current behaviour against the background of how he or she usually behaves. Failure to do so can result in physical disease being overlooked especially if atypical in presentation. Classic diagnostic mistakes have been described (for example, in hypoglycaemic states) attributable to a failure to make this distinction. In chronic conditions the personality change may be insidious and particularly difficult to recognize without information about the patient's earlier behaviour for comparison. The behavioural effects of chronic phenobarbitone treatment can be of this type. Patients forget how well they used to feel until reminded by a sense of improved well-being when the drug is discontinued.

The risk of such errors is increased where the behaviour in question is annoying or offensive, as in attention-seeking devices or 'hysteria' – a troublesome and ambiguous term which carries with it serious risk of inadequate patient care. Also as noted on page 25.3, hysterical symptoms can occur in organic disease of the nervous system, sometimes before neurological signs have developed. The symptoms of hysteria include motor and sensory dysfunction, attacks of altered behaviour, amnesia, fugue states, trances, and pseudo-dementia. Even extreme forms of hysterical behaviour do not exclude organic pathology and the underlying condition may be difficult to discern in the complexity of the situation. As the basic neurological condition may only declare itself long after the onset of the symptoms of hysteria, repeated assessment is required. This is particularly the case if no psychological cause can be identified, or if the behaviour is out of character.

The more usual forms of behavioural change in organic reactions are anxiety and depression. These are usually without specific diagnostic significance as far as the underlying disorder is concerned. However, some more specific relationships do occur. As discussed later (see page 25.38), some of the drugs used in general medicine can affect mood, notably hypotensive agents (which commonly cause depression), corticosteroids, or antiparkinsonian drugs. Phenomena associated with anxiety including panic attacks and depersonalization, are part of the wide variety of symptoms that occur in seizures of temporal lobe origin. These phenomena can also be salient features of disturbance caused by hypoglycaemia or phaeochromocytoma. Other interesting and more specific relationships between personality and organic states include obsessive-compulsive features seen in some postencephalitic patients, and hyposexuality associated with seizures originating in the temporal lobe. The constellation of behaviours which constitute the frontal lobe syndrome has been mentioned earlier. Inadequate attention to details of the mental state can lead to a diagnosis of depression when, in fact, the patient shows signs of apathy from a frontally placed lesion. Similarly, excitement due to frontal lobe involvement in organic disease may be diagnosed erroneously as hypomania. It is worth restating the general principle that personality change (whatever its nature) occurring without obvious environmental cause, and especially (though not only) in adult life, should be suspected of being a sign of physical disorder.

Schizophrenia and related psychoses

The diagnosis of schizophrenia is most convincingly made in the presence of 'first rank' symptoms, namely, certain types of auditory hallucinations, passivity feelings, and primary delusions in a setting of clear consciousness. Most schizophrenic patients show no convincingly abnormal physical signs or other evidence to suggest definite organic pathology. However, the association of schizophrenia with various disorders of the central nervous system does exceed chance expectation. This applies especially to epilepsy, cerebral trauma, cerebral tumours, some forms of encephalitis, and basal ganglia disorders. Although these 'organic schizophrenias' have the same range of clinical features as other cases of schizophrenia, they differ from the latter in the absence of a family history and in an ultimate outcome which is partly determined by the underlying cause.

Chronic amphetamine abuse can also produce a clinical picture like that of (strictly defined) schizophrenia. A similar clinical state has been described with the abuse of cannabis or LSD ingestion. The psychotic states of childhood (namely, early infantile autism, late-onset psychosis, and disintegrative psychoses) sometimes have a clear organic basis, especially the last of these conditions. In the elderly late paraphrenia is often associated with sensory deficits. Psychotic states can be induced at any age by prolonged sensory deprivation of the kind sometimes encountered after operations on the eyes, or with intensive care.

Paranoid symptoms are not confined to schizophrenia, they are seen in many organic states. Acute organic paranoid reactions (with delusions of persecution occurring in clear consciousness) occur after acute physical illness such as myocardial infarction, cerebro-vascular accidents, and pneumonia, especially in late middle age and in the elderly; and as a result of alcohol abuse.

Recognition of organic reactions in children and mentally handicapped patients

Compared with adults, younger patients may present special problems in the recognition of cerebral disease when the initial presentation is mainly or wholly behavioural. Because of developmental changes, it is less easy to speak of personality and to identify a significant change of behaviour. However, developmental delay in infants, especially loss of skills or abilities, should raise serious questions about organic pathology. Deterioration in performance at school, or the onset of behaviour seen as strange by other children, may be the first sign of an organic process as in some cases of subacute sclerosing panencephalitis or neurodegenerative disorders of a metabolic type. The development of physical signs or the onset of seizures provides confirmation of an organic process in these cases.

Although a 'brain-damaged syndrome' has been described in children, it is inappropriate, implying a more uniform clinical picture than really exists. Although behavioural change and altered intellectual level are common following brain damage, individual differences of a constitutional nature produce a variety of reactions which may be also related to the child's social circumstances or to the site and extent of the damage. Although restlessness and impulsiveness are common complications, they are not inevitable. Indeed, some young patients with brain damage are chronically inert.

The early recognition of organic reactions may be at least as difficult in intellectually handicapped adult patients as it is in children. Unusual or unpredictable behaviour may be part of the basic handicapping condition, and changes in ability or personality are likely to be more difficult to determine. As in young children, the subnormal patient's limited powers of self-expression will tend to hide organic changes of a subjective nature. Nevertheless, the same basic principles of diagnosis apply as in other patients, particularly the need to take note of unexplained behavioural change, especially in adult life when relatively set patterns of behaviour can be expected to have established themselves.

Deterioration of behaviour in a mentally handicapped person

There are several possible explanations when a mentally handicapped patient's mental state and general condition deteriorate. First patients may have developed a physical disorder, the presence and nature of which may be difficult to judge because of their inability to communicate effectively. This may be a particular problem with the severely retarded who may not be able to convey their discomfort or distress until the problems are advanced. Second, the patient may become emotionally upset or develop a psychiatric disorder. Mentally handicapped persons are particularly subject to psychiatric disorder, but its presentation may be atypical. Third, some forms of retardation may be progressive. For example, an Alzheimer type of dementia occurs in patients with Down's syndrome. The Sturge–Weber syndrome and tuberous sclerosis are also associated with progressive intellectual impairment.

Careful physical and psychological assessment is required when a handicapped patient shows deterioration in behaviour or general condition. A gentle reassuring approach is particularly needed to allay the patient's anxieties when faced with new people or situations. This is especially so when attendance at a medical outpatient clinic or admission to a general hospital is needed. If the patient's reaction in these circumstances is difficult to contain,

advice on management or practical help may be available on request from the Community Handicap Team who know the patient.

References

Benson, D. F. and Blumer, D. (eds) (1975). *Psychiatric aspects of neurologic disease*. Grune and Stratton, New York.

Lishman, W. A. (1978). *Organic psychiatry. The psychological consequences of cerebral disorder*. Blackwell Scientific Publications, Oxford.

Pearce, J. (1984). *Dementia. A clinical approach*. Blackwell Scientific Publications, Oxford.

Rutter, M. and Hersov, L. (eds) (1977). *Child psychiatry. Modern approaches*. Blackwell Scientific Publications, Oxford.

Whitty, C. W. M. and Zangwill, O. L. (eds) (1977). *Amnesia. Clinical psychological and medicolegal aspects*, 2nd edn. Butterworth, London.

Psychogeriatrics

R. A. MAYOU

In old age there are no psychiatric problems that are not seen in younger patients, but organic mental disorders are particularly common. In general, elderly patients can be given the same treatment as young people, but they have some particular needs that require separate description. When treating elderly patients the doctor should always bear in mind the frequent co-existence of physical and psychiatric conditions. He or she should know the general principles of social care, and the range of available residential and domiciliary services. This section begins with a review of psychiatric syndromes as they affect the elderly, and continues with a review of the general principles of assessment and treatment.

Psychiatric syndromes

Acute organic syndromes (delirium, acute confusional state)

Acute organic syndromes are common in the elderly, especially in those who are predisposed by pre-existing dementia, sensory impairment or advanced age. In people with these vulnerabilities, severe psychiatric symptoms may be precipitated by minor infections, drugs, exacerbations of chronic medical illness such as heart failure. Frequently impaired consciousness is not immediately obvious; hence doctors need to be specially vigilant not to dismiss the poor cognitive function of an acute organic syndrome as a manifestation of normal ageing nor to misdiagnose it as dementia.

The underlying physical cause should be sought and treated promptly. Nurses should aim to minimize confusion and distress by giving repeated explanation and reassurance, preferably from a few nurses or other people familiar to the patient. In hospital, a well-lit side room is more suitable than a noisy general ward. It may be helpful to prescribe small amounts of a hypnotic at night and, if behaviour is disturbed, a phenothiazine or haloperidol by day.

Dementia

Dementia occurs in 5–10 per cent of people aged over 65 years, and 20 per cent of those aged over 80 years. The commonest causes are senile dementia of the Alzheimer type (SDAT) and multi-infarct dementia (see previous chapter on Organic Mental States). Less common causes include neoplasms, infections, and metabolic disorders.

The assessment of dementia in the elderly follows the general principles described on page 25.15. Treatable causes should be sought systematically (see Table 1) but the intensity of the investigation will obviously depend upon the patient's age and general physical state.

Medical and social care, which should be planned with the relatives, family doctor, and social services, should avoid an excessive

Table 1 Investigation of an organic mental disorder

Haemoglobin, ESR and full blood count
Biochemical screen
Urinalysis and culture
Chest and skull X-ray
Syphilis serology
Thyroid function
Vitamin B_{12}
ECG and EEG
CT scan (if any suspicions of focal pathology)

Table 2 Causes of paranoid symptoms in the elderly

Acute and chronic organic mental syndromes
Depressive disorder
Paranoid personality
Schizophrenia and paranoid states

burden on families. It will sometimes be possible to organize help so that patients can continue to live in their own homes, especially if they are not alone, but many will need sheltered residential care. The very severely demented require long-term nursing in hospital.

Depressive disorders

Depressive disorders are common in later life. The incidence of first illnesses is highest between the ages of 50 and 65 years, and becomes low only after the age of 80 years. The incidence of suicide, usually associated with depression, increases with age. There is evidence that many treatable depressive disorders in the elderly are not detected in general practice or in general hospitals.

The clinical features are as described in the chapter on depressive disorder, but are often more striking than in younger people. For example, depressive delusions and hallucinations are frequently seen. A small proportion of retarded patients present with 'pseudo-dementia'; that is, difficulty in concentrating and remembering which may lead to a mistaken diagnosis of dementia.

The treatment of depressive disorders in the elderly generally follows that for young people on page 25.9. However, some special points should be noted. It is especially important to be aware of the risk of suicide. Antidepressants should be used cautiously starting with a third or a half of the normal adult dosage, and gradually increasing to normal adult dosages. Amitriptyline and imipramine are widely used, but there are advantages in prescribing mianserin because it has fewer anticholinergic side effects and is probably less cardiotoxic. Electroconvulsive therapy (ECT) is not contraindicated by advanced age, but if the patient becomes confused after treatment then applications should be given at longer intervals.

Although most patients show an excellent response to treatment with antidepressant drugs or ECT, about 15 per cent never completely recover. The relapse rate is high.

Mania

Mania accounts for between 5 and 10 per cent of affective illnesses in old age. The clinical picture nearly always combines depressive and manic symptoms, and the condition is frequently recurrent. As in younger patients lithium prophylaxis is valuable but considerable care is required, especially if renal function is impaired or the patient is being treated with diuretics.

Paranoid syndromes

Paranoid syndromes are common in the elderly. Most are secondary to organic or affective disorder, the rest being due to paranoid schizophrenia or occurring in paranoid personalities (Table 2). Many are chronic illnesses which first appeared earlier in life, others are first illnesses. These late onset illnesses, sometimes referred to as 'late paraphrenia', are especially common in women, in people living alone, and in those who are socially isolated either because of deafness or as a result of their personalities. Although these later onset disorders usually have a chronic course, the personality is relatively well preserved compared with younger patients.

Treatment is as described in the sections on schizophrenia, and drug treatment, most patients requiring long-term antipsychotic

medication. The dosage is usually about half that for younger adults.

Neurosis, personality disorder, and substance abuse

In later life, the incidence of new cases of neurosis declines and referral for neurosis to a psychiatrist is uncommon. However, the frequency of consultation with the general practitioner does not fall, presumably because many cases are chronic or recurrent. Neurotic syndromes in the elderly are usually of the mixed kind with symptoms of anxiety and depression. Hypochondriacal symptoms are often present.

Personality disorder causes many problems for elderly patients and their families. Paranoid traits may become exaggerated with age, and abnormal personality is one of the causes of the 'senile squalor syndrome' in which old people become withdrawn, isolated, and neglectful of themselves.

Alcoholism is an increasingly common cause of psychiatric and social problems among old people. The elderly may also become dependent on prescribed drugs such as benzodiazepines and hypnotics, and may suffer withdrawal symptoms when medication is changed.

The treatment of neurosis and personality disorder follows the general principles outlined on pages 25.2–25.7. However, in elderly people there is a greater need to treat concurrent physical illness and to deal with social problems.

General considerations

Assessment

It is helpful to see elderly patients in their own homes. Adequate assessment requires a thorough investigation of medical and social as well as psychiatric problems. Contact should also be made with any services already involved. In taking a history, the clinician needs to elicit the following: time and mode of onset of symptoms; previous medical and psychiatric history; the patient's living conditions and financial position; the patients' ability to look after themselves; any odd or undesirable behaviour that may cause difficulties with other people, the attitudes of the family and close friends, and their willingness and ability to help; other services already involved.

A thorough physical examination should be carried out, including a neurological assessment. There should always be a systematic assessment of cognitive functions, including memory, orientation, and everyday behaviour. The patient may need to be admitted to hospital or day care to allow more systematic observation of the functions.

Treatment

Treatment differs only in emphasis from that described for younger patients. There is necessarily a greater concern with physical care and with the provision of social services to enable a full life without undue burden on the family. Whenever possible, treatment at home is to be preferred because the elderly generally function best there.

The use of drugs

Great caution is necessary in prescribing psychotropic drugs for the elderly. It is essential to use simple regimes of a minimum number of drugs and to start with small doses. However, provided that the patient's mental and physical state is carefully observed, it is usually possible to increase dosages to effective levels without causing undesirable side-effects.

Haloperidol is the drug of choice for the control of the symptoms of organic mental disorders and for other acute disturbances of behaviour. It is less likely than phenothiazines to cause hypotension and oversedation but more likely to cause extrapyramidal symptoms, though in practice the latter is seldom a problem.

Phenothiazines such as chlorpromazine and thioridazine are valuable for the control of agitation and the symptoms of psychotic illnesses. It is important to avoid oversedation and to be alert for other side effects (hypotension, extrapyramidal symptoms, anticholinergic).

Benzodiazepines are useful for anxiety caused by short-term stress. Temazepam (or another short-acting benzodiazepine) is the hypnotic of choice. Chlormethiazole and chloral hydrate are alternatives.

Psychological treatment

Whilst interpretive psychotherapy is rarely indicated in the elderly, simple discussion and counselling are as necessary as they are with younger patients. Joint interviews with the spouse can also be helpful.

Behavioural methods are useful for helping patients with problems in eating, continence or social skills. If the patient can be maintained in well-ordered and suitably stimulating surroundings, psychological treatment of this kind can be surprisingly effective.

Social measures

Good care of the elderly infirm depends on a knowledge of all the available domiciliary and residential services. Well-organized practical and flexible help to the patient and family can often prevent hospital admission and enable the leading of a contented life in familiar surroundings. There is always a need to provide support for relatives so that they are not overwhelmed by excessive responsibilities. Day care or occasional hospital admission may be valuable.

References

Birren, J. E. and Sloan, R. B. (1981). *Handbook of mental health and aging*. Prentice Hall, Englewood Cliffs, New Jersey.
Levy, R. and Post, F. (1982). *The Psychiatry of late life*. Blackwell Scientific Publications, Oxford.

The patient who has attempted suicide

H. G. MORGAN

The form of behaviour to be discussed in this chapter may be defined as a deliberate act of self-harm not leading to death, whether involving physical means, drug overdosage, or poisoning, and carried out in the knowledge that it was potentially harmful and in the case of drug overdosage that the amount taken was excessive. The term 'non-fatal deliberate self-harm' (DSH) is preferable to alternatives such as 'attempted suicide' or 'parasuicide', because a conscious wish to die appears to be present in only a minority of these patients. After the event only a third of women and a half of men admitted to hospital because of DSH claim that they had wanted to die, even fewer (25 per cent) have expected to do so, and by the next day only 10–20 per cent regret having failed to kill themselves. Because only a minority are in fact failed suicides, the assessment and management of these patients encompasses a much wider remit than that of suicide risk.

Description

Epidemiology

DSH is most frequent in young adults, and it occurs more often in females than males at all ages except in the elderly. In the last 25 years the incidence of DSH has increased rapidly in countries throughout the western hemisphere, and in the United Kingdom

DSH now constitutes about 20 per cent of all emergency medical admissions to hospital. It is most common in social classes IV and V and tends to be concentrated in those parts of urban areas where social problems abound, particularly in local authority housing estates and city centres where the annual incidence in teenage and young adult females may reach 1.6 per cent.

Method of self-harm

The most frequent method is some kind of drug overdosage (95 per cent); self-injury, usually in the form of laceration, accounts for most of the remainder, either as the sole method or with drug overdosage. Psychotropic drugs (tranquillizers, antidepressants or sedatives) are involved in about half of all cases, and these drugs are commonly obtained through medical prescription. In teenagers the most commonly used agents are analgesics such as salicylates and paracetamol, usually obtained without prescription at chemists' shops. Poisons and gassing are each used in less than 1 per cent of cases. Alcohol intake within the previous six hours has been reported in 50–66 per cent of men and 25–45 per cent of women admitted to hospital because of DSH.

Psychological correlates

Personality disorder with its attendant chronic social disruption is seen in 25–50 per cent of persons admitted to hospital because of DSH and many of these people also have long-standing problems caused by alcohol abuse. Florid psychotic mental illness is found in only a small minority (12 per cent). Each episode of DSH is usually accompanied by marked anxiety and depressive symptoms. These symptoms generally subside rapidly after the event, but they usually persist unchanged in patients who have harmed themselves in the context of a depressive illness.

Social correlates

Some kind of upsetting life event appears to precipitate DSH in about two-thirds of cases. Most commonly this takes the form of disharmony with a person who is important to the patient. Other factors seen less frequently include problems concerned with work, financial matters, or physical health. Lack of close support and a sense of loneliness is reported by about half of all patients admitted to hospital because of deliberate self-harm.

Causes

In many cases the deliberate self-harm seems to be an impulsive act by a vulnerable person who has become emotionally upset in response to some disturbing event; and the intention is either to seek temporary oblivion or achieve some change in the situation, perhaps by appealing to others through an act which highlights the degree of personal distress. In such cases conscious suicidal intent is generally absent and even when present tends to be transient and barely enters into the conscious reasoning of the person concerned. However, it is necessary to remember that an important minority of patients who survive an episode of DSH are in fact failed suicides. In these patients suicide risk is likely to continue after the event, so that the reliable identification of this group is an important part of the assessment of a patient after DSH.

The reasons for the dramatic increase in the incidence of DSH since the early 1960s are complex. Changes in the attitudes of society to suicide and non-fatal self-harm seem to be important with an increase in the fashion of using DSH for its effect as an appeal to others. Changes in the prescribing of psychotropic drugs may also be important for there has been a marked increase in the quantity of prescriptions for these drugs during the period in which the incidence of DSH has increased. Also the types of drug used in DSH reflect quite clearly the general pattern of medical prescribing. The risk of DSH during treatment with psychotropic drugs is probably increased when medication is used merely to relieve symptoms without any attempt being made to resolve any concomitant upsetting life events.

Assessment

Adequate assessment of DSH requires full and reliable information and whenever possible other relevant informants should be interviewed as well as the patient. A detailed evaluation of social and interpersonal factors is necessary as well as a clinical assessment. Some patients are unwilling to discuss suicidal ideas openly, a few are suspicious because of psychotic ideas; and the aggressive behaviour of others may have arisen from a toxic confusional state due to the overdose of drugs. Some patients also show a marked reluctance to discuss personal matters. Good interview technique is needed to surmount these problems.

There are certain well-recognized risks attendant upon DSH and these should be evaluated without delay. The main immediate risks are: physical complications, a further episode of DSH, or suicide. There may also be risks to dependent children or other family members, which should be recognized and dealt with urgently.

Physical complications

Physical treatment is discussed in Sections 6 and 14. In this account only a few obvious points need be considered. First aid treatment is of the utmost importance particularly for the unconscious patient before transfer to hospital, maintenance of an adequate airway being a paramount consideration. Only a few (4 per cent) DSH patients need to be admitted to an intensive care unit, and less than a quarter are unconscious for more than 24 hours. Few specific antidotes are available and effective care for most overdose patients depends almost entirely upon good nursing and appropriate physiotherapy. These patients can cause considerable disruption in a medical ward and may evoke a degree of hostility from doctors and nurses. The provision of a special ward for overdoses sometimes reduces this problem, although it can be argued that treatment in the general medical ward with effective collaboration between physician, psychiatrist, and nurse is a better approach to management.

Suicide risk

Most DSH patients are interviewed in the hospital ward as soon as they are able to discuss matters fully and clearly, usually a day or so after the event. The detection of the minority of DSH patients who are failed suicides is an important immediate objective. It is a difficult and uncertain task, but it is helped by the fact that the social and clinical correlates of completed suicide tend to be different from those of patients whose deliberate self-harm does not have a fatal outcome. The risk of subsequent suicide is greater when: the overdose was massive with a serious risk to life; lacerations are deep, extensive and involve vital points; a potentially lethal agent such as a firearm was used; precautions were taken to succeed or avoid discovery; and the episode was carefully planned. Suicide risk also correlates with increasing age, male sex, loss of spouse or other relative through bereavement, separation, divorce, unemployment, incapacitating physical disability (especially terminal illness in the elderly), social isolation, and alienation. Increased suicide risk is also associated with certain types of psychiatric illness; of these, depressive illness is of paramount importance and its clinical features should be sought carefully in every case (see below). Other high-risk conditions include chronic alcoholism, drug addiction, schizophrenia, and the early stages of an organic brain syndrome. Epilepsy complicated by mood disorder is also important, especially when it occurs in the setting of an impulsive angry personality. Extreme care should be exercised when prescribing drugs for such patients.

Interviewing suicidal people

Continued suicidal motivation may not be easy to assess by interview and it is necessary to be aware of the potential pitfalls and ways of circumventing them. Assessment should ideally be performed without interruption in a quiet situation where the patient is able to talk in private without feeling hurried. The patient may show varying amounts of depression, despair, anger or frustration but may be reluctant to talk about personal feelings. There may also be reluctance to discuss the act of self-harm because this provokes guilt, shame, and the fear of adverse consequences. Assessment of the mental state should be directed particularly to the detection of the characteristic clinical features of depressive illness. These include overt depression of mood, tearfulness, disorders of thinking such as poor concentration, ideas of futility, and morbid self-blame; as well as 'biological' changes such as insomnia, poor appetite, and weight loss.

If the patient appears despairing and hopeless, it is appropriate to mention this in a sympathetic and reassuring way at an early stage in the interview. Such a comment can be an important first step in overcoming the feelings of isolation and alienation which are so characteristic of suicidal people. Discussion of suicidal ideas should be entered upon carefully. It is best to ask first about future plans and hopes; suicidal persons may be unable to see any future for themselves or indeed for others close to them. Discussion can then move to the present by asking how important the patient feels it is to go on living, and whether it is difficult to continue from day to day in the face of the identified difficulties. Following this sequence of discussion it is relatively easy to introduce the topic of suicide itself, and to ask whether this has been considered or planned. Continuing suicidal ideas after an episode of DSH must of course always be taken seriously.

There is no evidence that open discussion will in any way increase the risk of suicide: indeed the most common error is failure to enquire about such risk adequately. However, the enquiry must be made appropriately: a brusque, challenging, and unsympathetic approach is hazardous as it is liable to induce dangerous impulsive behaviour in a tense angry patient.

There may be marked fluctuations in the degree of overt distress shown by suicidal people, and some who are still at risk may at times appear free from symptoms. This is particularly likely in those who are admitted to hospital and thereby removed from the life problems causing despair. Those with continued suicidal intent often show anger and resentment towards either their situation or other people, and they may appear unco-operative and unreasonable as well as depressed and despairing. When the clinical picture is of this mixed kind it is important not to underestimate the suicide risk.

The majority (70 per cent) of those who commit suicide turn to others for help and communicate their suicidal ideas openly before killing themselves. It is therefore wrong to believe that people who talk about suicidal ideas never kill themselves. It is also rash to dismiss such comments as mere threats or manipulation, unless the patient is well known to the doctor and such an interpretation is wholly consistent with previous behaviour. Even then such a judgement can be mistaken.

A high proportion of individuals who have severe suicidal intent are ambivalent about ending their lives and may temporarily recover hope. This may lead an unsuspecting interviewer into a false sense of optimism. Occasionally a person at serious risk of suicide conceals the fact because of the belief that no help is likely to be effective. When a person who denies suicidal ideas has behaved in an inconsistent manner, such as having left a suicide note, or having engaged in life-endangering behaviour, particular care should be taken not to accept this denial too readily.

Non-fatal repetition

Another risk which requires immediate assessment is that of a further act of self-harm that is not fatal. The patient may talk openly about wishing to repeat the act of DSH and this statement should never be dismissed lightly, particularly when upsetting life events which led up to the episode are still present or have even been made worse by it, for example, by increasing the hostility of other people. Other correlates of non-fatal repetition include a long history of psychiatric disturbance suggestive of personality disorder, abuse of alcohol or drugs, and a previous history of DSH or of psychiatric treatment.

Management

During the initial period in an accident and emergency department or medical ward the emphasis of treatment is upon physical complications. Nevertheless the risks of suicide and non-fatal repetition should not be forgotten. The degree of risk should be decided in every case and if any doubt exists psychiatric advice should be obtained immediately. Once the risk is decided it should be clearly understood by all those concerned with the patient's care. Particular attention should be given to preventing access to hazards such as open stairs or windows: it is the hospital's responsibility to ensure that such patients are nursed only in situations where their safety can be reasonably assured. The number of nursing staff available is important and the needs should be reviewed frequently. Patients who have taken drug overdoses may be noisy and unco-operative because of confusion induced by drugs or disinhibition due to concomitant alcohol intake, often compounded by personality difficulties. As a result such people are not always the most welcome of the patients who are nursed in medical wards.

A minority (20 per cent) of DSH patients require admission to a psychiatric ward, usually because of florid mental illness, continuing risk of self-harm, or a worsening social situation. A very small number (1 per cent) may have to be admitted under a compulsory legislative provision because the immediate risk of suicide is very serious, and the patient is mentally ill and unwilling to accept help. In the United Kingdom this situation most commonly involves a Section 2 Assessment Order of the *Mental Health Act* 1983. This requires an application by (or on behalf of) the nearest relative together with two medical recommendations, one of which must be made by a recognized specialist in psychiatry.

In many hospitals about half of all cases of DSH are given appointments for subsequent outpatient treatment but only half of these patients actually attend. About a quarter are immediately returned to and remain in the care of their general practitioners.

Suicide risk

In the year after an episode of DSH about 2 per cent of patients commit suicide. While the initial detailed examination of the situation can be an immense relief to the suicidal person, ongoing management is required in an attempt to reduce the continuing risk. There should be a mutually agreed contract between patient and doctor, with clearly defined goals and explicit aims of treatment. The concern, sympathy, and non-judgemental attitudes of the therapist and a refusal to share the patient's feeling of despair are of great importance.

When a serious depressive disorder is the underlying cause of the suicidal intent, antidepressant medication may be needed, or even ECT. However, psychotropic drugs alone are never an adequate safeguard against the risk of suicide. Indeed there is evidence that persons who commit suicide have often been prescribed such drugs for long periods although in dosages too low to be effective. When a serious risk of suicide is present, the necessary degree of observation should be clearly understood by all members of staff. Those patients who are at the most serious risk of suicide may need a special nurse in attendance at all times and may have to be nursed in bed in a ward area which can provide physical security. When the risk is less severe it may be sufficient to ensure that the patient stays on the ward at all times, usually in night clothes, and is observed at regular agreed intervals.

Sometimes a psychiatrist has to support a suicidal person as an outpatient over a long period, especially when intensive treatment in hospital has not produced a complete resolution of the problems, for example, when there are intractable social or interpersonal difficulties. In such cases it is very important to use a clearly defined contractual approach as this helps to avoid overdependency on the therapist.

'Hotline' contact for vulnerable individuals can be useful, either with the medical services or one of the voluntary agencies such as the Samaritans. Although it is known that some of the clients of the Samaritan organization are persons at high risk of suicide, there has been considerable debate whether this organization prevents suicide to a significant degree. However, it is clear that the Samaritans are in contact with people who are in a serious crisis and who by the usual criteria are at risk of suicide. The principle of befriending is sound and voluntary initiative of this kind from the community should be strongly encouraged.

Prevention of non-fatal repetition

During the year after an episode of DSH about a quarter of patients repeat one or more non-fatal acts of self-harm. The great majority of repeats occur within the first year, particularly within the first three months. There may be a single further episode; or more than one. Repetition may be one more event in a chronic pattern of DSH, or it may cluster around acute episodes of stress. In some ways DSH behaviour seems to be self-perpetuating, in that the likelihood of an episode is greater when the person has made one or more previous attempts. This is one reason why patients seen after the first overdose should be encouraged to accept further help in the hope that this will prevent the development of a repetitive pattern of DSH. Nevertheless, it is disappointing that the provision of intensive psychiatric and social work after DSH has not been shown to have a significant effect on the rate of repetition of non-fatal DSH, even though life difficulties are reduced by such treatment. In planning treatment it is advisable to take into account the style of help the patients prefer: some wish to attend their general practitioner, others think psychiatric help more relevant to their problems. Treatment should include several strategies in order to encourage as many patients as possible to accept it. Situational and interpersonal difficulties need to be treated as well as personal problems.

When an overdose of prescribed medication has been taken it is essential to consider carefully whether the drug should be continued. It may be inappropriate to give further supplies, but occasionally there is a certain degree of physical and psychological dependence on the drug and sudden withdrawal may lead to acute anxiety and agitation. This reaction may occur even with minor tranquillizers when they have been prescribed over a long period of time in high dosage. In such cases it may be necessary to continue the treatment, giving small amounts at any one time. Major tranquillizers used in the long-term treatment of schizophrenia should of course not be stopped without psychiatric advice. The general practitioner should be telephoned whenever possible before any patient is discharged from hospital after an episode of DSH.

Primary prevention

The most important aspect of prevention is probably the role of psychotropic drugs prescribing as a factor leading to DSH. Most patients who take non-fatal drug overdoses do so when experiencing distressing situations. Psychotropic drugs prescribed for such people do not treat their fundamental problems: the difficulties continue, repeated prescriptions become almost inevitable, and when a further crisis occurs the scene is set for an overdose with the available medication. For this reason great care should be exercised in prescribing psychotropic drugs, especially for young adults in high-risk social areas. When drugs are considered essential, the course should be planned carefully, the duration should be finite, and adequate personal counselling made available.

References

Hawton, K. and Catalan, J. (1982). *Attempted suicide*. Oxford University Press, Oxford.

Kreitman, N. (1977). *Parasuicide*. Wiley, London.

Morgan, H. G. (1979). *Death wishes? The understanding and management of deliberate self-harm*. Wiley, London.

—— (1982). Deliberate self-harm. In *Recent advances in psychiatry*, Vol. 4 (ed. K. Granville-Grossman). Churchill Livingstone, Edinburgh.

The alcoholic patient

D. H. GATH

Many patients are admitted to general hospital wards with physical illnesses largely caused by alcohol. Recent studies in several industrial countries found that between 10 and 25 per cent of patients in medical wards had alcohol problems. These figures were obtained by special screening of patients for problem drinkers, and there can be no doubt that in ordinary hospital practice many such patients are missed.

Similarly in primary medical care (general practice), it has been shown that in a practice population of 2500 patients there are likely to be about 20 patients with a serious drinking problem, of whom only two or three will be known as such to the general practitioner.

Physicians should be constantly alert not to miss any patients with alcohol problems for two reasons. First, detection may provide an opportunity for treatment, which can sometimes alleviate deep suffering in the patient and family, and may prevent further decline in health and social well being. Secondly, there is strong evidence that over the past 25 years in many industrial countries there has been a steady rise in rates of alcoholism and of alcohol-related damage, such as deaths from cirrhosis of the liver, admissions to mental hospital for alcoholism, and legal offences like public drunkenness and drunken driving. Excessive drinking has been reported amongst many more women than previously and particularly amongst teenagers, many of whom will be dependent on alcohol in their twenties.

To avoid missing alcoholic patients in the medical wards or general practice, the physician should know what the main clinical features of alcoholism are, and how to elicit them. If the patient is to be helped either directly or by advice on specialist referral, the physician needs to be informed about the causes and treatment of alcoholism.

The term alcoholism is widely used, but with much uncertainty about its meaning. For practical purposes the term can be applied to all patients who cause serious harm to themselves or other people through excessive drinking. Three subgroups can be recognized: patients who drink harmfully but without being dependent on alcohol; those with the syndrome of alcohol dependence; and chronic alcoholics.

Excessive drinkers with problems but without dependence

The first group of problem drinkers can be recognized mainly by their drinking pattern and evidence of social damage.

The drinking pattern changes as life becomes more and more centred on alcohol. At first, more time is spent in social drinking and in consuming stronger and more frequent drinks. Then drinking is done not so much for pleasure as to relieve tension and to perform adequately at work or socially. Drinkers become preoccupied with finding alcohol, and drink surreptitiously with increasing worry or guilt. At the same time they find they can drink more without becoming drunk.

With this drinking pattern, social damage nearly always develops, usually in the form of marital disharmony, declining efficiency at work, financial problems or clashes with the law.

Physical disabilities are not so common, but symptoms of gastritis such as anorexia, nausea or retching should always suggest alcoholism. Psychological symptoms are usually mood changes, mainly depression and anxiety; these may have led to the heavy drinking originally, but they are aggravated by alcohol, not relieved.

Heavy drinkers often experience memory blanks (wrongly called blackouts) for the previous evening, especially if quick drinking had led to a rapid rise in blood alcohol.

It is important that excessive drinking of this kind should be recognized, because if it is not checked it will lead to dependence.

The syndrome of alcohol dependence

Alcohol becomes a drug of dependence when there is a compulsion to take it on a continuous or periodic basis. The dependence induced has both psychological and physiological elements, but the distinction need not be made in practice.

For the dependent drinker, alcohol takes priority over everything else, including health, family, home, career, and social life. As life centres increasingly on the need to relieve or avoid withdrawal symptoms, responsibilities at home and work are evaded, and behaviour becomes dishonest and deceitful.

Memory lapses may become longer and more frequent, affecting the day as well as the previous night. Eventually recollection of whole days may be lost, and amnesia may be combined with inexplicable wanderings (fugue). Whilst not pathognomonic of alcohol dependence, these are grave warning signs.

The diagnostic features of the dependence syndrome are:

Subjective awareness of compulsion to drink Dependent drinkers are aware of being unable to control drinking in a reasonable way and of being unsure that they can stop drinking once started. If they try to give up alcohol, they may experience craving for it.

Increased tolerance Dependent drinkers may be relatively unaffected by blood levels of alcohol that would incapacitate a normal drinker. They may then maintain that alcohol is no problem to them, but this is a false argument since tolerance is an important sign of increasing dependence.

Withdrawal symptoms Withdrawal symptoms occur in people who have been drinking heavily for years and who maintain a high intake of alcohol for weeks at a time. The symptoms follow a drop in blood alcohol level, and characteristically appear on waking in the morning.

The earliest and commonest feature is acute tremulousness affecting the hands, legs, and trunk, often known as the shakes. The sufferer may be unable to sit still, hold a cup steadily, or do up buttons. He or she is agitated and easily startled, and often dreads facing people or crossing the road. Nausea, retching, and sweating are frequent. If alcohol is taken, these symptoms may be relieved quickly; if not, they may last several days.

As withdrawal progresses, misperceptions and hallucinations may occur, usually only briefly. Objects appear distorted in shape, or shadows seem to move; disorganized voices, shouting or snatches of music may be heard. Later there may be epileptic seizures, and finally after about 48 hours delirium tremens may develop (described below).

Relief drinking Since they can only stave off withdrawal symptoms by further drinking, many dependent drinkers take a drink on waking in the morning. In most cultures, early morning drinking is diagnostic of dependency.

With increasing need to stave off withdrawal symptoms during the day, the drinker typically becomes secretive about the amount consumed, hides bottles or carries them in a pocket. Rough cider and cheap wines may be drunk regularly to obtain the most alcohol for the least money.

The dependence syndrome generally becomes established in men in the mid-forties, and in women a few years later, but it also occurs in the teens and late life. Once established, its usual course is inexorable advance; if unchecked, it progresses destructively to the stage of chronic alcoholism.

Chronic alcholism

Chronic alcoholics are those patients whose brains and other organs have been irreversibly damaged by alcohol, with effects that persist even after drinking has ceased (see next section). The physical and mental symptoms may lead to greater social isolation, which may in turn lead to increased drinking. At the same time tolerance becomes reduced, and the previously heavy drinker may now become incapacitated by a small amount of alcohol.

Alcohol-related damage

For the diagnosis and assessment of the alcoholic patient, an understanding of the concept of alcohol-related damage is important. The damage incurred through excessive drinking may be physical, psychological or social.

Physical damage

Alcohol may lead to physical damage in several ways: through a direct toxic effect on certain tissues, as in the liver; malnutrition, mainly deficiency of protein and vitamin B; increased susceptibility to infection; and trauma, such as head injury.

The physical complications of alcoholism are numerous. Only the neuropsychiatric conditions will be described here, the others being presented elsewhere. However, it should be stressed that alcohol may harm every bodily system. In the alimentary system, for example, alcohol-related disorders include peptic ulceration, cirrhosis of the liver, oesophageal varices, and acute pancreatitis. Examples in other systems include peripheral neuropathy, cerebellar degeneration, myopathy, cardiomyopathy, anaemia, vitamin deficiency, poorly controlled diabetes mellitus, hypoglycaemia, pneumonia, tuberculosis, and foetal damage. The list could be greatly extended.

Neuropsychiatric complications

These include forms of brain damage due to vitamin deficiencies and to the direct toxic action of alcohol, such as the following.

Dementia There is a loss of general intellectual capacity, with impairments of memory, judgement, grasp of new ideas, and abstract thinking. Disturbances of mood and behaviour usually accompany the intellectual deficits.

Korsakoff's psychosis There is gross impairment of memory for recent events, though not necessarily for events in early life (Section 21). Consciousness is normal. To compensate for the disabling loss of short-term memory, the patient may invent fanciful experiences (confabulation).

Wernicke's encephalopathy There is full consciousness but there may be difficulty in concentrating and slowness in answering questions, together with ophthalmoplegia, diplopia, and nystagmus, and disturbances of gait and balance.

Other neuropsychiatric complications may be induced by alcohol withdrawal, including epileptic seizures and delirium tremens.

Delirium tremens This occurs in people with a history of excessive drinking over several years. There is a dramatic and rapidly changing picture of disordered mental activity, with clouding of consciousness, disorientation in time and place, and impairment of recent memory. Perceptual disturbances include misinterpretations of sensory stimuli, and vivid hallucinations which are usually visual, but sometimes in other modalities.

There is severe agitation, with restlessness, shouting and evident fear. Insomnia is prolonged. The hands are grossly tremulous and sometimes pick up imaginary objects, and truncal ataxia occurs. Autonomic disturbances include sweating, fever, tachycardia, raised blood pressure, and dilation of pupils. Blood testing shows leucocytosis, a raised ESR, and impaired liver function. Dehydration and electrolyte disturbance are characteristic.

The condition lasts three to four days, with nocturnal exacerbation of symptoms. It often ends with deep prolonged sleep from which the patient awakens with no symptoms and little or no memory of the delirious period.

Psychological damage

Mention has already been made of changes in behaviour resulting from the compulsion to drink, particularly the increasing self-centredness and lack of consideration for others, and the decline in standards of conduct.

Several other psychological changes are associated with excessive drinking including the following.

Impaired psychosexual function Sexual impotence and delayed ejaculation are common. These difficulties may be worsened when drinking leads to marital estrangement, or if the wife develops a revulsion for intercourse with an inebriated partner.

Pathological jealousy Partly as a result of their own sexual difficulties, alcoholics may hold the delusional conviction that their partner is unfaithful, although there is no foundation for this. They may go to extraordinary lengths to detect the supposed lover. They repeatedly cross-question the wife, and suspect all her actions. Doctors should be aware of this condition, as it can be dangerous and may lead to murder.

Alcoholic hallucinosis This is a feature of advanced alcoholism. In full consciousness, the patient recurrently hears voices talking about him or her, typically in obscene language. The experience is quite different from the fleeting and disorganized hallucinations that occur with alcoholic tremulousness or delirium tremens. The condition may clear up when drinking stops, though it sometimes persists despite abstinence.

Suicidal behaviour In many countries, suicide rates amongst alcoholics are far higher than in non-alcoholics of the same age. Thus in various parts of the United Kingdom, the risk of suicide is about 80 times greater in alcoholics.

Alcohol contributes to many instances of attempted suicide (as distinct from accomplished suicide); this should always be borne in mind when assessing self-poisoning or self-injury patients.

Social damage

Excessive drinking is liable to cause profound disruption in the family and in society at large.

Marital tension is virtually inevitable, and the divorce rate high. Wives of heavy drinkers often consult the family doctor complaining of anxiety or depression. Many women admitted to hospital because of self-poisoning blame their husband's drinking.

The home atmosphere is often highly detrimental to the children, because of quarrelling and violence, or a poor parental model. The children are at risk of developing neurotic or behaviour disorders or poor performance at school, disabilities which may persist into adult life.

The heavy drinker often progresses through declining efficiency at work, repeated sacking, and a slide into lower grade jobs, to final unemployment.

Excessive drinking is associated with crime, mainly petty offences such as larceny, but also fraud, sexual offences, and crimes of violence.

In the United Kingdom, a third of drivers killed on the roads have blood alcohol levels above the statutory limit; around the hours of midnight, the figure rises to 50 per cent; and on Saturday night to 75 per cent.

Diagnosis and assessment of the alcoholic patient

Attention may first be drawn to alcoholic patients if they develop withdrawal symptoms on admission to a medical ward. This may occur in patients with no recognized history of intoxication or excessive drinking. Florid delirium tremens is usually obvious, but milder forms may mimic the delirium of pneumonia or postoperative confusional state.

Otherwise, in clinical medicine alcoholic patients are liable to escape detection. This is because, understandably, they are often unable to admit to themselves or anyone else that they have such a shaming and frightening diagnosis as alcoholism. Despite this concealment, the physician should be able to identify the condition because of its great potential dangers.

The first requirement is an attitude of constant vigilance, particularly in relation to the many medical illnesses known to be associated with alcoholism (see preceding section). Peptic ulcers, for example, may receive intensive treatment including surgery, whilst underlying alcoholism remains undetected.

In general practice, gastritis is a common complaint, although the most frequent presentation is some kind of social problem, such as marital or financial difficulties.

Complaints of anxiety and depression or general malaise should always lead to enquiry about drinking, and psychotropic drugs should never be prescribed without taking a drinking history.

Drink problems should be considered if patients have a history of accidents or a family history of alcoholism. The same applies to the high-risk occupational groups, which include people working in the drink trade or catering, seamen, business executives, and commercial travellers, doctors, actors, and entertainers.

Occasionally patients openly volunteer that they have a drink problem. More often they give a hint, which may be slight but still calls for full exploration. A general question as to how much they drink is likely to be answered with evasion or denial, and so of little value. Usually the picture can be built up gradually by a series of questions as to where, what, and how much the patient drinks throughout a typical day. Enquiry can begin with how the patient feels on waking up, and whether a morning drink is taken; what the pattern of drinking is at mid-day, and so on through the day. Similarly, tactful enquiry should be made about social effects of drinking, such as declining efficiency at work, missed promotion, accidents, lateness, absences, and extended meal breaks. The patient should be asked about difficulties in relationships with the wife and children.

In this way, patients may be led step by step to recognize and accept that they have a serious drinking problem which they have previously denied.

Once this stage is reached, the doctor should be in a position to enquire about the typical features of dependency, and the full range of physical, psychological, and social disabilities described in preceding sections.

The causes of alcoholism

It is generally agreed that alcoholism is not caused by a single factor, but by multiple interacting factors.

Biological factors

There is some evidence from adoption studies that genetic factors may play a part, but nothing is known about the possible extent or mode of inheritance.

Biochemical studies have focussed on the metabolism of alcohol and glucose, neuro-transmitter substances such as catecholamines, and brain amino acids such as gamma amino butyric acid, proline, and aspartic acid. So far there is no conclusive evidence that these or other biochemical factors play a causal role.

Psychological factors

In clinical practice, alcoholism is commonly found to be associated with certain kinds of personality. The main characteristic is difficulty in coping with the demands of life, which may result from chronic anxiety, or a pervading sense of inferiority, or self-indulgent tendencies due to a pampered upbringing. However, many people with personality problems of this kind do not resort to excessive drinking, and there is no scientific evidence that any personality traits are specific determinants of alcoholism. It is most likely that certain attributes of personality simply increase the risk in relation to other causal factors.

Psychiatric illness plays a relatively small part in the aetiology of pathological drinking, but should always be borne in mind, as it may be treatable. Patients with depressive illness may turn to alcohol in the mistaken hope that it will alleviate low mood. Those with anxiety states, including phobias of public places and social encounters, are at risk. Alcoholism occasionally occurs in patients with brain disease or schizophrenia.

Social factors

There is extensive evidence from international studies that rates of alcoholism and alcohol-related diseases are closely linked with changes in the national *per capita* consumption of alcohol. If there is a small rise in the average consumption per person, the number of casualties is likely to rise disproportionately.

Average consumption within the nation is partly affected by the availability of alcohol, which is determined by economic factors, licensing regulations, and other formal controls. The social customs and mores of different countries also contribute, as shown by the low rates of alcoholism amongst Jews, Mormons, and Moslems.

Aspects of treatment

If the patient acknowledges that he or she has a drinking problem, a first step has been taken towards treatment. The next step should be to make a thorough and detailed assessment of the whole drinking problem, including a drinking history and a systematic appraisal of any medical, psychological or social complications. It is often valuable to include the family in this initial assessment. An intensive exploration of this kind offers two advantages. First, it may help the patient to gain a new recognition and understanding of the problems, a process which may be therapeutic in itself. Second, it provides the basis for a treatment plan.

Treatment may be undertaken by a psychiatrist or specialized psychiatric unit, by the general practitioner or hospital physician, or by other agencies. Whoever provides treatment, it is essential to formulate an explicit treatment plan, which should be worked out with the patient and tailored to the individual needs. It should not deal with the drinking problem in isolation, but with whatever physical, psychological or social problems accompany it.

Specific goals should be defined, which require the patient to take some responsibility for realizing them. One of the main goals will be the control of drinking. For patients with the dependence syndrome, control means total abstinence, whilst for non-dependent drinkers it may mean drinking in moderation. (Recently some clinicians have advocated moderate drinking as the best goal even for severely dependent patients, but the majority regard total abstinence as essential.)

Other goals will be concerned with health, marriage, job, and social adjustment. These goals should be realistic and graded in difficulty. For some patients, full recovery of personal functioning will be realistic, whilst for others staying out of prison will be more appropriate.

Withdrawal from alcohol

For patients with the dependence syndrome, withdrawal from alcohol is usually managed in hospital. In the less severe cases, it may be carried out at home if suitable care is available. Sedatives are usually required to alleviate withdrawal symptoms. They should be used with *great care* particularly in patients with associated alcoholic liver disease (see page 12.250). Chlormethiazole edisylate capsules containing 192 mg in an oily base are given in 3–4 divided doses daily. The following regime is recommended: initially 2–4 caps, repeated if necessary; day 2, 9–12 caps; day 3, 6–8 caps; day 4, 4–6 caps. The dose is then gradually reduced over days 5–7. In severely confused patients who cannot tolerate oral therapy chlormethiazole can be given as an i.v. infusion, 40–100 ml, initially as an 0.8 per cent solution over 5–10 min. with the infusion rate then adjusted according to response. A modified chlormethiazole regime for patients with liver disease is described on page 12.250. *It is extremely dangerous to administer chlormethiazole intravenously in patients with severe liver disease.* Alternatively, chlordiazepoxide may be used starting with 10 mg 3 times daily and increasing up to 100 mg daily in divided doses. Chlordiazepoxide may also be given by deep slow i.m. injection in doses of 50–100 mg followed, if necessary, by 25–100 mg 3–4 times daily.

Vitamin supplements are often given, and in some countries anticonvulsants, glucose, and magnesium infusions are added.

Psychiatric treament

Referral to a psychiatrist is often appropriate, depending on the patient's attitudes, needs, and motivation. Thus, for the newly diagnosed alcoholic, psychiatric referral may both test and reinforce motivation. For other patients inpatient care may be needed to manage physical or psychiatric disorders, to provide an alcohol-free environment, or to offer specialized treatment techniques for changing drinking behaviour.

The most widely used techniques are various forms of group therapy. These are usually practised in specialized units which have an experienced and closely knit staff of psychiatrists, nurses, social workers, and clinical psychologists. Regular meetings are attended by about 10 patients and one or more members of staff. Patients learn to cope by observing their own problems mirrored in other alcoholics. They gain confidence and self-esteem as members of the group jointly strive to reorganize their lives without alcohol.

If group therapy is not available, or not acceptable to the patient, individual psychological support may be provided by a psychiatrist or social worker. The usual aim is to help the patient to cope with problems in day-to-day living without the crutch of excessive drinking. Discussion takes place in an atmosphere of tolerance and acceptance, and the enthusiasm of the therapist is important.

Psychological treatment of alcoholism also includes behavioural techniques. Aversion therapy was introduced over 30 years ago, but is rarely used now because it is disagreeable and its results disappointing. It has been replaced by other methods which aim to teach patients useful skills such as how to cope with feelings of tension, how to refuse a drink, or how to gauge their own blood levels.

Drug treatment plays a relatively small part in the management of alcoholism. Antidepressants or tranquillizers may be needed occasionally, but are ineffective in long-term management.

Disulfiram (antabuse) is sometimes prescribed as a deterrent to impulsive drinking. After taking disulfiram the patient may resist the temptation to drink so as to avoid unpleasant flushing of the face, headache, choking sensations, rapid pulse, and feelings of anxiety. The drug is not without risk, and has unpleasant side-effects. Treatment with disulfiram should not be started until at least 12 hours after the last ingestion of alcohol. On the first day the patient is given four tablets each of 200 mg and told not to take any alcohol whatever. The dosage is then reduced by one tablet a day over three days, the maintenance dose being half to one tablet a day.

Citrated calcium carbimide is used in the same way. Compared with disulfiram, it is more rapidly absorbed and excreted, it induces a milder reaction with alcohol and has fewer side-effects. It is given orally in a dose of 50 mg once or twice daily.

Drugs of this kind have a limited use for a small group of patients. They should not be used as a sole treatment, but as an adjunct to other measures.

Treatment by the general practitioner or general physician

Alcoholism may be treated effectively by clinicians other than psychiatrists, especially when psychiatric referral or specialized techniques are unacceptable to the patient. The usual form of treatment is individual supportive therapy as described above, often involving other members of the family. The general practitioner is particularly well placed to offer this kind of treatment.

Alcoholics Anonymous (AA)

This is a self-help organization which has the goals of stopping drinking and remaining abstinent by following a system known as the Twelve Steps. Members usually attend group meetings twice weekly on a long-term basis. In crisis they can obtain immediate help by telephone.

AA does not appeal to all problem drinkers as the meetings involve confession of problems and sometimes emotional arousal. But the organization is of great value to some alcoholics, and anyone developing a drink problem should be encouraged to try it.

Rehabilitation and after care

On completing the early stages of treatment, most alcoholic patients need continuing contact with a helping agency for a year or two afterwards. Job training may be needed, and patients without social support may have to live in special hostels.

Prognostic factors

The following characteristics in patients give a favourable prognosis:

(a) Good insight into the nature of their problems.

(b) Social stability in the form of a fixed abode, family support, and ability to keep a job.

(c) Ability to control impulsiveness, to defer gratification, and to form deep emotional relationships.

Evaluation of treatment

There is still much uncertainly about the efficacy of treatment. Most evalutive studies deal with patients referred to hospitals for treatment of the dependence syndrome. The consensus view seems to be that about 60 per cent of these patients will show substantial improvement at 12 month follow-up. Probably less than half of these will have remained abstinent, but they will have achieved worthwhile gains in drinking behaviour, health, marriage, work, social life or avoidance of crime. These are modest results, but good enough to justify a constant effort to detect alcoholic patients and to offer them treatment.

References
Hore, B. (1976). *Alcohol dependence*. Butterworths, London.
Royal College of Psychiatrists Special Committee on Alcoholism (1979). *Report on alcohol and alcoholism.* Tavistock Publications, London.
World Health Organisation (1977). *Alcohol-related disabilities.* Offset Publication No. 32. WHO, Geneva.

Drug addiction

M. MITCHESON

Introduction

This chapter encompasses the non-therapeutic consumption of psychoactive drugs other than alcohol and nicotine. The dividing lines between use, misuse, and abuse of drugs are necessarily somewhat arbitrary. Even with medical prescription, some patients consume drugs in a manner which constitutes abuse; whilst some prescribing of psychotropic drugs, which is based on expedience rather than known pharmacological actions, can be regarded as medical misuse. The older terms addiction and habituation have been abandoned in favour of the overall term 'drug dependence' defined by the World Health Organization (WHO) as: 'a state, psychic and sometimes also physical, resulting from the interaction between a living organism and a drug, characterized by behavioural and other responses that always include a compulsion to take the drug on a continuous or a periodic basis in order to experience its psychic effects, and sometimes to avoid the discomfort of its absence'.

In terms of the medical or social response to drug consumption it is useful to recognize three overlapping categories.

Type 1: The intermittent consumption of drugs for their psychic effect without development of tolerance, or physical withdrawal effects other than a brief hangover; much consumption of this type is not strictly drug dependence within the WHO classification, since the compulsion to use is usually absent.

Type 2: The daily consumption of drugs, or combinations of drugs, often by injection, with the object of obtaining a psychic effect, tolerance usually develops and may promote the consumption of other drugs with different pharmacological actions to maintain a noticeable psychic effect; use must be daily if withdrawal symptoms are to be avoided.

Type 3: The daily consumption, usually by mouth, of a regular dose without noticeable behavioural change; often the drugs are obtained with a medical prescription, and often dependence has been started by prescribing; the motivation to continue is primarily that of avoiding the psychological or physical withdrawal symptoms. The consumer is more likely to be middle aged or elderly than in type 2.

Type 1 only involves the medical profession when the use of the drugs is itself illegal, when intoxication results in illegal activity (e.g. driving under the influence of alcohol), when there is inadvertent overdose, or when panic reactions occur. Although types 2 and 3 fall within the definition of true dependence, the approach in the United Kingdom has been to condemn type 2 but condone type 3 subject to some disapproval. Indeed for the older patient in particular it is often considered acceptable to sanction type 3 consumption with maintenance prescriptions. The basis of much medical management of drug dependence is to try to convert type 2 drug consumption to type 3. Indeed this is the aim of the maintenance treatment of opiate users.

Prevalence of dependence

Little is known for certain about the prevalence of different types of drug dependence. In the United Kingdom in 1983 the number of opiate addicts known to the Home Office was 10 235; double the figure for 1980. This is likely to be an underestimate of the true number, by at least a factor of five. There is no reliable information about the extent of dependence on other drugs.

Causes of dependence

There can be no single cause for such a complex pattern of behaviour as drug dependence. There is general agreement that for dependence to occur there must be: (*a*) a susceptible consumer to whom (*b*) drugs are available in (*c*) a social setting which acquiesces with or even coerces towards drug use. It is obvious that in different circumstances the relative importance of these factors will vary, and that factors that may be important in preventing drug dependence may be of less importance in rehabilitating the individual patient. There is evidence that the attitudes of the majority in a society towards the consumption of psychotropic drugs may help to promote the abuse of drugs by a minority. Also, the medical professional should note its responsibility to prevent dependence both by avoiding overprescribing and by resisting the desires within society to seek and receive a pharmacological panacea for any pain, unhappiness or embarrassment.

When confronted with a drug user, it is difficult to decide in retrospect whether psychological difficulties have been a factor in the initial drug taking. Certainly many type 2 drug users report a severely disorganized family background and unhappiness during childhood, and may have displayed behavioural disturbances such as school truancy or adolescent criminality before taking drugs. Yet some addicted patients offer no such history of early disturbance, while many of those with such a history have brothers and sisters similarly affected but without drug problems; and many people with similar backgrounds never become dependent on drugs. Patients undergoing treatment often report a high level of depressive symptoms and social anxiety, for which they claim their drug taking provides at least symptomatic relief. However, these symptoms may be the consequence of drug dependences rather than the cause. It seems likely that patients who come from subcultures with a high incidence of drug abuse will display relatively fewer personality difficulties than those from a subculture where the use is less common. In the former, drug dependency presumably results more from cultural factors and the ready availability of drugs.

Recognition of the drug dependent patient

Clinicians are sometimes consulted by patients who openly declare that they are dependent on drugs. It is important to try to corroborate the history by asking about the duration of the drug taking, and the cost and source of the drugs; by checking the story for internal consistency; and by seeking verification from independent informants whenever possible. Physical examination for evidence of self injection and complications of drug taking should always be undertaken.

Other patients make no mention of drug dependency, but ask for the prescription of controlled drugs for the relief of pain, such as renal colic or dysmenorrhoea. The clinician should be specially wary in the case of temporary patients. Again the doctor should examine for signs of self injection, and should bear in mind that some addicts make up injections from tablets of Diconal (dipipanone hydrochloride, cyclizine hydrochloride), Palfium (dextromoramide, as tartrate), or Ritalin (methylphenidate hydrochloride), and from barbiturates formulated as capsules, especially Tuinal (quinalbarbitone sodium, amylobarbitone sodium) and Nembutal (pentobarbitone sodium).

Urine testing will provide confirmatory evidence of the nature of the drugs taken in the preceding 24 hours, provided that the sample is known to be from the patient and not someone else. The duration and degree of drug use cannot be established from urine analysis.

Management

The physician must not take a punitive or moralistic approach to drug misusers who require professional help. To accept and assist a drug user as a patient is not to condone drug taking, nor is it incompatible with explicit advice about the disadvantages of misusing drugs. Some physicians who avoid clinical responsibility for such patients may be uncertain about the procedures to adopt, and some fear exploitation by patients. However, doctors will encounter drug-dependent patients in several settings: incidentally in the course of managing an illness unrelated to drug dependence; in the treatment of drug-related complications such as cellulitis, pneumonia, serum hepatitis, or accidents; or in the treatment of acute drug effects, overdose, withdrawal symptoms, intoxication, or adverse reactions to psychedelic drugs. Long-term prescribing or rehabilitation are more likely to involve general practitioners, psychiatrists or, in larger cities, the staff of specialist drug-dependence services. Long-term prescribing is a contentious subject.

Careful and sympathetic history taking, a clear management policy, and the obtaining of specialist advice before making a commitment to prescribing will usually ensure that any necessary medical or surgical treatment can be provided without difficulty. If the patient already has maintenance prescriptions, it is usually appropriate to continue the same dose while treating other disorders. However, it is essential to verify with the usual medical attendant a patient's claim about the maintenance prescription and to supply this in divided doses to avoid accidental overprescribing in cases where the patient may have been disposing of part of the regular prescription to others. When the patient has been supporting a drug habit from illegally obtained drugs, it may still be necessary to provide short-term maintenance or a reducing dose to cover withdrawal. Guidance about appropriate dosage is given below.

Rehabilitation

Many drug takers have great difficulty in re-establishing themselves within normal society after they have been cured of their pharmacological drug dependence. This is a reflection of several of the factors discussed under Causation, some of which may have preceded drug taking, while others may be consequent upon the gradual social alienation associated with heavy drug consumption, psychological dependence upon drugs to control emotional distress, and the changes in brain function resulting from regular consumption of psychoactive drugs. There is no agreement about the relative value of long-term supportive maintenance compared with drug-free programmes. This reflects the difficulty of providing treatment to these patients and ambivalence about the propriety of prescribing drugs for what may not be strictly medical purposes, as well as the diversity of the drug users. Some dependent patients may be helped, particularly in the early stages, by simple measures with outpatient support. Some with more severe problems have sufficient resources to benefit from the confrontational treatment in a therapeutic community. Some who receive maintenance drugs achieve a degree of social stability, but others continue heavy drug abuse deteriorating both medically and socially. Long-term maintenance users may request an increase in dose, citing increasing tolerance as the reason; it is necessary to be clear that physiological withdrawal does not result from tolerance, unless the patient has covertly increased the regular dose from alternative sources. Also, opiate-dependent patients confronted by an emotionally stressful situation may seek an increased dose for purposes of tranquillization. If it seems reasonable to respond to the request by increasing the dose, this should be only for a clearly specified and limited time.

Probably, outcome depends as much on the person's previous resources as it does on treatment. When personality factors predominate, rehabilitation must concentrate on intrapsychic problems; and when social factors are prominent, more attention must be given to social reorganization, educational opportunities, development of work skills etc. Specialist treatment is not available in all parts of the United Kingdom. It is most readily available in the London metropolitan area which has the largest number of recorded drug takers, a variety of non-statutory agencies working with drug takers, and 13 drug clinics based in hospitals. Other large metropolitan areas usually have some specialist services. Information about treatment facilities, both statutory and non-statutory, in the United Kingdom may be obtained from the Standing Conference on Drug Abuse (1–4 Hatton Place, Hatton Garden, London EC1).

The government has accepted that there should be a specialized unit in each health region, and a psychiatrist identified as having a special concern regarding dependence in each district.

Opiates and other centrally acting major analgesics

The paradigm of the group is morphine, the principal active alkaloid in opium, but diacetyl morphine (heroin) is approximately twice as potent as morphine as a drug of addiction and has attained worldwide notoriety as a drug of abuse. Most natural derivatives and synthetic substitutes are liable to abuse and these include the less potent opiates such as codeine, and synthetic analogues such as dihydrocodeine which are contained in some of the traditional liquid preparations for diarrhoea and coughs. As mentioned above, drug-dependent persons often seek tablets of drugs in this group, ostensibly for treatment of physical illness, and then take them by injection – a practice which is even more hazardous than the self administration of preparations intended for injection.

Restrictions on the prescribing of opiates

In the United Kingdom, only specially licensed doctors are legally permitted to prescribe heroin, dipipanone, and cocaine to an addict for maintenance of addiction. Any doctor is permitted to prescribe heroin or cocaine for the treatment of physical illness including terminal illnesses. Any doctor may (1985) prescribe to addicts opiates other than heroin, dipipanone or cocaine, as well as stimulants or barbiturates. However, unlicenced doctors should avoid such prescribing to addicts except in an emergency and, if possible, should first obtain specialist advice; otherwise they may be liable to run into difficult management problems.

In the United Kingdom there is a central index of opiate addicts, but there is no formal procedure of registration. Any doctor attending an opiate addict is required to notify the latter's name to: The Chief Medical Officer, The Drugs Branch, Home Office, 50 Queen Anne's Gate, London SW1.

Maintenance treatment

Maintenance prescribing is accepted generally in the USA and in some parts of the United Kingdom. In the former country the patient is expected to attend a clinic and drink a daily dose of liquid methadone under supervision, limited take-home privileges being permitted to those of proven stability. In the United Kingdom some long-term patients still receive a maintenance prescription of injectable drugs but new patients are likely to be offered only oral methadone in a liquid preparation formulated to discourage attempts to inject it (methadone mixture drug tariff formula (DTF), containing 1 mg methadone hydrochloride per 1 ml). This preparation must not be confused with the cough mixture properly referred to as methadone linctus. The usual maintenance dose is between 20 and 70 mg per day: the higher dose should never be given on the first occasion except to a person known to be heavily addicted.

As indicated above, restriction on the prescribing of heroin, dipipanone, and cocaine do not (in 1985) apply to the prescribing of methadone including injections, or the other controlled opiate drugs. If no special drug clinic is available and a doctor feels obliged to undertake opiate prescribing, this should be confined to the methadone mixture DTF and each prescription limited to one or two days' supply.

Withdrawal

Withdrawal symptoms, while rarely threatening the life of someone in reasonable health, cause much mental anguish and usually result in determined efforts to obtain further supplies. Symptoms of opiate withdrawal vary between individuals. The only consistent symptoms are restlessness and insomnia. The classical syndrome includes muscle and joint pains; rhinorroea and lacrimation; abdominal cramps, vomiting, and diarrhoea due to increased intestinal activity; piloerection; pupillary dilation; raised pulse rate and disturbance of temperature control. These features may begin about six hours after the last dose of heroin, reach a peak after about 36–48 hours and then decline. After methadone, symptoms may begin after about 36 hours, reach a peak after three to five days and continue somewhat longer though less dramatically than after heroin or morphine alone.

Withdrawal may be accomplished humanely in a well-motivated person by prescribing any drug of the opiate group and reducing the dose over two to four weeks. Methadone mixture DTF is convenient and less likely to be abused than the alternatives. The initial dose depends upon the patient's usual consumption but normally lies within the range 20 to 70 mg in 24 hours; in the case of very heavy use a first day's supply of 100 mg may be needed. The dose should be reduced by between 20 and 30 per cent every two to three days according to the patient's response. If outpatient withdrawal is attempted, dose reduction should be smaller and the intervals longer to minimize the patient's temptation to seek supplementary supplies. Nevertheless, a clear time limit must be set at the outset to prevent the patient turning withdrawal into maintenance.

When the daily intake of heroin is not very great, patients can be withdrawn by using a combination of Lomotil (each tablet contains diphenoxylate hydrochloride 2.5 mg with atropine sulphate 0.025 mg) and chlormethiazole. The usual regimen is Lomotil two tablets four times daily for three days followed by one tablet for two days together with chlormethiazole 500 mg, one tablet morning and midday and two at night for three days followed by one by day and one at night for two days. Since chlormethiazole can be abused, this should only be carried out during inpatient care. The alpha-adrenoreceptor agonist, clonidine, has been advocated in order to decrease sympathetic overactivity occurring during withdrawal. Blood pressure must be monitored because of the drug's hypotensive effects. The usual adult daily dose for this purpose is in the range 0.1 to 0.3 mg t.d.s.

Sedatives, tranquillizers, and hypnotics

This is a large and varied group of drugs often consumed other than in accord with good medical practice. At present most problems are still encountered with the barbiturates, but they are now more carefully prescribed and other drugs in the group are being abused, especially chlormethiazole, glutethamide, and the very widely prescribed but technically safer benzodiazepines. Barbiturates and methaqualone are controlled drugs under the *Misuse of Drugs Regulations*. With barbiturates, tolerance develops less rapidly than with opiates, but it presents a particular danger since tolerance to intoxication and sedation occurs to a greater extent than dose tolerance to the depressant effects on the vital centres, thus increasing the risk of an inadvertent fatal overdose. Barbiturates are also commonly marketed in capsules and these can be dissolved and self injected. Taken in this way they are extremely irritant producing abscesses and cellulitis when injected subcutaneously; if inadvertently injected intra-arterially, they can cause severe tissue damage and even necrosis requiring amputation. Acute intoxication with barbiturates may be associated with amnesic episodes ('blackouts').

Although the benzodiazepines are abused to some extent, they do not present such acute problems as the barbiturates. The tablets are less convenient for self injection; the safety margin in the ratio of sedation of higher functions to depression of vital centres is greater; and animal experiments support the clinical experience that repeated and compulsive overadministration is less easily established than it is with the barbiturates. However, a true physical dependence with severe withdrawal symptoms does occur and some patients experience a withdrawal after prolonged clinical use.

Withdrawal

Because the withdrawal syndrome for sedative drugs is potentially more serious than for other psychoactive drugs, it is preferable to undertake withdrawal in hospital. Mild symptoms of insomnia, anxiety, restlessness, and anorexia may progress to vomiting, hypotension, pyrexia, tremulousness, and in severe cases, to major epileptic convulsions and/or an organic confusional state with disorientation and hallucinations. The syndrome is, of course, similar to delirium tremens associated with severe dependence on alcohol. The traditional immediate management of withdrawal requires the administration of sufficient pentobarbital in divided doses to maintain the patient in a balanced state between intoxication and withdrawal. This is followed by a progressive reduction by 50–100 mg daily, provided withdrawal symptoms are not manifest. Some recommend instead a short-acting benzodiazepine such as lorazepam for withdrawal, while chlormethiazole which has been used for withdrawal from alcohol, might also be used in withdrawal from drugs of this group. However, considerable caution should be exercised before prescribing any short-acting drug, for they are much sought after for their abuse potential. For this reason a regimen using short-acting drugs is only suitable for patients in hospital. For outpatients, the use of phenobarbitone has been recommended; although this is less flexible because the blood levels cannot be adjusted rapidly, it seems to be abused rarely.

The first step in withdrawal is to work out the patient's average and usual daily dosage, paying attention to all the drugs in this group which are being taken, including alcohol and benzodiazepines. For every 100 mg of a shorter acting barbiturate or its equivalent, a daily dose of 30 mg phenobarbitone should be given in divided doses, up to a maximum of 300 mg daily (exceptionally 400 mg). This is reduced progressively over ten days to three weeks, the patient being assessed at least every second or third day. Provided the patient has no history of epilepsy before drug

abuse, and has not been receiving antiepileptic medication (such as phenytoin) while abusing sedatives, this reduction programme generally provides an acceptable compromise when inpatient withdrawal facilities are not available. However, when larger doses of phenobarbitone may be required, inpatient treatment is essential. Major tranquillizers of the phenothizine group are contraindicated in the management of this withdrawal syndrome as these lower the fit threshold.

Management of long-term dependence

Patients who have been taking drugs of this group in a controlled manner over a long period (type 3) should be transferred to the safest drug in the group – currently a benzodiazepine. Withdrawal of drugs in stable patients can usually be achieved eventually, provided adequate time can be made available to help the patient cope with the withdrawal anxiety and insomnia; these symptoms are likely to affect not only the patient but other members of the household.

Prevention

Prevention of dependence is far less onerous than its cure. The prescriber of sedative drugs should explain to the patient that long-term daily consumption leads not only to a state of psychic dependence, but also to the development of tolerance, so that the drug becomes less effective with the symptom for which the patient requests treatment. Prescribing of sedatives should, therefore, be for a limited period and wherever possible the patient should be counselled to use these intermittently and not daily – a principle that the majority of patients seem to grasp more easily than some of their medical advisers! Management of overdose is described in Section 6. The long-term rehabilitation of heavy sedative abusers is similar to that of primary opiate abusers, and multiple drug abuse is the rule.

Stimulants

Stimulants liable to misuse include cocaine, the amphetamines, amphetamine-like drugs such as phenmetrazine and methylphenidate, and also stimulant anorectics such as diethylpropion and fenfluramine. Amphetamines are an effective stimulant and temporary euphoriant in some depressions, but the incidence of dependence is extremely high and the tendency to increase the dose is so frequent that they have largely been abandoned from psychiatric practice. Although some advocate their use in the management of the hyperkinetic syndrome of childhood, and there are still advocates for their intermittent prescription to suppress appetite as adjuncts to dietary restriction, the sole remaining agreed medical indication for these drugs is in the management of narcolepsy. This is not unknown to persons with a predilection for amphetamines, so patients claiming to suffer from narcolepsy should be received with some caution. Stimulants may be consumed orally, sniffed into the nostrils for more rapid mucosal absorption (especially cocaine) or injected intravenously. The United Kingdom experienced a minor epidemic of methylamphetamine injection during 1968, which terminated when the drug was withdrawn from the retail pharmaceutical market. The stimulants most likely to be injected now are cocaine and illicitly manufactured amphetamine sulphate.

In a blind trial, users could not distinguish between small intravenous doses of amphetamine and cocaine. In larger doses and with regular consumption, both drugs can produce a paranoid delusional illness with hallucinations including, characteristically, tactile hallucinations perceived as bugs crawling under the skin. Regular high dose (type 2) users also exhibit repetitive, stereotyped behaviour such as the making of detailed drawings, obsessive tidying or compulsive dismantling of equipment. Periods of very high intravenous use are generally interspersed with self medication with sedatives or opiates to terminate the 'run'. Chronic (type 3) consumption of oral stimulants in moderate dose is seen in many older patients originally prescribed amphetamine during the 1950s and early 1960s, who seem unable to cope with the withdrawal depression. Maintenance may be a viable course with these latter patients but short prescription periods and careful supervision, often in conjunction with a single nominated dispensing pharmacy, is advisable. Monoamine oxidase inhibitors which have some stimulant effect have been used in the management of the withdrawal depression among such patients. They must be used with extreme caution since the concomitant consumption of amphetamines with monoamine oxidase inhibitors is potentially fatal due to hypertension. The intermittent (type 1) hedonistic consumption of these drugs is probably quite common, and where the price is sufficiently high as is currently the case with illegal cocaine, then complications and dependence are the exception. Treatment of acute overdose requires sedation, and management of hyperpyrexia and cardiac arrythmias which may have caused death amongst athletes. Most toxic symptoms, including the paranoid psychoses, resolve rapidly without the use of tranquillizers as the drug is eliminated; the use of major tranquillizers in particular can confuse the differential diagnosis from acute paranoid schizophrenia. A urine sample should be taken within 24 hours of admission and analysed for amphetamine and cocaine whenever the diagnosis of amphetamine psychosis is remotely possible.

Psychedelics

The term psychedelic refers to the ability of these drugs to produce alterations of mood and perception. Unfortunately, the original meaning of the term has been lost through its association with pop culture, but it is still to be preferred to the alternatives of hallucinogenics or psychotomimetics since consumption of these drugs does not usually produce true hallucinations and causes conditions clearly similar to psychoses even less often.

By far the commonest of the drugs in this group likely to be encountered in the United Kingdom is lysergide (LSD). Consumers who believe they are consuming similar substances such as mescalin or DMT have often been sold lysergide in disguised form. A certain amount of consumption of hallucinogenic mushrooms containing psilocylin occurs. Anticholinergic drugs such as atropine and the veterinary anaesthetic phencyclidine (PCP) do not appear to be a significant problem ouside North America. Lysergide has been used in some psychotherapies, particularly to promote the re-experience of early childhood events. The dose of lysergide used in psychotherapy was in the range 200–500 μg: in street use it is usually in the range 50–200 μg. Lysergide has some sympathomimetic effects, particularly noted by the consumer as an increased heart rate, which may give rise to anxieties about possible cardiac illness. Even in overdose, severe physiological reactions do not apparently occur. Accidents have resulted from delusional behaviour during the lysergide experience. The evidence is against the probability of any chromosomal or teratogenic abnormalities resulting from consumption of conventional doses.

The mental effects develop during a period of two hours following lysergide consumption and generally last from 8 to 14 hours. The subject experiences an increased perception of various stimuli and there may be confusion between sensory modalities (synesthesia), whereby, for example, sounds are perceived visually or movements are heard. Objects may seem to merge with others or to move rhythmically. The subject's own body image may be distorted and there is often a loosening of ego boundaries so that the subject may seem to observe themselves from outside. A person who is not prepared for such an experience, or who is lacking in tangible supports, may panic and fear that sanity is being lost. Possibly, publicity designed to dissuade persons from taking lysergide may actually increase the incidence of such adverse reactions. Increasing sophistication among users who are now more likely to take precautions such as ensuring support and avoiding the use of lysergide when already in a state of psychic distress, has probably resulted in a reduction of adverse reactions. Similarly, increasing

experience by both medical and informal helpers has enabled many such reactions to be coped with by repeated reassurance, rather than having recourse to powerful tranquillizing drugs and hospitalization.

The management of the adverse reaction

The principles of management are to assist the person to relate the experience to the drug; to divert them from frightening thoughts towards immediate and real events; and only to prescribe tranquillizers when it is not feasible to undertake this time-consuming 'talking down' process. If a drug is given, a minor tranquillizer such as diazepam is to be preferred. Phenothiazines may be used in severe cases of lysergide intoxication but are contraindicated when anticholinergic drugs have been taken. It is uncertain whether long-term ill effects occur after taking lysergide because it is difficult to distinguish spontaneously occurring psychiatric disorder from that which may have resulted from taking the drug. Moreover, the young adults who are most likely to consume lysergide are the age group in which schizophrenia is most frequent. There have been cases of a close temporal connection between the development of a schizophrenic disorder and the recent consumption of lysergide. Psychiatrists sometimes attribute schizophrenic symptoms to lysergide taken a considerable time previously, however, such connections are extremely dubious. One long-term effect which can occur is a flashback; that is, the recurrence of psychedelic experiences even when the drug has not been taken recently, usually in a situation which produces intense anxiety. Occasionally such events are distressing and may require treatment, including a minor tranquillizer.

Cannabis

Cannabis is derived from the plant *Cannabis sativa*, and is consumed either as the dried vegetative parts in the form known as marijuana or 'grass', or as the resin secreted by the flowering tops of the female plant. The former is commoner in North America and southern Africa, the latter in Asia and Europe. In North Africa and Asia cannabis products are consumed by some social classes in a manner somewhat akin to alcohol in western society. In North America and Europe the use is usually prohibited by law, but the widespread consumption of cannabis by young adults has resulted either in a reduction of the maximum penalty or at least in a diminution of the actual penalties imposed for simple use. Severe penalties are available against anyone convicted of supplying the drug. Most consumption is of type 1, namely, occasional and intermittent recreational use; and the vast majority of such users do not apparently take any other illegal drug, although alcohol consumption may be higher than among non-users of cannabis.

No serious side effects have been proven amongst intermittent users. Like many drugs, cannabis, although not proved to be teratogenic, has not been proved to be safe when taken in the first three months of pregnancy. Inhaled cannabis smoke irritates the respiratory tract and is potentially carcinogenic. Heavy doses may possibly affect immune responses and sex hormone production. On the positive side, cannabis seems to be useful in counteracting the nausea and vomiting produced by radiation therapy and may have some value in the treatment of glaucoma.

The psychoactive effects for which cannabis is consumed are variable and depend on dose, the person's expectations, and the setting. Users experience a general sense of intoxication and may report heightened enjoyment of music and an increased appetite for food. Cannabis also exaggerates existing moods, so that as well as increasing hilarity in a humorous situation, it can potentiate depression or anxiety. Very occasionally, the latter comes to medical attention and then usually responds to simple reassurance. Continued heavy use may interfere with intellectual activity but the evidence for this is conflicting. Such consumption is the exception but may be regarded as constituting a dependence problem.

Volatile inhalants

Recently adolescents, often those too young to be able to purchase alcohol, have caused concern by the practice of sniffing volatile solvents, particularly those incorporated in glues. Inhalation of these substances has occurred over a period of 200 years and there are many curious accounts of similar practices in Victorian society. The toxic effects of the chemicals inhaled are not usually serious to the young person. However, the mode of inhalation can on occasion be extremely dangerous, particularly if the user adopts any or all of the following practices: putting a plastic bag over the head to increase the concentration of inhalant, with a very real risk of the bag being stuck to the face; sniffing in small, secret places such as broom cupboards or lavatories, where there is an increased risk of asphyxia; heating containers in order to promote the vaporization of the substances which are often explosive; substituting other, more dangerous substances, such as inhalation of butane from pressurized containers, which cause acute asphyxi-

ation. This is the cause of a small but significant number of deaths in adolescents. The majority of adolescents who inhale these substances do so occasionally and without long-term ill effects. A number seem to become dependent on the practice and may require treatment.

References

Department of Health and Social Security (1982). *Treatment and rehabilitation*. Report of the Advisory Council on the Misuse of Drugs. HMSO London.
—— (1984). *Guidelines of good clinical practice in the treatment of drug misusers*: Report of the Medical Working Group on Drug Dependence. Department of Health and Social Security, London.
Jaffe, J. H. (1982). Drug addiction and drug abuse. In *The pharmacological basis of therapeutics*, (eds L. S. Goodman, and A. Gilman), 6th edn. Macmillan, New York.
—— and Martin, W. R. (1982). Opioid analgesics and antagonists. In *The pharmacological basis of therapeutics*, (eds L. S. Goodman and A. Gilman), 6th edn. Macmillan, New York.
Schuckit, M. A. (1984). *Drug and alcohol abuse*, 2nd edn. Plenum Press, New York.

THE RELATIONSHIP BETWEEN PSYCHIATRIC DISORDERS AND PHYSICAL ILLNESS

Psychological factors and the presentation and course of illness

R. A. MAYOU

Psychological and social influences are major determinants of the presentation of illness to doctors. They may also have a primary role in the onset and course of physical illness, partly through direct physiological mechanisms, and partly by affecting the patient's compliance with medical advice. This section begins with the psychosocial aspects of presentation and compliance, and goes on to consider the aetiological significance of psychological and social factors in the onset and course of illness.

Presentation and consultation

The term 'illness behaviour' has been used to cover all the psychological and social influences that affect the ways in which 'symptoms are perceived, evaluated, and acted upon'. One aspect of 'illness behaviour' is consultation with doctors. It is apparent that many consultations, even among people with serious physical illness, are mainly determined by personality or by social circumstances. Thus, some people with minor or chronic physical complaints consult doctors only at times of stress (for example, students about to take examinations). In contrast, others are very reluctant to consult doctors and this may result in dangerous delay in diagnosis (for instance, of breast cancer). In addition to such differences between individuals, broader cultural patterns of illness behaviour have been described. For example, one study in New York contrasted the dramatic accounts of symptoms given by Italian Americans with the more stoical response of Anglo-Saxons.

A particularly important practical aspect of illness behaviour is failure to comply with medical advice, since this severely limits the effectiveness of all forms of treatment. For example, numerous reports indicate that the rate of compliance with long-term medication is rarely more than 50 per cent. Poor compliance is related to the nature of the treatment (side-effects and complicated regimens) as well as attitudes and understanding.

Observations on the significance of illness behaviour emphasize

the need for doctors to understand the psychological and social determinants of consultation and compliance; so that they can encourage attendance of those who need care and ensure that they obtain the maximum benefit from medical treatment. There is much research evidence to show that compliance is greater when there is a good relationship between patient and doctor, and the patient's role in treatment is explained clearly.

Psychological causes of physical illness

It is widely accepted that stress, emotional reactions, and social circumstances can affect both the onset and course of medical illnesses. From 1930 onwards, the work of Freud and Pavlov, as well as research on the autonomic nervous system led to the development of *psychosomatic* medicine, which proposed specific associations between types of unconscious conflict or personality, and particular illnesses. It was assumed that stress-induced physiological processes were particularly important in the aetiology of seven psychosomatic illnesses: hypertension, asthma, rheumatoid arthritis, thyrotoxicosis, peptic ulcer, ulcerative colitis, and neurodermatitis.

Despite a vast literature between the years of 1930 and 1950, few experts would now deny that these ideas hindered real progress. It is now obvious that there can have been no justification for elaborate theories based on retrospective clinical experience with highly selected patients. However, many doctors – and patients – still believe that emotional factors play a major part in a number of medical conditions. Since the methodological difficulties are very considerable there is still little research which satisfies the basic requirements for satisfactory prospective study using standardized measures.

Current theories are concerned with multiple causes of physical illness and make no attempt to identify a special group of psychosomatic illnesses. Instead, it is proposed that psychosocial factors play a part in the onset and course of many medical conditions. There are two main approaches to research: (a) the investigation of physiological responses to stress in normal subjects, patients, and animals; (b) epidemiological study of the association between psychological and social variables, and the onset and relapse of physical illness. There can be no doubt that stress and mental state can effect hormonal, immunological, and other processes, and these mechanisms have been seen as contributing, along with constitutional and physical risk factors, to the onset of disease in predisposed target organs. It remains an open question as to whether there are some idiosyncratic patterns of physiological response to stress which are especially pathogenic. The second approach, epidemiology, has provided considerable evidence that social and psychological functions may predispose to and precipitate a number of physical conditions, even though precise interpretation of statistical association is both difficult and controversial. There is stronger evidence for the effects of psychological and social variables on the course of the illness than at its onset.

The example of ischaemic heart disease

The most convincing evidence for the significance of psychological and social influence as a primary cause of physical illness relates to ischaemic heart disease, most particularly acute myocardial infarction. Research has outlined associations between psychological variables on the one hand, and blood lipids, autonomic control of the cardiovascular system, and even coronary artery spasm on the other. Research of a different kind has provided prospective evidence that several aspects of stress appear to predispose to and precipitate infarction. Interest has focussed on what has been called type A personality, a rather ill-defined group of traits characterized by ambition, 'time urgency', and hostility. Several large prospective studies have shown that type A subjects are significantly more likely to suffer heart attacks than those who are type B. There are, however, problems in interpreting current evidence and determining the clinical significance of psychosocial influences as primary risk factors. The most useful test of type A hypotheses is to attempt to modify the behaviour and examine the effect on heart disease. One recently completed study appears to have shown that intensive psychological intervention can modify type A behaviour in survivors of infarction, and that this results in a significant reduction in subsequent cardiac mortality and morbidity.

Clinical applications

An understanding of psychological aetiology is of importance to clinicians only in so far as it has practical consequences either for prevention of illness or for the care of patients. The original psychosomatic theories led to conclusions about the need for psychotherapy to change the supposed psychodynamic causes of illness, but such treatments have had no demonstrable benefit. The current more modest awareness that non-specific psychological distress affects the onset and course of a number of illnesses has more practical implications for prevention and treatment.

Prevention

Primary prevention requires health education and social policies intended to change attitudes and encourage healthier lifestyles. The great practical difficulties are evidenced by the resistance to propaganda about even such well-defined physical risk factors as smoking, diet, and lack of exercise. Although it is even more difficult to modify ways in which people cope with stress, this could be a useful part of multiple risk factor modification in selected high-risk groups.

Modification of the course of illness

Even though there are many uncertainties about the significance of stress in the onset and course of physical illness, it seems sensible to attempt to modify the emotional factors which may be associated with poor outcome. This does not mean psychotherapy for all patients, but the use of simple psychological methods with the minority of problem patients who are most likely to benefit. Straightforward discussion will often suggest simple practical steps which patients can take to improve their lives and reduce tension and worry. It is essential that discussion should centre on what the patient finds unpleasantly stressful rather than assumptions of others that certain ways of life are inherently harmful. Clinical

experience and the findings referred to above of the benefits of large-scale educational programmes to change behaviour type A are encouraging.

Conclusions

Disenchantment with earlier psychosomatic theories has been replaced by a more cautious belief that, as yet, ill-understood psychological and social factors can affect the onset and course of many illnesses. The application of these ideas to primary prevention are, at present, limited but in established illness simple psychological management may improve the medical outcome. In view of the continuing controversies about psychosomatic theories, it is reassuring to the clinician that commonsense efforts to encourage patients to avoid unnecessary stress and make their lives more satisfactory can improve patients' ability to cope with physical illness and may improve its prognosis.

Reference

Friedman, M., Thoresen, C. E., Gill, J. J. et al. (1984). Alteration of type A behavior and reduction in cardiac recurrences in post-myocardial infarction patients. Am. Heart J. 108, 237–248.

Emotional reactions to disorders

R. A. MAYOU

Attention has already been drawn to the frequency of emotional disorders amongst patients in medical wards. There can be no doubt that many of these disorders occur as psychological reactions to physical illness. When the physical illness is brief, any emotional disorder usually clears up quickly, but it may persist in certain vulnerable people. When the physical illness is chronic, the emotional reaction may improve over time or may persist unchanged, depending on the degree of physical handicap and the patient's capacity to adapt. These reactive conditions are described separately here because they can often be treated effectively with simple psychological measures in the medical ward.

Acute physical illness

Acute physical illness, especially if severe, is as likely to cause anxiety and depression as any other form of stress. It may also have considerable effects on social and family life and the whole range of psychological and social consequences of illness is often referred to as 'illness behaviour'. However, a minority of people show remarkably little distress or awareness of their illness. This *denial* is an example of a variety of *defence mechanisms*, the psychological processes which are used as ways of dealing with anxiety. Another example is displacement in which anger is often directed against the doctor and the hospital. Although denial can be maladaptive, leading to non-compliance with treatment or delay in consulting, it is usually a helpful way of enabling patients to live with unpleasant implications of illness or treatment.

In addition to psychological impact, illness has effects on behaviour, and individuals adjust by what are often referred to as 'coping strategies'. These may be adaptive such as seeking information, tackling problems and making use of help from others. They can also be maladaptive, examples being disregarding medical advice, blaming others, and excessive invalidism.

Most psychological reactions to acute illness are of moderate severity but in a minority of cases they are more severe and a small proportion need psychiatric assessment and treatment, as described in earlier sections. The severity of reactive emotional symptoms is determined by an interaction between (a) the nature of the stress, (b) the personality of the individual, and (c) social circumstances.

Physical illnesses as stressors

Physical illnesses may be stressful in many ways. Factors commonly leading to depression include: physical discomfort, such as pain or nausea; disfigurement or mutilation, as in mastectomy or limb amputation; and loss of function, such as sexual activity, social life, mobility or earning capacity. Factors commonly leading to anxiety include: threatened rather than actual loss, such as the possible future loss of working capacity or sexual function; and life-threatening illnesses such as cancer or myocardial infarction. The experience of being in hospital presents innumerable sources of anxiety which have been well documented by research. They include undergoing preparation for ward procedures or the operating theatre: lack of privacy when washing, dressing, weeping, seeing doctors or relatives; and the presence of some other patients, especially those whose behaviour is disturbed, or who have unsightly conditions, or appear to be dying.

It is important to recall that depression may be directly induced by demonstrable organic pathology, including, for example: brain diseases, such as tumours, vascular lesions and degenerations; endocrine disorders, such as Cushing's syndrome; and changes in brain metabolism occurring in a range of physical illnesses (see next chapter). Depression may also occur as a sequel to infectious diseases such as influenza and glandular fever, and may be induced by medication, and examples are reserpine, levodopa, the atropine group, or hypotensive agents and drugs used in the chemotherapy of malignant disease.

The individual personality

The impact of the stresses of illness depends largely on the patient's personality, particularly the capacity to cope with adversity of one kind or another. There are exceptions, but generally the patients who cope best with illness are those who have previously met life's challenges resourcefully and without breaking down emotionally. The impact of illness also depends upon how the meaning of illness is perceived, a process which is highly subjective and individual. Thus, the same physical illness may be perceived by one patient as a loss, by another as a gain, another as a threat and another as a punishment.

Certain types of people are particularly vulnerable to emotional distress when faced by physical illness. Those who take great pride in their physical fitness, such as athletes or body-builders, are especially prone to anxiety or depression on becoming physically ill. Obsessional patients find it difficult to tolerate uncertainty; they may become disturbed in the face of any uncertainty as to diagnosis, treatment or prognosis. On the other hand, people who enjoy dependency may welcome physical illness.

Social circumstances

Social circumstances are important determinants of emotional reactions to any physical illness. For example, the patient's difficulties are likely to be increased if he or she is poorly housed, living alone, and short of money. Social difficulties may also occur as direct consequences of the physical illness, in the form of reductions in social life, leisure activity, domestic skill, and earning capacity.

An important social factor is the capacity of the family to cope with the patient's physical disability. In some families there is resentment of the patient's dependence, or an increase in tension and irritability; whilst in other families there may be a remarkable improvement in the quality of relationships.

These three sets of factors – the physical illness, the patient's personality, and the social environment – react with one another and with the patient's emotional state in a reciprocal network of cause and effect. For example, physical disability leads to depressed mood, which leads to greater restriction of activity, which in turn leads to worse depression of mood; both sets of factors can result in increased family problems, which then aggravate the emotional disorder yet further.

Chronic physical illness

Chronic emotional reactions are understandably common in association with chronic physical illnesses, particularly when the latter cause substantial physical handicap. Examples of such handicapping illnesses are strokes and rheumatoid arthritis. Even with these disabling conditions, some patients experience only an initial emotional reaction, and then go on to make a surprisingly good psychological adaptation. The *clinical features* of chronic emotional reactions are similar to those described earlier in this section. There may be a state of chronic demoralization, with persistent low-level anxiety, depressed mood, irritability, reduced energy, and poor concentration. Alternatively, in more severe cases, the clinical features may be those of a depressive disorder or anxiety neurosis. With all these emotional states, the patient often leads a more restricted life than the physical status requires.

The same three groups of factors also play an important part in the *aetiology* of chronic emotional reactions as have been described for acute illness: the features of the physical illness, the patient's personality, and the social environment.

Chronic physical illnesses may be persistently stressful for several reasons. For example, they may cause frequent pain (rheumatoid arthritis); or limitation of movement (multiple sclerosis); or they may draw attention to the patient (colostomy, deformity, epilepsy). Their treatment may be complex and challenging (management of diabetes mellitus, renal dialysis), or may cause unpleasant side-effects (radiotherapy or chemotherapy).

As explained above, a patient's response to physical illness is greatly influenced by personality. Some patients may go into psychological and social decline, whilst others with an equal intensity of physical disability may achieve a marked improvement in their psychological and social life. In all these cases reactions to illness may be shaped by the processes described earlier: perception of the meaning of illness, psychological defences, and the adoption of coping strategies. Generally patients who adapt well to chronic physical illness are those who seek information about their illness, make suitable plans for their future life, and are able to continue family life without distortion of relationships. Such patients are to be contrasted with those who are overcautious, inflexible, and passively helpless.

Treatment

Emotional reactions to a physical illness are often precipitated or aggravated through the patient being uncertain and uninformed about that illness. Hence psychological support in the form of explanation together with appropriate reassurance is particularly important in the treatment of such reactions. These techniques are described in the section on psychological treatment. At this point it should be stressed that explanation can help only if it is suitably worded to the patient's intelligence and background. Technical language should be avoided, as should any implication that the illness is too complex for explanation to a non-expert. It is usually a mistake for the clinician to do all the talking. The patient should be encouraged to ask questions, as this will indicate how much detail should be given. For some patients, full explanations are acceptable, whilst others prefer to disregard aspects of their illness. Hence the explanation should be adapted to any cues given by the patient.

References

Creed, F. and Pfeffer, J. M. (1982). *Medicine and psychiatry: a practical approach.* Pitman, London.
Lipowski, Z. J. (1985). *Psychosomatic medicine and liaison psychiatry.* Plenum Publishing Co., New York.
Mechanic, D. (1978). *Medical sociology,* 2nd edn. Free Press, Glencoe.

Specific conditions giving rise to mental disorder

W. A. LISHMAN

Mental disorder can figure prominently in a number of medical conditions which compromise brain function. Its recognition and management will often be crucial to the patient's progress, and treatment may need to be specifically directed towards it. Not infrequently, moreover, the psychiatric components may be the initial manifestation of the underlying medical illness with the risk that the latter may be overlooked.

A strict concordance between type of pathology and type of mental disorder cannot be expected. Common forms of reaction by way of clouding of consciousness, dementia, or the well-known syndromes of focal cerebral disorder may result from divers affections of the brain. Affective disorder, or neurotic or psychotic developments, may owe much to the patient's inherent propensities no matter what the causative pathology. We still find, nevertheless, that certain forms of mental disturbance emerge with special frequency in certain situations as will be stressed below. Where such associations occur they can clearly be of diagnostic importance.

Neurological conditions which implicate the central nervous system directly will be considered first, then metabolic and toxic disorders which disturb brain function by way of their systemic effects. With all such conditions it will be necessary to bear in mind that both physiogenic and psychogenic components may be operative in contributing to the mental disorder; some aspects may owe their origin directly to the induced disturbance of cerebral function, whereas others may represent a reaction to the physical defects and discomforts occasioned by the illness.

Neurological conditions

Cerebral tumours

Brain tumours not unnaturally lead to a high incidence of mental disturbances. Clouding of consciousness is largely due to raised intracranial pressure, cognitive defects to local brain compression and destruction. Affective changes and alterations of personality may be attributable to a variety of additional processes such as brain distortion, oedema, and vascular derangements. Hallucinatory experiences can represent focal epileptic disturbances, or result from local brain irritation without evidence of paroxysmal activity. Much in the mental picture may also derive from the patients' premorbid personality and the situation in which he finds himself. Awareness of his plight, when retained, can profoundly influence the nature of his response.

Fast-growing malignant tumours show an especially high incidence of mental changes; multiple metastatic deposits cause the most florid disturbances of all. It is with slow-growing tumours, however, that the mental features may for a very considerable time be the sole manifestation, especially when they are situated in neurologically silent regions of the brain. Frontal meningiomas, for example, have proved to be particularly liable to be overlooked, as shown by autopsy surveys in mental hospital populations. Some of the more characteristic presentations of tumours in specific locations will therefore be briefly described.

Frontal lobe tumours

Frontal lobe tumours can present with symptoms indicative of dementia. Deterioration of intellect and memory may be accompanied by aspontaneity, slowing, and inertia, extending even to states of akinesis. Euphoria and irritability are common, and lack of insight usually marked. Changes in disposition and habitual behaviour are another characteristic form of presentation. Irresponsibility, childishness and lack of social restraint are the alterations stressed most frequently. A tendency towards facetiousness and indifference to the feelings of others may give a particular stamp to the overall picture. Disinhibition can occasionally lead to striking lapses of conduct or sexual indiscretions. With all of this neurological signs may remain in abeyance, likewise, evidence of raised intracranial pressure when the tumour is slow in evolution.

Temporal lobe tumours

Temporal lobe tumours show prominent dysphasic disturbances when the dominant lobe is affected. Apart from this there may be similar features to frontal lobe tumours. Disturbances of affect and personality are sometimes profound. Focal epileptic seizures are common and may display a wealth of psychic symptomatology. Complex hallucinatory experiences include formed auditory and visual hallucinations, the latter sometimes being confined within a hemianopic field. Olfactory and gustatory hallucinations arise from the uncinate region and can be the first indication of the tumour. Special interest attaches to the observation that a schizophrenia-like psychosis appears to be particularly common with temporal lobe tumours. Very occasionally this too can be the initial manifestation.

Parietal and occipital lobe tumours

Such tumours show in general a much lower incidence of mental changes than the above. With the parietal lobes, however, there may be features of dysphasia, dyspraxia, visuospatial agnosia or topographical disorientation. Puzzling pictures of unilateral inattention or neglect, and complex and elaborate body image disturbances, can at first sight suggest hysteria. With posterior parieto-occipital lesions there may be complex disturbances of visual recognition, including inability to recognize faces (prosopagnosia) and the rare visual object angosia.

Diencephalic tumours

Diencephalic tumours occasionally present with a highly characteristic amnesic syndrome when implicating the region of the third ventricle, reminiscent in all respects of Korsakoff's psychosis. Confabulation may be much in evidence. Thalamic tumours sometimes show an early and severe dementia. Lesions involving the posterior hypothalamus and upper mesencephalon may manifest somnolence and hypersomnia, or the striking syndrome of 'akinetic mutism'. Disturbances of endocrine control, appetite, and thermoregulation may or may not be present. Marked swings of mood and abrupt outbursts of temper have been described as characteristic of diencephalic tumours. With pituitary tumours dullness and apathy are said to be more common.

Quite apart from these more or less characteristic pictures one must beware of the patient who, in the earliest stages of the lesion, reacts by the development of quasi-neurotic symptoms. Depression and anxiety may be much in evidence before definite indications of the tumour are present. Elaborate neurotic developments may occasionally emerge, including hypochondriacal, phobic, and hysterical features. When no adequate precipitants for such developments can be discerned, and when premorbid adjustment has seemed to be relatively stable, screening tests for intracranial pathology will often be indicated. Even minor complaints of difficulty with thinking, headache or visual disturbance will always require comprehensive evaluation.

Strokes

The disablement resulting from stroke is often a mixture of physical and mental problems, the latter being sometimes directly attributable to brain damage and sometimes representing a reaction to the handicaps imposed. The mental sequelae can in either event be the most incapacitating aspects for patients. Moreover they can constitute a barrier to optimal recovery from the physical disabilities with which they must cope. Adams and Hurwitz deserve credit for highlighting this situation, and alerting physicians to the need for comprehensive evaluation of the patient's mental status when disablement persists and progress is slow.

Perhaps foremost among the 'mental barriers to recovery' is *depression*. This will often be reactive to the patient's disability and frustrations, the dependence on others and the forced imposition of the invalid role. The response to the disablement will be strongly influenced by the person's premorbid make up, and the social and financial aspects of the situation. Others may experience depression of an endogenous type, sometimes precipitated by strokes of a relatively minor nature. Adequate treatment will therefore often require appraisal of multiple contributory factors in addition to the prescribing of antidepressant medication.

Cognitive defects may pose grave handicaps to rehabilitation, even when less immediately obvious than the hemiplegia or other neurological sequelae. It is rare for a truly global dementia to follow a single cerebrovascular accident; more commonly there will be focal deficits of higher cortical function depending on the site and size of the infarction. Defects of communication are particularly distressing for the patient. Even minor comprehension problems can seriously retard progress, likewise diminished grasp or poor span of attention. Apraxic disturbances may persist as an obstacle well after motor paralysis has cleared.

Disturbed awareness of the self or of space is commoner after right hemisphere lesions than left. Neglect of the left half of external space may be accompanied by left sensory inattention, neglect or unawareness of body parts. In anosognosia there is lack of concern or seeming total unawareness of the disability, usually a left hemiplegia. In the early stages this may extend even to verbal denial, or rarely to more florid pictures in which the paralysed limbs are disowned or attributed to another person.

An organic *change of personality* can be particularly troublesome, overshadowing on occasion the intellectual defects. Querulous irritability and lack of co-operation may owe much to a 'reduction of margins' – the patient can adapt to a strictly circumscribed routine, but new demands call forth anxiety or even hostility. Frank 'catastrophic reactions' may be elicited when confronted with tasks or social demands beyond their capacity to cope. An accentuation of paranoid traits, or the devlopment of rebellious aggressive attitudes may sometimes be released.

In the longer term one may need to attempt to counter *unhelpful modes of adaptation* to persisting disabilities. These will be founded much more in premorbid personality than in the brain damage sustained. On the one hand there may be unrealistic strivings for independence, with denial of limitations and refusal of simple help. Other patients, by contrast, may succumb to invalidism to an unnecessary degree, exploit their disabilities, and make unrealistic demands on those around them. The long-term care of survivors from stroke can thus sometimes require on-going skilful help both for the patient and the family.

Epilepsy

The associations between epilepsy and mental disorder are numerous and complex. Considerable strides have been made in clarifying the interrelationships that obtain, though large areas of ignorance remain.

It is now clear, after long historical dispute, that the great majority of epileptic patients remain mentally normal. A liability to seizures need carry no implications *per se* for intellectual impairment, personality difficulties or predisposition to mental illness. Much depends, however, on the presence or absence of brain damage underlying the seizures; and it seems probable that the damage responsible for temporal lobe epilepsy carries special risk for certain psychiatric developments.

In those epileptics who suffer mental symptoms, this component can have seriously adverse effects on their life adjustment, often proving more disabling than the fits themselves. In some patients, moreover, the liability to seizures is exacerbated during emotional crises or periods of instability. Attention to aspects of psychological welfare can thus be an indispensable part of management.

In reviewing the mental disorders associated with epilepsy it is useful first to consider phenomena occurring in close association with the seizures themselves, than the problems that may be encountered in the interictal period.

Ictal and peri-ictal mental symptoms

These symptoms include complex disturbances which can feature as part of the aura preceding the actual seizure. Temporal lobe epilepsy is important in this respect. Peculiar disturbances of thinking, memory or awareness may usher in the fits: mental clouding, 'forced thoughts', distortion of time sense, panoramic memory, or feelings of derealization, depersonalization or *déjà vu*. Distortions of perception or hallucinations of sight, hearing, taste or smell may figure prominently. Sudden affects of intense anxiety, dread or ecstasy may occur. When the ensuing seizure is mild or abortive such complex auras may raise the possibility of a primary psychiatric illness.

Again, in seizures which implicate the temporo-limbic system the convulsion proper may be replaced by a 'psychomotor attack', with a period of profoundly disturbed behaviour lasting for minutes, hours, or occasionally longer. In psychomotor 'automatisms', most of which are brief, quite complex behaviour may be carried out, albeit in a somewhat dazed or muddled manner. On recovery there is virtually always complete amnesia for what has transpired. Differentiation may be required from periods of intoxication, outbursts of aggression or spells of hysterical dissociation. The abruptness of onset and termination will often provide the most important clue to the epileptic basis. Longer lasting fugue states, with aimless wandering, may very occasionally be encountered. In psychomotor 'twilight states' the patient becomes withdrawn for hours or even days, experiencing a wealth of bizarre ideation and vivid hallucinations. Distinction from a brief schizophrenic episode may sometimes be difficult until the epileptic basis is recognized.

A not uncommon conditon in children, occasionally appearing in adults as well, is the picture of 'petit mal status'. Sometimes for several hours the patient remains in a deeply obtunded state, slowed in thinking and clumsily inco-ordinated, while the electroencephalogram is dominated by continuous runs of three per second spike and wave activity.

Other disturbances follow in the wake of seizures, before full return of consciousness and awareness of the environment. In the postepileptic acute confusional state the patient may become dangerously restless and combative (postepileptic 'furor'). Postepileptic automatisms and twilight states show features similar to those described above. Prolonged psychotic episodes ('paranoid hallucinatory states') with a wealth of schizophrenia-like symptomatology may again lead to diagnostic error, unless the preceding fit is known and the element of clouding of consciousness detected.

Interictal psychiatric problems

These include cognitive and personality difficulties and occasional psychotic developments. To the extent that brain damage is responsible for the seizures there may be difficulties with memory and learning, sometimes obvious but sometimes only revealed on special testing. In children very frequent episodes of petit mal may seriously disrupt schooling despite lack of any coarse brain lesion. We are now much more aware than formerly that anticonvulsant drugs, when in toxic dosage or unfavourable combinations, can lead to difficulty in concentration, memory, and intellectual function generally. Hence the importance of careful review of medications and the estimation of serum concentrations in patients who complain of mental lethargy or perform below expected levels.

Personality problems may derive in large part from overprotective attitudes during development, or as a reaction to the profound social and occupational difficulties which the epileptic patient must face. Attitudes of dependency and insecurity may be engendered in this way. Depression, anxiety, and low self-esteem are common as with other chronically disabling conditions. Other personality traits, such as explosive irritability and aggressiveness, appear to be closely tied to the underlying brain damage and to be especially common in patients with temporal lobe epilepsy. Improvement here can follow temporal lobectomy, or emerge when the seizures are brought under control with medication. This strongly suggests that subclinical seizure discharges within the damaged brain regions may also contribute significantly to the personality dysfunction. Attention has likewise been drawn to the sexual difficulties which patients with temporal lobe epilepsy may suffer, and which may also respond to removal of the epileptic focus – hyposexuality with generally diminished libido, or, much more rarely, abnormalities such as fetishism or transvestism.

Psychotic illness, while relatively rare, is commoner than expectation in epileptic patients. In addition to the clearly organic psychoses, mentioned above, affective and schizophrenia-like illnesses may occur with full preservation of consciousness. The latter have been comprehensively evaluated in recent years, appearing to be closely tied to epileptic foci within the temporal lobes, and perhaps especially associated with foci in the left dominant lobe. Evidence of predisposition to schizophrenia, by way of a family history or schizoid premorbid personality, is mostly lacking in such patients. A chronic paranoid schizophrenia is the common picture, usually with onset a decade or more after the onset of the epilepsy.

Other neurological conditions

Parkinson's disease

Parkinson's disease is noteworthy for the high incidence of associated depression. The affective disturbance often outstrips what might be expected as a result of the patient's physical disability, and appears to be commoner than with equivalently disabling conditions. Moreover, appropriate treatment for severe depression, including electroconvulsive therapy, may sometimes lead to dramatic alleviation of the motor incapacities as well as improving mood.

Cognitive impairment in Parkinson's disease has been the subject of debate. Many patients remain mentally intact, though a significant proportion develop mental slowing and memory difficulties. A picture of global dementia is perhaps commoner than chance expectation, though given adequate time the patient may prove less impaired than was evident at first sight. The term 'subcortical dementia' has been coined to describe such a picture, which perhaps owes a good deal to lack of activating inputs to the cortex from lower centres. There is increasing evidence, however, that the incidence of an Alzheimer-type cortical pathology may also be increased in the presence of Parkinson's disease.

Multiple sclerosis

In *multiple sclerosis* it has proved hard to uphold earlier views that a cheerful euphoria is the predominant mental change. Reactive depression, often severe in degree, characterizes a high proportion of patients. Euphoria, when present, is closely tied to evidence of impaired intellectual function. Cognitive impairment has itself emerged as commoner than suspected, and may sometimes be severe in degree when large numbers of plaques affect the cerebral hemispheres.

Other conditions

Other associations of interest include the high incidence of psychiatric abnormalities in the early stage of *Wilson's disease*. A variety of behavioural abnormalities may figure prominently, and schizophrenia-like psychoses are probably commoner than chance. Schizophrenia-like psychoses may also feature in the course of *Schilder's disease, Friedreich's ataxia*, and *narcolepsy*. In the latter condition the influence of strong emotions in precipitating cataplectic attacks is well known; but there is evidence that psychological stresses can influence the timing and frequency of the attacks of somnolence as well. Emotional disturbances can aggravate *myasthenia gravis* in a noteworthy manner and adversely affect prognosis. *Dystrophia myotonica* carries a high incidence of personality abnormalities, especially a marked reduction of initiat-

ive, contributing to severe social deterioration among affected family members.

Endocrine and metabolic disorders

The influence of many endocrine and metabolic disorders on the mental state illustrates the importance of the correct biochemical milieu for the proper functioning of the central nervous system. There will usually, but not inevitably, be evidence of the primary provoking illness when mental symptoms are pronounced. With certain disorders the forms of mental disturbance encountered are reasonably characteristic, or at least have a characteristic colouring; much variability exists from case to case, however, and a good deal will obviously depend on the patient's mental constitution. This is particularly so where non-organic psychiatric developments are concerned.

Hypothyroidism

Hypothyroidism is characterized as clearly by mental as by physical manifestations. In both cretinism and myxoedema the mental symptoms are reversible by early treatment, but unfortunately the typical stigmata may sometimes be overlooked. With myxoedema the patient may receive a mistaken diagnosis of intractable depression or early presenile dementia for quite some time.

Slowing of mental and motor activity is almost invariable in myxoedema. Apathy rather than depression is the common mental picture. The paucity of complaints from the patients themselves may increase the risk of delay in reaching the diagnosis. A feeling of mental befuddlement is accompanied by memory and intellectual failure, or at least a strong impression of such. In the later stages dementia may be very closely simulated. Psychotic developments are not uncommon, but lack specific features apart from the organic colouring often lent to the mental state. Delusions of persecution may be gross and bizarre, and agitation severe. Florid hypochondriacal developments may sometimes emerge. Replacement therapy stands an excellent chance of success if instituted early, though additional measures by way of psychotropic medication or electroconvulsive therapy may be needed with severe psychotic disorders.

Hyperthyroidism

In hyperthyroidism the patient's overarousal and distractibility is again characteristic. Heightened tension leads to startle responses and intolerance of frustration. When well developed the picture can easily be mistaken for a primary anxiety state, and differentiation can be difficult when biochemical results are equivocal. Sometimes the disturbance extends to extreme anxiety with histrionic disturbed behaviour, or frank hypomanic illness. The rare 'apathetic hyperthyroidism', by contrast, shows inertia proceeding even to stupor, and may be mistaken for depression. Very occasionally an acute organic psychosis is seen, usually in association with a thyroid crisis, though this is rarer now than formerly owing to more satisfactory means of treatment. It may still occasionally be manifest while excessive thyroid activity is being brought under control. Transient schizophrenia-like psychoses have also been reported in such a situation.

Hypopituitarism and hypoadrenalism

In both hypopituitarism and hypoadrenalism psychiatric symptoms are almost universal in some degree. A general air of indifference is accompanied by withdrawal, anergia, and defective memory and concentration. Somnolence and a self-neglectful appearance may be striking. Early dementia may be suspected, especially since the picture is slow in evolution, or depressive neurosis or neurasthenia. Crises of adrenal failure may be accompanied by acute confusional states or stupor; sometimes they are heralded by a period of mounting irritability and apprehension.

Pituitary failure was sometimes mistaken for anorexia nervosa before tests of pituitary function were available. Both show amenorrhoea and loss of weight, but in pituitary failure the distinctive psychopathological reaction to food is lacking. Moreover, *severe* weight loss is rare before the terminal stages of hypopituitarism, and appetite is sometimes quite well preserved.

Cushing's syndrome

Cushing's syndrome is marked by the frequency and severity of the depression that may accompany it. This appears to be considerably more common than could be explained as a reaction to the discomforts of the disease, and may owe much to the excess of endogenously produced steroids. A significant proportion of patients develop a clear cut depressive psychosis, often with prominent paranoid features. Strangely the euphoric reactions encountered with exogenously administered steroids appear to be uncommon in Cushing's syndrome.

Other pictures include emotional lability with overreaction to stimuli, unco-operative behaviour, or sudden outbursts of restless disturbed behaviour. States of apathy verging on stupor may be seen. Rare cases have been reported in which a schizophrenia-like psychosis is the dominant manifestation; here interest lies in the observation that, as with the depressive reactions, treatment directed at the endocrine disorder can bring gratifying relief even when psychotropic medication has failed.

Phaeochromocytoma

The episodic disturbances seen with phaeochromocytoma may sometimes be falsely diagnosed as attacks of acute anxiety if the marked elevation of blood pressure is overlooked. Attacks may occasionally be provoked by excitement or other emotional precipitants, adding to the ease of the mistake. Attacks usually last from several minutes to several hours. Intense fear is often present from the start, along with palpitations, dizziness, tremulousness, and sweating. The fear may amount to an overwhelming conviction of impending death. In the wake of attacks there are sometimes transient periods of excitability and confusion.

Acromegaly

With acromegaly, apathy and lack of initiative are often present from an early stage. Lability of mood may be a feature. Difficulty with recent memory is sometimes seen. Some patients become depressed, touchy, and irritable in reaction to their discomforts and disfigurements, while others show little concern even when the disease is advanced. It is unclear how far such features depend on metabolic changes or on basal brain compression.

Parathyroid disorder

Parathyroid disorder has come under closer scrutiny with regard to its mental effects. Here it is interesting to see that maintenance of the serum calcium within quite close limits is important for emotional stability and mental functioning; it appears to be the altered concentration of this ion, rather than the level of circulating parathormone, that is responsible for mental symptoms. In both hypoparathyroidism and hyperparathyroidism depression can be a marked and early feature. Anergia and irritability accompany it in hyperparathyroidism ('fatigued depression'), with organic mental symptoms developing at higher levels of serum calcium. Acute confusional or stuporose states accompany crises of the metabolic derangement. Presentations with the picture of dementia have been reported.

'Pseudoneurosis' is described in hypoparathyroidism, with temper tantrums in children and depressive withdrawal in adults. Even commoner are symptoms of difficulty with concentration, mild confusion, and emotional lability. In postoperative cases, where biochemical changes are likely to be abrupt, there may be transient severe acute delirious states.

In pseudohypoparathyroidism and pseudo-pseudohypoparathyroidism intellectual impairment is by far the most common psy-chiatric abnormality, occurring in approximately half of reported cases.

Gonadal dysfunction

With regard to gonadal dysfunction, Turner's syndrome and Klinefelter's syndrome have aroused psychiatric interest. An issue has been how far observed psychological abnormalities might reflect the gonadal dysfunction itself, or derive more directly from the abnormal sex chromatin constitution. In *Turner's syndrome* (XO) mental subnormality was once regarded as common, though it now seems probable that verbal intelligence at least is normally distributed. A large verbal–performance discrepancy on intelligence tests seems characteristic, however, with special difficulties in visuo-spatial functions. In some respects this can be seen as an accentuation of the usual female as opposed to male pattern of differential cognitive abilities. *Klinefelter's syndrome* (XXY) has proved to be associated with more pervasive abnormalities, ranging from personality problems to psychotic illness. Defects of intelligence, generally mild but occasionally severe, have emerged as commoner than chance expectation, likewise disorders of personality and behaviour. The impairment of drive, passivity, and diminished libido may be determined in large measure by the hormonal defects and respond to replacement therapy. But other aspects may be related in some fashion to the chromosomal abnormalities. Thus when Klinefelter patients are compared with patients suffering from hypogonadism due to other causes, a higher incidence of mental illness, personality defect, and intellectual impairment has repeatedly been observed. Moreover, the abnormalities of behaviour are often manifest prior to puberty. An increased incidence of electroencephalographic abnormalities suggests that some form of minimal brain maldevelopment could be a contributory factor.

Diabetes mellitus

Surprisingly there seem to have been few comprehensive surveys of psychiatric disorder in diabetes mellitus. The most conspicuous complications are in relation to impending episodes of diabetic coma, when listlessness, irritability, and confusion may figure prominently, or in relation to hypoglycaemic attacks as described below. Other psychiatric aspects may, however, command attention. Diabetic children and adolescents sometimes cause grave concern in relation to the proper control of their condition, if rebellious and non-conformist to regimens. The relationship between emotional disturbance and liability to ketosis has not been properly clarified despite several intensive studies, but it seems probable that significant interactions do exist.

The later complications of diabetes include a somewhat increased incidence of cerebrovascular accidents and probably of dementia. Lesser grades of cognitive impairment also appear to be not uncommon. Atherosclerosis may be chiefly responsible, or repeated encephalopathies due to hypoglycaemic or ketotic episodes. Understandable depressive reactions may occur in response to physical complications of the disease.

Hypoglycaemia

Hypoglycaemia from any cause can lead to behavioural disturbance. With insulinomas there are typically transient and recurrent attacks, sometimes over very long periods of time before the diagnosis is made. Such episodes may be interpreted as psychopathic or dissociative behaviour, intoxication, or psychomotor epilepsy. Attacks can start suddenly, or with a gradual build up of weakness, ataxia, and confusion. Precipitating factors by way of exercise or recent fasting will not always be evident. Early symptoms are irritability, anxiety, and panic, or a detached feeling akin to depersonalization. As the episode develops childish disinhibited behaviour may be released. Foolhardy aggressive behaviour is common and the patient may become noisy and combative.

Clouding of consciousness may not always be evident to lay observers, though some degree of motor inco-ordination is usual. Progression to coma is rare except in the most severe attacks. On recovery amnesia is usually complete for all that has taken place.

A rarer variant seen with insulinomas consists of the gradual evolution of failing intellect and progressive organic change of personality. Such a development often proves to be irreversible.

Cerebral anoxia

Cerebral anoxia may lead to mental changes akin to hypoglycaemia. When gradual in development, as at high altitudes, there is a decline in concentration, fatigue, irritability, and foolish irrational behaviour. Insight may be markedly impaired, with dangerous results. Judgement and short-term memory are affected. In the many medical conditions which contribute to cerebral anoxia such features can become conspicuous and disabling.

After carbon monoxide poisoning the patient may occasionally be left with severe cognitive impairment and extrapyramidal disabilities. An unexplained feature is the latent interval of several days or weeks which may be interposed between recovery from coma and the onset of mental and neurological sequelae. The motor disabilities usually clear completely, but after severe exposure cognitive difficulties may persist. Memory impairments have been reported in a high proportion of cases at follow up, also a change of personality towards impulsiveness, moodiness, and aggression.

Uraemia

Uraemia is frequently accompanied by mental torpor, listlessness, and drowsiness. Difficulties with concentration and mental effort are characteristically episodic. With more severe degrees memory becomes obviously impaired and periods of disorientation and confusion appear. Episodes of acute delirium sometimes punctuate the course, with apprehension, bewilderment, and fleeting hallucinations. Depression can be marked and require treatment with antidepressants.

Sometimes such mental features may be the presenting abnormality; and occasionally an unsuspected uraemia proves to be aggravating an otherwise mild dementing illness in the elderly. The precise mechanisms responsible for the mental changes are uncertain. Electrolyte imbalance and disturbed osmolality seem likely to play a greater part than the elevated levels of blood urea *per se*. Drugs which have accumulated to toxic levels are also strongly incriminated in many cases.

Renal dialysis

Renal dialysis may bring a further range of mental complications. Rapid reduction of the blood urea can lead to headache, muscle twitching, fits, and transient confusion, sometimes progressing to coma ('dialysis disequilibrium syndrome'). Too rapid shifts in intracellular and extracellular biochemical components appear to be responsible, with resultant cerebral oedema. Marked cognitive deterioration was also sometimes observed in patients maintained on dialysis for considerable periods of time ('dialysis encephalopathy'). Their brain aluminium concentration was found to be increased, the aluminium apparently being derived from the water used as dialysate. Since taking steps to circumvent the problem this syndrome has now virtually disappeared. Much commoner than these specific complications are states of anxiety and depression, especially early in the course of dialysis. These will often require careful psychiatric management if the patient is to make a successful adjustment.

Electrolyte imbalances

Electrolyte imbalances from many causes may similarly dictate important mental symptoms. Depending on the underlying condition the metabolic dynamics will often be complex, disturbance in one aspect of electrolyte balance having repercussions on others. Hyponatraemia is associated with lassitude, weakness, and irritability, later with mental confusion. Hypokalaemia leads to apathy, lethargy, and sometimes profound confusion. Muscle weakness in the latter condition may extend to flaccid paralysis, raising the possibility of conversion hysteria. Disturbances in calcium balance have already been described in connection with parathyroid dysfunction above. Various pictures have been attributed to hypomagnesaemia and the situation remains controversial; depression, disorientation, delirium, and stupor have at various times been regarded as characteristic. In alkalosis of metabolic origin there is frequently dulling of perception and memory, and ultimately marked confusion, in addition to the well-known tetanic changes. Such states may be induced by overbreathing in markedly anxious patients. Metabolic acidosis, including that due to carbon dioxide retention in respiratory disease, leads to mental dulling, drowsiness, and progressive impairment of consciousness. Papilloedema may be observed as a result of raised intracranial pressure.

Hepatic disorder

The neuropsychiatric features of hepatic disorder have been highlighted by Sherlock and co-workers. A fluctuating subacute or chronic organic reaction involves both mental and motor features, these two aspects characteristically waxing and waning together. The condition may persist for years, sometimes with long complete remissions, or it may become a chronic continuing source of disability. The aetiological role of nitrogenous substances derived from the alimentary canal is shown by the ameliorating effect which can follow dietary protein restriction and other supportive medical measures.

Impairment of consciousness is present during episodes of the disorder. Warning signs include a fixed staring appearance and reduction of spontaneous movements. Hypersomnia is an early feature. At this stage flapping tremor of the outstretched hands or facial grimacing may be revealed. Progression occurs to periods of marked confusion, perplexity, and forgetfulness, accompanied by dysarthria, ataxia, rigidity, hyperreflexia, and clonus. Rapid changes in level of consciousness are accompanied by delirium, with hallucinations mainly in the visual modality. Confabulation may be much in evidence. Gross mental abnormalities, and even episodes of coma, may remit abruptly and spontaneously.

Swings of mood are common, or a fatuous change of personality reminiscent of frontal lobe disorder. Functional neurotic or psychotic disturbances may sometimes be prominent, owing much to the premorbid personality.

Acute intermittent porphyria

Acute intermittent porphyria is a rare but important cause of mental symptoms. During relapses of the disorder the abdominal or neuropathic phenomena are often accompanied by marked emotional disturbance. The latter can sometimes dominate the picture. Emotional lability is common, with histrionic demonstrative behaviour. Confusion may progress to a restless delirium, leading on to coma. Psychotic developments sometimes resemble schizophrenia, and paranoid reactions are not uncommon. Depression can be severe.

Repeated episodes of this nature may have conspired to give the impression of a severe personality disorder or functional psychotic illness before the underlying metabolic disease is uncovered. Contrary to earlier views there is no strong evidence for the emotional precipitation of attacks, and little to suggest that victims of the disorder are inherently mentally unstable.

Vitamin deficiencies

The vitamin deficiencies best known for their mental effects are those of thiamine and nicotinic acid. Experimental observations on volunteers maintained on vitamin B-deficient diets have shown how prominently mental symptoms can develop. Depression, emotional instability, and quarrelsomeness accompany the lassitude and anorexia. Vague somatic complaints are coupled with nervousness and apprehension. Forgetfulness and difficulty with thinking can be marked. Thiamine deficiency has proved to be particularly closely associated with such changes, though similar features are frequently encountered as prodromes to pellagra.

More severe chronic thiamine deficiency leads to the classical picture of beriberi in which central nervous system involvement is rare. Acute depletion, however, leads to the fulminating syndrome of Wernicke's encephalopathy, with Korsakoff's psychosis as a common residual defect (Section 21). The close dependence of the mental features in Wernicke's encephalopathy on thiamine deficiency is shown by the efficacy of prompt replacement therapy, which relieves the confusion and impairment of consciousness as well as the neurological manifestations. Replacement early in the course of Korsakoff's psychosis also meets with success in reversing or ameliorating the memory difficulties in a substantial proportion of cases.

In established pellagra florid psychiatric manifestations can appear. Disorientation and confusion sometimes progress to wild excitement and outbursts of violent behaviour. Depression is often conspicuous, and a paranoid hallucinatory psychosis can develop. Such pictures again respond to nicotinic acid, often in dramatic fashion.

Acute and severe nicotinic acid depletion, as in the case of thiamine, can lead to encephalopathy with delirium extending to stupor. Extrapyramidal rigidity and grasping and sucking reflexes are described as characteristic, likewise gastrointestinal disturbances accompanying the mental symptoms. The picture has been reported in elderly malnourished patients as well as alcoholics, also in patients maintained for some time on intravenous fluids. Replacement therapy can again be dramatic in reversing the situation.

Vitamin B_{12} and folic acid deficiency have been incriminated occasionally in leading to memory failure, confusional states, and dementia, usually in association with a megaloblastic anaemia but sometimes before haemopoiesis is obviously affected. Replacement therapy has been reported to have a definite effect where such pictures are concerned. A much broader range of mental disturbances has also, on slender grounds, been attributed to vitamin B_{12} deficiency in patients with pernicious anaemia: depression, neurotic symptoms, and even functional psychotic illness. There is a lack of critical evidence, however, to support a causal relationship where non-organic psychiatric disorders are concerned. Depression probably represents a reaction to the non-specific effects of the anaemia. Other mental symptoms are likely to be coincidental, or determined by matters of special predisposition in a person who feels physically unwell.

Folate deficiency of dietary origin is common among the elderly, and perhaps particularly so in those with organic psychosyndromes. Here it is hard to determine how far the mental condition is the cause or the consequence of the folate deficiency, though a seemingly definite response to replacement may occasionally be seen. Depression in association with low serum folate has also appeared to be helped. Epileptic patients maintained on phenobarbitone, phenytoin or primidone are also prone to low levels of serum and red cell folate, and this has emerged as especially common in those who are mentally disturbed. Some investigations have reported improvement in drive and energy, powers of concentration and stability of mood on giving folic acid in such a situation, though in other reports the response has been disappointing.

Drug-induced mental states

Many drugs, whether prescribed or self-administered, can produce toxic effects on the central nervous system and lead to psychiatric disturbance. The number involved is legion, likewise the variety of their effects and actions.

Drugs of abuse fall into the broad categories of sedatives, stimulants, hallucinogens, and narcotics. All are taken on account of their immediate psychological effects. Strangely, with the exception of alcohol, there is very little information about possible long-term adverse effects of such substances on mental functioning, and what evidence there is, is largely circumstantial.

Barbiturates
Addiction to barbiturates is associated with increasing tolerance so that ultimately enormous quantities may be consumed. The recognition of chronic intoxication is of great importance since other medical conditions may be closely simulated. States of fluctuating confusion follow ingestion or injection, with slurred speech, ataxia, and tell-tale nystagmus. The usual mood change is towards euphoria, though irritability and uninhibited behaviour may be marked. Withdrawal effects are similar to those of alcohol, with epileptic fits and delirium. Such features, punctuating the course over a long period of time, may give the essential clue to the addiction in patients suspected of obscure neurological disease, dementia or severe personality disorder. Epilepsy may itself be regarded as the primary diagnosis, with the result that further barbiturates are prescribed.

Analogous withdrawal effects may be seen with glutethimide, meprobamate, methaqualone, and other sedative drugs. Bromide intoxication is still very occasionally seen in patients consuming large amounts of proprietary 'cough cures' and 'nerve tonics'.

Amphetamine
Abuse of amphetamine and related stimulant drugs leads to hyperarousal and restless overactivity. The most remarkable effect on the mental state, however, is the not infrequent development of an acute paranoid psychosis. This can be hard to differentiate from an acute schizophrenia at initial presentation. Distinguishing features of some value are the acuteness of onset, the brisk and predominantly fearful affective response, and the presence of visual as well as auditory hallucinations. Persistence of the paranoid features for more than a week after the urine is free from amphetamines makes it very likely that an endogenous schizophrenia is afoot.

Hallucinogens
Hallucinogens such as lysergic acid (LSD-25) or mescaline can lead to the most dramatic mental states of all. LSD carries the special hazard that it can be administered without the subject's knowledge. Perceptual distortions, vivid hallucinations in many modalities, and striking alterations of body image typically occur without detectable clouding of consciousness. In this last respect the toxic states produced by hallucinogens differ markedly from those of most other agents. Occasionally severely adverse reactions ensue, even in habitual users, leading to hospital presentations – acute panic reactions or explosive outbursts of anger or paranoia. The acting out of impulses can lead to dangerous situations, such as running amok or attempting to leap from heights. Both brief and long-lasting schizophrenia-like psychoses may be precipitated probably owing much to premorbid vulnerability. An interesting phenomenon occasionally encountered is the 'flashback' effect, in which abnormal experiences induced during acute ingestion – vivid images or perceptual distortions – recur intermittently for several weeks or months thereafter.

Cannabis (marijuana)
Cannabis intoxication leads usually to a mildly euphoric state, often with slight impairment of consciousness and distortion of time sense. Fragmentation of thinking and hallucinations may occur, but the latter generally lack the profusion and vividness of those following LSD. With more severe intoxication waves of ecstasy, perplexity, and terror may be experienced along with depersonalization and derealization. Spontaneous recurrences of cannabis effects can apparently occur after discontinuation of the drug, much as with LSD.

It remains controversial how commonly seriously adverse effects can follow with cannabis. Acute disturbances include episodes of panic or hysterical dissociation, lasting for several minutes or hours. Schizophrenia-like reactions and confusional states with markedly paranoid colouring have been described. Chronic continuing effects, ascribed to possible central nervous system damage after excessive usage over long periods of time, include an insidious change of personality ('amotivational syndrome'), also progressive social and intellectual decline. Chronic psychotic developments akin to schizophrenia have been reported. With all such syndromes definitive evidence of the role of cannabis has been hard to obtain, and matters of special selection and special vulnerability have probably been operative in most series of cases reported to date.

Narcotic drugs

Drugs such as heroin and morphine are usually without the florid psychiatric effects of the drugs already described. A state of drowsy euphoria is the usual aftermath of administration. It is important to be aware, however, that poly drug abuse is now extremely common, so that addicts may come to display a variety of the pictures outlined above.

Among prescribed drugs many are prone to lead to disorientation and confusion, sometimes as an idiosyncratic response to normal dosage but more commonly as a result of accumulation to toxic levels. Such reactions are commoner in the elderly and the severely debilitated. With some medications mood disorder is the predominant change, and some may lead to functional psychotic developments.

Antiparkinsonian drugs

These drugs are notorious for their liability to disturb mental function. Anticholinergic drugs such as benzhexol, benztropine or procyclidine can produce transient disorientation, confusion, agitation, and visual hallucinations even in quite small dosage. Amantadine may induce similar symptoms. Levodopa has been associated with a much wider range of effects, from acute confusional states to severe affective disorder. Such mental complications may set in abruptly, sometimes after months of successful treatment, and appear to be distinctly commoner in patients with a previous psychiatric history. Florid psychotic developments may occur, with or without impairment of consciousness. Depression is sometimes severe. More subtle long-term changes, with insidious impairments of judgement and memory have also been described.

Antihypertensive drugs

These drugs were early incriminated in leading to mood disturbance. Rauwolfia-induced depression served as a direct stimulus to biochemical research into naturally occurring affective disorders. Methyldopa has a similar, though less marked propensity to depression, its most troublesome effects being tiredness, drowsiness, and weakness of the limbs. Many consider it best avoided, however, when there is a past history of depressive illness. A large number of other antihypertensive agents also share this problem, perhaps the least troublesome being the postganglionic sympathetic blockers such as guanethidine, bethanidine, and debrisoquine. The liability of these to produce impotence is, however, a serious drawback. Moreover, when a patient is both hypertensive and significantly depressed it must be remembered that tricyclic antidepressants antagonize their hypotensive action. In such a situation a change of medication to a thiazide diuretic or propanolol is often the treatment of choice, accepting the small risk that propanolol may aggravate the depression.

Digitalis toxicity

This has long been the subject of debate. Claims incriminating the drug in producing mental symptoms in a high proportion of patients must be set in the context of the disturbed renal function and cerebral anoxia which may figure prominently in patients with heart disease. Nevertheless it seems very probable that even pure digitalis preparations contribute to mental symptoms in a large number of patients. Confusion, disorientation, and transient hallucinations have frequently been reported. States of weakness, apathy, and depression may on occasion owe much to the drug, likewise excitement, agitation, and disturbed nocturnal sleep.

Diuretics

These can lead to profound mental changes by virtue of electrolyte imbalance, particularly potassium depletion. Depression, apathy, confusion, and muscular weakness may respond to correction of the situation.

Psychotropic drugs

Common psychotropic drugs can themselves have adverse mental effects, especially in high dosage and in the elderly. Antidepressants, both tricyclics and monoamine oxidase inhibitors, quite frequently lead to episodes of impaired memory and orientation, and occasionally to severe transient confusion with hallucinatory experiences. Diazepam has been shown to impair mental function more commonly than was suspected, and a well-marked withdrawal syndrome, including convulsions, can follow its abrupt termination. The 'neuroleptic malignant syndrome' is a rare but important complication of treatment with phenothiazines, butyrophenones or thioxanthines, requiring their abrupt termination. It presents acutely with extrapyramidal features, pyrexia, autonomic disturbances, and fluctuating impairment of consciousness progressing to coma. A fatal outcome can be expected in up to 20 per cent of cases, usually from cardiorespiratory or renal failure.

Salicylates

Salicylate intoxication produces a characteristic picture in which tinnitus, tremor, and hyperventilation become prominent. Confusion, agitation, and amnesia may progress to stupor. Paranoia, hallucinations, and disturbed combative behaviour have been described. There are indications that chronic analgesic abuse over long periods of time may ultimately produce an organic dementia, phenacetin being especially incriminated in this regard.

Steroids

Steroid therapy has proved to be frequently associated with mental disturbance. Cortisone and ACTH perhaps carry greater risk than prednisone or prednisolone. The usual reaction consists of mild mood changes only, and more often euphoria than depression. When given in high dosage for long periods, however, more striking changes may emerge. These are very variable in manifestations. Severe apathy or depression may be encountered as with Cushing's disease, or more rarely excitability, elation, and mania. Thinking can become disordered and incoherent, leading to a frank confusional psychosis. Psychotic developments with visual and auditory hallucinations, derealization, and impaired capacity for sequential thought have been reported, also states of immobility and negativism verging on catatonia.

Severe reactions of this nature generally subside within a few weeks when the steroids can be withdrawn. Sometimes, paradoxically, they may emerge shortly after the dose has been lowered. In many cases it can be hard to separate direct toxic actions of the steroids from the effects of the medical condition for which they were given, for example, in collagen diseases which may implicate the central nervous system. This may explain why severe psychotic responses seen on one occasion may fail to reappear when the drug is restarted later. Premorbid vulnerability in the individual concerned is also likely to play a part in many of the pictures encountered.

Other drugs

Other drugs which have attracted attention on account of their psychiatric effects include hyoscine (scopolamine), which, instead of sedation, may lead to paradoxical reactions with excitement and agitation. Acute confusion and incoherence are often accompanied by vivid hallucinations, especially in the visual modality, and constant plucking and picking movements. Such states generally subside completely within 24 hours. During antituberculous therapy isoniazid may lead to prolonged organic psychotic reactions, cycloserine to confusion, depression, and schizophreniform illness.

Other conditions leading to mental disorder

Other important medical situations which can lead to mental disorder include the collagen diseases, malignancy, and postoperative psychiatric complications.

Systemic lupus erythematosus

In this, cerebral involvement leads to mental symptoms in a high proportion of patients. Very occasionally these can be the presenting feature. The commonest picture is of an acute organic reaction accompanying relapses of the condition, often recurrent and usually brief in duration. Steroids can be incriminated in some but not all examples. Chronic organic defects, with memory impairment, emotional lability, and personality change are occasionally seen and can gravely complicate medical management. States of fluctuating anxiety and severe depression are usually reactive in nature, but sometimes seem independent of the degree of physical disability. Affective and schizophrenia-like psychoses have also been described.

Mental changes, chiefly organic in nature, can also figure prominently in periarteritis nodosa, thrombotic thrombocytopenic purpura and temporal arteritis. Severe depression as well as confusion may accompany the latter condition.

Malignant disease

This not infrequently turns out to be responsible for states of confusion and disorientation of obscure aetiology. Depressive illness has also been reported from the earliest or even the presymptomatic stages of the disease. Metabolic disturbance will sometimes prove to underlie such developments, though the precise aetiological mechanisms often remain uncertain. Particular interest attaches to those tumours which secrete hormone-like substances, also to the 'remote' effects of cancer on the central nervous system. Thus carcinomas, particularly of the lung, may cause disturbance of cerebral function in the absence of any metastatic deposits, usually in association with well-marked degenerative changes within the brain. Prolonged and fluctuating confusional states, marked deterioration of memory ('limbic encephalopathy') and pictures of dementia have been reported, with or without accompanying neurological features.

Postoperative psychiatric complications

These complications can often be traced to one or more of the provoking factors outlined in the sections above. Infective processes or electrolyte disturbances may underlie confusional states; or the drugs administered may prove to be responsible. Acute delirious episodes in the immediate postoperative phase may be attributable to cerebral anoxia or hypotension sustained during anaesthesia. It is always important to beware, however, of the patient in whom an ingravescent dementia was concealed up to the time of operation, and who now is unable to adapt to the abrupt change in circumstances and environment; much that appears to be new by way of disorientation and disturbed behaviour may be traced by a careful history to pre-existing impairments.

The patient who becomes severely depressed, or displays a marked psychotic reaction postoperatively, will often be found to be reacting adversely on account of special premorbid emotional vulnerabilities. Certain operations are associated with a particularly high incidence of adverse emotional reactions; major procedures such as open heart surgery and renal transplantation clearly pose special stresses which must be taken into account.

References

Adams, G. F. and Hurwitz, L. J. (1963). Mental barriers to recovery from strokes. *Lancet* **ii**, 533–537.

Boller, F., Mizutani, T., Roessmann, U. and Gambetti, P. (1980). Parkinson disease, dementia, and Alzheimer disease: clinicopathological correlations. *Ann. Neurol.*, **7**, 329–335.

Davison, K. and Bagley, C. R. (1969). Schizophrenia-like psychoses associated with organic disorders of the central nervous system: a review of the literature. In *Current problems in neuropsychiatry* (ed. R. N. Herrington.). British Journal of Psychiatry Special Publication No. 4. Headley Bros., Ashford, Kent.

Hécaen, H. and Ajuriaguerra, J. de (1956). *Troubles mentaux au cours des tumeurs intracraniennes*. Masson, Paris.

Lishman, W. A. (1978). *Organic psychiatry. The psychological consequences of cerebral disorder*. Blackwell Scientific Publications, Oxford.

Michael, R. P. and Gibbons, J. L. (1963). Interrelationships between the endocrine system and neuropsychiatry. *Int. Rev. Neurobiol.* **5**, 243–302.

Shader, R. I. (1971). Psychiatric effects of non-psychiatric drugs. *Sem. Psych.* **3**, 401–492.

Smego, R. A. and Durack, D. T. (1982). The neuroleptic malignant syndrome. *Arch. int. Med.* **142**, 1183–1185.

Summerskill, W. H. J., Davidson, E. A., Sherlock, S. and Steiner, R. E. (1956). The neuropsychiatric syndrome associated with hepatic cirrhosis and an extensive portal collateral circulation. *Q. J. Med.* **25**, 245–266.

Sexual problems associated with physical illness

K. E. HAWTON

Disorders of sexual function may be associated with a wide range of physical illnesses because of direct interference with the anatomical or physiological mechanisms by pathological processes or medication, or because of psychological reactions to physical disorders or treatments. Often sexual problems result from a combination of physical and psychological factors. In addition, illness may bring to light pre-existing sexual problems.

Detection of sexual problems depends upon asking appropriate questions about sexual function because patients are usually reluctant to raise the topic themselves. Unfortunately this aspect of history taking is often neglected because doctors feel embarrassed or do not know when to include these enquiries. Almost every physical illness is likely to have some effect on sexual function, whether this be due to impairment of sexual interest because of general debility, or to more direct effects of pathological processes on sexual arousal and performance. Often sexual function returns to normal after resolution of the physical condition. However, there are several medical conditions which may result in permanent impairment of sexual function, either because of the nature of the pathological process or because they result in a drastic change in lifestyle. Some of the more important of these conditions are considered below.

Medical conditions causing sexual problems

Endocrine disorders

Diabetes mellitus

Effects of diabetes on male sexual function are widely recognized. The major complication is erectile dysfunction which occurs in 40–50 per cent of male diabetics. It is not closely related to the duration of diabetes and is sometimes the presenting symptom which brings the endocrine disorder to notice. Transient erectile difficulty may occur during episodes of poor diabetic control.

Neuropathy affecting pelvic autonomic nerves was until recently regarded as the usual cause of chronic erectile dysfunction in diabetes. Now at least as much significance is attributed to vascular abnormalities. Erectile failure is more likely where there is symptomatic evidence of peripheral neuropathy (numbness, paraesthesiae, burning pains, and limb weakness) or autonomic neuropathy (e.g. postural hypotension and bladder dysfunction), and where retinopathy is present. Psychological factors are also relevant.

Failure of ejaculation is a less common complication and in some cases is due to retrograde ejaculation resulting from neuropathic involvement of the sympathetic nerves responsible for closure of the internal sphincter of the bladder at the moment of ejaculation.

Diabetes has surprisingly little effect on female sexuality, the only difficulty, reported by a minority of women, being impairment of vaginal lubrication. This is probably the result of similar pathology to that which causes erectile dysfunction.

Hypogonadism

Testicular production of androgens may be impaired in hypogonadal states associated with disorders such as Kleinfelter's syndrome, undescended testes, mumps in adulthood, hepatic cirrhosis, and neoplastic disease. Although hypogonadism occurring in adulthood will lead to sexual problems in some men, others suffer little or no reduction in sexual drive or erectile performance. Investigation of the hypogonadal male will reveal elevated serum gonadotrophins (FSH and LH) and low testosterone.

Pituitary disease

Hypopituitarism may impair sexual function because of reduced gonadotrophin production. Hyperprolactinaemia may be accompanied by erectile dysfunction particularly where serum prolactin levels are very high and testosterone levels are reduced.

Cardiovascular disorders

Sexual problems are particularly common in patients with cardiac disease, especially those with angina or who have suffered myocardial infarction. Sexual activity usually ceases for at least four weeks after myocardial infarction. Some patients never resume sexual relations in spite of a return to other normal activities. For some patients the frequency of activity may be reduced compared with the pre-infarct level. In some men erectile and ejaculatory difficulties occur; less is known about the consequences for women who have had infarcts. Impairment of sexual function may be due to chest pain, fear of relapse, loss of desire, and depression. In addition the spouse may fear relapse or feel guilty about expressing his or her sexual needs. Inadequate medical advice may contribute to such difficulties.

The physiological effects of sexual activity in patients who have suffered myocardial infarction are modest, being similar to those found with regular daily activities such as driving a car or climbing a flight of stairs. Since it is also known that the risk of sudden death during sexual activity with a regular partner is extremely low, it appears that most patients with ischaemic heart disease should be able to enjoy normal sexual relations without risk. However, it should be noted that individuals who suffer from cardiovascular disorders are at increased risk of sexual dysfunction resulting from abnormalities of the pelvic vasculature.

Neurological disorders

Involvement of any of the neurological mechanisms responsible for sexual arousal and response are likely to cause sexual problems. Erection is primarily mediated by parasympathetic activity in S2–4 under the control of a sacral erection centre. Another centre in the thoraco-lumbar portion of the cord influences erectile response via sympathetic fibres. Both centres are moderated by facilitatory and inhibitory influences from the brain and act in unison to produce erections.

Ejaculation occurs in two phases, *emission* of semen to the posterior urethra, and *expulsion* by muscular contraction. Emission results from sympathetic activity mediated by a lumbar ejaculation centre. The process of emission stimulates another ejaculation centre in the sacral cord, and expulsion then occurs because of the resulting activation of motor nerves. Both centres are moderated by cerebral influences. Although the neurological pathways controlling female sexual response are less well understood, they are assumed to correspond to those in the male.

The localization of higher centres which control sexual arousal and response are obscure but thalamic, hypothalamic, and limbic systems appear to be involved.

The effects of peripheral nerve damage were indicated when considering diabetic neuropathy.

Spinal cord damage

Disturbed spinal cord function likely to affect sexual response may occur with injury, tumours, multiple sclerosis, inflammatory processes, and congenital defects such as spina bifida. The results of such damage depend on whether the lesion is complete or incomplete and whether it affects upper or lower motor neurones. Broadly speaking, erection is more likely to return the higher the cord lesion, and ejaculation more likely to return the lower the lesion. If disturbed sexual function continues for more than six months after an injury, it is then unlikely to resolve. Although orgasm usually returns with ejaculation the sensation is often altered. Interference with spinal autonomic pathways often causes sterility due to elevation of testicular temperature. Electrically induced ejaculation shortly after injury can be used to produce semen which can be deep frozen and stored for possible use later in artificial insemination.

Little is known concerning the effects of spinal cord damage on female sexual function, except that total transection of the cord causes absence of orgasm.

The psychological sequelae of physical disablement and the attitudes of staff towards spinal injury patients are important determinants of subsequent sexual adjustment. Details of rehabilitation of disabled patients with impaired sexual function are provided by Heslinga (1974).

Damage to higher neurological centres

Focal cerebral lesions usually only cause sexual problems where there is paralysis, or when the frontal regions are damaged resulting in disinhibition. Hypothalamic, limbic, and temporal lobe lesions may cause erectile dysfunction. Hyposexuality is often found in patients with epilepsy, particularly temporal lobe epilepsy.

Other conditions

Sexual function may be disrupted by many other conditions including gastrointestinal disorders, particularly where an ileostomy or colostomy is necessary, diseases of the genital organs (e.g. hypospadias and Peyronie's disease), painful arthritides, respiratory conditions which limit exercise tolerance, and renal disease especially if dialysis is necessary. Chronic alcohol abuse may cause erectile dysfunction due to peripheral neuropathy or hypogonadism.

The effects of medication

Many drugs used in the general hospital can affect sexual interest and function. The effects of some of the more important drugs are summarized in Table 1. In men, broadly speaking, drugs which have sympathetic inhibitory activity are likely to impair ejaculation, and those with parasympathetic inhibitory activity are likely to disrupt erectile function. Far less is known about the effects of medication on female sexuality.

Some drugs, especially anticonvulsants such as phenytoin and carbamazepine, increase plasma hormone binding globulin thus causing a reduction in *free* testosterone. This may explain the impairment of sexual interest in some individuals (of both sexes) with epilepsy. Oral contraceptive users more often experience impaired sexual interest than non-users. At present it is uncertain if this is due to direct effects of the hormone constituents, depressive side-effects, or interference with androgen production.

Sexual problems due to psychological reactions to physical illness

Sexual problems often occur because of the adverse reactions of an individual to illness, the reactions of the partner, the nature of their relationship, or the attitudes of doctors to the condition.

Reactions of the individual

A patient may develop a sexual problem following an illness because of anticipation, albeit unjustifiable, that the illness would impair sexual capacity. The possibility of sexual activity causing relapse or even sudden death may concern the patient who has had a myocardial infarction. Harm or pain may be feared by the patient with an ostomy. Severe illness, particularly where disfiguring surgery has been necessary, may cause an individual to doubt his or her attractiveness to the partner and to fear rejection. Sexual interest is usually impaired in depression which is a common sequel to illness, especially if this has caused chronic pain or a major change in lifestyle.

The partner's reaction

A patient's partner may also fear the potential consequences of sexual activity. There may be guilt about sexual desires which appear to conflict with concern for the patient's physical health. Consequent restrictions on sexual activity may cause resentment and friction.

The nature of the relationship

How couples adjust to the effects of illness depends particularly on their previous sexual relationship. Poor adjustment is likely when there are inhibitory attitudes and difficulty discussing sex. Physical illness brings some partners closer together. For others it results in alienation because of resentment about changes in roles necessitated by disability or because the afflicted partner is found unattractive due to bodily change or depression.

Attitudes of the medical profession

The ways in which the implications of physical illness are dealt with by medical personnel may be important determinants of subsequent sexual adjustment. Discussion of the sexual aspects of disease is often avoided because of embarrassment, lack of concern, or inadequate information. Advice concerning sexual activity should be part of general rehabilitation counselling. Cursory discussion may be unhelpful because it will tend to leave patients to decide for themselves the likely nature of future sexual activity, and this may be based on ill-conceived notions about the effects of illness.

Management and prevention of sexual problems related to illness

Once the physician is aware of the effects of illness on sexual functioning, management and prevention are often a matter of common sense and do not require special training.

Assessment

Advice should be based on adequate assessment of the individual patient and the likely effects of the illness. If a sexual dysfunction is already established, the relative contributions of organic, pharmacological, and psychological factors must be considered.

The nature of the dysfunction should be clarified first, particularly what aspect of sexuality (interest, arousal or orgasm) is primarily affected. In cases of erectile dysfunction it should be established whether or not erections occur under any circumstances (e.g. on wakening, with masturbation). Careful enquiry concerning medication and possible alcohol abuse is always necessary.

During physical examination of a man, the physician should be alert to signs of hypogonadism (e.g. female hair distribution,

Table 1 Drugs which can affect sexuality

Drug group	Examples	Reported effects on sexual function		
		Interest	Arousal	Orgasm
Anticholinergic	Probanthine		Erectile dysfunction	
Antidepressants	Tricyclics		Erectile dysfunction	Delayed ejaculation or orgasm
	MAOIs		Erectile dysfunction	Delayed ejaculation or orgasm
Antihypertensives				
Central acting	Methyldopa	Reduced	Erectile dysfunction	Delayed ejaculation
Ganglion blockers	Hexamethonium		Erectile dysfunction	Failure of ejaculation or retrograde ejaculation
Alpha-blockers	Indoramin			Inhibited emission
Beta-blockers	Propranolol	Reduced	Erectile dysfunction	
Adrenergic blockers	Guanethidine		Erectile dysfunction	Failure of ejaculation or retrograde ejaculation
Anti-inflammatory	Indomethacin	Reduced		
Anti-parkinsonian	L-dopa	Increased		
Diuretics	Thiazides		Erectile dysfunction	
	Spironolactone	Reduced (may cause gynaecomastia)	Erectile dysfunction	
	Androgens	Increased in females		
	Corticosteroids	Reduced	Erectile dysfunction	Delayed ejaculation
	Oestrogens	Reduced (males)	Erectile dysfunction	Delayed ejaculation
Major tranquillizers	Thioridazine	Reduced	Erectile dysfunction	Retrograde ejaculation
	Chlorpromazine	Reduced	Erectile dysfunction	

breast development, testicular atrophy). Blood pressure, peripheral pulses, deep reflexes and sensation in the lower limbs should be tested. In some centres nocturnal penile tumescence recording is available, diminution or absence of erection during REM sleep suggesting, but not confirming, organic aetiology for erectile dysfunction. Possible vascular disorder of the genitals can be investigated by penile blood pressure measurement, corpus cavernosography, and other radiological studies of the pelvic vasculature. Local neurological causes of erectile dysfunction may be confirmed by testing of sacral nerve evoked potentials. When an abnormality of sex hormone production is suspected, serum testosterone, LH, and prolactin should be measured. Possible diabetes mellitus must be investigated by a glucose tolerance test.

In assessing psychological factors, enquiry should be made about the patient's previous sexual adjustment, current anxieties (especially about his or her illness), and the partner's sexual adjustment, attitude to the problem, and willingness to help in overcoming it. Usually it is essential to interview the partner.

Treatment

Having precisely clarified the nature of the problem, the physician should explain it in simple terms to the patient and the partner. The relative contributions of both physical and psychological factors, such as anxiety, unjustified expectations, and communication difficulties, must be made clear. Advice should then be given as clearly as possible and might usefully be supplemented by written information. If irreversible physical damage to sexual anatomy has occurred, then alternative forms of sexual behaviour may be suggested. A useful general principle is to encourage a couple to re-establish their sexual relationship gradually, perhaps starting with general caressing, in order to establish a relaxed atmosphere before fully resuming their sexual relationship. When doctors feel unable to provide such advice themselves then responsibility might be delegated to a suitably trained non-medical member of the team.

Hormone replacement therapy will be required for patients with hypogonadism. Most testosterone preparations, except testerone undecanoate, are poorly absorbed by the gut and should therefore be given parenterally. LHRH can be provided for patients with hypopituitarism, and bromocriptine sometimes restores erectile dysfunction resulting from hyperprolactinaemia.

Currently there is considerable enthusiasm in the United States for the use of penile implants in men with permanent erectile dysfunction of organic aetiology. Although various types of prosthesis are available, they are basically either semi-rigid or inflatable (via a small reservoir of fluid implantation in the lower abdomen under the rectus fascia). While clearly of benefit to some patients, especially young men with erectile dysfunction resulting from, for example, diabetes, Peyronie's disease, or priapism, they are not without drawbacks and potential complications. These include cost, risk of infection, and disappointment because implants do not improve genital sensation. Implantation of a prosthesis should be both preceded and followed by counselling of the man and his partner.

A further recent development in the treatment of organic erectile dysfunction is the injection into the corpus cavernosum of an alpha adrenergic blocker (e.g. phenoxybenzamine), which causes erections even when the nerve or blood supply to the penis is severely impaired. Such treatment might be significant in future in the management of erectile dysfunction resulting from diabetes mellitus.

Referral to a specialist in sexual medicine

This may be necessary for patients whose difficulties result from complex psychological factors, or who have failed to respond to simple counselling. They must be carefully prepared for such referral to ensure attendance. Sexual problems resulting from either psychological causes, or psychological complications of physical disorders, are often helped by sex therapy. In this approach both partners are seen together and a graduated series of homework assignments suggested including, first, non-genital caressing, later, genital caressing and, finally, resumption of sexual intercourse. Psychological barriers which are interfering with the relationship are identified by careful exploration, information about sexuality is provided when ignorance is an important factor, and particular emphasis is placed on helping partners communicate freely with each other about their sexual anxieties and needs. The results of sex therapy are reasonable, with as many as two-thirds of patients deriving considerable benefit.

Prevention

The physician should be particularly concerned with preventing sexual problems consequent on physical illness. Here, awareness of disorders likely to cause sexual difficulties, and willingness to offer appropriate advice are essential. Myocardial infarction provides a good example. The patient can be reassured that sexual intercourse is no more stressful than other moderate physical activity and that it is probably best to resume this aspect of the relationship gradually after about four to six weeks. Sexual activity is best avoided soon after a heavy meal, drinking alcohol, or when tired or anxious. The male superior position should not be used initially because of the extra energy expenditure involved in supporting body weight. If angina occurs during sexual intercouse, this may be prevented by taking a coronary vasodilatory ten minutes beforehand. Both partners should be present when such advice is being provided. Undoubtedly physicians can do much to prevent sexual problems after physical illness.

References

Bancroft, J. (1983). *Human sexuality and its problems.* Churchill Livingstone, Edinburgh.

Friedman, J. H. (1978). Sexual adjustment of the postcoronary male. In *Handbook of sexology* (eds J. LoPiccolo and L. LoPiccolo) pp. 373–386. Plenum Press, New York.

Hawton, K. (1985). *Sex therapy: a practical guide.* Oxford University Press, Oxford.

Heslinga, K. (1974). *Not made of stone.* C. C. Thomas, Illinois.

Higgins, G. E. (1978). Aspects of sexual response in adults with spinal-cord injury: a review of the literature. In *Handbook of sexology* (eds J. LoPiccolo and L. LoPiccolo), pp. 387–410. Plenum Press, New York.

Krane, R. J., Siroky, M. B. and Goldstein, I. (1983). *Male sexual dysfunction.* Little, Brown, Boston.

Emotional reactions in the dying and the bereaved

D. H. GATH

Until 20 years ago, there was little systematic knowledge about the emotional problems of the dying and the bereaved. Clinicians were seldom closely involved in such problems, and those who were involved had to rely on their own experience and insight.

In recent years, research has considerably increased our understanding of the emotional aspects of dying and bereavement. For example, there is strong evidence to refute the old belief that dying patients do not wish to talk about their condition or their feelings. It is now established that the emotional distress of the dying patient, which was probably made worse by the old 'conspiracy of silence', can often be alleviated by open communication.

Given the willingness to do so, both the hospital doctor and the general practitioner are well placed to prevent and relieve the emotional suffering of the dying and the bereaved. To achieve this, they need some knowledge of the common emotional symptoms and their causes, and of the principles of treatment.

The dying patient

Our concern here is with patients whose dying is prolonged due to conditions such as cancer or progressive renal failure, rather than those who die rapidly as a result of acute or subacute illnesses.

Frequency and nature of emotional symptoms

In dying patients the commonest emotional symptoms are depression and anxiety, which usually occur together but sometimes separately.

Findings of several surveys agree that these symptoms occur with some severity in 40–50 per cent of patients dying in hospital. They are considerably more frequent in such patients than in other patients suffering from serious but non-fatal physical illnesses.

The features of depression are unpleasant feelings of sadness and misery, with tearfulness, loss of interest, and of the capacity for enjoyment, disturbed sleep and unpleasant dreams, loss of appetite, morbid preoccupations, and social withdrawal. Suicidal inclinations are common, particularly if the depression is severe, or if there are self denigration and ideas of worthlessness. In a study of 102 patients dying in hospital, nine were found to have significant suicidal inclinations.

Anxiety is a mood of unease and restlessness characterized by fear or sometimes panic. In dying patients, as in others, anxiety sometimes manifests as irritable or demanding behaviour, or over-talkativeness.

The syndromes of depression and anxiety are described in more detail on pages 25.8 and 25.2, respectively.

Two other reactions are common in dying patients; guilt and anger. Guilt may occur alone or with depression. It is commonly focussed on such ideas as being a nuisance to relatives, being forced to abandon the family, or causing offence through incontinence or an unsightly wound.

Anger may be overt or concealed, and is often associated with depression. It is usually directed towards relatives, hospital staff, the clergy or God, and may lead to strained relationships between the patient and those around him or her.

Most of these emotional symptoms can be helped, at least in part, if their causes are recognized and understood.

The causes of emotional symptoms in the dying patient

The causes of emotional symptoms can be grouped under three headings: physical, psychological, and problems in communication. Consideration should also be given to defence mechanisms which may influence emotional symptoms.

Physical causes of emotional symptoms

In dying patients, one of the most important causes of emotional distress is physical distress.

It is obvious, but needs to be emphasized, that dying patients frequently suffer physical distress, such as pain, nausea, vomiting, and dyspnoea. In a study comparing dying patients with seriously ill non-dying patients, physical distress was found to be significantly more frequent and intense in the dying, but more likely to go unrelieved.

In the same study, it was found amongst the dying patients that emotional distress was greater in those who had physical distress, particularly if the latter was of long duration. A particularly strong association was found between dyspnoea and anxiety.

Physical factors may cause emotional symptoms in other ways. For example, patients with potentially fatal organic brain disease may experience distortions of consciousness, thinking or perception; they may then fear insanity, a prospect that may seem worse than death.

It should be remembered that medication for physical illness may cause emotional symptoms, as in the case of depression induced by steroids (see page 25.39).

Psychological causes of emotional symptoms

Surveys have revealed a number of psychological causes of emotional symptoms, most of which are readily understandable.

For example, depression in dying patients can be understood as mourning over many losses. Such patients frequently report being saddened by a sense of loss, particularly the impending loss of family or friends, of a role in society, or life itself.

Anxiety is commonly evoked by threats (as perceived by the patient) of two main kinds. The first is the possibility of physical distress. Thus patients commonly fear that they will have to undergo intolerable physical suffering which cannot be relieved, and that they will lose self control. Similarly, fears may be directed towards possible disfigurement, or urinary or faecal incontinence.

The second perceived threat may not be so obvious, but is nonetheless common. It is the possibility of being abandoned by other people, such as relatives, friends or medical staff. The fear of isolation and loneliness through abandonment is often strong, and is aggravated by the fear of being a burden to other people through increasing disability.

Feelings of anger are sometimes justifiably evoked by neglect or mismanagement by relatives or medical staff. More often anger is irrational, and is an expression of the patient's feelings of helplessness and frustration.

The extent to which these emotional reactions emerge in the individual patient will be considerably determined by the previous personality, and particularly by any earlier capacity to withstand stressful events.

These reactions are usually less frequent and less intense in elderly patients; in one survey the degree of anxiety and depression was found to be twice as great in patients under the age of 50 years as in those over 60 years. It is perhaps understandable that older patients may be more reconciled to losses. Also it has been shown that young adults are particularly likely to be disturbed by the prospect of leaving dependent children.

Problems in communication

Recent research has shown that difficulties in communication are a much greater cause of emotional distress than was formerly recognized. These difficulties occur because other people are uncertain how to talk to dying patients, and so withdraw from them, leaving them feeling isolated. It is as if the patient is walled-off by a barrier of non-communication, the conspiracy of silence.

It is particularly distressing when patients and their families feel unable to communicate openly with one another. This usually occurs because each is uncertain what the other knows about the diagnosis and prognosis. They draw back from one another, and the resulting loss of intimate contact is frightening and painful to patients. It also prevents them from discussing future plans realistically.

In the absence of good communication, an impending death may cause marital strain, particularly if the marriage has been disturbed in the past. The partner may be subjected to irrational outbursts of anger, and so feel puzzled, hurt or guilty. A dying husband who has been an active bread-winner may show a bewildering resentment to his wife as she takes on that role. A dying wife may make her husband feel rejected by turning more to her parents for support.

Psychological defence mechanisms

People facing adversity may use various defence mechanisms to ward off distressing thoughts and feelings. These mechanisms are unconscious in the sense that they are not recognized by the patient.

Defence mechanisms are almost universal in dying patients. Clinicians should be able to recognize them, and to determine whether they are adaptive or not. If they are adaptive, they lessen distress in the patient without ill-effects. If maladaptive, they may impair communication between the patient and the doctor or family. For example, excessive use of the mechanism of denial may lead the patient to make unrealistic plans for the future, leaving the relatives in doubt whether to collude or to retreat in some way.

Denial
Denial, a defence against anxiety evoked by danger or the threat of it, is probably the commonest mechanism used by the dying patient.

This mechanism sometimes operates in stages. For example, information about a fatal illness may produce in the patient an initial crisis of shock, anger, and depression. This may be followed by a phase of denial, in which there is relative calm. Subsequently denial may diminish, although still operating from time to time as the patient meets further signs of the progress of the disease.

Denial may lead the patient's behaviour to surprise the hospital staff. Thus dying patients who appear to have accepted the reality of their illness may later behave as if they knew nothing about it. They may repeatedly ask for information, as if for the first time. In this way, they may be able to assimilate information gradually without being overwhelmed by it.

Dependency
For the dying patient, a degree of dependency on other people is inevitable and appropriate. However, some patients show exaggerated dependency, relinquishing more responsibility than is appropriate to the stage of the illness. This may go to extreme lengths, the patient reverting to child-like or infantile behaviour (regression).

Refusal to be dependent also occurs, the patient stubbornly resisting help although obviously needing it.

Displacement
Sometimes dying patients deal with powerful emotions by displacing them onto other people. As already described, they may unreasonably direct anger against medical staff or relatives. Whilst this may help the patient to feel less disturbed the recipient of the anger may be distressed.

Principles of treatment

The treatment of emotional distress in the dying patient should be directed towards its three main causes: physical, psychological, and distorted communications.

The treatment of physical factors
Since much emotional distress is determined by physical distress, it is essential that physical symptoms such as pain, nausea, vomiting, and dyspnoea should be adequately treated with appropriate medication.

Dying patients not infrequently report that their physical discomfort has been inadequately relieved, so it is important to allow them the time and opportunity to explain their needs.

The treatment of psychological factors
For the treatment of psychological factors a basic requirement is to establish a good relationship with patients, such that they feel free to talk about their illness and feelings. Understandably, many doctors have reservations about entering into a close relationship with dying patients, largely because the latter are themselves a source of anxiety. However, if doctors can recognize and come to terms with their own anxiety, if they have some knowledge of the psychology of dying, and if they are willing to follow rather than lead during discussions, then they are in a good position to help the dying patient.

In the psychological treatment of dying patients, a fundamental principle is to leave most of the talking to them. If doctors are willing to listen compassionately, patients will usually be encouraged to talk of their feelings and problems as soon as they realise they will not be brushed aside.

Letting patients talk has several advantages. First, it makes them feel valued and accepted rather than abandoned. Second, by allowing them to set the pace on any potentially disturbing subject, it avoids causing them distress. Third, by listening to the cues offered by patients, the clinician can gauge when to offer any intervention.

This principle applies to the common issue of whether to tell dying patients their diagnosis and prognosis. There is good evidence that this need not be such a difficult issue as previously supposed. Whereas it was once thought that many patients did not know they were dying, it is now known that about 80 per cent become aware of their prognosis, whether they are told it or not. The important step for the doctor is to discover what the individual patient already knows, and how much more he or she really wants to know. This assessment can usually be made quietly and without causing distress. If the patient is not ready or willing to be told certain information about approaching death, it is probably best to withhold it, since forceful disclosure may be more harmful than evasion. On the other hand, if the patient sincerely wants to know the prognosis, it is probably best to tell it, since prevarication is likely to cause distrust. Research has shown that the majority of patients want to be told their prognosis, and appreciate frank discussion with the doctor.

On learning of a fatal prognosis, patients are often distressed and shocked for a few days, but then appear to come to terms with it. At this stage, they may be considerably helped by a mutual discussion of plans for their treatment.

If patients are given the chance to talk openly, they may obtain welcome relief from depression, anxiety, guilt or anger. Mourning over impending losses may be helped simply by discussion. If fear of physical distress is made explicit, it can be reduced by reassurance that pain can and will be relieved. Guilt and anger may be lessened by recognizing their origins in, for example, not being able to care for oneself and the family. Once a good relationship has been made with the dying patient, psychological management becomes a realistic goal.

The treatment of distorted communications
The danger of social isolation for the dying patient has already been described. It is possible to prevent such isolation by promoting better communications between the patient and those around him or her, especially hospital staff and the family. For example, if a clinician has made a good relationship with a patient, he or she may be able to facilitate intimate contact and support from the family. This can be done by preventing complications which arise if the patient and family are unsure who knows what about the prognosis and what the other's feelings are. Problems of this kind are sometimes best handled by seeing the family separately, and then together with the patient. Many kinds of family problem can arise when a member is dying. A common example is that of families who try to take over the patients' responsibilities in the mistaken belief that they are sparing them anxiety. It is often more helpful to encourage patients to preserve their role in the family.

Psychiatric medication
This is only indicated when anxiety or depression persists despite psychological and social support. Anxiolytics or antidepressants should be prescribed as for other patients (pages 25.51, 25.48–25.49).

In assessing the indications for antidepressants, it may be difficult to use signs such as sleep disturbance, or loss of appetite, which may be affected by the primary illness. In such cases, severity of depressed mood may be the best guide.

In dying patients, it is difficult to achieve any valid assessment of the efficacy of psychotropic drugs, but the general impression is that they do help.

Indications for psychiatric referral
Most emotional problems of dying patients can be treated by the general practitioner or hospital doctor. Psychiatric referral is

sometimes appropriate, the main indications being: emotional distress that remains severe despite adequate treatment as described above; baffling and incomprehensible behaviour; long-standing personality problems that impair the patient's ability to cope with dying; long-standing communication problems that may call for intensive treatment involving relatives.

Emotional reactions in the bereaved

Grief is the normal response to the loss of a loved person. Although it is experienced at some time by most people, many of its features are not widely recognized or understood. The psychology of grief was only recently clarified by psychiatric surveys of bereaved people in the United States of America and the United Kingdom, which showed that three patterns of reaction can be identified: typical grief, which has characteristic emotional and physical symptoms; atypical grief, in which symptoms are the same but more intense or prolonged; and psychiatric illness.

It is important for clinicians to have some knowledge of the features of grief. This is because they are likely to meet large numbers of bereaved people, whose plight can be helped by informed understanding. Amongst these numbers will be some who need active treatment for the symptoms of grief, especially those with atypical grief or psychiatric illness. In general practice, the rates of consultation for both emotional and physical symptoms are increased about three-fold in bereaved people for up to six months after the loss.

Typical grief

After bereavement there is usually a stage of non-reaction, followed by the full reaction.

Stage 1. Non-reaction

This stage usually lasts a few hours or days, and sometimes up to two weeks. The patient is largely free from distress and acts as if nothing has happened, apparently not realizing fully that the death has occurred. Sometimes the lack of distress goes as far as emotional blunting or numbness, an inability to experience any emotion.

With the realization that the death has occurred, the full reaction supervenes.

Stage 2. Full reaction

The intensity of the reaction usually begins to diminish within one to four weeks of its onset, becoming considerably less by six to ten weeks, and minimal or absent by six months. However, for several years after bereavement, there may be occasional brief recurrences of grief prompted by reminders such as anniversaries.

The features of typical grief can be described under three headings: (*a*) psychological changes; (*b*) social changes; and (*c*) physical symptoms.

Psychological changes

These include the following changes: depressed mood, preoccupation with memories, perceptual disturbances, and behavioural anomalies.

Depressed mood The bereaved person experiences many of the features of depression described in preceding sections (see pages 25.8–25.9). Typically they include sorrow, tearfulness, pessimism or despair, loss of interest in work, a sense of futility, self neglect, and anorexia. Three symptoms call for special comment: guilt, insomnia, and suicidal inclinations. Guilt is highly characteristic in grief, the bereaved persons accusing themselves of neglecting the deceased, or reproaching themselves for minor omissions. Insomnia is also common, occurring with some severity in up to 80 per cent of bereaved people.

Suicidal inclinations are more frequent than in non-bereaved people; they are usually associated with self-reproachful ideas of being responsible for the death, or with the belief that life now has little to offer.

Preoccupation with memories There may be intense preoccupation with memories of the dead person. Visual mental pictures of the deceased are sometimes experienced with unusual clarity and persistence, and in sleep there may be vivid dreams which are usually comforting rather than frightening. These preoccupations are sometimes accompanied by a tendency to talk about the lost person at great length, or to idealize them and disregard their faults.

Perceptual disturbances Perceptual misinterpretations (illusions) are very common. A stranger may be fleetingly misidentified as the dead person, or an ill-defined sound may be misinterpreted as their voice. Hallucinations (perceptions in the absence of an external stimulus) occur in the form of seeing or hearing the dead person, but are much less common. They are sometimes comforting, though they may lead to fear of insanity. Up to 50 per cent of bereaved people experience the feeling that the dead person is present, though not perceived. This is usually described as comforting.

Behavioural anomalies Restlessness and disorganized overactivity are frequent. Some bereaved people wander repeatedly from home, as if attempting to escape from distressing memories. Others do the opposite, returning to places associated with the deceased, such as their old haunts, or the hospital where the person died, or the cemetery. Other practices include clinging to the dead person's belongings, common examples being keeping all their clothes hanging in the wardrobe, talking to the deceased as if present, or even making them a cup of tea; and adopting the lost person's behaviour, such as the way of walking (identification).

Social changes

Bereavement usually affects social behaviour. Commonly there is withdrawal from social contact, and sometimes rejection of consolation. For someone recently widowed, meeting married couples at a social gathering may be a painful reminder of loss.

The bereaved sometimes show a disconcerting loss of warmth and compassion to other people. Resentment, irritability or open hostility may be shown to relatives, friends, doctors, clergymen or God. Not uncommonly doctors are accused of neglect and may be threatened with legal action, or even assaulted.

Grief usually impairs working capacity. Absence from work is generally no more than two weeks, but sometimes greatly prolonged.

Physical symptoms

The most common physical symptoms are those of autonomic disturbance occurring in bouts lasting 20 min to an hour. They include tightness in the throat, choking sensations with shortness of breath, sighing, and an empty feeling in the abdomen. These bouts are often precipitated by reminders, such as receiving sympathy or hearing the deceased mentioned.

Other common physical symptoms are headaches, blurred vision, anorexia, and weight loss, and lack of muscular power.

Episodes of major illnesses such as rheumatoid arthritis or ulcerative colitis have often been reported as following closely on bereavement, but these are difficult to evaluate because of lack of controlled studies.

Atypical grief

Atypical grief occurs mostly (80–90 per cent of cases) in women. Its features are the same as those of typical grief, but are of greater duration and intensity.

Compared with typical grief, atypical grief is more likely to lead to consultation with the general practitioner or to psychiatric referral.

Stage 1. Non-reaction

In atypical grief the stage of non-reaction is often prolonged beyond the upper limit of two weeks usually found in typical grief. The onset of distress may be delayed for several weeks, during which there may be no sense of loss, some overactivity, and even a sense of well being.

Stage 2. Full reaction

Whereas in typical grief the reaction is usually minimal within six months of the loss, in atypical grief it may last much longer, up to two years or more.

In atypical grief the mood is sometimes severely depressed, with uncontrollable crying and marked agitation. All the features described under typical grief occur, usually with greater severity. Marked insomnia is common. Suicidal inclinations and behaviour are more frequent than in typical grief. Three features are particularly characteristic: strong guilt and self-blame; difficulty in accepting the fact of the loss; and identification with the dead person in the form of adopting their symptoms.

Social behaviour is also more severely affected. Social isolation may be extreme, the bereaved person becoming totally inaccessible to family and friends. Resentment and anger may be marked, amounting to furious hostility with bitter accusations of neglect. Absence from work may continue well beyond the typical upper limit of two weeks.

Psychiatric illness

Amongst both widows and widowers, during six months after the spouse's death the risk of admission to a psychiatric hospital is six times greater than amongst married people of the same age and sex. Of the bereaved patients admitted to hospital in this way, about two-thirds suffer from depression. The others suffer from neurotic reactions which are not specific to bereavement but can follow any adversity; these reactions include hypochondriasis, phobia of serious illness or death, and obsessional preoccupations. Relapse into alcoholism also occurs, and rarely hypomania. Psychiatric illnesses that follow bereavement have a better prognosis than those which do not; they are, for example, less likely to lead to chronic disability.

Mortality and bereavement

The frequency of death due to suicide is greater amongst bereaved than amongst non-bereaved people of the same age and sex. The risk remains elevated during the first year after the loss, and is greater in males.

Death from other causes is also more frequent amongst the bereaved. In a Welsh semirural community, a survey was made of 903 relatives of 371 men and women who had died. During the first year after bereavement, the death rate was nearly six times greater amongst bereaved close relatives than amongst non-bereaved controls. Spouses were most at risk, especially widowers. After the first year, death rates fell sharply and were not significantly higher than in controls.

These findings were supported by another study, a nine-year follow-up of 4486 widowers. Mortality rates were again higher in the first year, falling to normal thereafter. The greatest increase in mortality was found amongst widowers dying from coronary thrombosis and other arteriosclerotic and degenerative heart disease. The reasons for these findings are not clear, but it is possible that the emotional effects of bereavement, and concomitant endocrine changes, may have contributed to the increased mortality.

Counselling the bereaved

Most people cope with grief without the provision of special care. Occasionally additional measures are needed, the main indications being abnormally severe or prolonged grief, especially with excessive guilt or self blame. These are more likely if there has been a very traumatic bereavement, or a highly ambivalent relationship with the deceased. Lack of supportive friends or relatives may be another indication.

Help can be provided in the form of counselling, which has the broad aims of supporting the bereaved person through the period of mourning, and of helping to accept unaccustomed feelings, to readjust to an environment in which the deceased is missing, and to establish new patterns of conduct and new relationships.

The first step in counselling is to befriend the bereaved person and to encourage him to talk freely about his grief. Reassurance is then given about the psychological and physiological accompaniments of grief, together with encouragement to review the lost relationship, to take stock of the present way of life, and to start exploring new directions.

Counselling is provided by professionals such as doctors, nurses, social workers, and psychologists, and by trained voluntary workers from organizations such as Cruse.

In the management of a bereaved patient, the role of the doctor can be summarized as assessing the need for special measures, using the guidelines given above; and, if indicated, providing counselling himself or else referring to an appropriate agency. Patients who are psychiatrically ill after bereavement may need psychotropic medication or other measures (see next chapter).

References

Bloch, S. (1980). Psychological management of the dying patient. *Med. Int.* **36**, 1837–1841.

Granville-Grossman, K. (1971). Grief. In *Recent advances in clinical psychiatry*, Vol. 1, pp. 180–190. Churchill-Livingstone, Edinburgh.

Stedeford, A. (1979). Psychotherapy of the dying patient. *Br. J. Psychiat.* **135**, 7–14.

ASPECTS OF TREATMENT

Psychopharmacology in medical practice

P. J. COWEN

Pharmacological treatment plays a major and undisputed role in the management of schizophrenia and severe affective illness, conditions most practitioners treat comparatively rarely. Psychotropic drugs are widely prescribed to patients with less serious psychiatric disorders but for these conditions alternative treatments are available (see page 00000) and the role of pharmacotherapy more difficult to define. In general, psychotropic medication should be prescribed for specific psychiatric syndromes, and not as a prop to help people in difficulties. When prescribing, the doctor should consider three problems: factors affecting the dosage, compliance, and the risk of deliberate overdosage. Each of these general problems will be considered briefly before reviewing specific groups of drugs.

Most psychotropic drugs are highly lipophilic and are well absorbed from the gastrointestinal tract. They are metabolized by the liver to water-soluble derivatives, which are eliminated by the kidney. In patients with hepatic or renal impairment the half-life of psychotropic drugs will be prolonged. Where psychotropic medication is added to other drug treatment the possibility of drug interaction must be considered. Alcohol potentiates the sedative effects of many psychotropic agents and should be avoided during treatment. Sudden discontinuation of psychotropic drugs, particularly tranquillizers and antidepressants, can cause withdrawal symptoms such as reduced sleep and anxiety. Where possible, therefore, medication should be reduced gradually under supervision.

In psychotropic drug prescribing, compliance is an even greater problem than in general therapeutics. Psychoactive drugs frequently have unpleasant side effects, and while side effects are experienced early in treatment, several days may elapse before a therapeutic response is evident. In addition, patients may not see the need for treatment, or believe that it can help them. Careful explanation, supplemented by written instructions, will help ensure that necessary medication is taken.

Particularly in depressed patients the risk of deliberate overdose must be assessed. There can be few experiences more dispiriting for the practitioner than to learn that medication prescribed to help a patient has been used in a suicide attempt. If such a risk is present medication should be dispensed in small amounts or entrusted to a relative.

Antidepressant drugs

Tricyclic antidepressants

Pharmacology

Tricyclic antidepressants inhibit the neuronal uptake of 5-hydroxytryptamine and noradrenaline, which would be expected to enhance the function of these neurotransmitters in the brain. However, it seems likely that the antidepressant effect of these drugs is associated with adaptive changes in brain monoamine receptors consequent upon the blockade of neurotransmitter uptake, so the net effect of the drugs on synaptic function is uncertain.

Principal drugs

These are amitriptyline, clomipramine, desmethylimipramine, dothiepin, doxepin, imipramine, nortriptyline, and protriptyline.

Indications and use

The indicators for the prescription of antidepressant medication have been described (page 25.9). Tricyclic antidepressants are the mainstay of drug therapy for a depressive disorder and should be the first choice of treatment for most patients.

Most depressed patients, particularly those with sleep disturbance and anxiety, should be treated with a sedative tricyclic antidepressant such as amitriptyline. Patients with a significant degree of retardation can be prescribed a less sedating preparation such as imipramine or desmethylimipramine. In order to obtain tolerance to side effects it is usual to begin treatment at a low dose, for example 50 mg amitriptyline at night, and to increase the amount over about 10 days to the usual therapeutic dose, which ranges between 75 and 200 mg amitriptyline at night. Because tricyclic antidepressants have long half-lives a single daily dose is appropriate, and if the whole of this daily dose is taken at night the sedative effect will help sleep. Patients should be warned about side effects (see below) because this helps to ensure compliance in the early stages of treatment. They should also be informed that a therapeutic response may not appear for up to three weeks. If treatment is successful it is usual to continue the antidepressant for 3–6 months, though the dose can be reduced while the patient's clinical state is monitored.

Table 1 Some side effects of tricylic antidepressants

Central nervous system	Sedation, psychomotor impairment, muscle weakness, muscle twitching, seizures, delirium, mania
Cardiovascular system	Tachycardia, postural hypotension, cardiac arrhythmias
Gastrointestinal system	Dry mouth, dyspepsia, nausea, constipation, paralytic ileus
Genitourinary system	Difficulty passing urine, retention of urine, failure of erection and ejaculation
Occular	Blurring of vision, precipitation of glaucoma
Other	Sweating, peripheral oedema, hepatitis, skin rash, blood dyscrasias, weight gain

Side effects and interactions (Table 1)

The main side effects of tricyclic antidepressants are attributable to blockade of muscarinic cholinergic receptors. Thus patients frequently experience dry mouth, blurring of vision, constipation, and difficulty in passing urine; sexual function in men is often impaired. In patients with closed angle glaucoma an acute rise in intraocular pressure may occur. Tricyclic antidepressants block α_1-adrenoceptors. In the central nervous system this blockade gives rise to drowsiness and psychomotor impairment, while peripherally, postural hypotension may result, especially in the elderly.

The most serious side effect of tricyclic antidepressants is cardiotoxicity. This is partly attributable to anticholinergic effects but the drugs also have direct effects on cardiac muscle. This effect is most problematic in cases of overdose, where serious and fatal arrhythmias may occur. However, there are also risks to patients with pre-existing cardiac disease, and a recent myocardial infarction is a contraindication to tricyclic antidepressants. With other cardiac disorders the situation must be carefully weighed; if a tricyclic antidepressant is to be used, doxepin is probably safest. Tricyclic antidepressants also lower seizure threshold and while spontaneous seizures are occasionally reported, difficulties are more likely to arise in patients with pre-existing epilepsy. Rarely these drugs have been associated with cholestatic hepatitis and blood dyscrasias.

Tricyclic antidepressants antagonize the hypotensive effects of adrenergic neurone blockers and clonidine but can be safely combined with thiazides and β-blockers. Because of their blockade of monoamine uptake, tricyclic antidepressants potentiate the cardiovascular effects of systemically administered noradrenaline and adrenaline, which may cause problems with certain local anaesthetic preparations.

Newer antidepressants

Principal drugs

These are lofepramine and mianserin.

Indications and use

The newer antidepressant drugs described here are less anticholinergic and cardiotoxic than the tricyclic antidepressants and should therefore be prescribed for patients in whom such side effects are contraindicated. In addition, the newer drugs are better tolerated than tricyclics, and can be tried in patients unable to take the full therapeutic dose of a tricyclic agent. Finally, in patients where the risk of overdose cannot be minimized the newer antidepressants should be preferred because of their low acute toxicity. The major disadvantage of the newer drugs is that they are less well tested in clinical practice and both their therapeutic effectiveness and long-term toxicity have yet to be fully evaluated. The newer antidepressants are also far more expensive than conventional tricyclic antidepressants.

Mianserin

Mianserin is a quadracyclic compound with sedative properties which does not block monoamine uptake. It does, however, antagonize the presynaptic α_2-adrenoceptor and might in this way increase noradrenaline transmission. Mianserin also blocks α_1-adrenoceptors and commonly causes drowsiness and sometimes postural hypotension. The dosage range is wide from 30 to 120 mg or greater, and as with tricyclic antidepressants the entire daily dose can be given at night. Some cases of aplastic anaemia and agranulocytosis have been associated with the use of mianserin though it is not yet clear if the incidence of this complication is higher than that seen with tricyclic antidepressant therapy.

Lofepramine

Lofepramine is a tricyclic drug which has little anticholinergic or cardiotoxic effect. It is a relatively selective inhibitor of noradrenaline uptake. The usual dose is up to 210 mg daily. Lofepramine is not sedating.

Monoamine oxidase inhibitors (MAOIs)

Pharmacology

MAOIs block the enzyme monoamine oxidase (MAO), which deaminates the neurotransmitters, noradrenaline, 5-hydroxytryptamine, and dopamine. Similarly to the tricyclic antidepressants, adaptive changes in central monoamine receptors may be the link between the acute pharmacological properties of MAOIs and their therapeutic effects.

Principal drugs

These are isocarboxazid, phenelzine, and tranylcypromine.

Indications and use

A few years ago MAOIs fell into relative disuse because some studies showed them to be less effective than tricyclic antidepressants in the treatment of depressive disorders, and also because they were implicated in dangerous interactions with certain drugs and foodstuffs (see below). However, recently MAOIs have begun to be used more frequently, and with a proper appreciation of their risks they can be useful drugs.

MAOIs are rarely used as a first choice of antidepressant except where a patient is known to have responded to them in the past. They are accordingly usually reserved for subjects who have failed to respond to tricyclic antidepressants or electroconvulsive therapy. Some workers believe that MAOIs are especially effective in depressions characterized by high levels of anxiety and histrionic behaviour.

Phenelzine and tranylcypromine are the two most commonly prescribed MAOIs. The usual therapeutic range of dose for phenelzine is between 30 and 90 mg daily. As with tricyclic antidepressants, patients should be warned about side effects and informed that a therapeutic effect from MAOIs may not be apparent for 3–4 weeks. Once a response is obtained it is usually necessary to continue the drug for some months, albeit at a reduced dosage.

Side effects and interactions

MAOIs may cause the following side effects. Central nervous system: dizziness, muscular twitching, insomnia, confusion, mania. Cardiovascular: tachycardia, postural hypotension, hypertension. Other: dry mouth, blurred vision, impotence, peripheral oedema, hepatocellular damage, leucopenia.

The major hazard of MAOI treatment is through interaction with indirect sympathomimetics, that is, agents which release noradrenaline from nerve endings. The usual source of the interaction is tyramine in certain foodstuffs, especially cheese and meat extracts. Tyramine is usually metabolized by MAO in the gut wall and liver but in patients taking MAOIs large amounts may enter the systemic circulation, resulting in hypertension and even cerebrovascular accidents. Similar adverse effects have been reported when sympathomimetic drugs such as amphetamine or ephedrine are administered to patients taking MAOIs. Since the latter drug or its derivatives are frequently present in cold cures, patients must be warned against self medication. Hypertensive episodes resulting from interaction of sympathomimetic drugs and MAOIs are best treated with an α-adrenoceptor blocking drug such as phentolamine. If this is unavailable, intramuscular chlorpromazine is an alternative. MAOIs also produce important interactions with other commonly used drugs including opiates, insulin and oral hypoglycaemics, and thiazide diuretics. Except in special circumstances combination with tricyclic antidepressants is best avoided.

From the foregoing it will be apparent that MAOIs should only be prescribed to patients capable of adhering to the necessary dietary restrictions. Written instructions listing prohibited foods should be provided. No additional medication should be given until the possibility of adverse drug interaction has been excluded. If MAOI treatment is stopped the dietary and pharmacological precautions should be continued for two weeks until new MAO has been synthesized.

Lithium

Pharmacology

Lithium is a cation usually administered in the form of the salt, lithium carbonate. In the body lithium is handled similarly to sodium and its psychotropic effects may depend on changes in excitability of neuronal membranes.

Indications and use

The main use of lithium is in the prophylaxis of recurrent affective disorders, especially manic depressive illness. Lithium is also used in the acute treatment of mania but is less immediately effective than antipsychotic medication.

The excretion of lithium from the body is critically dependent on the kidney and since there is little margin between therapeutic plasma levels of lithium (0.4–1.2 mmol/l) and those causing toxicity (>1.5 mmol/l) the introduction of lithium therapy should be preceded by a clinical and laboratory assessment of renal function. Renal function tests should include urine analysis, and estimations of plasma creatinine, urea, and electrolytes. A creatinine clearance test should be performed if there is any suggestion of impaired renal function.

Patients should initially be treated with 400–800 mg daily of lithium carbonate in two divided doses. Slow release formulations of this drug are available but their pharmacokinetics *in vivo* are very similar to those of the standard preparation. Dosage should be adjusted in 200–400 mg steps every 4–5 days on the basis of plasma lithium estimations obtained approximately 12 hours after the last dose. Recently it has been suggested that an adequate plasma level for the prophylactic effects of lithium lies between 0.4 and 0.8 mmol/l. Higher concentrations, up to 1.2 mmol/l, have been advocated for the treatment of acute mania. Most patients achieve adequate plasma levels on dosages of lithium carbonate between 800 and 1600 mg daily, and following this the lithium requirement is usually remarkably stable. In the absence of clinical indications it is usually sufficient to check lithium levels monthly, and repeat renal function tests every six months. Lithium can also cause hypothyroidism (see below), so thyroid function tests should be performed prior to treatment and at six-monthly intervals thereafter.

Side effects and interactions (Table 2)

Many patients suffer from a fine tremor, and nausea and diarrhoea may occur, especially at the start of treatment. Some degree of

Table 2 Some side effects of lithium

Central nervous system	Drowsiness, lethargy, headache, memory impairment, fine tremor
Cardiovascular system	Conduction defects (rare). T-wave flattening or inversion in ECG
Gastrointestinal system	Nausea, vomiting, diarrhoea
Genitourinary system	Increased thirst and polyuria, nephrogenic diabetes insipidus
Endocrine system	Hypothyroidism ($\downarrow$ T_4 $\uparrow$ TSH), hyperglycaemia, hyperparathyroidism
Other	Leucocytosis, skin rash, weight gain
Signs of toxicity (plasma level >1.5 mmol/l)	Nausea, vomiting, coarse tremor, drowsiness, dysarthria, seizures, coma, renal failure, cardiovascular collapse

thirst and polyuria is often present and a few patients develop nephrogenic diabetes insipidus. These latter effects are probably caused by lithium blocking the effect of ADH on the renal tubule. Most patients taking lithium have a demonstrable impairment of tubular concentrating ability though this is rarely of clinical significance. Glomerular function is usually not affected by lithium though following lithium toxicity, glomerular damage and interstitial fibrosis have been reported. Whether long-term use of lithium within therapeutic plasma concentrations results in irreversible renal damage is uncertain.

Up to 80 per cent of the lithium filtered by the renal glomerulus is reabsorbed by the proximal renal tubule. Conditions such as diarrhoea and excessive sweating, which decrease body sodium, result in increased lithium reabsorption by the renal tubule leading to elevated plasma lithium concentrations. In the same way, prescription of diuretics may well produce lithium toxicity unless the dose of lithium is reduced and plasma concentrations carefully monitored.

Lithium toxicity usually appears at plasma level of 1.5 mmol/l or greater. Early signs are coarse tremor, drowsiness, and dysarthria. High plasma concentrations (>2.5 mmol/l) lead to central nervous system depression, seizures, coma, and death. Toxic plasma lithium levels can also be associated with irreversible renal damage and cardiovascular collapse.

Plasma lithium levels may also be increased by concomitant administration of steroids or non-steroidal anti-inflammatory drugs. An interaction of lithium with succinylcholine has been reported, suggesting that the neuromuscular blockade produced by the latter drug may be prolonged in some patients.

Lithium reduces the production of thyroid hormone by the thyroid gland although in most patients an increase in pituitary TSH production allows an adequate compensation. Sometimes a goitre is apparent. Where patients have a limited thyroid reserve hypothyroidism may supervene but if it is considered necessary to continue lithium treatment thyroxine replacement therapy may be added.

Antipsychotic drugs

Pharmacology

Antipsychotic drugs, also known as major tranquillizers or neuroleptics, are a group of agents of varied structure which have in common the ability to block dopamine receptors in the central nervous system. It is likely that the antipsychotic effect of major tranquillizers is caused by blockade of dopamine receptors in mesolimbic and mesocortical brain regions. However, while the dopamine receptor blockade occurs within hours of drug administration, a useful clinical response may not occur for days, and sometimes weeks after the start of treatment.

Principal drugs

These are chlorpromazine, haloperidol, flupenthixol, fluphenazine, pimozide, sulpiride, thioridazine, and trifluoperazine.

Indications and use

Antipsychotic drugs are used mainly in the treatment of schizophrenia. They are also used to treat mania, and sometimes given to depressed patients who have psychotic symptoms, or who are particularly agitated. Antipsychotic drugs are also used in the management of disturbed behaviour arising from other causes, for example, organic illness, but their use as non-specific tranquillizing agents should be limited because of potentially serious side effects.

Dosage requirements of antipsychotic drugs vary considerably from patient to patient and also within the same patient at different stages of the illness. Generally for a young person with an acute psychosis, up to 1200 mg a day of chlorpromazine may be necessary, this dose being achieved gradually over the first two weeks, while sedative and hypotensive side effects decrease. In patients with cardiovascular disease, treatment with haloperidol in doses up to 60 mg daily is safer. All antipsychotic drugs are subject to first pass metabolism so parenterally administered medication produces a proportionately greater effect. If a patient has responded to an antipsychotic drug it is usual to continue the medication for a number of months into remission. Frequently it is necessary to administer medication on a long-term basis to prevent relapse, in which case a long-acting intramuscular preparation has the advantage of requiring less compliance and also more certain absorption. Flupenthixol decanoate or fluphenazine decanoate are the preparations most commonly used.

Side effects and interactions

The most common side effects seen with antipsychotic agents are those caused by dopamine receptor blockade in the basal ganglia (Table 3). Early in treatment patients may exhibit acute dystonias or akathisia, which is a sense of subjective motor restlessness. Subsequently symptoms of Parkinsonism may develop. All these disorders may be treated by a reduction in dose of the antipsychotic drug or the introduction of anticholinergic medication, for example, benztropine. However, anticholinergic drugs should not be prescribed routinely with antipsychotic medication because of the risk of abuse for their euphoriant effects. Later in treatment a further movement disorder may develop, known as tardive dyskinesia. This consists of involuntary repetitive movements, usually of the tongue and lips though other parts of the body may be involved. Tardive dyskinesia is thought to be due to supersensitivity of postsynaptic dopamine receptors in the basal ganglia; there is no good treatment for it and anticholinergic medication tends to make the movements worse. If possible, the antipsychotic drug should be stopped but this decision is often difficult because of the risk of relapse of the psychiatric disorder.

A further adverse reaction to antipsychotic drugs which involves the basal ganglia and probably the hypothalamus is the rare but important neuroleptic malignant syndrome, characterized by fever and muscle rigidity. This disorder may occur at any stage of neuroleptic treatment and has an appreciable mortality (> 15 per cent). There is no specific treatment but intensive care support is usually needed. Some workers recommend in addition the use of the muscle relaxant, dantrolene sodium, together with the dopamine agonist, bromocriptine.

Antipsychotic drugs, especially chlorpromazine and thioridazine, can produce a variety of autonomic side effects due to blockade of muscarinic receptors and α_1-adrenoceptors. These include: drowsiness, psychomotor impairment, delirium, tachycardia, postural hypotension, blurring of vision, precipitation of glaucoma, dry mouth, constipation, urinary hesitancy and retention, and impaired erection and ejaculation. Other side effects include: endocrine: elevated prolactin levels, amenorrhoea, and galactorr-

Table 3 Extrapyramidal disorders and antipsychotic drugs

Disorder	Description	Treatments employed
Dystonic reaction	Involuntary muscle contraction, especially face and jaw, occulogyric crisis	1 Benztropine (1–2 mg i.m. or i.v.) 2 Diazepam (10 mg i.v.)
Akathisia	Sense of subjective motor restlessness, continual pacing	1 Reduce dose of neuroleptic 2 Benztropine (1–6 mg daily) 3 Diazepam (10–30 mg daily)
Parkinsonism	Rigidity, bradykinesia, tremor	1 Reduce dose of neuroleptic 2 Benztropine (1–6 mg daily)
Tardive dyskinesia	Choreoathetoid movements, especially tongue, lips and jaw	1 Withdraw neuroleptic 2 Trial of tetrabenazine
Neuroleptic malignant syndrome	Fever, muscular rigidity, coma, death	1 Discontinue neuroleptic 2 Intensive care support

hoea; skin: rashes, pigmentation, and photosensitivity (especially phenothiazines); other: precipitation of seizures, hypothermia (especially chlorpromazine), cardiac conduction disorders (rare), weight gain, cholestatic hepatitis, leucopenia, and retinitis pigmentosa (thioridazine in daily dosage > 800 mg).

Antipsychotic drugs potentiate the effects of other central sedatives. They may delay the hepatic metabolism of tricyclic antidepressants and antiepileptic agents leading to increased plasma level of these latter drugs. The hypotensive properties of chlorpromazine and thioridazine may enhance the effects of antihypertensive drugs. However, phenothiazines have been reported to antagonize the hypotensive effect of adrenergic neurone blockers.

Anti-anxiety agents and hypnotics

Benzodiazepines

Pharmacology
Benzodiazepines enhance the action of the neurotransmitter, GABA, in the central nervous system, by binding to a specific benzodiazepine receptor located in a complex with a GABA receptor and a chloride ion channel. The pharmacological effects of benzodiazepines are attributed to facilitation of GABA transmission in various brain regions.

Principal drugs
These are chlorazepate, diazepam, flurazepam, lorazepam, lormetazepam, nitrazepam, temazepam, and triazolam.

Indications and use
The benzodiazepines have supplanted the barbiturates in the management of anxiety and insomnia, and are the most widely prescribed psychotropic drugs in the world. It seems likely that they are overprescribed. For most anxiety-related conditions alternative therapies are available (see page 25.3) and it is recommended that drug treatment of anxiety and insomnia should be limited to a few weeks' duration. The major indication for the use of benzodiazepines is to help patients in a crisis when anxiety and insomnia are causing functional impairment and reducing ability to cope. Patients should be instructed that treatment will be of short duration to help them manage their immediate difficulties.

All benzodiazepines have hypnotic and anxiolytic properties.

The main distinction of clinical use is their length of action. Derivatives with a 3-hydroxy group such as temazepam are metabolized by the liver to inactive glucuronides and tend to have short half-lives; such drugs are suitable hypnotics because of their lack of hangover effect and may also be used to treat anxiety on an infrequent 'as required' basis. Other benzodiazepines, for example, diazepam, have long half-lives and are metabolized to active compounds. These drugs may be used for the continuous treatment of anxiety throughout the day, given either as a single dose at night or in the more traditional regime of thrice daily.

Side effects and interactions
Benzodiazepines have a remarkably low toxicity. Their side effects are usually extensions of their clinical effects and include the following: drowsiness, psychomotor impairment, dizziness, ataxia, and paradoxical aggression (rare). Benzodiazepines potentiate other central sedatives, particularly alcohol. The effects of benzodiazepines are potentiated by cimetidine.

Patients who have taken clinical doses of a benzodiazepine for more than a few months may show a withdrawal syndrome when the medication is stopped. In some respects this syndrome resembles an anxiety state but perceptual disturbances and dysphoria may also occur. It is thus apparent that benzodiazepines can cause physical dependence and although the withdrawal syndrome is less severe than that seen following barbiturates, patients frequently find it extremely difficult to stop their medication. A gradual reduction is usually best. Generally, withdrawal from a long-acting benzodiazepine is easier than from a short-acting preparation. If patients taking short-acting benzodiazepines have difficulties withdrawing, a switch to a long-acting preparation may be helpful.

Chlormethiazole
The vitamin B_1 derivative, chlormethiazole, is sometimes used as an hypnotic in the elderly, mainly because of its short half-life (4–5 hours). Pharmacologically, chlormethiazole resembles the barbiturates more than the benzodiazepines, though, as yet, there are no reports of elderly patients becoming dependent on it. It is also used in short courses in alcohol withdrawal states (longer courses of treatment for alcoholic patients should be avoided because there is a risk of dependency). Chlormethiazole can cause serious respiratory depression in overdose, especially if combined with alcohol.

Other drugs
In the treatment of anxiety, MAOIs and tricyclic antidepressants may be helpful for patients who suffer from panic attacks. In addition, β-adrenoceptor blocking drugs are sometimes useful in patients with generalized anxiety who have marked somatic symptoms.

References
Bassuk, E. L., Schoonover, S. C. and Gelenberg, A. J. (1984). *The practitioner's guide to psychoactive drugs*, 2nd edn. Plenum Medical Book Company, New York.

Charney, D. S., Menkes, D. and Heninger, G. R. (1981). Receptor sensitivity and the mechanism of action of antidepressant treatment. *Arch. Gen. Psychiat.* **38**, 1160–1180.

Committee on the Review of Medicines (1980). Systematic review of the benzodiazepines. *Br. Med. J.* **1**, 910–912.

Crammer, J., Barraclough, B. and Heine, B. (1982). *The use of drugs in psychiatry*, 2nd edn. Gaskell, London.

Gelder, M., Gath, D. and Mayou, R. (1983). *The Oxford textbook of psychiatry*, pp. 516–575. Oxford University Press, Oxford.

Grahame-Smith, D. G. and Cowen, P. J. (1985). *Psychopharmacology*, Vol. 2. Excerpta Medica, Amsterdam.

Johnson, D. A. W. (1982). The long-acting depot neuroleptics. In *Recent advances in clinical psychiatry* (ed. K. Granville-Grossman), pp. 243–260. Churchill Livingstone, New York.

Johnson, F. N. (ed.) (1980). *Handbook of lithium therapy*. MTP Press, Lancaster.

Marsden, C. D. and Jenner, P. (1980). The pathophysiology of extrapyramidal side-effects of neuroleptic drugs. *Psychol. Med.* **10**, 55–72.

Paykel, E. S. and Coppen, A. (eds) (1979). *Psychopharmacology of affective disorders*. Oxford University Press, Oxford.

Pertusson, H. and Lader, M. (1981). Withdrawal from long-term benzodiazepine treatment. *Br. Med. J.* **283**, 643–645.

Snyder, S. H., Bannerjee, S. P., Yamamura, H. I. and Greenberg, D. (1974). Drugs, neurotransmitters and schizophrenia. *Science* **184**, 1243–1253.

Tyrer, P. (ed.) (1982). *Drugs in psychiatric practice*. Butterworth, London.

Psychological treatment

M. G. GELDER

Psychological treatment varies in complexity between the simple support and explanation which form a part of every kind of good medical care, and elaborate forms of psychotherapy carried out by specialist psychotherapists. The present account is restricted to an outline of the kinds of psychological treatment most likely to be of value for patients encountered by physicians. These treatments are: supportive therapy, crisis intervention, and certain behaviour therapies. Brief mention will also be made of dynamic psychotherapies. The simplest of these psychological measures can be carried out by the physician, some of the others can be given by another member of the medical team – usually a social worker – while the rest require referral to a psychiatrist or clinical psychologist. A fuller account will be found in the *Oxford textbook of psychiatry*.

The value of listening and giving information

The psychological help required by most anxious or depressed patients seen in medical practice is no more than an opportunity to express their worries and ask questions about the illness and its likely effect on their lives. Cartwright (1964) interviewed 739 patients who had been in hospitals in 12 randomly selected areas of England and Wales. Ninety per cent of these patients said they would have liked a better explanation of what was wrong, and 60 per cent wanted more information about such things as the purpose of medication, the results of tests, the length of time they might be off work, and whether any lasting disability was to be expected. Failures of communication arise both because the patients are too frightened to ask, and because doctors do not give enough time to finding out what patients want to know. Also physicians often underestimate the patient's capacity for understanding medical matters, while at the same time giving explanations in unnecessarily technical language.

Before *giving information*, it is important to find out what patients know already, what they want to know, and what particular aspects of the illness or its treatment cause them most worry. While this is being done, patients should feel that they have the undivided attention of the doctor, and that their concerns are being taken seriously. Because patients when anxious remember little of what they have been told, important points should be repeated or put in writing to be read later. A brief interview arranged in private surroundings will be more valuable than a longer time spent in a place where there are distractions and the risk of being overheard.

Apart from its value in putting the patient at ease, this stage of listening and finding out helps to ensure that the doctor does not give an account of the illness or its treatment which appears to contradict an explanation given previously by another doctor. It also directs attention to the points that will need most explanation. As explained in the section on transcultural psychiatry (pages 25.57–25.59) difficulties in communication are greatest when the

patient and doctor come from different countries, but it would be wrong to think that they are confined to these circumstances. Time spent in finding out what the patient knows and believes is also likely to improve co-operation with treatment.

Reassurance is important, but premature reassurance can destroy a patient's confidence in the doctor. Reassurance should be offered only after finding out the patient's concerns in some detail and it should be realistic and truthful. The purpose of reassurance is to dispel unnecessary fears, and to help the patient appreciate and make use of remaining assets; it is not concerned with making light of real problems. Of course, listening and reassurance are not only needed by the patients; many relatives need them as well. Indeed it is not uncommon to find that a patient's emotional upset does not subside until the relative's anxieties have been dispelled.

Supportive treatment

As explained above listening and explanation can relieve many of the psychological problems encountered in physically ill patients, but some patients require more help than this. Supportive treatment is used to help a person through a temporary crisis such as that of an acute physical illness, or to relieve prolonged distress resulting from chronic illness. Doctors may carry out the treatment themselves or ask social workers or suitably trained nurses to do it. Supportive treatment is not just an extension of everyday comfort and befriending: a few simple rules have to be followed especially those which are intended to reduce the patient's dependency on the doctor.

The therapist's main role in supportive treatment is that of listener. By listening, patients are allowed to express their feelings and in this way diminish them. The therapist also helps patients to clarify their ideas about their predicament by putting them into words, and helps patients think more clearly about their problems by prompting or asking questions. The therapist may also give advice but as far as possible encourages patients to work out their own solutions to their difficulties. However serious the disability caused by illness, emphasis should be placed on the best ways of making use of the patient's remaining assets.

An important part of supportive treatment is the regulation of the intensity of the relationship between patient and doctor. Over-intense relationships breed dependency, which may result in unnecessary distress for the patient and unreasonable demands upon the doctor. These problems are greatest in people with dependent personalities and after prolonged treatment. Undue dependency is less likely if two simple rules are followed. First an appropriate relationship should be maintained which while sympathetic and concerned is clearly a professional approach distinct from that of a friend. Second, the doctor should watch carefully for, and if necessary comment upon, the early signs of dependency such as attempts to prolong interviews unduly or other inappropriate ways of claiming the doctor's personal attention. Most of these problems can be avoided by stressing, from the beginning, the team work involved in the patient's treatment so that feelings of dependency are directed to the whole group of staff involved with the patient's care and not to an individual.

Crisis intervention

Physicians are most likely to make use of crisis intervention for patients who have taken deliberate drug overdoses. Usually the treatment will be carried out by a psychiatrist, social worker, or a specially trained psychiatric nurse. The aim of crisis intervention is not only to help a person cope with the immediate problems, it is also intended to bring about longer term changes so that the patient will cope with problems more effectively on a subsequent occasion. Treatment has three stages. First patients are encouraged to talk about the crises so that they become calmer. In the second stage patients are helped to think constructively about alternative ways of dealing with the problems which led to the crises. In doing this it is often helpful to encourage patients to list the problems on paper, and construct for each problem a series of alternative actions that they could take to resolve them. This approach helps to emphasize that it is the patient not the doctor, who can most usefully bring about these changes. In the third stage, patients are encouraged to choose between the alternative courses of action, carry one out, and talk over the results. These activities are presented as experiments in which an attempt that turns out to be unsuccessful is seen not as a failure but as an opportunity for learning how to do better on the next occasion. This no-failure approach is particularly important for people who habitually avoid facing difficulties and easily feel defeated. In both the second and third stages of treatment it is important to emphasize that the patient is learning a general approach that can be used for future problems, and not just a way of resolving those involved in the present crisis.

Behaviour therapy

Behavioural treatments are intended to control the symptoms of emotional disorders rather than deal with the original causes. (There are some exceptions to this general statement, but they need not concern the physician.)

Although many behavioural techniques are complex and require special training, the general principles of treatment are simple, and familiar to physicians because they resemble the principles used in rehabilitation from physical illness. These principles are: first that complicated problems need to broken down into manageable parts; second that a graduated approach should be used; and third that patients should practise the treatment techniques in their own time – they cannot rely entirely on the progress made in the course of their sessions with the therapist. For the disorders encountered by physicians, the most relevant forms of behaviour therapy are concerned with reducing anxiety and it is these forms which will be discussed here.

Relaxation training

This is the simplest technique for reducing anxiety. Physicians who wished to arrange these exercises for a chronically anxious patient might obtain them from an occupational therapist or a physiotherapist working with them, or the patient could be referred to a clinical psychologist or psychiatrist. Relaxation training can reduce anxiety that is of mild to moderate degree, producing in successful cases changes equivalent to those brought about by standard doses of anxiolytic drugs. However, relaxation is less effective for severe anxiety. Even for mild anxiety it may be difficult to persuade patients to practise relaxing regularly. This poor compliance with treatment can often be overcome by teaching relaxation to a group of patients who meet regularly and compare progress.

Anxiety management

This is a more elaborate procedure designed to improve compliance with treatment and to deal with aspects of the anxiety syndrome other than the autonomic arousal and muscle tension which are the target of relaxation training. In anxiety management, relaxation is combined with procedures directed to the worrying thoughts that preoccupy anxious patients and add to their anxiety. Simple procedures are used, so that patients can practise them on their own. These procedures are: activities which patients can use to distract themselves from worrying thoughts; and an explanation of the true nature of the anxiety symptoms which can be thought about when the worrying ideas are present, for example, an explanation that the patient's palpitations are a normal part of a fear response and not caused by heart disease. These simple measures have been shown in clinical trials to reduce anxiety significantly, but it is not certain to what extent these effects are specific. However, even if due mainly to placebo effects, the treatment is a useful alternative to the prolonged use of anxiolytic drugs.

Exposure treatment

This is used for phobic anxiety neuroses in which patients habitually avoid situations that provoke anxiety. Patients are encouraged to enter these situations repeatedly, on each occasion remaining until the anxiety symptoms have died away. This simple procedure is usually combined with some of the anxiety management techniques described above. Exposure is generally effective even in long-standing phobic disorders.

Response prevention

This technique is used to treat obsessional rituals. Like exposure, it is a simple procedure, but usually an effective one. The patient is encouraged strongly to control the ritual by voluntary effort for a period of an hour or more, first in circumstances in which the urge to perform the ritual is weak and then in situations in which the urge becomes progressively stronger (e.g. for hand-washing rituals, increasing degrees of dirtiness). The method usually succeeds when the patients' own efforts at control have failed, because patients seldom persist long enough or frequently enough to set in train the processes of relearning which terminate the condition.

Behavioural management

This method, also known as *contingency management*, is based on the principle that if an abnormal behaviour persists it is being reinforced by certain of its consequences, and that if these consequences can be altered the behaviour should change. The physician is most likely to make use of the method in the care of demented patients who are noisy or restless, or have problems with feeding or continence. While, in part, these disorders are clearly related to organic pathology, part is often due to inadvertent reinforcement by relatives or staff who pay extra attention to patients when their behaviour is abnormal. By training these other people to reward normal behaviour by immediate attention while avoiding as far as possible the rewarding of abnormal behaviour, worthwhile improvement can often be achieved.

Other kinds of behaviour therapy are described briefly in *The Oxford textbook of psychiatry* and more fully in specialist monographs.

Dynamic psychotherapy

In the past these methods were quite widely advocated, especially in the United States, for the treatment of 'psychosomatic' disorders. Controlled evaluation has not confirmed the original claims, although there is some evidence that psychotherapy can contribute to the treatment of selected patients with particular conditions. For these reasons, only a brief account of the treatment will be given here.

Dynamic psychotherapy is intended to modify emotional reactions and patterns of responding to other people. It does so in two main ways: by examining the patient's emotional reactions and other responses in the course of the treatment sessions; and by seeking connections between these present responses and events in childhood and adolescence. This kind of treatment may be performed with one patient at a time (individual psychotherapy) or with several patients together (group psychotherapy). In the latter, patients have the opportunity to learn from their responses to other patients as well as from their responses to the therapist. The technical procedures vary somewhat according to the training of the therapist (whether Freudian, Jungian etc.) but these variations have not been shown to affect the outcome.

Physicians who think that one of their patients might benefit from dynamic psychotherapy should seek the advice of a psychiatrist. They should consider doing this when a chronic or recurrent medical disorder appears to be exacerbated by anxiety, suppressed anger or other emotional problems, and when these emotions appear to arise more from the personality of the patient than from the circumstances of his or her life. There is some evidence that, chosen in this way, selected patients with respiratory disorders, eating disorders, and (possibly) ulcerative colitis gain a measure of added benefit when appropriate medical management is combined with psychotherapy.

References

Cartwright, A. (1964). *Human relations and hospital care*. Routledge and Kegan Paul, London.
Rimm, D. C. and Masters, J. C. (1979). *Behaviour therapy: techniques and empirical findings*. Academic Press, New York.
Rosser, A. M. and Guz, A. (1981). Psychological approach to breathlessness and its treatment. *J. Psychosomat. Res.* **25**, 439–447.

Psychiatric emergencies

R. A. MAYOU

All doctors need to be confident that they can manage acute psychiatric disturbance, in which there is rarely time either to make a detailed assessment or to obtain specialist help. Such management calls for the ability to recognize and treat primary psychiatric disorders, and also to distinguish between psychiatric and medical conditions since significant medical problems often underlie acute organic mental states. This section covers not only serious emergencies but also less dramatic problems, encountered in casualty departments or elsewhere in the general hospital, that require immediate decisions about management.

Successful management depends greatly on the clinical interview, in which the aim is first to establish a good relationship with the patient, and then to elicit information and make observations of the patient's behaviour and mental state. The pressures of an emergency often make this approach difficult, but nevertheless time can be saved and mistakes avoided if the doctor remains composed. Many emergencies become less urgent and bewildering if dealt with in a calm and deliberate way. Before seeing the patient, it is useful to obtain as much information as possible both from medical notes and from informants such as relatives, other physicians, nursing staff or the police.

General considerations

A number of problems that arise regularly in medical practice will be considered first. These are: the acutely disturbed patient, the violent patient, and the drug treatment of these emergencies; the stupose patient; the patient who refuses treatment for medical illness, and the patient who refuses treatment for mental disorder.

The disturbed patient

Table 1 lists some of the many causes of disturbed behaviour. The list includes several important physical causes that are easily missed, especially if the known history leads to an overhasty diagnosis of psychiatric, alcohol or drug problems.

Doctors should try as far as possible to take a history, observe behaviour and perform a physical examination. They should

Table 1 Some causes of disturbed behaviour

Anxiety, fear
Alcohol or drug abuse and withdrawal
Personality disorder
Acute organic (delirium, confusional state), e.g.
  Side effects of treatment
  Hypoglycaemia
  Epilepsy (postictal, status)
  Head injury
  Encephalitis and meningitis
Dementia
Schizophrenia and paranoid psychoses
Affective disorder: depression and mania

Table 2 Management of violence

1 Ensure adequate help and medication immediately available
2 Make sure you can retreat rapidly. Do not take risks
3 Do not let the patient feel trapped
4 Listen to the patient, talk calmly, and do not argue
5 Do not try to restrain patient in any way unless you have adequate support
6 If there are medical indications for restraint, act quickly and effectively but with minimum force

approach the patient in a friendly manner. At the beginning of the interview time spent in listening and reassuring is usually well spent. Many disturbed patients are frightened or angry; once these feelings are understood and taken seriously by the doctor, such patients can usually be reassured. Often the interview will then proceed relatively smoothly, but sometimes tranquillizing medication is necessary (see below). Once the disturbed behaviour has settled, full physical examination and appropriate investigations should be carried out.

The violent patient

If the patient's disturbed behaviour includes violence or the likelihood of violence, the doctor should be sure that adequate but unobtrusive support is available before approaching him (see Table 2). The doctor should always be ready to listen, sympathize, and compromise. Extreme caution is, of course, required with any patient thought to possess any kind of offensive weapon and in such cases it is often best to ask the police to intervene. Staff should always avoid attempting single-handed restraint or engaging in any behaviour suggesting that physical contact (e.g. a physical examination) is intended unless the purpose has been clearly understood and agreed by the patient.

If restraint cannot be avoided, it should be accomplished quickly by an adequate number of people using the minimum of force. Medication such as parenteral haloperidol or chlorpromazine should always be available, and is usually effective. The use of such medication may provide the only way to carry out a physical examination or obtain further information.

Emergency drug treatment of disturbed or violent patients

For a patient who is moderately frightened, diazepam (5–10 mg) may be useful. For a more disturbed patient, rapid calming is best achieved with 5–10 mg of haloperidol intramuscularly, repeated if necessary every half hour or every hour up to 60–100 mg in 24 hours. Chlorpromazine (75–150 mg intramuscularly) is a useful alternative to haloperidol, but more likely to cause hypotension. Once the patient is calm regular but flexible doses of haloperidol, probably three to four times a day, should be started, preferably as syrup or tablets. The exact dosage depends on the patient's weight and physical strength, and on the initial response to the drug. Careful nursing observations are necessary during tranquillization. Extrapyramidal side effects may require treatment.

Stupor

Stupor may be due either to neurological or psychiatric conditions. Thorough neurological examination and assessment is always necessary, even if the patient has a history of psychiatric disorder. A psychiatric diagnosis should be made only when tests of cerebral hemisphere and brain stem function have been found to be normal. Information from other informants is essential to establish the onset, nature, and cause of the condition. The most common psychiatric causes of stupor are severe depressive disorder, hysteria, and schizophrenia (catatonia). Since a patient in stupor stops eating or drinking, energetic management is necessary.

The patient who refuses medical treatment

Patients may be unwilling to accept medical advice for many reasons. Most commonly it is because they are angry or frightened, or do not understand what is happening; only very occasionally is the cause a mental illness that interferes with the patient's ability to make an informed decision. Only this small minority require referral to a psychiatrist. For the rest, the doctor should explain the proposed treatment and why it is needed, and should try to relieve any anger or anxiety that is preventing the patient from understanding. If this is done, it is usually possible to agree a reasonable plan of medical care although a degree of compromise may be needed. However, it has to be accepted that some patients will refuse treatment even after full and rational discussion, and it is, of course, a fundamental right of a conscious, mentally competent, adult to do so. When this happens doctors should keep a proper record of what they have tried to do, and whenever possible should ask the patient to sign a declaration of refusal to accept medical advice.

The patient who refuses treatment for psychiatric disorder

If a patient has a mental illness that impairs the ability to give informed consent, it may be appropriate for the doctor to seek legal powers of compulsory assessment and treatment. In England and Wales, provision for such action is made in the *Mental Health Act* 1983, and other countries have a comparable legislation. The doctor must be familiar with the local legislation and its application to clinical practice.

Powers for compulsory treatment of a mental disorder do not give a right to treatment of any concurrent physical disorder. However, in many countries, it is accepted that the doctor in charge of the patient does have the right to give immediate treatment in life-threatening *emergencies* without the patient's consent. If doctors have to do this they should if possible obtain opinions from other medical and nursing colleagues and the patient's relatives. They should keep detailed records of the reasons for their decision.

Successful treatment of any concurrent psychiatric disorder often results in the patient being able to give informed consent for the treatment of the physical illness at a later stage.

Psychiatric syndromes as causes of emergencies

Organic disorders

Disorders of behaviour and thinking due to acute or chronic organic mental disorders are usually easily recognized. (The main features are summarized in Table 3.) However, in the absence of a clear history or obvious physical signs, a functional psychiatric illness may be diagnosed in error. Doctors should always be suspicious that odd, out-of-character behaviour is a sign of an organic mental disorder, and they should be prepared to undertake full physical examination and assessment. In any patient who is exhibiting disturbed behaviour and who is elderly or has a physical illness, it is wise to assume that an organic mental disorder is likely until proved otherwise. Careful psychiatric assessment including observations of behaviour may reveal fluctuating disorientation, or cognitive functions that seem impaired as judged by what is known of the patient's normal functioning.

As explained in the section on organic mental disorders, treatment is primarily medical. Also, confused patients require consistent nursing care, with repeated reassurance and explanation from a few familiar nurses. It may be useful to nurse the patient in a single room with some light at night. Regular visits from close family and friends are helpful. Modest dosages of a benzodiazepine hypnotic or a tranquillizer (haloperidol or a phenothiazine) are valuable in the management of agitation, restlessness, and disturbed behaviour. Regular but flexible dosage regimes are preferable to the intermittent treatment of crises.

Table 3 Organic mental states

Acute (delirium)	Dementia
Onset usually acute	Onset often insidious
Consciousness clouded and fluctuating	Consciousness not clouded
Disorientation and memory disturbance	Loss of intellectual abilities
Perceptual disturbance (misinterpretation, hallucination, illusion)	Memory disorder
Incoherent speech	Disturbance of higher cerebral function
Increased or decreased motor activity	
Evidence of underlying physical condition	

Table 4 Causes of acute anxiety

General and phobic anxiety neurosis
Fear of physical illness and its treatment
Post-traumatic
Alcohol withdrawal
Drug intoxication and withdrawal
Specific medical illness, e.g. thyrotoxicosis, hypoglycaemia
Hyperventilation
Agitated depression

Table 5 Somatic symptoms without physical cause

(a) Hypochondriacal symptoms
   Transient fear of illness responding to reassurance
   Somatic symptoms of a primary psychiatric disorder: especially anxiety neurosis, depressive disorder, hysteria, schizophrenia
   Hypochondriacal personality

(b) Simulated symptoms
   Malingering
   Munchausen syndrome
   Specific simulated symptoms

States of acute anxiety

Table 4 lists some of the common causes of acute anxiety. Most of these causes are easily recognized. Mild anxiety is best treated by sympathetic discussion, encouragement, and reassurance. When anxiety is a response to acute stress, benzodiazepines can be helpful either as night sedatives or as anxiolytics. However, the prescription of these drugs should not be prolonged after the emergency has passed.

Somatic symptoms without physical cause

Somatic symptoms (Table 5) without significant physical cause are very common in all medical practice. Some of these patients also have an undoubted physical illness and are often said to have 'functional overlay'. Such cases may present as emergencies. Mild cases usually respond to authoritative reassurance after thorough history taking and examination. Major and persistent problems also require proper history taking and examination, but it is a mistake to order unnecessary investigations or seek repeated specialist advice in the hope that this will satisfy (or get rid of) a demanding patient. In a minority of cases in which an underlying psychiatric disorder is suspected, psychiatric assessment and, if necessary, treatment should be arranged. Patients whose hypochondriasis is related to their personalities require consistent, firm but yet sympathetic management over long periods.

Hysteria

Acute onset conversion or dissociative symptoms such as paralyses, sensory impairments, and amnesias are occasionally seen as emergencies. Such symptoms should always be taken seriously and require full medical examination and appropriate special investigations. The doctor should always bear in mind that some cases originally diagnosed as hysteria are later found to have physical illness, and that physical illness can occur in patients with a history of recurrent hysterical symptoms. Once hysteria is suspected, the exclusion of organic disorder must be accompanied by a search for a psychological explanation of the patient's symptoms. Admission to hospital may be necessary for further assessment and for treatment.

Hysteria of acute onset often recovers quickly. Resolution is helped by thorough assessment and sympathetic reassurance, and by avoiding anything that might reinforce the symptoms. The patient should not be confronted but rather given face-saving opportunities for improvement. As with other forms of neurotic disorder, psychological treatment directed to underlying emotional difficulties is important.

Simulated illness

Malingering is the faking of illness for obvious rewards (e.g. to obtain narcotics, take time off work, or gain compensation). Such cases are not uncommon in emergency departments. Suspicions should be raised by inconsistencies in the patient's account of the symptoms and of previous medical treatment, and vagueness about addresses and the names of doctors and other informants. The diagnosis can be confirmed only by the patient's confession, and careful history taking and gentle confrontation are often effective in securing this.

The Munchausen syndrome, and the simulation of particular symptoms such as bleeding and pyrexia, differ from malingering in bringing no obvious external reward for the fabrication of symptoms. Although the grosser syndromes of recurrent faking and pathological lying are notably resistant to all forms of psychological treatment, patients exhibiting them should be confronted tactfully and offered referral to a psychiatrist. Patients with less extreme and more specific forms of simulated illness are somewhat more likely to respond to psychological treatment.

Alcohol problems

There are numerous physical and psychiatric disorders that arise directly from abuse of alcohol (see page 25.23). In addition, injuries and social problems arising from drunkenness may present as physical emergencies. In such cases thorough physical assessment is always required.

Emergency departments should have a clear and positive management policy for such cases. There should be a procedure for managing noisy drunks, and, for those who subsequently show interest, advice on stopping drinking and rapid access to specialist services. Facilities for withdrawing alcohol ('detoxification') should also be available.

Acute withdrawal symptoms of tremor, nausea, and sweating occur 6–8 hours after stopping drinking or reducing alcohol intake. The much less common syndrome of delirium tremens (page 25.23) occurs 48–72 hours after stopping or reducing alcohol. Definite signs of delirium tremens are always an indication for hospital care; it is important to be aware of the dangers of fits, hyperthermia, and circulatory failure. In less severe cases withdrawal can be managed outside hospital but the abrupt discontinuance of alcohol usually requires tranquillizers, dispensed daily so as to avoid overdoses or other misuse. It is important to be flexible about dosage, adjusting it to the clinical state. Diazepam is valuable, in a basic regime of 10 mg four times/day for three days; 10 mg three times/day for two days; 5 mg twice/day for two days. Many doctors prefer chlormethiazole despite the considerable risk of dependence which contraindicates its use outside hospital. A basic regime is: 1.5 g three times/day for two days; 1 g three times/day for two days; 0.5 g three times/day for one day.

Drug dependence

Doctors should have a policy of refusing to prescribe addictive drugs to unknown patients who present themselves as needing emergency supplies. The management of withdrawal is described on pages 25.27 and 25.28. Any suspicion of drug misuse should lead to a careful history and physical examination, with efforts to check the genuineness of the history, and testing of urine and blood for the presence of drugs. Management depends on the nature of the drug and the circumstances of consultation (see pages 25.25–25.30).

Overnight hospital admission is required for drug-dependent patients who are brought to hospital after an overdose or who are disturbed enough to require care. For the latter, reassurance and the prescription of non-controlled drugs is often an effective temporary measure in relieving the patient's anxiety about withdrawal symptoms.

Post-traumatic states

Survivors of major accidents and people who have suffered bereavement or other emotional shocks may be dazed, numbed or distressed and present as emergencies. They require sympathy and reassurance, and help with immediate practical problems. A minor tranquillizer or night sedative can be helpful.

A particular problem is the management of victims of rape or other sexual assault. Apart from treating injuries, doctors should record any evidence that may be needed for subsequent legal proceedings. They should give the victim advice about possible venereal disease or pregnancy, and should provide support and reassurance. With the victim's permission, they should talk to her relatives or close friends. Some hospitals have special services for rape victims.

Reference

Rund, D. A. and Hulzher, J. C. (1983). *Emergency psychiatry*. C. V. Mosby, St Louis.

TRANSCULTURAL PSYCHIATRY

J. LEFF

Problems of psychiatric diagnosis in patients from developing countries arise less from the existence of unusual conditions in these countries than from difficulties in the diagnosis of familiar ones. These difficulties arise because psychiatric diagnosis depends mainly on information obtained in an interview and this is a form of negotiation between doctor and patient which is strongly influenced by the expectations of both parties. When doctor and patient come from different countries, their expectations may be so different that negotiation between them can be invalidated. Because these expectations are unspoken, misunderstandings arise particularly easily. This account begins by considering ways in which the expression of emotions and other psychological phenomena are affected by cultural influences; and then considers the expectations patients have of their doctors; and the expectations doctors have of patients. Finally, implications for practice are considered.

Factors affecting the patient

Cultural influences on the communication of distress

Distress is communicated by verbal and non-verbal means. There is evidence from ethnological studies of a high degree of consistency across cultures in the non-verbal expression of the major emotional states. However, these studies have assessed the recognition of 'pure emotions', whereas the majority of patients exhibit mixed emotional states. In clinical practice, doctors do not achieve a high reliability in assessing patients' emotional state from their non-verbal behaviour.

The verbal expression of emotional distress is inevitably limited by the vocabulary of words describing emotion available to the patient. In many African, Oriental, and Amerindian languages, words are lacking for the key emotions of anxiety and depression. In their place, phrases are used that refer directly to the bodily experiences that accompany emotional disturbances. For example, in one African language, Yoruba, the phrase used for anxiety translates as 'the heart is not at rest', while that for depression translates as 'the heart is weak'. It appears that in much of the developing world emotional distress is experienced largely in terms of its somatic accompaniments, which dominate the vocabulary of emotion in these cultures. It has been postulated (Leff, 1981) that as industrialization and urbanization have transformed the structure and values of traditional cultures, the focus has shifted from the group to the individual. With the greater value ascribed to the uniqueness of the individual there has been an increasing emphasis on introspection leading to a 'psychologizing' of emotional experience. The consequence has been an expansion of the vocabulary of words describing emotion and an increasing differentiation of emotional states. This process has occurred unevenly throughout the world. Thus, conversion hysteria (the bodily expression of emotional distress *par excellence*) has virtually disappeared from western countries, but still constitutes around 20 per cent of outpatient consultations for neurosis in developing countries.

The 'psychologizing' of emotions has also occurred unevenly within western societies, where it is linked with education and social status. The more highly educated patients and those in the upper socio-economic strata are more likely to express their emotional distress in psychological terms, complaining directly to the doctors of anxiety and depression. Those of lower education and socio-economic status are more likely to present their distress to their doctors as somatic symptoms. This poses the difficult problem of how to distinguish this form of presentation of emotional distress from physical disease.

It has been shown that in England a general practitioner, even when trained in psychiatry, misses about one-third of the cases of neurotic disorder presenting at the surgery. This proportion is greater in developing countries, where a somatic presentation of emotional distress is much more common. Tseng (1975) found that 70 per cent of patients with documented psychological disorders who visited the psychiatry clinic at the National Taiwan University Hospital initially presented with physical symptoms. A study of primary health care facilities in Colombia, India, Sudan, and the Philippines identified neurotic illnesses in 14 per cent of patients (Harding *et al.*, 1980). The majority of these patients presented a physical symptom, such as headache, abdominal pain, cough or weakness, so that it is hardly surprising that the health workers missed two-thirds of the cases of psychiatric disorder. This problem is partly attributable to the close resemblance between the somatic expression of emotional distress and the symptoms of physical disease. Another major contribution is derived from the mismatch between the expectations of doctors and those of their patients.

Cultural relativity of delusions and hallucinations

A person's cultural milieu includes many ideas and beliefs about the world, some explicit others implicit. When doctors are consulted by a patient belonging to a different cultural group who is expressing unusual beliefs, they should decide whether these beliefs are shared by other members of that group. Only then can they label the beliefs as pathological. This essential proviso is incorporated in the definition of a delusion, which includes a phrase 'inconsistent with the patient's educational and cultural background'. To give an example of the application of this exemption clause, the belief that neighbours are capable of causing misfortune by the use of magic is widespread throughout the developing world. Indeed this notion still persists in Southern Europe: for instance, a belief in the 'evil eye' is common in Greece, even amongst educated people. Consequently, a doctor hearing a patient from the Third World complaining that the neighbours are working black magic against him or her, would not be justified in jumping to the conclusion that the patient was expressing a delusion.

A more exotic example is provided by the condition known as *koro* which affects individuals in Southeast Asia and occasionally takes an epidemic form. The male sufferer develops a belief that his penis is shrinking and that it will disappear into his abdomen with fatal results. To prevent this happening, he may tie his penis to a rock or persuade his relatives to hold on to it in relays. Koro has been classified as a culture-bound psychosis. However, it is clear that the sufferer's relatives share the belief in the shrinking penis and its fatal outcome. This belief is widespread throughout the area in which koro occurs, and stems from the local myth that ghosts have no genitals. These considerations invalidate the labelling of the idea as a delusion, and the application of the term 'psychosis' to the condition.

It is not only beliefs that have to be judged in relation to culture, perceptual experiences should also be considered in this way. In many parts of the world, including the West, a belief in the existence of spirits persists, and normal people report sensory experiences which they attribute to spirits. In some societies the experience of hallucinations is actually sought by a variety of methods, indeed among the Xhosa people the experiencing of auditory and visual hallucinations appears to have status value. It is likely that in cultures where attitudes to such perceptual experiences are positive, the threshold for their appearance will be low. In such a milieu, accounts of hearing or seeing things which the doctor would regard as non-existent cannot be accorded the same pathological significance as in a western culture. Even within western countries people vary in the readiness with which they report hallucinations, and these variations are linked with socio-cultural factors. Schwab (1977) conducted a survey in Florida and found that people from the lowest socio-economic stratum were five times more likely to report hallucinations that those from the highest, while blacks were almost twice as likely to report hallucinations than whites. Religious affiliation also seemed to exert an influence, the extremes being represented by members of the Church of God, a fifth of whom reported hallucinations, and the Jews, of whom none did.

Faced with a bewildering variety of subcultures, each with its own system of beliefs and thresholds for hallucinatory experiences, how is the doctor to judge what is abnormal? It is clear that unless the doctor practises in a culturally homogeneous and isolated area, he or she is unlikely to become sufficiently familiar with the various cultural backgrounds of the patients to make informed judgements. In case of doubt the most sensible course is to ask the opinion of an informant from the patient's cultural group on the abnormality of the experiences reported or beliefs expressed by the patient.

Patients' concepts of illness

Patients' concepts of illness are formed in part by the folk culture in which they have lived. These concepts are important determinants of the patients' willingness to follow the doctor's advice once a diagnosis has been made. The framework of knowledge with which patients come to the consultation is very rarely explored by doctors, but it has an important effect on the patient's understanding of the doctor's explanation and on the likelihood that the prescribed treatment regime will be adhered to. Patients whose preformed ideas are consistent with the doctor's advice will feel more committed to follow this advice than those whose ideas are in conflict with those of the doctor. In a recent survey of general practice, only about one in ten patients of Anglosaxon origin did not appear committed to the doctor's hypothesis about the significance of their complaints, whereas this was true of a quarter of patients with other ethnic backgrounds. The least commitment to the prescribed regime was shown by West Indian and Irish patients (Health Education Studies Unit, 1982). In general the greater the cultural difference between doctor and patient, the smaller the overlap between their concepts of illness, and the less the likelihood that the patient will follow the doctor's advice.

In western countries, the doctor's concepts of disease are highly technical and esoteric, and are rarely shared with the patients. By contrast, in non-western countries theories of illness embedded in the folk culture are shared by traditional healers and their clients. As a result, the treatments prescribed by healers are understood and followed by clients. For example, in many traditional cultures psychiatric illnesses are ascribed to possession by spirits. The healer identifies the spirit or spirits involved and either conducts a propitiatory ritual or prescribes one for the client's social group to undertake. Either way it is not solely the client who is involved in consultation or treatment, but the kinfolk and wider social circle. The inclusion of the client's social group helps to combat the isolation that often afflicts psychiatric patients in the West.

In most developing countries people have a choice between consulting a traditional healer or a doctor trained in western medicine. This choice is strongly influenced by folk categories of illness. In a large variety of traditional cultures a dichotomy is maintained between native illnesses which are considered to have been sent by others and believed to respond to native treatments only, and European illnesses which appear spontaneously and are cured by European treatments. The illnesses in each category vary

somewhat from culture to culture. For instance, the Zulu assign measles, malaria, and smallpox to the European category, while the Yoruba include smallpox with madness as illnesses that emanate from a god, *Shopanna*, and do not repond to western methods of treatment.

Western scientific theories about disease have had little effect in displacing traditional theories in the Third World. Healers and their clients in traditional societies have retained their theories of illness intact, and have managed to do this by reclassifying certain conditions as belonging to the western system rather than to their own. This applies particularly to illnesses which western medicine has been conspicuously successful in treating or preventing, such as the epidemic diseases. Western methods of treating psychiatric illnesses in their acute stage are probably not dramatically more effective than traditional techniques, while the idea of prevention by taking maintenance drugs for long periods of time is totally alien to patients schooled to expect a one-time cure. It is hardly surprising, therefore, that psychiatric conditions are viewed as remaining firmly within the category of native illnesses. Clearly this results in the traditional healer being the first choice for consultation about psychiatric complaints. Thus the clientele of psychiatric facilities in the Third World must be composed largely of the healers' failures.

Patients' expectations of doctors

In western countries doctors are of higher social status than most of their patients, and even when they are not the doctors still wield authority by virtue of the power their professional skills and knowledge confer. In developing countries, social structure is generally more hierarchical and the doctor's position more authoritarian. In this type of relationship, the doctor tends to ask all the questions while the patient responds dutifully and shrinks from questioning the doctor's diagnosis or treatment. Paradoxically though, it is in the developing world that the traditional healer flourishes, and he is not expected to ask many questions. In particular, healers who practise divination are expected to know the nature of the client's problem by virtue of clairvoyant powers. As a result, some patients from a developing country, when consulting a western-trained physician, are disappointed when they encounter a barrage of probing questions. This is particularly true of a psychiatric consultation in which the diagnosis is most often elucidated by a careful verbal examination of the patient. Conversely, the western-trained physician may react with frustration and irritability to the passivity and reserve of a patient from the Third World.

Factors affecting the doctor

Doctors' expectations of what they will be presented with by their patients are strongly influenced by their own concepts of disease. These concepts provide a structure within which they organize patients' complaints and make sense of them. Doctors' initial efforts in a consultation are directed towards making a diagnosis. To this end they reformulate patients' complaints in terms of symptoms, discarding as unimportant anything that does not fit. The cluster of symptoms is then matched against an array of disease concepts for goodness of fit. These concepts are instilled during the doctors' training, but may be modified by subsequent experience of clinical practice.

Even some experienced psychiatrists maintain idealized concepts of disease. Thus many continue to regard anxiety and depressive neuroses as clearly differentiated even though more than 70 per cent of British patients exhibit a mixture of the symptoms considered characteristic of each type of neurosis. The problem is greater with patients from developing countries who present their emotional distress in the form of somatic complaints. The doctor then has to discount the usual clinical significance of these bodily symptoms in order to appreciate the emotional disorder they signal. This is the more difficult because the patients are not necessarily aware of a disturbance of their emotions. Even in a western country, patients commonly complain of, say, a churning feeling in their stomach on awakening, and strenuously deny any experience of anxiety or depression even when this is vigorously suggested by the doctor. Nevertheless their physical symptoms respond well to psychotropic drugs. In a non-western country the patient expects a doctor to take physical symptoms at their face value. A psychological explanation given by the doctor is most unlikely to be accepted, because the patient lacks concepts of illness that match the doctor's concepts of disease.

Implications for medical practice

The increasing migration of people from the Third World to the West results in most western doctors being consulted by patients whose cultural background is quite alien to their own. Emotional distress is more often presented by such patients in the form of somatic symptoms, for which costly and unnecessary laboratory investigations are commonly undertaken. How can the doctor avoid such mismanagement? First an awareness of the possible significance of physical complaints by a client from a different culture will help. This entails the doctor modifying expectations that emotional distress will be presented in psychological terms. Second, it is an advantage to know that the range of physical symptoms signifying distress is much wider in Third World patients than in western clients. Typical symptoms of African sufferers are creeping feelings in the skin, pains all over the body, generalized weakness, and a feeling of having an expanded head. Indian equivalents are watering of the eyes, belching a lot after eating, nocturnal emissions, and difficulty in passing water. Third, a careful history will often reveal the characteristic features suggesting the correct diagnosis. Thus somatic symptoms that are worse on waking in the morning and improve during the day are a good pointer to a depressive illness. Impaired concentration, and

poor sleep and appetite in the absence of reported depressed mood, add support to the diagnosis of depressive disorder. In the case of anxiety, an account of episodic somatic symptoms is suggestive, particularly if excessive sweating is a prominent feature. Physical symptoms occurring in particular situations suggest phobic anxiety which may present in a purely somatic form. Thus faintness or giddiness occurring only when the patient is out of doors, or only when alone, strongly suggest phobic neurosis.

Finally, the doctor should attempt to find out the patient's views about the significance of the problem, any ideas about action or prevention, and fears of social and psychological consequences. Ideally, in presenting the diagnosis and management, doctors should try to integrate medical and lay frameworks of knowledge by explaining their views in relation to those of the patient. Inevitably this will occupy extra time, but in the long run it will save on wasted prescriptions and unheeded advice.

References

Harding, T. W., De Arango, M. V., Baltazar, J., Climent, C. E., Ibrahim, H. H. A., Ladrido-Ignacio, L., Srinavasa Murthy, R. and Wig, N. N. (1980). Mental disorders in primary health care: a study of their frequency and diagnosis in four developing countries. *Psychol. Med.* **10**, 231–241.

Health Education Studies Unit (1982). *Final report on the patient project.* Health Education Council, London.

Katon, W. and Kleinman, A. (1981). Doctor–patient negotiation and other social science strategies in patient care. In *The relevance of social science for medicine* (eds L. Eisenberg and A. Kleinman). Reidel, London.

Leff, J. (1981). *Psychiatry around the globe.* Dekker, New York.

Schwab, M. E. (1977). A study of reported hallucinations in a South-eastern county. *Men. Hlth Soc.* **4**, 344–354.

Tseng, W. S. (1975). The nature of somatic complaints among psychiatric patients – the Chinese case. *Compreh. Psychiat.* **16**, 237–245.

SECTION 26
SPORTS MEDICINE

SPORTS MEDICINE

A. YOUNG

Introduction

Man moves by muscular activity. Good clinical practice demands an understanding of exercise physiology. Indeed, the acute and chronic effects of exercise should be an integral part of the syllabus in every medical specialty. It would be both futile and inappropriate to try to cover all the medical aspects of exercise in a single chapter. This one will not deal with the health benefits of exercise in general. Instead, it will concentrate specifically on aspects of recreational exercise, or sport.

The increasing availability of leisure time and the growth of sports participation mean that sports medicine is now an important part of western medical practice. It includes topics ranging from the enhancement of elite performance to ensuring safe participation despite the presence of disease or disability. The particular topics to be considered in this chapter are sudden cardiac death, the management of sport-related injuries, and the clinical physiology of endurance sports.

Sudden cardiac death

Frequency

Sudden death during sport tends to attract the attention of the press but is, in fact, very rare. Vigorous exercise carries only a very small absolute risk; a study from Rhode Island gives a figure of approximately 1 death per 7600 middle-aged joggers, half of whom had a premortem diagnosis of ischaemic heart disease. Nevertheless, this was still seven times the death rate during sedentary activities. A recent Seattle study supports these figures (Table 1) but also puts the increased risk during exercise into perspective. Among habitually vigorous men, the overall risk of sudden cardiac death, i.e. both during and not during vigorous activity, was only 40 per cent of that among sedentary men. Moreover, the risk of vigorous physical activity (whether sporting or non-sporting) was about 10 times as great among habitually inactive men as among the habitually most active group. Thus, vigorous physical activity carries a transiently increased risk of sudden cardiac death which is greatest in those who are habitually least active and which is outweighed in those who are habitually most active by a decreased overall risk.

Table 1 The relative risk of sudden cardiac death during vigorous physical activity by middle-aged men with no clinically recognized coronary heart disease

Source	Habitual frequency of high-intensity exercise	Overall (24 hour) incidence of sudden cardiac death (per 10^8 person-hours)	Relative risk during high-intensity exercise	
			Mean	95% confidence limits
Thompson et al. (1982)	High or very high	Not known	3.5	2–13
Siscovick et al. (1984)	Very high	5	5	2–14
	High	6	13	5–32
	Low	14	56	23–131
	Nil	18	—	—

Prevention

Exercise electrocardiography has been advocated as a screening procedure for all middle-aged sportsmen. Those who support such a course admit that an appreciable number of those at risk would not be identified but point out that, among asymptomatic men, subsequent overt coronary disease is 10–20 times more common in those with an abnormal exercise ECG. The other side of the coin, however, is that, among asymptomatic men, more than 70 per cent of those with an abnormal exercise ECG will have arteriographically normal coronary arteries, normal thallium perfusion scintigraphy, and will not develop overt coronary disease within the next 5 years. To have a chance of postponing the death of one asymptomatic middle-aged jogger per year, one would have to perform at least 15 000 tests, 10 per cent of which would be abnormal. This implies at least 1000 false-positives, an epidemic of iatrogenic cardiac handicap.

Medical evaluation is not a prerequisite for exercise training unless there are symptoms suggestive of myocardial ischaemia, strongly positive risk factors for coronary disease, a family history of premature sudden death, or a personal history of exercise-induced syncope. Instead, anyone unaccustomed to vigorous exercise should be taught that its intensity should at first be modest and should then increase only gradually. The exercising public should also be taught how to recognize symptoms suggestive of underlying cardiac disease and to seek medical advice should they occur.

Sports injuries

Direct soft-tissue trauma

Many sports put the participants at risk of direct trauma to muscle, tendon, ligament, and subcutaneous tissues by contact with the ground, the opponent, a ball or an opponent's bat or stick. Strict enforcement of the rules, a properly prepared playing surface, and tuition in the skills of the sport will prevent some of these injuries but they can never be completely avoided.

Acute treatment

Much of the pain and disability resulting from soft-tissue trauma is due not to the injury itself but to bleeding in and around the damaged tissues. Extravasated blood causes pain and limitation of movement at first by a space-occupying effect, then by causing local inflammation. Later, rehabilitation is hindered by fibrotic adhesions. Acute management concentrates on preventing this sequence of events.

The prevention of bleeding depends on ice, compression, and elevation (mnemonic 'ICE'). The local application of cold for 10–20 min will induce vasoconstriction and has the added benefit of relieving pain. Venous hydrostatic pressure at the site of injury is reduced by elevation of the injured limb for 2–24 hours. Extravasation of blood is limited by a compression bandage applied immediately the ice is removed, and maintained for 2–24 hours. Consider the contrast with the usual sequence of events after injury. After encouraging further bleeding by attempting to play on, the injured player retires from the game and maintains vasodilation by soaking in a hot bath. This is followed by a couple of hours standing, or at best sitting, enjoying a drink of vasodilating alcohol. Then he wonders why the sprained ankle is swollen, stiff, and painful the next day. Elevation is not only the simplest of the three measures to implement, it is probably also the most important and the most neglected.

Recovery is faster if a non-steroidal anti-inflammatory agent is administered, in full dosage, for the first 3–5 days after soft-tissue injury. There may be an advantage in starting treatment with a double strength 'loading' dose but this has not been demonstrated in a trial. It would be hard to justify such a practice in a patient with a history of dyspepsia. Indeed, this would be a relative contraindication to the use of an anti-inflammatory, even in normal dosage, to treat an acute injury.

Muscle and tendon Acute management follows the standard general guidelines. Prompt orthopaedic advice should be obtained if there is complete or substantial (say over 50 per cent) rupture. A palpable defect is an indication for orthopaedic referral, although not necessarily for surgery.

The patient with a large inter- or intramuscular haematoma should be immobilized for 24–48 hours, if necessary by admission to hospital. Compression and immobilization of the elevated limb can be achieved by a padded compression bandage or by the evacuation of air from a flexible bag of polystyrene beads fitted snugly around it. On the rare occasions when decompression is required, this can be done with a large bore needle under ultrasonographic guidance.

Ligament and joint The same general guidelines apply. Complete rupture (as indicated by joint instability or subluxation) requires orthopaedic referral. It may be possible to demonstrate instability only by stress X-rays taken under anaesthesia. Orthopaedic advice should also be obtained if there is any block to knee movement, implying the possibility of meniscal injury.

The accumulation of fluid within the first hour after injury implies haemorrhage, most often due, in the knee, to partial or complete tears of the anterior cruciate ligament and/or a meniscus. Prompt orthopaedic referral is indicated, with a view to early arthroscopy; some anterior cruciate tears are operable if diagnosed sufficiently early. Remember that a torn joint capsule (e.g. a torn collateral ligament) may accompany the cruciate ligament injury and will allow blood to escape from the knee joint, making the haemarthrosis less obvious.

Rehabilitation
Absolute rest is usually inappropriate after the first 24 hours. The indiscriminate use of plaster casts and similar devices is to be deprecated. Rather than immobilization, it is better to think in terms of selective, graded, and protected activity. A hinged brace may be helpful, allowing free movement within a predetermined range and plane.

The first aim is to preserve maximal movement and strength without disturbing the soft, new scar forming across the deficit in the torn tissue. As the scar matures, it is necessary to stimulate remodelling of its randomly oriented collagen into the organized orientation which will give maximal mechanical strength in the direction of future imposed stresses. This requires the regular controlled application of gradually increasing tension in the same direction(s). Isometric muscle contractions should be started 24 hours after injury, gradually increasing in intensity. Passive movement should begin at the same time, gradually increasing in range and progressing to forceful but controlled stretch.

Before return to competition can be permitted, balance and co-ordination skills, both conscious and unconscious, must be relearned. This requires the careful introduction of controlled dynamic activity, increasing gradually in both intensity and complexity. Especially in the case of severe ligament injuries, the 'relearning' of skills may depend, in part, on the regeneration of sensory nerve endings.

It is not clear why some muscle haematomata should ossify (myositis ossificans). Rebleeding, due to overvigorous activity, may be a factor; activity should be kept within the limits imposed by pain.

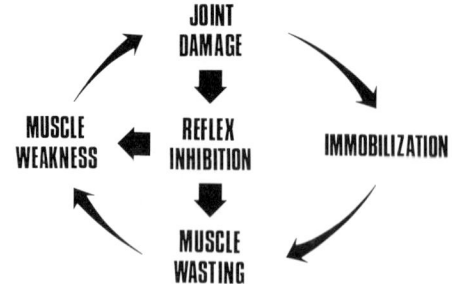

Fig. 1 'Vicious circles', of joint damage and muscle weakness. (Reproduced from Stokes and Young, 1984, *Clin. Sci.* **67**, 7, by permission of The Biochemical Society.)

Joint injury and muscle weakness Rehabilitation may be complicated by severe weakness of muscles acting across damaged joints. This is due partly to atrophy and partly to reflex inhibition of anterior horn cells by afferent stimuli arising in and around the joint (Fig. 1).

Ultrasound scanning and computerized tomography have shown that thigh muscle atrophy after knee injury is so localized to the quadriceps that its severity cannot be predicted accurately from measurements of thigh circumference. It is not unusual for the quadriceps to shrink by 30–50 per cent. There is a widespread belief that vastus medialis is more susceptible to atrophy than the rest of the quadriceps. This is not supported by the evidence; the atrophy is merely more obvious. It is also often said that vastus medialis is active only in the last 15° of extension. This too is false, although its activity is especially important towards full extension since it maintains patellar alignment. Inability to achieve full voluntary knee extension against gravity reflects quadriceps weakness and a mechanically disadvantageous position, not selective weakness of vastus medialis. Despite its severity, quadriceps wasting may be explained entirely by shrinkage of muscle fibres; simultaneous scans and biopsies suggest that there is no reduction in the number of muscle fibres. Full recovery of muscle mass should, therefore, be possible.

Reflex inhibition of quadriceps may be a very potent phenomenon. Even in the absence of perceived pain, a maximal effort may achieve only 10 per cent of the muscle's normal maximal activation. The experimental infusion of sterile saline into a normal subject's knee has a similar effect. Substantial inhibition may be produced by the infusion of as little as 20 ml, a volume which is barely detectable clinically. Even with a normal knee, patients may suffer quadriceps weakness and wasting as a result of inhibitory afferent stimuli arising in a periarticular lesion. This can be demonstrated by measuring the maximal surface EMG activity generated by voluntary efforts before and after infiltration of the suspected inhibitory source with local anaesthetic.

The fact that the quadriceps may be severely inhibited in the absence of any perceived pain has considerable implications for the resumption of full sporting activity. Even an apparently trivial knee effusion may weaken the quadriceps sufficiently to increase greatly its susceptibility to further injury. A similar argument probably applies at other joints.

Overuse injuries
Growing public enthusiasm for sport, and for distance running in particular, has increased the frequency with which stress fractures and friction syndromes (peritendinitis, tenosynovitis, and periostitis) are encountered in everyday practice (Fig. 2). To differentiate between them one must establish not only the pain's site, nature, distribution, speed of onset, and persistence after exercise, but also its timing in each stride, the effect of different speeds, terrains, and gradients, and the separate effects of joint angle and weight-bearing.

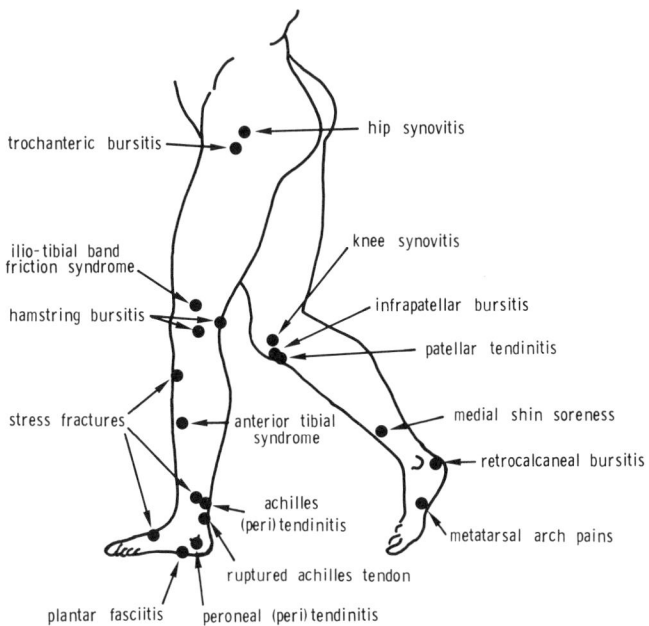

Fig. 2 Common sites of exercise injuries in joggers and runners. (Reproduced from Young, 1983, in *Preventive medicine in general practice*, eds M. Gray and G. Fowler, Oxford University Press, p. 160.)

In the recreational athlete the explanation is usually 'too much too soon'. In the experienced elite performer it is 'too much, too long, and too often'. Other factors may be a change of footwear, terrain or running speed. Overuse injuries are treated by rest, relief of local inflammation and the gradual reintroduction of controlled and protected activity. If recurrence is to be prevented, it is important also to ensure that the future training load is controlled more carefully and adjusted more gradually. For example, changes from endurance running to sprinting, or from road to track must be gradual. Shoes should be examined for the adequacy of arch support and heel-cushioning. The squash racket's handle should be thickened to prevent further strains of the common extensor origin. The swimmer's arm action should be analysed to reduce impingement of rotator cuff tendons on the coraco-acromial arch. The road runner should be advised to interpose the occasional run on grass.

Stress fracture
The repeated application of stress to a bone may result in a 'fatigue' or 'stress' fracture. The commonest sites are the tibia, the distal fibula, and the 2nd and 3rd metatarsals. Femoral stress fractures are also encountered, neck and shaft fractures being about equally common. There is no history of acute trauma, there need not be any pain at rest, and X-rays may at first appear normal. Later, however, the X-ray may show callus formation (Fig. 3). A bone scintigram may be necessary to confirm the diagnosis when the X-ray is negative. A simpler 'bed-side' test is the sharp pain produced by insonation of the suspect area of bone with a physiotherapist's ultrasound applicator. This may be particularly useful in order to distinguish between a tibial stress fracture and medial shin soreness. The latter is a common complaint, probably due to periostitis, presenting as localized pain and tenderness on the medial edge of the distal tibial shaft, requiring a shorter period of rest than a stress fracture and responding to oral anti-inflammatories, local steroid injection, and local ultrasound.

The immediate aims of treatment are to avoid complete fracture and to allow the bone to mend. This requires abstinence from running (Table 2). Weight-bearing should be avoided if it is painful. Casting is rarely required. Stress fractures of the femoral neck do not usually require internal fixation but orthopaedic advice should be obtained. Strength and endurance should be maintained by iso-

metric exercises and by a change of activity, for example, to cycling (for metatarsal or fibular fractures) or to swimming.

Friction syndromes
The local inflammatory response to overuse may be evident, with pain, swelling, discolouration, warmth, and palpable (or even audible) crepitation. Sometimes, however, examination may reveal little or nothing. Re-examination immediately after a provocation run may then be helpful.

There are few patients in whom the problem cannot be resolved by an oral non-steroidal anti-flammatory drug, possibly a local injection of steroid, 1–2 weeks relative rest, stretching, isometric strengthening, and the gradual resumption of activity. (Note that injection into the substance of a tendon should usually be avoided less it predispose to rupture.) Stretching is important to prevent local fibrosis and adhesions, especially within a stenosed tendon sheath. Surgical decompression is occasionally required to relieve

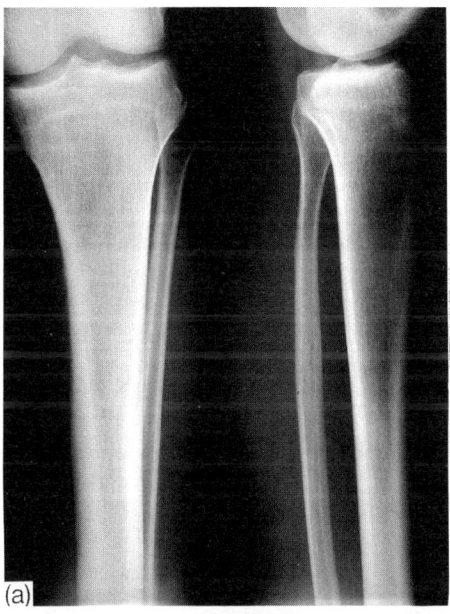

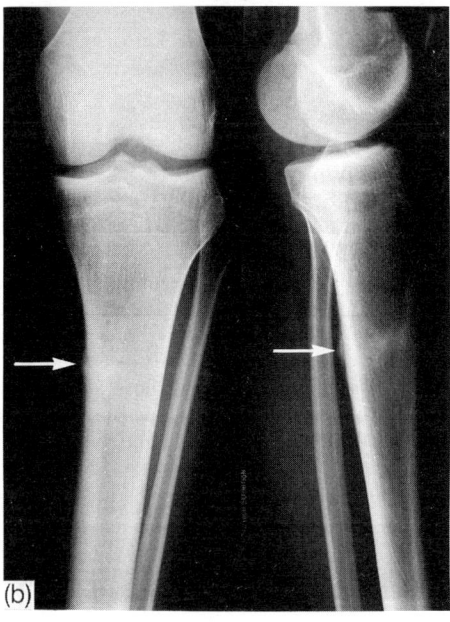

Fig. 3 (a) A normal X-ray does not exclude the possibility of a stress fracture. (b) A further X-ray 2 weeks later may show evidence of callus formation. (Reproduced from Young and Green, 1985, *Update* **30**, 1132.)

Table 2 Stress fracture: recommended periods of abstinence from running

Metatarsal	2–4 weeks
Fibula	3–4 weeks
Tibial shaft	4–6 weeks
Proximal tibia	8–10 weeks
Femur	3–4 months
Others	Individual

From Orava, 1980, *Br. J. Sports Med.* **14**, 40–44.

achilles peritendinitis, synovitis of the extensor tendons of the oarsman's forearm, or ilio-tibial band friction.

The ilio-tibial band friction syndrome seems to cause unnecessary diagnostic difficulty, sometimes even being mistaken for a lesion of the lateral meniscus. Tendoperiostitis develops where the ilio-tibial band passes over the lateral femoral epicondyle and also has a small insertion into it. The pain usually starts after 1 or 2 miles and becomes steadily worse. It may radiate proximally to the thigh or distally to the tibia. Running downhill, in heavy boots, in a tight circle, or with the foot inverted (e.g. to relieve a blister) may all be precipitating factors. Pain usually subsides rapidly after exercise but may still be felt for a day or two when using stairs. The diagnosis is confirmed by passively flexing the knee while maintaining thumb pressure over the lateral femoral epicondyle; tenderness is observed between 30° and 60° of flexion, as the ilio-tibial band passes between the bony prominence and the examining thumb.

Enthesitis

Inflammation at a tendon's point of insertion into bone (e.g. tennis elbow) is the result of repeated partial tears and subacute local inflammation. The principles of management include a combination of those for a tendon tear and for an overuse injury.

Endurance sports

Aerobic fitness

Aerobic exercise is exercise whose oxygen requirements, after the initial adjustment period, are met in full while it is being performed. It can be continued, therefore, for periods upwards of 5 min. During a bout of aerobic exercise there are increases in pulmonary ventilation, cardiac output, and muscle blood flow so that the transport of oxygen from the atmosphere to the working muscles can be maintained at a level sufficient to meet the muscles' requirements. Repeated bouts of aerobic exercise produce adaptations throughout the oxygen transport system so that the oxygen demands of future exercise can be met with less disturbance of the resting state. This improvement in the homoeostasis of the oxygen transport system is associated with a reduced subjective perception of exertion.

It seems highly likely that regular vigorous aerobic activity can contribute to the prevention of coronary heart disease. There is no doubt that it improves exercise performance and exercise tolerance both in health and even in the presence of angina pectoris, intermittent claudication or chronic airflow obstruction, making the performance of ordinary everyday activities significantly easier. It improves glucose tolerance, contributes to weight control, and may even promote a sense of well-being and 'positive health'. These health benefits depend on the 'training' exercise being repeated regularly and being more vigorous than that encountered in everyday life. To induce a training effect, there must be overload. Hence the medical value of sport.

Measurement

The physiologist's traditional measure of aerobic fitness is the aerobic power or maximal oxygen uptake ($\dot{V}O_2$ max), i.e. the greatest rate at which a person can utilize atmospheric oxygen during

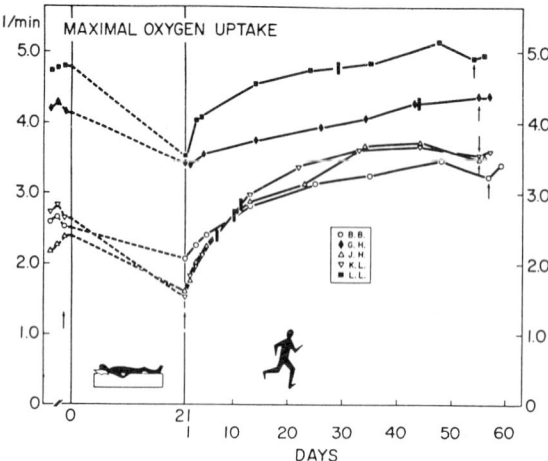

Fig. 4 Changes in maximal oxygen uptakes of five subjects before and after bed rest and at various intervals during training. (Reproduced from Saltin *et al.*, 1968, *Circulation* **38**, Suppl. VII, by permission of the author and the American Heart Association.)

continuous exercise. Aerobic training increases $\dot{V}O_2$ max: inactivity, such as bed rest, reduces it. These changes are quite rapid; 10–30 per cent changes may occur within a few weeks and, in extreme cases, a 100 per cent change may occur within 2–3 months of a major change in habitual physical activity (Fig. 4).

Most current tests of aerobic fitness, whether based on a treadmill, step-test or cycle ergometer, depend on measuring $\dot{V}O_2$ max, or some index from which it can be predicted. Even tests which measure the rate of heart rate recovery after exercise are indirect indicators of $\dot{V}O_2$ max. A typical $\dot{V}O_2$ max for a 20-year-old man might be 45 ml/kg/min. An elite endurance athlete might have a value of 70–80 ml/kg/min. Less than half of the difference between these values can be ascribed to the effects of training. The rest reflects the elite performer's congenital advantage over the average person.

The ability to sustain exercise at a fixed submaximal proportion of $\dot{V}O_2$ max is probably a more sensitive indicator of an individual's state of training (i.e. the extent to which he or she has realized their personal potential for aerobic fitness). Aerobic 'capacity' is more sensitive to training than aerobic 'power'. The time for which exercise can be sustained at, say, 75 per cent $\dot{V}O_2$ max may increase by 200–500 per cent when $\dot{V}O_2$ max has only increased by 5–20 per cent. The improvements in performance experienced by the recreational runner or jogger probably owe more to improvement in this 'endurance' aspect of aerobic fitness than to any increase in $\dot{V}O_2$ max. For the elite performer its importance is that he may be able to utilize 75–85 per cent of his $\dot{V}O_2$ max throughout most of a marathon instead of 60–70 per cent when only moderately trained. Other than by testing subjects to exhaustion, this aspect of aerobic fitness can be assessed by measuring the percentage of $\dot{V}O_2$ max that can be attained without stimulating anaerobic glycolysis, i.e. without significant accumulation of lactate. For example, a recreational runner's preparation for a marathon produced no change in his $\dot{V}O_2$ max but the work-rate corresponding to a blood lactate of 2 mM increased from 75 per cent to 82 per cent of his $\dot{V}O_2$ max and the running speed corresponding to 2 mM improved from 8.2 mph (7 min 19 s per mile) to 9.0 mph (6 min 40 s per mile) (Professor C. Williams, personal communication).

Central mechanisms

Maximal oxygen uptake is closely linked with maximal cardiac output. Since training produces little change in maximal heart rate (if anything, it reduces it), the increase in $\dot{V}O_2$ max with training is closely related to the increase in stroke volume. Not only does the heart get bigger, ventricular emptying during exercise becomes more complete. The trained person can achieve a greater cardiac ouput (and therefore a greater oxygen uptake) at any given heart rate.

Peripheral mechanisms

Trained muscles are better able to extract oxygen from their blood supply. The size and number of mitochondria and the density of muscle capillaries are increased, with the result that diffusion distances and capillary flow velocities are reduced. Thus the trained muscle requires a smaller total blood flow to achieve the same rate of oxygen consumption. The larger mitochondrial fraction is associated with a substantially increased muscle content of oxidative enzymes, ensuring that the muscle can utilize the enhanced availability of oxygen. These, incidentally, are the mechanisms behind the improvement in walking distance which the patient with stable intermittent claudication can achieve by training; the total blood supply to the claudicating muscle is not increased, only the muscle's ability to extract oxygen from it.

These changes are strictly local; they are more pronounced in the muscles, and even in the individual muscle fibres, which were used most during the training exercise. After one-legged training an exercise test with the trained leg shows the expected increase in $\dot{V}O_2$ max, in stroke volume, and in power output at a fixed submaximal heart rate. During exercise with the untrained leg, however, these indices remain close to their control values. Similarly, arm training reduces the heart rate response to arm work but not to leg work, whereas leg training reduces the heart rate response to leg work but not to arm work.

It is not long since the pendulum swung from central to peripheral factors as chief determinants of the upper limit to the training-induced improvement in $\dot{V}O_2$ max. The apparent dominance of peripheral factors, however, has now been challenged by recent experiments in which maximal exercise was performed by a limited mass of muscle. These have shown that muscle is capable of an oxygen uptake (per unit muscle mass) much greater than that achieved in whole body exercise. The current consensus is that the increase in $\dot{V}O_2$ max with training is limited by the improvement possible in circulatory haemodynamics, that is, by the increase in cardiac output and by its improved distribution. The prime role of the peripheral adaptations is believed to be metabolic. The release of energy by oxidation of fat 'costs' more oxygen than by oxidation of carbohydrate. The peripheral adaptations allow greater use of lipid oxidation as a source of energy during prolonged exercise, sparing the relatively limited glycogen stores and postponing fatigue. The shorter capillary–mitochondrion diffusion distance may facilitate free fatty acid uptake. The enzymes required for translocation of free fatty acids into the mitochondria and for their β-oxidation are increased. The increased capillary density also means that lipoprotein lipase activity is increased, possibly allowing greater utilization of circulating triglycerides during exercise. (Increased lipoprotein lipase activity may also explain the apparently 'cardioprotective' increase in the proportion of high density/low density lipoproteins seen in those undertaking regular vigorous aerobic exercise.)

Carbohydrate metabolism

Glycogen loading

Carbohydrate is stored in the body as glycogen, usually about 100 g in the liver and 350 g in muscle. The quadriceps glycogen of trained volunteers is completely depleted after about 90 min of strenuous pedalling. The availability of muscle glycogen becomes limited during the second half of a marathon ('hitting the wall'). The runner then relies more on fat as the fuel and is unable to sustain the same high percentage of $\dot{V}O_2$ max. (In a 24 hour run, power output falls to about 50 per cent $\dot{V}O_2$ max.)

It has been known for over 50 years that a low, or high, carbohydrate diet can substantially reduce, or increase, the time for which submaximal exercise (say about 70 per cent $\dot{V}O_2$ max) can be continued. More recently, it has been shown that the time to

exhaustion when pedalling depends on the quadriceps' initial glycogen content. Furthermore, if exercise to exhaustion is followed by 2–3 days on a diet rich in carbohydrate, the muscle glycogen store is not only restored but shows a 'rebound' effect, reaching double its normal concentration. A classical study used one-legged pedalling to demonstrate that glycogen depletion and rebound super-repletion are both confined to the muscle which has been exercised.

The marathon-running fraternity has been rather uncritical in its adoption of a pre-race regimen involving exhaustive exercise followed by 3 days on a low carbohydrate diet and then 3 days on a high carbohydrate diet. The low carbohydrate period is probably unnecessary. Moreover, the typical elite marathon runner probably exhausts the muscle glycogen at least twice a week and will usually start a race with a supranormal muscle glycogen concentration, without any dietary manipulation. It is probably sufficient for the endurance athlete to taper training for 2–4 days before the race and to eat a diet rich in carbohydrate (and with a correspondingly reduced protein content). Complex carbohydrate is preferred since slow absorption encourages glycogen storage rather than incorporation into fat.

Additional glucose

Before exercise There is a strong temptation to consume sugar or glucose just before the start of endurance exercise. This is not a good idea, however, as it suppresses fatty acid mobilization and so hastens exhaustion of muscle glycogen. Fatty acid mobilization depends not only on circulating adrenaline (high levels before and during a race) but also on the progressive suppression of insulin release as the exercise proceeds. The latter mechanism is inhibited by the absorption of a carbohydrate load just before the start of the exercise. Easily digestible carbohydrate should be consumed no later than 3 hours before the start.

Pre-exercise caffeine, as strong coffee, may enhance endurance performance by its lipolytic effect, increasing the availability of fatty acids to muscle. For many people, however, any benefit is more than counterbalanced by the disadvantages of its diuretic effect. Laboratory findings cannot always be applied in real life.

During exercise Endurance is improved by the ingestion of glucose in the later stages of prolonged exercise, for example, after the first hour of a marathon. This does not cause secretion of insulin, perhaps because of the high circulating level of adrenaline. The effectiveness of oral glucose depends also on the rate of gastric emptying and the rate of intestinal absorption. The higher the carbohydrate concentration of the fluid, the slower the stomach empties. To try and give a high concentration of glucose may be counterproductive. During heavy exercise the maximal rate of gastric emptying is about 25 ml/min. Moreover, an overfull stomach empties more slowly. Thus, to try and give a large volume of dilute glucose solution may also be counterproductive. It seems best to take small frequent drinks of a solution containing no more than 5 g of glucose/100 ml water.

Some exercise-induced 'abnormalities'

Amenorrhoea

Oligomenorrhoea and amenorrhoea are commoner among distance runners than among non-exercising women. Contributory factors include low body weight, loss of body fat, and perhaps also the emotional stresses associated with a time-consuming training schedule and with competition. It seems clear, however, that exercise itself has an independent effect. Weekly mileage correlates positively with the prevalence of amenorrhoea and negatively with the length of the luteal phase of the menstrual cycle. In some individuals, menstruation may be restored by an injury-induced break from exercise even if weight gain is carefully avoided. The most telling evidence, however, comes from a prospective study in which 28 previously untrained women followed a 2 month programme of progressive training. Abnormalities of luteal function were as common among those who allowed their weight to fall as among those who deliberately maintained a constant weight, affecting over 60 per cent of both groups of women. Even in the constant weight group, nearly half the women lost the 'surge' of luteinizing hormone (LH). Nevertheless, there is also an interaction with weight loss; both delay of the menses and loss of the LH surge were commoner in the weight-loss group.

When consulted by the amenorrhoeic runner, it is as well to remember that runners are susceptible to all the other causes of amenorrhoea. Pregnancy was the commonest reason for withdrawal from the 1984 London marathon during the 4 months before the event. If pregnancy testing is negative and menstruation does not resume when mileage is temporarily reduced, full investigation is essential (page 10.85).

A shortened luteal phase is unlikely to be harmful, and is also unlikely to be detected without specific assessment. Should this progress to loss of ovulation but continuing oestrogen production, however, there is a theoretical risk of endometrial hyperplasia and adenocarcinoma by the action of oestrogen on an endometrium unprotected by progesterone. Cyclical treatment with a progesterone analogue might be justifiable, under specialist guidance.

Exercise-induced hypogonadism may be even more pronounced, so that oestrogen levels are suppressed. Since the urogenital epithelium is oestrogen dependent, this may increase the likelihood of urethritis and atrophic vaginitis. More important, there is also the possibility of bone atrophy, analogous to the acceleration of calcium loss after the normal menopause. Despite the fact that regular exercise can slow bone loss in elderly women, there is the paradoxical possibility that hypooestrogenic amenorrhoea induced by severe exercise may accelerate bone loss in young women. Cyclical administration of an oestrogen and a progestagen has been advocated but, until the topic is better understood, should not be started without specialist advice.

Finally, it is reassuring to note that exercise-induced amenorrhoea appears to cause no impairment of future fertility.

Anaemia

Iron-deficiency anaemia impairs the aerobic exercise performance of untrained men. In well-trained endurance athletes, although total body haemoglobin is increased, haemoglobin concentration, serum iron, serum ferritin, transferrin saturation, and bone-marrow haemosiderin are all lower than normal. Haematocrit may be 5–10 per cent less than in matched controls.

'Sports anaemia' has usually been attributed to iron deficiency, perhaps because of iron losses in sweat or in repeated bouts of haemoglobinuria. New data suggest that this is not the case. It is suggested that prolonged running results in a slight increase in intravascular haemolysis. The resulting haemoglobin–haptoglobin complex is taken up by hepatocytes. This shift in red cell catabolism from the reticulo-endothelial system to hepatocytes may explain the reduced haemosiderin content of the distance runner's bone-marrow. The 'anaemia' itself, it is suggested, is a normal, but apparently unfavourable, physiological response to prolonged periods of high intensity exercise with a high degree of oxygen extraction from haemoglobin. This would increase the concentration of 2,3-DPG in red cells, shifting the oxyhaemoglobin dissociation curve to the right. This in turn may lead to erythropoietin production being reduced, so that the oxygen delivery capacity of arterial blood remains constant. There is no reason to treat 'sports anaemia' with iron.

Rhabdomyolysis

(See also Section 18)

'Physiological' The high levels of creatine kinase (CK) and other muscle proteins in plasma for several days after strenuous exercise, such as marathon running (Fig. 5), are due to leakage of protein from skeletal muscle. They may be associated with microscopic mechanical disruption of muscle cells, especially after

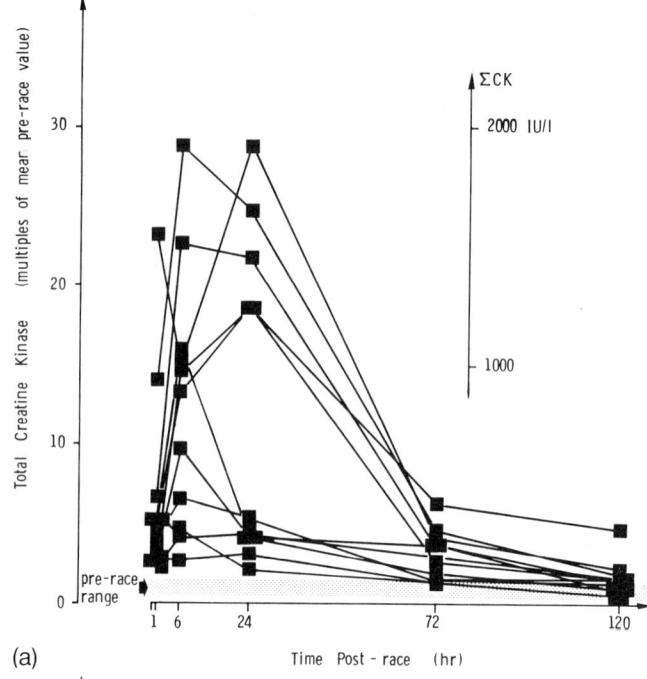

(a)

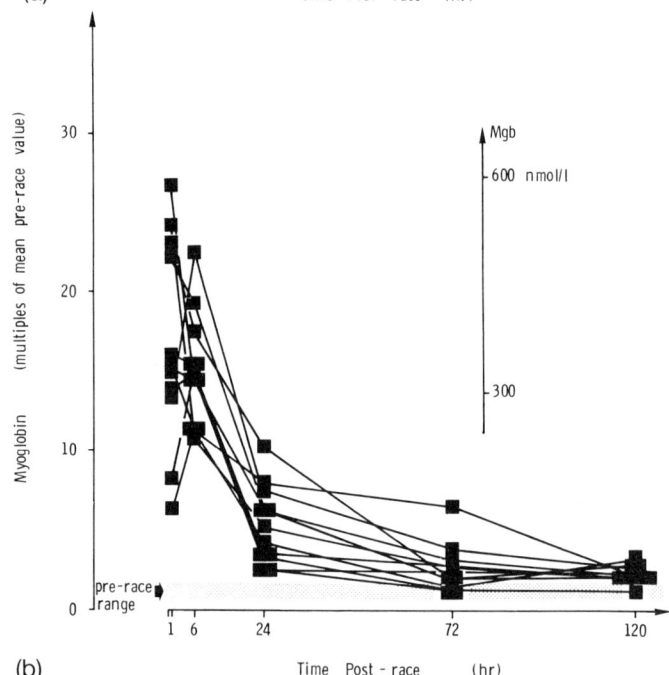

(b)

Fig. 5 Changes in (a) serum total CK and (b) plasma myoglobin in young men who had completed a marathon (running times: mean = 194 min, range = 163–280 min). (Data of Young *et al.*, 1984, *Eur. J. Clin. Invest.* **14**, 2(II), 58.)

downhill running or other exercise involving lengthening of active muscles ('eccentric' contractions). There is no evidence that marathon running damages a healthy, well-perfused myocardium, despite the fact that post-race plasma levels of CK, myoglobin, aspartate transaminase, lactate dehydrogenase, and tropomyosin normally rise to the same extent as after myocardial infarction. Increased circulating levels of the so-called 'cardiac-specific' isoenzyme CK-MB, of the ratio of CK-MB to total CK, and of the cardiac-specific LDH isoenzyme may be adequately explained by the increased proportion of these isoenzymes in endurance-trained muscles.

In the rare instance of a collapsed marathon runner who

requires admission to hospital, it may prove difficult to decide whether there is myocardial damage, especially if the normal electrocardiogram shows apparent abnormalities. The acute-phase protein response to marathon running is small but after longer distances it too may resemble the response to a small myocardial infarction. For the future, the radioimmunoassay for cardiac troponin-I may be able to distinguish between 'physiological' rhabdomyolysis and myocardial damage. In the meantime, however, the certain identification of myocardial injury or ischaemia in a marathon runner requires scintigraphic demonstration of technetium pyrophosphate uptake by myocardium or abnormalities of thallium perfusion imaging.

Major Catastrophic exertional rhabdomyolysis is rare, but may be life-threatening, as the release of large amounts of myoglobin causes acute tubular necrosis. Predisposing factors include dehydration, hyperthermia, and repeated eccentric contractions. The rapid and forceful eccentric quadriceps contractions which provide the decelerating force in squat jumps explain why this exercise has given its name to the potentially lethal exercise-induced rhabdomyolysis sometimes seen in military recruits undergoing their initial training ('squat jump syndrome'). Downhill running produces more muscle damage than uphill running.

An inborn deficiency of carnitine palmityl transferase may result in the very rare syndrome of recurring bouts of severe, exercise-induced rhabdomyolysis.

The patient will be nauseous, vomiting, and ill. The muscles may be swollen, tender, aching, and weak and there may be anuria or the passage of small quantities of 'Coca-cola' urine. Urine will be positive for 'blood' on strip-testing; microscopy will show no red cells but perhaps some pigment casts. Plasma creatine kinase levels will be hugely elevated, perhaps 100 times the upper limit of normal. The damaged muscle tissue takes up calcium and releases phosphate, creatine, and purines. The result is that, for a given degree of renal failure, the plasma calcium is unusually low and plasma levels of potassium, phosphate, creatinine, and urate are unusually high. Hospitalization and cardiac monitoring are mandatory, forced alkaline diuresis may facilitate myoglobin excretion, and the hyperkalaemia must be controlled. In some cases a period of dialysis is required (see Section 18).

Popular marathons and mass runs

The developed countries have seen an enormous upsurge in interest in endurance running, with fields of many hundreds or even thousands participating in events over courses from 10 km up to the full marathon distance of 26 miles 385 yards (42.2 km). In Britain, the number of full marathons per year has increased tenfold in 10 years. The increase in the number of participants per event has been even greater, reaching an average of about 1000 per full marathon. The corollary is that a very high proportion of participants are non-elite, inexperienced, and possibly underprepared. In half-marathons, not only are the numbers even bigger (more than 25 000 in the Great North Run), a higher proportion may be ill-prepared but set to 'have a go'. The experienced runners' training enables them to meet the homoeostatic challenges of prolonged running. They also know how to prevent undue strain or 'decompensation' when doing so, using pace judgement and technical knowledge, and 'listening to their bodies'. This may not be true for the participants in a mass run.

It is essential, therefore, that mass running events should have enough medical and paramedical personnel, trained and equipped to deal with hypovolaemia, hyperthermia, and hypothermia, and (in diabetic runners) hypoglycaemia. Local hospitals are unlikely to have to admit more than one or two runners, but must be party to the overall planning. Their staff must be warned of the biochemical derangements which are 'normal' after prolonged exercise, and should also be reminded of the essentials of management of exertional heat injury and acute rhabdomyolysis.

The positioning of medical facilities requires considerable care

and thought. The police and ambulance services must be asked to help plan for the occasional need for rapid evacuation (of a collapsed runner or of a local resident). The size and positioning of first aid posts and medical stations must take account of the stages of the race where most of the problems will arise, of the probable frequency of problems at each stage, and of the sheer numbers involved. Less than 0.1 per cent are likely to need detention in a race medical area but, with a field of 20 000, there may be 20 such 'collapses'. In order to ensure sufficient spare capacity, it is recommended that there should be provision for a 0.75 per cent collapse rate, including one intensive care bed per 10 000 runners.

Treatment for relatively trivial problems (blisters, cramps, chafing) will be required for only about 1 per cent but there should be provision, at the finish area, for a 5 per cent treatment rate plus first aid posts every 2–2½ miles around the course. These posts must also be able to cope with a 5–10 per cent (probably 5 per cent) contact rate, for non-medical 'treatments' such as new shoelaces, safety pins or encouragement/sympathy.

Medical responsibility for a mass run is not something to be undertaken lightly or at the last minute. The medical director must be involved in every stage of planning. For example, medical advice sheets should be sent to each entrant with the notification that their entry has been accepted. A sample advice sheet and fuller guidance on staffing numbers, preparation, and disposition are available elsewhere (Tunstall-Pedoe, 1984).

Hypovolaemia

Trained runners may lose as much as 5 or 6 per cent of body weight in the course of a marathon, representing perhaps 3–4 litres of fluid. Under hot conditions, fluid losses may be even greater. Maximal muscle blood flow and adequate cerebral blood flow are maintained, despite the reduction in plasma volume, by cutaneous and splanchnic vasoconstriction. There comes a point, however, when these mechanisms can no longer compensate for the loss of blood volume and may even cease to operate. This is especially likely when venous return is no longer maintained by the pumping action of the leg muscles. Relaxation of compensatory vasoconstriction may occur as much as 20 min after the finish, resulting in collapse if fluid losses have not been adequately restored in the meantime. (There is an analogy with the way that vasoconstriction can maintain blood pressure in the face of severe haemorrhage but may then suddenly fail just when all seems well.) The main medical post should be placed sufficiently beyond the finish line that the incoming tide of runners does not hinder staff carrying a shocked and collapsed runner from the clothing claim area. The organization of the finish area must be adequate for large numbers of athletes finishing together so that they are not required to stand still, queuing to pass the finish marshalls or to collect their clothes. (In the Great North Run, the peak period sees 500 runners per minute finishing together.)

Adequate fluid replacement during the run is, of course, the best way to prevent hypovolaemic collapse. The medical director is responsible for ensuring that the organizers provide sufficient drink stations and that the runners are educated in their importance. Runners should be fully hydrated at the start and should take additional fluid early in the race, before they feel thirsty. Water or a dilute glucose solution is recommended.

Hypovolaemia predisposes to hyperthermia (see below). The impaired physical performance of hypovolaemia may predispose to hypothermia (see below). Hypovolaemic collapse may both simulate and accompany either hypothermia or hyperthermia. Every confused or collapsed runner, with or without signs of peripheral circulatory collapse, must have their rectal temperature recorded.

Hypovolaemic collapse usually responds well to rest, leg elevation, and oral rehydration. Intravenous fluid is rarely required but is indicated in the confused or deteriorating patient or if fluid losses continue (by vomiting or diarrhoea, the result perhaps of overintense splanchnic vasoconstriction).

Hyperthermia

(See also Section 6.)

The rate of heat production while running is high; 75 per cent of the energy expended is converted to heat. When running fast, the rate of heat production may be greater than the body's capacity to dissipate heat. There are numerous, well-documented examples of rectal temperatures of 40–42 °C at least 10 min after running, even under rather mild environmental conditions and especially in the shorter events (10 km to half-marathon).

Sweating is the most important avenue of heat dissipation. Anything which impedes sweat loss will increase the risk of hyperthermia, for example, still or humid atmospheric conditions, excess clothing, or dehydration. Other predisposing factors may include a high ambient temperature, lack of fitness, obesity, age extremes, inadequate heat acclimatization, recent illness (e.g. cold or 'flu), previous history of heat stroke, or a susceptibility to malignant hyperthermia.

The prevention of heat injury depends, therefore, on education of participants and organizers and on adequate fluid replacement. The American College of Sports Medicine (1975) has provided guidelines, including the recommendation that an event should be cancelled if environmental conditions are such that WGPT >28 °C. (WGPT = 0.7 wet bulb temperature + 0.2 globe temperature + 0.1 dry bulb.) In the United Kingdom, where summer temperatures are lower than is usual in North America, runners will be less acclimatized and the cancellation threshold should probably be lower.

Runners and first aiders alike should be taught to recognize the early warnings of hyperthermia, such as piloerection, chilling, throbbing head, unsteadiness, nausea, and cessation of sweating. These need not be present, however, and the runner may continue to sweat profusely while deteriorating and developing a staggering gait, mental disturbance, and slurred speech. Even the unconscious patient with cold, clammy skin may well be hyperthermic. A rectal temperature is mandatory in any collapsed, confused or fitting runner.

The essentials of treatment are intravenous fluid replacement and heat loss. In order to promote the loss of heat by evaporation, the patient is shaded, stripped, wetted, and fanned. Cold water and cold air should not be used, as they would promote cutaneous vasoconstriction, impeding core-to-surface heat transfer. Both water and air should be applied at room temperature. Immersion in cold water is contraindicated but ice packs may be applied over major vessels in groins and axillae. These measures should be reduced when the rectal temperature is between 38 and 38.5 °C, lest there should be an overshoot into hypothermia.

Serious complications are managed along the lines described elsewhere in this book, e.g. rhabdomyolysis (see above and Section 18), acute tubular necrosis (Section 18), hepatic necrosis (Section 12), disseminated intravascular coagulation (Section 19) or haemorrhage (with hypoprothrombinaemia, hypofibrinogenaemia or thrombocytopenia) (Section 19).

Hypothermia

(See also section 6.)

Heat loss may outstrip heat production. Even in the same race, one runner may have a rectal temperature of >40 °C and another <36 °C. Factors predisposing to hypothermia include a low ambient temperature, rain, wind, ectomorphy, slow running speed, and inadequate clothing. Hypothermia is most likely to develop in the runners who are slowest over the second half of a marathon. Runners should be educated against setting off too fast; fatigue reduces the rate of metabolic heat production and increases the likelihood of hypothermia, especially if clothing has been discarded earlier in the race. A water- and windproof top layer which is light enough to be carried (e.g. a large polythene bag) may be a valuable preventive measure.

The hypothermic runner may present with impaired speech, thought or co-ordination. Rectal temperature must be measured; values below 36 °C require observation and below 34 °C demand close attention. Treatment is by removing wet clothing, thorough drying, dressing in adequate dry clothing and a reflective foil blanket, and warm drinks. The foil blanket used alone provides totally inadequate protection to runners who have finished and will not prevent post-race hypothermia if runners are denied immediate access to warm, dry clothing.

References

American College of Sports Medicine (1975). Position statement on prevention of heat injuries during distance running. *Med. Sci. Sport* **7**, vii–ix.

Åstrand, P. O. and Grimby, G. (eds) (1986). Physical activity in health and disease. *Acta. med. scand.* Suppl. (in press).

Bar-Or, O. (1983). *Pediatric sports medicine for the practitioner: from physiologic principles to clinical applications*. Springer-Verlag, New York.

Bullen, B. A., Skrinar, G. S., Beitins, I. Z., von Mering, G., Turnbull, B. A. and McArthur, J. W. (1985). Induction of menstrual disorders by strenuous exercise in untrained women. *N. Engl. J. Med.* **312**, 1349–1352.

Hallberg, L. and Magnusson, B. (1984). The etiology of 'sports anaemia'. *Acta. med. scand.* **216**, 145–148.

O'Donoghue, D. H. (1976). *Treatment of injuries to athletes* 3rd edn. W. B. Saunders, Philadelphia.

Siscovick, D. S., Weiss, N. S., Fletcher, R. H. and Lasky, T. (1984). The incidence of primary cardiac arrest during vigorous exercise. *N. Engl. J. Med.* **311**, 874–877.

Smith, A. *et al.* (eds) (1984). *Exercise, health and medicine: proceedings*. The Sports Council, London.

Stokes, M. and Young, A. (1984). The contribution of reflex inhibition to arthrogenous muscle weakness. *Clin. Sci.* **67**, 7–14.

Thomas, G. S., Lee, P. R., Franks, P. and Paffenbarger, R. S. (1981). *Exercise and health: the evidence and the implications*. Oelgeschlager, Gunn and Hain, Cambridge, Mass.

Thompson, P. D. (1982). Cardiovascular hazards of physical activity. In *Exercise and sport sciences reviews* Vol. 10, (ed. R. L. Terjung), pp. 208–235. Franklin Institute Press, Philadelphia.

Tunstall-Pedoe, D. (ed.) (1984). Popular marathons, half marathons, and other long distance runs: recommendations for medical support. *Br. med. J.* **288**, 1355–1359.

Uhl, G. S., Kay, T. N. and Hickman, J. R. (1981). Computer-enhanced thallium scintigrams in asymptomatic men with abnormal exercise tests. *Am. J. Cardiol.* **48**, 1037–1043.

Vinger, P. F. and Hoerner, E. F. (eds) (1981). *Sports injuries: the unthwarted epidemic*. John Wright P. S. G., Boston.

SECTION 27
MEDICINE IN OLD AGE

MEDICINE IN OLD AGE

F. I. CAIRD

Introduction

The medicine of old age requires separate treatment because special knowledge and skill is needed for the optimal management of many elderly patients. Disease processes occur against the background of age-related changes in all body systems. These changes, either singly or through interactions between them, result in impairment of homeostatic mechanisms, and in altered reactions to disease and to its treatment.

Altered reactions to disease manifest themselves in several ways. The elderly frequently fail to report illness, sometimes because of a misappreciation of the possible significance of symptoms, which they (and all too often their doctors) attribute to ageing. The symptoms of acute illness are often non-specific, so that common events such as confusion, falls, and incontinence, may each be due to a wide variety of diseases in several systems. Modification of symptoms may alter the presentation of disease, so that, for instance, conditions that are painful in middle-age may produce little or no pain in the elderly, though their relative silence is not evidence of lesser seriousness. Further major problems result from the multiplicity of pathological processes which may be found in the same individual. Multiple pathology may be due to chance, to the interaction of disorders in different body systems, or to the coexistence of disease processes with a common single cause (e.g. many years of cigarette smoking causing chronic airways obstruction, bronchial carcinoma, ischaemic heart disease, and peripheral vascular disease, all evident simultaneously in the same patient).

Nowhere are these differences more important than in the drug therapy of the elderly patient. Alterations in pharmacokinetics and pharmacodynamics result from age-related physiological changes and from disease processes. The physical and psychological consequences of disease, together with social factors such as isolation, make it very difficult for elderly people to comply accurately with drug regimens, particularly those involving multiple drugs and dose schedules. These vital facts must never be ignored in practice, though they receive little attention in many textbooks.

The optimum management of elderly patients also requires knowledge and skills related to rehabilitation, and the best use of hospital- and community-based medical and social resources. Rehabilitation is often regarded as an uninteresting aspect of medical care, best left to paramedical personnel, but to be effective it necessitates a detailed knowledge of the natural history of a wide range of medical conditions, together with the ability to organize and motivate a rehabilitation team. The best use of hospital-based resources includes an appreciation of the value of the Day Hospital, and of the indications for the use of and the limitations of community-based social services and voluntary resources. These are likely to vary considerably between systems of medical care in different countries, and also between different areas in the same medical care system, so that local knowledge is of great importance.

Finally, a vital part of a geriatrician's work, though not unduly time consuming, is the care of those elderly patients who cannot be discharged from hospital because of the severity of their disabilities. Maintenance of the standards of their environment and of nursing morale, and organizational skill and experience are important aspects of this, as is judgement in knowing what and when to treat and not to treat.

The physiology of ageing

Anatomical and physiological changes are described in almost every body system. They mostly begin in early or middle life, but their magnitude and practical importance vary considerably.

Central to an appreciation of the significance of many age-related physiological changes is the fact that body composition begins to alter at about the age of 40, with steady progression thereafter. There is a decline in lean body mass, and with it a fall in oxygen consumption, very largely attributable to a reduction in muscle bulk. Since body weight remains constant, or even increases slightly with age (at least until extreme old age), there must be an increase in body fat. This change in body composition may have important practical importance in pharmacokinetics, and is the background against which age-related changes in nutrition and in cardiovascular, respiratory, and renal function, and the tests for them, must be set.

The blood volume falls with age, and there is a slight decline in haemoglobin concentration, more evident in women than men, so that in elderly women a haemoglobin concentration in the range 11.5–11.9 g/dl is not evidence of anaemia. The structure and composition of red cells and the dynamics of haemopoiesis remain unaltered. The white cell count falls slightly, the principal decrease being in the lymphocyte count, but the platelet count and function are unaltered.

Normal values for the elderly for some common biochemical measurements are given in Table 1. The concentrations of major electrolytes are unaffected by age except for a tendency for the mean serum calcium to decline. Before the menopause, serum calcium concentrations are lower in women than men, and after that age higher; this probably reflects the loss at the menopause of the restraining influence of oestrogens on parathyroid activity. There is a very small reduction in serum albumin concentration, which is not clinically significant in healthy elderly people; the greater reduction in many elderly in hospital is due to the effects of disease, and not to ageing.

The principal anatomical alterations in the cardiovascular system include an increase in the amount of fibrous tissue in the skeleton of the heart and in the myocardium and valves, an accumulation of lipofuscin in the myocardial fibres (a change of no evident functional significance), and a decrease in the elasticity of

Table 1 Normal values for biochemical measurements in old age

	Men	Women
(i) Ranges (mean ± s.d.)		
Total protein (g/l)	71 ± 5	71 ± 5
Albumin (g/l)	40 ± 4	42 ± 4
Globulin (g/l)	32 ± 6	30 ± 5
Serum calcium (mmol/l)	2.4 ± 0.1	2.5 ± 0.1
Serum phosphate (mmol/l)	0.99 ± 0.16	1.09 ± 0.19
Serum urate (mmol/l)	0.32 ± 0.07	0.30 ± 0.09
(ii) Upper limits of normal		
Serum urea (mmol/l)	10	10
Serum creatinine (μmol/l)	160	160
Serum cholesterol (mmol/l)	9	12
Serum bilirubin (μmol/l)	23	20
(iii) Values unchanged from those for middle age		
Serum sodium, potassium, magnesium, chloride, bicarbonate		

the aorta and its main branches, accompanied by an increase in their diameter and length. Interpretation of changes in cardiovascular function in old age is made difficult by the very high prevalence of unequivocal heart disease (at least 50 per cent). There is no doubt of a minor decline of resting heart rate, and of greater changes in intrinsic heart rate (i.e. the heart rate after combined sympathetic and parasympathetic blockade), and in maximum heart rate on exercise; these changes probably relate to a decrease in the number of pacemaker cells in the sinoatrial node, and to alterations in their reactivity to sympathetic and parasympathetic stimuli. Cardiac output at rest falls with age, approximately in proportion to the reduction in basal oxygen consumption, so that the mean arteriovenous oxygen difference is unaltered. Pulmonary vascular pressures are unchanged (except for a slight rise on exercise), as is pulmonary blood volume. The mean systemic arterial pressure rises in most, but not all populations; it cannot therefore be a true age change, but according to one hypothesis may, in a proportion of elderly hypertensives, represent the response of susceptible people to excessive salt intake. The rate of rise with age of systolic arterial pressure is greater than that of diastolic; this increase in pulse pressure is an expression of the reduced elasticity of the aortic compression chamber.

The interpretation of respiratory function changes with age is complicated by the high prevalence of cigarette smoking. Total lung volume does not alter, but vital capacity falls and residual volume increases with age, so that over the age of about 60 the critical closing volume exceeds the functional residual volume. Ventilatory capacity falls with age, at a lesser rate in non-smokers than smokers. Ventilation–perfusion inequality increases slightly, probably mainly as a result of increasing inequality of ventilation. These changes in lung function reflect a decrease in elasticity of the lungs and in respiratory muscular strength, but their overall consequences are minimal in terms of their effects upon the blood gases, doubtless because they do not exceed the age-related changes in oxygen consumption and carbon-dioxide production.

Age changes in renal function are well documented. The glomerular filtration rate falls by approximately 1 per cent per year over the age of 40, as do tubular reabsorptive and secretory capacities. These changes exceed the decline in lean body mass, so that serum urea and creatinine concentrations rise. The response to an acid load is impaired, and the maximum rate of secretion of hydrogen ion falls; changes in blood pH in response to an acid load are thus greater in magnitude and longer in duration than in younger people. The response to antidiuretic hormone is reduced, and water conservation thus less efficient. The mechanism of these alterations is unknown, but the characteristic sclerosis of glomeruli with associated tubular atrophy may be due to hyperfiltration damage related to a persistently high dietary protein intake. These changes of renal function with age are particularly important in the field of pharmacokinetics.

In the gastrointestinal tract, gastric atrophy becomes increasingly common as age advances, perhaps as a true age change, or as a consequence of progressive autoimmune damage to the gastric mucosa. Minor atrophic changes in the mucosa of the small bowel are described, and there is evidence of slight impairment of absorption of some nutrients. Reduction in the motility of the large bowel may be age-related, or may reflect such factors as the high frequency of diverticular disease or chronic purgative abuse.

Age-related changes in hepatic mass and cellular structure are probably unimportant, and changes in hepatic function, as measured by conventional tests such as serum bilirubin and hepatic enzymes, are also minor. Reduction in the hepatic metabolism of some drugs is, however, well documented.

The major changes with age in the bony skeleton are discussed in Section 17. It is uncertain whether the virtually universal occurrence of osteoarthritic changes in many joints is an effect of age, the response of joints to time-related wear and tear, or a disease process unrelated to age. Each of the three explanations is probably important in some patients and some joints.

In the endocrine system, apart from the obvious changes in ovarian function at the menopause, there are minor declines in circulating thyroid hormone levels, a reduction in the rate of secretion of insulin in response to raised blood sugar levels, and a decline in insulin sensitivity (i.e. in glucose disposition per unit of circulating insulin at a given blood glucose). The release of antidiuretic hormone in response to osmotic loads increases, perhaps in association with reduced renal responsiveness, but thirst is reduced in the elderly. There is little evidence of any abnormality of parathyroid, adrenal, or pituitary function in old age. The response of the adrenals and of ACTH secretion to stress is essentially unaltered.

Age changes in the nervous system are among the most important, because of their great significance in the psychology of ageing, and in the production of disorders of movement. Their anatomical basis is complex and as yet imperfectly understood. The numbers of neurones fall in some parts of the nervous system (e.g. the motoneurones of the spinal cord, the Purkinje cells of the cerebellum, and the cells of the substantia nigra and neocortex, the last to a variable degree in different cortical areas), but there are no changes in other parts (e.g. many clearly defined brain-stem nuclei). Anatomical abnormalities of the neurones that remain are also described, including the accumulation of lipofuscin and loss of dendrites and dendritic spines in cortical neurones. The anatomical basis of alterations in cortical function may thus be not only a reduction in number of neurones, but also in connections between them. There is a reduction in peripheral nerve-conduction velocities, both motor and sensory, differing in different nerves, and reflecting a fall-out of larger fibres.

Central autonomic nuclei (e.g. the intermediolateral cell column in the spinal cord) and first- and second-order autonomic neurones outside the central nervous system show a fall in cell numbers. Changes in autonomic function include alterations in heart rate (see above), and a striking frequency of abnormalities of temperature regulation. The threshold for appreciation of skin-temperature changes may increase by as much as ten-fold. This may be an important reason for old peoples' inability to recognize temperature change, and thus to respond by appropriate behaviour to falls in environmental temperature. There may also be failure of cutaneous vasoconstriction in response to cold, and of vasodilatation and sweating in response to increasing body temperature, the last perhaps due to reduction in the number of sweat glands. Failure of vasoconstriction is clearly important in reducing the response to falling core temperature, and thus making hypothermia more likely. The impairment of vasomotor and sudomotor response to heat will increase the likelihood of heatstroke.

Failure of the blood pressure to respond to postural change is also important. Baroreceptor responses are blunted, perhaps as a result of sclerotic changes in the carotid sinus, and there may in addition be failure of central and perhaps peripheral vasoconstrictor responses to falling blood pressure.

Age changes in the eye and ear are well documented. Decrease in elasticity of the lens begins very early in life, but only becomes symptomatic in the fifth decade, when presbyopic hypermetropia results from failure of accommodation, which is probably due to changes both in the lens itself and in its capsule and suspensory ligaments. High-tone deafness (presbyacusis) has several mechanisms, and is perhaps a true age change, though there is little doubt of the importance in many individuals of prolonged exposure to industrial and non-industrial noise. Impaired vestibular function is also described.

Clinical assessment of the elderly patient

The process of history taking requires modification in the elderly. More time and considerably more patience are required to obtain an adequate history from an elderly patient who is deaf, and perhaps suffers from impairment of memory. Questions need to be simple and straightforward. It is frequently only possible to establish that a symptom exists though its duration is uncertain, or the converse – that something whose nature is uncertain has been amiss for a definite time. The duration of symptoms and the sequence of their development are often more important than their precise nature. If there is temporary or permanent impairment of memory, it is essential to take a history from some other person – a relative, or someone who has been caring for the patient.

Systematic enquiry should follow the usual lines. The past history is more important in the elderly, because there is more of it; medical records of previous illnesses may constitute vital evidence. An accurate drug history covering as much of the past as possible, and for non-prescribed as well as prescribed drugs, is essential. A clear account of the time scale of drug therapy and of the dates of starting and stopping individual drugs will go far to clarify the complexities of symptoms due to drugs, and to their withdrawal – both common in the elderly. A dietary history is on occasions of importance, though it is difficult without dietetic help to identify other than the grossest deficiencies. An accurate account of psychiatric symptoms is vital, since deterioration in mental state is the commonest factor limiting the possibility of investigation or of rehabilitation in physical disease.

A detailed account of the patient's social circumstances is essential, and of the physical and emotional environment at home. Such knowledge is vital if physical rehabilitation is to be effective in re-establishing the patient at home; this can best be obtained by visiting the house itself. No assessment is complete without information on what relatives the patient has, where they live, and what they are able to contribute to his or her welfare. It is essential to decide what supporting community services the patient requires and is receiving, and to know what are available locally, and how best to obtain them.

Principles of drug therapy in old age

Appropriate drug therapy remains one of the most important aspects of the medicine of old age, since drugs are more often prescribed for the elderly, multiple pathology is a standing temptation to polypharmacy, and the adverse effects of drugs increase with age both for individual drugs, and also to a large extent with the age-related increase in the number of drugs per patient. It has been calculated that 10 per cent of admissions of elderly patients to hospital in the United Kingdom are drug-induced, and likely therefore to be iatrogenic.

Understanding of alterations in drug kinetics with age is advancing rapidly, but there are at present few clear demonstrations of altered pharmacodynamics. Drug absorption is in general little affected by age, though a substantial increase in the absorption of levodopa, probably due to reduced dopa decarboxylase in the gastric mucosa, is an important exception. The bioavailability of drugs such as propranolol, which are extensively degraded in the liver, may be greatly increased by a reduction in their first-pass metabolism. The protein-binding of drugs bound to serum albumin may be reduced in sick, elderly people, in whom serum albumin concentrations are frequently low, and the ease with which one drug displaces another from albumin may be increased. There is, however, little evidence that these changes are of major practical importance.

The volume of distribution of some drugs is reduced; that of digoxin may be correlated with reduced muscle Na–K ATPase. That of others (e.g. diazepam) is increased. The fall in lean body mass and body water might be expected to reduce the volume of distribution of water-soluble drugs, and the increase in body fat to increase that of fat-soluble drugs, but other factors, at present poorly understood, may well play a greater part. Changes in the volume of distribution make it difficult to interpret changes in plasma half-time as a measure of drug elimination; this is most satisfactorily expressed in terms of clearance. The effects of age on other aspects of drug distribution are poorly understood. Thus the apparent increase in sensitivity of the elderly brain to nitrazepam, which is not explained by any change in its plasma kinetics, may be due to alterations in the blood–brain barrier.

Alterations in drug elimination are undoubtedly the most important pharmacokinetic differences so far demonstrated. The age-related fall in glomerular filtration rate is accompanied by a parallel decrease in the elimination of drugs principally excreted by this route (e.g. digoxin), but in this instance and others, additional, disease-related reduction in glomerular filtration is also very important. Drugs principally eliminated by renal tubular secretion (e.g. the penicillins and aminoglycosides) share in this reduction in rate of elimination; this may be important when high urinary concentrations of antibiotic are required in the treatment of urinary-tract infections, and in the case of the aminoglycosides is responsible for the relation of ototoxicity to age, because toxic serum concentrations follow standard adult doses given to the elderly. The situation with regard to drugs eliminated by the liver varies. The elimination rates of some decline with age, but of others do not. It is not yet clear whether different effects of age on different drug-metabolizing enzyme systems determine these differences, but obviously delayed elimination, and in certain cases delayed formation of active metabolites, will prolong the duration of action of some drugs.

There are few well-documented examples of age-related differences in pharmacodynamics. The effect of warfarin on the synthesis of clotting factors is increased in the elderly. Some at least of the cardiac effects of sympathomimetic amines and beta blockers are reduced, perhaps because of a reduction in the number and/or sensitivity of beta adrenergic receptors. In practice this may be cancelled out by the increased bioavailability of some beta blockers and consequent higher serum levels. No age effect on alpha adrenoceptors has been shown.

Other factors not strictly kinetic or dynamic may alter the response of the elderly to drugs. The chronic administration of thiazide and related diuretics produces little change in whole-body potassium in the middle-aged, but in the elderly is a prime cause of potassium depletion. The difference lies in the substantially lower dietary potassium intake of normal old people, in whom diuretic-induced urinary potassium loss can easily exceed intake and make depletion inevitable. Potassium supplements should therefore always accompany diuretic therapy in the elderly, or potassium-sparing drugs be used.

The compliance of elderly patients with prescribed drug therapy is imperfect, though perhaps not much more so than that of the middle-aged. The most satisfactory way of improving compliance is to reduce to a minimum the demands on the patient. Complex drug regimens are inappropriate. Simplicity of prescribing, clear instruction, reinforced by written indications of what is required, and appropriate packaging and labelling are important practical matters often thought beneath the attention of doctors. They can do much to improve compliance, and (always provided prescription is correct) ensure the maximum benefit at the minimum risk.

Rehabilitation

The principles of geriatric medicine are well illustrated by the approach to rehabilitation. This necessitates a realistic view of the patient and his or her psychological state, diseases and disabilities, an organized setting, a co-ordinated method of management, and an appreciation of a large number of points of detail. Though there may be little scientific evidence that rehabilitation as at present conducted affects eventual outcome (e.g. in stroke), it is unlikely that all its effects are psychological, while the consequences of a lack of rehabilitation (e.g. contractures and unnecessary immobility) are obvious.

The basic tool of rehabilitation of the elderly is a team of medical, nursing, and paramedical personnel, each with a special role. The co-ordination of the activities of the group usually falls to the doctor, though he may well not be the most important member of the team at a particular time during the rehabilitation of a particular patient. Nurses have a central place because they spend much the most time with the patient, and are thus the best placed both to gather and to transmit information. The functions of the paramedical members of the team (physiotherapist, occupational therapist, speech therapist, and social worker) are the assessment of the patient's disability in terms of their own discipline, treatment by appropriate techniques, and the counselling of patient and relatives. The physiotherapist's principal concern is mobility, the occupational therapist's are the activities of daily living, the provision of aids, and the adaptation of the home environment to the patient's disabilities. The speech therapist is concerned with communication disorders and their treatment; the function in counselling relatives is especially important. The social worker is concerned with the social and family problems presented by illness and disability.

The objectives of a rehabilitation programme for an individual rest on a detailed assessment of the patient's current disabilities in terms of function. Particular attention must be paid to mental state, since the most important barriers to recovery are mental rather than physical. Also essential are an appreciation of the likely natural course of the patient's illness, of its complications and how to prevent them, and of any relevant social factors which may assist or hinder rehabilitation, together with appropriate drug therapy. Each patient requires an individual rehabilitation programme, and each member of the team must know what is expected. The programme must be flexible, and take into account the unforeseen. It must be regularly reviewed in the light of the patient's progress, and no irretrievable action should ever be taken which might prevent the patient from benefiting from unanticipated improvement.

The operation of these principles can be illustrated by three common examples encountered in everyday geriatric hospital practice: rehabilitation in *acute physical illness*, *following stroke*, and in *Parkinson's disease.*

Rehabilitation in *acute illness* in the elderly should begin immediately on admission to hospital. The patient and his or her relatives should be made aware that discharge is anticipated, and the expectation, on the part of either, of prolonged or even permanent hospitalization must be prevented. When the patient is fit to get out of bed, the natural history of the illness and the time course of recovery require consideration, and the presence of complications should be assessed, including, in particular, pressure lesions of the skin and postural hypotension. Prevention of the former is an important immediate aspect of rehabilitation, since a full-thickness pressure sore will retard rehabilitation by many weeks; its prevention takes a few hours. Postural hypotension may be due to drugs, to biochemical disorders, or to bed rest itself. The patient's mental state requires assessment, with particular attention being paid to intellectual impairment, the presence of depression, and the adequacy of morale. Disability must be assessed in functional terms (e.g. the ability to feed, dress, maintain continence, and walk), and must be seen against the state preceding the acute illness. A target date for discharge should be set, and arrangements made with relatives and community services to ensure that support is available on the day of discharge and immediately thereafter. When the drug regimen has been reduced to the minimum necessary, it should be explained in detail, and the patient given the responsibility for it, supervised by the nursing staff or ward pharmacist. Active teaching of the patient in hospital may be of limited long-term benefit, but can hardly be disadvantageous or more dangerous than its omission.

Rehabilitation after *stroke* presents problems of greater complexity. A detailed neurological and functional assessment is the essential starting point, beginning with a determination of mental state and of problems of communication (deafness and language disorders), with particular attention to receptive dysphasia. In the upper limb, motor function can be most simply assessed from fine finger movements. If these return within three weeks, reasonable

recovery of upper limb function is likely. Important proprioceptive loss and the phenomena of neglect and denial imply a poor prognosis for functional recovery, though both tend to improve over a period of three to four months. Prevention of dislocation of the shoulder is important, since this is the prime cause of the painful, stiff shoulder of the hemiplegic. In the acute stage the arm should be rested with the elbow supported, and when the patient is sitting the arm should be in a sling, to prevent the effect of gravity on the shoulder. In the lower limb, power can be simply tested by asking the patient to lift the leg off the bed. If it can be held for 10 to 15 seconds, the patient should be able to stand, though disorder of balance or instability of the knee may remain important problems. The prevention of contracture of the knee and of pressure sores on the heel of the affected leg are essential. Sitting and standing balance must be assessed, since it is counterproductive to ask a patient who cannot sit unsupported to stand, or one who cannot stand unsupported to walk.

The functions of the members of the rehabilitation team are essentially as outlined above. The nursing staff are concerned with the maintenance of morale, the prevention of incontinence, and the organization of the patient's immediate environment. The physiotherapist is concerned with balance and walking, with whatever aid is appropriate. With further improvement, independence in activities of daily living (especially dressing) is the responsibility of the occupational therapist. The speech therapist will play a major part with those suffering from dysphasia, particularly in the serial assessment of improvement of language function. Finally, the social worker will be concerned with the problems of relocation and re-establishment at home.

The rehabilitation of the patient with *Parkinson's disease* illustrates other principles. Mental state is the principal determinant of the likelihood of benefit from drug therapy. Depression may be extremely difficult to diagnose, but responds well to antidepressant therapy. Proper drug therapy has a central role in rehabilitation. Initial doses of levodopa should be small, and increase in dose gradual, to a modest final dose; this will minimize the likelihood of adverse effects such as psychiatric disorder, dyskinesia, and postural hypotension. Many elderly patients in whom levodopa is thought to have failed have been given too large an initial dose with too large and too frequent increments. Such a regimen can result in the patient being denied highly effective treatment. Anticholinergic drugs should be used with caution; the place of bromocriptine and newer drugs has yet to be evaluated in the elderly.

The restoration of mobility is largely a function of proper drug therapy, but the physiotherapist can encourage confidence in walking, and the proper use of walking aids. The occupational therapist can provide appropriate aids to daily living (e.g. for feeding, in the kitchen and bathroom, and in the toilet); a visit to the patient's home is essential to determine which aids will be of benefit. Newly developed techniques of speech therapy are of value. The social problems of families of patients with Parkinson's disease who face prolonged disability often complicated by the psychiatric effects of the disease and its drug therapy, may require the assistance of a sympathetic social worker or voluntary organisation.

Psychiatric disorders in old age

Nowhere is the importance of psychiatry in medicine more evident than in old age. Correct assessment of the mental state of an elderly patient is always of the first importance. An accurate diagnosis is essential if those conditions that can be remedied are to be treated, and in the others the difficulties faced by patient and relatives properly appreciated and managed.

A clear and simple classification of mental disorders in old age is of value:

1. Brain failure: acute, chronic, and acute-on-chronic;
2. Disorders of mood: depression, hypomania;

Table 2 Some causes of brain failure in old age

1. Structural damage to the brain: e.g. cerebral infarction, cerebral haemorrhage, cerebral tumour (primary or secondary), Alzheimer's disease, subdural haematoma
2. Disorders of the cerebral circulation: e.g. carotid insufficiency, systemic hypotension, congestive cardiac failure
3. Metabolic brain disorders: e.g. hypoxia, uraemia, dehydration, electrolyte disorder, thyroid disease, hypoglycaemia, vitamin deficiency (of vitamin B_{12} or folate)
4. Epilepsy
5. Drug toxicity: e.g. poisoning with barbiturates, phenothiazines, alcohol, digitalis, etc.

Table 3 Severity of chronic brain failure

Mild impairment: there is definite impairment of memory and calculating ability; such patients are often unable to manage to live alone, and are in need of some degree of supervision

Moderate impairment: there is in addition disorientation for time, place or person; such patients can live at home with others, but if their behaviour is disturbed, institutional care may be needed

Severe impairment: there is in addition difficulty with self-care, in particular initially difficulty with dressing; some also have difficulty in walking, and/or incontinence of urine; such patients need devoted attention to continue to live outside hospital

3. Other disorders: anxiety states, paranoid states, personality disorders etc.

The term 'brain failure' is of value because by leaving the way open for detailed classification (where possible) on the basis of aetiology, it removes obstructions to investigation and treatment resulting from the inadequacies of conventional terminology. 'Acute brain failure' is synonymous with the terms 'delirium', and 'acute' or 'toxic confusional state', which give rise to difficulty when 'confusion' refers to both a symptom and a diagnosis. 'Chronic brain failure' is synonymous with dementia of senile or other origin, and with 'senile psychosis', with the important proviso that irreversibility is not part of the concept. Patients with chronic brain failure not infrequently develop superadded acute brain failure (acute-on-chronic brain failure). The analogy between acute and chronic brain failure and acute and chronic respiratory or renal failure, and the relationship between them, is intentional. A classification of the causes of brain failure is given in Table 2.

Acute brain failure may be recognized when an old person in previously good mental health suddenly becomes disturbed, confused, restless, and disoriented, and is obviously ill. There are often rapid fluctuations in mental state from apathy and inattention to comparative lucidity and reasonable rapport, and insight is often preserved. Recognition of acute brain failure should lead to a vigorous search for possible causes, with emphasis on the detection of focal neurological signs, cardiac or respiratory failure, a wide range of biochemical disorders, infection in a variety of possible sites, and drug toxicity. Only when the cause is recognized and treated will the patient's mental state improve.

In chronic brain failure there is by contrast a long history, usually of many months, of initial failure of memory, especially for recent events, gradually developing impairment of judgement and slowing of intellectual capabilities, loss of interest in the surroundings and in previous pursuits, wandering or aimless and inappropriate behaviour, blunting of emotional responses, reduction in emotional control, and lack of insight. Assessment requires detailed enquiry from relatives about how the patient spends his or her time, and about such manifestations as restlessness, wandering, and aggressive behaviour. Observation of the patient's appearance and behaviour during examination provides valuable information; physical examination may show neurological abnormalities depending on the cause. Simple psychometric tests are valuable, especially those which include simple tests of recent and remote memory, calculation, and general knowledge of current affairs; these are more satisfactory than detailed formal tests, which are often poorly standardized for the elderly.

A simple classification of the severity of intellectual impairment is of value, in part because it can provide guidance to the type of care the patient is likely to require. One such is given in Table 3. The management of chronic brain failure rests on alteration and simplification of the environment so that the sufferer can cope with it. This implies a need for supervision to maintain socially acceptable behaviour. Drug therapy has little place, though insomnia and nocturnal restlessness can be controlled with hypnotics, of which chlormethiazole is perhaps the most satisfactory.

Disturbed behaviour by day is best treated with small doses of thioridazine, with haloperidol and sulthiame as valuable alternatives.

The disorder of mood commonly encountered in later life is depression. Distinction between endogenous and reactive types is seldom useful or possible. Depression in the elderly is often atypical and the diagnosis difficult. It depends on the demonstration of its cardinal features, such as loss of energy and interest, and a gloomy and despondent outlook on life and the future, with disturbance of sleep and appetite, and complaints of constipation and loneliness. This last symptom must be distinguished from the state of being alone. Bizarre and repeated physical complaints are also common, either shifting from one system to another, or persistent and unvarying. Such hypochondriasis must be clearly distinguished from the manifold, organically determined physical symptoms of multiple pathology. Apparent impairment of cognitive capabilities, and incontinence due to apathy, are not uncommon, and must be distinguished by their setting from those due to brain failure. The patient who for no apparent reason, and in the absence of intellectual impairment, fails to rehabilitate, should always be suspected of being depressed, though the less easily definable state of failure of morale may be responsible. Examination may show apathy, poverty of movement and expression, inattention and difficulty in maintaining rapport, and a dejected appearance. Multiple physical symptoms, and the words used to describe them, combine with the general impression that nothing is right with the patient or his world. Specific questions on feelings of loneliness and thoughts of suicide are essential.

The depressed elderly patient usually responds reasonably to antidepressant drugs, of which mianserin is probably the most satisfactory, since the risk of major side-effects seems less than that of tricyclics. Treatment should be continued for three months, and the effects of discontinuance observed; some patients may require therapy indefinitely. The severely depressed patient with life-threatening reduction in food and fluid intake should not be denied the benefits of electroplexy; considerable risks may need to be taken in the presence of cardiac or cerebrovascular disease, but can be justified by the more rapid relief of suffering and the reduction in threat to life.

Much less common than depression is hypomania, in which restlessness and overactivity are distinguished from those occurring in acute brain failure by the lack of clouding of consciousness.

Chronic anxiety states rarely arise *de novo* in old age, and most elderly patients so afflicted have suffered for many years. Anxiety developing more acutely is often a manifestation of an agitated, depressive illness. The treatment of anxiety symptoms is difficult; simple support is safer than drug therapy.

Paranoid symptoms are not uncommon in the elderly. They may occur in the early stages of brain failure, in depressive illnesses, and by themselves as the principal manifestation of paraphrenia. In this condition they may be relatively mild and of fluctuating intensity, or persistent and severe. Limited and restricted delusional syndromes, present for years without affecting the patient's life-style or behaviour, are best left untreated, but when delusions result in behaviour which disturbs others, then treatment with phenothiazines is of great value, though sometimes difficult to maintain because one of the patient's delusions may be that the doctor is trying to poison him.

Some old people whose psychiatric state cannot be called normal defy precise categorization. They have shown persistently odd behaviour throughout their lives, have antagonized and driven away all their relatives and friends, and are in consequence solitary, isolated, and difficult. They may live in self-inflicted squalor which brings them to the attention of neighbours and local authority agencies. They may not be intellectually impaired, and are neither paranoid, depressed, nor anxious. The term eccentric is as good as any. Recognition is not difficult, but treatment is, since correction of the squalor and disarray in which they live is only of brief benefit.

Cardiovascular disease

The symptoms of heart disease in old age are not infrequently modified. Cardiac pain is often slight; angina may be manifest as a need to stop walking, and the pain of cardiac infarction may be absent, or be overshadowed by other symptoms, such as confusion. Breathlessness may be replaced by fatigue, which may reflect reduced cardiac output without great increase in pulmonary vascular volumes or pressures; decreased sensory input from the respiratory muscles, heart, and pulmonary vasculature may also be relevant.

Interpretation of cardiovascular signs must also be modified in the elderly. Reduction in hand blood flow may suppress the signs of increased cardiac output in anaemia or cor pulmonale. Decreased elasticity of the central arterial tree increases pulse pressure, and may mask the peripheral signs of aortic stenosis. The venous pressure is usually more easily visible through the thin skin of an elderly neck, but compression of the left innominate vein between an enlarged aorta and the back of the sternum may result in asymmetrical elevation of the venous pressure, that in the left jugular and subclavian veins being higher than that in the right, a difference abolished by deep inspiration. The true central venous pressure should thus be determined from the right jugular venous system, or after inspiration. The cardiac apex may be difficult to feel, and its site may be displaced by thoracic kyphoscoliosis, but the powerful and prolonged impulse of left ventricular hypertrophy, the diffuse impulse of left ventricular dilatation, and the increased left parasternal pulsation of right ventricular hypertrophy can usually be identified. The elderly heart shows no abnormal auscultatory findings, apart from the frequent presence of a soft ejection systolic murmur. The significance of an abnormal third or fourth heart sound remains unchanged, as do the signs of mitral and tricuspid valvular disease.

The proper recognition of cardiac failure rests upon the demonstration of breathlessness, elevation of the venous pressure in all phases of respiration, bilateral pulmonary signs (of oedema or effusion), hepatic enlargement (rather than mere downward displacement), and sacral or symmetrical ankle oedema. The diagnosis of left heart failure is more difficult, but nocturnal breathlessness, Cheyne–Stokes respiration, and evidence of left heart disease should be present. Accurate diagnosis, both of cardiac failure and of its underlying cause, is of great importance, since proper treatment is extremely rewarding, and the drugs used are certainly ineffective, and possibly dangerous, in patients who do not have cardiac failure.

Cardiac failure should initially be treated along the same lines as in the young: rest, digitalis and diuretics. The entirely proper enthusiasm for the active and early mobilization of the elderly has obscured the fact that in cardiac failure physical rest is essential. The patient should initially be nursed in bed or in a chair. Once signs of cardiac failure have disappeared, and weight loss following diuretic therapy has ceased, gradual mobilization may begin, initially with walking to the toilet, and then with longer distances on the flat within the house or ward.

Digitalis therapy (see page 13.101) is essential in patients with atrial fibrillation and an uncontrolled ventricular response, and may be valuable in those with atrial fibrillation and a slow ventricular rate, and those with sinus rhythm, at least for the first few weeks. Digitalization should be begun with a single oral dose of 0.5 or 0.75 mg, followed by a maintenance dose appropriate to the patient's renal function. If the blood urea is less than 10 mmol/l and creatinine less than 170 μmol/l, the initial maintenance dose should be 0.25 mg/day; if renal function is more obviously impaired, 0.125 mg/day is more appropriate. Digoxin in a dose of 0.0625 mg/day does not produce therapeutic serum levels unless the glomerular filtration rate is less than 10 ml/min. These simple rules, applied with flexibility, will enable the maximum benefit to be obtained from digoxin with the minimum risk of toxicity.

Digitalis therapy should be continued indefinitely in patients with atrial fibrillation in whom the ventricular rate rises to above 80 b/min in the absence of digitalis, but can be discontinued after three months in patients in sinus rhythm, particularly when cardiac failure has been precipitated by an event such as myocardial infarction, and there is spontaneous improvement in myocardial function.

Diuretic therapy poses particular problems. Increased urine volumes may result in retention of urine in elderly men, and in incontinence in either sex. Normal bladder function is usually restored when cardiac failure has resolved and mental state and mobility have improved. Potassium depletion is frequent (see pages 18.18 and 18.30), and potassium supplements should be given, or potassium-sparing agents used.

The place of vasodilator agents and inhibitors of angiotensin-converting enzyme in the treatment of cardiac failure in the elderly has not been clarified; at present they should be used cautiously, and only when other measures have failed.

Paroxysmal cardiac dysrhythmias are increasingly recognized as causes of syncope and falls. Common findings in routine ECGs, such as frequent ventricular ectopic beats or left bundle-branch block, are difficult to interpret in this context. If a dysrhythmia has not been demonstrated at the time of a syncopal episode, the most useful measure is 24-hour ECG monitoring, but even then it may be difficult or impossible to be certain of the association between brief episodes of dysrhythmia and the patient's symptoms. The combination of syncope and complete heart block, right bundle-branch block, or the sick sinus syndrome, is an indication for cardiac pacing whatever the age of the patient, since the quality of life is much improved and its length perhaps increased. When the symptoms are those of cardiac failure a decision is more difficult, but temporary pacing to see if symptoms are improved is justifiable. Elderly patients tolerate cardiac pacing extremely well, and the expectation of life of octogenarians paced for complete heart block has been shown to be restored to normal.

There are relatively few indications for anticoagulant therapy in the elderly. Systemic embolism, whether following myocardial infarction, or complicating atrial fibrillation, is certainly such an indication, but treatment need not exceed six months. Venous thrombosis is not by itself an indication; therapy must be confined to those with iliofemoral thrombosis or pulmonary embolism. Three months treatment is then probably rational. Heparin is rarely necessary, and warfarin should be given in smaller doses than in middle-age, since it produces a greater effect in the elderly. The usual contra-indications to anticoagulant therapy should always be observed.

The treatment of high blood pressure in the elderly over the age of 80 remains controversial. The increase in arterial pressure with age makes it difficult to determine the level at which high blood pressure should be regarded as in need of treatment. High blood pressure is associated with an increased risk of stroke, at least under the age of 80, and is also a risk factor for ischaemic heart disease and cardiac failure. Elderly patients with established stroke may not benefit from treatment of hypertension, but patients who have recovered from cardiac failure may do so. It is probably best to regard as in need of treatment a sustained pressure of over 160/90 mmHg in a patient under the age of 80. The object of treatment should be to reduce blood pressure to approximately 160/90 mmHg over two to three months. It is best to begin with a thiazide diuretic, and if this proves inadequate, a beta-blocker should be added; but the reverse sequence is also reasonable. In neither case should doses be large. The side-effects of thiazide diuretics in doses used for the treatment of hypertension are small; the undoubted risks of development of diabetes and gout may be ignored, although if either develops it will require treatment, and the thiazide should be discontinued. The bioavailability of some beta-blockers is increased in the elderly and their rate of elimination decreased; this is approximately compensated for by a reduction in sensitivity of the myocardium to beta-block-ade, so that the effectiveness of a given dose varies relatively little with age. The clinical impression is that methyldopa adversely affects brain-damaged elderly patients. Calcium antagonists (e.g. nifedipine), vasodilators (e.g. prazosin) and angiotensin-convert-ing enzyme inhibitors (e.g. captopril or enalapril) have not yet been fully evaluated in the elderly. Other hypotensive drugs (in particular reserpine and sympatholytic and ganglion-blocking drugs) should not be used.

Orthostatic hypotension is a common phenomenon in the elderly. A drop of 20 mmHg or more in systolic pressure on standing is found in 15 per cent of those aged 65–74, and in 25 per cent over that age. This drop is usually asymptomatic, but if the fall in systolic pressure is substantial or the standing systolic pressure is 110 mmHg or less, and autoregulation of cerebral blood flow is impaired, then orthostatic syncopal symptoms are likely. The great majority of cases are due to injudicious drug therapy, particularly with thiazides, tricyclic antidepressants, phenothiazines, benzodiazepines, levodopa, or combinations of drugs. Orthostatic hypotension may develop if bed rest is prolonged, and may obstruct rehabilitation following acute illness. In the small proportion of cases not due to drugs, primary age- or disease-related changes in the autonomic nervous system may be responsible; the complete Shy–Drager syndrome (see Section 21) is a distinct rarity. The recognition of orthostatic hypotension depends on a careful history indicating that the cerebral circulation is impaired immediately after rising from bed or chair. It is confirmed by taking the blood pressure in the standing as well as the lying position; if this is a routine, most cases of so-called 'vertebrobasilar insufficiency' will be found to have a simple and usually easily remediable cause. Management begins with reduction or discontinuance of the causal drug. Reduction in levodopa dosage will usually lead to a satisfactory compromise between improvement in Parkinsonism and incapacitating orthostatic hypotension. When drug therapy is not implicated, or orthostatic hypotension does not disappear when apparently causal drugs are discontinued, treatment with fludrocortisone 0.1–0.3 mg/day should be combined with tight full-length elastic stockings, and advice on the gradual achievement of the standing position from lying.

Bone disease (see Section 17)

Bone disease is common in the elderly. Three conditions require consideration – osteoporosis, osteomalacia, and Paget's disease.

So-called 'senile' osteoporosis presents problems of great difficulty. Cross-sectional studies of bone mass measured *in vivo* and direct determination of the calcium content of bone at autopsy clearly indicate that there is a progressive loss of bone mass with age, beginning at around the age of 30. The rate of decline of bone mass is probably approximately equal whatever its intial value, so that bone mass at its peak in the third decade is the principal determinant of that in old age. Bone mass in women is less at all ages than in men. Longitudinal studies suggest that for 5–10 years following the menopause the rate of decline in bone mass increases, and can be reduced by oestrogen administration. Bone loss in cortical and cancellous bone may proceed at different rates.

Whether reduced bone mass in old age may be regarded as purely age-related or as a disease is therefore debatable.

The most important manifestation of the decline in bone mass is a reduction in the mechanical strength of bone and an increase in tendency to fracture. Fractures at four sites show an exponential increase in incidence with age: the proximal femur, the neck of the humerus, the distal radius, and the vertebrae. The first three involve cortical, and the last cancellous bone. It remains uncertain whether the relation of these fractures to age is solely due to age-related bone loss, to an age-related increase in frequency of falls, or to both. The greater frequency of these fractures in women could be explained by their lesser bone mass, or their greater tendency to fall.

Understanding of the mechanisms of age-related bone loss is imperfect and its prevention therefore problematical. Numerous mechanisms have been proposed, including:

1. Age-related reduction in calcium absorption, perhaps due to reduction in vitamin D intake combined with persistent excess of urinary calcium excretion.
2. Increasing relative parathyroid activity, particularly following menopausal loss of the restraining activity of oestrogens on parathormone effects on bone; but can oestrogen-related bone loss be important in men? Oestrogen therapy of the menopause may prevent bone loss, but increase carcinogenesis in the breast and reproductive tract.
3. Simple vitamin D deficiency is improbable since age-related bone loss occurs in populations in which vitamin D deficiency, especially that due to lack of exposure of sunlight, does not occur.
4. Loss of bone matrix associated with age-changes in collagen would seem essentially incapable of prevention in our present state of knowledge.

Osteomalacia is common in the elderly in northern climates, especially among the housebound, who suffer from sunlight deprivation, and often a reduced dietary vitamin D intake in addition. Its manifestations cover a wide spectrum, from asymptomatic biochemical changes, to backache, diffuse bone pain, proximal-muscle weakness, mental changes, and fractures. The diagnosis should always be suspected in elderly patients with these features. Radiological evidence in the form of Looser's zones is usually lacking, but isotope bone scanning may reveal areas of increased uptake at the characteristic sites of pseudofractures. Biochemical changes are difficult to interpret because of age-related changes in serum calcium and alkaline phosphate (see Table 2). There is also a substantial overlap in serum vitamin D concentrations between undoubted normality and undoubted vitamin D deficiency. The single most satisfactory diagnostic measure is a therapeutic trial of vitamin D. Alfacalcidol (1α-hydroxycholecalciferol) in a dose of 1 μg/day should be given, and also calcium supplements. If osteomalacia is the diagnosis, bone and other symptoms will disappear within a few days, the serum calcium will rise, and the alkaline phosphatase begin to fall.

The prevention of osteomalacia is difficult. In continuing-care institutions, exposure to relatively small doses of ultraviolet light has been shown to produce as substantial an effect on serum vitamin D concentrations as considerable daily oral supplements, but there are possible hazards to both patients and staff from overdosage. Replacement of butter by margarine, or taking the opportunity of every possibility of exposure to sunlight, are simpler and safer methods, at least for elderly patients in institutions.

Paget's disease of bone shows a substantial increase in prevalence with age. It is often asymptomatic and discovered on radiographs taken for other reasons, or as a result of finding an elevated bone alkaline phosphatase. The sites commonly affected may produce physical signs, in particular increased warmth over exposed bones. The presence of such signs, together with a raised alkaline phosphatase, and increased urine hydroxyproline excretion, are the best evidence of disease activity. Patients with multifocal active disease may show evidence of a high cardiac output, and

Table 4 Proposed guidelines for diagnosis of diabetes mellitus and impaired glucose tolerance (stated in terms of venous whole blood, true glucose measurements, following a 75 g oral glucose load where appropriate)

---

1 Diabetes mellitus (DM) is diagnosed when:
    (*a*) The fasting blood glucose concentration equals or exceeds 7 mmol/l (126 mg/dl) on more than one occasion
    (*b*) The blood glucose concentration two hours after a 75 g oral glucose load equals or exceeds 10 mmol/l (180 mg/dl) irrespective of the fasting concentration
2 Impaired glucose tolerance (IGT) exists when the two-hour blood glucose concentration falls between 7 and 10 mmol/l. Action with IGT depends upon individual circumstances

---

rarely, cardiac failure may result. Treatment with calcitonin or diphosphonates should be considered when there is bone pain or a high cardiac output. Both will respond to treatment, but pain due to involvement of joint surfaces is unlikely to improve, as also are deafness due to auditory-nerve compression or neurological signs due to platybasia; a shunt procedure should be considered for the latter.

Metabolic and endocrine disorders

Diabetes mellitus (see page 9.51)

The definition and thus the diagnosis of diabetes become more difficult with advancing age. Glucose tolerance, whether tested orally or intravenously, shows a steady decline, and the incidence of newly discovered frank diabetes rises with age. The mean decline in glucose tolerance is such that if standard diagnostic criteria, adequate for middle age, are applied to those over the age of 70, more than 50 per cent of the elderly would be 'diabetic'. Severe glucose intolerance accompanied by symptoms of diabetes leaves no doubt that the patient should be treated as diabetic, but asymptomatic mild impairment of glucose tolerance can scarcely be regarded in the same sense. Help with resolution of these difficulties is provided by recent revision of the blood glucose criteria for the diagnosis of diabetes, the introduction of the concept of impaired glucose tolerance (Table 4), and the measurement of glycosylated haemoglobin in doubtful cases (normal values vary from laboratory to laboratory but seem unaffected by age). If diabetes is diagnosed according to the criteria shown, almost all symptomatic elderly patients will be diagnosed as diabetic. The category of impaired glucose tolerance includes many elderly people, but follow-up of this group suggests neither a much greater excess risk of the development of true diabetes nor of its specific complications, but rather of an increased susceptibility to atherosclerotic vascular disease.

The factors influencing the age-change in glucose tolerance are poorly understood. Obesity is probably less, and diabetogenic drugs more important than has been thought. Genetic factors remain as important as in younger people, and the diabetes-promoting influence of multiparity persists in women at least to the age of 80. The probable mechanism of the impairment of glucose tolerance with age is a combination of reduction both in the effectiveness of the action of insulin and in insulin secretion in response to hyperglycaemia.

The clinical presentation of diabetes in old age is very different from that at younger ages. Many are diagnosed as a result of routine testing during a medical or surgical illness, some because of the development of disorders associated with diabetes (e.g. peripheral vascular disease, cataract), and relatively fewer because of classical symptoms such as weight loss, polyuria, and pruritus vulvae. A small proportion present with life-threatening metabolic decompensation.

The management of newly discovered diabetes in old age is based in diet, oral hypoglycaemic agents, and insulin. Its most important aspect is the education of the patient and of those caring for him in the nature of the condition and the objectives of treatment. Dietary treatment should be advised for every old person in whom a definite diagnosis of diabetes is made. Reduction in carbohydrate intake to 120–150 g/day, with maintenance of normal protein intake, is usually all that is needed. Advice should be simple, flexible, and repeated, should allow adequate variety to take account of the individual's own preferences, and should avoid setting inappropriate dietary patterns.

Oral hypoglycaemic agents should be used if dietary therapy does not result in reduction in hyperglycaemia within a few weeks. Tolbutamide, glibenclamide, and glibornuride are probably to be preferred. Limitation of dosage and prompt discontinuance if food intake falls are important to prevent hypoglycaemia. The combination of a sulphonylurea and metformin is often appropriate; phenformin should not be used because of the much greater risk of lactic acidosis.

In elderly patients with acutely disordered diabetes, insulin should not be withheld. In the long term, it should be given to those in whom oral therapy fails, and there is also a small group of thin, elderly men whose diabetes is insulin-dependent from the first; it should never be thought that such diabetes does not or cannot occur in old age. Single daily injections of insulin are preferable to multiple. Regular urine testing is necessary, and the fact that the renal threshold for glucose rises slightly with age should not deter one from this necessary discipline. Many elderly diabetics, especially those on insulin, benefit from the support and advice available by regular attendance at a diabetic clinic.

Approximately one case in six of diabetic ketosis occurs in patients over the age of 60. Ketosis is usually precipitated by infection, but multiple causes are common. The degree of metabolic decompensation is often greater in the elderly. Vigorous rehydration and insulin therapy are essential, but the mortality remains high. Non-ketotic hyperosmolar coma is virtually confined to the elderly, but how this state arises is far from clear. Treatment with large amounts of intravenous fluid and small doses of insulin produces slower improvement than in ketosis, but mortality, mostly due to arterial occlusion, is substantial.

The evidence for a relationship between control of diabetes and the developments of complications in old age is not entirely satisfactory. Good control retards the development of complications, but cannot be relied upon to prevent progression of established lesions. In the elderly glucose intolerance (and presumably therefore poorly controlled diabetes) is more important than for instance hypercholesterolaemia as a risk factor for cardiac failure, intermittent claudication, and stroke, but less important than cigarette smoking in respect of intermittent claudication or raised blood pressure in respect of cardiac failure or stroke.

The specific complications of diabetes occur more frequently in the elderly than in the young. The majority of patients blind from diabetes are over the age of 60. The prognosis of diabetic retinopathy in old age is less favourable than in middle-age, but photocoagulation remains effective treatment for some macular lesions. Cataract extraction is three or four times more common in elderly diabetics than in non-diabetics, though the visual indications for operation are the same. The results of operation are excellent, except when there is visual impairment due to retinopathy. The neurological complication of diabetes particularly associated with old age is amyotrophy. Its clinical recognition is important because of its generally good prognosis and the need to avoid unnecessary investigation. The principal emphasis in the management of foot lesions is on preventive measures such as simple foot hygiene, proper footwear, avoidance of damaging extremes of heat and cold, and if necessary attendance at a chiropody clinic.

Hypothyroidism

Most cases of hypothyroidism in old age are of autoimmune origin. Classical clinical presentations probably only occur in a quarter of patients. Signs and symptoms such as cold intolerance, hair loss, voice change, and coarsening of the skin, are all less common than an insidious decline in general health and mobility, and pyschiatric manifestations, in particular depression. Hypothyroid coma, sometimes associated with severe headache and fits, and hypothermia (sometimes precipitated by phenothiazines), are less common but important presentations. The most useful physical signs are change in voice and delayed relaxation of tendon reflexes.

Cautious initial replacement therapy is advisable, beginning with thyroxine 25 μg/day, particularly if heart disease coexists. Adequacy of treatment may be established by a fall in serum TSH to normal; doses of 100–150 μg/day are usually adequate. Relapse due to discontinuance of treatment is regrettably frequent, and the responsible doctor must ensure that lifelong treatment is in fact lifelong. Poor compliance may necessitate supervision by a relative, neighbour, or visiting nurse. It has recently been shown that five times the daily dose given once a week is both safe and effective.

Hyperthyroidism

Hyperthyroidism is less common in old age than hypothyroidism, but perhaps even more likely to present in an atypical manner, so that a high index of suspicion is required if this important (because so easily treatable) condition is to be diagnosed. Weight loss, anorexia, and gastrointestinal and cardiovascular symptoms predominate. Cardiac failure, usually with atrial fibrillation, is the most important cardiac presentation, and proximal myopathy is not infrequent. The eye signs and goitre are less common in the elderly, and apathy or depression may be prominent. Untreated hyperthyroidism in old age is a serious threat to life. Treatment is best begun with carbimazole, followed, when thyroid function has returned to normal, by radioiodine. In mild cases radioiodine alone will be adequate but the correct dose is difficult to determine, and the patient may remain undertreated for months. Lifelong follow-up is necessary, because whether or not a dose of radioiodine sufficient to abolish thyroid function is used, hypothyroidism is a common sequel.

Disorders of temperature regulation

The elderly often show evidence of disordered thermoregulation, and are thus particularly liable to be sensitive to extremes of environmental temperature. Peripheral and central failure of appreciation of temperature can lead to defective behavioural responses, and there are also abnormal peripheral responses to changes in core temperature. This multiplicity of mechanisms involved in old age makes it difficult to classify disorders of thermoregulation satisfactorily.

Hypothermia (see page 6.94)

This may develop when reduced awareness of change in skin temperature, overall impairment of intellectual capacity, severe physical illness, inappropriate drug therapy, or a combination of these, lead to failure of normal behavioural responses to falling environmental temperature. The old person will fail to put on extra clothes, to close the windows, or to ensure that the fire is functioning. Failure of physiological mechanisms of heat conservation results in loss of vasoconstrictive skin responses, and absence of shivering.

Most elderly patients with hypothermia present after a period of two or three days of relatively cold weather, but it is entirely possible for hypothermia to develop in hospital in mid-summer at United Kingdom latitudes, especially if disease or drugs play an important part. The fall in central temperature occurs over 24–48 hours, and its principal manifestations are progressive ataxia and slowing of cerebration, leading to stupor and finally coma. On clinical examination the skin on unexposed surfaces such as the axilla, chest, and abdomen feels cold to touch. The pulse is slow, unless severe physical illness has raised it towards normal, and the blood pressure is low or difficult to record. Cerebration is slow, but may be remarkably accurate even in the presence of a considerable reduction in body temperature. Tendon reflexes are normal unless there is associated hypothyroidism. The diagnosis is made by recording the rectal temperature; this should be done without delay on all occasions when the oral temperature is recorded as 35 °C or less. The principal investigation likely to alert the clinician to the diagnosis is the electrocardiogram, which characteristically shows bradycardia with prominent J-waves. In severe hypothermia there is often slow atrial fibrillation with a slow ventricular response.

Hypothermia in the elderly carries a high mortality, related to its cause in the individual case (if due to drugs the patients usually recover; if due to severe physical illness the patients frequently die), also to its severity, and its complications (particularly pneumonia and pancreatitis). Its management is difficult. There is no rational basis for the use of steroids, while intravenous fluids are dangerous because they may produce pulmonary oedema; intravenous glucose is not metabolized, since insulin is ineffective in the hypothermic state. A slow rise in body temperature should be produced by exposing the patient to a relatively high ambient temperature of 27 °C; this cannot rationally be combined with the use of a thermal blanket, since this is as effective against heat gain as heat loss. Improvement is shown by an increase in rectal temperature and pulse rate, a maintained blood pressure, and improvement in conscious level. If hypothyroidism is suspected liothyronine (triiodothyronine) should be given, but only when the central temperature has risen to normal.

The elderly patient who has recovered from hypothermia should be regarded as at risk from a further episode, and relatives and social agencies should be mobilized to ensure maintenance of an adequate temperature in the home.

Hyperthermia

This may be an equal hazard. An increase in mortality in continuing-care wards and in the elderly at home has been recognized during heat waves. The absence of appropriate behavioural responses is probably as important as impairment of physiological responses. The paramount need is to collect elderly people at risk into environments that can be kept cool. There is little useful guidance about the management of grossly raised body temperatures in the elderly, except to maintain fluid intake.

References

Anderson, W. F. and Williams, B. O. (1983). *Practical management of the elderly* 4th edn. Blackwell Scientific Publications, Oxford.
Birren, J. E. and Sloane, R. B. (eds) (1980). *Handbook of mental health and aging.* Prentice Hall, Englewood Cliffs, N. J.
Brocklehurst, J. C. (ed.) (1984). *Textbook of geriatric medicine and gerontology* 3rd edn. Churchill Livingstone, Edinburgh.
Caird, F. I. (ed.) (1982). *Neurological disorders in the elderly.* Wright-PSG. Bristol.
——, Kennedy, R. D. and Williams, B. O. (1983). *Practical rehabilitation of the elderly.* Pitman, London.
Coakley, D. (ed.) (1980). *Acute geriatric medicine.* Croom Helm, London.
Hodkinson, M. (1984). *Clinical biochemistry of the elderly.* Churchill Livingstone, Edinburgh.
Martin A. and Camm, A. J. (eds) (1984). *Heart disease in the elderly.* John Wiley and Sons, Chichester.
O'Malley, K. (ed.) (1984). *Clinical pharmacology and drug treatment of the elderly.* Churchill Livingstone, Edinburgh.
Platt, D. (ed.) (1982). *Geriatrics I and II.* Springer-Verlag, Berlin.
Rowe, J. W. and Besdine, R. W. (1982). *Health and disease in old age.* Little, Brown and Co, Boston.

SECTION 28
TERMINAL CARE

TERMINAL CARE

C. M. SAUNDERS

I conceive it the office of the physician not only to restore the health but to mitigate pains and dolours; and not only when such mitigation may conduce to recovery but when it may serve to make a fair and easy passage.

FRANCIS BACON

Definition

'Terminal care refers to the management of patients in whom the advent of death is felt to be certain and not too far off and for whom medical effort has turned away from (active) therapy and become concentrated on the relief of symptoms and the support of both patient and family' (Holford 1973, slightly adapted). Many diseases have a terminal phase and patients suffering from them need treatment suited to their condition. Doctors, however, are often unwilling to make such a judgement except in the various forms of malignant disease. These may have a comparatively long terminal phase, needing much skill and support if relief is to be given. Like most discussions on terminal care this chapter will mainly have malignant disease in mind but many of the symptoms to be treated and much of the general management will be relevant to other situations. What is being researched and taught in the hospices and continuing care units is gradually spreading into the general field (Ford and Pincherle, 1978).

On making decisions

A patient needs appropriate treatment at all stages of the illness. If it is appreciated that palliative and terminal care both involve skilful and effective treatment and that the direction is not only one-way, doctors find it less difficult to discontinue active therapy. Palliative treatment to combat persistent disease is often rigorous but it may give good returns in active living or make curative treatment possible once again. If it is no longer effective, the alternative is not merely custodial care. During the past decade or so it has become clear that to practice competent care for the dying is a demanding and rewarding experience. It may give not only added quality to the life remaining but also at times add considerably to its length.

Doctors are committed to giving such appropriate treatment to their patients, not to every manoeuvre that may be technically possible. 'The prolongation of life should not in itself constitute the exclusive aim of medical practice, which must be concerned equally with the relief of suffering' (Parliamentary Assembly of the Council of Europe, 1976).

These two main aims must be balanced as the physician aims to act in the best interests of each patient. The doctor's activities may otherwise merely add to suffering (Cassell, 1982).

A patient has a right to refuse treatment and to have this decision respected, provided the patient is mature and lucid. If unconscious, a document drawn up previously giving the patient's general wishes may give the clinician some guidance in making decisions. The relatives of patients have no right to make decisions on their behalf unless they are incompetent. Even then, they may only act in the best interests of the patient.

To ease the pains of death has always been one of the commitments of medical practice and if, to ease such pain, a doctor must take measures which may hasten death, this is permissible provided the doctor's aim is only the relief of pain. This reflects the so-called double effect theory and was incorporated into English law in one of the few decided cases in this area (R. v Bodkin Adams 1957. Quoted by Kennedy, 1984).

The doctor may not embark on any conduct with the primary intention of causing the patient's death and if a terminally ill patient expresses a desire to commit suicide a doctor may not in law facilitate the suicide (*Suicide Act* 1961). To do so would be a criminal offence.

The overlapping of the arrows in Fig. 1 indicates that skilled control of the problems of advanced and terminal disease does not necessarily have to wait until all other treatment is abandoned: indeed its successful use may make that treatment more effective. When the clinician is involved with both chemotherapy and with the control of pain and nausea, it will be easier to recognize diminishing returns to the former and to discontinue it without either party feeling that now no treatment is being given. To accept a situation when treatment is directed to the relief of symptoms and the alleviation of general distress will no longer mean an implicit 'there is nothing more that I can do' but an explicit 'everything possible is being done.' Our concern and interest in the field brings us to the dying person with ever renewed concern and a positive attitude that is often transferred without words. It can do much to lift the feeling of helplessness from the situation and help the patient to die with a sense of worth to the end (Vanderpool, 1978).

The question of truth

Those who are close to a patient with a terminal illness have to consider the questions, spoken and unspoken, that this person is asking. Over the past 20 years doctors in the United Kingdom have become more inclined to tell cancer patients the truth of their diagnosis and to consider the demands made upon their time and understanding by the continuing communication that is needed if morale is to be sustained (Brewin, 1977). A patient can hardly be expected to go through modern cancer management without being given some explanation and some control over what is being done to the disease and to his or her life. Feelings of helplessness and hopelessness and unquestioning acceptance have been shown to have adverse effects upon prognosis. These can only be exacerbated by poor rapport, silence, and evasions.

There are undoubtedly some patients who do not wish to face the truth and who will continue to push it out of their minds. Denial, as well as a fighting spirit, have been shown to correlate with recurrence-free survival and, whatever we do or say, many patients are able to maintain their choice in the matter. Aitken-Swan and Easson (1959) reported follow-up interviews with 231 patients who had been told their diagnosis, reassured that the

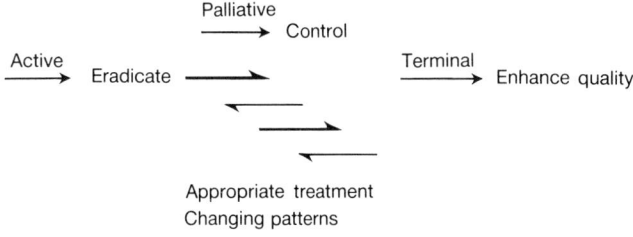

Fig. 1 Appropriate treatment-changing patterns.

disease was early and that treatment should cure them. They found that two-thirds of the patients were glad to have known the truth, 7 per cent resented the consultant's frankness, and 19 per cent denied that they had been told at all.

Two recent studies (Novack et al., 1979; Spencer-Jones, 1981) found that about half their patients wished to be informed concerning their illness. However, some who asked later denied knowledge while others, who did not ask, subsequently revealed their awareness. We must be ready for changes in our patients' knowledge and attitude. From many years of hospice experience and our own studies we believe that truth is likely to seep gradually into the consciousness of most patients. It happens as they watch and listen to other patients, as they remember previous illness and deceptions in the family and as they notice their own changing condition and the avoidances and evasions of those around them. Sometimes there is the more dramatic sighting of notes, the blood request form, or the like. If honest discussion has already been put out of court, how much support and reassurance can then be given?

To be told of a threatening diagnosis at the stage when treatment with hopes of a cure can be offered is hardly the same as a discussion of the disease when it has reached its terminal stage. Yet the earlier policy of at least a guarded truth will make it easier for both patient and doctor to adjust to the new conditions. The patient is then more ready to believe when told that the symptoms can be controlled and that any crisis will be dealt with. 'Implicit in the doctor–patient relationship is that the patient will not be abandoned if things go wrong' (Lancet, 1980).

We believe that when time is available for unhurried discussion most people are glad of the opportunity to express their deeper fears but they may need our help in initiating such discussions. They feel themselves at a disadvantage when faced with the doctor's greater knowledge and tendency to speak from a height. Many people need greatly to talk about their deteriorating condition with someone who is concerned and who is also confident that this part of life is important and that when symptoms are controlled it can still be lived creatively. Such discussion may take several brief sessions which are often interspersed with apparently contradictory optimism. But we all spend time reading holiday brochures and complicated menus that we know we will never undertake.

Those who continue to use denial to protect themselves should not be assaulted by truths they are neither willing nor able to handle. Some of them will do well, living from day to day, and their families are likely to go along with their lack of realism, often with considerable relief. Their choice is to be respected and seems to be the usual approach in a number of countries where this topic has been discussed.

There is evidence that in the United Kingdom a more open approach is appreciated as a patient nears death. In 1963 Hinton carried out a controlled study of a group of dying patients in the wards of a London teaching hospital. This paper showed that 50 per cent of his 102 dying patients already had a shrewd idea of the severity of their illness when he first interviewed them and that 'awareness of dying grew so that three out of every four spoke of this possibility or certainty.' These patients had often not been 'told' and the ward staff were often unaware that they had such knowledge. Later he studied 80 patients dying in four different settings, two where the policy was to avoid any discussion of unpalatable truth and two which encouraged attempts at more honest communication. The latter groups were less anxious and depressed and welcomed the greater openness. Although, as he points out, no general principle can tell us what we must say to an individual patient yet it can give us guidelines and encourage us not to take automatically the easy path of evasion (Hinton, 1979).

When patients express unrealistic fears we can provide reassurance and when they can share with us their realistic apprehensions concerning dependence and loss we can help them to express the grief they feel. When we have been honest in the past our reassurances that pain will not be allowed to escape control and that death itself will be peaceful are more likely to be accepted. Above all, more open awareness enables families to tackle this crisis of their lives together (Stedeford 1981a, b).

Terminal symptoms

Pain

The greatest fear of all is the fear of pain and all too often this fear has been justified. Terminal pain is frequently treated ineptly and the view of the public that death from cancer is likely to be accompanied by unremitting distress continues to be confirmed. The vast majority of these patients (and many of those with other diseases) could be given good relief by the competent use of narcotic analgesics and their adjuvants. Such treatment is denied them because of misconceptions concerning the use and effectiveness of these drugs; yet experience in many countries during the past two decades has shown that terminal pain can be thus relieved often over long periods without impairment of the patient's alertness or personality. An adequate analysis of the sometimes complex causes of terminal distress will lead to appropriate treatment, in some cases with specific measures such as radiotherapy, chemotherapy, and nerve blocks, but for most patients by the right use of the pharmacology now available which, used as part of a general approach, will maintain quality of life to the end for the patient.

The nature of pain

A series of pictures painted by patients at St Christopher's hospice illustrated how they saw the pain with which they presented. The feeling of being impaled by a red hot nail; of being totally isolated from the world by the encircling 'muscles of tension' with nothing but a hypodermic to pierce through them; the sudden jabs on movement and the implacable heaviness of pain were all illustrated vividly. So too were the conviction that one was some kind of scrap heap or was at the mercy of the demolition squad, suffering blow after blow.

These paintings expressed feelings that are common to many patients dying of cancer. The somewhat artificial division of such pain into separate areas helps the therapist to decide whether the analysis is adequate. Patients use such phrases as 'It was all pain', 'The pain was all around me,' 'You can't think about anything else.' It is no exaggeration to term such suffering 'total pain' but it may help to divide it into physical, emotional, social, and spiritual components. The pain which causes an animal to remain motionless while an injured part heals is a total 'feeling state.' Wall (1979) suggests that pain is better classified as a need state than as a sensation, serving more to promote healing than to avoid injury. Terminal pain is certainly a need state but it rarely promotes healing and has no built in meaning for those who suffer it. Rather it traps the patient in a situation for which there is no comforting explanation and to which there is no foreseeable end. This is a radically different pain from the postoperative pain which has been researched by many workers from Beecher (1960) onwards and which forms a large part of teaching hospital experience. Such pain is easily understood by the patient and we can ask considerable endurance of people who can expect recovery and who are coming through an event limited in time. Pain as a protective reflex is equally purposeful and comprehensible.

A few patients have suffered so greatly from 'total pain' before admission to the Hospice that they have attempted suicide. More might well have taken this step were they not convinced that this would be especially hurtful to their families, adding feelings of guilt and rejection to the losses of bereavement.

Case history Mr H G aged 73 years, had surgery for carcinoma of the stomach, followed by six courses of chemotherapy. He developed severe pain which was not relieved in spite of increasing

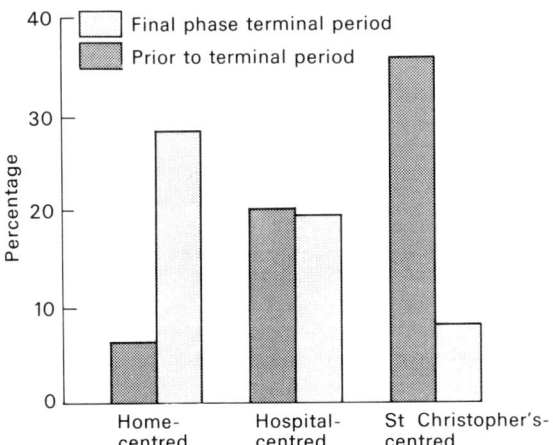

Fig. 2 Proportions of patients with severe and mostly continuous pain (Dr C. M. Parkes, by permission).

doses of analgesics until, in June 1978, he twice attempted to kill himself; first with an overdose of dextromoramide, which by this time he was taking hourly and later by slashing his wrists. On transfer to the Hospice he said 'the pain was driving me crazy.'

His pain was controlled within 48 hours by oral morphine which was given four hourly. His comment after 12 hours was 'last night's sleep was a gift.' The dose was increased in the following three weeks from 30 to 60 mg four hourly and chlorpromazine 25–50 mg was used as an adjuvant. As soon as his pain was controlled he no longer wished to end his life but as the disease progressed he became increasingly weak and dyspnoeic. During his last few days he had occasional episodes of confusion but he was still able to walk to the toilet the day before he died. He was free from pain.

A determined clarification of the responsibility for symptom control between the family doctor and the two hospitals involved and its vigorous pursuit at the time Mr H G was still being given chemotherapy should have been able to relieve a pain which the hospice did not find difficult to control. He should have had such relief for the full nine months of his advancing illness and not merely during the final three weeks. Referral to a pain clinic for consideration of a coeliac axis block might have been considered at an earlier stage but oral morphine given regularly with continual dose assessment and diamorphine given intramuscularly during his last 24 hours were sufficient to control his pain without impairment of his affect or alertness.

Incidence

Parkes' study from which Fig. 2 is taken was carried out during 1967–72. It showed that among 276 married patients under the age of 65 years who died of cancer in two London boroughs, 49 were still under active treatment at the time of death, and that while the length of time after the end of such treatment varied greatly, the median length of terminal care was nine weeks. Parkes divided these patients into home based, including in this group all who died within a week of final hospital admission, hospital based and St Christopher's based (Parkes, 1978).

The amount of preterminal and terminal pain reported by their next-of-kin afterwards is shown in Fig. 2. Although retrospective studies based on family memories are likely to be biased by confused and confusing feelings such as guilt at allowing patients to go into hospital, rationalization at not bringing them home, and projection of the angry feeling so common in bereavement, Woodbine (1982) showed that unrelieved terminal pain is still all too common. He interviewed 97 patients identified by their doctors as dying of their malignancy, 63 at home and 34 in hospital; 34 per cent of both groups reported moderate or severe pain in the 24

hours prior to interview, despite a variety of drugs. He comments that the medications written up only rarely included the narcotic analgesics and that of the 29 patients with pain only four 'received strong pain drugs on the day of interview.'

Another paper has shown how much pain goes unrecognized in a general teaching hospital where nurses accept the presence of unrelieved pain in patients too readily, as indicated by the practice of confining enquiry about pain to drug rounds and by ignoring non-verbal communication (Hunt *et al.*, 1977). However, Parkes has recently compared matched pairs of patients from his first study with others in the same area ten years later. He reports 'pain and distress in the patient is no longer a major problem in either setting' (general hospital or hospice) (Parkes and Parkes, 1984). Progress may be patchy but it is taking place.

Analysis

It is revealing to find out how many patients with terminal disease are surprised to find a doctor who will listen to the story of their suffering. While they appreciate the care and concern that have been focussed on the signs of their disease they frequently say that it is the first time that anyone has paid attention to its most troublesome aspects. As we listen to each patient and to the family, we are assessing the nature of the pain on the physical level, identifying its nature, sites, and possible causes but also analysing its implications for the patient, with family background and culture, past experience, and present anxieties taken into account.

An analysis of past history, accurate elucidation of present symptoms, a competent and thorough clinical examination, and appropriate investigations are still demanded at this stage of the disease. It is not, as before, to make a diagnosis of the nature of the disease but rather to diagnose the causes of the symptoms produced by the now incurable disease.

Once we know why a patient has pain or vomiting, is breathless or confused, we can give more effective treatment for the distress. Terminal suffering should be approached as an illness in itself, one that will respond to rationally based treatment.

Baines analysed the causes of pain in the first 100 patients with malignant disease on admission to St Christopher's Hospice in 1980. The results are shown in Table 1.

In no case was the cause thought to be purely psychogenic, though it was realized that depression and anxiety, family, financial, and spiritual problems frequently lower the thresholds for pain and thus increase the total pain experience.

With such an analysis it is possible to attempt a rational treatment of cancer pain, treatment which does not simply involve the

Table 1 Causes of pain in 100 patients with malignant disease on admission to St Christopher's Hospice in 1980. Of the 100 patients 82 were suffering from pain, with 114 separate causes

Type of pain	Number of patients
Visceral pain due to involvement of abdominal or pelvic organs	29 (including 7 with liver pain)
Bone pain	17
Soft tissue infiltration	10
Nerve compression	9
Secondary infection	6
Pleural pain	4
Colic due to bowel obstruction	4
Lymphoedema	3
Headaches due to increased intracranial pressure	3
Pain in paralysed limb(s)	3
Generalized aches and pains	3
Non-malignant causes (bedsores, constipation, piles, post-thoracotomy pain, indigestion, arthritis, corneal ulcer, gangrene)	17 (including 7 with bedsores)
Cause unknown	6

From Baines (1981).

prescription of strong analgesics (Table 2) (Baines, 1981). In no case was the cause thought to be purely psychogenic but, as with pain, it was acknowledged that anxiety could worsen the symptom. Having studied the causes it became possible to offer rational treatment.

Baines (1985) has recently summarized her observations concerning terminal intestinal obstruction (confirmed by limited autopsy). Symptom control was achieved by medication for some patients with automated subcutaneous narcotics and anti-emetics with anti-spasmodics as required. Patients were able to move about freely or to be treated at home. None were treated with intravenous fluids and nasogastric suction.

The treatment of symptoms other than pain

Although pain is the symptom most feared by patients and their families and most frequently discussed in lectures on terminal care it is probably not the most difficult to control. Nausea and vomiting, for example, may be particularly difficult to relieve and the assiduous detail with which they can be tackled has also been presented by Baines (Fig. 3, Tables 3–6). The fine details of her paper illustrate the methodical approach which will lead to the successful control of most of the symptoms with which we have to deal. As she notes, however, our prime duty in caring for the dying is to give relief as soon as possible, even when we do not fully understand the pathology. 'The greatest principle of symptom control must be "get moving and do it" ' (Baines, 1981).

Referral to other disciplines

The radiotherapy and oncology departments and the pain clinic are likely to be called on most often, although the help of many of the specialities of a general hospital may be needed.

Palliative radiotherapy may be helpful during the last weeks of a patient's life, provided it is applied skilfully. It must be given without delay, with the minimum number of treatments, and its benefit must have been carefully balanced against the price the patient has to pay in terms of the time and trouble involved. Its aim is to relieve symptoms with the lowest possible dose in the fewest possible treatments and with the minimum of side effects. It may have

an important part to play in the relief of pain from bone metastases and for many sites may be given on the day the patient is first seen in the department so that only one visit is necessary. Pelvic and vertebral metastases will need a fractionated course of treatment. The bone and joint pains of patients in the late stages of leukaemia respond to irradiation and the painful joints of hypertrophic pulmonary osteoarthropathy may be relieved by treating a primary bronchial carcinoma. Irradiation of a collapsing cervical or dorsal verebra should be considered as a prophylatic measure against possible incontinence and paralysis. A collapse causing paralysis is an emergency calling for immediate treatment or decompression if the patient's condition warrants this. Nerve root pain due to vertebral collapse and the severe pain of nerve plexus involvement is difficult to control by radiotherapy; this is a place for nerve-blocking procedures although analgesics and high-dose corticosteroids may also be used with benefit.

Radiotherapy may also be considered for the relief of haemoptysis, haematuria, or vaginal bleeding, all very disturbing to the patient and the family. It may be used to control fungation and discharge and to control cough and dyspnoea by treating either the primary tumour or mediastinal and other lymph-nodes (Bates 1984).

Regular rounds with a radiotherapist or oncologist are an essential for a hospice or continuing care unit, not only to discuss the patients selected by the terminal care team but also to review others who could benefit. Such rounds have taken place regularly at St Christopher's Hospice. Initially, they identified some 5 per cent of the total patient population as still likely to benefit. Such patients are now frequently discussed by telephone with the radiotherapist and this liaison is as straightforward as that of the continuing care unit which is part of the general hospital.

A similar exercise was carried out in developing a closer link with a pain clinic. A series of rounds reviewed all patients in the 62 Hospice beds. As the Hospice patients have a median stay of 10–12 days many patients were too ill to be considered but 5 per cent were thought likely to benefit. Various procedures were carried out on most of these patients, the majority with good, lasting relief. Others were treated as out patients or on a brief admission. Such co-operation between pain clinics and hospices is necessary and increasing (Baxter, 1984)

Table 2 Rational plan for the treatment of cancer pain

Cause of pain	Primary treatment	Secondary treatment	To consider
Visceral from involvement of abdominal or pelvic organs	Analgesics	Low-dose steroids may help	Coeliac axis block for abdominal pain Intrathecal block for pelvic pain
Bone pain Direct spread Distant metastases	1. Palliative radiotherapy 2. Non-steroidal antiinflammatory drugs 3. Immobilization cervical collar pinning	Analgesics	Nerve block; low-dose steroids may help
Soft tissue infiltration	Analgesics	Low-dose steroids	Nerve block
Nerve compression	Analgesics	High-dose steroids	Nerve block
Secondary infection 1. Deep	Systemic antibiotics including metronidazole if possibility of anaerobes; local surgery	Analgesics	Nerve block
2. Superficial	Systemic antibiotics; local applications e.g. povidone iodine	Analgesics	Topical local anaesthetics
Pleural pain	Antibiotics if appropriate	Analgesics	Intercostal block
Colic due to bowel obstruction	Faecal softeners, anti-spasmodics, e.g. Lomotil	Analgesics	
Lymphoedema	Intermittent positive pressure machine	Analgesics	High-dose steroids may help; diuretics rarely do
Headaches from raised intracranial pressure	High dose steroids*; raise head out of bed	Avoid opiate analgesics if possible	Diuretics may help
Pain in paralysed limb(s)	Physiotherapy and regular movement of limb(s) by nurses	Non-steroidal anti-inflammatory drugs	Muscle relaxants

* Steroid refers to glucocorticosteroids; low-dose steroids to prednisolone 15–30 mg daily or dexamethosone 2–4 mg daily; high-dose steroids to dexamethasone 8–16 mg daily. The dose should be gradually reduced when possible. From Baines (1981), by permission.

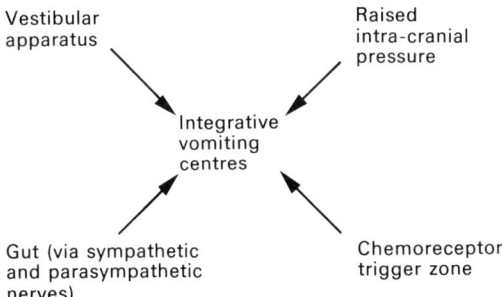

Fig. 3 The integrative vomiting centres in the midbrain can be stimulated in four ways, as shown. During the act of vomiting the glottis closes, the soft palate rises, and the abdominal muscles contract. During the sensation of nausea the stomach relaxes and there is reverse peristalsis in the duodenum. Anti-emetic drugs act at different sites in these pathways (Table 3).

Table 3 Anti-emetic drugs act at different sites

Group	Examples	Site of action
Phenothiazines	Chlorpromazine, prochlorperazine, perphenazine	Chemoreceptor trigger zone
Butyrophenones	Haloperidol	Chemoreceptor trigger zone
Metoclopramide	Metoclopramide	1. Chemoreceptor trigger zone 2. Upper gut; increases gastric peristalsis, relaxes pyloric antrum
Antihistamines	Cyclizine, promethazine	Integrative vomiting centre
Anticholinergic drugs	Hyoscine	Integrative vomiting centre

From Baines (1981).

Table 4 Postulated causes of nausea and vomiting in 35 patients. Of the 100 patients studied 65 had no problem with nausea or vomiting

Cause	Number of patients
Obstruction	
Oesophageal	3
High (pylorus, duodenum, jejunum)	2
Low (ileum, large bowel)	5
Constipation	1
Gross ascites	1
Biochemical changes	
Hypercalcaemia	5
Liver failure	5
Uraemia	3
Gastric irritation (including gastric bleeding)	6
Raised intracranial pressure	3
Drugs	1
With coughing	1
Cause unknown	6

From Baines (1981).

On the use of analgesics for terminal pain

While there is no need to resort automatically to strong analgesics when a patient approaches the terminal stages of the illness, pain must be relieved as soon as it becomes a matter for complaint. We may have to elicit such a complaint for these patients often underestimate our interest in their pain or the possibility of relief.

The essential first step is the careful taking of the history, the prerequisite of all effective work in this field and a therapeutic tool in itself. Adequate relief must be given from the beginning of the patient's downhill course for he or she should become accustomed to expect freedom from discomfort rather than its constant presence. The impact of pain is greatly influenced by past experience of pain and in turn it creates the expectation of future pain. If fear is aroused, it will immediately enhance pain by tension and once it has become established pain is likely to need larger doses for its relief. The dramatic ease that may be given by an injection naturally enhances any tendency to rely upon drugs and oral medication should be the norm. Crises should be anticipated and prevented wherever possible.

Mild pain

The relief of mild terminal pain can usually be achieved with weak analgesics and these may be sufficient throughout an entire illness. A well-tried remedy in which a patient has built up confidence over the months may be used later as a standby to supplement more powerful medication.

Aspirin and the newer non-steroidal anti-inflammatory drugs have long been used for all types of bone and joint pain in terminal disease. The work that has clarified the mechanisms of their action has endorsed years of trust in their effectiveness and in the view of many hospice doctors aspirin is still the most useful remedy for mild pain in terminal illness. Its dangers are not great in proportion to the number of patients who will benefit and are acceptable in this situation. Although gastric upset is not uncommon, it can usually be avoided by a sensible routine for taking medication, by trying different presentations of this valuable and versatile drug and by the use of antacids. It is important to discover a patient's preferences and idiosyncrasies. Paracetamol is a useful alternative.

There are many drugs for this pain. In spite of recent evidence of its potential dangers dextropropoxyphene, with or without paracetamol or aspirin (as Distalgesic, Doloxene or Darvon) continues to be widely used. It may benefit those patients who feel that aspirin is too 'ordinary' to be of help to them now and as these preparations need a doctor's prescription and come in unaccustomed forms and colours they may be expected to bring with them some placebo response.

We must be aware of the importance of factors other than pure drug action. Enthusiasm, careful instructions and the doctor's own confidence often do more to relieve terminal pain than any drugs. It is because enthusiastic interest is so often denied to the patient with terminal cancer that this pain becomes so fraught with misery.

The use of mild analgesics may be combined with small doses of one of the psychotropic drugs. When these were being introduced during the 1950s doctors working in terminal care found them a more useful addition to their pharmacopeia than the new analgesics. Drugs of the phenothiazine group are not always used with the discrimination they warrant. They may remove nausea, ease anxiety, help to control confusion, and calm restlessnesss. We certainly do not use them as a routine but they may enhance the effect of analgesics. While we await more definitive studies we rely mainly on clinical experience in making our choice between them. An effective anti-emetic with little sedative effect such as prochlorperazine may be added to any analgesic at this stage. For the more anxious patient chlorpromazine is still the best all purpose drug in this group and is often sufficient as a night sedative. This will usually be prescribed in what to psychiatrists would be very small doses, for example 10–12.5 mg three times daily or four hourly as a starting dose.

A syrup preparation is easily swallowed and is less likely to be refused by the suspicious and paranoid who are sometimes adept at removing their pills after the nurse with the drug round has disappeared.

The benzodiazepines have virtually replaced the barbiturates

Table 5

Cause	Primary treatment	Role and type of anti-emetic
Obstruction		
Oesophageal due to carcinoma of oesophagus or enlarged mediastinal glands	Radiotherapy; insertion of oesophageal tube	No use
High (pylorus or duodenum)	Consider nasogastric tube; steroids occasionally help	Metoclopramide may help
Low (ileum or large bowel)	Faecal softeners	Anti-emetics acting on vomiting centre
Constipation	Enema, suppositories aperients	Should not be needed
Gross ascites	Paracentesis with/without cytotoxic drug; diuretics may help	Anti-emetics acting on vomiting centre
Biochemical changes		
Hypercalcaemia	Steroids; may need injection at first; use low maintenance steroids or effervescent phosphate	Anti-emetics acting on CTZ* or vomiting centre
Liver failure, uraemia	Do not modify diet; steroids occasionally help	Anti-emetics acting on CTZ or vomiting centre
Gastric irritation		
Carcinoma of stomach	Cimetidine	Anti-emetics acting on gut or vomiting centre
Peptic ulcer		
Raised intracranial pressure		
Cerebral tumour	High-dose steroids; raise head of bed; diuretics occasionally help	Anti-emetics acting on vomiting centre
Drugs		
Opiate	Stop the drug if possible	Anti-emetics acting on CTZ or vomiting centre
Cytotoxic drugs		
Digoxin		
Anxiety	Emotional support; tranquillizers	

CTZ = chemoreceptor trigger zone. From Baines (1981).

with which anxiety and tension in terminal illness were usually treated 25 years ago. Diazepam may be a valuable addition to a regimen. It has also helped many relatives of dying patients to keep going so long as the dose prescribed was not too high or prolonged.

The place of the tricyclic antidepressants in the field of terminal pain control is being studied as the evidence so far is mostly anecdotal (Walsh, 1985). Both patients and family members may occasionally need them for frank depression, but sorrow should not be confused with depression; it is the appropriate reaction to the situation and calls for a listener rather than drugs.

Moderate pain

Moderate pain may be relieved by one of a number of analgesics but alone and in combination codeine is a well-known standby and serves as a standard. There are a number of drugs that appear to be equianalgesic in studies but vary in their clinical effectiveness, e.g. dihydrocodeine will help one patient and render another intractably constipated. Mixed preparations are usually to be avoided. It is better to discover a patient's own best combination of drugs.

In our view there is little place for the use of pentazocine or pethidine in terminal care. Neither are potent oral analgesics and both are comparatively short-acting. Pentazocine has the additional drawback of an unacceptably high proportion of patients experiencing psychotomimetic side-effects. Dextromoramide is more potent but relatively short-acting. It is useful, however, as a cover for a painful episode when given as a supplement to other regular medication.

Papaveretum and opium are frequently combined with aspirin and are given for moderate pain, often over long periods, in radiotherapy departments and some of the hospices. They may be the only oral opiates available in some countries. Oral morphine is most valuable when used to control moderate pain in small doses (such as 5–10 mg oral morphine). They should usually be given on

a four-hourly routine at the dose needed to give uninterrupted relief. There is no constant pattern of dose increase and patients are often successfully maintained on the same dose for weeks or months. Nor is there any problem in reducing the dose or withdrawing the narcotic altogether if pain control is later achieved by other means. Slow release morphine (MST Continus) is establishing its value and the simple twice daily regimen is welcome to many. However, accurate titration in a changing situation is less easy than with four-hourly morphine in solution.

Analgesics by suppository are valuable in home care. In our hands morphine by this route has not been as effective as oxycodone pectinate (Proladone.) Used at eight- or sometimes six-hourly intervals it may make home care a possibility for patients who can take nothing by mouth. Chlorpromazine and prochlorperazine suppositories may be added for patients with nausea and/or vomiting and should always be considered if a patient's injection sites become painful.

Severe pain

Case history The wife of a patient with severe pain from far advanced cancer is told by the houseman that the opiates are 'dangerous drugs' and that the patient will become addicted if he is given them 'too soon.'

He is finally written up for injections of morphine but the doses are spaced out beyond the effectiveness of the dose selected and frequently arrive late so that he is constantly in pain and waiting for relief. He is always anxious. A decision to try an oral mixture is made on a Friday, the dose given is ineffective and the houseman does not know what to do as no instructions have been left. The patient has a miserable weekend with greatly increased pain. Near the end of his life he is still anxiously clock watching as he waits for the next injections. At this point they are altered and become heavily sedative and he never again speaks clearly to his wife, who, like him, had been told till then that there were weeks or months ahead.

Table 6

Symptom	Comment	Therapy
Gastrointestinal		
Anorexia	Very common, may accompany taste change. Distressing to the family consider subliminal nausea	Suitable portions of food, note cultural choices, relax family pressures. Mouth care gluco corticosteroids
Dry mouth	Common, often drug induced note: thirst=symptom=unpleasant dehydration=metabolic state= frequently asymptomatic at this stage. Intravenous fluids and nasogastric tubes are generally not justifiable or acceptable	Mouth care, review drugs, suitable sweets etc. to suck, artificial saliva occasionally helpful. Narcotics usually relieve thirst, ice or choice of drinks always available
Sore mouth	Watch for thrush (common) or aphthous ulceration (uncommon). Ill fitting dentures are socially unacceptable and great misery	Nystatin may also be needed prophylatically; amphotericin, dental assistance, vitamin supplements usually disappointing, persistent mouth care, local anaesthetic gels, carbenoxolene pellets, hydrocortisone lozenges
Dysphagia	Note local lesion causing pain, treat if possible. Mediastinal obstruction, extrinsic or intrinsic, may still benefit from radiotherapy or oesophageal tube	Mouth care, local anaesthetic gels, adequate analgesia, drugs as suppositories or automated narcotic administration preferred to regular injections. Ice cream, liquidizer etc.
	'Splinting' by local fibrosis or tumour may give total dysphagia	Temporary palliation may be achieved with corticosteroids (Carter *et al.*, 1982)
Nausea and/or vomiting	See Tables 4 and 5	
Hiccup	Distressing and exhausting	Chlorpromazine, metoclopramide
Constipation	Extremely common, poor intake, debility, drugs, dehydration, immobility all contribute	Increase fluids if possible, bran if tolerated (rarely), combination of stool softener with bowel stimulant e.g. Dorbanex, suppositories, enemas
	Prevent rather than treat	Manual removals etc. are less acceptable than prevention and may be exhausting
Diarrhoea	Rule out constipation with overflow. May occur with tumours of gut, with incomplete obstruction, after radiotherapy, antibiotics, infections. Steatorrhoea with carcinoma of pancreas	Anti-diarrhoeal drugs, e.g. codein phosphate, Lomotil, adequate protection, specific treatment when indicated. Pancreatic replacements
Rectal discharge	After palliative colostomy with poor anal control is very distressing	Consider local radiotherapy, prednisolone retention enemas usually more effective than suppositories
Tenesmus	May require direct questioning to elicit	Gluco corticosteroids may reduce peritumour oedema. Consider coeliac axis block
Itch	May be severe with jaundice, Hodgkin's disease	Rule out sensitivities, cholestyramine if tolerated, antihistamines, testosterone calomine lotion with phenol crotamiton (Eurax), topical steroids
	May be caused by dryness of skin	Avoid soap, use emulsifying ointment in bath
Respiratory symptoms		
Dyspnoea	Common	Reassurance, windows, fan, positioning, physiotherapy
	Often associated with anxiety rarely associated with anaemia decreased capacity more often than increased demand, obstructive, e.g. mediastinal nodes sometimes associated with bronchospasm.	Oxygen little help and easily leads to dependence, diazepam. Bronchodilators, steroids, treat cardiac failure as appropriate
	Tumour spread, lymphangitis carcinomatosa, pleural effusion cardiac failure	Calibrated doses of narcotics *are not* lethal and give good relief. Anxiolytics
	Supervening infections with intractable cough	Antibiotics may be considered, narcotics preferred for most patients at this stage
Terminal respiratory distress	Must be controlled	Narcotics with tranquillizers until adequate dose is reached even if this may hasten death

Table 6—cont.

Symptom	Comment	Therapy
Terminal airway secretions	Distressing to family and other patients if not to the patient	Add hyoscine (Scopolamine) 0.4–0.6 mg to the injections
Cough	Exhausting, interrupts sleep	Linctus with hot drinks may still give relief even if on narcotics
	Haemoptysis is frightening, sputum may become offensive	Radiotherapy if possible, consider antibiotics, mucolytics and decongestants may be worth trying, narcotics orally and by injection terminally
Urinary symptoms		
Frequency	Common, cause of much anxiety and distress	Emepromium sometimes helps, treat infections
Incontinence	One of the greatest fears, identify causes and treat appropriately when possible	Catheterize with routine to prevent infection which leads to pain, leakage and blockage
Retention	Uncommon, may be drug induced	Review drugs, bethanechol chloride is occasionally effective, catheterization usually necessary with precautions against later infections
Central nervous system		
Depression and anxiety	See Section 25	
Confusion	Common, variety of aetiological factors require careful evaluation, some can be corrected but differential diagnosis often difficult/impossible may be drug induced, biochemical	Specific treatment if possible review drugs and doses reality reinforcement, social interaction, imaginative nursing care, psychiatrist may rarely be needed, phenothiazines if indicated
	Toxic, tumours, arteriosclerotic, psychogenic	For restlessness and agitation staff have preferences and patients idiosyncrasies, dexamethazone should be considered for tumours and their withdrawal planned according to effect
Insomnia	Not well tolerated, rarely a problem in a hospice where good symptom control and time to talk should be given, nightmares may make patients afraid to go to sleep	Physical and mental comfort rituals, alcohol, warm drinks, hypnotics, tricyclic antidepressants single dose nocte, narcotics to maintain pain control with increase of evening and/or midnight dose
Fungating tumours	Need not be offensive	Treat infections
	Radiotherapy should be considered especially for haemorrhage, infection is often anaerobic	Metronidazole ± broad spectrum antibiotics topical sprays clean with Eusol : paraffin 1:2–4, povidone iodine 4%, non-adhesive dressings, deodorant pads and fans
Decubitus ulcers	Fairly common, especially in older patients	Prevent with mobilization physiotherapy, positioning, etc. sheepskins, air or water beds, Spenco mattresses, local preference for dressings lotions, protective creams etc. oxygen, ultraviolet light

With acknowledgement to Mount (1978) and Baines (1984).

Similar stories continue to be repeated because misconceptions concerning the use of the strong analgesics deny relief to many patients. Fear of producing tolerance and psychological dependence is prevalent, repeated escalations of dose are anticipated, and both patients and doctors fear a time when nothing can be effective. It is thought that there is no middle road between a patient in pain and one heavily sedated and because no proper standard of pain relief with unaffected sensorium exists in the clinician's mind, he accepts these alternative as inevitable.

For many years those involved with the care of large numbers of patients with severe terminal pain have believed that nothing could replace the opiates and have known that they could be given without such problems. Although new understanding of pain mechanisms and of its chemistry may alter our approach and give us new tools during the next decade, patients need relief now and should expect the knowledge of how to give it to them from any doctor. No foreseeable number of hospices or pain clinics is going to reach the majority of the terminally ill many of whom are at present suffering pain and other physical distress, nor would it be right that such units or teams should undertake the care of all these patients as an exclusive speciality. Skill and confidence in handling analgesics and their adjuvants must become part of general medical education, and whoever treats these patients must know when to begin with narcotic drugs, what routine to establish, what other medications to combine with them and what drugs or manoeuvres to consider for the occasional patient who has a marked persistent intolerance to opiates (Twycross, 1984; Twycross and Lack, 1983).

When to begin

When terminal pain escapes control with moderate analgesics or when the patient finds he has to swallow more than two pills to obtain relief it is time for the smaller dose of a stronger drug. Vigorous effort must be made again to identify the cause of the increased pain and consider any specific treatment that may be available and appropriate. The clinical team should be as ready to consider the various measures for pain control as to discuss different forms of active treatment and to record plans for pain relief in the notes.

Any continuing problems must be reviewed constantly but there is no need to deny a patient relief of severe pain while its detailed aetiology is investigated. Adequate relief must be given as soon as possible. We believe that the drug of choice is still oral morphine, the most versatile and flexible available. If pain is relieved later by other means, it can easily be discontinued. Physical signs of withdrawal are rare and will be avoided by tapering the dose over several days. If this fact were more widely recognized, this drug might less often be withheld from those with non-malignant terminal disease causing severe pain who might benefit.

Routine for pain prevention

The typical pain of terminal cancer is constant in character, although it may have exacerbations such as on movement. Constant pain calls for constant control, not a desperate switch-back between bouts of pain and periods of somnolent relief. 'In our hospital the patients *earn* their morphine' (a medical student). Pain itself is the strongest antagonist to the drugs given to suppress it and it is of cardinal importance that neither its presence nor its threat should act against relief. If a patient has to ask for an analgesic, it will act as a reminder each time of the dependence on the drug and on the person who supplies it. If it is given regularly and at a dose that covers the extra period of relief that may be required should a dose be delayed, then pain can be forgotten and the self-perpetuating spiral of misery and dependence is not initiated. Continual expectations of the recurrence of pain with narcotic orders 'when required' is the route to iatrogenically induced dependence (Saunders, 1963).

Vere's series of diagrams (Figs. 4–8) illustrate how the regular giving of oral narcotics prevents pain breakthrough by keeping the plasma drug concentration continuously in the patient's own effective zone and below the level of toxicity. Oral doses, yielding a more rounded peak than intravenous administration, facilitate this. Doses should be regularly spaced, including a night dose for many patients, who will prefer being woken for a dose rather than by pain some time later. If injections are necessary because of nausea and vomiting, the same routine should be maintained.

Many years of experience have shown that tolerance is very rarely a clinical problem and that when it occurs it has usually been induced by unnecessary, automatic dose increase. Should a patient's pain break through and a larger dose is needed, the effective zone has shifted and this is as true for respiratory depression and other side effects as for analgesia. In a recent series of 20 hospice patients on high-dose narcotics, all 12 of whom had a history of chronic bronchitis and eight of whom were dying of carcinoma of bronchus, only one had an elevated PCO_2 level and only one was severely hypoxic (Walsh, 1984a). Titration of the dose rather than the employment of standard doses and oral administration may thus allow tolerance to the respiratory depressant effect of morphine while continuing to provide pain relief. Sequential increases in oral doses are usually in increments of 5 mg for doses of less than 20 mg, then to 30 mg, 45 mg, and 60 mg, and there-

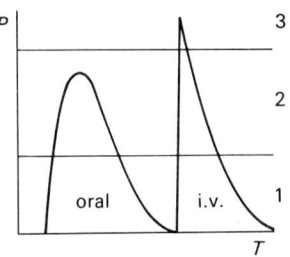

Fig. 5 Oral and intravenous plasma concentration–time curves. For symbols see Fig. 4 (Vere, 1978, by permission).

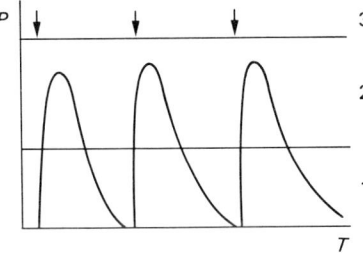

Fig. 6 Doses spaced too widely to maintain analgesia. Larger doses at the same frequency would only risk toxicity. For symbols see Fig. 4 (Vere, 1978, by permission).

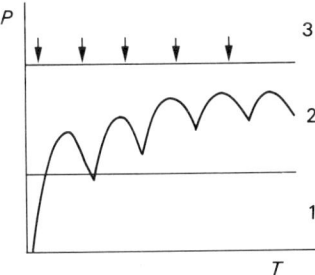

Fig. 7 Doses spaced at satisfactory intervals to maintain analgesia. For symbols see Fig. 4 (Vere, 1978, by permission).

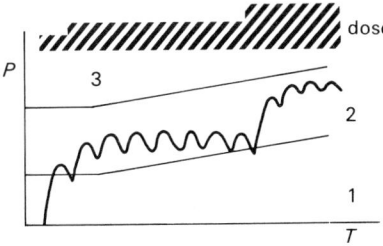

Fig. 8 The effects of tolerance. For symbols see Fig. 4 (Vere, 1978, by permission).

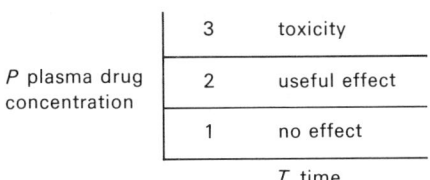

P plasma drug concentration	3	toxicity
	2	useful effect
	1	no effect
	T time	

Fig. 4 Plasma concentration zones in relation to drug effects. The same symbols are used in Figs. 5–8 (Vere, 1978, by permission).

after each increase is usually in the range of 20–30 mg. The maximum effective dose is ill-defined but in our practice doses higher than 90 mg or a reduction of the interval to three hourly are seldom needed. As Twycross and Wald (1976) have shown (Fig. 9) tolerance seems to level off in most cases and usually ceases to operate after a few weeks. Psychological dependence does not occur and whilst physical dependence may develop, it does not prevent the downward adjustment of the dose of narcotic when considered clinically possible. Many hospices are now using automated narcotic administration together with anti-emetics in their

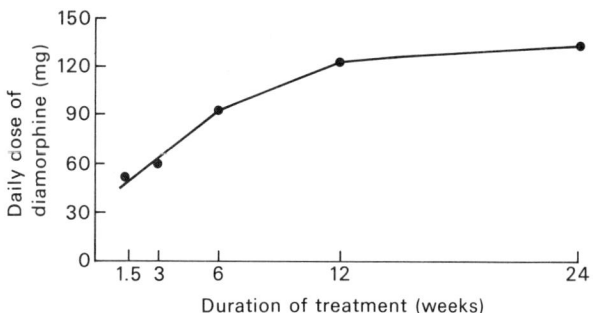

Fig. 9 418 patients admitted consecutively with advanced cancer were grouped according to survival following the start of treatment with diamorphine; group median final daily dose of diamorphine is shown plotted against group median duration of treatment (Twycross, 1977, by permission).

wards for patients with intractable vomiting and find that this (together with pain) is well controlled. Reduction in the doses needed as well as a return to oral medication have been found possible. This method is of great value in home care. Occasionally, epidural morphine may however be considered.

In many centres phenothiazines are routinely given with an oral narcotic solution. The usual practice is to dispense these separately and to keep the dose relatively stable while altering the narcotic. It is the increase in the drugs of the phenothiazine group that usually causes the over-sedation too often seen in general wards. Other adjuvant medication should also be added individually and only one drug change should be made at a time. A degree of polypharmacy is indicated for many of these patients but this must be carefully monitored and regularly reviewed.

The majority of the kinetic work conducted on morphine so far has been on single-dose profiles. These studies are of doubtful relevance to advanced cancer patients with multisystem disease, receiving opiates repeatedly. The pharmacokinetic study most commonly quoted (Brunk and Delle, 1974) showed 30 per cent relative bioavailability of oral morphine. This followed single-dose oral administration (tablet formulation) and showed low levels of plasma-free morphine, high plasma and urine-conjugated morphine levels, and an apparent increased tendency to normorphine formation after oral administration. These data have been interpreted as explaining the poor analgesic efficacy of oral morphine in clinical studies such as that of Beecher *et al.*, (1953). Recent work using radioimmunoassay has shown that when a suitable extraction procedure is employed (Grabkinski *et al.*, 1983) the apparent mean morphine plasma levels measured are about 30 per cent lower than those revealed by methods without this procedure confirming that a significant error in apparent plasma levels is produced by cross-reacting metabolites. Amongst 23 advanced cancer patients the apparent 'trough' concentrations of morphine in plasma were pre-extraction 80 ng/ml (95 per cent CI, 64–96 ng/ml) and post-extraction 26 ng/ml (95 per cent CI, 20–33 ng/ml), both calculated to 10 mg morphine base. These values are higher than would be predicted from data available from single-dose morphine pharmacokinetic studies and confirm that repeated oral morphine administration is an effective method of drug delivery. Recent pharmacokinetic data (Sawe *et al.*, 1981) confirm that dosage of aqueous morphine must be individualized because of between-individual variations in metabolism. Definitions of changes in morphine metabolism during chronic repeated administration awaits the result of further studies (Walsh, 1984b).

The last hours Many patients become somewhat drowsy and confused in their last hours. Medication commonly has to be given by injection at this time. Some people require less narcotic and may become relatively over-sedated but on the other hand patients who develop terminal restlessness may have increased pain with decreased ability to convey this to others. It is usually wise to give the intramuscular equivalent to the previous oral doses on a regular basis and increase the dose if indicated. Some patients develop jerking or twitching movements and, although they may not be aware of this, their visitors will be disturbed. Diazepam 5–10 mg added to the routine injection should give control. Fluid may accumulate in the lungs during the last hours and give rise to the 'death rattle.' If we prepare for this comparatively common occurrence and prescribe ahead for injections of hyoscine 0.4–0.6 mg together with the opiate an experienced nurse will detect the first signs and this injection added as required will usually prevent this distress for the family and other patients.

Terminal, confused restlessness must be controlled with adequate sedation, especially in home care. Chlorpromazine is usually the phenothiazine of choice at this stage but methotrimeprazine is more sedative and it is rare for an adequate dose (25–50 mg) to be ineffective. This should be repeated till control is achieved. Hyoscine itself is also a strong sedative when used with an opiate at this stage.

Which opiate?

Twycross was invited to test the fairly common clinical impression that diamorphine (heroin) was the opiate of choice. In a series of studies in St Christopher's Hospice a cross-over trial between morphine and diamorphine showed that given regularly at individually optimized doses in an elixir with cocaine and a phenothiazine, there was no clinically observable difference. As diamorphine is not available in most countries this was an important finding. The Hospice, which had previously used only diamorphine, changed its practice in 1977 and morphine is now prescribed for all oral narcotic medication (up to 80 per cent of all doses of narcotic given). Only a minority of patients receive doses above 30 mg morphine orally (equivalent to 15 mg by injection). Because of its greater solubility, diamorphine is retained for the subcutaneous and intramuscular injections most patients need in their final 24–48 hours. The dose is scaled down as a start in the ratio oral morphine: injected diamorphine 3:1. The number of patients needing the larger doses and therefore larger volume is small and morphine would be an acceptable alternative for all but a small minority (oral to injected morphine 2:1). Other more soluble opiates such as hydromorphone would be alternatives. These drugs should be used subcutaneously or intramuscularly, never as intravenous boluses to an existing line when tolerance develops rapidly with alternating toxicity and restlessness. Continuous i.v. or s.c. administration can be satisfactory alternatives.

Experience shows that when regularly administered oral morphine is used as the narcotic therapy of choice in this setting there will only infrequently be the need to broaden the armamentarium to include other agents. The only other strong analgesics likely to be prescribed in St Christopher's are phenazocine and dextramoramide. Phenazocine is given when a patient dislikes the morphine solution or prefers a tablet (5 mg are equivalent to 25 mg morphine). Methadone is rarely prescribed. There is no problem of cumulation with morphine or diamorphine but the fate and excretion of methadone is more complex. Although it has been widely used for ambulant and fitter groups of patients, life-threatening cumulation may occur among the frail and elderly.

The Brompton Cocktail Mixtures under this and other titles and containing different amounts of one or more of the narcotic drugs are widely used; frequently hospital staff do not know what their own mixture contains and little discrimination is used. Melzack *et al.* (1979) compared a formula containing alcohol and cocaine to a simple aqueous solution of morphine in a double blind study and, like Twycross (1979), showed that cocaine in the mixture added no sustained effect. We conclude that morphine in water or chloroform water (the traditional English vehicle for mixtures) is as effective as the previously popular mixtures and that the latter should be discontinued in view of confusions concerning the strength of the narcotic dose.

A solution is normally to be preferred to tablets: the dose can be titrated accurately to the patient's need and may be increased without enlarging the volume taken. A patient whose dose for pain control progresses from one to three or four tablets is reminded on each drug round of that increase.

Alcohol was omitted from the St Christopher's mixture without a controlled trial but is used separately as it enhances normal social interchange for the patients in a way open to not other tranquillizer. Like other diversions, a drink shared with family or friends may act as a potent reliever of all forms of pain.

No one drug and no routine method is the whole answer to the control of terminal pain. Regular giving is not a panacea, it is a pattern into which other treatments and a general approach should be integrated. Success in pain control is easier to achieve when realistic goals are set. A patient needing opiates for pain relief should usually be sleeping well within the first day or two. It is possible, especially with bone pain, that pain on movement may be more difficult to abolish and with a few patients this may never be fully achieved if supplementary treatment with non-steroidal anti-inflammatory drugs, radiotherapy or nerve blocks are not possible or successful. However, once nights are good and rest during the day is pain free, most of these patients will accept some change in their level of activity. The few we have encountered with apparent opiate insensitivity have taxed us all and further studies are much needed in this area as in other aspects of opiate metabolism. Other reasons for continued distress are discussed below.

Mental pain

It is rare to find among the results of investigations and examinations with which a patient's notes are filled any comment on the feelings or estimation of the patient's insight into what is happening.

These may well be the main problems and greatly exacerbate the total pain and undermine the patient's capacity to cope with increasing weakness. Any illness causes anxiety and one that becomes more serious in spite of a variety of treatments until it is patently life threatening will engender many fears. Patients tend to be left alone with these fears and receive only reassurances which they suspect are false or which have no relation to the anxiety they are facing. Mental suffering is likely to be enhanced by any physical distress; the doctor can do much to relieve the one as the other is tackled. Competent symptom control brings support at a deep level, demanding time with the patient and the close contact often denied at this stage; isolation adds to the feeling of failure and the obscure sense of guilt suffered by many dying patients.

Fears of parting, of what will happen to dependants, of pain and of failing to cope are all realistic fears, common among dying patients. Although the complexity of the problems faced by many are daunting, it need not make us feel helpless. Dying is not a psychiatric illness and does not usually call for specialized skills in counselling. Those who distance themselves, feeling they can bring nothing but a lack of comprehension, do not realize that it is their attempt to understand and not success in doing so that eases the patient's loneliness.

Nurses are closer to their patients than most doctors and are likely to hear more of a patient's questions and fears. Team consultations are essential if we are to reach helpful understanding. Social workers can listen in a unique way, for they are not involved with therapy and have been trained to act as the recipients of unacceptable feelings and projected angers; these are better expressed than buried only to appear in a different guise. Contact with physiotherapists offers more than the pleasure of assisted movement or even the joy of tackling the stairs again, with the consequent reward of the weekend home. It is well known that the interested ward orderly may know more than anyone of matters which patients do not feel able to share with the professionals who surround them and we must not forget that boredom may be a major component of mental pain and a good gossip, like other distractions, the best way to relieve it.

The psychotropic drugs may help in bringing the burden of the illness within a particular patient's compass and they are widely used. Their prescription as adjuvants to analgesics has been discussed above. The narcotic group of drugs are themselves powerful 'tranquillizers' and some of their effectiveness stems from this fact. Most dying patients are likely to have a drug of the phenothiazine group prescribed. The tricyclic group of drugs are used empirically, though less frequently. A patient with an endogenous or severe reactive depression stands out in a ward of dying patients and to a lesser extent so does one who has developed a chronic pain syndrome. These problems do not arise with most patients who die of malignant disease but are an occasional challenge that may need specialist advice.

Most people will finally accept the approach of death as they accept other forms of loss, although the faint hope of the unexpected recovery or remission is common until near the end and is not to be discouraged. Hope in different forms can exist all through such illness, gradually changing its content. This grows out of the realistic facing of problems and helps the patient to accept the responsibility of living the life that remains. It is patients who are persistently unable to accept losses of all kinds through a protracted illness who test the courage of all around them as well as their own. Isolation only makes this suffering harder to bear and those who feel they have little to give must still keep coming.

Social pain

When an illness has a foreseeable end most families will come to grips with the situation and will wish to look after a dying relative at home as long as possible. Although the trend is for a higher proportion of cancer deaths to occur in hospital, prolongation of life by the newer treatments frequently means that much of this extra time is spent at home. Only a minority will require heavy nursing for any length of time but there may be a prolonged period of emotional strain for patient and family alike. If they can be helped to handle this, it may be an important time for them all for it enables the survivors to prepare for parting and to make some restitution for the failures of the past. Old tensions may become acute but even at this stage, often because it is the final stage, reconciliation is not uncommon and many people make this a remarkably fruitful time. The dependence of the sick person often strengthens attachment and many people cope heroically with the heavy burden of care.

Others cannot handle the emotions involved and some families have such complicated problems that the help of a caseworker may be essential (Earnshaw-Smith, 1982). Financial burdens are often heavy, especially for those who have prolonged time off work but patients should be included in all discussions and plans as they should be involved as far as possible in normal family life. Patients who are kept in the dark about family finances and various practical matters will have the added burden of fancying they have hurt or offended others because of the barriers thus erected. One can understand the strong desire to keep all worries from patients, yet this protectiveness frequently leads to crippling tensions, and it is sad since patients are likely to come to know the truth by other means. To keep an unshared secret from an intimate inevitably impairs communication and can add greatly to the sum of the patients' distress.

Admission may bring comfort for the patient and reduction of anxiety for the family which must not be bought at the cost of feelings of guilt. The family must be reassured that they have done what they could and that professional help is now needed on a full-time basis. The ward staff must not take over care in such a way as to exclude the family, who may not easily be involved with much of the physical care of the patient. They can contribute greatly to security and peace by their mere presence and this should be made possible and explicit. They are present as of right at this time, both cared for and caring. The social worker and the chaplain may be much involved with those who react aggressively to their pain or are overwhelmed by their feelings but every member of staff should be able to give some recognition, even though brief, to the family that is maintaining its last watch with a dying member.

The long pain of the family's bereavement is part of terminal pain. They will begin to grieve their imminent parting during the illness but the real letting go and approach to the new situation will rarely happen before the patient dies. The final watch and the witnessing of a peaceful death may be very important for some families; others cannot remain by the bedside. Staying there may not be possible or advisable and care must be taken to protect them from feelings of guilt and responsibility. Ward staff are all too familiar with the desolation of the final moment of parting and the empty numbness that follows it but do not always appreciate how greatly their supporting presence can help.

Some families ask for sedatives but this is probably mistaken. Grief needs to be expressed at this point and drugs may inhibit this natural and eventually healing reaction. There is no ground for prescribing tranquillizers or antidepressants to the bereaved as a routine. Parkes believes that such drugs should be reserved for the potentially suicidal and for those who, despite all efforts to help, remain in a state of chronic agitation or depression. A mild hypnotic may be needed for those who sleep remains disturbed.

The bereaved family comes slowly to full realization of what has happened and after often intense inner struggle and dejection is eventually ready to build a new life. This may take many months and is felt like a sort of illness which is finally healed. Abnormal, unresolved grief needs skilled help.

The whole process of bereavement is not often seen by clinicians other than family doctors but we should all accept two responsibilities. Firstly, to see that others are alert to identifying and helping those who are especially at risk in their loss, and secondly, to do all that is possible to ease the memories of the final phase for those who live on (West, 1984).

Most dying people show remarkable endurance and those who spend time close to them find that this helps to reduce their own fears of death. The dying have a good heritage to leave which is not always recognized or received. Parkes writes of his admiration for many of the people who have shared their grief with him and finds that counselling the bereaved makes it easier to recognize bereavement as an acceptable part of life (Parkes, 1984).

Spiritual pain

Not many people are likely to express the suffering of their doubts and griefs in religious terms. Nevertheless, feelings of failure, regret, and meaninglessness are spiritual needs and liaison with a priest or minister of the patient's choice may then be important. The ward sister is often the person with whom the hospital chaplain has the most to do but contact with the doctor may be essential.

Consultation concerned with the patient's needs rather than medical information is required and is most effective when it is personal, informal, and continuing. It would be unwarranted intrusion to suggest such a contact when there is no understanding or willingness on the part of the patient but in spite of the gap that seems to exist between minister or priest and people we will often be surprised how welcome such a visit can be. We may all have to face these questions from our patients and need to remain as a listener when we feel there are no answers to give that could bring help.

Staff pain

The supporters themselves frequently need supporting, especially during their first weeks in terminal care. Its demands cause pain and bewilderment at times to all in this field and the closer the staff are to the weakness of the patients and the grief of the families, the more they too will suffer the pangs of bereavement. Many will find they are suffering a process of numbness and exhaustion, protest, anger, and depression and will need to share this if they

are to find their way through. The resilience of those who continue to work in this field is won by a full understanding of what is happening and not by a retreat behind a technique.

Efficiency is always comforting. The giving of effective relief to all types of pain makes this an extremely rewarding field. Nevertheless, if we are to remain for long near the suffering of dependence and parting we need to develop a basic philosophy and search, often painfully, for meaning in even the most adverse situations. We have to gain enough confidence in what we are doing and enough freedom from our anxieties to listen to another's distress. In this coming together we may see something of the achievement that good terminal care can make possible.

References

Aitken-Swan, J. and Easson, E. C. (1959). Reactions of cancer patients on being told their diagnosis. *Br. Med. J.* **1**, 779–783.
Baines, M. (1981). Principles of symptom control. In *Hospice – the living idea* (eds C.M. Saunders, D. Summers and N. Teller). Arnold, London.
—— (1984). Control of other symptoms. In *The management of terminal malignant disease* 2nd edn (ed. C. Saunders), pp. 100–132. Arnold, London.
—— (1985). Medical management of intestinal obstruction in patients with advanced malignant disease. *Lancet*.
Bates, T. (1984). Radiotherapy in terminal care. In *The management of terminal malignant disease* 2nd edn (ed. C. Saunders), pp. 133–138. Arnold, London.
Baxter, R. (1984). Specialized techniques for the relief of pain. In *The management of terminal malignant disease* 2nd edn (ed. C. Saunders), pp. 91–99. Arnold, London.
Beecher, H. K. (1960). Quantitive effect of drugs. Oxford University Press, New York.
Beecher, H. K., Keats, A. S., Mosteller, F. and Lasagna L. (1953). The effectiveness of oral analgesics (morphine, codeine, acetylsalicylic acid) and the problem of placebo 'reactors' and 'non-reactors'. *J. Pharmacol. Exp. Ther.* **109**, 393–400.
Brewin, T. B. (1977). The cancer patient: communication and morale. *Br. Med. J.* **ii**, 1623–1627.
Brunk, S. F. and Delle, M. (1974). Morphine metabolism in man. *Clin. Pharmacol. Ther.* **16**, 51–57.
Carter, R. L., Pittam, M. R. and Tanner, N. S. B. (1982). Pain and dysphagia in patients with squamous carcinomas of the head and neck: the role of perineural spread. *J. R. Soc. Med.* **75**, 598–606.
Cassell, E. J. (1982). The nature of suffering and the goals of medicine. *New Engl. J. Med.* **306**, 639–645.
Council of Europe (1976). Recommendation 779 on the Rights of the Sick and Dying. 27th ordinary session, January.
Earnshaw-Smith. E. (1982). Emotional pain in dying patients and their families. *Nursing Times* **78**, 1865–1867.
Ford, G. R. and Pincherle G. (1978). Arrangements for terminal care in the NHS (especially for cancer patients). *Health Trends* **10**, 73–76.
Grabkinski, P. Y., Kaiko, R. F., Walsh, T. D., Foley K. M. and Houde R. W. (1983). Morphine radioimmunoassay specificity before and after extraction of plasma and cerebrospinal fluid. *J. pharm. Sci.* **72**, 27–30.
Hinton, J. (1963). The physical and mental distress of the dying. *Q. J. Med.* **32**, 1–20.
—— (1979). Comparison of places and policies for terminal care. *Lancet* i, 29–32.
Holford, J. M. (1973). Terminal care. Care of the dying. Proceedings of a National Symposium held 29 November 1972. HMSO, London.
Hunt, J. M., Stollar, T. D., Littlejohns, D. W., Twycross, R. G., and Vere, D. W. (1977). Patients with protracted pain: a survey conducted at the London Hospital. *J. Med. Ethics* **3**, 61–73.
Kennedy, I. McC. (1984). The law relating to the treatment of the terminally ill. In *The management of terminal malignant disease* 2nd edn (ed. C. Saunders), pp. 227–231. Arnold, London.
Lancet, (1980). In cancer, honesty is here to stay, **ii**, 245.
Melzack, R., Mount B. M. and Gordon, J. M. (1979). The Brompton mixture versus morphine solution given orally: effects on pain. *Can. Med. J.* **120**, 435–439.
Mount, B. (1978). Palliative care of the terminally ill. *Ann. R. Coll. Phys. Surg. Can.* **XX**, 201–208.
Novack, D.H., Clumer R., Smith R. L. *et al.* (1979). Changes in physicians attitudes towards telling the patient. *J. Am. Med. Assoc.* **241**, 897–900.

Parkes, C. M. (1978). Home or hospital? Patterns of care for the terminally ill cancer patient as seen by surviving spouses. *J. R. Coll. Gen. Pract.* **28**, 19–30.

—— (1984). Psychological aspects In *The management of terminal malignant disease* 2nd edn (ed. C. Saunders), pp. 43–63. Arnold, London.

—— and Parkes, J. (1984). 'Hospice' versus 'hospital care – re-evaluation after 10 years as seen by surviving spouses. *Post Med. J.* **60**, 120–124.

Saunders, C. M. (1963). The treatment of intractable pain in terminal cancer. *Proc. R. Soc. Med.* **56**, 191–197.

Sawe, J., Dahlstrom, B., Paalzow, L. and Rane, A., (1981). Morphine kinetics in cancer patients. *Clin. Pharmacol. Ther.* **30**, 629–635.

Spencer-Jones, J. (1981). Telling the right patient. *Br. Med.J.* **283**, 291–292.

Stedeford, A. (1981a). Couples facing death. I. Psychological aspects. *Br. Med. J.* **283**, 1033–1036.

Stedeford, A. (1981b). Couples facing death. II. Unsatisfactory communication. *Br. Med. J.* **283**, 1098–1101.

Twycross, R. G. (1977). Choice of strong analgesic in terminal cancer: diamorphine or morphine? *Pain: J. Int. Assoc. Study Pain* **3**, 93–104.

—— (1979). Effect of cocaine in the Bromptom Cocktail. In *Advances in pain research and therapy*, Vol. 3 (eds J. J. Bonica and D. Albe-Fessard), pp. 927–932. Raven Press, New York.

—— and Wald, S. J. (1976). Long term use of diamorphine in advanced cancer. In *Advances in pain research and therapy*, Vol. 1 (eds J. J. Bonica and D. Albe-Fessard), pp. 653–661. Raven Press, New York.

—— (1984). Relief of pain. In *The management of terminal malignant disease* 2nd edn (ed. C. Saunders), pp. 64–90. Arnold, London.

—— and Lack, S. A. (1983) *Symptom control in far advanced cancer. Pain relief*. Pitman, London.

Vanderpool, H. Y. (1978). The ethics of terminal care. *J. Am. Med. Assoc.* **239**, 10, 850–852.

Vere, D. W. (1978). Pharmacology of morphine drugs used in terminal care. In *Topics in therapeutics*, Vol. 4 (ed. D. W. Vere), pp. 72–83. Pitman, London.

Wall, P. D. (1979). On the relation of injury to pain. *Pain* **6**, 253–264.

Walsh, T. D. (1984a). Opiates and respiratory function in advanced cancer. *Recent results in cancer research* **89**, 115–117.

—— (1984b). Oral morphine in chronic cancer pain. *Pain* **18**, 1.

—— (1986). Controlled study of imiprimine and morphine in chronic pain due to advanced cancer. In *Proceedings of the American Society of Clinical Oncology* Vol. 5, March 1983, p. 237.

West, T. W. (1984). In patient management of advanced malignant disease. In *The management of terminal malignant disease* 2nd edn (ed. C. Saunders), pp. 154–169. Arnold, London.

Woodbine, G. (1982). The care of patients dying from cancer. *J. R. Coll. Gen. Pract.* **32**, 685–689.

APPENDIX
NORMAL OR REFERENCE VALUES
FOR BIOCHEMICAL DATA

NORMAL OR REFERENCE VALUES FOR BIOCHEMICAL DATA

A.M. GILES AND B. D. ROSS

Classification of laboratory results

Values are presented in the following format; for individual tests see general text.

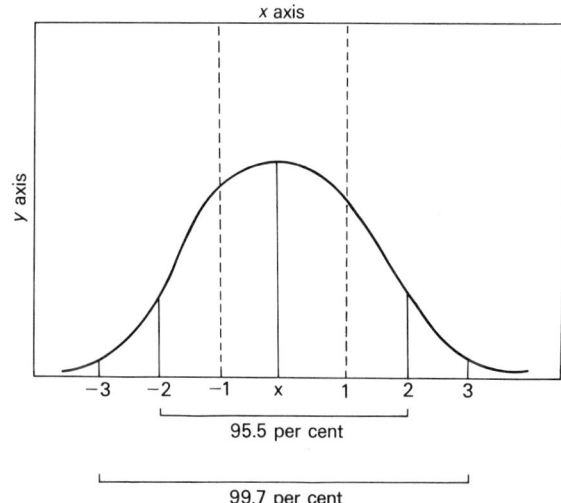

Fig. 1 Normal or Gaussian distribution curve.

Introduction

The precise quantitation of substances in easily accessible body fluids is an integral part of the clinical assessment of patients. The results are used in screening for disease as well as in diagnosis, and monitoring the response to therapy in established disease. Much diagnostic weight rests on single determinations and patterns of biochemical tests. To this end it is important to consider biological variations between healthy individuals, inherent variations in laboratory methods, and the errors of sampling and hospital practice which can influence every determination. The first (and the last) are the provinces of the physician ordering the test. The second is the concern of the laboratory which provides quality control and reference values for the test.

Normal range and 'abnormal' results

Clinical diagnostic decisions may depend equally upon finding a 'normal' or an 'abnormal' result for any test requested. The physician should be clear as to the meaning of these terms. An important task of the clinical chemist is therefore to provide relevant sets of reliable reference data. Customarily, laboratory test results are interpreted by comparison to traditional but often inadequately defined 'normal' values. The wide belief that biological data assume a Gaussian distribution is inappropriate. Most biological data are not symmetrically distributed and require statistical tools which assume other kinds of distribution or are independent of distribution form.

Normal range

In most texts, the normal range is defined as the mean $\pm$ 2 s.d. (Fig. 1). This is, however, not the commonest method applied to clinical chemistry tests. Many of the values most quoted in clinical practice are in fact 'ranges' in a skew-distribution calculated to include 95 per cent of values obtained from a 'healthy' population. By whatever criteria it is obtained, the normal range is compounded of both physiological variation and the irreducible analytical error. More elaborate statistical handling of human biochemical data is available for individual tests, but is not generally required in making a diagnosis. By way of warning however, it will readily be appreciated that if this criterion of health (viz. biochemical results within 95 per cent limits for the given value), is applied to multiple tests in any individual then with a battery of say 12 tests only 50 per cent of 'normal' individuals will be found to be 'healthy'.

In conclusion, the use of the following tables of normal values for biochemical tests must therefore include an appreciation of the limitations in 'normal' values of analytical variation and differences between methods of analysis, as well as the differences of sex, age, and sampling inherent in such an operation. The physician should constantly bear in mind the need to see individual results of laboratory tests in their clinical context.

Throughout the tables values are given in SI units; for conversion to mg%, multiply by molecular weight (MW) $\times 10^{-1}$.

Table 1 Everyday tests

Determination	Sample†	SI units	Conventional units
Alcohol	B or P	Legal limit (UK) < 17.4 mmol/l	< 80 mg/dl
α-Amylase	P	0–180 Somogyi units/dl	
Albumin	P	35–50 g/l	3.5–5.0 g/dl
Albumin—pregnancy	P	25–38 g/l	2.5–3.8 g/dl
Anion gap $(Na^+ + K^+) - (HCO_3^- + Cl^-)$*	P	12–17 mmol/l	
Barbiturate Short acting Medium acting Long acting	B	Possibly fatal if: > 35 μmol/l > 105 μmol/l > 215 μmol/l	 > 0.8 mg/dl > 2.4 mg/dl > 5.0 mg/dl
Bilirubin*	P	3–17 μmol/l	0.2–1.0 mg/dl
Bromsulphthalein retention	P	< 5% dye remains	
Bicarbonate*	P	24–30 mmol/l	24–30 mEq/l
Bicarbonate—pregnancy	P	20–25 mmol/l	20–25 mEq/l
Calcium (ionized)	P	1.0–1.25 mmol/l	4.0–5.0 mg/dl
Calcium (total)	P	2.12–2.65 mmol/l	8.5–10.6 mg/dl
Calcium (total)—pregnancy	P	1.95–2.35 mmol/l	7.8–9.4 mg/dl
Chloride	P	95–105 mmol/l	95–105 mEq/l
Copper	P	12–26 μmol/l	76–165 μg/dl
Creatinine	P	70–150 μmol/l	0.7–1.7 mg/dl
Creatinine—pregnancy	P	24–68 μmol/l	0.27–0.76 mg/dl
Cholesterol‡	P	3.9–7.8 mmol/l	150–300 mg/dl
Glucose (fasting)*	P	4.0–6.0 mmol/l	72–108 mg/dl
Iron	S	M 14–31 μmol/l F 11–30 μmol/l	78–174 μg/dl 62–168 μg/dl
Total iron-binding capacity (TIBC)	S	54–75 μmol/l	302–420 μg/dl
Lead (indicative of excessive exposure) Adults Children	B	0.3–1.8 μmol/l 1.8–3.9 mmol/l 1.8–3.0 mmol/l	6.2–37.2 μg/dl 37–81 μg/dl 37–62 μg/dl
Lithium	P	(therapeutic) 0.5–1.5 mmol/l (toxic) > 2.0 mmol/l	0.5–1.5 mEq/l > 2.0 mEq/l
Magnesium	P	0.75–1.05 mmol/l	1.5–2.1 mEq/l
Osmolality	P	278–305 mosm/kg	
Phenylalanine	P	(infants) 42–73 μmol/l	0.69–1.2 mg/dl
Phosphate (inorganic)*	P	0.8–1.45 mmol/l	2.48–4.5 mg/dl
Potassium*	P	3.5–5.0 mmol/l	3.5–5.0 mEq/l
Protein (total)*	P	60–80 g/l	6.0–8.0 g/dl
Sodium	P	135–145 mmol/l	135–145 mEq/l
Urea	P	2.5–6.7 mmol/l	15–40 mg/dl
Urea—pregnancy	P	2.0–4.2 mmol/l	12–25 mg/dl
Urea nitrogen		1.16–3.12 mmol/l	7.0–18.7mg/dl
Uric acid*	P	M 210–480 μmol/l F 150–390 μmol/l	3.5–8.0 mg/dl 2.5–6.5 mg/dl
Uric acid—pregnancy	P	100–270 μmol/l	1.7–4.5 mg/dl

These values are age-dependent.
* See Table 3.
† B = Whole blood: S = Serum: P = Plasma: U = Urine.
M = Male.   F = Female.
‡ Figures refer to current distribution in the United Kingdom. Desirable upper limit 5.9 mmol/l (228 mg/100 ml).

Table 2 Blood gases

	SI units	Conventional units
Arterial carbon dioxide ($PaCO_2$)	4.7–6.0 kPa	35.0–45.0 mm Hg
Mixed venous CO_2 ($PvCO_2$)	5.5–6.8 kPa	41.0–51.0 mm Hg
Arterial oxygen (PaO_2)	12.0–14.5 kPa	90.0–109 mm Hg
Mixed venous oxygen (PvO_2)	4.0–6.0 kPa	30.0–45.0 mm Hg
Newborn PaO_2	5.33–8.0 kPa	40.0–60.0 mm Hg
For every year over 60 subtract	0.13 kPa	1.0 mm Hg
Arterial pH	7.38–7.44	
Base excess	± 2 mmol/l	
Carboxyhaemoglobin Nonsmoker Smoker Toxic at Coma at	 <2% 3–15% >15% >50%	

Table 3 Paediatric normal ranges

	Sample	SI units	Conventional units
Alkaline phosphatase (p-nitrophenylphosphate method at 37°C)	P		
Birth		150–600 i.u./l	21–85 KA/dl
6 months–2 years		250–1000 i.u./l	35–141 KA/dl
3 years–10 years		250–800 i.u./l	35–113 KA/dl
11 years–17 years		250–1000 i.u./l	35–141 KA/dl
Bicarbonate	P		
Infants		18–22 mmol/l	18–22 mEq/l
Older children		20–26 mmol/l	20–26 mEq/l
Bilirubin	P		
First week of life		100–200 μmol/l (total)	6–11.6 mg/dl
After first week of life and throughout childhood		2–14 μmol/l (total) 0.4 μmol/l (direct)	0.11–0.8 mg/dl 0.02 mg/dl
β-Carotene	S		
< 1 year (upper limit falls with age up to $3\frac{1}{2}$ years)		1.3–6.3 μmol/l	69–338 μg/dl
$3\frac{1}{2}$ years onwards		1.9–2.8 μmol/l	102–150 μg/dl
Creatinine	P		
Cord blood		57–100 μmol/l	0.6–1.13 mg/dl
0–2 weeks		42–71 μmol/l	0.47–0.80 mg/dl
2–26 weeks		33–61 μmol/l	0.37–0.69 mg/dl
26–52 weeks		28–53 μmol/l	0.32–0.60 mg/dl
2 years		30–51 μmol/l	0.33–0.57 mg/dl
4 years		34–56 μmol/l	0.38–0.63 mg/dl
6 years		36–65 μmol/l	0.40–0.70 mg/dl
8 years		39–70 μmol/l	0.44–0.80 mg/dl
10 years		42–74 μmol/l	0.47–0.83 mg/dl
12 years		49–81 μmol/l	0.55–0.90 mg/dl
Creatinine clearance	U and P		
3–13 years		94–142 ml/min per 1.73 m^2	
Creatinine kinase (method—CK Boehringer at 37° C)	P		
Neonates		75–400 U/l	
Infants 3–12 months		10–145 U/l	
Children 1–6 years		20–130 U/l	
6–15 years		15–130 U/l	
Total protein	P		
1st month		51 g/l (mean)	
1st year		61 g/l (mean)	
Childhood		61–78 g/l	
Boys 7–16 years		66–82 g/l	
Girls 7–16 years		67–83 g/l	

	Sample	IgG (i.u./l)	IgG (g/l)	IgA (i.u./l)	IgA (g/l)	IgM (i.u./l)	IgM (g/l)
Immunoglobulins	S						
Newborn		100–200	8.66–19.05	0–2	0–0.03	0–20	0–0.17
1 month		55–150	4.76–12.99	0–12	0–0.20	10–35	0.09–0.30
2 months		30–120	2.60–10.39	2–22	0.03–0.36	10–60	0.09–0.52
3 months		25–108	2.17–9.35	2–35	0.03–0.57	15–90	0.13–0.78
6 months		25–105	2.17–9.09	5–45	0.08–0.74	25–135	0.22–1.17
9 months		30–110	2.60–9.53	10–60	0.16–0.98	35–170	0.30–1.47
1 year		40–122	3.46–10.57	12–68	0.20–1.11	40–200	0.35–1.73
2 years		48–138	4.16–11.95	15–80	0.25–1.31	45–205	0.39–1.78
5 years		63–160	5.46–13.86	25–117	0.41–1.92	50–220	0.43–1.91
10 years		70–180	6.06–15.59	40–175	0.66–2.87	60–240	0.52–2.08
15 years		72–190	6.24–16.45	55–208	0.90–3.41	60–270	0.52–2.34

	Sample	SI units	Conventional units
Parathormone	S		
Cord blood			39–390 ng/l
6th day			125–410 ng/l
4–36 weeks			120–380 ng/l
1–6 years			170–462 ng/l
8–10 years			130–630 ng/l
11–13 years			95–840 ng/l
14–16 years			145–590 ng/l
Inorganic phosphate	P		
Newborn		1.20–2.78 mmol/l	3.7–8.6 mg/dl
Young children		1.29–1.78 mmol/l	4.0–5.5 mg/dl
15 years girls		0.9–1.38 mmol/l	2.8–4.3 mg/dl
17 years boys		0.83–1.49 mmol/l	2.6–4.6 mg/dl

(over the age of 7 years there is a steady fall to reach adult levels at 15–17 years)

Table 3 Paediatric normal ranges—*cont.*

	Sample	SI units	Conventional units
Potassium	P		
Newborn		Up to 6.6 mmol/l	
Older than 1 month–6 years		4.1–5.6 mmol/l	
Boys 7–16 years		3.3–4.7 mmol/l	
Girls 7–16 years		3.4–4.5 mmol/l	
Uric acid (uricase/alcohol dehydrogenase method)	P		
Childhood		0.06–0.24 mmol/l	1.0–4.0 mg/dl
Uric acid (will rise until adulthood—further during puberty in boys but not in girls)			
Boys 16 years		0.23–0.46 mmol/l	3.8–7.7 mg/dl
Girls 16 years		0.19–0.36 mmol/l	3.2–6.0 mg/dl
Thyroid stimulating hormone outside neonatal period	S	0.5–5.0 mU/l	0.5–5.0 μU/ml
Hydroxymethyl mandelic acid (VMA)	U		
6 months		0.3–21.0 μmol/24 h	0.05–4.15 mg/24 h
6 months–6 years		1.5–21.0 μmol/24 h	0.3–4.15 mg/24 h
6–11 years		6.9–30.7 μmol/24 h	1.4–6.0 mg/24 h
11 years–adult		16.1–48.4 μmol/24 h	3.2–9.6 mg/24 h
17-Hydroxycorticosteroids	U		
5 months–1 year		4–24 μmol/24 h	1.1–6.9 mg/24 h
2–5 years		4–38 μmol/24 h	1.1–10.9 mg/24 h
5–10 years		2–22 μmol/24 h	0.57–6.4 mg/24 h
10–14 years		14–50 μmol/24 h	4.0–14.5 mg/24 h
17-Oxosteroids	U		
Newborn		Up to 7 μmol/24 h	Up to 2.0 mg/24 h
4 weeks–1 year		Up to 2 μmol/24 h	Up to 0.58 mg/24 h
1–5 years		Up to 6 μmol/24 h	Up to 1.73 mg/24 h
6–10 years		Up to 10 μmol/24 h	Up to 2.88 mg/24 h
11–17 years		Up to 32 μmol/24 h	Up to 9.22 mg/24 h
Osmolality (maximal urinary)	U		
1 week old		Up to 633 mmol/kg H_2O	
1 month old		Up to 896 mmol/kg H_2O	
1 year old		Up to 1362 mmol/kg H_2O	
2–16 years		1127 ± 256 mmol/kg H_2O	
Glycosaminoglycan/ creatinine ratio	U		
(Alcian blue 8GX assay)		mg/mmol creatinine	mg/g creatinine
1 month		22–41	194–362
1–3 months		9–39	80–345
3–6 months		11–35	97.3–310
6–12 months		4–31	35–274
1–2 years		6–22	53–195
2–3 years		9–20	80–177
3–5 years		6–16	53–142
5–7 years		6–12	53–106
7–9 years		4–11	35–97
9–11 years		4–11	35–97
11–13 years		2–10	17.6–88.5
13–15 years		2–8	17.6–70.8
18–50 years		1–5	8.8–44.2

Table 4 Diagnostic enzymes

Enzyme	Method	Sample	Normal range	Enzyme	Method	Sample	Normal range
Acid phosphatase	Kind/King 37 °C			Glutathione reductase	37 °C	B	7.8 ± 1.09/g Hb at 37 °C
total		S	1–5 i.u./l (or m.i.u./ml)	5′-Nucleotidase		P	3–17 i.u./l
prostatic		S	0–1 i.u./l	Cholinesterase		P	2.25–7.0 i.u./l
Alkaline phosphatase*	Bessey–Lowry 37 °C	P	Adult 30–300 i.u./l				

		% Inhibition with	
Cholinesterase	Method	Fluoride	Dibucaine
Normal homozygote	$Ch_1{}^U Ch_1{}^U$	40–50	82–88
Abnormal homozygote	$Ch_1{}^D Ch_1{}^D$	70–81	14–30
	$Ch_1{}^F Ch_1{}^F$	30–35	60–73
Abnormal heterozygote	$Ch_1{}^U Ch_1{}^D$	44–60	60–68
	$Ch_1{}^U Ch_1{}^F$	37–41	70–79
	$Ch_1{}^D Ch_1{}^F$	47–52	59–63

Remaining Table 4 left column entries:

Enzyme	Method	Sample	Normal range
Alanine-amino transferase (ALT)	Boehringer German OPT 37 °C	P	5–35 i.u./l
Aspartate-amino transferase (AST)	Boehringer German OPT 37 °C	P	5–35 i.u./l
α-Amylase	Cassaway 37 °C	P	0–180 Somogyi units/dl
Creatine kinase (CPK)	Boehringer German NAC activated 37 °C	P	F 25–170 i.u./l M 25–195 i.u./l
Gamma-glutamyl transpeptidase (γGT)	Szasz 37 °C	P	F 7–33 i.u./l M 11–51 i.u./l
Aldolase	Beisenherz et al. 37 °C	P	0.5–7.6 i.u./l
α-Hydroxybutyric dehydrogenase	Elliot and Wilkinson 37 °C	P	53–144 i.u./l
Lactate dehydrogenase	German OPT 37 °C	P	240–525 i.u./l
Lactate dehydrogenase	AM Blue 610	P	70–170 i.u./l

Urinary N-acetyl-β-D-glucosaminidase (NAG)
(in normal urine age 10–59)

1. 4-Methylumbelliferyl substrate (final conc. 0.2 mM)
   mean ± s.d.   5.51 ± 2.35 μmol 4 MU/h per mmol creatinine
   upper limit of normal 10.2 μmol 4 MU/h per mmol creatinine

2. Ω-Nitrostyryl substrates (MNP-NAG; 2-methoxyl 1-4-(2′-nitrovinyl)-phenyl-N-acetyl-β-D-glucosaminide)
   Mean ± s.d.   12.5 ± 6.1 μmol MNP/h per mmol creatinine
   upper limit of normal 24.7 μmol MNP/h per mmol creatinine

3. p-Nitrophenyl NAG
   Norak et al. (1981) Clin. Chem. **27**, 1180;
   mean 3.2 ± 1.3 activity NAG U/g creatinine

* See Table 3.

Table 5 Hormones

	Sample	SI units	Conventional units
ACTH	P	3.3–15.4 pmol/l	< 10–80 pg/ml
Adrenaline	U	< 100 nmol/day	11–49 μg/24 h
Aldosterone	P	100–500 pmol/l	4–18 ng/dl
Aldosterone	U	10–50 nmol/24 h	4–18 mg/24 h
Angiotensin II	P	5–35 pmol/l	5.2–36.0 pg/ml
Antidiuretic hormone (ADH)	P	0.9–4.6 pmol/l	1–5 ng/l
Calcitonin	P	< 27 pmol/l	< 100 ng/l
Catecholamines	U	< 2.6 μmol/24 h	< 440 μg/24 h
Cortisol (free)	U	< 280 nmol/24 h	< 10.0 μg/24 h
Cortisol	P	a.m. 280–700 nmol/l p.m. 140–280 nmol/l	10–25.3 μg/dl 5–10 μg/dl
FSH	P/S	2–8 U/l	2–8 m.i.u./ml
Gastrin	P	< 40 pmol/l	< 80 ng/l
Glucagon	P	< 50 pmol/l	< 17.7 ng/dl
Growth hormone	P	< 20 mU/l	< 20 μU/ml
HCG	S	< 5 i.u./l	< 5 m.i.u./ml
Insulin (fasting)	P	< 15 mU/l (NB age)	< 15 μU/ml
Insulin C-peptide	P	0.5–2.5 μg/l (undetectable in hypoglycaemia)	
Luteinizing hormone	P	3–8 U/l	3–8 m.i.u./ml
LH (pre-menopausal)	P	6–13 U/l	6–13 m.i.u./ml
Neurotensin	P	< 100 pmol/l	
Oestrogens (total)			
Non-pregnancy < 10 years	U	0.5 nmol/24 h	0.14 μg/24 h
Follicular phase	U	20–150 nmol/24 h	5.7–43.2 μg/24 h
Mid-cycle	U	60–300 nmol/24 h	17.3–86.5 μg/24 h
Luteal phase	U	45–290 nmol/24 h	12.9–83.5 μg/24 h
Post-menopausal	U	10–55 nmol/24 h	2.88–15.8 μg/24 h
Male	U	5–40 nmol/24 h	1.44–11.5 μg/24 h
Oestrogens (total) in pregnancy		Mean	
Gestation week 25	U	65 μmol/24 h	18.7 mg/24 h
26	U	69 μmol/24 h	19.9 mg/24 h
27	U	74 μmol/24 h	21.3 mg/24 h

Table 5 Hormones—*cont.*

	Sample	SI units	Conventional units
28	U	79.5 μmol/24 h	22.9 mg/24 h
29	U	85.4 μmol/24 h	24.6 mg/24 h
30	U	91.3 μmol/24 h	26.3 mg/24 h
31	U	97.9 μmol/24 h	28.2 mg/24 h
32	U	105 μmol/24 h	30.2 mg/24 h
33	U	112.5 μmol/24 h	32.4 mg/24 h
34	U	120.5 μmol/24 h	34.7 mg/24 h
35	U	129 μmol/24 h	37.1 mg/24 h
36	U	139 μmol/24 h	40.0 mg/24 h
37	U	149 μmol/24 h	42.9 mg/24 h
38	U	159 μmol/24 h	45.8 mg/24 h
39	U	170 μmol/24 h	48.9 mg/24 h
40	U	183 μmol/24 h	52.7 mg/24 h
Parathormone*	P	< 0.1–0.73 μg/l	0.1–0.73 ng/ml
Pancreatic polypetide (PP)	P	< 200 pmol/l	< 830 ng/l
Progesterone	P	M < 5 nmol/l	< 1.6 ng/ml
		F 15–77 nmol/l	4.7–24 ng/ml
Prolactin	P	M < 450 U/l	< 450 m.i.u./ml
		F < 600 U/l	< 600 m.i.u./ml
Renin activity		Recumbent 1.2–2.4 pmol/ml/h; Erect after 30 min 3.0–4.3 pmol/ml/h; depends on diuretics, salt, intake, etc.	4.8–9.6 μg/dl/h
Somatostatin	P	< 100 pmol/l	< 16.3 ng/dl
Steroids			
17-Oxogenic*	U	M 28–80 μmol/24 h	8–23 mg/24 h
		F 21–66 μmol/24 h	6–19 mg/24 h
17-Oxosteroids (neutral)*	U	M 17–76 μmol/24 h	5–22 mg/24 h
		F 14–59 μmol/24 h	4–17 mg/24 h
Testosterone			
Male		14–42 nmol/l	0.48–1.46 ng/dl
Female		1–2.1 nmol/l	0.035–0.07 ng/dl
TSH*	P	< 6 mU/l	< 6 m.i.u./ml
TBG	P	7–17 mg/l	
Thyroxine (T_4)	P	70–140 nmol/l	5.4–10.7 μg/dl
Free thyroxine	P	9–22 pmol/l	0.7–1.7 ng/dl
Tri-iodothyronine	P	1.2–3.0 nmol/l	1.85–4.62 ng/ml
Vasoactive intestinal polypeptide (VIP)	P	< 30 pmol/l	< 100 ng/l

Care should be taken in infants and children in the interpretation of normal ranges.
* See paediatric range.

Table 6 Tumour markers

	Sample	Normal range
Alpha-fetoprotein	S	< 10 ku/l
Carcino-embryonic antigen (CEA)	S	< 10 μg/l (but < 20 μg/l is still not necessarily indicative of malignancy)

Table 7 Vitamins and related tests

Vitamins	Sample	SI units	Conventional units
β-Carotene*	S	0.9–5.6 μmol/l	48–300 μg/dl
Vitamin A	S	0.7–1.7 μmol/l	20–50 μg/dl
Thiamin (B$_1$)	P	> 40 nmol/l	> 1 μg/dl
Riboflavine (B$_2$)	P	Free < 21.3 nmol/l	< 0.8 μg/dl
	P	Total < 85.0 nmol/l	< 3.2 μg/dl
Pyridoxine (B$_6$)	S	> 178 nmol/l	> 30 ng/ml
Folate	S	4.8–6.4 nmol/l	2.1–28 μg/l
Vitamin B$_{12}$	S		170–925 ng/l
Ascorbate	B	34–68 μmol/l	0.6–1.2 mg/dl
Vitamin D	S	23.8–111 nmol/l	12–56 ng/ml
Vitamin D metabolites			
25-OHD		12.5–125 nmol/l	5–50 ng/ml
24,25 (OH)$_2$ D$_3$		1.25–7.5 nmol/l	0.5–3.0 ng/ml
1,25 (OH)$_2$ D$_3$		50–100 pmol/l	20–40 pg/ml
Red cell transketolase	B	40–90 i.u./l	40–90 m.i.u./ml
Red cell folate	B	0.36–1.44 μmol/l	160–640 g/l

* See paediatric table.

Table 8 Intermediary metabolities (after overnight fast)

	Age 21–40 years	SI units	Age 41–60 years	SI units	Age 61–75 years	SI units
Glucose	75.2–98.8 mg/dl	4.18–5.9 mmol/l	71.6–108 mg/dl	3.98–6.02 mmol/l	73–109 mg/dl	4.06–6.07 mmol/l
Lactate	3.56–10.72 mg/dl	0.396–1.191 mmol/l	3.69–10.22 mg/dl	0.411–1.136 mmol/l	4.15–8.73 mg/dl	0.461–0.97 mmol/l
Pyruvate	0.023–0.14 μg/dl	0.027–0.164 mmol/l	0.025–0.126 μg/dl	0.029–0.144 mmol/l	0.029–0.10 μg/dl	0.034–0.117 mmol/l
Alanine	1.63–4.2 mg/dl	0.184–0.477 mmol/l	1.83–4.0 mg/dl	0.206–0.449 mmol/l	1.51–3.42 mg/dl	0.170–0.385 mmol/l
Glycerol	0.25–0.93 mg/dl	0.028–0.102 mmol/l	0.28–0.85 mg/dl	0.031–0.093 mmol/l	0.30–1.28 mg/dl	0.033–0.139 mmol/l
NEFA	1.59–18.6 mg/dl	0.06–0.70 mmol/l	5.32–19.9 mg/dl	0.20–0.75 mmol/l	3.99–23.6 mg/dl	0.15–0.89 mmol/l
3-Hydroxybutyrate	0.05–3.48 mg/dl	0.005–0.335 mmol/l	0.10–2.25 mg/dl	0.010–0.217 mmol/l	0.13–6.46 mg/dl	0.013–0.621 mmol/l
Acetoacetate	0.1–1.46 mg/dl	0.010–0.146 mmol/l	0.07–1.60 mg/dl	0.007–0.160 mmol/l	0.09–2.82 mg/dl	0.009–0.282 mmol/l
Total ketone bodies		0.016–0.441 mmol/l		0.024–0.304 mmol/l		0.024–0.840 mmol/l
Triglyceride	27.4–222 mg/dl	0.31–2.51 mmol/l	47.8–195 mg/dl	0.54–2.20 mmol/l	46.9–226 mg/dl	0.53–2.56 mmol/l
Insulin		1.8–15.0 m.i.u./l		2.0–13.2 m.i.u./l		1.9–12.3 m.i.u./l.

Values from one Unit; Newcastle/Southampton.
Alberti (1978). *Clin. Chem.* **24**, 1571.

Table 9 Lipids and lipoproteins

	Sample	SI units	Conventional units
Cholesterol*	P	3.9–7.8 mmol/l	150–300 mg/dl
Triglyceride	P	0.55–1.90 mmol/l	48.6–168 mg/dl
Phospholipid	S	2.9–5.2 mmol/l	9.0–15.6 mg/dl
Non-esterified fatty acids	S	M 0.19–0.78 mmol/l	5.05–20.9 mg/dl
		F 0.06–0.9 mmol/l	1.59–23.9 mg/dl
Fatty acids			
Total		3.16–18 mmol/l	100–500 mg/dl
Free		0.36–1.25 mmol/l	10–35 mg/dl
Lipoproteins (as cholesterol)			
VLDL	S	0.128–0.645 mmol/l	4.9–24.8 mg/dl
LDL	S	1.55–4.4 mmol/l	59.6–169 mg/dl
HDL	S	0.9–1.93 mmol/l	34.6–74.2 mg/dl
Lipoprotein x		Undetectable in normals	

* Desirable upper limit 5.9 mmol/l (228 mg/dl).

Table 10 Proteins and immunoproteins

	Samples	Normal range
Total protein	P	60–80 g/l
Albumin	P	35–50 g/l
Globulin fractions		
α_1-globulin	S	2–4 g/l
α_2-globulin	S	5–9 g/l
β-globulin	S	6–11 g/l
γ-globulin	S	7–17 g/l
α_1-antitryspin	S	1.3–3.28 g/l
α_2-haptoglobin	S	0.3–2.0 g/l
α_2-caeruloplasmin	S	20–40 mg/100 ml
β_1-transferrin	S	1.2–2.0 g/l
Immunoglobulins*		
IgG		7.2–19 g/l
IgA		0.8–5.0 g/l
IgM		0.5–2.0 g/l
Complement C$_3$		0.69–1.3 g/l
C$_4$		0.12–0.27 g/l
Caeruloplasmin	P	20–40 mg/100 ml
β_2-microglobulin	S	1.1–2.4 mg/l
	U	4–370 μg/l
		or 30–370 μg/24 h
Fibrinogen	P	2–4 g/l
Fibrinogen degradation products	S	Less than 0.8 μg/l

* See paediatric table'.

Table 11 Trace elements and metals

	Sample	SI units	Conventional units
Arsenic (neutron activation)	B		0.004 μg/g
Bromine	S	46.3 μmol/l $\pm$ 18.8	3.7 $\pm$ 1.5 μg/ml
Cadmium (neutron activation)	U	89–116 nmol/l	10–13 μg/l
Cadmium (whole blood)	B	26.7–480 nmol/l	3–54 ng/ml
Cadmium	S	22.2 nmol/l $\pm$ 15.1 nmol/l	1.5 $\pm$ 1.7 ng/ml
Chromium	B	94.2–183 nmol/l	4.9–9.5 ng/ml
Chromium—male	U	38–519 nmol/24 h	2–27 μg/24 h
Chromium—female	U	115–192 nmol/24 h	6–10 μg/24 h
Chromium—dry weight	Hair		> 500 ng/g
Cobalt	S	8.82 nmol/l $\pm$ 7.3 nmol/l	0.52 $\pm$ 0.43 ng/ml
	U	3.39–17.0 nmol/24 h	0.2–1.0 μg/24 h
Copper	P	12–26 μmol/l	76–165 μg/dl
Cyanide	S		
non-smokers		0.15 μmol/l	0.004 mg/l
smokers		0.22 μmol/l	0.006 mg/l
Gold	S	20–203 pmol/l	2–20 pg/ml
Iron			
Male	S	M 14–31 μmol/l	78–174 μg/dl
Female	S	F 11–30 μmol/l	62–168 μg/dl
Manganese	B	0.15 μmol/l $\pm$ 0.05 μmol/l	8.4 $\pm$ 2.7 μg/l
Molybdenum (neutron activation)	U	0.26–2.6 nmol/24 h	25–250 μg/24 h
Silver	S	8.34 nmol/l $\pm$ 3.7	0.9 $\pm$ 0.4 ng/ml
Zinc	P	6–25 μmol/l	39–163 μg/dl
	U	2.1–11.0 μmol/24 h	137–720 μg/24 h

Table 12 Urinary values

	SI units	Conventional units
Calcium	2.5–7.5 mmol/24 h	100–300 mg/24 h
Copper	0.2–1.0 μmol/24 h	13–64 μg/24 h
Iron		< 1.0 mg/24 h
Lead	< 0.39 μmol/24 h	< 80 μg/24 h
Magnesium	3.3–4.9 mmol/24 h	80–120 mg/24 h
Phosphate (inorganic)	15–50 mmol/24 h	0.5–1.5 g/24 h
Potassium	40–120 mmol/24 h	1.56–4.78 g/24 h
Sodium	100–250 mmol/24 h	2.3–5.7 g/24 h
Creatinine*	9–17 mmol/24 h	1.0–1.9 g/24 h
Amylase		8000–30 000 Wohlegmuth U/24 h
		35–260 Somogyi units/dl
Ascorbic acid	34–68 μmol/l	6–12 mg/l
Glucose	0.06–0.84 mmol/l	1.1–15.1 mg/dl
Hydroxy-indole acetic acid (5 HIAA)	16–73 μmol/24 h	3–14 mg/24 h
Oxalate	< 450 μmol/24 h	< 40 mg/24 h
Urate	2–6 mmol/24 h	0.3–1.0 g/24 h
Urea	250–500 mmol/24 h	15–30 g/24 h
Urobilinogen	Up to 6.7 μmol/24 h	Up to 4 mg/24 h
Zinc	2.1–11.0 μmol/24 h	137–720 μg/24 h
δ-Amino laevulinic acid	0.8–46 μmol/24 h	0.1–6 mg/24 h
Coproporphyrin	51–351 nmol/24 h	34–234 μg/24 h
Porphobilinogen	0.9–8.8 μmol/24 h	0.18–1.76 mg/24 h
Uroporphyrin	0–49 nmol/24 h	0–41 μg/24 h
β_2-Microglobulin	4–370 μg/l	
Osmolality†	350–1000 mosm/kg	
Cortisol	60–1500 nmol/l	2–54 μg/dl
Hydroxymethylmandelic acid	16–48 μmol/24 h	3.2–9.5 mg/24 h
24-hour urinary excretion		
Protein		Up to 150 mg/24 h
Pregnancy		Up to 300 mg/24 h
Albumin		Up to 25 mg/24 h
Creatinine		
Male	9.0–17.0 mmol	1.0–1.9 g/24 h
Female	7.5–12.5 mmol	0.8–1.4 g/24 h
Pregnancy	8.0–13.5 mmol	0.9–1.5 g/24 h
Uric acid*	Up to 5.0 mmol	Up to 0.84 g/24 h
Pregnancy (except late)	Up to 7.0 mmol	Up to 1.17 g/24 h
Cystine	0.04–0.42 mmol	9.6–100 mg/24 h

* On self-selected British diet; partially influenced by diet.
† Range of young adults, declines with age—see text.

Table 13 Faecal values

	SI units	Conventional units
Fat (on normal diet)	11–18 mmol/l	3–5 g/24 h
Nitrogen	70–140 mmol/24 h	1–2 g/24 h
Urobilinogen	50–500 μmol/24 h	30–300 mg/24 h
Coproporphyrin	0.018–1.2 μmol/24 h	0.012–0.832 mg/24 h
Protoporphyrin	0–4 μmol/24 h	0–2.09 mg/24 h

Table 14 Amniotic and cerebrospinal fluid

	SI units	Conventional units
Amniotic fluids		
Palmitate	> 50 μmol/l at fetal maturity	
Lecithin/ sphingomyelin ratio	< 1.8	
CSF		
Glucose	3.3–4.4 mmol/24 h	59–79 mg/dl
Protein	0.15–0.40 g/l	
Chloride	122–128 mmol/l	mEq/l
Lactate	Up to 2.8 mmol/l	Up to 25.2 mg/dl

Table 15 Functional tests

Fat absorption
  100 g fat load: an increase of 1.0 mmol/l (90 mg/100 ml) either 2 or 4 hours after load from the fasting level (esterified fatty acids). Significantly abnormal if increase is < 0.55 mmol/l (50 mg/dl)
Xylose absorption
  25 g dose xylose: normal urine excretion should be greater than 4 g/5 h period. Children only: normal plasma xylose > 1.6 mmol/l, 1 hour after 25 g (or 1 g/kg) xylose
Creatinine clearance
  Normal: 90–120 ml/min

  Calculation: $\dfrac{\text{Urine creatinine (mmol/l)} \times \text{vol/min}}{\text{Plasma creatinine (mmol/l)}}$

Renal functional capacity
  GFR   Male age 20   105–170 ml/min per 1.73 m^2
              age 50   95–138 ml/min per 1.73 m^2
              age 70   70–110 ml/min per 1.73 m^2
          Female age 20 104–158 ml/min per 1.73 m^2
              age 50   90–130 ml/min per 1.73 m^2
              age 70   74–114 ml/min per 1.73 m^2
  Maximum concentrating ability   800/1200 mosm/kg
  Minimum urinary pH   5.3 (after acid load)
Ischaemic lactate test
  Fasting lactate: 0.5–1.5 mmol/l (4.5–13.5 mg/dl)
  Immediate post-exercise: approximately 5 mmol/l (45 mg/dl)
  25 minutes post-exercise: return to normal
  Type V glycogen storage disease—no response to exercise
Dexamethazone-suppression of adrenal cortex
  1. Dose: 0.5 mg 6 hourly
     Plasma cortisol < 150 nmol/l
     Urine cortisol < 50 nmol/24 h
     Most patients with Cushing's syndrome give greater levels than stated, irrespective of aetiology
  2. Dose: 2 mg 6 hourly
     Pituitary-dependent Cushing's plasma and urine often gives values less than 50% of basal. Other aetiologies greater than 50% of basal
  3. Overnight dexamethasone suppression—dose 2 mg at midnight: Plasma cortisol at 9 a.m. < 200 nmol/l
Depot Synacthen (zinc)—dose 1 mg i.m.
  Normal cortisol > 900 nmol/l at 4–6 hours:
  ACTH deficient may only reach this value at 24 hours or even after further injections
  Addison's: < 10% increment over basal at any of these times, even after further injections

Short Synacthen—dose 0.25 mg i.m.
  plasma cortisol > 600 nmol/l or double basal
Response to insulin hypoglycaemia (pl glucose < 2.2 mmol/l)
  pl cortisol > 600 nmol/l or double basal
Plasma ACTH response to metyrapone
  ACTH at 0900 hours < 80 ng/l, at 2400 hours < 40 ng/l
  After metyrapone: rise in pituitary-dependent Cushing's between 6 and 12 hours of test to > double the basal level (not always present by this criterion)
  NB Basal levels depend on age, sex, and body weight
Growth hormone
  (i) Fasting < 20 mU/l
  (ii) Glucose suppression: 60 min, 90 min, 120 min, <5 mU/l
  (iii) Insulin hypoglycaemia, arginine or Bovril—peak > 20 mU/l
Glucose and insulin
  Overnight fasting glucose 3.0–5.0 mmol/l
  Overnight fasting plasma insulin 2–13 mU/ml (mean 5 mU/ml)
  If fasting plasma glucose > 7.0 mmol/l diagnosis of diabetes certain and GTT unnecessary
  If random plasma glucose > 10.0 mmol/l highly suggestive of diabetes
Criteria for normal 50 g oral GTT (various standards)
  Fasting glucose < 5.0 mmol/l
  60 min glucose < 9.0 mmol/l
  120 min glucose < 6.5 mmol/l
  GTT results rise with age; samples after glucose rise by approximately 0.55 mmol/l per decade, after the age of 50
  (Alternative dose 75 g)
Criteria for normal i.v. GTT
  Expressed as 'K value' = % fall of plasma glucose in 1 minute
  $K = \dfrac{0.693}{t_{\frac{1}{2}}} \times 100$
  $t_{\frac{1}{2}}$ = time in minutes for plasma glucose to fall by 50% from 10 minute level
  $K < 0.9$ = diabetic
  K 0.9–1.1 = borderline
  $K > 1.1$ = normal
Hypoglycaemia
  If plasma glucose < 2 mmol/l, plasma insulin should not exceed 1.5 mU/ml

Table 16 Therapeutic drugs

	Sample	SI units	Conventional units
Ethosuximide	P	283–708.3 μmol/l	40.0–100 μg/ml
Carbamazepine	P	33.9–50.8 μmol/l	8.0–12.0 μg/ml
Primidone	P	22.9–55.0 μmol/l	5.0–12.0 μg/ml
Phenobarbitone	P	64.6–172.2 μmol/l	15.0–40.0 μg/ml
Phenytoin	P	39.6–79.3 μmol/l	9.97–19.9 μg/ml
Epilim	P	0.3–0.7 mmol/l	43.0–101 μg/ml
Aminophylline	P		10–20 μg/ml (adult)
			5–10 μg/ml (paediatric)

Index

Pages in **bold** refer to principle discussions in text. 'vs' denotes differential diagnosis.

Abbreviations

ACTH	Adrenocorticotrophic hormone (corticotrophin)	GBM	Glomerular basement membrane
ADH	Antidiuretic hormone	hCG	human chorionic gonadotrophin
ADP	Adenosine diphosphate	MCTD	Mixed connective tissue disease
AIDS	Acquired immune deficiency syndrome	NMR	Nuclear magnetic resonance
ARDS	Adult respiratory distress syndrome	SIADH	Syndrome of inappropriate antidiuretic hormone secretion
ATP	Adenosine triphosphate	SLE	Systemic lupus erythematosus
CRF	Corticotrophin releasing factor	TTP	Thrombotic thrombocytopenic purpura
CT	Computerized tomography		

Fusobacterium necrophorum 5.225, 5.227, 5.228, 5.229, 5.379
fusospirochaetosis, *see* Vincent's angina

G

gadolinium 13.48
Gaisbock's syndrome 19.154
gait 17.7, 17.16
galactokinase deficiency **9.7**
galactorrhoea **10.110**, 10.120, 11.17
  drug-induced **10.121**
  hyperprolactinaemia with 10.20, 10.88, 10.110
galactosaemia **9.7**
  gene frequency 4.13
galactose 9.6–9.8
  congenital malabsorption 18.82
galactose 1-phosphate, accumulation 9.7
galactose 1-phosphate uridyl transferase deficiency, *see* galactosaemia
α-galactosidase A deficiency(Fabry's disease) 21.129, 21.208
galactosyl ceramide lipidosis 9.33, **9.34**
gallamine, action 22.2
gallbladder 12.198–12.206
  cancer of, epidemiology **4.103**
  congenital absence 12.267
  congenital deformities 12.267
  in diabetes mellitus 9.88
  dilation, in pancreatic cancer 12.193
  disease, obesity and 8.41–8.42, 8.60
  gallstones in, *see* cholelithiasis; cholecystitis; gallstones
  inflammation, *see* cholecystitis
  in opisthorchiasis 5.580, 5.582
  pain 12.17, 12.201
  removal, in acute pancreatitis treatment 12.188
gallium-67 19.173
gallstones 12.198
  acute pancreatitis and 12.183, 12.188
  bile pigment **12.200**
  cholecystitis due to 12.201, 12.202
  cholesterol 12.195, **12.200**
  in Crohn's disease 12.274
  detection by ultrasound, cholecystography 12.5
  dissolution 12.201
  formation 12.200
  after ileal resection 12.108
  ileus 12.201
  natural history of 12.201
  in obesity 8.41–8.42, 8.60
  in paroxysmal nocturnal haemoglobinuria 19.55
  in pregnancy 12.274
  recurrence 12.201
  'silent' 12.201
  treatment 12.201
gamete formation 4.2
gamma-aminobutyric acid(GABA), in isoniazid overdose 6.37
  benzodiazepine action 25.51
gamma camera 18.13, 18.14, 18.90
gammaglobulin,
  in idiopathic thrombocytopenic purpura 19.223
  in infections 5.9
  in Kawasaki disease 24.3
  replacement therapy 4.77

gammaglobulin (*cont.*):
  see also immunoglobulin
gamma-glutamyl synthetase deficiency 19.143
gamma-rays 6.130
ganglioglioma 21.174
ganglion blockers 16.91
  in pregnancy 11.52
  sexual problems 25.42
  stellate 6.35
ganglioneuroblastoma 12.57
ganglioneuroma 21.174
ganglioside neuraminidase deficiency 9.36
gangliosidosis 9.33, **9.34–9.36**, 21.207–21.208
gangosa 5.334
gangrene,
  alveolar 9.44
  of digit 16.35
  foot, in diabetes mellitus 9.89
  Fournier's 5.228
  gas, *see* gas gangrene
  Meleney's synergistic 5.195, 5.229
  in peripheral arterial disease in diabetics 13.190
  in polycythaemia vera 19.38
  in primary thrombocythaemia 19.44
  in Rocky Mountain spotted fever 5.346
  streptococcal 5.170
  synergistic 20.67
  in tourniquet use after snake bites 6.73, 6.74
  venous 19.235
  vibrating tools associated 6.156, 6.160
Ganjam virus 5.130, **5.131**
Ganser syndrome 25.4
gap junctions, myocardial cell 13.1
Gardnerella vaginalis 5.380, 5.445–5.446
Gardner's syndrome 12.154, 20.80
gargoylism 9.36, 17.30
gas,
  bubbles in decompression sickness 6.124
  combustion, pollution from **6.138–6.139**
  inert, narcosis 6.123
  inspired, distribution and mixing tests 15.33
  noxious occupational 6.146
  used in diving 6.123
gas exchange, pulmonary 13.326–13.327, 13.328, 15.7, 15.25, **15.27–15.29**
  in adult respiratory distress syndrome 15.164
  impairment in respiratory failure 15.167
  tests of **15.33–15.34**
gas gangrene 5.31, 5.51, **5.273–5.274**, 22.13
  of bowel 5.276
gasoline, *see* petrol
gastrectomy,
  chronic pancreatitis vs 12.191
  in gastric carcinoma 12.149
  gut hormones after 12.56
  partial,
    barium studies after 12.2
    dumping after 12.76
    in gastric ulcer treatment 12.76
    haemolysis in 19.147
    iron malabsorption after 19.86
    osteomalacia after 10.66, 17.18
    sequelae 12.76
    vitamin B$_{12}$ deficiency 19.99
  total 12.109, 19.99
gastric acid,
  in duodenal ulcer aetiology 12.64

gastric acid (*cont.*):
  in enteropathogen colonization 12.164
  in gastric ulcer aetiology 12.66
  hypersecretion 12.64
    after small intestinal resection 12.108
    in Zollinger–Ellison syndrome 12.58, 12.68
  hypersecretion(acid rebound) 12.72
  hyposecretion 12.66
  secretion 12.52, 12.61–12.63, 12.77, 12.78, 12.81
    histamine role 12.61–12.62, 12.73
  see also gastric secretion
gastric adenocarcinoma 12.80, 12.86
gastric aspiration 6.5, 6.26
gastric atrophy 12.79, 12.81, 20.17
  in aged 27.2
  in iron deficiency 19.85
  in pernicious anaemia 19.97, 19.98
  vitamin B$_{12}$ deficiency 19.104
gastric bypass, in obesity 8.50
gastric carcinoma,
  cimetidine in possible aetiology of 12.74
  diagnosis by radiology 12.2
  gastric ulcers vs 12.70, 12.75
  in hypogammaglobulinaemia 12.88
  in immunodeficiency 4.77
  see also stomach, carcinoma
gastric contents, aspiration, in pregnancy 11.15, 11.28
gastric crisis 5.395
gastric dilation, acute, in anorexia nervosa 8.35
gastric distension, satiety sign 8.46
gastric emptying 12.40
  accelerated **12.47**, 12.109
  delayed 12.16, **12.46**, 12.48
  in duodenal ulcer aetiology 12.64–12.65
  in endurance sports 26.5
  in iron overdosage 6.38
  motilin role 12.53
  neurotensin role 12.53
  in pregnancy 11.41, 11.51
  rapid, in chronic pancreatitis 12.190
  rate 12.63
  time 7.5, 7.10, 7.12
gastric incontinence **12.47–12.48**
gastric inhibitory polypeptide(GIP) **12.53**, 12.55, 12.56
gastric juice 12.61, 12.63
gastric lavage,
  in cardiovascular drug overdose 6.32, 6.33, 6.34
  contraindications, precautions, adverse effects 6.5
  emesis vs in acute poisoning 6.6
  in poisoning 6.5, 6.42, 6.43
  in respiratory drug overdose 6.36
gastric manometry 12.43
gastric mucosa 12.77, **12.78**
gastric mucus 12.63, 12.66
gastric outlet obstruction, causes 12.46, 12.70
gastric pepsin **12.63**, 12.78
gastric plication, in obesity 8.50
gastric secretion 12.61–12.64, 12.72, 12.78
  abnormal, in chronic pancreatitis 12.189
  inhibitor, in pancreatic extract administration 12.191, 12.196
  see also gastric acid
  tests 19.104
gastric stasis **12.46**
gastric surgery, malabsorption after **12.109**
gastric ulcer 12.66–12.70
  in Africa 12.281
  chronic gastritis with 12.82

gastric ulcer (*cont.*):
  gastric carcinoma and 12.70, 12.75, 12.148
  medical treatment **12.70–12.75**
  radiology 12.3
  rebleeding 12.22
  treatment 12.75–12.77
gastrin 12.12, **12.52–12.53**, 12.55, 12.62, 12.78, 19.104
  in chronic gastritis aetiology 12.85
  measurements, in duodenal ulcer 12.66
  secretion 10.55, 12.81
  after small intestinal resection 12.108
  in Zollinger–Ellison syndrome 12.58, 12.68
gastrinomas 4.129, **12.58–12.59**
  in Zollinger–Ellison syndrome 12.58, 12.68
gastrin-releasing peptide(GRP) 12.62
gastritis **12.77–12.86**
  acute 12.78–12.79
  acute erosive 12.78, 12.81, 12.84
  acute haemorrhagic 12.79, 12.84, 12.86
  acute infectious 12.84
  acute phlegmonous 12.84
  in Africa 12.281
  biliary 12.45
  chronic 12.79–12.80
  chronic atrophic 12.79–12.80, 12.81
    gastric carcinoma and 12.148
    in Southeast Asia 12.280
  chronic cystic 12.80
  chronic hypertrophic 12.82
  chronic superficial 12.79
  classification 12.78–12.83
  diseases associated 12.82
  follicular 12.80
  giant hypertrophic 12.80, 12.82
  management 12.86
  metaplasia 12.80–12.81
  in pernicious anaemia 19.98
  post-surgical 12.82
  prevalence 12.84
  prognosis 12.86
  types A, B 12.82, 12.85
  ulcer-associated 12.82
gastrocnemius rupture 16.88
gastrodisciasis **5.592**
Gastrodiscoides hominis 5.579, 5.581, 5.591
gastroenteritis 12.18, 12.19
  acute, occupational causes 6.151
  arthritis with 16.18
  cataracts due to 23.18
  eosinophilic **5.558**
  in infancy 5.14
  E.coli in **5.213–5.214**
  in measles 5.91–5.92
  Reiter's disease after 16.17, 16.18, 16.17, 16.18
  staphylococcal 5.170
  see also enteritis
gastroenteropathy, in infants 12.90
Gastrografin enema 12.143
gastrointestinal bleeding **12.21–12.22**
  in acute pancreatitis 12.185, 12.186, 12.187
  in acute renal failure 18.130
  acute upper **12.21**
  angiography in 12.4
  assessment 12.21
  causes and frequency 12.21
  in cirrhosis 12.231
  course, prognosis, mortality 12.22
  diagnostic procedures 12.22
  in haemorrhagic gastritis 12.84
  management 12.21–12.22, 12.86
  in oesophageal varices 12.242–12.243
  after renal transplantation 18.155
  in skin diseases 20.17
  surgery indications 12.22

H

N

Q

R

V